HEMATOLOGY

BASIC PRINCIPLES AND PRACTICE

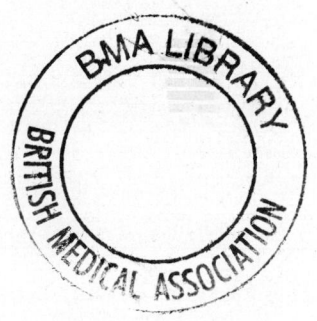

SEVENTH EDITION

HEMATOLOGY

BASIC PRINCIPLES AND PRACTICE

Ronald Hoffman, MD

Albert A. and Vera G. List Professor of Medicine
Tisch Cancer Institute
Hematology-Oncology Section
Department of Medicine
Icahn School of Medicine at Mount Sinai
New York, New York

Edward J. Benz, Jr., MD

President and CEO Emeritus, Dana-Farber Cancer Institute
Richard and Susan Smith Distinguished Professor of
Medicine, Professor of Pediatrics, Professor of Genetics
Harvard Medical School
Director and Principal Investigator Emeritus, Dana-Farber/
Harvard Cancer Center
Boston, Massachusetts

Leslie E. Silberstein, MD

Professor of Pathology (Pediatrics)
Harvard Medical School
Director, Joint Program in Transfusion Medicine
Boston Children's Hospital
Brigham and Women's Hospital
Boston, Massachusetts

Helen E. Heslop, MD, DSc (Hon)

Dan L. Duncan Chair
Professor of Medicine and Pediatrics
Director, Center for Cell and Gene Therapy
Baylor College of Medicine
Houston Methodist Hospital and Texas Children's Hospital
Houston, Texas

Jeffrey I. Weitz, MD

Professor of Medicine and Biochemistry and Biomedical
Sciences
McMaster University
Executive Director
Thrombosis and Atherosclerosis Research Institute
Canada Research Chair in Thrombosis
Heart and Stroke Foundation J. F. Mustard Chair in
Cardiovascular Research
Hamilton, Ontario, Canada

John Anastasi, MD

Associate Professor, Department of Pathology
University of Chicago, Pritzker School of Medicine
Director, Section of Hematopathology
Clinical Hematology Laboratory
University of Chicago Medical Center
Chicago, Illinois

Mohamed E. Salama, MD

Professor of Pathology and Clinical Hematology
The University of Utah School of Medicine
Chief of Hematopathology and Vice President
ARUP Reference Laboratories
Salt Lake City, Utah

Online Updates Editor
Syed Ali Abutalib, MD

Assistant Director
Hematology and Bone Marrow Transplant
Leader, Hematology Program Development
Cancer Treatment Centers of America
Chicago, Illinois

ELSEVIER

ELSEVIER

1600 John F. Kennedy Blvd.
Ste 1800
Philadelphia, PA 19103-2899

Notices

Knowledge and best practice in this field are constantly changing. As new research and experience broaden our understanding, changes in research methods, professional practices, or medical treatment may become necessary.

Practitioners and researchers must always rely on their own experience and knowledge in evaluating and using any information, methods, compounds, or experiments described herein. In using such information or methods they should be mindful of their own safety and the safety of others, including parties for whom they have a professional responsibility.

With respect to any drug or pharmaceutical products identified, readers are advised to check the most current information provided (i) on procedures featured or (ii) by the manufacturer of each product to be administered, to verify the recommended dose or formula, the method and duration of administration, and contraindications. It is the responsibility of practitioners, relying on their own experience and knowledge of their patients, to make diagnoses, to determine dosages and the best treatment for each individual patient, and to take all appropriate safety precautions.

To the fullest extent of the law, neither the Publisher nor the authors, contributors, or editors, assume any liability for any injury and/or damage to persons or property as a matter of products liability, negligence or otherwise, or from any use or operation of any methods, products, instructions, or ideas contained in the material herein.

Previous editions copyrighted 2013 by Saunders, an imprint of Elsevier Inc., 2009, 2005, 2000, 1995, and 1991 by Churchill Livingstone, an imprint of Elsevier, Inc.

Library of Congress Cataloging-in-Publication Data

Names: Hoffman, Ronald, 1945- editor.
Title: Hematology : basic principles and practice / [edited by] Ronald
    Hoffman, Edward J. Benz, Jr., Leslie E. Silberstein, Helen E. Heslop,
    Jeffrey I. Weitz, John Anastasi, Mohamed Salama.
Other titles: Hematology (Hoffman)
Description: 7th edition. | Philadelphia, PA : Elsevier, [2018] | Includes
    bibliographical references and index.
Identifiers: LCCN 2017003035 | ISBN 9780323357623 (hardcover : alk. paper)
Subjects: | MESH: Hematologic Diseases–diagnosis | Hematologic
    Diseases–therapy | Blood Physiological Phenomena
Classification: LCC RC633 | NLM WH 120 | DDC 616.1/5–dc23 LC record available at
https://lccn.loc.gov/2017003035

Content Strategist: Kayla Wolfe
Content Development Manager: Lucia Gunzel
Publishing Services Manager: Patricia Tannian
Senior Project Manager: Cindy Thoms
Book Designer: Ryan Cook

Printed in China

Last digit is the print number: 9   8   7   6   5   4   3   2   1

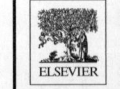

To the numerous authors who have toiled to create the chapters that constitute this book. Their energy and perseverance are emblematic of their continued commitment to the value of scholarship and education in medicine. The work of each of these authors enhances our knowledge of hematology, which ultimately leads to improved care for patients with blood disorders. To my wife, Nan, and my children, Michael, Judith, Daniel, and Margot, who continue to support my efforts and help me maintain a firm footing in life. To President Barack Obama who has created a country in which I am happy to live and who will always be my role model. To the members of my laboratory and clinical trials groups who make it a pleasure to come to work each day. This edition would not have happened without the continued support of the staff at Elsevier, especially Lucia Gunzel, who has made each edition significantly better and who provides the good cheer that allows us to complete this book. I would also like to acknowledge my colleagues at the Icahn School of Medicine at Mount Sinai School who continue to value the contribution that this book represents. Last, but not least, our loyal readers, who have made this book a success for more than 25 years and continue to value and use it in a manner that enhances their professional pursuits.

Ronald Hoffman, MD

To my wife, Peggy, for your support, inspiration, and partnership; to our children, Tim, Jenny, Julie, and Rob, for your understanding; to our grandchildren for delighting us during this phase of our lives; to my mentors, Art Parde, Arthur Nienhuis, Bernie Forget, and David Nathan, for your support and guidance; to Addy Donnelly and Amy Thorp, for your incredible skill, patience, and good humor throughout this project; and to the many patients and volunteers whose willingness to participate in clinical research made much of the knowledge conveyed by this book possible.

Edward J. Benz, Jr., MD

To my friends and family for their love and support; to my mentors, Eugene M. Berkman and Robert S. Schwartz, who have provided me with invaluable guidance; to my colleagues at the University of Pennsylvania and Harvard, who have helped me develop academic transfusion medicine programs; and to the trainees who make this endeavor enjoyable and worthwhile.

Leslie E. Silberstein, MD

To my family, friends, and all of my present and former colleagues and trainees for their support and encouragement; to all my mentors in hematology who have provided guidance, in particular, Michael Beard and Malcolm Brenner.

Helen E. Heslop, MD

To my wife, Julia, for her love and unwavering support: I would be lost without her; to my children, Daniel and Kyle, for their understanding and encouragement; to Gwen, for extending our family; to my colleagues for providing me with an environment for learning and growth; and to my trainees, for making this all worthwhile.

Jeffrey I. Weitz, MD

To my respected clinical colleagues with appreciation for trusting me with the diagnostic material from their patients; to my esteemed teachers, Jim Vardiman, Diana Variakojis, and from long ago, C. Robert Valeri, for your many lessons focused on things at both ends of the microscope; and to my awesome trainees; it is always a great pleasure to watch you grow to appreciate the serious, yet amazing, nature of our work.

John Anastasi, MD

I wish to express my appreciation to my family. I am grateful for the support, love, and inspiration from Nahla, Youssef, and Farah.

Mohamed E. Salama, MD

CONTRIBUTORS

Omar Abdel-Wahab, MD
Assistant Member in the Human Oncology and Pathogenesis Program, Attending Physician, Leukemia Service, Department of Medicine, Memorial Sloan Kettering Cancer Center, New York, New York
Stem Cell Model of Hematologic Diseases

Janet L. Abrahm, MD
Professor of Medicine, Harvard Medical School; Division of Adult Palliative Care, Department of Psychosocial Oncology and Palliative Care, Dana-Farber Cancer Institute; Division of Palliative Medicine, Department of Medicine, Brigham and Women's Hospital, Boston, Massachusetts
Palliative Care

Sharon Adams, MT, CHS (ABHI)
Supervisor, HLA Laboratory, Department of Transfusion Medicine, NIH Clinical Center, Bethesda, Maryland
Human Leukocyte Antigen and Human Neutrophil Antigen Systems

Adeboye H. Adewoye, MD
Director, Clinical Research Hematology-Oncology, Gilead Sciences, Inc, Foster City, California
Pathobiology of the Human Erythrocyte and Its Hemoglobins

Carl Allen, MD, PhD
Associate Professor of Pediatrics, Baylor College of Medicine, Houston, Texas
Infectious Mononucleosis and Other Epstein-Barr Virus-Associated Diseases

Richard F. Ambinder, MD, PHD
Professor of Oncology, Johns Hopkins School of Medicine, Baltimore, Maryland
Virus-Associated Lymphomas

Claudio Anasetti, MD
Blood and Marrow Transplantation, Moffitt Cancer Center, Tampa, Florida
Unrelated Donor Hematopoietic Cell Transplantation

John Anastasi, MD
Associate Professor, Department of Pathology, University of Chicago, Pritzker School of Medicine; Director, Secton of Hematopathology, Clinical Hematology Laboratory, University of Chicago Medical Center, Chicago, Illinois
The Pathologic Basis for the Classification of Non-Hodgkin and Hodgkin Lymphomas

Julia A. Anderson, MBChB, MD
Consultant Hematologist, Department of Clinical and Laboratory Hematology, Royal Infirmary of Edinburgh, Edinburgh, Scotland; Honorary Senior Lecturer, College of Medicine and Veterinary Medicine, University of Edinburgh, Edinburgh, Scotland
Hypercoagulable States

Joseph H. Antin, MD
Professor of Medicine, Harvard Medical School; Chief, Stem Cell Transplantation, Dana-Farber Cancer Institute, Boston, Massachusetts
Allogeneic Hematopoietic Stem Cell Transplantation for Acute Myeloid Leukemia and Myelodysplastic Syndrome in Adults

Asok C. Antony, MD, MACP
Chancellor's Professor of Medicine, Indiana University School of Medicine, Indianapolis, Indiana
Megaloblastic Anemias

David J. Araten, MD
Assistant Professor, New York University School of Medicine, New York VA Medical Center, Division of Hematology, Laura and Isaac Perlmutter Cancer Center, New York University Langone Medical Center, New York, New York
Complement and Immunoglobulin Biology Leading to Clinical Translation

Philippe Armand, MD, PhD
Associate Professor of Medicine, Medical Oncology, Dana-Farber Cancer Institute, Boston, Massachusetts
Immune Checkpoint Blockade in Hematologic Malignancies

Gillian Armstrong, PhD
The EMMES Corporation, Rockville, Maryland
Investigational New Drug–Enabling Processes for Cell-Based Therapies

Scott A. Armstrong, MD, PhD
Chairman, Department of Pediatric Oncology, Dana-Farber Cancer Institute; Associate Chief, Division of Hematology/Oncology, Boston Children's Hospital; David G. Nathan Professor of Pediatrics, Harvard Medical School, Boston, Massachusetts
Pathobiology of Acute Lymphoblastic Leukemia

Donald M. Arnold, MD, MSc
Associate Professor of Medicine, Michael G. DeGroote School of Medicine, McMaster University; Associate Medical Director, Canadian Blood Services, Hamilton, Ontario, Canada
Diseases of Platelet Number: Immune Thrombocytopenia, Neonatal Alloimmune Thrombocytopenia, and Posttransfusion Purpura

Andrew S. Artz, MD, MS
Associate Professor of Medicine, Section of Hematology/Oncology, University of Chicago, Chicago, Illinois
Hematology in Aging

Farrukh T. Awan, MD, MS
Associate Professor of Medicine, Division of Hematology, The Ohio State University, Columbus, Ohio
Chronic Lymphocytic Leukemia

Trevor P. Baglin, MB, PhD
Consultant Hematologist, Hematology, Addenbrookes Hospital, Cambridge University Teaching Hospitals, Cambridge, United Kingdom
Regulatory Mechanisms in Hemostasis

Don M. Benson, Jr., MD
Associate Professor of Clinical Internal Medicine, Department of Internal Medicine, Division of Hematology, The Ohio State University Comprehensive Cancer Center, Columbus, Ohio
Natural Killer Cell Immunity

Edward J. Benz, Jr., MD
President and CEO Emeritus, Dana-Farber Cancer Institute;
Richard and Susan Smith Distinguished Professor of Medicine,
Professor of Pediatrics, Professor of Genetics, Harvard Medical
School, Director and Principal Investigator Emeritus, Dana-Farber/
Harvard Cancer Center, Boston, Massachusetts
Anatomy and Physiology of the Gene
Pathobiology of the Human Erythrocyte and Its Hemoglobins
*Hemoglobin Variants Associated With Hemolytic Anemia, Altered
Oxygen Affinity, and Methemoglobinemias*

Nancy Berliner, MD
Chief, Division of Hematology, Medicine, Brigham and Women's
Hospital; Professor of Medicine, Harvard Medical School, Boston,
Massachusetts
Anatomy and Physiology of the Gene
Granulocytopoiesis and Monocytopoiesis

Govind Bhagat, MD
Professor of Pathology and Cell Biology, Division of
Hematopathology, Columbia University Medical Center, New York,
New York
T-Cell Lymphomas

Nina Bhardwaj, MD, PhD
Director, Immunotherapy, Hess Center for Science and Medicine;
Professor of Medicine, Division of Hematology and Oncology,
Mount Sinai, Tisch Cancer Institute, New York, New York
Dendritic Cell Biology

Ravi Bhatia, MBBS, MD
Professor of Medicine, Director, Division of Hematology/
Oncology, Deputy Director, University of Alabama at Birmingham
Comprehensive Cancer Center, Birmingham, Alabama
Chronic Myeloid Leukemia

Smita Bhatia, MD, MPH
Professor, Division of Pediatric Hematology/Oncology, Vice Chair,
Department of Pediatrics, Director, Institute of Cancer Outcomes
and Survivorship, University of Alabama at Birmingham School of
Medicine, Associate Director, University of Alabama at Birmingham
Comprehensive Cancer Center, Birmingham, Alabama
Late Complications of Hematologic Diseases and Their Therapies

Mihir D. Bhatt, MD, FRCPC
Clinical Scholar, Pediatric Hematology/Oncology, McMaster
University, Hamilton, Ontario, Canada
Disorders of Coagulation in the Neonate

Vijaya Raj Bhatt, MD
Assistant Professor, Internal Medicine, Division of Oncology and
Hematology, University of Nebraska Medical Center, Omaha,
Nebraska
Mantle Cell Lymphoma

Menachem Bitan, MD, PhD
Director, Pediatric Blood and Marrow Transplantation and
Immunotherapy Program, Department of Pediatric, Hematology/
Oncology, Tel-Aviv Sourasky Medical Center, Tel-Aviv, Israel
*Interactions Between Hematopoietic Stem and Progenitor Cells and the
Bone Marrow: Current Biology of Stem Cell Homing and Mobilization*

Craig D. Blinderman, MD, MA
Director, Adult Palliative Care Service, Department of Medicine,
Columbia University Medical Center, NewYork-Presbyterian
Hospital; Associate Professor of Medicine, Department of Medicine,
Columbia University, New York, New York
Pain Management and Antiemetic Therapy in Hematologic Disorders

Catherine M. Bollard, MBChB, MD
Associate Professor, Department of Pediatric Hematology Oncology,
Baylor College of Medicine, Houston, Texas
Malignant Lymphomas in Childhood

Benjamin S. Braun, MD, PhD
Associate Professor of Pediatrics, University of California, San
Francisco, San Francisco, California
*Myelodysplastic Syndromes and Myeloproliferative Neoplasms in
Children*

Malcolm K. Brenner, MD, PhD
Professor and Fayez Sarofim Chair, Center for Cell and Gene
Therapy, Baylor College of Medicine, Methodist Hospital,
Houston, Texas
T Cell Therapy of Hematologic Diseases

Gary M. Brittenham, MD
James A. Wolff Professor of Pediatrics and Professor of Medicine,
Department of Pediatrics, Columbia University College of
Physicians and Surgeons; Attending Pediatrician, Pediatrics,
Children's Hospital of New York, New York, New York
Pathophysiology of Iron Homeostasis
Disorders of Iron Homeostasis: Iron Deficiency and Overload

Robert A. Brodsky, MD
Professor of Medicine and Oncology, Director, Division of
Hematology, The Johns Hopkins University School of Medicine,
Baltimore, Maryland
Paroxysmal Nocturnal Hemoglobinuria

Myles Brown, MD
Director, Center for Functional Cancer Epigenetics, Dana-Farber
Cancer Institute; Professor, Department of Medicine, Harvard
Medical School, Boston, Massachusetts
Epigenetics and Epigenomics

Hal E. Broxmeyer, PhD
Distinguished Professor of Microbiology and Immunology, Indiana
University School of Medicine, Indianapolis, Indiana
Cytokine/Receptor Families and Signal Transduction

Kathleen Brummel-Ziedins, PhD
Associate Professor of Biochemistry, University of Vermont,
Burlington, Vermont
Molecular Basis of Blood Coagulation

Andrew M. Brunner, MD
Massachusetts General Hospital Cancer Center, Instructor in
Medicine, Harvard Medical School, Boston, Massachusetts
Pathobiology of Acute Myeloid Leukemia
Hematologic Manifestations of Malignancy

Francis K. Buadi, MD
Assistant Professor of Medicine, College of Medicine, Cons-
Hematology, Mayo Clinic, Rochester, Minnesota
Immunoglobulin Light Chain Amyloidosis (Primary Amyloidosis)

Birgit Burkhardt, MD, PhD
Pediatric Hematology and Oncology, University Hospital Münster,
Münster, Germany
Malignant Lymphomas in Childhood

Melissa Burns, MD
Instructor in Pediatrics, Harvard Medical School, Boston,
Massachusetts
Pathobiology of Acute Lymphoblastic Leukemia

John C. Byrd, MD
Professor of Medicine, Division of Hematology, The Ohio State
University, Columbus, Ohio
Chronic Lymphocytic Leukemia

Paolo F. Caimi, MD
Seidman Cancer Center, Division of Hematology and Oncology, Case Comprehensive Cancer Center, University Hospitals, Case Medical Center, Cleveland, Ohio
Pharmacology and Molecular Mechanisms of Antineoplastic Agents for Hematologic Malignancies

Michael A. Caligiuri, MD
JL Marakas Nationwide Insurance Enterprise Foundation Chair of Cancer Research, Director, Comprehensive Cancer Center, Department of Internal Medicine, Division of Hematology, The Ohio State University Comprehensive Cancer Center, Columbus, Ohio
Natural Killer Cell Immunity

Michelle Canavan, MB, PhD
Specialist Registrar in Geriatric Medicine, University Hospital Limerick, Limerick, Ireland
Stroke

Alan B. Cantor, MD, PhD
Associate Professor of Pediatrics, Division of Pediatric Hematology/Oncology, Boston Children's Hospital and Dana-Farber Cancer Institute, Harvard Medical School, Boston, Massachusetts
Thrombocytopoiesis

Manuel Carcao, MD, MSc
Hematologist, Division of Haematology/Oncology; Department of Paediatrics, Senior Associate Scientist, Child Health Evaluative Sciences, Research Institute; The Hospital for Sick Children, Associate Professor of Pediatrics, University of Toronto, Toronto, Ontario, Canada
Hemophilia A and B

Michael C. Carroll, PhD
Professor of Pediatrics, Harvard Medical School; Senior Investigator, Program in Cellular and Molecular Medicine, Boston Children's Hospital, Boston, Massachusetts
Complement and Immunoglobulin Biology Leading to Clinical Translation

Shannon A. Carty, MD
Assistant Professor, Division of Hematology/Oncology, Department of Medicine, University of Michigan, Ann Arbor, Michigan
T-Cell Immunity

Jorge J. Castillo, MD
Physician, Hematologic Malignancies, Dana-Farber Cancer Institute; Assistant Professor, Harvard Medical School, Boston, Massachusetts
Waldenström Macroglobulinemia/Lymphoplasmacytic Lymphoma

Anthony K.C. Chan, MBBS, FRCPC, FRCPath
Professor of Pediatrics, McMaster University, Hamilton, Ontario, Canada
Disorders of Coagulation in the Neonate

John Chapin, MD
Assistant Professor of Medicine, Weill Cornell Medicine; Assistant Attending Physician, Hematologic Oncology, NewYork-Presbyterian Hospital, New York, New York
Thalassemia Syndromes

April Chiu, MD
Associate Attending, Memorial Sloan Kettering Cancer Center, Hematopathology Service, Departments of Pathology and Laboratory Medicine, New York, New York
Hodgkin Lymphoma: Clinical Manifestations, Staging, and Therapy

John P. Chute, MD
Professor of Medicine and Radiation Oncology, Division of Hematology/Oncology, Broad Stem Cell Research Center, University of California, Los Angeles, Los Angeles, California
Hematopoietic Stem Cell Biology

David B. Clark, PhD
President, Platte Canyon Consulting, Inc., Shawnee, Colorado; Chairman, The Coalition for Hemophilia B, New York, New York
Preparation of Plasma-Derived and Recombinant Human Plasma Proteins

Thomas D. Coates, MD
Professor of Pediatrics and Pathology, University of Southern California Keck School of Medicine; Division Head for Hematology, Children's Center for Cancer and Blood Diseases, Children's Hospital Los Angeles, Los Angeles, California
Disorders of Phagocyte Function

Christopher R. Cogle, MD
Professor of Medicine, Hematology-Oncology, University of Florida, Gainesville, Florida
Regulation of Gene Expression, Transcription, Splicing and RNA Metabolism

Nathan T. Connell, MD, MPH
Instructor in Medicine, Harvard Medical School, Hematology Division, Brigham and Women's Hospital, Boston, Massachusetts
The Spleen and Its Disorders

Elizabeth Cooke, RN, MN, AOCN, PMHNP-BC
Nurse Practitioner, City of Hope National Medical Center, Duarte, California
Psychosocial Aspects of Hematologic Disorders

Sarah Cooley, MD
Associate Professor of Medicine, Department of Medicine, Division of Hematology, Oncology, and Transplantation, University of Minnesota; Associate Director, Cancer Experimental Therapeutics Initiative, Masonic Cancer Center, Minneapolis, Minnesota
Natural Killer Cell-Based Therapies

Paolo Corradini, MD
Professor of Hematology; Chairman, Department of Oncology and Hemato-oncology, University of Milano, Milan, Italy
T-Cell Lymphomas

Mark A. Creager, MD
Director, Heart and Vascular Center, Dartmouth-Hitchcock Medical Center, Anna Gundlach Huber Professor of Medicine, Geisel School of Medicine at Dartmouth, Lebanon, New Hampshire
Peripheral Artery Disease

Richard J. Creger, PharmD
Clinical Associate Professor of Medicine, Case Western Reserve University School of Medicine, Cleveland, Ohio
Pharmacology and Molecular Mechanisms of Antineoplastic Agents for Hematologic Malignancies

Caroline Cromwell, MD
Assistant Professor of Hematology/Oncology, Mount Sinai Hospital, New York, New York
Hematologic Changes in Pregnancy

Mark A. Crowther, MD, MSc, FRCPC
Professor of Medicine and Pathology and Molecular Medicine, Medicine, McMaster University, Hamilton, Ontario, Canada
Hematologic Manifestations of Renal Disease

Melissa M. Cushing, MD
Director, Transfusion Medicine and Cellular Therapy, Weill Cornell Medical College, New York, New York
Principles of Red Blood Cell Transfusion

Corey Cutler, MD, MPH, FRCP(C)
Associate Professor, Harvard Medical School; Department of Medical Oncology, Dana-Farber Cancer Institute, Boston, Massachusetts
Allogeneic Hematopoietic Stem Cell Transplantation for Acute Myeloid Leukemia and Myelodysplastic Syndrome in Adults

Chi V. Dang, MD, PhD
Professor and Director, Abramson Cancer Center, University of Pennsylvania, Philadelphia, Pennsylvania
Control of Cell Division

Nika N. Danial, PhD
Associate Professor of Medicine, Dana-Farber Cancer Institute, Harvard Medical School, Boston, Massachusetts
Cell Death

Sandeep S. Dave, MD, MS
Associate Professor of Medicine, Department of Medicine, Division of Hematologic Malignances, Duke University School of Medicine, Durham, North Carolina
Origin of Non-Hodgkin Lymphoma

James A. DeCaprio, MD
Professor of Medicine, Medical Oncology, Dana-Farber Cancer Institute; Professor of Medicine, Brigham and Women's Hospital; Professor of Medicine, Harvard Medical School, Boston, Massachusetts
Control of Cell Division

Mary C. Dinauer, MD, PhD
Fred M. Saigh Distinguished Chair of Pediatric Research, Pediatrics, Pathology and Immunology, Washington University School of Medicine, St. Louis, Missouri
Disorders of Phagocyte Function

Shira Dinner, BA, MD
Assistant Professor, Northwestern University, Division of Hematology/Oncology, Robert H. Lurie Comprehensive Cancer Center, Chicago, Illinois
Acute Lymphoblastic Leukemia in Adults

Reyhan Diz-Küçükkaya
Professor of Medicine and Hematology, Istanbul Bilim University Faculty of Medicine, Department of Internal Medicine, Division of Hematology, Istanbul, Turkey
Acquired Disorders of Platelet Function

Roger Y. Dodd, PhD
Executive Scientific Officer, Medical Office, American Red Cross, Holland Laboratory, Rockville, Maryland
Transfusion-Transmitted Diseases

Michele L. Donato, MD, FACP
Director, Adult Blood and Marrow Transplantation, John Theurer Cancer Center, Hackensack, New Jersey
Practical Aspects of Hematologic Stem Cell Harvesting and Mobilization

Kenneth Dorshkind, PhD
Vice-Chair of Research, Department of Pathology and Laboratory Medicine, David Geffen School of Medicine, University of California, Los Angeles, Los Angeles, California
B-Cell Development

Gianpietro Dotti, MD
Professor, Center for Cell and Gene Therapy, Baylor College of Medicine, Houston, Texas
T-Cell Therapy of Hematologic Diseases

Yigal Dror, MD, FRCP(C)
Division of Haematology/Oncology, Head, Haematology Section, Director, Marrow Failure and Myelodysplasia Program, Senior Scientist, Program in Genetics and Genome Biology, Research Institute, The Hospital for Sick Children, Institute of Medical Sciences, University of Toronto, Toronto, Ontario, Canada
Inherited Bone Marrow Failure Syndromes

Kieron Dunleavy, MD
Attending Physician and Investigator, Lymphoid Malignancies Branch, National Cancer Institute, Bethesda, Maryland
Diagnosis and Treatment of Diffuse Large B-Cell Lymphoma and Burkitt Lymphoma

Christopher C. Dvorak, MD
Associate Professor and Chief, Pediatric Allergy, Immunology, and Bone Marrow Transplant, University of California, San Francisco, San Francisco, California
Myelodysplastic Syndromes and Myeloproliferative Neoplasms in Children

Benjamin L. Ebert, MD, PhD
Professor of Medicine, Division of Hematology, Brigham and Women's Hospital; Director, Joint Leukemia Center, Dana-Farber/Brigham and Women's Cancer Center, Harvard Medical School, Boston, Massachusetts
Pathobiology of the Human Erythrocyte and Its Hemoglobins
Hemoglobin Variants Associated With Hemolytic Anemia, Altered Oxygen Affinity, and Methemoglobinemias
Myelodysplastic Syndromes

Michael J. Eck, MD, PhD
Professor of Cancer Biology, Dana-Farber Cancer Institute; Professor of Biological Chemistry and Molecular Pharmacology, Harvard Medical School, Boston, Massachusetts
Protein Architecture: Relationship of Form and Function

John W. Eikelboom, MBBS, MSc, FRACP, FRCPA, FRCPC
Associate Professor of Medicine, Division of Hematology and Thromboembolism, McMaster University, Hamilton, Ontario, Canada
Acute Coronary Syndromes

Narendranath Epperla, MD, MS
Fellow, Hematology and Oncology, Medical College of Wisconsin, Milwaukee, Wisconsin
Thrombotic Thrombocytopenic Purpura and the Hemolytic Uremic Syndromes

William B. Ershler, MD
Scientific Director, Hematology, Institute for Advanced Studies in Aging, Falls Church, Virginia
Hematology in Aging

William E. Evans, PharmD
ALSAC Chair in Pharmacogenomics, St. Jude Children's Research Hospital; Professor of Pediatrics and Clinical Pharmacy, University of Tennessee Colleges of Medicine and Pharmacy, Memphis, Tennessee
Pharmacogenomics and Hematologic Diseases

Stefan Faderl, MD
Chief, Division of Leukemia, John Theurer Cancer Center, Hackensack, New Jersey
Clinical Manifestations and Treatment of Acute Myeloid Leukemia

James L.M. Ferrara, MD, DSc
Ward-Coleman Professor of Cancer Medicine, The Tisch Cancer Institute, Icahn School of Medicine at Mount Sinai, New York, New York
Graft-versus-Host Disease and Graft-versus-Leukemia Responses

Alexandra Hult Filipovich, MD
Professor of Pediatrics, Bone Marrow Transplantation and Immune Deficiency, Cincinnati Children's Hospital Medical Center/University of Cincinnati, Cincinnati, Ohio
Histiocytic Disorders

Martin Fischer, PhD
Molecular Oncology, University of Leipzig Medical School, Leipzig, Germany; Department of Medical Oncology, Dana-Farber Cancer Institute, Department of Medicine, Brigham and Women's Hospital and Harvard Medical School, Boston, Massachusetts
Control of Cell Division

James C. Fredenburgh, PhD
Scientist, Research Associate, McMaster University, Hamilton, Ontario, Canada
Overview of Hemostasis and Thrombosis

Kenneth D. Friedman, MD
Medical Director, BloodCenter of Wisconsin; Associate Professor, Departments of Internal Medicine and Pathology, Medical College of Wisconsin, Milwaukee, Wisconsin
Thrombotic Thrombocytopenic Purpura and the Hemolytic Uremic Syndromes

Ephraim Fuchs, MD, MBA
Professor of Oncology and Immunology, Sidney Kimmel Comprehensive Cancer Center at Johns Hopkins, Baltimore, Maryland
Haploidentical Hematopoietic Cell Transplantation

Stephen J. Fuller, MB BS, PhD, FRACP, FRCPA
Senior Lecturer, Medicine, Sydney Medical School, The University of Sydney, Sydney, New South Wales, Australia
Heme Biosynthesis and Its Disorders: Porphyrias and Sideroblastic Anemias

David Gailani, MD
Professor of Pathology, Microbiology, and Immunology, Professor of Medicine, Medical Director, Clinical Coagulation Laboratory, Department of Pathology, Microbiology, and Immunology, Vanderbilt University Medical Center, Nashville, Tennessee
Rare Coagulation Factor Deficiencies

Jacques Galipeau, MD, FRCP(C)
Don and Marilyn Anderson Professor of Oncology, Assistant Dean for Therapeutics Discovery and Development, Director, Program for Advanced Cell Therapy, University of Wisconsin in Madison, Madison, Wisconsin
Mesenchymal Stromal Cells

Patrick G. Gallagher, MD
Professor of Pediatrics, Pathology, and Genetics, Yale University School of Medicine, New Haven, Connecticut
Red Blood Cell Membrane Disorders

Karthik A. Ganapathi, MD, PhD
Assistant Professor, Department of Laboratory Medicine, University of California, San Francisco, San Francisco, California
T-Cell Lymphomas

Lawrence B. Gardner, MD
Associate Professor of Medicine, Associate Professor of Biochemistry and Molecular Pharmacology, New York University School of Medicine, New York, New York
Anemia of Chronic Diseases

Adrian P. Gee, PhD
Professor of Pediatrics and Medicine, Center for Cell and Gene Therapy, Baylor College of Medicine, Houston, Texas
Graft Engineering and Cell Processing

Stanton L. Gerson, MD
Director, Case Comprehensive Cancer Center, Case Western Reserve University, University Hospitals Seidman Cancer Center, Cleveland, Ohio
Pharmacology and Molecular Mechanisms of Antineoplastic Agents for Hematologic Malignancies

Morie A. Gertz, MD, MACP
Chair and Seidler Professor of Medicine, Mayo Clinic, Rochester, Minnesota
Immunoglobulin Light Chain Amyloidosis (Primary Amyloidosis)

Patricia J. Giardina, MD
Professor of Clinical Pediatrics, Weill Cornell Medicine; Attending Pediatrician, Pediatrics, NewYork-Presbyterian Hospital, New York, New York
Thalassemia Syndromes

Christopher J. Gibson, MD, PhD
Dana-Farber Cancer Center, Boston, Massachusetts
Myelodysplastic Syndromes

Karin Golan, PhD
Postdoctoral Fellow, Department of Immunology, Weizmann Institute of Science, Rehovot, Israel
Interactions Between Hematopoietic Stem and Progenitor Cells and the Bone Marrow: Current Biology of Stem Cell Homing and Mobilization

Todd R. Golub, MD
Professor of Pediatrics, Harvard Medical School; Chief Scientific Officer, Broad Institute of MIT and Harvard; Charles A. Dana Investigator, Dana-Farber Cancer Institute, Boston, Massachusetts
Genomic Approaches to Hematology

Matthew J. Gonzales, MD
Institute for Human Caring, Providence Health & Services, Torrance, California
Psychosocial Aspects of Hematologic Disorders

Jason Gotlib, MD, MS
Professor of Medicine, Medicine/Hematology, Stanford University School of Medicine, Stanford, California
Eosinophilia, Eosinophil-Associated Diseases, Eosinophil Leukemias, and the Hypereosinophilic Syndromes
Mast Cells and Mastocytosis

Stephen Gottschalk, MD
Professor of Pediatrics, Baylor College of Medicine, Center for Cell and Gene Therapy, Baylor College of Medicine, Texas Children's Hospital, Houston Methodist Hospital, Houston, Texas
Infectious Mononucleosis and Other Epstein-Barr Virus-Associated Diseases

Marianne A. Grant, PhD
Assistant Professor of Medicine, Department of Medicine, Beth Israel Deaconess Medical Center, Harvard Medical School, Boston, Massachusetts
The Blood Vessel Wall

Timothy A. Graubert, MD
Director, Hematologic Malignancies, Massachusetts General Hospital Cancer Center; Professor of Medicine, Harvard Medical School, Boston, Massachusetts
Pathobiology of Acute Myeloid Leukemia

Xylina T. Gregg, MD
Hematology and Oncology, Practicing Physician, Utah Cancer Specialists, Salt Lake City, Utah
Red Blood Cell Enzymopathies

John G. Gribben, MD, DSc, FMedSci
Professor of Medical Oncology, Barts Cancer Institute, Queen Mary University of London, London, United Kingdom
Clinical Manifestations, Staging, and Treatment of Follicular Lymphoma

Dawn M. Gross, MD, PhD, FAAHPM
Division of Palliative Medicine, University of California, San Francisco, San Francisco, California
Psychosocial Aspects of Hematologic Disorders

Tanja A. Gruber, MD, PhD
Associate Member of Oncology, St. Jude Children's Research Hospital, Memphis, Tennessee
Acute Myeloid Leukemia in Children

Joan Guitart, MD
Associate Professor, Department of Dermatology, Northwestern University Medical School; Northwestern Memorial Hospital, Chicago, Illinois
T-Cell Lymphomas

Sandeep Gurbuxani, MBBS, PhD
Associate Professor, Department of Pathology, The University of Chicago, Chicago, Illinois
Acute Lymphoblastic Leukemia in Adults

Shiri Gur-Cohen, PhD
Immunology Postdoctoral Fellow, Weizmann Institute of Science, Rehovot, Israel
Interactions Between Hematopoietic Stem and Progenitor Cells and the Bone Marrow: Current Biology of Stem Cell Homing and Mobilization

Alejandro Gutierrez, MD
Assistant Professor of Pediatrics, Division of Hematology/Oncology, Boston Children's Hospital and Dana-Farber Cancer Institute, Harvard Medical School, Boston, Massachusetts
Pathobiology of Acute Lymphoblastic Leukemia

Mehdi Hamadani, MD
Associate Professor of Medicine, Division of Hematology and Oncology, CIBMTR and Medical College of Wisconsin, Milwaukee, Wisconsin
Indications and Outcomes of Allogeneic Hematopoietic Cell Transplantation for Hematologic Malignancies in Adults

Parameswaran N. Hari, MD, MS
Armand Quick William Stapp Professor of Hematology, Division of Hematology Oncology, Medical College of Wisconsin, Milwaukee, Wisconsin
Indications and Outcomes of Allogeneic Hematopoietic Cell Transplantation for Hematologic Malignancies in Adults

John H. Hartwig, MD
Professor, Department of Medicine, Brigham and Women's Hospital, Harvard Medical School, Boston, Massachusetts
Megakaryocyte and Platelet Structure

Suzanne R. Hayman, MD
Assistant Professor of Medicine, College of Medicine, Cons-Hematology, Mayo Clinic, Rochester, Minnesota
Immunoglobulin Light Chain Amyloidosis (Primary Amyloidosis)

Catherine P.M. Hayward, MD, PhD
Professor of Pathology and Molecular Medicine and Medicine, McMaster University; Hematologist, Division of Hematology and Thromboembolism, Hamilton Health Sciences and St. Joseph's Healthcare; Head, Coagulation, Hamilton Regional Laboratory Medicine Program, Hamilton, Ontario, Canada
Clinical Approach to the Patient with Bleeding or Bruising

Robert P. Hebbel, MD
Regents Professor and Clark Professor, Department of Medicine, Division of Hematology-Oncology-Transplantation, Director, Vascular Biology Center, University of Minnesota Medical School, Minneapolis, Minnesota
Pathobiology of Sickle Cell Disease

Helen E. Heslop, MD
Dan L. Duncan Chair, Professor of Medicine and Pediatrics, Director, Center for Cell and Gene Therapy, Baylor College of Medicine, Houston Methodist Hospital and Texas Children's Hospital, Houston, Texas
Overview and Historical Perspective of Current Cell-Based Therapies
Overview and Choice of Donor of Hematopoietic Stem Cell Transplantation

Christopher Hillis, MD
Assistant Professor, Department of Oncology, McMaster University, Hamilton, Ontario, Canada
Hematologic Manifestations of Liver Disease

Christopher D. Hillyer, MD
Professor, Department of Medicine, Weill Cornell Medical College; President and Chief Executive Officer, New York Blood Center, New York, New York
Transfusion of Plasma and Plasma Derivatives: Plasma, Cryoprecipitate, Albumin, and Immunoglobulins

Karin Ho, MD
Assistant Professor of Surgery, Northwestern Medicine, Feinberg School of Medicine, Chicago, Illinois
Disorders of Coagulation in the Neonate

David M. Hockenbery, MD
Full Member, Clinical Research, Fred Hutchinson Cancer Research Center; Professor, Internal Medicine, University of Washington, Seattle, Washington
Cell Death

Ronald Hoffman, MD
Albert A. and Vera G. List Professor of Medicine, Tisch Cancer Institute, Hematology-Oncology Section, Department of Medicine, Icahn School of Medicine at Mount Sinai, New York, New York
Progress in the Classification of Hematopoietic and Lymphoid Neoplasms: Clinical Implications
The Polycythemias
Essential Thrombocythemia
Primary Myelofibrosis

Kerstin E. Hogg, MBChB, MD, MSc
Assistant Professor, Department of Medicine, McMaster University, Hamilton, Ontario, Canada
Hypercoagulable States

Shernan G. Holtan, MD
Assistant Professor, University of Minnesota, Minneapolis, Minnesota
Complications after Hematopoietic Cell Transplantation

Hans-Peter Horny, MD
Professor, Institute of Pathology, Ludwig Maximilian University of Munich, Munich, Germany
Mast Cells and Mastocytosis

Yen-Michael S. Hsu, MD, PhD
Assistant Professor, Pathology and Laboratory Medicine, Weill Cornell Medical College, New York, New York
Principles of Red Blood Cell Transfusion

Zachary R. Hunter, MA
Department of Pathology and Laboratory Medicine, Boston University School of Medicine, Boston, Massachusetts
Waldenström Macroglobulinemia/Lymphoplasmacytic Lymphoma

James A. Huntington, PhD
Professor, Department of Hematology, University of Cambridge, Cambridge, United Kingdom
Regulatory Mechanisms in Hemostasis

Camelia Iancu-Rubin, PhD
Associate Professor, Medicine, Hematology, and Medical Oncology, Icahn School of Medicine at Mount Sinai, New York, New York
Essential Thrombocythemia

Ali Iqbal, BHSc, MD
Internal Medicine, McMaster University, Hamilton, Ontario, Canada
Hematologic Manifestations of Renal Disease

David E. Isenman, PhD
Professor Emeritus, Departments of Biochemistry and Immunology, University of Toronto, Toronto, Ontario, Canada
Complement and Immunoglobulin Biology Leading to Clinical Translation

Sara J. Israels, MD
Professor, Department of Pediatrics and Child Health, Senior Scientist, Research Institute in Oncology and Hematology, University of Manitoba, Winnipeg, Manitoba, Canada
Molecular Basis of Platelet Function

Joseph E. Italiano, Jr., PhD
Associate Professor of Medicine, Brigham and Women's Hospital; Associate Professor, Harvard Medical School; Assistant Professor, Surgery-Vascular Biology Program, Children's Hospital Boston, Boston, Massachusetts
Megakaryocyte and Platelet Structure

Elaine S. Jaffe, MD
Head, Hematopathology Section, Laboratory of Pathology, National Cancer Institute, Bethesda, Maryland
The Pathologic Basis for the Classification of Non-Hodgkin and Hodgkin Lymphomas

Iqbal H. Jaffer, MBBS, PhD
Resident, Division of Cardiac Surgery, Thrombosis and Atherosclerosis Research Institute, McMaster University, Hamilton, Ontario, Canada
Antithrombotic Drugs
Hematologic Problems in the Surgical Patient: Bleeding and Thrombosis

Sundar Jagannath, MBBS
Professor of Medicine, The Tisch Cancer Institute, Icahn School of Medicine at Mount Sinai, New York, New York
Plasma Cell Neoplasms

Ulrich Jäger, MD
Professor, Department of Medicine I, Head, Division of Hematology and Hemostaseology, Medical University of Vienna, Comprehensive Cancer Center, Vienna, Austria
Autoimmune Hemolytic Anemia

Nitin Jain, MD
Assistant Professor, Department of Leukemia, The University of Texas MD Anderson Cancer Center, Houston, Texas
Acute Lymphoblastic Leukemia in Adults

Paula James, MD, FRCPC
Professor, Department of Medicine, Division of Hematology, Queen's University, Kingston, Ontario, Canada
Structure, Biology, and Genetics of Von Willebrand Factor

Sima Jeha, MD
Director, Leukemia/Lymphoma Developmental Therapeutics, Regional Director, East and Mediterranean Region, International Outreach Program, St. Jude Children's Research Hospital, Memphis, Tennessee
Clinical Manifestations and Treatment of Childhood Acute Lymphoblastic Leukemia

Michael B. Jordan, MD
Professor of Pediatrics, Immunology and Bone Marrow Transplantation and Immune Deficiency, Cincinnati Children's Hospital Medical Center/University of Cincinnati, Cincinnati, Ohio
Histiocytic Disorders

Cassandra D. Josephson, MD
Professor of Pathology and Pediatrics, Director of Clinical Research, Director of Transfusion Medicine Fellowship Program, Department of Pathology, Center for Transfusion and Cellular Therapies, Emory University School of Medicine; Medical Director, Pathology Department, Blood and Tissue Services, Children's Healthcare of Atlanta, Atlanta, Georgia
Pediatric Transfusion Medicine

Moonjung Jung, MD
Instructor in Clinical Investigation, The Rockefeller University, New York, New York
Neutrophilic Leukocytosis, Neutropenia, Monocytosis, and Monocytopenia

Leo Kager, MD
Associate Professor of Pediatrics, St. Anna Children's Hospital, Department of Pediatrics, Medical University Vienna, Children's Cancer Research Institute, Vienna, Austria
Pharmacogenomics and Hematologic Diseases

Taku Kambayashi, MD, PhD
Associate Professor, Division of Tranfusion Medicine and Therapeutic Pathology, Department of Pathology and Laboratory Medicine, Perelman School of Medicine at the University of Pennsylvania, Philadelphia, Pennsylvania
Tolerance and Autoimmunity

Jennifer A. Kanakry, MD
Clinical Head of the Experimental Transplantation and Immunology Branch, National Cancer Institute, National Institutes of Health, Bethesda, Maryland
Virus-Associated Lymphomas

Hagop M. Kantarjian, MD
Chairman, Department of Leukemia, The University of Texas MD Anderson Cancer Center, Houston, Texas
Clinical Manifestations and Treatment of Acute Myeloid Leukemia

Jason Kaplan, MD
Assistant Professor of Medicine (Hematology and Oncology), Northwestern University, Feinberg School of Medicine, Chicago, Illinois
T-Cell Lymphomas

Matthew S. Karafin, MD, MS
Associate Medical Director, BloodCenter of Wisconsin; Assistant Professor, Department of Pathology, Medical College of Wisconsin, Milwaukee, Wisconsin
Transfusion of Plasma and Plasma Derivatives: Plasma, Cryoprecipitate, Albumin, and Immunoglobulins

Aly Karsan, MD
Professor of Pathology and Laboratory Medicine, University of British Columbia; Hematopathologist/Senior Scientist, British Columbia Cancer Agency, Vancouver, British Columbia, Canada
The Blood Vessel Wall

Randal J. Kaufman, PhD
Director, Degenerative Diseases Research, Sanford-Burnham-Prebys Medical Discovery Institute, La Jolla, California
Protein Synthesis, Processing, and Trafficking

Richard M. Kaufman, MD
Medical Director, Adult Transfusion Service, Department of Pathology, Brigham and Women's Hospital; Associate Professor of Pathology, Harvard Medical School, Boston, Massachusetts
Clinical Considerations in Platelet Transfusion Therapy

Frank G. Keller, MD
Associate Professor of Pediatrics, Emory University School of Medicine, Atlanta, Georgia
Hematologic Manifestations of Childhood Illness

Kara M. Kelly, MD
Waldemar J. Kaminski Endowed Chair of Pediatrics, Pediatric Oncology, Roswell Park Cancer Institute, University at Buffalo School of Medicine and Biomedical Sciences, Buffalo, New York
Malignant Lymphomas in Childhood

Craig M. Kessler, MD
Professor of Medicine and Pathology, Department of Medicine, Director, Division of Coagulation, Georgetown University Medical Center, Washington, DC
Inhibitors in Hemophilias

Nigel S. Key, MB, ChB, FRCP
Harold R. Roberts Distinguished Professor, Medicine and Pathology and Laboratory Medicine, Chief, Section of Hematology, Division of Hematology/Oncology, Director, University of North Carolina Hemophilia and Thrombosis Center, Co-Director, Thrombosis and Hemostasis Program, McAllister Heart Institute, University of North Carolina, Chapel Hill, North Carolina
Hematologic Problems in the Surgical Patient: Bleeding and Thrombosis

Alla Keyzner, MD
Assistant Professor of Hematology/Oncology, Icahn School of Medicine at Mount Sinai, New York, New York
Primary Myelofibrosis

Alexander G. Khandoga, MD
Department of Cardiology, German Heart Center Munich, Munich, Germany
Chemokines and Hematopoietic Cell Trafficking

Arati Khanna-Gupta, MSc, PhD
VP, Research and Development (Oncology), MedGenome Labs Pvt. Ltd, Bangalore, India
Granulocytopoiesis and Monocytopoiesis

Eman Khatib-Massalha, MSc, PhD Student
Immunology, Weizmann Institute of Science, Rehovot, Israel
Interactions between Hematopoietic Stem and Progenitor Cells and the Bone Marrow: Current Biology of Stem Cell Homing and Mobilization

Harvey G. Klein, MD
Chief, Transfusion Medicine, National Institutes of Health, Bethesda, Maryland; Adjunct Professor, Departments of Medicine and Pathology, The Johns Hopkins School of Medicine, Baltimore, Maryland
Hemapheresis

Birgit Knoechel, MD, PhD
Assistant Professor of Pediatrics, Harvard Medical School; Department of Pediatric Oncology, Dana-Farber Cancer Institute, Broad Institute of MIT and Harvard, Boston, Massachusetts
Genomic Approaches to Hematology

Orit Kollet, PhD
Immunology, Weizmann Institute, Rehovot, Israel
Interactions Between Hematopoietic Stem and Progenitor Cells and the Bone Marrow: Current Biology of Stem Cell Homing and Mobilization

Barbara A. Konkle, MD
Associate Chief Scientific Officer, Bloodworks Northwest; Professor of Medicine, Hematology, University of Washington, Seattle, Washington
Inhibitors in Hemophilias

Dimitrios P. Kontoyiannis, MD
Frances King Black Endowed Professor, Infectious Diseases, Deputy Head, Division of Internal Medicine, The University of Texas MD Anderson Cancer Center, Houston, Texas
Clinical Approach to Infections in the Compromised Host

John Koreth, MBBS, DPhil
Associate Professor, Harvard Medical School, Department of Medical Oncology, Dana-Farber Cancer Institute, Boston, Massachusetts
Allogeneic Hematopoietic Stem Cell Transplantation for Acute Myeloid Leukemia and Myelodysplastic Syndrome in Adults

Gary A. Koretzky, MD, PhD
Francis C. Wood Professor of Medicine, Division of Rheumatology, Abramson Family Cancer Research Institute, University of Pennsylvania, Philadelphia, Pennsylvania
T-Cell Immunity

Dipak Kotecha, MD, PhD
Clinician Scientist in Cardiovascular Medicine, Institute of Cardiovascular Sciences, University of Alabama at Birmingham, Birmingham, Alabama; Adjunct Research Fellow, Monash Centre of Cardiovascular Research and Education, Monash University, Melbourne, Australia
Atrial Fibrillation

Marina Kremyanskaya, MD, PhD
Assistant Professor, The Tisch Cancer Institute, Icahn School of Medicine at Mount Sinai, New York, New York
The Polycythemias
Essential Thrombocythemia
Primary Myelofibrosis

Anju Kumari, PhD
Postdoctoral Fellow, Department of Immunology, Weizmann Institute of Science, Rehovot, Israel
Interactions Between Hematopoietic Stem and Progenitor Cells and the Bone Marrow: Current Biology of Stem Cell Homing and Mobilization

Timothy M. Kuzel, MD, FACP
Professor of Medicine, Chief, Division of Hematology, Department of Internal Medicine, Rush University Medical Center, Chicago, Illinois
T-Cell Lymphomas

Ralf Küppers, MD
Professor, Institute of Cell Biology (Cancer Research), University of Duisburg-Essen Medical School, Essen, Germany
Origin of Hodgkin Lymphoma

Martha Q. Lacy, MD
Professor of Medicine, Myeloma, Amyloidosis, Dysproteinemia Group, Mayo Clinic, Rochester, Minnesota
Immunoglobulin Light Chain Amyloidosis (Primary Amyloidosis)

Elana Ladas, PhD, RD
Assistant Professor of Nutrition, Columbia University, New York, New York
Integrative Therapies in Patients with Hematologic Diseases

Wendy Landier, PhD, CRNP
Associate Professor, Department of Pediatrics, Division of Pediatric Hematology/Oncology, Institute for Cancer Survivorship and Outcomes, School of Medicine, University of Alabama at Birmingham, Birmingham, Alabama
Late Complications of Hematologic Diseases and Their Therapies

Kfir Lapid, PhD
Postdoctoral Fellow, University of Texas Southwestern, Dallas, Texas
Interactions Between Hematopoietic Stem and Progenitor Cells and the Bone Marrow: Current Biology of Stem Cell Homing and Mobilization

Tsvee Lapidot, PhD
Professor, Incumbent of the Edith Arnoff Stein Professorial Chair in Stem Cell Research, Department of Immunology, Weizmann Institute of Science, Rehovot, Israel
Interactions Between Hematopoietic Stem and Progenitor Cells and the Bone Marrow: Current Biology of Stem Cell Homing and Mobilization

Peter J. Larson, BS, MD
Director, Global Clinical Strategy, Biological Products, Research Triangle Park, North Carolina
Transfusion Therapy for Coagulation Factor Deficiencies

Marcel Levi, MD, PhD
Professor of Medicine, University College London Hospitals, University College London, London, United Kingdom
Disseminated Intravascular Coagulation

Russell E. Lewis, PharmD
Associate Professor, Infectious Diseases, Department of Medical and Surgical Sciences, University of Bologna, Bologna, Italy
Clinical Approach to Infections in the Compromised Host

Howard A. Liebman, MA, MD
Professor of Medicine and Pathology, Department of Medicine, Hematology, Keck School of Medicine, University of Southern California, Los Angeles, California
Hematologic Manifestations of HIV/AIDS

David Lillicrap, MD, FRCPC
Professor of Pathology and Molecular Medicine, Queen's University, Kingston, Ontario, Canada
Hemophilia A and B

Wendy Lim, MD, MSc, FRCPC
Associate Professor of Medicine, McMaster University, Hamilton, Ontario, Canada
Venous Thromboembolism
Hematologic Manifestations of Liver Disease

Judith C. Lin, MD
Assistant Professor of Hematology-Oncology, Mount Sinai Hospital, New York, New York
Approach to Anemia in the Adult and Child

Robert Lindblad, MD, FACEP
Chief Medical Officer and Director of Safety and Regulatory Affairs, The EMMES Corporation, Rockville, Maryland
Investigational New Drug–Enabling Processes for Cell-Based Therapies

Gregory Y.H. Lip, MD, FRCP, FACC, FESC
Professor of Cardiovascular Medicine, Institute of Cardiovascular Sciences, University of Birmingham, Birmingham, United Kingdom
Atrial Fibrillation

Jane A. Little, MD
Associate Professor in Hematology/Oncology, Department of Medicine, Case Western Reserve School of Medicine, Cleveland, Ohio
Anemia of Chronic Diseases

Jens G. Lohr, MD, PhD
Assistant Professor of Medicine, Harvard Medical School; Department of Medical Oncology, Dana-Farber Cancer Institute; Department of Medicine, Brigham and Women's Hospital, Broad Institute of MIT and Harvard, Boston, Massachusetts
Genomic Approaches to Hematology

José A. López, MD
Chief Scientific Officer, Research Institute, Bloodworks Northwest; Professor of Medicine and Biochemistry, University of Washington, Seattle, Washington
Acquired Disorders of Platelet Function

Francis W. Luscinskas, PhD
Professor of Pathology, Brigham and Women's Hospital, Boston, Massachusetts
Cell Adhesion

Jaroslaw P. Maciejewski, MD, PhD
Chairman and Professor of Medicine, Department of Translational Hematology and Oncology Research, Taussig Cancer Center, Cleveland Clinic, Cleveland, Ohio
Aplastic Anemia
Acquired Disorders of Red Cell, White Cell, and Platelet Production

Navneet S. Majhail, MD, MS
Director, Blood and Marrow Transplant Program, Cleveland Clinic; Professor, Cleveland Clinic Lerner College of Medicine, Cleveland, Ohio
Complications After Hematopoietic Cell Transplantation

Olivier Manches, PhD
Research Assistant, Division of Hematology and Oncology, Tisch Cancer Institute, Mount Sinai, New York, New York
Dendritic Cell Biology

Robert J. Mandle, PhD
President, Biosciences Research Associates, Inc., Cambridge, Massachusetts
Complement and Immunoglobulin Biology Leading to Clinical Translation

Kenneth G. Mann, PhD
Professor Emeritus, Biochemistry and Medicine, College of Medicine, University of Vermont, Burlington, Vermont; Chairman, Haematologic Technologies Inc., Essex Junction, Vermont
Molecular Basis of Blood Coagulation

Catherine S. Manno, MD
Pat and John Rosenwald Professor and Chair, Department of Pediatrics, New York University School of Medicine, New York, New York
Transfusion Therapy for Coagulation Factor Deficiencies

Andrea N. Marcogliese, MD
Associate Professor, Pathology & Immunology and Pediatrics, Section of Hematology Oncology, Baylor College of Medicine, Houston, Texas
Resources for the Hematologist: Interpretive Comments and Selected Reference Values for Neonatal, Pediatric, and Adult Populations

Guglielmo Mariani, MD
Faculty of Science and Technology, University of Westminster, London, United Kingdom
Inhibitors in Hemophilias

Francesco M. Marincola, MD
Chief Research Officer, Research Branch, Sidra Medical and
Research Center; Professor of Medicine, Weill Cornell Medical
College, Doha, Qatar
Human Leukocyte Antigen and Human Neutrophil Antigen Systems

John Mascarenhas, MD
Associate Professor of Medicine, The Tisch Cancer Institute, Icahn
School of Medicine at Mount Sinai, New York, New York
The Polycythemias
Essential Thrombocythemia
Primary Myelofibrosis

Steffen Massberg, MD
Professor of Cardiology, German Heart Center Munich, Technical
University of Munich, Munich, Germany
Chemokines and Hematopoietic Cell Trafficking

Rodger P. McEver, MD
Member and Chair, Cardiovascular Biology Research Program,
Oklahoma Medical Research Foundation, Oklahoma City,
Oklahoma
Cell Adhesion

Emer McGrath, MB, PhD
Brigham and Women's Hospital, Massachusetts General Hospital,
Harvard Medical School, Boston, Massachusetts
Stroke

Matthew S. McKinney, MD
Instructor in Medicine, Department of Medicine, Division of
Hematologic Malignancies, Duke University School of Medicine,
Durham, North Carolina
Origin of Non-Hodgkin Lymphoma

Rohtesh S. Mehta, MD, MPH, MS
Assistant Professor of Medicine, Stem Cell Transplantation and
Cellular Therapy, The University of Texas MD Anderson Cancer
Center, Houston, Texas
*Unrelated Donor Cord Blood Transplantation for Hematologic
Malignancies*

William C. Mentzer, MD
Professor Emeritus, Pediatrics, University of California, San
Francisco, San Francisco, California
Extrinsic Nonimmune Hemolytic Anemias

Giampaolo Merlini, MD
Director, Amyloidosis Research and Treatment Center, Foundation
IRCCS Policlinico San Matteo, Department of Molecular
Medicine, University of Pavia, Pavia, Italy
Waldenström Macroglobulinemia/Lymphoplasmacytic Lymphoma

Reid Merryman, MD
Clinical Fellow, Dana-Farber/Partners CancerCare Hematology/
Oncology Fellowship Program, Boston, Massachusetts
Immune Checkpoint Blockade in Hematologic Malignancies

Marc Michel, MD
Department of Internal Medicine, National Referral Center for
Adult Immune Cytopenias, Henri Mondor University Hospital,
Assistance Publique Hopitaux de Paris, Creteil, France
Autoimmune Hemolytic Anemia

Anna Rita Migliaccio, PhD
Professor, The Tisch Cancer Institute, Icahn School of Medicine
at Mount Sinai, New York, New York; Professor of Biological and
Neurological Sciences, Alma Mater University, Bologna, Italy
Biology of Erythropoiesis, Erythroid Differentiation, and Maturation

Jeffrey S. Miller, MD
Professor of Medicine, Division of Hematology, Oncology, and
Transplantation, University of Minnesota, Minneapolis, Minnesota
Natural Killer Cell-Based Therapies

Martha P. Mims, MD, PhD
Professor and Chief, Section of Hematology Oncology, Internal
Medicine, Baylor College of Medicine, Houston, Texas
*Lymphocytosis, Lymphocytopenia, Hypergammaglobulinemia, and
Hypogammaglobulinemia*

Traci Heath Mondoro, PhD
Alternate Representative Branch Chief, NHLBI Translational Blood
Science and Resources Branch, Division of Blood Diseases and
Resources, National Heart, Lung, and Blood Institute, National
Institutes of Health, Bethesda, Maryland
Investigational New Drug–Enabling Processes for Cell-Based Therapies

Paul Moorehead, MD
Section of Pediatric Hematology/Oncology, Janeway Children's
Health and Rehabilitation Centre; Clinical Assistant Professor,
Discipline of Pediatrics, Faculty of Medicine, Memorial University,
St. John's, Newfoundland and Labrador, Canada
Hemophilia A and B

Luciana R. Muniz, MD
PhD Student, Icahn School of Medicine at Mount Sinai, Division
of Hematology and Oncology, Tisch Cancer Institute, New York,
New York
Dendritic Cell Biology

Nikhil C. Munshi, MD
Associate Director, Jerome Lipper Multiple Myeloma Center, Dana-
Farber Cancer Institute; Physician, Hematology/Oncology and
Medicine, Boston VA Healthcare System; Associate Professor of
Medicine, Harvard Medical School, Boston, Massachusetts
Plasma Cell Neoplasms

Vesna Najfeld, PhD
Professor of Pathology and Medicine, Director, Tumor
CytoGenomic Laboratory, Icahn School of Medicine at Mount
Sinai, New York, New York
*Conventional and Molecular Cytogenomic Basis of Hematologic
Malignancies*
The Polycythemias
Essential Thrombocythemia
Primary Myelofibrosis

Lalitha Nayak, MD
Assistant Professor in Hematology and Oncology Medicine, Case
Western Reserve University School of Medicine, Cleveland, Ohio
Anemia of Chronic Diseases

Ishac Nazy, PhD
Associate Professor of Medicine, Michael G. DeGroote School of
Medicine, McMaster University, Hamilton, Ontario, Canada
*Diseases of Platelet Number: Immune Thrombocytopenia, Neonatal
Alloimmune Thrombocytopenia, and Posttransfusion Purpura*

Anne T. Neff, MD
Professor of Medicine, Cleveland Clinic Lerner College of
Medicine; Staff Physician, Cleveland Clinic Foundation, Cleveland,
Ohio
Rare Coagulation Factor Deficiencies

Paul M. Ness, MD
Director, Transfusion Medicine, The Johns Hopkins Hospital;
Professor of Pathology and Medicine, The Johns Hopkins
University School of Medicine, Baltimore, Maryland
Principles of Red Blood Cell Transfusion

Luigi D. Notarangelo, MD
Director, Research and Molecular Diagnosis Program on
Primary Immunodeficiencies, Professor of Pediatrics and
Pathology, Children's Hospital, Harvard Medical School, Boston,
Massachusetts
Congenital Disorders of Lymphocyte Function

Sarah H. O'Brien, MD, MSc
Associate Professor of Medicine, The Ohio State University,
Pediatric Hematology/Oncology, Pediatrics, Investigator, Center for
Innovation in Pediatric Practice Research, Nationwide Children's
Hospital, Columbus, Ohio
Hematologic Manifestations of Childhood Illness

Owen A. O'Connor, MD, PhD
Associate Professor of Medicine, Director, Lymphoid Development
and Malignancy Program, Herbert Irving Comprehensive Cancer
Center, Columbia University; Chief, Lymphoma Service, College
of Physicians and Surgeons, Presbyterian Hospital, Columbia
University Medical Center, New York, New York
T-Cell Lymphomas

Martin O'Donnell, MD, PhD
Associate Clinical Professor, Divisions of General Internal Medicine
and Hematology and Thromboembolism, Department of Medicine,
McMaster University, Hamilton, Ontario, Canada
Stroke

Amanda Olson, MD
Assistant Professor, Stem Cell Transplantion and Cellular Therapy,
The University of Texas MD Anderson Cancer Center, Houston,
Texas
*Unrelated Donor Cord Blood Transplantation for Hematologic
Malignancies*

Stuart H. Orkin, MD
David G. Nathan Professor of Pediatrics, Dana-Farber/Boston
Children's Cancer and Blood Disorders Center, Howard Hughes
Medical Institute, Harvard Medical School, Boston, Massachusetts
Hematopoietic Stem Cell Biology

Menaka Pai, BSc, MSc, MD, FRCPC
Associate Professor of Medicine and Associate Member of Pathology
and Molecular Medicine, McMaster University; Consultant
Hematologist, Hamilton Regional Laboratory Medicine Program,
Hamilton, Ontario, Canada
Laboratory Evaluation of Hemostatic and Thrombotic Disorders

Sung-Yun Pai, MD
Associate Professor of Pediatrics, Department of Medicine,
Children's Hospital Boston; Department of Pediatric Oncology,
Dana-Farber Cancer Institute, Boston, Massachusetts
Congenital Disorders of Lymphocyte Function

Michael Paidas, MD
Professor of Obstetrics, Gynecology, and Reproductive Sciences,
Yale University, New Haven, Connecticut
Hematologic Changes in Pregnancy

Sandhya R. Panch, MD, MPH
Staff Clinician, Cell Therapy Section, Department of Transfusion
Medicine, National Institutes of Health, Bethesda, Maryland
Hemapheresis

Reena L. Pande, MD, MSc
Associate Physician, Cardiovascular Division, Brigham and
Women's Hospital, Boston, Massachusetts
Peripheral Artery Disease

Thalia Papayannopoulou, MD
Professor of Medicine, Division of Hematology, University of
Washington, Seattle, Washington
Biology of Erythropoiesis, Erythroid Differentiation, and Maturation

Rahul Parikh, MD
Radiation Oncologist, Rutgers Cancer Institute of New Jersey, New
Brunswick, New Jersey
Hodgkin Lymphoma: Clinical Manifestations, Staging, and Therapy

Effie W. Petersdorf, MD
Professor of Medicine, University of Washington; Member, Fred
Hutchinson Cancer Research Center, Seattle, Washington
Unrelated Donor Hematopoietic Cell Transplantation

Shane E. Peterson, MD
Attending Physician, Emergency Medicine, Mount Sinai Health
System, New York, New York
Pain Management and Antiemetic Therapy in Hematologic Disorders

Stefania Pittaluga, MD, PhD
Staff Clinician, Hematopathology Section, Laboratory of Pathology,
Center for Cancer Research, National Cancer Institute, Bethesda,
Maryland
*The Pathologic Basis for the Classification of Non-Hodgkin and
Hodgkin Lymphomas*

Doris M. Ponce, MD
Assistant Professor of Medicine, Adult Bone Marrow
Transplantation, Memorial Sloan-Kettering Cancer Center, New
York, New York
*Unrelated Donor Cord Blood Transplantation for Hematologic
Malignancies*

Laura Popolo, PhD
Professor, Department of Biosciences, University of Milan, Milan,
Italy
Protein Synthesis, Processing, and Trafficking

Josef T. Prchal, MD
Professor, Division of Hematology and Hematologic Malignancies,
Department of Internal Medicine, University of Utah, Salt Lake
City, Utah
Red Blood Cell Enzymopathies

Ching-Hon Pui, MD
Member, Chair, Department of Oncology, Co-Leader,
Hematological Malignancies Program; Fahad Nassar Al-Rashid
Chair of Leukemia Research, American Cancer Society; Professor,
St. Jude Children's Research Hospital, Memphis, Tennessee
*Clinical Manifestations and Treatment of Childhood Acute
Lymphoblastic Leukemia*

Pere Puigserver, PhD
Professor of Cell Biology, Dana-Farber Cancer Institute; Associate
Professor of Cell Biology, Harvard Medical School, Boston,
Massachusetts
Signaling Transduction and Metabolomics

Janusz Rak, MD, PhD
Jack Cole Chair in Pediatric Hematology/Oncology, Professor,
Department of Pediatrics, McGill University, The Research Institute
of the McGill University Health Centre, Montreal Children's
Hospital, Montreal, Quebec, Canada
Vascular Growth in Health and Disease

Carlos A. Ramos, MD
Associate Professor, Department of Medicine, Hematology-
Oncology Section, Baylor College of Medicine; Center for Cell and
Gene Therapy, Baylor College of Medicine, Houston Methodist
Hospital and Texas Children's Hospital, Houston, Texas
Marginal Zone Lymphomas (Extranodal/MALT, Splenic, and Nodal)

Jacob H. Rand, MD
Professor, Department of Pathology and Laboratory Medicine, Weill Cornell Medical College, New York, New York
The Antiphospholipid Syndrome

Margaret L. Rand, PhD
Professor, Departments of Laboratory Medicine & Pathobiology, Biochemistry, and Paediatrics, University of Toronto; Senior Associate Scientist, Translation Medicine, Research Institute; Associate Scientific Staff, Division of Haematology/Oncology, The Hospital for Sick Children, Toronto, Ontario, Canada
Molecular Basis of Platelet Function

Dinesh S. Rao, MD, PhD
Assistant Professor of Pathology and Laboratory Medicine, David Geffen School of Medicine at University of California, Los Angeles, Los Angeles, California
Overview and Compartmentalization of the Immune System

Farhad Ravandi, MD
Professor of Medicine, Leukemia, The University of Texas MD Anderson Cancer Center, Houston, Texas
Hairy Cell Leukemia

David J. Rawlings, MD
Director, Center for Immunity and Immunotherapies, Seattle Children's Research Institute; Chief, Division of Immunology, Department of Pediatrics, University of Washington School of Medicine, Seattle, Washington
B-Cell Development

Pavan Reddy, MD
Associate Division Chief, Hematology and Oncology, Co-Director, Hematologic Malignancies and Bone Marrow Transplant Program, University of Michigan Cancer Center, Ann Arbor, Michigan
Graft-versus-Host Disease and Graft-versus-Leukemia Responses

Mark T. Reding, MD
Associate Professor of Medicine, Division of Hematology, Oncology, and Transplantation, Director, Center for Bleeding and Clotting Disorders, University of Minnesota Medical Center, Minneapolis, Minnesota
Hematologic Problems in the Surgical Patient: Bleeding and Thrombosis

Andreas Reiter, MD
Faculty of Medicine in Mannheim, Department of Hematology and Oncology, University of Heidelberg, Mannheim, Germany
Eosinophilia, Eosinophil-Associated Diseases, Eosinophil Leukemias, and the Hypereosinophilic Syndromes

Lawrence Rice, MD
Professor of Medicine, Weill Cornell Medical College; Chief of Hematology, Department of Medicine, Houston Methodist Hospital, Houston, Texas
Neutrophilic Leukocytosis, Neutropenia, Monocytosis, and Monocytopenia

Matthew J. Riese, MD, PhD
Assistant Professor, Division of Hematology/Oncology, Department of Medicine, Medical College of Wisconsin; Associate Investigator, Blood Research Institute, BloodCenter of Wisconsin, Milwaukee, Wisconsin
T-Cell Immunity

Arthur Kim Ritchey, MD
Professor of Pediatrics, Vice-Chair for International Affairs, Pediatrics, University of Pittsburgh School of Medicine, Pediatric Hematology/Oncology, Children's Hospital of Pittsburgh of UPMC, Pittsburgh, Pennsylvania
Hematologic Manifestations of Childhood Illness

David J. Roberts, MBChB, D Phil
Consultant Haematologist, National Health Service Blood and Transplant, John Radcliffe Hospital; Professor of Haematology, Nuffield Department of Clinical Laboratory Sciences, University of Oxford, Oxford, United Kingdom
Hematologic Aspects of Parasitic Diseases

Elizabeth Roman, MD
Assistant Professor of Pediatrics, New York University School of Medicine, New York, New York
Transfusion Therapy for Coagulation Factor Deficiencies

Cliona M. Rooney, PhD
Professor of Pediatrics, Section of Hematology-Oncology, Department of Molecular Virology and Microbiology, Department of Pathology and Immunology, Baylor College of Medicine, Houston, Texas
Infectious Mononucleosis and Other Epstein-Barr Virus-Associated Diseases

Steven T. Rosen, MD
Provost and Chief Scientific Officer, City of Hope Medical Center, Duarte, California
T-Cell Lymphomas

David S. Rosenthal, MD
Professor of Medicine, Emeritus, Harvard Medical School; Past Medical Director, Leonard P. Zakim Center for Integrative Therapies, Dana-Farber Cancer Institute, Boston, Massachusetts
Integrative Therapies in Patients with Hematologic Diseases

Marlies P. Rossmann, MD, PhD
Stem Cell Program and Division of Hematology/Oncology, Children's Hospital Boston, Howard Hughes Medical Institute and Harvard Medical School; Department of Medical Oncology and Department of Pediatric Oncology, Dana-Farber Cancer Institute, Harvard Medical School, Boston, Massachusetts; Department of Stem Cell and Regenerative Biology and Harvard Stem Cell Institute, Harvard University, Cambridge, Massachusetts
Hematopoietic Stem Cell Biology

Antal Rot, MD
Professor, Chair of Biomedical Sciences, The University of York, Heslington, York, United Kingdom
Chemokines and Hematopoietic Cell Trafficking

Scott D. Rowley, MD
Member, Adult Blood and Marrow Transplantation Program, John Theurer Cancer Center, Hackensack University Medical Center, Hackensack, New Jersey; Director, Bone Marrow and Stem Cell Transplant Program, Lombardi Comprehensive Cancer Center, MedStar Georgetown University Hospital, Washington, DC; Professor of Medicine, Georgetown University School of Medicine, Washington, DC
Practical Aspects of Hematologic Stem Cell Harvesting and Mobilization

Jeffrey E. Rubnitz, MD, PhD
Member, Oncology, St. Jude Children's Research Hospital, Memphis, Tennessee
Acute Myeloid Leukemia in Children

Natalia Rydz, MD
Clinical Assistant Professor, Division of Hematology and Hematologic Malignancies, University of Calgary, Calgary, Alberta, Canada
Structure, Biology, and Genetics of Von Willebrand Factor

Mohamed E. Salama, MD
Professor of Pathology and Clinical Hematology, The University of Utah School of Medicine, Chief of Hematopathology and Vice President, ARUP Reference Laboratories, Salt Lake City, Utah
Progress in the Classification of Hematopoietic and Lymphoid Neoplasms: Clinical Implications
Primary Myelofibrosis

Steven Sauk, MD, MS
Radiology Chief Resident, Mallinckrodt Institute of Radiology, Washington University School of Medicine, St. Louis, Missouri
Mechanical Interventions in Arterial and Venous Thrombosis

Yogen Saunthararajah, MB
Staff, Professor of Medicine, Cleveland Clinic and Lerner College of Medicine, Case Western Reserve University, Cleveland, Ohio
Sickle Cell Disease: Clinical Features and Management

William Savage, MD, PhD
Associate Medical Director, Transfusion Medicine, Brigham and Women's Hospital, Boston, Massachusetts
Transfusion Reactions to Blood and Cell Therapy Products

David Scadden, MD
Gerald and Darlene Jordan Professor of Medicine, Chair and Professor, Department of Stem Cell and Regenerative Biology, Co-director, Harvard Stem Cell Institute, Harvard University, Cambridge, Massachusetts; Director, Center for Regenerative Medicine, Massachusetts General Hospital, Boston, Massachusetts
Hematopoietic Microenvironment

Kristen G. Schaefer, MD
Assistant Professor of Medicine, Harvard Medical School; Senior Physician, Division of Adult Palliative Care, Department of Psychosocial Oncology and Palliative Care, Dana-Farber Cancer Institute; Division of Palliative Medicine; Department of Medicine, Brigham and Women's Hospital, Boston, Massachusetts
Palliative Care

Fred Schiffman, MD
Sigal Family Professor of Humanistic Medicine, Vice-Chair, Department of Medicine, Warren Alpert Medical School, Brown University, Providence, Rhode Island
Hematologic Manifestations of Malignancy
The Spleen and Its Disorders

Robert Schneidewend, DO, MS
Hematology and Oncology Fellow, Medical College of Wisconsin, Milwaukee, Wisconsin
Thrombotic Thrombocytopenic Purpura and the Hemolytic Uremic Syndromes

Stanley L. Schrier, MD
Professor of Medicine (Hematology), Stanford University School of Medicine, Stanford, California
Extrinsic Nonimmune Hemolytic Anemias

Edward H. Schuchman, PhD
Genetic Disease Foundation, Francis Crick Professor and Vice Chairman for Research, Genetics and Genomic Sciences, Icahn School of Medicine at Mount Sinai, New York, New York
Lysosomal Storage Diseases: Perspectives and Principles

Bridget Fowler Scullion, BS, PharmD, BCOP
Director of Clinical Pharmacy Services, Department of Pharmacy, Dana-Farber Cancer Institute, Boston, Massachusetts
Pain Management and Antiemetic Therapy in Hematologic Disorders

Kathy J. Selvaggi, MD, MS
Chair, Division of Palliative Care, Butler Memorial Hospital, Butler, Pennsylvania
Pain Management and Antiemetic Therapy in Hematologic Disorders

Keitaro Senoo, MD
Arrhythmia Care Center, Kouseikai Takeda Hospital, Kyoto, Japan
Atrial Fibrillation

Montaser Shaheen, MD
Associate Professor, Department of Internal Medicine, University of Arizona, Tucson, Arizona
Cytokine/Receptor Families and Signal Transduction

Beth H. Shaz, MD
Chief Medical and Scientific Officer, New York Blood Center; Adjunct Assistant Professor, Department of Pathology and Cell Biology, Columbia University Medical Center, New York, New York
Human Blood Group Antigens and Antibodies
Transfusion of Plasma and Plasma Derivatives: Plasma, Cryoprecipitate, Albumin, and Immunoglobulins

Samuel A. Shelburne, MD, PhD
Assistant Professor, Department of Infectious Diseases, Infection Control, and Employee Health, The University of Texas MD Anderson Cancer Center, Houston, Texas
Clinical Approach to Infections in the Compromised Host

Elizabeth J. Shpall, MD
Ashbel Smith Professor of Medicine, Medical Director, Cell Therapy Laboratory, Director, Cord Blood Bank, Deputy Chair, Department of Stem Cell Transplantation and Cellular Therapy, The University of Texas MD Anderson Cancer Center, Houston, Texas
Unrelated Donor Cord Blood Transplantation for Hematologic Malignancies

Susan B. Shurin, MD
Senior Adviser, Center for Global Health, National Cancer Institute, Bethesda, Maryland
The Spleen and Its Disorders

Deborah Siegal, MD, MSc, FRCPC
Assistant Professor, Medicine, McMaster University, Hamilton, Ontario, Canada
Venous Thromboembolism

Leslie E. Silberstein, MD
Professor of Pathology (Pediatrics), Harvard Medical School; Director, Joint Program in Transfusion Medicine, Boston Children's Hospital, Brigham and Women's Hospital, Boston, Massachusetts
Overview and Historical Perspective of Current Cell-Based Therapies

Lev Silberstein, MD, PhD
Instructor, Harvard Medical School; Center for Regenerative Medicine, Massachusetts General Hospital, Boston, Massachusetts
Hematopoietic Microenvironment

Roy L. Silverstein, MD
John and Linda Mellowes Professor and Chair, Department of Medicine, Professor of Physiology and Cell Biology, Medical College of Wisconsin; Senior Investigator, Blood Research Institute, BloodCenter of Wisconsin, Milwaukee, Wisconsin
Atherothrombosis

Steven R. Sloan, MD, PhD
Blood Bank Medical Director, Laboratory Medicine, Director, Pediatric Transfusion Medicine, Joint Program in Transfusion Medicine, Boston Children's Hospital; Assistant Professor of Pathology, Harvard Medical School, Boston, Massachusetts
Pediatric Transfusion Medicine

Franklin O. Smith, MD
Vice President, Medical Affairs Medpace, Professor of Medicine and Pediatrics, University of Cincinnati College of Medicine, Cincinnati, Ohio
Myelodysplastic Syndromes and Myeloproliferative Neoplasms in Children

James W. Smith, BSc, MT
Assistant Professor of Medicine, Michael G. DeGroote School
of Medicine, Technical Director, Ontario Provincial Platelet
Immunology Laboratory, McMaster University, Hamilton, Ontario,
Canada
*Diseases of Platelet Number: Immune Thrombocytopenia, Neonatal
Alloimmune Thrombocytopenia, and Posttransfusion Purpura*

Katy Smith, MBChB, BSc
Lymphoma Service, Memorial Sloan Kettering Cancer Center, New
York, New York
Hodgkin Lymphoma: Clinical Manifestations, Staging, and Therapy

David P. Steensma, MD
Associate Professor of Medicine, Dana-Farber Cancer Institute,
Boston, Massachusetts
Myelodysplastic Syndromes

Martin H. Steinberg, MD
Professor of Medicine, Pediatrics, Pathology, and Laboratory
Medicine, Boston University School of Medicine, Boston,
Massachusetts
Pathobiology of the Human Erythrocyte and Its Hemoglobins

Wendy Stock, MD
Anjuli Seth Nayak Professor of Medicine, Director, Leukemia
Program, Section of Hematology/Oncology, University of Chicago,
Chicago, Illinois
Acute Lymphoblastic Leukemia in Adults

Jill R. Storry, MSc, PhD
Clinical Immunology and Transfusion Medicine, University and
Regional Laboratories, Lund, Sweden
Human Blood Group Antigens and Antibodies

Susan L. Stramer, PhD
Vice President, Scientific Affairs, Biomedical Services, American
Red Cross, Gaithersburg, Maryland
Transfusion-Transmitted Diseases

Ronald G. Strauss, MD
Professor Emeritus, Pathology and Pediatrics, University of Iowa
College of Medicine, Iowa City, Iowa; Associate Medical Director,
LifeSource, Institute for Transfusion Medicine, Chicago, Illinois
Principles of Neutrophil (Granulocyte) Transfusions

David F. Stroncek, MD
Chief, Cell Processing Section
Department of Transfusion Medicine, National Institutes of Health
Clinical Center, Bethesda, Maryland
Human Leukocyte Antigen and Human Neutrophil Antigen Systems

Justin Taylor, MD
Hematology/Oncology Fellow, Omar Abdel-Wahab Lab, Memorial
Sloan Kettering Cancer Center, New York, New York
Stem Cell Model of Hematologic Diseases

Swapna Thota, MD
Fellow, Department of Hematology and Oncology, Taussig Cancer
Institute, Cleveland, Ohio
Acquired Disorders of Red Cell, White Cell, and Platelet Production

Steven P. Treon, MD, MA, PhD
Professor, Department of Medicine, Harvard Medical School;
Director, Bing Center for Waldenström's Macroglobulinemia, Dana-
Farber Cancer Institute, Boston, Massachusetts
Waldenström Macroglobulinemia/Lymphoplasmacytic Lymphoma

Anil Tulpule, MD
Associate Professor of Medicine, Keck School of Medicine of the
University of Southern California, Los Angeles, California
Hematologic Manifestations of HIV/AIDS

Roberto Ferro Valdes, MD
University of Nebraska Medical Center, Omaha, Nebraska
Mantle Cell Lymphoma

Peter Valent, MD
Professor, Department of Internal Medicine I, Division of
Hematology and Hemostaseology, Medical University of Vienna,
Vienna, Austria
*Eosinophilia, Eosinophil-Associated Diseases, Eosinophil Leukemias,
and the Hypereosinophilic Syndromes*
Mast Cells and Mastocytosis

Suresh Vedantham, MD
Professor of Radiology and Surgery, Mallinckrodt Institute of
Radiology, Washington University School of Medicine, St. Louis,
Missouri
Mechanical Interventions in Arterial and Venous Thrombosis

Gregory M. Vercellotti, MD
Professor of Medicine, University of Minnesota, Minneapolis,
Minnesota
Pathobiology of Sickle Cell Disease

Michael R. Verneris, MD
Professor of Pediatrics, Division of Pediatric Hematology, Oncology,
and Transplantation, University of Minnesota, Minneapolis,
Minnesota
Natural Killer Cell-Based Therapies

Elliott P. Vichinsky, MD
University of California, San Francisco Benioff Children's Hospital
Oakland; Adjunct Professor, University of California, San Francisco,
San Francisco, California
Sickle Cell Disease: Clinical Features and Management

Ulrich H. von Andrian, MD
Mallinckrodt Professor of Immunopathology, Department of
Microbiology and Immunobiology, Immune Disease Institute
and Division of Immunology, Harvard Medical School, Boston,
Massachusetts
Chemokines and Hematopoietic Cell Trafficking

Julie M. Vose, MD, MBA
Professor, Department of Internal Medicine, Chief, Division of
Oncology and Hematology, University of Nebraska Medical Center,
Omaha, Nebraska
Mantle Cell Lymphoma

Andrew J. Wagner, MD, PhD
Medical Oncologist, Center for Sarcoma and Bone Oncology;
Associate Chief Medical Officer, Dana-Farber Cancer Institute;
Associate Professor, Department of Medicine, Harvard Medical
School, Boston, Massachusetts
Anatomy and Physiology of the Gene

Ena Wang, MD
Research Chief, Translational Medicine, Research Branch, Sidra
Medical and Research Center, Doha, Qatar
Human Leukocyte Antigen and Human Neutrophil Antigen Systems

Jia-huai Wang, PhD
Associate Professor of Medical Oncology, Dana-Farber Cancer
Institute, Boston, Massachusetts
Protein Architecture: Relationship of Form and Function

Theodore E. Warkentin, MD
Professor, Departments of Pathology and Molecular Medicine and Medicine, Michael G. DeGroote School of Medicine, McMaster University; Regional Director, Transfusion Medicine, Hamilton Regional Laboratory Medicine Program; Hematologist, Service of Clinical Hematology, Hamilton General Hospital, Hamilton Health Sciences, Hamilton, Ontario, Canada
Thrombocytopenia Caused by Platelet Destruction, Hypersplenism, or Hemodilution
Heparin-Induced Thrombocytopenia

Melissa P. Wasserstein, MD
Associate Professor, Departments of Pediatrics and Genetics, Albert Einstein College of Medicine; Chief, Division of Pediatric Genetic Medicine, The Children's Hospital at Montefiore, New York, New York
Lysosomal Storage Diseases: Perspectives and Principles

Ann Webster, PhD
Director, Mind/Body Program for Cancer, Department of Psychiatry, Benson-Henry Institute for Mind/Body Medicine at Massachusetts General Hospital, Boston, Massachusetts
Integrative Therapies in Patients With Hematologic Diseases

Daniel J. Weisdorf, MD
Professor of Medicine, University of Minnesota, Minneapolis, Minnesota
Complications After Hematopoietic Cell Transplantation

Jeffrey I. Weitz, MD
Professor of Medicine and Biochemistry and Biomedical Sciences, McMaster University, Executive Director, Thrombosis and Atherosclerosis Research Institute, Canada Research Chair in Thrombosis, Heart and Stroke Foundation J. F. Mustard Chair in Cardiovascular Research Hamilton, Ontario, Canada
Overview of Hemostasis and Thrombosis
Hypercoagulable States
Acute Coronary Syndromes
Antithrombotic Drugs
Hematologic Problems in the Surgical Patient: Bleeding and Thrombosis

Connie M. Westhoff, PhD
Executive Scientific Director, Immunohematology and Genomics, New York Blood Center, New York, New York
Human Blood Group Antigens and Antibodies

Allison P. Wheeler, MD, MSCI
Assistant Professor of Pathology, Microbiology, and Immunology and Pediatrics, Vanderbilt University, Nashville, Tennessee
Rare Coagulation Factor Deficiencies

Page Widick, MD
Chief Medical Resident, Internal Medicine, Brown University, Providence, Rhode Island
Hematologic Manifestations of Malignancy

James S. Wiley, BSc, MD, FRACP, FRCPA
Principal Research Fellow, Florey Institute of Neuroscience and Mental Health, University of Melbourne, Parkville, Victoria, Australia
Heme Biosynthesis and Its Disorders: Porphyrias and Sideroblastic Anemias

Basem M. William, MD
Assistant Professor, Department of Internal Medicine, Division of Hematology, The Ohio State University Wexner Medical Center, Columbus, Ohio
Pharmacology and Molecular Mechanisms of Antineoplastic Agents for Hematologic Malignancies

David A. Williams, MD
Senior Vice President and Chief Scientific Officer, Boston Children's Hospital; President, Dana-Farber/Boston Children's Cancer and Blood Disorders Center; Leland Fikes Professor of Pediatrics, Harvard Medical School, Boston, Massachusetts
Principles of Cell-Based Genetic Therapies

Wyndham H. Wilson, MD, PhD
Senior Investigator, Lymphoid Malignancies Branch, National Cancer Institute, National Institutes of Health, Bethesda, Maryland
Diagnosis and Treatment of Diffuse Large B-Cell Lymphoma and Burkitt Lymphoma

Joanne Wolfe, MD, MPH
Associate Professor of Pediatrics, Harvard Medical School; Division Chief, Pediatric Palliative Care, Department of Psychosocial Oncology and Palliative Care, Dana-Farber Cancer Institute; Director, Pediatric Palliative Care, Department of Medicine, Children's Hospital Boston; Associate Professor of Pediatrics, Harvard Medical School, Boston, Massachusetts
Palliative Care

Lucia R. Wolgast, MD
Assistant Professor of Pathology, Albert Einstein College of Medicine; Director, Clinical Laboratories; Associate Director, Hematology Laboratories, Department of Pathology, Montefiore Medical Center, New York, New York
The Antiphospholipid Syndrome

Deborah Wood, BS MT (ASCP)
Project Manager, The EMMES Corporation, Rockville, Maryland
Investigational New Drug–Enabling Processes for Cell-Based Therapies

Jennifer Wu, MD, PhD
Instructor, Department of Pediatrics, Harvard Medical School, Dana-Farber/Boston Children's Cancer and Blood Disorders Center, Boston, Massachusetts
Epigenetics and Epigenomics

Joachim Yahalom, MD
Member and Professor, Radiation Oncology, Memorial Sloan Kettering Cancer Center, New York, New York
Hodgkin Lymphoma: Clinical Manifestations, Staging, and Therapy

Donald L. Yee, MD, MS
Associate Professor of Pediatrics, Baylor College of Medicine, Houston, Texas
Resources for the Hematologist: Interpretive Comments and Selected Reference Values for Neonatal, Pediatric, and Adult Populations

Anas Younes, MD
Chief, Lymphoma Service, Memorial Sloan Kettering Cancer Center, New York, New York
Hodgkin Lymphoma: Clinical Manifestations, Staging, and Therapy

Neal S. Young, MD
Chief, Hematology Branch, National Heart, Lung, and Blood Institute; Director, Center for Human Immunology, Autoimmunity, and Inflammation, National Institutes of Health, Bethesda, Maryland
Aplastic Anemia

Michelle P. Zeller, MD
Assistant Professor, Michael G. DeGroote School of Medicine, McMaster University; Medical Officer, Canadian Blood Services, Hamilton, Ontario, Canada
Diseases of Platelet Number: Immune Thrombocytopenia, Neonatal Alloimmune Thrombocytopenia, and Posttransfusion Purpura

PREFACE

This is the seventh edition of *Hematology: Basic Principles and Practice.* This textbook has, over the last 30 years, become a staple for many students of hematology. It is our intent that this seventh edition continue to fill this role. The goal of this venture has always been, and continues to be, the creation of a volume of information that summarizes the overall body of knowledge known as hematology. In this time of online publishing and rapid publication, as well as the availability of numerous search engines that provide algorithms to assist with patient care, the value of *Hematology: Basic Principles and Practice* to our readership is even greater than in the past. Currently, there is a trend to use content-lite vehicles that provide condensed forms of information to the hematology community. From our perspective, this bullet point–directed strategy of education dealing with complex science and medicine represents a serious misstep that ultimately diminishes the hematology community's opportunity to achieve excellence in research and patient care. This edition provides a compilation of chapters that summarizes an in depth analysis of hematology. These chapters have been created by luminaries in their respective fields and have been critically evaluated by the editorial team. We all understand that the medical literature changes by the hour, but practice-changing advances are relatively few. These chapters provide a solid foundation with which the readership can assess the significance of the most recent advances in hematology. From these carefully crafted and edited chapters the readership can *rapidly* gain access to a comprehensive body of knowledge that will serve as a platform to better appreciate the rapidly evolving literature in hematology science and practice. Cryptic summaries of complex issues that underlie hematology cannot be critically evaluated with a series of bullet points. Medicine and science are more nuanced and require a commitment by the target audience to appreciate where a particular field is and where it is going. Of course, the use of this textbook requires an initial time commitment on the part of the reader that ultimately will lead to significant rewards. In the long run the examination of these chapters is an investment in your intellectual development and educational pursuits. To some, this approach might be considered "old school," but we believe it really shows prudence and respect for this incredibly challenging field. It makes hematology challenging and exciting again. The editorial team for the sixth edition has remained intact and includes Drs. Ronald Hoffman, Edward Benz, Leslie Silberstein, Helen Heslop, Jeffrey Weitz, and John Anastasi. For this seventh edition, Dr. Mohammed Salama has joined our team. Dr. Salama is Professor of Pathology and Chief of Hematopathology at the University of Utah School of Medicine. He has helped to improve the quality of the photomicrographs that play a prominent role in many of our chapters. Additionally, Dr. Salama has developed a virtual microscopy system that will allow the readers to better examine relevant histopathology of a number of blood disorders. We believe this system will be useful to our readership in order to better appreciate the critical aspects of hemato-pathology needed to practice modern hematology. Dr. Syed Abutalib has also joined our group and will serve as the editor responsible for monthly updates. Dr. Abutalib is a hematologist and medical oncologist at the Midwestern Regional Medical Center in Zion, Illinois. Syed is in clinical practice and a full-time clinician. He has an intense interest and extensive track record in medical education. Our editorial team felt that a full-time practitioner would be best suited to determine which updates would be of greatest importance to our readership. Several updates will be provided monthly to the readership, and these will be vetted by the other editors working with Dr. Abutalib. These efforts will provide a path by which we can continue to expand and improve the content provided within the text after the time of publication. With this mechanism in place we have become a book that can change and evolve over time. Please utilize these updates to better evaluate the the massive wave of new information that we all encounter.

After the completion of this seventh edition we still feel this book is a work in progress. We are still seeking and considering the best ways to provide timely information to our readership, and we remain humbled by the complexity of this task in this age of rapid communication. We will continue to modify this book and have enjoyed the challenges we have encountered in its preparation. Over the years, we have added additional members to our editorial team to create a book that we can be proud of and that we have certainty will be of use to our readership. We hope that this seventh edition meets our joint expectations and the growing needs of our readership.

Ronald Hoffman, MD
Edward J. Benz, Jr., MD
Leslie E. Silberstein, MD
Helen E. Heslop, MD
Jeffrey I. Weitz, MD
John Anastasi, MD
Mohammed E. Salama, MD
Syed Abutalib, MD

CONTENTS

PART I

MOLECULAR AND CELLULAR BASIS OF HEMATOLOGY 1

1. **Anatomy and Physiology of the Gene** 3
Andrew J. Wagner, Nancy Berliner, and Edward J. Benz, Jr.

2. **Epigenetics and Epigenomics** 17
Jennifer Wu and Myles Brown

3. **Genomic Approaches to Hematology** 25
Jens G. Lohr, Birgit Knoechel, and Todd R. Golub

4. **Regulation of Gene Expression, Transcription, Splicing, and RNA Metabolism** 37
Christopher R. Cogle

5. **Protein Synthesis, Processing, and Trafficking** 45
Randal J. Kaufman and Laura Popolo

6. **Protein Architecture: Relationship of Form and Function** 59
Jia-huai Wang and Michael J. Eck

7. **Signaling Transduction and Metabolomics** 68
Pere Puigserver

8. **Pharmacogenomics and Hematologic Diseases** 79
Leo Kager and William E. Evans

PART II

CELLULAR BASIS OF HEMATOLOGY 93

9. **Hematopoietic Stem Cell Biology** 95
Marlies P. Rossmann, Stuart H. Orkin, and John P. Chute

10. **Stem Cell Model of Hematologic Diseases** 111
Justin Taylor and Omar Abdel-Wahab

11. **Hematopoietic Microenvironment** 119
David Scadden and Lev Silberstein

12. **Cell Adhesion** 127
Rodger P. McEver and Francis W. Luscinskas

13. **Chemokines and Hematopoietic Cell Trafficking** 135
Antal Rot, Steffen Massberg, Alexander G. Khandoga, and Ulrich H. von Andrian

14. **Interactions between Hematopoietic Stem and Progenitor Cells and the Bone Marrow: Current Biology of Stem Cell Homing and Mobilization** 145
Eman Khatib-Massalha, Kfir Lapid, Karin Golan, Orit Kollet, Shiri Gur-Cohen, Menachem Bitan, Anju Kumari, and Tsvee Lapidot

15. **Vascular Growth in Health and Disease** 152
Janusz Rak

16. **Cytokine/Receptor Families and Signal Transduction** 163
Montaser Shaheen and Hal E. Broxmeyer

17. **Control of Cell Division** 176
Martin Fischer, Chi V. Dang, and James A. DeCaprio

18. **Cell Death** 186
Nika N. Danial and David M. Hockenbery

PART III

IMMUNOLOGIC BASIS OF HEMATOLOGY 197

19. **Overview and Compartmentalization of the Immune System** 199
Dinesh S. Rao

20. **B-Cell Development** 210
Kenneth Dorshkind and David J. Rawlings

21. **T-Cell Immunity** 221
Shannon A. Carty, Matthew J. Riese, and Gary A. Koretzky

22. **Natural Killer Cell Immunity** 240
Don M. Benson, Jr. and Michael A. Caligiuri

23. **Dendritic Cell Biology** 247
Olivier Manches, Luciana R. Muniz, and Nina Bhardwaj

24. **Complement and Immunoglobulin Biology Leading to Clinical Translation** 261
David J. Araten, Robert J. Mandle, David E. Isenman, and Michael C. Carroll

25. **Tolerance and Autoimmunity** 285
Taku Kambayashi

PART IV

DISORDERS OF HEMATOPOIETIC CELL DEVELOPMENT 295

26. **Biology of Erythropoiesis, Erythroid Differentiation, and Maturation** 297
Thalia Papayannopoulou and Anna Rita Migliaccio

27. **Granulocytopoiesis and Monocytopoiesis** 321
Arati Khanna-Gupta and Nancy Berliner

28. **Thrombocytopoiesis** 334
Alan B. Cantor

29. **Inherited Bone Marrow Failure Syndromes** 350
Yigal Dror

30. **Aplastic Anemia** 394
Neal S. Young and Jaroslaw P. Maciejewski

31. **Paroxysmal Nocturnal Hemoglobinuria** 415
Robert A. Brodsky

32. Acquired Disorders of Red Cell, White Cell, and Platelet Production   425
Jaroslaw P. Maciejewski and Swapna Thota

PART V
RED BLOOD CELLS   445

33. Pathobiology of the Human Erythrocyte and Its Hemoglobins   447
Martin H. Steinberg, Edward J. Benz, Jr., Adeboye H. Adewoye, and Benjamin L. Ebert

34. Approach to Anemia in the Adult and Child   458
Judith C. Lin

35. Pathophysiology of Iron Homeostasis   468
Gary M. Brittenham

36. Disorders of Iron Homeostasis: Iron Deficiency and Overload   478
Gary M. Brittenham

37. Anemia of Chronic Diseases   491
Lalitha Nayak, Lawrence B. Gardner, and Jane A. Little

38. Heme Biosynthesis and Its Disorders: Porphyrias and Sideroblastic Anemias   497
Stephen J. Fuller and James S. Wiley

39. Megaloblastic Anemias   514
Aśok C. Antony

40. Thalassemia Syndromes   546
John Chapin and Patricia J. Giardina

41. Pathobiology of Sickle Cell Disease   571
Robert P. Hebbel and Gregory M. Vercellotti

42. Sickle Cell Disease: Clinical Features and Management   584
Yogen Saunthararajah and Elliott P. Vichinsky

43. Hemoglobin Variants Associated With Hemolytic Anemia, Altered Oxygen Affinity, and Methemoglobinemias   608
Edward J. Benz, Jr. and Benjamin L. Ebert

44. Red Blood Cell Enzymopathies   616
Xylina T. Gregg and Josef T. Prchal

45. Red Blood Cell Membrane Disorders   626
Patrick G. Gallagher

46. Autoimmune Hemolytic Anemia   648
Marc Michel and Ulrich Jäger

47. Extrinsic Nonimmune Hemolytic Anemias   663
William C. Mentzer and Stanley L. Schrier

PART VI
NON-MALIGNANT LEUKOCYTES   673

48. Neutrophilic Leukocytosis, Neutropenia, Monocytosis, and Monocytopenia   675
Lawrence Rice and Moonjung Jung

49. Lymphocytosis, Lymphocytopenia, Hypergammaglobulinemia, and Hypogammaglobulinemia   682
Martha P. Mims

50. Disorders of Phagocyte Function   691
Mary C. Dinauer and Thomas D. Coates

51. Congenital Disorders of Lymphocyte Function   710
Sung-Yun Pai and Luigi D. Notarangelo

52. Histiocytic Disorders   724
Michael B. Jordan and Alexandra Hult Filipovich

53. Lysosomal Storage Diseases: Perspectives and Principles   740
Edward H. Schuchman and Melissa P. Wasserstein

54. Infectious Mononucleosis and Other Epstein-Barr Virus–Associated Diseases   747
Carl Allen, Cliona M. Rooney, and Stephen Gottschalk

PART VII
HEMATOLOGIC MALIGNANCIES   761

55. Progress in the Classification of Hematopoietic and Lymphoid Neoplasms: Clinical Implications   763
Mohamed E. Salama and Ronald Hoffman

56. Conventional and Molecular Cytogenomic Basis of Hematologic Malignancies   774
Vesna Najfeld

57. Pharmacology and Molecular Mechanisms of Antineoplastic Agents for Hematologic Malignancies   849
Stanton L. Gerson, Paolo F. Caimi, Basem M. William, and Richard J. Creger

58. Pathobiology of Acute Myeloid Leukemia   913
Andrew M. Brunner and Timothy A. Graubert

59. Clinical Manifestations and Treatment of Acute Myeloid Leukemia   924
Stefan Faderl and Hagop M. Kantarjian

60. Myelodysplastic Syndromes   944
Christopher J. Gibson, Benjamin L. Ebert, and David P. Steensma

61. Allogeneic Hematopoietic Stem Cell Transplantation for Acute Myeloid Leukemia and Myelodysplastic Syndrome in Adults   970
John Koreth, Joseph H. Antin, and Corey Cutler

62. Acute Myeloid Leukemia in Children   981
Tanja A. Gruber and Jeffrey E. Rubnitz

63. Myelodysplastic Syndromes and Myeloproliferative Neoplasms in Children   994
Franklin O. Smith, Christopher C. Dvorak, and Benjamin S. Braun

64. Pathobiology of Acute Lymphoblastic Leukemia   1005
Melissa Burns, Scott A. Armstrong, and Alejandro Gutierrez

65. **Clinical Manifestations and Treatment of Childhood Acute Lymphoblastic Leukemia** 1020
Sima Jeha and Ching-Hon Pui

66. **Acute Lymphoblastic Leukemia in Adults** 1029
Shira Dinner, Sandeep Gurbuxani, Nitin Jain, and Wendy Stock

67. **Chronic Myeloid Leukemia** 1055
Ravi Bhatia

68. **The Polycythemias** 1071
Marina Kremyanskaya, Vesna Najfeld, John Mascarenhas, and Ronald Hoffman

69. **Essential Thrombocythemia** 1106
John Mascarenhas, Camelia Iancu-Rubin, Marina Kremyanskaya, Vesna Najfeld, and Ronald Hoffman

70. **Primary Myelofibrosis** 1125
John Mascarenhas, Vesna Najfeld, Marina Kremyanskaya, Alla Keyzner, Mohamed E. Salama, and Ronald Hoffman

71. **Eosinophilia, Eosinophil-Associated Diseases, Eosinophilic Leukemias, and the Hypereosinophilic Syndromes** 1151
Peter Valent, Andreas Reiter, and Jason Gotlib

72. **Mast Cells and Mastocytosis** 1170
Jason Gotlib, Hans-Peter Horny, and Peter Valent

73. **The Pathologic Basis for the Classification of Non-Hodgkin and Hodgkin Lymphomas** 1187
Elaine S. Jaffe, Stefania Pittaluga, and John Anastasi

74. **Origin of Hodgkin Lymphoma** 1204
Ralf Küppers

75. **Hodgkin Lymphoma: Clinical Manifestations, Staging, and Therapy** 1212
Katy Smith, April Chiu, Rahul Parikh, Joachim Yahalom, and Anas Younes

76. **Origin of Non-Hodgkin Lymphoma** 1230
Matthew S. McKinney and Sandeep S. Dave

77. **Chronic Lymphocytic Leukemia** 1244
Farrukh T. Awan and John C. Byrd

78. **Hairy Cell Leukemia** 1265
Farhad Ravandi

79. **Marginal Zone Lymphomas (Extranodal/Malt, Splenic, and Nodal)** 1277
Carlos A. Ramos

80. **Clinical Manifestations, Staging, and Treatment of Follicular Lymphoma** 1288
John G. Gribben

81. **Mantle Cell Lymphoma** 1298
Vijaya Raj Bhatt, Roberto Ferro Valdes, and Julie M. Vose

82. **Diagnosis and Treatment of Diffuse Large B-Cell Lymphoma and Burkitt Lymphoma** 1309
Kieron Dunleavy and Wyndham H. Wilson

83. **Virus-Associated Lymphoma** 1318
Jennifer A. Kanakry and Richard F. Ambinder

84. **Malignant Lymphomas in Childhood** 1330
Kara M. Kelly, Birgit Burkhardt, and Catherine M. Bollard

85. **T-Cell Lymphomas** 1343
Owen A. O'Connor, Govind Bhagat, Karthik A. Ganapathi, Jason Kaplan, Paolo Corradini, Joan Guitart, Steven T. Rosen, and Timothy M. Kuzel

86. **Plasma Cell Neoplasms** 1381
Nikhil C. Munshi and Sundar Jagannath

87. **Waldenström Macroglobulinemia/Lymphoplasmacytic Lymphoma** 1419
Steven P. Treon, Jorge J. Castillo, Zachary R. Hunter, and Giampaolo Merlini

88. **Immunoglobulin Light Chain Amyloidosis (Primary Amyloidosis)** 1432
Morie A. Gertz, Francis K. Buadi, Martha Q. Lacy, and Suzanne R. Hayman

PART VIII
COMPREHENSIVE CARE OF PATIENTS WITH HEMATOLOGIC MALIGNANCIES 1445

89. **Clinical Approach to Infections in the Compromised Host** 1447
Samuel A. Shelburne, Russell E. Lewis, and Dimitrios P. Kontoyiannis

90. **Psychosocial Aspects of Hematologic Disorders** 1462
Matthew J. Gonzales, Dawn M. Gross, and Elizabeth Cooke

91. **Pain Management and Antiemetic Therapy in Hematologic Disorders** 1473
Shane E. Peterson, Kathy J. Selvaggi, Bridget Fowler Scullion, and Craig D. Blinderman

92. **Palliative Care** 1488
Kristen G. Schaefer, Janet L. Abrahm, and Joanne Wolfe

93. **Late Complications of Hematologic Diseases and Their Therapies** 1496
Wendy Landier and Smita Bhatia

PART IX
CELL-BASED THERAPIES 1513

94. **Overview and Historical Perspective of Current Cell-Based Therapies** 1515
Leslie E. Silberstein and Helen E. Heslop

95. **Practical Aspects of Hematologic Stem Cell Harvesting and Mobilization** 1517
Scott D. Rowley and Michele L. Donato

96. **Investigational New Drug–Enabling Processes for Cell-Based Therapies** 1531
Robert Lindblad, Traci Heath Mondoro, Deborah Wood, and Gillian Armstrong

97. **Graft Engineering and Cell Processing** 1537
Adrian P. Gee

98. **Principles of Cell-Based Genetic Therapies** 1549
David A. Williams

99. Mesenchymal Stromal Cells 1559
Jacques Galipeau

100. T-Cell Therapy of Hematologic Diseases 1568
Gianpietro Dotti and Malcolm K. Brenner

101. Natural Killer Cell-Based Therapies 1575
Sarah Cooley, Michael R. Verneris, and Jeffrey S. Miller

102. Immune Checkpoint Blockade in Hematologic
Malignancies 1583
Reid Merryman and Philippe Armand

PART X
TRANSPLANTATION 1589

103. Overview and Choice of Donor of Hematopoietic Stem
Cell Transplantation 1591
Helen E. Heslop

104. Indications and Outcomes of Allogeneic Hematopoietic
Cell Transplantation for Hematologic Malignancies in
Adults 1596
Mehdi Hamadani and Parameswaran N. Hari

105. Unrelated Donor Hematopoietic Cell
Transplantation 1608
Effie W. Petersdorf and Claudio Anasetti

106. Haploidentical Hematopoietic Cell
Transplantation 1617
Ephraim Fuchs

107. Unrelated Donor Cord Blood Transplantation for
Hematologic Malignancies 1633
Rohtesh S. Mehta, Amanda Olson, Doris M. Ponce,
and Elizabeth J. Shpall

108. Graft-versus-Host Disease and Graft-versus-Leukemia
Responses 1650
Pavan Reddy and James L.M. Ferrara

109. Complications after Hematopoietic Cell
Transplantation 1669
Shernan G. Holtan, Navneet S. Majhail, and
Daniel J. Weisdorf

PART XI
TRANSFUSION MEDICINE 1685

110. Human Blood Group Antigens and Antibodies 1687
Connie M. Westhoff, Jill R. Storry, and Beth H. Shaz

111. Principles of Red Blood Cell Transfusion 1702
Yen-Michael S. Hsu, Paul M. Ness, and
Melissa M. Cushing

112. Clinical Considerations in Platelet Transfusion
Therapy 1715
Richard M. Kaufman

113. Human Leukocyte Antigen and Human Neutrophil
Antigen Systems 1721
Ena Wang, Sharon Adams, David F. Stroncek, and
Francesco M. Marincola

114. Principles of Neutrophil (Granulocyte)
Transfusions 1738
Ronald G. Strauss

115. Transfusion of Plasma and Plasma Derivatives:
Plasma, Cryoprecipitate, Albumin, and
Immunoglobulins 1744
Matthew S. Karafin, Christopher D. Hillyer, and
Beth H. Shaz

116. Preparation of Plasma-Derived and Recombinant
Human Plasma Proteins 1759
David B. Clark

117. Transfusion Therapy for Coagulation Factor
Deficiencies 1769
Elizabeth Roman, Peter J. Larson, and Catherine S. Manno

118. Hemapheresis 1781
Sandhya R. Panch and Harvey G. Klein

119. Transfusion Reactions to Blood and Cell Therapy
Products 1792
William Savage

120. Transfusion-Transmitted Diseases 1803
Susan L. Stramer and Roger Y. Dodd

121. Pediatric Transfusion Medicine 1821
Cassandra D. Josephson and Steven R. Sloan

PART XII
HEMOSTASIS AND THROMBOSIS 1829

122. Overview of Hemostasis and Thrombosis 1831
James C. Fredenburgh and Jeffrey I. Weitz

123. The Blood Vessel Wall 1843
Marianne A. Grant and Aly Karsan

124. Megakaryocyte and Platelet Structure 1857
Joseph E. Italiano, Jr. and John H. Hartwig

125. Molecular Basis of Platelet Function 1870
Margaret L. Rand and Sara J. Israels

126. Molecular Basis of Blood Coagulation 1885
Kathleen Brummel-Ziedins and Kenneth G. Mann

127. Regulatory Mechanisms in Hemostasis 1906
James A. Huntington and Trevor P. Baglin

128. Clinical Approach to the Patient with Bleeding or
Bruising 1912
Catherine P.M. Hayward

129. Laboratory Evaluation of Hemostatic and Thrombotic
Disorders 1922
Menaka Pai

130. Acquired Disorders of Platelet Function 1932
Reyhan Diz-Küçükkaya and José A. López

131. Diseases of Platelet Number: Immune
Thrombocytopenia, Neonatal Alloimmune
Thrombocytopenia, and Posttransfusion
Purpura 1944
Donald M. Arnold, Michelle P. Zeller, James W. Smith,
and Ishac Nazy

132. **Thrombocytopenia Caused by Platelet Destruction, Hypersplenism, or Hemodilution** 1955
Theodore E. Warkentin

133. **Heparin-Induced Thrombocytopenia** 1973
Theodore E. Warkentin

134. **Thrombotic Thrombocytopenic Purpura and the Hemolytic Uremic Syndromes** 1984
Robert Schneidewend, Narendranath Epperla, and Kenneth D. Friedman

135. **Hemophilia A and B** 2001
Manuel Carcao, Paul Moorehead, and David Lillicrap

136. **Inhibitors in Hemophilias** 2023
Guglielmo Mariani, Barbara A. Konkle, and Craig M. Kessler

137. **Rare Coagulation Factor Deficiencies** 2034
David Gailani, Allison P. Wheeler, and Anne T. Neff

138. **Structure, Biology, and Genetics of Von Willebrand Factor** 2051
Paula James and Natalia Rydz

139. **Disseminated Intravascular Coagulation** 2064
Marcel Levi

140. **Hypercoagulable States** 2076
Julia A. Anderson, Kerstin E. Hogg, and Jeffrey I. Weitz

141. **The Antiphospholipid Syndrome** 2088
Jacob H. Rand and Lucia R. Wolgast

142. **Venous Thromboembolism** 2102
Deborah Siegal and Wendy Lim

143. **Mechanical Interventions in Arterial and Venous Thrombosis** 2113
Steven Sauk and Suresh Vedantham

144. **Atherothrombosis** 2122
Roy L. Silverstein

145. **Stroke** 2133
Emer McGrath, Michelle Canavan, and Martin O'Donnell

146. **Acute Coronary Syndromes** 2142
John W. Eikelboom and Jeffrey I. Weitz

147. **Atrial Fibrillation** 2152
Dipak Kotecha, Keitaro Senoo, and Gregory Y.H. Lip

148. **Peripheral Artery Disease** 2159
Reena L. Pande and Mark A. Creager

149. **Antithrombotic Drugs** 2168
Iqbal H. Jaffer and Jeffrey I. Weitz

150. **Disorders of Coagulation in the Neonate** 2189
Mihir D. Bhatt, Karin Ho, and Anthony K.C. Chan

PART XIII

CONSULTATIVE HEMATOLOGY 2201

151. **Hematologic Changes in Pregnancy** 2203
Caroline Cromwell and Michael Paidas

152. **Hematologic Manifestations of Childhood Illness** 2215
Arthur Kim Ritchey, Sarah H. O'Brien, and Frank G. Keller

153. **Hematologic Manifestations of Liver Disease** 2238
Christopher Hillis and Wendy Lim

154. **Hematologic Manifestations of Renal Disease** 2244
Mark A. Crowther and Ali Iqbal

155. **Hematologic Manifestations of Malignancy** 2247
Page Widick, Andrew M. Brunner, and Fred Schiffman

156. **Integrative Therapies in Patients with Hematologic Diseases** 2253
David S. Rosenthal, Ann Webster, and Elana Ladas

157. **Hematologic Manifestations of HIV/AIDS** 2262
Howard A. Liebman and Anil Tulpule

158. **Hematologic Aspects of Parasitic Diseases** 2278
David J. Roberts

159. **Hematologic Problems in the Surgical Patient: Bleeding and Thrombosis** 2304
Iqbal H. Jaffer, Mark T. Reding, Nigel S. Key, and Jeffrey I. Weitz

160. **The Spleen and Its Disorders** 2313
Nathan T. Connell, Susan B. Shurin, and Fred Schiffman

161. **Hematology in Aging** 2328
Andrew S. Artz and William B. Ershler

162. **Resources for the Hematologist: Interpretive Comments and Selected Reference Values for Neonatal, Pediatric, and Adult Populations** e1
Andrea N. Marcogliese and Donald L. Yee
Chapter 162 can be found online at ExpertConsult.com

Index 2333

VIRTUAL MICROSCOPE SLIDE LIST

To view the slides, please go to ExpertConsult.com.

	Chapter	Chapter Title	Slide Label
	49	Lymphocytosis, Lymphocytopenia, Hypergammaglobulinemia, and Hypogammaglobulinemia	Sarcoidosis
	52	Histiocytic Disorders	Rosai-Dorfman
	54	Infectious Mononucleosis and Other Epstein-Barr Virus–Associated Diseases	Infectious Mononucleosis
	70	Primary Myelofibrosis	Myelofibrosis with Extramedullary Hematopoiesis in the Liver
	76	Origins of Non-Hodgkin Lymphomas	Follicular Lymphoma
	79	Clinical Manifestations and Treatment of Indolent Lymphomas: Marginal Zone Lymphomas (Extranodal/Malt, Splenic, and Nodal)	Splenic Marginal Zone Lymphoma
	81	Mantle Cell Lymphoma	Mantle Cell Lymphoma
	82	Diagnosis and Treatment of Diffuse Large B-Cell Lymphoma and Burkitt Lymphoma	Burkitt Lymphoma
	82	Diagnosis and Treatment of Diffuse Large B-Cell Lymphoma and Burkitt Lymphoma	T Cell Rich B Cell Lymphoma
	83	Virus-Related Lymphomas	Plasmablastic Lymphoma Oral Cavity, HIV+

MOLECULAR AND CELLULAR BASIS OF HEMATOLOGY

ANATOMY AND PHYSIOLOGY OF THE GENE

Andrew J. Wagner, Nancy Berliner, and Edward J. Benz, Jr.

Normal blood cells have limited life spans; they must be replenished in precise numbers by a continuously renewing population of progenitor cells. Homeostasis of the blood requires that proliferation of these cells be efficient yet strictly constrained. Many distinctive types of mature blood cells must arise from these progenitors by a controlled process of commitment to, and execution of, complex programs of differentiation. Thus, developing red blood cells must produce large quantities of hemoglobin but not the myeloperoxidase characteristic of granulocytes, the immunoglobulins characteristic of lymphocytes, or the fibrinogen receptors characteristic of platelets. Similarly, the maintenance of normal amounts of coagulant and anticoagulant proteins in the circulation requires exquisitely regulated production, destruction, and interaction of the components. Understanding the basic biologic principles underlying cell growth, differentiation, and protein biosynthesis requires a thorough knowledge of the structure and regulated expression of genes because the gene is now known to be the fundamental unit by which biologic information is stored, transmitted, and expressed in a regulated fashion.

Genes were originally characterized as mathematical units of inheritance. They are now known to consist of molecules of deoxyribonucleic acid (DNA). By virtue of their ability to store information in the form of nucleotide sequences, to transmit it by means of semiconservative replication to daughter cells during mitosis and meiosis, and to express it by directing the incorporation of amino acids into proteins, DNA molecules are the chemical transducers of genetic information flow. Efforts to understand the biochemical means by which this transduction is accomplished have given rise to the discipline of molecular genetics.

THE GENETIC VIEW OF THE BIOSPHERE: THE CENTRAL DOGMA OF MOLECULAR BIOLOGY

The fundamental premise of the molecular biologist is that the magnificent diversity encountered in nature is ultimately governed by genes. The capacity of genes to exert this control is in turn determined by relatively simple stereochemical rules, first appreciated by Watson and Crick in the 1950s. These rules constrain the types of interactions that can occur between two molecules of DNA or ribonucleic acid (RNA).

DNA and RNA are linear polymers consisting of four types of nucleotide subunits. Proteins are linear unbranched polymers consisting of 21 types of amino acid subunits. Each amino acid is distinguished from the others by the chemical nature of its side chain, the moiety not involved in forming the peptide bond links of the chain. The properties of cells, tissues, and organisms depend largely on the aggregate structures and properties of their proteins. The central dogma of molecular biology states that genes control these properties by controlling the structures of proteins, the timing and amount of their production, and the coordination of their synthesis with that of other proteins. The information needed to achieve these ends is transmitted by a class of nucleic acid molecules called RNA. Genetic information thus flows in the direction DNA → RNA → protein. This central dogma provides, in principle, a universal approach for investigating the biologic properties and behavior of any given cell, tissue, or organism by study of the controlling genes. Methods permitting direct manipulation of DNA sequences should then be universally applicable to the study of all living entities. Indeed, the power of the molecular genetic approach lies in the universality of its utility.

One exception to the central dogma of molecular biology that is especially relevant to hematologists is the storage of genetic information in RNA molecules in certain viruses, notably the retroviruses associated with T-cell leukemia and lymphoma, and the human immunodeficiency virus. When retroviruses enter the cell, the RNA genome is copied into a DNA replica by an enzyme called *reverse transcriptase*. This DNA representation of the viral genome is then expressed according to the rules of the central dogma. Retroviruses thus represent a variation on the theme rather than a true exception to or violation of the rules.

ANATOMY AND PHYSIOLOGY OF GENES

DNA Structure

DNA molecules are extremely long, unbranched polymers of nucleotide subunits. Each nucleotide contains a sugar moiety called deoxyribose, a phosphate group attached to the 5′ carbon position, and a purine or pyrimidine base attached to the 1′ position (Fig. 1.1). The linkages in the chain are formed by phosphodiester bonds between the 5′ position of each sugar residue and the 3′ position of the adjacent residue in the chain (see Fig. 1.1). The sugar–phosphate links form the backbone of the polymer, from which the purine or pyrimidine bases project perpendicularly.

The haploid human genome consists of 23 long, double-stranded DNA molecules tightly complexed with histones and other nuclear proteins to form compact linear structures called *chromosomes*. The genome contains 3 billion nucleotides; each chromosome is thus 50 to 200 million bases in length. The individual genes are aligned along each chromosome. The human genome contains about 30,000 genes. Blood cells, similar to most somatic cells, are diploid. That is, each chromosome is present in two copies, so there are 46 chromosomes consisting of approximately 6 billion base pairs (bp) of DNA.

The four nucleotide bases in DNA are the purines (adenosine and guanosine) and the pyrimidines (thymine and cytosine). The basic chemical configuration of the other nucleic acid found in cells, RNA, is quite similar, except that the sugar is ribose (having a hydroxyl group attached to the 2′ carbon rather than the hydrogen found in deoxyribose) and the pyrimidine base uracil is used in place of thymine. The bases are commonly referred to by a shorthand notation: the letters A, C, T, G, and U are used to refer to adenosine, cytosine, thymine, guanosine, and uracil, respectively.

The ends of DNA and RNA strands are chemically distinct because of the 3′ → 5′ phosphodiester bond linkage that ties adjacent bases together (see Fig. 1.1). One end of the strand (the 3′ end) has an unlinked (free at the 3′ carbon) sugar position and the other (the 5′ end) has a free 5′ position. There is thus a polarity to the sequence of bases in a DNA strand: the same sequence of bases read in a 3′ → 5′ direction carries a different meaning than if read in a 5′ → 3′ direction. Cellular enzymes can thus distinguish one end of a nucleic acid from the other; most enzymes that "read" the DNA sequence tend to do so only in one direction (3′ → 5′ or 5′ → 3′ but not

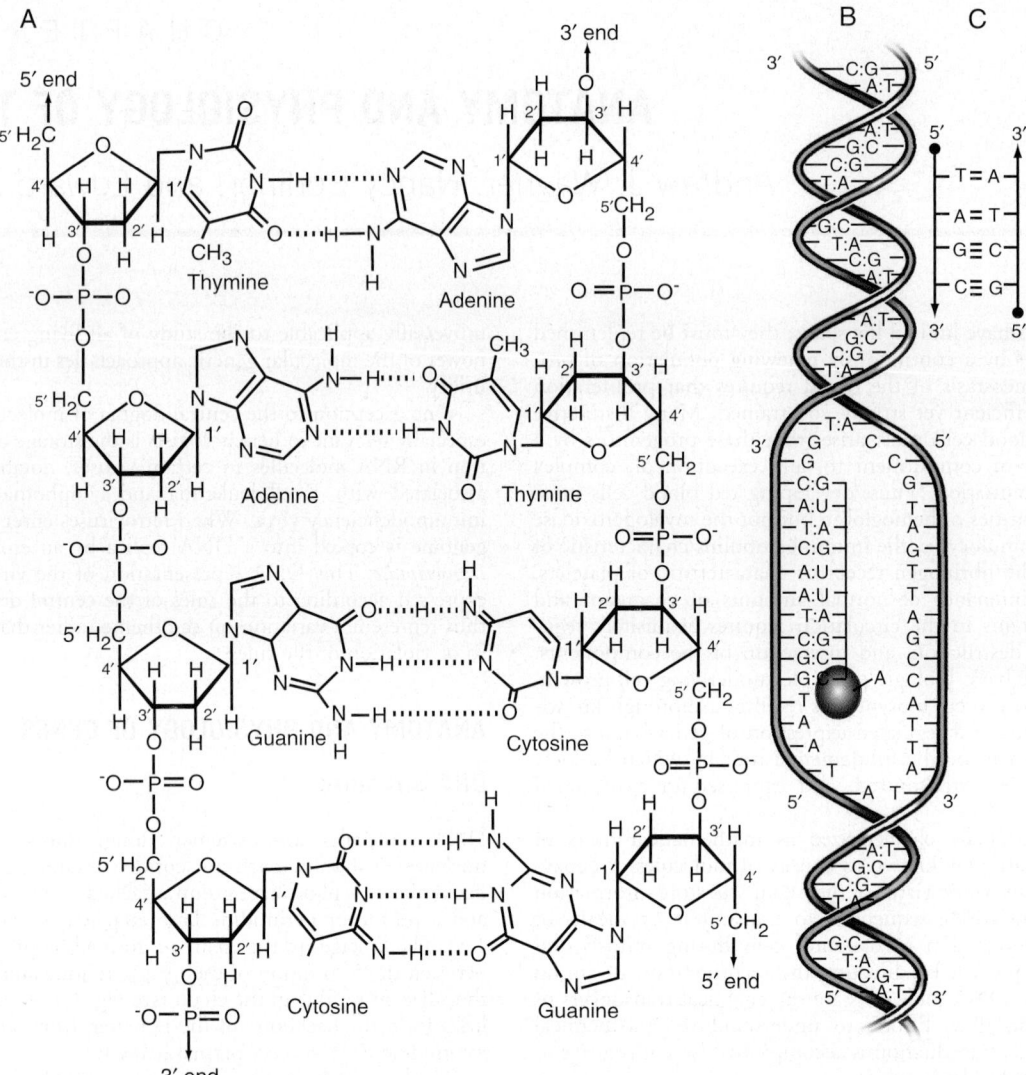

Fig. 1.1 STRUCTURE, BASE PAIRING, POLARITY, AND TEMPLATE PROPERTIES OF DNA. (A) Structures of the four nitrogenous bases projecting from sugar phosphate backbones. The hydrogen bonds between them form base pairs holding complementary strands of DNA together. Note that whereas A–T and T–A base pairs have only two hydrogen bonds, C–G and G–C pairs have three. (B) The double helical structure of DNA results from base pairing of strands to form a double-stranded molecule with the backbones on the outside and the hydrogen-bonded bases stacked in the middle. Also shown schematically is the separation (unwinding) of a region of the helix by mRNA polymerase, which is shown using one of the strands as a template for the synthesis of an mRNA precursor molecule. Note that new bases added to the growing RNA strand obey the rules of Watson–Crick base pairing (see text). Uracil (U) in RNA replaces T in DNA and, like T, forms base pairs with A. (C) Diagram of the antiparallel nature of the strands, based on the stereochemical 3′ → 5′ polarity of the strands. The chemical differences between reading along the backbone in the 5′ → 3′ and 3′ → 5′ directions can be appreciated by reference to (A). *A*, Adenosine; *C*, cytosine; *G*, guanosine; *T*, thymine; *U*, uracil.

both). Most nucleic acid–synthesizing enzymes, for instance, add new bases to the strand in a 5′ → 3′ direction.

The ability of DNA molecules to store information resides in the sequence of nucleotide bases arrayed along the polymer chain. Under the physiologic conditions in living cells, DNA is thermodynamically most stable when two strands coil around each other to form a double-stranded helix. The strands are aligned in an "antiparallel" direction, having opposite 3′ → 5′ polarity (see Fig. 1.1). The DNA strands are held together by hydrogen bonds between the bases on one strand and the bases on the opposite (complementary) strand. The stereochemistry of these interactions allows bonds to form between the two strands only when adenine on one strand pairs with

thymine at the same position of the opposite strand, or guanine with cytosine—the Watson–Crick rules of base pairing. Two strands joined together in compliance with these rules are said to have "complementary" base sequences.

These thermodynamic rules imply that the sequence of bases along one DNA strand immediately dictates the sequence of bases that must be present along the complementary strand in the double helix. For example, whenever an A occurs along one strand, a T must be present at that exact position on the opposite strand; a G must always be paired with a C, a T with an A, and a C with a G. In RNA–RNA or RNA–DNA double-stranded molecules, U–A base pairs replace T–A pairs.

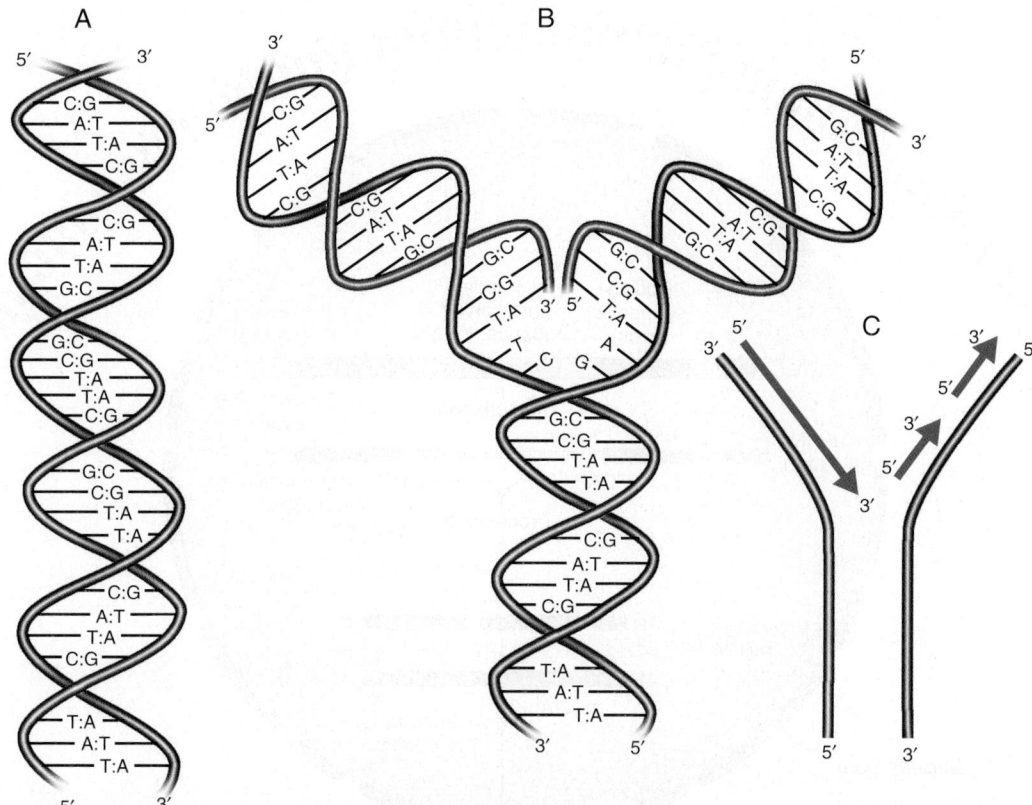

Fig. 1.2 SEMICONSERVATIVE REPLICATION OF DNA. (A) The process by which the DNA molecule on the left is replicated into two daughter molecules, as occurs during cell division. Replication occurs by separation of the parent molecule into the single-stranded form at one end, reading of each of the daughter strands in the 3′ → 5′ direction by DNA polymerase, and addition of new bases to growing daughter strands in the 5′ → 3′ direction. (B) The replicated portions of the daughter molecules are identical to each other *(red)*. Each carries one of the two strands of the parent molecule, accounting for the term *semiconservative replication*. Note the presence of the replication fork, the point at which the parent DNA is being unwound. (C) The antiparallel nature of the DNA strands demands that replication proceed toward the fork in one direction and away from the fork in the other *(red)*. This means that replication is actually accomplished by reading of short stretches of DNA followed by ligation of the short daughter strand regions to form an intact daughter strand.

STORAGE AND TRANSMISSION OF GENETIC INFORMATION

The rules of Watson–Crick base pairing apply to DNA–RNA, RNA–RNA, and DNA–DNA double-stranded molecules. Enzymes that replicate or polymerize DNA and RNA molecules obey the base-pairing rules. By using an existing strand of DNA or RNA as the template, a new (daughter) strand is copied (transcribed) by reading processively along the base sequence of the template strand, adding to the growing strand at each position only that base that is complementary to the corresponding base in the template according to the Watson–Crick rules. Thus, a DNA strand having the base sequence 5′-GCTATG-3′ could be copied by DNA polymerase only into a daughter strand having the sequence 3′-CGATAC-5′. Note that the sequence of the template strand provides all the information needed to predict the nucleotide sequence of the complementary daughter strand. Genetic information is thus stored in the form of base-paired nucleotide sequences.

If a double-stranded DNA molecule is separated into its two component strands and each strand is then used as a template to synthesize a new daughter strand, the product will be two double-stranded daughter DNA molecules, each identical to the original parent molecule. This semiconservative replication process is exactly what occurs during mitosis and meiosis as cell division proceeds (Fig. 1.2). The rules of Watson–Crick base pairing thus provide for the faithful transmission of exact copies of the cellular genome to subsequent generations.

EXPRESSION OF GENETIC INFORMATION THROUGH THE GENETIC CODE AND PROTEIN SYNTHESIS

The information stored in the DNA base sequence achieves its impact on the structure, function, and behavior of organisms by governing the structures, timing, and amounts of protein synthesized in the cells. The primary structure (i.e., the amino acid sequence) of each protein determines its three-dimensional conformation and therefore its properties (e.g., shape, enzymatic activity, ability to interact with other molecules, stability). In the aggregate, these proteins control cell structure and metabolism. The process by which DNA achieves its control of cells through protein synthesis is called *gene expression*.

An outline of the basic pathway of gene expression in eukaryotic cells is shown in Fig. 1.3. The DNA base sequence is first copied into an RNA molecule, called *premessenger RNA*, by messenger RNA (mRNA) polymerase. Premessenger RNA has a base sequence identical to the DNA coding strand. Genes in eukaryotic species consist of tandem arrays of sequences encoding mRNA (exons); these sequences alternate with sequences (introns) present in the initial mRNA transcript (premessenger RNA) but absent from the mature mRNA. The entire gene is transcribed into the large precursor, which is then

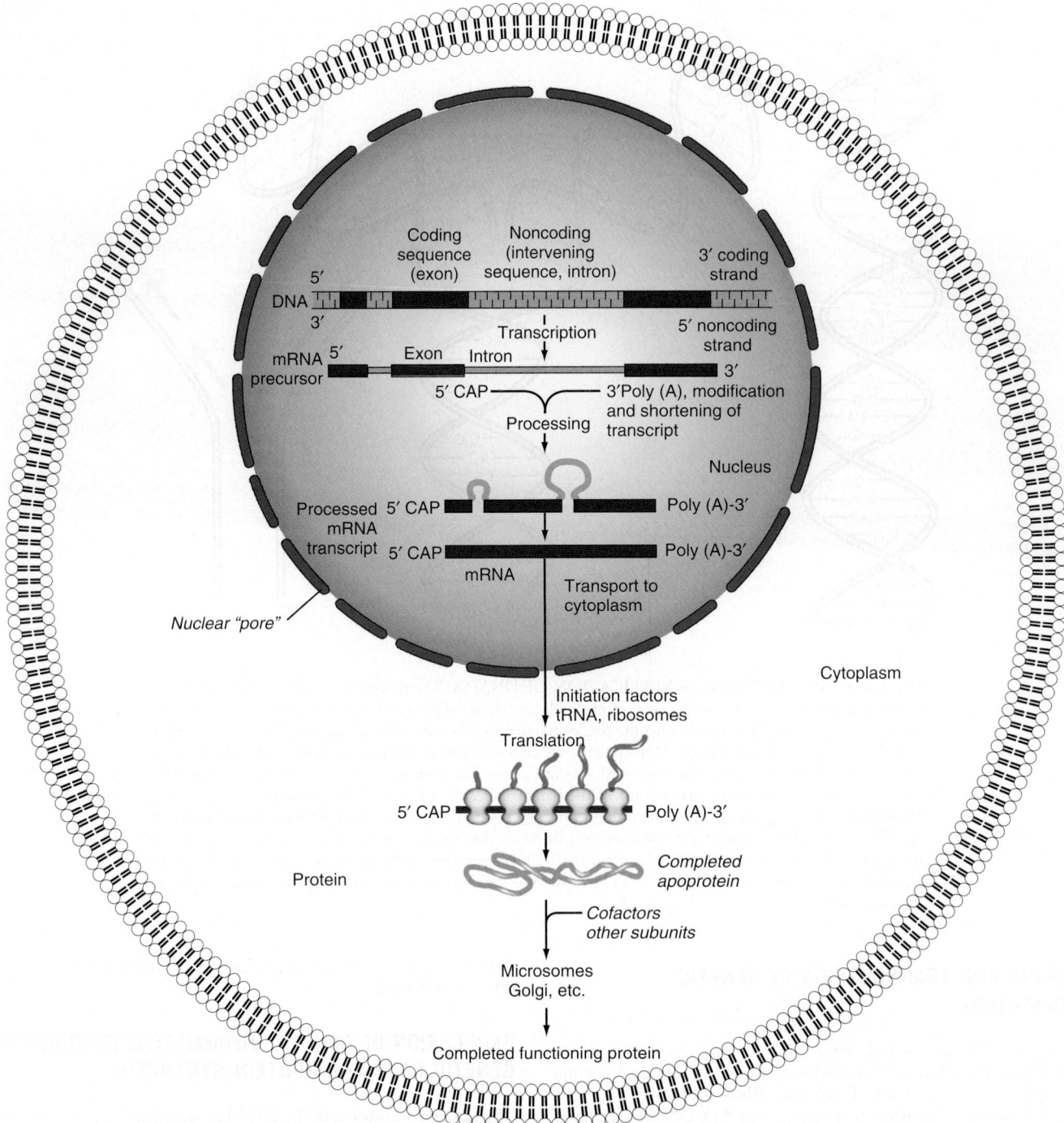

Fig. 1.3 SYNTHESIS OF mRNA AND PROTEIN—THE PATHWAY OF GENE EXPRESSION. The diagram of the DNA gene shows the alternating array of exons *(red)* and introns *(shaded color)* typical of most eukaryotic genes. Transcription of the mRNA precursor, addition of the 5'-CAP and 3'-poly (A) tail, splicing and excision of introns, transport to the cytoplasm through the nuclear pores, translation into the amino acid sequence of the apoprotein, and posttranslational processing of the protein are described in the text. Translation proceeds from the initiator methionine codon near the 5' end of the mRNA, with incorporation of the amino terminal end of the protein. As the mRNA is read in a 5' → 3' direction, the nascent polypeptide is assembled in an amino → carboxyl terminal direction.

further processed (spliced) in the nucleus. The introns are excised from the final mature mRNA molecule, which is then exported to the cytoplasm to be decoded (translated) into the amino acid sequence of the protein by association with a biochemically complex group of ribonucleoprotein structures called *ribosomes*. Ribosomes contain two subunits: the 60S subunit contains a single, large (28S) ribosomal RNA molecule complexed with multiple proteins, and the RNA

component of the 40S subunit is a smaller (18S) ribosomal RNA molecule.

Ribosomes read mRNA sequence in a ticker tape fashion three bases at a time, inserting the appropriate amino acid encoded by each three-base code word or codon into the appropriate position of the growing protein chain. This process is called *mRNA translation*. The glossary used by cells to know which amino acids are encoded by each

TABLE
1.1 **The Genetic Code^a Messenger RNA Codons for the Amino Acids**

Alanine	Arginine	Asparagine	Aspartic Acid	Cysteine
5'-GCU-3'	CGU	AAU	GAU	UGU
GCC	CGC	AAC	GAC	UGC
GCA	CGA			
GCG	CGG			
	AGA			
	AGG			

Glutamic Acid	Glutamine	Glycine	Histidine	Isoleucine
GAA	CAA	GGU	CAU	AUU
GAG	CAG	GGC	CAC	AUC
		GGA		AUA
		GGG		

Leucine	Lysine	Methionine	Phenylalanine	Proline^c
UUA	AAA	AUG^b	UUU	CCU
UUG	AAG		UUC	CCC
CUU				CCA
CUC				CCG
CUA				
CUG				

Serine	Threonine	Tryptophan	Tyrosine	Valine
UCU	ACU	UGG	UAU	GUU
UCC	ACC		UAC	GUC
UCA	ACA			GUA
UCG	ACG			GUG
AGU				
AGC				

Chain Termination^d
UAA
UAG
UGA

^{a}Note that most of the degeneracy in the code is in the third base position (e.g., lysine, AA [G or C]; asparagine, AA [C or U]; valine, GUN [where N is any base]).
^{b}AUG is also used as the chain-initiation codon when surrounded by the Kozak consensus sequence.
^{c}Hydroxyproline, the 21st amino acid, is generated by posttranslational modification of proline. It is almost exclusively confined to collagen subunits.
^{d}The codons that signal the end of translation, also called nonsense or termination codons, are described by their nicknames *amber* (UAG), *ochre* (UAA), and *opal* (UGA).
A, Adenosine; C, cytosine; G, guanosine; T, thymine; U, uracil.

DNA codon is called the *genetic code* (Table 1.1). Each amino acid is encoded by a sequence of three successive bases. Because there are four code letters (A, C, G, and U), and because sequences read in the 5' → 3' direction have a different biologic meaning than sequences read in the 3' → 5' direction, there are 4^3, or 64, possible codons consisting of three bases.

There are 21 naturally occurring amino acids found in proteins. Thus more codons are available than amino acids to be encoded. As noted in Table 1.1, a consequence of this redundancy is that some amino acids are encoded by more than one codon. For example, six distinct codons can specify incorporation of arginine into a growing amino acid chain, four codons can specify valine, two can specify glutamic acid, and only one each methionine or tryptophan. In no case does a single codon encode more than one amino acid. Codons thus predict unambiguously the amino acid sequence they encode. However, one cannot easily read backward from the amino acid sequence to

decipher the *exact* encoding DNA sequence. These facts are summarized by saying that the code is degenerate but not ambiguous.

Some specialized codons serve as punctuation points during translation. The methionine codon (AUG), when surrounded by a consensus sequence (the Kozak box) near the beginning (5' end) of the mRNA, serves as the initiator codon signaling the first amino acid to be incorporated. All proteins thus begin with a methionine residue, but this is often removed later in the translational process. Three codons, UAG, UAA, and UGA, serve as translation terminators, signaling the end of translation.

The adaptor molecules mediating individual decoding events during mRNA translation are small (40 bases long) RNA molecules called *transfer RNAs* (tRNAs). When bound into a ribosome, each tRNA exposes a three-base segment within its sequence called the *anticodon*. These three bases attempt to pair with the three-base codon exposed on the mRNA. If the anticodon is complementary in sequence to the codon, a stable interaction among the mRNA, the ribosome, and the tRNA molecule results. Each tRNA also contains a separate region that is adapted for covalent binding to an amino acid. The enzymes that catalyze the binding of each amino acid are constrained in such a way that each tRNA species can bind only to a single amino acid. For example, tRNA molecules containing the anticodon 3'-AAA-5', which is complementary to a 5'-UUU-3' (phenylalanine) codon in mRNA, can only be bound to or charged with phenylalanine; tRNA containing the anticodon 3'-UAG-5' can only be charged with isoleucine, and so forth.

Transfer RNAs and their amino acyl tRNA synthetases provide for the coupling of nucleic acid information to protein information needed to convert the genetic code to an amino acid sequence. Ribosomes provide the structural matrix on which tRNA anticodons and mRNA codons become properly exposed and aligned in an orderly, linear, and sequential fashion. As each new codon is exposed, the appropriate charged tRNA species is bound. A peptide bond is then formed between the amino acid carried by this tRNA and the C-terminal residue on the existing nascent protein chain. The growing chain is transferred to the new tRNA in the process, so that it is held in place as the next tRNA is brought in. This cycle is repeated until completion of translation. The completed polypeptide chain is then transferred to other organelles for further processing (e.g., to the endoplasmic reticulum and the Golgi apparatus) or released into the cytosol for association of the newly completed chain with other subunits to form complex multimeric proteins (e.g., hemoglobin) and so forth, as discussed in Chapter 5.

mRNA METABOLISM

In eukaryotic cells, mRNA is initially synthesized in the nucleus (see Figs. 1.3 and 1.4). Before the initial transcript becomes suitable for translation in the cytoplasm, mRNA processing and transport occur by a complex series of events including excision of the portions of the mRNA corresponding to the introns of the gene (mRNA splicing), modification of the 5' and 3' ends of the mRNA to render them more stable and translatable, and transport to the cytoplasm. Moreover, the amount of any particular mRNA moiety in both prokaryotic and eukaryotic cells is governed not only by the composite rate of mRNA synthesis (transcription, processing, and transport) but also by its degradation by cytoplasmic ribonucleases (RNA degradation). Many mRNA species of special importance in hematology (e.g., mRNAs for growth factors and their receptors, proto-oncogene mRNAs, acute-phase reactants) are exquisitely regulated by control of their stability (half-life) in the cytoplasm.

Posttranscriptional mRNA metabolism is complex. Only a few relevant details are considered in this section.

mRNA Splicing

The initial transcript of eukaryotic genes contains several subregions (see Fig. 1.4). Most striking is the tandem alignment of exons and

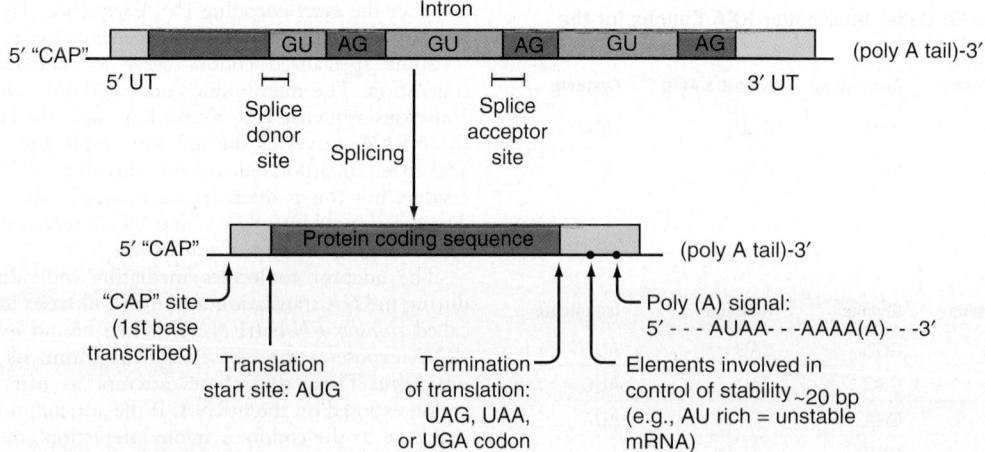

Fig. 1.4 ANATOMY OF THE PRODUCTS OF THE STRUCTURAL GENE (mRNA PRECURSOR AND mRNA). This schematic shows the configuration of the critical anatomic elements of an mRNA precursor, which represents the primary copy of the structural portion of the gene. The sequences GU and AG indicate, respectively, the invariant dinucleotides present in the donor and acceptor sites at which introns are spliced out of the precursor. Not shown are the less stringently conserved consensus sequences that must precede and succeed each of these sites for a short distance.

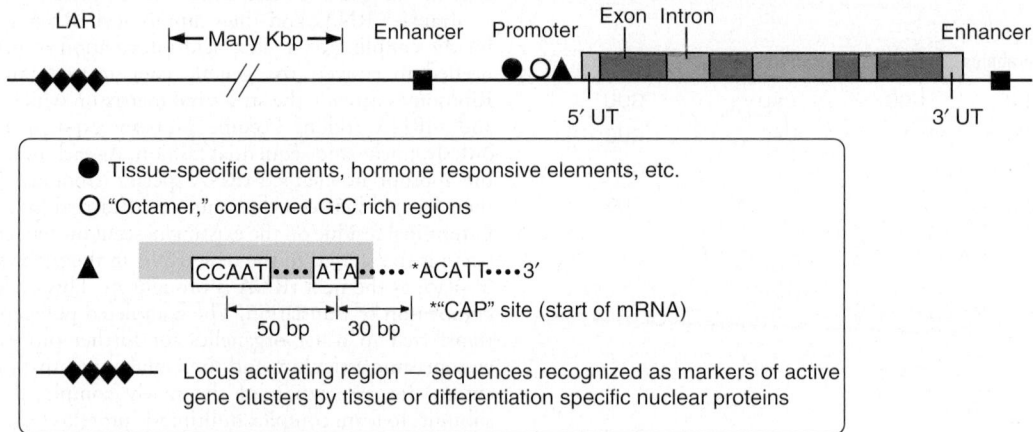

Fig. 1.5 REGULATORY ELEMENTS FLANKING THE STRUCTURAL GENE. *(*For more information refer to suggested readings from Jones B; Kumar A et al; Waddington S et al.)*

introns. Precise excision of intron sequences and ligation of exons is critical for production of mature mRNA. This process is called mRNA splicing, and it occurs on complexes of small nuclear RNAs and proteins called snRNPs; the term *spliceosome* is also used to describe the intranuclear organelle that mediates mRNA splicing reactions. The biochemical mechanism for splicing is complex. A consensus sequence, which includes the dinucleotide GU, is recognized as the donor site at the 5′ end of the intron (5′ end refers to the polarity of the mRNA strand coding for protein); a second consensus sequence ending in the dinucleotide AG is recognized as the acceptor site, which marks the distal end of the intron (see Figs. 1.4 and 1.5). The spliceosome recognizes the donor and acceptor, and forms an intermediate lariat structure that provides for both excision of the intron and proper alignment of the cut ends of the two exons for ligation in precise register.

mRNA splicing has proved to be an important mechanism for greatly increasing the versatility and diversity of expression of a single gene. For example, some genes contain an array of more exons than are actually found in any mature mRNA species encoded by that gene. Several different mRNA and protein products can arise from a single gene by selective inclusion or exclusion of individual exons from the mature mRNA products. This phenomenon is called *alternative mRNA splicing*. It permits a single gene to code for multiple mRNA and protein products with related but distinct structures and

functions. The mechanisms by which individual exons are selected or rejected are complex and highly context-specific, varying among different cell types, differentiation stages, and physiologic states. For present purposes, it is sufficient to note that important physiologic changes in cells can be regulated by altering the patterns of mRNA splicing products arising from single genes.

Many inherited hematologic diseases arise from mutations that derange mRNA splicing. For example, some of the most common forms of the thalassemia syndromes and hemophilia (see Chapters 40 and 135) arise by mutations that alter normal splicing signals or create splicing signals where they normally do not exist (activation of cryptic splice sites). Conversely, mutations altering key protein factors that modulate alternative splicing pathways are known to contribute to the pathogenesis of bone marrow dyscrasias (see Chapters 58 and 60).

Modification of the Ends of the mRNA Molecule

Most eukaryotic mRNA species are polyadenylated at their 3′ ends. mRNA precursors are initially synthesized as large molecules that extend farther downstream from the 3′ end of the mature mRNA molecule. Polyadenylation results in the addition of stretches of 100 to 150 A residues at the 3′ end. Such an addition is often called the *poly-A tail* and is of variable length. Polyadenylation facilitates rapid early cleavage of the unwanted 3′ sequences from the transcript and is also important for stability or transport of the mRNA out of the nucleus. Signals near the 3′ extremity of the mature mRNA mark positions at which polyadenylation occurs. The consensus signal is AUAAA (see Fig. 1.4). Mutations in the poly-A signal sequence have been shown to cause thalassemia (see Chapter 40).

At the 5′ end of the mRNA, a complex oligonucleotide having unusual phosphodiester bonds is added. This structure contains the nucleotide 7-methyl-guanosine and is called *CAP* (see Fig. 1.4). The 5′-CAP enhances both mRNA stability and the ability of the mRNA to interact with protein translation factors and ribosomes.

5′ and 3′ Untranslated Sequences

The 5′ and 3′ extremities of mRNA extend beyond the initiator and terminator codons that mark the beginning and the end of the sequences actually translated into proteins (see Figs. 1.4 and 1.5). These so-called 5′ and 3′ untranslated regions (5′ UTRs and 3′ UTRs) are involved in determining mRNA stability and the efficiency with which mRNA species can be translated. For example, if the 3′ UTR of a very stable mRNA (e.g., globin mRNA) is swapped with the 3′ UTR of a highly unstable mRNA (e.g., the c-myc gene), the c-myc mRNA becomes more stable. Conversely, attachment of the 3′ UTR of c-myc to a globin molecule renders it unstable. Instability is often associated with repeated sequences rich in A and U in the 3′ UTR (see Fig. 1.4). The UTRs in mRNAs coding for proteins involved in iron metabolism mediate altered mRNA stability or translatability by binding iron-laden proteins and thus govern iron storage and turnover (see Chapter 35).

Transport of mRNA From Nucleus to Cytoplasm: mRNP Particles

An additional potential step for regulation or disruption of mRNA metabolism occurs during the transport from nucleus to cytoplasm. mRNA transport is an active, energy-consuming process. Moreover, at least some mRNAs appear to enter the cytoplasm in the form of complexes bound to proteins (mRNPs). mRNPs may regulate stability of the mRNAs and their access to translational apparatus. Some evidence indicates that certain mRNPs are present in the cytoplasm but are not translated (masked message) until proper physiologic signals are received.

GENE REGULATION

Virtually all cells of an organism receive a complete copy of the DNA genome inherited at the time of conception. The panoply of distinct cell types and tissues found in any complex organism is possible only because different portions of the genome are selectively expressed or repressed in each cell type. Each cell must "know" which genes to express, how actively to express them, and when to express them. This biologic necessity has come to be known as *gene regulation* or *regulated gene expression*. Understanding gene regulation provides insight into how pluripotent stem cells determine that they will express the proper sets of genes in daughter progenitor cells that differentiate along each lineage. Major hematologic disorders (e.g., the leukemias and lymphomas), immunodeficiency states, and myeloproliferative syndromes result from derangements in the system of gene regulation. An understanding of the ways that genes are selected for expression thus remains one of the major frontiers of biology and medicine.

EPIGENETIC REGULATION OF GENE EXPRESSION

Most of the DNA in living cells is inactivated by formation of a nucleoprotein complex called *chromatin*. The histone and nonhistone proteins in chromatin effectively sequester genes from enzymes needed for expression. The most tightly compacted chromatin regions are called *euchromatin*. Heterochromatin, less tightly packed, contains actively transcribed genes. Activation of a gene for expression (i.e., transcription) requires that it become less compacted and more accessible to the transcription apparatus. These processes involve both *cis*-acting and *trans*-acting factors. *Cis*-acting elements are regulatory DNA sequences within or flanking the genes. They are recognized by *trans*-acting factors, which are nuclear DNA–binding proteins needed for transcriptional regulation.

DNA sequence regions flanking genes are called *cis*-acting because they influence expression of nearby genes only on the same chromosome. These sequences do not usually encode mRNA or protein molecules. They alter the conformation of the gene within chromatin in such a way as to facilitate or inhibit access to the factors that modulate transcription. These interactions may twist or kink the DNA in such a way as to control exposure to other molecules. When exogenous nucleases are added in small amounts to nuclei, these exposed sequence regions become especially sensitive to the DNA-cutting action of the nucleases. Thus, nuclease-hypersensitive sites in DNA have come to be appreciated as markers for regions in or near genes that are interacting with regulatory nuclear proteins.

Methylation is another structural feature that can be used to recognize differences between actively transcribed and inactive genes. Most eukaryotic DNA is heavily methylated; that is, the DNA is modified by the addition of a methyl group to the 5 position of the cytosine pyrimidine ring (5-methyl-C). In general, whereas heavily methylated genes are inactive, active genes are relatively hypomethylated, especially in the 5′ flanking regions containing the promoter and other regulatory elements (see "Enhancers, Promoters, and Silencers"). These flanking regions frequently include DNA sequences with a high content of Cs and Gs (CpG islands). Hypomethylated CpG islands (detectable by methylation-sensitive restriction endonucleases) serve as markers of actively transcribed genes. For example, a search for undermethylated CpG islands on chromosome 7 facilitated the search for the gene for cystic fibrosis.

DNA methylation is facilitated by DNA methyltransferases. DNA replication incorporates unmethylated nucleotides into each nascent strand, thus leading to demethylated DNA. For cytosines to become methylated, the methyltransferases must act after each round of replication. After an initial wave of demethylation early in embryonic development, regulatory areas are methylated during various stages of development and differentiation. Aberrant DNA methylation also occurs as an early step during tumorigenesis, leading to silencing of tumor suppressor genes and of genes related to differentiation. This finding has led to induction of DNA demethylation as a target in cancer therapy. Indeed, 5-azacytidine, a cytidine analog unable to be methylated, and the related compound decitabine, are approved by the United States Food and Drug Administration for use in myelodysplastic syndromes, and their use in cases of other malignancies is being investigated.

Although it is poorly understood how particular regions of DNA are targeted for methylation, it is becoming increasingly apparent that this modification targets further alterations in chromatin proteins that in turn influence gene expression. Histone acetylation, phosphorylation, and methylation of the N-terminal tail are currently the focus of intense study. Acetylation of lysine residues (catalyzed by histone acetyltransferases), for example, is associated with transcriptional activation. Conversely, histone deacetylation (catalyzed by histone deacetylase) leads to gene silencing. Histone deacetylases are recruited to areas of DNA methylation by DNA methyltransferases and by methyl–DNA-binding proteins, thus linking DNA methylation to histone deacetylation. Drugs inhibiting these enzymes have been demonstrated to be active anticancer agents and continue to be the focus of ongoing studies. The regulation of histone acetylation and deacetylation appears to be linked to gene expression, but the roles of histone phosphorylation and methylation are less well understood. Current research suggests that in addition to gene regulation, histone modifications contribute to the "epigenetic code" and are thus a means by which information regarding chromatin structure is passed to daughter cells after DNA replication occurs.

ENHANCERS, PROMOTERS, AND SILENCERS

Several types of *cis*-active DNA sequence elements have been defined according to the presumed consequences of their interaction with nuclear proteins (see Fig. 1.5). Promoters are found just upstream (to the 5′ side) of the start of mRNA transcription (the CAP). mRNA polymerases appear to bind first to the promoter region and thereby gain access to the structural gene sequences downstream. Promoters thus serve a dual function of being binding sites for mRNA polymerase and marking for the polymerase the downstream point at which transcription should start.

Enhancers are more complicated DNA sequence elements. Enhancers can lie on either side of a gene or even within the gene. Enhancers bind transcription factors and thereby stimulate expression of genes nearby. The domain of influence of enhancers (i.e., the number of genes to either side whose expression is stimulated) varies. Some enhancers influence only the adjacent gene; others seem to mark the boundaries of large multigene clusters (gene domains) whose coordinated expression is appropriate to a particular tissue type or a particular time. For example, the very high levels of globin gene expression in erythroid cells depend on the function of an enhancer that seems to activate the entire gene cluster and is thus called a *locus-activating region* (see Fig. 1.5). The nuclear factors interacting with enhancers are probably induced into synthesis or activation as part of the process of differentiation. Chromosomal rearrangements that place a gene that is usually tightly regulated under the control of a highly active enhancer can lead to overexpression of that gene. This commonly occurs in Burkitt lymphoma, for example, in which the MYC proto-oncogene is juxtaposed and dysregulated by an immunoglobulin enhancer.

Silencer sequences serve a function that is the obverse of enhancers. When bound by the appropriate nuclear proteins, silencer sequences cause repression of gene expression. Some evidence indicates that the same sequence elements can act as enhancers or silencers under different conditions, presumably by being bound by different sets of proteins having opposite effects on transcription. *Insulators* are sequence domains that mark the "boundaries" of multigene clusters, thereby preventing activation of one set of genes from "leaking" into nearby genes.

TRANSCRIPTION FACTORS

Transcription factors are nuclear proteins that exhibit gene-specific DNA binding. Considerable information is now available about these nuclear proteins and their biochemical properties, but their physiologic behavior remains incompletely understood. Common structural features have become apparent. Most transcription factors have DNA-binding domains sharing homologous structural motifs (cytosine-rich regions called zinc fingers, leucine-rich regions called leucine zippers, and so on), but other regions appear to be unique. Many factors implicated in the regulation of growth, differentiation, and development (e.g., homeobox genes, proto-oncogenes, antioncogenes) appear to be DNA-binding proteins and may be involved in the steps needed for activation of a gene within chromatin. Others bind to or modify DNA-binding proteins. These factors are discussed in more detail in several other chapters.

REGULATION OF mRNA SPLICING, STABILITY, AND TRANSLATION (POSTTRANSCRIPTIONAL REGULATION)

It has become increasingly apparent that posttranscriptional and translational mechanisms are important strategies used by cells to govern the amounts of mRNA and protein accumulating when a particular gene is expressed. The major modes of posttranscriptional regulation at the mRNA level are regulated alternative mRNA splicing, control of mRNA stability, and control of translational efficiency. As discussed elsewhere (see Chapter 5), additional regulation at the protein level occurs by mechanisms modulating localization, stability, activation, or export of the protein.

A cell can regulate the relative amounts of different protein isoforms arising from a given gene by altering the relative amounts of an mRNA precursor that are spliced along one pathway or another (alternative mRNA splicing). Many striking examples of this type of regulation are known—for example, the ability of B lymphocytes to make both IgM and IgD at the same developmental stage, changes in the particular isoforms of cytoskeletal proteins produced during red blood cell differentiation, and a switch from one isoform of the *c-myb* proto-oncogene product to another during red blood cell differentiation. Abnormalities in mRNA splicing due to mutations at the splice sites can lead to defective protein synthesis, as can occur in β-globin, leading to a form of β-thalassemia. The effect of controlling the pathway of mRNA processing used in a cell is to include or exclude portions of the mRNA sequence. These portions encode peptide sequences that influence the ultimate physiologic behavior of the protein, or the RNA sequences that alter stability or translatability.

The importance of the control of mRNA stability for gene regulation is being increasingly appreciated. The steady-state level of any given mRNA species ultimately depends on the balance between the rate of its production (transcription and mRNA processing) and its destruction. One means by which stability is regulated is the inherent structure of the mRNA sequence, especially the 3′ and 5′ UTRs. As already noted, these sequences appear to affect mRNA secondary structure, recognition by nucleases, or both. Different mRNAs thus have inherently longer or shorter half-lives, almost regardless of the cell type in which they are expressed. Some mRNAs tend to be highly unstable. In response to appropriate physiologic needs, they can thus be produced quickly and removed from the cell quickly when a need for them no longer exists. Globin mRNA, on the other hand, is inherently quite stable, with a half-life measured in the range of 15 to 50 hours. This is appropriate for the need of reticulocytes to continue to synthesize globin for 24 to 48 hours after the ability to synthesize new mRNA has been lost by the terminally mature erythroblasts.

The stability of mRNA can also be altered in response to changes in the intracellular milieu. This phenomenon usually involves nucleases capable of destroying one or more broad classes of mRNA defined on the basis of their 3′ or 5′ UTR sequences. Thus, for example, histone mRNAs are destabilized after the S-phase of the cell cycle is complete. Presumably this occurs because histone synthesis is no longer needed. Induction of cell activation, mitogenesis, or terminal differentiation events often results in the induction of nucleases that destabilize specific subsets of mRNAs. Selective stabilization of mRNAs probably also occurs; α-globin mRNA, for example, is stabilized by the protective binding of a specific stabilizing protein to a nuclease target sequence in its 3′ UTR.

The amount of a given protein accumulating in a cell depends on the amount of the mRNA present, the rate at which it is translated into the protein, and the stability of the protein. Translational efficiency depends on a number of variables, including polyadenylation and presence of the 5′ cap. The amounts and state of activation of protein factors needed for translation are also crucial. The secondary structure of the mRNA, particularly in the 5′ UTR, greatly influences the intrinsic translatability of an mRNA molecule by constraining the access of translation factors and ribosomes to the translation initiation signal in the mRNA. Secondary structures along the coding sequence of the mRNA may also have some impact on the rate of elongation of the peptide.

Changes in capping, polyadenylation, and translation factor efficiency affect the overall rate of protein synthesis within each cell. These effects tend to be global rather than specific to a particular gene product. However, these effects influence the relative amounts of different proteins made. mRNAs whose structures inherently lend themselves to more efficient translation tend to compete better for rate-limiting components of the translational apparatus, but mRNAs that are inherently less translatable tend to be translated less efficiently in the face of limited access to other translational components. For example, the translation factor eIF-4 tends to be produced in higher amounts when cells encounter transforming or mitogenic events. This causes an increase in overall rates of protein synthesis but also leads to a selective increase in the synthesis of some proteins that were underproduced before mitogenesis.

Translational regulation of individual mRNA species is critical for some events important to blood cell homeostasis. For example, as discussed in Chapter 35, the amount of iron entering a cell is an exquisite regulator of the rate of ferritin mRNA translation. An mRNA sequence called the *iron response element* is recognized by a specific mRNA-binding protein but only when the protein lacks iron. mRNA bound to the protein is translationally inactive. As iron accumulates in the cell, the protein becomes iron bound and loses its affinity for the mRNA, resulting in translation into apoferritin molecules that bind the iron.

Tubulin synthesis involves coordinated regulation of translation and mRNA stability. Tubulin regulates the stability of its own mRNA by a feedback loop. As tubulin concentrations rise in the cell, it interacts with its own mRNA through the intermediary of an mRNA-binding protein. This results in the formation of an mRNA–protein complex and nucleolytic cleavage of the mRNA. The mRNA is destroyed, and further tubulin production is halted.

These few examples of posttranscriptional regulation emphasize that cells tend to use every step in the complex pathway of gene expression as points at which exquisite control over the amounts of a particular protein can be regulated. In other chapters, additional levels of regulation are described (e.g., regulation of the stability, activity, localization, and access to other cellular components of the proteins that are present in a cell).

SMALL INTERFERING RNA AND MICRO RNA

Another posttranscriptional mechanism of gene silencing utilizes so-called "small RNAs". One such process is carried out by small interfering RNAs (siRNAs): short, double-stranded fragments of RNA containing 21 to 23 bp (Fig. 1.6). The process is triggered by perfectly complementary double-stranded RNA, which is cleaved by Dicer, a member of the RNase III family, into siRNA fragments. These small fragments of double-stranded RNA are unwound by a helicase in the RNA-induced silencing complex (RISC). The antisense strand anneals to mRNA transcripts in a sequence-specific manner and in doing so brings the endonuclease activity within the RISC to the targeted transcript. An RNA-dependent RNA polymerase in the RISC may then create new siRNAs to processively degrade the mRNA, ultimately leading to complete degradation of the mRNA transcript and abrogation of protein expression.

Although this endogenous process likely evolved to destroy invading viral RNA, the use of siRNA has become a commonly used tool for evaluation of gene function. Sequence-specific synthetic siRNA may be directly introduced into cells or introduced via gene transfection methods and targeted to an mRNA of a gene of interest. The siRNA will lead to degradation of the mRNA transcript, and accordingly prevent new protein translation. This technique is a relatively simple, efficient, and inexpensive means to investigate cellular phenotypes after directed elimination of expression of a single gene. The 2006 Nobel Prize in Physiology or Medicine was awarded to two discoverers of RNA interference, Andrew Fire and Craig Mello.

Micro RNAs (miRNAs, or MIRs) are 22-nucleotide small RNAs encoded by the cellular genome that alter mRNA stability and protein translation. These genes are transcribed by RNA polymerase II and capped and polyadenylated similar to other RNA polymerase II transcripts. The precursor transcript of approximately 70 nucleotides is cleaved into mature miRNA by the enzymes Drosha and Dicer. One strand of the resulting duplex forms a complex with the RISC that together binds the target mRNA with imperfect complementarity. Through mechanisms that are still incompletely understood,

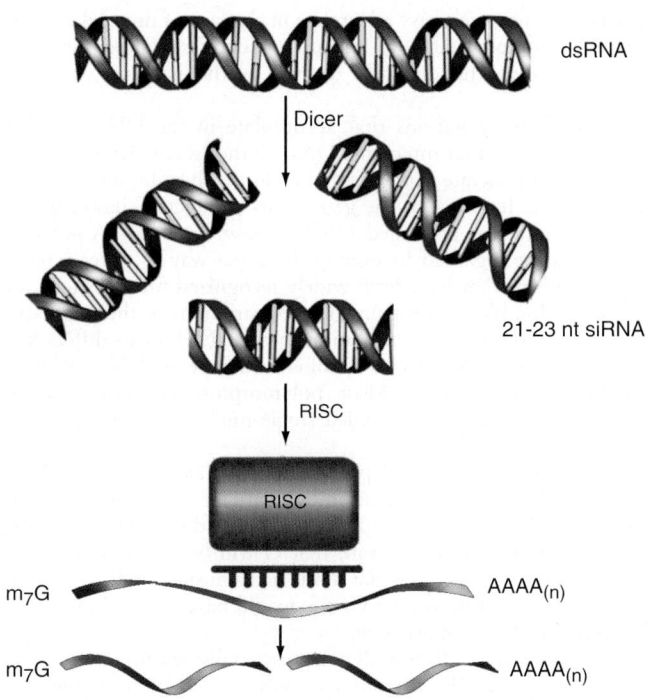

Fig. 1.6 mRNA DEGRADATION BY siRNA. dsRNA is digested into 21- to 23-bp siRNAs by the Dicer RNase. These RNA fragments are unwound by RISC and bring the endonucleolytic activity of RISC to mRNA transcripts in a sequence-specific manner, leading to degradation of the mRNA. *dsRNA*, Double-stranded RNA; *mRNA*, messenger RNA; *RISC*, RNA-induced silencing complex; *siRNA*, small interfering RNA.

miRNA suppresses gene expression, likely either through inhibition of protein translation or through destabilization of mRNA. miRNAs appear to have essential roles in development and differentiation, and are aberrantly regulated in many types of cancer cells. The identification of miRNA sequences, their regulation, and their target genes are areas of intense study.

ADDITIONAL STRUCTURAL FEATURES OF GENOMIC DNA

Most DNA does not code for RNA or protein molecules. The vast majority of nucleotides present in the human genome reside outside structural genes. Structural genes are separated from one another by as few as 1 to 5 kilobases or as many as several thousand kilobases of DNA. Almost nothing is known about the reason for the erratic clustering and spacing of genes along chromosomes. It is clear that intergenic DNA contains a variegated landscape of structural features that provide useful tools to localize genes, identify individual human beings as unique from every other human being (DNA fingerprinting), and diagnose human diseases by linkage. Only a brief introduction is provided here.

The rate of mutation in DNA under normal circumstances is approximately $1/10^6$. In other words, one of 1 million bases of DNA will be mutated during each round of DNA replication. A set of enzymes called *DNA proofreading enzymes* corrects many but not all of these mutations. When these enzymes are themselves altered by mutation, the rate of mutation (and therefore the odds of neoplastic transformation) increases considerably. If these mutations occur in bases critical to the structure or function of a protein or gene, altered function, disease, or a lethal condition can result. Most pathologic mutations tend not to be preserved throughout many generations because of their unfavorable phenotypes. Exceptions, such as the hemoglobinopathies, occur when the heterozygous state for these mutations confers selective advantage in the face of unusual environmental conditions, such as malaria epidemics. These "adaptive" mutations drive the dynamic change in the genome with time (evolution).

Most of the mutations that accumulate in the DNA of *Homo sapiens* occur in either intergenic DNA or the "silent" bases of DNA, such as the degenerate third bases of codons. They do not pathologically alter the function of the gene or its products. These clinically harmless mutations are called *DNA polymorphisms*. DNA polymorphisms can be regarded in exactly the same way as other types of polymorphisms that have been widely recognized for years (e.g., eye and hair color, blood groups). They are variations in the population that occur without apparent clinical impact. Each of us differs from other humans in the precise number and type of DNA polymorphisms that we possess. Most polymorphisms represent single-nucleotide changes and are called single-nucleotide polymorphisms (SNPs).

Similar to other types of polymorphisms, DNA polymorphisms breed true. In other words, if an individual's DNA contains a G 1200 bases upstream from the α-globin gene, instead of the C most commonly found in the population, that G will be transmitted to that individual's offspring. Note that if one had a means for distinguishing the G at that position from a C, one would have a linked marker for that individual's α-globin gene.

Occasionally, a DNA polymorphism falls within a restriction endonuclease site. (Restriction enzymes cut DNA molecules into smaller pieces but only at limited sites, defined by short base sequences recognized by each enzyme.) The change could abolish the site or create a site where one did not exist before. These polymorphisms change the array of fragments generated when the genome is digested by that restriction endonuclease. This permits detection of the polymorphism by use of the appropriate restriction enzyme. This specific class of polymorphisms is thus called *restriction fragment length polymorphisms* (RFLPs).

RFLPs are useful because the length of a restriction endonuclease fragment on which a gene of interest resides provides a linked marker for that gene. The exploitation of this fact for diagnosis of genetic diseases and detection of specific genes is discussed in Chapters 2 and 3; Fig. 1.7 shows a simple example.

RFLPs have proved to be extraordinarily useful for the diagnosis of genetic diseases, especially when the precise mutation is not known. Recall that DNA polymorphisms breed true in the population. For example, as discussed in Chapter 135, a mutation that causes hemophilia will, when it occurs on the X chromosome, be transmitted to subsequent generations attached to the pattern (often called a framework or haplotype) of RFLPs that was present on that same X chromosome. If the pattern of RFLPs in the parents is known, the presence of the abnormal chromosome can be detected in the offspring.

Genomic technologies (see Chapters 2 and 3) have made it possible to characterize SNPs scattered across the entire genome, whether or not they alter restriction endonuclease sites. SNP analysis is gaining momentum as a means for characterizing genomes. The advent of highly efficient, speedy, and increasingly cheap genome sequencing technologies now permits one to identify SNPs almost at will, and is rapidly replacing the use of RFLPs. The principles of choosing the right comparison populations and of the "breeding true" through generations, however, remain important principles in interpreting the results.

An important feature of the DNA landscape is the high degree of repeated DNA sequence. A DNA sequence is said to be repeated if it or a sequence very similar (homologous) to it occurs more than once in a genome. Some multicopy genes, such as the histone genes and the ribosomal RNA genes, are repeated DNA sequences. Most repeated DNA occurs outside genes, or within introns. Indeed, 30% to 45% of the human genome appears to consist of repeated DNA sequences.

The function of repeated sequences remains unknown, but their presence has inspired useful strategies for detecting and characterizing individual genomes. For example, a pattern of short repeated DNA

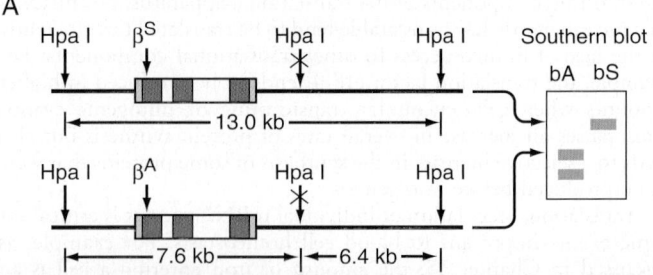

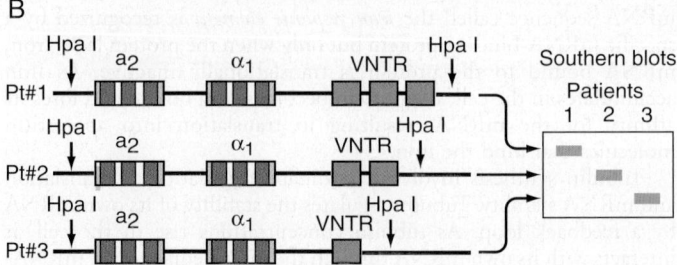

Fig. 1.7 TWO USEFUL FORMS OF SEQUENCE VARIATION AMONG THE GENOMES OF NORMAL INDIVIDUALS. (A) Presence of a DNA sequence polymorphism that falls within a restriction endonuclease site, thus altering the pattern of restriction endonuclease digests obtained from this region of DNA on Southern blot analysis. (Readers not familiar with Southern blot analysis should return to examine this figure after reading later sections of this chapter.) (B) A variable-number tandem repeat (VNTR) region (defined and discussed in the text). Note that individuals can vary from one to another in many ways according to how many repeated units of the VNTR are located on their genomes, but restriction fragment length polymorphism differences are in effect all-or-none differences, allowing for only two variables (restriction site presence or absence).

sequences, characterized by the presence of flanking sites recognized by the restriction endonuclease Alu-1 (called "Alu repeats"), occurs approximately 300,000 times in a human genome. These sequences are not present in the mouse genome. If one wishes to infect mouse cells with human DNA and then identify the human DNA sequences in the infected mouse cells, one simply probes for the presence of Alu repeats. The Alu repeat thus serves as a signature of human DNA.

Classes of highly repeated DNA sequences (tandem repeats) have proved to be useful for distinguishing genomes of each human individual. These short DNA sequences, usually less than a few hundred bases long, tend to occur in clusters, with the number of repeats varying among individuals (see Fig. 1.6). Alleles of a given gene can therefore be associated with a variable number of tandem repeats (VNTR) in different individuals or populations. For example, there is a VNTR near the insulin gene. In some individuals or populations, it is present in only a few tandem copies, but in others, it is present in many more. When the population as a whole is examined, there is a wide degree of variability from individual to individual as to the number of these repeats residing near the insulin gene. It can readily be imagined that if probes were available to detect a dozen or so distinct VNTR regions, each human individual would differ from virtually all others with respect to the aggregate pattern of these VNTRs. Indeed, it can be shown mathematically that the probability of any two human beings sharing exactly the same pattern of VNTRs is exceedingly small if approximately 10 to 12 different VNTR elements are mapped for each person. A technique called *DNA fingerprinting* that is based on VNTR analysis has become widely publicized because of its forensic applications.

There are many other classes of repeated sequences in human DNA. For example, human DNA has been invaded many times in its history by retroviruses. Retroviruses tend to integrate into human DNA and then "jump out" of the genome when they are reactivated, to complete their life cycle. The proviral genomes often carry with them nearby bits of the genomic DNA in which they sat. If the retrovirus infects the DNA of another individual at another site, it will insert this genomic bit. Through many cycles of infection, the virus will act as a transposon, scattering its attached sequence throughout the genome. These types of sequences are called *long interspersed elements*. They represent footprints of ancient viral infections.

KEY METHODS FOR GENE ANALYSIS

The foundation for the molecular understanding of gene structure and expression is based on fundamental molecular biologic techniques that were developed in the 1970s and 1980s. These techniques allow for the reduction of the multibillion nucleotide genome into smaller fragments that are more easily analyzed. Several key methods are outlined here.

Restriction Endonucleases

Naturally occurring bacterial enzymes called *restriction endonucleases* catalyze sequence-specific hydrolysis of phosphodiester bonds in the DNA backbone. For example, EcoRI, a restriction endonuclease isolated from *Escherichia coli*, cleaves DNA only at the sequence 5′-GAATTC-3′. Thus, each DNA sample will be reproducibly reduced to an array of fragments whose size ranges depend on the distribution with which that sequence exists within the DNA. A specific six-nucleotide sequence would be statistically expected to appear once every 4^6 (or 4096) nucleotides, but in reality, the distance between specific sequences varies greatly. Using combinations of restriction endonucleases, DNA several hundred million base pairs in length can be reproducibly reduced to fragments ranging from a few dozen to tens of thousands of base pairs long. These smaller products of enzymatic digestion are much more manageable experimentally. Genetic "fingerprinting," or restriction enzyme maps of genomes, can be constructed by analyzing the DNA fragments resulting from digestion. Many enzymes cleave DNA so as to leave short, single-stranded overhanging regions that can be enzymatically linked to other similar fragments, generating artificially recombined, or recombinant, DNA molecules. These ligated gene fragments can then be inserted into bacteria to produce more copies of the recombinant molecules or to express the cloned genes. While still useful in a number of contexts, restriction enzyme analysis is increasingly being supplanted by direct DNA sequence analysis.

DNA, RNA, and Protein Blotting

There are many ways that a cloned DNA sequence can be exploited to characterize the behavior of normal or pathologic genes. Blotting methods deserve special mention because of their widespread use in clinical and experimental hematology. A cloned DNA fragment can be easily purified and tagged with a radioactive or nonradioactive label. The fragment provides a pure and highly specific molecular hybridization probe for the detection of complementary DNA (cDNA) or RNA molecules in any specimen of DNA or RNA. One set of assays that has proved particularly useful involves Southern blotting, named after Dr. E. Southern, who invented the method (Fig. 1.8). Southern blotting allows detection of a specific gene, or region in or near a gene, in a DNA preparation. The DNA is isolated and digested with one or more restriction endonucleases, and the resulting fragments are denatured and separated according to their molecular size by electrophoresis through agarose gels. By means of capillary action in a high-salt buffer, the DNA fragments are passively transferred to a nitrocellulose or nylon membrane. Single-stranded DNA and RNA molecules attach noncovalently but tightly to the membrane. In this fashion, the membrane becomes a replica, or blot, of the gel. After the blotting procedure is complete, the membrane is incubated in a hybridization buffer containing the radioactively labeled probe. The probe hybridizes only to the gene of interest and renders radioactive only one or a few bands containing complementary sequences. After appropriate washing and drying, the bands can be visualized by autoradiography.

Digestion of a DNA preparation with several different restriction enzymes allows a restriction endonuclease map of a gene in the human genome to be constructed. Southern blotting has thus become a standard way of characterizing the configuration of genes in the genome.

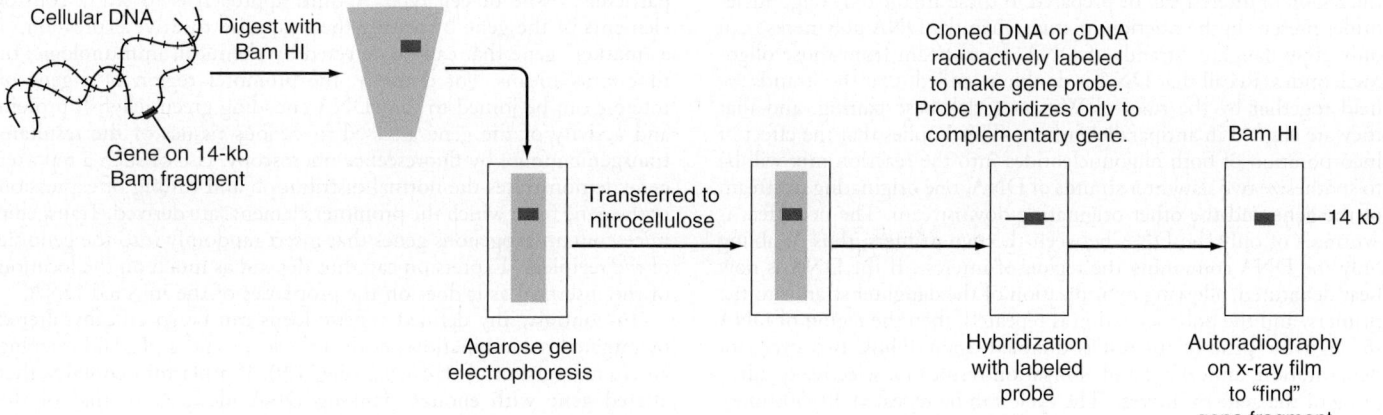

Fig. 1.8 SOUTHERN GENE BLOTTING. Detection of a genomic gene *(red)* that resides on a 14-kilobase Bam HI fragment. To identify the presence of a gene in the genome and the size of the restriction fragment on which it resides, genomic DNA is digested with a restriction enzyme, and the fragments are separated by agarose gel electrophoresis. Human genomes contain from several hundred thousand to 1 million sites for any particular restriction enzyme, which results in a vast array of fragments and creates a blur or streak on the gel; one fragment cannot be distinguished from another readily. If the DNA in the gel is transferred to nitrocellulose by capillary blotting, however, it can be further analyzed by molecular hybridization to a radioactive cDNA probe for the gene. Only the band containing the gene yields a positive autoradiography signal, as shown. If a disease state were to result in loss of the gene, alteration of its structure, or mutation (altering recognition sites for one or more restriction enzymes), the banding pattern would be changed. *cDNA,* Complementary DNA.

Northern blotting represents an analogous blotting procedure used to detect RNA. RNA cannot be digested with restriction enzymes (which cut only DNA); rather, the intact RNA molecules can be separated according to molecular size by electrophoresis through the gel (mRNAs are 0.5 to 12 kilobases in length), transferred onto membranes, and probed with a DNA probe. In this fashion, the presence, absence, molecular size, and number of individual species of a particular mRNA species can be detected.

Western blotting is a similar method that can be used to examine protein expression. Cellular lysates (or another source of proteins) can be electrophoresed through a polyacrylamide gel so as to separate proteins on the basis of their apparent molecular sizes. The resolved proteins can then be electrically transferred to nitrocellulose membranes and probed with specific antibodies directed against the protein of interest. As with RNA analysis, the relative expression levels and molecular sizes of proteins can be assessed with this method.

Polymerase Chain Reaction

The development of the polymerase chain reaction (PCR) was a major breakthrough that has revolutionized the utility of a DNA-based strategy for diagnosis and treatment. It permits the detection, synthesis, and isolation of specific genes and allows differentiation of alleles of a gene differing by as little as one base. It does not require sophisticated equipment or unusual technical skills. A clinical specimen consisting of only minute amounts of tissue will suffice; in most circumstances, no special preparation of the tissue is necessary. PCR thus makes recombinant DNA techniques accessible to clinical laboratories. This single advance has produced a quantum increase in the use of direct gene analysis for diagnosis of human diseases. Indeed, PCR analysis combined with direct DNA sequencing technologies have largely supplanted restriction enzyme mapping and blotting strategies for many research and diagnostic applications.

The PCR is based on the prerequisites for copying an existing DNA strand by DNA polymerase: an existing denatured strand of DNA to be used as the template and a primer. Primers are short oligonucleotides, 12 to 100 bases in length, having a base sequence complementary to the desired region of the existing DNA strand. The enzyme requires the primer to "know" where to begin copying. If the base sequence of the DNA of the gene under study is known, two synthetic oligonucleotides complementary to sequences flanking the region of interest can be prepared. If these are the only oligonucleotides present in the reaction mixture, then the DNA polymerase can only copy daughter strands of DNA downstream from those oligonucleotides. Recall that DNA is double stranded, that the strands are held together by the rules of Watson–Crick base pairing, and that they are aligned in antiparallel fashion. This implies that the effect of incorporation of both oligonucleotides into the reaction mix will be to synthesize two daughter strands of DNA, one originating upstream of the gene and the other originating downstream. The net effect is synthesis of only the DNA between the two primers, thus doubling only the DNA containing the region of interest. If the DNA is now heat denatured, allowing hybridization of the daughter strands to the primers, and the polymerization is repeated, then the region of DNA through the gene of interest is doubled again. Thus, two cycles of denaturation, annealing, and elongation result in a selective quadrupling of the gene of interest. The cycle can be repeated 30–50 times, resulting in a selective and geometric amplification of the sequence of interest to the order of 2^{30} to 2^{50} times. The result is a millionfold or higher selective amplification of the gene of interest, yielding microgram quantities of that DNA sequence.

PCR achieved practical utility when DNA polymerases from thermophilic bacteria were discovered; when synthetic oligonucleotides of any desired sequence could be produced efficiently, reproducibly, and cheaply by automated instrumentation; and when DNA thermocycling machines were developed. Thermophilic bacteria live in hot springs and other exceedingly warm environments, and their DNA polymerases can tolerate 100°C (212°F) incubations without substantial loss of activity. The advantage of these thermostable polymerases is that they retain activity in a reaction mix that is repeatedly heated to the high temperature needed to denature the DNA strands into the single-stranded form. Microprocessor-driven DNA thermocycler machines can be programmed to increase temperatures to 95°C to 100°C (203°F to 212°F) (denaturation), to cool the mix to 50°C (101°F) rapidly (a temperature that favors oligonucleotide annealing), and then to raise the temperature to 70°C to 75°C (141.4°F to 151.5°F) (the temperature for optimal activity of the thermophilic DNA polymerases). In a reaction containing the test specimen, the thermophilic polymerase, the primers, and the chemical components (e.g., nucleotide subunits), the thermocycler can conduct many cycles of denaturation, annealing, and polymerization in a completely automated fashion. The gene of interest can thus be amplified more than a millionfold in a matter of a few hours. The DNA product is readily identified and isolated by routine agarose gel electrophoresis. The DNA can then be analyzed by restriction endonuclease, digestion, hybridization to specific probes, sequencing, further amplification by cloning, and so forth.

USE OF TRANSGENIC AND KNOCKOUT MICE TO DEFINE GENE FUNCTION

Recombinant DNA technology has resulted in the identification of many disease-related genes. To advance the understanding of the disease related to a previously unknown gene, the function of the protein encoded by that gene must be verified or identified, and the way changes in the gene's expression influence the disease phenotype must be characterized. Analysis of the role of these genes and their encoded proteins has been made possible by the development of recombinant DNA technology that allows the production of mice that are genetically altered at the cloned locus. Mice can be produced that express an exogenous gene and thereby provide an in vivo model of its function. Linearized DNA is injected into a fertilized mouse oocyte pronucleus and reimplanted in a pseudopregnant mouse. The resultant transgenic mice can then be analyzed for the phenotype induced by the injected transgene. Placing the gene under the control of a strong promoter that stimulates expression of the exogenous gene in all tissues allows the assessment of the effect of widespread overexpression of the gene. Alternatively, placing the gene under the control of a promoter that can function only in certain tissues (a tissue-specific promoter) elucidates the function of that gene in a particular tissue or cell type. A third approach is to study control elements of the gene by testing their capacity to drive expression of a "marker" gene that can be detected by chemical, immunologic, or functional means. For example, the promoter region of a gene of interest can be joined to the cDNA encoding green jellyfish protein and activity of the gene assessed in various tissues of the resultant transgenic mouse by fluorescence microscopy. Use of such a reporter gene demonstrates the normal distribution and timing of expression of the gene from which the promoter elements are derived. Transgenic mice contain exogenous genes that insert randomly into the genome of the recipient. Expression can thus depend as much on the location of the insertion as it does on the properties of the injected DNA.

In contrast, any defined genetic locus can be specifically altered by targeted recombination between the locus and a plasmid carrying an altered version of that gene (Fig. 1.9). If a plasmid contains that altered gene with enough flanking DNA identical to that of the normal gene locus, homologous recombination can occur, and the altered gene in the plasmid will replace the gene in the recipient cell. Using a mutation that inactivates the gene allows the production of a null mutation, in which the function of that gene is completely lost. To induce such a mutation, the plasmid is introduced into an embryonic stem cell, and the rare cells that undergo homologous recombination are selected. The "knockout" embryonic stem cell is then introduced into the blastocyst of a developing embryo. The resultant animals are chimeric; only a fraction of the cells in the animal contain the targeted gene. If the new gene is introduced into some of the germline cells of the chimeric mouse, then some of the offspring of that mouse will carry the mutation as a gene in all of

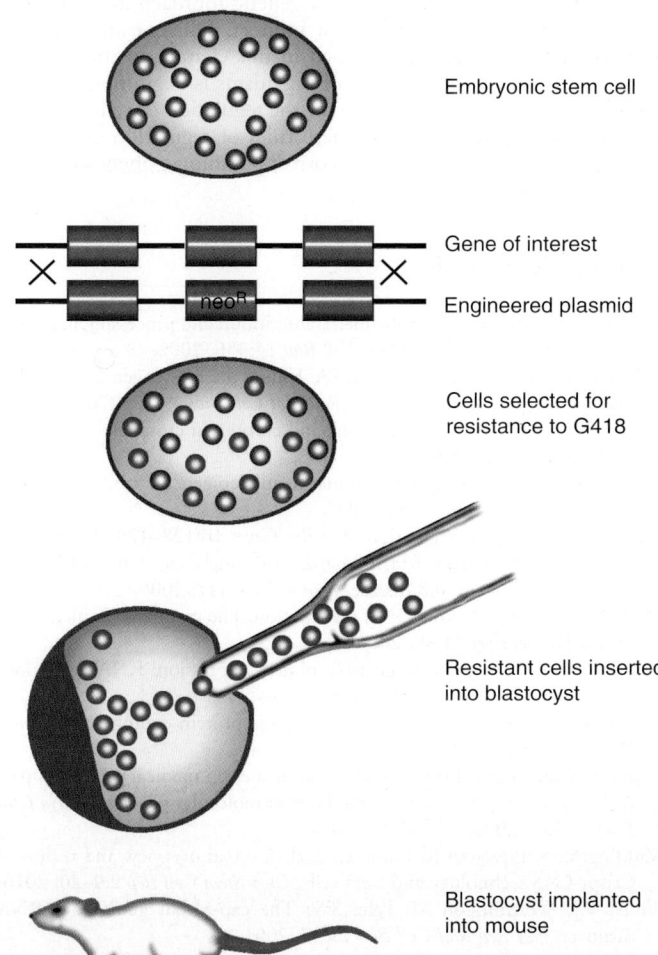

Embryonic stem cell

Gene of interest

Engineered plasmid

Cells selected for
resistance to G418

Resistant cells inserted
into blastocyst

Blastocyst implanted
into mouse

Fig. 1.9 GENE "KNOCKOUT" BY HOMOLOGOUS RECOMBINA-
TION. A plasmid containing genomic DNA homologous to the gene of
interest is engineered to contain a selectable marker positioned so as to disrupt
expression of the native gene. The DNA is introduced into embryonic stem
cells, and cells resistant to the selectable marker are isolated and injected into
a mouse blastocyst, which is then implanted into a mouse. Offspring mice
that contain the knockout construct in their germ cells are then propagated,
yielding mice with heterozygous or homozygous inactivation of the gene of
interest.

their cells. These heterozygous mice can be further bred to produce
mice homozygous for the null allele. Such knockout mice reveal the
function of the targeted gene by the phenotype induced by its
absence. Genetically altered mice have been essential for discerning
the biologic and pathologic roles of large numbers of genes implicated
in the pathogenesis of human disease.

DNA-BASED THERAPIES

Gene Therapy

The application of gene therapy to genetic hematologic disorders is
an appealing idea. In most cases, this would involve isolating hematopoietic stem cells from patients with diseases with defined genetic
lesions, inserting normal genes into those cells, and reintroducing the
genetically engineered stem cells back into the patient. A few candidate diseases for such therapy include sickle cell disease, thalassemia,
hemophilia, and adenosine deaminase–deficient severe combined
immunodeficiency. The technology for separating hematopoietic

stem cells and for performing gene transfer into those cells has
advanced rapidly, and clinical trials have begun to test the applicability of these techniques. Despite the fact that gene therapy has progressed to the enrollment of patients in clinical protocols, major
technical problems still need to be solved. Presently, there are only
few (but increasing, such as severe combined immunodeficiency
syndromes, Wiskott–Aldrich disease, and others) proven therapeutic
successes from gene therapy.

Progress in this field continues rapidly and is likely to accelerate
as a consequence of the development of "gene editing" technologies.
Among these, "CRISPR" is the most prominent current example. It
is based on the discovery of enzyme systems used by microorganisms
to excise foreign DNA sequences (e.g., integrated viral genomes) from
the host genome. These systems can be adapted to insert, replace, or
delete, in principle, any desired DNA sequence in its naturally occurring position in the host genome. For example, one could excise the
mutation causing sickle cell anemia and replace it with the normal
DNA sequence in the β-globin gene of a patient's hematopoietic stem
cells, and then re-introduce them into the patient's bone marrow
without introducing any foreign DNA. This exciting technology is
rapidly moving toward clinical trials. The scientific basis for gene
therapy and the clinical issues surrounding this approach are discussed
in Chapter 98.

Antisense Therapy

The recognition that abnormal expression of oncogenes plays a role
in malignancy has stimulated attempts to suppress oncogene expression to reverse the neoplastic phenotype. One way of blocking mRNA
expression is with antisense oligonucleotides. These are single-
stranded DNA sequences 17 to 20 bases long, having a sequence
complementary to the transcription or translation start of the mRNA.
These relatively small molecules freely enter the cell and complex to
the mRNA by their complementary DNA sequence. This often
results in a decrease in gene expression. The binding of the oligonucleotide may directly block translation and clearly enhances the rate of
mRNA degradation. This technique has been shown to be promising
in suppressing expression of *bcr-abl* and to suppress cell growth in
chronic myelogenous leukemia. The technique is being tried as a
therapeutic modality for the purging of tumor cells before autologous
transplantation in patients with chronic myelogenous leukemia.

FUTURE DIRECTIONS

The elegance of recombinant DNA technology and its successor
technologies of genomics, epigenomics, and proteomics resides in the
capacity they confer on investigators to examine each gene as a discrete physical entity that can be purified, reduced to its basic building
blocks for decoding of its primary structure, analyzed for its patterns
of expression, and perturbed by alterations in sequence or molecular
environment so that the effects of changes in each region of the gene
can be assessed. Purified genes can be deliberately modified or
mutated to create novel genes not available in nature. These provide
the potential to generate useful new biologic entities, such as modified live virus or purified peptide vaccines, modified proteins customized for specific therapeutic purposes, and altered combinations of
regulatory and structural genes that allow for the assumption of new
functions by specific gene systems.

Purified genes facilitate the study of gene regulation in many ways.
First, a cloned gene provides characterized DNA probes for molecular
hybridization assays. Second, cloned genes provide the homogeneous
DNA moieties needed to determine the exact nucleotide sequence.
Sequencing techniques have become so reliable and efficient that it
is often easier to clone the gene encoding a protein of interest and
determine its DNA sequence than it is to purify the protein and
determine its amino acid sequence. The DNA sequence predicts
exactly the amino acid sequence of its protein product. By comparing
normal sequences with the sequences of alleles cloned from patients

known to be abnormal, such as the globin genes in the thalassemia or sickle cell syndromes, the normal and pathologic anatomy of genes critical to major hematologic diseases can be established. In this manner, it has been possible to identify many mutations responsible for various forms of thalassemia, hemophilia, thrombasthenia, red blood cell enzymopathies, porphyrias, and so forth. Similarly, single base changes have been shown to be the difference between many normally functioning proto-oncogenes and their cancer-promoting oncogene derivatives.

Third, cloned genes can be manipulated for studies of gene expression. Many vectors allowing efficient transfer of genes into eukaryotic cells have been perfected. Gene transfer technologies allow the gene to be placed into the desired cellular environment and the expression of that gene or the behavior of its products to be analyzed. These surrogate or reverse genetics systems allow analysis of the normal physiology of expression of a particular gene, as well as the pathophysiology of abnormal gene expression resulting from mutations.

Fourth, cloned genes enhance study of their protein products. By expressing fragments of the gene in microorganisms or eukaryotic cells, customized regions of a protein can be produced for use as an immunogen, thereby allowing preparation of a variety of useful and powerful antibody probes. Alternatively, synthetic peptides deduced from the DNA sequence can be prepared as the immunogen. Controlled production of large amounts of the protein also allows direct analysis of specific functions attributable to regions in that protein.

Finally, all of the aforementioned techniques can be extended by mutating the gene and examining the effects of those mutations on the expression of or the properties of the encoded mRNAs and proteins. By combining portions of one gene with another (chimeric genes) or abutting structural regions of one gene with regulatory sequences of another, the researcher can investigate in previously inconceivable ways the complexities of gene regulation. These activist approaches to modifying gene structure or expression create the opportunity to generate new RNA and protein products whose applications are limited only by the collective imagination of the investigators.

The most important impact of the genetic approach to the analysis of biologic phenomena is the most indirect. Diligent and repeated application of the methods outlined in this chapter to the study of many genes from diverse groups of organisms is beginning to reveal the basic strategies used by nature for the regulation of cell and tissue behavior. As our knowledge of these rules of regulation grows, our ability to understand, detect, and correct pathologic phenomena will increase substantially.

SUGGESTED READINGS

Bentley D: The mRNA assembly line: Transcription and processing machines in the same factory. *Curr Opin Cell Biol* 14:336, 2002.

Dykxhoorn DM, Novina CD, Sharp PA: Killing the messenger: Short RNAs that silence gene expression. *Nat Rev Mol Cell Biol* 4:457, 2003.

Fischle W, Wang Y, Allis CD: Histone and chromatin cross-talk. *Curr Opin Cell Biol* 15:172, 2003.

Grewal SI, Moazed D: Heterochromatin and epigenetic control of gene expression. *Science* 301:798, 2003.

Jones B: Layers of gene regulation. *Nat Rev Genet* 16:128–129, 2015.

Kloosterman WP, Plasterk RHA: The diverse functions of microRNAs in animal development and disease. *Dev Cell* 11:441, 2006.

Klose RJ, Bird AP: Genomic DNA methylation: The mark and its mediators. *Trends Biochem Sci* 31:89, 2006.

Kumar A, Garg S, Garg N: Regulation of gene expression: RNA regulation. *Rev Cell and Mol Med* 1–59, 2014.

Lee TI, Young RA: Transcription of eukaryotic protein-coding genes. *Annu Rev Genet* 34:77, 2000.

Tefferi A, Wieben ED, Dewald GW, et al: Primer on medical genomics, part II: Background principles and methods in molecular genetics. *Mayo Clin Proc* 77:785, 2002.

Waddington S, Privolizzi R, Karda R, et al: A broad overview and review of Crispr-CAS technology and stem cells. *Curr Stem Cell Rep* 2:9–20, 2016.

Wilusz CJ, Wormington M, Peltz SW: The cap-to-tail guide to mRNA turnover. *Nat Rev Mol Cell Biol* 2:237, 2001.

CHAPTER 2

EPIGENETICS AND EPIGENOMICS

Jennifer Wu and Myles Brown

Epigenetics can be defined as inheritance of variation above and beyond changes in the DNA sequence. In other words, epigenetics comprises the study of how cells sharing the same exhaustive DNA blueprint can appear and function so distinctly as white blood cells, hepatocytes, neurons, and so forth. Whereas the genome contains all of an organism's vital information, a cell's epigenome dynamically filters and organizes that information into highly coordinated programs of gene expression.

Within the nucleus, DNA interacts with a variety of proteins to form chromatin, which can be broadly classified as highly compacted and transcriptionally silent (heterochromatin) versus loosely compacted and transcriptionally active (euchromatin). Heterochromatin comprises two distinct classes of DNA: (1) noncoding, often repetitive, "structural" DNA of centromeres and telomeres (constitutive heterochromatin), and (2) gene-encoding and gene-regulatory "functional" DNA that is selectively rendered inactive in different cell types (facultative heterochromatin). When euchromatin is described as loosely compacted, the information content of its DNA is readily accessible to binding the protein and RNA machinery that regulate gene expression. The aim of the study of epigenetics and chromatin therefore is to describe and understand the chromatin dynamics that orchestrate the four-dimensional symphony of molecular and cellular biology from the (seemingly) one-dimensional score that is the genome.

The information contained within chromatin can be grossly divided into two main categories: (1) the structural genes themselves, which are transcribed and translated into proteins or act as functional RNAs, and (2) gene-regulatory regions, which control the timing and amount of transcription (Fig. 2.1A). The information contained in transcribed and translated regions can be interpreted using the "genetic code," wherein the DNA sequence of the gene specifies, through a messenger RNA (mRNA) intermediate, the amino acid sequences of resulting proteins. Although there is no genetic code for functional RNAs that are not translated into proteins, some, such as ribosomal RNA and transfer RNA genes, have well understood functions. There are in addition a number of other types of functional RNA genes whose functions are only partially elucidated. Transcribed regions comprise approximately 3% of the genome. In contrast, the information contained in gene-regulatory regions is the "epigenetic code," which has yet to be fully deciphered and is based on the accessibility of those regions to dynamic protein–DNA interactions, the identity of those interacting proteins, and the identity of the gene(s) whose expression is being modulated.

The most dramatic example of chromatin compaction is the condensation that occurs during mitosis, making individual chromosomes visible by light microscopy and allowing segregation of replicates equally among daughter cells. A condensed or compacted chromosome is folded many times upon itself and is highly protein bound, affording little or no access to genomic information and remaining transcriptionally silent (Fig. 2.1B). Contrast this with the "decondensed" chromatin state that is necessary for DNA replication during the synthesis phase of the cell cycle. DNA replication requires unfolding of chromatin, disruption of its protein–DNA interactions, and "unzipping" the double helix to allow every base in the genome to be copied. When not dividing, cells maintain their chromatin in intermediate states of compaction. Actively transcribed genes and their associated regulatory chromatin regions are "open" and "accessible" insofar as the underlying protein–DNA interactions are readily modified and disrupted to accommodate binding of transcription factors, cofactors, RNA polymerases, and the totality of functional components underlying gene expression.

It is important to remember some key differences between genomic and epigenomic research. Whereas the genome is an essentially unvarying feature of every cell in an organism (with the important exception of T and B cells that rearrange and mutate their antigen receptor genes), the epigenome of each cell within that organism is unique. Moreover, epigenomes are fluid throughout a cell's life span, integrating intrinsic cellular "identity" with contextual signals to specify a program of gene expression. Finally, the mechanics of DNA replication and cell division necessarily disrupt the protein–DNA interactions that comprise the epigenome. How cells reestablish their epigenetic identity after cell division is not well understood.

FUNCTIONAL CHROMATIN DOMAINS

Regulatory, noncoding DNA regions can have a variety of different functions (illustrated in Fig. 2.1A), variously classified as promoters, enhancers/silencers, superenhancers, and insulators. Promoters are typically located within 1 to 2 kb of the transcriptional start site (TSS) of a gene. At a minimum, RNA polymerase II–dependent promoters contain binding sites for the general transcription factors TATA box-binding protein (TBP) and transcription factor IIB (TFIIB), which form the core of the transcriptional complex. Transcription factor binding sites within the promoter modulate gene expression by recruiting histone-modifying enzymes and transcriptional coactivators or corepressors.

An enhancer/silencer is a short (50- to 1500-bp) region of DNA that can be bound by transcription factors to increase/decrease the likelihood that transcription of a particular gene will occur. Enhancers/silencers can act both in *cis* (within a chromosome) and rarely in *trans* (between chromosomes), can be located up to 1 Mb away from the gene, and can be upstream or downstream from the TSS. Promoters physically interact with their associated enhancers or silencers via three-dimensional chromatin "looping" facilitated by Mediator and cohesin protein complexes (Fig. 2.1D). Genes may be regulated by several enhancers/silencers, and each enhancer/silencer may modulate expression of one or more genes. A superenhancer is a cluster of physically and functionally associated enhancers that regulates genes critical for cell identity. Superenhancers are marked by high levels of enhancer-associated histone modification and bind high levels of cell type–specific and lineage-defining transcription factors (known as "master" transcription factors).

Insulators help to restrict the set of genes that can be modulated by an enhancer by blocking the physical interactions between enhancers and promoters. Insulators are bound by cohesin and CTCF proteins and form boundaries between silenced and active genes. Clusters of insulators separate heterochromatin from euchromatin, and the segments of active chromatin bounded by these clusters are known as topologic domains—genomic regions within which regulation occurs.

DNA METHYLATION

Methylation of cytosine by DNA methyltransferases (DNMTs) occurs at 60% to 90% of CpG dinucleotides in the mammalian genome. Methylated DNA is bound by methyl-CpG-binding domain

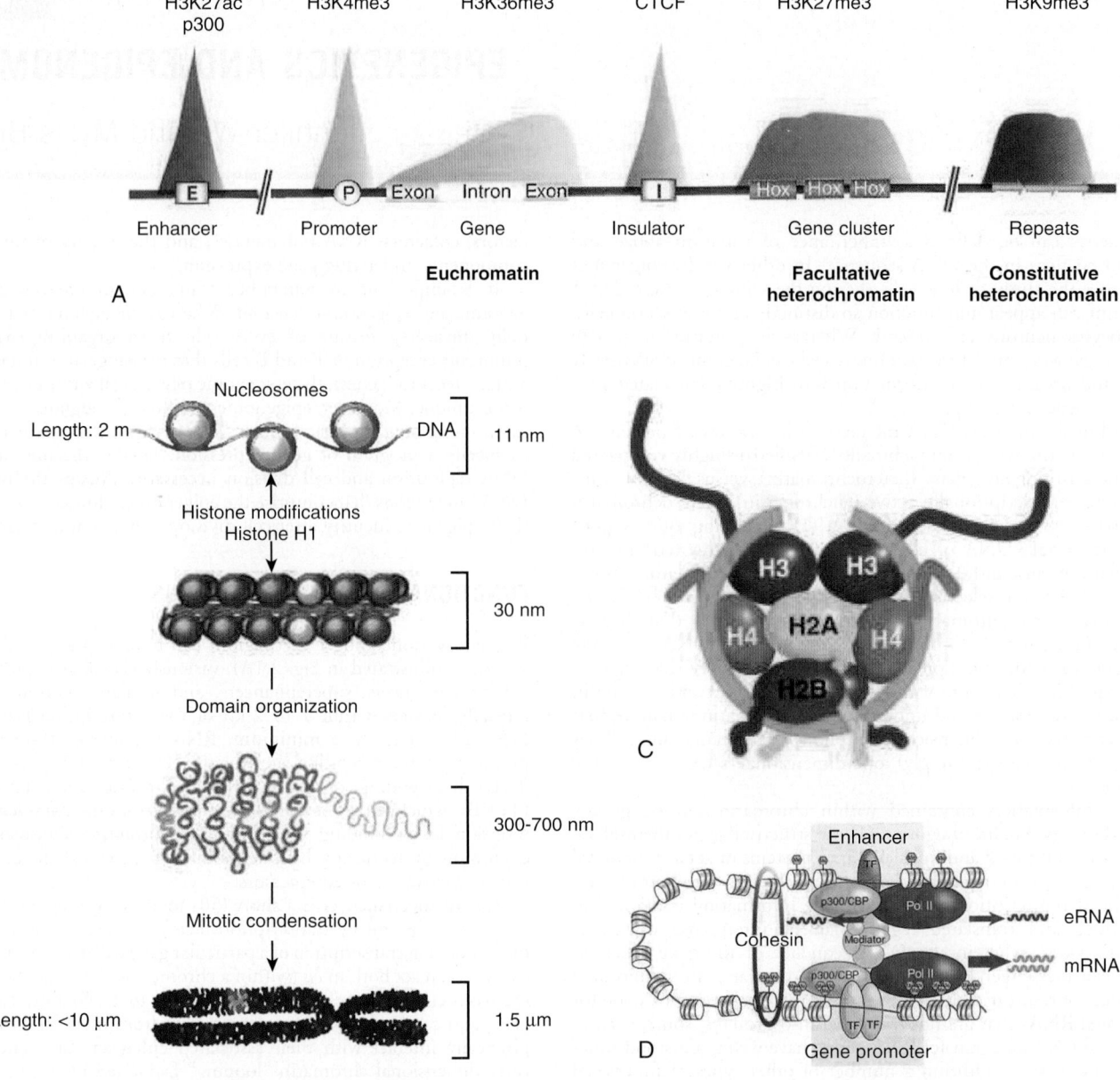

Fig. 2.1 CHROMATIN STRUCTURE. (A) Functional chromatin domains and their characteristic histone modifications and protein-binding features. (B) Higher-order chromatin structure, from least condensed *(top)* to most condensed *(bottom)*. (C) Schematic of nucleosome with DNA *(light blue)* wrapped around histone octamer (H2A, H2B, H3, H4) having protruding histone tails. (D) Three-dimensional chromatin looping brings enhancers into close proximity with promoters via interactions with cohesin and Mediator protein complexes. *eRNA,* Enhancer RNA; *mRNA,* messenger RNA; *TF,* transcription factor.

proteins (MBDs) that recruit histone-modifying enzymes and chromatin remodeling proteins, resulting in highly condensed heterochromatin. Methylation of promoter regions thereby represses transcription. Patterns of DNA methylation are replicated during DNA synthesis and cell division and can be used to distinguish cell types and stages of differentiation.

The genome-wide pattern of DNA methylation, known as the methylome, has been characterized for a wide variety of tissues. Approximately 75% of the methylome is consistent across all cell types. The remaining 25% is differentially hypo- or hypermethylated in a cell type–specific manner. Cell type–specific hypomethylated regions are enriched for nucleosomes with modifications associated with active regions and transcription factor–binding sites, whereas cell type–specific hypermethylation is associated with transcription factor silencing during differentiation. Aberrant DNA methylation is an extremely common feature of cancers, where hypermethylation of tumor suppressor genes and hypomethylation of oncogenes may play important roles in oncogenesis and tumor progression.

HISTONES AND HISTONE VARIANTS

Histones H2A, H2B, H3, and H4 are known as the core histones, and histones H1 and H5 are known as the linker histones. The core histones all exist as dimers, and the four dimers come together to form one octameric nucleosome core. The smallest unit of chromatin structure is the nucleosome, consisting of 147 bp of DNA double helix wrapped around the core histone octamer (Fig. 2.1C). Linker histones, primarily H1, bind the nucleosome at the entry and exit sites of the DNA and allow the formation of higher-order structure. Histone N-terminal domains are rich in lysine and arginine residues that are subject to a variety of posttranslational modifications (see later).

In addition to these major histones, dozens of minor histone variants have been identified and are highly evolutionarily conserved. Some minor variants have very specific roles in chromatin regulation. For example, histone H3–like centromere protein A (CENPA) is associated with centromeres. H2A.Z is associated with the promoters and enhancers of actively transcribed genes. Histone H3.3 is associated with the body of actively transcribed genes. Phosphorylated H2A.X is found in regions around double-stranded DNA breaks and recruits DNA repair machinery.

COVALENT HISTONE MODIFICATIONS

Histones undergo a variety of posttranslational modifications (including methylation, acetylation, phosphorylation, SUMOylation,

citrullination, ubiquitination, and ADP-ribosylation) that alter their interactions with DNA and nuclear proteins (Fig. 2.2). Histone-modifying enzymes are broadly classified as "writers," such as histone methyltransferases (HMTs) and histone acetyltransferases (HATs) that add functional groups, or "erasers," such as histone demethylases (HDMs) and histone deacetylases (HDACs). DNA-binding proteins contain a variety of "reader" protein domains (including bromodomains, chromodomains, tudor domains, SANT domains) that have increased affinity for modified histones. In this way, covalently modified histones constitute a "histone code" that is a defining feature of the dynamic epigenome. Each of the eight histones in a nucleosome can harbor multiple covalent modifications, giving the histone code tremendous combinatorial complexity.

Trimethylation of H3 lysine 4 (H3K4me3) and trimethylation of H3 lysine 36 (H3K36me3) are both associated with transcriptional activation. H3K4me3 occurs at the promoter of active genes, and the degree of trimethylation is broadly correlated with transcriptional activity of the gene. H3K36me3 is deposited by the lysine methyltransferase KMT2A (also known as MLL1) component of the Mediator complex and occurs in the body of active genes. H3K36me3 associates with elongating RNA polymerase II, thus marking actively transcribed genes. Mono- and dimethylation of H3 lysine

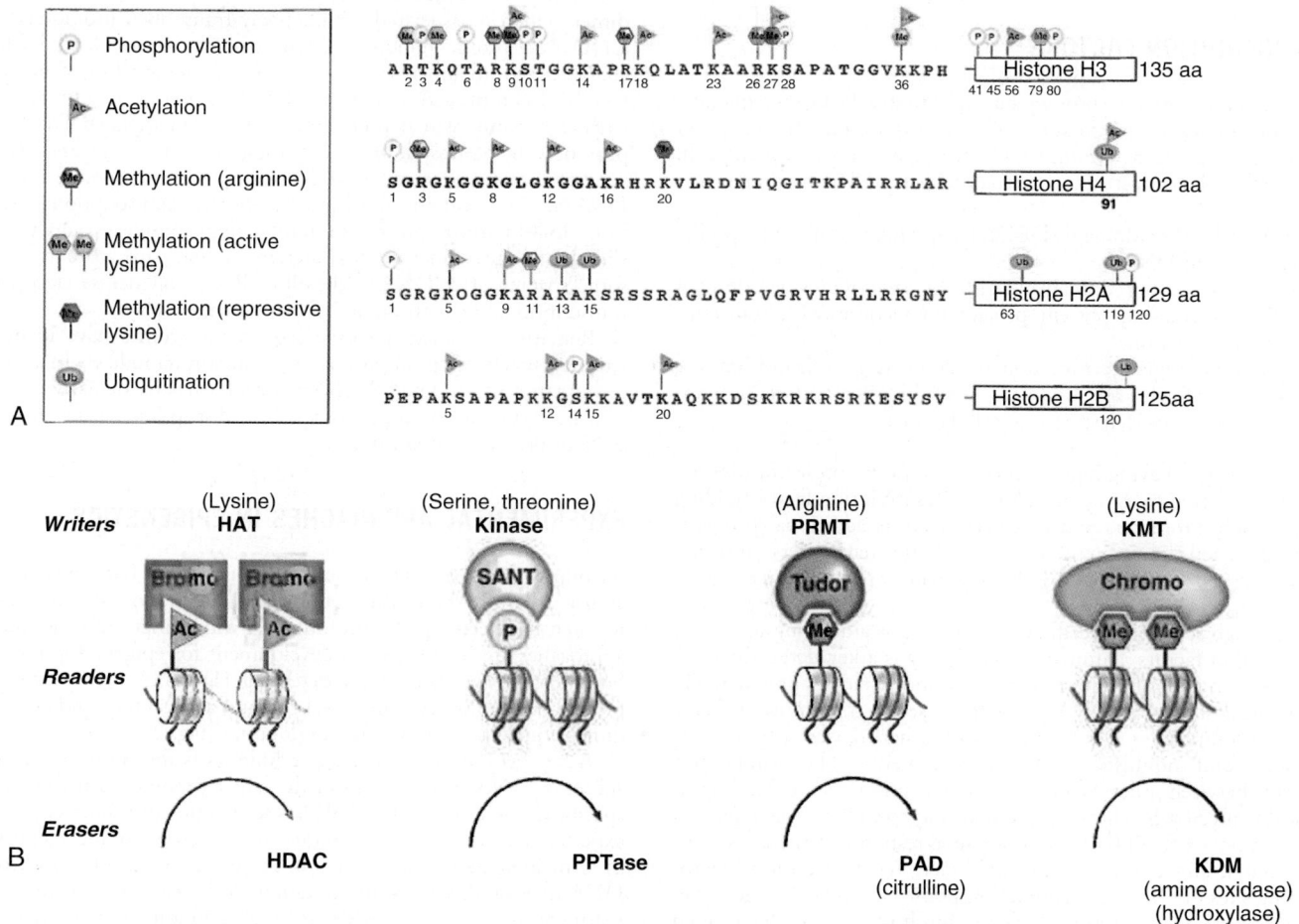

Fig. 2.2 HISTONE MODIFICATIONS AND HISTONE-MODIFYING ENZYMES. (A) The N-terminal tails of core histones contain lysine (K), arginine (R), serine (S), and threonine (T) residues that are common targets for a variety of posttranslational modifications, including methylation (Me), acetylation (Ac), phosphorylation (P), and ubiquitination (Ub). (B) Histone-modifying enzymes can be broadly classified as either "writers" or "erasers" based upon addition or removal of functional groups, respectively. Moreover, many DNA-binding proteins contain "reader" protein domains (bromodomains, SANT domains, tudor domains, or chromodomains) having increased affinity for acetylated, phosphorylated, methylarginine, and methyllysine modified nucleosomes, respectively. *HAT,* Histone acetyltransferase; *HDAC,* histone deacetylase; *KDM,* lysine demethylase; *KMT,* lysine methyltransferase; *PAD,* peptidylarginine deiminase; *PPTase,* protein phosphatase; *PRMT,* protein arginine methyltransferase.

4 (H3K4me1/2) and acetylation of H3 lysine 27 (H3K27ac) are marks of active enhancers, and the degree of H3K27ac is broadly correlated with enhancer activation. H3K27ac is the enhancer mark most commonly used to define superenhancers.

Several histone modifications are particularly associated with repressed genes: trimethylation of H3 lysine 27 (H3K27me3), di- and trimethylation of H3 lysine 9 (H3K9me2/3), and trimethylation of H4 lysine 20 (H4K20me3). H3K27me3 is deposited at both promoters and enhancers by the polycomb repressive complex 2 (PRC2) and mediates recruitment of PRC1, resulting in chromatin condensation and transcriptional repression. H3K9me2/3 and H4K20me3 are both highly associated with heterochromatin. H3K9me2/3 serves as a binding site for heterochromatin protein 1 (HP1). HP1 recruits additional histone-modifying enzymes, including the lysine methyltransferases KMT5B and KMT5C that produce H4K20me3.

Stem cells harbor promoters marked by both activating H3K4me3 and repressive H3K27me3. Upon cellular differentiation, these "bivalent" or "poised" promoters are rapidly converted to either an activated or a repressed state.

The Aurora B kinase phosphorylates histone H3 at serine 10 (phospho-H3S10), triggering chromosome condensation during mitosis. Phosphorylation of H2B at serine 14 (phospho-H2BS14) mediates chromatin condensation during apoptosis.

TRANSCRIPTION FACTORS

A transcription factor is a protein that binds to specific DNA sequences and contributes to modulation of gene expression. Transcription factors are the key determinants of the epigenetic state of the cell. They are modular in structure and contain the following domains:

- A DNA-binding domain (DBD), having high affinity for specific sequences of DNA
- A *trans*-activating domain (TAD) or *trans*-repressive domain (TRD), mediating protein–protein interactions with transcriptional coregulators
- An optional signal-sensing domain (SSD) (e.g., a ligand binding domain), which can modulate DNA-binding and/or protein-binding activity in response to cellular cues

DNA sequences having high affinity for transcription factor binding are often referred to as *response elements*. Transcription factor binding to accessible promoters and enhancers recruits additional proteins, such as coactivators/corepressors, chromatin remodelers, histone-modifying enzymes, and RNA polymerases, to modulate gene expression.

Although sequence-specific DNA binding is a defining feature of transcription factors, chromatin accessibility is a key determinant of transcription factor binding. Most transcription factors preferentially bind nucleosome-free DNA. In many cases, a transcription factor needs to compete for DNA binding with other transcription factors, histones, and nonhistone chromatin proteins. The competitive balance between nucleosome and transcription factor binding is critically affected by chromatin remodeling complexes (see later). In practice, only a small fraction of potential response elements is actually bound, and many experimentally detected transcription factor binding sites (TFBS) lack canonical response elements. The genome-wide pattern of transcription factor binding can be determined experimentally using chromatin immunoprecipitation (ChIP) and next-generation sequencing (ChIP-Seq; see later) and is known as the transcription factor cistrome.

Different cell types typically express both common and distinct transcription factors. Moreover, the cistrome of a transcription factor differs among cell types, reflecting differences in chromatin accessibility and helping to define active promoters and enhancers. Master transcription factors are a special subset of lineage-defining transcription factors having expression restricted to specific cell types and demonstrating very high binding at superenhancers.

CHROMATIN REMODELERS

Chromatin remodeling alters the position, occupancy, or histone composition of a nucleosome within chromatin. Adenosine triphosphate (ATP)-dependent changes in nucleosome position and occupancy are mediated by the multisubunit chromatin remodeling complexes, which fall into four families: switch/sucrose nonfermentable (SWI/SNF), imitation SWI (ISWI), chromodomain helicase DNA binding (CHD), and INO80. ATP-independent changes in nucleosome position and occupancy can occur in response to transcription factor binding or through the action of histone chaperones that can deposit, remove, or exchange histones. Each of these activities alters the accessibility of DNA to transcription factors and other DNA-binding proteins.

Complexes in the SWI/SNF family include the Brg1/Brm-associated factor (BAF) complex, polybromo-associated BAF (PBAF) complex, and Williams syndrome transcription factor *including* nucleosome assembly complex (WINAC). They contribute to transcriptional regulation and DNA repair. In addition to nucleosome sliding, SWI/SNF complexes have been implicated in chromatin looping as well as in eviction of H2A/H2B dimers from the nucleosome. Members of the INO80 family of complexes participate in transcription and DNA repair, but they can also catalyze the exchange of histones from the nucleosome structure. For example, SRCAP can exchange the H2A/H2B histone dimer for a variant H2A.Z/H2B dimer, which is associated with actively transcribed promoters. The CHD nucleosome remodeling family is the largest, and its best-characterized member is the nucleosome remodeling deacetylase (NURD) complex. A subset of NURD complexes incorporates the MBD2 subunit, which preferentially binds methylated DNA, and promotes the repression of genes through its remodeling and HDAC activities. Many alternative NURD complexes incorporate different DNA-binding proteins and can contribute to transcriptional activation. ISWI family chromatin remodeling complexes catalyze the sliding of nucleosomes in short increments and participate in nucleosome spacing after DNA replication, RNA polymerase elongation, transcriptional regulation, and DNA damage repair.

Remarkably, cancer genome sequencing studies have identified frequent inactivating mutations in chromatin remodelers in a variety of human cancers. The SWI/SNF complex has particularly emerged as a powerful tumor suppressor whose disruption occurs in nearly 20% of primary human tumors.

EXPERIMENTAL APPROACHES IN EPIGENETICS

As dramatically as high-throughput sequencing has impacted the ability to understand the genome, its facilitation of epigenomic research has been equally profound. A wide variety of experimental approaches are in use and in development for epigenomic research, but most are predicated on detecting (1) DNA methylation, (2) protein–DNA interactions, (3) chromatin accessibility, and (4) three-dimensional chromatin structure/looping (Fig. 2.3).

A key feature of all of these techniques is the ability to isolate a subset of DNA sequences from the larger genome on the basis of a specific chromatin feature. This has several practical implications for experiments. First, many techniques rely on cross-linking agents such as formaldehyde to covalently link proteins to each other and to the DNA they bind. Cross-linking rapidly kills cells and "freezes" chromatin. Second, all of these experimental techniques involve fragmenting chromosomes into much smaller pieces, either by physical disruption (sonication) or by endonuclease treatment. Third, the chromatin subset of interest is extracted and enriched by immunoprecipitation, isolation of chromatin fragments of specific sizes, and/or sequence-specific amplification via polymerase chain reaction (PCR). Finally, DNA is isolated from this chromatin subset and subjected to next-generation sequencing.

A common technique for determining the genome-wide methylome is bisulfite-sequencing. Treatment of DNA with bisulfite converts cytosine residues to uracil but leaves 5-methylcytosine (5mC)

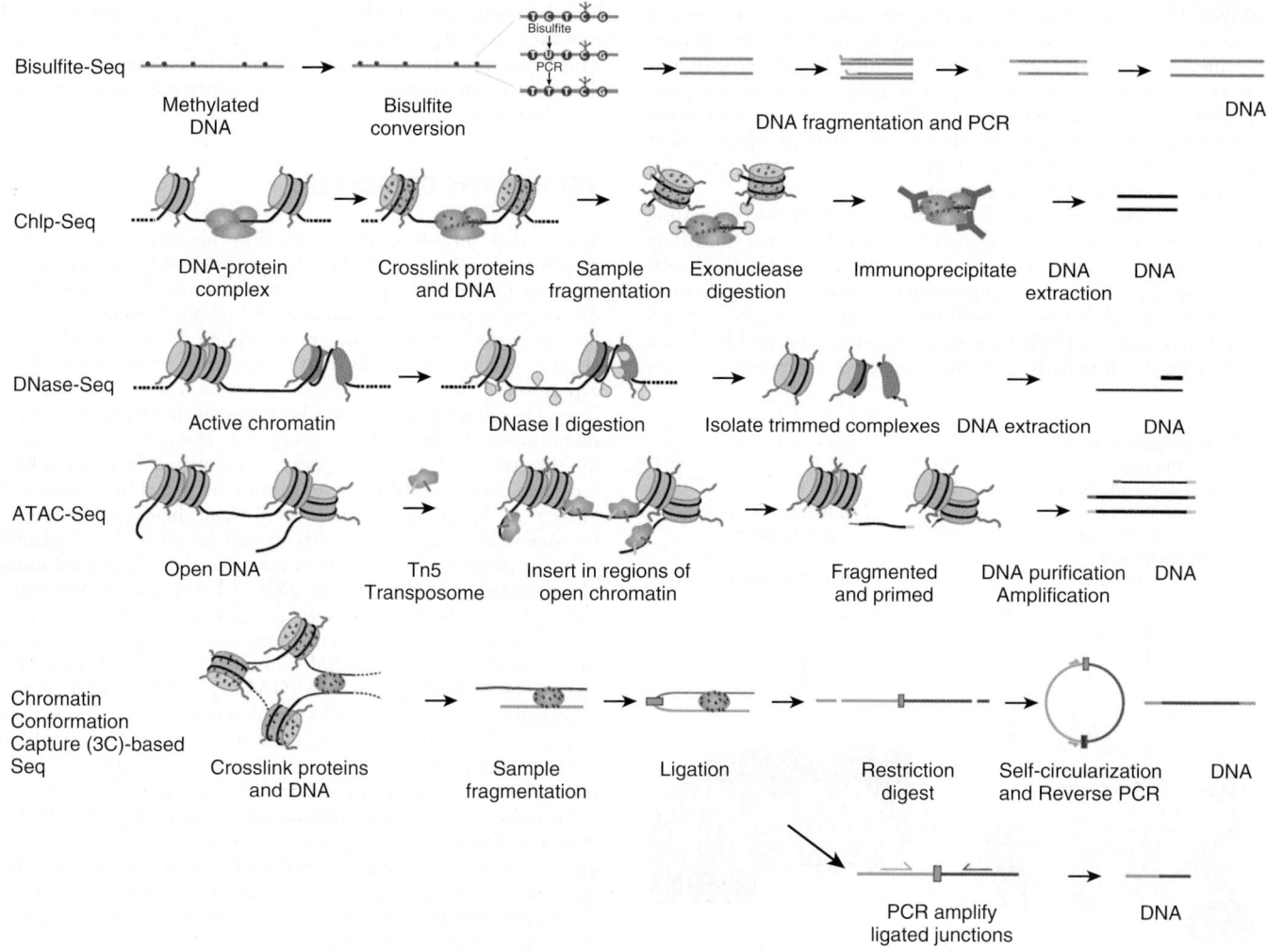

Fig. 2.3 EXPERIMENTAL TECHNIQUES IN EPIGENOMICS. Schematic representations of bisulfite sequencing (Bisulfite-Seq), chromatin immunoprecipitation sequencing (ChIP-Seq), DNase I sequencing (DNase-Seq), assay for transposase-accessible chromatin with high-throughput sequencing (ATAC-Seq), and chromatin conformation capture–based (3C-based) experimental techniques. *PCR,* Polymerase chain reaction.

residues unaffected. Comparing results of bisulfite-treated and bisulfite-untreated DNA sequencing permits genome-wide differentiation of methylated and unmethylated cytosines. Alternatively, methylated DNA immunoprecipitation sequencing uses an antibody recognizing 5mC to enrich for methylated segments of the genome before next-generation sequencing.

DNA binding by transcription factors, transcriptional machinery, structural proteins, and covalently modified histones can all be mapped in genome-wide fashion using ChIP-Seq. ChIP-Seq typically requires cross-linking of proteins to DNA using formaldehyde or other chemical fixation techniques. Chromatin is then fragmented, antibodies are used to enrich for a protein of interest, and the associated DNA fragments are then identified by next-generation sequencing. ChIP-Seq is the most versatile technique in epigenomic research. For example, genome-wide maps of histone modifications (such as H3K27ac or H3K36me3), active RNA polymerase II, insulator protein CTCF, superenhancer-associated Mediator complex, and transcription factors can all be accomplished via ChIP-Seq using different antibodies.

DNase-Seq and assay for transposase-accessible chromatin sequencing (ATAC-Seq) are two common techniques used to assess genome-wide chromatin accessibility. DNase-Seq exposes native chromatin to cleavage by the DNase I endonuclease, the activity of which is inversely related to protein binding by DNA. Chromatin

regions most sensitive to DNase I cleavage are termed *DNase hypersensitive sites* (DHSs) and are highly enriched for transcriptionally active and gene-regulatory segments of the genome. ATAC-Seq is an alternative measure of chromatin accessibility based upon susceptibility of chromatin regions to the activity of a hyperactive transposase. Transposase activity is highest in nucleosome-free regions, and ATAC-Seq typically identifies transcriptionally active and gene-regulatory regions largely similar to those identified by DNase-Seq. Importantly, DNase-Seq and ATAC-Seq provide genome-wide snapshots of active chromatin regions without regard to the involved transcription factors or chromatin regulators.

Chromosome conformation capture (3C) techniques aim to identify three-dimensional chromatin loops, such as those bringing promoters in close proximity to enhancers. All 3C-based methods begin with chromatin cross-linking. Following DNA fragmentation, a random DNA ligation step is performed to generate circular DNA molecules. Sequencing these DNA loops yields fragment pairs that, although separated by many kilobases in linearly organized DNA, are physically approximated in functional chromatin. 3C-based methods have tremendous potential to map enhancers to the genes whose activity they modulate.

The fundamental challenge in epigenomic research is integrating the results of many different experiments to understand how myriad chromatin features interact in regulating transcription and cellular behavior (Fig. 2.4). Thus, interpreting the epigenetic code requires measuring transcriptional activity in addition to chromatin features. Measurement of global transcript levels by mRNA sequencing (RNA-Seq) is now the most common technique used to study gene expression, but interest is growing in the related genomic run-on sequencing (GRO-Seq) technique. GRO-Seq measures active transcription rather than total cellular transcript level and therefore holds promise for improved correlation with epigenomic data.

Several collaborative research consortia are dedicated to generating and curating genome-wide epigenetic data for public use, including the National Human Genome Research Institute (NHGRI) ENCODE and Roadmap Epigenomics projects. These resources include results of histone modifications and transcription factor ChIP-Seq, DNase-Seq, DNA methylation sequencing, and RNA-Seq experiments for hundreds of human cancer cell lines and primary human tissues, respectively. The most versatile and widely available tool for visualizing epigenomic data is the UCSC Genome Browser, which incorporates easy access to ENCODE, Roadmap, and other data sources for integrative analysis of epigenomic and gene expression data (Fig. 2.5).

MECHANISMS OF DISEASE

The mechanisms of disease described in this chapter are not strictly epigenetic, insofar as they are all predicated on changes in genome sequence or structure (genetic mutations). Nonetheless, insights into disease pathogenesis and development of novel therapeutic targets have been vastly informed by understanding the ways in which these genetic changes drive aberrant chromatin regulation and gene expression.

Sickle cell anemia has long been known to result from a point mutation in the hemoglobin beta gene. The severity of this often life-threatening hemoglobinopathy is attenuated in patients having increased expression of the fetal gamma hemoglobin variant, a trait known as hereditary persistence of fetal hemoglobin (HFPH). Genome-wide association studies in patients with HFPH identified frequent single-nucleotide polymorphisms (SNPs) in a small number of noncoding regions near the *BCL11A* gene on chromosome 2. Subsequent studies have elegantly demonstrated that these SNPs are located in erythroid-specific enhancers modulating *BCL11A* expression. The HFPH-associated SNPs diminish binding of transcription factors GATA-binding protein 1 (GATA1) and T-cell acute lymphocytic leukemia protein 1 (TAL1), which results in decreased expression of *BCL11A*. Because *BCL11A* is required for efficient silencing of fetal hemoglobin expression, patients with sickle cell anemia having these common variant SNPs demonstrate elevated fetal hemoglobin throughout adulthood and are often protected from the most severe manifestations of the disease. Just as sickle cell anemia is among the most striking examples of disease caused by a point mutation in the coding region of a gene, these *BCL11A* enhancer SNPs demonstrate the power of gene-regulatory elements to modulate the sickle cell disease phenotype.

Chromosomal translocations that result in aberrant expression of oncogenes or leukemogenic transcription factors are another common mechanism of disease. The classical example of this is Burkitt lymphoma, in which t(8;13) translocations juxtapose the highly active immunoglobulin heavy chain enhancers and the *c-myc* oncogene, driving myc overexpression and oncogenic transformation of mature B cells. Similarly, many different translocations have been identified in T-cell acute lymphoblastic leukemia (T-ALL) whereby

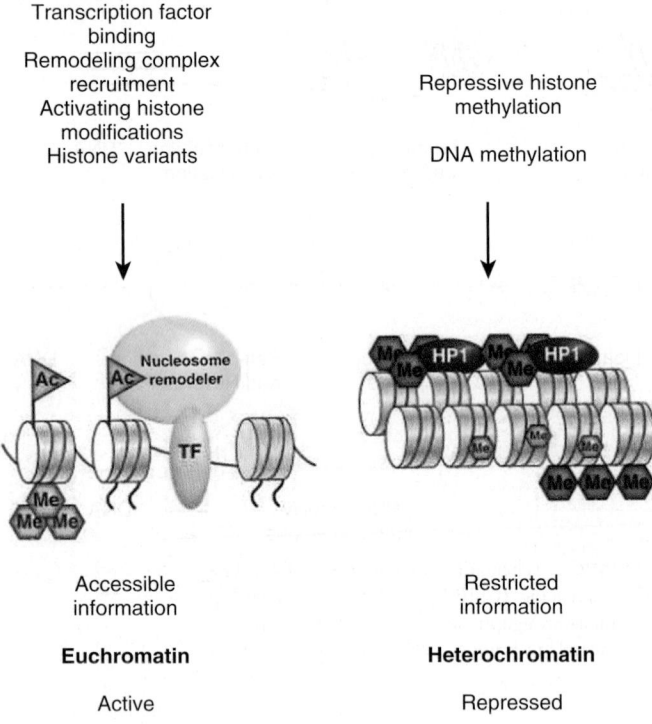

Fig. 2.4 DNA–PROTEIN INTERACTIONS IN EUCHROMATIN AND HETEROCHROMATIN.

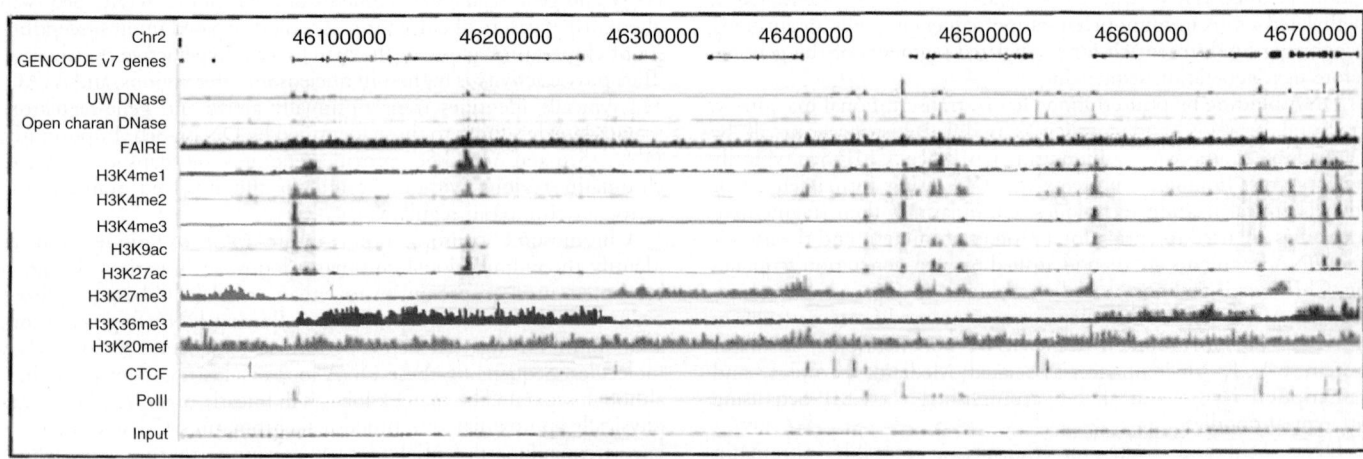

Fig. 2.5 VISUALIZING THE EPIGENOMIC LANDSCAPE. Sample of a UCSC Genome Browser representation of a 700-kb segment of chromosome 2 in the lymphoblastoid human cell line GM12878. Integration of publicly available, genome-wide data for a variety of epigenomic experiments is the cornerstone of efforts to decode the epigenome.

overexpression of master transcription factors such as *TAL1, LIM domain only 1 (LMO1), LMO2,* and *HOX11* is driven by chromosomal rearrangements involving the T-cell receptor loci.

An alternate mechanism driving *TAL1* overexpression in T-ALL has recently been described in which small genomic insertions (2–18 bp) upstream of the *TAL1* coding region introduce novel binding sites for the myeloblastosis (MYB) transcription factor. This aberrant MYB binding recruits additional transcription factors Runt-related transcription factor 1 (RUNX1), GATA3, and TAL1, as well as the HAT CREB-binding protein (CBP), and forms a superenhancer driving leukemogenic *TAL1* overexpression.

Many different translocations resulting in fusion of the mixed-lineage leukemia *(MLL1/KMT2A)* gene, located on chromosome 11q23, with over 70 different partner proteins have been identified in infant ALL and therapy-associated acute myeloid leukemia (AML). The mechanisms underlying the leukemogenic nature of these translocations have been elucidated only recently. Leukemogenic MLL1 fusion proteins fuse the N-terminal targeting domain with a transcription elongation factor such as ENL or AF9. The resulting fusion protein drives overexpression of common MLL1 targets by recruiting the DOT1L complex (having H3K79 methyltransferase activity) and the positive transcription elongation factor b (P-TEFb) complex (containing CDK9 and phosphorylating RNA polymerase II). Moreover, a subset of leukemogenic MLL1 fusions can inhibit the transcriptional repressive activity of PRC1. In summary, MLL translocations in ALL and AML define a paradigm of leukemia development based upon transcriptional dysregulation through aberrant targeting and control of transcription elongation activity.

As noted earlier, inactivating mutations in components of chromatin remodeling complexes such as SWI/SNF have been identified in a wide variety of human cancers. For example, researchers in a recent study found mutations in the ARID1A subunit of SWI/SNF in 17% of patients with Waldenström macroglobulinemia, and patients with ARID1A mutations had more aggressive disease features. In addition to their nucleosome remodeling activities, chromatin remodeling complexes contribute to three-dimensional chromatin structure, participate in DNA damage repair, modulate transcription factor binding, and recruit histone-modifying enzymes. Precisely how disruption of these many chromatin regulatory activities contributes to disease is an extremely active area of research.

In addition to these epigenetic contributions to disease development, much interest has evolved in potential epigenetic mechanisms of resistance to existing cancer therapies. One example of this is resistance of T-ALL to γ-secretase inhibitors (GSIs), used to target abnormal *NOTCH1* activation. Treatment of T-ALL cell lines with GSIs in vitro kills a large proportion of cells, but it leaves behind a "persister" population of GSI-resistant cells. If GSI treatment is removed, these persister cells revert to their prior GSI-sensitive state, suggesting an epigenetic mechanism of drug resistance. A screen of chromatin regulators required for persister cell viability identified the bromodomain-containing 4 protein (BRD4), a key factor in activating transcriptional elongation. This study and many others have ignited broad interest in other potential epigenetic mechanisms of therapy resistance as well as BRD4 as a specific therapeutic target.

EPIGENETIC THERAPIES

Epigenetic therapies are among the most active areas of preclinical and clinical cancer research because of their potential to specifically target chromatin-mediated disease mechanisms and the expectation that these therapies will have fewer side effects than conventional cytotoxic chemotherapies. As seen in Table 2.1, several classes of drugs have emerged, and the rationales for their ongoing development are briefly discussed next.

The first class of epigenetic drugs to show significant clinical benefit is the DNMT inhibitors, particularly 5-azacytidine and its analogue decitabine. As discussed earlier, abnormal DNA methylation is a common feature of many cancers. However, azacytidine is

TABLE 2.1	Emerging Epigenetic Therapies	
Class	**Target**	**Disease**
DNA Methylation Inhibitors	DNMTs	MDS, AML
Histone-modifying enzymes		
HMT inhibitors	DOT1L, EZH2, nonspecific	MLL-rearranged leukemias, NHL, MDS, AML
HDAC inhibitors	HDAC6, nonspecific	MM, CLL, lymphoma
HMT activators	SIRT1, SIRT5	MM
HDM inhibitors	KDM1A	AML
BET Bromodomain Inhibitors	BRD4, nonspecific	Hematologic malignancies

AML, Acute myeloid leukemia; BET, bromodomain and extra-terminal motif; CLL, chronic lymphocytic leukemia; DNMTs, DNA methyltransferases; HDAC, histone deacetylase; HDM, histone demethylase; HMT, histone methyltransferase; MDS, myelodysplastic syndrome; MLL, mixed-lineage leukemia; MM, multiple myeloma; NHL, non-Hodgkin lymphoma.

beneficial primarily in treating myelodysplastic syndromes and AML. The theoretical basis for this therapeutic effect is reactivation of key tumor suppressor genes by disruption of DNA methylation at their promoters. However, this mechanism has not yet been confirmed in azacytidine-treated patients, and alternate mechanisms of action are under investigation.

By far the largest class of epigenetic therapies is inhibitors of histone-modifying enzymes. Drugs inhibiting HMTs and HDACs are most prevalent, though several compounds that activate HDACs or inhibit HDMs are also being developed. For example, inhibitors of the H3K79 methyltransferase DOT1L are in clinical trials for MLL-rearranged leukemias. Alternatively, inhibitors of the H3K27 methyltransferase EZH2 (the catalytic component of the PRC2 complex) are being tested in non-Hodgkin lymphoma. Specific inhibitors of HDAC6 are being used in trials for multiple myeloma, and drugs having broad HDAC inhibitory activity are in ongoing trials for a wide variety of hematologic malignancies.

The newest class of epigenetic therapies includes the bromodomain and extra-terminal motif (BET) bromodomain inhibitors. As discussed briefly earlier, bromodomains are an extremely common feature of DNA-binding proteins and preferentially recognize acetylated chromatin. The abundance of bromodomain-containing DNA-binding proteins makes development of substrate-specific drugs extremely challenging. However, initial clinical trials using BET bromodomain inhibitors having broad binding specificity have been very promising in a wide variety of advanced hematologic and non-hematologic malignancies. The likely therapeutic targets of these drugs are the transcriptional machinery itself, though many additional mechanisms plausibly contribute.

FUTURE DIRECTIONS

Interpreting the epigenetic code holds great potential for bridging the gaps between the molecular biology of the genome, cellular biology, and physiology of health and disease. The application of next-generation sequencing technology and development of novel techniques to interrogate chromatin have produced a profusion of new epigenetic data. Collaborative epigenomic projects such as ENCODE and the Epigenome Roadmap, as well as genomics efforts such as the 1000 Genomes Project and The Cancer Genome Atlas, make these vast data widely available to researchers. The substantial challenge remains integrating and interpreting these data to generate novel insights into human health and disease. Substantial collaboration between biomedical scientists, computational biologists, and physicians will be necessary to design, execute, and analyze projects with high relevance to medical progress.

SUGGESTED READINGS

Allis CD, Jenuwein T, Reinberg D, et al, editors: *Epigenetics*, Cold Spring Harbor, NY, 2007, Cold Spring Harbor Laboratory Press.

Bauer DE, Kamran SC, Lessard S, et al: An erythroid enhancer of *BCL11A* subject to genetic variation determines fetal hemoglobin level. *Science* 342:253, 2013.

Chadwick LH: The NIH Roadmap Epigenomics Program data resource. *Epigenomics* 4:317, 2012.

Chaidos A, Caputo V, Karadimitris A: Inhibition of bromodomain and extra-terminal proteins (BET) as a potential therapeutic approach in haematological malignancies: emerging preclinical and clinical evidence. *Ther Adv Hematol* 6:128, 2015.

Clarke L, Zheng-Bradley X, Smith R, et al: The 1000 Genomes Project: data management and community access. *Nat Methods* 9:459, 2012.

ENCODE Project Consortium: A user's guide to the Encyclopedia of DNA Elements (ENCODE). *PLoS Biol* 9:e1001046, 2011.

Karolchik D, Barber GP, Casper J, et al: The UCSC Genome Browser database: 2014 update. *Nucleic Acids Res* 42:D764, 2014.

Knoechel B, Roderick JE, Williamson KE, et al: An epigenetic mechanism of resistance to targeted therapy in T cell acute lymphoblastic leukemia. *Nat Genet* 46:364, 2014.

Mansour MR, Abraham BJ, Anders L, et al: An oncogenic super-enhancer formed through somatic mutation of a noncoding intergenic element. *Science* 346:1373, 2014.

Stratton MR, Campbell PJ, Futreal PA: The cancer genome. *Nature* 458:719, 2009.

Slany RK: The molecular mechanics of mixed lineage leukemia. *Oncogene* 35:5215, 2016.

Treon SP, Xu L, Yang G, et al: MYD88 L265P somatic mutation in Waldenström's macroglobulinemia. *N Engl J Med* 367:826, 2012.

The Cancer Genome Atlas Research Network, Weinstein JN, Collisson EA, et al: The Cancer Genome Atlas Pan-Cancer analysis project. *Nat Genet* 45:1113, 2013.

CHAPTER 3

GENOMIC APPROACHES TO HEMATOLOGY

Jens G. Lohr, Birgit Knoechel, and Todd R. Golub

The publication of the initial draft sequence of the human genome in 2001 heralded a new era of biomedical research. Just as molecular biology changed the face of research in the 1970s and 1980s, genomics has promised a novel perspective into the biologic basis of human disease. Genomics involves the systematic study of biologic systems, typically focusing on aspects of the genome (e.g., DNA and its derivatives RNA and protein). However, a major tenet of genomic research involves *hypothesis-generating* data collection as opposed to *hypothesis-testing* experimentation. The latter has formed the basis of biomedical research, whereby existing knowledge and insight guide the testing of a particular hypothesis. In contrast, genome-based research tends to make few prior assumptions, favoring unbiased data generation and analysis as a path to discovery. Clearly, both approaches are powerful and essential, and both should continue at full force in the future. Although still associated with substantial cost, sequencing approaches such as whole genome and whole exome DNA sequencing or whole-transcriptome RNA sequencing have become available at most academic institutions, either through in-house services or through a number of commercial providers. Large-scale national and multinational genomic profiling efforts such as The Cancer Genome Atlas have led to the establishment of repositories of genomic variants for the most common malignancies. Next-generation sequencing approaches are being integrated into clinical routine and are used as both prognostic and predictive biomarkers. The latter are proving particularly useful as more drugs become available that target specific genomic variants (e.g., BRAF inhibitors targeting *BRAF* V600E mutations). The assignment of a particular therapeutic agent to a specific genomic finding has gained momentum over the past several years and was recently termed *precision medicine*.

However, with the ability to generate data of unprecedented scale, including sequencing of the whole genome, comes the challenge of data analysis. This has driven an entirely new generation of computer scientists to focus on new approaches to genomic data analysis, leading to new methods of pattern recognition and large-scale data processing. Translating these data into useful knowledge that provides biologic insight and clinical utility is an ongoing challenge.

This chapter describes the principles underlying common genomic approaches in the study of hematologic and other diseases, focusing more on concepts than on technical detail. Undoubtedly, there will be continuous acceleration of the pace of use of genomic approaches in clinical research and clinical care in the years ahead.

PRINCIPLES OF GENOMIC APPROACHES

Measurements and Perturbations

A common feature of many genomic approaches is the systematic nature of the approach (e.g., interrogating *all* kinases for their potential role in a particular biologic system). A more traditional approach would be to first determine (on the basis of prior knowledge) the kinase (or kinases) most likely to be important and then develop highly validated assays for that particular kinase. On one hand, a strength of the traditional approach is that the quality of the final assay is often high, given the attention paid to the one (or a couple of) kinase(s) of interest. On the other hand, such an approach is limited by the quality of the initial hypothesis. In contrast, a genomic approach would be more systematic and comprehensive, attempting to screen all kinases for the phenotype of interest. Although this is compelling, it also comes with an important limitation—the quality of the assay for each kinase's activity may not be uniformly high. For example, a screen for kinase phosphorylation as a surrogate for kinase activity has been reported. Such an approach is limited by the sensitivity and specificity of kinase-directed antibodies, which can be enormously variable across kinase family members.

Although genomics is most commonly associated with systematic *observational* studies, the same principles can also be applied to *perturbational* studies (i.e., systematic modulation of proteins followed by a phenotypic read-out). In this manner, all genes within a particular class (e.g., kinases) can be mutated, knocked down (e.g. by RNA interference), or completely knocked out (e.g., by genome editing), and the phenotypic consequence of each can be assessed. A number of genomic perturbational technologies have been developed recently, most notably the discovery of clustered regularly interspaced short palindromic repeats (CRISPR)/CRISPR-associated protein 9 (Cas9)-mediated genome editing, as described later. Use of these perturbational technologies in combination with high-throughput sequencing will yield great insight into the biology of hematologic diseases in the years ahead.

Importance of Sample Acquisition

Acquisition of the appropriate samples for a genomic experiment is arguably the most crucial step for the generation of a dataset expected to be rich with biologic information. This is particularly true for gene expression analysis, in which a number of processes may affect data quality. Because gene expression is a dynamic process that can be affected by any type of cellular manipulation, RNA abundance measurements are potentially complicated by changes that occur between the time that the biopsy is taken and the time that the RNA is isolated from the specimen. In general, the highest-quality RNA is obtained if, as soon as possible after harvesting a sample, cells are dissolved in a solution such as TRIzol reagent that inactivates RNase enzymes and the sample is stored at −80°C until RNA can be extracted. Procedures for measuring gene expression in formalin-fixed, paraffin-embedded (FFPE) tissues (in which messenger RNA [mRNA] is degraded to less than 100 nucleotides) have been used, but the lack of robustness of these methods may preclude routine clinical implementation.

Another extremely important but complicated issue is the complexity of cell types (e.g., tumor cells, normal cells of the same lineage, stromal cells, immune cells) present in the sample. This may be less of an issue for bone marrow samples taken from patients with newly diagnosed leukemia, in whom the number of blasts often approaches 90% or greater. In the relapsed leukemia setting (where the percentage of blast cells may be low) or in other tumor types, however, the admixture of multiple cell types may be vexing for gene expression studies. Multiple methods are available for enrichment and selection of cells of interest from a biopsy sample; these methods include flow cytometry, immunomagnetic bead sorting, and laser-capture microdissection. All have the benefit of enrichment of the cell of interest but also increase the amount of processing time and sample manipulation. Although in principle "contaminating," nonmalignant cells may reflect informative aspects of the tumor environment, the high degree of sample-to-sample variability makes such interpretations challenging. A promising new approach to the problem of cell-type heterogeneity involves analyzing cells at the single-cell level, as described later.

At the level of DNA analysis (as opposed to RNA analysis), the admixture of nonmalignant cells within a tumor may not obscure the presence of mutations in the tumor cells, even if those cells represent a minority population. However, the detection of mutations in a subset of cells within a sample requires extra depth of sequencing beyond what would be required to sequence, for example, a normal diploid genome. Thus it becomes critical to have a rough estimate of the purity of a given sample so that the appropriate genomic approach can be used subsequently.

Analytical Considerations

Unsupervised learning approaches (often referred to as *clustering*) have become an important part of the discovery process in genomic analysis. This type of analysis involves grouping samples solely on the basis of data obtained without regard to any prior knowledge of the samples or the disease. Thus one can obtain the predominant "structure" of the dataset without imposing any prior bias. For example, unsupervised learning approaches have been used to cluster leukemia or lymphoma samples on the basis of their gene expression profiles with the goal of uncovering the most robust classification schemes. Clustering algorithms can also cluster genes that have a similar expression profile in a gene expression dataset. There are a number of methods for clustering genes and samples, all of which have computational strengths and weaknesses. Comparison of the clustering methods is beyond the scope of this chapter, but suffice it to say that

all of these methods identify major associations within a given dataset if the signature is strong and robust. Great care must be taken in the interpretation of clustering results because clusters with distinct gene expression profiles may be caused not only by biologically important distinctions but also by artefacts of sample processing. Unsupervised learning methods that have been used include hierarchical clustering, principal component analysis, nonnegative matrix factorization, *k*-means clustering, and *t*-distributed stochastic neighbor embedding.

Supervised learning approaches are best suited for comparing data between two or more classes of samples that can be distinguished by some known property (or class distinction), such as biologic subtype or clinical outcome. For example, to determine the gene expression differences between different leukemia subtypes with distinct genetic abnormalities, one would use a supervised approach (Fig. 3.1). The same genes might be clustered together on the basis of unsupervised approaches already described, but they might also be obscured by a more dominant gene expression signature that is unrelated to the distinction of interest. For example, if there were another major signature within the data (i.e., a stage of differentiation signature), the differences that the investigator was searching for might be lost. A number of metrics can be used to identify genes that are differentially expressed between two groups of samples, all of which are best suited to identification of genes that are uniformly highly expressed in one group. Although the different metrics may generate slightly different lists of gene expression differences, if the gene expression difference is robust, all should give comparable results.

With the ability to generate large-scale genomic datasets come a number of analytical issues that are unique to what has come to be known as "big data." In particular, when the number of features

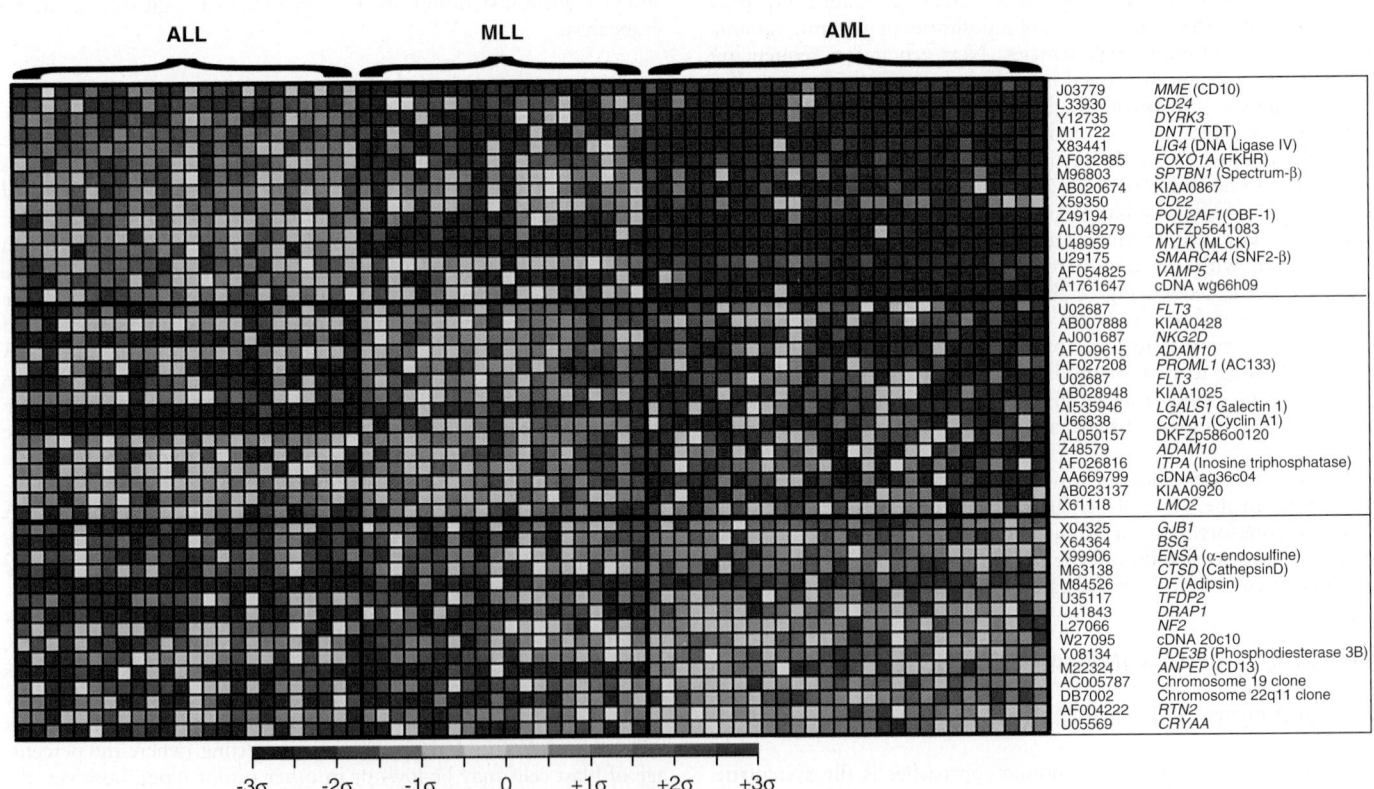

Fig. 3.1 COMPARISON OF GENE EXPRESSION IN ACUTE LYMPHOBLASTIC LEUKEMIA (ALL), MIXED-LINEAGE LEUKEMIA (*MLL*)-REARRANGED ALL (DESIGNATED *MLL),* AND ACUTE MYELOGENOUS LEUKEMIA (AML) SAMPLES USING A SUPERVISED LEARNING APPROACH. Gene expression in leukemia samples was analyzed using Affymetrix microarrays containing 12,600 unique probe sets. Genes that are highly expressed in one type of leukemia relative to the other two are shown. Each column represents a patient sample, and each row represents a gene. *Red* represents relative high-level expression and *blue* relative low-level expression. *(From Armstrong SA, Staunton JE, Silverman LB, et al: MLL translocations specify a distinct gene expression profile that distinguishes a unique leukemia. Nat Genet 30:41, 2002.)*

analyzed in an experiment (e.g., the expression of each of 22,000 mRNA transcripts) exceeds the number of samples (e.g., 50 patients with a particular type of lymphoma), there is potential for finding patterns in the data simply by chance. The more features analyzed and the fewer the number of samples, the more likely such a phenomenon is to be encountered. For this reason, the use of nominal *p*-values to estimate statistical significance of an observed observation is generally discouraged. Rather, some approach to correcting for multiple hypothesis testing is in order. (In the present example, 22,000 hypotheses are effectively being tested.) In the absence of such penalization, the significance of observations is likely to be grossly overestimated. Indeed, such misinterpretations of data were at the root of many of the early uses of gene expression profiling data in biomedical research.

Related to the challenges with high-dimensional data described, special considerations of pattern-matching algorithms must be made. With the availability of high-dimensional gene expression profiling data in the late 1990s came a flood of computational innovation from computer scientists looking to find biologically meaningful patterns amid biologic data. With that early wave of computational analysis came the realization that with often limited numbers of samples (compared with the number of features analyzed) comes the possibility of "overfitting" a computational model to a particular dataset—that is, defining a pattern (e.g., a spectrum of genes that are differentially expressed) that is correlated with a phenotype of interest (e.g., survival) in an initial dataset but then does not predict accurately when applied to an independent dataset. This failure to reproduce initial findings was variously attributed to technical defects in the genomic data itself, insufficiently complex algorithms, and the possibility that perhaps the most important features were not being analyzed in the first place (e.g., noncoding RNAs). In fact, however, nearly all of the early failures of pattern recognition algorithms to validate when applied to new datasets were attributable to overfitting of the models to an initial, small dataset. The solution to this problem is to ensure that discovery datasets are sufficiently large to avoid overfitting and to insist that, before any clinical or biologic claims are made, the model be tested on completely independent samples.

NEXT-GENERATION SEQUENCING TECHNOLOGY

Beginning around 2006, a number of new approaches to DNA sequencing burst onto the scene. These technical advances have transformed the field of genomics and will likely equally transform the diagnostics field in the years to come. A number of novel sequencing approaches have been commercialized, and their details are beyond the scope of this chapter. However, they differ fundamentally from traditional Sanger sequencing, which has been the mainstay for the past several decades. First, and most well recognized, is the dramatically lower cost of current sequencing methods compared with Sanger sequencing. Costs have dropped by nearly 1 million–fold compared with the sequencing of the first human genome. This drop in cost has transformed genome sequencing from the work of an entire community over the course of more than a decade (the initial sequencing of the human genome took 15 years and approximately $3 billion) to a routine experiment that can be done for hundreds of samples by major sequencing centers in the course of a week in 2016. These exponential cost reductions have come about not through dramatic drops in reagent costs but rather through dramatic increases in data output. A single lane on a modern sequencer generates vastly more data than a lane of conventional sequencing. This is relevant because to realize the lower costs of contemporary sequencing, large-scale projects must be undertaken. That is, devoting a single lane of sequencing to the sequencing of a plasmid, for example, is *more* expensive with current technologies than with traditional Sanger sequencing; the cost savings are realized only when large data outputs are required (e.g., the sequencing of entire genomes or of isolated genes across large numbers of patients).

When executed and analyzed properly, next-generation sequencing technologies can yield nearly perfect fidelity of sequence. At the same time, the error rates for any given sequencing read can be as high as 1%, depending on the sequencing platform. How can these two statements both be correct? Although a 1% error rate (99% accurate) may seem low, when taken in the context of sequencing all 3 billion bases of the human genome, that would in principle result in 30 million errors! Thankfully, this is not the case, because most sequencing errors are idiosyncratic—that is, they are not a function of a particular DNA sequence. The consequence of this is that by simply resequencing the same region multiple times and taking the consensus read, such idiosyncratic errors are lost; it is highly unlikely for them to occur over and over again at the same spot.

For normal, diploid genomes, sequencing is typically done at least 30-fold over (referred to as *30× coverage*). The consensus obtained by observing a given nucleotide 30 times is generally sufficient for rendering the correct read of that nucleotide. However, things get more complicated when dealing with (1) tumors containing gene copy number alterations (e.g., aneuploidy or regions or gene deletion or amplification) or (2) admixture of normal cells within the tumor sample. To compensate for copy number variation and normal cell contamination seen in most samples, typical cancer genome sequencing projects aim for a depth of coverage of at least 100×. Sequencing for diagnostic purposes may require even greater depth of coverage. In addition, the analysis of samples containing only rare tumor cells (e.g., 10%) would require ultradeep sequencing; otherwise, any tumor-specific mutations would likely become false negatives. Importantly, the frequency of cancer-associated mutations in studies performed using traditional Sanger sequencing methods may have been underestimated because of the lack of power to detect mutations in tumors with significant normal cell contamination. Whereas Sanger sequencing delivers the *average* allele observed in a sample, next-generation sequencing methods deliver a *distribution* of observed alleles, allowing for mutant alleles to be identified even if they represent a minority population.

Future of Sequencing Technologies

No one could have predicted the dramatic advances that have come to DNA sequencing technologies over the past decade. Costs have dropped dramatically, and it is predicted that costs will continue to drop, although less precipitously. The cost of whole-genome sequencing was estimated to be $1000 in 2016; however, this cost can be achieved only when sequencing many samples from large cohorts of patients, not on an individual sample-by-sample basis. Also, in addition to sequence *generation,* there is a high cost associated with sequence *analysis.* The cost of storage of genome sequence and analysis may exceed the cost of generating the data in the first place, and a detailed analysis is far from straightforward. Nevertheless, it is likely that, over the decade ahead, genome sequencing will become a routine component of both clinical research and routine clinical care.

DNA-LEVEL CHARACTERIZATION

Somatic Versus Germline Events

It is important to recognize the fundamental difference between *germline* variants and *somatic* variants in genome sequences. Germline variants are present in all cells of the body (with the exception of rare mosaicism), and these variants can contribute to the risk of future disease. Germline variants can be common (i.e., seen in ≥5% of the human population), or they can be rare (in principle, unique to a single individual). Each individual also carries de novo variants that are present in neither of the individual's parents' genomes. It has been demonstrated recently by genetic analyses of large populations that aging individuals without evidence of hematologic disease acquire mutations over time in genes that are associated with leukemia. This observation has been named *clonal hematopoiesis of indeterminate potential.* This indicates that expansion of particular clones occurs that is associated with an increased risk of myeloid and lymphoid neoplasia. Similarly, monoclonal gammopathy of undetermined significance and monoclonal B-cell lymphocytosis are characterized by clonal expansion of lymphoid clones that are usually associated with multiple myeloma and chronic lymphocytic leukemia, respectively. Because only a minority of individuals go on to develop a clinically symptomatic neoplasm, an important goal is to identify additional variants that promote the development of overt malignancy. Also of great interest is the question of the extent to which hematologic diseases (whether malignant or otherwise) are caused by germline genetic variation. Although it is clear that certain disorders (e.g., hemophilia) have a highly penetrant, Mendelian basis, it is less certain whether genetic variation substantially contributes to diseases that have been historically considered "sporadic" in the large majority of cases, such as multiple myeloma.

In contrast, mutations present in tumors but absent in the normal cells from that individual are referred to as *somatic*. Somatic mutations are thought to be a major driver of cancer behavior. However, all somatic mutations are not causal *drivers* of cancer. Indeed, the majority of somatic mutations observed in any individual tumor are likely passenger mutations—that is, they play no functional role in the pathogenesis of the tumor but rather were present in a cell that subsequently acquired a driver mutation that resulted in the cell's clonal outgrowth. The proportion of passengers to drivers differs dramatically from tumor type to tumor type. For example, tumors associated with tobacco (e.g., lung cancer) or sunlight exposure (e.g., melanoma) have very high mutation frequencies, with the majority of the observed mutations being "passengers." In contrast, many hematologic malignancies (e.g., acute myeloid leukemia) have relatively low mutation rates, and some cancers such as infant leukemias have extraordinarily low rates, with only a handful of protein-coding somatic mutations seen per patient.

Distinguishing passenger mutations from driver mutations is a major focus of cancer genome research. The complete delineation of the biologically important mutations in cancer requires both large-scale sequencing studies (enabling the identification of recurrent mutations) and the functional characterization of observed mutations.

Point Mutations

The most common type of genetic variants (both germline and somatic) are single-nucleotide variants (SNVs), also known as point mutations. As more individuals are sequenced and deposited into databases, it is becoming possible to catalog all common SNVs in the human population. Still, it is estimated that every individual will harbor 50 to 100 coding mutations not present in any database. For these reasons, it is particularly important to compare the somatic genome of a tumor with its matched normal germline sequence; otherwise, "private" germline variants may be mistaken for somatic mutations.

Certain patterns of point mutation are characteristic of particular environmental exposures. For example, G>T/C>A transversions are characteristic of tobacco-associated lung cancer, and C>T/G>A transitions are characteristic of ultraviolet radiation–associated skin cancers. Most hematologic malignancies lack a particular pattern of mutation, although B-cell lymphomas demonstrate a characteristic pattern of hot spots of mutations caused by activation-induced, adenosine deaminase–mediated.

Although not as common as point mutations, small somatic insertions or deletions (referred to collectively as *indels*) are also observed in tumors. These generally consist of the loss or gain of one or a few nucleotides that, when they occur within protein-coding regions, result in translational frameshifts that generally yield loss-of-function alleles.

Copy Number

Gains (amplifications) or losses (deletions) of genetic material at specific loci are recognized as playing an important role in the pathophysiology of disease. Trisomy 21, for example, predisposes individuals to transient myeloproliferative disorders and acute megakaryoblastic leukemia. Deletions at the *RB1* locus encoding the retinoblastoma gene or deletions of the *TP53* gene encoding the p53 tumor suppressor predispose individuals to the development of solid cancers, although only rarely to hematologic malignancies. In a landmark set of studies, it was shown that tumors from patients who inherit a mutant copy of the retinoblastoma tumor suppressor gene often have deletions of the remaining allele. This process has been termed *loss of heterozygosity,* and the search for genetic loci showing loss of heterozygosity in tumor samples has identified a number of genes that are involved in critical cellular processes and are important for cancer progression. Similarly, amplification of genomic loci can play an important role in oncogenesis and cancer biology. For example, amplification of the *ERBB2* (*HER2*) oncogene in human breast cancer predicts a poor prognosis, and ERBB2 has been shown to be an important therapeutic target in this disease.

The search for gains and losses of genetic material can be carried out using a number of techniques that require various levels of expertise and allow assessment of genomic integrity at various resolutions. The first method developed to assess genomic integrity, *cytogenetic analysis,* is still used today, but it allows identification only of abnormalities that encompass large regions of the genome. Nevertheless, cytogenetic analysis has provided tremendous insight into the pathophysiology of disease, particularly for leukemogenesis. Cytogenetic analysis remains a key part of the diagnostic workup for new cases of leukemia. It is likely, however, that over time it will be replaced by next-generation sequencing methods that have the ability to detect point mutations, deletions/insertions, copy number changes, and chromosomal translocations, all at high resolution.

More recently developed methods for assessing copy number variation include comparative genomic hybridization (CGH) and high-density single-nucleotide polymorphism (SNP) arrays. Although CGH and SNP arrays are falling out of favor, massively parallel genome sequencing can be used for copy number variant detection. Special note should be made of the analysis of copy number data. At the level of the individual sample (e.g., a tumor), one can easily visualize regions of aberration using tools such as the Integrative Genomics Viewer (IGV) (Fig. 3.2). Although this type of analysis highlights those aberrations in a *particular* sample, it does not reflect copy number abnormalities that are commonly observed across a *collection* of samples. Such recurrent copy number gains or losses tend to indicate biologically important events as opposed to copy number aberrations that simply reflect genomic instability but do not contribute to cancer pathogenesis (and therefore are nonrecurrent). To identify statistically significant regions of copy number abnormalities, algorithms such as the genomic identification of significant targets in cancer (GISTIC) method can be applied, yielding a plot of regions of amplification and deletion that are commonly observed in a set of samples (as shown in Fig. 3.3 for 24 patients with multiple myeloma).

Rearrangements

Chromosomal rearrangements (including balanced and unbalanced translocations, inversions, and more complex aberrations) are particularly important in the hematologic malignancies. Translocations were among the very first genomic defects to be discovered in cancer because cytogenetic analysis of metaphase chromosome spreads was feasible for the acute leukemias long before more technically advanced methods became available. Two basic types of translocations are common: those that result in fusion proteins involving two distinct genes and those that result in overexpression of an otherwise structurally normal gene. Translocations resulting in fusion transcripts (e.g., *ETV6/RUNX1* in acute lymphoblastic leukemia [ALL]) generally involve chromosomal breakage within intronic regions of the two genes, with in-frame fusion being a result of the normal process of RNA splicing. In contrast, translocations resulting in overexpression typically involve the juxtaposition of a coding region next to a highly active promoter or enhancer region such as an immunoglobulin

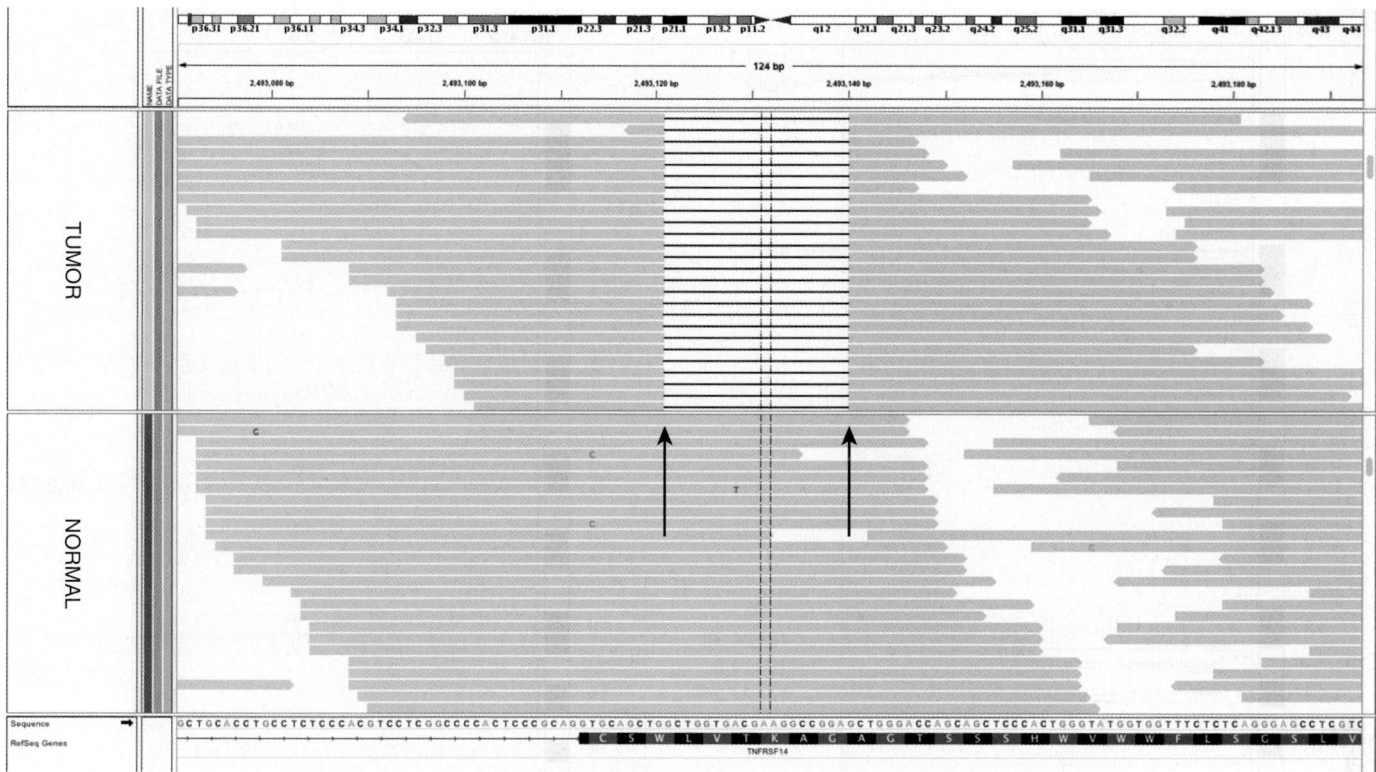

Fig. 3.2 GENOME DELETION IN A PATIENT WITH DIFFUSE LARGE B-CELL LYMPHOMA (DLBCL). Genome sequencing of a patient with DLBCL revealed a clear region of genome deletion within the *TNFRS14* gene, as visualized in the Integrative Genomics Viewer. The *gray bars* indicate the extent of the sequence read, with this region being interrogated multiple times. The *white block* in the middle (bracketed by *arrows*) indicates the region of genome deletion captured by all of the reads in the tumor but in none of the reads from the matched normal DNA sample (*bottom portion* of figure).

region in B cells. For example, in follicular lymphoma, translocations frequently involve juxtaposition of the antiapoptotic gene *BCL2* to the immunoglobulin heavy chain enhancer region, leading to massive overexpression of *BCL2* RNA and protein.

Translocations are best detected by either whole-genome sequencing or RNA sequencing (RNA-Seq), although their detection requires advanced computational analysis to distinguish them from artefactual errors in aligning sequence reads to a reference genome. For reasons that remain unclear, some tumors contain few, if any, translocations, but others contain hundreds, often involving multiple complex rearrangements. A particularly interesting phenomenon, termed *chromothripsis*, involves extensive complex genome rearrangements thought to occur via a single "big bang" genomic catastrophe (Fig. 3.4). It has been speculated that chromothripsis may represent a mechanism by which a cell can acquire multiple oncogenic events required for cellular transformation in a single event rather than in a stepwise manner.

SEQUENCING APPROACHES TO EPIGENOMICS

Sequencing approaches to epigenomics include chromatin immunoprecipitation followed by sequencing (ChIP-Seq), micrococcal nuclease (MNase) sequencing, DNAse sequencing (DNAse-Seq), bisulfite sequencing and assay for transposase-accessible chromatin with high-throughput sequencing (ATAC-Seq). Although the majority of information encoded in the genome is thought to emanate from its primary DNA sequence, the importance of epigenetic gene regulatory mechanisms has become increasingly evident over the past few years. Epigenetic modifications play a critical role in the regulation of transcription, DNA repair, and replication. For example, DNA methylation can occur, particularly in CpG-rich regions of the genome, and such methylation can lead to the silencing of gene expression at that locus. Widespread methylation appears frequently in cancer and may serve as an important mechanism of silencing tumor suppressor genes. Massively parallel sequencing, coupled with bisulfite sequencing approaches, allows for genome-wide assessment of DNA methylation in development and disease. DNA methylation is an effective mechanism of silencing genes, for example, as is required to specify cell type, but with relatively few dynamic changes over time. In contrast, open chromatin regions may be analyzed by technologies that are based on sequencing of DNA regions that are accessible for certain DNA-cutting enzymes such as DNase, micrococcal nuclease, or transposase that preferentially cut at open chromatin regions. Several large-scale profiling efforts (e.g., through the National Institutes of Health ENCODE project) have used these technologies to annotate cancer cell lines and normal human and murine tissues, including hematopoietic subsets.

Modifications to histones are orchestrated and tightly regulated by a group of enzymes called *chromatin regulators*. Perhaps one of the most striking results derived from genome-wide sequencing analyses in cancer is the frequency of somatic mutations in chromatin regulators, which account for up to 25% of all cancer drivers. Detailed mechanistic analysis of epigenetic modifications and the contribution of individual chromatin regulators to these modifications have long been hindered by a lack of effective technologies. With the use of next-generation sequencing techniques combined with chromatin immunoprecipitation, it is now possible to comprehensively investigate the molecular mechanisms of epigenetic alterations and define their disease relevance. ChIP-Seq can be used to map histone modifications that are associated with actively transcribed regions, repressed regions, or regions found at distal regulatory elements. Optimized technologies now allow for ChIP-Seq with small input of samples or with FFPE samples, which has significant implications for translating this technology to approaches for the analysis of clinical specimens.

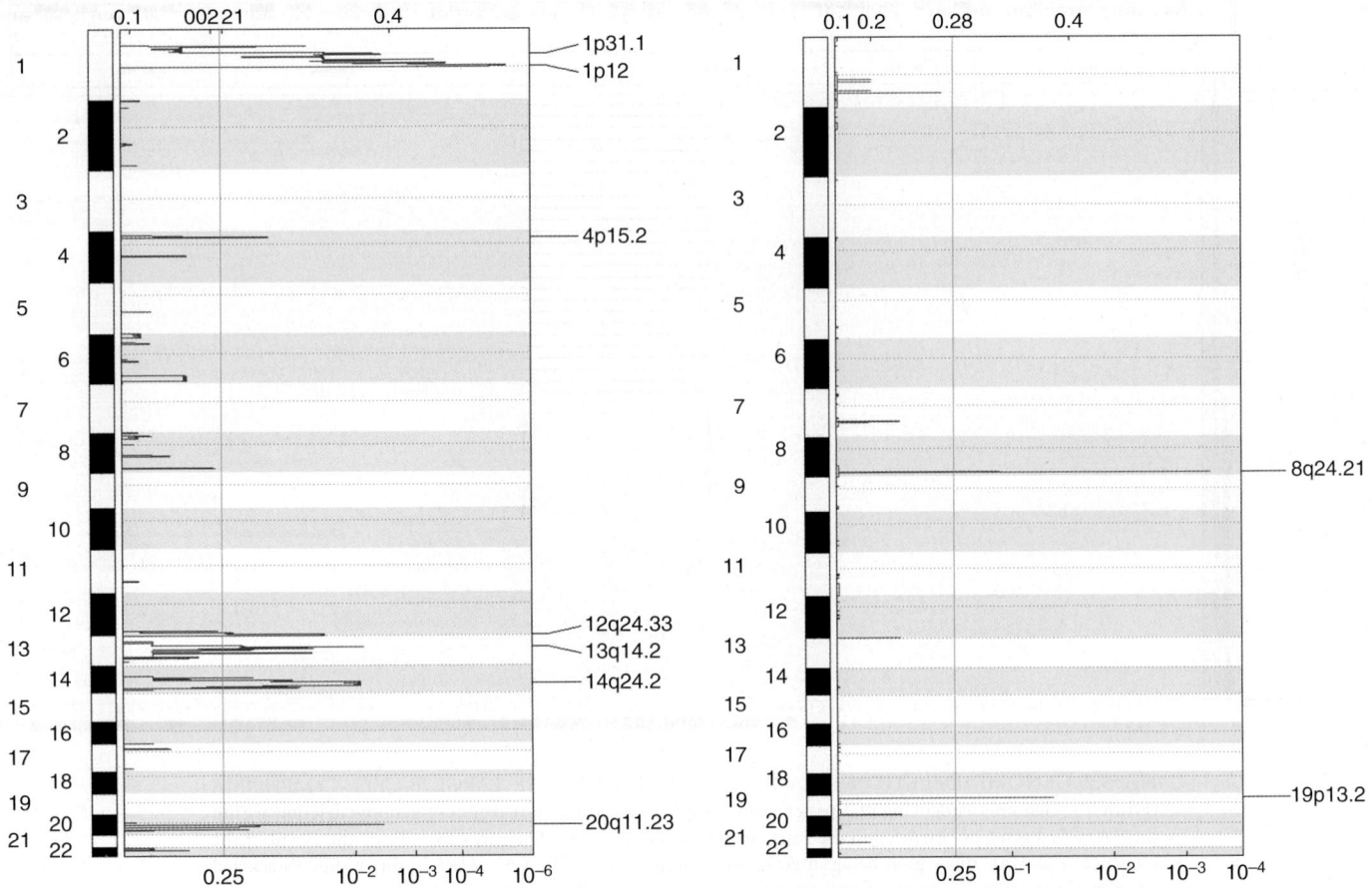

Fig. 3.3 RECURRENT COPY NUMBER ABERRATIONS IN MULTIPLE MYELOMA. Output of the genomic identification of significant targets in cancer (GISTIC) algorithm indicates recurrent regions of gene copy number gain and loss. Recurrent gains are shown in *red* (including the *MYC* gene at 8q24), and recurrent losses are shown in *blue* (including the *RB* gene at 13q14). The height of each peak indicates the statistical significance of the event (a function of frequency and the rate expected by chance).

RNA-LEVEL CHARACTERIZATION

mRNA Profiling

The most well-developed and widely used genomic technology is genome-wide expression profiling of protein-coding RNAs (mRNAs). Since the late 1990s profiling has been done using an array format in which sequence-specific probes are immobilized onto a solid surface (or are synthesized in situ). mRNA is isolated from a sample of interest (e.g., a tumor biopsy or a cell line). The mRNA is then labeled in some fashion, often with a fluorescent tag, and the extent of hybridization of the mRNA to the array is captured by a laser-scanning device. This technology enables the interrogation of all 22,000 or so mRNAs in the human and mouse transcriptomes.

Expression profiling of FFPE tissues deserves special mention because formalin fixation causes the degradation of mRNAs into fragments of only about 80 nucleotides in length. Conventional array-based profiling approaches therefore do not work well, particularly those that involve labeling of the mRNAs by priming of the 3′ polyadenylation tail; however, approaches have been developed that allow for the profiling of FFPE-derived tissues. These include modification of standard arrays involving the use of 3′-biased probes for each mRNA transcript, such that even degraded mRNAs can be profiled. Although it is likely that any method applied to FFPE samples will yield noisier data than frozen samples, the ability to analyze archived material, particularly those samples with long-term clinical outcome data, will prove invaluable. Array-based approaches do not give absolute quantitation, but often this is not required.

Rather, researchers wish to compare the expression level of a gene (or genes) in one sample with another (or one group of samples with another). Most gene expression profiling thus requires the *relative* assessment of expression across a set of samples, and absolute quantitation (e.g., number of mRNA copies per cell) is neither possible nor in most cases necessary.

More recent sequencing-based approaches to expression profiling (RNA-Seq), however, provide the opportunity to provide a count of the number of transcripts in a given sample. In addition, RNA sequencing allows for the profiling of previously unknown genes (i.e., those not previously recognized to encode a transcript) as well as of alternative splice forms of known mRNAs. Furthermore, gene fusions within coding regions and SNVs can be detected simultaneously with gene expression. One advantage of hybridization-based (microarray) methods is that they effectively measure both abundant and non-abundant transcripts. RNA sequencing, however, favors abundant transcripts. The consequence of this is that, in order to capture less abundant mRNAs, deep sequencing is required, resulting in increased costs.

Noncoding RNA Profiling

Although the focus within the family of RNAs is often on those that code for proteins, a wealth of noncoding RNAs exist in mammalian cells. Two major classes of noncoding RNAs are short RNAs, known as *microRNAs* (miRNAs), and *large intergenic noncoding RNAs* (lincRNAs), as described later.

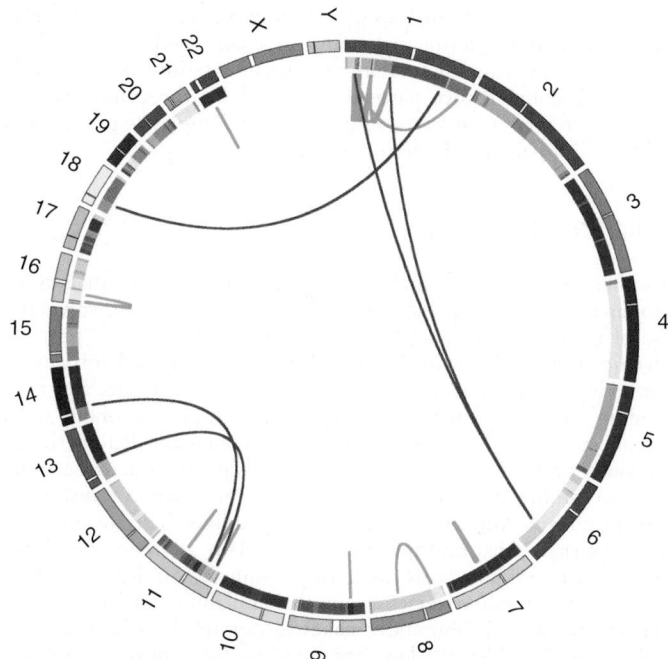

Fig. 3.4 CHROMOTHRIPSIS. Circos plot showing the extensive genomic rearrangements in a glioblastoma tumor. Each of the human chromosomes is displayed around the circle of the plot. *Purple lines* indicate rearrangements between different chromosomes, and *green lines* indicate intrachromosomal rearrangements. In this tumor, chromosome 1p has nearly 100 chromosomal rearrangements, indicative of a single-step genomic catastrophe mechanism known as *chromothripsis.*

miRNAs are small (approximately 22-nucleotide) RNAs that do not encode for proteins but bind to mRNA transcripts to regulate translation and mRNA stability. Several hundred miRNAs are thought to exist in the human genome. In *Caenorhabditis elegans,* zebrafish, and other model organisms, miRNAs play a critical role in development through regulation of translation of key proteins. In mammalian cells, a role for miRNAs has been recognized in the regulation of cellular differentiation. Not only are many miRNAs differentially expressed across hematopoietic lineages, but several miRNAs have also been demonstrated to play key functional roles in hematopoietic lineage specification and differentiation. Moreover, the expression or function of several miRNAs is altered by chromosomal translocations, deletions, or mutations in leukemia. In addition, members of the protein complex (including the protein DICER) that process the maturation of miRNAs from longer RNA forms have been implicated in malignancy.

Noncoding lincRNAs are approximately 1000 nucleotides in length and number approximately 5000 in the human genome. The widespread existence of lincRNAs was only discovered in 2009, and their function remains largely unknown. However, recent evidence suggests that they may play important roles in establishing and maintaining cell fate and may play key roles in regulation of the epigenome. Their role in the pathogenesis of disease is heavily investigated. Interestingly, lincRNAs appear to have exquisite tissue-specific patterns of expression, suggesting that they may have diagnostic potential. Evidence is also mounting that some RNAs encode short peptide sequences (less than 100 amino acids), which may eventually require reclassification from lincRNA to protein-coding RNA.

SINGLE-CELL RNA AND DNA SEQUENCING

Next-generation sequencing applications in hematology and oncology have typically focused on interrogating *populations* of cells. Although computational methods have been developed to decipher the relative contribution of individual genetic subclones to the entire tumor, these approaches usually have limited resolution and are not able to detect very small subclones that comprise few tumor cells. Several novel technologies have been developed that allow DNA and RNA sequencing of *single* tumor cells as well as of single cells from the tumor microenvironment. Advances in microfluidic approaches make it possible to generate RNA sequencing data from thousands of cells simultaneously, and several different technological concepts have emerged for highly parallel sample preparation. For example, the entire sample processing workflow, from isolating single cells to generating sequencing libraries, can be generated in multiwell plates in order to perform multiple reactions at the same time. This can be done with typical multiwell plates, or the entire experimental workflow can take place in a fully integrated microfluidic "lab on a chip." Another approach uses microdroplet technology. To this end, a single cell is packaged into an emulsion droplet, and thousands of droplets are generated. Although the single cells are segregated into individual droplets, a molecular barcoding step takes place with which every RNA molecule in each cell is labeled with a unique molecular tag. After this step, the droplets are dissolved and RNA sequencing preparation is performed in a single tube. The barcodes can later be used to precisely assign each RNA molecule to the correct cell, making it possible to determine the gene expression profile of each single cell.

These technologies currently enable sequencing of thousands of single cells simultaneously, but that number will undoubtedly increase with rapid progress in technology development. Having a methodology in hand that allows RNA sequencing with single-cell resolution is particularly useful to precisely define the composition of the tumor microenvironment in addition to the tumor itself. These novel technologies and their ability to successfully sequence even minimal amounts of DNA and RNA are not only useful for sequencing tumor tissue with single-cell resolution but also empower "blood biopsy" approaches. This approach is based on the discovery that various types of tumor-derived material can be detected in the blood of patients with cancer, including circulating tumor cells (CTCs), circulating tumor DNA, or cell-free DNA (cfDNA), as well as various types of circulating microvesicles, such as exosomes and apoptotic bodies. There is increasing evidence that interrogation of these materials from the blood provides a representation of the tumor simply by drawing a vial of blood. In some cancers, the entire genome or the entire exome can be reproduced by genomic sequencing of cfDNA or CTCs. Because blood draws are safer, less complicated, and less expensive than tissue biopsy, and because they can easily be done at many time points, there is great interest in genomic approaches to blood-derived materials, including DNA and RNA sequencing.

PROTEIN-LEVEL CHARACTERIZATION

Unlike the characterization of DNA and RNA, which has become routine, the systematic, genome-wide characterization of proteins remains extremely technically challenging. Not long ago, comparative proteomic experiments consisted largely of the comparison of single proteins across various conditions or samples. However, a number of new advances in technology have made for a dramatic acceleration of the pace at which the abundance of proteins can be measured and their posttranslational modification (e.g., phosphorylation) can be assessed.

Mass Spectrometry

The workhorse of proteomics remains mass spectrometry. The fundamental principles of mass spectrometry have not changed over the years, but technical advances (the details of which are beyond the scope of this chapter) have led to increased ability to detect proteins in complex mixtures. Previously, extensive biochemical fractionation of the proteome was required to render mixtures of proteins sufficiently limited in number and with sufficient abundance to be reliably detected and identified. Such fractionation required extensive time, expertise, and instrumentation as well as a large amount of starting material, all of which tended to make systematic proteomic experiments difficult to perform routinely. However, newer instruments and methods allow for the analysis of significantly more complex mixtures, with increased sensitivity and speed. Sequence assignment confidence, especially for modified peptides, has also been markedly improved owing to the increase in both resolution and mass accuracy. For example, in mammalian cells, it is possible to confidently detect more than 8000 unique proteins and more than 15,000 phospho-peptides in a few days using a single instrument. Efforts to perform proteome-wide analysis of complex samples such as cells and tissues without extensive fractionation represent one end of the spectrum; proteomic analysis with single-cell resolution represents the other end. Although these methods (single-cell Western blot analysis and flow cytometry for intracellular proteins) can currently interrogate only one or a few analytes at the same time, these methods will evolve with ongoing technological progress.

Reverse Phase Lysates

An attractive alternative to mass spectrometry involves the use of *reverse phase protein arrays* (RPPAs). RPPAs involve the robotic spotting of minute amounts of total cell protein lysates onto glass slides (thus creating an array of lysates derived from different samples) (Fig. 3.5). The slides can then be probed with antibodies against particular proteins of interest, including phosphorylation-specific antibodies. The advantage of RPPAs is that only a tiny amount of cellular material is required, and hundreds of samples can be tested on a single array. The downside is that the method requires the availability of high-quality antibodies that are both sensitive and specific for the protein of interest. Unfortunately, such high-quality antibodies are available for only a minority of human proteins. In addition, RPPAs

are not suitable for the analysis of large numbers of proteins, because each protein to be interrogated requires a separate slide. Nevertheless, RPPA remains a useful tool in the armamentarium of proteomic research and may prove particularly useful for the comparison of proteins of interest across a large panel of samples (e.g., across a collection of patient samples or cell lines).

Bead-Based Profiling

Another proteomic method involves the multiplexed analysis of protein abundance or phosphorylation. Phosphorylation involves the use of microspheres (beads). In this approach, a different protein-specific antibody is coupled to beads of distinct color. A mixture of antibody-coupled beads is then mixed with protein lysate, and then binding events are detected with a labeled secondary antibody (e.g., antiphosphotyrosine antibody). Multiple analytes are thereby simultaneously profiled in a single sample. This approach was successfully used to profile the tyrosine phosphorylation status of nearly all protein tyrosine kinases across a panel of cell lines. The advantage of this approach is that multiple proteins (as many as 100 or more) can be assessed simultaneously in a single sample. Similar to RPPA, however, the method depends on the availability of high-quality antibodies, and this limitation makes the approach difficult to generalize broadly. Nevertheless, the method may prove useful for interrogating particular classes of proteins, such as kinases, for which suitable antibodies exist.

METABOLITE-LEVEL CHARACTERIZATION

Beyond nucleic acid and protein characterization, systematic profiling of small-molecule metabolites has also recently become possible. Such unbiased approaches to the assessment of metabolite levels have yielded new insights into the pathogenesis of metabolic diseases such as diabetes. In addition, the discovery of mutations in metabolic enzymes in acute myeloid leukemia has spurred interest in the metabolic consequences of these mutations on the "metabolome." Metabolite profiling is at present not routinely used in biomedical research, but it is likely that the years ahead will see a significant surge in its use.

FUNCTIONAL GENOMICS

Although the bulk of genomic research takes the form of observational studies (i.e., determining the spectrum of mutations in a tumor), functional approaches to genomic research are increasingly becoming feasible. Several discoveries have led to technologies that allow gene-specific perturbation. Zinc finger nucleases, transcription activator–like effector *nucleases* (TALENs), RNA interference (RNAi), and random chemical mutagenesis with agents such as *N*-ethyl-*N*-nitrosourea have been used to functionally perturb genes. For example, RNAi technology made it possible to knock down the expression of all genes in a given cell line and measure the consequences. This approach has been used most extensively in the area of cancer, where the complete set of genes that are essential for the survival of a cancer cell line was identified via genome-wide RNAi screens (Fig. 3.6). In addition to loss-of-function RNAi screens, it has become possible to perform systematic gain-of-function screens by overexpressing a library of complementary DNAs and then selecting for a phenotype of interest. Zinc finger nucleases and TALENs are much more precise genomic tools that enable genetic mutations, insertions, and deletions. Although very powerful, all of these approaches have substantial disadvantages. Although RNAi is technically relatively easy to perform, it enables "knockdown" of genes but not complete "knockout" in most cases. It can be associated with off-target effects (i.e., perturbation of random genes that are not intended to be targeted). Insertion of precise genetic defects, such as single-nucleotide variants, is not possible with RNAi but can be done

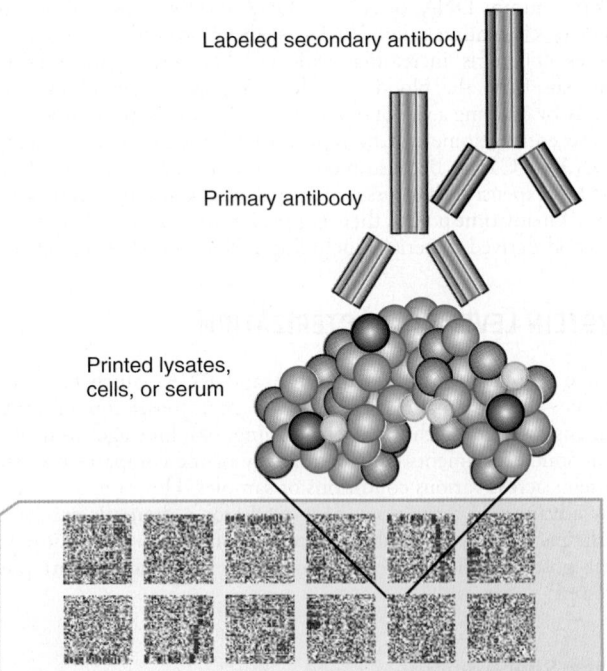

Labeled secondary antibody

Primary antibody

Printed lysates, cells, or serum

Fig. 3.5 REVERSE PHASE PROTEIN ARRAYS (RPPAs). Schematic illustrating the concept of RPPA. Cellular lysates derived from patient samples or cell lines are robotically spotted onto a glass slide. Next, a primary antibody specific for a protein of interest is added to the slide, with the antibody sticking to the array in proportion to the abundance of the protein in question. To visualize the antibody-binding event, a secondary antibody that recognizes the primary antibody (generally fluorescently labeled) is added, and the slide is examined by microscopy or using a laser-scanning instrument.

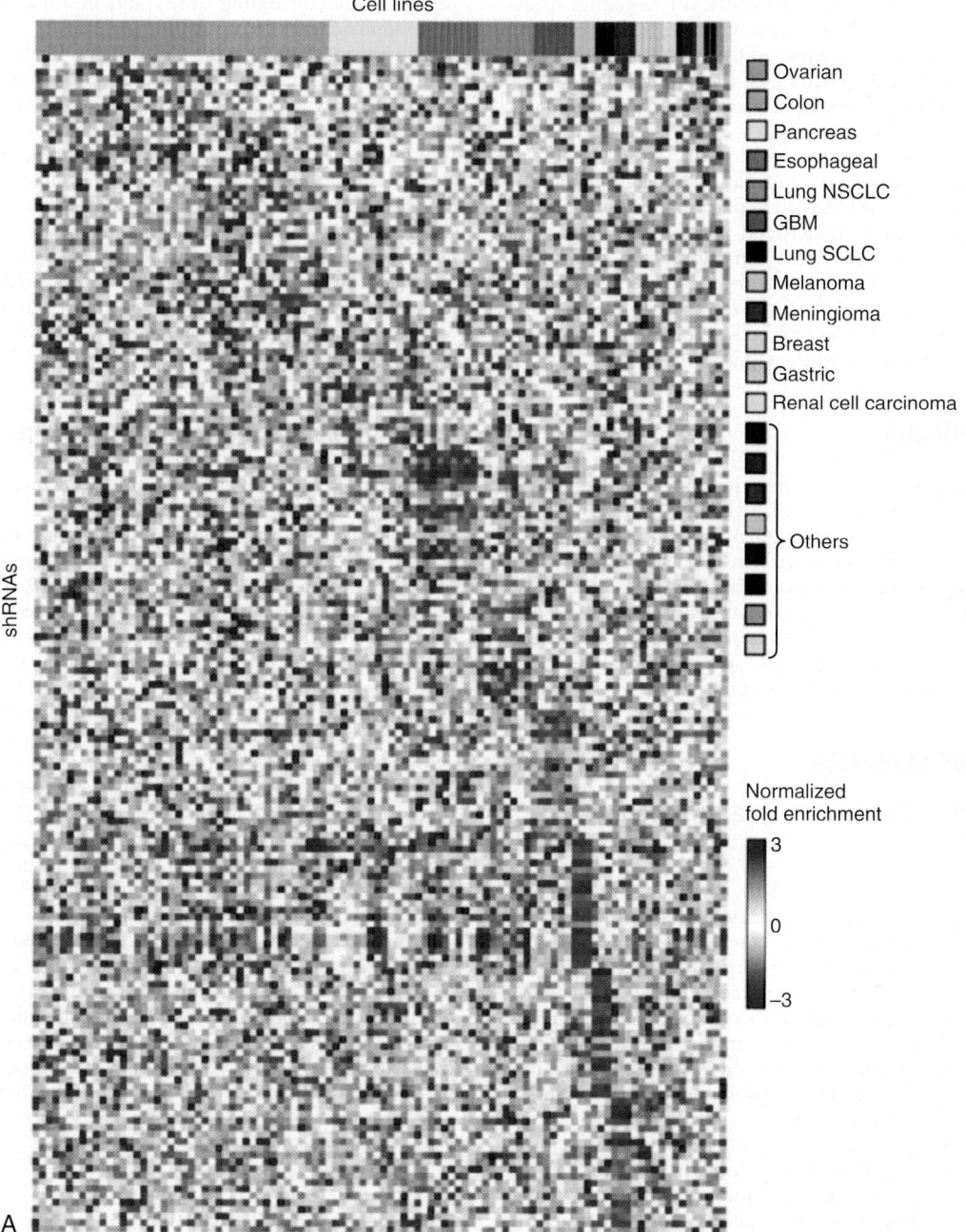

Cell lines

shRNAs

- ☐ Ovarian
- ☐ Colon
- ☐ Pancreas
- ☐ Esophageal
- ☐ Lung NSCLC
- ☐ GBM
- ☐ Lung SCLC
- ☐ Melanoma
- ☐ Meningioma
- ☐ Breast
- ☐ Gastric
- ☐ Renal cell carcinoma
- } Others

Normalized fold enrichment

3

0

−3

A

Fig. 3.6 SYSTEMATIC RNA INTERFERENCE SCREENS. Lineage-specific dependencies are illustrated in this heatmap of differentially antiproliferative short hairpin RNAs (shRNAs) in cell lines from individual cancer lineages in comparison with all others. The top 20 shRNAs that distinguish each lineage from the others are displayed. *GBM,* Glioblastoma multiforme; *NSCLC,* non–small cell lung cancer; *SCLC,* small cell lung cancer. *(From Cheung HW, Cowley GS, Weir BA, et al: Systematic investigation of genetic vulnerabilities across cancer cell lines reveals lineage-specific dependencies in ovarian cancer.* Proc Natl Acad Sci U S A *108:12372, 2011.)*

with zinc finger nucleases and TALENs. However, these latter two technologies are difficult to perform and expensive. In hematology and cancer research in general, all of these technologies have largely been superseded by the recent development of the transformative CRISPR/Cas9 technology. CRISPR/Cas9 technology combines the strengths of all of these approaches: The technology is relatively easy to use and allows precise and efficient editing of the genome. The method can be used to introduce specific genetic alterations in eukaryotic cells, and the consequences of these alterations can be identified by genomic approaches. CRISPR tools have been developed using programmable transcription factors that may activate targeted genes, or alternatively genes can be silenced without causing

double-stranded DNA breaks. The method can be used in cells from different species, and it can be used to create mouse models of human diseases faster and more efficiently than are possible with well-established homologous recombination to generate genetically engineered mouse models, allowing genetic modification of multiple loci at the same time. In 2015, another nuclease, Cpf1, was discovered with properties different from those of Cas9, including a different DNA cutting pattern, and requiring fewer components. Progress in this field is being made at a rapid pace, and the technology will undoubtedly develop rapidly. Although immensely powerful, there are several drawbacks of the technology that have to be addressed in the coming years, such as a genomic copy number bias that causes a gene-independent cell response to CRISPR/Cas9 targeting. Moreover, the ability to express Cas9 or related nucleases is not consistent across cell types. As with every genome-editing technology, off-target effects exist, which may lead to editing of the wrong gene. Because of the ease of use, libraries have been created targeting the entire protein-coding region of the genome (i.e., exome), as well as many noncoding regions of the genome, which will allow scientists to perform comprehensive functional genetics. The combination of genomics with CRISPR/Cas9-mediated perturbation provides an unprecedented opportunity to understand the consequences of the genetic defects encountered in patients. In addition to pointing to new potential therapeutic targets for cancer, screens using these technologies hold the promise of identifying genetic predictors of gene dependency. Such predictors will be key for the translation of these in vitro approaches to use in the clinic.

PHARMACOGENOMICS

The use of the genome to study drug response deserves special mention and is the subject of an entire chapter of this book (see Chapter 8). As the cost of genome sequencing continues to fall, it will become increasingly feasible to perform population-scale genetic studies to identify genetic determinants of drug toxicity and response. Although some examples of such pharmacogenomic markers have been discovered (e.g., genetic predictors of antimetabolite chemotherapy), the field awaits truly large-scale, systematic studies of large numbers of patients with known drug response data.

CLINICAL USE OF GENOMICS

Sequencing-Based Diagnostics and Precision Medicine

With the falling cost of genome sequencing and streamlined workflows, next-generation sequencing has entered into routine clinical diagnostic use. Sequencing panels that target the genes commonly mutated in cancer are available at many academic centers and are actively being used to triage patients to specific treatments. Genomic variants in such a "precision medicine" approach either suggest a therapeutic agent that directly targets the variant itself (e.g., a BRAF inhibitor in a patient with a *BRAF* V600E mutated neoplasm) or inform therapeutic decisions that are less directly related (e.g., not using epidermal growth factor receptor inhibitors in colon cancers harboring *KRAS*-activating mutations). Similarly, genomic variants may predict an individual's response to immunotherapy. In particular, it has been observed that tumors with high mutation burden tend to have more favorable responses to programmed death 1/programmed death ligand 1 (PD1/PDL1) blockade than in patients whose tumors have fewer mutations, presumably reflecting a lower neoantigen load.

Compared with RNA-based analysis, DNA-based diagnostics have the advantage of being more definitive in that one is looking, for example, for the presence of a mutation (an A, G, C, or T) as opposed to a relative abundance of a particular transcript or transcripts, the latter being confounded by an admixture of cell types within tumors or tissues. Because modern sequencing approaches allow for allele separation, the admixture of tumors with normal cells can be addressed at the DNA level simply by increasing the depth of sequencing coverage, as described earlier. Whether single-cell RNA sequencing approaches (which combat the issue of cellular heterogeneity) have the potential to be introduced into the routine clinical setting remains to be determined. Currently, their technical complexity precludes routine use. Similarly, if the cost of sequencing continues to drop, this will likely give way to more systematic approaches that include whole exome sequencing and whole-genome sequencing rather than just sequencing a limited number of loci. However, the pace of technology advancement will likely outstrip understanding of clinical utility and financial reimbursement by health insurance payers, so demonstrating utility and measurable patient benefit of these approaches is of utmost importance.

Sequencing-based diagnostics will also likely have an increasingly important role in nonmalignant conditions, such as blood-clotting disorders, in which it will become possible to systematically resequence all genes in the coagulation cascade, thereby identifying either common or highly rare sequence variants that might explain or predict disease. The widespread use of germline sequencing to predict disease also raises a large set of ethical questions that must be addressed, particularly those relating to children and family members of individuals undergoing sequence analysis. Whether whole-genome sequencing will become a routine part of health care in the future remains to be determined, but it is almost certain that much of the current diagnostic approach to medicine will eventually be supplanted by DNA-level analysis.

Minimal Residual Disease Diagnostics

Combination therapies using multiple therapeutic agents have been a great success in hematologic malignancies. For instance, childhood ALL has been associated with very high cure rates for a long time. The therapy of multiple myeloma has been transformed over the last 15 years with the advent of many new therapeutic agents. Both of these are examples of diseases for which deep remissions can be achieved, and therefore the ability to detect minimal residual disease (MRD) is of increasing importance. Traditional approaches to detect MRD include quantitative PCR, as is used for the detection of the Bcr-Abl fusion in patients with chronic myeloid leukemia undergoing treatment with tyrosine kinase inhibitors, or multiparametric flow cytometry, which is used for MRD detection in multiple myeloma. Deep next-generation sequencing of T-cell receptors and B-cell receptors is now being used to detect MRD in B-cell and T-cell malignancies. This sequencing approach targets a limited number of genomic regions that are involved in VDJ recombination of the T-cell and B-cell receptors, thus allowing identification of monoclonal B and T cells, which define the malignant tumor cells. Because these regions are sequenced many times over (i.e., with great "depth"), malignant clones can be detected even if they occur with a frequency of only 1 in 10^5 to 10^6. The advances in sequencing of very small cell numbers down to the single-cell level, as described earlier, allow for comprehensive detection of genomic alterations as well as interrogation of transcriptional profiles. Combining these sequencing approaches with highly sensitive cell isolation and cell-sorting technology holds great promise to better characterize what types of tumor cells remain viable at the stage of MRD.

Expression-Based Diagnostics

It has been over a decade since the first proof-of-principle studies were published demonstrating the possibility of using gene expression profiling to classify diseases such as cancer. Those studies raised the possibility that such promising gene expression signatures might be further validated and then implemented in the routine clinical setting as powerful diagnostic tests. The reality is that few such transitions to clinical practice have been made. One of these is the Oncotype Dx Breast Cancer Assay test, which consists of a tumor gene expression signature of 21 genes capable of determining the requirement for chemotherapy in women with early-stage breast cancer. This test has now become part of the standard of care at many cancer centers in the United States.

One should ask, however, why, despite thousands of papers being published on potential diagnostic applications of gene expression profiling, so few have progressed to routine clinical implementation. There are likely several reasons to explain the slow pace of advancement. First, to develop truly valid diagnostic tests, the test must be applied to large numbers of patients with known clinical outcomes, and in many cases, such cohorts of patients simply do not exist, making validation challenging. Second, because gene expression signatures are based on relative transcript abundance (as opposed to, for example, genome sequencing), it is subject to technical variation such as stromal admixture of tumors that can distort a diagnostic signature. Third, although the academic publishing system tends to reward *initial* discoveries (which are often published in high-profile journals), the essential follow-up *validation* studies tend to be valued less, and therefore investigators do not have an incentive to follow up on their initial observations. Fourth, the economics of molecular diagnostics have in general not been favorable, thus discouraging companies from making major investments in the validation and commercialization of promising diagnostic tests. It is likely that diagnostic tests will command more of a premium in the future as a mechanism to use expensive therapeutics only in patients likely to benefit, but the time required for this to evolve is uncertain.

However, the potential utility of clinically relevant gene expression signatures has regained interest with the progress and greater availability of sophisticated RNA sequencing technology. Whether RNA sequencing provides data sufficiently robust to be used in clinical routine remains to be established.

FUTURE DIRECTIONS

The field of genomics has matured greatly over the past decade. Major analytical advances have made it possible to analyze and interpret complex datasets beyond what was previously possible. In addition, dropping costs have made it possible to generate data at a scale that was never before imaginable. DNA sequencing is now routine at many academic centers and is increasingly being used to drive precision medicine by suggesting potential therapies based on individual patients' genetic profiles. Nevertheless, such approaches are still in their infancy; the majority of patients do not receive direct benefit from such precision medicine approaches. The future will also hold an explosion of functional genomic studies, particularly using genome editing methods such as CRISPR/Cas9. With deep genomic, transcriptomic, and epigenetic data already available for the most common hematologic and malignant diseases, and with new data being generated at an ever-increasing rate, there will be great opportunity for diagnostic and therapeutic development. The integration of genomic and other high-throughput sequencing approaches into clinical research and routine clinical care will continue to be one of the greatest challenges and opportunities in medicine in the decade ahead.

SUGGESTED READINGS

Alizadeh AA, Eisen MB, Davis RE, et al: Distinct types of diffuse large B-cell lymphoma identified by gene expression profiling. *Nature* 403:503, 2000.

Armstrong SA, Staunton JE, Silverman LB, et al: MLL translocations specify a distinct gene expression profile that distinguishes a unique leukemia. *Nat Genet* 30:41, 2002.

Bernstein BE, Kamal M, Lindblad-Toh K, et al: Genomic maps and comparative analysis of histone modifications in human and mouse. *Cell* 120:169, 2005.

Beroukhim R, Getz G, Nghiemphu L, et al: Assessing the significance of chromosomal aberrations in cancer: methodology and application to glioma. *Proc Natl Acad Sci USA* 104:20007, 2007.

Boyd SD, Marshall EL, Merker JD, et al: Measurement and clinical monitoring of human lymphocyte clonality by massively parallel VDJ pyrosequencing. *Sci Transl Med* 1:12ra23, 2009.

Buenrostro JD, Giresi PG, Zaba LC, et al: Transposition of native chromatin for fast and sensitive epigenomic profiling of open chromatin, DNA-binding proteins and nucleosome position. *Nat Methods* 10:1213, 2013.

Cabili MN, Trapnell C, Goff L, et al: Integrative annotation of human large intergenic noncoding RNAs reveals global properties and specific subclasses. *Genes Dev* 25:1915, 2011.

Carter SL, Cibulskis K, Helman E, et al: Absolute quantification of somatic DNA alterations in human cancer. *Nat Biotechnol* 30:413, 2012.

Cheung HW, Cowley GS, Weir BA, et al: Systematic investigation of genetic vulnerabilities across cancer cell lines reveals lineage-specific dependencies in ovarian cancer. *Proc Natl Acad Sci USA* 108:12372, 2011.

Cong L, Ran FA, Cox D, et al: Multiplex genome engineering using CRISPR/Cas systems. *Science* 339:819–823, 2013.

Dryja TP, Cavenee W, White R, et al: Homozygosity of chromosome 13 in retinoblastoma. *N Engl J Med* 310:550, 1984.

Du J, Bernansconi P, Clauser KR, et al: Bead-based profiling of tyrosine kinase phosphorylation identifies SRC as a potential target for glioblastoma therapy. *Nat Biotechnol* 27:77, 2009.

Emmert-Buck MR, Bonner RF, Smith PD, et al: Laser capture microdissection. *Science* 274:998, 1996.

Garraway LA, Lander ES: Lessons from the cancer genome. *Cell* 153:17, 2013.

Hanahan D, Weinberg RA: Hallmarks of cancer: the next generation. *Cell* 144:646, 2011.

Hoshida Y, Villanueva A, Kobayashi M, et al: Gene expression in fixed tissues and outcome in hepatocellular carcinoma. *N Engl J Med* 359:1995, 2008.

Jaiswal S, Fontanillas P, Flannick J, et al: Age-related clonal hematopoiesis associated with adverse outcomes. *N Engl J Med* 371:2488, 2014.

Jinek M, Chylinski K, Fonfara I, et al: A programmable dual-RNA-guided DNA endonuclease in adaptive bacterial immunity. *Science* 337:816–821, 2012.

Johannessen CM, Boehm JS, Kim SY, et al: COT drives resistance to RAF inhibition through MAP kinase pathway reactivation. *Nature* 468:968, 2010.

Lohr JG, Kim S, Gould J, et al: Genetic interrogation of circulating multiple myeloma cells at single-cell resolution. *Sci Transl Med* 8:363ra147, 2016.

Lohr JG, Adalsteinsson VA, Cibulskis K, et al: Whole-exome sequencing of circulating tumor cells provides a window into metastatic prostate cancer. *Nat Biotechnol* 32:479, 2014.

Macosko EZ, Basu A, Satija R, et al: Highly parallel genome-wide expression profiling of individual cells using nanoliter droplets. *Cell* 161:1202, 2015.

Mardis ER, Ding L, Dooling DJ, et al: Recurring mutations found by sequencing an acute myeloid leukemia genome. *N Engl J Med* 361:1058, 2009.

Melo SA, Luecke LB, Kahlert C, et al: Glypican-1 identifies cancer exosomes and detects early pancreatic cancer. *Nature* 523:177, 2015.

Miyamoto DT, Zheng Y, Wittner BS, et al: RNA-Seq of single prostate CTCs implicates noncanonical Wnt signaling in antiandrogen resistance. *Science* 349:1351, 2015.

Morin RD, Mendez-Lago M, Mungall AJ, et al: Frequent mutation of histone-modifying genes in non-Hodgkin lymphoma. *Nature* 476:298, 2011.

Nik-Zainal S, van Loo P, Wedge DC, et al: The life history of 21 breast cancers. *Cell* 149:994, 2012.

Paiva B, Vidriales MB, Cerveró J, et al: Multiparameter flow cytometric remission is the most relevant prognostic factor for multiple myeloma patients who undergo autologous stem cell transplantation. *Blood* 112:4017, 2008.

Paweletz CP, Charboneau L, Bichsel VE, et al: Reverse phase protein microarrays which capture disease progression show activation of pro-survival pathways at the cancer invasion front. *Oncogene* 20:1981, 2001.

Ramsköld D, Luo S, Wang YC, et al: Full-length mRNA-Seq from single-cell levels of RNA and individual circulating tumor cells. *Nat Biotechnol* 30:777, 2012.

Robinson JT, Thorvaldsdóttir H, Winckler W, et al: Integrative genomics viewer. *Nat Biotechnol* 29:24, 2011.

Rowley JD: The critical role of chromosome translocations in human leukemias. *Annu Rev Genet* 32:495, 1998.

Satija R, Farrell JA, Gennert D, et al: Spatial reconstruction of single-cell gene expression data. *Nat Biotech* 33:495–502, 2015.

Schwarzenbach H, Hoon DSB, Pantel K: Cell-free nucleic acids as biomarkers in cancer patients. *Nat Rev Cancer* 11:426, 2011.

Shaffer AL, Emre NC, Lamy L, et al: IRF4 addiction in multiple myeloma. *Nature* 454:226, 2008.

Shipp MA, Ross KN, Tamayo P, et al: Diffuse large B-cell lymphoma outcome prediction by gene-expression profiling and supervised machine learning. *Nat Med* 8:68, 2002.

Shivdasani RA: MicroRNAs: regulators of gene expression and cell differentiation. *Blood* 108:3646, 2006.

Slamon DJ, Leyland-Jones B, Shak S, et al: Use of chemotherapy plus a monoclonal antibody against HER2 for metastatic breast cancer that overexpresses HER2. *N Engl J Med* 344:783, 2001.

Stephens PJ, Greenman CD, Fu B, et al: Massive genomic rearrangement acquired in a single catastrophic event during cancer development. *Cell* 144:27, 2011.

Van der Maaten L, Hinton G: Visualizing data using t-SNE. *J Mach Learn Res* 9:2579, 2008.

Vogelstein B, Papadopoulos N, Velculescu VE, et al: Cancer genome landscapes. *Science* 339:1546, 2013.

Wang TJ, Larson MG, Vasan RS, et al: Metabolite profiles and the risk of developing diabetes. *Nat Med* 17:448, 2011.

Yeoh EJ, Ross ME, Shurtleff SA, et al: Classification, subtype discovery, and prediction of outcome in pediatric acute lymphoblastic leukemia by gene expression profiling. *Cancer Cell* 1:133, 2002.

REGULATION OF GENE EXPRESSION, TRANSCRIPTION, SPLICING, AND RNA METABOLISM

Christopher R. Cogle

INTRODUCTION TO GENE REGULATION IN HEMATOLOGY

The function of a cell is governed by the sum of the specific proteins expressed. Protein expression is most commonly regulated at the level of gene transcription into RNA, which is then processed and translated. The life of a cell is the life of its RNA. Therefore, to understand how a cell behaves, one must understand the expression of a gene through RNA.

Transcription of DNA into RNA controls cellular differentiation, proliferation, and apoptosis in all differentiating cell systems, but especially in hematopoiesis. For example, through regulation of transcription, hematopoietic stem cells maintain a balance between quiescence and differentiation to mature blood cell types. Regulation of transcription is also necessary for erythroid progenitors to produce vast quantities of hemoglobin, for myeloid cells to generate granules of immune responses, for lymphocytes to control immunoglobulin levels, and for platelets to regulate levels of thrombotic receptors.

Aberrant gene expression can result in hematologic disorders such as lymphomas, leukemias, and myelodysplastic and myeloproliferative syndromes, as will be discussed later. Understanding the process behind RNA synthesis is also crucial for the diagnosis and treatment of hematologic disorders. Converting genetic information contained in the DNA sequence of a gene into a finished protein product is a complex process consisting of several steps, with each step involving distinct regulatory mechanisms. Beginning with the basics of gene structure, this chapter will present the foundation necessary to understand the process of gene expression through RNA synthesis and processing, including transcription, splicing, posttranscriptional modification, and nuclear export. Subsequent chapters will present regulation of protein translation and posttranslational modifications.

The first step of gene expression is transcription, where RNA polymerases decode the DNA using specific start and stop signals to synthesize RNA. In the subsequent step, splicing removes portions of the RNA that do not code for protein. Next, the spliced RNA is modified for export out of the nucleus and into the cytoplasm, where ribosomes translate the RNA into protein products.

HOW GENES ARE ORGANIZED IN DNA

The gene is the fundamental unit for storage and expression of genetic information. Genes are made up of nucleotide sequences of DNA, and are transferred to daughter cells during mitosis (and meiosis in gametes) via semi-conservative replication. Each cell in the human body contains about 25,000 genes, which are distributed unevenly across the 46 individual chromosomes found within the nucleus. Chromosomes are dense DNA–protein complexes that are made up of individual linear DNA helices packed tightly together by specific protein repeats. Unwound completely and stretched out, the largest chromosome is about 1 m in length, demonstrating that the cell, to even exist, must be an expert at packaging.

Only 1% to 2% of human DNA actually serves as genes, which are the templates for protein production. Most genes are broken down into separated coding sections known as *exons* (Fig. 4.1). These exons are separated from each other by intervening, noncoding sequences known as *introns*. Genes also have other noncoding DNA, typically short sequences near or within genes that function as regulatory sequences critical for controlling gene expression. Together these regulatory sequences determine in which cell, at what time, and in what amount the gene is converted into the corresponding protein.

In order for transcription to begin, RNA polymerase must attach to a specific DNA region at the beginning of a gene. These regions, known as *promoters,* contain specific nucleotide sequences and response elements. These provide a secure initial binding site on the gene for RNA polymerase. RNA polymerase often requires other proteins called *transcription factors* for proper recruitment to a given gene. Not all transcription factors are activating; some may inhibit RNA polymerase, and repress gene expression by attaching to specific promoters and blocking binding of RNA polymerase. Promoters can additionally function together with other more distant regulatory DNA regions (termed *enhancers, silencers, boundary elements,* or *insulators*) to direct the level of transcription of a given gene. Unlike RNA polymerase, transcription factors are not limited to the promoter region, but can be directed by these other regulatory DNA sequences to either promote or repress transcription. The minimum essential transcription factors needed for transcription to occur are termed *basal transcription factors* and include transcription factor (TF) IIA, TFIIB, TFIID, TFIIE, TFIIF, and TFIIH. These ubiquitous proteins bind to the recognition sequence in the promoter, forming a transcription initiation complex that recruits the RNA polymerase. Basal transcription factors cannot by themselves increase or decrease the rate of transcription but may be linked to activators by coactivator proteins that can.

The promoter is a regulatory sequence located near the start of the gene, to provide the exact start site recognized by the transcription machinery where conversion of the DNA template into intermediary molecules begins. The promoter contains the consensus sequence to bind the transcription factors and then the RNA polymerase needed to initiate transcription. The best known example of this sequence is the TATA box sequence, TATAAA, which binds RNA polymerase and associated transcription factors. However, more than 80% of mammalian protein-coding genes are driven by TATA-less promoters, which contain different recognition sequences—often GC boxes. The GC promoters are repeats of guanine and cytosine nucleotides, frequently have multiple transcriptional start sites, and require alternative transcription factors, like Specificity Protein 1 (Sp1).

Genes can have more than one promoter. This results in different-sized mRNAs, depending on how far the promoter is from the 5′ end of the gene. The binding strength between a promoter and the transcription factors determines the avidity of RNA polymerase binding, and subsequently of transcription. Some genetic diseases are associated with mutations in promoters, such as β-thalassemia, which can involve single nucleotide substitutions, small deletions, or insertions in the β-globin promoter sequence. The promoter mutations in β-thalassemias result in decreased RNA polymerase binding to the transcriptional start site, and thereby reduce β-globin gene expression.

Globin gene expression in erythroid cells is also dependent on another regulatory unit: the enhancer. Unlike promoters, which are situated close to the start site of the gene, enhancers can be positioned

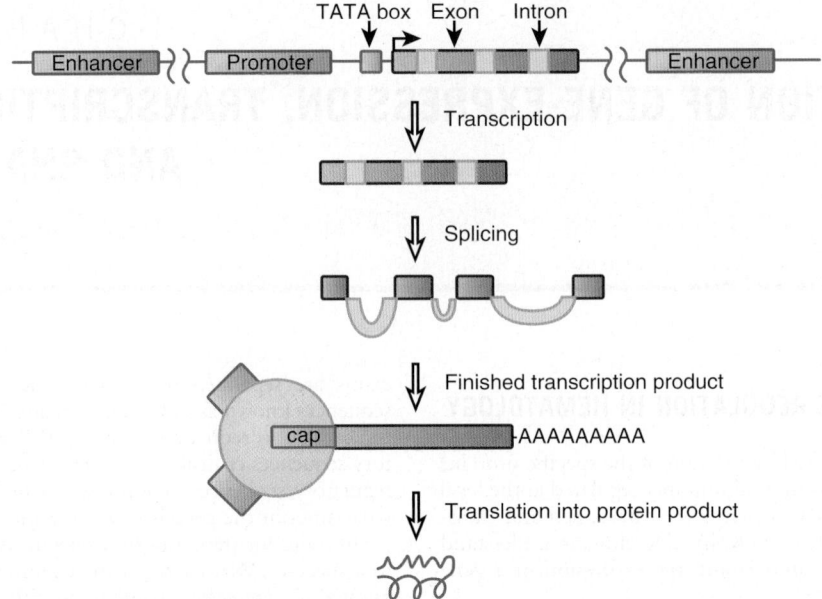

Fig. 4.1 OVERVIEW OF GENE TRANSCRIPTION FROM DNA TO RNA AND THEN TRANSLATION FROM RNA TO PROTEIN. Protein synthesis requires multiple processes and regulatory steps including transcript of DNA into RNA, splicing and posttranscription modification of RNA, translation of RNA into protein, and posttranslational protein modification.

far from either side of the gene, or even within it. This means that there may be several signals determining whether a certain gene can be transcribed. In fact, multiple enhancer sites may be linked to one gene, and each enhancer may be bound by more than one transcription factor. Whether or not such a gene is transcribed is the sum of the activity of these transcription factors bound to the different enhancers. Enhancers can compensate for a weak promoter by binding activator transcription factors. For instance, regulation of gene expression during T-lymphocyte differentiation requires multiple activating transcription factors, such as lymphocyte enhancer factor (LEF-1), GATA-3, and ETS-1, binding to the T-cell receptor alpha gene (TCRA) enhancer.

Transcription factors can also influence multiple genes in coordination, like the globin family. Enhancers are often the major determinant of transcription of developmental genes in the differing lineages and stages of hematopoiesis. They can also inhibit transcription of specific genes in one cell type while at the same time activating it in another cell type. When gene sequences routinely negatively regulate gene transcription, they are termed *silencers*, not enhancers. Another type of DNA regulatory sequence is called *insulators*. These define borders of multigene clusters to prevent activation of one set of genes from affecting a nearby set of genes in another cluster.

TRANSCRIPTION OF GENES

The first phase of gene expression occurs when the RNA polymerase synthesizes RNA from a DNA gene template, which, as described in the previous section, is called *transcription*. The encoded material on the transcribed gene determines the kind of RNA synthesized. For example, proteins are coded for by messenger RNA (mRNA), which will later undergo the process of translation. Alternatively, the transcribed gene may encode transfer RNA (tRNA), which carries specific amino acids to the ribosome for incorporation into the growing protein chain during translation. Another type of RNA synthesized from genes in DNA is ribosomal RNA (rRNA), which serves as the backbone of ribosomes and interacts with tRNA during translation. Ribosomes catalyze the formation of proteins using the mRNA as the code and the tRNA to obtain the amino acids to build the proteins. Each amino acid is attached to the previous one by hydrolysis and aminotransferase activity residing within the ribosome.

Transcription of the different classes of RNAs in eukaryotes is carried out by three different RNA polymerase enzymes. RNA polymerase I synthesizes the rRNAs, except for the 5S species. RNA polymerase II synthesizes the mRNAs and some small nuclear RNAs (snRNAs) involved in RNA splicing. RNA polymerase III synthesizes 5S rRNA and tRNAs.

The most intricate controls of eukaryotic genes are those that govern the expression of RNA polymerase II–transcribed genes, the genes that encode mRNA. Most eukaryotic mRNA genes contain a basic structure consisting of alternating coding exons and noncoding introns, and have one of two major types of basal promoters, as defined earlier. These protein-coding genes also can have a variety of transcriptional regulatory domains, such as the enhancers or silencers mentioned previously. In addition to management of gene expression by the binding strength of the RNA polymerase promoters at the beginning of a given gene, the interaction between activator and inhibitor transcription factor proteins binding to the given promoter also exerts regulatory action on transcription.

To initiate transcription, the RNA polymerase must bind to the promoter sequence. However, as mentioned earlier, this can only happen with help from gene-specific transcription factors that mediate RNA polymerase binding to the promoter. These transcription factors are sequence-specific DNA binding proteins that can be modified by cell signals. Many transcription factors, such as signal transducer and activator of transcription (STAT) proteins, require phosphorylation in order to bind DNA. Because transcription factors can be targeted by kinases and phosphatases, phosphorylation can effectively integrate information carried by multiple signal transduction pathways, thus providing versatility and flexibility in gene regulation. For example, the Janus kinase (JAK)–STAT pathway is widely used by members of the cytokine receptor superfamily, including those for granulocyte colony-stimulating factor (G-CSF), erythropoietin, thrombopoietin, interferons, and interleukins. Normally, ligand-bound growth factor receptors lead to JAK2 phosphorylation, which then activates STAT, also by phosphorylation. Activated STAT then dimerizes, translocates to the hematopoietic cell nucleus, binds DNA, and promotes transcription of genes for hematopoiesis. Alteration of JAK2, such as a V617F mutation, results in a constitutively active kinase capable of driving STAT activation. This leads to constitutive transcription of STAT target genes, and results in myeloproliferative disorders such as polycythemia vera.

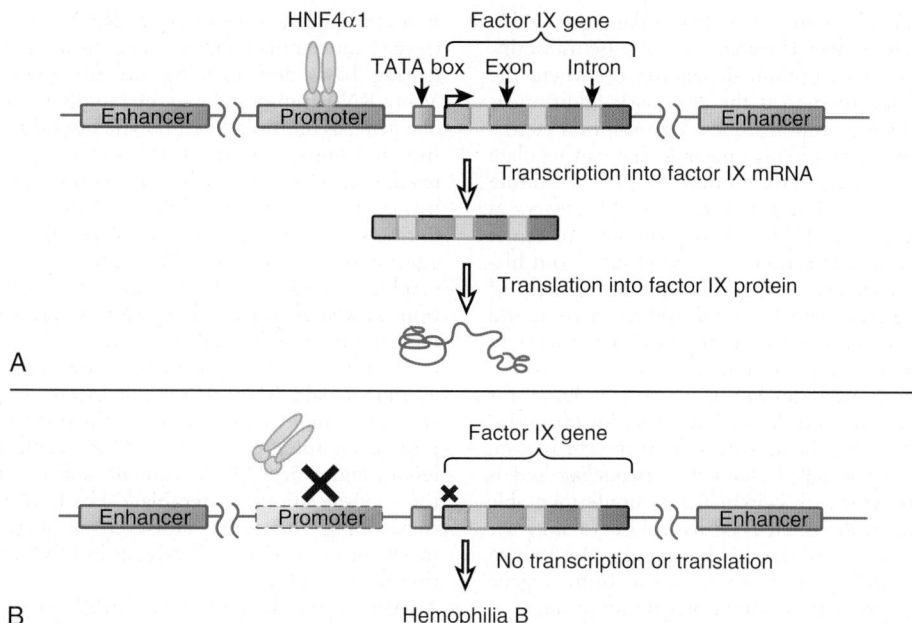

Fig. 4.2 ROLE OF TRANSCRIPTION FACTOR BINDING SITES IN THE REGULATION OF EUKARYOTIC GENE EXPRESSION. (A) Schematic diagram of a eukaryotic promoter showing transcription factor binding sites in the promoter region before the factor IX gene, the TATA box, and the start site of transcription *(red ×)*. Not shown are histones, coregulators, mediators, or chromatin remodeling complexes. (B) Effect of a mutation in the HNF4α1 binding site on expression of the blood coagulation gene factor IX.

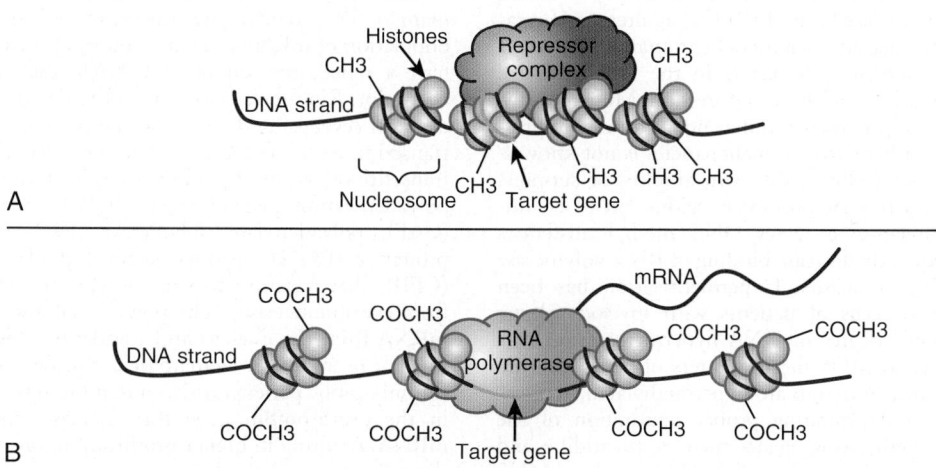

Fig. 4.3 CHROMATIN STRUCTURE. (A) The nucleosome is the fundamental unit of chromatin and is made up of DNA coiled around histone proteins. In a condensed state, the DNA is tightly wrapped around histone complexes and target genes are inaccessible to transcription machinery. (B) Histones and DNA can be epigenetically modified by acetylation and methylation, rendering the target genes more accessible to transcription machinery.

Mutations in promoter sequences that result in decreased transcription factor binding, and therefore less RNA polymerase binding, result in decreased gene expression. One of the best examples of a mutation in a transcription factor binding site associated with a human disease is in the factor IX gene. The transcription factor HNF4α is required to bind to the factor IX promoter before this gene can be transcribed. Patients with a mutation in the HNF4α binding site can develop hemophilia B, an X-linked recessive bleeding disorder primarily affecting males (Fig. 4.2).

The ability of transcription factors and RNA polymerases to access specific promoters and transcribe genes is also regulated by the packaging of DNA into discrete packets by proteins generically termed *chromatin*. Chromatin can package DNA tightly or loosely, and this regulates the availability of a gene for transcription. Several

factors affect the openness of chromatin, and therefore regulate availability of the DNA to transcription factors and RNA polymerases. There are two types of chromatin: euchromatin and heterochromatin. *Euchromatin* refers to loosely packaged DNA, where RNA polymerases can freely bind to DNA and genes are actively transcribed. *Heterochromatin* refers to tightly packaged DNA, protected from transcription machinery, sequestering genes away from transcription. The basic unit of chromatin is the nucleosome, which contains eight histone proteins packaging 146 base pairs of DNA wound 1.7 times around the histone complex (Fig. 4.3).

These histones can be extensively modified to regulate the accessibility of the DNA to the transcriptional apparatus. Histones can be chemically modified by acetylation, methylation, phosphorylation, or ubiquitination. In general, acetylation opens the nucleosome to increase transcription, while phosphorylation marks damaged DNA. Histone methylation can either open chromatin to increase transcription, or close it to repress transcription, depending on where the histone is methylated. Ubiquitination is the enzymatic addition or removal of the ubiquitin moiety from histones. Transcription factors can themselves recruit histone-modifying enzymes that can regulate transcription. In hematopoiesis, transcription factors including GATA-1, ELKF, NF-E2 and PU.1 recruit histone acetyltransferases (HATs) and histone deacetylases (HDACs) to promoters of target genes, leading to addition or subtraction of acetyl groups from histones, thereby affecting chromatin structure and the openness of DNA to transcription. A gene essential to erythroid maturation and survival, GATA-1, for instance, directly recruits HAT complexes to the β-globin locus to stimulate transcription activation.

Chromatin usually tightly packages DNA, which is essential for the cell to have a functional size and shape. Therefore, for transcription to take place, the DNA must be unwound from the chromatin. This process of unpackaging is called *chromatin remodeling* and is mediated by a family of proteins with switch/sucrose nonfermentable SWI/SNF domains. These proteins use ATP hydrolysis to shift the nucleosome core along the length of the DNA, a process also known as *nucleosome sliding*. By sliding nucleosomes away from a gene sequence, SWI/SNF complexes can activate gene transcription.

SWI/SNF proteins also contain helicase enzyme activity, which unwinds the DNA by breaking hydrogen bonds between the complementary nucleotides on opposite strands. By unwinding the DNA into two single strands, the DNA can then be read by RNA polymerases in the direction 3' to 5'. A new antiparallel RNA strand, 5' to 3', is produced by RNA polymerases to mirror the coding strand of the DNA, with the exception of all thymine nucleotides replaced by uracil nucleotides. SWI/SNF proteins have the ability to utilize Brahma (BRM) or Brahma-related gene 1 (BRG1) as alternative catalytic subunits with ATPase activity to remodel chromatin. The SWI/SNF complex has been shown to be active in the DNA damage response and is also responsible for tumor suppression. More recently, BRM and BRG1 have been proposed as independent tumor suppressors; however, their role in hematologic malignancies is not known.

DNA itself can be chemically modified to amplify or suppress transcription. CpG sites with gene promoter regions can be chemically modified by methylation enzymes DNA methyltransferases (DNMTs), which subsequently decrease binding of RNA polymerase and associated transcription factors. Hypermethylation has been observed in bone marrow cells of patients with myelodysplastic syndromes (MDS) and the degree of DNA hypermethylation correlates with disease stage. In MDS the promoters of genes that are important for myeloid differentiation are hypermethylated, repressing their transcription, and inhibiting proper maturation of the myeloid lineages. Hypomethylating agents such as azacitidine and decitabine can induce remission and prolonged survival in MDS patients. The regulation of gene expression by modification of chromatin or DNA itself is termed *epigenetic*, as it alters cell function without altering the nucleotide sequence of the DNA.

Such epigenetic modifications are crucial to the behavior of hematologic diseases. Mutation of the DNMT3 genes may have indirect effects on gene expression without altered DNA methylation, as have been observed in 20% of acute myeloid leukemia (AML) cases and are correlated with poor clinical outcome. The Ten-Eleven-Translocation oncogene member, TET2, which plays a role in DNA methylation and therefore epigenetic stability, is mutated in AML, MDS, chronic myelomonocytic leukemia (CMML), and other myeloproliferative neoplasms (MPNs). Another recurring observation in blood malignancies is aberrant histone methylation, for example at H3K27, seen in myelodysplasia. This is associated with altered gene expression affecting cell cycle, cell death, and cell adhesion pathways.

Before a final mRNA product is made that can be translated, several proofreading regulatory steps must take place. The RNA polymerase may not even clear the promoter and slip off, producing truncated transcripts. Once the transcript reaches approximately 23 nucleotides, the RNA polymerase no longer slips off, and full

transcript elongation can occur. RNA polymerase then continues to traverse the template DNA strand, using ATP while complementarily pairing bases and forming the phosphodiester–ribose backbone. Many RNA transcripts may be rapidly produced from a single copy of a gene, as multiple RNA polymerases may be transcribing the gene simultaneously, spaced out from one another. An important proof-reading mechanism during elongation allows the substitution of incorrectly incorporated bases, usually by permitting short pauses during which the appropriate RNA editing factors can bind. RNA editing mechanisms in mRNAs include nucleoside modifications of cytidine to uridine (C-U) and adenosine to inosine (A-I) by deamination, as well as nucleotide insertions and additions without a DNA template by proteins called *editosomes*.

Another repair mechanism is transcription-coupled nucleotide excision repair, where RNA polymerase stops transcribing when it comes to a bulky lesion in one of the nucleotides in the gene. A large protein complex excises the DNA segment containing the bulky lesion, and a new DNA segment is synthesized to replace it, using the opposite strand as a template. The RNA polymerase then resumes transcribing the gene. However, in general, RNA proofreading mechanisms are not as effective as in DNA replication, and transcription fidelity is lower.

After a gene is transcribed, mRNA is modified to protect it and target it for translation to protein. These modifications include capping and polyadenylation. Capping occurs shortly after the start of transcription, when a modified guanine nucleotide is added to the 5' end of the mRNA. This terminal 7-methylguanosine residue is necessary for proper attachment to the ribosome during translation. It also protects the RNA from endogenous ribonucleases that degrade uncapped RNA, which is often viral in origin.

RNA polymerases do not terminate transcription in an orderly manner. They tend to be processive, yet the cell cannot tolerate a population of mRNAs that are enormous in size. Therefore, mRNAs have a signal, the sequence AAUAA, that defines the end of the transcript. Ribonucleases cut mRNAs shortly after that signal, and a chain of several hundred adenosine residues is added to that free 3' transcript end. Synthesis of this poly(A) tail and termination of transcription requires binding of specific proteins, including cleavage/polyadenylation specificity factor (CPSF), cleavage stimulation factor (CstF), polyadenylate polymerase (PAP), polyadenylate binding protein 2 (PAB2), cleavage factor I (CFI), and cleavage factor II (CFII), that function to catalyze cleavage and protect the mRNA from exoribonucleases. The poly(A) tail also assists in export of the mRNA from the nucleus and translation. Mutations in the poly(A) signal can result in hematologic disease. For example, there are thrombophilic patients with a mutation in the polyadenylation signal in the prothrombin gene that increases the stabilization of this mRNA, resulting in higher prothrombin protein levels and increased thrombosis.

RNA SPLICING

Before the mRNA can be translated into protein, introns must be removed and the exons re-connected (Fig. 4.4). This process, termed splicing, requires a series of reactions mediated by the spliceosome, a complex of small nuclear ribonucleoproteins (snRNPs). The types of snRNPs in the spliceosome determine the mechanism of splicing. Canonical splicing, also called the *lariat pathway*, utilizes the major spliceosome and accounts for more than 99% of splicing. The major spliceosome is composed of the nuclear active snRNPs U1, U2, U4, U5, and U6 along with specific accessory proteins, U2AF and SF1. This complex recognizes the dinucleotide GU at the 5' end of an intron, and an AG at the 3' end. Intermediately a lariat structure forms, connecting these ends, providing for both excision of the intron and proper alignment of the ends of the two bordering exons to allow precise ligation. When the intronic flanking sequences do not follow the GU-AG rule, noncanonical splicing removes these rare introns with different splice site sequences using the minor spliceosome. The same U5 snRNP is found in the minor spliceosome, in

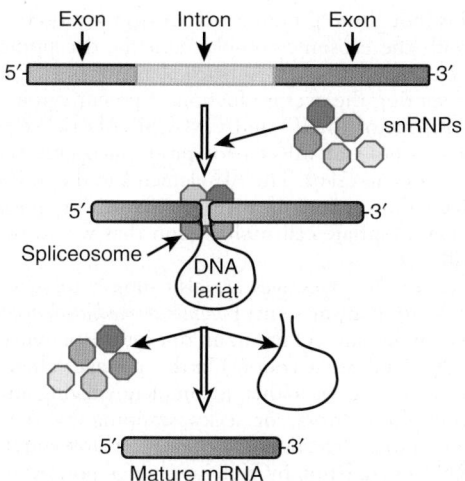

Fig. 4.4 RNA SPLICING. Introns from pre-mRNA are removed by snRNPs, which form a protein complex called a spliceosome. The spliceosome loops introns into a lariat, excises them, and then joins exons. The mature mRNA is then ready for further posttranscriptional processing. *snRNP*, Small nuclear ribonucleoprotein.

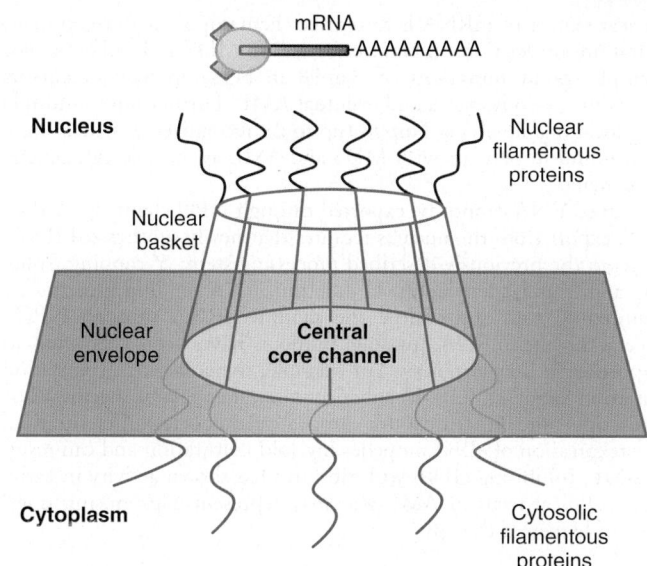

Fig. 4.5 NUCLEAR EXPORT OF RNA THROUGH NUCLEAR PORE COMPLEXES. The central core of the nuclear pore complex consists of a ring structure embedded in the nuclear envelope. Radiating in toward the nucleus is a nuclear basket that extends filamentous proteins in surveillance for mRNA. The central ring structure also radiates cytosolic protein filaments, which act to facilitate release of cargo into the cytoplasm.

addition to the unique yet functionally similar U11, U12, U4atac, and U6atac. Furthermore, there are splicing mechanisms, including tRNA splicing and self-splicing, that function without any spliceosome.

Splicing is central to proper gene expression, and therefore is required for appropriate hematopoietic development. One of the best examples of inappropriate splicing leading to hematologic disease is β-thalassemia, where there are a number of different mutations that occur in the GU-AG splicing signals, resulting in aberrant β-globin mRNAs. Abnormal splicing can also lead to AML and other hematologic disorders. Translocated in liposarcoma (TLS) is a protein that recruits splicing complexes to mRNAs, and it is involved in the TLS–ERG fusion oncogene in t(16;21) in AML. This fusion of TLS with the transcription factor ERG alters the splicing profile of immature myeloid cells, blocking the expression of genes required for proper differentiation.

Trans-splicing is a form of splicing that joins two exons that are not within the same mRNA transcript. Some trans-splicing events occur when the intron splice donor sites are not filled by spliceosomes. They can lead to mRNAs displaying exon repetitions or chimeric fusion RNAs, which can mimic the presence of a chromosomal translocation in normal cells. For example, specific chimeric fusion mRNA seen in acute leukemias, such as MLL-AF4, BCR-ABL, TEL-AML1, AML1-ETO, PML-RAR, NPM-ALK, and ATIC-ALK, have been found in blood cells of healthy individuals with normal chromosome karyotype. Interestingly, these individuals do not develop leukemia, indicating that these fusion oncoproteins must be heritable (in DNA) and that they must occur in the appropriate hematopoietic precursor cell for leukemogenesis.

Alternative splicing can enhance the versatility and diversity of a single gene. By alternatively excising different introns along with the intervening exons, a wide range of unique proteins of differing sizes can be generated. These alternative proteins, termed *isoforms,* come from one gene that generates a variety of mRNA with varying exon composition. Alternative splicing is common, and essential for the proper function of almost all hematopoietic cells. For example, B cells are able to produce both IgM and IgD at the same developmental stage using alternative splicing. Additionally, erythrocytes use alternative splicing to produce differing isoforms of cytoskeletal proteins. However, alternative splicing does not always give beneficial results. The mutations in the splicing signals in the β-globin gene mentioned earlier for β-thalassemia result in abnormal alternative splicing. In addition, in patients with chronic myelogenous leukemia (CML) resistance to tyrosine kinase inhibitor therapy has been linked to alternative splicing of the BCR-ABL transcript.

Because RNA splicing is central to proper gene expression, mutations in spliceosomes can result in MDS and other related hematologic disorders. Mutations in the RNA spliceosome splicing factor 3b, subunit 1 (SF3B1) has been observed in 68% to 75% and 81% of RARS and RARS-T patients, respectively. The molecular consequences of altered SF3B1 splicing activity are yet to be determined.

Additional spliceosomal mutations that are associated with MDS include U2 small nuclear RNA auxiliary factor I (U2AF1) and serine/arginine-rich splicing factor 2 (SRSF2). U2AF1 is a subunit of the U2AF heterodimer, which is also composed of a 65-kDa subunit (U2AF2). While U2AF2 contacts the pyrimidine site, U2AF1 interacts with the AG splice acceptor of the target intron. Mutations in the U2AF1 gene are associated with a number of myeloid malignancies and occur in 8.7% to 11.6% of de-novo cases of MDS.

SRSF2 is a member of the serine/arginine-rich pre-mRNA splicing factors. SRSF2 appears to play an important role in the acetylation/phosphorylation processes of RNA splicing and may be vital to alternative mRNA splicing. Mutations in the SRSF2 gene are associated with MDS and related diseases, particularly CMML. Frequencies of mutations in CMML have been reported to occur in up to 47% of patients. While the overall consequences of these spliceosomal mutations are not fully understood, they each contribute to the overall survival outcomes of MDS and other hematologic disorders.

NUCLEAR EXPORT OF RNA

The nuclear envelope serves as a major regulator of gene expression by controlling the flow of RNA to the cytoplasm for translation. Nuclear pore complexes (NPCs) inserted within the nuclear envelope regulate the transport of molecules in and out of the nucleus. Ions, small metabolites, and proteins under 40 kDa passively diffuse across NPC channels. However, larger proteins and mRNA are transported through NPCs via energy-dependent (GTP) and signal-mediated processes that require chaperoning transport proteins.

NPCs are composed of three major parts: (1) a central core containing a 10-nm channel, (2) a nuclear basket that can dilate in response to large cargoes, and (3) flexible fibrils that extend from the central core into the cytoplasm (Fig. 4.5). These large NPCs are composed of nucleoporins (Nups). Demonstrating how crucial nuclear export of mRNA is for correct hematopoietic development, mutations or deletions in Nups can result in MDS and leukemia. For example, point mutations of Nup98 in hematopoietic precursors results in myelodysplasia and eventual AML. Furthermore, multiple translocations involving Nup98 (up to 29 recognized partners) have been found in patients with MDS and AML as the sole cytogenetic abnormality.

Naked RNA cannot be exported through NPC channels. Rather, RNA export from the nucleus requires that newly synthesized RNAs undergo the previously described processing steps: 5′ capping, splicing, and 3′ polyadenylation. In addition, RNA binding proteins are required to fold and shuttle the modified RNA through NPCs. Several of these RNA binding proteins have been identified as important in hematopoiesis. For example, the eukaryotic translation initiation factor 4E (eIF4E) enhances nuclear export of specific RNA transcripts and is critical for proper granulocyte differentiation. Overexpression of eIF4E impedes myeloid maturation and can result in AML. Inhibiting eIF4E with ribavirin has shown activity in early-phase clinical trials of AML and may represent a promising novel class of leukemia therapy.

RNA METABOLISM

RNA does not live forever, and that is a good thing. In mammalian cells, mRNA lifetimes range from several minutes to days. The limited lifetime of mRNA enables a cell to alter protein synthesis in response to its changing needs. The stability of mRNA is regulated by the untranslated regions (UTRs) of mRNA. UTRs are sections of the mRNA before the start codon (5′) and after the stop codon (3′) that are not translated. These regions govern mRNA half-life, localization, and translational efficiency. Translational efficiency—both enhancement and inhibition—can be controlled by UTRs. Both proteins and small RNA species can bind to either the 5′ or 3′ UTRs, and these can either regulate translation or influence survival of the transcript. There are several fascinating mechanisms by which this occurs, and these will be described later. UTR sequence regulation of mRNA survival is essential for proper hematopoietic differentiation. The best example of this is globin synthesis, where its mRNA is quite stable because of UTR sequences. This long half-life meets the needs of reticulocytes to synthesize globin for up to 2 days after terminally mature erythroblasts lose the ability to make new mRNA.

Some of the elements contained in UTRs form a characteristic secondary structure that alters the survival of the mRNA transcript. One class of these mRNA elements, the riboswitches, directly bind the small molecules that their mRNA encodes enzymes that regulate its synthesis. For example, the mRNA for several enzymes in the cobalamine pathway has riboswitches that bind adenosylcobalamine, and this regulates the survival of these mRNAs. Thus, in states of high cobalamine, there is decreased survival of the mRNA for enzymes used in this synthetic pathway.

Another class of UTR secondary structures that regulate stability is exemplified by the prothrombin 3′ UTR. This mRNA is constitutively polyadenylated at seven or more positions, and the 3′ UTR folds into at least two distinct stem-loop conformations. These alternate structures expose a consensus binding site for trans-acting factors, like heterogeneous nuclear ribonucleoprotein 1 (hnRNP-I), polypyrimidine tract-binding protein-1 (PTB-1), and nucleolinin, with translational regulatory properties. Another type of 3′ UTR regulatory sequence involves selenocysteine insertion sequence (SECIS) elements. These represent another stem-loop RNA structure found in mRNA transcripts that serve as protein binding sites on UTR segments that direct the ribosome to translate the codon UGA as selenocysteines rather than as a stop codon. An example of this regulation can be found in selenoprotein P in plasma.

Another class of UTR binding site that affects the stability of the mRNA is the AU-rich elements (AREs). AREs are lengths of mRNA consisting mostly of adenine and uracil nucleotides. These sequences destabilize those transcripts attached to them through the action of riboendonucleases that stimulate poly(A) tail removal. Loss of the poly(A) tail is thought to promote mRNA degradation by facilitating attack by both the exosome complex and the decapping complex. Rapid mRNA degradation via AU-rich elements is a critical mechanism for preventing the overproduction of potent cytokines such as tumor necrosis factor (TNF) and GM-CSF. AU-rich elements also regulate the synthesis of mRNA for proto-oncogenic transcription factors like c-Jun and c-Fos. The AU elements in the mRNA of these genes mediate destruction of their transcripts in quiescent cells, preventing inappropriate cell proliferation that would occur if Fos/Jun were still active.

Eukaryotic mRNA messages are also subject to surveillance for accuracy by a mechanism termed *nonsense-mediated decay* (NMD). The NMD complex surveys the transcript for the presence of premature stop codons (nonsense codons) in the message. These premature stop codons can arise via either incomplete splicing mutations in DNA, transcription errors, or leaky scanning by the ribosome, causing frame shifts. Detection of a premature stop codon by NMD triggers mRNA degradation by 5′ decapping, 3′ poly(A) tail removal, or endonucleolytic cleavage.

Translational efficiency can be regulated by cellular factors that bind mRNA in a sequence-specific manner. Iron metabolism is an excellent example of how cells coordinate uptake and sequestration of an essential metabolite in response to availability. Transferrin is a plasma protein that carries iron. Receptors for transferrin (TfR) are expressed on cells requiring iron for maturation, such as erythroid progenitor cells. They mediate internalization of transferrin loaded with iron into the cytoplasm through receptor-mediated endocytosis. When a cell becomes iron deficient, a Kreb cycle enzyme, aconitase, is structurally altered, becoming an iron-responsive protein (IRP) so that it can bind to iron-responsive elements (IREs) in the UTR of transferrin receptor (TfR) mRNA (Fig. 4.6). UTR binding leads to stabilization of the TfR mRNA transcript, thus allowing greater availability for translation, which results in increased protein expression. However, when a cell has sufficient iron, aconitase is not altered, and TfR mRNA becomes unstable and prone to degradation. Therefore, in that situation, TfR receptor expression is low and the fewer receptors import less iron.

MICRO-RNA

In the last two decades another powerful mechanism of regulation of gene expression at the RNA level has been discovered. In this mechanism small RNA molecules, termed *micro-RNA* (miRNA), bind to complementary sequences on target mRNA transcripts. This binding results in either degradation or inhibition of translation, and consequent silencing of gene expression. There are roughly 1000 miRNA molecules coded in the human genome, indicating how robust this regulatory mechanism is. These miRNAs usually contain 18 to 25 nucleotides, and each miRNA has the potential to target about 500 genes. Conversely, an estimated 60% of all mRNAs have one or more sequences that are predicted to interact with miRNAs. This principle, often termed *RNA interference* (RNAi), has also been very useful in the laboratory, allowing investigators to repress the expression of specific genes to study artificially induced phenotypes. In these studies, small interfering RNAs (siRNA) are synthetically created to bind to homologous sequences within specific mRNAs. These are then transfected into cells, where they mediate destruction of their target mRNA through endogenous ribonucleases. Repression of gene expression in this manner has become known as "gene knock-down," and is widely used to define the function of genes by assessing what function the cell lacks in the absence of the expression of the target gene.

miRNAs are produced from transcripts that form stem-loop structures, whereas siRNAs are produced from long double-stranded RNA (dsRNA) precursors (Fig. 4.7). Similarly, both miRNAs and siRNAs are processed in the nucleus by a multiprotein complex called the RNA-induced silencing complex (RISC), which contains the RNase III enzyme Dicer, DGCR8, and Argonaute. The specificity of miRNA and siRNA interactions with their target mRNAs mediates

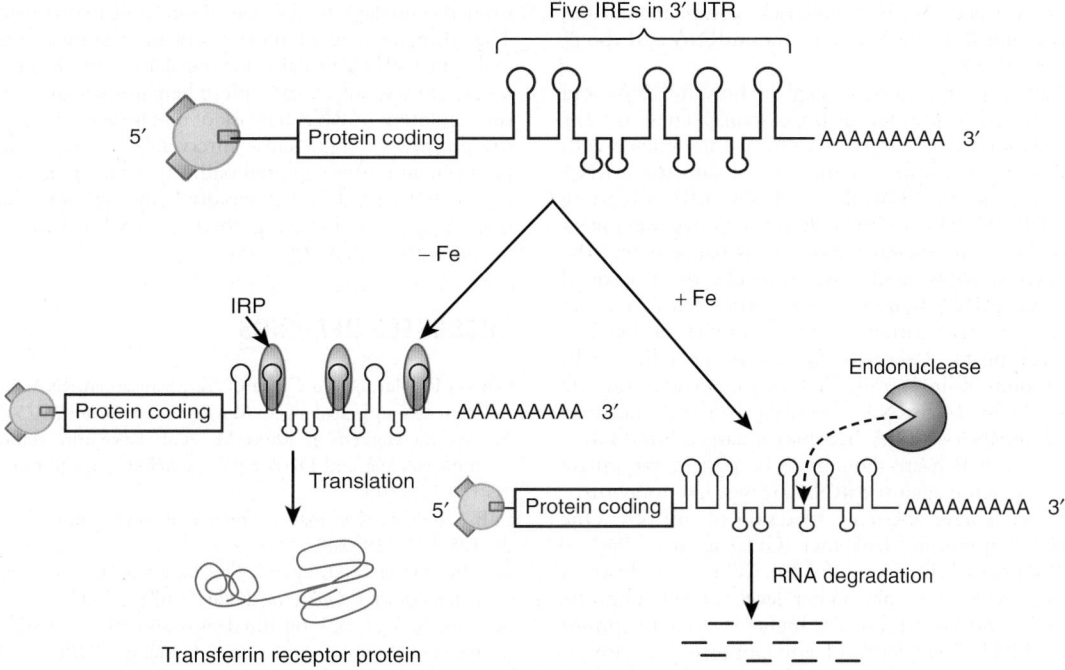

Fig. 4.6 CONTROL OF TRANSFERRIN RECEPTOR GENE EXPRESSION. The transferrin receptor mRNA has five IREs in the 3′ end of its UTR. In an iron-deficient state (−Fe), IRPs bind to IREs and stabilize the mRNA transcript for translation into protein product. In an iron-replete state (+Fe), IRPs are downregulated and the transferrin receptor mRNA is susceptible to endonucleases. Endonuclease cleavage of mRNA leads to RNA degradation and reduced availability of the transcript for protein production. *IRE*, Iron-responsive element; *IRP*, iron-responsive protein; *UTR*, untranslated region.

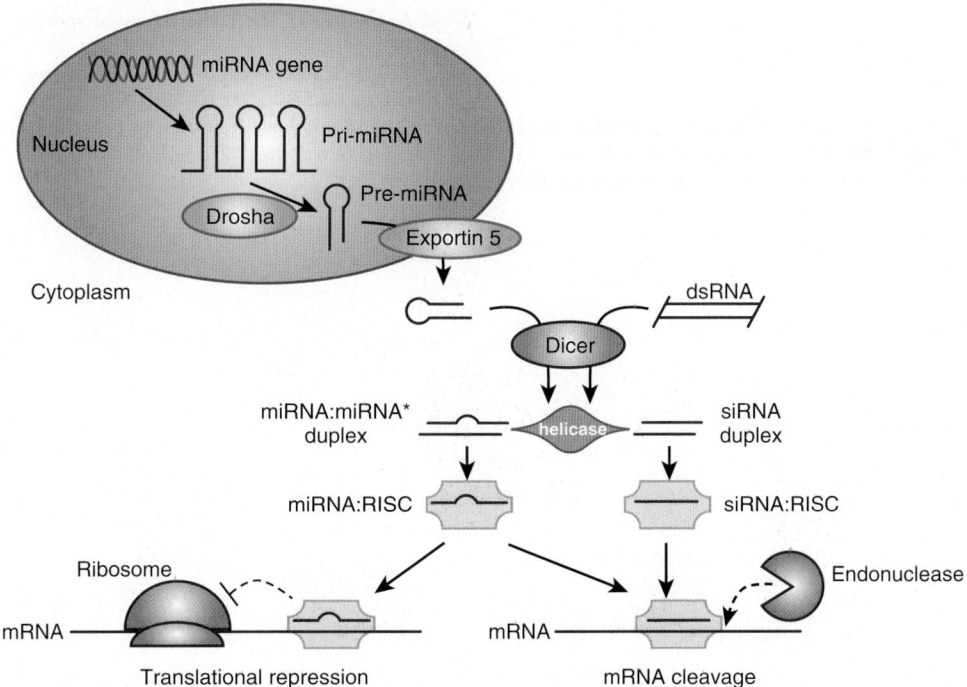

Fig. 4.7 RNA INTERFERENCE AND CONTROL OF GENE EXPRESSION. The stem-loop of the pri-miRNA gene transcript is first cleaved through the action of the Class 2 ribonuclease III enzyme called Drosha, which takes place in the nucleus and generates the pre-miRNA. In the siRNA pathway the duplex RNAs are cleaved into 22 to 25 nucleotide pieces through the action of the enzyme Dicer in the cytosol. Processed miRNA stem-loop structures are transported from the nucleus to the cytosol via the activity of exportin 5. In the cytosol the processed miRNA stem-loop is targeted by Dicer, which removes the loop portion. The nomenclature of the mature miRNA duplex is miRNA:miRNA*, where the miRNA* strand is the nonfunctional half of the duplex. Ultimately, fully processed miRNAs and siRNAs are engaged by the RISC, which separates the two RNA strands. The active strand of RNA derived either from the miRNA or siRNA pathway is complementary or antisense to a region of the target mRNA. RNA interference results in blockade of translation by ribosomes and/or degradation of mRNA. *Pre-miRNA*, Recursor miRNA; *Pri-miRNA*, primary miRNA; *RISC*, RNA-induced silencing complex; *siRNA*, small interfering RNA.

how they regulate gene expression. For example, the specificity of miRNA targeting is ruled by Watson–Crick complementarities between positions 2 and 8 at the 5′ end of the miRNA and the 3′ UTR of their target mRNAs.

Two models have been proposed to explain how miRNAs and siRNAs interfere with the expression of target genes. These models are: directed degradation of the target mRNA, or interference with the translation of a target mRNA. In the case of directed mRNA degradation, the proposed model involves miRNA–mRNA binding and recruitment of RISC, which ultimately leads to degradation of the target mRNA. In the interference model it is believed that the interaction of miRNA, RISC, and mRNA blocks the ribosomal machinery along the mRNA transcript, preventing translation yet sparing the mRNA from degradation. This latter model was hypothesized based on work on the *Caenorhabditis elegans* gene lin-14. In this example the amount of lin-14 mRNA does not decrease, but the protein product of the lin-14 mRNA is reduced. In the degradation model, the paired miRNA–mRNA becomes a target for double-stranded ribonucleases, which are thought to be part of the innate immune system as a defense against dsRNA viruses, like rotavirus.

Various disease states have aberrant expression of miRNA. One example in chronic lymphocytic leukemia (CLL) is the *miR-15a/miR16-1* cluster (located on chromosome 13q). When this cluster is deleted in B lymphocytes, there are higher levels of antiapoptotic proteins such as BCL2 and MCL1, but also higher levels of the tumor suppressor protein TP53. High levels of antiapoptosis yet with an intact TP53 tumor suppressor pathway could explain why 13q deletions in CLL are associated with an indolent form of the disease. Patterns of miRNA expression are correlated with disease progression in CML, although it is not clear whether these changes are causative or epiphenomena. An example of the prognostic information that can be provided by changes in miRNA levels is miR328, whose expression levels fall significantly when CML begins to progress to blast crisis.

SUMMARY

In summary, control of gene expression is a highly regulated process with several steps including: (1) DNA transcription into RNA, (2) splicing of mRNA into translatable transcripts, (3) modifying the mRNA transcripts for stability, (4) packaging the mRNA for export from the nucleus to the cytoplasm, and (5) regulation by miRNA. The ultimate goal of most posttranscriptional modifications is to make the mRNA available for translation into proteins. Perturbations in any of these steps can result in hematologic disease. However, while the regulation of RNA has risk of disease at every step, it also possesses the promise of therapeutic intervention. Indeed, RNA metabolism has been an under-explored pathway for drug development in hematology, but that deficit is rapidly being overcome as more attention is being paid to targeting aberrant RNA pathways in an effort to restore normal gene expression.

SUGGESTED READINGS

Garzon R, Marucci G, Croce C: Targeting microRNAs in cancer: rationale, strategies and challenges. *Nat Rev Drug Discov* 9:775–789, 2010.

Kowarz E, Merkens J, Karas M, et al: Premature transcript termination, trans-splicing and DNA repair: a vicious path to cancer. *Am J Blood Res* 1:1–12, 2011.

Li B, Carey M, Workman J: The role of chromatin during transcription. *Cell* 128:707–719, 2007.

Rice K, Hormaeche I, Licht J: Epigeneic regulation of normal and malignant hematopoiesis. *Oncogene* 26:6697–6714, 2007.

Schwartz S, Ast G: Chromatin density and splicing destiny: on the cross-talk between chromatin structure and splicing. *EMBO J* 29:1629–1636, 2010.

Siddiqui N, Borden K: mRNA export and cancer. *Wiley Interdiscip Rev RNA* 3:13–25, 2012.

Valencia-Sanchez M, Liu J, Hannon G, et al: Control of translation and mRNA degradation by miRNAs and siRNAs. *Genes Dev* 20:515–524, 2006.

Visconte V, Makishima H, Maciejewski JP, et al: Emerging roles of the spliceosomal machinery in myelodysplastic syndromes and other hematologic disorders. *Leukemia* 26:2447–2454, 2012.

Ward A, Cooper T: The pathobiology of splicing. *J Pathol* 220:152–163, 2010.

Ward A, Touw I, Yoshimura A: The Jak-Stat pathway in normal and perturbed hematopoiesis. *Blood* 95:19–29, 2000.

Zhang Y: Transcriptional regulation by histone ubiquitination and deubiquitination. *Genes Dev* 17:2733–2740, 2003.

PROTEIN SYNTHESIS, PROCESSING, AND TRAFFICKING

Randal J. Kaufman and Laura Popolo

The final step in the transfer of the genetic information stored in DNA into proteins is the translation of the intermediary messenger molecules, mRNAs (see Chapter 1). Protein synthesis occurs in the cytoplasm and generates a great variety of products endowed with a wide spectrum of functions. The complete set of proteins produced by a cell is called the *proteome* and is responsible for the remarkable diversity in cell specialization that is typical of metazoan organisms. To be functional, proteins need to be properly folded, assembled, often modified and transported to the final destination. The cell has in its interior several membrane-bound compartments, termed *organelles,* such as the mitochondria, the peroxisomes, the nucleus and the endoplasmic reticulum to which the proteins may be targeted. Since each compartment serves a particular purpose, protein transport is crucial to maintain the identity and functions of each organelle. Intracellular physiology depends on the proper and coordinated functioning of the organelles. In many cases protein folding and processing are coupled with protein trafficking so that the targeting process is unidirectional and irreversible.

This chapter briefly describes how proteins are synthesized and then focuses on their processing and delivery to their appropriate destinations within the cell. An understanding of the machines that catalyze protein folding, assembly, processing, and targeting is relevant to the study of hematology providing a basis for an explanation of how malfunctions in these processes can cause hematologic disorders.

PROTEIN SYNTHESIS

Among the biosynthesis of macromolecules occurring in a cell, protein synthesis is the most important in quantitative terms. It is a highly energy-consuming process and proceeds through a mechanism that has been conserved during evolution. Proteins are synthesized by the joining of amino acids, each of which has characteristic physico-chemical properties (see Table 5.1 for single letter designations). Peptide bonds are created by the condensation of the α-carboxyl group (COOH) of one amino acid with the α-amino group (NH$_2$) of another. The free NH$_2$ and COOH groups of the terminal amino acids define the amino- or N-terminal end and the carboxyl- or C-terminal end of the resulting polypeptide chain, respectively. In many cases multiple polypeptide chains assemble into a functional protein. For example, hemoglobin is formed by four polypeptide chains, two α-globin chains and two β-globin chains that assemble with heme, an iron-containing prosthetic group, to yield the functional protein designed to deliver molecular oxygen to all cells and tissues.

The whole process of protein synthesis is orchestrated by a large ribonucleoprotein complex, called the *ribosome.* The ribosome 80S (S stands for Svedberg unit, and refers to the rate of sedimentation) is typical of mammalian cells and is constituted by a large subunit of 60S and a small one of 40S. Additional components are messenger RNAs (mRNAs), transfer RNAs (tRNAs), amino acids, soluble factors, ATP and GTP. Activation of amino acids by coupling to their cognate tRNAs occurs before polypeptide chain initiation. This crucial function is carried out by 20 different aminoacyl-tRNA synthetases, one for each amino acid, which generate aminoacyl-tRNAs at the expense of ATP and operate a quality control on the coupling reaction. Eukaryotic mRNA molecules typically contain a 5'-untranslated region (5' UTR), a protein coding sequence that begins with the initiation codon AUG and ends with one of three stop codons (UAA, UAG, UGA), and a 3'-untranslated region (3' UTR). The 5'-end carries a 7-methylguanosine structure called a "cap" (m^{7}GpppN mRNA) whereas the 3'-end is polyadenylated. These modifications are required to protect the mRNA from degradation, for export out of the nucleus, and for efficient recruitment of ribosomes for translation. Once in the cytoplasm, the 40S ribosomal subunit binds to the cap and then scans the mRNA toward the 3'-end until a translation start codon is encountered, usually the first AUG (underlined) located in a nucleotide context optimal for translation initiation which is called the Kozak consensus sequence (A/GNNAUGG). The assembly of the 60S subunit with the 40S produces an 80S ribosome. A special tRNA specific for methionine, called the initiator (tRNA$_i^{Met}$) is required for the initiation of protein synthesis at the initiation codon. Aminoacyl-tRNAs ferry amino acids to the ribosome for joining together in sequence as the ribosome moves toward the 3'-end of the mRNA. The codons in the mRNA interact by base-pairing with the anticodon of the tRNAs so that amino acids are incorporated into the nascent polypeptide chain in the right order. Translation is terminated when the ribosome encounters a stop codon where the polypeptide is released. Typically, multiple ribosomes are engaged in the translation of a single mRNA molecule in a complex termed a polyribosome or polysome.

Protein synthesis is divided into three phases: initiation, elongation and termination. Each phase requires a set of soluble proteins (or factors) which transiently associate with the ribosomes and are called initiation, elongation and termination (or release) factors that are termed eIFs, eEFs, and eRFs, respectively, where the prefix "e" indicates their eukaryotic origin. Many soluble factors required for protein synthesis belong to the G-protein (guanine nucleotide-binding proteins) superfamily which are regulatory molecules that promote unidirectionality of important cellular processes such as hormone and growth factor signaling, membrane trafficking and neurotransmission. Dysfunctions of G-proteins are involved in human diseases, including cancer.

REGULATION OF mRNA TRANSLATION

There are two major general regulatory steps in mRNA translation that are mediated by the initiation factors eIF2 and eIF4. All cells regulate the rate of protein synthesis through reversible covalent modification of eIF2, a soluble factor required for the binding and recruitment of the Met-tRNA$_i^{Met}$ to the 40S ribosomal subunit.

eIF2 is a heterotrimeric G-protein that can exist in an inactive form bound to GDP or an active form bound to GTP. The eIF2-GTP/Met-tRNA$_i^{Met}$ ternary complex binds to the 40S subunit. Joining of the 60S subunit triggers hydrolysis of GTP to GDP and thus converts eIF2 to the inactive form whereas the opposite reaction is catalyzed by a guanine nucleotide exchange factor (GEF) called eIF2B. Phosphorylation regulates eIF2 function. In reticulocytes, which primarily synthesize hemoglobin, heme starvation inhibits the synthesis of α- and β-globin chains by activating a protein kinase, called hemin-regulated inhibitor (HRI) that specifically phosphorylates the α subunit of eIF2. The phosphorylated form of eIF2 binds more tightly than usual to eIF-2B, so that eIF-2B is sequestered and not available for the exchange reaction. Thus, eIF2 molecules remain in the GDP-bound form and translation of globin mRNA comes to a halt. In this manner, globin chains are not synthesized in the

Organelle	Signal Location[a]	Example

TABLE 5.1   Examples of Sorting Signals

Organelle	Signal Location[a]	Example
Posttranslational Uptake		
Nucleus	Internal	SP**KKKRK**V*E* (import; NLS of SV40 large T antigen)
		KR-spacer (PAATKKAGQ)-**KKKK** (import; bipartite NLS of nucleoplasmin)
		LQLPPL*E*RLTL*D* (export; NES of HIV-1 rev)
Mitochondrion	N-terminal	MLGI**R**SSV**K**TCF**K**PMSLTS**KR**L (iron-sulfur protein of complex III)
Peroxisomes	C-terminal	**K**ANL (PTS1, human catalase)
	N-terminal	**R**LQVVLG**H**L (PTS2, human 3-ketoacyl-CoA thiolase)
Cotranslational Uptake		
ER	N-terminal	MMSFVSLLLVGILFWAT*EAE*
		QLT**K**C*E*VFQ (ovine lactalbumin)

ER, Endoplasmic reticulum; HIV, human immunodeficiency virus; NES, nuclear export signal; NLS, nuclear localization signal; PTS1, peroxisomal targeting signal-1; PTS2, peroxisomal targeting signal-2; SV40, simian virus 40.
[a]Acidic residues (negatively charged) are in italic type; basic residues (positively charged) are in bold type. Amino acids: A, alanine; C, cysteine; *D*, aspartic acid; *E*, glutamic acid; F, phenylalanine; G, glycine; **H**, histidine; I, isoleucine; **K**, lysine; L, leucine; M, methionine; N, asparagine; P, proline; Q, glutamine; **R**, arginine; S, serine; T, threonine; V, valine; W, tryptophan; Y, tyrosine.

5′ UTR respectively. In iron-starved cells, the binding of IRPs to IREs results in the stabilization of Tfr mRNA and inhibition of translation initiation of ferritin mRNA. Conversely, when iron is abundant, IRPs have a lower affinity to IREs and as a result Tfr mRNA is degraded whereas ferritin mRNA translation is stimulated. In this manner, cells can coordinately regulate iron uptake and iron sequestration in response to the changes in iron availability.

Among the cellular factors that modulate translation, noncoding small RNAs called micro-RNAs (miRNAs) are currently intensely studied.[1] miRNAs are single stranded RNAs of 20–22 nucleotide in length that result from the nuclear processing of double-stranded RNA precursors. miRNAs regulate translation by three molecular mechanisms: translation repression, mRNA degradation, and miRNA-mediated mRNA decay. miRNAs anneal to the 5′-end, but even more frequently to the 3′-end of the target mRNA, and block translation by inhibiting eIF4F or ribosome scanning of the 5′ UTR, keeping in mind that mRNA circularizes because of interaction of proteins that bind the 5′ and 3′ UTRs. Base pairing at the 3′-end can also lead to deadenylation of the mRNA and degradation or to endonucleolytic cleavage of the mRNA. Degradation of mRNA takes place in specialized cytoplasmic organelles, called P-bodies, that are rich in enzymatic machinery for RNA degradation. Interestingly, miRNAs contribute to the fine regulation of processes such as apoptosis, cell proliferation, hematopoietic differentiation and in cancer progression.

Finally, another destiny of mature mRNAs is to remain silent in the cytoplasm. In oocytes or during the first stages of embryogenesis, latent mRNAs are present and they are quickly translated as the appropriate signal is triggered.

PROTEIN FOLDING

As the polypeptide emerges from the ribosome, it must fold to become a mature functional protein. The conformation of a protein is dictated primarily by the primary structure. Some proteins can spontaneously acquire their mature three-dimensional conformation as they are synthesized in the cell and can even fold in a test tube by a self-assembly process. However, most polypeptides require assistance from other protein for proper folding. These proteins are *molecular chaperones* that either directly assist folding reactions and/or prevent aberrant interactions, such as aggregation that can occur in a densely packed environment as the cytosol of eukaryotic cells (protein concentration of 200–300 mg/mL). Most molecular chaperones are heat-shock proteins (Hsps) and in particular are members of the Hsp70 family. Chaperones bind to short sequence protein motifs, in many cases containing hydrophobic amino acids. By undergoing cycles of binding and release (linked to ATP hydrolysis), chaperones help the nascent polypeptide to find its native conformation, one aspect of which is hiding hydrophobic sequence motifs in the protein interior so that they no longer contact the hydrophilic environment of the cytosol. Some properly folded protein monomers are assembled with other proteins to form multisubunit complexes. The population of chaperones that assist folding and assembly in the cytosol is distinct from those that operate within the endoplasmic reticulum (ER) or mitochondria.

PROTEIN MODIFICATIONS

Proteins often need to be modified to become functional or be localized to the correct site. More than a hundred protein modifications were identified in mammals. These modifications can take place during synthesis of the polypeptide (cotranslational) or after synthesis (posttranslational) and can also be reversible or irreversible. Most of the reversible modifications are carried out by enzymes that catalyze the transfer of a chemical group from a donor molecule to the target amino acid and counterpart enzymes catalyze the opposite reaction. In contrast, proteolytic cleavage of precursor proteins to generate

absence of heme, which is required for assembly of functional hemoglobin. This mechanism of translational inhibition is of more general significance because eIF2 is a target of phosphorylation by additional protein kinases that cause translational arrest in response to different conditions of cell stress, such as amino acid starvation, glucose starvation, and viral infection. Overall, eIF2 phosphorylation is a central event mediated by four protein kinases activated by different stress conditions to inhibit protein synthesis and has been termed the *integrated stress response*.

A second major control point of general protein synthesis is mediated by the eIF4F protein complex that binds the cap (eIF4E) and uses an ATP-dependent RNA helicase (eIF4A) activity and its stimulatory subunit (eIF4B) to unwind structural elements in the 5′-end of mRNA to make it accessible for 40S ribosome subunit binding. The eIF4E subunit binds the 5′-cap structure and is the least abundant factor regulating translation in mammalian cells. eIF4E forms a complex with the RNA helicase eIF4A and eIF4G, another crucial factor that binds mRNA and recruits the 40S ribosomal subunit. Increased levels of eIF4E stimulate protein synthesis. The cap-binding activity of eIF4E is inhibited by eIF4E-binding proteins (eIF4EBPs) which prevent assembly of the eIF4F complex. The activity of eIF4EBP is regulated by phosphorylation mediated by the protein kinases AKT (also named PKB) and TOR. Since phosphorylated eIF4BP cannot bind eIF4E, eIF4EBP phosphorylation stimulates translation initiation since it permits eIF4G binding and recruitment of the 40S subunit. Extracellular factors, such as insulin, activate signaling pathways that stimulate protein synthesis through this mechanism. Insulin also activates eIF2B exchange activity and in the long term also increases the cellular ribosome content.

The efficiency of mRNA translation can also be modulated by cellular factors that bind mRNA in a sequence-specific manner. An example of this mode of regulation is the control of iron metabolism in animal cells. Key players of this system are (i) the **i**ron-**r**esponsive **e**lement (IRE), a hairpin structure that is formed in the untranslated regions of the mRNAs and (ii) **i**ron **r**egulatory **p**roteins that bind IRE (IRPs). In the transferrin receptor (Tfr) mRNA and ferritin mRNA, IREs are located in the 3′ UTR and

mature products is irreversible. Here are some features of the most common protein modifications:

- *Acetylation*: ribosome-associated Met-aminopeptidases and acetylases cotranslationally cleave off the N-terminal methionine and acetylate the second residue if it is small (Gly, Ala, Ser, Thr, Cys. Pro or Val). Approximately 90% of human proteins are N-acetylated (acetyl group: $COCH_3$). In general, the N-terminal residue affects the lifetime of a protein.

Another type of *acetylation* is posttranslational and occurs on the α-amino group of the side chain of lysine. This modification abolishes the positive charge of this amino acid. The N-terminal tails of histones, are targets of acetylation that is carried out by histone acetyl transferases (HATs) and is reversed by histone deacetylases (HDACs). The degree of histone acetylation increases transcriptional activity by relaxing chromatin structure.

- *Methylation*: is the reversible addition of a methyl group (CH_3) to lysine or arginine residues. This modification abolishes the positive charge and increases the hydrophobicity of the protein. Histone methylation by histone methyltransferases affects transcriptional activity by modifying the accessibility to DNA either positively or negatively.

Other processing reactions add anchors to the proteins for membrane association. Among the most important of these modifications are:

- *Myristoylation*: is the attachment of a 14-carbon myristoyl group to the N-terminal glycine residue of a protein. This modification is co- or posttranslational, irreversible and allows the association of the target protein with membranes or with other proteins or lipids.
- *Prenylation:* involves the attachment of the 15 carbon farnesyl group or 20 carbon geranyl group to acceptor proteins that harbor at the C-terminus the CAAX consensus sequence (C = cysteine, AA = any aliphatic amino acid except alanine, X = any amino acid). AAX is first removed by a CAAX protease and the prenyl group is attached to the side chain of cysteine that is finally also methylated by a prenylcysteine methyltransferase that uses *S*-adenosylmethionine. This complex modification occurs on RAS protein family members and variants involving CC or CXC elements at the C-terminus take place on the RAB protein family that is involved in signaling pathways that control intracellular membrane traffic (see later). Lack of prenylation on these otherwise soluble proteins leads to lack of membrane association and generates severe phenotypes.

Other modifications are crucial to regulate protein function:

- *Phosphorylation*: is the transfer of a phosphate group from ATP to target amino acids in a protein (serine, threonine or tyrosine with a ratio of occurrence of 1000:100:1). It can be reversed by the action of protein phosphatases that remove the phosphate group. It has been estimated that the human genome encodes about 500 protein kinases and 100 protein phosphatases. The catalytic or biologic activity of many enzymes is transiently regulated by reversible phosphorylation. Another role of phosphorylation emerged from studies on intracellular signaling pathways. Phosphorylation of a protein substrate can create an interaction site (or docking site) to bind another protein. Interestingly, many pairs of docking sites that bind specific small protein domains to promote protein–protein interaction have been identified. An example is the SH2 domain of the c-Src protein kinase and other signal-transducing proteins that recognizes specific phosphotyrosine in other proteins. About 111 SH2 domains are found in proteins encoded by the human genome.
- *Sulfation*: this modification occurs at tyrosine residues and is catalyzed by tyrosyl-protein sulfotransferases (TPST) which are membrane-associated enzymes of the *trans*-Golgi network. An

---

BOX 5.1 Protein γ-Carboxylation: A Rare Posttranslational Modification Crucial for Life

γ-Carboxylation of glutamic acid residues in the Gla domain serves to coordinate calcium ions and is essential for the proper biologic activity of factors involved in blood coagulation. These factors are prothrombin, factors VII, IX and X which are involved in the coagulant response, and protein C and S which play roles in an antithrombotic pathway that limits coagulation. Bone proteins osteocalcin and matrix Gla protein also require processing by γ-carboxylation for full activity.

This posttranslational modification is catalyzed by γ-glutamyl carboxylase, an endoplasmic reticulum (ER) membrane protein. Its obligate cofactor, reduced vitamin K, is produced by the action of vitamin K-epoxide reductase (VKOR) which converts oxidized vitamin K to the reduced form. The activity of VKOR is inhibited by warfarin, a potent anticoagulant compound. γ-Carboxylase homozygous null mutants manifested dramatic effects on development with partial midembryonic loss and postnatal hemorrhage. Similar effects were observed in prothrombin or factor V-deficient mice. Thus, the results of these studies have suggested that the functionally critical substrates for γ-carboxylation are primarily restricted to components of the blood coagulation cascade. These results highlight the importance of a rare protein modification for blood coagulation.

---

unusual nucleotide, a 3′-phosphoadenosine 5′-phosphosulfate (PAPS), is the universal sulfate donor for TPST-catalyzed reactions. Addition of sulfate occurs almost exclusively on secreted or membrane proteins and is believed to play a role in the modulation of protein-protein interactions. This protein modification is critical in the processes of blood coagulation, various immune functions, intracellular trafficking, and ligand recognition by several G protein-coupled receptors. Notably, coagulation factors V and VIII, the gut peptides gastrin and cholecystokinin are modified by sulfation.

- *γ-Carboxylation:* this modification converts glutamate into γ-carboxyglutamate that is found in several components of the coagulation pathway, as well as in a number of other proteins. This modification is carried out by the enzyme γ-glutamyl carboxylase (GGCX) that requires vitamin K as an essential cofactor. The formation of modified glutamate residues is crucial for the process of blood coagulation and is described in more detail in Box 5.1.
- *Ubiquitination:* this posttranslational modification results from the sequential activity of three enzymes, the first activates a small protein of 76 amino acids named *ubiquitin*, the second transfers ubiquitin to ubiquitin ligase that links ubiquitin to lysine residues present in target proteins and then other ubiquitin molecules to ubiquitin lysine residues (polyubiquitination). Seven lysine residues in ubiquitin may serve as sites of linkage in formation of a polyubiquitin chain. Initially discovered as a mechanism to regulate protein degradation via the proteasome, in recent years, ubiquitination was described to regulate different cellular processes including DNA repair, vesicle trafficking, and inflammation. According to the pattern of modification of the target proteins (monoubiquitinated, polyubiquitinated) different processes can be triggered (see next section).
- *Sumoylation:* this modification belongs to a group of ubiquitin-like proteins (Ubl) that are added to proteins via posttranslational reactions. The small peptide SUMO (**s**mall **u**biquitin-related **mo**difier) is among the best characterized Ubl and over 50 proteins are modified by SUMO addition.
- *Proteolysis:* this modification consists in the cleavage of the polypeptide chain at a specific site during its maturation (proinsulin to insulin), or occurs upon secretion of its inactive form (zymogen) to prevent potential toxic effects of the processed protein in the cell (digestive proteases) or because proteolysis is regulated as occurs for coagulation factors that are secreted into the blood in an inactive form and are activated by proteolysis at sites of damaged blood vessels. Proteolysis can take place in more than one site to generate smaller products as for instance in the maturation of hormones starting from a larger precursor. Proteolytic

processing of propolypeptides into their mature forms occurs after the Arg-Xxx-Lys-Arg motif and is mediated by the general protein processing protease FURIN. FURIN is expressed in all cell types and removes propeptides from many proteins, including clotting factors, growth factors, and proteases, and is responsible to convert these proteins into their functional forms. Other members of the proprotein convertase (PC) family cleave after pairs of dibasic amino acids (for example Lys-Arg) and are expressed in specific cell types, such as neuroendocrine cells. The PCs are responsible for cleavages that occur to generate many hormones, such as insulin, glucagon, and adrenocorticotropic hormone.

Other modifications such as *N*-glycosylation, *O*-glycosylation and attachment of a glycosylphosphatidylinositol (GPI) anchor will be discussed in a separate section.

Finally, proteins can also be susceptible to nonenzymatic modifications that take place under particular conditions, such as during oxidative stress or in the presence of excess glucose in the blood as in the case of hemoglobin glycation.

PROTEIN DEGRADATION

The level of a protein in the cell results from the balance between its synthesis and degradation and a protein's half-life can vary from minutes to hours. Moreover, the cell eliminates proteins that contain mutations that cause protein misfolding. Such misfolded proteins are marked for destruction and then degraded to avoid toxic effects of their accumulation. The breakdown of these molecules is achieved in two major phases. First, the molecules are tagged with *ubiquitin,* which is covalently linked to the substrate protein as described earlier. Second, the tagged molecules are ferried to an ATP-dependent protease complex called the 26S proteasome, a multi-subunit molecular machinery specialized in protein destruction. Peptides and amino acids derived from protein disposal are recycled.

Since its first discovery in carrying out the disposal of damaged and misfolded proteins, protein ubiquitylation was found associated to an increasing number of specific regulatory events involving a selective degradation of key regulatory proteins. Thus, ubiquitylation is responsible for regulating a wide array of cellular processes including differentiation, tissue development, induction of inflammatory responses, antigen presentation, cell cycle progression and programmed cell death also named apoptosis (Chapter 18 will review cell death). In addition, according to the pattern of modification of the target proteins (monoubiquitination, polyubiquitination) different proteins can trigger DNA repair (monoubiquitination of N-terminal tails in histones) or be subjected to endocytosis (monoubiquitination of surface receptors).

SORTING FROM THE CYTOSOL INTO OTHER COMPARTMENTS

Most proteins are synthesized on free polysomes and remain in the cytosol. These include enzymes involved in many metabolic and signal transduction pathways, proteins required for mRNA translation or assembly of the cytoskeleton. Other proteins are imported from the cytosol into organelles including the nucleus, the mitochondrion, and the peroxisome (Fig. 5.1).

In general, there are two types of protein trafficking. In one type, the protein crosses a lipid bilayer. The polypeptide crosses the membrane in an unfolded state through an aqueous channel composed of proteins. In the second type, the protein does not traffic across a lipid bilayer and is exemplified by trafficking into the nucleus or from the endoplasmic reticulum (ER) to the Golgi compartment. In these cases, proteins and protein complexes are transported in their folded/assembled state.

The trafficking events are governed by sorting signals (i.e., short linear sequences or three-dimensional patches of particular amino acids) and by their cognate receptors (see some examples in Table

5.1). The first sorting decision occurs after approximately 30 amino acids of the nascent polypeptide are extruded from the ribosome. If the nascent polypeptide lacks a "signal sequence," most often found near the amino-terminal end, the translation of the polypeptide is completed in the cytosol. Then the protein either remains in the cytosol or is posttranslationally incorporated into one of the indicated organelles (see Fig. 5.1). If the protein does contain an amino-terminal signal sequence it is imported co- or posttranslationally into the ER or mitochondrion. Trafficking of proteins from the ER to the Golgi compartment and lysosomes occurs via vesicle budding and fusion events (see Fig. 5.1).

Targeting of Nuclear Proteins

One of the distinctive features of all eukaryotic cells is that the genome is contained in an intracellular compartment called the *nucleus*. The nucleus is bounded by a double membrane that forms the nuclear envelope (NE) (see Fig. 5.1). The outer nuclear membrane is continuous with the ER and has a polypeptide composition distinct from that of the inner membrane. About 3000 nuclear pore complexes (NPCs) perforate the NE in animal cells. Although NPCs allow unrestricted, bidirectional movement of molecules smaller than 40,000 Daltons, traversal of larger molecules across NPCs is tightly regulated. NPCs are approximately 120 nm in external diameter and comprise approximately 50 different proteins (nucleoporins), arranged in a complex cylindrical structure with an octagonal symmetry. Nucleoporins constitute the scaffold of the NPC and are arranged in rings. In the inner ring, nucleoporins containing repeats of two hydrophobic amino acids, phenylalanine and glycine (FG-repeats), seem to be essential for the movement of the cargo-carrier complexes and for creating a selectivity barrier against the diffusion of nonnuclear proteins. The FG-nucleoporin filaments protrude toward the inner core of the NPC and the weak hydrophobic interactions between the FG-repeats and the cargo-carrier complexes mediate the passage of molecules.

NPCs are capable of importing and exporting molecules or complexes, provided that the molecules have an exposed nuclear localization signal (NLS) or nuclear export signal (NES). These signals are not always easy to predict. In Table 5.1 some of the best-known signals are listed. The function of these signals in importing or exporting a protein was analyzed by critically testing both the effects of amino acid substitutions on transport and the capability of the signal to target in or out of the nucleus an attached reporter protein. The nuclear localization signals are not cleaved off as occurs for other signals (see later) and thus can function repetitively. Candidates exposing signals for nuclear import (i.e., transcription factors, coactivators or corepressors, DNA repair enzymes, ribosomal proteins and mRNA processing factors, etc.) or export (ribosomal subunits, mRNA-containing particles, tRNAs, etc.) are transported through the NPC in association with soluble carrier proteins, called karyopherins (also called importins, exportins or transportins), which function as shuttling receptors for different protein cargos. According to the direction of transport, they are divided into two groups: (i) importins, if they bind their cargo on the cytoplasmic side of the NPC and release it on the other and (ii) exportins if they bind the cargo in the nucleus and release it in the cytoplasm.

Ran is a small Ras-like GTPase, belonging to the G-protein superfamily, that controls both the docking of carrier proteins with their cargo and the directionality of transport through cycles of GTP binding and hydrolysis. Fig. 5.2 exemplifies a cycle of import into the nucleus. An importin binds the cargo in the cytosol and then associates with Ran-GDP for trafficking into the nucleus where a Ran-GEF (guanine-nucleotide exchange factor) catalyzes GTP exchange for GDP on Ran that triggers cargo release. The importin-Ran-GTP complex is transported back to the cytoplasm where the conversion of GTP to GDP is stimulated by a Ran-GAP protein (GTPase-activating protein) that causes dissociation of Ran from the importin which can initiate a new cycle. The movement of cargo from the nucleus to the cytoplasm occurs by formation of a Ran-GTP-exportin-cargo

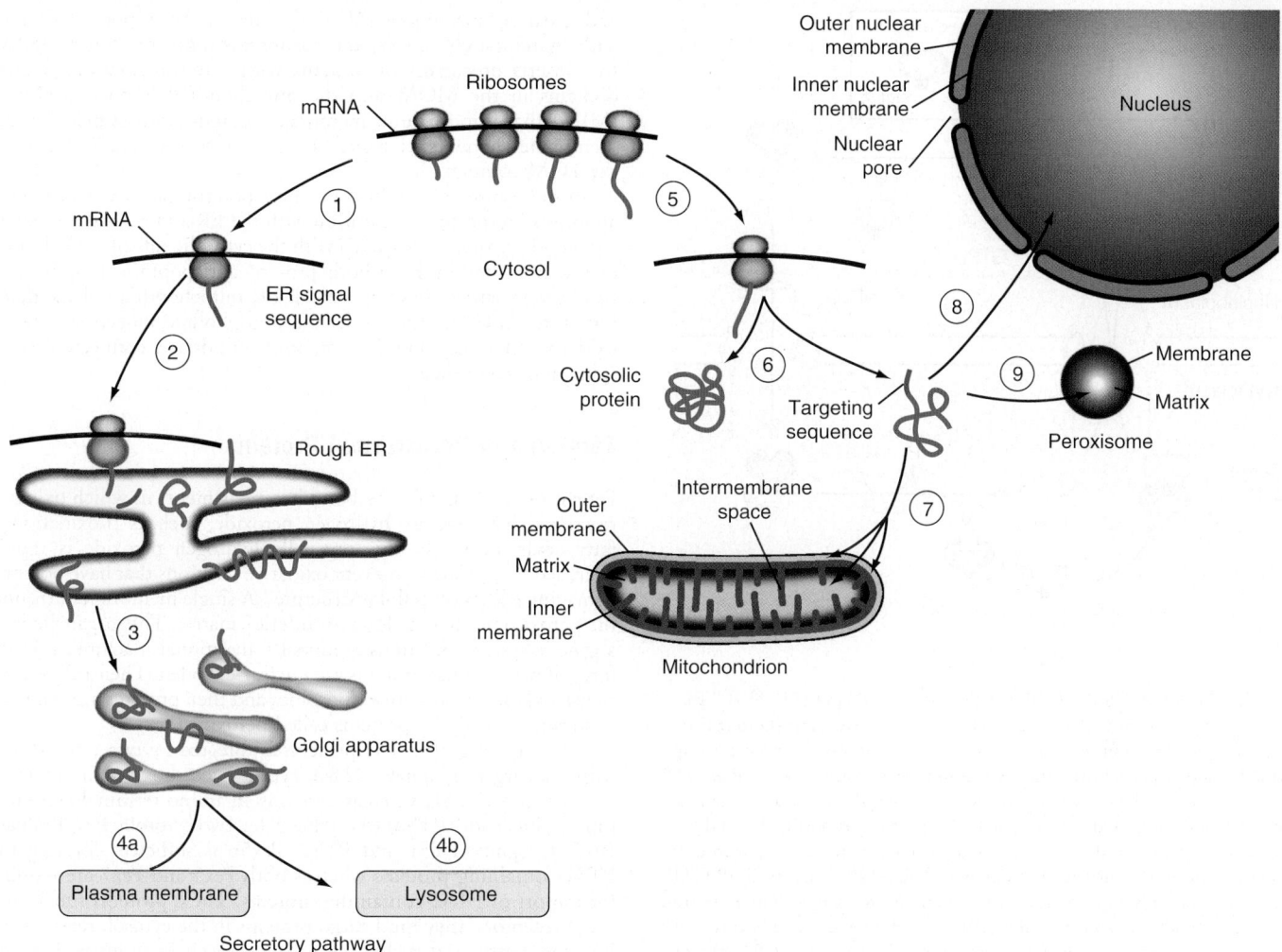

Fig. 5.1 SORTING OF PROTEINS FROM THE CYTOSOL TO DIFFERENT DESTINATIONS. *Left:* steps *1* to *4a* and *4b* depict the sorting of proteins destined to organelles of the secretory pathway, endoplasmic reticulum (ER), Golgi, plasma membrane, lysosome or extracellular space. *Right:* steps *5* and *6*: synthesis of a cytosolic protein; steps *7*, *8* and *9*: sorting of proteins to mitochondrion, the nucleus and the peroxisome.

complex that is transported to the cytoplasm where Ran-GAP triggers the hydrolysis of GTP. The conformational change of the exportin releases the cargo in the cytoplasm. The different localization of Ran-GEF and Ran-GAP and the continuous transport of Ran-GDP in the nucleus create an asymmetry that is important for the directionality of the process. In conclusion, karyopherins possess a cargo-binding domain but also binding domains for nucleoporins and Ran-GTPase.

Interestingly, there are remarkable examples of regulation of protein transport into the nucleus. NFκB, a nuclear factor for the transcriptional enhancer of the κ light chain in B lymphocytes, is a key element of the stress response. This factor is normally retained in the cytoplasm by interaction with IκB. The TNF-α dependent phosphorylation of IκB releases NFκB that exposes an NLS and migrates into the nucleus where it activates transcription of several target genes. For the glucocorticoid receptor (GR), which is localized in the cytoplasm, the binding to the lipophilic ligand exposes an NLS which is recognized by an importin and allows translocation into the nucleus where GR activates genes by binding to GR-responsive-elements in their promoter regions.

Targeting of Mitochondrial Proteins

The mitochondrion is an essential cellular compartment in eukaryotes. Although it contains a genome organized in a circular DNA

molecule and independent transcriptional/translational machinery, 98% of the approximately 1500 proteins that constitute the mitochondrial proteome are encoded by nuclear DNA and are imported from the cytosol after their synthesis. A small number of highly hydrophobic proteins is encoded by mitochondrial DNA and synthesized inside the organelle by a translational machinery of bacterial origin using organelle-transcribed mRNAs.

Like nuclei, mitochondria have two membranes: the outer membrane (MOM) contacts the cytosol whereas the inner membrane (MIM) forms numerous invaginations named *cristae* where the enzymes that synthesize ATP through reactions of the electron transport chain and oxidative phosphorylation reside. Where the MOM is permeable to small molecules (less than 5 kDa) and ions, the inner membrane is highly impermeable, a property essential to create an electrochemical gradient necessary to drive the synthesis of ATP. The space enclosed by the two membranes is the intermembrane space (IMS) and the space enclosed by the inner membrane is the *matrix*. Protein transport into mitochondria appears to be unidirectional, as no proteins are known to be exported from mitochondria. A remarkable exception is represented by apoptosis. Upon this condition, there is a mitochondrial permeability transition that permits release of cytochrome c and other factors from the IMS to the cytosol that trigger an intracellular pathway leading to death. Posttranslational translocation and sorting of nuclear-encoded proteins into the various mitochondrial subcompartments are achieved by the concerted action of translocases.

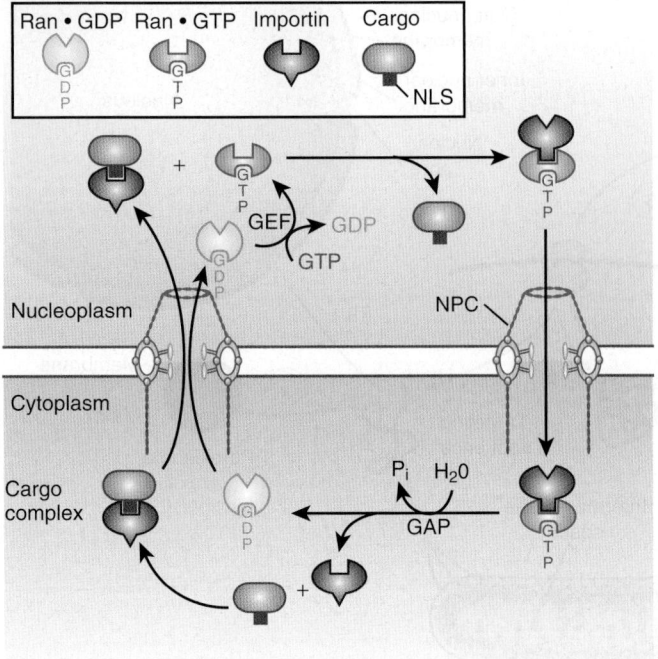

Fig. 5.2 MECHANISM OF PROTEIN IMPORT INTO THE NUCLEUS. The figure shows the different localization of Ran-GAP and Ran-GEF that regulate the direction of nuclear transport. A Ran-GTP-exportin-cargo complex is transported from the nucleus to the cytoplasm where a Ran-GAP stimulates the GTPase activity of Ran. Ran-GDP dissociates from the complex and induces the release of the cargo from exportin. Ran-GDP is transported back to the nucleus by association with an importin-cargo complex and in the nucleus the activity of a Ran-GEF triggers GDP-GTP-exchange and this induces the dissociation of the cargo from importin. Ran-GTP binds an exportin-cargo complex and another cycle begins. *GAP*, GTPase-activating protein; *GDP*, guanosine diphosphate; *GEF*, guanine nucleotide exchange factor; *GTP*, guanosine triphosphate; *NLS*, nuclear localization signal, *NPC*, nuclear pore complex. *(Adapted from Lodish H, Berk A, Matsudaira P, et al: Molecular cell biology, ed 5, New York, 2003, W.H. Freeman.)*

Precursor proteins usually have one of two targeting signals: (1) an amino-terminal presequence that is generally between 10 and 80 amino acids long and forms an amphipathic α-helix, which is rich in positively charged, hydrophobic and hydroxylated amino acids (Table 5.1); or (2) a less well-defined, hydrophobic targeting sequence distributed throughout the protein. The translocase of the outer membrane (TOM) complex functions as a single entry point of incoming precursors into the mitochondria and is crucial for the biogenesis of the organelle and for the viability of eukaryotic cells. Preproteins translocate through the TOM complex in an N-to-C direction in an unfolded state. TOM translocase is a heteromolecular protein complex whose central component is Tom40, an essential protein that forms the protein-conducting channel. After crossing the outer membrane, proteins segregate according to their signals and recognize two distinct translocases of the inner membrane (TIM23 and TIM22). Presequence-containing proteins are directed to the TIM23 complex that mediates transport across the inner membrane, a process which requires the electrochemical membrane potential and the ATP-driven action of the matrix heat shock protein 70 (mtHsp70). Once in the matrix, the presequence is often cleaved by a mitochondrial processing peptidase (MPP). Proteins with internal targeting signals are guided to the TIM22 complex. Membrane insertion at the TIM22 complex is also dependent on the membrane potential. Other machineries of protein sorting are the intermembrane space import

and assembly machinery (MIA) that drives the import of proteins with cysteine-rich motifs, the sorting/assembly machinery (SAM) that inserts precursors of proteins with a transmembrane β-barrel domains in the MOM and the mitochondrial import machinery (MIM) that import outer membrane proteins with α-helical transmembrane segments after their recognition by the Tom70 subunit of the TOM complex.[2]

In the context of cell biology, mitochondria play relevant roles in apoptosis, in the communication with the ER and in oxidative stress. Among the proteins associated with the cytosolic side of MOM, those of the Bcl-2 family have both pro- or antiapoptotic functions. In addition, recent studies unveiled an ER-mitochondria linkage that is important in Ca^{2+} homeostasis and phospholipid biogenesis whereas oxidative stress generated in the mitochondria is connected to cell aging and senescence.

Targeting of Peroxisomal Proteins

Peroxisomes are membrane-bound compartments in which oxidative reactions that generate hydrogen peroxide, such as β-oxidation of fatty acids, occur. In this organelle hydrogen peroxide is rapidly degraded by catalase to prevent oxidative reactions that have potential damaging effects on cellular structures. A single membrane surrounds the peroxisome that encloses an interior matrix. This organelle lacks a genetic system and transcriptional/translational machinery. Therefore, all peroxisomal proteins are nuclear-encoded. Their mRNAs are translated on cytosolic-free ribosomes and then proteins are imported posttranslationally by proteins called peroxins (Pex).[3]

The targeting of matrix proteins is directed by two types of peroxisomal targeting signals (PTSs). Type 1 is a carboxyl-terminal tri- or tetra-peptide (PTS1) whereas type 2 is an amino-terminal peptide of nine amino acids (PTS2) (see Table 5.1). Two cytosolic Pex, Pex5 and Pex7, recognize PTS1 and PTS2. Pex5p is sufficient for targeting PTS1-containing proteins whereas both Pex5 and Pex7 are required for import of PTS2-containing proteins. These proteins function as cargo receptors; they bind cargo proteins in the cytosol, release them into the matrix and cycle back to the cytosol. In humans, Pex5 has two isoforms, Pex5S and Pex5L. The latter has an additional exon that is required for binding of Pex7 to Pex5. Matrix proteins cross the membrane in a folded state, or even as oligomers. Other peroxins are involved in the import of peroxisomal membrane proteins (PMPs). Pex3, Pex16 and Pex19 are thought to be involved in the formation of the peroxisomal membrane and/or insertion of PMPs in the peroxisomal membrane. Experimental evidence suggests the existence of two routes by which PMPs can reach peroxisomes, one direct route and one via the ER. Some PMPs are targeted to peroxisomes by Pex19 and others are not. The PMP binds Pex19, a soluble recycling receptor/chaperone, to form a cargo-receptor complex that docks on Pex3 in the peroxisomal membrane and then membrane insertion occurs. The indirect targeting via the ER involves only some PMPs, Pex3 for example, and so far, has been demonstrated only in yeast where the Sec61 translocon is required. Other Pex proteins are involved in ubiquitination. Ubiquitination of the receptors has been proposed to function in concert with ATPases associated to diverse activities (AAA+ ATPases) that move proteins across membrane using an ATP-dependent mechanism that resembles the retrotranslocation of misfolded proteins from ER lumen to the cytosol and in recycling the receptors to the membrane surface.

One consequence of the existence of two different mechanisms for protein import is that when the import of matrix proteins is defective, membrane ghosts of peroxisomes persist in the cells. In contrast, when the import of membrane proteins is impaired, neither normal peroxisomes nor membrane ghosts are present. Defects in *PEX3* underlie Zellweger syndrome that is characterized by the presence of empty peroxisomes and abnormalities in the brain, liver, and kidney that cause death shortly after birth. Other syndromes in peroxisome biogenesis were identified and their occurrence underlines the essential role of these organelles for human metabolism and development.[4]

COTRANSLATIONAL PROTEIN TRANSLOCATION INTO THE ENDOPLASMIC RETICULUM

The ER is an extensive membranous network that is continuous with the outer nuclear membrane and is the site for the synthesis of the massive amounts of lipid and protein used to build the membranes of most cellular organelles. The ER comprises three interconnected domains: rough ER, smooth ER, and ER exit sites. The rough ER is so called because it is studded with bound ribosomes that are actively synthesizing proteins. Cells specialized in protein secretion, such as cells of the exocrine glands and plasma cells are rich in rough ER. The smooth ER lacks ribosomes, is not very abundant in most cells (except hepatocytes), and is thought to be the site of lipid biosynthesis and of cytochrome P450–mediated detoxification reactions. Finally, ER exit sites are specialized areas of the ER membrane where transport cargo is packaged into transport vesicles en route to the Golgi apparatus.

Nascent secretory proteins are marked for translocation into the ER by the presence of an amino-terminal signal sequence (see Table 5.1). This sequence has a length of about 15–30 amino acids and displays no conservation of amino acid sequence, although it contains a hydrophobic core flanked by polar residues that preferentially have a short side chain in proximity to the cleavage site. As the signal sequence emerges from the ribosome, it is recognized by the signal recognition particle (SRP), a ribonucleoprotein, and this binding induces a temporary arrest in translational elongation (Fig. 5.3). The docking of ribosomes to the ER occurs by interaction of the SRP with the SRP receptor. Upon binding of GTP to both the SRP and its receptor, the ribosome and the nascent chain are transferred to the Sec61 translocon complex allowing translation to resume. Preproteins translocate through the Sec61 complex in an N-to-C direction. As the nascent polypeptide emerges from the luminal side of the translocon, its signal sequence is cleaved by signal peptidase.

In the absence of specific targeting sequences, proteins that completely translocate into the ER lumen traffic through bulk flow to the cell surface. In contrast, proteins that have specific targeting signals may be localized to the lumen of the ER, the Golgi compartment, or lysosomes. Other proteins that reside in membranes of the cell contain topologic sequences called transmembrane domains that consist of ~20 largely apolar amino acids. When a transmembrane domain enters the translocon, the polypeptide is released laterally from the Sec61 channel into the lipid bilayer. Membrane proteins can assume different topologies according to the number and type of TM domains.

PROTEIN TRAFFICKING WITHIN THE SECRETORY PATHWAY

Proteins that enter the ER are transported towards the plasma membrane through the secretory pathway (Fig. 5.4). Specific signals cause resident proteins to be retained in the ER, Golgi or plasma membrane. Proteins may also be targeted from the Golgi compartment to lysosomes or from the plasma membrane to endosomes (see Fig. 5.4, pathways 8 and 9). Initially the study of this complex protein trafficking took advantage of the use of yeast genetics to isolate temperature-sensitive mutants (*sec*) that were defective at different stages of the secretory pathway. The subsequent characterization of *SEC* genes, thanks to the advent of DNA recombinant techniques, made possible the isolation of the counterparts in mammalian cells and the beginning of molecular and biochemical investigation of protein secretion. Many genes encoding products involved in secretion are strikingly conserved from yeast to mammals, indicating the importance of this pathway for the life of a eukaryotic cell.

Transport through the secretory pathway is mediated by vesicles. Different sets of structural and regulatory proteins control the fusion of the appropriate vesicles with the target membrane. Sorting motifs dictate the selective incorporation of cargo proteins into these vesicles and their delivery to the intended destination. A major question in cell biology today is how the identity of the compartments of the secretory pathway is maintained while allowing unimpeded transit of other nonresident proteins.

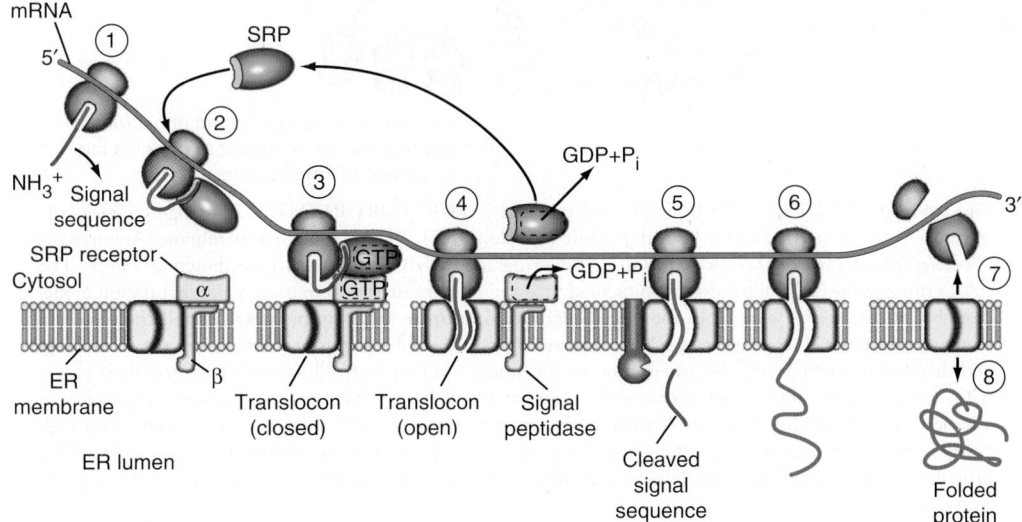

Fig. 5.3 SYNTHESIS OF PROTEINS SORTED FOR IMPORT IN THE ENDOPLASMIC RETICULUM. The figure depicts the main steps of the cotranslational translocation of a secretory protein into the endoplasmic reticulum (ER). *Steps 1* and *2*: the signal sequence of the emerging polypeptide binds the signal recognition particle (SRP) to induce a translation arrest. *Steps 3* and *4*: the binding of the SRP-nascent polypeptide-ribosome complex to the SRP-receptor triggers GTP hydrolysis on both SRP and the SRP-receptor. The translocon channel (Sec61p) opens and translation resumes. SRP is recycled. *Step 5*: the polypeptide chain elongates and emerges on the luminal side of the ER where a signal peptidase removes the signal sequence. *Steps 6, 7* and *8*: the synthesis of the polypeptide proceeds until the end of translation and the protein assumes its native conformation (concurrent glycosylation is not shown). The ribosome dissociates and its subunits are released.

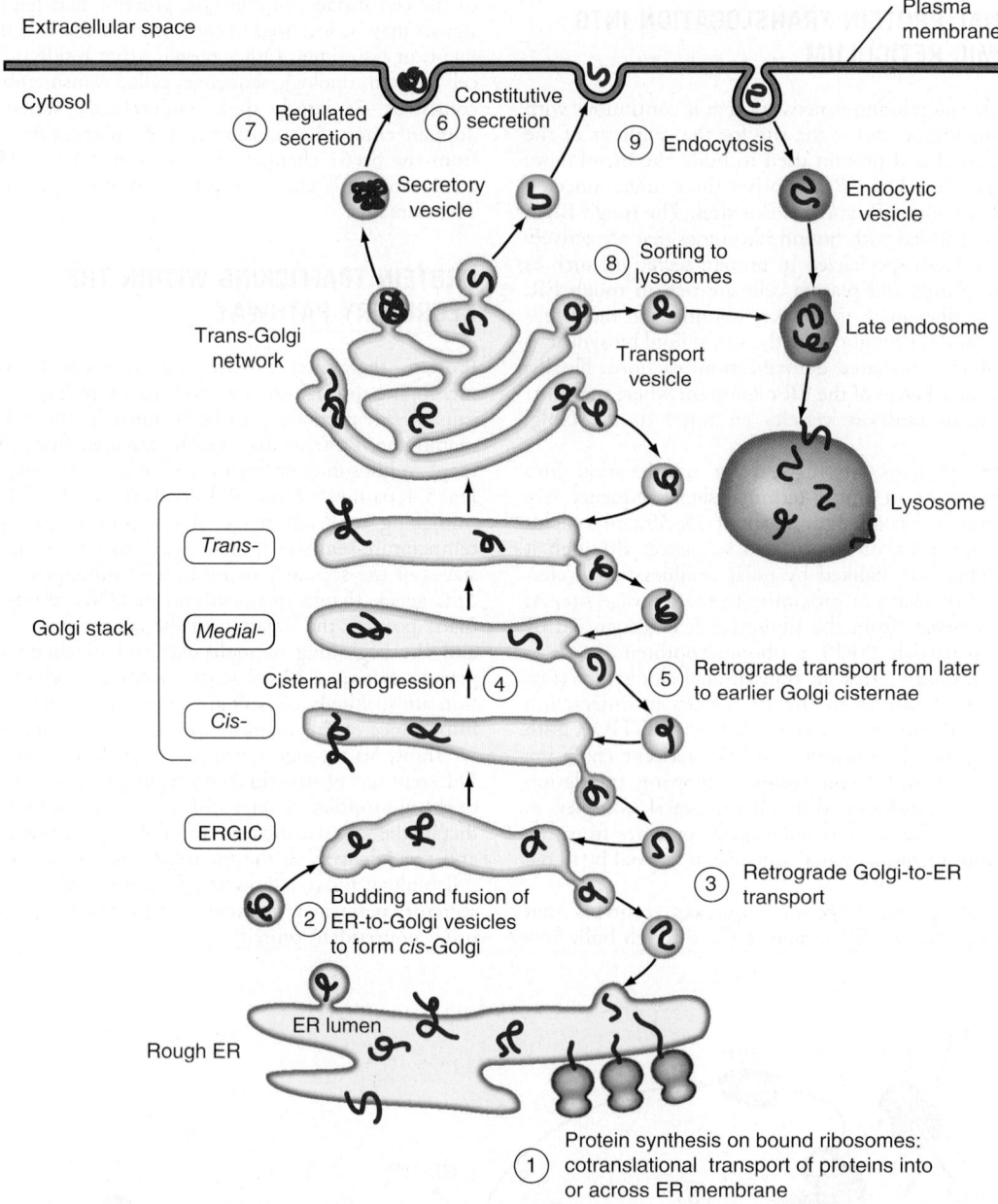

Fig. 5.4 PROTEIN TRAFFICKING THROUGH THE SECRETORY PATHWAY. The figure depicts the secretory pathway starting from the endoplasmic reticulum (ER) *(1)* to the plasma membrane. Anterograde *ER-Golgi intermediate compartment* (ERGIC) and retrograde ERGIC-ER transport are shown *(2 and 3)*. The transit through the Golgi apparatus is represented according to the cisternae progression and maturation model described in the text *(4 and 5)*. In the *trans*-Golgi the constitutive secretory pathway *(6)* and the regulated secretory pathway *(7)* separate. In specialized secretory cells, selected proteins are sorted from the *trans*-Golgi and diverted to secretory vesicles where proteins are stored until an extracellular signal triggers their fusion with the plasma membrane and release of the content in the extracellular space (regulated exocytosis). In addition, at the *trans*-Golgi proteins destined to the lysosome are sorted and delivered to the organelle through vesicles *(8)*. The endocytotic pathway *(9)* mediates the internalization of membrane or soluble extracellular proteins and their targeting to the lysosome or the recycling of some proteins to the cell surface (not shown in the figure).

PROCESSING OF PROTEINS IN THE ENDOPLASMIC RETICULUM

Protein Folding in the Lumen of the ER

Protein chaperones facilitate protein folding in the ER, but amino acid posttranslational modifications such as asparagine(*N*)-linked-glycosylation and disulfide bond formation are also involved. Proteins start to fold cotranslationally by interaction with a host of chaperones, among which is the Hsp70 family member BiP. In addition, there are folding catalysts that increase the rate of protein folding. For example, the proper pairing and formation of disulfide bonds is catalyzed by oxidoreductases, such as protein disulfide isomerase (PDI), that also shuffle nonnative disulfide bonds. In the current model, the oxidation of two thiols produces a disulfide bond (S–S) in the substrate protein and concomitantly reduces two thiols within PDI which return to the oxidized state by another thiol-disulfide exchange catalyzed by

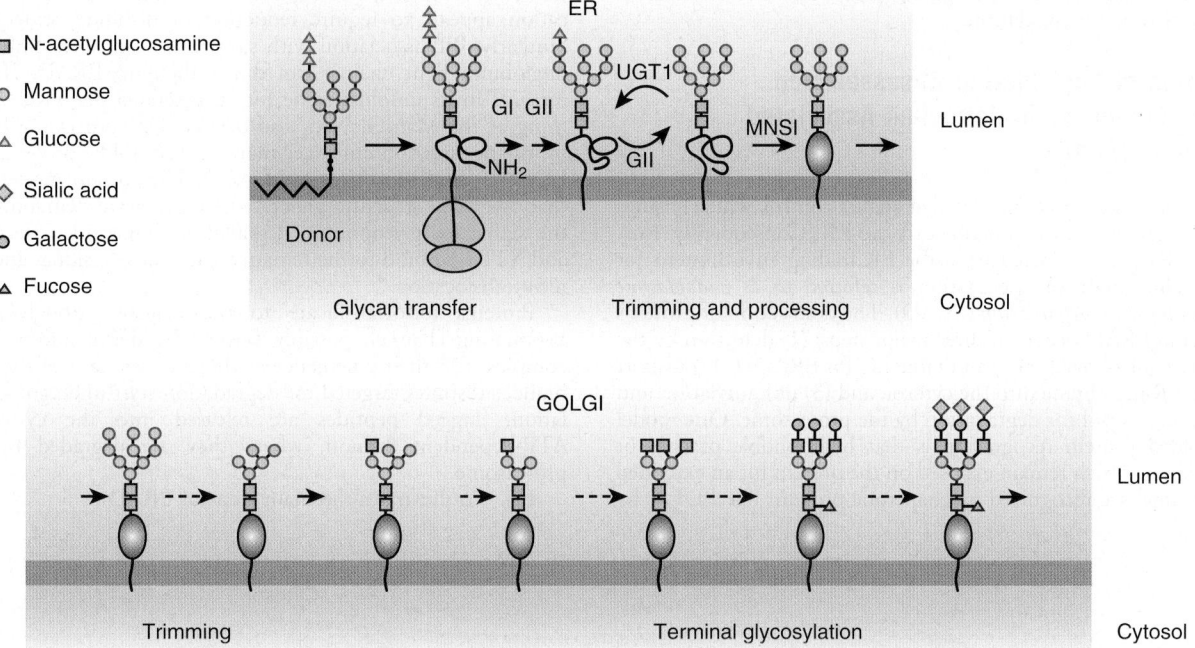

N-acetylglucosamine
Mannose
Glucose
Sialic acid
Galactose
Fucose

Fig. 5.5 *N*-GLYCOSYLATION OF PROTEINS. In the lumen of the endoplasmic reticulum (ER), a core oligosaccharide, $Glc_3Man_9GlcNac_2$, is transferred from a lipid-linked precursor (dolichol donor) to the asparagine residue in an N-X-S/T motif in the nascent polypeptide chain. The terminal glucose residues are removed by GI and GII and cycles of reglucosylation by UGT1 (UGGT1) can occur (*curved arrows*). When the protein is folded, one mannose is trimmed by ER-mannosidase I and the protein is transported to the Golgi. Core oligosaccharides are further trimmed by mannosidases to produce the $Man_5GlcNac_2$ unit. Further elaboration is catalyzed by glycosyltransferases that add various sugars and create branches. Bi, tri and tetra antennary chains are generated. In the figure, only one pathway of terminal glycosylation is shown. (*Modified from Helenius A, Aebi M: Intracellular function of N-linked glycans.* Science *291:2364, 2001.*)

ERO1, a membrane associated oxidoreductase. ERO1 returns to the oxidized state by transfer of electrons to molecular oxygen via its cofactor flavin adenine dinucleotide (FAD). In contrast to the highly reducing environment of the cytosol where disulfide bonds do not typically form, the lumen of the ER is very oxidizing so that disulfide bonds formation is favored.

Protein Modifications in the ER

Most proteins that enter the secretory pathway are modified by *N*-glycosylation (Fig. 5.5). This process starts with the transfer of a core oligosaccharide from a lipid-linked dolichol donor to an asparagine residue within the consensus sequence N-X-S/T of a nascent polypeptide (X can be any amino acid except for proline). The N-linked oligosaccharide is composed of a glucose3-mannose9-*N*-acetylglucosamine2 unit ($Glc_3Man_9GlcNac_2$). The oligosaccharide is transferred to the asparagine residue by an ER oligosaccharyltransferase (OST) that is composed of a catalytic subunit (STT3A or STT3B) and a set of accessory subunits. Further processing of the terminal sugars occurs in the ER and after the polypeptide transits the Golgi compartment (see Fig. 5.5). Many blood proteins, for example immunoglobulins, antiproteases, coagulation factors, and many membrane proteins of the cell are glycosylated.

Although glycan chains are often not required for the enzymatic activity of glycoproteins, they are important for the physical properties they confer and for many physiologic functions. Glycans protect proteins from protease digestion and heat denaturation, confer hydrophilicity and adhesive properties to the proteins, and mediate interaction with other proteins or receptors. A remarkable example is the hormone erythropoietin that requires a particular complex type of *N*-glycan chains for its biologic function to stimulate erythropoiesis.

In the recent years several studies have revealed the importance of protein *N*-glycosylation in promoting folding. The addition of glycan chains may prevent aggregation or provide steric influences that affect polypeptide folding and disulfide bond formation and also mediate interaction with specific chaperones. In mammalian cells, N-linked oligosaccharides are also used as signal for monitoring protein folding and trafficking. They are ligands for a complex chaperone system composed of the lectin chaperones calnexin (CNX) and calreticulin (CRT), Erp57 (an oxidoreductase), two α-glucosidases (GI and GII) and one folding sensor (UGGT1) endowed with reglucosylation activity (UDP-glucose:glycoprotein glucosyltransferase). GI removes the most terminal glucose and diglucosylated polypeptides associated with malectin, an ER resident lectin. Then, GII removes the second terminal glucose residue to form a monoglucosylated N-linked chain (see Fig. 5.5) that is a ligand for CNX and CRT. CNX and CRT associate with the thiol-disulfide oxidoreductase ERP57 which promotes proper rearrangement of disulfide bonds. Then the remaining glucose residue is removed by GII. UGGT1 recognizes and reglucosylates N-linked oligosaccharides on proteins that have not completed the folding process. The addition of glucose residues allows reassociation with the CNX/CRT chaperone system for another attempt for the polypeptide to attain its proper conformation.[5]

Besides N-core glycosylation and oxidative folding, the ER is also site of other protein modifications. A remarkable one is γ-carboxylation of glutamic acid residues. Although this is a rather rare modification, it is crucial for the functionality of specific proteins, such as the coagulation factors VII, X, IX and prothrombin, and is essential for life as described earlier (see Box 5.1). Another modification is the attachment of a GPI to the C-terminal end of protein with concomitant release of the GPI signal peptide. The GPI attachment promotes membrane association.

Destruction of Misfolded or Misassembled Proteins: Endoplasmic-Reticulum Associated Degradation (ERAD)

In the ER, proteins undergo a so-called quality control, which ensures that only correctly folded proteins exit the ER. Consequently, misfolded proteins are extracted from the ER folding environment for disposal. This mode of degradation is referred to as *endoplasmic reticulum-associated degradation* (ERAD). The destruction of proteins that undergo ERAD occurs in three major steps: (1) detection by the ER quality control machinery and targeting for ERAD, (2) transport across the ER membrane into the cytosol, and (3) ubiquitylation and release in the cytosol for degradation by the proteasome. One model for misfolded protein recognition is that hydrophobic patches or sugar moieties, which remain exposed on the protein for an extended period of time, are recognized by chaperone proteins like PDI or by

the CNX/CRT chaperone system. In a number of cases retrotranslocation appears to require reduction of disulfide bridges by PDI. Similarly, BiP association with substrates (e.g., unassembled immunoglobulin light chains) can direct them to ERAD. If a protein remains in its unfolded state for an extended period of time, trimming of the $Man_8GlcNac_2$ also occurs. This processing is catalyzed by ER-degradation enhancer mannosidase α-like proteins EDEM1, EDEM2, EDEM3 (Htm1p in yeast). The current model postulates that *N*-glycan structure generated by extensive demannosylation is the signal for glycoprotein degradation. ER-resident lectins (OS-9 and XTP3-B) bind to the remaining mannose residues and assist the retrotranslocation.

Proteins retrotranslocate to the cytosol through a protein-conducting channel, possibly formed by derlin and/or the Sec61 complex. On their emergence at the cytosolic face of the ER membrane, substrates targeted for degradation start undergoing ubiquitylation. Tagged peptides are released into the cytosol in an ATP-dependent fashion, where they are degraded by the 26S proteasome.

Fig. 5.6 illustrates the main steps of ERAD.

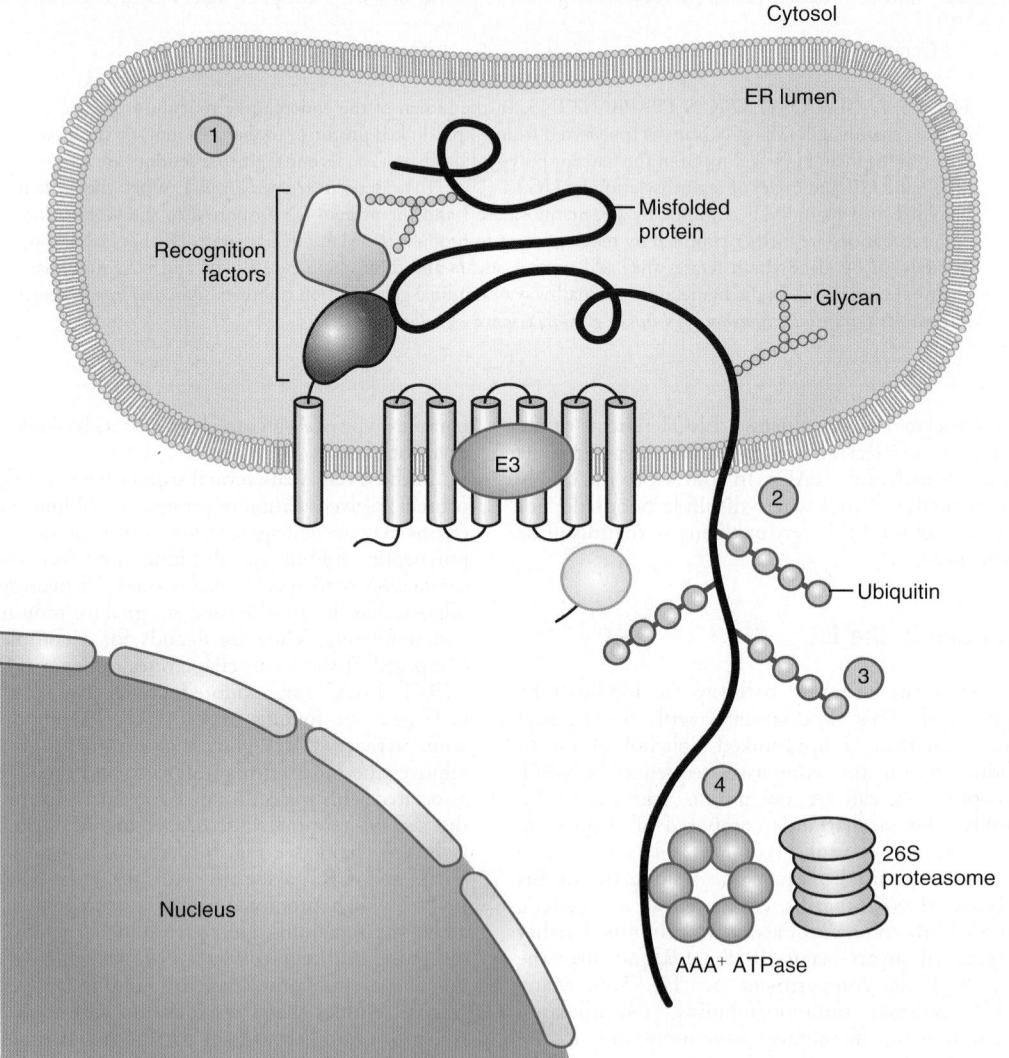

Fig. 5.6 ENDOPLASMIC RETICULUM–ASSOCIATED PROTEIN DEGRADATION (ERAD). The figure depicts the steps in the degradation of misfolded proteins in the ER. *Step 1*: Recognition factors, some of which are lectins, and ubiquitin ligases of the ER membrane cooperate in recognizing substrate proteins. *Step 2*: proteins are exported into the cytosol. *Step 3*: on the cytosolic face of the ER, the protein is ubiquitinated by an ER ligase. *Step 4*: the substrate is removed from the membrane by the AAA+ ATPase Cdc48 and directed to the 26S proteasome. *(From: Hirsch C, Gauss R, Horn SC, Neuber O, Sommer T: The ubiquitylation machinery of the endoplasmic reticulum.* Nature *458:453, 2009.)*

The Unfolded Protein Response

The ER monitors the amount of unfolded protein in its lumen. When that number exceeds a certain threshold, ER sensors activate a signal transduction pathway. The set of responses activated by this pathway is called the unfolded protein response (UPR). A number of cellular insults disrupt protein folding and cause unfolded protein accumulation in the ER lumen. The UPR is an adaptive response signaled through three ER-localized transmembrane proteins PERK, IRE1, and ATF6. These proteins function as sensors through the properties of their ER-luminal domains and trigger a concerted response through the function of their cytosolic domains. The activation of the sensors results in a complex response aimed to (i) limit accumulation of unfolded protein through reducing protein synthesis, (ii) increasing the degradation of unfolded protein, and (iii) increasing the ER protein folding capacity.

IRE1 is conserved in all eukaryotic cells and has protein kinase and endoribonuclease activities that, upon activation, mediate unconventional splicing of a 26-base intron from the XBP1 mRNA to produce a basic Leucine Zipper (bZip) potent transcription factor. ATF6, upon accumulation of unfolded protein in the ER lumen, is transported to the Golgi compartment where it is cleaved by two proteases, S1P and S2P. These enzymes release a cytosolic fragment of ATF6 containing a bZip-transcription factor that migrates to the nucleus to activate gene transcription. S1P and S2P are two important Golgi proteases as they are also involved in the regulation of cholesterol metabolism. Finally, PERK-mediated phosphorylation of eIF2α attenuates general mRNA translation; however, paradoxically, it increases translation of the transcription factor ATF4 mRNA to also induce transcription of UPR genes. If the UPR adaptive response is not sufficient to correct the protein folding defect, the cells enter apoptotic death.

ER is now regarded as a sensor of perturbations of cell homeostasis.[6,7] Activation of the UPR and defects in UPR are known to be important factors that contribute to many disease processes ranging from metabolic disease, neurologic disease, infectious disease, and cancer (reviews on cancer and on UPR and diseases under the section Suggested Readings).

Control of Exit From the Endoplasmic Reticulum

On achieving transport competence, proteins are granted access to higher-ordered membrane domains termed ER exit sites. At ER exit sites, membrane-bound and soluble proteins are concentrated into transport vesicles for trafficking to a network of smooth membranes called the *ER-Golgi Intermediate Compartment* (ERGIC, see Fig. 5.4). COPII complex, composed of coat proteins, concentrate and package the protein cargo into vesicles. COPII binds to cargo molecules either directly, if they span the membrane, or through intermediate cargo receptors and then provides some of the force that causes vesicle budding, thereby linking cargo acquisition to vesiculation.

ER resident proteins are selectively sequestered in the ER both for the absence of export signals and to the presence of ER retention signals. Soluble luminal ER resident are retained through a C-terminal ER tetrapeptide retention motif KDEL. Frequently, transmembrane proteins have either a C-terminal dilysine motif KKXX or an N-terminal diarginine motif XXRR, or variants thereof for transmembrane proteins. However, it is more accurate to indicate ER localization signals as "retrieval motifs" because proteins bearing these signals can transiently escape from the ER into the ERGIC, from which they are returned to the ER through the retrograde vesicular transport (see Fig. 5.4).

For the KDEL motif of luminal ER proteins, a specific retrieval receptor has been identified, first in yeast and then in mammals. The KKXX motif has been shown to interact directly with the COPI coat protein complex that is involved in retrograde transport from the ER to the Golgi. Retrograde transport also serves to replenish the vesicle components lost as a result of anterograde (forward) transport. In conclusion, selective protein exit from the ER is achieved by monitoring/regulating (1) transport competence of nascent proteins, (2) capture of cargo in transport vesicles, and (3) protein retention/retrieval for ER-localized proteins.

INTRAGOLGI TRANSPORT AND PROTEIN PROCESSING

Organization of the Golgi Apparatus

The Golgi complex comprises a stack of flattened, membrane-bound cisternae that is highly dependent on microtubules for structural integrity. The stack of cisternae can be subdivided into three parts referred to as *cis, medial,* and *trans* with the *cis* and *trans* sides facing the ER and the plasma membrane, respectively (see Fig. 5.4). Both the *cis* and *trans* faces are associated with tubulovesicular bundles of membranes. The ERGIC comprises the bundle on the *cis* side of the Golgi stack and is the site where incoming proteins from the ER are sorted into those directed for anterograde or for retrograde transport. The tubulovesicular bundle at the *trans* side is the *trans-Golgi* network (TGN, see Fig. 5.4).

A major feature of the Golgi is polarity. The processing events are temporally and spatially ordered because the processing enzymes have a characteristic distribution across the Golgi stack. In the Golgi, different types of modifications take place as for example proteolytic processing, protein *O*-glycosylation and elaboration of N-linked chains, phosphorylation or sulfation of oligosaccharides, and sulfation of tyrosines.

The importance of protein glycosylation for human biology is underlined by the identification of many inherited human disorders that are caused by defects in these processes and cause clinical manifestations in members of families as described in Box 5.2.

Retention of Resident Golgi Proteins

Extensive analysis has failed to reveal a clear retention motif enabling subdomain-specific retention of resident Golgi proteins. Two possible models have been proposed. One *model is retention by preferential interaction with membranes of optimal thickness.* It is based on the finding that the transmembrane domains of Golgi proteins are shorter than transmembrane domains of plasma membrane proteins. These differences should allow a preferential interaction with the Golgi membrane lipid bilayer that is thinner than that of plasma membrane. The other model is *kin-recognition/oligomerization.* It postulates that proteins of a given subdomain of the Golgi membrane can aggregate

---

BOX 5.2 **Human Glycosylation Disorders**

In humans, the three main glycosylation pathways are the *N*- and *O*-glycosylation and the glycosylphosphatidylinositol (GPI) anchoring. About 2% of the human genome encodes glycosylation reactions. Moreover, glycosylation pathways intersect with glucose, lipid, and isoprenoid metabolism, expanding the number of players involved in these key protein modifications. Nearly 70 inherited glycosylation disorders have been identified so far and this number is steadily increasing because of the progress in the technology of DNA sequencing and in mapping mutations.[8] The characterized mutations combined to the biochemical lesion and to the clinical manifestations are classified in the CDG (congenital disorders of glycosylation) database. Mutations affect almost every organ and some proved to block embryo development in animal models of disease. Abnormalities in *N*-glycosylation cause severe myasthenic syndromes caused by hypoglycosylation of the acetylcholine receptor that affects the signal transmission at the neuromuscular plaque. Other cause neurologic disorders. Complications also arise from secondary effects caused by ER stress consequent to poor glycosylation. *O*-Glycosylation defects are associated mainly to severe muscular dystrophy (Walker-Warburg syndrome) whereas lack of the first step of GPI synthesis provokes paroxysmal nocturnal hemoglobinuria, a well-known hematologic disorder that results in erythrocyte lysis.

into large detergent-insoluble oligomers as a way of minimizing lipid-protein contact. This would prevent the entry of proteins into the vesicles and thus their traffic to more distal cisternae. There is evidence in support of both models.

Protein Trafficking to and Through the Golgi Apparatus

Cargo proteins exit the ER in COPII-coated vesicles that enter the ERGIC and are ultimately delivered to the *cis*-Golgi either in vesicles or along extended tubules. However, the mechanism whereby cargo proteins move across the Golgi complex from *cis* to *trans* remains controversial. Two models have been proposed. The vesicular transport model contends that anterograde transport occurs in vesicles or tubules that traffic cargo in an anterograde direction. The second suggests that there is a cisternal progression and maturation. This alternative model proposes that Golgi cisternae are not fixed structures but move forward from the *cis* side to the *trans* side generating an anterograde movement. As cisternae mature, resident Golgi proteins that belong to more *cis*-like cisternae must be selectively pinched off in vesicles and trafficked back to the *cis* side of the Golgi stack. This would occur by COPI-mediated retrograde vesicular transport (see Fig. 5.4). Although which of these models is correct is currently unclear, a majority of the experimental data supports the cisternal maturation model. In particular, technical progress in live-cell imaging provided evidence supporting a very dynamic nature of this organelle as expected by the progression/maturation model.

SORTING EVENTS AT THE *TRANS*-GOLGI NETWORK

Overview

The TGN is an important site of intracellular sorting, where proteins bound for lysosomes or regulated secretory vesicles are separated from those entering the constitutive pathway leading to the plasma membrane (see Fig. 5.4, pathways 6, 7 and 8). The secretion process is called exocytosis. The molecular basis for diversion of proteins into lysosomes and regulated secretory granules are described later.

Sorting Into Lysosomes

Lysosomes are acidic (pH of approximately 5.0–5.5), membrane-bound organelles containing numerous hydrolytic enzymes designed to degrade proteins, carbohydrates, and lipids. Soluble hydrolases are selectively marked for sorting into lysosomes by phosphorylation of their *N*-linked oligosaccharides that creates the mannose-6-phosphate sorting signal (M6P). On arrival at the TGN, the M6P-modified hydrolase is bound by a cargo receptor, the M6P-receptor (M6P-R), which delivers it first to a "late endosomal compartment," where the low pH releases the hydrolase from the M6P-R. Subsequently, the hydrolase is delivered to the lysosome, and the M6P-R is recycled from the endosomes through retromer-coated vesicles to the TGN to be reused (for simplicity the endosome to Golgi transport is not represented in Fig. 5.4).

The motif responsible for targeting M6P-R to lysosomes is YSKV and is recognized by all three distinct adaptor protein (AP) complexes (AP-1, -2, and -3) that contribute to delivery of cargo to lysosomes by linking cargo acquisition to vesiculation. Cargo recruitment occurs in a manner similar to that described for the COPI- and COPII-dependent vesicles, except that the cytosolic coat complex is clathrin. In addition to luminal hydrolases, lysosomes also contain a wide array of membrane proteins that are targeted to lysosomes via one of two consensus motifs: (1) YXXe, where X is any amino acid and e is any amino acid with a bulky hydrophobic side chain and (2) a leucine-based motif (LL or LI). Trafficking of these membrane-bound proteins to lysosomes is indirect, proceeding first to late endosomes or the plasma membrane before their retrieval to lysosomes. Failure to accurately target lysosomal hydrolases underlies two well-known human diseases, Hurler syndrome and I-cell disease. *Hurler syndrome* is caused by a mutation in a hydrolase responsible for breakdown of glycosaminoglycans that prevents the hydrolase from acquiring the mannose-6-phosphate (M6P) modification, consequently preventing targeting to lysosomes. Similarly, in *I-cell diseases* undigested material accumulates in lysosomes because a mutation in the enzymes that create the M6P modification, causes missorting of lysosomal hydrolases.

Autophagy: A Lysosomal Degradation Pathway

Autophagy, the most common name for *macroautophagy*, consists in the capture and degradation of cellular components and organelles. Cellular material is sequestered inside double-membrane vesicles, called autophagosomes, and degraded upon fusion with lysosomal compartments. Raw precursors are then recycled for new biosyntheses. Constitutive autophagy serves to demolish damaged organelles or cytosolic components and contributes to the maintenance of cell homeostasis.

Autophagy is also stress responsive. It accelerates the catabolism of cellular components to sustain the demand of energy in adverse conditions and promotes cell survival. From yeast to human cells, starvation typically activates autophagy. Yeast has been a useful model microorganism to identify the first autophagy genes (ATG) that allowed the subsequent isolation of the mammalian counterparts. Atg proteins are involved in the basic mechanism of autophagy on which a complex regulation has been superimposed in mammals to respond to a wider variety of hormonal, environmental and intracellular signals. An increasing body of evidence suggests that autophagy plays an important role in development and cell differentiation by facilitating cell and tissue remodeling. Remarkably, the basis for erythrocyte maturation into reticulocytes, which involves mitochondria loss, remained mysterious for decades, but is now known to be partly dependent on autophagy (mitophagy).

Defects in constitutive autophagy compromise fitness of an organism. As a consequence, defective autophagy increases susceptibility to tumorigenesis, neurodegenerative disorders, liver disease, aging, inflammatory diseases and defective host defense against pathogens. However, recent evidence suggests autophagy provides a survival advantage for tumor cells in a hostile microenvironment. Thus, autophagy is regarded as a target for tumor prevention and cancer therapy.

Sorting Into Regulated Secretory Granules

In regulated secretion proteins are condensed into stored secretory granules that require an appropriate stimulus for release from the cell (see Fig. 5.4, pathway 7). After budding from TGN, the granule proteins are concentrated (up to 200-fold in some cases) by selective removal of extraneous contents from clathrin-coated vesicles. Mature secretory granules are thought to be stored in association with microtubules until the stimulation of a surface receptor triggers their exocytosis. One example of stimulus-induced exocytosis is the binding of a ligand to the T-cell antigen receptor (TCR) complex on a cytotoxic T lymphocyte. Conjugation of a cytotoxic T cell with its target causes its microtubules and associated secretory granules to reorient toward the target cell. Subsequently, the granules are delivered along microtubules until they fuse with the plasma membrane, releasing their contents for lysis of the target cell. Following release of the granule contents, the granule membrane components are internalized and transported back to the TGN, where the granule can be refilled with cargo proteins.

ENDOCYTIC TRAFFIC

Overview

Substances are imported from the cell exterior by a process termed *endocytosis* (see Fig. 5.4, pathway 9). Endocytosis also serves to recover the plasma membrane lipids and proteins that are lost by ongoing secretory activity. There are three types of endocytosis: (1) phagocytosis (cell eating), (2) pinocytosis (cell drinking) and (3) receptor-mediated endocytosis. Defects in endocytosis can underlie human diseases. For example, patients with familial hypercholesterolemia (FH) have elevated serum cholesterol because of mutations in the low-density lipoprotein (LDL) receptor that prevents the endocytic uptake of LDL and its catabolism in lysosomes.

Phagocytosis

During *phagocytosis*, cells are able to ingest large particles (greater than 0.5 μm in diameter) which serves not only to engulf and destroy invading bacteria and fungi but also to clear cellular debris at wound sites and to dispose of aged erythrocytes. Primarily, specialized cells, including macrophages, neutrophils and dendritic cells, execute phagocytosis. Phagocytosis is triggered when specific receptors contact structural triggers on the particle, including bound antibodies, complement components as well as certain oligosaccharides. Then actin polymerization is stimulated, driving the extension of pseudopods, which surround the particle and engulf it in a vacuole called phagosome. The engulfed material is destroyed when the phagosome fuses with a lysosome, exposing the content to hydrolytic enzymes. In addition, phagocytosis is a means of "presenting" the pathogen's components to lymphocytes, thus eliciting an immune response.

Pinocytosis

Pinocytosis refers to the constitutive ingestion of fluid in small pinocytotic (endocytic) vesicles (0.2 μm in diameter) and occurs in all cells. Following invagination and budding, the vesicle becomes part of the endosome system that is described later. The plasma membrane portion that is ingested returns later through exocytosis. In some cells, pinocytosis can result in turnover of the entire plasma membrane in less than 1 hour.

Receptor-Mediated Endocytosis

Receptor-mediated endocytosis is a means to import macromolecules from the extracellular fluid. More than 20 different receptors are internalized through this pathway. Some receptors are internalized continuously whereas others remain on the surface until a ligand is bound. In either case, the receptors slide laterally into coated pits that are invaginated regions of the plasma membrane surrounded by clathrin and pinch off to form clathrin-coated vesicles. The immediate destination of these vesicles is the endosome.

The endosome is part of a complex network of interrelated membranous vesicles and tubules termed the *endolysosomal system*. The endolysosomal system comprises four types of membrane-bound structures: early endosomes (EEs), late endosomes (LEs), recycling vesicles, and lysosomes. It is still a matter of debate whether these structures represent independent stable compartments or one structure matures into the next. The interior of the endosomes is acidic (pH about 6). Endocytosed material is ultimately delivered to the lysosome, presumably by fusion with LE. Lysosomes also digest obsolete parts of the cell in a process called autophagy.

During the formation of clathrin-coated vesicles, clathrin molecules do not recognize cargo receptors directly but rather through the adaptor proteins, that form an inner coat. The AP-2 components bind both clathrin and sorting signals present in the cytoplasmic tails of cargo receptors close to the plasma membrane. These internalization motifs are: YXXϕ (where ϕ is a hydrophobic amino acid), as a most common motif, and the NPXY signal that was first identified in the LDL receptor. For receptors that are internalized in response to ligand binding, the internalization signal may also be generated by a conformational change induced by the binding of the ligand. Through the specificity of the AP-2 complex, the capture of a unique set of cargo receptors is linked to vesiculation resulting in concentration of the cargo. The coated pit pinches off from the plasma membrane by the action of a GTP-binding protein, dynamin, which forms a ring around the neck of each bud and contributes to the vesicle formation. After release and shedding of the clathrin coat, the vesicle fuses with the EE compartment.

SPECIFICITY OF VESICULAR TARGETING

As described earlier, COPI-, COPII-vesicles transport material early in the secretory pathway whereas clathrin-coated vesicles transport material between the plasma membrane and Golgi. Coating proteins assemble at specific areas of the membrane in a process controlled by the coat-recruitment GTPases: Arf1 is responsible for the assembly of COPI coats and clathrin coats at Golgi membranes whereas Sar1p is responsible for COPII coat assembly at the ER membrane. In yeast, the process of vesiculation in the transport from the ER to Golgi has been dissected at a molecular level. On the cytosolic face of the ER membrane, Sar1p is activated by the ER localized GEF Sec12p. Sar1-GTP assembles with the Sec23-Sec24 complex whose Sec24 subunit binds directly or through a membrane receptor to specific signals displayed by the cargo. This prebudding cargo complex recruits the outer layer Sec13-Sec31 complex leading to coat polymerization, membrane deformation and COPII-vesicle formation.

Clathrin-coat assembly at the plasma membrane is also thought to involve a GTPase but its identity is unknown. These regulatory proteins also ensure that membrane traffic to and from an organelle are balanced.

After budding, vesicles are transported to their final destination by diffusion or motor-mediated transport along the cytoskeletal network (microtubules or actin). The molecular motors kinesin, dynein and myosin have been implicated in this process. The vesicles undergo an uncoating process before fusion with the correct target membrane. Both transport vesicles and target membranes display surface markers that selectively recognize each other.

Three classes of proteins guide the selectivity of transport vesicle docking and fusion: (i) complementary sets of vesicles SNAREs, v-SNAREs, (soluble NSF association protein receptor) and target membrane SNAREs (t-SNAREs) that are crucial for the fusion, (ii) a class of GTPases, called Rabs, and (iii) protein complexes called tethers that, together with Rabs, facilitate the initial docking of the vesicles to the target membrane.

Rab GTPases function as the master regulators of membrane traffic but are themselves regulated by factors that control their activation by GEFs or their inactivation by GAP, proteins that stimulate the intrinsic GTPase activity.

CONCLUSIONS

The mechanisms regulating protein synthesis, processing, degradation and transport are under intense investigation. Protein motifs and their cognate receptors have been identified for many intracellular sorting and processing reactions. Studies are now directed to elucidate these processes at a molecular level by resolution of the three dimensional structures of the proteins involved in protein processing and trafficking. The future challenge will be to find ways of exploiting this knowledge to intervene in the numerous disease states that result from errors in these processes.

SUGGESTED READINGS

Amm I, Sommer T, Wolf DH: Protein quality control and elimination of protein waste: the role of the ubiquitin-proteasome system. *Biochim Biophys Acta* 1:182–2014, 1843.

Bagola K, Mehnert M, Jarosch E, et al: Protein dislocation from the ER. *Biochim Biophys Acta* 3:925–2011, 1808.

Breitling J, Aebi M: N-linked protein glycosylation in the endoplasmic reticulum. *Cold Spring Harb Perspect Biol* 5(8):a013359, 2013.

Cao SS, Kaufman RJ: Unfolded protein response. *Curr Biol* 22(16):R622–R626, 2012.

Cao SS, Kaufman RJ: Endoplasmic Reticulum Stress and Oxidative Stress in Cell Fate Decision and Human Disease. *Antioxid Rredox Signal* 21:396–413, 2014.

Dancourt J, Barlowe C: Protein sorting receptors in the early secretory pathway. *Annu Rev Biochem* 79:777–802, 2010.

Fabian MR, Sonenberg N, Filipowicz W: Regulation of mRNA translation and stability by microRNAs. *Annu Rev Biochem* 79:351–379, 2010.

Freeze HH: Understanding human glycosylation disorders: biochemistry leads the charge. *J Biol Chem* 288(10):6936–6945, 2013.

Fujiki Y, Yagita Y, Matsuzaki T: Peroxisome biogenesis disorders: molecular basis for impaired peroxisomal membrane assembly: in metabolic functions and biogenesis of peroxisomes in health and disease. *Biochim Biophys Acta* 1822(9):1337–1342, 2012.

Hershey JW, Sonenberg N, Mathews MB: Principles of translational control: an overview. *Cold Spring Harb Perspect Biol* 4(12):2012.

Hong W, Lev S: Tethering the assembly of SNARE complexes. *Trends Cell Biol* 24(1):35–43, 2014.

Kim PK, Hettema EH: Multiple Pathways for Protein Transport to Peroxisomes. *J Mol Biol* 427(6PA):1176–1190, 2015.

Pfeffer SR, Novick PJ: Membrane traffic. *Curr Opin Cell Biol* 22(4):419–421, 2010.

Shrimal S, Cherepanova NA, Gilmore R: Cotranslational and posttranslocational N-glycosylation of proteins in the endoplasmic reticulum. *Semin Cell Dev Biol* 2014.

Sommer T, Wolf DH: The ubiquitin-proteasome-system. *Biochim Biophys Acta* 1843(1):1, 2014.

Tannous A, Pisoni GB, Hebert DN, et al: N-linked sugar-regulated protein folding and quality control in the ER. *Semin Cell Dev Biol* 41:79, 2015.

Wang M, Kaufman RJ: The impact of the endoplasmic reticulum protein-folding environment on cancer development. *Nat Rure Rev Cancer* 14(9):581–597, 2014.

Wente SR, Rout MP: The nuclear pore complex and nuclear transport. *Cold Spring Harb Perspect Biol* 2(10):a000562, 2010.

Wenz LS, Opalinski L, Wiedemann N, et al: Cooperation of protein machineries in mitochondrial protein sorting. *Biochim Biophys Acta* 1853(5):1119–1129, 2015.

REFERENCES

For the complete list of references, log on to www.expertconsult.com.

CHAPTER 6

PROTEIN ARCHITECTURE: RELATIONSHIP OF FORM AND FUNCTION

Jia-huai Wang and Michael J. Eck

Previous chapters have outlined the central dogma of molecular biology: the storage of genetic information in DNA and its regulated transcription into messenger RNA and eventual translation into proteins. In this chapter, we briefly outline the chemical structure of proteins and their posttranslational modifications. We explain how the properties of the 20 amino acids of which proteins are composed allow these polymers to fold into compact, functional domains and how particular domains and motifs have been assembled, modified, and reused in the course of evolution. Finally we describe a sampling of proteins and domains of relevance to the hematologist and explore briefly how point mutations, chromosomal translocations, and other genetic alterations may modify protein structure and function to cause disease.

AMINO ACIDS AND THE PEPTIDE BOND

Proteins are linear polymers of the 20 naturally occurring amino acids, linked together by the peptide bond. All of the amino acids share a common core or backbone structure and differ only in the "side chain" emanating from the central "α-carbon" of this core. The common backbone elements include an amino group, the central α-carbon, and a carboxylic acid group. Peptide bonds are formed by reaction of the carboxylic acid of one amino acid with the amino group of the next amino acid in the chain. This reaction is templated and catalyzed by the ribosome and leads to the release of water formed by the loss of an –OH group from the carboxylic acid of one amino acid residue and a hydrogen atom from the amino group of the next residue in the chain. Coupling of multiple amino acids together via the peptide bond produces the repeating main-chain structure of the polypeptide chain, composed of the amide (NH) nitrogen, alpha carbon (Cα), and carbonyl carbon (CO), followed by the amide nitrogen of the next amino acid in the chain (Fig. 6.1A). The resonant, partial double-bond character of the peptide bond prevents rotation about this bond; thus the five main-chain carbon, nitrogen, and oxygen atoms of each peptide unit lie in a plane. The conformational flexibility in the polypeptide chain is conferred by rotation about the bonds on either side of the α-carbon atom; these bond angles are referred to as phi and psi angles. The angle of the N–Cα bond is the phi angle (Φ), and that of the Cα–CO bond is the psi angle (ψ).

The *primary structure* or primary sequence of a protein refers to the order in which various residues of the 20 amino acids are assembled into the polypeptide chain, and this sequence is critically important for determining the three-dimensional fold and thus function of the protein. It is the diverse chemical structure and physicochemical properties of the 20 amino acid side chains that guide the three-dimensional fold of proteins and also provide for the enormous repertoire of protein function, from catalysis of myriad chemical reactions to immune recognition, to establishment of muscle and skeletal structure.

The amino acids can be divided into general classes based on the physicochemical properties of their side chains, and in particular their propensity to interact with water. *Hydrophobic* amino acids have aliphatic or aromatic side chains and include alanine, valine, leucine, isoleucine, proline, methionine, and phenylalanine. The hydrophobic amino acids predominate in the interior of proteins, where they are sequestered from water. They tend to pack against each other via *van der Waals* interactions, which contribute to the overall stability of folded protein domains. By contrast, *hydrophilic,* or *polar,* amino acids (including serine, threonine, tyrosine, asparagine, glutamine, cysteine, and tryptophan) are often exposed on the surface of proteins, where they can form *hydrogen bonds* with each other, with the protein main chain, and with water or ligand molecules. Hydrogen bonding refers to the attractive interaction of a proton covalently bonded to one electronegative atom (usually a nitrogen or oxygen in proteins) with another electronegative atom. Hydrogen bonds are an important contributor to the stability of proteins and to the specificity of protein–protein and protein–ligand interactions. *Charged* amino acids are also polar and are important participants in hydrogen bonding. Hydrogen bonds between negatively charged (acidic) and positively charged (basic) amino acids, also termed *salt bridges,* are also important components of protein stability and protein–protein interactions. The acidic amino acids are aspartate and glutamate, and the basic amino acids are lysine, arginine, and histidine. Histidine merits special mention, as it is the only amino acid whose side chain can be protonated or unprotonated, and therefore charged or uncharged, around physiologic ranges of pH. For this reason, histidine is part of many enzyme-active sites. For example, in the serine proteases of the coagulation cascade, an active site histidine acts as a general base, accepting and then releasing a proton in sequential steps of the enzymatic reaction. It is also important to note that some of the polar amino acids are *amphipathic*; in other words, they have both polar and hydrophobic character. This dual nature of threonine, lysine, tyrosine, arginine, and tryptophan makes them well suited for participating in protein–protein interactions, where they may be alternately exposed to solvent or buried upon formation of a complex.

Protein Secondary Structure

The alternating pattern of hydrogen bond–donating amide groups and hydrogen bond–accepting carbonyl groups gives rise to repeating elements of protein structure that are stabilized by hydrogen bonds between these main-chain groups. These *secondary structure* elements include α-helices and β-sheets. In an α-helix, the main chain adopts a right-handed helical conformation in which the carbonyl oxygen of the ith residue in the polypeptide chain accepts a hydrogen bond from the amide nitrogen of the $(I+4)^{th}$ residue (see Fig. 6.1B). The pattern may repeat for only a few residues, forming a single turn of β-helix, or for more than 100 residues, forming dozens of turns of helix. There are 3.6 residues per turn of helix, and the pitch or rise of the helix is 1.5 Å per residue or 5.4 Å per turn. The side chains of residues in an α-helix project outward, away from the central axis of the helix. Often a polar side chain will "cap" the end of a helix by forming a hydrogen bond with the otherwise unpartnered amide or carbonyl group at the N- or C-terminal end of the helix.

In a β-sheet secondary structure, the protein backbone adopts an extended conformation and two or more strands are arranged side by side, with hydrogen bonds between the strands. The strands can run in the same direction (parallel β-sheet) or antiparallel to one another.

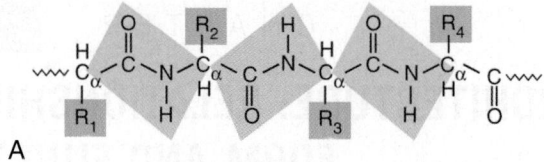

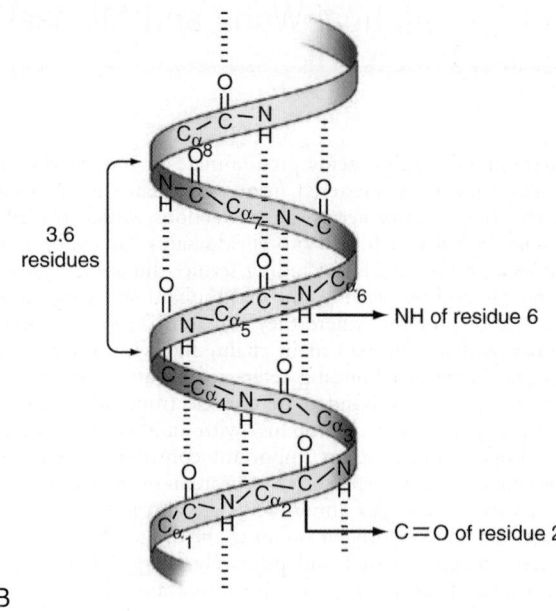

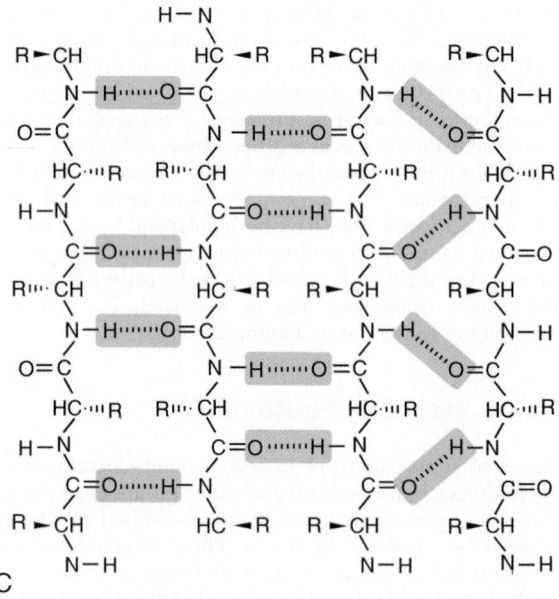

Fig. 6.1 (A) Diagram showing a polypeptide chain where the main-chain atoms are represented as peptide units, linked through the Cα atoms. Each peptide unit is a planar, rigid group *(shaded in pink)* and has two degrees of freedom; it can rotate around the Cα–CO bond and the N–Cα bond. The peptide bonds are depicted in the trans conformation: adjacent Cα carbons and their side chains *(highlighted in blue)* on opposite sides of the N–C bond. This is the preferred configuration for most amino acids, as it minimizes steric hindrance. (B) The α-helix. The hydrogen bonds between residue *n* and residue *n* + 4, which stabilizes the helix, are shown as *dashed lines*. (C) Schematic drawing of a mixed β-sheet. The first three β-strands are antiparallel to one another, whereas the last two β-strands are parallel. The hydrogen bonds that stabilize their structures are highlighted.

Mixed sheets with both parallel and antiparallel strands are also possible (see Fig. 6.1C). In β-sheets, the side chains of a given strand extend alternately above and below the plane defined by the hydrogen-bonded main chains. Other common types of secondary structure include a variant of the helix with an *I* + 3 hydrogen bonding pattern (the 3_{10} helix) and specific types of β-turns, short segments connecting other elements of secondary structure that are stabilized by intrachain hydrogen bonds. Although any of the amino acids can be found within α-helices or β-sheets, the special characteristics of proline and glycine merit mention. The cyclic structure of proline means that it lacks an amide proton; thus it introduces an irregularity in hydrogen bonding. For this reason it is infrequently found in α-helices, but if present it will introduce a "kink" stemming from its constrained structure. Glycine lacks a side chain—it has only a second hydrogen atom on its α-carbon—and therefore has less steric restriction and can adopt a wider range of backbone phi and psi angles. This added flexibility means that it tends to disfavor regular secondary structure.

Because proteins are large and complicated structures, they are typically illustrated with "ribbon" diagrams that trace the path of the polypeptide backbone. In such representations helices are drawn as helical coils or cylinders, and β-strands as elongated rectangles with an arrow as a guide to the direction of the protein chain from its amino- to carboxy-terminal end. Specific side chains of amino acids of functional interest can then be added to illustrate a particular feature.

Disulfide Bonds and Posttranslational Modifications

The covalent structure of proteins is commonly modified in structurally and functionally important ways beyond the linear coupling of amino acids via the peptide bond. Regulated proteolysis can be considered a posttranslational modification and can serve an important regulatory role, as in the cleavage of prothrombin in the blood-clotting cascade. The structure of cell-surface and extracellular proteins is often stabilized by *disulfide bonds*, covalent bonds formed between the thiol groups of spatially juxtaposed cysteine residues. In general, disulfide bonds are not found in intracellular proteins, where the reducing environment disfavors their formation. Disulfide bonds can form between cysteines within the same polypeptide chain, stabilizing the fold of the polypeptide backbone, or they may covalently join two different polypeptide chains, such as the heavy and light chains of immunoglobulins. In addition to their role in disulfide bond formation, cysteine residues often contribute to protein stability via their participation in metal ion coordination, in particular zinc, which is often bound by conserved sets of cysteine and histidine residues in small protein domains.

A number of functional groups are appended to proteins to regulate their function, localization, protein interactions, and degradation. Examples of these posttranslational modifications (PTMs) include phosphorylation, glycosylation, ubiquitination, methylation, acetylation, and lipidation.[1] PTMs occur at distinct amino acid side chains or peptide linkages; they are most often mediated by enzymatic activity and can occur at any step in the "life cycle" of a protein. As discussed below, a number of protein domains have evolved to recognize and bind specifically to proteins labeled by a particular PTM. Protein *phosphorylation*, most commonly on serine, threonine, or tyrosine residues, is one of the most important and well-studied posttranslational modifications. Phosphorylation is mediated by protein kinases and can activate or deactivate many enzymes through conformational changes and as such plays a critical role in the regulation of many cellular processes including cell cycle, growth, apoptosis, and signal transduction pathways. Protein *glycosylation* encompasses a diverse selection of sugar-moiety additions to proteins that ranges from simple monosaccharide modifications to highly complex branched polysaccharides. Glycosylation has significant effects on protein folding, conformation, distribution, stability, and activity. Carbohydrates in the form of asparagine-linked (N-linked) or serine/threonine-linked (O-linked) oligosaccharides are major structural components of many cell surface and secreted proteins, and also of many viral proteins. Protein *methylation* on arginine or lysine residues is carried out by methyltransferases with *S*-adenosyl methionine (SAM) as the primary methyl group donor. Methylation is an important mechanism of epigenetic regulation, as histone methylation and demethylation influence the availability of DNA for transcription. *N-acetylation*, the transfer of an acetyl group to the amine nitrogen at the N-terminus of the polypeptide chain, occurs in a majority of eukaryotic proteins. Lysine acetylation and deacetylation is an important regulatory mechanism in a number of proteins. It is best characterized in histones, where histone acetyl transferases (HATs) and histone deacetylases (HDACs) regulate gene expression via modification of histone tails. Many cytoplasmic proteins are also acetylated, and therefore acetylation seems to play a greater role in cell biology than simply transcriptional regulation.[2] *Lipidation* is a modification that targets proteins to membranes in organelles, vesicles, and the plasma membrane. Examples of lipidation include *myristoylation, palmitoylation,* and *prenylation.* Each type of modification gives proteins distinct membrane affinities, although all types of lipidation increase the hydrophobicity of a protein and thus its affinity for membranes. In N-myristoylation, the myristoyl group (14-carbon saturated fatty acid) is transferred to an N-terminal glycine by N-myristoyltransferase. The myristoyl group does not always permanently anchor the protein in the membrane; in a number of proteins the N-terminal myristoyl group has been observed to pack into the protein core. N-myristoylation can therefore act as a conformational localization switch, in which protein conformational changes influence the availability of the handle for membrane attachment.

The Domain Structure of Proteins

In general, the minimal biologically functional unit of protein three-dimensional structure is the protein *domain*. Domains are locally compact and semi-independent units of usually contiguous polypeptide chain. The common size of a domain is between 100 and 200 amino acid residues, although much larger and smaller domains are also frequently observed. Protein domains are composed of closely packed secondary structure elements—α-helices, β-sheets, or a combination of both—and the loops that connect them. Domains are stabilized by hydrophobic interactions among these elements and typically have very hydrophobic central cores, with more hydrophilic amino acids extending from their surface. Alternating patterns of hydrophobic residues in secondary structure elements are a reflection of the role of hydrophobicity in driving protein folding and stability. Helices are often amphipathic and pack in a folded domain such that their hydrophobic face is buried in the domain interior and their hydrophilic face is exposed on the surface. Likewise, β-sheets often have a buried hydrophobic face and an exposed hydrophilic face. The importance of the hydrophobic core to the stability of protein domains is highlighted by the fact that point mutations that introduce polar or charged residues into the protein interior often cause misfolding and thus a loss of function. Although these general characteristics are shared by protein domains that are found in an aqueous environment, such as that on the cytosol or on the cell surface, membrane-embedded proteins have very different properties reflective of their residence in the lipid bilayer. Several common domain structures representing different categories with regard to their secondary structure composition are shown in Fig. 6.2.

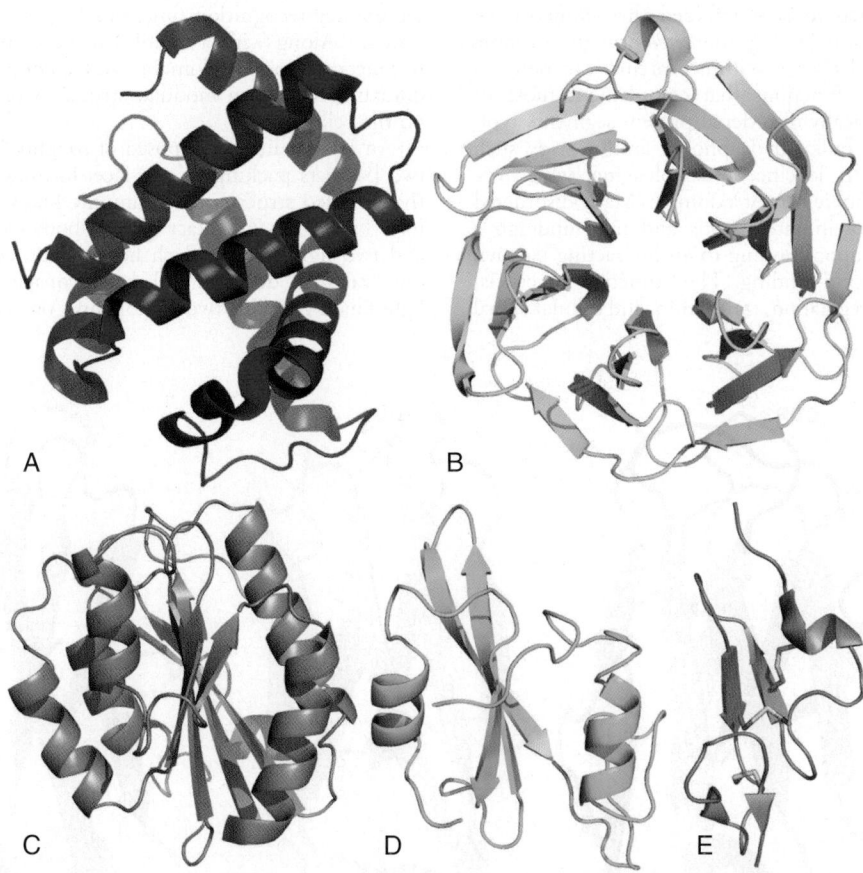

Fig. 6.2 SEVERAL COMMON DOMAIN STRUCTURES. (A) The α-globin domain of hemoglobin is all α-helical (Protein Data Bank [PDB] entry 2MHB). (B) The β-propeller domain is an all β-strand structure found in many extracellular matrix and cell surface proteins (PDB entry 1NPE). (C) The integrin "I" domain is composed of alternate β-strands and α-helices (PDB entry 1ID0). (D) The SH2 (Src homology-2) domain is found in proteins involved in tyrosine kinase signaling and is also a mixed α/β fold (PDB entry 1FMK). (E) The EGF (epidermal growth factor) domain is found in many extracellular matrix proteins and cell adhesion molecules. Its structure is stabilized by 3 to 4 disulfide bonds (PDB entry 1UZJ).

Deciphering this basic protein building block is key for understanding the structure and evolution of proteins. Kinetically, the domain structure of a protein may simplify the folding process into a step-wise course.[3] Thus a long amino acid sequence may fold into multiple domains rapidly and correctly. For many proteins, individual domains fold in a cotranslational manner; from the N-terminal region, a growing nascent polypeptide chain immediately begins to fold domain-by-domain during translation from the ribosome in a very efficient manner.[4] Genetically, it was long suspected that the exon structure of genes was correlated with the domain structure of proteins.[5] Subsequent multigenome analysis did find a strong correlation between domain organization and exon–intron arrangement in genomic DNA. The exon–domain correlation facilitates extensive exon shuffling events during evolution,[6] although it is not necessarily always one-exon/one-domain. This mechanism ensures that a stable and functionally efficient domain can be repeatedly used as a module assembled into many proteins with shared functions. A well-known early example is the nucleotide-binding domain identified in various dehydrogenases; its robust alternate β-strand–α-helix–β-strand fold provides a common structural unit for these enzymes.[7]

Recent computational approaches demonstrate that almost all the growing number of known sequences come from new combinations of various domains, and more than 70% of all sequences can be partially modeled from known structures with homologous domains.[8] This has been reflected in the human genome sequence.[9] Impressive progress has already been made in computational protein prediction and design, principally based on the known structural elements.[10]

Importantly, not all protein sequences fold into a compact domain. Depending on computational methods used, 35% to 50% of the human proteome is estimated to lack a folded three-dimensional structure. Nevertheless, these *intrinsically disordered* proteins (or more often, intrinsically disordered regions within proteins) can perform critically important biologic functions that complement those of structured proteins.[11] Intrinsically disordered protein segments typically contain relatively few bulky hydrophobic amino acids such as tryptophan, phenylalanine, leucine, and isoleucine, which are required to form the hydrophobic core of a domain. Many disordered regions mediate protein–protein interactions and may undergo a disorder-to-order transition upon binding to an interacting partner, a process dubbed folding-upon-binding. They function in crucial areas such as transcriptional regulation, translation, and cellular signal transduction.[12] Unstructured segments are well suited for protein interactions controlled by posttranslational modifications. For example, sites of tyrosine phosphorylation are typically unstructured and therefore accessible for modification, but after phosphorylation they become ordered upon phosphorylation-dependent binding to a partner protein.

Most proteins are composed of multiple domains, which may confer multiple functions, couple a targeting function to a catalytic function, or provide for allosteric regulation. In the following sections we highlight the structure of a few proteins and domains and that are of central and recurring importance in hematology in order to illustrate the relationship between domain architecture and function. We discuss representative examples from the extracellular space (the immunoglobulin domain), from intracellular signaling (protein kinase domain), and from the cell membrane (G protein–coupled receptors and the vitamin K receptor).

The Immunoglobulin Domain and Variations

As implied by its name, the immunoglobulin (Ig) domain was first recognized in antibodies.[13] A detailed discussion on antibody biology can be found in Chapter 24. The human genome project has identified the Ig superfamily (IgSF) as the largest superfamily in human genome, due to its extensive usage in a more recently developed immune system in vertebrates.[9] In fact, the Ig domain is an evolutionarily ancient structural unit that can be found in *Caenorhabditis elegans*.[14] Although Ig-like domains also exist in a few intracellular proteins, they are found predominantly in the extracellular space and are the most abundant structural unit found in cell surface receptors, serving key recognition functions in both the immune and nervous systems. Along with a handful of other modular domains such as fibronectin type III domains and epidermal growth factor (EGF) domains, they form modular structures of most receptor molecules on the cell surface.[15]

An Ig domain is composed of roughly 100 residues, folding into two β-sheets packing face-to-face, forming a β-barrel. This distinctively folded structure is commonly known as the immunoglobulin fold (Fig. 6.3A). An intact IgG antibody consists of two heavy chains and two light chains. Each heavy chain contains four Ig domains, one "variable" domain, and three "constant" domains; whereas each light chain contains two Ig domains, one constant and one variable.

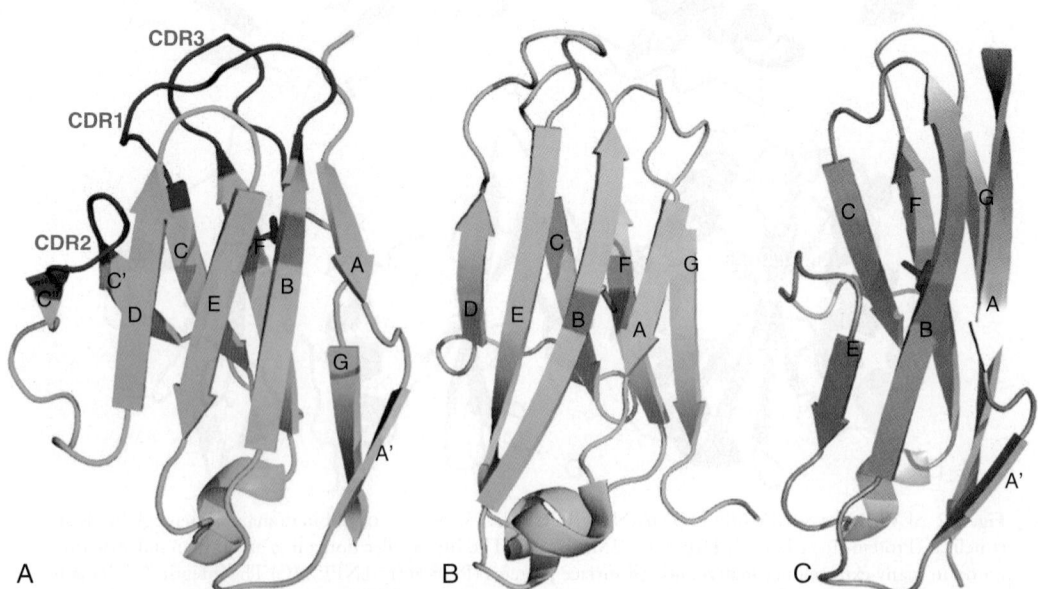

Fig. 6.3 Ig DOMAIN ARCHITECTURE. (A) V-set Ig domain (Protein Data Bank [PDB] entry 3IDG). (B) C-set Ig domain (3IDG). (C) I-set Ig domain, which can be described as a truncated V-set domain (PDB entry 2V5M). Disulfide bonds are highlighted in *orange*.

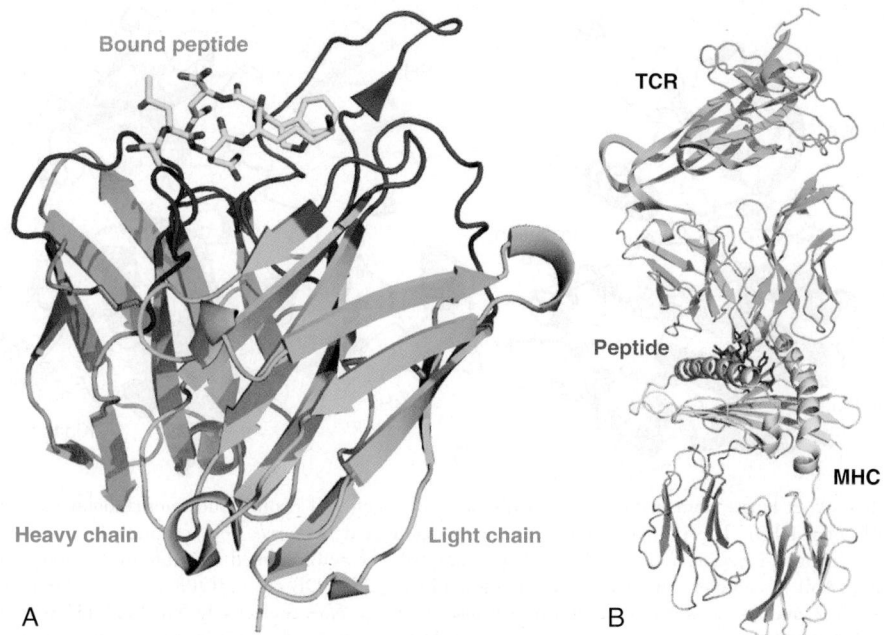

Fig. 6.4 (A) Structure of an HIV-neutralizing antibody in complex with an antigenic peptide. Complementarity-determining region of the heavy and light chains are shown in *red* and *purple*, respectively. Note that only the two variable domains of the antibody are shown (drawn from Protein Data Bank [PDB] entry 3IDG). (B) Structure of an antigenic peptide bound to a major histocompatibility complex (MHC) molecule in complex with T-cell receptors (TCR) (PDB entry 2CKB).

The variable and constant Ig domains differ somewhat in structure and are correspondingly classified as V-set and C-set Ig folds. A V-set Ig domain has β-strands A, B, E, and D on one sheet and A', G, F, C, C', and C'' strands on the other (Fig. 6.3A), whereas a C-set Ig domain lacks A', C', and C'' strands on either edge (Fig. 6.3B). In both, the two sheets are linked together by a conserved disulfide bond between the B and F strands (as reviewed by Williams et al[16]). Within variable domains, hypervariable sequences are found in three connecting loops at one end of the domain. These loops are termed complementarity-determining regions or CDRs (Fig. 6.3A). In the intact antibody, the CDRs of the heavy and light chains combine to make up the antigen-binding site. Fig. 6.4A depicts how the CDRs of an HIV-neutralizing antibody form an antigen-binding pocket that recognizes an antigenic peptide from an HIV surface protein.[17] A similar structural platform is used in cellular immunity by T-cell receptors (TCR), which, distinct from antibodies, recognize an antigenic peptide along with the MHC (major histocompatibility complex) molecule that presents the peptide on the infected cell surface. In this case, CDR3 loops of the variable domains of TCR play a key role in antigen recognition, whereas germline-encoded CDR1 and CDR2 loops are responsible for contacting the polymorphic region of the MHC molecule, with CDR1 also taking part in peptide binding.[18,19] Fig. 6.4B illustrates a typical structure of a TCR in a complex with an antigenic peptide bound to the MHC molecule. An extensive discussion on the role of these proteins in cellular immunity can be found in Chapter 21.

A number of variations on the Ig fold are found in other cell surface receptors. These Ig-like domains include the topologically similar fibronectin type III domains[20] and the domains of cadherins, which also assume the same strand topology.[21] The fibronectin domains and cadherins lack the disulfide bridge found in the Ig domain, which demonstrates the thermodynamic robustness of the immunoglobulin fold.

Further variations are found in modular cell surface receptors, which often have a V-set Ig-like domain at their N-terminus, positioned to extend from the plasma membrane for ligand-binding, serving a role analogous to antigen-recognition. By contrast, "I-set" Ig-like domains (see Fig. 6.3C) usually function as one of the building blocks lined up in tandem to present the ligand-binding V-set domain on the cell surface. This can be seen in many immune receptors such as CD2[22] and CD4.[23] There are also many receptors that are exclusively composed of I-set domains, including immune receptor ICAM-1 (intercellular adhesion molecule-1),[24] neuroreceptors NCAM,[25] and Dscam.[26,27] Thus the I-set variant is the most abundant Ig-like domain and plays a critical biologic role in cell surface receptors.

The Protein Kinase Domain

Protein kinases catalyze the transfer of a phosphate group from ATP to specific sites on target proteins. More than 500 protein kinases have been identified in the human genome; approximately 90 of these are tyrosine kinases, the remainder specifically phosphorylate serine or threonine residues. Both ser/thr and tyrosine kinases share a conserved bi-lobed protein fold, composed of a smaller N-terminal subdomain (N-lobe) and larger C-terminal subdomain (C-lobe).[28] The active site cleft, including the site for binding the substrate ATP, is found at the interface between the N- and C-lobes. The phosphate-coordinating "P-loop" is a portion of the β-sheet in the N-lobe that coordinates the triphosphate moiety of ATP. The activity of protein kinases is typically regulated by phosphorylation on a loop in the C-lobe termed the activation loop or A-loop. In the absence of phosphorylation the A-loop may play an inhibitory role, sometimes blocking binding of ATP in the active site; or it may be disordered altogether. Upon autophosphorylation, or phosphorylation in trans by an upstream activating kinase the activation loop rearranges to adopt a characteristic hairpin conformation that creates the site for docking of the polypeptide segment that will become phosphorylated. Activation loop phosphorylation may also induce other structural rearrangements required for catalytic activation, in particular a reorientation of a helix within the N-lobe (known as the C-helix) that brings a glutamic acid residue into proper position within the active site (see Fig. 6.5A).

Deregulated tyrosine kinases are the cause of a number of hematologic malignancies. Two general classes of tyrosine kinases can be

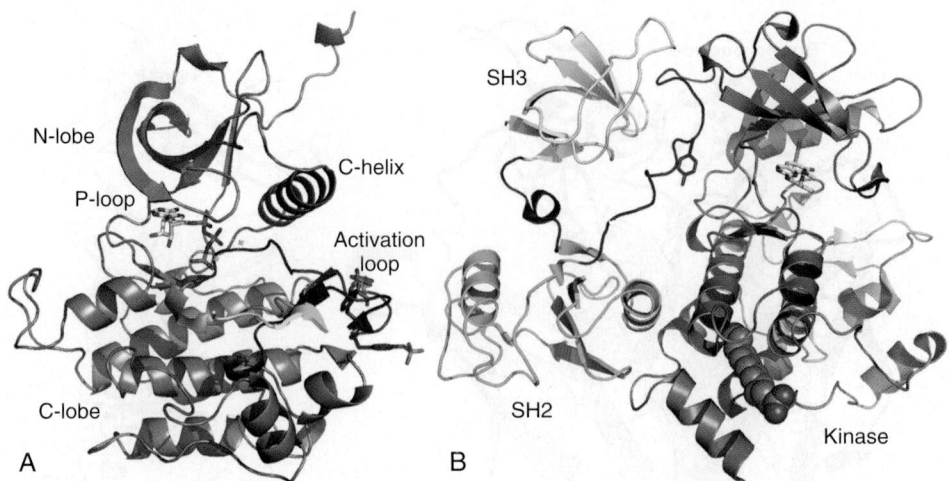

Fig. 6.5 (A) A kinase domain in complex with an ATP analog and peptide substrate (Protein Data Bank [PDB] entry 1IR3). The phosphate-binding loop is highlighted in *purple*, the activation loop is *red*, the substrate peptide is *yellow*, and the ATP analog is *gray*. (B) The autoinhibited structure of Abelson tyrosine kinase (c-Abl) in complex with the kinase inhibitor PD166326 (PDB entry 1OPK). The Src-homology-3 (SH3), SH2, and kinase domains are shown in *yellow, green,* and *blue,* respectively. The SH2–kinase-domain linker and the SH3–SH2 connector are shown in *red.* The myristate is shown in *orange spheres* in the C-lobe of the kinase.

defined: receptor and nonreceptor tyrosine kinases. Receptor tyrosine kinases are transmembrane proteins with an extracellular ligand-binding domain—often composed of Ig-like domains as described above, a single transmembrane domain, and the cytoplasmic tyrosine kinase domain. They are typically activated by dimerization upon binding of ligands to their extracellular region, which induces autophosphorylation and activation of their catalytic domains inside the cell.[29] Chromosomal translocations that underlie a number of human leukemias fuse a tyrosine kinase domain to an oligomerization domain from an otherwise unrelated protein, often the dimerization domain of a transcription factor, to generate a constitutively dimeric, and therefore constitutively active, kinase. Examples of such oncogenic translocations include the fusion of the dimerization domain of an ETS-family transcription factor to a Jak-family tyrosine kinase in the leukemogenic Tel-Jak2 fusion,[30] and the fusion of the oligomerization domain of nucleophosmin with the tyrosine kinase domain of ALK in the NPM-ALK fusion in anaplastic large cell lymphoma.[31] These translocations are further described in Chapters 56 and 73, respectively.

Perhaps the best characterized kinase translocation is the BCR–Abl fusion protein produced by the (9:22) chromosomal translocation in chronic myelogenous leukemia (see also Chapter 67). Treatment of this disease with imatinib, a specific inhibitor of Abl, has established a paradigm for targeted therapy in cancer.[32] Abl is a nonreceptor tyrosine kinase that contains Src-homology 3 and 2 (SH3 and SH2) domains in addition to its tyrosine kinase domain. Additionally, the normal Abl protein is myristoylated at its N-terminus. In the normal protein, the N-terminal region including the myristoyl-group and adjacent sequences and the SH3 and SH2 domains assemble with the kinase domain to lock it in an inactive conformation (Fig. 6.5B).[33] These interactions are released to activate the kinase when the phosphotyrosine-binding SH2 domain and proline motif-binding SH3 domains bind their cognate ligands in a target protein.[34] Upon activation the myristoyl group may also be released from its docking site in the C-lobe of the kinase to promote membrane localization of the protein.[35] Thus in its normal state the various domains of Abl comprise an exquisite signaling switch that is regulated by appropriate binding interactions; in the absence of the proper targeting interactions the kinase is maintained in an inactive state by the intramolecular associations of its domains. In the oncogenic BCR–Abl fusion protein, this regulatory control is lost because the N-terminal regulatory region including the myristoylation site is truncated and replaced with unrelated sequences from the BCR protein. Interestingly, the vacant myristate pocket in BCR–Abl is the target of recently developed allosteric inhibitors of BCR–Abl, which may synergize with ATP-site inhibitors.[36]

Membrane Proteins

Membrane proteins account for 20% to 30% of all gene products in most genomes, and they are the targets of 50% of modern drugs.[37] Proteins embedded in or transversing the lipid bilayer mediate exchange of information and materials across membrane barriers. They are architecturally and functionally diverse. Single-pass transmembrane proteins have functional extracellular and/or intracellular domains connected by a single membrane-spanning helix; for example, the receptor tyrosine kinases described previously and cell adhesion molecules such as ICAM-1 and VCAM-1, which are anchored to the endothelial surface of blood vessels for leukocyte recruitment via a single transmembrane helix.

By contrast, integral membrane proteins typically have much of their mass embedded within the lipid bilayer, with multiple membrane-spanning segments connected by cytoplasmic and extracellular loops. Historically, integral membrane proteins have been difficult to study at a structural level. However, innovations in membrane protein crystallization and protein engineering have made such studies more tractable, allowing elucidation of many important structures at near-atomic resolution. Most membrane-embedded proteins are predominately helical, although β-strand membrane proteins also occur. Diverse ion channels and G-protein–coupled receptors (GPCRs) are integral membrane proteins. One of the largest and most complicated membrane protein complexes characterized to date is that of mitochondrial complex I. This huge proton-pumping machine features 82 transmembrane helices, accounting for approximately half of its molecular mass.[38]

GPCRs are the largest family of membrane proteins—more than 800 have been identified in the human genome. GPCRs mediate fundamental signal transduction processes touching virtually every aspect of human physiology, from vision, taste, and smell to cardiovascular, endocrine, immunologic, and reproductive functions. Not surprisingly, they represent an important class of drug target. The conserved domain structure of GPCRs includes seven transmembrane helices that pack together across the lipid bilayer.[39,40] They form a

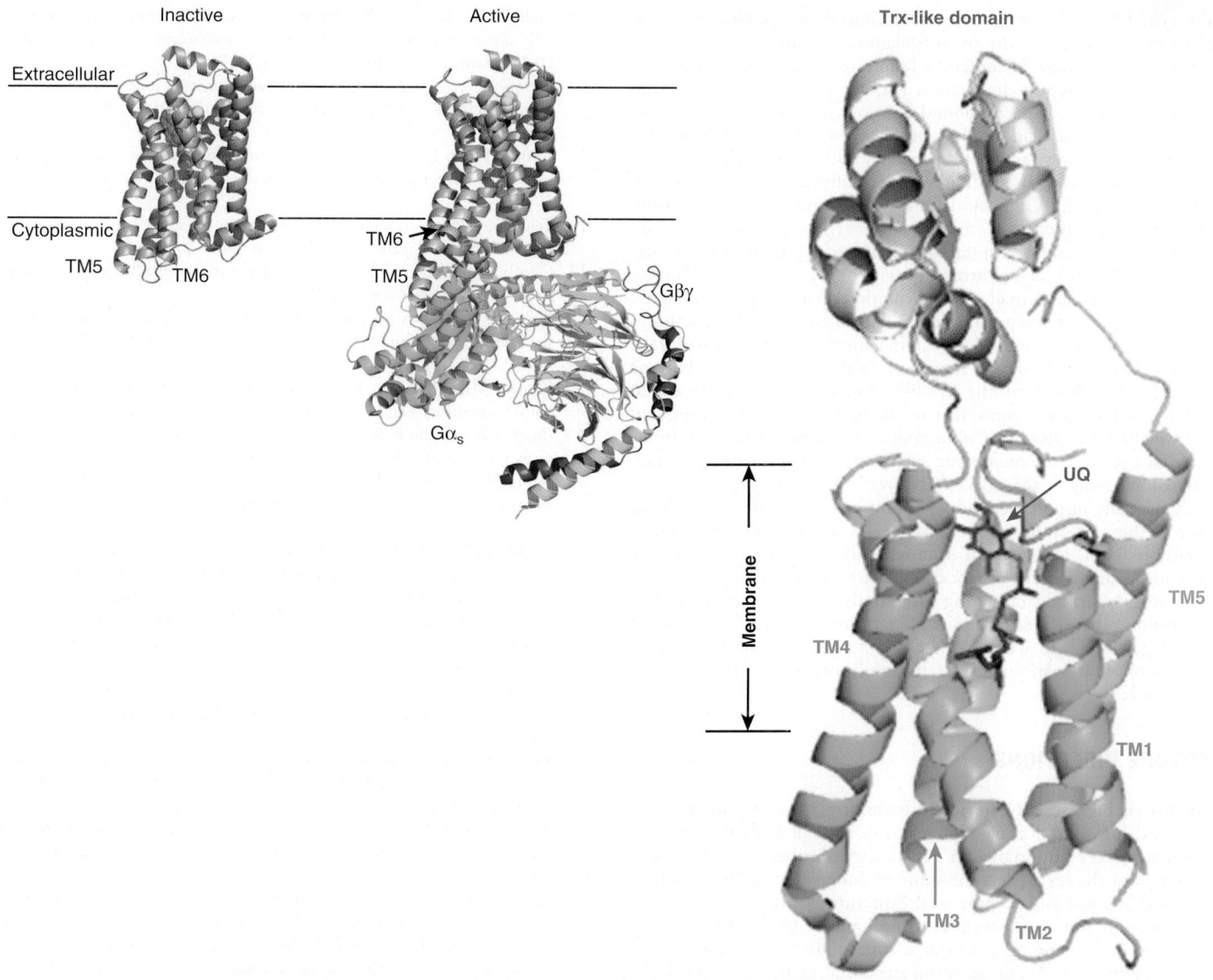

Fig. 6.6 (A) Structures of the β2 adrenergic receptor (β2AR) in the inactive *(left)* and active *(right)* conformations. Like all GPCRs, β2AR contains seven transmembrane helices. The inactive structure was determined
with the antagonist carazolol bound in the ligand binding site, whereas the active structure was determined
in complex with the tight-binding agonist BI-167107 (ligands are shown as *yellow spheres*). Agonist binding
induces conformational changes on the cytoplasmic face of the receptor, including reorientation of the sixth
transmembrane helix (TM6) and lengthening of TM5, which in turn promote binding of the heterotrimeric
Gαβγ complex. Interactions with the receptor are mediated by the Gαs subunit *(green)*. This interaction
induces exchange of GDP for GTP in the Gαs subunit, and promotes dissociation of βγ complex (shown in
cyan and *magenta* for β and γ, respectively). Illustration is drawn from Protein Data Bank (PDB) entries 2RH1
and 3SN6 for the inactive and active structures, respectively. T4 lysozyme fusion partners and a nanobody
that was engineered to facilitate crystallization are not illustrated. (B) Structure of a bacterial homolog of the
human vitamin K epoxide reductase (VKOR). VKOR is expected to bind vitamin K in a pocket homologous
to that formed by four conserved transmembrane helices *(green)* that is occupied by a ubiquinone *(magenta)*
in this structure. Warfarin inhibits VKOR by displacing vitamin K from this pocket. See text for further details.
(Illustration drawn from PDB entry 3KP9, www.rcsb.org, accessed June 1, 2016.)

ligand-binding cleft that opens to the extracellular space. The cleft
can vary dramatically in size and shape in different GPCRs, as some
receptors recognize small molecules (for example, the β2-adrenergic
receptor), whereas others have protein ligands (for example, chemokine receptors).

Structural studies of the β2-adrenergic receptor have recently
revealed its mechanism of transmembrane signal transduction via the
heterotrimeric G-protein Gαsβγ (Fig. 6.6A). Binding of the agonist
in the extracellular-facing cleft induces key conformational changes
in the cytoplasmic region, in particular a large movement of the sixth

transmembrane helix and an extension of the cytoplasmic end of the
fifth transmembrane helix. These alterations promote binding to the
Gα-subunit of Gαsβγ. In binding Gα, the agonist-bound receptor
functions as a guanine–nucleotide exchange factor (GEF), inducing
exchange of GDP for GTP. GTP-bound Gα dissociates from the βγ
heterodimer to activate adenyl cyclase, whereas the free βγ component
signals to Ca²⁺ channels. The inactive and active β2-adrenergic receptor structures are illustrated in Fig. 6.6A.

Membrane proteins can also fulfill catalytic roles; they operate
not only in the plasma membrane but in every lipid membrane in

the cell. One example of interest is vitamin K epoxide reductase (VKOR), the target of the anticoagulant drug warfarin (see Chapter 125). VKOR resides in the endoplasmic reticulum membrane, and catalyzes a key step in the vitamin K cycle: regeneration of vitamin K hydroquinone. This compound is a cofactor for the enzyme that converts glutamic acid residues in the N-termini of vitamin K–dependent clotting factors to γ-carboxy glutamate (Gla) residues. This posttranslational modification is required for interaction of these proteins with Ca^{2+}, and thus for their function in coagulation. Although the structure of the human enzyme has not been elucidated, the structure of a homologous bacterial protein was recently described.[41] In this crystal structure (Fig. 6.6B), the bacterial homologue of VKOR is naturally fused to a thioredoxin (Trx)-like domain, which supplies reducing equivalents. The core of VKOR structure is a four-helix bundle embedded in the membrane (transmembrane helices TM1–TM4, shown in green), with a fifth transmembrane helix (TM5) linked to the Trx-like domain on the extracellular surface (topologically equivalent to the luminal side of ER-resident mammalian VKOR). The ubiquinone compound has its quinone ring located near the membrane surface with its isoprenyl tail intercalated into the V-shaped cleft between TM2 and TM3. All the enzymatically important residues are on or close to the extracellular side of the membrane, adjacent to the Trx-like domain, providing a plausible path for electron transfer.[41] Interestingly, mapping of mutations that confer resistance to warfarin onto the bacterial structure reveals striking clustering around the ligand-binding pocket, confirming that it is also the site of warfarin binding. This pocket is not large enough to accommodate both vitamin K and warfarin, an indication that warfarin exerts its inhibitory effect by displacing vitamin K.[41]

FUTURE DIRECTIONS

In this chapter, we have reviewed basic principles of protein structure and introduced a few representative protein folds that recur in proteins of key importance in hematology. Further examples found throughout the text reflect the value of understanding the structural foundations of biologic processes. Structure is key for understanding macromolecular function at a mechanistic level, and by extension for understanding pathogenic mutations and mechanisms of drug action. Increasingly powerful structural methods, in particular in cryo-electron microscopy,[42,43] promise to bring ever larger and more complicated proteins and macromolecular complexes into focus.

REFERENCES

1. Walsh C: *Posttranslational modification of proteins: expanding nature's inventory*, Englewood, CO, 2006, Roberts and Co. Publishers.
2. Glozak MA, Sengupta N, Zhang X, et al: Acetylation and deacetylation of nonhistone proteins. *Gene* 363:15, 2005. doi: 10.1016/j.gene.2005.09.
3. Richardson JS: The anatomy and taxonomy of protein structure. *Adv Protein Chem* 34:167, 1981.
4. Kolb VA, Makeyev EV, Sirin AS: Co-translational folding of an eukaryotic multidomain protein in a prokaryotic translation system. *J Biol Chem* 275:16597, 2000.
5. Gilbert W: Why genes in pieces? *Nature* 271:501, 1978.
6. Liu M, Grigoriev A: Protein domains correlate strongly with exons in multiple eukaryotic genomes–evidence of exon shuffling? *Trends Genet* 20:399, 2004.
7. Rossmann MG, Moras D, Olsen KW: Chemical and biological evolution of nucleotide-binding protein. *Nature* 250:194, 1974.
8. Levitt M: Nature of the protein universe. *Proc Natl Acad Sci USA* 106:11079, 2009.
9. Lander ES, Linton LM, Birren B, et al: Initial sequencing and analysis of the human genome. *Nature* 409:860, 2001. doi: 10.1038/35057062.
10. Das R, Baker D: Macromolecular modeling with rosetta. *Annu Rev Biochem* 77:363, 2008.
11. Oldfield CJ, Dunker AK: Intrinsically disordered proteins and intrinsically disordered protein regions. *Annu Rev Biochem* 83:553, 2014. doi: 10.1146/annurev-biochem-072711-164947.
12. Dyson HJ, Wright PE: Intrinsically unstructured proteins and their functions. *Nat Rev Mol Cell Biol* 6:197, 2005. doi: 10.1038/nrm1589.
13. Bork P, Holm L, Sander C: The immunoglobulin fold. Structural classification, sequence patterns and common core. *J Mol Biol* 242:309, 1994.
14. Teichmann SA, Chothia C: Immunoglobulin superfamily proteins in Caenorhabditis elegans. *J Mol Biol* 296:1367, 2000.
15. Chothia C, Jones EY: The molecular structure of cell adhesion molecules. *Annu Rev Biochem* 66:823, 1997.
16. Williams AF, Davis SJ, He Q, et al: Structural diversity in domains of the immunoglobulin superfamily. *Cold Spring Harb Symp Quant Biol* 54(Pt 2):637, 1989.
17. Zwick MB, Komori HK, Stanfield RL, et al: The long third complementarity-determining region of the heavy chain is important in the activity of the broadly neutralizing anti-human immunodeficiency virus type 1 antibody 2F5. *J Virol* 78:3155, 2004.
18. Wang JH, Reinherz EL: The structural basis of alphabeta T-lineage immune recognition: TCR docking topologies, mechanotransduction, and co-receptor function. *Immunol Rev* 250:102, 2012. doi: 10.1111/j.1600-065X.2012.01161.x.
19. Rudolph MG, Stanfield RL, Wilson IA: How TCRs bind MHCs, peptides, and coreceptors. *Annu Rev Immunol* 24:419, 2006.
20. Parker MJ, Dempsey CE, Hosszu LL, et al: Topology, sequence evolution and folding dynamics of an immunoglobulin domain. *Nat Struct Biol* 5:194, 1998.
21. Boggon TJ, Murray J, Chappuis-Flament S, et al: C-cadherin ectodomain structure and implications for cell adhesion mechanisms. *Science* 296:1308, 2002.
22. Jones EY, Davis SJ, Williams AF, et al: Crystal structure at 2.8 A resolution of a soluble form of the cell adhesion molecule CD2. *Nature* 360:232, 1992.
23. Wu H, Kwong PD, Hendrickson WA: Dimeric association and segmental variability in the structure of human CD4. *Nature* 387:527, 1997.
24. Yang Y, Jun CD, Liu JH, et al: Structural basis for dimerization of ICAM-1 on the cell surface. *Mol Cell* 14:269, 2004.
25. Cunningham BA, Hemperly JJ, Murray BA, et al: Neural cell adhesion molecule: structure, immunoglobulin-like domains, cell surface modulation, and alternative RNA splicing. *Science* 236:799, 1987.
26. Meijers R, Puettmann-Holgado R, Skiniotis G, et al: Structural basis of Dscam isoform specificity. *Nature* 449:487, 2007.
27. Sawaya MR, Wojtowicz WM, Andre I, et al: A double S shape provides the structural basis for the extraordinary binding specificity of Dscam isoforms. *Cell* 134:1007, 2008.
28. Taylor SS, Kornev AP: Protein kinases: evolution of dynamic regulatory proteins. *Trends Biochem Sci* 36:65, 2011.
29. Lemmon MA, Schlessinger J: Cell signaling by receptor tyrosine kinases. *Cell* 141:1117, 2010.
30. Golub TR, McLean T, Stegmaier K, et al: The TEL gene and human leukemia. *Biochim Biophys Acta* 1288:M7, 1996.
31. Barreca A, Lasorsa E, Riera L, et al: Anaplastic lymphoma kinase in human cancer. *J Mol Endocrinol* 47:R11, 2011.
32. Druker BJ: Translation of the Philadelphia chromosome into therapy for CML. *Blood* 112:4808, 2008.
33. Nagar B, Hantschel O, Young MA, et al: Structural basis for the autoinhibition of c-Abl tyrosine kinase. *Cell* 112:859, 2003.
34. Nagar B, Hantschel O, Seeliger M, et al: Organization of the SH3-SH2 unit in active and inactive forms of the c-Abl tyrosine kinase. *Mol Cell* 21:787, 2006.
35. Hantschel O, Nagar B, Guettler S, et al: A myristoyl/phosphotyrosine switch regulates c-Abl. *Cell* 112:845, 2003.
36. Zhang J, Adrián FJ, Jahnke W, et al: Targeting Bcr-Abl by combining allosteric with ATP-binding-site inhibitors. *Nature* 463:501, 2010. doi: 10.1038/nature08675.
37. Overington JP, Al-Lazikani B, Hopkins AL: How many drug targets are there? *Nat Rev Drug Discov* 5:993, 2006. doi: 10.1038/nrd2199.

38. Zickermann V, Wirth C, Nasiri H, et al: Structural biology. Mechanistic insight from the crystal structure of mitochondrial complex I. *Science* 347:44, 2015. doi: 10.1126/science.1259859.

39. Rosenbaum DM, Rasmussen SG, Kobilka BK: The structure and function of G-protein-coupled receptors. *Nature* 459:356, 2009. doi: 10.1038/nature08144.

40. Katritch V, Cherezov V, Stevens RC: Structure-function of the G protein-coupled receptor superfamily. *Annu Rev Pharmacol Toxicol* 53:531, 2013. doi: 10.1146/annurev-pharmtox-032112-135923.

41. Li W, Schulman S, Dutton RJ, et al: Structure of a bacterial homologue of vitamin K epoxide reductase. *Nature* 463:507, 2010. doi: 10.1038/nature08720.

42. Scheres SH: Beam-induced motion correction for sub-megadalton cryo-EM particles. *Elife* 3:e03665, 2014. doi: 10.7554/eLife.03665.

43. Grigorieff N: Direct detection pays off for electron cryo-microscopy. *Elife* 2:e00573, 2013. doi: 10.7554/eLife.00573.

CHAPTER 7

SIGNALING TRANSDUCTION AND METABOLOMICS

Pere Puigserver

Hematopoiesis is a cellular process in which self-renewing stem progenitor cells differentiate into mature blood cells, which carry out specific biologic functions. These functions include oxygen delivery, clot formation, and defense of the host from infection. Homeostasis of the whole hematopoietic system in vivo requires a tight control of systems and networks governing proliferation, cell fate, cell death, differentiation, cell–cell interaction, and migration. Imbalance in or dysregulation of these processes results in pathologic alterations. For example, uncontrolled cell proliferation is a signature of leukemias, and defective lymphocyte differentiation can lead to immunodeficiency. A better understanding at the molecular level of these biologic events will help to identify new therapeutic targets for the design of better drugs to treat hematologic diseases.

Because of the diversity in cellular types and their respective, specific biologic functions, hematopoietic cells respond to a broad array of extrinsic and intrinsic signals transduced through signaling and metabolic pathways. It is therefore important to recognize that these pathways serve to ultimately define a specific functional response in a given cell type. These regulatory signals (Table 7.1) can be general, such as growth factors (e.g., insulin growth factor [IGF], fibroblast growth factor [FGF]), or amino acids that control proliferation, or highly specific, such as the antigen signaling response in immune cells or 2,3-diphosphoglycerate in erythrocytes. Importantly, the action of these signals, as well as their integration inside the cell, is needed to accomplish a specific cellular task (either a physiologic or cellular fate decision). Moreover, as will be discussed later in this chapter, these signals also serve to tightly control metabolites in hematopoietic cells, defining a metabolomic profile involved in processes such as anaerobic glycolysis for energy generation in red blood cells.

Extrinsic cellular signals, often polypeptides, are recognized by plasma membrane receptors that trigger a phosphorylation cascade (using tyrosine and/or serine/threonine residues) that propagates through the cytoplasm and cellular organelles, including the nucleus. Thus, the sequential activation of this cascade occurs in a temporal and spatial manner to define the specific biologic response. In general, there are two types of signals (Fig. 7.1): (1) signals that transduce immediate- or short-term biologic outputs without changes in gene expression, and (2) signals that transduce medium- and long-term biologic outputs with changes in gene expression. In the first case, for example, chemoattractants induce the phosphatidylinositol 3-kinase (PI3K) and Cdc42 pathways to rapidly establish neutrophil polarity. One example in the second case is the signaling transduced through Frizzled (Fz) receptors and the transcription factor T-cell–specific transcription factor (TCF)-1 necessary for T-cell development. In both cases, the signals transduced are amplified through a series of physical interactions and chemical modifications on proteins, the most common being phosphorylation, but others such as ubiquitination, acetylation, and sumoylation also play important roles.

In this chapter, a general survey of the different key signaling and changes in metabolite profiles that operate in hematopoietic cells will be reviewed. The goal is to provide the molecular basis by which signals are transduced and control fundamental cellular processes in different lineages of the hematopoietic system.

SIGNALING TRANSDUCTION

Hematopoietic cells use general signaling transduction pathways that are common to most cell types. The specificity in these signaling transduction pathways is often established at the beginning of the pathway's activation; for example, by specific antigen-binding or ligand–membrane receptor complexes (Table 7.2), and at downstream targets including transcription of the specific genes that will serve to define a particular biologic response (see Fig. 7.1). Here we will review these general signaling transduction pathways, illustrating some of the specific components of hematopoietic cells.

Receptor Tyrosine Kinases, Phosphoinosite-3-Kinase, and Mitogen-Activated Protein Kinase Pathways

Receptor Tyrosine Kinases

Receptor tyrosine kinases (RTKs) are enzyme-linked receptors localized at the plasma membrane containing an extracellular ligand-binding domain, a transmembrane domain, and an intracellular protein–tyrosine kinase domain. In general, the ligands for RTKs are proteins such as IGF, epidermal growth factor (EGF), platelet-derived growth factor (PDGF), and FGF. Ephrins that bind to Eph receptors also form a large subset of RTK ligands. Colony-stimulating-factor 1 (CSF-1), which is important for macrophage function, is another example of an RTK ligand. RTKs can function as monomers or multimeric subunits assembled at the plasma membrane that, upon ligand binding, cause oligomerization or conformational changes followed by tyrosine (trans)-phosphorylation in the kinase activation loop. Activation of RTKs results in phosphorylation of additional sites in the cytoplasmic part of the receptor, leading to docking of protein substrates, which initiates the intracellular signaling cascade. These substrates bind to RTK-phosphorylated tyrosines through Src Homology domain-2 (SH2) or phosphotyrosine-binding (PTB) domains. Examples of these types of proteins are insulin receptor substrates or the p85 regulatory subunit of PI3K. RTKs recruit, assemble, and phosphorylate different proteins including adaptors and enzymes.

There are mechanisms to terminate ligand-induced RTK activity through cellular processes including receptor-mediated endocytosis and/or through a family of regulated protein tyrosine phosphatases (PTPs), some of which are transmembrane and have extracellular domains, suggesting the possibility of ligand-mediated regulation. Interestingly, there is also intracellular regulation of PTPs through negative-feedback loops to attenuate the signal or direct control through reactive oxygen species (ROS) (see later discussion).

Phosphatidylinositol-3-Kinase Pathway

One of the key signaling components associated with RTKs is the phosphatidylinositol-3-kinase (PI3K) signaling transduction pathway. This pathway is also activated by cytokine receptors and G-protein–coupled receptors (GPCRs). Among the many functions of this pathway in hematopoietic cells, the IL-3–dependent survival

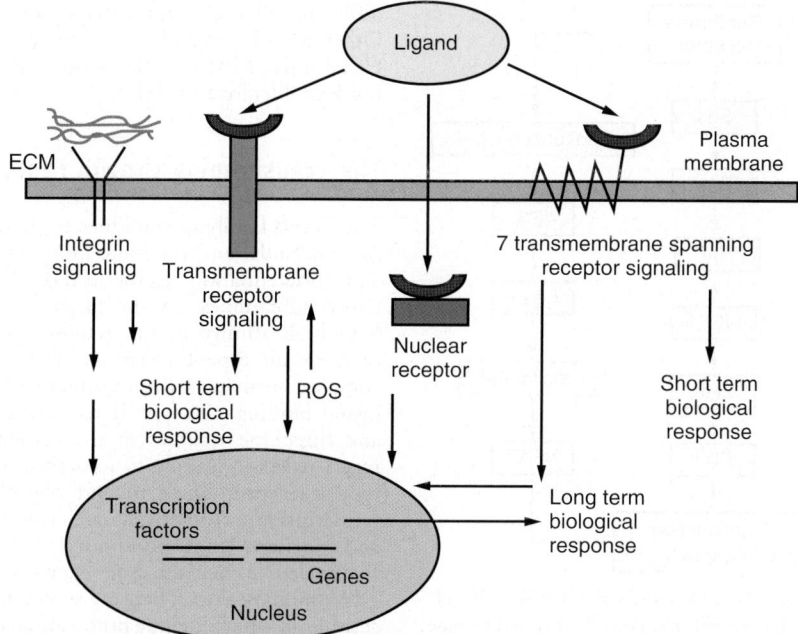

Fig. 7.1 EXAMPLES OF LIGANDS AND RECEPTORS THAT TRANSDUCE BIOLOGIC RESPONSES. Signals can originate from fixed ligands (e.g., the extracellular matrix, ECM) or soluble ligands that are not membrane permeable and bind to extracellular regions of transmembrane receptors. Membrane-permeable ligands bind to intracellular receptors, such as the nuclear receptor family. Signals can also originate from within the cell, such as increases in ROS levels. These signals cause short-term biologic outputs without changes in gene expression, or transduce medium- and long-term biologic outputs with changes in gene expression. *ECM,* Extracellular membrane; *ROS,* Reactive oxygen species.

TABLE 7.1   Signals in the Hematopoietic System

Types of Ligands	Examples
Peptide or Protein	
Soluble	Growth factors or cytokine
ECM	Fibronectin, collagen
Cell surface bound	ICAM, Kit ligand
Small organics	Thyroid hormone
Nucleotides	
Soluble	ADP
DNA	Double-strand breaks
Lipids	Eicosanoids, LPA
Gases	H_2O_2, nitric oxide[a]

[a]Function in hematopoietic system not well defined.
ADP, Adenosine diphosphate; ECM, extracellular matrix; ICAM, intercellular adhesion molecule; LPA, lipopolysaccharide.

TABLE 7.2   Receptors in the Hematopoietic System

Types of Receptors	Examples	Types of Ligands
RTK	Insulin, Kit, Fms	Kit ligand, M-CSF
RSK	TGFβ receptors	Activin, BMPs, TGF-β
GPCR	Thrombin receptor, CXC, CC receptors	Thrombin chemokines
PTK-associated MIRR	Cytokine receptors BCR/TCR/FcR	Epo, interleukins, IFN peptide/MHC, Fc domains
TNF family	Fas, TNFR, CD40	Fas, TNF, CD40L
Notch	Notch	Delta-serrate-LAG-2
Frizzled family	Wnt receptors	Wnts
Toll receptors	TLR1-10	Bacterial DNA, LPS
RPTP	CD45	Unknown
Nuclear receptors	AR, RAR	Testosterone, retinoids
Adhesion receptors	Integrins	Fibronectin, collagen

AR, Androgen receptor; BCR, B-cell antigen receptor; BMP, bone morphogenetic protein; CC, CXC, types of chemokine receptors; CD40L, ligand for CD40; Epo, erythropoietin; FcR, receptors for Fc portion of antibodies; GPCR, G protein–coupled receptor; LPS, lipopolysaccharide; M-CSF, macrophage colony-stimulating factor; MIRR, multichain immune recognition receptor; RAR, retinoic acid receptor; RPTP, receptor protein-tyrosine phosphatase; RSK, receptor serine kinase; RTK, receptor tyrosine kinase; TCR, T-cell antigen receptor; TGFβ, transforming growth factor β; TNF, tumor necrosis factor.

of these cells largely depends on activation of the PI3K pathway. PI3K is a heterodimeric complex formed of a regulatory and a catalytic subunit. The regulatory protein subunits are encoded by isoforms (which include p85α and p85β) that contain SH3-binding domains that mediate binding to activated RTKs. This binding allows additional recruitment and activation of the PI3K catalytic subunits (p110α, p110β and p110*). At the plasma membrane, activated PI3K phosphorylates phosphoinosite-2 (PIP2) at position 3 of the inositol to produce PIP3. In addition, Ras, a small GTP-binding protein and potent oncogene, also activates PI3K. PTEN, an important lipid phosphatase and tumor suppressor, dephosphorylates PIP3, counteracting PI3K and decreasing the intensity of the pathway. Accumulation of PIP3 at the plasma membrane recruits several pleck-strin homology domain (PHD) containing proteins, among them PDK and AKT serine/threonine kinases, which are key components

in transducing PI3K signaling. Activated AKTs target different protein substrates for initiation of a biologic response. For example, the Bad protein, phospho-Bad, does not bind Bcl-2 and functions as an antiapoptotic mechanism, promoting cell survival. Another key target of AKTs are the Forkhead transcription factors (FoxOs)

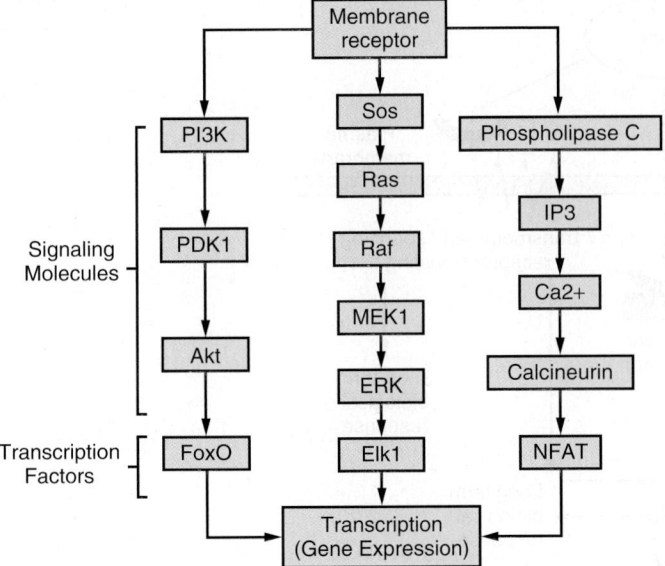

Fig. 7.2 EXAMPLES OF SIGNALING/TRANSCRIPTIONAL PATHWAYS PROGRAMMING GENE EXPRESSION. Proteins involved in gene expression are a common target of many signaling pathways, and receptors often stimulate multiple pathways that can regulate common and distinct transcription factors. In the examples shown here, production of PtdIns-3,4,5-P3 by PI3K leads to the activation of the serine/threonine kinase Akt. Akt phosphorylates and inactivate FoxO transcription factors. Ras is activated by the guanine nucleotide exchange factor Sos. Ras activation initiates a cascade of serine/threonine kinase activity: Ras activates Raf, Raf phosphorylates and activates Mek1, and Mek1 phosphorylates and activates Erk. Phosphorylation of the transcription factor Elk1 by Erk activates gene expression. Increased intracellular calcium is also a common signaling event. Activation of phospholipase C leads to hydrolysis of PtdIns-4,5-P2 and production of IP3. IP3 binds to its receptor, leading to intracellular calcium release and then extracellular calcium influx. Calcium activates the serine phosphatase calcineurin, which dephosphorylates NFAT proteins, allowing them to enter the nucleus and stimulate transcription. *FoxO,* Forkhead transcription factors; *IP3,* inositol triphosphate; *NFAT,* nuclear factor of activated T cells; *PI3K,* phosphatidylinositol 3-kinase; *Sos,* Son of Sevenless.

(Fig. 7.2). When phosphorylated by AKT, phospho-FoxOs are sequestered and inactive in the cytoplasm through direct binding to 14-3-3 proteins. Dephosphorylated FoxOs, on the other hand, activate gene expression associated with stress resistance and cell growth arrest. Another major component downstream of Akt is mammalian target of rapamycin (mTOR, a kinase that belongs to the PI3K-related protein kinase family), which is involved in metabolism, growth, and proliferation. Akt phosphorylates TSC2, which forms a complex with TSC1, decreasing its GTPase-activating protein (GAP) activity for the small GTPase Rheb; as a consequence, the increases in GTP-Rheb activate mTORC1 (one of the mTOR complexes). Among the key downstream targets of mTOR are S6K and 4EBP1, which control protein translation. mTOR can also be activated independently of RTKs through nutrients including branched chain amino acids. Interestingly, mTORC1 inhibitors such as rapamycin are used as immunosuppressants in organ transplantation.

MAPK/ERK Pathway

Activated RTKs recruit docking proteins, such as Grb2 and SOS, that allow binding of GTP to Ras to become active and trigger a kinase signaling cascade. Ras activates RAF kinase that, in turn, triggers a series of MEKs, which finally activate MAPK or Erk kinases. Erk phosphorylates many proteins involved in cell growth including ribosomal S6K, which is involved in protein translation, and AP-1 and c-myc transcription factors, which increase many

different cell cycle and antiapoptotic-related genes (see Fig. 7.2). Other MAPKs include the stress-activated kinases JNK and p38. Constitutive MAPK in hematopoietic stem cells is known to induce myeloproliferative disorders.

The Transforming Growth Factor-β Pathway

The TGFβ family of cytokines contains two subfamilies: the TGFβ/Activin/Nodal and the bone morphogenetic protein (BMP)/growth and differentiation factor (GDF)/Müllerian-inhibiting substance (MIS) subfamilies. At the plasma membrane TGFβ ligands bind with high affinity to the ectodomain of type II receptors, which then recruit type I receptors. This forms a large ligand–receptor complex involving a ligand dimer and four receptor subunits. Upon ligand binding, the type II receptor phosphorylates multiple serine and threonine residues in the cytoplasmic GS-rich region of the type I receptor, leading to its activation. The phosphorylated TGFβ type I receptor binds to and phosphorylates Smad2 and Smad3 transcription factors, which are critical mediators of TGFβ signaling and function. Upon phosphorylation, Smad proteins translocate to the nucleus to activate gene expression through binding to specific DNA-binding sites. There are several mechanisms to terminate Smad activation, which include proteasomal degradation and dephosphorylation. TGFβ-1 has been shown to be associated with active centers of hematopoiesis and lymphopoiesis in the developing fetus.

Signaling Through Receptors Associated With Protein-Tyrosine Kinases

Here, three different types of receptors and their signaling are included: (1) cytokine receptors; (2) multichain immune recognition receptors; and (3) integrin receptors.

Cytokine Receptors and Janus-Activated Kinase Signaling

The cytokine receptor superfamily mediates many of the central specific responses in hematopoietic cells. Ligands for these receptors include interleukins, thrombopoietin, erythropoietin, and so on. Cytokine receptors possess a conserved extracellular region (cytokine receptor homology domain [CDH]) and several structural modules, including extracellular immunoglobulin or fibronectin type III–like domains, transmembrane domains, and intracellular homology regions. Based on the divergence of the CHD, cytokine receptors are classified into two classes: class I and class II receptors. Class I receptors contain two pairs of cysteines linked through a disulfide bond and a C-terminal WSXWS motif within the CHD. This class is further subdivided into three families: IL-2R, IL-3R, and IL-6R. All three receptor families share similar receptor chains. The class I cytokine receptors are formed by one chain containing two motifs (Box 1 and Box 2), which transduce signaling through binding to Janus-activated kinase (JAK; see later discussion). Also included in this class are the homomeric receptors that form homodimers upon ligand binding. Examples of these receptors include the erythropoietin, thrombopoietin, prolactin, and growth hormone receptors. Class II receptors also have two pairs of cysteines but lack the WSXWS motif found in class I receptors. There are pools of 12 class II receptor chains that are capable of forming a total of 10 receptor complexes. This class is functionally divided into antiviral receptors (three receptor complexes that bind interferons) and non-antiviral receptors, which bind to several interleukins such as IL-10 and IL-20.

The oligomeric structures of cytokine receptors are complex and cannot be generalized. Cytokine binding often induces oligomerization, which activates protein tyrosine kinases in the JAK family that are constitutively associated with the Box 1 and 2 motifs of the cytokine receptor. Oligomerization brings JAKs in close enough proximity to transphosphorylate on Tyr residues. This activates JAK, which results in the phosphorylation of other cytokine receptors as well as other substrate proteins. Among these substrates, the signal transducer and activator of transcription (STAT) family of transcription factors are pivotal to JAK-mediated cytokine signaling. STATs are phosphorylated on Tyr residues by JAKs upon cytokine binding to the receptor. Phospho-STATs homo- or hetero-dimerize, and translocate to the nucleus to activate gene expression. STATs are also phosphorylated on a serine residue via MAPK, which serves to strengthen the intensity of the signal. As part of the cytokine signaling attenuation, STATs induce genes encoding for suppressors of cytokine signaling proteins (SOCS), which bind to phospho-tyrosine residues of the cytokine receptor and JAK through SH2-binding domains.

JAK inhibitors, based on their ability to block cytokine signaling, are used in allergic and rheumatoid arthritis disease therapy.

Multichain Immune Recognition Receptors

This family of receptors include antigen receptors in B and T lymphocytes, activating receptors in natural killer (NK) cells, and immunoglobulin E (IgE) and Fc receptors. This class of receptors contains different integral membrane subunits that bind the ligand at the cell surface and transduce the signal. Ligand binding induces oligomerization of receptor subunits that contain immunoreceptor tyrosine-based activation motifs (ITAMs) within their cytoplasmic domains. These domains become phosphorylated on tyrosine residues upon receptor activation. These phosphotyrosines are involved in activation of a series of protein tyrosine kinases containing SH2 domains that include Src (Src family kinase [SFK]), Syk (Syk or ZAP-70), and Tec (Btk, Itk, Rlk), which mediate immune signaling through downstream pathways that include MAPK, calcium signaling, and NF-κB, among others. In Tec kinases, additional downstream targets include enzymes such as phospholipase C γ (PLCγ). The precise mechanism of this activation is not completely understood, and in some cases, such as T-cell receptors, a protein tyrosine phosphatase (-CD45, which counteracts the action of SFKs) is regulated upon ligand binding.

The activities of some of these receptors are the basis of immunotherapy in cancer. For example, programmed death-1 (PD-1) mediates tumor-induced immunosuppression. Cancer cells express the PD-1 ligand, which activates the PD-1 receptor present in tumor-infiltrated lymphocytes, suppressing the immune response. Blockade of PD-1 activation with monoclonal antibodies has been successful in treating several human tumors such as melanoma. Mechanistically, T cells are activated through the T-cell receptor upon binding of major histocompatibility complex (MHC) plus peptides on an antigen-presenting cell (APC; in this case in the tumor cell), and binding of APC CD80/86 to T cell CD28. Activation of the T-cell receptor increases expression of PD-1 to suppress the immune/inflammatory response. Cancer cells activate this pathway, upregulating the PD-1 ligand to promote survival and suppress the immune-mediated death of tumor cells.

Integrin Signaling

Integrin receptors are involved in cell adhesion, migration, survival, and growth. This signaling is central in hematopoietic cell function, for example, at places of inflammation or infection, where integrins trigger a cascade by which leukocytes exit the vasculature. Interestingly, these receptors signal bidirectionally through the plasma membrane in pathways referred to as *inside-out* and *outside-in signaling*. Integrins are a class of receptors that comprise heterodimeric type I transmembrane proteins consisting of α and β subunits. These subunits contain a large extracellular domain, a single transmembrane domain, and a short cytoplasmic tail. There are 18 α and 8 β subunits that are associated and form 24 different integrins with different affinities for ligands. Most of the ligands are ECM proteins containing one of the two motifs: arginine–glycine–aspartate (RGD) or leucine–aspartate–valine (LDV). Examples of integrin ligands are ICAM-1, which is present at the plasma membrane of antigen-presenting cells and binds to the integrin receptor LFA-1 to promote cell–cell adhesion.

Ligand binding to the extracellular domain induces clustering of integrins, allowing separation of the different subunits cytoplasmic portions forming interactions with cytoskeleton proteins involved in actin polymerization (outside-in signaling). Signals arising from the cellular interior, including phosphorylation, can also separate these cytoplasmic domains and can affect ligand binding (inside-out). Ligand binding to integrin receptors also signals to protein tyrosine kinases such as the SFKs and focal adhesion kinase (Fak). This part of the signaling is not completely understood, but appears to involve a domain in the β-integrin tail (NPXY motif) that binds talin, which in turn recruits paxillin that binds Fak, which, once activated, phosphorylates SFKs to mediate integrin response.

Tumor Necrosis Factor Receptors and Signaling

Tumor necrosis factor receptors (TNFRs) influence inflammation, innate immunity, lymphoid organization and T-cell responses. There are approximately 19 different ligands for TNFR that mediate cellular responses through 29 TNFRs. TNFRs are a family of single-membrane-spanning proteins that contain an extracellular TNF-binding region and a cytoplasmic tail. As in the case of other cytokine receptors, ligand binding causes oligomerization and the formation of a mature receptor complex that is required to transduce the signal. TNFRs fall into three classes: (1) death domain (DD) containing receptors (fatty acid synthase, TNFR1, and DR3), which activate the caspase cascade via the DD-initiating extrinsic apoptotic pathway; (2) decoy receptors, which lack a cytoplasmic tail and therefore cannot transmit the signal, making these receptors ligand sequesters; and (3) TNFR-associated factor (TRAF) receptors such as TNFR2, which lack the DD-recruiting TRAF proteins. In general, TRAFs are associated with either proapoptotic or survival pathways through activation of the NF-κB family of transcription factors and MAPK signaling (Erk, JNK, and p38). TRAFs activate NF-κB through ubiquitin-mediated degradation of their inhibitor IκBα, which retains NF-κB inactive in the cytoplasm. This process is initiated by phosphorylation of IκBα by the IκBα kinase (IKK) complex, mainly by the IKK-β catalytic subunit, and requires a regulatory subunit (also known as NEMO). Upstream of IKKs are other kinases including NF-κB-inducing kinase (NIK), which binds to TRAFs. Nuclear-activated NF-κB modulates gene expression, which mediates TNF biologic responses.

Toll-Like Receptors and Signaling

Toll-like receptors (TLR) play essential roles in the innate immune response. Ten TLRs have been identified and can be grouped into two classes based on their extracellular domain: (1) TLRs with leucine-rich repeats; and (2) TLRs with immunoglobulin domains. The ligands for TLRs are diverse and include the different constituent components of the microorganism, such as lipopolysaccharides and heat shock proteins (which bind to TLR2 and TLR4). Host defense against microorganisms mainly relies on signals originating from the TIR (Toll/IL-1) intracellular domain (a domain present in TLRs and IL-1Rs). The TLR signaling pathway is similar to the one triggered by the IL-1R. Ligand binding induces TLR multimeric receptor complexes, recruiting adaptor proteins such as MyD88, which contains a TIR domain and a death domain, that in turn binds to the IL-1R-associated kinase (IRAK). IRAK is activated by phosphorylation and then associates with TRAF6, leading to activation of mainly two different pathways, JNK and NF-κB to activate the innate immune response, including release of inflammatory cytokines.

Wnt Signaling

Wnt proteins are lipid-modified, secreted proteins of approximately 400 amino acids that bind to Wnt cell surface transmembrane receptors, called Frizzled (Fz), to initiate the canonical Wnt signaling transduction pathway. At the plasma membrane, binding of Wnt ligands to Fz receptors connect through direct binding to several intracellular proteins including Disheveled (Dsh), glycogen synthase kinase-3β (GSK3β), Axin, and adenomatous polyposis coli (APC), inhibiting proteasome-mediated degradation of the transcriptional protein β-catenin. This degradation is regulated through GSK3β-mediated phosphorylation of β-catenin. As a consequence, β-catenin accumulates in the cytoplasm and translocates to the nucleus, where it interacts with transcription factors such as lymphoid enhancer-binding factor 1 (LEF)/TCF to modulate gene expression.

Notch Signaling

Notch ligands are plasma single-pass transmembrane proteins named Delta-like and Jagged. Thus, cells expressing the ligands are adjacent to cells expressing the Notch receptors, which are also transmembrane proteins. The Notch receptor interacts with a Notch ligand on a contacting cell; this interaction produces Notch receptor cleavage, which releases the Notch intracellular domain (NICD). The NICD translocates to the nucleus where it binds to several DNA-binding proteins including CBF1/Suppressor of Hairless/LAG-1 (CSL). As a result of this interaction between NICD and CSL, changes in Notch target genes occur. In contrast to the other signaling pathways discussed in this chapter that mainly function through phosphorylation, there is no amplification from the initial Notch ligand binding to the receptor. Moreover, this core pathway is modulated through auxiliary proteins that influence the response to the Notch ligand. Among these proteins are acute myeloid leukemia 1 (AML1), discoidin domain receptor family (DDR1), NECD, Notch extracellular domain, and CBF1-interacting protein.

Hedgehog Signaling

Hedgehog (Hh) signaling is a ligand-dependent signaling pathway. There are three different protein ligands—Sonic, Desert, and Indian—that are secreted and produce an N-terminal active fragment. Indian appears to be highly expressed in hematopoietic tissue. These ligands bind to Patch transmembrane receptors and are internalized, and Smoothened (a GPCR member) translocates to the plasma membrane of the primary cilium and promotes activation of the Gli family of zinc finger transcription factors. Hg targets include genes involved in differentiation, apoptosis, and the cell cycle. Abnormal activation of Hh signaling occurs in hematologic malignancies and maintains stem cell expansion. Because these cells are resistant to conventional chemotherapy, Hh antagonism is considered a plausible target in these malignancies.

Nuclear Hormone Receptor Superfamily

Nuclear hormones include steroid hormones (sex hormones, glucocorticoids, and mineralocorticoids), sterol hormones (vitamin D and its derivatives), thyroid hormones, and retinoids. These hormones are lipophilic and need carrier proteins to be transported in the blood. Due to this hydrophobicity, they can diffuse across the plasma membrane to reach the receptor proteins inside the cells, either in the cytoplasm or in the nucleus. These receptors are called the nuclear hormone receptor (NHR) superfamily. What distinguishes this receptor family from those discussed previously is their ability to directly bind to DNA and coordinate gene expression, which effectively makes them a form of transcription factor. NHRs contain a central DNA-binding domain, which targets the receptor to DNA sequences known as hormone response elements. In addition, the C-terminal part of the receptor contains a ligand-binding domain where the ligand or hormone binds. Upon ligand binding, NHRs control the expression of diverse sets of genes related to the hormonal response. Based on the types of ligands that they can bind, NHRs can be

grouped into four classes: (1) steroid receptors, which include receptors for glucocorticoids, mineralocorticoids, progesterone, androgen, and estrogen; (2) retinoid X receptor heterodimers, such as thyroid receptor, retinoic acid receptor, vitamin D receptor, and peroxisome proliferator-activated receptors; (3) dimeric orphan receptors, such as COUPTF or HNF4; and (4) monomeric orphan receptors, such as NGFI. The cognate ligands for orphan receptors have yet to be identified.

G Protein–Coupled Receptor and Chemokine Signaling

GPCR Signaling

The GPCR superfamily comprises a large collection of proteins, with approximately 2000 annotated genes in the human genome (~10% of the entire genome). GPCRs are involved in a large array of physiologic functions, including platelet aggregation and leukocyte chemotaxis. GPCRs are single polypeptides with seven-pass transmembrane domains containing both cytoplasmic and extracellular regions. Ligands for GPCRs are very diverse and include proteins or peptides, amino acids, lipids, and nucleotides that bind at the cell surface where GPCRs are localized. In spite of its vast size and variety of activational ligands, the GPCR superfamily relies upon three main intracellular signaling cascades for communicating receptor activation: the cyclic adenosine monophosphate (cAMP)/protein kinase A (PKA), the phosphatidylinositol/phospholipase C, and the Rho GTPase-based cascades.

GPCRs are coupled to a heterotrimeric G protein formed from three unique subunits (α, β, and γ) that are membrane bound. The G-α subunit contains a GTPase domain, which is capable of hydrolyzing GTP to GDP. When bound to GDP, the complex is functionally inactive, with the G-α subunit remaining tightly associated with the other subunits of the GPCR complex. Upon ligand binding to the GPCR, structural conformational changes produce the release of GDP from the heterotrimeric complex, allowing GTP to bind to the G-α subunit. In this GTP-bound form, the G-α subunit dissociates from the G-β and G-γ subunits with which it interacts. The G-α subunit then proceeds to interact with its downstream cognate targets to affect a particular signal response, depending upon the GPCR and the specific G-α subunit isoform. Among these second-messenger effectors are the cAMP/PKA pathway, ion channels, Rho GTPase, MAPK, PI3K, and inositol-3-phosphate/diacylglycerol (InsP3/DAG) pathways. In the case of the cAMP pathway, adenylate cyclase is downstream of different GPCRs (e.g., adrenergic receptors) and is activated by GTP-bound G-α. Adenylate cyclase converts ATP to cAMP, a freely diffusible second-messenger molecule. A key effector of intracellular cAMP is PKA, an inactive tetrameric protein complex consisting of two regulatory and two catalytic subunits. Binding of cAMP to the regulatory subunits causes release and activation of the catalytic subunits, which phosphorylate different cellular targets. Among them are the transcription factor cAMP-responsive element (CREB) and several ion channels. In addition to adenylate cyclase, there are other common effectors downstream of GPCRs, such as phospholipase C, a plasma membrane–bound enzyme that cleaves phosphatidyl inositol (PIP2) into two products and messengers: inositol triphosphate (IP3) and diacyl glycerol (DAG). IP3 can diffuse through the cytoplasm and bind receptors in the endoplasmic reticulum, resulting in calcium release to the cytoplasm. Importantly, calcium propagates the signaling cascade through different proteins such as calcineurin and nuclear factor of activated T cell (NFAT) transcription factors (see Fig. 7.2), which are involved in, for example, IL-2 gene expression. DAG at the plasma membrane binds and activates, in conjunction with calcium, protein kinase C (PKC), which will phosphorylate other downstream targets. Rho guanine nucleotide exchange factor (RhoGEF) is also a target for some G-α subunits. Binding of the G-α subunit to Rho allosterically activates it, causing GTP to be preferentially bound. This, in turn, allows RhoGEFs to activate Rho kinase, which is involved in the cytoskeletal reorganization necessary for changes in cell shape and motility.

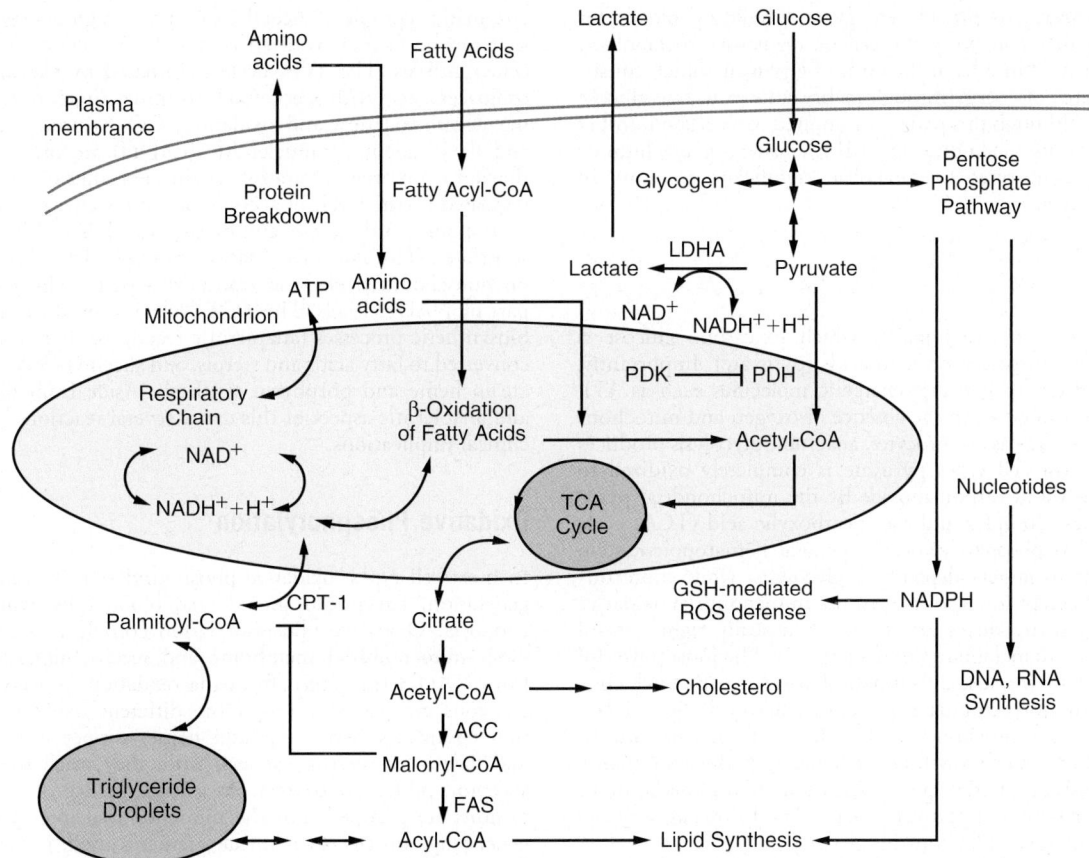

Fig. 7.3 INTEGRATION OF CENTRAL METABOLIC PATHWAYS. The metabolic fluxes within anabolic and catabolic routes are controlled by different signals including metabolite concentrations. These metabolic pathways are localized in different cellular compartments to adequately provide cellular energetic and nutrient homeostasis necessary for growth and survival. See text for further details. *ACC*, Acetyl-CoA carboxylase; *CoA*, coenzyme A; *FAS*, fatty acid synthase; *LDHA*, lactate dehydrogenase A; *PDH*, pyruvate dehydrogenase; *PDK*, pyruvate dehydrogenase kinase; *ROS*, reactive oxygen species; *TCA*, tricarboxylic acid.

Chemokine Signaling

Chemokines mediate cell migration in immune surveillance, inflammation, and development. There are nearly 50 human chemokines divided into four families (CXC, CC, C, and CX3C) on the basis of the pattern of internal cysteine residues; thus C stands for cysteine and X/X3, one or three noncysteine amino acids. Expression of some of these chemokines is induced by inflammatory signals such as TNFα, interferon-γ, trauma, or microbial infection. There are approximately 20 signaling chemokine receptors and they are all GPCR receptors, thus the chemokine acts as a ligand, and activation of the chemokine receptor follows the principles described previously. The major downstream effectors are cAMP and calcium messengers. Interestingly, some of the chemokine receptors also bind HIV viral proteins.

cGAS–cGAMP–STING Signaling Pathway

The presence of cytoplasmic DNA, through infection or DNA damage, activates innate immune responses. A mechanism of sensing this misplaced DNA is through the cGAS–cGAMP–STING signaling pathway. Cytosolic DNA binds and activates the cGAS enzyme (cGAMP synthase), which produces a second messenger, the cyclic dinucleotide 2′,3′-cGAMP, using ATP and GDP as substrates. 2′,3′-cGAMP is a high-affinity ligand for STING, an endoplasmic reticulum membrane protein that undergoes several structural conformations. 2′,3′-cGAMP bound to STING binds to the protein kinase TBK1, which phosphorylates IRF3; in addition, activated

STING signals to IKK to phosphorylate and degrade IκBα, which sequesters NFκB in the cytoplasm. Both phosphorylated and dimerized IRF3 and NFκB translocate to the nucleus to activate expression of type I interferons and other cytokines.

METABOLOMICS AND CONTROL OF HEMATOPOIETIC CELL METABOLISM

There are three important general pathways by which metabolism impacts cellular function and the metabolomic state (Fig. 7.3): (1) activity of catabolic routes that supply energy in the form of ATP, such as glycolysis or oxidative phosphorylation; (2) activity of anabolic routes that synthesize molecules that are used for cellular growth or a specific function; and (3) changes in metabolites that control intrinsic and extrinsic cellular activities. This regulation is intimately connected to signaling transduction, as most of the pathways described in the previous section directly control cellular metabolism and metabolite levels. Here, this part of the review will cover the main metabolic pathways and new metabolomic research, taking into consideration their implications in hematopoietic cells.

Glucose Metabolism

Hematopoietic cells have different types of glucose transporters; for example, activation of T cells causes dramatic increases in Glut1 expression in order to maintain immune homeostasis. Once transported into the cell, glucose is metabolized through different biochemical pathways to provide energy and building blocks for macromolecules that constitute the cell or regulatory metabolites. Glucose can be stored in cells in the form of glycogen, which constitutes a rapid source of energy through its breakdown to free glucose (glycogenolysis), although this pathway is limited to a certain number of hematopoietic cells. Chemotaxins (FMLP, C5ades arg, arachidonic acid) activate granulocytes to catabolize significant amounts of endogenous glycogen.

Glycolysis

Glycolysis is a series of reactions by which six-carbon glucose is converted into two three-carbon keto-acids (pyruvate). Importantly, these oxidative reactions generate energetic molecules such as ATP and NADH, and can occur in the absence of oxygen and mitochondria. In some cells, such as erythrocytes, anaerobic glycolysis produces lactate, but in most cell types pyruvate is completely oxidized to acetyl coenzyme-A and carbon dioxide by the mitochondrial pyruvate dehydrogenase complex and the tricarboxylic acid (TCA) cycle coupled to oxidative phosphorylation. In general, hematopoietic stem cells are thought to largely depend on glycolysis, while more differentiated cells, except for erythrocytes, use mitochondrial oxidative metabolism. Glycolytic fluxes are under intrinsically tight control through intermediate metabolites in the pathway. The most powerful control is exerted by fructose 2,6-bisphosphate (F-2,6-BP), which is generated by phosphofructokinase 2. F-2,6-BP allosterically activates phosphofructokinase, providing a "feed-forward" mechanism of stimulation. Activation of growth factor signaling pathways potently stimulate glycolysis at different points, including phosphorylation of phosphofructokinase 2 and pyruvate kinase. The PI3K pathway is a major signaling pathway that controls glycolysis.

Interestingly, in erythrocytes, 1,3-diphosphoglycerate can be diverted from glycolysis to synthesize 2,3-diphosphoglycerate (2,3-DPG) via the enzyme diphosphoglycerate (Rapoport–Laubering shunt). 2,3-DPG is an important metabolite that regulates oxygen binding to hemoglobin; thus increased levels of 2,3-DPG (e.g., under hypoxic conditions) allow hemoglobin to release oxygen under low partial oxygen tensions.

Pentose Phosphate Pathway

The pentose phosphate pathway (PPP) derives from glycolysis in the cytoplasm. The first enzyme in this pathway is glucose-6-phosphate dehydrogenase (G6PDH) and produces NADPH, a substrate utilized for lipogenesis and glutathione regeneration by glutathione reductase. The regulation of NADPH production through G6PDH is through NADPH-mediated product inhibition. The PPP is also important in generating ribose-5 phosphate, which is a precursor for nucleotide synthesis in proliferating cells. Interestingly, G6PDH deficiency leads to low levels of NADPH, which is essential for controlling reactive oxygen species (ROS) through glutathione reductase. It is one of the most common erythrocyte enzymopathies and these cells cannot prevent oxidative damage in critical molecules such as heme, causing overall irreparable damage to the cell at a much higher rate than normal, particularly in response to certain environmental triggers such as drugs and stress. The damaged erythrocytes are removed from circulation in the spleen and destroyed by macrophages at an elevated rate, leading to anemia. This enzymopathy occurs in areas with high malarial burden, in part because the mutated recessive allele confers malarial resistance. This resistance is because red blood cells with low G6PDH activity, when infected with the parasite, are continuously removed from the circulation.

Tricarboxylic Acid or Krebs Cycle

A major route for pyruvate oxidation is conversion to acetyl-CoA, a reaction catalyzed by the mitochondrial pyruvate dehydrogenase enzymatic complex. Acetyl-CoA is a high-energy intermediate that can be further oxidized by the TCA cycle or utilized for fatty acid synthesis. The TCA cycle is initiated by the condensation of oxaloacetic acid with acetyl-CoA, forming citrate. In reactions involving decarboxylation and oxidation, CO_2 is produced and NADH and flavin adenine dinucleotide (FADH) are produced for use in the mitochondrial respiratory chain. The flux of the TCA cycle is regulated by the levels of acetyl-CoA and oxaloacetic acid, which are entry points in the cycle, and by the availability of NAD^+ and FAD^+ substrates. The rate of oxidation through the TCA cycle depends on mitochondrial electron transport activity, which is governed in part by NADH levels. The TCA cycle also produces metabolites for biosynthetic processes (anaplerotic reactions). For example, citrate is converted to fatty acids and sterols, and succinyl CoA is an intermediate in heme and porphyrin synthesis. Aside from the bioenergetic and anaplerotic aspect of this cycle, several reactions have important clinical implications.

Oxidative Phosphorylation

In most cell types, oxidative phosphorylation is dominant on ATP generation. Exceptions include red blood cells, which lack mitochondria. Oxidative phosphorylation complexes are located at the inner mitochondrial membrane and receive high-energy electrons from NADH (produced from the oxidation of acetyl-CoA). These electrons are passed through the different oxidative phosphorylation complexes (which contain heme, copper iron–sulfur groups, and flavins as electron carriers) until they reach the final electron acceptor, molecular oxygen. As a consequence of electron transfer, protons are pumped into the mitochondrial intermembrane space, generating an electrochemical gradient used to synthesize ATP. There are five oxidative phosphorylation complexes: complex I (NADH–CoQ reductase complex), complex II (succinate–CoQ reductase complex), complex III ($CoQH_2$–cytochrome c reductase complex), complex IV (cytochrome C oxidase complex), and complex V (ATP synthase complex). In general, hematopoietic stem cells are located in low-oxygen niches and largely depend on glycolysis instead of oxidative phosphorylation to maintain ATP levels. The differentiation process is associated with increases in mitochondria, which allow for the generation of ATP through the respiratory chain. For example, this occurs in quiescent T cells that are in a catabolic phase, producing ATP mainly through oxidative phosphorylation. Upon stimulation, activated T cells shift towards an anabolic phase, relying upon a high rate of glycolysis for ATP generation. Mitochondrial DNA encodes for several oxidative phosphorylation subunits and mutations in this DNA produce mitochondrial diseases. Interestingly, anemia, a symptom associated with patients having Pearson syndrome, is caused by accumulation of mutated mitochondrial DNA in sideroblasts. This suggests that hematopoietic cell-specific respiration defects can be responsible for anemia by inducing abnormalities in erythropoiesis during development.

Reactive Oxygen Species Metabolism

Reactive oxygen species (ROS) are chemically reactive small molecules with oxygen in different oxidation states, such as partially reduced oxygen ions and peroxides. The three major species are superoxide, hydrogen peroxide, and hydroxyl radicals. The major cellular sites for ROS production are the mitochondria and NADPH oxidase, a plasma membrane or phagosome-bound enzyme. Approximately 85% of cellular ROS is a subproduct of normal oxidative phosphorylation. Superoxide is the initial ROS produced in the electron transport chain, and it is transformed to hydrogen peroxide by the enzyme superoxide dismutase. Hydrogen peroxide is the substrate of catalase or glutathione peroxidase, which reduces it to water. Hydrogen peroxide, however, is also converted to hydroxyl radicals, the most reactive oxygen species, in a Fenton reaction with ferrous iron. NADPH oxidase catalyzes the NADPH-dependent reduction of oxygen into the superoxide anion.

ROS cause cellular damage through oxidation and chemical modifications of proteins, lipids, and DNA. Nuclear and mitochondrial DNA can be oxidized, producing strand breaks. Intracellular levels of ROS are regulated through different signaling transduction pathways. Growth factor–mediated signaling increases ROS levels, for instance. Conversely, ROS also affect this signaling through modulation of protein tyrosine phosphatases that contain cysteine-sensitive residues that modulate their enzymatic activity and regulate the biologic responses associated with this signaling.

ROS are particularly deleterious to hematopoietic stem cells because of their effect on genomic stability and survival. In phagocytic cells (neutrophils, macrophages, or eosinophils), NADPH oxidase is responsible for the oxidative burst that is triggered upon phagocytosis of pathogens. Superoxide generated by NADPH oxidase is rapidly converted to other ROS, which, in cooperation with pH-sensitive proteases, are responsible for killing the microorganisms in the phagosome vacuole.

Recently, gain-of-function mutations of isocitrate dehydrogenase 1 and 2 (IDH1 is cytoplasmic and is unrelated to the TCA cycle; IDH2 is the TCA mitochondrial form) have been found in 20% of acute leukemia patients. IDH1 and IDH2 are highly homologous but distinct (in structure and function) from the NAD^+-dependent heterotrimeric IDH3 enzyme that is part of the TCA cycle producing NADH to the respiratory chain. The cellular function of the NADP-dependent IDH1/2 enzymes is not clear but they are part of glucose, fatty acids, and glutamine metabolism, and contribute to the maintenance of cellular reduction–oxidation balance. In three identified mutations, the enzyme undergoes a change in its normal physiologic catalytic reaction (i.e., oxidative decarboxylation of isocitrate to produce α-ketoglutarate and CO_2 while converting NAD[P] to NAD[P]H) and instead produces 2-hydroxyglutarate, which is now considered to be a protoncometabolite. The mechanism appears to be linked to competition with α-ketoglutarate for the active site of ketoglutarate-dependent dioxygenases, such as TET2, which functions as a cytosine demethylase.

Lipid Metabolism

Fatty acids and triglycerides (the storage form of fatty acids) constitute an energetic reserve in the body. Most of the cells are able to synthesize fatty acids, but there are essential fatty acids such as linoleic acid, α-linoleic, and arachidonic acid that cannot be synthesized. Arachidonic acid is made from linoleic acid, and is the precursor for prostaglandins, thromboxanes, and leukotrienes that participate in different pathways such as the inflammatory response. Drugs that block the enzyme cyclo-oxygenase and prostaglandin synthesis such as acetaminophen, ibuprofen, and acetylsalicylate provide pain relief. Fatty acids can directly mediate transcriptional responses, acting as ligands for peroxisome proliferator-activated receptors, a family of nuclear hormone receptors. In addition, there are specific GPCR receptors such as GPR40 and GPR120 activated by medium- or long-chain fatty acids. GPR43 is activated by short-chain fatty acids and is highly abundant in leukocytes.

Fatty Acid Synthesis

In the mitochondrial matrix acetyl-CoA is generated from pyruvate and is the precursor for fatty acid synthesis. Acetyl-CoA cannot cross the mitochondrial membrane; thus acetyl-CoA condenses with oxaloacetate (first reaction in the TCA cycle) to form citrate, and is exchanged into the cytoplasm through TCA translocases. Once in the cytoplasm, citrate is converted to acetyl-CoA by ATP citrate lyase. The rate-limiting reaction of fatty acid synthesis is the carboxylation of acetyl-CoA to form malonyl CoA, which is catalyzed by acetyl-CoA carboxylase (ACC). Malonyl CoA is a potent inhibitor of fatty acid oxidation. ACC is allosterically regulated by citrate to

form active enzyme polymers, which are depolymerized by the end product of fatty acid synthesis: long-chain fatty acids. Growth factors positively control ACC dephosphorylation. Catecholamines, on the other hand, result in the phosphorylation and inhibition of ACC via PKA. Fatty acids are synthesized in the cytoplasm by a multifunctional enzyme, fatty acid synthase (FAS). Two of these functional domains are the acyl carrier protein and the condensing enzyme (CE). After completion of the different rounds of synthesis, the palmityl group is transferred to CoASH. In macrophages, lipopolysaccharide (LPS) activates lipogenesis through activation of sterol regulatory element–binding protein (SREBP), a key transcriptional mediator of cholesterol and fatty acid synthesis.

Fatty Acid Oxidation

Fatty acids are "charged" before oxidation to form acyl-SCoA, a cytoplasmic reaction catalyzed by the enzyme fatty acyl-CoA synthetase. Fatty acid β-oxidation, however, occurs in the mitochondrial matrix and charged fatty acids must first be conjugated to carnitine in order to cross the mitochondrial membrane. This transport is carried out by the carnitine acyltransferases I and II. These enzymes constitute a rate-limiting step for β-oxidation of fatty acids and are allosterically regulated by malonyl CoA, allowing the cell to avoid a futile cycle of fatty acid synthesis and breakdown. Inside the mitochondria, acyl-CoA undergoes a cycle of reactions removing acetyl-CoA from the main chain. This acetyl-CoA is then processed through the TCA cycle.

Cholesterol

Cholesterol is an important component of cellular membranes and a substrate for the production of steroid hormones. Free cholesterol is tightly controlled in cells through synthesis, storage, and transport. Excess cholesterol in cells is secreted through reverse cholesterol transport or stored in the cytoplasm as cholesterol ester, produced by Acy-CoA:cholesterol acyltransferase located in the endoplasmic reticulum. Cholesterol is transported in the plasma by lipoproteins including chylomicrons and very low-density lipoprotein (VLDL). The main sources of cellular cholesterol for hematopoietic cells are the cholesterol-rich lipoprotein, low-density lipoprotein (LDL), and de novo synthesis from acetyl-CoA. The rate-limiting step for cholesterol synthesis is catalyzed by HMG-CoA reductase, the direct target of cholesterol-lowering statin drugs, and converts hydroxymethylglutaryl CoA to mevalonic acid. Cellular cholesterol levels are sensed in the endoplasmic reticulum through the SREBP transcription factor, which directly controls most the enzymes in cholesterol synthesis as well as LDL transport. Excess of LDL becomes oxidized and taken by macrophages, a main cause of atherosclerosis. The SREBP pathway is also important for T-cell activation under antigenic challenge, as its activation favors cholesterol synthesis and transport, which is used for membrane biogenesis and cell proliferation in the activated T cell.

Amino Acid Metabolism

The major sources of amino acids derive from the diet or protein breakdown. Nonessential amino acids are synthesized from carbon skeletons using different metabolic pathways. Amino acids conjugated to tRNA are used in protein synthesis; however, in excess they can be used for energy production. In addition, amino acids are necessary for the synthesis of other compounds. For example, tryptophan catabolism constitutes a route for de novo NAD^+ synthesis in a pathway that is important in leukocytes for the replenishment of NAD^+ levels after oxidative stress. Interestingly, different metabolites derived from tryptophan catabolism via the kynurenine pathway play a role in immune tolerance. Plasma amino acids are transported in cells against a concentration gradient. Amino acid transporters are specific for neutral (small and larger), basic, and acidic amino acids.

Depending on the cell type and specific state (growth, hypoxia, fasting, and so on) intracellular amino acids are used in anabolic or catabolic pathways.

Most of the regulation of amino acid metabolism is achieved through substrate fluxes affecting specific enzyme kinetics. However, there are two major regulatory pathways that involve amino acid sensing mechanisms and metabolic control. (1) General control nonrepressed 2 (GCN2) is a protein kinase that senses amino acid deficiency through direct binding to uncharged tRNA. GCN2 controls the transcription factor ATF4, affecting different enzymes of amino acid metabolism. (2) mTOR is a protein kinase activated in response to increased amino acid concentrations (particularly branch chain amino acids). mTOR controls many aspects involved in protein synthesis, inhibition of protein degradation, and amino acid biosynthetic enzymes. The high asparagine requirement of certain acute lymphoblastic leukemias has resulted in the use of asparaginase to deplete circulating levels of asparagine. Limited amounts of asparagine result in activation of GCN2 in leukemic cells, and reduce their proliferation and viability rates.

Biosynthesis of Nonessential Amino Acids

Nonessential amino acids are synthesized by most of the cells, including hematopoietic lineages. Nonessential amino acids are mainly synthesized from glucose (alanine, arginine [from the urea cycle in hepatic cells], asparagine, aspartate, cysteine, glutamate, glutamine, glycine, proline, and serine), except for tyrosine, which is synthesized from phenylalanine. The rest of the nine amino acids are essential and the body needs to obtain these from the diet. Serine, glycine, and cysteine are synthesized from glycolytic intermediates. Serine synthesis has recently been found to be increased and necessary in stem cells. For some hematopoietic cells, the synthesis of cysteine and glycine is of elevated importance owing to their use in the synthesis of the tripeptide glutathione. Aspartate and asparagines are synthesized by transamination of oxaloacetate by glutamate and amide transfer from glutamine, respectively. Glutamate, glutamine, proline, and arginine are formed from the TCA cycle intermediate α-ketoglutarate.

Amino Acid Catabolism

Two central reactions in amino acid catabolism are the generation of ammonia through transamination (catalyzed by amino transferases) and oxidative deamination (catayzed by glutamate dehydrogenase) in which the α-amino group of the different amino acids is transferred to α-ketoglutarate to form glutamate, which undergoes the release of free NH_3. Free ammonium is added to glutamate to generate glutamine, which is then exported into the circulation to the liver, where it then enters the urea cycle. The urea cycle only occurs in the liver and has two purposes: (1) to get rid of free ammonium; and (2) to supply arginine. Interestingly, one of the enzymes of the urea cycle, arginase (which converts arginine to ornithine) is expressed in immune cells. Myeloid cell arginase depletes arginine and suppresses T-cell immune response, and is an important mechanism of inflammation associated with immunosuppression. Arginase is viewed as a promising strategy in the treatment of cancer and autoimmunity. Arginine is also essential for the differentiation and proliferation of erythrocytes.

Nucleotide Metabolism

Nucleotides are involved in a diverse array of cellular functions including (1) energy metabolism (ATP, NAD^+, $NADP^+$, and FAD^+ and their corresponding reduced forms); (2) units of nucleic acids (NTPs are substrates for RNA and DNA polymerases); and (3) physiologic mediators such as adenosine, ADP (which is critical in platelet aggregation), cAMP and cGMP (second messenger molecules), and GTP (which participates in signal transduction via GTP-binding proteins).

Most of the regulatory pathways that are associated with nucleotide synthesis and degradation are strictly controlled by regulatory components of the cell cycle machinery. The amount of intracellular nucleotides has to reach certain levels in order for the cell to proceed through the S-phase checkpoint. In addition, several of the key cell cycle regulators, including the c-myc oncogene (which is translocated in certain myelomas), directly increase the expression of most of the key enzymes associated with nucleotide synthesis.

Nucleotide Synthesis

There are two pathways for the synthesis of nucleotides, salvage and de novo. The salvage pathway uses free bases via a reaction with phosphoribosyl pyrophosphate (PRPP) and generation of nucleotides. De novo pathways synthesize pyrimidines and purine nucleotides from amino acids, carbon dioxide, folate derivatives, and PRPP. Importantly, both salvage and de novo pathways depend on PRPP, which is produced from ATP and ribose-5-phosphate (generated in the pentose phosphate pathway) by PRPP synthetase, an enzyme that is inhibited by metabolic markers of low-energy AMP, ADP, and GDP to avoid nucleotide synthesis in these conditions. In general, PRPP levels are low in postmitotic cells but high in proliferating cells. Folate is essential in nucleotide biosynthesis, and lack of folate in the diet can lead to anemia due to inhibition of proliferation of red blood cell precursors.

Nucleotide Degradation

Nucleotidases and nucleosidases initially participate in purine nucleotide degradation. For example, adenosine is deaminated to produce inosine, which, after ribose is removed, generates hypoxanthine, which is used by xanthine oxidase to form uric acid. Immune cells have potent nucleotide salvage pathways, and a lack of adenosine deaminase causes severe combined immune deficiency (SCID) syndrome. SCID is associated with a large accumulation of dATP in immune cells, which, through a negative-feedback mechanism on ribonucleotide reductase, blocks production of dNTPs and results in a failure to replicate DNA.

Introduction to Metabolomics

Analytical measurements of blood metabolites such as glucose, urea, and cholesterol is part of clinical biochemistry to track diseases. Along these lines and facing the new era of personalized medicine emerges metabolomics, which evaluates metabolism with a comprehensive and quantitative analysis of all metabolites, as well as its impact on cell biology, and aims to discover novel biomarkers or targets for therapy. Recent technical innovations in mass spectrometry and nuclear magnetic resonance (NMR) have allowed the measurement of many metabolites simultaneously. These advances, in combination with metabolite flux analysis with isotopic tracers, have provided new information on many metabolic processes. The use of metabolomics also offers a tool to identify metabolic enzymes as drug targets, as they are poised for inhibition with small-molecule drugs and possess allosteric sites that can be utilized to alter catalytic activity.

A major effort in metabolomics has been the identification of biomarkers for diseases and therapeutic targets. As an example, metabolomics was used to analyze plasma from diabetic patients showing increases in branch chain amino acids before hyperglycemia. Another example comes from the combination of genome-wide sequencing analysis and metabolomics: sequence analysis of acute myeloid leukemias was able to identify IDH1 or IDH2 mutations in 20% of patients. Metabolomics analysis revealed accumulation of a noncanonical metabolite, 2-hydroxyglutarate, which promotes the tumorigenic process (see following discussion). In general, there are two different metabolomic approaches: targeted, which measures

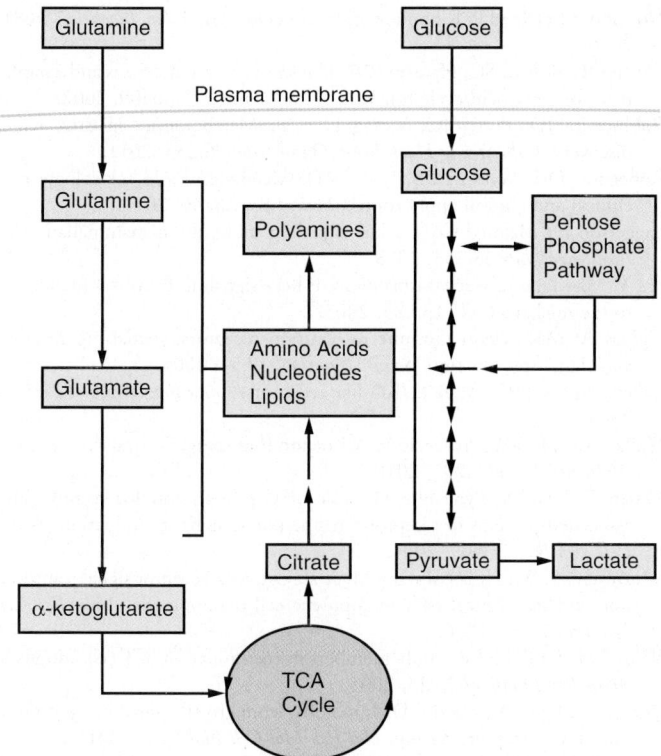

Fig. 7.4 METABOLITE PROFILING UPON T-CELL ACTIVATION. Metabolomic analysis has revealed that glycolytic fluxes and glutaminolysis are increased during activation of T cells. Polyamines that are required for T-cell proliferation are synthesized from glutamine. See text for further details. *TCA*, Tricarboxylic acid.

known and specific metabolites; and nontargeted, which includes analytical measurements of unknown metabolites.

Metabolomics of Glucose Metabolism

Systematic and simultaneous quantitative targeted polar metabolite analysis of glucose metabolic pathways using metabolomic and flux measurement techniques has introduced new basic and clinically relevant information in hematology (Fig. 7.4). For example, increases in glucose metabolism signatures measuring serum metabolite linked to glycolysis and the TCA cycle have been correlated with a prognostic risk score in AML patients.

Metabolic reprogramming or switches are crucial for T-cell activation. Quiescent naive T cells obtain most of their ATP from mitochondrial oxidative phosphorylation for energy, whereas activated T cells switch to glycolytic, glutaminolysis, and anabolic metabolism to promote clonal expansion that appears to be dependent on the transcription factor Myc. Moreover, metabolomic signatures have revealed that Th1, Th2, and Th17 cell lineages and T effectors exhibit an increased glycolytic metabolism. However, regulatory T cells and CD8[+] memory T cells depend more on mitochondrial oxidative phosphorylation. In addition, T cells are exposed to different nutrient environments, from high nutrient levels in the lymphoid organs to a more restricted nutrient availability in the effector sites such as tumors or infection. Under these conditions metabolic reprogramming through mTOR and AMP kinases control and maintain survival and immune function of T cells.

Metabolomics of Lipid Metabolism

Nonpolar metabolomics has provided metabolite profiles linked to lipid metabolism. In the case of fatty acids, de novo fatty acid synthesis is necessary for differentiation of T helper 17. Bioactive lipids have also been profiled in different types of blood cells. For example, sphingosine-1-phosphate is stored in erythrocytes, and is found highly elevated in the blood of sickle cell disease patients owing to increased erythrocyte sphingosine kinase 1.

Metabolomics of Nucleotide Metabolism

Measurements of the different polar metabolites in nucleotide metabolism are linked to particular stages of cell growth. For example, unbiased metabolomics has identified that pyrimidine starvation is a mechanism for specific types of cell death in multiple myeloma cells.

Metabolomics of Amino Acid Metabolism

Metabolomic studies have revealed that activated T cells reprogram their metabolism from fatty acid and pyruvate oxidation, and the TCA cycle, to aerobic glycolysis, the PPP, and glutaminolysis, and metabolic fingerprint similar to tumor cells. In particular, glutamine is used to increase polyamine biosynthesis, which is essential for T-cell proliferation, a process controlled by the transcription factor Myc.

SUMMARY AND PERSPECTIVES

This short review summarizes the central signaling and metabolic pathways that play a pivotal role in all the processes executed by hematopoietic cellular systems. In normal physiologic conditions these pathways are regulated and operating to achieve homeostatic cellular functions in healthy individuals. In pathologic conditions, however, dysregulation or failure of these pathways leads to diseases of lymphohematopoietic tissues. To a large extent, the main components and regulatory circuitries of these pathways have been elucidated, but the challenge for the future is to fully integrate them and identify therapeutic targets that will enable the development of effective treatments for these diseases. New technologies in metabolomics are promising for the identification of biomarkers that can be used in personalized medicine, as well as new therapeutic targets including metabolic enzymes.

SUGGESTED READINGS

Abram CL, Lowell CA: The ins and outs of leukocyte integrin signaling. *Annu Rev Immunol* 27:339, 2009.

Aggarwal BB: Signaling pathways of the TNF superfamily: a double-edged sword. *Nat Rev Immunol* 3:745, 2003.

Bolanos JP, Almeida A, Moncada S: Glycolysis: a bioenergetic or a survival pathway? *Trends Biochem Sci* 35:145, 2010.

Brown MS, Goldstein JL: The SREBP pathway: regulation of cholesterol metabolism by proteolysis of a membrane-bound transcription factor. *Cell* 89:331, 1997.

Buck MD, O'Sullivan D, Pearce EL: T cell metabolism drives immunity. *J Exp Med* 212:1345, 2015.

Cai X, Chiu YH, Chen ZJ: The cGAS-cGAMP-STING pathway of cytosolic DNA sensing and signaling. *Mol Cell* 54:289, 2014.

Cairns RA, Mak TW: Oncogenic isocitrate dehydrogenase mutations: mechanisms, models and clinical opportunities. *Cancer Discov* 3:730, 2013.

Chan DI, Vogel HJ: Current understanding of fatty acid biosynthesis and the acyl carrier protein. *Biochem J* 430:1, 2010.

Engelman JA, Luo J, Cantley LC: The evolution of phosphatidylinositol 3-kinases as regulators of growth and metabolism. *Nat Rev Genet* 7:606, 2006.

Evans DR, Guy HI: Mammalian pyrimidine biosynthesis: fresh insights into an ancient pathway. *J Biol Chem* 279:33035, 2004.

Fritsche K: Fatty acids as modulators of the immune response. *Annu Rev Nutr* 26:45, 2006.

Gordon MD, Nusse R: Wnt signaling: multiple pathways, multiple receptors, and multiple transcription factors. *J Biol Chem* 281:22429, 2006.

Hamanaka RB, Chandel NS: Mitochondrial reactive oxygen species regulate cellular signaling and dictate biological outcomes. *Trends Biochem Sci* 35:505, 2010.

Hurlbut GD, Kankel MW, Lake RJ, et al: Crossing paths with Notch in the hyper-network. *Curr Opin Cell Biol* 19:166, 2007.

Irvine DA, Copland M: Targeting hedgehog in hematologic malignancy. *Blood* 119:2196, 2012.

Kim C, Ye F, Ginsberg MH: Regulation of integrin activation. *Annu Rev Cell Dev Biol* 27:321, 2011.

Kolch W: Coordinating ERK/MAPK signaling through scaffolds and inhibitors. *Nat Rev Mol Cell Biol* 6:827, 2005.

Lemmon MA, Schlessinger J: Cell signaling by receptor tyrosine kinases. *Cell* 141:1117, 2010.

Levine AJ, Puzio-Kuter AM: The control of the metabolic switch in cancer by oncogenes and tumor suppressor genes. *Science* 330:1340, 2010.

Lunt SY, Vander-Heiden MG: Aerobic glycolysis: meeting the metabolic requirements of cell proliferation. *Annu Rev Cell Dev Biol* 27:441, 2011.

Mangelsdorf DJ, Thummel C, Beato M, et al: The nuclear receptor superfamily: the second decade. *Cell* 83:835, 1995.

McDermott DF, Atkins MB: PD1 as a potential target in cancer therapy. *Cancer Med* 2:662, 2013.

Mitin N, Rossman KL, Der CJ: Signaling interplay in Ras superfamily function. *Curr Biol* 15:R563, 2005.

Munder M: Arginase: an emerging player in the mammalian immune system. *Br J Pharmacol* 15:638, 2009.

Norlund P, Reichard P: Ribonucleotide reductases. *Annu Rev Biochem* 75:681, 2006.

Owen OE, Kalhan SC, Hanson RW: The key role of anaplerosis and cataplerosis for citric acid cycle function. *J Biol Chem* 277:30409, 2002.

Rabinowitz JD, Purdy JG, Vastag L, et al: Metabolomics in drug target discovery. *Cold Spring Harb Symp Quant Biol* 76:235, 2011.

Robertson DG, Watkins PB, Reily MD: Metabolomics in toxicology: preclinical and clinical applications. *Toxicol Sci* 1:S146, 2011.

Saggerson D: Malonyl-CoA, a key signaling molecule in mammalian cells. *Annu Rev Nutr* 28:253, 2008.

Shi Y, Massague J: Mechanisms of TGF-beta signaling from cell membrane to the nucleus. *Cell* 113:685, 2003.

Sigalov A: Multi-chain immune recognition receptors: spatial organization and signal transduction. *Semin Immunol* 17:51, 2005.

Takeda K, Kaisho T, Akira S: Toll-like receptors. *Annu Rev Immunol* 21:335, 2003.

Wallace DC, Fan W, Procaccio V: Mitochondrial energetics and therapeutics. *Annu Rev Pathol* 5:297, 2010.

Waters C, Pyne S, Pyne NJ: The role of G-protein coupled reeptors and associated proteins in receptor tyrosine kinase signal transduction. *Semin Cell Dev Biol* 15:309, 2004.

Watowich SS, Wu H, Socolovsky M, et al: Cytokine receptor signal transduction and the control of hematopoietic cell development. *Annu Rev Cell Dev Biol* 12:91, 1996.

Watts TH: TNF/TNFR family members in costimulation of T cell responses. *Annu Rev Immunol* 23:23, 2005.

Zoncu R, Efeyan A, Sabatini DM: mTOR: from growth signal integration to cancer, diabetes and ageing. *Nat Rev Mol Cell Biol* 12:21, 2011.

CHAPTER 8

PHARMACOGENOMICS AND HEMATOLOGIC DISEASES

Leo Kager and William E. Evans

A fundamental hypothesis pursued in genetics is that heritable genetic variation (i.e., genotypes or haplotypes) translates into inherited phenotypes (e.g., disease risk, drug response). On the basis of this hypothesis, one aim of medical genetics and pharmacogenomics is to understand the myriad associations between inherited genotypes and specific phenotypes of disease or drug response, with the ultimate goal of better defining the risk for, or outcome of, diseases and the response to specific medications. In cancer, disease prognosis and treatment response can be affected by both inherited (germline) and acquired (somatic) genome variation, and both types of genome variation have been shown to alter the effects of certain medications. Many seminal discoveries in medical genetics were made in the course of investigating hematologic disorders, as exemplified by the fact that the most prevalent monogenic disorders, the hemoglobinopathies, affect approximately 7% of the world's population. Pharmacogenomics also has a long tradition in hematology; one of the first documented clinical observations of inherited differences in drug effects was the relationship between hemolysis after antimalarial therapy and the inherited glucose-6-phosphate dehydrogenase (G6PD) activity in erythrocytes.[1]

In the pregenomic era, efforts concentrated on mapping highly penetrant monogenic (Mendelian) loci for both specific diseases and drug-metabolizing pathways that influence the effects of medications. Completion of the Human Genome Project and the development of arrays for genome-wide single-nucleotide polymorphism (SNP) and DNA methylation analyses, "next-generation" DNA sequencing technologies (whole-exome sequencing [coding regions only] and whole-genome sequencing [coding and noncoding regions]) have enabled relatively inexpensive and essentially agnostic genome-wide approaches to identify genomic variants that predispose to diseases and/or modify drug responses and/or contribute to heterogeneity of monogenetic disorders and complex diseases that are polygenetic in nature.[2] In addition to genome sequence variation, epigenetic differences are increasingly recognized as important for the development of diseases and contribute to differences in the pharmacologic effects of many medications, referred to as *pharmacoepigenomics*.[3] This chapter provides a brief overview of pharmacogenomics and pharmacoepigenomics, using selected examples to illustrate its current and potential impact on the treatment of hematologic diseases.

VARIATION IN THE HUMAN GENOME

The genome-wide systematic identification of heritable (i.e., germline) and acquired (i.e., somatic) variants, and the functional analysis of genes, their variants, their expression, and their related products (i.e., proteins) have revolutionized the study of many diseases, the development of new medications, and the optimization of drug therapy. Genomics increasingly enable clinicians to make intelligent and reliable assessments of a person's risk for acquiring a particular disease, to identify drug targets, and to explain interindividual differences in the effectiveness and toxicity of medications.[2]

The Human Genome Project and subsequent projects such as the International HapMap Project, the 1000 Genomes Project, and the ENCODE Project have unveiled many types of variations within the 3 billion base pairs (bp) of the human haploid genome (Table 8.1); the spectrum ranges from single-base-pair differences to large chromosome events. Variations encompass SNPs, insertions or deletions of chromosomal DNA, and structural variants (SVs; genomic

rearrangements that affect >50 bp of sequence). Comparisons among human genomes showed that they differ more as a consequence of structural variation than as a result of single-nucleotide variation. For practical purposes, the term *sequence variation* is mainly used herein. *Polymorphisms* are defined as common inherited variations in DNA sequence that are typically, although somewhat arbitrarily, defined as the least common allele having a frequency of 1% or more in the population.

SINGLE-NUCLEOTIDE POLYMORPHISMS

The most common and important inherited sequence variations are SNPs, positions in the genome where individuals have inherited a nucleotide that differs from the most common sequence ("wild-type") at the position in the genome. Many efforts are underway to catalogue these variants, because a comprehensive SNP catalog offers the possibility to pinpoint important variants in which nucleotide changes alter the function or expression of a gene that influences diseases or response to medications. The main public database is the "Database of Short Genetic Variations" (dbSNP; a repository of genetic variations less than 50 bp in length) and a growing number of SNPs (currently about 88 million validated) has recently been driven largely by the International HapMap Project and the 1000 Genomes Project (see Table 8.1).

SINGLE-NUCLEOTIDE POLYMORPHISMS AND PHENOTYPES

SNPs are present in exons, introns, promoters, enhancers, and intergenic regions. To elucidate the relationship between SNPs and phenotypes of interest, initial efforts have concentrated mainly on SNPs that are likely to alter the function or expression of a gene. However, only a small portion of the identified SNPs lie within coding regions; only about half of those SNPs cause amino acid changes in expressed proteins, and only a subset of those alter the function of the encoded protein ("damaging SNPs"). SNPs that cause amino acid changes are referred to as *nonsynonymous SNPs* (nsSNPs), and are the main sequence variants underlying most of the highly penetrant inherited monogenic diseases currently known, such as hemoglobinopathies. The likelihood that nsSNPs will result in disease or functional changes in drug metabolism or transport depends on the localization and nature of the amino acid change within the encoded protein; software algorithms have been developed to "predict" whether a certain amino acid change is likely to have a major or minor effect on protein function (i.e., "damaging" versus "non-damaging").

Although it is intuitively obvious that amino acid substitutions have the potential to change the function of a protein, gene expression also can be affected by SNPs positioned in regulatory sequences or intronic regions. For example, a "silent" or synonymous SNP has been identified that affects protein folding and function of an important drug transporter, namely ATP-binding cassette transporter ABCB1, and this variant has the potential to influence the intracellular accumulation of drugs that are substrates for ABCB1 (a transporter out of cells).[4] Moreover, SNPs in the promoter region can alter the regulatory promoter function and the gene's expression, thereby influencing drug effects. Using a genome-wide association study (GWAS), the rs924607 TT polymorphism in the promoter

TABLE 8.1	A Selection of Relevant Websites	
Genomic Variants	**Description**	**Address**
National Human Genome Research Institute (NHGRI)	Website of the NHGRI with the aim to improve human health by genome research	http://www.genome.gov/
GenBank	NIH genetic sequence database—an annotated collection of all publicly available DNA sequences	http://www.ncbi.nlm.nih.gov/genbank/
The 1000 Genomes Project	A deep catalogue of human genetic variation	http://www.1000genomes.org/
dbSNP	Repository of all types of short genetic variations <50 bp in length	http://www.ncbi.nlm.nih.gov/SNP/
dbVar	Archive of large-scale genomic variants (generally >50 bp) such as insertions, deletions, translocations and inversions	http://www.ncbi.nlm.nih.gov/dbvar/
ClinVar	Archive of reports of the relationships among human variations and phenotypes	http://www.ncbi.nlm.nih.gov/clinvar/
Database of genomic variants (DGV)	Catalogue of human genomic structural variation	http://dgv.tcag.ca/dgv/app/home
The Encyclopedia of DNA Elements (ENCODE)	Project to identify all functional elements in the human genome sequence	http://www.genome.gov/10005107
Roadmap Epigenomics Project	Public resource of human epigenomic data	http://www.roadmapepigenomics.org/
International HapMap Project	Public resource to find genes associated with human disease and response to pharmaceuticals	http://hapmap.ncbi.nlm.nih.gov/
Pediatric Cancer Genome Project	Decodes the genomes of more than 600 childhood cancer patients	http://www.pediatriccancergenomeproject.org/site/
Pharmacogenomics	**Description**	**Address**
Pharmacogenomics Knowledge Base	Most comprehensive website on pharmacogenomics	http://pharmgkb.org
Clinical Pharmacogenetics Implementation Consortium (CPIC)	Provides guidelines that enable the translation of genetic laboratory test results into actionable prescribing decisions for specific drugs (see Table 8.2)	https://www.pharmgkb.org/page/cpic
U.S. Food and Drug Administration— Pharmacogenomic Biomarkers	Contains a list of FDA-approved drugs with pharmacogenomic information in their labeling	http://www.fda.gov/drugs/scienceresearch/researchareas/pharmacogenetics/ucm083378.htm
Cytochrome P450 Homepage	Comprehensive data collection on cytochrome P450	http://drnelson.uthsc.edu/CytochromeP450.html
Human CYP Allele Nomenclature Committee	Unified allele designation system, and database of CYP alleles and their associated effects	http://www.cypalleles.ki.se/
The UCSF-FDA TransPortal	A public drug transporter database	http://dbts.ucsf.edu/fdatransportal/

region of the gene encoding a centrosomal protein 72 kD (*CEP72*) was recently found to be significantly associated with vincristine-induced peripheral neuropathy in children with acute lymphoblastic leukemia (ALL), and in vitro experiments have shown that the *CEP72* promoter rs924607 TT polymorphism creates a binding site for a transcriptional repressor leading to lower expression of CEP72 mRNA and increased sensitivity of neurons and ALL cells to vincristine.[5]

In addition, diverse classes of small to long noncoding RNAs (ncRNAs) have emerged as important regulators of gene expression and genome stability. For example, micro-RNAs (miRNAs) are small (19- to 22-nucleotide–long), single-stranded RNA molecules that can influence cellular mRNA levels or impair translation after binding to miRNA binding sites at the target gene's 3′-untranslated region. SNPs in miRNA binding sites or in the sequence encoding miRNAs have the potential to alter binding and function of miRNAs, respectively. Indeed, a so-called miRSNP, which is defined as a functional SNP that can interfere with miRNA function, had been reported to affect the expression of the antifolate target dihydrofolate reductase, thereby influencing antifolate pharmacodynamics.[6]

Collectively, these examples demonstrate that SNPs in functionally different genomic regions can influence drug disposition and response.

HAPLOTYPES, LINKAGE DISEQUILIBRIUM, AND HAPMAP

Combinations of SNPs are commonly inherited together in the same region of DNA, forming haplotypes. Genome-wide haplotypes can be constructed by linkage disequilibrium (LD) analysis. LD analysis is a statistical measure of the extent to which particular alleles or SNPs at two loci are associated with each other in the population, and LD occurs when haplotype combinations of alleles or SNPs at different loci occur more frequently than would be expected from random association. SNPs and alleles of interest are presumably inherited together if they are physically close to each other (usually <50 kilobases [kb]), producing strong LD. Therefore SNPs that are in LD with a disease phenotype or response-to-drug phenotype can *mark* the position on the chromosome where a susceptibility gene is located, even though the SNP itself may not be the cause of the phenotype.

By studying millions of SNPs in hundreds of individuals from geographically diverse populations, the international HapMap consortium created genome-wide maps of haplotypes (see Table 8.1). The HapMap project has revealed a block-like structure of LD, as well as the existence of areas of low or high recombination rate, and this has helped to identify so-called tagging (tag) SNPs. Such tagging SNPs can be used to predict with high probability the alleles at other co-segregating "tagged" SNPs, and the number of identified tag SNPs varies considerably among populations of different ancestry. Of note, common SNPs are also in LD with other common variants in the human genome (e.g., structural variants [SVs]).

STRUCTURAL GENOMIC VARIANTS

SVs are balanced or unbalanced changes in DNA content, and encompass alterations ranging from submicroscopic sequence variants greater than 50 bp to larger, sometimes cytogenetically visible, variants. Unbalanced DNA alterations that change the number of base pairs in comparison with a reference genome are as frequent as or even more common than SNPs, and include copy number variants (CNVs) or smaller insertions/deletions (indels). Balanced variations such as inversions and translocations are less common. Many efforts focus on the identification, validation, and mapping of these variants, and the major catalogs are the Database of Genomic Variants (DGV) and the Database of Genomic Structural Variation (dbVAR; see Table 8.1). CNVs are found in a wide spectrum of genomic regions; therefore, many pharmacologically relevant genes can be affected by these variants. Indeed, CNVs have been described to influence activity of some of the most important drug-metabolizing enzymes, such as cytochrome P450 enzymes and glutathione S-transferases.[7]

SOMATIC GENOMIC VARIANTS

Genomic instability is a hallmark of cancer cells. Nonrandom genetic abnormalities, including aneuploidy (gains and losses of whole chromosomes) and structural rearrangements that often result in the expression of chimeric fusion genes (e.g., BCR–ABL1), can be found in the majority of hematologic malignancies. These acquired (somatic) genomic variations can differ significantly from inherited (germline) genomic variations and can, for example, create allele-specific copy number differences between normal host cells and cancer cells. Such differences can have pharmacologically relevant consequences. Indeed, it was shown that the cellular acquisition of additional chromosomes in leukemia cells—for example, the gain of additional chromosomes 21 in hyperdiploid ALL (>50 chromosomes)—can cause discordance between germline genotypes and leukemia cell phenotypes, which are important when these discordant genotypes/ phenotypes influence the disposition of antileukemic agents. Moreover, somatic deletions of genes encoding proteins that regulate the stability of the DNA mismatch repair enzyme mutS Homolog 2 (MSH2) have been identified in approximately 11% of children with newly diagnosed ALL. These deletions in ALL cells have been shown to cause DNA mismatch repair deficiency and increased resistance to thiopurines, representing another genomic mechanism by which leukemia cells can acquire MSH2 deficiency and mercaptopurine (MP) resistance.[8]

CATALOGUES OF GENOMIC VARIANTS, GENOTYPING PLATFORMS, AND GENOME-WIDE ASSOCIATION STUDIES

Cataloguing the pattern of genome variation in diverse populations is fundamental in understanding areas of human phenotypic diversity such as interindividual and interethnic differences in drug responses; increasingly detailed maps of human genomic variation are provided in public databases (see Table 8.1). Information from these maps has been used to design high-throughput genotyping platforms (e.g., SNP chips), thereby providing tools to interrogate the relationship between genetic variation across the human genome and important phenotypes such as disease or response to medications in a relatively unbiased (agnostic) fashion.[2]

SNP catalogues have been used in GWASs to pinpoint genes important to diseases and drug responses, and in the past few years more than 2000 robust associations with more than 300 complex diseases and traits have been identified.[9]

Variation in the Human Epigenome

Epigenetics encompasses inherited and acquired changes in gene function that cannot be explained by alterations in sequence of nucleic acids. The epigenome is a complex layer of regulatory information that is superimposed on the genome (*epigenetics* literally means "above genetics"), with major mechanisms that contribute to epigenetic variation including DNA methylation, DNA hydroxymethylation, and various histone modifications such as histone acetylation and methylation. As in medical genetics, many seminal discoveries in medical epigenetics were made during investigations of hematologic diseases, and the myelodysplastic syndrome is considered a prototypical example of an epigenetic disease. In contrast to stable sequence variants, the epigenetic cellular state is principally malleable and can be influenced by environmental factors such as diet and toxin exposure. Of note, the expression of genes that encode important drug-metabolizing enzymes (e.g., cytochrome P450) and drug transporters (e.g., solute carrier family) have been shown to be altered via intrinsic and extrinsic factors that modify the epigenetic signature, thereby influencing the disposition and effects of drugs.[3] Moreover, the dynamic nature of epigenetics provides a mechanism to modulate the expression of genes that influence drug sensitivity, and so-called "epidrugs" (i.e., drugs that influence gene expression via epigenetic mechanisms) have already been successfully incorporated into the treatment of hematologic diseases (e.g., hypomethylating agents such as decitabine and vidaza for myelodysplastic syndrome, and histone deacetylase inhibitors such as vorinostat and romidepsin for cutaneous T-cell lymphomas).[3]

Major efforts are ongoing to generate detailed epigenomic maps to provide a basis for understanding cellular processes, the pathogenesis of diseases, and alterations in drug responses, such as the Encyclopedia of DNA Elements (ENCODE) and the Epigenomics Roadmap (see Table 8.1).

GENETIC VARIATIONS INFLUENCING DRUG RESPONSE: PHARMACOGENETICS–PHARMACOGENOMICS–PHARMACOEPIGENOMICS

Pharmacogenomics is a major element of the recently announced U.S. President's Precision Medicine initiative. Mostly empiric approaches are used to select drug therapy for most patients and most diseases, despite the fact that there is great heterogeneity in the way people respond to medications, in terms of both host toxicity and treatment efficacy. Unfortunately, for almost all medications, interindividual differences are the rule, not the exception, and these differences result from the interplay of many variables, including genetics and environment. Variables influencing drug response include pathogenesis and severity of the underlying disease being treated; drug interactions; the patient's age, sex, nutritional status, and renal and liver function; the presence of concomitant illnesses; and other components of treatment. In addition to these clinical variables, both inherited and acquired (e.g., somatic mutations in cancers) genome variation can influence the disposition and effects of medications, including many used to treat hematologic diseases. Clinical observations of inherited differences in drug effects (based on family studies and twin studies) were first documented in the 1950s, and the concept of pharmacogenetics was defined initially in 1959 by Friedrich Vogel as "the study of the role of genetics in drug response." The number of recognized clinically important pharmacogenetic traits grew steadily in the 1970s; the elucidation of the molecular genetics underlying these traits began in the late 1980s and 1990s, with their translation to molecular diagnostics to guide drug therapy being well underway in the 2000s. The study of pharmacogenetics began with the analysis of genetic variations in drug-metabolizing enzymes and how those variations translate into inherited differences in drug effects. Subsequently, the field has incorporated genome-wide approaches to identify networks of genes that govern the clinical response to drug therapy (i.e., pharmacogenomics). The terms *pharmacogenetics* and *pharmacogenomics*, however, are generally considered to be synonymous for all practical purposes. With the recognition that epigenetic modification affects gene expression and can contribute to variability in drug effects, the field of pharmacoepigenomics has gained additional attention and importance.

Overall, pharmacogenomics can be viewed as a broad strategy to establish models of drug disposition and effects by integrating information from genome sequencing, functional genomics, high-throughput molecular analyses, pharmacokinetics (e.g., drug metabolism and disposition), and pharmacodynamics (treatment response). Approaches to establish pharmacogenomic models include candidate gene analyses (which focus on the analysis of single genes or sets of functionally related genes in pathways thought to be important for the medicine under study) and more agnostic genome-wide analyses. Pharmacogenomic models can be used to maximize efficacy and reduce toxicity of existing medications, as well as to identify novel therapeutic targets.

Comprehensive reviews on pharmacogenomics and epigenomics are available elsewhere.[1–3,6,7] Herein, clinically relevant examples are provided to illustrate the potential of pharmacogenomics and epigenomics to improve current drug therapy for hematologic disorders, to prevent hematologic toxicity, and perhaps to identify novel targets for developing new therapeutic approaches in hematology.

OPTIMIZATION OF DRUG THERAPY

Drug effects are typically determined by the interplay of several gene products that influence the pharmacokinetics and pharmacodynamics of medications. Pharmacokinetics entails characterization of the absorption, distribution, metabolism, and excretion (ADME) of medications. Pharmacodynamics is the relationship between the pharmacokinetic properties of drugs and their pharmacologic effects, either desired or adverse. The ultimate goals of pharmacogenomics and pharmacoepigenomics in this context are to elucidate the inherited determinants for drug disposition and response to select medications and dosages on the basis of each patient's inherited ability to metabolize, eliminate, and respond to specific drugs. A model of how polygenic variables can determine drug response is illustrated in Fig. 8.1.

GENETIC VARIATIONS THAT INFLUENCE DRUG DISPOSITION

Drug Metabolism

There are many enzymes involved in drug metabolism, which are often categorized into phase I reactions that involve oxidation, reduction, or hydrolysis of medications, and phase II enzymes that conjugate drugs via acetylation, glucuronidation, sulfation, or methylation. Although phase I metabolism often inactivates medications, this is not always the case, as exemplified by codeine's activation by cytochrome P450 CYP2D6 and clopidogrel's activation via CYP2C19. Phase II conjugation generally makes medications more water soluble and therefore more readily excreted in the urine, but some phase II conjugates have pharmacologic effects. Although the liver is generally considered the major organ for drug metabolism, phase I and phase II metabolic enzymes are found in many other tissues, including the kidney, intestinal tract, lung, brain, spleen, erythrocytes, and lymphocytes.

Essentially all genes encoding drug-metabolizing enzymes with more than 30 families of enzymes in humans exhibit genetic variation, many of which translate into functional changes in the proteins encoded. Inheritance of genes containing sequence variations that

alter the function of enzymes they encode, as well as CNVs or epigenetic signatures that alter the expression of functionally relevant genes, can influence either drug activation or inactivation, and ultimately determine the extent of drug effects. This is most evident when polymorphic genes encode enzymes that are involved in crucial pathways of elimination or activation of the administered medication. It should also be recognized that genetic polymorphism in genes that encode the protein targets of medications (e.g., VKORC1, the target of warfarin) can also have a significant influence on drug effects.

The focus of this chapter is to provide examples that are relevant to hematologists to illustrate the potential impact of genome variation on the effects of medications. We discuss enzymes involved in inactivation of the antileukemic agent MP, as well as genes encoding the enzyme (CYP2C9) that metabolizes active warfarin and the gene that encodes its target (VKORC1). These examples therefore involve both phase I (CYP2C9) and phase II (thiopurine S-methyltransferase [TPMT]) drug-metabolizing enzymes and the target of the most widely prescribed anticoagulant. Our examples include both inherited genome variations (*CYP2C9, TPMT, NUDT15,* and *VKORC1*) and somatically acquired genome variants (*NT5C2*) that have been shown to alter drug effects in humans. This is a rapidly evolving component of "precision medicine," thus providing an understanding of their relevance and potential is of greater value than attempting a current and comprehensive literature review.

Thiopurines and Inherited Variants in *TPMT* and *NUDT15*, and Acquired Somatic Variants in *NT5C2*

MP is metabolized by numerous enzymes, either to activate it to thioguanine nucleotides (TGNs) or to inactivate it via methylation or dephosphorylation of TGNs. Although there is genetic polymorphism in enzymes involved in MP activation (e.g., hypoxanthine phosphoribosyltransferase 1 [HPRT1]), there is little evidence that genetic polymorphisms in these enzymes play an important role in controlling the pharmacologic effects of MP, with the exception of patients who inherit HPRT1 deficiency, an X-linked disease that occurs in approximately 1 in 350,000 Caucasian males (Lesch–Nyhan syndrome). In contrast, genetic polymorphisms in two enzymes involved in the inactivation of thiopurines (MP, and the MP prodrug azathioprine and thioguanine) increase the accumulation of their active TGNs, thereby increasing the risk of hematopoietic toxicity; TPMT and NUDT15 (nucleoside diphosphate linked moiety X-type motif 15). Inherited variants in TPMT were first discovered in the 1990s, with two major inactive variant alleles accounting for the majority of inherited TPMT deficiency in major world populations studied to date (*TPMT*3C* [rs1800460] for persons of Asian and African ancestry, and *TPMT*3A* [rs1142345 and rs1800469] for persons of European ancestry). *TPMT*3A, TPMT*3C,* and *TPMT*2* (rs1800462) account for more than 95% of the clinically relevant TPMT variants; variant *TPMT* alleles encode unstable proteins. Patients who are heterozygous (5% to 10% of persons) are about five times more likely to develop hematologic toxicity, whereas patients who inherit two variant alleles (1 in 300 persons) will all develop hematologic toxicity if treated with conventional doses of thiopurines.[10]

It has been recognized for many years that patients of Asian ancestry develop more hematologic toxicity than patients of European or African ancestry, yet the frequency of nonfunctional *TPMT* alleles is lower in Asians. Important new insights were recently provided by the identification of variant alleles of *NUDT15* in South Korean patients with inflammatory bowel disease who developed hematologic toxicity while receiving azathioprine therapy.[11] The *NUDT15* variant was very strongly related to thiopurine hematopoietic toxicity. In a GWAS of children with ALL receiving MP therapy, both TPMT and NUDT15 were significantly related to thiopurine intolerance in U.S. children.[12] Together, these studies show that genetic polymorphisms in both of these genes influence thiopurine tolerance, and that *TPMT* variants are more common in patients of European and African

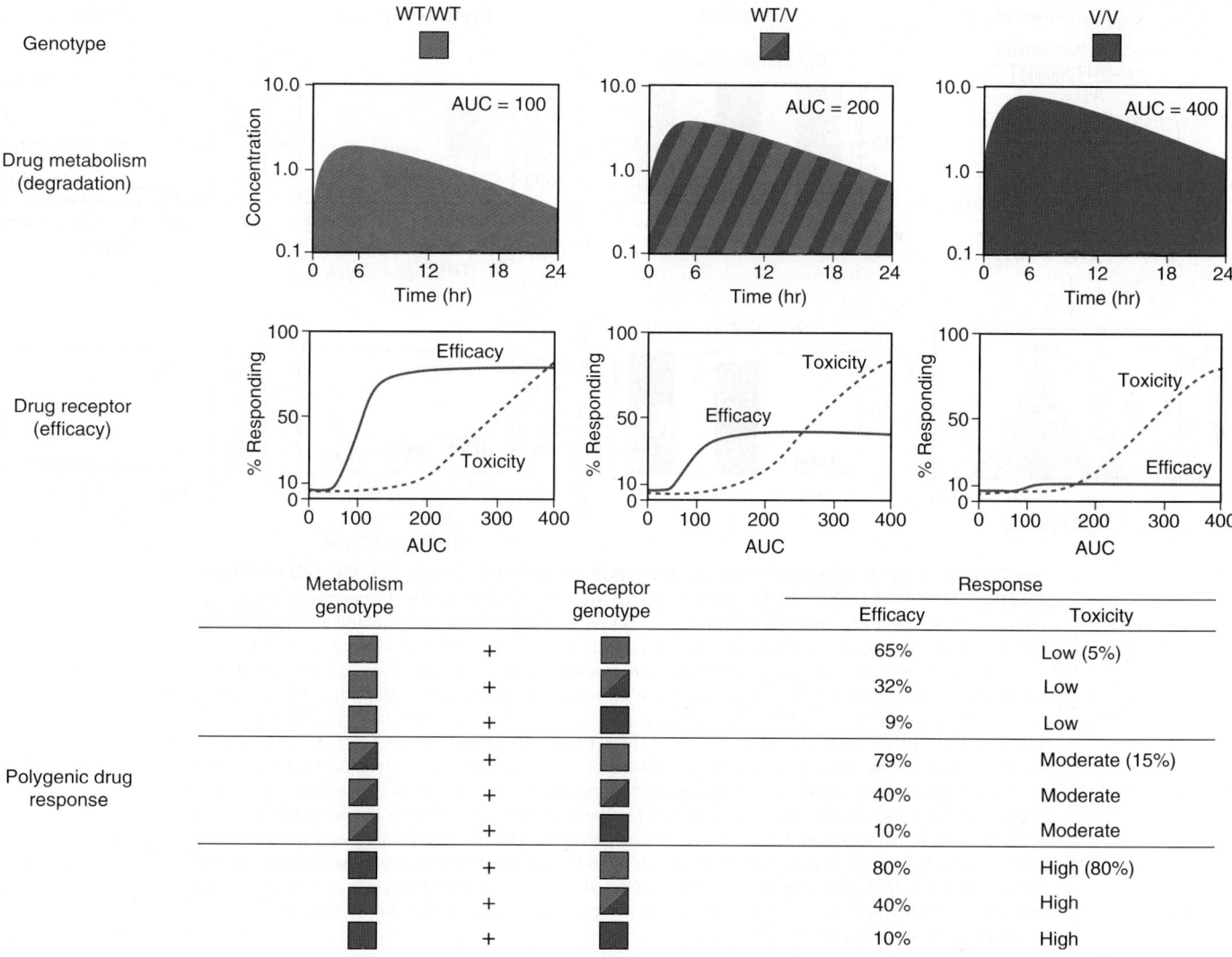

Fig. 8.1 POLYGENIC DETERMINANTS OF DRUG RESPONSE. The potential effects of two genetic variants are illustrated. One genetic variant involves a drug-metabolizing enzyme *(top)*, and the second involves a drug receptor *(middle)*. Differences in drug clearance (or the AUC) and receptor sensitivity are depicted in patients who are either homozygous for the wild-type allele (WT/WT) or heterozygous for one wild-type and one variant allele (WT/V), or have two variant alleles (V/V) for the two genetic variants. At the *bottom* are shown the nine potential combinations of drug metabolism, drug-receptor genotypes, and the corresponding drug-response phenotypes, which were calculated with data from the *top*. The therapeutic indexes (efficacy-to-toxicity ratios) ranged from 13 (65%:5%) to 0.125 (10%:80%). *AUC,* Area under the plasma concentration–time curve; *V,* variant; *WT,* wild-type. *(Courtesy Evans WE, McLeod HL: Pharmacogenomics: drug disposition, drug targets, and side effects.* N Engl J Med *348:538, 2003. Copyright 2003 Massachusetts Medical Society. All rights reserved.)*

ancestry, whereas *NUDT15* variants are much more common in Asians.[12]

In addition, it was recently discovered that somatic mutations in the *NT5C2* gene (encoding 5′-nucleotidase, cytosolic II) are relatively common in ALL cells at the time of disease relapse, conferring resistance to MP.[13,14] The mechanisms by which each of these genetic polymorphisms or somatic mutations influence the pharmacologic effects of thiopurine medications and the appropriate dosage adjustments for such patients are discussed in greater detail in the following section.

Inherited Variants in TPMT and NUDT15, and Their Influence on Thiopurine Hematopoietic Toxicity

The prodrugs MP and thioguanine (TG) are among the agents that constitute the backbone of treatment for childhood ALL. Childhood ALL studies have shown that all "homozygous" TPMT-deficient patients experience dose-limiting hematotoxicity, and some

experience life-threatening hematotoxicity if given conventional doses of thiopurines.[10] In TPMT-deficient patients, the thiopurine dose must be reduced to 10% to 15% of the conventional dose to avoid severe hematopoietic toxicity. Although many patients with one nonfunctional TPMT allele can tolerate essentially full doses of thiopurines (dependent on starting dose and other therapy), thiopurine-intolerant heterozygous patients typically require a 30% to 50% dose reduction. Multivariate analyses have demonstrated that children who have ALL and at least one *TPMT*-variant allele tend to respond well to MP therapy (i.e., 75 mg/m² per day), and may experience better leukemia control than is obtained in those who have two wild-type *TPMT* alleles. Most importantly, in the St. Jude Total protocols prospective MP dose adjustments (i.e., reduced doses in heterozygotes) were associated with less toxicity without compromise in treatment efficacy.[10]

In children in whom MP dose was adjusted according to *TPMT* genotypes, a sequence variant in inosine triphosphatase (*ITPA*) was

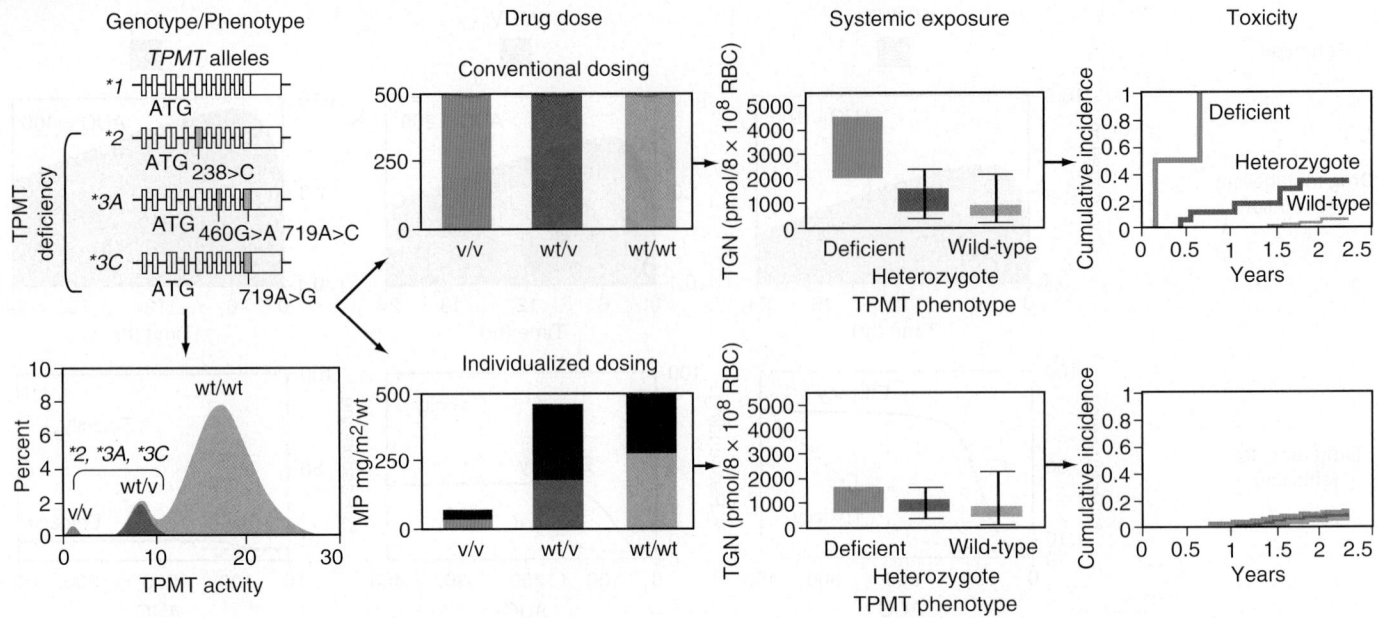

Fig. 8.2 GENETIC POLYMORPHISM OF THIOPURINE METHYLTRANSFERASE AND ITS ROLE IN DETERMINING TOXICITY TO THIOPURINE MEDICATIONS. Under "Genotype/phenotype" *(far left)* are depicted the predominant TPMT mutant alleles that cause autosomal-codominant inheritance of TPMT activity in humans. As shown in the graphs under "Drug dose", "Systemic exposure", and "Toxicity", when uniform (conventional) dosages of thiopurine medications (e.g., azathioprine, MP, thioguanine) are administered to all patients, TPMT-deficient patients accumulate markedly higher (10-fold) cellular concentrations of the active TGNs, and TPMT-heterozygous patients accumulate approximately twofold higher TGN concentrations, which translates into a significantly higher frequency of toxicity *(far right)*. As depicted in the bottom row of graphs, when genotype-specific dosages of thiopurines are administered, comparable cellular TGN concentrations are achieved, and all three TPMT phenotypes can be treated without acute toxicity. In the two graphs under "Drug dose", the *solid* or *striped* portion of each bar depicts the mean MP doses that were tolerated in patients who presented with hematopoietic toxicity; the *stippled* portion depicts the mean dosage tolerated by all patients in each genotype group, not just those patients presenting with toxicity. *MP*, Mercaptopurine; *TGN*, thioguanine nucleotide; *TPMT*, thiopurine S-methyltransferase; *v*, variant; *wt*, wild-type. *(Courtesy Evans WE: Thiopurine S-methyltransferase: a genetic polymorphism that affects a small number of drugs in a big way.* Pharmacogenetics *12:421, 2002.)*

identified as a risk factor for febrile neutropenia, illustrating that when treatment is adjusted for the most penetrant genetic polymorphism, less penetrant polymorphisms can emerge as clinically important.[10] *TPMT* genotypes do not fully explain all variability in MP sensitivity, and "trans" effects of SNPs that affect TPMT activity in patients with wild-type *TPMT* genotypes have recently been discovered in the protein kinase C and casein kinase substrate in neurons 2 (*PACSIN2*) gene. More importantly, GWAS investigations have identified germline variants in the nucleoside diphosphate-linked moiety X-type motif 15 (*NUDT15*) gene, which predisposed patients to azathioprine-related hematopoietic toxicities during treatment of Crohn disease or MP therapy for ALL: *NUDT15* variants were especially common in East Asians and in Hispanics with high Native American ancestry.[11,12]

The TPMT genotype is the strongest genetic factor for MP effects in patients of European and African ancestry, and in 2004 the U.S. Food and Drug Administration (FDA) added information about TPMT testing for determining the appropriate dosage of MP. Evidence suggests that *TPMT* genotyping before initiation of MP treatment can be cost effective in children with ALL. By using the *TPMT* genotype to individualize thiopurine therapy, clinicians can now diagnose inherited differences in drug response, thereby preventing serious toxicities. Guidelines for TPMT genotype and thiopurine dosing are available from the Clinical Pharmacogenetics Implementation Consortium (CPIC); these guidelines are periodically updated at the Pharmacogenomics Knowledge Base (PharmGKB)[10] (also see Table 8.1, box on Relevance to Clinical Hematology, and Fig. 8.2). There are no consensus guidelines for using *NUDT15* variants to

adjust thiopurine dosages, but they are likely to be forthcoming as these early findings are replicated.

Relevance to Clinical Hematology

MP Dosage Adjustment Based on TPMT Genotypes in Acute Lymphoblastic Leukemia

MP is a mainstay of treatment of childhood ALL. However, conventional doses of this prodrug can induce severe hematotoxicity in patients who have impaired thiopurine metabolism in hematopoietic tissues owing to less stable TPMT enzyme variants. The three major variant alleles (*TPMT*2*, *TPMT*3C*, and *TPMT*3A*) encoding the variant proteins can quickly be determined by commercially available Clinical Laboratories Improvement Act–certified molecular diagnostics or in special laboratories (e.g., Prometheus Labs, CA, USA) using samples obtained from peripheral blood before MP therapy. In patients with two nonfunctional alleles (1 out of 300), MP dosage must be reduced to 10% to 15% of conventional 75 mg/m² per day dosages. Patients with one variant allele (5% to 10% of the population) can tolerate MP at full dosage; however, in intolerant patients, a dose reduction of 50% often is required.[10]

Although inherited variants in *NUDT15* are strongly associated with thiopurine intolerance,[11,12] precise dosage adjustments to avoid toxicity without compromising treatment efficacy based on *NUDT15* genotype have not yet been defined owing to its relatively recent discovery.

Thiopurines and Somatic Variants in *NT5C2*

To explore molecular mechanisms for drug resistance in childhood ALL, two study groups recently sequenced the transcriptomes and whole exomes of diagnostic, remission, and relapse samples from ALL patients.[13,14] In B-cell precursor (BCP)-ALL up to 10% and in T-ALL up to 19% of the relapse samples had mutations in the *NT5C2* nucleotidase. The NT5C2 nucleotidase can inactivate the thiopurines MP and TG. Remarkably, six of the identified variants in NT5C2 increased the enzyme activity of the variant proteins (up to 48-fold), thereby protecting ALL blast cells against thiopurine-induced apoptosis. Of note, no resistance to other antileukemic agents was observed when the variant proteins were expressed in cell lines. Maintenance therapy with the antimetabolites MP and methotrexate is an essential element for successful ALL therapy, and one can speculate that resistance to MP can give rise to early relapse of ALL. Indeed, a significant association of activating *NT5C2* variants and early ALL relapse was found.[13,14] Novel strategies are necessary to overcome this drug resistance phenotype in the subset of patients with *NT5C2* mutations, and such strategies may help to further improve outcome in ALL by avoiding inappropriate drug levels at the target site (e.g., by using drugs that are not inactivated via NT5C2 or by design of small molecules that inhibit NT5C2 function).

Inherited Genome Variants in Cytochrome P450 Enzymes

The cytochrome P450 (CYP) superfamily is a system of phase I enzymes involved in the metabolism of endogenous substances and exogenous compounds (e.g., drugs, environmental chemicals). In humans the CYP enzymes are encoded by more than 57 genes, and the majority of these genes are polymorphic. Updated information regarding the nomenclature and properties of the variant alleles with links to the dbSNP database is available at the human CYP allele website (see Table 8.1).

On the basis of patient genotype (diplotype) CYP variant alleles, individuals are often categorized into one of four major predicted drug metabolism phenotypes: poor metabolizers (having two loss-of-function alleles), intermediate metabolizers (being deficient in one allele), extensive metabolizers (having two copies of functional alleles), and ultrarapid metabolizers (having three or more functional gene copies due to gene duplications, or two increased-activity alleles, or one functional allele plus one increased activity allele).

Different populations of metabolizers have been linked to different types of variants in the coding region of CYP genes (i.e., SNPs that alter the amino acid encoded, thereby altering protein function or stability); SNPs in intronic regions, which can alter CYP gene mRNA expression; CNVs (e.g., gene deletions, gene duplications) of CYP genes; or differences in the methylation at CpG islands in promoter and 5′ regions, which alter expression of CYP genes.

Many pharmacologically relevant variants in CYP genes have been identified. The focus here is on the variants in *CYP2C9*, which have been shown to influence the metabolism of an extensively prescribed medication: warfarin.

CYP2C9, VKORC1, and Warfarin

In the United States, the oral vitamin K antagonist warfarin is still widely used to prevent thromboembolic events in patients with chronic conditions such as atrial fibrillation, and the drug is prescribed to more than 1 million persons annually. A narrow therapeutic index with a risk for serious hemorrhage and interindividual variability in response to warfarin necessitate individualization of treatment, which has been based primarily on monitoring prothrombin time via international normalized ratio (INR) testing. Compared with the therapeutic INR range (i.e., 2–3), INR greater than 4 is associated with a 25-fold higher risk of bleeding in elderly patients treated with warfarin, and the percentage time in therapeutic range (PTTR) is a widely accepted read-out for treatment effect. Complications from inappropriate warfarin dosing remain among the most common reasons for hospitalization due to adverse drug reactions.

Pharmacologically, warfarin is a racemic mixture of *R*- and *S*-enantiomers that differ in their patterns of metabolism and in their potency of pharmacologic effects, with *S*-warfarin being more potent. Warfarin dose requirements can be influenced by both modifiable (e.g., compliance, dietary vitamin K intake, therapeutic level surveillance) and nonmodifiable factors (e.g., age, gender, genetics). Candidate gene studies initially demonstrated that the *CYP2C9* genotype influences warfarin clearance, and alters oral anticoagulant dose requirements and bleeding risks. CYP2C9 is the principal CYP2C isoenzyme in the human liver, and it is involved in the oxidative metabolism and inactivation of *S*-warfarin.[15]

The two most common *CYP2C9* variants with diminished enzyme activities are *CYP2C9*2* (rs1799853) and *CYP2C9*3* (rs1057910). Approximately 35% of Caucasians have one or two of these variant alleles; the *2 and *3 variants are virtually nonexistent in Africans and Asians (95% express the wild-type genotype [i.e., extensive metabolizers]).

Compared with the wild-type genotype (*CYP2C9*1/*1*), patients with two nonfunctional variants have a reduction of enzyme activity to approximately 12% for *CYP2C9*2/*2* and approximately 5% for *CYP2C9*3/*3*. Therefore, the required dose of warfarin is lowest in homozygous carriers of the *CYP2C9*3* variant (e.g., dose reduction of about 1.6 mg/day) and intermediate in homozygote carriers of the *CYP2C9*2* variant (e.g., dose reduction of about 1 mg/day).[15]

An important finding was the identification of a novel mechanism underlying warfarin resistance—the discovery of sequence variants in the warfarin target gene *VKORC1*, which encodes the vitamin K epoxide reductase complex 1. This complex regenerates reduced vitamin K for another cycle of catalysis, which is essential for the posttranslational γ-carboxylation of vitamin K–dependent clotting factors. A common noncoding variant (-1639G>A, rs9923231) was shown to be significantly associated with warfarin dose requirements. Patients with the -1639 AA genotype require lower initial warfarin doses (e.g., dose reduction of up to 3 mg/day) when compared with individuals with the -1639 GG variant. As the -1639G>A polymorphism affects a VKORC1 transcription factor binding site, the functional effect of the variant is thought to be related to decreased VKORC1 transcription, leading to lower protein expression. There are major differences in the distribution of VKOCR1 haplotypes among ethnic groups, and this may explain interethnic differences in coumarin requirement.[15] GWAS in patients treated with warfarin showed two major signals in and around *VKORC1* and *CYP2C9*, and identified a much weaker association with *CYP4F2*. The CYP2F4 enzyme catalyzes vitamin K oxidation, and the V433M variant (rs2108622) was identified to require increased warfarin dosing. Overall, *VKORC1* explains approximately 25% of the variance in coumarin dose requirement, *CYP2C9* explains about 15%, and *CYP4F2* explains about 3%.[15]

In 2010 the FDA updated the label on warfarin, providing *VKORC1* and *CYP2C9* genotype-specific ranges of doses, and suggested that *VKORC1* and *CYP2C9* genotypes be taken into consideration when the drug is prescribed. Additionally, dosing algorithms are available online (e.g., from the International Warfarin Pharmacogenetics Consortium [IWPC]), including genetic and nongenetic information that can help to optimize the warfarin starting dose (see CPIC Guidelines: Table 8.2).

The results of two large randomized trials, which have prospectively evaluated the benefit of genotype-guided warfarin dosing, have recently been reported. Whereas the European Pharmacogenetics of Anticoagulant Therapy (EU-PACT) trial demonstrated that pharmacogenetic-guided dosing is superior to a fixed-dosing regimen for achieving therapeutic INRs, the U.S. Clarification of Optimal Anticoagulation Through Genetics (COAG) study failed to demonstrate an improvement in PTTR with genotype-guided dosing compared with the algorithm-guided dosing control arm. Potential reasons for the differences include differences in the algorithmic strategies and control arms, as well as ethnic heterogeneity. In summary, the results of these trials and recent metaanalyses indicate

TABLE 8.2   CPIC Recommendations on Medications Whose Adverse Effects Have Been Associated With Variability in Candidate Genes and Manifest Predominantly as Hematologic Abnormalities (see Table 8.1, CPIC website)

Adverse Drug Reaction	Drug(s) That Cause ADR	Important Genetic Variant(s)	CPIC Recommendation
Myelosuppression	6-Mercaptopurine 6-Thioguanine azathioprine	TPMT*2 (rs1800426), *3A (rs1800460 + rs1142345), *3C (rs1142345)	Start with reduced doses for patients with one nonfunctional TPMT allele, or drastically reduced doses for patients with malignancy and two nonfunctional alleles; adjust dose based on degree of myelosuppression and disease-specific guidelines. Consider alternative nonthiopurine immunosuppressant therapy for patients with nonmalignant conditions and two nonfunctional alleles
Bleeding risk	Clopidogrel	CYP2C19*17 (rs12248560)	Recommends an alternative antiplatelet therapy (e.g., prasugrel, ticagrelor) for poor or intermediate CYP2C19 metabolizers if there is no contraindication
Myelosuppression (mucositis, neurotoxicity)	5-Fluorouracil (5-FU)	Dihydropyrimidine dehydrogenase: DPYD*2A (rs3918290), *13 (rs55886062), DPYD rs67376798 A (on the positive chromosomal strand)	For fluoropyrimidines (i.e., 5-FU, capecitabine, or tegafur) recommends an alternative drug for patients who are homozygous for DPYD nonfunctional variants, as these patients are typically DPD deficient. Consider a 50% reduction in starting dose for heterozygous patients (intermediate activity)
Bleeding risk	Warfarin and other coumarin derivatives	CYP2C9*2 (rs1799853), CYP2C9*3 (rs1057910), VCORC1 (rs9923231)	The best way to estimate the anticipated stable dose of warfarin is to use the algorithms available on http://www.warfarindosing.org
Acute hemolytic anemia	Rasburicase and other drugs (see Ref. 20 and 21 for a full list of drugs)	Deficient or deficient with chronic nonspherocytic hemolytic anemia (CNSHA). A male carrying a class I, II, or III allele, a female carrying two deficient class I–III alleles (see text for more details)	Rasburicase is contraindicated in G6PD-deficient patients with or without CNSHA. In patients with a negative or inconclusive genetic test results an enzyme activity test is recommended prior to rasburicase treatment to determine whether a patient is G6PD deficient

that pharmacogenetic-guided warfarin dosing is more accurate than standard fixed, but not algorithm-guided, dosing. Neither the EU-PACT nor the COAG trial were powered for clinically relevant endpoints, such as bleeding and thromboembolic events, and the currently ongoing randomized Genetics Informatics Trial (GIFT) of Warfarin to Prevent Deep Venous Thrombosis will assess the clinical outcome benefit of pharmacogenetic-guided warfarin dosing.[15]

Alternative anticoagulants (e.g., dabigatran, apixaban, rivaroxaban, and edoxaban) have been developed; for example, the dosing of dabigatran, which acts as a direct thrombin inhibitor, is not influenced by these genetic polymorphisms, which makes this drug a potential alternative for patients in whom heredity is associated with extreme variations in warfarin effects.

DRUG TRANSPORTERS

Although passive diffusion is thought to account for tissue distribution of some drugs and their metabolites, there is a growing body of evidence that membrane transporters play an important role in drug disposition and effects. Membrane transporters are highly expressed in epithelial cells, and move drugs and other xenobiotics across the gastrointestinal (GI) tract into systemic circulation and across hepatic and renal tissue into the bile and urine, respectively, for excretion. They also distribute drugs into and out of "therapeutic sanctuaries" such as the brain and testes, and transport them into and out of sites of action, such as leukemia cells.

The two multi-specific drug transporter superfamilies encompass the adenosine triphosphate (ATP)-binding cassette (ABC) and the solute carrier (SLC) transporters.[16] Whereas SLC transporters largely, but not exclusively, mediate cellular uptake, the ABC drug transporters mainly efflux substrates from cells. The function, substrate specificity, and organ distribution among different transporters vary

and comprehensive drug transporter databases are available elsewhere (see Table 8.1). There is also a growing body of data on the endogenous functions (e.g., transport of metabolites, antioxidants, signaling molecules, and hormones) of ATP and SLC transporters, and a number of hematologic diseases were identified to be caused by variants in these transporters (e.g., variants in SLC19A2 in thiamine-responsive megaloblastic anemia, variants in SLC11A2 in sideroblastic anemia, variants in SLC4A1 in hereditary spherocytosis type 4 and southeast Asian ovalocytosis, and variants in ABCG5 and ABCG8 in mitochondriopathies with large platelets and ovalocytes). Herein we provide one selected example on how variants in a drug transporter (i.e., SLCO1B1) have been identified to influence the disposition and toxicity of the antileukemic drug methotrexate (MTX).

SLCO1B1 and Methotrexate

The solute carrier organic anion-transporter family member 1B1 (SLCO1B1) gene, for example, encodes an organic anion transporter 1B1 (OATP1B1) that is located primarily on the sinusoidal face of human hepatocytes. OATP1B1 mediates the hepatic uptake of many endogenous compounds (e.g., bilirubin) and xenobiotics such as HMG-CoA reductase inhibitors (e.g., simvastatin) from sinusoidal blood, resulting in their net excretion from blood, likely via biliary excretion. A common sequence variant in the coding region of SLCO1B1 (rs4149056) decreases the transport activity of the encoded protein and results in markedly increased plasma concentrations of drugs that are eliminated from the blood via hepatic uptake. Using GWAS, correlations have been established between variants in SLCO1B1 and myopathy after treatment with the HMG-CoA reductase inhibitor simvastin.[9]

In the field of hematology, a GWAS identified the rs4149056 variant to be significantly associated with MTX clearance and GI toxicity; this association was robustly confirmed with five different MTX treatment regimens in more than 1000 pediatric ALL patients.[17] Deep sequencing of *SLCO1B1* identified additional rare (minor allele frequency of <1%) "damaging" nsSNPs that had larger effect sizes than the common "damaging" nsSNPs.[18] SLCO1B1, however, is associated with hepatobiliary excretion, which is a relatively minor path for MTX elimination (<30%). Therefore, the overall contribution of *SLCOB1B* variants to explaining interindividual variability in MTX pharmacokinetics is approximately 12% to 15%, and the major genetic contributors remain largely unknown.

GENETIC VARIATIONS INFLUENCING DRUG TARGETS

To exert their pharmacologic effects most drugs interact with specific target proteins, such as receptors, enzymes, or proteins involved in signal transduction, cell cycle control, or other cellular events. Molecular studies have revealed that many of the genes encoding these drug targets exhibit genetic variations, which can alter the sensitivity of these targets to specific medications (e.g., *VKORC1* and warfarin effects).

The following section illustrates this, focusing on somatic genetic variants in chronic myeloid leukemia (CML) cells that alter the targets of tyrosine kinase inhibitors (TKIs).

BCR–ABL1 and Tyrosine Kinase Inhibitors

Somatic genome variants caused by major structural variants, such as the t(9;22) chromosomal translocation producing the *BCR–ABL1* fusion gene, are major mechanisms underlying many forms of hematopoietic malignancies. The increased tyrosine kinase activity of the BCR–ABL1 protein (encoded by the chimeric BCR–ABL1 or "Philadelphia [Ph] chromosome") is the driving oncogenic event in the majority of patients with CML and in a subset of patients with ALL (Ph-ALL). This realization resulted in the development of specific TKIs. The treatment of CML was revolutionized with the introduction of the first TKI imatinib, a small-molecular-weight drug that binds to ABL1, thereby leading to inhibition of tyrosine phosphorylation of proteins involved in signal transduction. Imatinib was shown to induce durable remissions in CML patients, which led to a paradigm shift in cancer treatment—that is, a more targeted therapy instead of the nonspecific inhibition of rapidly dividing cells.

Although most patients with CML have a favorable outcome when treated with imatinib, some patients eventually fail on therapy, mainly as a result of acquired point mutations in the target kinase ABL1 that induce drug resistance. Of note, the second-generation TKIs nilotinib and dasatinib can successfully inhibit the majority of these mutation proteins that confer resistance to imatinib. However, one relatively common variant, the T315I or "gatekeeper" variant, confers resistance to all three drugs.[19] To overcome the resistance mechanisms of the T315I variant, ponatinib, which has activity against all known single amino acid *ABL1* mutations including T315I, was designed and successfully tested in clinical trials, and its use was first approved by the FDA in 2012 for patients with CML resistant to other TKIs. However, ponatinib was temporarily suspended in 2013 due to serious vascular adverse events (VAEs; i.e., arterial and venous thromboembolic events, arterial hypertension), and VAEs are now recognized as also limiting the use of second-generation TKIs. Moreover, the strong selective pressure of ponatinib has led to the emergence of TKI resistance due to so-called "compound mutations" in ABL1.[19] Compound mutations are multiple-point variants occurring in the same *BCR–ABL1* allele, and this drug-resistance mechanism is different to the emergence of multiple clones with different mutations. In a recent investigation, computed modeling and in vitro proliferation studies were used to analyze the impact of compound mutations in *BCR–ABL1* on TKI resistance. Molecular dynamic simulations showed, for instance, that the compound mutation Y253H/E255V induced a shift in the P-loop of the ABL1 kinase, obstructing the ponatinib binding site, resulting in resistance to ponatinib. Moreover, it was found that additional acquisition of an E255V variant in T315I-positive CML confers resistance to ponatinib.[19]

As second- and third-generation TKIs have a risk for VAEs, especially in older patients with preexisting vascular disease, TKI selection based on cardiovascular risk factors and mutational *BCR–ABL1* status is of utmost importance to guide CML therapy. Upfront and repeated monitoring of the mutational status of patients with BCR–ABL1-positive leukemias can help select appropriate TKIs and tailor TKI treatment, and also has the potential to provide new insights into mechanisms underlying selection of resistant clones during TKI therapy.

ADVERSE DRUG EFFECTS PRESENTING AS HEMATOLOGIC DISORDERS

Adverse drug reactions (ADRs) constitute a major clinical problem, and strong evidence indicates that ADRs account for approximately 5% of all hospital admissions and increase the length of hospitalization by approximately 2 days. Although the factors that determine susceptibility to ADRs are unclear in most cases, there is increasing interest in the role of genetic predisposition to these ADRs; the possibility of a genetic test to identify patients at risk for rare but serious adverse effects would be of great clinical value. Based on the clinical relevance of ADRs, the FDA has provided advice on the use of certain biomarkers (e.g., variants in *TPMT*, *UGT1A1*, *CYP2C9*, *CYP2C19*) to avoid serious adverse drug effects; a full list of these biomarkers is available on the FDA website (see Table 8.1).

CPIC recommendations on medications whose adverse effects have been associated with variability in candidate genes and manifest predominantly as hematologic abnormalities are listed in Table 8.2. In the following section, we provide information on genetic variants in G6PD that can cause acute hemolytic anemia (AHA) after administration of certain drugs.

Glucose-6-Phosphate Dehydrogenase Deficiency and Rasburicase

Occurrence of AHA after mass administration of the antimalaria drug primaquine (PQ) was first documented in some U.S. soldiers in Korea. The so-called "PQ sensitivity syndrome" was more common among African Americans, and clinically identical to "favism" (i.e., AHA after ingestion of fava beans). The underlying biochemical (Fig. 8.3) and genetic (variants in *G6PD*) causes of the clinical phenotype (i.e., AHA after PQ and fava beans) were identified, and the disease was named G6PD deficiency.[20] The severity of AHA in individuals with G6PD deficiency after treatment with drugs that induce oxidative stress is influenced by host and environmental factors (Fig. 8.3).

The *G6PD* gene is localized on Xq28, and currently more than 180 genetic variants have been identified, most of which are missense mutations resulting in single-amino acid substitutions, thereby affecting G6PD stability.[20] Complete loss of G6PD is lethal; the very rare, more complex variants, for instance, in-frame deletions in exon 10, which affect important regions within the enzyme-like the substrate binding site, can cause severe transfusion-dependent chronic nonspherocytic hemolytic anemia (CNSHA). Variants have been divided into five classes based on enzyme activity in red blood cells (RBCs) and clinical presentation: class I (CNSHA, activity <10%), class II (no CNSHA, activity <10%), class III (no CNSHA, >10% to 60%), class IV (normal activity; variants G6PD B and G6PD A); class V (higher activity). It is estimated that about 5% of the world's population have G6PD deficiency, and almost all of these individuals have class II or III variants.[21]

Drugs that have the potential to cause oxidative stress in erythrocytes, which results in AHA in G6PD-deficient patients, have been recently classified into two groups: (1) predictable hemolysis (i.e., AHA can be expected in a G6PD-deficient patient after

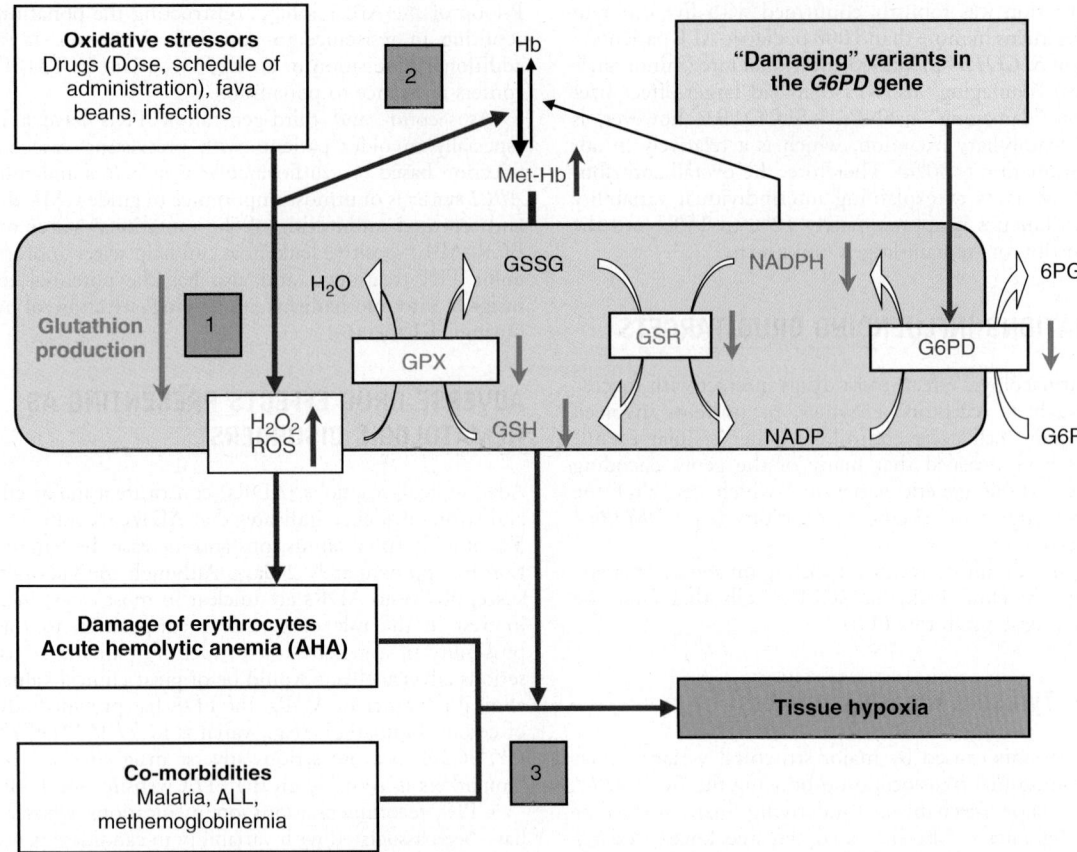

Fig. 8.3 Damaging variants in the G6PD gene lead to G6PD deficiency in red blood cells, which, under oxidative stress (1), leads to depletion of glutathione (with low cellular NADPH and GSH pools causing low activity of GPX [the enzyme that detoxifies H_2O_2]) and subsequent loss of protection against oxidation of proteins, with precipitation of denaturized hemoglobin leading to AHA, and (2) oxidation of hemoglobin iron with formation of methemoglobin (MetHb is converted back to Hb via an NADPH-dependent reaction; as the cellular NADPH pool is low, MetHb accumulates), resulting in methemoglobinemia. The severity of AHA and tissue hypoxia in individuals with G6PD deficiency after treatment with drugs that induce oxidative stress is influenced by host factors such as genetic variants in G6PD and (3) comorbidities such as malaria, methemoglobinemia, and ALL, as well as environmental factors (i.e., drugs, their dose, and schedule of administration). *6PG,* 6-Phosphogluconolactone; *AHA,* acute hemolytic anemia; *ALL,* acute lymphoblastic leukemia; *G6P,* glucose 6-phosphate; *G6PD,* glucose-6-phosphate dehydrogenase; *GPX,* glutathione peroxidase; *GSH,* glutathione; *GSR,* glutathione reductase; *GSSG,* glutathione disulfide; H_2O_2, hydrogen peroxide; *NADP(H),* nicotinamide adenine dinucleotide phosphate; *ROS,* reactive oxygen species.

administration of the drug) and (2) possible hemolysis (i.e., AHA may or may not occur, related to dosage and administration of the drug, comorbidities).[20] Drugs with predictable hemolysis include, for instance, the antimalaria drug PQ and the recombinant urate oxidase rasburicase. A comprehensive list of drugs is provided in two exhaustive recent reviews,[20,21] and we focus on rasburicase herein.

Rasburicase is used in the prophylaxis and treatment of hyperuricemia, and the most important indications are tumorlysis (e.g., in patients with hyperleukocytosis leukemia or lymphoma) or after acute renal failure in infants. Rasburicase catalyzes the cleavage of uric acid, thereby producing hydrogen peroxide. Normally, hydrogen peroxide is promptly inactivated via glutathione peroxidase (GPX). In individuals with G6PD deficiency, however, the activity of GPX is markedly reduced due to impaired glutathione metabolism, and rasburicase induces AHA and often significant methemoglobinemia. This can cause severe tissue hypoxia, especially in patients with leukemia who have already reduced RBC counts, and fatalities have been reported after rasburicase administration in ALL patients with G6PD deficiency (Fig. 8.3).[21]

The FDA and the European Medicines Agency (EMA) have contraindicated the use of rasburicase in individuals with G6PD deficiency. However, tumorlysis syndrome (TLS) is also a life-threatening condition, and one must carefully balance the risk of reversible severe AHA and methemoglobinemia, which can be treated via RBC transfusions, and the risk of renal failure and hyperkalemia in TLS. Online enzyme activity testing before the use of rasburicase (i.e., providing results within 1 h) is an ideal but not commonly achievable scenario. More information on available genetic and activity test options is provided in the recently published CPIC guidelines (Table 8.2).[21]

Of interest are the results of a recent pharmacoepigenetic investigation, in which it was shown that histone deacetylase inhibitors (HDACis) can selectively reinstate enzyme activity in G6PD-deficient erythroid precursors in vitro by boosting *G6PD* gene transcription.[22] Whether administration of the epidrug HDACi sodium butyrate can also increase G6PD activity in patients with G6PD deficiency to levels that protect their erythrocytes from oxidative damage by rasburicase or other oxidative stressors, and if such an approach is not associated with severe side effects, remains to be proven. However, the ability of HDACi to increase the transcription of a subset of active genes, like *G6PD*, would offer a novel and appealing therapeutic approach, especially for the subset of patients with severe forms of enzymopathies, such as CNSAH class I G6PD deficiency.

DRUG DEVELOPMENT

Optimizing the selection and dosage of medications is a principal goal of pharmacogenomics. Another important application is in drug development, which is evolving in parallel with improved insights into the mechanisms by which medications exert their pharmacologic effects. Such improved insights into the mechanism(s) of drug action in target cells can help elucidate mechanisms that confer drug resistance (e.g., inactivation of thiopurines via NT5C2), and they will facilitate the development of strategies to further enhance efficacy. This knowledge can be used as a basis to engineer drugs that amplify treatment effects or bypass resistance mechanisms, or both.

Here we focus on examples to show how insights from pharmacogenomic investigations have helped to develop novel strategies to further improve outcome in subgroups of children with ALL who still have a poor outcome despite intensive treatment with current multiagent risk-adapted therapies (so-called high-risk ALL [HR-ALL]). Although excellent outcomes with 5-year event-free survival of higher than 85% can be achieved in childhood ALL in more developed countries, ALL is still a leading cause of death from disease in children older than 1 year, and treatment of children with HR-ALL remains one of the greatest challenges in pediatric oncology. HR-ALL features include the resistance of leukemia cells to steroids and multidrug therapy (clearance of leukemia blasts in the peripheral blood, bone marrow, and sanctuary sites), and the presence of certain genetic alterations in leukemia cells—for instance, mixed-lineage leukemia rearrangements (MLL-R), the BCR–ABL1 fusion gene (Ph-ALL), and the recently identified so-called "Ph-like ALL."[23,24]

The introduction of TKIs in the treatment of Ph-ALL has led to a significant improvement in outcome, as demonstrated by results from the Children's Oncology Group (COG) AALL0031 trial. The following sections focus on further examples of the development of novel approaches to treat infants, children, and adolescents with HR-ALL.

Identification of Novel Therapies for MLL-Rearranged Infant ALL

Infants (age <1 year) with BCP-ALL have long been recognized to have very poor outcomes when treated with ALL standard therapy. The identification that transcriptome profiles separate infant ALL from ALL and acute myeloid leukemia (AML), and that infant ALL blast cells are highly sensitive to cytarabine in vitro, provided the rationale to establish an ALL/AML hybrid treatment concept. Indeed, Interfant-99 hybrid therapy resulted in better, but still poor, outcomes, and further improvements of infant ALL therapy are needed. Of note, the pharmacokinetics of many conventional antileukemia drugs differ between infants and older children, and recently an intensive induction therapy concept (with intensive dosing of standard ALL medications) in the COG AALL0631 trial had to be modified because of a high rate of fatal toxicities during this treatment phase. Therefore, the unique drug metabolism profile in infants (i.e., developmental pharmacology) needs to be considered when planning future infant ALL trials and novel, less toxic therapies are needed.

About 80% of infants with ALL have rearrangements of the *MLL* gene (MLL-R) at 11q23 and MLL translocations. Recently, next-generation sequencing approaches were used in a Pediatric Cancer Genome Project investigation and identified that infant MLL-R ALL has one of the lowest frequencies of somatic mutations of any as yet sequenced cancer, with a mean of 1.3 nonsilent mutations.[25] Wild-type *MLL* is a histone methyltransferase that targets lysine 4 on histone 3 (H3K4), and leukemias carrying MLL-R (i.e., BCP-ALL in infants and older age groups, and AML in adults) can be considered as prototypical cancers driven by dysregulated epigenetic mechanisms. *MLL* rearrangements lead to the loss of the catalytic methyltransferase domain, with subsequent in-frame fusion to one

of 70 known translocation partners. The resulting chimeric oncoproteins interact with another methyltransferase—DOT1-like histone H3K79 methyltransferase (DOT1L)—which then methylates lysin 79 in the globular region of histone H3 (H3K79) at MLL target genes, causing aberrant gene expression and leukemogenesis. Inhibition of DOT1L has emerged as an attractive concept for therapeutic intervention in MLL-R leukemias, and in vitro and animal studies have shown that the recently designed small molecular inhibitors of DOT1L selectively target MLL-R leukemia cells.[26] A phase I trial (NCT01684150) for the clinical evaluation of the epidrug EPZ-5676 was initiated for patients older than 18 years with MLL-R leukemias, and if this approach proves to be successful, it remains primed for testing in infants with MLL-R ALL.

A different approach focuses on targeting the class III receptor tyrosine kinase (RTK) FMS-like tyrosine kinase-3 (FLT3). Using genome-wide gene expression analyses, the *FLT3* wild-type gene was identified as being overexpressed in MLL-R ALL. FLT3 inhibitors have been shown to inhibit growth in cells that overexpress FLT3.[27] The COG AALL0631 trial investigates the combination of the FLT3 inhibitor lestaurtinib given after induction therapy in combination with an intensive chemotherapy backbone in children with MLL-R infant ALL, and this approach may also help to improve outcomes in this poor prognostic ALL subtype.

Identification of Novel Therapies for "BCR–ABL1-like" ALL

In contrast to the prognostically favorable BCP-ALL subtypes ETV6-RUNX1, TCF3-PBX1, and hyperdiploid ALL (which account for almost 50% of childhood ALL cases), BCP-ALL with the *BCR–ABL1* (or Philadelphia [Ph]) fusion gene responds poorly to conventional ALL therapy, and patients with Ph-ALL belong to the HR-ALL group. Ph-ALL is rare in children (1–15 years, 4.2%), but is more common in adolescents (16–20 years, 5.9%) and young adults (21–39 years, 22%); and this is a contributor to the overall poor prognosis of adolescents and young adults (AYAs) with ALL.

In 2009, genome-wide trancriptome analyses identified a subtype of HR-BCP-ALL that has a gene expression profile similar to that of Ph-ALL.[23,24] In contrast to Ph-ALL, leukemia cells in the identified subtype did not harbor the *BCR–ABL1* fusion gene; therefore this HR-ALL subtype has been named Ph-like ALL. Ph-like ALL is more common, but has the same age distribution pattern as Ph-ALL (i.e., 1–15 years, 11.9%; 16–20 years, 20.6%; 21–39 years, 27.4%). It was speculated that genetic alterations that can influence tyrosine kinase signaling pathways similar to those downstream of BCR–ABL1 might be involved in the pathogenesis of Ph-like ALL. Indeed, kinase-activating alterations (fusions, deletions, or point mutations) were recently identified in a comprehensive analysis, which included transcriptome, whole-genome, and whole-exome sequencing in 91% of 154 patients with Ph-like ALL.[28]

This large-scale investigation corroborated and extended previous findings in Ph-like ALL and identified two major subgroups, distinguished by the type of cytokine receptor or kinase alterations. For example, 60% of adolescents with Ph-like ALL had rearrangements in the lymphoid signaling receptor gene *CRLF2* (encoding cytokine receptor-like factor 2) and concomitant mutations in *JAK1* or *JAK2* (which encode the Janus kinases [JAKs]). These rearrangements (e.g., the frequently observed *PAX5–JAK2* fusion), when ectopically expressed in cell lines, activated JAK-STAT signaling and conferred cytokine-independent proliferation that can be suppressed by the JAK2 inhibitor ruxolitinib in vitro. The second major subgroup within the Ph-like ALL cohort was identified to have fusions that involve the nonreceptor Abelson-related (ABL)-class kinase genes (e.g., *ABL1* and *ABL2*), as well as activated oncogenic signaling pathways and cellular proliferation that is potentially inhibited by TKIs such as dasatinib. Other less frequently observed targetable alterations affect the *NTRK3* gene, which encodes the neurotrophic tyrosine kinase receptor type 3, and *ETV6* (ets variant 6)–*NTRK3* fusions have been shown to respond to the ALK inhibitor crizotinib in vitro. The in vitro results with the TK, JAK2, and ALK inhibitors were confirmed in mouse xenograft models, when patient-derived Ph-like ALL cells were exposed to respective inhibitors based on the genetic profile of the leukemia cells.[28]

In summary, this provides evidence that kinase-activating genetic alterations are biologically relevant drivers in Ph-like ALL, and that the genetic signature can help to select drugs such as TKIs, JAK2 or ALK inhibitors. However, rapid molecular profiling is needed to identify potentially actionable mutations in patients with Ph-like ALL, and additional prospective trials are needed to establish their benefit in the clinical setting. In contrast to children, outcomes in ALL have not improved significantly during recent decades in the AYA cohort; and as Ph-like ALL is the most common subtype in AYAs, the introduction of signaling pathway inhibitors may be an attractive strategy to improve outcome in these patients who have been therapeutically neglected for too long.

FUTURE DIRECTIONS

Pharmacogenomics has already proven to be an important approach to improve drug therapy, and as of March 2015 the FDA has included information on pharmacogenomic biomarkers in the labels of more than 130 medications. A full list of these medications and further details are available on the FDA's website (see Table 8.1). There is, however, a relatively slow pace of translating pharmacogenomics into clinical practice. Laboratory tests (e.g., liver and kidney function tests) are widely used to adjust drug dosages, but even though technology for testing relevant pharmacogenomic biomarkers is widely available, simple, robust, and inexpensive genotyping tests are rarely used to optimize drug therapy. As of 2015 only five institutions in the United States are routinely performing "preemptive genotyping" for pharmacogenomic traits to guide the optimal selection of medications and their dosage. Because genotyping at the time of prescribing is compromised by the relatively long delay until genotype results are available, prospective genotyping early in a person's life or at the time of initial illness is a more efficient and cost-effective approach. In addition, because a person's germline genotype does not change over a lifetime, it only needs to be done once. As genotyping becomes faster and cheaper, it is anticipated that this issue may no longer be an obstacle. In addition, educative and legislative initiatives, and the implementation of user-friendly decision-support systems (e.g., as realized in the "Clinical implementation of pharmacogenomics—PG4KDS protocol" at St. Jude Children's Research Hospital)[29] will help to make pharmacogenomic biomarkers a routine part of clinical care.

The recent unprecedented gain of insights into the human genome and genomic variations among individuals has already changed the practice of medicine. High-throughput technologies, such as hybridization-based microarray approaches and next-generation sequencing technologies, are available for genome-wide analyses of genomic variants, gene expression patterns, epigenetic patterns, and proteomic and metabonomic profiles. Moreover, sophisticated methods have been developed to integrate these data in order to uncover genotype–phenotype interactions, and some of the most important methods are metadimensional and multistaged analyses.[30] The recent application of these genome-wide tools has already yielded novel insights into drug actions and led to important drug discoveries.

Moreover, these tools are being used to elucidate differences between genomes of normal cells and cancer cells (e.g., the Pediatric Cancer Genome Project; see Table 8.1), and this knowledge has the potential to illuminate paths toward novel prognostic markers (those that can be used for risk stratification in clinical trials) and/or novel therapeutic targets (those that can be used to discover new medications).

Once novel candidate genes have been identified via GWA studies, functional investigations such as systematic mutagenesis, RNA interference, and genome-wide CRISPR/Cas9 knockouts or enhancement of gene expression, use of overexpression systems (cDNA, open-reading frame and miRNA expression libraries), and

chemistry-based approaches to biologic pathway perturbations are likely to accelerate the discovery of pharmacogenomics mechanisms. The outputs of such studies will advance understanding of the pharmacology of existing medications and will help to identify genes and pathways involved in drug resistance and novel therapeutic targets.

One important consideration in modern medicine is that clinically useful approaches must also be cost effective. About a decade ago, the cost for the first full human genome sequence was approximately US$3 billion; this cost is now (2015) about US$1000. The markedly lower cost for robust genotyping points to an exciting future for genomics and pharmacogenomics research and translation, suggesting that the current approach to selecting medications (often "trial and error") will continue to evolve into more scientific-based methods for selecting the optimal medications and doses for individual patients—with genomics playing an increasing role in such therapeutic decisions. As pharmacoggenomics research expands the number of robust associations between genome variation and drug response, the challenges of successful clinical translation and implementation will be hurdle that will need to be overcome for precision medicine is to become a reality.[31]

REFERENCES

1. Evans WE, Relling MV: Moving towards individualized medicine with pharmacogenomics. *Nature* 429(6990):464–468, 2004.
2. Chhibber A, Kroetz DL, Tantisira KG, et al: Genomic architecture of pharmacological efficacy and adverse events. *Pharmacogenomics* 15(16):2025–2048, 2014.
3. Ivanov M, Barragan I, Inglman-Sundberg M: Epigenetic mechanisms of importance for drug treatment. *Trends Pharmacol Sci* 35(8):384–396, 2014.
4. Hunt RC, Simhadri VL, Indoli M, et al: Exposing synonymous mutations. *Trends Genet* 30(7):308–321, 2014.
5. Diouf B, Crews C, Lew G, et al: Association of an inherited genetic variant with vincristine-related peripheral neuropathy in children with acute lymphoblastic leukemia. *JAMA* 313(8):815–823, 2015.
6. Rukov JL, Wilentzik R, Jaffe I, et al: Pharmaco-miR: linking microRNAs and drug effects. *Brief Bioinform* 15(4):648–659, 2014.
7. He Y, Hoskins JM, McLeod HL: Copy number variants in pharmacogenetic genes. *Trends Mol Med* 17(5):244–251, 2011.
8. Diouf B, Cheng Q, Krynetskaia N, et al: Somatic deletions of genes regulating MSH2 protein stability cause DNA mismatch repair deficiency and drug resistance in human leukemia cells. *Nat Med* 17(10):1298–1303, 2011.
9. Manalio TA: Bringing genome-wide association findings into clinical use. *Nature Rev Genet* 14:549–558, 2013.
10. Relling MV, Gardner EE, Sandborn WJ, et al: Clinical Pharmacogenetics Implementation Consortium guidelines for thiopurine methyltransferase genotype and thiopurine dosing: 2013 update. *Clin Pharmacol Ther* 93(4):324–325, 2013.
11. Yang SK, Hong M, Baek J, et al: A common missense variant in NUDT15 confers susceptibility to thiopurine-induced leucopenia. *Nat Genet* 46(9):1017–1020, 2014.
12. Yang JJ, Landier W, Yang W, et al: Inherited NUDT15 variant is a genetic determinant of mercaptopurin intolerance in children with acute lymphoblastic leukemia. *J Clin Oncol* 2015. doi: 10.1200/JCO.2014.59.4671.
13. Tzoneva G, Perez-Garcia A, Carpenter Z, et al: Activating mutations in the NT5C2 nucleotidase gene drive chemotherapy resistance in relapsed ALL. *Nat Med* 19(3):368–371, 2013.
14. Meyer JA, Wang J, Hogan LE, et al: Relapse specific mutations in NT5C2 in childhood acute lymphoblastic leukemia. *Nat Genet* 45(3):290–294, 2013.
15. Pirmohamed M, Kamali F, Daly AK, et al: Oral anticoagulation: a critique of recent advances and controversies. *Trends Pharmacol Sci* 36(2):153–163, 2015.
16. Nigam SK: What do drug transporters really do? *Nat Rev Drug Discov* 14:29–44, 2015.

17. Ramsey LB, Panetta JC, Smith C, et al: Genome-wide study of methotrexate clearance replicates SLCO1B1. *Blood* 121(6):898–904, 2013.

18. Ramsey LB, Bruun GH, Yang W, et al: Rare versus common variants in pharmacogenetics: SLCO1B1 variation and methotrexate disposition. *Genome Res* 22:1–8, 2012.

19. Zabriskie MS, Eide CA, Tantravahi SK, et al: BCR–ABL1 compound mutations combining key domain positions confer clinical resistance to ponatinib in Ph chromosome-positive leukemia. *Cancer Cell* 26:428–442, 2014.

20. Luzzatto L, Seneca E: G6PD deficiency: a classic example of pharmacogenomics with on-going clinical implications. *Br J Haematol* 164:469–480, 2014.

21. Relling MV, McDonagh EM, Chang T, et al: Clinical pharmacogenetics implementation consortium (CPIC) guidelines for rasburicase therapy in the context of G6PD deficiency genotype. *Clin Pharmacol Ther* 96(2):169–174, 2014.

22. Makarona K, Caputo VS, Costa JR, et al: Transcriptional and epigenetic basis for restoration of G6PD enzymatic activity in human G6PD-deficient cells. *Blood* 124(1):134–141, 2014.

23. Den Boer ML, van Slegtenhorst M, De Menezes RX, et al: A subtype of childhood acute lymphoblastic leukemia with poor treatment outcome: a genome-wide classification study. *Lancet Oncol* 10:125–134, 2009.

24. Mullighan CG, Su X, Zhang J, et al: Deletion of IKZF1 and prognosis in acute lymphoblastic leukemia. *New Engl J Med* 360:470–480, 2009.

25. Andersson AK, Ma J, Wang J, et al: The landscape of somatic mutations in infant MLL-rearranged acute lymphoblastic leukemias. *Nat Genet* 47(4):330–337, 2015.

26. Neff T, Armstrong SA: Recent progress toward epigenetic therapies: the example of mixed lineage leukemia. *Blood* 121(24):4847–4853, 2013.

27. Annesley CE, Brown P: The biology and targeting of FLT3 in pediatric leukemia. *Front Oncol* 4:263, 2014. doi: 10.3389/fonc.2014.00263. eCollection 2014.

28. Roberts KG, Li Y, Payne-Turner D, et al: Targetable kinase-activating lesions in Ph-like acute lymphoblastic leukemia. *N Engl J Med* 371:1005–1015, 2014.

29. Hoffman JM, Haidar CE, Wilkinson MR, et al: PG4KDS: a model for the pre-emptive implementation of pharmacogenetics. *Am J Med Genet C Semin Med Genet* 166C:45–55, 2014.

30. Ritchie MD, Holzinger ER, Li R, et al: Methods of integrating data to uncover genotype-phenotype interactions. *Nat Rev Genet* 16:85–97, 2015.

31. Relling MV, Evans WE: Pharmacogenomics in the clinic. *Nature* 526:343–350, 2015.

CELLULAR BASIS OF HEMATOLOGY

CHAPTER 9

HEMATOPOIETIC STEM CELL BIOLOGY

Marlies P. Rossmann, Stuart H. Orkin, and John P. Chute

Hematopoietic stem cells (HSCs) are characterized by their unique ability to self-renew and give rise to the entirety of the blood and immune system throughout the lifetime of an individual.[1–3] HSCs are very rare cells, representing approximately one in 100,000 bone marrow (BM) cells in the adult.[4] The concept of the existence of an HSC that is capable of reconstituting hematopoiesis in vivo was first introduced more than 60 years ago, when Jacobson et al[5] demonstrated that lead shielding of the spleen protected mice from otherwise lethal γ-irradiation.[5] Subsequently, Jacobson and colleagues[6] demonstrated that similar radioprotection of mice could be achieved via shielding of one femur. Shortly thereafter, it was demonstrated that intravenous injection of BM cells also provided radioprotection of lethally irradiated mice.[7] Interestingly, investigators initially hypothesized that the radioprotected spleen or BM provided soluble factors that mediated radiation protection.[8,9] However, subsequent experiments by Nowell et al[10] and Ford et al[11] critically demonstrated that transplanted BM cells provided radioprotection directly via cellular reconstitution of the blood system. The historical significance of these studies cannot be overestimated because they provided the basis for not only the ultimate isolation and characterization of HSCs but also for the field of hematopoietic cell transplantation.

Subsequent landmark studies by Till and McCulloch[12] demonstrated that transplantation of limiting doses of BM cells gave rise to myeloid and erythroid colonies in the spleens of irradiated recipient mice. Importantly, Till and McCulloch showed that the numbers of colonies detected in recipient mice was proportional to the numbers of BM cells injected into the irradiated mice, suggesting that a particular population of hematopoietic cells was capable of reconstituting hematopoiesis in vivo.[12–14] The clonogenic nature of a subset of BM cells was definitively shown when these investigators irradiated BM cells and then transplanted the cells into lethally irradiated mice. Persistent chromosomal aberrations were demonstrated in spleen colonies in recipient mice.[15] It was subsequently shown that cells within the spleen colonies were radioprotective of lethally irradiated mice and contained myeloid, erythroid, and lymphoid cells.[12,16] Taken together, these data strongly suggested the presence of hematopoietic stem or progenitor cells that were capable of in vivo engraftment and generation of multilineage progeny from a small number of parent cells.[17]

EMBRYONIC ORIGIN OF HEMATOPOIETIC STEM CELLS

Mammalian hematopoiesis occurs in several waves, which are separated temporally and spatially and produce different cell types: a transient first "primitive" is followed by a "prodefinitive" and then a "definitive" wave, which is lasting through life.[18–20] While most of the evidence is derived from the mouse, data from humans, albeit limited, point to a very comparable hematopoietic program.[21,22]

During embryogenesis, the hematopoietic cells of the first, primitive wave are formed when cells from the epiblast that constitute the prospective mesoderm ingress and migrate through the primitive streak between the endoderm and ectoderm, both in the embryo proper and in the extraembryonic yolk sac (YS). In the latter, mesodermal cells aggregate to form blood islands surrounded by visceral endodermal cells on mouse embryonic day (E) 7–7.5. The close proximity of erythroid cells and vascular endothelium in YS blood islands, their origin from mesoderm and their simultaneous differentiation led to the proposal of a common precursor, the hemangioblast,

over a century ago.[23,24] In support of this hypothesis, a spontaneous zebrafish mutant, *cloche* (named for its bell-shaped heart because of the loss of endothelium), lacks both vasculature and hematopoietic cells but no other mesodermal lineages such as cardiac progenitors.[25,26] The gene mutated in *cloche* was recently cloned and encodes a PAS (PER-ARNT-SIM)-domain-containing basic helix-loop-helix (bHLH) transcription factor (*npas4l*), which belongs to the same class that also includes the aryl hydrocarbon receptor and HIF-1α.[26a] Also, mice lacking FLK1 (VEGFR2, a receptor for vascular endothelial growth factor), expressed on endothelial (progenitor) cells, fail to develop both vascular endothelium and blood islands during embryogenesis.[27,28] Indeed, gene tracing studies in mouse and human embryonic stem cell cultures identified a progenitor with both hematopoietic and endothelial potential.[29–31]

Primitive hematopoiesis encompasses the generation of primarily large erythroid cells and primitive macrophages.[32–34] Following this initial wave, beginning at mouse E8.25, erythromyeloid progenitors are generated as prodefinitive progenitors.[35,36] Both waves arise transiently in the YS during a time comparable to the first trimester in humans,[37] but the cells lack the capacity for self-renewal and multilineage differentiation present in definitive HSCs. The first definitive HSCs capable of long-term, multilineage reconstitution of irradiated adult recipient mice appear at E10.5 in the intraembryonic region encompassing the aorta, gonads, and mesonephros (AGM), in particular in hematopoietic intraaortic clusters in the ventral wall of the dorsal aorta.[20,38–40] Then, within a remarkably short period of 1.5 days during embryonic development virtually all HSCs are born that will replenish the hematopoietic system throughout fetal and adult life.[41,42] Several complementary studies using lineage tracing experiments in both mice and zebrafish have demonstrated that within the dorsal aorta, hemogenic endothelial cells (ECs) are the direct precursors of definitive HSCs.[42–47] In a process known as endothelial-to-hematopoietic transition, HSCs bud off the hemogenic endothelium to form intraaortic hematopoietic clusters from which they are released into circulation. Interestingly, while the AGM gives rise to HSCs, it is not the site of hematopoietic differentiation.[48] Rather, HSCs colonize the fetal liver where they expand and then differentiate ([49] and references therein).

Evidence from studies in mice suggests that some adult hematopoiesis also occurs at sites other than the AGM. By E12 the fetal liver contains more HSCs than can be accounted for by HSCs generated in the AGM alone.[50] Quantitative analysis of HSC distribution showed that both YS[50] and placenta[51,52] generate definitive HSC that migrate to the liver and other hematopoietic sites.[53] Lastly, a c-Myb- and thus HSC-independent cell lineage that emerges between E8.5 and E9.5 in the YS has recently been shown to give rise to YS macrophages and later on to tissue macrophages in brain (microglia), liver (Kupffer cells), and skin (Langerhans cells).[54]

DEFINITION AND CHARACTERIZATION OF HEMATOPOIETIC STEM CELLS

Phenotype

Murine HSCs

The HSC is the most well-defined somatic, multipotent stem cell in the body. With the emergence of antibody technology and flow

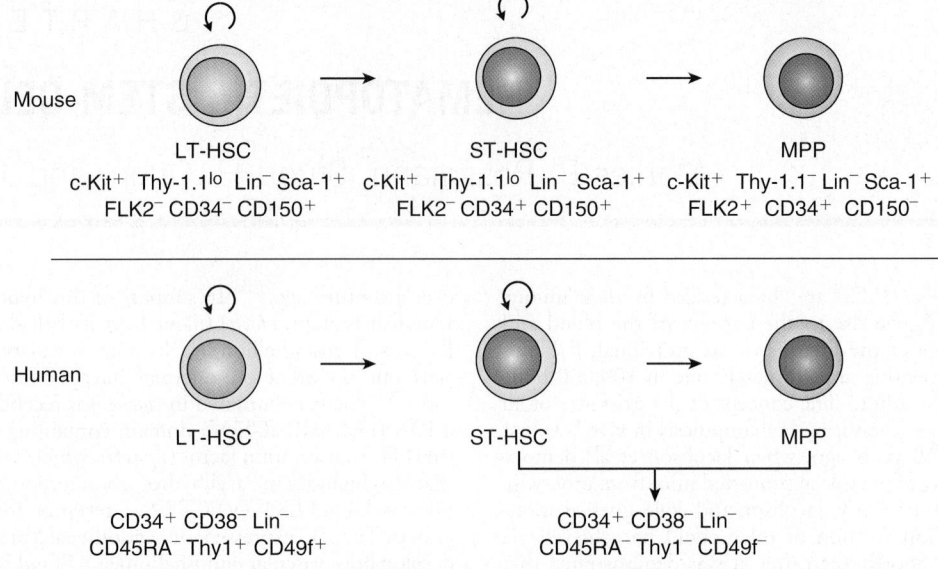

Fig. 9.1 PHENOTYPE OF MURINE AND HUMAN HEMATOPOIETIC STEM CELLS (HSCs). Long-term HSCs (LT-HSCs), short-term HSCs (ST-HSCs), and multipotent progenitor cells (MPPs) have precise cell surface markers that discriminate them from more committed progenitor cells. *(Adapted from Prohaska SS, Weissman I: Biology of hematopoietic stem and progenitor cells. In Appelbaum F, Forman SJ, Negrin RS, Blume K, editors: Thomas' hematopoietic cell transplantation, UK, 2008, Wiley-Blackwell, p 36-63.)*

cytometry[17,55,56] and coupled with in vitro and in vivo functional assays,[57–62] biologists have developed reproducible methods to analyze and isolate murine and human HSCs with a high level of enrichment. In mice, Weissman and colleagues were able to show that antibody-based depletion of BM cells expressing myeloid, B cell, T cell, and erythroid cells along with positive selection for cells expressing c-Kit, Sca-1, and Thy-1.1[lo] ("KTLS" cells), allowed for enrichment for HSCs to approximately one of 10–30 cells as measured by the capacity to provide long-term, multilineage hematopoietic reconstitution in a competitively transplanted, lethally irradiated congenic mouse.[58,63–66] Because Thy-1.1 is not expressed in many strains of mice,[64] additional markers were developed, including FLK2 (FLT3), the absence of which was shown to substantially enrich for murine long-term (LT)-HSCs.[67,68] Similarly, it has been demonstrated that the isolation of murine BM c-Kit+Sca-1+Lin− (KSL) cells based upon the lack of expression of CD34 (34−KSL) enriches for HSCs with long-term reconstituting capability at the level of one of 5–10 cells (Fig. 9.1).[69]

An alternative and effective method for isolating BM HSCs involves the use of intravital dyes, Hoechst 33342 (Ho33342) and Rhodamine 123 (Rh123).[70–74] HSCs, unlike more committed progenitor cells, efficiently efflux these dyes such that HSCs display low-intensity staining for these dyes.[74,75] Li and Johnson[73] demonstrated that HSCs capable of long-term, multilineage repopulation in lethally irradiated mice were significantly enriched in the Rh123[lo]Sca-1+Lin− cells, but Rh123[hi]Sca-1+Lin− cells possessed little repopulating activity. Similarly, McAlister et al[72] showed that isolation of Ho33342[lo] BM mononuclear cells significantly enriched for both the potential to produce colony-forming units in the spleen (CFU-S) on day 14 and cells capable of radioprotection and multilineage reconstitution in lethally irradiated mice. A subsequent and important refinement in the use of Ho33342 to isolate HSCs was made by Goodell et al,[74] who showed that a Ho33342 side population (SP) can be identified via the emission of Ho33342 at two wavelengths, which yields a tail profile on flow cytometric analysis. Importantly, isolation of Ho33342 SP cells has been shown to yield variable enrichment for HSCs compared with 34−FLT3−KSL cells, and this may be caused by the sensitivity of the assay to variations in staining techniques and batch-to-batch differences in Ho33342 dye.[76–78] However, Matsuzaki et al[79] demonstrated that transplantation of

single Ho33342 SP 34−KSL cells into lethally irradiated C57BL/6 mice yielded donor cell multilineage engraftment greater than 1% in more than 95% of transplanted mice. Therefore, the combination of Ho33342 SP cells with 34−KSL markers provides a basis for isolation of highly enriched LT-HSCs from mice.[55,76–78]

A major advance in this field involved the discovery by Kiel et al[80] that the surface expression of CD150, a member of the signaling lymphocyte activation molecules (SLAM) family, significantly enriched for murine BM HSCs. It was also shown that the absence of CD41 and CD48 on CD150+ cells enriches further for the HSC population and that approximately half of CD150+CD41−CD48− or CD150+CD48−KSL cells reconstitute lethally irradiated mice competitively transplanted with limiting numbers of cells.[80] Taken together, isolation of SLAM- and KSL-enriched BM cells has become a reproducible and efficient strategy to isolate murine LT-HSCs with maximal enrichment (see Fig. 9.1).[81]

Although this chapter focuses on the phenotypic and functional characterization of HSCs, increasing evidence suggests that a subset of adult T-cell progenitors may possess myeloid potential.[82–84] Using various methodologies, Bell et al[83] and Wada et al[82] first reported that adult T-cell thymic progenitors possessed myeloid differentiation potential. However, a subsequent study using in vivo transplantation models did not confirm the myeloid potential of adult T cells.[84] More recently, De Obaldia et al reported that the majority of resident granulocytes in the mouse thymus were derived from early thymic progenitors.[85] Mechanistically, it has also been shown that the transcription factor, HES1, constrains myeloid gene expression in T-cell progenitors via repression of C/EPB-α.[86] Taken together, these data suggest that a population of common lymphoid progenitors (CLPs) may indeed possess myeloid differentiation potential.[85,86] Recent studies have also clarified the nature of CLPs and have dissected this population further into an all-lymphoid progenitor cell (ALP), which retains full lymphoid potential and thymic seeding capability, and B lymphoid progenitor cells (BLPs), which is restricted to the B-cell lineage.[87] Whereas ALPs are characterized by the lack of surface expression of LY6D, BLPs demonstrate expression of LY6D and upregulate the B-cell-specific factors, EBF1 and PAX5.[87] The phenotypic markers of the hematopoietic hierarchy through myeloid and lymphoid differentiation are shown in Fig. 9.2.

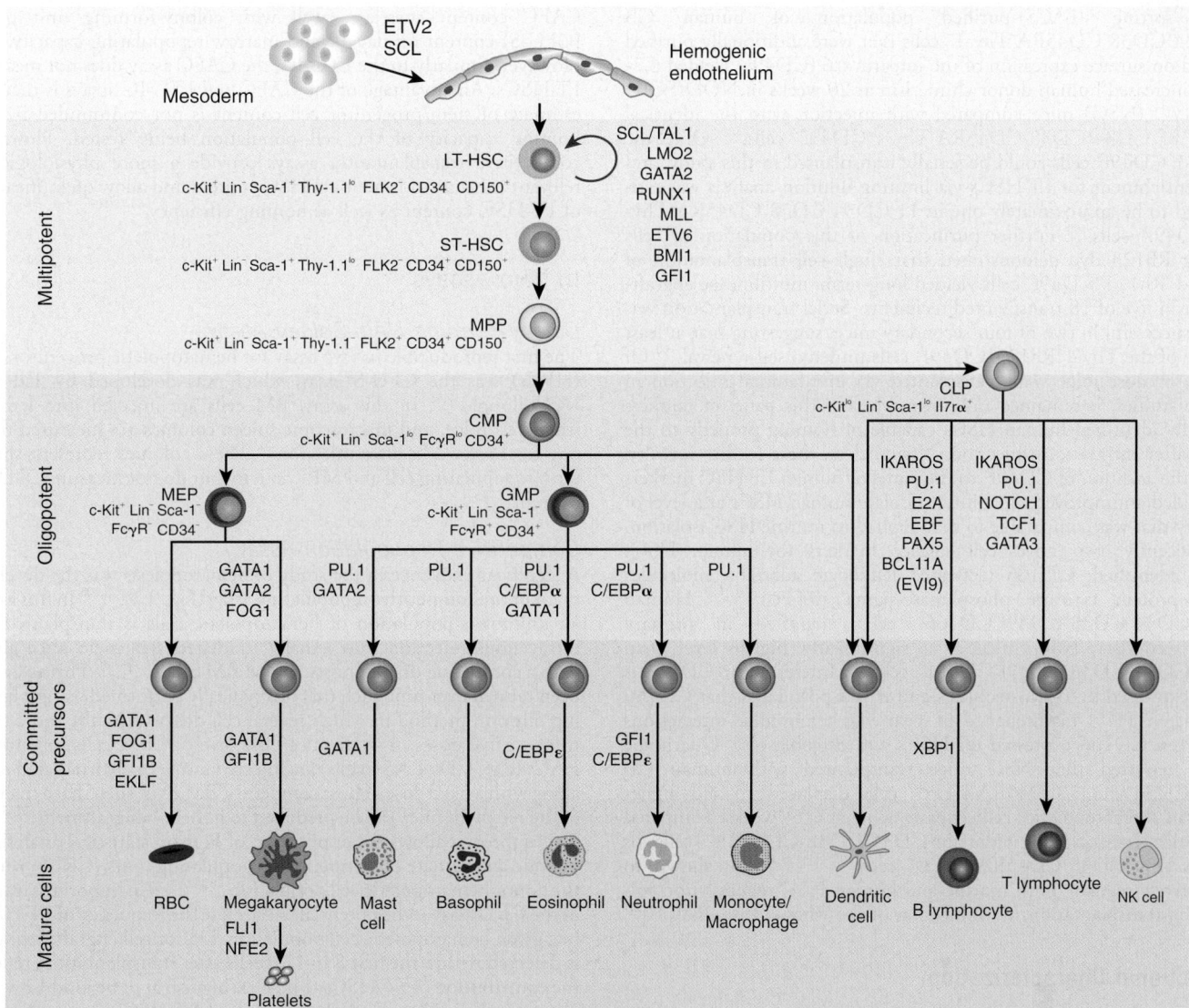

Fig. 9.2 HEMATOPOIETIC CELLULAR HIERARCHY. The phenotypes of murine hematopoietic stem cells (HSCs) and oligopotent progenitor cells, as well as transcription and epigenetic factors critical for specification and differentiation of HSCs are shown. *CLP,* common lymphoid progenitor; *CMP,* common myeloid progenitor; *GMP,* granulocyte-macrophage progenitor; *LT-HSC,* long-term HSC; *MEP,* megakaryocytic-erythroid progenitor; *NK,* natural killer; *RBC,* red blood cell; *ST-HSC,* short-term HSC. *(Adapted from Prohaska SS, Weissman I: Biology of hematopoietic stem and progenitor cells. In Appelbaum F, Forman SJ, Negrin RS, Blume K, editors:* Thomas' hematopoietic cell transplantation, *UK, 2008, Wiley-Blackwell, p 36-63; Orkin SH, Zon LI: Hematopoiesis: an evolving paradigm for stem cell biology.* Cell *132, 631-644, 2008; Voehringer D: Protective and pathological roles of mast cells and basophils.* Nat Rev Immunol *13, 362-375, 2013.)*

Human HSCs

Significant progress has also been made in the phenotypic characterization of human HSCs via flow cytometric analysis combined with in vivo transplantation assays in immune-deficient mice.[88,89] Of particular note, although murine HSCs can be characterized by the absence of CD34 expression on the cell surface, human HSCs are primarily enriched using CD34 surface expression, and this provides the basis for confirming sufficient HSC content to allow for successful hematopoietic cell transplantation in patients.[17,90,91] There is also some controversy in this area because some investigations have suggested that LT-HSCs can be isolated from CD34⁻ human hematopoietic cells.[92–95] Of note, only a small percentage (<0.1%) of CD34⁺ human hematopoietic cells possess the capacity to engraft following intravenous injection into nonobese diabetic/severe combined immune deficient (NOD/SCID) mice.[4,89] Further enrichment of human HSCs has been demonstrated via negative selection for surface expression of CD38 and depletion of lineage surface markers.[89,96,97] Thy-1 (CD90) surface expression also enriches for multilineage colony-forming ability and in vivo reconstituting capacity of human hematopoietic cells.[17,98] Majeti et al showed that the Lin⁻CD34⁺CD38⁻CD45RA⁻Thy-1⁺ population in human cord blood (CB) was enriched at the level of one in 10 cells for LT-HSCs.[98] The authors also showed that candidate multipotent progenitor cells (MPPs) were demarcated by the Lin⁻CD34⁺CD38⁻CD45RA⁻Thy-1⁻ population, suggesting that the loss of Thy-1 reflects the transition of LT-HSCs to short-term (ST)-HSCs/MPPs.[17,98]

CD49f⁺ Human HSCs

Although it is possible to enrich murine BM HSCs to the level of nearly single-cell purity using various combinations of cell surface markers, isolation of human BM HSCs to the same level of purity has not been readily achieved.[74,80,99] However, Notta et al demonstrated that intrafemoral injection of a fluorescence-activated cell sorting (FACS)-purified population of human CB CD34$^+$CD38$^-$CD45RA$^-$Thy-1$^+$ cells that were additionally purified based on surface expression of the integrin α6 (CD49f) yielded 6.7-fold increased human donor chimerism at 20 weeks in NOD/SCID IL2Rγ$^{-/-}$ (NSG) mice compared with injection with the identical dose of CD34$^+$CD38$^-$CD45RA$^-$Thy-1$^+$CD49f$^-$ cells.[100] Only the Thy-1$^+$CD49f$^+$ cells could be serially transplanted in this study, and the enrichment for LT-HSCs via limiting dilution analysis was estimated to be approximately one in 11 CD34$^+$CD38$^-$CD45RA$^-$Thy-1$^+$CD49f$^+$ cells.[100] Further purification of this population of cells using Rh123 dye demonstrated that single-cell transplantation of Thy-1$^+$Rh123^{lo}CD49f$^+$ cells yielded long-term, multilineage engraftment in five of 18 transplanted recipients. Serial transplantation was also successful in two of four secondary mice, suggesting that at least some of the Thy-1$^+$Rh123^{lo}CD49f$^+$ cells undergo self-renewal.[100] Of note, because mice were transplanted via intrafemoral injection in these studies, it remained unknown whether this panel of markers equally identified human HSCs capable of homing properly to the BM after intravenous injection. Nonetheless, these studies revealed that the addition of CD49f$^+$ to the panel of human LT-HSC markers provided an improved capability to isolate human HSCs at a level of purity that was comparable to that applied to murine HSC isolation.

Recently, two novel cell surface markers for human HSCs were identified, CD166 (activated leukocyte adhesion molecule) and protein tyrosine phosphatase-sigma (PTPσ).[101,102] Human Lin$^-$CD34$^+$CD38$^-$CD49f$^+$CD166$^+$ cells engrafted in primary and secondary NSG mice at a significantly higher level than Lin$^-$CD34$^+$CD38$^-$CD49f$^+$CD166$^-$ cells.[101] Interestingly, CD166 is also expressed by BM osteoblasts and it was postulated that CD166 mediated HSC maintenance in vivo via hemophilic interactions between CD166 expressed on HSCs and osteoblasts.[101] Quarmyne et al reported that NSG mice transplanted with human CB Lin$^-$CD34$^+$CD38$^-$CD45RA$^-$PTPσ$^-$ cells displayed 15-fold higher human hematopoietic cell engraftment at 16 weeks compared to mice transplanted with Lin$^-$CD34$^+$CD38$^-$CD45RA$^-$ cells or Lin$^-$CD34$^+$CD38$^-$CD45RA$^-$PTPσ$^+$ cells.[102] PTPσ was shown to negatively regulate both murine and human HSC repopulation following transplantation, via inhibition of the RhoGTPase, RAC1.[102]

Functional Characterization

In Vitro Assays

The colony-forming cell (CFC) assay does not measure HSC content but rather committed myeloid progenitor cell content via a 14-day assay for colonies within methylcellulose media that is supplemented with specific growth factors.[78] The CFC assay measures colony-forming unit-granulocyte/macrophage (CFU-GM), burst-forming unit-erythroid (BFU-E) and CFU-granulocyte/erythroid/macrophage/megakaryocyte (CFU-GEMM). The CFU-GEMM, or CFU-mix colonies, represent a more immature progenitor cell population. B- and T-cell progenitor cell content can also be measured via in vitro assays but requires specialized coculture conditions, which are described elsewhere.[78,103,104]

The long-term culture-initiating cell (LTC-IC) assay is a 6-week in vitro assay in which BM cells are cocultured with murine stromal cells for four weeks followed by replating of the entire culture system into methylcellulose and additional two-week assay for colony formation.[78,105] The LTC-IC, unlike the CFC, measures a more immature stem/progenitor cell population, although the results of the LTC-IC are inherently dependent and limited by technical variabilities in stromal coculture experiments.[78] Importantly, the LTC-IC population lacks long-term repopulating cells because transplantation of LTC-ICs into mice in a competitive transplantation assay does not result in any long-term reconstitution.[78,88,89]

The cobblestone area-forming cell (CAFC) assay also involves coculture of HSCs with preestablished stromal cell monolayers and relies on microscopic quantification of cobblestone-forming cells embedded underneath the stromal layer.[105,106] It has been shown that

CAFC content correlates well with colony-forming unit-spleen (CFU-S) content on day 12 and marrow repopulating capacity.[78,105] However, similarly to the LTC-IC, the CAFC assay does not measure LT-HSCs. An advantage of the CAFC and LTC-IC assays is that the estimate of stem/progenitor cell content is not confounded by the homing capacity of the cell population being tested. However, competitive transplantation assays provide a more physiologically relevant measure of functional HSC content and allow quantification of LT-HSC content as well as homing efficiency.[64,78,107]

In Vivo Assays

Colony-Forming Unit–Spleen Assay

The first reproducible in vivo assay for hematopoietic progenitor cells (HPCs) was the CFU-S assay, which was developed by Till and McCullough.[12,88] In this assay, BM cells are injected into lethally irradiated mice, and macroscopic spleen colonies are measured from one to three weeks after injection.[78] These colonies represent short-term repopulating cell and MPP activity but do not measure LT-HSC content.[4,78]

Competitive Repopulation Assay

A significant advance in the study of hematopoiesis was the development of the competitive repopulating assay (Fig. 9.3).[78,108] In this assay, an unknown population of hematopoietic cells is transplanted via intravenous injection into lethally irradiated syngeneic mice along with a competing dose of host-derived BM cells.[78,109,110] This assay has been refined over time such that it is typically performed using a limiting dilution method in which several cell doses (typically more than three to five doses; $n = 10$ mice/dose level) of BM cells or purified HSCs (e.g., CD34$^-$KSL cells) are injected into lethally irradiated mice along with a fixed dose of host competitor BM cells, such that a fraction of the recipient mice can be predicted to have nonengraftment.[78,111,112] This approach allows the application of Poisson statistical analysis to provide an estimate of competitive repopulating units (CRUs) within the donor hematopoietic cell population.[78,111–113] An important feature of the CRU assay is the potential to estimate the frequency of LT-HSCs in a given hematopoietic cell population. Donor cell engraftment that is detected within the first 8 to 12 weeks after transplantation, reflects the contribution of ST-HSCs, which extinguish at or beyond 12 weeks posttransplant. Therefore, the number of LT-HSCs cannot be convincingly estimated until more than 12–20 weeks posttransplantation.[78,114] Dykstra et al[115] showed that competitive transplantation of single, phenotypic HSCs results in stable donor cell engraftment in lethally irradiated mice beyond 16 weeks, and retroviral marking of HSCs revealed that stable donor-derived hematopoiesis was not observed in recipient mice until six months posttransplant.[114]

A commonly used and rigorous approach to estimate the presence of LT-HSCs is the performance of secondary, tertiary, and quaternary HSC transplants.[78] This approach is based on the principle that a singular feature of primitive LT-HSCs is the capacity to serially reconstitute multilineage hematopoiesis in vivo without exhaustion.[78,116–118] In this method, whole BM is typically collected from primary recipient mice and then injected, along with host competitor BM cells, into lethally irradiated syngeneic mice. Donor cell repopulation is then measured at 12–20 weeks posttransplantation. Serial transplantation assays have the limitation of being potentially confounded by variables such as homing efficiency of the donor cells.[78,119,120] Therefore, as pointed out by Purton and Scadden[78] in an excellent review of this subject, serial transplantation assays may be better suited to studies of wild type hematopoietic cell populations as opposed to mutant mice-derived hematopoietic cells, which may have alterations in homing or engraftment mechanisms independent of HSC content.[78] Utilization of whole BM avoids issues regarding the fidelity of phenotypic markers of HSCs in mutant mice and is perhaps more broadly feasible than FACS-isolated HSC populations at some centers.[78,121–124] However, the use of purified HSCs avoids the potential confounding effects of accessory cells contained within the BM graft on donor cell repopulation and allows for precise

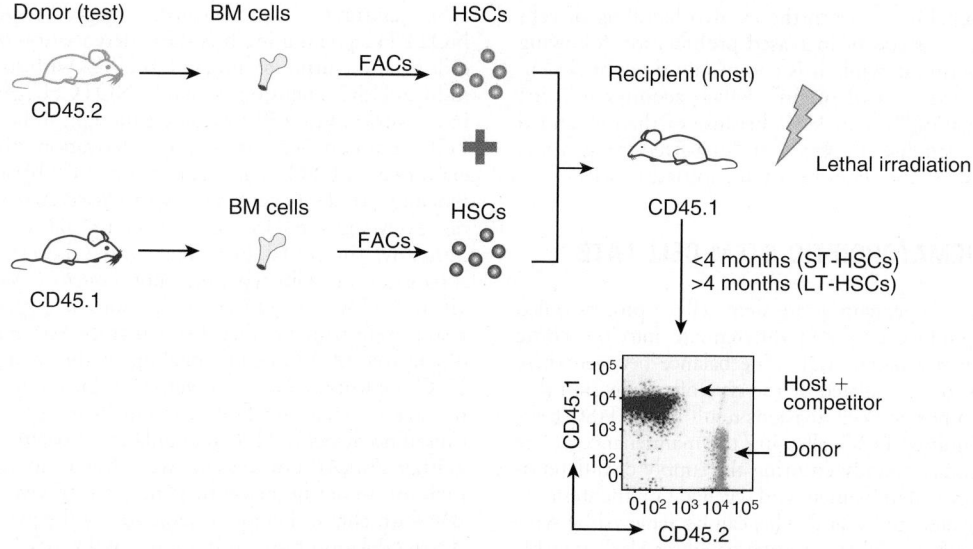

Fig. 9.3 COMPETITIVE REPOPULATION ASSAY. Bone marrow (BM) cells from donor mice carrying the CD45.2 allele are sorted by fluorescence-activated cell sorting (FACS) and transplanted with an excess of BM cells from CD45.1 mice into lethally irradiated CD45.1 recipient mice. In general, three to four months posttransplantation, peripheral blood cells are analyzed by flow cytometry to identify the fraction of donor CD45.2 BM cells that, if present, must have homed to and engrafted the myeloablated recipient mouse. While short-term hematopoietic stem cells (ST-HSCs) do not persist in the recipient mouse after four months, long-term (LT)-HSCs are defined by their presence in the recipient mouse after four months and the ability to repopulate secondary, tertiary, and quaternary recipients. *(Adapted from http://stemcellassays.com/2011/11/experimental-bone-marrow-transplantation-101-%E2%80%93-part-2-congenic-mouse-model/.)*

determination of effects of growth factors on HSC content in vitro compared with unmanipulated BM.[103,125] Lastly, Poisson statistical analysis and estimation of CRU frequency is based on particular criteria for "positive" donor engraftment in recipient mice, typically 0.1–1% multilineage donor engraftment.[103,126] Therefore, the estimation of CRU frequency can be substantially altered depending on what criteria for engraftment are established. Given the limitations of flow cytometric analysis for accurate multilineage engraftment of hematopoietic cells, it is recommended that greater than 1% multilineage engraftment is used as a criterion for evidence of donor cell repopulation using the competitive repopulating assay.[78]

Clonal Dynamics of HSCs

Historically, the transplantation assay, in which prospectively purified cell populations are transplanted into myeloablated recipients, has served as the "gold standard" for testing BM compartments for HSC potential. A single HSC can reconstitute the entire hematopoietic system of the host under optimal conditions.[63,69,80,115,127] Based on initial transplantation studies, HSCs have been fitted into a simple linear branching hierarchy.[128] Such a hierarchical model assumes that all HSCs have similar developmental potential and, when committed to differentiate, can give rise to both a myeloid and lymphoid progenitor with equal probability. However, tracking experiments with individual retrovirally marked HSCs have revealed extensive heterogeneity within the HSC pool,[114,116,129,130] which was subsequently confirmed by limiting dilution transplantation.[63,127,131–135] Several models have been put forth to explain how diversity in HSC functionality is generated. These are broadly separated into instructive and intrinsic regulation models. According to the instructive models, each HSC is provided with slightly different cues from the microenvironment in which it resides.[136–138] On the other hand, intrinsic regulation of HSC heterogeneity is either completely unpredictable (stochastic)[139–142] or "programmed" (deterministic).[135,143]

The development of methods to obtain highly purified HSCs by FACS has permitted single-cell transplants that address the basis of heterogeneity.[115,127,144–146] These studies demonstrate the existence of myeloid and lymphoid "biased" HSCs and that long-term repopulation is dependent on sustained myeloid reconstitution, irrespective of a contribution to the lymphoid compartment. HSCs may also differ in their response to extrinsic signals such as transforming growth factor-β1 (TGF-β1).[145,147] A striking observation is the stable propagation of HSC "heterogeneity" upon secondary transplantation.[115,148,149] This finding argues for some intrinsic regulation in which all HSCs in a clone follow a predetermined fate that is preset earlier in development.

Hematopoiesis as analyzed by transplantation is generally oligoclonal, that is, only few of the transplanted HSC clones contribute to multilineage repopulation.[114,116,150,151] These results have argued for a "clonal succession" model of stem cell activation which posits that a small number of HSCs are sequentially activated from a pool of otherwise noncycling quiescent cells, but that these HSCs exhaust and are replaced over time.[114,152,153] In contrast, the "clonal stability" model states that many or all HSCs have a low but constant cell cycle activity allowing them to continuously contribute to an organism's blood life-long. Support for this model is derived from experiments showing that after transplantation a few HSC clones persist for a long time.[139,154,155] HSCs could also show both models' behaviors as other studies have shown that HSCs may reversibly switch between the quiescent and self-renewal state in a homeostatic environment or when challenged by injury, respectively.[156–158]

A general limitation to transplantation approaches is their dependence on HSCs that home to and engraft a niche, proliferate rapidly and tolerate the stress imposed by the engraftment and an unbalanced cytokine milieu in myeloablated niches. Novel studies have recently explored endogenous, unperturbed hematopoiesis in the mouse and demonstrated that steady-state hematopoiesis appears to rely predominantly on rather long-lived progenitors rather than HSCs.[159,160] These studies argue for the dominant contribution of MPPs or ST-HSCs to hematopoiesis in the untransplanted mouse. Thus, in contrast to the transplantation setting, native hematopoiesis is highly polyclonal, supported by the successive recruitment of thousands of clones and as such fits the clonal succession model.

Why more restricted progenitors, such as ST-HSCs or MPPs, cannot repopulate the hematopoietic system after transplantation is unknown but presumably relates to the ex vivo handling of cells for transplantation or the stress of increased proliferation following transplantation. Furthermore, while it is commonly thought that in myeloid malignancies the "cell of origin", which acquires the first cancer-promoting mutation[161] is an HSC because of their extended lifespan, these recent studies suggest that long-lived progenitors might be equally suitable candidates for tumor-initiating cells.[160]

REGULATION OF HEMATOPOIETIC STEM CELL FATE

HSCs have the capacity to generate more stem cells, a process called self-renewal, and to produce cells that differentiate into the entire spectrum of mature hematopoietic cells. The balance between these fate choices is thought to be regulated by the type of cell division that HSCs undergo.[162] Asymmetrical cell divisions result in one HSC (self-renewal) and one committed HPC, allowing the maintenance of the stem cell pool while concomitantly ensuring the supply of differentiated cells. However, during development and regeneration the stem cell pool must have the capacity to expand. This can be achieved by symmetrical cell divisions, which will lead to two daughter HSCs capable of self-renewing. Another outcome of symmetric division would be two HPCs, diminishing and ultimately exhausting the HSC pool. The fate decision governing this balance between self-renewal and differentiation is regulated by cell-intrinsic including transcriptional and epigenetic mechanisms that are intertwined with cell-extrinsic mechanisms from the microenvironment or by the action of systemic factors.

Extrinsic Regulation

The past three decades have yielded substantial progress in the discovery and characterization of intrinsic and extrinsic mechanisms that regulate HSC self-renewal and differentiation. Despite this, the translation of these discoveries into the development of translatable methods to expand human HSCs ex vivo or therapeutics to induce HSC expansion in vivo has proven to be difficult. Therefore, further dissection of the mechanisms governing HSC function continues to be a high priority. The following pathways are extrinsically controlled and reflect unique mechanistic targets for the development of therapeutics to amplify the human HSC pool.

NOTCH Signaling

The NOTCH signaling pathway has been shown to have an important role in regulating the development of the central nervous system, eye, muscle, hematopoietic system, and germline, among others.[163,164] To date, four NOTCH receptors have been identified (NOTCH1–4) as well as five ligands for Notch receptors (JAGGED1 and 2 and DELTA1, 3, and 4).[165] Ligand receptor interaction on HSCs induces two NOTCH cleavage steps, the last of which is mediated by γ-secretase and releases the constitutively active NOTCH-intracellular domain (NICD). The NICD then translocates to the nucleus, interacts with the DNA-binding protein RBPJ (recombination signal binding protein for immunoglobulin kappa J region) and initiates transcription of target genes such as the transcription factors HES1 and HES5 (mammalian homologues of Drosophila hairy and Enhancer of split).[166–169] Depending on the specific NOTCH ligand, different NOTCH receptors and thus different NOTCH target genes are activated, leading to diverse cellular outcomes. For example, NOTCH1 activation by Delta1 and 4 is required for T-cell differentiation while it inhibits differentiation of the B-cell lineage. Jagged2- or Delta1-mediated activation of NOTCH2 inhibits myeloid differentiation and induces the generation of LT-HSCs and MPPs.[167,170]

Activation of NOTCH signaling is sufficient to induce ex vivo HSC expansion. Retroviral expression of the Notch1 ICD in murine HSCs leads to the generation of an immortal, cytokine-dependent cell line with multilineage in vivo repopulating capacity,[171] and immobilized Delta1 promotes a several-log expansion of murine

HSC cultures.[172] Furthermore, Jagged2-mediated activation of NOTCH signaling inhibits the differentiation of human CB CD34+ cells,[173] and culture of human CB HSCs with soluble human Jagged1 induces HSC expansion ex vivo.[174] NOTCH ligands that are expressed in the surrounding BM niche are thought to be critical in promoting HSC maintenance through the activation of NOTCH receptors expressed on HSCs. For example, BM osteoblasts express Jagged1 and blocking NOTCH activation with a γ-secretase inhibitor significantly decreases murine HSC expansion in BM osteoblast cocultures.[175] Similarly, sinusoidal ECs that express NOTCH ligands stimulate expansion of wild-type but not Notch1−/−Notch2−/− LT-HSCs in vitro.[176] However, although deletion of Jagged1, Notch1, or Rbpj results in impaired embryonic hematopoiesis in the mouse, the physiologic role of NOTCH signaling in the maintenance of the adult HSC pool in vivo is controversial.[175] Deletion of Jagged1 was shown to have no effect on HSC content in mice,[177] and deletion of Rbpj caused no defect in HSC repopulating capacity.[178] Interestingly, while neither Notch1 nor Notch2 were found to be required for HSC function under homeostatic conditions in vivo,[170,177] challenging the BM with chemotherapy or radiation in the presence of a conditional Notch2 deletion resulted in more rapid myeloid differentiation at the expense of HSC self-renewal.[170]

In keeping with the evidence obtained from mouse studies that activation of NOTCH signaling can induce HSC expansion, Delaney et al[179] showed that serum-free culture of human CB progenitor cells with immobilized Delta1 plus cytokines for three weeks yielded a 5.3-fold increase in human hematopoietic cell engraftment in transplanted NOD/SCID mice. This group subsequently completed a phase I clinical trial showing that transplantation of CB cells, which had been expanded with immobilized Delta1 along with an unmanipulated CB unit shortened the time interval to neutrophil recovery (median, 16 days) compared with a cohort that received two unmanipulated CB units (median, 26 days).[180] Of note, in this phase I study, the unmanipulated CB cells demonstrated dominant engraftment by day 80 after transplant and in seven of eight reported recipients, ex vivo expanded CB cells were not detectable in recipients by day 40 posttransplant.[180] The extinction of the Delta1-expanded CB units might be explained by T-cell depletion as donor CB CD8+ T cells of a successful graft have been shown to mediate the rejection of the other CB unit in the setting of double CB transplantation.[181]

WNT Signaling

WNT signaling is initiated by the interaction of WNT ligands with the so-called Frizzled/LRP (lipoprotein receptor-related protein) cell surface receptor complex. In the absence of ligand binding, the WNT signal transducer β-catenin is phosphorylated by kinases such as glycogen synthase kinase-3 beta (GSK-3β), leading to its rapid degradation. Upon activation of the canonical WNT pathway, β-catenin is no longer phosphorylated and thereby stabilized, translocates into the nucleus and interacts with transcription factors of the T-cell factor/lymphoid enhancer factor (LEF/TCF) family to regulate expression of target genes.[182] Several lines of evidence implicate WNT signaling in the regulation of HSC self-renewal and differentiation. First, WNT proteins have been shown to be expressed at sites of embryonic and fetal hematopoiesis, and WNT ligands, receptors and LEF/TCF transcription factors are expressed by adult HSCs as well as the BM microenvironment.[183,184] Second, ample evidence suggests that activation of WNT signaling is capable of promoting HSC expansion, at least in vitro.[185–189] Using mice transgenic for human BCL2 enabling HSCs to survive in the presence of stem cell factor (SCF) alone,[190,191] it was shown that BM KTLS cells treated with purified WNT3A protein or transduced with active β-catenin ex vivo resulted in their expansion and multilineage reconstitution of competitively transplanted recipients.[185,189] In a related study, treating immune-deficient recipient mice with a GSK-3β inhibitor after transplantation of lineage-depleted human CB HSCs increased their engraftment and repopulating capacity, which was accompanied by faster recovery from posttransplant cytopenia.[192] Importantly,

WNT-mediated maintenance of the HSC pool was demonstrated to depend on intact NOTCH signaling,[193] suggesting a deterministic role for the NOTCH pathway in controlling the effects of WNT signaling on the undifferentiated HSC pool.[194] On the other hand, HSCs from mice engineered to conditionally express a stable form of β-catenin were blocked in differentiation and failed to self-renew leading to their exhaustion.[195,196] These results raise the possibility that the prior report of HSC expansion in response to β-catenin overexpression may have been affected by the use of *Bcl2* transgenic mice.[185] Alternatively, WNT signaling might have a more pronounced role in vitro than in the more complex in vivo setting.[188]

Some WNT ligands, e.g., WNT5A, are able to activate pathways other than the canonical WNT pathway, depending on the particular WNT receptor context.[197] In vivo activation of noncanonical WNT signaling via systemic administration of WNT5A was shown to induce a greater than threefold increase in human CB HPC repopulation in NOD/SCID mice.[186] More recent studies have demonstrated noncanonical WNT signaling in the BM niche to be required for HSC maintenance in vitro and in vivo.[198,199] Interestingly, it was shown that *Wnt5a* expression is increased in ageing LT-HSCs. Induction of *Wnt5a* in young mice induced ageing-associated HSC phenotypes, including apolarity, decreased repopulation capacity and myeloid bias. Conversely, knocking down *Wnt5a* in old mice attenuated HSC ageing.[200]

Although activation of WNT signaling can induce HSC expansion, it is uncertain whether WNT signaling is indispensable for normal hematopoiesis to occur. Conditional deletion of β-catenin in adult BM progenitors did not impair their ability for multilineage reconstitution.[201] In support of these results, hematopoietic cell ablation of porcupine, a membrane-bound *O*-acyl transferase essential for WNT ligand secretion and receptor interaction, had no effect on proliferation, differentiation, and self-renewal of adult HSCs in vivo.[202] Conversely, embryonic conditional knockout of β-catenin caused a deficiency in self-renewal of murine LT-HSCs,[203] and HSCs derived from *Wnt3a*$^{-/-}$ mice failed to repopulate secondary recipients,[204] suggesting that WNT signaling might have different roles in embryonic versus adult HSCs.

TGF-β and Hedgehog Signaling

The TGF-β pathway represents a signaling mechanism that can be activated by members of the TGF-β superfamily including TGF-β, activins and bone morphogenetic proteins (BMPs).[205] Each of these ligands binds to a specific receptor heterodimer composed of a type I and II receptor, leading to the phosphorylation of a subset of the receptor-regulated SMAD proteins (R-SMADs: SMAD1, 2, 3, 5, and 8). Thus activated R-SMADs then form a complex with the common SMAD SMAD4, and translocate into the nucleus to co-regulate target gene transcription. Another class of SMADs, inhibitory SMADs (SMAD6 and 7) block TGF-β family signaling by binding to R-SMADs.

TGF-β is one of the most potent inhibitors of HSC proliferation in vitro, and neutralization of TGF-β releases HSCs from quiescence.[206–208] It has been suggested that TGF-β mediates cell cycle inhibition in HSCs via upregulation of cyclin-dependent kinase inhibitors, p21, p27 and p57, as well as downregulation of cytokine receptors.[209–213] The role of TGF-β in vivo appears to be more complex. TGF-β likely functions as a negative hematopoietic regulator in vivo as supported by the observation that deletion of TGF-β1 results in extensive myelopoiesis in mice[214] as well as defective homing of HSCs.[215] Moreover, HSCs from mice with a conditional deletion of the TGF-β type II receptor show increased cell cycling and impaired repopulation capacity.[216] Conversely, TGF-β type I receptor null mice display normal HSC self-renewal and regeneration in vivo, although these HSCs exhibited increased proliferation in vitro.[217,218] The discrepancies between different knockout phenotypes could be caused by differences in expression levels of the TGF-β receptors in HSCs and thus different in vivo importance.[209] Still, TGF-β is considered a critical signal for HSC quiescence also in vivo.[209]

BMP signaling is required for mesoderm formation and patterning, and BMPs are key regulators for the hematopoietic specification from mesoderm across different species (reviewed in[205]). BMP4 has been shown to modulate adult human HSC maintenance and proliferation in a concentration-dependent manner, with high BMP4 levels extending the survival of hematopoietic repopulating cells in ex vivo cultures.[219] However, in vivo, BMP signaling does not seem to be required for adult HSC function as determined in mouse knockouts for its signal transducers, SMAD1 and 5.[205] On the other hand, complete inhibition of the SMAD network has demonstrated the importance of SMAD proteins in regulating HSC self-renewal in vivo. Conditional deletion of *Smad4* in mice led to a significantly reduced ability of HSCs to repopulate primary and secondary recipients.[220] Also, retrovirus-mediated overexpression of the inhibitory *Smad7* promoted HSC self-renewal in vivo.[221] Taken together, these results have been interpreted to indicate that SMAD4 positively regulates HSC self-renewal independently from its role as a mediator of SMAD pathway signaling. This hypothesis is supported by evidence demonstrating that SMAD proteins can activate WNT signaling,[222,223] which has been shown to promote HSC expansion as discussed earlier.

As in other species and developmental contexts,[224,225,226] an intersection between BMP4 and Hedgehog signaling has been described in the human hematopoietic system. Hedgehog proteins play an essential role in the embryonic development of a wide variety of organs, and, like BMPs, they are required for mesoderm patterning.[227,228] Culture of human CB progenitor cells with Sonic Hedgehog (SHH), one of three human Hedgehog proteins,[229,230] promoted the expansion of cells capable of multilineage repopulation in NOD/SCID mice.[231] The addition of Noggin an endogenous inhibitor of BMP4, blocked the effect of SHH on CB stem cell proliferation in vitro, whereas Hedgehog inhibition did not block BMP4-induced hematopoietic stem and progenitor cell (HSPC) proliferation, suggesting that BMP4 acts downstream of *SHH* in the regulation of human HSC growth.[231] Several other studies suggest that hedgehog signaling regulates HSC growth. Mice heterozygous for the Hedgehog antagonist Patched1 (*Ptc1*) were shown to have an expanded HSC compartment[232] and their fetal HSCs exhibited increased colony-forming potential in serial plating assays.[233] Interestingly, while conditional deletion of the Hedgehog effector Smoothened (*Smo*) resulted in a profound loss of LT-HSCs in the embryo,[234] conditional deletion of *Smo* or pharmacologic inhibition of Hedgehog had no effect on HSC content or hematopoiesis in adult mice.[235,236] Thus, Hedgehog signaling during embryogenesis might be required for certain aspects of HSC function important in adult life.[237]

CXCL12–CXCR4 Signaling

CXCL12 is a chemokine that is expressed by BM osteoblasts, ECs, and perivascular stromal cells in the BM microenvironment and regulates the homing and retention of HSCs.[238–240] Expression of CXCL12 or its receptor, CXCR4, is necessary for HSC maintenance in vivo.[239–241] Recently, Ding et al reported that deletion of *Cxcl12* from perivascular stromal cells or vascular ECs depleted HSCs in mice, whereas depletion of *Cxcl12* from nestin$^+$ mesenchymal cells or osteoblasts had no effect on HSC numbers.[239] Greenbaum et al also showed that deletion of *Cxcl12* in *Prx1*-expressing perivascular stromal cells led to HSC depletion,[242] confirming the importance of CXCL12 signaling in the perivascular niche for HSC maintenance. A more detailed review of CXCL12-CXCR4 signaling in the context of the BM microenvironment, as well as a comprehensive review of HSC-HSC niche signaling interactions[243] are presented in Chapter 11.

INTRINSIC PATHWAYS

Transcription Factors

Transcription factors are proteins that bind specific sequences of DNA within promoter or enhancer regions to regulate the process of transcribing DNA into RNA.[244] Because the intrinsic phenotype or state of a cell is the result of its gene expression, it is governed by the concerted action of transcription factors (guided by the epigenetic landscape discussed further below). The balance between self-renewal and differentiation of HSCs is intricately regulated by transcription factors of many different classes.[245] Several general principles have emerged. First, given the relative limited number of transcription factors, they are used at multiple stages in development, such that they may be required in HSCs and also subsequently in lineage differentiation.[18] Second, the balance between self-renewal and lineage commitment is thought to be regulated, at least in part, by the antagonism of lineage-specific transcription factors. To promote a given lineage, transcription factors need to actively counteract factor(s) supporting other cell fates. Third, and most relevant to clinical situations, most hematopoietic transcription factors are subject to somatic mutation and/or chromosomal translocation in one or more hematopoietic malignancies. Thus, malignancy can be viewed as a disruption of normal development. Fig. 9.2 depicts key transcription factors within the hematopoietic hierarchy, and Table 9.1 summarizes main roles of critical transcription factors in HSPCs and hematologic malignancies.

TABLE 9.1   Roles of Critical Transcription and Epigenetic Factors in Hematopoietic Stem and Progenitor Cells (HSPCs) and Hematologic Malignancies

	Requirement in HSPCs[a]	Type of Alteration	Disease	Reference
Transcription Factor				
SCL (TAL-1)	Mesoderm-endothelial/ hematopoietic lineage transition; MegE lineage differentiation	Chromosomal translocations involving *TCR* genes; *SIL–TAL1* fusion gene; aberrant expression for other reasons	T-ALL	245, 263, 533
LMO2	Primitive erythropoiesis; generation and maintenance of definitive HSCs	Chromosomal translocations involving *TCR* genes; interstitial deletion; aberrant expression for other reasons	T-ALL (B-cell lymphoma; B-ALL; X-SCID gene therapy associated T-cell leukemia)	533, 534
GATA2	EHT; HSC survival and self-renewal; MegE, mast cell, monocyte lineage differentiation	Mutations	MonoMAC, MDS, AML, CMML, Emberger syndrome	535
RUNX1 (AML1, CBF-α)	Formation of intraaortic clusters and HSCs during EHT; lymphopoiesis	*RUNX1-ETO* chromosomal translocations; mutations	AML	536, 299, 288
CBF-β (CBFB)	Emergence of HSCs from HE (in complex with RUNX1)	*CBF-β-MYH11* chromosomal translocations	AML	288, 537, 538
E2A (TCF3)	Maintenance of adult LT-HSC; LMPP, CLP, early thymocyte progenitor, pro-B-cell differentiation	*E2A-PBX1* chromosomal translocations; mutations	Pre-B-cell ALL; T-cell lymphoma	245, 539
ETV6 (TEL)	Maintenance/survival of adult LT-HSCs	*ETV6-RUNX1* chromosomal translocations; mutations	Pre-B-cell ALL; immature adult T-ALL	299, 539, 297, 540
MYB (C-MYB)	Self-renewal and multilineage differentiation of adult LT-HSCs	Chromosomal translocation involving TCRβ; duplication	T-ALL	541–543
EVI1	Generation of definitive HSCs; Self-renewal of adult LT-HSCs	Aberrant expression; Chromosomal translocations involving *RUNX1* and *ETV6*	AML; MDS, CML blast crisis	246, 544
Epigenetic Factor				
MLL	Generation of definitive HSCs; adult HSC quiescence and self-renewal	Chromosomal translocations involving *AF4, AF9, ENL, AF10, ELL, AF6*, etc. (79)	ALL, AML	545, 546
DNMT3A	HSC differentiation	Mutations	AML, T-cell leukemia and lymphoma, MDS	348
TET2	HSC differentiation	Mutations, *IDH1/2* mutations	CMML, AML, MDS, T-cell lymphoma, DLBCL	547, 548
ASXL1	HSC differentiation	Mutations	CMML, AML, MDS	549, 359, 550

[a]Data from complete or conditional knockout studies in mice

AML, acute myeloid leukemia; B-ALL, B-cell acute lymphoblastic leukemia; CML, chronic myeloid leukemia; CMML, chronic myelomonocytic leukemia; DLBCL, diffuse large B-cell lymphoma; EHT, endothelial-to-hematopoietic transition; HE, hemogenic endothelium; HSC, hematopoietic stem cell; HSPCs, hematopoietic stem and progenitor cells; LMPP, lymphoid primed multipotent progenitors; MDS, myelodysplastic syndrome; MegE, megakaryocyte/erythrocyte; MLL, mixed-lineage leukemia; MonoMAC, monocytopenia and *Mycobacterium avium* complex infections; SIL, SCL interrupting locus; T-ALL, T-cell acute lymphoblastic leukemia; X-SCID, X-linked severe combined immunodeficiency.

Transcription Factors Required for the Specification of HSCs

As one of the few transcription factors known to be essential for the mesoderm-hemangioblast transition, the ETS class protein ETV2 is expressed in a subset of FLK1[+] cells with enhanced endothelial and hematopoietic potential and downregulated thereafter.[246,247] Together with the forkhead transcription factor FOXC2, it cooperatively induces the FLK1[+] mesoderm by stimulating the expression of key endothelial and hematopoietic genes such as *Flk1, vascular endothelial (VE)-cadherin, Tie2, Scl* and *Notch4*.[248]

Before the emergence of HSCs, the bHLH protein SCL is required for the specification of the bipotent hemogenic endothelium within the hemangioblast during embryonic development.[249] Its knockout in mice, as well as that of its binding partner LIM domain protein *Lmo2*,[250–252] results in the lack of hematopoiesis with early embryonic lethality,[253–256] and an absence of adult HSCs.[257,258] SCL expression is regulated by three hematopoiesis-specific enhancers, one of which comprises an ETS/ETS/GATA motif that binds ETS transcription factors FLI1 and ELF1 as well as GATA2, revealing the transcriptional cascade at the top of the hematopoietic hierarchy.[259] Interestingly, once emerged, HSCs require either SCL or the closely related bHLH factor LYL1 for function and survival.[260–262] Elevated expression of *SCL* and/or *LMO2*, as well as *LYL1* is found in 35–65% of T-cell acute lymphoblastic leukemia (T-ALL), mostly because of chromosome translocations but also, in the case of *SCL*, intragenic deletions.[263]

GATA2, a zinc finger transcription factor, is expressed before HSC emergence in the paraaortic splanchnopleura and later in the AGM.[264] GATA2 has been shown to be essential for the production of cells belonging to all lineages in definitive (or adult) hematopoiesis.[265,266] Interestingly, it functions to preserve the pool of immature HSPCs by preventing the differentiation of hematogenic precursor cells.[267] Thus, reduction of *GATA2* expression or activity is a prerequisite for HSC commitment. Heterozygous germline mutations in *GATA2* are the cause of several previously known clinical syndromes: MonoMAC (monocytopenia and *Mycobacterium avium* complex infections),[268,269] which are also described as combined dendritic cell, monocyte, B and natural killer lymphoid or DCML deficiency.[270,271] Individuals with MonoMac almost invariably progress to a distinct form of myelodysplastic syndrome (MDS) and in 14% and 8% to acute myeloid leukemia (AML) and chronic myelomonocytic leukemia (CMML), respectively.[272] Familial myelodysplastic and AML syndrome[273] as well as Emberger syndrome (primary lymphedema with predisposition to AML)[274] also belong to this group, and in some cases are caused by the identical *GATA2* mutation.

The core-binding protein RUNX1 and its obligate binding partner CBF-β are both required for the transition from hemogenic endothelium to definitive HSCs.[275–278] *Runx1* expression is upregulated during the endothelial-to-hematopoietic transition (EHT) in the hemogenic endothelium, probably by GATA2, the ETS transcription factors FLI1 and PU.1 and the SCL complex (SCL, LMO2, LDB1).[279] RUNX1 then induces expression of other critical transcription factors such as GFI1 and GFIB which in turn downregulate the endothelial markers TIE2, VE-cadherin and KIT.[280] In addition, RUNX1 causes rapid global reorganization of transcription factors such as SCL, FLI1 and C/EBPβ which is critical for the EHT and hematopoietic fate.[281] RUNX1 is also required to antagonize the effects of the homeobox transcription factor HOXA3, a negative regulator of specification of the hemogenic endothelium. HOXA3 represses a cascade of transcription factors that promote hemogenesis while at the same time inducing a set of genes critical for maintaining endothelial character.[282] *RUNX1* and *CBF-β* are the most common target of chromosomal translocations in acute leukemia. In particular, translocations resulting in *RUNX1-ETO* and *CBF-β-MYH11* cumulatively account for 15% of AML.[283] Consistent with the fact that neither *RUNX1-ETO*[284] nor *CBF-β-MYH1*[285] induce leukemia by themselves in mouse models but rather require additional mutations, next-generation sequencing studies have identified both as preleukemic lesions.[286,287] In addition, mutations in *RUNX1* are observed in patients with various hematologic diseases including MDS, CMML, ALL, de novo and therapy-related AML and the autosomal dominant preleukemic syndrome familial platelet disorder with predisposition to AML (FPD/AML).[288]

Transcription Factors Required for HSC Homeostasis

Many transcription factors from different protein classes that play a role in setting up the hematopoietic hierarchy are necessary for HSC self-renewal in competitive transplantation assays.[1] For example, SCL is expressed much higher in LT-HSCs compared to ST-HSCs, and promotes their quiescence,[289] which preserves the LT-HSC pool.[290] In HSCs as well as differentiating progenitors, SCL exists in different complexes most of which include GATA2 (or GATA1 in the erythroid lineage), E2A and the non-DNA binding adaptor proteins LMO2 and LDB1.[279,291] Loss of any of these SCL partners leads to defects in HSC maintenance.[255,262,292–294] Apart from GATA2 and LMO2, also deregulation of E2A causes hematologic malignancies. Six percent of all pediatric ALLs, in particular pre-B cell ALL (23%) are caused by a chromosomal translocation that fuses the *E2A* gene with *PBX1* (pre-B-cell leukemia homeobox 1),[295,296] which encodes an important HOX interacting factor discussed later.

The ETS-related transcriptional repressor TEL/ETV6 is specifically required for HSC survival but not their emergence.[297] Like E2A, also ETV6 is involved in chromosomal translocations; the *ETV6-RUNX1* is the most common fusion gene in pediatric cancers, found in 22% of childhood ALL (of the pre-B-cell subtype).[298] In contrast to the translocation generating the *E2A-PBX1* fusion gene most of the *ETV6-RUNX1* fusions seem to originate in utero.[299]

Another transcription factor associated with human malignancies, *EVI1*, is specifically expressed in LT-HSCs. When overexpressed in mice *Evi1* boosts LT-HSC self-renewal, whereas its heterozygous loss leads to marked reduction of their self-renewal capacity.[300] Aberrant expression of *EVI1* isoforms is observed in 8–11% of AML,[301,302] and 28% of mixed-lineage leukemia (MLL)-rearranged AML,[303] and usually associated with a poor prognosis.[302] Furthermore, its translocation with *ETV6* or *RUNX1* is associated with progression to blast crisis in chronic myeloid leukemia (CML).[304,305]

The HOX Cluster in HSC Self-Renewal

Homeobox (HOX) genes encode homeodomain-containing transcription factors critical for embryonic patterning, organized into four paralogous clusters (A, B, C, and D) on four chromosomes.[306] Because of limited DNA sequence specificity and selectivity, HOX proteins function through interaction with DNA-binding cofactors, in particular, PBX and/or myeloid ectopic insertion site (MEIS) family members.[307,308] At least 22 of the 52 HOX genes (none from the HOXD cluster) are expressed in mouse and human HSPCs and are subsequently downregulated to permit lineage commitment.[309] Therefore, continuous HOX expression generally blocks differentiation and leads to rapid expansion of preleukemic HSPCs. In mice, overexpression of *HOXA10* has been shown to block myeloid and lymphoid differentiation leading to AML.[310] This is also the case for *Hoxa9*, in particular conjunction with *Meis1* or the *E2A-Pbx1* fusion gene.[311–313] *HOXA9* overexpression belongs to a gene signature that distinguishes AML from ALL, and in AML patients highly correlates with treatment failure.[314]

A number of leukemic chromosomal translocations, either directly or indirectly, lead to the overexpression of HOX genes. The nuclear pore complex protein NUP98 was first implicated in hematologic malignancies by the discovery of *NUP98-HOXA9* fusions in AML.[315,316] Approximately half of all *NUP98* translocations involve HOX genes, most commonly *HOXA9* in AML, MDS, CML and CMML, but also *HOXA11* and *HOXA13* as well as their paralogues in the B and C cluster.[317,318] While the overall prevalence of these fusions is low, they are associated with a poor prognosis.[319]

In normal HSPCs, the expression of HOX genes is regulated by MLL1,[320] as part of a multiprotein complex that regulates the chromatin structure at HOX clusters.[321,322] MLL1 fusion proteins in *MLL1*-rearranged leukemias further induce the transcription of specific HOX genes including *HOXA5*, *HOXA9* and *HOXA10*.[323,324] Indeed, HOX gene overexpression is essential for MLL1-fusion induced leukemogenesis as demonstrated by the dependence of transplanted AMLs induced by both *MLL1-ENL* and *MLL1-AF4* rearrangements on *HOXA9*.[325,326]

Transcription Factor Networks

Transcription factors act within larger multiprotein complexes. In the setting of hematopoiesis, transcription factors often act positively to sustain their own expression, while simultaneously acting to cross-regulate other transcription factors, thereby establishing complex transcriptional networks. With the advent of genome-wide molecular studies, networks can be constructed computationally. Examples include a core heptad regulatory network consisting of SCL, LYL1, LMO2, ERG, FLI1, GATA2 and RUNX1 bound to over 1,000 genes in HSPCs[327,328] or a regulatory module composed of GATA1, GFI1 and GFI1B with a potentially important role in specifying early lymphoid cells.[329] Also, profiling of transcription factors in single HSPCs combined with computational lineage progression analysis suggests a role for GATA2 in driving a network that specifies megakaryocytic and erythroid from lymphomyeloid lineage cells.[330] As these constructed networks become more mature, in silico methods will predict developmental outcomes that can be tested experimentally by modulation of one or multiple transcription factors in a direct manner.[331] A comprehensive understanding of how gene regulatory networks are perturbed in hematologic malignancies may lead to new therapeutic approaches based on restoring normal regulatory patterns.

Epigenetic Regulation of HSC Self-Renewal

Epigenetic regulation leads to a "stably heritable phenotype resulting from changes in a chromosome without alteration in the DNA sequence".[332] Epigenetic modifications include DNA methylation, covalent histone modification, chromatin remodeling and mechanisms involving noncoding RNAs which will be discussed further later. By modifying chromatin structure and accessibility, epigenetic mechanisms regulate the expression of genes involved in determining the balance between self-renewal and lineage commitment of HSCs, ultimately leading to all hematopoietic cell types. Epigenetic dysregulation has been implicated in the pathogenesis of virtually all hematologic malignancies.[333,334] In contrast to genetic mutations, epigenetic alterations are in principle reversible, making epigenetic modifiers attractive targets for the innovative treatment of hematologic malignancies. Fig. 9.2 depicts key epigenetic factors within the hematopoietic hierarchy, and Table 9.1 summarizes main roles of critical epigenetic factors in HSPCs and hematologic malignancies.

DNA methylation plays a critical role in HSC self-renewal and commitment.[335–338] Through recruitment of multiprotein complexes, methylated DNA results in transcriptional repression of nearby genes. In mammalian cells, DNA methylation occurs at cytidines, mostly in the context of CpG dinucleotides, dispersed throughout the genome and clustered (as CpG islands) within gene promoters. In a number of hematologic cancers, for example, the progression from MDS to AML, promoter CpG islands become hypermethylated and the affected genes, including tumor suppressor genes silenced.[339] Furthermore, subgroups of AML can be defined by unique DNA methylation profiles, which can be used to stratify AML patients with respect to their overall survival.[340] The family of DNA methyltransferases includes the de novo DNA methyltransferases DNMT3A and DNMT3B that establish methylation whereas another family member, DNMT1, maintains DNA methylation.[341,342] DNA methylation is required for HSCs to differentiate. Conditional knockout

of *Dnmt3a*, further pronounced by ablation of *Dnmt3b*, leads to an accumulation of self-renewing HSCs in the BM which lose their differentiation capacity upon serial transplantation.[343,344] Next-generation sequencing studies have identified *DNMT3A* mutations in most hematologic malignancies, in particular in patients with cytogenetically normal AML (over 30%),[345] where they can be detected as preleukemic lesions,[286,346] and T-ALL (16%[347]; for a complete list see[348]). In contrast, *DNMT1* mutations have been rarely found in AML.[334]

Recently it was discovered that DNA methylation is in fact reversible,[349,350] owing to the activity of ten-eleven translocation (TET) proteins (TET1, TET2, and TET3), which iteratively oxidize 5-methylcytosine present in methylated CpG dinucleotides.[351] Mice deficient for *Tet2*, the only TET expressed in the BM, show enhanced self-renewal of HSCs and develop a CMML-like disease.[352–354] *TET2* is mutated in 49% of CMML[355] and up to 23% of AML[356–358] patients. Interestingly, gain-of-function mutations in isocitrate dehydrogenase 1 and 2 (*IDH1/2*) that indirectly impair TET2 function are mutually exclusive with *TET2* mutations in AML. *IDH1* and *2* are found mutated in 13–33% of AML cases and lead to similar methylation profiles as *TET2* mutations.[359,360–363] IDH1/2 enzymes catalyze the conversion of isocitrate to α-ketoglutarate (α-KG), but mutated IDH1/2 further convert α-KG to 2-hydroxyglutarate, which inhibits the α-KG dependent TET2 enzyme.[364,365]

The effects of histone modifications are combinatorial in nature, and there is crosstalk between DNA methylation and histone modifications.[366] Histones have protruding flexible and charged NH_2-termini ("tails") that can be posttranslationally modified in various ways, by methylation, acetylation, phosphorylation, ubiquitination and sumoylation, to name but a few.[367] Many histone modifications have been implicated in HSC self-renewal by knockout or overexpression of chromatin regulators that function as their "writers", "readers" or "erasers" (for a recent list, see[368]). Recurrent mutations of CREBBP and/or and EP300, members of the histone acetyltransferase family that activate transcription, have been detected in several lymphoma types,[369] and 18% of relapsed pediatric ALL patients exhibit mutations in the enzymatic domain of CREBBP, which are thought to contribute to drug resistance.[370]

Unlike histone acetylation, methylation of histones can have activating or repressive effects, dependent on the context and the targeted histone residue. With respect to active marks, most epigenetic studies have focused on lysine methylation carried out by lysine methyltransferases (KMTs) and removed by lysine demethylases (KDMs). The large multidomain KMT *MLL1* is essential for the generation of definitive HSCs in the mouse,[371] likely through its regulation of HOX cluster genes.[320] The *MLL1* locus has been found to be frequently involved in chromosomal translocations in up to 70% of infant and childhood AML and ALL and in 5–10% of adult leukemia,[372] generally associated with a poor prognosis.[373] 85% of *MLL1* translocations involve six proteins (AF4, AF9, ENL, AF10, ELL, and AF6), of which MLL1-AF4 in ALL and MLL1-AF9 in AML are most common.[374] Many MLL1 fusion partners belong to the super elongation complex (SEC); when fused to MLL1 the aberrantly recruited SEC bypasses the normal transcription initiation-to-elongation checkpoints leading to high expression of MLL1-regulated genes such as HOX, WNT and leukemic stem cell target genes.[375] Furthermore, almost all fusion proteins aberrantly recruit another KMT, DOT1L, which by methylating H3K79 induces the expression of MLL1 target genes sufficient for leukemogenesis such as *HOXA9* and *MEIS1*.[311] In addition, MLL1 fusion proteins provoke a global loss of DNA methylation in AMLs.[376] In fact, *Dnmt1* haploinsufficiency, while not perturbing normal HSC function, significantly delays leukemia progression in the *MLL-AF9* AML mouse model.[377]

At many lineage-specifying promoters in HSCs, epigenetic activators are balanced with repressive complexes, namely the polycomb repressive complex 1 (PRC1) and PRC2. The latter typically comprises the catalytically active EZH2, as well as EED and SUZ12, and is responsible for di- and trimethylation of H3K27, a repressive histone mark that is then "read" and maintained by PRC1 through histone H2A ubiquitination.[378,379] EZH2 also recruits DNA methyl-transferases to its target genes, thereby enhancing its repressive effect.[380] Overexpression of *Ezh2* in mice enhances LT-HSC self-renewal by silencing differentiation genes[381,382] and causing a shift to the expression of proliferation genes.[383] EZH2 has been described with either tumor suppressive or oncogenic roles, depending on the cellular context. *EZH2* gain-of-function mutations, resulting in overall "hyper-trimethylation", occur in 7.2% and 21.7% of follicular lymphoma and diffuse large B-cell lymphoma, respectively. Loss-of-function mutations have been observed in 12% of myelodysplastic/myeloproliferative neoplasms and 18% of T-ALL cases but are rare in de novo AML (1–2%). PRCs do not bind to DNA directly but require the interaction with other proteins such as ASXL1. *ASXL1* is mutated in 6–30% of AML and 43% of CMML.[359] These mutations hinder ASXL1 from recruiting PRC2 to and thus repressing target genes such as *HOXA9*.[384]

Regulation of HSCs by Noncoding RNAs

Sequencing the human genome revealed that less than 1.5% of the DNA encodes proteins[385] but, remarkably, subsequent analyses discovered that still 76% of the genome is transcribed into RNA.[386] Many noncoding RNAs (ncRNAs) are enriched in HSCs compared to hematopoietic progenitors.[387] ncRNAs other than ribosomal RNAs and transfer RNAs are arbitrarily categorized into long ncRNAs (lncRNAs) and short ncRNAs if >200 or <200 nucleotides long, respectively. Among the short ncRNAs, microRNAs (miRNAs) are ~22-nucleotide regulatory ncRNAs that repress gene expression predominantly by binding to the 3′ untranslated region of protein-encoding mRNAs leading to their destabilization.[388] A miRNA can target large numbers of mRNAs, and a single mRNA can be regulated by multiple miRNAs.[389] HSCs depend on miRNA function for their survival as demonstrated by the finding that deletion of *Dicer* or *Ars2*, both essential factors for miRNA biogenesis results in HSC apoptosis and BM failure.[390,391] More than 100 different miRNAs are specifically expressed during hematopoiesis, preferentially targeting and fine-tuning expression of transcription factors and their upstream activators.[392] Hematologic malignancies show characteristic changes in their miRNA expression profiles. For example, ALL samples can be classified into subtypes according to their miRNA expression patterns.[393]

Numerous miRNAs are specifically enriched in HSPCs, including miR-155,[394] miR-125a,[391] miR-125b,[395–397] miR-29a,[398] miR-126, and miR-130a.[399] Overexpression of the miRNA cluster miR-99b/let7e/125a or miR-125a alone is capable of expanding the HSC pool in mice,[391,395,400] potentially by inhibiting apoptosis of HSCs mediated by the proapoptotic gene *Bak1*, which is a miR-125a target.[391] In addition, several miRNAs have been implicated in regulating HPC differentiation, including miR-155 (lymphoid and myeloid development),[394,401] miR-223 (myeloid development)[402,403] and the miR-181/miR-150/miR-17-92 cluster (lymphoid development).[404–407] The example of miR-155 shows that, like transcription factors, some miRNAs are repurposed during hematopoietic ontogeny.[408]

Most of the miRNAs conferring a competitive advantage to the engrafted BM have been implicated in malignant transformation, and are therefore called oncomiRs.[409] Overexpression of miR-125 family members causes myeloid and lymphoid malignancies in mice[395,397,400,410,411] and they are upregulated in chromosomal translocations leading to MDS/AML and B-cell ALL.[412–414] oncomiRs contribute to leukemic phenotypes by different mechanisms such as expediting cell cycle transitions,[398] targeting tumor suppressors such as TET2,[415] or dysregulating the balance between lineage-specific transcription factors.[401] miR-155, the first miRNA shown to be sufficient to cause lymphoblastic leukemia or high-grade lymphoma in a transgenic mouse model,[416] is overexpressed in B-cell lymphomas[417] and AML.[418,419] miR-196, which is upregulated specifically during the transition from quiescent LT-HSCs to ST-HSCs, targets several of its neighboring HOX genes important for self-renewal such as *HOXA9*.[408,420–423] Like HOX genes, miR-196b is transcriptionally

regulated by MLL and highly induced in MLL-rearranged leukemias, contributing to an unfavorable prognosis.[422,424] In this context, miR-196 has been shown to be necessary for *MLL-AF9* dependent immortalization of BM cells.[424] miRNAs can also function as tumor suppressors, exerting their function by targeting oncogenes. For example, the miRNA cluster miR-15a/miR16-1 is deleted or epigenetically silenced in 68% of chronic lymphoid leukemia patients,[425] resulting in the upregulation of its target oncogene *BLC2*.[426]

In contrast to miRNAs, little is known about the expression of lncRNAs in HSPCs and only a few lncRNAs have been further functionally characterized. Several recent studies have compiled lists of lncRNAs expressed in HSCs, some of which are downregulated in more differentiated progeny[338,387] and in leukemic cells.[427] Knockdown of a lncRNA specifically expressed in mouse BM LT-HSCs increased self-renewal of HSCs in vivo and abolished recruitment of the transcription factor E2A, essential for the development of multi-lineage HPCs,[292] to chromatin.[428] HSCs from female mice depleted for *Xist* lncRNA (responsible for X chromosome inactivation) were shown to have maturation defects and to be compromised in their repopulation capacity.[429] Furthermore, all *Xist* mutant female mice developed highly aggressive mixed myeloproliferative neoplasms/MDS.[429] With those relatively few studies the overall relevance of lncRNAs for the pathogenesis of hematopoietic diseases is not yet well understood.

HEMATOPOIETIC STEM CELL METABOLISM

The role of oxidative and nonoxidative glucose metabolism in regulating HSC and HPC function has recently been elucidated.[430] Wang et al reported that deficiencies in either lactate dehydrogenase A (LDHA) or the M2 isoform of pyruvate kinase (PKM2), two enzymes which catalyze the fermentation of glucose to lactate, result in differential effects on HSC and progenitor cell function.[430] Deletion of *Ldha* inhibited normal HSC and progenitor cell function, whereas deficiency in *Pkm2* impaired progenitor cell function without affecting HSCs.[430] The authors further showed that deficiency of either *Ldha* or *Pkm2* inhibited leukemia initiation, suggesting that these metabolic enzymes may be therapeutically useful in targeting leukemia.[430] Separately, Ito et al demonstrated that the loss of peroxisome proliferator-activated receptor δ (PPAR-δ) or inhibition of mitochondrial fatty acid oxidation induced the loss of HSC maintenance.[431] Interestingly, this PPAR-δ-FAO axis was considered to serve as a "metabolic switch" which regulated HSC symmetric versus asymmetric division.[431] The tumor suppressor gene, *Lkb1*, which encodes a serine/threonine kinase that regulates phosphorylation of AMP-activated protein kinase, was also shown to be essential for HSC maintenance.[432] *Lkb1* inactivation was shown to deplete quiescent HSCs associated with depletion of all hematopoietic subpopulations, coupled with mitochondrial defects, depletion of ATP and alterations in lipid and nucleotide metabolism.[432]

Not surprisingly, the metabolic state of HSCs is influenced by the hypoxic microenvironment in which HSCs reside.[433,434] Specifically, hypoxia contributes to the maintenance of quiescent HSCs which have high expression of HIF-1α and rely primarily on anaerobic glycolysis, rather than oxidative phosphorylation, to produce ATP.[434–436] The therapeutic importance of understanding the cellular metabolic state of HSCs was recently highlighted by Liu et al,[437] who showed that treatment of HSCs with alexidine dihydrochloride, a selective inhibitor of the mitochondrial phosphatase PTPMT1, reprogrammed HSC metabolism from aerobic to glycolysis, resulting in increased HSC maintenance in culture. Alterations in HSC metabolism have also been described with aging, thereby impacting HSC function. Mohrin et al recently reported that SIRT7, a histone deacetylase which regulates the expression of the mitochondrial master regulator, nuclear respiratory factor 1, was reduced in aging HSCs.[438] SIRT7 inactivation was shown to increase mitochondrial folding stress and compromise the regenerative capacity of HSCs, suggesting that alterations in the mitochondrial unfolded protein response contribute to HSC aging.[438]

TABLE 9.2	Soluble Proteins and Small Molecules That Regulate Hematopoietic Stem Cell Self-Renewal	
Growth Factor	Function in HSC Self-Renewal	Reference[a]
NOTCH ligands	Sufficient, not necessary	167, 171–173, 177, 178
WNT proteins	Sufficient, ? necessary	185, 189, 201, 203
BMPs	? Sufficient, SMAD4 necessary	220
SCF	Necessary, not sufficient	439
TPO	Necessary, not sufficient	440
CXCL12	Necessary	239, 242
RAR-γ	Necessary	117
ANGPTL	Sufficient	441, 442
PGE$_2$	Sufficient	445, 448
PTN	Necessary, sufficient	107, 454
AHR antagonist	Sufficient	456

[a]References are representative, not all-inclusive.
AHR, aryl hydrocarbon receptor; ANGPTL, angiopoietin-like protein; BMP, bone morphogenetic protein; CXCL12, C-X-C motif chemokine 12; HSC, hematopoietic stem cell; PGE$_2$, prostaglandin E$_2$; PTN, pleiotrophin; RAR-γ, retinoic acid receptor γ; SCF, stem cell factor; TPO, thrombopoietin.
Adapted from Zon L: Intrinsic and extrinsic control of haematopoietic stem cell self-renewal. *Nature* 453:306, 2008, with permission.

NOVEL GROWTH FACTORS FOR HEMATOPOIETIC STEM CELLS AND CLINICAL TESTING

Several novel proteins and small molecules have been reported to promote potent expansion of murine or human HSCs in culture (Table 9.2).[107,439,440] Moreover, leveraging insights into the mechanisms which regulate HSC self-renewal and differentiation, several different approaches to expand human CB HSCs have been tested in early clinical trials. Zhang et al[441] reported the discovery of the proteins angiopoietin-like 2 (ANGPTL2) and ANGPTL3 in a fetal liver stromal cell line and demonstrated that the addition of ANGPTL2 or ANGPTL3 to cytokine cultures supported a 24- to 30-fold expansion of human BM cells capable of long-term repopulation in NOD/SCID mice. Subsequently, Zhang et al[442] demonstrated that the addition of ANGPTL5 and insulin-like growth factor binding protein 2 (IGFBP2) to the combination of SCF, TPO, and FGF1 supported up to a 20-fold increase in human CB cells capable of 8-week engraftment in NOD/SCID mice. Of note, because the addition of ANGPTL5 and IGFBP2 did not substantially increase total cell expansion compared with SCF, TPO, and FGF1 alone, it remains possible that treatment with ANGPTL proteins or IGFBP2 may enhance the homing of HSCs in immune-deficient transplant models.[442] Because of their potency in expanding human CB HSCs in preclinical models, ANGPTL proteins represent attractive targets for translation into the clinic. Recently, several ANGPTL proteins, including ANGPTL2 and ANGPTL5 have been found to bind and activate the immune-inhibitory receptor human leukocyte immunoglobulin-like receptor B2 (LILRB2).[443] Interestingly, studies in zebrafish and human cells indicate that ANGPTL2, through its interaction with LILRB2, leads to cleavage and activation of the NOTCH receptor, ultimately inducing MYC target genes stimulating HSPC formation and expansion.[444]

North et al[445] reported that prostaglandin E$_2$ (PGE$_2$) positively regulates HSC formation in the zebrafish model. These authors also demonstrated that short-term (2-hour) treatment of murine HSCs with PGE$_2$ produced a two- to threefold increase in donor cell repopulation in transplanted mice compared with mice transplanted with untreated cells.[445] Subsequently, Goessling et al[446] showed

that PGE$_2$ modulates WNT signaling via regulation of β-catenin degradation and PGE$_2$/WNT activation regulated both hematopoietic regeneration in the zebrafish and long-term HSC repopulation in mice. Hoggatt et al[447] also showed that short-term exposure to PGE$_2$ promoted the enhanced homing and repopulation of human CB HSCs in immune-deficient mice caused by increased CXCR4 expression on PGE$_2$-treated CB HSCs. Ex vivo treatment with PGE$_2$ was subsequently shown to increase human CB CFC content and engraftment capacity after transplant into immune-deficient mice, and PGE$_2$-treated BM cells were also found to provide more than one year of multilineage reconstitution in a nonhuman primate model.[448] Based on these encouraging results, a phase I clinical trial was undertaken, in which one unmanipulated CB unit and a second CB unit that was cultured for two hours in the presence of 16,16-dimethyl PGE$_2$ (dmPGE$_2$) were transplanted into adult patients after nonmyeloablative conditioning. dmPGE$_2$-treated CB cells resulted in accelerated neutrophil recovery (17.5 days versus 21 days) and long-term engraftment in 10 of 12 patients.[449]

Recently, screening strategies in human cells have been successfully used to identify novel growth factors, developmental factors and chemical compounds, for HSCs. Himburg et al identified pleiotrophin (PTN), a heparin binding growth factor, from a gene expression analysis of human brain-derived endothelial cells (ECs) that support human HSC expansion in vitro.[450–453] Treatment of murine BM HSCs with PTN produced a 10-fold expansion of long-term repopulating HSCs in culture, and systemic administration of PTN to irradiated mice caused a 20-fold increase in the recovery of BM LTC-ICs in vivo.[107] Mechanistically, PTN signaling caused the upregulation of PI3K/AKT signaling and *Hes1* expression in HSCs, suggesting that activation of these signaling cascades may contribute to PTN-mediated HSC expansion.[107] Mice lacking *Ptn* had 11-fold less BM HSC content than their wild-type littermates.[454] Interestingly, LT-HSC content, as measured in tertiary and quaternary transplants, was increased in chimeric mice with *Ptn* deletion in the BM microenvironment compared with wild-type mice.[455] Taken together, these results suggest that PTN regulates BM HSC expansion and regeneration, and in the context of constitutive *Ptn* knockout, *Ptn* loss in hematopoietic cells may dominate over effects of *Ptn* loss in the niche.[109,455] Further studies will be necessary to resolve these questions and define the potential therapeutic efficacy of PTN. Boitano et al[456] described a screening approach of more than 100,000 heterocyclic compounds for the capacity to maintain human CD34$^+$ cells in culture for five days. This screen yielded the discovery of the purine derivative StemRegenin 1 (SR1), which was shown to promote the expansion of human CB repopulating cells in vitro.[456] Three-week cultures of human CB CD34$^+$ cells with thrombopoietin, SCF, FLT3 ligand, interleukin-6 (IL-6), and SR1 promoted a 17-fold increase in SCID-repopulating cells compared with the progeny of cultures containing thrombopoietin, SCF, FLT3 ligand, and IL-6 alone.[456] SR1 appears to mediate its effects via inhibition of the aryl hydrocarbon receptor. Aryl hydrocarbon receptors are expressed by HSCs, but the downstream signaling mechanism through which SR1 mediates HSC expansion remains unknown.[456] Recently, Dahlberg et al reported that the combination of SR1 with the NOTCH ligand, Delta$^{\text{Ext-IgG}}$, caused a threefold increase in human CB-derived myeloid repopulation in NSG mice at two weeks compared to CB cells cultured with Delta$^{\text{Ext-IgG}}$ or SR1 alone.[457] Preliminary results from a phase I trial of transplantation with SR1-treated CB cells have demonstrated the feasibility and safety of this approach.[458]

In a recent analysis of growth factors elaborated by an AGM-derived stromal cell line, Wohrer et al reported that nerve growth factor and collagen 1, when added to a defined serum-free medium containing SCF and IL-11, produced fourfold expansion of murine long-term repopulating HSCs in seven-day cultures compared to SCF and IL-11 alone.[459,460] Separately, treatment of human CB HSCs with a pyrimidoindole derivative, UM171, was shown to promote a 13-fold expansion of CB cells capable of repopulating NSG mice at 20 weeks posttransplantation.[461] Although the mechanism of action of UM171 has not been elucidated, preliminary analyses suggested that UM171 inhibited erythroid and megakaryocytic differentiation of human HSCs in culture. Jaroscak et al[462] tested the combination of FLT3 ligand, a GM-CSF/IL-3 fusion protein, and erythropoietin in a continuous perfusion culture system as a means to expand human CB cells before transplant. Similarly, Shpall et al[463] tested the capacity of SCF, granulocyte colony-stimulating factor (G-CSF), and mega-karyocyte growth and differentiation factor to expand human CB cells that were then transplanted into adult CB transplant recipients. An alternative approach to cytokine-based expansion of human CB cells was suggested by Peled et al[464–466] who demonstrated a 159-fold increase in human CD34+ cells after seven-week culture with a copper chelator, tetraethylenepentamine (TEPA), and cytokines. Subsequently, de Lima et al[467] reported the safety and feasibility of culturing human CB cells with TEPA and SCF, FLT3 ligand, IL-6, and throm-bopoietin followed by transplantation into patients in a phase I/II clinical trial. Although each of these clinical trials has shown the feasibility of transplanting ex vivo–cultured CB cells, none demonstrated substantial acceleration in hematopoietic cell engraftment in CB transplant recipients compared to historical controls. However, the TEPA plus cytokine strategy is being tested further in a phase II/III study in several countries, including the United States.[166]

Several other clinical trials have recently indicated progress toward the clinical expansion of human CB HSCs for therapeutic purposes. De Lima et al reported a median time to neutrophil engraftment of 15 days in recipients of one unmanipulated CB unit plus CB cells cultured with mesenchymal stromal cells, compared to 24 days in historical controls, although long-term donor hematopoiesis derived almost exclusively from the unmanipulated cord blood unit.[468] Lastly, Horwitz et al reported that transplantation of one unmanipulated CB unit and the progeny of 21-day culture of human CB cells with nicotinamide produced earlier neutrophil recovery (13 versus 25 days for historical controls) and dominant engraftment from the nicotinamide-treated CB unit in eight of 11 treated patients.[469]

GENERATING HEMATOPOIETIC STEM CELLS FROM PLURIPOTENT STEM CELLS AND BY REPROGRAMMING OF SOMATIC CELLS

Globally more than 50,000 patients per year receive allogeneic and autologous HSC transplantations as treatments for congenital and acquired hematopoietic diseases and other malignancies.[470] At present, the only cell sources for HSC transplantations are BM, CB, or mobilized peripheral blood. However, insufficient numbers, shelf-life concerns as well as immunologic incompatibility leading to graft-versus-host disease, even in human leukocyte antigen-matched grafts, limits their availability.[471,472] One option to generate more HSCs is by expanding existing HSCs in vitro as described earlier. Despite substantial efforts, this has proven difficult; because of their tendency to differentiate in culture, the expansion of HSCs is not very efficient and does often not lead to fully functional HSCs in terms of their migratory behavior and long-term multilineage reconstitution potential.[461,473,474]

The observation in 1981 that embryonic stem cells (ESCs) could be derived from mouse or, later, human blastocysts[475–477] fueled experiments to differentiate HSCs from ESCs. In 2006, the discovery that mouse or human fibroblasts could be reprogrammed to induced pluripotent stem cells (iPSCs) by retroviral transduction with the same four factors, OCT3/4, SOX2, KLF4, and c-Myc,[478,479] opened the door for the possibility of autologous stem-cell based therapies in the clinic.[480,481] Since its first report this technology has been constantly modified[482] and is allowing the generation of iPSC lines from patients with a variety of blood disorders (references in[483]). This approach presents a new opportunity for disease modeling and drug screening.

Numerous methods for directed differentiation of HSCs from ESCs or more recently iPSCs have been developed, but so far none yield long-lived cells with full HSC functionality. In a recent study, inducible expression of five transcription factors, HOXA9, RORA, ERG, SOX4, and MYB imparted human ESC- and iPSC-derived progenitors with short-term myeloid and erythroid engraftment potential.[483] This and similar approaches are characterized by the lack of robust lymphoid potential, likely because these progenitors are developmentally still too immature.[484]

In light of the obstacles in generating HSCs from ESCs or iPSCs, approaches to directly reprogram somatic cells into HSCs, or trans-differentiate them to hematopoietic cells are being explored as alternative strategies. The concept of direct reprogramming was first demonstrated with the conversion of embryonic fibroblasts into contracting myocytes by just the transcription factor MyoD.[485] Pluripotency-related factors are upregulated during endogenous reconstitution of mouse hematopoiesis after irradiation.[486] Thus, studies successfully reprogramming human skin fibroblasts directly into HSPC-like cells used the pluripotency factors OCT4 or SOX2 together with a specific cytokine cocktail.[486,487] While these cells engrafted, they again lacked lymphoid potential. In contrast to these examples of indirect lineage conversion via a less differentiated state, direct lineage conversion (or transdifferentiation) attempts have included the enforced expression of transcription factors critical for normal hematopoiesis.[488] In analogy to the HSC-producing hemogenic endothelium, human umbilical-vein ECs cultured on an artificial vascular niche and overexpressing four transcription factors (FOSB, GFI1, RUNX1 and PU.1) yielded serially transplantable hematopoietic colonies.[489] However, these cells did not differentiate into T cells. In another approach demonstrating the benefit of the niche, lymphoid or myeloid progenitors were transduced with a transcription factor cocktail (HLF, LMO2, PBX1, PRDM5, RUNX1T1 and ZFP37) and matured in irradiated mice to yield serially transplantable HSCs producing all lineages.[490] Despite this progress in mice, fully functional human HSCs have not yet been generated in vitro. In addition, future studies will have to focus on strategies to avoid the risk of malignant transformation inherent in any directed differentiation or cellular reprogramming method.[491]

HEMATOPOIETIC STEM CELL REGENERATION

Although much is now known about the intrinsic and extrinsic mechanisms that regulate adult HSC self-renewal and differentiation,[1,166,188] the process through which HSCs regenerate after injury (e.g., chemotherapy or radiation) remains less well understood. Successful delineation of the mechanisms that control HSC regeneration has significant therapeutic potential because a large proportion of patients with cancer receive myelosuppressive or myeloablative therapy during the course of their disease. Signaling through the BMP and WNT signaling pathways has been shown to be necessary for hematopoietic regeneration to occur in zebrafish after sublethal irradiation.[492] These authors further demonstrated that SMAD and TCF, the downstream effectors of BMP and WNT signaling, respectively, couple with master regulators of myeloid and erythroid differentiation (C/EBPα and GATA1) to drive lineage-specific regeneration.[492] In a murine model of hematopoietic injury, Congdon et al[493] showed that Wnt10b expression is increased in BM stromal cells in response to irradiation, and WNT signaling is activated in BM HSCs after irradiation. As discussed earlier, in a zebrafish model, activation of WNT signaling during hematopoietic regeneration is modulated by PGE2.[446] WNT reporter activity was responsive to PGE2 treatment, and the effect of Wnt8 toward enhancing hematopoietic recovery after sublethal irradiation was inhibited by administration of indomethacin, a PGE2 antagonist.[446] NOTCH signaling has also been implicated in the regulation of hematopoietic regeneration after stem cell transplantation.[279] Deletion of Notch2, but not Notch1, was shown to delay myeloid reconstitution in mice after stem cell transplantation.[170] These data suggest that the BMP, WNT, and NOTCH pathways are attractive mechanistic targets for strategies to augment hematopoietic regeneration after myelosuppressive therapy.

Additional signaling pathways have been implicated in regulating hematopoietic regeneration. Deletion of plasminogen (Plg), a fibrinolytic factor, was shown to prevent HPC proliferation and recovery after 5-fluorouracil (5-FU)-induced myelosuppression in mice.[494] Conversely, activation of PLG by administration of tissue plasminogen activator promoted HPC proliferation and differentiation after myelosuppression, and this effect was dependent on matrix metallopeptidase 9–mediated release of c-Kit ligand.[494] Similarly, Trowbridge et al[232] reported that mice that were heterozygous for the hedgehog receptor *Ptc1*, displayed earlier recovery of hematopoiesis after 5-FU-induced myelosuppression compared with wild-type littermate mice. Hedgehog binding blocks PTC1-mediated inhibition of SMO, thereby promoting downstream Hedgehog signaling. Therefore, heterozygous *Ptc1* mice have enhanced Hedgehog signaling, and these results implicate Hedgehog signaling as positively regulating short-term hematopoietic regeneration after injury. However, this acceleration in hematopoietic recovery in mice heterozygous for *Ptc1* occurred at the expense of LT-HSCs, which were exhausted in these mice.[232] Genetic studies have similarly demonstrated that the homozygous deletion of *Ship* in mice (SH2-containing inositol phosphatase) is associated with increased loss of HSCs after 5-FU exposure compared with heterozygous *Ship* deletion.[495] In a similar model of 5-FU-mediated myelosuppression, Nemeth et al[496] reported that mice deficient in the high-mobility group box 3 (*Hmg3b*) DNA binding protein exhibited more rapid recovery of phenotypic HSCs compared with wild-type mice. The enhanced recovery of the stem/progenitor pool in *Hmgb3*-deficient mice was associated with activation of WNT signaling, again suggesting that activation of the WNT pathway may accelerate HSC recovery after myelosuppression. Of note, expression of a constitutively active form of the signal transducer and activator of transcription 3 (*Stat3*) in HSCs increases their regenerative capacity after transplant into lethally irradiated mice.[497] In this study, it was not determined whether alteration in *Stat3* expression affected HSC regeneration after myelosuppression (e.g., 5-FU or irradiation).[497]

At the cellular level, increasing evidence suggests an important role for BM ECs in promoting hematopoietic regeneration after myelotoxic stress.[498–501] Genetic deletion or antibody-based inhibition of VEGFR2, which is expressed by sinusoidal BM ECs, was shown to delay both BM vascular and hematopoietic recovery after total-body irradiation (TBI).[499] Systemic infusion of syngeneic or allogeneic ECs has also been shown to significantly accelerate the recovery of both the HSC pool and overall hematopoiesis in mice after high-dose TBI.[501,502] Salter et al[501] and Butler et al[176] further demonstrated that hematopoietic regeneration after irradiation is dependent on VE-cadherin-mediated vascular reorganization because administration of a neutralizing anti-VE-cadherin antibody caused significant delay in hematologic recovery in mice after TBI. While the precise mechanisms through which BM ECs regulate HSC regeneration in vivo remain unclear, it was shown that systemic administration of PTN, a heparin binding growth factor that is secreted by both BM and brain ECs, causes a rapid increase in recovery of the HSC pool in mice after high-dose TBI.[107] Taken together, these studies suggested that the BM vascular niche may be an important reservoir for the discovery of growth factors and membrane-bound proteins that mediate HSC regeneration. Additional studies have further validated the important role of the BM vascular niche in regulating HSC regeneration following myelosuppressive injury. Deletion of the proapoptotic proteins, BAK and BAX, from *Tie2*-expressing BM ECs was shown to protect HSCs from radiation-induced depletion in mice, independent of HSC-autonomous effects.[503] Furthermore, Doan et al reported that EGF is expressed by BM ECs after TBI and that systemic administration of EGF improved HSC regeneration and survival after TBI.[503] EC-specific deletion of the NOTCH ligand, Jagged1, has also been shown to cause delayed white blood cell recovery and decreased survival in mice following sublethal TBI.[504] Interestingly, recent studies have suggested several novel mechanisms through which HSC regeneration can be augmented following radiation-induced myelotoxicity, including augmentation of the thrombomodulin-activated protein C pathway,[505] administration of the bactericidal/permeability-increasing protein (rBPI$_{21}$),[506] activation of nuclear factor erythroid-2-related factor 2[507] or Ras/MEK/ERK signaling in HSCs.[508] Interestingly, it was also recently shown that both HSCs and leptin receptor-expressing BM stromal

cells secrete Angiopoietin 1 (ANGPT1) and that deletion of *Angpt1* in these cell populations accelerated vascular and hematopoietic recovery in mice after irradiation.[509] Taken together, these studies reveal the remarkable complexity and orchestration of molecular responses to myelotoxicity and also suggest several potential pathways that can potentially be exploited for the therapeutic regeneration of HSCs.

Lastly, the effect of age on the capacity for HSCs to regenerate after myelosuppressive challenge remains an important question.[510] Clinical studies have confirmed the impaired reconstitutive capacity of HSCs from older patients in autologous stem cell transplant settings.[511] Not surprisingly, older mice with defects in DNA damage repair mechanisms (nucleotide excision repair, nonhomologous end-joining) and telomere maintenance displayed severe defects in their capacity to reconstitute hematopoiesis after transplantation into lethally irradiated recipient mice compared with age-matched control subjects that retained the DNA repair and telomerase genes.[512] Furthermore, Flach et al recently showed that aging HSCs display heightened levels of replication stress during cell cycling as a result of decreased expression of mini-chromosome maintenance replicative helicase components and altered DNA replication forks.[513] Therefore, therapeutic targeting to accentuate these DNA repair and replication mechanisms may facilitate the recovery of the functional HSC pool after myelosuppression and may lessen the oncogenic risk incurred via repeated exposure to DNA-damaging therapies (e.g., alkylators and irradiation).[512,513] Interestingly, prolonged fasting has been shown to ameliorate chemotherapy-induced HSC damage and age-dependent myeloid bias in mice, associated with reduction in IGF1 levels.[514] Further research into the HSC-autonomous and extrinsic mechanisms which regulate HSC aging and HSC regeneration during aging should be prioritized going forward and will hopefully yield therapeutic avenues to reverse some aspects of hematopoietic aging.

HEMATOPOIETIC STEM CELLS AND MALIGNANCY

Similar to the HSC at the apex of the hematopoietic hierarchy, an entity termed a leukemic stem cell (LSC) has been proposed to drive tumorigenesis because of its ability to self-renew and reinitiate leukemia upon transplantation in an experimental setting (e.g., mouse transplant; Fig. 9.4).[515–517] A clonal origin of a hematopoietic malignancy was first demonstrated for CML where the presence of the characteristic Philadelphia chromosome in myeloid, erythroid, megakaryocytic and B-lymphoid cells suggested a common origin,[518–520] which was later proven by molecular analysis.[521] Genetic analyses in a case of CML also provided the first proof for another important concept in cancer, that of clonal evolution (see Fig. 9.4),[522] which had already been hypothesized for solid tumors.[516] This model posits that a subclone within the initial LSC-derived clone acquires additional genetic or epigenetic alterations that convey a growth advantage and lead to heterogeneity within the tumor.[515] Whereas the HSC pool itself does not expand during progression of chronic phase CML to blast crisis, granulocyte-macrophage progenitors (GMPs) with increased expression of the continuously active tyrosine kinase fusion protein BCR-ABL and high self-renewal capacity driven by activation of nuclear β-catenin are amplified.[523] Thus, the LSC may differ from the tumor-initiating "cell of origin".[161,523] While in CML the tumor-initiating HSC maintains the chronic phase of the disease, subsequent genetic events arising in the GMPs give rise to LSCs sustaining the blast crisis.

The first cancer stem cell to be identified in any malignancy was the LSC in AML.[517,524] CD34$^+$CD38$^-$ cells but not CD34$^+$CD38$^+$ cells derived from all known AML subtypes (except for the AML subtype M3) repopulated secondary NOD/SCID recipient mice and fully reproduced AML.[524,525] Next-generation sequencing efforts have revealed the clonal evolution in primary and relapsed AML.[287,334,345,526–529] While healthy and AML genomes contain hundreds of exonic mutations,[287] as few as two key somatic "driver" mutations enable clonal expansion of a cell that takes along all the background "passenger" mutations.

STEM CELL MODEL OF HEMATOLOGIC DISEASES

Justin Taylor and Omar Abdel-Wahab

CELL OF ORIGIN STUDIES IN HEMATOLOGIC MALIGNANCIES

One of the prevailing models of cancer development proposes that a cancer is initiated and maintained through the function of cancer stem cells (CSCs), which represent a rare population of cells within a cancer that have an indefinite proliferative potential and are ultimately responsible for the generation of the bulk of cancer cells. This so-called cancer stem cell hypothesis has been best studied in hematopoietic malignancies. The ability to purify hematopoietic cells more easily than cells from other tissues, combined with the well-defined cell-surface markers of hematopoietic cells, has allowed the prospective isolation of nearly every hematopoietic cell subset from humans as well as mice.

The CSC hypothesis proposes that cancers are organized into hierarchical populations like normal tissues. At the apex of hierarchy are largely quiescent long-lived CSCs with marked self-renewal capacity that sustain the disease and give rise to the majority of the bulk cancer cells that constitute the disease. While identification of a single normal hematopoietic cell subset as the target of the malignant transformation and the cellular reservoir for disease has been possible for a variety of myeloid leukemias and lymphomas, pinpointing a single cell as the target of malignant transformation has not yet proven possible for other hematopoietic malignancies. In this chapter, we will discuss efforts to identify the malignant stem cell for each of the common forms of myeloid and lymphoid leukemias.

ACUTE MYELOID LEUKEMIA

The first evidence of a stem cell origin of malignancy came from studies in 1997 performed by Blair et al[1] as well as Bonnet and Dick[2] into acute myeloid leukemia (AML). These studies demonstrated that most leukemia cells were unable to proliferate extensively and that only a subset of cells was consistently clonogenic. In these studies a small subset of human Thy1−CD34+CD38− AML cells (0.2–1.0%) was identified and shown to be the only cells capable of transferring human AML to immunodeficient mice. In humans, normal hematopoietic stem cells (HSCs) reside in the lineage-negative (Lin−) CD34+CD38−CD90+CD45RA− compartment and generate multipotent progenitors with lymphomyeloid potential (LMPPs) defined as Lin−CD34+CD38−CD90−CD45RA− cells, as well as more committed myeloid progenitors that are present in the CD34+CD38+ compartment.[3] Among the myeloid progenitors, the common myeloid progenitors (CMPs), granulocyte–macrophage progenitors (GMPs), and megakaryocyte-erythroid progenitors (MEPs) can be discriminated based on differential expression of CD123 (IL3RA), CD110 (MPL), and CD45RA.

The initial observation that AML leukemia-initiating cells (LICs) reside within the CD34+CD38− compartment suggested that AML HSCs are rare cells that most closely resemble normal HSCs sharing a common limited immunophenotype and being in rare populations (Fig. 10.1). However, subsequent data have suggested that this conclusion is an oversimplification and that the cell of origin of any myeloid malignancy is likely dictated by a combination of the specific genetic and epigenetic alterations present in the individual patient as well as the cells in which these alterations occur. For example, the aforementioned earliest studies of LICs in AML relied on their transplantation into immunodeficient nonobese diabetic/severe combined immunodeficient (NOD/SCID) mice (see box on Evolution of Immunodeficient Mouse Models) to assay the ability of a defined population of AML cells to give rise to AML in vivo. However, using more immunodeficient xenotransplant models, primary human cells from both CD34+CD38− and CD34+CD38+ compartments have been shown to have LIC activity. In addition, work by Vyas and colleagues has revealed that two expanded populations, both with LIC activity, exist in CD34+ AML (Fig. 10.1).[4] One population shares the immunophenotype of normal LMPPs and the other mirrors the GMP population. The LMPP-like leukemic stem cell (LSC) population can give rise to the GMP-like LSC population but either can give rise to AML in immunocompromised mice in vivo.

As described in the box on Functional Evaluation of Cell-of-Origin In Vivo, the leukemogenic effects of specific oncogenes directly depend on the specific oncogene as well as the target cell of expression. Based on these facts, consistent LICs may be most easily defined for specific genetically defined subsets of leukemias (such as specific chronic leukemias defined by specific translocations or point mutations) but are much more difficult to define for normal karyotype AML. For example, expression of the AML1-ETO fusion transcript, generated by the common t(8;21) translocation in AML, can be detected not only in leukemic cells but also in normal HSCs from patients in clinical remission from AML.[8] However, these AML1-ETO–expressing HSCs are not leukemic and can differentiate into myeloid and erythroid cells in vitro in a manner similar to HSCs without the AML1-ETO fusion transcripts (Fig. 10.1). Similarly, analysis of mice expressing the AML1-ETO fusion from the endogenous Aml1 locus in vivo has revealed that AML1-ETO–expressing HSCs have aberrant self-renewal capacity but do not develop overt leukemia unless additional genetic abnormalities are present. These data strongly suggest that acquisition of additional genetic abnormalities in a subset of HSCs or their progeny is required to give rise to overt leukemia. In these studies the HSCs bearing the AML1-ETO fusion reside within the Lin−CD34+CD38− subpopulation that is also the immunophenotype of normal human HSCs, suggesting that the initiating lesion must occur in a cell with an immunophenotype of normal HSCs. However, leukemic cells from 30% to 40% of patients with AML do not express CD34, and LICs from some patients with AML can actually be CD34−. Interestingly, prior work evaluating the location of the PML-RARA transcript present in acute promyelocytic leukemia (APL) revealed that the PML-RARA translocation is actually present in CD34−CD38+ populations and not in CD34+CD38− HSC-enriched populations[9] (Fig. 10.1). These data clearly reveal that there is enormous heterogeneity in the cell-of-origin of AML.

Advancement in techniques to map genetic alterations in cancer have allowed for much finer tracking of somatic mutations in AML and other hematopoietic malignancies with a normal karyotype. It is now believed that an average of five coding mutations is present in adults with de novo AML. Several groups have now studied the occurrence of somatic mutations in bulk AML cells and the remaining seemingly nonaffected HSCs. This work has clearly shown that the HSC compartment in patients with AML contains HSCs with none of the mutations found in the AML as well as HSCs with various combinations of genetic alterations similar to that present in the bulk malignant cells (Fig. 10.1). These latter HSCs are now understood to be "preleukemic stem cells" that initiate AML and can

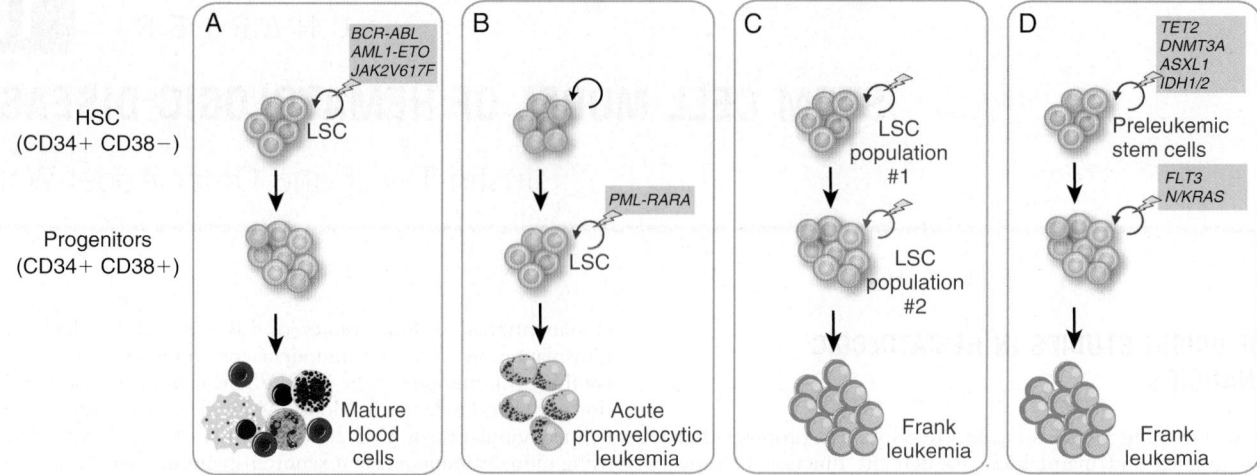

Fig. 10.1 SCHEMATIC MODELS DEPICTING THE ORIGIN OF LEUKEMIC STEM CELLS (LSCs) IN VARIOUS MYELOID MALIGNANCIES. (A) Genetic evidence from some forms of acute and chronic myeloid leukemias reveals that the inciting genetic event occurs in a cell type in which normal hematopoietic stem cells (HSCs) are enriched (lineage-negative (Lin−)CD34+CD38−). For example, the *AML1-ETO* and *BCR-ABL* translocations found in acute myeloid leukemia (AML) and chronic myelogenous leukemia (CML) are present in HSCs. In addition, the *JAK2*V617F mutation is present in HSCs. However, presence of these mutations alone may not be sufficient to generate overt AML and may be associated with aberrant self-renewal (as is the case with *AML1-ETO*) or chronic myeloproliferation (as with *BCR-ABL* and *JAK2*V617F) alone. (B) In contrast, other forms of AML appear to be generated due to acquisition of genetic alterations in a cell type more differentiated than HSCs. For example, *PML-RARA* translocations occur in Lin−CD34+CD38+ cells in patients with acute promyelocytic leukemia (APL). (C) In addition, in a proportion of patients with de novo non-APL AML, LSC activity may be present in a cell with an immunophenotype distinct from HSCs. In some cases, multiple populations of LSCs may be present, each with a distinct immunophenotype as shown. (D) Finally, most recently it has been proposed that genetic alterations may occur in a proportion of HSCs in patients with AML and that confer aberrant self-renewal properties to these cells. Further stepwise accumulation of genetic alterations then occurs in these preleukemic HSCs results in an overt malignant phenotype. As shown, mutations associated with the preleukemic HSCs include genes affecting DNA methylation and chromatin state whereas mutations associated with frank leukemia include genetic alterations associated with increased cell proliferation.

also be identified in remission samples, indicating that they are able to survive induction chemotherapy (see box on Preleukemic Stem Cells).[11–13] Many of the mutations that occur in preleukemic HSCs confer growth properties that allow them to outcompete normal HSCs and presumably lead to relapse. Interestingly, mutations occurring in preleukemic HSCs are enriched in genes regulating DNA methylation, chromatin modifications, and the cohesion complex while genetic alteration activating signaling are often present in more downstream overt malignant cells and absent from preleukemic HSCs.

MYELODYSPLASTIC SYNDROMES

Much as in AML, tracking major chromosomal abnormalities allowed earlier investigators to establish that clonal hematopoiesis in MDS originated in HSCs. Studies performed in 2000 identified deletion of the long arm of chromosome 5 (del(5q)) in the HSCs of patients with del(5q)-MDS. Moreover, del(5q) CD34+CD38− cells possessed MDS-initiating potential based upon in vitro and in vivo stem cell assay. Systems subsequently improved phenotypic identification of HSCs have allowed investigators to focus on Lin−CD34+CD38−CD90+CD45RA− cells as candidate CSCs in MDS. These studies showed that in patients with del(5q)-MDS, 99% of Lin−CD34+CD38−CD90+CD45RA− cells contained del(5q) and that they were molecularly and functionally distinct from clonally involved GMPs and MEPs.[20] By gene expression profiling and principle component analysis of RNA sequencing data, the three cell populations were shown to be distinctively different, with the Lin−CD34+CD38−CD90+CD45RA− cells selectively expressing genes

The earliest studies of cancer stem cells in acute myeloid leukemia (AML) suggested that AML is initiated by genetic alterations that take place in hematopoietic stem cells (HSCs). Alternatively, however, there is clear evidence that some leukemias may be initiated by mutations arising in more committed progenitors that provide these cells with aberrant self-renewal capacity that they otherwise lack. Numerous studies have attempted to directly address each of these possibilities through selective expression of specific oncogenes in isolated HSCs, common myeloid progenitors (CMPs), granulocyte–macrophage progenitors (GMPs), and even more mature myeloid cells (Figure). Such experiments have been most thoroughly performed using expression of mixed lineage leukemia (MLL) fusion oncoproteins. *MLL* encodes an epigenetic enzyme required for normal hematopoiesis due to its role in maintenance of *HOX* gene expression. Translocation events fusing the N-terminus of MLL to over 50 different C-terminal partners are common in both AML and acute lymphoblastic leukemia (ALL). Overexpression of the *MLL-ENL*

fusion oncoprotein in self-renewing HSCs as well as myeloid progenitor populations with more restricted self-renewal potential including CMPs and GMPs result in the rapid onset of AML in vivo.[10] Similar results have been seen with retroviral overexpression of a different MLL fusion oncoprotein, *MLL-AF9* as well as an unrelated AML-associated fusion, *MOZ-TIF2* (Figure). In contrast, overexpression of *BCR-ABL* is only able to transform HSCs but not committed downstream progenitors. These results unequivocally demonstrate (1) the ability of an MLL fusion oncoprotein to convert a myeloid progenitor cell population that is distinct from an HSC to acquire leukemogenic self-renewal activity and (2) that the cell-of-origin where a genetic alteration is expressed may regulate the resultant ability for a malignant disease to develop. It is also important to note that when the MLL-AF9 fusion is expressed under endogenous regulatory control, *Mll-Af9* transforms HSCs but not GMPs. These data clearly reveal that the dosage of oncogene expression may also regulate cellular transformation.

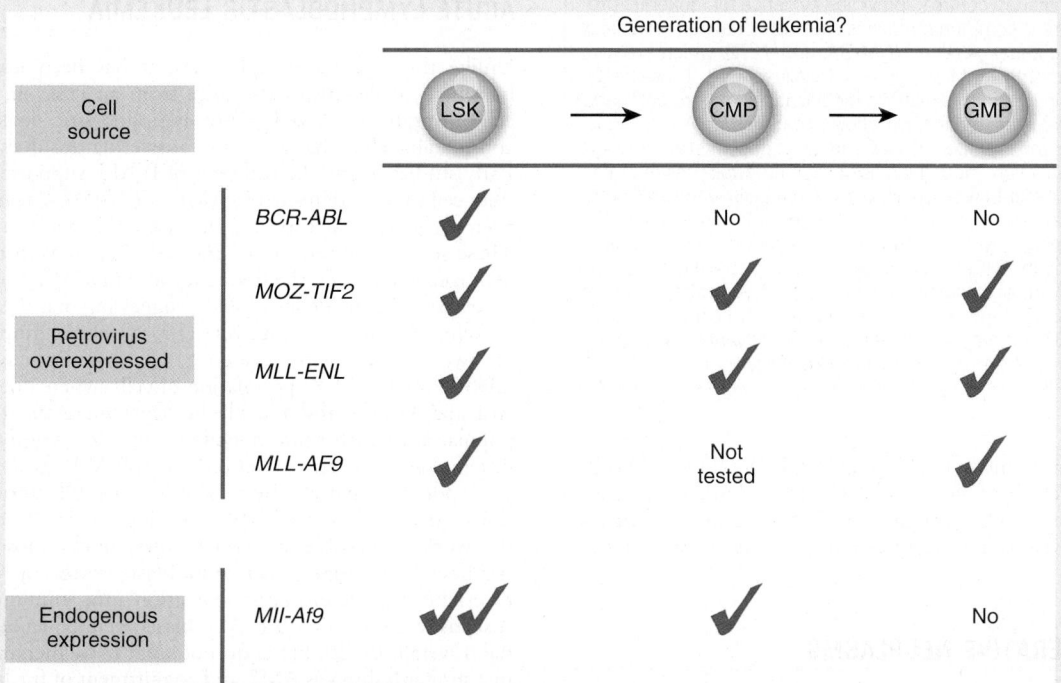

Cell source		LSK	→	CMP	→	GMP
		Generation of leukemia?				
Retrovirus overexpressed	*BCR-ABL*	✓		No		No
	MOZ-TIF2	✓		✓		✓
	MLL-ENL	✓		✓		✓
	MLL-AF9	✓		Not tested		✓
Endogenous expression	*Mll-Af9*	✓✓		✓		No

Pink Box 10.1 Figure LEUKEMIC CELL-OF-ORIGIN DEPENDS ON THE GENETIC ALTERATION, THE CELLULAR CONTEXT, AND GENE DOSAGE. Schematic of experiments testing the leukemogenic effects of retroviral overexpression of a number of leukemogenic fusions in hematopoietic stem and progenitor cell populations from mice followed by their transplantation into recipient mice. Populations studied include the hematopoietic-stem cell enriched LSK cell population as well as the common myeloid progenitor (CMP) and granulocyte–macrophage cell progenitor population. While retroviral overexpression of MLL-AF9 transforms LSK cells, CMP, and GMP populations, expression of MLL-AF9 from its endogenous locus efficiently transforms LSK cells but is only able to transform a proportion of CMP cells and unable to transform GMPs.

characteristic of normal HSCs. These candidate stem cells were the only cells able to sustain long-term generation of MDS myeloid progenitors in vitro that was never observed in GMPs, MEPs, or CMPs. Moreover, patients with del(5q)-MDS were found to have residual del(5q) clones in the CD34+CD38−CD90+ stem cell compartment during clinical remission.[21] Over time, most of these patients experienced expansion of the clone, leading to cytogenetic and clinical progression.

The evidence for an MDS-initiating stem cell is not limited to isolated del(5q)-MDS, which may be a unique disease entity given its distinct clinical features. In fact, recent studies have shown that recurrent driver mutations occur at the HSC level in a broad panel of low to intermediate risk MDS and that the 5q deletion preceded any other identifiable recurrent driver mutations in isolated

del(5q)-MDS. The same was observed with *SF3B1* in MDS with ringed sideroblasts, where *SF3B1* mutations are thought to be early and potentially initiating events. Targeted screening for mutations in a large number of genes known to be frequently mutated in MDS and other myeloid malignancies on bulk bone marrow from patients with MDS was performed. After identifying the mutations specific to each patient, the different cell compartments (HSC, GMP, or MEP) were purified and the screen for mutations was repeated. It was hypothesized that if progenitor cells acquired self-renewal capacity allowing them to persist long enough for the mutations to be responsible for the MDS phenotype, then the mutations would be identifiable in progenitors but not within upstream HSCs. However, all of the mutations in MDS patients have been traced back to the HSC compartment (Lin−CD34+CD38−CD90+CD45RA− cells) and

Hematopoietic stem cells (HSCs) are rare (~1–2 per 10^8 bone marrow cells) and quiescent cells that rarely divide. However, all blood cells originate from progenitor cells that in turn originate from HSCs and thus HSCs must replicate/self-renew to continue the cycle. Mutations in HSCs can therefore occur during cell division and accumulate, sometimes speeding self-renewal divisions and leading to clonal hematopoiesis. Although able to confer a growth advantage to clones derived from mutated HSCs, these single mutations alone are not sufficient to transform cells, resulting in an overt malignant phenotype. Because growth promoting gene mutations are common in cancer, it is thought that HSCs with mutations that cause clonal hematopoiesis might exist as preleukemic stem cells in patients with leukemia for months to years prior to diagnosis. Cooperative driver mutations are then acquired that cause cancer to develop. Recent publications have reported that somatic mutations causing clonal hematopoiesis exist in healthy persons and increase in frequency with age.[14–16] The risk of a hematologic malignancy is higher in patients with clonal hematopoiesis compared with matched controls, providing evidence for leukemic predisposition. The most common mutations causing clonal hematopoiesis were found in the genes ASXL1, DNMT3A, and TET2, which are also known to be recurrently mutated in myeloid malignancies. These genes encode proteins involved in epigenetic modifications of chromatin and DNA. Functional experiments have shown that DNMT3A and TET2 actually increase the number of HSCs in the bone marrow through impaired differentiation and increased self-renewal, respectively. Studies of a few patients with preleukemic stem cells who went on to develop leukemia were able to show that at least in some cases, the leukemia developed only after acquisition of another driver mutation such as mutations in FLT3.[17] Additionally, different somatic mutations drive distinct patterns of clonal hematopoiesis, such as mutations in the splicing factors SF3B1 and SRSF2, which exclusively occur in patients over the age of 70 and may only confer a growth advantage under the selection pressures of an aging hematopoietic system.[18,19]

all of the mutations found in the Lin⁻CD34⁺CD38⁻CD90⁺CD45RA⁻ MDS initiating cells have also been identified in downstream GMPs and MEPs.[20] These findings suggest that MDS is propagated by a stem cell that develops and acquires mutations at an early stage in the disease.

MYELOPROLIFERATIVE NEOPLASMS

The translocation between chromosomes 9 and 22, the so-called Philadelphia chromosome, is the hallmark of CML and gives rise to the BCR-ABL oncogene and its constitutively active protein tyrosine kinase product p210$^{BCR-ABL}$. In patients with CML, there is a clonal expansion of HSCs and the BCR-ABL translocation can be detected in HSCs from patients with CML as well as all myeloid as well as even committed lymphoid cells generated by these HSCs (Fig. 10.1). This data clearly identifies chronic phase CML as a stem cell disorder in which the target cell of transformation is a HSC. This is a finding that has direct therapeutic implications as ABL kinase inhibitors, which are used clinically for CML, do not consistently eradicate the quiescent BCR-ABL–positive CML LICs.

In contrast to the chronic phase of CML where the normal HSC appears to be the target cell-of-origin, transformation of CML to the myeloid blast crisis appears to be associated with expansion of a more committed myeloid progenitor population (which consists mostly of GMPs) rather than expansion of the HSC population. The GMPs from blast crisis patients with CML actually have the ability to serially replate in vitro, a proxy of aberrant self-renewal capacity not seen in normal GMPs. These data suggest that disease progression from chronic phase to myeloid blast crisis occurs due to aberrant acquisition of self-renewal potential within the committed GMP population, a possibility which has been directly studied in animal models (Pink Box 10.2).

The other chronic myeloproliferative neoplasm besides CML in which a specific genetic alteration is present in nearly 100% of

patients is polycythemia vera (PV); a single mutation results in the substitution of phenylalanine for valine at codon 617 of the Janus kinase 2 (JAK2) tyrosine kinase in nearly every patient. Targeted sequencing of JAK2 in patients with PV showed that the JAK2V617F mutation is present in cells with an HSC phenotype[22] (Fig. 10.1). Moreover, HSCs from patients with PV are skewed toward the erythroid lineage at the HSC level already and there is also an expansion of the CMP pool, suggesting that expression of the JAK2V617F mutation affects HSC and progenitor cell populations. Interestingly, early efforts to study the effects of JAK inhibition in PV revealed that JAK inhibition exhibited inhibitory effects on the erythroid potential of PV HSCs but did not result in preferential eradication of JAK2V617F-mutant HSCs versus normal HSCs. Thus this finding of an HSC origin for PV has direct therapeutic implications, as curative eradication of the disease would require therapy that eliminates rare quiescent bone marrow–based HSCs.

ACUTE LYMPHOBLASTIC LEUKEMIA

Unlike the myeloid malignancies, it has been less clear whether lymphoid malignancies also arise from an HSC or have a different cell-of-origin. In B-cell acute lymphoblastic leukemia (B-ALL), considerable effort has gone into answering this question (Fig. 10.2). Early studies in specific subtypes of B-ALL supported a preleukemic stem cell such as identified in AML. TEL/AML-1 rearranged ALL has been particularly well studied and is associated with a good prognosis. These studies showed that TEL/AML-1 alone is insufficient for leukemogenesis. In fact, the frequency of TEL/AML-1 in healthy infants far exceeds the incidence of ALL, suggesting that the development of leukemia requires a second hit. This is evident from studies of pairs of twins, both with evidence of a preleukemic TEL/AML-1 CD34⁺CD38⁻CD19⁺ population of cells, where one twin developed ALL and the other did not. The healthy twin retained the preleukemic population, which showed evidence of self-renewal and hierarchical differentiation. Later studies of high-risk ALL showed that leukemogenic potential may also be present in more differentiated cell populations, such as CD34⁻CD19⁺ cells (Fig. 10.2). Recent extension of this work to B-ALL cases with a variety of chromosomal abnormalities have found that even mature blasts expressing CD20 were able to establish leukemia upon transition into immunodeficient mice. Also, as many as 1 in 40 B-ALL blasts retained leukemogenic potential. Overall, B-ALL blasts do not seem to be hierarchically arranged in a similar fashion as AML and engraftment of further differentiated CD34⁻ blasts can give rise to both CD34⁻ and CD34⁺ populations in vivo.[23] Together, these data suggest that B-ALL arises in a committed lymphoid progenitor rather than only a small population of cells accumulating mutations and retaining stem cell properties, and that most or even all of the leukemic blasts retain the ability to propagate the malignancy.

In contrast to TEL/AML-1, those patients with ALL carrying the BCR-ABL fusion protein have much worse clinical outcomes. However, like TEL/AML-1, BCR-ABL is also thought to be a primary mutation that is necessary but not sufficient for ALL transformation. Interestingly, the two BCR-ABL transcripts, P190 and P210, caused by different break points in the t(9;22) translocation, show distinct patterns of HSC and committed B-cell progenitor involvement. In most cases, the P190 BCR-ABL originates in a CD34⁺CD38⁻CD19⁺ progenitor cell while P210 BCR-ABL originates in a multipotent HSC. When purified P210 BCR-ABL HSCs were transplanted into NOD/SCID mice, they exclusively reconstituted normal, BCR-ABL–negative multilineage hematopoiesis.[24] These data suggest that the purified HSC also contained normal HSCs that outcompeted the P210 BCR-ABL HSCs, which are not the leukemia stem cells. In contrast, more committed CD19⁺ P210 BCR-ABL–positive cells resulted in leukemic reconstitution upon transplantation into NOD/SCID mice that was enhanced following secondary transplant. These data complement recent findings suggesting that the primary BCR-ABL translocation in CML originates in HSCs, yet the leukemic transformation in blast crisis results in an LSC with a committed

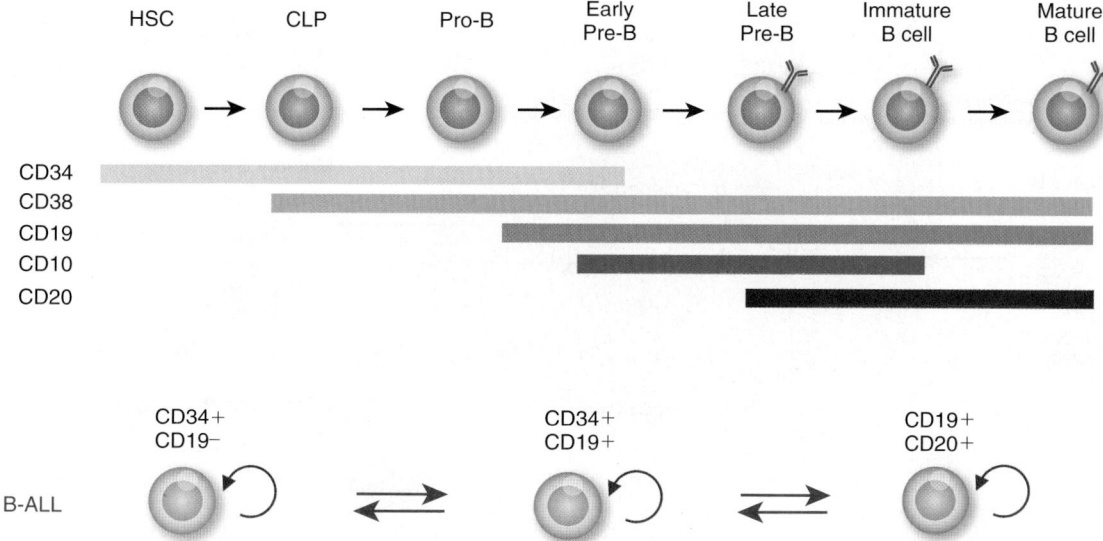

Fig. 10.2 STAGES OF NORMAL EARLY B-CELL DIFFERENTIATION AND SCHEMATIC OF LEUKEMIC STEM CELLS IN B-CELL ACUTE LYMPHOBLASTIC LEUKEMIA (B-ALL). Based on several studies testing the ability of human B-ALL blasts to engraft in immunodeficient mice, it appears that multiple blast populations in B-ALL are able to establish the disease in immunodeficient mice. For example, $CD34^+CD19^+$ blasts as well as $CD34^-CD19^+$ blasts from individual patients have been shown to be able to transplant leukemia in vivo and to give rise to $CD34^+$ and $CD34^-$ leukemic cells. Thus B-ALL does not appear to follow a hierarchical model in which blasts with a more mature immunophenotype lose their stem cell capacity as has been seen in some cases of acute myeloid leukemia.

progenitor cell phenotype. This begs the question whether P210 BCR-ABL–positive ALL represents de novo ALL or CML in lymphoid blast crisis.

MATURE B-CELL MALIGNANCIES

The classification of mature B-cell malignancies based on their histology and immunophenotypic resemblance to a particular stage of lymphoid differentiation has led to the theory that each lymphoma subtype originates within lymphocytes at distinct differentiation stages (Fig. 10.3). Another model predicts that cells acquire initial alterations at early stages, even at the HSC level, that may drive clonal expansion or resistance to apoptosis and that these cells then develop additional complementary alterations at a later stage that lead to overt malignancy. Recent studies have identified novel lymphoid associated mutations and alterations across large panels of lymphomas, creating the opportunity to define the clonal architecture and cell-of-origin in lymphoma subtypes.

CHRONIC LYMPHOCYTIC LEUKEMIA

Chronic lymphocytic leukemia (CLL) is a B-cell malignancy marked by the accumulation of clonal mature B cells in the lymph node, bone marrow, and/or blood. In nearly all cases, CLL is preceded by a preleukemic monoclonal B cell lymphocytosis (MBL), though not all cases of MBL continue on to CLL. The precise cell within B-cell development that gives rise to CLL has been debated for decades and two recent studies have implicated HSCs in the pathogenesis of CLL. Kikushige et al investigated the cellular origin of CLL by isolating distinct subpopulations of cells and assaying their ability to initiate disease in immunodeficient mice. Only the $CD34^+CD38^-CD90^+$ fraction engrafted and this population, known to be highly enriched in HSCs, gave rise to both lymphoid and myeloid hematopoiesis. Interestingly, these engrafted mice showed an increased proportion of polyclonal B cells and a population of monoclonal B cells expressing CD5, akin to MBL.[25] Further examination determined that they

had different variable, joining and diversity segments (VDJ) rearrangement patterns compared to the prior CLL. The finding of aberrant HSCs in CLL suggest that they are primed to generate MBL cells, which are likely to accumulate additional mutations that eventually results in a clonal CLL disorder.

In a different approach, Damm et al investigated whether molecular alterations present in CLL cells could be traced to cells in the earliest stages of hematopoietic development before committed B-cell development. In fact, acquired mutations were detected in HSCs in the majority of the patients with CLL studied.[26] These findings support a preleukemic phase and the clinical implications imply that treatments with true curative intent in CLL might require approaches other than those focused solely on cell-surface antigens restricted to B cells or B-cell receptor signaling pathways.

HAIRY CELL LEUKEMIA

Hairy cell leukemia (HCL) is a chronic lymphoproliferative disorder characterized as a mature B-cell malignancy based on the expression of CD19, surface immunoglobulin, and the clonal rearrangement of immunoglobulin heavy and light chain genes. At the same time, HCL cells also express cell surface markers not present on normal B cells, including CD103 and CD11c, which are typically expressed by dendritic cells and monocytes. In addition, patients with HCL have long been known to have clinical features disparate from most mature B-cell malignancies, including the absence of lymph node involvement and frequent splenomegaly due to extramedullary hematopoiesis (EMH). Recent identification of BRAFV600E mutations in nearly 100% of patients with classic HCL provided genetic insight into the pathogenesis of HCL and a clonal marker to track the origin and propagation of HCL. The BRAFV600E mutation was found in purified (Lin$^-$) $CD34^+$ $CD38^-CD90^+CD45RA^-$ HSCs in primary samples from patients with HCL. These aberrant HSCs were also able to recapitulate BRAFV600E-mutant hematopoiesis after transplantation into NOD/SCID/gamma-null (NSG) mice. Additionally, conditional knock-in mice were generated expressing BRAFV600E in either HSCs or $CD19^+$ cells. Those mice with BRAFV600E HSCs

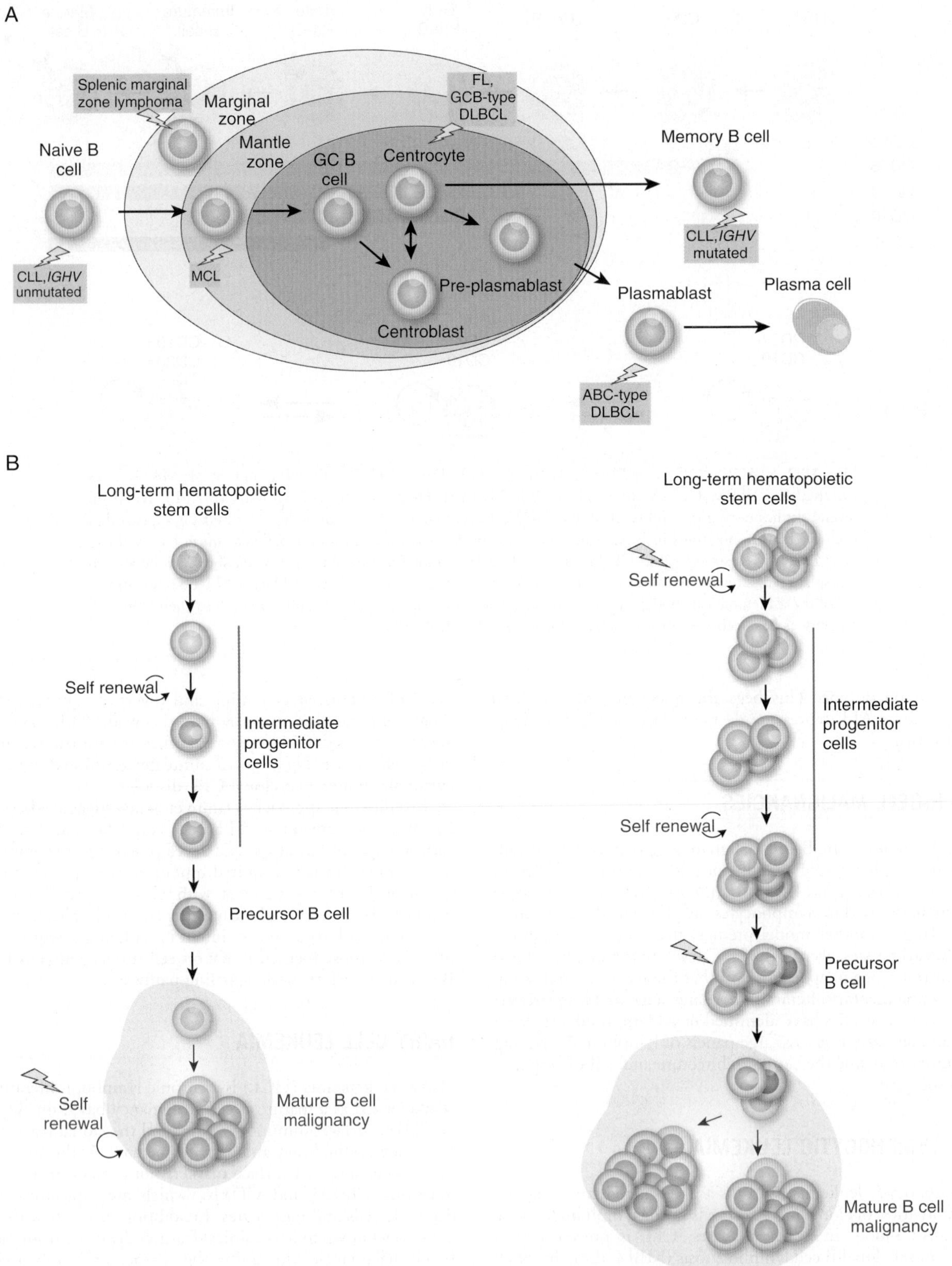

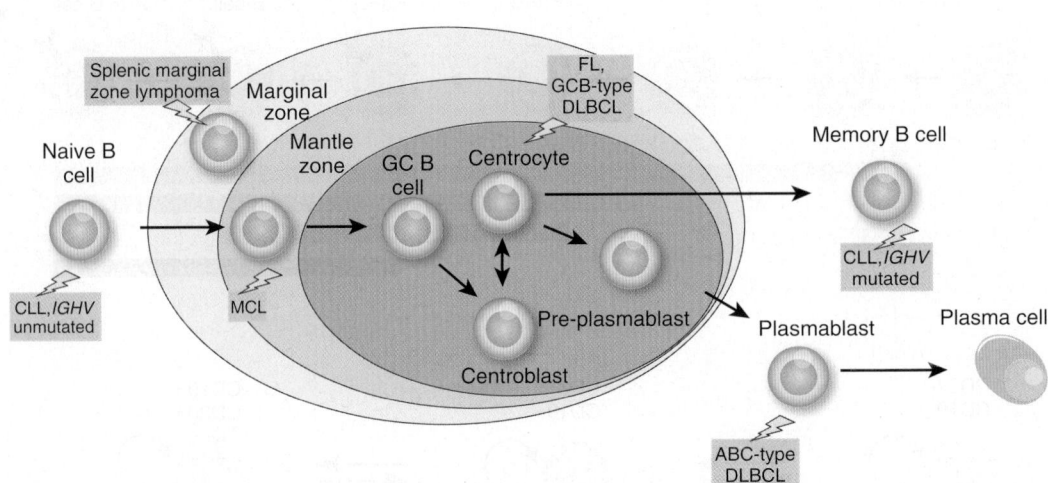

Fig. 10.3 MODELS OF LYMPHOMA ONTOGENY. (A) The conventional model of lymphoma classifies lymphomas based on differentiation of mature peripheral B cells. This model is based on the presence of somatic hypermutation as well as immunophenotypic and gene expression analyses comparing the malignant cells to normal B-cell counterparts. (B) At the same time, mature B cells are derived from precursor B cells and earlier progenitor and hematopoietic stem cells (HSCs). In the conventional model (*left*), it is assumed that cells more primitive than the peripheral B cell depicted in (A) are not involved with the lymphoma disease process. However, there is increasing evidence that HSCs and/or more intermediate progenitors may harbor aberrancies directly linked to mature B-cell malignancies. *ABC DLBCL,* Activated B-cell–like diffuse large B-cell lymphoma; *CLL,* chronic lymphocytic leukemia; *FL,* follicular lymphoma; *GCB,* germinal center B cell–like DLBCL; *MCL,* mantle cell lymphoma.

showed an HCL-like phenotype of anemia, thrombocytopenia, and EMH; however, no phenotypic hairy cells were seen. In contrast, mice with BRAFV600E expression limited to lineage committed B cells did not have reduced survival or an overt phenotype. These data suggest that HCL is initiated within the HSC compartment but that the development of additional genetic alterations occurring along the course of hematopoiesis may be necessary to give rise to HCL cells. Indeed, in patients with genetic alterations in addition to BRAFV600E in HCL cells, these additional mutations were not found in the BRAF-mutated HSCs.[27]

DIFFUSE LARGE B-CELL LYMPHOMA

High-resolution genomic analyses of a large number of human diffuse large B-cell lymphoma (DLBCL) samples identified copy number gain of chromosome 3q27.2 to be associated with the worst prognosis and the aggressive activated B-cell (ABC) disease subtype. The transcription factor BCL6 is likely the target oncogene affected by this copy number alteration at this locus given its propensity to be targeted by other alterations in DLBCL such as translocations and point mutations, which were mutually exclusive from the 3q27.2 gain. Other roles for BCL6 have been described in normal hematopoiesis and myeloid leukemia stem cells, prompting inquiries into whether BCL6 expression in HSCs has a role in the origins of DLBCL. This hypothesis was tested by the generation of a mouse model that expressed BCL6 only in HSCs, under the control of a stem cell–specific promotor so that BCL6 was no longer expressed by the differentiated progeny. These mice developed a form of lymphoma that resembled DLBCL with an ABC phenotype that did not overexpress BCL6.[28] This led to a proposed model of "hit-and-run" oncogenesis, wherein BCL6 expression in hematopoietic precursors is sufficient to produce DLBCL without requiring sustained overexpression.

FOLLICULAR LYMPHOMA

The most common subtype of lymphoma is follicular lymphoma (FL), which is so named because histologically the lymph node follicle B cell is affected. These aberrant B cells carry a hallmark translocation between chromosomes 14 and 18, resulting in juxtaposition of the immunoglobulin heavy chain gene (IGH) and the antiapoptotic protein BCL-2, thus driving overexpression of BCL2 and resistance to programmed cell death. This malignancy usually follows an indolent course and is more common in elderly patients. It has been shown that up to 25% of healthy individuals harbor BCL-2/IGH rearranged cells, yet do not have disease, indicating that the hallmark lesion is not sufficient to cause lymphoma and that additional genetic mutations must be required for lymphomagenesis. As in other hematologic malignancies, newer sequencing technologies have allowed identification of novel recurrent mutations in FL and some researchers have begun investigating the timing of those mutations. By taking the opportunity presented by an unfortunate but rare occurrence of donor-derived FL after hematopoietic stem cell transplantation, investigators have shown that some of these genetic mutations occur in hematopoietic precursors prior to the cells in which the BCL-2/IGH rearrangement occurs.

Hematopoietic stem cell donors are screened for signs and symptoms of malignancy but are not currently subjected to genetic testing for premalignant conditions. Often the donor is a brother or sister due to the 25% chance of being a complete HLA-match and the willingness of a sibling to donate. This inherently means that a sibling donor is at slightly higher risk of having a malignancy given their close relationship to someone with cancer (i.e., the recipient), yet it is still a rare occurrence that donor cells will transfer a malignancy to the recipient after stem cell transplantation. In the case mentioned previously,[29] the donor and the recipient both developed FL 7 years after the transplant. Both patients' FL had exactly identical BCL-2/IGH rearrangement breakpoints and the same VDJ recombination, indicating that they were derived from the same mutation. The

recipient had received a donor-lymphocyte infusion (DLI) 7 years prior, which also harbored the same BCL-2/IGH and VDJ rearrangements, thus confirming the donor-derived source. There was no sample left of the original stem cell transplant to test but the BCL-2/IGH rearrangement was not present in the cells other than CD19+ mature B cells in the DLI sample. However, there were mutations known to occur in lymphoma present in the CD34+CD10−CD19− population that includes multipotent progenitors and HSCs.[30] These alterations presumably contributed to the development of FL prior to the acquisition of the hallmark translocation and occur in progenitors of the follicle B cell. These findings provide evidence of a possible role of stem cell progenitors in the development of mature B-cell malignancies.

CONCLUSION

The stem cell model of hematologic diseases has implications beyond a theoretical construct for the pathogenesis of disease. Not only does this model support stem cell transplant and gene therapy as curative treatments in some cases, but also has much broader application in the management of hematologic malignancies. Most of our current standard therapies are based on the principle of interrupting DNA replication in rapidly dividing cancer cells, yet stem cells are quiescent and spend little time in active cell cycle. Many of the new and developing therapies are targeted at cell surface markers or mutated genes whose expression may be restricted to the most mature malignant cells and may be lacking in the premalignant or malignant stem cells. It remains to be seen whether the same challenges will face immune response checkpoint modulators, but one could consider the possibility that neoepitopes recognized by activated T cells might have differential expression on different cell populations.

Remarkable progress has been made in the field of CSCs in hematologic malignancies due to the evolution of immunodeficient mouse models and the improvement of sequencing technologies that have allowed the mapping of clonal evolution and studies of mutational ontogeny. There are controversies from inside and outside of the field as to whether stem cells should be defined phenotypically, molecularly, or functionally but as the evidence accumulates there is broad agreement on the stem cell model of hematologic diseases.

REFERENCES

1. Blair A, Hogge DE, Ailles LE, et al: Lack of expression of Thy-1 (CD90) on acute myeloid leukemia cells with long-term proliferative ability in vitro and in vivo. *Blood* 89:3104–3112, 1997.
2. Bonnet D, Dick JE: Human acute myeloid leukemia is organized as a hierarchy that originates from a primitive hematopoietic cell. *Nat Med* 3:730–737, 1997.
3. Majeti R, Park CY, Weissman IL: Identification of a hierarchy of multipotent hematopoietic progenitors in human cord blood. *Cell Stem Cell* 1:635–645, 2007.
4. Goardon N, et al: Coexistence of LMPP-like and GMP-like leukemia stem cells in acute myeloid leukemia. *Cancer Cell* 19:138–152, 2011.
5. Doulatov S, Notta F, Laurenti E, et al: Hematopoiesis: a human perspective. *Cell Stem Cell* 10:120–136, 2012.
6. Rongvaux A, et al: Development and function of human innate immune cells in a humanized mouse model. *Nat Biotechnol* 32:364–372, 2014.
7. Cosgun KN, et al: Kit regulates HSC engraftment across the human-mouse species barrier. *Cell Stem Cell* 15:227–238, 2014.
8. Miyamoto T, Weissman IL, Akashi K: AML1/ETO-expressing nonleukemic stem cells in acute myelogenous leukemia with 8;21 chromosomal translocation. *Proc Natl Acad Sci USA* 97:7521–7526, 2000.
9. Turhan AG, et al: Highly purified primitive hematopoietic stem cells are PML-RARA negative and generate nonclonal progenitors in acute promyelocytic leukemia. *Blood* 85:2154–2161, 1995.
10. Cozzio A, et al: Similar MLL-associated leukemias arising from self-renewing stem cells and short-lived myeloid progenitors. *Genes Dev* 17:3029–3035, 2003.

11. Corces-Zimmerman MR, Hong WJ, Weissman IL, et al: Preleukemic mutations in human acute myeloid leukemia affect epigenetic regulators and persist in remission. *Proc Natl Acad Sci USA* 111:2548–2553, 2014.

12. Jan M, et al: Clonal evolution of preleukemic hematopoietic stem cells precedes human acute myeloid leukemia. *Sci Transl Med* 4:149ra118, 2012.

13. Shlush LI, et al: Identification of pre-leukaemic haematopoietic stem cells in acute leukaemia. *Nature* 506:328–333, 2014.

14. Busque L, et al: Recurrent somatic TET2 mutations in normal elderly individuals with clonal hematopoiesis. *Nat Genet* 44:1179–1181, 2012.

15. Jaiswal S, et al: Age-related clonal hematopoiesis associated with adverse outcomes. *N Engl J Med* 371:2488–2498, 2014.

16. Genovese G, et al: Clonal hematopoiesis and blood-cancer risk inferred from blood DNA sequence. *N Engl J Med* 371:2477–2487, 2014.

17. Shih AH, et al: Mutational cooperativity linked to combinatorial epigenetic gain of function in acute myeloid leukemia. *Cancer Cell* 27:502–515, 2015.

18. Xie M, et al: Age-related mutations associated with clonal hematopoietic expansion and malignancies. *Nat Med* 20:1472–1478, 2014.

19. McKerrell T, et al: Leukemia-associated somatic mutations drive distinct patterns of age-related clonal hemopoiesis. *Cell Rep* 10:1239–1245, 2015.

20. Woll PS, et al: Myelodysplastic syndromes are propagated by rare and distinct human cancer stem cells in vivo. *Cancer Cell* 25:794–808, 2014.

21. Tehranchi R, et al: Persistent malignant stem cells in del(5q) myelodysplasia in remission. *N Engl J Med* 363:1025–1037, 2010.

22. Jamieson CH, et al: The JAK2 V617F mutation occurs in hematopoietic stem cells in polycythemia vera and predisposes toward erythroid differentiation. *Proc Natl Acad Sci USA* 103:6224–6229, 2006.

23. McClellan JS, Majeti R: The cancer stem cell model: B cell acute lymphoblastic leukaemia breaks the mould. *EMBO Mol Med* 5:7–9, 2013.

24. Notta F, et al: Evolution of human BCR-ABL1 lymphoblastic leukaemia-initiating cells. *Nature* 469:362–367, 2011.

25. Kikushige Y, et al: Self-renewing hematopoietic stem cell is the primary target in pathogenesis of human chronic lymphocytic leukemia. *Cancer Cell* 20:246–259, 2011.

26. Damm F, et al: Acquired initiating mutations in early hematopoietic cells of CLL patients. *Cancer Discov* 4:1088–1101, 2014.

27. Chung SS, et al: Hematopoietic stem cell origin of BRAFV600E mutations in hairy cell leukemia. *Sci Transl Med* 6:238ra271, 2014.

28. Green MR, et al: Transient expression of Bcl6 is sufficient for oncogenic function and induction of mature B-cell lymphoma. *Nat Commun* 5:3904, 2014.

29. Weigert O, et al: Molecular ontogeny of donor-derived follicular lymphomas occurring after hematopoietic cell transplantation. *Cancer Discov* 2:47–55, 2012.

30. Weigert O, Weinstock DM: The evolving contribution of hematopoietic progenitor cells to lymphomagenesis. *Blood* 120:2553–2561, 2012.

CHAPTER 11

HEMATOPOIETIC MICROENVIRONMENT

David Scadden and Lev Silberstein

EVOLUTION OF THE NICHE CONCEPT

In 1868, Ernest Neumann first suggested that blood cells are being replenished throughout postnatal life, and this proposal led to the attempts to localize the place of hematopoiesis. His hypothesis that blood cell production takes place in the bone marrow (BM) was experimentally validated by selective lead shielding of limbs in irradiated animals almost a century later. Notably these and other studies showed that differentiation pathways of immature blood cells are determined by their location and are different between the spleen and the BM. Based on this difference between BM and spleen, Schofield first proposed that there is a specialized place or niche where stem cells reside and are governed. He succinctly posed in 1978 that "stem cell is seen in association with other cells which determine its behavior."

Trentin further clarified how different sites affected hematopoietic stem/progenitor cell (HSPC) differentiation. Although both spleen and marrow support multiple cell lineages (erythropoietic and granulocytopoietic, for example), the ratios of differentiating cells were distinct: spleen favored erythropoiesis, but BM predominantly supported granulopoiesis. This controlling influence of the surrounding cells was further illustrated by implanting BM stroma into the spleen and showing that hematopoietic cells abruptly changed from erythropoiesis to granulopoiesis at the spleen–BM demarcation. These observations suggest that immature differentiating progenitors require interactions with other specific cell types in a defined *micro*environment.

This chapter reviews the current knowledge of the hematopoietic microenvironment during development and in postnatal life in normal hematopoiesis and in myelodysplasia and leukemia. The opportunities for therapeutic manipulation of the niche in the treatment of these disorders are also discussed. For the related topics on stem cell mobilization, hematopoietic cytokines and the role of microenvironment in lymphoid malignancies, plasma cell disorders, and myeloproliferative conditions, readers are referred to other chapters of this book.

HEMATOPOIETIC MICROENVIRONMENT DURING DEVELOPMENT

In mammals, hematopoiesis during development takes place in distinct extraembryonic and embryonic sites. Sequentially, it moves from the yolk sac to the aorta-gonad-mesonephros (AGM) region, fetal liver, placenta, and BM (for details, see Chapter 26).

The first definitive adult HSPCs emerge from the floor of the dorsal aorta, more precisely from AGM region in midgestation mouse embryo, and the HSPC clusters appear in close association with the aortic endothelium.[1] Recent reports indicate that phenotypically defined HSPCs (Sca1$^+$ c-kit §$^+$ CD41$^+$) arise directly from ventral aortic endothelial cells and that fluid shear stress may be important for this process.[2] Although direct cellular interactions during the emergence of hematopoietic stem cells (HSC) in the embryo remain to be dissected, bone morphogenetic protein 4 (BMP4), fibroblast growth factor (FGF), transforming growth factor (TGF), and vascular endothelial growth factor (VEGF)-Flk1 signaling pathways are involved in early mouse hematopoiesis.

Recently placenta has been identified as a hematopoietic organ during development. Placenta is known to produce hormones that influence vascularization and therefore may affect blood cell production because hematopoiesis and vasculogenesis are tightly coupled.[3]

The hematopoiesis-promoting factors may be either produced by the placental trophoblast cells or enter via maternal circulation. Hematopoietic progenitors appear in the placenta at E9, but their number declines by E13. The cells and local factors providing placental hematopoietic support are currently unknown, but mesenchymal/stromal cells have been suggested as candidates. Placental microenvironment is thought to be geared toward supporting the expansion or maturation of HSPCs without their concomitant differentiation.

In the fetal liver, the HSPCs are first detected on day 9 of mouse embryonic development, and large expansion of the HSPCs occurs between days 12 and 15 before migration to the bone on day 18. Stromal cell lines obtained from the fetal liver are able to support primitive hematopoietic cells in ex vivo cultures. Some of these cells (termed *myelosupportive stroma*) are able to differentiate in vitro into mesenchymal components (osteoblasts, chondrocytes, and adipocytes). Although the nature of fetal liver cells participating in the HSPC niche remains enigmatic, recent studies point to a nonhematopoietic hepatic population that express Dlk-1, a member of deltalike family of cell surface transmembrane proteins, and stem cell factor, and can be prospectively isolated based on the expression of these molecules.[4] These cells express angiopoietin ligand 3 and CXCL12, and in combination with stem cell factor, thrombopoietin, FGF1 and FGF2, and either angiopoietin ligand 2 or 3 are able to produce more than 30-fold expansion of the murine HSPCs in culture.

Despite the differences in the hematopoietic microenvironment between the sites of fetal and adult hematopoiesis, the key components of the molecular milieu are likely to be shared, as evidenced by successful (although limited) engraftment of HSPCs across developmental barriers. For example, AGM- or fetal liver–derived HSPCs are able to engraft in the adult BM. Notably, they have a competitive advantage over their BM-derived counterparts, with the long-term repopulating ability exceeding that of the BM by fivefold. Vice versa, BM HSPCs engraft in fetal liver when transplanted in utero, although at low efficiency (<5% for the whole BM and 0.43% for highly enriched HSPCs), which may be partly attributable to the absence of pretransplant conditioning.[5]

Multilineage hematopoiesis during development occurs largely by the virtue of sequential HSPC migration from the AGM region to the fetal liver and the BM, as opposed to de novo HSPC generation. Failure of migration to the "next niche," as exemplified by the targeted disruption of the guanine-nucleotide–binding protein stimulatory α-subunit (GS-α), calcium-sensing receptor, or CXCL12/CXCR4 axis (discussed in detail in Chapter 14 on HSPC migration) leads to severe impairment in hematopoiesis. This suggests even in the absence of cell-intrinsic HSPC defects, proper progression of blood cell production throughout development critically depends on the ability of the HSPC to sequentially move to the appropriate microenvironmental compartments.

ADULT BONE MARROW MICROENVIRONMENT

Niches for Hematopoietic Stem and Progenitor Cells

Location of the HSPC Niche

In mammals, BM is a major site of hematopoiesis throughout life. The niche preserves and dynamically regulates the HSPC pool by providing signals required for maintenance, quiescence and retention of HSPCs in the BM. However, the location of HSPC niche within the marrow has been a subject of controversy.[6] The endosteal surface has long been considered the zone in which HSPCs are preferentially located. In the setting of irradiation conditioning, this has been directly demonstrated by intravital imaging studies, which allow dynamic assessment of the interaction between transplanted HSPC and the niche. Currently, in vivo imaging is limited to calvarial BM, an area in the mouse skull where the bone is very thin, thus permitting penetration of the laser beam into the BM cavity. Using this technique and simultaneous multicolor fluorescent labeling of osteolineage cells (OLCs), HSPCs, and the vasculature, studies showed that in irradiated recipients, transplanted HSPCs home closest to the endosteal surface and individual OLCs as compared with more differentiated progenitors, and that they are "anchored" to their niches at least through 72 hours.[7] Preferential localization of primitive hematopoietic cells to the endosteal surface under the homeostatic conditions has been also demonstrated, although this analysis was performed using immunostaining of histologic BM sections of either femoral bones or the sternum.[8]

However, other studies performed under steady state (not transplant) conditions indicate that most HSPC are located in the central marrow in a perivascular position, thus arguing in favor of more primitive mesenchymal cells and endothelial cells governing the niche.

Deletion of a key niche factor, such as stem cell factor (kit-ligand), from either endothelial or perivascular cells leads to decrease in the HSPC number further supporting the notion of a perivascular niche.[9] Although the debate about location of the HSPC niche, and consequently, cell types that serve as niche participants, continues it is important to bear in mind that HSPCs themselves are molecularly and functionally heterogeneous, and that several distinct niches may coexist to support this heterogeneity, particularly under different conditions such as the stress of transplantation.

Cellular Components of the HSPC Niche

Over recent years, animal studies revealed marked complexity in cellular and molecular organization of the HSPC BM niche. Major cellular components of the HSPC niche and the factors that they produce (summarized in Table 11.1) are discussed later.

Osteolineage Cells

OLCs are a heterogeneous population of mesenchymal cells that line the endosteal surfaces of flat and trabeculated bones at the interface between the bone and the BM and become embedded within the bone matrix upon terminal differentiation. OLCs are thought to originate from mesenchymal stem cells (MSCs) and gradually progress from the early immature progenitors that express OLC-specific transcription factors Runx2 and osterix to mature osteoblasts

TABLE 11.1	HSPC Niche Factors and Their Cellular Sources	
Factor	Source	Effect
Membrane-bound SCF	Lepr+ perivascular cells, Tie2+ endothelial cells	Maintenance of HSC in the bone marrow (Ding et al, 2012)
CXCL12	Lepr+ perivascular cells, Tie-2+ endothelial cells	Retention of HSC in the bone marrow (Ding and Morrison, 2013)
	Prx-1+ osteoprogenitors	Retention of HSC, myeloid and lymphoid progenitors in the bone marrow (Ding and Morrison, 2013; Greenbaum et al, 2013)
	Osx+ osteoprogenitors and Col-2.3+ osteoblastic cells	Retention of lymphoid progenitors in the bone marrow (Ding and Morrison, 2013; Greenbaum et al, 2013)
Notch signaling (Jagged1)	VE-cadherin+ endothelial cells, osteoblastic cells (in PPR model)	Maintenance of HSC and regeneration posttransplantation (Poulos et al, 2013)
		Expansion of HSC and progenitors (Calvi et al, 2003)
Wnt signaling (Canonical)	Col-2.3+ osteoblastic cells (Wnt inhibitor DKK1)	Maintenance of HSC and quiescence (Fleming et al, 2008)
Wnt signaling (Noncanonical)	N-cadherin+ osteoblastic cells	Maintenance of HSC and quiescence (Sugimura, 2012)
E-Selectin	CD-31+ endothelial cells	Promotion of HSC cycling (Winkler et al, 2012)
Pleiotrophin	VEGFR3+/VE-cadherin+ endothelial cells and CXCL12 perivascular cells	Maintenance of HSC and retention in the bone marrow (Himburg et al, 2012; Himburg et al, 2010)
Thrombopoietin	Alkaline phosphatase+ osteoblastic cells	Maintenance of HSC and quiescence (Qian et al, 2007; Yoshihara et al, 2007)
Osteopontin	Osteoblastic and other microenvironmental cells	Negative regulation of HSC numbers and maintenance of quiescence (Nilsson et al, 2005; Stier et al, 2005)
TGF-β	Nonmyelinating Schwann cells, megakaryocytes	HSC quiescence (Yamazaki et al, 2011)
Angiopoietin-1	Osteocalcin+ osteoblasts	Promotion of HSC quiescence (Arai et al, 2004)
Robo-4 ligand(s) (Slit2[a])	Bone marrow stromal cells ([a]Slit2 identified at the mRNA level)	Promotion of HSC homing to the bone marrow (Smith-Berdan et al, 2011; Smith-Berdan et al, 2012)
Junction adhesion molecule B (JamB)	Osteoblasts, MSCs, endothelial cells	HSC adhesion and quiescence (Archangeli Blood, 2011)
CXCL4	Megakaryocytes	Promotion of HSC quiescence

Updated and modified from Kfoury Y, Mercier F, Scadden DT: Snapshot: the hematopoietic stem cell niche. Cell 3;158(1), 2014.

expressing extracellular matrix (ECM) protein osteocalcin and eventually to osteocytes.

Several lines of in vivo evidence support a functional role of the OLCs in regulation of primitive hematopoietic cells. In the studies providing the first experimental evidence for a mammalian niche in vivo, mice with genetically modified OLCs had an increase in the number of activated OLCs and a corresponding increase in the number of HSPCs.[10,11] This effect was associated with an increased trabecular bone area and an elevated number of trabecular osteoblasts that expressed the Notch ligand Jagged 1. When the OLCs were depleted, there was a reduction in the BM cellularity and migration of hematopoiesis to the extramedullary sites. Thus, OLCs play a role in regulation of HSPC pool size. In addition, OLCs participate in controlling HSPC quiescence through contributing to production of CXCL12, Angiopoietin 1, thrombopoietin, paninhibitor of canonical Wnt signaling Dickkopf1 (Dkk1), noncanonical Wnt ligands and ECM protein osteopontin. Finally, OLCs govern HSPC localization by controlling their egress into blood and return to the BM, a process that forms the basis for clinical peripheral blood stem cell collection for transplantation. When mature OLCs are deleted from bone, there is an increase in the number of circulating progenitors and a decrease in the mobilization of HSPC with granulocyte colony-stimulating factor (G-CSF) indicating that OLC-derived signals retain primitive hematopoietic cells in the marrow. Following G-CSF–induced mobilization, the OLCs in the trabecular bone adapt a flattened morphology with short projections, which is associated with HSPC egress from the niche. Similar changes are seen after treatment with nonsteroidal antiinflammatory drugs (NSAIDs), which are known to enhance G-CSF–induced HSPC mobilization. When CXCL12, a major HSPC chemoattractant and retention factor, is deleted from the osteoprogenitors using osterix-Cre promoter, increased HSPC mobilization is also observed. Thus, OLCs participate in the BM niche by regulating HSPC number, quiescence and retention in the BM space.

Despite the evidence presented earlier, several studies have argued against the role of OLCs in the niche, citing the absence of HSPC changes either in genetic models associated with reduced OLC number or following OLC-specific deletion of HSPC regulators such as kit-ligand or CXCL12. Several experimental factors are likely to account for this discrepancy, including developmental adaptation when the genetic modification is present throughout the ontogeny, or inability of genetic tools to target a specific subset within the OLC compartment that serves as a nodal point of the HSPC regulation: several studies suggest that immature OLCs are important for the niche function, whereas mature OLCs are dispensable.

Endothelial Cells

Endothelial cells are known to secrete hematopoietic cytokines and express several adhesion molecules such as E-selectin, P-selectin, vascular cell adhesion molecule 1 (VCAM-1), and intercellular adhesion molecule 1 (ICAM-1) which have been shown to participate in cellular interactions within HSPC niche. The existence of vascular niche for the HSPCs has been suggested by in vivo imaging studies showing early homing of transplanted BM progenitors to specific subdomains of the vascular tree as well as by histologic assessment of the BM using CD150 antibody when HSPCs were found to be in a close proximity to the BM sinusoids.

Endothelium-derived factors have diverse effects on HSPCs in vivo. For example, E-selectin (which is expressed exclusively in the endothelial cells) negatively regulates HSPC quiescence; consequently, HSPCs from E-selectin knockout (KO) mice are more quiescent and resistant to irradiation.[12] On the other hand, endothelial-specific deletion of stem cell factor or CXCL12 lead to the respective reduction of the HSPC pool and loss of repopulating capacity. Similar changes are seen upon endothelial-specific deletion of Notch ligand Jagged 1, which in contrast to E-selectin, promotes HSPC quiescence. The heparin-binding growth factor, pleiotrophin, which is produced

by sinusoidal endothelial cells also plays a role in the retention and self-renewal of HSPC in BM.[13]

Perivascular Cells

The observation that HSPCs colocalize with the marrow vasculature raised the possibility that perivascular cells may also play a role in the HSPC regulation by the niche. So far, three types of perivascular cells have been characterized: CXCL 12-abundant reticular cells (CAR cells), nestin-GFP^{dim}/leptinR$^+$ MSCs and nestin-GFP^{bright}/NG2$^+$ pericytes.

CAR cells were identified in a mouse model in which GFP was driven by *CXCL12* promoter. Similar to the other components of the niche, CAR cells are found in a close proximity to HSPCs. It is likely that they are genetically and phenotypically related to nestin-GFP^{low} cells (see later) because their ablation also severely impaired adipogenic and osteogenic differentiation of nonhematopoietic BM cells in addition to reducing the number of HSPCs. Notably, the effect of deletion was not limited to HSPCs but also affected mature lineages, such as lymphoid cells, indicating a wider role for these cells in hematopoietic support.

MSCs are located in the perisinusoidal BM space and have been initially defined by low expression of green fluorescent protein (GFP) driven by gene regulatory elements of intermediate filament protein Nestin (nestin-GFP^{low}).[14] Nestin-GFP^{low} cells express the genes associated with HSPC retention in the niche (*Cxcl12*, *VCAM-1*), which are downregulated upon G-CSF mobilization. Selective deletion of Nestin-positive cells in mice resulted in 50% reduction in the number of long-term HSPCs and their relocation to the spleen, although it is not clear whether this effect was mediated directly by Nestin-positive cells or through their more differentiated downstream progeny. Subsequent studies revealed that a population that largely overlaps with nestin-GFP^{low} cells can be also defined by expression of leptin receptor. Specific deletion of known HSPC regulators (stem cell factor, CXCL12) specifically from MSCs using Cre-recombinase driven by leptin receptor gene regulatory elements lead to reduction in the HSPC number and long-term repopulating capacity, further delineating the functional significance of MSCs in the HSPC niche.

Careful analysis of HSPC distribution within BM sections led to discovery of another perivascular cell subset (termed nestin-GFP^{high}), which is closely associated with arterioles.[15] Cell deletion experiments demonstrated the role for nestin-GFP^{high} in maintaining HSPC quiescence. Interestingly, nestin-GFP^{high} cells are preferentially found close to the endosteum leading to a model that denotes the endosteal surface as a quiescent niche and central BM (where nestin-GFP^{low} form the niches around sinusoidal vessels) as a proliferative niche, with the two being involved in a dynamic interaction with each other.

Adipocytes

An observation that adipocyte-rich vertebrae in mice contained significantly fewer cycling HSPCs compared with adipocyte-poor thoracic vertebrae led to the discovery of their role in HSPC regulation.[16] In a genetic mouse model of lipoatrophy (i.e., a condition with reduced adipocyte number), posttransplant hematopoietic recovery was accelerated, although a concomitant increase in trabecular bone could have contributed to this result.

Osteoclasts

Osteoclasts are BM-derived cells that are located in close proximity to stem cell–rich endosteum and play a critical role in bone remodeling. During stress and G-CSF–induced mobilization, the activity of the osteoclasts increases and is accompanied by secretion of proteolytic enzymes and reduction in the endosteal niche components, as evidenced by downregulation of the osteopontin expression by the

OLCs.[17] Conversely, inhibition of the osteoclasts leads to reduced HSPC and progenitor egress.

Bone Marrow Macrophages

During experiments investigating the mechanisms of G-CSF–induced HSPC mobilization, it was noted that in addition to previously reported reduction in the endosteal OLCs, BM macrophages were also decreased in number. In vivo depletion of this cell population by clodronate administration produced the same result.[18] It therefore appears that macrophages play a critical role in supporting the OLC niche compartment. A similar role for the macrophages, but with regard to supporting nestin-GFP^low MSCs, has been suggested by another study that used clodronate-mediated macrophage ablation. Again, this resulted in HSPC egress from the BM, perhaps through the effect on nestin-GFP^low, which showed a marked downregulation of genes responsible for HSPC retention in the niche (see earlier discussion). Thus, macrophages appear to function at a level of regulation upstream of OLCs and nestin-GFP^low cells.

Megakaryocytes

Megakaryocytes are the most recent addition to a growing list of niche cell types and appear to be directly involved in regulation of HSPC quiescence, as shown by cell deletion studies. This effect is mediated by CXCL4, also known as platelet factor 4, and TGF-β.[19] Overall, only 20% of immunophenotypically defined HSPCs are associated with megakaryocytes, and were spatially distinct from HSPCs that are located near the arterioles, suggesting the existence of specific megakaryocytic niche. The above findings also illustrate a feedback mechanism, by which mature hematopoietic cells may regulate HSPC number.

EXTRINSIC REGULATION OF THE HEMATOPOIETIC STEM CELL NICHE

Sympathetic Innervation

Sensory and autonomic innervation of the BM is critical for its ability to respond to hematopoietic stress. Increase in sympathetic tone promotes HSPC mobilization and downregulates the components of the endosteal niche, mainly through the activation of β_2-adrenergic receptor.[20] Nestin-positive cells express both β_2 and β_3 receptors and act as another mediator between sympathetic signaling and HSPCs, again facilitating egress from the BM. In a mouse model of streptozotocin-induced diabetes, diabetic autonomic dysfunction was shown to disrupt this regulatory circuit, alter the function of Nestin-positive cells, and lead to impaired G-CSF-induced HSPC mobilization, providing a biologic explanation for a higher frequency of peripheral blood stem cell mobilization failure in diabetic patients. The sympathetic nervous system is also involved in regulation of HSPC egress from the BM as governed by circadian rhythms, a remarkable discovery based on a chance observation that continuous exposure to light (because of a broken light switch in the animal house) significantly altered the number of HSPCs mobilized after G-CSF administration. Thus, sympathetic niche innervation is essential for relaying and integrating extrinsic signals, and acts as a responsive and finely tuned tool, which regulates HSPC traffic between peripheral blood and the BM.

Not only sympathetic nerves, but also the glial cells that surround them can regulate HSPC behavior in the marrow, as exemplified by the studies of nonmyelinating Schwann cells.[21] These cells ensheathe sympathetic nerves, come into contact with HSPCs and are responsible for activation of the latent form of TGF-β. Denervation experiments lead to significant reduction in the number of glial cells and associated increase in HSPC cycling.

Hypoxia

The niche for quiescent HSPCs is thought to be hypoxic. These observations are based on studies that use an intracellular marker of reducing equivalents, pimonidazole, or direct measurement of oxygen tension in the BM using intravital microscopy. By direct measurement of oxygen, it is apparent that the absolute level of Po$_2$ in the BM is quite low (<32 mmHg) and reduces to ~10 mmHg deeper into the marrow space.[22] The vascular network in the marrow is extensive and it appears that the low Po$_2$ levels reflect high consumption by the action of hematopoiesis.

Hypoxia is associated with upregulation of stromal cell–derived factor 1 (SDF-1) expression in the endosteal region and HSPC traffic to the BM; in contrast, hyperbaric oxygen (exposure to 100% oxygen under increased atmospheric pressure) mobilizes HSPC and progenitors away from the BM. Hypoxic responses in the HSPCs are mediated through a family of hypoxia-inducible factors (HIFs). The best-studied species of HIFs is HIF1-α, which induces SDF-1 expression and directs metabolic circuits within HSPCs toward anaerobic metabolism. HIF1-α also stimulates secretion of VEGF, thereby promoting bone formation and angiogenesis. HIF1-α affects HSPC function, as HIF1-α deletion from HSPCs leads to HSPC exhaustion.

What is a physiologic role of hypoxia? Firstly, hypoxia is believed to protect HSPCs in the niche from oxidative stress. Indeed, HSPCs within the niche contain a lower level of reactive oxygen species. Moreover, it appears that hypoxic conditions are beneficial for the HSPC function because culturing human BM HSPCs under lower oxygen tension leads to an increase in their ability to engraft and repopulate nonobese diabetic/severe combined immune deficient (NOD/SCI) mice. Finally, hypoxia may also protect the HSPC pool from exhaustion by promoting cell cycle quiescence. Of note, when radiation or cytotoxic chemotherapy are used, the Po$_2$ levels in marrow go dramatically higher, raising the question of whether Po$_2$ levels participate in the hematopoietic regenerative response to injury.

LYMPHOID NICHES

BM is the site of *B-cell lymphopoiesis*. Several cell types involved in the HSPC niche also participate in formation of the lymphoid niches. Interestingly, B-cell niches correspond to maturation stages of the lymphoid cells: OLCs, osteoclasts, and CAR cells are necessary for the less mature stages of development, whereas interleukin-7 (IL-7) secreting cells and sinusoidal endothelial cells are important for more differentiated cells. These observations come from targeted deletion of each supporting cell population using genetic means and analyzing the effect on B-cell homeostasis. For example, deletion of the OLCs leads to a considerable decrease in pre–pro and pro-B cells. This process appears to be mediated by the heterotrimeric G protein α subunit because its deletion in the OLCs leads to 60% decrease in the percentage of B-cell precursors in the BM. A similar phenotype is seen upon deletion of CAR cells.

Naive recirculating B and T cells are located in the perisinusoidal space and colocalize with dendritic cells, which are thought to deliver supportive signals, because as their deletion leads to significant decrease in B-cell number and reduction in IgM production after immunization.

Plasma cells are the product of terminal differentiation of B cells after antigen exposure. In vitro and in vivo studies showed that plasma cells receive multiple extrinsic survival signals, including CXCL12, IL-6, BAFF (B-cell activating factor of the TNF family), and APRIL (a proliferation-inducing ligand), which may account for their longevity. Mice deficient in CXCR4 displayed impaired homing of plasmablasts, illustrating the involvement of CXCL12–CXCR4 axis in plasma cell trafficking. Eosinophil- and megakaryocyte-derived APRIL and BAFF appear to regulate the number of plasma cells, which is greatly reduced upon eosinophil or megakaryocyte deletion.

The majority of long-lived *memory T cells* reside in the BM and appear to require a close contact with IL-7 secreting stromal cells to ensure that they remain quiescent in the absence of antigen stimulation. The BM also contains a large proportion of *regulatory T cells,* which have recently been found to exclusively protect HSPCs and early progenitors from rejection after allogeneic transplantation, arguing that the endosteal surface acts as an immune privileged site. Surprisingly, BM harbors specific niche cells (osteocalcin+ OLCs) which provide instructive cues to T-competent progenitors that migrate from the BM to the thymus, since deletion of the osteocalcin-expressing cells leads to decreased intrathymic T-cell precursors and impaired generation of mature T-cells in the presence of normal thymic function. Specific OLCs therefore appear to be important in T-lymphopoiesis. Their damage in the settings of conditioning for transplantation or graft-versus-host disease (GVHD) may compromise the ability of BM to provide the early T-lineage cells for thymocyte and ultimately, T-cell production.[23]

ERYTHROID NICHES

Erythroblastic islands were first described by a French hematologist Marcel Bessis more than 50 years ago and consist of developing erythroblasts surrounding a central macrophage. They are present in the BM, fetal liver, and the spleen and in in vitro long-term BM cultures. The number of erythroblasts per island ranges from 10 cells observed in sections of rat femur to 5 to 30 erythroblasts seen in human BM. Some islands are located adjacent to the BM sinusoids, and the others are scattered throughout the BM cavity. Within erythroid islands, the macrophage functions as a "nurse cell" providing iron to the developing erythroblasts and phagocytosing the extruded nuclei at the end of erythroid differentiation.

Adhesion between maturing erythroblasts and central macrophage is mediated by several molecules, including erythroblast macrophage protein (Emp via homophilic binding), α4β1 integrin (VCAM-1), and αv integrin (ICAM-4); antibody-mediated blockade of each of these molecule results in disruption of the islands. The most striking effect is seen with the blockade of Emp, which causes significant increase in proliferation, maturation, and apoptosis of maturing erythroblasts in vitro. Of note, Emp-null fetuses die in utero from severe anemia.

In addition to interaction within macrophages, maturing erythroblasts adhere to ECM proteins, fibronectin, and laminin for the maturation to proceed. Fibronectin protects erythroblasts from apoptosis, partly through antiapoptotic bcl-xL, and laminin is thought to localize reticulocytes to sinusoids as the initial step before their release into circulation.

MEGAKARYOCYTIC NICHES

Megakaryocytes localize to BM endothelial cells in vivo and release platelets into the marrow intravascular–sinusoidal space or the lung capillaries. Although CXCL12 induces platelet production by megakaryocytes if preceded by migration through endothelial cells, this is not observed in the absence of endothelial cells, suggesting that megakaryocyte interaction with specific molecules present on the endothelial cells is necessary for thrombopoiesis. FGF4 and CXCL12 enhance the interaction of megakaryocytes with endothelial cells and restore thrombopoiesis in mice deficient in thrombopoietin or its receptor c-mpl. Thus, chemokine-mediated localization of megakaryocytes within a specific vascular microenvironment is necessary for their maturation and platelet production.

HUMAN BONE MARROW MICROENVIRONMENT

Because direct mechanistic studies of human BM microenvironment cannot be undertaken, the bulk of our knowledge comes from experiments in xenotransplantation models. These initially involved fetal sheep and heavily irradiated or nude mice as recipients, but only very low level of human hematopoietic engraftment was observed. The discovery of SCID mice led to development of two powerful models. The first, known as SCID-hu mouse, was generated by engrafting human thymus and fetal liver. This model was most informative for the study of human lymphoid development and is still used for testing novel HIV drugs. The second model, hu-SRC (for SCID-repopulating cell), through the pioneering work of John Dick and colleagues, enabled investigation of human HSPC engraftment and differentiation. Further modifications of the SCID model led to generation of NOD/SCID–IL2 receptor γ chain knock-out (NSG) strain, which supports robust normal human multilineage (myeloid and lymphoid) hematopoietic engraftment, as well as engraftment of acute myeloid leukemia (AML) and acute lymphoblastic leukemia (ALL) cells from patients. The sensitivity of the transplant assay is further increased by direct intrafemoral injection into the BM cavity; remarkably, in NSG recipients, human hematopoietic engraftment can be detected after intrafemoral transplantation of a single highly purified human HSPC. Further advance in the field of xenotransplantation is the development of mouse strains that express several human hematopoietic cytokines, thereby enabling support of innate immune cells (myeloid and NK cells).

Similar to mouse HSPCs, human HSPCs transplanted into mouse recipients preferentially traffic to the trabecular bone and home next to the endosteal surface.[24] They are guided to their niches by the CXCL12–CXCR4 pathway and cell adhesion molecules such as very late antigen-4 (VLA-4), very late antigen-5 (VLA-5), and lymphocyte function-associated antigen-1 (LFA-1); of note, CXCL12 is expressed by human OLCs, mesenchymal stromal, Nestin-positive, and endothelial cells. CD44 and hyaluronic acid cooperate with CXCL12 in human HSPC homing. Recent experiments identified α6 integrin CD49f as a novel marker for human HSPCs, alluding to functional importance of HSPC anchorage within BM microenvironment.[25,26] The cellular components of the human HSPC niche are yet to be identified. One potential candidate is a population of mesenchymal subendothelial cells expressing CD146, which can be prospectively isolated from human BM.[26] These perivascular cells were able to establish both bone and hematopoietic microenvironment upon subcutaneous transplantation; had a documented self-renewal capacity; and produced angiopoietin 1, a cytokine known to induce HSPC quiescence. CD271 has been suggested as another marker for human hematopoiesis-supporting mesenchymal population; in addition to CD146+ perivascular cells, it labels CD146-endosteal population, which colocalizes with hematopoietic CD34+ cells in human BM.

The limitations of our knowledge of human hematopoietic microenvironment restrict our ability to accomplish in vitro stem cell expansion. The potential benefits of doing so are especially evident in the context of cord blood transplantation when the number of donor cells is small and in the setting of gene modified stem cells where gene transduction efficiencies are low. Several molecules have been tested. One of them is Sonic hedgehog protein, which has been shown to induce proliferation of primitive human hematopoietic cells when added to highly purified CD34+ CD38− lineage human cells; this effect translated into increased level of progenitor expansion in NOD/SCID mice. The aryl hydrocarbon receptor antagonist, SR-1 also appears to increase HSPC. An engineered Notch ligand Delta 1 and pleiotrophin have both been shown to increase HSPC. Prostaglandin E2 enhances murine HSPC localization in the BM after brief in vitro exposure. This resulted in a two- to threefold increase in the number of HSPCs compared with control (vehicle-exposed) cells. A phase 1 study in transplant recipients concurrently receiving PGE2-treated and vehicle-treated cord blood units showed that PGE2-treated cells generated durable multilineage engraftment and displayed greater efficacy, as evidenced by accelerated neutrophil recovery.[27] These results are encouraging but require validation in larger studies.

HEMATOPOIETIC MICROENVIRONMENT IN ACUTE LEUKEMIA AND MYELODYSPLASIA

Given a critical role of hematopoietic microenvironment in safeguarding cellular homeostasis in the BM, it is not surprising that alterations within it—either primary or induced by the presence of malignant cell population—have been proposed to contribute toward tumor initiation, maintenance, and resistance to treatment. Here, we will summarize the data related to the role of microenvironment in the pathogenesis of acute leukemia and myelodysplasia. For the review of this topic in other hematologic neoplasms, readers are referred to disease-specific chapters of this book.

Early in vitro studies alluded to significant contribution of nonhematopoietic BM cells (collectively termed *stroma*) to the pathogenesis of acute leukemia. For example, fibroblastic stromal cells from patients with AML were unable to support normal granulocytic-macrophage (GM) colony formation in contrast to those obtained from normal individuals. However, when the stromal cells were tested from patients in remission, they maintained growth of GM colonies similar to normal stroma. Strikingly, when the patients relapsed, this GM colony-supporting ability was lost. In another series of observations, when nonadherent cells from continuous marrow cultures or GM-CSF–dependent progenitor cell lines were cocultured with mouse stromal cells that had been previously irradiated, they developed factor-independence and multiple distinct karyotypic abnormalities; upon subcutaneous injection, these newly transformed cell lines produced granulocytic monomyeloid tumors that spread to spleen, lymph nodes, and BM. Although by no means definitive, these studies suggested that either the altered stromal cells may contribute to the emergence of leukemia, or leukemia itself may affect the nonhematopoietic compartment. Both of these hypotheses found confirmation in the later studies reviewed later.

Niche Contribution to Leukemia Development

The idea of "niche-induced oncogenesis," or contribution of the microenvironment to the emergence of malignant disease, stems from the clinical observation of donor-induced leukemia. In this condition, which has a reported incidence between 0.12% and 5%, the leukemic clone arises from an apparently normal donor hematopoietic cells after allogeneic BM transplantation.[28] Although the etiology is clearly multifactorial, damage to the BM microenvironment, either because of previous chemotherapy or pretransplant conditioning, may be an important contributing factor. In keeping with this notion, several experimental mouse models illustrate that microenviromental alterations, either alone or in conjunction with corresponding molecular lesions in the hematopoietic compartment, can play a critical role in the initiation of malignant disease. For example, the mice with deficiency of phosphatase and tensin homologue (PTEN) both in the microenvironment and HSPC developed a myeloproliferative disorder, but PTEN deficiency in HSPCs alone did not result in the disease. Similarly, widespread deletion of retinoblastoma protein or retinoic acid receptor led to the development of myeloproliferative disorder, in the latter case purely because of gene deletion in the microenvironment. Using a cell type-specific approach, it was found that targeted deletion of the microRNA processing enzyme Dicer 1 in immature OLCs resulted in development of myelodysplasia and acute leukemia associated with independent complex genetic changes.[29] The effect of Dicer-1 deletion was entirely attributable to the microenvironment because transplantation of Dicer 1-deleted BM into normal microenvironment resulted in reversal of the myelodysplastic phenotype. Remarkably, hematopoietic abnormalities were observed when Dicer-1 was deleted in very immature OLCs (osterix⁺) but not in those at a more mature differentiation stage (osteocalcin⁺). Deletion of Shwachman-Diamond-Bodian syndrome gene in immature OLCs recapitulated the key features of the Dicer-1 deletion phenotype and implicated their role in its pathogenesis. In another striking example, niche involvement in leukemia generation, mice carrying an OLC-specific mutation of constitutively activated beta-catenin developed AML. The leukemic process was microenvironment-dependent and mediated by Notch signaling. Genetic or pharmacologic inhibition of Notch signaling lead to reversal of the leukemic phenotype. The findings of this study are clinically relevant, as 38% of patients

with MDS and AML showed nuclear (activated) beta-catenin in osteoblasts.

Altogether, the above studies illustrate that perturbed BM microenvironment can act as a source of signals that promote malignant change in the hematopoietic compartment, and highlight their potential role as therapeutic targets.

Niche Alterations by Leukemia

Just as the microenvironment can contribute to disordered hematopoiesis, it can be disrupted and modified by leukemic cells leading to competitive advantage over normal counterparts. Visualization of BM niches by intravital microscopy studies revealed that primary ALL and AML blasts are able to downregulate CXCL12 expression in the BM, causing the egress of normal CD34⁺ HSPCs from the BM and impairment of normal hematopoiesis. This process was mediated by the stem cell factor (SCF) secreted by leukemic blasts and reversed upon SCF neutralization.[30] Similarly, in myeloproliferative disorders such as chronic myeloid leukemia (CML), it is thought that microenvironmental changes that are induced by malignant cells result in formation of self-reinforcing loop leading to preferential expansion of leukemic cells at the expense of their normal counterparts. Leukemia can also affect the niches indirectly, i.e., through perturbation of sympathetic innervation: both in CML and AML, "sympathetic neuropathy" promotes leukemogenesis through either reduction in quiescence-inducing nestin⁺ cells or altering their differentiation properties and frequency relative to nestin-GFP^high /NG2⁺ cells.[31] The "niche-modifying" ability of the leukemic cells in vivo is an area of ongoing investigation because it suggests that the leukemic niche can be molecularly distinct from the normal thus creating an opportunity for altering the leukemic niche as a means of reducing persistence of leukemia-initiating cells.

Therapeutic Targeting of Leukemic Niche

The CXCR4–CXCL12 pathway is critical for homing and subsequent adhesion of not only normal, but also leukemic stem cells (LSCs) to the BM microenvironment. Of note, the level of CXCR4 is elevated in patients with AML and is associated with a poor outcome. The presence of Flt3 internal tandem duplication (a poor prognostic factor in AML) is in turn associated with increased CXCR4 expression. Experimentally, treatment of NOD/SCID mice transplanted with primary human AML cells using a neutralizing antibody against CXCR4 reduced the leukemic burden. Follow-up studies confirmed the antileukemic effect of blocking CXCL12–CXCR4 axis using competitive antagonists of CXCR4 (AMD3100 and AMD3254) in mouse models of AML. These findings formed the basis for ongoing clinical trials of CXCR4 antagonist AMD3100 (Plerixafor) as a chemosensitizing agent in AML.[32] So far, these studies have confirmed safety and tolerability of this drug in combination with chemotherapy, but the effect on response rate and survival has not been demonstrated.

Another example of LSC niche dependence is a cell adhesion molecule CD44, which is present on the surface of leukemic cells and interacts with hyaluronan on the endosteal surface. Blocking the interaction between CD44 and hyaluronan using activating CD4 antibody had significant effect on LSC eradication and even cured some mice.[33] The therapeutic effect of the antibody was more marked when it was administered soon after injection of human leukemic cells compared with the animals with established disease, suggesting that it acts predominantly at the stage when LSCs engage their respective niches. It is also possible that some of the effect of the CD44 antibody was attributable to differentiation induction in the LSCs. Nevertheless, this study provided a proof-of-principle demonstration that LSCs interaction with the niche is required for their survival and leukemia progression and thereby raised the potential for targeting therapy.

Other molecular mediators of LSC–microenvironment interaction have also been identified. B4 integrin (also known as very late antigen 4),[34] mediates lodgment of leukemic cells in the BM and interacts with fibronectin to confer resistance to cytosine arabinoside-induced apoptosis. Integrin ligation triggers prosurvival pathways, and the blocking antibody leads to reduction in the level of leukemic burden and a modest prolongation of the lifespan in human AML-transplanted animals. Similar protective role for AML blasts has been observed for β1 and β2 integrins. IL-3 receptor α chain (CD123),[35] also contributes to LSC survival, at least partly through being involved in controlling LSC homing to the BM; CD123 blocking antibody demonstrated considerable antileukemic activity, which was also attributable to promoting immune-mediated destruction of leukemic cells. This idea that has been explored further in the studies of blocking a macrophage-associated molecule CD47. Expression of CD47 on LSCs appears to protect the LSCs from phagocytosis.[36] CD47 expression is associated with Flt3-ITD mutation and independently predicts worse prognosis. Mechanistically, CD47 acts as a "do not eat me" signal for the macrophages. Blocking CD47 antibody produces depletion of AML in xenotransplantation models and specific eradication of LSCs. Phase 1 study of CD47 antibody in hematologic malignancies and solid tumors is ongoing.

Emerging experimental evidence (using the chemical marker of hypoxia pimonidazole) suggests that leukemic BM niches are hypoxic and that leukemic cells adapt to hypoxic conditions. Although low oxygen tension in the leukemic niche remains to be directly demonstrated, the findings of overexpression of the key hypoxia-response factor HIF1-α in clusters of ALL cells, together with increased angiogenesis and production of VEGF by the ALL blasts support this hypothesis. Hypoxia-activated dinitrobenzamide mustard, PR-104, prolonged survival of NSG mice engrafted with ALL cell line Nalm-6 and lead to transient cytoreduction in some patients with refractory AML in a Phase 1 study. Although very preliminary, these results identify hypoxia as another potential avenue for niche-based antileukemic therapy.

FUTURE DIRECTIONS

Although the concept of specific microenvironment for different hematopoietic compartments was first proposed more than 100 years ago, it was not until recently that the existence of the "niches" has been experimentally proven and the molecular factors involved in cellular interactions have been discovered.

Our current knowledge of the hematopoietic microenvironment has been evolving in parallel and often leading that in other stem cell systems. It appears that fundamental components and molecular pathways are highly conserved among evolutionary diverse species, although their role in specific niches may vary. These include supporting stromal cells secreting soluble molecules regulating stem cell self-renewal (bone morphogenic protein and Wnt signaling), ECM proteins that serve as stem cell anchors (integrin ligands), blood vessels that are responsible for nutritional support and transit of stem cells in and away from the niche, and neural inputs for integrating signals from different systems. It is therefore likely that future studies in spatial and molecular organization of other stem cell niches will inform the knowledge of hematopoietic niches and vice versa.

With a rapidly increasing number of cell types known to be involved in hematopoietic niches (and the number of different cytokines they produce, which will inevitably follow), it will be important to use a "network" approach—similar to the one used for analysis of transcriptional networks—to understand how these multiple factors act in concert to control location, proliferation, and trafficking of HSPCs and more mature cells in the BM. It is possible that these factors work in combinatorial manner, ultimately creating a "niche code" that is designed to suit a specific physiologic situation.

A particularly notable development over the recent years has been our improvement in understanding of the role of microenvironment in initiation and maintenance of malignant disease, although many questions remain. We still know very little about the molecular mediators of "niche-induced oncogenesis" and those involved in microenvironment-induced chemoresistance. Recent advances in xenotransplantation assay using highly immunocompromised mouse strains for the study of normal and leukemic hematopoiesis, together with further molecular insights into biology of leukemic stem cells, will provide an opportunity to address these issues.

Therapeutic manipulation of the hematopoietic microenvironment remains an ultimate goal of ongoing research. Clearly, the effort of the next several years will be focused on translating the wealth of data obtained from the animal models into human biology and the clinic. This work has already started with the clinical trials of ex vivo HSPC expansion before cord blood transplantation. A number of clinical trials are also underway to examine the efficacy of niche-directed therapies in hematologic malignancies. Although the animal data suggest that targeting the niche alone is often insufficient to achieve cure, especially in an established disease, this approach has been successful in regaining leukemia chemosensitivity to commonly used agents and may become a valuable component of future treatment protocols, particularly in the setting of low tumor burden, such as minimal residual disease. Gaining a deeper insight into the molecular distinctions between normal and malignant niches will enable better understanding of "niche competition" between normal and leukemic populations and lead to development of novel approaches based on eradication of leukemic cells and fostering normal hematopoiesis through manipulation of niche-derived signals.

REFERENCES

1. Medvinsky AL, Samoylina NL, Muller AM, et al: An early pre-liver intraembryonic source of CFU-S in the developing mouse. *Nature* 364:64, 1993.
2. North TE, et al: Hematopoietic stem cell development is dependent on blood flow. *Cell* 137:736, 2009.
3. Gekas C, Dieterlen-Lievre F, Orkin SH, et al: The placenta is a niche for hematopoietic stem cells. *Dev Cell* 8:365, 2005.
4. Chou S, Lodish HF: Fetal liver hepatic progenitors are supportive stromal cells for hematopoietic stem cells. *Proc Natl Acad Sci U S A* 107:7799, 2010.
5. Peranteau WH, et al: CD26 inhibition enhances allogeneic donor-cell homing and engraftment after in utero hematopoietic-cell transplantation. *Blood* 108:4268, 2006.
6. Morrison SJ, Scadden DT: The bone marrow niche for haematopoietic stem cells. *Nature* 505:327, 2014.
7. Lo Celso C, et al: Live-animal tracking of individual haematopoietic stem/progenitor cells in their niche. *Nature* 457:92, 2009.
8. Nombela-Arrieta C, et al: Quantitative imaging of haematopoietic stem and progenitor cell localization and hypoxic status in the bone marrow microenvironment. *Nat Cell Biol* 15:533, 2013.
9. Ding L, Saunders TL, Enikolopov G, et al: Endothelial and perivascular cells maintain haematopoietic stem cells. *Nature* 481:457, 2012.
10. Calvi LM, et al: Osteoblastic cells regulate the haematopoietic stem cell niche. *Nature* 425:841, 2003.
11. Zhang J, et al: Identification of the haematopoietic stem cell niche and control of the niche size. *Nature* 425:836, 2003.
12. Winkler IG, et al: Vascular niche E-selectin regulates hematopoietic stem cell dormancy, self renewal and chemoresistance. *Nat Med* 18:1651, 2012.
13. Himburg HA, et al: Pleiotrophin mediates hematopoietic regeneration via activation of RAS. *J Clin Invest* 124:4753, 2014.
14. Mendez-Ferrer S, et al: Mesenchymal and haematopoietic stem cells form a unique bone marrow niche. *Nature* 466:829, 2010.
15. Kunisaki Y, et al: Arteriolar niches maintain haematopoietic stem cell quiescence. *Nature* 502:637, 2013.
16. Naveiras O, et al: Bone-marrow adipocytes as negative regulators of the haematopoietic microenvironment. *Nature* 460:259, 2009.
17. Kollet O, et al: Osteoclasts degrade endosteal components and promote mobilization of hematopoietic progenitor cells. *Nat Med* 12:657, 2006.

18. Chow A, et al: Bone marrow CD169+ macrophages promote the retention of hematopoietic stem and progenitor cells in the mesenchymal stem cell niche. *J Exp Med* 208:261, 2011.

19. Bruns I, et al: Megakaryocytes regulate hematopoietic stem cell quiescence through CXCL4 secretion. *Nat Med* 20:1315, 2014.

20. Katayama Y, et al: Signals from the sympathetic nervous system regulate hematopoietic stem cell egress from bone marrow. *Cell* 124:407, 2006.

21. Yamazaki S, et al: Nonmyelinating Schwann cells maintain hematopoietic stem cell hibernation in the bone marrow niche. *Cell* 147:1146, 2011.

22. Spencer JA, et al: Direct measurement of local oxygen concentration in the bone marrow of live animals. *Nature* 508:269, 2014.

23. Yu VW, et al: Specific bone cells produce DLL4 to generate thymus-seeding progenitors from bone marrow. *J Exp Med* 212:759, 2015.

24. Ninomiya M, et al: Homing, proliferation and survival sites of human leukemia cells in vivo in immunodeficient mice. *Leukemia* 21:136, 2007.

25. Notta F, et al: Isolation of single human hematopoietic stem cells capable of long-term multilineage engraftment. *Science* 333:218, 2011.

26. Sacchetti B, et al: Self-renewing osteoprogenitors in bone marrow sinusoids can organize a hematopoietic microenvironment. *Cell* 131:324, 2007.

27. Cutler C, et al: Prostaglandin-modulated umbilical cord blood hematopoietic stem cell transplantation. *Blood* 122:3074, 2013.

28. Flynn CM, Kaufman DS: Donor cell leukemia: insight into cancer stem cells and the stem cell niche. *Blood* 109:2688, 2007.

29. Raaijmakers MH, et al: Bone progenitor dysfunction induces myelodysplasia and secondary leukaemia. *Nature* 464:852, 2010.

30. Colmone A, et al: Leukemic cells create bone marrow niches that disrupt the behavior of normal hematopoietic progenitor cells. *Science* 322:1861, 2008.

31. Hanoun M, et al: Acute myelogenous leukemia-induced sympathetic neuropathy promotes malignancy in an altered hematopoietic stem cell niche. *Cell Stem Cell* 15:365, 2014.

32. Nervi B, et al: Chemosensitization of acute myeloid leukemia (AML) following mobilization by the CXCR4 antagonist AMD3100. *Blood* 113:6206, 2009.

33. Jin L, Hope KJ, Zhai Q, et al: Targeting of CD44 eradicates human acute myeloid leukemic stem cells. *Nat Med* 12:1167, 2006.

34. Matsunaga T, et al: Interaction between leukemic-cell VLA-4 and stromal fibronectin is a decisive factor for minimal residual disease of acute myelogenous leukemia. *Nat Med* 9:1158, 2003.

35. Jin L, et al: Monoclonal antibody-mediated targeting of CD123, IL-3 receptor alpha chain, eliminates human acute myeloid leukemic stem cells. *Cell Stem Cell* 5:31, 2009.

36. Majeti R, et al: CD47 is an adverse prognostic factor and therapeutic antibody target on human acute myeloid leukemia stem cells. *Cell* 138:286, 2009.

CHAPTER 12

CELL ADHESION

Rodger P. McEver and Francis W. Luscinskas

Cell adhesion is essential for the development and maintenance of multicellular organisms. Cell-to-cell and cell-to-matrix adhesion provide a mechanism for intercellular communication and to define the three-dimensional architecture of organs. The regulated nature of cell adhesion is particularly evident in the hematopoietic system, where blood cells routinely make transitions between nonadherent and adherent phenotypes during differentiation, and in response to stimuli in the circulation or extravascular space.

In the bone marrow (BM), hematopoietic stem cells reside in a specialized microenvironment called the *stem cell niche*, and their proliferation and differentiation are controlled not only by soluble growth factors but also by adhesion to stromal cells and matrix molecules (see Chapter 9 for more detailed discussion). Weakening of these adhesive interactions is required for mature blood cells to enter the circulation. Circulating erythrocytes normally remain nonadhesive until they become senescent and are finally cleared by the reticuloendothelial system (see Chapter 33 for more discussion). Other circulating blood cells often participate in regulated adhesive events during their lifespan. For example, prothymocytes adhere to thymic stromal cells where they undergo guided movement from the cortex to the medulla during maturation before reentering the circulation. T cells regularly stick to the specialized high endothelial venules of lymphoid tissues, migrate into these tissues for sampling of processed antigens, and then exit via the lymphatics to recirculate in the blood (see Chapter 13 for more discussion). During inflammation, specific classes of leukocytes roll at very low velocity on the endothelium that line all blood vessels, then adhere more tightly, and finally emigrate between endothelial cells into the tissues. There, neutrophils and monocytes phagocytose invading pathogens, and lymphocytes adhere to antigen-presenting cells, such as dendritic cells, B cells, and macrophages (see Chapter 123 for more discussion). During hemorrhage, platelets stick to exposed subendothelial matrix components, spread, and recruit additional platelets into large aggregates that serve as an efficient surface for thrombin and fibrin generation. This is discussed in more detail later in Chapter 124. Leukocytes also adhere to activated platelets and to other leukocytes, and platelets roll on the endothelium. When activated, endothelial cells increase expression of molecules that affect the adhesiveness of platelets or leukocytes. Tight contacts between adjacent endothelial cells also regulate access of blood cells to the underlying tissues.

ADHESION MOLECULES

Cells adhere through noncovalent bond formation between macromolecules on cell surfaces with macromolecules on other cell surfaces or in the extracellular matrix (ECM). These interactions involve either protein–protein or protein–carbohydrate recognition. Although some adhesion molecules are expressed only by blood or endothelial cells, most also are synthesized by other cells. Many adhesion molecules can be grouped into families according to related structural and functional features.

EXTRACELLULAR MATRIX PROTEINS

The ECM provides structural and mechanical support for many tissues and spatial cues that enable cell–cell communication and signaling. The principal constituents of the ECM are adhesive proteins and proteoglycans. The major proteins are collagens, von Willebrand factor (vWF), thrombospondin, elastin, fibronectin, laminin, and vitronectin. These proteins are large and often highly extended, and consist of multiple domains with different binding functions. In some proteins such as fibronectin, alternative splicing can increase diversity by producing molecules with variable numbers of domains. In addition, stretching of fibronectin can expose cryptic binding sites. The many binding domains allow adhesive proteins to interact with each other as well as with cell-surface receptors, resulting in multipoint contacts that stabilize matrix structure. One adhesive protein, fibrinogen, is found predominantly in plasma but also may be deposited in exposed subendothelial matrix after vascular injury. Fibronectin, vitronectin, thrombospondin, and vWF are located predominantly in the ECM but also are found in plasma in lower amounts. Several adhesive proteins also are stored in α-granules of platelets, where they are secreted after platelet activation at sites of vascular injury. Similarly, the endothelium stores adhesive proteins in cytoplasmic storage granules, called *Weibel–Palade bodies*, that are released upon injury or activation.

Proteoglycans contain protein cores to which are covalently attached many glycosaminoglycans—long linear polymers of repeating disaccharides. Most proteoglycans are in the ECM, but some are anchored on cell surfaces through a core protein that contains a membrane-spanning domain. Hyaluronan is a unique glycosaminoglycan that forms polymers with molecular masses up to several million daltons that are not covalently attached to a protein. Hyaluronan forms noncovalent interactions with globular domains on the protein core of proteoglycans and with a small molecule called *link protein*. The resultant hyaluronan–proteoglycan complexes can become very large, contributing to the structural stability of the matrix and function as space fillers during embryonic development. Hyaluronan can also bind to cell-surface receptors and is also abundantly produced during wound healing.

INTEGRINS

Integrins are a broadly distributed group of cell-surface adhesion receptors that consist of noncovalently associated α- and β-subunits (Fig. 12.1 and Table 12.1). There are 18 α-chains and eight β-chains that pair in many, but not all, of the possible combinations. All blood cells have several different integrins. The four β2 integrins, each paired with a unique α-subunit, are expressed only by leukocytes, and the αIIbβ3 integrin (glycoprotein IIb–IIIa [GPIIb–IIIa]) is expressed only by megakaryocytes and platelets. Multidomain adhesive proteins of the ECM are ligands for many integrins. Integrins are unusual adhesion molecules because they usually reside in an inactive state on the cell surface until they receive an activating signal. Some integrins bind to specific domains of several different proteins, and some adhesive proteins bind to several different integrins. These interactions generally mediate cell–matrix and cell–cell adhesion. A unique feature of integrins is transmission of signals in both directions across the cell plasma membrane. Integrin binding to matrix informs the interior of the cell (outside-in), and intracellular signals or conditions inside cells transmit signals outward (inside-out) that regulate binding to matrix or to adhesion receptors on the surface of adjacent cells. Force can also regulate integrin adhesive function.

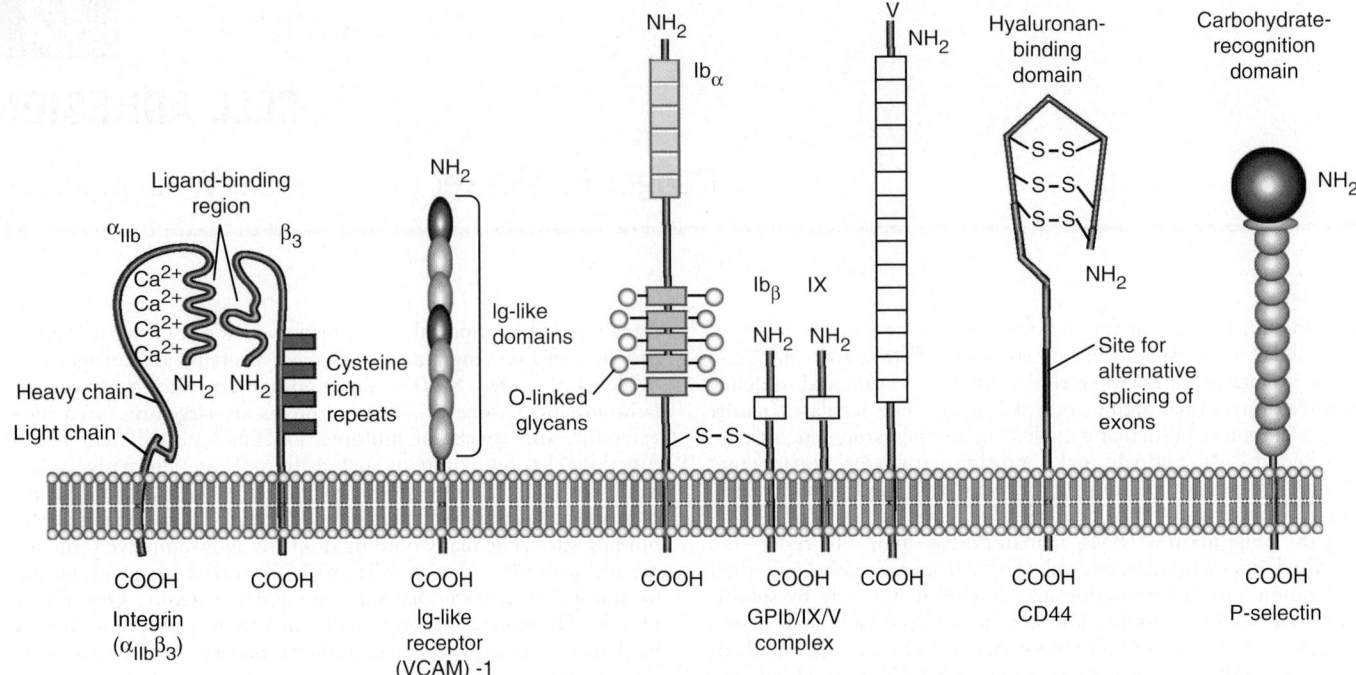

Fig. 12.1 SCHEMATIC DIAGRAMS OF SEVERAL TYPES OF CELL SURFACE ADHESION RECEPTORS. Integrins consist of noncovalently linked α- and β-subunits, both of which contribute to ligand binding. The platelet αIIbβ3 integrin is illustrated at *far left*. Ig-like receptors contain a variable number of Ig homology domains, of which some bind ligands and others extend the ligand-binding domains from the membrane. Shown *second from left* is VCAM-1, which contains seven Ig domains; the two domains that bind to integrins are *shaded*. The platelet GPIb–IX–V complex, depicted in the *middle diagram*, consists of several leucine-rich protein subunits. CD44, illustrated next, contains an amino-terminal (*N*-terminal) domain that binds to hyaluronan. Each of the selectins contains an *N*-terminal carbohydrate recognition domain that binds sialylated and fucosylated oligosaccharides on specific cell-surface GP ligands. Illustrated at *far right* is P-selectin, the largest of the three selectins. *GP*, Glycoprotein; *Ig*, immunoglobulin; *VCAM-1*, vascular cell adhesion molecule-1.

TABLE 12.1	Integrins on Blood Cells			
Integrin Designation	**Other Name(s)**	**Expressed by**	**Ligand(s)**	**Function(s)**
α₁β₁	VLA-1	Leukocytes, other cells	Collagens, LM	Adhesion to ECM
α₂β₁	VLA-2 GPIa/IIa	Leukocytes, platelets, other cells	Collagens, LM	Adhesion to ECM
α₃β₁	VLA-3	Leukocytes, other cells	Collagens, LM, FN	Adhesion to ECM
α₄β₁	VLA-4	Monocytes, lymphocytes, eosinophils	VCAM-1, FN	Adhesion to cells, ECM
α₅β₁	VLA-5 GPIc/IIa	Leukocytes, platelets, other cells	FN	Adhesion to ECM
α₆β₁	VLA-6 GPIc/IIa	Leukocytes, platelets, other cells	LM	Adhesion to ECM
α₉β₁		Neutrophils	VCAM-1	Adhesion to ECs
αLβ₂	LFA-1 CD11a/CD18	Leukocytes	ICAM-1, -2, -3	Leukocyte aggregation and adhesion
αMβ₂	MAC-1 CR3 CD11b/CD18	Neutrophils, monocytes	ICAM-1, FIB, CR for iC3b	Neutrophil aggregation and adhesion to ECs
αXβ₂	P150,95 CD11c/CD18	Neutrophils, monocytes	CR for iC3b	Adhesion to ECs
αDβ₂	CD11d/CD18	Eosinophils, monocytes, lymphocytes	VCAM-1, ICAM-3	Adhesion to leukocytes and to ECs
αIIbβ₃	GPIIb/IIIa	Platelets	FIB, FN, vWF, VN, TSP	Platelet adhesion and aggregation
αVβ₃	VN receptor	Platelets, ECs	FIB, FN, vWF, VN, TSP, collagens	Platelet adhesion, angiogenesis
α₄β₇	LPAM-1	Lymphocytes	VCAM-1, MAdCAM-1, FN	Lymphocyte adhesion to ECs and ECM

CR, Complement receptor; EC, endothelial cell; ECM, extracellular matrix; FIB, fibrinogen; FN, fibronectin; GP, glycoprotein; LFA-1, leukocyte function-associated antigen; LM, laminin; LPAM-1, lymphocyte Peyer patch adhesion molecule; MAdCAM-1, mucosal addressin cell adhesion molecule-1; TSP, thrombospondin; VCAM-1, vascular cell adhesion molecule-1; VLA, very late-appearing antigen; VN, vitronectin; vWF, von Willebrand factor.

The application of tension to integrins can increase ligand binding, and a reduction in tension lessens integrin adhesiveness. Cell–cell interactions result from integrin recognition of cell-surface members of the immunoglobulin superfamily. Binding of fibrinogen to $\alpha IIb\beta 3$ integrins on adjacent platelets creates a molecular bridge that promotes platelet aggregation. Furthermore, fibrinogen simultaneously binds to the $\alpha M\beta 2$ integrin on leukocytes and to an immunoglobulin-like receptor on endothelial cells, promoting leukocyte adhesion to the endothelium.

IMMUNOGLOBULIN-LIKE RECEPTORS

Immunoglobulin superfamily members contain a variable number of disulfide-stabilized motifs similar to those in antibodies, which are linked to transmembrane and cytoplasmic domains (Table 12.2; see also Fig. 12.1). The immunoglobulin-like motif provides a framework on which specific recognition structures for other proteins can be added. Some of these motifs also recognize glycoconjugates. The immunoglobulin-like molecules, intercellular adhesion molecule 1 and 2 (ICAM-1 and ICAM-2), and vascular cell adhesion molecule 1 (VCAM-1), expressed on endothelial cells, as well as ICAM-3, expressed on leukocytes, mediate cell–cell contact through recognition of specific integrins on leukocytes. ICAM-4, expressed on erythroid precursors, binds to integrins on stromal cells of BM, which may regulate erythropoiesis. ICAM-5 is restricted to neural tissues. The immunoglobulin-like GPVI on platelets promotes cell activation by binding to collagen exposed on damaged blood vessels. Interactions between immunoglobulin-like molecules help to mediate adhesion between T cells and antigen-presenting cells. Thus, whereas the immunoglobulin-like molecules CD8 and CD4 on T cells bind to the conserved membrane-proximal domains of class I and class II major histocompatibility complex (MHC) proteins, respectively, the α- and β-chains of the T-cell receptor (TCR) bind to the polymorphic antigen-presenting domain. In addition, the immunoglobulin-like proteins CD2 and CD28 on T cells bind to the immunoglobulin-like

protein leukocyte function-associated antigen-3 (LFA-3) and B7-1 (CD80) and B7-2 (CD86), respectively, on antigen-presenting cells. The immunoglobulin-like receptor, platelet and endothelial cell adhesion molecule-1 (PECAM-1; CD31) uses homotypical interactions to promote contacts between adjacent endothelial cells and to mediate adhesion of leukocytes to platelets and endothelium. The immunoglobulin-like junctional adhesion molecules (JAMs), expressed on endothelial and epithelial cells and leukocytes, regulate endothelial and epithelial cell junctions, paracellular permeability, and leukocyte trafficking between endothelial and epithelial cells by homotypical interactions or by heterotypical interactions with integrins. JAM-A, the founding member of this family, functions as a homodimer and transmits intracellular signals critical for its function in regulation of endothelial and epithelial permeability.

OTHER ADHESION RECEPTORS THAT MEDIATE PROTEIN–PROTEIN INTERACTIONS

Cadherins are cytoskeletally linked type 1 transmembrane proteins that mediate cell–cell contact in many organs through homotypical binding to cadherins on adjacent cells (Table 12.3). Cadherins have not been described on blood cells but are found on endothelial cells, where, similar to PECAM-1 and JAMs, they help form cell junctions and participate in the process of leukocyte migration across endothelial cell-to-cell borders, termed *diapedesis* or *transendothelial migration*. Cadherins are also expressed in the epithelium and help form cell-to-cell junctions.

The GPIb–IX–V complex on platelets consists of leucine-rich protein subunits (see Fig. 12.1). Under conditions of high shear stress such as those found in arterial circulation, this complex promotes the initial platelet adhesion to injured vessels by binding to vWF exposed in the subendothelium. It also may assist interactions with other platelets or with endothelial cells by binding to P-selectin, which normally binds to glycoconjugates, and it may assist platelet adhesion to leukocytes by binding to the integrin $\alpha_m\beta_2$.

TABLE 12.2	Immunoglobulin-Like Receptors			
Name	**Other Name**	**Expressed by**	**Ligand**	**Function(s)**
ICAM-1		Macrophages, EC, other cells	$\alpha_M\beta_2$, $\alpha_L\beta_2$, FIB	T-cell responses, leukocyte adhesion to EC
ICAM-2		EC	$\alpha_L\beta_2$	Leukocyte adhesion to EC
ICAM-3		Leukocytes	$\alpha_L\beta_2$	T-cell responses, leukocyte aggregation
ICAM-4		Erythroid precursors	$\alpha_4\beta_1$, $\alpha_V\beta_3$, $\alpha_{IIb}\beta_3$	Regulate erythropoiesis
GPVI		Platelets	Collagen	Platelet adhesion and activation
PECAM-1	CD31	Leukocytes, platelets, EC	PECAM-1	EC junctions, leukocyte transmigration, cell signaling
VCAM-1		Activated EC, smooth muscle cells	$\alpha_4\beta_1$, $\alpha_4\beta_7$	Mononuclear cell adhesion to EC
MAdCAM-1		EC of Peyer patches	$\alpha_4\beta_7$	Lymphocyte homing
Siglecs		Leukocyte subsets	Sialylated glycans	Regulates B-cell activation, innate immunity?, hematopoiesis?
JAMs		EC	JAMs, $\alpha_L\beta_2$, $\alpha_4\beta_1$	EC junctions, leukocyte transmigration
CD2		T cells	LFA-3[a]	T-cell responses
CD4		T cells	Class II MHC[a]	T-cell responses
CD8		T cells	Class I MHC[a]	T-cell responses
CD3	T-cell receptor	T cells	Antigen on MHC[a]	T-cell responses
CD28	Costimulatory molecule	T cells	B7-1 (CD80)	T-cell responses

[a]LFA-3 and classes I and II MHC molecules are also immunoglobulin-like receptors.
ICAM-1, -2, -3, -4, Intercellular adhesion molecules; JAM, junctional adhesion molecule; MHC, major histocompatibility complex; PECAM-1, platelet and endothelial cell adhesion molecules-1. For other abbreviations, see Table 12.1 footnotes.

TABLE 12.3 Other Adhesion Receptors

Name	Other Name	Expressed by	Ligand	Function(s)
Cadherins		EC, many other cells	Homotypic binding	Formation of EC junctions
GPIb/IX/V		Platelets	vWF	Platelet adhesion to ECM under shear
CD36	GPIV	Platelets, many other cells	Collagens, TSP	Platelet adhesion to ECM
CD44		Leukocytes, other cells	Hyaluronan, serglycin	Lymphopoiesis, lymphocyte activation
DC-SIGN		Dendritic cells	Mannosylated glycans, other glycans	Regulate T-cell–dendritic cell interactions, recognize pathogens
NK cell receptors		NK cells	MHC molecules	Recognition of virus-infected or other foreign cells

DC-SIGN, Dendritic cell-specific ICAM-3 grabbing nonintegrin; MHC, major histocompatibility complex; NK, natural killer. For other abbreviations, see Table 12.1 footnotes.

TABLE 12.4 Selectins

Name	Other Name	Expressed by	Ligand	Ligands Expressed by	Function(s)
P-selectin	CD62P GMP-140 PADGEM	Thrombin-activated platelets and ECs, cytokine-activated ECs	PSGL-1, GPIbα	Leukocytes, platelets	Leukocyte adhesion to activated ECs and platelets
E-selectin	CD62E ELAM-1	Cytokine-activated ECs	PSGL-1, other sialylated and fucosylated GPs	Leukocytes	Leukocyte adhesion to activated ECs
L-selectin	CD62L LECAM-1 LAM-1	Leukocytes	PSGL-1, also GlyCAM-1, CD34, and other mucins on ECs of lymph nodes	Leukocytes, ECs or lymph nodes	Leukocyte adhesion to other leukocytes; lymphocyte homing to lymph nodes

The selectins bind to sialylated, fucosylated, and (in some cases) sulfated oligosaccharides on specific glycoproteins, of which only some have been identified.
EC, Endothelial cell; ELAM-1, endothelial leukocyte adhesion molecule-1; Gly-CAM-1, glycosylation-dependent cell adhesion molecule-1; GMP-140, granule membrane protein-140; LAM-1, leukocyte adhesion molecule-1; LECAM-1, leukocyte endothelial cell adhesion molecule-1; PADGEM, platelet activation-dependent granule external membrane protein; PSGL-1, P-selectin glycoprotein ligand-1. For other abbreviations, see Table 12.1 footnotes.

CD36 is a receptor with at least two membrane-spanning domains that is expressed on many cell types. On platelets, it has been implicated as a receptor for collagen and for thrombospondin; both interactions could facilitate adhesion to the subendothelial matrix at sites of hemorrhage.

LECTIN ADHESION RECEPTORS

CD44 is an unusual transmembrane GP expressed to variable degrees on many subsets of leukocytes (see Fig. 12.1). It has a membrane-distal domain that is structurally related to link protein of the ECM, and similar to link protein, can bind to hyaluronan. CD44 also binds to serglycin, a proteoglycan secreted by hematopoietic cells. The hyaluronan-binding function of CD44 may modulate a number of leukocyte responses. The most clearly demonstrated function is in lymphopoiesis, where maturation of lymphocyte precursors requires contacts with BM stromal cells bearing surface hyaluronan. CD44–hyaluronate interactions also may promote lymphocyte entry to and transit through organized lymphoid tissues. The membrane-proximal regions of CD44 are structurally diverse because of the insertion of variable numbers of domains through alternative splicing. These insertions may regulate the ability of CD44 to bind hyaluronan and may mediate postbinding events that affect cell signaling.

The selectins are a group of three receptors that terminate in a membrane-distal carbohydrate-recognition domain related to those in Ca^{2+}-dependent (C-type) animal lectins such as the hepatic asialoglycoprotein receptor (see Figs. 12.1 and 12.2). L-selectin is expressed on leukocytes, E-selectin on cytokine-activated endothelium, and P-selectin on macrophages, platelets, and endothelial cells exposed to secretagogues such as thrombin or histamine (Table 12.4). The selectins mediate leukocyte adhesion to platelets, endothelium, or other

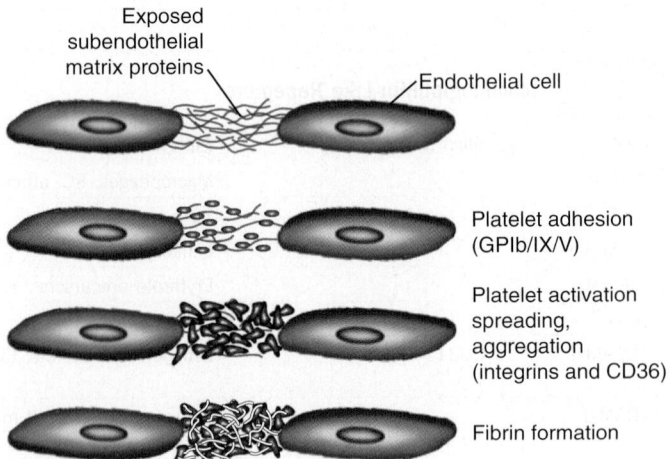

Fig. 12.2 PLATELET ADHESION AND AGGREGATION. In response to arterial injury under high shear forces, platelets rapidly adhere to the subendothelial matrix of injured vessels. The initial contacts are made between GPIb–IX–V on platelets and von Willebrand factor (vWF) in the matrix. These molecular interactions help activate platelets, thereby increasing the affinity of several platelet integrins for other adhesive matrix proteins such as fibronectin, laminin, and collagen. GPVI further activates platelets by binding to collagen. CD36 also interacts with both collagen and thrombospondin. Fibrinogen cross-links activated platelets into aggregates by binding to α$_{IIb}$β$_3$ integrins. The platelet plug then serves as an efficient surface for generation of thrombin and fibrin. *GP*, Glycoprotein.

leukocytes through Ca^{2+}-dependent interactions of the carbohydrate-recognition domains with cell-surface carbohydrates on apposing cells. High-affinity binding appears to require specific carbohydrate structures displayed on a limited number of membrane GPs. The best-characterized GP ligands for selectins are mucins, which have large numbers of clustered, sialylated *O*-linked oligosaccharides. Site-specific construction of *O*-glycans with specific sialylated, fucosylated, and (in some cases) sulfated moieties is required for these mucins to bind optimally to selectins. In the case of one mucin, P-selectin GP ligand-1 (PSGL-1), sulfation of tyrosine residues near a specific *O*-glycan is required for binding to P- and L-selectin.

Dendritic cells and related macrophages express a novel group of C-type lectins, of which the best characterized is dendritic cell-specific ICAM-3-grabbing nonintegrin (DC-SIGN). DC-SIGN binds to particular oligosaccharides on ICAMs, thereby regulating T-cell and dendritic cell function during antigen presentation. It also binds to glycans on a variety of pathogens, which may have critical roles in innate immunity. Natural killer cells express a different group of proteins, with some containing membrane-distal C-type lectin-like domains (e.g., NKG2D). Although these receptors are important for interactions of natural killer cells with target cells, they may bind to proteins rather than to glycoconjugates.

Siglecs are a subgroup of membrane proteins of the immunoglobulin superfamily that bind to carbohydrates instead of to proteins (see Table 12.2). The first two amino-terminal (*N*-terminal) domains appear to be necessary and sufficient for carbohydrate recognition. The *N*-terminal domain is a V-type structure that includes an unusual disulfide bond that is not found in the more common C-type immunoglobulin domains. Siglecs bind well to sialylated glycans on some but not all GPs. Different siglecs preferentially recognize sialic acid that is linked α2,6-, α2,8-, or α2,3- to an underlying galactose residue. Most siglecs have immune receptor tyrosine-based inhibitory motifs and transmit inhibitory signals. Siglecs can form *cis* interactions with other GPs on the same cell or *trans* interactions with GPs on another cell. The best-characterized example is CD22, which negatively regulates B-cell activation when it engages sialylated GPs. Sialoadhesin, expressed on BM macrophages, may regulate hematopoietic cell differentiation.

LIGAND BINDING VERSUS CELL ADHESION

As with all noncovalent macromolecular interactions, adhesion molecules bind to each other with equilibrium affinities that are defined by their association and dissociation rates. However, the efficiency of cell adhesion is not simply a function of the solution-phase equilibrium affinities of adhesion molecules for one another. Adhesion molecules in cell membranes and matrix are limited primarily to two dimensions, and even low-affinity molecular interactions may stabilize adhesion if there is time for sufficient bonds to form along the plane of cell contact. The efficiency of cell attachment and the ensuing strength of adhesion reflect multiple factors that dictate the probability of formation of bonds between adhesion molecules on cell or matrix surfaces. The kinetics of bond formation and dissociation are especially important for certain kinds of cell adhesion. Furthermore, interactions between cell adhesion molecules are subjected to force, which affects the lifetimes of adhesive bonds. This is particularly true in the circulation, where platelets and leukocytes must rapidly adhere to the blood vessel wall and withstand forces applied by the wall shear stresses of flowing blood. Other factors that affect bond formation include the number of adhesion molecules on a cell or matrix surface, the distance the binding domain of an adhesion receptor protrudes from the cell membrane, the lateral mobility of receptors, receptor dimerization, and the clustering of receptors on microvilli or other membrane domains. Cell adhesion can be further stabilized by events that occur after the initial interactions of adhesion molecules. For example, the cytoplasmic domains of many adhesion molecules bind to cytoskeletal components, allowing clustering of receptors into surface patches that strengthen adhesion, thereby promoting cell spreading or migration.

TABLE 12.5	Regulation of Adhesion Receptors	
Mechanism	**Example**	
Synthesis	Erythroid precursor synthesis of α$_5$β$_1$	
	Lymphocyte synthesis of CD44	
	Cytokine-induced synthesis of E-selectin, P-selectin, ICAM-1, and VCAM-1 by endothelial cells	
Surface expression	Proteolytic cleavage of L-selectin from leukocytes	
	Redistribution of P-selectin from granule membranes to plasma membrane of platelets and endothelial cells	
	Endocytosis of P- and E-selectin on endothelial cells	
Ligand affinity	Activation-induced increased affinity of many integrins for their ligands	
	Activation-induced increased affinity of CD44 for hyaluronan	

For abbreviations, see Table 12.1 footnotes.

REGULATION OF ADHESION RECEPTORS

To prevent inappropriate interactions of cells with each other or with the ECM, the expression and function of adhesion receptors must be tightly controlled. Three primary control mechanisms are used: (1) the rate of synthesis of the receptor, (2) the time during which the receptor is displayed on the cell surface, and (3) the binding affinity or avidity of the receptor for ligands (Table 12.5). All of these mechanisms are used to control interactions of blood and vascular cells.

REGULATION OF SYNTHESIS

The synthesis of many adhesion receptors is regulated. Erythroid precursors synthesize integrins that mediate their interactions with stromal cells and with ECM in the BM. As the precursors mature, synthesis ceases, resulting in loss of expression of cell-surface integrins by the time a mature erythrocyte enters the circulation. Lymphocyte precursors synthesize CD44 during differentiation in the BM, stop synthesis before release, and resume synthesis during maturation in the thymus. On exposure to antigens, immunologically naive lymphocytes synthesize increased amounts of several adhesion receptors and chemokine receptors during their conversion to the effector phenotypes; this process presumably allows these cells to become more adhesive in response to a subsequent antigenic challenge. Endothelial cells in postcapillary venules of the peripheral vasculature express very low, if any, levels of adhesion molecules that bind leukocytes. When exposed to inflammatory cytokines such as tumor necrosis factor-α and interleukin-1 (IL-1) or bacterial endotoxin, endothelial cells transiently increase synthesis of E- and P-selectin, ICAM-1, and VCAM-1, resulting in an adhesive surface for leukocytes.

REGULATION OF SURFACE EXPRESSION

The surface expression of some adhesion receptors is tightly controlled. L-selectin is present on the plasma membrane of leukocytes, where it is available to bind to ligands on the endothelial cell surface. Stimulation of the leukocyte causes L-selectin to be shed into the plasma by proteolytic cleavage. P-selectin is constitutively synthesized by megakaryocytes (where it is incorporated into platelets) and by endothelial cells. Rather than being directly delivered to the plasma membrane, it is sorted into secretory storage granules: the α granules of platelets and the Weibel–Palade bodies of endothelial cells. On stimulation of these cells by agonists such as thrombin, P-selectin is rapidly transported to the cell surface during fusion of granule membranes with the plasma membrane. When they are on the surface of the endothelium, both E-selectin and P-selectin are internalized and delivered to lysosomes for degradation. The cytoplasmic domain of

P-selectin contains signals that direct sorting into secretory granules, internalization through coated pits of the plasma membrane, and movement from endosomes to lysosomes; the latter two signals are probably also present in the cytoplasmic domain of E-selectin. The net result of these events is to control the duration of exposure of E- and P-selectin on the endothelium, where they can mediate adhesion of leukocytes. Activation of leukocytes also mobilizes a pool of β₂ integrins from storage compartments to the plasma membrane, although some of these molecules are also constitutively expressed on the cell surface. Finally, platelet activation redistributes a portion of the GPIb–IX–V complexes from ligand-accessible positions on the plasma membrane to sequestered, invaginated membrane domains known as the *surface-connected canalicular system*. This process, which requires interactions of the cytoplasmic domain of GPIb–IX–V with the cytoskeleton, may serve to downregulate GPIb-mediated adhesion of platelets to immobilized vWF.

REGULATION OF BINDING AFFINITY

Regulation of binding affinity is an important control mechanism for other adhesion receptors. Many integrins are constitutively present on the cell surface but interact poorly with their ligands. Cell activation by a number of agonists induces conformational changes in integrins so that they effectively recognize their ligands. An example is the $\alpha_{IIb}\beta_3$ integrin, which requires platelet stimulation to bind fibrinogen; if this binding affinity were not regulated, circulating platelets would indiscriminately aggregate in the fibrinogen-rich plasma milieu. The cytoplasmic domains of integrins can exert both positive and negative influences on binding affinity. Binding of specific cytoplasmic proteins to these domains may propagate structural changes to the extracellular ligand-binding regions of the integrins. Three-dimensional structures of integrins suggest that the integrin "headpiece" that contains the ligand-binding site faces down toward the membrane in the inactive conformation and rapidly extends upward in a "switchblade"-like opening motion on activation. Low-affinity ligand binding may stabilize some active conformations of integrins, perhaps explaining why integrins on unactivated cells will sometimes bind to immobilized, multivalent adhesive proteins but not to the same proteins in solution. Cellular activation may also regulate the binding avidities of CD44, L-selectin, P-selectin, and some integrins through changes in membrane distribution engineered by interactions of their cytoplasmic domains with the cytoskeleton or with clathrin-coated pits.

CELL SIGNALLING THROUGH ADHESION MOLECULES

In addition to their roles in cell–cell and cell–matrix contacts, adhesion molecules may cause cell signaling through indirect or direct mechanisms. Proteoglycans in the ECM can sequester growth factors that can be released to bind to surface receptors on nearby cells. Some chemoattractants bind to proteoglycans on the surface of endothelial cells, where they can activate adherent leukocytes. Binding of adhesive ligands to cell-surface integrins, GPIb–IX–V, CD44, cadherins, CD36, PECAM-1, selectins, ICAM-1 and VCAM-1, and perhaps other receptors can directly trigger intracellular events. The consequences of such signaling include changes in affinity or avidity of other adhesion receptors for their ligands, shape change, secretion, proliferation, synthesis of cytokines and other molecules, and migration. In some cases, binding of a monovalent adhesive ligand to a receptor may induce a signal. More commonly, signaling requires cross-linking of several receptors through interactions with multivalent ligands in matrix or on apposing cells.

Many studies of adhesion receptor signaling have focused on integrins. Binding of the same ligand to different integrins can mediate different responses in the same cell. Furthermore, ligand binding to the same integrin expressed in different cells can result in different signals. These data suggest that very specific interactions occur between ligand-occupied integrins and intracellular components. The cytoplasmic domains of integrins are essential for initiating signaling.

Tyrosine kinases have been localized at the interaction zones between integrins, the cytoskeleton and several adaptor and effector molecules, and tyrosine phosphorylation of a number of proteins accompanies integrin-mediated cell signaling. Tyrosine phosphorylation initiates a cascade of signaling events, including the activation of serine/threonine kinases, which cause a variety of cellular responses. Ligand binding to integrins also results in generation of lipid second messengers, alkalization of the cytoplasm, and influxes of Ca²⁺.

COOPERATIVE INTERACTIONS BETWEEN SIGNALING AND ADHESION MOLECULES

Signaling and adhesion molecules frequently function cooperatively in sequential cascades to enhance the specificity of cell adhesion. Three examples of how these cooperative interactions facilitate blood cell responses are described next.

Platelet Adhesion and Aggregation

At sites of blood vessel injury in the arterial circuit, platelets rapidly tether to and then translocate or roll along the damaged vessel through reversible interactions of GPIb–IX–V receptors with immobilized vWF exposed in the subendothelial matrix of injured vessels (Fig. 12.3). These interactions are facilitated by arterial flow, perhaps because of complex effects of high wall shear stresses on the lifetimes of bonds between GPIb and vWF. An important feature of this initial reversible adhesive event is that prior activation of the platelets is not required. After adhesion, however, the interaction of immobilized vWF with GPIb receptors triggers intracellular signals that lead to platelet activation. These signals synergize with those produced by engagement of the collagen receptor GPVI. Platelet activation, in turn, increases the affinity of platelet integrins for collagen and fibronectin, which stabilizes adhesion. Binding of these ligands transduces signals that propagate further activation responses such as spreading, secretion of granule contents, and recruitment of additional platelets through cell–cell contact mediated by binding of fibrinogen to activated $\alpha_{IIb}\beta_3$ integrins. This adhesion cascade allows

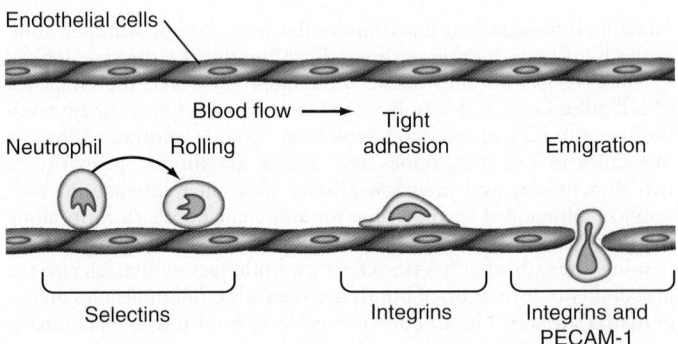

Fig. 12.3 NEUTROPHIL ROLLING, SPREADING, AND EMIGRATION. At sites of tissue injury or infection, neutrophils first roll on the endothelial cells in postcapillary venules. These transient adhesive interactions are mediated by activation-induced transcription-dependent expression of E- or P-selectin on the endothelial cell surface. E- and P-selectin bind to carbohydrate ligands on the neutrophil. These molecular bonds can form under the shear forces in the venular circulation. The rolling neutrophils are then activated by locally generated inflammatory mediators that increase the affinity of β₂ integrins for immunoglobulin-like receptors such as intercellular adhesion molecule-1 (ICAM-1) on the endothelium. These bonds slow rolling and then promote firm adhesion to the endothelium. Neutrophil migration between endothelial cells into tissues at the site of infection requires disengagement of old adhesive bonds and formation of new bonds among integrins, PECAM-1, and their respective ligands. *PECAM-1*, Platelet and endothelial cell adhesion molecule-1.

unstimulated platelets to home to the site of vascular injury and then be activated by locally generated mediators.

Neutrophil Rolling, Spreading, and Migration

Near sites of extravascular bacterial infections, neutrophils first tether to and roll on the endothelial surface of venules through the interactions of selectins with cell-surface carbohydrate ligands (Fig. 12.3). Little, if any, leukocyte adhesion occurs in nearby arterioles. Neutrophil rolling on the endothelium occurs under shear forces, just as platelets adhere to subendothelial matrix under shear forces, although the shear flow in postcapillary venules is lower than that in arterioles. Rolling requires a balance between the formation of selectin–ligand bonds at the leading edge of the cell and the dissociation of bonds at the trailing edge of the cell. Whereas shear forces affect the lifetimes of selectin–ligand bonds, lower forces prolong lifetimes (catch bonds) and higher forces shorten lifetimes (slip bonds). Catch bonds help explain why a minimum shear force is required to support leukocyte rolling, particularly through L-selectin. Just as the initial adhesion to vWF does not require prior activation of platelets, selectin-mediated rolling does not require prior activation of neutrophils. Instead, locally generated inflammatory mediators induce expression of E- or P-selectin on the endothelial cell surface. The requirement for activation of endothelial cells rather than leukocytes allows the latter to adhere to vessels only at the site of vessel inflammation. After being situated on the vessel wall through selectin-mediated contacts, however, the neutrophils become exposed to activators such as platelet-activating factor, a phospholipid signaling molecule, activated complement proteins, and interleukin-8 (IL-8), a potent chemoattractant cytokine or chemokine, both of which are presented on the surface of activated endothelial cells. These signals cooperate with others directed by engagement of selectin ligands and promote very slow rolling of neutrophils on the surface of activated endothelium. Neutrophil activation increases the affinity of β_2 integrins for immunoglobulin counterreceptors on the endothelial cell surface such as ICAM-1. Although flowing cells cannot form these bonds, neutrophils rolling on selectins can do so because of their slower velocities. The integrin–ICAM interactions further slow rolling and then arrest the cells on the endothelium. The leukocytes then migrate, presumably because of disengagement of integrin–ICAM bonds and redistribution of integrins to the leading edge of the cell, where new bonds form. Interactions of leukocytes with JAMs and PECAM-1 and other molecules at interendothelial cell junctions facilitate transendothelial migration of the neutrophils into the underlying tissues. Adhesion of leukocytes to the endothelium disrupts cytoskeletal tethers to the endothelial cadherins; this disruption leads to dissociation of homotypical cadherin interactions that normally prevent passage of leukocytes. Both the integrin- and the PECAM-1–mediated adhesive events may signal cytoskeletal redistributions in leukocytes that enhance migration toward chemotactic molecules released in the vicinity of the infection. When leukocytes enter in the tissues, integrin recognition of ECM protein ligands may trigger secretion of proteolytic enzymes and production of superoxide anions, both required for optimal bactericidal function.

Adhesion of T Cells to Antigen-Presenting Cells

The initial engagement of T cells with antigen-presenting cells requires that the TCR ($\alpha\beta$ TCR) recognize antigen presented by the polymorphic domain of MHC molecules (Fig. 12.4). Subsequent interactions include the binding of CD8 or CD4 to MHC class I or II molecules, respectively, plus the binding of CD2 to LFA-3 and CD28 binding to B7 molecules. These molecular contacts are all of low affinity but are highly specific because they first require specific antigen presentation to the appropriate T cell. The combination of these binding events triggers inside-out signals that increase the affinity of LFA-1 ($\alpha_L\beta_2$), a β_2 integrin on T cells, for its ligand ICAM-1 on antigen-presenting cells, strengthening and prolonging the length of time cells stably adhere. During this time, the T cell is further

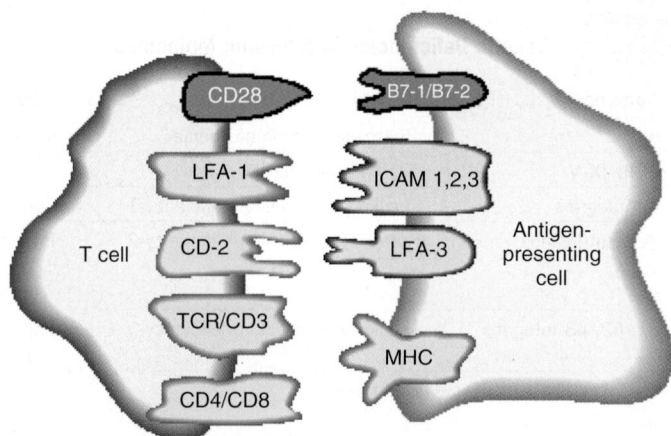

Fig. 12.4 ADHESION BETWEEN T LYMPHOCYTES AND ANTIGEN-PRESENTING CELLS. The initial contact is mediated by the TCR, or CD3, which binds with low affinity but high specificity to a specific antigen presented by a MHC molecule. Additional contacts, also of low affinity, are between CD4 (on helper cells) or CD8 (on cytotoxic cells) and MHC, and between costimulatory molecules CD2 and LFA-3 and CD28 and CD80 (B7-1) and CD86 (B7-2). These interactions signal the T cell to transiently increase the affinity of the β_2 integrin LFA-1 for ICAM-1 on the antigen-presenting cell. These bonds strengthen adhesion, and the costimulatory molecules transduce sustained and additional signals to the T cell that cause increased gene transcription, proliferation, and cytokine secretion. Not shown is the redistribution of these adhesion molecules into different regions of the contact zone as adhesion strengthens. Additional signals result from binding of β_1 integrins on the T cell to adhesive proteins in the extracellular matrix. *LFA-3*, Leukocyte function-associated antigen-3; *MHC*, major histocompatibility complex; *TCR*, T-cell receptor.

activated by a second or costimulatory signal delivered by T-cell CD28 binding to B7 molecules expressed by antigen-presenting cells. Together these interactions drive TCR-induced gene activation (IL-2 production) and cell proliferation and differentiation into different effector T cells that exit the secondary lymph node and migrate to immune reactions (see Chapter 21 for detailed discussion of T-cell–antigen-presenting cell activation).

The first principle of these three responses is that the initial adhesive event, although relatively limited, is highly specific. Thus, platelets bind to exposed subendothelial matrix in injured vessels, neutrophils bind to hyperadhesive endothelium near the site of infection, and T cells bind to cells presenting specific antigen in secondary lymph nodes. The second principle is that subsequent activation events strengthen cell adhesion and lead to further responses such as secretion, fibrin formation, cellular migration, and release of cytotoxic mediators or cell activation and proliferation. Activation often results from cooperative signaling by soluble agonists and by binding of ligands to adhesion receptors. Costimulation by multiple signals can amplify and provide specificity to cellular responses by mechanisms not always feasible for individual mediators. Thus, adhesion and cell signaling are highly interrelated processes.

The process of reversing cell adhesion, although less well understood, is equally important for the control of cell behavior. Some molecules such as the selectins can be proteolytically cleaved or internalized. The activation-induced increases in affinity of integrins and CD44 for their ligands are generally transient, but the mechanisms for return to the inactive conformation are obscure.

ALTERED EXPRESSION OF ADHESION MOLECULES

The highly regulated nature of adhesive events by hematopoietic cells suggests that defects in or excessive expression of adhesion molecules may contribute to the pathogenesis of disease. A variety of clinical observations support this hypothesis.

TABLE 12.6	Genetic Deficiencies in Adhesion Molecules			
Molecule	**Disease**	**Laboratory Finding(s)**		**Clinical Finding(s)**
$\alpha_{IIb}\beta_3$	Glanzmann thrombasthenia	Impaired platelet aggregation		Mucocutaneous bleeding
GPIb–IX–V	Bernard–Soulier syndrome	Impaired platelet adhesion to vWF		Mucocutaneous bleeding
β2 integrins	Leukocyte adhesion deficiency-1	Impaired adhesion of activated leukocytes to EC		Frequent infections
Selectin ligands	Leukocyte adhesion deficiency-2	Impaired fucose metabolism resulting in defective carbohydrate ligands for selectins, impaired rolling of leukocytes on venules		Frequent infections
β1, β2, β3 integrins	Leukocyte adhesion deficiency-3	Impaired platelet adhesion and aggregation and impaired adhesion of activated leukocytes to EC		Mucocutaneous bleeding and frequent infections

For abbreviations, see Table 12.1 footnotes.

Genetic Deficiencies in Adhesion Molecules

Genetic deficiencies in platelet adhesion receptors such as the GPIb complex (as in Bernard–Soulier syndrome) and the $\alpha_{IIb}\beta_3$ integrin (as in Glanzmann thrombasthenia) result in hemorrhagic symptoms similar to those in patients with thrombocytopenia (Table 12.6). Genetic deficiencies in the leukocyte β_2 integrins (as in leukocyte adhesion deficiency-1) are associated with frequent severe bacterial infections and a failure of neutrophils to enter the infected tissues. Similar symptoms are seen in patients with a congenital defect in fucose metabolism that prevents synthesis of the carbohydrate ligands for selectins (leukocyte adhesion deficiency-2). A recently identified set of patients has both hemorrhagic symptoms and life-threatening infections (leukocyte adhesion deficiency-3). The molecular mechanism is attributable to mutations in an intracellular protein kindlin-3, which binds to β_1, β_2, and β_3 integrin cytoplasmic tails upon cell activation. These patients have normal levels of integrin surface expression (see Table 12.6).

Dysregulated Expression of Adhesion Molecules

Inappropriate expression of adhesion molecules has been implicated in thrombotic and inflammatory disorders and in tumor metastasis. For example, erythrocytes from patients with sickle cell anemia adhere to each other, to leukocytes, and to the endothelium, contributing to vasoocclusive crises. These adhesive events may reflect, in part, the expression of integrins and selectin ligands not normally found on mature erythrocytes. Inappropriate adhesion and activation of platelets on exposed atherosclerotic plaques may contribute to thrombosis and acute ischemic coronary artery syndromes. Dysregulated expression of selectins on the endothelium of ischemic blood vessels during myocardial infarction or shock may contribute to neutrophil-mediated tissue necrosis after reperfusion of the vessel. Mediators released while the neutrophils are adherent in the reperfused vessels may activate integrin function, strengthening adhesion and generating further signals that release destructive oxygen radicals and proteases within the vasculature. Finally, malignant cells appear to use molecules normally used for adhesion of blood cells to promote metastatic spread through interactions with platelets, endothelial cells, and extravascular matrix.

These examples underscore the importance of proper regulation of adhesion molecule expression in the physiology of blood cells.

SUGGESTED READINGS

Alcaide P, Auerbach S, Luscinskas FW: Neutrophil recruitment under shear flow: It's all about endothelial cell rings and gaps. *Microcirculation* 16:43, 2009. Erratum in: *Microcirculation* 16:782, 2009.

Berndt MC, Shen Y, Dopheide SM, et al: The vascular biology of the glycoprotein Ib-IX-V complex. *Thromb Haemost* 86:178, 2001.

Cambi A, Koopman M, Figdor CG: How C-type lectins detect pathogens. *Cell Microbiol* 7:481, 2005.

Cao H, Crocker PR: Evolution of CC33-related siglecs: Regulating host immune functions and escaping pathogen exploitation? *Immunology* 132:18, 2010.

Chen J, Lopez JA: Interactions of platelets with subendothelium and endothelium. *Microcirculation* 12:235, 2005.

Dinauer MC: Disorders of neutrophil function: An overview. *Methods Mol Biol* 1124:501–515, 2014.

Fooksman DR, Vardhana S, Vasiliver-Shamis G, et al: Functional anatomy of T cell activation and synapse formation. *Annu Rev Immunol* 28:79, 2010.

Hickey MJ, Kubes P: Intravascular immunity: The host-pathogen encounter in blood vessels. *Nat Rev Immunol* 9:364, 2009.

Hogg N, Patzak I, Willenbrock F: The insider's guide to leukocyte integrin signalling and function. *Nat Rev Immunol* 11:416, 2011.

Hynes RO: Integrins: Bidirectional, allosteric signaling machines. *Cell* 110:673, 2002.

Kfoury Y, Scadden DT: Mesenchymal cell contributions to the stem cell niche. *Cell Stem Cell* 16:239, 2015.

Koppel EA, van Gisbergen KP, Geijtenbeek TB, et al: Distinct functions of DC-SIGN and its homologues L-SIGN (DC-SIGNR) and mSIGNR1 in pathogen recognition and immune regulation. *Cell Microbiol* 7:157, 2005.

McEver RP: Adhesive interactions of leukocytes, platelets, and the vessel wall during hemostasis and inflammation. *Thromb Haemost* 86:746, 2001.

McEver RP, Zhu C: Rolling cell adhesion. *Annu Rev Cell Dev Biol* 26:363, 2010.

Mendelson A, Frenette PS: Hematopoietic stem cell niche maintenance during homeostasis and regeneration. *Nat Med* 20:833, 2014.

Muller WA: Mechanisms of leukocyte transendothelial migration. *Annu Rev Pathol* 28:323, 2011.

Ponta H, Sherman L, Herrlich PA: CD44: From adhesion molecules to signalling regulators. *Nat Rev Mol Cell Biol* 4:33, 2003.

Ruggeri ZM: Platelet adhesion under flow. *Microcirculation* 16:58, 2009.

Shattil SJ, Kim C, Ginsberg MH: The final steps of integrin activation: The end game. *Nat Rev Mol Cell Biol* 11:288, 2010.

Sperandio M, Gleissner CA, Ley K: Glycosylation in immune cell trafficking. *Immunol Rev* 230:97, 2009.

Springer TA, Wang JH: The three-dimensional structure of integrins and their ligands, and conformational regulation of cell adhesion. *Adv Protein Chem* 68:29, 2004.

Tailor A, Cooper D, Granger DN: Platelet-vessel wall interactions in the microcirculation. *Microcirculation* 12:275, 2005.

Vestweber D, Winderlich M, Cagna G, et al: Cell adhesion dynamics at endothelial junctions: VE-cadherin as a major player. *Trends Cell Biol* 19:8, 2009.

Wang H, Lim D, Rudd CE: Immunopathologies linked to integrin signalling. *Semin Immunopathol* 32:173, 2010.

CHEMOKINES AND HEMATOPOIETIC CELL TRAFFICKING

Antal Rot, Steffen Massberg, Alexander G. Khandoga, and
Ulrich H. von Andrian

The mammalian immune system has evolved to mount multifaceted molecular and cellular microbicidal responses tailored and custom-adapted to eliminate an endless variety of infectious agents and, at the same time, remain tolerant to self-antigens. Accomplishing these tasks requires continuous movement of billions of motile immune cells that roam throughout the body along distinct nonrandom traffic routes from one tissue to another using blood and lymphatic vessels as avenues for rapid access. Migratory pathways characteristic for distinct immune cell subsets are integral parts of their functional make-up determined in the process of cell differentiation and activation. During development in the bone marrow (BM) or thymus, or following stimulation by antigens or pathogen-associated molecules, immune cells acquire the expression of characteristic repertoires of cell surface molecules that enable and restrict their migration to defined tissues and microenvironments. For example, naive lymphocytes largely disregard inflammatory tissue sites, but migrate efficiently into secondary lymphoid organs. Conversely, innate immune cells and antigen-experienced lymphocytes can respond to inflammation-induced traffic cues, although some subsets also enter noninflamed lymphoid and nonlymphoid target tissues.[1-4] Notably, not only mature leukocytes but also hematopoietic stem cells (HSCs) and progenitor cells, and other rare cell subsets recirculate throughout the body.[5-13] The characteristic trafficking routes of leukocyte subpopulations are determined by their expression of cell surface adhesion molecules and chemoattractant receptors. Chemoattractants are generated in target sites and signal through their cognate receptors on leukocytes to induce their emigration and directed locomotion within the tissues. Leukocyte chemoattractants include a number of lipid mediators, microbial factors, complement fragment 5a and, most importantly, members of the chemokine family. This chapter discusses chemokines as master navigation signals for leukocyte trafficking and then focuses on specific trafficking pathways that direct leukocyte subsets to distinct target tissues.

CHEMOKINES IN CONTROL OF LEUKOCYTE TRAFFICKING

Chemokines (a clipping blend of *chemo*tactic cyto*kines*) are critical molecular messengers in the complex cellular communication network used by the immune system. Almost 50 human chemokines have been identified to date (Table 13.1).[14-18] However, due to the existence of different splice variants and enzymatically processed forms the number of individual functionally distinct chemokine molecules is much higher. The two major subclasses of chemokines are designated CC- or CXC-, depending on the relative position of the two proximal to the N-terminus canonical cysteines, being either adjacent or separated by a single amino acid, respectively. XCL1 and XCL2, and CX3CL1 constitute two additional structural chemokine forms with one cysteine and three amino acids between the two canonical cysteines, respectively. CX3CL1 and another chemokine, CXCL16, are associated with a cell membrane via a long spacer sequence and anchored by a transmembrane domain; however, both these chemokines can be cleaved of their stalks and give rise to functional soluble molecules. All other chemokines are secreted proteins of 67 to 127 amino acids. Historically, chemokines have been grouped into functional subfamilies termed *inflammatory* and *homeostatic* chemokines. The former are induced by inflammatory

signals and control the recruitment of effector leukocytes in infection, inflammation, tissue injury, and malignancies, whereas the latter navigate leukocytes during hematopoiesis in the BM and in the thymus during initiation of adaptive immune responses in secondary lymphoid organs and in immune surveillance of healthy peripheral tissues. However, it is now clear that such functional distinction is largely blurred, as many "inflammatory" chemokines are produced under physiologic conditions and the expression of "homeostatic" chemokines is upregulated in inflammation.

Chemokine signals are transmitted through specific cell-surface G protein–coupled receptors (GPCRs) with seven transmembrane domains.[19-23] The human chemokine receptor repertoire identified at present consists of 20 different GPCRs (Table 13.2).[24] The tremendous specificity and plasticity of leukocyte homing and tissue localization is largely determined by the interactions of chemokines with their cognate receptors. Individual leukocyte subsets express characteristic fingerprints of chemokine receptors, and each chemokine receptor binds defined sets of chemokines, albeit with various binding affinities and resulting in a spectrum of downstream of responses, from agonism to antagonism.[25,26] Chemokine receptors function as allosteric molecular relays where chemokine binding to the extracellular portion modifies the tertiary structure of the receptor. This allows the intracellular domain of the engaged receptor to bind to and activate heterotrimeric G proteins. In response, the activated G proteins exchange GDP for GTP, and in the process dissociate into Gα and Gβγ subunits. The dissociated Gβγ subunits mediate most chemokine-induced signals by activating different phosphatidylinositol 3-kinase (PI3K) isoforms, leading to the formation of phosphatidyl-3,4,5-triphosphate (PIP_3). PI3K and its product PIP_3 then translocate to the pseudopod at the leading edge of migrating leukocytes, where they colocalize with the small GTPase Rac.[27-30] PIP_3 activates Rac through specific guanine nucleotide exchange factors.[31,32] Rac in turn acts through the downstream effectors p21-activated kinase and the Wiskott-Aldrich syndrome protein homologue WAVE, which stimulate actin-related protein 2/3. Together, this process induces focal polymerization, required for the development and forward extension of the pseudopod, a critical step in leukocyte chemotaxis.[33] The importance of PI3K-dependent signaling for leukocyte chemotaxis is evidenced by the lack of migration of myeloid leukocytes to chemokines in mice lacking PI3Kγ.[34-39] Notably, though, distinct signaling pathways or at least other PI3K isoforms appear to be involved in the trafficking of immune cells. For example, neutrophil and B-cell migration requires PI3Kδ[42-45], whereas T-cell chemotaxis is not impaired in PI3K-deficient mice, but depends on the Rac guanine exchange factor DOCK2.[40-42]

Different pathways have been identified that can terminate chemokine signaling through their GPCRs. The Gα subunit possesses an intrinsic GTPase activity to hydrolyze GTP. In a negative-feedback loop this GTPase activity allows the Gα subunits to reassociate with the Gβγ subunits, thereby restoring the heterotrimeric G protein to its inactive state. In addition, another class of molecules, known as regulators of G protein signaling (RGS), also modulates signaling through chemokine GPCRs. RGS are a large and diverse protein family initially identified as GTPase-activating proteins of heterotrimeric G protein Gα-subunits.[43,44] At least some RGS can also influence Gα activity through either effector antagonism by competing with effector molecules for GTP-bound Gα-subunits or by acting as

TABLE 13.1   Chemokines and Chemokine Receptors

Chemokine	Chemokine Receptor	Chemokine	Chemokine Receptor
CC Family		CCL25 (TECK)	CCR9[a], ACKR4[d]
CCL1 (I309)	CCR8[a]	CCL26 (eotaxin-3)	CCR3[a], CCR2[b]
CCL2 (MCP-1)	CCR2[a], ACKR1[d], ACKR2[d]	CCL27 (CTACK)	CCR10[a]
CCL3 (MIP-1α)	CCR1[a], CCR5[a], ACKR2[d]	CCL28 (MEC)	CCR3[a], CCR10[a]
CCL3L1 (MIP-1αP)	CCR1[a], CCR3[a], CCR5[a], ACKR2[d]	**CXC Family**	
CCL4 (MIP-1β)	CCR5[a], ACKR2[d]	CXCL1 (GROα)	CXCR2[a], ACKR1[d]
CCL4L1 (MIP-1β2)	CCR5[a], ACKR2[d]	CXCL2 (GROβ)	CXCR2[a], ACKR1[d]
CCL5 (RANTES)	CCR1[a], CCR3[a], CCR5[a], ACKR2[d], ACKR2[d]	CXCL3 (GROγ)	CXCR2[a], ACKR1[d]
CCL7 (MCP-3)	CCR1[a], CCR2[a], CCR3[a], CCR5[b], ACKR1[d], ACKR2[d]	CXCL4 (PF4)	CXCR3B[a]
CCL8 (MCP-2)	CCR1[a], CCR2[a], CCR3[a], CCR5[a], ACKR1[d], ACKR2[d]	CXCL5 (ENA-78)	CXCR2[a], ACKR1[d]
		CXCL6 (GCP2)	CXCR1[a], CXCR2[a], ACKR1[d]
CCL11 (eotaxin)	CCR2[b], CCR3[a], CCR5[a], CXCR3A[c], CXCR3B[c], ACKR1[d], ACKR2[d]	CXCL7 (NAP-2)	CXCR2[a], ACKR1[d]
CCL13 (MCP-4)	CCR1[a], CCR2[a], CCR3[a], ACKR1[d], ACKR2[d]	CXCL8 (interleukin-8)	CXCR1[a], CXCR2[a], ACKR1[d]
CCL14 (HCC1)	CCR1[a], CCR5[a], ACKR1[d], ACKR2[d]	CXCL9 (MIG)	CXCR3A[a], CXCR3B[a], CCR3[b]
CCL15 (HCC2, MIP-1δ)	CCR1[a], CCR3[a]	CXCL10 (IP-10)	CXCR3A[a], CXCR3B[a], CCR3[b]
CCL16 (HCC4)	CCR1[a], CCR2[a], CCR5[a]	CXCL11 (I-TAC)	CXCR3A[a], CXCR3B[a], CCR3[b], ACKR3[d]
CCL17 (TARC)	CCR4[a], ACKR1[d], ACKR2[d]	CXCL12 (SDF-1)	CXCR4[a], ACKR3[d]
CCL18 (PARC)	CCR1[a], CCR3[b]	CXCL13 (BCA-1)	CXCR5[a], ACKR4[d]
CCL19 (ELC)	CCR7[a], ACKR4[d]	CXCL14 (BRAK)	?
CCL20 (MIP-3β, LARC)	CCR6[a]	CXCL16 (SR-PSOX)	CXCR6[a]
CCL21 (SLC)	CCR7[a], ACKR4[d]	CXCL17	CXCR8
CCL22 (MDC)	CCR4[a], ACKR2[d]	**CX₃C Family**	
CCL23 (MPIF-1, SCYA23)	CCR1[a]	CX3CL1 (fractalkine)	CX3CR1[a]
CCL24 (Eotaxin-2)	CCR3[a]	**XC Family**	
		XCL1 (lymphotactin, SCM-1α)	XCR1[a]
		XCL2 (SCM-1β)	XCR1[a]

*For abbreviations, see Table 13.3.
[a]Agonistic interaction.
[b]Antagonistic interaction.
[c]Nonagonist–nonantagonistic interaction.
[d]"Atypical" receptor.

guanine nucleotide dissociation inhibitors.[43] To date, over three dozen genes have been identified within the human genome that encode proteins containing an RGS or RGS-like domain.

An additional mechanism of termination of chemokine signaling involves ligand-induced internalization of GPCRs from the cell membrane into intracellular vesicular compartments. Receptor internalization is triggered by intracellular domains of GPCRs associating with beta arrestins, which together with other potential intracellular effectors, is involved in G protein–independent signaling of GPCRs.[45] Internalized chemokines are targeted for lysosomal degradation, whereas GPCRs may be recycled onto the cell membrane.

In addition to GPCRs, most chemokines also bind to one or two of the four "atypical" chemokine receptors (ACKRs) identified to date.[46] Like GPCRs, these are serpentine membrane receptors with seven transmembrane domains. However, unlike GPCRs, ACKRs lack or have an altered DRYLAIV consensus motive in the second intracellular loop, which is required for G-protein coupling. Therefore upon chemokine binding ACKRs do not trigger signaling events characteristic of GPCRs and cannot mediate cell migration. However, ACKRs internalize chemokines and may target them either into lysosomes or alternatively into transcytotic pathways.[47] ACKRs may also transmit intracellular signals, independently of G proteins, for example, through triggering biochemical cascades downstream of beta arrestin or affect signaling through classical chemokine GPCRs

expressed by the same cell, possibly through receptor heterodimerization. Based on the chemokine-scavenging activity of ACKRs, it has been postulated that the main role of ACKRs is to reduce the overall chemokine levels in the tissues. However, because ACKRs are expressed in discrete and often sparse cellular microenvironments, they cannot affect chemokine availability in the tissues globally, but only at the immediate sites of their cellular expression. Thus, the key role of ACKRs may be only to determine in which tissue microenvironments chemokines may or may not exert their activities.[48] This is achieved either through chemokine scavenging or chemokine transport. Currently four ACKRs have been included in the nomenclature (Table 13.3) and shown to bind a broad range of chemokine ligands.[49]

Additional fine-tuning of chemokine communication is achieved by proteolytic cleavage and inactivation of chemokines, generating truncated chemokines with either increased or decreased receptor affinities and an altered spectrum of agonistic activities on different receptors. This adds a further layer of plasticity to the chemokine system. Proteases, such as dipeptidyl peptidase CD26, elastase, the ADAM (a disintegrin and metalloproteinase) family, as well as matrix metalloproteases (MMPs), have been implicated in the control of chemokine-mediated navigation of leukocyte trafficking.[50–53] MMPs are a family of more than 20 enzymes with important functions in matrix degradation. They also act on chemokines to regulate varied aspects of inflammation and immunity.[54] In fact, the ADAM family of disintegrins and metalloproteinases has been identified as

TABLE 13.2 Classical Chemokine Receptors

Receptor	Chemokine Ligands[a]	Cell Types
CC Family		
CCR1	CCL3 (MIP-1α), CCL5 (RANTES), CCL7 (MCP-3), CCL8 (MCP-1), CCL14 (HCC1), CCL15 (HCC2, MIP-1δ), CCL16 (HCC-4), CCL23 (MPIF)	T cells, monocytes, eosinophils, basophils
CCR2	CCL2 (MCP-1), CCL8 (MCP-2), CCL7 (MCP-3), CCL13 (MCP-4), CCL16 (HCC4)	Monocytes, dendritic cells (immature), memory T cells
CCR3	CCL11 (eotaxin), CCL13 (eotaxin-2), CCL7 (MCP-3), CCL5 (RANTES), CCL8 (MCP-2), CCL13 (MCP-4), CCL24 (eotaxin-2), CCL26 (eotaxin-3), CCL28 (MEC)	Eosinophils, basophils, mast cells, Th2, platelets
CCR4	CCL17 (TARC), CCL22 (MDC)	T cells (Th2), dendritic cells (mature), basophils, macrophages, platelets
CCR5	CCL3 (MIP-1α), CCL4 (MIP-1β), CCL5 (RANTES), CCL11 (eotaxin), CCL14 (HCC1), CCL16 (HCC4), CCL8 (MCP-2)	T cells, monocytes
CCR6	CCL20 (MIP-3β, LARC)	T cells (T regulatory and memory), B cells, dendritic cells
CCR7	CCL19 (ELC), CCL21 (SLC)	T cells, dendritic cells (mature), antigen-experienced B cells
CCR8	CCL1 (I309), CCL18 (PARC)	T cells (Th2), dendritic cells
CCR9	CCL25 (TECK)	T cells, IgA+ plasma cells
CCR10	CCL27 (CTACK), CCL28 (MEC)	T cells
CXC Family		
CXCR1	CXCL8 (interleukin-8), CXCL6 (GCP2)	Neutrophils, monocytes
CXCR2	CXCL8, CXCL1 (GROα), CXCL2 (GROβ), CXCL3 (GROγ), CXCL5 (ENA-78), CXCL6, CXCL7 (NAP-2)	Neutrophils, monocytes, microvascular endothelial cells
CXCR3-A	CXCL9 (MIG), CXCL10 (IP-10), CXCL11 (I-TAC)	Th1 helper cells, mast cells, mesangial cells
CXCR3-B	CXCL4 (PF4), CXCL9 (MIG), CXCL10 (IP-10), CXCL11 (I-TAC)	Microvascular endothelial cells, neoplastic cells
CXCR4	CXCL12 (SDF-1)	Widely expressed
CXCR5	CXCL13 (BCA-1)	B cells, T_{FH}
CXCR6	CXCL16 (SR-PSOX)	CD8+ T cells, natural killer cells, memory CD4+ T cells
CXCR8	CXCL17	Monocytes, T cells, neutrophils, dendritic cells
CX₃C Family		
CX₃CR1	CX3CL1 (fractalkine)	Macrophages, endothelial cells, smooth muscle cells
XC Family		
XCR1	XCL1 (lymphotactin), XCL2	T cells, natural killer cells

*For abbreviations, see Table 13.3.

TABLE 13.3 Atypical Chemokine Receptors

Receptor	Chemokine Ligands	Cell Types
ACKR1	CCL2 (MCP-1), CCL5 (RANTES), CCL7 (MCP-3), CCL8 (MCP-2), CCL11 (eotaxin), CCL13 (MCP-4), CCL14 (HCC1), CCL17 (TARC) CXCL1 (GROα), CXCL2 (GROβ), CXCL3 (GROγ), CXCL5 (ENA-78), CXCL6 (GCP-2), CXCL7 (NAP-2), CXCL8 (interleukin-8), CXCL11 (I-TAC)	Erythrocytes, blood endothelial cells, Purkinje neurons
ACKR2	CCL2 (MCP-1), CCL3 (MIP-1α), CCL4 (MIP-1β), CCL5 (RANTES), CCL7 (MCP-3), CCL8 (MCP-2), CCL11 (eotaxin), CCL13 (MCP-4), CCL14 (HCC1), CCL17 (TARC), CCL22 (MDC), CCL23 (MPIF-1, SCYA23), CCL24 (eotaxin-2)	Lymphatic endothelial cells, placenta syncytiotrophoblast, innate-like B cells, marginal zone B cells, dendritic cells, monocytes, tissue-resident mast cells, macrophages
ACKR3	CXCL11 (I-TAC), CXCL12 (SDF-1)	Blood endothelial cells in the brain, embryonic, and neonatal tissues, marginal zone B cells
ACKR4	CCL19 (ELC), CCL21 (SLC), CCL25 (TECK), CXCL13 (BCA-1)	Lymphatic endothelial cells lining the ceiling of the lymph node subcapsular sinus, thymic epithelial cells

BCA-1, B-cell chemoattractant 1; CTACK, cutaneous T cell–attracting chemokine; ELC, Epstein Barr virus–induced molecule 1 ligand chemokine; ENA, epithelial cell–derived neutrophil-activating peptide; GCP, granulocyte chemotactic protein; GRO, growth-regulated oncogene; HCC, hemofiltrate chemokine; IgA, immunoglobulin A; IP-10, interferon-inducible protein 10; I-TAC, interferon-inducible T-cell alpha chemoattractant; LARC, liver and activation-regulated chemokine; MCP, monocyte chemoattractant protein; MDC, macrophage-derived chemokine; MEC, mammary-enriched chemokine; MIG, monokine induced by interferon-γ; MIP, macrophage inflammatory protein; SDF-1, stromal cell–derived factor-1; SLC, secondary lymphoid-tissue chemokine; SR-PSOX, scavenger receptor for phosphatidylserine-containing oxidized lipids; TARC, thymus and activation-regulated chemokine; TECK, thymus-expressed chemokine; T_{FH}, follicular helper T cells.

the most relevant group of proteases implicated in the shedding of L-selectin, VCAM, as well as CX3CL1 and junctional adhesion molecule (JAM)-A, and thereby involved in facilitating the detachment of leukocytes.[55] In addition, chemokines such as CCL2, CXCL10, and CXCL12 are cleaved and inactivated by MMP-2 and MMP-9.[56,57] Apart from MMPs, proteases stored in neutrophil granules, in particular cathepsin G and elastase, inactivate chemokines such as CXCL12 and its receptor CXCR4 that regulate not only the migration of mature leukocytes but also the mobilization and homing of immature HSCs.[58,59] Hence, proteases by means of their chemokine-modifying properties must be regarded as integral components in the control of trafficking of mature leukocytes and their precursors.

In general, leukocyte trafficking can be classified into three distinct patterns of migration (1) entry into tissues from the circulation; (2) migration within tissues; and (3) exit from tissues. The following sections will discuss each of these steps in leukocyte trafficking.

LEUKOCYTE ENTRY INTO TISSUES

In order to leave the circulation and enter target tissues, leukocytes must engage in several sequential steps of adhesion to the endothelial cells, which most often take place in the venular segment of the circulatory tree.[27,60-65] Discrete individual adhesion steps are mediated by binding interactions of pairs of adhesion receptors and their counter-ligands expressed in trans-geometry by leukocytes and endothelial cells. The initial tethering of leukocytes to the endothelial cell is induced by adhesion molecules, which are able to rapidly bind their ligands with high tensile strength. The most important initiators of leukocyte tethering are selectins, expressed on leukocytes (L-selectin), endothelial cells (E- and P-selectin), and platelets (P-selectin). The most important selectin counter-ligands are sialomucins, which are decorated with oligosaccharides related to sialyl-Lewis[x], including P-selectin glycoprotein ligand (PSGL)-1 and the peripheral-node addressin (PNAd). Selectin-mediated adhesion bonds that are formed in the bloodstream are transient and do not allow prolonged, firm leukocyte arrest. As tethered leukocytes are pushed along the vessel wall by the blood flow, selectin bonds continuously dissociate at the upstream end of the cells and new ones form downstream, resulting in the slow rolling motion characteristic of leukocyte tethering. To undergo firm adhesion the rolling leukocyte must engage additional adhesion receptors that belong to the integrin family, particularly CD11a/CD18 (leukocyte function–associated antigen-1 [LFA-1]) and the α4 integrins, α4β1 (very late antigen [VLA]-4) and α4β7. Without exception, individual integrins are expressed by the subsets of leukocytes and their counter-ligands by the endothelial cells.

Whereas selectins are constitutively active, integrins first need to be activated to assume a high-affinity state that promotes efficient adhesion to endothelial ligands. Integrin activation is induced by chemoattractant signals that trigger a reversible change in integrin conformation (leading to enhanced ligand-binding affinity) or in integrin clustering (enhancing avidity), or both.[20] Some (but not all) chemokines presented on the luminal surface of microvascular endothelial cells can trigger rapid integrin activation and efficiently induce leukocyte arrest. The retention of chemokines on the vessel endothelium is mediated through binding to glycosaminoglycans (GAGs) in the luminal glycocalix. Chemokines that are produced in the extravascular space can be transported across the endothelial barrier to the luminal surface.[66] This process is triggered by chemokine binding to the atypical chemokine receptor ACKR1 (previously known as *Duffy antigen receptor for chemokines* [DARC]), which is also involved in luminal immobilization of chemokines.[47] ACKR1 expression by the endothelial cells characterizes only the venular but not the capillary or arterial segment of the circulatory tree.[67]

Chemokines signal through the Gα$_i$ subfamily of large heterotrimeric G proteins, which can be inhibited by pertussis toxin (PTX). Consequently, intravital microscopy studies have shown that lymphocytes treated with PTX undergo normal tethering and rolling

interactions in high endothelial venules (HEVs) in lymph nodes (LNs) and Peyer patches (PPs), but unlike control cells, the PTX-treated cells are unable to undergo integrin-dependent firm arrest. Chemokine receptor activation precipitates a cascade of intracellular signaling and adapter proteins, including Kindlin-3 and RAP-RAPL, which are involved in the so-called *inside-out signaling* that results in integrin activation. Modifications at the cytoplasmic tails of the integrin α and β chains are critical to regulate leukocyte adhesion to integrin ligands, such as the binding and spreading of neutrophils on intercellular cell adhesion molecule (ICAM)-1 and the complement C3 activation product, iC3b.[68] Once arrested, the adherent leukocytes rapidly polarize and slowly migrate within the vessel in random directions.[69-71] The intraluminal crawling is thought to be essential to enable leukocytes to find exit points within the vessel through which they can leave the vasculature.[27] A subset of monocytes crawl within uninflamed microvessels under steady-state conditions.[62,72,73] These patrolling monocytes are poised to provide immune surveillance of the endothelial cell surfaces and clear the intravascular debris,[73] but may also enter the extravascular space in response to damage and infection. Once emigrated, some monocyte cells may differentiate into macrophages or dendritic cells (DCs). In some tissues and organs, such as the intestine, monocyte emigration contributes throughout life to the replenishing of the resident macrophage pool.[72,74,75] In other tissues, macrophage and DC precursors home only during the embryonic period from either the liver or yolk sack, and the resident mature cells proliferate in situ to give rise to their progeny.[76,77]

The interactions between the β2-integrins LFA-1 and Mac-1 with endothelial ICAMs are required for intravascular adhesion and crawling. However, the specificity of these interactions differs between different leukocytes, such as neutrophils and monocytes.[69,72] Neutrophil luminal crawling is mainly mediated by Mac-1,[69] whereas monocytes and T cells use LFA-1.[1,72] Recent studies using blocking antibodies against Mac-1 and LFA-1 showed that crawling patterns of monocytes and neutrophils differ at steady state compared with those under inflammatory conditions; both LFA-1 and Mac-1 contribute to monocyte crawling; however, the LFA-1–dependent crawling in unstimulated venules becomes Mac-1 dependent upon inflammation. By contrast, Mac-1 alone is responsible for neutrophil crawling in both unstimulated and cytokine-stimulated venules.[78] This indicates that differences in monocyte and neutrophil crawling behavior result from involvement of different β2 integrins and consequently affect the next step of the leukocyte migration cascade: transendothelial migration.

Transendothelial migration or diapedesis is a critical event allowing leukocytes to cross the vascular wall and enter their target tissue. Two routes of leukocyte diapedesis have been observed: a paracellular route that dominates most extravasation processes, and a transcellular route reported for neutrophils and some T cells.[79-85] Both routes involve the action of apical and junctional endothelial ICAM-1, and, at least in some settings, vascular cell adhesion molecule-1 (VCAM-1). In inflammatory conditions, additional junctional endothelial ligands such as PECAM-1, vascular endothelial (VE)-cadherin, ESAM, CD99, CD99L2, and junctional adhesion molecule (JAMs) can contribute to leukocyte diapedesis.[80,86-92]

After penetration of the endothelial barrier, leukocytes may move further within the interstitium toward their target destinations in the tissue. This locomotion is considered to reflect in vivo chemotaxis, increased rate-directed cell locomotion driven by the putative gradients of chemoattractants.[93,94] Several signaling pathways have been proposed to be involved in this gradient-driven process, the most predominant being the PI3K pathway.[35] Thereby, leukocytes use an "internal compass" for sensing the direction of chemotactic gradients, and undergo polarization characterized by the formation of lamellipodia at the leading edge of the cell and an uropod at the trailing edge.[95,96] Chemokines released by a broad range of tissue cells, epithelial cells, stromal cells, mast cells, smooth muscle cells, fibroblasts, myocytes, and tissue-resident immune cells may form gradients and mediate the leukocyte chemotaxis in the interstitium. In this context, the spatiotemporal formation of chemokine gradients in the interstitial tissue may be supported by GAGs, which immobilize chemokines and, thus, determine the position and temporal persistence of chemokine gradients.[97,98] It has been shown that immobilized, substrate-bound chemokines are effective in inducing directed leukocyte migration, which is called *haptotaxis*.[99] It has also been suggested that efficient development of tissue chemokine gradients also requires, in addition to the free diffusion of chemokines from their cellular sources, scavenging of chemokines by their atypical chemokine receptors expressed by cells in apposition to chemokine sources.[100] Leukocytes moving within the interstitial tissue receive signals from neighboring cells as well as from the extracellular matrix, activate intracellular processes, release inflammatory mediators, and upregulate adhesion molecules and release enzymes.[101] Although neutrophils display enhanced expression of β1-integrins upon transmigration, it remains unclear whether integrins are relevant for interstitial leukocyte migration. According to this, the involvement of integrins seems to be rather different in 2D versus 3D settings. In contrast to 2D migration, the 3D tissue network confines and mechanically anchors cells from all sides so that they intercalate alongside and perpendicular to tissue structures. Importantly, 2D but not 3D leukocyte migration seems to be integrin dependent.[102] In this context, proteolytic enzymes (proteases) such as heparase, elastase, and matrix metalloproteinases (MMP-2 and MMP-9) provide for degradation of the components of the basement membrane and the ECM, and thus play an important role in leukocyte interstitial migration.[52,103]

All consecutively occurring steps of (1) leukocyte tethering and rolling, (2) exposure to a chemotactic stimulus, (3) firm arrest, (4) postadhesive strengthening and intraluminal crawling, (5) diapedesis, and (6) interstitial migration are essential for leukocytes to migrate to sites of inflammation. Accordingly, genetic defects in any of the molecules involved in either step lead to compromised host defenses. Patients with leukocyte adhesion deficiency (LAD) syndrome may have a genetic defect in β2 integrins (type 1) or in fucosylated selectin ligands (type 2), and neutrophils either cannot stop or cannot roll, respectively.[104–106] Type 3 LAD involves the deficiency of kindlin-3, a molecule regulating integrin activation and leukocyte adhesion reinforcement.[107,108] LAD syndrome is characterized by marked leukocytosis and frequent and severe soft-tissue infections.

Chemokine Control of Lymphocyte Homing to Secondary Lymphoid Organs

Migration of blood-borne lymphocytes to secondary lymphoid organs is the best-characterized example of leukocyte trafficking from the circulation into distinct target tissues.[2,4,109–114] Lymphocytes constantly survey secondary lymphoid organs, which include the spleen, tonsils, appendix, PPs, and LNs. Such homing allows lymphocytes to encounter antigen that may pose a threat to the organism. Antigens are collected and presented to T cells by DCs, in conjunction with signals by costimulatory molecules and cytokines. In contrast to the spleen, where the molecular mechanisms of leukocyte homing are still are not entirely clear and differ from all other lymphoid organs, the rules that govern homing of immune cells to LNs are well understood. Mature DCs, which have acquired antigen in peripheral tissues, and some memory cells reach the LNs through afferent lymph vessels.[115–117] In contrast, circulating T and B lymphocytes gain access to LNs and PPs through specialized postcapillary microvessels lined with cuboid endothelial cells that are known as *high endothelial venules* (HEVs).[118–121] HEVs in different secondary lymphoid organs express distinct patterns of trafficking molecules to serve as tethering platforms for defined subsets of lymphocytes. For example, HEVs in LNs express PNAd, whereas HEVs in PPs express mucosal addressin-cell adhesion molecule (MAdCAM-1). Other mucosa-associated lymphoid organs, such as mesenteric LNs, express both MAdCAM-1 and PNAd. Although T and B lymphocytes are recruited by similar multistep cascades to home to secondary lymphoid organs, the roles of individual traffic molecules are not necessarily identical, even when both subsets interact with the same microvessel.[2]

The first step in the homing cascade in LNs is mediated by L-selectin/CD62L expressed on all lymphocytes, except effector/memory cells. PNAd, an O-linked sulfated core 1 carbohydrate moiety that is exclusively found in HEVs, is the major endothelial L-selectin ligand.[122–126] Binding of L-selectin to PNAd initiates lymphocyte rolling in HEVs and slows down and marginates the free-flowing lymphocytes.[2,65,125] While the L-selectin–PNAd interaction is required, it is not by itself sufficient to promote firm leukocyte adhesion. The subsequent firm arrest of rolling T and B lymphocytes is mediated by the α4β1 integrin, β2-integrin CD11a/CD18 (LFA-1), CD11b/CD18 (Mac-1), and β7-integrin, which bind ICAMs, in particular ICAM-1 and ICAM-2, VCAM-1, or MAdCAM-1 on high endothelial cells.[125–130]

Chemokines that are presented in the lumen of HEV function as triggers of integrin activation.[131,132] On naive T cells integrin activation is primarily mediated by CCL21 (previously known as *SLC, TCA4, exodus 2,* or *6-C-kine*), which is constitutively expressed and secreted by HEVs. The secreted chemokine is noncovalently bound to GAGs on the surface of HEVs. Here it activates rolling lymphocytes through binding to CCR7, which is expressed on naive B and T cells. Another CCR7 ligand, CCL19 (previously termed *ELC* or *MIP3*β), also supports T-cell homing to LNs.[132] CCL19 is not expressed by high endothelial cells themselves. However, CCL19 and other chemokines may be released by extravascular cells in LNs or in tissues that discharge lymph to a local LN. Lymph-borne chemokines can be transported to the luminal aspect of HEVs. Correspondingly, chemokines, including CCL2, CCL19, and CCL21, injected under the skin of mice accumulate on the luminal surface of the HEV in draining LNs, where they promote integrin activation on rolling leukocytes bearing the cognate receptors.[133–135] In this context, endothelial heparan sulfate has been shown to be essential for controlling chemokine presentation on the endothelium and thereby for recruitment of lymphocytes and DCs to lymph nodes.[136]

B cells use largely the same trafficking molecules as naive T cells to home to LN. However, B-cell–HEV interactions are only moderately affected by the absence of CCR7 or its ligands.[137] Correspondingly, LNs of mice lacking CCR7 contain few T cells, while the B-cell compartment (and the memory T-cell compartment) is less affected.[138,139] Similar observations were made in *plt/plt* mice, which have a spontaneous genetic defect resulting in deletion of CCL19 and the HEV-expressed form of CCL21 (mice, unlike humans, have a second *ccl21* gene that is only expressed in lymph vessels of peripheral tissues), demonstrating that B cells are not absolutely dependent on CCR7 to adhere to HEVs.[137] In fact, rolling B cells can be induced to arrest in HEVs by either CCR7 agonists or by CXCL12 (previously called *stromal cell–derived factor [SDF-1]*α), the ligand for CXCR4.[140] An additional chemokine pathway involving CXCL13 (also called *BLC*) and its receptor CXCR5 has also been implicated in B-cell homing to secondary lymphoid tissues.[141] Of note, although B cells encounter several distinct integrin-activation signals in HEVs, B-cell homing to LNs is nonetheless less efficient than that of T cells. A likely reason is that the B cells express only approximately half the number of L-selectin molecules expressed on T cells, which greatly affects their ability to initiate the adhesion cascade in HEVs.[121,142]

The requirement for a sequence of distinct molecular steps that each leukocyte must undergo to arrest within microvessels explains why only certain leukocyte subsets gain access to lymphoid tissues, while others are excluded. Granulocytes, for example, express LFA-1 and L-selectin, but not CCR7. Consequently, although granulocytes can roll in HEVs (via L-selectin), these leukocytes do not perceive an integrin-activating stimulus and, therefore, fail to accumulate in LNs or PPs. Likewise, mature DCs express CCR7 and CD11a/CD18, but not L-selectin. Because these cells are thus incapable of rolling in HEVs, they fail to home to noninflamed LNs from the blood (although mature DCs readily access LNs via afferent lymph). Hence, the GPCR-mediated integration activation step is critical for imparting specificity to the process of lymphocyte homing to LN.

In HEVs of PPs, similar homing mechanisms are encountered as described earlier for LNs. However, the levels of L-selectin ligands (which are immunologically distinct from PNAd) expressed by HEVs in PPs are considerably lower when compared with LNs.[143,144] As a result, L-selectin itself is not sufficient to initiate a successful homing cascade for most lymphocytes in PPs.[143] Indeed, HEVs in PPs (and also in mucosa-associated LNs) additionally express MAdCAM-1, a ligand for the $\alpha4\beta7$ integrin.[143–145] The $\alpha4\beta7$ heterodimer, which comprises an $\alpha4$ integrin chain (CD49d) linked to the $\beta7$ integrin chain, is expressed at low levels by naive T and B cells, and is required for the successful homing of these cells in PP HEVs.[143] Following formation of an initial L-selectin–dependent tether, the $\alpha4\beta7$–MAdCAM-1 pathway stabilizes and slows the rolling lymphocytes without requiring chemokine activation. Once a chemokine signal has been transmitted, both $\alpha4\beta7$ and LFA-1 become activated and jointly mediate firm arrest.[143]

Of note, $\alpha4\beta7$ is strongly upregulated on gut-homing effector/memory lymphocytes, but completely absent on skin-homing memory T and B cells; these differential levels of $\alpha4\beta7$ integrin expression allow certain antigen-experienced lymphocyte subsets to acquire tissue selectivity.[146] The mechanisms underlying this specificity and plasticity of lymphocyte homing will be addressed later. Like in LNs, chemokines are essentially involved in promoting integrin activation and allowing firm lymphocyte arrest in HEVs of PPs. Thus, CXCR4, CXCR5, and CCR7 have been implicated in B-cell homing, while CCR7 seems exclusively responsible for T-cell homing. Interestingly, while T and B cells are recruited across the same HEVs in LNs, there is segmental segregation of T- and B-cell recruitment in PPs. HEVs supporting B-cell accumulation in PPs are concentrated in or near B follicles and present CXCL13, but not CCL21, whereas T cells preferentially accumulate in interfollicular HEVs (i.e., within the T-cell area), which express high levels of CCL21 but not CXCL13.

Trafficking of Leukocytes From Blood Into Nonlymphoid Tissues

As outlined previously, naive lymphocytes migrate most efficiently into secondary lymphoid organs, from which innate immune cells are excluded. However, both innate immune cells and subsets of lymphocytes can respond to inflammatory and/or activation signals by modulating the expression and/or activity of traffic molecules, which allows them to migrate to nonlymphoid tissues.[4] For example, in response to inflammatory stimuli, granulocytes, including neutrophils, eosinophils, and basophils, are rapidly recruited into the affected site and provide the first line of antimicrobial defense. Thereafter, additional immune cells, including monocytes, DCs, and effector as well as memory lymphocytes, may be recruited. Essentially, all of these different recruitment events depend on distinct multistep adhesion cascades.

Many of the inflammation-associated traffic molecules required for access into nonlymphoid tissues are shared by the different leukocyte subsets. The key receptors that initiate capture and mediate rolling of neutrophils, monocytes, natural killer cells, eosinophils, and effector T and B cells at peripheral sites of injury and inflammation are the three selectins, the leukocyte-expressed L-selectin as well as P- and E-selectin, which are induced on both acutely and chronically stimulated endothelial cells.[147–151] In addition, interactions between leukocytes involving PSGL-1 and L-selectin can also support the accumulation of immune cells in inflamed tissues.[150,152–154] Subsequent to rolling, firm arrest of leukocytes in nonlymphoid tissues involves integrins, including CD11a/CD18 (and its counter-ligand ICAM-1 and possibly also ICAM-2), VLA-4 (and its counter-ligand VCAM-1), as well as CD11b/CD18 (and its counter-ligand ICAM-1).[1,27,155] As discussed above for lymphoid tissues, chemoattractants, including chemokines and other GPCR agonists, such as formyl peptides, complement fragment 5a, and lipid mediators (e.g., PAF and LTB4), contribute essential integrin-activation signals for leukocytes at sites of inflammation. The molecular diversity of chemoattractants and their restricted temporal and spatial expression patterns combined with leukocyte subset-specific fingerprints of chemoattractant receptor expression provide

a crucial mechanism for the fine-tuning of the migratory cellular responses.[65,156,157]

In contrast, the migratory properties acquired by T and B lymphocytes in response to activation are diverse depending on the strength, the quality, and the context of the antigenic stimulus.[146] Specifically, antigen stimulation of naive lymphocytes results in the generation of effector and memory cells that express specific repertoires of trafficking molecules that guide them back to tissues containing the stimulatory antigen.[158–160] Thus, a cutaneous challenge generates preferentially a skin-tropic memory response, whereas orally ingested antigens induce preferentially gut-homing effector and memory cells. Recent studies have broadened our understanding of the molecular events that induce the generation of tissue-specific memory cells.

In addition to presenting antigen, DCs in different lymphoid organs are endowed with information characteristic for the tissue in which the antigen was obtained. DCs in mucosa-associated lymphoid tissues, but not other lymphoid organs, possess the enzymatic machinery to synthesize retinoic acid (RA) from vitamin Ab.[161] Exposure of activated T cells to RA induces the expression of gut-homing receptors (i.e., $\alpha4\beta7$ and CCR9) and suppresses skin-homing molecules.[159,162] In the absence of RA, T-cell stimulation induces few or no gut-homing molecules, but instead promotes the expression of P- and E-selectin ligands, as well as CCR4, which are needed for homing to the skin. Additionally, when activated T cells are exposed to IL-12 and high levels of vitamin D3, which is physiologically induced by sunlight in the skin, they upregulate CCR10, the receptor for the epidermal chemokine CCL27.[163] This organ-specific information can reprogram and "imprint" the tissue-tropic memory cells as they differentiate from naive lymphocytes.[160]

Like T cells, B-cell subsets also express homing receptors that permit their selective trafficking to specific tissues. For example, distinct B-cell subsets produce the immunoglobulin isotype IgA, which is present in secreted body fluids, including tears, breast milk, and mucus. IgA$^+$ B cells are characterized by their expression of CCR10.[164,165] The ligand for CCR10, MEC/CCL28, is expressed predominantly in mucosal tissues that secrete IgA.[166] Hence, CCR10 may function as a homing receptor that allows IgA-secreting B cells to migrate to tissues where IgA is required. A large subset among the IgA-secreting B cells are those in the small intestine, which in addition to CCR10 express the gut-homing receptors $\alpha4\beta7$ and CCR9. When naive B cells are activated in the presence of intestinal DCs, they upregulate not only these two traffic receptors, but also undergo class switching to IgA. This imprinting effect is dependent upon RA, which is sufficient to induce gut-homing receptors, but must be combined with DC-derived IL-5 or IL-6 to promote IgA class switching.[162] More than 50 different subtypes of lymphocytes have been characterized in human blood and it is likely that multiple similar associations between homing receptors, immunologic effector function, and tissue specificity will be revealed in future.

Migration of Hematopoietic Stem Cells to the Bone Marrow and Mobilization in the Niche

The BM is the principal site of hematopoiesis in the adult body. Correspondingly, most HSCs are lodged in the BM cavity. Within the BM, maintenance of HSCs and regulation of their self-renewal and differentiation is thought to depend on the specific microenvironment, which has historically been termed *stem cell niche*.[6,8,167–169] The central role of stem cell niches for HSC function has been recognized with the discovery that *Sl/Sl^d* (steel-Dickie) mice bearing a mutation in the gene encoding membrane-bound stem cell factor (SCF; also known as *KIT ligand*) show failure of BM HSC maintenance.[170] However, the exact localization as well as the composition of BM HSC niches and the molecular cross-talk that controls the retention of HSC within the niches are the subject of intense ongoing research.[171–174]

Notably though, not all HSCs reside within the BM. In fact, it has been known for almost four decades that a small amount of hematopoietic precursors are also present in peripheral blood.[10–13] Blood-borne HSCs continuously migrate back to the BM cavity, presumably to fill any vacant stem cell niches.[13] Although the exact physiologic relevance of blood-borne HSCs remains to be determined, the intrinsic capacity of HSCs to home to the BM compartment is the prerequisite for successful clinical BM and stem cell transplantation. Homing of HSCs to the BM is a rapid process, as intravenously injected murine and human progenitors are quickly cleared from the recipient's circulation.[13,175,176] Like mature lymphocytes, HSCs and hematopoietic progenitor cells (HPCs) interact through a multistep adhesion cascade with BM microvessels.[7,176–180] Initially, HPCs tether and roll along BM microvessels.[181,182] This process involves α4β7 integrin on HSCs/HPCs, which binds VCAM-1, as well as E- and P-selectin on BM sinusoidal endothelial cells, which bind α(1–3)-fucosylated ligands including CD44 and PSGL-1 on the surface of HPCs.[176] The subsequent firm arrest is mediated by activated α4β1 and VCAM-1, which is constitutively expressed in BM sinusoids. In addition to α4β1 integrin, the integrins α4β7, α5β1 and α6β1, and CD44 as well as JAM-B have recently been implicated in HSC homing to the BM.[180,183–186] Integrin-mediated adhesion is important for HSPC movement not only in adulthood but also during embryogenesis. Thus, HSPCs in the yolk sac, aorto-gonad-mesonephros region, and placenta express CD41 (GPIIb integrin encoded by the gene *Itga2b*). Expression gradually decreases during development, and adult HSPCs express little or no CD41.[7,187] In addition to CD41, β1 integrins tune the migration of fetal HSPCs. The use of chimeric mice generated with β1 integrin-deficient fetal HSPCs has revealed that fetal HSPCs lacking β1 integrins form and differentiate but they cannot colonize the follicular lymphoma, suggesting an essential role of β1 integrins in fetal HSPC trafficking. The role of the β2-integrins LFA-1 (CD11a/CD18) and Mac-1 (CD11b/CD18) is controversially discussed. Although some studies have reported their involvement in HSPC retention,[188,189] others have indicated that the effect of β2 integrins becomes apparent only in synergy with α4β1.[190]

The chemokine CXCL12, the ligand for CXCR4 expressed by most hematopoietic cells including HSCs, is thought to play a pivotal role in BM homing of HSCs. BM endothelial cells (in addition to immature osteoblasts and other stromal cells) constitutively express and secrete CXCL12.[177,191–194] However, alternate pathways appear to exist because fetal liver-derived mouse HSCs home to the BM of adult recipients independent of CXCR4,[195] and adult HSCs treated with a CXCR4 antagonist are still able to home sufficiently to the BM.[196] This indicates that HSCs may use different receptors and/or respond to distinct integrin-activation signals. In this context, the recent description of CXCR7, an alternate receptor for CXCL12, may explain some of the seemingly contradictory findings.[197]

Of note, the CXCL12/CXCR4 axis is not only involved in the homing process of HSCs to the BM, but (among others) has also been linked to the retention of HSCs within stem cell niches and to the regulation of the maturation of more committed HPCs (in particular, B-cell progenitor cells).[59,198–202] Correspondingly, disruption of the CXCL12/CXCR4 pathway leads to premature release of HPCs into the peripheral blood.[203,204] HPCs lacking CXCR4 accumulate in the circulation and fail to undergo normal lymphopoiesis and myelopoiesis, most likely because the cells do not receive the required maturation signals. Interestingly, upregulation of metalloproteinases (see earlier), which cleave and inactivate CXCR4 and CXCL12, has recently been implicated in HSC mobilization.[205–208] Mechanisms that modulate the CXCR4/CXCL12 axis are also thought to play a role in the coordinated mobilization of HPCs in response to cytokines that are used for this purpose in clinical practice.[58]

In addition to CXCL12, the egress from BM niches has been recently shown to be critically dependent on the nervous system. Thus, it was found that the mouse line exhibiting aberrant nerve conduction (UDP-galactose ceramide galactosyltransferase-deficient [Cgt−/−] mice) was characterized by the absence of HSPC egress from BM following granulocyte colony-stimulating factor (G-CSF) or fucoidan administration.[209] Interestingly, norepinephrine signaling–controlled bone CXCL12 downregulation and HSPC mobilization,

whereas administration of a beta(2) adrenergic agonist enhanced HSPC mobilization. Therefore, the sympathetic nervous system regulates the attraction of stem cells to their niche via transduction of circadian information from the central pacemaker in the brain, the suprachiasmatic nucleus, to the BM microenvironment.[210] Recent data show that circadian regulation is regulated by beta-2 and beta-3 adrenergic receptors (beta-ARs) expressed on HSCs, osteoblasts, and mesenchymal stem/progenitor cells. Moreover, beta(2)-ARs and beta(3)-ARs have specific roles in stromal cells and cooperate during progenitor mobilization.[211] Whereas activation of beta(3)-ARs downregulates Cxcl12, beta(2)-AR stimulation induces clock gene expression.[211] In addition, double deficiency in beta(2)-ARs and beta(3)-ARs compromises enforced mobilization. Therefore, these data demonstrate that HSC trafficking and hematopoiesis do not escape the circadian regulation that controls most physiologic processes. For the clinical settings, the timing of stem cell harvest or infusion may influence the yield or engraftment, respectively, and may result in better therapeutic outcomes.[210]

LEUKOCYTE MIGRATION WITHIN TISSUES

Trafficking Patterns of Lymphocytes

After a leukocyte has accessed a tissue, it must migrate to specific interstitial positions. As discussed earlier, homing typically requires that the blood-borne leukocyte completes a complex tissue- and subset-specific multistep adhesion cascade. One exception to this rule is the spleen, where most blood-borne lymphocytes can leave the circulation even in the absence of multiple traffic molecules. However, chemokines are essential in all lymphoid organs, including the spleen, to guide the newly arrived lymphocytes to their proper position within the organ.

Multiphoton intravital microscopy was used as a tool to decipher the mechanisms that control the extravascular traffic patterns of homed lymphocytes within lymphoid and nonlymphoid tissues.[212–220] For example, imaging experiments have shown that T cells that have entered an LN move incessantly within the paracortex (T-cell area). Here, they query the resident DCs for the presence of antigens that activate their T-cell receptor. B cells that home to LNs migrate to the more superficial B-cell–rich follicles, where they may detect antigens presented by follicular DCs. Activated B cells that encounter antigens then move to the margins of the B- and T-cell zones.[215] Here, they can receive help from antigen-specific CD4 T cells. Analogous specific microenvironments for T and B cells also exist in the other lymphoid tissues.

Migration of T Cells to T Zones Within Secondary Lymphoid Organs

After homing to secondary lymphoid organs, T cells migrate within the T zones. They engage in highly motile amoeboid movement (average speed ~12 μm/min) and undergo multiple brief encounters with resident DCs.[221–223] In this context, the fibroblastic reticular cell (FRC) network regulates naive T-cell access to the paracortex and also supports and defines the limits of T-cell movement within this domain.[224,225] As a consequence of high T-cell motility, it has been estimated that every DC in an LN touches as many as 5000 naive T cells within 1 hour. When T cells encounter a specific antigen, they progressively decrease their motility, become activated, and form long-lasting stable conjugates with DCs. Finally, antigen-experienced T cells start to proliferate and resume their rapid migration while contacting DCs only briefly.[223,226]

The positioning and high motility of T cells in the T-cell area is dependent on CCR7 and its ligands CCL19 and CCL21.[110,138,139,212,227,228] Both ligands are abundantly expressed in T zones by radiation-resistant stromal cells. Notably, ectopic expression of CCL21 induces the formation of LN-like structures in the pancreas of mice.[229] The expression of CCL19 and CCL21, but also of CXCL13, which attracts B cells to B-cell follicles (see later), by lymphoid stromal cells is strongly dependent on the cytokine lymphotoxin (LT)–α1β2 heterotrimer signaling via the LT β receptor.[230–232] Correspondingly, mice deficient in LT have no morphologically detectable LNs or PPs.[233] Moreover, CCL21 and CXCL13 have been shown to be transiently downregulated by a mechanism controlled by the cytokine interferon-γ. This modulation alters the localization of lymphocytes and DCs within responding lymphoid tissues. As a consequence, priming of T-cell responses to a second distinct pathogen after chemokine modulation became impaired. Therefore, transient chemokine modulation may help orchestrate local cellularity, thus minimizing competition for space and resources in activated lymphoid tissues.[234,235]

The differential ability of T-cell subsets to migrate in response to interstitial chemokine gradients is also an important determinant of immunologic memory.[236] For example, LNs harbor not only naive T cells, but also a major subset of antigen-experienced cells, the central memory T cells (T_{CM}). In steady-state LNs, both T-cell subsets localize in the deep T-cell area and interact dynamically with antigen-presenting DCs. However, upon entry of a lymph-borne virus into an LN, virus-specific T_{CM} relocalize rapidly toward the outermost LN regions where virally infected cells are concentrated. This rapid peripheralization of T_{CM} is coordinated by a cascade of cytokines and chemokines, particularly ligands for CXCR3 that diffuse from the outer cortex toward the T-cell area. Antiviral T_{CM} express high levels of CXCR3 and are responsive to the virus-induced chemokine gradient. By contrast, naive T cells do not express CXCR3 and remain initially sequestered in the T-cell zone. This delayed T-cell response in nonimmune hosts allows more time for the viral infection to spread than in immune individuals. Thus, early antigen detection afforded by intranodal chemokine guidance of T_{CM} is essential for efficient antiviral memory.[236]

Positioning of B Cells Within Secondary Lymphoid Organs

Similar to T cells, B cells enter secondary lymphoid organs from the blood to search for their specific antigens.[237] As previously outlined, the homing and entry of B cells into secondary lymphoid organs such as the LNs and PPs depends on chemokine/receptor interactions that finally result in firm integrin-mediated adhesion on the surface of HEVs. This adhesion is followed by cell movement into lymphoid tissue.[140,234,238,239] After entering secondary lymphoid organs, the naive B cells travel to B cell–rich areas, the B-cell follicles. This migration depends on the presence of CXCR5 on the surfaces of B cells and the localized expression of CXCL13 by follicular stromal cells.[109,232,239] Follicular B cells are also highly motile, migrating on a network of follicular DCs (FDCs), a process that is thought to be necessary to ensure optimal surveillance of the FDC for surface-displayed antigen. After a period of random migration within follicles, those B cells that have not encountered a cognate antigen return to the circulation via the lymph or, in case of the spleen, via the blood. In contrast, B cells that become stimulated by antigen relocate to the B–T boundary area to receive help from T cells, which is necessary for further differentiation. To achieve this repositioning, activated B cells rapidly upregulate CCR7. This permits their chemotaxis toward CCR7 ligands expressed in the T cell–rich zones of the secondary lymphoid organs.[215] Real-time imaging revealed that antigen-stimulated follicular B cells initially reduce their migration velocity upon antigen exposure. About 6 hours later the activated B cells move toward the follicle border with the T cell–rich zone and undergo highly dynamic interactions with helper T cells during the following several days.[215]

In the spleen, a subpopulation of "innate" B cells is present in the marginal zone (MZ) immediately adjacent to the marginal sinus that surrounds the white pulp cords. The exact extent to which chemokine-induced attraction and adhesion affect the positioning of MZ B cells is still unclear. However, recent studies indicate that the localization of B cells in the MZ is dependent upon interactions of αLβ2 and α4β1 on MZ B cells with their ligands (ICAM-1 and VCAM-1, respectively).[240,241] As with follicular B cells in LN, antigen encounter of MZ B cells causes their rapid repositioning to the B-T boundary area. The retention of naive B cells in the MZ and their relocalization to the B-T boundary area upon antigen encounter is thought to involve signaling though the phospholipid sphingosine-1 phosphate (S1P) and its receptor $S1P_1$.[242]

LEUKOCYTE EXIT FROM TISSUES

Although the coordinated role of adhesion molecules and chemokines governing lymphocyte entry into tissues has been examined in great detail, less is known about the exit of these cells from tissues. The final sections of this chapter will discuss examples of emerging research on the diverse mechanisms that regulate exit of distinct leukocyte subsets from tissues.

Reprogramming Dendritic Cells to Exit Tissues Toward Secondary Lymphoid Organs

Lymphocyte homing remains without consequence unless lymphocytes encounter DCs that present their cognate antigen. DCs capture and present antigen to T cells more efficiently than any other antigen-presenting cell. In general, two routes of antigen delivery to LNs have been described to date. (1) Antigenic material becomes lymph borne and is taken up by DCs that reside in the LN a priori; (2) antigen is acquired by DCs that reside in peripheral tissues and then transport the material to the draining LN. DCs constitutively patrol all tissues and engulf microorganisms, dead cells, and cellular debris. In the absence of inflammatory stimuli, the cells remain in an immature state that is only weakly immunogenic and often stimulates T-cell tolerance, rather than activation. However, multiple signals associated with infection or tissue damage can induce DC maturation. Immature DCs express a variety of chemokine receptors, including as CCR1, CCR5, and CCR6, which are believed to result in the constitutive homing of immature DCs into tissues, particularly sites of inflammation where ligands for these receptors are abundant.[4,115,243–245] After exposure to a maturation stimulus, such as Toll-like receptor agonists (e.g., lipopolysaccharide, bacterial lipoproteins, peptidoglycans or CpG dinucleotides), which often originate from infectious pathogens,[246,247] DCs lose CCR1, CCR5, and CCR6, while expression of GPCRs for lymphoid chemokines, in particular CCR7 and CXCR4, are upregulated.[248] Lymphatic endothelial cells in peripheral tissues express CCL21, the ligand for CCR7.[249] The loss of chemokine receptors that keep the DCs within the tissue together with the increased expression of CCR7 results in the exit of the mature DCs via the lymphatic drainage system.[138,250] Recently, using a microfluidic device that allows rapid establishment of stable gradients in three-dimensional matrices, it was shown that CCL21 is a more potent directional cue for DC migration than CCL19.[251] DC migration into the draining lymphatics also requires β2 integrin binding to ICAM-1 expressed by lymphatic endothelial cells. Moreover, JAM-A, which is expressed by DCs and the lymphatic endothelium, also affects DC migration to lymph nodes, because the absence of JAM-A expression by DCs facilitates their migration to lymph nodes.[117,252] The expression and activation of β1-integrins, which mediate the interaction of DCs with extracellular matrix components, might favor retention of DCs in the periphery.[117]

While traveling to the draining LN, DCs upregulate the expression of molecules for efficient antigen presentation and T-cell stimulation, and begin to generate chemokines and other cytokines that allow them to attract and stimulate T cells.[250,253,254]

Egress of Lymphocytes From Secondary Lymphoid Organs

When naive lymphocytes do not encounter antigen on antigen-presenting DCs after a period of random walk, they exit secondary lymphoid organs through efferent lymph vessels or, in the case of the spleen, by directly returning to the blood. Several adhesion receptors have been implicated in the egress of lymphocytes into lymphoid sinusoids, including PECAM-1 (CD31); the mannose receptor, which interacts with L-selectin; and common lymphatic endothelial and vascular endothelial receptor 1 (CLEVER-1).[255]

We still have very limited information about the signals that determine the dwell time of lymphocytes in secondary lymphoid organs (~12–24 hours for T cells). However, the recent observation that the egress of both T and B cells from LNs can be prevented by the immunosuppressant molecule FTY720 has revealed some of the principal mechanisms underlying lymphocyte egress. FTY720 is a synthetic derivative of myriocin, a metabolite of the fungus *Isaria sinclairii*, which has been used in Chinese traditional medicine. FTY720 induces lymphocyte sequestration in LNs and causes profound lymphopenia. In animal models of transplantation and autoimmunity FTY720 causes immunosuppression, and it has recently been shown to exert significant therapeutic effects in a placebo-controlled clinical trial of relapsing multiple sclerosis.[256–258] Although lymphocyte sequestration in LNs and lymphopenia in response to FTY720 have been reported some time ago, the underlying molecular mechanisms were uncovered only recently.[114] Upon in vivo administration FTY720 becomes rapidly phosphorylated and then binds to four of the five known S1P receptors ($S1P_1$ and $S1P_{3-5}$).[109,259–261] Naive B and T cells express substantial levels of $S1P_1$, and it appears to be this receptor that plays a predominant role in lymphocytes egress from lymphoid tissues into the efferent lymph vessels. Studies using gene-targeted mice have shown that T lymphocytes deficient in $S1P_1$ cannot exit secondary lymphoid organs (and in the case of T cells, also the thymus).[262,263] Reports using FTY720 and $S1P_1$-selective agonists also supported a role for $S1P–S1P_1$ signaling in the regulation of lymphocyte egress from secondary lymphoid organs. Notably, $S1P_1$ receptors not only regulate lymphocyte exit from tissues but also modulate lymphocyte homing capacity.[120]

The sphingolipid S1P is abundant in blood and lymph, while low levels of S1P are maintained within lymphoid tissues. This S1P gradient is established by the action of the S1P degrading enzyme S1P lyase.[264–266] Based on these findings, it has been proposed that S1P gradients between blood, lymphoid tissue, and lymph fluid together with cyclical ligand-induced modulation of $S1P_1$ on recirculating lymphocytes regulates lymphocyte egress and determines the lymphoid organ transit time of lymphocytes.[6,267] Indeed, recent observations support that concept by showing that $S1P_1$ on lymphocytes is downregulated in the blood, upregulated in lymphoid organs, and downregulated again in the lymph.[265] Notably, CD69, which is rapidly induced when T cells become activated, negatively regulates $S1P_1$ and thus promotes lymphocyte retention in lymphoid organs.[268,269]

Besides chemokines, other factors are also involved in the migration patterns of lymphocytes. By combining confocal, electron, and intravital microscopy, it has been found that the FRC network regulates naive T-cell access to the paracortex, whereas a distinct follicular DC network served as the substratum for movement of follicular B cells.[225] These results highlight the central role of stromal microanatomy in orchestrating cell migration within the LN.

Although the mechanism of HSPC homing into the BM is well investigated, little is known about the signals regulating the exit of HSPCs out of tissues other than the BM. HSPCs arrive in peripheral organs via blood, but leave them predominantly via the draining lymphatics.[6,270] Interestingly, it has been shown that, as on lymphocytes, S1P and S1P receptors mediate the egress of HSPCs from peripheral tissues.[6–8] The inhibition of $S1P–S1P$ receptor signaling decreases the number of HSPCs in tissue-draining lymph due to impaired egress from the tissue. Stress signals that mimic an infection (induced by administration of a Toll-like receptor [TLR]4 agonist) reduce $S1P1$ expression on HSPCs, leading to prolonged retention in peripheral organs, and thus providing necessary time for HSPCs to differentiate into immune cells that are required to eliminate the danger. Tuning of HSPC retention in peripheral tissues could support innate immune responses by fostering a local and versatile supply of effector cells.

SUMMARY

In this chapter we have outlined three distinct aspects of leukocyte trafficking: (1) leukocyte entry into tissues from the circulation; (2) migration within tissues; and (3) exit from tissues. Migration of leukocytes throughout the body is essential for the development of lymphocyte subsets and underpins their functions in immune surveillance and responses of effective adaptive immunity. The molecular reactions involved in leukocyte migration are tightly regulated and involve chemoattractants and adhesion molecules. Leukocyte migration is characterized by a considerable plasticity and specificity, because different leukocyte subsets express unique patterns of traffic molecules that enable their navigation into and within target tissues. Our expanding knowledge of the mechanisms that control leukocyte trafficking will likely influence the development of multiple therapeutic strategies, including the use of stem cells, cell immunotherapy of cancer, and autoimmune, inflammatory, and infectious diseases.

SUGGESTED READINGS

Alon R, Shulman Z: Chemokine triggered integrin activation and actin remodeling events guiding lymphocyte migration across vascular barriers. *Exp Cell Res* 317:632, 2011.

Arcangeli ML, Frontera V, Bardin F, et al: JAM-B regulates maintenance of hematopoietic stem cells in the bone marrow. *Blood* 118:4609, 2011.

Bachelerie F, Ben-Baruch A, Burkhardt AM, et al: International Union of Basic and Clinical Pharmacology. [corrected]. LXXXIX. Update on the extended family of chemokine receptors and introducing a new nomenclature for atypical chemokine receptors. *Pharmacol Rev* 66(1):1–79, 2014.

Bain CC, Bravo-Blas A, Scott CL, et al: Constant replenishment from circulating monocytes maintains the macrophage pool in the intestine of adult mice. *Nature Immunol* 15(10):929–937, 2014.

Carlin LM, Stamatiades EG, Auffray C, et al: Nr4a1-dependent Ly6C(low) monocytes monitor endothelial cells and orchestrate their disposal. *Cell* 153(2):362–375, 2013.

Chi H: Sphingosine-1-phosphate and immune regulation: trafficking and beyond. *Trends Pharmacol Sci* 32(1):16–24, 2011.

Griffith JW, Sokol CL, Luster AD: Chemokines and chemokine receptors: positioning cells for host defense and immunity. *Annu Rev Immunol* 32:659, 2014.

Haessler U, Pisano M, Wu M, et al: Dendritic cell chemotaxis in 3D under defined chemokine gradients reveals differential response to ligands CCL21 and CCL19. *Proc Natl Acad Sci USA* 108(14):5614–5619, 2011.

Hashimoto D, Chow A, Noizat C, et al: Tissue-resident macrophages self-maintain locally throughout adult life with minimal contribution from circulating monocytes. *Immunity* 38(4):792–804, 2013.

Hoeffel G, Wang Y, Greter M, et al: Adult Langerhans cells derive predominantly from embryonic fetal liver monocytes with a minor contribution of yolk sac-derived macrophages. *J Exp Med* 209(6):1167–1181, 2012.

Kannagi R, Ohmori K, Chen GY, et al: Sialylated and sulfated carbohydrate ligands for selectins and siglecs: involvement in traffic and homing of human memory T and B lymphocytes. *Adv Exp Med Biol* 705:549–569, 2011.

Muller WA: Mechanisms of leukocyte transendothelial migration. *Annu Rev Pathol* 6:323–344, 2011.

Nibbs RJ, Graham GJ: Immune regulation by atypical chemokine receptors. *Nature Reviews Immunol* 13(11):815–829, 2013.

Nomiyama H, Osada N, Yoshie O: A family tree of vertebrate chemokine receptors for a unified nomenclature. *Dev Comp Immunol* 35(7):705–715, 2011.

Obinata H, Hla T: Sphingosine 1-phosphate in coagulation and inflammation. *Semin Immunopathol* 34:73, 2011.

Robert P, Canault M, Farnarier C, et al: A novel leukocyte adhesion deficiency III variant: kindlin-3 deficiency results in integrin- and nonintegrin-related defects in different steps of leukocyte adhesion. *J Immunol* 186(9):5273–5283, 2011.

Schajnovitz A, Itkin T, D'Uva G, et al: CXCL12 secretion by bone marrow stromal cells is dependent on cell contact and mediated by connexin-43 and connexin-45 gap junctions. *Nat Immunol* 12(5):391–398, 2011.

Schulte D, Kuppers V, Dartsch N, et al: Stabilizing the VE-cadherin-catenin complex blocks leukocyte extravasation and vascular permeability. *EMBO J* 30(20):4157–4170, 2011.

Spiegel S, Milstien S: The outs and the ins of sphingosine-1-phosphate in immunity. *Nat Rev Immunol* 11(6):403–415, 2011.

Sun H, Wu Y, Qi J, et al: The CC' and DE loops in Ig domains 1 and 2 of MAdCAM-1 play different roles in MAdCAM-1 binding to low- and high-affinity integrin alpha4beta7. *J Biol Chem* 286(14):12086–12092, 2011.

Sung JH, Zhang H, Moseman EA, et al: Chemokine guidance of central memory T cells is critical for antiviral recall responses in lymph nodes. *Cell* 150(6):1249–1263, 2012.

Ulvmar MH, Hub E, Rot A: Atypical chemokine receptors. *Exp Cell Res* 317(5):556–568, 2011.

Ulvmar MH, Werth K, Braun A, et al: The atypical chemokine receptor CCRL1 shapes functional CCL21 gradients in lymph nodes. *Nature Immunol* 15(7):623–630, 2014.

Umemoto E, Hayasaka H, Bai Z, et al: Novel regulators of lymphocyte trafficking across high endothelial venules. *Crit Rev Immunol* 31(2):147–169, 2011.

Zhi L, Kim P, Thompson BD, et al: FTY720 blocks egress of T cells in part by abrogation of their adhesion on the lymph node sinus. *J Immunol* 187(5):2244–2251, 2011.

Zlotnik A, Yoshie O: The chemokine superfamily revisited. *Immunity* 36(5):705–716, 2012.

REFERENCES

For the complete list of references, log on to www.expertconsult.com.

INTERACTIONS BETWEEN HEMATOPOIETIC STEM AND PROGENITOR CELLS AND THE BONE MARROW: CURRENT BIOLOGY OF STEM CELL HOMING AND MOBILIZATION

Eman Khatib-Massalha, Kfir Lapid, Karin Golan, Orit Kollet, Shiri Gur-Cohen, Menachem Bitan, Anju Kumari, and Tsvee Lapidot

The hallmarks of hematopoietic stem and progenitor cells (HSPCs) are their migration, bone marrow (BM) homing, and repopulation potential. These primitive cells are continuously released at low levels from the BM to the circulation as part of steady-state homeostasis, and at accelerated rates during stress hematopoiesis situations such as injury or inflammation as part of host defense and repair mechanisms. Migration of hematopoietic stem cells from the blood, across the endothelial vasculature to their BM niches, requires active navigation, a process termed *homing*. The ability of HSPCs to home to the BM is the first and essential step for clinical transplantation. Physiologic stress caused by bleeding, injury, or infection induces massive proliferation and differentiation of HSPCs in the BM, which is accompanied by increased progenitor cell egress and recruitment to the circulation. This process is mimicked in clinical mobilization protocols, to increase the HSPC pool in the circulation and to harvest stem cells for clinical transplantation protocols. The transplanted stem cells actively home to the recipient BM and repopulate it by extensive proliferation and differentiation, while maintaining their self-renewal potential and motility capacity, enabling them to egress back to the circulation. These processes involve the stromal chemokine SDF-1 (also termed CXCL12) and its major receptor CXCR4, which regulate stem cell motility and proliferation, as well as their adhesion, retention, and quiescence. HSPC mobilization can be clinically induced by a variety of cytokines, such as the myeloid cytokine granulocyte colony-stimulating factor (G-CSF), the CXCR4 antagonist AMD3100, and by DNA-damaging chemotherapy drugs, such as cyclophosphamide (Cy).

HSPCs in the BM continuously replenish the blood with new maturing myeloid and lymphoid immune cells with a finite life span throughout life. Some of the circulating leukocytes are short lived, in particular neutrophils, which rapidly age within a few hours and home back to the BM across the physical blood–BM barrier, resulting in their apoptotic cell death. SDF-1/CXCR4 signaling is also involved in neutrophil retention in the BM, while the CXCL2/CXCR2 signaling pathway is involved in neutrophil trafficking from the BM to the circulation.

This chapter discusses recent findings concerning the biology of HSPCs and mature leukocyte (especially neutrophil) homing and mobilization, emphasizing the major roles of the SDF-1/CXCR4 and CXCL2/CXCR2 signaling cascades in their dynamic retention and mobilization.

HEMATOPOIETIC STEM AND PROGENITOR CELL HOMING

Migration of HSPCs from the circulation and their extravasation across the physical barrier of the blood vessels to the BM require an active navigation, a process termed homing. HSPC homing is the critical first step leading to successful clinical engraftment in the ablated BM of transplanted recipients, which is the predominant physiologic site of hematopoiesis.[1]

The BM endothelium is the first anchoring site for homing cells, exposing them to presented adhesion molecules and stimulating chemokines. The small blood vessels in both human and murine BM, the sinusoids, in which transendothelial migration is thought to take place, are composed of specialized cell structures that regulate cell trafficking.

The homing process is initiated by a SDF-1/CXCR4 guiding signal, leading to firm adhesion and docking to the vascular sinusoidal wall (Fig. 14.1), which induces cytoskeleton rearrangement and activation of integrins (e.g., VLA-4) and metalloproteinases (e.g., MMP-2/9). These cellular alterations are followed by transmigration across the physical BM–blood endothelial cell and extracellular matrix barriers (reviewed by Lapidot et al[2]).

HSPCs are localized and anchored in special stromal niches via adhesion interactions, which provide them with signals that prevent their motility, proliferation, and uncontrolled differentiation. Stromal CXCL12 abundant reticular (CAR) cells express the highest levels of SDF-1, which is essential for murine stem cell quiescence and maintenance; they serve as stem cell niche cells. While murine stem cell homing can be investigated in genetically matched recipient mice without rejection of donor cells, functional preclinical immune-deficient animal models have been developed to study human stem cell homing and engraftment.

Mechanisms Regulating HSPC Homing: The Essential Role of the SDF-1/CXCR4 Axis

As discussed by Cottler-Fox et al,[2a] SDF-1/CXCR4 interaction and downstream signaling have been implicated in retention, migration, homing, and mobilization of HSPCs during steady-state homeostasis, as well as during injury (reviewed by Lapidot et al[2]). Both human and murine BM stromal cells, including endothelial cells and endosteal bone-lining osteoblasts, express and secrete high levels of SDF-1, observed in regions rich in HSPCs.

Concomitantly, the expression of CXCR4 on circulating HSPCs is very dynamic and allows their direct chemoattraction toward high levels of SDF-1 found in the BM endothelium, thus facilitating the homing process (see Fig. 14.1). CXCR4-dependent homing is also observed in aging neutrophils, which express high levels of CXCR4 and migrate back to the BM across the mechanical barrier in order to engage cell death. Genetic overexpression of CXCR4 or cytokine-induced increased surface expression of CXCR4 (e.g., by hepatocyte growth factor [HGF]) enhanced the homing capacity of transplanted human HSPCs, while Kollet et al[2b,2c] showed that administration of neutralizing anti-CXCR4 antibodies impaired the homing of immature human CD34[+] stem and progenitor cells to the BM of transplanted immunodeficient mice. Given the important clinical challenge of improving HSPC engraftment and repopulation, upregulation of CXCR4 expression is a promising approach.

Murine BM stem cell niches contain a rare population of mesenchymal stem and progenitor cells (MSPCs), which express the highest levels of SDF-1 in the BM microenvironment. Depletion of stromal-supporting niche cells results in defective hematopoiesis and

Homing of transplanted HSPC

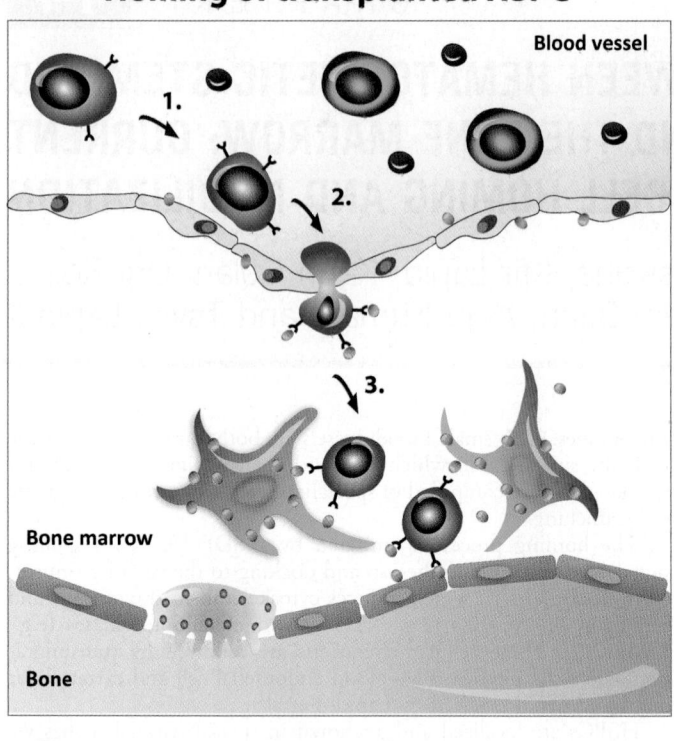

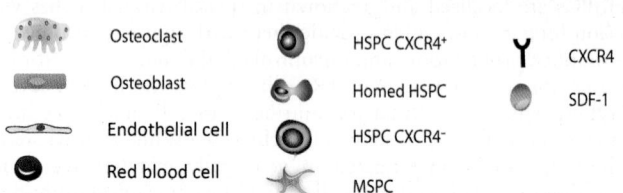

	Osteoclast		HSPC CXCR4+		CXCR4
	Osteoblast		Homed HSPC		SDF-1
	Endothelial cell		HSPC CXCR4-		
	Red blood cell		MSPC		

Fig. 14.1 HOMING OF TRANSPLANTED HEMATOPOIETIC STEM AND PROGENITOR CELLS TO THE BONE MARROW. Following transplantation, navigating HSPCs from the circulation roll and adhere *(1)* to BM endothelial cells. This process is followed by transendothelial migration across the physical blood–BM barrier *(2)*. HSPCs interact with MSPCs via surface SDF-1/CXCR4 signaling, which is a key regulator of stem cell homing and adhesion to the BM-supportive niche, an essential process for HSPC lodgment and retention *(3)*. *BM*, Bone marrow; *HSPC*, hematopoietic stem and progenitor cell; *MSPC*, mesenchymal stem and progenitor cell.

reduced homing of transplanted HSPCs to the BM, demonstrating the crucial role of SDF-1 in homing of HSPCs.[3]

Administration of high doses of SDF-1 induce cell survival and quiescence, whereas low doses promote cell motility, proliferation, and migration (reviewed by Lapidot and Kollet[4]). Accordingly, Cashman et al showed that in vivo treatment with high doses of SDF-1 increased engraftment of human repopulating cells (reviewed by Lapidot and Kollet[4]).

A single injection of human SDF-1 to nonirradiated $\beta 2m^{null}$ NOD/SCID mice increased homing of transplanted human mobilized peripheral blood and cord blood (CB) CD34+ cells to the murine BM. It was found that the noncleaved active form of SDF-1 can cross the BM endothelium to the BM in a CXCR4-dependent manner. This increase in SDF-1 level in the BM functionally enhances the homing capacity of transplanted human CD34+ progenitors of NOD/SCID mice (reviewed by Lapidot et al[2]). According to this data, enhanced CXCR4 expression as well as inhibition of SDF-1 degradation is important to enable a stable chemotactic response, directing the homing of HSPCs to the BM.

Another important cytokine regulating progenitor cell homing is stem cell factor (SCF; also termed c-Kit ligand), which plays an important role in hematopoiesis. Prestimulation of human or murine HSPCs with SCF improved their in vivo homing abilities through

increased migration and adhesion via very late antigen (VLA)-4 and VLA-5 integrins. Moreover, the homing of murine progenitor cells to the BM of mice deficient in P- and E-selectin was impaired, demonstrating the crucial role of adhesion interactions for proper homing, allowing HSPC rolling on the BM endothelium and retention in their stromal supportive niches. Interestingly, SDF-1 is not the only chemoattractant factor for HSPC homing; previous studies have shown that the chemoattractant lipid sphingosine-1-phosphate (S1P) has a role in inducing murine HSPC homing to the BM by increasing progenitor adhesion to stromal cells.[5] S1P, together with SDF-1, was indeed reported to have a synergistic effect on the migration of hematopoietic progenitor cells; however, this finding was later refuted by Ryser et al, showing no additive effect when both chemoattractants are added to the same plate. In contrast, this group showed that overexpression of $S1P_1$ (S1P receptor) on immature human CD34+ cells strongly reduces their migration toward a gradient of SDF-1 and in vivo homing via inhibition of CXCR4 signaling (reviewed by Golan et al[6]).

Taken together, manipulation of SDF-1 levels in the target organ and CXCR4 on the surface of transplanted stem cells can be used to navigate stem cells in vivo. Enhanced SDF-1 production by BM stromal cells after host preconditioning, crossing the blood–BM barrier, and activation of the adhesion machinery are required for HSPC attachment to BM-supporting niches, allowing their subsequent self-renewal and differentiation (see Fig. 14.1).

HEMATOPOIETIC STEM AND PROGENITOR CELL MOBILIZATION: A DYNAMIC MULTIFACETED PROCESS

HSPCs are actively retained in the BM via adhesion interactions with their stromal microenvironment. In the BM, they undergo extensive proliferation and differentiation, giving rise to all mature leukocyte and erythrocyte reservoirs, and replenishing the blood with new cells. Interestingly, in addition to mature leukocytes, low levels of HSPCs are also released to the blood as part of steady-state homeostasis. During stress situations and upon demand of accelerated hematopoiesis, HSPC egress is dramatically augmented in a process termed *recruitment*.[7] Enhanced HSPC egress occur as part of host defense and repair mechanisms following various stress situations, such as inflammation (mimicked by lipopolysaccharides [LPS]; endotoxins found in the outer membrane of Gram-negative bacteria, or endotoxin administration), bleeding, and administration of cytotoxic agents, such as chemotherapy.

Stem and progenitor cell recruitment is achieved by clinical mobilization protocols, such as repeated G-CSF stimulations, which are used to expand the HSPC pool and to harvest the cells from the blood for clinical transplantation.

Stress-induced HSPC recruitment and mobilization is a complex process involving essential motility mechanisms, activities of various cytokines, chemoattractants (e.g., SDF-1), proteolytic enzymes, and other extrinsic factors that enable detachment of HSPCs from their BM niches. These BM niches prevent HSPC migration and proliferation via adhesion interactions, and therefore disconnecting such interactions are essential for HSPC motility, leading to their egress. Recent evidence for the involvement of other cellular players, such as neutrophils, macrophages, and osteoblasts, in the regulation of stress-induced HSPC recruitment will be discussed.

This part of the chapter summarizes insights regarding mechanistic aspects of mobilization, as well as recent data on steady-state and rapid HSPC mobilization mechanisms. Currently, new rapid mobilization protocols using CXCR4 antagonists, such as AMD3100, together with G-CSF, lead to higher levels of HSPC mobilization.[8]

The SDF-1/CXCR4 Axis in Hematopoietic Stem and Progenitor Cell Mobilization

As noted earlier in this chapter (in the section Mechanisms Regulating HSPC Homing: The Essential Role of the SDF-1/CXCR4

Axis), SDF-1 has important roles in HSPC homing, retention, survival, and quiescence. Impairment SDF-1 or CXCR4 levels in murine embryos results in multiple lethal defects, including lack of stem cell seeding of the BM.[9] In order to circumvent lethality, conditional knock-out models were established. Induced deletion of CXCR4 in the hematopoietic system of the adult mouse or ablation of SDF-1 in the BM stroma led to severely reduced BM cellularity and hematopoietic stem cell (HSC) numbers, as well as impaired repopulation capacity.[10] Conditional deletion of CXCR4 or SDF-1 also results in dramatically increased HSPC numbers in the peripheral blood and spleen,[10] suggesting that blocking CXCR4 hampers their retention in the BM. Selective chemical antagonists of CXCR4, such as AMD3100, were originally developed to block CXCR4-mediated HIV infection, without any success in blocking in vivo infection. Nevertheless, serendipitous research shows that upon AMD3100 administration, mouse and human HSPCs undergo rapid mobilization within hours[11] and the mobilized HSPCs demonstrate increased repopulation potential in vivo.

AMD3100 synergistically augments G-CSF–induced mobilization. AMD3100 is the only chemokine receptor antagonist utilized clinically for inducing mobilization, either alone or in combination with G-CSF administration.[11] AMD3100 has been shown to be an effective mobilizing agent in murine and human clinical models,[12] which are known to be poor mobilizers in response to G-CSF. Mechanistically, AMD3100-induced SDF-1 release from BM stromal cells to the circulation, together with an inhibitory effect in vivo, induces rapid mobilization of HSPCs.

The essential role of SDF-1/CXCR4 signaling in HSPC retention can be inferred from the observations that following G-CSF administration, SDF-1 levels in the BM are transiently increased followed by their downregulation at both protein[7,13] and mRNA levels, enabling transient and local SDF-1 gradients toward the blood. In addition, CXCR4 upregulation is observed in immature murine BM cells following G-CSF treatment, as well as on immature human CD34$^+$ cells and primitive CD34$^+$CD38$^-$ cells resident in the BM of G-CSF–treated chimeric mice.[7] Blocking CXCR4 or SDF-1 reduces G-CSF–induced mobilization, thus demonstrating an essential role for SDF-1/CXCR4 in mobilization of murine progenitors.[7]

Christopherson et al reported that, compared with continuous SDF-1 expression in the BM, SDF-1 in the peripheral blood is short-lived and is prone to proteolysis by proteases, such as CD26, and metalloproteases, for example MMP-9 (reviewed by Lapidot et al[2]). SDF-1 can directly activate the metalloprotease MMP-9, which in turn cleaves and degrades this chemokine, participating in the enhanced migration capacity and recruitment of HSPCs to the periphery.[14] These observations suggest that SDF-1 levels in the peripheral blood are dynamically regulated during homeostasis in addition to its major role in retention of HSPCs in the BM. Repetitive daily administrations of SDF-1 for 5 consecutive days induce murine HSPC mobilization.[15] Hampering SDF-1/CXCR4 signaling in the BM results in loss of retention, because active SDF-1/CXCR4 signaling is required for stem cell adhesion and quiescence in the BM.

The Dynamics of Hematopoietic Stem and Progenitor Cell Niches and Bone Marrow Microenvironment During Mobilization

Coupling of bone degradation and bone formation, carried out by monocyte-derived osteoclasts and MSPC-derived osteoblasts, respectively, is part of the complex process of bone remodeling. Noteworthy, osteoblasts and osteoclasts maintain bone equilibrium by also acting in the endosteum in the vicinity of HSPCs.[16] Thus the endosteal stem cell niche is dynamically altered during bone remodeling, affecting HSPC function and maintenance. Furthermore, accumulating evidence supports dynamic alteration of the HSPC microenvironment upon stress-induced mobilization procedures. G-CSF or cyclophosphamide injections, as part of a clinically oriented HSPC mobilization procedure, lead to the disappearance or altered morphology of bone-lining osteoblasts, resulting

in their reduced function, which is also associated with reduced transcription of SDF-1.[17,18] Of interest, upon G-CSF administration, osteoblasts rapidly expand, promoting HSPC proliferation prior to their apoptosis, which in turn enables loss of HSPC retention. The importance of BM stromal cells in the retention of HSPCs can be illustrated, for example, by the conditional deletion of the cell cycle regulator Retinoblastoma protein (Rb). Absence of Rb in the murine hematopoietic system, as well as in the BM stroma, is sufficient to increase the numbers of circulating HSPCs, in addition to a myeloproliferative-like disease and extramedullary hematopoiesis.[17]

Involvement of Monocytes/Macrophages

Chow et al (2011) found that depletion of mononuclear phagocytes in mice is sufficient to mobilize HSPCs, suggesting that BM macrophages promote retention of HSPCs in the BM (reviewed by Ludin et al[18]). Because macrophages play a crucial role in osteoblast growth and survival, it has been proposed that their depletion mobilizes HSPCs by disruption of the osteoblastic niche.[19] By using a variety of approaches to abrogate monocytes and macrophages from the BM, previous studies have reported that G-CSF-stimulated recruitment of HSPCs to the peripheral blood is dependent on direct activation of the monocyte lineage (Chow et al, 2011, and Christopher et al, 2011, reviewed by Ludin et al[18]). Christopher et al (2011) supported the important role of BM-resident macrophages in regulating the osteoblastic niche by utilizing chimeric mice that expressed the G-CSF receptor only in CD68$^+$ macrophages. Upon G-CSF administration, HSPC mobilization and SDF-1 downregulation in the BM were completely restored in these chimeric mice (reviewed by Ludin et al[18]). BM-resident macrophages may therefore regulate SDF-1 production by BM osteoblasts and other stromal cells, which generate factors that are yet to be determined. Of interest, cholesterol efflux pathways within mouse BM-resident macrophages are necessary to mediate this function, as a lack of cholesterol transporters in macrophages and dendritic cells leads to osteoblast suppression, elevated plasma G-CSF levels, and reduction in SDF-1 production in the BM, including by MSPCs.[20] As a result, these mice demonstrated increased numbers of circulating HSPCs and extramedullary hematopoiesis.[20] Intriguingly, Ludin et al (2012) has demonstrated the existence of an additional type of BM-resident myeloid niche cell that regulates the maintenance of primitive murine HSPCs. These rare, activated αSMA$^+$ monocytes/macrophages, which are located near small blood sinuses, produce high levels of prostaglandin E$_2$ (PGE$_2$) in a COX2-dependent manner; they apparently act to protect the HSPC pool from exhaustion in steady state and upon stress by direct intercellular contact and reactive oxygen species (ROS) inhibition, preventing stem cell migration and differentiation (reviewed by Ludin et al[18]). BM monocytes/macrophages emerge as central players in driving HSPC retention, probably via osteoblast maintenance, stromal SDF-1 expression, and PGE$_2$ production; however, other immune cells of the innate immune system play additional roles, as discussed later.

Bioactive Lipid-Induced Mobilization

Other potential chemoattractants responsible for egress of HSPCs into the peripheral blood include heat-resistant bioactive lipids, in particular S1P, which was previously shown by Ratajczak et al (2010) to directly induce chemoattraction of human and murine HSPCs (reviewed by Golan et al[6]). Alvarez et al (2007) showed that S1P is a bioactive lipid implicated in cell migration, survival, proliferation, and angiogenesis, as well as immune and allergic responses (reviewed by Golan et al[6]). Human and murine HSPCs, and BM stromal and endothelial cells have been shown to express functional S1P receptors, which also cross-talk with SDF-1/CXCR4 signaling, affecting migration, adhesion, homing, mobilization, development, and engraftment capacities. It is proposed that S1P is a crucial chemoattractant for BM-residing HSPCs, increasing ROS levels and leading to recruitment of HSPCs to the circulation (reviewed by Golan et al[6]). Accordingly, S1P concentrations in the plasma were rapidly increased following both G-CSF and AMD3100 treatments in mice, as well as expression of its receptor S1P$_1$ on HSPCs (reviewed by Golan et al[6]). By utilizing mice with reduced S1P levels, or lacking the S1P$_1$ receptor, Golan et al (2012) showed a reduced capacity to mobilize upon G-CSF or AMD3100 treatments.[5] Bendall et al (2013) found that manipulation of the S1P/S1P$_1$ axis may be used to improve clinical mobilization protocols. As suggested by Bendall and colleagues, activation of S1P$_1$ by a specific agonist during AMD3100 administration led to increased levels of mobilized stem cells that are harvested for BM transplantation (reviewed by Golan et al[6]). Furthermore, S1P was shown to induce SDF-1 secretion from BM MSPCs and endothelial cells, followed by SDF-1 release from the BM to the peripheral blood, adding another regulatory aspect for HSPC mobilization (reviewed by Golan et al[6]). Altogether, recent data suggest that additional chemoattractive compounds, such as S1P, mediate egress and recruitment of HSPCs from the BM to the circulation by regulating the SDF-1/CXCR4 axis.

The Dynamic Brain–Bone–Blood Triad

The *brain–bone–blood triad* is composed of the nervous system, bone-lining osteoblasts, and the hematopoietic system. The nervous system, a major regulator of the mammalian body that interacts with the immune system directly as well as indirectly, influences both bone- and blood-forming stem and progenitor cells. The mammalian nervous system regulates the immune system during homeostasis as well as acute physiologic conditions, for example, during mental stress as part of the "fight-or-flight" response.[21] The importance of the nervous system for HSPC mobilization has been determined by establishing mice lacking catecholaminergic activity, which display an inability to induce HSPC mobilization by G-CSF.[22] Adrenergic stimulation suppresses bone-lining osteoblasts, causing a significant reduction in SDF-1 production and leading to detachment of HSPCs from their BM niches. Katayama et al (2006) showed that G-CSF administration in mice lacking catecholaminergic activity does not result in osteoblast suppression, BM SDF-1 downregulation or subsequent HSPC mobilization. Concomitantly, Spiegel et al (2008) have also shown a role for the nervous system in hematopoiesis, not only indirectly through its effects on bone-lining osteoblasts,[22] but also through a direct effect on HSPC (reviewed by Spiegel et al[23]). In this regard, it was demonstrated that primitive human progenitor cells express β$_2$ adrenergic receptors as well as dopamine receptors. These receptors are upregulated during G-CSF-induced mobilization of immature human CD34$^+$ cells, as well as on primitive CD34$^+$CD38$^-$ cells, suggesting a role of sympathetic stimulation in inducing HSPC mobilization. β$_2$-Adrenergic stimulation by norepinephrine administration in mice results in increased numbers of circulating HSPCs, while administration of β$_2$-adrenergic antagonists reduced peripheral blood numbers[8] (reviewed by Spiegel et al[23]). Interestingly, there are daily oscillations of circulating murine HSPCs, peaking 5 h after the initiation of light in parallel to reduced BM SDF-1 levels.[24] Thus the physiologic egress of BM HSPCs into the circulation is not random but follows daily circadian oscillations. These oscillations are dependent on the sympathetic neurotransmitter, norepinephrine, through the β$_3$-adrenergic receptors expressed by BM stromal cells, leading to downregulation of SDF-1 in the BM, and subsequently reducing HSPC BM retention.[24] Although all players of the brain–bone–blood triad are linked and mutually regulated, much is unknown with regard to the specific molecular mechanisms of this dynamic regulation (reviewed by Spiegel et al[23]).

Involvement of Bone Marrow Neutrophils in Stem and Progenitor Cell Mobilization

Neutrophils are the most abundant myeloid leukocytes in mammals and are an essential component of the innate immune system, as they are the first line of defense upon pathogen infiltration. During steady-state homeostasis, mobilization of neutrophils from the BM occurs at a dramatic rate of about 10^{11} cells in humans and 10^7 in mice per day, and they are characterized by a very short life span of about 12 h in mice. At baseline, the great majority (>98% in mice) of neutrophils are located in the BM, given a reservoir of neutrophils to respond to stress conditions such as infections (reviewed by Day and Link[25]). During the acute phase of inflammation, neutrophils are the first leukocytes to migrate from the circulation to sites of infection following a gradient of inflammatory stimuli, where they eradicate the pathogens and are eventually cleared by macrophages. During homeostasis, neutrophils are maintained through a balance between their production in the BM, release through the endothelial barrier to the circulation, and clearance from the circulation.[26] Neutrophils are key regulators of HSPC mobilization via HGF secretion, ROS signaling, and proteolytic enzymes. The chemokine CXCL2 is a potent chemoattractant of neutrophils, and it is known to play a crucial role in the emigration of activated neutrophils from the BM, indirectly inducing HSPC mobilization. In addition, the major mediators of neutrophil driving power for HSPC mobilization are proteolytic enzymes (e.g., MMP9), which are released by activated neutrophils into the BM microenvironment and periphery. These proteolytic enzymes interfere with the SDF-1/CXCR4 retention signal that preserves HSPCs in their BM niches,[13] enabling their subsequent recruitment from the BM to the blood. The requirement of neutrophils and G-CSF–induced HSPC mobilization was supported by a study in 2012 showing that G-CSF mediated neutrophil expansion in the BM of mice. In addition, G-CSF induced apoptosis of MSPCs and osteoblasts through increased ROS production and reduced expression of retention factors in the BM, including SDF-1.[27] Depletion of activated neutrophils in mice by administration of neutralizing antibodies led to attenuation of G-CSF–mobilization effects.[27] Although ROS generation in neutrophils is critical during eradication of pathogens and is involved in the apoptotic processes, it also serves as a common signaling mediator. Except for ROS generation in activated neutrophils, ROS signaling is a key intrinsic cellular mechanism during HSPC differentiation and recruitment to the periphery. Dar et al (2011) demonstrated that inhibition of ROS by the antioxidant *N*-acetyl cysteine could preferentially attenuate AMD3100-induced mobilization of murine HSPCs,[8] suggesting that ROS signaling is involved in rapid HSPC motility and egress. Tesio et al (2011) found that granulocytes (e.g., neutrophils), activated by repeated G-CSF stimulations, release HGF. HGF in turn binds to its receptor c-Met on the HSPCs themselves, triggering mTOR/ROS signaling as part of the HSPC mobilization process (reviewed by Ludin et al[18]). It is therefore not surprising that blocking c-Met, mTOR, or ROS leads to inhibition of G-CSF–induced HSPC mobilization, while HGF administration induces their mobilization. Of note, Dar et al (2011) showed that inhibition of ROS by *N*-acetyl cysteine not only reduces AMD3100-induced mobilization of HSPCs, but also reduces the induction of SDF-1 release by BM stromal and endothelial cells.[8] These studies identified a cross-talk between SDF-1/CXCR4 via ROS signaling, which is essential for HSPC egress and mobilization[8] (reviewed by Ludin et al[18]). Collectively, results taken from different studies support the claim that neutrophils are key elements in G-CSF–induced HSPC mobilization, as shown by HGF secretion, release of proteolytic enzymes, suppression of osteoblasts, and increased ROS generation. The mechanism of HSPC and neutrophil mobilization is summarized in Fig. 14.2.

Neutrophil Retention and Egress: The Essential Role of SDF-1/CXCR4 and CXCL2/CXCR2 Signaling

Accumulating evidence suggests that the SDF-1/CXCR4 axis regulates neutrophil retention. SDF-1 is a chemoattractant not only for HSPCs, but also for many hematopoietic cell types, including neutrophils. BM neutrophils and neutrophil precursors express low but visible levels of surface CXCR4 and high intracellular levels, suggesting an internalization of CXCR4 in vivo (reviewed by Day

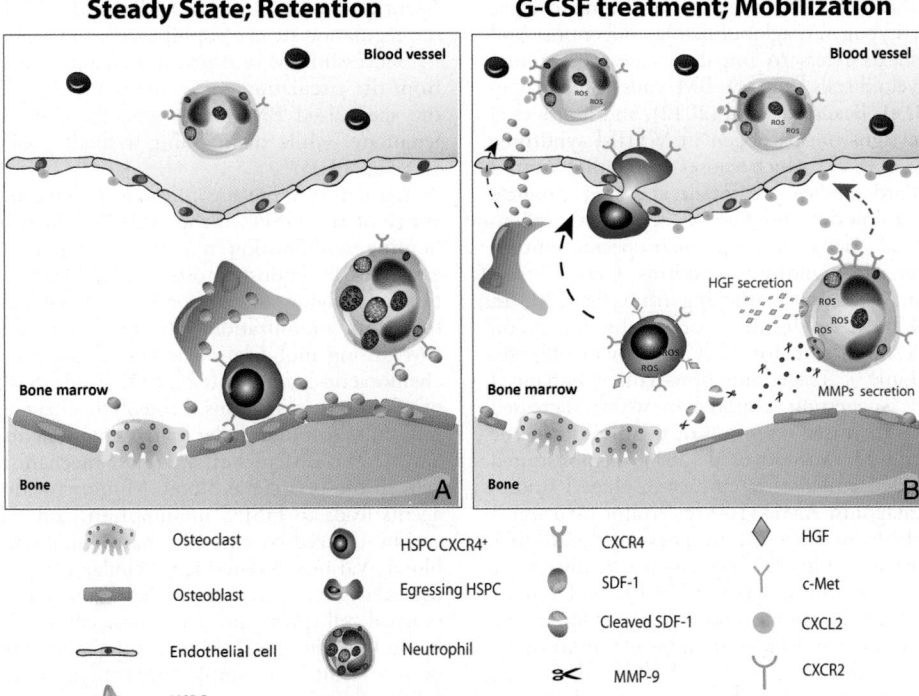

Fig. 14.2 NEUTROPHILS AND HEMATOPOIETIC STEM AND PROGENITOR CELL RETENTION AND MOBILIZATION FOLLOWING G-CSF TREATMENT. (A) During steady state, HSPCs are localized in specific bone marrow (BM) stromal niches associated with MSPCs and osteoblasts via SDF-1/CXCR4-induced adhesion and retention. The balance between the chemokine stromal SDF-1 and endothelial CXCL2 favors neutrophil retention, with only a small fraction of neutrophils released to the blood. (B) Repeated G-CSF administration increases SDF-1 secretion from MSPCs, leading to HSPC mobilization to the blood. G-CSF also alters the balance of BM chemokines by increasing endothelial CXCL2 expression and decreasing SDF-1 expression by BM osteoblasts and other stromal cells, leading to neutrophil activation and mobilization to the blood. The activated neutrophils in the BM secrete ROS, HGF and proteolytic enzymes (e.g., MMP-9), which interfere with retention signals. These inflammatory signals induce detachment of HSPCs from BM MSPCs and osteoblasts, leading to their enhanced proliferation, differentiation, and mobilization to the circulation. *HGF*, Hepatocyte growth factor; *HSPC*, hematopoietic stem and progenitor cell; *MMP-9*, matrix metalloproteinase-9; *MSPC*, mesenchymal stem and progenitor cell; *ROS*, reactive oxygen species.

and Link[25]). Previous studies have shown neutrophilia and impaired neutrophil mobilization in response to G-CSF in mice carrying a myeloid-specific deletion of CXCR4. In addition, conditional deletion of SDF-1 is also related to neutrophilia. Finally, treatment with AMD3100 in humans or mice results in rapid neutrophil mobilization.[11] Another major player in neutrophil activation and egress is the chemokine CXCL2 (also termed macrophage inflammatory protein 2 [MIP-2]), which is known to play an essential role in their egress from the BM to the circulation or to sites of inflammation (reviewed by Day and Link[25]). CXCL2 is expressed by endothelial cells and megakaryocytes in the BM, and induces neutrophil egress by binding to its correspondent receptor CXCR2 on neutrophils. It has been demonstrated that neutrophils in CXCR2-deficient mice are retained in the BM, leading to a myelokathexis-like phenotype (reviewed by Day and Link[25]). These data provide strong evidence that CXCL2/CXCR2 signaling plays a major role in neutrophil egress from the BM to the circulation. Under steady-state conditions, the balance of SDF-1 and CXCL2 chemokines favors neutrophil retention in the BM, with a relatively small population of neutrophils egressing to the circulation (reviewed by Day and Link[25]). On the contrary, under stress situations (e.g., infections) the expression of inflammatory cytokines, in particularly G-CSF, is upregulated and leads to massive neutrophil egress into the circulation. Link et al (2005) showed that after G-CSF administration there is a suppression of osteoblasts, resulting in decreased SDF-1 expression in the BM (reviewed by Day and Link[25]). In addition, G-CSF causes cleavage of surface CXCR4

on neutrophils, disrupting SDF-1/CXCR4 signaling, which leads to their mobilization.[28] G-CSF administration also elevates CXCL2 expression by BM endothelial cells, increasing the interaction between CXCL2 and CXCR2, followed by activation of neutrophils and egress to the circulation. Taken together, administration of G-CSF alters the balance of chemokine production in the BM by stromal and endothelial cells, thereby regulating neutrophil mobilization from the BM (see Fig. 14.2). There is evidence for cross-talk between CXCR4 and CXCR2, and disruption of one signaling pathway may enhance another chemokine's receptor signaling. Martin et al (2003), Suratt et al (2004), and Wengner et al (2008) showed that pharmacologic blockade of CXCR4 signaling results in enhanced CXCR2 ligand-induced neutrophil mobilization in mice (reviewed by Day and Link[25]). Previously, Eash et al (2009) demonstrated that neutrophils lacking both CXCR4 and CXCR2 receptors exhibit increased neutrophil egress, similar to mice lacking only the CXCR4 receptor in neutrophils. In accordance, administration of CXCL2 does not induce neutrophil mobilization in mice lacking CXCR4 expression in neutrophils (reviewed by Day and Link[25]).

WHIM Syndrome

WHIM syndrome is an autosomal-dominant combined immunodeficiency disease caused by mutations in the receptor CXCR4, resulting in increased BM retention and severe reduction in circulating neutrophils. The term *WHIM* is an acronym for the main signs of the syndrome: warts, hypogammaglobulinemia, infections, and myelokathexis; myelokathexis refers to impaired egress of mature neutrophils and other myeloid cells from the BM, causing neutropenia. Al Ustwani et al (2014), Beaussant et al (2012), and Dotta et al (2011) reported that the signature pathogen in WHIM syndrome is human papillomavirus (HPV), which causes warts that cannot be controlled with standard medical treatment and may progress to cancer. Prophylactic antibiotics and G-CSF are often used to reduce the frequency of infections; however, their specific efficacy has not been established. This syndrome confirms a crucial role for CXCR4 signaling in neutrophil trafficking from the BM. In the majority of cases, WHIM syndrome is caused by truncation mutations in a domain important for CXCR4 downregulation (reviewed by Day and Link[25]). These mutations confer enhanced responsiveness to SDF-1, suggesting a model in which increased CXCR4 signaling leads to increased retention of neutrophils in the BM. Dale et al (2011) and McDermott et al (2011) demonstrated safety and preliminary evidence of clinical efficacy in phase I studies of the specific CXCR4 antagonist AMD3100 (plerixafor [Mozobil]) in WHIM syndrome, which increases the numbers of neutrophils in the circulation (reviewed by Link[29]). Spontaneous remission or cure of WHIM syndrome has been reported in 2015. McDermott et al (2015) describe chromothripsis (chromosome chattering) in one patient with WHIM syndrome that deleted one copy of chromosome 2, including deletion of the disease allele $CXCR4^{R334X}$ in a single HSC. Because CXCR4 regulates stem cell quiescence and the cell cycle, this led to their increased proliferation and differentiation due to a missing copy of CXCR4. This clone took over the BM and resorted normal immune function, which resulted in cure of the disease. This study suggests that partial CXCR4 inactivation might enhance clinical BM repopulation in transplanted patients.[30]

CONCLUDING REMARKS

This chapter discusses the mechanisms and pathways involved in the regulation of HSPC homing, egress, and mobilization, emphasizing the major roles of the SDF-1/CXCR4 axis in the regulation of these complex interactive processes. In addition, this chapter discusses the essential role of SDF-1/CXCR4 and CXCL2/CXCR2 signaling in the regulation of neutrophil egress and retention.

Successful BM reconstitution requires directed stem cell migration from the circulation across the blood–BM barrier, and lodgment in the specialized BM niches wherein stem cells proliferate and differentiate, while maintaining a small pool of primitive stem cells (see Fig. 14.1).

Currently, there are multiple hypotheses regarding the defined entity of the HSPC niche. SDF-1, which has a prominent role in homing, mobilization, retention, and quiescence of HSPCs, is highly expressed by endosteal osteoblasts, MSPCs, and other stromal cell types, implying the importance of regulating the niche in order to induce mobilization. The retention capacity of HSPCs in the BM during mobilization is altered due to several signaling events, chemotactic gradients (e.g., SDF-1 and S1P), as well as breakdown of adhesion interactions. Proteolytic enzymes that degrade adhesion molecules or extracellular matrix components, thus promoting adherence to the BM niches, are a key mechanism that enables egress of cells to the peripheral blood. Mimicry of this process by mobilizing agents leads to HSPC mobilization, and therefore such procedures can be utilized to clinically harvest repopulating HSPCs from the blood. Various BM-resident cellular players, including neutrophils, osteoclasts, and osteoblasts, play significant roles in mediating physiological cell egress and stress-induced mobilization to the peripheral blood (see Fig. 14.2). Mutual interactions and effects between these players result in a complex microenvironmental niche that regulates HSPC function, retention, and migration. Suppression of osteoblasts, MSPCs, or both, resulting in decreased SDF-1 expression in the BM, seems to be a major mechanism by which detachment of HSPCs is enabled as part of their recruitment to the peripheral blood. Hence, BM niches are dynamic and undergo alterations on demand, directly affecting hematopoiesis and motility. Additionally, there exist significant data implying a major contribution of innate immunity in mobilizing HSPCs (e.g., by neutrophils; see Fig. 14.2). This interplay is evident by studies showing activation of neutrophils upon administration of mobilizing agents, such as G-CSF. Disruption of CXCR4 signaling is an important mechanism by which neutrophils and HSPCs are mobilized into the circulation under stress conditions. CXCL2 is a secondary chemokine that, together with SDF-1, controls neutrophil trafficking from the BM.

Relevance to Clinical Hematology

Optimal HPSC migration from the BM to the circulation (mobilization) for donor cell transplant harvest and from the recipient blood into the BM (homing) for stem cell lodgment is an essential prerequisite for successful BM reconstitution in clinical transplantation. As discussed in this chapter, experimental systems involving human and murine HSPCs enable dissection of these migration processes to identify regulatory mechanisms to improve clinical settings. Current understanding of HSPC biology reveals that these cells home to the BM homeland, where they proliferate and differentiate, giving rise to multilineage hematopoietic cells while maintaining a small pool of primitive stem cells. The majority of HSPCs remain confined to the BM cavity in a nonmotile mode, adjacent to niche-supportive cells that preserve them in a quiescent, nonproliferative mode, but a very low level of primitive progenitors and stem cells also continuously egress to the circulation as part of homeostasis. The levels of these rare migrating HSPCs are dramatically enhanced during alarm situations caused by injury and inflammation as part of the host defense and repair mechanism. The physiologic process of enhanced HSPC recruitment from the BM has been used clinically to accelerate stem and progenitor cell migration to the circulation. Thus collection of HSPCs from the donor's peripheral blood, rather than from their BM, became the most common clinical protocol for BM transplantation (BMT).

Clinical BMT has gained immense success within the past four decades in the treatment of malignant hematologic diseases and immunodeficiency states by providing long-term immune recovery after high-dose chemotherapy. The basic premise in BMT is either using a patient's own stem cells (i.e., autologous BMT), which are used primarily as stem cell support for myeloma or lymphoma while undergoing intensive chemotherapy; or alternatively, allogeneic BMT, performed for the most part in the setting of marrow-infiltrating malignancies such as leukemia, which uses donor stem cells infused to a patient, thus capitalizing on the graft-versus-leukemia effect, which affords a significant reduction in relapse rate. One of the major clinical obstacles facing BM transplant experts today is the mobilization of the so-called "difficult mobilizers," who fail to mobilize the required amount of CD34 progenitors. Known risk factors for insufficient numbers of HSPCs after mobilization include older age, previous failed mobilization, heavy BM infiltration by tumor cells, and previous chemotherapy and radiotherapy, to name just a few. Several strategies have attempted to address this clinical problem using optimized current mobilization protocols, among them high-dose G-CSF regimens, erythropoietin, SCF, and chemomobilization achieved by chemotherapy treatment combined with G-CSF. Despite the wide gamut of therapeutic strategies used, most of them have either failed to show a clear advantage compared with standard mobilization regimens or were associated with substantial adverse effects (chemomobilization). With the recent introduction of the CXCR4 antagonist AMD3100 (also termed plerixafor [Mozobil]), there is renewed optimism in the management of difficult-to-mobilize patients. AMD3100 mediates rapid secretion of SDF-1 from BM stromal cells and its release to the circulation, resulting in CD34+ progenitor mobilization. Treatment with AMD3100 exhibits marked synergism with G-CSF, suggesting their different and complementary mechanisms of action to induce HSPC mobilization. Several studies have shown its success in mobilization of previously failed myeloma in non-Hodgkin lymphoma and Hodgkin lymphoma patients.

REFERENCES

1. Lapidot T, Kollet O: The brain-bone-blood triad: traffic lights for stem-cell homing and mobilization. *Hematology Am Soc Hematol Educ Program* 2010:1–6, 2010.

2. Lapidot T, Dar A, Kollet O: How do stem cells find their way home? *Blood* 106:1901–1910, 2005.

2a. Cottler-Fox MH, Lapidot T, Petit I, et al: Stem cell mobilization. *Hematology* 419–437, 2003.

2b. Kollet O, Petit I, Kahn J, et al: Human CD34+CXCR4- sorted cells harbor intracellular CXCR4, which can be functionally expressed and provide NOD/SCID repopulation. *Blood* 100:2778–2786, 2002.

2c. Kollet O, Spiegel A, Peled A, et al: Rapid and efficient homing of human CD34+CD38-/lowCXCR4+ stem and progenitor cells to the bone marrow and spleen of NOD/SCID and NOD/SCID/B2mnull mice. *Blood* 97:3283–3291, 2001.

3. Méndez-Ferrer S, Michurina TV, Ferraro F, et al: Mesenchymal and haematopoietic stem cells form a unique bone marrow niche. *Nature* 466:829–834, 2010.

4. Lapidot T, Kollet O: The essential roles of the chemokine SDF-1 and its receptor CXCR4 in human stem cell homing and repopulation of transplanted immune-deficient NOD/SCID and NOD/SCID/B2m(null) mice. *Leukemia* 16:1992–2003, 2002.

5. Golan K, Vagima Y, Ludin A, et al: S1P promotes murine progenitor cell egress and mobilization via S1P 1-mediated ROS signaling and SDF-1 release. *Blood* 119:2478–2488, 2012.

6. Golan K, Kollet O, Lapidot T: Dynamic cross talk between S1P and CXCL12 regulates hematopoietic stem cells migration, development and bone remodeling. *Pharmaceuticals (Basel)* 6:1145–1169, 2013.

7. Petit I, Szyper-Kravitz M, Nagler A, et al: G-CSF induces stem cell mobilization by decreasing bone marrow SDF-1 and up-regulating CXCR4. *Nat Immunol* 3:687–694, 2002.

8. Dar A, Schajnovitz A, Lapid K, et al: Rapid mobilization of hematopoietic progenitors by AMD3100 and catecholamines is mediated by CXCR4-dependent SDF-1 release from bone marrow stromal cells. *Leukemia* 25:1286–1296, 2011.

9. Nagasawa T, Hirota S, Tachibana K, et al: Defects of B-cell lymphopoiesis and bone-marrow myelopoiesis in mice lacking the CXC chemokine PBSF/SDF-1. *Nature* 382:635–638, 1996.

10. Tzeng YS, Li H, Kang YL, et al: Loss of Cxcl12/Sdf-1 in adult mice decreases the quiescent state of hematopoietic stem/progenitor cells and alters the pattern of hematopoietic regeneration after myelosuppression. *Blood* 117:429–439, 2011.

11. Liles WC, Broxmeyer HE, Rodger E, et al: Mobilization of hematopoietic progenitor cells in healthy volunteers by AMD3100, a CXCR4 antagonist. *Blood* 102:2728–2730, 2003.

12. Broxmeyer HE, Orschell CM, Clapp DW, et al: Rapid mobilization of murine and human hematopoietic stem and progenitor cells with AMD3100, a CXCR4 antagonist. *J Exp Med* 201:1307–1318, 2005.

13. Lévesque JP, Hendy J, Takamatsu Y, et al: Disruption of the CXCR4/CXCL12 chemotactic interaction during hematopoietic stem cell mobilization induced by gcsf or cyclophosphamide. *J Clin Invest* 111:187–196, 2003.

14. Kollet O, Shivtiel S, Chen YQ, et al: HGF, SDF-1, and MMP-9 are involved in stress-induced human CD34 + stem cell recruitment to the liver. *J Clin Invest* 112:160–169, 2003.

15. Kollet O, Dar A, Shivtiel S, et al: Osteoclasts degrade endosteal components and promote mobilization of hematopoietic progenitor cells. *Nat Med* 12:657–664, 2006.

16. Kollet O, Dar A, Lapidot T: The multiple roles of osteoclasts in host defense: bone remodeling and hematopoietic stem cell mobilization. *Annu Rev Immunol* 25:51–69, 2007.

17. Walkley CR, Shea JM, Sims NA, et al: Rb regulates interactions between hematopoietic stem cells and their bone marrow microenvironment. *Cell* 129:1081–1095, 2007.

18. Ludin A, Gur-Cohen S, Golan K, et al: Reactive oxygen species regulate hematopoietic stem cell self-renewal, migration and development, as well as their bone marrow microenvironment. *Antioxid Redox Signal* 21:1605–1619, 2014.

19. Winkler IG, Sims NA, Pettit AR, et al: Bone marrow macrophages maintain hematopoietic stem cell (HSC) niches and their depletion mobilizes HSCs. *Blood* 116:4815–4828, 2010.

20. Westerterp M, Gourion-Arsiquaud S, Murphy AJ, et al: Regulation of hematopoietic stem and progenitor cell mobilization by cholesterol efflux pathways. *Cell Stem Cell* 11:195–206, 2012.

21. Benschop RJ, Rodriguez-Feuerhahn M, Schedlowski M: Catecholamine-induced leukocytosis: early observations, current research, and future directions. *Brain Behav Immun* 10:77–91, 1996.

22. Katayama Y, Battista M, Kao WM, et al: Signals from the sympathetic nervous system regulate hematopoietic stem cell egress from bone marrow. *Cell* 124:407–421, 2006.

23. Spiegel A, Kalinkovich A, Shivtiel S, et al: Stem cell regulation via dynamic interactions of the nervous and immune systems with the microenvironment. *Cell Stem Cell* 3:484–492, 2008.

24. Méndez-Ferrer S, Lucas D, Battista M, et al: Haematopoietic stem cell release is regulated by circadian oscillations. *Nature* 452:442–447, 2008.

25. Day RB, Link DC: Regulation of neutrophil trafficking from the bone marrow. *Cell Mol Life Sci* 69:1415–1423, 2012.

26. Christopher MJ, Link DC: Regulation of neutrophil homeostasis. *Curr Opin Hematol* 14:3–8, 2007.

27. Singh P, Hu P, Hoggatt J, et al: Expansion of bone marrow neutrophils following G-CSF administration in mice results in osteolineage cell apoptosis and mobilization of hematopoietic stem and progenitor cells. *Leukemia* 26:2375–2383, 2012.

28. Christopher MJ, Liu F, Hilton MJ, et al: Suppression of CXCL12 production by bone marrow osteoblasts is a common and critical pathway for cytokine-induced mobilization. *Blood* 114:1331–1339, 2009.

29. Link DC: Regulation of hematopoiesis by CXCL12 / CXCR4 signaling. In *Targeted therapy of acute myeloid leukemia*, 2015, pp 593–605.

30. McDermott DH, Gao J-L, Liu Q, et al: Chromothriptic cure of WHIM syndrome. *Cell* 160:686–699, 2015.

VASCULAR GROWTH IN HEALTH AND DISEASE

Janusz Rak

HEMOSTATIC, HEMATOPOIETIC, AND VASCULAR SYSTEMS AS A FUNCTIONAL CONTINUUM

Although specific demands of practice, concepts, and methodologies define the unique scope of current hematology, the underlying biologic processes do not occur in isolation. Thus it is increasingly obvious that diseases affecting bone marrow and peripheral blood are closely intertwined with the state of the vascular system,[1] which acts as a niche, conduit, and regulator of many of these events.[2] This is exemplified by the anatomic proximity and interactions among several related cellular populations, including hematopoietic progenitors, their derivatives, endothelial cells and their precursors, platelets, perivascular tissues, and other components involved in blood vessel formation, repair, homeostasis, and patency.[2,3] The remarkable recent progress in understanding the molecular mechanisms involved in communication between these cells increasingly informs medical practice and drug discovery efforts.[2,4,5] For instance, agents designed to block vascular growth (antiangiogenics) in solid tumors also elicit hematologic perturbations,[6] and are being considered for treatment of hematopoietic malignancies.[7] Indeed, hematopoietic, hemostatic, and vascular compartments can be viewed as a functional continuum, both in health and in disease.

CONSTITUENTS OF THE VASCULAR SYSTEM

The hematopoietic and vascular systems emerge from a common progenitor cell (hemangioblast) early during embryogenesis. Subsequently, the vascular lineage evolves to form a network of channels that integrate, control, and reflect the structure and function of the tissues (parenchyma) and organs that they supply.[8] Local characteristics of the vascular system are superimposed on a more general, hierarchical branching pattern (arborization) and arteriovenous directionality essential for the function of the circulation. Structurally, distinct lymphatics emerge from the venous system to return extravascular (interstitial) fluid and extravasated cells to the venous circulation.[2]

Blood vessels are not only the essential supply routes of nutrients and oxygen to tissues (parenchyma), but also conduits of long-range regulatory signals (hormonal/endocrine), and an important source of paracrine cues that act on surrounding cells in a perfusion-independent (angiocrine) manner.[2,9,10] The latter influence may constitute a regulatory niche to either stimulate or inhibit the activity of parenchymal cells, including subsets of normal and cancer stem cells.[11,12] Postnatal tissue maturation imposes a quiescent phenotype throughout the vascular system, a state that is only rarely and transiently interrupted by posttraumatic tissue regeneration, wound healing, vascular repair, or cyclic changes in reproductive organs. This quiescent state may be chronically compromised in certain pathologies (inflammation, hyperplasia, or cancer), which can lead to unscheduled or abnormal vascular growth.[2] Out of several forms of such growth, vasculogenesis, angiogenesis, and vascular remodeling stand out as fundamentally important and distinct. In vasculogenesis, endothelial progenitor cell self-assembly results in the formation of new vascular channels (e.g., during embryogenesis). In contrast, angiogenesis is a process whereby preexisting vascular channels are extended to form additional capillary loops (e.g., during tissue

remodeling and in cancer). Structural changes leading to enlargement or shrinkage of such structures are referred to as vascular remodeling.[2]

Cells Involved in Vascular Growth

Specialized endothelial cells (ECs) constitute the crucial structural and functional element of the adult vasculature. ECs create antithrombotic luminal surfaces within all blood vessels, produce an active interface between the blood and the surrounding tissues, control the transmural flux of fluids and macromolecules (permeability), and are the key component of vascular growth processes (see Chapters 122 and 123). Such growth not only involves cessation of the quiescent state in subsets of resident endothelial cells, but is also associated with multiple systemic events, such as release of cytokines into the circulation and mobilization of cells from the bone marrow, including endothelial progenitor cells (EPCs), hematopoietic stem cells (HSCs), and myeloid (bone marrow-derived) cells (BMDCs).[2] These cells serve as surveillance and regulatory mechanisms that control and coordinate the responses of the peripheral vasculature (Fig. 15.1).[13] In established blood vessels the functionality of the endothelial tube is dependent on the support of the abluminal basement membrane, which is shared between these cells and one or more layers of contractile mesenchymal cells of the blood vessel wall (mural cells). Among those cells, sparse networks of pericytes (PCs) are associated with capillary endothelium, while continuous sheaths of smooth muscle cells (SMCs) cover the pre- and post-capillary vascular segments (arterial and venous, respectively).[2] The thickness and complexity of the vessel wall differ between veins and arteries, and increase with vascular hierarchy, so much so that the multilayered walls of large arteries contain their own capillary networks (vasa vasorum). The growth of the vasa vasorum can be induced in and contributes to the formation of atherosclerotic plaques, a process also involving metabolic abnormalities and increasingly well-characterized molecular pathways.[14] Blood vessel integrity and growth are also dependent on platelets and the hemostatic system (tissue factor, thrombin, thrombin receptor/PAR-1, the fibrinolytic system, and other effectors), all of which play important roles in the regulation of vascular continuity, patency, and permeability.[2] Coagulation proteases not only regulate clot formation upon injury, but also elicit signals within the surrounding vascular, inflammatory, and parenchymal cells, thereby modulating the related biologic responses and gene expression patterns.[9,15]

Molecular Regulators of Vascular Responses

The state of the vascular networks is controlled by a web of intercellular communications, which are executed by soluble growth factors, adhesion molecules, extracellular matrix (ECM) molecules, cell–cell contacts, the hemostatic system, various proteases, and the intercellular exchange of molecules (proteins, mRNA, and microRNA). A part of this circuitry entails the emission/uptake of extracellular vesicles (EVs), including exosomes.[2,16,17] Of the involved mediators, some are essential for vascular growth and homeostasis, while others play more pleiotropic and context-dependent roles (Table 15.1).[1,2]

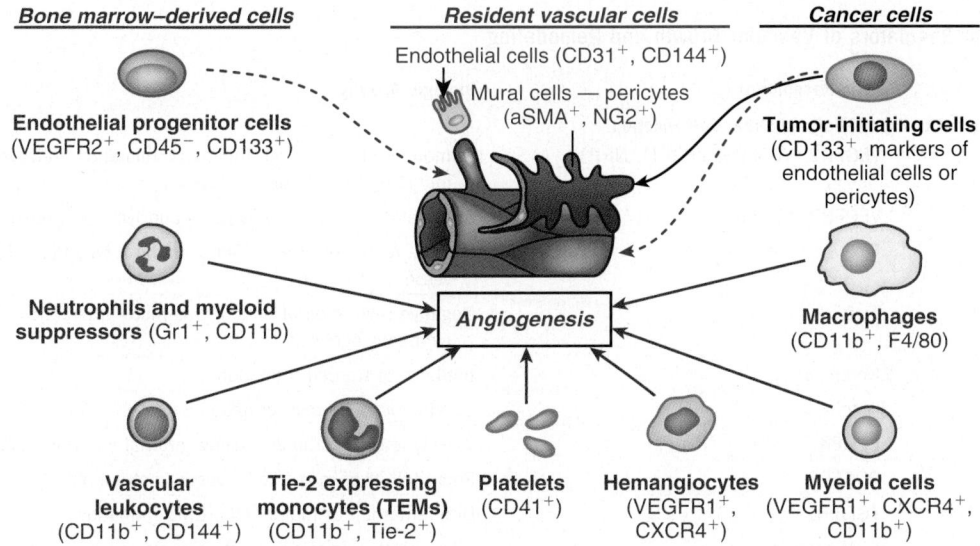

Fig. 15.1 CELL POPULATIONS INVOLVED IN VASCULAR GROWTH AND TUMOR ANGIOGEN-ESIS. Cells involved in blood vessel formation include endothelial cells, their progenitor cells, mural cells (pericytes), several populations of bone marrow–derived cells, as well as angiogenic fibroblasts, platelets, cancer cells, stem cells, and immune effectors not included in this diagram (based on Carmeliet and Jain[2], Kerbel[4], and De Palma and Naldini[13]). *VEGFR,* Vascular endothelial growth factor receptor.

Vascular Endothelial Growth Factors

Vascular endothelial growth factor-A (VEGF-A), which is also known as VEGF or vascular permeability factor (VPF), is indispensable for vascular development.[2,3,5] VEGF is the key member of a larger family of related polypeptides, which includes VEGF-B, VEGF-C, VEGF-D, VEGF-E, VEGFR-F, and placental growth factor (PlGF).[2] Upon dimerization, these factors bind to their tyrosine kinase receptors (RTKs/VEGFRs), including VEGFR1/Flt-1, VEGFR2/KDR/Flk-1, and VEGFR3/Flt-4, often in conjunction with their neuropilin coreceptors (NRP1, NRP2),[2] as depicted in Fig. 15.2. For instance, VEGF-A interacts with VEGFR2, VEGFR1, and VEGFR3, while PlGF is selective for VEGFR1. The distribution of different VEGFRs on vascular (VECs) and lymphatic (LECs) endothelial cell subsets, as well as among EPCs, hematopoietic, myeloid, and certain tumor cells, defines the known biologic activities of various VEGF ligands. The effects of VEGF include stimulation of endothelial mitogenesis, migration, survival, morphogenesis, and vascular permeability (e.g., through formation of intercellular gaps or transcellular structures know as *fenestrae*).[3] The signaling activity of VEGFR2 is crucial for these processes, whereas VEGFR1 is often expressed as a soluble splice variant (sFlt-1) that neutralizes VEGF (acts as VEGF "sink"), thereby inhibiting angiogenesis.[2]

VEGF activity is also regulated by splicing of the corresponding mRNA, which results in the generation of several protein isoforms, including VEGF121, VEGF145, VEGF165, VEGF189, and VEGF206 (designations based on the number of amino acids).[2,5] These variants differ in their cell association, solubility, and their ability to bind heparinoids or to interact with neuropilins, all of which define the formation of extracellular gradients and related biologic responses. In this regard, VEGF165 is an especially potent inducer of angiogenesis (Fig. 15.3). VEGF-C and VEGF-D stimulate the growth of lymphatics (lymphangiogenesis) via activation of VEGFR3, while VEGF-B and PlGF interact with VEGFR1 and are involved in vascular pathologies and inflammation.[2]

Platelet-Derived Growth Factors

This family of VEGF-related growth factors consists of four members: PDGF-A, PDGF-B, PDGF-C, and PDGF-D, the homo- or heterodimers of which interact preferentially with one of the three known cellular RTKs, namely PDGFRα, PDGFRβ, and PDGFRγ, each endowed with different cellular functions. For example, PDGF-BB is expressed by endothelial cells and mediates their capacity to attract mural cells harboring PDGFRβ.[2]

Prokineticins

This group of factors consists of the endocrine gland vascular endothelial growth factor/prokineticin 1 (EG-VEGF/PK1) and the protein 8/prokineticin 2 (Bv8/PK2) secreted by *Bombina variegata,* both of which interact with their respective G-protein–coupled receptors on endothelial cells (PK-R1 and PK-R2). These mediators induce VEGF-like effects in endothelial cells and may render tumors resistant to VEGF inhibition.[5]

Angiopoietins and Tie Receptors

Angiopoietins (Ang1, 2, and 4) interact with the Tie2/TEK receptor (RTK), which is preferentially expressed by endothelial cells and some myeloid cells (see Figs. 15.1 and 15.2). A related orphan receptor, known as Tie1, remains poorly characterized and likely acts by modulating Tie2 activity.[2] Ang1 emanates from perivascular tissues and serves as the main Tie2 agonist to stabilize endothelial–mural cell interactions and to promote endothelial cell survival, vascular quiescence, and the nonpermeable state. Ang2, which is produced by VEGF-stimulated endothelium, exerts the opposite effect and stimulates pericyte detachment, permeability, vascular growth, or regression, as well as lymphangiogenesis.[2]

Notch Pathway

Delta-like (Dll1, 3 and 4) and Jagged (1 and 2) are membrane-bound ligands that activate Notch receptors (Notch 1–4) on adjacent cells. During vascular development and growth Dll4 and Jagged 1 are expressed by subsets of endothelial and mural cells, respectively, and regulate their distinct functions within the capillary outgrowths

TABLE 15.1	Molecular Regulators of Vascular Growth and Remodeling	

Regulator	Main Receptor(s)	Biologic Activity
Angiogenic Effectors Central to Endothelial and Mural Cell Function		
VEGF-A/VEGF	VEGFR2 (VEGFR3, VEGF1), NRP1	Stimulator of angiogenic functions, migration and survival of ECs, including formation of tip cells
VEGF-C	VEGFR3 (VEGFR2)	Stimulator of angiogenesis (ECs) and lymphangiogenesis (LECs)
Ang 1	Tie2	Positive regulator of endothelial–mural interactions, EC survival, and vessel maturation
Ang 2	Tie2	Negative regulation of endothelial–mural interactions, stimulator of lymphangiogenesis
Dll4	Notch	Inhibitor of tip cell formation
Jag1	Notch	Stimulator of tip cell formation
EphrinB2	EPHB4	VEGFR internalization/signaling, arterial identity, tube formation
PDGF-B	PDGFRβ	Recruitment of mural cells, vessel maturation
TGFβ1	TGFβRII	Differentiation of mural cells, ECM formation
Integrins (αv, β1, β5)	ECM proteins	EC survival, migration morphogenesis
Stimulators Involved in Pathologic Angiogenesis		
PIGF	VEGFR1	Stimulates angiogenesis by interaction with ECs and BMDCs
Acidic FGF (FGF-1)	FGFRs 1–4	Stimulator of EC mitogenesis, survival, and angiogenesis
Basic FGF (FGF-2)	FGFRs 1–4	Stimulator of EC mitogenesis, survival, and angiogenesis
FGF-3	FGFRs 1–4	Stimulator of EC mitogenesis, survival, and angiogenesis
FGF-4	FGFRs 1–4	Stimulator of EC mitogenesis, survival, and angiogenesis
IL-8	CXCR1	Stimulator of ECs and inflammatory cells
IL-6	IL-6R	Stimulator of inflammatory angiogenesis
TNFα	TNFR1 (p55)	EC stimulator and VEGF inducer
Bv8	GPCR	Stimulator of endocrine and tumor ECs
PD-ECGF/TP	Unclear	Stimulator of angiogenesis
Angiogenin	170-kDa receptor	Stimulator of angiogenesis and tRNAse
MMP9	ECM proteins	Matrix metalloproteinase that breaks down the ECM and releases angiogenic growth factors
Endogenous Angiogenesis Inhibitors		
Inhibitor	*Biologic Activity*	
TSP-1	Interacts with the CD36 receptor, integrins, and other proteins, causing growth inhibition and apoptosis of angiogenic ECs	
Endostatin	Proteolytic fragment of collagen XVIII with antiangiogenic activity	
Angiostatin	Proteolytic fragment of plasminogen with antiangiogenic activity	
Tumstatin	Proteolytic fragment of collagen IV alpha 3 chain	
sFlt-1/sVEGFR1	Soluble splice variant of VEGFR1 neutralizing VEGF and blocking VEGFR2 signaling	
VEGF165b	Splice variants of VEGF with antiangiogenic activity	
PEX	Inhibitor of EC invasion and MMP activity	
IFNα (β)	Inhibits release of angiogenic growth factors	

Ang (1,2), Angiopoietin; Bv8, *Bombina variegata* protein; Dll4, delta-like 4; FGF, fibroblast growth factor; GPCR, G-protein-coupled receptor; IFN, interferon; IL-6, interleukin 6; IL-8, interleukin 8; Jag1, Jagged 1; MMP9, matrix metalloproteinase 9; PD-ECGF/TP, platelet-derived endothelial cell growth factor/thymidine phosphorylase; PDGF, platelet-derived growth factor; PIGF, placenta growth factor; TNFα, tumor necrosis factor alpha; TSP-1, thrombospondin 1; VEGF, vascular endothelial growth factor. See text and references for details.[2]

(sprouts), as depicted in Figs. 15.2 and 5.3.[5] Dll1 is also involved in circumferential vascular enlargement (arteriogenesis; Fig. 15.4).[2]

Ephrins and Eph Receptors

The arterial or venous identity of endothelial cells in the evolving microcirculation is preprogrammed by the expression of transmembrane guidance molecules, especially ephrin B2 and its EPHB4 receptor. Bidirectional signals emanating from these molecules, together with mechanosensory cues, govern the arteriovenous vascular arborization that is essential for, and maintained by, proper blood flow.

Other ephrins are implicated in endothelial–pericyte interactions, and communication between blood vessels and tumor cells. They may also cooperate in VEGFR2 endocytosis and signaling.[2]

Vascular Integrins, Cadherins, and Cell Adhesion Molecules

Quiescent endothelial cells are anchored to the basement membrane, a structured layer of ECM composed mainly of laminin and collagen type IV. In contrast, growing (angiogenic) endothelial cells are surrounded by provisional ECM containing fibrin, vitronectin, fibronectin, and

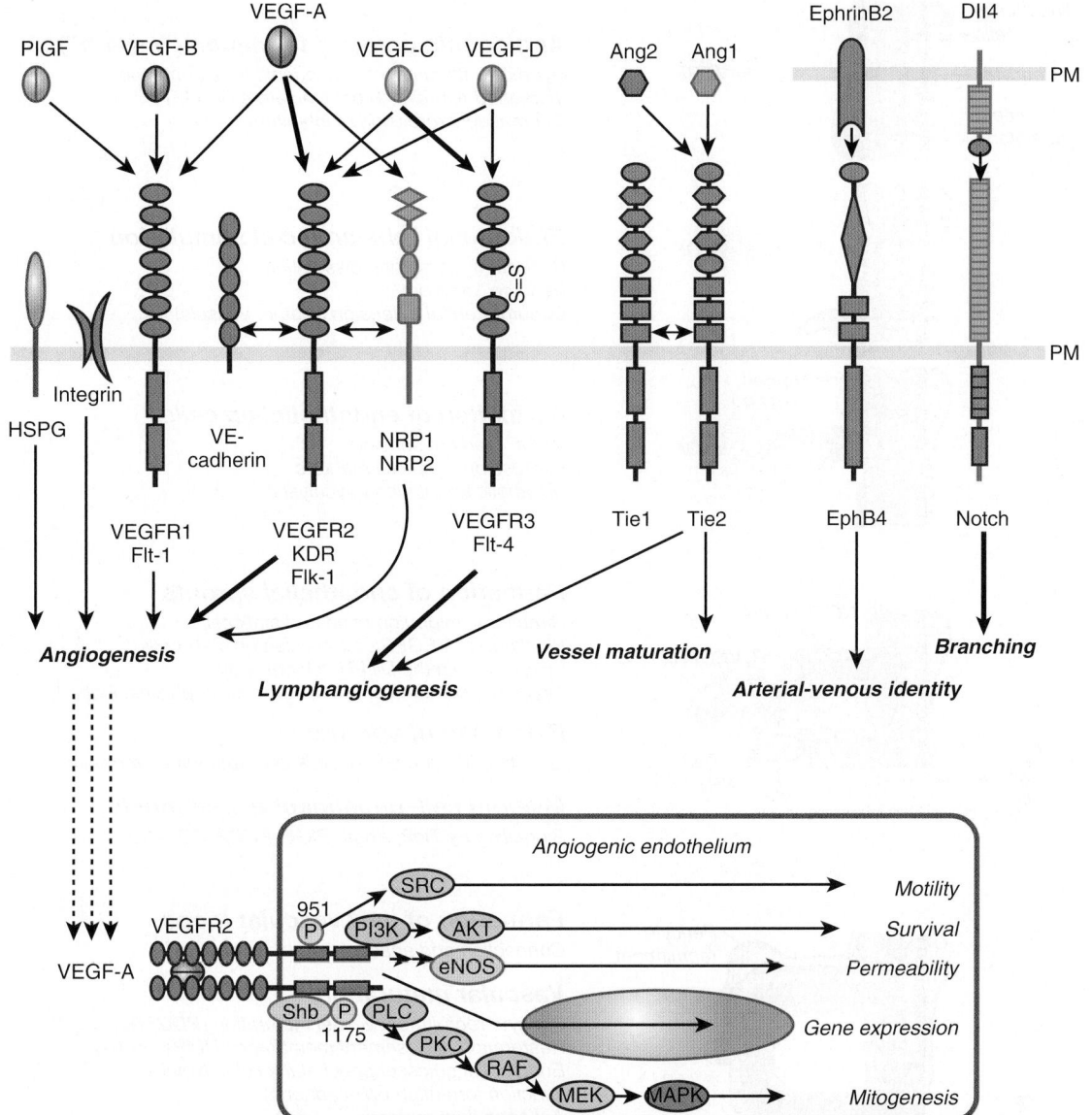

Fig. 15.2 ELEMENTS OF THE SIGNALING CIRCUITRY INVOLVED IN BLOOD VESSEL FORMATION AND TUMOR ANGIOGENESIS. Receptors and co-receptors involved in angiogenic, lymphangiogenic, and regulatory signaling. *Bottom panel:* Outline of signaling pathways and their effector mechanisms downstream of VEGF-A/VEGF. *Dll4,* Delta-like 4; *eNOS,* endothelial nitric oxide synthase; *HSPG,* heparan sulfate proteoglycan; *MAPK,* mitogen-activated protein kinase; *NRP,* neuropilin; *PI3K,* phosphatidylinositol 3-kinase; *PLC,* phospholipase C; *PlGF,* Placental growth factor; *PKC,* protein kinase C; *PM,* plasma membrane; *VE-cadherin,* vascular endothelial cadherin; *VEGF,* vascular endothelial growth factor; *SRC,* Rous sarcoma virus-related proto-oncogene.

partially degraded collagens. Growth factors upregulate the expression of dimeric integrin receptors (αvβ3, αvβ5, α1β1, α2β1, α4β1, α5β1), which recognize specific motifs in ECM molecules (often the RGD sequence). Angiogenic growth factor receptors require integrin interactions for their signaling function, while integrin αvβ3 is one of several antiangiogenic targets under investigation.[2,4]

Vascular endothelial cadherin (VE-cadherin/CD144) is selectively expressed by endothelial cells and contributes to their barrier function, homotypic adhesion, and growth regulatory signals. Other cadherins, as well as claudins (e.g., endothelial claudin 5) and connexins, contribute to homo- and heterotypic endothelial cell interactions, and the formation of gap and tight junctions, as well as transmission of intercellular signals.[2] On the other hand, interactions between endothelium and circulating immune, myeloid, inflammatory, and progenitor cells, and platelets are mediated by selectins (e.g., P- L- and E-selectin), integrins (α4β1/VLA4), and members of the immunoglobulin family of cell adhesion molecules (ICAM-1/2

and VCAM1), all of which play distinct roles in the regulation of angiogenesis and vascular homeostasis.[2,5]

Proteases

Proteases regulate remodeling, growth, and invasion of new blood vessels; liberation of ECM-bound angiogenic growth factors; generation of regulatory peptides (e.g., angiogenesis inhibitors); clotting and fibrinolysis; intracellular signaling; and numerous other steps involved in vascular maintenance and remodeling. For example, matrix metalloproteinases (MMPs) and their tissue inhibitors (TIMPs 1–4) participate in the controlled ECM/basement membrane breakdown that is required for invasiveness of the angiogenic endothelium.[2,18] The key enzymes in this group include: MMP-1, MMP-2, MMP-9, and MMP-14, coagulation factors (VIIa and thrombin) and their receptors (tissue factor and PAR-1), plasminogen activators (uPA)

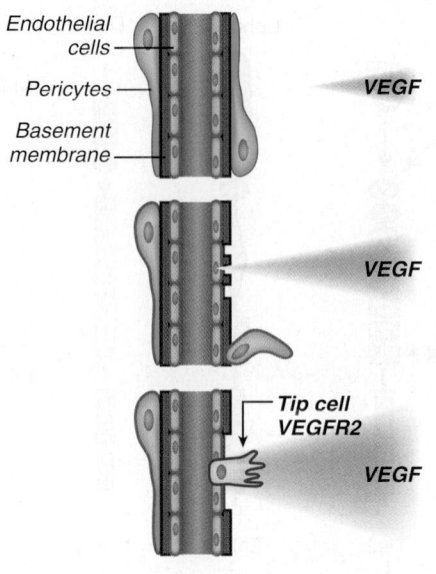

Angiogenic gradient formation ("switch")
Hypoxia, inflammation, oncogenic transformation
Increased expression of stimulators (VEGF)
Decreased expression of inhibitors

Endothelial (phalanx) cell stimulation
Basement membrane dissolution
Pericyte "drop out"
Circumferential extension (mother vessels)

Formation of endothelial tip cells
VEGF gradient sensing
Expression of tip cell markers
Metabolic adaptation (glycolysis)

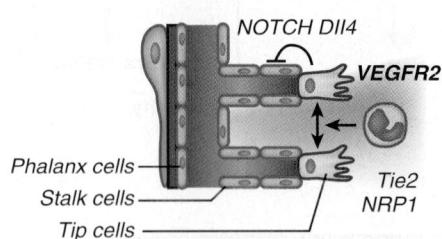

Formation of endothelial sprouts
Directional migration of tip and stalk cells
Blockade of VEGFR2 expression on stalk cells
by tip cells via the Dll4/Notch pathway
Tip guidance (semaphorins, neuropilins, plexins, Robo4)

Extension of sprouts
Growth and migration of stalk cells and lumen formation

Myeloid cell–dependent anastomosis
Signalling by Tie2, Ang2, PlGF, PHD2, SDF-1α

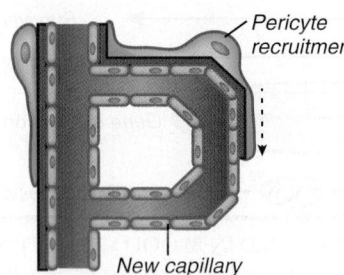

Formation of new vascular loops
Connection and anastomosis of sprouts

Vascular maturation
Pericyte recruitment/vessel maturation (PDGFRb, Ang1)
Restoration of basement membrane (TIMPs, PAI-1)
Endothelial quiescence–phalanx cells (Notch)
Junction formation (VE-cadherin)
Anticoagulant surfaces

Blood flow
Resolution of hypoxia

Fig. 15.3 SPROUTING ANGIOGENESIS. The change in balance between angiogenesis stimulators and inhibitors (angiogenic switch) and especially the gradient of VEGF leads to sprouting angiogenesis. This process begins with changes in the vessel wall (endothelial phalanx cells), resulting in the formation of enlarged mother vessels, endothelial tip cells, proliferating stalk cells, capillary loops, and eventually anastomoses, as depicted (details in the text and in Carmeliet and Jain[2]). *Ang,* Angiopoietin; *Dll4,* delta-like 4; *PAI-1,* plasminogen inhibitor; *TIMP,* tissue inhibitor of MMP; *VEGF,* vascular endothelial growth factor; *VEGFR,* vascular endothelial growth factor receptor.

and their inhibitors (PAI-1), members of the disintegrin and metalloproteinase domain, and thrombospondin motif-containing families (ADAM and ADAMTS).

Angiogenesis Stimulators and Inhibitors

In addition to "professional" angiogenesis regulators, a number of molecules with more pleiotropic biologic activity serve as stimulators or inhibitors of vascular growth, either directly or indirectly (e.g., as inducers of VEGF). Examples of these diverse effectors are listed in Table 15.1 and include certain cytokines (FGF1, FGF2, HGF, TGFβ), chemokines (IL-8/CXCL8, SDF-1/CXCL12), secreted ECM proteins (TSP1, TSP2), proteolytic ECM fragments (tumstatin, angiostatin),

phospholipids (sphingosine 1 phosphate [S1P]), and several other entities.[1] The effects of angiogenesis regulators are mediated by intracellular signaling pathways, including GTP-ases (Ras), kinases (src, Akt, PKC), transcription factors (ERG, HIF, MYC), microRNA species (miR17-92, miR155), and other effectors (see Fig. 15.2).[2]

PROCESSES INVOLVED IN BLOOD VESSEL FORMATION

The vascular system is programmed to rapidly respond to changes in the microenvironment. Although these responses may be provoked by local factors (e.g., tissue injury or hypoxia), they are regulated at several levels, including locally, regionally, and systemically, and with the involvement of perivascular, vessel wall–associated, circulating,

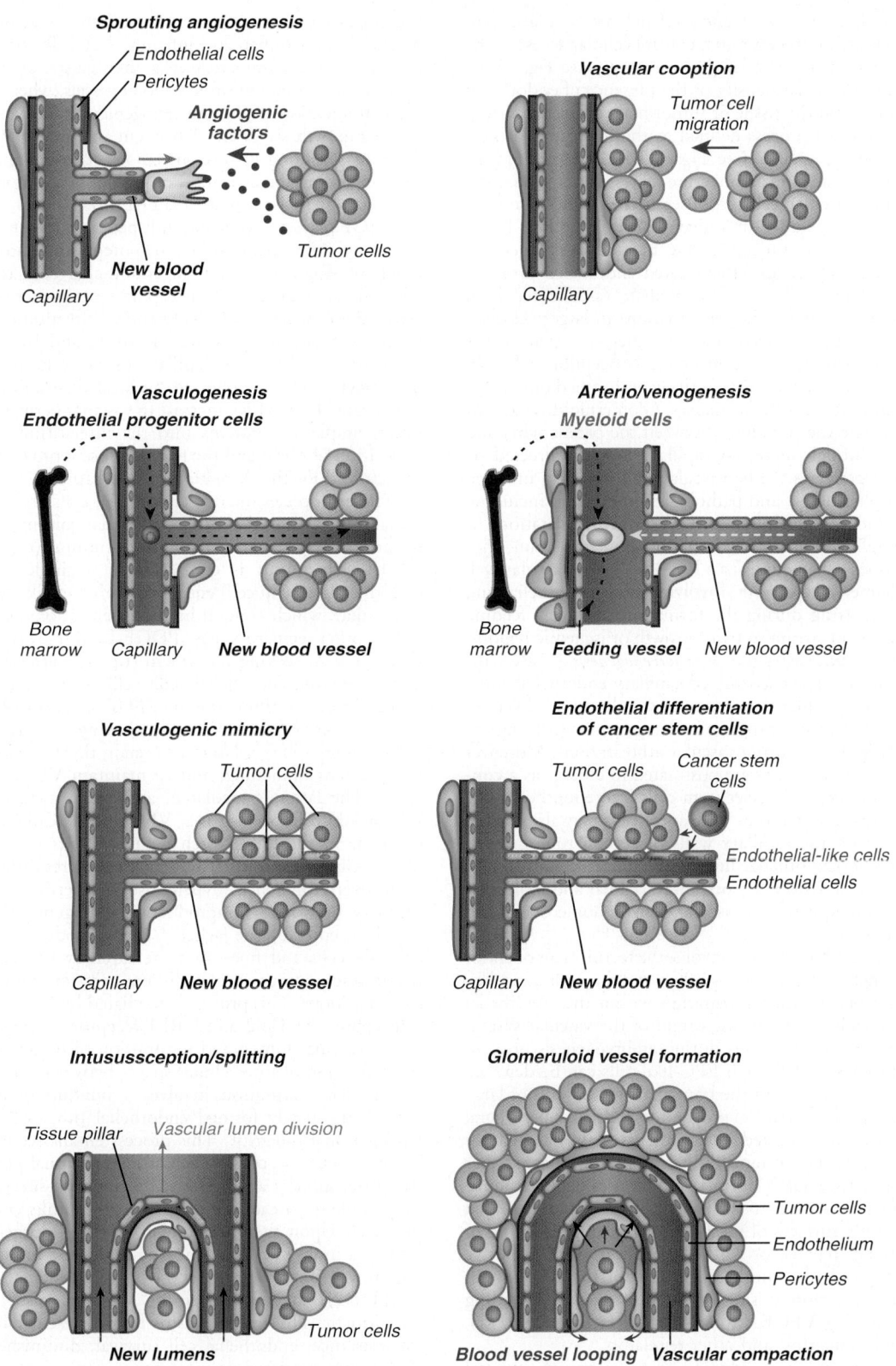

Fig. 15.4 PROCESSES OF VASCULAR GROWTH AND REMODELING IN CANCER. Neoplastic growth can serve as a paradigm for cellular programs regulating the proximity between parenchymal (cancer) cells and the vascular lumen[2,24] (see text for details). *Angiogenesis,* Recruitment of new capillary vessels through paracrine effects of angiogenic factors on endothelial cells of the preexisting vasculature; *Vascular cooption,* recruitment of cancer cells to the proximity of preexisting blood vessels; *Vasculogenesis,* recruitment of bone marrow–derived endothelial progenitor cells (EPCs) to the sites of vascular growth or repair (although EPC are essential during embryogenesis, postnatally their role is more limited as they lodge in, and contribute to, fragments of the newly formed vascular wall, or participate in the repair at sites of endothelial denudation); *Arterio/venogenesis,* retrograde circumferential enlargement and remodeling of feeding vessels that supply expanding capillary networks with blood, a process involving bone marrow derived myeloid cell recruitment through tissue-related stimuli and shear forces; *Vasculogenic mimicry,* contribution of cancer cells to the vascular wall involving adoption of some endothelial-like features; *Endothelial differentiation (or trans-differentiation) of cancer stem cells,* certain types of multipotential tumor-initiating (stem) cells may activate programs of endothelial or pericytic transdifferentiation and form segments of the newly formed vasculature[22,23]; *Intussusception,* division of the vascular lumen into smaller tubes by ingrowth of external tissue pillars; *Glomeruloid vessel formation,* formation of bundles of vascular loops through forces (arrows) generated by endothelial, pericyte, and parenchymal cell interactions.[2,4,20,24]

and bone marrow–derived cells.[2] Cancer-related neovascularization exemplifies the diversity of processes that control cellular access to the perfused vascular space and the related terminology (see Fig. 15.4). Indeed, an increase in vascular density or the presence of endothelial structures or blood within the tissue or tumor mass is not necessarily related to angiogenesis,[1] a process defined as the formation of new capillaries from preexisting ones (see Figs. 15.1, 15.3, and 15.4). Instead, the vascular density and architecture represent a combination of parenchymal and vascular cell responses to metabolic demands and regulatory circuits operative in a given context (see Fig. 15.4). As mentioned earlier, these processes may include vasculogenesis, recruitment, and assembly of undifferentiated endothelial progenitor cells (EPCs).[2,4] These cells may also mediate vascular repair in response to endothelial damage (i.e., denudation) in larger vessels.[19] Extravascular tissues may actively increase their vascular access through processes of vascular cooption or intussusception, whereby blood vessels may respectively become actively ensheathed or divided (split) by advancing external cellular masses. Glomeruloid vessels, or tufts, may also increase the proximity between the parenchyma and the vascular space through increased capillary looping directed by forces generated by pericytes.[20] The vascular wall may also undergo different forms of physiologic and pathologic remodeling, including circumferential lumen enlargement through growth, dilatation, or both. This is exemplified by capillary mother vessel formation prior to the onset of proper angiogenesis (see Fig. 15.3). The vascular wall thickening and diameter expansion, involving both endothelial and mural cells, and occurring during the formation of larger "feeding vessels" (or collaterals) upstream to tissue growth or ischemic regions, is often referred to as *arteriogenesis* or *arterio/venogenesis*.[18,21] Recruitment of pericytes to the newly assembled capillary endothelial tubes signifies the process of vascular maturation or stabilization.[18] Distinct mechanisms also regulate the programmed regression (pruning) of superfluous capillaries (e.g., during vascular arborization). Moreover in cancer, new vascular structures are postulated to emerge as a consequence of differentiation of cancer stem cells into endothelial-like or pericyte-like cellular populations.[22,23] Cancer cells may also replace endothelial cells within the capillary walls of certain tumor types, giving rise to a pseudoendothelial lining (vasculogenic mimicry).[24] Each of these processes is driven by specialized cellular and molecular circuitry, and plays a unique role in vascular growth, homeostasis, and pathology, as outlined briefly below[2,4,5,24] (see Fig. 15.4).

Vasculogenesis and vascular repair involve the recruitment of endothelial precursors, such as angioblasts or EPCs, and their self-assembly, differentiation, and/or structural integration within the endothelial lining. Vasculogenesis is central to the origin of the vascular system (primary capillary plexus formation) during embryogenesis prior to the onset of angiogenesis.[8] Although EPC-like cells can be detected during postnatal life, especially in the bone marrow, in walls of large vessels, and as circulating endothelial progenitors (CEPs) in peripheral blood, they have a more restricted role, which is mainly regulatory and reparative in nature. For instance, EPCs may accumulate at sites of angiogenesis, but they rarely form complete vascular segments. However, EPCs may contribute to the endothelialization of denuded luminal surfaces, inner surfaces of vascular grafts, damaged lining of larger vessels (vascular repair), or to the recanalization of occlusive thrombi.[19] Several molecular mechanisms control the recruitment of EPCs and their retention at sites of vascular growth, including high levels of circulating VEGF, stromal-derived factor 1 (SDF-1), expression of certain integrins, and other regulators.[2,4]

Angiogenesis occurs under conditions of tissue growth, wound repair, inflammation, hypoxia, or proliferative disease (e.g., cancer). The new vascular structures emerge from preexisting endothelial channels mainly through a mechanism known as *sprouting angiogenesis* (see Fig. 15.3). In this case, the triggering event involves the formation of a gradient of proangiogenic activity around hypoxic or activated cells. The resulting cascade of responses within the wall of the nearest capillary begins with local capillary distension to form an enlarged mother vessel. Although high concentrations of VEGF are sufficient to induce these changes,[3] the underlying molecular events usually involve a more global shift in levels of multiple angiogenesis inhibitors and stimulators

("angiogenic switch").[1] Some of these factors may upregulate VEGF in parenchymal, stromal, and inflammatory cells, or act directly on the endothelium. Inflammatory cells often cluster at sites of angiogenesis prior to the formation of new blood vessels, where they contribute to the consolidation of the proangiogenic microenvironment, or trigger vascular growth via VEGF-dependent and independent mechanisms.[2,5] Efficient sprouting involves metabolic reprogramming of endothelial cells, including the activation of glycolysis and upregulation of phosphofructokinase isoenzyme 3 (PFKFB3).[25]

VEGF plays a central and indispensable role in normal angiogenic sprouting. After exposure to this potent stimulator, there is upregulation of Ang2 expression in endothelial cells residing within the continuous monolayer of the capillary or mother vessel wall (phalanx cells). Endothelial Ang2 blocks tonic activation of the Tie2 receptor by the constitutive presence of Ang1, and by disrupting the key mechanism maintaining capillary structure leads to the detachment of pericytes. This is followed by local dissolution of the basement membrane (by MMPs), increase in vascular permeability, and extravasation of plasma proteins into the interstitium. The extravascular deposition of fibrin and the formation of a provisional ECM provide the scaffold for the formation of new capillaries.[2]

These processes liberate endothelial cells and initiate their directional migration in the form of a cellular column (angiogenic sprout) toward the source of the angiogenic stimulus (e.g., VEGF-expressing cells). Each sprout is composed of a single, specialized leading endothelial cell (tip cell) equipped with hair-like, sensing projections (filopodia), which contain high concentrations of VEGFR2 and are rich in other regulators (e.g., PDGF-B, SDF-1, Apelin, and Dll4). In their gradient-seeking movement, tip cells are followed by a cohort of proliferating endothelial stalk cells, which express VEGFR1 and Notch. Stronger stimulation by VEGF results in VEGFR2-dependent upregulation of Dll4 in tip cells, allowing them to instruct their stalk cell counterparts (via Notch) to retain their phenotype, refrain from independent branching, and to maintain VEGF signaling at lower levels. The latter is mediated, at least in part, by upregulation of soluble VEGFR1, acting as a "VEGF sink." Consequently, exogenous blockade of the Dll4/Notch pathway leads to excessive generation of tip cells and sprouts (from stalk cells), resulting in the formation of an overly branched, hyperdense, nonperfused, and dysfunctional capillary network ("nonproductive angiogenesis").[26] Stimulation of Notch receptor by the Jagged 1 ligand modulates the effects of Dll4 on stalk cells and fine-tunes the capillary branching patterns. The neighboring sprouts eventually connect (anastomose) to form new capillary loops. This process is mediated by interaction with myeloid cells expressing Tie-2 and NRP1 receptors.[27] Subsequent generation of the vascular lumen and resumption of blood flow occur through the formation of intercellular spaces between endothelial stalk cells.[2]

Vascular maturation involves a buildup of a mural cell layer around the newly formed endothelial tube, which is essential for its functional integrity.[2] This process entails secretion of PDGF-BB by endothelial tip cells, which attracts regional pericytes; a source of structural support and vessel-stabilizing, pro-survival Ang1 activity.[28] S1P regulates N-cadherin, which further links endothelial cells and pericytes. Upon their attachment to the endothelial tube, pericytes assume a more mature phenotype under the influence of transforming growth factor beta 1 (TGFβ1).[28] Endothelial prolyl hydroxylase 2 (PHD2), an oxygen-sensing enzyme, also regulates pericyte recruitment. These mechanisms restore vascular integrity, mechanical resistance, endothelial cell survival, diminished dependence on VEGF, and restricted permeability.[2]

Lymphangiogenesis and lymphatic dilatation represent key responses of specialized lymphatic endothelial cells (LECs) to external stimuli. LECs express distinct molecular markers (VEGFR3, Prox-1, LYVE-1) and respond to VEGF-C, VEGF-D, VEGF, and Ang2 (which acts as a Tie2 agonist in LECs and a Tie2 antagonist in their blood vessel counterparts—VECs). Even though LECs exhibit up to 98% molecular similarity to VECs and originate from vascular endothelium, they form separate networks of thin-walled vessels that serve as conduits for the collection of interstitial fluid and cells, including inflammatory cells and metastatic cancer cells.[29]

Vasculogenic mimicry and endothelial differentiation of cancer stem cells are processes whereby nonendothelial cells adopt endothelial-like phenotypes and line vascular channels.[30] Vasculogenic mimicry occurs during normal placentation and in tumors, such as melanoma, or mouse teratoma, and results in positioning of parenchymal cells (e.g., cancer cells) within the layer of endothelium or around blood-containing channels. Such cells may adopt some of the morphologic and antigenic attributes of proper endothelium.[24] In human glioblastoma, cancer stem cells were reported to undergo a more profound endothelial or pericytic transdifferentiation, including the expression of corresponding lineage markers and some contribution to the vascular wall. The scope and functional role of these processes remain unclear and controversial.[22,23,30]

Vascular cooption occurs when cancer cells actively adopt a growth and invasion pattern around preexisting blood vessels.[31] This process is observed in highly vascular organs, such as the lungs and brain, resulting in a nonangiogenic form of tumor neovascularization. Coopted vessels may undergo secondary structural alterations, which may result in their remodeling, formation of occlusive thrombi, and regression that can lead to ischemia.[32]

MECHANISMS TRIGGERING ANGIOGENESIS

Vascular growth may occur in response to hypoxia, metabolic stress, expression of growth factors, emission of inflammatory mediators, or after activation of the coagulation system or malignant transformation. These mechanisms are interdependent and often converge upon the regulation of the VEGF gene,[2] but may also involve additional (or alternative) complex networks of molecular effectors. Although angiogenic responses may be morphologically similar, they exhibit context-dependent degrees of regulatory and functional redundancy.[5] The most studied in this regard is the regulation of VEGF, which is transcriptionally controlled by dimeric hypoxia-inducible factors 1 and 2 (HIFs). Normally, the HIF alpha subunit (HIF-1α) is constitutively degraded by a pathway involving oxygen-dependent prolyl and aspargyl hydroxylases, von Hippel–Lindau (VHL) ubiquitin ligase, and the proteasome.[33] Hypoxia blocks this process, resulting in elevated HIF activity and VEGF production by parenchymal, stromal, and inflammatory cells. Several other mechanisms of proangiogenic, hypoxic responses have also been described (e.g., NFκB, EGR1).[33] Likewise, the exposure of cells to growth factors (EGF, FGF, HGF) and inflammatory cytokines (IL-6) may upregulate VEGF, and some of these effectors may also directly stimulate endothelial cells.[2] Activation of oncogenes (e.g., ras) and loss of tumor suppressors (VHL) lead to upregulation of VEGF and may also affect other angiogenic growth factors in cancer cells, even under conditions of normoxia.[9] Oncogenic transformation also shuts down some of the angiogenic inhibitors, contributes to coagulopathy (through upregulation of tissue factor and thrombin receptors), and enhances proangiogenic cellular vesiculation (biogenesis and emission of extracellular vesicles loaded with vascular mediators). Indeed, oncogenic pathways often mimic, distort, or exacerbate the effects of hypoxia, inflammation, or microenvironmental stress.[9]

THERAPEUTIC IMPLICATIONS OF ANGIOGENESIS IN HEMATOLOGY

Vascular events associated with cancer, hemangioma, or vascular malformations have the potential to trigger hematologic consequences, either spontaneously or during therapeutic angiogenesis or antiangiogenesis. These linkages are poorly understood, but often include one or more of the following factors: (1) endothelial cell activation associated with intravascular upregulation of procoagulant tissue factor, adhesion molecules, and other mediators; (2) disruption of vascular wall continuity; (3) recruitment of inflammatory cells; (4) enhanced vascular permeability resulting in the extravasation and activation of circulating coagulation factors; (5) platelet activation; (6) contact between procoagulant cell surfaces (e.g., metastatic cancer cells) and

circulating blood; (7) flow perturbations and stasis; (8) indirect external effects (e.g., indwelling catheters or administration of chemotherapy); and (9) shedding of procoagulant, anticoagulant, or bioactive extracellular vesicles (microparticles), and soluble factors into blood.[9] A better understanding of blood vessel–directed therapies and their capacity to modulate or exacerbate some of these events represents an emerging challenge in hematology (see Chapter 149).

Therapeutic Inhibition and Stimulation of Angiogenesis

Excessive, protracted, or aberrant activation of vascular growth may represent a correlative and/or a causative factor in several pathologies (often referred to collectively as *angiogenesis-related diseases*).[1] These include chronic inflammation, certain forms of blindness, metabolic diseases, atherosclerosis, and cancer.[1] In some of these disorders (e.g., macular degeneration, certain malignancies) antiangiogenic therapies, especially inhibitors of the VEGF pathway (Table 15.2), already represent the standard of care. Numerous clinical trials are ongoing to explore other agents and indications.[2]

Conversely, pathology may also arise due to insufficient angiogenesis, arteriogenesis, or regulatory/repopulating activity of bone marrow–derived cells, as is the case in the myocardium postinfarction, in limb ischemia, and in other hypovascular states, especially in the elderly. In these disorders, stimulation of vascular growth may provide a therapeutic benefit, notably through delivery of angiogenic cells (EPCs), growth factors (VEGF, FGF), or gene therapy vectors into the affected site. Several such (proangiogenic) strategies are under investigation.[2]

Tumor Angiogenesis and Antiangiogenesis

The disorganized signaling cues during tumor angiogenesis may produce highly abnormal, leaky, tortuous, prothrombotic, and poorly perfused vasculature (vessel "abnormalization"), which may contribute to aberrant hemostasis.[2] Antiangiogenic agents may cause further perturbations by selective destruction of tumor-associated endothelial cells or by inhibition of their stimulatory circuitry.[1] Several classes of antiangiogenic compounds have been evaluated to date, including derivatives of natural angiogenesis inhibitors (e.g., endostatin or tumstatin), inhibitors of proangiogenic signaling pathways (antibodies, small-molecule agents), and agents that block proangiogenic inflammatory pathways (e.g., thalidomide analogs). Anticancer drugs may also be administered in low but frequent doses (metronomic chemotherapy) to target endothelial immune and regulatory cells preferentially (Table 15.2).[1,4,34]

Bevacizumab (Avastin), a humanized monoclonal anti-VEGF antibody, was the first antiangiogenic agent to be approved (in 2004) for cancer treatment, and the drug is now used to treat colorectal, lung, kidney, and recurrent brain tumors.[2,34] Several tyrosine kinase inhibitors (TKIs) with anti-VEGFR or multikinase activity (sunitinib, sorafenib, pazopanib) are also in common use, as are inhibitors of oncogenic pathways that drive the production of VEGF.[9] The latter include inhibitors of epidermal growth factor receptor (EGFR) and HER2 (cetuximab and transtuzumab, respectively), and other oncogene inhibitors.[9] These VEGF/VEGFR antagonists are mostly used in combination with chemotherapy, which suggests that they serve as chemosensitizers or mediators of vascular normalization.[2,4] Studies are underway to develop drugs that specifically target pathologic angiogenesis (e.g., blockers of PlFG), or established tumor blood vessels (e.g., vascular disrupting agents [VDAs]).[4]

The overall objectives of antiangiogenic therapy in cancer are at least threefold: (1) to induce tumor hypovascularity, thereby causing hypoxic damage to cancer cells; (2) to deprive cancer (stem) cells of the paracrine growth stimulation and support rendered by angiogenic endothelial cells (anti-angiocrine effect)[9,10]; and (3) at lower doses, to induce vessel "normalization," resulting in the improved tumor perfusion associated with increased sensitivity to chemotherapy and radiation.[2]

TABLE 15.2 Blood Vessel–Targeting Therapeutics

Drug	Type	Target	Stage of Development
Targeted Agents Designed to Obliterate Defined Angiogenic Pathways			
Bevacizumab (Avastin)	Neutralizing huMoAb	VEGF	Approved for human use
Ramucirumab (Cyramza)	Neutralizing huMoAb	VEGFR2	Approved for human use
Sunitinib (Sutent)	TKI	VEGFR1-3, PDGFRα/β, KIT, FLT3, RET, CSF1R	Approved for human use
Sorafenib (Nexavar)	TKI	VEGFR2–3, C-Raf, B-Raf, VEGF-C, FLT3, FGFR1, PDGFβ, KIT, p38	Approved for human use
Pazopanib (Votrient)	TKI	VEGFR1-3, PDGFRα/β, KIT, FGFR1,3,4, FMS,	Approved for human use
Vandetanib (Caprelsa)	TKI	VEGFR2, EGFR, RET	Approved for human use
Axitinib (Inlyta)	TKI	VEGFR1–3, PDGFR, KIT	Approved for human use
Regorafenib (Stivarga)	TKI	VEGFR-1, -2, -3, TIE2, PDGFR, FGFR, KIT, RET, RAF, BRAF, BRAFV600E	Approved for human use
Cabozantinib (Cometriq)	TKI	VEGFR2, MET, RET	Approved for human use
VEGF-trap Ziv-aflibercept (Zaltrap)	Soluble "VEGFR-body"	VEGF-A, -B, PlGF	Approved for human use
Cilengitide	Cyclic peptide	αvβ3/β5 integrin	In clinical trials
Agents With Direct Antiangiogenic Activity			
Endostar	Protein fragment	Unclear	In human use (China)
ABT510	Peptide	Endothelial CD36	Investigational agent
2ME2	Sterol	HIF-1α, tubulin	Investigational agent
TNP470 (Lodamin)	Small molecule (slow release)	Complex activity	Investigational agent
Indirect-Acting Agents Designed to Block Oncogenic Pathways Driving Angiogenesis			
Trastuzumab (Herceptin)	Neutralizing huMoAb	HER-2	Approved for human use
Cetuximab (Erbitux)	Neutralizing huMoAb	EGFR	Approved for human use
Gefitinib (Iressa)	TKI	EGFR	Approved for human use
Erlotinib (Tarceva)	TKI	EGFR	Approved for human use
Lapatinib (Tykerb)	TKI	EGFR, HER-2	Approved for human use
Imatinib (Gleevec)	TKI	ABL, PDGFRβ, KIT	Approved for human use
PF00299804	TKI	Irreversible pan-Erb inhibitor	In development
Tipifarnib	FTI	Ras, farnesylated proteins	In clinical development
Agents With Antiangiogenic and Non-antiangiogenic Activities			
Chemotherapy (metronomic)	Various agents (CTX, VBL, TMZ, TAX)	Stress response pathways, DNA, cytoskeleton	Under clinical exploration
Celecoxib (Celebrex)	Small molecule	COX-2	Under clinical exploration
Thalidomide and analogues (Lenalidomide)	Small molecule	Inflammatory pathways	Approved in multiple myeloma, under investigation
Antivascular Agents/Vascular-Disrupting Agents			
ASA404	Flavonoid	EC survival	Clinical trials
CA4P	Tubulin binding	Tubulin assembly	Clinical trials
AVE8062	Tubulin binding	Tubulin assembly	Clinical trials
ABT-751	Tubulin binding	Tubulin assembly	Clinical trials
OXi4503	Tubulin binding	Tubulin assembly	Early clinical trials

2ME2, 2-Methoxyestradiol; CTX, cyclophosphamide; EC, endothelial cell; EGFR, epidermal growth factor receptor; FTI, protein farnesyltransferase inhibitor; huMoAb, humanized monoclonal antibody; TAX, paclitaxel; TKI, tyrosine kinase inhibitor; TMZ, temozolomide; VBL, vinblastin; VEGFR, vascular endothelial growth factor receptor. See text and references for more details[2,34] (http://www.angio.org/).

Angiogenesis and Antiangiogenesis in Hematopoietic Malignancies

The vascular bone marrow stroma plays a pivotal role in leukemogenesis.[7] Indeed, angiogenesis, increased vascular density, and increased levels of angiogenic growth factors have all been observed in the bone marrow of patients with hematopoietic malignancies.[7] VEGF may play multiple roles in this context, including as (1) vascular growth stimulator; (2) paracrine growth factor for leukemic stem cells[7]; and (3) inducer of angiocrine interactions between these cells and the endothelium.[10] Consequently, a wide spectrum of antiangiogenic agents, including VEGF antagonists (bevacizumab, sorafenib, sunitinib, cediranib), are under investigation for the treatment of hematologic disorders, such as acute myelogeneous leukemia, chronic myelogeneous leukemia, acute lymphoblastic leukemia, myelodysplastic syndrome, non-Hodgkin lymphoma, multiple myeloma, and others.[7] Additional agents with antiangiogenic activity have also been explored, including bortezomib and antiinflammatory antiangiogenics (thalidomide and lenalidomide), some of which are already in human use in hematologic malignancies (e.g., in mantle cell lymphoma, multiple myeloma, and myelodysplastic syndrome; see Medinger and Mross[7] for review, also Chapter 55).

Hematologic Complications Associated With Blood Vessel–Directed Agents

Manipulation of endothelial and mural cells in the course of pro- and antiangiogenic therapy creates the potential for side effects.[35] The most extensive clinical experience is in the area of cancer, where some toxicities (e.g., hypertension, proteinuria, fatigue, hypothyroidism) have been observed in this setting, along with hematologic side effects, mainly thrombosis and/or bleeding. While cancer patients are prone to thrombosis,[36] antiangiogenic therapy increases the risk of venous thromboembolism or arterial thrombosis.[6] The risk varies depending on the agent and the type of cancer, and is exacerbated by accompanying chemotherapy or hormonal therapy.[36] Thrombosis is of particular concern in patients with multiple myeloma who receive thalidomide derivatives in combination with anthracyclins and dexamethasone. In this case the reported risk of thrombosis may be as high as 75%.[36] Bevacizumab may increase the risk of arterial thrombosis up to twofold in patients with solid tumors, especially in the elderly with additional risk factors. These estimates are variable, however (0.9% to 19.4% according to different studies), and drug specific, because small-molecule tyrosine kinase inhibitors acting on VEGFR are less likely to trigger venous thromboembolism (0% to 3%; also see Chapters 126 and 149).[36]

Bleeding complications were also recorded with several of these agents, ranging from minor to life threatening.[37] In general, however, antiangiogenic agents are relatively well tolerated, and their side effects are usually manageable with careful monitoring and standard supportive care.[6]

SUMMARY

The functional integration of the vascular system, bone marrow, and circulating blood results in a high degree of biologic interdependence in health and disease (Fig. 15.5). While this may not always be

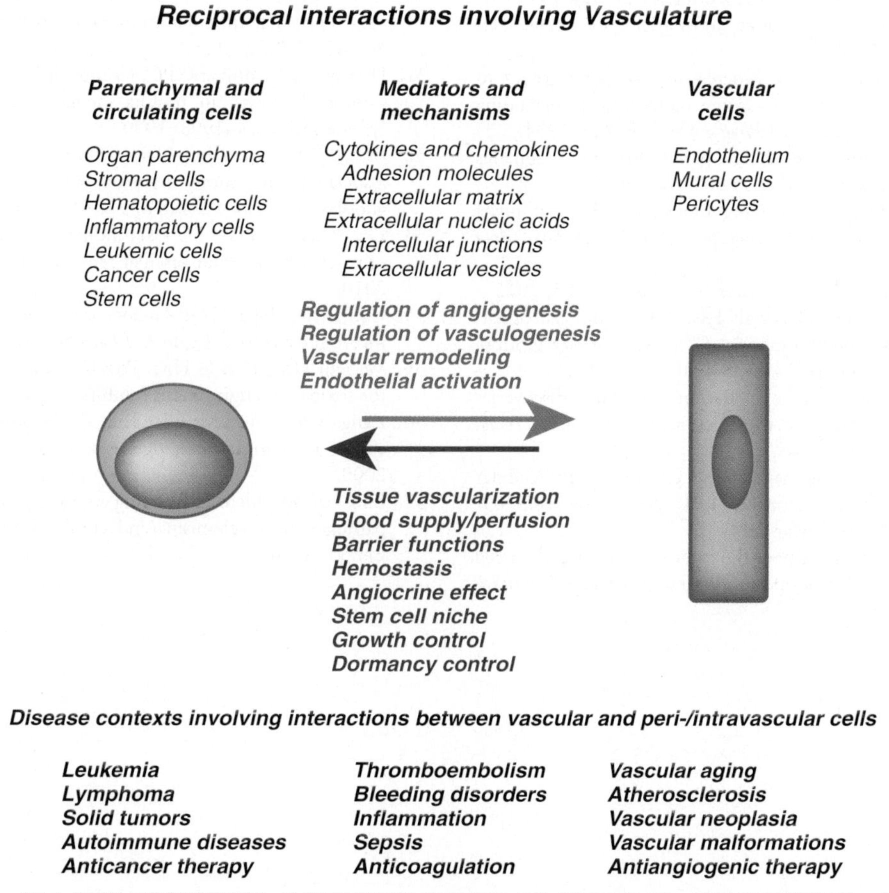

Reciprocal interactions involving Vasculature

Parenchymal and circulating cells	Mediators and mechanisms	Vascular cells
Organ parenchyma	Cytokines and chemokines	Endothelium
Stromal cells	Adhesion molecules	Mural cells
Hematopoietic cells	Extracellular matrix	Pericytes
Inflammatory cells	Extracellular nucleic acids	
Leukemic cells	Intercellular junctions	
Cancer cells	Extracellular vesicles	
Stem cells		

Regulation of angiogenesis
Regulation of vasculogenesis
Vascular remodeling
Endothelial activation

Tissue vascularization
Blood supply/perfusion
Barrier functions
Hemostasis
Angiocrine effect
Stem cell niche
Growth control
Dormancy control

Disease contexts involving interactions between vascular and peri-/intravascular cells

Leukemia	Thromboembolism	Vascular aging
Lymphoma	Bleeding disorders	Atherosclerosis
Solid tumors	Inflammation	Vascular neoplasia
Autoimmune diseases	Sepsis	Vascular malformations
Anticancer therapy	Anticoagulation	Antiangiogenic therapy

Fig. 15.5 THE RECIPROCAL INTERDEPENDENCE OF VASCULAR, NONVASCULAR, AND BLOOD CELLS IN HOMEOSTASIS AND DISEASE. In multicellular organisms blood flow connects all constituent cells to each other and to the external environment (oxygen supply, nutrition, regulation, migration). The ubiquitous presence of blood vessels, vascular cells, circulating cells, soluble mediators, and blood components defines and integrates multiple functions of organs and tissues in health and disease. Examples of processes, disease states, and therapies that epitomize this web of relationships are described in this chapter.

clinically obvious, the existence of these subtle links necessitates a greater consideration of blood vessel–regulating processes in the pathogenesis and therapy of hematologic disorders.

REFERENCES

1. Folkman J: Angiogenesis: an organizing principle for drug discovery? *Nat Rev Drug Discov* 6:273–286, 2007.
2. Carmeliet P, Jain RK: Molecular mechanisms and clinical applications of angiogenesis. *Nature* 473:298–307, 2011.
3. Dvorak FH, Rickles FR: Malignancy and hemostasis. In Coleman RB, Marder VJ, Clowes AW, et al, editors: *Hemostasis and thrombosis: Basic principles and clinical practice*, Philadelphia, 2006, Lippincott Company Williams & Wilkins, p 851.
4. Kerbel RS: Tumor angiogenesis. *N Engl J Med* 358:2039–2049, 2008.
5. Ferrara N: Role of myeloid cells in vascular endothelial growth factor-independent tumor angiogenesis. *Curr Opin Hematol* 17:219–224, 2010.
6. Hurwitz HI, Saltz LB, Van CE, et al: Venous thromboembolic events with chemotherapy plus bevacizumab: a pooled analysis of patients in randomized phase II and III studies. *J Clin Oncol* 29:1757–1764, 2011.
7. Medinger M, Mross K: Clinical trials with anti-angiogenic agents in hematological malignancies. *J Angiogenes Res* 2:10, 2010.
8. Ciau-Uitz A, Monteiro R, Kirmizitas A, et al: Developmental hematopoiesis: ontogeny, genetic programming and conservation. *Exp Hematol* 42:669–683, 2014.
9. Rak J: Ras oncogenes and tumour vascular interface. In Thomas-Tikhonenko A, editor: *Cancer genome and tumor microenvironment*, New York, 2009, Springer, p 133.
10. Butler JM, Kobayashi H, Rafii S: Instructive role of the vascular niche in promoting tumour growth and tissue repair by angiocrine factors. *Nat Rev Cancer* 10:138–146, 2010.
11. Rak JW, Hegmann EJ, Lu C, et al: Progressive loss of sensitivity to endothelium-derived growth inhibitors expressed by human melanoma cells during disease progression. *J Cell Physiol* 159:245–255, 1994.
12. Ghajar CM, Peinado H, Mori H, et al: The perivascular niche regulates breast tumour dormancy. *Nat Cell Biol* 15:807–817, 2013.
13. De Palma M, Naldini L: Tie2-expressing monocytes (TEMs): novel targets and vehicles of anticancer therapy? *Biochim Biophys Acta* 1796:5–10, 2009.
14. Lusis AJ: Genetics of atherosclerosis. *Trends Genet* 28:267–275, 2012.
15. Ruf W, Disse J, Carneiro-Lobo TC, et al: Tissue factor and cell signalling in cancer progression and thrombosis. *J Thromb Haemost* 9(Suppl 1):306–315, 2011. doi: 10.1111/j.1538-7836.2011.04318.x.
16. Welti J, Loges S, Dimmeler S, et al: Recent molecular discoveries in angiogenesis and antiangiogenic therapies in cancer. *J Clin Invest* 123:3190–3200, 2013.
17. Rak J: Extracellular vesicles - biomarkers and effectors of the cellular interactome in cancer. *Front Pharmacol* 4:21, 2013. doi: 10.3389/fphar.2013.00021. [Epub; 2013 Mar 6:21].
18. Nagy JA, Dvorak HF: Heterogeneity of the tumor vasculature: the need for new tumor blood vessel type-specific targets. *Clin Exp Metastasis* 29:657–662, 2012.
19. Xu Q: The impact of progenitor cells in atherosclerosis. *Nat Clin Pract Cardiovasc Med* 3:94–101, 2006.
20. Dome B, Hendrix MJ, Paku S, et al: Alternative vascularization mechanisms in cancer: Pathology and therapeutic implications. *Am J Pathol* 170:1–15, 2007.
21. Heil M, Schaper W: Arteriogenic growth factors, chemokines and proteases as a prerequisite for arteriogenesis. *Drug News Perspect* 18:317–322, 2005.
22. Cheng L, Huang Z, Zhou W, et al: Glioblastoma stem cells generate vascular pericytes to support vessel function and tumor growth. *Cell* 153:139–152, 2013.
23. Rodriguez FJ, Orr BA, Ligon KL, et al: Neoplastic cells are a rare component in human glioblastoma microvasculature. *Oncotarget* 3:98–106, 2012.
24. Welti J, Loges S, Dimmeler S, et al: Recent molecular discoveries in angiogenesis and antiangiogenic therapies in cancer. *J Clin Invest* 123:3190–3200, 2013.
25. Ghesquiere B, Wong BW, Kuchnio A, et al: Metabolism of stromal and immune cells in health and disease. *Nature* 511:167–176, 2014.
26. Thurston G, Noguera-Troise I, Yancopoulos GD: The Delta paradox: DLL4 blockade leads to more tumour vessels but less tumour growth. *Nat Rev Cancer* 7:327–331, 2007.
27. Fantin A, Vieira JM, Gestri G, et al: Tissue macrophages act as cellular chaperones for vascular anastomosis downstream of VEGF-mediated endothelial tip cell induction. *Blood* 116:829–840, 2010.
28. Gaengel K, Genove G, Armulik A, et al: Endothelial-mural cell signaling in vascular development and angiogenesis. *Arterioscler Thromb Vasc Biol* 29:630–638, 2009.
29. Tammela T, Alitalo K: Lymphangiogenesis: Molecular mechanisms and future promise. *Cell* 140:460–476, 2010.
30. Ricci-Vitiani L, Pallini R, Biffoni M, et al: Tumour vascularization via endothelial differentiation of glioblastoma stem-like cells. *Nature* 468:824–828, 2010.
31. Holash J, Maisonpierre PC, Compton D, et al: Vessel cooption, regression, and growth in tumors mediated by angiopoietins and VEGF. *Science* 284:1994–1998, 1999.
32. Brat DJ, Van Meir EG: Vaso-occlusive and prothrombotic mechanisms associated with tumor hypoxia, necrosis, and accelerated growth in glioblastoma. *Lab Invest* 84:397–405, 2004.
33. Rey S, Semenza GL: Hypoxia-inducible factor-1-dependent mechanisms of vascularization and vascular remodelling. *Cardiovasc Res* 86:236–242, 2010.
34. Cook KM, Figg WD: Angiogenesis inhibitors: current strategies and future prospects. *CA Cancer J Clin* 60:222–243, 2010.
35. Verheul HM, Pinedo HM: Possible molecular mechanisms involved in the toxicity of angiogenesis inhibition. *Nat Rev Cancer* 7:475–485, 2007.
36. Zangari M, Fink LM, Elice F, et al: Thrombotic events in patients with cancer receiving antiangiogenesis agents. *J Clin Oncol* 27:4865–4873, 2009.
37. Elice F, Rodeghiero F: Bleeding complications of antiangiogenic therapy: pathogenetic mechanisms and clinical impact. *Thromb Res* 125(Suppl 2):S55, 2010.

CHAPTER 16

CYTOKINE/RECEPTOR FAMILIES AND SIGNAL TRANSDUCTION

Montaser Shaheen and Hal E. Broxmeyer

CYTOKINE/RECEPTOR FAMILIES AND SIGNAL TRANSDUCTION

Cytokines are secreted biologically active molecules that regulate cell growth and metabolism and cellular interactions through their specific binding to defined receptors and the subsequent induction of intracellular signaling. Cytokines are classified based on the primary structural features of the extracellular domains of their receptors.[1] Most of what is known of cytokine actions and their intracellular signaling is based on the effects of purified natural or recombinant cytokines on either a factor-dependent cell line or an isolated population of primary target cells. It is however, becoming clear that cytokines can be functionally modified in vivo by specific enzymes, and these modifications, which are not usually taken into consideration when analyzing intracellular signaling can elicit different signaling events. Moreover, it has also recently become clear that removing cells from the body for analysis can change their metabolism and activity, and perhaps how these cells may signal in response to intact or enzyme-truncated cytokines.

Class or type I cytokines (often referred to as hematopoietins) regulate development, differentiation, and activation of hematopoietic and immune cells. Their receptors are type I membrane proteins with an N-terminal extracellular and C-terminal intracellular orientation. Type I cytokine receptors include those for colony stimulating factors (CSFs), interleukins (ILs), erythropoietin (EPO), thrombopoietin (TPO) (Fig. 16.1), and hormones such as growth hormone (GH) and leptin.

Class II cytokines consist of type I interferons (IFNs), which include 16 members that are produced by almost every nucleated cell with approximately 20% to 60% sequence identity including 12 subtypes of IFN-α, IFN-β, IFN-ϵ, IFN-κ, and IFN-ω. Type I IFNs initiate signaling by binding to the same receptor composed of two subunits called IFNAR1 and IFNAR2. Type II IFN consists of the single IFN-γ, which signals through a heterodimeric receptor composed of IFNGR1 and IFNGR2. Type III IFNs include IFN-λ1 (IL-29), IFN-λ2 (IL-28A), and IFN-λ3 (IL-28B). Some place the IL-10 family of cytokines (IL-10, IL-19, IL-20, IL-22, IL-24, IL-26) within this group. Type III IFN receptor is composed of IL-10Rβ and IL-28R (Fig. 16.2).

The structural similarities of type I cytokines were not initially recognized. Cloning of their receptors, however, revealed significant homology in that the extracellular regions contain a common domain with four conserved cysteines (C4) in the N-terminal segment and a tryptophan-serine doublet near the C-terminal end.[2] Mutagenesis studies revealed an essential structural role for these amino acids in maintaining the tertiary structure of the receptor without being involved in cytokine interactions. There is a 200 amino acid region evolutionarily derived from a tandem of two ancestral fibronectin-like domains, which has been named the hematopoietin receptor domain or cytokine-binding homology region (CHR) because it mediates the interactions with cytokines. The α receptors of IL-2 and IL-15 of the γc family are atypical cytokine receptors in that they do not contain a CHR, but rather they contain sushi domains. Two conserved Box 1/Box 2 regions are located in the proximal intracytoplasmic segment (Fig. 16.3). By contrast, type II cytokine receptors contain two cysteine doublets (C2-C2) located in the C-terminal end of both fibronectin-derived domains. They retain Box 1/2 regions but lack the tryptophan-serine-x-serine-tryptophan motif. Both types of receptors bind ligands that display common spatial four α-helix bundle organization and use intracellular signaling mediators of the Janus kinase (JAK) and signal transducer and activator of transcription (STAT) families. In this regard type I and II cytokine receptors represent a homogeneous structural group of proteins. However, sequence homology is observed in a limited number of cases, such as for the GH/prolactin (PRL) family and for the IL-6 family. Nonetheless, evidence of the common derivation of cytokines can be observed in the common four-helix bundle structure, in addition to the similar intron-exon relationship and the clustering observed for certain cytokine genes such as genes of the IL-4 family.[3] The receptors can be composed of dimers of a single chain (granulocyte-CSF receptor (G-CSFR), EPO receptor (EPOR), TPO receptor (c-MPL), or can be heterodimeric with a common signaling subunit and a unique ligand-binding chain. These heterodimeric receptors can be grouped into families based on whether they share the common β-chain (granulocyte–macrophage [GM]-CSFRα, IL-3Rα, IL-5Rα), or those that share the gp130 receptor (IL-6Rα, leukemia inhibitory factor (LIF) receptor β, ciliary neurotrophic factor receptor α, IL-11Rα IL-12R, IL-23R, oncostatin M receptor α, Ciliary Neurotrophic Factor Rα [NTFRα]) and those that share the common γ-chain (IL-2Rα, IL-2Rα, IL-4Rα, IL-7Rα, IL-9Rα, IL-13Rα, IL-15Rα and IL-21Rα;) (see Fig. 16.1). Cytokine binding triggers receptor homodimerization (e.g., G-CSFR[4]) or heterodimerization/oligomerization of receptor subunits (e.g., GM-CSFR) or it induces a conformational change in preformed receptor dimers (EPOR) resulting in the activation of the JAKs (Fig. 16.4). Unlike other receptors with intrinsic enzyme activity (e.g., receptor tyrosine kinases [RTK] such as Flt3 and c-Kit), most cytokine receptors are constitutively associated with kinases. These cytoplasmic kinases comprise the four members of the JAK family: JAK1, JAK2, and Tyk2, which bind to a wide range of receptors, whereas JAK3 binds to only one receptor, the common gamma chain (γc).[5] This binding is mediated by interactions between the 4.1, ezrin, radixin, moesin (FERM) domain of JAK (Fig. 16.5), and the Box 1 membrane proximal intracytoplasmic region of the receptor. Upon ligand binding, JAKs come into juxtapositioning and phosphorylate themselves and their associated receptors. Mutagenesis studies have shown that there are distinct regions of individual phosphorylated receptors that transmit signals for cell survival, proliferation, differentiation, and/or activation via interaction with adaptor molecules. Phosphorylation of certain residues generates docking sites for the Src homology 2 (SH2) domains of the STATs. Once bound to the receptor/JAK complex, STATs themselves become phosphorylated, which induces a conformational change that generates active STAT dimers via reciprocal phosphotyrosine and SH2 domain interaction (see Fig. 16.4). The dimers translocate to the nucleus, where they bind to DNA sequences in the promoters of target genes to activate transcription.

Other posttranslational modifications beside tyrosine phosphorylation occur. These include acetylation, sumoylation and ubiquitylation that modulate cytokine signaling through modifying protein-protein or protein-DNA interactions and protein stability. Multiple mechanisms exist to attenuate cytokine signaling, which ensures controlled cellular responses to cytokines and prevents pathologic hyperactivation. Because the signaling is mediated by extensive phosphorylation, phosphatases have emerged as important negative regulators. Examples of these include the SH2 containing phosphatase (SHP) proteins. Other regulators have been identified including protein inhibitors of activated STAT (PIAS), suppressor of cytokine signaling (SOCS) proteins and cytokine inducible

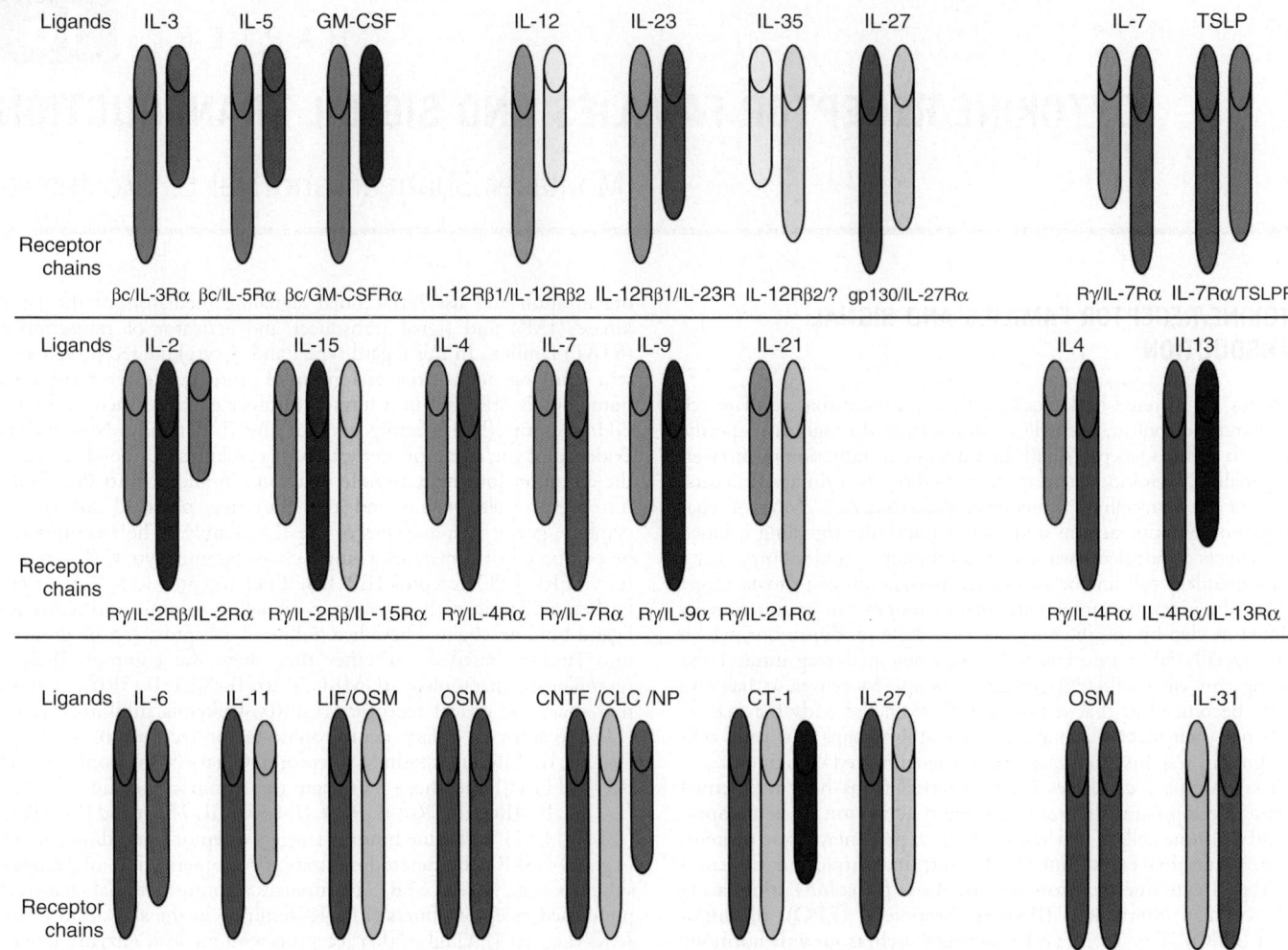

Fig. 16.1 CLASS OR TYPE I CYTOKINES (OFTEN REFERRED TO AS HEMATOPOIETINS) REGULATE DEVELOPMENT, DIFFERENTIATION, AND ACTIVATION OF HEMATOPOIETIC AND IMMUNE CELLS. Simple depiction of type 1 cytokine receptor subfamilies. IL-3R, IL-5R, and GM-CSFR share a common βc chain that place them in one group. IL-12 family members include four cytokines. IL-12 and IL-23 share the IL12Rβ1 unit, while IL-12 and IL-35 share the IL-12Rβ2 unit. IL-27 share the gp130 with the IL-6 family. Multiple cytokines (IL-2, IL-4, IL-7, IL-9, IL-15, IL-21) share the common Rγ chain, which is mutated in a subset of patients with SCID. IL-4R shares a subunit with IL-13R. Both IL-4 and IL-13 drives Th2 response. IL-7R shares one subunit with the thymic stromal lymphopoietin (TSLP). This sharing of receptor subunit may explain why deletion of the gene encoding IL-7R affects the lymphoid system more severely than deleting the IL-7 gene. The IL-6 family includes multiple cytokines that all have the signal transducer gp130. Deleting gp130 results in embryonic lethality. Some IL-6 family members activate more than one receptor. Oncostatin M (OSM) can work through a heterodimer receptor consisting of gp130 with OSMRβ or gp130 with leukemia inhibitory factor-receptor (LIF-R). Ciliary neurotrophic factor (CNTF), cardiotrophin-like cytokine (CLC), and neuropoietin (NP) engage the receptor composed of gp130, LIFR and CNTFR. Cardiotrophin-1 (CT-1) uses a receptor composed of gp130, LIF-R and another, yet to be identified subunit. IL-27 shares gp130 with its specific receptor unit. IL-31 receptor is composed of gp130 like receptor (GPL) and OSMRβ.

SH2-domain-containing proteins (CIS). We will discuss the proposed mechanisms of inhibition of these proteins in some detail later. Expression of receptors is also regulated at the level of gene transcription, protein translation, internalization, and degradation.

MODELS OF LIGAND-RECEPTOR BINDING AND ACTIVATION

Cytokines usually bind with high affinity to their cognate receptors, although low-affinity binding has been documented. The presence and the density of the receptors determine biologic responses in hematopoietic stem and progenitor or more mature cell populations.[6] The crystal structures of cytokines bound to the receptors have been illustrated for multiple cytokine families. For most cytokine-receptor couples, more than one cytokine molecule engages more than one receptor unit at one time to form a complex. For example, two IL-6 molecules aggregate with four receptor chains to form a hexameric and interlocking assembly mediated by a total of 10 symmetry-related, thermodynamically coupled interfaces (Fig. 16.6).[7] The assembly of this hexameric complex occurs sequentially: IL-6 is first engaged by IL-6Rα and then is presented to gp130 in the proper geometry to facilitate a cooperative transition into the high-affinity, signaling-competent hexamer. This structure also reveals that gp130

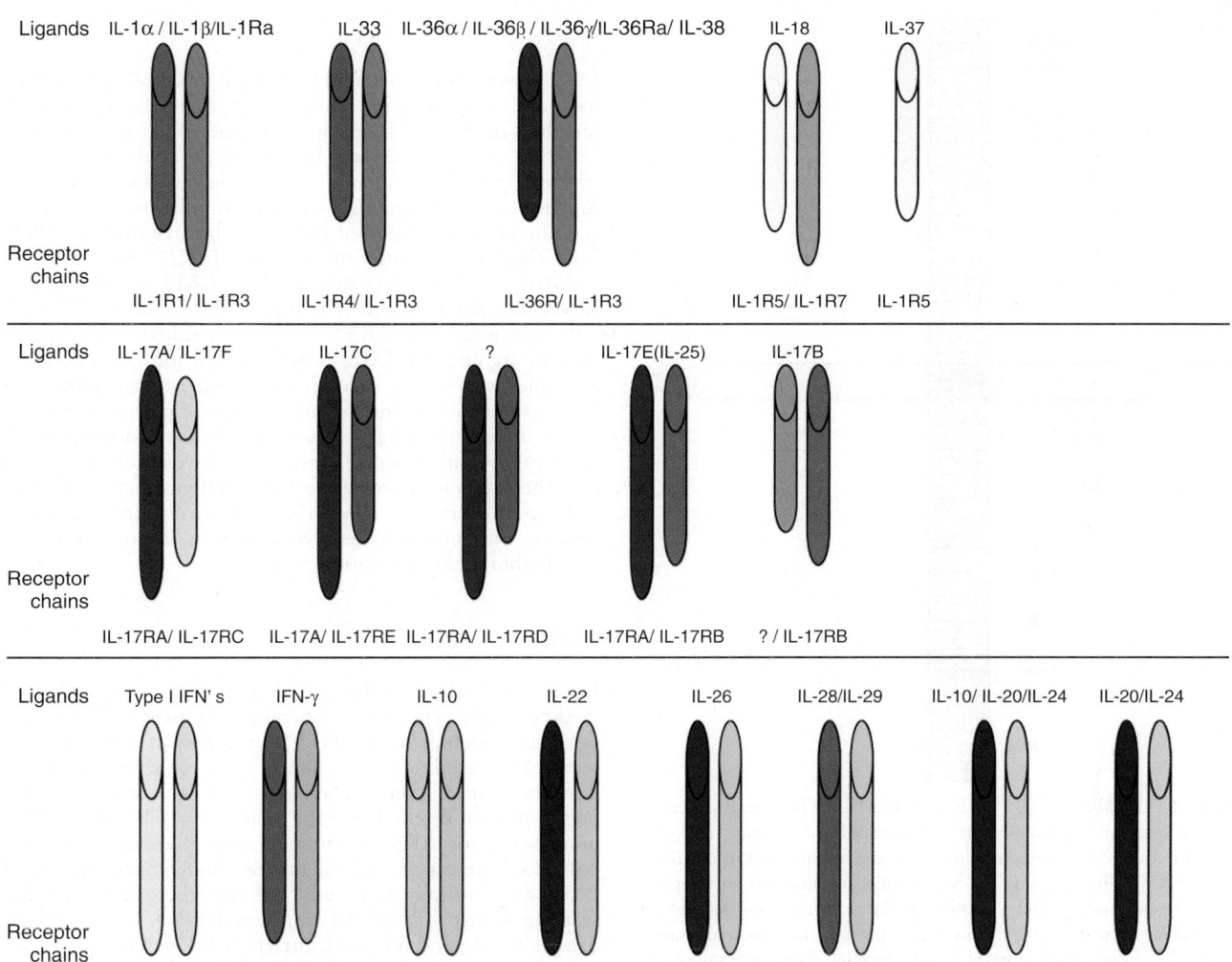

Fig. 16.2 SCHEMATIC DIAGRAMS OF IL-1, IL-17, AND TYPE II CYTOKINE FAMILY MEMBERS AND RECEPTORS. IL-1 family and receptors. The IL-1 family is associated with acute and chronic inflammation and plays an essential role in the host response to infection. IL-1α and IL-1β share the same receptor. IL-33 and the IL-36 subfamily share with IL-1 and the IL-1R3 receptors *(top panel)*; IL-17 family and receptors. IL-17 secretion defines the Th17 cells that mediate host defensive mechanisms to various infections and that are involved in the pathogenesis of many autoimmune diseases. The five IL-17 receptors are not homologous to any known receptors and show considerable sequence divergence. They harbor extracellular domains composed of fibronectin type III domains and cytoplasmic SEF–IL-17R domains that show loose homology to toll–IL-1R domains *(middle panel)*; and type II cytokine receptor family. These include receptors for IFNs and the IL-10 family *(lower panel)*.

is bent such that the membrane-proximal domains of gp130 are close together at the cell surface, enabling activation of intracellular signaling. Variation in the receptor bend angles suggests a possible conformational transition from open to closed states upon ligand binding.[8] Reconstruction of full-length JAK1 in conjunction with gp130/IL-6/IL-6Rα complex reveals a three-lobed structure of JAK1 possessing extensive intersegmental flexibility that likely facilitates allosteric activation (Fig. 16.7).[9] Single-particle imaging of the gp130/IL-6/IL-6Rα/Jak1 holocomplex shows JAK1 associated with the membrane proximal intracellular regions of gp130, abutting the would-be inner leaflet of the cell membrane. JAK1 association with gp130 appears to be enhanced by the presence of a membrane environment. Mutated JAK proteins can transmit a signal independent of the receptor, but a recent line of investigation revealed that manipulating the receptor by surrogate ligands, such as diabodies to mimic dimeric receptor-ligand system, can attenuate the mutant JAK2 downstream signaling, which may have therapeutic implications.

It has been debated how the 16 human type I IFN molecules signal through the same receptors, IFNAR1 and IFNAR2, yet they can evoke different physiologic effects. Structural analysis of this family in complexes with this single receptor complex indicates that the receptor-ligand cross-reactivity is enabled by conserved receptor-ligand "anchor points" interspersed among ligand-specific interactions that "tune" the relative IFN-binding affinities, in an apparent extracellular "ligand proofreading" mechanism that modulates biologic activity.[10] This differential binding leads to variable conformational change in the receptor complex resulting in different STAT phosphorylation profiles, receptor internalization rates, and downstream gene expression patterns.

Signaling networks are typically measured in either their basal (minimum) or hyperstimulated (maximum) states, but there is a cytokine signal "dynamic range," in which the responsiveness of cell outcomes to incremental changes in signal activation is more important for biologic outcome than signal strength per se.[11]

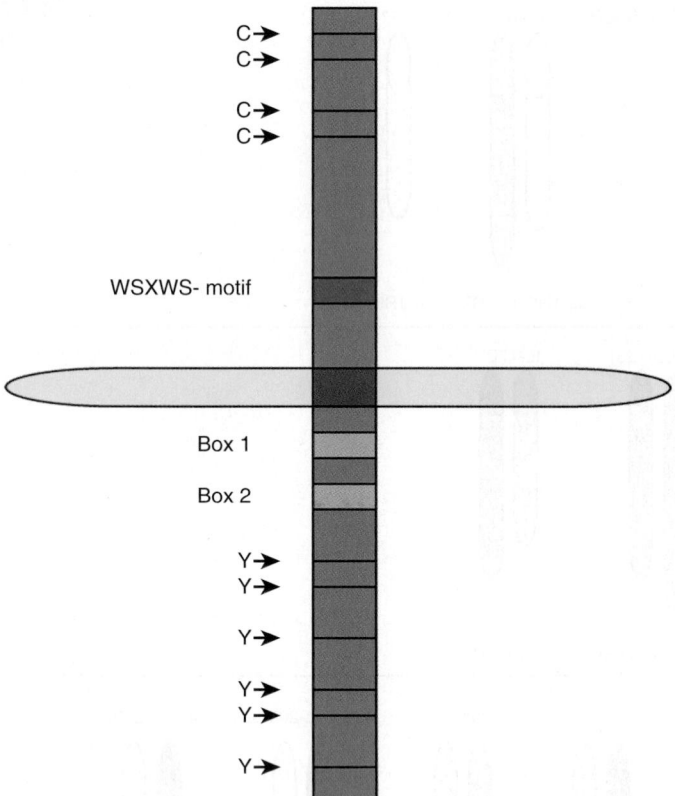

C→
C→

C→
C→

WSXWS- motif

Box 1

Box 2

Y→
Y→

Y→

Y→
Y→

Y→

Fig. 16.3 CYTOKINE RECEPTOR SUPERFAMILY. The general structure of cytokine receptor superfamily. In the extracellular cytokine receptor module, four conserved cysteine residues exist and are involved in disulfide bonds. A WSXWS (Tre, Ser, any, Tre, Ser) motif that is essential for receptor processing, ligand binding, and activation of the receptor is also located in the extracellular domain. In the intracellular portion, two short domains termed *Box 1* and *Box 2* are important for JAK binding. Tyrosine residues are present on the intracellular part to be phosphorylated upon receptor activation.

Janus Kinases

JAK proteins are tyrosine kinases of approximately 1000 amino acids. They have clear nonredundant in vivo functions defined by analysis of gene deletion in mice, and mutations of JAK3 or Tyk2 in humans that lead to primary immunodeficiency syndromes (severe combined immunodeficiency [SCID] and autosomal-recessive hyperimmunoglobulin E syndrome [AR-HIES], respectively).[5] In addition, somatic mutations of JAKs are seen in human neoplastic conditions. The following is a brief description of JAK functions in cytokine signaling. Fig. 16.5A depicts the general structure of the JAK proteins.

JAK1

JAK1 is widely expressed and associates with the IFN receptors and receptors that use gp130 or the γc. JAK1$^{-/-}$ mice have grossly normal nonlymphoid organogenesis[12]; however, they die perinatally of a poorly characterized defect that may be neurologic. It is believed that this morbid phenotype is caused by the failure of cytokine signaling that promotes neuronal cell survival via gp130. Defective cytokine signaling is observed with class II cytokine receptors (IFNs), IL-2, IL-6, and IL-7 families. JAK1$^{-/-}$ mice manifest a SCID phenotype, consistent with the fact that JAK1 binds to the ligand-specific receptor subunit of γc-. Somatic JAK1 activating mutations have been described in occasional cases of acute leukemia and solid tumors.

JAK2

JAK2 is widely expressed and is involved in signaling by single chain hormone receptors, the common β chain family, and certain members of the class II receptor cytokine family. JAK2 deficiency is lethal at day 12.5 caused by failure of erythropoiesis,[13] which explains the lack of reports of individuals with germline loss-of-function JAK2 mutations. Receptor stimulation by EPO induces tyrosine phosphorylation of JAK2, which is required for EPO function. Defective responses of cells from JAK2$^{-/-}$ mice also reveal its essential role in the signaling of IL-3, GM-CSF, IL-5, TPO, and IFN-γ, but not IL-6 and IFN-α/β.[14] Transfer of JAK2$^{-/-}$ fetal liver cells into irradiated JAK3$^{-/-}$ recipients resulted in normal thymic subsets, arguing that JAK2 is not essential for T cell development. Multiple groups have identified acquired activating mutations in JAK2 as the etiology for virtually all cases of polycythemia vera, and in a significant percentage of cases of essential thrombocythemia and primary myelofibrosis. JAK2 mutations have also been described in other hematopoietic neoplasms. JAK2 inhibitors have shown efficacy at least in decreasing spleen size and constitutional symptoms in patients with myeloproliferative neoplasms irrespective of whether they harbor a JAK2 mutation.

JAK3

In contrast to the ubiquitous expression of the other JAKs, JAK3 is predominantly expressed in hematopoietic tissues. JAK3 selectively associates with only the γc, which is a component of multiple cytokine receptors. Accordingly, mutation of γc or JAK3 results in a SCID disorder in man, characterized by a lack of T and NK cells, with preservation of B cells, hence the designation T$^-$B$^+$NK$^-$ SCID. Mice homozygous for JAK3 null mutation show severe defects in lymphoid cells. B cell precursors in bone marrow, thymocytes, and both T and B cells are drastically decreased,[15] although these defects can improve as aging occurs.[16] Peripheral lymph nodes, NK cells, dendritic epidermal T cells, and intestinal intraepithelial gamma delta T cells are absent in these mice. Normal numbers of bone marrow hematopoietic progenitor cells with a similar capability to generate myeloid and erythroid colonies as wild-type mice indicates specific defects in lymphoid progenitor cells. Thymus progenitors are severely deficient. This phenotype is attributable to failure of IL-7 and IL-2 signaling, which explains the T-cell deficiency while the absence of natural killer cell development has been attributed to the impairment in IL-15 signaling. There is an increased apoptotic rate in the lymphocytes generated in these mice, and this is consistent with the identified function of JAK3 in regulating Bcl-2 and Bax.

Activation of JAK3 because of gain-of-function mutations is found in human hematologic malignancies, including acute megakaryoblastic leukemia and cutaneous T-cell lymphoma.

Given the essential role of JAK3 in cytokine signaling through γc and given its limited tissue expression, inhibition of JAK3 activity has emerged as a promising strategy for immunosuppression in autoimmune disorders and immune rejection.

Tyk2

Tyk2 was the first JAK family member identified that plays a role in cytokine signaling. Tyk2 was discovered as an essential component in a screen for mutants in IFN-α signaling.[17] Type I IFN receptors require Tyk2 and JAK1, while IFN-γ signaling depends on the combination of Tyk2 and JAK2. The combination of Tyk2 with JAK2 is not only required for IFN-γ signaling but also for the differentiation of IFN-γ-producing Th1 cells from naive Th cells. Lymphocyte development and proliferation are not affected in Tyk2-deficient mice, but signaling by cytokines that are important for host defense is impaired. The IL-12 receptor (IL-12R) is associated with Tyk2 and JAK2 and activates mainly the transcription factor STAT4. IL-12 signaling is markedly impaired in the absence of Tyk2, and

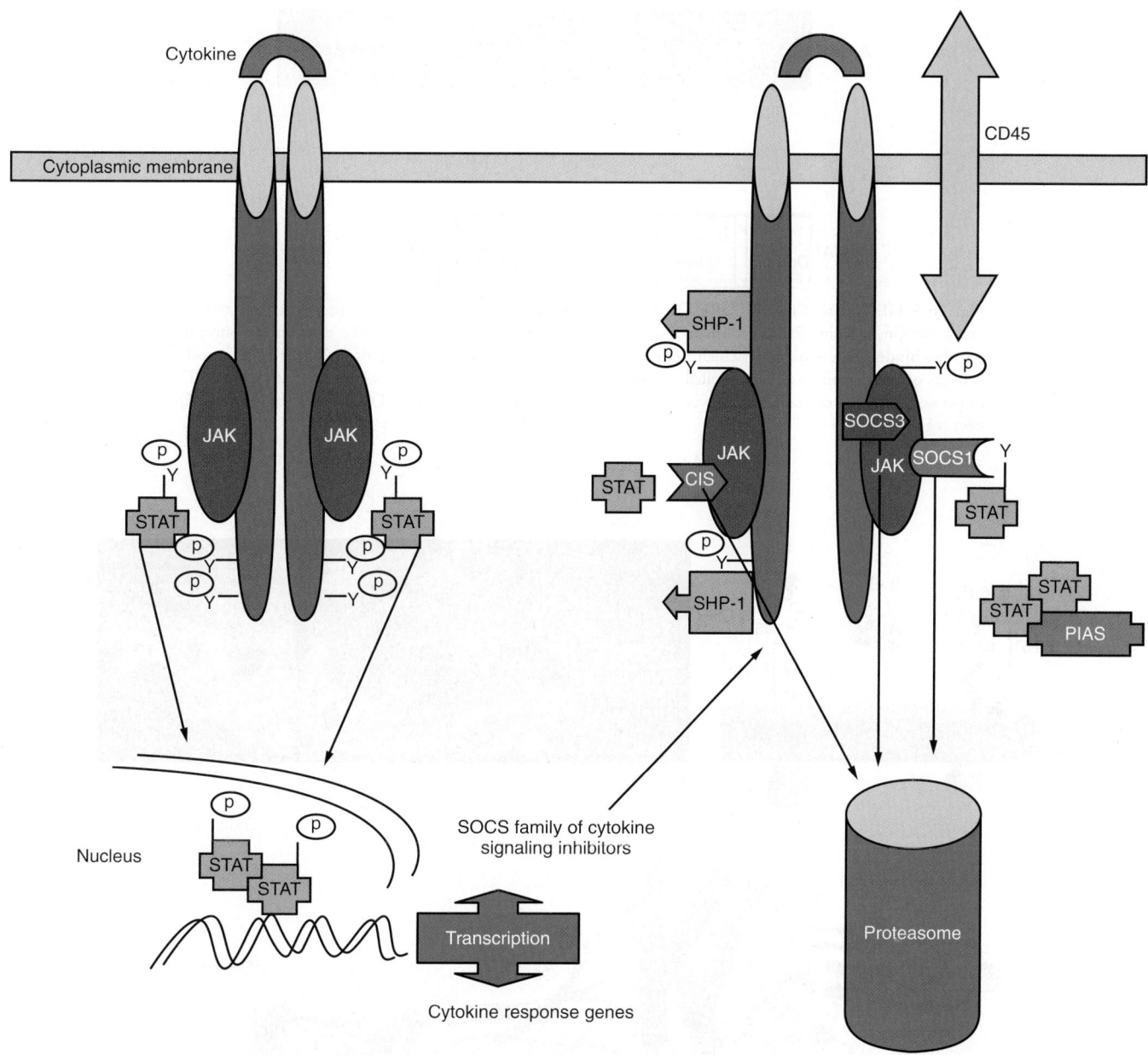

Fig. 16.4 CYTOKINE RECEPTOR SIGNALING. A general depiction of signal transduction by cytokine receptor superfamily. Ligand binding leads to dimerization or oligomerization of the receptor, which brings into proximity the associated JAKs, which phosphorylate tyrosine residues on the receptor and JAKs. This phosphorylation creates docking sites for proteins containing SH2 domains such as STATs. The later heterodimerize or homodimerize and translocate to the nucleus where they affect transcription of target genes. Several mechanisms exist to reverse this cytokine-activated state. STATs trigger a negative feedback loop by inducing transcription of suppressors of cytokine signaling (SOCSs). There are eight SOCS members. SOCS1 interacts directly with JAK1 and inhibits its catalytic activity. CIS (another SOCS) binds the receptor and blocks binding and phosphorylating of STATs. SOCS3 binds the receptor before inhibiting JAK. SOCS proteins contain SOCS box that leads to proteosomal degradation of the SOCS associated molecules. SHP-1 is a tyrosine phosphatase that negatively regulates the cytokine transduction process by dephosphorylating JAKs and the cytokine receptors. CD45 is a transmembrane phosphatase that inactivates JAKs. PIAS family members interact with STAT dimers and inhibit their functions as described in the main text.

downstream activation of STAT3 and STAT4 is clearly reduced, resulting in the inability of IFN-γ production by T cells. Both STAT3 and STAT1 activation by type I and type II IFNs are reduced in Tyk2-deficient mice, although at high concentrations IFN-α can fully transduce its signal in the absence of Tyk2. IL-10 signaling is essentially normal. Because of all the above, Tyk2-deficient mice are susceptible to viral and bacterial infections.[18] This susceptibility can be explained not only by impaired Th1 lineage development, but also

impaired Th17 differentiation. Since IL-4 is essential in generating Th2 cells, and since its signaling is independent of Tyk2, there is no disruption of Th2 in Tyk2-deficient mice. Th2 cell differentiation can however be inhibited by Tyk2-mediated signals occurring in response to IL-12 or IFNs. As anticipated, Th2-induced diseases such as allergic bronchitis are enhanced in the background of Tyk2 deficiency. One example is a mouse asthma model where pronounced lung inflammation is observed because of an enhanced Th2 response

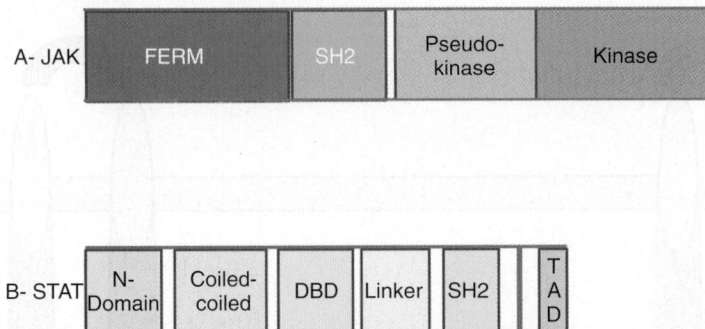

Fig. 16.5 GENERAL STRUCTURE OF JAK AND STAT PROTEINS. (A) JAK protein consists of 4.1, ezrin, radixin, moesin (FERM) domain (which modulates the kinase activity), SH2 domain for phospho-tyrosine binding, pseudokinase (which can exert inhibitory function), and kinase domain. (B) STAT protein consists of a N-terminus domain, coiled-coil domain for protein interaction, DNA binding domain (DBD), linker domain, SH2 domain, a conserved tyrosine, and trans-activation domain (TAD), which binds transcription regulators.

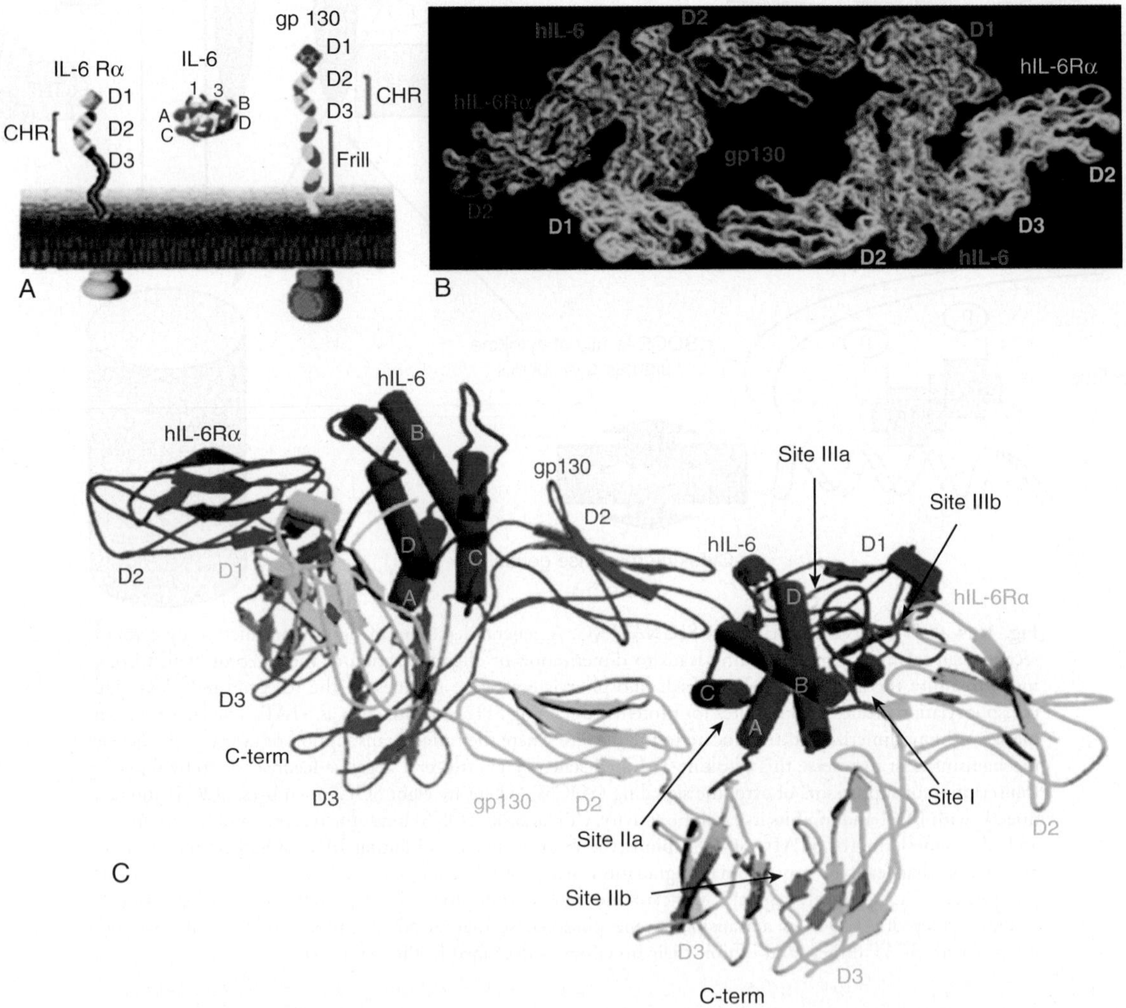

Fig. 16.6 IL-6 COMPLEX STRUCTURE. (A) The complex is a hexamer consisting of IL-6, the IL-6 α-receptor (IL-6Rα), and the shared signaling receptor gp130. (B) 3.65 angström–resolution shows a hexameric, interlocking assembly mediated by a total of 10 symmetry-related, thermodynamically coupled interfaces. (C) Assembly of the hexameric complex occurs sequentially: IL-6 is first engaged by IL-6Rα and then presented to gp130 to activate the downstream signaling. *(Reproduced with permission from Boulanger MJ et al: Hexameric structure and assembly of the interleukin-6/IL-6 alpha-receptor/gp130 complex. Science 300:2101–2104, 2003.)*

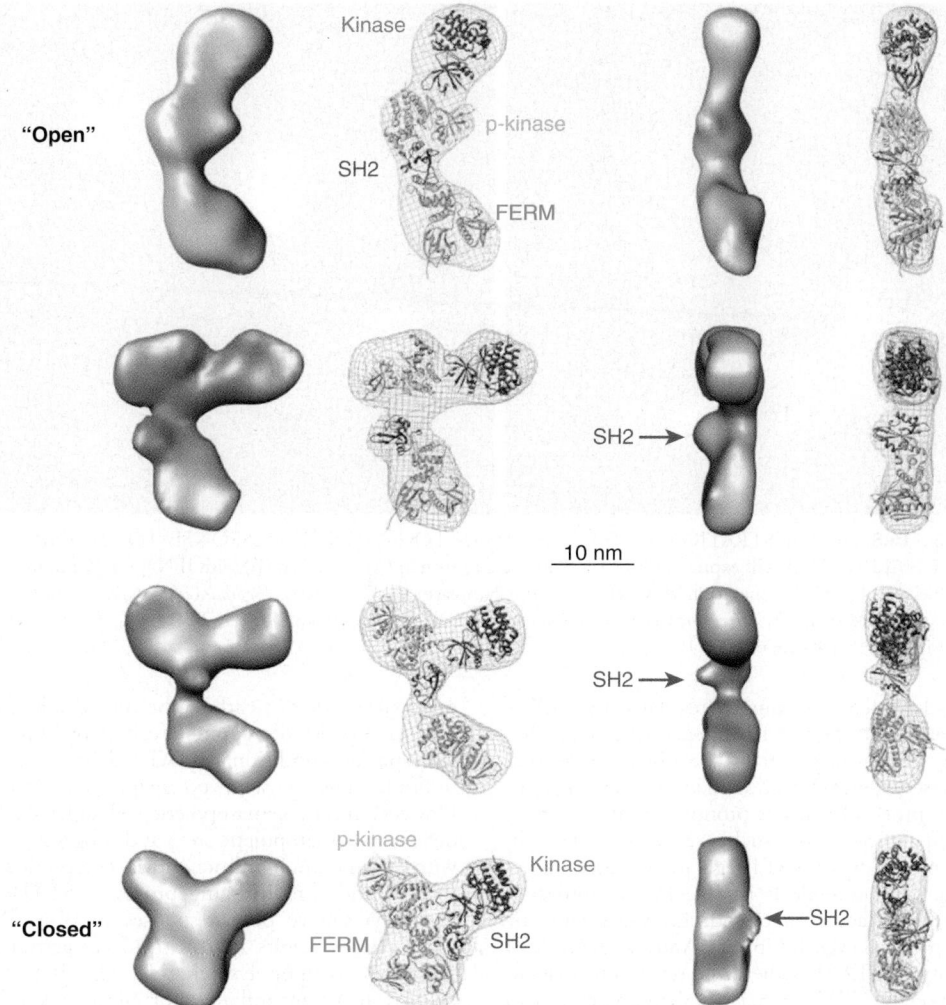

Fig. 16.7 THREE-DIMENSIONAL REPRESENTATION OF JAK1 SHOWING IT FORMING THREE LOBES. It switched in vitro from an open to a closed conformation. The orientations of the reconstructions in the left column represent the particles face-on, while the orientations to the right are rotated 90 degrees, reflecting the flatness of the surface on which JAK1 is lying. It is uncertain whether the open or the closed conformation what represents the active state. *FERM,* 4.1, ezrin, radixin, moesin; *SH2,* Src homology 2. *(Reproduced with permission from Lupardus PJ et al: Structural snapshots of full-length Jak1, a transmembrane gp130/ IL-6/IL-6Rα cytokine receptor complex, and the receptor-Jak1 holocomplex.* Structure *19:45–55, 2011.)*

associated with an increase of IL-4 production, increased immunoglobulin E (IgE) levels, and recruitment of eosinophils.

Signal Transducers and Activators of Transcription

There are seven STAT family members that share similar structure, but mediate distinct biologic functions.[18] Fig. 16.5B shows the general structure of the STATs. STAT1, for example, harbors an N-terminal domain, followed by α-helical coiled-coil and DNA-binding domains and a linker that connects to the C terminus. The C terminus contains an SH2 domain, followed by a short region containing a tyrosine residue, which is critical for the activation by JAK-mediated phosphorylation, and a transactivation domain that is the most divergent region within the STAT family. STAT proteins can be tyrosine phosphorylated by receptor-associated JAKs, by growth factor RTK, or by non-RTK. Latent STATs diffuse freely in the cytoplasm. Upon STAT phosphorylation and dimerization with a partner, the dimer quickly translocates to the nucleus (Fig. 16.8). This is achieved through an active process mediated by the nuclear transport machinery. For example, phosphorylated STAT1 transport is facilitated by the importin-α5/importin-β1 heterodimer.[19] This nuclear movement culminates in DNA binding and transcriptional

activity. For example, IFN-γ binding to its receptor leads to tyrosine phosphorylation of STAT1. The STAT1 dimer was originally called the IFN-γ activated factor. It recognizes a DNA sequence termed the IFN-γ activated sequence, which contains an inverted repeat of GAAA residues spaced by two to four nucleotides. Later, we briefly discuss the biologic activities of STAT proteins largely inferred from gene targeting experiments.

STAT1

STAT1 mediates IFN signaling. STAT1-deficient mice do not have significant developmental abnormalities, but display a complete lack of responsiveness to either IFN-α or IFN-γ and are highly sensitive to infection by microbial pathogens and viruses.[20] The induction of IFN-inducible genes is disrupted. A missense mutation of *Stat1* was initially identified in a patient suffering from atypical mycobacterial infections, similar to individuals with mutations of IFNGR subunits. However, this *Stat1* mutation was not associated with susceptibility to viral infections. Since then, other families have been described with mutations in STAT1 that lead to viral and mycobacterial infections. Families with muco-cutaneous candidiasis with STAT1 mutations have been reported.[21] These families have defective Th1 and Th17

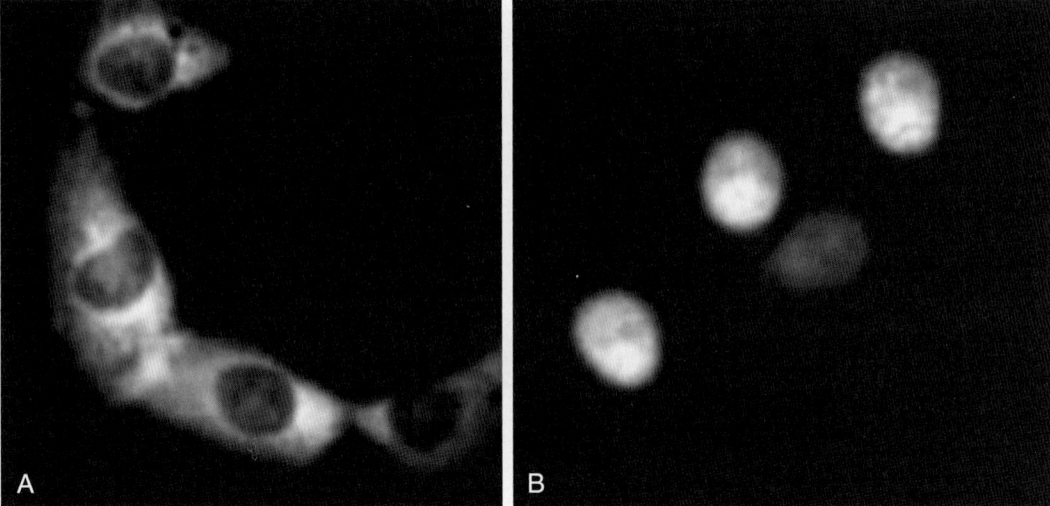

Fig. 16.8 DEMONSTRATION OF STAT PROTEIN LOCATION IN RESPONSE TO CYTOKINE SIGNALING. U3A cells expressing STAT1–GFP were untreated (A) or treated (B) with IFN-γ for 30 minutes. One can observe the migration of STAT1 from the cytoplasm to the nucleus. *(Reproduced with permission from McBride KM et al: Nuclear export signal located within the DNA-binding domain of the STAT1 transcription factor. EMBO J 19:6196–6206, 2000.)*

responses. Not all IFN-dependent signaling is regulated by STAT1 since, as there is a large number of STAT1-independent genes that are induced by IFN-γ, which may explain the observations that STAT1$^{-/-}$ mice are less susceptible to infection than mice lacking both IFN-γ and IFN-α/β receptors. Other, less pronounced defects have been described in STAT1-deficient mice such as a subtle decrease in bone marrow erythroid progenitors. STAT1 regulates other cytokine/growth factor signaling. One example is its role in the inhibitory activity of fibroblast growth factor on chondrocytes mediated by transcriptional activation of cell cycle inhibitors. Another example of IFN-independent activity of STAT1 is the more severe impairment of natural killer cells caused by STAT1 deficiency than observed with deficiencies of both IFN-γ and IFN-α/β receptors.

Because IFNs have antineoplastic activities, a role for STAT1 in tumor suppression has been suspected, and indeed, STAT1-deficient mice have a higher incidence of tumor formation in response to chemical carcinogens and also on a background of P53 deletion. However, given the involvement of STAT1 in other cellular pathways such as myc regulation and apoptosis, it cannot be concluded with certainty that this tumor-promoting phenotype is completely caused by the lack of immune surveillance.

STAT2

The main function of STAT2 is to mediate IFN-α/β signaling. STAT2 is constitutively associated with a non-STAT protein, IFN regulatory factor 9 (IRF-9). Tyrosine phosphorylated STAT1-STAT2-IRF-9 multimeric complex is called the IFN stimulated gene factor 3. This complex binds to a specific DNA sequence in type I IFN induced genes called the IFN stimulated response element. Because of the impaired IFN-α/β responsiveness, STAT2 knockout mice are susceptible to viral infections.[22] As it is the case with STAT1-deficient mice, STAT2-deficient mice are viable and develop normally. The absence of STAT2 results in reduced tyrosine phosphorylation and activation of STAT1 because of the fact that STAT2 facilitates recruitment and activation of STAT1 by the IFN-α/β receptor complex.

STAT3

STAT3 mediates signaling from multiple cytokines. It was originally cloned as an acute-phase response factor, activated by IL-6. Murine embryos deficient in STAT3 die at postcoital day 7.5. One potential explanation for this early embryonic death is failure of extraembryonic trophoblast development caused by impaired LIF signaling. Cell line specific conditional STAT3 deletions have been reported for multiple lineages with no major developmental abnormalities.[23] However, mouse hematopoietic-cell targeted STAT3 deletion leads to defects in hematopoietic stem and progenitor cells that are associated with dysfunction in mitochondria, overproduction of reactive oxygen species, and a rapid aging process.[24] STAT3-deficient T cells and hepatocytes have poor responses to IL-6. Deletion of STAT3 in macrophages results in constitutively activated cells and increased sensitivity to lipopolysaccharide. This is attributed to the role for STAT3 in the antiinflammatory responses induced by IL-10. CD4$^+$ T cells can differentiate into the Th17 cells whose development and function are critically dependent on STAT3. These cells produce the inflammatory cytokine IL-17, and they are responsible for recruitment and activation of neutrophils and other inflammatory cells. Th17 cells can be generated from naive CD4$^+$ T cells by IL-6 and TGF-β but can also produce another cytokine IL-21, which promotes IL-17 production in an autocrine-paracrine manner. Another cytokine, IL-23, also acts to expand and maintain Th17 cells. The importance of IL-23 signaling in inflammation is exemplified by recent discoveries that polymorphisms in *IL23R* are associated with increased risk of inflammatory bowel disease, ankylosing spondylitis, and psoriasis. IL-6, IL-21, and IL-23 all activate STAT3 by binding to their cognate receptors. The importance of STAT3 in Th17 cell development and function is appreciated in patients with Job syndrome, an autosomal-dominant disorder caused by STAT3 mutations, who fail to make Th17 cells (Chapter 21).

STAT3 deficiency in multiple types of T cells results in decreased IL-21 production, which is required for hematopoietic progenitor proliferation. STAT3 promotes optimal Th2 cell differentiation and cytokine production in the presence of activated STAT6.

Selective targeting of the STAT3b isoform has been reported and such mice exhibit diminished recovery from endotoxic shock. STAT3 deletions in other cell lineages have been described. For example, Stat3 deletion in mammary glands results in a delay in involution after weaning, arising from a decrease in apoptosis. STAT3-deficient epidermal cells show defective wound healing and in vitro migration of epidermal cells.

STAT3 is activated in multiple tumor types. This activation enhances tumor cell survival mediated by multiple mechanisms including enhanced levels of prosurvival genes (e.g., *Bcl-2* and *Bcl-X$_L$*). STAT3 is also frequently activated in cells that are transformed by a variety of oncogenes (e.g., *v-src* and *BCR-abl*). The enforced expression of a constitutively active STAT3 homodimer is sufficient to transform immortalized fibroblasts. STAT3 inhibitors are in early clinical trials for advanced malignancies.

STAT4

STAT4 is predominantly activated in response to IL-12, which drives T-helper cell differentiation towards the Th1 and Th17 pathways. The phenotype of STAT4-deficient mice is very similar to that of mice lacking IL-12. IL-12 promotes differentiation of naive CD4+ T cells to Th1 cells, which produce IFN-γ and augment cell-mediated immune responses. Th1 cells are critical in host defense against intracellular pathogens and tumors and in the pathogenesis of autoimmune diseases. Thus the phenotype of STAT4-deficient mice includes impaired Th1 differentiation, IFN-γ production, and cell-mediated immunity.[25] IL-12-, IL-12 receptor-, and STAT4-deficient mice have increased susceptibility to infection with intracellular organisms. STAT4-deficient mice are resistant to autoimmune diseases characterized by a Th1 response. A common haplotype of *STAT4* gene has been shown to be associated with susceptibility to rheumatoid arthritis, systemic lupus erythematosis, and primary Sjögren syndrome.[26] In acute sepsis, STAT4 deficiency is associated with improved survival, whereas STAT4$^{-/-}$ mice had *increased* lethality in a noninfectious sepsis model. It appears that STAT4 may have either proinflammatory or antiinflammatory effects, depending upon context.

STAT4 is also activated by IL-23. In addition, in humans, but not in mice, IFN-α/β induces STAT4 phosphorylation. This is notable because IFN-α/β can promote Th1 differentiation in humans and not in mice. This has been attributed to STAT4/STAT2 dimer being recruited to the human type I IFN receptor via the carboxy terminus of STAT2. STAT4 also mediates IFN-γ production by dendritic cells and macrophages induced by IL-12, which may explain the mechanisms by which dendritic cells (DC) promote Th1 differentiation.

STAT6

STAT6 is primarily activated by IL-4 and IL-13. STAT6-deficient mice lack most of the physiologic functions associated with IL-4, in particular the ability of IL-4 to induce the in vitro differentiation of Th2 cells.[25] STAT6 is critically involved in several distinct aspects of allergic inflammatory disease, like airway hyperresponsiveness, eosinophilic infiltration, and responses of mast cells. B cells of STAT6-deficient mice cannot undergo class switching to produce IgE against helminthes and allergens. As expected, STAT6$^{-/-}$ mice have impaired expulsion of helminthic parasites and reduced pathology in models of asthma. STAT6$^{-/-}$ mice have increased lethality, inflammation, and cytokine production in a noninfection induced model of endotoxemia, but reduced lethality and enhanced clearance of bacteria in an infection model.

STAT6 induces expression of GATA3, which is considered the Th2 cell master regulator. Transgenic mice expressing IL-4 or constitutively active STAT6 are characterized by the development of spontaneous allergic inflammation. Certain chemokines such as CCL11, CCL17 CCL22, and CCL26 have been reported to be regulated in a STAT6-dependent manner and are involved in allergic disorders. Although a number of pathways, including the mitogen-activated protein kinase and the phosphoinositide-3-kinase pathways, are involved in signal transduction because of IL-4, IL-4–induced T cell differentiation appears to occur almost exclusively via STAT6. IL-4 also antagonizes Th1 responses through STAT6. In fact, residual STAT4-independent Th1 differentiation becomes apparent in doubly deficient STAT4/STAT6 knockout mice. A study of murine mast cells demonstrated IL-15–inducible STAT6 phosphorylation, involving Tyk2, although IL-15 was less potent than IL-4.[27]

Functional deletion of STAT4 or STAT6 led to the determination that Th1 cells regulate hematopoietic progenitor cell homeostasis mediated by the production of oncostatin M.[28]

STAT5

The genes encoding STAT5A and STAT5B are juxtaposed, and the transcriptional start sites are within 10 kb of each other. Although *Stat5a* and *Stat5b* gene promoters might share certain regulatory elements, lineage specific expressions have been reported. The highly related STAT5 proteins (A and B) are activated in response to a variety of cytokines and tyrosine kinase receptors. Mice lacking STAT5A,[29] STATB,[30] or STAT5A/B,[31] display distinct phenotypes suggesting discrete functions for these proteins. STAT5A deficiency results in the loss of PRL-dependent mammary gland development, which is necessary for lactation. STAT5B-deficient mice are sexually dimorphic with growth retardation. In contrast, a good portion of STAT5A/B double knockout mice die within a few weeks of birth, are infertile with defective corpus luteum development, and have defective mammary gland development. Both male and female STAT5A/B-deficient mice are small with smaller fat pads and reduced levels of insulin-like growth factor-1 (IGF-1). STAT5A/B double knockout mice have hypocellular bone marrows, lymphopenia, neutrophilia, and modest anemia and thrombocytopenia. Moreover, the hematopoietic progenitors of STAT5A/B-deficient have defective bone marrow repopulating potential. Myeloid development is grossly normal in STAT5A/B knockout mice, but in vitro cytokine dependent proliferation, survival, and migration of myeloid cells are impaired. With respect to T- and B-cell development, complete deletion of the STAT5A/B locus results in severely impaired lymphoid development and differentiation with abrogated T-cell receptor γ rearrangement and survival of peripheral CD8+ T. In other words, complete STAT5 deficiency results in SCID, similar in lymphoid phenotype to deficiencies of IL-7R, γc, and JAK3. Deficiency of both STAT5A and STAT5B results in loss of CD4+ regulatory T (Treg) cells that express the transcription factor Foxp3, whereas constitutive activation of STAT5B enforces Foxp3-positive Treg cell development, bypassing the requirements for upstream cytokine or costimulatory signals to activate Foxp3 transcription. STAT5 deficiency abrogates transformation by Tel-JAK but not by v-Abl or BCR-abl. Mutations in the *Stat5b* gene has been documented in a few patients with severe growth retardation. Loss of functional STAT5B is associated with severe IGF-1 deficiency, indicating that this pathway is responsible for most of the GH-induced IGF-1 production.

Negative Regulators of Cytokine Signaling

Whereas the JAK-STAT pathway activation is important for homeostasis, its inactivation prevents excessive responses to cytokine stimulation. In addition to protein tyrosine phosphatases (PTPs), other factors are involved in downregulating this pathway as discussed later.

Src-Homology 2 Containing Phosphatase 1 (PTPN6)

The expression of SHP-1, a cytoplasmic phosphotyrosine phosphatase is limited to the hematopoietic system. SHP-1 was identified as the protein encoded by the mutated locus (Hcph) in the *moth-eaten* (*me*) mice.[32] These mice that are characterized by reduced SHP-1 display severe immunologic dysfunction; enhanced proliferation of macrophages and neutrophils in the lungs, which leads to pneumonitis; and patchy dermatitis that results in the "moth-eaten" phenotype. SHP-1 associates with cytokine receptors and dephosphorylates JAK kinases. For example, it downregulates EPO-induced signaling by binding to the EPOR and dephosphorylating JAK2 associated with it. SHP-1 also dephosphorylates JAK1, because IFN-α–induced phosphorylation of JAK1 is enhanced in SHP-1–deficient macrophages. SHP-1 also interacts with JAK3. This interaction may explain the activation of JAK3/STAT3 pathway in some cases of ALK (+) anaplastic large cell lymphoma where SHP-1 appears to be suppressed by promoter methylation. The expression of an inactive SHP-1 in the cytokine-dependent cell line Ba/F3 increased the proliferative response to IL-3, STAT5 phosphorylation, and cell survival following IL-3 withdrawal.

Consistent with the negative role of SHP-1 on the JAK/STAT pathway, silencing of SHP-1 by promoter methylation is often associated with various kinds of leukemia and lymphomas, myeloma, and acute myeloid leukemia. On the other hand, in a limited number of cases, SHP-1 has been described to have a positive role in promoting JAK/STAT signaling. For example, epidermal growth factor– and IFN-γ–induced STAT activation was suppressed by expressing a catalytically inactive form of SHP-1 in HeLa cells, while this pathway was essentially unaffected by the expression of wild-type SHP-1. There is no known molecular explanation for this observation.

Src-Homology 2 Containing Phosphatase 2 (PTPN11)

SHP-2 is a protein-tyrosine phosphatase that is widely expressed, with high levels of expression in hematopoietic cells. It contains two tandem SH2 domains (N-SH2 and C-SH2), a PTP domain and a C-terminal tail. SHP-2 has low basal enzymatic activity caused by autoinhibition of the PTP domain by the N-SH2 domain. SHP-2 directly or indirectly (via adaptor proteins) associates with activated receptor protein tyrosine kinases or cytokine receptors via its two SH2 domains. Binding of SH2 domains to phosphotyrosine sites of these receptors alters the conformation of the N-SH2 domain, releasing its binding to PTP domain and causing catalytic activation.[32] Despite being a phosphatase, SHP-2 promotes activation of the Ras and ERK pathway by cytokines. Its catalytic activity is required for cytokine activation of phosphatidylinositol 3-kinase pathway. SHP-2 plays an essential role in hematopoietic cell development. Embryonic lethality is observed at day 8.5 in mice with a truncated version of SHP-2 because of severe defects in gastrulation and mesodermal patterning. Complete loss of SHP-2 causes embryonic death in the periimplantation period and SHP-2 is required for trophoblast stem cell survival. HSCs from SHP-2 haploinsufficient mice display a competitive repopulating defect. Embryonic stem (ES) cells lacking SHP-2 exhibit severely decreased differentiation to erythroid and myeloid progenitors in vitro and fail to contribute to erythroid and myeloid lineages in chimeric mice derived from SHP-2$^{-/-}$ ES cells and wild-type embryos. SHP-2 loss-of-function causes an early block of lymphocyte development before Pro-T and Pro-B stages. The exact mechanisms by which SHP-2 regulates cytokine signaling and hematopoiesis are uncertain. SHP-2 both enhances and inhibits the JAK/STAT pathway depending on the context. It functions as a negative regulator of the IFN-stimulated JAK1/STAT pathway and it dephosphorylates STAT1 and STAT5. At the same time SHP-2 is required for optimal JAK2 activation.

Activating germline mutations of *PTPN11* (the gene encoding for SHP-2 protein) are seen in patients with Noonan syndrome while loss-of-function mutations are seen in patients with LEOPARD syndrome. Both are congenital disorders associated with abnormal hematopoiesis. Somatic activating mutations are seen in approximately 35% of patients with juvenile myelomonocytic leukemia. PTPN11 mutations are also seen in patients with myelodysplastic syndrome, acute lymphoblastic leukemia, and acute myelogenous leukemia. These gain-of-function mutations induce hyperactivation of the Ras pathway, which results in growth factor and cytokine independent proliferation and survival of hematopoietic progenitor cells (HPCs). Increased SHP-2 expression has also been observed in acute leukemia cells, suggesting a potential role in leukemogenesis.

CD45, PTP1B, TC-PTP, PTPRT, and PTP-BL

CD45 is a receptor-like tyrosine phosphatase highly expressed by hematopoietic cells. CD45 was identified as a JAK family phosphatase. CD45 is able to dephosphorylate all JAKs in murine cells, and dephosphorylate JAK1 and JAK3 in human cells. Targeted disruption of the CD45 gene leads to enhanced cytokine and IFN-receptor-mediated activation of JAKs and STAT proteins. The removal of CD45 also increases erythroid colony formation and antiviral activity, which is consistent with the fact that CD45 negatively regulates EPO and IFN signaling. Inactivating mutations occur in patients with T-cell acute lymphoblastic leukemia. The Src family kinase members Lck and Lyn are key substrates for CD45 in T and B lymphocytes, respectively. CD45 positively regulates T cell receptor-mediated signaling through the activation of Src-family kinases.

PTP1B (PTP1B or PTPN1) and T-cell PTP (TC-PTP or PTPN2) are closely related PTP, sharing 74% homology in their catalytic domain. PTP1B is expressed in many tissues and TC-PTP is ubiquitously expressed with particularly high expression in hematopoietic tissues. PTP1B is involved in multiple signaling pathways by down-regulating several tyrosine kinases. For example, PTP1B-deficient mice display increased insulin sensitivity. Increased phosphorylation of JAK2, Tyk2, STAT3, and STAT5 has been observed in PTP1B-deficient embryonic fibroblasts. TC-PTP targets multiple STAT and JAK proteins in addition to growth factor receptors for dephosphorylation. TC-PTP–deficient mice develop anemia, lymphadenopathy and splenomegaly and die at early age. These mice display excessive inflammation and demonstrate increased numbers of bone marrow, HSCs and HPCs. Other phosphatases such as PTP-receptor type T (PTPRT) and PTP-Basophil like (PTP-BL) and the adapter protein LNK have also been implicated in cytokine signaling. LNK mutations have been reported in patients with myeloproliferative neoplasms including essential thrombocythemia and primary myelofibrosis (Chapters 69 and 70).

Protein Inhibitors of Activated STAT

PIAS3 was the first family member to be identified as a repressor of STAT3 activity.[33] Three additional family members PIAS1, PIASy (or PIAS4), and PIASx (or PIAS2) were later identified with high sequence homology. Other proteins with weak homology (hZIMP7 and hZIMP10) have been reported. PIAS1 was identified as a STAT1-interacting protein and subsequently found to inhibit STAT1-mediated transcriptional activation. The PIAS family members PIASx and PIASy were identified based on sequence similarity to PIAS1 and have been shown to inhibit STAT1 and STAT4, respectively. PIAS proteins have been shown to affect the function of many different proteins, with particular effects on gene transcription.

PIAS proteins contain a domain known as SP-RING (Fig. 16.9) with structural similarity to ubiquitin E3 ligase RING fingers. PIAS binds the protein modifier SUMO (small ubiquitin-like modifier) and recruits the E2 SUMO ligase UBC9, which transfers SUMO to target proteins, particularly to transcription factors such as STATs. PIAS1, PIAS3, and PIASx sumoylate STAT1 at Lys-703, close to the site at which it is phosphorylated by JAKs (Tyr-701). A mutation of Lys-703 results in an increased response to IFN-γ.

Thus the binding of PIAS to STAT results in the inhibition of STAT-mediated gene activation. PIAS1 and PIAS3 inhibit STAT DNA binding activity, while PIASy and PIASx repress STAT1 and STAT4-mediated gene activation without affecting DNA binding. PIAS proteins also act by recruiting other corepressor molecules. One example is the inhibition of natural regulatory T-cell differentiation by PIAS1 through chromatin-based epigenetic repression. Sumoylation may affect nuclear localization of proteins as is the case for the transcriptional factor LEF1, where LEF1 sumoylation by PIASy results in its sequestration into nuclear bodies hindering its transcriptional activity. Given its impact on STAT1 and IFN signaling, PIAS1 has a tangible role in innate immunity. The antiviral activity of IFNs is significantly increased in PIAS−/− cells. In addition, PIAS−/− mice have increased protection against bacterial and viral infection.

Suppressor of Cytokine Signaling

The SOCS family consists of eight proteins that antagonize the signaling of STAT proteins. STATs activate the transcription of genes

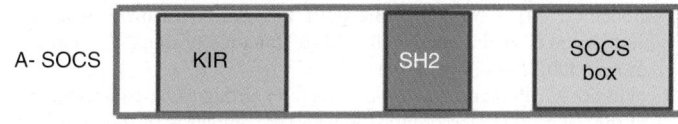

A- SOCS

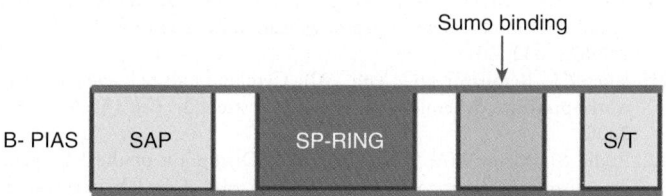

Sumo binding

B- PIAS

Fig. 16.9 THE GENERAL STRUCTURE OF A SOCS AND A PIAS PROTEIN. (A) SOCS protein has a central SH2 domain, an amino-terminal domain of variable length and divergent sequence that contains a kinase inhibitory region (KIR), and a carboxy-terminal 40-amino-acid SOCS box. (B) PIAS protein contains a SAP (SAFA/B, ACINUS, PIAS) domain that is present in other chromatin associated proteins. PIAS proteins that are SUMO E3 ligases contain a conserved SP-RING domain that shares sequence similarity to RING domains of ubiquitin E3 ligases. This domain recruits the SUMO E2 ligase (UBC9).

encoding the SOCS family as a negative feedback regulation.[34] For example, expression of SOCS3 is activated by several transcription factors, including STAT1, STAT3, and mitogen-activated protein kinase p38, while expression of SOCS1 is dependent on the production of IFN regulatory factor-1, a STAT1-inducible transcription factor. Each SOCS has two major domains, an SH2 domain and a SOCS box that mediates a complex formation with elongins B and C, a cullin, and Rbx2, to form an E3 ubiquitin ligase (see Fig. 16.9). SOCS proteins function in a negative feedback loop to inhibit cytokine signaling by binding to either phospho-JAK or phospho-receptor through SH2 domain, and thus competing with the STAT proteins or directly inhibiting JAK activity, and also by targeting the receptor complex for ubiquitylation and subsequent proteasome-mediated degradation. Gene targeting studies have delineated the distinct in vivo functions of SOCS proteins. For example, SOCS1-/- mice die as neonates from an inflammatory disease caused by dysregulated IFN signaling, and which presents as lymphopenia, infiltration of macrophages, and T cells into the liver and other organs, and fatty degeneration of the liver.[35] SOCS3 deletion results in an embryonic lethality at 10 to 16 days because of a defect in placental formation likely from excess LIF1 signaling associated with marked erythrocytosis.[36] In addition, the in vitro proliferative capacity of high proliferative progenitor cells is greatly increased.

CYTOKINE-RECEPTOR INTRACELLULAR SIGNALING IN THE CONTEXT OF IN VIVO

Physiology/Pathology

Targeted gene deletions of JAKS, STATS, and other intracellular signaling molecules have highlighted the embryonic and hematopoietic requirements of these signaling molecules (Table 16.1). However, most information on intracellular signaling is achieved ex vivo using full-length cytokines in either natural or recombinant forms. However, in vivo these cells are not isolated, but rather are present in an environment with many other cell types, containing numerous other molecules including enzymes that have the capability of modifying the structure, and potentially also the functional capacity of these cytokines and other growth factors.[37,38] One example

TABLE 16.1	Consequence of Deficiencies in Genes of Intracellular Signaling Molecules
Signal Transduction Molecule	**Phenotype of Deficient Mice**
JAK1	Perinatal mortality, defects in IL-6, IL-2, and cytokine receptor type II families
JAK2	Embryonic lethality caused by defective definitive hematopoiesis. Defects in TPO, IL-2 family, IL-3 and IFN-γ signaling
JAK3	Immunodeficiency because of absent common γ chain signaling. JAK3 expression is restricted to the hematopoietic system
Tyk2	Reduced responses to IFN-α/β, IL-12, and unexpectedly IFN-γ
STAT1	Complete lack of responsiveness to either IFN-α/β or IFN-γ and high sensitivity to infections by viruses and other microbial pathogens. Normal response to other cytokines such as growth hormone (GH), IL-10, and epidermal growth factor
STAT2	Lack of responsiveness to IFN-α/β; susceptibility to viral infections
STAT3	Early embryonic lethality before gastrulation STAT3 ± mice demonstrate decreased HSC/HPCs
STAT4	Defective Th1 response caused by defective IL-12 signaling
STAT5a	Defective mammary gland development and lactogenesis; GM-CSF and follicular lymphoma signaling is impaired but no gross hematopoietic abnormalities
STAT5B	Disrupted sexual dimorphism of body growth rates. Defective GH signaling
STAT5A/B	Anemic embryos of the double knock-outs with apoptotic erythroid progenitors because of impaired EPO signaling. Adult mouse erythrocyte red blood cell number is normal. Loss of GH and prolactin signaling. Infertile females. Severe impairment of IL-2 induced T-cell responses
STAT6	Defective Th2 response with eliminated IL-4 signaling
SHP-1	Natural mutation in *moth-eaten* mice results in hair loss, immunodeficiency, autoimmune disorders, enhanced SDF-1 chemotactic activities, enhanced hematopoietic progenitor proliferation in response to cytokines such as GM-CSF
CD45	Enhanced cytokine and IFN-receptor-mediated activation of JAKs and STATs
SOCS1	Neonatal lethality probably because of excessive IFN-γ responses, with hematopoietic infiltration of multiple organs, lymphopenia, and fatty liver degeneration
SOCS2	Gigantism caused by GH and/or IFG-1 excessive signaling
SOCS3	Embryonic lethality with placental defect likely because of LIF1 excess signaling Erythrocytosis in embryos

This table outlines the phenotypes of mice deficient in the major signaling molecules that directly interact with the cytokine receptors.
The phenotypes range from significant embryonic lethality because of hematopoietic impairment to less remarkable defects in other organ systems. Please refer to the main text for more details on the functions of these molecules. GM-CSF, Granulocyte-macrophage colony-stimulating factor; HPC, hematopoietic progenitor cell; HSC, hematopoietic stem cell; JAK, Janus-activated kinase; LIF, leukemia inhibitory factor; STAT, signal transducer and activator of transcription.

of such an enzyme modifying effect is that of dipeptidylpeptidase 4 (DPP4). This enzyme has the capability to truncate amongst a plethora of growth factors: GM-CSF, G-CSF, IL-3, EPO, and TPO. The DPP4-truncated GM-CSF manifest less or no activity, yet is able to compete by increased receptor-binding capacity to block the functional activity of the full-length GM-CSF. A similar effect is noted for DPP4-truncated IL-3, and DPP4 truncated-GM-CSF and -IL-3 can reciprocally block the stimulating activity of each other through common receptor-mediated events.[39] Moreover, the full-length and DPP4 truncated-GM-CSF and -IL-3 each trigger qualitatively, in addition to quantitatively, different intracellular signaling events in terms of proteins, phosphorylated proteins, and microRNAs produced. There is a large and clearly not yet comprehensive list of biologically active molecules with putative DPP4 truncation sites,[37,38] and the signaling events elicited by these truncated molecules should be taken into account in terms of the effects of different cytokines on normal and abnormal cell growth.

To add another layer of complexity to the emerging knowledge of cytokine induced receptor-mediated intracellular signaling is the state of the cell itself. It is now becoming clear that once a cell is removed from its in vivo hypoxic environment to that of ambient air, which is defined here as normoxic (~21% O_2), a phenomenon termed extraphysiologic oxygen shock/stress (EPHOSS) is initiated and changes the metabolism of hematopoietic stem and progenitor cells, and likely other cell types through an axis encompassing the mitochondrial permeability transition pore-cyclophilin D-p53, which also involves hypoxia inducing factor-1α and the hypoxamir microRNA 210.[40,41] Thus the intracellular signaling that one detects by assessing the effects of a cytokine on a cell collected and processed under ambient-air (normoxia) may not exactly mimic how that cytokine might signal in a cell in its in vivo hypoxic environment. Those differences in cascades in signaling molecules may manifest differently under physiologic and pathologic conditions. Ambient air induced EPHOSS, as compared with the in vivo hypoxic environment, results in differences in hematopoietic stem and progenitor numbers and activity. Cyclophilin D-/- and p53-/- have EPHOSS protective effects, while hypoxia inducing factor 1α-/- and microRNA 210-/- abrogate the protective effects achieved by the harvesting and processing cells under hypoxic conditions.[40]

How cytokine-receptor signaling is influenced by enzyme truncated cytokines/growth factors, such as seen with DPP4 truncated proteins,[37-39] and consideration of the in vivo hypoxic condition cells are usually bathed in will have to be assessed for more detailed and potentially greater physiologic and pathologic understanding of intracellular signaling and its modification for clinical advantage.[40,41] Also, how multiple cytokines signal together under these conditions and with that of synthesized small molecules currently being used for ex vivo expansion of hematopoietic stem cells should be considered.[42,43] It may be that such evaluations will be critical for the development of more efficacious treatments for cancer and related hematologic disorders.

REFERENCES

1.* Boulay J, O'Shea J, Paul W: Molecular phylogeny within type I cytokines and their cognate receptors. *Immunity* 19:159–163, 2003.

2. Bazan J: Structural design and molecular evolution of a cytokine receptor superfamily. *Proc Natl Acad Sci USA* 87:6934–6938, 1990.

3. Boulay JL, Paul WE: The interleukin-4 family of lymphokines. *Curr Opin Immunol* 4:294–298, 1992.

4. Horan T, Wen J, Narhi L, et al: Dimerization of the extracellular domain of granuloycte-colony stimulating factor receptor by ligand binding: a monovalent ligand induces 2:2 complexes. *Biochemistry* 35:4886–4896, 1996.

5. Ghoreschi K, Laurence A, O'Shea J: Janus kinases in immune cell signaling. *Immunol Rev* 228:273–287, 2009.

6. McKinstry WJ, Li CL, Rasko JE, et al: Cytokine receptor expression on hematopoietic stem and progenitor cells. *Blood* 89:65–71, 1997.

7. Boulanger MJ, Chow DC, Brevnova EE, et al: Hexameric structure and assembly of the interleukin-6/IL-6 alpha-receptor/gp130 complex. *Science* 300:2101–2104, 2003.

8. Skiniotis G, Boulanger MJ, Garcia KC, et al: Signaling conformations of the tall cytokine receptor gp130 when in complex with IL-6 and IL-6 receptor. *Nat Struct Mol Biol* 12(6):545–551, 2005.

9. Lupardus PJ, Skiniotis G, Rice AJ, et al: Structural snapshots of full-length Jak1, a transmembrane gp130/IL-6/IL-6Rα cytokine receptor complex, and the receptor-Jak1 holocomplex. *Structure* 19:45–55, 2011.

10. Thomas C, Moraga I, Levin D, et al: Structural linkage between ligand discrimination and receptor activation by type I interferons. *Cell* 146:621–632, 2011.

11. Janes KA, Reinhardt HC, Yaffe MB: Cytokine-induced signaling networks prioritize dynamic range over signal strength. *Cell* 135:343–354, 2008.

12. Rodig SJ, Meraz MA, White JM, et al: Disruption of the Jak1 gene demonstrates obligatory and nonredundant roles of the Jaks in cytokine-induced biologic responses. *Cell* 93:373–383, 1998.

13. Neubauer H, Cumano A, Müller M, et al: Jak2 deficiency defines an essential developmental checkpoint in definitive hematopoiesis. *Cell* 93:397–409, 1998.

14. Parganas E, Wang D, Stravopodis D, et al: Jak2 is essential for signaling through a variety of cytokine receptors. *Cell* 93:385–395, 1998.

15. Nosaka T, Van Deursen JM, Tripp RA, et al: Defective lymphoid development in mice lacking Jak3. *Science* 270:800–802, 1995.

16. Thomis DC, Gurniak CB, Tivol E, et al: Defects in B lymphocyte maturation and T lymphocyte activation in mice lacking Jak3. *Science* 270:794–797, 1995.

17. Velazquez L, Fellous M, Stark GR, et al: A protein tyrosine kinase in the interferon alpha/beta signaling pathway. *Cell* 70:313–322, 1992.

18. O'Shea JJ, Gadina M, Schreiber RD: Cytokine signaling in 2002: new surprises in the Jak/Stat pathway. *Cell* 109(Suppl):S121–S131, 2002.

19. Reich NC: STAT dynamics. *Cytokine Growth Factor Rev* 18:511–518, 2007.

20. Meraz MA, White JM, Sheehan KC, et al: Targeted disruption of the Stat1 gene in mice reveals unexpected physiologic specificity in the JAK-STAT signaling pathway. *Cell* 84:431–442, 1996.

21. van de Veerdonk FL, Plantinga TS, Hoischen A, et al: STAT1 mutations in autosomal dominant chronic mucocutaneous candidiasis. *N Engl J Med* 365:54–61, 2011.

22. Park C, Li S, Cha E, et al: Immune response in Stat2 knockout mice. *Immunity* 13:795–804, 2000.

23. Akira S: Roles of STAT3 defined by tissue-specific gene targeting. *Oncogene* 19:2607–2611, 2000.

24. Mantel C, Messina-Graham S, Moh A, et al: Mouse hematopoietic cell-targeted STAT3 deletion: stem/progenitor cell defects, mitochondrial dysfunction, ROS overproduction, and a rapid aging-like phenotype. *Blood* 120:2589–2599, 2012.

25. Wurster AL, Tanaka T, Grusby MJ: The biology of Stat4 and Stat6. *Oncogene* 19:2577–2584, 2000.

26. Remmers EF, Plenge RM, Lee AT, et al: STAT4 and the risk of rheumatoid arthritis and systemic lupus erythematosus. *N Engl J Med* 357:977–986, 2007.

27. Masuda A, Matsuguchi T, Yamaki K, et al: Interleukin-15 induces rapid tyrosine phosphorylation of STAT6 and the expression of interleukin-4 in mouse mast cells. *J Biol Chem* 275(38):29331–29337, 2000.

28. Broxmeyer HE, Bruns H, Zhang S, et al: Th1 cells regulate hematopoietic progenitor cell homeostasis by production of oncostatin M. *Immunity* 16:815–825, 2002.

29. Liu X, Robinson GW, Wagner KU, et al: Stat5a is mandatory for adult mammary gland development and lactogenesis. *Genes Dev* 11(2):179–186, 1997.

30. Udy GB, Towers RP, Snell RG, et al: Requirement of STAT5b for sexual dimorphism of body growth rates and liver gene expression. *Proc Natl Acad Sci USA* 94(14):7239–7244, 1997.

31. Teglund S, McKay C, Schuetz E, et al: Stat5a and Stat5b proteins have essential and nonessential, or redundant, roles in cytokine responses. *Cell* 93(5):841–850, 1998.

32. Neel BG, Gu H, Pao L: The 'Shp'ing news: SH2domain-containing tyrosine phosphatases in cell signaling. *Trends Biochem Sci* 28:284–293, 2003.

33. Chung CD, Liao J, Liu B, et al: Specific inhibition of Stat3 signal transduction by PIAS3. *Science* 278(5344):1803–1805, 1997.

34. Wormald S, Hilton DJ: The negative regulatory roles of suppressor of cytokine signaling proteins in myeloid signaling pathways. *Curr Opin Hematol* 14:9–15, 2007.

35. Marine JC, Topham DJ, McKay C, et al: SOCS1 deficiency causes a lymphocyte-dependent perinatal lethality. *Cell* 98:609–616, 1999.

36. Marine JC, McKay C, Wang D, et al: SOCS3 is essential in the regulation of fetal liver erythropoiesis. *Cell* 98:617–627, 1999.

37. Broxmeyer HE, Hoggatt J, O'Leary HA, et al: Dipeptidylpeptidase 4 negatively regulates colony stimulating factor activity and stress hematopoiesis. *Nat Med* 18:1786–1796, 2012.

38. Ou X, O'Leary HA, Broxmeyer HE: Implications of DPP4 modification of proteins that regulate stem/progenitor and more mature cell types. *Blood* 122:161–169, 2013.

39. O'Leary HA, Mantel C, Lai X, et al: DPP4 (CD26) Truncation of GM-CSF and IL-3 alters their signaling and functional activity in normal and leukemic hematopoietic stem and progenitor cells. *Blood* 122:1206, 2013.

40. Mantel CR, O'Leary HA, Chitteti BR, et al: Enhancing hematopoietic stem cell transplantation efficacy by mitigating oxygen shock. *Cell* 161:1553–1565, 2015.

41. Broxmeyer HE, O'Leary HA, Huang X, et al: The importance of hypoxia and EPHOSS for collection and processing of stem and progenitor cells to understand true physiology/pathology of these cells ex-vivo. *Curr Opin Hematol* 22:273–278, 2015.

42. Iancu-Rubin C, Hoffman R: Role of epigenetic reprogramming in hematopoietic stem cell function. *Curr Opin Hematol* 22:279–285, 2015.

43. Fares I, Rivest-Khan L, Sauvageau G: Small molecule regulation of normal and leukemic stem cells. *Curr Opin Hematol* 22:309–316, 2015.

CHAPTER 17

CONTROL OF CELL DIVISION

Martin Fischer, Chi V. Dang, and James A. DeCaprio

THE CELL DIVISION CYCLE

The mammalian cell cycle is divided into four phases: mitosis (M), DNA synthesis (S), and the gap phases G_1 and G_2 (Fig. 17.1). Mitosis is recognized when cells visibly undergo cell division and chromatin becomes condensed, sequentially progressing through prophase, metaphase, anaphase, and telophase. The G_1 phase occurs immediately after mitosis has been completed and ends when DNA synthesis begins. During S phase, cells duplicate their entire genome by DNA replication. G_2 occurs after DNA synthesis has been completed and before chromosomal condensation in mitosis. Although the duration of the S, G_2, and M phases is relatively constant for most mammalian cells, there can be a large degree of variability in the duration of G_1. Among the earliest observations regarding the generation time for cells, it was shown that by varying the growth conditions, the length of a cell division cycle could change, with the length of G_1 responsible for most of this variability. Although cells progress through S, G_2, and M phases in relatively invariable time periods, the length of the G_1 phase is highly variable, and this variability is dependent at least in part on the presence of growth factors.

Quiescence and Differentiation

Quiescence (G_0) is a nonproliferative state in which viable cells have left the cell cycle and may remain for prolonged periods. Quiescent cells may be difficult to distinguish morphologically from cells in a prolonged G_1 phase, but they can be distinguished by different markers. Terminally differentiated cells, such as neutrophilic granulocytes, muscle cells, and neurons, have irreversibly exited the cell cycle during the process of differentiation and are examples of cells that have irreversibly entered G_0. Other cells, including stem cells, reversibly enter G_0 and may be induced to reenter the cell cycle with appropriate stimuli, such as growth factors. Differentiation provides the organism with a supply of cells to execute specific and specialized functions. In some cell types, such as muscle and nerve cells, differentiation and proliferation are mutually exclusive fates, and cells undergo "terminal differentiation." In other cell types, such as those of the hematopoietic lineage, proliferation may continue after cells acquire differentiated characteristics. For example, erythroblasts, myeloblasts, and megakaryoblasts are committed to particular differentiation pathways and possess lineage-specific markers yet continue to proliferate. T and B lymphocytes are fully differentiated and express antigen-specific receptors but can be induced to proliferate when appropriately stimulated.

G_1 Phase

G_1, which occupies the period or gap between M and S phases, is the interval between the completion of one round of cell division and initiation of the next. Its duration is the most variable, can be prolonged depending on the cell type, and is subject to regulation by environmental factors such as the availability of growth factors and nutrients. It is the period of cell growth, and as a first approximation, the amount of time a cell spends in G_1 is inversely related to its rate of proliferation. A certain increase in mass usually is required before the cell initiates the next S phase. When conditions are unsuitable for proliferation (e.g., because of insufficient nutrients or absence of mitogens), cells arrest in G_1, and those that are already in S, G_2, or M phase usually complete the round to which they have been committed and arrest only when they reach G_1 again. For example, when the 40S ribosomal protein S6 is missing, cells stop proliferation. If cell size or mass were not regulated, S phase entry might cause cells to become progressively smaller or be at risk for DNA replication errors as a result of insufficient substrates. Cell size regulation is intimately linked to ribosome biogenesis and nutrient-sensing systems, central to which are the phosphoinositide 3-kinase (PI3K) and target of rapamycin (TOR) pathways. Notably, when the MYC transcription factor is missing, cells slow their growth and often do not enter S phase. MYC regulates *cyclin* and *cyclin-dependent kinase (CDK)* genes as well as genes involved in ribosome biogenesis and translation.[1] In aggregate, studies of a variety of cell systems indicate that cell size regulation is linked to cell proliferation, except in specialized cells that undergo endoreplication or in embryos shortly after fertilization, when G_1 is virtually undetectable, and there is no cell enlargement. As a result, the original mass of egg cytoplasm is partitioned among thousands of cells within a few hours without a noticeable increase in size.

S Phase

S phase is the period of wholesale DNA synthesis during which the cell replicates its genetic content; a normal diploid somatic cell with a 2N complement of DNA at the beginning of S phase acquires a 4N complement of DNA at its end. (Recall that N = 1 copy of each chromosome per cell [haploid]; 2N = 2 copies [diploid].) The duration of S phase may vary from only a few minutes in rapidly dividing, early embryo cells to a few hours in most somatic cells. Early embryo cells generally "live off" the accumulated stores of maternal RNA and proteins present in the egg and are transcriptionally silent, whereas cells in later development and mature organisms must actively transcribe subsets of their genes to survive and maintain specialized functions. The longer time required for the latter to complete S phase probably allows these cells to coordinate DNA replication with transcription and to preserve higher-order gene and chromatin structural information that influences gene expression for transmission to progeny cells.

G_2 Phase

G_2 is the period or gap between S and M phases when cells have finished replicating their DNA, are preparing to divide, and have a 4N DNA content. For most cells entering S phase, passage through G_2 is "automatic," and the duration of G_2 is fixed, except under unusual circumstances. For example, G_2 duration can be extremely short and is essentially undetectable in rapidly proliferating, early embryonic cells.

M Phase

Mitosis, or M phase, is the period of actual nuclear and cell division during which the duplicated chromosomes are divided equally between two progeny cells. It is obvious microscopically as the period of chromosome condensation and segregation, nuclear division

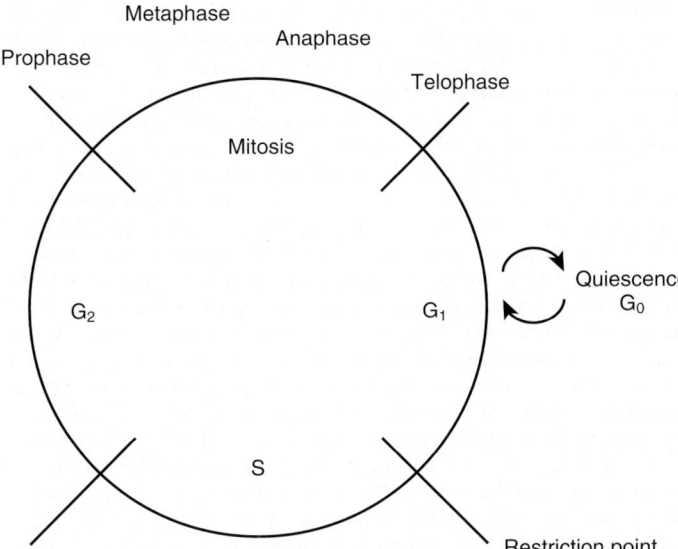

Fig. 17.1 THE CELL DIVISION CYCLE. The mammalian cell cycle is divided into four phases that include mitosis (M), DNA synthesis (S), and the gap phases G_1 and G_2. Mitosis is subdivided into prophase, metaphase, anaphase, and telophase. Quiescence (G_0) is a nonproliferative state in which viable cells have left the cell cycle and may remain for prolonged periods. A particularly important point in G_1 is the restriction point, or R, which occurs near the G_1–S boundary. After the cell passes the G_1/S restriction point, it is committed to cell cycle progression.

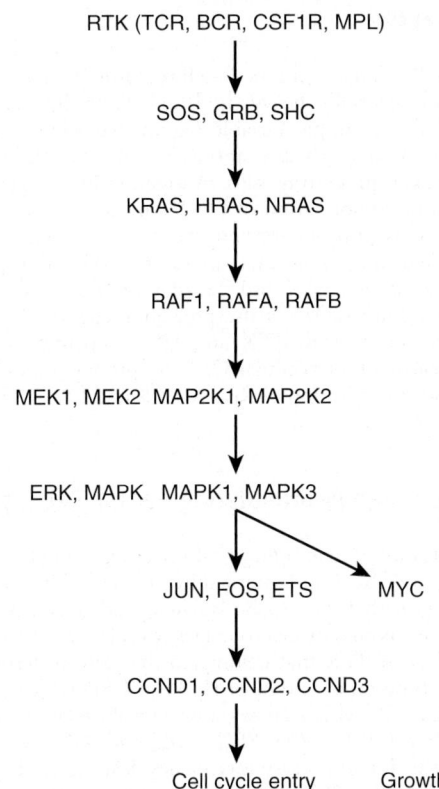

Fig. 17.2 SIGNALING PATHWAYS, SUCH AS THE RAS–MITOGEN-ACTIVATED PROTEIN KINASE (MAPK) PATHWAY, CONTROL CELL CYCLE ENTRY. Cells scan their environment with the help of cell surface receptors such as receptor tyrosine kinases (RTKs). When RTKs become activated by ligand-stabilized dimerization, they can induce signaling pathways. The RAS-MAPK signaling pathway plays a particularly important role in proliferation. RAS GTPases are activated by many receptors, such as T-cell receptors (TCRs), B-cell receptors (BCRs), and colony-stimulating factor 1 receptor (CSF-1R), and recruit MAPK complexes. These complexes are formed by scaffolds, such as kinase suppressor of RAS (KSR), binding to the three-tier MAPK module that comprises RAF, mitogen-activated protein kinase kinase (MEK), and extracellular signal–regulated kinase (ERK). When activated by RAS (H-RAS, K-RAS, N-RAS), the MAPKKK RAF (RAF-1, A-RAF, B-RAF) phosphorylates the MAPKK MEK (MEK1, MEK2), which in turn phosphorylates the MAPK ERK (ERK1, ERK2). Activated ERK kinases phosphorylate the transcription factors MYC and activator protein 1 (JUN/FOS), leading to transcription activation of cyclin D1, CDK4, and CDK6. Monophosphorylation of retinoblastoma protein (RB) by cyclin D-CDK4/6 is required for cells to leave quiescence and enter the cell cycle.

(karyokinesis), and physical separation of the two daughter cells (cytokinesis). A cell entering M phase has a 4N DNA content and finishes as two cells, each with an identical 2N complement of DNA. The complex sequence of changes that take place allows mitosis to be subdivided into prophase, prometaphase, metaphase, anaphase, and telophase. *Prophase* is the period of chromatin/chromosome condensation, centrosome separation/migration to opposite poles, and nuclear membrane breakdown. The centrosomes are microtubule organization centers that eventually give rise to the bipole mitotic spindle apparatus that will separate the sister chromatids of each duplicated chromosome. During *prometaphase,* chromosomes attach to microtubules of the mitotic spindle, so that sister chromatids become attached to opposite poles. In *metaphase,* the condensed chromosomes align at the equatorial plate. The cohesive "bond" between sister chromatids of duplicated chromosomes is dissolved, allowing *anaphase,* the period of sister chromatid separation, to proceed. On reaching their poles, nuclear membranes form to envelop each of the two separated sets of chromosomes, which also begin to decondense, marking *telophase* and karyokinesis. This is soon followed by cytokinesis and exit from mitosis. Following mitosis, cells reenter G_1, and for approximately 3 hours they are capable of leaving the cell cycle into quiescence when growth factors and nutrients are missing. Once past this point, cells are no longer sensitive to mitogen withdrawal and can commit to another round of cell division.

SIGNALING

To decide whether to proliferate, cells scan their environment with the help of cell surface receptors such as receptor tyrosine kinases (RTKs) that bind extracellular ligands and activate signaling pathways. RTKs become activated by ligand-stabilized dimerization that allows autophosphorylation. The intracellular phosphotyrosine residues are recognized by SH2 (Src homology 2) or PTB (phosphotyrosine-binding) protein domains, leading to the recruitment of signaling effectors and formation of signaling complexes. In turn, these complexes permit activation of signaling pathways, such as RAS–mitogen-activated protein kinase (MAPK), PI3K, and phospholipase Cγ

(PLCγ). Together, these signaling pathways stimulate cell proliferation (Fig. 17.2).

T-Cell Receptor

Activation of T cells occurs upon ligation of the T-cell receptor (TCR) by major histocompatibility complex molecules in antigen-presenting cells.[2] The TCR and its coreceptors CD4 and CD8 have no intrinsic enzymatic activity. Instead, the associated non–RTK LCK binds to cytoplasmic domains of TCR coreceptors CD4 and CD8, and their activation leads to phosphorylation of immunoreceptor tyrosine-based activation motifs (ITAMs) in CD3. Phosphorylated CD3 recruits the tyrosine kinase ZAP70, leading to a cascade of phosphorylation events that in turn activates LAT (linker for activation of T cells) complexes. The LAT signalosome triggers the release of intracellular Ca^{2+} and production of diacylglycerol (DAG). The latter activates RAS-MAPK and protein kinase C (PKC)–nuclear factor κB (NFκB) signaling pathways.

B-Cell Receptor

Every normal B cell has a unique B-cell receptor (BCR) consisting of pairs of immunoglobulin heavy (IgH) and light (IgL) chains. Each IgH and IgL has a unique variable region that allows the BCR to recognize and bind to diverse antigens, both soluble and on the surface of antigen-presenting cells. Antigen-induced aggregation of BCR leads to phosphorylation of ITAMs by the Src family tyrosine kinase LYN. This phosphorylation event initiates the assembly of intracellular signaling molecules, including SYK, PLCγ2, Bruton tyrosine kinase (BTK), VAV, and the adaptor B-cell linker (BLNK). The BCR coreceptor CD19 is also phosphorylated by LYN, leading to the recruitment of PI3K, BTK, and AKT.[3] Together, this signaling leads to the release of intracellular Ca^{2+} and production of DAG, and ultimately leads to activation of RAS-MAPK and PKC–NFκB signaling pathways.

Macrophage Colony-Stimulating Factor Receptor

The known ligands of macrophage colony-stimulating factor 1 receptor (CSF-1R) are CSF-1 and interleukin (IL)-34.[4] CSF-1 was the first hemopoietic growth factor to be isolated, and it can promote the growth of pure colonies of macrophages from bone marrow progenitors. CSF-1R is an RTK that belongs to the platelet-derived growth factor family. Binding of CSF-1 or IL-34 to CSF-1R leads to dimerization of CSF-1R, which allows autophosphorylation. Numerous proteins, such as GRB2, SOS, SFK, CBL, and p85, are recruited to the intracellular domain phosphotyrosines, leading to the activation of the PI3K-AKT and RAS-MAPK pathways, among others.

RAS Pathway to Cyclin D

The RAS-MAPK pathway is evolutionarily conserved and controls many fundamental processes, including cell proliferation. RAS GTPases are activated by many receptors, such as TCR, BCR, and CSF-1R, and recruit MAPK complexes. These complexes are formed by scaffolds, such as KSR (kinase suppressor of RAS), binding to the three-tier MAPK module that comprises RAF, mitogen-activated protein kinase (MEK), and extracellular signal–regulated kinase (ERK). When activated by RAS (H-RAS, K-RAS, N-RAS), the MAPKKK RAF (RAF-1, A-RAF, B-RAF) phosphorylates the MAPKK MEK (MEK1, MEK2), which in turn phosphorylates the MAPK ERK (ERK1, ERK2). The principal function of RAS in cell cycle induction is to inactivate retinoblastoma protein (RB), relieving cells from its growth-inhibitory actions.[5] The RAS-MAPK signaling pathway is required to induce complexes of cyclin D1 and CDK4/CDK6. Activated ERK kinases phosphorylate the transcription factors MYC and activator protein 1, leading to transcription activation of cyclin D1, CDK4, and CDK6. Notably, PI3K-AKT and PKC–NFκB pathways cooperate with RAS-MAPK in activating cyclin D1. Monophosphorylation of RB by cyclin D–CDK4/6 is required for cells to leave quiescence and enter the cell cycle. Given the important functions of RAS-MAPK signaling in cell proliferation, it is not surprising that cancer hijacks this pathway: K-RAS, N-RAS, and B-RAF are frequently mutated in cancer, leading to constant activation of the RAS-MAPK pathway.

CYCLINS AND CDKS

The 2001 Nobel Prize in Physiology or Medicine was awarded for discoveries concerning the control of the cell cycle: Leland Hartwell, Tim Hunt, and Paul Nurse discovered CDKs and cyclins that regulate the cell cycle. Identification and subsequent functional analysis of the factors and cofactors involved in mammalian cell cycle regulation have led to the current view that progression through the cell division cycle is driven by CDKs. CDKs are serine/threonine protein kinases that play an essential role in promoting the cell division cycle.[6] There

are many cyclins and CDKs, but only a limited number directly contribute to promoting cell cycle entry and progression (Fig. 17.3). Typically, the cyclin component binding to the CDK activates the kinase activity. Additionally, the cyclin component provides specificity to the substrate. During G_1 phase, cyclin D (cyclin D1, D2, or D3) binds to either CDK4 or CDK6. The principal targets of cyclin D–CDK4/6 are RB and the RB-related protein p130, which become monophosphorylated by cyclin D–CDK4/6.[7] Unphosphorylated and monophosphorylated RB can bind to the activating E2F (E2F1–E2F3) transcription factors and block E2F-dependent gene expression. In accordance with the important functions of cyclin D–CDK4/6 complexes in leaving quiescence and entering the cell cycle, they are frequently found overexpressed or mutated in some cancers. At the G_1- to S-phase transition, E-type cyclins (E1 and E2) bind to and activate CDK2, which promotes multiple phosphorylation (hyperphosphorylation) of RB and dissociation of RB from E2F. Consequently, E2F-dependent gene expression is enabled, leading to the expression of genes that encode for proteins required for DNA replication. Cyclin A binds to CDK2 at the end of S phase and promotes entry into mitosis. CDK2 bound to cyclin E and cyclin A can phosphorylate multiple targets that contribute to DNA replication and cell cycle progression during S and G_2 phases. Finally, cyclin B (B1 and B2) associates with CDK1 (CDC2) and contributes to phosphorylation of many cellular proteins, driving cells through mitosis.

Control of cyclin-CDK activity occurs at many levels. First is the appearance and disappearance of different cyclins at specific phases of the cell cycle, which dictates the cyclin–CDK complexes that can form in each phase. Regulation at this level is a result of highly regulated synthesis and degradation of cyclin messenger RNA (mRNA) and protein at different points in the cell cycle. A second level of regulation is afforded by posttranslational modification of CDK kinases, which is often necessary to activate their function. Cyclin B–CDK1 complexes, for example, are initially inhibited by WEE1 kinase and are activated by CDC25C phosphatase when cells enter mitosis. A third level of regulation is provided by proteins that inhibit the activity of CDK kinases or cyclin-CDK complexes (see later).

Additional kinases and substrates that contribute to cell cycle progression include DDK (Dbf4-dependent kinase), PLK (polo-like kinase), and Aurora kinases. The DDK CDC7, together with cyclin E–CDK2, coordinates the initiation of DNA replication. The polo-like kinase PLK1 activates, among others, CDC25C and deactivates WEE1, leading to active cyclin B–CDK1 complexes that drive mitosis, and PLK4 regulates centriole biogenesis during mitosis. Aurora kinases coordinate mitotic progression through phosphorylation of multiple proteins that function in chromosome segregation and cytokinesis.

CDK INHIBITORS

Sharp control of CDK activity is achieved by two major classes of small polypeptide CDK inhibitors: the INK4 family (inhibitors of CDK4) comprising p16 (INK4A), p15 (INK4B), p18 (INK4C), and p19 (INK4D); and the CIP/KIP (CDK-interacting protein/kinase inhibitor protein) family that comprises p21 (CDKN1A), p27 (CDKN1B), and p57 (CDKN1C).[8] All members of the INK4 family specifically bind to CDK4 and CDK6, inhibiting their kinase activity by competing with their association with cyclin D. In contrast, CDK inhibitors of the CIP/KIP family bind to cyclin–CDK complexes and disturb their activities.

The first inhibitor to be identified and cloned in mammalian cells was p21 (CIP1, CDKN1A), which binds several different cyclin–CDK complexes. The proteins p27 (Kip1) and p57 (Kip2) were subsequently identified as CDK inhibitors with structural and functional similarities to p21. The regulation of p21 expression sheds light on its function[9]: Expression is transcriptionally induced by p53, the tumor suppressor protein activated by DNA damage, and induction of p21 expression provides a mechanism for halting cell proliferation after DNA damage to allow time for damage assessment and repair.

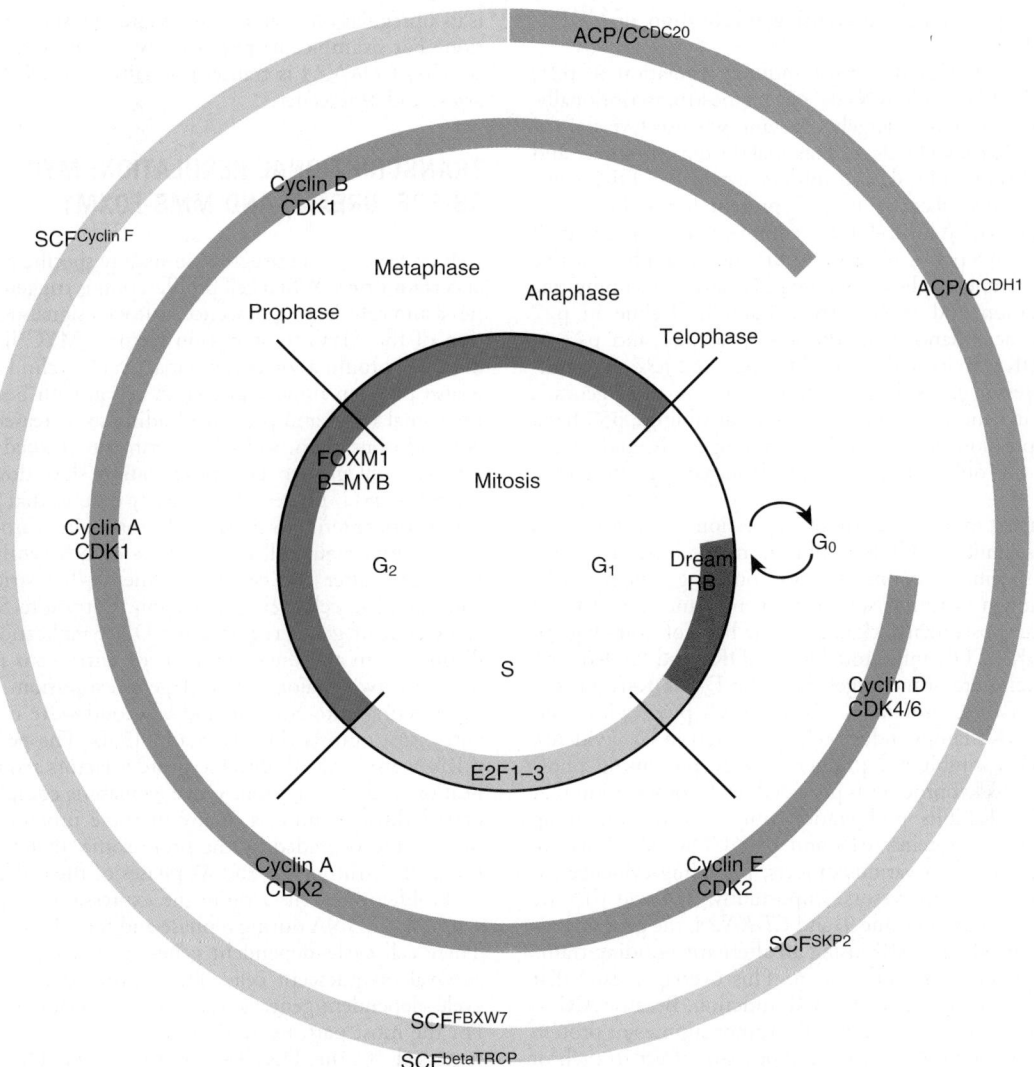

Fig. 17.3 A MULTILAYERED NETWORK CONTROLS THE CELL CYCLE. Many proteins that carry out important functions during the cell cycle are encoded by genes that display a periodic expression pattern during the cell cycle. In G_0 and early G_1, dimerization partner, RB-like, E2F, and multivulval class B (DREAM) and retinoblastoma protein (RB) complexes repress the expression of cell cycle genes. In late G_1 and S phases, RB releases the activating E2F transcription factors that upregulate G_1/S cell cycle genes encoding for important proteins in the process of DNA replication. When S phase is completed, E2F7 and E2F8 will replace E2F1–E2F3 and serve to repress the expression of the G_1/S genes. In G_2 and mitosis, B-MYB and FOXM1 transcription factors bind to the MuvB core and promote the expression of G_2/M genes that encode important proteins for cell division. These transcription factors, as well as many other important cell cycle effectors, are controlled through phosphorylation by cyclin–cyclin-dependent kinase (CDK) complexes. Cyclin D-CDK4/6 complexes promote cell cycle entry and progression through G_1 phase. Cyclin E–CDK2 complexes stimulate S-phase entry and progression, and cyclin A–CDK2 complexes facilitate S-phase completion. Cyclin A–CDK1 complexes promote G_2 phase progression and cyclin B–CDK1 complexes regulate mitosis. These proteins are targets of an additional layer of cell cycle control that mediates their proteasomal degradation. anaphase-promoting complex/cyclosome (APC/C)^{CDH1} becomes activated in anaphase and promotes exit from mitosis, and ensures proper G_1-phase progression. Skp, Cullin, F-box–containing complex SCF^{SKP2} functions in late G_1 and early S phase, whereas SCF$^{\beta TRCP}$ and SCF^{FBXW7} are active throughout S phase. SCF$^{cyclin\,F}$ stimulates mitosis entry, and APC/C^{CDC20} promotes progression through mitosis. Importantly, SCF, APC/C, and cyclin-CDK complexes also regulate each other, and all these complexes contain effector proteins that are transcriptionally regulated by RB-E2F and MuvB complexes. This multilayered network ensures precise control of the cell cycle.

The p21 protein also can be expressed in cells lacking functional p53, indicating that p53-independent pathways of expression exist. These other pathways may account for increased p21 expression in other circumstances associated with cell cycle arrest, such as senescence and terminal differentiation. p21 inhibits cell cycle progression primarily through the inhibition of CDK2 activity: RB pocket proteins lose their hyperphosphorylated state, leading to the formation of RB-E2F and DREAM (dimerization partner, RB-like, E2F, and multivulval class B) complexes and downregulation of cell cycle genes. Interestingly, p21 promotes the formation of cyclin D–CDK4/6 complexes, and the resulting RB monophosphorylation is required for RB function in the DNA damage response program.[7] Inversely, cyclin

D-CDK4/6 can sequester p21, preventing inactivation of CDK2-containing complexes.

In marked contrast with the transcriptional regulation of p21, regulation of p27 (KIP1, CDKN1B) occurs posttranscriptionally, such that mRNA levels remain largely constant, whereas levels of the protein change. p27 protein levels are maximal during quiescence and early G_1, and p27 protein binds and inhibits cyclin E–CDK2 complexes. The progressive decrease in p27 protein levels during G_1 allows for activation of cyclin E–CDK2 complexes that are required for the transition into S phase. Notably, to the end of G_1 phase, active cyclin E–CDK2 complexes phosphorylate p27, causing its ubiquitin-mediated degradation and leading to a dramatic decline in p27 protein levels. In accordance with the ability of p21 and p27 to inhibit cyclin-CDK activity and cell cycling, *p21* and *p27* are candidate tumor suppressor genes, but silencing or loss of these genes is very uncommon in cancers. Unlike its ubiquitous siblings, p57 has a tissue-specific expression pattern during embryogenesis, and in the adult, and it is the only CDK inhibitor required for embryonic development.

Striking diversity in the pattern of expression of *INK4* genes suggests that this family of CDK inhibitors might have cell type–specific or tissue-specific functions. The two founding members, p16 and p15, were cloned as tumor suppressor genes, and the p18 and p19 proteins were subsequently cloned on the basis of homology to p16 and p15. INK4 CDK inhibitors block CDK4 and CDK6, and as RB family proteins are prime targets of cyclin D–CDK4/6 kinase; phosphorylation of these proteins is crucial for G_1 progression, and inhibitors of the INK4 family induce cell cycle arrest in G_1. Evidence that INK4 proteins inhibit cell proliferation by preventing phosphorylation of RB pocket proteins is provided by the observation that p16 overexpression inhibits proliferation only of cells containing functional RB pocket proteins. p16 and p15 CDK inhibitors are inactivated by mutations in various cancers, providing evidence for their function as tumor suppressors. Importantly, p16 and p15 are neighboring genes on chromosome 9, and *CDKN2A*, the gene encoding for p16, also encodes for ARF using an alternative reading frame that produces a totally different protein. This overlap means that inactivating mutations affect p16 and ARF function. Because ARF is a positive regulator of p53 expression and a tumor suppressor protein in its own right, attribution of a tumor suppressor effect to each of these two genes is difficult. An interesting aspect of p16 expression is its upregulation in aging tissues and in response to oncogene activation. For example, in response to continuously high RAS or E2F activity, *CDKN2A* is transcriptionally induced, leading to cell cycle arrest and senescence.

TRANSCRIPTIONAL REGULATION: MYC, RB-E2F, DREAM, AND MMB-FOXM1

Cell cycle entry and progression require specific genes to be expressed at certain times. When cell proliferation is triggered by growth conditions and cells leave quiescence, mitogen signaling leads to the activation of the MYC transcription factor.[10] MYC has the capability to drive cell proliferation because it activates cyclin D and CDK4/6, and it also plays an important role in cell growth because it upregulates ribosomal RNA and proteins, leading to increased ribosome biogenesis and translation. Indeed, experiments showed that when MYC is missing, cell growth and proliferation slow down and cells arrest primarily in G_1 phase. MYC activity ensures that cells reach a certain size before entering S phase and progressing through the cell cycle.

The two main cell cycle events—DNA synthesis and mitosis—take place after the cell passes the G_1/S restriction point and is committed to cell cycle progression. Entry into S phase requires the expression of genes required for DNA replication. These genes are distinct from the ones required for entry into mitosis. In general, there are two major waves of gene expression, one occurring just before entry into S phase and a second wave occurring just before entry into mitosis (Fig. 17.3 and 17.4). The periodic expression of mRNA produces the specific protein factors required for DNA replication and cell division. Once S phase is completed and cells have passed through mitosis, many of these protein factors are ubiquitinated and degraded by the proteasome, thereby ensuring one-way progression through S and M phases of the cell cycle.

Proliferating cells require the expression of specialized genes for synthesis of DNA during S phase and for cell division during mitosis. These cell cycle–dependent genes are not typically required for the survival of quiescent cells. The expression of more than 1000 cell cycle–dependent genes is nearly absent during quiescence in G_0 cells. For the most part, expression of these cell cycle–dependent genes is repressed by the DREAM complex. The DREAM complex is a multisubunit protein complex that binds to promoters of cell

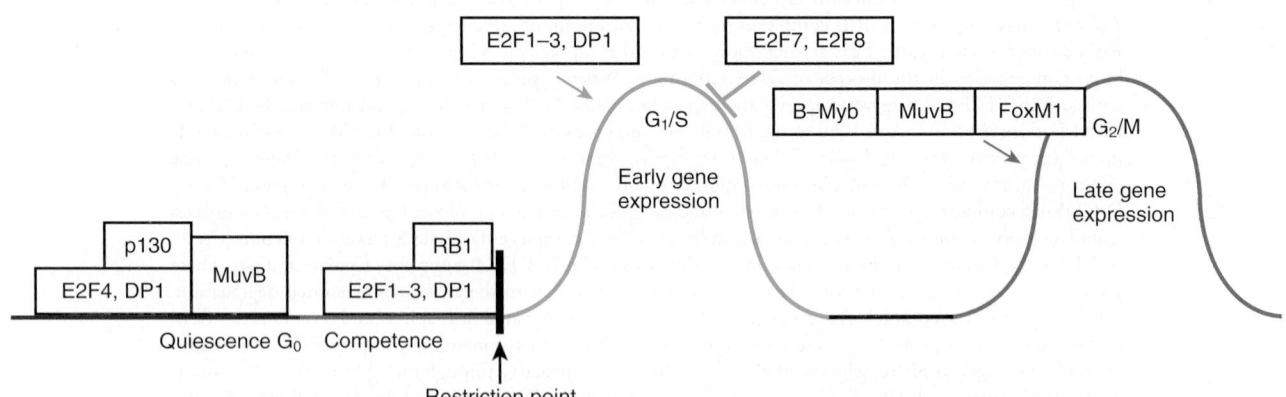

Fig. 17.4 TRANSCRIPTION CONTROL OF G_1/S AND G_2/M CELL CYCLE GENES. There are two major waves of gene expression, one occurring just before entry into S phase and a second wave just before entry into mitosis. The dimerization partner, RB-like, E2F, and multivulval class B (DREAM) complex represses both early and late cell cycle gene expression during quiescence (*magenta line*). Retinoblastoma protein (RB) binds to the activating E2F transcription factors (E2F1–E2F3) and blocks E2F-mediated activation of S-phase genes. In late G_1 phase and S phase, the activating E2Fs dimerize with dimerization partner 1 (DP1) or DP2, bind to the promoters of genes required for DNA synthesis through E2F promoter elements, and promote their expression. During late S phase, E2F7 and E2F8 will replace E2F1–E2F3 and serve to repress the expression of the G_1/S genes when DNA synthesis is completed. The B-MYB transcription factor binds to the MuvB core when p130, E2F4, and DP are released from the DREAM complex. The B-MYB–MuvB (MMB) complex recruits FOXM1 to promote the expression of genes in late G_2 phase and M phase.

cycle–regulated genes and contributes to their repression.[11] The DREAM complex is comprised of the RB-like protein p130 (RBL2), E2F4 or E2F5, DP1 or DP2, and the 5-component MuvB complex containing LIN9, LIN37, LIN52, LIN54, and RBBP4. Whereas the DREAM complex contributes to the expression of both S phase– and M phase–specific genes, the RB protein specifically represses S phase–specific genes.[12] RB binds to the activating E2F transcription factors (E2F1–E2F3) and blocks E2F-mediated activation of S-phase genes. S- and M-phase genes possess distinct promoter elements that mediate binding of RB-E2F and DREAM complexes. E2F promoter elements can be found in S-phase genes and specifically mediate binding of E2F transcription factors. In contrast, M-phase genes possess cell cycle genes homology region (CHR) promoter elements that specifically mediate binding of the MuvB complex.

When a quiescent cell is stimulated to enter the cell cycle, it begins to express cyclin D that binds to CDK4 or CDK6 and is capable of monophosphorylating RB. In late G_1 phase, Cyclin E–CDK2 complexes multiphosphorylate the monophosphorylated RB, leading to the release of the activating E2F transcription factors.[7] The activating E2Fs dimerize with DP1 or DP2, bind to the promoters of genes required for DNA synthesis through E2F promoter elements, and promote their expression during late G_1 phase and S phase. These G_1/S genes encode many of the factors required for DNA replication. During late S phase, E2F7 and E2F8, which are E2F targets themselves, will replace E2F1–E2F3 and serve to repress the expression of the G_1/S phase genes when DNA synthesis is completed.[13]

Cyclin D–CDK4/6 and cyclin E–CDK2 are also capable of phosphorylating p130, thereby enabling the release of p130 from the DREAM complex. The B-MYB (MYBL2) transcription factor is encoded by a G_1/S gene and binds to the MuvB core when p130, E2F4, and DP are released from the DREAM complex.[11] The newly formed MMB (B-MYB–MuvB) complex does not contain any E2F transcription factor and thus binds exclusively to genes that possess CHR promoter elements. These genes are highly expressed in late G_2 phase and M phase, and encode for proteins that carry out essential functions in mitosis. The MMB complex recruits FOXM1, a third transcription factor, to promote the expression of these G_2/M genes. Notably, *FOXM1* is a G_2/M gene itself, and together with the important role of FOXM1 in promoting the expression of G_2/M genes, *FOXM1* has emerged as one of the most robust biomarkers for stratifying high-risk and low-risk cancers.[14] The B-MYB and FOXM1 factors are ubiquitinated and destroyed by the proteasome during late mitosis, resulting in decrease in expression of the G_2/M genes when a cell exits mitosis. Therefore the DREAM complex represses all cell cycle genes during quiescence, with the G_1/S cell cycle genes being activated by E2F1–E2F3 and the G_2/M late cell cycle genes being activated by B-MYB–MuvB–FOXM1.

Together, proliferation signals will enable MYC-dependent gene expression that contributes to the growth in size of the cell, whereas the E2F and B-MYB/FOXM1-dependent gene expression induces genes required for DNA replication during S phase and cell division during mitosis.

UBIQUITINATION

Cells employ a variety of mechanisms to control the cell division cycle, ensuring one-way progression through S and M phases of the cell cycle. Cell cycle genes are cell cycle–dependently expressed at certain times, and cyclin-CDK complexes drive the cell cycle through the control of the cell cycle transcription machinery and regulation of critical events in S and M phases. The mRNA of many cyclins and CDKs is also cell cycle–dependently regulated, and in addition, cyclin-CDK activity is regulated by CDK inhibitors. Yet, cells employ an additional layer of cell cycle control through the timed destruction of essential cell cycle proteins, including cyclins, CDKs, and cell cycle transcription factors (Fig. 17.3). Two ubiquitin ligases, the Skp, Cullin, F-box–containing complex (SCF) and the anaphase-promoting complex/cyclosome (APC/C), are responsible for the specific ubiquitination of many of these cell cycle proteins.[15]

The SCF complex consists of the three invariable components RBX1, CUL1, and SKP1. RBX1 is a RING finger protein that functions as an E3 ubiquitin ligase, CUL1 is a scaffold protein, and SKP1 is an adaptor protein. In addition to the three invariable components, one variable coactivator, known as an F-box protein, binds through its F-box motif to SKP1 and is responsible for substrate recognition. Approximately 70 putative F-box proteins have been identified in humans, and at least 4 of them are thought to be involved in cell cycle control: SKP2, FBXW7, β-transducin repeats-containing proteins (β-TRCP), and cyclin F. The SCF complex mediates degradation of cell cycle proteins during the progression from late G_1 phase through S phase until the onset of mitosis. Important substrates include cyclin D and cyclin E; the transcriptional regulators MYC, E2F1, and p130; the CDK inhibitors p27 and p21; and WEE1 kinase. WEE1 kinase deactivates cyclin B–CDK1 complexes. Degradation of these important cell cycle regulators allows for proper S-phase entry and completion, and onset of mitosis.

The APC/C complex consists of several invariable components, and the central ones are structurally similar to the SCF complex components. APC11 is a RING-finger protein related to RBX1, and APC2 is a scaffold protein related to CUL1. Similar to the SCF complex, APC/C contains a variable coactivator that confers substrate specificity. Two of such variable coactivators function in the cell cycle: CDC20 and CDH1. APC/C^CDC20 mediates the degradation of substrates during mitosis, whereas APC/C^CDH1 functions primarily in G_1 phase. Key substrates of APC/C^CDC20 are cyclin A and cyclin B. With the onset of anaphase, activation of APC/C^CDH1 leads to the degradation of CDC20, PLK1, and Aurora kinases.

Similar to the other cell cycle control systems, SCF and APC/C are controlled within the cell cycle, in part by their own substrates. Most important, SCF and APC/C can regulate each other. The cell cycle protein FBXO5 (EMI1) functions as an inhibitor of APC/C^CDC20 and is sent to proteasomal degradation by SCF^β-TRCP when mitosis starts, and SCF^cyclin F mediates degradation of CDH1. Similarly, ubiquitination of CDC20 and cyclin F by APC/C^CDH1 leads to their destruction when cells exit mitosis. Further regulation occurs on the transcriptional level because substrate-specific components of SCF and APC/C are encoded by cell cycle–regulated genes, including *SKP2*, *FBXO5*, *Cyclin F*, and *CDC20*.

DNA REPLICATION

The initiation of DNA replication represents a commitment to cell proliferation, and is a central event in the growth and division of all organisms.[16] The assembly of replication machineries is coordinated by multiple proteins, which ensure that DNA synthesis begins at the correct chromosomal locus. Strict regulation of initiation is crucial to viability because inappropriate replication start is linked to genetic instability, including alterations in gene copy number and DNA damage. DNA replication starts with the assembly of prereplication complexes (pre-RCs) at multiple DNA replication origins during the G_1 phase. At the transition from G_1 to S phase, the replicative helicase is activated, leading to a change from pre-RCs to preinitiation complexes, which unwind DNA and initiate DNA synthesis. The recognition of pre-RC sites is known as replication origin licensing, and the activation of DNA synthesis is known as origin firing. Separation of these two steps is critical for preventing rereplication within the same cell cycle.

Replication origin licensing in G_1 phase involves sequential assembly of different proteins. The origin recognition complex (ORC) consists of the subunits ORC1–ORC6 and binds initially to replication origins. Then, CDC6 and CDT1 are recruited to the ORC, leading to the recruitment of the minichromosome maintenance (MCM) complex, which consists of six subunits: MCM2–MCM7. The MCM complex is a helicase that forms a double hexamer and encircles double-stranded DNA. Together, the inactive assembly of ORC, CDC6, CDT1, and MCM are known as the pre-RC. Notably, the Meier-Gorlin syndrome, a form of primordial dwarfism, is linked to mutation or depletion of ORC1, which impairs cell cycle progression.

During the transition from G_1 to S phase, the MCM complex is phosphorylated by CDC7 and cyclin E–CDK2, leading to the recruitment of CDC45 and the four-protein DNA replication complex GINS. Together, CDC45, MCM, and GINS represent the CMG complex, and dissociation of the two MCM hexamers enables the formation of two preinitiation complexes at a replication origin. Cyclin E–CDK2 phosphorylates Treslin (TICRR) and RECQL4 that, with TOPBP1 and MCM10, facilitate the formation of the preinitiation complex. After replication origins are licensed, ORC1 phosphorylation by cyclin A–CDK1 inhibits rebinding of ORC1 to replication origins, and CDT1 is blocked by Geminin (GMNN) and sent to proteasomal degradation by SCF^{SKP2} to prevent relicensing during S phase.

In S phase, initiation of DNA replication by CDK2 promotes helicase activation, which leads to unwinding of DNA and recruitment of DNA polymerases alpha (POLA), delta (POLD), and epsilon (POLE), together with PCNA (proliferating cell nuclear antigen) and RFC (replication factor C). The MCM complex translocates from replication origins to unwind double-stranded DNA, whereas POLA binds to single-stranded DNA and initiates DNA synthesis on both the leading and lagging strands by providing an RNA primer and synthesizing the first bases of DNA. POLE and POLD elongate these primers with a base substitution error rate of approximately 10^{-5}. When they occasionally incorporate a false nucleotide, it is usually removed by an exonuclease associated with these DNA polymerases. This so-called proofreading, together with DNA mismatch repair mechanisms, leads to mutation rates of as low as 10^{-9} per base and per cell division cycle.

An immediate consequence of DNA replication is the disruption of chromatin in front of the replication fork, which results in release of parental histones. When the replication fork has passed, chromatin is rapidly reassembled onto old as well as newly replicated DNA, and in the reassembled chromatin, half of the histones are recycled from the parental chromatin, whereas the other half are newly synthesized. Then, the multiprotein complex cohesin mediates cohesion between replicated sister chromatids in S phase, which is essential for chromosome segregation in M phase.

In addition to DNA replication, the centrosome also needs to be replicated to allow the formation of two daughter cells.[17] The centrosome is the major microtubule-organizing center and consists of two centrioles. Phosphorylation by cyclin E–CDK2 promotes the formation of one procentriole at each centriole. During S and G_2 phases, procentrioles elongate until they reach the length of the older centrioles. In early M phase, the two centrosomes separate to promote cytokinesis.

MITOSIS

The decision to enter mitosis is mediated by a network of proteins that regulate activation of the cyclin B–CDK1 complex. In principle, a feedback system between CDK1, WEE1/CDC25C, and the CDK1-counteracting phosphatases generates a bistable switch, leading to robust directionality that prevents cells from going back and forth between G_2 and M phases. Cyclin B and CDK1 levels increase in late S phase and G_2 phase, and the activity of newly made cyclin B–CDK1 complexes is blocked through phosphorylation by WEE1. Activation of the cyclin B–CDK1 complex is the key to cell entry into mitosis and occurs just before mitosis through the action of CDC25C, causing dephosphorylation of CDK1. The activities of WEE1 and CDC25C are themselves regulated with phosphorylation, inhibiting WEE1 function and enhancing CDC25C function. Once a small amount of cyclin B–CDK1 is activated, it can phosphorylate CDC25C and create a self-amplifying feedback loop that generates more active cyclin B–CDK1 from the large preexisting stock of inactive complex. What starts this sequence of events by initially phosphorylating and activating CDC25C is unclear, but PLK1 is a candidate kinase that can phosphorylate WEE1, CDC25C, and

cyclin B, leading to nuclear localization of cyclin B and CDC25C. Cyclin B–CDK1 can phosphorylate serine/threonine residues in many cellular proteins that are essential for mitosis. Phosphorylation of lamins by cyclin B–CDK1 promotes nuclear lamina disassembly and envelope breakdown, which occurs during prophase. Phosphorylation of some kinesin motor proteins that function in spindle assembly, such as KIF11 and CENPE, by cyclin B–CDK1 increases their efficiency of microtubule binding and increases processive motility along microtubules. Other kinesins that function in midzone formation, such as KIF23, are blocked in their activity by cyclin B–CDK1–mediated phosphorylation.

After chromosome condensation, centrosome separation, and nuclear envelope breakdown during prophase, chromosomes become attached to microtubules of the mitotic spindle apparatus in prometaphase. Kinetochores were originally called *centromeres* because they are located at the center of chromosomes. They are formed by centromere proteins during G_2 phase and prophase and link chromosomes to the mitotic spindle apparatus, so that sister chromatids become attached to opposite poles. In metaphase, the chromosomes align at the equatorial plate, and cyclin B–CDK1 levels start to decline by APC/C^{CDC20}-mediated degradation of cyclin B. The APC/C^{CDC20} further targets securin (PTTG1) and thereby activates separase (ESPL1), which cleaves the cohesin complexes linking sister chromatids. Once CDK1 activity is low, APC/C^{CDH1} becomes active and removes CDC20, PLK1, and Aurora kinases, as well as the mitotic cyclins and CDKs.

In anaphase, the spindle midzone forms between the separating chromosomes by coordinated actions of the microtubule cross-linker PRC1, the kinesin KIF4, and the multiprotein complexes centralspindlin and CPC (chromosomal passenger complex).[18] Centralspindlin consists of the kinesin KIF23 and the Rho GTPase RACGAP1, and the CPC consists of Aurora kinase B, the scaffold INCENP, survivin (BIRC5), and CDCA8. Phosphorylation by CPC promotes recruitment of centralspindlin to the spindle midzone through KIF23 and allows for multimerization and accumulation of centralspindlin, which in turn promotes localization of the RhoGEF ECT2 (epithelial cell transforming 2) to microtubules. ECT2 then fuels RhoA, which promotes the recruitment of effector contractile ring proteins. As the ring closes, the spindle midzone is remodeled to form the densely packed telophase midbody, which organizes the intracellular bridge. At this time in telophase, nuclear membranes form to envelop each of the two separated sets of chromosomes, which also begin to decondense. This is soon followed by the abscission event near the midbody, which completes mitosis.

CELL CYCLE CHECKPOINTS

Competence

Cells require the presence of nutrients and growth factors to switch from quiescence to a state of proliferation. When cells sense that conditions are suitable for proliferation, they leave quiescence into G_1 phase and become competent to enter the cell cycle. G_1 has been subdivided into segments and regulatory points based largely on the study of the proliferative response of cells to sequential application of different growth factors, nutrients, and metabolic inhibitors. From the standpoint of cell cycle regulation, a particularly important point in G_1 is the restriction point, or R, which occurs near the G_1–S boundary. The period after mitosis, when cells can enter quiescence, is termed G_1pm (postmitosis), and the period between quiescence and S phase is termed G_1ps (pre-DNA synthesis)[19] (Fig. 17.5). Notably, nearly all of the variability in the length of G_1 can be accounted for by the G_1ps interval. Experiments have shown that, to leave quiescence and to enter the cell cycle, cells require growth signals either continuous for several hours during G_1 or, alternatively, as two discrete pulses of approximately 1 hour in duration and with a pause of several hours in between.[20] To become competent for cell cycle entry, initial activation of the MAPK pathway by mitogen signals is required that in turn activates essential metabolic programs.

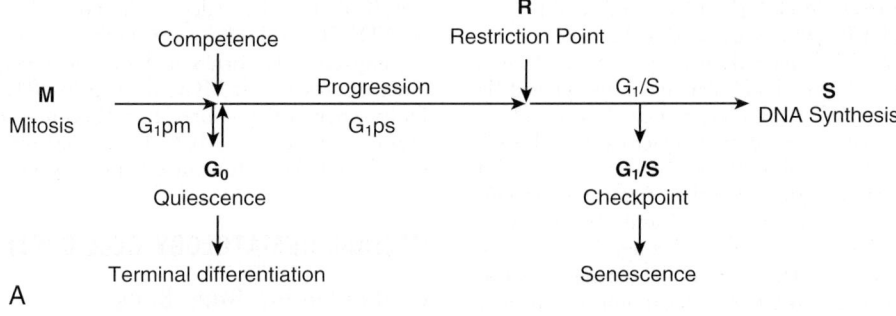

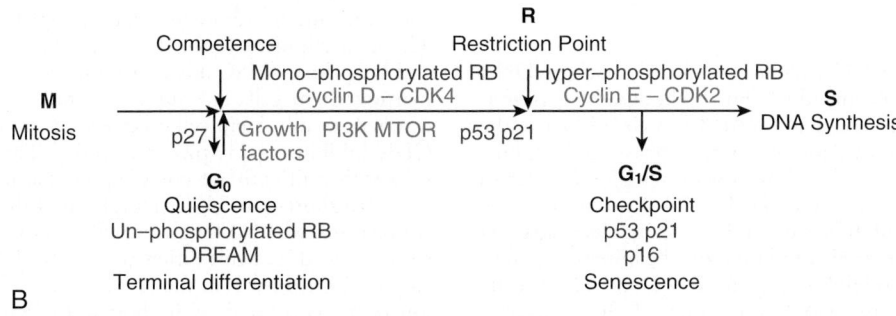

Fig. 17.5 CHECKPOINTS OF CELL CYCLE ENTRY. (A) Quiescence is a nonproliferative state in which viable cells have left the cell cycle and may remain for prolonged periods. In contrast, terminally differentiated cells have irreversibly exited the cell cycle during the process of differentiation. When cells sense that conditions are suitable for proliferation, they leave quiescence into G_1 phase and become competent to enter the cell cycle. G_1 has been subdivided into segments, and a particularly important point is the restriction point, or R, which occurs near the G_1–S boundary. The period after mitosis, when cells can enter quiescence, is termed G_1pm (postmitosis), and the period between quiescence and S phase is termed G_1ps (pre-DNA synthesis). When DNA damage is recognized in G_1, the G_1/S checkpoint becomes activated, which blocks cells from S-phase entry, although they may have passed the restriction point. If damage is not repaired in a timely manner, cells will enter senescence, where they remain viable but not capable of reentering the cell cycle. (B) During quiescence, the cyclin-dependent kinase (CDK) inhibitor p27 prevents cyclin-CDK activity, and dimerization partner, RB-like, E2F, and multivulval class B (DREAM) and retinoblastoma protein (RB) bind and repress cell cycle genes. When prompted by growth signals, cells enter the competent state. Activation of RAS–mitogen-activate protein kinase and phosphoinositol 3-kinase (PI3K) signaling pathways is followed by activation of cyclin D–CDK4/6, leading to monophosphorylation of RB. The progressive decrease in p27 protein levels during G_1 allows for activation of cyclin E–CDK2, which multiphosphorylate the monophosphorylated RB, leading to the release of the activating E2F transcription factors. When DNA damage is recognized in G_1, p53 becomes activated, and the p53 target gene *p21* promotes cell cycle arrest at the G_1/S transition through inhibition of cyclin E–CDK2 and activation of RB. Also, p16 can become activated by oncogenic stress, which leads to inhibition of cyclin D–CDK4/6 and activation of the G_1/S checkpoint. If stress signaling is not relieved, cells will enter a senescent state. *MTOR*, Mammalian target of rapamycin.

However, this initial increase in MAPK activity does not lead to induction of MYC and cyclin D; it leads only to the presence of growth signals several hours later that activate the PI3K pathway and MYC. Functions of MYC include transcriptional activation of *CDK4* and *Cyclin D*, as well as downregulation of CDK inhibitors. The following increase in cyclin D–CDK4 complex activity leads to phosphorylation of the principal target RB during G_1 phase.

Restriction Point

In 1974, Arthur Pardee published the first report on the restriction point, and defined it as a point at which cells become committed to entering S phase, regardless of subsequent availability of growth factors or essential nutrients.[21] He also correctly predicted that cancer cells undergo changes that lose the dependency on growth factors and are not dependent on the restriction point. In the four decades that have passed since the initial description of the restriction point, many important insights have been gained that revealed the signaling events that contribute to proliferation and growth. In addition to the key

contributions of signaling by MAPK, PI3K, and MYC to enable cell growth, it also became clear that there are restraining activities that can inhibit cell cycle entry and progression. As mentioned earlier, cyclin D levels increase during the progression phase of G_1, and cyclin D–CDK4/6 complexes monophosphorylate RB, which restricts the activating E2F transcription factors.[7] Later in G_1, cyclin E levels increase, and cyclin E binds specifically to CDK2. This leads to RB hyperphosphorylation and release of the activating E2Fs, enabling E2F-dependent gene expression. Once past this point, growth factors are no longer required for S-phase entry. Therefore expression and activation of cyclin E–CDK2 resulting in the hyperphosphorylation of RB enables a cell to pass the restriction point and become committed to cell cycle entry.

G_1/S Checkpoint

The G_1/S DNA damage checkpoint can be viewed as a point in the cell cycle when the cell has become fully committed to enter into S phase and past the restriction point, but is unable to enter S phase because cyclin E–CDK2 and cyclin D–CDK4 are inactivated by p21 and p16, respectively, and RB remains capable of binding to and repressing the activating E2Fs, thereby decreasing levels of factors required for DNA synthesis. In G_1, DNA damage is recognized by ataxia-telangiectasia mutated (ATM) kinase, which in turn phosphorylates histone variant H2AX to recruit repair factors and CHEK2 kinase.[22] CHEK2-mediated phosphorylation activates p53 and inactivates CDC25A, which is required for the activation of cyclin E–CDK2 complexes. The p53 target genes *p21* and *BTG2* further promote cell cycle arrest at the G_1/S transition through inhibition of cyclin E–CDK2 and activation of RB. If the DNA damage or stress signals are repaired, cells can exit the G_1/S checkpoint and reenter the cell cycle.

S-Phase Checkpoint

Under conditions that put DNA replication at risk, such as DNA damage or nucleotide depletion, the S-phase checkpoint gets activated. Ataxia telangiectasia and Rad3-related protein (ATR) is the main kinase that senses DNA damage during S phase, and it phosphorylates CHEK1 kinase, which in turn activates p53. Similar to the G_1/S checkpoint, inhibition of cyclin E–CDK2 is central to the S-phase checkpoint. The inhibition of CDK2 activity blocks loading of CDC45 onto replication origins and prevents the initiation of new origin firing. In addition to inhibiting cyclin E–CDK2, p21 directly interacts with PCNA to stop DNA replication. If the damage is repaired, cells continue DNA replication and cell cycle progression.

G$_2$/M Checkpoint

The G_2/M checkpoint prevents cells from initiating mitosis when DNA damage occurs during G_2, or when cells progress into G_2 with some unrepaired damage inflicted during previous S or G_1 phases. The G_2/M checkpoint also involves DNA damage recognition by ATM and ATR kinases and subsequent p53 activation through CHEK1 and CHEK2 kinases, and it ultimately requires activation of the p21 CDK inhibitor. If p21 is missing, both G_1/S and G_2/M checkpoints are abolished. In addition to p21, p53 induces GADD45A and 14-3-3 (SFN), which contribute to G_2/M cell cycle arrest. 14-3-3 removes essential mitotic regulators from the nucleus and thereby promotes G_2/M arrest. Moreover, inhibition of cyclin-CDK activity through p21 induces DREAM and RB-E2F complexes, which in turn repress the transcription of the cell cycle machinery.[12]

Senescence

If damage is not repaired timely, cells will enter a senescent state in which they remain viable but not capable of reentering the cell cycle. Telomere shortening, which signals cell aging, also is recognized as a type of DNA damage and can trigger senescence.[23] RB is key in establishing the senescent state, which is activated downstream of p53 and the CDK inhibitors p16 and p21. During senescence, cells have committed to proliferation and presumably have passed the restriction point. In contrast to quiescence, senescent cells are unable to reenter the cell cycle in response to external stimuli, such as growth signals.

Spindle Assembly Checkpoint

The spindle assembly checkpoint (SAC) involves the MAD (mitotic arrest deficient) proteins MAD1, MAD2, BUBR1 (MAD3), and BUB1.[24] To complete mitosis, the cell strictly requires the activity of cyclin B–CDK1. The main effector of the SAC is the mitotic checkpoint complex (MCC), which consists of MAD2, BUBR1, and BUB3 and binds to CDC20, the substrate-specific cofactor of the APC/C that mediates degradation of cyclin B and securin. Inhibition of CDC20 prolongs prometaphase until all chromosomes have become correctly orientated on the metaphase plate. Unattached kinetochores recruit MCC through BUB1, leading to active MCCs. Only when kinetochores have become correctly attached to the mitotic spindle is the MCC deactivated, which in turn activates APC/C^{CDC20} and allows for mitosis progression.

SPECIAL HEMATOLOGY CELL CYCLE FEATURES

Hematopoietic Stem Cells

Hematopoietic stem cells (HSCs) are characterized by their ability to execute multiple cell fate choices, including self-renewal, quiescence, and differentiation into the many different mature blood cell types. The stem cell niche forms the essential microenvironment for HSCs, and the primary HSC niche in adult organisms is located in the bone marrow. Stem cells are quiescent until prompted to proliferate by external stimuli. Stem cell quiescence is achieved largely through the CDK inhibitors p21, p27, and p57.[25] The pool of HSCs contains subsets that differ in self-renewal potential and cell division frequency. So-called short-term HSCs rapidly enter the cell cycle upon mitogen stimulation, whereas long-term HSCs exit quiescence later. A recent study showed that this difference is achieved at least in part through varying CDK6 levels in the HSC subsets.[26] The absence of CDK6 in long-term compared with short-term HSCs results in a delay in quiescence exit, and the cumulative effect of this delay limits proliferation of these cells and ultimately preserves long-term integrity of the HSC pool.

Endoreplication

A special type of cell cycle progression is featured in the differentiation of cells that have high metabolic profiles required for synthesis of specific proteins, such as plasma proteins produced by hepatocytes, or for the production of platelets by megakaryocytes (MKs). Thrombopoietin (TPO) is the major regulator that directs the growth and development of MKs from HSCs.[27] TPO binds to the MK-specific receptor MPL, leading to MPL dimerization and activation of JAK2 (Janus kinase 2). Initially, this signaling leads to endoreplication and accumulation of DNA content of up to well over 128N before proceeding to final maturation and proplatelet formation. Endoreplication requires impaired cyclin B–CDK1 kinase activity, which is achieved through upregulation of the CDK inhibitor p21 and induction of the APC/C subunit CDH1 after S-phase completion.[28] MK endoreplication also requires the prevention of active RhoA through downregulation of ECT2. During S phase, cyclin E–CDK2 inactivates CDH1 to allow for proper DNA replication. As a result of the following CDK1 inhibition, mitosis is completely bypassed after DNA replication. Inhibition of CDK1 and RhoA and activation of ACP/C^{CDH1} promote bypass of mitosis and entry into the next G_1 phase.

REFERENCES

1. Dang CV: MYC, metabolism, cell growth, and tumorigenesis. *Cold Spring Harb Perspect Biol* 5:a014217, 2013.
2. Smith-Garvin JE, Koretzky GA, Jordan MS: T cell activation. *Annu Rev Immunol* 27:591, 2009.
3. Harwood NE, Batista FD: Early events in B cell activation. *Annu Rev Immunol* 28:185, 2010.
4. Stanley ER, Chitu V: CSF-1 receptor signaling in myeloid cells. *Cold Spring Harb Perspect Biol* 6:a021857, 2014.
5. Coleman ML, Marshall CJ, Olson MF: RAS and RHO GTPases in G_1-phase cell-cycle regulation. *Nat Rev Mol Cell Biol* 5:355, 2004.
6. Malumbres M, Barbacid M: Cell cycle, CDKs and cancer: a changing paradigm. *Nat Rev Cancer* 9:153, 2009.

7. Narasimha AM, Kaulich M, Shapiro GS, et al: Cyclin D activates the Rb tumor suppressor by mono-phosphorylation. *Elife* 3:e02872, 2014.

8. Besson A, Dowdy SF, Roberts JM: CDK inhibitors: cell cycle regulators and beyond. *Dev Cell* 14:159, 2008.

9. Abbas T, Dutta A: p21 in cancer: intricate networks and multiple activities. *Nat Rev Cancer* 9:400, 2009.

10. Kress TR, Sabò A, Amati B: MYC: connecting selective transcriptional control to global RNA production. *Nat Rev Cancer* 15:593, 2015.

11. Sadasivam S, DeCaprio JA: The DREAM complex: master coordinator of cell cycle-dependent gene expression. *Nat Rev Cancer* 13:585, 2013.

12. Fischer M, Grossmann P, Padi M, et al: Integration of TP53, DREAM, MMB-FOXM1 and RB-E2F target gene analyses identifies cell cycle gene regulatory networks. *Nucleic Acids Res* 44:6070, 2016.

13. Bertoli C, Skotheim JM, de Bruin RAM: Control of cell cycle transcription during G_1 and S phases. *Nat Rev Mol Cell Biol* 14:518, 2013.

14. Gentles AJ, Newman AM, Liu CL, et al: The prognostic landscape of genes and infiltrating immune cells across human cancers. *Nat Med* 21:938, 2015.

15. Teixeira LK, Reed SI: Ubiquitin ligases and cell cycle control. *Annu Rev Biochem* 82:387, 2013.

16. Fragkos M, Ganier O, Coulombe P, et al: DNA replication origin activation in space and time. *Nat Rev Mol Cell Biol* 16:360, 2015.

17. Nigg EA, Stearns T: The centrosome cycle: centriole biogenesis, duplication and inherent asymmetries. *Nat Cell Biol* 13:1154, 2011.

18. Green RA, Paluch E, Oegema K: Cytokinesis in animal cells. *Annu Rev Cell Dev Biol* 28:29, 2012.

19. Zetterberg A, Larsson O: Kinetic analysis of regulatory events in G_1 leading to proliferation or quiescence of Swiss 3T3 cells. *Proc Natl Acad Sci USA* 82:5365, 1985.

20. Zwang Y, Sas-Chen A, Drier Y, et al: Two phases of mitogenic signaling unveil roles for p53 and EGR1 in elimination of inconsistent growth signals. *Mol Cell* 42:524, 2011.

21. Pardee AB: A restriction point for control of normal animal cell proliferation. *Proc Natl Acad Sci USA* 71:1286, 1974.

22. Kastan MB, Bartek J: Cell-cycle checkpoints and cancer. *Nature* 432:316, 2004.

23. Muñoz-Espín D, Serrano M: Cellular senescence: from physiology to pathology. *Nat Rev Mol Cell Biol* 15:482, 2014.

24. Lara-Gonzalez P, Westhorpe FG, Taylor SS: The spindle assembly checkpoint. *Curr Biol* 22:R966, 2012.

25. Cheung TH, Rando TA: Molecular regulation of stem cell quiescence. *Nat Rev Mol Cell Biol* 14:329, 2013.

26. Laurenti E, Frelin C, Xie S, et al: CDK6 levels regulate quiescence exit in human hematopoietic stem cells. *Cell Stem Cell* 16:302, 2015.

27. Machlus KR, Italiano JE: The incredible journey: from megakaryocyte development to platelet formation. *J Cell Biol* 201:785, 2013.

28. Fox DT, Duronio RJ: Endoreplication and polyploidy: insights into development and disease. *Development* 140:3, 2013.

CELL DEATH

Nika N. Danial and David M. Hockenbery

Cell death is a highly organized fundamental activity that is equally complex in regulation as cell division and differentiation. In the physiologic contexts of embryonic development and tissue renewal, or as a pathologic response to cell injury and infectious pathogens, cell deaths are orchestrated for multiple purposes that benefit the organism. These include maintenance of epithelial barrier function, destruction of microbes, adaptive immune responses, recycling of biologic macromolecules, intracellular signaling, and preservation of genomic integrity. The majority of mammalian cell deaths have morphologic and biochemical features of apoptosis (Fig. 18.1), a self-inflicted death program encoded in the genetic material of all cells (Fig. 18.2). Necrosis, an alternative mechanism of cell death, occurs in the aftermath of extreme cellular insults and could be viewed as a failure of cellular homeostasis. Recently, a programmed pathway of necrosis, referred to as necroptosis, has been identified. Although cells contain their own death apparatus, cell death in multicellular organisms is exquisitely sensitive to the consent of neighboring cells. As might be expected, the internal cell death machinery is tightly interwoven with other essential cell pathways. Investigations of cell death have also informed our understanding of living cells; for example, the recognition that cellular remodeling shares some pathways with apoptotic cell death.

PHYSIOLOGIC CELL TURNOVER

An adult human loses approximately 10^{11} cells/day, with skin, intestine, and hematopoietic tissues accounting for the majority. Apoptotic cell death in the adult occurs most clearly in the context of cyclically renewing (endometrium, breast, hair follicle) tissues. Homeostatic mechanisms in skin and intestine balance generation of new cells with loss of terminally differentiated cells, principally by nonapoptotic mechanisms. In the intestinal epithelium, terminally differentiated enterocytes migrate onto the epithelium surface and are extruded as viable cells, triggered by cellular crowding. Keratinocytes in the external layer of skin undergo a process of cornification to form an epithelial barrier before being shed.

Neutrophils recruited to sites of inflammation undergo apoptosis upon removal of the inflammatory stimulus. Apoptotic neutrophils are unable to degranulate, and reprogram macrophages to an anti-inflammatory phenotype when phagocytosed (termed *efferocytosis*). This clearance mechanism is specialized to apoptotic neutrophils, as necrotic neutrophils and opsonized cells trigger macrophages to secrete inflammatory cytokines. Apoptotic cell death of anucleate platelets controls platelet lifespan, and in the absence of the anti-apoptotic protein BCL-X$_L$, platelets survive 24 h compared with 5 days in wild-type mice.

Reversible physiologic cell deaths also provide a reserve production capacity for functionally mature cells. The glycoprotein hormone erythropoietin (EPO) is produced by kidney mesangial cells and stimulates excess red blood cell production in proportion to the demand for blood oxygen-carrying capacity. The EPO receptor is expressed on committed erythrocyte precursors (erythroid colony-forming units and proerythroblasts). Growth factors, in general, also generate survival signals. The primary in vivo effect of EPO is to rescue erythroid precursors from physiologic death. The EPO-responsive erythroid compartment in the bone marrow and spleen is maintained at a constant size and rate of cell proliferation under various demands (hypoxia, hypertransfusion), despite widely differing production rates of mature erythroid cells. The raison d'être appears to be to overproduce erythroid colony-forming units and proerythroblasts at low altitudes, with excess cells removed prior to the erythroblast stage. This scheme provides a rapidly accessible reserve under conditions of higher demand.

A final physiologic application for apoptosis is as a mechanism for selection of specific cell phenotypes. A well-known example occurs in the adaptive immune system following clonal diversification of T- and B-lymphocyte antigen receptors by gene recombination and error-prone DNA replication. Positive and negative clonal selection to match T-cell receptors to cognate class I and class II histocompatibility antigens on accessory cells and elimination of many receptors reacting with self-antigens takes place in the thymus. Affinity maturation of immunoglobulin-bearing B cells takes place in germinal centers of lymphoid organs. In each case, cells run through a gauntlet of near-death experiences, with death and survival signals directly linked to the binding properties of the antigen receptor on individual cells.

EXECUTIONERS OF APOPTOSIS

Caspases

The central effectors of apoptosis are a family of cysteine proteases known as caspases (cysteinyl aspartate–specific protease).[1] All caspases are aspartases with a four residue recognition sequence P4–P1 (Fig. 18.3). A serine protease that also recognizes aspartic acid motifs, granzyme B, is similarly involved in cytolytic T-cell killing. Often only one or two caspase cleavage sites are found in a variety of cellular proteins, in many cases members of the same complex or biochemical pathway, leading to limited digestion of substrate proteins. Proteins truncated by caspase cleavage frequently exhibit altered functions, demonstrating that caspases can act as signaling proteases. The number of identified caspase substrates is over 1500.[2]

While no single caspase substrate has been identified that is obligate for cell death, some progress has been made in attributing biochemical and morphologic features of apoptotic death to proteolysis of specific substrates. Caspase-mediated cleavage and activation of Rho-associated kinase-1 (ROCK1) stimulates actin–myosin contractility, leading to membrane blebbing and fragmentation of the nucleus weakened by cleavage of nuclear lamins. DNA fragmentation is mediated by an endonuclease, DNA fragmentation factor 40 (DFF40), also known as caspase-activated DNAse (CAD), which is activated following caspase-mediated degradation of an inhibitory binding partner, ICAD/DFF45. Extracellular release of ATP, a "find-me" signal for macrophages, is triggered by caspase-mediated cleavage of a C-terminal inhibitory domain from Pannexin 1 channels, and outer plasma membrane leaflet exposure of phosphatidylserine, an "eat-me" signal for efferocytosis, follows caspase-mediated inactivation of ATP11C flippase activity.

In the intracellular battle between survival and proapoptotic factors, caspases can also swing the advantage toward death by altering the balance of forces. The mitochondrial survival proteins BCL-2 and BCL-X$_L$ are subject to N-terminal cleavage by caspases. Not only does N-terminal truncation eliminate a survival function, but the cleaved versions also behave as proapoptotic factors. Activation

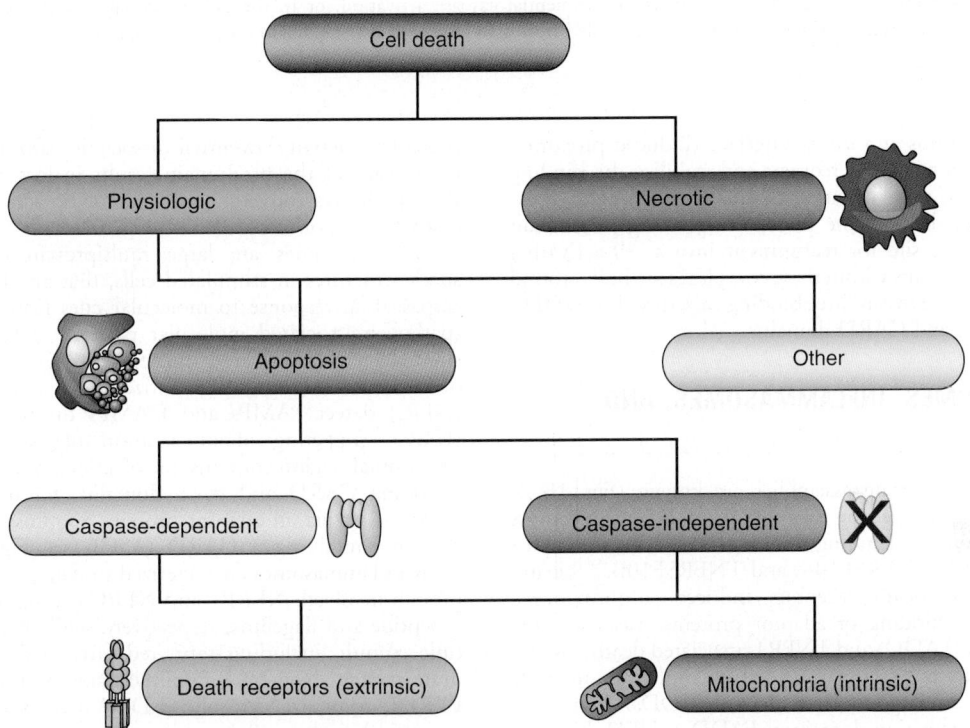 Apoptosis	Necrosis
Cell shrinkage and fragmentation	Cell swelling and lysis
Nuclear condensation	Karyolysis
Internucleosomal DNA fragmentation	Random DNA breaks
Loss of asymmetry of phospholipids in plasma membrane bilayer	Loss of plasma membrane integrity
Detachment and engulfment by phagocytes	Recruitment of inflammatory cells

Fig. 18.1 MORPHOLOGIC FEATURES ASSOCIATED WITH APOPTOSIS AND NECROSIS.

of a proapoptotic BCL-2 family member, BID, also features caspase-mediated processing to a truncated factor, tBID, which then traffics to its mitochondrial site of action.

ACTIVATION OF PROCASPASES

Caspases are expressed in healthy cells as zymogens with low-to-absent protease activity, with association as homodimers and proteolytic processing into large and small subunits required for strong activation (Fig. 18.4). Downstream or executioner caspases (caspase-3, -6, and -7) exist as preformed dimers.[1] Cleavage of a flexible interchain connector between subunits facilitates the movement of surface loops to form an open active site. Processing of procaspases occurs immediately after aspartate residues within caspase recognition motifs. Subsite specificities are distributed among caspases so that many caspase zymogens must be processed in *trans* by a different caspase, creating a hierarchy of proteolytic activation. Apical (initiator) caspases (caspase-2, -8, -9, -10) have limited proteolytic (including autocatalytic) activity at high concentrations without a requirement

Fig. 18.2 CLASSIFICATION OF CELL DEATH PATHWAYS.

	P4	P3	P2	P1
Caspase-6, -8, -9, -10	L/V	E	X	D
Caspase-2, -3, -7	D	E	X	D
Caspase-1, -4, -5	W	E	H	D

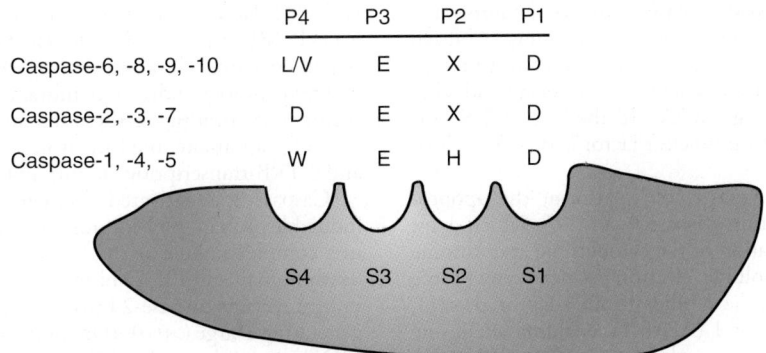

Fig. 18.3 SUBSTRATE SPECIFICITY OF CASPASES. Subject specificity of caspases is determined by the geometry of specificity binding pockets S4–S1, recognizing peptide side chains numbered P1–P4 on the acyl side of a scissile peptide bond. All caspases require Asp in the S1 pocket.

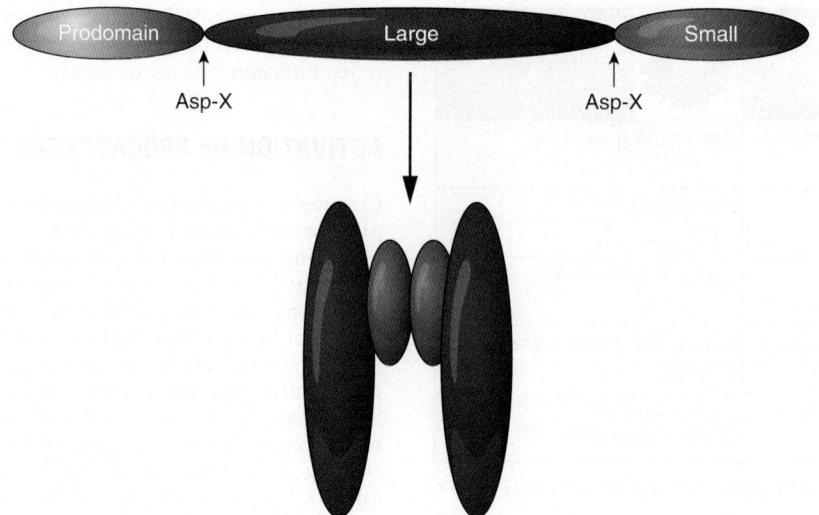

Fig. 18.4 MATURE CASPASES ARE FORMED BY PROTEOLYTIC PROCESSING OF PROCASPASES TO DIVIDE LARGE AND SMALL SUBUNITS AND REMOVE N-TERMINAL PEPTIDES. Caspase substrate motifs at cleavage sites enable sequential caspase activation, or in the case of initiator caspases, autoactivation. Caspase dimers are assembled from two large and two small subunits. *Asp,* Aspartate.

for processing. Interactions at a dimer interface (induced proximity or induced conformation model) reorient and stabilize the binding pocket conformation of these caspases. Normally monomeric, these zymogens are distinguished by the presence of a long prodomain that serves as a docking site for recruitment into a self-activating complex. Protein associations within these complexes are built around homomeric interactions between three binding cassettes, death (DD), death effector (DED), and CARD domains.

DISCS, APOPTOSOMES, INFLAMMASOMES, AND PIDDOSOMES

Four distinct caspase-activating assemblies are known (Fig. 18.5). Caspase-8 and -10 are engaged by a family of cell surface receptors known as death receptors, including tumor necrosis factor receptor 1 (TNFR1), Fas/CD95, TNFRSF10A, and TNFRSF10B.[3,4] Ligand binding to trimerized death receptors induces conformational changes that promote binding of adaptor proteins, Fas-associated death domain protein (FADD) and TNFR1-associated death domain protein (TRADD), to the cytoplasmic tail of the death receptor by dimerization of homologous death domains (DDs) from each molecule. A second interaction domain in FADD, a DED, binds to a similar DED in the prodomain of caspase-8/10, leading to caspase dimerization and localized autocatalysis. The prodomain of caspase-8/10 is severed during processing, dispersing active caspases to cellular substrates. Analysis of unprocessed caspase-8 dimers demonstrated that active sites can be formed in the absence of processing, stabilized by hydrophobic interactions at the dimer interface. The death receptor, FADD, and caspase complex is known as the death-inducing signaling complex (DISC) (see Fig. 18.5A). In the case of TNFR1, additional complexes are involved in nuclear factor kappa-B (NFκB) signaling and necroptosis.

The second caspase-activating assembly platform, the apoptosome, is specialized for activating caspase-9 and -7, which have CARD-type prodomains. Formation of the cytoplasmic apoptosome is initiated by release of the soluble electron carrier, cytochrome c, from mitochondria. Cytochrome c binds to an adaptor protein, apoptotic protease activating factor 1 (APAF-1), enabling adenosine triphosphate (ATP)/dATP-dependent oligomerization of APAF-1 in a heptameric wheel and exposure of its own CARD domain (see Fig. 18.5B). Docking of caspase-9 to the apoptosome through CARD–CARD interactions is both necessary and sufficient for

proteolytic activity. Eventual dissociation from the apoptosome due to cleavage of the prodomain results in loss of proteolytic activity. Both pathways converge with proteolytic activation of caspase-3 by caspase-8, -9, or -10.

Inflammasomes are large multiprotein complexes, visible as speck structures in stimulated cells, that are dedicated to activating caspase-1 in response to molecular cues from infectious pathogens (pathogen-associated molecular patterns [PAMPs]) or endogenous signals (danger-associated molecular patterns [DAMPs]).[5] A family of nucleotide-binding oligomerization domain (Nod)-like receptors (NLRs) detect PAMPs and DAMPs through leucine-rich repeats (LRRs), triggering oligomerization of Nod domains. A third, N-terminal, region contains one of several protein interaction motifs, including CARD and pyrin domains, for direct interaction with caspase-1 or via an adaptor protein, apoptosis-associated speck-like protein containing a CARD (ASC) (see Fig. 18.5C). The three NLR inflammasomes characterized to date are named after the NLR protein involved. NLRP1 and NLRC4 recognize bacterial muramyl dipeptide and flagellins, respectively, while NLRP3 recognizes multiple stimuli, including saturated fatty acids, bacterial RNA, and urate crystals. Non-NLR family inflammasome proteins, AIM2 and PYRIN, recognize cytosolic dsDNA and modified Rho GTPases, respectively. The inflammasome scaffold is postulated to trigger caspase-1 activity according to the induced proximity model. An inflammatory cell death termed *pyroptosis* is initiated by inflammasome activation. Inflammasome activation may also be triggered by viral PAMPs. RNA viruses are recognized by retinoic acid-inducible gene-1 (RIG-I) and RIG-I-like-receptor (RLR) helicases, which oligomerize upon binding viral RNA and translocate to the interface between mitochondrial membranes and mitochondria-associated membranes. Binding to the mitochondrial antiviral signaling protein (MAVS), a tail-anchored membrane adaptor protein, activates IRF3 and NFκB transcription of antiviral responses.[6]

Caspase-2 is activated following genotoxic damage via a p53-inducible protein, p53-induced protein with a death domain (PIDD), in a complex known as the PIDDosome. Similar to death receptors, death domains in PIDD bind to an adaptor protein, RAIDD, which in turn recruits caspase-2 through death effector domain interactions, generating a large (>670 kDa) multiprotein complex (see Fig. 18.5D). PIDD also activates NFκB downstream of DNA damage responses through competing interactions with the receptor-interacting protein 1 (RIP1) serine/threonine kinase and I-kappa-B kinases (IKK) scaffold, NFκB essential modulator (NEMO).

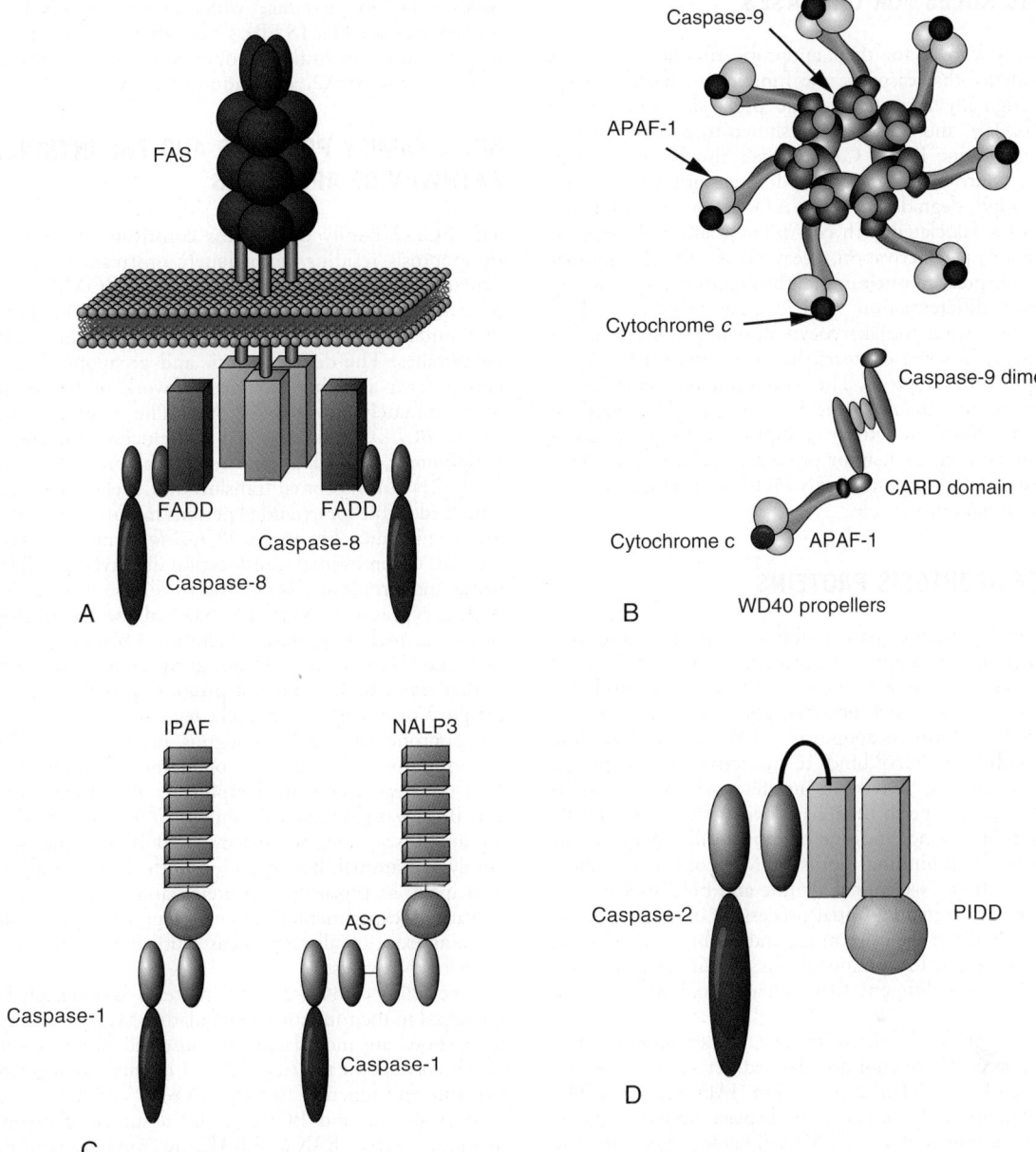

Fig. 18.5 CASPASE ACTIVATION PLATFORMS. (A) DISC (death-inducing signaling complex) is assembled after binding of ligand (Fas) to death receptor (CD95) at the cell surface. Protein interaction domains (death domain [DD] and death effector domain [DED]) mediate associations among death receptor, initiator caspase (caspase-8), and adaptor protein (FADD). (B) Apoptosome resembles a seven-spoked disc, with procaspase-9 molecules bound at the hub extending above one surface and APAF-1 adaptors aligned as spokes, presenting CARD interaction domains at the hub and WD40 propellers bound to cytochrome *c* at the rim. (C) Inflammasomes are multiprotein complexes containing either ICE-protease activating factor (IPAF) or NACHT, LRR, and PYD containing proteins (NALPs) as adaptor proteins that recruit caspase-1 and contain oligomerization domains. IPAF binds procaspase-1 through its CARD domain, while NALP-based inflammasomes recruit procaspase-1 indirectly through ASC-1, which possesses a pyrin domain for NALP binding and a CARD domain for caspase-1 recruitment. (D) The PIDDosome is a molecular platform consisting of the DD-containing p53-inducible protein PIDD, which binds another DD-containing protein RIP-associated Ich-1/CED homologous protein with death domain (RAIDD). RAIDD recruits procaspase-2 through DD-based interactions. *ASC-1*, Apoptosis-associated speck-like protein containing a CARD-1; *APAF-1*, apoptosis protease-activating factor-1; *CARD*, caspase activation and recruitment domain; *IPAF*, ICE-protease activating factor; *NALP*, NACHT, LRR, and PYD containing proteins; *PIDD*: p53-induced protein with a death domain.

NONAPOPTOTIC ROLES FOR CASPASES

Although justifiably known for their apoptotic functions, there is accumulating evidence that caspases also function in healthy cells.[7] Caspase-1 was originally identified as the processing enzyme for interleukin 1β (IL-1β), and subsequently shown to process another proinflammatory cytokine IL-18. Caspases can also be involved in negative-feedback control of erythroblast differentiation by mature erythroblasts through degradation of GATA-1. Several dramatic structural alterations associated with cell differentiation also appear to require transient caspase activation. Cleavage of a limited number of caspase substrates precede nuclear and chromatin changes during terminal erythroid differentiation, and caspase inhibitors block proplatelet formation from megakaryocyte and macrophage differentiation. Caspase-8, in some contexts, has a prosurvival function, inhibiting necroptosis or apoptosis. The more limited caspase activation in these instances may involve some degree of compartmentalization in space or time. Since the activity of unprocessed apical caspases requires persistent binding to adaptor proteins, this constraint may allow for localized, limited caspase activity under some circumstances consistent with a nonapoptotic role.

INHIBITORS OF APOPTOSIS PROTEINS

The only known endogenous caspase inhibitor in mammalian cells is a member of the inhibitor of apoptosis proteins (IAPs) family. IAPs were originally described in insect viruses as viral proteins produced during cellular infection to block host cell apoptosis.[8] In mammalian cells, X-linked inhibitor of apoptosis (XIAP) is the only fully validated caspase inhibitor. XIAP binds to the active sites of specific caspases[4,8] to block catalytic activity or interferes with dimerization (caspase-9). IAPs contain one to three baculovirus IAP repeat (BIR) domains that coordinate zinc, and one or more additional protein-interaction domains. IAP-binding motifs (IBMs) consist of a short peptide sequence with an N-terminal alanine and bind to a surface groove on certain BIR domains. Initial processing of caspase-3, -7, and -9 generates an IBM at the N-terminal end of the short subunit, providing an anchor point for additional physical interactions with IAP proteins. XIAP uses different BIR domains to bind IBMs of specific caspases.

Two proteins normally localized in the mitochondrial intermembrane space, second mitochondria-derived activator of caspase (SMAC)/Diablo and Omi/HtrA2, can bind IAPs via an NH$_2$-terminal IBM sequence and competitively displace bound caspases. Whereas the NH$_2$-terminus of active SMAC/Diablo is generated by removal of a presequence during mitochondrial import, Omi/HtrA2 is a stress-activated serine protease that is cleaved by autoprocessing. Cytoplasmic translocation of SMAC/Diablo and Omi/HtrA2 during apoptosis provides an additional mechanism for caspase activation.

CORE APOPTOSIS PATHWAYS

In mammals, the execution of apoptosis downstream of death signals is governed by two molecular programs that terminate in caspase activation, which may be linked in certain cell types. The extrinsic pathway operates downstream of death receptors, such as Fas and other members of the TNF receptor family, which recruit DISC upon ligand binding. This complex, in turn, recruits and activates caspase-8 and -10, leading to activation of other downstream caspases. The second program, also known as the *intrinsic pathway*, is marked by the involvement of mitochondria.[9–12] Besides their role in biosynthesis, calcium buffering, and ATP production, mitochondria participate in apoptosis by releasing factors such as cytochrome *c*, a component of the mitochondrial electron transport chain. The permeabilization of the outer mitochondrial membrane (MOMP) and release of apoptogenic factors marks the "point of no return" in the intrinsic pathway of apoptosis, and is exquisitely regulated by BCL-2 family proteins. Once released, cytochrome *c* is assembled with APAF-1 and caspase-9

to form the "apoptosome," which in turn triggers downstream effector caspases (see Fig. 18.5B). Other apoptogenic factors released from mitochondria, including apoptosis-inducing factor (AIF), SMAC/Diablo, Omi/HtrA2, and endonuclease G, augment apoptosis.

BCL-2 FAMILY PROTEINS AND THE INTRINSIC PATHWAY OF APOPTOSIS

The BCL-2 family of proteins constitutes a critical control point in apoptosis residing immediately upstream to irreversible cellular damage, where the members control MOMP.[9–13] Several BCL-2 proteins reside at subcellular membranes, including the mitochondrial outer membrane, the endoplasmic reticulum (ER), and nuclear membranes. The different anti- and proapoptotic members of this family form a highly selective network of functional interactions that ultimately governs MOMP. The founding member of this family, *BCL-2*, was discovered as the defining oncogene in follicular lymphomas, located at one reciprocal breakpoint of the t(14;18) (q32;q21) chromosomal translocation. Cells transduced with *BCL-2* remained viable for extended periods in the absence of growth factors. Transgenic mice bearing a *BCL-2-Ig* mini-gene recapitulating the t(14;18) chromosomal translocation displayed B-cell follicular hyperplasia and progressed over time to diffuse large B-cell lymphomas. BCL-2 expression specifically blocked the morphologic features of apoptosis, including plasma membrane blebbing, nuclear condensation, and DNA cleavage. Importantly, unlike other oncogenes known at that time, BCL-2 did not promote proliferation, defining a new category of oncogenes, namely regulators of cell death.[10] The first proapoptotic BCL-2 homologous protein to be identified, BAX, coimmunoprecipitated in stoichiometric amounts with BCL-2. *BAX*-transfected cells died rapidly in the absence of growth factor and BAX was subsequently shown to be capable of directly triggering apoptosis. Since the discovery of BCL-2 and BAX, the BCL-2 family in mammals has expanded, with several family members acting principally as prosurvival proteins and others hastening cell death in various experimental systems (Fig. 18.6). Homologs of BCL-2 proteins exist in all metazoans studied to date, as well as several animal DNA viruses.

The ability of BCL-2 family proteins to selectively bind each other is integral to their function in regulating MOMP and apoptosis. These interactions are modulated by conserved homology domains (BH), which correspond to α-helical and connecting segments that dictate structure and function (see Fig. 18.6).[9–13] All antiapoptotic members, such as BCL-2 and BCL-X$_L$, and a subset of proapoptotic family members, such as BAX and BAK, are "multidomain" proteins sharing sequence homology within 3–4 BH domains. The "BH3-only" subset of proapoptotic molecules, including BCL-2 antagonist of cell death (BAD), BID, BCL-2 interacting mediator of cell death (BIM), NOXA, and p53 upregulated modulator of apoptosis (PUMA), show sequence homology only within a single α-helical segment, the BH3 domain, which is also known as the critical death domain required for binding to "multidomain" BCL-2 family members. BCL-2 family interactions ultimately regulate mitochondrial intramembranous oligomerization of BAX/BAK, which is the prime mechanism of MOMP. BAX and BAK are absolutely required to execute death by all apoptotic signals that activate the intrinsic pathway, nominating these molecules as the requisite gateway to the mitochondrial apoptotic machinery.

A combination of genetic, biochemical, and structural studies has begun to unravel the molecular mechanism underlying regulation of MOMP by BCL-2 proteins (Fig. 18.7). BH3-only molecules are upstream sentinels that selectively respond to proximal death and survival signals to regulate BAX/BAK oligomerization.[9–12] However, their apoptotic activity is suppressed unless activated by transcriptional and posttranslational mechanisms in a tissue- and signal-specific manner.[10,12] For example, the activation of NOXA and PUMA is under direct transcriptional regulation by p53, a finding that is consistent with their roles as specialized death sentinels during DNA damage. On the other hand, cytosolic BID is activated upon cleavage by caspase-8, and the apoptotic activity of BAD is regulated

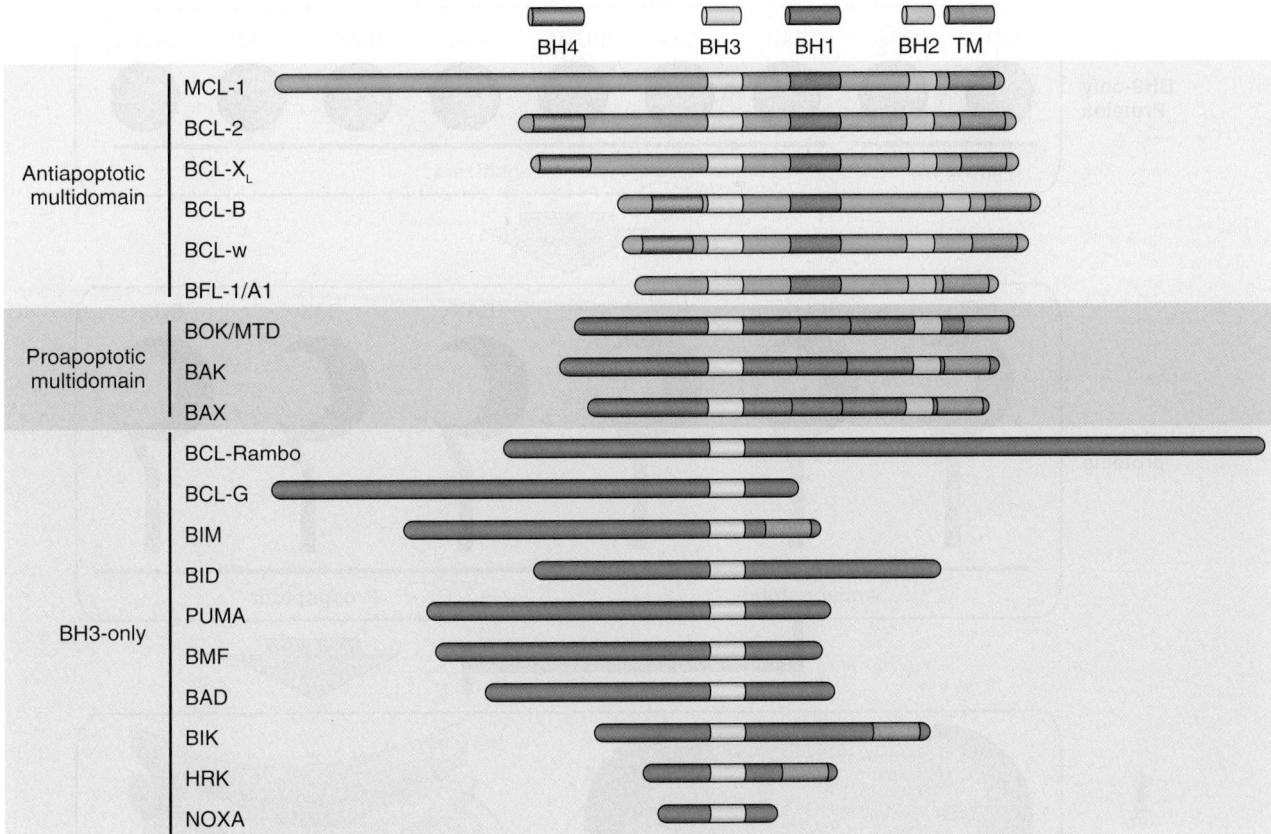

Fig. 18.6 CLASSIFICATION OF THE BCL-2 FAMILY ACCORDING TO CONSERVED DOMAINS. BH1–3 domains form a surface hydrophobic groove capable of binding BH3 domains of other family members. C-terminal hydrophobic sequences function to target and/or anchor BCL-2 family proteins to intracellular lipid membranes. *BAD,* BCL-2 antagonist of cell death; *BAK,* BCL-2 antagonist/killer; *BAX,* BCL-2–associated x protein; *BCL,* B-cell lymphoma; *BID,* BH3 interacting domain death agonist; *BIK,* BCL-2–interacting killer; *BIM,* BCL-2–interacting mediator of cell death; *BMF,* BCL-2–modifying factor; *BOK,* BCL-2–related ovarian killer; *HRK,* harakiri; *MCL-1,* myeloid cell leukemia sequence 1; *PUMA,* p53 upregulated modulator of apoptosis; *TM,* transmembrane domain.

by phosphorylation. Thus the large number of "BH3-only" members is indicative of specialization, rather than redundancy. The unique localizations, protein associations, and mechanisms of activation for the individual BH3-only proteins suggest that each acts as a sentinel for distinct damage signals, thereby increasing the range of inputs for endogenous death pathways.

The proapoptotic activity of BH3-only proteins is associated with exposure of the hydrophobic face of their BH3 helix, which binds the hydrophobic groove of multidomain dimerization partners. Certain BH3-only proteins such as BAD and NOXA, which are known as "sensitizers" or "de-repressors," bind and inhibit antiapoptotic partners. Other BH3-only proteins such as BIM, BID, and PUMA, known as "activators," can directly bind and trigger BAX/BAK oligomerization (Fig. 18.8). Activator BH3-only proteins can also bind and inhibit antiapoptotic BCL-2 proteins. Antiapoptotic proteins inhibit apoptosis by engaging activator BH3-only proteins and by inhibiting BAX/BAK oligomerization[11] (see Fig. 18.8). Activation of BH3-only proapoptotic proteins in response to death stimuli can eventually counter the neutralizing function of antiapoptotic BCL-2 proteins. The complex and selective molecular interactions between the multidomain anti- and proapoptotic molecules also involve both cytosolic and membrane conformers of select family members, each of which is under distinct regulatory mechanisms, including binding affinities, on/off rates, and association with membrane lipids and/or other binding proteins.[9] For example, membrane-inserted conformers of BCL-2, which are defective in oligomerization, can in turn bind membrane-embedded BAX/BAK, inhibiting their oligomerization.[9]

BCL-2 FAMILY PROTEIN AND THE ENDOPLASMIC RETICULUM GATEWAY TO APOPTOSIS

Apart from cytochrome *c* release, the control of Ca^{2+} dynamics at the ER by BCL-2 family proteins also affects the threshold for apoptosis.[9,14] This is consistent with the ability of multiple members of this family to localize to the ER. ER Ca^{2+} content is a chief determinant of the amount of Ca^{2+} that can be released in the cytosol and thus constitutes an important regulator of Ca^{2+} signals known to control myriad cellular functions, including survival/death. The ER Ca^{2+} dynamics directly affect the function of mitochondria as these organelles are in close proximity and mitochondria take up Ca^{2+} released by the ER. Ca^{2+} stimulates important enzymes in the tricarboxylic acid (TCA) cycle, and influences oxidative phosphorylation and ATP synthesis by mitochondria. Supraphysiologic levels of Ca^{2+}, however, can prompt the opening of a large mitochondrial inner-membrane conductance channel known as the *permeability transition pore*, which can eventually cause the swelling and rupture of mitochondria.

Cells overexpressing BCL-2 or deficient for both BAX and BAK show lower levels of ER Ca^{2+} and consequently lower Ca^{2+} entry into the mitochondrion. Lower ER Ca^{2+} content in these cells is associated with a higher rate of ER Ca^{2+} leak. Consequently, Ca^{2+}-mobilizing death stimuli specifically require the function of BAX and BAK at the ER. ER Ca^{2+} content and inhibition of inositol 1,4,5-trisphosphate receptor (IP3R)-mediated Ca^{2+} release is an important component of the prosurvival effect of antiapoptotic BCL-2 proteins, which is reversed by the proapoptotic members of the family. Modulation of

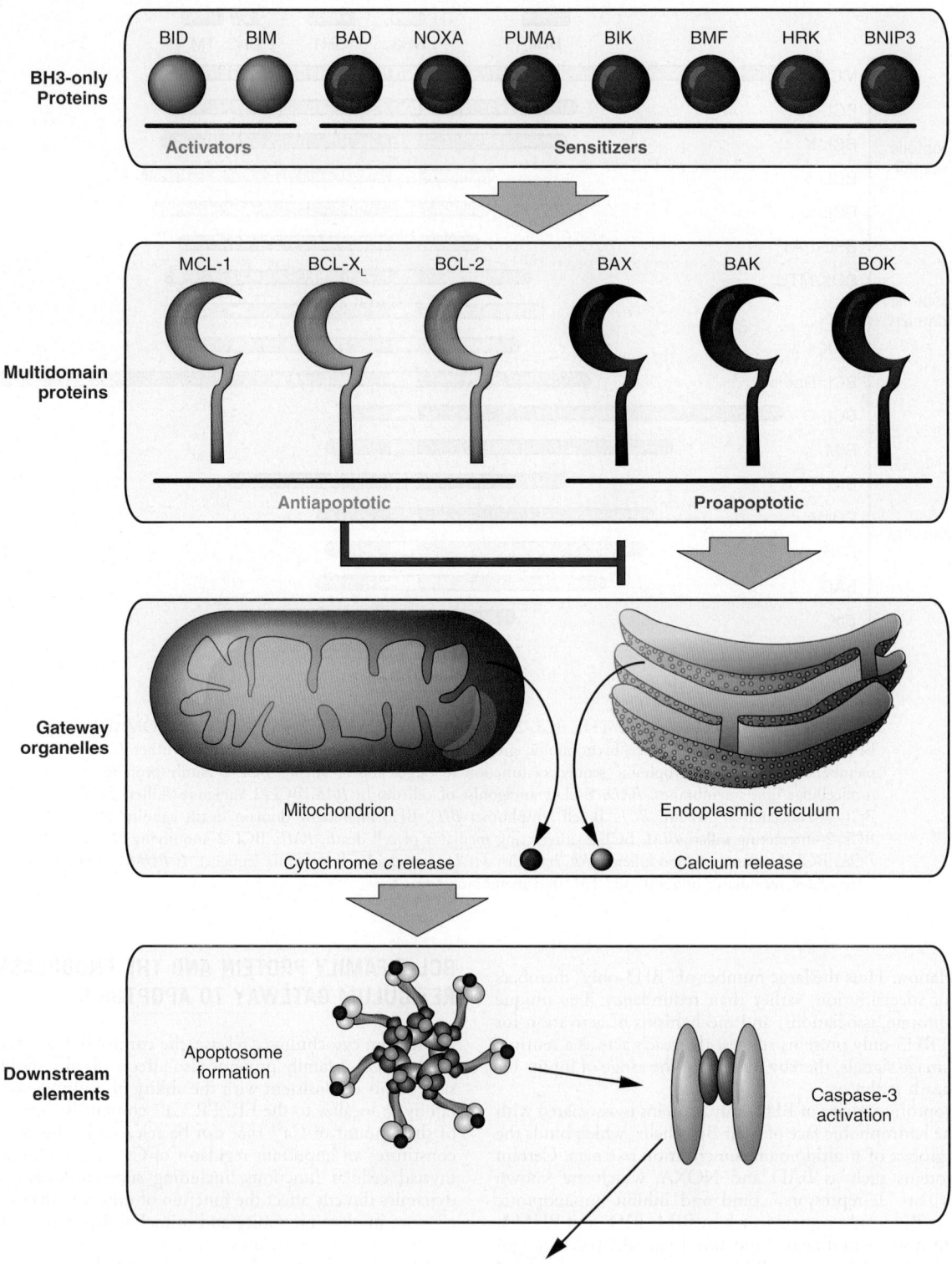

Fig. 18.7 SCHEMATIC REPRESENTATION OF THE INTRINSIC APOPTOTIC PATHWAY IN WHICH A BH3-ONLY MOLECULE SERVE AS UPSTREAM SENTINELS THAT SELECTIVELY RESPOND TO SPECIFIC DEATH SIGNALS. BH3-only molecules ultimately regulate BAX and BAK activation directly or indirectly. This process is in turn inhibited by antiapoptotic BCL-2 family members. BAX and BAK serve as gateways to apoptosis, regulating both cytochrome *c* release from the mitochondria and Ca^{2+} release from the endoplasmic reticulum (ER). See Fig. 18.6 for definition of abbreviations.

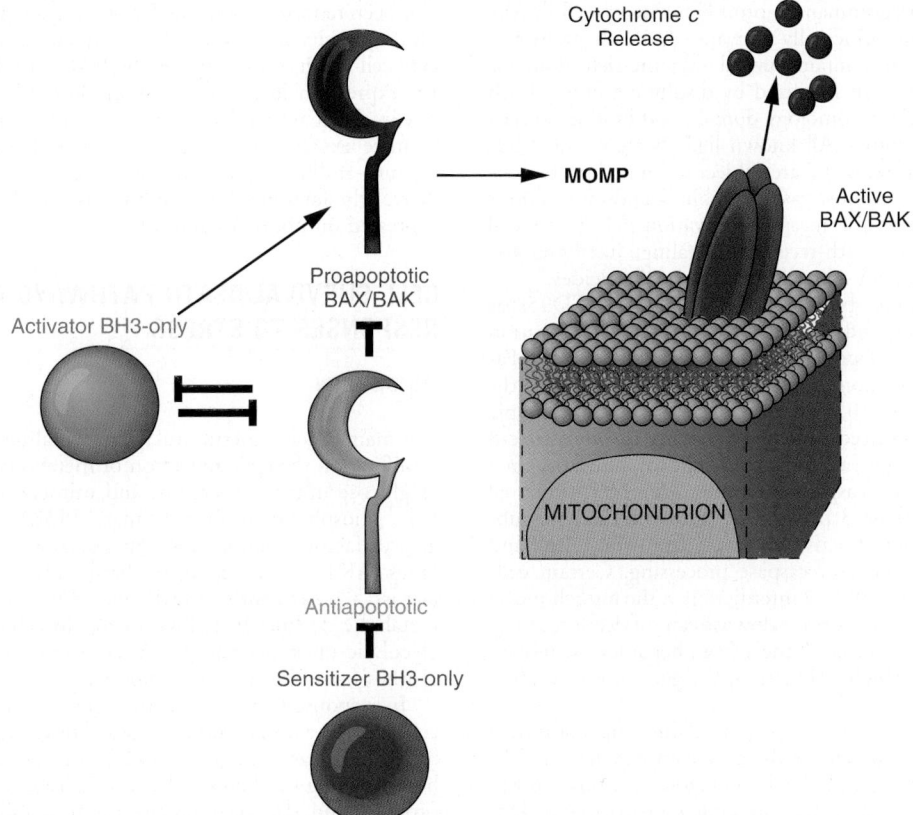

Fig. 18.8 REGULATION OF BAX AND BAK OLIGOMERIZATION. BAX/BAK activation is directly triggered by activator BH3-only proteins (BCL-2–interacting mediator of cell death, BH3-interacting domain death agonist, and p53 upregulated modulator of apoptosis) and is inhibited by antiapoptotic BCL-2 family members. Sensitizer BH3-only proteins do not activate BAX and BAK directly, but lower the threshold for apoptosis by binding antiapoptotic members and releasing activators to trigger BAX and BAK oligomerization. BAX and BAK are activated when the number of activator molecules exceeds the neutralizing capacity of antiapoptotic proteins. *BAK*, BCL-2 antagonist/killer; *BAX*, BCL-2–associated x protein; *MOMP*, permeabilization of the outer mitochondrial membrane.

ER Ca^{2+} content by BCL-2 proteins is mediated, at least in part, by their direct or indirect modulation of IP3R and sarcoplasmic/ER calcium ATPase (SERCA).

NONAPOPTOTIC ROLES FOR BCL-2 FAMILY PROTEINS

Biochemical evidence indicates that the network of protein–protein interactions for select BCL-2 proteins extends to a number of non-BCL-2 protein partners that endow them with homeostatic roles beyond regulation of apoptosis.[15–18] These functions include, but are not limited to, mitochondrial energy and nutrient metabolism, calcium signaling, cell cycle checkpoints, and DNA damage response. The BH3-only protein BAD binds and directly activates glucokinase (hexokinase IV), the product of the maturity-onset diabetes of the young (*MODY*) 2 gene, known for its tissue-restricted regulation of glucose homeostasis through the control of glucose-stimulated insulin secretion by islet β-cells as well as hepatic glucose utilization and storage. The GK-dependent effect of BAD on glucose homeostasis is independent of its apoptotic function and is determined by the phosphorylation state of its BH3 domain, which enables it to activate GK while simultaneously inhibiting its apoptotic function.[17] The BH3-only protein BID, on the other hand, is a downstream substrate for DNA damage checkpoint kinases ATM/ATR, and plays a role in intra-S phase checkpoint separate from its role in apoptosis. In addition, several BCL-2 family proteins have been implicated in the regulation of mitochondrial electron transport chain activity in healthy cells that have not been stressed with any apoptotic signals.[17]

For example, proteolytic processing of MCL-1 produces an isoform that targets to mitochondria and regulates oxidative phosphorylation, in part by influencing the assembly of mitochondrial respiratory chain complexes in higher order complexes known to regulate the efficiency of carbon substrate oxidation and ATP production. This MCL-1 isoform does not have antiapoptotic activity. The above findings are but three examples of an emerging notion that BCL-2 family members are an integral component of cellular homeostatic pathways and carry functions separate from their capacity to regulate apoptosis. Understanding the precise molecular mechanisms underlying these functions and how they can be independently manipulated is critical for effective targeting of these proteins in disease settings.

DEATH RECEPTOR SIGNALING AND THE EXTRINSIC PATHWAY OF APOPTOSIS

Death receptors are expressed on many cell types, especially in the immune system, where they have apoptotic and nonapoptotic functions, dependent on cell context.[19] The cytoplasmic sequences of members of the death receptor superfamily all contain the death domain (DD 80 aa) protein-interaction motif. Once clustered by receptor–ligand interaction, the DD serves to nucleate the formation of DISC for initiator caspases (caspases-8 and -10) with distinct protein interaction motifs in their long prodomains.

There are six mammalian death receptors (TNFR1, Fas, DR3, DR4 [TRAILR1], DR5 [TRAILR2], and DR6). Signaling through

TNFR1 and DR3 is predominantly proinflammatory, while the remaining death receptors principally activate cell death pathways. The extracellular segments contain several cysteine-rich domains forming an extended structure stabilized by disulfide bonds. Death receptor ligands share a TNF homology domain and bind as trimers to the corresponding receptors. All known ligands are expressed as type II transmembrane proteins and are subject to limited proteolysis generating soluble forms. In most cases, soluble ligands are inferior to membrane-bound forms for receptor activation. Thus cell–cell contacts are necessary for death-receptor signaling, justifying the characterization of subsequent apoptotic deaths as "fratricides."

In the simplest example, binding of Fas ligand to CD95/Fas receptor triggers clustering and allosteric conformational activation of a trimeric receptor. An adaptor protein, FADD, binds at the Fas cytoplasmic domain using homotypic DD associations. Similarly, procaspase-8 (or procaspase-10) is bound to FADD by homotypic DED interactions. The induced proteolytic activity of procaspase-8 associated with the DISC appears to be sufficient for autoprocessing in *trans* of neighboring procaspase molecules. An NH_2-proximal cleavage separates the caspase-8 prodomain from the catalytic subunits, allowing untethering of active caspase-8 from the DISC and initiation of a cascade of effector caspase processing. Certain cells (e.g., thymocytes) can bypass BCL-2 interdiction at the mitochondria and activate sufficient effector caspases downstream of death receptor signaling to kill cells (type I cells). Others (e.g., hepatocytes) rely on an amplification loop in which BID cleavage triggers mitochondrial apoptosis (type II cells).

Superimposed on this three-component model are additional factors that can substitute for one of the core components. FLICE/caspase-8 inhibitory protein (FLIP) is homologous to caspase-8 but devoid of protease activity (the active site cysteine is replaced). Different splice forms of FLIP retain the DED motif and compete with caspase-8 for binding to FADD. The long splice variant of FLIP, $FLIP_L$, forms heterodimers with caspase-8. Caspase-8 bound to $FLIP_L$ has catalytic activity, but is processed inefficiently and remains associated with the DISC. Importantly, the caspase-8–$FLIP_L$ heterodimer is unable to cleave caspase-3 or BID. Thus FLIP can either suppress caspase-8 activation or allow local activity. Moreover, $FLIP_L$ is also a substrate for caspase-mediated cleavage in the DISC. The cleaved product may assist with the recruitment of RIP1 kinase to the DISC, promoting activation of NFκB and MAP kinases. Rapid turnover of FLIP explains the sensitization of death receptor–induced apoptosis by protein synthesis inhibition.

Recent evidence indicates that the signaling output of TNFR1 and other death receptors arises from distinct complexes.[19] The TNFR1-bound complex triggers NFκB/MAPK signaling. Alternatively, a cytosolic complex lacking the TNFR1 is established following deubiquitination of RIPK1 kinase by the CYLD deubiquitinase and ubiquitin-editing functions of A20. This complex, designated the ripoptosome, is capable of apoptosis signaling via caspase-8. Notably, NFκB upregulates expression of FLIP to inhibit ripoptosome-triggered apoptosis. In the absence of caspase-8 (or presence of caspase inhibitors), a third complex known as the necrosome promotes necroptosis, a programmed necrosis pathway characterized by cell swelling and rupture.[20] This requires association with another RIP kinase family member, RIPK3. Curiously, deletion of both caspase-8 and RIPK1/RIPK3 are synthetically viable in mice, indicating that the embryonic lethality associated with caspase-8 is due to RIPK1/RIPK3-dependent necroptosis.[19] The downstream target of RIPK1/RIPK3 in necroptosis, the pseudokinase mixed lineage kinase domain-like protein (MLKL), oligomerizes after phosphorylation by RIPK3 and promotes plasma membrane permeabilization. Caspase-8 suppresses necroptosis by cleaving RIPK1 and RIPK3. Necrostatin 1, a small-molecule RIP1 kinase inhibitor, is a potent inhibitor of necroptosis.[20]

Two arenas where death receptors have physiologic roles involve lymphocytes. Activation-induced cell death upon antigen restimulation involves Fas receptor signaling. Fas ligand (FasL) and Fas are induced during T-cell activation downstream of Lck and NFκB. Engagement of Fas on one cell by Fas ligand on a second cell triggers apoptosis. Autocrine suicide from FasL and Fas on the same cell have

also been reported. Thus the Fas–FasL system provides an upper limit on the density of activated T cells at sites of inflammation. Lymphocyte cell death is also directed by FasL expression on dissimilar cells. Fas expression in germinal center B-lymphocytes appears to play a role in eliminating cells bearing self-reactive surface immunoglobulin, as mice expressing Fas only on T-lymphocytes acquire high levels of auto-antibodies. In this case, FasL expression on T cells may deliver the fatal blow. T-lymphocytes can also be eliminated by FasL expressed on nonlymphoid cell types.

CELL SURVIVAL/DEATH PATHWAYS AND ADAPTIVE RESPONSES TO STRESS

Autophagy

The main function of survival factor signaling is to support growth and proliferation through activation of metabolism, including regulation of glucose uptake, glycolysis, and mitochondrial membrane potential.[21] Phosphatidylinositol 3-kinase (PI3K) activation downstream of growth factor receptors, including activation of the serine/threonine kinase AKT, is essential for mediating the metabolic effect of growth factors. Consequently, growth factor withdrawal is associated with metabolic decline, including a drop in cellular ATP levels, blunted glycolytic rates, decrease in O_2 consumption, inhibition of protein synthesis, and induction of apoptosis.

In response to such metabolic stress and nutrient starvation, the cell activates a homeostatic pathway known as autophagy (from Greek meaning to eat ["phagy"] oneself ["auto"]). Autophagy is primarily a housekeeping mechanism that normally serves to degrade long-lived proteins and damaged organelles. It involves the formation of a double-membrane vesicle termed the autophagosome, which engulfs cytoplasmic cargo followed by fusion with the lysosome and subsequent degradation of internal contents. Autophagy is best known as a response to starvation, where the recycling of proteins and organelles supplies required nutrients to the cell.[22,23] This process is regulated by an evolutionarily conserved set of proteins that ultimately orchestrate the recruitment of protein/organelle cargo to vesicles that will deliver their contents to lysosomes. Autophagy serves multiple functions, including tissue remodeling during development in addition to survival in the face of nutrient starvation or other environmental stress.[22,23]

The survival signaling pathway and autophagy are hard wired to preserve the cellular bioenergetic balance. Survival signaling inhibits autophagy. Downstream of AKT, the mammalian target of rapamycin (mTOR) kinase (a mechanistic target of rapamycin) serves as a nutrient sensor that is activated by high levels of ATP, glucose, or amino acids, and in turn stimulates protein synthesis and inhibits autophagy. In the presence of growth factors and extracellular nutrients, mTOR inhibits autophagy through inactivation of unc-51 like autophagy activating kinase 1 (ULK1), an autophagy-related serine/threonine kinase that is important for autophagy induction. During nutrient starvation, the activity of mTOR is inhibited by adenosine monophosphate-activated protein kinase (AMPK), another nutrient sensor kinase that is activated when the ratio of AMP to ATP increases during metabolic stress. AMPK activates autophagy by inhibiting mTOR and phosphorylating ULK1. Upon cellular metabolic decline and nutrient starvation, breakdown of organelles and proteins in autophagosomes produces amino acids and metabolites that can then feed into the mitochondrial TCA cycle, sustaining the production of $FADH_2$ and NADH, ensuring that the flow of electrons through the mitochondrial respiratory chain complexes remains uninterrupted. The bioenergetic benefits of autophagy are temporary until the metabolic stress is eliminated (e.g., growth factor or oxygen availability). Inactivation of autophagy during metabolic decline and nutrient stress leads to apoptosis, unless apoptosis is inactivated (e.g., BAX/BAK deficiency), in which case cell death occurs through necrosis. Whether autophagy is primarily a means of cellular survival or, under certain contexts, can promote cell death, is the subject of intense investigation. Current findings support the notion that autophagy is primarily a self-limiting survival pathway and a temporary adaptive response during metabolic stress, which can promote cell death if not terminated.

The interrelationship among apoptosis, autophagy, and necrosis carries significant relevance in tumor settings where defects in the apoptotic pathway (e.g., overexpression of BCL-2 or BAX, or BAK deficiency) and abnormal upregulation of proliferation (e.g., constitutive activation of the PI3K/AKT pathway) are common. Prior to vascularization, malignant cells in the center of tumors are exposed to hypoxia and metabolic stress. Here, autophagy meets the bioenergetic demands of tumor cells until vascularization supplies oxygen and nutrients. When exposed to hypoxia and nutrient limitation, such apoptosis-resistant tumor cells cannot undergo autophagy due to constitutive activation of AKT. They revert instead to necrosis, which through inflammation and stimulation of cytokine and chemokine production has been proposed to initiate a cellular repair program analogous to wound healing, further promoting proliferation and angiogenesis. Indeed, necrotic tumors are known to have poor prognosis. The above findings also explain, in part, why defects in autophagy are tumorigenic despite the notion that autophagy is primarily a survival pathway during metabolic stress.

Unfolded Protein Response

Protein stress responses also link into apoptotic pathways. These highly conserved mechanisms provide feedback fidelity control of protein folding, glycosylation, and secretory pathways in the ER and other subcellular compartments. Multiple inputs (amino acid deficiency, glucose deprivation, calcium dysregulation, redox poise) trigger this pathway via their effects on ER protein folding.

Three protein sensors, protein kinase-like ER kinase or EIF2AK3 (PERK), activating transcription factor 6 (ATF6), and inositol requiring transmembrane kinase/endonuclease 1 or ERN1 (IRE1), are triggered in response to unfolded proteins within the ER, and activate a homeostatic process that reduces production of new client proteins for the ER folding machinery, helps refold misfolded proteins, and degrades protein aggregates.[14,24] The activity of these sensors is normally held dormant due to association with the ER chaperone BiP (HSPA5). During the unfolded protein response (UPR), BiP is bound and sequestered by unfolded proteins, leading to derepression of each UPR sensor. PERK is activated by dimerization and autophosphorylation to subsequently phosphorylate the translation initiation factor eIF2α, leading to inhibition of general protein translation and selective increase in ATF4 translation. The transcription factor ATF4, in turn, increases the expression of select chaperones and antioxidant defense genes. ATF6 is activated upon translocation to the Golgi and undergoes subsequent proteolytic cleavage to a fragment that translocates to the nucleus and binds the UPR response element found in the promoters of target genes. Another UPR sensor, the bifunctional protein kinase IRE1, is activated by dimerization and transphosphorylation, leading to stimulation of its inherent endoribonuclease activity and processing of mRNA encoding the basic leucine zipper transcription factor X-box binding protein 1 (XBP1). XBP1, together with ATF6, regulates transcription of additional genes required for UPR, including chaperones, folding enzymes, protein disulfide isomerase, ER-associated degradation components, and autophagy genes. Increased ER-associated degradation components and autophagy help clear unfolded proteins, protein aggregates, and damaged organelles. Increased ER biogenesis is also part of the UPR transcriptional program ensuring sufficient ER mass matches the protein quality control response. This process is especially important for the differentiation of B-lymphocytes to antibody-secreting plasma cells. If the integrated outcome of these signaling pathways does not salvage the ER load of unfolded and aggregated proteins, these same UPR sensors can engage the intrinsic pathway of apoptosis.[14,24] TP53 and CHOP/GADD153, a transcription factor induced by ATF4, initiate an ER stress-associated transcription program that is marked by changes in expression levels of several BCL-2 family members, death receptors such as Fas and DR5, and attenuation of the AKT

survival pathway. In addition, recruitment of the adaptor protein TRAF2 to IRE1 may further sensitize cells to ER-stress mediated apoptosis through activation of ER-linked caspases or c-Jun-terminal kinase.

Emerging evidence from multiple experimental systems indicates that select protein modulators of UPR can be both prosurvival or prodeath depending on the extent of ER damage or the duration of UPR. The discovery of BAX and BAK association with IRE1 and modulation of its downstream effectors, such as XBP1, suggest cross-talk between BCL-2 family proteins and UPR.[14] Interestingly, the role of BAX and BAK in UPR is distinct from their function at mitochondria. How BAX and BAK modulate IRE1 activity/signaling and whether they execute a direct role or an accessory function during each of the adaptive/protective or apoptotic phases of UPR and ER stress remain to be determined.

Oncogene-Induced Apoptosis

Hyperactivity of mitogenic oncogenes such as Myc, adenovirus E1A, and Ras triggers a common pathway of p53 accumulation via stabilization of the ARF tumor suppressor protein. p14ARF (or p19ARF in mice) is encoded by an alternative reading frame in the p16INK4a locus. ARF inhibits Mdm2, the p53 E3 ubiquitin ligase, and also exhibits p53-independent functions, including binding to Myc and E2F transcription factors, inhibiting transactivation of target genes. The nature of the oncogenic stress leading to induction of ARF is still poorly understood, but may involve DNA replication or nucleolar stress.

CLINICAL APPLICATIONS

Abnormal regulation of cell death pathways is believed to contribute significantly to several diseases associated with excess cell number or function (e.g., neoplasia, autoimmune disorders) or accelerated cell loss (marrow failure syndromes, neurodegenerative diseases). The clearest supporting evidence is linkage to an altered gene sequence or epigenetic alteration, followed by mechanism testing in cellular/animal models. As previously discussed, *BCL-2* gene rearrangement is associated with t(14;18) in follicular B-cell lymphomas, leading to transcriptional activation and high expression levels. Mutations in the Bax coding region are found in approximately 50% of colorectal and gastric cancers associated with mismatch repair defects, representing frame-shift mutations at a poly(G)8 tract in the coding region.

One of the anticipated benefits of basic research on cell death pathways is the ability to selectively manipulate cell survival or cell death through rational drug design. Members of the BCL-2 protein family, p53, and caspases have been targets of intensive efforts at drug discovery and design. Two small-molecule inhibitors of BCL-2 and related antiapoptotic proteins (BCL-X$_L$ and MCL-1) have advanced to phase I–II clinical trials for chronic lymphocytic leukemia, Hodgkin and non-Hodgkin lymphoma, acute myelogenous leukemia, multiple myeloma, and myelofibrosis.[25,26] These and several other inhibitors in late preclinical development bind to the hydrophobic groove in a similar manner to proapoptotic BH3 peptides, and are understood to act by preventing antiapoptotic proteins from sequestering proapoptotic proteins in the BCL-2 family. In addition, a broad-spectrum oxamyl dipeptide caspase inhibitor has completed phase II trials in treatment-resistant hepatitis C and orthotopic liver transplantation.[27]

As targeted drugs against individual members of the BCL-2 antiapoptotic protein family enter clinical trials, a rapid and accurate cellular assay known as BH3 profiling has been developed to predict their efficacy in primary cancer cells.[28]

SUMMARY

Apoptosis is an evolutionarily conserved, highly regulated mechanism for maintaining cell and tissue homeostasis in multicellular organisms.

Numerous signals are capable of modulating cell death. After a death stimulus, the signal is propagated and amplified through the activation of caspases, culminating in the ordered disassembly of the cell. The process may transpire through an intrinsic, mitochondria-dependent pathway, or an extrinsic pathway depending on the death signal and cell type involved. The BCL-2 family of proteins is situated upstream of irreversible cell damage in the apoptotic pathway, providing a pivotal checkpoint in the fate of a cell after a death stimulus. The proapoptotic molecules BAX and BAK undergo allosteric conformational activation to permeabilize mitochondria upon receipt of a death stimulus. BH3-only members connect distinct upstream signal transduction pathways with the common, core apoptotic pathway. The distribution and responsiveness of the BH3-only members suggests that they function as sentinels for recognizing cellular damage. This model would explain how seemingly diverse cellular injuries converge on a final common pathway of cell death.

REFERENCES

1. Pop C, Salvesen GS: Human caspases: activation, specificity, and regulation. *J Biol Chem* 284:21777–21781, 2009.
2. Poreba M, Strozyk A, Salvesen GS, et al: Caspase substrates and inhibitors. *Cold Spring Harb Perspect Biol* 5:a008680, 2013.
3. Dickens LS, Powley IR, Hughes MA, et al: The 'complexities' of life and death: death receptor signalling platforms. *Exp Cell Res* 318:1269–1277, 2012.
4. Mace PD, Riedl SJ: Molecular cell death platforms and assemblies. *Curr Opin Cell Biol* 22:828–836, 2010.
5. Lamkanfi M, Dixit VM: Mechanisms and functions of inflammasomes. *Cell* 157:1013–1022, 2014.
6. Park S, Juliana C, Hong S, et al: The mitochondrial antiviral protein MAVS associates with NLRP3 and regulates its inflammasome activity. *J Immunol* 191:4358–4366, 2013.
7. Yi CH, Yuan J: The Jekyll and Hyde functions of caspases. *Dev Cell* 16:21–34, 2009.
8. Gyrd-Hansen M, Meier P: IAPs: from caspase inhibitors to modulators of NF-kappaB, inflammation and cancer. *Nat Rev Cancer* 10:561–574, 2010.
9. Chi X, Kale J, Leber B, et al: Regulating cell death at, on, and in membranes. *Biochim Biophys Acta* 1843:2100–2113, 2014.
10. Danial NN, Korsmeyer SJ: Cell death: critical control points. *Cell* 116:205–219, 2004.
11. Moldoveanu T, Follis AV, Kriwacki RW, et al: Many players in BCL-2 family affairs. *Trends Biochem Sci* 39:101–111, 2014.
12. Youle RJ, Strasser A: The BCL-2 protein family: opposing activities that mediate cell death. *Nat Rev Mol Cell Biol* 9:47–59, 2008.
13. Czabotar PE, Lessene G, Strasser A, et al: Control of apoptosis by the BCL-2 protein family: implications for physiology and therapy. *Nat Rev Mol Cell Biol* 15:49–63, 2014.
14. Urra H, Dufey E, Lisbona F, et al: When ER stress reaches a dead end. *Biochim Biophys Acta* 1833:3507–3517, 2013.
15. Bonneau B, Prudent J, Popgeorgiev N, et al: Non-apoptotic roles of Bcl-2 family: the calcium connection. *Biochim Biophys Acta* 1833:1755–1765, 2013.
16. Danial NN, Gimenez-Cassina A, Tondera D: Homeostatic functions of BCL-2 proteins beyond apoptosis. *Adv Exp Med Biol* 687:1–32, 2010.
17. Gimenez-Cassina A, Danial NN: Regulation of mitochondrial nutrient and energy metabolism by BCL-2 family proteins. *Trends Endocrinol Metab* 26:165–175, 2015.
18. Hardwick JM, Chen YB, Jonas EA: Multipolar functions of BCL-2 proteins link energetics to apoptosis. *Trends Cell Biol* 22:318–328, 2012.
19. Oberst A, Green DR: It cuts both ways: reconciling the dual roles of caspase 8 in cell death and survival. *Nat Rev Mol Cell Biol* 12:757–763, 2011.
20. Yuan J, Kroemer G: Alternative cell death mechanisms in development and beyond. *Genes Dev* 24:2592–2602, 2010.
21. DeBerardinis RJ, Lum JJ, Hatzivassiliou G, et al: The biology of cancer: metabolic reprogramming fuels cell growth and proliferation. *Cell Metab* 7:11–20, 2008.
22. Galluzzi L, Pietrocola F, Levine B, et al: Metabolic control of autophagy. *Cell* 159:1263–1276, 2014.
23. White E: The role for autophagy in cancer. *J Clin Invest* 125:42–46, 2015.
24. Walter P, Ron D: The unfolded protein response: from stress pathway to homeostatic regulation. *Science* 334:1081–1086, 2011.
25. Anderson MA, Huang D, Roberts A: Targeting BCL2 for the treatment of lymphoid malignancies. *Semin Hematol* 51:219–227, 2014.
26. Manion MK, Fry J, Schwartz PS, et al: Small-molecule inhibitors of Bcl-2. *Curr Opin Investig Drugs* 7:1077–1084, 2006.
27. Linton SD, Aja T, Armstrong RA, et al: First-in-class pan caspase inhibitor developed for the treatment of liver disease. *J Med Chem* 48:6779–6782, 2005.
28. Chonghaile TN, Roderick JE, Glenfield C, et al: Maturation stage of T-cell acute lymphoblastic leukemia determines BCL-2 versus BCL-XL dependence and sensitivity to ABT-199. *Cancer Discov* 4:1074–1087, 2014.

IMMUNOLOGIC BASIS OF HEMATOLOGY

OVERVIEW AND COMPARTMENTALIZATION OF THE IMMUNE SYSTEM

Dinesh S. Rao

The immune system is critical to the survival of humans and other mammals, keeping at bay a seemingly endless variety of pathogenic organisms that are encountered continuously in the course of life. It is a complex, multilayered system that has evolved over millions of years. From its earliest evolutionary incarnation in invertebrate species as a system of cells that ingests and destroys pathogens, the human immune system has evolved a variety of functions, including the ability to discriminate between highly related biochemical structures that differentiate harmful pathogens from harmless antigens. It also plays an increasingly recognized role in the clearance of dead cells and tissues, promotion of wound healing, and recognition of transformed cells. Disorders that are the consequence of immune under- or overactivity are found in all areas of medicine. Methods of manipulating the immune system in the areas of infectious disease, transplantation biology, autoimmunity, and tumor immunology are active frontiers of medical research and drug development.

Conceptually, the immune response may be divided into innate and adaptive systems (Table 19.1). The innate system is evolutionarily the oldest, with many components found in invertebrate species. Activated early in an immune response, the innate immune system is responsible for a rapid response mediated by cells with invariant pathogen recognition receptors. Pathogen–receptor binding results in the immediate activation of specific protective humoral and cellular responses. In contrast, cells of the adaptive system are responsible for development of long-term immunity against specific pathogens. In general, recurrent infections or infections by pathogens that escape the innate immune system result in the expansion of populations of pathogen-specific lymphocytes and the formation of immunologic memory. Although superficially separate, there is extensive cross-talk between the innate and adaptive immune systems, such that pathogens that activate one lead to the recruitment and activation of the other.

The innate and adaptive immune systems have been characterized in depth at the cellular and molecular levels. The principal goal of these systems is defense against pathogens seeking entry through one of four anatomic sites: the respiratory, gastrointestinal, and genitourinary tracts and the skin. Consequently, immune function has to be understood in terms of the anatomy of these four entry points and their relation to lymphatics, blood vessels, and lymphoid organs. This chapter provides an introduction to the molecular and cellular components of innate and adaptive immunity with an overview of their anatomic relationships.

THE INNATE IMMUNE SYSTEM

Pathogen Recognition Receptors and Pathogen-Associated Molecular Patterns

As the first responders to a pathogenic insult, the cells of the innate immune system use surface receptors, known as pathogen (or pattern) recognition receptors (PRRs), that recognize common molecular motifs, known as pathogen-associated molecular patterns (PAMPs), on various types of pathogens.[1] PAMPs are molecular motifs common to bacteria, fungi, and some viruses but not viable mammalian cells. They frequently are characterized by a repeating pattern of hydrophobic or charged molecules. Common PAMPs include lipopolysaccharide (LPS, or endotoxin of gram-negative bacteria), peptidoglycans and teichoic acids (gram-positive and negative bacteria), mannans (fungi), single-stranded (ss) or double-stranded (ds) RNA (viruses), dsDNA (viruses or necrotic/apoptotic cells), and as most recently discovered, bacterial pigments.[2] PAMPs are thus integral structural motifs within various pathogens, and these common motifs are recognized by the PRRs (Table 19.2). PRRs are germline encoded and constitutively expressed, key features that distinguish them from the receptors expressed by cells of the adaptive immune system. PRRs may be transmembrane proteins expressed on the surface of bone marrow (BM)-derived effector cells, while others are soluble receptors found both intra- and extracellularly. They are also produced by epithelial cells in the gut, bronchial airways, renal tubules, uterus, skin, and endothelial cells in the liver.[3] As such, they are poised to act at the four major portals of pathogen entry.

Pathogen recognition molecules or receptors encompass several different structural families (see Table 19.2). Two PRR families—peptidoglycan receptor proteins (PGRPs) and the Toll-like receptors (TLRs)—were first identified in *Drosophila* and only later demonstrated in vertebrate organisms.[4] In humans, four PGRPs have been identified and are secreted by neutrophils, hepatocytes, and epithelial cells on mucous membranes and defend against gram positive and gram-negative organisms. Ten TLRs have been identified; their ligands include bacterial lipopeptides (TLR1, TLR2, TLR6), peptidoglycans (TLR2), LPS (TLR2, TLR4), fungal saccharides (TLR2, TLR6), ds- and ssRNA (TLR3, TLR7, TLR8), flagellin (TLR5), and dsDNA and CpG DNA fragments (TLR9).[3,5] The TLRs are type I transmembrane proteins that contain leucine repeats extracellularly that bind to their cognate PAMPs and intracellular domains that mediate signaling. Other PRR families include the C-type lectins (including the mannose-binding lectin [MBL] and pulmonary surfactant proteins), dectin-1, macrophage scavenger receptors, RIGI-like receptors (RLRs), NOD-like receptors (NLRs), and the aryl hydrocarbon receptor (AhR).[6] These families include extracellular PRRs, transmembrane and intracellular (cytosolic) PRRs. The cytosolic PRRs are thought to be important in recognition of intracellular pathogens such as viruses and bacteria. The RLRs recognize RNA viruses via their RNA helicase enzymatic activity; the twenty different NLRs recognize a variety of PAMPs, non-PAMP particles, and cellular stresses, and the AhR binds to bacterial pigments. Hence the innate immune system has evolved a number of strategies to recognize common structural motifs and thereby initiate the immune response.

Consequences of PRR–PAMP Engagement: Phagocytosis, the Cytokine Response, and Priming the Adaptive Immune Response

PRR–PAMP ligation triggers immune and inflammatory responses in three stages. In the first stage, the "professional" innate immune cells, including monocytes, macrophages, and neutrophils, facilitate clearance of pathogens. This process is initiated by pathogen binding directly to PRRs on the surfaces of these cells followed by internalization, or the opsonization of pathogens bound by a soluble PRR, which are subsequently recognized by receptors on a

TABLE 19.1	Human Innate Versus Adaptive Immune System	
Feature	**Innate**	**Adaptive**
Response time	Hours to days	>5 days
Expression	Constitutive	Induced by pathogen exposure
Shaped by pathogen exposure	No	Yes
Approximate number of gene products involved in direct pathogen recognition	10^2–10^3	10^{10}–10^{14}
Clonal response	No	Yes
Found in invertebrate species	Yes	No

phagocytic cell. Internalized pathogens are destroyed by a combination of hydrolytic and oxidation reactions within vacuoles inside the phagocytic cells. Phagocytosis also triggers the release of bactericidal or bacteriostatic molecules from intracellular granules into the tissue. These products (e.g., lysozyme, lactoferrin, myeloperoxidase, antimicrobial peptides, nitrous oxide, and superoxide radicals) are toxic to pathogens and induce a local inflammatory response that can lead to tissue injury. Other molecules released, including elastase and collagenase, participate in tissue injury and wound healing.[7,8]

The second stage is cytokine production, which is responsible for initiating, amplifying, and maintaining the innate and adaptive immune response. The signaling pathways involved within the cell vary by PRR, but activation of NFκB (nuclear factor κ-light-chain-enhancer of activated B cells) is a central event in almost every aspect of the immune response. Other signaling pathways that are activated include the caspases, IRF3/5/7, MyD88, and other kinase cascade pathways. Also involved in the downstream activation and regulation of the immune response are novel small RNA molecules, known as microRNAs. These small RNA molecules can regulate the expression of critical proteins that can be effectors of the immune response (e.g., microRNA-155), and certain microRNAs seem to be key in reigning in overactivity of the immune system (e.g., microRNA-146a).[9] Downstream of these signaling pathways, cytokines, which include interleukins, interferons (IFNs), and chemokines, are synthesized and secreted. Interleukins, which are produced by monocytes, macrophages, lymphocytes, or certain epithelial cells, can amplify the innate and initiate the adaptive immune responses. IFNs, produced by virtually every cell type, propagate antiviral and antitumor responses by activating T cells and natural killer (NK) cells. Chemokines are produced primarily by cells of the innate immune system and function dually as chemoattractants (i.e., recruiting cells) and cytokines (i.e., activating cells). Members of the tissue necrosis factor family mediate the sepsis response and cell death and participate in the development of lymphoid organs. A simplified organization of some of the better-characterized cytokines by biologic effects is presented in Table 19.3, and a more detailed discussion of some cytokines can be found in Chapter 16.

Finally, activation of the adaptive immune response occurs. Both by the production of cytokines, which activate lymphocytes, and by the processing, transport, and presentation of antigens directly to T cells (primarily done by dendritic cells [DCs]), PRRs and cells of the innate immune system are essential for the development of adaptive immune responses. The biology of T cells, B cells, and DCs is discussed in detail in Chapters 20 to 23.

IMMUNE DEFICIENCY CONDITIONS CAUSED BY MUTATIONS IN THE INNATE IMMUNE SYSTEM

Mutations of several components within the innate immune system have been identified. These include mutations in PRRs, downstream signaling components and cytokines. For instance, 10 different MBL haplotypes have been identified with serum levels varying by up to 1000-fold. Low levels can be associated with increased severity of infections with encapsulated organisms in immunocompromised or chronically infected hosts. Mutations in TLR3 have been associated with increased susceptibility to encephalitis caused by DNA viruses.[10] Many different mutations of signaling intermediates and cytokines, such as Myd88 and components of IL-12, have also been identified, and lead to susceptibility to streptococcal infections and mycobacterial infections, respectively. However, it should be noted that the complete lack of certain key components of the innate immune system is incompatible with life, as evidenced by experiments in mice. Hence many of the genetic changes found in patients with mild phenotypic changes are better viewed as phenotypic variants, rather than as disease-causing mutations.

INNATE IMMUNITY AND TISSUE HOMEOSTASIS

Pathogen recognition molecules or receptors and cells of the innate immune system also play roles in normal tissue homeostasis. Specific PRRs are involved in the clearance of serum clotting factors, hormones, lysosomal hydrolases, and senescent cells, and in wound healing.[11] The class A scavenger receptor on macrophages is involved in the internalization of oxidized low-density lipoprotein, the development of atherosclerosis, and the clearance of apoptotic T cells in the thymus.[12] The immune system is actively involved in surveillance against transformed or cancerous cells, much of it via interfaces between the innate and adaptive immune systems (IFN-γ, γδ T cells, NK cells, and cytotoxic T lymphocytes [CTLs]).

ADAPTIVE IMMUNE RESPONSE

In juxtaposition to the innate immune system, which is characterized by rapid, fixed, and broad responses to pathogens, the adaptive immune system has evolved to respond to pathogens in a remarkably specific and long-lasting manner. This is accomplished by the generation of a receptor repertoire far more diverse than that represented by PRRs, and the amplification of populations of pathogen-specific cells as a consequence of pathogen exposure (i.e., generation of specific immunologic memory). The two key receptors, those encoding the T-cell receptor (TCR) and the B-cell receptor/immunoglobulin (BCR/Ig), are generated by somatic rearrangements and mutations in TCR and BCR/Ig genes during T- and B-cell development. This process results in a remarkable diversification and amplification of the repertoire of pathogen-specific recognition molecules (see Table 19.1). Indeed, the number of possible pathogen detection motifs encoded by the TCR and BCR/Ig following genetic rearrangement vastly outnumber the number of known pathogenic organisms by many orders of magnitude.

The activation of the adaptive immune system depends on the initial recognition of a pathogenic insult by the innate immune system. This initial response triggers the production of cytokines that activate resident DCs, which then phagocytize and process the antigens by cleaving them into small peptides. These peptides are then presented on the DCs' surfaces bound to major histocompatibility complex (MHC) molecules. Recognition of the processed antigens by the TCR leads to activation of T cells, which in turn activate B cells, thus initiating the adaptive immune response. This antigen presentation step may occur at the site of pathogen exposure, or it may require the migration of antigen-containing DC from the point of pathogen entry through lymphatic channels to lymphoid tissues. In addition, activation of innate immune cells leads to changes in vascular permeability, and lymphocyte adhesion. These steps result in local inflammation and the recruitment of additional lymphocytes to the site of pathogen entry, hence localizing all the correct cellular players to the site of infection. DCs, B cells, and T cells are discussed in depth in Chapters 20 to 23.

TABLE 19.2 Human Pathogen Recognition Receptors

Receptor	Location	Ligands or PAMPs	Features
TLRs (leucine-rich protein)	Leukocytes and some epithelial cells in bronchial airways, urogenital tract, and gut	Cell wall components of gram-positive and gram-negative bacteria (peptidoglycans and lipopeptides), viral dsDNAs, ds- and ssRNAs, bacterial flagellin, and other pathogen-derived molecules	A family of 10 different proteins (TLR1–TLR10) found as transmembrane proteins on the surface of cells or internal endosomes or as free cytosolic proteins; trigger cell activation and cytokine response
CD14 (leucine-rich protein)	Soluble and membrane-bound forms found on monocytes, macrophages, and endothelial cells	LPS from gram-negative bacteria	Binding of LPS on the cell surface forms a complex, including TLR4, which results in cytokine production and the sepsis response
Serum MBL (C-type lectin)	Soluble protein found in serum and lymphatic fluid	Pathogen-derived carbohydrate structures containing mannose, fucose, or N-acetylglucosamine	Secreted by hepatocytes; binding to pathogen triggers complement activation and assembly of the membrane attack complex
Pulmonary surfactant proteins (C-type lectin)	Soluble proteins found extracellularly on pulmonary mucosal surfaces	Carbohydrate structures or lipid motifs on viral, bacterial, or fungal pathogens and inhaled irritants, including pollens	Secreted by alveolar type II cells and nonciliated bronchiolar epithelial cells; binding to pathogen induces opsonization and leukocyte activation (including alveolar macrophages)
Macrophage mannose receptor (C-type lectin)	Surface of monocytes and macrophages	Pathogen-derived carbohydrate structures similar to MBP	Ligand binding results in phagocytosis and monocyte or macrophage activation
NKG2 (C-type lectin)	Surface of NK cells	Carbohydrates on HLA molecules or other host molecules	Involved in recognition and destruction of virally infected or transformed host cells
Dectin-1 (C-type lectin)	Surface of macrophages, neutrophils, and DCs	β-Glucan structures on fungi and plants	Binding results in cell activation, cytokine production, and internalization of pathogen
Class A scavenger receptors (SR-A I/II/III) (scavenger receptor family)	Monocytes, macrophages, and epithelial cells	Modified, cell wall components of gram-positive and gram-negative organisms	Phagocytosis of nonopsinized particles and macromolecules triggers macrophage activation and cytokine release; plays a role in the generation of atherosclerotic plaques and diabetic nephropathy
MARCO (scavenger receptor family)	More restricted macrophage populations than SR-A, including alveolar, peritoneal, and thymic macrophage populations	Similar to SR-A, including silica particles	Phagocytosis of nonopsinized particles and macromolecules triggers macrophage activation and cytokine release
RIG-I like receptors (RLRs) (RIG-I, Mda-5)	Cell cytoplasm	dsRNA	Bind to dsRNA produced during intracellular replication of certain classes of viruses
CRPs and serum amyloid P (Pentraxins)	Serum proteins	Bind to and affect clearance or activation of host proteins (C1q and DNA fragments) as well as constituents of some pathogenic organisms	Secreted by the liver during early acute-phase response and influence clearance and complement activation of recognized macromolecules
Peptidoglycan recognition proteins	Soluble proteins found intracellularly in leukocyte granules or synthesized by the liver and secreted into the serum	Peptidoglycan structures	Direct bacteriocidal or bacteriostatic activity by interfering with bacterial peptidoglycan wall biosynthesis
NOD-LRR receptor family (NLR) (includes NOD, NALP, CIITA, IPAF, and NAIP proteins)	Soluble intracellular proteins	NOD1 and NOD2 bind bacterial peptidoglycan; PAMPs for other proteins not identified	Survey intracellular compartment for intracellular pathogens, binding to bacterial wall fragments produced either during bacterial proliferation or lysozomal degradation; ligand binding triggers activation of NFκB inflammation pathway
$\alpha_v\beta_3$ (integrin)	Epithelial cells	*Trypanosome cruzi*	Binding induces opsonization and cell activation
CD11b/CD18 (also CR3) (integrin)	Monocytes, macrophages, and epithelial cells	LPS, constituents of *Mycobacterium tuberculosis*, yeast saccharides (including zymosan)	Binding induces opsonization and cell activation
Sialic acid–binding immunoglobulin-like lectins (Siglecs)	Surface receptors on monocytes, macrophages, NK cells, and myeloid cells	Sialylated complex carbohydrates (found on endogenous proteins and some pathogenic organisms)	Role for binding and phagocytosis of pathogenic organisms proposed

CIITA, Class II transcription activator; CRP, C-reactive protein; DC, dendritic cell; HLA, human leukocyte antigen; IPAF, ICE-protease activating factor; LDL, low-density lipoprotein; LPS, lipopolysaccharide; MARCO, macrophage receptor with collagenous domain; MBL, mannose-binding lectin; MBP, mannose-binding protein; NAIP, neuronal apoptosis inhibitory protein; NALP, NACHT-, LRR-, and PYD-containing proteins; NFκB, nuclear factor κ-light-chain-enhancer of activated B cells; NK, natural killer; NLR, NOD-like receptor; NOD-LRR, nucleotide-binding oligomerization domain leucine-rich repeats; PAMPs, pathogen-associated molecular patterns; SR-A, scavenger receptor type A; TLR, Toll-like receptor.

TABLE 19.3	The Cytokines	
Cytokines and Cellular Targets	**Examples**	**Biologic Consequences**
Interleukins		
Monocyte and macrophages, endothelial cells	IL-1, IL-2, IL-6, IL-10, IL-13, IL-16, TNF-α	Local inflammation, cell recruitment, hepatic acute phase reaction, sepsis response
B cells	IL-2, IL-4, IL-6, IL-7, IL-9, IL-14	Recruitment, activation, differentiation of B cells
T cells (type 1 cytokines)	IFN-$\alpha/\beta/\gamma$, IL-2, IL-12, IL-15	T helper(T_H)1 response: defense against intracellular pathogens
T cells (type 2 cytokines)	IL-4, IL-5, IL-6, IL-10, IL-13	T_H2 response: defense against parasitic infections
Neutrophils, epithelial cells	IL-17, IL-22	T_H17 response: defense against extracellular pathogens; mucosal inflammation and release of antimicrobial peptides, neutrophil recruitment, and autoimmunity
Interferons		
T cells and NK cells	IFN-α, IFN-β, IFN-γ	Upregulate activity of T cells and NK cells against virally infected cells and malignant cells
Tissue Necrosis Factors		
All cells except erythrocytes	TNF-α, TNF-β	Pyrexia, tissue hyperemia, capillary leak, sepsis/shock syndrome, enhancement of target cell effector functions, expansion of lymphoid compartments
Chemokines		
Monocytes and macrophages, granulocytes, dendritic cells, lymphocytes	MCPs, eotaxin, TARC, MDC, MIPs, RANTES, PF4	Recruit and activate cells of innate and adaptive immune system to specific sites of pathogen exposure, inflammation, or tissue damage
Hematopoietic Growth Factors		
Hematopoietic cells in marrow and peripheral compartments	G-CSF, GM-CSF, M-CSF, SCF	Maintenance, growth, and differentiation of hematopoietic cells

G-CSF, Granulocyte colony-stimulating factor; GM-CSF, granulocyte-macrophage colony-stimulating factor; IFN, interferon; IL, interleukin; MCP, macrophage/monocyte chemotactic protein; M-CSF, macrophage colony-stimulating factor; MDC, macrophage-derived chemokine; MIP, macrophage inflammatory protein; PF4, platelet factor 4; RANTES, regulated on activation, normally T cell expressed and segregated chemokine; SCF, stem cell factor; TARC, thymus and activation–regulated chemokine; TNF, tumor necrosis factor.

CELLS OF THE INNATE AND ADAPTIVE IMMUNE SYSTEMS

Traditionally, cells of the immune system were designated as being either innate or adaptive immune cells: the cells of the innate immune system included granulocytes, monocytes/macrophages, and dendritic cells, while the major cells of the adaptive immune system were lymphocytes, including B cells, T cells, and NK cells. Through the years, it has been discovered that several subsets of lymphocytes have innate immune cell–like properties, and hence this traditional distinction has been blurred somewhat. Nonetheless, it remains conceptually useful to understand the function of these cells as contributing to innate or adaptive immunity. For the most part, immune cells are generated in the BM and may undergo subsequent maturation steps in the periphery. Innate cells such as monocytes mature in tissues where they may become resident, while lymphocytes undergo maturation at specific sites: thymus, lymph node, and spleen. In general, innate immune cells are short-lived, whereas antigen-specific lymphocytes are long-lived and provide long-term protection. In addition to these BM-derived cells, additional cells, such as epithelial cells with pathogen clearance functions, are also involved in the immune response.

B Cells

B cells were first described approximately 50 years ago as being the cells in the bursa of chickens that were the likely source of antibody production.[13] Many different subsets of B cells have been described based on their stage of maturation and their presumed function in the immune response. Surface expression of BCR/Ig marks a mature B cell, and these generally express CD19 and CD20. The majority of B cells are B2 B cells, which undergo activation by T cells via an antigen-specific mechanism, and are the cornerstone of the adaptive immune response. A second subset, known as B1 B cells, are best described in mice and have distinctive properties. These cells can secrete antibodies in the absence of T cell–mediated stimulation, and are sometimes considered a portion of the innate immune system. Other subsets of B cells include plasma cells, which are specialized secretory cells that produce, on a per-cell basis, incredibly high levels of secreted immunoglobulins, and long-lived memory B cells, which carry a memory of a prior pathogen in the highly specific BCR/Ig that they express.

T Cells

After emerging from the BM compartment, T cells develop further into $\alpha\beta$ T-cell or $\gamma\delta$ T-cell populations (further discussed in Chapter 21). The $\alpha\beta$ T cells are the most abundant subset and include CD3$^+$CD8$^+$ and CD3$^+$CD4$^+$ T-cell populations. CD3$^+$CD8$^+$ T cells, which develop into CTLs, are involved in defense against virally infected or transformed cells. CD3$^+$CD4$^+$ T cells can be further subdivided into T helper (TH)1 cells (stimulate development of CTLs), TH2 cells (stimulate isotype switching and antibody production in B cells), TH17 cells (induce or enhance tissue damage secondary to autoimmune or infectious processes), and T-regulatory (Treg) cells (control or limit autoimmune responses). A recently recognized anatomic subset of CD4$^+$ T cells, T-follicular helper cells (TFH), are found in germinal centers of activated LNs and constitute the most common cell of origin for T-cell lymphoma.[14] $\gamma\delta$ T cells are CD3$^+$ T cells that can develop in the thymus and the gut. Thought to function in innate immunity, $\gamma\delta$ T cells represent only 1% to 5% of circulating T cells but up to 50% of the T cells in certain epithelial sites (e.g., skin and intestinal tract). Carrying a TCR of poorly defined specificity, γδ T cells respond to bacterial and viral infections and possibly malignant transformation.

NK Cells

Natural killer cells are a distinct lymphocyte subset and comprise approximately 10% of the circulating lymphocyte population. NK cells are identifiable by their CD3⁻CD56⁺ phenotype. They function in defense against virally infected cells and transformed cells through the generation of cytotoxic cytokines, direct cytolytic activity, and antibody-dependent cellular cytotoxicity. Although traditionally included as a subset of lymphocytes, like B1 B cells and γδ T cells, NK cells seem to bridge the adaptive and innate immune systems. These cells carry invariant receptors, including both activating and inhibitory receptors. The activating receptors such as CD94/NKG2s, and natural cytotoxicity receptors (NCRs), lead to the generation of cytotoxic cytokines and direct cytolytic activity. NK cells also have inhibitory receptors, including the killer cell Ig-like receptors (KIRs), which allow for suppression of NK cell activity, generally through ligation of a self-molecule (classical major histocompatibility class I molecules). Hence the balance between activating and inhibitory signals allows NK cells to function in clearance of infected, damaged, or cancerous cells, and to function in immune system surveillance.

Monocytes, Macrophages, and Dendritic Cells

Monocytes develop in the BM and then circulate through the blood and lymphatics with an average half-life of 1 to 3 days before migrating into tissues and maturing into macrophages.[15] Macrophages can be found in all tissues, particularly at points of entry for pathogens such as the skin, respiratory tract, gastrointestinal tract, and genitourinary tract. Tissue-specific macrophage populations include Kupffer cells (liver), alveolar macrophages (lung), osteoclasts (bone), microglia (central nervous system), and type A lining cells (synovia), which can be identified morphologically and by surface immunophenotype. Macrophages function at many levels in the immune response, with their traditional role being in phagocytosis, cytolytic granule release, and antigen presentation. More recently, their role as cytokine secreting cells and in coordinating the immune response has been appreciated.

Dendritic cells are specialized antigen-presenting cells (APCs). Similar to macrophages, DCs are found at points of pathogen entry, including the skin and mucosal surfaces, and locations of lymphocyte proliferation, such as germinal centers (GCs). Their main role is to present processed antigens to T-helper cells, but they are also known to activate the cytotoxic T-cell response. DC biology is described further in Chapter 23.

Granulocytes

Granulocytes can be further subclassified into neutrophils, basophils, and eosinophils by the types of cytoplasmic granules that they contain. Neutrophils mature in the BM, and large pools of neutrophils are found there, with significant numbers also found in the lung, spleen, and liver. The recruitment of neutrophils from these reservoirs into the circulation and inflamed tissues can occur within hours of exposure to bacterial products such as endotoxin. Neutrophils can be triggered to their effector function via PAMP-PRR ligation. Neutrophils have multiple functions, including the direct killing of foreign organisms via phagocytosis or release of toxic enzymes from granules, release of PRRs, and the formation of neutrophil extracellular nets (webs of degraded nucleic acids and histones), which trap organisms. Neutrophils can also recruit and activate the cells of the adaptive immune system (lymphocytes and DCs).

The basophilic leukocytes—mast cells and basophils—have several structural and functional similarities. They are key mediators of immediate allergic and inflammatory responses, with mast cells being more predominant in tissues and basophils in circulation. Both cell types express FcεR, which induces rapid degranulation when triggered by aggregated IgE, and have granules containing histamine, platelet-activating factor, and bioactive proteoglycans. Degranulation can be rapid, producing anaphylaxis, or sustained, inducing a more sustained inflammatory response. Mast cells and diseases related to mast cells are discussed in Chapter 72.

Eosinophils are found predominantly in tissues, with a smaller fraction found in circulation. The eosinophilic granules of this subset contain hydrolytic enzymes that may be damaging to invading pathogens and host tissues. Eosinophil activation also triggers leukotriene production and the release of an array of cytokines. A role in allergic responses and defense against helminth pathogens has long been presumed consequent to the eosinophilia characteristic of these conditions; however, the true physiologic function of eosinophils remains elusive. Although traditionally thought of as part of the innate immune system, eosinophils may be viewed as effector cells of the adaptive immune system because they can be acutely triggered by a B-cell product (IgE) and their development in part depends on T cells. Disorders of eosinophils are discussed in Chapter 71.

Non–Bone Marrow–Derived Cells Involved in Immune Function

Populations of non-BM–derived cells function in innate immunity. Renal tubular cells and epithelial cells in the gut, bronchial airways, reproductive organs, and dermis express PRRs. In these cells, the receptors function in pathogen clearance or by triggering pathogen-dependent inflammatory responses. Bronchial airway cells secrete pulmonary surfactants and antimicrobial peptides, creating a localized antimicrobial barrier. Liver endothelial cells use several PRRs, including the Fcγ, scavenger, and mannose receptors, to clear particular serum proteins and pathogens. The functions of these cells dovetail with those of the leukocytes in pathogen defense and tissue homeostasis.

ANATOMY OF THE IMMUNE SYSTEM

An array of soluble mediators and a repertoire of immune cells mediate the host response to microbial pathogens, to tumors, to self-antigens in autoimmunity, and to foreign antigens in graft rejections. Where do these cells and mediators come from, and where do these interactions take place?

Immune Cell Development: Primary and Secondary Lymphoid Organs

The organs and tissues of the immune system are divided into the primary (or *generative*) *lymphoid organs* and *secondary* (or *peripheral*) *lymphoid organs*. The *primary lymphoid organs* consist of the BM and thymus and are the sites where cells of the innate and adaptive immune system are generated and produced. The *secondary lymphoid organs* include the spleen, LNs, and epithelial- and mucosa-associated lymphoid tissues such as Peyer patches in the small intestine. These secondary lymphoid tissues are the anatomic site for coordination of the adaptive immune response.

Most immune cells arise in the BM (discussed in detail in Chapters 9, 20, 21, and 27). The cellular components of the innate immune response—neutrophils, eosinophils, basophils, and monocytes—leave the BM as mature, functional cells. In contrast, the cellular components of the adaptive immune response require further development and refinement of function in specific anatomic sites. T-cell precursors leave the BM and migrate to the thymus, where they develop their antigen receptor, the TCR. Following acquisition of a functional TCR, the T cells undergo further refinement of function in the periphery, where they can adopt various fates. Although B cells leave the BM with a functional BCR/Ig, they require further maturation

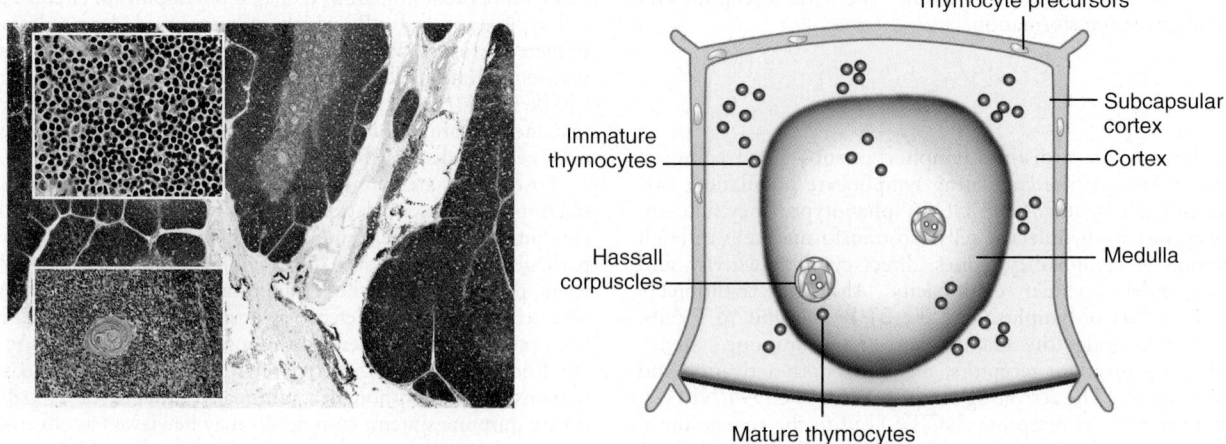

Fig. 19.1 ANATOMY OF THE THYMUS. The human thymus *(left)* is composed of lobules, each separated by a thin capsule. Immediately under the capsule is a narrow zone called the *subcapsular cortex* that surrounds the larger zone of the cortex, the darkly staining region. In the center of each lobule is the medulla, the lighter staining region. In the medulla, nests of epithelial cells called *Hassall corpuscles (inset)* are visible. T-cell precursors *(right, morphology shown in inset 2 on left)* arising in the bone marrow migrate through the blood and enter the thymus as immature cells. During maturation in the cortex, most of the immature thymocytes fail to produce functional T-cell receptors (TCRs) and die. Cells that produce functional TCRs are positively selected to survive and migrate to the thymic medulla. Mature, naive T cells exit the medulla to the peripheral circulation.

following interaction with T cells and antigen in secondary lymphoid organs, such as the spleen or LNs.

T-Cell Maturation

T-cell precursors mature into functional T cells in the thymus (Fig. 19.1).[16] The thymus is composed of developing T lymphocytes, DCs, epithelial cells, and mesenchymal components, collectively referred to as the thymic stroma. The thymic stroma arises primarily from the third and fourth pharyngeal pouches during fetal development, and is then populated by waves of lymphocyte precursors emigrating from the BM. The stromal meshwork is essential for thymic T-cell development, as evidenced by patients with DiGeorge syndrome, otherwise known as 22q11 deletion (del22q11) syndrome. These patients have a failure of involution of the third and fourth pharyngeal pouches and consequent absence of thymic stroma, consequent to the deletion of developmentally critical genes. Although patients with DiGeorge syndrome have T-cell precursors in the BM, they have no recognizable thymus and have markedly reduced numbers of mature T cells in the peripheral circulation and in tissues. As discussed in "Secondary Lymphoid Tissue," the observation that most patients with DiGeorge syndrome do have small numbers of circulating mature T cells suggests that extrathymic sites in these patients may partially substitute for the thymus in promoting T-cell maturation.

The thymus is divided histologically into two general zones, the cortex and the medulla, although further distinctions in zonal properties of resident thymocytes have been noted.[17] Early T-cell precursors leave the BM, circulate in the blood, and selectively home to the thymus, entering to populate the subcapsular cortex. At this site, TCR rearrangement begins, and maturing thymocytes move into and through the cortex, continuing to proliferate. Interactions among TCRs expressed by developing T cells and self-peptide/MHC-I complexes presented by resident thymic cortical and medullary epithelial cells (cTECs and mTECs) mediate the process known as selection.[17] A large fraction of thymocytes, however, fail to express a functional TCR and are never able to interact with cTECs; as a result, these cells do not receive critical survival signals from cTECs and thus undergo programmed cell death. T cells that do express a functional TCR undergo one of two fates—positive selection or negative selection. In positive selection, thymocytes that have successfully assembled

a TCR with low to intermediate affinity for self-peptide–MHC complexes are selected to survive and mature. In negative selection, thymocytes bearing TCRs with a high affinity undergo apoptosis. Hence the two extremes of TCR signal strength, absence and high affinity, lead to an identical fate, apoptosis, while intermediate levels allow the cell to survive and become part of the T-cell repertoire.[18]

T cells that survive the selection process in the cortex proceed to the medulla, where they commit to a particular T-cell lineage (CD4 or CD8) and undergo further negative selection by interactions with mTECs that express tissue-specific antigens promiscuously.[17] Negative selection by the mTECs is partially regulated by the transcription factor termed *autoimmune regulator* (AIRE). AIRE deficiency results in inadequate deletion of self-reactive T cells and manifests clinically as autoimmune polyendocrinopathy–candidiasis–ectodermal dystrophy in humans (APECED).[19]

Only 1% to 3% of the initial thymic progenitor cells succeed in surviving the selection process and thus emigrate from the thymus as non–self-reactive, functional CD4 or CD8 cells. This remarkably complex process hinges on the special anatomic organization of the thymus and leads to the establishment of a T-cell repertoire capable of directing the adaptive immune response against a broad range of antigens. The development of T cells is further elaborated in Chapter 21.

B-Cell Maturation

Although there are parallels between T- and B-cell development, important differences exist. For example, B cells have a functional BCR/Ig by the time they leave the BM, which is discussed in Chapter 20. Nonetheless, they have not yet encouraged antigen, and these naive B cells traffic to *secondary lymphoid tissues,* where cells of the adaptive immune system encounter non–self-antigens and become activated. Briefly, naive cells enter primary follicles in the cortex of the secondary lymphoid tissue.[20] When B cells in primary follicles encounter antigens that are recognized by their surface BCR/Ig, this is presented to T cells bearing receptors for non–self-antigens. The T cells become activated and in turn provide signals to the B cells, leading them to proliferate and to activate the DNA-editing enzyme, activation-induced deaminase (AID).[21] This enzyme causes double-stranded breaks in the DNA, which allows for two concurrent processes: class switch recombination (CSR) and somatic hypermutation (SHM) of immunoglobulin genes. CSR allows the B cell to express a secreted Ig with unique properties, by replacing the constant region of the BCR/Ig with a different constant region via DNA recombination. SHM can sometimes lead to advantageous mutations that can allow a BCR to have higher affinity for a pathogenic antigen. These B cells, bearing a higher-affinity BCR than the B-cell clone that they derived from, are positively selected to proliferate.

When B-cell proliferation begins, the primary follicle becomes a secondary follicle. The secondary follicle has two general regions: (1) a GC filled with proliferating B cells, some T cells, macrophages, and DC; and (2) the surrounding mantle zone of nonproliferating B cells that have not encountered an antigen they recognize. The GC can be further divided into dark and light zones, depending on the stage of proliferation, as discussed later in "Systemwide Surveillance."

ENCOUNTERS WITH ANTIGEN: THE INFLAMMATORY RESPONSE

A primary function of the immune system is to protect against microbial pathogens. The most common sites for microbes to breach the protective barriers of epithelium are the skin and the respiratory, gastrointestinal, and genitourinary tracts. These tissues directly encounter the outside world and possess complex, multifaceted mechanisms for dealing with antigens. It should be noted, however, that there is a vast array of nonpathogenic microbes that live in close proximity to these epithelial barriers, and an emerging body of scientific work points to the importance of these commensal organisms for maintaining immune homeostasis.[22,23]

To defend against pathogenic organisms, these barriers contain many components of the innate immune system, including macrophages and DCs. Some tissues have specialized or unique populations of macrophages and DCs, although these cells have many common features in different tissues. Macrophages provide a critical first line of defense against pathogens by directly phagocytizing microorganisms. Macrophages also send the first signals that recruit granulocytes from the circulation into the tissues (Fig. 19.2). These signals include cytokines, nitrous oxide, and leukotrienes that cause vasodilatation,

endothelial cell activation, leukocyte adhesion to endothelial cells at the inflammatory site, and diapedesis of leukocytes into the tissues (see Chapter 13). The resulting exudate fluid at the site of vasodilatation is also rich in plasma proteins that participate in innate immunity, such as complement and PRRs. Hence the soluble and cellular components of the innate immune system provide the first line of defense at the tissues where pathogens invade.

The epithelial barriers also contain resident lymphocytes and plasma cells. The lymphoid cells respond to cytokines secreted by resident macrophages, such as IL-2, which stimulates T-cell proliferation. The ability of macrophages to secrete mediators that cause vasodilatation and recruitment of granulocytes, as well as initiate T-cell activation, illustrates the interplay between innate and adaptive immunity and underscores the point that the innate and adaptive immune systems work in concert in host defense. Resident T cells and plasma cells in the tissue can respond to antigen, with local activation of antigen-specific effector T cells and increased antibody secretion, respectively, so that the adaptive immune response is stimulated locally after pathogens are sensed by the innate immune system.

SYSTEMWIDE SURVEILLANCE: THE ROLE OF LYMPHATIC CIRCULATION

Lymphatics are an essential component of the vascular system (Fig. 19.3). Even in the absence of inflammation, a fraction of the fluid component of blood continually leaves the capillary bed during circulation caused by the pressure drop between the arterial and venous sides. This fluid bathes the tissues of the body picking up antigens and cells and then drains into lymphatic channels that interdigitate in every capillary bed.

At sites of inflammation, the amount of fluid and cells draining into the local lymphatics increases because of changes in the vascular tone and permeability mediated by macrophage- and neutrophil-derived chemokines, lipid mediators, and oxygen radicals. This exuded fluid, along with antigen-loaded DCs, T cells, and cytokines, drains from the tissues back through the lymphatic channels.

Lymphatic fluid eventually returns to blood circulation via the thoracic duct, which drains into the vena cava. However, before

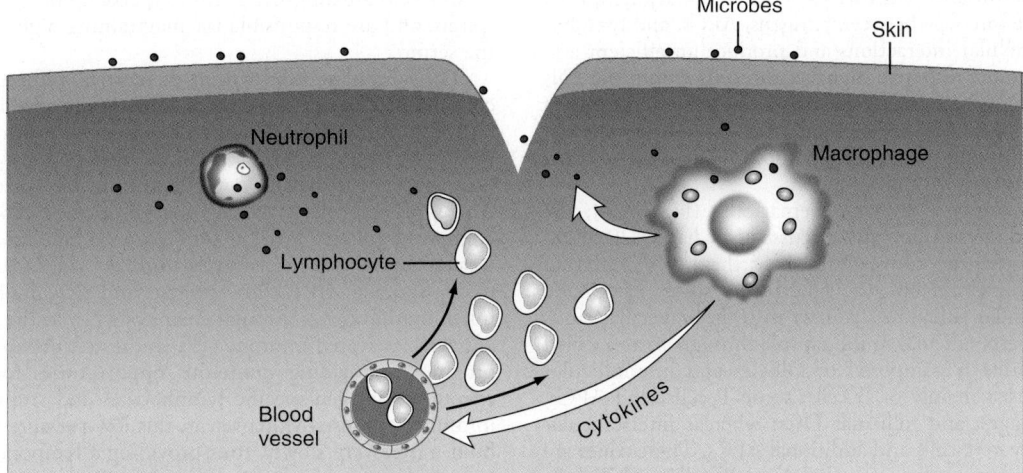

Fig. 19.2 ENCOUNTERS WITH ANTIGEN. The immune system evolved primarily to protect against invading microorganisms that penetrate the epithelial coverings of the body. In this schematic, microbes entering through a break in the skin epithelium are phagocytosed by resident macrophages as the first line of defense in innate immunity. The macrophages can secrete products that are directly microbicidal, as well as cytokines and other mediators that cause vasodilatation and endothelial cell separation, to allow influx of soluble mediators and inflammatory cells such as neutrophils and lymphocytes into the skin. Neutrophils, as a component of innate immunity, can also directly kill microorganisms, typically by releasing granular contents. Lymphocytes responding to microbial antigens proliferate and contribute to the adaptive immune response against microbes.

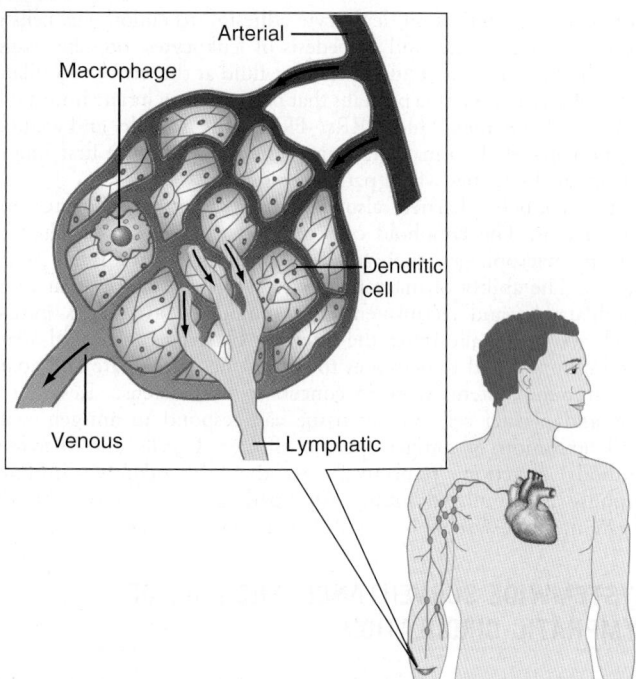

Fig. 19.3 LYMPHATIC DRAINAGE IS A CRITICAL PART OF IMMUNE SURVEILLANCE. As shown in Fig. 19.2, fluid and cells leave the vasculature at sites of inflammation. Hydrostatic pressure across the capillary bed continually drives transudation of fluid from the blood into tissues. The extravasated fluid, along with antigen-presenting cells (APCs) such as macrophages and dendritic cells, collects in lymphatics *(inset)*. Lymphatics drain past series of lymph nodes *(dark ovals)*, affording the APCs the opportunity to migrate to lymph nodes and stimulate lymphocytes in the nodes. Fluid in lymphatics passing through chains of lymph nodes eventually collects in the thoracic duct, which returns the fluid to the vascular circulation by draining into the vena cava.

returning to the venous circulation, lymphatic fluid travels through the secondary lymphoid tissues and undergoes sampling for foreign antigens, thus providing a mechanism of systemic immune surveillance. The organization and structure of these secondary lymphoid tissues create a close interface between antigens, APCs, and lymphocytes to optimize cellular interactions and produce an efficient and robust adaptive immune response. Signals from cells within the LNs can also expand the lymphatic vessel network, again resulting in increased drainage of DCs and antigens into the LNs. The movement of lymphatic fluid through secondary lymphoid tissue is an essential component of the adaptive immune system.

Lymph node anatomy is shown schematically (Fig. 19.4); the anatomy of LNs and the spleen is also discussed in Chapter 20. Fluid and cells gain entry to the convex surface of the LN via afferent lymphatic vessels that drain into the subcapsular sinus. Lymphatic fluid in the subcapsular sinus then courses into the trabecular sinus network that runs perpendicular to the capsule through an area called the cortex. The cortex is composed of follicles and interfollicular zones. Follicles consist mainly of B cells, some T cells, and APCs, including macrophages, and follicular DCs; whereas interfollicular zones consist mainly of T cells and additional APCs. These zones are separate but contiguous compartments where B cells and T cells initially encounter antigen. In the follicles, additional processing of antigens may be carried out by local APCs, such as follicular DCs. The net effect of the antigenic exposure is the proliferation of antigen-specific lymphocytes; and this proliferation further increases lymphatic drainage to the LN. In this way, LNs are a primary site for the refinement and amplification of antigen-specific adaptive immune responses.

Follicles are functionally characterized as either primary or secondary follicles. Primary follicles are composed of nonproliferating naive B cells that have yet to encounter antigen recognized by their surface BCR/Ig complex. Recognition of an antigen by the BCR/Ig leads to B cell activation. A complex set of interactions between the B cell, T cell, and APCs leads to the activation and proliferation of B cells carrying an antigen-specific BCR. A fraction of these activated proliferating B cells form GCs, which are surrounded by a mantle zone of naive B cells, which together comprise a secondary follicle (Fig. 19.5).

Germinal centers are classically divided into two compartments, denoted as the dark and light zone based on their appearance under light microscopy (see Fig. 19.5, inset). Dark zones are located adjacent to the T-cell areas, and contain a high density of proliferating B cells termed *centroblasts,* which are large cells with a high nuclear:cytoplasmic ratio, and do not express surface BCR/Ig. The light zone has a lower cellular density secondary to the presence of an extensive loose network of follicular DCs, and this imparts the "light" appearance.[24] B cells in the light zone are termed *centrocytes,* which in contrast to the centroblasts, are small B cells expressing surface BCR/Ig. Some of these cell types, such as centrocytes and centroblasts, are discussed in Chapter 73 in the context of lymphoid malignancies.

Within the germinal center, the series of sequential shuttling and reentry of B cells into the dark and light zones is termed the GC reaction, or the B-cell selection process. The cyclic reentry model proposes that centroblasts in the dark zone undergo cell division and SHM of variable light-chain genes mediated by AID. Next, they reexpress BCR/sIg and exit the cell cycle, migrating into the light zone to interact with antigen-presenting follicular DCs and TFH cells. In light zones, B cells with increased affinity for antigen are preferentially selected for survival by receiving vital signals from TFH cells; in contrast, B cells with impaired or absent antigen binding undergo apoptosis and clearance by resident macrophages, known as tingible body macrophages.[25] Selected centrocytes in the light zone are thought to return to the dark zone to undergo further rounds of proliferation, affinity maturation, and selection to improve the affinity of B-cell repertoire. Positively selected GC B cells eventually leave the GC, differentiating into memory B cells or plasma cells possessing somatically mutated immunoglobulin genes that encode for a high-affinity BCR/Ig. The modified capability of these selected B cells to generate a fast, highly specific humoral immune response upon a second encounter with the same pathogen forms the mechanistic basis of humoral memory. Memory B cells may circulate through secondary lymphoid organs and colonize the splenic marginal zone. Plasma cells are long-lived cells that take up residence in the BM and spleen, and are responsible for maintaining high levels of Ig seen in the serum.

The lymphatic fluid within the cortical trabecular sinus network continues to drain toward the medullary sinus, which lies deep to the cortex, forming the central part of the LN, known as the *hilum.* The medullary sinus contains additional APCs, some T cells, and numerous plasma cells that have migrated from the cortex to the medulla. There, plasma cells may leave the LN in the lymphatic fluid via the efferent lymphatic vessel at the hilum, to take up residence in other tissues. Lymphatic fluid travels through additional LNs on the way to the thoracic duct; thus antigens and cells draining from sites of inflammation travel through chains of LNs. In the lymphatic system, antigens, activated immune cells, and cytokines are kept in anatomic proximity, providing numerous opportunities for the antigens to encounter antigen-specific lymphocytes and stimulate the adaptive immune response. Moreover, in this low-pressure system, lymphatic fluid moves very slowly, thus providing a temporal as well as spatial opportunity for immune system activation.

In addition to lymphatic fluid, blood must also travel through LNs to provide oxygen and nutrients and to deliver new B and T cells that have not yet encountered antigen. Arterial blood enters the LN at the hilum, where arterioles arborize toward each follicle. Anatomically, the direction of blood flow is opposite to that of the lymphatic fluid, which drains toward the hilum. Naive T cells leave the blood to enter LNs through specialized vessels called *postcapillary venules,* which arise from follicular capillary beds, and travel through the T cell–rich interfollicular zones. Naive T cells exit from these

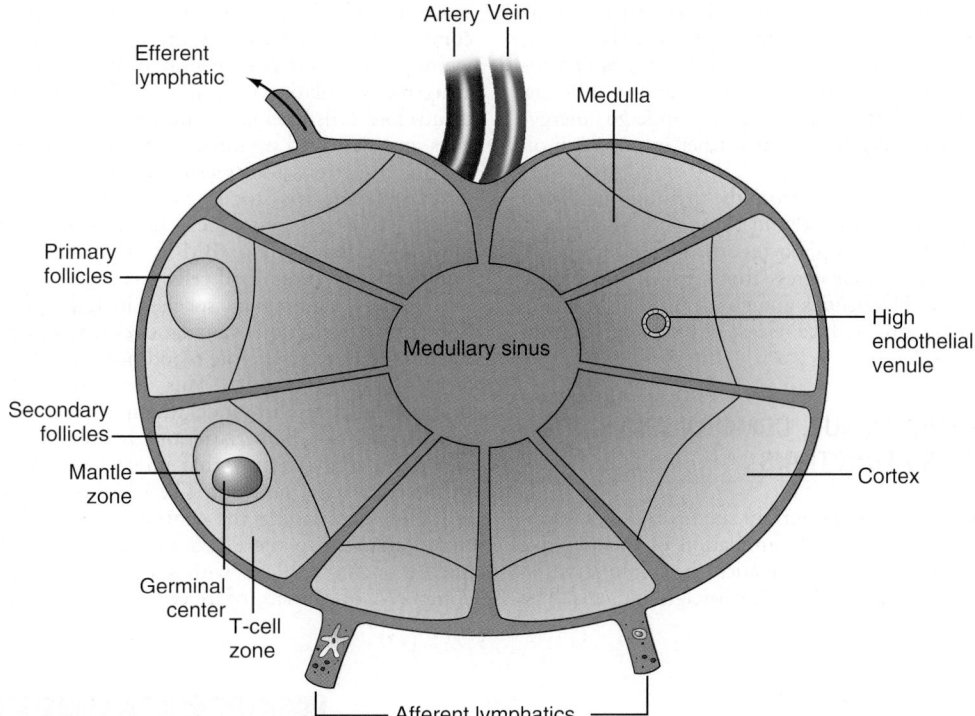

Fig. 19.4 LYMPH NODE ANATOMY. The lymph node is surrounded by a capsule. Afferent lymphatics draining tissues enter the node on the convex side into the capsule. Fluid and cells drain through the node and collect in the medullary sinus, where the fluid leaves the node through efferent lymphatics to rejoin the lymphatic circulation. The outer rim of the node is called the *cortex* and contains primary follicles composed of naive, nonproliferating B cells that have not encountered antigens, and secondary follicles with proliferating B cells in the germinal center. The germinal center can be subdivided into dark and light zones. Each lymph node is supplied with blood by the arterial circulation. Arterioles expand into a meshwork of capillaries within each follicle, and venous blood drains back out of the node. Naive T cells in the peripheral circulation can exit the blood and enter the lymph node through the high endothelial venules.

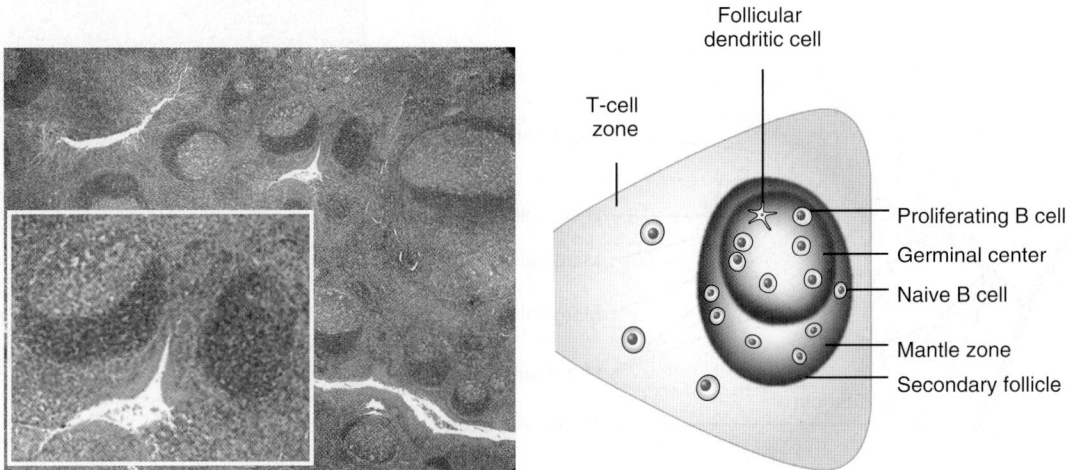

Fig. 19.5 B-CELL PROLIFERATION IN FOLLICLES AND GERMINAL CENTERS. B cells primarily populate the lymphoid follicles. A section of lymph node *(left)* demonstrates numerous secondary follicles. Adjacent to the follicles are the T cell–rich zones of the paracortex. Secondary follicles contain germinal centers filled with proliferating B cells, scattered T cells, and specialized antigen-presenting cells called follicular dendritic cells. The germinal center is surrounded by a mantle zone populated by naive B cells. Within each germinal center, are dark zones and light zones *(inset)*. The schematic of a section of lymph node *(right)* demonstrates a secondary follicle with a germinal center and a mantle zone. Scattered T cells can be found in the germinal center and are typically helper T cells that stimulate B-cell proliferation.

postcapillary venules, and upon antigenic recognition, remain in the node to proliferate and differentiate. If the naive T cells do not encounter antigens they recognize, the cells drain by means of lymphatic fluid back to the blood and repeat their route in a different LN until they become resident lymphocytes or undergo anergy-mediated cell death (refer to Chapter 21 for further information on T-cell immunity).

Egress of lymphocytes from LNs and from the thymus is regulated by a specialized lipid produced in lymphoid tissue and is known as sphingosine-1-phosphate (S1P). Lymphocytes express S1P receptor-1 (S1P$_1$) receptors that facilitate their egress from tissues into blood. Novel immunosuppressive therapeutics antagonizing S1P are being developed; these S1P antagonists reduce release of lymphocytes from lymphoid tissues into blood.

SECONDARY LYMPHOID TISSUE: COMMON AND UNIQUE ANATOMY AND FUNCTIONS

In addition to LNs, the spleen is an important site for B-cell development and for antigen presentation and stimulation of the adaptive immune system.[26–28] Lacking afferent lymphatics, the spleen serves to sample blood, rather than lymphatic fluid for foreign antigens. The spleen is divided into two functionally and morphologically distinct compartments, the white pulp and the red pulp (Fig. 19.6). The white pulp is composed mainly of lymphoid cells and is the site of antigenic stimulation of B and T cells. The red pulp consists mainly of myeloid cells, including macrophages that ingest opsonized antigens and damaged erythrocytes from the systemic circulation. The red pulp functions also as a site of extramedullary hematopoiesis early in fetal life and is a storage site for iron, erythrocytes, and platelets. Extramedullary hematopoiesis in the spleen may also occur postnatally in patients whose BM is incapable of producing adequate numbers of mature blood cells.

In many mammalian species, including humans, splenic blood flows through a unique vascular circulation that ensures the interposing of blood (and therefore blood-borne antigens) with the lymphoid areas of the white pulp. This has been best characterized in the murine model. In this model, the splenic white pulp consists of three compartments—the periarteriolar lymphoid sheath (PALS), follicles, and the marginal zone—that interact with blood through an open sinusoidal arterial network. The PALS is the spleen's T-cell zone and is found surrounding the central artery. Follicles in the spleen are found adjacent to the PALS and are capable of generating primary and secondary follicles with GCs as in LNs. The marginal zone, composed of subsets of B cells and macrophages, surrounds the

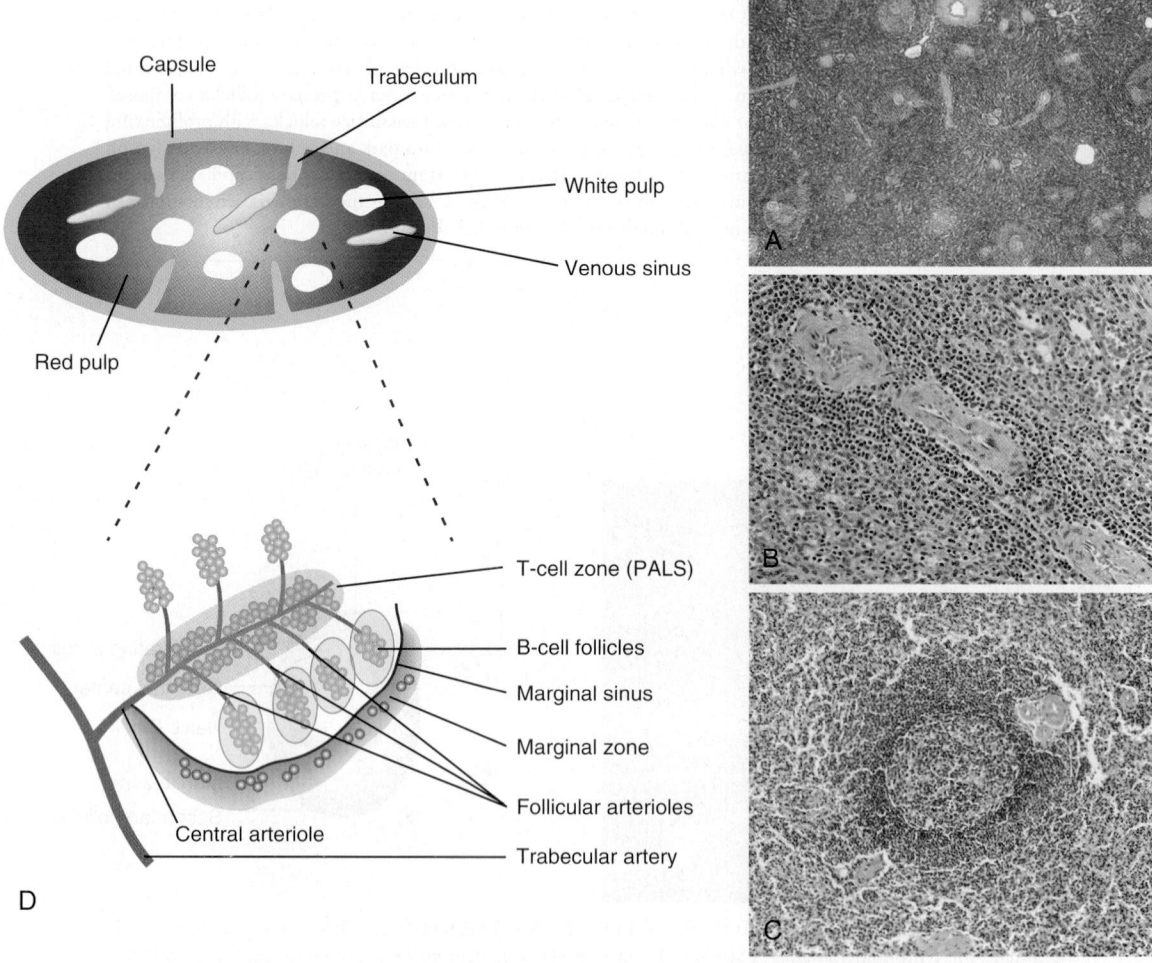

Fig. 19.6 ANATOMY OF THE SPLEEN. The spleen consists broadly of red pulp and white pulp (A). The red pulp is the site of myeloid cells (B) that ingest and remove opsonized antigens and damaged red blood cells from the circulation. The white pulp consists of lymphoid cells, with a periarteriolar T-cell sheath and mixed B- and T-cell follicles (C). In addition to lymph nodes, this is a major site for antigen-dependent B-cell maturation and activation. The schematic of splenic anatomy (D) demonstrates how the microscopic architecture is integrated into spleen to yield a site for the interaction of the innate and adaptive immune systems.

follicles in the spleen and serves as the major route of entry of blood-borne antigens and lymphocytes from the blood into the white pulp. Unlike other organs that have a closed vascular circulation in which blood travels from arterial to venous circulation through capillary beds, branches of the splenic artery penetrate the white pulp, forming an open sinusoidal network termed the *marginal sinuses*. From the marginal sinuses, blood filters through the white pulp regions of the spleen and encounters resident B and T cells. Following this encounter, the blood is drained via branches of the splenic vein, but an efferent lymphatic circulation also collects and drains the spleen. Beyond the white pulp, the splenic artery sends additional branches into the red pulp for further blood antigen surveillance and filtration that is accomplished by macrophages.

In addition to LNs and the spleen, there are numerous other sites of secondary lymphoid tissue.[29] A critical part of the secondary lymphoid system is the mucosa-associated lymphatic tissue (MALT). As the name implies, the MALT is in physical proximity with the mucosa (i.e., the epithelium and associated connective tissue that line the surfaces of the body). MALT is found at sites where antigens most commonly breach these epithelial barriers: the gastrointestinal, respiratory, and genitourinary tracts. In some tissues, the MALT forms relatively large structures that can be clearly distinguished histologically, such as the Peyer patches in the ileum and in the lymphoid tissue under the epithelium of the appendix. In these sites, perhaps because of the constant stimulation by microbial pathogens in the intestine, the MALT resembles lymphatic tissue in the spleen and LNs, with well-demarcated primary and secondary follicles that contain primarily B cells and intervening T cell–rich zones.

In other tissues, such as the genitourinary tract and the salivary glands, the microscopic anatomy of the MALT may not be as well defined as seen in Peyer patches; but the stromal tissue underlying the epithelium contains numerous lymphocytes and APCs. These sites provide an additional compartment of secondary lymphoid tissue where antigens can accumulate, be processed, and be presented to lymphocytes to stimulate an adaptive immune response.

Whereas the MALT constitutes a lymphoid population beneath the surface epithelium, a separate population of lymphocytes, primarily T cells, traffics directly through the epithelium in certain tissues, such as the gastrointestinal tract. These intraepithelial lymphocytes (IELs) include $\alpha\beta$ T cells and $\gamma\delta$ T cells, and comprise 1 in every 5 to 10 cells in the intestinal epithelium. Because the lining of the intestine is the largest organ surface area of the body, IELs are one of the largest T-cell populations. These IEL T cells are composed of different subpopulations, some of which are conventional T cells that recognize foreign antigens; others are regulatory T cells that limit the extent of an immune response and maintain immune homeostasis, a critical function in the antigen-rich milieu of the gut.[30]

SUGGESTED READINGS

Akira S, Uematsu S, Takeuchi O: Pathogen recognition and innate immunity. *Cell* 124:783, 2006.

Belardelli F, Ferrantini M: Cytokines as a link between innate and adaptive antitumor immunity. *Trends Immunol* 23:201, 2002.

Borregaard N: Neutrophils, from marrow to microbes. *Immunity* 33:657, 2010.

Bottazzi B, Doni A, Garlanda C, et al: An integrated view of humoral innate immunity: pentraxins as a paradigm. *Annu Rev Immunol* 28:157, 2010.

Cheroutre H: IELs: Enforcing law and order in the court of the intestinal epithelium. *Immunol Rev* 206:114, 2005.

Gowthaman U, Chodisetti SB, Agrewala JN: T cell help to B cells in germinal centers: Putting the jigsaw together. *Int Rev Immunol* 29:403, 2010.

Greaves DR, Gordon S: The macrophage scavenger receptor at 30 years of age: Current knowledge and future challenges. *J Lipid Res* 50:S282, 2009.

Josefowicz SZ, Lu LF, Rudensky AY: Regulatory T cells: mechanisms of differentiation and function. *Annu Rev Immunol* 30:531, 2012.

Misch EA, Hawn TR: Toll-like receptor polymorphisms and susceptibility to human disease. *Clin Sci* 114:347, 2008.

Papayannopoulos V, Zychlinsky A: NETs: A new strategy for using old weapons. *Trends Immunol* 30:513, 2009.

Sansonetti PJ: To be or not to be a pathogen: That is the mucosally relevant question. *Mucosal Immunol* 4:8, 2011.

Steinman L: A brief history of T(H)17, the first major revision in the T(H)1/T(H)2 hypothesis of T cell-mediated tissue damage. *Nat Med* 13:139, 2007.

Trinchieri G, Sher A: Cooperation of Toll-like receptor signals in innate immune defence. *Nat Rev Immunol* 7:179, 2007.

Turvey SE, Hawn TR: Towards subtlety: Understanding the role of Toll-like receptor signaling in susceptibility to human infections. *Clin Immunol* 120:1, 2006.

van de Vosse E, van Dissel JT, Ottenhoff THM: Genetic deficiencies of innate immune signalling in human infectious disease. *Lancet Infect Dis* 9:688, 2009.

Villasenor J, Benoist C, Mathis D: AIRE and APECED: Molecular insights into an autoimmune disease. *Immunol Rev* 204:156, 2005.

Walker JA, Barlow JL, McKenzie AN: Innate lymphoid cells—how did we miss them? *Nat Rev Immunol* 13:75, 2013.

REFERENCES

For the complete list of references, log on to www.expertconsult.com.

CHAPTER 20

B-CELL DEVELOPMENT

Kenneth Dorshkind and David J. Rawlings

B lymphocytes are the subset of white blood cells specialized to synthesize and secrete immunoglobulin (Ig). Their name derives from the finding that the avian *bursa* of Fabricius is a site of B-cell production. However, B-cell production in mammals takes place in the bone marrow (BM). Following their production in that organ, newly generated B lymphocytes migrate into secondary lymphoid organs such as the spleen where they undergo final maturation. At this point, the mature B cells may remain in the spleen or relocate via the circulation to additional tissues such as lymph nodes, where they are poised to respond to antigenic challenge.

This chapter will focus on adult B-cell development and the regulation of that process, although we briefly discuss fetal B lymphopoiesis and its distinguishing features. We then outline B-cell maturation in secondary lymphoid tissues. The information presented provides a basis for understanding abnormalities of B-cell development such as leukemia, lymphoma, and immunodeficiency states, which are discussed in other chapters. Studies in mice have contributed much to what is known about B-cell development and have served as a basis for understanding human B lymphopoiesis. Thus, although we emphasize the human literature as much as possible, frequent reference to findings in mice are made.

STAGES OF B-CELL DEVELOPMENT

As a result of advances in the development of monoclonal antibodies to leukocyte cell surface antigens and in flow cytometry, it is possible to resolve various stages of murine and human B-cell development from the hematopoietic stem cell (HSC) to newly produced, surface IgM-expressing B cells (Fig. 20.1).

Murine B-Cell Development

As the progeny of murine HSCs differentiate, they generate lymphoid-primed multipotent progenitors (LMPPs). LMPPs, defined by their lineage negative (Lin⁻) CD117 (c-kit)⁺ Sca-1⁺ Flt3⁺ phenotype, lack erythroid and megakaryocyte potential but can generate all other lymphoid and myeloid cells. A subset of LMPPs includes early lymphoid progenitors (ELPs), which express the *Rag1* gene (discussed later). ELPs are the precursors of Lin⁻ c-kit^low Sca-1^low CD127⁺ (interleukin-7 receptor α) common lymphoid progenitors (CLPs). Lin⁻ indicates that the cells lack expression of determinants present on mature myeloid, erythroid, and lymphoid lineage cells. CLPs then mature through pre-pro-B-, pro-B-, pre-B-, and B-cell stages of development that can be phenotypically resolved based on their expression of various cell surface and cytoplasmic determinants, as shown in Fig. 20.1.[1]

Human B-Cell Development

Various stages of human B-cell development can also be phenotypically identified.[2] A population of human Lin⁻ CD10⁻ CD62L^hi cells appears to be the human LMPP counterpart, whereas CLPs are CD34⁺ CD45RA⁺ CD10⁺ IL-7R⁺. As in the mouse, CLPs sequentially generate pro-B, pre-B, and B cells.[3,4] Human pro-B cells can be identified based on their expression of CD10, CD34, and CD19.

μ Heavy chain protein is detected in the cytoplasm of pre-B cells that no longer express CD34. Finally, when Ig light chain expression occurs, the cells become surface IgM-expressing B cells. Developing and mature B lineage cells also express additional cell surface determinants, which include CD20, CD21, CD22, CD24, CD38, and CD40, several of which are linked to critical intracellular signaling pathways. Antibodies against the CD20 determinant (rituximab) are in widespread clinical use for the treatment of lymphoma and, increasingly, autoimmune diseases.

B LINEAGE SPECIFICATION AND COMMITMENT

As differentiation of HSCs and other immature precursors into the B lineage occurs, genetic programs that promote B lymphopoiesis are activated while those used by non-B lineage cells are silenced. This results in gradual "specification" of progenitors towards the B-cell lineage. For example, cells at the CLP stage of development are destined to generate B cells, but they retain limited T and myeloid potential. Because of this, CLPs can be thought of as B lineage "specified." However, by the time the pro-B-cell stage has been reached, the cells can only generate B lymphocytes and are "committed" to the B-cell lineage. The processes of specification and commitment are dependent on the regulated expression of a network of transcription factors and other regulatory molecules in developing B lineage cells.[5]

Transcriptional Regulation of B-Cell Development

The generation of lymphoid cells from HSCs is critically dependent on expression of the Ets family member PU.1. Mice in which *Sfpi1*, the gene encoding PU.1, is not expressed produce erythroid and megakaryocytic but not monocytic, granulocytic, and lymphoid cells. As a result of this severe defect, PU.1 knock-out mice die during the fetal period or within a few days after birth. PU.1 regulates a number of early events as precursors become B lineage specified. These include the expression of Flt3, which is expressed on LMPPs, the CD45R(B220) cell surface determinant, and IL-7Rα. However, deletion of *Sfpi1* at the CLP stage of development has no negative effect on B-cell development, indicating that PU.1 expression is not required once B-cell specification has occurred.

Further specification toward the B-cell lineage is dependent on the expression of additional transcription factors that include early B-cell factor (EBF) and the E2A-encoded splice variants E12 and E47. Each of these DNA-binding proteins regulates the expression of a variety of B-lineage target genes. For example, Ebf1 regulates the expression of Igα, VpreB, λ5, and Pax5, and represses genes associated with alternative lineage fates. That EBF and E2A expression play a critical role in B lymphopoiesis has been demonstrated by the fact that mice in which they are not expressed exhibit an almost complete block in B-cell development at the pro-B-cell stage.

Ebf1- and E2A-expressing progenitors can still exhibit some non-B lineage potential, indicating that the expression of these DNA-binding proteins does not result in absolute commitment of cells to the B lineage. Instead, this is dependent on expression of the Pax5 transcription factor.[6] Phenotypically identifiable B-cell precursors are present in *Pax5* knock-out mice, and when placed under appropriate

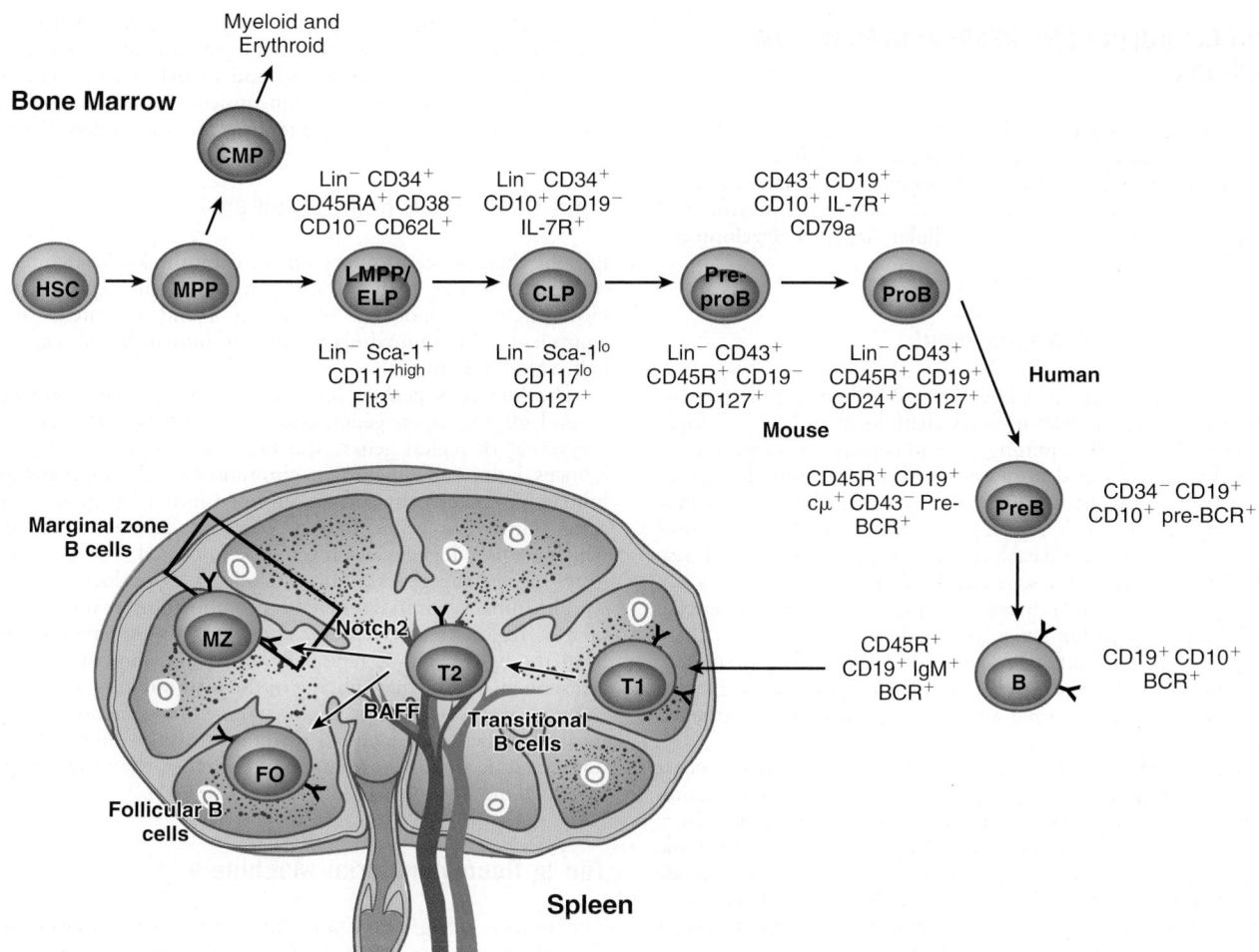

Fig. 20.1 HEMATOPOIESIS WITH AN EMPHASIS ON B-CELL DEVELOPMENT. Stages of human and mouse B-cell development and selected cell surface and cytoplasmic determinants that can be used to distinguish various stages of differentiation are shown. Note that there are additional cell surface and molecular determinants that can be used to define the various stages of development. After leaving the bone marrow, newly produced B cells migrate to the spleen and mature through transitional cell stages into marginal zone or follicular B cells. *CLP*, Common lymphoid progenitor; *CMP*, common myeloid progenitor; *ELP*, early lymphoid progenitor; *FO*, follicular B cell; *HSC*, hematopoietic stem cell; *LMPP*, lymphoid-primed multipotential progenitor; *MPP*, multipotential progenitor; *MZ*, marginal zone B cell; *T1*, transitional 1 B cell; *T2*, transitional 2 B cell.

conditions, they can differentiate into myeloid, T, and natural killer (NK) cells. However, if the gene encoding Pax5 is introduced into *Pax5*-deficient precursors, this developmental promiscuity is no longer observed. Thus a critical function of Pax5 is to suppress non-B lineage potential. For example, Pax5 may repress myeloid growth factor receptors, such as those for macrophage colony-stimulating factor, and inhibit the T-cell potential of lymphoid-restricted progenitors by antagonizing expression of Notch1, a cell-surface receptor whose stimulation activates signaling pathways required for commitment to the T-cell lineage. In addition to regulating commitment to the B-cell lineage, continued Pax5 expression is necessary to maintain lineage fidelity even in relatively mature B cells.

Many additional transcription factors, such as Ikaros, Satb1, Foxo1, IRF4, IRF8, c-Myb, Gfi1, Miz-1, Bcl6, and Bach2, function at various times during B-cell development. For example, IRF4 is involved with Ig recombination and the attenuation of the IL-7 signaling pathway, thus promoting the transition from the pre-B to B-cell stages of maturation (discussed later). IRF8, along with PU.1, regulates EBF expression. Ikaros plays a role in regulating expression of key B lineage genes such as IL-7Rα and EBF, and promoting B lineage commitment. c-Myb has been shown to synergize with PU.1 to activate IL-7 receptor gene transcription. Focused reviews should be consulted for a full discussion of these and additional transcriptional regulators of B lymphopoiesis.

MicroRNAs

MicroRNAs (miRNAs) are RNA molecules, 19 to 23 nucleotide long, that are processed from longer RNA precursors. miRNAs are biologically active as RNA molecules and act post-transcriptionally, either by promoting degradation of mRNA targets or by blocking their translation. However, like transcriptional regulators, a single miRNA can potentially regulate many targets to provide coordinated and simultaneous regulation of a network of genes.

Mice with conditional deletion of Dicer, an enzyme necessary for miRNA synthesis, in pro-B cells do not develop B lymphocytes, indicating the importance of miRNA regulatory mechanisms during B-cell differentiation. Work is now ongoing to identify the role of specific miRNAs at specific stages of B-cell development. For example, germ line deletion of miR-17–92 cluster blocks pro-B-cell maturation.[7]

IMMUNOGLOBULIN GENE REARRANGEMENT AND EXPRESSION

The defining feature of a B lymphocyte is its expression of cell surface Ig, which is formed by two heavy chains and two light chains, each of which is encoded by multiple gene segments. The process of Ig gene rearrangement occurs in a step-wise manner as murine and human B cells mature through the cellular stages of development just described.[8,9]

Heavy Chain Gene Rearrangement

The initial Ig rearrangement events during B-cell development occur at the heavy chain locus. The Ig heavy chain locus includes multiple variable (V), diversity (D), joining (J), and constant (C) region gene segments that are separated from one another by introns. The genes that encode Ig heavy chain protein are located on human chromosome 14 (Fig. 20.2). The V region genes are located at the 5′ end of the Ig heavy chain locus, and each consists of approximately 300 base pairs. These genes, which are separated by short intron sequences, are organized into seven families based on sequence homology. There are about 25 human D region genes located 3′ to the V region. These also are grouped into families, and at least 10 have been described. Downstream of the D region are six human J region genes. Finally, 10 C region genes representing alternative Ig isotypes are arranged in tandem.

The transcription of the unrearranged heavy chain locus occurs prior to actual Ig gene recombination. This results in the production of developmentally regulated transcripts of unrearranged Ig genes, referred to as germline or sterile transcripts. Multiple species of sterile transcripts have been described, and some could conceivably encode proteins. A mechanistic link between transcription and Ig gene rearrangement has been hypothesized. For example, transcription might make unrearranged Ig genes accessible to both RNA polymerase and V(D)J recombinase, the germline transcripts could function in the rearrangement reaction, or transcription could alter structural characteristics of DNA, making the recombination signal sequences, described later, better targets for recombination.

The initial event during heavy chain gene rearrangement occurs as early as the CLP stage and juxtaposes a D region segment to a J segment. Although in theory any D region gene can join with equal frequency to any J region gene, there may be preferential utilization of selected D and J region genes at various times during fetal and adult B-cell development. The next recombination event involves the rearrangement of a V region gene to the D–J complex, and this occurs at the pro-B-cell stage of development. Evidence suggests that biased usage of J proximal V genes occurs in the newly generated repertoire of neonatal mice and humans. The heavy chain C region remains separated from the rearranged VDJ complex by an intron, and this entire sequence is transcribed. RNA processing subsequently leads to deletion of the intron between the VDJ complex and the most proximal C region genes. After translation, μ heavy chain protein is expressed in the cytoplasm of pre-B cells (Fig. 20.2).

The E2A-encoded transcription factors are particularly important for Ig gene recombination and mediate their effects via binding to specific promoter sequences located 5′ of each heavy chain V region and one or more heavy chain enhancer regions located 3′ of the J region genes and downstream from the CH region genes (see Fig. 20.2). Before Ig gene rearrangement, E12 and E47 proteins may be in an inactive state owing to their heterodimeric association with another protein known as *Id*. In this configuration, DNA binding by E12 and E47 does not occur. Thus, successful transition from the pro-B- to pre-B-cell stage is dependent on cessation of Id expression. This conclusion is consistent with the fact that mice expressing an Id transgene have a complete block in B-cell differentiation.

Each pro-B cell has two Ig heavy chain genes, but only one of these encodes heavy chain protein in any given cell. This phenomenon is known as *allelic exclusion*. One theory for how this occurs

is that functional Ig rearrangements are rare, so the chance that two functional rearrangements will occur in an individual cell is extremely low. An increasingly accepted, second model of allelic exclusion is that the expression of heavy chain protein from a successfully rearranged allele inhibits rearrangements at the other heavy chain allele.

Light Chain Gene Rearrangement

Ig light chain protein can be encoded by the kappa (κ) or lambda (λ) genes. Greater than 90% of murine B cells express κ protein. However, the proportions of human κ and λ proteins are more equivalent, with approximately 60% of human B cells expressing κ light chain protein.

The human κ gene is located on chromosome 2 and includes around 40 Vκ region genes, clustered in up to seven families, five functional Jκ region genes, and one Cκ region gene. The human λ locus is located on human chromosome 22. Approximately 30 human Vλ genes exist and are grouped into 10 families. There are seven human Cλ genes, four of which are functional and three of which are pseudogenes. Each Cλ gene is located 3′ of a respective Jλ gene. Light chain genes do not include D region loci.

The initial event in light chain recombination involves the joining of a V region to a J region. The VJ complex remains separated from the light chain C region by an intron, the entire complex is transcribed, and further splicing of the intron results in formation of a mature V–J–C transcript. Light chain rearrangements in mice occur initially at the kappa locus. If rearrangements at the first κ allele are unsuccessful, attempts are made to rearrange the second κ gene. If this fails, the λ locus is used.

The Ig Recombinatorial Machinery

The process of Ig heavy and light chain gene rearrangement is dependent on enzymes that delete intronic sequences and join coding segments of DNA. The enzymes that mediate these functions act through recognition of recombination signal sequences that are located 3′ of each heavy chain V region exon, 5′ of each heavy chain J segment, and 5′ and 3′ of each heavy chain D region gene. Fig. 20.2 shows the association of these recognition sequences with the various heavy chain exons. Each recombination signal sequence consists of conserved heptamer and nonamer sequences separated by nonconserved DNA segments of 12 or 23 base pairs. During Ig gene recombination, these recognition sequences form loops of DNA, which in turn bring the coding exons in apposition to one another. These noncoding loops are subsequently deleted and degraded.

The expression of two highly conserved proteins, referred to as recombinase-activating genes-1 (RAG-1) and RAG-2, is required for heavy and light chain gene recombination.[10] Mice and humans in whom *Rag* genes are not expressed do not generate B or T cells. Results from cell-free systems that measure V(D)J recombination indicate that RAG proteins are involved in cleavage of DNA at recombination signal sequences and the subsequent joining of coding sequences to one another. In addition to the RAG proteins, general DNA repair enzymes, those encoded by the Ku complex of genes in particular, also play a critical role in Ig heavy chain gene recombination.

Generation and Selection of the Primary B-Cell Repertoire

For the organism to mount an effective humoral immune response, an array of Igs with unique antigen-binding specificities, together referred to as the *Ig repertoire*, must be generated. Several mechanisms have evolved to ensure that this occurs.

First, heavy and light chain proteins can be encoded by multiple germline V, J, and, in the case of the heavy chain, D region genes, and the combinatorial diversity among them is enormous. Second, nucleotides not encoded in the germline can be added to D–J and

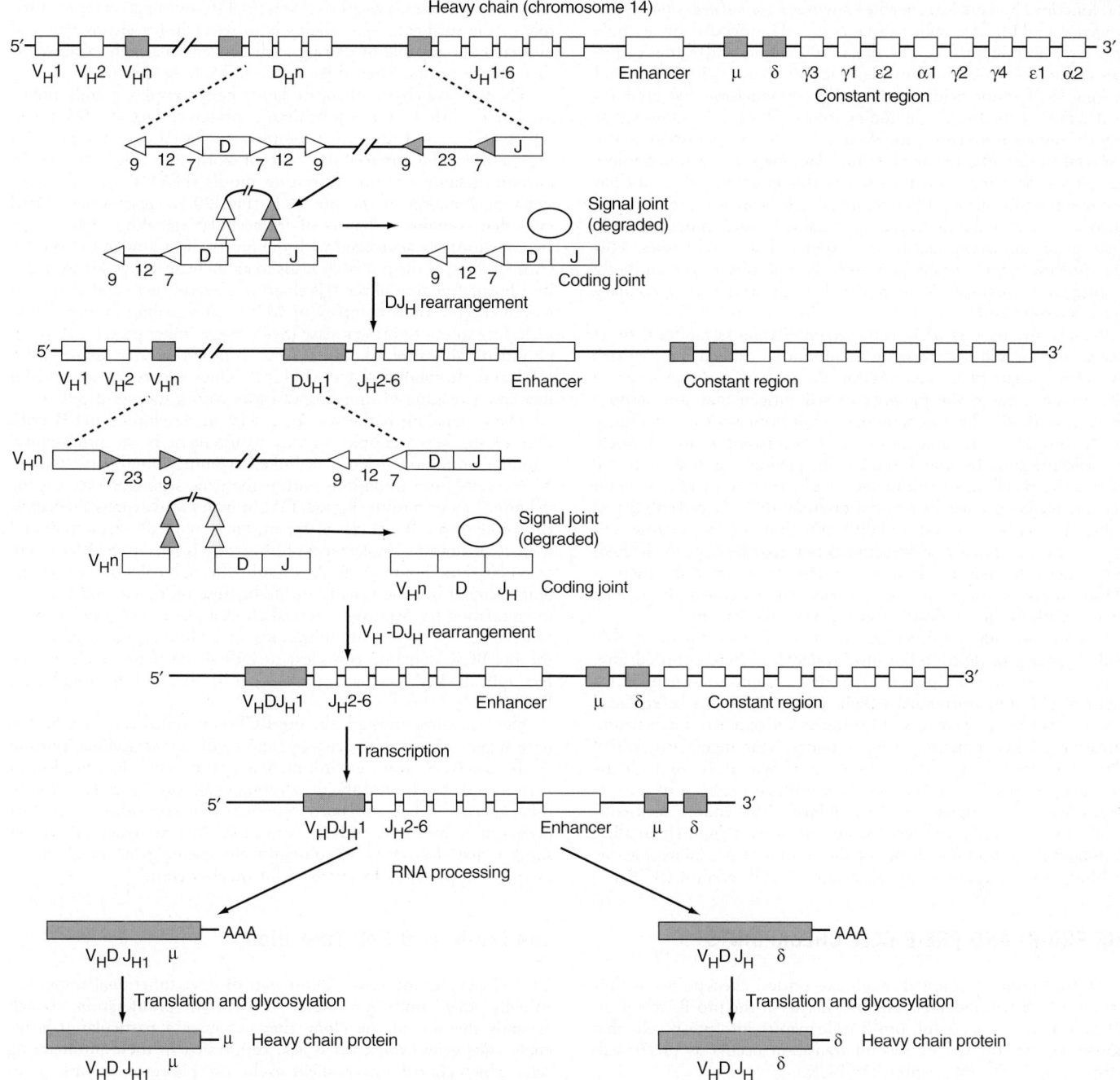

Fig. 20.2 REARRANGEMENT AND EXPRESSION OF THE HUMAN IMMUNOGLOBULIN HEAVY CHAIN GENE. The figure shows the Ig heavy chain gene and the signal sequences 3′ of each V region locus, 5′ and 3′ of each D region locus, and 5′ of each J region locus. These consist of heptamer and nonamer sequences separated by either 12 or 23 base pairs. During immunoglobulin (Ig) recombination, a signal sequence of 12 base pairs can only join to another of 23 base pairs (the so-called 12–23 rule). As shown in the figure, initial heavy chain gene rearrangements form coding joints between D and J regions, as well as signal joints that are ultimately degraded. Subsequently, the joining of the V region gene to the DJ complex occurs. After a successful rearrangement, the VDJ complex, the μ intron, and portions of the constant regions are transcribed. RNA processing and differential splicing results in formation of an mRNA molecule that is then translated. In the example shown, the rearranged VDJ complex and the constant region, with the μ and δ C region genes, is transcribed. After RNA processing and translation, a particular B cell could then express μ protein, δ protein, or both.

VDJ junctions by a nuclear enzyme known as *terminal deoxynucleotidyl transferase* (TdT). Two splice variants of TdT, encoded by a single gene, have been identified. The short (509-amino acid) variant catalyzes the addition of nontemplated nucleotides at coding joints and the long (529-amino acid) form is a 3′–5′ exonuclease that catalyzes the deletion of nucleotides at coding joints. Third, DNA joints that form during recombination are often imprecise and can occur at any of several nucleotides in the germline. Although out-of-frame joints that cannot be transcribed may result, this junctional diversity has the potential to generate different amino acid sequences, resulting in added diversity of the Ig repertoire. Finally, somatic mutation of V region genes can occur, usually in secondary lymphoid tissues. This latter process, which results in an increased affinity of the antibody for antigen, is discussed in more detail in the section on secondary B-cell development.

Because the process of Ig gene recombination is random, some B cells that are self-reactive may be produced. Several mechanisms have been proposed to account for the fate of such self-reactive cells. In some cases, the presence of self-antigen may not activate self-reactive B cells. This scenario may result from weak B-cell affinity for the antigen or the autoantigen may be present at an extremely low concentration. In other instances, interaction of antigen with the autoreactive B cell may result in anergy. The level of membrane Ig on such anergic B cells may be reduced up to 20-fold, the cell's ability to proliferate may be impaired, and differentiation into Ig-secreting cells may be blocked. Finally, self-reactive B cells may be clonally deleted. Clonal deletion may result from cytolysis by other cells, such as BM macrophages, or autoreactive B cells may undergo a physiologic change resulting in cell death after receptor engagement.[11]

The recognition of self-antigen by a B cell may not necessarily result in anergy or deletion but instead may lead to receptor editing. In this process, which represents the most common mechanism for negative selection, rearranged κ light chain alleles can be replaced by secondary rearrangements of upstream Vκ genes to downstream, unrearranged Jκ segments. These secondary rearrangements, which may delete the primary VκJκ complex or separate it from Cκ by inversion, are possible because of the continual presence of unrearranged Vκ regions upstream of the joined VκJκ coding segments. Finally, unsuccessful rearrangements of the initial κ light chain allele are followed by rearrangements of the second allele, increasing the likelihood of generating a less self-reactive B-cell receptor (BCR).

THE PRO-B- AND PRE-B-CELL CHECKPOINTS

B-cell progenitors progress through two critical checkpoints as they mature into B lymphocytes. The first occurs at the pro-B- to pre-B-cell transition. If successful, pro-B cells mature into pre-B cells that express the pre-BCR. The second transition occurs as pre-B cells mature into B cells that express the BCR.

The Pro-B- to Pre-B-Cell Transition

The key event during the pro-B- to pre-B-cell transition is the rearrangement and expression of the Ig heavy chain genes. It is important to recognize that not all pro-B cells successfully navigate this transition. The principal reason for this is that not all Ig gene recombination events are successful. For example, Ig heavy chain gene rearrangements are productive in only around one-third of pro-B cells. Those cells with nonproductive Ig gene rearrangements undergo apoptosis and are eliminated from the BM by resident macrophages and stromal cells.

However, if Ig heavy chain recombination is productive and μ heavy chain protein is expressed, it appears on the surface of the pre-B cells in association with two additional molecules referred to as the surrogate light chains. The surrogate light chain proteins, Vpre-B and λ5, are encoded by genes located on chromosome 16 in mice and on chromosome 22 in humans, and are noncovalently linked to one another. λ5 in turn is covalently linked to the CH1 domain of

the μ heavy chain via a carboxyl-terminal (C-terminal) cysteine. One role of the surrogate light chains is to select heavy chains that will ultimately be capable of pairing with conventional light chains.[12] If this does not occur, then these cells will likely be deleted.

The μ heavy chain–surrogate light chain complex is additionally associated with two transmembrane proteins, Igα (CD79a) and Igβ (CD79b), and the entire complex is referred to as the *pre-BCR* (Fig. 20.3). The intracellular tails of both Igα and Igβ contain immunoreceptor tyrosine activation motifs (ITAMs) critical to the signaling function of the pre-BCR (Fig. 20.3, *upper panel*). Lipid rafts that contain mediators of intracellular signaling such as Lyn are constitutively associated with the pre-BCR in human pre-B cells. Cross-linking of the pre-BCR leads to an increase in Lyn kinase activity, phosphorylation of the Igβ chain, and recruitment and activation within the pre-BCR complex of additional signaling intermediates, including spleen tyrosine kinase (Syk), B-cell linker protein (BLNK), phosphatidylinositol 3-kinase (PI3K), Bruton's tyrosine kinase (Btk), VAV, and phospholipase C-γ (PLCγ2). These events lead to calcium flux and activation of signaling cascades within the pre-B cell.

These signaling pathways are crucial in developing pre-B cells. One of the best examples of this requirement is the prototypical humoral immunodeficiency, X-linked agammaglobulinemia (XLA). XLA results from mutations within the gene segments that encode the nonreceptor tyrosine kinase, Btk. In males who express a defective Btk protein, pre-B-cell clonal expansion is markedly depressed, and there is an almost complete loss of immature B cells in the BM and in secondary lymphoid organs. As a result, affected males develop recurrent bacterial infections early in life because of a profound decrease in circulating Ig. A nearly identical clinical phenotype also has been observed in persons with mutations in additional components of the pre-BCR signaling complex, including the μ heavy chain, λ5, Igα, Igβ, the key B-cell adaptor protein BLNK, and the lipid kinase PLCγ2.

How signaling through the pre-BCR is initiated is unclear. It has been suggested that this occurs by binding of the extracellular portion of the pre-BCR to an environmental ligand. The identification of such ligands has been difficult, although galectin-1 may function in this capacity. It has also been proposed that constitutive signaling occurs after pre-BCR surface expression. Recent structural studies suggest that the pre-BCR constitutively assembles as an oligomer, providing a potential mechanism for this behavior.[13,14]

The Pre-B- to B-Cell Transition

Pre-BCR-expressing cells exhibit two distinct functional responses. Initially they undergo several rounds of proliferation, which expands the size of the clone that expresses a particular μ-heavy chain. *Rag* gene expression is also suppressed in these proliferating cells, which contributes to allelic exclusion. However, at some point these pre-BCR-expressing cells exit the cell cycle and reactivate the recombinatorial machinery so that light chain gene recombination can commence.

Recent studies indicate that a highly regulated balance between signaling through the IL-7 receptor (discussed later) and the pre-BCR ensures that proliferation and Ig recombination are mutually exclusive events. IL-7 receptor signaling stimulates cell proliferation and inhibits light chain gene rearrangements.[14] In contrast, pre-BCR signaling represses proliferation, likely through activation of the RAS–extracellular-signal-regulated kinase (ERK) pathway as well as via limiting PI3K activity through BLNK-mediated signals.[14] This in turn leads to the expression of transcription factors, including E2A, IRF4, and PAX5, that induce cell cycle exit, RAG expression, and light chain gene recombination. These events are strongly influenced by the movement of developing B-cell progenitors through various niches wherein they are exposed to different environmental signals including, most notably, transiting from a setting of high to low IL-7 availability (Fig. 20.4).

Once the recombinatorial machinery is reactivated, light chain gene rearrangement and expression occurs. As with heavy chain

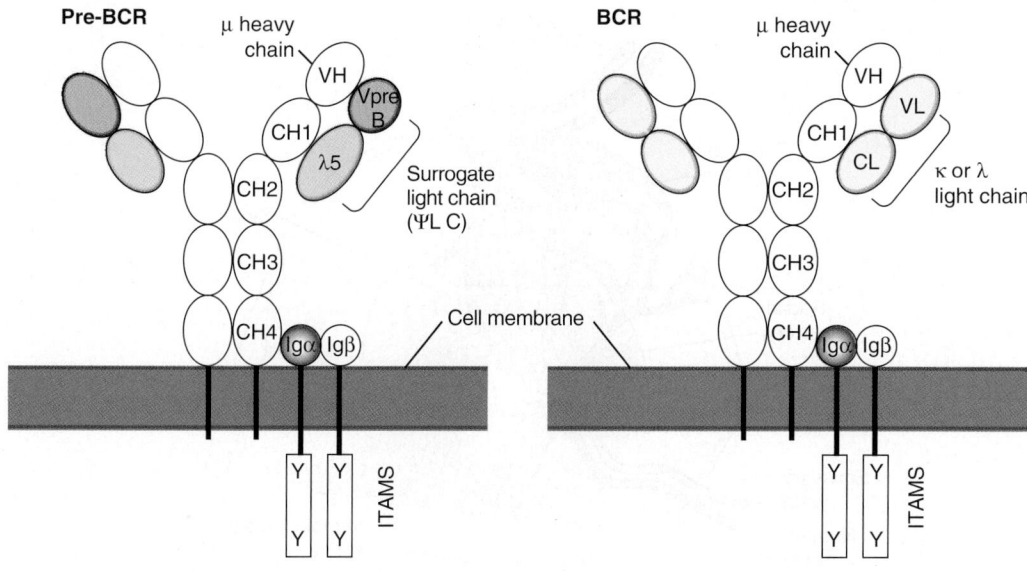

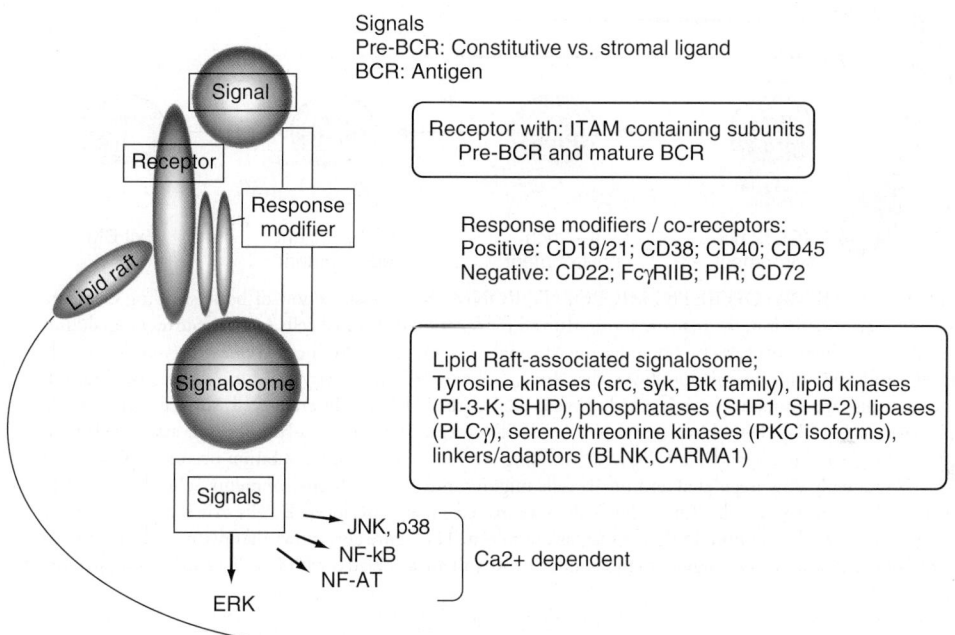

Fig. 20.3 THE PRE-B-CELL RECEPTOR AND B-CELL RECEPTOR AND ASSOCIATED SIGNAL-ING INTERMEDIATES. *Top,* μ-Heavy chain protein in pre-B cells is associated with the surrogate light chains v-pre-B and λ5 *(left)* to form the pre-BCR. In newly produced B lymphocytes, μ-heavy chain is associated with conventional light chains *(right)* to form the BCR. Associated with heavy chain in both pre-B and B cells are two additional transmembrane proteins, Ig-α and Ig-β, that contain ITAMs critical to the signaling function. Expression of the pre-BCR (or possibly its binding to a stromal ligand) or binding of antigen to the mature BCR, respectively, initiates the assembly of a lipid raft, BCR-associated "signalosome" composed of multiple signaling molecules, ultimately leading to transcriptional events that promote cell proliferation, survival, and differentiation *(bottom).* *BCR,* B-cell receptor; *ERK,* extracellular signal-regulated kinase; *Ig,* immunoglobulin; *ITAM,* immunoreceptor tyrosine activation motif; *JNK,* Janus kinase; *NFκB,* nuclear factor kappa–light-chain enhancer of activated B cells; *NFAT,* nuclear factor of activated T cells; *PKC,* protein kinase C; *PLCγ,* phospholipase C-γ; *SHIP,* src homology 2-containing inositol phosphatase; *SHP,* src homology-containing protein tyrosine phosphatase.

recombination, functional light chain gene rearrangements do not occur in all pre-B cells. However, when they are successful, the heavy and light chains assemble and are expressed on the surface of a newly produced B lymphocyte as the B-cell receptor.

Events that disrupt the pre-B-cell transition including, for example, activating lesions in IL-7 receptor subunits or downstream mediators, significantly enhance the risk for development of pre-B acute lymphoblastic leukemia; an improved understanding of these changes will likely provide new therapeutic targets to inhibit leukemia cell growth.[15]

The B-Cell Receptor

Once light chain expression occurs, a complete Ig molecule is expressed on the surface of the newly produced B cells. All newly

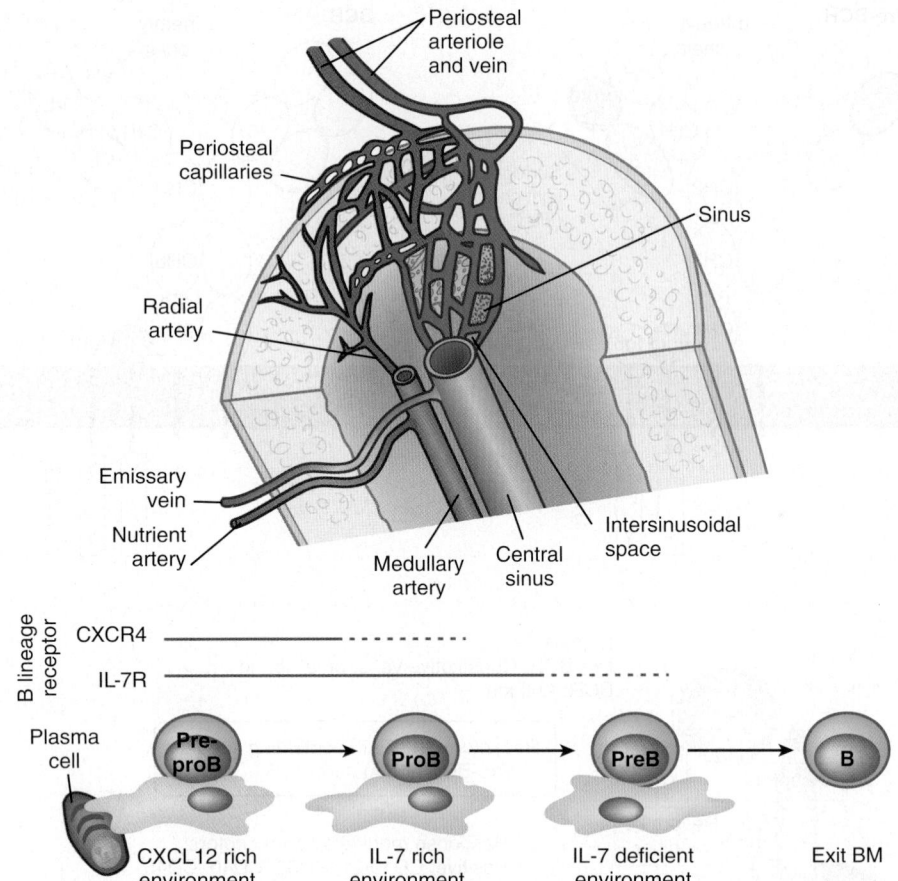

Fig. 20.4 THE HEMATOPOIETIC MICROENVIRONMENT. Cross-section of bone showing elements of the medullary circulation, the marrow sinusoids, and the location of stromal cells *(top)*. (Courtesy Dorshkind K: Regulation of hematopoiesis by bone marrow stromal cells and their products. *Annu Rev Immunol* 8:111, 1990. Reproduced with permission from the *Annual Review of Immunology.*) During their maturation, B lineage cells are thought to migrate between niches that deliver different cell surface and soluble signals *(bottom)*. CXC-chemokine receptor 4 (CXCR4)-expressing pre-pro-B cells are associated with C-X-C motif chemokine ligand 12 (CXCL12)-secreting stromal cells. As differentiation occurs, expression of CXCR4 is gradually downregulated and pro-B cells migrate into IL-7–rich environments. The IL-7 receptor is downregulated on pre-B cells. Once the BCR is expressed, newly produced B cells exit the bone marrow and migrate to secondary lymphoid tissues such as the spleen. The figure also shows that plasma cells generated in secondary lymphoid organs migrate to the bone marrow and are associated with CXCL12-expressing stromal cells.

produced B lymphocytes express IgM, but others may coexpress cell surface IgD (see Fig. 20.2). This occurs because the primary heavy chain transcript includes the rearranged VDJ heavy chain complex, the μ and δ C regions, and the intron separating these exons. If RNA processing results in association of the Cμ region with the VDJ complex, the B cell expresses IgM. Alternatively, if the Cμ exon is deleted along with the heavy chain intron, the VDJ complex and the Cδ exon become contiguous and the B cell expresses IgD.

The complex of cell surface Ig, along with Igα and Igβ, is referred to as the BCR (Fig. 20.3). The cytoplasmic tail of the Ig heavy chain is relatively short, and, as noted earlier, both Igα and Igβ contain an ITAM in their intracellular tails that that is required for signal transduction following antigen binding to the BCR. Antigen engagement initiates assembly of a lipid raft, BCR-associated "signalosome," composed of multiple signaling molecules that include tyrosine kinases, serine/threonine kinases, lipid kinases, lipases, phosphatases, and linkers and adaptors. This signalosome mediates a cascade of intracellular signals that includes the initiation of calcium influx. Additional calcium-dependent and -independent downstream signals that include the mitogen-activated protein (MAP) kinase cascade (c-jun N-terminal kinase [JNK], p38, ERK) and activation of key transcription factors that include JUN, c-fos, nuclear factor of activated T cells (NFAT), and nuclear factor kappa-B (NFκB) in turn

mediate transcriptional events leading to cell proliferation, survival, and differentiation. The level and duration of receptor activation and hence transcriptional output are further modified by a series of cell surface coreceptors or "response modifiers" that bind to complement or to receptors on the surface of stromal cells, activated T cells, or other populations present in secondary lymphoid organs.

THE HEMATOPOIETIC MICROENVIRONMENT

Hematopoiesis takes place in the intersinusoidal spaces of the medullary cavity in association with several types of nonhematopoietic cells that together form the hematopoietic microenvironment (Fig. 20.4). For example, HSCs are associated with niches that include osteoblasts as well as endothelial cells that line the sinusoids present in the intersinusoidal spaces. These nonhematopoietic supporting cells, also referred to collectively as stromal cells, support blood cell development via direct cell-to-cell interactions and through the secretion of various soluble mediators.[16]

Several cell surface determinants that mediate adhesion between developing B lineage cells and the stroma have been described. Both murine and human pre-B cells express the very late antigen 4 (VLA-4) integrin that interacts with a stromal cell ligand identified as vascular cell adhesion molecule-1 (VCAM-1). VLA-4 also promotes binding to fibronectin, an extracellular matrix protein. CD44 on developing B lineage cells has been implicated in mediating stromal cell–lymphocyte interactions in the mouse through binding to stromal cell–derived hyaluronate. These intercellular interactions presumably would allow B cells to receive proliferative or developmental signals (or both) from stromal cells. The stromal cells may not be passive populations that constitutively provide these signals. Instead, the binding of the B-lineage cell may stimulate the stromal cell in turn to produce such differentiation or growth-potentiating activities. Various cytokines that regulate the growth, differentiation, and/or survival of B lineage cells have also been described and include C-X-C motif chemokine ligand 12 (CXCL12; SDF1), Flt3 ligand, stem cell factor, IL-7, Wnt family members, transforming growth factor beta (TGF-β) family members, and thymic stromal lymphopoietin (TSLP).[17]

A full discussion of these and additional factors that regulate B-cell development is beyond the scope of this chapter. However, the focus can be narrowed considerably when only those with obligate effects on B-cell development are considered. In this regard, the critical B lymphopoietic cytokine in mice is IL-7, which binds to the IL-7 receptor (IL-7R). The IL-7R is formed by the IL-7 receptor α chain and the common cytokine γ chain. The Janus kinases (JAKs) JAK3 and JAK1 are associated with the γc and IL-7Rα, respectively, and are critical for IL-7 receptor-mediated signaling. When IL-7 binds to the IL-7 receptor, these JAKs are phosphorylated, and this in turn recruits signal transducer and activator of transcription 5A (STAT5A) and STAT5B. The STAT molecules can then translocate to the nucleus where they act as transcriptional activators. In addition to stimulating the growth and survival of developing B lineage cells, IL-7 signaling also potentiates the recombination of a VH region gene segment to an already rearranged DJH complex. The requirement for IL-7 in murine B-cell development is demonstrated by studies showing a block in B-cell development at approximately the pro-B-cell stage in IL-7 and IL-7 receptor knock-out mice.[14]

Developing B-cell progenitors are exposed to IL-7 and other signals, and this is thought to occur as they traffic through different niches in the BM (Fig. 20.4). The most immature B-cell progenitors express the CXC-chemokine receptor 4 (CXCR4) receptor and associate with stromal cells that express high levels of its ligand, CXCL12. CXCL12 induces focal adhesion kinase (FAK) phosphorylation in pro-B cells, and this in turn is thought to promote VLA-4-mediated adhesion to VCAM-1 expressing stroma. As maturation occurs, pro-B cells migrate towards IL-7-producing stromal cells. Ultimately, pre-B cells dissociate from the IL-7-rich environment. As discussed earlier, this movement away from IL-7-expressing niches may be associated with their reduced proliferation, induction of *Rag* gene expression, and Ig light chain recombination. Finally, newly produced B cells exit the BM.[18]

IL-7 in Humans

The precise role of IL-7 during human B-cell development is unclear. Human CD34+CD19+ pro-B cells proliferate in response to IL-7, but human B lymphopoiesis may not be dependent on IL-7, because B cells are present in patients whose B lineage cells express a mutated IL-7Rα chain. In addition, B cells are present in patients with X-linked severe combined immunodeficiency; these individuals have mutations in the gene encoding the cytokine common γ chain, which is part of the receptor for IL-7.[19] Other receptors that could compensate for the loss of IL-7 receptor signaling have not been identified.

Systemic Factors

In addition to regulation by microenvironmental factors, there is a growing appreciation that systemic factors, and those of endocrine origin in particular, also regulate B-cell development. For example, B-cell development in mice is dependent on the integrity of the pituitary–thyroid axis because mice deficient in the production of thyroid hormone or expression of the thyroid hormone receptor exhibit suppressed BM B lymphopoiesis. Whether or not these events also occur in human B lymphopoiesis has not been established. It also has been demonstrated that hormones can negatively affect B-cell development. In particular, increased levels of estrogens occurring during pregnancy inhibit lymphopoiesis.

FETAL B-CELL DEVELOPMENT

Most knowledge of fetal hematopoiesis is based on studies in mice. It has long been recognized that some blood cells in that species are generated prior to the appearance of HSCs in an early wave of hematopoiesis that occurs in tissues such as the yolk sac. It has traditionally been thought that this pre-HSC wave of development is restricted to the production of erythroid and selected myeloid cells. However, emerging data suggest that B- and T-cell potential is also associated with this early wave of hematopoiesis.[20,21] The contribution of B cells generated in this pre-HSC phase to the adult immune system remains to be determined. HSCs are generated at embryonic day 10.5 of murine gestation, and their B lineage progeny can be detected several days thereafter in fetal liver, BM, and spleen.

Studies of human fetal B-cell development are limited. Hematopoiesis initiates in the human yolk sac at 3 weeks of gestation, pre-B cells are present in human fetal liver by week 8 of gestation, and surface IgM+ cells are detectable at week 9. IgM-expressing cells have also been observed in additional human fetal tissues that include the omentum, the peritoneal cavity, and the spleen.

B-1 B Cells in Mice

The B cells that are produced in adult BM and that constitute the majority of B cells in the spleen and lymph nodes are often referred to as B-2 B cells. This nomenclature serves to contrast them with another functionally distinct population of mature B cells that are referred to as B-1 B cells. B-1 B cells are best characterized in mice, where they constitute around 5% of total B lymphocytes. Murine B-1 B cells preferentially localize in serous cavities and can be distinguished by their unusual phenotype that includes high levels of sIgM, low levels of sIgD, and CD11b, a determinant expressed on myeloid cells. B-1 B cells can be further subdivided into B-1a B cells that are CD5+ and B-1b B cells that do not express this determinant. Antibodies from B-1 B cells, at least in mice, are required for protection against pathogens such as *Streptococcus pneumoniae*.

B-1 B cells are generated most efficiently from precursors that arise in the fetus. Thus, although HSCs from fetal liver can efficiently generate both B-1 and B-2 B cells, those from the adult primarily produce B-2 B lymphocytes. These observations support the long-held view that B-1 cells are a distinct B-cell lineage preferentially derived from fetal precursors.[22] The description of a phenotypically identifiable B-1 B-cell–specified progenitor that is preferentially generated in the fetus provided strong support for this view.

The regulation of B-1 and B-2 development is distinct, providing further support for the conclusion that these are distinct B-cell populations. For example, although B-2 B-cell development is blocked in IL-7-deficient mice, B-1 development can occur. More recently, the preferential generation of B-1 B cells from fetal progenitors has been linked to the expression of the Lin28b miRNA binding factor by fetal HSCs and B lineage progenitors. Adult HSCs are Lin28b−, but ectopic Lin28b expression in adult hematopoietic stem/progenitor cells results in their ability to generate B-1 B cells, and B-1a B cells in particular.[23]

B-1 B Cells in Humans

B-1a B cells in mice are CD5+, and many studies have claimed to have identified human B-1 cells based on simultaneous expression of

CD5 and sIgM. These reports must be viewed with caution because CD5 is not a B-1–restricted determinant. Thus the identification of B-1 B cells in humans has proven elusive. However, a CD20$^+$ CD27$^+$ CD43$^+$ CD70$^-$ population of cord blood B cells that has properties consistent with their being classified as human B-1 cells was recently described.[24] The further characterization of human B-1 B cells and studies to define their origin remain areas of active investigation.

SECONDARY LYMPHOID COMPARTMENTS

Newly produced B cells are functionally immature, and they complete their final differentiation steps in peripheral, also referred to as secondary, lymphoid tissues. These events in the mouse occur in the spleen. During this process, the BM-derived surface IgM$^+$ B cells transit through transitional stages of development before generating marginal zone (MZ) or follicular (FO) B cells (Fig. 20.1). MZ B cells are rapidly recruited in the immune response and play a critical role in the response to T-independent antigens. FO B cells are poised to respond to T-dependent antigens, which, as their name implies, require help from T cells. The localization of MZ and FO B cells in distinct anatomic sites and their intraorgan migration during the response to antigenic stimulation is governed by a variety of cytokines and chemokines.[25,26]

Transitional B Cells

Two stages of transitional B-cell development have been defined. The most immature transitional cells, referred to as transitional 1 (T1) B cells, localize at the outer edge of the periarterial lymphoid sheath (PALS; see Figs. 20.1 and 20.5). The PALS in mice is occupied by a considerable number of T cells, but in humans few T cells are present in this region. T1 B cells give rise to a more mature population of splenic B cells, referred to as transitional 2 (T2) cells. Each of these transitional cell stages can be phenotypically distinguished.

The T1 and T2 populations respond differentially to developmental stimuli, and a considerable degree of selection occurs during the T1 to T2 transition. For example, T1 cells with BCR specificities for blood-borne self-antigens are deleted by negative selection. Positive selection via BCR signaling must occur, and if it does not, the T2 cells will die by neglect. The survival of T2 cells, but not T1 cells, is also dependent on the B-cell growth factor BAFF (BLyS, TALL-1, THANK, zTNF4), which is produced by the splenic microenvironment. A fraction of T2 cells are no longer in the G0 phase of the cell cycle, suggesting they are in a more activated state than is the case for T1 cells.

Various signals determine whether T2 cells mature into MZ or FO B cells.[26] Weak signaling through the BCR along with engagement of the Notch2 receptor promotes entry into the MZ B-cell compartment. There is a marked depletion of MZ B cells when the Notch2 pathway is blocked. Self-reactive B cells are enriched within the MZ population, suggesting that weak self-antigens may play an important role in their generation. This feature may permit them to respond rapidly to cross-reactive epitopes on pathogens. BCR signals, along with activation of the alternative NFκB pathway, are required for T2 cells to mature into an FO B cell. It is estimated based on murine studies that only 1% to 3% of splenic transitional B cells develop into mature, naive B cells.

MZ B Cells

MZ B cells localize at the outer limit of the splenic white pulp in an area known as the *marginal zone* (see Fig. 20.5). This region also contains macrophages and dendritic cells. MZ B cells play a role in T-independent responses elicited by polymeric antigens, such as polysaccharides, that are composed of repetitive antigenic epitopes. On antigen binding, MZ B cells undergo rapid proliferation and maturation into plasma cells that secrete low-affinity IgM and IgG3

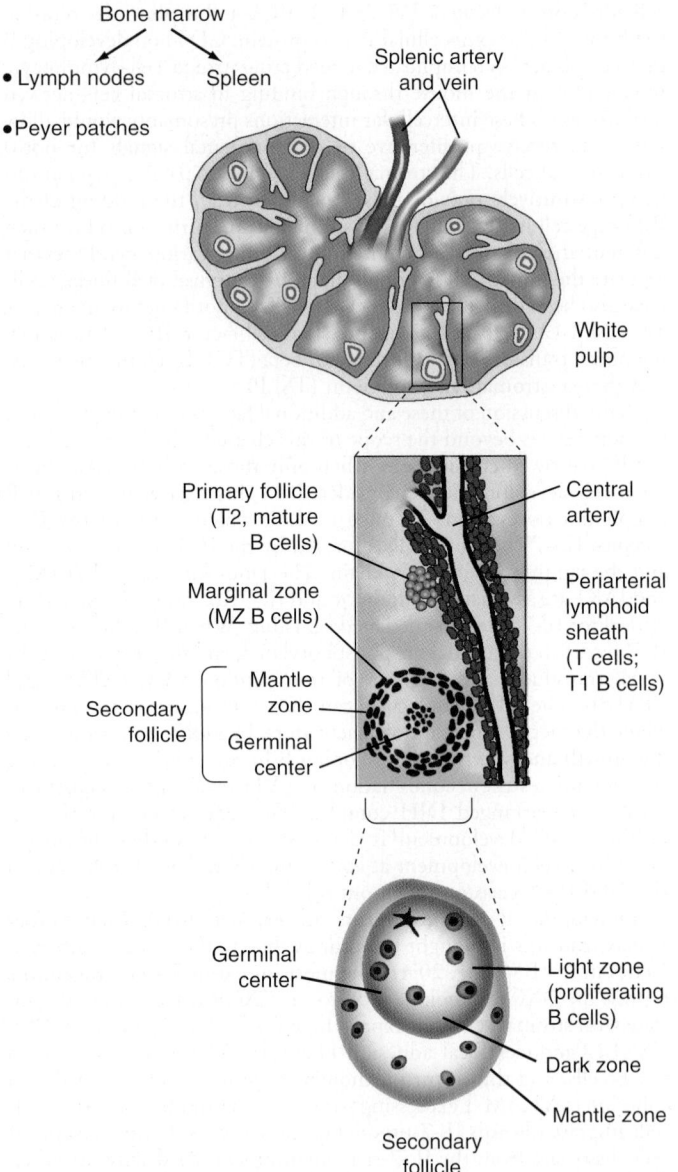

Fig. 20.5 ORGANIZATION OF B CELLS IN SECONDARY LYMPHOID ORGANS WITH EMPHASIS ON THE SPLEEN. *MZ*, Marginal zone.

antibodies that provide a first line of defense. The rapid response of MZ B cells to antigen has led to the idea that this effector population, similar to B-1 B cells, constitutes a key element of the innate immune response to bacterial and other selected pathogens. In view of this, it is not surprising that many of the properties of MZ B cells overlap with those of B-1 B cells.

Human MZ B cells are heterogeneous and include a large proportion of CD27$^+$ IgM$^+$ unswitched memory B cells with somatically mutated Ig heavy chains. The origin of this cell population is unclear but is presumed to be antigen driven yet may not require T-cell help. Although MZ B cells in rodents appear to be a static, nonrecirculating population, cells with a CD27$^+$ IgM$^+$ phenotype are clearly present in human peripheral blood as well as other lymphatic tissues. However, it remains unclear if these circulating memory cells can reenter the splenic MZ.

The poor response of infants to some types of T-independent antigens correlates with the fact that the MZ is not fully formed until the age of 1 to 2 years. In addition, splenectomized individuals are more susceptible to infection with some bacteria, owing to the deficient antibody response to capsular polysaccharides.

FO B Cells and Germinal Centers

When mature, naive FO B cells are generated, they recirculate and take up residence in various lymphoid tissues that include lymph nodes, intestinal Peyer patches, and the spleen itself. Within these tissues, mature naive cells localize in clusters of B lymphocytes, and each such cluster is termed a *primary follicle* (see Fig. 20.5). Within these regions, the FO B cells are poised to respond to antigen and undergo the germinal center reaction described later. Although some B cells in the MZ can respond to T-dependent antigens, most B cells that do so are the mature, naive FO B cells located in these sites.

After their binding of a T-dependent antigen (as soluble antigen, indirectly via presentation by a local antigen-presenting cell, or as an immune complex) mature, naive B cells in primary follicles undergo a blastogenic response. Some of these cells will immediately mature into plasma cells that secrete low-affinity IgM to provide a rapid initial response to infection. In response to T-cell help, however, other B cells undergo further proliferation and differentiation. The histologic appearance of the follicle changes as these events evolve. The nonresponsive B cells form an outer mantle zone surrounding the proliferating, antigen-responsive B cells in a central germinal center.

Germinal center B cells are shielded from soluble antigens and are exposed only to a unique set of antigens presented by follicular dendritic cells. Two regions can be distinguished within the germinal center of the secondary follicle. At one pole, the cycling B-cell blasts are referred to as *centroblasts* and form the dark zone. The other pole, referred to as the *light zone*, consists of nonproliferating cells referred to as *centrocytes* (Fig. 20.5). Some of these centrocytes go on to become memory B cells, which constitute about 40% of all B cells and are responsible for the relatively rapid response observed on secondary exposure to the same antigen. Others mature into short- or long-lived plasma cells that secrete high-affinity Ig. Plasma cells migrate to the BM where they associate with stromal cells secreting the chemokine CXCL12 and APRIL, a TNF-receptor cytokine similar to BAFF, that supports plasma cell survival (Fig. 20.4).

Immunoglobulin Class Switching and Affinity Maturation

After the initial low-affinity IgM response that helps to keep a developing infection in check, germinal center B cells can undergo three distinct modifications that can increase the affinity of the Ig for antigen.

Ig class switching involves deletions of germline DNA resulting in religation of the VDJ complex to downstream heavy chain C region genes, such as γ3, γ1 γ2b, γ2a, ε, and α. These DNA deletions are believed to occur at or near nucleotide sequences called *switch regions* that are located in the intron 5′ to each CH exon. These class-switching events are highly regulated, secondary-differentiation events that occur in spleen and lymph nodes and are potentiated by helper T cells and their secreted products. Note that Ig class switching is distinct from the previously discussed differential splicing events that allow the newly produced B cell to express the same VDJ complex associated with either the μ or δ heavy chain C regions.[27]

B cells may also undergo receptor editing. Receptor editing usually involves modifications of the existing light chain, in which an upstream V region segment joins to a downstream J region gene. As a result, the genetic region encoding the originally expressed light chain is deleted. For this process to occur, RAG-1 and RAG-2 expression is required. It has been proposed that B cells in germinal centers might reactivate *Rag* gene expression to mediate events such as receptor editing. However, that this occurs has been questioned. Instead, receptor editing in splenic B cells may be limited to a small subset of recent immature BM immigrants that enter germinal centers before their *Rag* expression has been extinguished.

Somatic hypermutation provides a third means to increase antibody affinity. During this process, single-nucleotide exchanges, deletions, and mutations are introduced into the genes encoding the antibody-binding regions of the Ig receptor. A B-cell-specific gene that encodes activation-induced cytidine deaminase (AID), which is expressed in germinal center B cells, has been identified. AID is a putative RNA-editing enzyme that acts as a cytidine deaminase and has been shown to be indispensable for somatic hypermutation and class switch recombination.[27,28]

These events are dependent on signals delivered to the antigen-responsive B cells by antigen-specific T-follicular helper (Tfh) lymphocytes that migrate into the germinal center from the PALS. Tfh cells mediate their effects on B cells through the secretion of cytokines as well as through direct intercellular contacts, and these stimuli result in B-cell growth, differentiation, and Ig class switching. For example, CD40 is a T-cell–surface glycoprotein encoded by a member of the tumor necrosis gene family, and its ligand is expressed on B cells. CD40 ligand knock-out mice do not form germinal centers, and humans who do not express CD40 ligand have X-linked hyper IgM immunodeficiency. Another key T-cell costimulatory signal includes the cytokine IL-10, which is secreted by T cells in response to their activation via the "inducible costimulator" (ICOS). Humans lacking expression of ICOS on T cells have adult-onset common variable immune deficiency, leading to a severe deficit in generation of class-switched and memory B cells.

There are two unintended consequences of affinity maturation. One is that autoreactive clones may be inadvertently generated. The other is the development of B-cell lymphoma. Lymphomagenesis results in part from the fact that vigorous B-cell proliferation, combined with the changes at the DNA level that lead to molecular alterations, may promote malignant transformation.[28] Numerous studies have assigned B-cell lymphomas to each of the normal B-cell counterparts described earlier. Events that limit differentiation of immature or activated mature B cells can also promote malignant transformation. Importantly, many genetic lesions leading to B-cell lymphoma directly affect the BCR signaling cascade, and improved understanding of these signaling events may lead to new therapies. These include application of Btk-specific small-molecule inhibitors in a broad range of human lymphomas.[29]

EFFECTS OF AGING ON B-CELL DEVELOPMENT AND FUNCTION

Studies of both rodents and humans have demonstrated that the quality of the immune response is diminished with age. Such declines are not incompatible with life, but they may become a factor when the individual is required to mount an immune response to a novel pathogen, respond to vaccination, or when considering the use of BM derived from older donors.[30]

The production of B cells from HSCs is severely attenuated with age, and the frequency and number of CLPs, pro-B cells, and pre-B cells is significantly reduced in the BM of old mice. Similar age-related reductions in B lymphopoiesis also occur in humans. B-cell progenitors from young and old mice have been compared, and this has revealed that expression of the *Ink4a* and *Arf* genes increases with age and is a factor that contributes to the diminished proliferation and increased apoptosis of aging B-cell progenitors.

In addition to declines in primary B lymphopoiesis, which reduces the number of newly generated naive B cells that are produced, senescence also affects mature B cells resident in peripheral lymphoid tissues. For example, in addition to an accumulation of memory B cells in the spleen of old mice, the Igs they produce are less protective because of low titer and affinity. Some of these defects may be intrinsic to the B cells but others may be secondary to age-related defects in T cells.

Although the molecular changes that underlie the aging of HSCs and B lineage cells are being delineated, the events that trigger the aging process are incompletely defined. One possibility is that HSCs and lymphoid progenitors are genetically programmed to age. An alternative hypothesis is that these age-related events occur secondary to changes in the local and systemic environments.

REFERENCES

1. Hardy RR, Kincade PW, Dorshkind K: The protean nature of cells in the B lymphocyte lineage. *Immunity* 26:703–714, 2007.
2. Sanz E, Munoz-A N, Monserrat J, et al: Ordering human CD34⁺CD10⁻ CD19⁺ pre/pro-B-cell and CD19⁻ common lymphoid progenior stages in two pro-B-cell development pathways. *Proc Natl Acad Sci USA* 107:5925–5930, 2010.
3. Blom B, Spits H: Development of human lymphoid cells. *Annu Rev Immunol* 24:287–320, 2006.
4. Ichii M, Oritani K, Kanakura Y: Early B lymphocyte development: similarities and differences in human and mouse. *World J Stem Cells* 66:421–431, 2014.
5. Pang S, Carotta S, Nutt S: Transcriptional control of pre-B cell development and leukemia prevention. *Curr Top Microbiol Immunol* 381:189–213, 2014.
6. Cobaleda C, Schebesta A, Delogu A, et al: Pax5: the guardian of B cell identity and function. *Nat Immunol* 8:463–470, 2007.
7. de Yebenes V, Bartolome-Izquierdo N, Ramiro A: Regulation of B-cell development and function by microRNAs. *Immunol Rev* 253:25–39, 2013.
8. Schatz D, Ji Y: Recombination centres and the orchestration of V(D)J recombination. *Nat Rev Immunol* 11:251–263, 2011.
9. Perlot T, Alt F: Cis-regulatory elements and epigenetic changes control genomic rearrangements of the IgH locus. *Adv Immunol* 99:1–32, 2008.
10. Schatz D, Swanson P: V(D)J recombination: mechanisms of initiation. *Annu Rev Genet* 45:167–202, 2011.
11. Yarkoni Y, Getahun A, Cambier J: Molecular underpinning of B-cell anergy. *Immunol Rev* 237:249–263, 2010.
12. Mårtensson I, Keenan R, Licence S: The pre-B-cell receptor. *Curr Opin Immunol* 19(2):137–142, 2007.
13. Reth M, Neilsen P: Signaling circuits in early B-cell development. *Adv Immunol* 122:129–175, 2014.
14. Clark M, Mandal M, Ochiai K, et al: Orchestrating B cell lymphopoiesis through interplay of IL-7 receptor and pre-B cell receptor signalling. *Nat Rev Immunol* 14:69–80, 2014.
15. Buchner M, Swaminathan S, Chen Z, et al: Mechanisms of pre-B-cell receptor checkpoint control and its oncogenic subversion in acute lymphoblastic leukemia. *Immunol Rev* 263:192–209, 2015.
16. Morrison S, Scadden D: The bone marrow niche for haematopoietic stem cells. *Nature* 505:327–334, 2014.
17. Nagasawa T: Microenvironmental niches in the bone marrow required for B-cell development. *Nat Rev Immunol* 6:107–116, 2006.
18. Beck T, Gomes A, Cyster J, et al: CXCR4 and a cell-extrinsic mechanism control immature B lymphocyte egress from bone marrow. *J Exp Med* 211:2567–2581, 2014.
19. Giliani S, Mori L, de Saint Basile G, et al: Interleukin-7 receptor alpha (IL-7R alpha) deficiency: cellular and molecular bases. Analysis of clinical, immunological, and molecular features in 16 novel patients. *Immunol Rev* 203:110–126, 2005.
20. Kobayashi M, Shelley W, Seo W, et al: Functional B-1 progenitor cells are present in the hematopoietic stem cell-deficient embryo and depend on Cbfβ for their development. *Proc Natl Acad Sci USA* 111:12151–12156, 2014.
21. Böiers C, Carrelha J, Lutteropp M, et al: Lymphomyeloid contribution of an immune-restricted progenitor emerging prior to definitive hematopoietic stem cells. *Cell Stem Cell* 13:535–548, 2013.
22. Kantor AB, Herzenberg LA: Origin of murine B cell lineages. *Annu Rev Immunol* 11:501–538, 1993.
23. Yuan J, Nguyen C, Liu X, et al: Lin28b reprograms adult bone marrow hematopoietic progenitors to mediate fetal-like lymphopoiesis. *Science* 335:1195–1200, 2012.
24. Rothstein T, Griffin D, Holodick N, et al: Human B-1 cells take the stage. *Ann N Y Acad Sci* 1285:97–114, 2013.
25. Cyster J: B cell follicles and antigen encounters of the third kind. *Nat Immunol* 11:989–996, 2010.
26. Pillai S, Cariappa A: The follicular versus marginal zone B lymphocyte cell fate decision. *Nat Rev Immunol* 9:767–777, 2009.
27. Matthews A, Zheng S, DiMenna L, et al: Regulation of immunoglobulin class-switch recombination: choreography of noncoding transcription, targeted DNA deamination, and long-range DNA repair. *Adv Immunol* 122:1–57, 2014.
28. Pavri R, Nussenzweig M: AID targeting in antibody diversity. *Adv Immunol* 110:1–26, 2011.
29. Young R, Shaffer A, Phelan J, et al: B-cell receptor signaling in diffuse large B-cell lymphoma. *Semin Hematol* 52(2):77–85, 2015.
30. Montecino-Rodriguez E, Berent-Maoz B, Dorshkind K: Causes, consequences and reversal of immune system aging. *J Clin Invest* 123:958–965, 2013.

CHAPTER 21

T-CELL IMMUNITY

Shannon A. Carty, Matthew J. Riese, and Gary A. Koretzky

INTRODUCTION

Thymus-derived (T) lymphocytes play an essential role in the immune response to pathogens and against host cells that have undergone malignant transformation. T cells are critical regulators of other arms of the immune system via soluble mediators they produce and through direct interactions between ligands on the T-cell surface and receptors on other immune cells. This chapter first reviews T-cell activation after engagement by specific antigens and describes how signals delivered by the antigen receptors shape the repertoire of mature T cells in secondary lymphoid organs. We then discuss how different populations of mature T cells exert their effector functions. Because homeostasis of the immune system requires not only that T cells become activated under appropriate conditions but also that their activity be curtailed once the pathogenic challenge has been met, we describe several means by which T-cell activation is terminated. Finally, we review recent therapeutic advances that make use of our understanding of the molecular basis for T-cell activation.

T-CELL ACTIVATION

T-cell activation begins when the T cell encounters a specific antigen that engages and then initiates signal transduction through the T-cell antigen receptor (TCR). Unlike B cells that respond to soluble antigens, T cells are stimulated by small peptides presented on the surface of other cells. These peptides are incorporated into the binding groove of proteins of the major histocompatibility complex (MHC, known in humans as human leukocyte antigen [HLA] complexes) through a process called *antigen presentation*. Thus the ligand for the TCR is a peptide surface that is generated from both amino acids in the antigenic peptide and residues found in the MHC molecules themselves. Engagement of peptide–MHC complexes by the TCR induces a series of intracellular biochemical events that culminate in T-cell activation. Although T cells make use of many of the same biochemical pathways used by other cells for activation, there are a number of molecules unique to immune cells that are critical for T-cell activation. This section discusses TCR signal transduction, focusing on immune cell-specific molecular events.

Antigen Presentation: Creating the Ligand for the T-Cell Receptor

Invading pathogenic bacteria and viruses use different strategies to survive within infected hosts. Many bacteria, such as the pathogens *Staphylococcus, Streptococcus,* and various enteric Gram-negative bacilli, survive in the extracellular milieu, whereas viruses and other bacteria, such as *Listeria,* survive inside host cells. Successful elimination of pathogens in each of these locations requires distinct responses from the host. T cells play a central role in the control of extracellular and intracellular pathogens; however, the subset of T cells differs for each type of pathogen, with T cells expressing the cell surface marker CD4 most important for the response against extracellular pathogens and those expressing the CD8 marker essential for control of intracellular organisms. Stimulated CD4$^+$ T cells act on other cells of the immune system by producing cytokines, soluble mediators that elicit a variety of cellular responses important for clearance of extracellular

pathogens, whereas CD8$^+$ T cells function largely by directly lysing host cells that have become infected with an intracellular organism. It is therefore critical for antigens derived from extracellular sources to stimulate CD4$^+$ T cells and for antigens derived from within the cell to stimulate CD8$^+$ T cells. Whether a particular antigenic peptide activates a CD4$^+$ versus a CD8$^+$ T cell is determined by which MHC proteins present the peptide to the TCR.

Class II MHC proteins are found on cells of the innate immune system known as "professional" antigen-presenting cells (APCs) as well as B cells and the thymic epithelium. Professional APCs include dendritic cells (DCs) and various tissue macrophages, which engulf extracellular organisms (often after these are coated with host antibodies), host cells that have undergone apoptosis (programmed cell death), and cellular debris through an endocytic pathway that brings the ingested material into contact with degradative enzymes. The peptides that are formed in these reactions are bound to the MHC class II proteins for presentation to T cells. The MHC class II complex is a dimer consisting of a single α chain and a single β chain. Both α and β contribute to peptide binding and interaction with the TCR. As they are being synthesized within the cell, MHC class II complexes bind invariant chain (Ii), a protein that directs the newly formed MHC proteins into an acidic vesicle. During this trafficking event, a portion of the Ii occupies the peptide-binding site. Once the MHC class II protein reaches the acidic vesicle, Ii is proteolyzed by cathepsin S, leaving behind a small fragment that remains lodged within the peptide-binding cleft of the MHC class II complex. This fragment is termed *the class II–associated invariant chain peptide (CLIP)*. The MHC class II–containing vesicles then fuse with other vesicles containing the peptide fragments from the endocytosed particles. There, CLIP is replaced with a peptide, thus stabilizing the MHC class II complex and allowing it to be transported to the cell surface, where it interacts with CD4$^+$ T cells (Fig. 21.1).

All cells of the body are at risk of being infected with intracellular pathogens or becoming transformed. Because protection against such challenges requires a CD8$^+$ T-cell response, all nucleated cells in the body express class I MHC, the protein complex that presents antigen to CD8$^+$ T cells. Like class II MHC, class I MHC is a protein dimer. However, in contrast to class II, only the α chain of class I MHC is variable. This α chain is associated with β$_2$ microglobulin, which stabilizes the complex but plays no direct role in antigen presentation. During its assembly in the endoplasmic reticulum (ER), the MHC class I complex comes into contact with peptides derived from proteins being translated in the cell. During protein synthesis, small amounts of protein are modified by ubiquitinylation. This serves as a targeting sequence, directing the modified protein to the proteasome, where it is degraded into small peptide fragments. These fragments are transported back into the ER by the transporters associated with antigen processing (TAP-1 and TAP-2), where they become available for binding to the newly synthesized MHC class I complexes. Peptide association completes the folding and assembly of MHC class I, which is then transported to the cell surface, where it can be recognized by CD8$^+$ T cells.

T cells can respond to antigenic peptides only if these peptides fit into the binding pocket of either MHC class I or MHC class II. Although a large number of peptides are able to bind to a specific MHC complex, the diversity of antigen presentation is enhanced through expression of three different MHC class I alleles (in humans, HLA A, B, and C) and class II alleles (in humans, HLA DR, DP,

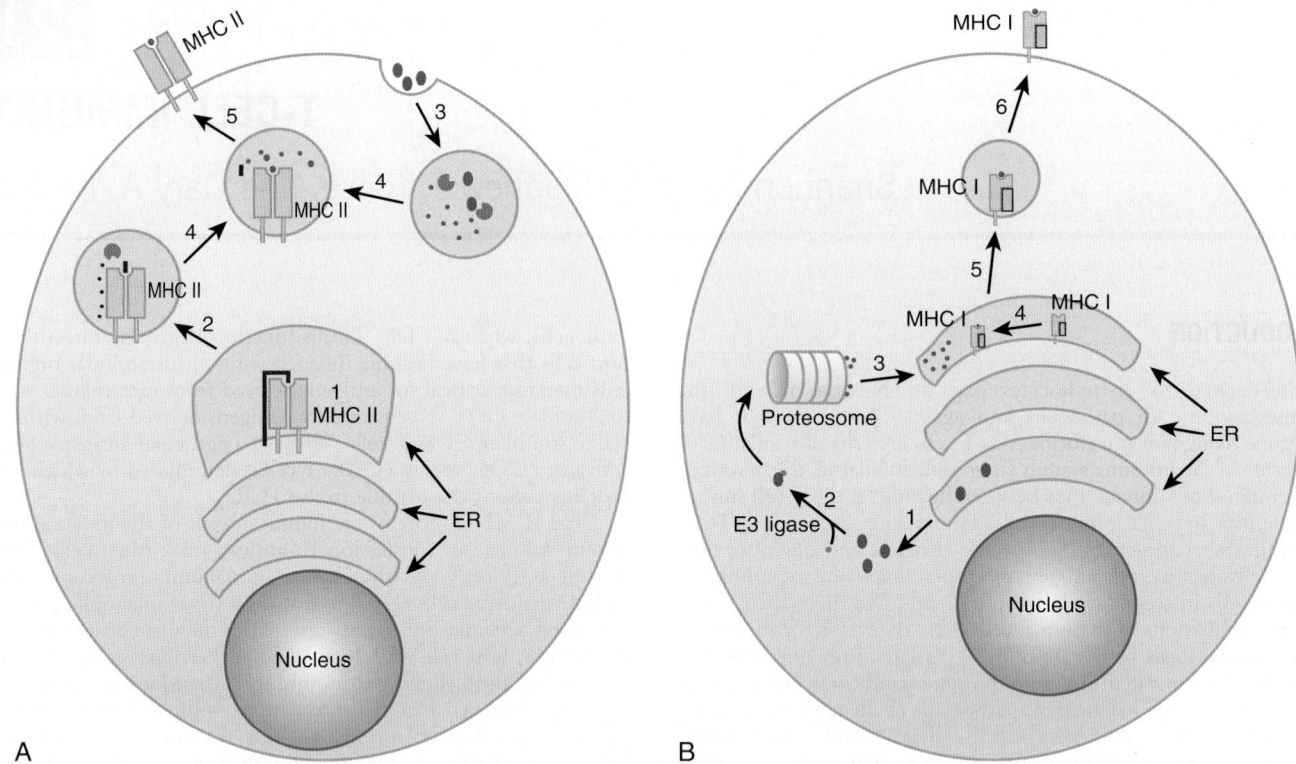

Fig. 21.1 ANTIGEN PRESENTATION. Presentation of peptides by major histocompatibility complex (MHC) class I and class II molecules occurs by different mechanisms. (A) Processing and presentation of class II peptides are limited to specialized antigen-presenting cells (APCs). *(1)* MHC class II molecules are synthesized in the APC endoplasmic reticulum (ER) in conjunction with a stabilizing protein known as *invariant chain* (Ii) *(purple)*. *(2)* After transport into intracellular vesicles, proteases degrade Ii chain, leaving only the class II-associated invariant chain peptide (CLIP) in the antigen presentation cleft of the class II molecule. *(3)* Peptides for MHC class II molecules are generated from extracellular proteins that are endocytosed from the surrounding milieu and degraded by proteases in intracellular vesicles after vesicle acidification. *(4)* Class II peptides are exposed to MHC molecules after fusion of peptide-containing vesicles and vesicles containing CLIP-loaded MHC class II complexes. After exposure to peptide, CLIP is replaced with a peptide derived from the ingested materials, and the vesicle moves to the plasma membrane, depositing the peptide-loaded class II molecule at the cell surface *(5)*. (B) All nucleated cells are capable of processing and presenting MHC class I peptides. Peptides for MHC class I molecules are generated from intracellular proteins that are synthesized in the ER *(1)* and transported into the cytosol. *(2)* A fraction of these cytosolic proteins become ubiquitinated by E3 ubiquitin ligases that target their proteolysis by the proteosome. Resultant peptides are subsequently transported back into the ER *(3)* and loaded onto MHC class I molecules *(4)*. Peptide-loaded MHC class I molecules bud into vesicles *(5)* that fuse with the plasma membrane *(6)*, resulting in cell surface expression.

and DQ). To increase the spectrum of peptides any particular cell may present even further, MHC alleles are always codominantly expressed. Thus any individual expresses a large number of different class II dimers on its APCs and class I dimers on all nucleated cells, providing excellent protection against potential pathogenic organisms. It is possible, however, that even with this degree of potential for antigen presentation, pathogens may evolve that do not possess unique proteins with sequences to fit into the MHC grooves. To circumvent this problem, the MHC locus evolved to be highly polymorphic, thus providing enormous diversity within the population for antigen presentation, ensuring that some individuals will express MHC dimers that can present antigens from virtually any pathogen. Interestingly, predominant MHC alleles exist in different parts of the world, suggesting that there is local pressure, perhaps based upon prevailing microorganisms, that shapes selection of MHC expression.

Neither MHC class I nor MHC class II distinguishes foreign from host peptides as they fill their peptide binding grooves. Because MHC class II samples all ingested antigens and class I is stabilized by a sampling of all proteins produced by the cell, the majority of the MHC complexes are filled with self-peptides. The T cell must distinguish self from nonself to ensure that a response is directed only

against that which is foreign. Control over what antigens elicit a T-cell response is accomplished through selection of a population of T cells expressing appropriate TCRs (see T-Cell Development section later).

The T-Cell Receptor Complex

The TCR is a multimolecular complex with separate components able to bind ligand or to transduce an activating signal to the cell. The peptide–MHC binding regions of the TCR consist of an α/β heterodimer in the majority of T cells, and the related γ/δ heterodimer in a smaller subset of T cells. α and β as well as γ and δ consist of variable and constant regions. Similar to antibodies (see Chapter 20), the variable regions of the TCR antigen-binding proteins arise from rearranging gene segments that are imprecisely joined during T-cell development. This process allows for an extraordinarily diverse repertoire of potential antigen reactivity, although there are in total only several hundred genes that make up the α, β, γ, and δ loci. The germline configurations of the α and β loci are different, such that the α-chain locus comprises about 70 variable (V) segments, 60 joining (J) segments, and 1 constant (C) segment, whereas the β-chain locus

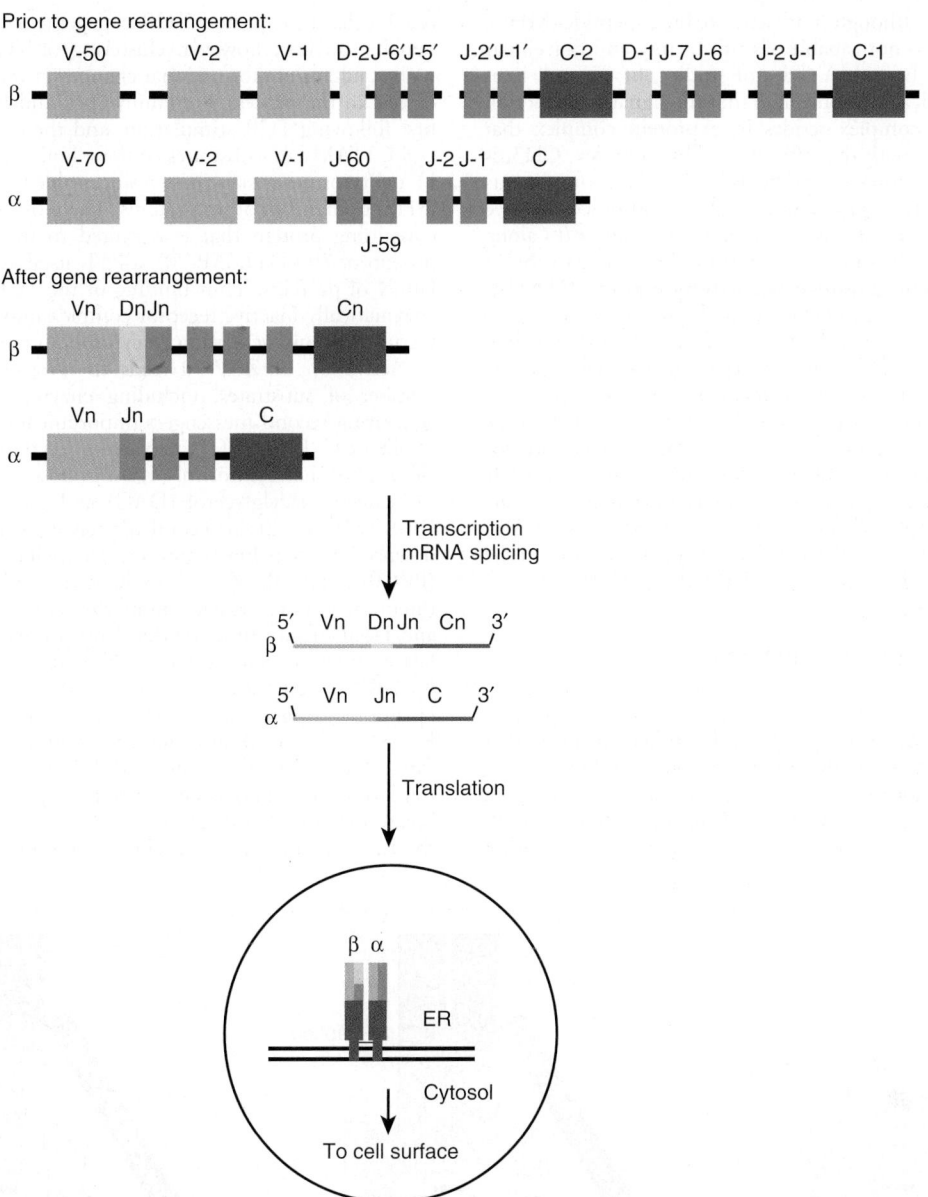

Fig. 21.2 GENERATION OF DIVERSITY OF THE T-CELL ANTIGEN RECEPTOR. To generate the diverse repertoire of antigen receptors needed for protective T-cell immunity, the genetic loci encoding the two proteins of the T-cell antigen receptor (TCR) undergo multiple rearrangements to form the mature α and β chains. For the β chain, DNA recombination occurs between a variable (V) segment, a diversity (D) segment, and a joining (J) segment to create, along with remaining joining segments and a constant region, a messenger RNA (mRNA) transcript. This transcript is spliced to remove intervening joining regions, creating the final mature β chain mRNA. For the α chain, recombination takes place between a V segment and a J segment, with the insertion of additional nucleotides between the recombined segments. As with the β chain, mRNA processing removes intervening J segments to permit translation of the mature α chain. After translation, β chains and α chains pair to form the TCR heterodimer that is transported to the cell surface. Note that peptide-binding regions of the TCR are generated from the recombined V(D)J segments of the TCR gene. *ER,* Endoplasmic reticulum.

comprises 50 V regions, 2 diversity (D) segments, 13 J segments, and 2 C regions. Greater diversity is generated by the addition of nucleotides between the V and J gene segments on α chains and the V, D, and J segments in β chains during the formation of the mature TCR. In total, it has been calculated that approximately 10^{18} different TCRs can be created from these segments, although the functional population is much smaller because of the requirements for selection during maturation in the thymus (see T-Cell Development section later). Thus, once it has completed its developmental program, an individual T cell expresses a unique TCR encoded by a combination of gene segments that have been altered and rearranged (Fig. 21.2). The T cells circulating through the lymphatics, lymph nodes, and spleen possess sufficient diversity for nearly all pathogens encountered to express an antigenic sequence recognized by a circulating T cell, which will then expand in number to combat that pathogen.

Soon after identification of the genes encoding TCR α and β, gene transfer studies in cell lines provided definitive proof that the α/β heterodimer contains all of the information necessary for peptide–MHC binding and that it is this protein complex that confers specific antigen reactivity on a particular T-cell clone. It also became apparent that although sufficient to bind peptide–MHC, the α/β heterodimer was not capable of transmitting an intracellular signal once ligand was bound. A series of studies, first in cell lines and then in mouse models, demonstrated that the signal transduction function of the TCR complex resides in a protein complex that associates noncovalently with the α/β dimer. This complex, CD3, is required both for stable expression of the ligand-binding components of the TCR and for signal transduction. CD3 is composed of three subunits, δ, ε, and γ, expressed as heterodimers (γ/ε and δ/ε) along with the ζ subunit, which is present as a homodimer. Each subunit contains immunoreceptor tyrosine-based activation motifs (ITAMs), a stretch of amino acids with discretely placed tyrosine residues: one ITAM in δ, ε, and γ and three ITAMS in ζ. The ITAM tyrosines are key for the CD3 and ζ chains to transduce signals and are inducibly phosphorylated upon engagement of the α/β TCR chains by peptide–MHC. Upon their phosphorylation, the ITAMs become docking sites for other proteins that initiate the signaling cascade for T-cell activation. Notably, the CD4 or CD8 protein also plays a role in mediating signal transduction. These coreceptors bind both the appropriate MHC complex (MHC I for CD8, MHC II for CD4) and, via their cytoplasmic tails, the signaling molecule Lck, one of the kinases capable of phosphorylating the ITAMs (Fig. 21.3).

T-Cell Receptor Signal Transduction

Once the genes were cloned for each TCR complex component, it became clear that, unlike many other cell surface receptors that transduce activating signals, neither the ligand-binding domains nor the CD3 proteins of the complex have intrinsic enzymatic function. Engagement of the TCR by the peptide–MHC was found to result in the rapid activation of protein tyrosine kinases (PTKs) within

the T cells. Exactly how TCR engagement initiates PTK activation remains unclear; however, clustering of TCRs on the cell surface with resultant conformational changes in the CD3 proteins appears critical in the process. Src family (Lck and Fyn) PTKs are activated first following TCR stimulation, and the tyrosines within the CD3 and ζ ITAMs are substrates of these kinases. Phosphorylation of the ITAM tyrosines makes these residues able to bind to Src homology 2 (SH2) domains of other proteins. The most important SH2 domain-containing protein that is recruited to the ITAMs is ζ-associated protein of 70 kDa (ZAP-70), a PTK itself and a member of the Syk family of proteins. Thus binding of the TCR by ligand converts an enzymatically inactive receptor complex into an active PTK through recruitment and activation of cytosolic proteins.

Activation of ZAP-70 leads to tyrosine phosphorylation of a number of substrates, including enzymes that catalyze reactions generating second messengers important for T-cell activation. Phospholipase Cγ1 (PLCγ1) is activated by its tyrosine phosphorylation to cleave phosphatidylinositol-(4,5)-bisphosphate (PIP$_2$) into the second messengers diacylglycerol (DAG) and inositol-(1,4,5)-triphosphate (IP$_3$). DAG is a lipid second messenger that binds to and activates downstream signaling components, including protein kinase C θ (PKCθ) and the Ras guanine exchange factor RasGRP. PKCθ, a serine/threonine kinase, regulates numerous effectors of gene transcription and T-cell effector function development, including the transcription factors nuclear factor κB (NFκB) and activator protein 1 (AP-1). RasGRP is responsible for activating the small molecular weight guanosine triphosphate (GTP)-binding protein Ras by enhancing Ras release of GDP, allowing it to assume its activated GTP-bound form. Active Ras collaborates with PKC family members to stimulate transcription of new genes by activating mitogen-activated protein kinase (MAPK) family members. IP$_3$ mobilizes calcium stores from the ER. This increase in calcium is important for enzyme function,

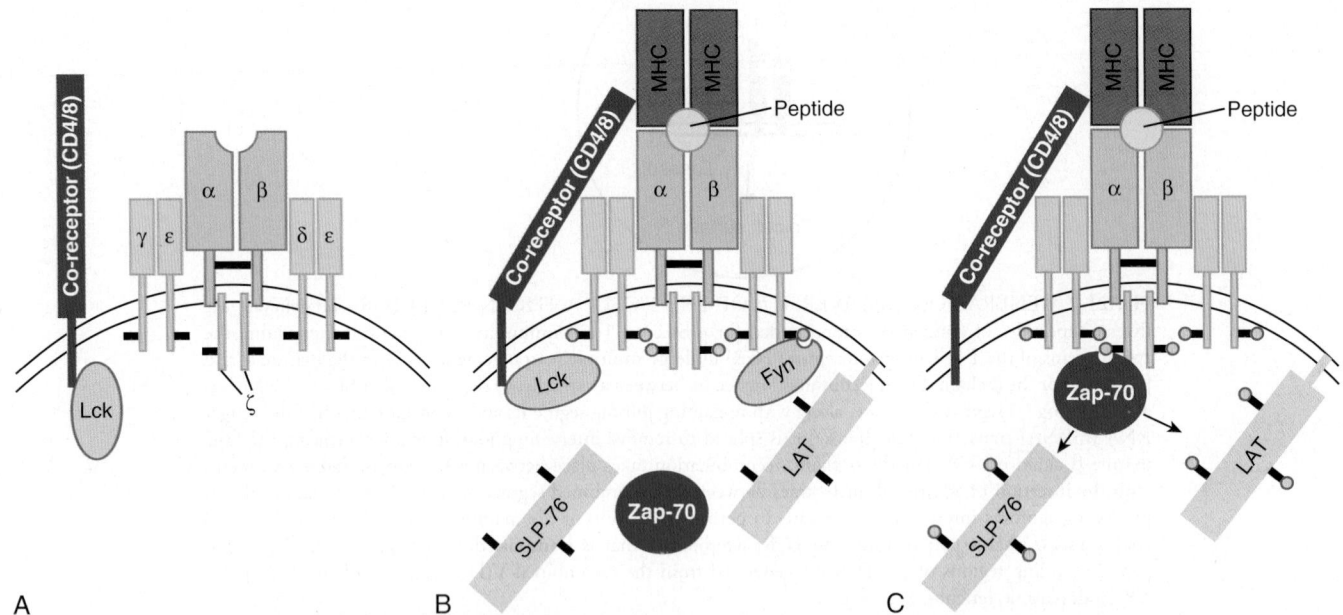

A   B   C

Fig. 21.3 PROXIMAL T-CELL RECEPTOR SIGNAL TRANSDUCTION. Binding of major histocompatibility complex (MHC) and peptide to the T-cell antigen receptor (TCR) and corresponding coreceptor (CD4 for MHC class II complexes and CD8 for MHC class I complexes) results in a series of molecular events that culminate in T-cell activation. (A) At rest, the TCR exists in a complex with CD3 that consists of heterodimers between δ, ε, or γ (δ/ε, δ/ε, ζ/ζ) chains (*olive, left* or *right* of the TCR) and homodimers of ζ chains (*olive, between* TCR chains). (B) Initially after ligand binding, the Src family kinases Lck (associated with CD4 and CD8) and Fyn (cytoplasmic) phosphorylate immunoreceptor tyrosine-based activation motifs (ITAMs) of CD3 and ζ (*black lines*). Note that the transmembrane adapter protein linker of activated T cells (LAT) is and the cytosolic adapter protein SH2 domain-containing leukocyte protein of 76 kDa (SLP-76) are not phosphorylated. (C) ITAMs serve as docking sites for the kinase ζ-associated protein of 70 kDa (Zap-70) that subsequently phosphorylates the adapter proteins LAT and SLP-76, which nucleate the complex containing signaling proteins.

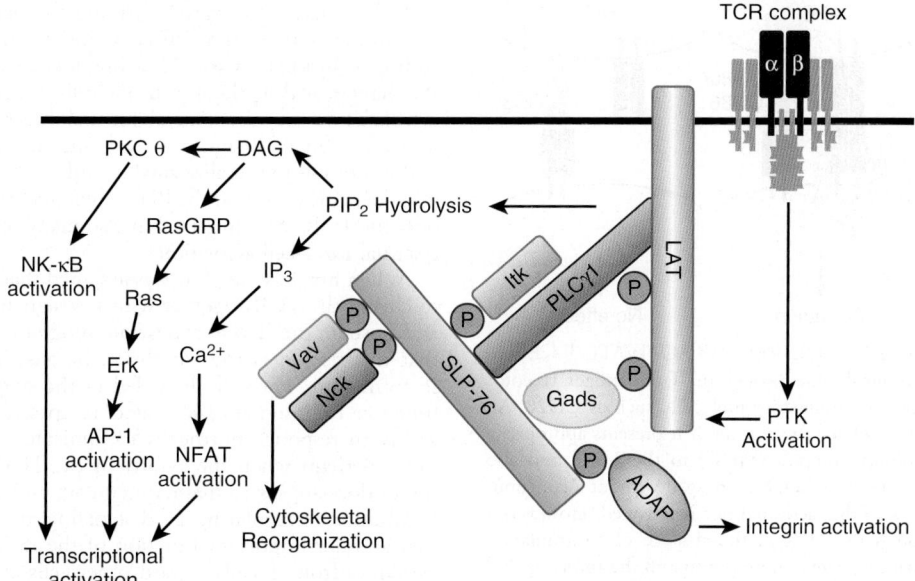

Fig. 21.4 INTEGRATION OF T-CELL RECEPTOR SIGNALS BY ADAPTER PROTEINS. Following engagement of the T-cell antigen receptor (TCR) and activation of protein tyrosine kinases, several hematopoietic-specific adapter proteins are phosphorylated, enabling the formation of a multimolecular signaling complex. The transmembrane adapter protein linker of activated T cells (LAT) recruits SH2 domain-containing leukocyte protein of 76 kDa (SLP-76) through the growth factor receptor-bound protein 2 (Grb2) family member Grb2-related adaptor downstream of Shc (Gads). This SLP-76 nucleated complex associates with phospholipase Cγ1 (PLCγ1), inducible T-cell kinase (Itk), Vav1, and degranulation-promoting adapter protein (ADAP). After phosphorylation by Itk, PLCγ1 catalyzes the cleavage of phosphatidylinositol-(4,5)-bisphosphate (PIP$_2$) into inositol 1,4,5-trisphosphate (IP$_3$) and diacylglycerol (DAG). IP$_3$ induces calcium flux from the endoplasmic reticulum, leading to activation of the transcription factor nuclear factor of activated T cells (NFAT). DAG binds and activates proteins important in signaling such as protein kinase Cθ (PKCθ), a kinase whose substrates initiate the activation of the transcription factor nuclear factor κB (NFκB), and Ras guanine exchange factor (RasGRP), a Ras-activating protein that induces activation of extracellular signal-regulated kinase (Erk) and formation of the transcription factor activator protein 1 (AP-1). Apart from transcriptional changes, T cells also undergo cytoskeletal changes after TCR stimulation mediated in part by Vav1, an activating protein for the actin-modulating protein Rac1, and activation of cell surface integrins, mediated in part by the adapter protein ADAP. *PTK,* Protein tyrosine kinase.

most notably the phosphatase calcineurin that dephosphorylates nuclear factor of activated T cells (NFAT), allowing it to translocate to the nucleus and transactivate genes necessary for T-cell proliferation, such as the gene encoding interleukin 2 (IL-2).

Although early TCR signal transduction studies demonstrated the importance of TCR-initiated PTK activity for T-cell activation, it took longer to unravel how this PTK activation drove the many critical second-messenger cascades. This mechanism was elucidated with the identification and characterization of adapter proteins, which possess modular domains important for intermolecular interactions. Two central adapters in the TCR signaling pathway are linker of activated T cells (LAT) and SH2 domain-containing leukocyte protein of 76 kDa (SLP-76). LAT is a transmembrane protein with seven cytoplasmic tyrosines that are phosphorylated by the PTKs activated by the TCR. SLP-76 is a cytosolic adapter protein that is also phosphorylated by these PTKs. Because these tyrosine phosphorylation events create docking sites for other proteins with SH2 domains, once the TCR is engaged, SLP-76 and LAT nucleate a large complex of signaling molecules at the membrane, in the vicinity of the activated TCR. This cluster of molecules initiates the signaling cascades that are integrated to result in T-cell activation. Key proteins in this complex are Vav1, a guanine nucleotide exchange factor important for cytoskeletal reorganization; inducible T-cell kinase (ITK), a member of the Tec family of PTKs (a third family of PTKs essential for T-cell activation); adhesion and degranulation-promoting adapter protein (ADAP), an adapter that is a key regulator of integrins to promote T-cell interactions with other cells; PLCγ, the enzyme described earlier that initiates both

the calcium and Ras/MAPK pathways in T cells; and growth factor receptor-bound protein 2 (Grb2) and Son of Sevenless (SOS), two proteins, like RasGRP, capable of activating Ras (Fig. 21.4).

For T-cell immunity to be effective, T cells must possess TCRs that are exquisitely sensitive to specific antigen. Because the TCR is generated through random reassortment and alteration of gene segments, it is impossible to prevent generation of TCRs that have the potential to respond to self-antigens. Although the developmental program of T cells in the thymus provides a mechanism to eliminate most potentially self-reactive T cells (see T-Cell Development section later), this process is not 100% effective. Hence mechanisms exist to prevent mature T cells from responding against normal host tissues. One such mechanism is the requirement for T cells to receive two signals to become activated, one mediated by the TCR and the second through a costimulatory receptor. Although several different T-cell molecules can provide this costimulatory function, the best studied is the surface protein CD28. This additional requirement for T-cell activation helps to prevent autoimmunity because the ligands for CD28 (CD80 and CD86) are upregulated on APCs only in the presence of "danger signals" generated largely by bacterial and viral components or in the setting of cellular stress. (The mechanism of how bacterial and viral components signal through Toll-like receptors to activate APCs is described in Chapter 23.)

For CD28 engagement to provide the second signal for T-cell activation, it must also initiate signal transduction pathways (Fig. 21.5). CD28 signaling not only augments those signals stimulated by the TCR (described earlier) but also delivers independent signals. The interaction between CD28 and its ligands triggers the activation of

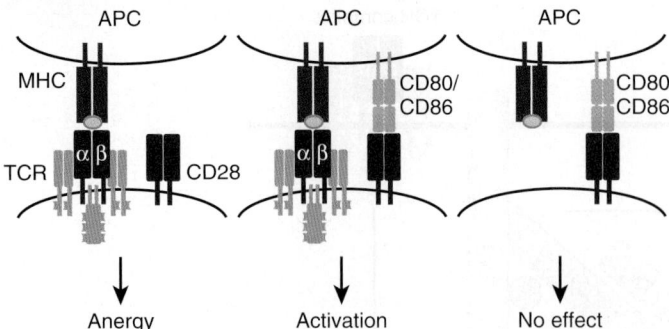

Fig. 21.5 TWO SIGNALS ARE REQUIRED TO ACTIVATE T CELLS. T-cell activation requires two signals, one through the T-cell antigen receptor (TCR) and one mediated by a costimulatory molecule, such as CD28. An antigen-presenting cell (APC) will activate a T cell if it presents appropriate peptide–major histocompatibility complex (MHC) to the T cell and also expresses a ligand to engage CD28. If CD28 is engaged without a concomitant TCR signal, the T cell is neither activated nor inactivated. However, if a T cell is stimulated through the TCR in the absence of costimulation through CD28, then it becomes anergic, unresponsive to the initial as well as subsequent stimulations.

phosphatidylinositol 3-kinase (PI3K), a protein that phosphorylates PIP_2 to form phosphatidylinositol-(3,4,5)-trisphosphate (PIP_3). Although the formation of PIP_3 induces broad changes within cells, the PIP_3 effector pathways that have been studied most intensively include two serine/threonine kinases: Akt, a PIP_3-binding protein responsible for regulating the metabolism of T cells to favor cell division, and $PKC\theta$, a protein required for cytokine production in T cells that is dependent upon PIP_3 generation for full activation. The importance of CD28 costimulation of T cells goes beyond its requirement for T-cell activation because engagement of the TCR in the absence of CD28 signaling induces an impaired functional state within T cells termed *anergy* (see Anergy section later in this chapter).

Although CD28 is the prototypical and best studied costimulatory receptor, a multitude of other costimulatory molecules are expressed on T cells and regulated in a spatiotemporal manner in response to environmental cues, including CD27, inducible costimulator (ICOS), and 4-1BB. These costimulatory molecules bind an array of ligands on other cells (primarily APCs). Stimulation of individual costimulatory molecules can uniquely influence T-cell activation, effector function, and survival. One of the mechanisms by which distinct costimulatory molecules play unique roles in T-cell responses is likely due to the differential activation of discrete signaling pathways through their intracellular signaling domains. For instance, ICOS contains a binding motif that recruits the more active subunit of PI3K, leading to enhanced AKT signaling compared with CD28 activation.

Spatial Coordination of T-Cell Receptor Signal Transduction: The Immunologic Synapse

As the biochemical signaling events that occur following TCR engagement by peptide–MHC became known, investigators sought to define the topography of the activation events. Sophisticated imaging technologies were applied to visualize the contact site between the APC and the T cell, and this interaction was modeled by visualizing the contact between key receptors on T cells and ligands fixed to a solid support. These studies revealed a stepwise reorganization of the T-cell membrane at the contact site called the *immunologic synapse* (IS). The first step in IS formation is an interaction between integrins on the surface of the T cell and their ligands on the APC that brings the T cell and APC into close proximity. If a productive interaction occurs between the TCR and peptide–MHC, the next event is clustering of TCRs in the central portion of the developing IS (the so-called central supramolecular activation complex [cSMAC])

with the activated integrins forming the peripheral supramolecular activation complex (pSMAC), a ring around the clustered TCRs. Although ligands on the APC initially direct the formation of the IS, changes within the T cell, including reorganization of the actin cytoskeleton, are also critical for stabilization of this structure. As sophistication of imaging in real time has advanced and with the advent of tools to visualize smaller and smaller numbers of molecules, it has become clear that the IS is a dynamic structure that includes not only the TCR and integrins but also many of the signaling molecules essential for T-cell activation.

When first described, it was assumed that the purpose of the IS is to cluster the TCR together with key signaling molecules to initiate and sustain the T-cell activation program. Recent work indicates that this notion is too simplistic, because TCR signaling precedes IS formation. These findings led to the suggestion that the IS may function to internalize activated receptors, thus terminating their ability to respond. Further work indicates that under other conditions, perhaps when the avidity of the TCR for its ligand is lower, the IS does appear to maintain contact and allow signaling to occur. In addition to regulating TCR signaling, more recent studies suggest that another important function of the IS is to focus the release of cytokines from T cells toward other cells of the immune system or materials from the lytic granules of cytotoxic T cells toward their targets, thus enhancing the ability of T cells to exert their appropriate effector functions.

T-Cell Proliferation

The number of naive T cells potentially responsive to any particular peptide antigen (the precursor frequency of the responding population) is quite small, yet a large number of antigen-specific T cells are required to combat pathogens. Accordingly, a consequence of TCR plus costimulatory receptor engagement is the clonal expansion of an activated T cell. One outcome of the second-messenger cascades stimulated by the TCR and CD28 is the production of IL-2, an essential cytokine for T-cell proliferation. Another outcome of TCR signaling is upregulation of the high-affinity receptor for IL-2, thus making the activated T cell able to respond to local concentrations of this cytokine. Signaling through the IL-2 receptor is necessary for the proliferative response. Similarly to the TCR, the IL-2 receptor makes use of cytoplasmic PTKs (in this case members of the Janus kinase [JAK] family) to initiate a cascade of second messengers that lead ultimately to T-cell proliferation. The details of IL-2 and other cytokine receptor signaling are provided in Chapter 16.

T-CELL DEVELOPMENT

Protective T-cell immunity requires populating the secondary lymphoid organs with a large number of mature T cells. Unlike most hematopoietic cells that complete the transition from progenitors to mature cells in the bone marrow, T cells develop primarily in the thymus. This population collectively must possess a diverse TCR repertoire capable of recognizing the enormous number of foreign antigens that will be encountered over life. Because the TCR binds antigenic peptide plus amino acid residues of self-MHC molecules, it is essential that only cells with a TCR able to recognize self-MHC, albeit with limited affinity, be exported from the thymus to the periphery. It is also critical, however, that the population of peripheral T cells be restricted to those that respond to foreign antigens, and cells possessing TCRs recognizing self-peptides plus MHC must not be allowed to complete their developmental program. Ensuring that only those cells with an appropriate TCR mature in the thymus relies heavily on many of the same TCR signal transduction events described earlier.

Of the T-cell lineages, those expressing the $\alpha\beta$ TCR cells are the best studied and most numerous. However, $\gamma\delta$ T cells, another population that possesses an antigen receptor generated through combinatorial rearrangement of gene segments, as well as natural killer (NK) T cells, a subtype of lymphocytes that has characteristics of both T and NK cells (see Chapter 22), are also generated in the thymus. It has become clear recently that additional small populations of T cells possessing unique characteristics are also produced in the thymus. This chapter focuses primarily on αβ T cells and touches briefly on γδ T-cell development.

Early T-Cell Development

Identifying T-cell progenitors is an area of intense investigation because developing tools to manipulate these cells has great therapeutic potential for increasing the speed at which T-cell repopulation may occur following hematopoietic stem cell transplant. A population of bone marrow–derived thymic settling progenitors (TSPs) that can give rise to mature T-cell populations has been identified. As these cells enter the thymus at the corticomedullary junction, they develop into double-negative (DN) T cells, characterized by lack of expression of the CD4 or CD8 coreceptors (Fig. 21.6). As these early T cells progress though the DN stage, they are further subdivided into DN1, DN2, DN3, and DN4 stages on the basis of the cell surface receptors they express. During DN1, TSPs lose the ability to differentiate into non-T lineages and begin to proliferate in the deep cortex of the thymus. As these early thymocytes progress to the DN2 phase, they begin to express T cell–specific markers, such as Thy-1 (CD90), CD24, and CD25, and initiate TCR gene rearrangement at the TCR-γ, TCR-δ, and TCR-β loci. Throughout the DN1 to DN3 stages, as the cells migrate from the cortex to the subcapsular zone,

interactions between Notch receptors on the developing T cells and specific Notch ligands collaborate with signaling through the IL-7 cytokine receptor to regulate lineage commitment and developmental progression.

During the DN3 stage, rearrangement of TCR-γ, TCR-δ, and TCR-β loci occurs with maximal efficiency, and initial expression of the TCR proteins these genes encode occurs. From this time onward in T-cell development, the proliferation and survival of the developing thymocytes depend on TCR signals. Two key checkpoints must be passed for full T-cell development to occur. First, upon productive rearrangement of the TCR-β locus, the TCR-β protein forms a "pre-TCR" complex with an invariant cytosolic protein designated *pre-Tα*. This complex engages the TCR signaling machinery, including the PTKs Lck, Fyn, and Syk (a ZAP-70-related PTK) and the adapters SLP-76 and LAT, to initiate the TCR signaling cascade. The resultant biochemical second messengers suppress rearrangement of the other β allele resulting in "allelic exclusion," or silencing of the nonrearranged allele, to ensure each T cell expresses only one TCR specificity. These signals also induce continued T-cell development by promoting rearrangements at the α locus, maintaining cellular survival, initiating a proliferative burst, and inducing expression of CD4 and CD8. For effective signaling to occur, the rearranged β locus must encode a protein that folds correctly and pairs with pre-Tα. Because the rearrangement of the genes that eventually make up the β chain is a random process, it is often the case that the rearranged allele encodes a dysfunctional protein. In this circumstance, signaling does not occur, and the cell initiates rearrangement at the other β chain allele. Again, if this does not result in a functional protein, no

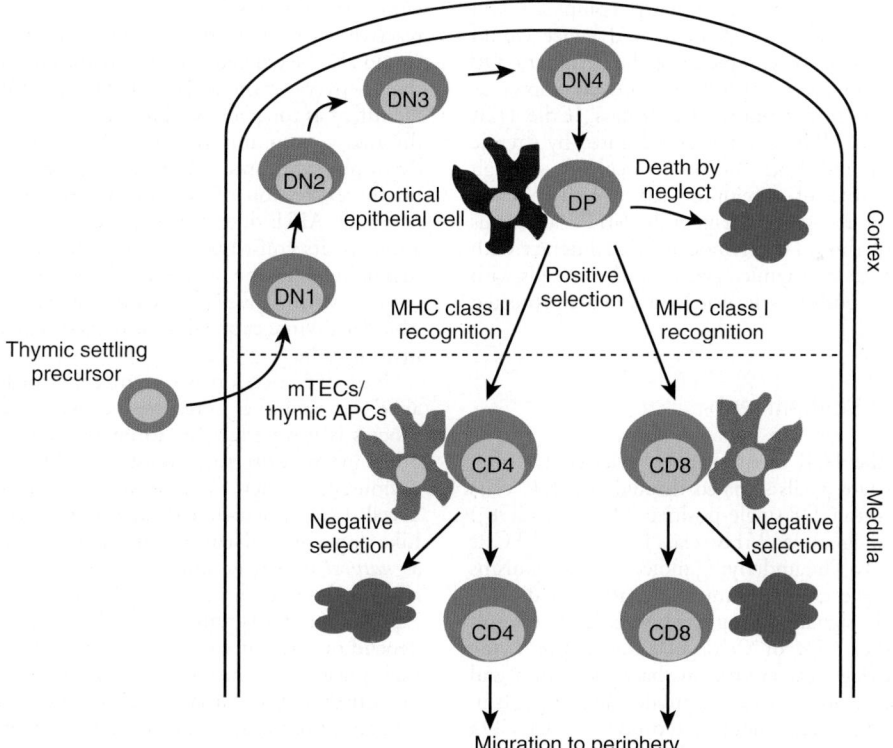

Fig. 21.6 T-CELL DEVELOPMENT IN THE THYMUS. Thymic settling precursors (TSPs) from the bone marrow enter the thymus at the corticomedullary junction. These hematopoietic precursors develop into double-negative (DN) thymocytes, at which time they lose the ability to differentiate into non-T lineages, express T-cell markers, and begin T-cell antigen receptor (TCR) gene rearrangement. Developing αβ thymocytes pass through the β-selection checkpoint before progression to the double-positive (DP) stage to ensure that the rearranged TCR proteins are able to transduce signals. DP thymocytes undergo positive selection if their TCR is able to recognize self-MHC molecules; otherwise, they undergo "death by neglect." Negative selection occurs in the thymic medulla, when cells bearing TCRs that bind with strong avidity to self-MHC with self-peptide undergo apoptosis, thereby promoting central tolerance. Mature CD4 single-positive (SP) and CD8 SP cells then emigrate to the periphery. *APC,* Antigen-presenting cell; *mTEC,* medullary thymic epithelial cell.

signaling occurs, and the cell undergoes apoptosis. In other cells, a similar rearrangement process occurs in the γ and δ loci. Productive rearrangements of these gene families create a functional, mature γδ TCR that also associates with the TCR signaling complex to propagate signals to trigger further cellular development.

Although the determining factors that result in either γδ or αβ T-cell development have not been fully elucidated, several molecular events are thought to contribute. The expression of a TCR gene rearrangement product likely plays a role in lineage determination because there is evidence suggesting that developing thymocytes with a functional γδ TCR are often excluded from the αβ cell fate. However, TCR expression is not the only factor in determining lineage fate; cytokine signals and TCR signal strength may also play a role. Experiments have shown that DN2 thymocytes distinguished according to IL-7 receptor expression differentiate into αβ or γδ T cells, with DN2 cells expressing high IL-7 receptor levels preferentially developing into γδ T lymphocytes and those with lower expression more likely to differentiate into the αβ lineage. Other studies have suggested that the strong signals propagated by the γδ TCR in comparison to those of the pre-TCR complex may promote γδ lineage commitment.

Positive Selection

Developing αβ T cells that have passed the first checkpoint demonstrating functional β-chain rearrangement transition into the double-positive (DP; CD4+CD8+) stage and complete TCR-α rearrangement to produce a mature αβ TCR heterodimer. The stochastic nature of TCR gene rearrangements guarantees that a significant proportion of cells expressing TCR-αβ complexes will not be able to interact with self-MHC proteins and hence would not be stimulated by peptide–MHC complexes in the periphery. DP thymocytes therefore undergo a series of tests, collectively known as *positive* and *negative selection,* to determine TCR fitness. If the TCR is not stimulated via peptide–MHC complexes presented by thymic APCs, the developing cell undergoes "death by neglect" through apoptosis. Approximately 90% of developing αβ DP thymocytes express a TCR that cannot recognize self-peptide–MHC and thus die by neglect. In contrast, those DP thymocytes that interact with self-peptide–MHC complexes on thymic cortical epithelial cells with sufficient strength pass this "positive selection" test and are protected from apoptosis.

CD4 and CD8 Lineage Commitment

The MHC specificity of the TCR on a positively selected DP thymocyte influences lineage fate. Cells signaled through a MHC class I–restricted TCR develop into CD8 single-positive (SP; CD4−CD8+) cells, and those that receive signals via MHC class II–restricted TCRs develop into CD4 SP T cells. The underlying molecular mechanisms governing CD4/CD8 lineage choice is much debated. Predicated on the thought that TCR signals during positive selection result in the termination of either *CD4* or *CD8* gene transcription, the two classical models of lineage fate are the stochastic selection and instructive models. In the stochastic selection model, TCR signals in a positively selected DP thymocyte randomly terminate either CD4 or CD8 expression. In the instructive model, certain TCR signal qualities, such as strength or duration of signal, direct termination of mismatching coreceptor expression. More recently, a kinetic signaling model has emerged. It proposes that CD4 or CD8 lineage fate is determined by TCR signal duration. Experimental models continue to be tested to fully elucidate the mechanisms underlying lineage fate.

Among the many proteins that are involved in CD4 or CD8 lineage choice are key transcription factors. One such example is T-helper-inducing POZ/Krüppel-like factor (Th-POK), a zinc finger protein that is expressed exclusively in CD4+ T cells and not in CD8+ T cells. In transgenic mice, expression of this protein forces the majority of positively selected thymocytes to adopt CD4+ T cell fate,

even those with MHC class I–restricted TCRs. In addition, mice with a spontaneous mutation in *Th-POK* lack virtually all CD4+ T cells, indicating that its expression is necessary for CD4+ T-cell development. Another important factor is RUNX3, a member of the Runx transcription factor family. As DP thymocytes differentiate, RUNX3 regulates CD8+ T-cell differentiation by silencing *CD4* transcription, promoting the initiation of *CD8* gene transcription and downregulating *Th-POK* expression. Additional studies have identified a network of key transcription factors and signaling proteins important for lineage choice in the thymus, underscoring the complexity of this stage of T-cell development.

Negative Selection

Although positive selection ensures that the random combinatorial rearrangement of gene segments results in a TCR that recognizes antigen presented by self-MHC proteins, until this point in T-cell development, there is no guard against the emergence of T cells that possess TCRs with high reactivity against self-peptides in the MHC binding pockets. Thus, to prevent autoimmunity, there must also be a mechanism to eliminate developing T cells with TCRs expressing these potentially autoreactive specificities. This process is called *negative selection*. Negative selection occurs primarily in the thymic medulla, where thymocytes serially interact with medullary thymic epithelial cells (mTECs) and other thymic APCs including DCs. At this stage, if thymocytes with TCRs engage peptide–MHC complexes with high affinity, a strong TCR signal initiates apoptosis. Whereas it is easy to see how this model allows for deletion of developing thymocytes with reactivity against self-antigens generated within the thymus itself, it was difficult to imagine how cells with reactivity against antigens known to be expressed outside the thymus would also be deleted. An explanation for how this occurs came from the discovery of the autoimmune regulator (AIRE) protein. Initially identified as the gene product mutated in a rare human autoimmune disorder, autoimmune polyendocrinopathy-candidiasis-ectoderm dystrophy syndrome (APECED), AIRE was later found to be essential for the expression of peripheral tissue-specific antigens by mTECs. Although AIRE does not regulate thymic expression of all peripheral antigens, its contribution to the elimination of autoreactive cells is highlighted by the widespread, multiorgan autoimmunity seen in patients with APECED. Identifying additional mechanisms responsible for thymic expression of tissue-specific genes is an area of active investigation.

Negative selection is one mechanism for development of "tolerance" or immune unresponsiveness to self-antigens; however, the process is not perfect in eliminating all self-reactive T cells. Hence, other means exist to promote self-tolerance after T cells leave the thymus. One such mechanism relies on development of regulatory T cells (Tregs), which actively interfere with effector T-cell function. Like conventional αβ T cells, a subset of Tregs (previously known as *natural* or *nTregs* and more recently designated *thymic* or *tTregs*) also develops in the thymus. Tregs are characterized by the surface expression of CD4 and CD25 (the α chain of the IL-2 receptor) and depend on the transcription factor *forkhead box protein 3 (FoxP3)* for their lineage commitment. The gene encoding FoxP3 was originally identified as the causal mutation in a rare, and frequently fatal, human autoimmune disease called *immunodysregulation, polydendocrinopathy, and enteropathy, X-linked (IPEX) syndrome.* A mutation in the mouse gene for *FoxP3* causes a similar disease (*scurfy* mice). These naturally occurring loss-of-function mutations demonstrate the necessity for Tregs in maintaining self-tolerance. In the thymus, development into a tTreg is enhanced in cells that have high-affinity TCR-peptide-MHC interactions, suggesting that these cells develop specifically to counter autoreactive responses. The exact mechanism that drives these cells to adopt a Treg fate and avoid negative selection during development is being investigated.

The path of developing γδ thymocytes contrasts with that of αβ T-cell development, which is likely related to the function of mature γδ T cells. In the periphery, γδ T cells reside in secondary

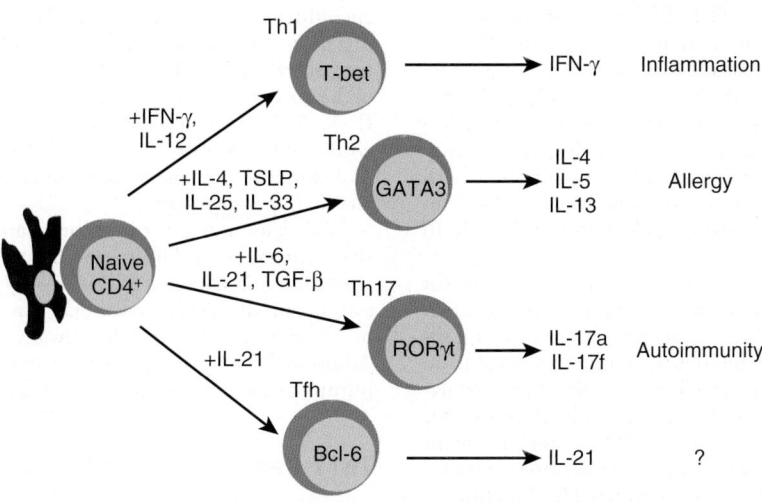

Fig. 21.7 DIFFERENTIATION OF CD4⁺ T HELPER SUBSETS. When activated, CD4$^+$ T cells differentiate into distinct, functionally mature effector subsets. Various factors, including the cytokine milieu, promote the expression of signature transcription factors and effector molecules. CD4$^+$ helper subsets are defined largely by their cytokine production driven by these key transcription factors. Th1 cells are induced by interferon γ (IFN-γ) and interleukin 12 (IL-12), express the transcription factor T-bet, and produce IFN-γ. IL-4 is the primary cytokine that promotes Th2 differentiation. Th2 cells are characterized by expression of GATA3 and production of IL-4, IL-5, and IL-13. Naive CD4$^+$ cells that are activated in the presence of IL-6 and IL-21 differentiate into Th17 cells, typified by the expression of retinoic acid receptor–related orphan receptor γt (ROR-γt) and production of the IL-17 family of cytokines. T follicular helper (Tfh) cell differentiation is mediated by IL-21. These cells are characterized by the transcription factor B cell lymphoma 6 protein (Bcl-6) and production of IL-21. If CD4$^+$ helper differentiation and activity are not adequately controlled, imbalanced responses can lead to pathologic conditions.

lymphoid organs with conventional αβ T cells but also are enriched in epithelial tissues of various organs, such as the skin, intestinal epithelium, reproductive tract, and lung. In these distinct settings, the TCR diversity of the γδ T cells is more restricted, suggesting that these subsets may preferentially recognize ligands expressed at these anatomic locations during times of infection or tissue damage.

T-CELL FUNCTION

As T cells leave the thymus, they circulate to secondary lymphoid tissues. Before interaction with their cognate antigen, these cells are designated naive T cells. As naive T cells migrate through peripheral lymphoid organs, composed primarily of the spleen, lymph nodes, and mucosa-associated lymphoid tissue, they sample various peptide–MHC complexes on APCs. These APCs include cells residing in the secondary lymphoid organs as well as those in tissues that sample their local environment and then migrate to the secondary lymphoid organs, hence concentrating antigen in these locations. If a naive T cell does not encounter its specific antigen, it leaves the lymphoid tissue via the lymphatic system to reenter the bloodstream and repeat this process.

When a naive T cell recognizes its cognate antigen on an APC, a program of proliferation and differentiation transforms the naive T cell into an effector T cell, now primed to respond rapidly upon encountering its corresponding antigen in the tissues. One important difference between naive and activated T cells is the cell surface expression of chemokine receptors and integrins. These receptors direct the cell to the appropriate tissue where the effector T cell is needed. Thus, as a part of the T-cell activation process, those receptors that direct the naive T cell in its pathway recirculating between the lymphatic organs and blood vessels are altered for those that direct the activated cell to the tissues, so that the effector T cell reaches the site of pathogen challenge.

CD4$^+$ and CD8$^+$ T cells undergo analogous differentiation processes to acquire functional maturity but play distinct roles in the adaptive immune response to infection. Naive cells of both lineages are activated through peptide-MHC interaction with their TCRs, and their differentiation is influenced by a combination of signals, including TCR signal strength, costimulation by ligands that interact with other T-cell surface receptors, and the local cytokine environment during antigen encounter. Integration of these signals promotes expression of signature transcription factors and key effector molecules, which allow the mature cell to perform its individualized function. Activated CD8$^+$ T cells possess the machinery to induce death in host cells that express the appropriate peptide within the binding groove of MHC class I (see later), whereas CD4$^+$ T cells exert their functions through the production of cytokines or by interacting with other immune cells through direct cell–cell contact following restimulation of their TCR by peptide presented by class II MHC. These so-called helper functions marshal and activate other cells of the immune system (Fig. 21.7). Until they encounter peptide–MHC, naive CD4$^+$ T cells have the potential to develop into one of several effector subsets, including Th1, Th2, Th17, and T follicular helper (Tfh) cells. Additional subsets have been defined recently, but these remain less well characterized and are not discussed in this chapter.

Th1 Cells

Th1 cells activate macrophages, NK cells, and CD8$^+$ T cells to combat intracellular pathogens. Th1 cells also stimulate immunoglobulin class switching in B cells for the production of immunoglobulin G2a (IgG2a) antibodies that optimize clearance of viruses and extracellular bacteria (see Chapter 20). During priming of naive CD4$^+$ T cells, several factors combine to promote differentiation along the Th1 pathway, including characteristics of the antigen, costimulatory signals from the presenting APC, and the cytokine microenvironment.

Several cytokines are implicated in Th1 differentiation, but the two most critical are interferon γ (IFN-γ) and IL-12. IFN-γ produced by innate immune cells promotes Th1 differentiation by activating signal transducer and activator of transcription 1 (STAT1), a key signaling molecule that regulates T-bet, one of the signature transcription factors associated with Th1 cells. IL-12, produced by activated APCs and other innate immune cells, acts through a separate STAT4-dependent pathway to promote IFN-γ production. IL-12 also signals to upregulate its own receptor and the IL-18 receptor, thereby allowing IL-18 to act in concert with IL-12 to promote IFN-γ production, thus creating a "feedforward" cycle to amplify the Th1 response.

T-bet, a T-box family member, is the key transcription factor associated with Th1 differentiation and function. T-bet-deficient T cells are defective in their ability to differentiate into Th1 cells either in vitro or in vivo, and T-bet-deficient mice are unable to control *Leishmania major* infection, a well-characterized intracellular pathogen model that depends on the characteristic Th1 cytokines for pathogen clearance. Whereas T-bet is considered the "essential" factor that directs Th1 lineage determination, other transcription factors, such as Runx3 and Hlx, are important for optimal Th1 function.

Once differentiated, Th1 effector cells are characterized by production of proinflammatory cytokines such as IFN-γ and tumor necrosis factor-α (TNF-α) that stimulate macrophages, NK cells, and CD8$^+$ T cells to promote pathogen clearance. It is clear, however, that Th1 function must be balanced. Evidence from both animal models and human patients indicates that overexuberant Th1 responses drive inflammatory conditions and may lead to tissue destruction.

Th2 Cells

Th2 cells are critical for the immune response against extracellular parasites, such as helminths, through production of IL-4, IL-5, and IL-13. At initial sites of parasitic infection, epithelial cells of the target organs, including the skin, lungs, and intestines, and resident cells of the innate immune system sense parasite-derived products and produce Th2-inducing cytokines, including thymic stromal lymphopoietin (TSLP), IL-4, IL-25, and IL-33. These cytokines then act on innate immune cells, including basophils and DCs, as well as directly on naive CD4$^+$ cells to promote Th2 differentiation.

Recent work has provided insight into how cytokine signaling, particularly IL-4 signaling, promotes Th2 differentiation. Through interaction with its receptor, IL-4 activates STAT6. STAT6 plays a vital role in Th2 differentiation, as evidenced by the profound reduction in development of this lineage in *Stat6*-deficient mice. STAT6 activation leads to its nuclear translocation and subsequent induction of the transcription factor GATA3, which, like T-bet for Th1 cells, is considered the master regulator of Th2 differentiation. GATA3 regulates Th2 cytokine production by binding and activating the "Th2 locus," which includes the genes encoding IL-4, IL-5, and IL-13. When GATA3 function is abrogated, Th2 differentiation is virtually absent both in vitro and in vivo. In mature differentiated Th2 cells, GATA3 deficiency results in loss of IL-5 and IL-13 production. GATA3 is both necessary and sufficient for Th2 differentiation because forced expression either by retroviral constructs or transgenic expression promotes Th2 differentiation and represses Th1 differentiation. Repression of Th1 development occurs at least partially through GATA3-dependent inhibition of STAT4, thus interfering with *Ifng* gene transcription.

TCR signal strength also is involved in determining if a naive T cell will differentiate into a Th1 or Th2 cell. Studies in mice using altered peptide ligands that have decreased affinity for particular TCRs and experiments using limiting doses of antigen have demonstrated that diminished TCR stimulation promotes Th2 cell differentiation. Differences in costimulation also affect Th2 pathway differentiation. Mice deficient in CD28 or its ligand have a more pronounced defect in Th2 responses, suggesting that these molecules may play a greater role in promoting Th2 differentiation than Th1 differentiation.

IL-4 produced by mature Th2 cells acts in a positive feedback loop to promote further Th2 cell differentiation in naive T cells as they encounter antigen. Th2-derived IL-4 also mediates IgE class switching in B cells. Soluble IgE binds to and crosslinks its high-affinity receptor FcϵRI on basophils and mast cells, promoting production of histamine and serotonin as well as several cytokines, including IL-4, IL-13, and TNF-α. IL-5 produced from Th2 cells recruits eosinophils, whereas Th2-derived IL-13 promotes both the expulsion of helminths during parasitic infection and also the induction of airway hypersensitivity.

Th2 responses are critical for immunity against extracellular parasites, but excessive Th2 responses are associated with the pathologic conditions of allergy and airway hypersensitivity. The increase in asthma in the developed world has been linked to an imbalance of Th subsets with skewing toward "Th2-ness" in the population. Additional work is necessary to more firmly establish a molecular immunologic link to the epidemiology of these diseases.

Th17 Cells

The original description of Th1 and Th2 cells, indicating that not all mature CD4$^+$ T cells were alike, led to the search for other CD4$^+$ subsets. Studies exploring the role of IL-23 in experimental autoimmune disease models found IL-23 to be critical for the generation of an IL-17-producing CD4$^+$ T-cell population, designated Th17 cells. Extensive analyses of IL-17 and the cells that produce this cytokine demonstrate that Th17 cells are important for the control of extracellular bacterial and fungal infections. With excessive activity, however, these cells also appear to play an important role in autoimmune diseases through the production of proinflammatory cytokines, including IL-17A, IL-17F, IL-21, and IL-22.

Although IL-23 is a key regulator of Th17 cells, the IL-23 receptor is not expressed on naive CD4$^+$ cells and hence could not explain the differentiation of cells into the Th17 subset. Subsequent studies demonstrated that the combination of transforming growth factor-β (TGF-β) with either IL-16 or IL-21 induces Th17 differentiation. The cytokines that are key mediators of Th17 differentiation and survival, including IL-6, IL-21, and IL-23, all activate STAT3. The critical role of this STAT family member was demonstrated in murine studies, when its deletion abrogated the ability of T cells to undergo Th17 differentiation. In humans, the importance of STAT3 was highlighted when it was identified as the genetic mutation present in many patients with hyper-IgE syndrome (HIES, or Job syndrome). HIES is a rare immunodeficiency syndrome characterized by recurrent staphylococcal skin abscesses, elevated serum IgE, and pneumatocele-forming pneumonias. Patients with HIES with STAT3 mutations have an impaired ability to form Th17 cells, which may explain part of their immunodeficiency. STAT3 regulates expression of many cytokine and cytokine receptor genes involved in Th17 generation or function, including IL-17A, IL-17F, IL-21, IL-21R, and IL-23R.

STAT3 is also important for induction of the signature Th17 transcription factor ROR-γt, which is a member of the retinoic acid–related orphan receptor (ROR) family. In naive CD4$^+$ cells, ROR-γt induces IL-17 gene transcription and promotes expression of the IL-23 receptor. Overexpression of ROR-γt induces Th17 differentiation, but deficiency of ROR-γt only partially affects Th17 cells in vivo because of expression of the related transcription factor ROR-α, which is also expressed in T cells and is induced by IL-6/TGF-β in a STAT3-dependent manner. Cells deficient in both ROR-γt and ROR-α lose the ability to undergo Th17 differentiation, both *in vitro* and *in vivo*.

Th17 cells are induced during the response to extracellular bacteria and fungi, including *Klebsiella pneumoniae*, *Bacteroides* species, and *Candida albicans*. Indeed, some patients with chronic mucocutaneous candidiasis have been shown to have mutations in IL-17F and the IL-17 receptor genes. Excessive Th17 cell function also plays a role in autoimmune diseases, such as rheumatoid arthritis, psoriasis, and Crohn disease, and therapies targeting the IL-17/IL-23 axis have been approved or are under active clinical investigation for treating these disorders.

Tfh Cells

In addition to Th1, Th2, and Th17 subsets, naive CD4$^+$ cells develop other functions dependent on the cytokines produced. Examples include recently described Th9, Th22, and Tfh cells. This latter subset enhances the humoral immune response by providing help to B cells during germinal center reactions. Tfh cells express high levels of CXCR5, the receptor for the chemokine CXCL13. The expression of CXCR5 permits differentiating Tfh cells to migrate from the T-cell zone to the CXCL13-rich B cell follicle, thereby allowing Tfh cells to interact with B cells and exert their function. In addition to CXCR5 expression, other signals, such as TCR signal strength and costimulatory molecules, are important for Tfh differentiation. A study using adoptive transfer of naive CD4$^+$ cells expressing high- and low-affinity transgenic TCRs demonstrated that high-affinity TCR interactions preferentially developed into the Tfh subset. Tfh cells have higher expression of multiple costimulatory molecules, including CD40L, ICOS, and OX40, than other T helper subsets. Because costimulatory molecules enhance B cell differentiation, the higher expression of these molecules on Tfh cells is hypothesized to positively correlate with the enhanced ability to facilitate B cell antibody production. It appears that the expression of costimulatory molecules on Tfh cells is important not only for their function but also for their development and/or maintenance, because both mice and humans deficient in ICOS have fewer Tfh cells with reduced germinal center formation.

Similarly to other CD4$^+$ helper subsets, Tfh programming depends on a signature transcription factor, in this case B-cell lymphoma 6 protein (Bcl-6). In Tfh cells, Bcl-6 acts as a transcriptional repressor. Studies employing complementary methods of T cell–specific Bcl-6 deficiency and overexpression demonstrated that Bcl-6 expression in T cells is both necessary and sufficient for Tfh differentiation in vivo.

CD4$^+$ Th Plasticity

Although CD4$^+$ T helper differentiation was classically thought to be a model of lineage specification and differentiation, it is clear that there is more plasticity in the CD4$^+$ Th subsets than was originally appreciated. Traditionally, Th subsets are associated with a signature cytokine(s) and transcription factor. However, recent data demonstrate CD4$^+$ Th cells can express more than one cytokine, particularly in vivo, and even the "master regulators" can be coexpressed in the same cell. The mechanisms that underlie this plasticity and its functional relevance are areas of active investigation.

CD8$^+$ Cytotoxic T Cells

The principal function of CD8$^+$ cytotoxic T cells (CTLs) is to kill host cells that have been infected with pathogens or that have undergone deleterious changes, such as malignant transformation. Like CD4$^+$ cells, naive CD8$^+$ cells initially encounter peptide antigen and MHC on the surface of APCs in the secondary lymphoid organs. However, unlike CD4$^+$ cells that are stimulated by class II MHC alleles on the APCs, CD8$^+$ cells are engaged by class I MHC plus peptide. For many years it remained unclear how APCs, which acquire peptide antigens largely by engulfing materials generated outside the cell, are able to present MHC class I–restricted peptides, which typically are generated within the cell (see earlier). This mystery was solved with the description of "cross-presentation," a mechanism by which APCs present engulfed antigens on both class I and class II alleles. Thus, tissue-resident phagocytic cells ingest virally infected or malignantly transformed host cells, degrade the ingested material, and present the peptide antigens in the binding grooves of both class I and class II MHC alleles. These activated phagocytic cells then migrate to the

lymph nodes, where they encounter recirculating naive CD8$^+$ cells. TCR engagement of foreign peptide–MHC class I complexes triggers activation of the CD8$^+$ T cells and initiates CTL differentiation. As part of its activation program, the CTL changes its expression of integrins and chemokine receptors so that it can leave the circulation and enter the tissues, looking for host cells displaying the same antigen that induced CTL activation by the APC in the lymph node.

Once an appropriate target cell is identified in the tissues, the CTL is again stimulated through its TCR, this time by the peptide–MHC class I combination on the target cells. A structure similar to the IS forms between the CTL and the target cell. The CTL contains specialized granules that are transported to the contact site between the CTL and target. These granules are modified lysosomes that contain effector proteins, including perforin, granzymes, and granulysin. Perforin facilitates the entry of the granzymes into the cytosol of the target cell. The granzyme family, consisting of granzyme A, granzyme B, granzyme H, granzyme K, and granzyme M, are proteases that degrade host cell proteins. Granzyme B is the best-studied family member and is known to cleave caspase 3, activating a proteolytic cascade leading to DNA degradation and apoptosis of the target cell (Fig. 21.8). Granzyme B also promotes cell death in a caspase-independent manner through cleavage of the proapoptotic protein Bid, promoting its migration to and disruption of the outer mitochondrial membrane, resulting in the release of cytochrome c. CTLs also produce cytokines, including IFN-γ, TNF-α, and IL-2. IFN-γ acts to inhibit viral replication in the affected tissues and also induces increased class I MHC expression, thus improving the ability of cells to stimulate the TCR on CTLs. IFN-γ synergizes with TNF-α for macrophage activation.

The transcription factors important for CD8$^+$ T-cell effector differentiation include two members of the T-box family, T-bet and Eomesodermin (Eomes). Initially identified as the master Th1-determining transcription factor in CD4$^+$ cells, T-bet also plays an essential role in CD8$^+$ effector cell differentiation. Recent work has shown that T-bet expression is highest in short-lived effector cells and lower in CD8$^+$ T cells destined to become memory cells (see later), suggesting that a gradient of T-bet expression controls the balance between different CD8$^+$ effector fates. Eomes cooperates with T-bet in CTL function, and cells deficient in both factors are unable to generate CTLs in response to viral infection.

MATURATION OF T CELL–MEDIATED IMMUNITY

T-Cell Memory

The activation of naive T cells does not complete their maturation process; instead, it is the starting point for the changes that result in T cell–mediated immunity. At the initiation of an infection, individual antigen-specific T cells become activated and expand robustly to combat the pathogen. As the pathogen is eradicated, the large population of activated T cells must contract dramatically to ensure homeostasis of the immune system. However, a discrete but relatively small population of antigen-specific T cells persists. These long-lived T cells have properties distinct from naive or activated T cells, including self-renewal through homeostatic proliferation and the ability to rapidly proliferate and regain effector function upon reexposure to antigen. These are the cardinal features of cell-mediated immunologic memory.

Immunologic memory refers to the observation that after an initial exposure and mounting of an effective immune response to a pathogen, subsequent interactions with that pathogen elicit rapid and robust T-cell activation, with more efficient clearance of the pathogen. Memory is the foundation of vaccination because immunization with pathogen-specific antigens induces a memory response so that first exposure of the host to the intact pathogen results in a rapid, effective response, thus abrogating signs and symptoms of the infection.

Within days of infection, subsets of activated effector CD8$^+$ T cells can be identified with different cell fates: those that are terminally differentiated and those that have the potential to develop

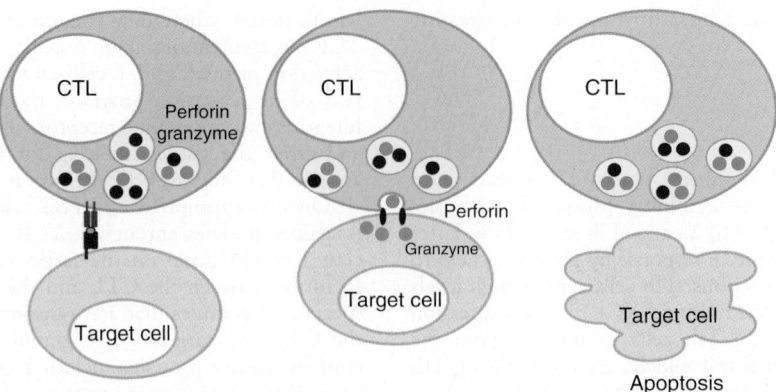

Fig. 21.8 CD8+ CYTOLYTIC FUNCTION. Cytotoxic CD8+ T cells function primarily to kill host cells that have been infected by intracellular pathogens or that have undergone malignant transformation. After naive CD8+ cells encounter peptide–major histocompatibility complex (MHC) class I plus costimulation in secondary lymphoid organs, these activated cytotoxic T lymphocytes (CTLs) leave the circulation and enter the tissues. There, upon interaction with a target expressing that same peptide–MHC class I, a CTL forms a lytic synapse, similar to the immunologic synapse, with the target. Cytoplasmic granules containing perforin and granzymes congregate at the synapse, and granule contents are exocytosed into the cleft between the CTL and its target cell. Perforin molecules facilitate entry of the cytolytic molecules into the target cells, and granzymes act to promote apoptosis of the target cell.

into memory cells. How memory cells develop from naive T cells is a subject of ongoing debate, and several models have been proposed. In one model, memory T cells are thought to develop from a broad pool of activated effector T cells, with most effector cells undergoing apoptosis and others surviving to provide memory. A second model suggests that when activated, naive T cells randomly differentiate into either effectors or memory cells. Recent studies using single-cell adoptive transfer experiments demonstrate that individual naive CD8+ T cells have the ability to differentiate into a heterogeneous pool of short-lived effector and long-lived memory cells, likely in response to differences in antigen specificity and duration of stimulation, precursor frequency, and the inflammatory environment.

Different subsets of memory cells are observed after resolution of infection. The two main classes are effector memory and central memory T cells. Effector memory T cells, characterized by loss of expression of lymph node homing molecules CD62L and CCR7, rapidly produce cytokines in response to restimulation with previously encountered antigen, thereby allowing for rapid responses to invading pathogens. These cells preferentially reside in nonlymphoid tissues, such as lung and intestinal mucosa, which are frequently sites of pathogen entry. In contrast, central memory cells express high levels of CD62L and CCR7, are more prevalent in lymphoid tissues, and mount a robust proliferative response after reencountering antigen.

As with differentiation of naive T cells into efficient effectors, cytokines play an important role in memory T-cell development and maintenance. IL-2 is essential for initial memory cell differentiation, whereas IL-7 and IL-15 are crucial for memory cell persistence. Other signals, such as the strength of antigenic and inflammatory signals during T-cell activation, also influence memory cell development and maintenance. An important consideration for memory development is cell–cell interactions because CD4+ T cells are required during initial priming of CD8+ cells for development of fully functional CD8+ memory cells. A number of infectious disease models have demonstrated that in the absence of CD4+ T-cell help, fewer CD8+ memory T cells are maintained, and those that do persist are of the central memory phenotype.

Although great progress has been made in elucidating the molecular underpinnings of immunologic memory, much remains to be learned. Recent data have emerged on the importance of the cellular metabolic state in the control of memory T-cell differentiation. As CD8+ T cells are activated, they transition from using primarily oxidative phosphorylation to generate basal energy in the quiescent state to using glycolysis during the effector phase and then back to using oxidative phosphorylation as memory cells. In experimental models,

manipulations of the cell's metabolic profile can influence effector function and memory differentiation. As additional discoveries are made, it is anticipated that new approaches will develop to improve T-cell responses to vaccines against infectious agents, to promote T-cell recall responses to pathogens that today result in chronic infections, and to harness host T-cell responses to combat tumors.

T-Cell Exhaustion: An Aborted T-Cell Response

Under most circumstances, acute infection results in the expansion of T lymphocytes specific for the inciting pathogen, clearance of the pathogen, and the development of memory T cells able to clear that pathogen more effectively upon reexposure of the host. However, some pathogens cannot be efficiently cleared from infected hosts and persist throughout the lifetime of the organism, despite the formation of pathogen-specific T cells. Examples of such pathogens include human immunodeficiency virus and hepatitis viruses B and C. These persistent infections result in chronic antigen exposure, which, instead of continuing to induce maximal productive T-cell responses, leads to the generation of "exhausted" T cells that have reduced ability to kill and produce cytokines in response to infection. The development of T-cell memory and the exhaustion response are initiated in similar ways, with the formation of cells that are capable of responding to antigen challenge through proliferation and the secretion of cytokines. However, during exhaustion, the persistence of pathogen causes T cells to become increasingly less responsive to stimulation. At early time points in this process, exhausted CD8+ T cells lose the ability to secrete IL-2 or TNF-α and cannot induce cytolysis of infected host cells. At later time points, CD8+ T cells become completely unresponsive and ultimately undergo apoptosis. The induction of exhaustion is thought to represent a functional adaption that permits some degree of control of chronic infection while limiting immune-induced tissue damage.

Concurrent with the loss of functional responses, exhausted cells upregulate inhibitory cell surface receptors. The best studied of these inhibitory receptors is programmed death 1 (PD-1), which binds its ligands, PD-L1 and PD-L2, expressed on activated macrophages and other APCs. Engagement of PD-1 dampens the T-cell response, likely by recruiting phosphatases that oppose the PTKs necessary for T-cell activation. PD-1 is normally expressed on T cells after initial activation, presumably as a means to prevent excessive responses, and is then downregulated as T cells acquire a memory phenotype after the pathogen clearance. Exhausted T cells, however, continue to express this inhibitory receptor. Early during exhaustion, PD-1 blockade reversed T-cell exhaustion in experimental models; however, other inhibitory receptors become expressed as exhaustion continues. Blockade of PD-1 with these other receptors has been shown to improve T-cell responsiveness, even at later stages of exhaustion. Therapeutic targeting of the PD-1 axis and other key inhibitory receptors is an exciting new avenue for immunotherapy against malignancies (see later) and chronic infections.

INHIBITION OF T CELL–MEDIATED IMMUNITY

Efficient signaling through the TCR and other cell surface molecules is required for initial T-cell activation. Similarly, appropriate maturation of the T-cell response to generate effector and memory cells is critical for adequate responses to pathogens. However, because of the potential for activated T cells to damage host tissues, an integral aspect of the immune system is also to negatively regulate T-cell activities. The mechanisms for inhibiting T-cell responses are critical for the prevention of inappropriate activation of naive T cells at the initiation of an immune response, for limiting the robustness of an appropriate T-cell response as effector cell functions are developed, and for terminating the T-cell response once an antigenic challenge has been met. This section discusses examples of how T-cell activation is modulated at each of these three critical steps of T-cell immunity.

Prevention of Inappropriate Initiation of T-Cell Responses

Given the enormous power of immune effector cells to damage tissues, it is essential that the immune system be nonreactive (tolerant) to self. As described earlier, T-cell tolerance is achieved centrally through the requirement to pass selection checkpoints during thymic development. However, negative selection in the thymus is not sufficient to eliminate all cells with potential autoreactivity, and some T cells bearing TCRs that may respond to self-antigens are exported from the thymus to the periphery. Mechanisms are in place to prevent these cells from becoming active effectors as they encounter antigen. Two such mechanisms are anergy, a process by which T cells limit their own responsiveness based upon engagement of particular cell surface receptors (a cell-intrinsic path to inactivation), and the action of Treg cells, which instruct potential effectors to remain quiescent.

Anergy

One means of limiting T-cell responses against host tissues is a process of self-inactivation termed *anergy*. As noted earlier, T cells require signaling through both the TCR and costimulatory receptors such as CD28 to become activated (Fig. 21.5). Stimulation of the TCR alone in the absence of adequate costimulation produces T cells that fail to secrete IL-2 or upregulate high-affinity receptors for this cytokine and hence fail to clonally expand. Cells that have been rendered anergic fail to respond to subsequent stimulation, even if ligands for both the TCR and CD28 or other costimulatory receptors are available. This two-signal requirement ensures that only APCs activated by pathogens or other "danger signals" can initiate an immune response, because ligands for costimulatory receptors, such as CD80 and CD86, for CD28 are upregulated only in activated APCs. Thus, under circumstances of pathogen invasion, APCs present peptide antigens to T cells in addition to CD28 ligands. In the absence of an immune challenge, APCs express only low levels of CD80 or CD86. If a T cell encounters an APC that presents a stimulatory peptide–MHC complex but lacks sufficient expression of CD28 ligands, the T cell does not become activated. In this situation, the absence of ligands for CD28 implies that there is no "danger" and that the antigen being recognized is derived from a self-protein. The result of such an encounter leaves the T cell in an anergic state, refractory to

activation even in the face of subsequent TCR stimulation by an activated APC.

The role of anergy in human immunology remains unclear, as investigators have largely used in vitro model systems and/or animal models. However, several lines of evidence indicate that there are self-antigen–reactive T cells that remain quiescent in normal human hosts. The biochemical basis of anergy also remains incompletely understood, but intriguing models suggest that an imbalance between the strength of Ras versus calcium signaling may be crucial. In this paradigm, it is the activation of calcium-dependent transcription factors, such as NFAT, in the absence of transcription factors activated by Ras signaling, such as AP-1, that confers an anergic state. Although anergy is classically thought to persist indefinitely, under some circumstances there is apparent plasticity, as exposure of T cells to high concentrations of IL-2 can improve functional responses in previously anergic cells. Thus the physiologic importance of anergy in limiting endogenous T-cell activation and preventing autoimmunity and whether there are times when anergy must be reversed for appropriate immune responses are areas of active investigation.

Regulatory T Cells

Tregs are a subset of CD4+ T cells that suppress the proliferation and cytokine production of activated T cells whose TCRs have been engaged by peptide–MHC, even in the presence of costimulation. Hence, as opposed to anergy, which operates in a cell-intrinsic fashion, Tregs block responsiveness in *trans*, by modulating responses of other cells. Tregs arise in two ways: "thymic" Tregs (tTregs) that acquire function during development in the thymus (described earlier) and "inducible" Tregs (iTregs) that are generated through the differentiation of naive CD4+ T cells in the periphery. Both tTregs and iTregs are characterized by expression of the key transcription factor FoxP3 and by surface expression of CD25, a subunit of the IL-2 receptor.

As noted, there are multiple steps and checkpoints that occur during development of T cells in the thymus. After reaching the DP stage, T cells test their TCR for reactivity against peptide–MHC complexes presented by thymic APCs and epithelial cells. Cells bearing TCRs with no reactivity undergo apoptosis (failed positive selection) as do cells with very strong TCR reactivity (through negative selection). Only cells whose TCRs have moderate affinity for peptide–MHC continue to mature. Within this continuum of permitted reactivity, those cells with TCRs exhibiting the highest affinity for peptide–MHC are induced to express FoxP3 and develop into Tregs. In the periphery, these cells respond to TCR stimulation by diminishing the response of "conventional" T effector cells, thus downregulating immune responses.

iTregs act similarly to tTregs, but these cells do not leave the thymus poised to have suppressive function. Instead, these cells arise from naive T cells that encounter antigen in the secondary lymphoid structures. Similarly to other CD4+ subsets, iTregs are induced on the basis of prevailing cytokine conditions and which receptor-ligand interactions predominate during this initial antigen encounter. Regardless of whether they arise in the thymus or are induced in the periphery, Tregs exert their immunosuppressive functions on a variety of immune cells, including CD4+ and CD8+ T cells, DCs, B cells, macrophages, and NK cells, within their microenvironment. Tregs mediate these immunosuppressive effects through the secretion of suppressor cytokines such as IL-10 and TGF-β, the consumption of local concentrations of IL-2, and the induction of apoptosis or cell cycle arrest through direct cell-to-cell contact (Fig. 21.9).

Limiting T-Cell Responses After Stimulation by Foreign Antigen

Even when stimulated appropriately to combat an invading pathogen, it is essential to limit T-cell activation. Unchecked T-cell effector functions present a danger to the host through production of

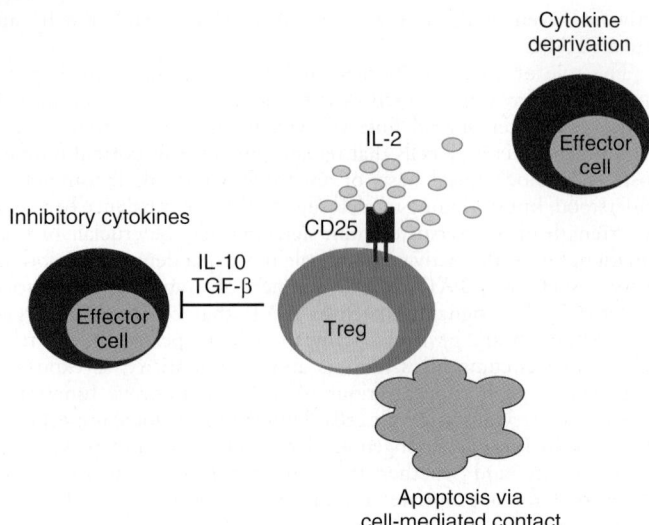

Fig. 21.9 T-REGULATORY CELL ACTIONS. T-regulatory cells (Tregs) act to suppress other T cells through a multitude of mechanisms, including the secretion of suppressor cytokines interleukin 10 (IL-10) and transforming growth factor β (TGF-β), consumption of local concentrations of IL-2, and induction of cell cycle arrest or apoptosis.

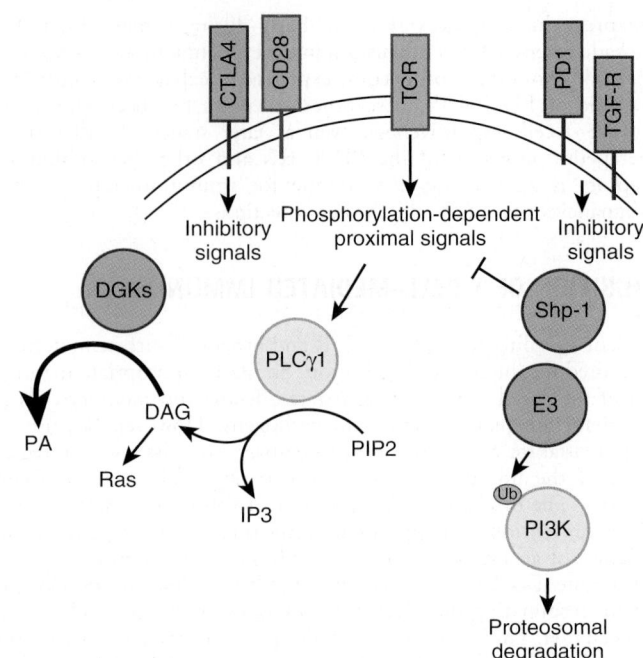

Fig. 21.10 INHIBITORY PATHWAYS IN T CELLS. Negative influences on T cells and T-cell antigen receptor (TCR) signaling take place at multiple levels within T cells and are crucial for the prevention of autoimmunity. Examples (indicated in *red*) include the protein tyrosine phosphatase SH2 domain-containing phosphatase-1 (SHP-1) that opposes early phosphorylation events mediated by kinases after TCR activation, E3 ubiquitin ligases such as Casitas b-lineage lymphoma-b (Cbl-b) that ubiquitinate key signaling mediators, such as phosphatidylinositol 3-kinase (PI3K), resulting in proteosome-mediated degradation and diacylglycerol kinases (DGKs), which terminate TCR signaling by metabolizing signaling intermediates such as diacylglycerol (DAG). Cytotoxic T-lymphocyte antigen-4 (CTLA-4), a T-cell surface receptor upregulated after activation, also induces T-cell inhibition, both by sequestering CD80/CD86 away from the activating costimulatory molecule CD28 and by transducing its own inhibitory signals after CD80/CD86 binding. Other well-established inhibitory T-cell surface receptors are programmed death 1 (PD-1), which is expressed under prolonged antigenic stimulation or "exhaustion," and the transforming growth factor β receptor (TGF-β-R), a receptor for one a cytokine key for regulatory T cell–mediated suppression. *IP₃*, Inositol 1,4,5-trisphosphate; *PA*, phosphatidic acid; *PIP₂*, phosphatidylinositol-(4,5)-bisphosphate; *PLCγ1*, phospholipase Cγ1.

proinflammatory cytokines that recruit other cells of the immune system and through direct damage of self-tissues. T-cell effector functions are limited by modulating the T-cell activation pathways through activation of signaling molecules that counter the second messengers stimulated by TCR engagement, through inducible expression of cell surface receptors that compete with activating receptors on the T cell, or by targeting key activating proteins for destruction, thus limiting their ability to promote T-cell effector function. Additionally, the local environment in which the T cell exists may change, with cell extrinsic factors (e.g., inhibitory cytokines) becoming available to dampen T-cell responses (Fig. 21.10).

Limitation of T-Cell Activity From Cell-Intrinsic Components

Protein Tyrosine Phosphatases

As noted earlier, the most proximal known biochemical event to occur following engagement of the TCR by peptide–MHC results is activation of PTKs, including Lck and Zap-70, enzymes central to the T-cell activation program. Thus one means by which to limit TCR signaling is to oppose the activating PTKs with deactivating protein tyrosine phosphatases, reversing the phosphorylation events that drive T-cell activation. Several such phosphatases have now been identified, including SH2 domain-containing phosphatase 1 (SHP-1) and protein tyrosine phosphatase, nonreceptor type 1 (PTPN1). Although the direct targets of these phosphatases have yet to be demonstrated conclusively, there is increasing evidence in murine systems that they are important for control of T-cell activation as well as for regulating the function of other cells of the immune system. Experiments show that, compared with wild-type cells, SHP-1-deficient T cells demonstrate enhanced proliferation and cytokine production after stimulation. These cells also show prolonged phosphorylation of TCR signaling molecules, consistent with a role for SHP-1 in reversing these events. Overexpression of SHP-1 within T cell lines inhibits TCR-mediated signaling events. Furthermore, SHP-1 is recruited into the IS after engagement of the TCR, thus providing an appropriate physical localization for SHP-1 to directly engage targets of the TCR-stimulated PTKs. SHP-1 inhibitory activity appears to be crucial in vivo because mice that lack functional SHP-1 develop fatal autoimmunity, likely secondary to alterations of

function of both innate and adaptive immune cells. There is accumulating evidence that other phosphatases are also critical for interfering with T-cell activation, both in animal models and more recently in studies of patients. Polymorphisms in the genes encoding several protein tyrosine phosphatases, including CD45 and *PTPN22*, align with susceptibility to human immune-mediated disorders. These intriguing findings are being pursued actively by researchers in a number of laboratories to uncover the molecular basis of how these phosphatases exert their control on immune cell function.

CTLA-4

A second strategy to limit T-cell activity is through the induced expression and activation of inhibitory cell surface receptors, such as cytotoxic T lymphocyte antigen-4 (CTLA-4). As discussed earlier, activation of T cells requires two independent signals, one through the TCR and a second through a costimulatory receptor such as CD28. Several days after initial T-cell activation, however, another member of the CD28 superfamily, CTLA-4, becomes upregulated on T cells. CTLA-4 differs from CD28 in that, instead of serving as an essential costimulatory receptor, engaged CTLA-4 actively interferes with T-cell activation. Moreover, CTLA-4 binds CD80 and CD86 with much higher affinity than CD28, thus sequestering these key ligands away from CD28. The importance of CTLA-4 in controlling immune reactions was highlighted in the study of CTLA-4-deficient mice, which were found to die as a result of autoimmune disease at 3 to 4 weeks of age. Targeting CTLA-4 with blocking antibodies to augment T-cell responses is a new therapeutic strategy for human cancer treatment (see later). Conversely, providing soluble CTLA-4 to patients with autoimmunity has been shown to be effective at blocking T-cell activation, presumably by acting as a competitive antagonist and interfering with the ability of CD28 to bind to its ligands, resulting in an anergizing signal to T cells.

E3 Ubiquitin Ligases

TCR signaling is also limited through the targeted destruction of proteins required for TCR signal transduction. E3 ubiquitin ligases are a class of proteins that target intracellular proteins for degradation by the proteasome, the large multisubunit cytosolic complex essential for protein turnover. In T cells, several E3 ubiquitin ligases target components of TCR signal transduction for degradation after TCR activation. These include Casitas b-lineage lymphoma-b (Cbl-b), c-Cbl, and Itch, among many others. As with other negative modulators of TCR signaling, genetic deletion of E3 ubiquitin ligases, either alone or in combination, results in dysregulation of immune function or the development of frank autoimmune disease in mice. The targeted degradation of crucial signaling modulators after T-cell activation thus serves as an additional physiologic mechanism to limit T-cell responses.

Diacylglycerol Kinases

Intrinsic cellular components limit T-cell activity through degradation of second messengers of T-cell signal transduction, such as metabolism of diacylglycerol (DAG) by diacylglycerol kinases (DGKs). As described earlier, engagement of the TCR results in the activation and recruitment of PLCγ1 that cleaves PIP_2 into the second messengers DAG and IP_3. DAG levels are regulated in T cells through the activity of DGKs that metabolize DAG to terminate its ability to transduce signals. Two DGK isoforms, DGK-α and DGK-ζ, are important for limiting TCR signaling, as deletion of either in mice results in enhanced proliferation and cytokine production after TCR stimulation. Moreover, deletion of DGK-α leads to impaired induction of T-cell anergy. Mice deficient in either isoform of DGK do not develop overt autoimmune disease, likely because of some biochemical redundancy between the isoforms, and, in the case of DGK-z, enhanced numbers of tTregs. However, enhanced functional responses to viral infection and tumors have been reported in DGK-deficient T cells, defining an important role for DGKs in limiting immune responses.

Limitation of T-Cell Activity From Cell-Extrinsic Components

Extrinsic factors also help limit the function and activation state of T cells. The predominant influences of T cells in this respect are inhibitory cytokines that bind cell surface receptors and influence transcriptional changes that favor decreased activation. Two cytokines that serve as a paradigm for understanding cytokine-mediated inhibition of T cells are IL-10 and TGF-β.

IL-10 is a major negative regulator of immune effector function. Its central role is underscored by the fact that pathogenic viruses, such as cytomegalovirus and Epstein-Barr virus, use homologs of IL-10 to subvert immunologic activity and create environments more favorable for viral spread and replication. IL-10 is produced by both innate and adaptive immune cells in response to activation. As with other cytokines, binding of IL-10 to the IL-10 receptor induces

signaling through JAKs, resulting in the nuclear translocation of STAT proteins and the implementation of a transcriptional program that results in decreased expression of inflammatory cytokines and in antagonism of crucial signaling molecules.

IL-10 exerts broad changes within the immune system. In monocytes, IL-10 decreases the production of inflammatory mediators and antigen presentation. In T cells, the effects of IL-10 are generally inhibitory, resulting in decreased capacity for proliferation and a decreased capacity to secrete cytokines. These effects vary by T-cell subtype, however, as IL-17 secretion by Th17 cells is not impaired in the presence of IL-10. As in other proteins important in the negative regulation of T cells, *IL10* germline deletion often results in fatal autoimmunity, in this case a gastrointestinal disease resulting from the inability to control inflammation caused by commensal bacteria.

TGF-β is a pleiotropic inhibitor that acts as a potent immunosuppressor. As noted, TGF-β is important both in its capacity to upregulate the transcription factor FoxP3, required for the generation of Tregs, and in inducing more global changes that favor immunosuppression. TGF-β binds its cell surface receptor complex and subsequently induces the phosphorylation, activation, and nuclear transport of intracellular Smad proteins. Effector Smad proteins exert their effects by directly coordinating transcriptional programs that inhibit immune responsiveness. Like IL-10, TGF-β acts on numerous cell types. It has been shown to inhibit the differentiation of effector Th cells; induce the conversion of naive T cells into Tregs; suppress the proliferation and production of IL-2 by T cells; and inhibit the activity of macrophages, DCs, and APCs. Mice lacking TGF-β1 develop autoimmune-mediated multiorgan failure and die shortly after birth, underscoring the important role that this molecule plays in attenuating immune reactions.

Terminating Immune Responses After Pathogen Clearance

The simplest way in which T-cell responses end following clearance of a pathogenic challenge is by the removal of antigen, which limits the perpetuation of T-cell activation and abrogates the recruitment of new effector cells. Effector functions of those T cells that were stimulated to respond to the pathogen challenge also diminish as the inhibitory mechanisms described earlier exert their effects. However, homeostasis of the immune system also requires that the majority of those T cells that emerged from the clonal expansion of antigen-stimulated cells (at its peak representing several percent of the hosts' T-cell pool) be eliminated, retaining only a small population of memory T cells responsive to the inciting antigens. Elimination of the expanded population occurs through activation-induced cell death (AICD).

AICD is initiated when CD95 (also called Fas), a T-cell surface receptor present on the activated effector cells, is engaged by its ligand (CD95 ligand), expressed on multiple immune cells, including the activated cells themselves. CD95 is a member of the TNF family of receptors and, when stimulated, recruits the adapter molecule Fas-activating via death domain (FADD). FADD creates a multimolecular complex that triggers the activation of several intracellular caspases that induce DNA damage and apoptosis of the effector T cell. During T-cell activation, both CD95 and CD95 ligand are upregulated on the surface of the cell, and all of the machinery is present to initiate AICD. Hence the default pathway for activated T cells is apoptosis, an event that is blocked when T cells are appropriately stimulated to respond to antigen. Once antigen is cleared and the stimulatory events cease, AICD takes over, reducing the expanded population of cells (Fig. 21.11).

Experiments of nature have taught us much about the biology and importance of both CD95 and CD95 ligand. Loss of these proteins as well as components of their signaling machinery results in the human disease autoimmune lymphoproliferative syndrome (ALPS). ALPS is characterized by massive enlargement of lymphoid organs, autoimmune cytopenias, and an increased risk of hematologic malignancy.

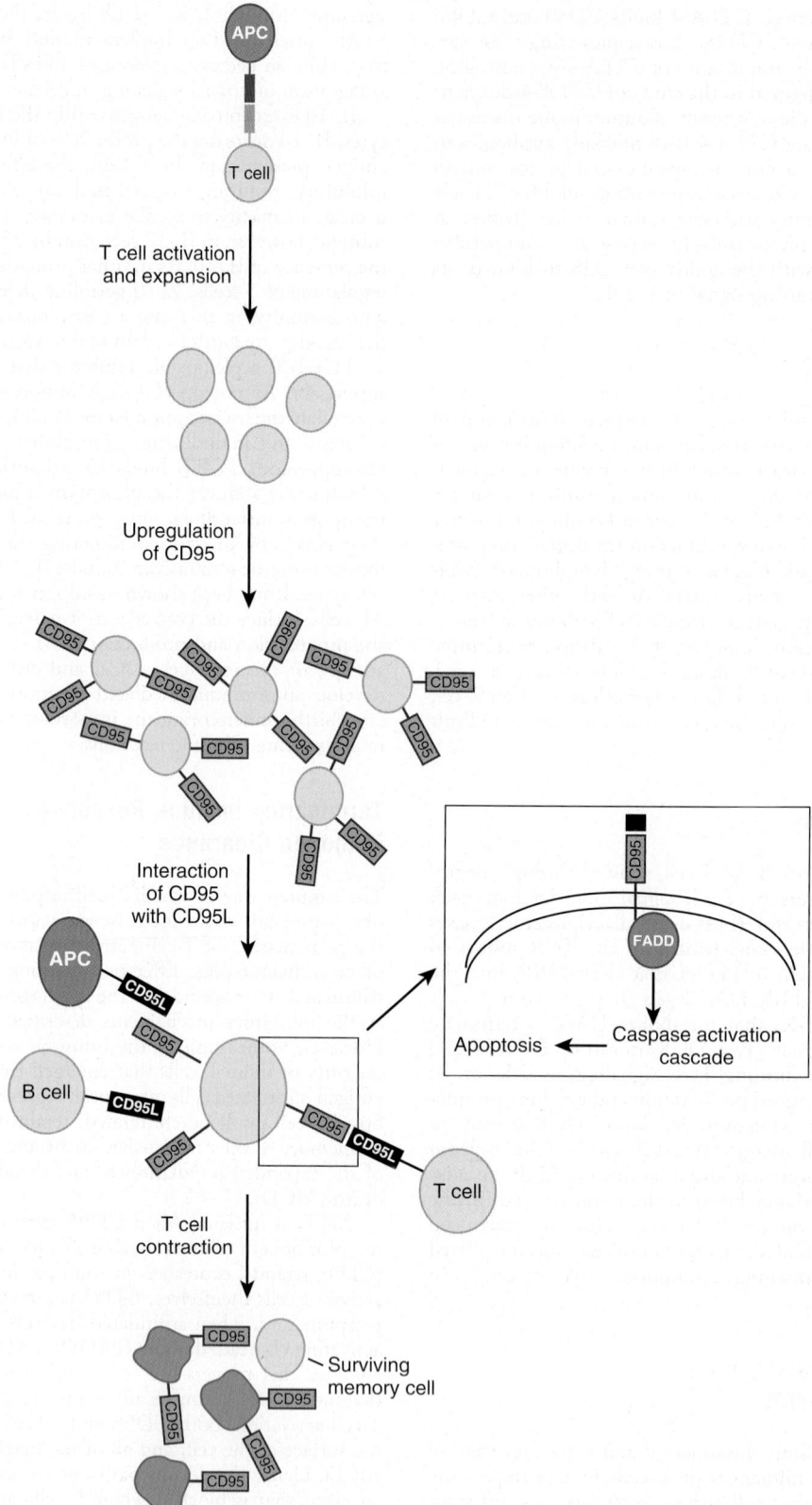

Fig. 21.11 CD95-DEPENDENT ACTIVATION-INDUCED CELL DEATH. After T-cell activation and resultant expansion, T cells begin to upregulate the cell death receptor CD95. The ligand for CD95, CD95L, is expressed on many cell types, including antigen-presenting cells (APCs), B cells, and the activated T cells themselves. Binding of CD95 to CD95L triggers recruitment of the adapter protein Fas-activating via death domain (FADD), resulting in activation of caspases and the induction of cell death through apoptosis. The process of CD95 upregulation and apoptosis leads to contraction of activated T-cell populations.

THERAPEUTIC MANIPULATION OF T CELL–MEDIATED IMMUNITY

A comprehensive description of the myriad ways in which the manipulation of T cells has led to important clinical advances is beyond the scope of this chapter. Thus only a subset of the ways in which an enhanced understanding of the molecular basis for T cell–mediated immunity has resulted in changes in clinical practice is described here. Many human diseases are related to T-cell dysfunction, both in cases of overexuberant immune responses, as in autoimmune diseases and rejection of transplanted organs, and in insufficient immune responses, as in the case of some chronic infections and in uncontrolled malignancy. Here, we briefly address T-cell responses in graft rejection and in malignancy as paradigms for how T-cell immunity can be modulated therapeutically.

Modulating T Cells to Permit Allograft Transplantation

The success of solid organ transplant depends greatly on the ability to control the immune response of the recipient against the donor organ. Donor tissues express foreign MHC alleles and other proteins to which endogenous T cells have not been exposed (and therefore tolerized against) during thymic development, and thus these tissues serve as potential targets for T cell–mediated immunity. Initially, the only medications capable of permitting graft survival were high-dose steroids, medications with potent effects in essentially all organ systems and with severe side effects not limited to the immune system. Subsequently, however, several classes of medications were identified that act more specifically on T cells, first cyclosporine and subsequently tacrolimus and sirolimus. These agents target the IL-2 axis: cyclosporine and tacrolimus inhibit IL-2 transcription, and sirolimus inhibits mammalian target of rapamycin (mTOR), which is critical for facilitating IL-2 signal transduction. Because T cells, depending on the treatment modality, are unable to either produce IL-2 or respond to IL-2, they fail to proliferate, despite conditions favorable for stimulation, leading to impaired T cell–mediated immunity and improved survival of transplanted organs.

Cyclosporine and rapamycin were originally identified in screens of compounds that interfered with immune cell function, and their mechanism of action was discerned only after much of the basic biology of T-cell activation was understood. Other agents currently in use in the clinic were designed precisely because of insights that emerged from studies probing the molecular basis of immune cell function. For example, antibodies directed against CD3 are potent T-cell inhibitors and are now used in the setting of acute solid organ transplant rejection. Similarly, blocking the IL-2 receptor with monoclonal antibodies prevents IL-2 receptor signaling and thus abrogates division of stimulated T cells, thereby quelling T cell–mediated immune destruction.

Given the importance of costimulation for T-cell activation and the success in interfering with CD28 signaling in various autoimmune disorders, recent studies have demonstrated efficacy in transplantation with blockade of the CD28/CD80-CD86 interaction using soluble CTLA-4 as a competitive inhibitor of the interaction between CD28 and CD80/CD86. A soluble CTLA-4 fusion protein has recently been approved in the setting of transplant rejection. Additional studies are in progress to examine ways in which modulation of other costimulatory receptors, alone or in combination with soluble CTLA-4, may be used to preserve allografts. As our understanding of how different T-cell subsets are induced is becoming more precise, new therapeutics are on the horizon that are being designed to redirect immune responses by changing the balance of the various effector subsets that emerge as the recipient responses to the transplanted organ. Additional agents directed against receptors and signaling molecules discovered to be key for T-cell activation are currently being tested for clinical efficacy and safety and likely will soon be available to block T-cell responses in the setting of solid organ transplant.

Manipulating T Cells to Improve Activity Against Malignancy

In contrast to the need to impede immune responses in organ transplant, in the setting of malignancy, the desire is to intervene to enhance T-cell activity. T cells face several hurdles in their response to spontaneous malignancy. First, they must recognize peptides and proteins that are unique to tumor tissue. These include oncogenic mutant proteins, fusion proteins that may have formed during the course of tumor development or aberrantly expressed embryonic proteins that result from altered transcription often found in malignant tissue. Second, T cells must overcome the lack of costimulation provided by tumor cells. Because tumor cells originate from normal host tissue, they fail to generate the bacterial or viral products crucial for activating APCs. Third, T cells must overcome the generally immunosuppressive microenvironment within tumor tissue, which may include an abundance of TGF-β, Tregs, immunosuppressive macrophages, and/or the induction of an anergy-like state.

The first broadly successful approach to enhance T cell–mediated responses to tumors also makes use of the biology of CTLA-4. In this case, however, instead of using soluble CTLA-4 as an agent to inhibit T-cell responses by interfering with costimulation, antibodies against CTLA-4 are being used as a means to block the ability of CTLA-4 expressed on activated T cells to inhibit T-cell function. Preliminary studies have shown that CTLA-4 blocking antibodies may prolong T-cell activation in response to malignancy, and their use has resulted in long-term disease remission in approximately 15% of patients with metastatic melanoma, an otherwise uniformly fatal disease. Some antibodies against CTLA-4 may also function by depleting Tregs from immune organs and the tumor microenvironment. Whether CTLA-4 antibodies mediate their effect by inducing the expansion of newly activated tumor-specific cells or by reversing the immunosuppressive microenvironment on existing cells continues to be studied; however, one major concern of using antibodies against CTLA-4 has been the generation of severe autoimmune colitis in a significant fraction of patients.

The initial success achieved by blocking CTLA-4 on the surface of T cells led to the search for other molecules that might similarly be targeted with blocking antibodies. One obvious candidate molecule is PD-1, the inhibitory receptor present on activated and exhausted T cells. Because many, if not all, patients with cancer have circulating T cells capable of binding tumor antigen, albeit with limited responsiveness, it was speculated that relieving exhaustion of tumor-specific T cells with antibodies that block PD-1 would permit improved T-cell responses against malignancy. In fact, therapies targeting PD-1 and its ligand have demonstrated profound activity in patients with malignancy, with overall survival rates as high as 35% in patients with advanced melanoma, and activity in cancers previously thought to be poor targets for immune-based therapy, such as Hodgkin lymphoma, lung and bladder cancers. Surprisingly, in studies described to date, autoimmune disease occurs much less frequently in patients treated with antibodies targeting PD-1 versus those targeting CTLA-4. The biologic basis of this finding is unclear, but it suggests that PD-1 and other "immune checkpoint" receptors, such as Lag-3 and Tim-3, represent superior targets to boost T cell–mediated activity against tumors. In ongoing research, investigators are evaluating how best to integrate PD-1 blocking strategies into existing cancer treatment regimens.

In addition to targeting inhibitory receptors on T cells to augment antitumor responses, studies are underway to engineer T cells to more effectively activate effector T-cell responses against malignancies. Knowledge gained through fundamental studies of proximal signaling events important for T-cell activation has led investigators to engineer chimeric antigen receptors (CARs), which permit direct activation of T cells by tumor cells. These "designer" molecules have a modular structure: an extracellular binding domain for antigens on tumor cells, transmembrane domains from CD8a or other cell surface proteins, cytoplasmic signaling components of the ζ chain of the TCR complex, and a costimulatory domain(s)

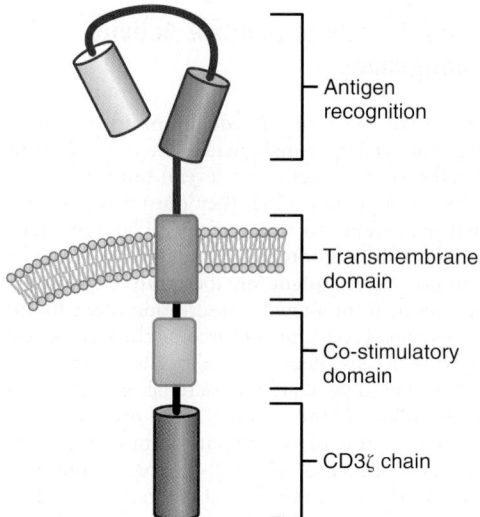

Antigen recognition

Transmembrane domain

Co-stimulatory domain

CD3ζ chain

Fig. 21.12 DESIGN OF A CHIMERIC ANTIGEN RECEPTOR T CELL. The modular design of successful chimeric antigen receptors (CARs) uses the knowledge gained through the study of fundamental properties of antigen recognition and signaling pathways in immune cells. The extracellular antigen recognition domain is typically derived from a single-chain variable fragment of an antibody specific for an antigen expressed by the tumor cells. This domain is coupled to a transmembrane domain, which has been derived from either CD8 or CD28 molecules. The CAR transmits an activation signal through the costimulatory domains and the CD3ζ chain to intracellular T cell signaling pathways. The costimulatory domain contains one (or more) signaling domains derived from costimulatory molecules, including CD28, CD27, 4-1BB, and ICOS (inducible costimulator). This costimulatory domain significantly augments signaling from the CD3ζ chain and has been shown to improve CAR T-cell function, proliferation, and persistence.

containing other key activating receptors (Fig. 21.12). T cells are removed from patients, genetically engineered to express CARs, and reintroduced into patients with the anticipation that these T cells will engage the tumor through the CAR, resulting in T-cell activation. These activated T cells, when effective, generate robust antitumor responses, bolstering antitumor immunity sufficiently to eliminate the cancer.

Generation of optimal CAR constructs is currently the subject of intensive investigation. Two important considerations in the generation of CARs are the identification of tumor antigens for CAR binding and the selection of signaling domains to combine with the TCR ζ chain to facilitate T-cell activation. One of the most well-studied tumor antigens selected for CAR-T-cell therapy is CD19, a cell surface costimulatory receptor found exclusively on B cells. In patients with refractory B cell leukemias and lymphomas, treatment with CD19-directed CAR-T cells have demonstrated striking success, with a significant proportion of patients achieving complete and durable remission. As predicted from selection of CD19 as the cellular target, these patients also develop B-cell aplasia and hypogammaglobulinemia resulting from the elimination of healthy B cells by CAR-T cells; however, this long-term side effect can be effectively managed by antibody infusions or coupling CAR-T-cell therapy with subsequent bone marrow transplantation. Identification of appropriate target antigens for CAR-T cells is a key challenge because many tumor antigens may also be expressed on normal tissues and "on-target, off-tumor" effects of CAR-T cells could potentially lead to unacceptable toxicity. These concerns will require careful evaluation of each CAR targeting domain for both efficacy against the tumor and potential deleterious effects on normal tissues.

Apart from identifying the best targets for CARs, much effort has also been placed on optimal construction of the CAR signaling domains. First-generation CARs, which contain only the ζ chain of the TCR complex, led to suboptimal antitumor responses. The

incorporation of an additional intracellular signaling domain derived from costimulatory molecules, such as CD28 or 4-1BB, into second-generation CARs augmented CAR-T-cell activation and antitumor efficacy, and third-generation CARs include signaling domains from two costimulatory receptors. Currently, most CARs adhere to the second-generation model. Which intracellular costimulatory domains will work best in CARs and how many costimulatory domains are required for optimal T-cell activation and antitumor efficacy are under active investigation. Other outstanding questions in the biochemistry of CARs concern the optimal number of functional ITAMs present in ζ chain domains and the length and composition of the transmembrane hinge domain and interdomain junctions. Defining the biochemistry and signal transduction of CARs should permit broadening its use to more common malignancies.

The examples presented here are only a small subset of novel approaches in use or being tested to modulate immune cell function based upon our understanding of the molecular basis of T-cell activation. It is anticipated that as more is learned about the molecules and pathways critical for control of T cell–mediated immunity, additional new agents with greater efficacy and improved safety profiles will become available for clinical use. The advent of these new therapeutics and their potential to improve treatments for serious human diseases underscore the importance of continued efforts to understand the mechanisms of T-cell development and function.

SUGGESTED READINGS

Anderson MS, Venanzi ES, Klein L, et al: Projection of an immunological self shadow within the thymus by the Aire protein. *Science* 298:1395, 2002.

Chan AC, Iwashima M, Turck CW, et al: ZAP-70: a 70 kd protein-tyrosine kinase that associates with the TCR zeta chain. *Cell* 71:649, 1992.

Clements JL, Yang B, Ross-Barta SE, et al: Requirement for the leukocyte-specific adapter protein SLP-76 for normal T cell development. *Science* 281:416, 1998.

Crotty S: Follicular helper CD4 T cells (TFH). *Annu Rev Immunol* 29:621, 2011.

Day CL, Kaufmann DE, Kiepiela P, et al: PD-1 expression on HIV-specific T cells is associated with T-cell exhaustion and disease progression. *Nature* 443:350, 2006.

Dembić Z, Haas W, Weiss S, et al: Transfer of specificity by murine alpha and beta T-cell receptor genes. *Nature* 320:232, 1986.

Dustin ML, Depoil D: New insights into the T cell synapse from single molecule techniques. *Nat Rev Immunol* 11:672, 2011.

Gill S, June CH: Going viral: chimeric antigen receptor T-cell therapy for hematologic malignancies. *Immunol Rev* 2631:68, 2015.

Huang F, Gu H: Negative regulation of lymphocyte development and function by the Cbl family of proteins. *Immunol Rev* 224:229, 2008.

Irving BA, Weiss A: The cytoplasmic domain of the T cell receptor zeta chain is sufficient to couple to receptor-associated signal transduction pathways. *Cell* 64:891, 1991.

Kremer JM, Westhovens R, Leon M, et al: Treatment of rheumatoid arthritis by selective inhibition of T-cell activation with fusion protein CTLA4Ig. *N Engl J Med* 349:1907, 2003.

Love PE, Bhandoola A: Signal integration and crosstalk during thymocyte migration and emigration. *Nat Rev Immunol* 11:469, 2011.

Monks CR, Freiberg BA, Kupfer H, et al: Three-dimensional segregation of supramolecular activation clusters in T cells. *Nature* 395:82, 1998.

Postow MA, Callahan MK, Wolchok JD: Immune checkpoint blockade in cancer therapy. *J Clin Oncol* 33:1974, 2015.

Rieux-Laucat F, Le Deist F, Fischer A: Autoimmune lymphoproliferative syndromes: genetic defects of apoptosis pathways. *Cell Death Differ* 10:124, 2003.

Rudd CE, Taylor A, Schneider H: CD28 and CTLA-4 coreceptor expression and signal transduction. *Immunol Rev* 229:12, 2009.

Sakaguchi S, Ono M, Setoguchi R, et al: Foxp3+CD25+CD4+ natural regulatory T cells in dominant self-tolerance and autoimmune disease. *Immunol Rev* 212:8, 2006.

Sallusto F, Lanzavecchia A, Araki K, et al: From vaccines to memory and back. *Immunity* 33:451, 2010.

Singer A, Adoro S, Park JH: Lineage fate and intense debate: myths, models and mechanisms of CD4- versus CD8-lineage choice. *Nat Rev Immunol* 8:788, 2008.

Smith-Garvin JE, Koretzky GA, Jordan MS: T cell activation. *Annu Rev Immunol* 27:591, 2009.

Vang T, Miletic AV, Arimura Y, et al: Protein tyrosine phosphatases in autoimmunity. *Annu Rev Immunol* 26:29, 2008.

Vyas JM, Van der Veen AG, Ploegh HL: The known unknowns of antigen processing and presentation. *Nat Rev Immunol* 8:607, 2008.

Waterhouse P, Penninger JM, Timms E, et al: Lymphoproliferative disorders with early lethality in mice deficient in Ctla-4. *Science* 270:985, 1995.

Webber A, Hirose R, Vincenti F: Novel strategies in immunosuppression: issues in perspective. *Transplantation* 91:1057, 2011.

Williams MA, Bevan MJ: Effector and memory CTL differentiation. *Annu Rev Immunol* 25:171, 2007.

Zhang W, Sommers CL, Burshtyn DN, et al: Essential role of LAT in T cell development. *Immunity* 10:323, 1999.

Zhu J, Paul WE: Peripheral CD4+ T-cell differentiation regulated by networks of cytokines and transcription factors. *Immunol Rev* 238:247, 2010.

CHAPTER 22

NATURAL KILLER CELL IMMUNITY

Don M. Benson, Jr. and Michael A. Caligiuri

Natural killer (NK) cells are large, granular lymphocytes comprising about 10% to 15% of the peripheral circulation.[1,2] First characterized by their ability to lyse targets independent of activating or initiating stimuli,[3] NK cells are a critical cellular component of the innate immune system. In addition, NK cells secrete cytokines that help to marshal and shape the innate and adaptive immune response to infection and malignant transformation. There has been a recent surge of interest in NK cells as new discoveries in both the laboratory and the clinic have characterized the crucial contributions of NK cells in shaping the early immune response.[4] NK cells play a key role in maintaining host defense, as exemplified in human NK cell deficiency syndromes (which carry increased susceptibility to overwhelming viral, intracellular, and atypical mycobacterial infections)[5] and in animal models of NK cell deficiency (e.g., such mice are particularly susceptible to developing cancer).[6,7] This chapter reviews current understanding of NK cell biology, the role of NK cells in human diseases, and the recent clinical applications of NK cells in cancer therapy.

FUNDAMENTAL BIOLOGY

Natural Killer Cell Subsets

NK cells are phenotypically recognized by surface expression of CD56 (also called *neural cell adhesion molecule*) and the absence of the T cell–specific surface antigen CD3 as well as the T-cell receptor.[8,9] Based on the intensity of CD56 surface expression, two functional subsets (so-called CD56^{bright} and CD56^{dim}) of NK cells may be discriminated from one another. CD56^{dim} NK cells comprise 85% to 90% of the NK cells in peripheral circulation and are potent mediators of cytotoxicity. About 10% to 15% of NK cells in the circulation are CD56^{bright}, and upon activation, this subset is capable of robust cytokine and chemokine production.[2] Fig. 22.1 graphically represents the NK subsets described later, and Table 22.1 summarizes major surface antigens associated with each NK cell subset.

CD56^{dim} Natural Killer Cells

CD56^{dim} NK cells have exquisite cytolytic properties and are able to kill infected as well as tumor cell targets without prior sensitization.[10] They constitutively express the interleukin-2/15 (IL-2/IL-15) receptor (R) β- and common γ-receptor chains, which together form a receptor complex through which cells may respond to stimulation by either IL-2 or IL-15.[11,12] CD56^{dim} NK cells can lyse tumor cell targets through at least three distinct mechanisms. First, they can execute cytotoxicity through granule exocytosis of perforin and granzyme.[13,14] Second, cytotoxicity can be mediated through Fas ligand and tumor necrosis factor (TNF)-related apoptosis-inducing ligand associated with production of cytokines, including interferon-γ (IFN-γ), TNF-α, and granulocyte macrophage colony-stimulating factor.[15] Third, CD56^{dim} NK cells can mediate antibody-dependent cytotoxicity (ADCC) via the high-density surface expression of CD16 (the FcγRIII receptor).[2,16] Freshly isolated, unstimulated CD56^{dim} NK cells have intrinsically greater cytotoxicity against NK-sensitive targets such as the K562 cell line in vitro compared with the CD56^{bright} NK cells.[17]

Other antigens are differentially expressed by CD56^{dim} NK cells and provide insight into their functional role in the immune response. For example, CD56^{dim} NK cells also exhibit relatively high surface density expression of killer immunoglobulin-like receptors (KIRs). NK cell KIR expression appears important in preventing autoimmunity and in surveying against malignant transformation.[16,18]

Both CD56^{dim} and CD56^{bright} NK cells express modest levels of chemokine (C-X-C motif) receptor 3 (CXCR3). However, in contrast to CD56^{bright} NK cells, CD56^{dim} NK cells display relatively abundant surface expression levels of CXCR1, CXCR4, and CX3CR1.[19] CXCR1 binds IL-8, and CXCR4 binds stromal cell–derived factor 1 (SDF-1). These cytokines are associated with local inflammatory response; for example, IL-8 levels are increased in the setting of acute viral infections,[20] and IL-8 and SDF-1 levels are increased with solid[21,22] and hematopoietic malignancies.[23,24] Thus expression of these chemokine receptors allows NK cells to traffic to local areas of inflammatory response to mediate antiviral and antitumor activity.

CD56^{bright} Natural Killer Cells

CD56^{bright} NK cells play more of an immunoregulatory role. CD56^{bright} NK produce a multitude of cytokines and chemokines, have a relatively high proliferative capacity, reside primarily in the parafollicular T cell–rich region of secondary lymphoid tissue (SLT), and have modest cytolytic granules, KIR, and FcγRIII expression (see Table 22.1).[10] CD56^{bright} NK cells are unique among cytotoxic effector cells in their constitutive expression of the high-affinity IL-2Rαβγ complex, making them responsive to picomolar concentrations of IL-2 released by activated T cells in the parafollicular T cell–rich region of SLT.[25] As noted, CD56^{bright} NK cells comprise only about 10% of the circulating NK population but predominate almost to the exclusion of the CD56^{dim} NK subset in SLT.[2,26] This likely results from their selective expression of a number of receptors that assist in homing cells to and retaining cells in SLT (e.g., CCR7 and CD62L).[10]

The ability of CD56^{bright} NK cells to produce an abundant variety of cytokines and chemokines compared with the CD56^{dim} subset likely relates more to the differential expression of both negative and positive regulators of cytokine/chemokine production and less to constitutive expression of cytokine-activating receptors. For example, CD56^{bright} NK cells have little or no expression of two negative regulators of cytokine/chemokine production, namely SHIP-1 (Src homology 2 domain-containing inositol 5-phosphatase 1) and HLX (H2.0-like homeobox 1),[27,28] but CD56^{dim} NK cells lack constitutive expression of a positive regulator of cytokines called *SET*.[29]

NATURAL KILLER CELL DEVELOPMENT

NK cells are prototypic, founding members of a population of cells referred to as *innate lymphoid cells* (ILC).[30] Three populations of ILC have been described based on differential expression of specific transcription factors and cytokine production, and NK cells are believed to arise from group 1 ILCs, which are characterized by T-bet and EOMES expression.[31] Acquisition of the IL-15 receptor (CD122) is likely a first step toward NK cell differentiation from CD34$^+$ hematopoietic stem cells and a subsequent common lymphoid precursor cell. Moreover, IL-15 is required for NK cell

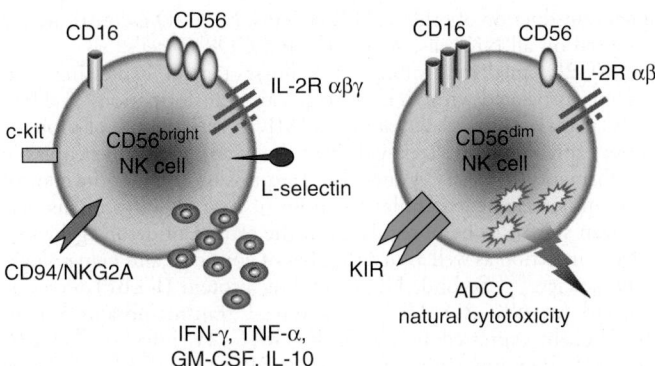

Fig. 22.1 SIMPLIFIED REPRESENTATION OF NATURAL KILLER CELL SUBSETS. CD56^bright cells have immunoregulatory function, whereas CD56^dim cells have cytolytic function. *ADCC,* Antibody-dependent cellular cytotoxicity; *GM-CSF,* granulocyte macrophage-colony stimulating factor; *IFN,* interferon; *IL,* interleukin; *KIR,* killer immunoglobulin-like receptor; *R,* receptor; *TNF,* tumor necrosis factor. *(Modified from Cooper MA, Fehniger TA, Caligiuri MA: The biology of human natural killer cell subsets.* Trends Immunol *22:633, 2001.)*

TABLE 22.1	Human Natural Killer Cell Subsets Display Different Repertoires of Surface Antigens	
Antigen	**CD56^dim**	**CD56^bright**
CD16 (FcγRIIIa)	+++	–/+
KIR	+++	–/+
CXCR1	+	–
CXCR3	++	–
CX3CR3	+	–
CXCR4	++	–
CD94	–	++
NKG2A	–/+	+
NKG2D	+	+
c-kit	–	+
CCR7	–	++
CD2	++	+++
CD62L (L-selectin)	+	++
CD44	+	++

KIR, Killer immunoglobulin-like receptor.
Modified from Cooper MA, Fehniger TA, Caligiuri MA: The biology of human natural killer cell subsets. *Trends Immunol* 22:633, 2001.

development in mice and humans,[32,33] and the NK cell maturation process appears to occur outside the bone marrow.[2,34] Freud et al identified a CD34^dim CD45RA^+ α₄β₇^bright cell to be the only CD34^+ subset in SLT.[26] Found within the parafollicular T cell–rich region of SLT in the same region as the CD56^bright NK cell, this CD34^dim CD45RA^+ α₄β₇^bright cell can differentiate into a CD56^bright NK cell in the presence of IL-15.[22] Five novel, discrete stages of NK cell development were characterized in situ within the same parafollicular region of SLT, each by their differential expression of CD34, CD117, and CD94.[30,35,36] As development proceeds along this continuum, cells acquire the ability to secrete cytokines (e.g., IFN-γ), display natural cytotoxicity, and lose the ability to differentiate into dendritic cells, T cells, or both. This orderly development in SLT from a CD34^+ subset to CD56^bright NK cells suggests that CD56^dim NK cells represent a terminally differentiated NK stage that follows CD56^bright NK development and exit into the periphery. The acquisition of phenotypic markers occurs in a progressive, orderly manner: (1) CD161; (2) CD56, CD94, NKp46, and NKG2D;

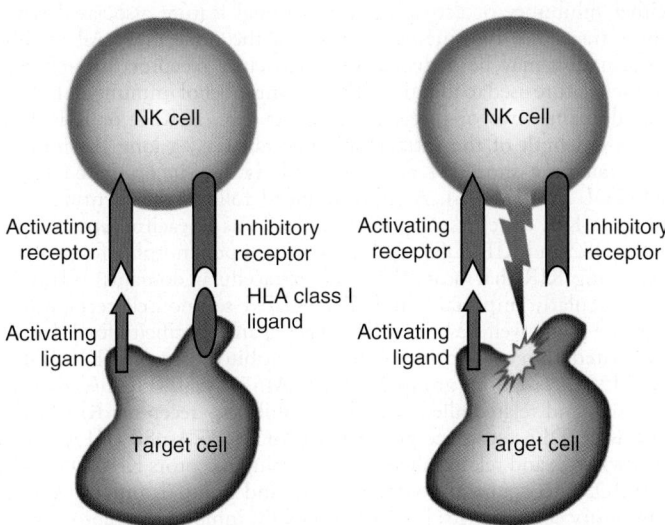

Fig. 22.2 SIMPLIFIED REPRESENTATION OF NATURAL KILLER CELL CYTOTOXICITY MEDIATED THROUGH THE BALANCE OF ACTIVATING AND INHIBITORY SIGNALING IN RESPONSE TO LIGANDS ON POTENTIAL TARGETS. The target cell on the left is spared, but the target cell on the right is lysed. *HLA,* Human leukocyte antigen; *NK,* natural killer. *(Modified from Farag SS, Fehniger TA, Ruggeri L, et al: Natural killer cell receptors: new biology and insights into the graft-versus-leukemia effect.* Blood *100:1935, 2002.)*

and (3) CD16 and KIR. CD94 expression may mark a functional intermediary step between C56^bright and CD56^dim human NK cells.[37] The abundance of CD56^dim NK cells in blood versus SLT and their loss of both CD117 (c-kit) expression and proliferative capacity, along with their acquisition of KIR, FcRγRIII, and cytolytic granules, are all consistent with this notion.[2] CD57 has been identified as a surface marker of terminally differentiated NK cells.[38]

NATURAL KILLER CELL RECEPTORS

NK cells, as opposed to B and T lymphocytes, do not undergo clonotypic gene rearrangement in order to express antigen receptors; however, through the expression of a complex repertoire of surface molecules, NK cells may efficiently determine nonself from self and rapidly initiate an appropriate response.[39] NK cell receptors may be activating or inhibitory—in other words, binding of the receptor to its ligand expressed on a target cell either activates or suppresses a functional NK response. Such receptors fall into three general categories: those that are members of the immunoglobulin-like superfamily (KIR), one type that belongs to the C-type lectin receptor (CTLR) superfamily,[40] and finally NK cell–specific receptors. The complex function of these receptor subsets is a matter of ongoing research; however, a model by which NK cell receptors KIR may recognize particular features of major histocompatibility complex (MHC) class I alleles (e.g., human leukocyte antigen A [HLA-A],[41] HLA-B,[42] HLA-C[43]) or recognize other surface antigens on target cells has been developed.[44,45] Fig. 22.2 is a simplified, schematic representation of current understanding of the ability of NK cells and their receptors to survey the immune system.

Killer Immunoglobulin-Like Receptors

KIRs provide one method by which NK cells recognize self from nonself to mediate the appropriate cytotoxic response. There are at least 15 KIRs identified on chromosome 19q13.4.[18,44,45] Structurally, KIRs contain two or three extracellular immunoglobulin-like domains and recognize MHC class I proteins.[18,41,42] KIRs may be either inhibitory or activating, a functional feature associated with the intracellular tyrosine-based motif of the molecule.[18] All of this information may be deduced for a particular receptor through the nomenclature used to identify KIRs. The number of immunoglobulin-like domains (two or three) is expressed (e.g., KIR2D or KIR3D), and the length of the intracytoplasmic tail (i.e., a long [L] inhibitory tail or a short [S] activating tail) is also incorporated (e.g., KIR2DL or KIR2DS). A suffix numeral follows the identification of some KIR to represent polymorphic forms of each receptor (e.g., KIR2DS2 and KIR2DS3, each indicating a polymorphic form of an activating KIR that bears the same extracellular domains). HLA-C is particularly important in KIR-mediated self/nonself recognition because many well-described KIR have ligand specificity for HLA-C associated antigens. For example, the inhibitory receptor KIR2DL1 (CD158a) recognizes group 2 HLA-C Asn77Lys80 (HLA-Cw2, w4, w5, w6, and related alleles), and the inhibitory receptors KIR2DL2 and KIR2DL3 recognize group 1 HLA-C Ser77Asn80 (HLA-Cw1, w3, w7, w8, and related alleles).[45] Activating receptors KIR2DS1 and KIR2DS2 recognize the same group 2 and group 1 antigens as the inhibitory counterparts; however, generally, inhibitory receptors bind with greater avidity or attraction for a corresponding HLA antigen than activating receptors.[46] Complementary activating and inhibitory KIRs recognize the same cognate extracellular domains on target cells; thus, if an NK cell expresses both activating and inhibitory KIR for an identical ligand, the cell will generally be inhibited from killing.

The KIR family is likely not all-inclusive for human classical type I HLA allotypes; for instance, only one inhibitory KIR directed against HLA-A (KIR3KL2) and none toward HLA-B alleles have been found.[45] Additionally, specific KIRs may have particular roles in maintaining host immunity in unique settings. For example, KIR2DL4 recognizes the nonclassical HLA-G molecule that is expressed only on fetal extravillous trophoblasts that invade the maternal decidua during pregnancy.[47] Controversy surrounds the exact nature of this KIR; however, KIR2DL4 is likely not clonally distributed as are other KIRs but is present on the surfaces of most mature NK cells.[48] Interestingly, despite having an inhibitory intracellular signaling moiety, KIR2DL4 serves to promote IFN-γ secretion but not cytolytic activity.[48] It is possible that this KIR functions to facilitate immune tolerance to developing fetuses.[49]

C-Type Lectin Receptors

CTLRs, located on human chromosome 12p.12.3, share a common subunit (CD94) covalently bonded to one of four closely related gene products of the NKG2 family.[50,51] CTLRs represent a second type of NK cell receptor–mediating killing and include NKG2A (and splice variant B), NKG2C, NKG2E (and splice variant H), and NKG2F.[51] NKG2D, which does not bind CD94 and shares little sequence homology to other NKG2 proteins, is discussed later. All but one of the CTLRs are activating and expressed on NK cells and cytotoxic T lymphocytes. CD94/NKG2A is inhibitory and is expressed on NK cells, as well as on cytotoxic T lymphocytes, where they serve to regulate CD8[+] T-cell antiviral responses.[52] CD94/NKG2A specifically recognizes the nonclassical HLA-E class I molecule.[53] Interestingly, HLA-E specifically presents leader peptides from other HLA receptor antigens; thus sensitivity to HLA-E provides a mechanism for NK cells to sense functional overexpression of class I MHC molecules on cell surfaces. As with KIR, binding between CD94/NKG2A and HLA-E is more avid than binding of activating CTLRs to other epitopes; however, unlike KIR, the target antigens for activating and inhibitory CTLR are not the same.[54]

NKG2D is a CTLR; however, it has only modest sequence homology with other members of the NKG2 family and does not associate with CD94.[53] NKG2D exists as a homodimer and does not have inherent signaling capability, but rather signals via the PI3K pathway as recruited through DAP10Wu or KAP10.[55] This unique signal transduction arrangement renders NKG2D signaling privileged from inhibitory, intracellular intermediaries that modulate signal transduction of other CTLR systems. NKG2D is constitutively expressed on all NK cells, γδ T cells, and CD8[+] T cells.[56]

NKG2D mediates killing of cellular targets expressing two antigens associated with viral or neoplastic transformation.[45,57] First, MHC class I chain–related antigens (MICs) are a family of proteins whose expression correlates with heat shock and viral and neoplastic transformation.[56,58] MICA and MICB expression is under the control of promoter elements similar to those of heat shock proteins and has been shown to be upregulated in the setting of cytomegalovirus (CMV) infection as well as in a number of epithelial and hematologic malignancies.[58,59] Second, UL16 binding protein (ULBP) serves as a ligand for NKG2D. UL16 is a type I transmembrane protein ubiquitously expressed in the setting of CMV infection.[60] UL16 binds MICB and two other proteins, ULBP-1 and ULBP-2.[61] (These latter proteins have α_1 and α_2 domains but lack an α_3 domain as MIC and MHC class I molecules have; furthermore, they are expressed via a glycosylphosphatidyl inositol anchor and thus have no requirement for β_2 microglobulin.) In binding MICB, ULBP-1, and ULBP-2, CMV-produced UL16 counteracts cell surface expression of these NKG2D ligands, thus providing a mechanism of immune evasion from NK cell surveillance and cytotoxicity.[62] In a similar fashion, some human tumors downregulate expression of NKG2D ligands or release soluble forms of such (e.g., MICA or ULBPs) as a mechanism of immune escape from NK cells.[63–65] Although ULBPs are expressed more ubiquitously than MIC proteins, some tissues with high mRNA levels express no protein, implying important posttranscriptional control of these antigens.[61] IL-15 stimulation enhances the NK cell NKG2D-mediated response to tumors expressing ULBP.[66]

Other Activating Natural Killer Receptors

A third family of NK receptors that mediate cell killing are called *natural cytotoxicity receptors* (NCRs).[59,67] In addition to NKG2D, NCRs comprise an important family of activating NK cell receptors involved in the process of target recognition and elimination. NCRs include three receptors called *NKp46* and *NKp30*, which are exclusively and constitutively expressed on NK cells, and *NKp44*, which is expressed after IL-2 stimulation on NK and some γδ T cells.[59,67,68] Infectious, pathogen-specific ligands for NCR have been identified that recognize and engage various virus-specific hemagglutinin and hemagglutinin-neuraminidase.[69] B7-H6 has been identified as a ligand for NKp30 and a number of other endogenous ligands, and bacterial and parasite-derived proteins have been described in some settings as NCR ligands as well.[70–73]

ADAPTIVE IMMUNE PROPERTIES OF NATURAL KILLER CELLS

Recent findings regarding NK cell biology are blurring the functional borders between the innate and adaptive arms of the immune system. Although NK cells have traditionally been dichotomized in the innate immune system, emerging data suggest that NK cells demonstrate sophisticated adaptive properties and do not interact in an invariant manner in the microenvironment.[74]

Natural Killer Cell Education

The potential for NK cell autoreactivity exists because some NK cells may lack inhibitory receptors, but others may express activating receptors for self ligands. This can occur because the receptor array that individual NK cells express occurs largely at random and because ligands to these receptors are inherited independently.[75] Potentially autoreactive NK cells are not clonally deleted but rather rendered hyporesponsive. For example, NK cells lacking inhibitory receptors for self MHC are unresponsive to self cells.[76] In a complementary manner, humans who lack MHC class I expression do not experience NK cell–mediated autoimmunity. By comparison, through an

MHC-dependent processing termed *licensing,* NK cells that express receptors for self MHC exhibit greater responsiveness to stimulation; however, their effector function against normal cells is blocked by engagement of inhibitory receptors for self MHC.[77] Whether responsiveness is determined by interaction with cells expressing ligands for NK cell receptors (so-called arming) or hyporesponsiveness is induced via encounters with normal cells lacking MHC ligands ("disarming" or "anergy") is unclear; however, experimental data suggest that persistent stimulation results in hyporesponsiveness but persistent stimulation with concomitant inhibition leads to NK cell responsiveness.[78,79] Studies such as these and others suggest that NK cells may be sensitive to changes in the microenvironment and may modulate responsiveness to stimuli.

Natural Killer Cell Memory

Immunologic memory has long been reserved as a process of the adaptive immune system; however, recent data suggest that NK cells possess a form of memory as well. This idea was first demonstrated in a recombinase-activating gene 1 (RAG-1)-deficient mouse lacking T and B cells. Hapten-induced hypersensitivity was mediated by NK cells in this model, and "memory" NK cells were described as residing in the liver and bearing Thy1 and CXCR6 on their surfaces.[80]

This concept has also been demonstrated in the setting of viral infection in mice with vesicular stomatitis virus, HIV-1, influenza, and murine CMV (MCMV).[80,81] In regard to MCMV, for instance, Ly49H[+] NK cells recognize MCMV m157 glycoprotein, resulting in NK cell–mediated control of the disease. These Ly49H[+] NK cells preferentially expand in the setting of infection and contract after infection is controlled. However, "memory" NK cells could be detected months after infection, and, upon restimulation, these NK cells exhibited augmented cytotoxicity and cytokine production against MCMV.[81] Although a unique marker of memory is unclear, these NK cells stably express KLRG1, a cadherin-recognizing inhibitory receptor, and could be detected 2 months after infection control even in adoptive transfer models.[81]

A third demonstration of functional NK cell memory has been reported whereby human NK cells preactivated after brief exposure to IL-12, IL-15, and IL-18. These cells showed an enhanced response to restimulation up to 3 weeks later that also was retained in dividing NK cells.[82] This subset was associated with CD94, NKG2A, NKG2C, and CD69 expression and lacked KIR and CD57.

THE ROLE OF NATURAL KILLER CELLS IN HUMAN DISEASE

NK cell deficiencies are rare; however, such conditions provide insight into the role NK cells play in response to infectious pathogens, autoimmune disorders, and the development of malignancy. Selective NK cell deficiency has not been associated with a particular Mendelian disorder[83]; however, studies have shed new light on the genetic mechanisms responsible for proper NK development and function. Many syndromes have been linked to increased susceptibility to infection, and others may predispose to autoimmune disease.

Natural Killer Deficiency Syndromes Linked to Increased Infectious Risks

The first gene directly implicated in NK deficiency was *FCGR3A,* which codes for FcγRIIIa (*CD16*) expressed on NK cells. A "T → A" substitution at position 230 leads to coding of a lysine residue at position 48, normally a histidine. Although the protein expressed appears phenotypically normal, patients present with increased susceptibility to severe and disseminated herpes simplex virus (HSV) infections.[84] Other patients present with progressive Epstein-Barr virus and varicella infections.[85] Patients have variable deficits in NK cytotoxicity

and responsiveness to cytokine stimulation. Population studies have subsequently suggested that the H48 allele may be necessary but not sufficient to produce clinical disease.[86]

Clinical examples of patients entirely lacking any CD56[+] lymphocyte subsets have been reported. The first report was of a young patient who presented with life-threatening varicella infection. She subsequently developed CMV pneumonia and cutaneous HSV infection. Analysis of her lymphocyte subsets demonstrated a striking and selective absolute absence of CD56[+] or CD16[+] cells.[5] The patient went on to develop aplastic anemia and died as a result of complications of stem cell transplant.[86] A second patient who presented with disseminated *Mycobacterium avium* went on to die as a result of disseminated varicella.[87] Other patients have been described with an isolated deficiency of CD56[+]/CD3[−] lymphocytes but with normal or even increased populations of CD56[+]/CD3[+] cells. One such patient presented with severe, recurrent human papilloma virus–related condylomatous disease.[88] Although the genetic mechanisms of these diseases remain unknown, they highlight the functional role of NK cells in providing immunity toward infectious pathogens.

NK cell deficiencies have been described as a component of other disease processes affecting multiple hematopoietic and immune lineages. The genetic deficiencies responsible for many of these disorders have been described and can be found in Table 22.2.

The Role of Natural Killer Cells in Autoimmunity

Interestingly, NK cells have been implicated in both the regulation and the pathogenesis of autoimmune disorders. For example, in a murine experimental autoimmune encephalomyelitis model of multiple sclerosis in which disease is induced with myelin oligodendrocyte glycoprotein (MOG), NK depletion leads to enhanced T-cell response to MOG. Similarly, in human multiple sclerosis, NK cells have been implicated in the maintenance of disease remission.[89] NK cells have also been shown to control inflammation in an experimental model of autoimmune colitis.[90] NK cells may exert this effect through recognition and elimination of T cells activated against autoantigens.[91]

There are also examples of NK cells promoting autoimmune disorders. For instance, experimental evidence supports the idea that NK cells may promote development of type 1 diabetes mellitus through targeted elimination of pancreatic islet β cells after viral infection.[92] This pathobiology may be mediated via an as yet unidentified NKp46 ligand located in the insulin granules.[73,93] Other studies suggest that NK cells can promote humorally mediated autoimmune diseases such as myasthenia gravis through potentiation of autoreactive B cells.[94] Synoviocytes of patients with rheumatoid arthritis (RA) have been shown to express abnormally high levels of MICA, the previously described ligand for NKG2D.[95,96] In fact, NK cells present in acute RA joint effusions may perpetuate this autoimmune inflammatory response.[97]

Finally, NK cell receptor polymorphisms have been implicated in the pathogenesis and progression of autoimmune disease. For example, a T → G substitution at position 559 in the FcγRIIIa (*CD16*) gene leads to a phenylalanine-to-valine substitution at residue 176 of the FcγRIIIa protein.[98] Although the receptors are expressed similarly on the cell membrane, the V/V homozygous state is associated with a higher affinity for immunoglobulin G (IgG) binding than the F/F state. The low binding state (F/F) is associated with lupus nephritis.[99] Others have confirmed this observation by genetic linkage studies in patients with systemic lupus erythematosus.[100] Another polymorphism in the FcγRIIIa receptor (158V/F) has been associated with RA in certain ethnic groups.[101] This mutation may also be associated with the development of subcutaneous rheumatoid nodules in patients with established RA.[101] Because CD16 is expressed on a number of immune cells, the specific role of NK cells contributing to pathology is unclear; however, as discussed later, these polymorphisms have also been linked to an enhanced response to monoclonal antibody therapy for cancer.

TABLE 22.2   Human Disorders Characterized in Part by Natural Killer Cell Deficiency

Disease	Gene		Protein	Cell Count	Cytotoxicity	ADCC	Cytokine Response
X-linked SCID	1.1.1.1.1.1.1.1	IL2Rg	Common γ-chain	Low/absent	Low/absent	N/A	Reduced
Autosomal recessive SCID	1.1.1.1.1.1.1.2	JAK3	Janus kinase 3	Low/absent	Low/absent	N/A	n/a
Bloom syndrome	1.1.1.1.1.1.1.3	BLM	Bloom helicase	Normal	Low	N/A	Normal
Chediak-Higashi syndrome	1.1.1.1.1.1.1.4	LYST	Lysosome trafficking regulator	Normal	Absent	Absent	Reduced
Xeroderma pigmentosum	1.1.1.1.1.1.1.5	XPAG	DNA repair enzymes	Normal	Low	N/A	Normal
Familial erythrophagocytic lymphohistiocytosis	1.1.1.1.1.1.1.6	PFP1	Perforin	Normal	Absent	Absent	Reduced/absent
X-linked lymphoproliferative syndrome	1.1.1.1.1.1.1.7	SH2-DIA	SLAM-associated protein	Normal	Absent	Normal	Normal
Paroxysmal nocturnal hemoglobinuria	1.1.1.1.1.1.1.8	PIG-A	Phosphatidylinositol glycan class A	Low	Absent	Normal	Reduced/absent
von Hippel–Lindau syndrome	1.1.1.1.1.1.1.9	NKTR	Tumor recognition molecule	Normal	Absent	Normal	Reduced
Wiskott-Aldrich syndrome	1.1.1.1.1.1.1.10	WASP	WAS protein	High	Low	Low/normal	n/a
X-linked agammaglobulinemia	1.1.1.1.1.1.1.11	BTK	Bruton tyrosine kinase	Normal	Low	Low	n/a
Ectodermal dysplasia with immunodeficiency	1.1.1.1.1.1.1.12	IKBKG	NEMO	Normal	Low	Low/normal	Reduced
Common variable immunodeficiency	TACI		TNF receptor family member	Low	Low/normal	Low/normal	Normal

ADCC, Antibody-dependent cytotoxicity; N/A, not applicable; NEMO, nuclear factor-κB essential modulator; SCID, severe combined immunodeficiency; SLAM, signaling lymphocyte-activation molecule; TNF, tumor necrosis factor.
Modified from Orange J: Human natural killer cell deficiencies and susceptibility to infection. *Microbes Infect* 4:1545, 2002.

THE THERAPEUTIC POTENTIAL OF NATURAL KILLER CELLS

On one hand, T lymphocytes depend on recognition of tumor-specific antigens to effect an antitumor immune response, an approach limited by the inability to identify such targets for the vast majority of nonviral neoplasms. NK cells, on the other hand, have long been recognized as being capable of antitumor rejection independent of such tumor antigens. As the understanding of how NK cells identify and eliminate targets has advanced, novel roles for the application of NK in clinical anticancer therapy have been defined. Three general approaches have been developed.

First, with therapeutic intent, direct infusion of NK cells into patients has been performed.[102] This strategy was developed on the basis of observations such as that in the allogeneic peripheral blood stem cell transplant setting, where higher doses of transplanted NK cells have been associated with better outcomes as evidenced by reductions in posttransplant infections as well as reduction in nonrelapse mortality.[103] Several studies have shown this approach to be safe and associated with at least a modicum of effectiveness in the autologous setting.[104,105] Trials of direct NK cell infusion have been reported in the allogeneic setting, one correlating successful transfer and expansion of haploidentical NK cells with hematologic remission of leukemia.[106] This field has grown in terms of NK cell sources for expansion and infusion[107] as well as in pairing NK cell therapy with combinatorial strategies to enhance efficacy.[108]

Second, NK cells have been successfully expanded in vivo in patients with cancer through the exogenous administration of recombinant human cytokines, such as low-, intermediate-, or high-dose IL-2.[109–113] The first-in-human trial of IL-15 was associated with a greater than 10-fold expansion of NK cells; however, in contradistinction to studies with IL-2, virtually no change in the regulatory T-cell population was observed in parallel with IL-15.[114] A novel superagonist form of IL-15 is also in clinical development.[115] The tumor nonspecificity of these strategies is being explored by concomitantly administering a tumor-specific monoclonal antibody whose Fc portion can bind to CD16 expressed on the cytokine-expanded NK cells, thus initiating a process called *antibody-dependent cellular cytotoxicty.*[112,116,117]

A third methodology under development to enhance the antitumor response of NK cells is based on the emerging understanding of KIR biology.[118] More than 25 years ago, an inverse relationship was reported between expression of MHC class I molecules on target cells and the ability of NK cells to kill such targets successfully.[39] As this "missing self" model was further characterized, three principal, common HLA class I allele specificities were identified that serve as ligands for three specific NK cell–inhibitory KIR receptors. These have been termed *group 1* HLA-C alleles expressing Asn80 (e.g., HLA-Cw1, w3, w7, w8, and related alleles), *group 2* HLA-C alleles expressing Lys80 (e.g., HLA-Cw2, w4, w5, w6, and related alleles), and HLA-Bw4 alleles (e.g., HLA-B27). As one's NK receptor repertoire, including inhibitory KIRs, is dictated during development by the HLA class I genotype, ultimately every NK cell expresses at least one inhibitory KIR specific to self HLA class I molecules.[18] Moreover, allogeneic targets sensitive to NK cytotoxicity are identified by their lack of self MHC class I–inhibitory KIR ligands.

These principles have been applied in a number of therapeutic settings. Perhaps most dramatically, Aversa and colleagues[119] demonstrated an impressive improvement in survival after allogeneic stem cell transplant–based therapy for patients with acute myeloid leukemia. Donor-versus-recipient NK cell alloreactivity has been shown to contribute to enhanced survival in this setting, as well as to improve engraftment and protec against graft-versus-host-disease.[120,121] In a series of patients receiving haploidentical grafts with a median follow-up of 4 years, 68% of patients without NK alloreactivity had relapsed disease, but only 15% of patients with NK alloreactivity relapsed.[120] Similarly, KIR mismatch has been shown to improve outcome after reduced-intensity chemotherapy followed by allogeneic stem cell transplant in patients with multiple myeloma.[109,122] Fig. 22.3 shows how mismatching KIR epitopes facilitate NK-mediated tumor cytotoxicity in a haploidentical setting.

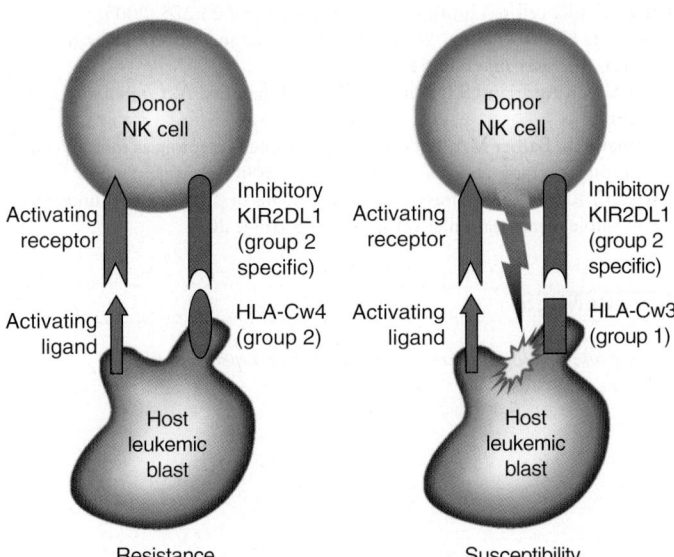

Fig. 22.3 SIMPLIFIED REPRESENTATION OF HAPLOTYPE-MISMATCHED ALLOGENEIC STEM CELL TRANSPLANT FOR ACUTE MYELOID LEUKEMIA: PROPER MAJOR HISTOCOMPATIBILITY COMPLEX CLASS I MISMATCH CAN LEAD TO DONOR NATURAL KILLER CELL KILLING HOST LEUKEMIC BLASTS. As the human leukocyte antigen C (HLA-C) ligand binds to the natural killer (NK) cell inhibitory killer immunoglobulin-like receptor (KIR) on the left, the inhibitory signal interrupts the activation signal, and no killing occurs. However, when the HLA-C ligand does not bind the NK inhibitor KIR on the right, no inhibitory signal is sent, and tumor killing occurs. *(Modified from Farag SS, Fehniger TA, Ruggeri L, et al: Natural killer cell receptors: new biology and insights into the graft-versus-leukemia effect.* Blood *100:1935, 2002.)*

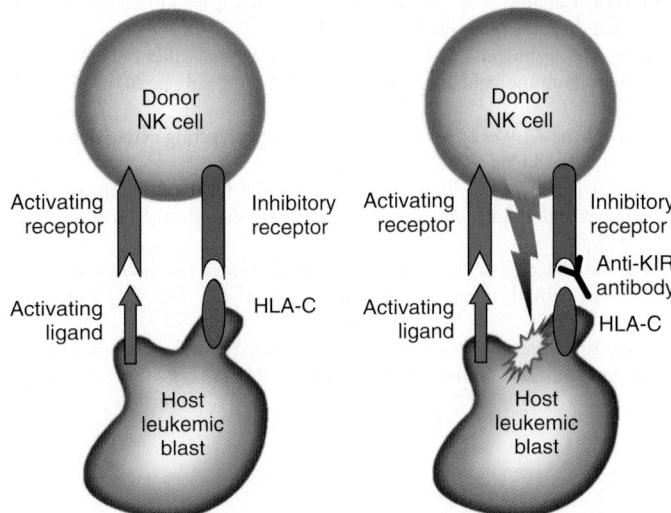

Fig. 22.4 SIMPLIFIED REPRESENTATION SHOWING THE GENERAL EQUILIBRIUM BETWEEN ACTIVATING AND INHIBITORY SIGNALING THAT FAVORS NO KILLING. General equilibrium favoring no killing is shown on the left. The introduction of an antibody to the inhibitory receptor tips this balance toward activation and elimination of the target cell, as shown on the right. *HLA-C,* Human leukocyte antigen C; *KIR,* killer immunoglobulin-like receptor; *NK,* natural killer. *(Modified from Farag SS, Fehniger TA, Ruggeri L, et al: Natural killer cell receptors: New biology and insights into the graft-versus-leukemia effect.* Blood *100:1935, 2002.)*

Others have extended on these transplantation-based findings by manipulating the relationship between NK receptors and MHC class I receptors by means of monoclonal antibodies. For example, a murine model lends support to the notion that tumor expression of MHC class I molecules becomes engaged by inhibitory NK cell receptors and thus mediates NK tolerance.[123] When antibody fragments were introduced to disrupt this ligand–receptor interaction, increased NK cytotoxicity and decreased tumor growth were observed. Furthermore, adoptive transfer of murine NK cells pretreated with an antibody to block inhibitory NK receptor expression into leukemia-bearing mice led to enhanced survival as compared with transfer of untreated NK cells. These findings support the notion that blocking inhibitory NK receptors may be beneficial in increasing the efficacy of cancer immunotherapy.[123,124] Phase I clinical trials of anti-KIR antibodies have been completed in humans, and combinatorial trials are now underway.[125,126] Fig. 22.4 demonstrates this principle.

In complementary fashion, other approaches have sought to enhance activating NK receptors, such as NKG2D. One group has created a novel bivalent protein (ULBP2-BB4) that recognizes NKG2D and CD138, a protein overexpressed in a number of malignancies, including multiple myeloma. Although such an approach is limited by knowledge of particular tumor antigens, the concept of enhancing NK function was demonstrated in this model through increases in NK cytokine secretion as well as abrogation of tumor cell growth in the presence of the molecule.[127] Bispecific killer cell engager molecules as well as engineered chimeric antigen receptor–expressing NK cells are now in development for a variety of malignancies.[128–130] Finally, the use of monoclonal antibodies directed against tumor cell antigens has significantly advanced treatment of some malignancies. For example, treatment with the monoclonal, IgG, chimeric anti-CD20 antibody rituximab (just one of over 300 monoclonal antibodies either in development or already in clinical use) has been shown to improve survival of patients with non-Hodgkin lymphoma. As discussed, genotypic, single-nucleotide polymorphisms in the

FcγRIIIA (CD16) receptor expressed on NK cells and other immune cells may convey functional differences in the receptor that have clinical consequences. Patients with the V/V homozygous state at residue 176 have a higher affinity for the Fc portion of the rituximab, and these patients show enhanced clinical response to the antibody.[131] Such a finding supports the notion that enhanced ADCC function in CD16-bearing cells, including NK cells, is one key mechanism of action of rituximab and suggests that antibody-mediated cancer therapies could be advanced by enhancing NK cell numbers and cytotoxic potential in vivo.

FUTURE DIRECTIONS

NK cells are a critical cellular component of innate immunity. Rapid secretion of powerful immunomodulatory cytokines and chemokines support the role of NK cells as "first responders" to immune insults, facilitating mobilization and tailoring of the innate and adaptive immune response. Potent natural cytotoxicity, unrestricted by classical antigen presentation, and costimulation required for adaptive immune cells suggest that NK cells have an important, complementary role to that of cytotoxic T lymphocytes, which provide antigen-specific cytotoxicity and lasting memory. Further understanding of the functional differences between CD56[dim] and CD56[bright] subsets, their cytotoxicity and cytokine receptor expression, and their developmental biology will certainly shed more light on the therapeutic potential for NK cells in the pathogenesis, prevention, and treatment of human disease.

SUGGESTED READINGS

Becknell B, Caligiuri MA: Interleukin-2, interleukin-15, and their roles in human natural killer cells. *Adv Immunol* 86:209, 2005.

Borrego F, Masilamani M, Marusina AT: The CD94/NKG2 family of receptors: From molecules and cells to clinical relevance. *Immunol Res* 35:263, 2006.

Caligiuri MA: Human natural killer cells. *Blood* 112:461, 2008.

Colucci F, Caligiuri MA, Di Santo JP: What does it take to make a natural killer? *Nat Rev Immunol* 3:413, 2003.

Cooper MA, Fehniger TA, Turner SC: Human natural killer cells: A unique innate immunoregulatory role for the CD56^{bright} subset. *Blood* 97:3146, 2001.

Djeu JY, Jiang K, Wei S: A view to a kill: Signals triggering cytotoxicity. *Clin Cancer Res* 8:636, 2002.

Farag SS, Fehniger TA, Ruggeri L, et al: Natural killer cell receptors: New biology and insights into the graft-versus-leukemia effect. *Blood* 100:2002, 1935.

Freud AH, Yokohama A, Becknell B, et al: Evidence for discrete stages of human natural killer cell differentiation in vivo. *J Exp Med* 203:1033, 2006.

Jie HB, Sarvetnick N: The role of NK cells and NK cell receptors in autoimmune disease. *Autoimmunity* 37:147, 2004.

Lanier L: NK cell recognition. *Annu Rev Immunol* 23:225, 2005.

Orange J: Human natural killer cell deficiencies and susceptibility to infection. *Microbes Infect* 4:1545, 2002.

Paust S, von Andrian UH: Natural killer cell memory. *Nat Immunol* 12:500, 2011.

Sentman CL, Barber MA, Barber A, et al: NK cell receptors as tools in cancer immunotherapy. *Adv Cancer Res* 95:249, 2006.

Vivier E, Raulet DH, Moretta A, et al: Innate or adaptive immunity? The example of natural killer cells. *Science* 331:44, 2011.

REFERENCES

For the complete list of references, log on to www.expertconsult.com.

CHAPTER 23

DENDRITIC CELL BIOLOGY

Olivier Manches, Luciana R. Muniz, and Nina Bhardwaj

Dendritic cells (DCs) are a sparsely distributed population of bone marrow (BM)–derived mononuclear cells that exist in an "immature" form in virtually all tissues in the body.[1] DCs serve as professional antigen-presenting cells (APCs) with an extraordinary capacity to stimulate naive T lymphocytes (as well as B, natural killer [NK], and NK T cells) and initiate primary immune responses. In their immature state, DCs detect and capture "danger signals" originating from microorganisms or their macromolecular constituents in their resident tissues. Upon encountering such danger signals, DCs undergo a complex series of events leading to their "maturation."[1] Maturation of DCs is characterized by migration of DCs to draining lymph nodes and by processing and presentation of antigens in the context of antigen-presenting molecules such as major histocompatibility complex (MHC) and CD1 to naive T, B, and NK cells. This chapter provides a snapshot of the current understanding of DC function as well as the potential clinical applications of DCs as immunotherapeutic agents in diseases such as cancer, HIV, and autoimmunity.[2]

DENDRITIC CELL SUBSETS AND DEVELOPMENT

Extensive research has demonstrated that DCs exist in many "flavors."[3,4] However, understanding of DC differentiation and the different DC subsets is complicated by the heterogeneity of data obtained from in vitro human and mouse studies as well as in vivo animal studies and limited in vivo human studies. In this chapter, we will concentrate on human DCs with little reference to murine models. Readers are encouraged to seek additional information in several comprehensive reviews.[5–14]

Most studies on the developmental origin of human DC subsets have used in vitro culture systems. The CD34+ hematopoietic progenitor cells (HPCs) and blood monocytes are commonly used as precursor cells for generating DCs in culture in vitro for both research and immunotherapeutic purposes. Monocytes, obtained by simple adherence of HPCs to plastic, when exposed to a combination of granulocyte-macrophage colony-stimulating factor (GM-CSF) and interleukin-4 (IL-4), yield immature DCs (imDCs) that are comparable to some degree with tissue interstitial DCs. Maturation of these different DCs can be induced by the addition of various stimuli. Recently it was shown that monocyte-derived DCs (moDCs) constitute a subset of DCs that are not equivalent to blood DCs but resemble more inflammatory DC subsets 15 (Fig. 23.1). Pre-DCs and imDCs, similar to other cell types in the immune system, are continuously produced at a steady rate and in a pathogen-independent manner from CD34+ hematopoietic stem cells (HSCs) within the BM. Fms-like tyrosine kinase-3 ligand (Flt3L) and granulocyte colony-stimulating factor (G-CSF) represent the key DC growth and differentiation factors.[15] The development of stromal cell culture systems comprising HSCs cultured with BM mouse stromal cells and stem cell factor, GM-CSF, and Flt3L have led to the identification of a definitive pre-DC that gives rise to DC subsets found in the blood.[15a,16,17]

Recent studies have shown that DCs originate from human granulocyte monocyte dendritic cell precursors, which sequentially develop into monocyte dendritic cell precursors, which subsequently give rise to a common dendritic cell progenitor (hCDP) that is restricted to produce the three major subsets of DCs: 2 classical DC (cDCs) subsets, DC1 (CD141+) and DC2 (CD1c+) and the plasmacytoid DCs (pDCs). Prior studies suggesting that DCs can arise from other multilineage sources may not be inconsistent, because these are generally speaking heterogeneous populations. In addition, hCDP can also give rise to pre-cDC progenitors in human cord blood, BM, blood, and peripheral lymphoid organs. These pre-cDCs sustain the CD1c+ and CD141+ DC subsets, indicating that pDCs and cDCs arise during hematopoiesis from progenitors with already distinct and restricted lineage potential.[16-18,18a] Moreover, these pre-cDC precursors in the blood can either be uncommitted or display early commitment towards DC1 and DC2 development (pre-DC1 and pre-DC2 phenotypes). Furthermore, Flt3-L given systemically to humans has been shown to increase the pre-cDC pool.[17,19] Altogether, these studies confirmed that there is a sequential pathway of DC development that involves progenitors which display increasing restricted commitment to give rise to the 3 major DC subsets.

The 3 DC subsets not only can be distinguished phenotypically, but also through molecular signatures. DC1 DCs, as briefly described above, are phenotypically described by their expression of CD141, XCR1 and CADM1; DC2s express CD1c and SIRPα; and pDCs express CD123. On the molecular level, DC1s express IRF8, Batf3, Zbtb46 and Flt3; DC2s express ETS2, ID2, ZBTB46 IRF4 and Flt3, while pDCs, as expected, express IRF7, TCF4, Spi-B and IL-3RA.[16] In addition to the committed DC subsets, pre-cDCs are also known to express specific markers such as CD45RA, CD123 (at low/intermediate levels), CD135, CD116, CD117 and CX3CR1 and these can be used in the sorting of these precursors for DC1 and DC2 development.[19]

Under different culture systems, the CD34+ HSCs have been shown to give rise to CD34+CLA+ and CD34+CLA− populations (skin homing receptor cutaneous lymphocyte-associated antigen [CLA]), which differentiate to phenotypically distinguishable CD11c+CD1a+ and CD11c+CD1a− imDCs, respectively.[20] The former migrate into the skin epidermis and differentiate into Langerhans cells, and the latter localize to the skin dermis and other tissues and become interstitial imDCs.[21] The human Langerhans cell DC subset has distinct markers, including the presence of Birbeck granules, the expression of CD1a, and langerin, a member of the C-type lectin family of receptors involved in the uptake of pathogens.[22]

In contrast to the blood "myeloid DCs" derived from pre-cDCs, the "plasmacytoid DCs" contain "lymphoid" mRNA transcripts for pre–T-cell α-chains, germline IgK, and Spi-B and are also called *interferon (IFN) type I-producing cells*. These latter cells display a distinct plasma cell morphology, contain abundant endoplasmic reticulum (ER), and express high levels of IL-3αR but lack myeloid antigens, including CD11c and most lineage markers. pDCs are found in the peripheral blood, thymus, and many lymphoid tissues. The production of extraordinarily high levels of IFN type I by pDCs is unique to this cell type, and it may be important for initiating a strong antiviral innate response and may promote maturation of bystander CD11c+ cDCs to protect them from the cytopathic effect of viruses.[22-25] It is hypothesized that human cDCs and pDCs have evolved to recognize and respond to different pathogens in unique ways owing to their complementary expression of receptors for pathogen-associated molecular patterns (PAMPs) (see Antigen Acquisition section), capacity to secrete either IFN type I or IL-12, antigen presentation, and migration into secondary lymphoid organs. As mentioned, pDCs secrete high amounts of IFN-α upon viral infection but no IL-12

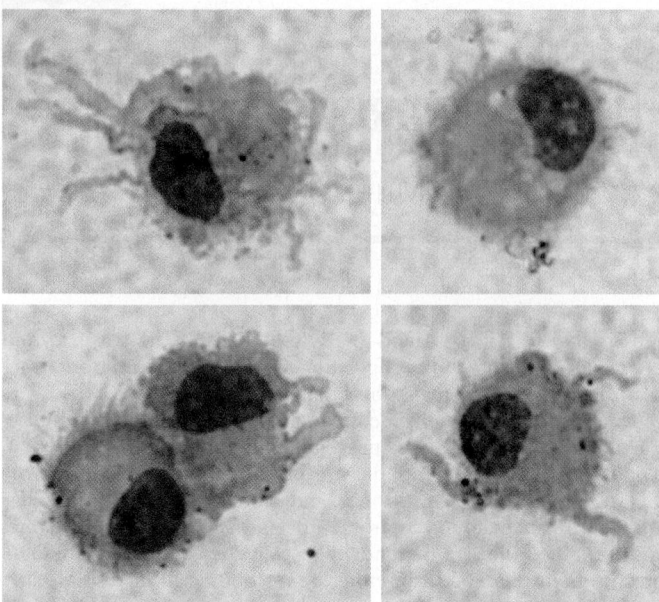

Fig. 23.1 EXAMPLES OF MONOCYTE-DERIVED MATURE DENDRITIC CELLS. The mononuclear cells were enriched by adherence; were cultured with interleukin-4 (IL-4) and granulocyte colony-stimulating factor for 6 days; and underwent maturation with IL-1, IL-6, tumor necrosis factor-α, and prostaglandin E$_2$ for 24 hours.

and display poor antigen capture and presentation capacity. Upon activation, pDCs differentiate into cells bearing characteristics similar to those of activated cDCs (i.e., with a dendritic morphology, high expression of MHC class II molecules, and the capacity to prime naive T cells),[26,27] but they express low levels of CD11c and lack typical myeloid markers. The functional properties of these latter pDC-derived DCs are still to be investigated thoroughly,[28] although they may differ from cDCs, especially in their cross-presentation[29] or T-cell skewing capacities. Thus, whereas DCs derived from pDCs upon culture with IL-3 and activation by CD40L preferentially prime naive CD4$^+$ T cells toward a type 2 T helper (Th2) cell profile, DCs derived from pDCs by viral and/or Toll-like receptor (TLR) stimulation prime toward a Th1 profile in an IFN-α–dependent and IL-12–independent pathway.[24] Upon activation, immature cDCs migrate through afferent lymph from nonlymphoid tissues to the T-cell–rich areas of lymph nodes. pDCs, which also migrate into T-cell areas of secondary lymphoid tissues, do so through high endothelial venules of lymph nodes and marginal zone of the spleen, likely using CCR7 and CD62L.[30] Both activated blood cDCs and pDCs can migrate in response to lymph node–homing chemokines (CCL19 and CCL21) through expression of CCR7. Although cDCs can be found in virtually every peripheral tissue as well as in lymphoid organs, pDCs seem to display a more restricted distribution. They can be found mostly in the T-cell area of lymphoid organs (lymph node, tonsils, spleen, thymus, BM, and Peyer patches), blood, and some peripheral tissues (liver, nasal mucosa). While cDCs and pDCs express a similar array of chemotactic receptors (e.g., CCR2, CCR5, CXCR2, CXCR4), pDCs do not respond to a number of inflammatory chemokines. However, they accumulate in inflamed tissues, such as in systemic lupus erythematosus (SLE) and contact dermatitis, probably through their expression of ChemR23 and CXCR4.

This division of DCs into cDC and pDC subsets is likely to be an oversimplified view of DC heterogeneity. For example, splenic DCs are heterogeneous with regard to expression of CD4, CD11b, and CD11c, but most of the thymic DCs are CD11c$^+$ but lack other myeloid markers, thereby not fitting into either of the classical categories of cDCs and pDCs in blood.[31]

An important role for CD103$^+$ (αE integrin) has recently been uncovered. CD103$^+$ DCs reside in the intestinal mucosa and play a crucial role in tolerance to commensal bacteria and food antigens.

These cells originate in the lamina propria and migrate to the mesenteric lymph nodes, where they drive the differentiation of gut-homing FoxP3$^+$ regulatory T cells (Tregs) by producing retinoic acid (RA) from dietary vitamin A.

In addition, the BDCA3$^+$ (DC1 CD141$^+$) DC subset has been found to be the equivalent of murine CD8α$^+$ DCs, and are involved at cross-presenting antigens to CD8$^+$ T cells. They express the chemokine receptor XCR1 and the DC NK lectin group receptor 1 C-type lectin, a sensor for necrotic cells, and specifically β-actin, and they mediate the phagocytosis of dead cells. They also express basic leucine zipper transcriptional factor ATF-like-3 (BATF3) and INF regulatory factor-8 (IRF8), which may be essential for their development. BDCA3$^+$ DCs express high levels of TLR3 and TLR8, and, upon stimulation by TLR3 agonists (e.g., polyinosinic-polycytidylic acid [poly(I:C)]), they secrete high amounts of IL-12 and IFN-β, both Th1-skewing cytokines. These combined characteristics make them attractive targets for DC-based vaccines in cancer and chronic immune diseases.

Although Langerhans cells and microglia seem to be capable of self-renewal in ectodermal tissues, epidermis, and brain, other DCs arise from blood-borne precursors from BM as described earlier. Recent studies of human immunodeficiencies have highlighted the transcription factors directing the development of DCs and have emphasized their role in defense against microbial pathogens. Thus in DC, monocyte, B, and NK lymphoid deficiency (DCML), blood and interstitial DCs are absent along with monocytes and pDCs. The DCML is attributable to GATA-binding factor 2 mutations, a transcription factor involved in the homeostasis of HSCs. Patients with DCML deficiency have increased susceptibility to *Mycobacteria* spp., fungi, and viruses. Another DC deficiency syndrome is caused by IRF8 mutations. The autosomal recessive K108E mutation leads to defects in peripheral cDCs, pDCs, and monocytes, with increased susceptibility to *Mycobacteria* spp., other intracellular bacteria, and viruses, and it is accompanied by a myeloproliferative syndrome. The dominant sporadic mutation T80A induces a specific loss of CD1c$^+$ DCs, with increased susceptibility to mycobacterial infection but otherwise a normal life expectancy.

It seems that whereas cDC differentiation is dependent on the transcription factor Ikaros, pDC development is dependent on the Ets family transcription factor Spi-B and probably PU.1. A recent study also described an important role for the upregulation of basic helix–loop–helix transcription factor (E-protein) E2-2 in developing pDCs, and E2-2–deficient hematopoietic progenitors do not produce pDCs.[33] Studies in mice described the conversion of BM pDCs into cDCs upon viral infection, again highlighting the complexity and plasticity of DC development.[34]

The migration of myeloid DCs and plasmacytoid pre-DCs from the BM can be increased by administration of Flt3L up to 50-fold for pre-DCs and 15-fold for pDCs.[35,36] G-CSF is also known to increase the number of pDCs in the circulation. With the advent of newer technologies, it has also become feasible to generate large numbers of DC subsets in vitro.

THE CONCEPT OF MATURATION

In their resting state, imDCs are primed to acquire antigens in situ through a variety of receptors and mechanisms. Upon encountering pathogens or other "activating stimuli," DCs undergo a complicated series of phenotypic and functional changes referred to here as *activation* and *maturation*, respectively.[1] The process of DC activation is an intricate differentiation process under tight control that is closely associated with antigen acquisition. It is induced by various stimuli (Table 23.1) or danger signals (e.g., signs of pathogenic infection or cell injury), including cytokines (e.g., IFN type I, tumor necrosis factor α [TNF-α], and IL-1), microbial products (e.g., lipopolysaccharide [LPS], flagellin), intracellular products (e.g., heat shock proteins [HSPs]), growth factors (e.g., thymic stromal lymphopoietin [TSLP]), immune complexes, and T-cell molecules (e.g., CD40). The process of activation is characterized by upregulation of adhesion

TABLE 23.1   **Agents That Cause Dendritic Cell Maturation**[a]

Agent Property	Molecules
Stimulatory agents	TNF family members (TNF-α, CD40L, FasL, TRANCE)
	TLR ligands (dsRNA, LPS, imiquimod, CpG ODNs)
	Growth factors (TSLP)
	Interferons (IFN-α)
	Adhesion molecules (CECAM-1 [CD66a])
	Costimulatory molecules (LIGHT, B7-DC)
	Receptors (FcR via Ag-Igs; TREM-2 via Dap-12)
	Viruses or microbes (influenza, bacteria, bacterial products)
	Chemokines (MCP, MIP1α, RANTES, IP10, IL-8, MDC, TARC)
	Chemokine receptors (CCR7 and loss of CCR2 and CCR5)
Inhibitory agents	Drugs (rapamycin, FK506, cyclosporine A, dexamethasone, IVIg)
	Chemokines (IL-10)
	Viruses (EBV, vaccinia, canarypox, HSV)
	Others (2 microglobulin)
Survival signals	CD40L, TRANCE, B7-DC, Bcl-2
Cell–cell interaction	Activated cells (CD4 and CD8 cells [via CD40L])
	NK cells, NK T cells
	Vδ1+, γδT cells

[a]Maturation is a complex process tightly linked to antigen acquisition and the surrounding microenvironment. See text for more details.
Ag-Igs, Antigen–immunoglobulin immune complexes; Bcl-2, B-cell lymphoma 2; CCR, chemokine (C-C motif) receptor; CECAM-1, carcinoembryonic antigen-related cell adhesion molecule-1; CpG ODNs, CpG oligodeoxynucleotides; dsRNA, double-stranded RNA; EBV, Epstein-Barr virus; FcR, Fc receptor; HSV, herpes simplex virus; IFN, interferon; IL, interleukin; IP10, interferon-γ–induced protein 10; IVIg, intravenous immunoglobulin; LIGHT, homologous to lymphotoxins, exhibits inducible expression, and competes with HSV glycoprotein D for herpesvirus entry mediator, a receptor expressed by T lymphocytes; LPS, lipopolysaccharide; MCP, macrophage/monocyte chemotactic protein; MDC, macrophage and dendritic cell precursor; MIP1α, macrophage inflammatory protein 1α; NK, natural killer; RANTES, regulated on activation, normal T expressed and secreted; TARC, thymus and activation-regulated chemokine; TNF, tumor necrosis factor; TRANCE, TNF-related activation-induced cytokine; TREM-2, triggering receptor expressed on myeloid cells 2; TSLP, thymic stromal lymphopoietin.

and costimulatory molecules such as CD54, CD80, CD86, MHC class I and II molecules, cytokines (e.g., TNF-α, IL-12, IL-18), and chemokines (e.g., RANTES [regulated on activation, normal T expressed and secreted], MIP-1α [macrophage inflammatory protein 1α], IP-10 [interferon-γ–induced protein 10]). The latter enable the recruitment of T cells, monocytes, and other DCs into the local environment. In their mature state, DCs express markers, which distinguish them from imDCs such as CD83 (a molecule involved in thymic T-cell selection and DC–DC interactions) and DC-LAMP, a lysosomal protein. Maturation also changes the migratory properties of DCs. They express CCR7 and acquire responsiveness to the chemokines CCL19 and CCL21 that are expressed in the T-cell areas of lymph nodes where mDCs generate immune responses. Concomitantly, DCs downregulate their receptors for CCL3, CCL4, and CCL5, which are secreted at sites of inflammation; reduce their capacity for phagocytosis, macropinocytosis, antigen uptake, and processing; but acquire potent immunostimulatory ability through enhanced T-cell–DC immune synapse formation, production of immunoproteosomes, and upregulation of unique DC-specific costimulatory molecules such as B7-DC.[37] However, although increased expression of costimulatory molecules and migration to secondary lymphoid organs often correlate with their capacity to prime CD4 and CD8 immunity, activated DCs may also induce

tolerization of T cells, such as when CD4+ T-cell help is missing[38,39] or on activation by inflammatory cytokines in the absence of TLR engagement,[40] and they can potentially induce the generation of Tregs. Some stimuli, such as TSLP, can induce phenotypic maturation of DCs without concomitant secretion of proinflammatory cytokines such as IL-12, IL-6, TNF-α, or IL-1.[41] Therefore DC maturation is more appropriately used in a functional sense, with mDCs being defined as able to prime naive T-cell responses. What makes a phenotypically activated DC capable of priming instead of tolerizing a T cell appears multifactorial and dependent on factors such as the state of the microenvironment and the DC subset in question, although this remains to be clearly defined.

Recent work has shed some light on the intricate transcriptional modifications that DCs undergo upon stimulation and activation. This study was focused on mapping genetic variants that contribute to variation of gene expression in DCs and how these associate with response to stimuli such as LPS, influenza virus, and IFN-β. The researchers in this study identified a gene signature that can be instructive of variation in the response to stimuli in a larger cohort of samples. In genome-wide association studies of inflammatory diseases such as psoriasis, multiple sclerosis, Crohn disease, and leprosy, regions closest to the susceptibility loci were enriched in DC-specific genes and in genes induced by LPS or influenza stimulation of DCs. Thus DC pathogen-sensing mechanisms that lead to their activation are potentially implicated in the pathogenesis of inflammatory diseases. These studies underscore the importance of high-throughput and integrative approaches in the analysis of DC-mediated responses.[42]

ANTIGEN ACQUISITION AND DENDRITIC CELL ACTIVATION

DCs have a remarkable ability to process and present antigens restricted by MHC and CD1 molecules. The processing is tightly associated with DC activation. imDCs sample their environment through several mechanisms, including micropinocytosis, macropinocytosis, receptor-mediated endocytosis, and phagocytosis. They display an array of surface receptors, which facilitate acquisition of antigens and pathogens and at the same time induce differentiation into activated DCs. An important class of receptors is the pattern recognition receptors (PRRs), which recognize PAMPs expressed by many microorganisms. PRRs serve as an important link between innate and adaptive immunity because they directly mature DCs while also inducing the production of a variety of cytokines and chemokines. PRRs consist of several groups of receptors, including secreted molecules (e.g., MBL, CRP, SAP, LBP), cell surface molecules (e.g., CD14, macrophage mannose receptor [MMR], MSR, MARCO),[43] and intracellular molecules (e.g., RIG-I and MDA5, which are RNA helicases involved in the recognition of nucleic acids upon viral infection; stimulator of interferon genes [STING], DAI, and AIM2 [absent in melanoma 2], which recognize intracellular DNA[44]; nucleotide-binding oligomerization domain-like [NOD] receptors, which recognize peptidoglycan subcomponents or other bacterial molecules; inflammatory caspases, such as caspase-1 and caspase-5, which form an intracellular complex with NALP1 or NALP2 and NALP3 called the *inflammasome* that recognizes bacterial RNA and other danger signals and induces the production of the proinflammatory cytokines IL-1β and IL-18) (Table 23.2). TLRs, which constitute another group of PRRs, are expressed by imDCs and mediate activation by microbial components such as peptidoglycan, LPS, flagellin, and unmethylated CpG DNA motifs. Ligation of the TLRs results in the activation of Rel family members, particularly the transcription factor nuclear factor κB (NFκB), c-Jun N-terminal kinase, and p38 mitogen-activated protein kinase, leading to the initiation of the maturation process.[45,46] TLRs are unevenly distributed among DCs, with myeloid DCs expressing TLRs 2, 3, 4, 5, 7, and 8 and pDCs strongly expressing TLRs 7 and 9 (Table 23.3). Another important feature of some TLRs is their capacity to induce secretion of IFN type I for antiviral defense and immune regulation.

Antigen Recognition and Uptake Receptors Expressed by Dendritic Cells[a]

Receptor	Antigenic Ligand
C-type lectins (DC-SIGN, MMR, DEC-205)	Mannosylated molecules, viruses, bacteria, fungi
FcγR (CD32, CD64)	Immune complexes, antibody-coated tumor cells
CD1 a, b, c, d	Bisphosphonate moieties in *Mycobacterium tuberculosis*, BCG, and *Listeria monocytogenes*; lipid and glycolipid foreign and self-antigens
Integrins ($\alpha_v\beta_5$, CR3, CR4)	Opsonized antigens, apoptotic cells
Scavenger receptors (CD36, LOX-1)	Opsonized antigens, apoptotic cells, heat shock proteins
TLRs and other PRRs	TLRs 2–8 (myeloid DC) peptoglycans, endotoxin, flagellin TLR 7 (plasmacytoid DC) bacterial DNA; RIG-I, MDA5, STING, DAI, AIM2, PKR, NOD proteins
HSP-R (CD91)	Heat shock proteins
Aquaporins	Fluids

[a]The table lists some of the receptors expressed by DCs that are involved in antigen acquisition. The antigen receptor repertoire dictates that range of antigens captured by the DC. Ligation of some of these receptors induces DC maturation.
AIM2, Absent in melanoma 2; BCG, bacillus Calmette-Guérin; DAI, DNA-dependent activator of IFN-regulatory factors; DC, dendritic cell; DC-SIGN, dendritic cell–specific intercellular adhesion molecule-3-grabbing nonintegrin; HSP-R, heat shock protein receptor; MDA5, melanoma differentiation-associated protein 5; NOD, nucleotide oligomerization domain; PKR, protein kinase R; PRR, pattern recognition receptor; RIG-1, retinoid-inducible gene I; STING, stimulator of interferon genes; TLR, Toll-like receptor.

Toll-Like Receptors Expressed by Dendritic Cells[a]

mDC	pDC	Ligand(s)
TLR1	TLR1	?
TLR2		Peptidoglycan (*Staphylococcus aureus*) Lipoproteins and lipopeptides from several bacteria Glycophopshotidylinositol anchors from *Trypanosoma cruzi* Lipoaminomannan from *Mycobacterium tuberculosis* Zymosan (yeast)
TLR3		Double-stranded RNA (e.g., poly[I:C])
TLR4		LPS + MD-2, taxol, hsp60 (?), heparan sulfate (?), RSV, fibronectin
TLR5		Flagellin (*Salmonella typhimurium, Listeria* spp.)
TLR6	TLR6	? or undergoes dimerization with TLR2
	TLR7	Imiquimod (Aldara), R-848 (resiquimod), single-stranded RNA
TLR8	TLR8	Imiquimod (Aldara), R-848 (resiquimod), single-stranded RNA
	TLR9	CpG ODNs, DNA from bacteria and viruses, chromatin-IgG complexes
	TLR10	?

[a]Toll-like receptors (TLRs) can form heterodimeric receptor complexes consisting of two different TLRs or homodimers (as in the case of TLR4). The TLR4 receptor complex requires supportive molecules (MD-2) for optimal response to its ligand lipopolysaccharide (LPS). A common feature of the TLR receptors is the cytoplasmic Toll/IL-1 receptor (TIR) domain that serves as a scaffold for a series of protein–protein interactions that result in the activation of a unique signaling module consisting of MyD88; interleukin-1 receptor associated kinase (IRAK) family members; and Tollip, which is used exclusively by TIR family members. Subsequently, several central signaling pathways are activated in parallel, the activation of nuclear factor κB (NFκB) being the most prominent event of the inflammatory response. Recent developments indicate that, in addition to the common signaling module MyD88/IRAK/Tollip, other molecules can modulate signaling by TLRs, especially of TLR4, resulting in differential biologic responses to distinct pathogenic structures. TLR2 is also involved in cross-presentation.
CpG ODNs, CpG oligodeoxynucleotides; IgG, immunoglobulin G; poly(I:C), polyinosinic-polycytidylic acid; RSV, respiratory syncytial virus.

cDCs express TLRs 3 and 4, mediating recognition of viral double-stranded RNA and LPS, respectively, and on triggering secrete low amounts of IFN-β through a signaling pathway using the adaptor Toll/IL-1 receptor domain-containing adapter-inducing IFN-β and the transcription factor IRF3. Although cDCs can also induce IFN type I through RIG-I and MDA-5 upon viral infection, pDCs seem to rely mostly on a specialized MyD88-dependent signaling pathway, allowing them to secrete very high amounts of IFN-α upon triggering of TLRs 7 and 9. This is because of their constitutive high expression of IRF7, a crucial IFN-α gene transcription factor, and because of a specialized spatiotemporal regulation of TLR7 and TLR9 signaling, allowing IRF7 to interact with MyD88 docked onto TLRs in the endosomal membrane.[47]

The inflammasome consists of a family of PRRs that induce IL-1 and IL-18 secretion. IL-1β secretion can be triggered through the NLRP3, NLRC4, and NLRP1 inflammasomes, as well as by the DNA sensor AIM2.[48] Activation of the inflammasome occurs through activation of the nucleotide-binding domain, leucine-rich repeat-containing proteins (NLRs). NLRs are composed of three domains: at the N-terminus a pyrin domain, a caspase recruitment domain, or a baculovirus inhibitory repeat domain; the central domain is the nucleotide-binding domain responsible for dNTPase activity and oligomerization; and the leucine-rich repeat domain at the C-terminus.[49] Activation of the inflammasome leads to caspase-1–mediated processing of pro-IL-1 and pro-IL-18 for IL-1β or IL-18 secretion and inflammatory cell death (pyroptosis and pyronecrosis). The inflammasome can be activated by sterile (non-microbial) activators of both host (adenosine triphosphate [ATP], uric acid crystals, amyloid-β) and microenvironment (alum, silica, asbestos) origin. It can also be activated by pathogen-derived products, including PAMPs. Microbial activators include pore-forming toxins, RNA and DNA, flagellin, β-glucans, and zymosan. The

best-studied inflammasome is the NLRP3 inflammasome, whose activation requires two signals: the first upregulates NLRP3 and pro-IL-1β, and the second induces the assembly of the inflammasome complex.[48] This can occur via various mechanisms: generation of reactive oxygen species (ROS), possibly by the phagosomal NADH (nicotinamide adenine dinucleotide) oxidase, release of cathepsin B upon phagolysosomal destabilization, and pore formation at the plasma membrane through the P2X7 receptor, allowing K+ efflux.[50] Inflammasome components can be found in human DCs, with some found in both pDC and cDC subsets (e.g., NLRP3, ASC, and pro-caspase-1), whereas other molecules are expressed only in cDCs or moDCs in steady state and upon TLR priming (e.g., IL-1 and IL-18).[51]

C-type lectins are calcium-dependent, carbohydrate-binding proteins with a broad range of biologic functions, many of which are involved in immune responses. They are well represented on DCs and include the following: DC-SIGN, responsible for binding of HIV-1, HIV-2, simian immunodeficiency virus, Ebola viruses, dengue virus, *Candida* spp., *Leishmania* spp.; BDCA2, potentially responsible for delivering tolerogenic signals; BDCA4/neuropilin-1, capable of binding vascular endothelial growth factor (VEGF); langerin, responsible for uptake and processing of antigens in Langerhans cells; DEC-205 (CD205), involved in the uptake and processing of antigens in MIIV (vesicles enriched for MHC class II molecules and proteases such as the cathepsins that mediate antigen processing and MHC class II peptide complex formation), as well as the generation of tolerogenic signals; and MMR, involved in the processing of microbial organisms.

Other receptors expressed by DCs include FcR, which is involved in cross-presentation of immune complexes and antibody-opsonized dead cells; integrins such as $\alpha_v\beta_5$, scavenger receptor CD36, and Mer family tyrosine kinases for phagocytosis of apoptotic cells and lipoxygenase-1 or CD91 for uptake of HSPs; complement receptors that play a role in uptake of opsonized microbes and apoptotic cells; receptors for viruses (e.g., CD4, CCR5, and CXCR4 for HIV and CD46 for measles virus); and the CD1 family of receptors that activate CD4, CD8, $\gamma\delta$T cells, and NK T cells through binding and processing of antigens such as sphingolipids, sulfatides, glycosphingolipids, glycosylphosphatidylinositol (GPI)-anchored mucin-like glycoproteins (GPI mucins), glycoinositolphospholipids, and their phosphatidylinositol moieties. Altogether, these various receptors provide substantial avenues for DCs to efficiently capture multitudes of antigens in their environment.

Antigen capture is tightly coupled to DC activation and antigen presentation, and triggering of TLR or exposure to inflammatory cytokines first induces a transient increase in the macropinocytic uptake followed by a nearly complete downregulation of the uptake process. Furthermore, it has been suggested that TLR engagement also enhances microbe-loaded phagosome maturation, potentially discriminating between nonimmunogenic antigens (apoptotic cells) and microbial antigens at the antigen-processing level.[52]

ANTIGEN PROCESSING

DCs are highly efficient in processing and presenting antigens via their MHC or CD1 molecules and presenting those to other immune cells such as CD4 and CD8 T cells. Depending on the antigens the DCs encounter, the presentation pathway will differ, as described in detail later.

Major Histocompatibility Complex Class I Antigen Presentation (Endogenous Route)

The process of antigen processing and presentation to CD8+ T cells begins with degradation of proteins synthesized within the cytoplasm, either as mature proteins or as neosynthesized defective proteins (defective ribosomal products), into oligopeptides by the ubiquitin–proteasome pathway. Misfolded proteins are also a source of antigenic peptides after retrotranslocation from the ER to the cytosol through the ER-associated degradation pathway. Subsequently, aminopeptidases cleave N-terminal precursors into peptides of appropriate length for presentation on MHC class I molecules. Antigen processing via this route is regulated through activation of the catalytically active subunits of the proteasome, the PA28 proteasome activator, and leucine aminopeptidase, which are upregulated by IFN.[53] mDCs in particular express immunoproteosomes containing the active site subunits latent membrane protein 2 (LMP2), LMP7, and MECL-1, which can enhance antigen processing.[54] After transport into the ER through the transporter associated with antigen processing (Fig. 23.2), long peptides are further trimmed by ER aminopeptidase-1 to 8-mer or 9-mer peptides for loading onto MHC class I molecules.

DCs also have the capacity to acquire antigens exogenously and process them for presentation on MHC class I molecules. This phenomenon, referred to as *cross-presentation,* allows the immune system to recognize antigens that are not otherwise presented or that may not access DCs directly (e.g., tumor cells, viruses). DCs can acquire

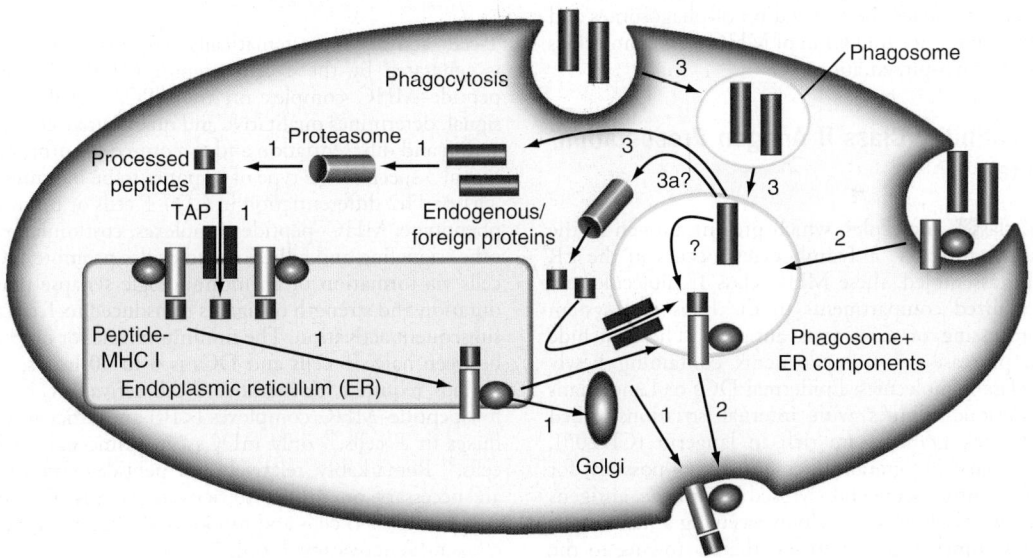

Fig. 23.2 PATHWAYS FOR MAJOR HISTOCOMPATIBILITY COMPLEX (MHC) CLASS I PRESENTATION. The classical pathway for MHC class I presentation *(1)* involves degradation of endogenous or viral antigens into peptides by the proteasome, followed by transport into the endoplasmic reticulum (ER). After further trimming in the ER, the peptides are loaded onto newly synthesized MHC class I molecules, and the peptide–MHC class I complexes are transported to the plasma membrane. Two main pathways of cross-presentation *(2, 3)* have been described that allow presentation of exogenous antigens in association with MHC class I molecules. Antigens endocytosed or phagocytosed can be cleaved into peptides by proteases and loaded onto recycling MHC class I molecules within the same phagosome or on the cell surface (vacuolar pathway) *(2)*. Alternatively, antigens may escape from the phagosome and enter the cytosol (phagosome-to-cytosol pathway) *(3)* to be processed via the classical MHC class I pathway. It has been suggested recently that elements of the ER can be associated with phagosomes, allowing transfer of antigens into the cytosol by the ER-associated degradation pathway and degradation by the phagosome-associated proteasome *(3a)*. The importance of each pathway *(2, 3)* for cross-presentation in vivo as well as the precise mechanisms and the locations of antigen processing in each model are under investigation. *TAP,* Transporter associated with antigen processing.

such antigens in the form of apoptotic cells, apoptotic microparticles, necrotic cells, antibody-opsonized cells, immune complexes, and HSPs (intracellular chaperones for antigenic peptides, which are released by necrotic cells).[55,56] DCs even acquire antigens via phagocytosis of particles released from intracellular vesicles (referred to as *exosomes*).[57] Finally, DCs may even nibble bits of live cells to acquire antigens.[58] This phenomenon of cross-presentation is especially efficient in, if not unique to, DCs compared with other APCs. Evaluation of freshly isolated lymphoid organ-resident human DCs has confirmed that these cells also have the capacity to cross-present soluble antigens similarly to their blood counterparts.[59]

Mechanistically, cross-presentation occurs via two major pathways: the cytosolic and the vacuolar pathways.[60] In the first, antigens are transferred to the cytoplasm, which is followed by processing by the proteasome and loading onto newly formed MHC class I molecules (phagosome-to-cytosol pathway), with a possible recruitment of the ER machinery for antigen processing and MHC class I loading (see Fig. 23.2).[61-64] This pathway is sensitive to proteasome inhibitors, suggesting that proteins access the cytosol and are degraded by proteasomes, but whether the peptide loading occurs via the classical MHC I pathway or in endocytic compartments remains to be determined.[64,65] The vacuolar pathway is resistant to proteasome inhibitors and sensitive to inhibitors of lysosomal proteolysis, and it is known to be cathepsin S–dependent, thus indicating that both antigen processing and loading onto MHC class I molecules may occur in endocytic compartments (see Fig. 23.2).[66,67] The relative contribution of the cytosolic and vacuolar pathways is still unclear, but some evidence suggests the predominant use of the cytosolic pathway.[65] Currently, it is known that specific DC subsets are more efficient at cross-presentation, with the resident CD8α+ and the migratory CD1013+ DCs being the most efficient.[68,69] In humans, the proposed CD8α homologue cells—the CD141+ (BDCA3+) DCs—are specialized at cross-presentation.[70-73] Finally, in recent years, it has been described that TLR signaling can influence the maturation of phagosomes and also can have an effect on the accumulation of MHC class I molecules in the phagosomes for cross-presentation.[74]

Major Histocompatibility Class II Antigen Presentation (Exogenous Route)

Assembly of MHC class II molecules, which present antigen in the form of short peptides to CD4+ T lymphocytes, occurs in the ER of DCs. After being assembled, these MHC class II molecules are transported to specialized compartments in the lysosomal system involved in the processing of exogenous antigens. These include MIIVs, which are protease-rich compartments containing newly synthesized MHC class II molecules. Epidermal DCs or Langerhans cells contain cytoplasmic tubules with internal striations called *Birbeck granules*. Birbeck granules are rich in langerin (CD205), a C-type lectin necessary for granule formation and possibly for capture of pathogens.[75] After being endocytosed by imDCs, antigens are partially retained within lysosomes. Upon receiving a maturation signal, the pH of lysosomes decreases to less than 5 (owing to the activation of a vacuolar H+-ATPase). Concomitantly, there is antigen degradation caused by activation of proteases such as cathepsins. Cystatin C, a protein that blocks the activity of cathepsin S, is also degraded, thereby allowing the degradation of invariant chain peptide (Ii chain), which normally blocks access of antigenic peptides to MHC class II molecules. These changes occur in late endosomes and lysosomes (the MIIV compartment). After antigenic peptide is bound to MHC class II molecules, it exits the lysosomes through the formation of long tubular structures, which simultaneously deliver costimulatory molecules such as CD86 to the cell surface.[76,77]

DCs handle internalized antigens in a specialized way unlike other phagocytic cells such as macrophages, which degrade most of the internalized material, leaving only limited amounts of antigenic peptides for presentation onto MHC molecules. On the contrary, internalized antigens in cDCs are preserved for longer times, thereby allowing their transport by maturing DCs to secondary lymphoid organs, where actual presentation occurs. mDCs display higher levels of proteolysis than imDCs do, allowing appropriate degradation of the antigens for loading onto MHC molecules. These differences are accounted for by several features unique to DCs, such as low levels of lysosomal proteases in immature stages compared with macrophages, expression of protease inhibitors (cystatin C), regulation of lysosomal pH (and hence activity of proteases) by regulation of the acidifying V-type H+-ATPase activity, and consumption of H+ upon reaction with superoxide radicals generated by NADPH (nicotinamide adenine dinucleotide phosphate) oxidase NOX2 in maturing DCs.[78] During maturation, trafficking of MHC class II molecules to the surface is dramatically increased, probably because of degradation of Ii chain (containing endosome-lysosome targeting signal) in acidic compartments, leading to transport of MHC class II molecules via the constitutive secretory pathway to the cell membrane.

In addition to direct presentation of intracellular antigens and cross-presentation of internalized material, DCs can acquire preformed MHC class I molecules in complex with antigens from other cells by the process of trogocytosis (transfer of cell-membrane patches or individual proteins between cells) or through gap junctions, in a process termed *cross-dressing;* this allows rapid presentation without processing of antigens. It has been suggested that memory CD8 T cells are preferentially activated by this mode of presentation in contrast to naive T cells.[79] It further provides a mechanism for antigen transfer between DC populations, which can be exploited for vaccine design. Thus it has been shown that ex vivo loaded DCs sometimes do not directly activate host CD8+ T cells, which rather requires transfer of peptide–MHC complexes from vaccine DCs to resident DCs for efficient priming.[80]

T-CELL ACTIVATION

T-cell activation systematically requires three signals. Signal 1 is generated by the T-cell receptor (TCR) after engagement by a peptide–MHC complex on the APC. Signal 2, or costimulatory signal, determines qualitative and quantitative elements of T-cell activation and differentiation and is required for priming of naive T cells. Signal 3 specifies the type of response to be mounted, inducing either Th1 or Th2 differentiation in CD4 T cells or promoting a regulatory phenotype. MHC–peptide complexes, costimulatory molecules, and other signaling and adhesion molecules promote DC contact with T cells via formation of an immunologic synapse that determines the duration and strength of signals transduced to T cells, leading to their subsequent activation. The minimum time for productive interaction between naive T cells and DCs is 6 to 30 hours, with shorter time periods required for memory T-cell activation.[81,82] Although only a few peptide–MHC complexes (<10) are sufficient to trigger calcium fluxes in T cells,[83] only mDCs can prime naive CD4 and CD8 T cells.[84] Remarkably, relatively few peptide–MHC complexes (<200) are necessary on mDCs to activate T cells. Compared with other APCs, such as B cells and monocytes, DCs are up to 1000-fold more efficient at activating T cells.[85]

Costimulatory molecules include the CD80 and CD86 members of the B7 family, which ligate to CD28 on T cells, and members of the TNF family, such as CD40 (Table 23.4).[12] Notably, one new member of the B7 family, B7-DC, is unique to DCs and stimulates naive T cells highly efficiently.[86] Other molecules play inhibitory roles upon encountering their receptor on T cells. For example, programmed cell death ligand 1 (PD-L1) on DCs interacts with programmed cell death protein 1 (PD-1) on T cells to downregulate T-cell responses. Inducible costimulator ligand (ICOSL) is present on both DCs and B cells and is critical for germinal center formation and immunoglobulin class switching.

Signal 3 determines the skewing of the T-cell response such that T cells may terminally differentiate either toward IFN-γ–producing CD4+ T cells (Th1 cells), which eradicate intracellular pathogens (bacteria or viruses), or into Th2 cells producing IL-4, IL-5, and IL-13, which promote elimination of extracellular infections.

TABLE 23.4 **Costimulatory Molecules Involved in the Interaction Between Dendritic Cells and T Cells (Signal 2)[a]**

Dendritic Cell	T Cell	Signal
B7 Family		
B7-1(CD80)/B7-2(CD86)	CD28	Activating
B7-1(CD80)/B7-2(CD86)	CTLA-4	Inhibitory
B7-H1(PDL1)/B7-DC(PDL2)	?	Activating
B7-H1(PDL1)/B7-DC(PDL2)	PD-1	Inhibitory
B7-H2 (B7h; B7PR1; ICOSL)	ICOS	Activating
B7H3	?	Activating
B7H4 (B7S1; B7x)	?	Inhibitory
TNF Receptor Family		
4–1BBL	4–1BB	Activating
CD27L	CD27	Activating
OX40L	OX40	Activating
LIGHT	LIGHT-R	Activating
Cytokines		
IL-2	IL-2R	T-cell proliferation
IL-12	IL-12R	T-cell proliferation
IL-18		

[a]T-cell activation requires two signals. The T-cell receptor interaction with a peptide–MHC complex (signal 1) is accompanied by signal 2, delivered by one of the mechanisms listed in this table. Formation of the immunologic synapse between a dendritic cell and a T cell determines the fate of the lymphocyte. The number of identified costimulatory molecules responsible for signal 2 is increasing steadily.
CTLA-4, Cytotoxic T-lymphocyte antigen 4; IL, interleukin; LIGHT, homologous to lymphotoxins, exhibits inducible expression, and competes with HSV glycoprotein D for herpesvirus entry mediator, a receptor expressed by T lymphocytes; PD-1, programmed cell death 1; TNF, tumor necrosis factor.

Additionally, cytokines such as IL-12 for Th1 or IL-4 for Th2 differentiation are crucial determinants of initiation or amplification of Th responses. It has been suggested that DCs express the Notch ligands δ or Jagged under Th1 or Th2 conditions, respectively, and that these ligands promote differentiation of naive T cells toward one or the other Th profile.[87] Thus, whereas factors and pathogens, which stimulate DC maturation and IL-12 production, promote Th1 responses (e.g., *Escherichia coli*), inducers of IL-4 production prime Th2 responses (e.g., *Porphyromonas gingivalis*).

Furthermore, the Th1-polarizing capacity of DCs depends on a number of variables that include the expression of certain transcription factors, the microenvironment, exposure to various maturation stimuli, the kinetics of maturation, and the antigen dose. For example, expression by DCs of the transcription factor T-bet, which controls IFN-γ expression in CD4[+] T cells, appears to be required for optimal development of Th1 responses.[88] Epithelial DCs in the respiratory tract may by default induce Th2 responses upon production of factors such as TSLP by epithelial cells.[41] The duration of DC activation and antigen dose also determines the direction of T-cell skewing. Prolonged activation causes IL-12 depletion and results in "exhausted DCs."[37] DCs presenting low amounts of antigen skew toward Th2, whereas high doses skew toward Th1, which in turn depends on the maturation state of the DCs and consequences of environmental exposure.[89,90]

Since 2005, new CD4 T-cell lineages have been discovered. These include Th9, Th22, and Th17, which is the best characterized of the three.[91–94] Named *Th17* because of their characteristic secretion of IL-17, this lineage of cells is implicated in several chronic inflammatory disorders. The IL-12 family member IL-23 and transforming growth factor-β (TGF-β) are involved in the generation of Th17 cells.[91] LPS-stimulated DCs secrete inflammatory cytokines, notably IL-6, and in combination with TGF-β seem to divert differentiation of Tregs into Th17 cells.[95,96] TGF-β upregulates the expression of the pivotal transcription factor retinoic acid–related orphan receptor-γt

(RORγt) in a concentration-dependent manner, but high TGF-β concentration favors Treg development over Th17 differentiation, partly through Foxp3-inhibitory interaction with RORγt.[97] On one hand, the pathogenic role of Th17 cells may depend on the cytokine milieu in which they are differentiated or expand, and DC-derived IL-23 or IL-1β could contribute to enhanced pathogenicity of Th17 cells. On the other hand, Th17 cells display heightened levels of the IL-10 receptor and are more susceptible to IL-10–mediated regulation, a cytokine secreted by DCs upon ligation of some TLRs (e.g., TLR2, TLR4). Moreover, the pathogenic role of Th17 is also controlled in the intestine.[98] Therefore the flexibility of DC activation and cytokine secretion profile may affect the pathogenic potential of developing Th17 cells.

The recently described Th9 cells are defined by their secretion of IL-9. Their development relies on several molecules, including signal transducer and activator of transcription 6 (STAT6) (downstream of the IL-4 receptor), needed to suppress T-bet (Th1 transcription factor) and TGF-β–induced Foxp3 expression, as well as IRF4 and STAT5, which directly activate the *Il9* promoter.[92] Furthermore, TGF-β was shown to redirect Th2 cells into Th9 cells.[99] These cells have been associated with both protective and pathogenic roles and have been identified as contributors to human atopic disease and inflammatory bowel disease (IBD); however, they are also known to mediate antihelminth infections and have antitumor activity.[100] Recently, Th9-derived IL-9 was shown to inhibit both mouse and human melanoma cell growth, highlighting an antitumor role.[101,102]

Th22 cells are characterized by their secretion of IL-22, and they have been associated with autoimmune diseases such as psoriasis, SLE, and allergies.[94] They are closely related to Th17 cells, but the details of this relationship are not very well described. Th22 can modulate antimicrobial pathways in the intestine and skin, and IL-22 was shown to regulate the expression of genes involved in antimicrobial defense (e.g., the Reg family of antimicrobial proteins) in these two tissues.[103,104]

It is important to note that T-cell priming depends on mDCs because imDCs may induce immunosuppressive or Tregs.[105,106] In fact, antigen presentation by imDCs in vivo is an important pathway by which tolerance is maintained at both the CD4 and CD8 T-cell levels, either through the induction of Tregs or through the deletion of autoreactive T cells.[107] Nevertheless, recent data suggest that, in some conditions, mDCs can also induce the generation of CD4+CD25+ Tregs.[108,109]

CD8+ T cells[105] and generation of effective CD8 memory cells in turn require CD4 T-cell help.[110–112] This help is provided through activation of DC via CD40L–CD40 interactions and the production of cytokines such as IL-2, although some studies have suggested that when cytotoxic T-lymphocyte precursor frequencies are high, priming of CD8 T-cell responses may be CD4 T-cell–independent. In these cases, though, memory generation is likely to be hampered because of the absence of IL-2 during priming,[113] and primed T cells may commit fratricide through expression of tumor necrosis factor-related apoptosis-inducing ligand (TRAIL),[114] or they may become functionally tolerant upon receiving signals through the inhibitory receptor PD-1.[115]

Evidence is accumulating that pDCs, which were believed to play a role only in the innate immune response because of their ability to produce high levels of IFN type I, can present viral and tumor antigens to initiate both CD4[+] and CD8[+] T-cell responses.[116] pDCs mature in response to certain viral infections (e.g., influenza and HIV), thereby providing an important link between innate and adaptive arms of the immune response. Similarly to their myeloid counterparts, however, pDCs display plasticity, even inducing immunosuppressive responses depending on their microenvironment or the stimuli to which they are exposed.[117] Genetic depletion of pDCs, using transgenic mice expressing diphtheria toxin receptor under the control of BDCA2 promoter, has allowed dissecting precisely the role of pDC in antiviral responses. In the case of vesicular stomatitis virus infection, depletion of pDCs resulted in decreased specific CD8[+] T-cell responses, but depletion of pDCs during lymphocytic choriomeningitis virus (LCMV) did not affect the magnitude of the

LCMV-specific CD8+ T-cell response. This suggests that pDCs may be required to enhance weak cytotoxic T-cell responses.[118] A recent study targeting Siglec-H by conditional genetic ablation specifically induced specific pDC depletion and demonstrated a complex role of pDCs. Siglec-H and pDCs depleted pDC-suppressed, antigen-specific CD4+ T-cell responses in vivo, but they were required to enhance the CD8+ T-cell response to soluble and microbial antigens.[119]

B-CELL ACTIVATION

In addition to affecting T-cell function, DCs can also influence B-cell proliferation, isotype switching, and plasma cell differentiation.[120] DCs produce factors that activate and induce B-cell proliferation (B-Lys and APRIL).[121] Furthermore, DCs stimulate antibody responses in a T-cell–independent manner against polysaccharide antigens. The initial interactions between B cells and DCs occur in the T-cell area of lymph nodes and in the germinal centers of lymph nodes or splenic red pulp (or both). Importantly, antigen-exposed cDCs possess a specialized nondegradative pathway that allows them to present internalized antigens in their native state for the engagement of B-cell receptors on B cells. This is mediated by endocytosis of antigenic immune complexes through the inhibitory Fc receptor FcγRIIB and recycling of the endocytic vesicle to the surface without antigen degradation.[122] The follicular DCs, which are present in germinal centers of lymph nodes and which constitute a different class of DCs, participate in the maintenance of B-cell memory by formation of multiple antigen–antibody complexes and continuous stimulation of B cells. The antigen–antibody complexes may remain in the lymph node for an extended period of time (up to months or years).

NATURAL KILLER CELL ACTIVATION

The interactions between DCs and NK cells are complex and further underscore a role of DCs as a link between innate and adaptive immunity.[8] Direct interactions between NK cells and mDCs can result in NK-cell activation as well as the potentiation of their cytolytic activity, and, conversely, NK cells can induce further DC maturation. NK cells and DCs can form an immune synapse, probably helping directional and confined secretion of cytokines as well as facilitating receptor–ligand interactions with one another. Activated NK cells induce DCs through both cell contact (involving NKp30) and TNF-α and IFN-γ secretion. In turn, activated DCs secrete IL-12/IL-18, IL-15, and IFN-α/β, which enhance IFN-γ secretion, proliferation, and cytotoxicity of NK cells. In some conditions, NK cells can lyse DCs through NKp30, although mDCs are protected from cytolysis. This might represent a form of "cellular editing" whereby immature and tolerogenic DCs (tDCs) are cleared by NK cells in the course of an ongoing immune response.[123]

It is thus possible that DC and NK cells play complementary roles in sensing pathogens, such that DCs could be the first to detect microbes through their expression of PRRs (TLRs, NOD proteins), whereas NK may become activated in the absence of overt inflammation but in the presence of ligands for activating NK-cell receptors, such as in the setting of tumors (which frequently lose MHC class I expression or express NKG2D ligands, such as MHC class I polypeptide-related sequences A and B). In both situations, either DCs or NK cells could create an inflammatory environment and induce the integrated activation of other cell types. Thus, in mice, infection by murine cytomegalovirus (CMV) induces pDCs to secrete high levels of IFN-α/β, but CD8α+ DCs are the major producers of IL-12, and resistance to the virus is associated with expansion of Ly49H+ NK cells, driven by IL-12/IL-18.

The interaction between NK cells and DCs is likely to take place early during the course of an immune response. This allows DCs to exploit the ability of NK cells to kill tumor or virus- or parasite-infected cells and to cross-present this material to T cells.[124]

ACTIVATION OF OTHER ELEMENTS OF THE IMMUNE SYSTEM

DCs have proven to be quite versatile in their ability to interact with many constituents of the immune system. For example, they can activate NK T cells by presentation of the synthetic ligand α-galactosyl ceramide on CD1, inducing the production of cytokines such as IFN-γ and resistance to tumors.[125] CD1-restricted γδT cells, which respond to microbial antigens from *Mycobacterium tuberculosis* and other organisms, induce maturation of resting DCs and also induce IL-12 production. This pathway and the IFN-γ secretion by activated γδT cells provide the immune system with a source of activated APCs, which can polarize Th1 responses.[126]

In summary, the influence of DCs on other cell types of the immune system is broad and integrative (Fig. 23.3). Future studies will ascertain the interplay between the myriad host cells and the innate and adaptive immune responses.

TOLERANCE AND AUTOIMMUNITY

DCs play a pivotal role in the balance between immunity and tolerance. DCs are important in the induction of both central and peripheral tolerance. In the former, DCs play a role in deletion of autoreactive T cells in the thymus. In the latter, imDCs in their steady state induce T-cell deletion, anergy, or generation of Tregs, which interfere with IL-2 production and proliferation of effector T cells against self.[127]

In the thymus, medullary thymic epithelial cells (mTECs) are the major population responsible for inducing central tolerance. Autoreactive T cells in the thymus are negatively selected upon recognition of self-antigens, which are expressed at low levels by mTECs via their expression of autoimmune regulator (AIRE) transcription factor. AIRE induces the release of stalled RNA polymerase II to promote the ectopic expression of these self-antigens.[128] Thymic DCs contribute to negative selection in that they can cross-present the self-antigens from mTECs to T cells in the thymus. DCs acquire antigen from apoptotic debris of mTECs, a consequence of normal turnover of the cells,[129] or they can acquire intact antigens via antigen transfer from mTECs,[130] a process that may occur by tunneling nanotubes,[131] trogocytosis,[58] or trafficking of mTEC-derived exosomes.[132] In this context, AIRE was also reported to control the transfer of antigen from mTECs to DCs.[133] Additionally, circulating DCs from the periphery have also been shown to migrate to the thymus and play a role in negative selection by inducing clonal deletion of autoreactive T cells or Treg development.[134]

In the periphery, how DCs induce tolerance is still an area of active investigation, although a number of possible mechanisms have been identified. These processes are critical because they limit harmful immune responses to antigens that may not have been available during thymic selection, or from autoreactive T cells that may have escaped central tolerance.[135] In the steady state, antigen delivery via the endocytosis receptor DEC-205 in imDCs was shown to induce T-cell tolerance, highlighting a function of DCs as promoters of naive peripheral T-cell deletion.[136] Using a genetic approach, Probst and colleagues showed that antigen expression in steady-state DCs also induced strong CD8+ T-cell tolerance to immunodominant antigens and that this effect was dependent on negative costimulation via inhibitory receptors of the CD28 family, such as PD-1 and cytotoxic T lymphocyte–associated protein 4 (CTLA-4).[127,137]

Production of indoleamine 2,3-dioxygenase (IDO) has been proposed to account for some of the tolerogenic potential of DCs.[138] IDO is an enzyme that degrades the indole moiety of tryptophan and other molecules and induces the production of immunoregulatory metabolites known as *kynurenines*. Local depletion of tryptophan and increases in proapoptotic kynurenines affect T-cell proliferation and survival. Induction of IDO in DCs has been postulated as one means by which deletional tolerance occurs.[138] DC-derived IDO can promote T-cell tolerance by mechanisms that may or may not depend

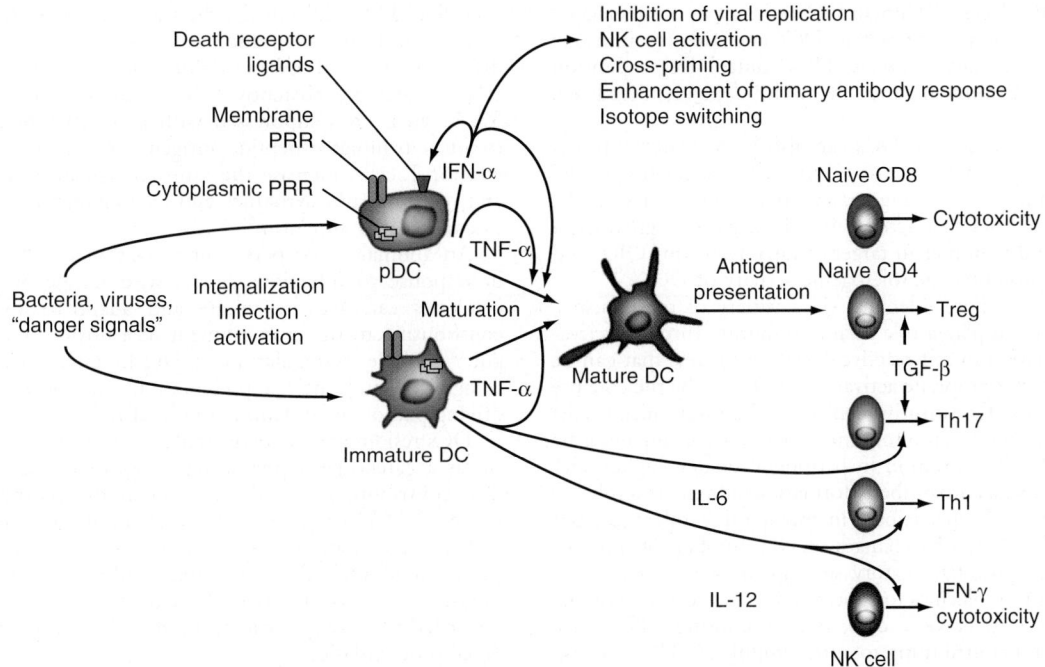

Fig. 23.3 DENDRITIC CELLS (DCs) LINK INNATE AND ADAPTIVE IMMUNITY. Through the expression of pattern recognition receptors (PRRs), such as Toll-like receptors, DCs act as sensors of pathogen intrusion. Upon signaling by PRRs, DCs secrete cytokines and express receptors, allowing stimulation of the innate immune system. Interferon-α (IFN-α) or interleukin-12 (IL-12) stimulates natural killer (NK) cell activation while also inducing the expression of death receptor ligands (tumor necrosis factor–related apoptosis-inducing ligand, or TRAIL) on DCs, harnessing them for direct killing of infected cells. They take up antigens through direct infection or phagocytosis, undergo a complex program of maturation by upregulating the expression of costimulatory and major histocompatibility complex (MHC) molecules, migrate to the secondary lymphoid organs, and stimulate naive T cells. They secrete cytokines, skewing the type of response induced toward Th1, Th2, regulatory T cell (Treg), or Th17 differentiation; inducing the generation of cytotoxic CD8 T cells; or participating in the generation of antibody responses. *pDC,* Plasmacytoid dendritic cell; *TGF,* transforming growth factor.

on IDO's catalytic activity. Moreover, expression of death-inducing ligands such as FasL or perforin may render DCs capable of killing activated T cells and exerting an immunoregulatory role.[136,139,140]

In addition to T-cell deletion and anergy, DCs contribute to peripheral tolerance largely via induction or Tregs. tDCs are known to promote Tregs via secretion of particular stimuli, such as TGF-β or RA, and the maintenance of Treg numbers was shown to be dependent on tDC expression of costimulatory molecules CD80 and CD86.[141] Tregs are CD4+ or CD8+ in nature and express CD25, CTLA-4, lymphocyte activation gene 3 (LAG3), Helios, and the transcription factor Foxp3 (a member of the Forkhead transcription factor family). These cells exert their tolerogenic effects either via cell contact or through release of immunosuppressive cytokines such as IL-10[142] or TGF-β, preventing proliferation and cytotoxicity of activated CD4 or CD8 T cells, and can also inhibit TLR-mediated maturation of cDCs but not pDCs.[143] Tregs are fundamental to the maintenance of the tolerogenic potential of DCs, and Foxp3+ Treg depletion studies highlighted the role of these cells in preserving DCs in a nonmature state. Furthermore, this effect was mediated by direct TCR–MHC class II interactions between Tregs and DCs.[144,145] Also, pDCs activated through TLR7 or TLR9 upregulate the expression of IDO and can induce the generation of Tregs from naive CD4+ T cells.[146]

There are several mechanisms by which Tregs are thought to exert their suppressive functions on DCs. One example is Treg-induced downregulation of CD70 expression in DCs, which is essential for the tolerogenic role of these cells.[147] Another mechanism of suppression by Tregs is via their coinhibitory molecules, such as CTLA-4 and LAG3. CTLA-4 from Tregs was shown to induce downregulation of CD80 and CD86 on DCs, whereas LAG3 was shown to suppress DC

activation via direct binding to MHC class II molecules.[148,149] Finally, DCs are also targeted by TGF-β–dependent suppression; however, whether this is a Treg-mediated suppression is still unclear.[150]

Altogether, these properties of DCs make them attractive candidates for inducing tolerance in the setting of transplantation or autoimmunity. Indeed, injection of antigen-pulsed imDCs in vivo induces antigen-specific IL-10–producing CD8+ Tregs, which supplant their IFN-γ–producing effector cell counterparts.[105,151]

DCs may also be actively rendered tolerogenic via a number of mechanisms. Resting imDCs acquire self-antigens through phagocytosis of apoptotic bodies formed as a consequence of physiologic cell turnover. In the absence of a maturation signal, these DCs induce tolerance to such self-antigens.[152] Some studies have suggested that ligation of specific receptors on DCs, such as complement receptors CR3 and CR4, by apoptotic cells or apoptotic microparticles inhibit their maturation, thereby ensuring the delivery of a tolerogenic rather than stimulatory signals.[153] Others include MER, CD91/calreticulin, CD36/α$_v$β$_5$, and CD44.[154] External factors such as steroids, IL-10, and TGF-β may also compromise DC immunostimulatory function by inhibiting their full maturation.[155] For example, DCs isolated from tumor environments are poorly immunostimulatory because of the presence of immunosuppressive cytokines or the induction of costimulatory molecules, such as PD-L1, which deliver negative signals.[156] Moreover, there may exist distinct tDC subsets. A particular DC subset was identified in normal mice that were CD11c^{low}/CD45RB^{high}, secreted IL-10 after activation, and induced tolerance through induction of Tregs.[157] In mice, pDCs have recently been shown to induce tolerance against a vascularized cardiac allograft upon administration of a tolerizing regimen.[158] After capturing pDC alloantigens from the graft, they migrated to peripheral lymph nodes and induced specific Tregs.[158] Human DC deficiencies are associated with a loss of Tregs, and it seems that DCs and Tregs reciprocally control each other's expansion, where DCs control Treg expansion and Tregs control DC numbers through an Flt3-dependent feedback loop.

The tolerogenic function of DCs can also be regulated intrinsically by signaling molecules such as NFκB, a key regulator of DC function; A20, a ubiquitin-editing enzyme that is implicated in the degradation of molecules that activate NFκB, negative regulators of NFκB (CD31), and mammalian target of rapamycin (mTOR); and β-catenin, which promotes the tolerogenic activity of DCs.[159–164]

Although DCs promote tolerance via a variety of mechanisms, they are also known to play a role in autoimmunity through activation and differentiation of self-reactive T cells, a process that can be triggered either by inappropriate activation of DCs or by the collapse of negative regulation. Constitutive depletion of DCs in mice results in a syndrome resembling autoimmunity that was accompanied by increased CD4+ T-cell infiltration in peripheral tissues, higher Th1 and Th17 cell numbers, autoantibody formation, and neutrophilia.[165] In the steady state, DCs participate in maintaining tolerance, but this balance can be altered by changes in DC number, phenotype, and function.[166] In proinflammatory settings, or when there is an absence of regulatory molecules to control DCs, they can potentially present self-antigens to naive T cells, thus promoting self-reactive T-cell activation and contributing to autoimmunity.[167] DCs are also believed to be important for the induction of the chronic phase of autoimmune diseases. Some of these conditions are discussed in more detail later.

DCs from patients with SLE exhibit altered CD40, CD86, and Fcγ receptor expression[168] and have altered PD-L1 expression, which can modulate T-cell suppression.[169] Activated cDCs (possibly through immune complexes or cell-derived microparticles) may promote lupus pathogenesis by presenting RNA-associated proteins and chromatin to self-reactive T cells.[170] In mouse models of SLE, activated DCs also enhance B-cell proliferation, IL-6 and IFN-γ secretion, and antinuclear antibody production.[171,172] IFN-α produced by pDCs is thought to contribute to the autoimmune response in SLE.[173–176] pDCs can be activated through TLR7 and TLR9 by immune complexes containing RNA and DNA, respectively, from dead cells and induced to secrete high amounts of IFN-α. This can further promote the differentiation of monocytes into activated cDCs, thus enhancing presentation of self-antigens, increasing the cytotoxicity of CD8 and NK cells, and promoting plasma cell differentiation and subsequent generation of pathogenic autoantibodies. Several host factors can convert self-DNA into triggers of pDC activation. For example, the antimicrobial peptide LL-37 forms large aggregates with self-DNA released from dying cells, protecting it from extracellular nuclease digestion, and is taken in pDCs for induction of type I IFN. LL-37 has been found to be overexpressed in psoriatic skin, and the gene encoding LL-37 is the most upregulated in the blood of patients with lupus.[177]

A role of cDCs during disease onset is also strongly suggested in arthritis, multiple sclerosis, diabetes, and atherosclerosis.[178–180] The similarity between outcomes of microbial infection and autoimmunity suggests that TLRs or PRRs triggered by microbial molecules on DCs induce their maturation and secretion of cytokines and chemokines. This may cause DCs to upregulate presentation of self-antigens in instances such as apoptosis or necrosis induced directly by pathogens or antimicrobial immune response. Endogenous ligands such as extracellular matrix breakdown products (heparan sulfate and hyaluronate), molecules released from necrotic cells (high-mobility group box 1 protein [HMGB1], uric acid, or even endogenous nucleic acids), fibronectin, and HSPs, which can activate TLRs on cDCs, may also contribute to the generation of autoimmune responses.[181]

In rheumatoid arthritis (RA), DCs migrate into the synovium, where they produce proinflammatory molecules that concentrate in the vicinity of T cells, thereby possibly contributing to overall inflammation. DCs are hypothesized to regulate the production of autoantibodies in RA, and a correlation between DC numbers and concentration of anticitrullinated peptide antibodies in RA sera has

been found.[182] Additionally, the transfer of mature, collagen-pulsed DCs is sufficient to induce arthritis in a mouse model through induction of local inflammation and priming of autoreactive T cells.[183] DCs are currently being used to "tolerize" patients with RA in vivo. DCs suppressed with a NFκB inhibitor and exposed to four citrullinated peptide antigens were recently shown to reduce effector T cells, increase the ratio of regulatory to effector T cells, and reduce serum cytokines and chemokines and a T-cell response to citrullinated vimentin.[184]

An anomalous or persistent activation of DCs in the intestine in response to infectious agents with release of proinflammatory cytokines can activate innate and adaptive immune cells, thus contributing to the establishment of a noxious environment in the gut.[185,186] The dysregulation of DC function (related to pathogen recognition and antigen presentation) was shown to be critical in driving pathologic inflammation in IBD.[185]

DCs residing at the perivascular space of the blood–brain barrier act as a gatekeepers, presenting antigens to migrating T cells and thus contributing to inflammation in the central nervous system (CNS).[187,188] However, experimental autoimmune encephalomyelitis (EAE) can be induced in the absence of DCs, and the conditional depletion of DCs does not affect pathogenic Th priming in this model.[189,190] Thus DCs contribute to the onset of EAE, but they are not strictly necessary for it, and other APCs might promote harmful T-cell differentiation.

DCs play a tolerogenic role in preventing type 1 diabetes,[191] but they can promote it if, in an activated state, they cross-present β-cell antigens to T cells, initiating pathogenic T-cell differentiation.[192] A distinct subset of AIRE+ DCs was described to express antigen insulin derived from β-cells, suggesting a role for tDCs in controlling activation of insulin-reactive T cells.[193]

Overall, DCs play an important role in the development of autoimmune disease, either via direct activation of self-reactive T cells or indirectly because of the proinflammatory environment that they can create with secretion of cytokines and reduction of Tregs. When considering treatment approaches for these autoimmune diseases, there is a need to identify and define the balance between regulatory and pathogenic DC roles.

SUBVERSION OF DENDRITIC CELL FUNCTION BY PATHOGENS AND TUMORS

Several pathogens have evolved different mechanisms to inhibit DC functions, allowing them to downregulate specific immune responses and hence persist in the host. Numerous viruses, such as measles, vaccinia, herpes simplex, smallpox, and LCMV, can impair antigen presentation by infected cells through different mechanisms. Thus human CMV induces downmodulation of MHC class I or class II molecules and can inhibit activated T cells through secretion of a virally encoded IL-10 homolog. Directly targeting DCs allows viruses to impair the generation and quality of the antiviral immune responses. In mice, CMV has been shown to trigger paralysis of infected DCs, preventing them from secreting IL-12 or IL-2 upon TLR4 triggering, impairing their capacity to mature, and eventually rendering them unable to prime an effective T-cell response.[194] Some viral products interfere with IFN-α secretion pathways, such as the E6 oncoprotein of human papillomavirus, inhibiting transactivation of IRF3 or IRF7, or NS3/4A inhibiting RIG-I- and MDA5-mediated activation of IRF3.

It is now well documented that in HIV-infected patients not only are the number of pDCs and cDCs in blood reduced, but cDCs are also less efficient at stimulating primary T-cell responses and may generate IL-10–secreting T cells with a potential regulatory role. DCs, such as Langerhans cells, may be the first cells to encounter HIV in mucosal tissues and may mediate the spread of virus to CD4+ T cells in lymphoid organs. Formation of virions and release from the cell surface are counteracted by tetherin, an IFN-regulated restriction factor that retains virions at the cell surface. The Vpu accessory protein antagonizes tetherin activity to allow virion release. cDCs can mediate transinfection of CD4$^+$ T cells through the formation of an infectious synapse, carrying the virus with or without infection of the DCs themselves. DCs express the coreceptors CD4, CCR5, CXCR4, and the C-type lectin DC-SIGN necessary for binding or entry of HIV. HIV can infect DCs, but its replication is not as efficient as in CD4$^+$ T cells because of expression of the viral restriction factor SAMHD1, a deoxynucleoside triphosphate triphosphohydrolase. SAMHD1 functions to reduce cellular dNTP pools, thus reducing reverse transcription, although its restriction activity may be separate from its trihydrolase activity.[195] Under permissive conditions, however, HIV can induce the production of the cyclic dinucleotide cyclic guanosine monophosphate-adenosine monophosphate (cGAMP) via the cytosolic sensor cGAMP synthase (cGAS), suggesting that cGAMP can bypass the block of innate immune responses against HIV.[196] Under these conditions, HIV induces type I IFN production in monocyte-derived DCs that is dependent upon activation of the STING pathway. Recent studies have shown that polyglutamine binding protein 1 (PQBP1) directly binds to reverse-transcribed HIV-1 DNA and interacts with cGAS to generate cGAMP, which in turn primes an IRF3-dependent innate response.[197] Virions formed in cGAMP-expressing cells have the capacity to trigger a STING-dependent antiviral program in newly infected cells. Indeed, cGAMP-loaded lentiviruses are able to activate DCs, revealing a new way by which innate immunity can be transferred between cells.[198] The cGAS pathway is the only signaling pathway triggered by HIV in monocyte-derived DCs thus far. TLR7 and TLR8 do not appear to play a role in this respect.[199]

The viral envelope protein gp120 can bind to CD4 and C-type lectins such as DC-SIGN and mannose receptor, but the contribution of each receptor to binding and internalization may vary, depending on the particular type of DC encountered by HIV. Thus, although DCs are not the main reservoir of HIV, the virus can "highjack" DCs to mediate its spread to CD4$^+$ T cells from mucosal tissues to lymphoid organs. Nevertheless, although cDCs are only minimally activated by HIV, pDCs can become infected and strongly activated by HIV, causing them to secrete high amounts of IFN-α and other antiviral molecules. This can inhibit the replication of HIV in CD4$^+$ T cells, suggesting that the two subsets play different and opposing roles during HIV infection. However, pDCs may also function to downregulate the response by secreting TRAIL.[200,201] Furthermore, the continuous secretion of IFN-α by pDCs stimulated by HIV may be detrimental to the host by participating to chronic immune activation and CD4$^+$ T-cell depletion.

Tumors also evolve mechanisms to negate the functionality of DCs. For example, the number of cDCs (but not pDCs) is reduced in the blood of patients with cancer, and these numbers of DCs are restored upon surgical removal of the tumor, indicating a systemic defect orchestrated by the tumor cells. Moreover, increased numbers of imDCs are found in blood and tumor tissue, also displaying an impaired response to activation stimuli. A subset of immature myeloid cells, composed of immature macrophages, DCs, granulocytes, and myeloid cells at early stages of differentiation, accumulate in the secondary lymphoid organs and tumors of tumor-bearing mice and presumably humans. These myeloid suppressor cells are endowed with suppressive activity toward antitumor T cells through various mechanisms, such as regulation of arginine metabolism and release of ROS. In some tumors, IDO-expressing pDCs are found in significant numbers, thereby decreasing availability of tryptophan and generating tryptophan catabolites. IDO-expressing pDCs can activate intratumoral (IT) Tregs. It seems that tumors impair early myeloid, and in particular DC, differentiation at a systemic level by secreting soluble factors such as VEGF, macrophage colony-stimulating factor, IL-6, and IL-10. Macrophage-derived IL-10, for example, blocks IL-12 production by DCs and prevents the induction of tumor-specific CD8$^+$ T cells.[202] Many tumors constitutively express activated STAT3, a transcription factor partially implicated in the production of these cytokines, the constitutive activation of which also impairs the secretion of proinflammatory cytokines. STAT3 is also responsible for abnormal differentiation of hematopoietic precursor cells,

suggesting that inhibition of its activity may be a promising route to restoring DC function in cancer. The tumor microenvironment (TME) thus profoundly affects the function of infiltrating DCs and T cells, and it has recently been shown that overexpression of matrix metalloproteinase-2 (MMP-2) conditions DCs to produce low levels of IL-12 and to express OX40L, which biases antitumor CD4$^+$ T cells toward suboptimal Th2 differentiation.[203] This pathway has been shown to involve the interaction of MMP-2 and TLR2 on DCs.[204] There can also be a failure of recruitment of DCs into the TME. For example, upregulation of a tumor-intrinsic WNT/β-catenin signaling pathway is associated with poor T-cell infiltration into the TME of melanoma tumors.[205] These tumors are defective in CCL4 production, leading to a failure to locally recruit CD103/CD8α-lineage DCs, the murine equivalent of human CD141$^+$ DCs. CD103$^+$ DCs are critical for the induction of T-cell immunity, and increased frequencies of these cells are correlated with improved clinical outcomes.[206]

Immunotherapeutic Strategies and Clinical Trials

The past decade has seen increasing interest in clinical applications of DCs by harnessing the growing knowledge about DC biology. It is becoming apparent that any effective vaccine must activate and induce antigen presentation by DCs, the most potent cells at stimulating T-cell immunity. A number of clinical trials (mostly phases I and II) have been completed describing the use of DCs in cancer immunotherapy (e.g., non-Hodgkin lymphoma, malignant melanoma, multiple myeloma, prostate cancer, renal cell carcinoma, breast cancer) and in the immunotherapy of human pathogens such as HIV. Most of these studies have relied on monocyte-derived DCs, but a few have used DCs prepared from CD34$^+$ HPCs. A critical issue is antigen delivery to the DCs and the type of DC, with the nature of the antigen and the vehicle for delivery probably being decisive. DCs can be pulsed with defined antigens in the form of human leukocyte antigen–binding antigenic peptides or whole proteins or the whole assortment of tumor antigens upon phagocytosis of dying or opsonized autologous tumor cells. Artificial fusion of DCs with tumor cells allows the generation of hybrid cells with characteristics of DCs but expressing the whole set of tumor antigens as well. Because autologous tumor cells are not always available from patients with advanced disease, allogeneic tumor cells of the same histologic origin expressing shared tumor antigens are also used for loading DCs.

DCs themselves can also be genetically modified through transfection. However, DCs are terminally differentiated nondividing cells and often challenging to transfect. Methods using RNA electroporation and infection by recombinant viruses (lentivirus, poxvirus, herpes virus, and adeno-associated virus) lead to foreign transgene expression in DC. Another strategy is to target DCs in situ using antibodies recognizing DC-specific molecules, such as DEC-205, as demonstrated in mouse models[207] and more recently in patients with cancer.[208] A phase II trial that involved priming by a recombinant vaccinia virus encoding prostate-specific antigen and the "tricom" CD80, intercellular adhesion molecule-1), and lymphocyte function–associated antigen 3 and boosting by a fowlpox virus gave promising clinical results in patients with prostate cancer. GM-CSF was injected at the same time to further amplify immune stimulation. This vaccine was designed to mimic antigen presentation by DCs, even in an incomplete way, and induce significant overall survival benefit.[209] A phase III study using this approach is currently underway.

Because the activation state of antigen-presenting DCs is a determining factor in shaping the ensuing immune response, genetic engineering of DCs or triggering activating receptors also allows enhancing their secretion, migration, and antigen presentation capacity. Thus DCs can be activated by artificial TLR ligands (e.g., R848, which is a ligand for TLR7; unmethylated CpG oligonucleotides, which are ligands for TLR9; or inflammatory cytokines, such as type I IFNs, IL-1β, IL-6, or TNF-α) that can be used in a clinical setting to activate DCs before injection or even in vivo.[210] DCs can also be transfected for immunostimulatory molecules, such as cytokine genes (e.g., IL-2, IL-12), or inhibitory small interfering RNA for molecules dampening DC activation (e.g., suppressor of cytokine signaling 1 [SOCS1]).

The first U.S. Food and Drug Administration–approved, cell-based antitumor vaccine, Sipuleucel-T (Dendreon, Seattle, WA), comprising a partially enriched preparation of blood APCs pulsed with a recombinant fusion protein of human prostatic acid phosphatase and GM-CSF and given intravenously, is approved for the treatment of castration-resistant prostate cancer.[211] The vaccine resulted in modest improvement in overall survival, indicating a need to further improve DC-based vaccines in the clinic. Several trials tested over the past two decades have established that DC vaccines are safe, and evidence of their immunogenicity is not in dispute. However, there remains no standardized protocol for their ex vivo manipulation. The optimal source of DCs (monocyte-derived, circulating differentiated DCs, DCs derived from CD34+ progenitors), antigen loading, maturation stimulus, and route of delivery are still in contention, and, until appropriately compared, it is difficult to reconcile studies that have addressed these variables.[212]

To improve immunogenicity, DC vaccines are being manipulated in novel ways. For example, they are being loaded through electroporation with RNA that encodes tumor-associated antigens[213] or costimulatory molecules (CD40L, CD70, and constitutively active TLR4) or delivered directly into lymph nodes to improve access to secondary lymphoid organs or even intratumorally.[214] Because skin injections of DCs result in just a small percentage of cells migrating to draining nodes, investigators are preconditioning the vaccine site to stimulate local production to enhance their migration to draining lymph nodes.[215] DC–tumor cell hybrids are also being explored as immunogens. With newer methods to readily expand CD34+ HPCs from blood, the concept of using these progenitors to derive large numbers of more immunogenic DC subsets (e.g., CD141+ DCs) is a future target. The ability to use the CRISPR (clustered regularly interspaced short palindromic repeats)/Cas9 system for gene editing may further facilitate manipulation of DCs, such as to prevent expression of inhibitory molecules or cytokines to improve their effectiveness in vivo or to preferentially drive CTL differentiation. Flt3L is being used to systemically increase the pre-cDC pool and/or to target DCs in vivo using cancer antigens fused to monoclonal antibodies targeting DC surface receptors (e.g., DEC-205).[208] This approach is also being tested in combination with decitabine and the IDO inhibitor INCB024360, which suppresses Treg generation. Other receptor targets under consideration for DC targeting include CD40, mannose receptor, DC-SIGN, DCIR, Clec9A, and XCR1.

Indirect approaches to targeting DCs include the use of vaccines that employ tumor cells expressing GM-CSF (GVAX), which are demonstrating evidence of immunogenicity and clinical activity in vivo, viral or bacterial vectors that can infect and mDCs (vaccinia virus, *Listeria monocytogenes* constructs), implantable scaffolds that recruit DCs through expression of TLR agonists and GM-CSF,[216] and exosomes derived from DCs (dexosomes).

Altogether, DC interventions have clear immunologic and in some cases small clinical impact. Beyond Sipuleucel-T, however, no other DC-based vaccine has reached approval in the clinic. The outcomes of phase III trials that are testing DCs' immunogenicity in renal cancer and glioblastoma multiforme are pending. Ultimately, DCs may be more effective when given as immune prevention after tumor resection or in the neoadjuvant setting, where early studies suggest they may have impact.[217]

Novel approaches to target DCs in situ include the concept of IT vaccination. IT injection of the CpG oligonucleotide (PF-3512676) in low-grade B-cell lymphoma, thus targeting TLR9 on pDCs and B cells, has led to complete and partial clinical in several patients with induction of tumor-specific CD8 T-cell responses.[218,219] Tumor regression was observed in injected and distant tumor sites. IT approaches are being tested with other immune modulators, such as poly(I:C), a TLR3 and MDA5 agonist,[220] and in combination with antibodies that target checkpoint molecules, such as CTLA-4 and PD-1. Oncolytic viruses are gaining momentum when they are

delivered either IT or systemically. The rationale is that they destroy cancer cells, making them available to be recognized by the immune system. They can be engineered to prevent replication in normal cells. The herpes simplex virus (HSV)-based product talimogene laherparepvec (T-VEC), which is an HSV-engineered oncolytic virus that also expresses GM-CSF (to attract and differentiate DCs) improved the durable response rate in advanced unresectable melanoma (16.3% in the treated group versus 2.1% in subjects receiving only GM-CSF; $p < 0.001$).[221] T-VEC is now being tested in combination with ipilimumab or pembrolizumab (anti-PD-1), and early results of the T-VEC and ipilimumab trial appear to be showing synergistic activity. T-VEC has now been approved for the treatment of unresectable melanoma.

Anticancer vaccination can be used in synergy with chemotherapy and radiotherapy. The rationale is that chemotherapy and radiotherapy trigger tumor cell death, which provides a source of tumor antigens to DCs while inducing exposure of immunogenic molecules on tumor cells[222] (Fig. 23.4). Thus anthracycline-treated tumor cells expose the ER chaperones calreticulin and ERp57 because of induction of an ER stress response and potentiate dying tumor cell phagocytosis. Death of tumor cells as a result of radiotherapy is also accompanied by release of nonhistone chromatin-binding nuclear protein HMGB1, which can trigger TLR4 and, in response to taxanes, ATP, which, upon binding to P2RX7 on APCs, potentiates inflammasome activation and IL-1β release. Finally, cyclophosphamide can cause, through release of tumor-associated nucleic acids, induction of type I IFN.[222] Increased uptake of tumor antigen in the context of maturation signals strongly enhances cross-presentation and cross-priming of tumor antigens by DCs.

Thus far, DC vaccines have not met the desired endpoints in clinical studies (i.e., tumor regression) in the majority of patients, despite clear evidence that DC vaccination can induce measurable cellular or humoral immune responses in patients with cancer.[223–226] It is likely that, to achieve significant clinical responses upon vaccination for cancer, combining DC vaccination with other strategies will improve the therapeutic outcome. For example, some strategies are aimed at depleting or inactivating Tregs (using a toxin targeting CD25, a molecule expressed by Tregs, or cyclophosphamide), alleviating T-cell anergy (using antagonistic CTLA-4 or PD-1), and differentiating myeloid suppressor cells into nonimmunosuppressive cells (by injection of RA derivative ATRA [all-*trans* retinoic acid]), injection of common γ-chain cytokines such as IL-7, which have potent effects on T-cell survival and function, or adoptive immunotherapy of in vitro activated T cells.[227,228] Irradiation of the tumor tissue conditions it for enhanced migration of APCs and T cells, augments MHC class I expression on tumor cells, and induces apoptotic cell death, thus augmenting delivery of tumor antigens to DCs.[229–231] The identification of specific surface receptors regulating DC–T-cell interaction and T-cell activation and differentiation allowed use of targeting antibodies functioning as immune modulators. Thus agonistic antibodies targeting glucocorticoid-induced TNF receptor (GITR), OX40, CD137, or CD40 or cytokines potently enhancing cytotoxic T-cell responses, such as IL-15, can be harnessed to enhance vaccine-induced antitumor immune responses. Researchers in ongoing trials are testing DCs in combination with antibodies that inhibit checkpoint molecules (e.g., CTLA-4, PD-1), radiation, cytokines (IL-7), and drugs (e.g., enzulutamide [for prostate cancer] and agents that reduce Tregs [cyclophosphamide, temozolomide]), among other strategies.

In the authors' opinion, DC immunotherapy will be most efficacious when coadministered with one or more additional interventions and when the tumor burden is low. The timing of vaccination is probably also crucial, and frequent immunizations may dramatically improve clinical efficacy.[232] In the setting of HIV infection, a recent study of a small group of chronically infected individuals showed that vaccination with DCs loaded with chemically inactivated virus allows stabilization and even suppression of viral load for an extended period of time without any other treatment.[233] Vaccination with DCs holds great promise in cancer and infectious diseases, but its potential is likely to be best exploited in combination with other strategies manipulating other arms of the immune system.

A. Compromised immunity in advanced cancer

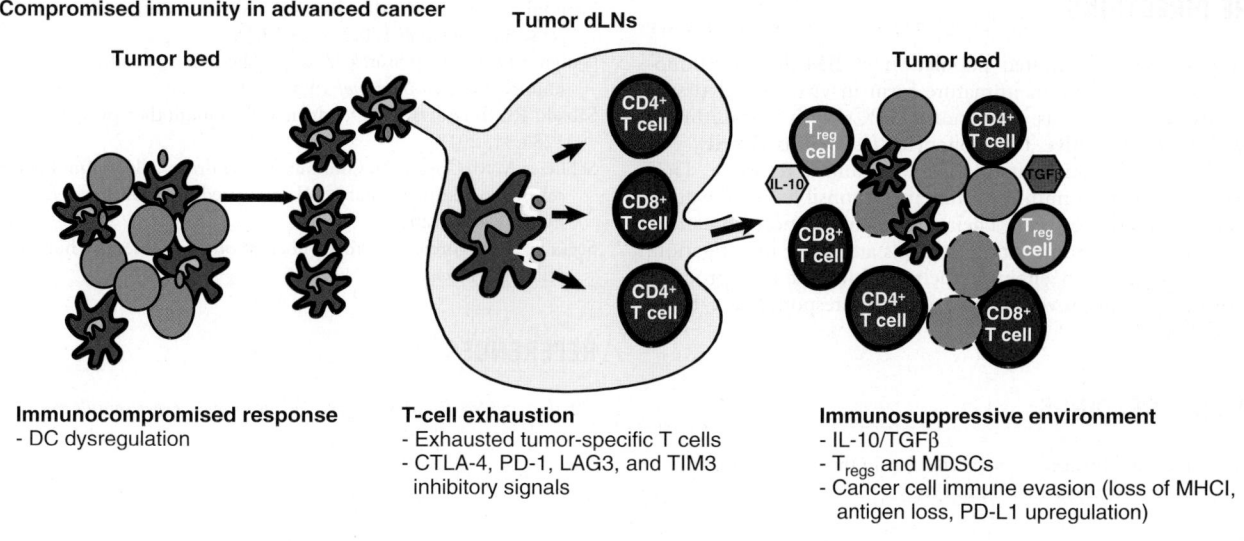

Immunocompromised response
- DC dysregulation

T-cell exhaustion
- Exhausted tumor-specific T cells
- CTLA-4, PD-1, LAG3, and TIM3 inhibitory signals

Immunosuppressive environment
- IL-10/TGFβ
- Tregs and MDSCs
- Cancer cell immune evasion (loss of MHCI, antigen loss, PD-L1 upregulation)

B. Cancer vaccines

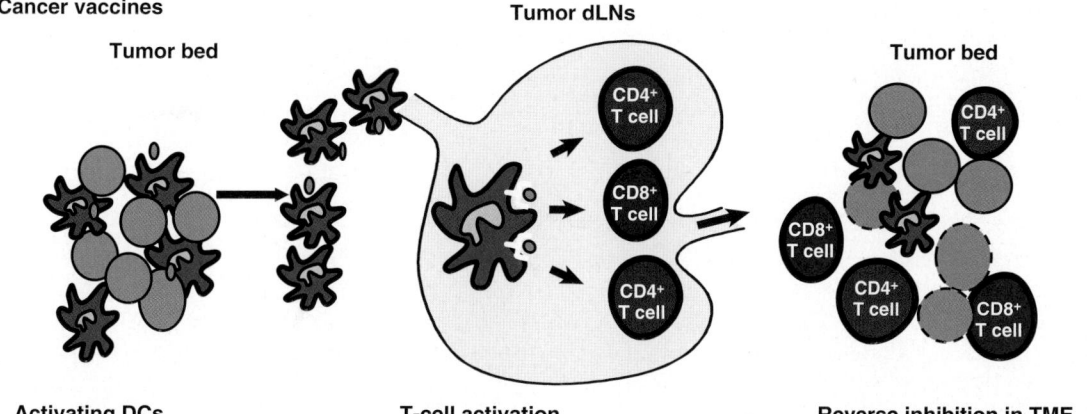

Activating DCs
- DC-based or targeted vaccines and adjuvants
- DC mobilizing agents
- Anti-CD40 mAbs

T-cell activation
- Cytokines - IL-2, IL-7 and IL-15
- IDO inhibitors
- Anti-CD27, CD134, CD137

Checkpoint blockade
- Anti-CTLA-4, Anti-PD-1, Anti-PD-L1

Reverse inhibition in TME
- Immunogenic cell death induction (XRT and chemotherapy)
- Anti-VEGF mAbs
- Anti-tumor specific mAbs (Anti-CD20, Ab-drugs congugates, etc.)

Fig. 23.4 ROLES OF CANCER VACCINES. In advanced tumor settings, tumor immunity is compromised in several ways (A). The dendritic cells (DCs) in the tumor are deregulated, and there is also evidence of T-cell exhaustion mediated by inhibitory signals such as cytotoxic T lymphocyte–associated protein 4 (CTLA-4), programmed cell death protein 1 (PD-1), lymphocyte activation gene 3 (LAG3), and T-cell immunoglobulin and mucin domain containing-3 (TIM3). In the tumor bed, there is an immunosuppressive environment with secretion of interleukin-10 (IL-10) and transforming growth factor-β (TGF-β) as well as the presence of immunosuppressive cells such as regulatory T cells (Tregs) and myeloid-derived suppressor cells (MDSCs). The goal of cancer vaccines is to improve antitumor immunity (B), and this can be achieved with numerous approaches, such as DC activation and recruitment into tumors (with the use of DC-based or targeted vaccines) and T-cell activation or checkpoint inhibitor blockade (anti-CTLA-4, anti-PD-1, or anti-PD-L1). Additionally, to reverse inhibition in the tumor microenvironment (TME), methods to induce immunogenic cell death (x-ray therapy [XRT] and chemotherapy) and to target tumor-specific peptides can be implemented. *dLNs,* Draining lymph nodes; *IDO,* indoleamine 2,3-dioxygenase; *mAbs,* monoclonal antibodies; *MHCI,* major histocompatibility complex class I; *VEGF,* vascular endothelial growth factor.

Although DCs are considered the most potent cells in inducing T-cell responses, they can also function as tolerizing cells, a function that can be harnessed against autoimmune diseases and in a transplant setting. Thus it is possible to differentiate in vitro maturation-resistant imDCs or differentially activated DCs using biologic agents such as IL-10, TGF-β, or the fusion protein CTLA-4-Ig, as well as pharmacologic agents such as corticosteroids, cyclosporine, rapamycin, mycophenolate mofetil, vitamin D₃, or prostaglandin E₂ or inhibitors of NFκB.[184] The clinical relevance of some of these strategies is being evaluated in autoimmune diseases such as RA. Another way to dampen pathologic immune responses is to use antagonists for TLRs or other innate immune sensors participating in amplifying damaging responses. Thus, because the role of DNA–immune complexes has been established as important in the etiology of SLE, synthetic inhibitory oligodeoxyribonucleotides have been developed that can prevent or inhibit activation through TLR9 on pDCs and B cells and block SLE in animal models. Finally, significant challenges remain with respect to DC-based immunotherapy, including the applicability of preclinical models to humans as well as regulatory and funding hurdles.

FUTURE DIRECTIONS

DCs are a sparsely distributed population of BM-derived mononuclear cells that exist in an immature form in virtually all tissues in the body. DCs serve as professional APCs with extraordinary capacity to stimulate naive T lymphocytes (as well as B cells, NK cells, and NK T cells) and initiate primary immune response. They link innate and adaptive immunity and are responsible for activation and inhibition of effector cells. Their clinical applications in cancer, transplantation, and chronic viral infections are under investigation. Promising approaches to enhance their recruitment and promote their activation to improve adaptive immune responses are being tested in the clinic.

SUGGESTED READINGS

Bhardwaj N: DCs and NK cells: critical effectors in the immune response to HIV-1. *Nat Rev Immunol* 11:176, 2011.

Cerboni S, Gentili M, Manel N: Diversity of pathogen sensors in dendritic cells. *Adv Immunol* 120:211, 2013.

Ganguly D, Haak S, Sisirak V, et al: The role of dendritic cells in autoimmunity. *Nat Rev Immunol* 13:566, 2013.

Sabado RL, Bhardwaj N: Dendritic cell immunotherapy. *Ann N Y Acad Sci* 1284:31, 2013.

Schlitzer A, McGovern N, Ginhoux F: Dendritic cells and monocyte-derived cells: Two complementary and integrated functional systems. *Semin Cell Dev Biol* 41:9, 2015.

Segura E, Amigorena S: Cross-presentation in mouse and human dendritic cells. *Adv Immunol* 127:1, 2015.

REFERENCES

For the complete list of references, log on to www.expertconsult.com.

COMPLEMENT AND IMMUNOGLOBULIN BIOLOGY LEADING TO CLINICAL TRANSLATION

David J. Araten, Robert J. Mandle, David E. Isenman, and Michael C. Carroll

This chapter is divided into four parts. The first part details the current understanding of the activation and biology of the complement system and how it links innate and adaptive immunity. The second part focuses on immunoglobulins and their importance in protecting against disease. The third part discusses immunoglobulins as therapeutic agents, and the fourth part discusses therapies, including monoclonal antibodies, that target the complement system.

THE COMPLEMENT SYSTEM: AN OVERVIEW

Complement refers to a family of distinct proteins that play a pivotal role in host defense against infection. In the 1880s, the serum factors involved in host response to pathogens were placed into two categories based on sensitivity to heat. Whereas the heat-stable component, antibody, was recognized as being specific for the invading pathogen and arose after immunization, the heat-labile (>56°C [133°F]) fraction displayed nonspecific killing activity. The heat-labile fraction acted to complement the antibody-mediated lytic killing of targeted organisms.[1–3]

In addition to its lytic role in the effector arm of the antibody response, the complement system serves several other functions. First, components of the complement system are involved in clearance of targeted microorganisms by the process of opsonization. *Opsonization* is the coating of a particle with proteins that facilitate phagocytosis of the particle by tissue macrophages and activated follicular dendritic cells (FDCs) as well as binding by receptors on peripheral blood cells.[4,5] Second, complement promotes inflammation by releasing small peptide fragments from complement proteins. These peptides cause mast cell degranulation, smooth muscle contraction, and directed migration (chemotaxis) of motile cells to sites of inflammation.[6,7]

Complement can be activated via three distinct pathways: classical, lectin, and alternative. Although all depend on different molecules for their initiation, eventually they converge to generate the same set of effector molecules. Each of these pathways is described here (Fig. 24.1).

Classical Pathway

The classical pathway (CP), so called because it was the earliest studied arm of the complement system, directly links the innate and acquired immune systems. There are nine proteins in the CP. As a matter of terminology, each CP component protein is designated with an uppercase C followed by a number. Fragments of these proteins generated by cleavage during the complement cascade are designated with a lower-case letter suffix (e.g., C3a, C3b). In general, the smaller product arising from a proteolytic activation step is given the fragment designation "a," and the larger product is designated "b." The sole exception to this rule is for the naming of the C2 proteolytic activation fragments, where, for historical reasons, the larger fragment is C2a and the smaller one is C2b.

C1, the first component of the CP, binds and is activated by the Fc portion of the antibody molecule. C1q is a macromolecule complex composed of three individual protein subunits: C1q, C1r, and C1s.[8–12] The largest of these subunits, C1q, is an 18-chain molecule with six copies each of three chains: A, B, and C.

Structurally, C1q consists of a central core with six radiating arms. Each arm possesses a triple helical structure similar to collagen that is capped at the end with a head region consisting of a quaternary assembly of the globular domains from each of chains A, B, and C. C1q, largely through ionic interactions, links the C1 complex to the antibody molecule. In addition to its capacity for binding to antibody molecules, C1q possesses the capability to bind directly to the surfaces of some microorganisms and apoptotic cells, not unlike mannan-binding lectin (MBL; see lectin pathway discussion, later).

Associated with C1q are two molecules each of C1r and C1s. In unactivated C1, C1r and C1s are proenzyme serine esterases. Upon binding of C1q with an array of target-associated immunoglobulin G (IgG) Fc regions, or directly to surface molecules of the pathogen, a conformational change occurs that leads to reciprocal autoactivation of the associated C1r molecules. The active form of C1r then cleaves its associated C1s to generate an active serine protease.

Activated C1s is responsible for cleaving C4 and C2, the next two proteins in the complement pathway. Cleavage of C4 yields two fragments: C4a and C4b. C4b possesses a highly reactive thioester group that allows it to bind covalently to molecules in the immediate vicinity of its active site. Only a small proportion of the C4b produced binds to proteins or carbohydrates on the targeted surface; the rest is inactivated by reaction with water in the surrounding milieu. This helps to prevent inadvertent C4b binding to surrounding host cells.

C2, the next substrate in the CP cascade, is susceptible to cleavage by C1s. Upon association with C4b, C2 is cleaved by activated C1s into two fragments: C2a and C2b. C2a, which is now an active serine protease, remains bound to C4b, thereby confining it to the targeted surface. C4b2a is termed the *C3 convertase,* an enzymatic complex that is responsible for binding and cleaving C3, the next component in the cascade. The function of the C3 convertase is to cleave large numbers of C3 molecules to produce C3b and C3a. Nascently activated C3b, similar to C4b, also possesses a highly reactive thioester bond, allowing a portion of the nascent C3b to covalently bind to the targeted surface (opsonization of the target) and thereby mark it for phagocytosis. The activated thioester in the bulk of the nascent C3b becomes water hydrolysed and can no longer bind to a target. By contrast, all of the C3a fragment remains in solution, where it initiates a local inflammatory response.

An Ig-independent mechanism for activation of C1q has been identified.[13] The lectin protein Sign R1, which is expressed on a subset of macrophages within the outer marginal zone sinus of the spleen, is capable of capturing to the surface of the marginal zone macrophage both C-polysaccharide–containing bacteria and C1q. The recruited C1 becomes activated and propagates the CP to deposit C3b on the captured bacterium. Recently, Sign R1 was identified on the surface of resident dendritic cells (DC) in draining lymph nodes and shown to be important in capture and transport of inactivated influenza virus.[13a] This novel pathway provides an alternative innate recognition of pathogens leading to activation of the CP of complement.

Lectin Pathway

Before continuing with the discussion of the complement cascade at the point of C3 cleavage by convertase, we turn our attention to the

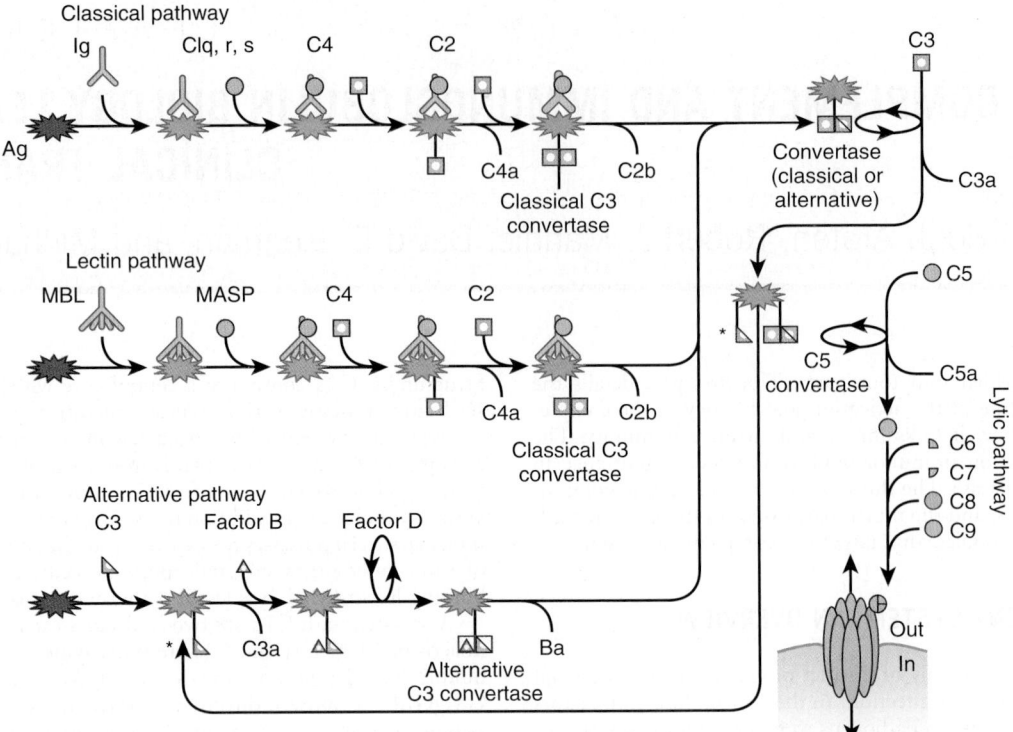

Fig. 24.1 SCHEMATIC OVERVIEW OF THE COMPLEMENT CASCADE. Classical, lectin, and alternative pathways commence from the left side of the figure, leading to the converging point of C3 activation *(top right)*. In every subsequent proteolytic step, the position of the new addition to the antigen complex is shown in *black* for clarity. From the central C3 activation step downward, the C3 amplification loop through the alternative pathway is indicated by *asterisks*. The lytic pathway is initiated with the formation of C5 convertase and leads to the assembly of the C5–C6–C7–C8–C9 membrane attack complex, which interferes with the target's structural integrity by penetrating the cellular membrane *(bottom right)*. *MASP,* Mannan-binding lectin–associated serine protease; *MBL,* mannan-binding lectin.

other two complement-activating pathways: the lectin pathway (LP) and the alternative pathway (AP). What will become evident is that all of these pathways converge at C3.

The lectin pathway is a relatively recently described pathway for complement activation.[15,16] MBL, similar to C1q, is a triple helical structure with collagen-like arms (most commonly three or four) coupled to C-type lectin globular domains, which form carbohydrate recognition domains that bind repeating polysaccharides present on the surfaces of many microorganisms. MBL attaches to the terminus of polymeric carbohydrate chains in the following order: mannose > GlcNAc > fucose > glucose. The greatest avidity appears to be for repeating mannose-based structural patterns typical of microbial surfaces. On vertebrate cells, these sugars are not as dense as on microbial surfaces, thus decreasing the avidity of the MBL-binding interaction, and furthermore, they often are covered by sialic acid residues, thus limiting recognition by MBL. The MBL-associated serine proteases MASP-1 and MASP-2, whose domain architecture is similar to C1r and C1s, predominantly bind as homodimeric zymogens to separate MBL oligomers. Upon MBL binding to polysaccharides on a pathogen surface, MASP-1 and MASP-2 become activated. The mechanism of activation has recently been clarified and is distinctly different from the conformational distortion-based intracomplex mechanism described above for the C1 activation. Although it had originally been thought that MASP-2 was capable of autoactivating itself when MBL bound to its target, and that MASP-1 played a non-essential and ill-defined augmentary role,[14] under physiological conditions autoactivated MASP-1 has now been firmly established to be the obligatory activator of MASP 2.[16a,16b] Although the relationship between MASP-1 and MASP-2 parallels that of C1r to C1s in the C1 activation mechanism, what is decidedly different is that MASP-1 autoactivation is intercomplex, as is MASP-2

activation by autoactivated MASP-1. Specifically, it is the juxtaposition through clustering of the MBL–MASP-1 and MBL–MASP-2 complexes brought about by MBL binding to the target surface that leads to the intercomplex autoactivation of MASP-1, and the subsequent cleavage of MASP-2 by autoactivated MASP-1 on a neighboring complex.[16c] Activated MASP-2 acts similar to C1s, cleaving C4 and C2 and thereby forming a C3 convertase, C4b2a, as found in the CP.[17] Besides its role in cleaving zymogen MASP-2, activated MASP-1 also cleaves C2, but not C4. Nevertheless, given the approximately 24-fold higher serum concentration of MASP-1 relative to MASP-2, this would ensure the efficiency of C2 activation on C4b deposited near an MBL-MASP2 complex.

While MBL was the microbial pattern recognition molecule initially identified in the lectin pathway, ficolins H-, M- and L- are collagen triple helix-containing paralogues of MBL in serum, which also associate with MASP-1and MASP-2[17a] and which undergo activation in a similar manner to the MBL-MASP complexes.[16c] The globular regions of the respective ficolin chains bear a fibrinogen-like domain fold and they recognize acetyl groups, be they on carbohydrate (e.g., N-acetylglucosamine), or non carbohydrate entities (e.g., N-acetyl-glycine or acetylcholine).[17a]

MBL serum concentration can differ by up to 1000-fold among individuals, with those having low circulating MBL apparently more vulnerable to infections. MBL insufficiency appears to be a particular risk factor for infections in infants and individuals undergoing chemotherapy or immunosuppression treatment.[18]

Gene-targeted knock-out mouse models deficient in MBL components have been described. In general, in pathogenic microbe infection models, such as *Candida albicans* or *Staphylococcus aureus,* MBL knock-out mice showed increased susceptibility to systemic infection and relatively much higher mortality compared to wild type.[19,20]

Alternative Pathway

The AP may represent one of the earliest forms of innate immunity. Unlike the CP or LP pathway, the AP can be fully activated in the absence of specific pathogen binding by a "recognition" equivalent to C1q or MBL.[21] In fact, the AP is always "on" at a low level. In addition, the AP forms and uses the distinct C3 convertase C3bBb.[22]

Complement C3 is a two-chain protein with an apparent molecular weight of approximately 200 kDa. The crystal structure of native C3, shown as a domain-colored ribbon model in Fig. 24.2A, identified 13 distinct domains, including the thioester domain (TED), which contained the covalent binding site.[23] In the native molecule, the intramolecular thioester bond, formed between the side chains of cysteine and glutamine residues within the sequence CGEQ, is buried within a hydrophobic interface formed between the TED and MG8 domains, which is nevertheless close to the protein's surface. The subsequent determination of the atomic structure of the activated form of C3 (i.e., C3b) demonstrated a dramatic shift in the location of the TED.[24,25] Proteolytic cleavage releases the C3a anaphylatoxin peptide, and the TED becomes fully exposed to engage potential targets (see structure-based depiction of C3b in Fig. 24.2B). Thus the dramatic shift in structure also exposes potential binding sites for factor B of the AP and competing sites for regulators of C3b, such as factor H (FH), membrane cofactor protein (MCP), complement receptor type 1 (CR1), and decay accelerating factor (DAF; all described later in this section). At a low so-called "tickover" level, the thioester bond undergoes spontaneous hydrolysis, forming $C3(H_2O)$. This conformationally altered C3b-like form of C3 (see Fig. 24.2B) allows for binding to factor B, a plasma protein. Factor B is a serine protease that is approximately 30% identical to C2. The binding of

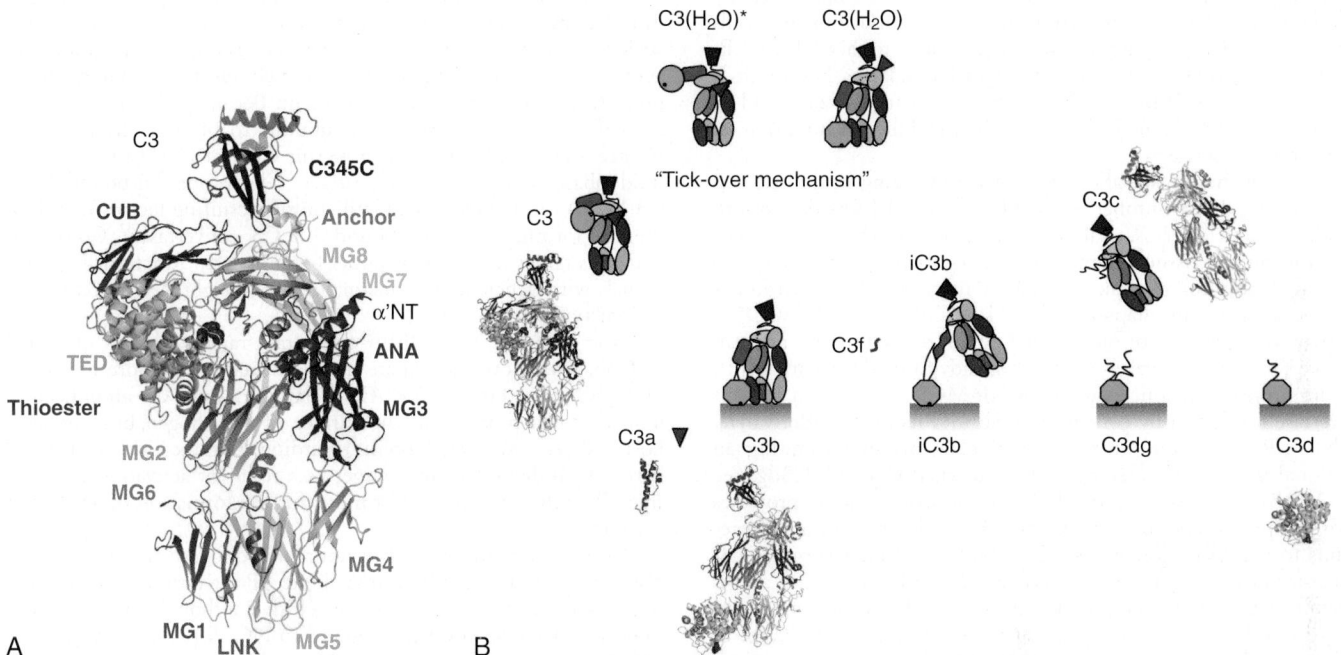

Fig. 24.2 THE STRUCTURE OF NATIVE C3, ITS CONFORMATIONAL INTERMEDIATES, AND ITS CLEAVAGE FRAGMENTS. (A) Ribbon diagram representation of the x-ray crystal structure of native C3 indicating the 13 domains (*bold lettering*, color-coded the same as the domain) of which it is composed. (B) Structure-based cartoon representation of the conformational states of intact C3, as well as its cleavage fragments. Where these cartoons are derived from x-ray structures, those structures are depicted as ribbon diagrams adjacent to the cartoon. The remaining cartoons are based on electron micrograph images,[27] as well as established biochemical data. In all cases, the domain colors in the cartoons correspond to those in the ribbon diagrams. Proteolytic activation of C3 to C3b results in an approximate 90-Å downward movement of the thioester domain (TED), a significant repositioning of the CUB (complement C1r/C1s, urchin EGF, bone morphogenic protein 1), and a flipping of the positions macroglobulin 7 (MG7) and MG8 domains. The reorientation of these domains creates binding sites for ligands of C3b that were not present in the native molecule. The reactive thioester produced during this conformational transition is capable of binding a portion of the C3b molecules covalently to a target surface (*gray-shaded boxes*). Subsequent cleavage of C3b by factor I releases a small C3f fragment and results in a reorientation of the C3c portion of the molecule relative to C3d/TED within iC3b, a molecule that remains bound to the target. This reorientation relative to C3b relieves the steric blockage by MG1 of a portion of the binding site for CR2/CD21, as iC3b is an equivalent ligand to C3dg and C3d with respect to CR2 binding. C3dg and C3c are the products of an additional cleavage by factor I within the CUB domain. A noncomplement protease removes an N-terminal segment from C3dg, yielding the still target-associated C3d fragment. The remaining "squiggle" on C3d represents 16 residues at its C-terminus that are sufficiently flexible that they were not visible in the x-ray crystal structure of C3d. Although the thioester in native C3 is protected from the solvent, native C3 is in conformational equilibrium with a stable conformational intermediate, $C3(H_2O)^*$, in which the thioester become susceptible to hydrolysis. Although the equilibrium strongly favors the native state, if hydrolysis of the thioester in $C3(H_2O)^*$ occurs, it cannot reform, and the molecule undergoes a unidirectional conformational change to the $C3(H_2O)$ stage, which adopts both a C3b-like conformation and functional profile. This conformational transition of intact C3 is the basis of the "tick-over mechanism" for alternative pathway initiation. (*Modified from P. Gros, Utrecht University; contains elements previously published in Gros P, Milder FJ, Janssen BJ: Complement driven by conformational changes.* Nat Rev Immunol 8:48, 2008.)

factor B by C3(H$_2$O) allows factor D, another protease, to cleave factor B to form Ba and Bb. Bb remains associated with C3(H$_2$O) to form the C3(H$_2$O)Bb complex. Factor D appears to function as a serine protease in its native state but can cleave factor B only when bound to C3. Recently, there has been an interesting connection found between factor D and MASP-1, a component of the LP. It was found that a *MASP-1/MASP-3* knockout mouse (the proteins MASP-1 and MASP-3 are alternative splice products of the same gene) completely lacked AP functionality. Upon further investigation, it was determined that the secreted factor D in this mouse possessed a five-residue propeptide at its amino terminus. Removal of this propeptide from factor D by the addition of MASP-1 resulted in restoration of AP functionality.[26]

C3(H$_2$O)Bb is an enzymatic complex capable of cleaving native C3. This complex is a fluid-phase C3 convertase. Although it is formed only in small amounts, it can cleave many molecules of C3. Much of the C3b produced in this process is inactivated by hydrolysis, but some attaches covalently to the surface of host cells or pathogens. C3b bound in this way is able to bind factor B, allowing its cleavage by factor D to yield Ba and Bb. The result is the formation of C3bBb, a C3 convertase akin to C4b2a found in the classical and MBL pathways, with the capability of initiating an amplification cascade.

In light of the nonspecific nature of C3b binding in the AP, it is not surprising that a number of complement regulators exist both in the plasma and on host cell membranes to prevent complement activation on self-tissues. Some of these regulatory components are mentioned now for the sake of clarity; more detailed attention is provided later in this chapter (Table 24.1). CR1 and DAF (CD55) compete with factor B for binding to C3b on the cell surface and can displace Bb from a convertase that has already formed.[28] Factor I (FI), a serum protease, in concert with CR1 or MCP (CD46) can prevent convertase formation by converting C3b into its inactive derivative, iC3b.[29] CR1 is unique among the FI cofactors in facilitating an additional proteolytic cleavage of iC3b to yield C3c and C3dg (see Fig. 24.2B). Trimming of the latter by noncomplement proteases yields the proteolytic limit fragment C3d, which structurally corresponds to the TED domain (see Fig. 24.2B). Another complement regulatory protein found in the plasma is FH. FH binds C3b and is able to compete with factor B and displace Bb from the convertase. In addition, FH acts as a cofactor for FI to convert C3b to iC3b. In addition to interaction sites for C3b, FH possesses two distinct binding sites for polyanionic molecules, particularly various sulfated glycosaminoglycans (e.g., heparan sulfate) or arrays of sialic acid (e.g.,

from membrane surface glycoproteins) found on host surfaces in contact with blood plasma. Although these polyanion binding sites are not required for FH to regulate fluid phase AP C3 convertase, they are required for its activity on surface-bound C3bBb. In fact, this is the basis for FH being able to discriminate between AP C3 convertase adventitiously deposited on host tissue versus that deposited on a microbial surface because the latter do not possess either the sulfated glycosaminoglycans or the sialic acid arrays.[30,31]

Pathogen surfaces are normally not afforded the protection offered by these regulators. Persistence of the C3bBb convertase on microbial surfaces may additionally be favored by the positive regulator properdin (factor P). This positive modulation of the AP by properdin has traditionally been thought to be attributable to its ability to prolong the lifetime of the AP C3 convertase by forming a C3bBbP complex. This mechanism is still valid, but recently, evidence has been presented that properdin, which circulates predominantly as a homotrimer, may also be able to recognize AP targets directly. Specifically, it has been shown to bind to microbial surfaces, such as to *Neisseria gonorrhoeae* or yeast cell walls, that are known AP activators, but not to strains of *Escherichia coli* that are known to be nonactivators of the AP of complement. Because it is a homotrimer, even if factor P uses two of its subunits to bind to the microbial surface, one is still left that can recruit C3b, or C3(H$_2$O), from the fluid phase to the microbial surface. The properdin-bound C3b/C3(H2O) can then act as a platform for recruiting factors B and D, thereby forming a surface-bound AP C3 convertase.[32] Consistent with this target recognition model for properdin functionality, individuals with deficiencies in factor P have a heightened susceptibility to infection with *Neisseria*.[33]

After forming, the C3bBb convertase rapidly cleaves more C3 to C3b, which can participate in the formation of more molecules of C3bBb convertase. The AP thereby activates an amplification loop that can proceed on the surface of a pathogen but not on a host cell. An additional point regarding amplification by the AP is that C3b deposited on a target as a result of activation of either the CP or the LP can act as a nidus for the formation of an AP C3 convertase.

Although specific antibody is not required for AP activation, many classes of immunoglobulin can facilitate AP activation.[34] The mechanism by which this occurs remains elusive, although some evidence indicates that C3b covalently bound to IgG displays a reduced rate of inactivation to iC3b by factors H and I.[35] However, in contrast to CP activation, which requires Fc, AP activation can occur with F(ab)′$_2$ fragments.

An instructive demonstration for the role of antibody in continuing the AP cascade, with possible ramifications for human disease, comes from a murine model of rheumatoid arthritis. Mice do not spontaneously develop rheumatoid arthritis.[36] However, a murine model has been developed in which expression of antibodies specific for the ubiquitously expressed cytoplasmic protein glucose-6-phosphate can cause joint destruction reminiscent of human rheumatoid arthritis. Interestingly, the disease state, through complement-mediated joint destruction, can occur even if the specific antibodies are of isotypes incapable of fixing complement through the CP. The response may be localized to the joints because of the absence of complement cascade regulators on cartilage.

C3, C5, and the Membrane Attack Complex

The formation of the C3 convertase, C4b2a (CP and LP) and C3bBb (AP), is the point at which the three pathways converge (see Fig. 24.1). The function of these complexes is to convert C3 to C3a and C3b. C3 is the most abundant complement protein in plasma, occurring at a concentration of 1.2 mg/mL, and up to 1000 molecules of C3b can bind in the vicinity of a single C3 convertase.[37]

The covalent attachment of C3b to either C4b2a or C3bBb converts this enzyme into a trimeric complex (C5 convertase) capable of binding and cleaving C5 into C5a and C5b. Mechanistically, the "adduct" C3b molecule increases the binding affinity of the

TABLE 24.1	Control Proteins of the Classical and Alternative Pathways
Name	**Role in the Regulation of Complement Activation**
C1 inhibitor (C1INH)	Binds to activated C1r, C1s, removing it from C1q
C4-binding protein (C4BP)	Binds C4b, displacing C2a; cofactor for C4b cleavage by factor I
Complement receptor 1 (CR1)	Binds C4b, displacing C2a, or C3b displacing Bb; cofactor for FI
Factor H (FH)	Binds C3b, displacing Bb; cofactor for factor I
Factor I (FI)	Serine protease that cleaves C3b and C4b: aided by factor H, MCP, C4BP, or CR1
Decay-accelerating factor	Membrane protein that displaces Bb from C3b and C2a from C4b
Membrane cofactor protein	Membrane protein that promotes C3b and C4b inactivation by factor I
CD59	Prevents formation of membrane attack complex on autologous cells expressed on membranes

C5 convertase for its substrate C5 such that its Michaelis constant (K_M) is now well below the physiologic concentration of C5 in plasma.[38] C5b is the initiating component of the membrane attack complex (MAC). The MAC is a multiprotein complex whose components are C5b, C6, C7, C8, and multiple C9s.[39,40] The constituent components of the MAC associate in the numeric order C5b–C6–C7–C8–C9.

The MAC, when viewed by electron microscopy, resembles a cylinder that possesses a hydrophobic outer face and a hydrophilic central core. If assembled near a lipid bilayer, such as a cell or the bacterial membrane of a gram-negative strain, the MAC can associate with and insert into the lipid bilayer. Such insertion can be thought as "punching holes" into the membrane, allowing for passage of water and small ions into the cell. Osmotic equilibrium is thereby lost, leading to eventual lysis of the targeted cell or bacterium. C5b678 are sufficient to form small pores in the target membrane. The role of C9 appears to be to enlarge the channel through multiple C9 polymerization, thereby causing more rapid loss of membrane function and lysis. Deficiencies in complement components C5 to C9 have only been associated with increased susceptibility to *Neisseria* species–based infections, such as gonorrhea and bacterial meningitis. Also, the extended cell wall peptidoglycan layer of gram-positive strains of bacteria make them resistant to the lytic arm of complement. It can be concluded from these observations that the requirement for MAC is limited in host protection.

Complement Receptors and Their Role in Immune Complex Clearance and Activation

As described in the previous section, complement can act by the direct lysis of targeted cells. Another important function of complement in host protection is facilitating the uptake and destruction of pathogens by phagocytic cells. This occurs by the specific recognition of C3b/C4b–coated (opsonized) particles by complement receptors.[41,42]

The best characterized complement receptor for the uptake of C4-coated immune complexes is CR1 (CD35). CR1 binds C4b/C3b–bearing immune complexes. CR1, similar to most proteins that bind activation products of C4 and C3 molecules, shares a structural motif known as the short consensus repeat (SCR). Each short consensus repeat consists of approximately 60 amino acids. CR1 in humans is composed of 30 linked short consensus repeats. CR1 possesses three binding sites for C4b and two for C3b.

CR1 is expressed on a wide variety of cell types in humans, including erythrocytes, macrophages, polymorphonuclear leukocytes, B cells, monocytes, and FDCs. The role of CR1 expression on B cells and FDCs in activating and maintaining the adaptive immune response is detailed subsequently. For now, the focus is on the other cell types that express CR1.

Because CR1 is not directly associated on its cytoplasmic side with any intracellular signaling molecules, binding of C3b by CR1 expressed on phagocytic cells is not in itself capable of inducing endocytosis of the C3b-opsonized target. A secondary signal is required to induce phagocytosis. This second signal can be provided by IgG binding to the phagocyte's Fc receptor, by carbohydrates commonly found on bacterial surfaces, or by exposure of the phagocytic cell to the appropriate cytokines. In addition, some phagocytic cells, such as macrophages, are activated by binding of C5a through C5a receptor (C5aR, [CD84]) (see Biologic Activity of C3a and C5a, later). What these secondary ligands have in common is that they all bind to receptor domains that are the ligand recognition units of a cell signaling molecule or complex.

The largest pool of CR1-expressing cells is erythrocytes.[43] Erythrocytes bearing opsonized material are removed from the circulation presumably to prevent deposition in tissue sites such as the renal glomerulus. Erythrocytes bearing opsonized material traverse the sinusoids of the liver and spleen, where they come into close contact with fixed phagocytic cells. These phagocytic cells affect the transfer of opsonized material from the erythrocyte onto their own membranes. The transfer of complexes is enhanced by cleavage of C3b to iC3b by FI, as iC3b is a poor ligand for CR1, but is a good ligand for CRIg, a complement receptor of the Ig superfamily present on tissue-resident phagocytic cells (see later for further discussion of CRIg).

Given its central position in the complement cascade, the presence of C3b is tightly regulated. This regulation is brought about by cleaving C3b into inactive derivatives that cannot participate in forming an active convertase. One of the conformationally altered inactive derivatives of C3b, iC3b (see Fig. 24.2B), can act as an opsonin in its own right for complement receptors CR2 (CD21), CR3 (CD11b/CD18), and CR4 (CD11c/CD18). CR3 binds iC3b and plays a major role in inducing phagocytosis but probably not activation in the absence of a second signal (e.g., Fc receptor or pattern recognition receptor). CR4 also binds iC3b-opsonized particles, resulting in direct endocytosis. Although its role as a phagocytic receptor is not well characterized, CD11c is the major marker for DCs. It is important to understand the functional importance of this complement receptor on DC and how it participates in uptake of antigen for presentation to T lymphocytes.

CR2 expressed on B cells augments cognate antibody receptor signaling (see later section). This receptor recognizes targets that are coated with iC3b, as well as the subsequent degradation products C3dg and C3d, all of which remain covalently bound to the target (see Fig. 24.2B). CR2 is the only complement receptor that recognizes C3d/TED on its own as its ligand. However, the CR2 binding site on TED only becomes accessible after degradation of C3 to at least the iC3b stage. Activation of complement plays a contributing role in producing a strong antibody response. An interesting aside is that CR2 is the cell surface receptor on human B cells that is recognized by the Epstein-Barr virus.[44]

CRIg is a recently described complement receptor that plays an important role in the clearance of C3b opsonized complexes by phagocytic cells of the liver.[45] It is also expressed on subsets of macrophages, but less is known about this role. The recent cocrystallization of C3b and CRIg revealed binding to the C3b β chain, which is in contrast to all other known C3-interacting partners, in which binding to the activated C3 occurs via the α chain.

Biologic Activity of C3a and C5a

The role of the complement fragments C3a and C5a in the immune response is to produce localized inflammation.[46] C3a and C5a are anaphylatoxins and are structurally similar to chemokines. When produced in large amounts or injected systemically, they induce a generalized circulatory collapse and shock-like syndrome similar to that seen in a systemic allergic reaction involving IgE antibodies.[47]

Of the two fragments, C5a is the most stable and possesses the best characterized and possibly highest specific biologic activity. Both C3a and C5a induce smooth muscle contraction and increased vascular permeability. C5a and C3a also act on endothelial cells lining blood vessels to induce adhesion molecule expression.[48,49] In addition, C3a and C5a can activate the mast cells that populate submucosal tissues and line vessels throughout the body to release histamine, tumor necrosis factor α (TNF-α), and protease.[6] The changes induced by C3a and C5a recruit antibody, complement, and phagocytic cells to the site of infection, thereby hastening the adaptive immune response. C5a also induces the upregulation of CR1 and CR3 on the surfaces of these cells. C5a is the only complement chemotactic agent for neutrophils, macrophages, and basophils. By contrast, both C3a and C5a possess chemotactic activity for mast cells.[50] Although a similar fragment, C4a, is produced in the course of C4 activation, its physiologic relevance as an anaphylatoxin is highly questionable. First, human C4a binds to neither C3aR nor C5aR, the two well-characterized complement anaphylatoxin receptors, and a specific C4a-binding entity has not been identified. Second, anaphylatoxin activity for human C4a has only been reported on guinea pig targets, but even there, it is two to three orders of magnitude less potent than human C3a.[50]

Regulation of Complement Activation

Activation of the complement system must be tightly regulated to prevent autologous tissue damage (see Table 24.1).[51] Some of the proteins involved in regulating complement action have been described (see Alternative Pathway, earlier). In addition to these regulators, a number of other checkpoints limit the scope and target of complement activation.

As a result of binding to antibody or pathogen, conformational changes to C1q induce the enzymatic activity of C1r and C1s. Both of these enzymes are regulated by the C1 inhibitor (C1-INH). C1-INH is a member of a family of *ser*ine protease *in*hibitors termed *serpins*.[52] Serpins provide a bait sequence that mimics the active site of the substrate. When C1r or C1s proteolytically attacks this sequence, the net result is that their respective active site serine hydroxyls become permanently covalently bound to the C1-INH bait site, thereby destroying their proteolytic activity. C1-INH works in a similar fashion in regulating the activated MASP proteases of the LP. Finally, C1-INH is also responsible for preventing spontaneous fluid-phase activation of C1 in plasma, but this activity can be overridden by immune complexes.

Although C1 is capable of cleaving multiple C4 molecules, only approximately 10% of the produced C4b clusters about the targeted antigen.[53] The rest is released into the fluid phase. C4b in the fluid phase is rapidly bound by C4 binding protein (C4bp), which is a cofactor for FI. Factor I cleaves C4b into two fragments, C4c and C4d, which are quickly cleared from the circulation.

In addition to their FI cofactor activities, the soluble regulators C4bp and FH, respectively, promote the dissociation of the CP (C4b2a) and AP (C3bBb) C3 convertases into their constituent components. This decay-dissociation is unidirectional because neither C2a nor Bb can reassociate on its own with their respective C3 convertase subunits. The membrane-bound regulators CR1 and DAF similarly possess decay-accelerating functionality toward both the CP and AP C3 convertases. The importance of CR1 or CR1-like molecules in curbing the complement response can be witnessed in a rather unexpected condition. Complement receptor 1–related gene (*Crry*) is a murine homologue of the human *CR1* gene, although its near-ubiquitous tissue distribution more closely resembles that of MCP (a somewhat more distant homologue).[54,55] Mice lacking Crry are unable to properly regulate C3. Crry-deficient mice spontaneously abort because of C3-dependent injury to the fetus. This presumably is the result of uncontrolled C3 deposition on the placenta. This observation in mice sheds light on the possibility that defective MCP (or perhaps CR1) plays a role in recurrent fetal loss manifest in patients with antiphospholipid syndrome.

Biologic Consequences of Complement Cascade Deficiencies

The important role of the complement system in preventing disease is witnessed in cases in which components of the system are absent either because of random mutation in the human population or by design in gene-targeted "knock-out" mice. Some complement cascade deficiencies have been described. This section focuses on the biologic consequences of deficiencies in complement cascade activation that have profound biologic consequences followed by a discussion on deficiencies in complement regulatory proteins.

Homozygous deficiencies in C1q, the most common form of C1 deficiency in humans, is a powerful susceptibility factor for the development of systemic lupus erythematosus (SLE).[56,57] Patients lacking C1q nearly always present with SLE. They have increased susceptibility to viral and bacterial infections, but it is not nearly as pronounced as in C3 deficiency (see later discussion). C1q knock-out mice show increased mortality, with up to 25% of mice having histologic evidence of glomerulonephritis.

C4 in humans is encoded by two separate loci giving rise to two distinct protein products, C4A and C4B.[58] Complete C4 deficiency correlates with a 75% prevalence of SLE in humans. However, at least in certain human populations, the absence, or even haploinsufficiency, of C4A, but not C4B, is associated with elevated risk for development of autoimmune diseases such as SLE and other lupus-like autoimmune disease. The reason for the protective effect of C4A is not settled, but it is worth noting that the one indisputable functional difference between C4A and C4B is in the nature of the covalent bond formed upon target deposition. Whereas C4A transacylates onto amino group nucleophiles, forming amide bonds, C4B shows a strong preference for forming ester linkages to hydroxyl group nucleophiles. The approximately threefold greater propensity of C4A, relative to C4B, to bind to amino group–rich C1-bearing IgG aggregates,[59] as would be present in immune complexes in need of complement-dependent clearance, is one possible reason for the association of C4A null states with SLE. Finally, as with C1q, mice deficient in C4 are predisposed to SLE-like disease.

C2 deficiency appears to be relatively benign.[60] Humans lacking C2 appear to have a normally functioning immune system, although autoimmune disorders and, less commonly, infections are observed with increased frequency.

In light of the central role of C3 in the complement cascade, it is not surprising that C3 deficiency has dire consequences for the host organism. Of all known cases of C3 deficiency among humans, no patients have been reported as disease free. Infectious complications, predominantly pyogenic in nature, occur frequently and recurrently. *Streptococcus pneumoniae* and *Neisseria meningitidis* are the major pathogens reported. In addition, SLE, vasculitic syndromes, and glomerulonephritis have been documented in up to 21% of C3-deficient patients. Mice deficient in C3 show, similar to humans, greatly increased susceptibility to streptococcal infection and death.[61] The 50% lethal dose (LD_{50}) is 50-fold less for C3-deficient mice than for C3-sufficient control subjects. This may be attributable in large part to the inability of mice deficient in C3 to effectively opsonize the bacteria. Moreover, the deficient mice have an impaired humoral response (see later section).

Biologic Consequences of Complement Regulatory Protein Deficiencies

Deficiencies in C1-INH have been observed in the human population.[62] C1-INH deficiency can be inherited as an autosomal dominant trait or can result from autoantibodies that recognize C1-INH, blocking its function.[52] The inherited form of this deficiency is the cause of hereditary angioedema. Patients with hereditary angioedema experience chronic spontaneous complement activation leading to the production of excess cleaved fragments of C4 and C2. The biochemical cause of angioedema in these patients is not definitively elucidated. One line of reasoning points to excess production of C2 kinin and bradykinin. The peptide C2 kinin is a breakdown product of C2a after cleavage of C2. This peptide causes extensive swelling; the most dangerous is local swelling in the trachea, which can lead to suffocation. Bradykinin, which has similar actions to C2 kinin, is also produced in an uncontrolled fashion in this disease as a result of the lack of inhibition of another plasma protease, kallikrein, which is activated by tissue damage and is regulated by C1-INH. Although C1 is unregulated in patients with hereditary angioedema, large-scale cleavage of C3 is prevented by C4 and C2 control mechanisms and by regulation of C3 convertase formation on host cells. An increased risk of infection is not associated with C1-INH deficiency. This disease can be fully corrected by infusion of purified C1-INH.

Acquired C1-INH deficiency may be associated with lymphoproliferative disorders and in most cases represents development of an autoantibody that binds to and neutralizes C1-INH. In two examined cases, autoantibodies abrogate C1-INH activity by preventing formation of the C1s–C1-INH complex. However, after the complex formed, the autoreactive antibodies had no effect on C1-INH function. To date, there is no uniform, fully effective therapy for these patients.

The role of FI in complement cascade regulation can be witnessed in patients with FI deficiency.[63] In the presence of a cofactor protein,

FI cleaves C3b, producing iC3b, the inactive form of C3b. iC3b is incapable of reacting with factor B to form the AP C3 convertase, thereby preventing uncontrolled AP activation. In the absence of FI, unrestrained C3 consumption occurs secondary to accelerated spontaneous AP turnover. Patients with FI deficiency have recurrent infections caused by pyogenic organisms, including meningococcal meningitis.

Likewise, mice deficient in the central protein FH exhibit unrestrained C3 activation via the AP, leading to near depletion of serum C3. An important outcome of the failure to regulate C3 activation is glomerulonephritis. Strikingly, mice deficient in FH develop a disease resembling the human disorder membrane glomerulonephritis. The phenotype of the mice confirms the general notion that the AP is always "on" and that failure to regulate activated C3 results in consumption of circulating C3 and tissue injury.

Another example of the importance of FH regulation are reports of genetic association between variant alleles of FH and the human diseases age-related macular degeneration (AMD) and atypical hemolytic uremic syndrome (aHUS). Whereas AMD is a fairly common condition—indeed, it is the leading cause of blindness in the Western world—it has been the elucidation of the etiology of the much rarer aHUS condition (two cases per million) that has led to a fuller appreciation of the diverse ways through which dysregulation of the AP of complement can give rise to severe pathology. Classically, HUS is a clinical triad of microangiopathic hemolytic anemia, thrombocytopenia, and acute renal failure. The disease is characterized by a precipitating injury of endothelial cells. In contrast to the fairly common classical form of HUS, which is diarrhea-associated and is usually caused by a Shiga toxin–secreting pathogen, the atypical form of HUS is nondiarrheal and is caused by genetic predisposition. Even haploinsufficiency of variants of FH, MCP, and FI resulting from either loss of expression—or more commonly, loss of regulatory

function—results in disease pathology. In addition, gain-of-function variants of factor B have been described that either form the AP C3 convertase more efficiently than wild-type factor B or are more resistant to decay-dissociation by FH or DAF. Finally, several C3 variants have been described in aHUS patients that are gain of function in the sense that as C3b there is decreased binding affinity for MCP and FH and thus AP C3 convertases formed with this C3b as subunit would have a prolonged lifetime relative to wild-type C3b.[64,65]

Because FH mutations account for at least 30% of reported aHUS cases and approximately 70% of these are caused by missense mutations in SCR domains 19 and 20, the molecular basis of this disease association has been intensively investigated, and the findings of these studies are best understood in the context of a structure-based domain model[66] of FH bound to C3b on a nonactivator (i.e., host) surface (Fig. 24.3). FH consists of 20 SCR domains, where some domains in the middle of the molecule appear to play mainly a structural role, likely allowing the molecule to bend back on itself, but domain clusters near the ends mediate specific functions. SCRs 1 to 4 bind to C3b and mediate both decay-accelerating and FI-cofactor functionalities. Indeed, FH(SCR1–4) on its own is able to regulate a fluid-phase AP C3 convertase, but it cannot do so for surface-bound AP C3 convertases. For regulation of the latter, there are three additional binding interactions that become relevant. Two of these are located within SCRs 19 to 20, specifically, a site localized mainly to SCR19 binds to the C3d/TED domain of the surface-bound C3b molecule, and a site within SCR20 binds to surface-associated polyanions such as sulfated glycosaminoglycans or sialic acid arrays. The aHUS-associated missense mutations found within SCRs 19 to 20 affect one or other of these two binding functions and lead to dysregulation of the AP C3 convertase at the surface of host tissue. In particular, complement-mediated damage to the kidney basement membrane is often a hallmark of aHUS. As a tissue devoid of the membrane-associated complement regulators MCP, DAF, or CR1, but rich in sulfated glycosaminoglycans, the functionality of the soluble AP regulator FH becomes even more crucial for host protection and likely explains the high incidence of missense mutations within SCRs 19 to 20 in aHUS patients. Interestingly, missense mutations in FH SCRs 19 to 20 do not result in systemic C3 consumption, as would be the case for complete deficiencies of FH. This is because SCRs 1 to 4 of the mutant molecule are still capable of regulating spontaneously formed AP C3 convertases in the fluid phase.

In addition to the polyanion binding site in FH SCR 20, there is also one in SCR 7. This SCR is the site of an amino acid polymorphism in FH (tyrosine to histidine at residue 402, Y402H) that is a significant risk factor for AMD but interestingly does not correlate with disease susceptibility for aHUS. Heterozygotes and homozygotes for H402 are respectively 2.7-fold and 7.4-fold more at risk for AMD than homozygous Y402 individuals, and this single polymorphism can account for up to 50% of the risk of AMD.[67,68] Two significant functional differences have been observed for the Y402 and H402 variants of FH. First, the affinity and specificity for a spectrum of sulfated glycosaminoglycans is different for the two variants of FH. Secondly, the affinity of the H402 variant of FH for C-reactive protein (CRP), an acute-phase protein that binds to damaged tissue, is substantially lower than that of the Y402 variant. It is notable that the Bruch's membrane of the macula, similar to the kidney basement membrane, is devoid of membrane-associated complement regulators and so is highly dependent on FH for local AP regulation. Indeed, the spectrum of sulfated glycosaminoglycans found on the Bruch's membrane appear to be more dependent on the polyanionic binding site in SCR 7 for the interaction than that in SCRs 19 to 20 because even with non-AMD eye tissue, there is preferential binding of the Y402 variant to the Bruch's membrane.[69] Thus the lower binding affinity of the H402 FH variant, coupled with a possible age-related change in the biosynthesized spectrum of sulfated glycosaminoglycans on Bruch membrane, could account for the dysregulation of the AP in the macula with the ensuing inflammation of the macula seen in AMD patients. There may also be a contribution from the differential binding of the FH variants to CRP present on the particulate debris

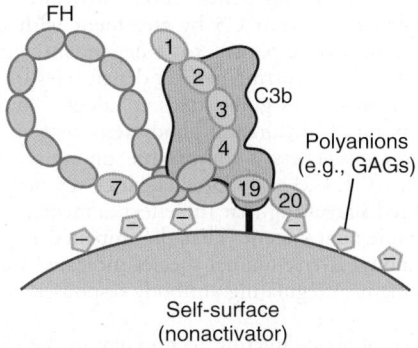

Fig. 24.3 A STRUCTURE-BASED MODEL OF THE FACTOR H (FH)–MEDIATED REGULATION OF THE ALTERNATIVE PATHWAY ON HOST CELLS BEARING ADVENTITIOUSLY DEPOSITED C3b. Whereas the depicted interaction of FH domains SCR(1–4) with C3b is sufficient to prevent C3b in solution from becoming a subunit of an AP C3 convertase, for surface-bound C3b, at least two additional interactions are necessary. The first is the interaction indicated between FH SCR19 and the thioester domain (TED)/C3d domain of the C3b molecule. The second is between FH SCR20 and cell surface–associated sulfated glycosaminoglycans (GAGs) or arrays of sialic acid containing glycans, in both cases denoted by *pentagons with an internal minus sign.* Mutations affecting either the C3d binding site or the polyanion binding site within FH SCR(19–20) lead to alternative pathway dysregulation and the disease atypical hemolytic uremic syndrome (aHUS). There is an additional polyanion binding site in SCR7, which appears to be important for regulating the alternative pathway on some host surfaces, most particularly Bruch's membrane in the eye because the SCR7 Y402H polymorphism is a risk factor for AMD. *(Adapted from Kajander T, Lehtinen MJ, Hyvärinen S, et al: Dual interaction of factor H with C3d and glycosaminoglycans in host-nonhost discrimination by complement.* Proc Nat Acad Sci U S A *108:2897, 2011; reproduced with permission of the National Academy of Science.)*

(drusen) residing in between the retinal pigment epithelium and the Bruch's membrane.

The MAC is one mechanism used by the host to rid itself of certain microorganisms. Host cells are protected from MAC-mediated lysis by CD59 (protectin), a membrane-bound protein. CD59 performs its function by inhibiting the binding of C9 to the C5b–C6–C7–C8–C9 complex. CD59 and DAF are linked to the cell surface by a phosphoinositol glycolipid (PIG) tail. One of the enzymes involved in the synthesis of PIG tails is encoded on chromosome X. Mutation of this gene leads to a failure to synthesize PIG tails and with it an inability to express CD59 or DAF on the cell surface.[61–72] Lack of CD59 and DAF expression on host cell surfaces is the cause of paroxysmal nocturnal hemoglobinuria. This disease is characterized by episodes of chronic intravascular hemolysis and propensity to thrombosis.

Autoimmunity and Complement Deficiencies

There exists a strong correlative relationship between the lack of certain components of the complement system (i.e., C1 and C4) and autoimmune disease, particularly SLE. Two general nonmutually exclusive hypotheses have been put forward to explain the increased incidence of SLE among complement deficient individuals: the clearance hypothesis and the tolerance hypothesis.[57,73,74] The clearance hypothesis is based on the known role of the CP of complement in binding to foreign antigens and transporting them to the liver and spleen for degradation and removal from the circulation. Thus defects in clearance of apoptotic cells or debris would lead to inappropriate accumulation of self-antigen and overstimulation of self-reactive lymphocytes.

The tolerance model proposes that innate immunity protects against SLE by delivering lupus autoantigens to sites where immature B lymphocytes are tolerized, thereby eliminating a source of autoreactive antibody molecules. SLE is characterized by high-affinity antibodies specific for autoantigens such as double-stranded DNA (dsDNA), ribonuclear proteins, and histones. Validation of the model comes in part from studies with human B cells demonstrating that self-reactive B cells are eliminated or anergized at two major checkpoints, bone marrow (BM) and spleen. Thus counterselection of potentially pathogenic B cells is an active process and most likely involves components of innate immunity.

Recent studies in a mouse model (strain 564 Igi) in which the B cells express an Ig receptor specific for the lupus antigen SSB/LA suggests a third possible explanation for why C4 is critical for protection against SLE. Accordingly, this hypothesis suggests that C4-dependent defects in clearance of immune complexes leads to a loss of tolerance of certain autoreactive B cells. Thus accumulation of immune complexes composed of lupus antigens that bear DNA or ribonucleoprotein (RNP) ligands that trigger Toll-like receptors (TLRs) TLR 7 and TLR 9 may induce myeloid cells to release excess type I interferon (IFN-α). In a feed-forward loop, IFN-α release induces increased sensitivity of TLR 7 and 9 receptors, in particular on B cells, such that the combined effects of engagement of DNA or RNP self-antigen and increased TLR 7 and 9 leads to escape of B-cell tolerance.[74a,74b]

The first part of this section familiarized the reader with the general aspects of the complement system. The remainder of this section focuses on the role of the complement system in the initiation and propagation of the adaptive immune response and begins with a description of natural antibody.

Natural Antibody

Natural antibody, in contrast to antibody secreted in response to active immunization, is continuously released, mostly by the B1 subpopulation of lymphocytes. Predominantly IgM but also IgA and IgG3 (in mice), natural antibodies tend to be polyreactive, with low-affinity binding for antigens such as nuclear proteins, DNA, and

phosphatidylcholine, which are common structures among both pathogens and host tissue. These antibodies rarely show evidence of somatic mutation. It has been speculated that the variable region genes that predominate among natural antibodies have been selected evolutionarily for their ability to recognize pathogens and act as a rapid response to infection, thereby acting as a stop gap to provide sufficient time for the adaptive immune response to form. Natural antibody mediates its protective effects via the CP of complement.

IgM natural antibody is important in initiating the CP, leading to enhanced humoral immunity. In addition to its role in protecting against pathogens, natural antibody protects against lupus-like disease based on studies in mice. Thus, similar to C1q and C4, deficiency in IgM predisposes to an SLE-like phenotype.

Complement Links Innate and Adaptive Immune Responses

One of the critical functions of CP complement is providing a bridge between innate and acquired immune systems. The process is achieved through attachment of complement products to the antigen or pathogen, either directly to the surface or via antibody (see earlier section). This complement "tag" consists of breakdown products of C3 (i.e., C3b, C3dg, and C3d) that facilitate recognition of pathogens by the immune system. The recognition phase is mediated principally through complement receptors CD21 (CR2) and CD35 (CR1). This section details complement-dependent mechanisms of immune detection and humoral responses to thymus (T)-dependent antigens.

Soluble Complement Mediators of Antibody Responses

The first clue that complement is important in regulating B-lymphocyte responses came from the observation that B lymphocytes bind activated C3 fragments.[75] Soon thereafter, it was noted that mice depleted of serum C3 by treatment with cobra venom factor had diminished responses to T-dependent antigens.[76] The discovery of naturally occurring genetic deficiencies in C3, C4, and C2 in species as diverse as guinea pigs,[77,78] dogs,[79] and humans[80,81] allowed description of impaired antibody responses as well. Because the impaired responsiveness is comparable among animals deficient in CP activators (C4, C2) and C3-deficient or C3-depleted animals, a model emerged suggesting that the effect is mediated through the CP of the complement system. That the impaired responsiveness is comparable among diverse animal species indicated the importance of CP complement in regulating antibody responses to T-dependent antigens.

The advance of gene-targeting technology in the murine system led to development of engineered strains devoid of various components of CP complement. C1q-, C4-, and C3-deficient mouse strains generate reduced antibody responses to T-dependent antigens.[82–85] Furthermore, these strains fail to switch Ig isotypes normally, suggesting that germinal center responses are impaired.[84] Germinal centers are microanatomic structures whose purpose is to provide for increasing affinity of serum antibody for antigens (affinity maturation), isotype switching, and development and differentiation of memory B lymphocytes and plasma cells.[86] Consistent with this theory, immunized complement-deficient mice produce fewer and smaller germinal centers compared with immunized wild-type mice.[84] Importantly, humoral responses in each of the C1q-, C4-, and C3-deficient strains can be rescued by transplantation of wild-type BM.[56,87,88] Therefore BM-derived cells can produce sufficient complement to reconstitute antibody responses to T-dependent antigens administered intravenously.

It is suggested that the CP potentiates antibody responses through involvement of immune complex formation. The implication is that natural antibodies or specific IgM released early in the response by B cells responding to antigen recognize and bind pathogens, thereby activating the CP. In support of this model, genetically engineered mice producing only membrane IgM (i.e., with gene-targeted deletion of secretory signals) produce significantly reduced antibody responses to T-dependent antigens.[89] A second mechanism for initial CP activation on the antigen, which may be relevant to a subset of antigens bearing a repeating epitope, involves binding of the antigen by B cells through the surface IgM of two or more B-cell receptors (BCRs). The cross-linking and distortion that is imparted to the Fc$_\mu$ regions of adjacent BCRs is sufficient to activate the CP at the B-cell surface. Indeed, this mechanism does not work if the BCR μ-chain contains a mutation that abolishes C1q binding.[90] Finally, a third permutation of these mechanisms may apply to monovalent soluble T-dependent antigens. The antigen is first captured by the BCR, creating an antigen array on the B-cell surface, to which low-affinity natural repertoire IgM can bind by virtue of avidity effects and initiate the CP.[91] As illustrated by these examples, immune complex formation is only important for initiating the CP, leading to the deposition of C3 activation products on the antigen or immune complex. Indeed, antigens directly conjugated to C3b or C3d fragments are more potent immunogens compared to unconjugated antigen.[92,93] Furthermore, the magnitude of the immune response is directly influenced by the number of C3d fragments conjugated to the antigen.[92] Therefore activated products of complement component C3 act as a natural adjuvant in driving efficient antibody responses.

Complement Receptors and Antibody Responses

B-Lymphocyte Coreceptors

The effects of complement-coated antigens on antibody responses are mediated primarily through complement receptors CD21 and CD35. CD21 and CD35 are expressed predominantly on B lymphocytes and FDCs.[94,95] CD35 is also found on polymorphonuclear cells, macrophages, mast cells, and DCs.[94] CD21 and CD35 are encoded for by separate yet closely linked genes in humans.[96] In mice, CD21 and CD35 originate from the same locus (Cr2) and are generated by alternative splicing events at the RNA level.[97,98]

Two novel sets of experiments demonstrated that CD21 and CD35 are important in regulating B-lymphocyte responses to T-dependent antigens. In the first set of experiments, antibodies specific for both CD21 and CD35 or CD35 alone were administered to immunized mice.[99–102] In the second set of experiments, a soluble form of CD21 was administered to immunized mice, thereby competing for C3d-coupled antigen interactions.[103] In both sets of experiments, treatment impaired antibody responses. In the first approach, the antibody that specifically blocked the interaction of C3d with CD21 was much more effective at blocking antibody responses compared with anti-CD35 antibody treatment, which blocked only the binding of C3b to CD35. This suggested that although both receptors contribute, CD21 is more important in regulating antibody responses.[100]

Because CD21 and CD35 are found on B lymphocytes and FDCs, two important cell types for humoral responses, two nonmutually exclusive models are proposed for their function. In the first model, CD21 augments antibody responses through activity as a coreceptor on B lymphocytes[104] (Fig. 24.4A). The second model proposes that CD21/CD35 on FDCs trap and focus antigen such that B lymphocytes can efficiently cross-link their antigen receptor to become activated[105] (Fig. 24.4B).

As is apparent from the schematics in Fig. 24.4A–B and as will be elaborated upon further in the ensuing discussion, the key ligand receptor–receptor interaction mediating the linkage between complement and the adaptive humoral immune system is that between the C3d fragment that is covalently coupled to antigen and CD21 (CR2) present on B cells and FDC. The extracellular region of CD21 is composed of 15 or 16 SCR domains (because of the usage of alternative splice sites for exon 11), but the C3d binding site is confined to the two N-terminal–most SCR domains.[106] In what is an instructive lesson on the need to have concordance between x-ray crystallographic

structures and biochemical data, the nature of this important interface had been hotly debated for a decade because of discrepancies between a structure of the CR2(SCR1-2):C3d complex published[107] in 2001 with both preexisting and subsequent biochemical data in the literature. A 2011 de novo structure of this complex,[108] depicted in Fig. 24.4C, appears to have resolved the issue because the interactions seen in the new structure are fully supported by the biochemical data in the literature. For example, the biochemical data suggesting that there should be multiple ionic bonds mediating the binding is fully rationalized in terms of the five such bonds seen in the structure between a very negatively charged interface on a concave face of C3d that is remote from the covalent attachment site and positively charged lysine and arginine side chains from CR2 sticking down and interacting with oppositely charged residues on the C3d interface, as can be appreciated in Fig. 24.4C.

As a coreceptor, engagement of CD21 by complement-coupled antigen on the surface of a B lymphocyte, in combination with membrane Ig (BCR) cross-linking, would lower the threshold of signal through the BCR required to activate the cell.[104] Accordingly, naive B lymphocytes bear low-affinity receptors for antigen; therefore, especially under conditions of limiting antigen, as would be the case during initial encounter with a microbial pathogen, additional signaling by the CD21 coreceptor is required for efficient activation. This was demonstrated in vitro by culturing B lymphocytes with cognate antigen, either uncoupled or coupled to C3d. By measuring intracellular Ca^{2+} levels as a measure of cell activation, it was estimated that 100- to 1000-fold less C3d-conjugated antigen was required to activate B lymphocytes compared with unconjugated antigen.[92]

The opportunity to test the importance of CD21 and CD35 as B-lymphocyte coreceptors in vivo came from studies using mice with targeted disruption in the Cr2 locus. Importantly, Cr2-deficient mice have impaired humoral responses similar to C1q-, C4-, and C3-deficient mice (Fig. 24.5).[109–111] Using embryonic stem cells with a disrupted Cr2 locus, Croix et al[112] used blastocyst complementation of Rag2$^{-/-}$ mice, such that chimeric mice expressed CD21/CD35 on FDCs but not on B lymphocytes. These chimeric mice displayed impaired antibody responses to the T-dependent antigen NP-KLH compared with control subjects. Therefore CD21/CD35 on B lymphocytes is important for normal antibody responses. Although CD21/CD35 on FDC is on its own, insufficient for normal antibody responses, as discussed in the next section, CD21/CD35 on FDC does have a specific role in the memory response of B cell–mediated immunity.

The covalent attachment of complement to antigen engages CD21 as a complex with CD19/CD81 and BCR on the cell surface (see Fig. 24.4A).[104,113,114] Dual binding of CD21/CD19/CD81 with BCR generates a stronger signal compared with BCR engagement alone.[104] If the combined signal is sufficient, the B lymphocyte is activated. If insufficient, then the B lymphocyte is likely eliminated by apoptosis.[87,115–119] The major ligand-binding receptor within the CD21/CD19/CD81 complex is CD21. The major role of CD19 is in initiating a signaling cascade within the cell.[120] CD81 is a tetraspanning molecule that stabilizes the complex within the membrane. After coligation of the BCR with the CD21/CD19/CD81 complex, CD81 gets S-palmitoylated on a cysteine side chain, and this in turn mobilizes the coligated complexes to a special compartment of the plasma membrane known as a lipid raft. Localization to this compartment facilitates prolonged intracellular signaling because the compartment is rich in signal-propagating phosphokinases but is relatively devoid of the regulatory phosphatases.[121] Absence of any of the CD21/CD19/CD81 components adversely affects antibody responses to T-dependent antigens, although the degree of impairment varies.[109,122–124]

Focusing Antigen on Follicular Dendritic Cells

The second role of complement receptors CD21 and CD35 in regulating humoral responses is that they permit FDCs to trap antigen (Fig. 24.6).[105,125] FDCs concentrate in regions of ongoing immune

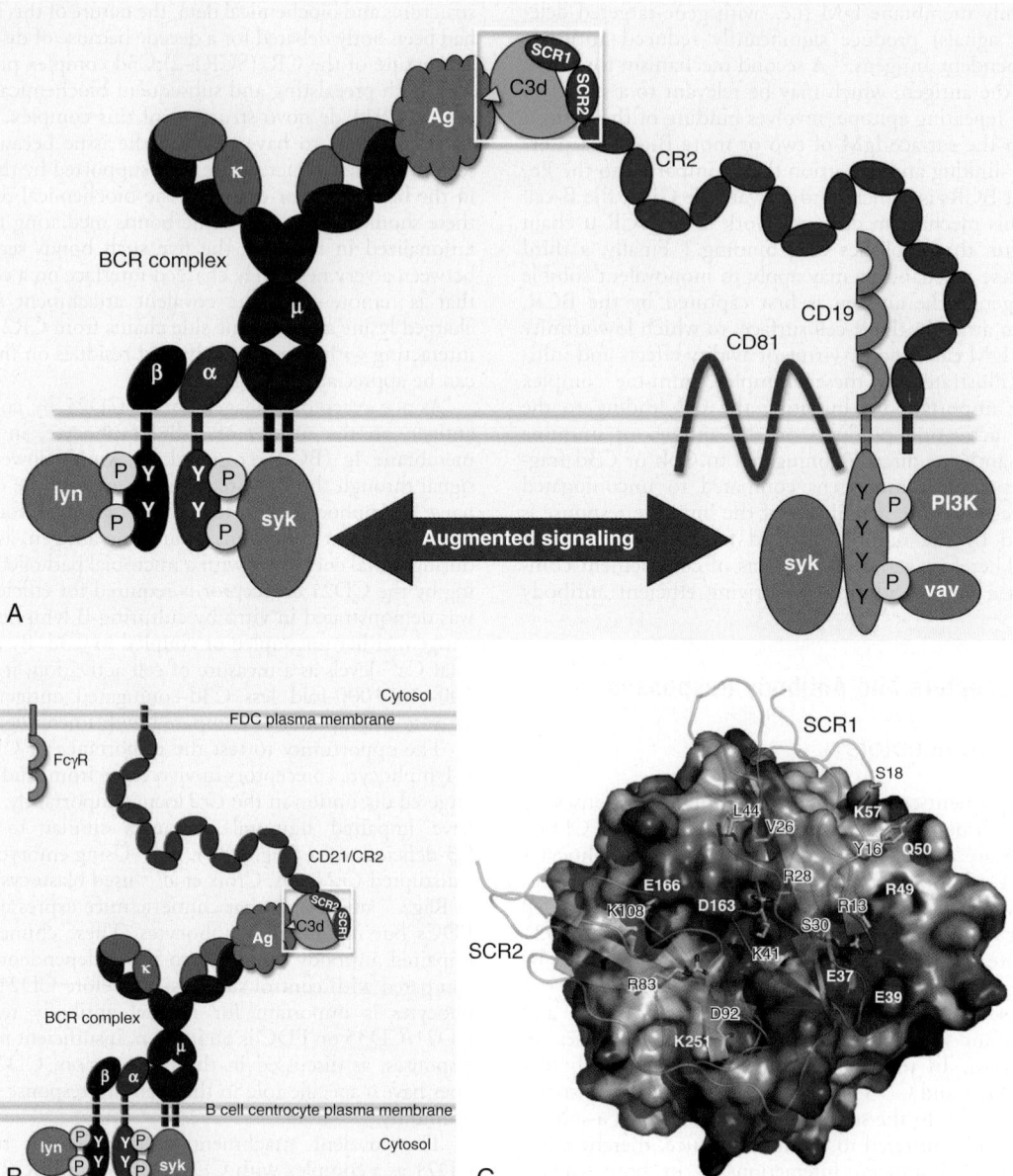

Fig. 24.4 COUPLING OF C3D TO ANTIGEN ALTERS ITS FATE IN B-CELL RESPONSE. (A) Coligation of the B-cell receptor (BCR) with the CD19/CD21/CD81 complex by antigen coated with C3d regulates essential functions for naïve B-cell activation. The *boxed area* indicates the key binding interaction between CD21/CR2(SCR1-2), and the C3d fragment that is covalently bound *(yellow triangle)* to the antigen recognized by this B cell's BCR. (B) C3d-coated antigens are also captured on the surface of the follicular dendritic cells (FDCs) by CD21, allowing for efficient stimulation of previously antigen-engaged B-cell centrocytes in the germinal centers during the process of affinity maturation and the generation of memory B cells. (C) The structure of the CR2(SCR1-2):C3d complex as a surface representation of C3d colored for electrostatic potential (*red,* negative; *blue,* positive) and an overlayed, semitransparent, ribbon diagram of CR2(SCR1–2) showing stick models of the side chains of some of the interacting residues. Note the charge complementarity for many of the interacting amino acids. *(C, Reproduced with permission from van den Elsen JM, Isenman DE: A crystal structure of the complex between human complement receptor 2 and its ligand C3d.* Science 332:608, 2011.*)*

responses, such as germinal centers, and they appear necessary for antibody responses. Germinal centers (see earlier section) promote somatic hypermutation within Ig heavy- and light-chain genes along with isotype switching and production of memory B lymphocytes and plasma cells. They can be divided into two regions, dark zone and light zone. To gain entry into the dark zone, B lymphocytes are activated by receiving above threshold signals from the CD21/CD19/CD81 and BCR in combination with costimulation from helper T lymphocytes.[126–128] Within the dark zone, activated B lymphocytes divide and mutate their Ig receptor genes.[127–130] After several rounds

of proliferation in the dark zone, B lymphocytes enter the light zone, where they are subjected to selection on antigen deposited on FDCs (i.e., clonal selection).[131,132] The selection of high-affinity B lymphocyte clones into memory B-lymphocyte and plasma cell pools ensures future protection against repeat antigen exposure.

How antigen is retained on FDCs, both for primary B-lymphocyte responses and for long-term memory responses, is subject to intense research. However, supporting evidence indicates that complement receptors on FDCs are important in both short- and long-term B-lymphocyte responses. Papamichail et al[105] demonstrated that

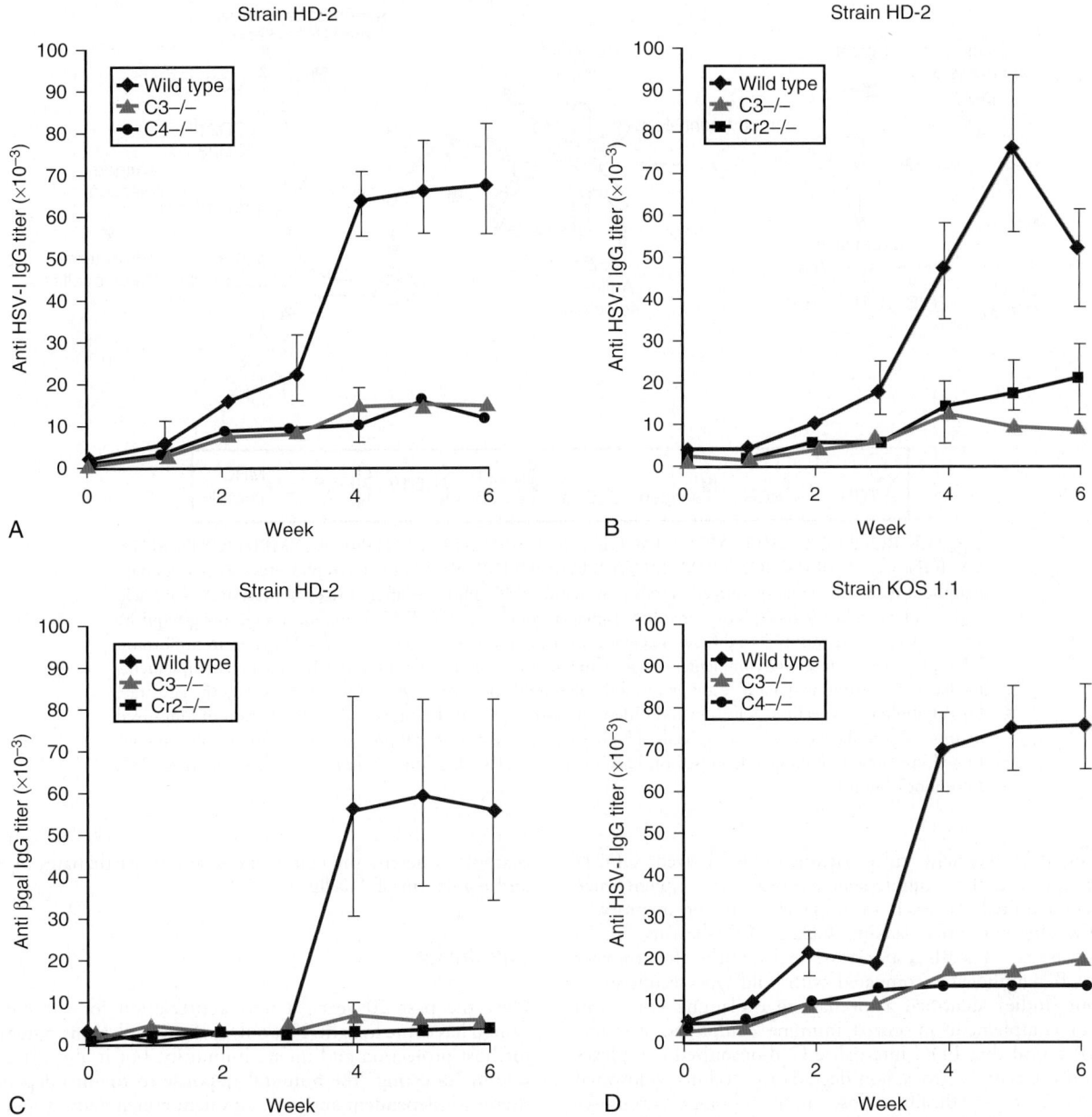

Fig. 24.5 Classical pathway complement and complement receptors CD21/CD35 are required for the humoral response to replication-defective HD-2 virus or replication-sufficient KOS1.1 wild-type (WT) virus. Mice were injected at days 0 and 21 with 2×10^6 plaque-forming units of replication-defective (A–C) or replication-sufficient (D) virus, HD-2, and KOS1.1, respectively. Antibody titers were determined by enzyme-linked immunosorbent assay. Mean titer ± SD represents at least five mice analyzed in two separate experiments. (A) Deficiency in either C3 or C4 results in an impaired secondary humoral response to infectious herpes simplex virus (HSV). (B) Cr2$^{-/-}$ mice have an impaired secondary response similar to mice deficient in C3. (C) Humoral response to recombinant virus-expressed heterologous protein (β-galactosidase) is also impaired in mice deficient in C3 or CD21/CD35. (D) Secondary humoral response to replication-sufficient HSV-1 (strain KOS1.1) depends on complement C3 and C4. *(From Da Costa XJ, Brockman MA, Alicot E, et al: Humoral response to herpes simplex virus is complement-dependent. Proc Nat Acad Sci U S A 96:12708, 1999; reproduced with permission of the National Academy of Science.)*

retention of antigen–IgG immune complexes on FDCs was reduced upon depletion of C3 using cobra venom factor. Therefore it appears that immune complex deposition on FDCs is complement dependent. In addition, antibody production in vitro using FDCs demonstrates that antibody production is dependent on CD21/CD35.[133]

Availability of *Cr2*-deficient mice has shed light on the importance of FDC-derived CD21/CD35 on humoral responses. Because FDCs are radioresistant, it was possible to generate chimeric mice that restricted CD21/CD35 expression to B lymphocytes by BM transplantation. Ahearn et al[109] made chimeric mice with *Cr2*-deficient

FDCs by transplanting wild-type BM (B-lymphocyte *Cr2*$^{+/+}$) into lethally irradiated *Cr2*-deficient recipient mice (FDC-*Cr2*$^{-/-}$). After secondary challenge with antigen, the chimeric mice failed to sustain high-level antibody production, suggesting that CD21/CD35 on FDCs is important for recall or memory responses. Fang et al[134] came to a similar conclusion regarding the importance of CD21/35 expression on FDC for a strong immune response.

CD21/CD35 do appear important for persistence of antibody titers, normal frequencies of memory B lymphocytes and plasma cells, and affinity maturation. Adoptively transferring memory B

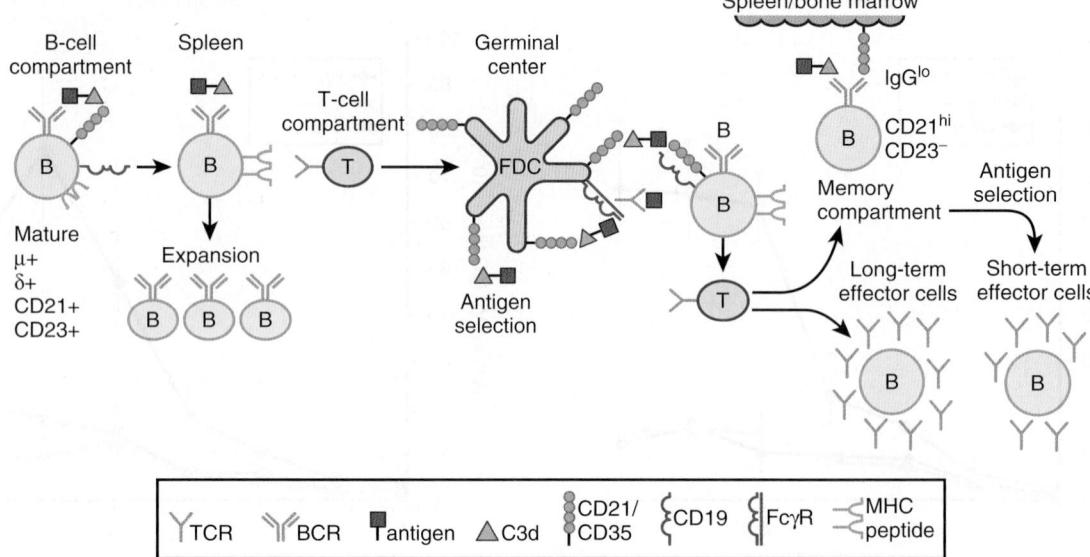

Fig. 24.6 ROLE OF COMPLEMENT-TAGGED ANTIGEN IN DIRECTING B-LYMPHOCYTE ACTIVATION AND FORMATION OF MEMORY B LYMPHOCYTES. Mature B lymphocytes survey secondary lymphoid tissues in search of antigen. Survival of mature B lymphocytes after antigen contact and T-cell help within splenic follicles depends on coreceptor signals through CD21/CD35. Lymphocytes receiving requisite signals expand and continue to differentiate within germinal centers, where CD21/CD35 is again important. B lymphocytes not receiving complement–ligand interactions in germinal centers die. In addition, complement-mediated deposition may localize antigen to follicular dendritic cells (FDCs), thereby providing the substrate for B-lymphocyte selection. Selection and differentiation in germinal centers lead to production of long-lived memory B lymphocytes and effector cells. The lifespan of memory B lymphocytes may also depend on continued interaction of antigen deposited on FDCs with CD21/CD35 in the spleen and in bone marrow. *IgG,* Immunoglobulin G.

lymphocytes into recipient mice lacking FDC-derived CD21/CD35 demonstrated that complement receptors on recipient mice stroma were required for each of these elements of memory.[115] Importantly, chimeric mice lacking CD21/CD35-bearing FDCs had severely impaired recall responses several months after transfer of memory B lymphocytes compared with wild-type recipients.[115] More recent studies identified a mechanism explaining long term retention of complement-opsonized immune complexes. Heesters et al (2013) found that FDC internalize C3d-opsonized complexes via the CD21 receptor into a non-degradative cycling endosomal compartment that periodically exposes intact immune complexes on the cell surface for recognition by cognate B cells.[115a,115b] These studies suggest that CD21/CD35 on FDCs have an important role in long-term storage of antigen, thereby facilitating B-lymphocyte memory.

Complement and T-Cell Immunity

The complement system is important not only in humoral immunity; it also enhances responses by both CD4 and CD8 T cells.[135] Studies with influenza in C3-deficient mice first identified an important role for C3 in both the CD8 and CD4 response to infectious virus.[136] Although the mechanism is not clear, given the importance of DC in uptake and presentation of antigen, one likely role is C3 opsonization of virus. Moreover, the anaphylatoxins C3a and C5a released during complement activation stimulate cytokine releases by mast cells via their respective complement receptors. Studies of mice deficient in C3a receptor identified reduced responsiveness of a subset on CD4 T cells.[137] Likewise, C5a receptor appears to play an important role in the lung in T cell–dependent allergic responses.

T-cell responses are also "tuned down" via complement receptor. Interestingly, cross-linking of the CD46 complement receptor via C3b on activated CD4 T cells induces differentiation to a T-regulatory phenotype.[138] Further investigation on this topic will reveal additional

examples whereby the complement system participates in activation and regulation of T cells.

Conclusion

Over the past 20 years, a new appreciation for the complement system has come to light. Not only is the complement system required for host protection and innate immunity, but it also plays a critical role in "directing" the humoral response to thymus-dependent and thymus-independent antigens. Covalent attachment of split products of C3 (i.e., C3d) alters the fate of antigen and targets it to FDC within the lymphoid compartment. Other studies are uncovering additional roles for complement in the regulation of self-reactive B cells. The next decade will likely witness a similar revolution on our understanding of how complement participates in protection against autoimmune diseases such as SLE.

IMMUNOGLOBULINS

Properties and Structure

The mammalian immune system responds to the almost unlimited array of antigens by producing antibodies that react specifically with the molecules that induced their production. During the immune response, the structure of the inducing antigen is imprinted on the immune system, and subsequent challenges with the same or structurally related molecule(s) causes a more rapid rise in antibody levels to much greater concentrations than were achieved after the primary antigenic challenge. Thus the hallmarks of the humoral immune system include induction, specific protein interaction, and memory.

Antibodies belong to the family of proteins called the *immunoglobulins*. The basic structure of all immunoglobulins consists of a monomer that contains four polypeptide chains: two identical heavy (H) chains and two identical light (L) chains covalently linked by disulfide bonds (Fig. 24.7).[139] The x-ray crystallographic structure of a monomeric immunoglobulin, specifically a mouse IgG2a monoclonal antibody (mAb), is shown depicted in both ribbon and space-filling models in Fig. 24.8.[140] Depending on the angle between the constituent Fab (fragment antigen-binding) monomers, an immunoglobulin monomer consists of a Y- or T-like structure. The size of the Fab arms is 80 × 50 × 40 Å, and the size of base, called the Fc (fragment crystallizable) region, is approximately 70 × 45 × 40 Å according to the x-ray structure models. The Ig molecule exhibits considerable flexibility. In electron microscopic, low-angle x-ray scattering, transient electric birefringence, and resonance energy transfer studies, the angle between the Fab domains has been observed to vary from 0 to 180 degrees. All antibodies have two identical combining sites for each antigen located at the ends of the Fab domains.

Fab and Fc represent functional domains in immunoglobulins. They were discovered by performing limited proteolytic digestion of the molecule. Both the H and L chains contribute amino acids that constitute the antigen-binding site in Fab. The monovalent Fab fragment will bind to, but will not precipitate, multivalent antigens, in contrast to native IgG. A fragment can be prepared, called F(ab')₂, that is devoid of Fc but still precipitates antigen. This form of immunoglobulin consists of two Fabs disulfide bonded at a part of the molecule called the *hinge region*. The hinge region is the part of the Ig molecule that is responsible for the molecular flexibility exhibited by all immunoglobulins. The other major function of immunoglobulins, binding to specific receptors on cells and certain effector proteins such as C1q, is associated with binding site(s) also found in Fc. The Fc region of IgG, one of the classes of

immunoglobulin, also interacts with protein A, an immune evasion molecule on the cell walls of *S. aureus*. When bound to protein A, the binding of IgG to host effector molecules such as C1q is sterically interfered with.

The chain structure of immunoglobulins explains neither antibody structural diversity nor antibody binding to antigen. The discovery of variable and constant regions of amino acid sequence formed the basis for understanding both phenomena. Thus in the L chain, the 100 or so amino acids in the amino-terminal half of the protein (variable region [V_L]) vary among antibody molecules, but in the second half (constant region [C_L]), there is virtual complete

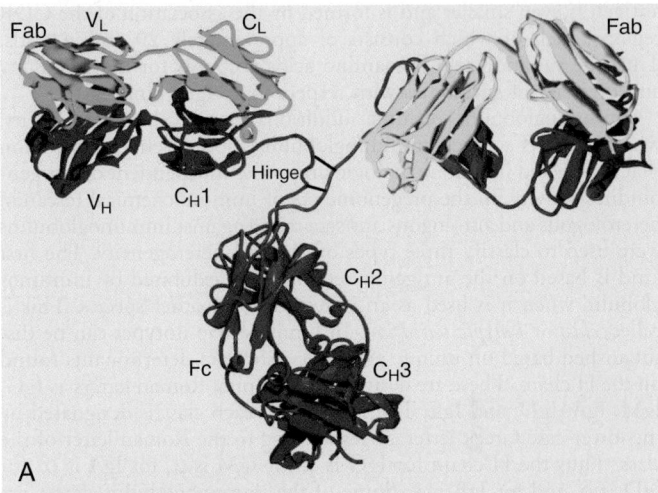

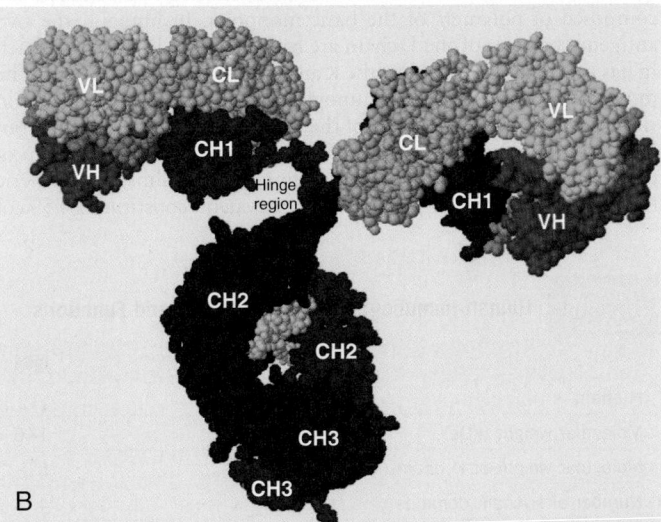

Fig. 24.8 X-RAY CRYSTALLOGRAPHIC STRUCTURE OF AN INTACT IgG MOLECULE shown as a ribbon diagram (A), or a space-filling model (B). The structure is that of a mouse immunoglobulin G2a (IgG2a) monoclonal antibody (protein data base [PDB] file 1IGT) and it was the first intact IgG to have its structure determined. (A) The two-layer β-sandwich characteristic of the "immunoglobulin fold" is clearly visible within each of the constituent domains of the γ-heavy chains *(blue and red)* and κ-light chains *(green and yellow)*, respectively. *Black lines* indicate the positions of inter-heavy chain disulfide bonds in the hinge region. (B) The constant domains of the heavy chains and light chains are in various shades of *blue,* and the glycan chain lining a region between apposing C_H2 domains is in *white.* The variable regions are colored according to the genetic segment encoding them. *Dark green* denotes the polypeptide region encoded by the V segment of V_H and *orange* the DJ segment of V_H. *Light green* denotes the polypeptide encoded by the V segment of V_L and *yellow* that encoded by the J segment of V_L. *(A, Modified from http://proteopedia.org/wiki/index.php/Image:Opening_1igt.png; **B** from http://www.imgt.org/IMGTeducation/Tutorials/IGandBcells/_UK/3Dstructure/Figure2.html.)*

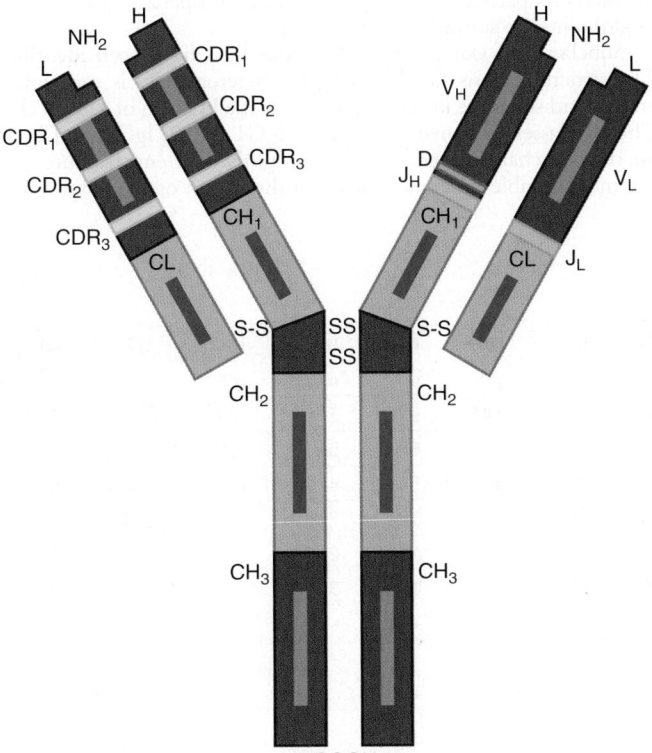

Fig. 24.7 DIAGRAMMATIC REPRESENTATION OF THE STRUCTURAL FEATURES OF AN IMMUNOGLOBULIN G (IgG) MOLECULE. NH_2 indicates the N-terminus and COOH the C-terminus. V_H, C_{H1}, V_L, and C_L homology domains are shown as *boxes*. Only the disulfide linkages that join H and L chains are shown. *Left,* Approximate boundaries of the complementarity-determining region (CDR) regions in the V_L and V_H regions. *Right,* Sequences encoded by V_H, D, J_H, V_L, and J_L segments in the V_H and V_L regions.

correspondence in amino acids, position for position, to the carboxy-terminus. The H chains exhibit a similar pattern and can be divided likewise into V_H and C_H1, C_H2, and C_H3. Comparison of the amino acid sequence of many V_Ls has revealed that whereas certain parts of the variable region exhibit excess variability, others are less variable. The former regions are called *hypervariable* or *complementarity-determining regions* (CDRs). The latter framework regions function as a structural scaffold to support the CDRs. Antigen binding is mediated by six CDRs, three in each of the V_H and V_L domains. The combining site for antigen is a trough, cavity, or even flat surface composed of parts of the hypervariable regions of both the H and L chains. It is a small region, representing only 25% of the antibody V region. The region that interacts directly with the epitope on the antigen is even smaller and is formed by the association of the CDR regions, each of which consists of approximately 20 amino acids. Thus the variation in a few amino acids accounts for the specificity and diversity of antibodies with respect to antigen binding.[141]

Immunoglobulins exhibit additional physical heterogeneity, which imparts to each immunoglobulin a special effector function that is reflected in unique biologic properties independent of antigen-binding activity. In the pregenome era of immunochemical research, heterologous and autologous antisera raised against immunoglobulins were used to classify three types of physical heterogeneity. The first kind is based on the antigenic heterogeneity exhibited by immunoglobulin when it is used as an immunogen in other species. This is called *class* or *isotypic variation*. In humans, five isotypes can be distinguished based on unique antigenic (isotypic) determinants found on the H chain. These are designated by capital Roman letters as IgG, IgM, IgA, IgD, and IgE. The H chain of each class is designated by the lower-case Greek letter corresponding to the Roman letter of the class. Thus the H chain for IgG is γ, for IgM is μ, for IgA is α, for IgD is δ, and for IgE is ε. Some of the immunoglobulin classes are composed of polymers of the basic monomer. In humans, the two antigenic varieties of the L chain are kappa (κ) and lambda (λ). Each Ig has two identical L chains; the κ and λ are shared by all classes. The monomeric form of any immunoglobulin is described by its chain structure. The molecular mass of the immunoglobulins can vary from 150 to 1000 kDa. This variation is attributable to polymerization of the basic monomer form. None of the immunoglobulins are polymeric forms of another class. IgG is the most prevalent, constituting 75% of

the total Ig in blood. It is present in normal adults at concentrations of 600 to 1500 mg/dL. IgG is designated $\gamma 2\kappa 2$ or $\gamma 2\lambda 2$. It is the only class of Ig that crosses the placenta (Table 24.2).[142]

The isotype IgM is predominantly a pentamer consisting of five monomeric units disulfide linked at the C-terminus of the H chain. Each monomer of IgM is 180 kDa because of the presence of an additional C_H domain, specifically the $C\mu 2$ domain, which replaces the hinge segment. The complete protein has a sedimentation coefficient of 19 S, which corresponds to a molecular mass of 850 kDa. IgM is designated $(\mu 2\kappa 2)_5$ or $(\mu 2\lambda 2)_5$. IgM also contains a 15-kDa protein called the *J chain*. In the current structural model of IgM, the J chain forms a disulfide-bonded clasp at the C-terminus of two H chains (Fig. 24.9).[139]

The structure of the other isotypes of immunoglobulins are summarized as follows. The isotype IgA has a variable number of monomeric units and is designated $(\alpha 2\kappa 2)_n$ or $(\alpha 2\lambda 2)_n$, where n = 1–5. Serum IgA constitutes 20% of the total serum immunoglobulin, and 80% of this is monomeric. The remainder exists as polymers, where n = 2–5. The other form of IgA is found in external secretions such as saliva, tracheobronchial secretions, colostrum, milk, and genitourinary secretions. Secretory IgA consists of four components: a dimer of two monomeric molecules, a 70-kDa secretory component that binds noncovalently to the IgA dimer, and the 15-kDa J chain that is believed to form a disulfide-bonded clasp at the C-terminus of the H chains (see Fig. 24.9). The isotype IgD has a molecular mass of 180 kDa. Its serum concentration is very low, approximately 3 mg/dL. IgD apparently functions as a membrane molecule, being associated on mature but unstimulated B cells in association with IgM. IgE is the homocytotropic or reaginic Ig and mediates immediate hypersensitivity. It has a molecular mass of 180 kDa and, similar to IgM, has four C domains. The Fc portion of IgE binds strongly to a receptor on mast cells, FcεR, and this is how this immunoglobulin exerts its particular activity. The overall properties of the immunoglobulins are summarized in Table 24.2.

Subclasses of isotypes IgG, IgA, and IgM have been identified. The structural basis for this antigenic heterogeneity is variation in amino acid sequence in the Fc portion of the H chain of a given class. The subclasses of human IgG, called IgG1, IgG2, IgG3, and IgG4, are the best characterized. Each has a slightly different structure, with the most notable differences being in the length of the hinge and in

TABLE 24.2   **Human Immunoglobulins: Properties and Functions**

	IgG1	IgG2	IgG3	IgG4	IgM	IgA1	IgA2	IgD	IgE
H chain	$\gamma 1$	$\gamma 2$	$\gamma 3$	$\gamma 4$	μ	$\alpha 1$	$\alpha 2$	δ	ε
Molecular weight (kDa)	146	146	170	146	970	160	160	194	199
Molecular weight of H chain (kDa)	51	51	60	51	65	56	52	70	73
Number of H-chain domains	4	4	4	4	5	4	4	4	5
Carbohydrate (%)	2–3	2–3	2–3	2–3	12	7–11	7–11	9–14	12
Hinge inter-heavy chain disulfides	2	5	11	2	NA	2	1	1	NA
Serum concentration (mg/dL)	900	300	100	50	150	300	50	3	0.005
Classical pathway complement fixation	++	+	+++	−	+++	−	−		
Alternative pathway complement activity			−			+	+		−
Placental transfer	+	+	+	+	+				−
Binding to mononuclear cells	+	−	+					−	−
Binding to mast cells and to basophils	−	−	−	−	−			−	+++
Reaction with protein A from *Staphylococcus aureus*	+	+	−	+				−	−
Half-life (days)	21	20	7	21	10	6	6	3	2
Distribution (% intravascular)	45	45	45	45	80	42	42	75	50
Fractional catabolic rate (% Intravascular pool catabolized/day)	7	7	17	7	9	25	25	37	71
Synthetic rate (mg/kg/day)	33	33	33	33	33	24	24	0.4	0.002

Data from Golub ES: *Immunology: A synthesis*. Sunderland, MA, 1987, Sinaur.

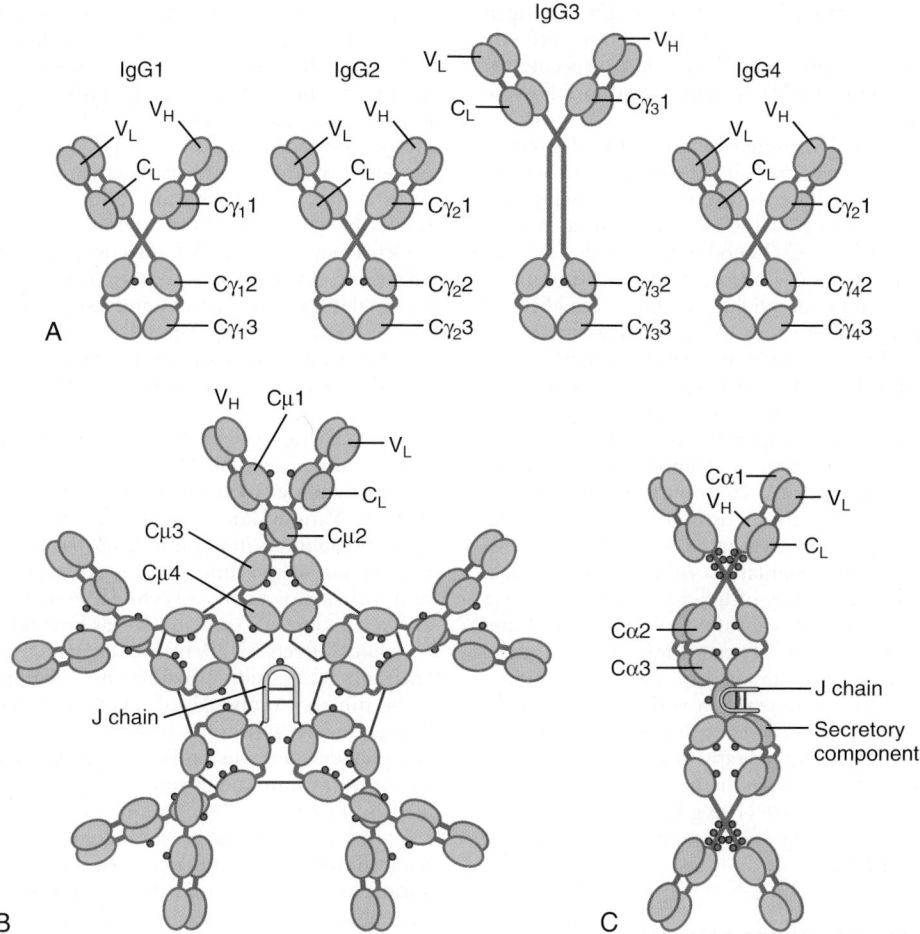

Fig. 24.9 (A) Structure of the four subclasses of human immunoglobulin G (IgG). Constant region domains are indicated by C_nN, where n is the subclass and N is the domain. (B) Structure of human IgM. The J chain is shown in the model as disulfide linked to two μ-chains. Other models have been proposed. *Filled circles* indicate carbohydrate. (C) Structure of human secretory IgA. This model shows the possible arrangement of the two IgA monomers in relation to the secretory component and J chain. As the IgA molecule passes through the epithelial cells, the secretory components are synthesized and attached covalently to the Fc domain of the α-chains that have previously been joined to the J chain with disulfide links. Light chains are shown in *blue*, heavy chains in *purple*, disulfide bonds as *gray lines*, and carbohydrates as *red circles*. (*From Turner M:* Molecules which recognize antigens. *In Roitt DK, editor:* Immunology, *London, 1989, Gower, p 51.*)

the number of interchain disulfide bonds (see Fig. 24.9 and Table 24.2). IgG1 constitutes 70% of the total IgG and IgG2 20%. IgG3 and IgG4 constitute 8% and 2%, respectively, of the total IgG. The subclasses of IgG exhibit different catabolic rates and bind differentially to cell-associated Fc receptors (FcγR) and to C1q. Specifically, IgG2 does not bind to the FcγRs and IgG4 binds about 10-fold less well than do IgG1 and IgG3. For C1q binding, the rank order of affinities is IgG3 > IgG1 > IgG2 ≫ IgG4. Despite the most obvious sequence differences among the human IgG isotypes being in their hinge regions, studies using engineered domain-swapped chimeric molecules have demonstrated that it is the more subtle amino acid sequence differences within the respective Cγ2 domains that account for the differences in binding to C1q and to the FcγRs. Transport across the placenta is mediated by the Fc-neonatal receptor (FcRn) and for this functional activity IgG2 crosses the placenta slightly more slowly than the other three subclasses. The other known subclasses of Ig isotypes are associated with IgM (IgM1 and IgM2) and IgA (IgA1 and IgA2). The properties and function of these subclasses are less well known.

The second type of variation is called *allotypic variation*. It is attributable to genetically controlled antigenic determinants found on both the H and L chains. Although each human has all immunoglobulin isotypes, an individual has only one form of each allotype on his or her immunoglobulin molecules. Allotypes are codominantly expressed, but an individual B lymphocyte secretes only one of the parental forms. This phenomenon is called *allelic exclusion*.

The third type of variation is attributable to antigenic determinants that are unique to each particular antibody molecule produced by an individual. These markers are called *idiotypic determinants,* and they are associated with a single species of antibody. The antiidiotypic antibodies that recognize a particular idiotype will not react with any other immunoglobulins in the donor other than the purified antibody that was used to raise the antiidiotype antibody. In most cases, the immune response to an antigen results in a mixture of several antibodies, each of which has identical binding specificity but distinct idiotypic determinants. Thus there can be many idiotypes for a given antigenic specificity, which has been interpreted as being a reflection of physical heterogeneity in or near the antibody combining site, for example, in the variable region domains. In some species (notably certain strains of mice), the response to antigen results in a predominant idiotype on all antibodies of a given specificity. Because this quality is inherited, the idiotypes are called major, cross-reactive, or public. Some public idiotypes have been found in certain species (again, most notably mice) to be genetically linked to allotypes. Three kinds of antiidiotype antibodies have been described, those that function as an internal image of the original antigen by mimicking the antigen structure, those that recognize antibody combining site-associated idiotypes, and those that are specific for framework-associated determinants. The internal image antiidiotypic antibodies are of clinical interest.

Every immunoglobulin is a glycoprotein, and the critical glycan is attached to the H chain in the Fc domain at the conserved asparagine at position 297 (Asn297). This single, N-linked glycan is essential for maintaining an open conformation of the two H chains as it lines the opposing faces of the pair of C_H2 subdomains of Fc (see Fig. 24.8B). The core structure of the N-linked glycan is a biantennary heptapolysaccharide containing N-acetylglucosamine plus additional sugars (fucose, galactose), with bisecting N-acetylglucosamine and sialic acid variably present. Effector functions depend on the Asn297-linked glycan and are influenced by its structure.[143] Deglycosylated IgG does not interact effectively with Fcγ receptors (FcγRs) and cannot support in vivo effector responses, including antibody-dependent cell-mediated cytotoxicity or complement-dependent cytotoxicity.[144] Individual glycoforms contribute to modulating inflammatory responses and have disease association. For example, glycosylation differs in patients with rheumatoid arthritis[145] or vasculitis[146] compared with the normal population. Addition of sialic acid to the N-linked glycan reduces binding of IgG to FcγRs and reduces in vivo cytotoxicity. Regulation of sialylation of IgG contributes to the antiinflammatory homeostasis of serum IgG. Upon antigen challenge, reduced sialic acid–IgG can mediate immune clearance and protective immunity through interaction with subclass-specific FcγRs. Kaneko et al[147] have proposed that the protective effect of intravenous immunoglobulin (IVIg) therapy is attributable to the minor fraction of sialylated IgG species in the total IVIg preparation and that the high doses required (1–3 g/kg body weight) for antiinflammatory activity could be significantly reduced by increasing the percentage of sialylated IgG.

THERAPEUTIC USE OF IMMUNOGLOBULIN

IVIg

IgG was one of the first plasma proteins prepared in a purified state as a therapeutic drug for treatment of clinical disorders. It remains, along with albumin and α-proteinase inhibitor, the most widely used therapeutic plasma derivative and is currently the major plasma product on the global market. Polyvalent human immunoglobulin preparations have been used to reconstitute humoral immunity in agammaglobulinemic patients for more than three decades. Until 30 years ago, intramuscular treatment was the mode of administration. Intramuscular preparations caused severe adverse reactions when injected intravenously.[148–150] The most serious were anaphylactoid reactions and were probably complement mediated. Efforts to reduce anticomplementary activity and the prekallikrein activator activity were initiated in the early 1980s and safer IVIg preparations became available.

Intravenous immunoglobulin is prepared from pooled human plasma pools of 3000 to 50,000 L. The World Health Organization requires more than 1000 donors per lot. The majority of IVIg is produced by cold ethanol fractionation procedures,[151,152] with filtration and polishing chromatography steps added to increase yield and decrease pathogen transmission.[153,154] Gamunex (Talecris Biotherapeutics) is produced from cold ethanol fractionation followed by caprylate precipitation and chromatograpy.[153,155] This is the first significant change in commercial IVIg production in 20 years. IVIg contains concentrated IgG with normal plasma ratios of IgG1 and IgG2, lower percentages of IgG3 and IgG4, and only trace amounts of IgA and IgM. It retains the antibody repertoire, reflecting the combined immunologic experience of the donors.[156,157] Hyperimmune IVIg is purified from donor plasma selected for high titer toward a specific pathogen. Prophylaxis for cytomegalovirus and respiratory syncytial virus are two approved clinical applications.[157,158]

The availability of safe IVIg preparations and the fortuitous observation that IgG treatment of a patient with thrombocytopenia and IgG deficiency increased the patient's platelet count began an intense period of clinical use of IVIg for indications other than primary immune deficiency. In 1990, the National Institutes of Health sponsored a Consensus Development Conference, which produced the first consensus statement on IVIg clinical indications.[159] As a result, six disease indications—primary immunodeficiency, Kawasaki syndrome, chronic lymphocytic leukemia, human immunodeficiency virus (HIV) infections during childhood to prevent infections, BM transplantation to prevent graft-versus-host disease or bacterial infections in adults, and idiopathic purpura—were approved by the Food and Drug Administration (FDA) for labeling and marketing. The licensed indications remain unchanged, but off-label uses include more than 100 conditions (for further discussion, see Chapter 116).[160,161]

The experience with IVIg clinical development has been largely empiric and anecdotal. The mechanisms for patient benefit or harm are poorly understood, especially for high-dose immune modulation therapy. Various known and some yet undiscovered functions of immunoglobulins in immune homeostasis may contribute, including modulation of the function and expression of Fc receptors, interaction with complement and cytokine systems, antiidiotypic antibodies, and regulation of T-cell and B-cell function.[162–164]

Many effects of IVIg are explained by mechanisms beyond antigenic recognition of pathogens. IVIg preparations contain up to 30% dimers composed of idiotype–antiidiotype antibody pairs. These dimers appear to be very effective as a sink for activated complement and can inhibit complement activation.[165] Benefit for treatment of immune thrombocytopenia purpura seems to be mediated by Fc-receptor blockade of the reticuloendothelial cell salvage receptor, also known as FcRn, combined with an antiidiotypic neutralization of antiplatelet antibody that together eliminates antiplatelet antibody from the blood. Other indications of antibody neutralization can be seen in IVIg treatment of myasthenia gravis. The dramatic success of IVIg in treating Kawasaki syndrome may be attributable to several mechanisms, including antiidiotypic neutralization of antiendothelial antibodies, inhibition of cytokine production and function, and elimination of causative superantigens.[166,167] IVIg inhibits B-cell activation and autoantibody production by enhancing CD8+ suppressor T-cell function. Cell-mediated immunity is also affected.[162] As mentioned earlier, Kaneko et al[147] ascribe much of the effect of IVIg to a small fraction of it that is sialylated. A 2011 report from this group suggests a mechanism for the way that sialylated IgG in IVIg downmodulates the inflammatory response of the immune system.[168] They suggest that the sialylated IgG Fc region binds to DC-SIGN, a molecule on the surface of "regulatory" myeloid cells, including DCs. In response to DC-SIGN ligation by sialylated IgG, these cells secrete the cytokine IL-33, which in turn stimulates IL-4 production by basophils. IL-4 upregulates the synthesis of the "inhibitory" class of FcγR on effector macrophages, namely FcγRIIB. Because ligation of this class of FcγR by immune complexes actually results in the recruitment of regulatory phosphatases, which shut down intracellular signaling cascades, the net effect is to increase the activation threshold required to initiate inflammation by these effector cells.

Adverse Events Related to Intravenous Immunoglobulin Infusion

Adverse events associated with IVIg can be characterized as (1) early systemic events, (2) infectious disease transfer, and (3) high-dose treatment-related adverse effects.[149]

Early Systemic Events

Common transfusion-related early events are listed in Table 24.3. Most early events are self-limiting and infusion rate dependent.

TABLE 24.3	Early Systemic Adverse Events Associated With Intravenous Immunoglobulin Infusion	
Fever	Rash or urticaria
Chills	Chest tightness
Sore throat	Dyspnea
Face flush	Wheezing
Tachycardia	Low or high blood pressure
Palpitations	Shock
Lumbar pain	Anxiety
Abdominal pain	Nervousness
Nausea	Headache
Vomiting	Migraine
Shaking	Anaphylaxis
Fatigue	Malaise
Myalgia	Leukopenia

Premedication with steroids, aspirin, or other nonsteroidal antiinflammatory drugs often decreases symptoms. Prophylaxis with propranolol can be effective for induced migraine. Aseptic meningitis is a rare early event, is observed 1 to 2 days postinfusion, is unrelated to infusion rate, and can be treated with intravenous steroids and analgesics.[149,169]

The frequency of reported adverse events varies considerably, ranging from 10% to 85%.[149,159,170–172] There are many reasons for this high variability in reporting, including (1) differences in product,[154,170,173] (2) infusion rate, (3) dose and frequency of dosing, (4) patient population, and (5) relative experience of patient and physician. Both patients and physicians become steeled to the adverse events, and because incidents are not life threatening and often respond to prophylaxis medication, they are ignored as "normal." Nonetheless, these events are common and affect health and quality of life of patients.[160,170]

Infectious Disease Transfer

A few early preparations of IVIg transmitted hepatitis C virus. Manufacturers have added viral inactivation and partitioning steps, and current licensed products are safe with respect to HIV, hepatitis C virus, hepatitis B virus, and other blood-borne pathogens (see Chapter 116).[174] The industry has responded to the threat of prions with process validation,[171,175] donor screening, donor testing, inventory management (look back), and plasma pool testing.

High-Dose Treatment–Related Adverse Events

Intravenous immunoglobulin treatment for immune modulation of neurologic diseases requires doses of 1 to 2 kg/kg body weight or two to five times the dose recommended for replacement therapy. Adverse events with high-dose administration include those listed in Table 24.3 and occasionally thromboembolic events, renal complications, and anemia.[149,172,176–179] Thromboembolic events include deep venous thrombosis, pulmonary embolism, myocardial infarction, and stroke. Thromboembolic events and renal failure seem to be independent of infusion rate. The cause of thromboembolic events is not known. Dalakas[180] has suggested that increased serum viscosity plays a role. Factor XIa has also been identified in IVIg preparations.[173] Factor XIa could directly lead to shortening of coagulation time and risk of thrombosis. Renal complications are rare but result in high morbidity and mortality. Whether IgG, contaminants, or excipients are responsible is not clear. Of the 88 renal adverse events reported to the FDA, 90% were stabilized with sucrose.[149,169] Whether the adverse events observed with IVIg treatment of neurologic diseases are related to a preexisting medical condition or the high doses required for treatment is not clear.

Passive Immunization and Monoclonal Antibody Therapy

Passive immunization in the broadest sense represents the transfer of antibodies to a human recipient who is unable to produce the antibody due to the acuity of an infection, immunodeficiency, or immune tolerance to the target antigen. The use of plasma from patients who have recovered from Ebola virus to treat those acutely ill with the infection[181] is an example of the simplest form of antibody transfer, where neither the antigenic epitope nor the sequence of the antibodies are known, and there is no purification step. Indeed, the pathogen need not be identified; it is only necessary that antibodies can clear the infection.

With the use of intravenous immunoglobulin (described earlier) to normalize IgG levels in patients with inherited immunodeficiencies (e.g., CVID or X-linked hypogammaglobulinemia) or chronic lymphoproliferative disorders, the goal is to provide a wide range of IgG immunoglobulins specific for antigens encountered by the general population, using a product purified from plasma donated by a large pool of healthy donors. Specialized IVIg products have also been developed that are enriched for antibodies that recognize specific pathogens by prescreening donors. Examples include VariZIG (for varicella), Cytogam (CMV), HBIG (hepatitis B) as well as products for rabies, botulinum toxin, and tetanus.

Immunized animals once served as the major source of therapeutic immunoglobulins; indeed, the modern medical era can be traced to the late 1800s, when serum from horses immunized with diphtheria toxin was first used therapeutically. The antigen used to immunize the animal need not be infectious: antivenom products can be used to treat bites from coral snakes, pit vipers, black widow spiders, and scorpions. Some of these products are treated with proteolytic enzymes to produce Fab fragments, such as crotalidae polyvalent immune FAB (Crofab). Digibind is another such Fab product, derived from sheep immunized with digoxin bound to human albumin, as used to treat digoxin overdoses.

When the intended antigen is of human origin, there is the challenge that human plasma donors are likely to be tolerant to the antigen. A notable exception is the Rh-D antigen, which, being genetically polymorphic, is immunogenic to Rh-negative individuals, and human-derived anti-Rh preparations can be used to prevent sensitization during pregnancy and also as a treatment for immune thrombocytopenic purpura. However, apart from this special case, targeting human antigens generally requires a sensitized animal, a prominent example being antithymocte globulin (ATG), which induces lymphopenia as a treatment for aplastic anemia or as part of an immunosuppressive regimen in organ transplantation.

Polyclonal antibodies can be advantageous in some cases (especially for ATG and antivenin) but the epitopes recognized and the biologic activity may be variable between different lots of the product. In retrospect, then, it is not surprising how Kohler and Milstein's technique for the generation of monoclonal antibodies[182] quickly revolutionized medical diagnostics and almost all of biomedical research. Monoclonal antibodies as therapies came more slowly, and there were initial concerns about the generation of "HAMA" (human antimouse antibodies). However, now there are modifications to partially or fully replace mouse sequences with human sequences (Fig. 24.10A). Furthermore, fully human antibodies can be generated using mice that are lacking mouse immunoglobulin genes and are transgenic for the human sequences.[183] Using mice with a germline knockout for the gene encoding the antigen of interest can enable the generation of antibodies that have been previously difficult to obtain.[183,184] Four fully human monoclonal antibody products (ranibizumab, adalimumab, belimumab, and ramacirumab) now on the market were developed by an alternative method, phage display (Fig. 24.10B).[185–189]

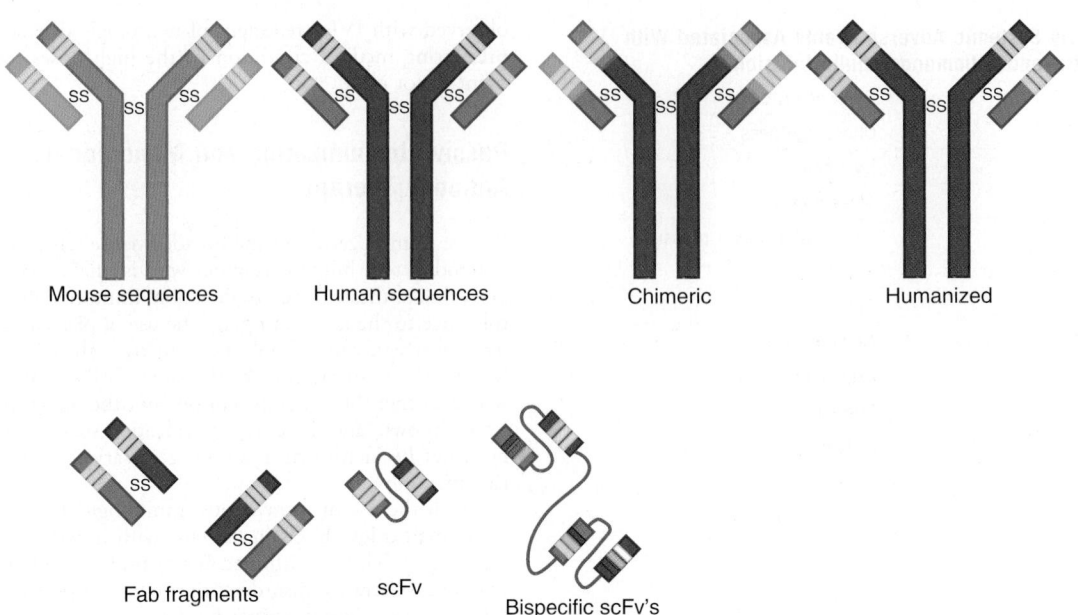

Mouse sequences   Human sequences   Chimeric   Humanized

Fab fragments   scFv   Bispecific scFv's

A

Fig. 24.10 GENERATION, STRUCTURE, AND MODIFICATION OF MONOCLONAL ANTIBOD-IES. To generate monoclonal antibodies, based on the technique of Kohler and Milstein,[182,190] first, a mouse is immunized repeatedly with the antigen, using an adjuvant. After verification of an antibody response, the spleen is removed. Polyethylene glycol is then used to fuse isolated splenic lymphocytes with a mouse nonsecretory myeloma cell line carrying a mutation in the X-linked *Hgprt* gene, which is essential for the purine salvage pathway. The mutation ensures that the myeloma cell line will not grow in HAT (hypoxanthine, aminopterin, thymidine) media. Normal cells can survive despite the presence of aminopterin, which disrupts the de novo purine synthesis pathway, because they have an intact purine salvage pathway and can use hypoxanthine. (Because aminopterin interferes with folate metabolism, which also affects pyrimidine synthesis, provision of thymidine is required.) Fusions (hybridomas) between the lymphocytes and the myeloma cell line can grow in HAT only if they have incorporated an X chromosome with the normal *Hgprt* gene from the mouse lymphocyte, restoring the purine salvage pathway. Unfused lymphocytes, on the other hand, have no stimulus to grow. Hybridomas growing in HAT are then cloned by limiting dilution (e.g., in 96-well plates); some of these hybridomas will have retained the chromosomes containing the rearranged immunoglobulin light and heavy chain of the original lymphocyte. Because these genes are now present in a plasma cell with the cellular apparatus for immunoglobulin secretion, immunoglobulin expressed by the original mouse lymphocyte will now be secreted into the media. The supernatant of each hybridoma clone must be screened for the presence of the desired antibody. (A) Modifications of immunoglobulins derived from monoclonal antibody technology. Chimeric mAbs contain the mouse variable region and retain the human constant regions. Humanized antibodies retain only the mouse sequences from the CDRs, which recognize antigens. Fabs are also shown, which lack the constant region of the heavy chain. scFVs (single chain variable fragments) contain only the N-terminal sequences of the heavy and the light chain required for antigen recognition. Because they no longer have any disulfide bond to connect the heavy and the light chain, a linker peptide must be introduced. In the example shown, the carboxy terminus of the light chain is linked to the amino terminus of the heavy chain. The structure of a bispecific scFv is also shown, which can engage two separate ligands simultaneously, bringing together two separate cell types (e.g., immune effector cells with malignant target cells).

Monoclonal antibodies can affect target cells by activation-induced cell death, blockage of ligand-receptor interactions, activation of complement, antibody-dependent cell-mediated cytotoxicity, and uptake of antibody-coated cells in the reticuloendothelial system. To increase cytotoxicity, immunoglobulins can be conjugated to toxins (e.g., brentuximab vedotin, targeting CD30; trastuzumab emtansine, targeting human epidermal growth factor receptor 2 [HER2]; and gemtuzumab ozogamicin, targeting CD33) or radionuclides (e.g., ibritumomab tiuxetan or I131-tositumomab). Obinutuzumab (for chronic lymphocytic leukemia [CLL]) has been glycoengineered such that its Fc moiety has increased affinity for Fc receptors. A chimeric molecule consisting of bispecific single chain variable antibody sequences (scFvs) has been developed (blinatumomab), to engage cytotoxic CD3+ T cells with CD19 expressing acute lymphoblastic leukemia (ALL) cells. mAbs targeting blood cells have impacted practically every hematologic condition including lymphoma and

autoimmune diseases (rituximab), CLL (rituximab, obinutuzumab, ofatumumab), Hodgkin disease (brentuximab and pembrolizumab[191]), acute myeloid leukemia (AML) (gemtuzumab[192–194]), myeloma (daratumumab and elotuzumab), and allogeneic transplantation (alemtuzumab[195]). In addition to surface molecules, mAbs can target plasma components—in theory, any protein. Vascular endothelial growth factor (VEGF), TNF-α (and other cytokines) are prominent examples, as well as C5 (described later). Omalizumab is a special case of a humanized IgG immunoglobulin molecule that targets a whole class of immunoglobulin: IgE.[196] Targeting plasma proteins may increase their clearance from the circulation and inhibit protein–protein interactions or ligand-receptor binding.

The side effects of any monoclonal or polyclonal antibody therapy depends on the source of the antibody, the target, and the dose. The administration of human-derived IVIg, which involves a very large dose of immunoglobulin, is typically preceded by acetaminophen and

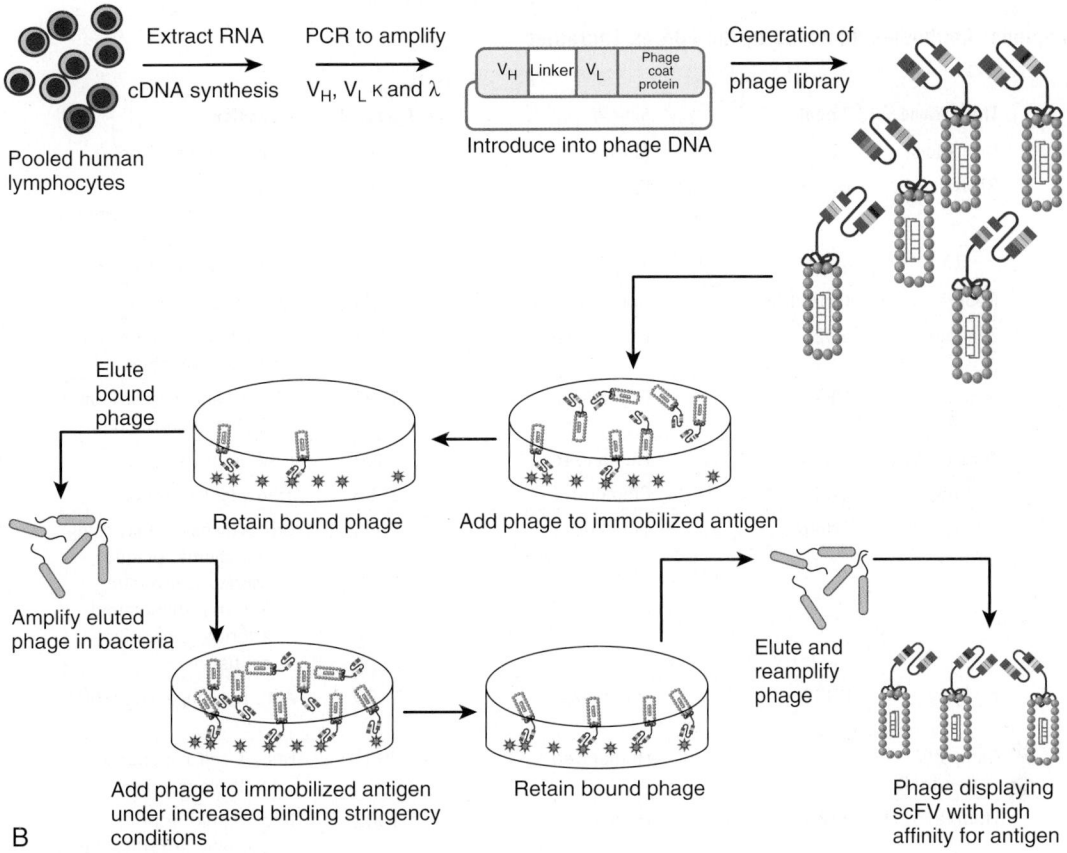

Fig. 24.10, cont'd (B) Isolation of human scFVs by phage display.[185,188,189] This is a newer technique that does not require mouse immunization. First, a library of human variable chain sequences is generated by amplification of cDNA from pooled human lymphocytes. These sequences are then cloned into the DNA of a filamentous phage, such that one of the phage coat proteins is linked to the scFv. Each phage displays a different scFv, and a critical step is to ensure the diversity of the scFvs contained in the library (typically 10^9 to 10^{10} unique clones are desirable). The phage expressing an scFv can be captured by an immobilized antigen (on a plate, or on the surface of a cell) and the retained phage can be recovered and amplified in bacteria. The phage obtained from this step can be further purified in one or more additional capture steps, and at the end, a phage expressing an scFv highly specific for antigen can be recovered, allowing the human immunoglobulin sequences that recognize the antigen to be determined.

diphenhydramine to prevent infusional reactions, as described earlier. For products derived from animal serum, anaphylactoid reactions are commonly seen, requiring premedication regimens that include high dose steroids, for example, for equine ATG administration. When the patient later makes an antibody response against horse proteins, this can result in immune complex deposition, leading to serum sickness, characterized by fever, rash, and arthritis. Purified chimeric, humanized, or human monoclonal antibodies will typically not result in these reactions. Rather, side effects are dependent, typically, on "on target" effects. A notable example of this are the febrile infusion reactions that occur with the initial use of rituximab caused by the lysis of CD20-expressing (malignant and nonmalignant) B cells and the immunosuppressive effects of drugs targeting TNF-α, C5, and integrins. However, a true "off target" side effect, could, theoretically, occur if a mAb were to cross-react with unintended epitopes on plasma proteins or extracellular surface proteins.

The overall half-life of IgG is approximately 20 days[197]; when targeting an abundant surface protein or rapidly produced plasma protein, the half-life may be shorter. Most monoclonal antibodies are administered less often than weekly; based on their affinity constants, doses required are generally high enough that they must be given by intravenous rather than subcutaneous injection, with some exceptions. As of 2016, 52 monoclonal antibodies have been approved by the FDA (Table 24.4). The naming of monoclonal antibodies follows a convention[198] such that the first syllable is coined by the company

developing the drug, the second syllable indicates the use (e.g., "ci," for "cardiovascular," "li" for "immune system," "tu" for "tumor") and the penultimate syllable indicates whether the antibody is derived from mouse sequences ("–omab"), chimeric mouse-human sequences ("–ximab"), more fully humanized molecules ("–zumab"), or fully human sequences ("–umab"). For example, ce*tu*ximab is a **chimeric** antibody used to treat *tumors*, whereas ecu*li*zumab is a **humanized** antibody that targets the *immune* system.

DRUGS TARGETING THE COMPLEMENT SYSTEM

Eculizumab

The humanized anti-C5 mAb, eculizumab (Soliris), represents an interesting link between the previous sections of this chapter. Eculizumab has already dramatically affected the management of patients with both paroxysmal nocturnal hemoglobinuria (PNH) (see Chapter 31) and atypical hemolytic uremic syndrome (see Chapter 134), with more indications likely to come.

C5 is an attractive target because it is essential for all three pathways of complement activation and it is present in a considerably lower circulating concentration than C3 (by a factor of about 10.[199]) Furthermore, congenital absence of C5 and other downstream members of the MAC results in a predisposition mainly to

TABLE 24.4   Monoclonal Antibodies Approved by the FDA as Therapies

Generic Name	Trade Name	Target	Source	Year Approved	Indication	Route of Administration
Muromonab-CD3	Orthoclone	CD3	Murine	1986	Transplant rejection	Intravenous
Rituximab	Rituxan	CD20	Chimeric	1994	Lymphoma, CLL, microscopic polyarteritis nodosa, Wegener, rheumatoid arthritis	Intravenous
Abciximab	ReoPro	GPIIb/IIIa	Chimeric Fab	1994	Angioplasty	Intravenous
Daclizumab	Zenapax	CD25	Humanized	1997	Transplant rejection (no longer available)	Intravenous
Trastuzumab	Herceptin	HER-2	Humanized	1998	Breast cancer, gastric and GE junction tumors	Intravenous
Palivizumab	Synagis	RSV	Humanized	1998	RSV prophylaxis	Intramuscular
Basiliximab	Simulect	CD25	Chimeric	1998	Transplant rejection	Intravenous
Infliximab	Remicade	TNF-α	Chimeric	1998	Crohn disease, ankylosing spondylitis, plaque psoriasis, psoriatic arthritis, rheumatoid arthritis, ulcerative colitis	Intravenous
Gemtuzumab ozogamicin	Mylotarg	CD33	Humanized	2000	AML (no longer available)	Intravenous
Alemtuzumab	Campath/ Lemtrada	CD52	Humanized	2001	CLL, T-cell lymphoma, multiple sclerosis	Intravenous or subcutaneous
Adalimumab	Humira	TNF-α	Human	2002	Rheumatoid arthritis, psoriatic arthritis, Crohn disease	Subcutaneous
Ibritumomab tiuxetan	Zevalin	CD20	Mouse radioconjugate	2002	Lymphoma	Intravenous
Omalizumab	Xolair	IgE	Humanized	2003	Severe (allergic) asthma, idiopathic urticaria	Subcutaneous
Tositumomab-I131	Bexxar	CD20	Mouse radioconjugate	2003	Lymphoma (no longer available)	Intravenous
Cetuximab	Erbitux	EGFR	Chimeric	2004	Colon cancer, head and neck cancer,	Intravenous
Natalizumab	Tysabri	α4β1	Humanized	2004	Multiple sclerosis, Crohn disease	Intravenous
Bevacizumab	Avastin	VEGF	Humanized	2004	Colon, renal, cervical, ovarian, and lung cancer	Intravenous
Ranibizumab	Lucentis	VEGF	Humanized Fab	2006	Wet AMD, diabetic macular edema, macular edema following retinal vein occlusion	Intravitreal
Panitumumab	Vectibix	EGFR	Human	2006	Colorectal cancer	Intravenous
Eculizumab	Soliris	C5	Humanized	2007	PNH, aHUS	Intravenous
Certolizumab pegol	Cimzia	TNF-α	Humanized Fab	2008	Crohn disease, psoriatic arthritis	Subcutaneous
Canakinumab	Ilaris	IL-1b	Human	2009	Cryopyrin-associated periodic syndromes, familial cold urticaria, systemic onset juvenile chronic arthritis, Muckle-Wells syndrome	Subcutaneous
Golimumab	Simponi	TNF	Human	2009	Rheumatoid and psoriatic arthritis, ankylosing spondylitis	Subcutaneous

TABLE 24.4 Monoclonal Antibodies Approved by the FDA as Therapies—cont'd

Generic Name	Trade Name	Target	Source	Year Approved	Indication	Route of Administration
Ustekinumab	Stelara	IL-12/23	Human	2009	Psoriatic arthritis, plaque psoriasis	Subcutaneous
Ofatumumab	Arzerra	CD20	Human	2009	CLL	Intravenous
Denosumab	Prolia/Xgeva	RANK-L	Human	2010	Bone metastases, osteoporosis	Subcutaneous
Tocilizumab	Actemra	IL-6 receptor	Humanized	2010	Rheumatoid arthritis, systemic juvenile idiopathic arthritis	Intravenous
Bretuximab vedotin	Adcetris	CD30	Chimeric conjugate	2011	Hodgkin, anaplastic large cell lymphoma	Intravenous
Belimumab	Benlysta	BLyS	Human	2011	Systemic lupus	Intravenous
Ipilimumab	Yervoy	CTLA-4	Human	2011	Melanoma	Intravenous
Raxibacumab	From CDC	Anthrax protective antigen	Human	2012	Inhalational anthrax	Intravenous
Pertuzumab	Perjeta	HER2	Humanized	2012	Breast cancer	Intravenous
Obinutuzumab	Gazyva	CD20	Humanized	2013	CLL	Intravenous
Ado trastuzumab emtansine	Kadcyla	HER2	Humanized, conjugated	2013	Breast cancer	Intravenous
Nivolumab	Opdivo	PD1	Human	2014	Melanoma, lung cancer	Intravenous
Blinatumomab	Blincyto	CD19; CD3	Mouse	2014	ALL	Intravenous continuous infusion
Pembrolizumab	Keytruda	PD1	Humanized	2014	Melanoma	Intravenous
Ramucirumab	Cyramza	VEGFR2	Human	2014	Gastric, GE junction, and lung cancer	Intravenous
Vedolizumab	Entyvio	α4β7 integrin	Humanized	2014	Crohn disease, ulcerative colitis	Intravenous
Siltuximab	Sylvant	IL-6	Chimeric	2014	Multicentric Castleman disease	Intravenous
Dinutuximab	Unituxin	Ganglioside GD2	Chimeric	2015	Neuroblastoma	Intravenous
Evolocumab	Repatha	PCSK9	Human	2015	Hypercholesterolemia	Subcutaneous
Idarucizumab	Praxbind	Dabigatran	Humanized Fab	2015	Reversal of anticoagulation effect of dabigatran	Intravenous
Alirocumab	Praluent	PCSK9	Human	2015	Hypercholesterolemia	Subcutaneous
Necitumumab	Portrazza	EGFR	Human	2015	Squamous non-small cell lung cancer	Intravenous
Mepolizumab	Nucala	IL-5	Humanized	2015	Asthma	Subcutaneous
Daratumumab	Darzalex	CD38	Human	2015	Myeloma	Intravenous
Secukinumab	Consentyx	IL-17a	Human	2015	Plaque psoriasis, psoriatic arthritis, ankylosing spondylitis	Subcutaneous
Elotuzumab	Empliciti	SLAMF7	Humanized	2015	Myeloma	Intravenous
Ixekizumab	Taltz	IL-17	Humanized	2016	Psoriasis	Subcutaneous
Reslizumab	Cinqair	IL-5	Humanized	2016	Asthma with eosinophilic phenotype	Intravenous
Obiltoxaximab	Anthim	Anthrax protective antigen	Humanized	2016	Inhalational anthrax	Intravenous

aHUS, Atypical hemolytic uremic syndrome; AMD, age-related macular degeneration; AML, acute myeloid leukemia; ALL, acute lymphoblastic leukemia; CLL, chronic lymphocytic leukemia; EGFR, epidermal growth factor receptor; GE, gastroesophageal; IL, interleukin; PNH, paroxysmal nocturnal hemoglobinuria; RSV, respiratory syncytial virus; TNF, tumor necrosis factor.

N. meningitidis infections[200,201] but not to other infections. In contrast, inherited mutations in C3 result in a broader spectrum of infections as well as autoimmunity. Eculizumab is derived from the sequence of an immunoglobulin from a mouse hybridoma, generated by immunizing mice with purified human C5, followed by screening of thousands of clones. The antibody secreted by the selected clone, m5G1.1mAb, could inhibit complement activation at a 0.5:1 ratio (as expected given the bivalency of IgG) in a standard hemolytic assay.[202-204] The CDRs were cloned and grafted onto the respective human light and heavy chain sequences. An IgG2/IgG4 hybrid was chosen for the constant regions, because IgG2 binds Fc receptors minimally, and IgG4 activates complement minimally, given that these were two functions not desired for this particular drug.[205] The humanized antibody retains the affinity of the mouse antibody, with a dissociation constant (K_d) of 120 pM. It has a half-life in humans of approximately 11 days, and it has been suggested that a minimum trough level of 35 μg/mL is required for sustained inhibition of terminal complement in humans.[206] Although there is currently only one laboratory that offers serum drug level testing, testing for CH50, which is inhibited by eculizumab, is widely available and predicts clinical responses.[207]

Early development of eculizumab focused on testing the drug (and in some cases a related single chain variant) in patients with rheumatoid arthritis, lupus, coronary bypass, myocardial infarction, and membranous nephritis.[208-211] The strategy of therapeutically inhibiting terminal complement in PNH was validated by a pilot study, a randomized study, and an open label study of eculizumab, where dramatic reductions in the serum hemolytic activity, lactate dehydrogenase, visible hemoglobinuria, and transfusion requirements—as well as improvements in male erectile dysfunction and esophageal spasms—were shown after a series of loading doses of 600 mg weekly for 4 weeks followed then by 900 mg, repeated every 2 weeks.[212-214] While these studies were dramatic enough for drug approval in 2007, the question could have arisen as to whether correction of anemia and amelioration of transfusion requirements was an outcome important enough to justify the risk of meningococcal infection, a potentially fatal outcome, whose incidence was not known at the time. However, that same year, it was reported that the use of eculizumab dramatically decreased the rate of thromboses,[215] which are often recurrent,[216] and which represent the most important predictor of mortality. Survival curves in treated patients are now similar to age-matched controls.[217] Whereas pregnancies had been fraught with thrombotic complications, there is now evidence that not only is eculizumab safe for the fetus, but it also may be instrumental in reducing maternal mortality.[218] The effect of eculizumab on thrombosis points to a role for complement (e.g., activation of CD59-deficient platelets derived from the PNH clone) among the proposed mechanisms to explain hypercoagulability in PNH.

Neisseria infections, as seen in patients with inherited deficiencies of terminal complement, have indeed been seen in patients treated with eculizumab, sometimes despite immunization[219]; the risk may be ~1% per year. All patients on eculizumab can now be vaccinated with a new quadrivalent meningococcal B vaccine (Trumenba or Bexsero) in addition to one of the quadrivalent a,c,w,y vaccines (e.g., Menactra, Menomune, Menveo). All patients must be instructed to report to an emergency room for blood cultures and immediate empiric treatment with antibiotics (e.g., ceftriaxone) in the event of any fever over 100.0°F or 37.7°C. Patients should also carry with them a letter from their physician explaining their condition (or wear an alert bracelet) and should carry on their persons at all times an antibiotic that covers meningococcal infection, such as azithromycin or ciprofloxacin. Interestingly, meningococcal infections in hypocomplementemic patients are a bit less fulminant than in normal hosts, and generally do not result in central nervous system (CNS) infections but rather septicemia, such that lumbar punctures are rarely required for patients on eculizumab—and should never delay empiric treatment with antibiotics. As for adults who have been splenectomized, practices vary such that in the United Kingdom, all patients on eculizumab are treated prophylactically with penicillin, whereas in the United States, there is more of a concern for the

emergence of resistant strains. It is possible to monitor antibody titers and the CDC is now recommending a booster of the a, c, w, y conjugate vaccine at 2 months for those with complement deficiency.

Patients with PNH may fail to respond to eculizumab because of (1) underlying aplastic anemia; (2) rapid drug clearance, as manifested by a nonsuppressed CH50 level, or a low eculizumab level on day 14 of the treatment cycle; (3) the Arg885His polymorphism in the C5 gene, as seen in about 3% of the Japanese population, such that the drug does not recognize the C5 protein at all[220]; or (4) extravascular hemolysis, caused by opsonization of C3d-coated red cells in the reticuloendothelial system.

The latter as described by Risitano et al[236] is most interesting, reflecting a mechanism that has been "unmasked" by eculizumab. Despite blockade at the C5 level, the PNH red cell is still lacking CD55, which normally functions to inhibit the classical and alternative C3 and C5 convertases.[221] The PNH red cell is also lacking CD59, which may inhibit not only the MAC formation, but also the deposition of C3d on the red cell in the setting of loss of CD55.[222] Indeed, in some patients on eculizumab, C3d deposition on the red cell can be demonstrated by the direct antiglobulin test or by flow cytometry; such cells would have been lysed by the MAC in untreated patients. Opsonization by C3d can account for persistently elevated reticulocyte counts, the requirement for occasional transfusions, and progressive iron overload in some patients on eculizumab. Polymorphisms in the *CR1* gene, which affect levels of expression of this complement-regulating gene, may predict which patients have a partial versus complete response to eculizumab.[223]

Atypical hemolytic uremic syndrome (aHUS) (see Chapter 134), a different complement-mediated disorder, is the other FDA-approved indication for eculizumab. aHUS is characterized by thrombocytopenia, hemolysis, an elevated lactate dehydrogenase (LDH), microangiopathy, and dysfunction of many organs, but particularly the kidneys. Other entities with similar presentations that need to be distinguished include thrombotic thrombocytopenia purpura (TTP), malignant hypertension, Shiga toxin–producing *E. coli* (STEC), calcineurin inhibitors (and other medications), lupus, and the antiphospholipid antibody syndrome, the latter two being potential triggers for aHUS itself. The disease is recognized by schistocytes on the peripheral smear, an elevated LDH, and a disintegrin and metalloproteinase with thrombospondin motifs 13 (ADAMTS 13) level (drawn before empiric pheresis) that is not significantly decreased, and a variable and often subadequate response to plasmapheresis. Compared with TTP, the degree of thrombocytopenia is not as severe, there are fewer schistocytes, but the degree of renal insufficiency is often much more severe. aHUS is genetically complex, in that it can result from inherited mutations in the genes encoding the inhibitory complement factors H, I, membrane cofactor protein (CD46) or thrombomodulin—or gain of function mutations in the effector complement factors B or C3. Autoantibodies against factor H can produce a similar syndrome, and in a substantial proportion, no mutation is ever found. The inheritance is typically dominant with incomplete penetrance.[224]

The FDA granted approval to eculizumab for the treatment of aHUS based on two single arm studies reporting rapid improvement in thrombocytopenia, typically by day 7, and a more gradual improvement in the renal function, in many cases, allowing for discontinuation of dialysis.[225,226] As in PNH, where eculizumab only masks an underlying defect, relapses have been seen upon drug discontinuation.[227] Since recurrences after renal transplantation are common in aHUS, initiation and maintenance of eculizumab before and after transplant may be critical for maintaining graft function. Since undertreatment would be more serious here than in PNH, the recommended dose in aHUS is higher.

There is a growing literature on successful "off label" use of eculizumab, for example, for catastrophic antiphospholipid antibody syndrome,[228] cold agglutinin disease,[229] HUS due to Shiga toxin–associated *E. coli*,[230] antibody-mediated renal graft rejection and dense deposit disease,[231] calcineurin inhibitor-induced thrombotic microangiopathy,[232] Devic neuromyelitis optica,[233] myasthenia

TABLE 24.5   FDA-Approved Complement Inhibitors and Some New Drugs Under Development

Company/Reference	Drug/Class	Target	Structure/Derivation	Route	Biochemical Data	Stage
Alexion	Eculizumab	C5	Humanized monoclonal antibody	Intravenous	K_d = 120 pM	FDA approved for PNH and aHUS
ViroPharma, CSC Behring	C1 esterase inhibitor: plasma derived	C1 esterase	Human protein	Intravenous		FDA approved for hereditary angioedema
Pharming-Salix	C1 esterase inhibitor: recombinant	C1 esterase	Protein analogue, produced in rabbits	Intravenous		FDA approved for hereditary angioedema
Alexion (Taligen)	TT30	C3 convertase	Factor H-CR2 fusion	Intravenous/ subcutaneous	IC_{50} = 0.5 μM	Human studies
Norvartis	LFG 316	C5	mAb	Intravenous/ intravitreal		Human studies
Amyndas, Apellis, Potentia	Compstatin analogues	C3/C3b	Cyclic peptide/ phage display	Intravitreal, subcutaneous, inhaled	IC_{50} = 62 nM, K_d for C3b = 2.3 nM	Human studies
Volution Akari	Coversin	C5	Peptide/tick saliva	Subcutaneous	Maximal inhibition at 10 μg/mL	Human studies
Achillion	Small molecule	Complement factor D	X-ray crystallography	Oral	K_d <1 nm, IC_{50} = 17 nm (protease inhibition)	Preclinical studies
Amyndas	Mini Factor H	C3 convertase	Derived from factor H		IC_{50} = 0.22 μM (for C3 deposition)	Preclinical studies
Alnylam	ALN-CC5	C5 RNA	RNAi conjugate	Subcutaneous		Preclinical studies
Lindofer et al	3E7/H17	C3b	mAb		100% blockage of lysis at 1 μM	Preclinical studies
Ra Pharmaceuticals	several	C5	Cyclic peptide	Subcutaneous	K_d 2.6 nM, IC_{50} 8.1 nm (% RBC lysis)	Preclinical studies

aHUS, Atypical hemolytic uremic syndrome; IC_{50}, half maximal inhibitory concentration; K_d, dissociation constant; PNH, paroxysmal nocturnal hemoglobinuria; RBC, red blood cell.

gravis,[234] and lupus nephritis.[235] Other possible uses under investigation include Guillain-Barré syndrome and thrombocytopenia refractory to platelet transfusion.

New Directions and New Anticomplement Therapies

While eculizumab is likely to find additional indications, there is also a plethora of additional agents and targets under investigation—but there will be challenges. Particularly, in targeting complement proteins upstream from C5, there may be a predisposition to a broader range of infections, and possibly also to autoimmune diseases, as seen in patients with genetic deficiencies of C3. Furthermore, C3 may be harder to inhibit because it circulates at considerably higher concentrations than C5. While PNH provides the most convenient clinical endpoint for the efficacy of any new complement inhibitor, it is no longer ethical to randomize patients with a large PNH clone to an arm that contains neither eculizumab nor anticoagulation, at least for long term. Possible approaches could be to investigate new drugs in patients with PNH with inadequate responses to eculizumab (or in those who have the Arg885His polymorphism in the C5 gene), or to conduct a noninferiority study.

Potential targets of new anticomplement drugs include C5, C3, factor B, and factor D. In addition to monoclonal antibodies, fusion proteins, cyclic peptides, small molecules, RNAi conjugates, and soluble complement receptors are examples of approaches under investigation[236] (Table 24.5). Among those already introduced to human subjects include TT30, a fusion of a fragment of complement inhibitor factor H and the iC3b/C3d binding domain of complement receptor 2 (CR2); this is intended to direct the factor I cofactor activity and decay-accelerating activity of factor H to the site of complement activation on the surface of the red cell.[237] Compstatin analogues are circular peptides that are specific for C3 and C3b, originally identified by phage display. There is now a phase I study of the compstatin analogues APL-2 in patients with PNH[238] and POT-4 in age-related macular degeneration.[239] A new anti-C5 mAb has been investigated in humans with macular degeneration in several studies (see Table 24.5), and recently, coversin,[240] a peptide derived from ticks, has been examined for its effect on C5 complement activity in healthy volunteers.[241] It is possible that these new complement inhibitors will need to be used in combination with other drugs for maximal efficacy.

SUGGESTED READINGS

Ahearn JM, Fischer MB, Croix D, et al: Disruption of the Cr2 locus results in a reduction in B-1a cells and in an impaired B cell response to T-dependent antigen. *Immunity* 4:251, 1996.

Bayary J, Dasgupta S, Misra N, et al: Intravenous immunoglobulin in autoimmune disorders: An insight into the immunoregulatory mechanisms. *Int Immunopharmacol* 6:528, 2006.

Carroll MC: The complement system in regulation of adaptive immunity. *Nat Immunol* 5:981, 2004.

Carter RH, Fearon DT: CD19: Lowering the threshold for antigen receptor stimulation of B lymphocytes. *Science* 256:105, 1992.

Dalakas MC: Mechanisms of action of IVIG and therapeutic considerations in the treatment of acute and chronic demyelinating neuropathies. *Neurology* 59:S13, 2002.

Fischer MB, Goerg S, Shen L, et al: Dependence of germinal center B cells on expression of CD21/CD35 for survival. *Science* 280:582, 1998.

Gros P, Milder FJ, Janssen BJ: Complement driven by conformational changes. *Nat Rev Immunol* 8:48, 2008.

Helmy KY, Gorgani NN, Kljavin NM, et al: CRIg: A macrophage complement receptor required for phagocytosis of circulating pathogens. *Cell* 124:915, 2006.

Hillmen P, Hall C, Marsh J, et al: Effect of eculizumab on hemolysis and transfusion requirements in patients with paroxysmal nocturnal hemoglobinuria. *N Engl J Med* 350:552–559, 2004.

Hillmen P, Muus P, Duhrsen U, et al: Effect of the complement inhibitor eculizumab on thromboembolism in patients with paroxysmal nocturnal hemoglobinuria. *Blood* 110(12):4123–4128, 2007.

Hopken UE, Lu B, Gerard NP, et al: The C5a chemoattractant receptor mediates mucosal defence to infection. *Nature* 383:86, 1996.

Jordan SC, Vo AA, Peng A, et al: Intravenous gammaglobulin (IVIG): A novel approach to improve transplant rates and outcomes in highly HLA-sensitized patients. *Am J Transplant* 6:459, 2006.

Kang YS, Do Y, Lee HK, et al: A dominant complement fixation pathway for pneumococcal polysaccharides initiated by SIGN-R1 interacting with C1q. *Cell* 125:47, 2006.

Kelsoe G: Life and death in germinal centers (redux). *Immunity* 4:107, 1996.

Kemper C, Chan AC, Green JM, et al: Activation of human CD4+ cells with CD3 and CD46 induces a T-regulatory cell 1 phenotype. *Nature* 421:388, 2003.

Kohler G, Milstein C: Continuous cultures of fused cells secreting antibody of predefined specificity. *Nature* 256:495–497, 1975.

Kopf M, Abel B, Gallimore A, et al: Complement component C3 promotes T-cell priming and lung migration to control acute influenza virus infection. *Nat Med* 8:373, 2002.

Legendre CM, Licht C, Muus P, et al: Terminal complement inhibitor eculizumab in atypical hemolytic-uremic syndrome. *N Engl J Med* 368:2169–2181, 2013.

Minard S, Papa SM, Campiglio M, et al: Biologic and therapeutic role of HER2 in cancer. *Oncogene* 29:6570, 2003.

Nixon A, Sexton D, Lander R: Drugs derived from phage display: from candidate identification to clinical practice. *MAbs* 6:73–85, 2014.

Thiel S, Vorup-Jensen T, Stover CM: A second serine protease associated with mannan-binding lectin that activates complement. *Nature* 386:506, 1997.

van den Elsen JM, Isenman DE: A crystal structure of the complex between human complement receptor 2 and its ligand C3d. *Science* 332:608, 2011.

REFERENCES

For the complete list of references, log on to www.expertconsult.com.

CHAPTER 25

TOLERANCE AND AUTOIMMUNITY

Taku Kambayashi

The role of the immune system is to eliminate potential threats invading the organism from the environment and from those that are generated within the organism. Examples of environmental threats include pathogens and toxins, whereas internal threats include neoplastic transformation and inadvertently formed toxic metabolites. To function properly, the immune system must be able to balance the capacity to mount a response against true threats that may pose harm to the organism, while being tolerant to those that should be ignored including commensals, inert environmental antigens, and antigens that are derived from normal self. A complex and multilayered approach has evolved to successfully handle this problem. However, hypersensitivity reactions, in which this balance is upset, are remarkably common in the population. Autoimmunity is a subset of such hypersensitivity reactions, whereby the immune system loses tolerance to a particular self-derived antigen and starts to attack the organism itself. The diversity and variable severity of such diseases most likely reflects the various approaches the immune system takes to regulate self-directed responses and thereby the various points at which this multilayered system can break down. The normal functions that prevent autoimmune disease are collectively known as *self-tolerance mechanisms*.

Autoimmune diseases are relevant to hematology at several levels, as autoimmune responses can be directed towards the hematopoietic system. For example, autoimmune hemolytic anemia (AIHA) and idiopathic thrombocytopenic purpura (ITP) are diseases in which antibodies are spontaneously made against red blood cells (RBCs) and platelets, respectively. In some cases, the RBC and platelet autoantibodies are not generated spontaneously but are induced by transfusion: these include posttransfusion purpura (PTP) and possibly AIHA associated with transfused thalassemia. Other hematopoietic components such as the bone marrow (BM) and neutrophils are targeted in aplastic anemia and in autoimmune neutropenia, respectively. However, the target does not necessarily have to be a cellular component. In acquired thrombotic thrombocytopenic purpura (TTP), an autoantibody is generated against an enzyme known as a disintegrin and metalloproteinase with thrombospondin motifs, member 13 (ADAMTS13), which results in the accumulation of ultra large von Willebrand factor (UL-VWF) fragments that lead to microangiopathic hemolytic anemia (MAHA). Finally, although not a classic autoimmune disease, graft-versus-host disease (GVHD), a common complication of allogeneic stem cell transplantation whereby allogeneic donor T cells attack recipient tissues, shares many features with autoimmune syndromes.

An important principle in understanding the etiology of autoimmune diseases is that no special mechanism, cell, antibody type, or reaction is specific to autoimmune diseases. Rather, the pathogenesis involves the inappropriate or dysregulated triggering of the normal mechanisms of immunity. Therefore an understanding of autoimmune disease induction and pathogenesis requires a firm grounding in the basic immune cell functions and interactions, which can be found in the preceding chapters.

SELF-REACTIVE LYMPHOCYTES: ORIGIN AND CONTROL

One challenge that the adaptive immune system faces is the immense variety of molecules that it needs to specifically mount responses against. How can the immune system generate an antibody that specifically binds to one pathogen but not another? How can the immune system generate a T cell that can specifically kill a pathogen-infected cell while sparing noninfected cells? To mount responses with such specificity, the receptors that activate adaptive immune cells (T and B cells) must be created with enormous diversity. The B-cell receptor (BCR) and T-cell receptor (TCR) genes are encoded in pieces (V, D, and J segments) that rearrange in the DNA of precursor lymphocytes to ultimately form a complete gene (VDJ recombination). This process allows for many possible gene segment combinations (e.g., 4000 different ones for the human immunoglobulin [Ig] heavy chain alone), and in addition, small deletions and random additions at the sites where the pieces are joined together create additional diversity. Inevitably, autoreactive lymphocytes are formed as a consequence of this rather random process of TCR and BCR generation. Hence diversity is generated at the expense of creating autoreactive lymphocytes. There are two implications of this process for self-tolerance. First, it is impossible to prevent the assembly of a self-reactive receptor by filtering these out of the germline gene repertoire. Second, a developing lymphocyte cannot be considered autoreactive until the assembly process is complete and the BCR or TCR is expressed. Thus autoreactive lymphocytes are produced every day, and it is at this key developmental stage—when the BCR or TCR is first expressed by the cell—that the immune system can first eliminate these potentially harmful cells. For B cells, this occurs in the BM, the primary central lymphoid organ (Fig. 25.1); for T cells, it occurs in the thymus (Fig. 25.2). The process is thus termed *central tolerance* and is described in further detail later.

Regulation: Central Tolerance

Clonal Deletion: B Cells

The classic experiments of Nossal and Pike were the first to demonstrate that developing autoreactive B cells can be eliminated in the BM.[1] The details of this process remained murky until the Goodnow[10] and Nemazee groups each developed a BCR transgenic mouse system for the study of self-tolerance.[2] These mice have been genetically altered to carry the preformed Ig variable (V) genes that encode a specific autoantibody. The presence of this preformed transgene short circuits and prevents the normal rearrangement process at the natural Ig gene loci. Thus each B cell in the animal expresses only the transgene and has the same specificity. By choosing a target antigen that is carried by only some strains of mice (e.g., the polymorphic major histocompatibility complex [MHC] class I genes used by Nemazee), it is possible to render the transgenic B cells autoreactive when crossed onto one strain (Fig. 25.3) but not autoreactive in a different strain. The results of such systems were dramatic. A complete loss or deletion of the B cells was demonstrated in the strain of mice that had the autoantigen, but perfectly good expression of the B cells was observed when the autoantigen was absent. Furthermore, it was shown that this deletion occurred at the immature B-cell stage, just when the cells first express their BCR. It has been since discovered that deletion is just the final step in controlling autoreactive B cells. B cells that have completed H- and L-chain rearrangement and then recognize self-antigen while still immature in the BM may actually undergo a second round of V gene rearrangement. This most likely occurs at the L-chain loci, which are particularly suited to secondary V to J rearrangements.

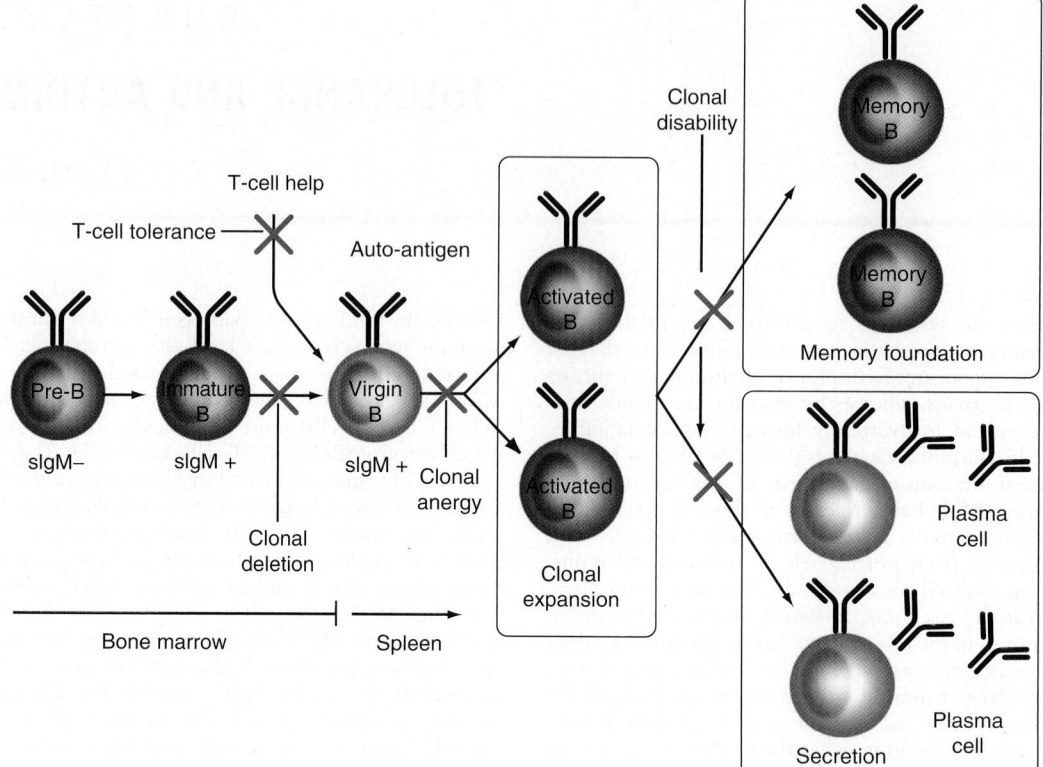

Fig. 25.1 STAGES AT WHICH SELF-TOLERANCE CAN BLOCK B-CELL DEVELOPMENT. *Arrows* indicate the normal pathway of development. *X* indicates where these differentiation steps can be interrupted for self-reactive B cells as a consequence of encountering self-antigen. Each *X* is labeled with the type of self-tolerance it represents. The clonal disability steps are somewhat more hypothetical than the earlier steps. See text for details. *sIgM*, Surface immunoglobulin M.

This process has been termed *receptor editing*.[3,4] Evidently, a cell has a certain period of time in which to produce a second L-chain rearrangement that will inactivate the cell's self-reactivity. If this does not occur, the cell fails to mature and is eventually eliminated. More recently, evidence has been accumulating that autoreactive B cells are similarly filtered out of the human repertoire. Polyreactive and antinuclear B cells are progressively eliminated during the progression of B-cell development.

Clonal Deletion: T Cells

In many respects, clonal deletion of T cells is similar to that of B cells.[5,6] Because of the randomness of VDJ recombination, T cells with overtly self-reactive TCRs are formed during their development in the thymus. However, the process is slightly more complicated in T cells; unlike B cells, T cells do not directly recognize antigens but do so in the context of MHC molecules. MHC molecules are specialized proteins that bind to and present short peptide sequences on the cell surface. The source of the peptide could be endogenous (intracellular self-proteins) or exogenous (endocytosed proteins or intracellular infection). It is this peptide determinant that needs to push an antigen-specific T cell over its activation threshold. As the number of contact sites of the TCR with a particular peptide sequence is limited, the interaction of the TCR and the MHC–peptide complex cannot be dictated by the peptide alone and is dependent in part by affinity of the TCR to the self-MHC molecule itself. Thus selection of T cells in the thymus with appropriate TCRs first involves the selective survival of T cells that display sufficient affinity to self MHC molecules, a process called *positive selection*. Because T cells that bind too strongly to self-derived MHC–peptide complexes are also contained within positively selected thymocytes, T cells bearing

TCRs that are too reactive with these complexes are eliminated by a process called *negative selection* (see Fig. 25.2). Evidence for this two-step selection process comes from experiments similar to those performed in B cells, where transgenic mice with T cells bearing a single TCR specific for an MHC class I molecule are crossed to different MHC backgrounds.[5] When such mice are crossed to an MHC background that does not bind well to the transgenic TCR, the T cells fail to be positively selected and die by neglect. However, when crossed to an MHC background that reacts too strongly with the TCR or when crossed to mice that express the cognate peptide, the transgenic T cells are purged by negative selection. Similar results were seen in another TCR transgenic system in which all T cells were specific to a male-derived antigen (H-Y).[6] Although T cell development was normal in H-Y TCR transgenic female mice, T cells were deleted at an immature stage in the thymus of H-Y TCR transgenic male mice. Thus positive and negative selection in the thymus generate a diverse repertoire of useful T cells containing a variety of TCRs that recognize self-MHC but not strong enough to cause self-reactivity and hence autoimmunity.

Limitations of Central Tolerance[7]

Although mechanisms to eliminate self-reactive B and T cells during development are clearly critical for the viability of an animal, they only account for part of the overall system that protects against autoimmunity. There are many reasons to believe that central tolerance cannot and should not be perfectly efficient. One is that the ability to tolerate self must be balanced against the ability to efficiently respond to a wide variety of foreign antigens. Each cell that is eliminated in the interest of self-tolerance is one that cannot respond to a potential foreign antigen. Thus one might imagine

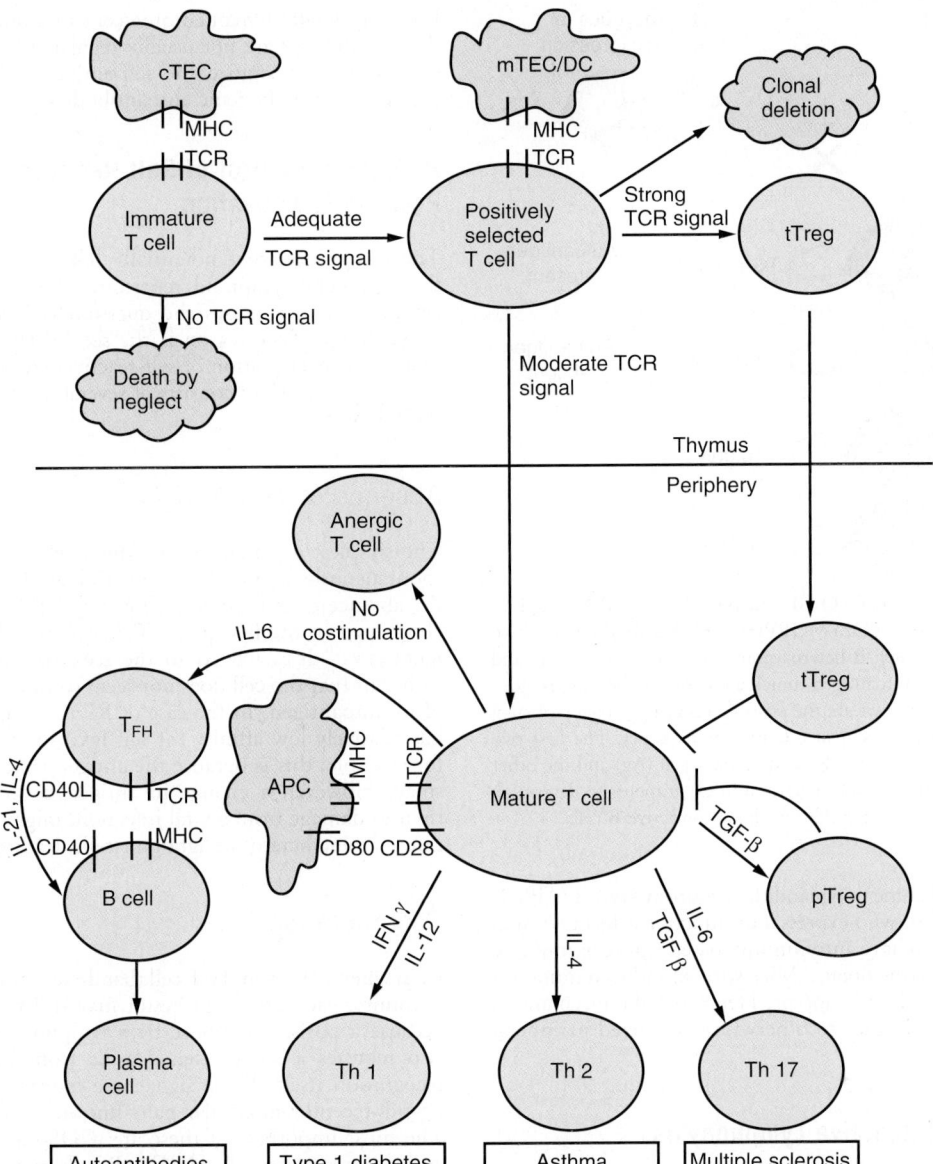

Fig. 25.2 T-CELL TOLERANCE MECHANISMS. Immature T cells are positively selected by cortical thymic epithelial cells (cTEC) for sufficient affinity to self major histocompatibility complex (MHC)–peptide complexes in the thymus. Positively selected T cells that react too strongly with self-MHC/peptide complexes presented by medullary thymic epithelial cells (mTEC) or dendritic cells (DC) are clonally deleted or alternatively adopt a thymic Treg (tTreg) phenotype. T cells with moderate affinity to self-MHC–peptide complexes enter the periphery as mature T cells. A mature T cell that encounters its cognate antigen presented by an antigen presenting cell (APC) in the absence of costimulation will become unresponsive (anergy). In the presence of costimulation, CD4⁺ T cells can differentiate into a T helper (Th)1, Th2, Th17, T follicular helper (Tfh), or peripheral Treg (pTreg) cell depending on the cytokine milieu as depicted. Tfh cells can potentially provide help to autoreactive B cells for their differentiation into plasma cells that produce autoantibodies. Both tTregs and pTregs can suppress mature T-cell activation. Examples of hypersensitivities that are associated with each Th phenotype are depicted.

that it is advantageous to allow some (weakly) self-reactive cells to escape these purging mechanisms. A second way to view this same problem is that even if it were desirable to have complete elimination of self-reactive lymphocytes, it would be impossible. It is unlikely that during development, each B or T cell will be exposed to a sufficient quantity of each and every self-antigen in the body to be functionally tested for self-reactivity. Furthermore, some antigens are tissue specific, such as thyroglobulin, and are unlikely to be found in the circulation at appreciable quantities.

This could be a particularly challenging task for negative selection of T cells, as the self-peptide determinants are processed from intracellular proteins (either endogenously expressed or acquired exogenously by macropinocytosis/phagocytosis). Thus one might imagine that it would be difficult to tolerize developing T cells to peptides derived from proteins that are not expressed in the thymus. To deal with this issue, a mechanism exists by which many peripheral tissue proteins are "ectopically" expressed in the thymus. These self-proteins are expressed in specialized thymic epithelial cells concentrated in the thymic medulla (medullary thymic epithelial cells [mTEC]). A gene known as Aire (autoimmune regulator) is required for the expression of a large number of these peripheral tissue proteins.[7] The importance of Aire in tolerance induction is exemplified

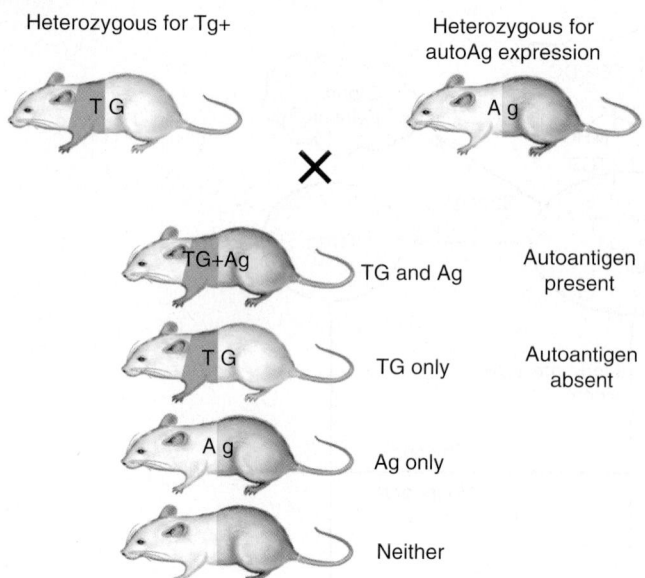

Heterozygous for Tg+

Heterozygous for autoAg expression

TG and Ag — Autoantigen present

TG only — Autoantigen absent

Ag only

Neither

Fig. 25.3 MATING STRATEGY TO GENERATE TRANSGENIC MICE WITH AND WITHOUT A POLYMORPHIC AUTOANTIGEN. Two mice are crossed, each of which is heterozygous, one for the transgene and the other for a polymorphic autoantigen (much as people can be heterozygous for blood group antigens). Shown are the possible resulting progeny of such a cross, each of which would occur at one-fourth frequency. The first two types of mice, one with transgenic (TG) and autoantigen (Ag) and the other control with TG and not the Ag, are compared in experiments to determine how autoantigen affects the development of the autoreactive B cells.

by patients with autoimmune polyglandular syndrome-type I (APS-1, also known as APECED), who express a dysfunctional form of Aire. People with the condition have autoimmune-based failure of multiple endocrine and nonendocrine organs. Mice with an induced mutation of Aire also display a similar phenotype. Hence specific mechanisms enhance thymic T-cell tolerance to otherwise sequestered peripheral antigens.

Persistence of Self-Reactive Lymphocytes

Despite mechanisms to expose developing B and T cells to a wide variety of self-antigens, central tolerance is nevertheless incomplete. Thus self-reactive cells nonetheless exist in peripheral lymphoid organs of normal animals. It has been observed for some time that many immune responses are accompanied by transient antiself antibody responses. For example, rheumatoid factor (RF) with specificity for self-IgG often accompany strong secondary immune responses to foreign proteins or viruses. The simplest explanation for such phenomena is that the B cells that make these autoantibodies already exist in the peripheral lymphoid compartment but are quiescent until they receive the proper stimulus.

Transgenic mouse models similar to those described earlier have provided the most convincing evidence of the existence of such B cells. One of particular relevance to hematology was generated by Honjo et al.[8] These workers isolated the V genes that came from an actual anti-RBC autoantibody originally obtained from an NZB mouse with AIHA and created a BCR transgenic mouse. Although central deletion was seen in most of the transgenic mice studied, many also had some residual autoreactive B cells in the spleen and lymph nodes, and some otherwise normal mice even developed frank AIHA. These results were interpreted as follows: central tolerance is not completely efficient even in a nonautoimmune mouse, and some autoreactive B cells can be stimulated to cause disease. Shlomchik et al, also using a transgenic approach, demonstrated that an RF autoantibody that was isolated from a diseased mouse was not subject to self-tolerance when expressed in a normal BALB/c mouse.[9] These

B cells generally remained quiescent in a normal animal, suggesting that B cells that are not usually regulated by self-tolerance (perhaps because they recognize the self-antigen only weakly) may be the precursors of pathogenic autoantibodies in disease.

Peripheral Control of Self-Reactive Lymphocytes: Preventing Activation

The recognition that potentially self-reactive lymphocytes exist in the peripheral lymphoid repertoire of normal individuals, despite central tolerance, raises the question of why they do not usually cause disease. One reason is the second layer of immune tolerance that prevents activation of self-reactive lymphocytes that exist in the periphery. This layer consists of several facets, which are described in the following sections.

Absence of Self-Antigen

The simplest explanation for why a self-specific lymphocyte is not spontaneously activated in the peripheral lymphoid compartment is the absence of self-antigen. This may be the reason why it was not eliminated in the first place. This situation has been termed clonal ignorance.[10] It is related to the scenario described for RF B cells earlier in that the cell does not seem to care about the concentration of its autoantigen. In the case of RF though, this is because the cell has relatively low affinity for self-IgG; in the case of thyroglobulin, for example, this is because the antigen concentration is vanishingly small. However, a change in antigen concentration, such as after thyroid damage from a viral infection, might then precipitate activation of these heretofore ignorant cells, leading to autoimmunity.

Costimulation

Even when a B cell and a T cell that do recognize the same self-antigen encounter each other, the result may still not be activation. This is because a positive response by a lymphocyte to antigen encounter also requires a second signal aside from the stimulus of antigen recognition itself. These signals are transmitted through a series of ligand–receptor molecular pairs known as costimulatory molecules. The most important of these are: CD80 and CD86 (expressed on antigen presenting cells [APCs], B cells, macrophages, and dendritic cells) and CD28 (expressed on T cells). In order for T cells to expand and differentiate into effector cells, the APC must provide costimulatory signals to the T cell. The lack of costimulatory signals leads to a state of unresponsiveness (anergy) and is characterized by the reduced ability of T cells to proliferate and to secrete interleukin (IL)-2 upon TCR stimulation.[11] The discovery of this important step in T-cell activation has led to the development of therapeutics that block costimulatory signals, in an attempt to induce an anergic state in autoreactive T cells.

Another important pair is CD40 (expressed on B cells, macrophages, and dendritic cells) and CD40 ligand (CD40L, expressed on T cells and missing in patients with X-linked immunodeficiency/hyper-IgM syndrome).[12] CD40 stimulation is especially important for B cells, as it is for other APCs as well. Other significant costimulatory molecules in T–B interactions include ICOS and ICOS-L, which are critical for germinal center responses and isotype switching.

In general, for proper transmission of this second signal, one or the other of the lymphocytes must have been previously activated. This concept generates a paradox in that if one lymphocyte must already be activated, how is it possible to start an immune response at all? In general, mounting an immune response is dependent on inflammation, as this is a powerful inducer of these same costimulatory molecules. Thus in the presence of ongoing inflammation, such as would occur with infection or trauma, immune responses are much easier to start. Indeed, recent evidence suggests an important role in systemic autoimmunity for Toll-like receptors (TLRs), which recognize molecules specific to pathogens and induce costimulatory molecules and immune system activation. Ligands for TLRs include lipopolysaccharide (TLR4), bacterial DNA enriched for CpG dinucleotides (TLR9), and single-stranded and double-stranded RNA (TLR7 and TLR3). TLRs can be activated by infection and may provide a mechanism by which some infections can trigger autoimmunity. However, in the right context some self (as opposed to pathogen) molecules, such as DNA found in chromatin, a target for systemic lupus erythematosus (SLE) autoantibodies, can also activate TLRs (TLR9 in the case of DNA).[13] Third, certain "professional" APCs, such as dendritic cells, may constitutively express these costimulatory molecules at moderate levels and can start the cascade, for example, by activating T cells, which is then amplified by T–B interactions.[14] In summary, there are two main functions of costimulatory requirements: (1) they focus the interactions between two antigen-specific T and B cells and limit nonspecific interactions, and (2) they restrict immune responses in the absence of inflammation. Both of these features of costimulation tend to prevent the activation of self-reactive lymphocytes that exist in peripheral lymphoid organs. For B cells, this means that tolerance in the T-cell compartment alone will prevent many self-reactive B cells from being activated.

Even with antigen sequestration and costimulatory regulation, mechanisms that prevent the activation of self-reactive lymphocytes are incomplete at best. For example, it seems likely during infection or trauma that antiself responses could initiate because costimulatory molecules will be nonspecifically induced. Furthermore, during infection and tissue damage, self-proteins that ordinarily are sequestered can be released. This leads to activation of the ignorant cells circulating in the body. In fact, (usually) self-limited autoimmune responses after infection are well known, such as poststreptococcal glomerulonephritis or postmycoplasmal cold agglutinins. Although these syndromes can cause serious clinical problems, they are self-limited, unlike autoimmune diseases such as SLE.

Tolerance of Germinal Center B Cells

Fig. 25.1 indicates that there are yet other stages of B-cell development at which one could imagine that self-tolerance should occur. The most important of these is during the germinal center reaction. After initial activation and expansion of antigen-activated B cells, the genes that encode the antibody receptor molecule undergo a process of random mutation. This process known as *somatic hypermutation* or *affinity maturation* allows editing of the template antibody molecule in an attempt to increase affinity of the antibody against the immunizing antigen. The B cells that have mutated their antibodies then compete for the same antigen in the germinal center for selection of B cells expressing higher affinity antibodies. However, a side effect of any random process, just as in the receptor rearrangement itself, is the potential to create novel antiself specificities.[15] This problem is dealt with because T and B cells are dependent on each other for activation. Germinal centers contain a recently characterized specialized T-cell subset known as T follicular helper cells (Tfh).[16] For germinal center B cells to survive, they must incorporate an antigen through its BCR, then process and present the antigen on MHC class II molecules. Only B cells that have incorporated the relevant antigen and can interact with antigen-specific Tfh cells are allowed to survive and differentiate into memory B cells or plasma cells.[16] It is evident that for this to occur, B and Tfh cells specific for the same self-antigen must be in the same place at the same time. If such cells are rare, then the requisite coexistence of two such cells will happen very infrequently, minimizing the chance of starting an autoimmune reaction. A second consequence of T–B interdependence is that specific inefficiencies of central tolerance in one limb can be compensated for in the other. For example, T cells are probably very efficiently purged of cells that react with thymus-specific antigens, but B cells are probably not. However, antithymus B-cell responses are unlikely even though many thymus-specific B cells probably circulate; the cognate

T cell with specificity for the same self-antigen simply does not exist. Thus the generation of B cells expressing antiself antibodies in the germinal center is largely avoided by the lack of T-cell help for the self-antigen.

Control of Self-Reactive Lymphocytes: Downregulation

The difference between transient autoimmune responses and chronic severe autoimmunity may lie in the third layer of protection against autoimmunity: downregulation of ongoing responses. Again, this layer is a normal part of the immune system, functioning to regulate both normal and autoimmune responses. Initially, in a normal response to a viral pathogen, there is clonal expansion of lymphocytes specific for viral antigens. This process leads ultimately to the elimination of the pathogen, which was traditionally thought of as the signal to stop an immune response. However, when the pathogen is eliminated, in the absence of any other regulatory mechanism, there would be many residual cells that had been responding to the pathogen. Although a few such cells could be retained to provide immunologic memory, most of these are no longer useful in the short term. In addition to unnecessarily filling the lymphoid compartment, these cells may be a risk for causing autoimmunity. For example, there is a possibility that lingering B cells will contribute to the generation of newly autoreactive B cells by virtue of random somatic hypermutation. Thus elimination of most of the reactive B cells regardless of specificity would mitigate this problem.

Several pathways for the removal of such postexpansion cells have been elucidated. One seems to be an inborn program that causes cells to undergo apoptosis after a certain amount of proliferation. Particularly important in this program in lymphocytes are the Bcl2-inhibitable pathways that are activated in large part by the pro-apotoic protein Bim. In B cells, CD40 signaling in concert with BCR stimulation and cytokines (IL-4 and IL-21 provided by Tfh cells) rescue these cells from this self-destructive fate, allowing these cells to become long-lived memory cells or plasma cells. There are also active mechanisms such as Fas and FasL that signal cells to apoptose. Generally, when Fas is ligated by FasL, the cell expressing Fas is triggered to die by apoptosis.[17] Fas and FasL are not expressed at high levels on unstimulated resting lymphocytes. On activation, T cells express both Fas and FasL, whereas B cells express Fas.[18] Thus, after a certain degree of activation and proliferation, a T cell (expressing FasL) encountering an activated B cell (expressing Fas) may actually kill that B cell. There are likely other ligand pairs, particularly those in the tumor necrosis factor (TNF) family that may serve similar functions, both for B and T cells.

Another method of downregulating immune function is the acquisition of inhibitory receptors. For example, CTLA4 is an inhibitory receptor expressed on activated T cells,[19] and when ligated by CD80 or CD86, causes inactivation of the receptive T cell. CD80 and CD86 send a positive signal to naive T cells by ligating CD28; however, CTLA4 has higher affinity for CD80/86 allowing it to outcompete binding of CD80/86 to CD28. Thus the same ligand can promote activation early on in the immune response while, through a change in the receptive T cell, it can inhibit activation at a later time. An analogous receptor pair of the B7 family is PD-1, an inhibitory receptor similar to CTLA-4, and its ligands PD-L1 and PD-L2. PD-1 is expressed on a number of activated lymphocytes and its ligands are constitutively and inducibly expressed on a variety of parenchymal cells and hematopoietic cells. Absence of these molecules leads to exaggerated immune responses and autoimmunity.[20] These examples underscore the careful means by which the immune system regulates and dampens activation presumably to prevent excessive immune responses and autoimmunity.

Control of Self-Reactive Lymphocytes: Channeling the Type of Effector Response

A final layer of protection against self-inflicted immune damage involves channeling of responses so that they are less harmful.

Depending on the context, only certain effector functions will effectively eliminate certain pathogens. For example, antibodies will not be effective against intracellular pathogens. By analogy, only certain effector functions may cause autoimmune disease, depending on the circumstances. Based on their cytokine secreting profile, T-helper (Th) cell responses can be divided into multiple subsets including Th1, Th2, and Th17 cells that in turn lead to very different effector functions (see Fig. 25.2). The propensity to make these various types of responses depends on a number of factors including the cytokine milieu, costimulation, genetics, route of antigen exposure, and dose of antigen.[21] Intriguingly, in certain murine models of autoimmunity such as the nonobese diabetic (NOD) model, experimental manipulations that shift responses away from Th1 and toward Th2 are highly protective against disease. This is also relevant to B-cell autoimmunity per se because, through the use of different isotypes of Ig, different effector functions can occur. The cytokines secreted by Th1 and Th2 cells have profound effects on the isotypes of immunoglobulins that are produced during a response. Thus, not only is the T-cell component of the response channeled in this way, but the humoral response is also influenced. Th17 cells, which are important for responses to extracellular bacteria as well, have been recognized as important pathogenic cells in several autoimmune diseases. These include mouse models of multiple sclerosis, collagen-induced arthritis, and inflammatory bowel disease. Thus genetic predisposition or environmental factors that drive Th-cell differentiation to a particular Th subset may enhance the chances of developing certain autoimmune diseases that are associated with that type of response.

Control of Self-Reactive Lymphocytes: Regulatory T Cells

As described earlier, one fate of a developing thymocyte that binds too strongly to a self-MHC–peptide complex in the thymus, is its elimination by negative selection. An alternative fate for such a T cell is the adoption of a suppressive phenotype and differentiation into a specialized subset called regulatory T cells, which dampen immune responses (see Fig. 25.2).[22] As they are selected by recognition of self-peptide–MHC complexes in the thymus, thymically derived regulatory T cells are activated upon encounter with their self-derived cognate antigen in the periphery and can subsequently inhibit autoreactive immune responses. Regulatory T cells are characterized by their expression of the lineage-determining transcription factor Foxp3 and the high-affinity IL-2 receptor CD25. In the most extreme case, the importance of these cells is underscored by a rare and fatal inherited autoimmune disorder, IPEX (immune dysregulation, polyendocrinopathy, enteropathy, and X-linked inheritance), that lacks functional Foxp3 and hence regulatory T cells. The absence of functional regulatory T cells in these patients leads to a fatal systemic autoimmune syndrome within 1 year of age, unless bone marrow transplantation is performed. Similar observations have been made in Scurfy mice and in mice genetically engineered to lack Foxp3.[23] Interestingly, the autoimmune syndrome that develops in patients lacking Aire (APECED, as described earlier) likely involves defective regulatory T-cell generation, because the adoptive transfer of specific regulatory T cells prevents the onset of autoimmunity in Aire-deficient mouse models.

In cases that are less extreme than Foxp3 or Aire deficiency, perturbance in the homeostasis, development, or expansion of regulatory T cells could still predispose individuals to develop autoimmune diseases. Increasing regulatory T cells in patients with autoimmune diseases could be therapeutically beneficial, as expansion of regulatory T cells have been shown to prevent autoimmune syndromes such as inflammatory bowel disease, type I diabetes, and autoimmune encephalomyelitis in murine models. Furthermore, they can also be used to prevent transplantation rejection and bone marrow transplant-associated GVHD. Regulatory T cells inhibit the activation of other T cells through multiple mechanisms including the secretion of suppressive cytokines (IL-10, transforming growth factor

[TGF]-β, and IL-35), competition for survival factors (costimulation and cytokines), and by direct cell–cell contact. Thus regulatory T cells represent a major peripheral tolerance mechanism to prevent aberrant autoreactive T-cell activation.

BREAKDOWN OF SELF-TOLERANCE IN AUTOIMMUNE DISEASES

Presumably, for autoimmune diseases and autoantibody production to occur, one or more of the multilayered mechanisms to prevent autoimmunity must fail. Surprisingly, the precise nature of these failures is not well understood. The mechanisms of failure are likely different for the various autoimmune diseases and perhaps even for different patients with similar syndromes. Moreover, it seems likely both from phenomenologic and genetic studies that failures at several levels are required to generate clinically significant autoimmunity.

This chapter is not meant to review the nature of autoimmune diseases; however, before considering the likely points at which self-tolerance mechanisms break down, it is useful to review some basic concepts about these diseases. Grossly, autoimmune diseases have often been divided into organ-specific and systemic autoimmune syndromes. This classification is useful, but as these diseases are becoming better understood, the dividing lines are blurring; pathogeneses of all these diseases are likely to have much in common. In particular, systemic autoimmune diseases are actually much more specific in their antigenic targets than is commonly realized. Table 25.1 shows the types of autoantibodies commonly found in several systemic autoimmune diseases. Certain autoantibodies are diagnostic for specific autoimmune diseases, such as anti-Sm in SLE. Thus Sm is a specific target in SLE, but patients with autoimmune diseases, such as rheumatoid arthritis (RA), do not respond to this autoantigen. In fact, only 30% of all patients with SLE make anti-Sm, meaning that the other 70% are tolerant of their own Sm despite having a systemic autoimmune disease. Another salient feature of most human autoimmune diseases is adult onset. Both the selective nature of disease and its late onset argue against gross defects in the basic central tolerance mechanisms as being the cause.

Instead, these considerations suggest that most clinical autoimmune diseases are likely to arise from defects in the later stages

TABLE 25.1	Patterns of Autoantibody Expression in Systemic Autoimmune Diseases			
Autoantigen/ Autoimmune Diseases (% of Patients With Autoantibody)	Systemic Lupus Erythematosus	Rheumatoid Arthritis	Scleroderma	Sjögren Syndrome
dsDNA	40			
ssDNA	70			
Histones	70			
Sm	30			
nRNP	30			
Ro (SS-A)	35			60
La (SS-B)	15			40
IgG (RF)	20	90		10–20
Scl-70 (Topo I)			70	
Centromere			70	

dsDNA, Double-stranded DNA; nRNP, native ribonucleoprotein; Scl-70, scleroderma 70-kDa antigen (topoisomerase I); Sm, Smith ribonucleoprotein; ssDNA, single-stranded DNA. Blank space indicates rarely or never detected.
From Tan EM: Antinuclear antibodies: Diagnostic markers for autoimmune diseases and probes for cell biology. *Adv Immunol* 44:93, 1989.

of self-tolerance, such as preventing the activation of autoreactive cells or downregulating them when they are activated. Because in no case is the primary cause of a polygenic autoimmune disease known, it cannot be excluded that subtle defects in the earlier stages, including central tolerance, may also play a role; in fact, for some diseases, recent data suggest that there is a role for more "leaky" central self-tolerance. However, it does seem clear that a gross defect in central tolerance would lead to a severe syndrome of congenital autoimmunity.

Genetic and Environmental Factors Contributing to Autoimmunity

Genetic Factors

Both genetic and environmental factors help to explain why autoimmunity occurs in some individuals and not others.[24] The most well-known genetic factor is the major histocompatibility complex, known as human leukocyte antigen (HLA) in humans. Many different autoimmune diseases are more or less associated with specific genotypes at this polymorphic locus. Among these are ankylosing spondylitis (HLA-B27), insulin-dependent diabetes mellitus (HLA-DR3/4), RA (HLA-DR4), and to some degree SLE (HLA-DR2/3). It should be emphasized that although individuals with these genotypes are relatively more prone, most will not develop the autoimmune disease. How certain HLA genes predispose to autoimmunity is not very clear, but some recent advances have been made. For example, a potential structural and mechanistic explanation of how certain HLA-DR4 alleles may predispose individuals to developing RA has been proposed. One important diagnostic/prognostic indicator of RA is the development of antibodies against citrullinated peptides. It is thought that the citrullination of self-peptides protect them from proteolytic degradation, thereby enhancing its presentation of MHC molecules and hence autoreactivity. A recent study has shown that among HLA-DR4 alleles, ones that have the highest predisposition to RA (HLA-DRB1-04:01 or HLA-DRB1-04:04) can only bind citrullinated Vimentin peptide, whereas the more protective HLA-DR4 allele HLA-DRB1-04:02 is more permissive and can bind to the uncitrullinated peptide as well.[25] Thus restricting antigen presentation of this citrullinated peptide would lead to more exposure to this epitope, which could predispose to development of RA.

Inheritance patterns of all systemic autoimmune diseases suggest that multiple genes, in addition to the HLA locus, contribute to susceptibility. Such genes are beginning to be identified in human and in animal models. Interestingly, risk alleles have been identified for a number of the same genes in more than one autoimmune disease; these include CTLA-4, STAT-4, PTPN-22, TNFAIP3, and IRF-5, all of which are known to regulate inflammation. Interestingly, most of them seem to have direct effects on B-cell function or activity. Table 25.2 lists categories of genes that are likely involved in genetic predisposition to autoimmune disease, drawing from both human and murine studies. Note that these include genes involved in the processes of antigen sequestration, T–B collaboration, and immune response downregulation that were discussed earlier as key features of the self-tolerance mechanisms that normally prevent autoimmune disease. In ongoing work, the precise nature of defects in these genes may be defined; these include noncoding polymorphisms that affect expression levels in addition to structural alleles. This will in turn permit screening for defects in human autoimmune disease patients with the ultimate goals of aiding diagnosis, providing insights into pathogenic mechanisms, and guiding patient-specific therapies.

Although human genetic studies and animal models suggest multigenic inheritance, there are certain instructive cases in which single-gene defects play a major role. A well-studied example of mutations in these genes is the lpr/lpr mouse, which carries an inactivated murine Fas.[17] The gld mutation, which inactivates murine Fas ligand (FasL),[18] has a very similar phenotype to the lpr/lpr mouse. Both of these mutations lead to an age-dependent autoimmune syndrome with autoantibody profiles that remarkably resemble human SLE, presumably, as a result of failure to eliminate postactivation T and B cells by the Fas-based mechanism. Exactly how defects in the apoptotic Fas pathway lead to autoimmunity has yet to be elucidated. Interestingly, a rare syndrome in humans with incomplete penetrance, called autoimmune lymphoproliferation syndrome (ALPS), has been traced to mutations in human Fas. Patients with ALPS develop polyclonal expansion of their lymphocytes and often display autoimmune cytopenias and less commonly SLE. The phenotypes of mutations in the Fas pathway illustrate two important points. They demonstrate the critical nature of the late downregulatory controls in preventing autoimmune disease. They also point out pathways in which less severe mutations might be discovered that account for human disease.

A final category of genes regulates the clearance of self-antigens and dead cells, which is particularly important in systemic autoimmune diseases such as SLE. These include complement components C4, C3, and C2, C1q, and genes such as *MER*, which plays a role in signaling for the uptake of apoptotic fragments by macrophages. Evidently, when self-antigens are not cleared promptly after cell death, they can become targets of the immune system, leading to autoimmunity to intracellular components such as chromatin.

As noted, TLRs can recognize some of these molecules when they are present in high concentrations, thus providing proinflammatory signals. In murine models of lupus, it has been demonstrated in vivo that TLR9 is required to generate antichromatin autoantibodies and that TLR7, which recognizes RNA, is required for the generation of autoantibodies to RNA-related antigens.[26] Indeed, a mutant mouse with a double dose of TLR7 develops spontaneous lupus with high levels of RNA antibodies. Stimulation of these TLRs on specialized plasmacytoid dendritic cells leads to release of abundant type I interferon, which itself may be causally linked to lupus in mice

TABLE 25.2	Genes Involved in Regulation of Autoimmune Responses	
Category	**Types of Genes[a]**	**Known Examples[b]**
Central and peripheral deletion and anergy	Receptor signaling, MHC genes, receptor V genes	CD45, PTPN22, HLA (certain types), CD3, CD4, CD8, CD28/B7
Initiation of response	Receptor signaling, costimulatory molecules, adhesion molecules	BLK, STAT-4, IRF5, ITGAM, PTPN22, FcγRII
Downregulation of response	Apoptosis genes, interleukins, negative costimulatory molecules	Fas, TNF, CTLA4, CD40, CD3, TNFAIP3, CD28/B7
Channeling of response	Interleukins, interleukin receptors	STAT-4, IL-4, IL-10, IL-12, IFN-γ
Autoantigen metabolism and apoptosis	Complement components, apoptosis signaling	C1q, C2, C4, DNAse I, MER

[a]Indicates some of the categories of genes that may be involved in regulating autoimmunity at the indicated step.
[b]Some genes in the categories of genes that may be involved in regulating autoimmunity are indicated in the left column. Some have also been directly shown to play a role in autoimmunity.
BLK, B-lymphocyte kinase; CTLA, cytotoxic T-lymphocyte activation; IFN, interferon; IL, interleukin; IRF, interferon response factor; MER, C-mer tyrosine kinase; MHC, major histocompatibility complex; PTP, posttransfusion purpura; STAT, signal transducers and activators of transcription.

and humans. These findings highlight a genetic basis for recognizing self-molecules in autoimmune diseases and suggest new therapeutic targets that are currently being explored.

Environmental Factors

Environment plays a role that is at least as important as genetics. This is illustrated by the fact that concordance rates among identical twins, even raised in the same household, are surprisingly low. Only 20% of twins of patients with RA also get RA. There are many examples of environmental factors causing either chronic or transient autoimmune diseases. There are postinfectious syndromes such as postmycoplasmal cold agglutinin disease. The pattern of incidence of multiple sclerosis suggests a viral etiology, although no causative virus has ever been convincingly demonstrated. Another category of infectious associations includes postviral myocarditis, which follows certain coxsackievirus infections. It is sometimes conceptually difficult to draw a line between viral damage and consequent immune system damage; however, if sensitization to self-antigens occurs as a consequence of viral infection and these later are pathogenic targets independent of viral antigens, it seems reasonable to consider the syndrome as autoimmune.

Infections are not the only source of environmental stimuli for autoimmunity. Toxins, such as mercury, cause autoimmunity in animal models. Another form more familiar to those in hematology is drug-induced autoimmunity, as in AIHA. Drugs such as procainamide that cause lupus-like syndromes are particularly prominent examples. Despite these specific examples, the environmental factors that play a role in promoting common autoimmune diseases such as RA or SLE are unknown.

Examples in Hematology: Epitope Spreading in Posttransfusion Purpura

One potential way to break self-tolerance may be particularly relevant to syndromes found in hematology and is worthy of elaboration. This is a form of environmental stimulation, albeit iatrogenic. In PTP, transfusion with allogeneic platelets that contain a platelet-specific antigen (e.g., HPA-1a) lacking in the recipient leads to rapid destruction of the transfused platelets and antibody formation (in this case, anti-HPA-1a antibodies) to the foreign platelet antigen.[27] However, several days later, the recipient becomes severely thrombocytopenic owing to a paradoxical destruction of the recipient's own platelets. Although how such destruction of self-platelets occurs secondary to destruction of allogeneic platelets is controversial, the best explanation is the development of an autoimmune response. How does this response get stimulated? The probable pathway bears significant parallels to one demonstrated in mice a number of years ago by Janeway and colleagues.[28] These workers immunized normal mice with human cytochrome c, which differed slightly from endogenous murine cytochrome c. The mice made both an antibody response and a T-cell response to the human cytochrome c; however, because the human and mouse cytochromes are so similar, the antibody response (but not the T-cell response) cross-reacted with murine cytochrome c. Presumably this reflected activation of ignorant B cells with specificity for self-cytochrome c (and also human). However, several weeks later, if the mice were given a dose of self-cytochrome c, now both a vigorous B-cell and T-cell antiself response ensued. These authors suggested that priming with the cross-reactive antigen first induced self-reactive B cells, which in turn could then break tolerance in anergic or ignorant self-reactive T cells.

How does this relate to PTP? Fig. 25.4 illustrates the author's hypothetic adaptation of this mechanism to the platelet transfusion situation. The foreign platelets actually share many common antigens with the host, as well as differ at the HPA-1a locus. The foreign antigenic difference allows ignorant self-specific B cells (as well as HPA-1a–specific B cells) to interact with helper T cells that

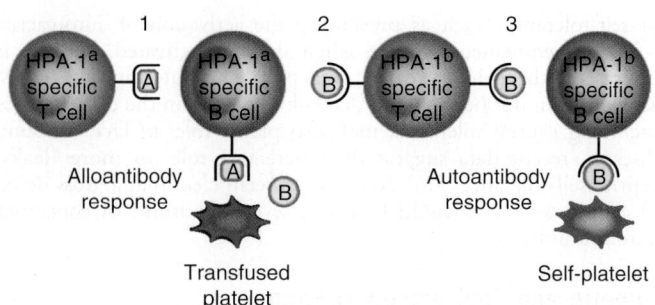

Fig. 25.4 EPITOPE SPREADING AS A POSSIBLE AUTOIMMUNE MECHANISM FOR POSTTRANSFUSION PURPURA (PTP). Events are depicted as progressing from left to right. An HPA-1b person is transfused with an HPA-1a/b platelet product. An alloantibody response ensues as an HPA-1a–specific B cell recognizes the platelet, becomes activated to secrete antibody, and presents the HPA-1a antigen to an anti-HPA-1a T cell (step 1). In addition, the activated B cell may now activate a previously ignorant anti-HPA-1b–specific T cell to initiate an autoimmune response (step 2). The activated B cell acquired the self-HPA-1b antigen as a passenger on the HPA-1a/b allogeneic platelet. This autoreactive T cell can then activate an ignorant anti-HPA-1b B cell to make an autoantibody response (step 3) in response to autologous platelets. Note that the sensitization involved in steps 1 and 2 may take place in a primary response during the first transfusion or exposure and that step 3 may take place in a clinically noticeable way only after a secondary exposure to homologous platelets.

are specific for the foreign HPA-1a antigen and become activated. Moreover, these activated B cells can then present self-platelet antigens along with costimulatory signals to self-reactive T cells. When this happens, the immune response can perpetuate even in the absence of the foreign platelets. This is exactly what is seen in PTP, in which a delayed response continues to eliminate self-platelets for many days after the disappearance of the transfused platelets. Thus a foreign platelet is analogous to foreign cytochrome c in having a few different antigens along with many shared antigens. In the same way as shown experimentally with cytochrome c, it is hypothesized that the few foreign antigens existing on the same particle (in the case of cytochrome c, it is the same molecule) allow spreading of autoimmunity from a foreign antigen to self-antigens. The key events are the activation of ignorant B cells that cross-react with both self and foreign molecules and then the activation of T cells that are specific for self by these B cells.

It is reasonable to question how such antiself responses are ever stopped once started. PTP, for example, is a self-limited syndrome. In fact, the answer is not known; however, both downregulation of antigen as the platelet count falls to near zero, and the natural mechanisms that cause apoptosis of responding lymphocytes probably play a role. Regulatory T cells could also help bring the response under control. In the absence of an autoimmune-prone host who has mutations affecting the downregulation of immune responses, these autoimmune reactions will remain transient. It is speculated that when similar events—for example, a response to a viral DNA-binding protein that eventually spreads to allow for responses to self-DNA and chromatin, as in SLE—occur in people who do have genetically based problems in downregulating such responses, a chronic autoimmune syndrome can be induced.

IMPLICATIONS AND THERAPY

The significance of this issue to hematology ranges from syndromes such as AIHA and ITP to iatrogenically induced autoimmunity as in PTP. A basic understanding of the mechanisms of self-tolerance and their breakdown in autoimmune disease raises the possibility of many types of specific therapeutic interventions. One of the clearest would be to identify initiating factors, such as infections, and to prevent or treat them. A second approach would be to reset tolerance. If the system can be set back to the state before that event, the disease could be cured. At present, it is unclear how to do this; however, an autologous or even allogeneic hematopoietic stem cell transplant may have the desired effect. In fact, this sort of radical therapy has been tried in selected cases of severe SLE and seems to have some efficacy. Another promising area is in channeling the immune response, particularly as the steering mechanisms are becoming better understood at the molecular level. A third area is to design more specific modulators of inflammation, including interfering with costimulatory signals. These latter approaches have seemed promising in various animal models, although issues with unexpected effects on clotting have arisen in clinical trials of CD40L inhibition.

Current therapy is much more crude and typically involves general nonspecific immunosuppression either with steroids or cytotoxic drugs. Although these therapies can be effective, they have numerous undesirable side effects, not the least of which is increased susceptibility to infection caused by immunosuppression. More promising are drugs such as monoclonal antibodies that inhibit the effects of specific cytokines such as TNF-α, which have proven successful in modifying progression of RA, inflammatory bowel disease, and psoriasis. Additionally, the injection of cytokines themselves could also be effective at treating autoimmunity. For example, IL-2 administration has been shown to expand regulatory T cells and ameliorate disease in multiple autoimmune mouse models including type I diabetes and multiple sclerosis. In human clinical trials, IL-2 was shown to be effective in reducing chronic GVHD. It would be interesting to see if IL-2 and other therapies aimed at expanding regulatory T cells will be an effective treatment for autoimmune disorders.

Reciprocally, therapies for autoimmune diseases in humans have in turn taught us new aspects of autoimmune disease pathogenesis. A prime example of this is rituximab, which is a monoclonal antibody that targets the CD20 antigen and hence depletes CD20+ B cells. Rituximab was originally developed to treat CD20+ B cell malignancies,[29] but during clinical trials it was unexpectedly found that cancer patients with concomitant RA showed improvement in their RA symptoms. This was surprising given that RA was thought to be predominantly driven by T cells rather than by B cells. This finding prompted clinical trials using rituximab for the treatment of a number of autoimmune diseases. These include autoimmune diseases that are clearly antibody-mediated (e.g., ITP, AIHA, TTP, pemphigus vulgaris) but also include those that have less well-defined involvement of autoantibodies (e.g., vasculitides, multiple sclerosis, RA, type I diabetes).[30] Although one might predict that rituximab attenuates autoimmunity by reducing autoantibody production by B cells, this appears to not always be the case. For example, although clinically effective, rituximab only decreases levels of RF but not of anticitrullinated peptide antibodies in RA patients. Similarly, antineutrophil cytoplasmic antibody (ANCA) levels are not decreased in patients with ANCA-associated vasculitides treated with rituximab despite clinical efficacy. In fact, it is somewhat puzzling why rituximab would reduce circulating antibodies at all, given that CD20 is expressed on mature B cells but not on plasma cells, which provide the long-lasting source of autoantibodies in chronic autoimmunity. Chronic treatment of patients with rituximab depletes memory and activated B cells that repopulate the pool of plasma cells that are turning over, which may explain why circulating antibody levels can be decreased. However, B-cell depletion by rituximab is most likely effective in many of these autoimmune disorders because of the antibody-independent functions of B cells including cytokine production and antigen presentation.

The therapeutic approaches discussed earlier, although a result of modern biotechnology and our understanding of immunopathogenesis, still targets effector function of the immune system and does not modify the root cause of disease. Therapies should ultimately be directed toward either prevention or else specific downregulation of ongoing responses. Future work will include continuing to define how self-tolerance is imposed and how it is broken in disease, what the critical triggers and autoantigens are, and how to

use immunomodulation to treat autoimmune diseases on the basis of a better understanding of the pathogenesis.

REFERENCES

1. Nossal GJ, Pike BL: Mechanisms of clonal abortion tolerogenesis. I. Response of immature hapten-specific B lymphocytes. *J Exp Med* 148:1161, 1978.
2. Nemazee DA, Burki K: Clonal deletion of B lymphocytes in a transgenic mouse bearing anti-MHC class I antibody genes. *Nature* 337:562, 1989.
3. Gay D, Saunders T, Camper S, et al: Receptor editing: an approach by autoreactive B cells to escape tolerance. *J Exp Med* 177(4):999–1008, 1993.
4. Tiegs SL, Russell DM, Nemazee D: Receptor editing in self-reactive bone marrow B cells. *J Exp Med* 177(4):1009–1020, 1993.
5. Sha WC, Nelson CA, Newberry RD, et al: Positive and negative selection of an antigen receptor on T cells in transgenic mice. *Nature* 336(6194):73–76, 1988.
6. Kisielow P, Bluthmann H, Staerz UD, et al: Tolerance in T-cell-receptor transgenic mice involves deletion of nonmature CD4+8+ thymocytes. *Nature* 333(6175):742–746, 1988.
7. Anderson MS, Venanzi ES, Klein L, et al: Projection of an immunological self shadow within the thymus by the aire protein. *Science* 298(5597):1395–1401, 2002.
8. Okamoto M, Murakami M, Shimizu A, et al: A transgenic model of autoimmune hemolytic anemia. *J Exp Med* 175(1):71–79, 1992.
9. Shlomchik MJ, Zharhary D, Saunders T, et al: A rheumatoid factor transgenic mouse model of autoantibody regulation. *Int Immunol* 5(10):1329–1341, 1993.
10. Goodnow CC: Transgenic mice and analysis of B-cell tolerance. *Annu Rev Immunol* 10:489–518, 1992.
11. Mueller DL, Jenkins MK, Schwartz RH: Clonal expansion versus functional clonal inactivation: a costimulatory signalling pathway determines the outcome of T cell antigen receptor occupancy. *Annu Rev Immunol* 7:445–480, 1989.
12. Allen RC, Armitage RJ, Conley ME, et al: CD40 ligand gene defects responsible for X-linked hyper-IgM syndrome. *Science* 259(5097):990–993, 1993.
13. Leadbetter EA, Rifkin IR, Hohlbaum AM, et al: Chromatin-IgG complexes activate B cells by dual engagement of IgM and Toll-like receptors. *Nature* 416(6881):603–607, 2002.
14. Inaba K, Witmer-Pack M, Inaba M, et al: The tissue distribution of the B7-2 costimulator in mice: abundant expression on dendritic cells in situ and during maturation in vitro. *J Exp Med* 180(5):1849–1860, 1994.
15. Shlomchik MJ, Aucoin AH, Pisetsky DS, et al: Structure and function of anti-DNA autoantibodies derived from a single autoimmune mouse. *Proc Natl Acad Sci USA* 84(24):9150–9154, 1987.
16. Crotty S: T follicular helper cell differentiation, function, and roles in disease. *Immunity* 41(4):529–542, 2014.
17. Watanabe-Fukunaga R, Brannan CI, Copeland NG, et al: Lymphoproliferation disorder in mice explained by defects in Fas antigen that mediates apoptosis. *Nature* 356(6367):314–317, 1992.
18. Suda T, Takahashi T, Golstein P, et al: Molecular cloning and expression of the Fas ligand, a novel member of the tumor necrosis factor family. *Cell* 75(6):1169–1178, 1993.
19. Tivol EA, Borriello F, Schweitzer AN, et al: Loss of CTLA-4 leads to massive lymphoproliferation and fatal multiorgan tissue destruction, revealing a critical negative regulatory role of CTLA-4. *Immunity* 3(5):541–547, 1995.
20. Keir ME, Butte MJ, Freeman GJ, et al: PD-1 and its ligands in tolerance and immunity. *Annu Rev Immunol* 26:677–704, 2008.
21. Zhu J, Yamane H, Paul WE: Differentiation of effector CD4 T cell populations (*). *Annu Rev Immunol* 28:445–489, 2010.
22. Asano M, Toda M, Sakaguchi N, et al: Autoimmune disease as a consequence of developmental abnormality of a T cell subpopulation. *J Exp Med* 184(2):387–396, 1996.
23. Fontenot JD, Gavin MA, Rudensky AY: Foxp3 programs the development and function of CD4+CD25+ regulatory T cells. *Nat Immunol* 4(4):330–336, 2003.

24. Wakeland EK, Liu K, Graham RR, et al: Delineating the genetic basis of systemic lupus erythematosus. *Immunity* 15(3):397–408, 2001.

25. Scally SW, Petersen J, Law SC, et al: A molecular basis for the association of the HLA-DRB1 locus, citrullination, and rheumatoid arthritis. *J Exp Med* 210(12):2569–2582, 2013.

26. Christensen SR, Shupe J, Nickerson K, et al: Toll-like receptor 7 and TLR9 dictate autoantibody specificity and have opposing inflammatory and regulatory roles in a murine model of lupus. *Immunity* 25(3):417–428, 2006.

27. Mueller-Eckhardt C: Post-transfusion purpura. *Br J Haematol* 64(3):419–424, 1986.

28. Lin RH, Mamula MJ, Hardin JA, et al: Induction of autoreactive B cells allows priming of autoreactive T cells. *J Exp Med* 173(6):1433–1439, 1991.

29. Maloney DG, Grillo-Lopez AJ, White CA, et al: IDEC-C2B8 (Rituximab) anti-CD20 monoclonal antibody therapy in patients with relapsed low-grade non-Hodgkin's lymphoma. *Blood* 90(6):2188–2195, 1997.

30. Gurcan HM, Keskin DB, Stern JN, et al: A review of the current use of rituximab in autoimmune diseases. *Int Immunopharmacol* 9(1):10–25, 2009.

PART IV

DISORDERS OF HEMATOPOIETIC CELL DEVELOPMENT

DISORDERS OF HEMATOPOIETIC
CELL DEVELOPMENT

BIOLOGY OF ERYTHROPOIESIS, ERYTHROID DIFFERENTIATION, AND MATURATION

Thalia Papayannopoulou and Anna Rita Migliaccio

The production of erythroid cells is a dynamic and exquisitely regulated process. The mature red cell is the final phase of a complex but orderly series of genetic events that initiates when a multipotent stem cell commits to the erythroid program. Expression of the erythroid program occurs several divisions later in a greatly amplified population of erythroid cells, which have a characteristic form and structure, maturation sequence, and function. These maturing cells are termed *erythroid precursor cells* and *reticulocytes*. Terminally differentiated cells have a finite life span, and they are constantly replenished by influx from earlier compartments of progenitor cells that are irreversibly committed to express the erythroid phenotype. During ontogeny, successive waves of erythropoiesis occur in distinct anatomic sites. Erythroid cells developing in these sites have distinguishable phenotypes and intrinsic programs that are dependent on gestational time and their microenvironment. At each site, erythroid cells are in intimate contact with other cells (e.g., stromal cells, hematopoietic accessory cells, and extracellular matrix) comprising their microenvironment. Within this microenvironment, erythroid development is influenced by cytokines, which are either elaborated by microenvironmental cells or produced elsewhere and then entrapped in the extracellular matrix.

Knowledge of the properties of erythroid progenitor and precursor cells and their complex interactions with the microenvironment is essential for understanding the pathophysiology of erythropoiesis. Aberrations in the generation and/or amplification of fully mature and functional erythroid cells or in the regulatory influences of microenvironmental cells or their cytokines/chemokines form the basis for various clinical disorders, including aplasias, dysplasias, and neoplasias of the erythroid tissue.

ERYTHROID PROGENITOR CELL COMPARTMENT

The erythroid progenitor cell compartment, situated functionally between the multipotent stem cell and the morphologically distinguishable erythroid precursor cells, contains a spectrum of cells with a parent-to-progeny relationship, all committed to erythroid differentiation. A complete understanding of how erythroid commitment is achieved at the biochemical or molecular level is lacking, although some attempts at determining the molecular basis have been made.[1-4] Evidence from in vitro cultures of single multipotent progenitor cells allowed to differentiate in competent environments, as well as evidence obtained by studying the phenotype of leukemic cells, suggests that commitment to a specific hematopoietic lineage is accomplished not by acquisition of new genetic information but by restriction (probably on a stochastic basis) to specific programs from a wider repertoire available to pluripotent progenitor cells.[5,6] Molecular evidence supports this view.[6-8] Although all erythroid progenitor cells share the irreversible commitment to express the erythroid phenotype, the properties of these cells progressively diverge as the cells become separated by several divisions.

Erythroid progenitor cells are sparse (Table 26.1) and difficult to isolate in sufficient purity and numbers for study. For these reasons, the existence and characteristics of these cells were inferred from their ability to generate hemoglobinized progeny in vitro in clonal erythroid cultures (Fig. 26.1). Two classes of progenitors have been identified using this approach.[9] The first, more primitive class consists of the burst-forming unit-erythroid (BFU-E), named for the ability of BFU-E to give rise to multiclustered colonies (erythroid bursts) of hemoglobin-containing cells. BFU-E represent the earliest progenitors committed exclusively to erythroid differentiation and a quiescent reserve, with only 10% to 20% in cycle at any given time. However, once stimulated to proliferate in the presence of appropriate cytokines, BFU-Es demonstrate a significant proliferative capacity in vitro, giving rise to colonies of 30,000 to 40,000 cells, which become fully hemoglobinized after 2 to 4 weeks, with a peak incidence at 14 to 16 days. They have a limited self-renewal capacity; at least a subset of BFU-E is capable of generating secondary bursts upon replating. In contrast to this class of progenitor cells, a second, more differentiated class of progenitors consists of the colony-forming unit–erythroid (CFU-E). Most (60–80%) of these progenitors already are in cycle and thus proliferate immediately after initiation of culture, forming erythroid colonies within 7 days. Because CFU-E are more differentiated than BFU-E, they require fewer divisions to generate colonies of hemoglobinized cells, and the colonies are small (8–64 cells per colony).

Although the two classes of committed erythroid progenitors (BFU-E and CFU-E) appear distinct from each other, in reality progenitor cells constitute a continuum, with graded changes in their properties. Only progenitor cells at both ends of the differentiation spectrum have distinct properties. Perhaps the earliest cell with the potential to generate hemoglobinized progeny is an oligopotent progenitor, which is capable of giving rise to mature cells of at least one other lineage (granulocytic, macrophage, or megakaryocytic) in addition to the erythroid. This progenitor, a multilineage colony-forming unit (CFU) called a *colony-forming unit-granulocyte, erythrocyte, macrophage, megakaryocyte* (CFU-GEMM) or *common myeloid progenitor,* and the most primitive BFU-E have physical and functional properties that are shared by both pluripotent stem cells and progenitor cells committed to nonerythroid lineages. These properties include high proliferative potential, low cycling rate, response to a combination of cytokines, and presence of specific surface antigens or surface receptors (see Table 26.1). In contrast, the latest CFU-E have many similarities with erythroid precursor cells and little in common with primitive BFU-E. Their proliferative potential is limited, they cannot self-renew, they lack the cell surface antigens common to all early progenitors, and they are exquisitely sensitive to erythropoietin (EPO; see Table 26.1).

Although clonal erythroid cultures are indispensable for the study of erythroid progenitors, they do not faithfully reproduce the in vivo kinetics of red cell differentiation/maturation, and many maturing cells have a megaloblastic appearance and lyse before they reach the end stage of red cell development. In vivo, erythropoiesis probably occurs faster than predicted from culture data. For example, studies in dogs with cyclic hematopoiesis, a genetic stem cell defect leading to pulses of hematopoiesis, provide evidence that BFU-E mature to CFU-E over 2 to 3 days in vivo, although this process may require 5 to 6 days in canine marrow cultures.[14]

Erythroid progenitors can be cultured in serum-depleted media,[15,16] as well as in serum-containing media. The effects of recombinant growth factors can be studied in serum-depleted cultures without the complicating influences of multiple or unknown factors present in serum. Conditions that imitate lower oxygen pressures, found in

TABLE 26.1   Changes in General Properties During the Differentiation of Erythroid Progenitors

	CFU-GEMM (CMP)	BFU-E	CFU-E		CFU-GEMM (CMP)	BFU-E	CFU-E
General Features				HLA-DR (-DP, -DQ)	++	++	+
Self-renewal	++	+	0	EPO receptor	+	+	++
Differentiation potential	Multipotent	Erythroid committed	Erythroid committed	gp130	+	+	+
Cycling status % suicide with ^{3}H thymidine	15–20	30–40	60–80	Tumor necrosis factor receptor	+	+	++
				P67 laminin	–	+	–
Cell density (g/mL)	<1.077	<1.077	<1.077	EP-1[12]	+	+	++
Incidence/10^5 cells	2–5	40–120	200–600	23.6[a]	0	0	+
Circulate in blood	+	+	0	CD36	0	±	+
Growth Factor Response				Glycophorin A	0	0	+
EPO	+	+	++	ABH, Ii[b]	0	+	+
TPO	+	+	+	**Adhesion Molecules**			
KL	+	+	–	VLA4 (CD49d/CD29)	++	++	++
GM-CSF, IL-3	+	+	–	VLA5 (CD49e/CD29)	+	+	+
FL	+	0	0	CD41	+	+	
G-CSF, IL-6, IL-1	+	0	0	CD11a/CD18	+	+	
Insulin, insulin-like growth factor, activin	0	0	+	CD44	+	+	+
				HCAM[c]	+	+	
TGF-β1	–	–	++	**Transcription Factors**			
Hyper-IL-6	+	+	+	GATA2	++	+	–
Receptor/Antigen				GATA1	+	++	+++
CD34	++	++	–	SCL	+	+	+
CD33	+	+	0	EKLF	+	+	++
C-KIT	++	++	–	Myb	++	+	–
				Id1, Id2	++	+	–

[a]23.6 (SFL 23.6) is a monoclonal antibody reactive with CFU-E, erythroblasts, and erythrocytes.[13]
[b]ABH and Ii are blood group antigens.
[c]Presence of other cytoadhesion molecules (i.e., CD31, L-selectin, P-selectin, E-cadherin) has been described in progenitors (see text). However, the extent of their presence in BFU-E as compared to other cells is not clear.
BFU-E, Burst-forming unit-erythroid; CFU-E, colony-forming unit-erythroid; CFU-GEMM (CMP), colony-forming unit-granulocyte, erythrocyte, macrophage, megakaryocyte (common myeloid progenitor); EKLF, erythroid Krüppel-like factor; EPO, erythropoietin; FL, Flt-3 ligand; G-CSF, granulocyte colony-stimulating factor; GM-CSF, granulocyte-macrophage colony-stimulating factor; HCAM, homing-associated cytoadhesion molecule; HLA, human leukocyte antigen; IL, interleukin; KL, KIT ligand; SCL, stem cell leukemia; TGF, transforming growth factor; TPO, thrombopoietin.

bone marrow in vivo, favorably influence erythroid development in culture and may be advantageous.[17]

BFU-E are generated from multipotent or oligopotent progenitors within the marrow, and their survival and proliferation are dependent on the presence of cytokines, elaborated by either stromal cells or accessory cells within the microenvironment. A number of cytokines influence proliferation and/or survival of early progenitors. Among the cytokines, KIT ligand (KL, also known as *stem cell factor* [SCF]), which is produced by stromal cells, and interleukin (IL)-3, which is produced by a subset of T cells, alone and in synergy, have a profound proliferative effect on BFU-E and its progeny. Other cytokines, such as granulocyte-macrophage colony-stimulating factor (GM-CSF), IL-11, and thrombopoietin (TPO), stimulate a subset of BFU-E.[18–20] Cytokines exert their effects through interaction with specific receptors present on the BFU-E surface. The presence of such receptors also has been documented in the leukemic counterparts of normal BFU-E and in leukemic cell lines.[21] BFU-E in culture cannot survive for more than a few days in the absence of cytokines. If they are deprived of cytokines for more than 6 days, more than 80% of BFU-E are lost.[22] In addition to positive regulators (IL-3, GM-CSF, TPO, KL, and IL-11), substances with negative influences on BFU-E proliferation have been identified. They include tumor necrosis factor-α (TNF-α), tumor necrosis factor–related apoptosis-inducing ligand (TRAIL),

transforming growth factor-β (TGF-β), and interferon-γ (IFN-γ).[23–25] These negative regulators are responsible, at least in part, for the anemia associated with chronic inflammatory states. The effects of TNF-α and TRAIL are mediated through induction of apoptosis at specific stages of erythroid maturation. In the case of TRAIL, a complex system of signaling and decoy receptor isoforms determines the precise cell window susceptible to TRAIL-induced apoptosis.[25] TRAIL probably induces apoptosis by competing with EPO for activation of Bruton tyrosine kinase. Its effects are counteracted by KL[26,27] and protein kinase Cε[28] signaling. TRAIL is also involved in the pathobiology of the anemia associated with multiple myeloma (TRAIL is overproduced by the malignant plasma cells of these patients[29]) and myelodysplastic syndrome (MDS) (myelodysplastic erythroid progenitors overexpress the adaptor Fas-associated death domain of the TRAIL receptor[30]). On the other hand, the negative effects of TGF-β[31] are mainly achieved by accelerating cell differentiation, whereas data on mouse models of chronic exposure indicate that IFN-γ reduces the erythrocyte life span and inhibits erythropoiesis by promoting the expression of PU.1, a transcription factor that antagonizes GATA1, a master transcriptional regulator of erythropoiesis[32,33] (see Transcription Factors in Erythropoiesis).

In addition to the negative growth factors, overexpression of hepcidin, a key regulator of systemic iron homeostasis (see

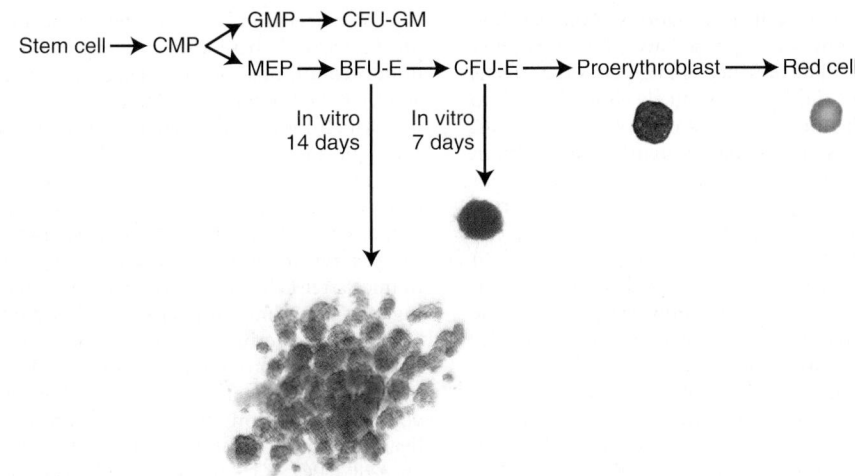

Fig. 26.1 CELLULAR MODEL OF ERYTHROID DIFFERENTIATION. Multipotent stem cells generate cellular compartments defined on the basis of their antigenic profile and restricted toward the myeloid differentiation pathway-defined common myeloid progenitor (CMP).[10,11] CMP in turn gives rise to granulocyte/macrophage progenitor (GMP) and megakaryocyte-erythroid progenitor (MEP), which probably correspond to the burst-forming unit-erythroid (BFU-E). Lastly, MEP generate cells capable of unilineage differentiation toward either the megakaryocytic (colony-forming unit-megakaryocyte [CFU-Mk], not shown) or the erythroid pathway (colony-forming unit-erythroid [CFU-E]). These cells occur infrequently in the marrow (approximately 0.3% of mononuclear cells) and are defined on the basis of clonogenic assays. If marrow is placed in semisolid medium (e.g., methylcellulose) to decrease cell motility, with appropriate nutrients and growth factors (e.g., transferrin, insulin, erythropoietin, and interleukin-3), CFU-E (after approximately 7 days) differentiate into small clusters of hemoglobinized or red cells termed *erythroid colonies*. Most BFU-E present in the inoculum differentiate to form multiclustered colonies of hemoglobinized cells, or erythroid bursts, by days 14 to 16. Each erythroid colony or burst derives from one BFU-E or CFU-E, respectively. *CFU-GM,* Colony-forming unit-granulocyte-macrophage.

Chapters 35 and 36), is involved in determining the anemia associated with chronic inflammation.[34] The increased hepcidin synthesis that occurs during inflammation traps iron in macrophages, decreases plasma iron concentrations, and causes iron-restricted erythropoiesis characteristic of the anemia of inflammatory states. Hepcidin deficiency induces iron overload in transgenic mice, whereas hepcidin excess induces iron accumulation in macrophages similar to observations in patients with chronic inflammation.[35] Hepcidin might inhibit proliferation of erythroid progenitors at low EPO concentrations.[36] The stringent need for iron during erythroid maturation led Dr. Clement Finch to first hypothesize the existence of signals released by mature erythroid cells that controls iron metabolism. This hypothesis has been recently confirmed by the identification of erythroferrone (ERFE), a protein released by erythroid cells that suppresses hepcidin expression in mice under conditions of stress.[37] ERFE-deficient mice fail to suppress hepcidin after hemorrhage and exhibit a delayed recovery after blood loss. Data in additional mouse models suggest that ERFE also contributes to recovery from anemia after inflammation.[38]

BFU-E and immediate progeny (but not CFU-E) are motile cells found in significant numbers in peripheral blood. As with BFU-E, the ability of stem cells and progenitor cells to circulate is physiologically important for the redistribution of marrow cells in cases of local damage to the microenvironment and for reconstitution of hematopoiesis after transplantation. The spectrum of BFU-E in circulation probably is narrower (consisting mostly of early, quiescent BFU-E) than that of BFU-E in the bone marrow; otherwise, their properties are similar to those of marrow BFU-E. The number of circulating BFU-E (along with other progenitors and stem cells) can increase to significant levels after cytokine/chemokine treatments and after chemotherapy, a finding that has been exploited for transplantation purposes.[39] At present, mononuclear cells contained in the blood from subjects mobilized with granulocyte colony-stimulating factor (G-CSF) are routinely used as a source of stem/progenitor cells in autologous and allogeneic transplantation,[40] alone or in combination with AMD3100, a CXCR4 inhibitor.[41] In addition to forming colonies in semisolid medium, hematopoietic progenitors from different sources can generate erythroid cells in liquid culture.[42] Liquid cultures do not allow progenitor cell enumeration but may generate more differentiated cells per progenitor cell than do semisolid cultures.[43,44] The number of erythroblasts generated in liquid cultures can be further increased by adding to the media glucocorticoid steroids,[43,45] which exert a reversible inhibition on proerythroblast maturation.[46,47] In theory this culture system may generate numbers of erythroid cells equivalent to 1 unit of blood from discarded stem cell sources (cord blood <50 mL and from buffy coats produced during the leukoreduction process of blood donations).[48–50] This recognition led to the belief that red blood cells generated ex vivo may one day be used for transfusion. Recently it has been demonstrated that red blood cells generated in vitro from mobilized CD34[pos] cells collected by apheresis have normal survival when transfused into an autologous recipient.[51] Although production of red blood cells in numbers required for transfusion is currently a challenging proposition (approximately 2.5 × 10^{12}), this first-in-man proof-of-principle has fostered great interest in studies addressing the various aspects of the complex process of making red blood cells in vitro to ultimately translate this approach into clinical transfusion practice.

Surface antigens of human BFU-E have been defined through the use of monoclonal antibodies.[52,53] The antibodies tested include two broad categories: antibodies raised against leukemic cells or cell lines with progenitor cell properties, and antibodies raised against normal, terminally differentiated red cells. Enrichment in BFU-E (or CFU-E) after labeling with these antibodies, or their loss after complement-dependent lysis, is considered indicative of the presence of test antigens on the BFU-E surface. Reactivities of BFU-E with several antibodies directed against defined surface antigens are listed in Table 26.1. Like other hematopoietic progenitors, BFU-E display human leukocyte antigen (HLA) class I (A, B, C) and class II (DP, DQ, DR) antigens on their surface. Class II antigens (especially the products of the DR locus), in contrast to class I, are variably expressed among BFU-E. This may relate to variations in their cycling status, because myeloid progenitors in S phase have relatively higher expression of class II antigens.[54] The presence of HLA class II antigens (DR and, to a lesser extent, DP and DQ) most likely allows BFU-E to recognize and interact with the immunoregulatory cells (e.g., T cells, monocytes), which also express class II determinants.[55] In addition to HLA antigens, several other antigenic structures are found on cells within the BFU-E compartment (see Table 26.1). The best representative of these is the CD34 antigen, which has been successfully exploited for isolation of BFU-E and other progenitors. CD34 is a highly O-glycosylated cell surface glycoprotein. It is expressed in all hematopoietic progenitors and vascular endothelial cells.[56] The role of CD34 in human hematopoiesis is not clearly defined. The numbers of all hematopoietic progenitors were reduced in CD34 "null" murine embryos and adult animals, but no other abnormalities were identified.[57] Expression of CD34 was low or absent in a population of adult long-term repopulating cells in mouse[58] and in man.[59] However, the clinical significance of this finding is not clear because of the fluctuating expression of CD34[60] and the difference in regulatory mechanisms of CD34 gene expression in mouse and human stem cells.[61] Furthermore, use of antibodies or conjugated ligands determined that BFU-E present in enriched progenitor preparations display receptors for KL, EPO, TPO, GM-CSF, IL-3, IL-6, and IL-11. However, the majority of BFU-E, in contrast to myeloid progenitors (colony-forming unit–granulocyte-macrophage [CFU-GM]), do not express the restricted hematopoietic phosphatase CD45RA.[62,63] Furthermore, BFU-E appears to share with late colony-forming unit–megakaryocyte (CFU-Mk) progenitors the expression of the TPO receptor (c-Mpl or TPO-R)[63,64] and glycoprotein IIb/IIIa (CD41), a marker of the divergence between definitive hematopoiesis and endothelial cells during development.[65,66]

As BFU-E mature to the CFU-E stage, they begin to express surface proteins characteristic of erythroblasts, the morphologically recognizable erythroid cells. For example, CFU-E expresses Rh antigens and the erythroid-specific sialoglycoprotein glycophorin A. Blood group antigens of the ABH Ii type are detectable in a subset of CFU-E. In contrast, CD34 molecules, class II antigens, and certain growth factor receptors (i.e., IL-3R, C-KIT) are greatly diminished or virtually absent at the CFU-E stage (see Table 26.1). The most important functional difference between BFU-E and CFU-E is the abundance of erythropoietin receptors (EPORs) on CFU-E and their dependence on EPO for cell survival. CFU-E, in contrast to BFU-E, cannot survive in vitro even for a few hours in the absence of EPO. Although greater than 80% of CFU-E have detectable EPORs,[67] only a small proportion of BFU-E have receptors[68,69] and can terminally differentiate in culture in the presence of EPO alone.[70] Direct binding studies show that the number of EPORs peaks at the CFU-E/proerythroblast level and progressively declines when cells mature further (see Table 26.1),[67] reflecting the declining influence of EPO. In addition to the abundance of EpoRs, erythroid progenitors are distinguished from other marrow progenitors by the presence of high levels of transferrin receptors (TfRs).[68,71,72] Peak levels of TfRs are seen on CFU-E and erythroid precursors, and lower levels are present on reticulocytes.[64,71] (For a detailed review of iron metabolism and heme synthesis in erythroid cells, see references 73–75).

In addition to the functional definition, the hemopoietic compartments in the marrow of a normal adult mouse have been prospectively identified on the basis of expression of specific cell surface antigens and subsequent differentiation in vitro and in vivo.[10] The Lin^neg IL-7R^neg Thy1^neg C-KIT^pos Sca1^neg fraction of the marrow of normal adult mice has been subdivided into three populations based on the expression of CD34 and CD16/CD32: CD16/CD32^low CD34^high representing the common myeloid progenitor (CMP), CD16/CD32^low CD34^low representing the megakaryocyte/erythroid progenitor (MEP), and CD16/CD32^high CD34^high representing the granulocyte/macrophage progenitor (see Fig. 26.1).[10] Many laboratories have also prospectively identified the corresponding human compartments.[11,76,77] In humans, the transition from CMP to MEP is characterized by loss of aldehyde dehydrogenase activity[78] and acquisition of c-Mpl expression.[79]

The correlation between phenotype and function of cells isolated on the basis of these antigenic expression profiles is not maintained under conditions of perturbed or stressed erythropoiesis. Stress activates the bone morphologic protein 4 (BMP4)/Hedgehog signaling, which induces the generation of erythroid progenitor cells with a unique phenotype, KIT^pos, CD71^pos, and TER-119^pos (TER-119 recognizes the murine equivalent of glycophorin A).[80,81] The expression on these cells of "true" markers of terminal erythroid maturation suggests that stress-specific erythroid progenitors may be related to the proerythroblasts with extensive proliferative potential generated in mice after EPO treatment or anemia challenge,[82,83] thereby indicating that stress may uncouple proliferation and differentiation programs during terminal erythroid maturation. The proliferation and differentiation programs are also during ontogenesis. The number of erythroblasts generated in vitro by embryonic/primitive (E7.5 yolk sac), embryonic/definitive (E8.5-9.5 yolk sac and E12.5 fetal liver), and adult/definitive murine erythroid progenitors in the presence of EPO, KL, and dexamethasone differ widely.[84] Embryonic/definitive proerythroblasts originating from a transient wave of early fetal erythropoiesis are capable of generating large numbers (10^{10}- to 10^{30}-fold expansion) of proerythroblasts that, because of their great expansion potential, were characterized as extensively self-renewing erythroblasts (ESREs). By contrast, under the same conditions, embryonic/primitive proerythroblasts failed to expand and adult/definitive proerythroblasts expanded only 10^2- to 10^5-fold. Interestingly, human erythroblasts generated in the presence of dexamethasone also express high levels of C-KIT and acquire self-renewal potential.[85] In addition to steroids, polymeric immunoglobulin A1 (IgA1) has also been shown to control erythroblast proliferation and to accelerate erythropoiesis recovery in anemia.[86] These observations challenge the notion that erythroblasts are capable of a limited (at most two to four) number of divisions.

More recently, erythroid cells have been derived in vitro from stem cell sources with unlimited proliferation potential such as human embryonic stem cells (hESCs) and induced pluripotent stem cells (iPSCs).[87] Seminal studies in 2008 from Hiroyama et al established that red blood cells generated from murine ESCs are functional in vivo because they protect mice from lethal hemolytic anemia.[88] Methods for generating red blood cells from hESCs have also been published, and the biologic properties of these hESC-derived red blood cells have been extensively characterized.[89,90] A number of groups have also published methods for generating red blood cells from iPSCs.[91,92] In general, independently of their origin, ESC- or iPS-derived erythroid cells express mostly embryonic and fetal globins. In addition, several investigators are exploring the feasibility of reprogramming somatic cells directly into erythroid cells, bypassing the pluripotent state and/or generating stem cells with unlimited expansion potential by epigenetic or genetic in vitro treatments.[93,94] In both cases, the modified cells generated erythroblasts that mature into circulating red cells when injected into immunodeficient NOD/SCID/γc^null mice.

ERYTHROID MORPHOLOGICALLY RECOGNIZABLE PRECURSOR CELL COMPARTMENT

The erythroid precursor cell compartment, also termed the *erythron*, includes cells that, in contrast to the erythroid progenitor cells (BFU-E and CFU-E), are defined by morphologic criteria. The earliest recognizable erythroid cell is the *proerythroblast*, which after four to five mitotic divisions and serial morphologic changes gives rise to mature erythroid cells. Its progeny include basophilic erythroblasts, which are the earliest daughter cells, followed by polychromatophilic and orthochromatic erythroblasts. Their morphologic characteristics reflect the accumulation of erythroid-specific proteins (i.e., hemoglobin) and the decline in nuclear activity (Fig. 26.2). The last mitotic division involves elimination of unwanted organelles (mitochondria, ribosomes and other intracytoplasmic organelles) by the autophagic machinery,[95] intense membrane trafficking,[96] and asymmetric partitioning of the remaining cell components between two morphologically distinct daughter cells: one nucleated, the pyrenocyte, and one

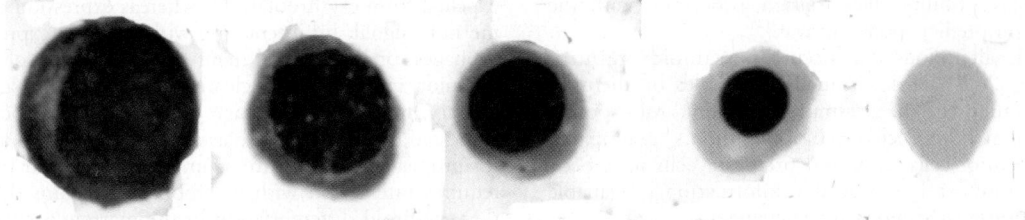

Fig. 26.2 ERYTHROID MATURATION SEQUENCE. As proliferation parameters (i.e., rates of deoxyribonucleic acid [DNA] and ribonucleic acid [RNA] synthesis) and cell size decrease, accumulation of erythroid-specific proteins (i.e., heme and globin) increases, and the cells adapt their morphologic characteristics. *(Modified from Granick S, Levere R: Heme synthesis in erythroid cells. In Moore CV, Brown EB, editors: Progress in hematology, Vol 4, Orlando, FL, 1964, Grune & Stratton, p 1.)*

enucleated, the reticulocyte. During this last mitosis, the inactive dense nucleus of the orthochromatic erythroblast moves to one side of the cell and is extruded, encased by a thin cytoplasmic layer, the pyrenocyte that is ingested by marrow macrophages. By contrast, the majority of the cytoplasm and plasma proteins form the reticulocyte that is released in the blood stream to further mature into red blood cell. Although all mammals have enucleated cells in their circulation, the evolutionary advantage of enucleation is not readily apparent. It may allow for more red cell deformability when traveling through the small vasculature, or it may minimize cardiac workload.

Maturation from proerythroblast to reticulocyte likely does not always adhere to a rigid sequence in which each division is associated with the production of two more differentiated and morphologically distinct daughter cells (i.e., basophilic erythroblast gives rise to two polychromatophilic ones). Rather, significant flexibility, both in the number and rate of divisions and in the rate of enucleation, may be allowed. Such deviations from the normal orderly maturation sequence may be dictated by the level of EPO or "stress" conditions. Thus in cases of acute demand for red cell production (because of blood loss or hemolysis), the kinetics of formation of new reticulocytes are significantly more rapid. Resulting red cells may be larger (i.e., with increased mean corpuscular volume). This has led to the concept of "skipped" divisions.[97] The orderly unilineage differentiation pathway shown in Fig. 26.1 is likely restricted to conditions of steady-state hematopoiesis. Similar to occurrences in the lymphoid system,[98] alternative routes are taken under conditions of "stress." Murine models have been developed to address phenotype-function cell relationships during recovery from acute and chronic erythroid stress. A model for acute stress is represented by the hemolytic anemia induced by phenylhydrazine treatment. Recovery from this acute anemia involves recruitment of the spleen as an additional erythropoietic site and is dependent on EPO. The amount of ^{3}H-thymidine incorporated by splenic erythroblasts produced in response to this stress initially represented the biologic assay for EPO.[99] Genetic evidence indicates that recovery from this hemolytic anemia is controlled by a receptor complex formed between the EPOR and a truncated version of the Stk receptor encoded by Fv2[s], a locus that also determines strain susceptibility to Friend virus infection.[100] An additional control on the response to acute erythroid stress in mice is exerted by the glucocorticoid receptor (GR), because mice in which this receptor is targeted recover poorly from phenylhydrazine treatment.[101] On the other hand, experimentally induced mutations in genes involved in the regulation of erythroid differentiation, such as signal transducer and activator of transcription 5 (STAT5[null100]) and GATA1[LOW101], or inability of response to reactive oxygen species (ROS) challenge (i.e., Foxo3 deficiency)[102] increase the rate of erythroblast apoptosis. The spleen is also recruited as a hemopoietic site in response to chronic erythroid stress.[103,104] Several studies in aggregate suggest that the erythron does not respond to stress only by amplifying the normal erythroid progenitor cell compartments (i.e., CMP, MEP, and CFU-E), but by generating alternative routes of differentiation, possibly through cooperation between EPOR and other receptors (e.g., Stk, GR, soluble KL, BMP4/Hedgehog pathway) specifically

recruited as part of the stress response.[82,83,105,106] Genetic heterogeneity in the control of gene expression of these receptors may add another layer of variability in recovery from anemia in humans.

The importance of GR in the control of stress erythropoiesis was established by studies in transgenic mice harboring a dimerization-defective GR (GR[dim/dim] mice).[107] These mice have normal steady-state erythropoiesis but were unable to increase red blood cell production in response to hypoxia. Gene deletion studies established that GR facilitates stress erythropoiesis in mice by blocking maturation of erythroid precursors and inducing a limited self-renewal state.[108] Although clinical observations indicating that the GR ligand such as dexamethasone stimulates erythropoiesis have been available since 1961,[109,110] the precise role of GR in human erythropoiesis is still unclear. Murine GR is not polymorphic, whereas human GR (GR/NR3C1 located in the 5q31-32 region of chromosome 5 and deleted in 5q-syndrome) contains several single-nucleotide polymorphisms (SNPs).[111–114] Because of this genetic diversity, human cells may express more than 260 isoforms with slightly or greatly different biologic activities. The most studied isoform is GRα, an isoform similar to the murine GR. Alternative splicing between exon 3-4 generates GRγ, an isoform containing an additional arginine in the DNA-binding domain that reduces the transactivation potential by half. An alternative splicing of exon 9 generates messenger RNA (mRNA) encoding the dominant-negative GRβ isoform.[114] It is debatable whether an isoform with dominant-negative action similar to GRβ exists in mice.[112,115] It is generally accepted that responses to GR ligands depend on the signal transduction potential of the GR isoforms expressed by different cells and tissues. Studies in human nonerythroid cell types have identified that GR isoform expression predicts the variegation of cellular response to dexamethasone in vitro.[116–118] Recently clinicians have established important correlations between GR haplotype and variability in patients' responses to glucocorticoids and in the development of glucocorticoid resistance in several disorders.[119] GR polymorphism and/or epigenetic changes are emerging as the leading cause for dexamethasone unresponsiveness or for development of dexamethasone resistance in patients with inflammatory and autoimmune diseases[120] (i.e., Crohn disease, systemic lupus) and in chronic depression.[119,121–123]

Similarly, several in vitro and in vivo studies suggest that variegation of GR isoform expression may also have biologic and clinical effects on terminal erythroid maturation. The numbers of erythroblasts generated by murine erythroid progenitors in response to dexamethasone is fairly consistent, whereas the number generated by human erythroid progenitors from different individuals may vary by 1 to 2 logs,[45,49] likely reflecting the genetic background of human GR. In addition, the frequency of the rs6198 SNP is greater than normal in patients with the Philadelphia-negative myeloproliferative neoplasm polycythemia vera (PV) (55%, $p = .0028$)[124] and primary myelofibrosis[125] and with Diamond-Blackfan anemia (DBA) (43%, $p = .03$),[124] suggesting that genetic conditions favoring GRβ expression may represent host genetic modifiers in diseases with altered terminal erythroid differentiation. A retrospective analysis of 499 patients with primary myelofibrosis (PMF) indicated that the rs6198

SNP represents a susceptibility allele that in association with the *JAK2*V617F mutation predicts poor survival.[125]

The morphologic alterations that occur as erythroid precursor cells mature (see Fig. 26.2) are determined by complex biochemical changes, which accommodate the accumulation of erythroid-specific proteins and the progressive decline in proliferation.[126] Compared with erythroid progenitor cells, erythroid precursor cells have been more accessible to study, and considerable information is available about their maturation-related biochemical changes.

The shape and deformability of the red cells are determined by the appropriate assembly of their membrane proteins with the cytoplasmic cytoskeleton. Red cells survive shear forces in the microvasculature because transmembrane complexes embedded in the lipid bilayer attach to the cytoskeleton, ensuring its flexibility. These complexes contain clinically relevant blood group antigens determined by genetic polymorphisms in proteins of these complexes.[127-129] The similarity between the amino acid sequence of the blood group antigens and that of proteins present on the surface of bacteria and the increased frequency of certain blood group antigens in regions with high incidence of malaria suggest that blood group antigens, in addition to ensuring appropriate membrane structure, may facilitate development of appropriate immunoreactivity toward opportunistic infections.

Most membrane cytoskeletal proteins (spectrin, glycophorin, band 3, band 4.1, and ankyrin) accumulate after the CFU-E stage (i.e., within the precursor cell compartment). Specifically, expression of membrane glycoproteins such as band 3 and band 4.1 is greatly enhanced at the later stages of erythroid maturation.[126,130,131] Likewise, the quantity of polylactosaminoglycan, a specific carbohydrate chain that carries blood group ABH and Ii antigenic determinants, is much higher in mature erythrocytes than in erythroblasts.[132] Whereas a linear, virtually unbranched polylactosamine structure is present in fetal and newborn erythroid cells (reflected by i antigenic reactivity), a branched polylactosaminyl structure is present in adult erythroblasts (reflected by I antigenic reactivity), and branching increases further as maturation progresses.[132,133] A correctly assembled cytoskeleton is important for the deformability and dynamic plasticity of red blood cells in circulation. A recently recognized player required for actin assembly in red cells, Rac GTPase, has been identified.[134] Glycophorins, especially glycophorin A, are expressed fully at the CFU-E or proerythroblast level just before expression of globin, and few changes occur during maturation.[53] In contrast, the membrane glycoproteins p105 and p95 decline during the later stages of maturation,[132] and yet other membrane glycoproteins, such as vimentin (an intermediate filament protein), are totally lost.[126] Loss of vimentin expression at the late erythroblastic stages most likely facilitates enucleation.

The process of erythroblast enucleation involves membrane remodeling,[96] chromatin condensation to form pyknotic nuclei, and formation of spindle-independent motors driving the separation of the reticulocyte from the pyrenocyte.[135] Partitioning of erythroblast plasma membrane components to reticulocytes is regulated by the degree of skeletal linkage[136] and by the Coimbra domain of band 3.[137] In fact, red cells from patients with homozygous band 3 Coimbra express reduced levels of multiple cell surface antigens which are all rescued in vitro by forced expression of normal band 3. Chromatin condensation may require DNA demethylation, since with maturation the total methylation state of the DNA greatly decreases down to barely detectable levels[138] and is mediated by the histone deacetylase (HDAC) 2,[139] suggesting that impairment of HDAC2 activity may contribute to the development of anemia observed in HDAC-based cancer treatments.

Nonmuscle myosin appears to represent the motor driving the separation between the reticulocyte and the pyrenocyte.[140] Reticulocytes are released in the blood, where they undergo extensive cytoplasmic remodeling to reduce the number of ribosomes and mitochondria and to become mature red cells. This process is mediated by autophagic machinery,[141] whereas engulfment of pyrenocytes, and subsequent degradation by macrophages, occurs only after pyrenocytes are totally disconnected from reticulocytes. Phosphatidylserine, the "eat me" flag for apoptotic cells, is also used for engulfment of pyrenocytes

expelled from erythroblasts,[142] whereas expression of CD47, the "eat me not" signal, by interacting with SIRP1α expressed by the macrophages, prevents engulfment and destruction of erythroblasts and reticulocytes.[143] The enucleation process is caspase independent[144] but erythroblast macrophage protein (EMP) dependent.[145] EMP is expressed by both erythroblasts and macrophages, and it is necessary for proper enucleation to occur.[145] The fact that proper enucleation requires interaction with macrophages explains the old observation that erythroid differentiation in the marrow occurs in discrete sites, the "erythroblastic islands," which are composed of erythroblasts surrounding a central macrophage. Presence of molecules enhancing adherence of erythroblasts to central macrophages are thought to be important mediators of the interaction of erythroblasts with macrophages. Several of these molecules have been described and summarized in recent reviews.[146-149] Among these are the VLA4 interacting with VCAM-1, the ICAM-4 on erythroblasts interacting with αv and α4 on macrophages, the CD163 on macrophages serving as the Hb-Hp binding receptor, or the Palladin on Macrophages with an unclear counter receptor on erythroblasts. In addition, direct contact soluble factors are secreted by macrophages and these may serve as either positive or negative regulators of erythroblast proliferation. Data from in vitro models of human stress erythropoiesis indicated that glucocorticoids may induce the generation of a "unique" macrophage that interacts with multiple erythroblasts, leading to the formation of "transient erythroblast islands" that promote erythroid proliferation instead of maturation (Falchi et al[150] and Video 26.1).

In addition to quantitative changes that occur during maturation, gradual switches in subunit composition of some cytoskeletal proteins occur. For example, exclusively erythroid subunits of α- and β-spectrin are displayed only in end-stage cells.[57] Likewise, multiple transcripts of ankyrin or protein 4.1 have been identified, and the ratios of these transcripts change during maturation.[151] Initial expression of many of these membrane components likely begins at the progenitor cell level. However, in these cells, final assembly may be discouraged because of the higher turnover of these proteins, which minimizes mutual interactions, or because of asynchrony in protein synthesis. Prevention of cytoskeletal assembly at these early stages may secure more membrane fluidity and cell motility needed during this proliferative phase of differentiation. Because molecular probes for many of the red cell cytoskeletal components have been developed, detailed information about the transcription and processing of most of these proteins is beginning to emerge.[131] For example, band 3, the major anion transport protein of human erythrocytes, is a key component of a multicomplex that also contains protein 4.2. Appropriate display of this protein complex on the cell membrane is dependent on critical interactions established between newly synthesized band 3 and protein 4.2 already at the proerythroblast stage.[152]

Expression of the majority of genes encoding cytoskeletal components is not restricted to red cells. Dissecting hemopoietic from nonhemopoietic consequences of abnormalities in these genes has been difficult, but the development of mouse models that mimic defects found in human diseases has been helpful in this respect.[153]

Gene activity during erythroid maturation is dominated by globin expression. Globin represents less than 0.1% of protein at the proerythroblast level but constitutes 95% of all protein at the reticulocyte level.[154] Globin expression has been extensively studied, and its gene regulation is well understood in molecular terms. Major steps in globin transcription and processing are known in considerable detail and are summarized elsewhere in this text (see Chapter 33). The globin type synthesized by adult precursors is hemoglobin A (HbA; $\alpha_2\beta_2$). In addition, two other minor globin components, HbA2 ($\alpha_2\delta_2$) and HbF ($\alpha_2\gamma_2$), are present. Of significant biologic interest are the low amounts of HbF that continue to be synthesized throughout life.

The small amount of HbF, which is present in all normal individuals, has the following characteristics.[155] (1) It is confined to a small fraction of red cells, called *F cells*, which are detected by sensitive immunofluorescence assays or acid elution techniques and usually constitute 2% to 5% of all red cells. Within each F cell, HbF or γ-globin constitutes 14% to 25% of total globin. (2) The number of F cells is genetically determined, and the gene(s) linked or nonlinked to the β-locus is responsible for F-cell formation. (3) F cells do not display other features of "fetalness" because their membrane components and enzymes are characteristically adult. (4) Synthesis of HbF peaks earlier than that of HbA, so the proportion of HbF is higher in immature cells compared with mature, fully hemoglobinized cells. (5) F cells and cells that contain only HbA are not derived from distinct stem cell populations but from a common adult stem cell. Whether the latter will form F or non-F (i.e., A) cells is determined at the BFU-E level and throughout the CFU-E level.[156] In vitro the great majority of BFU-E have the potential to express HbF, whereas in vivo only a very small proportion of red cells contain HbF. This potential appears to be lost during normal cell differentiation and maturation in vivo. This concept links the potential for HbF expression to the pathway of erythroid differentiation and thus may have implications for interpreting the reactivation of HbF that occurs in adults under diverse circumstances (e.g., after chemotherapy or with acute bleeding).[155] Many of these circumstances seem to influence HbF levels by directly or indirectly modifying the kinetics of the normal differentiation/maturation process,[157,158] or the result of changes in stress signaling molecules.[159] HbF levels in red cells can be increased by exposing the cells during maturation to chemical inhibitors of HDAC. This class of enzymes suppresses gene transcription by catalyzing deacetylation of histones, and consequently inducing chromatin condensation, and of transcription factors altering their DNA binding ability.[160] Therefore they can directly activate transcription of γ-globin genes in vitro and in vivo[161-163] and in a number of patients with β-thalassemia.[164,165] Recently new insights have been revealed about transcription factors that are responsible for the physiologic silencing of fetal Hb in adult life. Most prominent among these are BCL11A, KLF1, and c-Myb along with chromatin modifiers. These novel discoveries may be considered as therapeutic targets in the future.[166]

Synthesis of globin appears to be coordinated with synthesis of heme throughout erythroid maturation so that functional hemoglobin tetramers are formed rapidly and spontaneously after release of newly synthesized globins from polysomes. Information about the accumulation of heme and its synthetic intermediaries has been provided by crude biochemical approaches (see Fig. 26.2). However, now that the genes for several enzymes in the heme synthetic pathway (e.g., δ-5-aminolevulinic acid synthase, porphobilinogen deaminase, ferrochelatase) have been cloned, information about their regulation is rapidly emerging.[73,75]

An important role in coordinating heme and globin chain assembly during hemoglobin production is exerted by α-hemoglobin-stabilizing protein (AHSP). AHSP is a protein abundantly expressed in erythroid cells[167] whose function is to bind free α-chains, stabilizing their structure and limiting their ability to participate in chemical reactions that generate ROS.[168,169] In addition, AHSP binding increases the affinity of α-chains for β-chains, accelerating the formation of Hb tetramers. The essential role exerted by this gene in erythroid development has been demonstrated by the fact that its deletion in normal mice impairs red cell production. AHSP[null] red cells have a decreased half-life, contain Hb precipitates, and exhibit signs of oxidative damage.[167] The observation that double AHSP[null] β-thalassemic mutant mice have an exacerbated phenotype[170] suggests that AHSP is a gene modifier that, like the hereditary persistence of HbF mutations, ameliorates the phenotype of thalassemic patients. However, the search for AHSP polymorphisms that might correlate with milder clinical phenotypes in thalassemia has not provided consistent results. Gene mapping, direct genomic sequencing, and extended haplotype analysis did not reveal any mutation or specific association between haplotypes of AHSP in 120 β-thalassemic patients.[171] On the other hand, a polymorphism in the putative AHSP promoter leading to a threefold higher expression of the gene in reticulocytes has been observed in the normal population,[172] but the clinical consequences of this observation are unknown.

Crucial to the functional response of erythroid precursors is the expression of EPORs and TfRs. EPORs decrease progressively (from approximately 1000 to <300 receptors per cell) as proerythroblasts mature, and they are undetectable at the reticulocyte level.[67,173] Through these receptors, EPO exerts its proliferative influence on proerythroblasts and basophilic erythroblasts, but maturation beyond these stages can proceed in the absence of EPO.

TfRs are found in characteristic abundance in erythroid cells (300,000 to 800,000 TfRs per cell).[174] This composition reflects not only the proliferative needs of erythroid cells but also their extreme requirements for iron uptake for hemoglobin synthesis. For this reason, TfRs persist in maturing nondividing erythroblasts and in reticulocytes. TfRs belong to a large group of receptors that internalize their ligand through receptor-mediated endocytosis. This cycle allows for reuse both of the ligand (transferrin) for resaturation with iron and of the receptor for entering another route of endocytosis.[175] The density of TfRs decreases with maturation. After the reticulocyte stage, receptors appear to be shed as small lipid vesicles.[176] An inverse relationship exists between receptor density and iron availability. Deprivation of iron results in receptor induction, and excess iron results in receptor suppression.[175] However, the mechanisms that regulate the number of TfRs throughout the maturation of precursors (even within progenitors) are largely unknown. Erythroid precursor cells differ from nonerythroid cells not only by requiring a higher number and higher occupancy of TfRs, but also by displaying immunologically distinct receptor isoforms.[72] A second gene for transferrin receptor (TfR2) has been identified,[177] and monoclonal antibodies recognizing distinct receptor isoforms are useful in isolating erythroid cells from bone marrow.[12,72] TfR1 and TfR2 are members of a family of genes encoding at least seven different homologous proteins in primates.[178] TfR1 is a type II membrane glycoprotein that, as a cell surface homodimer, binds iron-loaded transferrin as part of the process of iron transfer and uptake. In addition to providing erythroid cells with the much needed iron directly, data in mouse models have recently indicated that expression of TfR1 on erythroid marrow cells may favor iron uptake also indirectly by establishing an ERFE-independent feedback mechanism that suppresses hepcidin expression in the liver.[179] TfR2 is expressed in two forms, membrane-bound (TfR2-α) and nonmembrane (TfR2-β), both of which bind transferrin with low affinity. The specific role of TfR2 in hematopoietic cells is unclear. TfR2 may also play a prominent role in the liver[180] as the key regulator of iron metabolism. In cells from 67 patients with de novo acute myeloid leukemia (AML), high levels of TfR2-α expression were correlated with better prognosis, and higher levels of both TfR2-α and TfR2-β were associated with longer survival, suggesting that TfR-independent iron uptake plays a role in in vivo proliferation of AML cells.[181] Recent data in TfR2-deficient mouse models suggest that this receptor may modulate erythroblast sensitivity to EPO.[182]

Maintenance of stable extracellular iron concentrations requires the coordinated regulation of iron transport into plasma from dietary sources in the duodenum, recycled senescent red cells in macrophages, and storage in hepatocytes. Diferric transferrin is present in the liver because of complex machinery involving the product of the hereditary hemochromatosis (HFE) gene (a protein of the major histocompatibility complex class I), TfR2, and the product of the hemojuvelin (HJV) gene (also known as HFE2). Given that the levels of TfR2 expression are exclusively regulated by holotransferrin, TfR2 expressed by hepatocytes is likely the first element of the iron sensory pathway in the liver.[183] Hepatocytes respond to iron sensing by modulating hepcidin expression and secretion. Hepcidin, a 25-amino acid disulfide-rich peptide, acts as a systemic iron regulatory hormone that regulates both dietary iron absorption by the enterocytes and iron recycling by the macrophages. Because ferroportin shuttles iron from the enterocytes to the macrophages and hepcidin is required for ferroportin internalization and degradation, decreased hepcidin expression blocks iron export in the two cell types.[184] Each gene involved in iron metabolism has a role in regulating the expression of the other genes. In particular, reduced expression of HEF, TfR2, and HJV reduces expression of hepcidin. It is not surprising then that mutations altering the function of all of these genes have been found to be associated with hereditary hemochromatosis. The most prevalent form of hereditary hemo-chromatosis (type 1; HFE1) involves mutations in HFE.[185] Most families with juvenile hemochromatosis (HFE2) have mutations in the *HJV* gene.[186] Homozygous nonsense[187] and single-point muta-tions causing methionine→lysine substitution at position 172 of the protein M172K[188] have been detected in the gene encoding TfR2 in patients with familial hemochromatosis HFE3. Autosomal dominant iron overload is associated with previously unrecognized ferroportin 1 mutations (p.R88T and p.I180T)[189] and with mutations in the divalent metal transporter 1 gene *DMT1*, which mediates apical iron uptake in duodenal enterocytes and iron transfer from the TfR endosomal cycle into the cytosol in erythroid cells.[190] The observation that targeted deletions of any of these genes (including TfR2) induce a hemochromatosis-like syndrome in mice provides proof of direct involvement of the mutations in disease development.[191–194] On the other hand, the finding that hepcidin is a gene modifier of the HEF[null] mouse model of hemochromatosis suggests that heterogeneity at the hepcidin locus mediates the low penetrance of the genetic disease.[195] In addition to its role in determining the pathobiology of hereditary hemochromatosis, hepcidin plays an important role in determining the anemia of chronic diseases. Based on the central involvement of hepcidin in iron regulation and its pathologic conditions, a hepcidin assay has been proposed as a useful tool for diagnosing iron disorders and monitoring their treatment. On the other hand, development of hepcidin agonists and antagonists may provide useful therapeutics for treatment of iron disorders.[196]

The patterns of TfR and glycophorin A expression during erythroid maturation have been exploited to define flow cytometric criteria that distinguish the different populations of erythroid precursors in mice and men. By coupling size and forward scatter (both progres-sively reduced) with CD71 (TfR) and TER-119, murine erythroid precursors were divided into the classes TER-119[med]CD71[high], TER-119[high]CD71[high], TER-119[high]CD71[med], and TER-119[high]CD71[low], which correspond to proerythroblasts and basophilic, chromatophilic, and orthochromatophilic erythroblasts, respectively.[103] However, such distinction is not conserved in all mouse strains. For example, in C57Bl/6 mice, CD71 expression levels remain constant during maturation.[197] CD44/glycophorin A expression provides a better flow cytometric definition of the maturation stage of murine erythro-blasts.[198] Although reduced levels of CD44 do not correlate with the maturation of human erythroblasts, it marks loss of proliferation potential of these cells.[150] Double CD71/glycophorin A staining is therefore still used as criteria to define human erythroblast precursors by flow cytometry. However, the pattern of CD71 expression during erythroid maturation presents a high level of donor variability. Given that downmodulation of CD36 expression during erythroid matura-tion is relatively independent of genetic variability, an alternative flow cytometric definition of erythroblast subclasses is proposed by the phenotype CD36[high]/glycophorin A[medium], CD36[high]/glycophorin A[high], and CD36[low]/glycophorin A[high], corresponding to basophilic, polychromatic, and orthochromatic erythroblasts, respectively.[199] Flow cytometric criteria for reticulocytes and red cells are instead provided by size (reticulocytes and red cells are distinctively smaller than erythroblasts) and by lack of reactivity for DNA (both reticulo-cytes and red cells) and RNA (reticulocyte only) staining.

ERYTHROPOIETIN AND EPOR

EPO, a 35-kDa glycoprotein,[200] is the physiologically obligatory growth factor for erythroid development. It is produced mainly in the kidney by peritubular cells.[201] A heme-containing protein senses oxygen need and then triggers the synthesis of EPO and its release into the bloodstream.[202,203] Through the interaction of EPO with receptor-bearing cells within the bone marrow, physiologic oxygen demands are translated into increased red cell production. Thus EPO is a true hormone, manufactured at one anatomic site and transported through the bloodstream to the site of activity.

According to the prevailing model of hematopoiesis, progeni-tor cells committed to erythroid differentiation (i.e., BFU-E) are generated in a stochastic fashion from pluripotent stem cells.[4,5] Neither EPO nor other lineage-restricted regulators play any role in determining lineage commitment. According to this model, EPO influences erythroid differentiation by rescuing (from apoptosis) cells that express EPOR and amplifying them further. Whether EPORs are present on all BFU-E (detectable only in a subset of BFU-E) is not clear.[69] Thus whether the presence of EPOR in BFU-E is synchronous with the initial commitment event or follows it, is not known. In addition to the permissive role of EPO ascribed by the stochastic theory, experiments in vivo, in anemic states, or after pharmacologic doses of EPO suggest that high levels of EPO hasten the transition from BFU-E to hemoglobin-synthesizing cells by decreasing either the number of divisions required for this transition[97] or the resting periods between cell divisions.[204] Autoradiographic studies of purified BFU-E populations indicate that EPORs increase as BFU-E mature to CFU-E, with the highest level observed at the CFU-E/proeryth-roblast boundary.[69] That the transition from BFU-E to CFU-E occurs under the influence of EPO suggests ligand (EPO)-induced receptor upregulation. Whether the magnitude of such upregulation is dependent on EPO dose and whether it can modulate the rate of entry of these cells into the maturing compartment is unclear.

BFU-E and CFU-E can be generated in vitro[205] and in vivo,[206] in the absence of EPO or EPOR (in EPO or EPOR[null] mice), but their survival and terminal maturation normally are dependent on EPO. For CFU-E, EPO seems to stimulate all the biochemical processes characterizing erythroid cells (i.e., heme synthesis, globin synthesis, and synthesis of cytoskeletal proteins). However, the necessity of EPO in these processes is not absolute. In vitro experiments showing complete maturation of BFU-E in the absence of EPO suggest that other factors or combinations of factors can influence red cell matura-tion. Activation of the gp130 signaling pathway by use of soluble IL-6 receptor and IL-6 leads to full terminal erythroid maturation (in the presence of stem cell factor and IL-3 but in the absence of EPO), suggesting some form of cross-circuiting in signaling pathways among hematopoietic growth factor receptors.[207,208] Furthermore, stimulation by TPO of erythroid colony formation from yolk sac cells in the absence of EPOR (in EPOR[-/-] embryos)[209] can be explained by the same reasoning and the finding of a very high proportion of bipotent erythroid/megakaryocytic progenitors in yolk sac carrying both EPO and TPO receptors (c-Mpl) compared to adult bone marrow.[63,210,211]

Whatever the precise mode of EPO action, it directly affects the number of CFU-E and the maturation of their progeny. This control is achieved by influencing CFU-E survival and not their cycling status.[212] CFU-E are irrevocably lost after one cycle of DNA synthesis if EPO is not present.[213]

With the availability of radiolabeled recombinant EPO and purified or enriched populations of progenitors and precursors, has come information about the characteristics of EPORs in erythroid cells. Direct binding studies have shown that a progressive decrease in the number of EPORs occurs as CFU-E and proerythroblasts mature to reticulocytes.[68,69,173] Pure reticulocyte populations show no detectable binding to EPO. The maturation-associated decline in the number of EPORs parallels the declining influence of EPO on erythroid cells during the terminal phase of maturation. The exquisite role of EPO in determining red cell numbers in the circulation has been clearly established by direct correlations between hematocrit and EPO plasma concentrations in individuals exposed to hypoxia and in patients with compromised kidney functions.[214] However, the variabilities around the mean of hematocrit and EPO plasma levels found in normal individuals under steady-state conditions are not correlated, indicating that other factors (sex and age) cooperate with EPO in determining the fluctuations in red cell mass under steady-state hematopoiesis.[215]

Cloning and expression of EPOR has allowed for a better understanding of the role of EPO in the regulation of erythroid development. The EPOR polypeptide is a 66-kDa membrane protein that is a member of the cytokine receptor superfamily.[216,217] Many of the structural features of the cell surface EPOR have been previously reviewed.[218] Like other members of the cytokine receptor superfamily, which includes the receptors for IL-3, GM-CSF, and IL-5, the EPOR polypeptide contains four conserved cysteine residues and a WSXWS motif in the extracellular region. Additional extracytoplasmic sequences of EPOR determine the specificity for EPO binding. The cytoplasmic region of EPOR does not contain a tyrosine kinase catalytic domain; instead it interacts with cytoplasmic tyrosine kinases. Cross-linking of radiolabeled EPO to cell surface EPOR results in formation of at least two major cross-linked protein complexes of 140 and 120 kDa.[219] The molecular composition of these complexes remains unsolved but suggests that EPOR contains additional subunits or accessory proteins.[220] The extracytoplasmic region of the EPOR polypeptide contains the EPO binding activity of the receptor.[221-223] Therefore additional EPOR subunits may provide other structural and functional elements of the receptor but are not required for high-affinity EPO binding. The extracytoplasmic region of the EPOR polypeptide has been crystalized.[224-226] The crystal structure confirms the dimeric structure of the activated receptor. Interestingly, small synthetic peptides are capable of inducing EPOR dimerization, suggesting a profitable avenue for EPO-mimetic and EPO-antagonist drug design.[227] EPO-mimetic agents are represented by polypeptides restricted to the portion of the protein that binds the receptor, by forms of the protein molecularly engineered to increase its glycosylation state and therefore its stability in vivo, or by dimeric forms of proteins obtained by genetic introduction of bridging sites or chemical cross-linking.[228] It is also possible that nonpeptide chemicals sharing the same stereo and electric properties of the receptor-binding domain of the protein might be identified. As shown for carbamylated EPO, modified isoforms may have biologic activity that partially differs from, and is possibly more effective than, the native protein,[229] especially with regard to the activity of the growth factor in nonhematopoietic tissues.[230] In addition to EPO mimetics, erythroid stimulating agents under development are represented by modulators of HIF-1α expression, IgA2, an immunoglobin that selectively increases under conditions of anemic stress[86] and TGF-β superfamily ligand traps.[231]

EPOR mRNA, originally isolated from murine erythroblast cell lines (MEL and HCD57)[200] and from a human erythroid cell line (OCIM1),[232] has been found in nonerythroid cells as well. EPO promotes the differentiation of megakaryocytes at physiologic concentrations of hormone, suggesting that megakaryocytes have functional cell surface EPORs. Rat and mouse placenta also have cell surface EPOR, detected by radiolabeled EPO cross-linking. EPO promotes a chemotactic effect on endothelial cells,[233,234] suggesting the presence of a cell surface receptor in these cells. Other studies suggest that EPOR is expressed in neural cells[235] and smooth muscle cells.[236] Adverse effects in cancer patients treated with EPO have been attributed to the effects of EPO on tumor cells.[237] The functional importance of EPOR expression in nonerythroid cells has been revealed by rescue experiments in EPOR[null] mice.[238] Because EPOR[null] mutant mice die of severe anemia between days 13 and 15 of embryonic development, the mutant embryos can be rescued by transgenic expression of EPOR under the control of the hemopoietic-specific GATA1 regulatory domain. Under steady-state conditions, the rescued animals are normal, because the gene is expressed only in erythroid cells. However, in comparison with normal mice, the increase in plasma EPO concentration in response to induced anemia was delayed in the rescued animals, suggesting that one of the major functions of EPOR expression in nonerythroid cells is fine-tuning the regulation of the response to stress.[238]

The existence of naturally occurring splice variants of the EPOR gene encoding EPOR polypeptides of variable length and activity has been shown.[239-242] The soluble secreted form of EPOR[243] binds EPO and thereby competes with the cell surface receptor isoform. The biologic function of alternative forms of the cell surface EPOR, including a truncated form of EPOR found in early progenitors,[244] remains unknown but may be related either to differential EPO signaling and responses (survival, proliferation, differentiation) at different stages in erythroid development or to the establishment of erythroid-specific versus myeloid-specific niches in the marrow microenvironment.

SIGNAL TRANSDUCTION BY EPOR

Considerable progress has been made in our understanding of EPOR-mediated signal transduction. Early studies demonstrated that stimulation of EPOR on primary erythroid cells resulted in increased calcium ion flux and increased globin mRNA synthesis.[245] Since the cloning of the EPOR polypeptide and its stable expression in heterologous cell systems, such as the Ba/F3 cell system,[246] considerable molecular insight has been gained.[247] For instance, it is now clear that EPO induces homodimerization of the EPOR polypeptide.[248,249] Following receptor dimerization at the cell surface, a series of tyrosine phosphorylation events occurs, resulting in a mitogenic signal and a differentiative signal.[250,251] Initial studies of the EPOR signal transduction pathway made use of mutant forms of EPOR stably expressed in the indicator cell line Ba/F3. Ba/F3 cells are a murine IL-3–dependent pro-B lymphocyte cell line. These cells can be readily transfected with the complementary DNA (cDNA) for EPOR, resulting in stable expression of the receptor on the cell surface. Expression of the full-length, wild-type EPOR polypeptide in these cells resulted in EPO-dependent growth and partial EPO-induced erythroid differentiation.[250,251] Expression of truncated forms of the EPOR polypeptide in these cells resulted in variable growth responses. For instance, truncation of the membrane proximal region of EPOR demonstrated a critical positive regulatory domain of EPOR required for mitogenesis.[246] Furthermore, truncation of the carboxy-terminal (C-terminal) 40 amino acids of EPOR resulted in increased EPO-dependent growth, suggesting that the C-terminal region contained a negative regulatory domain normally required for downmodulating EPOR mitogenic signals.[246]

The biochemical basis for these positive and negative regulatory domains has been elucidated. The membrane proximal positive regulatory region of EPOR binds constitutively to Janus-activated kinase 2 (JAK2),[252] a cytoplasmic tyrosine kinase necessary for erythroid differentiation, as evidenced by mice lacking the corresponding gene dying at an early embryonic stage.[253] Upon EPO binding to the receptor, the receptor dimerizes, resulting in activation of prebound JAK2. The JAK2 next tyrosine phosphorylates multiple signaling proteins in the cell, leading to various mitogenic and differentiative responses. The negative regulatory domain of EPOR is required for recruiting the phosphatase SHP1 to EPOR.[254] SHP1 binds to an activated tyrosine phosphate on the EPOR polypeptide and rapidly downregulates JAK2 activity and dephosphorylates the EPOR polypeptide. Failure to recruit the SHP1 phosphatase can result in increased EPOR signaling and a polycythemic state (see Alterations in EPOR and Its Signaling in Disorders of Erythropoiesis).

JAK2 is required for appropriate Golgi processing and cell surface expression of EPOR.[255] Once activated by EPO/EPOR binding on the cell surface, JAK2 initiates several events in EPOR-mediated signal transduction. JAK2 initially activates tyrosine phosphorylation of several tyrosine residues of the cytoplasmic tail of EPOR. These phosphorylated tyrosine residues next serve as docking sites for binding of other cytoplasmic effector proteins containing Src homology 2 (SH2) domains, such as the p85 subunit of phosphatidylinositol 3-kinase,[256] the adaptor protein Shc,[257,258] and STAT5.[259,260] (Examples of signal transduction proteins expressed in primary human erythroblasts are given in Table 26.2). Once these proteins have docked on EPOR, they become tyrosine phosphorylated and engage other downstream signaling events. In addition, JAK2 activates the Ras/Raf/MAPK (mitogen-activated protein kinase) pathway, further contributing to the EPO-induced mitogenic signal.[261,262] The molecular mechanism of Ras activation by JAK2 remains unknown but may entail direct binding of the proteins and tyrosine phosphorylation.[262]

Activation of the JAK2/STAT5 signaling pathway has been studied in considerable detail. Upon EPOR tyrosine phosphorylation, STAT5 protein binds to a specific phosphorylated tyrosine residue of the EPOR.[259,263] Binding is mediated by the SH2 domain of STAT5. Following EPOR binding, STAT5 itself becomes tyrosine phosphorylated at amino acid Y694.[264] Activated STAT5 then disengages from EPOR, undergoes homodimerization, and translocates to the cell nucleus, where it activates transcription of EPO-inducible

TABLE 26.2   Major Transcription Factors/Signaling Molecules Involved in the Control of Erythropoiesis

Transcription Factor	Binding Motif	Role in Hematopoiesis	Knock-Out Phenotype	Mutations/Human Disease
GATA1	(A/T)GATA(A/G)	↑ Erythroid differentiation	• No terminal erythropoiesis • Arrest in Mk development (with hyperproliferation)	Directly • X-linked thalassemia/thrombocytopenia • Leukemia (Down syndrome) • PMF Indirectly (targeted by other mutations) • DBA
GATA2	(A/T)GATA(A/G)	↑ Proliferation ↓ Differentiation	↓ Proliferative expansion of primitive and definitive erythropoiesis Absence of mast cells	Directly MonoMAC syndrome, MDS, AML Indirectly (targeted by other mutations) MDS
FOG-1	None	GATA1 cofactor	↓ Erythroid maturation Block in megakaryocytopoiesis	
EKLF	CACCC	Promotes terminal erythroid differentiation	Severe anemia β-Globin deficiency Impaired ability of macrophages to promote erythropoiesis	β-Thalassemia, Lu-negative blood phenotype, HPFH, Nan phenotype in mice
SCL	CANNTG (E-box)	Specification of hematopoiesis	Absence of prenatal hematopoiesis ↓ Erythro/Mk in adults	Translocation in T-cell ALL
LMO2	LIM domain		Absence of hematopoiesis	T-cell ALL
Myb	(T/C)AAC(G/T)G	↓ Definitive erythropoiesis	Block in definitive erythropoiesis	HPFH, Myb-GATA1 fusion gene in acute basophilic leukemia
Fli-1	Winged helix-turn-helix	Inhibition of GATA1 expression		
BKLF	CACC		Myeloproliferative disorder	
SHP1 (BKLF activated?)				Erythroleukemia Polycythemia vera
STAT5	GAS		Transient fetal anemia because of apoptosis of erythroid progenitors Mild anemia, exacerbated by stress in adult life	
PU.1	GGAA	↓ Erythropoiesis	Absence of myelomonocytic differentiation	
Id		Blocks terminal differentiation of all cell types		
FAK/IaPI-3 kinase (p85)		↓ Proliferation/differentiation	↓ Fetal erythropoiesis Perinatal death	
Gfi-1b	Zinc finger domain	↑ Proliferation (↑ GATA2)		
Sp3			↓ Fetal erythropoiesis Perinatal death	
NF-E2	TGAGTCA	Promotes terminal erythroid differentiation in vitro	Thrombocytopenia Absence of erythroid abnormalities (?)	

ALL, Acute lymphoblastic leukemia; AML, acute myeloid leukemia; BKLF, basic Krüppel-like factor; EKLF, erythroid Krüppel-like factor; FOG-1, Friend of GATA1; HPFH, hereditary persistence of fetal hemoglobin; LMO2, LIM domain only 2; MDS, myelodysplastic syndrome; SCL, stem cell leukemia; ↓ Erythro/Mk, decrease in erythropoiesis/megakaryocytopoiesis.

genes. Some EPO-inducible genes, such as *MYC* and *FOS*, are common to other hematopoietic growth factor signaling pathways. Other EPO-inducible genes are specifically expressed in erythroid cells and are not shared by other growth factor responses.[265]

Other signal transduction pathways downstream from cytokine receptors have been identified. For instance, EPO and IL-3 activate tyrosine phosphorylation of the signaling protein CBL and the subsequent binding and tyrosine phosphorylation of the signal protein CrkL.[266] The mechanism of activation of this pathway by EPOR is not known, and the relative role of this pathway in EPO-induced growth and erythroid differentiation remains largely unexplored. Inositide-specific phospholipases C (PLCs) and the protein kinase C (PKC) pathway also are involved in EPO signaling. PLCs catalyze hydrolysis of phosphatidylinositol 4,5-bisphosphate to generate diacylglycerol and inositol 3,4,5-bisphosphate, a well-known intracellular messenger for PKC activation and intracellular Ca^{2+} mobilization. PLCs are classified into four isoform families (α, β, γ, and δ), and each family has multiple isoforms.[267,268] The involvement of PLCs in erythroid differentiation was suggested by early studies demonstrating that stimulation of EPOR in primary erythroid cells results in increased calcium ion flux.[245] More recent studies demonstrated that primary erythroblasts express only some (i.e., PLC β_1, β_2, β_3, δ_1, γ_1, and γ_2) PLC isoforms. Among these, PLCβ_1 most likely is involved in EPO signaling, based on findings that its expression is induced within 6 hours of stimulation with the growth factor.[26,199,269] On the other hand, PKC represents a family of nine different serine-threonine kinases genes, encoding a total of 12 different isoforms, involved in the regulation of many cellular functions.[270] These enzymes exert their biologic functions as a cytoplasmic-nuclear shuttle of the transduction machinery and become phosphorylated, and hence activated, in response to a variety of stimuli. Human multipotent CD34+ progenitor cells express all of the PKC isoforms.[271,272] Commitment of these cells along the erythroid lineage requires suppression of PKCε.[271,273] PKCε exerts a positive control on erythropoiesis, because its inhibitors specifically impair the ability of erythroid cells to respond to EPO[274] and to phosphorylate EPOR, STAT5, GAB1, ERK1/2, and AKT.[275] It also is possible that different PKC isoforms are active at different ontogenic stages, because PKCα and PKCδ are differentially phosphorylated, and hence activated, during differentiation of neonatal and adult erythroblasts.[276]

EPO signaling activates also Lyn, a tyrosine kinase member of the Src family[277] physically associated with EPOR.[278] Lyn acts upstream to both the STAT5[278] and the PLCγ2/PI3K pathways.[279] Failure to activate Lyn prevents erythroid differentiation of the J2E cell line[277] and Lyn[null] mice have a phenotype remarkably similar to that of GATA1[LOW] mice (normal hematocrit in spite of reduced levels of GATA1, erythroid Krüppel-like factor [EKLF], and STAT5 expression because of development of extramedullary hematopoiesis in spleen).[280] In addition to STAT5 and PLCγ2/PI3K signaling, Lyn activates Liar, a Lyn-binding nuclear/cytoplasmic shuttling protein[281] specifically responsible for downregulating KIT expression in response to EPO.[282] In humans, Lyn is responsible for the phosphorylation of several membrane proteins, and failure to activate Lyn results in the formation of acanthocytic red cells, a diagnostic marker of chorea-acanthocytosis, a rare autosomal recessive neurodegenerative disorder.[283]

Erythroblasts generated under conditions of stress retain C-KIT expression. Several studies have investigated the relationship between KIT signaling and erythroid cell fate. In human and murine erythroid progenitors, KL induces rapid (within 15 minutes) ERK activation, which lasts only 1 hour.[284,285] In human erythroleukemic K562 and myeloid MO7e cells, the rapid KL-dependent ERK activation is associated with proliferation, whereas the late sustained ERK activation is responsible for differentiation.[286,287] Whether KL activates the STAT5 pathway in erythroid cells is controversial. Although KL was found to be unable to activate STAT5 in prospectively isolated human erythroid progenitor cells,[284] more recent single-cells fluorescence-activated cell sorter (FACS) analyses indicate that KL activates STAT5 in bipotent erythroid/megakaryocytic but not in myelomonocytic progenitor cells.[288] KL has also been described to activate the PI3K/AKT pathway in murine erythroid progenitors[285] and in human MO7e cells.[287] Finally, coexpression of KIT and EPOR deletion mutants in 32D cells have identified that KIT intracellular tyrosines play an essential role in EPOR cosignaling,[289] providing a mechanism for the signaling synergy observed between KL and EPO.

A critical question in the field of EPOR signal transduction is the mechanism of EPO specificity. Most, if not all, of the signal transduction pathways activated by EPOR (i.e., Ras/Raf/MAPK and JAK/STAT) are shared by other hematopoietic cytokine receptors, such as the receptors for IL-3, GM-CSF, and IL-5. How EPOR triggers a specific growth factor response resulting in erythroid differentiation is unclear. Several models are possible. First, EPOR may activate unique but unknown signaling pathways specific to EPOR and distinct from other cytokine receptors. Alternatively, EPOR may activate identical pathways, activated by other cytokine receptors. In the latter model, the specificity of the EPO signal is derived not from EPOR itself but from interactions with other developmentally programmed events in

the erythroid cell, such as expression of erythroid-specific transcription factors.

Activation of EPOR in the murine IL-3–dependent cell line Ba/F3 results in induction of both mitogenesis and globin accumulation.[173] In contrast, the murine IL-2–dependent cell line CTLL-2, when engineered to express the heterologous EPOR, grows in EPO but does not differentiate into globin-bearing cells. These data suggest that expression of EPOR is necessary for erythroid differentiation but not sufficient alone. Other erythroid-specific markers, such as GATA1 and NF-E2, or EKLF, are likely required for cells to differentiate down the erythroid pathway. Other cytokine receptors, such as IL-3R and IL-2R, do not drive β-globin synthesis in these cell lines. Taken together, these results suggest that EPOR generates a differentiation-specific signaling within the context of a proper transcriptional environment.

Regardless of the mechanism of cytokine specificity, each cytokine receptor activates a similar but not identical pattern of signaling events. For instance, EPOR shows a preferential activation of the JAK2/STAT5 pathway in cultured erythroid cells in vitro. In contrast, IL-2R shows preferential activation of the JAK1/JAK3/STAT6 pathway.[264,290,291] Interestingly, although EPO activates STAT5a and STAT5b in cultured cells, knockout of the STAT5a or STAT5b gene by homologous recombination results in a mouse phenotype with slightly impaired stem cell activity but apparently normal baseline erythroid development.[292,293] More extensive analysis of this phenotype has revealed that the mice experience increased apoptotic rates at erythroblast levels that are compensated by a cellular compensatory mechanism very similar to that described for GATA1[LOW] mutants,[103] involving expansion of hemopoietic progenitors in the marrow and recruitment of the spleen as an additional hemopoietic site. These results suggest that, in vivo, other STAT proteins are at least partially capable of substituting for STAT5 and functioning downstream of the EPOR. These findings emphasize the importance of in vivo studies in confirming the phenotypic relevance of in vitro studies.

Studies have suggested that EPO functions synergistically with other multilineage growth factors, such as KL and IL-3. EPO and KL function together, resulting in increased erythroid colony cell growth in methylcellulose culture. Studies with the EPOR polypeptide suggest a molecular mechanism for such synergy.[294] Activation of the KIT receptor by KL results in transphosphorylation of EPOR at the cell surface. A direct interaction between EPOR and the KIT receptor has been demonstrated.[295] Physical interaction between EPOR and the β common chain of the IL-3 receptor in erythroid cells has been demonstrated.[296] This interaction might be involved in the neuroprotective action exerted by EPO.[297] In fact, a carbamylated derivative of EPO prevents motoneuron degeneration in vitro and in vivo[297] and ameliorates recovery in several in vivo models of brain and heart injuries, such as chronic autoimmunoencephalomyelitis in mice,[298] radiosurgery- or ischemia-induced brain injury,[299] and myocardium ischemia-reperfusion injury[300] in rats. (For a review of the nonhematopoietic activity of EPO, see reference 301.) Taken together, these results suggest that receptor cross-talk at the cell surface may account, at least in part, for the physiologic interaction of some cytokines in controlling hematopoietic versus nonhematopoietic effects of EPO.

ALTERATIONS IN EPOR AND ITS SIGNALING IN DISORDERS OF ERYTHROPOIESIS

As discussed earlier, the normal role of EPO is to stimulate cell surface EPOR in developing erythroid cells. The latter cells respond to EPO via a proliferative and differentiation response. EPO-activated signal transduction of EPOR is quickly downregulated in the cell, and continuing presence of EPO is required for optimal differentiation.

In some cells, the EPOR may become constitutively activated. In these cases, erythroid progenitor cells are placed into a sustained proliferative state. Interestingly, these mechanisms underlie several murine and human examples of erythrocytosis (erythroid overproduction). Multiple mechanisms exist by which EPOR may become constitutively activated. First, the Friend spleen focus-forming virus of the Friend erythroleukemia complex encodes the glycoprotein F-gp55, which binds and activates murine EPOR.[302-304] F-gp55 appears to bind to EPOR via its transmembrane region. EPO and F-gp55 binding sites are discrete; tertiary complexes of EPOR, EPO, and F-gp55 have been detected on the surface of Friend virus-infected cells.[305] Second, EPOR can be constitutively activated by a point mutation (R129C) in the extracytoplasmic region of the polypeptide.[306] This mutation occurs in the "dimerization domain" of EPOR and results in constitutive homodimerization of the EPOR polypeptide, presumably through a disulfide bond. This mutation further underscores the importance of receptor dimerization in the initiation of a receptor signaling response. Third, EPOR can be constitutively activated in an autocrine manner. Murine erythroleukemia cell lines have been established that coexpress EPOR and EPO. A fourth mechanism of EPOR constitutive activation results from EPOR overexpression. For instance, some murine erythroleukemia cell lines have increased EPOR mRNA, resulting from spleen focus-forming virus proviral integration within the first intron of the murine EPOR gene.[307] Overexpression of the normal murine EPOR polypeptide may thereby contribute to oncogenesis.

Soon after the cDNA of mouse and human EPOR were cloned, the mouse and human genomic structures were identified. The gene for mouse EPOR was found to map to mouse chromosome 9,[308] whereas the human gene was found on human chromosome 19p.[309] Mapping of the EPOR genes led to their implication in various human disease states. For instance, studies demonstrated that a chromosomal breakpoint 3′ to the human EPOR gene results in increased EPOR expression.[310] The rearranged EPOR allele appears to encode a mutated EPOR polypeptide with increased activity, perhaps secondary to loss of the C-terminal negative regulatory domain.

EPOR plays a role in the rare congenital disease familial erythrocytosis. Familial erythrocytosis is a heterogeneous group of hereditary conditions characterized by an increase in red blood cell mass in the setting of low serum EPO levels. A few families that demonstrate autosomal dominant inheritance have been identified.[311] The linkage between the EPOR gene and familial erythrocytosis was first established by the observation that a mutant EPOR allele segregates with the disease in one familial erythrocytosis kindred. This allele contains a nonsense mutation in the coding region of the gene that results in synthesis of a truncated EPOR that lacks the negative regulatory domain of its C-terminal region.[312,313] Since that report, several other frameshift and deletion EPOR gene mutations, all encoding C-terminal–truncated forms of the protein providing EPO hypersensitivity and resulting in familial erythrocytosis, have been reported.[314-318]

Congenital polycythemia may arise not only from gene mutations leading to abnormal EPOR signaling but also from gene mutations altering EPO production. The T598T mutation in one of the genes controlling oxygen sensing (von Hippel-Lindau [VHL] gene), which leads to increased EPO production by the kidney, is associated with congenital erythrocytosis, the Chuvash polycythemia.[319,320] The C598T VHL mutation is endemic in Chuvashia, Russian Federation, and in the small island of Ischia, in southern Italy. The frequency of the mutation on this small island is higher than in Chuvashia (0.07% versus 0.02%), but the haplotype of Italian patients matches that identified in the Chuvash cluster, supporting a single-founder hypothesis.[321]

Acquired mutations in the EPOR signaling pathway have been identified in PV, essential thrombocythemia, and idiopathic myelofibrosis, a class of myeloproliferative neoplasm that lacks the Philadelphia chromosome (Ph) abnormality and therefore cannot be cured with inhibitors such as Gleevec, which are specific for the signaling pathway altered by the Ph abnormality. These diseases originate at the level of the pluripotent hematopoietic stem cell and are characterized by proliferation of one or more of the myeloid lineages but relatively normal hematopoietic cell maturation. Several investigators have reported a mutation in the JAK2 gene resulting in a valine→phenylalanine substitution at position 617 of the protein (JAK2V617F mutation) in patients with Ph-negative chronic proliferative disorders.[322-325] Since the early reports, the presence of

JAK2V617F in patients with Ph-negative myeloproliferative disorders has been confirmed by numerous publications. Depending on the study, JAK2V617F has been reported in 60% to 90% of patients with PV, 30% to 50% of patients with essential thrombocythemia (ET), and 30% to 60% of patients with PMF. The mutation is harbored at either the heterozygous or, by somatic recombination, the homozygous stage. It is detectable in all myeloid cells up to the clonal hematopoietic stem cells.[326] The mutation affects the domain of the protein that is not directly involved in signal transduction but is necessary to return the protein to its resting configuration after signaling. As a consequence, after its first engagement with EPO, EPOR signaling becomes constitutively activated. Because JAK2 is the earliest element of the EPOR pathway, it is conceivable that the high red cell numbers found in patients with PV carrying the JAK2V617F mutation is a direct consequence of constitutive EPO signaling in erythroid cells. The extent to which the downstream EPOR signaling pathway is altered as a consequence of this constitutive activation is a debatable issue. The observation that erythroblasts derived in vitro from patients with PV carrying the JAK2V617F mutation are highly resistant to TRAIL-induced apoptosis[327] suggests that the mutation exquisitely increases erythroblast survival. However, additional abnormalities induced by the presence of JAK2V617F are represented by hypersensitivity to insulin-like growth factor I[328] and increased EPOR recycling from the Golgi apparatus.[255] More difficult to understand is why the mutation is also present in some patients with ET and PMF. JAK2, in addition to EPOR, has an important role in transducing the signal from c-Mpl, the TPO receptor.[329] The protein has two opposing effects on the intracellular processing of the two receptors after growth factor stimulation: it favors EPOR recycling from the Golgi apparatus,[255] but it determines retention and degradation of c-Mpl in the cytoplasm.[330] As such, the JAK2V617F mutation should increase the number of EPOR on the surface of erythroid cells while reducing that of c-Mpl on megakaryocytes. This hypothesis explains why the mutation is found preferentially in PV. However, megakaryocytes originating from JAK2V617F stem cells might express a reduced number but constitutively active c-Mpl, so it can be argued that the mutation manifests itself prevalently in the erythroid or the megakaryocytic lineage, depending on genetic polymorphisms outside the JAK2 locus present in the population. This hypothesis is supported by the observation that mice transplanted with JAK2V617F hematopoietic stem cells develop either a PV- or an ET-like syndrome, depending on their genetic background[331] and/or level of JAK2V617F expression.[332,333] One of the genetic factors that may determine the phenotype expressed by JAK2V617F-positive myeloproliferative neoplasms may be represented by the GR locus. The blood mononuclear cells from PV patients, but not those from ET or PMF, express increased levels of the dominant negative GRβ isoform. Increased levels of GRβ are also expressed by the erythroblasts expanded in vivo from PV patients. The observations that these erythroblasts lack nuclear STAT5 activity, in spite of constitutive STAT5 phosphorylation induced by the presence of JAK2V617F mutation, and do not mature in response to EPO[124] suggest that constitutive inhibition of the EPO maturation signal provided by GRβ expression may confer a self-renewal state to PV erythroblasts, contributing to erythrocytosis. Expression of GRβ may be favored by the increased frequency of the rs6198 SNP, which stabilize GRβ mRNA observed in these patients.[124]

Studies on the biology and biochemistry of the JAK2V617F mutation are actively being pursued by many investigators. Furthermore, in JAK2V617F-negative PV or idiopathic erythrocytosis patients, several other gain-of-function mutations affecting JAK2 exon 12 with a distinct phenotype (idiopathic erythrocytosis) have been identified.[334] The identification of specific mutations and the availability of the crystal structures of EPO, EPOR, and JAK2 has allowed computer modeling to design targeted protein-signaling inhibitors for treatment of Ph-negative myeloproliferative neoplasms.[335] In as few as 9 years after the discovery of JAK2 mutations, JAK2 inhibitors have been designed, clinical trials with selected drugs conducted, and the drugs approved for clinical use by the U.S. Food and Drug Administration.[336] The observation that the genetic lesions found in

Philadelphia-negative MPN are heterogeneous have raised concerns whether *JAK2* mutations represent the primary transformation event in these diseases.[337] Mutations involving *Mpl, LNK, TET2, ASXL1, EZH2, IDH1/2, CBL,* and *IKZF1* have been observed in 3% to 20% of MPN patients,[338] and more recently Klampfl et al[339] and Nangalia et al[340] have identified novel mutations in exon 9 of the calreticulin (*CALR*) gene in the majority of ET and PMF patients who did not harbor *JAK2* or *MPL* mutations. CALR is a Ca^{2+} binding protein mostly localized in the endoplasmic reticulum that regulates Ca^{2+} homeostasis and chaperones other proteins to the nucleus and other cellular compartments. Unexpectedly, the results of a large clinical trial have recently identified that the JAK2 inhibitor ruxolitinib effectively reduced spleen size and disease manifestation both in JAK2-mutated and JAK2-nonmutated patients,[341] whereas the JAK2 inhibitor fedratinib reduced splenomegaly in two CALR-mutated patients.[342] These results suggest that mutations leading to development of MPN may occur along a unifying pathogenetic pathway including JAK2 that may be, therefore, targeted by inhibitors of this enzyme.[343]

HEMATOPOIETIC MICROENVIRONMENT

In invertebrates such as worms and sessile marine creatures, erythropoiesis occurs adjacent to peritoneal and endothelial cells. In premammalian species, the spleen is the primary site of erythropoiesis. With evolutionary advancement, the function gradually shifts to the liver and the sinusoidal cavities of bones.[9] These observations suggest that sufficient oxygen, a stagnated flow of blood to avoid dispersion of factors produced locally, and extensive and redundant surfaces for cell–cell interactions are essential to supporting red cell production. Similar sites support erythropoiesis during human development (see Ontogeny of Erythropoiesis). During both phylogeny and ontogeny, the liver and spleen are primarily erythropoietic organs; granulocytic cells dominate in the bone marrow.[9] Within the bone marrow, hematopoiesis is restricted to the extravascular space, where compact collections of cells are interspersed among venous sinuses. These sinuses originate adjacent to the endosteal bone surface and empty into a central longitudinal vein. Studies in mice demonstrate that BFU-E follows a bimodal distribution with peaks adjacent to the periosteum and midcavity, whereas CFU-E and later erythroid cells have a broad distribution with highest incidence toward the axis of the femur, adjacent to the central vein,[9,344] thus suggesting that the local anatomy (specialized niches?) influences the maturation of erythroid cells.

The bone marrow microenvironment consists of three broad components: stromal cells (e.g., fibroblasts, endothelial cells, mesenchymal stem cells and their diverse descendant progeny), accessory cells (monocytes, macrophages, megakaryocytes, T cells), and extracellular matrix (a protein–carbohydrate scaffold). In the bone marrow, although early studies described two distinct hematopoietic niches for hematopoietic stem cells/progenitor cells (i.e., the "endosteal" niche and the "endothelial or vascular niche" within the medulla), more recent studies suggest that this distinction may be artificial, because both cellular structures can be intimately associated in trabecular bone. Thus mesenchymal stem cell–derived osteoprogenitor cells and stromal reticular cells (nestin+ or leptinR+) are intimately associated with sinusoidal endothelium and seem to be pivotal organizers of the bone marrow niche.[345–347] Reciprocal communication of hematopoietic stem cells with cells/matrix in their bone marrow niche ensures both their quiescent state and self-renewal dynamics.

EPO, in addition to promoting erythropoiesis directly, enhances erythropoiesis indirectly by decreasing the interaction of hematopoietic stem cells with their niches, reducing the amount of trabecular bone[348] and downregulating CXCR4 expression, the receptor for CXCR12L/SDF1, on hematopoietic stem cells.[349]

Accessory cells are progeny of hematopoietic stem cells; hence after marrow transplantation these cells are of donor origin, whereas stromal cells remain mostly host derived.[350,351] Extracellular matrix molecules are synthesized and secreted by microenvironmental cells and include collagens (types I, III, IV, and V), glycoproteins (fibronectin, laminins, thrombospondins, hemonectin, and tenascin), and glycosaminoglycans (hyaluronic acid, chondroitin, dermatan, and heparan sulfate).[352,353] The production of extracellular matrix proteoglycans by mesenchymal stromal cells may be regulated by the Wnt pathway.[354]

Besides providing structure to the marrow space and a surface for cell adhesion, the microenvironment is important for hematopoietic cell homing, engraftment, migration, and the response to physiologic stress and homeostasis. Although the functional consequences of the microenvironment ultimately must be defined by in vivo studies in mice, dissection of the cellular components of the microenvironment, definition of the cytokines that are produced by individual cells, and the nature of cell–cell interactions have been aided by in vitro models. Long-term bone marrow cultures provide an experimental approach for such studies.[355,356] Under these in vitro conditions, murine hematopoiesis can be maintained for 8 to 10 months and human hematopoiesis for 2 to 3 months.[355] An adherent layer consisting of fibroblasts, adipocytes, and macrophages is a crucial component of the culture system. Progenitor cells adherent to stroma are generally quiescent (dormant), whereas those in the nonadherent cell compartment are in active cell cycle.[356,357]

In vitro studies have demonstrated that stromal cells, including endothelial cells and fibroblasts, elaborate cytokines such as GM-CSF, G-CSF, IL-1, IL-3, IL-6, IL-11, KL, Flt-3 ligand, activin A, and basic fibroblast growth factor, which influence, alone or in combination, the growth of adjacent marrow progenitors.[355–358] In addition to positive regulators of replication and differentiation, stromal cells elaborate factors such as TGF-β, TPO, CXCL12L, IFN-γ, and TNF-α, which exert a negative influence on proliferation and may help maintain a dormant (noncycling) state.[356,357,359–361] Because some regulators inhibit differentiation along certain lineages but not others, there is an intriguing possibility that lineage-specific regulation within the microenvironment can be achieved through negative, rather than positive, factors.[362] Several cytokines are expressed in a transmembrane form as well as a soluble (secreted) product. Others bind extracellular matrix, a mechanism that not only allows for high concentrations of a factor within the microenvironment that metabolically stabilizes these factors but also keeps them adjacent to developing progenitors.

Among the factors elaborated by stromal cells, KL has the most profound effect on erythropoiesis. Mice unable to synthesize KL die in utero because of severe anemia. Steel-Dickie (Sl^d) mice that are unable to make the membrane-restricted form of KL are viable but severely anemic, whereas other lineages in these animals are marginally affected or not affected by this defect.[363] The fact that erythropoiesis is abnormal, despite high levels of circulating EPO and the presence of soluble KL, suggests that normal erythroid differentiation and maturation require both a functional membrane-restricted KL/KIT and an EPO signaling pathway. Cross-phosphorylation of EPOR by KL may provide a basis for the predominantly erythroid effect.[295] Furthermore, data suggest that tyrosine cross-phosphorylation of EPOR is sustained longer when cells are cultured on steel stromal cells engineered to express the membrane-restricted form of KL than cells expressing the soluble form.[364]

The soluble form of KL is produced by proteolytic cleavage of membrane KL and is released in the circulation. Soluble KL effectively supports erythroid maturation in vitro[365] but is dispensable for steady-state erythropoiesis, because targeted mutant mice expressing exclusively the more stable membrane isoform of KL, KL2, lacking the major proteolytic cleavage site, have normal hematocrit values.[366] However, these mice recover poorly from radiation-induced anemia.[366] In wild-type mice, sublethal radiation induced a transient fourfold increase in KL in the serum (from <0.5 up to >2 ng/mL), reaching a peak after 7 days. In contrast, the proteolytic-cleavage mutant KL$^{KL2/KL2}$ mice did not release soluble KL into the serum after sublethal radiation, and survival was significantly diminished because of anemia. This phenotype is remarkably similar to that of mice lacking the dimerization domain of GR.[107] Recent data indicate that soluble KL specifically induce expression of GRα in human erythroid cells,[367] suggesting that soluble KL initiates the response to stress by priming erythroid cells to respond to glucocorticoids.

The pathway(s) that regulate erythropoiesis under conditions of acute or chronic anemia are starting to emerge.[368] In mice, stress induces the formation of an erythroid permissive microenvironment in the spleen and other extramedullary sites. In fact, recent evidence suggests that, in addition to increasing EPO production by the kidney, to raise the levels of soluble KL in the serum and to activate GR response, this pathway activates spleen-specific microenvironmental cues (BMP4/Hedgehog), which generate stress-specific hematopoietic compartments.[82,369] The identity of the hematopoietic stem cell niche in the spleen and the human equivalent of this cell are yet to be determined.

Besides cell–cytokine interactions, (paracrine) cell–cell adhesion and adhesion of cells to the extracellular matrix are important functions of the microenvironment.[370,371] Perhaps most studied are the β_1 integrins VLA4 and VLA5, which mediate the adherence of hematopoietic cells to stromal cells, fibronectin, or other components of the extracellular matrix.[371,372] In mice lacking β_1 integrins, hematopoietic stem cells fail to colonize the fetal liver during embryonic development,[373] and cells lacking α_4 integrin fail to contribute to normal hematopoiesis postnatally.[374] Conditional deletions of β_1 integrin or α_4 integrin during adult stage lead to mild anemia with increased ROS formation and decreased RBC survival in β_1-deficient mice and in impairment in erythroid stress response in both β_1- and α_4-deficient mice.[375] In addition to intrinsic effects on erythropoiesis, antibodies to VLA4 or to the vascular cellular adhesion molecule-1 (VCAM-1, a VLA4 ligand on endothelial cells) influence the retention of stem/progenitor cells in bone marrow and thereby impair their homing and lead to their mobilization in adult mice, in primates, and in MS patients.[376–380] In in vitro studies, hematopoietic progenitors bind to specific domains of fibronectin in a differentiation-dependent manner (long-term culture-initiating cell and day 12 colony-forming unit-spleen in mice adhere mainly through the heparin-binding domain and CS-1). BFU-E and other progenitor cells adhere to both the cell-binding (Arg-Gly-Asp-Ser [RGDS]) and heparin-binding domains, whereas CFU-E preferentially bind the RGDS sequence, and reticulocytes fail to adhere to fibronectin.[353,381–384] This differential binding could influence the proliferation and especially the maturation and survival of developing erythroid cells, particularly under stress,[385] as well as the migration of progenitor cells in and out of the bone marrow cavity.[374,376] Hematopoietic cytokines/chemokines present in the microenvironment can also modulate the affinity of $\beta1$ integrins for ligand,[386,387] adding complexity to the regulation of erythropoiesis within the marrow microenvironment.

Many observations suggest that hematopoietic progenitor cells at one stage of fetal development may not be supported by a hematopoietic microenvironment of a different ontogenetic stage. For example, cells present in the murine yolk sac are not able to repopulate adult recipients,[388] although they can repopulate newborn recipients with active fetal liver hematopoiesis.[389] Targeted disruption of CXCL12/SDF1, a member of the CXC chemokine family that is constitutively expressed by bone marrow stromal cells (i.e., reticular/endothelial cells or osteoblasts), leads to inhibition of marrow hematopoiesis, although fetal liver hematopoiesis is unaffected,[390] suggesting that this chemokine is important in maintaining normal bone marrow hematopoiesis. Other factors with distinct function on fetal versus adult hematopoiesis have also been described: Sox17 for fetal hematopoiesis[391] or TEL (translocation-ETS [E26 transformation-specific]-leukemia)[392] and Bmi-1 for adult hematopoiesis.[393] Accessory cells, such as stromal cells, in addition to secreting cytokines, express adhesion molecules, and they may influence marrow hematopoiesis by their nonrandom distribution in the marrow cavity. T cells (along with mast cells) are the only source of IL-3 and, through secretion of TNF-α and IFN-γ, may negatively affect erythropoiesis. In histologic sections of normal marrow, islands of maturing erythroblasts (erythroblastic islands) often surround a central macrophage, termed a *nurse cell*.[394] Adhesion may be mediated through the binding of VLA4 (on erythroid cells) to VCAM-1 (on central macrophages),[395] or through

several other molecules.[396] These molecular interactions have been identified as being critical for erythroblastic island integrity (see also Erythroid Morphologically Recognizable Precursors). EMP expressed on both erythroblasts and macrophages mediates cell–cell attachment through homophilic binding, and erythroblast intercellular adhesion molecule-4 (ICAM-4) links erythroblasts to macrophages by interacting with α_v integrin expressed in macrophages.[397–399] Mice with targeted deletion of EMP are severely anemic and die at an embryonic stage,[145] and ICAM-4[null] mice[398] have markedly reduced erythroblastic islands. Of interest, retinoblastoma (RB)-deficient macrophages do not bind RB[null] erythroblasts,[400] and failure of this interaction may mediate the defect in fetal liver erythropoiesis observed in RB[null] mice. RB normally stimulates macrophage differentiation by counteracting inhibition of Id2 (a helix-loop-helix protein) on PU.1, a transcription factor crucial in macrophage differentiation. In addition to the aforementioned pathways, macrophage CD163 can serve as an erythroblast adhesion receptor in erythroblastic islands, promoting erythroid proliferation and/or survival.[401] More studies addressing the specific interactions between macrophages and erythroid cells that promote erythroid differentiation are needed for definite conclusions regarding specialized "erythroid niches" and their complex function. Of note, tissue macrophages express RNA for EPO[402] and may also influence erythropoiesis through this mechanism.

The microenvironment is not only a passive surface for the adherence of progenitor cells; it exerts a crucial and interactive role in development and maturation. Some interactions are lineage (red cell) specific, whereas other interactions affect hematopoiesis more broadly. Stromal and accessory cells secrete cytokines and/or express them in a transmembrane form on their cell surface. Cytokines are retained via binding to components of the extracellular matrix. All components of the microenvironment are involved in adhesive interactions, some of which maintain quiescence (i.e., interactions of stem cells with endosteal surfaces[403,404]), whereas other cell–cell interactions or interactions of cells with matrix components induce proliferation and/or differentiation.[405–407] An individual progenitor cell, in an anatomic niche adjacent to certain stromal cells, accessory cells, and extracellular matrix molecules, likely responds to the sum of the signals that it uniquely receives. In this way, erythropoiesis, or the entire hematopoiesis, is influenced by the complexity of the ME interaction network.

ONTOGENY OF ERYTHROPOIESIS

During human development, distinct anatomic areas for production of erythroid cells are recruited sequentially, in a temporal succession that allows overlap (Fig. 26.3). In addition, parallel changes occur in the morphologic and functional properties of the erythroid cells themselves.

During the phase of embryonic erythropoiesis in the blood islands of yolk sac, aggregates of immature erythroid cells undergo maturation synchronously as a single cohort. Before their maturation is completed, they begin to circulate, and by gestational week 5 they are found in the vascular spaces of the rudimentary liver (Fig. 26.4). At about the same time, foci of immature erythroid cells emerge within the fetal liver as the fetal (or hepatic) phase of erythropoiesis commences.[408] From week 7 onward, the liver is progressively filled with erythroid precursors and becomes the dominant site of erythroid cell production until approximately gestational week 30. Although some red cell production can be found in the thymus, the spleen, or occasionally in the lymph nodes, these other sites are never dominant. However, recently placenta has been recognized as an important local erythropoietic site.[409] From month 6 onward, the cavities of long bones are invaded by vascular sprouts and become competent to support red cell development. Shortly after birth, all bone cavities are actively engaged in erythroid production, and the hepatic (fetal) phase of erythropoiesis comes to an end, as the final (adult) phase of erythropoiesis unfolds exclusively within the bone marrow.

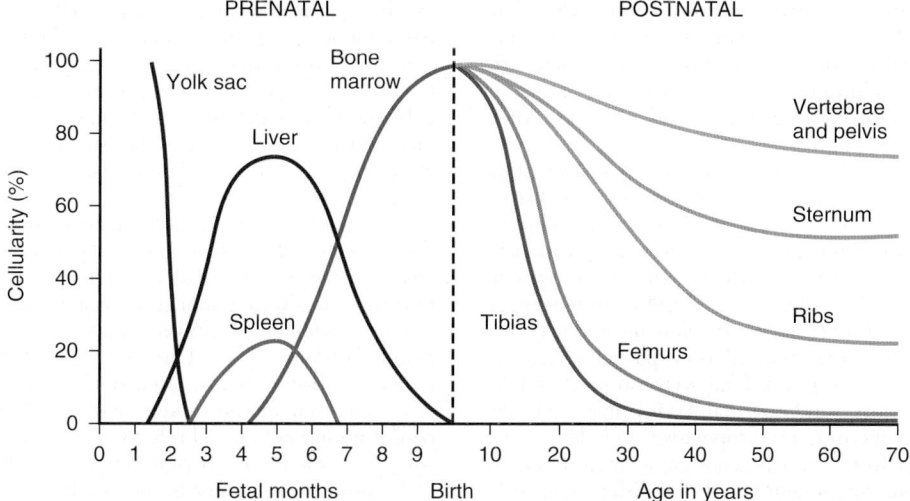

Fig. 26.3 SITES OF HEMATOPOIESIS DURING FETAL DEVELOPMENT AND AFTER BIRTH. Only erythroid cells and possibly lymphocytes are generated by the yolk sac and early embryo. Significant megakaryocytopoiesis and granulopoiesis develop at 4 to 5 months. After birth, hematopoiesis occurs in the sinusoidal cavities of the tibias, femurs, and axial skeleton. *(Modified from Erslev A, Gabuzda T:* Pathophysiology of blood, *ed 2, Philadelphia, PA, 1979, WB Saunders.)*

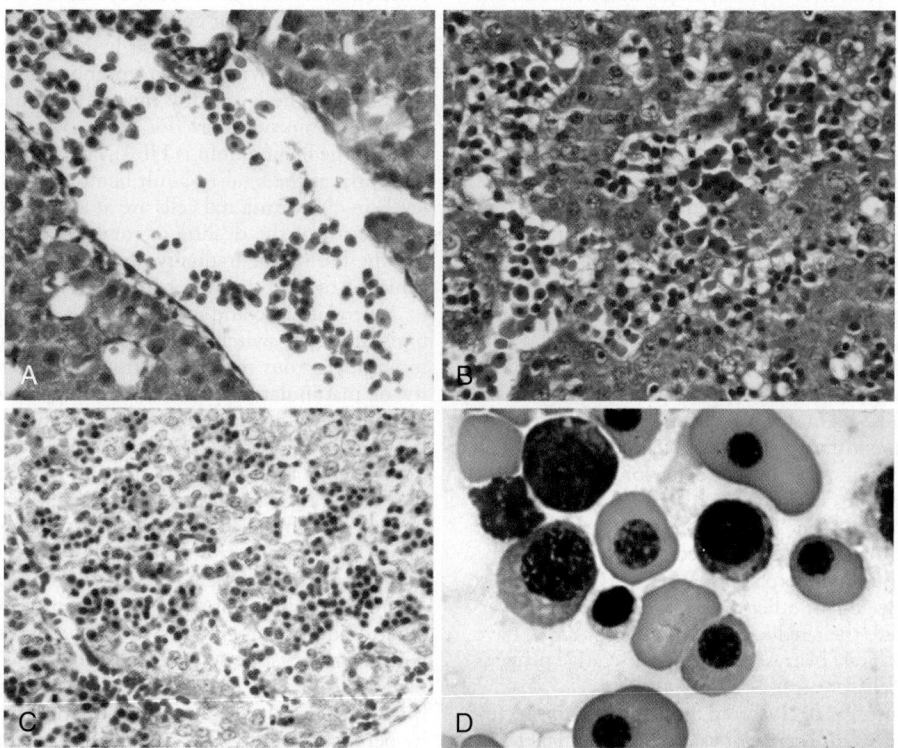

Fig. 26.4 EMBRYONIC/FETAL ERYTHROPOIESIS. (A) Section of an 8-mm embryo depicting a portion of hepatic parenchymal cells with embryonic erythroblasts present within primitive sinusoidal cavities. (B) At 6 to 8 weeks, discrete aggregates of definitive erythroblasts appear within the liver parenchyma, whereas mature embryonic erythroblasts persist in well-developed sinusoids. (C) Definitive erythroblasts are spread throughout the liver (100-day fetus). (D) Cytologic spread from disaggregated fetal liver cells of a 55-day embryo. Characteristic form of embryonic erythroblasts and immature (basophilic) definitive erythroblasts is shown. (A–C, Hematoxylin-eosin stain; D, Wright-Giemsa stain.)

In addition to the anatomic shifts in the sites of erythropoiesis are associated shifts in the phenotypic characteristics of erythroid cells. Embryonic erythroid cells (derived from the yolk sac) are large (approximately 200 μm), circulate as nucleated cells, and have a megaloblastic appearance (see Fig. 26.4). The fact that primitive erythroblasts of mammals, like erythroid cells of lower vertebrates, retain their nuclei at terminal stages of maturation may serve as an

example of embryonic recapitulation of the phylogenetic evolution of the erythroid system. However, a study has identified the presence of enucleated megaloblasts in the blood of the mouse embryo at late stages of development, indicating that the enucleation process predominantly in the fetal liver is at least partially at work.[410] Other studies using genetic reporter models further suggest that embryonic (primitive) cells represent a stable cell population that persists through the end of gestation.[411] Fetal erythroid cells (produced in the fetal liver and later in fetal bone marrow spaces) are smaller than embryonic cells (approximately 125 μm) but have a macrocytic appearance compared with adult normocytic red cells (approximately 80 μm). However, like adult cells, fetal erythroid cells eject their nuclei during maturation.

Apart from variations in size and morphologic characteristics, embryonic and fetal erythroid cells differ from each other and from their adult counterparts in several other characteristics, including hormonal or growth factor requirements, proliferative status, and transplantation potential. For example, whereas fetal erythropoiesis is under the control of EPO,[412] the extent of EPO's influence on embryonic erythropoiesis is disputed. Most convincing are the results of EPO/EPOR knockouts[206] that showed only partial effects on embryonic erythropoiesis, in contrast to fetal erythropoiesis. Single-lineage transcriptosome analyses indicate that TGF-β may represent a primary regulator of embryonic erythropoiesis.[413] Evidence suggests that precursor cells from the extraembryonic mesoderm are dependent on EPO for proliferation and erythroid differentiation.[414] EPO levels increase between weeks 9 and 32 of gestation, and fetuses respond to hypoxia or anemia with increased EPO as early as 24 weeks. Fetal erythroid progenitors when studied in vitro appear more sensitive to EPO and KL than adult progenitors. In contrast, their in vitro response to lymphokines (e.g., IL-3 or GM-CSF) is minimal compared to that of adult erythroid progenitors.[415,416] Of note, in the early stages of fetal liver erythropoiesis, mainly erythroid differentiation/maturation is promoted.[258] Progenitors committed to other lineages are abundant in the fetal liver, but few mature cells (granulocytes, megakaryocytes) from other lineages are seen. In addition to their heightened sensitivity to EPO, fetal erythroid progenitors and precursors are characterized by high proliferative potential and shorter doubling times than adult cells when cultured in vitro.[415,417] The dependency of stem/progenitor cells on KL changes during ontogeny. Although generation of repopulating stem cells (C-KIT$^+$/Sca1$^+$/Thy1^{lo}/Lin$^-$) and colony-forming unit–spleen is minimally affected during fetal life in mice that cannot produce KL, adult steel-Dickie (Sl/Sl^d) mutant mice (which produce only some soluble KL) display greatly impaired erythropoiesis and hematopoiesis, suggesting that the KL/C-KIT pathway plays a role in the recruitment and self-renewal behavior of adult stem cells in vivo.[418,419] The long-term transplantation potential is impaired in cells with mutations of C-KIT kinase activity.[419] Transplantable stem cells from the yolk sac, in contrast to fetal liver cells, cannot engraft adult recipients, because of altered homing behavior or inability of bone marrow to support their development,[389] as suggested by their engraftment in neonatal liver.[420] The homing properties of fetal stem cells transplanted into adult irradiated recipients were found to be inferior to those of their adult counterparts.[421] Whether this finding is related to their increased cycling or other reasons is unclear. However, fetal liver stem cells, despite their reduced homing potential,[421] have higher engraftment levels, likely because of their proliferative prowess compared to adult stem cells.[422]

The surface antigenic profiles of erythroid progenitors and precursors are distinct at each ontogenic stage. For example, HLA class I and class II antigens are not detected in embryonic erythroid progenitor cells but reach adult levels at approximately gestational week 9.[423] CD34$^+$ hematopoietic progenitors present in yolk sac express Mac-1 but are negative for stem cell antigen 1 (Sca-1), which is expressed in fetal and adult CD34$^+$ murine progenitor cells.[424] On the other hand, adult CD34$^+$ progenitors lack Mac-1 and AA4.1, which are expressed in fetal CD34$^+$ progenitor cells. Fetal BFU-E and CFU-E express similar levels of HLA class II antigens, whereas adult CFU-E are largely devoid of these antigens.[423,425] β$_1$ integrins, especially α$_4$β$_1$ and α$_5$, are expressed widely in all hemopoietic cells, including nucleated erythroid cells. However, in the latter, they display a differentiation-dependent, developmentally segregated pattern of expression, because they are absent in embryonic murine erythroblasts,[426] and among adult cells, stem/progenitor cells express them in a constitutively active form in contrast to more mature cells.[427–429] Fetal red cells display a straight, unbranched polylactosaminyl chain (i antigen)

on their surface, whereas in adult cells, this structure, which bears ABH blood group determinants, is highly branched (I antigen).[131] The enzymatic activity of several enzymes in the glycolytic pathway is greater in fetal than in adult red cells.[430] In contrast, carbonic anhydrase levels are very low during intrauterine and early neonatal life.[431] Distinct isozyme patterns for several enzymes (i.e., phosphoglycerate kinase, acetylcholinesterase) also distinguish fetal from adult red cells.[432,433]

The most widely studied changes during red cell ontogeny are the shifts or "switches" in globin types. Embryonic erythroblasts are characterized by their avid accumulation of iron, which is stored as ferritin[434] (0.3% to 1% of total protein) and by the synthesis of the unique hemoglobins Gower I ($\zeta_2\varepsilon_2$), Gower II ($\alpha_2\varepsilon_2$), and hemoglobin Portland ($\zeta_2\gamma_2$). The ζ- and ε-globin chains are embryonic α-like and β-like chains, respectively.[94] These three embryonic types of hemoglobin are most likely synthesized in succession, because the concentration of Gower I is highest in smaller embryos. Thus a switch from ζ- to α- and ε- to γ-globin gene production begins during the embryonic phase of erythropoiesis but is not complete until fetal erythropoiesis is well established. During the transition from yolk sac to fetal liver erythropoiesis (6 to 9 weeks), erythroid precursors within the fetal liver coexpress embryonic (ζ- or ε-) and fetal (α- or γ-) globin both in vivo and in vitro.[435,436] The predominant type of hemoglobin synthesized during fetal liver erythropoiesis is HbF ($\alpha_2\gamma_2$), with a high proportion of γ^G:γ^A (7 : 3). Adult HbA ($\alpha_2\beta_2$), which is detectable at the earliest stages of fetal liver erythropoiesis, is synthesized as a minor component throughout this period. However, HbA$_2$ ($\alpha_2\delta_2$), which is a minor hemoglobin in the adult, is undetectable in these early stages. From about gestational week 30 onward, β-globin synthesis steadily increases so that, by term, 50% to 55% of hemoglobin synthesized is HbA. By 4 to 5 weeks of postnatal age, 75% of the hemoglobin is HbA. This percentage increases to 95% by 4 months as the fetal-to-adult hemoglobin switch is completed. HbF levels in circulating red cells are at a plateau for the first 2 to 3 weeks (as a result of the decline in total erythropoiesis that follows birth), but the HbF level gradually declines so that normal levels (<1%) are achieved by 200 days after birth.[437]

Several in vitro and in vivo approaches have been used to study the basis of globin switching through development. Beyond its biologic interest, rigorous research in this area was propelled by the possibility of manipulating globin switching to increase HbF production in adults and ameliorate the clinical symptoms of disorders of the β-globin locus (e.g., sickle cell anemia, thalassemia). Transplantation experiments and ablative endocrine maneuvers in the sheep model have failed to provide convincing support for the effects of environmental or humoral factors on the switching process, although some modulation of the rate of switching was seen in these models.[438,439] Similar conclusions were reached with transplantation of human fetal liver cells to adult recipients.[440,441] The most important determinant of fetal-to-adult hemoglobin switching seems to be postconceptual age, with the sharpest period for transition between 30 and 52 weeks. The fetal-to-adult switch appears to be unaffected by the time at which birth occurs or by changes in the kinetics of erythropoiesis induced by perinatal hemolysis.[442] A delay in switching usually is observed in cases of general developmental retardation, in patients with certain chromosomal abnormalities (e.g., trisomy 13), and in diabetic infants because of increased circulating levels of α-aminobutyric acid, which directly affects HbF synthesis.[443] Integration of data from studies using in vitro and in vivo approaches indicates that developmental control of globin switching is intrinsic to erythroid cells. Stage-specific transcriptional forces with negative or positive influences (or both) on specific globin genes may provide the molecular basis for differential transcriptional activity during development. This view is favored by experiments in transgenic mice[444] and in heterokaryons (produced by fusion of human with mouse cells),[445] as well as by isolation of stage-specific transcription factors in other erythroid systems (e.g., avian).[446] Furthermore, because α-like and β-like globin genes are activated sequentially in the order of their location in chromosome 11 or 16, respectively, it is possible that polarity of the transcriptional activity and globin promoter competition for the locus control region and developmental stage–specific transcription factors contribute to this regulation.[447]

Recently genetic linkage and genome-wide association studies in individuals with increased levels of HbF or hereditary persistence of fetal hemoglobin (HPFH) syndromes have provided new and important insights in the control of fetal to adult globin switching.[448,449] Of interest, besides *cis* control of switching (deletions in β-globin cluster or mutations in the γ-globin gene promoters), *trans* control was revealed through direct and indirect interactions of γ-globin with molecules (controlled by loci unlinked to the β-globin cluster) exerting repressive fetal globin activity. These molecules were BCL11A, a transcription factor involved in juvenile leukemia, and HBS1L-Myb. The full-length BCL11A is expressed in adult but not fetal erythroid cells, and adult individuals with high hemoglobin F/BCL11A genotype have reduced expression of full-length BCL11A. Suppression of its expression reactivates HbF expression in adult erythroid cells in vitro,[450] and deletion of BCL11A interferes with fetal hemoglobin silencing during development and rescues the phenotype of a mouse model of sickle cell disease.[451] These observations have suggested that genome editing of BCL11A may represent a useful strategy to ameliorate the clinical picture of hemoglobinopathies.[452] Genome editing approaches based on new editing tools (zinc fingers, TALENS and Crisper/cas technology) are rapidly being developed and allow precise targeting either of BCL11A or its newly identified erythroid-specific enhancers.[166] Myb-HBS1L is downregulated in individuals with elevated HbF levels and overexpression of Myb inhibits γ-globin in human erythroleukemia cells. The levels of Myb were found to be controlled by micro-RNA 15a and 16-1 in patients with human trisomy 13 and high HbF levels.[453]

In addition to the above molecules with γ-globin repressive activity, recent data support a role of KLF1, the major erythroid transcriptional regulator, as suppressor of fetal globin gene. KLF1 mutations were found relatively more common in a thalassemia-endemic region and were associated with a milder β-thalassemia phenotype.[454] Valuable insights on the mechanism of KLF1 on the regulation of globin genes were obtained from families with haplo-insufficiency of KLF1 (missense mutations affecting DNA binding) and increased fetal hemoglobin levels.[455,456] However, this was not always the case, and a compound heterozygosity was required in other families for high HbF expression.[457] It appears that KLF1 targets genes such as *BCL11A*, *EPB4.9*, and *CD44*, which are very sensitive to KLF1 activity, whereas its effects on other genes like γ-globin, or *BCAM* (carrying the Lutheran blood group antigens) are variable. Collectively, it turned out that KLF1 has a critical role in globin gene switching both by directly activating β-globin and indirectly by suppressing γ-globin through its control of *BCL11A*.

Overall, genetic data account for approximately 70% of the HPFH phenotypes observed in human populations, suggesting that new factors are yet to be identified. In this context, it is of interest that three β[0]-thalassemia major patients who failed to engraft after stem cell transplantation became transfusion-independent because they expressed sustained levels of increased HbF in autologous red cells posttransplantation without evidence of any known HPFH genotypes.[458,459] From all of these studies, it has become apparent that switching is very complex, involving many players, *cis* and *trans*, with distinct and variable roles. The many models of globin switching proposed previously (i.e., the competitive model, the chromosome looping, the gene silencing) are not mutually exclusive and may complement each other.

In summary, throughout human development, waves of hematopoiesis are initiated sequentially in newly recruited sites. The first wave of erythropoiesis is seen in yolk sac between days 15 and 18 (7.5 days after conception in mice). In addition to erythroid cells, uncommitted progenitors and progenitors for nonerythroid cells are present in the yolk sac and are thought to be the source of cells colonizing the fetal liver.[211,460–462] However, in addition to yolk sac, foci of hematopoietic activity have been detected within the embryo around the developing aorta (in para-aortic-splanchnopleura [P-Sp] and aorto-gonad-mesonephros [AGM] area).[463–465] In fact, the P-Sp/AGM site in mice was shown to harbor progenitor cells before

circulation begins and 1 day before these cells are found in the yolk sac. Long-term repopulating cells after their transplantation in adult recipients were detected only in the AGM area, leading to speculation that this intraembryonic site is the main or only source of fetal liver colonization,[465] in contrast to earlier experiments implicating the yolk sac in that role.[460–462] Establishment of blood flow and the concentration of nitric oxide appear to play an important role in determining the number of definitive hematopoietic stem cells generated in the AGM region.[466] Presence of mesodermally derived hematopoietic cells in two distinct anatomic sites, one intraembryonic and the other extraembryonic, has been seen in explant studies of *Xenopus* and after analysis of chick–quail chimeras.[467] More recent experiments with human cells have led to similar conclusions.[468] Although the presence of progenitors for definitive hematopoiesis in two independent sites (extraembryonic and within the embryo proper) is indisputable, the extent to which these two sites contribute to fetal liver colonization has been a matter of dispute. The conclusion that only the AGM area contributes to fetal liver colonization was based on transplantation experiments in adult recipients and has been challenged.[389] Transplantation experiments using newborn mice with active fetal liver hematopoiesis as recipients showed that adult long-term repopulating cells are detectable in the yolk sac at day 9 postconception and are 37-fold greater in number than repopulating cells present in the P-Sp/AGM area at the same time. Therefore failure of yolk sac cells (or AGM cells before day 10 postconception) to engraft adult recipients may be caused by either compromised homing or impaired survival and proliferation within the adult bone marrow environment (because of positive regulators or inhibition by negative regulators). In light of this information, the 30-year-old theory that yolk sac colonizes the fetal liver has been revived.[460] A question that remains unanswered is whether stem cell activity 9 days postconception in yolk sac and P-Sp/AGM is generated autonomously and independently or is derived from a common precursor cell with migratory properties. Murine studies comparing newborn transplant outcomes before the onset of systemic circulation between the yolk sac site and the intraembryonic AGM site have emerged,[469] and these, together with the identification of placenta as an autonomous circulation-independent site with terminal erythroid maturation of primitive cells,[470] have added an additional layer of complexity.

A common precursor cell giving rise to erythroid cells with either yolk sac or fetal liver characteristics has been identified by culture of murine and human embryonic stem cells in vitro.[471,472] Environmental regulation of specification to the primitive or definitive lineage has been shown in *Xenopus*.[473] However, because BFU-E present in yolk sac, fetal liver, and fetal bone marrow have a definitive-like progeny and these progenitors were not present after ablation of core binding factor (CBF)-β[474] despite the presence of normal embryonic erythropoiesis, the derivation of embryonic erythroblasts from a distinct progenitor, not present in subsequent life, remains a viable hypothesis. Of further interest is the observation that deletion of Mdm2 and Mdm4, two critical negative regulators of p53, exerted distinct outcomes on primitive and definitive hematopoiesis. Whereas Mdm2 is required for primitive erythropoiesis, Mdm4 is required for massive expansion of definitive erythropoiesis in fetal liver and is dispensable for adult erythropoiesis. These data are also consistent with the distinct molecular control between fetal and adult cells[475] discussed earlier.

TRANSCRIPTION FACTORS IN ERYTHROPOIESIS

Lineage-specific transcription factors are widely believed to be responsible for regulating the expression of erythroid genes during both ontogeny and the course of erythroid differentiation. The majority of erythroid-specific transcription factors has been identified from cloning of breakpoints or translocations associated with human leukemias or from expression libraries obtained from erythroid cell lines. The precise role exerted by each of these factors in erythropoiesis was later clarified by painstaking experiments with somatic cell fusions and in transgenic mice.[445,476,477] Some of the major transcription factors implicated in the control of erythropoiesis are listed in Table 26.2.

Studies of mice with targeted gene disruption have provided key insights into the complex molecular pathways that regulate hematopoiesis in general and erythropoiesis in particular.[1,2] These studies, complemented by in vitro differentiation of mutated embryonic stem cells into different lineages, have provided clear evidence about distinct regulatory requirements of primitive (yolk sac) versus definitive (fetal liver and bone marrow) erythropoiesis, or of early versus late stages of erythroid differentiation. Because erythropoiesis is the first differentiated lineage in embryonic yolk sac hematopoiesis and the predominant lineage in fetal liver hematopoiesis, factors that affect hematopoiesis in general will disturb erythropoiesis during early stages of development and lead to lethality at different gestational days, depending on the defect. The time in development at which disruption of each specific gene manifests its phenotype is used to establish a hierarchical control among the different transcription factors. The earliest disruption of erythroid differentiation is observed in mice lacking the bHLH factor TAL1/SCL, which is encoded by a gene initially identified on the basis of its localization in a chromosomal breakpoint region frequently associated with T-cell acute leukemia.[478] SCL[null] embryos are bloodless and die very early, with abrogation of both yolk sac and fetal liver erythropoiesis.[479] Because of the requirement for SCL in the formation of the transcription complex with the nuclear protein Rbtn2/LMO2 rhombotin 2/LIM domain only 2 (Rbtn2/LMO2) and GATA1 (detailed later), it is not surprising that targeted disruption of Rbtn2 and LMO2 also produces a bloodless phenotype.[480]

Mice lacking expression of GATA2, a member of the GATA family of transcription factors, exhibit an early and severe quantitative defect in hematopoiesis that influences all lineages.[481] Other regulatory factors seem to totally spare embryonic (yolk sac) hematopoiesis and have a specific effect only on fetal liver hematopoiesis, with death occurring at later days (12.5 days postconception). In this category are the proto-oncogene c-Myb and the core-binding factors CBF-α_2/AML1 and CBF-β.[482-484] Embryonic erythropoiesis is spared in mice with targeted ablation of these genes. Both c-Myb, the cellular homologue of v-Myb proto-oncogene, and the heterodimeric transcription factor CBF are abundantly expressed early in normal myelolymphoid cells, with decreasing expression as differentiation proceeds. Their expression pattern and their functional influence on growth factor receptor genes (i.e., IL-3, GM-CSF, CSF1, T-cell antigen receptor [TCR] α, β) may underlie their importance in the development of all definitive hematopoietic lineages.[1]

Of paramount importance for adult erythropoiesis is the transcription factor GATA1, the founder of the GATA family of factors.[1] The GATA1 protein controls erythroid differentiation at several levels by controlling (in cooperation with GATA2) the proliferative capacity of erythroid progenitor/precursor cells, the apoptotic rate of erythroblasts, and the expression of lineage-specific genes. These effects are mediated through activation of expression of target genes by binding to specific sequences (WGATAR) present in the regulatory domains of virtually any erythroid gene, including EPOR and GATA1 itself. However, WGATAR binding sites are also present in genes specific for megakaryocytic, eosinophilic, mast cell, and dendritic lineages, as well as in genes expressed in testicular Sertoli cells. Insights into the specificity of GATA1 in erythroid differentiation have been provided by studies on the organization of WGATAR sites in erythroid-specific regulatory sequences. A minimal erythroid transcription-activation sequence that consists of a core-binding motif flanked by two canonical GATA1 binding sites has been identified. The core-binding motif is composed of one SCL binding site and one GATA binding site separated by 10 bp.[2] Different domains of the GATA1 protein are responsible for binding to the core and the flanking sequences. At least three functional domains in the GATA1 protein have been identified: two zinc finger domains (amino-terminal [N-terminal] finger [NF] and C-terminal finger [CF]) and an active N-terminal domain. The NF domain is required for association with Friend of GATA1 (FOG-1), a protein encoded by a gene identified using GATA1 as bait in the two-hybrid yeast assay.[485] FOG-1 contains 10

zinc finger domains, only the first of which is required for GATA1 binding. The function of its other nine zinc finger domains is not clear because they appear to be dispensable in structure-function studies, but they are well conserved in evolution. The GATA1-FOG-1 heterodimeric complex binds to the two flanking sites of the minimal erythroid transcription activation domain. Experimentally induced genetic mutations, such as GATA1[V205M], impairing GATA1-FOG-1 interaction in mice lead to impaired megakaryocytopoiesis and absence of definitive erythropoiesis, whereas primitive erythropoiesis is normal.[486] Rescue experiments indicate that GATA1[V205M] newborns are severely anemic with anisocytosis and spherocytosis with striking reduction mainly in the expression of genes encoding membrane proteins, whereas expression of other erythroid-specific genes, such as *Alas2*, was not affected.[487] These results indicate that DNA binding of the GATA1-FOG-1 complex is necessary for activation of a subset of GATA1 target genes in definitive erythroid cells but is dispensable for their activation in primitive erythroblasts. It should be emphasized that GATA1-FOG-1 interaction, while activating the expression of erythroid genes, inhibits target gene activation in testicular Sertoli cells.[488] This result provides insight into how one factor regulates more than one differentiation program by suggesting that its function, but not its expression, is different depending on the cellular context. (Whether GATA1-FOG-1 interaction inhibits erythroid gene expression in myelomonocytic cells has not been investigated.)

The CF domain, on the other hand, recognizes and binds to the GATA site localized in the core of the minimal erythroid transcription sequence 10 bp downstream to the SCL binding site. SCL and GATA1 bind simultaneously to their respective sites of the core as multimeric complexes formed by SCL/E47/LMO2 on the one hand and by GATA1/LMO2 on the other. Binding of the two complexes to the core is stabilized by Lbd1, which forms a physical bridge between them. The paramount importance of the CF finger for GATA1 function is proved by the fact that *GATA1* genes lacking the region encoding this domain are unable to rescue erythroid differentiation in GATA1[null] embryonic stem cells,[489] whereas minigenes containing only the CF of either GATA1 or GATA2 are sufficient to induce megakaryocytic differentiation of myeloid cell lines.[490] In addition to forming heterodimers with LMO2, CF can form complexes with Sp1 and PU.1, two factors essential for myelomonocytic differentiation. The GATA1-PU.1 complex is unable to bind DNA, so its function might be to establish either an erythroid- or a myeloid-permissive cellular environment depending on which factor is expressed at the highest concentration.[2] The presence of relatively higher concentrations of GATA1 would favor the formation of GATA1-LMO2 complexes leading to activation of erythroid-specific genes, whereas the presence of relatively higher concentrations of PU.1 would lead mainly to the formation of the transcriptionally inactive GATA1-PU.1 complexes.

Although early experiments on cell lines failed to identify any function for the N-terminal domain of GATA1,[490,491] knock-in experiments in mice indicated that this domain, although dispensable for primitive erythropoiesis, is required for appropriate production of definitive red cells.[489] A truncated *GATA1* gene lacking the N-terminal domain is 10 times less efficient than the full-length gene in rescuing erythroid differentiation in GATA1[null] mice.[489] This experiment suggests that interaction of the N-terminal domain of *GATA1* with a suitable partner(s) is required for optimal definitive erythropoiesis. Structure function studies have identified that interaction between the N-terminal domain of *GATA1* and the product of the retinoblastoma (RB) gene is essential for proper terminal erythroid maturation, providing a unifying mechanism for the similar phenotype of several GATA1 and RB mouse mutants and of human diseases associated with mutations in these two genes.[492]

In addition to all the evidence pointing to *GATA1* as exerting a predominant but ontogenetic-specific role in the control of erythroid differentiation, other evidence indicates that this gene exerts exquisite control in the differentiation of other hemopoietic lineages, such as megakaryocytes,[1] mast cells,[493] eosinophils,[494] and dendritic cells.[495] The mechanism used by one single factor in guiding differentiation along different lineages does not rely on specific domains in the

GATA1 protein itself. In fact, the structure of all the GATA proteins is so well conserved among different family members and in evolution that GATA1[null] embryonic stem cells are rescued not only by reintroduction of the *GATA1* gene itself but also by introducing any other member of the GATA family, such as GATA3.[496] The lineage-specific action of *GATA1* in regulating gene expression is achieved through the presence of lineage-specific regulatory sequences in the promoter regions of the target genes. Therefore the relative concentration of *GATA1*, as opposed to the levels of a few key regulatory partners, may establish a lineage-permissive microenvironment. Furthermore, the existence of lineage-specific regulatory sequences in the *GATA1* gene itself ensures that such concentrations are achieved only in the right cell. Although GATA1 is expressed in erythroid, megakaryocytic, mast, dendritic, and eosinophilic cells, its level of expression differs greatly among the various cell types, with erythroid cells expressing the most. Three DNase hypersensitive sites (HS) have been recognized within the 8 Kb upstream and the first intron of the murine *GATA1* gene, defined as HSI, HSII, and HSIII. Targeted deletion mutants in the mouse have shown that each of these sites functions as an enhancer in different cell types. HSI is required for GATA1 expression in megakaryocytes,[497] mast cells,[493] and also for upregulation of GATA1 expression during the process of antigen presentation in dendritic cells[498] and during the progression of erythroid maturation.[499] HSIII is capable of sustaining low levels of GATA1 expression in erythroid and dendritic cells. HSII, which is dispensable for erythroid and megakaryocyte expression, is absolutely required for gene expression in eosinophils.[494] All of the 317 bp of HSI are required for GATA1 expression in megakaryocytes, but only the first 5′ 62 bp are needed for erythroid-specific reporter activity.[500] The HSI region contains a canonical minimal erythroid activation sequence, and point mutations in the GATA site, but not in the E-box, abolish HSI function in both erythroid and megakaryocytic cells. Of note, GATA1 mRNA has an unusually long half-life (>9 hours). Two GATA1 bands, corresponding to the native and processed (acetylated and phosphorylated) forms of the protein, have been detected by Western blot analysis.[501] The processed form binds DNA with higher affinity than the native form. Furthermore, although the half-life of the native form is short (approximately 0.5 hour) and stabilized by EPO, the processed form is extremely stable (half-life >6 hours) and EPO-independent.[501] Because the cell cycle of hemopoietic cells in vivo is as short as 6 hours, erythroid cells accumulate GATA1 mRNA and protein as they proliferate. Because maturation is dependent on the levels of GATA1 expressed by cells, the cellular GATA1 content might represent the biologic clock that, by controlling the number of precursors, determines the cellular output of the differentiation process. This hypothesis suggests that EPO-induced GATA1 processing through the ubiquitin–proteasome pathway is an important element in the regulation of erythroid differentiation. On the other hand, the TRAIL-Bruton kinase death pathway has as an end point caspase 3, the protein specifically responsible for GATA1 cleavage. However, caspase 3 is unable to cleave GATA1 if the protein is complexed in the nucleus with the chaperone protein heat shock protein 70 (Hsp70). EPO-receptor signaling counteracts the apoptotic pathway by favoring Hsp70-GATA1 colocalization in the nucleus.[502] The equilibrium between TRAIL and EPO-dependent control on Hsp70 localization may be perturbed under pathologic conditions. As an example, defective nuclear localization of Hsp70 and increased GATA1 cleavage is associated with dyserythropoiesis in myelodysplastic disorders.[503] Similarly, by sequestering Hsp70, free α-globin promotes GATA1 degradation and induces ineffective erythropoiesis in β-thalassemia.[504] The biochemical studies detailing the link between EPO and TRAIL from one side and GATA1 from the other are consistent with additional data indicating that EPO signaling also induces GATA1 phosphorylation at Ser310 and that this phosphorylation plays an important role in regulating GATA1 function in erythroid cell lines.[505,506] Although GATA1 mutants expressing only the native form of GATA1 do not have a detectable erythroid phenotype under steady-state conditions,[507] more studies on the response of these mice to erythroid stress will clarify the role of GATA1 processing in stress erythropoiesis.

Another gene of the GATA family important for erythroid differentiation is *GATA2*. Both *GATA1* and *GATA2* are expressed early in multipotential progenitors; however, their expression ratios change as the cells differentiate (see Table 26.1),[508] suggesting that the ratio of these two factors may be important at specific stages of erythroid differentiation. Knock-out experiments with both of these genes have borne this out. Thus in contrast to *GATA2*, which is expressed at high levels in early cells and affects expansion of all hematopoietic lineages,[481] *GATA1* expression increases as differentiation advances and seems to be the obligatory factor required for survival and terminal differentiation of erythroid cells. In mice with targeted disruption of *GATA1*, erythropoiesis proceeds only up to the stage of proerythroblasts; these mice die early and fail to mature further.[509,510] Furthermore, transgenic mice with partial loss of function (knockdown alleles, GATA1[LOW]) of *GATA1* show that erythroid differentiation is dose-dependent with respect to *GATA1*.[499] High levels of GATA1 are necessary to form complexes with its cofactor FOG-1[485] and with the other proteins described earlier (LM02, SCL, or Hsp70) during terminal erythroid differentiation.

The realization that minute differences in transcription factor concentrations are required for lineage specification under physiologic conditions supports the idea that the differentiation system allows more flexibility in both the choice and the reversibility of pathway commitment toward a specific lineage. For example, a CFU-E was thought to have no other choice than to become an erythroid cell or to die.[6] More recently, experiments with forced expression of transcription factors in fully committed or even mature cells have demonstrated that the system has some degree of plasticity and that forced expression of *FOG*-1 into mast cells may turn them into erythroblasts,[511] whereas forced expression of *GATA1* into common myeloid progenitor cells induces their transdifferentiation into MEP.[512] (It is foreseen that future experiments will demonstrate that any cell type may be turned into an erythroblast by overexpression of an appropriate combination of transcription factors.) All of these manipulations were performed in vitro. Of interest, experimentally decreased expression of *GATA1* in progenitor cell compartments in vivo does not alter the frequency of individual compartments (i.e., does not decrease MEP by increasing the granulocyte/macrophage progenitor) but results in alternative differentiation pathways. Although the numbers of cells phenotypically recognizable as MEP in these animals are much higher than normal, MEP with reduced *GATA1* expression, unlike normal cells, also have the potential to differentiate into mast cells.[513]

Another factor with special importance in the erythroid lineage is the CACCC binding protein designated EKLF (also known as KLF1), which is expressed at all stages of erythropoiesis but binds preferentially to CACCC sites in the β-globin promoter. EKLF is a zinc finger protein that binds not only DNA, but also, after appropriate posttranslational modifications, is a key regulatory protein that modulates chromatin structure of the β-globin locus.[514] Mice lacking EKLF (EKLF[null]) die of a thalassemic-like defect because of severe deficiency of β-globin expression.[515] Microarray analysis of EKLF[null] erythroid cells and promoter-specific expression of reported genes in EKLF[null] cells have identified that the first GATA1-dependent molecular control of erythroid differentiation is followed by a second EKLF-dependent phase.[516,517] Primarily GATA1-dependent genes include, in addition to *EPOR* and those involved in the control of apoptosis, α- and δ-globin. EKLF-dependent genes, in addition to β-globin[518,519] and AHSP, are represented by those required for appropriate membrane assembly, such as β-spectrin, ankyrin, and band 3 (but not α-spectrin). These results are consistent with the notion that, in erythroid differentiation, activation of α-globin gene expression precedes that of β-globin[520] and that loss of GATA1 binding sites in the promoter of the gene is found in α-thalassemia,[521] in the Greek nondeletion HPFH (guanine to adenine at nucleotide position −117 of γ-globin),[522] and in δ-thalassemia (point mutation leading to G→A substitution at position +69 of the δ-globin gene),[523] whereas loss of EKLF binding site is present in other forms of HPFH. In addition to regulating globin gene expression directly, EKLF inhibits γ-globin expression indirectly by activating BCL11A expression.[524]

More recently, it has been identified that KLF1 promotes terminal erythroid maturation also in a noncell-autonomous fashion by regulating expression of DNase IIα, in the central macrophage of fetal liver erythroblastic islands thus facilitating digestion of the DNA of engulfed pyrenocytes, in the central macrophage of the erythroblastic island present in mouse fetal liver.[525,526]

Intrinsic control of erythroid differentiation also is exerted by genes that, until repressed, prevent terminal cell maturation. The most studied of these genes is ID1,[527] which as its name indicates, inhibits differentiation along almost all mesenchymal cell lineages, including the erythroid lineage.[528,529] ID1 appears to act between GATA1 and EKLF by preventing EKLF from executing its program.

Because common transcription factors are present in erythroid and megakaryocytic cells, and bipotent erythroid/megakaryocytic progenitors exist both in vitro (in the form of cell lines) and in vivo,[63] exciting insights regarding subtleties in the molecular control of these two lineages by the same transcription factors have surfaced. Modified gene-targeting strategy ("knockdown") of GATA1 uncovered a largely unanticipated role of this transcription factor in the control of proliferation and maturation of megakaryocytes.[499] In addition to GATA1, other important transcription factors essential for terminal megakaryocytic development are NF-E2[530] and its partner mafG.[531]

Nevertheless, the fact that several regulators are necessary for primitive (yolk sac), as opposed to definitive (fetal liver and bone marrow), erythropoiesis provides evidence that molecular control between these two hemopoietic sites is different and may include both ubiquitous and hematopoietic-specific factors. In fact, evidence suggests that GATA1 transcription is differentially regulated in yolk sac cells compared to fetal liver erythroid cells, with alternative promoter use and an additional intron element requirement for promoter activation in fetal liver cells.[532]

In addition to transcription factors/oncogenes influencing erythropoiesis, targeted ablation and naturally existing mutations of hematopoietic growth factor receptors, especially of the tyrosine kinase family, have disclosed important insights into the control of erythropoiesis. Whereas deletion of the vascular endothelial growth factor (VEGF)/flk-1 receptor affects both endothelial and hematopoietic development[533] through its presumed presence in the hemangioblast, the common endothelial/hematopoietic stem cell, mutations affecting the tyrosine kinase KIT receptor (present in hematopoietic cells) or of its ligand KL (present in stromal cells) seem to predominantly affect erythropoiesis in the fetal liver and the adult animal. Mice with KIT mutations (W mutations) leading to absence of or compromised kinase activity and steel mice with mutations of KL have disproportionate and severe reduction of the numbers of late erythroid progenitors, CFU-E, and differentiated erythroid precursors resulting in anemia.[534] Studies showing cross-phosphorylation of EPOR following activation of KIT/KL signaling may be relevant to the effect.[294] Mutations or targeted ablations of some downstream signaling substrates for KIT or other receptors (i.e., SHP2 phosphatase or gp130) seem to produce a hematopoietic picture not unlike the one produced by receptor mutations.[535,536]

Taken together, these studies have significantly expanded our understanding of the molecular basis of hematopoietic cell development in general and of erythropoiesis in particular. The emerging picture is that certain genes, such as SCL, are absolutely required for hematopoietic development, whereas other genes, such as GATA2, c-Myb, CBF, TEL, and some downstream signal transducing molecules such as gp30 and SHP2, are responsible for expansion and maintenance of a normal pool of fetal liver and adult hematopoietic progenitors. The participation of many of these molecules in multicomponent molecular complexes with protein/protein and protein/DNA interactions (i.e., LM02/Lbd1/SCL/E2A/GATA), during the early proliferative stages of hematopoiesis[537] may underlie their role in the proliferation and maintenance of immature progenitor/precursor pools in erythropoiesis. Other genes such as GATA1, its partner FOG-1, and EKLF are necessary to direct high levels of function of erythroid-specific genes in cells already committed to terminal differentiation. Thus a hierarchical requirement in the expression of

specific regulators during early versus late erythroid differentiation or during yolk sac versus fetal liver/adult erythropoiesis is demonstrated. However, this does not exclude the involvement of some factors (i.e., SCL, TEL) at both early and late stages of erythropoiesis. In fact, more recent studies on conditional knockouts have clarified that SCL exerts two different levels of control in the development of the hemopoietic system. First, SCL is required for the determination event that induces one (or few) mesenchymal cell(s) to become a hematopoietic stem cell(s) in the early embryos.[197] After this initial event has taken place, its presence becomes dispensable, as demonstrated by the fact that conditional SCL deletion in the adult animals impairs only erythropoiesis and megakaryocytopoiesis.[197,538]

With information from innovative applications of molecular approaches becoming available at a fast pace, the list of regulators with a biologic impact on hematopoiesis/erythropoiesis not only is continuously expanding but is starting to fill the gap between the individual transcription factors and the epigenetic control of erythroid cells. Actively expressed genes are localized in areas on the chromosome in an open configuration. The DNA switch from a closed to an open configuration is determined by the tightness of its binding to the histones by which it is surrounded.[539] A series of enzymes regulates the chromosome configuration state by modifying either the DNA (cytosine methylation mediated by specific methylases) or the histones (e.g., histone acetyltransferase [HAT] and deacetylase [HDAC], polycomb repressive complexes). HAT exerts a positive control (promoting the formation of an open configuration state), whereas methylases and HDAC exert a negative control (inducing a closed chromatin configuration state) on gene expression. Once the chromatin is in an open configuration state, appropriate enzymatic complexes (e.g., polymerases, spliceosomes) are recruited to the locus for appropriate expression to occur. Because of their ability to recognize specific DNA sequences, transcription factors play an important role in the recruitment of the epigenetic and/or transcriptional protein machinery to a specific locus. The link between epigenetic and transcriptional control of gene expression in erythroid cells is emerging. The first global methylation status of erythroid cells as they mature has been determined.[138] The relationship between chromatin architecture and transcription factor occupancy in the loci encoding key erythrocyte membrane proteins has been established.[540] In addition to binding GATA1, FOG-1 is also capable of binding NuRD, a complex that contains HDAC1.[541] The multicomplex GATA1/FOG-1/NuRD is responsible for appropriate activation/repression of several erythroid specific genes, including the GATA2-GATA1 switch occurring at early stages of erythroid development.[542] Recently, a complex formed by the class II HDAC HDAC5, GATA1, EKLF, and ERK was identified in human erythroblasts.[543] Based on the observation that this complex was not detected in megakaryocytes and that the function of class II HDAC is to chaperone other proteins to the nucleus, this novel complex was defined as nuclear remodeling shuttle erythroid (NuRSERY). By balancing the level of GATA1 and EKLF during terminal erythroid maturation, NuRSERY may represent at least one of the mechanisms that links the extrinsic (ERK phosphorylation by KL) to the intrinsic (transcription factor concentration) control of erythropoiesis.

Genome-wide analyses have recently detailed the sequence of epigenetic events that regulates the expression of erythroid specific genes during the process of terminal erythroid maturation. Erythroid-specific enhancers and promoters are already in an active configuration at the progenitor levels.[544,545] There is little difference in the enhancer activation profile of fetal and adult erythroid progenitors. Surprisingly this difference is related to binding of cofactors, such as the interferon regulatory factors 2 and 6 that are essential for activation of adult erythroid programs but not to binding of master erythroid regulators such as GATA1. During erythroid maturation, the expression of these genes is mainly regulated posttranscriptionally (mRNA stability and splicing and binding to the ribosome translational machinery). Erythroid-specific micro-[546,547] and long-[548,549] noncoding RNAs may play important roles in the posttranscriptional regulation of erythroid genes at late stages of maturation. This regulation may represent another layer of complexity. In fact, increased expression of LIN28B, by suppressing the biogenesis of the let-7 microRNA in adult CD34+ cells in vitro, upregulates HbF expression with production of fetal-like erythrocytes, thus presenting an additional target for increasing fetal Hb to ameliorate beta globin disorders.[550,551]

TRANSCRIPTIONAL AND POSTTRANSCRIPTIONAL IMPAIRMENT IN DISORDERS OF ERYTHROPOIESIS

The transcription factor found most frequently altered in inherited and acquired human diseases of the erythroid and megakaryocytic lineage is GATA1. The mutations often involve the region of the gene encoding the NF domain. Mutations in the GATA1 NF domain interrupting its interaction with FOG-1, such as V205M and G208S, are responsible for familial dyserythropoietic anemia and X-linked thrombocytopenia, respectively.[552,553] A different mutation at position 208 leading to G→A substitution is associated with dyserythropoietic anemia and macrothrombocytopenia.[554] Mutations in the NF terminal domain of GATA1 responsible for DNA binding, such as A216G[555] and D218G,[556] instead have been found to be associated with X-linked thalassemia and/or thrombocytopenia. The phenotype of X-linked thrombocytopenia was mimicked in mice by knock-in experiments of the mutant V205G GATA1 gene.[557] However, the same A216G mutation has been found associated with X-linked gray platelet syndrome, a mild bleeding disorder characterized by thrombocytopenia and large agranular platelet,[558] whereas a R216G mutation was identified in two families in which the X-linked thrombocytopenia and thalassemia phenotype was associated with a PMF phenotype (reticulin fibrosis and increased angiogenesis).[559] Furthermore, a mutation at codon 216 changing arginine to tryptophan (R216W) was detected in a 3-year-old boy with congenital erythropoietic porphyria, an autosomal recessive disorder usually because of mutations of the uroporphyrinogen III synthase gene (UROS). The boy also presented with microcytic anemia and red cell morphologic characteristics and a globin chain pattern compatible with β-thalassemia and increased HbF levels (59.5%).[560] The different phenotype expressed by patients carrying mutations either in the FOG-1 or the DNA binding portion of NF supported the notion that the two domains influence erythroid versus megakaryocytic maturation.[561] To clarify why mutations in the same codon may cause diseases with different phenotype, systematic analyses of disease-causing GATA1 mutations in murine gene complementation systems were performed.[562] These analyses revealed that mutations shown to impair DNA binding of GATA1 in vitro did not affect target gene occupancy in vivo but rather disrupted GATA1 association with partner proteins. More specifically, substitution at the same amino acid selectively inhibited TAL1 or FOG1 binding, producing distinct cell phenotype. However, this brilliant approach does not explain why the same mutation results in a different phenotype. It is possible that the phenotype induced by mutations in the GATA1 gene is extremely sensitive to genetic modifiers outside the GATA1 locus. This hypothesis has been demonstrated in mice in which the same mutation induces embryonic lethality, thrombocytopenia, or myelofibrosis, depending on the mouse background in which it is harbored.[563]

On the other hand, frameshift and splice mutations encoding GATA1s, a protein lacking the N-terminal domain, are not only associated with impaired erythropoiesis[564] but are also found in patients with megakaryocytic leukemia in Down syndrome,[565,566] in newborns with transient myeloproliferative syndromes,[567] and in one adult patient with megakaryocytic leukemia.[568] A mutation equivalent to that found in patients with acute megakaryoblastic leukemia and Down syndrome was created in mice by N-ethyl-N-nitrosourea mutagenesis screening. The reduced expression of the full-length GATA1 was not compensated in mice by expression of GATA1s. The mutation was embryonic lethal in hemizygous males and induced thrombocytopenia in heterozygous females.[569] However, when introduced in mice the GATA1s mutation increased proliferation of a "unique" fetal stem/progenitor cell extinguished in

adult life.[570] The association between a mutation of GATA1 and the development of leukemia supports the concept that GATA1 controls the proliferation of hematopoietic progenitors. Reduced GATA1 expression, by increasing progenitor cell proliferation, may predispose hematopoietic cells to leukemia by favoring accumulation of secondary mutations. These mutations may involve the GATA1 itself because transforming Myb-GATA1 fusion genes have been associated with reduced GATA1 levels in acute basophilic leukemia.[571,572] Alterations of hematopoietic proliferation appear to be achieved through quantitative, rather than structural, GATA1 alterations. The GATA1s protein is far less efficient than the full-length GATA1 in rescuing the phenotype of GATA1null embryonic stem cells,[489] and hypomorphic mutations in mice induce either leukemia[573] or a phenotype similar to idiopathic myelofibrosis,[574] depending on the severity of the reduction of expression. Interestingly, the reduced content of GATA1 in megakaryocytes, through an as yet unidentified molecular defect independent of JAK2V617F, distinguishes primary myelofibrosis from all the other myeloproliferative neoplasms in humans.[575] (For a more complete review on the role of GATA factors in hematologic diseases, see review article by Cantor[576].)

Point mutations in the EKLF/KLF1 gene have been associated with human diseases of terminal erythroid maturation (see Table 26.2). E325K substitution in the conserved residue of the zinc finger domain 2 is associated with congenital dyserythropoietic anemia and increased levels of embryonic globins, revealing a role of EKLF in repressing embryonic globin expression in humans.[577–579] Premature stop codons (L127X, K292X), point mutations in conserved residues of the zinc finger 1 (H299Y) and 2 (R328L, R328H, R331G), frameshift (X47 and X34), and hypomorphic mutations (deletion of the GATA1 binding site in the promoter region) have been associated with lack of Lutheran group antigen (Lu negative phenotype),[580] whereas neutral substitution (M39L), premature stop codon (K288X), and premature stop codon plus point mutations in the conserved residue of zinc finger 2 (S270X plus K332Q) have been associated with the HPFH phenotype with or without elevated zinc protoporphyrin.[455,457] Not all heterozygotes for EKLF mutations have increased HbF, and different levels are seen even with the same mutation. Hereditary spherocytosis has also been observed in mice carrying the spontaneous Nan mutation (E339D substitution in the conserved residue of zinc finger 2).[581]

Another disease associated with abnormalities in the molecular machinery of red cell differentiation is represented by DBA, a rare congenital red cell hypoplasia characterized by anemia, bone marrow erythroblastopenia (lack of late erythroid forms), and congenital anomalies. The disease is associated with heterozygous mutations in the ribosomal protein S19 gene (RPS19) in approximately 25% of probands.[582] In a large cohort of 172 new families with familial history of DBA, mutations affecting the coding sequence of RPS19 or splice sites were found in 34 cases (19.8%), whereas additional mutations in noncoding regions were found in eight patients (4.6%). Mutations included nonsense, missense, splice site, and frameshift mutations. More recently, de novo nonsense and splice-site mutations in another ribosomal protein, RPS24 (encoded by RPS24 [10q22-q23]), was identified in approximately 2% of RPS19 mutation-negative probands.[583] The molecular defect of other families is the subject of numerous investigations, and novel mutations in ribosomal genes already implicated in the disease or in new genes (such as RPL27)[584] are continuously discovered.

No correlation between the nature of mutations and the different patterns of clinical expression, including age at presentation, presence of malformations, and therapeutic outcome, has been documented. The lack of a consistent relationship between the nature of the mutations and the clinical phenotype implies that as yet unidentified factors modulate the phenotypic expression of the primary genetic defect in families with RPS19 mutations.[585] Two not mutually exclusive hypotheses have been proposed to explain the pathobiologic role of RPS19 (and RPS24) in the pathogenesis of the disease: (1) loss of unknown functions not directly connected with RPS19's structural role in ribosomes and (2) altered protein synthesis because of poor ribosome organization. The first hypothesis was suggested by findings based on a proteomic approach that identified numerous proteins bound to RPS19. In addition to FGF2, complement component 5 receptor 1, a nucleolar protein called RPS19 binding protein, and Pim-1, the other RPS19-binding proteins fall in the following Gene Ontology categories: NTPases (ATPases and GTPases; 5 proteins), hydrolases/helicases (19 proteins), isomerases (2 proteins), kinases (3 proteins), splicing factors (5 proteins), structural constituents of ribosome (29 proteins), transcription factors (11 proteins), transferases (5 proteins), transporters (9 proteins), DNA/RNA-binding protein species (53 proteins), other (1 dehydrogenase protein, 1 ligase protein, 1 peptidase protein, 1 receptor protein, 1 translation elongation factor), and 13 proteins with unknown function.[586] However, more recent studies have identified that RPS19 plays an essential role in the biogenesis and maturation of the 40S small ribosomal subunit in human cells[587,588] because of reduced gene expression of clustered ribosomal proteins owing to abnormal pre-mRNA processing.[589] Such a defective ribosomal gene expression results in alterations of the transcription, translation, apoptosis, and oncogenic pathways.[590] Expression of RPS19 mRNA and protein decreases during terminal erythroid differentiation.[591] A mouse model of the disease has been generated by disrupting the endogenous Rps19 gene.[592–594] Cellular models of the disease have been established by small interfering RNA (siRNA) technology against RPS19 protein.[595–597] These models are establishing that RPS19 deficiency is accompanied by an unanticipated activation of p53 and death of the erythroid cells. Treatment of RPS19[null] cells with dexamethasone prevents p53 activation and restores terminal erythroid maturation,[598] providing a molecular mechanism for the therapeutic effects exerted by dexamethasone in these patients. Alternatively, it has been proposed that dexamethasone may rescue defective protein synthesis in ribosomal-deficient erythroid cells by increasing expression of a subset of GR target genes (such as Zfp36l2, which controls RNA stability and/or translation and is required for BFU-E self-renewal).[599,600] Only 40% to 50% of DBA patients respond to steroids.[601] The mechanism underlying this lack of response has been the subject of recent investigation. The increased frequency of rs6198 GR SNP observed in these patients suggests that the failure to respond to steroids may be influenced by genetic and/or epigenetic modifications of the GR locus.

In addition to ribosomal defects, DBA has been recently associated with mutations in the GATA1 gene.[602,603] This discovery led to the identification that the ribosomal abnormalities observed in DBA reduces GATA1 translation.[604]

RSP19 deficiency and p53 activation is also observed in the 5q-MDS syndrome,[598] and p53 activation associated with reduced ribosomal gene dosage has been reported in low-risk MDS.[605] Whole-exome sequencing of MDS has recently uncovered mutations in genes involved in RNA splicing.[606,607] Whether these mutations also activate p53 has yet to be determined. These results suggest that defective mRNA splicing/translation may represent a unifying mechanism for the etiology of MDS. Interestingly, MDS has also been associated with mutations in GATA2. In fact, in spite of its importance in the early phases of erythroid maturation, GATA2 mutations have not been detected in erythroid diseases so far. However, a gain-of-function GATA2 mutation has been reported in one patient with chronic myelomonocytic leukemia[608] and loss-of-function GATA2 mutations have been systematically detected in patients with a rare genetic immunodeficiency distinguished by reduced levels of all the immune cells produced in the marrow (monocytes, dendritic, NK and B cells, MonoMAC syndrome)[609,610] (see Table 26.2). The marrow of these patients is hypocellular, with absent/reduced levels of multilymphoid and myeloid progenitor cells and dysplasia of the myeloid as well as the erythroid and megakaryocytic lineage. These patients may eventually develop MDS and AML. Mutations in the coding region of GATA2 have also been found in four patients with MDS without immunodeficiency.[611] In addition, quantitative alterations (reduced levels) in GATA2 expression, possibly secondary to the primary lesions, have been described in the CD34+ cells from patients with aplastic anemia[612] and in blasts from AML,[613] and although hypomorphic GATA2 mutations do not induce a strong phenotype in mice,[611] genome-wide analyses of transcriptional reprogramming

of mouse models of AML have identified GATA2 as one of the few key transcription factors whose expression is reduced in leukemic blasts.[613]

In conclusion, for a mechanism still to be identified, ribosomal deficiency may affect either GATA1 inducing DBA, or GATA2 inducing MDS deficiency. The different targets of the translational defect are reflected by the different agents that are effective in the two diseases. DBA is treated with glucocorticoids[601] that reduce p53, reducing apoptosis, and increase BFU-E possibly by activating ZFP36L2, while MDS is treated with lenalinomide,[614] which increases CFU-E[615] possibly by activating Wnt/TGF-β signaling.[616]

CELLULAR DYNAMICS IN ERYTHROPOIESIS

The primary function of the mature red cell, which is the end product of erythropoiesis, is to transport oxygen efficiently through the circulation to the tissues. To achieve this goal, the adult marrow must release approximately 3×10^9 new red cells or reticulocytes per kilogram per day.[617] This number of reticulocytes represents (1%) of the total red cell mass and is derived from an estimated 5×10^9 erythroid precursors per kilogram.[617] In addition to maintaining homeostasis (i.e., a stable hematocrit), the erythron must be able to respond quickly and appropriately to increased oxygen demands, either acute (e.g., following red cell loss) or chronic (e.g., with hypoxia from pulmonary disease or a right-to-left cardiac shunt). It is well established that EPO is responsible both for maintaining normal erythropoiesis and for increasing red cell production in response to oxygen needs. However, the overall marrow response is complex and requires not only the participation of erythroid cells responsive to EPO but also a structurally intact microenvironment and an optimal iron supply within the marrow.

EPO stimulation elicits two types of measurable responses: changes in proliferative activity (including improved survival) and changes in maturation rates. The first detectable response to increased serum EPO is amplification of CFU-E and erythroid precursors, cells that are extremely sensitive to EPO. Because all these cells virtually are already in cycle, increases in their numbers cannot be achieved by increasing their fraction in cycle. Either additional divisions are involved, or new cells are recruited to the CFU-E pool (from a pre–CFU-E pool). Additional divisions of CFU-E or precursor cells would increase their transit time within the marrow and potentially delay the delivery of new red cells to the periphery. Because a shortened maturation time has been observed instead and the proliferative potentials of CFU-E and proerythroblasts are finite, high levels of amplification cannot be achieved through this mechanism. Therefore such needs are met by influx into the CFU-E and precursor pools of newly differentiating cells from earlier progenitor compartments.

Such a surge of newly produced cells has been observed in prior experiments.[204,618,619] A rapid influx of fresh cells was particularly notable in polycythemic mice that were experimentally depleted of CFU-E and erythroid precursors at the time the stimulus was applied.[175,204] Because of the rapidity of response (i.e., within 24 hours in the polycythemic animals), it appeared that the orderly progression from BFU-E to CFU-E to proerythroblast had been compressed. Such acceleration of differentiation is possible through shortened intermitotic intervals, fewer mitotic divisions, or differentiation without divisions. This short-circuiting in differentiation requires high serum levels of EPO and adequate numbers of BFU-E (i.e., these conditions are met in a previously hypertransfused, polycythemic animal stimulated by EPO or in marrow suddenly recovering from acquired pure erythroid aplasia). Once CFU-E and precursors are expanded through this mechanism, most persisting erythropoietic demands can be met through this pool without excess input from pre–CFU-E pools. Thus acute demand for erythropoiesis is met by influx from pre–CFU-E pools through an accelerated differentiation and maturation sequence. Demonstration of such an event was seen in mice with conditional deletions of integrins using the EPOR-Cre model deleting at the post–CFU-E level.[620] In contrast, chronic demands (i.e., demands because of a chronic hemolytic anemia) are mainly satisfied through a greatly amplified late erythroid pool and with a minimum distortion in the differentiation sequence.[155,621] The fact that the kinetics of erythroid differentiation/maturation are different in acute versus chronic marrow regeneration is supported by differing qualitative changes in the newly formed red cells. An increase in i antigen and HbF expression as well as an increase in cells with higher mean corpuscular volumes is seen with an acute response, whereas these alterations are minimal or less pronounced with chronic responses.[155,622] When severe anemia persists from birth onward, erythroid production can increase up to 10-fold above baseline.[621] This is possible not only because of maximally expanded erythropoietic pools but also because the sites of active erythropoiesis may extend to include those that support red cell differentiation during fetal life. Thus although the marrow space in axial bones (vertebrae, pelvis, ribs, sternum, clavicles) is sufficient for normal erythropoiesis or for response to moderate anemia, the femur, humerus, spleen and/or liver, and (rarely) thymus may support red cell production in children with congenital hemolytic anemia (e.g., thalassemia major). Expanded erythropoiesis may lead to skeletal deformities, hepatosplenomegaly, or erythropoiesis in the soft tissues adjacent to bone.

Quantitative assessments of changes in erythroid progenitor cell pools in response to EPO stimulation can be made through cultures of bone marrow cells. Despite sampling errors, erythroid cultures can provide rough estimates of relative progenitor abundance within an aspirated marrow specimen and have shown consistent increases in the frequency of CFU-E in proportion to the level of EPO stimulation.[623,624] Conversely, with increases in the hematocrit or in polycythemic animals, a decrease in CFU-E frequency has been observed.[625,626] In contrast to CFU-E, the incidence of BFU-E was found to fluctuate less with either acute or chronic expansion of erythropoiesis, probably because a few BFU-E can generate several thousand cells. Furthermore, BFU-E can increase their fraction in cycle and thus increase the number of differentiated progeny without a significant change in their total numbers. Most BFU-E detectable in marrow or blood erythroid cultures probably represent a reservoir of progenitors not normally participating in day-to-day erythropoiesis. The parameters needed to maintain a healthy or appropriate BFU-E pool in hematopoiesis are not defined. That hematopoietic expansion is curtailed in mice with steel mutations and anemia develops in mice treated with anti-C-KIT antibody[627] suggests that adequate levels of normal KL may be crucial for early erythropoietic expansion.[205]

The rate of red cell production can also be accurately evaluated by ferrokinetic studies (i.e., study of iron incorporation into developing red cells). In addition, a marrow scan, typically with technetium Tc 99m, can document the extent of active erythropoiesis. However, these approaches are seldom necessary in clinical practice because estimates of erythropoiesis can be obtained from the reticulocyte index.[621] First, the observed percentage of reticulocytes is normalized to the hematocrit to calculate the total marrow output of reticulocytes. Alternatively, the absolute number of reticulocytes per microliter can be counted directly using fluorescent RNA labeling. However, because younger reticulocytes are prematurely released into the circulation under conditions of acute need, the total number of reticulocytes overestimates the true level of red cell production as measured by iron kinetics.[621] Therefore a second correction is made to account for the maturation of early circulating reticulocytes, or "shift" cells (polychromatophilic red cells), when present in the blood smear. The resulting reticulocyte index gives excellent estimates of effective red cell production.

Although the presence, density, or both of EPORs on developing erythroid cells determines the responses to EPO, other properties (e.g., surface antigens on BFU-E versus CFU-E versus end-stage red cells) may provide the basis for selective suppression of CFU-E versus BFU-E or selective immune destruction of red cells versus erythroblasts. For example, suppression of CFU-E or erythroblasts can occur in acquired pure red cell aplasia[628] or B19 parvovirus infection,[629] respectively, whereas BFU-E in both these conditions remain largely unperturbed. Thus the boundary from BFU-E to CFU-E and erythroblast may be biologically important for the pathophysiology of these disease states. Furthermore, in acquired hemolytic anemia,

selective destruction at a given stage of maturation (of red cells only or of both erythroblasts and red cells) can be observed depending on the type of antibody produced and the density of its antigen on maturing erythroid cells. Qualitative aberrations in the response of erythroid progenitors to cytokines or EPO may underlie the abnormalities of congenital erythroid hypoplasia (Diamond-Blackfan syndrome).[389] Analogous qualitative or functional defects can be observed in neoplastic erythropoiesis, because erythroid progenitors from patients with polycythemia vera and other myeloproliferative neoplasms have altered sensitivities to EPO.[630]

Detailed knowledge of the structural and functional properties of erythroid cells throughout their differentiation may provide significant insights into the pathogenesis of hematopoietic disorders affecting the red cell lineage.

SUGGESTED READINGS

Abdel-Wahab O, Levine R: The spliceosome as an indicted conspirator in myeloid malignancies. *Cancer Cell* 20:420, 2011.

Agarwal N, Gordeuk RV, Prchal JT: Genetic mechanisms underlying regulation of hemoglobin mass. *Adv Exp Med Biol* 618:195, 2007.

Andrews NC: Closing the iron gate. *N Engl J Med* 366:376, 2012.

Anstee DJ: The relationship between blood groups and disease. *Blood* 115:4635, 2010.

Baron MH, Isern J, Fraser ST: The embryonic origins of erythropoiesis in mammals. *Blood* 119:4828, 2012.

Bauer DE, Kamran SC, Orkin SH: Reawakening fetal hemoglobin: prospects for new therapies for the beta-globin disorders. *Blood* 120:2945, 2012.

Bianco P: Bone and the hematopoietic niche: a tale of two stem cells. *Blood* 117:5281, 2011.

Bieker JJ: Putting a finger on the switch. *Nat Genet* 42:733, 2010.

Bissels U, Bosio A, Wagner W: MicroRNAs are shaping the hematopoietic landscape. *Haematologica* 97:160, 2012.

Bowie MB, Kent DG, Copley MR, et al: Steel factor responsiveness regulates the high self-renewal phenotype of fetal hematopoietic stem cells. *Blood* 109:5043, 2007.

Bowman TV, Trompouki E, Zon LI: Linking hematopoietic regeneration to developmental signaling pathways: a story of BMP and Wnt. *Cell Cycle* 11:424, 2012.

Bresnick EH, Lee HY, Fujiwara T, et al: GATA switches as developmental drivers. *J Biol Chem* 285:31087, 2010.

Bunn HF: New agents that stimulate erythropoiesis. *Blood* 109:868, 2007.

Byon JC, Papayannopoulou T: MicroRNAs: allies or foes in erythropoiesis? *J Cell Physiol* 227:7, 2012.

Choesmel V, Bacqueville D, Rouquette J, et al: Impaired ribosome biogenesis in Diamond-Blackfan anemia. *Blood* 109:1275, 2007.

Crispino JD, Weiss MJ: Erythro-megakaryocytic transcription factors associated with hereditary anemia. *Blood* 123:3080, 2014.

Di Baldassarre A, Di Rico M, Di Noia A, et al: Protein kinase Calpha is differentially activated during neonatal and adult erythropoiesis and favors expression of a reporter gene under the control of the (A)gamma globin-promoter in cellular models of hemoglobin switching. *J Cell Biochem* 101:411, 2007.

Dore LC, Crispino JD: Transcription factor networks in erythroid cell and megakaryocyte development. *Blood* 118:231, 2011.

Fabriek BO, Polfliet MM, Vloet RP, et al: The macrophage CD163 surface glycoprotein is an erythroblast adhesion receptor. *Blood* 109:5223, 2007.

Flygare J, Aspesi A, Bailey JC, et al: Human RPS19, the gene mutated in Diamond-Blackfan anemia, encodes a ribosomal protein required for the maturation of 40S ribosomal subunits. *Blood* 109:980, 2007.

Fraser ST, Isern J, Baron MH: Maturation and enucleation of primitive erythroblasts during mouse embryogenesis is accompanied by changes in cell-surface antigen expression. *Blood* 109:343, 2007.

Ganz T, Nemeth E: Iron metabolism: interactions with normal and disordered erythropoiesis. *Cold Spring Harb Perspect Med* 2:a011668, 2012.

Ghinassi B, Sanchez M, Martelli F, et al: The hypomorphic Gata1low mutation alters the proliferation/differentiation potential of the common megakaryocytic-erythroid progenitor. *Blood* 109:1460, 2007.

Ginder GD: Epigenetic regulation of fetal globin gene expression in adult erythroid cells. *Transl Res* 165:115, 2015.

Hattangadi SM, Wong P, Zhang L, et al: From stem cell to red cell: regulation of erythropoiesis at multiple levels by multiple proteins, RNAs, and chromatin modifications. *Blood* 118:6258, 2011.

Higgs DR, Engel JD, Stamatoyannopoulos G: Thalassaemia. *Lancet* 379:373, 2012.

Kaneko H, Shimizu R, Yamamoto M: GATA factor switching during erythroid differentiation. *Curr Opin Hematol* 17:163, 2010.

Kerenyi MA, Orkin SH: Networking erythropoiesis. *J Exp Med* 207:2537, 2010.

Lambert LA, Mitchell SL: Molecular evolution of the transferrin receptor/glutamate carboxypeptidase II family. *J Mol Evol* 64:113, 2007.

Listowski MA, Heger E, Boguslawska DM, et al: microRNAs: fine tuning of erythropoiesis. *Cell Mol Biol Lett* 18:34, 2013.

Liu J, Mohandas N, An X: Membrane assembly during erythropoiesis. *Curr Opin Hematol* 18:133, 2011.

Maetens M, Doumont G, Clercq SD, et al: Distinct roles of Mdm2 and Mdm4 in red cell production. *Blood* 109:2630, 2007.

Migliaccio AR, Whitsett C, Papayannopoulou T, et al: The potential of stem cells as an in vitro source of red blood cells for transfusion. *Cell Stem Cell* 10:115, 2012.

Mohandas N, Gallagher PG: Red cell membrane: past, present, and future. *Blood* 112:3939, 2008.

Narla A, Ebert BL: Translational medicine: ribosomopathies. *Blood* 118:4300, 2011.

Orru S, Aspesi A, Armiraglio M, et al: Analysis of the ribosomal protein S19 interactome. *Mol Cell Proteomics* 6:382, 2007.

Palis J: Ontogeny of erythropoiesis. *Curr Opin Hematol* 15:155, 2008.

Paralkar VR, Weiss MJ: Long noncoding RNAs in biology and hematopoiesis. *Blood* 121:4842, 2013.

Paulson RF: Targeting a new regulator of erythropoiesis to alleviate anemia. *Nat Med* 20:334, 2014.

Phillips JD, Steensma DP, Pulsipher MA, et al: Congenital erythropoietic porphyria due to a mutation in GATA1: the first trans-acting mutation causative for a human porphyria. *Blood* 109:2618, 2007.

Ribeil JA, Zermati Y, Vandekerckhove J, et al: Hsp70 regulates erythropoiesis by preventing caspase-3-mediated cleavage of GATA-1. *Nature* 445:102, 2007.

Roy CN, Mak HH, Akpan I, et al: Hepcidin antimicrobial peptide transgenic mice exhibit features of the anemia of inflammation. *Blood* 109:4038, 2007.

Scott LM, Tong W, Levine RL, et al: JAK2 exon 12 mutations in polycythemia vera and idiopathic erythrocytosis. *N Engl J Med* 356:459, 2007.

Siatecka M, Bieker JJ: The multifunctional role of EKLF/KLF1 during erythropoiesis. *Blood* 118:2044, 2011.

Tober J, Koniski A, McGrath KE, et al: The megakaryocyte lineage originates from hemangioblast precursors and is an integral component both of primitive and of definitive hematopoiesis. *Blood* 109:1433, 2007.

Tubman VN, Levine JE, Campagna DR, et al: X-linked gray platelet syndrome due to a GATA1 Arg216Gln mutation. *Blood* 109:3297, 2007.

Wallace DF, Summerville L, Subramaniam VN: Targeted disruption of the hepatic transferrin receptor 2 gene in mice leads to iron overload. *Gastroenterology* 132:301, 2007.

Wilber A, Nienhuis AW, Persons DA: Transcriptional regulation of fetal to adult hemoglobin switching: new therapeutic opportunities. *Blood* 117:3945, 2011.

Zambidis ET, Sinka L, Tavian M, et al: Emergence of human angiohematopoietic cells in normal development and from cultured embryonic stem cells. *Ann N Y Acad Sci* 1106:223, 2007.

REFERENCES

For the complete list of references, log on to www.expertconsult.com.

CHAPTER 27

GRANULOCYTOPOIESIS AND MONOCYTOPOIESIS

Arati Khanna-Gupta and Nancy Berliner

GRANULOCYTOPOIESIS

Granulocytes (neutrophils, eosinophils, and basophils) are short-lived cells that are critical to both antimicrobial and inflammatory responses. The bone marrow (BM) produces granulocytes, especially neutrophils, at a prodigious rate to supply the baseline needs of circulating cells that survive in the peripheral blood only 3 to 24 hours. It also has the capacity to increase granulocyte production sharply in response to a wide range of stresses. The regulation of granulocyte production is controlled by a variety of cytokines that induce the myeloid differentiation program through the carefully orchestrated interaction of multiple general and myeloid-specific transcription factors. Understanding this intricate maturation sequence provides important insights into normal neutrophil responses to infectious, inflammatory, and allergic stresses, as well as into the dysregulation of differentiation contributing to myelodysplasia and leukemia.

Granulocyte Ontogeny

Stages of Neutrophil Differentiation

Granulocytes differentiate from early progenitors in the BM in a process that takes 7 to 10 days. The cells pass through several identifiable maturational stages, during which they acquire the morphologic appearance and granule contents that characterize the mature granulocyte.[1] The earliest identifiable granulocyte precursor is the myeloblast, a minimally granulated cell with scant cytoplasm and a prominent nucleolus (Fig. 27.1). Transition to the promyelocyte stage is associated with the acquisition of abundant primary granules. Primary granules are found in both granulocytes and monocytes and contain many of the proteins necessary for intracellular killing of microbes. The transition to the myelocyte stage is associated with the acquisition of secondary or "specific" granules, which give the characteristic staining pattern that differentiates neutrophils from eosinophils and basophils.

Neutrophil precursors account for approximately half of the cells in the BM of normal individuals, with a majority of these at the metamyelocyte stage and beyond. Promyelocytes and myelocytes represent the primary proliferative pool of granulocyte precursors in the BM. Beyond the myelocyte stage, cells mature as nondividing cells. Bands and segmented neutrophils constitute greater than 50% of the total granulocyte mass, primarily as a storage pool of mature cells in the BM. Only 5% of total neutrophils circulate in the periphery, where 60% are marginated in the spleen and on vessel walls. Mature neutrophils circulate in the peripheral blood for 3 to 24 hours and then migrate to the tissues, where they survive 2 to 3 days. Hence the peripheral neutrophil count reflects roughly 2% of the total neutrophil cell mass during approximately 1% of the neutrophil life span.

Biochemical events that accompany these physical changes include the sequential acquisition of primary granules and their content proteins (e.g., myeloperoxidase, lysozyme, neutrophil elastase [NE, also known as ELANE], defensins, myeloblastin), secondary granules and their content proteins (lactoferrin [LF], neutrophil collagenase (MMP8), neutrophil gelatinase [MMP9], neutrophil gelatinase-associated lipocalin [NGAL], transcobalamin 1), and tertiary granules containing neutrophil gelatinase (Table 27.1). The

progressive gain of these characteristics is accompanied by a loss of proliferative potential. This carefully coordinated process is disrupted in acute myeloid leukemias (AMLs), in which a block in the myeloid maturation pathway usually results in the circulation of immature blasts in the peripheral blood.

Markers of Granulocytic Maturation

Stem cells have been characterized primarily by their marrow repopulating potential, as outlined in Chapter 10. Early granulocytic progenitors form hematopoietic colonies in vitro, and their more differentiated progeny express specific cell surface proteins that are critically important to myeloid differentiation and function. They mediate both the adhesion of precursors within the BM and the vascular adhesion of mature neutrophils that is critical to normal neutrophil activation. Other proteins serve as receptors that recognize pathogens or as stimulatory peptides that facilitate activation of phagocytosis and killing of organisms. Appropriate expression of these surface proteins plays an important role in normal neutrophil function, and abnormalities of their expression are implicated in a wide range of diseases affecting the neutrophil compartment. For example, congenital abnormalities in the surface expression of integrin proteins are responsible for failure of neutrophil adhesion in leukocyte adhesion deficiency, whereas acquired abnormalities of expression of the same proteins are hypothesized to underlie the abnormal circulation of immature precursors in myeloproliferative neoplasms.[2] These markers also serve to help distinguish among the stages of myeloid commitment and maturation.

The phenotype of the early hematopoietic stem cells is CD34+/CD33-, with absence of lineage-specific markers. The common myeloid progenitor, colony-forming unit–granulocyte–erythrocyte–macrophage–megakaryocyte (CFU-GEMM), is characterized by the coexpression of CD33. CD33 is expressed at high levels on committed myeloid progenitors and on early precursors of both the granulocytic and monocytic lineages. Expression of CD33 wanes with granulocytic maturation, and it is absent or nearly absent beyond the myelocyte stage. CD33 is a member of the sialic acid–binding Ig-like lectins (siglecs), which generally mediate cell–cell interactions and cell signaling. The precise biologic function of CD33 itself is unknown.

Characteristic granulocyte markers acquired as the early myeloid progenitor cells become committed to the neutrophil lineage include CD45RA, myeloperoxidase (MPO), and CD38, all of which are expressed on the myeloblast. Further differentiation beyond the myelocyte stage is associated with acquisition of increased expression of CD16, CD11b/CD18 (Mac-1), and leukocyte alkaline phosphatase (LAP), all of which are expressed at high levels in mature neutrophils.

Neutrophil Granules and Their Content Proteins

The acquisition of granules and their content proteins is a critical part of the developmental program of the granulocyte.[3] Acquired at specific identifiable stages of neutrophil maturation, these intracellular and secretory organelles contain many of the requisite enzymes that mediate the oxidative and nonoxidative killing functions of the neutrophil (see Table 27.1).

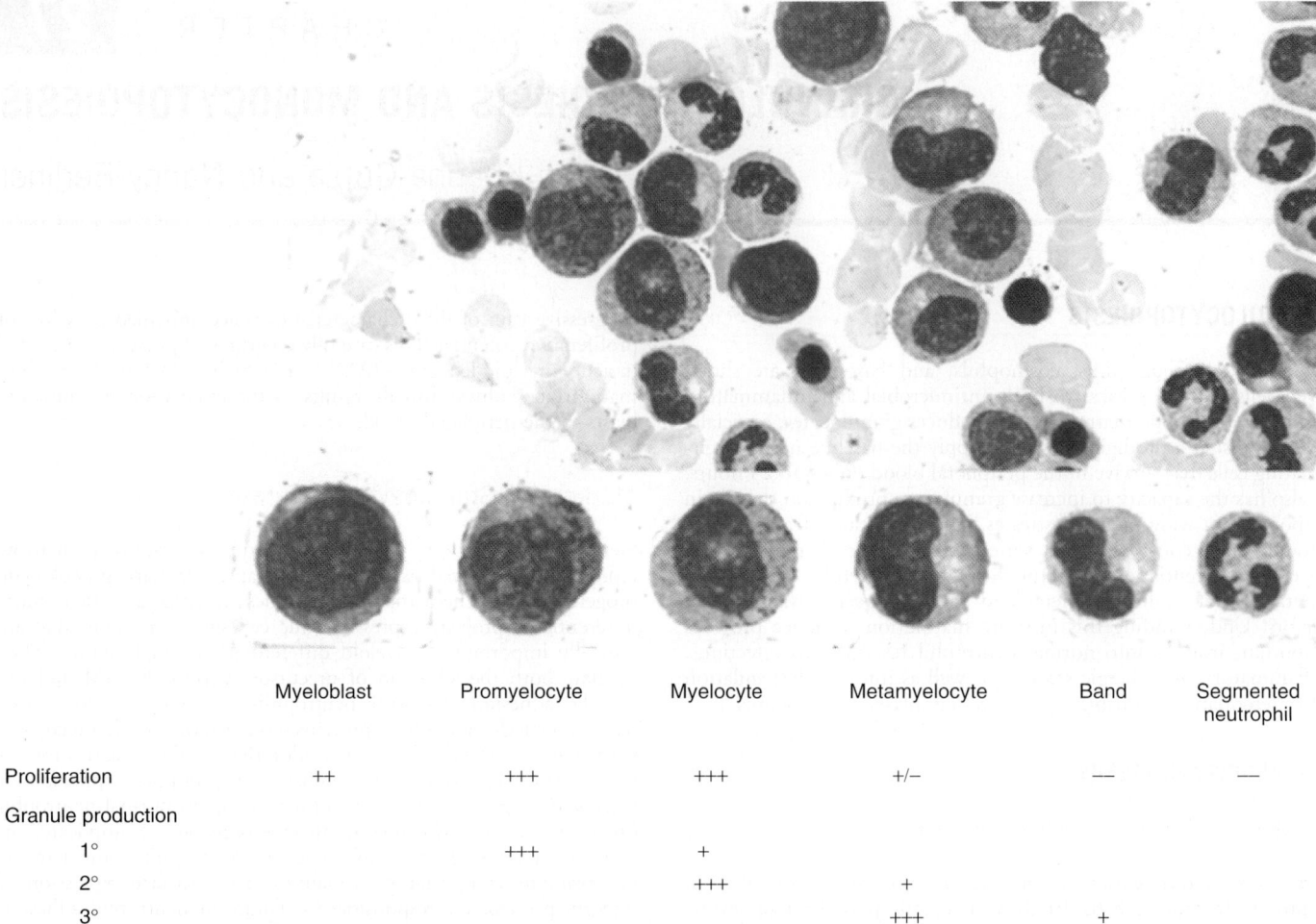

	Myeloblast	Promyelocyte	Myelocyte	Metamyelocyte	Band	Segmented neutrophil
Proliferation	++	+++	+++	+/−	—	—
Granule production						
1°		+++	+			
2°			+++	+		
3°				+++	+	

Fig. 27.1 NEUTROPHIL MATURATION STAGES WITH ASSOCIATED ACQUISITION OF STAGE-SPECIFIC GRANULES.

Primary (azurophilic) granules are acquired at the promyelocyte stage and contain a wide array of proteins, including myeloperoxidase, defensins, cathepsins, and ELANE. *Secondary* granules are secretory granules acquired at the transition to the myelocyte stage. Neutrophil secondary granules contain LF, the vitamin B_{12}-binding protein transcobalamin I, and the metalloproteinases (neutrophil collagenase and gelatinase), as well as NGAL. With the exception of gelatinase, which is also expressed by monocytes, expression of the secondary granule proteins is restricted within the hematopoietic lineage to neutrophils. Secondary granules and the synthesis of their contents therefore constitute a definitive marker of commitment to terminal neutrophil maturation. As discussed later, characteristic secondary granules are acquired at the same stage by eosinophils and basophils. *Tertiary* granules, containing primarily gelatinase, are formed during later stages of neutrophil maturation. *Secretory vesicles* are formed by endocytosis and contain plasma proteins.[4]

On stimulation, the neutrophil first mobilizes secretory vesicles, which contribute their membrane proteins, including abundant integrin receptors, to the plasma membrane. They may thus increase cellular adhesion by upregulating surface integrin expression in response to selectin stimulation or inflammatory mediators. Primary granules fuse with the phagosome and contribute to bacterial killing. Secondary and tertiary granules have a complex function. They are secretory granules, releasing the matrix-modifying metalloproteinase collagenase (MMP8) and gelatinase (MMP9) into the extracellular milieu, enhancing neutrophil penetration into sites of inflammation. The function of LF and transcobalamin I remains unconfirmed, but

they are hypothesized to contribute to the antimicrobial response by sequestering iron and cobalamin, respectively, away from infecting organisms. Secretion also results in the contribution of membrane proteins to the plasma membrane and is the source of the prominent upregulation of surface integrin receptor Mac-1 (CD11b/CD18) expression that occurs on neutrophil activation. Finally, they also fuse intracellularly with the phagosome to help promote bactericidal activity.

The fusion of azurophilic and peroxidase-negative granules allows for cross-exposure to their contents within the phagosome. These proteins are carefully sequestered in separate organelles, preventing premature activation and damage to the resting neutrophil; on fusion, the contents of the two granule subtypes cooperate in generating the antimicrobial response. Hydrogen peroxide, a by-product of nicotinamide adenine dinucleotide phosphate (NADPH) oxidase in the secondary granule, in combination with MPO from the primary granules, produces hypochlorous acid, a highly toxic microbicidal agent. In addition, both neutrophil gelatinase (MMP9) and neutrophil collagenase (MMP8) (secondary granule proteins) are produced as zymogens and are converted to their active forms by the action of ELANE released from the primary granules.

Current evidence largely supports the hypothesis that the content of the neutrophil granules is dictated primarily by the timing of synthesis of their respective content proteins. Studies have demonstrated that each distinct granule population is generated not by a sophisticated protein-sorting mechanism but rather by a highly regulated transcriptional process that results in sequential gene expression. For example, because myeloperoxidase and the other primary granule

TABLE 27.1	Neutrophil Granules: Major Classes and Contents	
Primary (Azurophilic)	**Secondary (Specific)**	**Tertiary**
Microbial Agents		
Lysozyme	Lysozyme	
Myeloperoxidase		
Defensins		
Cationic proteins		
Bactericidal permeability–increasing agent (BPI)		
Proteases		
Elastase	Collagenase	Gelatinase
Cathepsin G		
Other proteases		
Acid Hydrolases		
N-acetylglucuronidase		
Cathepsins B and D		
β-Glucuronidase		
β-Glycerophosphatase		
α-Mannosidase		
Other		
Kinin-generating enzyme		
C5a-inactivating factor	Lactoferrin	
Vitamin B_{12}–binding protein		
Plasminogen activator		
Cytochrome b[a]		
CD11/1B complex[a]		
Formyl peptide receptor[a]		
Histaminase[a]		
NGAL		

[a]These granule constituents are conventionally assigned to the secondary granule, but their exact compartment remains controversial. Some may be located in the tertiary granule or possibly in one of the other, heterogeneous small-granule populations.
Adapted from Boxer LA, Smolen JE: Neutrophil granule constituents and their release in health and disease. *Hematol Oncol Clin North Am* 2:101, 1988.

proteins are expressed between the promyelocyte and the myelocyte stages of neutrophil development, they are packaged into the primary granules. Secondary granule proteins such as LF, on the other hand, are expressed between the myelocyte and the metamyelocyte stages and hence are packaged into the secondary granules. Overexpression of the secondary granule protein NGAL in HL60 cells, a leukemic cell line that is arrested at the myeloblast stage of differentiation, resulted in its incorporation into primary granules, lending empiric support to the concept that gene expression and protein sorting into granules are coordinated events. This hypothesis may, however, be a somewhat oversimplified view of granule protein sorting, because there is some overlap of expression between certain primary and secondary granule protein genes. Whereas secondary granule protein gene transcription appears to be coordinately regulated, the sequence of primary granule protein gene expression is much less synchronous. The defensins are expressed later than the other primary granule proteins, and defensin transcription appears to be regulated by the same transcriptional regulatory pathway as for the secondary granule proteins gelatinase (MMP9) and LF.[5] Indeed, the defensins are the only primary granule proteins that are absent in patients with neutrophil-specific granule deficiency. This suggests that defensin regulation would predict targeting to the secondary granule.[6] Consequently, how defensins become directed exclusively to the primary granule remains unclear.

CONTROL OF GRANULOPOIESIS

Granulocytes arise from pluripotent hematopoietic stem cells by a process of commitment, proliferation, and differentiation. Stem cells are long-lived cells capable of both self-renewal and differentiation to lineage-specific–committed progenitors. The process governing the cell fate decision that takes a stem cell down the path to lineage commitment and the subsequent factors that regulate lineage-specific differentiation have been the subjects of intense study for many years. Three models of hematopoietic differentiation have been proposed to address the mechanism underlying lineage commitment and differentiation of the pluripotent stem cell. The first or *inductive* model proposes that lineage commitment and differentiation are the results of external stimuli (e.g., growth factors, stroma). A second model, the *stochastic* model, emphasizes intrinsic cellular factors as being critical to hematopoiesis; a third model combines the attributes of the first two. It appears likely that the transition from a stem cell to a committed progenitor is largely stochastic, although the subsequent maturation from progenitor to precursor to mature neutrophil requires cytokines. Controversy remains as to whether cytokines and the BM microenvironment play an instructive or a permissive role in influencing stem cell commitment and in inducing the proliferation and maturation of committed progenitors. As discussed subsequently, this complex issue has been elucidated in mice with homologous null mutations of specific cytokines and their cognate receptors, alone or in combination.

Cytokine Regulation of Myeloid Proliferation and Differentiation

Early progenitor cells express receptors for multiple cytokines, but expression becomes more restricted as the cell becomes committed to a specific lineage.[7] As a consequence of this broad range of cytokine receptor expression, early progenitors respond to combined growth factors, many of which show synergy of activity. The "early-acting" cytokines include the interleukins IL-1 and IL-6, stem cell factor (SCF), FLT3 ligand, and several others including granulocyte colony-stimulating factor (G-CSF) and thrombopoietin (TPO). IL-3 is important in directing the pluripotent stem cell toward the myelomonocytic lineage, giving rise to the mixed myeloid progenitor (CFU-GEMM). Subsequent stages leading to commitment- and lineage-restricted differentiation are governed by more "late-acting" cytokines (Fig. 27.2).

The major cytokines mediating neutrophil maturation are G-CSF and granulocyte–macrophage colony-stimulating factor (GM-CSF). G-CSF not only supports the survival and proliferation of developing myeloid cells at all stages of differentiation but also increases the functional activity of mature neutrophils. Although the major role of G-CSF is thought to be the induction of neutrophil proliferation and differentiation, the G-CSF receptor (G-CSFR) is expressed on a wide range of cell types. In addition to myeloid progenitors and precursors at all stages of neutrophil differentiation, G-CSFR is expressed on platelets, monocytes, lymphocytes, and several nonhematopoietic cells, including endothelial cells and placenta. The role of G-CSF as both an early- and late-acting cytokine is underscored by the successful use of G-CSF to mobilize early progenitors into the peripheral blood for stem cell collection and to speed neutrophil recovery following chemotherapy.

The G-CSFR is a member of the cytokine receptor superfamily that signals through activation of the JAK-STAT (Janus kinase-signal transducer and activator of transcription) pathway and the Ras pathway. Ligand binding induces homodimerization of the receptor, leading to a cascade of downstream phosphorylation events. Dimerization leads to phosphorylation of associated JAK kinases that in turn phosphorylate STAT1 and STAT3. In addition, the activated G-CSFR also phosphorylates mediators of the Ras–mitogen-activated protein (MAP) kinase pathway by tyrosine phosphorylation of Shc.[8]

The importance of G-CSF in myeloid proliferation and differentiation has been studied in G-CSF-null and G-CSFR-null mice. Mice lacking G-CSF or G-CSFR had markedly decreased myeloid

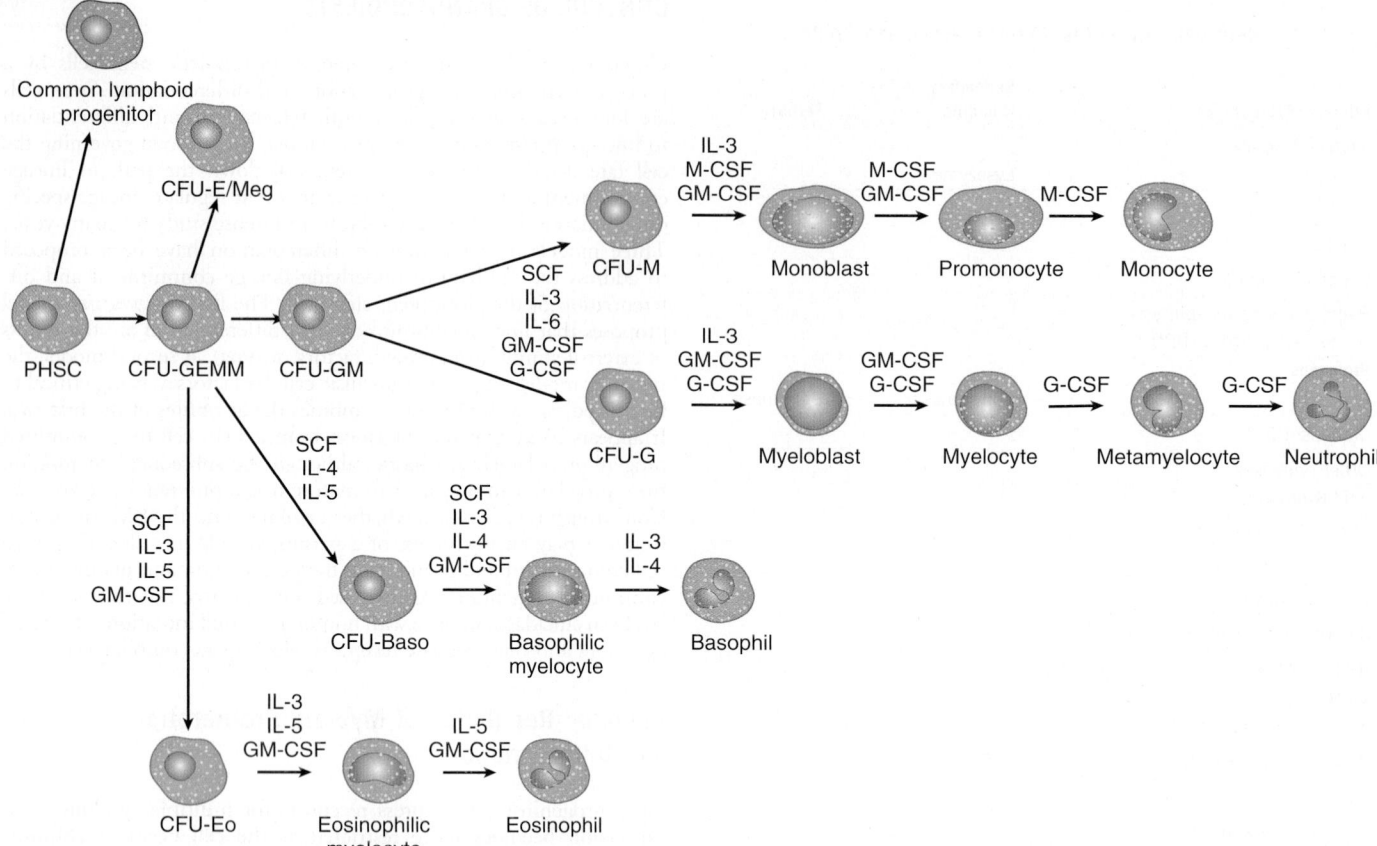

Fig. 27.2 CYTOKINE REGULATION OF GRANULOCYTIC PROGENITORS. *CFU-Baso,* Colony-forming unit-basophil; *CFU-E/Meg,* colony-forming unit-erythrocyte/megakaryocyte; *CFU-Eo,* colony-forming unit-eosinophil; *CFU-G,* colony-forming unit-granulocyte; *CFU-GEMM,* colony-forming unit-granulocyte/erythrocyte/macrophage/megakaryocyte; *CFU-GM,* colony-forming unit-granulocyte/macrophage; *CFU-M,* colony-forming unit-macrophage; *G-CSF,* granulocyte colony-stimulating factor; *GM-CSF,* granulocyte–macrophage colony-stimulating factor; *IL,* interleukin; *M-CSF,* monocyte colony-stimulating factor; *PHSC,* pluripotent hematopoietic stem cell; *SCF,* stem cell factor.

progenitors and impaired neutrophil production, with low circulating neutrophil counts. In addition, G-CSF-null mice had impaired mature neutrophil mobilization, and mature neutrophils from G-CSFR-null mice had increased susceptibility to apoptosis, supporting the role of the G-CSF pathway in sustaining the mobilization, survival, and function of mature neutrophils as well. However, despite all of these abnormalities, G-CSF/G-CSFR knock-out mice continued to make some neutrophils, suggesting that there are alternative overlapping cytokine pathways that support granulocyte development.

GM-CSF also induces proliferation and differentiation of myeloid precursors. The GM-CSFR is a heterodimeric protein composed of an α- and a β-subunit. The α-subunit binds GM-CSF. The β-subunit is shared by the GM-CSFR and the receptors for IL-3, IL-5, and IL-6. The β-subunit does not bind ligand but is necessary for the high-affinity ligand binding to the αβ-heterodimer of each receptor. Signaling through the GM-CSFR also depends on the JAK-STAT pathway, signaling through JAK2, and also serves to activate the Ras-MAP kinase pathway. Of interest, however, the GM-CSF-null mouse has no defect in hematopoiesis. Mice with null mutations in both G-CSF and GM-CSF had more profound neutropenia in the perinatal period but the same levels of neutrophils in adulthood as those for mice lacking G-CSF alone.

Transcriptional Regulation of Myeloid Differentiation

Lineage-specific maturation of committed hematopoietic progenitors is ultimately driven by transcription factors, which have been hypothesized to be the final common pathway leading to commitment and differentiation of the pluripotent stem cell.[9] The role of transcription factors in cellular proliferation, differentiation, and survival of the stem cell during hematopoiesis in the mammalian BM has been well established. Studies of the regulation of individual genes that show tissue- and stage-specific myeloid expression have implicated a small number of transcription factors that are responsible for directing both phenotypic myeloid maturation and the expression of functionally important myeloid genes. As described in detail later, this role is underscored by the observations in acute myeloid leukemia (AML), in which disruption of differentiation and defective myeloid-specific gene expression are linked to pathognomonic chromosomal translocations that result in the dysregulation of transcription factor expression.

Maturation of multipotent progenitor stem cells into specialized blood cells (lymphocytes, erythrocytes, neutrophils, monocytes, and eosinophils, among others) is regulated by a well-orchestrated interplay of transcription factors that are capable of instructing the expression of a specific set of genes within a specified lineage. Gene knock-out technology and overexpression studies, in conjunction with newer techniques that involve the use of multicolor fluorescence-activated cell sorting (FACS), have aided in delineating several transcription factors critical to the development of specific hematopoietic lineages. On the basis of these studies, critical transcription factors have been classified into two major categories. The first category includes factors such as stem cell leukemia transcription factor (SCL), GATA-2, and AML transcription factor-1 (AML-1) now known as Runx1, that influence differentiation to all of the hematopoietic lineages; the

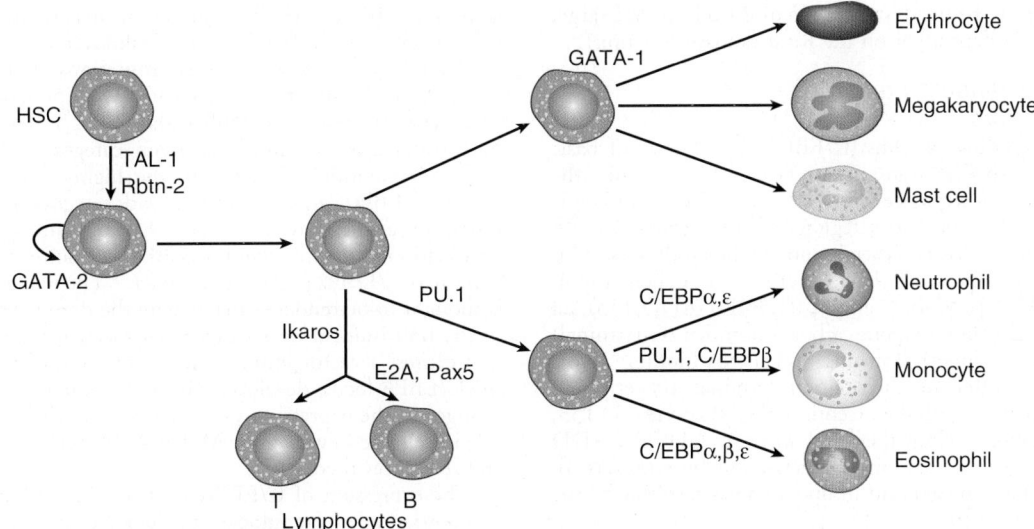

Fig. 27.3 SIMPLIFIED SCHEMA OF TRANSCRIPTIONAL REGULATION OF HEMATOPOIESIS. *C/EBP,* CCAAT enhancer-binding protein; *HSC,* hematopoietic stem cell; *SCL,* stem cell leukemia transcription factor.

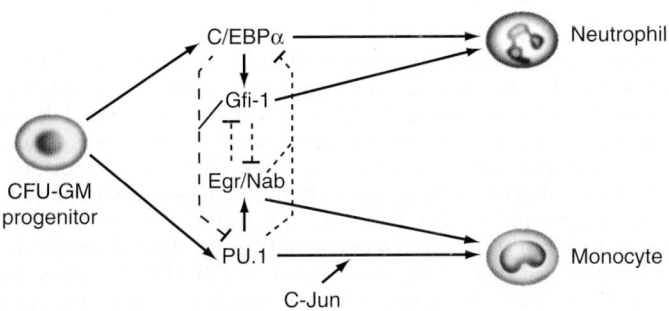

Fig. 27.4 TRANSCRIPTION FACTOR CROSS-TALK AFFECTING NEUTROPHIL AND MONOCYTE DEVELOPMENT.

second category comprises the master regulators of lineage development, including GATA-1, PU.1, and CCAAT enhancer-binding protein-α (C/EBPα). These factors not only promote lineage-specific gene expression but also suppress alternative lineage pathways. Fig. 27.3 summarizes the postulated role of several key transcription factors during hematopoietic development. Myeloid progenitors exhibit multilineage patterns of gene expression. Studies by Laslo et al[10] elegantly demonstrated that cell fate determination is dependent upon subtle changes in expression levels of transcription factors, which regulate differential lineage maturation. For example, levels of PU.1 expression are increased by Egr-1/Nab-2 in developing macrophages; at the same time, Egr-1 represses the expression of the neutrophil-specific Gfi-1 transcription factor, thereby simultaneously repressing the neutrophil development program (Fig. 27.4).

Transcription Factors Regulating Myeloid Differentiation and Myeloid-Specific Gene Expression

Runx1

AML-1 belongs to a family of highly conserved transcription factors that harbors a 128-amino-acid motif referred to as the Runt domain. The Runt domain functions in DNA binding, protein–protein interaction, ATP binding, and contributes to nuclear localization.[11] This family of transcription factors, also known as the core binding

factor (CBF) family, has been implicated in specification of cell fate and has a role in myeloid differentiation and lineage-specific granulocytic function.

Runx1 is the DNA-binding α-subunit of the CBF complex. Together with CBFβ, a widely expressed protein that enhances the DNA-binding affinity of the α-subunit, Runx1 binds the consensus DNA motif 5′ Pu ACCPuCA 3′ as a dimer. Disruption of the *Runx1* gene in mice results in embryonic lethality resulting from a failure of definitive hematopoiesis in the fetal liver. Although high levels of Runx1 expression have been reported in the early stages of myeloid differentiation, its expression levels decrease beyond the promyelocytic stage. In concordance with its pattern of expression, Runx1 has been implicated in regulating a number of genes expressed early in the myeloid development pathway, including GM-CSF, macrophage colony-stimulating factor (M-CSF) receptor, myeloperoxidase, ELANE, and IL-3, among others. In addition to activating lineage-specific myeloid markers, Runx1 has been shown to stimulate the G_1 to S transition in myeloid and lymphoid cell lines.

A significant percentage (10–20%) of human leukemias have been found to be associated with mutations in the *Runx1* gene. Most common of these is the t(8;21) translocation, which results in the Runx1-ETO (*e*ight *t*wenty-*o*ne oncoprotein) fusion protein. In Runx1-ETO, the Runt domain of Runx1 is fused in frame with the ETO transcriptional corepressor. The fusion protein is thought to function predominantly as a repressor that inhibits expression of genes that are normally activated by Runx1. For example, the tumor suppressor gene p14/p19(ARF), a critical Runx1 target gene that is necessary for the activation of p53 function, is normally activated by Runx1 but is repressed by Runx1-ETO. The mechanisms underlying Runx1 function through its target genes are not yet fully understood. Studies in sea urchins, however, have suggested that Runx1 regulates genes that contribute to chromatin architecture during cell proliferation. It has also been shown that Runx1 functions within a narrow window during development by assisting in the opening of chromatin associated with genes that are vital to hematopoietic development, and for the formation of transcription factor complexes on these genes.[12]

Studies involving mouse knock-in models of Runx1-ETO expression have indicated that the fusion protein alone is not sufficient to cause leukemia. These animals are more susceptible to mutagen-induced AML, however, suggesting that Runx1-ETO is part of a multistep process that contributes to leukemogenesis. Although the fusion partner of Runx1 (e.g., ETO) may contribute to the role of the Runx1 fusion protein in leukemogenesis, the primary cause of the disease is thought to be the dysregulation of Runx1-specific target genes that are directly dependent on the Runt domain of Runx1.

CCAAT Enhancer-Binding Protein Family of Transcription Factors

CCAAT enhancer-binding proteins (C/EBPs) are a family of basic region-leucine zipper (b-ZIP) transcription factors that recognize the consensus DNA-binding sequence 5′TKN NGYAAK3′ (Y = C or T; K = T or G) within the regulatory regions of target genes. C/EBP family proteins bind DNA as either homo- or heterodimers. This family of transcription factors, which plays a crucial role in hematopoiesis, includes C/EBPα,-β,-γ, -δ,-ε, and -ζ (CHOP-GADD 153), all of which contain highly homologous carboxyl-terminal (C-terminal) dimerization (leucine zipper) domains and DNA-binding (basic region) motifs but differ in their amino-terminal (N-terminal) transactivation domains—with the exception of CHOP-GADD 153, which lacks this domain altogether.[9] Of interest, CHOP-GADD 153 can dimerize with and inhibit transactivation by C/EBPα,-β, and -ε and is found at a breakpoint in liposarcomas resulting in the TLS-CHOP fusion protein.

With the exception of C/EBPε, which is expressed exclusively in the late stages of granulopoiesis and in T lymphocytes, the other C/EBP members are expressed in a wide variety of cells including liver, adipose tissue, lung, intestine, adrenal gland, and peripheral blood mononuclear cells and placenta. Both C/EBPβ and C/EBPδ are expressed at high levels in late-stage granulocytes. The C/EBP family members are known to exert pleiotropic effects in the tissues in which they are expressed. This may be because of their tissue- and stage-specific expression, their ability to dimerize with members of their own family and of the Fos/Jun and ATF/CREB families of transcription factors, and their ability to interact with other transcription factors such as nuclear factor-κB (NFκB) and specificity protein-1 (Sp-1).

The C/EBP factors have been implicated in regulating the differentiation of a variety of tissues. C/EBPα plays a role in adipocyte differentiation: Inhibition of C/EBPα blocks adipocyte differentiation, and overexpression of C/EBPα induces adipocyte differentiation. Regulation of constitutive hepatic genes as well as acute-phase response genes in the liver involves several C/EBP family members, in particular, C/EBPα. Modulation of myelomonocytic differentiation is also attributed to the activity of C/EBP family members. The importance of this family of transcription factors in myeloid differentiation has been demonstrated by the study of hematopoietic abnormalities observed in mice with targeted disruption of C/EBPα, -β, and -ε.

C/EBPα

C/EBPα has been postulated to be a master regulator of the granulopoietic developmental program. It is expressed at high levels throughout myeloid differentiation and has been shown to bind to the promoters of multiple myeloid-specific gene promoters regulating gene expression at many different stages of myeloid maturation. Although C/EBPα[-/-] mice die perinatally because of defects in gluconeogenesis that result in fatal hypoglycemia, they also have a selective early block in the differentiation of granulocytes without affecting either monocyte/macrophage maturation or the differentiation of other hematopoietic lineages. Myeloid cells of C/EBPα[-/-] mice lack G-CSFR, and it has been postulated that lack of mature neutrophils in these mice may be because of the lack of G-CSFR. However, the myeloid defect in C/EBPα[-/-] mice is more severe than that seen in G-CSFR[-/-] mice, suggesting that C/EBPα has additional functions vital to granulocytic maturation.

C/EBPα is a single exon gene, but it is expressed as two isoforms that arise from alternate translation start sites that give rise to a full-length C/EBPαp42 and a truncated dominant negative C/EBPαp30 isoform.[13] Translational control of C/EBPα isoform expression is orchestrated by a conserved upstream open reading frame (uORF) in the 5′ untranslated region (UTR). This region is thought to be responsive to the activities of the translation initiation factors eIF4E and eIF2 (reviewed by Khanna-Gupta[14]) such that an increase in the

activity of eIF2 or eIF4E results in an increase in expression of the shorter p30 isoform (reviewed by Calkhoven et al[13]).

Several groups have reported mutations in the *C/EBPα* gene in a subset of patients (~10%) with AML presenting with normal karyotypes (reviewed by Muller and Pabst[15]). These mutations can be broadly classified into two main categories. The first includes in-frame mutations clustered in the highly conserved C-terminus of the C/EBPα protein. The second category involves frameshift mutations at the N-terminus of C/EBPα resulting in the premature termination of the full length C/EBPαp42 isoform while keeping the truncated C/EBPα p30 protein intact.[16] The remaining C/EBPαp42 is thought to be rendered inactive by the dominant-negative activity of the p30 isoform by an unknown mechanism. In addition, mice that express a vector inducing overexpression of p30 C/EBPα from the C/EBPA locus, develop AML with complete penetrance.[17] Thus changes in the expression ratio of the two C/EBPα isoforms play a role in cell fate (reviewed by Muller and Pabst[15] and Kirstetter et al,[18] and references therein).

The expression of C/EBPα is associated with growth arrest and differentiation of granulocyte precursor cells. This block in proliferation is thought to occur via the interaction of C/EBPα with the cyclin-dependent protein kinases cdk2 and cdk4, resulting in a block in cell proliferation by inhibiting these cell cycle kinases. In addition, C/EBPα inhibits E2F-dependent transcription, which in turn contributes to inhibition of cell proliferation and induction of differentiation associated with C/EBPα-induced granulopoiesis.

C/EBPβ

Expression of C/EBPβ increases during myeloid maturation and is important for monocyte/macrophage gene expression and development. Mice lacking the *C/EBPβ* gene demonstrate reduced B-cell numbers and defects in macrophage activation and function, and they are more prone to microbial infections. The C/EBPβ knock-out studies reveal that this transcription factor is not essential for myeloid development per se, but knock-in of C/EBPβ into the C/EBPα locus of C/EBPα[-/-] mice rescues granulopoiesis. Several monocyte/macrophage-specific genes are activated by C/EBPβ, including the G-CSF receptor, lysozyme, CD11c, monocyte chemoattractant protein-1 (MCP-1), IL-6, IL-8, and nitric oxide synthase, among others. Similar to C/EBPα, multiple isoforms of C/EBPβ are generated from a single transcript through the use of three translation initiation sites and a leaky ribosome scanning mechanism. The shortest of these isoforms, initiated at the most 3′ AUG, results in the formation of LIP (*l*iver-enriched *i*nhibitory *p*rotein), which lacks the N-terminal activation domain present in full-length C/EBPβ and has been implicated as a negative regulator of C/EBPβ function. It has been suggested that the ratio of C/EBPβ to LIP may affect cellular proliferation and differentiation. The activity of C/EBPβ is regulated posttranscriptionally through protein–protein interactions and covalent modifications. For example, in early myeloid progenitor cells, C/EBPβ is found in an unphosphorylated state in the cytoplasm. However, on differentiation, C/EBPβ becomes phosphorylated and translocates to the nucleus.[19]

C/EBPβ in Emergency Granulopoiesis

Since they are very short-lived cells, neutrophils must be continuously produced in the BM under normal steady-state conditions. The large storage pool of neutrophils is sufficient to provide an immediate increase in circulating neutrophils in response to acute infection. However, if there is a severe or persistent demand for neutrophils related to a prolonged or particularly severe infection, a switch from steady-state to emergency granulopoiesis occurs to meet the increased demand for neutrophils. This marked de novo increase in neutrophil production is defined as "emergency granulopoiesis," and is critical for survival of the host. As a rule, the emergency granulopoiesis pathway follows three distinct steps, pathogen sensing and alerting the innate immune system of infection, triggering the molecular events that lead to increased neutrophil production in the BM and finally, restoration of steady-state conditions following clearance of the pathogen from the system (reviewed by Dao et al[1]).

Transcriptional Networks in Emergency Granulopoiesis

The role of transcription factors in emergency granulopoiesis has only recently begun to be addressed. In an elegant study, expression levels of C/EBP family members were measured in early granulocytic precursor cells following induction of emergency granulopoiesis with cytokines or *Candida albicans* infection. While expression levels of C/EBPα, C/EBPδ and C/EBPε were downregulated in the granulocytic precursor cells, C/EBPβ levels remained elevated, suggesting that C/EBPβ may play a role in emergency granulopoiesis.[3] While C/EBPα-null hematopoietic precursor cells are capable of generating neutrophils in substantial numbers upon cytokine stimulation[3–5] or upon infection with *C. albicans*,[3] C/EBPβ-null mice were unable to support emergency granulopoiesis in response to cytokines,[3,6] even though steady-state granulopoiesis remained unaffected. Based on these observations, it has been suggested that C/EBPα and C/EBPβ function specifically but antagonistically towards one another during steady-state and emergency granulopoiesis.[3] On the one hand, C/EBPα functions as a master regulator of steady-state granulopoiesis by limiting proliferation via inhibition of expression of the cyclin-dependent kinases, cdk2 and cdk4[7] and of c-Myc[8] and by promoting granulocytic differentiation. On the other hand, C/EBPβ drives emergency granulopoiesis largely because it does not block the expression of cdk2, cdk4, or c-Myc, thereby allowing proliferation of granulocytic progenitors and increasing neutrophil numbers during emergency granulopoiesis.

According to the current model, the switch from steady-state to emergency granulopoiesis is thought to be regulated by the increased levels of cytokines such as G-CSF and to a lesser extent GM-CSF and IL-6. These cytokines are known to be upregulated in response to pathogen invasion. G-CSF signaling involves activation of the JAK-signal transducer and activator of transcription (STAT) pathway. In particular, STAT3, a known regulator of granulopoiesis,[9] is activated in response to G-CSF, and together with C/EBPβ binds to the proximal promoter of c-Myc, thereby activating gene expression. This in turn suppresses binding of C/EBPα to the c-Myc promoter, resulting in C/EBPβ-mediated gene expression prevailing over that of C/EBPα, leading to increased cell cycle progression and c-Myc activation during emergency granulopoiesis.[10] In summary, emergency granulopoiesis is triggered by the very high levels of granulocytic cytokines (G-CSF in particular) in response to microbial infections, leading to the activation of the JAK-STAT pathway, which together with C/EBPβ stimulate granulocyte precursor proliferation and differentiation.

C/EBPγ

C/EBPγ is a ubiquitously expressed C/EBP family member that was first identified by its affinity for *cis*-regulatory sites in the Ig heavy chain promoter and enhancer. C/EBPγ contains a C/EBP-like b-Zip domain but lacks an N-terminal transactivation domain and can inhibit transcriptional activation of other C/EBP members in some cell types. Impairment of natural killer (NK) cytotoxic activity and of interferon-γ production has been reported in C/EBPγ[−/−]mice.

C/EBPδ

C/EBPδ is expressed at low or undetectable levels in several tissues of adult mice and humans. Expression has been shown to dramatically increase on induction with bacterial lipopolysaccharide and inflammatory cytokines, suggesting a role for C/EBPβ in acute-phase and inflammatory response. Double-knock-out experiments using C/EBPβ and C/EBPβ suggest a synergistic role for these two C/EBP family members in controlling terminal adipocyte differentiation. Of interest, both C/EBPβ and C/EBPβ are expressed during late neutrophil development and have been postulated to play roles in late neutrophil gene expression.

C/EBPε

CCAAT enhancer-binding protein ε (C/EBPε) is the most recently described C/EBP protein. The human *C/EBPε* gene resides on chromosome 14 and is transcribed by two alternative promoters, Pα (thought to function in mature neutrophils) and Pβ (thought to function in BM). A combination of differential splicing and alternate promoter usage results in four messenger RNA (mRNA) isoforms 2.6 kilobases and 1.3 to 1.5 kilobases in size, from which three proteins of 32.2 kDa, 27.8 kDa, and 14.3 kDa have been described. C/EBPε[−/−] mice produce hyposegmented granulocytes that are functionally defective. Late in life, these mice develop myelodysplasia. Absence of C/EBPε is thought to block the later steps in terminal differentiation of mature segmented granulocytes. Mutant mice usually survive 2 to 5 months and eventually succumb to low-pathogenicity bacterial infections. C/EBPε thus plays a crucial role in terminal granulocytic differentiation.

C/EBPε[−/−] mice have wild-type levels of the G-CSF receptor, and the defects manifested in these mice are confined to late-stage gene expression associated with the function of the mature neutrophil. It has been demonstrated that the ability of G-CSF to regulate myeloid differentiation is dependent on the induction of C/EBPε. Verbeek and colleagues demonstrated that the mRNA of several genes including p47 phox (a component of the neutrophil–NADPH oxidase complex), as well as the secondary granule protein (SGP) genes, are either absent or abnormal in the BM of C/EBPε[−/−] mice. These investigators further suggest that C/EBPε plays a critical role in the regulation of host antimicrobial defense.

Neutrophils from C/EBPε[−/−] mice have morphologic and biochemical features very similar to those observed in patients with neutrophil-specific SGD. SGD is an extremely rare congenital disorder that is characterized by frequent and severe bacterial infections. Patients with SGD have defects in neutrophil function including atypical nuclear morphology, impaired bactericidal activity, and abnormalities in neutrophil migration; they also lack both neutrophil and eosinophil secondary granule proteins. Sequence analysis of genomic DNA from two patients with SGD revealed mutations within the *C/EBPε* gene, resulting in the identification of a mutant protein lacking the dimerization and DNA-binding domains and hence transcriptional activity. Lack of functional C/EBPε activity has been postulated to underlie the observed pathology in these patients.

C/EBPζ

C/EBPζ-C/EBP homologous protein (CHOP) is a C/EBP family member that was originally isolated as the product of a gene induced in response to DNA-damaging agents. It has subsequently been shown to be induced by various extracellular or endoplasmic reticulum stresses. The basic region of CHOP is less well conserved than that of the other C/EBP family members, and CHOP does not seem to bind to canonical C/EBP *cis* elements. CHOP has been shown to interfere with the transcriptional activity of C/EBPβ in a manner dependent on its leucine zipper.

PU.1

PU.1 is a member of the Ets family of transcription factors and is expressed abundantly in B cells and macrophages. Expression of PU.1 has also been reported in granulocytes and eosinophils as well as in CD34[+] hematopoietic progenitor cells. High levels of PU.1 expression in fetal livers of mice preferentially direct macrophage development, whereas low levels of PU.1 result in B-cell development. C-Jun, another member of the b-Zip family of transcription factors, serves as a coactivator of PU.1 during macrophage development. It has been demonstrated that overexpression of c-Jun in myeloid progenitor cells results in macrophage development. Furthermore, downregulation of c-Jun by C/EBPα is necessary for granulocytic maturation and appears to be the mechanism through which C/EBPα blocks macrophage development. C/EBPα not only binds to the promoter of the c-*jun* gene and decreases its expression but also binds PU.1, thereby inhibiting its activity.

PU.1-binding sites have been reported in almost all myeloid-specific promoters reported to date, including those for M-CSF, GM-CSF, and G-CSF receptors, all of which play critical roles in myeloid cell development. PU.1 activity is modulated both by covalent modifications and by protein–protein interactions. For example, phosphorylation of PU.1 by casein kinase II or by JNK kinase leads to increased transcriptional activity.

Abrogation of PU.1 expression in PU.1$^{-/-}$ mice results in perinatal lethality accompanied by the absence of mature monocytes/macrophages and B cells and delayed and reduced granulopoiesis. Following in vitro differentiation, embryonic stem (ES) cells derived from PU.1$^{-/-}$ blastocysts fail to express mature myeloid cell markers, suggesting that PU.1 is not essential for the initial events associated with myeloid lineage commitment but is necessary for the later stages of development.

Growth Factor Independence-1 (Gfi-1)

The *Gfi-1* gene was first identified as a target of proviral insertion following infection with Moloney murine leukemia virus (MoMuLV) resulting in interleukin-2 (IL-2) factor independence in a rat lymphoma cell line (reviewed by van der Meer et al[20]). *Gfi-1* is a highly conserved gene that encodes a 55-kDa nuclear proto-oncogene that harbors six C_2H_2 type zinc finger domains at the C-terminus and a 20–amino acid stretch at the N-terminus known as the SNAG domain (reviewed by van der Meer et al[20]). The SNAG domain that appears to be conserved in the Snail/Slug family of proteins, has been shown to confer transcriptional repressor activity on Gfi-1. The human *Gfi-1* gene is located on chromosome 1p22 and its closely related paralog Gfi1b maps to chromosome 9q34. Gfi-1 is expressed at high levels in the thymus and BM while Gfi1B expression is confined to the BM and spleen. Homozygous knockout of Gfi-1B results in embryonic lethality at day E15, despite the fact that myelopoiesis is normal. Death in these mice has been attributed to a failure of erythropoiesis and megakaryopoiesis.

The essential role of Gfi-1 in neutrophil differentiation became apparent following two reports of gene disruption in mice. Gfi-1-null mice are severely neutropenic and eventually succumb to bacterial infections. In addition, these mice lack mature neutrophils and their granulocyte precursors are unable to differentiate into mature neutrophils upon induction with G-CSF. These cells also lack SGP expression reminiscent of C/EBP$^{-/-}$ granulocytes. Gfi-1$^{-/-}$ BM contains an atypical Gr1$^+$Mac1$^+$ myeloid precursor cell that appeared to share characteristics of both granulocyte and macrophage precursors. Ectopic expression of Gfi-1 in ex vivo sorted Gfi1$^{-/-}$ progenitor cells restores G-CSF–mediated neutrophil maturation to these cells. These observations provide evidence for the critical role of Gfi-1 in the neutrophil maturation program. Other studies have further demonstrated that Gfi-1 together with C/EBPε synergize to transactivate the promoters of late myeloid genes. This synergy is lost in a patient with SGD, who has a heterozygous substitution mutation in the C/EBPε gene and decreased levels of Gfi-1 in the BM.

Heterozygous dominant negative mutations in the *Gfi-1* gene have been described in two patients with SCN, underscoring the role of Gfi-1 in the neutrophil maturation pathway. It has been suggested that mutant Gfi-1 in these patients alters the expression of ELANE, mutations in which are commonly associated with SCN (see later). This observation confirms the vital role Gfi-1 plays in human granulopoiesis.

CCAAT Displacement Protein

CCAAT displacement protein/cut (CDP) is a ubiquitously expressed, highly conserved, homeodomain protein with extensive homology to the *Drosophila* cut protein. CDP has been shown to act as a repressor of developmentally regulated genes including the phagocyte-specific cytochrome heavy chain gene (gp91 phox), which is expressed exclusively in differentiating granulocytes (reviewed by Nepveu[21]). Overexpression of CDP in 32Dcl3 myeloid cells blocks G-CSF–induced expression of *SGP* genes without blocking phenotypical maturation. CDP therefore acts as a negative regulator of stage-specific expression of both early and late neutrophil-specific genes.

The CDP homeobox protein contains three highly conserved DNA-binding repeats referred to as *cut repeats* (CR1, CR2, CR3) and a homeodomain (HD), each of which is capable of recognizing and binding specific DNA motifs in target genes. This may explain why the CDP molecule as a whole does not have a well-defined consensus DNA-binding sequence. It has been demonstrated that the cut repeats cannot bind DNA as monomers but in combination

exhibit high DNA-binding affinity. It has further been suggested that CDP-binding activity is restricted to proliferating cells, in which CDP target genes are repressed. These targets are upregulated as cells undergo cell cycle arrest and terminal differentiation, in association with a decrease in CDP binding. Target genes of CDP include c-*myc*, c-*mos*, and the thymidine kinase (TK), cdk inhibitor p21(*WAF1/CIP1*), cystic fibrosis transmembrane conductance regulator (CFTR), transforming growth factor-β (TGF-β) type II receptor, gp91 phox, major histocompatibility complex (MHC) class I locus, and neutrophil *SGP* genes.

During myeloid differentiation, CDP binding has been shown to regulate genes that are expressed at widely disparate stages of differentiation. For example, it represses the *gp91 phox* gene, which is expressed at a much earlier time in myelopoiesis than is the case for the *LF* gene. The mechanism by which CDP mediates repression, and the means by which it modulates stage-specific gene expression at different stages of differentiation within a single lineage, are not fully understood. CDP is reported to have repressive activity associated with its ability to be displaced by a positive *trans*-acting factor involving the CR1 and CR2 cut repeats. However, other modes of repressive activity involving the two active repression domains within the C terminus of CDP have also been reported. CDP has been shown to function as a repressor of transcription via chromatin modification through recruitment of histone deacetylases (HDACs), consistent with the hypothesis that transcriptional silencing is associated with hypoacetylated histones. Both acetylation and phosphorylation of CDP are posttranscriptional modifications that have been postulated to regulate CDP function. Thus differential modification, by phosphorylation or acetylation, of CDP-DNA complexes binding the promoters of target genes could result in the observed differential repression exerted by CDP during neutrophil development.

ROLE OF DEVELOPMENTALLY IMPORTANT NEUTROPHIL-SPECIFIC GENES IN DISEASE

Our understanding of the role of neutrophil-specific genes has been enhanced by the study of mice in which targeted disruption of a gene results in phenotypically important defects in neutrophil differentiation and function. Similarly, the importance of these genes has been underscored by the analysis of naturally occurring genetic events within these genes that result in human disease. The links between some genes and the diseases induced by their dysfunction may be anticipated by their important roles in neutrophil differentiation and function, whereas the pathophysiologic link between others and the diseases they induce remain elusive (Table 27.2).

TABLE 27.2	Differentiation-Specific Genes Implicated in Neutrophil Disorders
Transcription Factors	
C/EBPα, PU.1, RARα, AML-1, and others in AML	
C/EBPε and Gfi-1 in specific granule deficiency	
Gfi-1 in neutropenia	
Granule and Functional Proteins	
Neutrophil elastase in Kostmann syndrome and cyclic hematopoiesis	
gp91 phox in chronic granulomatous disease	
Adhesion Molecules, Receptors	
Common β-chain of integrin receptors in LAD	
G-CSF receptor mutations in AML arising in patients with Kostmann syndrome	

AML, Acute myeloid leukemia; C/EBP, CCAAT enhancer–binding protein; G-CSF, granulocyte colony-stimulating factor; gp91 phox, glycoprotein 91 phagocyte NADPH oxidase; LAD, leukocyte adhesion deficiency.

Disruption of neutrophil transcriptional regulation is a recurring theme in the pathogenesis of leukemia. Nearly half of patients with AML have pathognomonic translocations resulting in the fusion of a transcription factor with a tissue-specific gene. These translocations have been shown to interfere with appropriate myeloid differentiation and emphasize the role of transcription factors in that process.

As discussed previously, the same transcription factors that are implicated in the induction of neutrophil differentiation also direct the expression of genes encoding neutrophil-specific functional proteins. The link between morphologic differentiation and synthesis of neutrophil functional proteins is illustrated by the demonstration that disruption of C/EBPε signaling results in SGD, associated with both morphologic abnormalities and increased infections attributable to neutrophil functional defects. It is intriguing that C/EBPε[-/-] mice share these abnormalities while also demonstrating a predilection for the development of myelodysplasia (i.e., myelodysplastic syndrome [MDS]). Although the development of MDS or AML has not been reported in patients with SGD, the deficiency is a rare disease described in fewer than a dozen patients, so a tendency to develop MDS/AML could easily be missed.

Other diseases have been linked to defects in functionally important neutrophil proteins. Abnormalities in integrin expression, notably, loss of the common β-chain of the integrin receptors, result in leukocyte adhesion deficiency, and absence of any of the components of the reduced nicotinamide adenine dinucleotide phosphate (NADPH) oxidase leads to chronic granulomatous disease.

Abnormalities in granule protein gene expression again underscore the complexity of the granulocyte functional program. Congenital absence of many individual granule proteins, including myeloperoxidase, LF, and transcobalamin, has been described. In the absence of the more global defects seen in SGD, which presumably reflect more complex abnormalities than simple protein deficiency, these defects tend to be incidental laboratory findings with minimal or no associated pathology.

One prominent exception to that observation is the association between point mutations in the gene encoding NE (ELA2; neutrophil elastase, ELANE) and SCN. The pathogenesis of SCN originally was sought in studies of G-CSFR, supported by the observation of a truncation mutation in G-CSFR in select patients with Kostmann syndrome (reviewed by Berliner[22]). It was later demonstrated that these were acquired mutations that may predispose the patient to secondary AML but did not constitute the pathologic basis for the neutropenia itself.

Severe Congenital Neutropenia and the Unfolded Protein Response (UPR)

SCN is a rare BM failure syndrome characterized by maturation arrest at the promyelocyte/myelocyte stage during neutrophil maturation in the BM (reviewed by Coffman[11] and Lichtinger[12]). Because of profound neutropenia, the disease was almost uniformly fatal as a result of bacterial infections before the advent of granulocyte colony stimulating factor (G-CSF) therapy (reviewed by Calkhoven et al[13]). In addition to having an increased risk of infections, patients with SCN treated with G-CSF also have an underlying predisposition for the later development of myelodysplastic syndrome/acute myelogenous leukemia (MDS/AML) (see Lichtinger et al[12] and references therein). Although originally described as an autosomal recessive disorder, SCN is genetically heterogeneous, with multiple modes of inheritance including autosomal recessive (30% of patients), autosomal dominant (60% of patients), X-linked, and sporadic. Pathogenic mutations associated with SCN have been identified in a number of genes including HAX1, ELANE (neutrophil elastase or NE, previously ELA2), GFI1, WAS, CSF3R, and G6PC3 (reviewed by Coffman[11]). Regardless of the mode of inheritance or gene mutation, newborns with SCN have severe neutropenia. In contrast, patients with cyclic neutropenia (CN) have regular and consistent oscillations of their circulating neutrophils, with a mean cycle of 21 days. Patients with CN tend to have milder symptoms that often manifest later in life.[14] In addition, CN responds well to lower doses of G-CSF and does not transform to MDS/AML. It has been hypothesized that rather than being two separate disease entities, SCN and CN represent two ends of the same disease spectrum.

Mutations in ELANE encoding neutrophil elastase (NE), a neutrophil primary granule protein, are the most common causes of both SCN (35–60%) as well as CN (80–100%).[11] To date, 73 distinct mutations of ELANE have been identified in patients with SCN and CN. Although some studies have suggested a correlation between ELANE mutations and disease severity, a clear genotype–phenotype connection has not been established.[12] While the role of ELANE mutations in contributing to CN remains unknown, two schools of thought have emerged in the literature with regard to SCN. The first suggests that ELANE mutations in SCN disrupt NE function by altering its enzymatic activity. The second suggests a structural rather than a functional perturbation of mutant ELANE, resulting in activation of a terminal UPR leading to a disruption of neutrophil maturation and an increase in apoptosis.[12,13] Many of the ELANE mutations yield proteins that share a potential propensity to misfold,[12,14] leading to misfolded ELANE protein accumulation and mislocalization in the cell, thus triggering the UPR with increased apoptosis in the granulocyte compartment.[13] It has been suggested that the UPR is not activated to the same degree in CN as in SCN, accounting for the milder phenotype associated with CN. Typically, the UPR is activated when a load of misfolded proteins entering the ER exceeds the cell's capacity to handle the protein load. The response to this cellular crisis involves (a) decreasing protein synthesis so as to reduce levels of the misfolded proteins; (b) increasing the transcriptional activation of UPR target genes, including ones that contribute to proper ER-protein folding such as chaperones (e.g., BiP); and (c) triggering ER-associated protein degradation (ERAD). If these measures are unsuccessful at reversing the ER stress, the cell is programmed to die. A moderate increase in levels of UPR-associated proteins has been observed in both mouse and human models of SCN.[12,13] The UPR hypothesis however, is unable to explain why pharmacologic doses of G-CSF alleviate the neutropenia of both CN and SCN, although it may reflect a prominent antiapoptotic effect of high doses of cytokine.[15]

Role of MicroRNAs in Controlling Gene Expression in Granulopoiesis

MicroRNAs (miRNAs) are 18- to 24-nucleotide-long noncoding RNAs that regulate eukaryotic gene expression in general, by binding to specific sites in the 3′ UTR of target genes and altering expression by destabilizing mRNA or blocking mRNA translation. miRNAs are encoded in the genome and are initially transcribed by RNA polymerase II as long primary transcripts referred to as primary miRNAs (pri-miRNAs). These transcripts are recognized and processed by a ribonuclease called Drosha into 60- to 80-nucleotide intermediates called precursor miRNAs (pre-miRNAs), which are then exported to the cytoplasm where a second ribonuclease termed Dicer cleaves pre-miRNAs to generate double-stranded 18- to 24-nucleotide-long miRNAs. The miRNAs are then incorporated into the RNA-induced silencing complex or RISC, a large protein complex that also contains the Argonaute or mRNA cleaving proteins. The miRNA guides the RISC complex to target complementary regions in the 3′ UTRs of mRNAs, leading to repression of translation or destabilization of the mRNA by deadenylation (reviewed by Manikandan et al[23]).

An increasing body of evidence implicates miRNA activity in mediating both normal and abnormal myelopoiesis (reviewed by Pelosi et al[24]). MiRNAs have been shown to activate or be activated by myeloid-specific transcription factors such as C/EBPα and Gfi-1. For example, mir-223 is thought to be a direct target of C/EBPα and its expression increases during granulopoiesis. Ablating mir-223 in mice results in the expansion of granulocyte precursor cells resulting from a cell autonomous increase in the number of

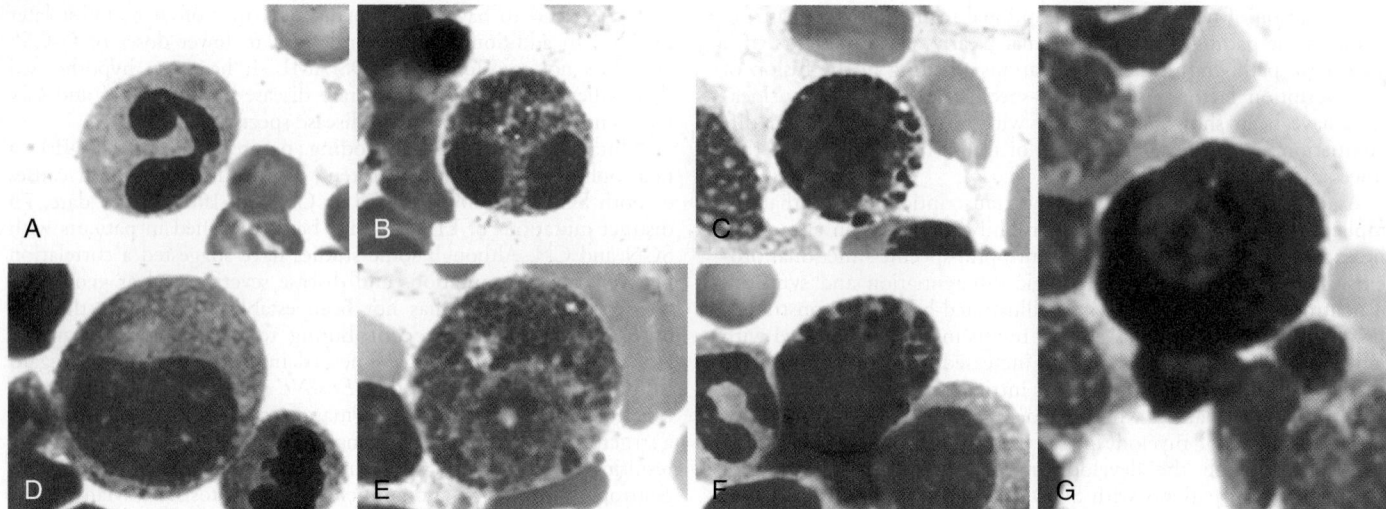

Fig. 27.5 NEUTROPHILIC, EOSINOPHILIC, AND BASOPHILIC GRANULOCYTES; THEIR MYELOCYTE PRECURSORS; AND MAST CELLS. Eosinophilic and basophilic granulocytes are always best viewed compared with neutrophilic granulocytes because staining can vary from laboratory to laboratory and even from case to case. When compared with a neutrophil (A), the eosinophil (B) has larger and more red/orange-colored and almost refractile granules than the pink and barely perceivable granules in the neutrophil. Mature eosinophils are also frequently bilobed, but neutrophils tend to have three or four lobes. The basophil (C) has dense, dark blue granules that frequently overlie the condensed and lobulated nucleus. The granules frequently obstruct the nucleus and are much larger than the primary granules of promyelocytes. The myelocyte stage of maturation is when the secondary granules first appear (D–F). In the neutrophilic myelocyte (D), the secondary granules first appear in the Golgi region and have been described as resembling the sunrise over the horizon, the "dawn of neutrophilia." The eosinophilic and basophilic myelocytes (E, F) are relatively infrequent in the bone marrow and are usually enumerated together with the mature forms. Mast cells (G) must be distinguished from basophils and basophilic myelocytes. Mast cells are larger and have quite numerous granules mostly in the cytoplasm. Mast cells have round nuclei, which are frequently obscured by the granules. A toluidine blue cytochemical reaction will be positive (metachromatic) in the granules of both basophils and mast cells. However, a mast cell tryptase immunostain used on a tissue section will be positive only in mast cells.

granulocytic progenitors.[25] In addition, overexpression of mir-223 in acute promyelocytic leukemia (APL) cells results in an enhanced capacity for granulocytic differentiation.[26] Mir-223 is thus thought to be a positive regulator of granulopoietic differentiation. In addition, mir-223 targets E2F1, a master cell cycle regulator, by inhibiting translation of its mRNA. Thus granulopoiesis appears to be regulated by a C/EBPα–miR-223–E2F1 axis, wherein miR-223 functions as a key regulator of myeloid cell proliferation associated with E2F1 in a mutual negative feedback loop.[27]

Eiring et al have demonstrated another role for miRNAs in granulopoiesis. They demonstrated that mir-328 is downregulated in CML patients in blast crisis. Restoration of mir-328 expression restores differentiation by interaction with both the C/EBPα translational inhibitor hnRNP-E2 and the mRNA for PIM1, a survival factor. The interaction with hnRNP-E2 leads to the release of C/EBPα mRNA from hnRNA-E2–mediated translational inhibition through an interaction that is independent of its seed sequence. Thus mir-328 appears to control cell fate by its ability to base pair with the 3′ UTR of target mRNAs (PIM1) as well as by acting as a decoy for hnRNP binding thus interfering with cell fate by releasing C/EBPα from translational inhibition.[28]

A role for mir-27 in granulopoiesis has also been documented. This miR targets the myeloid transcription factor Runx1, whose expression decreases during granulocytic differentiation in a mir-27 dependent manner. Anti-mir-27 treatment of immature myeloid progenitors resulted in an increase in the expression of Runx1 and impaired granulocytic differentiation.[29] In a separate study, the transcription factor Gfi-1 was shown to bind to the promoter of miR-196b and repress its expression, thereby promoting granulocytic maturation while repressing monocytic lineage development. Overexpression of

miR-196b blocked granulopoiesis in GMPs (granulocyte monocyte precursors).[30]

Thus, a growing number of feed-forward and feedback regulatory loops involving specific miRNAs and myeloid-specific transcription factors that determine lineage development and fate have been recognized in recent years, thereby underscoring a vital role of miRNAs in granulopoiesis.

EOSINOPHIL PRODUCTION

Eosinophil precursors constitute approximately 3% of BM progenitors, of which about two-thirds are myelocyte precursors and the remainder mature eosinophils. Eosinophilic myelocytes are large cells with a bilobed nucleus (Fig. 27.5). The characteristic specific granules of eosinophils contain major basic protein, eosinophil cationic protein, eosinophil peroxidase, and eosinophil-derived neurotoxin. Eosinophils also contain primary granules that contain Charcot-Leyden crystal protein. Mature eosinophils are released into the BM, where they circulate up to 18 hours before migrating to the tissues.

Eosinophils proliferate and mature under the influence of IL-3, IL-5, and GM-CSF. Evidence suggests that these cytokines are secreted by T cells as the stimulus to eosinophil production in many disorders associated with eosinophilia. Recent studies of idiopathic hypereosinophilic syndrome have described activating mutations in the platelet-derived growth factor receptor-α (PDGFR-α) that result in constitutive tyrosine kinase activation and eosinophil proliferation.

Transcriptional regulation of eosinophilic differentiation is mediated through PU.1 C/EBPα and -β. Because these same factors serve

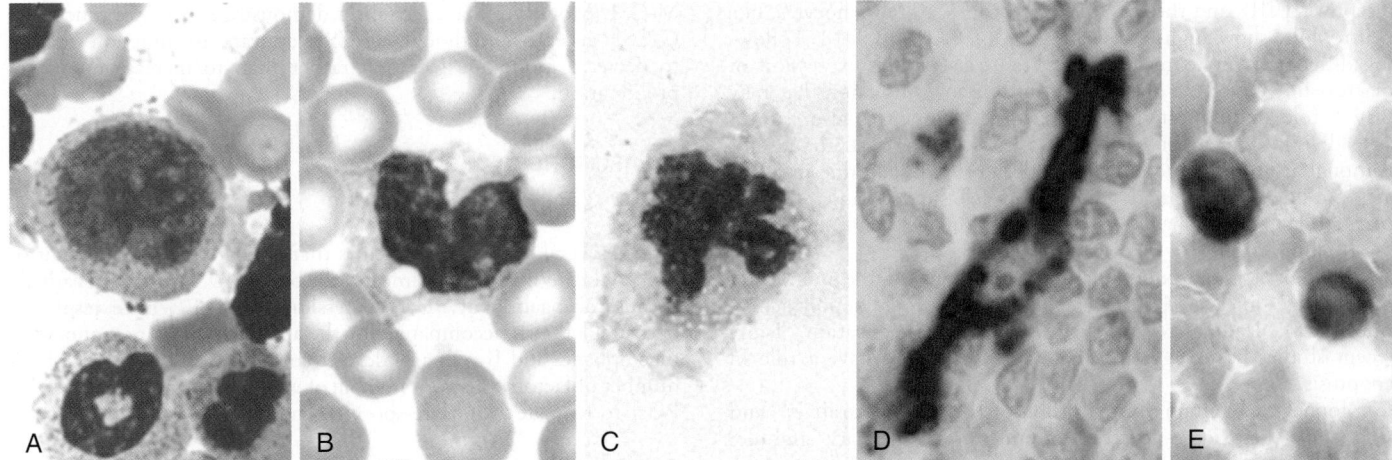

Fig. 27.6 A PROMONOCYTE, MONOCYTE, MACROPHAGE, AND HISTIOCYTE. Promonocytes are rare in the bone marrow (BM) (A) and are more frequently seen during recovery or during marrow regeneration after chemotherapy or other insult. They are typically slightly folded and have nucleoli. The cytoplasm is moderately abundant and blue/gray with very faint granules. Monocytes seen in the blood (B) typically have more folded or horseshoe-shaped nuclei and more abundant gray cytoplasm frequently with vacuoles and rare granules. The macrophage (C) is seen in body fluid specimens such as peritoneal fluid or cerebrospinal fluid and resembles the blood monocyte. Tissue histiocytes are fixed in the tissues and are seen on tissue sections. The histiocyte illustrated (D) is stained with CD68 and is from a lymph node. It likely represents a dendritic cell in a germinal center. Monocytes in the BM can be more easily enumerated with a nonspecific esterase cytochemical reaction such as alpha-naphthyl acetate esterase, which gives an orange/brown reaction product (E).

to induce myeloid differentiation, the modulation of the signals determining the choice between these two lineages is not well defined. It has been proposed that levels of GATA-1 may be important in determining whether C/EBP expression induces the eosinophilic or the myeloid maturation program.

BASOPHIL AND MAST CELL PRODUCTION

Basophils and mast cells mediate allergic responses, where they are the central cells involved in IgE-induced immune responses to parasites and other allergens. Both cell types are derived from BM precursors, but they have a very different ontogeny.

Basophils have a single lobed nucleus and characteristic intensely staining purple granules that may cover the nucleus (see Fig. 27.5). These granules contain glycosaminoglycans, predominantly heparin. Basophils differentiate from BM progenitors and are released from the BM as mature cells, where they circulate briefly, with a lifespan similar to that of neutrophils. Maturation is induced in response to IL-3, which serves both to induce basophilic differentiation and to mediate activation of mature basophils. Although IL-3 is the primary mediator of basophil development, studies of IL-3-null mice have demonstrated that it is not required for baseline production of basophils. It is, however, required for the induction of basophilia in response to parasitic infection. Other cytokines that influence basophil proliferation include GM-CSF, IL-5, and SCF.

Mast cells arise from BM precursors but are released into the circulation as immature cells. They circulate only briefly in the peripheral blood before migrating to the tissues, where they complete their maturation. There remains some question about whether mast cells and basophils arise from a common precursor. In vitro studies showed that adding SCF and IL-3 to cultured CD34+ cells results in an increased proliferation and maturation of both basophils and mast cells but did not establish a common progenitor cell for the two lineages. It is clear that SCF is especially effective in inducing mast cell proliferation; in fact, activating mutations in c-Kit, the SCF receptor, is the underlying molecular defect in most cases of systemic mastocytosis.

MONOCYTOPOIESIS

Monocyte Ontogeny

Stages of Monocyte Differentiation

Monocytes originate in the BM from promonocytes, which constitute approximately 3% of the total cells in the normal BM (Fig. 27.6). Promonocytes have round nuclei and basophilic cytoplasm. Differentiation occurs rapidly, with a maturation time of 50 to 60 hours, associated with two rounds of replication and morphologic maturation marked by progressive lobulation of the nucleus. Stress-induced release of monocytes occurs primarily through their premature release from the proliferating pool. Survival in the blood is short, approximately 8 to 72 hours. Monocytes then enter the tissues, where they develop into macrophages that may survive 2 to 3 months. Tissue-fixed macrophages are found in the lung (alveolar macrophages), the liver (Kupffer cells), the spleen, and the central nervous system (glial cells).

Monocytes may also serve as precursors to a subset of dendritic cells. Dendritic cells are professional antigen-presenting cells that arise from both myeloid and lymphoid precursor cells. The myeloid subset of dendritic cells arises from a precursor that can alternatively differentiate into macrophages. Similar cells have been generated for immunotherapy by exposing peripheral blood monocytes to GM-CSF and IL-4 in vitro.

Markers of Monocyte Maturation

Unique surface markers of monocyte maturation have been difficult to identify. In the mouse, the marker F4/80 was identified as a nearly universal marker of monocytes and macrophages; this antigen has been shown to be homologous to the human EGF module containing mucin-like hormone receptor 1. The function of this receptor is unknown, because the knock-out mouse has no phenotype. Monocyte precursor cells express the M-CSF receptor, lysozyme, the Fcγ receptor (II/III), and the scavenger receptor. Mature monocytes, like neutrophils, show high-level expression of CD11b/CD18. Following differentiation to macrophages, the cells acquire expression of macrosialin (CD68), a glycoprotein of unknown function that may play a role in lipoprotein metabolism. Macrophages also express sialoadhesin, a member of the sialic acid-binding receptor family. Although its precise function has not been proved, sialoadhesin mediates binding to sialic acid moieties on cell surfaces and probably plays a role in macrophage cell–cell interactions and cell–extracellular matrix interactions.

CD14 is a major functional surface protein of the monocyte/macrophage lineage. CD14 is the receptor for lipopolysaccharide (LPS), leading to monocyte/macrophage activation. More recent studies have suggested that CD14 may also have a role in apoptosis.

Monocytes contain both primary (peroxidase-positive) and secondary (peroxidase-negative) granules. The primary granules of monocytes, like those of neutrophils, contain myeloperoxidase. Secondary granule fusion with the membrane on stimulation of monocytes results in upregulation of Mac1 and p150, and is thought to play a role in adhesion and diapedesis of stimulated monocytes.

Control of Monocytopoiesis

Cytokine Regulation of Monocyte Proliferation and Differentiation

The effects of colony-stimulating factor 1 (CSF-1, also known as M-CSF), the primary regulator of mononuclear phagocyte production, are thought to be mediated by the high-affinity receptor tyrosine kinase CSF-1 receptor (CSF-1R). CSF-1R is encoded by the c-*fms* proto-oncogene. A total of five human or mouse mRNAs result from alternative splicing and the alternative use of the 3' untranslated region. This results in three isoforms of the CSF-1 protein: a secreted proteoglycan, a secreted glycoprotein, and a membrane-spanning cell surface proteoglycan have been described.

The phenotypes of Csf1-null mice and of mice harboring an inactivating mutation in the coding region of *CSF-1* (Csf1^{op}/Csf1^{op}) (osteopetrotic mice) are virtually identical; features include toothlessness, low body weight, low growth rate, and deficient tissue macrophages. In addition, the mutant mice have defects in both male and female fertility. Compared with their wild-type littermates, splenic erythroid burst-forming unit and high-proliferative-potential colony-forming cell levels in both Csf1^{op}/Csf1^{op} and Csf1$^-$/Csf1$^-$ mice were significantly elevated, consistent with a negative regulatory role for CSF-1 in erythropoiesis and in the maintenance and proliferation of primitive hematopoietic progenitors. The plasma CSF-1 levels in CSF receptor-null (Csf1R$^-$/Csf1R$^-$) mice was elevated 20-fold, in agreement with the previously reported clearance of circulating CSF-1 by CSF-1R-mediated endocytosis. Despite their overall similarity, several phenotypic characteristics of the Csf1R$^-$/Csf1R$^-$ mice were more severe than those of the Csf1^{op}/Csf1^{op} mice. The results suggest that all of the effects of CSF-1 are mediated via the CSF-1R, but that additional effects of the CSF-1R could result from CSF-1-independent activation.

Signaling through the CSF-1R appears to be critical for monocyte/macrophage development. Although little is known about the events that lead to stimulation of a monocyte/macrophage–specific array of genes, it is clear that several transcription factors, probably stimulated by M-CSF–related signaling, play vital roles in the development of this lineage. It should be noted, however, that the ability of phorbol esters to induce monocytic differentiation of myeloid cell lines through activation of the protein kinases Cα and Cδ suggests a role for the PKC pathway in monopoiesis.

IL-3, G-CSF, and tumor necrosis factor (TNF) have all been shown to synergize with M-CSF in the proliferation of macrophages. G-CSF has also been shown to induce the increased release of monocytes; this is an indirect effect dependent on the presence of

M-CSF. Monocytes have also been demonstrated to have functional G-CSF receptors, although G-CSF appears to function mainly to decrease monokine secretion rather than to increase monocyte proliferation.

Transcriptional Regulation of Monocyte Differentiation

Of the several transcription factors that regulate the development of the monocyte/macrophage lineage, the best is PU.1 (discussed earlier), because abrogation of PU.1 expression in PU.1$^{-/-}$ mice results in perinatal lethality accompanied by the absence of mature monocytes/macrophages and B cells and delayed and reduced granulopoiesis. A number of factors, the most notable of which is c-Jun, cooperate with PU.1 to regulate monocyte-specific genes.

c-Jun

The c-*jun* proto-oncogene encodes the transcriptional activator protein AP-1. As a member of the early response genes, c-*jun* is rapidly and transiently activated in response to external proliferative signals. The expression of c-Jun as well as related family members JunB and JunD is upregulated during monocytic differentiation. In addition, overexpression of c-Jun in M1, U937, or WEHI-B D$^+$ myeloid cell lines, as well as in myeloid progenitor cells, was found to result in partial monocytic differentiation. However, c-Jun$^{-/-}$ fetal liver cells are capable of reconstituting hematopoiesis in syngeneic recipients, suggesting that c-Jun is not required for myeloid development. This finding may reflect a compensatory role played by other Jun family proteins.

As discussed, c-Jun serves as a coactivator of PU.1 during macrophage development. Recent studies have revealed that downregulation of c-*jun* by C/EBPα is necessary for granulocytic maturation and appears to be the mechanism through which C/EBPα blocks macrophage development (see Fig. 27.4). C/EBPα not only binds to the promoter of the c-*jun* gene and decreases its expression but also binds to PU.1, thereby inhibiting its activity. Such transcription factor cross-talk resulting in subtle changes in the levels of transcription factors within a given lineage appears to be an emerging paradigm through which master regulators of lineage specification, such as C/EBPα and PU.1, direct lineage-specific development by directly upregulating lineage-specific genes as well as by blocking the progression of alternate lineages.

Other Transcription Factors Modulating Monocyte Development

Egr-1. Egr-1 belongs to a family of zinc finger transcription factors, and is expressed in a number of tissues and at various points in development including the terminal stages of macrophage and neutrophil differentiation. Egr-1 is necessary for monocytic differentiation of myeloid cell lines U937 and M1 and prevents factor-induced granulocytic differentiation of HL60 and 32Dcl3 cells. In addition, ectopic expression of Egr-1 in myeloid BM progenitors was found to result in an increase in the number of CFU-M at the expense of CFU-G. However, mice lacking Egr-1 develop normal numbers of macrophages, a phenomenon attributed to the possible compensatory effects of other Egr family members.

C/EBPβ. As discussed, expression of C/EBPβ increases during myeloid maturation and has been shown to be important for monocyte/macrophage gene expression and development.

MafB and c-Maf. The transcription factors MafB and c-Maf belong to a family of basic-leucine zipper (b-Zip) factors that bind DNA as dimers. The Maf proteins can dimerize with members of other b-Zip family proteins including c-Jun, fos, and NF-E2 in erythroid cells. Ectopic expression of MafB in myeloblasts directed their expression to macrophages, whereas overexpression of c-Maf in HL60 and U937 myeloid cells resulted in monocytic differentiation.

SUGGESTED READINGS

Bjerregaard MD, Jurlander J, Klausen P, et al: The in vivo profile of transcription factors during neutrophil differentiation in human bone marrow. *Blood* 101:4322, 2003.

Buck M, Chojkier M: Signal transduction in the liver: C/EBPβ modulates cell proliferation and survival. *Hepatology* 37:731, 2003.

Coffman J: Runx transcription factors and the developmental balance between cell proliferation and differentiation. *Cell Biol Int* 27:315, 2003.

D'Alo F, Johansen LM, Nelson EA, et al: The amino terminal and E2F interaction domains are critical for C/EBPα-mediated induction of granulopoietic development of hematopoietic cells. *Blood* 109:3163, 2003.

Hattori T, Ohoka N, Hayashi H, et al: C/EBP homologous protein (CHOP) up-regulates IL-6 transcription by trapping negative regulating NF-IL6 isoform. *FEBS Lett* 541:33, 2003.

Hock H, Hamblen M, Rooke H, et al: Intrinsic requirement for zinc finger transcription factor Gfi-1 in neutrophil differentiation. *Immunity* 18:109, 2003.

Horwitz M, Benson KF, Duan Z, et al: Role of neutrophil elastase in bone marrow failure syndromes: molecular genetic revival of the chalone hypothesis. *Curr Opin Hematol* 10:49–54, 2003.

Jafar-Nejad H, Bellen HJ: Gfi/Pag-3/senseless zinc finger proteins: a unifying theme? *Mol Cell Biol* 24:8803, 2004.

Jongstra-Bilen J, Harrison R, Grinstein S: Fcgamma-receptors induce Mac-1 (CD11b/CD18) mobilization and accumulation in the phagocytic cup for optimal phagocytosis. *J Biol Chem* 278:45720, 2003.

Keeshan K, Santilli G, Corradini F, et al: The transcription activation function of C/EBP(alpha) is required for induction of granulocytic differentiation. *Blood* 102:1267, 2003.

Khanna-Gupta A, Hong S, Zibello T, et al: Growth factor independence 1 (Gfi-1) plays a role in mediating specific granule deficiency (SGD) in a patient lacking a gene inactivating mutation in the C/EBP gene. *Blood* 109:4181, 2007.

Khanna-Gupta A, Zibello T, Sun H, et al: Chromatin immunoprecipitation (ChIP) studies indicate a role for CCAAT enhancer binding proteins alpha and epsilon (C/EBP alpha and C/EBP epsilon) and CDP/cut in myeloid maturation-induced lactoferrin gene expression. *Blood* 101:3460, 2003.

Laslo P, Spooner CJ, Warmflash A, et al: Multilineage transcriptional priming and determination of alternate hematopoietic cell fates. *Cell* 126:755, 2006.

Manz M, Boettcher S: Emergency granulopoiesis. *Nat Rev Immunol* 14:302, 2014.

Parfrey H, Mahadeva R, Lomas DA: Alpha$_1$-antitrypsin deficiency, liver disease and emphysema. *Int J Biochem Cell Biol* 35:1009, 2003.

Person RE, Li FQ, Duan Z, et al: Mutations in proto-oncogene GFI1 cause human neutropenia and target ELA2. *Nat Genet* 34:308, 2003.

Rangatia J, Vangala RK, Singh SM, et al: Elevated c-Jun expression in acute myeloid leukemias inhibits C/EBPalpha DNA binding via leucine zipper domain interaction. *Oncogene* 22:4760, 2003.

Tenen DG: Disruption of differentiation in human cancer: AML shows the way. *Nat Rev Cancer* 3:89, 2003.

Wehrle-Haller B, Imhof BA: Integrin-dependent pathologies. *J Pathol* 200:481, 2003.

REFERENCES

For the complete list of references, log on to www.expertconsult.com.

CHAPTER 28

THROMBOCYTOPOIESIS

Alan B. Cantor

Platelets, once regarded simply as "blood dust," are now recognized to play essential roles in hemostasis. Not only do they form a hemostatic plug and initiate thrombus formation in the event of vascular injury, but they also repair minute vascular damage that occurs on a daily basis. Platelets also participate in wound healing and angiogenesis via delivery of key growth factors to sites of vascular injury and interact with the innate immune system. Disorders associated with platelet production carry significant morbidity and mortality in humans because of hemorrhage, thrombosis, bone marrow (BM) fibrosis, BM failure, and/or hematologic malignancy. Platelets are generated from their precursor cells, megakaryocytes, via a complex process. For a long time, the extreme rarity of megakaryocytes significantly hampered studies aimed at understanding the molecular mechanisms underlying platelet biogenesis. However, the purification and cloning (in 1994) of thrombopoietin (TPO), the major megakaryocyte cytokine, has enabled considerable progress to be made. Recent application of whole exome and genome DNA sequencing has further stimulated discovery of new disease-associated genes involved in human thrombocytopoiesis. These new insights provide an important foundation for improved diagnosis and treatment of disorders of thrombocytopoiesis. This chapter reviews the current understanding of megakaryocyte biology and platelet production, highlighting connections with human disease.

MEGAKARYOCYTE BIOLOGY

Megakaryocyte Development

Although platelets were described as early as the 1840s, it was not until 1906, in a seminal study by James Homer Wright, that their origin from megakaryocytes was first recognized.[1] Megakaryocytes are large polyploid cells that reside predominantly within the BM during postnatal life. They are rare cells, constituting only about 0.1% of nucleated cells under normal steady-state conditions. They develop from common bipotential megakaryocyte-erythroid progenitor (MEP) cells, which are themselves derived from common myeloid progenitor (CMP) cells, and ultimately from totipotent hematopoietic stem cells (HSCs). Recent data suggest that megakaryocyte progenitor (MkP) cells can also develop in a more direct hierarchical fashion from HSCs. Once committed to the megakaryocytic lineage, MkPs undergo a series of dramatic maturational steps ultimately tailored to their final task of platelet production and release. These include changes in proliferative capacity, cell size, nuclear content, organelle biogenesis, membrane development, and cytoskeletal rearrangement. The large increase in cell size is linked to an unusual process termed *endomitosis,* in which cells replicate their DNA but fail to undergo cytokinesis. Mature megakaryocytes reach diameters of approximately 100 μm and contain DNA content as high as 128N. They contain a multilobulated nucleus enclosed by a single nuclear membrane. Their abundant cytoplasm is filled with ribosomes, platelet-specific granules, mitochondria, and complex intracellular membrane systems. Although megakaryocytes reside predominantly within the BM, they are also found in peripheral blood, spleen, and lung under normal conditions. These extramedullary megakaryocytes release platelets, but their contribu-tion to total thrombocytopoiesis is estimated to account for at most 7% to 15%.

Megakaryocyte Progenitors

Like other hematopoietic progenitor cells, MkPs can be cultured in vitro using semisolid media. Animal studies using these colony assays have allowed delineation of hierarchal developmental pathways of MkP maturation based on proliferative potential, DNA content, morphologic criteria, and gene expression pattern (Fig. 28.1). This pathway can be conceptually divided into three broad stages: proliferating MkPs, which contain normal DNA content (2N/4N), nonproliferating immature megakaryocytes (4N to 8N DNA content), and nonproliferating mature megakaryocytes (DNA content 8N to128N). Within the proliferating MkP compartment, the earliest detectable cell is the megakaryocyte high-proliferative-potential colony-forming cell (Mk-HPP-CFC), which is capable of generating macroscopically visible colonies containing a few thousand megakaryocytes. This corresponds to a proliferative capacity of ≈8 to 10 replicative cycles. These cells require IL-3 and simultaneous activation of the protein kinase C and cyclic adenosine monophosphate signaling pathway.

The burst-forming unit-megakaryocyte (BFU-Mk), which is thought to be a direct progeny of Mk-HPP-CFC, is more mature than the Mk-HPP-CFC, but retains a high degree of proliferative potential, developing "bursts" of individual colony-forming cells. These colonies contain approximately 100 to 500 megakaryocytes, representing ≈5 to 7 replicative cycles. In humans, BFU-Mk cells require mitogenic stimulation with IL-3 or granulocyte-macrophage colony-stimulating factor (GM-CSF) and synergistic signaling with stem cell factor (SCF; also called *kit-ligand*), interleukin (IL)-11, IL-1α, and TPO. They are also resistant to treatment in vitro with 5-fluorouracil.

The most mature proliferating cell is the colony-forming cell-megakaryocyte (CFU-Mk), which has very limited proliferative potential, representing only 2 to 5 cell divisions (4 to 32 megakaryocytes per colony). This progenitor responds to a variety of single growth factors, such as IL-3 and GM-CSF, and coregulators such as SCF, FMS-like tyrosine kinase-3 ligand, and TPO. They express early markers of differentiation such as glycoprotein IIb (GPIIb) and platelet factor 4 (PF4) before initiating endomitotic cell cycles.

Immature Megakaryocytes: Promegakaryoblasts

Promegakaryoblasts are transitional cells intermediate between proliferating progenitor cells and postmitotic, mature megakaryocytes. These cells are not readily observed morphologically in vitro or in BM specimens but may be identified by their expression of megakaryocyte-specific or platelet-specific markers, such as platelet peroxidase, platelet GPIIb/IIIa, and von Willebrand factor (vWF). They have DNA content levels intermediate between proliferating progenitors and mature megakaryocytes. Promegakaryoblasts respond to a variety of cytokines in vitro, including IL-3, SCF, IL-6, and TPO, to produce large polyploid megakaryocytes. At least three distinct subpopulations of promegakaryoblasts have been identified based on different physiochemical characteristics, morphology, antigen expression, and enzyme content.

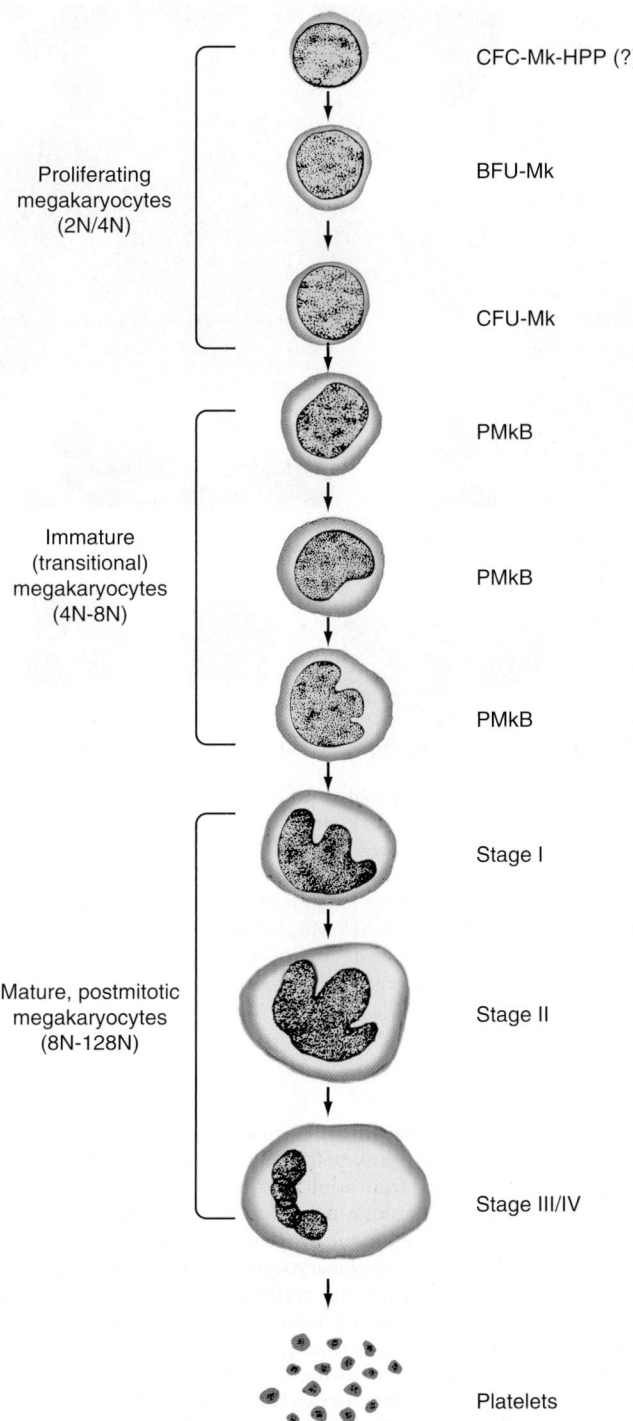

Fig. 28.1 CELLULAR HIERARCHY OF MEGAKARYOCYTE DEVELOPMENT. Megakaryocyte development can be conceptually divided into three stages: The proliferating progenitor cells, which have the typical 2N/4N DNA content; the immature megakaryocytes, which have an intermediate DNA content and are transitional between the progenitor cells and the more mature cells; and the mature, postmitotic cells, which have an 8N to 128N DNA content. *BFU-Mk,* Burst-forming unit-megakaryocyte; *CFU-Mk,* colony-forming unit-megakaryocyte; *CFC-Mk-HPP,* colony-forming unit-megakaryocyte high-proliferative potential; *PMkB,* promegakaryoblast.

Labels in figure: CFC-Mk-HPP (?); BFU-Mk; CFU-Mk; Proliferating megakaryocytes (2N/4N); PMkB; PMkB; PMkB; Immature (transitional) megakaryocytes (4N-8N); Stage I; Stage II; Stage III/IV; Mature, postmitotic megakaryocytes (8N-128N); Platelets

Mature Megakaryocytes

Morphologically recognizable megakaryocytes exist in at least four distinct maturation stages as defined morphologically (Fig. 28.2). The megakaryoblast (stage I) is characterized by a high nucleus-to-cytoplasm ratio and scanty basophilic cytoplasm, reflecting the large amount of protein synthesis occurring in these cells. The promegakaryocyte (stage II) is the cell in which the cytoplasmic volume and number of platelet-specific granules increase. The granular or "platelet shedding" megakaryocyte (stages III and IV) is the most mature cell. In reality, these stages likely represent a continuum.

Prospective Isolation of Megakaryocyte Progenitor Cells

The surface immunophenotype: c-kit(+)Sca-1(-)IL7Ralpha(-)Thy1.1(-)Lin(-)CD9(+)CD41(+)FcgammaR(lo) can be used to prospectively isolate murine clonogenic committed MkPs. This fraction represents approximately 0.01% of the total nucleated BM cells and gives rise to CFU-Mk and occasionally BFU-Mk in colony assays. The immunophenotype Lin(-)c-kit (+)Sca1(-)CD150 (+)CD41(+) has also been used to enrich for committed murine MkPs. Identification of a comparable set of surface markers for human MkPs has not been reported.

Structure of Mature Megakaryocytes

Mature megakaryocytes contain a large multilobulated polyploid nucleus often situated toward the periphery of the cell. They have abundant cytoplasm, which contains platelet-specific secretory granules, alpha (α-) granules and dense granules (Fig. 28.3).[2] The biogenesis of α-granules and dense granules begins in immature megakaryocytes, and both granule types develop concomitantly. α-Granules are 200 to 500 nm in diameter and have a dense center and fine granular matrix. Megakaryocytes synthesize many of the constituents of α-granules and target them to the granules. These include vWF, fibronectin, P-selectin, fibrinogen receptors, PF4, coagulation factor V, and plasminogen activator inhibitor-1, among others. In addition, some constituents, such as fibrinogen, are taken up by megakaryocytes via endocytosis and/or pinocytosis and stored in α-granules. It was once thought that α-granules were a homogeneous population of vesicles. However, it has become clear that there are distinct populations of α-granules containing different constituents, and that these can be differentially released during platelet activation.[3] Dense granules are 200 to 300 nm in diameter and consist of a halo encircling an electron opaque core. They contain many soluble hemostatic factors such as serotonin, catecholamines, adenosine, adenosine 5′-diphosphate, adenosine 5′-triphosphate, and calcium. Their limiting membranes contain glycoproteins such as αIIbβ3, glycoprotein Ib (GPIb), and P-selectin, which are also present in α-granules, as well as unique membrane proteins such as granulophysin. Multivesicular bodies serve as intermediates in the biogenesis of both α-granules and dense granules. It has been proposed that they constitute a sorting compartment between α-granule and dense granule components.

Mutations in the *NBEAL2* gene have recently been linked to gray platelet syndrome (OMIM 139090), a disorder of impaired platelet α-granule synthesis. This gene encodes a large BEACH domain containing protein that shares homology with the *LYST* gene product. LYST is involved in vesicular trafficking and is mutated in Chediak-Higashi syndrome (OMIM 214500), a disorder that includes impaired platelet dense granule biogenesis.

The megakaryocyte cytoplasm contains at least two complex membranous systems: the demarcation membrane system (DMS) and the dense tubular network (DTS) (see Fig. 28.3). The DMS consists of an extensive network of tubular and flattened membranous structures that interconnect with one another and communicate with the extracellular space. Whole cell patch-clamp studies in living rat

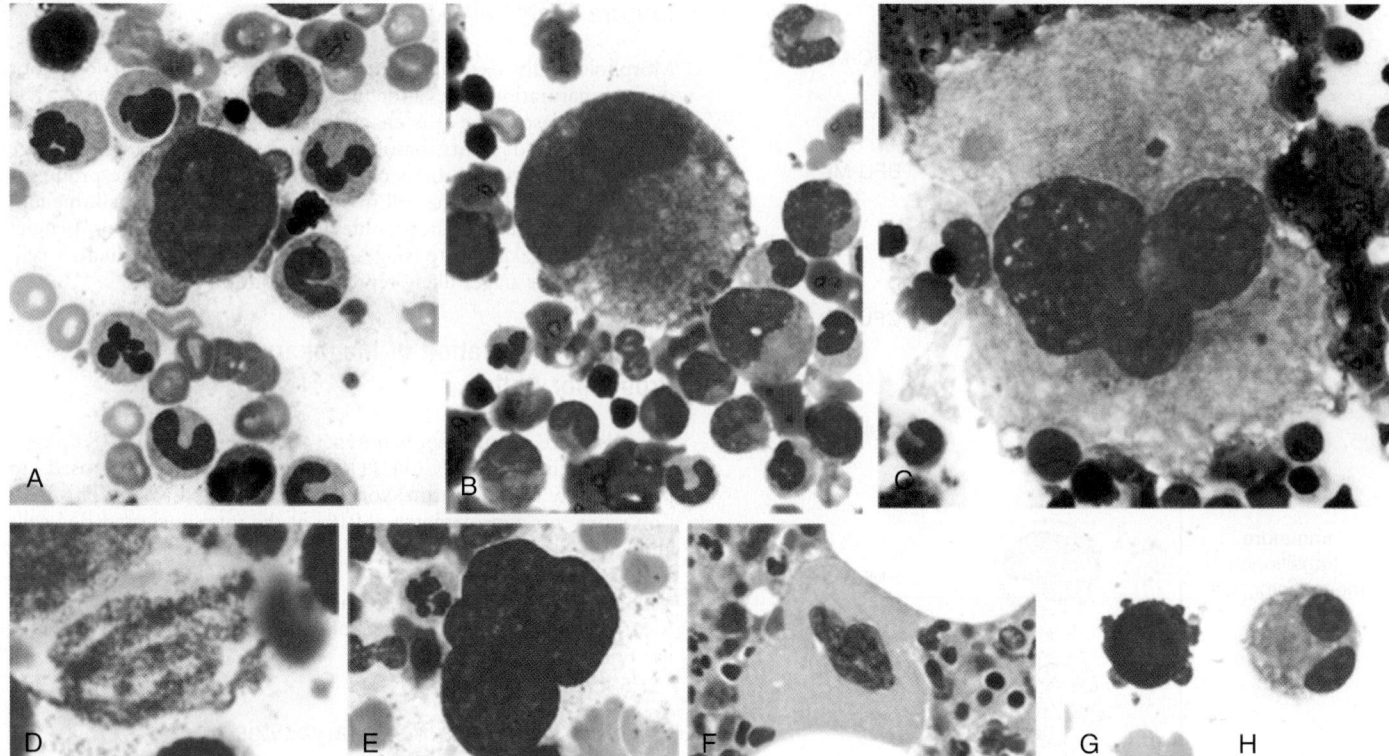

Fig. 28.2 MEGAKARYOCYTOPOEISIS AND MEGAKARYOCYTES. (A) Megakaryoblast (stage I) with intermediate ploidy level. Cytoplasm is scant. Note prominent cytoplasmic pseudopods. (B) Promegakaryocyte with early platelet production (stage II). (C) Mature, high-ploidy megakaryocyte (stage III or IV) with abundant cytoplasm. Note cells traveling through cytoplasm. This is referred to as *emperipolesis* and is not uncommonly seen in large megakaryocytes. (D) Portion of megakaryocyte cytoplasm in a long strand. Fragments of these can sometimes be seen in the blood and are referred to as *proplatelets*. (E) Megakaryocyte nucleus denuded of its platelets and cytoplasm. (F) Mature megakaryocyte seen in a tissue section of bone marrow biopsy. (G) Megakaryoblast from a patient with acute megakaryoblastic leukemia. Note cytoplasmic pseudopods. (H) Micromegakaryocyte from a patient with myelodysplasia. Note small, low-ploidy (2–4N) nucleus, but mature cytoplasm.

megakaryocytes show that they are electrophysiologically contiguous with the plasma membrane. The open canalicular system of platelets shares many features of the megakaryocyte DMS and may represent a remnant of this structure. The DMS serves as a vast membrane reservoir for proplatelet and platelet formation. The DTS of megakaryocytes is distinct from the DMS. Unlike the DMS, it fails to stain with surface membrane tracer dyes, indicating a lack of communication with the plasma membrane. The DTS is thought to be a site of platelet prostaglandin synthesis.

Ontogeny of Megakaryopoiesis

Hematopoiesis develops in distinct waves during embryonic development. In mammals, the first hematopoietic progenitors are found in blood islands of the yolk sac. These give rise to a distinct population of large erythrocytes, termed *primitive erythrocytes,* which express unique globin genes and retain their nucleus longer than adult-type or "definitive" erythrocytes. "Definitive" hematopoiesis arises later during embryogenesis from HSCs that develop de novo from the ventral aspect of the dorsal aorta in the aorto-gonad-mesonephros (AGM) region. These then seed the fetal liver, which serves as a major site of hematopoiesis during gestation. Eventually, hematopoiesis shifts to the BM (and spleen in mice), where it is sustained postnatally.

MkPs have been detected in yolk sac as early as embryonic day 7.5 (e7.5) of mouse development. They are capable of generating proplatelets and platelets after in vitro culture. Circulating platelets

have been detected in the mouse embryo as early as e10.5. Megakaryocytes cultured from early yolk sac have features somewhat distinct from those cultured from adult BM, such as lower modal ploidy, smaller size, different cytokine requirements, and faster kinetics of platelet generation. These unique progenitors disappear by e13.5. In addition, mixed erythroid-megakaryocyte colonies derived from the early yolk sac give rise to primitive erythrocytes. It has therefore been suggested that a separate wave of "primitive megakaryocytes," akin to "primitive erythrocytes," exists during early yolk sac stages of hematopoiesis. These rapidly maturing megakaryocytes may prevent hemorrhage from the developing vasculature until definitive hematopoiesis is available to provide a steady supply of platelets.

Several pieces of evidence suggest that fetal liver megakaryocytes also have unique features compared with adult BM–derived megakaryocytes.[4] This could be caused by either intrinsic differences in the progenitors, or possibly their interactions with a distinct microenvironment. Megakaryocytes that develop from murine neonatal liver progenitors after transplantation into myeloablated mouse recipients are smaller and have lower ploidy levels than those derived from transplanted adult BM. However, these differences are no longer apparent 1 month after transplant. In addition, several congenital disorders of megakaryopoiesis in humans, such as Down syndrome transient myeloproliferative disorder (DS-TMD) and thrombocytopenia with absent radii resolve spontaneously after the newborn period, suggesting specific effects on fetal megakaryocytopoiesis. It is possible that these differences account for the delayed platelet engraftment often observed when umbilical cord blood is used as a graft source for human stem cell transplantation.

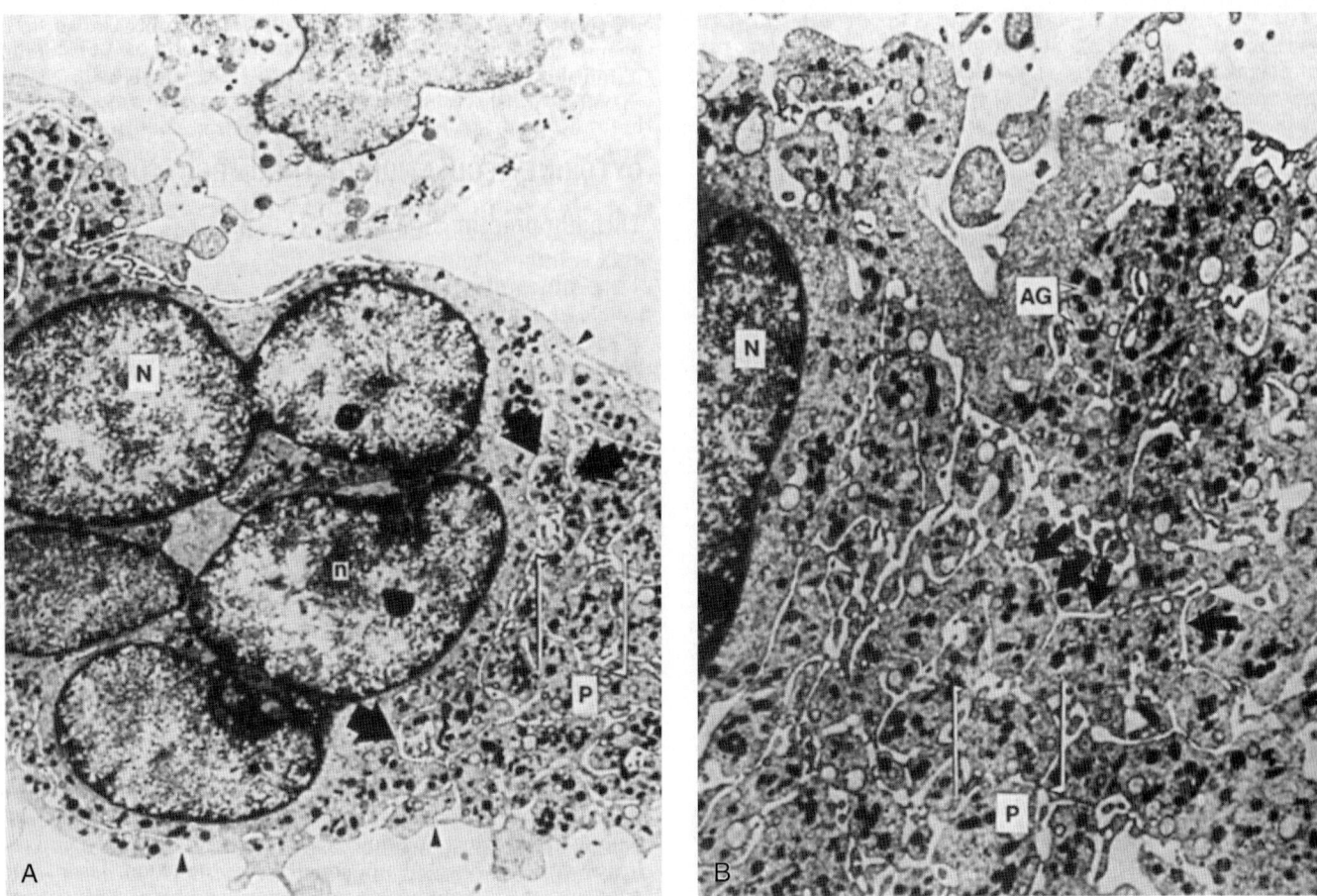

Fig. 28.3 MATURE HUMAN MEGAKARYOCYTE ULTRASTRUCTURE. (A and B) Transmission electron micrographs of two stage III and IV human megakaryocytes. Openings of the demarcation membrane system (*arrowheads*). *AG,* α-Granules; *n,* nucleolus; *N,* nucleus; *P,* a platelet field within the megakaryocyte cytoplasm. *(Courtesy Dr. Maryann Weller.)*

Platelet Biogenesis

It has been estimated that each megakaryocyte produces between a few hundred to several thousand platelets. The exact mechanism by which this occurs has been controversial, with several competing models proposed in the past. It was initially suggested that the DMS established platelet fields, which defined territories of prepackaged platelet contents. These fields would generate platelets directly upon breakdown of the megakaryocyte cytoplasm. However, prevailing evidence supports an alternate model in which platelets are released from dynamic megakaryocyte pseudopod extensions called *proplatelets*. This model was first proposed by Becker and DeBruyn[4a] in 1976 and supported by ultrastructural studies later in the 1980s. Italiano et al.[5] extended these earlier studies on proplatelet formation and platelet biogenesis using videomicroscopy of cultured murine megakaryocytes (see Chapter 124). These in vitro experiments demonstrate that platelet biogenesis begins with a reorganization of unique cortical microtubules within the megakaryocyte to produce large pseudopodia structures from one pole of the megakaryocyte. This spreads across the megakaryocyte, generating extensions that elongate into complex branching tubular proplatelet processes. During this time, organelles travel along microtubules within the shafts of the proplatelets and are loaded into the proplatelet tips where they are captured.[6] It is only at the tips of the proplatelet processes that platelets are shed. During proplatelet formation, extensive remodeling and branching occurs, allowing for marked amplification of proplatelet ends. This phenomenon likely accounts for the ability of each megakaryocyte to generate such a large number of platelets. The DMS serves as an extensive membrane reservoir for these processes.[7] Proplatelet formation is regulated by a pathway involving Rho GTPase proteins, Rho-associated kinase (ROCK), the *MYH9* gene product myosin IIA, and myosin light-chain kinase.[8] In vivo imaging studies suggest that murine megakaryocytes frequently release proplatelets into circulation. These are then subsequently processed into individual platelets.

Bone Marrow Spatial Cues and Megakaryocyte Maturation

There is mounting evidence that the proliferation and terminal maturation of MkPs occur in distinct spatial compartments within the BM (see Chapter 11). In a simplified model, the BM space can be conceptually divided into distinct regions, a space adjacent to the cortical bone (an "osteoblastic niche"), an intermediate zone, and a "vascular niche" containing sinusoidal vessels lined with specialized BM endothelial cells (BMECs). HSCs are thought to reside in a quiescent state adjacent to the bone. Under appropriate conditions, they are recruited to generate hematopoietic multipotent progenitor cells, which leave the osteoblastic niche, perhaps in part under the regulation of metalloproteinases such as MMP-9. The multipotent progenitors are then subject to expansion and lineage commitment under the influence of various cytokines and likely other signaling molecules. This is where TPO is postulated to affect MkP proliferation and survival. Rafii et al. have shown that the chemokines stromal derived factor-1 (SDF-1; also called CXCL12) and fibroblast growth factor-4 (FGF-4) promote migration and attachment of murine MkP cells (which express the receptor for SDF-1, CXCR4) to the vascular endothelium,

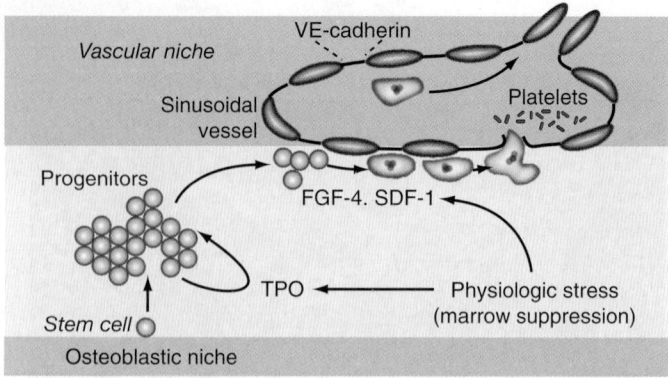

Fig. 28.4 MODEL OF TERMINAL MATURATION OF MEGAKARYO-CYTES AT THE BONE MARROW VASCULAR SINUSOID. Schematic diagram showing hematopoietic stem cells (HSCs) located predominantly adjacent to the cortical bone ("osteoblast niche"), megakaryocyte progenitors (MkPs) proliferating in the bone marrow space, and migration of progenitor cells to the vascular sinusoid ("vascular niche") under the influence of chemokines such as SDF-1 and fibroblast growth factor 4 (FGF-4). Once attached to the sinusoidal vascular endothelium, MkPs cease proliferating, undergo terminal maturation and proplatelet formation, and shed platelets into the vascular sinusoidal space. *TPO,* Thrombopoietin. *(Reproduced with permission from Avecilla ST, Hattori K, Heissig B, et al: Chemokine-mediated interaction of hematopoietic progenitors with the bone marrow vascular niche is required for thrombopoiesis.* Nat Med *10:64, 2004. Reproduced with permission.)*

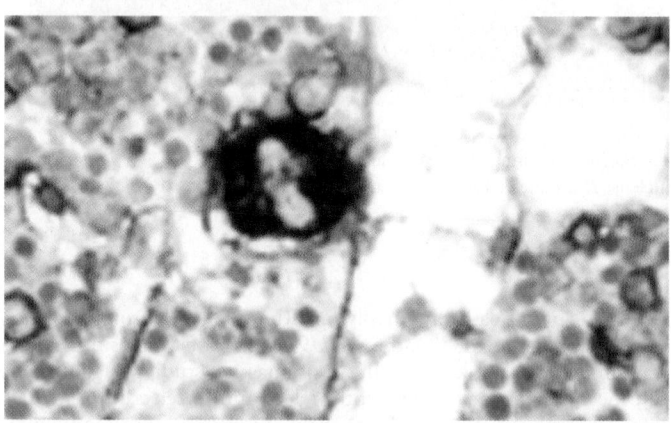

Fig. 28.5 MEGAKARYOCYTE ATTACHED TO SINUSOIDAL VASCULAR ENDOTHELIUM. Bone core biopsy with megakaryocyte (stained with CD31) attached to the endothelium of a sinusoidal vessel *(right).*

where they physically attach, mature, and produce intercalating pseudopod structures.[9] In fact, exogenous SDF-1 and FGF-4 restores thrombopoiesis in TPO$^{-/-}$ or TPO receptor (c-Mpl)$^{-/-}$ mice to near wild-type levels. This occurs in the absence of enhanced MkP proliferation and requires direct physical interaction with BMECs. Based on these findings, Rafii et al. have proposed a model in which MkPs proliferate in an immature developmental state (in response to TPO) in a nonvascular niche (Fig. 28.4). However, once the progenitors reach and adhere to the sinusoidal vessels in the vascular niche in response to chemokines (Fig. 28.5), proliferation ceases and terminal maturation and platelet release ensues. Work from other investigators supports this model. Multiple electron microscopic studies have captured megakaryocytes extending proplatelet processes through vascular endothelium and into BM sinusoids, and in vivo imaging studies have documented this process in living mice.[10] Isolated megakaryocytes can be induced to form proplatelets after adhering to bovine corneal endothelial cells-derived extracellular matrix or via binding of the megakaryocyte surface integrin αIIbβ3 to fibrinogen, which is present in BM vascular sinusoids. Conversely, culture of

megakaryocytes with BM stromal cells inhibits megakaryocyte differentiation. These mechanisms are likely in place to coordinate terminal megakaryocyte maturation with vascular access, facilitating the efficient delivery of platelets into circulation.

CYTOKINE REGULATION OF THROMBOCYTOPOIESIS

Thrombopoietin Signaling

Thrombopoietin

It has been estimated that an adult human produces nearly 2×10^{11} platelets per day, and this number can increase fourfold to eightfold during times of increased demand.[11] The regulation of this process has been the subject of intense investigation. Kelemen[11a] first used the term *thrombopoietin* in 1958 to describe a humoral substance responsible for enhancing platelet production following the onset of thrombocytopenia. However, it was not until 1994 that five independent groups succeeded in purifying and cloning the responsible cytokine, now known as TPO (previously referred to as *c-Mpl ligand, megakaryocyte growth and development factor [MGDF],* and *megapoietin).*[12] The gene for TPO is located on chromosome 3q27. It encodes a 30 kDa glycoprotein of 353 amino acids that can be divided into two structural domains: an amino terminal region with homology to human erythropoietin (EPO), and a carboxyl terminal region that contains multiple N- and O-linked oligosaccharides. The amino terminal 155 residues of human TPO share 21% sequence identity and 46% overall sequence similarity to human EPO. This region mediates binding to the TPO receptor (c-Mpl). The carboxyl region does not share sequence homology with any known protein. TPO is reported to enhance multiple stages of megakaryocyte maturation, including cell size, cell ploidy, and platelet production. The predominant sites of TPO production are the liver and kidney, which secrete it in a generally constitutive fashion. Expression of TPO has been detected by more sensitive methods in BM stroma and spleen in the setting of thrombocytopenia, although this likely accounts for only a minor fraction of total TPO production. Low-level expression has also been reported in the amygdala and hippocampus of the brain.

Thrombopoietin Receptor (c-Mpl)

The receptor for TPO (TPO receptor; c-Mpl) is the normal homologue of the oncogene *v-Mpl,* the transforming gene of murine myeloproliferative leukemia virus. It is a 635 amino acid protein that contains a number of distinct functional domains: a 25-amino acid signal peptide, a 465 amino acid extracellular domain, a 22-residue transmembrane domain, and an intracellular domain that contains two conserved motifs, termed Box 1 and Box 2 (Fig. 28.6). The extracellular domain contains of a distal region that negatively influences TPO signaling. It is a member of the type I cytokine receptor superfamily. Like the EPO receptor, it is thought to function as a homodimer. The TPO receptor is expressed on MkPs, as well as earlier multipotential progenitors, including MEPs, CMPs, and HSCs. TPO receptors are present on the surface of platelets at an estimated density of 20 to 200 receptors per platelet and bind TPO with an affinity of 200 to 560 pM. Binding of TPO to platelets plays an important role in the regulation of total body platelet mass by the TPO-TPO receptor system. Both TPO receptor$^{-/-}$ (c-Mpl$^{-/-}$) and TPO (TPO$^{-/-}$) knock-out mice contain ≈85% to 90% lower platelet and megakaryocyte numbers as compared with wild-type mice.[13,14] The structure of the megakaryocytes and platelets in these animals is normal, reinforcing the notion that TPO signaling plays an important role in expansion and development of MkPs, but not in terminal maturation and proplatelet release. In addition, the residual platelet production in these mice suggests alternate cytokine, or possibly cytokine-independent, pathways for thrombocytopoiesis. Interbreeding experiments of TPO receptor$^{-/-}$ mice with knock-out mice for IL-3, IL-6, IL-11, or leukemia inhibitory factor (LIF) or their

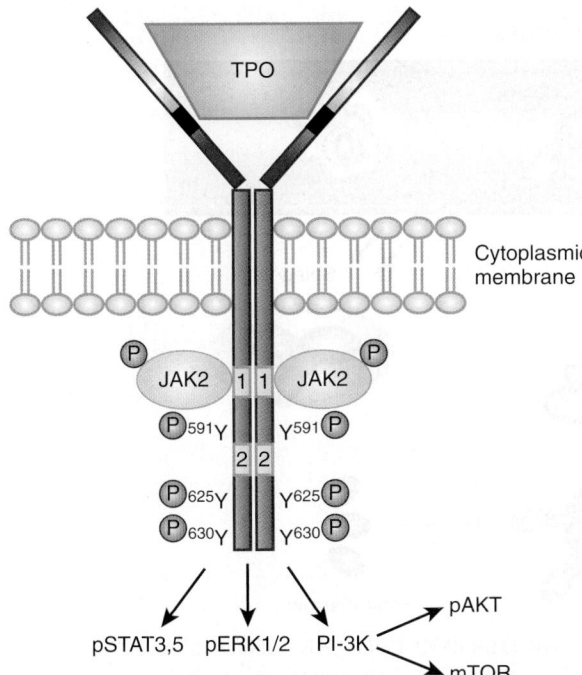

Cytoplasmic
membrane

Fig. 28.6 THE THROMBOPOIETIN RECEPTOR. Schematic diagram of the thrombopoietin (TPO) receptor depicted as a homodimer with TPO bound. Binding of JAK2 at Box 1 of the cytoplasmic tail is shown. Conformational changes in the TPO receptor upon TPO binding results in juxtaposition of the two cytoplasmic tails, as well as JAK2 autophosphorylation and JAK2-mediated phosphorylation of the c-Mpl cytoplasmic tail (Tyr[591], Tyr[625], and Tyr[630]). Activation of STAT, ERK, phosphoinositol-3 kinase (PI-3K)-Akt, and PI3K-mTOR signaling pathways then occurs. *(Reproduced with permission from Geddis AE: Megakaryopoiesis. Semin Hematol 47:212, 2010.)*

receptors, show that these other cytokines are not responsible for the residual platelet production.

TPO Receptor Downstream Signaling Pathways

The TPO receptor lacks intrinsic tyrosine kinase activity. Instead, ligand binding is thought to induce a conformational change in the homodimeric receptor and stimulates the cytoplasmic tyrosine kinase Janus-kinase 2 (JAK2), which binds to Box 1 of the cytoplasmic tail. This results in tyrosine phosphorylation of multiple targets, including signal transducers and activators of transcription (STATs), Shc adaptor protein, and the TPO receptor itself (Tyr[591], Tyr[625], and Tyr[630]). Additional signaling pathways activated upon TPO receptor engagement include the mitogen-activated protein kinase (MAPK) p38, p42/p44 extracellular signal-regulated kinase 1 (ERK1/ERK2), phosphoinositol-3-kinase-AKT (PI3K-AKT), and PI3K-Mammalian target of rapamycin (mTOR) signaling pathways.

Several of these downstream signaling pathways have been shown to be functionally important in TPO-mediated effects on megakaryocytopoiesis. Double STAT5a/STAT5b–deficient mice have impaired platelet production as well as defects in early multipotent progenitor cells. Moreover, megakaryocyte-selective overexpression of a dominant negative mutant STAT3 in transgenic mice reduces platelet recovery following 5-fluorouracil–induced myelosuppression. These findings suggest a functional role for STAT family members in thrombopoiesis.

Studies in primary megakaryocytes show a requirement for PI3-AKT signaling in TPO-induced cell cycling. This involves silencing of the Forkhead O family of transcription factors. Activation of the p42/p44-MAPK plays an important role in TPO-induced maturation and endomitosis. The mTOR signaling pathway is involved in

TPO-mediated megakaryocytic progenitor proliferation and possibly terminal megakaryocyte size determination, ploidy, and cellular maturation.

Negative Regulation of TPO Signaling

As with other receptor-mediated signaling processes, feedback mechanisms exist to limit or turn off the signal once initiated to avoid uncontrolled growth. Lnk, an adaptor protein implicated in immunoreceptor and cytokine receptor signaling negatively modulates TPO signaling in megakaryocytes. Overexpression of Lnk decreases TPO-dependent megakaryocyte growth and polyploidization in BM–derived cultures. Conversely, loss of Lnk expression by gene targeting results in increased numbers of megakaryocytes, accentuated megakaryocyte polyploidization, and a myeloproliferative disorder in mice.[15] This correlates with enhanced and prolonged TPO-mediated induction of STAT3, STAT5, AKT, and MAPK signaling pathways.

Following TPO binding, the TPO receptor is internalized and subsequently degraded. This process depends on dileucine repeats, and Tyr[591] and Tyr[625] within the TPO receptor cytoplasmic tail, and involves ubiquitinylation via the E3 ubiquitin ligase c-Cbl.

TPO Signaling in Hematopoietic Stem Cells

The TPO-TPO receptor signaling system is not only important for megakaryocyte proliferation and development, but also plays a role in HSCs survival, self-renewal, and expansion.[16] TPO receptor[−/−] HSCs compete poorly with wild-type HSCs, even at a ratio of 10:1, in murine BM competitive repopulation studies. The role of TPO signaling in HSC expansion is in part because of its activation of the homeobox domain containing transcription factor HOXA9, via a mechanism involving phosphorylation and nuclear translocation of its partner protein MEIS1.

Congenital Amegakaryocytic Thrombocytopenia

Biallelic mutations in the TPO receptor gene cause congenital amegakaryocytic thrombocytopenia (CAMT, OMIM 604498). In this disorder, megakaryocytes are absent or greatly diminished in number in the BM. Patients typically present shortly after birth with petechiae, bruising, or bleeding. Patients with severe CAMT are at high risk for developing progressive BM failure, typically within the first few years of life. This is consistent with a role of TPO signaling in maintaining HSCs and/or multipotential progenitor cells. Of interest, no mutations in the gene encoding TPO itself have been reported in patients with CAMT. It should also be noted that in contrast to the humans, TPO receptor[−/−] (as well as TPO[−/−]) mice do not develop BM failure states. The reason for this discrepancy is not known, but it highlights important differences between human and mouse hematopoiesis.

Essential Thrombocythemia

Essential thrombocythemia (ET) is a chronic myeloproliferative neoplasm associated with sustained excessive megakaryocyte hyperproliferation, thrombocytosis, and abnormal platelet function leading to either hemorrhage or thrombosis (see Chapter 69). In 2005, an acquired activating mutation in the JAK2 family (V617F JAK2) was identified by four independent groups in a large proportion (≈50%) of patients with ET. The identical mutation has also been identified in several other myeloproliferative neoplasms, including polycythemia vera (95% of patients) and primary myelofibrosis (50% of patients). How the identical mutation leads to distinct clinical entities is not well understood but may be related to the allelic dosage of the mutation. Mutations leading to constitutive activation of the TPO receptor or enhanced translation efficiency of the *TPO* gene have also been reported in rare cases of familial thrombocytosis. These two classes of disorders can be distinguished by measuring circulating TPO levels, which are elevated with mutations enhancing TPO mRNA translation

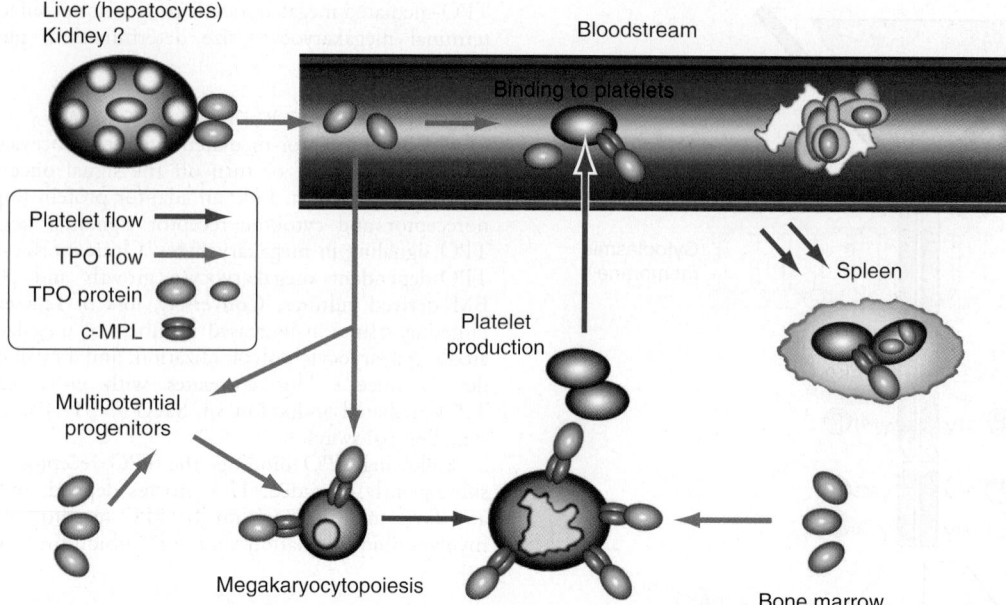

Fig. 28.7 REGULATION OF PLATELET COUNT BY THROMBOPOIETIN: THE "SPONGE" MODEL. TPO is secreted at a constitutive rate primarily from liver, and perhaps other sources such as the kidney, into the circulation. There it binds with high affinity to TPO receptors (c-Mpl) present on the surface of platelets. The TPO is then internalized by the platelets and degraded. Free TPO (i.e., TPO not bound to platelets) enters the bone marrow and stimulates megakaryocytopoiesis. Thus in the presence of high platelet counts, little free TPO is available to stimulate megakaryocytopoiesis. Conversely, low platelet numbers lead to increased free TPO and active megakaryocytopoiesis. The net result is preservation of total platelet mass.

efficiency, and decreased with mutations leading to constitutive TPO receptor activation. In 2013, somatic mutations involving exon 9 of the calreticulin (*CALR*) gene were identified in a large number of non-JAK2 mutated myeloproliferative neoplasms (67–88% of cases), particularly ET and primary myelofibrosis.[17] Theses mutations result in the generation of an altered protein containing a novel carboxyl terminal domain. Recently, three groups have shown that the mutant CALR leads to myeloproliferative neoplasms by activating C-Mpl and its downstream pathways (Chapters 69 and 70).

Regulation of Platelet Mass by Thrombopoietin

Platelet counts are typically held at a relatively fixed level in humans, ranging from 150,000 to 400,000/mm³. The maintenance of platelet number by the TPO-TPO receptor system involves an unusual homeostatic mechanism among hematopoietic cytokine-mediated regulation. This is sometimes referred to as the "sponge" model (Fig. 28.7). Unlike other cytokines, TPO is secreted predominantly in a constitutive manner, mostly from the liver and kidney. High affinity TPO receptors present on the platelet surface bind free TPO and internalize it, where it is degraded. Therefore, when platelet counts are low, less TPO is removed, and more is available to stimulate megakaryocytopoiesis in the BM. Conversely, when platelet counts rise above a given set point, they act as a "sink" for TPO, binding and destroying it before it can stimulate megakaryocytopoiesis in the BM. Thus total platelet mass is preserved, rather than absolute platelet number. This may explain the mild to moderate thrombocytopenia seen in certain disorders associated with large platelets, such as Bernard-Soulier syndrome.

Several pieces of evidence support this model. First, it has been known for over 40 years that the peripheral blood platelet count varies inversely with plasma TPO activity. Second, TPO receptor deficient mice (c-Mpl⁻/⁻) have elevated levels of circulating TPO, and this is reduced when the mice are transfused with washed platelets from normal mice. Third, in contrast to platelets from TPO receptor–deficient mice, platelets from normal mice bind purified radiolabeled TPO and degrade it. Fourth, TPO levels are low to intermediate in normal individuals and in those with idiopathic thrombocytopenic purpura (where the bound TPO is destroyed along with the platelets). However, following chemotherapy, or in individuals with aplastic anemia, levels are markedly elevated.

Although the model described above likely explains the predominant basal regulation of platelet number by the TPO-TPO receptor signaling system, overlying inducible mechanisms also probably exist. It has been shown that the *TPO* gene is transcriptionally activated in BM stroma and spleen during times of thrombocytopenia, although the degree to which this may contribute to total TPO levels is uncertain. In addition, IL-6 mediates upregulation of hepatic TPO mRNA transcripts in inflammation-related thrombocytosis. Recent work shows that binding of desialylated platelets to the hepatic Ashwell-Morell receptor triggers *TPO* gene transcription and protein production via a JAK 2/STAT3 pathway, linking platelet turnover directly to TPO production.[18]

Additional Cytokines Involved in Megakaryocytopoiesis

Although TPO is the major cytokine regulating megakaryocytopoiesis, other cytokines have been shown to be active in vitro, particularly during earlier stages of megakaryocyte development. These include SCF, IL-3, IL-6, IL-11, LIF, G-CSF, and EPO. None of these factors are megakaryocyte-specific, but act as synergistic coregulators with TPO. Only SCF and TPO have been shown to affect megakaryocyte development and platelet production in vivo using genetic ablation experiments in mice. No effects were seen with knockout of IL-3, IL-6, IL-11 receptor, or LIF.

Therapeutic Cytokine Stimulation of Megakaryocytopoiesis

Since the identification of TPO as a major activator of megakaryocyte growth and maturation, there has been considerable

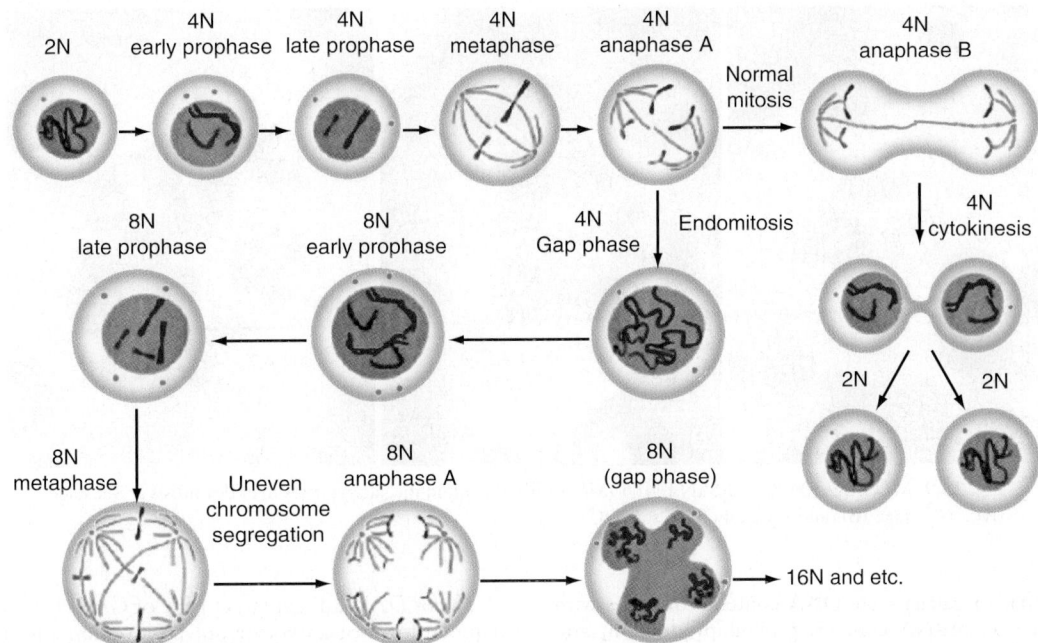

Fig. 28.8 THE ENDOMITOTIC CYCLE IN MEGAKARYOCYTES. Schematic diagram depicting stages of the cell cycle in cells undergoing endomitosis *(bottom left)* versus normal mitosis *(right)*. Endomitotic and mitotic cells share all stages of the cell cycle until anaphase A. Normal mitotic cells proceed through anaphase B and complete cytokinesis, yielding two daughter cells, each with 2N DNA content. In contrast, endomitotic cells fail to undergo anaphase B or cytokinesis, and proceed to the next cycle following a gap phase. Subsequent rounds produce multicentric spindles with uneven chromosome segregation. A single nuclear membrane *(shown in pink)* reforms after each round of endomitosis. Centrosomes are shown as *blue dots. (Reproduced with permission from Ravid K, Lu J, Zimmet JM, et al: Roads to polyploidy: the megakaryocyte example.* J Cell Physiol *190:7, 2002.)*

interest in developing recombinant forms of TPO for clinical use in the treatment of chemotherapy-related thrombocytopenia and immune-mediated thrombocytopenia. Small pilot studies using a polyethyleneglycol (PEG)ylated, truncated form of human TPO (PEG-MGDF) showed activity in stimulating megakaryocyte growth and maturation, resulting in elevated platelet counts. However, some recipients subsequently developed thrombocytopenia as a result of the generation of a neutralizing anti-TPO antibody that cross-reacted with endogenous TPO. The agent was therefore withdrawn from further testing. Since then, several nonimmunogenic thrombopoietic peptides and small, nonpeptide molecules have been developed. Romiplostim (formerly called *AMG 531*), a synthetic molecule consisting of an immunoglobulin Fc domain fragment linked to two identical peptide chains that activate the TPO receptor, stimulates platelet production and has been approved by the U.S. Food and Drug Administration (FDA) for the treatment of adults with chronic immune thrombocytopenia purpura (ITP). It is given intravenously or subcutaneously. Eltrombopag, an orally administered small molecule that binds to a portion of the TPO receptor distinct from the normal TPO binding site, also stimulates thrombopoiesis and is FDA approved for the treatment of chronic ITP. It has also been shown to improve trilineage hematopoiesis in refractory aplastic anemia, likely through its effect on HSC TPO receptor signaling pathways (Chapter 30).[19] Additional agents that stimulate the TPO receptor are also under development.

IL-11 has multiple effects on in vivo and in vitro megakaryocytopoiesis. It affects IL-3–dependent megakaryocyte colony formation and has a potent effect on megakaryocyte maturation. Administration of recombinant IL-11 to mice results in increased numbers of MkPs, increased megakaryocyte polyploidization, and increased peripheral platelet counts. Recombinant IL-11 has been approved for use in humans for the treatment of chemotherapy-induced thrombocytopenia.

ENDOMITOSIS

The Endomitotic Cell Cycle

Megakaryocytes derive their name from their large and complex nuclei. This arises from an atypical cell cycle, termed the *endomitotic* cell cycle (see comprehensive review by Ravid et al.[20]; Fig. 28.8). Like normal diploid cells, the cycle begins with a G1 phase, followed by S phase (DNA replication), and a G2 phase. The cells then enter M phase, but unlike normal diploid mitotic cells, fail to complete anaphase B, telophase, or cytokinesis. A cleavage furrow initially develops but then regresses. The cells then proceed directly to the next G1 phase and subsequent rounds of DNA replication. As DNA ploidy increases, multiple spindle poles and centrosomes form, but chromosome segregation is incomplete and asymmetric. During each endomitotic cell cycle (Fig. 28.9), the nuclear envelope breaks down and later reforms as a single nuclear membrane around all of the sister chromatids. The end result is a polyploid cell with a multilobulated nuclei encapsulated by a single nuclear membrane. Mature human megakaryocytes have been observed to reach ploidy levels as high as 128N. The term *endoreduplication* has at times been used erroneously to describe megakaryocyte polyploidization. *Endoreduplication* correctly refers to a cell cycle that involves DNA replication but no entry into M phase.

Role of Endomitosis in Thrombocytopoiesis

The reason that megakaryocytes undergo endomitosis is not known. It has been speculated that it provides a means for generating the abundant membrane, protein, biosynthetic cargo, and energy required for the dramatic final stages of proplatelet elaboration and platelet release. Several circumstantial pieces of evidence support this model.

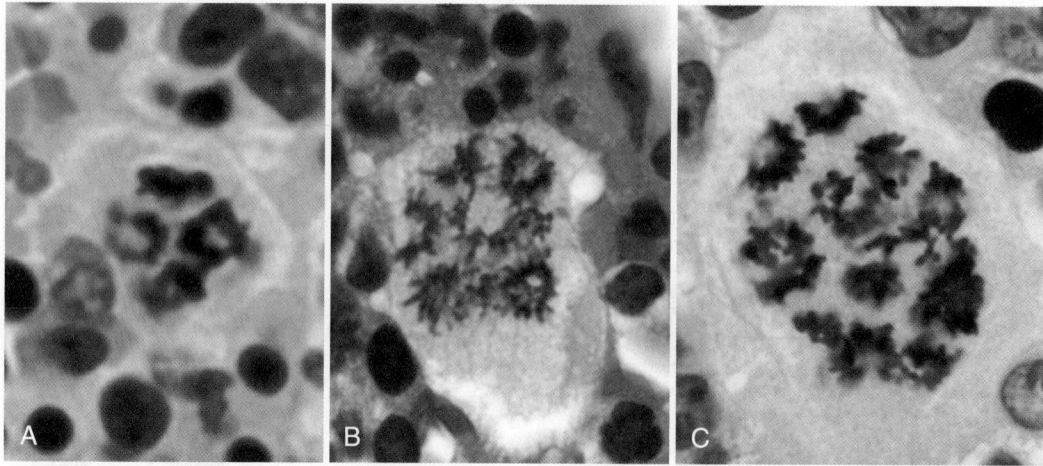

Fig. 28.9 MEGAKARYOCYTES IN ENDOMITOSIS. Polyploid megakaryocytes in endomitosis at 8N stage (A), 16N stage (B), and probably 32N stage (C).

First, it is known that megakaryocyte DNA content correlates with megakaryocyte cell size, mRNA content, protein production, and eventual numbers of platelets released. Second, an increased DNA content of megakaryocytes precedes increases in platelet count during recovery from acute thrombocytopenia. Third, increases in cytoplasmic volume and maturation occur predominantly, if not completely, in stage II and III megakaryocytes, which do not synthesize DNA. Fourth, in polyploid megakaryocytes (4N to 32N), all alleles of the genes studied (i.e., ITGA2B [GPIIb], VWF, ACTB [β-actin], HSPA1 [HSP70], MPL, FLI1, and ZFPM1 [FOG-1]) have been found to be transcriptionally active.

Mechanisms of Endomitosis in Megakaryocytes

The molecular mechanisms mediating endomitosis in megakaryocytes are incompletely understood. Studies investigating endomitosis have been hampered by the rarity of megakaryocytes, difficulty separating direct effects from general perturbations of cell maturation, complications associated with synchronizing the cell cycle, use of transformed cell lines, and potential differences between rodent and human megakaryocytes.

Cyclins and Cyclin-Dependent Kinases

Two classes of proteins control the cell cycle in mammalian cells. These are the cyclins, so named for their cyclical synthesis and degradation during the cell cycle, and cell division kinases (Cdks, also known as *cyclin-dependent kinases*). Together, these two families of proteins form a protein-kinase complex in which the regulatory unit is the cyclin and the catalytic unit is the Cdk. The role of these kinase complexes in cell cycle control is complex. At least seven members of the cyclin gene family and seven distinct *Cdk* genes have been identified.

Given the importance of cyclins and Cdks in controlling cell cycle, they have been the focus of considerable attention in investigations of the mechanisms underlying megakaryocyte endomitosis. The most compelling evidence probably exists for a role of the D-type cyclins in megakaryocyte endomitosis. The D-type cyclins are unique in that their activity can be modulated by extracellular mitogens. Megakaryocytes express cyclin D3 and, to a lesser extent, cyclin D1. Levels of both of these factors increase after treatment with TPO. Overexpression of cyclin D3 results in increased megakaryocyte ploidy in transgenic mouse models. Complexes of cyclin D3 and its major kinase subunit, Cdk2, show high kinase activity in polyploid cells. Antisense knockdown of cyclin D3 levels suppresses endomitosis and abrogates normal development of primary mouse megakaryocytes.

Cyclin D1 is a direct target gene of GATA1, a transcription factor required for megakaryocyte polyploidization and maturation. Overexpression of cyclin D1 in transgenic mice increases megakaryocyte modal ploidy compared with nontransgenic littermates, and the combination of cyclin D1 and Cdk4 kinase activity restores polyploidization of GATA1-deficient murine megakaryocytes. Conversely, enforced expression of p16^{ink4a}, a cell cycle inhibitor of Cdk4/6, blocks polyploidization in murine megakaryocytes. p16^{ink4a} is also potently repressed by GATA1.

Cyclin E$^{-/-}$ mice have impaired megakaryocytopoiesis with reduced modal ploidy. These mice also have defective trophoblast development, another tissue characterized by endomitosis. Cyclin B1/CDC2 is a mitotic cyclin complex. Yeast strains deficient in cyclin B1 or CDC2 undergo an additional round of DNA replication without cytokinesis. Several studies have shown that low levels of cyclin B1/CDC2 are required for progression of endomitosis in megakaryocytic cell lines. However, studies of primary megakaryocytes have shown normal cyclin B1 and CDC2 levels and functional mitotic activity during endomitosis.

Other Mitotic Kinases

Aurora-B kinase (also called *AIM-1 kinase*) is involved in late anaphase and cytokinesis, and mRNA transcript levels of Aurora-B kinase have been reported to decrease during polyploidization of primary megakaryocytes and megakaryocytic cell lines. This suggests that Aurora-B kinase may play a mechanistic role in megakaryocyte endomitosis. However, functional activity of Aurora-B kinase appears normal in late anaphase of endomitotic primary megakaryocytes, indicating that simple deficiency of Aurora-B kinase activation is an unlikely mechanism to explain endomitosis. Polo-like kinase (PLK-1) is a serine-threonine kinase required for assembly of the mitotic spindle, separation of chromosomes during anaphase, and exit from mitosis. PLK-1 mRNA and protein levels decrease during polyploidization of murine megakaryocytes, and enforced expression of PLK-1 in primary murine megakaryocytes impairs endomitosis. However, the effects of overexpression are modest, preferentially affect lower-ploidy megakaryocytes, and are complicated by alterations in cell cycle kinetics.

The Spindle Checkpoint

During mitosis of normal diploid cells, a spindle assembly checkpoint prevents progression of anaphase until all of the chromosomes are aligned with the mitotic spindle and each sister chromatid is properly attached to spindle microtubules originating from the opposing spindle pole. This ensures that each daughter cell receives the proper complement of chromosomes. The anaphase-promoting complex (APC) is a multisubunit protein complex with ubiquitin ligase activity that regulates chromosome segregation and anaphase progression by targeting key factors for degradation. Since some chromosomal missegregation occurs during megakaryocyte endomitosis, several groups have examined the expression levels and/or activity of certain APC components and associated factors. These studies have shown no significant difference in protein levels of the core APC protein CDC27 or the kinetochore-associated signaling protein hsMAD2 in primary murine megakaryocytes undergoing polyploidization compared with nonendomitotic precursors. Haploinsufficiency of BUBR1, a key component of the spindle checkpoint, perturbs megakaryocyte development and polyploidization in mice, but does not cause alterations in circulating platelet counts.

Microtubule Regulation

Microtubules play key roles in mitosis. Therefore factors that regulate their assembly have also been investigated as candidates involved in megakaryocyte endomitosis. Protein regulator of cytokinesis 1 (PRC-1) is involved in mitotic spindle elongation and cytokinesis. However, no differences in PRC-1 levels were detected in primary murine megakaryocytes undergoing polyploidization compared with nonendomitotic precursors. Stathmin is a microtubule-depolymerizing factor that plays an important role in regulation of the mitotic spindle. Levels of stathmin are inversely related to the level of ploidy of megakaryocytic cell lines and primary megakaryocytes. Inhibition of stathmin in K562 cells increases their propensity to undergo endomitosis when induced to differentiate into megakaryocytes, and overexpression of stathmin prevents the transition from mitotic to endomitotic cell cycles. Together, these findings support a possible role of stathmin in modulating endomitosis.

Contractile Ring Activity

Cytokinesis requires the assembly and activity of a contractile ring. The failure to complete cytokinesis during endomitotic cell cycles in megakaryocytes may involve functional defects in the Rho/Rock pathway.[21] Silencing of nonmuscle myosin heavy chain IIB (Myh10) by the transcription factor RUNX1 is also required for efficient megakaryocyte polyploidization.[22] Further studies will be required to fully dissect the molecular pathways involved in megakaryocyte endomitosis.

TRANSCRIPTIONAL CONTROL OF MEGAKARYOCYTOPOIESIS

Since platelets do not contain nuclei, all transcriptional regulation of platelet-specific genes must occur at the level of the megakaryocyte. Significant strides have been made in identifying key transcription factors involved in megakaryocyte development and platelet-specific gene expression. Importantly, mutations in a large number of these factors are linked to various human thrombopoiesis disorders providing significant new insights into the pathogenesis of these diseases (see box on Inherited Causes of Thrombocytopenia).

GATA Family Transcription Factors

GATA1

GATA transcription factors comprise a family of zinc finger proteins that bind the consensus DNA sequence (T/A)GATA(A/G). There are six known members of the GATA family in vertebrates. GATA1, GATA2, and GATA3 play roles predominantly, although not exclusively, within the hematopoietic system. GATA4, GATA5, and GATA6 are expressed in nonhematopoietic tissues and play diverse developmental roles within the cardiac, gastrointestinal, endocrine, and gonadal systems. Functionally important binding sites for GATA

factors have been identified in cis-acting regulatory elements of essentially every megakaryocytic and erythroid gene that has been studied. GATA1, the founding member of this family, is highly expressed in erythroid and megakaryocytic cells and, to a lesser extent, in eosinophils and mast cells. GATA1 plays an essential role in erythroid development, with loss of function resulting in blocked erythroid maturation and apoptosis of erythroid progenitor cells. GATA1 is also required for megakaryocyte maturation and growth control. Lineage-selective loss of GATA1 in megakaryocytes results in marked thrombocytopenia in mice with platelet counts of only ≈15% of wild-type littermates. Megakaryocytes are present in the mutant animals but have a disorganized DMS, paucity of platelet-specific granules, reduced expression of multiple megakaryocyte-specific genes (including *GPIbα, GPIbβ, PF4, c-Mpl,* and *p45 NF-E2*), and marked hyperproliferation as compared with wild-type mice. Gene expression studies of GATA1-deficient versus wild-type murine megakaryocytes have revealed a large number of potential GATA1 target genes, and many of these have been found to be bound by GATA1 in genome-wide chromatin occupancy studies. Mice containing reduced megakaryocyte-specific expression of GATA1 (GATA1low) develop myelofibrosis as they age, a frequent finding with disorders of MkP hyperproliferation. A GATA binding site mutation in the *GPIbβ* promoter has been described in a patient with Bernard-Soulier syndrome, which is characterized by deficiency of the GPIb/IX/V complex and a bleeding diathesis. Taken together, these findings suggest that GATA1 acts as master regulator of megakaryocyte maturation and proliferative control.

Friend of GATA

All vertebrate GATA factors contain two zinc fingers. The carboxyl zinc finger mediates high-affinity DNA binding, whereas the amino zinc finger stabilizes the DNA interaction at certain double GATA sites. The amino zinc finger also interacts with friend of GATA (FOG) proteins, a family of large multitype zinc finger transcriptional cofactors. This interaction occurs on the surface of the zinc finger opposite to its DNA binding surface. FOG-1 (also called zfpm1), the founding member, is expressed predominantly within erythroid and megakaryocytic cells. Knockout of FOG-1 in mice results in embryonic lethality caused by severe anemia from a block in erythroid maturation similar to that observed in GATA1⁻ mice. In addition, FOG-1⁻ᐟ⁻ mice have complete failure of megakaryocytopoiesis, establishing FOG-1 as the first identified transcription-associated factor selectively required to generate the entire megakaryocyte lineage. FOG-1's role in megakaryocyte and erythroid development requires direct physical interaction with GATA factors. The discrepancy between the relatively late block in megakaryocyte development seen in GATA1-deficient animals and the complete loss of megakaryocytopoiesis in FOG-1⁻ᐟ⁻ mice is explained by overlapping FOG-dependent roles of GATA1 and GATA2 during early stages of megakaryocytopoiesis.

X-Linked Dyserythropoietic Anemia and Thrombocytopenia Caused by GATA1 Mutations

Germline GATA1 mutations that impair binding to FOG-1 and/or DNA have been identified in several families with X-linked macrothrombocytopenia and/or anemia (GATA1 is located on the X chromosome in both humans and mice). The first case, reported by Nichols et al.,[22a] involved a woman with mild chronic thrombocytopenia who had two pregnancies with male offspring that were both complicated by severe fetal anemia and thrombocytopenia requiring in utero transfusions. BM examination after birth revealed marked dyserythropoiesis and an overabundance of immature-appearing, dysplastic megakaryocytes that share many of the features of GATA-1low murine megakaryocytes. Remarkably, sequencing of the *GATA1* gene from affected family members identified substitution of valine by methionine at codon 205 within the amino zinc finger. This mutation (GATA1^{V205M}) significantly impairs FOG-1 binding, but retains normal DNA affinity based on electromobility shift assays using synthetic oligonucleotides. This is consistent with the location of this residue on the surface of the zinc finger opposite the DNA binding face.

Several other GATA1 mutations have been linked to cases of familial X-linked macrothrombocytopenia with or without anemia. These substitutions all impair FOG-1 binding, although to different degrees. Substitution of glycine by serine at codon 208 (GATA1^{G208S}) results in moderate to severe thrombocytopenia and mild dyserythropoiesis, but no anemia. Substitution of the same residue by arginine (GATA1^{G208R}) results in thrombocytopenia with anemia and severe dyserythropoiesis. Similarly, substitution of aspartic acid by glycine at codon 218 (GATA1^{D218G}) leads only to thrombocytopenia, whereas substitution of this same codon by tyrosine (GATA1^{D218Y}) leads to severe thrombocytopenia, moderate anemia, and marked dyserythropoiesis. The severity of the phenotype appears to correlate with the degree of FOG-1 binding impairment, suggesting that megakaryocytic development is more sensitive to affinity changes in GATA1–FOG-1 interactions than is erythroid development.

X-Linked Thrombocytopenia and β-Thalassemia Caused by GATA1 Mutations

Mutations mapping to the DNA binding surface of the amino zinc finger of GATA1 have also been described (GATA1^{R216Q}). As expected, this reduces DNA affinity to double (palindromic) GATA sites but not to single GATA sites. FOG-1 binding is not substantially altered. Affected family members exhibit an X-linked β-thalassemia syndrome characterized by imbalance of alpha and beta globin chain synthesis, reticulocytosis and hemolysis. They also have mild to moderate thrombocytopenia. In vitro platelet aggregation studies are normal, but there is a prolonged bleeding time. Substitution of the same residue by tryptophan (R216W) produces thrombocytopenia, β-thalassemia intermedia, and congenital erythropoietic porphyria (CEP). The CEP is likely caused by dysregulation of the *GATA1* target gene uroporphyrinogen III synthase.

X-Linked Gray Platelet–Like Syndrome

Gray platelet syndrome (GPS) refers to a disorder of large platelets with absent or markedly reduced α-granules and/or α-granule proteins. Platelets from individuals with GATA1^{R261Q} share some features with classical GPS. Ultrastructural studies of platelets from a different family with GATA1-related X-linked macrothrombocytopenia (GATA1^{G208S}) also demonstrate hypogranular platelets that contain small vacuoles, likely representing membranes of empty α-granules. However, the GATA1 mutant platelets also possess unique features such as masses of dense tubular system channels, dense double membranes, and platelets within platelets, not seen in classical GPS, suggesting a more general disorder of platelet biogenesis.

GATA1 Mutations in Down Syndrome Transient Myeloproliferative Disorders and Acute Megakaryoblastic Leukemia

About 10% of children with DS (trisomy 21) are born with a TMD, which is characterized by an abundance of circulating erythromegakaryocytic precursor cells, pancytopenia, and in some cases, severe liver fibrosis. Remarkably, this myeloproliferation resolves spontaneously over the first few months of life. In about 20% to 30% of cases, DS–associated acute megakaryocytic leukemia (DS-AMKL) develops within a few years, sometimes preceded by a myelodysplastic phase. In 2002, Wechsler et al.[23] reported that DS-AMKL cells harbor acquired mutations in their *GATA1* gene. Since then, several groups have reproduced these findings and identified similar mutations

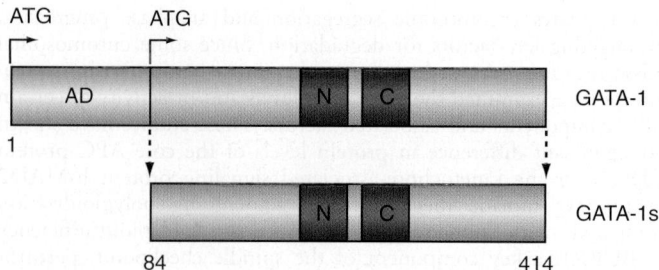

Fig. 28.10 GENERATION OF AN AMINO TERMINAL TRUNCATED ISOFORM OF GATA1 BY MUTATIONS ASSOCIATED WITH DS-TMD AND DS-AMKL. Schematic representation of full-length GATA1 is shown *(top)*; the truncated form (GATA1s) *(bottom)*. The amino terminal transcriptional activation domain, as defined by reporter assays in transiently transfected cells, is indicated *(AD)*. The amino *(N)* and carboxyl *(C)* zinc fingers are shown as *gray boxes*. In DS-TMD and DS-AMKL, mutations involving exon 2 of GATA1 (point mutations, deletions, insertions, and/or splice site mutations) lead to exclusive translation from a downstream in-frame methionine at codon 84, producing the amino terminal truncated GATA1 protein (GATA1s).

in DS-TMD cells. Although a wide spectrum of mutations have been found, including missense, deletion, insertion, and splice-site mutations, they all involve exon 2 (or rarely exon 3) and result in the same outcome: generation of an amino terminal truncated protein (loss of amino acids 1–83) because of translation initiation from a downstream ATG codon (Fig. 28.10). This removes a region that functions as a transcriptional activation domain in transient transfection reporter assays. The mutations are detectable in BM from DS-AMKL patients but disappear when patients enter remission, indicating a strong correlation between the mutated clone and the leukemic phenotype. Mutations involving exon 2 of *GATA1* are highly specific for DS-AMKL and DS-TMD, or AMKL with acquired trisomy 21. There is only one reported case of such a mutation in AMKL without trisomy 21, and no mutations have been detected in DS-acute lymphoblastic leukemia or a large number of healthy individuals.

Analysis of stored neonatal blood spots shows the coexistence of several different GATA1 mutations (all resulting in the generation of GATA1s) in patients who subsequently developed DS-AMKL, suggesting an oligoclonal expansion. In a few cases in which material was available, identical GATA1 mutations have been found in both the DS-TMD and DS-AMKL cells from the same patient. DS-AMKL cells often harbor additional genetic abnormalities, such as trisomy 8 or tetrasomy 21, not observed in DS-TMD cells. Acquisition of secondary loss-of-function mutations in member of the cohesin complex, and other epigenetic factors, is also common. Taken together, these findings support a clonal evolution model of DS-AMKL, with GATA1 mutations associated with an early initiating event.

Generation of knock-in mice that recapitulate the truncating GATA1 mutations show unexpected stage-specific effects on megakaryocytopoiesis. During fetal liver hematopoiesis, the mutant megakaryocytes markedly hyperproliferate, similar to what is observed for GATA1-deficient megakaryocytes. However, during adult-stage BM hematopoiesis, megakaryocytopoiesis and thrombocytopoiesis appear normal. This suggests that the fetal liver and BM cellular contexts interact differentially with the GATA1 truncated molecule. This may also explain the restriction of TMD to the neonatal period. A family has been described with members containing a germline *GATA1* gene splice site mutation (G332C) that results in exclusive production of the GATA1s protein product. Affected individuals exhibit a unique phenotype characterized by trilineage BM dysplasia, macrocytic anemia, and neutropenia. None of the family members has developed leukemia, suggesting that trisomy 21 plays a role in DS-TMD progression to DS-AMKL.

Of note, Calligaris et al.[23a] previously reported that GATA1s is produced naturally at low levels in erythroid cells. They proposed that this might serve a regulatory role during normal hematopoiesis by acting as a dominant negative molecule at specific times/environmental stimuli. Endogenous GATA1s has also been detected in normal mouse fetal liver megakaryocytes and adult human BM megakaryocytes. Thus it has been proposed that the ratio of GATA1 to GATA1s plays a role in developmental aspects of megakaryocytopoiesis and that acquired GATA1 mutations observed in DS-TMD and DS-AMKL, or germline mutations in the family described earlier, perturb hematopoiesis by altering this ratio.

E26 Transformation Specific (ETS) Family Transcription Factors

A common feature of megakaryocyte-specific genes is the presence of tandem binding sites for GATA and ETS family transcription factors in their promoters and enhancers. The ETS transcription factor family is composed of a diverse group of proteins that share a common ETS DNA-binding domain, which recognizes a GGAA core sequence. Over 30 different ETS factors have been identified, at least 10 of which (ELF1, ELF2, Fli-1, PU.1, TEL, GABPα, ETS1, ETS2, ELK4, ERG) are expressed in megakaryocytes. Functional studies have implicated several of these, including Fli-1, ETS1, ETV6 (TEL), ERG, and GABPα, in megakaryocytopoiesis.

Fli-1

The role of Fli-1 megakaryocytopoiesis is the best characterized of the ETS factors in terms of its functional role in megakaryocyte development. Fli-1[−/−] mice die during embryogenesis from hemorrhage, likely caused by both vascular defects and dysmegakaryocytopoiesis. Colony assays show an increased number of MkPs in Fli-1[−/−] embryos as compared with wild-type mice. However, the megakaryocytes from these colonies are small, contain a high nuclear/cytoplasmic ratio, and have hypolobulated nuclei, disorganized platelet demarcation membranes, and reduced number of α-granules. Expression of the late megakaryocyte marker gene *GPIX* is markedly reduced, whereas expression of the early genes, TPO receptor, and αIIb are normal or mildly reduced, consistent with a role of Fli-1 in late megakaryocyte maturation. Fli-1 is involved in the synergistic transcriptional activation of several megakaryocyte-specific genes by GATA1, FOG-1, and RUNX1. Different ETS factors act in a stage-specific manner during megakaryocytopoiesis, with GABPα predominantly regulating genes active during early stages of megakaryocytopoiesis and Fli-1 during later stages.

Fli-1 has been implicated in the lineage commitment of bipotent erythroid-MkP cells to the megakaryocyte pathway. Fli-1 expression is downregulated as bipotent cells commit to the erythroid lineage, and its overexpression in the bipotent human erythroleukemia cell line K562 enhances the expression of several megakaryocyte-specific genes and induces a megakaryocyte phenotype. In addition, functional cross-antagonism occurs between Fli-1 and the erythroid-specific transcription factor EKLF.

Paris-Trousseau syndrome (OMIM 188925) and Jacobsen syndrome (OMIM 147791) are overlapping contiguous gene-deletion disorders in humans involving the long arm of chromosome 11 (11q23). The constellation of findings in these syndromes includes severe congenital cardiac abnormalities, trigonocephaly, mental retardation, dysmorphogenesis of the hands and face, and macrothrombocytopenia. The etiology of the thrombocytopenia in these patients appears to be related to impaired platelet production, since platelet survival time is normal. Examination of BM reveals significant dysmegakaryocytopoiesis with an abundance of micromegakaryocytes and death of large numbers of megakaryocytes during terminal stages of maturation. Peripheral blood platelets contain giant α-granules, which are thought to arise from aberrant α-granule fusion during

prolonged residence in the BM. The minimal chromosome regions deleted in Paris-Trousseau and Jacobsen syndromes associated with thrombocytopenia includes the genes for the ETS factors *Fli-1* and *ETS-1*. Lentiviral expression of Fli-1 in CD34[+] cells from patients with Paris-Trousseau thrombocytopenia rescues megakaryocyte differentiation in vitro, providing evidence that it is deficiency of Fli-1 that is the cause of impaired thrombopoiesis in these patients. Of interest, Raslova et al.[23b] have shown that in normal individuals, expression of Fli-1 is mostly monoallelic in early megakaryocytic progenitors (CD41[+]/CD42[−] cells) but predominantly biallelic in later stages. They propose that the different populations of megakaryocytes seen in patients with Paris-Trousseau disorder arise from expression of the normal allele in the normally differentiating megakaryocytes, and the deleted allele (leading to complete loss of Fli-1 expression) in the dying population of megakaryocytes.

Germline heterozygous missense *Fli-1* gene mutations have recently been reported in patients with a familial platelet defect. Most of these mutations involve the DNA binding domain and abolish transcriptional activity. The small number of patients reported have presented with mild macrothrombocytopenia and a storage pool-type platelet defect.

ETS-Related Gene (ERG)

ERG is closely related to Fli-1. Mouse studies show that ERG and Fli-1 play compensatory roles in murine thrombopoiesis. The *ERG* gene is located on chromosome 21 in humans and has been suggested to play a role in DS-TMD and AMKL.

ETV6 (TEL)

Generation of a fusion protein between ETV6 and RUNX1 is the most frequent chromosome translocation in childhood pre-B cell acute lymphoblastic leukemia. Although ETV6 is required for the ontogeny of all definitive hematopoiesis, a conditional knock-out study of the *ETV6* gene in mice demonstrates its specific requirement for adult-stage megakaryocytopoiesis. Heterozygous germline ETV6 mutations have recently been described as a cause of autosomal dominant thrombocytopenia.[24] The mutations described to date involve either the DNA binding domain (and disrupt DNA interaction) or a common site in a linker region located between the DNA binding domain and the Pointed protein–protein interaction domain. Megakaryocytes from these patients are generally small and contain hypolobulated nuclei and underdeveloped cytoplasm. There is also variable red blood cell macrocytosis. Importantly, affected individuals have increased risk for the development of hematologic malignancies.

RUNX1

In 1999, Song et al. used positional cloning to identify the genetic cause of a rare dominant disorder characterized by thrombocytopenia, an aspirin-like functional platelet defect, and increased risk for developing acute myelogenous leukemia (FPD/AML; OMIM 601399).[25] They identified nonsense mutations, intragenic deletions, or missense mutations on one allele of the gene for RUNX1 (formerly called *AML-1* and *CBFA2*) that cosegregated with the disease in six separate pedigrees. These mutations all resulted in loss of function, indicating that haploinsufficiency of RUNX1 plays a causal role in this disorder. BM or peripheral blood from these patients were characterized by reduced megakaryocyte colony formation, indicating that RUNX1 dosage affects megakaryocytopoiesis.

RUNX1 is a member of an evolutionarily conserved family of transcription factors that share a conserved 128 amino acid domain in their amino half with homology to Drosophila *runt* gene. This region mediates binding to DNA (consensus [C/T]G[C/T]GGT), as well as to its heterodimeric binding partner CBF-β via protein-protein interactions. RUNX1 is the most frequently mutated transcription factors in human leukemia. In addition, acquired mutations in RUNX1 have been identified in significant number of patients with myelodysplastic syndrome, particularly those that progress to AML. Homozygous knockout of either RUNX1 or CBF-β in mice is embryonic-lethal because of a complete failure of definitive hematopoiesis. This is thought to arise from a defect in the ontogeny of HSCs in the AGM region. Conditional knockout of RUNX1 in adult hematopoiesis demonstrate a specific role of RUNX1 in megakaryocytopoiesis. BM deletion of RUNX1 in adult mice results in up to ≈80% reduction in peripheral blood platelet numbers, although no bleeding diathesis. BM megakaryocytes are small, lack lobulated nuclei, have poorly developed demarcation membranes, and reduced polyploidization. These findings are reminiscent of the abnormal "micromegakaryocytes" seen in humans with myelodysplastic syndromes and myelofibrosis. Paradoxically, there is an increase in in vitro megakaryocyte colony plating efficiency, suggesting an expansion of early MkPs. These effects are cell-autonomous. No defects are seen in the erythroid lineage. Reduced dosage of RUNX1's essential cofactor CBF-β also perturbs megakaryocytopoiesis in vivo. Taken together, these findings indicate a specific role of RUNX1/CBF-β in megakaryocyte terminal maturation.

NF-E2 p45

NF-E2 is a heterodimeric transcription factor composed of two basic region-leucine zipper (bZip) subunits: a hematopoietic-specific 45 kDa protein (p45) and a widely expressed 18 kDa subunit (p18). NF-E2 p45 is expressed in erythroid, megakaryocytic and mast cell lineages. In vitro studies implicated NF-E2 p45 as a critical factor for β-globin expression. Unexpectedly, NF-E2 p45$^{-/-}$ mice were found to have only mild perturbations of the erythroid lineage. However, these mice fail to produce platelets secondary to a maturational arrest in the megakaryocyte lineage, and succumb to hemorrhage in the neonatal period. Since the initial studies, NF-E2 p45 has been recognized as being a major regulator of terminal megakaryocyte maturation and platelet release. Notably, although NF-E2 p45$^{-/-}$ mice are severely thrombocytopenic, they have normal serum levels of TPO. In addition, megakaryocytes from these animals proliferate in vivo in response to TPO administration. These findings suggest that NF-E2 p45 regulates target genes independent of the action of TPO.

Several important target genes of NF-E2 p45 have been identified, including β-1 tubulin, 3β-hydroxysteroid dehydrogenase (3β-HSD), thromboxane synthase, caspase 12, and Rab27b. β-1 tubulin is a megakaryocyte-restricted isoform of β-tubulin that plays a key role in the marginal band structure of platelets and is essential for their discoid shape. Deficiency of β-1 tubulin leads to spherocytic platelets. Heterozygosity for a polymorphism (Q43P, because of the double nucleotide substitution AG>CC) in the human β1-tubulin gene is present in about 11% of individuals in a Caucasian Northern European population and correlates with a reduced risk for cardiovascular disease in humans. This may be caused by alterations in platelet structure and function. 3β-HSD catalyzes autocrine biosynthesis of estradiol within megakaryocytes and plays an important role in proplatelet formation.

p18 (also called mafK) is a member of a family of small maf proteins (mafF, mafG, mafK) related to the chicken v-maf oncoprotein. Knockout of mafK, and the related mafF, in mice has no discernable phenotypes, whereas deficiency of mafG leads to mild thrombocytopenia. Compound mafK::mafG null mice have profound thrombocytopenia, phenocopying NF-E2 p45 mice. This indicates functional redundancy of the small maf family members in megakaryocytopoiesis.

SCL (TAL1)

SCL (also known as TAL1) is a member of the basic helix-loop-helix member of transcription factors and is expressed predominantly in megakaryocytic and erythroid cells. Dysregulated expression of SCL because of chromosomal translocation is associated with certain cases of T-cell acute lymphoblastic leukemia. SCL forms obligate heterodimers with ubiquitously expressed E proteins (such as E12 and E47), which bind to E-box motifs (sequence CANNTG). It participates in multiprotein complexes that include E2A, GATA1, LMO2, LDB1, and the repressor ETO-2. SCL$^{-/-}$ mice die during embryogenesis as a result of failure of all hematopoiesis and defective vasculogenesis. However, conditional SCL knock-out models show a specific role for SCL in late stages of megakaryopoiesis and stress thrombopoiesis during adult hematopoiesis. SCL-null megakaryocytes have disorganized DMSs and a reduced number of platelet granules. SCL modulates thrombopoiesis, in part, by direct transcriptional activation of NF-E2 p45.

Gfi-1b

Gfi-1b (Gfi standing for "growth factor independent") is a member of a family of hematopoietic expressed zinc finger transcription factors that contain a unique amino terminal transcriptional repressor Snail/Gfi-1 (SNAG) domain. It represses target genes by recruitment of histone lysine methyltransferases. Knockout of Gfi-1b in mice results in embryonic lethality because of severe anemia. The fetal liver of mutant mice contains erythroid and megakaryocytic progenitors that are blocked in their maturation. Culture of these cells in the presence of TPO, in contrast to those from wild-type animals, generates only small colonies and the cells are acetylcholinesterase negative (a marker of maturing megakaryocytes in mice). They contain markedly reduced mRNA transcript levels of vWF, NF-E2 p45, c-Mpl, and GPIIb, compared with wild-type, suggesting a requirement for Gfi-1b in at least relatively early stages of megakaryocytopoiesis. Germline dominant negative Gfi1b gene mutations have recently been reported as a cause of familial gray platelet syndrome.[26] The patients have macrothrombocytopenia, platelet dysfunction, and red blood cell anisopoikilocytosis. Megakaryocytes from the patients are dysplastic-appearing with some having hypolobulated nuclei and others with multiple separated nuclei. All of the mutations described to date involve the carboxyl terminal zinc finger domain and result in truncated protein products.

HOX-Related Genes

Homeobox containing transcription factors (HOX factors) play central role in embryonic patterning and development. Several of these factors have specific functions in megakaryopoiesis. The best evidence is for MEIS1, a homeodomain protein belonging to the Transcription activator-like effector (TALE) subfamily. MEIS1 knock-out mice fail to produce megakaryocytes. Genome-wide chromatin occupancy studies show high enrichment for binding near megakaryocyte and platelet function-specific genes. Heterodimers of MEIS1 and the homeobox protein PBX1 have been shown to functionally regulate the PF4 gene in megakaryopoiesis.

Other HOX genes have also been implicated in megakaryopoiesis. Mutations in the HOXA11 gene cause a rare syndrome of congenital thrombocytopenia with radio-ulnar synostosis (CTRUS; OMIM #605432). The described mutations reduce DNA binding and lead to impaired in vitro megakaryocyte differentiation. There are also limited data suggesting a role for HOXA10 in murine megakaryopoiesis.

c-Myb

Carpinelli et al.[26a] performed an N-ethyl-N-Nitrosourea (ENU) mutagenesis screen in TPO receptor$^{-/-}$ mice to identify factors that might influence thrombopoiesis. They identified two independent loss-of-function alleles of the transcription factor c-Myb (substitution of valine for aspartic acid at residue 152 within the DNA binding domain and residue 384 within the leucine zipper domain). Both TPO receptor$^{-/-}$ and wild-type mice containing these mutations have supraphysiologic production of platelets as a result of excessive megakaryocytopoiesis, at the expense of erythroid and lymphocyte development. Megakaryocytes from these animals have a 200-fold increased sensitivity to GM-CSF, suggesting dysregulation of signaling pathways. Similar megakaryocytic hyperplasia and thrombocytosis occur in mice containing germline c-Myb mutations that disrupt binding the transcriptional coactivator p300. Thus c-Myb may play an important negative regulatory function in megakaryocytopoiesis and thrombocytopoiesis.

Megakaryocyte Enhancesome Complex

A number of biochemical and genome-wide chromatin occupancy studies have provided evidence for physical and functional interactions between a core set of megakaryocyte transcription factors that includes GATA1, GATA2, Fli-1, RUNX1, and SCL/TAL1.[27] This suggests that a specific "enhancesome complex" involving these factors drives megakaryocyte-specific gene expression. MEIS1, Gfi1b and NF-E2 p45 likely act independently of this complex.

MicroRNAs in Megakaryocytopoiesis

MicroRNAs (miRNAs) are a class of small (typically 19–25 nucleotide) noncoding RNAs that interact in a sequence-specific manner with mRNAs (typically in their 3′ untranslated region in mammals) and modulate gene expression through either enhanced mRNA decay or inhibiting translation. They play roles in development and differentiation by fine-tuning tissue-specific transcription factor expression. Each miRNA can have multiple target genes, and conversely, each mRNA can be subject to regulation by multiple miRNA species. In addition, the transcription of miRNAs themselves are mediated by RNA polymerase II and are subject to control by transcription factors. Therefore complex regulatory networks can exist between miRNAs and transcription factors. A number of miRNAs have been shown to influence thrombopoiesis.[28] miR-150 enhances megakaryocytopoiesis at the expense of erythropoiesis, suggesting a critical role in the cell fate decision of bipotent MEP cells. This is mediated, at least in part, via targeting the 3′-UTR of c-MYB mRNA transcripts. TPO signaling increases miR-150 levels. miR-155 inhibits megakaryocytopoiesis by targeting ETS1 and MEIS1 transcription factors. Other miRNAs have been implicated in controlling thrombopoiesis, but the evidence supporting a functional role is not as strong as for miR-150 and miR-155. miRNAs are also present in platelets. Further studies are needed to examine their potential role in platelet activation and function.

Relationship Between Megakaryocytes and HSCs

Megakaryocytes and HSCs share a striking number of similarities.[29] This includes common signaling pathways (TPO signaling), surface receptors (CD41, CD150, CXCR4, TPO receptor), and transcription factors (RUNX1, GATA2, TAL1, ETV6, and MEIS1). Recent work has also uncovered a close hierarchical developmental relationship between HSCs and megakaryocytes, where MkP cells can develop directly (or close to directly) from HSCs. Lastly, HSCs and megakaryocytes share a common niche at the BM vascular sinusoids, where they physically contact one another. One recent study also suggests that megakaryocytes are necessary for HSC function. The teleologic explanation for such a close relationship between HSCs and megakaryocytes remains to be elucidated.

Inherited Causes of Thrombocytopenia

Although the most common cause of thrombocytopenia is ITP, it is important to maintain a high index of clinical suspicion for inherited disorders of thrombocytopoiesis. This is a particular problem because ITP is essentially a diagnosis of exclusion, and many inherited disorders mimic the macrothrombocytopenia seen in ITP. Making the correct diagnosis early is paramount, since it may spare patients unnecessary treatment with corticosteroids, other immunosuppressants, and/or splenectomy. In addition, it may be important in guiding decisions about surveillance for myelodysplasia or leukemia, screening for additional associated clinical problems, and/or possible family planning. Obtaining a careful family history, and sometimes obtaining blood counts of first-degree relatives, is important in fully evaluating patients with chronic thrombocytopenia. Associated abnormalities may provide important clues to the presence of a nonimmune familial thrombocytopenia. For instance, associated erythroid abnormalities and/or an X-linked inheritance pattern (GATA1, FLNA, WASP mutations) (obligate female carriers may have dimorphic populations of platelets); leukocyte Döhle bodies, +/– nephritis, sensineural hearing loss, and early-onset cataracts (Myh9 mutations); family history of myelodysplasia or myeloid leukemia (RUNX1, ANKRD26, and ETV6 mutations); developmental delay, congenital cardiac anomalies, hand/face dysmorphogenesis (Paris-Trousseau/Jacobsen syndrome; Fli-1 [ETS-1] mutations); bleeding diathesis out of proportion to degree of thrombocytopenia (Bernard-Soulier syndrome). A superb review of inherited thrombocytopenias and an excellent diagnostic algorithm has been provided by Balduini et al.[30] Table 28.1 summarizes genes involved in normal thrombopoiesis that are known to be mutated in human platelet disorders.

| TABLE 28.1 | Genetic Causes of Human Thrombopoiesis Disorders |

Disease	Inheritance	Mutated Gene	Theme	Comments	Diagnosis
Thrombocytopenic *Large Platelets*					
MYH9-related disease	AD	*MYH9*	Cytoskeletal defect	Can include nephritis, sensorineural hearing loss, cataracts, Dohle bodies in granulocytes. Mild bleeding tendency.	Myh9 immunofluorescence; DNA sequencing
Paris-Trousseau; Jacobsen syndrome	AD	Large deletions at 11q23; likely *FLI1* or *ETS1* gene	Transcription factor	Cardiac and facial anomalies, ± developmental delay. Mks/platelets with giant alpha granules.	FISH
Bernard-Soulier syndrome	AR-AD	*GPIbα, GPIb*	Glycoprotein receptor for vWF	Giant platelets, bleeding diathesis in biallelic forms	Platelet aggregation (absent response to ristocetin); flow cytometry

Continued

| TABLE 28.1 | Genetic Causes of Human Thrombopoiesis Disorders—cont'd | | | | |

Disease	Inheritance	Mutated Gene	Theme	Comments	Diagnosis
Gray platelet syndrome	AD-AR XL	NBEAL2, GFI1b GATA1	Alpha granule defect	Giant "pale" platelets. Variable bleeding disorder. Mild red blood cell anisopoikilocytosis in some cases.	Platelet EM; DNA sequencing
Platelet-type vWD	AD	GPIba	Binds to vWF to easily	Platelet count decreases with stress	Ristocetin titration; vWF multimer analysis; vWF binding studies
Filamin-related thrombocytopenia	XL	FLNA	Cytoskeletal defect	Platelets small to large size	DNA sequencing
Tubulin-related thrombocytopenia	AD	TUBB1	Cytoskeletal defect	Giant platelets	DNA sequencing
GATA1-related disease	XL	GATA1	Transcription factor	Can also have anemia, β-thalassemia, and/or dyserythropoiesis	DNA sequencing
Thrombocytopenia associated with sitosterolemia	AR	ABCG5, ABCG8	Channel-opathy	Stomatocytes, possible anemia, tendon xanthomas, atherosclerosis	DNA sequencing
Normal-Size Platelets					
Thrombocytopenia with absent radii (TAR)	AR	RBM8A (1q21.1 del)	RNA binding protein	Bilateral radial aplasia ± other malformations. Thrombocytopenia often resolves by 12–24 mo.	X-ray; FISH (for microdeletion)
CAMT	AR	MPL	Cytokine receptor	Reduced Mks; can evolve into full BM failure	DNA sequencing; TPO levels
Familial platelet disorder with propensity to develop AML (FPD/AML)	AD	RUNX1 ETV6	Transcription factor	Associated platelet dysfunction; ~35% risk of developing MDS/leukemia. Red blood cell macrocytosis.	DNA sequencing
ANKRD26-related thrombocytopenia (THC2)	AD	ANRKD26	Cytoskeletal, signaling defect?	Associated platelet dysfunction; increased risk of leukemia	DNA sequencing
CTRUS	AD	HOXA11, MECOM (EVI1)	Transcription factor	Reduced Mks; cannot pronate distal arms; risk for BM failure and leukemia?	X-ray; DNA sequencing
CYCS-related thrombocytopenia	AD	CYCS	Cytochrome c		DNA sequencing
Small Platelets					
Wiskott-Aldrich syndrome	XL	WASP	Cytoskeletal defect	Severe immunodeficiency; eczema; platelet dysfunction	WASP western blot; DNA sequencing
X-linked thrombocytopenia	XL	WASP	Cytoskeletal defect	No or mild immunodeficiency; platelet dysfunction	WASP western blot; DNA sequencing
Nonthrombocytopenic Normal-Size Platelets					
Glanzmann thrombocythemia	AR	ITGA2B ITGB3	Integrin deficiency	Bleeding tendency	Platelet aggregation (absent response to all agonists except ristocetin); flow cytometry
Hermansky-Pudlak syndrome	AR	HPS1-8	Granule defect	Mild to moderate bleeding tendency. Oculocutaneous albinism, rotary nystagmus, pulmonary fibrosis. Higher frequency in Puerto Rico	Platelet EM; DNA sequencing
Chediak-Higashi syndrome	Autosomal	LYST	Granule defect	Bleeding tendency, immune dysfunction, partial albinism; can develop lymphoproliferative disorder	Platelet EM; DNA sequencing; flow cytometry?

AD, Autosomal dominant; *AR*, autosomal recessive; *BM*, bone marrow; *CAMT*, congenital amegakaryocytic thrombocytopenia; *CTRUS*, congenital thrombocytopenia with radio-ulnar synostosis; *EM*, electron microscopy; *FISH*, fluorescence in situ hybridization; *MDS*, myelodysplastic syndrome; *Mks*, megakaryocytes; *vWD*, von Willebrand disease, *vWF*, von Willebrand factor; *XL*, X-linked.

FUTURE DIRECTIONS

Although the molecular details regarding the regulation and generation of platelets remain to be fully elucidated, considerable progress has been made over the past few decades. This has been significantly facilitated by the isolation of TPO and its receptor. Important models of thrombocytopoiesis have now been tested rigorously in vivo, yielding new insights into the final stages of platelet formation and shedding. These studies highlight the efficient mechanisms that have developed to satisfy the demands for dynamic and high-output platelet production. Several important transcription factors have been identified that regulate different stages of megakaryocytopoiesis, and mutations in these, and other genes, have been linked to human disorders of thrombocytopoiesis. The role of miRNAs in controlling thrombopoiesis is beginning to be appreciated. Although mouse models have played important roles in the analysis of these genes, it is becoming clear that they do not always faithfully recapitulate human disease. In addition, several studies have documented important differences between rodent and human platelets, including differences in size, circulating numbers, and DMS ultrastructural features. Thus some caution must be exercised when extrapolating results of mouse studies to human thrombocytopoiesis. The advent of megakaryocyte in vitro differentiation systems using human CD34$^+$ cells, embryonic stem cells, and induced pluripotent cells are providing important tools for additional studies geared toward understanding and treating human disorders of megakaryocytopoiesis and thrombocytopoiesis.

REFERENCES

1. Wright J: The origin and nature of blood platelets. *Boston Med Surg J* 23:1906.
2. King SM, Reed GL: Development of platelet secretory granules. *Sem Cell Dev Biol* 13:293, 2002.
3. Italiano JE, Jr, Battinelli EM: Selective sorting of alpha-granule proteins. *J Thromb Haemost* 7(Suppl 1):173, 2009.
4. Liu ZJ, Sola-Visner M: Neonatal and adult megakaryopoiesis. *Curr Opin Hematol* 18:330, 2011.
4a. Becker RP, De Bruyn PP: The transmural passage of blood cells into myeloid sinusoids and the entry of platelets into the sinusoidal circulation; a scanning electron microscopic investigation. *Am J Anat* 145:183–205, 1976.
5. Italiano JE, Jr, Lecine P, Shivdasani RA, et al: Blood platelets are assembled principally at the ends of proplatelet processes produced by differentiated megakaryocytes. *J Cell Biol* 147:1299, 1999.
6. Richardson JL, Shivdasani RA, Boers C, et al: Mechanisms of organelle transport and capture along proplatelets during platelet production. *Blood* 106:4066, 2005.
7. Schulze H, Korpal M, Hurov J, et al: Characterization of the megakaryocyte demarcation membrane system and its role in thrombopoiesis. *Blood* 107:3868, 2006.
8. Chang Y, Aurade F, Larbret F, et al: Proplatelet formation is regulated by the Rho/ROCK pathway. *Blood* 109:4229, 2007.
9. Avecilla ST, Hattori K, Heissig B, et al: Chemokine-mediated interaction of hematopoietic progenitors with the bone marrow vascular niche is required for thrombopoiesis. *Nat Med* 10:64, 2004.
10. Junt T, Schulze H, Chen Z, et al: Dynamic visualization of thrombopoiesis within bone marrow. *Science* 317:2007, 1767.
11. Harker LA, Finch CA: Thrombokinetics in man. *J Clin Invest* 48:963, 1969.
11a. Cserhati I, Kelemen E: Acute prolonged thrombocytosis in mice induced by thrombocythaemic sera: a possible human thrombopoietin: a preliminary communication. *Acta Med Acad Sci Hung* 11:473–475, 1958.
12. Kaushansky K: The molecular mechanisms that control thrombopoiesis. *J Clin Invest* 115:3339, 2005.
13. Gurney AL, Carver-Moore K, de Sauvage FJ, et al: Thrombocytopenia in c-mpl-deficient mice. *Science* 265:1445, 1994.
14. Bunting S, Widmer R, Lipari T, et al: Normal platelets and megakaryocytes are produced in vivo in the absence of thrombopoietin. *Blood* 90:3423, 1997.
15. Bersenev A, Wu C, Balcerek J, et al: Lnk constrains myeloproliferative diseases in mice. *J Clin Invest* 120:2058, 2010.
16. Kimura S, Roberts AW, Metcalf D, et al: Hematopoietic stem cell deficiencies in mice lacking c-Mpl, the receptor for thrombopoietin. *Proc Natl Acad Sci USA* 95:1195, 1998.
17. Nangalia J, Massie CE, Baxter EJ, et al: Somatic CALR mutations in myeloproliferative neoplasms with nonmutated JAK2. *N Engl J Med* 369:2391, 2013.
18. Grozovsky R, Begonja AJ, Liu K, et al: The Ashwell-Morell receptor regulates hepatic thrombopoietin production via JAK2-STAT3 signaling. *Nat Med* 21:47, 2015.
19. Olnes MJ, Scheinberg P, Calvo KR, et al: Eltrombopag and improved hematopoiesis in refractory aplastic anemia. *N Engl J Med* 367:11, 2012.
20. Ravid K, Lu J, Zimmet JM, et al: Roads to polyploidy: the megakaryocyte example. *J Cell Physiol* 190:7, 2002.
21. Lordier L, Jalil A, Aurade F, et al: Megakaryocyte endomitosis is a failure of late cytokinesis related to defects in the contractile ring and Rho/Rock signaling. *Blood* 112:3164, 2008.
22. Lordier L, Bluteau D, Jalil A, et al: RUNX1-induced silencing of non-muscle myosin heavy chain IIB contributes to megakaryocyte polyploidization. *Nat Comm* 3:717, 2012.
22a. Nichols KE, Crispino JD, Poncz M, et al: Familial dyserythropoietic anaemia and thrombocytopenia due to an inherited mutation in GATA1. *Nat Genet* 24:266–270, 2000.
23. Wechsler J, Greene M, McDevitt MA, et al: Acquired mutations in GATA1 in the megakaryoblastic leukemia of Down syndrome. *Nat Genet* 32:148–152, 2002.
23a. Calligaris R, Bottardi S, Cogoi S, et al: Alternative translation initiation site usage results in two functionally distinct forms of the GATA-1 transcription factor. *Proc Natl Acad Sci USA* 92:11598–11602, 1995.
23b. Raslova H, Komura E, Le Couedic JP, et al: FLI1 monoallelic expression combined with its hemizygous loss underlies Paris-Trousseau/Jacobsen thrombopenia. *J Clin Invest* 114:77–84, 2004.
24. Zhang MY, Churpek JE, Keel SB, et al: Germline ETV6 mutations in familial thrombocytopenia and hematologic malignancy. *Nat Genet* 47:180, 2015.
25. Song WJ, Sullivan MG, Legare RD, et al: Haploinsufficiency of CBFA2 causes familial thrombocytopenia with propensity to develop acute myelogenous leukaemia. *Nat Genet* 23:166, 1999.
26. Monteferrario D, Bolar NA, Marneth AE, et al: A dominant-negative GFI1B mutation in the gray platelet syndrome. *N Engl J Med* 370:245, 2014.
26a. Carpinelli MR, Hilton DJ, Metcalf D, et al: Suppressor screen in Mpl-/- mice: c-Myb mutation causes supraphysiological production of platelets in the absence of thrombopoietin signaling. *Proc Natl Acad Sci USA* 101:6553–6558, 2004.
27. Tijssen MR, Cvejic A, Joshi A, et al: Genome-wide analysis of simultaneous GATA1/2, RUNX1, FLI1, and SCL binding in megakaryocytes identifies hematopoietic regulators. *Dev Cell* 20:597, 2011.
28. Edelstein LC, McKenzie SE, Shaw C, et al: MicroRNAs in platelet production and activation. *J Thromb Haemost* 11(Suppl 1):340, 2013.
29. Huang H, Cantor AB: Common features of megakaryocytes and hematopoietic stem cells: what's the connection? *J Cell Biochem* 107:857, 2009.
30. Balduini CL, Pecci A, Noris P: Diagnosis and management of inherited thrombocytopenias. *Semin Thromb Hemost* 39:161, 2013.

CHAPTER 29

INHERITED BONE MARROW FAILURE SYNDROMES

Yigal Dror

INTRODUCTION

Inherited bone marrow (BM) failure is defined herein as decreased production of one or more of the major hematopoietic lineages caused by germline mutations that were derived from the parents or occurred de novo (Table 29.1). Although outdated, the term "constitutional" has been used interchangeably with "inherited" and similarly implies that a genetic abnormality causes the BM dysfunction. The designation "congenital" has a looser connotation and refers to conditions that manifest early in life, often at birth, but does not imply a particular causation. Therefore "congenital BM failure" is not necessarily inherited and may be caused by a de novo gene mutation during early embryogenesis or by acquired factors such as viruses, drugs, or environmental toxins.

Hematopoiesis is an orderly but complex interplay of stem and progenitor cells, growth factors, BM stromal elements, and positive and negative cellular and humoral regulators. Thus BM failure can potentially occur at several critical points in the hematopoietic lineage pathways. With regard to inherited BM failure syndromes (IBMFSs), germline mutations interfere with orderly hematopoiesis and cause the BM failure. The discovery of specific, high-penetrance mutant alleles associated with discrete IBMFSs provides evidence for this. Many of these alleles are of genes that directly affect physiologic cell survival and function in pathways that are essential for normal hematopoiesis (e.g., DNA repair, telomere maintenance, ribosome biogenesis, microtubule stabilization, chemotaxis, signaling from hematopoietic growth factors, signal transduction related to hematopoietic cell differentiation, and granulocytic enzymes). Modifying genes, epigenetic processes, acquired factors, and chance effects may also be operative and interact with the mutant genes to produce overt disease with varying clinical expression. Hence the disorders listed in Table 29.1 are transmitted in a Mendelian pattern determined primarily by mutant genes with inheritance patterns of autosomal dominant, autosomal recessive, or X-linked types. Newly discovered IBMFSs may follow similar inheritance patterns or be multifactorial in origin caused by an interaction of multiple genes and a variety of exogenous or environmental determinants.

The incidence of the IBMFSs can be approximated from experience at large centers. Data from Children's Hospital Boston show that the IBMFSs comprise about 30% of cases of pediatric BM failure disorders, with Fanconi anemia (FA) cases leading the list. Data from the Canadian Inherited Marrow Failure Registry (CIMFR) suggest an incidence of about 65 cases diagnosed per million live births per year. Importantly, none of these syndromes is restricted to the pediatric age group. Patients with IBMFSs may be detected for the first time in adulthood. Reported cases include patients with FA, dyskeratosis congenita (DC), Diamond-Blackfan anemia (DBA), and Kostmann/severe congenital neutropenia (K/SCN) among others, whose condition first became evident when they reached adulthood.

INHERITED BONE MARROW FAILURE SYNDROME WITH PANCYTOPENIA

Fanconi Anemia

Background

FA is inherited in an autosomal recessive manner in 98% of cases. In about 2% of cases, it is transmitted in an X-linked recessive mode caused by a mutant *FA type B* gene.

Although the original report of FA in 1927 by Dr. Guido Fanconi described pancytopenia combined with physical anomalies in three brothers, a published summary in 2010 of more than 2000 FA cases has underscored the clinical variability of the condition. FA is a *genomic instability disorder* characterized by chromosomal fragility and breakage, a defect in DNA repair, progressive BM cell underproduction, peripheral blood cytopenias, developmental anomalies, and a strong propensity for hematologic and solid tumor cancers.

Patients with FA may present with either physical anomalies but normal hematology, or normal physical features but abnormal hematology, normal physical features *and* normal hematology, or physical anomalies and abnormal hematology (Fig. 29.1). There can also be sibling heterogeneity in presentation with discordance in clinical and hematologic findings, even in affected monozygotic twins. Using published information, the median age at diagnosis of FA is about 6.5 years with a reported range from birth to 49 years.

Epidemiology

The overall prevalence of FA is 1 to 5 cases per million with a carrier frequency of 1 in 200 to 300 in most populations. Data from the CIMFR showed a prevalence of 11.4 cases per million live births per year. It occurs in all racial and ethnic groups. Spanish Gypsies have the world's highest prevalence of FA with a carrier frequency of 1 in 64 to 1 in 70 for a common founder mutation. A founder effect has also been demonstrated in Afrikaners in South Africa in whom one specific mutation is common (frequency, 1 in 83), as well as in Ashkenazi Jews (1 in 89), Moroccan Jews, Tunisians, sub-Saharan African blacks, Indians, Israeli Arabs, Brazilians, and Japanese.

Genetics

Patients with FA show abnormal chromosome fragility that is readily seen in metaphase preparations of peripheral blood lymphocytes cultured with phytohemagglutinin (PHA) and enhanced by adding a DNA interstrand cross-linking agent, either mitomycin C (MMC) or diepoxybutane (DEB) (see Abnormal Chromosome Fragility section later). This feature was used to discover the first FA genes by complementation. A breakthrough in the search for FA genes evolved from the important observation that fusion of normal cells with FA cells (i.e., cell hybridization) resulted in correction of MMC hypersensitivity of the FA cells in a growth inhibition assay. Thus the cell hybridization corrected the abnormal FA chromosome fragility, a process known as *complementation*. It was further demonstrated that cell hybridization in several unrelated patients with FA could also produce the corrective effect on chromosomal fragility by complementation, which led directly to subtyping of patients into discrete complementation groups. A second method for complementation testing, which is currently used more often for research and clinical purposes, is retroviral transduction. The cDNA of each wild-type FA gene can be transfected into T cells from a newly diagnosed patient using retroviral vectors. If a specific wild-type FA gene corrects (complements) the abnormal chromosome breakage in the patient's T cells in culture on exposure to DEB, the mutant gene is identified. So far, 18 genetic groups (termed types A, B, C, D1, D2, E, F, G, I, J, L, M, N, O, P, Q, R, S) have been proposed, most of them on the

TABLE 29.1 Inherited Bone Marrow Failure Syndromes: Inheritance and Mutated Genes

Disorder	Inheritance	Gene
Fanconi anemia	AR	FANCA, FANCC, FANCD1/BRCA2, FANCD2, FANCE, FANCF, FANCG/XRCC9, FANCI, FANCJ/BRIP1, FANCL/PHF9, FANCM, FANCN/PALB2, FANCO/RAD51C, FANCP/SLX4, FANCQ/ERCC4, FANCR/XRCC2, FANCS/BRCA1
	XLR	FANCB
	AR	ERCC1/XPF (FA/XP/Cockayne)
Shwachman-Diamond syndrome	AR	SBDS
Dyskeratosis congenita	XLR	DKC1
	AD	TINF2, TERC, TERT
	AR	RTEL1, NOP10, NHP2, TCAB1, CTC1, TPP1
Congenital amegakaryocytic thrombocytopenia	AR	MPL
Lig4-associated aplastic anemia	AR	LIG4
Other inherited aplastic anemia	AR	ERCC6L2
Other inherited aplastic anemia	AR/AD	THPO
Reticular dysgenesis	AR	AK2
Cartilage-hair hypoplasia	AR	RMRP
Pearson syndrome	Maternal	mDNA
Familial thrombocytopenia with predisposition to AML	AD	CBFA2/ RUNX1
	AD	ETV6
Familial aplasia and myelodysplasia	AD	SRP72
Familial myelodysplastic syndrome (MonoMac syndrome, Emberger syndrome)	AD	GATA2
Seckel syndrome	AR	ATR/SCKL1, RBBP8/SCKL2, CENPJ/SCKL4, CEP152/SCKL5, CEP63/SCKL6, ATRIP/SCKL8
Schimke immunoosseous dysplasia	AR	SMARCL1
Rothmud-Thomson syndrome	AR	RECQL4
Li-Fraumeni syndrome	AD	TP53
Dubowitz syndrome	AR	NSUN2
Noonan syndrome	AD	PTPN11, SOS1, KRAS, NRAS, RAF1, BRAF, SHOC2, MEK1, CBL, RASA2, RIT1, MAP2K1, SOS2, LZTR1
Diamond-Blackfan anemia	AD	RPS7, RPS10, RPS17, RPS19, RPS24, RPS26, RPS27, RPS28, RPS29, RPL5, RPL11, RPL26, RPL27, RPL31, RPL35a
	XL	GATA1
Inherited sideroblastic anemia	XL	ALAS2
	XL	ABCB7
	AR	SLC19A2, GLRX5, PUS1, SLC25A38, YARS2, TRNT1
	Maternal	MT-ATP6
Congenital dyserythropoietic anemia type I	AR	CDAN1, C15ORF41
Congenital dyserythropoietic anemia type II	AR	SEC23B
Congenital dyserythropoietic anemia type III	AD	KIF23
Congenital dyserythropoietic anemia—unclassified	AR	KLF1
Kostmann/Severe congenital neutropenia	AD	ELA2, GFI1, JAGN1
	AR	HAX1, G6PC3, VPS45, TCIRG1
	XLR	WASP
Cyclic neutropenia	AD	ELA2
WHIM syndrome	AD	CXCR4
Glycogen storage diseases Ib	AR	G6PT/SLC37A4
Barth syndrome	XL	TAZ
Poikiloderma with neutropenia	AR	C16orf57
Neutropenia, immune deficiency and skeletal dysplasia and glycosylating defect	AR	PGM3
Cohen syndrome	AR	COH1/VPS13B
Dominant intermediate Charcot-Marie-Tooth	AD	DNM2

Continued

TABLE 29.1	Inherited Bone Marrow Failure Syndromes: Inheritance and Mutated Genes—cont'd	
Disorder	**Inheritance**	**Gene**
Thrombocytopenia absent radii syndrome	AR	*RBM8A*
Thrombocytopenia with radioulnar synostosis	AD	*HOXA11*
Familial autosomal dominant nonsyndromic thrombocytopenia	AD	*MASTL, ANKRD26, ACBD5, CYCS*
Familial platelet disorder with AML	AD	*CDC25C*
Thrombocytopenia with dyserythropoiesis	XL	*GATA1*
X-linked thrombocytopenia	XL	*WASP*
Mediterranean platelet disorder	AD	*GP1BA*
Familial thrombocytopenia	AD	*GFI1B*
Familial thrombocytopenia	AR	*FYB, SBF2*
Gray platelet syndrome	AR	*NBEAL2*
Epstein/Fechtner/Sebastian/May-Hegglin/Alport syndrome	AD	*MYH9*
Familial macrothrombocytopenia	AR	*FLNA, ABCG5, ABCG8, ACTN1, MYSM1, PRKACG*
Familial macrothrombocytopenia	AD	*TUBB1, ITGA2/ITGB3*
Stormorken syndrome (thrombocytopenia with anemia)	AD	*STIM1*

AD, Autosomal dominant; AR, autosomal recessive; IBMFSs, inherited bone marrow failure syndromes; UK, unknown; WHIM, warts, hypogammaglobulinemia, infections, and myelokathexis; X-L, X-linked recessive.
Modified from Dror Y: Inherited bone marrow failure syndromes: Genetic complexity of monogenic disorders. In *Genetic disorders*. InTech Open Access Publisher. Available at http://www.intechweb.org.

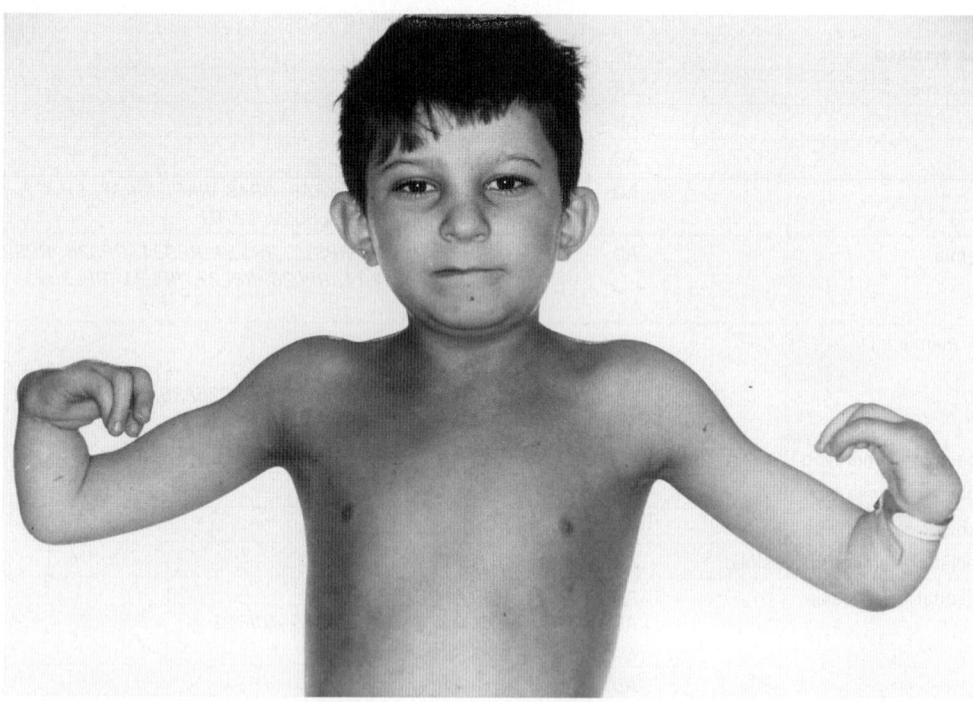

Fig. 29.1 CLASSIC PHENOTYPE OF FANCONI ANEMIA. The patient has pigmentary changes around the neck, shoulders, and trunk; short stature; absent radii and absent thumbs bilaterally; microcephaly; and low-set ears.

basis of somatic cell hybridization or retroviral transduction experiments, while others by targeted gene testing or exome sequencing.

The identification of complementation groups facilitated the cloning of the corresponding FA or *FANC* genes (see Table 29.1). The first gene, *FANCC* on chromosome 9q22.3, was discovered in 1992 in Toronto, and then the other genes, corresponding to each of the other complementation groups, were subsequently cloned:

FANCA, FANCB, FANCC, FANCD1/BRCA2, FANCD2, FANCE, FANCF, FANCG, FANCI, FANCJ/BACH1/BRIP1, FANCL, FANCM, FANCN/PALB2, FANCO/RAD51C, FANCP/SLX4, FANCQ/ECCR4, FANCR/EXCC2, and *FANCS/BRCA1.*

Of patients tested, up to 70% have mutant *FANCA,* 14% *FANCC,* 10% *FANCG,* 3% *FANCD1,* 3% *FANCD2,* 3% *FANCE,* and 2% or less for the others. Until recently, the most commonly used genetic investigation algorithms included FA complementation grouping to determine the genetic group, followed by targeted gene analysis (by Sanger sequencing and multiplex ligation-dependent probe amplification).

Genotype–Phenotype Correlations

The clinical severity of FA is only partly determined by the specific *FANC* gene involved and by the type of mutation. Patients with **FANCA** who are homozygous for null mutations and produce no protein tend to have an earlier onset of anemia and a higher propensity to leukemic transformation compared with patients with hypomorphic *FANCA* who produce protein, albeit abnormal. Compared with other **FANCC** mutations, *FANCC* IVS4+4A>T, commonly found in Ashkenazi Jews, is particularly severe and is linked with early-onset anemia, early BM failure, and severe physical anomalies, including some cases with physical features of VACTERL-H syndrome (a well-known malformation association, including vertebral, anal, tracheoesophageal, renal, and limb abnormalities). Of genetic-ethnic interest, the identical IVS4+4A>T mutation in Japanese patients with FA manifests with a *milder* phenotype than in Ashkenazi Jews. **FANCD1/BRCA2** and **FANCN/PALB2** mutations are both associated with a significant predisposition to develop solid tumors, acute myeloid leukemia (AML), and with a severe physical anomaly phenotype. The VACTERL-H cluster of anomalies is closely linked with biallelic mutations of *FANCD1/BRCA2* and *FANCB*. Null mutations of **FANCG** correlate with very severe manifestations compared with most other *FANC* mutations and correlate with early-onset anemia and BM failure, a higher incidence of AML, and severe physical anomalies. **FANCD2** and **FANCI** mutations also correlate with severe anomalies, and *FANCI* is associated with early-onset anemia.

Murine Models

Multiple FA mouse models have been generated in which targeted disruption of genes like *Fanca*, *Fancc*, *Fancd1*, *Fancd2*, *Fancg*, and *Fancn*. Knock-out mouse models largely do not recapitulate the hypocellularity and cytopenia that characterizes FA, with few exceptions (e.g., *Slx*$^{-/-}$ or combined *Fancc*$^{-/-}$/*Fancg*$^{-/-}$). However, these models provide insight into the various functions of the genes and the role of individual FA mutations. Consistent findings in some or all of the mice include impaired proliferation of BM hematopoietic progenitors, hypogonadism, impaired fertility, growth retardation, microphthalmia, development of cancers, hypersensitivity of BM progenitor cells to administered MMC, as well as to interferon-γ (INF-γ) or tumor necrosis factor-α (TNF-α) in vitro and in vivo. The phenotype of these mutant mice shows abnormal G_2/M progression of the cell cycle similar to patients with FA. Interestingly, double knockout of several *Fanc* genes together with genes that play a role in balancing oxidative stress and other genotoxic agents (e.g., Fancd2$^{-/-}$/Foxo3a, Fancc$^{-/-}$/Sod1$^{-/-}$, Fancd2$^{-/-}$/Aldh2$^{-/-}$) leads to a phenotype that is closer to the human FA disease. For example, *Fancc*$^{-/-}$/*Sod1*$^{-/-}$ mice develop hypocellular BM; *Fancd2*$^{-/-}$/*Foxo3a*$^{-/-}$ mice feature an initial expansion followed by a progressive decline of BM stem and progenitor cells, and *Fancd2*$^{-/-}$/*Aldh2*$^{-/-}$ develop low progenitors and leukemia.

Functions of FANC Proteins

DNA damage repair. Cells and cell lines from patients with FA are phenotypically similar regardless of the complementation group that they represent. A hypothesis was therefore formulated and subsequently substantiated that the various wild-type FANC proteins function in a common response pathway to repair DNA damage incurred during DNA replication.

There are three general steps in the FA DNA damage response pathway: (1) **Core complex**. Eight wild-type FANC proteins (FANCA, FANCB, FANCC, FANCE, FANCF, FANCG, FANCL, and FANCM) and four additional proteins (FAAP16, FAAP 20, FAAP24, and FAAP100) form a single large nuclear protein *core complex* as the first step. The *core complex* functions as a ubiquitin ligase of which FANCL is the catalytic subunit. (2) **ID2 complex**.

The activated *core complex* results in conversion of two downstream protein targets, FANCI and FANCD2 (called the *ID2 complex*), from unubiquitinated isoforms to monoubiquitinated isoforms. Monoubiquitination does not occur if the *core complex* upstream of the *ID2 complex* is not intact, and therefore FA cells from patients with upstream mutations do not show the monoubiquitinated FANCI/FANCD2. (3) **Downstream effector complexes**. In normal cells after monoubiquitination of the *ID2 complex,* the wild-type *core complex* translocates the monoubiquitinated *ID2 complex* to chromatin and localizes the *ID2 complex* to nuclear foci, where it probably forms a binding interface for single- and double-stranded DNA and downstream effector complexes with additional FANC proteins (FANCD1/BRCA2, FANCJ/BACH1/BRIP1, FANCN/PALB2, FANCO/Rad51C, FANCP/SLX4, FANCS/BRCA1) and other non-FA DNA repair proteins. There are three main DNA repair processes that the FA genes cooperate with: (1) excision repair that excises one DNA strand flanking the interstrand cross-link (via interaction between SLX4 and MUS81, SLX1, and others), (2) translesion synthesis that extend the uncut strand (via recruitment of translesion polymerase), (3) homologous recombination that is initiated after repair of the interstrand cross-link remnant possibly by ERCC4 and nucleotide excision repair protein, and involves interactions between FANCJ, FANCN, FANCO, FANCS/BRCA1, and RAD51. Other DNA-repair proteins such as MRE11-RAD50-NBS1, replication protein A, PCNA, and BLM are also involved in the later stages of the DNA repair response.

Cell Survival and Balancing Oxidative Stress. There are important protein–protein interactions between FA proteins and non-FA "binding partners" for cell survival. FANCC and FANCD2 form complexes with members of the signal transducer and activator of transcription (STAT) family of transcription factors in cytokine-mediated biologic responses. Secondly, heat shock proteins provide several cell survival functions, and FANCC protein specifically facilitates the antiapoptotic role of Hsp 70. FANCC also interacts with cdc2, PKR, and p53, suggesting that FANCC has other roles that are independent of DNA damage recognition and repair. GSTP1 is an enzyme that detoxifies byproducts of redox stress and xenobiotics and FANCC protein enhances GSTP1 activity in cells exposed to apoptosis inducers.

Previous studies suggested a role of oxidative stress in the evolution of BM failure and leukemia in FA. Reactive oxygen species (ROS) were shown to be elevated in FA cells, and high oxidative stress caused increased DNA damage, increased hematopoietic stem cell (HSC) senescence, and a decreased HSC pool, thereby leading to BM failure. Further, in vivo and in vitro studies demonstrated the ability of the antioxidant *N*-acetylcysteine to reduce DNA damage, reduce HSC senescence, and improve HSC reconstitution ability. Therefore it is possible that patients with FA are particularly sensitive to ROS-induced DNA damage because of impaired DNA repair mechanisms. This increased sensitivity may be caused, at least in part, by impaired detoxification of ROS and naturally produced aldehydes.

In the skin fibroblasts of patients with FA, *N*-acetylcysteine was able to reduce ROS levels and apoptosis as measured by activation of caspase-3 and PARP cleavage. In fancc$^{-/-}$ mice, *N*-acetylcysteine rescues hematopoietic colony formation that is impaired by spontaneous secretion of TNF-α. It also reduces TNF-α-mediated hematopoietic colony formation and HSC senescence and HSC reconstitution potential. Using a fancd2$^{-/-}$ mouse model, treatment with the antioxidant drug, resveratrol, has also been shown to preserve HSC quiescence, partially correct the abnormal cell cycle status and significantly improve the spleen colony-forming capacity of BM cells. Importantly, treatment of FA mice with *N*-acetylcysteine has been shown to reduce the accumulation of cytogenetic abnormalities (that are commonly seen in patients with FA who transform to MDS/AML). In one study the antioxidant, tempol, delayed cancer in tumor-prone fancd2$^{-/-}$/Trp53$^{+/-}$ mice. However, in another study neither *N*-acetylcysteine nor the antioxidant resveratrol had this property.

Pathophysiology

Wild-type FA proteins are part of a cluster of survival signaling molecules that protect against genotoxic insult and suppress apoptosis signaling. With inactivation of any of the known FA genes, the prosurvival benefit is lost. This underlies the phenotype of clinical FA but does not explain or unify the relationship among congenital anomalies, BM failure, the predisposition to cancer, and chromosome fragility.

Two theories of the pathophysiology of FA relate to either (1) a heightened sensitivity to oxygen, resulting in cell damage; or (2) defective DNA repair. The oxygen sensitivity phenotype of FA cells is characterized by overproduction of oxygen radicals, a deficient oxygen radical defense, a deficiency in superoxide dismutase, and poor cell growth at ambient oxygen, all producing shortened cell survival. A cardinal phenotype of FA cells is an abnormality in cell cycle distribution with an increased number of cells with 4N DNA content arising from a delay in the G_2/M or late S phase of the cell cycle. The strongest evidence supporting an oxygen metabolism deficiency in FA is a *reduction* of FA cells with 4N DNA content when grown at *low* oxygen levels and the unexpected appearance of 4N DNA content when normal cells are grown at *high* oxygen levels. Of note, some wild-type FA proteins play a role in redox-related functions. FANCC associates with NADPH (nicotinamide adenine dinucleotide phosphate), cytochrome P-450 reductase, and glutathione *S*-transferase, proteins with redox functions. FANCA and FANCG are redox-sensitive proteins that multimerize after H_2O_2 treatment, prompting the notion that the FA pathway may function in oxidative stress management.

The best evidence supporting the theory that the primary defect is in DNA repair relates to the critical role of wild-type FANC proteins in the DNA damage response pathway. Whereas clastogenic bifunctional cross-linker agents such as MMC and DEB induce chromosomal breakage in FA cells, monofunctional chemical agents do not, indicating that FA cells cannot repair interstrand cross-links. There were also experiments in the 1980s in which the frequency of mutations induced by 8-methoxypsoralen plus near-ultraviolet radiation at the *HPRT* locus was lower in FA cells than in control participants. These results indicated that FA cells cannot repair cross-links through the normal pathway involving mismatch repair, recombinational repair after bypass of the lesion, or both. Additional evidence for defective DNA repair in FA cells includes an accumulation of DNA adducts, a failure to arrest DNA synthesis in response to DNA damage, increased homologous recombination, defective nonhomologous end joining, abnormal induction of p53, and increased apoptosis.

The two theories for the pathophysiology of FA can be reconciled theoretically. It is possible that loss of any FA protein causes a transient increase of oxidative damage to which the repair machinery is particularly sensitive.

Hematopoietic Dysfunction

Hematologic abnormalities in FA are evident at the hematopoietic progenitor cell level in BM and peripheral blood. The frequencies of CFU-E (colony-forming unit-erythroid), BFU-E (burst-forming unit-erythroid), and CFU-GM (colony-forming unit-granulocyte macrophage) colony-forming cells are reduced fairly consistently in almost all patients after aplastic anemia ensues as well as in a few patients before the onset of aplastic anemia. Although FA BM cells show normal transcripts for the α and β chains of the GM-CSF (granulocyte macrophage colony-stimulating factor)/interleukin-3 (IL-3) receptor and for c-kit protein, there is a deficient proliferative response of CFU-GEMM (colony-forming unit granulocyte, erythrocyte, macrophage, megakaryocyte), BFU-E, and CFU-GM progenitors to GM-CSF plus stem cell factor (SCF) (c-kit ligand) or to IL-3 plus SCF. Because all hematopoietic lineages are affected, the basic defect is presumed to be at the HSC level. Cure of FA BM failure by HSC transplantation (HSCT) supports this view. Confirmatory data for defective stem cells in FA using long-term BM cultures were reported by one group but not confirmed by another.

Decreased colony numbers in these studies can be interpreted as the result of an absolute decrease in progenitors and/or progenitors that have faulty proliferative properties and cannot form colonies in vitro.

Additional factors are operative in FA BM failure. Telomeres, the nonencoding DNA at each end of chromosomes, shorten with each round of cell division in normal human somatic cells. Their length is a reflection of the mitotic history of the cell. Telomerase, a ribonucleoprotein reverse transcriptase that can restore telomere length, is variably present in hematopoietic progenitors. Leukocyte telomere length is significantly shortened in patients with FA but there is increased telomerase activity, suggesting an abnormally high proliferative rate of progenitors that ultimately leads to their premature senescence. In parallel, increased BM cell apoptosis has been demonstrated in patients with FA and in knock-out mouse models and is mediated by Fas, a membrane glycoprotein receptor containing an integral death domain. FA cells exposed to TNF-α, INF-γ, MIP-1α, Fas ligand, and double-stranded RNA undergo exaggerated apoptotic responses.

Studies of cytokines in patients with FA have shown varied abnormalities. Although FA fibroblasts showed no deficiencies in SCF or macrophage colony-stimulating factor (M-CSF) production, variability ranging from diminished production to augmentation of production of IL-6, GM-CSF, and G-CSF (granulocyte colony-stimulating factor) has been observed in different patients. A consistent finding that may relate directly to pathogenesis is diminished IL-6 production in patients with FA and markedly increased TNF-α generation.

Initial attempts to generate induced pluripotent stem cells (iPSCs) from patients with FA have been difficult since reprogramming causes increased DNA double-stranded break and the FA pathway needs to be activated. This barrier can be bypassed by either correcting the genetic defect before reprogramming or performing the reprogramming under hypoxic conditions. Successful reprogramming resulted in cells that recapitulate the hematopoietic defect and identify the early pathogenetic defect at the stage of hemoangiogenic progenitors.

Clinical Features

History and Physical Examination

The diagnosis of FA can readily be made based on signs and symptoms related to aplastic anemia and the presence of characteristic congenital physical anomalies. However, a study from the International Fanconi Anemia Registry (IFAR, Rockefeller University), which used confirmatory chromosomal breakage studies, showed that only 39% of patients with FA have both aplastic anemia and anomalies. The rest of the patients had aplastic anemia but no anomalies (30%), anomalies but not aplastic anemia (24%), or neither (7%).

Table 29.2 lists the characteristic physical abnormalities and their approximate frequency based on more than 2000 published case reports. The two most common anomalies are *skin hyperpigmentation* and *short stature,* each with a frequency of 40% of cases. Characteristically, the hyperpigmentation is a generalized brown melanin-like splattering that is most prominent on the trunk, neck, and intertriginous areas and that becomes more obvious with age. Café-au-lait spots are common alone or in combination with the generalized hyperpigmentation and sometimes with vitiligo or hypopigmentation. The skin pigmentation should not be confused with hemosiderosis-induced bronzing in transfusion-dependent patients who have not been adequately iron chelated. In those with short stature, most are less than the third percentile for height. In some patients, growth failure is associated with endocrine abnormalities. In one report, spontaneous overnight growth hormone secretion was abnormal in all patients tested, and 44% had a subnormal response to growth hormone stimulation. Approximately 40% of patients also have overt or compensated hypothyroidism, sometimes in combination with growth hormone deficiency.

Malformations involving the upper limbs are common, especially hypoplastic, supernumerary, bifid, or absent thumbs. Hypoplastic or

TABLE 29.2	Characteristic Physical Anomalies in More Than 2000 Published Case Reports of Patients With Fanconi Anemia	
Anomalies		**Approximate Frequency (%)**
Skin pigment changes or café-au-lait spots		40
Short stature		40
Upper limb anomalies (thumbs, hands, radii, ulnae)		35
Hypogonadal and genitalia changes (mostly male)		27
Other skeletal findings (head or face, neck, spine)		25
Eye, eyelid, or epicanthal fold anomalies		20
Renal malformations		20
Gastrointestinal or cardiopulmonary malformations		11
Ear anomalies (external and internal), deafness		10
Hips, legs, feet, toe abnormalities		5
CNS imaging anomalies		3

CNS, Central nervous system.
From Shimamura A, Alter BP: Pathophysiology and management of inherited bone marrow failure syndromes. *Blood Rev* 24:101, 2010.

absent radii are always associated with hypoplastic or absent thumbs in contrast to the thrombocytopenia with absent radii (TAR) syndrome in which thumbs are always present. Less often, anomalies of the feet are seen, including toe syndactyly, short toes, a supernumerary toe, clubfoot, and flat feet. Congenital hip dislocation and leg abnormalities are occasionally seen. Male patients often have gonadal and genital abnormalities, including an underdeveloped penis or micropenis, undescended, atrophic, or absent testes, hypospadias, phimosis, and an abnormal urethra. Female patients occasionally have malformations of the vagina, uterus, or ovary. Renal anomalies occur but require imaging for documentation. Ectopic, pelvic, or horseshoe kidneys are detected often, as are duplicated, hypoplastic, dysplastic, or absent organs. Occasionally, hydronephrosis or hydroureter is present.

Many patients have a *Fanconi facies,* and unrelated patients can resemble each other almost as closely as siblings. The head and facial changes vary but commonly consist of microcephaly, small eyes, epicanthal folds, and abnormal shape, size, or positioning of the ears (see Fig. 29.1). Anomalies in the tympanic membrane and middle ear ossicles are seen in almost 70% of patients, resulting in hearing loss in most affected patients. Approximately 10% of patients with FA have cognitive deficiencies.

Laboratory Manifestations

Peripheral Blood and Bone Marrow Findings

A cardinal feature is the gradual onset of BM failure usually in the first decade of life, with declining values in one or more hematopoietic lineages. Of 754 patients with FA followed prospectively by the IFAR, 80% had hematologic abnormalities other than acute leukemia or myelodysplastic syndrome (MDS). The cumulative incidence of BM failure by 40 years of age was 90%. Patients with *FANCC* mutations appeared to have the earliest onset of changes and the highest incidence (see Phenotype-Genotype Correlations section). Thrombocytopenia with red blood cell (RBC) macrocytosis usually develops initially, with subsequent onset of granulocytopenia and

then anemia. Severe BM aplasia eventually ensues in most cases, but the degree of pancytopenia is variable and evolves over a period of months to years. The development of aplastic anemia can be accelerated by intercurrent infections or by drugs such as chloramphenicol. Within families, there is a tendency for the hematologic changes to occur at approximately the same age in affected siblings.

The RBCs are macrocytic with mean corpuscular volumes (MCVs) often above 100 fL even before the onset of significant anemia. Erythropoiesis is characterized by increased fetal hemoglobin (HbF) levels. The increased HbF production has a heterogeneous distribution in contrast to most cases of hereditary persistent HbF. Ferrokinetic studies indicate that most patients have an element of ineffective erythropoiesis. The RBC lifespan may be slightly shortened, but this is a minor contributory factor to the anemia.

In the early stages of the disease, the BM may not be hypocellular and can even show erythroid hyperplasia, sometimes with dyserythropoiesis, myelodysplastic changes, and even megaloblastic-appearing cells. Dysplastic changes may be very prominent with nuclear–cytoplasmic dyssynchrony, hypolobulated megakaryocytes, and binucleated erythroid cells; the findings are difficult to distinguish from MDS. As the disease progresses, the BM becomes hypocellular and fatty, sometimes in a patchy manner, and shows a relative increase in lymphocytes, plasma cells, reticulum cells, and mast cells. When full-blown BM failure occurs, the morphology of the BM biopsy is identical to severe acquired aplastic anemia.

Abnormal Chromosome Fragility. A major finding in FA is abnormal chromosome breakage seen in metaphase preparations of peripheral blood lymphocytes cultured with PHA. The karyotype is characterized by chromatid breaks, rearrangements, gaps, endoreduplications, and chromatid exchanges. Cultured skin fibroblasts also show the abnormal karyotype, underscoring the systemic nature of the disorder. The abnormal lymphocyte chromosome patterns and the number of breaks per cell have no direct correlation with the hematologic or clinical course of individual patients.

Although the breakage is increased in these baseline lymphocyte cultures, it is strikingly enhanced by adding a bifunctional DNA interstrand cross-linking agent, such as DEB or MMC. This is the recommended diagnostic test for FA. Indeed, homozygous FA cells are hypersensitive to many oncogenic and mutagenic inducers such as ionizing radiation; SV40 viral transformation; and alkylating and chemical agents, including cyclophosphamide, nitrogen mustard, and platinum compounds, but DEB and MMC have supplanted them for diagnostic testing.

For a definitive diagnosis of FA, the IFAR has defined FA as being associated with increased numbers of chromosome breaks per cell occurring after exposure to DEB with a range of 1.06 to 23.9 compared with the normal control range of 0.00 to 0.10. Further supportive features are unusual chromosome abnormalities such as triradial and quadriradial figures. This pattern of abnormal chromosome breakage can also be used to make a prenatal diagnosis of FA (see later). DEB testing of heterozygote carriers is unreliable for diagnosis because there is overlap of results with normal individuals.

A scoring system was developed for the probability of an accurate diagnosis of FA using discriminating clinical and laboratory variables in patients enrolled in the IFAR whose diagnosis was confirmed by DEB-induced chromosomal breakage analysis. The scoring system was useful in proving that DEB-induced chromosomal breakage results could be correlated with common FA findings. DEB testing is considered by the IFAR to be the gold standard for diagnosis, but MMC testing is still used in many laboratories.

DEB and MMC also induce cell cycle arrest in G2/M in cultures of FA lymphocytes or fibroblasts leading to a resultant 4N DNA cellular content. This alteration can be detected by flow cytometry and has been used to diagnose FA. It requires sophisticated instrumentation and is not used as widely as the DEB or MMC chromosome breakage assay.

About 10% to 15% of patients with clinical FA do not show increased chromosome breakage when tested with DEB or MMC. These patients usually have hematopoietic cell somatic mosaicism as a result of a genetic correction in a stem cell, resulting in one normal allele. The mechanisms for this phenomenon include gene conversion events, back mutations, or compensatory deletions or insertions. The end result is mixed populations of somatic cells, some with two abnormal alleles and some with one. If FA is strongly suspected, a skin biopsy is performed to assess chromosomal breakage in cultured fibroblasts with DEB or MMC rather than in lymphocyte cultures.

Immunoblotting for FANCD2. Immunoblotting of the FANCD2 protein have been proposed as a diagnostic test for most cases of FA or as a tool to direct specific gene testing. In this assay, primary lymphocytes or fibroblasts are assayed for FANCD2 after exposure to MMC or radiation by immunoblotting, which distinguishes the unubiquitinated and monoubiquitinated forms. The testing is useful in three situations for screening FA mutations: (1) in patients with FA with diagnostic MMC-induced chromosomal breakage assays, FANCD2 null mutations are presumed if no full-length FANCD2 is detected by immunoblotting; (2) if FANCD2 is detected but is not monoubiquitinated, mutations of one of the upstream core complex genes are predicted; and (3) if FANCD2 is detected and is monoubiquitinated, a mutation of FANCD1/BRCA2, FANCJ/BACH1/BRIP1, FANCN/PALB2, FANCO/Rad51C, or FANCP/SLX4 is expected because all five localize downstream of FANCD2. Monoubiquitination of FANCD2 is normal in other BM failure syndromes and chromosomal breakage disorders. Nevertheless, with the development of relatively rapid and affordable molecular diagnostic tests such as next generation sequencing, this test is rarely required.

Other Findings. FA cells exposed to alkylating agents arrest in the G_2/M phase of the cell cycle. The transfected wild-type FA gene that reduces G_2/M arrested cells as determined by cell cycle kinetics using flow cytometry pinpoints the mutant gene.

Apparently, the majority of patients with FA have stable, elevated levels of serum α-fetoprotein expressed constitutively that are independent of liver complications and of androgen therapy. Levels are also unchanged after HSCT. The clinical utility of these findings is limited.

Ultrasonographic examination of the abdomen may reveal congenital anomalies of the kidneys and urogenital system. Echocardiography may reveal cardiac anomalies. Radiography and computed tomography (CT) can be informative in revealing bone, intestinal, or other anomalies; however, imaging using radiation should be minimized as much as possible because of the carcinogenic risk.

Predisposition to Malignancy

A major feature of the FA phenotype is the propensity to develop cancer. The chromosome fragility, the defects in DNA repair, the genomic instability, and the cellular damage that occur in patients with FA translate into a significant predisposition to develop a malignancy. Because there are at least 17 genes that are associated with FA and because alterations in the FA pathway are relevant to the pathogenesis of common types of cancers, the disorder is a critical human model of the genetic determinants of hematologic cancers and solid tumors.

FA is a member of two families of cancer predisposition syndromes. The first is composed of genetic disorders of DNA repair that include ataxia telangiectasia, xeroderma pigmentosum, and Bloom syndrome. The close relationship between FA and these syndromes is underscored by data showing convergence of signaling pathways in these conditions and the identification of *ERCC4* mutations in patients who manifest a complex phenotype of both xeroderma pigmentosum and FA. The second family of predisposition syndromes consists of other inherited BM failure disorders described herein, including Shwachman-Diamond syndrome (SDS) and DC, that show a propensity for malignant myeloid transformation or solid tumors.

The magnitude of the risk of developing malignancy in FA has been defined in several comprehensive reports: a Canadian population-based study of patients up to the age of 18 years, the IFAR prospective registry of 754 patients, a retrospective North American cohort survey of 145 cases, and a literature review of more than 2000 published cases. The median patient age for the development of all cancers in the literature review was 16 years of age, which is strikingly different from the median age of 68 years for the same types of cancer in the general population. It was apparent from the above reports that the crude risk of cancer in patients with FA is extraordinarily high: 5% to 10% for leukemia, about 5% for MDS, and 5% to 10% for solid tumors. The IFAR data indicate that by the age of 40 years, the cumulative incidence of leukemia and nonhematologic cancers is 33% and 28%, respectively. In a recently published study of the Canadian cohort, the cumulative risk of clonal and malignant myeloid transformation (clones, MDS and AML) by the age of 18 years was 75%.

Previous observations by the IFAR showed that the risk of developing MDS and AML was higher for patients in whom a prior clonal BM cytogenetic abnormality had been detected. Monosomy 7, rearrangement or partial loss of 7q, rearrangements of 1p36 and 1q24-34, and rearrangements of 11q22-25 are frequent recurring cytogenetic clonal changes. Additional data indicate a strong correlation in FA BM cells of chromosome 3q26q29 partial trisomies and tetrasomies and rapid progression to MDS or AML. When interpreting the significance of clonal cytogenetic abnormalities in patients with FA, note that clonal variation is frequent, including appearances of new clones, inability to detect established clones on repeat examination, and clonal evolution. In a study from France the investigators used SNP arrays to analyze whole marrow cells of patients with FA with MDS/leukemia. They identified a relatively high frequency of somatic *RUNX1* gene disruption compared with what is typically seen in patients with de novo MDS/leukemia. Similar to the literature review, the IFAR verified that the risk for developing hematologic and nonhematologic cancer in FA increased with advancing age, but the IFAR did not show an age-related plateau for the risks for MDS and AML, possibly because both diagnoses were analyzed together.

The literature review also identified 320 patients with other forms of cancer, 25 of whom had up to three separate types of solid tumors, and 14 additional cases of solid tumors who also had leukemia. None of these patients had received a bone marrow transplant (BMT) before developing cancer. The most frequent solid tumor reported was squamous cell carcinoma involving head and neck and upper and lower esophagus followed by the vulva or anus, cervix, and skin. There were additional cases of tongue and oral squamous cell carcinoma that occurred after HSCT. Liver tumors, benign and malignant, were second most frequent. Most of these hepatoma and adenoma patients had received prior androgen therapy for aplastic anemia. Androgen administration has therefore been implicated in liver tumor pathogenesis. In descending order of frequency, cancers were also reported in brain, kidney, breast, and adrenal gland. The IFAR 20-year prospective observational study and the North American cohort survey corroborated the literature review in terms of type of cancer, site, and risk.

Heterozygote Phenotype

Heterozygote carriers of *FANC* gene mutations do not develop peripheral blood cytopenias or aplastic anemia, and cell lines from heterozygote carriers do not show excessive chromosome fragility in culture when exposed to DEB or MMC. The mean chromosomal breakage level of lymphocytes from FA carriers tested in cultures with a clastogenic agent may be higher than controls, but individual carrier testing may show overlap with normal values and severely limits its diagnostic utility. Literature from the early 1980s describes congenital anomalies of the hand and the genitourinary system in relatives of patients with FA, and parents of children with FA may have short stature. FA carriers may have increased levels of HbF, decreased natural killer (NK) cell counts, and diminished reactivity to mitogen stimulation.

Monoallelic carriers for *FANCD1, FANCN, FANCJ, FANCS, FANCP,* and *FANCO* are at increased risk of developing cancer. Female carriers of *FANCD1/BRCA2* and *FANCS/BRCA1* have an increased risk of breast cancer ranging from 40% at age 80 years to a lifetime risk of about 80%, and of ovarian cancer with a risk of up to 20% at age 70 years. Male carriers have a 7% risk of breast cancer and a 20% risk of prostate cancer before age 80 years. Heterozygous mutations in *FANCP* and *FANCO* are also associated with breast and ovarian cancers. Mutant FANCN and FANCJ are low-penetrance breast cancer susceptibility alleles with about a twofold increased risk in carriers compared with the general population.

Differential Diagnosis

About 30% of patients with FA do not have physical anomalies, and such individuals may not be recognized until they present with aplastic anemia, MDS, AML, unilineage cytopenias, or macrocytic RBCs. Thus FA should be part of the differential diagnosis in children and adults with unexplained cytopenias; characteristic birth defects; a diagnosis of aplastic anemia, MDS, or AML in patients mainly up to the age of 40 years, but sometimes also older; unusual sensitivity to chemo- or radiotherapy; cancer typical of FA but at an atypical age such as cancer of the cervix when younger than 30 years; or squamous cell carcinoma of the head and neck when younger than 50 years of age. Any of these should prompt consideration of FA as the underlying problem. All patients with idiopathic aplastic anemia who are younger than 40 years should have chromosomal fragility testing. However, if the test was not performed at diagnosis, patients with "idiopathic" aplastic anemia who fail to respond to immunosuppressive therapy with antithymocyte globulin (ATG) and cyclosporine should be tested.

Although neutropenia is a consistent feature of **SDS**, anemia or thrombocytopenia (or both) is seen in more than 50% of patients and can be confused with FA. Because growth failure is also a manifestation of SDS, differentiating between the two disorders can initially be difficult. The major difference between them is that SDS is a disorder of exocrine pancreatic dysfunction that may or may not produce gut malabsorption. This can be confirmed by fecal fat analysis; by showing reduced levels of serum trypsinogen, serum isoamylase, or fecal elastase; and by reduced levels of fat soluble vitamins such as A, D, and E. Nowadays pancreatic stimulation studies using intravenous secretin or cholecystokinin and measuring enzyme secretion is rarely done. CT, ultrasonography, or magnetic resonance imaging (MRI) of the pancreas may also demonstrate fatty changes within the pancreas. Other skeletal distinguishing features found in some patients with SDS are short flared ribs, thoracic dystrophy at birth, delayed bone maturation, and metaphyseal dysostosis of the long bones. Chromosomes analyses do not show spontaneous breaks in SDS, and there is no increased breakage after clastogenic stress testing using DEB or MMC. Mutations in the *SBDS* gene can be demonstrated in 90% of patients with SDS.

DC shares some features with FA, including development of pancytopenia, a predisposition to cancer and leukemia, and skin pigmentary changes. However, the pigmentation pattern is somewhat different in DC and manifests with a lacy reticulated pattern affecting the face, neck, chest, and arms, often with a telangiectatic component. At some point, usually in the first decade of life, patients with DC also develop dystrophic nails of the hands and feet and, somewhat later, leukoplakia involving the oral mucosa, especially the tongue. Other findings seen only in DC and not in FA are teeth abnormalities with dental decay and early tooth loss, hair loss, and hyperhidrosis of the palms and soles. Chromosomal fragility with DEB testing is typically normal in patients with DC, who contrast sharply with patients with FA. Molecular analysis of the DC genes is positive in about three-quarters of the patients (see Table 29.1).

Congenital amegakaryocytic thrombocytopenia (CAMT) and **TAR syndrome** both manifest in the neonatal period with thrombocytopenia. Patients with CAMT develop impairment in other blood cell lineages soon after presentation. A neonatal hematologic presentation

is atypical for FA; fewer than 5% of patients are diagnosed during the first year of life. Neither CAMT nor the various thrombocytopenia syndromes above show chromosome fragility, which separates them from FA. Genetic testing is available for many of these disorders (see Table 29.1). In TAR syndrome, thumbs are always preserved and intact despite the absence of radii, but in FA, the thumbs are hypoplastic or absent when the radii are absent.

Seckel syndrome, or **"bird-headed dwarfism"** manifests with short stature, microcephaly, cognitive delay, sinopulmonary infections, and a predisposition to developing lymphomas, pancytopenia, and AML. Some patients may show increased chromosomal breakage in lymphocyte cultures with DEB or MMC and mimic FA. There are several genes that have been linked to Seckel syndrome: mutant *ATR* has been associated with Seckel Type 1, *RBBP8* with Type 2, *CENPJ* with Type 4, *CEP152* with Type 5, *CEP63* with Type 6, and *ATRIP* with Type 8. Genotyping will distinguish FA from Seckel syndrome.

Nijmegen breakage syndrome (NBS) is an autosomal recessive disorder caused by mutations in the *NBS1* gene and is characterized by stunted growth, microcephaly, a distinctive facies, café-au-lait spots, immunodeficiency, and a predisposition to lymphoid malignancy. Some patients resemble those with FA, have BM failure, and may show increased chromosome breakage in lymphocyte cultures with MMC. The genetic defect is a mutant *NBS1* gene whose wild-type protein product is involved in DNA repair. Because NBS can mimic and be confused with FA, genotyping is essential and diagnostic.

Cells from patients with **Bloom syndrome** show abnormal spontaneous breakage, but unlike FA cells, the breakage does not increase in vitro in response to DEB. **Ataxia telangiectasia** is characterized by sister chromatid exchange without hypersensitivity to DEB or BM failure.

Natural History and Prognosis

The most serious early consequence in most patients with FA is BM failure. The exceptions are patients with biallelic *FANCD1/BRCA2* mutations who have a cumulative probability of 97% of developing a malignancy by age 6 years, including AML, Wilms tumor, and medulloblastoma. Judging from the literature, the overall risk for patients with FA developing solid malignant tumors, liver tumors, acute leukemia, and MDS is at least 15%, but it is likely higher in older patients. Treatment for cancer imposes additional problems and probably increases the risk for additional cancers secondary to therapy. Thus the major causes of death in FA are sepsis and bleeding from BM failure, complications of HSCT, and progressive cancer or consequences of its treatment.

Despite these serious issues, the prognosis for patients with FA is improving. Based on a literature review of more than 2000 FA case reports, the median survival from 1927–1999 was 21 years. In contrast, the median survival from 2000–2009 was 29 years of age. Patients with FA are now predicted to reach adulthood because more than 80% of patients reach age 18 years or more. Earlier diagnosis, especially of mild cases, diagnosis of FA in young adults with AML or a solid tumor, comprehensive clinical and laboratory surveillance programs, timely therapeutic interventions, and HSCT are attributed to the improved outlook.

Therapy

Because of their clinical and psychosocial complexity, patients with FA should be supervised by a hematologist at a tertiary care center using a comprehensive and multidisciplinary approach. On the initial visit, the practitioner should take a detailed personal and family history, a careful physical examination with emphasis on physical anomalies, complete blood counts and chemistries, a BM biopsy for cellularity and morphology, an aspirate for additional morphology, cytogenetics, and an iron stain for ringed sideroblasts. DEB or MMC chromosome fragility testing on peripheral blood lymphocytes on patients and siblings should be arranged. If FA is confirmed by DEB or MMC testing, genetic diagnosis should be offered to the family. On a separate visit, imaging studies should be requested to search for internal anomalies. Imaging using radiation should be minimized as much as possible because of the carcinogenic risk. When all the results from the workup have been compiled, a follow-up visit with the patient and family is arranged to discuss the diagnosis, management options, and prognosis. A referral to a genetic counselor should ensue. High-resolution human leukocyte antigen (HLA) typing of the patient and immediate family members is recommended shortly after the diagnosis is established to determine potential matched-related donors in case HSCT becomes necessary.

If the patient is stable, has only minimal to moderate hematologic changes, and does not have transfusion requirements, a period of observation is indicated. During this time, subspecialty consultations (e.g., with orthopedic surgeons, urologists, gynecologists, and otolaryngologists) can be arranged. Blood counts should be monitored every 1 to 3 months to determine their stability. In a stable patient with mild cytopenias, blood counts can be monitored every 3 months, and BM evaluation should be performed annually. Falling counts, a clonal BM cytogenetic abnormality, or prominent multilineage dysplasia require more frequent clinic visits and blood and BM sampling to monitor for progression to severe aplastic anemia, MDS, or AML. Spectral karyotyping (SKY), fluorescent in situ hybridization (FISH), and comparative genomic hybridization of BM cells can enhance the diagnostic capability.

A surveillance program for solid cancers should be initiated at least annually. After the age of 10 years or 1 year after HSCT, the oral cavity should be examined every 6 months for signs of malignant change because the risk in untransplanted patients with FA is 700-fold that of the general population. Dentists, oral surgeons, or head and neck surgeons should be periodically recruited after the age of 10 years or after HSCT to screen for head and neck squamous cell carcinomas by rhinopharyngoscopy using a flexible endoscope. Beginning at age 13 years, all women with FA should undergo annual gynecologic screening because the relative risk of vulvar squamous cell carcinoma is 4000-fold higher and cervical cancer is 200-fold higher than that of the general population. Human papilloma virus (HPV) DNA can be detected in 84% of FA squamous cell carcinoma specimens from various anatomic sites. Although the role of HPV in FA carcinogenesis is controversial, quadrivalent HPV vaccine is still recommended for boys and girls with FA at 9 years of age as a possible preventive approach.

Growth should be serially documented, and when growth velocity or stature falls below expectations, endocrine evaluation is needed to identify growth hormone deficiency. Diabetes mellitus occurs more commonly in FA, and random glucose levels should be evaluated annually or biannually. Based on the degree of hyperglycemia found on initial testing, fasting glucose levels and glucose tolerance tests should be performed. Screening for hypothyroidism should also be performed annually.

Hematopoietic Stem Cell Transplantation

Hematopoietic stem cell transplantation is the only curative therapy for the hematologic abnormalities of FA: aplastic anemia, MDS, and AML. The best donor source is an HLA-matched sibling in whom thorough history, physical examination, blood counts, HbF, chromosome breakage testing, and ideally genetic testing have excluded a diagnosis of FA. Initial efforts to transplant patients with FA using standard preparative regimens and graft-versus-host disease (GVHD) prophylaxis were plagued by two serious and often lethal problems, severe cytotoxicity from chemotherapy and irradiation, and exaggerated GVHD. Reduced-intensity HSCT protocols that remain myeloablative for patients with FA were subsequently introduced and improved outcomes ensued. Research is constantly ongoing for the most effective strategies.

Absolute indications for a matched sibling donor HSCT are (1) severe underproductive cytopenias and transfusion dependency; (2) high-risk MDS with chromosomal clonal abnormalities like monosomy 7, partial trisomies and tetrasomies of 3q26q29 and

deteriorating counts, or a BM blast count of greater than 5%; or (3) overt AML. Decision to transplant for milder, relative indications should be made on a case-by-case basis.

Three caveats about transfusional supportive care before HSCT are (1) more than 20 exposures to blood products is a risk factor that adversely affects engraftment and survival posttransplant; (2) use of directed donations from family members may cause alloimmunization to an antigen that can increase the risk of graft rejection after a matched sibling donor or haploidentical related HSCT; and (3) single-donor apheresis platelets should be requested when required and the product should be leukodepleted and irradiated.

Most published studies for matched related donor HSCT have used one of the following protocols: (1) cyclophosphamide, ATG, and total-body irradiation (TBI); (2) fludarabine, cyclophosphamide, and ATG; or (3) cyclophosphamide alone. In several studies usage of radiation-containing regimens in the setting of FA and matched related donor HSCT was shown to be associated with higher toxicity and lower long-term overall survival than nonradiation regimens and have gradually been avoided. Fludarabine, a purine antimetabolite with potent immunosuppressive and myeloablative properties with minimal toxicity to other tissues, continues to gain favor as an effective adjunct to preparative regimens. Transplant centers usually intensify the cytoreductive regimen when the patient has MDS or AML. Disease-free survival data for TBI-based protocols vary between 64% and 89%. Disease-free survivals for non-TBI protocols are as high as 93% using cyclophosphamide alone. The risk of primary or secondary graft failure is 5% to 10%, and the risk of acute GVHD ranges from 8% using cyclosporine and methotrexate prophylaxis to 55% using cyclosporine alone.

Hematopoietic stem cell transplantation using HLA-mismatched related donors, matched or one-antigen mismatched unrelated donors, or cord blood carries a higher risk of complications and a lower disease-free survival than matched sibling donor HSCT. The best outcome predictors are recipients younger than 10 years old, recipient seronegativity for CMV, history of fewer than 20 exposures to blood products, and use of fludarabine in the cytoreductive regimen. Risk factors adversely affecting survival are an HLA-mismatched donor, an FA phenotype with three or more congenital malformations, and prior administration of androgen therapy. The latter factor might be related to the delay in transplant rather than the therapy itself. Indications for an alternate donor HSCT are identical to those for a matched sibling donor HSCT.

Provided that no extended family members are suitable BM or peripheral blood stem cell donors, unrelated BM donors are sought and identified by searching donor and umbilical cord blood registries. An acceptable unrelated donor should be fully matched by high-resolution typing for all HLA-A, B, C, and DRB1 antigens, a so-called 8/8 match. A second choice is a one-antigen mismatch in a BM donor. Matched or one-antigen mismatched banked umbilical cord blood is equally suitable to a one-antigen mismatched BM donor and is an option. The last choice is a two-antigen mismatched cord blood. Using cord blood cells from unrelated donors, engraftment and survival are comparable to related or unrelated BM, although engraftment is slower with cord blood. The incidence of acute and chronic GVHD is reduced with cord blood grafts even in one or two HLA antigen mismatched transplants. Three-year published survival rates after unrelated HSCT for FA range between 40% and 75%.

Haploidentical HSCT from a haploidentical related donor using CD34(+) positively selected cells with or without T cell-depletion and reduced-intensity regimens have gained interest because of the almost universal availability of such donors (parents). Data is still limited, but engraftment has been seen in most patients, and 5-year overall survival of up to 83% has been reported. Failures are mainly caused by graft rejection, acute and chronic GVHD, and infections.

Molecular technology has led to preimplantation genetic diagnosis (PGD) coupled with in vitro fertilization (IVF) and selection of HLA-matched embryos for implantation. This is an option for parents who have a child with FA and a defined *FANC* mutation but without a matched sibling donor. If the mother is fertile, eggs are harvested and fertilized with the father's sperm in vitro, resulting in a number of blastomeres. Using single-cell polymerase chain reaction (PCR) technology, isolated cells from several blastomeres can be tested for an HLA match and for absence of biallelic *FANC* mutation. The selected HLA-compatible normal blastomeres can then be transferred and implanted in utero, resulting in a successful pregnancy and subsequent birth of a matched unaffected sibling. Cord blood from the PGD-selected healthy infant sibling can be banked for an HSCT for the affected sibling. The notion of "designer babies" is still debated in ethical circles.

Despite the successes of HSCT in correcting the BM failure of patients with FA, there is a subset of survivors who develop cancers, particularly squamous cell carcinoma of the head and neck. These malignancies reflect the ongoing genetic susceptibility of FA nonhematopoietic tissue to cancer despite successful transplantation for aplastic anemia, MDS, or AML. Published data comparing cancer risks in transplanted and nontransplanted patients with FA show a 4.4-fold increase in age-specific hazard rate of squamous cell carcinoma in the transplanted cohort. The causes for the increased cancer risk above the baseline seen in patients with FA who have not been transplanted are not proven, but GVHD, especially chronic, and the preparative regimens of chemotherapy and irradiation are highly suspect. T-cell depletion has been introduced in some protocols to reduce GVHD, and irradiation has been reduced or eliminated in others to address this issue.

G-CSF mobilization and collection of peripheral blood CD34[+] cells from patients with FA before the onset of severe pancytopenia has not attained broad application. These cells in theory can be used as targets for gene therapy; however, their cryopreservation and infusion later when severe BM failure ensues or as an autologous rescue after chemotherapy in the event of leukemic transformation is unlikely to reconstitute the hematopoietic system or confer a survival benefit.

Androgens

Androgen therapy has been used to treat FA for decades. The overall response rate in the literature is about 50% heralded by reticulocytosis and a rise in hemoglobin within 1 to 2 months. If the other lineages respond to androgens, white blood cells increase next and then platelets, but it may take many months to achieve the maximum response. Accepted indications for treating with androgens are one or more of the following: hemoglobin level less than 8 g/dL or symptoms from anemia, platelet count less than 30,000/mm^3, and neutrophil count less than 500/mm^3. Oxymetholone, an oral 17-α alkylated androgen, is used most frequently at 1 to 5 mg/kg once a day. The author's practice is to start with 0.5 mg/kg/day and increase it monthly if there are no major side effects and an insufficient response. Although unproven, some clinicians add corticosteroids to offset androgen-induced growth acceleration and to prevent thrombocytopenic bleeding by promoting vascular stability. For this purpose, 5 to 10 mg of prednisone is given orally every second day. There are increasing data on the efficacy of the attenuated androgen, danazol, in FA; however, there are no comparative data with oxymetholone. Claims of reduced masculinizing side effects in female patients with FA treated with danazol compared with those treated with oxymetholone have not yet been substantiated in clinical trials. A maintenance danazol dose of 1 to 5 mg/kg/day is probably sufficient to maintain good blood counts in those who respond. A danazol clinical trial for FA at Children's Hospital Boston is underway. Another androgen, oxandrolone, is also in clinical trial for FA at Cincinnati Children's Hospital. If an injectable androgen is preferred to decrease the risk of liver toxicity and growth of hepatic tumors, nandrolone decanoate, 1 to 2 mg/kg/week, is given intramuscularly followed by the application of local pressure and ice packs to prevent the development of hematomas. When the response is deemed maximal or sufficient, the androgens should be slowly tapered but not stopped entirely.

Almost all patients relapse when androgens are stopped. The few who successfully discontinue treatment are often in the puberty age range when temporary "spontaneous hematologic remissions" have been observed to occur. Most patients on long-term androgens eventually become refractory to therapy as BM failure progresses. Potential side effects include masculinization, which is especially troublesome in female patients, and elevated hepatic enzymes, cholestasis, peliosis hepatis, and liver tumors. Five complications of androgen therapy require consideration.

1. *Peliosis hepatis* is a cystic dilation of hepatic sinusoids that fill with blood and can be life-threatening if they rupture. They may be clinically silent or produce right upper quadrant pain. Liver function test results are normal. Ultrasonographic examination is a safe way to diagnose the abnormality. The lesions may regress after stopping the androgens.
2. *Androgens also damage hepatocytes* nonspecifically. This may be manifest as cholestatic jaundice or elevated liver enzymes. Stopping androgen therapy usually leads to complete resolution. Hepatic cirrhosis may develop in patients on continued androgen therapy. If resolution of enzyme elevation does not occur after androgen withdrawal, a liver biopsy is indicated.
3. *Hepatocellular adenomas* are associated with androgen therapy. These are benign, noninvasive tumors. They can, however, rupture, leading to life-threatening bleeding. Patients with FA may develop these tumors rapidly, but they can be readily detected by imaging. The tumor may regress after stopping the androgens. If persistent, surgical resection or radiofrequency ablation may be necessary.
4. *Hepatocellular carcinoma* (HCC; hepatoma) occurs with androgen use, and some studies have suggested that patients with FA on treatment may be at increased risk for HCC. The HCC associated with androgens characteristically does not produce α-fetoprotein in serum, distinguishing it from de novo HCC. Patients developing HCC should discontinue androgen therapy.
5. Androgen therapy for patients with FA is recognized as an *adverse prognostic factor* for those receiving a transplant by a European study. Consequently, several investigators recommended that androgens be given to patients with FA only if a suitable donor cannot be identified. Unfortunately, comparative studies between androgen administration and HSCT from related or unrelated donors are not available, and are probably not feasible because of the rarity of the disease. The cause of the association is unknown but may be related to delay in HSCT rather than the drug itself.

Those receiving androgens should be evaluated serially with liver enzyme profiles every 2 to 3 months and ultrasonography of the liver every 6 to 12 months. If liver enzymes increase to above normal or if abnormalities appear on imaging, the androgen dose should be decreased or stopped.

Hematopoietic Growth Factors

Both G-CSF and GM-CSF can induce a neutrophil response in neutropenic patients with FA. G-CSF is indicated for a patient with recurrent or serious bacterial infection, especially if the neutrophil counts are less than 500/mm^3. In a published clinical trial of G-CSF in 12 patients with FA, all 12 had an increase in absolute neutrophil numbers, five had a significant increment in hemoglobin levels, and four had an increase in platelet counts. Concurrent with the impressive improvements in blood counts, 8 of 10 patients who finished 40 weeks of G-CSF treatment showed elevations in the percentage of BM and peripheral blood CD34[+] cells. The starting dose for subcutaneous G-CSF is 5 μg/kg/day, and after a neutrophil response occurs, the dose can be decreased to every second day or 2 to 3 times a week. Long-acting pegylated G-CSF has not been studied in FA.

In another published clinical trial, combination cytokine therapy consisting of subcutaneous G-CSF 5 μg/kg once daily with erythropoietin 50 units/kg administered subcutaneously or intravenously three times a week was given to patients with FA. Androgen therapy was added if the response was inadequate. Of 20 patients treated, 19 had improved neutrophil numbers, 6 had an increase in hemoglobin levels, and 4 achieved a sustained rise in platelets.

Because genomic instability and a marked predisposition to leukemia and cancer are features of FA, the wisdom of using granulopoietic growth-promoting cytokines on a long-term basis for FA is an issue. There may be a heightened risk of inducing or promoting expansion of a leukemic clone, especially one with monosomy 7. Therefore, before starting cytokine therapy, a baseline BM aspirate and biopsy is recommended and then repeated every 6 months to document changes in morphology and cytogenetics.

Genetic Counseling

Genetic counseling should be offered to all patients and families with FA. The discussion should include mode of transmission, risk of having the disease in family members, risk of recurrence in future pregnancies, available diagnostic tests during pregnancy, and PGD/IVF and selection of HLA-matched embryos who do not have FA as potential donors for HSCT. Screening of all first-degree relatives should be offered.

During pregnancy, the abnormal chromosome breakage pattern characteristic of FA can be used to make a prenatal diagnosis of FA as well as gene testing. Diagnostic testing can be performed on fetal amniotic fluid cells obtained at week 16 of gestation or on chorionic villus biopsy specimens at 9 to 12 weeks of gestation. A very high degree of prenatal diagnostic accuracy has been obtained by looking at both spontaneous and DEB-induced breaks in fetal tissue. DEB testing of heterozygote carriers is unreliable for diagnosis because there is overlap of results with normal individuals.

An updated manual for the management of patients with FA has been published by the Fanconi Anemia Research Fund (see www.fanconi.org for *Fanconi Anemia Guidelines for Diagnosis and Management*, 4th edition, 2014).

Future Directions

The premise for gene therapy in FA is based on the assumption that corrected hematopoietic cells would have a growth advantage. Strengthening this supposition are patients with FA with hematopoietic somatic mosaicism who show spontaneous disappearance of cells with the FA phenotype. These *mosaic* patients may show spontaneous hematologic improvement, suggesting that hematopoiesis was derived from stem cells with a normal phenotype. In the context of gene therapy, evidence suggests that even one genetically corrected HSC may be able to repopulate the BM of a patient with FA.

Despite encouraging preclinical studies more than a decade ago using retroviral vectors showing that wild-type *FANCC* and *FANCA* could be integrated into normal and FA CD34⁺ cells, the ensuing clinical trials in *FANCC* and *FANCA* patients using retrovectors were disappointing. A central problem was suboptimal wild-type gene integration into FA cells in culture. Because of the apoptotic phenotype and the sensitivity to oxidative stress, FA cells die rapidly in vitro before efficient gene transfer is accomplished. Changing the tissue culture conditions (e.g., usage of low oxygen condition) and introducing lentiviral vectors that can infect noncycling human cells were deemed the solutions, and the first clinical trial for FA group A has been opened. Ongoing research is directed at improving vector design, transduction methodology, and improved strategies for preparing HSCs. One caveat: a successful FA gene therapy protocol may correct BM failure and possibly the propensity for MDS and AML, but the predisposition for cancer in other tissues will continue unchecked.

Shwachman-Diamond Syndrome

SDS is an autosomal recessive multisystem disorder characterized by varying degrees of BM failure, a high risk of leukemia, and exocrine pancreatic insufficiency. Additional features may include short stature and skeletal abnormalities. The mutant gene responsible for this complex pleiotropic phenotype, termed *Shwachman-Bodian-Diamond syndrome (SBDS)*, has been identified and has been confirmed in 90% of patients with the classic presentation. SBDS seems to be multifunctional and promotes cell survival, ribosome biogenesis, mitotic spindle stability, and chemotaxis. To date, though, no unifying pathogenesis has been able to account for all of the multisystem features of SDS.

Epidemiology

SDS has been reported among all ethnic groups. Older studies suggested a higher incidence in males. However, recent data suggest an equal distribution between genders as expected from an autosomal recessive disorder. Based on data from the CIMFR, SDS is the third most common IBMFS with an incidence of 8.5 cases per million live births.

Pathobiology

The identification of *SBDS* on chromosome 7q11 was the entry point for studies on the molecular basis for SDS. The gene encodes a 250 amino acid protein product, which is a member of a highly conserved protein family of previously unknown function with putative orthologs in diverse species, including Archaea and eukaryocytes. Based on structural studies of the ortholog in Archaea and the human protein, the SBDS protein has three main domains (N-terminal, middle, and C-terminal) with predicted protein–protein, protein–DNA, and protein–RNA binding motifs.

There is an adjoining pseudogene *(SBDSP)* with 97% homology in its coding regions to *SBDS*. The common *SBDS* mutations are composed of sequences that are homologous to *SBDSP*. Hence these mutations are believed to result from gene recombination events in which *SBDSP1* acts as the donor. These recombinational events result in three common gene conversion mutations in exon 2 that account for 75% of *SDS* alleles: (1) a splice-site mutation, c.258+2T>C, which may either cause premature truncation of the SBDS protein by frameshift (p,C84fs3) or use an alternative splice site; (2) a nonsense mutation, c.183_184TA>CT that introduces an in-frame stop codon (p.K62X); and (3) an extended conversion mutation, c.183_184TA>CT and c.258+2T>C, encompasses both mutations. In the Toronto database of 210 SDS families, 89% of unrelated SDS individuals carry a gene conversion mutation on one allele, and 60% carry conversion mutations on both alleles. Thus the vast majority of patients are compound heterozygotes with respect to p.K62X and p.C84fsx3. Additional rare mutations in the *SBDS* gene have been identified in patients with SDS. These include dozens of insertion, deletion, and missense mutations that have not arisen from gene conversion events. Most *SBDS* mutations alter the N-terminal domain of the protein and lead to markedly reduced protein levels.

SBDS protein is essential for life because no patients with homozygous null mutations have been reported, and small levels of residual protein can usually be detected in patients with SDS. Furthermore, a complete loss of the protein in mice causes developmental arrest before embryonic day 6.5 and early lethality. SBDS seems to be multifunctional and play a role in several cellular pathways, including ribosomal biogenesis, cell survival, chemotaxis, mitotic spindle formation, and protection from cellular stress.

The SBDS protein phylogeny is shared with proteins that are enriched for RNA metabolism and/or ribosome-associated functions. The SBDS protein can be detected in human cell nuclei and cytoplasm. It concentrates in the nucleolus during G1 and G2. Synthetic genetic arrays of YHR087W, a yeast homolog of the N-terminal domain of SBDS, suggested interactions with several genes involved in RNA and rRNA processing. Loss of the protein in humans and yeast results in failure to remove eukaryotic initiation factor 6, eIf6 or its homologue in yeast, Tif6, from the ribosomal large subunit in the cytoplasm and impairs the assembly of the large and small ribosome subunits to form the mature ribosomes. SBDS directly interacts with the GTPase elongation factor-like 1 (EFL1). The interaction promotes eIF6 removal from the 60S subunit by a mechanism that requires guanosine triphosphate (GTP) binding and hydrolysis by EFL1. SBDS interacts with multiple proteins with diverse molecular functions; many of them are involved in ribosome biogenesis, such as RPL4, and DNA metabolism, such as RPA70.

SBDS is critical for cell survival. When *SBDS* is lost in SDS BM cells or in *SBDS*-knockdown K562 and HeLa cells, the cells undergo accelerated apoptosis. The accelerated apoptosis in BM cells and *SBDS*-knockdown cells seems to be through the Fas pathway and not through the Bax/Bcl-2/Bcl-XL pathway. SBDS deficiency in primary SDS cells and in *SBDS*-knockdown cells results in abnormal accumulation of functional Fas (transcript 1) at the plasma membrane level.

Interestingly, knocking down *SBDS* in CD34⁺ hematopoietic stem cells/early progenitors and in cell lines increased the levels of ROS, and antioxidants reduced Fas-mediated cell death and improved hematopoiesis from primary SDS cells. This suggests that *SBDS* balances the levels of ROS and thereby protects hematopoietic cells from cell death.

Patients with SDS have a defect in leukocyte chemotaxis. Consistent with this observation, the *SBDS* homologue in amoeba was found to localize to the pseudopods during chemotaxis. These observations suggest that the *SBDS* protein deficiency in SDS causes a chemotaxis defect in patients.

SBDS has been shown to colocalize to the mitotic spindle and bind microtubules and stabilize them. Its deficiency results in centrosomal amplification and multipolar spindles.

The pathophysiologic link between *SBDS* mutations and BM failure is still unclear. Initial studies in the 1970s and early 1980s showed reduced CFU-GM and BFU-E colony formation in most patients compatible with a defective stem cell origin of the BM failure. Recent investigations have characterized a much more extensive hematopoietic phenotype (Table 29.3). SDS BM has decreased numbers of CD34⁺ cells as well as an impaired ability for CD34⁺ cells to form multilineage hematopoietic colonies in vitro, confirming that they are intrinsically defective. Patients' BM cells overexpress Fas, the membrane receptor for Fas ligand, and show increased patterns of apoptosis after preincubation with activating anti-Fas antibody, pinpointing this as a central pathogenetic mechanism for the BM failure. Induction of differentiation (at least toward erythroid lineage) results in markedly accelerated apoptosis in SBDS-deficient cells, with only a minimal effect on proliferation. Importantly, oxidative stress is increased during differentiation of SBDS-deficient erythroid cells, and antioxidants enhance the expansion capability of both differentiating *SBDS*-knockdown K562 cells and colony production of SDS patient HSCs and progenitors. Erythroid differentiation also results in reduction of all ribosomal subunits and global translation. These studies indicate that when *SBDS* protein is deficient, several biologic pathways may be dysfunctional during hematopoietic cell development; this may be the cause of the high predilection for BM

failure in patients with SDS. A group from Boston used iPSCs from patients with SDS and demonstrated an alternative mechanism for cell death. During differentiation of iPSCs to promyelocytes protease levels are increased and apoptosis is enhanced. Supplementing the culture media with protease inhibitors provides a rescue.

Two other abnormalities have been identified in SDS. When the averages of telomere lengths adjusted for age are compared with those of control participants, a tendency toward shortening of telomeres is found in patient leukocytes, reflecting premature cellular aging. This may represent either an inherent defect in telomere maintenance or compensatory stem cell hyperproliferation. In addition to an inherent hematopoietic defect, it has also been shown that the BM stroma is markedly defective in terms of its ability to support and maintain normal hematopoiesis.

Clinical Features

The many clinical manifestations that occur in varying combinations are shown in Table 29.4. Most patients present in infancy with evidence of growth failure, feeding difficulties, diarrhea, and infections. Steatorrhea and abdominal discomfort are frequent. Approximately 50% of patients exhibit a modest improvement in pancreatic function and do not require further pancreatic enzyme replacement therapy. Hepatomegaly is a common physical finding in young children but typically resolves with age and does not have clinical significance.

Patients with SDS are particularly susceptible to bacterial and fungal infections, including otitis media, bronchopneumonia, osteomyelitis, septicemia, and recurrent furuncles. Overwhelming sepsis is a well-recognized fatal complication of this disorder, particularly early in life.

Short stature is a fairly consistent feature of the syndrome. When treated with pancreatic enzyme replacement, most patients show a normal growth velocity yet remain consistently below the third percentile for height and weight, indicating an intrinsic growth defect. The occasional adult achieves the 25th percentile for height. Although metaphyseal dysplasia is a common radiologic abnormality (44–77% of patients), particularly in the femoral head and the proximal tibia, in most patients it fails to produce any symptoms. Occasional patients have clinical joint deformities, resulting in pain, functional impairment, or cosmetic problems, necessitating surgery. Some patients present at birth with respiratory distress caused by thoracic dystrophy. Others may have asymptomatic short and flared ribs.

TABLE 29.3 Hematopoietic Phenotype in Shwachman-Diamond Syndrome

Decreased BM CD34⁺ cells
Decreased colonies from CD34⁺ cells
Abnormal telomere shortening of leukocytes
Increased apoptosis of BM cells
Apoptosis is mediated by Fas pathway
Impaired BM stromal cell function
Abnormal lymphoid immune function
Increased BM microvessel density
BM cell upregulation of specific oncogenes
Increased levels of reactive oxygen species
Accentuation of the ribosome biogenesis defects with reduced ribosome subunits, ribosomes, and polysomes
Accentuation of the protein translation defect

BM, Bone marrow.

TABLE 29.4 Clinical and Hematologic Features of Shwachman–Diamond Syndrome

Major Features	Patients (%)
Pancreatic insufficiency (decreased digestive enzymes)	86–100
Hematologic cytopenias	
Neutropenia	88–100
Thrombocytopenia	24–70
Anemia	42–66
Pancytopenia	10–44
MDS/AML	≈30
Other Features	
Short stature	50
Delayed bone maturation	100
Metaphyseal dysplasia	44–77
Rib cage anomalies	32–52
Hepatomegaly or elevated enzymes	<50
Poor oral health (caries, ulcers, tooth loss)	>50
Learning and behavioral problems	>50

AML, Acute myeloid leukemia; *MDS,* myelodysplastic syndrome.

The majority of patients have deficits in cognitive abilities at varying levels of severity. These include delayed language development, low intellectual ability, impaired visual-motor integration, and failure to achieve higher order language functioning and problem solving. About one-fifth of the children have behavioral challenges such as attention deficit hyperactivity disorder, pervasive developmental disorder, or oppositional defiant disorder.

Some additional clinical features are seen very infrequently in SDS. Endocrine abnormalities include insulin-dependent diabetes, growth hormone deficiency, hypogonadotropic hypogonadism, hypothyroidism, and delayed puberty. Cardiomyopathies have been noted in some cases. Urinary tract anomalies, renal tubular acidosis, and cleft palate also occur.

Laboratory Findings

Peripheral Blood and Bone Marrow Findings. Published data accurately represent the spectrum of hematologic findings (see Table 29.4). Neutropenia is present in almost all patients on at least one occasion. The neutropenia can be chronic or intermittent. Neutropenia has been identified in some patients with SDS in the neonatal period during an episode of sepsis. Anemia is recorded in about half of the patients. RBC MCV and HbF are elevated in 60% and 75% of the patients, respectively, after the age of 1 year. Whether this reflects stress hematopoiesis or ineffective erythropoiesis concomitant with chronic infections has not been clarified. The combination of isolated neutropenia and high MCV or high HbF after the first year of life is seen in up to 28% of patients with SDS and almost never in other IBMFSs. Reticulocyte responses are inappropriately low for the levels of hemoglobin in 75% of patients. Thrombocytopenia can be seen in about 40% of patients.

More than one lineage can be affected, and pancytopenia is observed in up to 65% of cases. The pancytopenia can be profound as a result of severe aplastic anemia (Fig. 29.2). However, BM biopsies and aspirates vary widely with respect to cellularity; varying degrees of BM hypoplasia and fat infiltration are the usual findings. BM with normal or even increased cellularity has also been observed, typically in young children. The severity of neutropenia does not always correlate with BM cellularity, nor is the severity of the pancreatic insufficiency concordant with the hematologic abnormalities.

SDS neutrophils may have defects in mobility, migration, and chemotaxis. There appears to be a diminished ability of SDS neutrophils to orient toward a gradient of N-formyl-methionyl-leucyl-phenylalanine. An unusual surface distribution of concanavalin A has also been reported that reflects a cytoskeletal defect in SDS neutrophils. Whatever the magnitude of the chemotaxis abnormality is in

vitro in SDS, neutrophil recruitment into abscesses or empyemas ensues robustly in vivo.

Immune Dysfunction. Impaired immune function can be significant in SDS and underlie recurrent infections even if adequate numbers of neutrophils are present. Patients have various B-cell abnormalities, including one or more of the following: low immunoglobulin G (IgG) or IgG subclasses, low percentage of circulating B lymphocytes, decreased in vitro B-cell proliferation, and lack of specific antibody production. Patients may also have T-cell abnormalities, including a low percentage of circulating T lymphocytes or subsets or NK cells, and decreased in vitro T-cell proliferation. Inverted CD4:CD8 ratios have also been described.

Exocrine Pancreatic Tests. The exocrine pancreatic pathology is caused by failure of pancreatic acinar development (Fig. 29.3). Pathologic studies reveal normal ductular architecture but extensive fatty replacement of pancreatic acinar tissue, which can be visualized by CT, ultrasonography, or MRI. Pancreatic function studies using

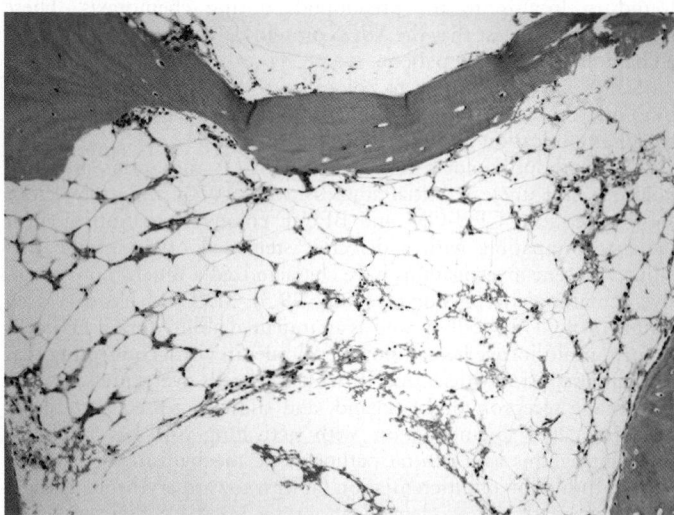

Fig. 29.2 BONE MARROW BIOPSY IN SEVERE SHWACHMAN-DIAMOND SYNDROME SHOWING STRIKING HYPOCELLULARITY, FATTY CHANGES, AND TRILINEAGE APLASIA. *(Courtesy Dr. Mohamed Abdelhaleem, Toronto.)*

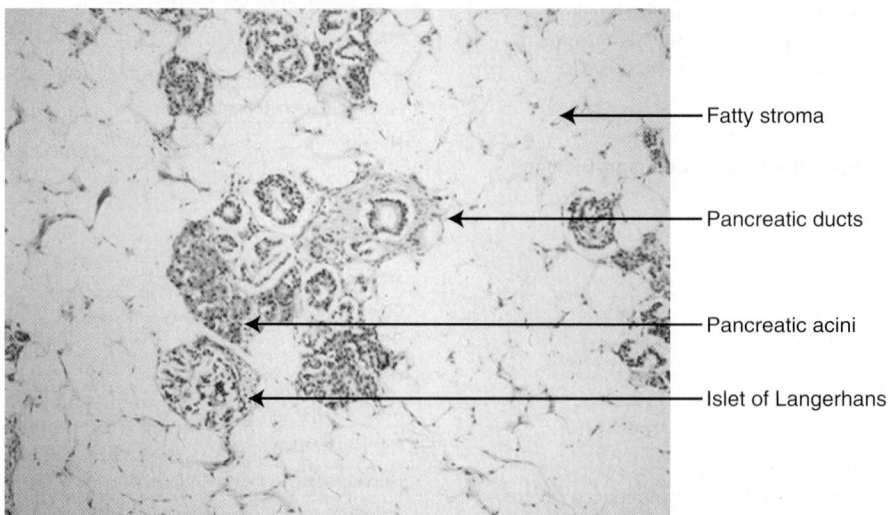

Fig. 29.3 PANCREATIC TISSUE PATHOLOGY IN SEVERE SHWACHMAN-DIAMOND SYNDROME. The two classic features, deficiency of acinar tissue and fatty replacement, are shown. Islets of Langerhans are intact. *(Provided by Dr. Peter Durie, Toronto.)*

intravenous secretin or cholecystokinin confirm the presence of markedly impaired enzyme secretion averaging 10% to 14% of normal but with preserved ductal function. Because of its invasive nature, this test has largely been replaced by measuring the levels of pancreatic enzymes in the serum.

During the first 3 years of life, serum trypsinogen is typically reduced and can be used for diagnostic purposes. Serum isoamylase levels are low in patients with SDS of all ages. However, normal children younger than 3 years have low isoamylase levels, so its measurement is not diagnostically useful at this age. Fecal elastase is another pancreatic enzyme that is reduced in SDS. Approximately 50% of patients exhibit a modest improvement in enzyme secretion with advancing age and normal fat absorption when assessed by 72-hour fecal fat balance studies. These patients do not require further pancreatic enzyme replacement therapy.

Imaging Studies. Radiographs of the bone are useful as a screening diagnostic test for SDS. Osteopenia is seen in most patients but rarely results in clinical osteoporosis. Metaphyseal dysplasia has been reported in about 50% of patients, particularly of the femoral heads, knees, humeral heads, wrists, ankles, and vertebrae. Rib cage abnormalities can be found in 30% to 50% of patients. These include a narrow rib cage, short ribs, flared anterior rib ends, and costochondral thickening. Digital abnormalities such as clinodactyly, syndactyly, and supernumerary thumbs have been reported but are rare. Spinal deformities, including kyphosis and scoliosis, have been reported.

Patients with SDS do not have macroscopic brain malformations by MRI testing. However, they may have a decreased global brain volume (both gray matter and white matter) and a smaller posterior fossa, cerebellar vermis, corpus callosum, brainstem, and occipitofrontal head circumferences compared with control participants. These anomalies might be the basis for the neurocognitive and neurobehavioral difficulties.

The French registry found cardiac anomalies in 11% of patients with SDS. These include dilated and nondilated cardiomyopathy, and structural malformations such as atrial septal defect, ventricular septal defect, coarctation of the aorta, and tetralogy of Fallot.

Circumferential strain as measured by echocardiography was found to be decreased by the U.S. SDS registry, suggesting systolic dysfunction.

Cancer Predisposition. SDS is characterized by a high propensity to develop MDS and leukemia, particularly AML. The published crude rate for MDS or AML (MDS/AML) in patients with SDS ranges from 8% to 33%. Data from the CIMFR and the French Severe Chronic Neutropenia Registry, the cumulative risk of MDS/AML by the age of 18 and 20 years, was 20% and 19%, respectively. The risk of leukemia in the French registry was 36% by the age of 30 years.

There is an increased frequency of BM clonal cytogenetic abnormalities as the sole evidence for a clonal disease in an otherwise hypocellular BM without excess blast counts or major prominent multilineage dysplasia. The incidence is roughly estimated to be 7% to 41% based on pooled published data. Isochromosome 7q [i(7q)], an extremely uncommon finding rarely described in MDS or AML in patients without SDS, was seen in 44% of patients with SDS. This high occurrence suggests that it is a fairly specific marker for SDS and might be related to the mutant gene on 7q(11). Other chromosome 7 abnormalities are seen in 33% of patients with SDS and include monosomy 7, i(7q) combined with monosomy 7 and deletions or translocations involving part of 7q. The prognostic significance of the cytogenetic changes requires prospective monitoring for clarification. Of the patients with i(7q), progression to advanced MDS with excess blasts or to AML has rarely been reported, but development of severe cytopenia and additional clones was described in three of four patients on long-term follow-up in the Canadian registry. Among a group of six patients with i(7q) from several hospitals in the United Kingdom, none progressed to advanced MDS/AML. In contrast, approximately 40% of patients with the other chromosomal 7 abnormalities progress to either advanced MDS or

to AML. Similarly, patients with SDS with del(20q) rarely evolve into advanced MDS/AML.

The pathophysiologic link between *SBDS* mutations and propensity to MDS and AML is unknown. It is possible that patients with SDS cells develop more frequent mutations caused by genomic instability, possibly because of mitotic spindle dysregulation or telomere shortening. It is also possible that impaired ribosome biogenesis and accelerated apoptosis cause a growth disadvantage for SDS BM cells, allowing for a growth advantage and expansion of malignant clones. Although molecular and cellular parameters do not distinguish patients with SDS with transformation from those with SDS without transformation, it is remarkable that all SDS BM demonstrates many characteristic features observed in MDS. These include impaired BM stromal support of normal hematopoiesis, increased BM cell apoptosis mediated by the Fas pathway, telomere shortening of leukocytes, increased BM neovascularization, high frequency of clonal cytogenetic abnormalities, and abnormal leukemia-related gene expression in BM progenitor cells, such as overexpression of the oncogenes *TAL1* and *LARG*.

The vast majority of the published cases of SDS-associated MDS/AML developed without previous G-CSF therapy. None of the six patients with SDS-associated MDS/AML from our institution were treated with G-CSF before transformation. However, it is still unclear whether G-CSF increases the risk of developing leukemia or promotes the expansion of existing malignant clones. Because G-CSF might increase neutrophil counts and prevent infections in SDS, a fraction of the reported patients with SDS-associated MDS/AML had been previously treated with G-CSF. For example, two of the 29 patients with SDS on the Severe Chronic Neutropenic International Registry who received G-CSF therapy developed MDS/leukemia.

The *SBDS* gene must play a critical role in preventing leukemic myeloid transformation because up to one-third of patients with SDS develop MDS/AML. To address whether an acquired mutant *SBDS* gene is associated with leukemic transformation in de novo AML, 77 AML BM samples at diagnosis or relapse were analyzed for *SBDS* mutations, and none were identified. To see if a subset of patients with previously undiagnosed SDS presented for the first time with AML, 48 AML BM samples were studied at remission, but no *SBDS* mutations were found. Patients with SDS who also have MDS/AML have common *SBDS* mutations, and a genotype–phenotype study of 21 patients with SDS with MDS/AML showed no relationship (Linda Ellis, RN, Toronto, personal communication). Thus the link between mutant *SBDS*; hematologic cancer; and upregulated oncogenes, including *LARG*, and *TAL1,* is undetermined.

Several cases of solid tumors have been described in SDS. These include two cases of pancreatic ductal adenocarcinoma, one brain frontal lobe B-cell lymphoma, one dermatofibrosarcoma protuberans and one breast cancer. However, more data are needed to determine whether the risk of solid tumors is higher than in the general population.

Differential Diagnosis

The introduction of genetic testing has improved the ability to diagnose the disorder and particularly has helped identify cases with an atypical presentation (Y. Dror, unpublished data). The diagnostic criteria include having at least two of the following: (1) chronic BM failure, (2) exocrine pancreatic insufficiency, (3) positive genetic testing results or a first-degree relative with SDS. Several syndromes with overlapping features have to be excluded.

The syndrome of refractory sideroblastic anemia with vacuolization of BM precursors, or **Pearson syndrome,** is clinically similar to SDS but characterized by very different BM morphology. Severe anemia requiring transfusions rather than neutropenia is often present at birth and by 1 year of age in all cases. In contrast to SDS, the major BM morphologic findings are ringed sideroblasts with decreased erythroblasts and prominent vacuolation of erythroid and myeloid precursors. The disorder shares clinical similarities with SDS because of exocrine pancreatic dysfunction. Malabsorption and severe failure to thrive occur in approximately half of cases within the first 12 months of life. Qualitative pancreatic function tests show depressed acinar function and reduced fluid and electrolyte secretion. Approximately 50% of reported patients die early in life from sepsis, acidosis, and liver failure; the others appear to improve spontaneously with reduced transfusion requirements. At autopsy, the pancreas shows acinar cell atrophy and fibrosis; fatty infiltration as seen in SDS is not a prominent feature. The need for long-term pancreatic enzyme replacement is unclear. These patients have a diagnostic deletion of mitochondrial deoxyribonucleic acid (mtDNA). mtDNA encodes enzymes in the mitochondrial respiratory chain that are relevant to oxidative phosphorylation, including the reduced form of nicotinamide adenine dinucleotide dehydrogenase (NADH), cytochrome oxidase, adenosine triphosphatase (ATPase), mitochondrial transfer ribonucleic acids (tRNAs), and mitochondrial ribosomal RNAs. The degree of heteroplasmy affects the disease expression. SDS shares some manifestations with FA such as BM dysfunction and growth failure, but patients with SDS can usually be distinguished because of malabsorption syndrome, fatty changes within the pancreatic body that can be visualized by imaging, and characteristic skeletal abnormalities not seen in patients with FA. In difficult cases with incomplete disease expression, the distinction relies on normal clastogenic stress-induced chromosome fragility testing and genetic testing of SDS and FA genes.

Atypical SDS cases with only little evidence of pancreatic changes can be difficult to distinguish from early-onset **dyskeratosis congenita** with no mucocutaneous manifestations. Establishing a diagnosis in such cases can be assisted by telomere length screening, which might show telomere shortening in SDS, but typically not in the very severe range seen in dyskeratosis congenita.

Prognosis

Because of the broad pleiotropy in SDS, the number of undiagnosed patients with mild or asymptomatic disease is unknown. Hence the overall prognosis may be better than previously thought. The majority of *SBDS* mutations represent hypomorphic alleles with reduced but variable protein expression. Also, there is phenotypic heterogeneity in patients carrying identical *SBDS* mutations. Therefore, until more information is forthcoming, the natural history and prognosis are not yet defined.

From a literature review, the projected median survival of patients with SDS was calculated as 35 years. During infancy, morbidity and mortality are mostly related to infections, thoracic dystrophy, and malabsorption. Later in life, the major problems are hematologic or complications related to their treatment. Cytopenias tend to fluctuate in severity but do not fully resolve spontaneously. The most common cause of death in late childhood or adulthood is related to MDS/AML.

Therapy

Patient management is ideally shared by a multidisciplinary team consisting of a hematologist and a gastroenterologist as core members and other subspecialists such as a dentist, an orthopedic surgeon, and a psychologist as required. The malabsorption component of SDS responds to treatment with oral pancreatic enzyme replacement with meals and snacks using guidelines similar to those for cystic fibrosis. Supplemental fat-soluble vitamins are also usually required. When monitored over time, approximately 50% of patients convert from pancreatic insufficiency to sufficiency because of spontaneous improvement in pancreatic enzyme secretion. This improvement is particularly evident after 4 years of age. A long-term plan should be initiated for early detection of severe cytopenias that require corrective action or malignant myeloid transformation. There are currently no data about the cost effectiveness of a specific leukemia surveillance program in SDS. However, it is generally accepted that it should include periodic blood counts with differentials and blood smears every 3 to 4 months, a clinical evaluation by a hematologist every 6

months, and BM testing every 1 to 3 years. The latter includes aspirates for smears and cytogenetics analyses. Concomitant BM biopsies are recommended when the patient's clinical status changes.

G-CSF

G-CSF given for profound neutropenia has been very effective in inducing a clinically beneficial neutrophil response. Data from the Severe Chronic Neutropenia International Registry (SCNIR) demonstrated that treatment with G-CSF results in a brisk neutrophil response in about 90% of patients. The response was sustained in some cases for more than 11 years (Beate Schwinzer, Hannover, Germany, personal communication).

Androgens

A smaller number of patients received androgens plus steroids for the treatment of FA, and improved BM function was also noted. Anecdotal cases treated with androgens alone, cyclosporine, or erythropoietin do not allow broad therapeutic conclusions. Few cases of patients who were treated with corticosteroids with some hematologic improvement were reported in the 1980s.

Blood Products and Other Supportive Care

Anemia and thrombocytopenia are managed with transfusions of RBCs or platelets when symptoms appear or prophylactically for profound cytopenias. Antifibrinolytic therapy with tranexamic acid can also be given for mild mucosal bleeding. Broad-spectrum antibiotics are indicated for febrile episodes and severe neutropenia.

Hematopoietic Stem Cell Transplantation

At present, the only curative option for severe BM failure in SDS is allogeneic HSCT. The indications for HSCT include BM failure with severe or symptomatic cytopenia, MDS with excess blasts (5–29%), or leukemia. Published data are limited and derived from case reports or small case series with a mix of sibling and matched unrelated donors. Two registries in Europe have provided additional information.

The European Group for Blood and Bone Marrow Transplantation (EBMT) Registry reported 26 transplanted patients with SDS. The indications included aplastic anemia ($n = 16$), MDS/AML ($n = 9$), or other ($n = 1$). Patients were transplanted with myeloablative conditioning regimens that included either busulfan or total-body irradiation. The majority of the donors were unrelated ($n = 19$). Eighty-one percent were engrafted. The incidence of grade III to IV GVHD was 24%; chronic GVHD was 29%. The overall survival was 65% at 1.1 years. Deaths were primarily caused by infections, GVHD, or major organ toxicities. Factors associated with adverse outcome included MDS/AML or usage of total-body irradiation.

The French Neutropenia Registry reported 10 transplanted patients with SDS. The indications included severe BM failure ($n = 5$) or MDS/leukemia ($n = 5$). Patients were conditioned with myeloablative regimens incorporating busulfan or total-body irradiation. Six received grafts from unrelated donors and four from a sibling donor. BM engraftment occurred in eight patients. The 5-year overall survival was 60%. Causes of death included infections related to neutropenia, GVHD, relapse, and transplant-related toxicity. Factors associated with adverse outcome included MDS/AML.

A note of caution is sounded regarding HSCT for SDS. Left ventricular fibrosis and necrosis without coronary arterial lesions has been reported in 50% of patients with SDS at autopsy, suggesting that there may be an increased risk of cardiotoxicity as well as other problems with the intensive preparatory chemotherapy used in HSCT. Indeed, published data emphasized that complications are more common in patients with SDS who receive chemotherapy or undergo transplantation than in non-SDS patients with aplastic anemia. Complications include cardiotoxicity, neurologic and renal complications, venoocclusive disease, pulmonary disease, posttransplant graft failure, and severe GVHD. The heightened risk for patients with SDS after transplantation can be explained in three ways: (1) the presence of the SDS BM stromal defect that is not corrected by the allograft and might be aggravated by the conditioning regimen; (2) increased sensitivity to chemotherapy and radiation, resulting in massive apoptosis in various organs; or (3) performing HSCT relatively late and at an advanced disease stage.

Results of reduced-intensity HSCT regimens have been published by two groups. In a study from Cincinnati published in 2008, six patients with severe cytopenia with or without clonal BM cytogenetic abnormalities and one patient with AML in remission were transplanted. The conditioning regimen included Campath-1H, fludarabine, and melphalan. Four patients received matched related MB, two received unrelated peripheral blood, and one had unrelated BM. All patients engrafted and were alive at a median follow-up of 548 (range, 93–920) days. In another study from Hannover, three patients received conditioning with fludarabine, treosulfan, and melphalan in addition to Campath-1H or rabbit ATG. Donor sources were matched sibling BM, matched unrelated BM, or 9/10 matched cord blood. The indications were severe BM failure (*n* = 2) and MDS (*n* = 1). The patients who received BM cells survived at 9 and 20 months posttransplant. The other patient died of idiopathic pneumonitis.

Future Directions

Mutant *SBDS* causes SDS in 90% of clinically diagnosed patients. The hunt for additional causative mutant genes in the other 10% is still underway. Identification of such gene(s) may expand our understanding of pathogenesis. Several other clinical and basic research questions in SDS must be addressed. First, the various biochemical functions of the *SBDS* gene require further study. How SBDS protein maintains normal hematopoiesis and protects from apoptosis as well as cancer is unclear. The natural history, and risk factors for the development of complications need to be determined. There is also a need to understand the mechanism for the heightened sensitivity of patients with SDS to chemotherapy and irradiation and to develop low-intensity regimens for HSCT. Research should continue on the efficacy of innovative drugs such as antiapoptotic agents in increasing the growth potential of HSCs and relieving the severity of cytopenia. Determining risk factors and molecular events during malignant myeloid transformation might prompt strategies for prevention and screening for complications.

Dyskeratosis Congenita

Background

DC is an inherited multisystem disorder of the mucocutaneous and hematopoietic systems in association with a wide variety of other somatic abnormalities. Originally, it was considered a dermatologic disease and was termed *Zinsser-Cole-Engman syndrome*. The traditional diagnostic ectodermal triad consists of reticulate skin pigmentation of the upper body, mucosal leukoplakia, and nail dystrophy. The skin and nail findings usually become apparent during the first 10 years of life, but the oral leukoplakia is observed later. These manifestations tend to progress as patients get older.

Hematologic manifestations were subsequently recognized to be a major component of the syndrome and are responsible for substantial morbidity and mortality. Indeed, the full diagnostic dermatologic triad is present only in about 46% of patients, but BM failure of varying severity is reported in up to 90% of cases. With the recent advances in understanding the molecular basis of the disease, patients with hematologic abnormalities but without dermatologic findings have been identified that dramatically changed the historical definition of the disease. Patients with DC also have a predisposition to develop solid tumors and MDS/AML.

Epidemiology

The estimated incidence of DC in childhood is about 4 cases per million per year. In older literature, most patients with DC were reported as males. However, with better understanding and broadening of the clinical spectrum of the disease and with more autosomal cases being identified, the proportion of males is much lower.

Pathobiology

Multiple genes have been associated with DC (see Table 29.1). DC genes encode components of the telomerase complex (*TERT*, *DKC1*, *TERC*, *NOP10*, and *NHP2*), T-loop assembly protein (*RTEL1*), telomere capping (*CTC1*), the telomere shelterin complex (*TINF2*), and the telomerase trafficking protein (*TCAB1*); all are critical for telomere maintenance. The **X-linked recessive** disease is a common form of DC. It was originally estimated to comprise as many as 75% of DC cases, but with the identification of more DC genes and more patients with autosomal dominant inheritance, the true incidence is approximately 30%. The X-linked disease is caused by mutations in *DKC1* on chromosome Xq28. *DKC1* encodes for the protein dyskerin. Dyskerin associates with the H/ACA class of RNA. Dyskerin binds to the 3′ H/ACA small nucleolar RNA-like domain of the *TERC* component of telomerase. This stimulates telomerase to synthesize telomeric repeats during DNA replication. Dyskerin is also involved in maturation of nascent rRNA. It binds to small nucleolar RNA through the 3′ H/ACA domain and catalyzes the isomerization of uridine to pseudouridine through its pseudouridine synthase homology domain. This might be the mechanism for impaired translation from internal ribosome entry sites seen in mice and human DC cells.

Several genes are mutated in families with **autosomal dominant** inheritance. *TINF2* is probably the most commonly mutated gene in this group and accounts for approximately 11% to 25% of the DC families. TINF2 protein is part of the shelterin protein complex that binds to and protects telomeres by allowing cells to distinguish between telomeres and regions of DNA damage. In the complex, TINF2 binds to TRF1, TRF2, POT1, TPP1, and RAP1.

Heterozygous mutations in *TERT* also results in autosomal dominant disease. *TERT* encodes for the enzyme component of telomerase. Telomerase is a ribonucleoprotein polymerase that maintains telomere ends by synthesis and addition of the telomere repeat TTAGGG at the 3′-hydroxy DNA terminus using the *TERC* RNA as a template.

Heterozygous mutations in the *TERC* gene are another cause of autosomal dominant DC. *TERC* encodes for the RNA component of telomerase and has a 3′ H/ACA small nucleolar RNA-like domain.

The **autosomal recessive** forms of DC are caused by biallelic mutations in *NOP10*, *NHP2*, *TERT*, or *TCAB1*. Interestingly, biallelic mutations in *TERT* and *TERC* have also been associated with a DC. In the latter families, parents might be affected with a milder disease. In the telomerase complex, the H/ACA domain of nascent human telomerase RNA forms a preribonucleoprotein with NAF1, dyskerin, NOP10, and NHP2. Initially, the core trimer dyskerin-NOP10-NHP2 forms to enable incorporation of NAF1, and efficient reverse transcription of telomere repeats. NOP10 and NHP2 also play an essential role in the assembly and activity of the H/ACA class of small nucleolar ribonucleoproteins that catalyze the isomerization of uridine to pseudouridine in rRNAs.

TCAB1 facilitates trafficking of telomerase to Cajal bodies. Mutations in this gene impair this trafficking activity and lead to misdirection of telomerase RNA to nucleoli; thereby preventing elongation of telomeres by telomerase.

DC with hemizygous mutations in the *DKC1* on the X chromosome, or heterozygous *TINF2* and biallelic *TERT* mutations can result in a severe form of DC called **Hoyeraal-Hreidarsson syndrome**. It is characterized by hematologic and dermatologic manifestations of DC in addition to cerebellar hypoplasia. Immune deficiency is common when this syndrome is caused by *DKC1* mutations. **Revesz syndrome** is a combination of classical manifestations of DC and exudative retinopathy. It is caused by mutations in *TINF2* and is an autosomal dominant form of the disease. *TINF2* mutations have also been found in children with severe **aplastic anemia** without physical anomalies. Biallelic mutations in *TERT* are also associated with a severe form of DC. However, heterozygosity for mutations in *TERT* is associated with a milder phenotype, late presentation, severe aplastic anemia without physical malformations, isolated pulmonary fibrosis, isolated hepatic fibrosis, or a combination of these clinical manifestations. Heterozygosity for mutations in *TERC* is associated with a milder phenotype, late presentation and severe aplastic anemia, or MDS without physical malformations. **Coats plus syndrome** is caused by mutations in the *CTC1* gene. It is characterized by retinal telangiectasia and exudates, intracranial calcification, leukodystrophy, brain cysts, osteopenia, gastrointestinal bleeding, and portal hypertension caused by the development of vasculature ectasias in the stomach, small intestine, and liver. Some patients with this disease have the additional manifestations of DC, which include sparse and gray hair, dystrophic nails, and anemia. Telomeres are short.

DC cells are characterized by very short telomeres. In several acquired and IBMFSs, telomeres are short compared with those from age-matched control participants. However, because the telomerase function is profoundly impaired in DC, the telomeres in this disease are very short (lower than the first percentile of the normal range). Shortening of telomeres results in cellular senescence, apoptosis ("cellular crisis"), or chromosome instability. However, some cells may survive the crisis by harboring compensatory genetic mutations that confer proliferative advantage and neoplastic potential.

DC is a chromosome "instability" disorder of a different type than FA. Results of clastogenic stress studies of DC cells are typically normal. There is no significant difference in chromosomal breakage between patient and normal lymphocytes with or without exposure to bleomycin, DEB, MMC, or γ-radiation. This contrasts sharply with FA cells and distinguishes one disorder from the other. However, metaphases of cultured patient peripheral blood cells, BM cells, and fibroblasts show numerous spontaneous unbalanced chromosome rearrangements such as dicentrics, tricentrics, and translocations. These are probably caused by short telomeres.

Most studies of the pathogenesis of the aplastic anemia in DC have shown a marked reduction or absence of CFU-GEMM, BFU-E, CFU-E, and CFU-GM. Long-term DC BM cultures have shown that hematopoiesis is severely defective in all patients with a low frequency of colony-forming cells. The function of DC BM stromal cells is normal in their ability to support growth of hematopoietic progenitors from normal BM, but generation of progenitors from DC BM cells seeded over normal stroma is reduced, suggesting that the defect in DC is of stem cell origin. Telomerase is activated in HSCs and might be necessary for HSC self-renewal capacity and prevention of senescence. The BM failure in this disorder may be a result of a progressive attrition and depletion of HSCs. This is supported by studies showing reduced number of CD34⁺/CD38⁻ in patients' bone marrows. Alternatively, the BM dysfunction may represent a failure of replication, maturation, or both.

iPSCs from patients with DC have been shown to have defects in telomere elongation during programming in a mechanism that is concordant with the mutated gene in the patients. In iPSCs from patients with heterozygous mutations in *TERT*, telomerase activity is directly affected. iPSCs from patients with mutant *DKC1* manifest reduced telomerase activity because of impaired telomerase assembly. iPSCs from a patient with *TCAB1* mutations are characterized by mislocalization of telomerase from Cajal bodies to nucleoli. It was also shown that extended culture of *DKC1*-mutant iPSCs leads to progressive telomere shortening and eventual loss of self-renewal. In contrast, another group studied telomerase reactivation and *TERC* regulation during reprogramming and showed that reprogramming restores telomere elongation in DC cells despite genetic lesions affecting telomerase. This group showed that *TERC* upregulation is a feature of the pluripotent state and that several telomerase components are targeted by pluripotency associated transcription factors.

Clinical Features

Clinical manifestations in dyskeratosis congenita often appear during childhood. The skin pigmentation and nail changes typically appear

first; mucosal leukoplakia and excessive ocular tearing appear later; and by the mid-teens, the serious complications of BM failure and malignancy begin to develop. In a portion of the patients, BM abnormalities appear before or without the skin manifestations.

The DC Registry data from England have detailed the prevalence of somatic abnormalities in families with classic DC. Cutaneous findings are a typical feature of the syndrome. Lacy reticulated skin pigmentation affecting the face, neck, chest, and arms is a common finding (89%). The degree of pigmentation increases with age and can involve the entire skin surface. There may also be a telangiectatic erythematous component. Nail dystrophy of the hands and feet is the next most common finding (88%) (Fig. 29.4). It usually starts with longitudinal ridging, splitting, or pterygium formation and may progress to complete nail loss. Leukoplakia usually involves the oral mucosa (78%), especially the tongue (Fig. 29.5), but may also be seen in the conjunctiva, anal, urethral, or genital mucosa. Hyperhidrosis of the palms and soles is common, and hair loss is sometimes seen. Eye abnormalities are observed in approximately 50% of cases. Excessive tearing (epiphora) secondary to nasolacrimal duct obstruction is common. Other ophthalmologic manifestations include conjunctivitis, blepharitis, loss of eyelashes, strabismus, and cataracts and optic atrophy. Abnormalities of the teeth, particularly an increased rate of dental decay and early loss of teeth, are common. Skeletal abnormalities such as osteoporosis with recurrent long bone fractures, avascular necrosis, abnormal bone trabeculation, scoliosis, and mandibular hypoplasia are seen in approximately 20% of cases. Genitourinary abnormalities include hypoplastic testes, hypospadias, phimosis, and urethral stenosis and horseshoe kidney. Gastrointestinal findings, such as esophageal strictures, hepatomegaly, or cirrhosis, are seen in 10% of cases. A subset of patients develops pulmonary fibrosis with reduced diffusion capacity or a restrictive defect. In fatal cases, lung tissue shows pulmonary fibrosis and abnormalities of the pulmonary vasculature. Hepatic fibrosis may also occur. Vasculopathy of the gut, kidneys, liver, chest, or other organs is seen in severe cases and may cause massive bleeding.

Laboratory Findings

Peripheral Blood, Bone Marrow, and Immunologic Findings

The incidence of cytopenias caused by BM failure has been reported in up to 90% of patients. Severe aplastic anemia occurs in about 50% of patients. When BM failure is evident, most patients already have physical manifestations of DC, but this is variable. The initial hematologic change is usually thrombocytopenia, anemia, or both followed by full-blown pancytopenia caused by aplastic anemia. The RBCs are often macrocytic, and the HbF can be elevated. It is noteworthy that early BM specimens and biopsies may be normocellular or hypercellular; however, with time, the cellular elements decline with a symmetric decrease in all hematopoietic lineages. Ferrokinetic studies at this point are consistent with aplastic anemia. Some patients with DC, particularly those with *DKC1* mutations, have immunologic abnormalities, including reduced immunoglobulin levels, reduced B- or T-lymphocyte numbers, and reduced or absent proliferative responses to PHA. Severe immunodeficiency necessitating HSCT has also been described.

On imaging studies, a small-sized cerebellum may give a clue to the diagnosis in patients with atypical presentations. Imaging of the skeleton usually shows nonspecific osteopenia.

Telomere length is a useful screening testing for DC. In the vast majority of patients, the telomeres are very short (i.e., lower than the first percentile adjusted to age).

Cancer Predisposition

Cancer develops in about 10% to 15% of patients, usually in the third and fourth decades of life. Similar to FA, patients with DC can develop solid tumors as well as MDS/AML. However, the incidence

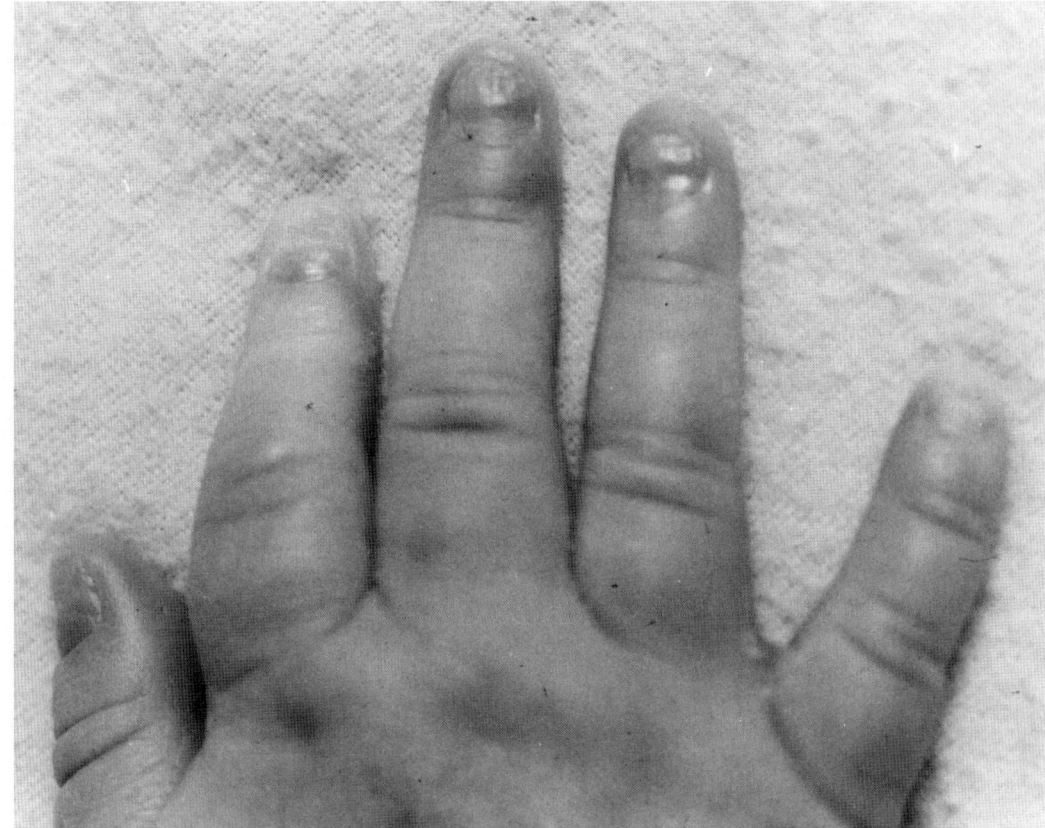

Fig. 29.4 DYSTROPHIC NAILS IN DYSKERATOSIS CONGENITA.

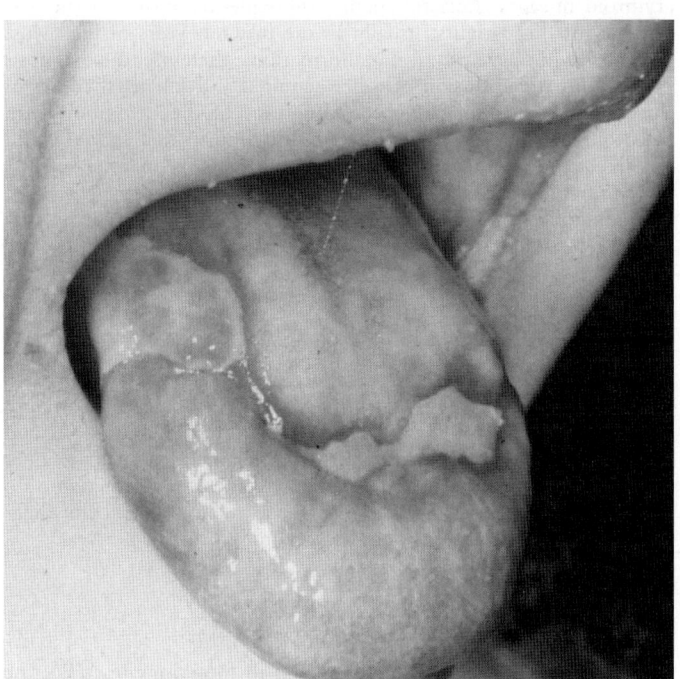

Fig. 29.5 LEUKOPLAKIA OF THE TONGUE IN DYSKERATOSIS CONGENITA.

multiple separate primaries in different sites involving the tongue and nasopharynx. Thus the sites of most of the cancers involve areas known to be abnormal in DC, such as mucous membranes and the gastrointestinal tract.

Differential Diagnosis

Several physical findings can be used to distinguish **FA** from DC. The following abnormalities are seen only in DC and not FA: nail dystrophy, leukoplakia, abnormalities of the teeth, hyperhidrosis of the palms and soles, and hair loss. Specific presentations of DC may have prominent overlap with other syndromes. The **Hoyeraal-Hreidarsson syndrome** variant of DC and the **Revesz syndrome** variant of DC are two examples. **The ataxia–pancytopenia syndrome** at least in some families is a variant of DC with mutations in *TINF2*. The spectrum of manifestations in **Coats plus syndrome** may lead to investigative workup towards inherited eye disorders and degenerative brain disease, but screening for DC by telomere length should be considered.

Natural History and Prognosis

In classical DC, nail dystrophy and skin pigmentation present first, often in the first 10 years of life. BM failure usually follows in the teenage years and twenties. The primary causes of death are hemorrhage secondary to thrombocytopenia or intestinal vascular anomalies, pulmonary fibrosis, sepsis from severe neutropenia, and complications after HSCT. In the patients who develop cancer or MDS/AML, the disease or its treatment can prove fatal. Pulmonary fibrosis can develop in 20% of cases and is typically progressive and culminates in death caused by respiratory failure. Considerable clinical heterogeneity exists even within the same family, and some patients live into their forties with only moderate nail changes and mild cytopenias.

of MDS/AML in DC is much lower than in FA. At the age of 50 years, the cumulative risk of solid cancers and MDS/AML is estimated as 40% and 3%, respectively. Most of the cancers are squamous cell carcinomas or adenocarcinomas, and the oropharynx and gastrointestinal tract are involved most frequently. Some patients have

The median survival in the cases reported in the past decade was estimated at 49 years.

Therapy

Androgens

Management of aplastic anemia is similar to treatment for FA. Androgens improve BM function in about 70% of patients. If a response is achieved and deemed to be sufficient or maximal, the minimal androgen dose to maintain this response should be considered. As in FA, patients typically become refractory to androgens as aplastic anemia progresses. Immunosuppressive therapy is not effective for this disorder, and a portion of the patients with DC are only diagnosed after failure to respond to immunosuppressive therapy for severe aplastic anemia. Since androgens have been shown to activate telomerase activity, the question whether they can alleviate symptoms related to nonhematologic complications of DC needs to be answered.

G-CSF

A small number of patients were reported who responded to G-CSF therapy with significant increases in absolute neutrophil counts (ANCs). Similarly, two other patients received GM-CSF therapy that resulted in improved neutrophil numbers. G-CSF with erythropoietin resulted in a trilineage hematologic response in one patient. G-CSF plus androgens has led to splenic peliosis and rupture in DC and is not recommended as a long-term treatment if a donor for HSCT is available. Although the reports are scanty, cytokine therapy appears to offer potential benefit, at least in the short term, especially for improving granulopoiesis.

Hematopoietic Stem Cell Transplantation

Publications focusing on HSCT in DC are mostly isolated case reports or a small series that limit one's ability to make meaningful correlations of the types of regimens, donors, and indications with outcome. The older literature consists of patients who received myeloablative regimens resulting in a median survival of approximately 3 years after HSCT. Causes of death include unusual complications related to DC that are not prevented by HSCT such as vascular lesions of the gut, kidneys, liver, and lung (≈50% of patients) and fibrosis involving the lung and liver (≤40% of patients). A recent review of the CIBMTR database identified 34 patients with DC who had been transplanted between 1981 and 2009. The overall 10-year survival among this group was 30%. Early posttransplant deaths were caused by graft failure and other transplant-related complications. Late mortality was related to pulmonary failure. These striking complications after HSCT probably reflect the natural history of the disease. However, it is not known whether HSCT can accelerate their course. These unusual complications, uniquely seen in DC, have not been reported in other IBMFSs such as FA.

DC is a disorder with chromosomal instability caused by flawed telomere maintenance. This might explain the hypersensitivity to irradiation and chemotherapy. The increased hypersensitivity of patients with DC to transplant conditioning can be related to the telomere shortening from DC combined with the accelerated telomere shortening that occurs after HSCT. Further, because of the high degree of mucocutaneous involvement, patients with DC may be more susceptible to endothelial damage, which occurs after HSCT as a result of various factors, including the conditioning regimen, cyclosporine A, infectious diseases, GVHD, and cytokine storm. The increased predisposition to posttransplant complications and the tendency to develop tumors highlight the need to avoid certain conditioning agents such as busulfan and irradiation and possibly reduce the intensity of the transplant preparative regiments.

The strategy of using low-intensity fludarabine-based protocols for HSCT has produced encouraging results for patients with DC. From 2002–2013, 25 patients were transplanted using reduced intensity protocols (mostly fludarabine-based). Overall, 20 of the 25 were reported alive at 10 to 212 months posttransplant. These regimens appear to be well tolerated and allow prompt engraftment without significant complications. However, the benefit in reducing the risk of nonhematologic disease-related complications, such as bleeding from vascular lesions and respiratory failure caused by pulmonary fibrosis, is not clear. Posttransplant deaths among published cases in which reduced intensity transplant regimens were incorporated include such complications. All the three Toronto patients reported in 2003 did develop these complications 7 to 14 years after transplant. Also, the role of these conditioning regimens in increasing the additive risk of cancer caused by HSCT is still to be determined.

Future Directions

So far, about 75% of the patients with DC can be genotyped. Clearly, there is a need to discover additional DC genes. Furthermore, the mechanism by which impaired activity, transport, and stability of telomerase and other ribonucleoprotein complexes influence HSC function requires clarification. The complete spectra of disorders and phenotypes caused by mutations in these genes are still to be defined. Effective therapies with reduced toxicity are necessary to prevent devastating complications such as BM failure, pulmonary fibrosis, and vascular anomalies. Last, there is a need for studies focusing on translating this genetic knowledge into gene therapy.

Congenital Amegakaryocytic Thrombocytopenia

Background

CAMT is an autosomal recessive syndrome that typically presents in infancy with isolated thrombocytopenia caused by reduced or absent BM megakaryocytes with preservation initially of granulopoietic and erythroid lineages. Aplastic anemia subsequently ensues in the vast majority of the patients, usually in the first few years of life. Most patients do not have physical malformations; therefore, the diagnosis depends on the exclusion of other acquired and inherited causes of thrombocytopenia in early life. Mutations of the thrombopoietin receptor, MPL, have been identified and confirm that sporadic and familial cases are inherited in an autosomal recessive manner. CAMT is a distinct genetic entity, but mutations in several other genes have been described in a number of inherited thrombocytopenias that must be considered in the differential diagnosis (Table 29.5).

Epidemiology

More than 100 cases have been reported in the literature. However, some patients might be reported more than once. On the other hand, with the recent identification of patients with MPL mutations and relatively late presentation, it is possible that the incidence is higher and includes a portion of the patients with aplastic anemia who do not respond to immunosuppressive therapy. The incidence of diagnosed cases is estimated at one case per million births per year.

Pathobiology

The defect in CAMT is directly related to mutations in MPL, the gene for the thrombopoietin receptor that maps to 1p34 in 94% of patients. Heterozygote carriers of the mutant gene have normal blood cell counts. Affected individuals have mutations in both alleles in either homozygous or compound heterozygous state. Mutations have been found throughout the MPL gene, including nonsense, missense, frameshift, and splicing mutations. The mutations cause either reduced cell surface receptor expression or defective TPO binding and receptor activation. A genotype–phenotype correlation has been identified in CAMT patients and two prognostic groups were established, types I and II.

TABLE 29.5   Miscellaneous Inherited Thrombocytopenia Disorders and Their Major Hematologic Features

Disorder	Genetics	Mutant Gene	Platelet Size[a]	Features
Amegakaryocytic thrombocytopenia	AR	*MPL*	Normal	± Physical anomalies
Thrombocytopenia absent radii	AR	*RBM8A*	Normal	Physical anomalies
MYH9-related thrombocytopenia: May-Hegglin anomaly	AD	*MYH9*	Large	Neutrophil inclusions
Fechtner syndrome	AD	*MYH9*	Large	Neutrophil inclusions, hearing loss, nephritis
Epstein syndrome	AD	*MYH9*	Large	No inclusions, hearing loss, nephritis
Sebastian syndrome	AD	*MYH9*	Large	Neutrophil inclusions
X-linked macrothrombocytopenia	X-L	*GATA1*	Large	Anemia, dyserythropoiesis, thalassemia
Wiskott-Aldrich syndrome	X-L	*WAS*	Small	Immune deficiency, eczema
X-linked thrombocytopenia	X-L	*WAS*	Small	No associated features
Thrombocytopenia and radio-ulnar synostosis	AD	*HOXA11*	Normal	Fused radius, limited range of motion
Familial platelet disorder/AML	AD	*AML1 (RUNX1; CBFA2)*	Normal	MDS, AML
Familial dominant thrombocytopenia	AD	*FLJ14813*	Normal	No associated features
Paris-Trousseau thrombocytopenia	AD	*FLI1* (hemizygous deletion)	Large	Dysmegakaryocytopoiesis, Jacobsen syndrome
Bernard-Soulier syndrome	AR	*GP1BA*	Large	No associated features
Bernard-Soulier carrier/Mediterranean macrothrombocytopenia	AD	*GP1BA*	Large	No associated features

[a]Platelet size: small, MPV <7 fL; normal, MPV 7-11 fL; large or giant, MPV >11 fL.
AD, Autosomal dominant; AML, acute myeloid leukemia; AR, autosomal recessive; MDS, myelodysplastic syndrome; MPV, mean platelet volume; X-L, X-linked recessive.

Type 1

Frameshift, nonsense and splicing mutations result in a complete loss of function of and signaling from the thrombopoietin receptor in type I by deletion of all or most of the intracellular domain. This causes persistently low platelet counts and a rapid progression to pancytopenia. Thrombopoietin plays a critical role in the proliferation, survival, and differentiation of early and late megakaryocytes. This clearly explains the thrombocytopenia. However, *MPL* is also highly expressed in HSCs and promotes their quiescence and survival. Thus MPL protein insufficiency may account for depletion of HSCs and pancytopenia. Evolution into severe aplastic anemia is particularly common in type I.

Type II

CAMT with missense and certain splicing mutations cause reduced expression of the protein, reduced localization to the plasma membrane (e.g., R102P in the extracellular domain), or an inability to bind thrombopoietin (e.g., F104S). Patients with these mutations have a milder course; a transient increase in platelet counts during the first years of life; and delayed onset, if any, of pancytopenia, indicating residual receptor function.

Serial studies of CAMT hematopoiesis using clonogenic assays have been informative. Initially, when the only hematologic abnormality is isolated thrombocytopenia, the numbers of hematopoietic progenitors are comparable to those of control participants, including the number of megakaryocyte precursors, CFU-MK (colony-forming unit megakaryocytes). As the disease evolves into aplastic anemia, the peripheral blood counts decline, and colony numbers from progenitors belonging to each myeloid lineage also decline in parallel. Stromal cells established in short- and long-term cultures of patient BM show normal proliferative activity and yield a "fertile" BM microenvironment for patient and control BM colony growth. The findings are consistent with current knowledge about *MPL* mutations, namely, that the central problem in CAMT is an intrinsic HSC defect rather than an abnormality of the BM milieu.

Other data demonstrate measurable numbers of CFU-MK progenitors in vitro from patients with CAMT when studied early in the disease in response to IL-3, GM-CSF, or a combination of both but defective CFU-MK colony formation in response to recombinant human thrombopoietin that fits with *MPL* mutations. Plasma thrombopoietin levels in patients with CAMT are always elevated and are among the highest seen in any patient population.

The pathogenesis of the associated neurologic abnormalities (see Clinical Features) is less understood; however, MPL is expressed in the neuronal cells and might be important for their development.

Clinical Features

Almost all patients present with a petechial rash, bruising, or bleeding during the first year of life. Most cases are obvious at birth or within the first 2 months. Most patients with proven *MPL* mutations have normal physical and imaging features, but isolated cases with anomalies have been identified. Many of the published cases with CAMT and physical malformation were not tested for *MPL* mutations. A patient in the CIMFR with an *MPL* mutation had a cystic fourth ventricle and Dandy-Walker malformation (Dror, unpublished data). The commonest anomalies in published phenotypic CAMT patients are neurologic, including varying degrees of cerebellar hypoplasia or agenesis, cerebral atrophy, cortical dysplasia and lissencephaly, and hypoplasia of the corpus callosum and brainstem. Facial malformations have also been described. Developmental delay is a prominent feature among those with physical malformations. Patients may also have microcephaly and an abnormal facies.

Congenital heart disease with a variety of malformations can be detected, including atrial septal defects, ventricular septal defects, patent ductus arteriosus, tetralogy of Fallot, and coarctation of the aorta. Some of these occur in combinations. Other anomalies include abnormal hips or feet, kidney malformations, eye anomalies, and cleft or high-arched palate. Some affected sibships manifested both normal and abnormal physical findings in the same family.

Laboratory Findings

Thrombocytopenia is the major laboratory finding with normal hemoglobin levels and white blood cell counts initially. Although there are usually measurable but reduced platelet numbers, peripheral

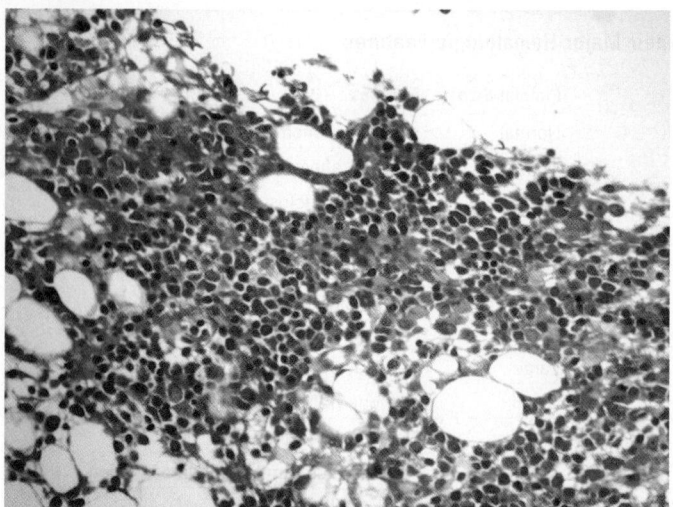

Fig. 29.6 LOW-POWER VIEW OF A BONE MARROW ASPIRATE FROM A NEWLY DIAGNOSED PATIENT WITH CONGENITAL AMEGAKARYOCYTIC THROMBOCYTOPENIA. The three findings are normal cellularity, normal granulopoiesis and erythropoiesis, and absent megakaryocytes. (*Photomicrograph prepared by Dr. Mohamed Abdelhaleem, Toronto.*)

blood platelets may be totally absent. Those that can be identified are of normal size and appearance. Similar to several other IBMFSs, RBCs may be macrocytic. HbF is increased in most but not all patients. BM aspirates and biopsies initially show normal cellularity with markedly reduced or absent megakaryocytes (Fig. 29.6). In patients who develop aplastic anemia, BM cellularity is decreased with fatty replacement, and the erythropoietic and granulopoietic lineages are symmetrically reduced.

Predisposition to Leukemia

Cases with CAMT have been reported with secondary clonal BM cytogenetic abnormalities such as monosomy 7 and trisomy 8, MDS, or AML. Several published cases clearly demonstrate a typical progression of thrombocytopenia, aplastic anemia, and clonal or malignant myeloid transformation. One boy with a normal physical appearance had amegakaryocytic thrombocytopenia from day 1 of life, developed aplastic anemia at 5 years of age, responded poorly to androgens and steroids, and then developed AML at age 16 years with death at age 17 years. A girl had thrombocytopenia at 2 months of age, pancytopenia at 5 months, and thereafter developed a preleukemic picture with clonal abnormalities involving chromosome 19. Another patient had thrombocytopenia at 6 months of age, developed progressive aplastic anemia over the next 2 years, acquired monosomy 7 in BM cells at 5 years of age, and then developed MDS with an activating *RAS* oncogene mutation in hematopoietic cells. Hence the current evidence indicates that CAMT is another IBMFS that is preleukemic. The risk or incidence of malignant conversion is difficult to determine because of the rarity of the disease and the paucity of published data, and because patients frequently require early HSCT.

Differential Diagnosis

If CAMT presents at birth or shortly after, it must be distinguished from other causes of severe neonatal thrombocytopenia, which most commonly are caused by severe systemic infections (e.g., by bacteria or viruses). Usually, these infectious etiologies are characterized by increased peripheral destruction of platelets or a combination of peripheral destruction and BM suppression. Congenital infections collectively designated as the **TORCH** (*Toxoplasma gondii*, **r**ubella, **c**ytomegalovirus, and **h**erpes simplex virus) **syndrome** should be considered.

Passive transplacental passage of IgG antiplatelet antibodies into fetal circulation can cause rapid destruction of fetal platelets. This occurs in two circumstances: a (1) **maternal autoimmune disease** such as idiopathic thrombocytopenic purpura or systemic lupus erythematosus and (2) in **neonatal alloimmune thrombocytopenia** by alloimmunization of the pregnant mother to fetal antigens inherited from father but absent in the mother. In the former situation, the mother has thrombocytopenia or a history of such; in the latter situation, the mother has a normal platelet count and serum antibodies to human platelet alloantigens.

Thrombocytopenia with absent radii syndrome is distinguished from CAMT because in TAR, the radii are absent. Peripheral blood chromosomes analysis is not associated with increased breakage with DEB or MMC clastogenic stress testing, which allows CAMT to be distinguished from **FA**. Increased platelet destruction also occurs in newborns with giant benign hemangiomas of skin, liver, or spleen, the so-called **Kasabach-Merritt syndrome.**

In an infant or young child with a CAMT clinical diagnosis but without mutant *MPL*, **other inherited forms of thrombocytopenia** should be addressed (see Table 29.5). These can generally be classified according to inheritance pattern (autosomal dominant, autosomal recessive, or X-linked recessive), size of the platelets (small, normal, large or giant), and presence or absence of associated clinical features. Identification of the specific mutant gene for each disorder confirms the diagnosis.

If CAMT presents beyond the neonatal age period, it must be distinguished from causes of peripheral platelet destruction such as in chronic immune thrombocytopenia purpura, acquired amegakaryocytic thrombocytopenia or aplastic anemia, other IBMFSs, MDS, and acute leukemias. The medical history of the patient and family, physical examination, and initial laboratory test results may help to exclude other disorders. However, a BM aspirate and biopsy will point to the diagnosis, and a *MPL* mutational analysis will confirm the diagnosis.

Therapy and Prognosis

Supportive treatment has been largely unsatisfactory to date, and the mortality rate from thrombocytopenic bleeding, complications of aplastic anemia, or malignant myeloid transformation has been very close to 100%. For that reason, HLA typing of family members should be performed as soon as the diagnosis is confirmed to determine if a matched related donor for HSCT exists. If not, a search for a matched unrelated donor or for a cord blood graft should ensue as soon as the severity of the clinical picture is appreciated. The need for transfusional support is a cogent indication.

Platelet transfusions should be used discretely. Platelet numbers should not be a sole indication; clinical bleeding is a more appropriate trigger for the use of platelets. Single-donor filtered platelets are preferred to multiple unfiltered random donor platelets to minimize sensitization, and if HSCT is a realistic possibility, all blood products should be free of cytomegalovirus and irradiated.

Androgens may induce a partial response, but the effect is short-lived. Androgens can be considered when HSCT is contraindicated or as a temporary measure until HSCT donor is available. Corticosteroids have been used for thrombocytopenia with no apparent efficacy.

Based on the in vitro augmentation of megakaryocyte progenitor colony growth in response to IL-3, a small phase I/II clinical trial was initiated for CAMT. IL-3 resulted in improved platelet counts in two of five patients and decreased bleeding and transfusion requirements in the other three. Prolonged IL-3 administration in two additional patients also resulted in platelet increments. This pilot study illustrates that IL-3 may have been an important adjunct to the medical management of CAMT, but it was not adopted broadly and is no longer commercially available. GM-CSF has a positive in vitro effect but not in vivo. Thrombopoietin has not been tried for the treatment of severe type I CAMT and would likely fail because endogenous thrombopoietin levels are markedly increased and the mutated thrombopoietin receptor is nonfunctional. Nevertheless, thrombopoietin agonists that bind to the transmembrane domain might prove efficacious, similar to the in vitro effect of LGD-4665 on cells carrying the F104S *MPL* mutation. LGD-4665 binds to the transmembrane domain of the MPL receptor. Initial application of such a strategy should be assessed as part of clinical trials because of a potential risk of developing hematologic malignancies.

CAMT can be cured by HSCT. Most of the recent published cases have had successful outcomes. Matched sibling donor sources are ideal even if the donor is a carrier with one mutant allele. Reduced-intensity conditioning regimens for CAMT have been successfully used in both related and unrelated donor setting. Such an approach was successful even in a case with monosomy 7 from the CIMFR who received BM from an unrelated donor. HSCT using T cell–depleted BM with relatively high CD34$^+$ cell numbers and enhanced T cell–specific immunosuppression in the transplant cytoreductive regimens that have also been successful.

Future Directions

Novel therapy that can activate the mutated thrombopoietin receptor may be suitable for some patients with CAMT. Alternatively, drugs that stimulate downstream targets of the receptor might be effective. The cellular consequences of specific gene mutations need to be further studied because this might help to develop novel strategies in patients who do not respond to such therapies. CAMT is also a candidate disease for gene therapy because restoration of wild-type *MPL* would provide in vivo selection of corrected HSCs.

Other Inherited Syndromes With Associated Pancytopenia

Bone marrow failure and cancer predisposition can occur as part of several specific other inherited syndromes and in familial settings that do not exactly correspond with the entities already described.

Down Syndrome

Down syndrome, or constitutional trisomy 21 (+21), has a unique association with aberrant hematologic abnormalities. Four related events can occur. In the neonatal period, a *transient myeloproliferative disorder* with large numbers of circulating blast cells has been observed in approximately 10% of these infants. The blasts show somatic *GATA1* mutations and apparently are clonal but, remarkably, disappear spontaneously over several weeks in most cases.

Second, in 20% to 30% of these transient cases, *true* acute megakaryoblastic leukemia (AMKL), also with *GATA1* mutations, appears later and requires treatment. Acute lymphoblastic and myeloblastic leukemias are also seen in Down syndrome, but AMKL is the most common form of myeloblastic leukemia and is estimated to be 500 times greater in children with trisomy 21 than in other children.

Third, the onset of AMKL is frequently preceded by an interval of MDS characterized by thrombocytopenia; abnormal megakaryocytopoiesis; megakaryoblasts in the BM; and an abnormal karyotype, commonly trisomy 8 or monosomy 7.

Fourth, a few patients have been reported with aplastic anemia. Of six trisomy 21 with aplastic anemia cases that we identified in the literature, three died of BM failure, two responded to androgen therapy, and one underwent HSCT.

Dubowitz Syndrome

This is an autosomal recessive disorder characterized by a peculiar facies, infantile eczema, small stature, and mild microcephaly. The face is small with a shallow supraorbital ridge, a nasal bridge at the same level as the forehead, short palpebral fissures, variable ptosis, and micrognathia. This is a rare disorder, and incidence rates for complications are difficult to establish; however, there appears to be a predilection to develop cancer as well as hematopoietic disorders in children with Dubowitz syndrome. Patients have developed acute leukemia, neuroblastoma, and lymphoma. Approximately 10% of patients also develop hematologic abnormalities varying from hypoplastic anemia to moderate pancytopenia and full-blown aplastic anemia. A homozygous splice-site mutation in the *NSUN2* gene has been identified in one family. The gene encodes a conserved RNA methyltransferase. Patient cells lack expression of the protein.

Seckel Syndrome

Sometimes called *bird-headed dwarfism,* patients with this autosomal recessive developmental disorder have marked intrauterine and postnatal growth failure, mental deficiency, severe microcephaly, a hypoplastic face with a receding forehead and chin, a prominent curved nose, and low-set or malformed ears. Some patients may show increased chromosomal breakage in lymphocyte cultures with DEB or MMC and mimic FA. About 25% of patients develop aplastic anemia or malignancies. There are possibly five genes linked to Seckel syndrome, all in different cytogenetic locations. There are several genes that have been linked to Seckel syndrome: mutant *ATR* has been associated with Seckel Type 1, *RBBP8* with Type 2, *CENPJ* with Type 4, *CEP152* with Type 5, *CEP63* with Type 6, and *ATRIP* with Type 8. The abnormal gene for Seckel 3 has been mapped to 14q21-q22. Genotyping will distinguish FA from Seckel syndrome.

Reticular Dysgenesis

Reticular dysgenesis is a combined immunodeficiency and BM failure disorder. It is characterized by severe lymphopenia and agranulocytosis. Anemia, thrombocytopenia and aplastic anemia may be evident. Immunologically, the disorder is a variant of severe combined immune deficiency in which cellular and humoral immunity are absent. A striking feature is absent lymph nodes and tonsils and an absent thymic shadow on radiographs. Because of profoundly compromised immunity, the syndrome presents early with severe infection at birth or shortly thereafter. BM specimens are hypocellular with markedly reduced myeloid and lymphoid elements. Clonogenic assays of hematopoietic progenitors consistently show reduced to absent colony growth, indicating that the disorder has its origins at the HSC level. The mode of inheritance is autosomal recessive caused by biallelic mutations in mitochondrial *AK2*. The only curative therapy is HSCT.

Schimke Immunoosseous Dysplasia

Schimke immunoosseous dysplasia is an autosomal recessive disorder caused by mutations in the chromatin remodeling gene *SMARCAL1* in 50% to 60% of patients. Patients manifest spondyloepiphyseal dysplasia with exaggerated lumbar lordosis and a protruding abdomen. They have pigmentary skin changes and abnormally discolored and configured teeth. Renal dysfunction can be problematic with proteinuria and nephrotic syndrome. Approximately 50% of patients have hypothyroidism and 50% have cerebral ischemia; 50% have anemia, 50% have neutropenia, 30% have thrombocytopenia, and 10% have aplastic anemia. Lymphopenia and altered cellular immunity are present in 80% of patients. Hematopoietic stem cell transplantation has been applied in five cases with severe BM failure/immunodeficiency; one of them survived.

Noonan Syndrome

Noonan syndrome (NS) is a developmental disorder characterized by the *Noonan facies* (hypertelorism, ptosis, short neck, low-set ears), short stature, congenital heart disease, and multiple skeletal and hematologic abnormalities. The literature describes several NS patients who developed amegakaryocytic thrombocytopenia and another who developed pancytopenia and a hypocellular BM. NS is an autosomal dominant disorder with genetic heterogeneity. So far, heterozygous germline mutations in one of 14 genes (*PTPN11, SOS1, KRAS, NRAS, RAF1, BRAF, SHOC2, MEK1, CBL, RASA2, RIT1, MAP2K1, SOS2,* and *LZTR1*) underlie the disorder in 75% of cases. These genes encode for proteins in the RAS-mitogen–activated protein kinases signal transduction pathway. A variant of neurofibromatosis type 1(NF1) caused by germline mutations in the *NF1* gene shares a phenotypic overlap disorder with NS, the so-called *neurofibromatosis–Noonan syndrome*. Remarkably, children with NS have an increased risk of juvenile myelomonocytic leukemia (JMML); however, in contrast to classical JMML, NS-associated myeloproliferative disorder has an aggressive course, and typically remits spontaneously within several months. The thrombocytopenia may persist after the myeloproliferative process improves. Of note, some of the mutated genes that cause NS (e.g., *PTPN11, KRAS,* and *NRAS*) are also found as somatic mutations in BM cells from children with JMML.

Cartilage-Hair Hypoplasia

Cartilage-hair hypoplasia (CHH) is an autosomal recessive syndrome characterized by metaphyseal dysostosis; short-limbed dwarfism; and fine, sparse hair. Additional skeletal findings include scoliosis, lordosis, chest deformity, and varus lower limbs. Aganglionic megacolon and other gastrointestinal abnormalities have been reported. Most cases in the literature are Finnish or Amish. Mutations in the noncoding RNA gene *RMRP* are seen in more than 80% of cases. Macrocytic anemia of varying severity is seen in the majority of patients. Most patients have mild and self-limited anemia, but some are severe and persistent, resembling DBA, and require RBC transfusions. Severe immunodeficiency can occur, often with the severe anemia. HSCT has been used successfully to reconstitute the immune system. Neutropenia has been reported in 25% of CHH cases and lymphopenia in 65%. Lymphomas and basal cell carcinoma also occur at an increased frequency.

Pearson Syndrome

Pearson syndrome is an inherited failure of BM and, in 30% of cases, impaired exocrine pancreatic function caused by acinar cell atrophy and fibrosis. Patients with Pearson syndrome have a maternally inherited diagnostic deletion of mtDNA that encodes enzymes that are critical to oxidative phosphorylation. The genetic deletion results in a syndrome of refractory anemia with ringed sideroblasts and prominent vacuolization of BM erythroid and myeloid precursors. Physical malformations are rarely observed. Severe anemia requiring transfusions is present within the first year of life, sometimes at birth. Pancytopenia may occur alone or in association with hepatic failure and a renal tubulopathy leading to lactic acidosis. The projected median survival time is 4 years. Anemia is managed with RBC and platelet transfusional support. Erythropoietin has been used for the anemia of renal failure. G-CSF is indicated for severe neutropenia. HSCT has been used in two cases with Pearson syndrome; both patients engrafted and achieved normal blood counts. One of the children survived at 3 years follow-up post-HSCT. The second patient developed acute myeloid leukemia 12 months post-HSCT and died. Interestingly, HSCT was associated not only with improved hematopoiesis, but also with resolution of lactacidemia and acidosis. Although HSCT was traditionally not recommended for the hematopoietic complications of Pearson syndrome because of their tendency to improve spontaneously in most cases, further studies are necessary to decipher HSCT role in this disease. The need for pancreatic enzyme replacement is unclear.

Unclassified Inherited Forms of Bone Marrow Failure

Bone marrow failure can cluster in families, but many of these cases cannot be readily classified into discrete diagnostic entities such as FA, SDS, or DC. In other cases, the patients manifest chronic BM shortly after birth or have physical malformations and most likely also have IBMFSs. The phenotype of these unclassified cases can be complex with varying combinations of cytopenias, macrocytosis, elevated levels of HbF, hypocellular BM, immunologic deficiency, physical malformations, and predisposition to leukemia. The BM failure might be the result of mutations in novel IBMFS genes or atypical presentations of classified syndromes. Complex interplay of mutations in multiple genes, modifying genes, epigenetic processes, acquired factors, and chance effects that may be specific to each affected cases cannot be excluded. Published examples of unclassified IBMFSs have been reviewed and divided into inheritance patterns, and then subdivided into cases with and without physical anomalies.

Using the Canada-wide database of the CIMFR, a unique study was launched on IBMFS cases that were deemed unclassifiable at study entry. Of 162 enrolled patients, 39 were registered as having an unclassified disorder. Although the hematologic phenotypes were similar to the classified syndromes in the registry (single- or multilineage cytopenia, severe aplastic anemia, MDS, AML, and cancer), the patients presented at an older age (median, 9 months versus median 1 month for classified), and the variation in clinical presentations was substantial. Grouping patients according to physical abnormalities and hematologic phenotype was not always sufficient to characterize or diagnose a condition because affected members from several families fit into different phenotypic groupings. It was difficult to formulate a sensible and cost-effective diagnostic workup based on the family histories and hematologic and physical findings. Compared with workups of classifiable syndromes, clastogenic chromosomal fragility testing and extensive genotyping efforts of the unclassified cases required use of several-fold higher specific diagnostic tests at a cost that was 4.5 times higher per evaluated patient. Despite these efforts and the huge, recent explosion of gene discovery, only 20% of unclassified patients were diagnosed with a specific syndrome, underscoring ongoing diagnostic limitations for these disorders.

Treatment of Unclassified Familial Forms of Bone Marrow Failure

Because these disorders are rare, broad conclusions about management are difficult to formulate. For full-blown aplastic anemia with a hypocellular, fatty BM or for MDS/AML, curative therapy with HSCT remains the first choice if a suitable donor is identified. In the familial cases, potential related stem cell donors must be thoroughly assessed clinically, hematologically, and by diagnostic laboratory testing to ensure that latent or masked BM dysfunction is not present. If a matched sibling donor is not available, an unrelated donor search should be initiated, and in the interim, principles of medical management with androgens and supportive care similar to other IBMFSs can be used.

INHERITED BONE MARROW FAILURE SYNDROMES WITH PREDOMINANTLY ANEMIA

Diamond-Blackfan Anemia

Background

DBA, previously called *congenital hypoplastic anemia*, is an inherited form of pure RBC aplasia. The syndrome is heterogeneous with respect to genetic causes, clinical and laboratory findings, in vitro data, and therapeutic outcome. DBA is the first disease to be identified as a *ribosomopathy*. It is also the best example of the ribosomopathies because except for *GATA1*, all currently known

DBA genes are components of the small or large ribosome subunits. Except for the rare cases with mutations in *GATA1*, all genetically proven cases show autosomal dominant inheritance with variable penetrance. Recessive inheritance was inferred in more than 30 families published in the literature that had affected siblings with normal parents, affected cousins, or consanguinity. However, these cases have not been confirmed as autosomal recessive. Some of these may be autosomal dominant with partial penetrance or arise from gonadal mosaicism.

Epidemiology

Based on data from a European registry of DBA patients, the estimated incidence of the disorder as assessed for France over a 13-year period was 7.3 cases per million live births. Data from the CIMFR show an incidence of 10.4 cases per million live births as assessed over a 9-year period. Although the majority of published patients are white, DBA has been recognized in several ethnic groups, including African blacks, Arabs, East Indians, and Japanese.

In terms of gender distribution, both sexes are equally affected. About 80% of DBA cases are sporadic.

Genetics

The discovery of 16 DBA genes (see Table 29.1) demonstrates heterozygosity for mutations in the respective genes consistent with autosomal dominant inheritance in most currently known genetic groups. Except for *GATA1*, all known DBA proteins are structural components of either the small or large ribosomal subunits.

In most DBA cases peripheral blood karyotype is normal. Discovery of a balanced reciprocal translocation t(x;19) in a sporadic female case of DBA and the identification of microdeletions on chromosome 19 in some other DBA patients led to the identification of the first DBA gene mutation. Subsequent studies revealed mutations in one allele for the gene in 25% of patients, and it is currently the most common known mutant DBA gene.

RPS19 protein is a component of the ribosomal 40S subunit. Multiple other genes encoding either the 40S small ribosome subunit or 60S ribosome subunit have been subsequently identified in DBA. The second most commonly mutated gene in DBA is *RPL5*. It is mutated in 12% to 21% of patients. Other mutated genes are *RPL11* (7–9% of patients), *RPS26* (10%), *RPS10* (4%), *RPS24* (2%), *RPL35a* (2%), *RPS17* (<1%), and *RPS7* (<1%). About 70% of patients with DBA can now be genotyped.

It is important to note that about 20% of patients with DBA have large deletion in one of the DBA genes rather than nucleotide-level mutations. Therefore metaphase cytogenetics and molecular karyotyping to detect microscopic and submicroscopic deletions, respectively, should be included in the genetic testing process if the sequencing of known DBA gene is negative.

Pathophysiology

Recent studies have shed light on the function of the RPS19 protein in ribosome biogenesis. RPS19 associates with the ribosomal subunit 40S. It is critical for normal maturation of rRNA because its deficiency causes defective cleavage of the pre-rRNA at the ITS1 sequence and abnormal maturation of the 40S subunit. This leads to accumulation of faulty pre-40S ribosome subunits.

Other ribosomal proteins that are mutated in DBA are also critical for ribosome biogenesis, For example, it has been shown that the yeast RPL11 is positioned at the intersubunit cleft of the large ribosome subunit central protuberance, thereby forming an intersubunit bridge with the small subunit protein S18. Mutations in this region such as F96 and A66 lead to halfmer formation. Mutations in *RPS24* also impair pre-rRNA processing of the 18S rRNA and decrease the production of the 40S ribosomal subunit. On the other hand,

depletion of RPL35A reduces the amount of the 60S subunit and of the mature 80S ribosomes.

The mechanism by which ribosomal protein gene mutations impairs RBC development remains unknown. In 25% of cases with mutant *RPS19,* the prevailing opinion is that the disorder results from protein haploinsufficiency. In support of this, two classes of *RPS19* mutations have been described: quantitative defects resulting in undetectable protein and hotspot mutations leading to loss of function. Additional links between *RPS19* and erythropoiesis have now been clearly established. Defective erythropoiesis ensues when *RPS19* is knocked down in cellular models. In addition, wild-type gene transfer corrects the defective erythropoiesis in *RPS19*-deficient DBA CD34+ cells resulting in a threefold increase in erythroid colony growth. In yeast, the introduction of *RPS19* mutations found in DBA results in a defect in the processing of pre-rRNA similar to that observed in DBA cells with decreased expression of *RPS19*.

A large body of evidence indicates that the erythroid progenitor compartment is intrinsically defective in DBA. A study from England showed that the frequency and clonogenicity of DBA early erythroid progenitors (defined by LinCD34+CD38+CD45RA−CD123−CD71+ CD41a−CD105−CD36−) and late erythroid progenitors (as defined by Lin−CD34+/−CD38+CD45RACD123−CD71+CD41a−CD105 +CD36+) are significantly decreased in DBA. Standard clonogenic assays for CFU-E and BFU-E progenitors consistently have shown reduced or absent colonies in most DBA patients and intermediate, normal, or occasionally increased numbers in the rest. The DBA erythroid progenitors are relatively insensitive to erythropoietin in vitro and to burst-promoting activity, but the hyporesponsiveness to erythropoietin can be corrected in some cases by the addition of glucocorticoids in vitro or by clinically administering prednisone.

The data underscore the fact that the intrinsic defect of DBA erythroid progenitors is an inability to respond normally to inducers of erythroid proliferation, differentiation, or both. Indeed, DBA CD34+ HSCs/early progenitors differentiate normally along megakaryocytic and granulocytic pathways in short-term cultures but aberrantly along the erythroid lineage. Accelerated programmed cell death (apoptosis) plays a central role in this pathogenesis as it does in many, if not all, inherited BM failure disorders. A role for induction of apoptosis by the Fas–Fas ligand system in DBA was suggested because of elevated serum soluble Fas ligand in patients compared with control participants. Based on the various patterns of erythroid colony growth seen with DBA patients, a model for the aberrant erythropoiesis was developed that proposes maturational arrest at varying sites along the differentiation pathway.

The combination of recombinant IL-3 and stem cell factor (SCF) increases the in vitro clonogenicity of DBA BM progenitors. The size and number of DBA BFU-E colonies are dramatically increased. The data on the effect of IL3, SCF, or GM-CSF as single agents is less conclusive. The human ligand for flt-3 apparently has no effect on DBA BM colony growth. However, addition of IL-9 to SCF, IL-3, and erythropoietin does potentiate DBA BFU-E growth.

There are significant age-related changes in erythroid and granulopoietic progenitors in DBA patients. Despite profound anemia, seven of 10 patients studied within 1 year of diagnosis had normal numbers of CFU-E and BFU-E that showed a normal response to cytokines. In contrast, 12 of 14 patients followed for more than 3 years had decreased erythroid progenitors and, in 7 cases, decreased CFU-GM. The data are consistent with the idea that the DBA defect involves other hematopoietic lineages and worsens with time.

Strong support for this conclusion comes from a detailed study that examined the interaction between DBA CD34+ cells and the hematopoietic microenvironment using long-term BM cultures. Stromal adherent layers from DBA patients did not show evidence of any morphologic, phenotypic, or functional abnormality, and the stroma sustained the proliferation of normal CD34+ cells. A major finding was an impaired capacity of DBA CD34+ cells in the presence of normal stromal cells to proliferate and differentiate along not only the erythroid pathway but also along the granulocytic–macrophage pathway. These results indicate an intrinsic defect of a hematopoietic progenitor with at least bilineage potential that places it earlier than previously suspected and that was only unmasked by testing in long-term cultures. This observation, however, is in keeping with the clinical observation that in addition to anemia, patients may have neutropenia and thrombocytopenia. These findings were extended with evidence in long-term culture initiating assays for a trilineage defect in DBA refractory to treatment. The data broaden the definition of DBA and explain generalized BM dysfunction and hypoplasia in some cases of DBA that have puzzled investigators for years.

The molecular mechanism that links ribosome protein haploinsufficiency to the erythroid defect is unclear. One hypothesis is that it is related to translation insufficiency. It is well known that during early stages of erythropoiesis, translation is increased. It is possible that the need for protein synthesis is not met during this critical developmental stage. A second hypothesis is that *ribosomal protein* gene mutations lead to accumulation of abnormal rRNA precursors as well as dysregulation of multiple ribosomal protein genes and protein expression as shown with *RPS19*. This leads to defective ribosome biogenesis, unassembled ribosome proteins, and cellular stress. Indeed, loss of ribosome proteins have been shown to increase the levels of S6 kinase phosphorylation via increased ROS, which in turn results in stimulating erythroid cell autophagy. A third hypothesis and the one considered most plausible is that defective ribosome biogenesis leads to activation of p53, thereby causing apoptosis and cell cycle arrest. A role of p53 is supported by a recent mouse model with mutations in *RPS19* that is characterized by RBC underproduction and small mouse size and by zebrafish models of *RPS19* inhibition that manifest impaired erythropoiesis and malformations. Activation of p53 may involve the interactions of MDM2 with specific ribosomal proteins such as RPL5, RPL11, and RPL23. These interactions may lead to dissociation of p53 from MDM2, impairment of p53 targeting to the proteosome, and prevention of proteosome degradation. However, these models do not explain how haploinsufficiency of RPL5 and RPL11 leads to p53 activation. Further, coinhibition of Tp53 activity in five different zebrafish models of ribosome protein knockdown rescued the morphologic malformations associated with the ribosome protein knockdown, but did not alleviate the erythroid aplasia. This suggests that ribosomal protein deficiency causes erythroid failure in a Tp53-independent manner.

Extraribosomal functions have been ascribed to various ribosomal protein genes that might mediate BM failure. Recently it has been shown that ribosome protein haploinsufficiency results in decreased GATA1 mRNA translation. This observation might be at least in part responsible for the erythropoietic defect as the defective erythropoiesis can be partially rescued by increasing GATA1 expression. Also, RPS19 has been shown to interact with a nucleolar protein S19-binding protein (S19BP), fibroblast growth factor 2, and the PIM-1 oncoprotein. PIM-1 is a ubiquitous serine-threonine kinase, the expression of which can be induced in erythropoietic cells by several growth factors, including erythropoietin. Thus there may be a possible link between erythropoietic growth factor signaling and RPS19.

The erythroid lineage is predominantly impaired in DBA for unknown reasons. Studies have shown that the heme exporter FLVCR1 is critical for CFU-E development. Knocking out FLVCR1 in mice causes impaired CFU-E development. A partial block in human FLVCR1 in CD34+ HSCs recapitulates the hematologic features of DBA, including CD36+/CD135a+ erythroid progenitor cell development but not myeloid cell development. Importantly, 55% to 95% of the *FLVCR1* transcript is alternatively spliced in DBA cells compared with 4% to 24% in normal immature erythroid cells. The spliced variants in DBA encode *FLVCR1* proteins that are defective in their cellular and surface expression and in their function. It is possible that expression of *FLVCR1* splicing variants leads to impaired export of intracellular iron and apoptosis because of accumulation of iron.

Patients with mutations in *RPL5* and *RPL11* are more likely to have multiple physical malformations. For example, thumb anomalies are seen in 56% and 39% of patients with *RPL5* and *RPL11* mutations, respectively, compared with 7% in patients who have *RPS19* gene mutations. Interestingly, cleft lip or palate was reported in 42% of patients with *RPL5* mutations compared with 6% and 0% of patients with *RPL11* and *RPS19* gene mutations, respectively.

Clinical Features

DBA registries with longitudinal data and a summary of published cases provide comprehensive information about clinical aspects of the disorder. Aside from findings associated with anemia, about half of infants at presentation look healthy and are normal physically. Unless the baby develops cardiac failure as a result of anemia, hepatosplenomegaly and edema are absent.

Pregnancy, birth history, or both are often abnormal. In a survey from the French and German DBA registries of 64 pregnancies in 26 women with DBA, complications were seen in 42 pregnancies (66%) and included abortion, preeclampsia, in utero fetal death, in utero growth retardation, retroplacental hematoma, and preterm delivery. Thirteen of 34 children born alive had DBA. Fetal DBA with hydrops fetalis has been reported. In current reports, more than 90% of cases present in the first 12 months of life; however, because of the availability of genetic testing, patients with mild to moderate phenotype are diagnosed later on in life. After diagnosis, family screening may identify the parents or older siblings as affected.

About 30% to 47% of patients present with one or more congenital anomalies. Most of these phenotypic abnormalities belong to the following categories: (1) craniofacial dysmorphism, including hypertelorism, microcephaly, microphthalmos, congenital cataract or glaucoma, strabismus, microretrognathism, and a high-arched palate or cleft palate; (2) prenatal or postnatal growth failure independent of steroid therapy; (3) neck anomalies, which may consist of a pterygium coli or the fusion of cervical vertebrae with flaring of the trapezius muscle (Klippel-Feil syndrome), giving a Turner syndrome appearance or there may also be the Sprengel deformity (congenital elevation of the scapula) as an isolated anomaly or a combination of the two anomalies; and (4) thumb malformations, such as bifid thumb (Fig. 29.7), duplication, subluxation, hypoplasia, or absence

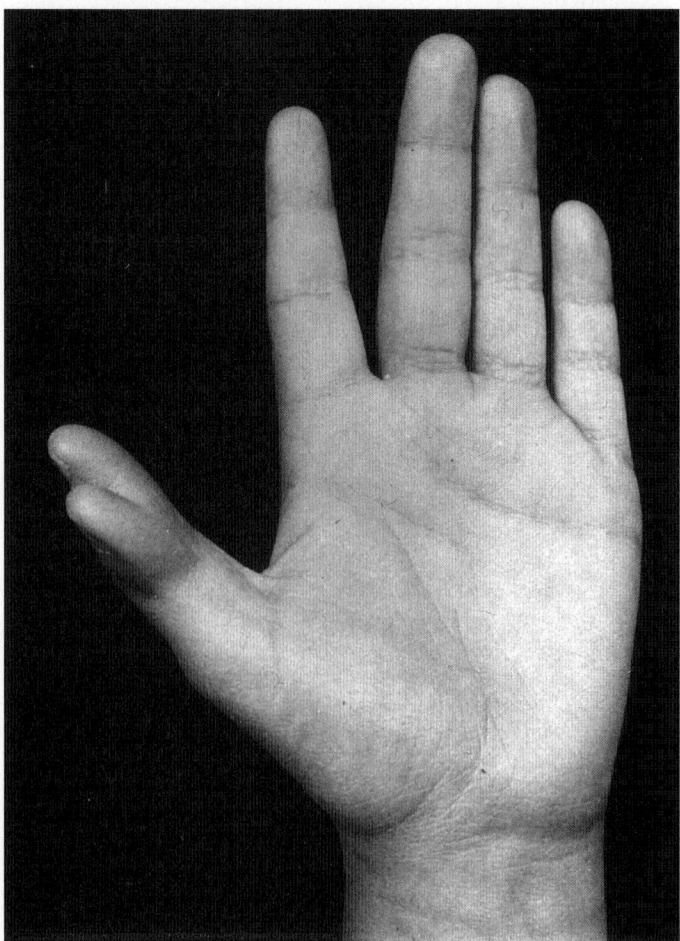

Fig. 29.7 BIFID THUMB IN DIAMOND-BLACKFAN ANEMIA.

of the thumb. There is a characteristic association of triphalangeal thumbs with DBA (Fig. 29.8) commonly referred to as "Aase syndrome II" or "Aase-Smith syndrome." In addition, some patients have a flat, hypoplastic thenar eminence, weak or absent radial pulses, or both, which probably represent variations of the thumb malformations.

Some patients have a characteristic facial appearance. The facies of individuals with DBA is said to consist of tow-colored hair, a snub nose, wide-set eyes, a thick upper lip, and an intelligent expression.

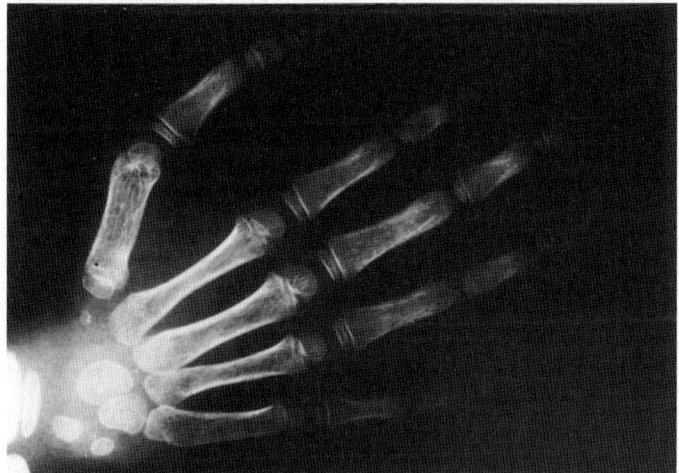

Fig. 29.8 RADIOGRAPH OF A TRIPHALANGEAL THUMB IN DIAMOND-BLACKFAN ANEMIA.

Another facies observed in two unrelated girls of markedly different ancestries consists of small heads, almond-shaped eyes with a slight antimongoloid slant, a "fish-like" smile, and a pointed chin. These patients resemble each other more than they resemble their own family members (Fig. 29.9A–B). Some patients with DBA have a phenotype indistinguishable from Treacher-Collins syndrome, a disorder of ribosome biogenesis caused by *TCOF1* mutations.

Various other anomalies are occasionally reported in association with DBA. There may be urogenital malformations, such as dysplastic or horseshoe kidneys, duplication of ureters, or renal tubular acidosis. There may also be congenital heart disease, mainly ventricular and atrial septal defects, or hypogonadism, ear malformations, mental retardation, congenital hip dislocation, or tracheoesophageal fistula.

Laboratory Findings

Peripheral Blood and Bone Marrow. The main hematologic findings in DBA are summarized in Table 29.6. The anemia is usually profound at the time of diagnosis. Hemoglobin levels average 6.5 g/dL in patients diagnosed in the first 2 months of life (range, 1.7–9.1 g/dL) and 4.0 g/dL (range, 1.8–7.4 g/dL) in those diagnosed later. In the vast majority of patients, the MCV is above the expected values for age. The peripheral blood smear may show, in addition to macrocytes, a mild degree of nonspecific anisocytosis and poikilocytosis. The aregenerative component of the anemia is reflected by the absence of both polychromasia and nucleated RBCs on the blood film. Decreased RBC production is confirmed by the absence of a reticulocyte response and by characteristic findings on BM examination.

In more than 90% of patients, the BM aspirate is normocellular, but erythroblasts are markedly decreased or absent. Proerythroblasts, if present, account for less than 3% of all nucleated elements, with a myeloid-to-erythroid ratio of 10 to 1 (Fig. 29.10). In 5% to 10% of

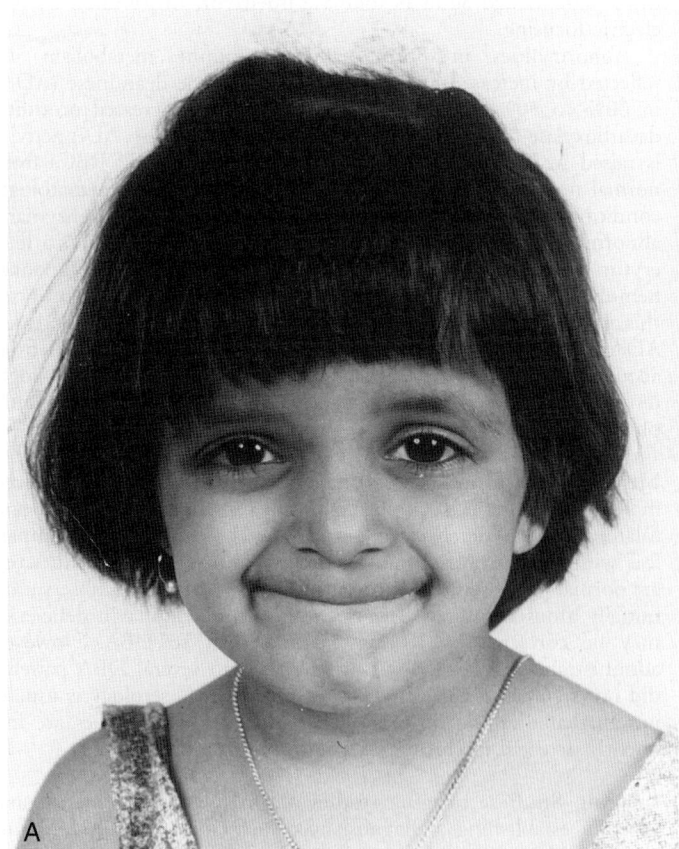

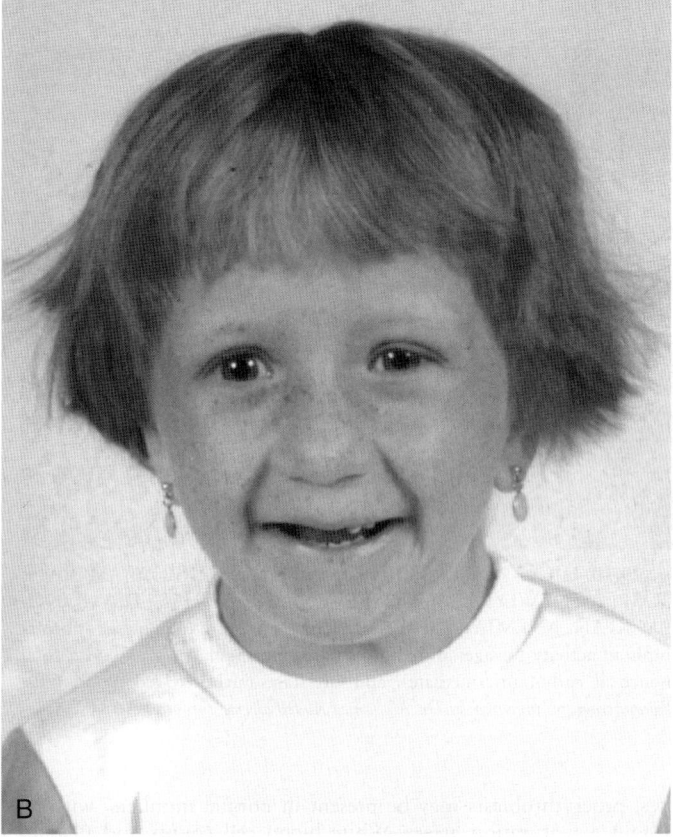

Fig. 29.9 SIMILAR DIAMOND-BLACKFAN FACIES IN TWO UNRELATED GIRLS OF DIFFERENT ANCESTRIES, CONSISTING OF A SMALL HEAD, ALMOND-SHAPED EYES WITH A SLIGHT ANTIMONGOLOID SLANT, A "FISH-LIKE" SMILE, AND A POINTED CHIN.

TABLE 29.6	Hematologic Features in Diamond-Blackfan Anemia at Diagnosis Based on Data on 21 Toronto Cases and on 41 Cases From the Canadian Inherited Marrow Failure Registry	

Hematologic Parameters	Laboratory Findings
Mean hemoglobin value (range)	
Newborns younger than 2 months of age	6.5 g/dL (1.7–9.1 g/dL)
Children 2 months of age or older	4.0 g/dL (1.8–7.4 g/dL)
High MCV for age after the age of 1 year	87%
Low reticulocyte for the degree of anemia	100% (usually markedly decreased to <1%)
Increased HbF for age after 1 year of age	100%
RBC adenosine deaminase activity	77%
RBC i antigen	Expression increased beyond first year of life
RBC enzymes	Fetal pattern
Neutropenia	31%
Thrombocytopenia	11%
BM cellularity	Normal or increased in 90%; mildly reduced in 10%
BM erythropoiesis	Markedly reduced/absent erythroid precursors in >90% of cases
BM myeloid and megakaryocytic lineages	Normal in 100% of the cases

BM, Bone marrow; HbF, fetal hemoglobin; MCV, mean corpuscular volume; RBC, red blood cell.

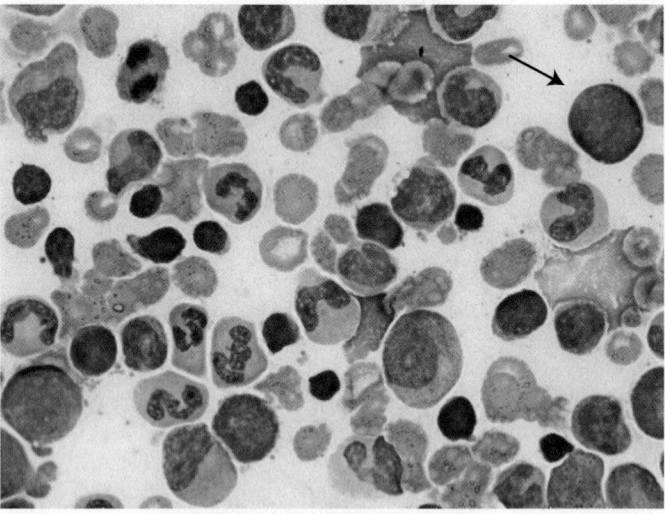

Fig. 29.10 HIGH-POWER VIEW OF A BONE MARROW ASPIRATE FROM A NEWLY DIAGNOSED INFANT WITH DIAMOND-BLACKFAN ANEMIA. The findings are active granulopoiesis; normal lymphoid activity for age; and an isolated pronormoblast *(arrow)* with total absence of early-, intermediate-, and late-stage nucleated red blood cells. *(Photomicrograph prepared by Dr. Mohamed Abdelhaleem, Toronto.)*

cases, proerythroblasts may be present in normal numbers, with or without a maturation arrest. White blood cell counts and platelet counts are usually normal at diagnosis, but platelets may be increased with normal function. Among DBA patients enrolled in the CIMFR mild to moderate neutropenia and thrombocytopenia occurred in

31% and 11% of patients, respectively, either at presentation or at follow-up. Progression of the single-lineage erythroid deficiency of DBA into pancytopenia and severe aplastic anemia is rare but occurs. Of 36 deaths reported to the American DBA Registry, one died from severe aplastic anemia.

Erythrocyte Findings. Erythrocytes in DBA express a number of fetal characteristics. The level of HbF is increased persistently even during remission. It remains at a level of about 10% after the age of 6 months and has a heterogeneous distribution in RBCs. The HbF has a specifically fetal amino-acid profile with a high glycine-to-alanine ratio (G-γ:A-γ). Similarly, the i antigen, which normally disappears from the erythrocyte surface by 1 year of age, is expressed at near fetal levels in older patients with DBA.

The precise cause of this fetal-like erythropoiesis is unclear. It is clearly distinct from the fetal erythropoiesis implicated in various types of leukemia, notably in juvenile myelomonocytic leukemia in which the fetal RBCs presumably arise from the leukemic clone. The situation in DBA may be analogous to that in other forms of BM failure and in the hematologic recovery phase after BMT. In all of these conditions, the fetal (or "stress") erythropoiesis may represent an accelerated recapitulation of RBC ontogeny in the face of an increased demand for new RBCs in peripheral blood.

Red blood cell enzymes often display an abnormal pattern of activity that reflects a fetal expression pattern of RBC glycolytic and hexose monophosphate shunt enzyme activities. Enzymes, such as enolase, glyceraldehyde-3-phosphate dehydrogenase, phosphofructokinase, and glutathione peroxidase, have increased activity in patients with DBA compared with those in normal children and adults and in patients with transient erythroblastopenia of childhood (TEC). For some enzymes, this increased activity is comparable to cord blood RBCs. In apparent contradiction, carbonic anhydrase isoenzyme B, which is not normally present in fetal RBCs, was detected in hemolysates from three patients with DBA. Also, the RBCs of two of the three patients had adult hexokinase isoenzyme distribution by isoelectric focusing.

Abnormalities in purine and pyrimidine metabolism are reflected by increased activity of RBC adenosine deaminase (ADA) in 60% to 90% of patients with DBA. Also, increased orotidine decarboxylase (ODC) activity is seen in some patients. ADA activity is raised in DBA erythrocytes but not in cord blood RBCs from normal newborns or from patients with any of several hematologic conditions associated with "stress" erythropoiesis. Thus this enzymatic abnormality cannot be simply attributable to a "reversion" to fetal erythropoiesis. Raised ADA activity may also be detected in some hemolytic anemias and acute leukemias, which limits the utility of this assay as a specific diagnostic marker for DBA. However, increased ADA activity does appear to be useful in differentiating DBA from acquired pure cell anemias such as TEC and for epidemiologic testing of DBA pedigrees to identify family members with a mild phenotype.

Miscellaneous Findings. Serum levels of various factors involved in RBC production, such as erythropoietin, iron, vitamin B_{12}, and folate, are appropriately elevated in DBA. These findings are compatible with any form of chronic hypoplastic anemia. Riboflavin levels are normal in the serum but not in the erythrocytes. This observation initially aroused interest because experimental riboflavin deficiency may be corrected by corticosteroids similar to DBA. However, administration of large doses of riboflavin to several DBA patients did not result in a hematopoietic response. RBC serology is usually unremarkable at the time of diagnosis, but alloantibodies are frequently detected in chronically transfused patients.

Imaging Studies. Imaging studies are frequently informative and assist in establishing a diagnosis. Skeletal radiography may define abnormalities suspected from physical examination, such as hypoplastic, absent, or extra phalanges. Ultrasound of the abdomen may reveal malformations such as of the urogenital system. Echocardiography may reveal undiagnosed cardiac defects.

TABLE 29.7	Distinguishing Features Between Diamond–Blackfan Anemia (DBA) and Transient Erythroblastopenia of Childhood (TEC)	
	DBA	**TEC**
Etiology	Genetic	Acquired
Immune mediated	None	Common
Family history	≈10%	Occasional siblings with concurrent TEC
Antecedent history	None	Viral infection
Age at diagnosis	90% by 1 year	6 months–4 years
Physical anomalies	≈50%	None
Neurologic findings	None	Occasional
Transfusion dependence	Yes, if steroid refractory	None
Course	Chronic	Full recovery
Risk of cancer	Increased	Not increased
Risk of MDS or leukemia	Increased	Not increased
Laboratory findings at diagnosis:		
RBC size	Macrocytic	Normocytic
HbF	Increased	Normal[a]
i Antigen	Increased	Normal[a]
RBC enzyme activities	Fetal levels	Adult levels
RBC adenosine deaminase	Increased in 40–90%	Normal

[a]During spontaneous recovery, values may be increased.
HbF, Fetal hemoglobin; MDS, myelodysplastic syndrome; RBC, red blood cell; TEC, transient erythroblastopenia of childhood.

Differential Diagnosis

The diagnosis of DBA is made if the patients have at least two of the following criteria (1) pure RBC aplasia as documented by normochromic-macrocytic anemia, relative reticulocytopenia, and normocellular BM with a selective deficiency of RBC precursors; (2) classical constellation of physical malformations; or (3) a first-degree relative with DBA or a mutation in a DBA gene.

In clinical practice, after excluding a viral etiology, particularly parvovirus B$_{19}$, **TEC** is usually the main diagnosis that is confused with DBA (Table 29.7). Both entities share the same morphologic findings in the BM. However, TEC is a self-limited disorder with an excellent prognosis and needs no specific therapy except for RBC transfusions in the most profoundly anemic patients. The definition of TEC includes the following features: (1) gradual onset of pallor in previously healthy children usually 1 to 4 years of age (85% of cases); (2) normochromic-normocytic anemia with varying reticulocytopenia unless recovery has already ensued; (3) BM erythroid hypoplasia (60% of cases) or aplasia (10% of cases) or a recovery picture (30% of cases); and (4) spontaneous recovery usually within 4 to 8 weeks without recurrence, with rare exceptions.

There are some additional important features of TEC. It can occur in siblings simultaneously and in seasonal clusters from June to October and from November to March. Of concern are the transient neurologic changes that can accompany TEC and that appear to be linked to the disorder. Affected children may have one or more of the following: hemiparesis, papilledema, abnormal extraocular movements, seizures, and unsteadiness of gait. The affected patients in the published reports recovered without sequelae, and the precise relationship of these neurologic changes to the pathogenesis of TEC has not been determined.

It was claimed initially that only the erythroid lineage was affected in TEC and all other hematopoietic lineages were normal. Nevertheless, significant neutropenia also occurs in many patients with TEC, being associated in some with hypocellular BM or with a granulopoietic maturational arrest. The neutropenia may be caused by a common pathogenetic mechanism that produces anemia. An unusual presentation of TEC as a leukoerythroblastic anemia has been recorded, possibly reflecting a recovery stage.

Although two cases of TEC were reported to be associated with detection of the parvovirus B19 genome, no data firmly incriminate other infectious agents in the etiology of TEC. Nevertheless, a history of a preceding viral-like illness can be obtained in more than half of the patients. The most plausible explanation proposed to date is that TEC is caused by transient immunosuppression of erythropoiesis and possibly of granulopoiesis in those with neutropenia. Increased numbers of CD10$^+$ lymphoid cells in BM of TEC patients might be an indication for such a mechanism. Most supportive evidence for this hypothesis comes from in vitro studies. Two reports described an inhibitory effect of TEC serum and fractionated IgG on erythroid colony growth that disappeared as TEC improved. An IgG inhibitor of erythropoiesis was discovered in one case and an IgM inhibitor in a second patient. A summary of other published studies suggests that more than 60% of TEC patients have autologous or allogeneic serum inhibitors of erythroid colony formation. Autologous or allogeneic cell-mediated immune suppression of erythropoiesis has also been identified in about 25% of cases. All of the in vitro studies have generated varying patterns of erythroid colony growth in TEC. Colony numbers can be normal, but reduced numbers of BFU-E and CFU-E progenitors have been recorded in 30% and 50% of cases, respectively.

TEC cases are not caused by DBA mutations. However, anemia in DBA may be mild, not present, or transiently exacerbated by viral infections. Therefore cases with transient anemia and reduced BM erythropoiesis should be carefully evaluated for the possibility of an underlying undiagnosed DBA and a period of follow-up with serial blood counts is recommended.

In summary, TEC has an autoimmune pathogenesis. The transient nature of TEC is similar to other autoimmune hematologic disorders of childhood such as immune thrombocytopenia purpura and some cases of autoimmune hemolytic anemia. The decreased activities of virtually all RBC enzymes in TEC compared with control participants probably relate to the aged population of peripheral blood erythrocytes being tested.

Regarding **viral causes** of non-DBA RBC aplasia, Epstein-Barr virus, hepatitis virus, human T-cell leukemia virus-1, and human immunodeficiency virus-1 have all been implicated and should be excluded if the etiology of the anemia remains unclear. Parvovirus B$_{19}$ stands out as a major causal agent of RBC aplasia in the context of an underlying chronic hemolytic anemia in infants and children with chronic congenital and acquired forms of immunosuppression. Fetuses are uniquely susceptible to parvovirus infection, and in utero transmission is a well-documented cause of nonimmune hydrops fetalis. Parvovirus infection should be ruled out in every case of childhood RBC aplasia by serial measurements of serum IgM and IgG and by BM examination for the characteristic giant pronormoblasts. Parvovirus may also be detected in BM by gene amplification using PCR and confirmed by direct in situ hybridization.

An important differential diagnosis is a milder form of **mitochondrial DNA deletion syndrome** or **Pearson syndrome**. This disorder can also present with macrocytic anemia and may mimic DBA. In a recent study, about 3% of patients with a clinical diagnosis of DBA, were eventually diagnosed with Pearson syndrome. In some of these cases erythroid hypoplasia was demonstrated with variable vacuolated progenitors and without ringed sideroblasts.

Rarely, the initial hematologic manifestation of several other IBMFSs such as **FA, DC**, and **congenital hair hypoplasia** is isolated macrocytic anemia. Specific screening testing for these conditions might be necessary.

Predisposition to Malignancy

DBA is associated with hematologic cancer and with solid tumors, albeit to a much lesser degree than FA, DC, SDS, and K/SCN. The link between DBA and hematologic cancer is more understandable from the data described herein that implicate an early pluripotent BM progenitor in the pathobiology of DBA. From published data up to 2011, 10 DBA patients developed AML, 2 developed MDS, 1 had acute lymphoblastic leukemia, 3 had Hodgkin lymphoma, and 1 had non-Hodgkin lymphoma. Regarding solid tumors, a predilection to osteosarcoma was reported in 6 of the 11 solid tumors. The other solid tumors included HCC, breast carcinoma, gastric carcinoma, vaginal melanoma, and malignant fibrous histiocytoma. Among patients enrolled in the American DBA Registry, the cumulative risk of solid tumors and leukemia by the age of 40 years was about 5%. Among patients enrolled in the CIMFR none developed clonal and malignant myeloid transformation during childhood. Therefore regular surveillance for detection of early MDS/leukemia in DBA is probably not indicated during childhood.

The published cases implicate several possible operative factors, including genetic predisposition, transfusional iron overload, use of androgens, immunosuppression from corticosteroids, thymic and skeletal irradiation during childhood as "therapy" for DBA in one case, and cyclophosphamide "treatment" in another. It is noteworthy that inhibition of ribosome protein genes in zebrafish is associated with the development of cancer.

Natural History and Prognosis

Historically the only treatment for DBA was blood transfusions. Without this, patients died of anemia. When corticosteroids were introduced as an effective therapy for DBA, all patients were assigned to one of the two therapeutic interventions, and the "natural history" of the disorder took on a different dimension.

A notable phenomenon is spontaneous remission that occurs in about 20% of cases that allows patients to discontinue whatever treatment they are receiving, either chronic transfusion therapy or corticosteroids. The American DBA Registry has actuarial data showing that 75% of these patients remit before their 10th birthday, and in most cases, the remission is sustained. It appears that an equal number of patients remit from either corticosteroids or transfusions. A relapse of DBA requires reintroduction of treatment.

The overall actuarial survival for DBA patients greater than 40 years of age is 75% ± 4.8%. For those in sustained spontaneous remission, it is 100%; for corticosteroid responders, it is 57% ± 8.9%; and for transfusion-dependent patients, it is 8.9%. Causes of death mostly relate directly to the development of cancer or its treatment, complications from corticosteroid-induced immunosuppression, HSCT–related complications, and transfusional hemosiderosis.

Therapy

In younger children and infants, it is important to determine whether the RBC aplasia is DBA or TEC (see Table 29.7). Until a firm diagnosis is established, the initial treatment in children is almost always transfusions. This allows the flexibility to complete the viral workup and other investigations and to await a spontaneous remission if the anemia is caused by TEC or another self-limited condition. Demonstration of a mutant DBA gene would clinch the diagnosis, but negative molecular analysis does not rule out this diagnosis.

If transfusions are used, it is recommended to aim for a moderate but not full correction of anemia so that erythropoiesis is not suppressed and recovery from TEC not delayed. In general, the nadir should not be less than 6 g/dL and should not allow the development of significant symptoms. Most patients with TEC usually recover within a few weeks after receiving only one transfusion. Occasionally, recovery from TEC is slow and may mimic DBA in chronicity. If there is confusion about the proper diagnosis, it is appropriate to withhold corticosteroids in favor of a further transfusion to allow more observation time.

Transfusions for Patients With Diamond-Blackfan Anemia

Before the first transfusion, it is recommended that a full RBC phenotype be performed on the patient. This information is valuable for prevention and management of alloantibody formation caused by sensitization. For patients in whom corticosteroids are either ineffective or excessively toxic, a regular program of RBC transfusions is usually required. During the course of this program, a small number of steroid-resistant patients may show responsiveness to corticosteroids when retreated or even proceed to a spontaneous transient or prolonged remission. If not, leukocyte-depleted packed RBCs are given monthly to keep the hemoglobin concentration at a level compatible with normal activity, usually above 9 g/L. CMV-negative packed cells should be used if HSCT is contemplated. Several complications may arise from transfusions such as blood-borne infections and sensitization, but the major long-term threat is iron overload, which causes delayed puberty, growth retardation, diabetes mellitus, hypoparathyroidism, and eventually liver cirrhosis and cardiac failure. These complications can be delayed and possibly prevented by the early administration of an iron chelator.

Two iron chelators are available in North America. The first, deferoxamine (Desferal), is administered by a battery-powered pump as a daily 12-hour subcutaneous infusion. It has been the main chelator used for the past four decades. Deferasirox (Exjade) is an effective oral iron chelator in patients with iron overload and is approved for children older than 6 years of age (>2 years of age in some countries). The initial dose is 20 to 30 mg/kg by mouth once daily. In a randomized trial of Desferal versus Exjade in patients with transfusional iron overload, the two chelators showed similar efficacy. In an international multicenter study in which the efficacy of Exjade was assessed in patients with anemia of various etiologies, 30 patients with DBA were included. Successful chelation was observed in 54% of DBA patients as defined by reduction of liver iron concentration by biopsy to less than 7 mg/g dry weight within 1 year. Given its oral route of administration, Exjade has been replacing Desferal as the iron chelator of choice if the former is not contraindicated.

There are uncertainties about the optimal age at which to start patients younger than 2 years old with transfusion-dependent anemia with Desferal therapy. There have been reports of abnormal linear growth and metaphyseal dysplasia in patients with thalassemia major treated with Desferal before the age of 3 years. This adverse event has prompted recommendations for starting Desferal later. However, a progressively rising serum ferritin level or, more accurately, excessive hepatic iron concentration obtained by FerriScan (using R2-MRI imaging technology) or biopsy after a period of regular transfusions would be an appropriate indication to commence chelation therapy. The daily starting subcutaneous infusion dose of Desferal should not exceed 50 mg/kg. Ascorbate supplementation should be considered if there is sustained loss of efficacy of deferoxamine, especially if tissue ascorbate concentrations are reduced.

Corticosteroids

Steroid responsiveness occurs in 50% to 75% of DBA patients. Upon administration of prednisone at a dose of 2 mg/kg/day in 2 or 3 divided doses, reticulocytosis is usually seen within 1 to 4 weeks and is followed by a rise in hemoglobin concentration. When the hemoglobin level reaches 9.0 to 10.0 g/dL, prednisone can be slowly tapered by reducing the number of daily doses. If a single daily dose of prednisone maintains the desired hemoglobin level, the dose can be doubled and given on alternate days, but this may not prevent significant steroid toxicity.

The dose of prednisone can be further reduced by small decrements on a weekly basis or more slowly until the minimal effective dose is determined. This dose is extremely variable. A few patients can be maintained on minute, nonpharmacologic doses, but other patients need large doses that preclude long-term therapy because of serious side effects such as Cushingoid features, pathologic fractures, cataracts, growth failure, diabetes, and avascular necrosis of the femoral or humeral heads. There is no known predictor of steroid responsiveness or any way to anticipate the type of individual responses. In general, a corticosteroid dose equivalent of prednisone, 0.5 mg/kg/day, is suggested as a maximum "maintenance" dose after the initial dose of 2 mg/kg/day. About one-third of patients can maintain a response at a low prednisone dose. The rest are usually managed with chronic RBC transfusions.

There are several patterns of response to corticosteroid therapy, some of which may occur at different times in the same patient. Most children who respond to steroids cannot be completely weaned off the medication and become steroid dependent. About one-third of these patients, however, enter steroid-free remission after a prolonged period of treatment. Between 1% and 5% of responders immediately enter a durable steroid-independent remission. However, late relapses, sometimes precipitated by an infectious illness or by hormonal changes such as in pregnancy or with the use of birth control pills, are common. In other cases, a progressive resistance to steroids occurs, requiring escalating doses of prednisone or alternative therapy. After a relapse, some patients are responsive to steroids again, but others are refractory to subsequent trials. Initial refractoriness to steroids is observed in 36% of cases. In more than 60% of patients, long-term steroid therapy is hampered by the development of resistance or by side effects of the treatment. In adolescent responders on long-term steroids, an option is to stop prednisone temporarily to allow a normal growth spurt. Infants with DBA on high doses of steroids are at risk for pneumocystis pneumonia and should be given prophylactic antibiotics.

Megadose steroid therapy for DBA patients who were refractory to conventional-dose prednisone has been reported to induce a sustained erythroid response leading to transfusion independence in 8 of 13 cases. Eleven had been treated with 100 mg/kg/day intravenously, and two additional patients had been treated with 30 mg/kg/day orally. Another report showed only a transient response in one of eight patients after intravenous treatment with 30 mg/kg/day and a sustained response after a higher dosage (100 mg/kg/day) in three of eight patients, but side effects were weight gain, oral moniliasis, increase in hepatic transaminases, transient hyperglycemia, and bacteremia related to a central venous catheter. A conclusive study of nine refractory DBA patients using megadose oral methylprednisolone showed no response in five cases and a partial or complete response in the other four during the initial 4 to 8 weeks of therapy, but all of these patients relapsed with a taper and became transfusion dependent. Thus none of the cases exhibited a clinically significant or durable response.

Cytokine Therapy

Because of the "corrective" effect on erythropoiesis by IL-3 in vitro, clinical trials were introduced for steroid-refractory and steroid-dependent DBA patients and for those in whom HSCT was considered too risky. The early enthusiasm generated by sustained remissions in some patients was tempered by the realization that IL-3 is effective in only a very small number of cases of steroid-refractory, transfusion-dependent DBA. Of 49 patients treated with IL-3 in a European multicenter compassionate-need study, only three children had a significant response with sustained remissions off therapy. A comparison of individual patient characteristics confirmed that patients who had never achieved significant in vivo erythropoiesis in response to steroids or during a spontaneous remission were highly unlikely to respond to IL-3. Thus the overall response rate in all published studies averaged 10–20%. Currently, there are no IL-3 or other growth factor clinical trials in North America for DBA. Serum erythropoietin levels are elevated in DBA, and attempts at treatment with high-dose erythropoietin have been ineffective.

Hematopoietic Stem Cell Transplantation

Hematopoietic stem cell transplantation is a therapeutic option for DBA, but the risks must be weighed against the benefits on a case-by-case basis. The fundamental issue centers on the defined mortality rate with HSCT when used for a nonlethal medical disorder, at least a disorder that is nonlethal in the short term. In steroid-responsive patients on low-dose maintenance, quality of life is not threatened by life-threatening complications. Thus in this setting HSCT is widely considered as not indicated. In properly transfused and adequately chelated patients who do not have severe thrombocytopenia, severe neutropenia, severe aplastic anemia or MDS/AML, HSCT is ultimately a choice made by the parents and patients. With the advances in the management of patients who need chronic transfusion (e.g., developing of oral chelators and MRI-based imaging of iron overload) the quality of life of these patients substantially improves; hence it is possible that HSCT for DBA patients will be applied less frequently in the future.

Experience has broadened since the first HSCT was performed for DBA in 1976. Preparative regimens, supportive measures, and GVHD management have progressively become more refined, thereby reducing the overall risks of the procedure. For consideration in the decision-making process, though, there are still lethal risks, including sepsis, fatal complications associated with chronic GVHD, graft failure, graft rejection, interstitial pneumonia, and cardiac failure. Results from the International Bone Marrow Transplant Registry show a 64% 3-year probability of overall survival of 61 transplanted DBA patients. The American DBA Registry and the Aplastic Anemia Committee of the Japanese Society of Pediatric Hematology report an 87.5% and an 85% survival, respectively, but express caution that alternative donors pose a much higher risk than matched sibling donors. From the American DBA Registry database, the survival rate for patients younger than the age of 10 years receiving matched related HSCT is greater than 90%. A report from the Italian Association of Pediatric Haematology and Oncology Registry from 2014 indicated 80.4% 5-year survival for HSCT from matched sibling donor and 69.9% for matched unrelated donor without statistically significant difference between the groups. Umbilical cord blood as a stem cell source has been used for DBA HSCT with favorable results.

Given the generally favorable results with related donors, this procedure can now be offered to patients approximately after the age of 5 years when no spontaneous remission is apparent. However, HSCT from an unrelated donor is not recommended unless the patient has severe thrombocytopenia, severe neutropenia, severe aplastic anemia, MDS, or leukemia or as part of a clinical trial.

This success with related donors has sparked interest in PGD with in vitro fertilization to "create" HLA-matched sibling donors without a mutated DBA gene, and a number of patients worldwide have been successfully transplanted using umbilical cord–derived stem cells from donors produced in this way. The religious, ethical, and economic questions generated by PGD to find a healthy matched donor for DBA and other inherited BM failure transplantations are ongoing.

Other Therapeutic Options

Based on the role of the DBA genes in ribosome biogenesis and global protein translation and in vitro studies aimed to stimulate translation in BM cells, a trial was performed in which the branched amino acid leucine was administered to a patient with DBA. The patient had an impressive response. Based on this, two leucine trials are ongoing in the United States and Europe. Leucine stimulates translation by enhancing the activation of translation initiation factors that regulate mRNA binding to the ribosomal complex and by activation of the ribosomal protein S6 kinase and the mTOR (mammalian target of rapamycin) pathway. Thus far, the efficacy of leucine has been documented in cellular models of DBA, in several ribosomal protein deficient zebrafish models and in a *RPS19*-knockdown mouse model where doxycycline-regulatable specific shRNA was used.

A number of uncontrolled therapeutic trials have been performed in steroid-refractory patients using various medications and treatments with varying anecdotal successes in a few patients. The medications include cyclosporine, metoclopramide, lenalidomide, androgens, riboflavin, vitamin B_{12}, folate, iron and other "hematinic" agents, 6-mercaptopurine, cyclophosphamide with antilymphocyte globulin, and antithymocyte globulin alone. There is a case report claiming efficacy of valproic acid for DBA and another report of an 8-month transfusion-free remission after rituximab therapy. Plasmapheresis has also been tried. Splenectomy, used in the past, shows no effect on erythropoiesis but may be helpful in transfused patients with proven hypersplenism.

Future Directions

Registries and DBA patient databases will continue to broaden our understanding of the genetic origins and epidemiology of DBA. Specimen collection and distribution to qualified research laboratories globally will identify the remaining DBA genes. Genetically based DBA diagnosis and pedigree analysis will underscore the broad dimensions of the DBA phenotype, from clinically silent to life-threatening severe. Genotype–phenotype correlations will facilitate HSCT donor selection, allow counseling for reproductive options, and be predictive of cancer risk. Deciphering the pathogenesis of BM failure and other disease manifestations using animal models and iPSCs may allow the development of effective erythropoietic stimulators for use in this disease.

Congenital Dyserythropoietic Anemias

Background

The designation *congenital dyserythropoietic anemia* (CDA) refers to a family of inherited refractory anemias characterized by BM erythroid multinuclearity, ineffective erythropoiesis, and secondary hemosiderosis. The ineffective erythropoiesis is reflected by BM erythroid hyperplasia, inappropriately low reticulocyte counts for the degree of anemia, and intramedullary RBC destruction. Splenomegaly and chronic or intermittent jaundice are additional features. Granulopoiesis and thrombopoiesis are normal. These disorders are genetically transmitted and result in anemia with a blunted erythropoietic response. Some patients, especially with CDA type I, have congenital anomalies.

Three classic forms of CDA have been described as well as a number of variants. An arbitrary classification used in practice for these three is based on the inheritance pattern, the peripheral blood and BM morphology, and the serologic findings in each case. The distinguishing features of the three types of CDA are as follows:

- Type I: Autosomal recessive; macrocytosis; megaloblastic erythroid precursor cells; 2% to 5% binucleated erythroid precursor cells; internuclear chromatin bridges involving polychromatic erythroblasts; negative acidified serum lysis test (Ham test) results.
- Type II: Autosomal recessive; normocytic RBCs; normoblastic erythroid precursor cells; 10% to 40% binucleated late normoblasts; positive acidified serum lysis test (Ham test) results.
- Type III: Autosomal dominant (or sporadic); macrocytosis; megaloblastic erythroid maturation; giant multinucleated erythroid precursors with up to 12 nuclei per cell; negative acidified serum lysis test (Ham test) results.

The designation "type IV" is defunct but was briefly used to classify cases of morphologic CDA type II with a *negative* Ham acidified serum test result. Because some of these were reclassified as CDA type II after retesting using a large panel of heterologous sera, "type IV" is no longer used as a category. There are also several other forms of CDA that are distinct from CDA types I, II, and III. Some of these variants have been identified in three or more families and have been tentatively classified phenotypically into CDA *groups* (not types) IV, V, VI, and VII (see later section, Other CDAs). Additional CDAs are associated with specific gene mutations other than those seen in CDA I and II. The growing number of variants underscores the complex nature of CDA and the current direction to reclassify these disorders accurately by genotype rather than by morphology.

Etiology, Genetics, Pathophysiology, and Clinical Features

CDA Type I

CDA I is inherited in an autosomal recessive manner. The disorder is caused by biallelic mutations in *CDAN1* or in *C15ORF41*. *CDAN1*

was identified in highly inbred Israeli Bedouins. The gene product, codanin-1, may be involved in nuclear envelope integrity, but this is uncertain, and little is known about pathogenesis. The functions of *C15ORF41* are unknown.

The onset of anemia, jaundice, and other symptoms may be noted at any age, especially in neonates. Eighty percent of infants in a recent large series required blood transfusions during the first month of life. Case with anemia in utero requiring intrauterine exchange transfusions at the third trimester have been reported. Affected patients often have some degree of icterus and splenomegaly.

CDA I can be associated with a variety of congenital anomalies. The following have been catalogued: patches of brown skin pigmentation, syndactyly in the feet, absence of phalanges and nails in the fingers and toes, an additional phalanx, duplication or hypoplasia of metatarsals, short stature, pigeon chest deformity, varus deformity of hips, flattened vertebral bodies, a hypoplastic rib, congenital ptosis, Madelung deformity of the wrist, and deafness. The pigmentation, syndactyly and absence of phalanges and nails are not common in CDA I patients but appear to be quite specific for this subtype. Dysmorphic features are seen in up to 65% of patients. Three siblings from a Bedouin family presented with neonatal pulmonary hypertension. In a French family, three siblings had sensorineural deafness and a lack of motile sperm cells.

Laboratory Abnormalities. The degree of anemia is usually mild to moderate (hemoglobin in the range of 6.6–11.6 g/dL), and RBCs appear macrocytic. Peripheral blood RBC morphology is characterized by anisocytosis and poikilocytosis, and occasionally Cabot rings are seen. Cabot rings appear to be unique to CDA I and are not seen in types II and III. White blood cells and platelets are normal. Examination of the BM reveals erythroid hyperplasia with some megaloblastic erythropoiesis and a small number of erythroblasts with dyserythropoietic features. The unique morphologic abnormality seen in CDA I is the presence of chromatin bridges between nuclei of two separate erythroblasts, a reflection of impaired cellular division (Fig. 29.11). This internuclear bridging of erythroblasts seen with light microscopy is also a common feature in MDS. Electron microscopy reveals additional abnormalities that include widening of the nuclear membrane pore space with cytoplasmic invagination into the nucleus, separation of nuclear chromatin, and chromatin condensation, all of which give the general appearance of a spongy nucleus (Fig. 29.12). Dyserythropoiesis seems limited mostly to more mature RBC precursors. In contrast to CDA II, there are no unique serologic features.

The defect in CDA I is at the stem cell level. The numbers of CFU-E and BFU-E colonies are normal but contain a mixture of normal and abnormal cells when examined by electron microscopy. This suggests that the abnormality is expressed variably in the mature progeny of each stem cell. Erythroid precursors also demonstrate S phase arrest and morphologic features of apoptosis. In some CDA I patients, hemoglobin A_2 levels are increased. Also, some cases show unbalanced globin chain synthesis. Patients do not have thalassemia, and the cause of these findings is not known.

CDA Type II (HEMPAS)

CDA II is commonly known as HEMPAS, an acronym for hereditary erythroblastic multinuclearity with a positive acidified serum test. It is inherited in an autosomal recessive manner. The disorder is caused by biallelic mutant *SEC23B*. The wild-type gene encodes the SEC23B component of the coat protein (COP) II complex. COP II vesicles transport secretory proteins from the endoplasmic reticulum to the Golgi complex. Mutations result in misglycosylation and an impaired clearance of endoplasmic reticulum cisternae past a given point during erythroid differentiation. The mutations in *SEC23B* are localized along the entire coding sequence of the gene, in splicing sites and in regulatory regions, no case with biallelic mutations has been described, suggesting an essential role of the gene.

A significant body of knowledge has been accumulated about the pathogenesis of CDA II. At the stem cell level, in vitro culture of CDA II erythroid progenitors produces CFU-E and BFU-E

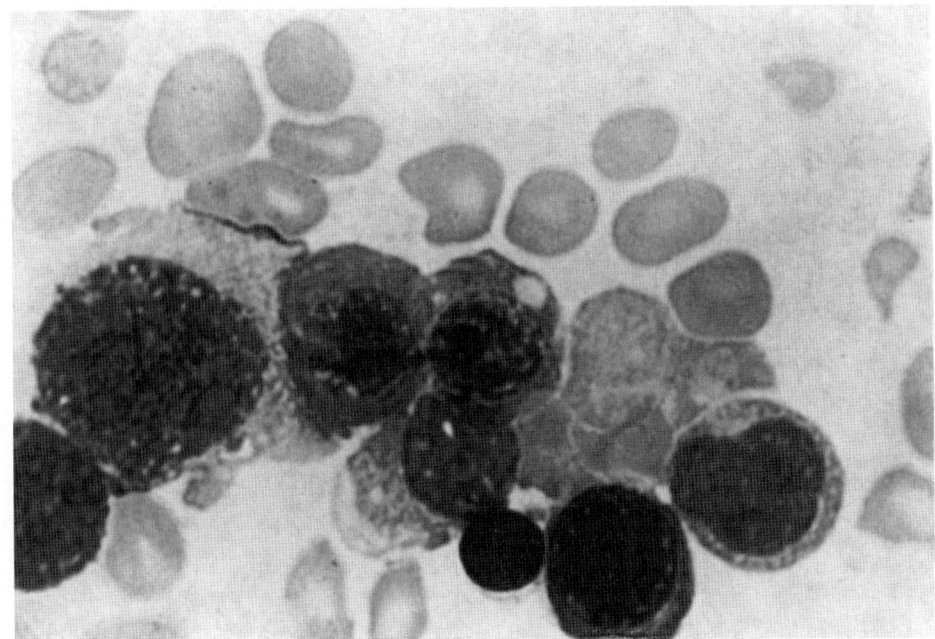

Fig. 29.11 BONE MARROW FROM PATIENT WITH CONGENITAL DYSERYTHROPOIETIC ANEMIA TYPE I. Erythroblasts are connected by internuclear bridges between two cells. *(Provided by Dr. Jean Shafer, Rochester, NY.)*

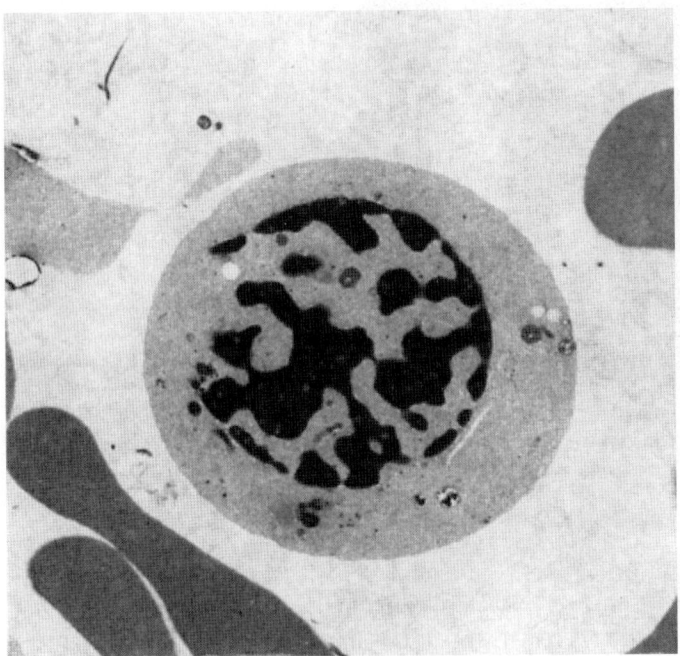

Fig. 29.12 ELECTRON MICROSCOPY OF BONE MARROW FROM CONGENITAL DYSERYTHROPOIETIC ANEMIA TYPE I. Note the "spongy" appearance of the nucleus resulting from uneven chromatin with cytoplasmic invagination into the nucleus. *(Provided by Dr. Raoul Fresco, Maywood, IL.)*

Additional data suggested that the IgM antibody responsible for hemolysis in the acidified-serum lysis test (Ham test) recognized an abnormal glycolipid structure sharing homology with i and I antigens. Thus a variety of data predicted and confirmed that abnormalities in the glycosylation pathway were involved in the etiology of CDA II.

The two major defects in the CDA II glycosylation enzymatic pathway are a deficiency of α-mannosidase II and of N-acetylglucosaminyl transferase II. A third defect in a CDA II variant is deficient levels of the membrane-bound form of galactosyl transferase. All three of these enzymatic deficiencies lead to abnormal oligosaccharides on major erythrocyte proteins such as the anion transporter Band 3 that could cause disruption of the structural network of erythrocytes and their precursors, thereby leading to their premature demise. Defective glycosylation on the RBC surface may also affect the regulation of complement on the surface of erythrocytes. Enhanced functional activity of the alternative pathway C3 convertase and of the membrane attack complex may result from the improper glycosylation of glycophorin A, which has been proposed to serve as a complement regulatory protein. These abnormalities are not a consequence of quantitative or functional deficiencies of the complement regulatory proteins CD55 or CD59.

Laboratory Abnormalities. There is overlap of some clinical and laboratory manifestations between CDA I and CDA II, but there are three major differences. The first is that the magnitude of anemia is usually more severe, and patients, especially children, often require RBC transfusions. Peripheral blood RBCs are usually normocytic but show anisocytosis and poikilocytosis (Fig. 29.13). The second difference is that the BM in CDA II reveals greater numbers of abnormal erythroblasts with binuclearity in up to 35% of late erythroblasts, as well as multinuclearity and abnormal lobulation (Fig. 29.14). These nuclear abnormalities are seen only in the late erythroblasts, not in basophilic erythroblasts. Karyorrhexis is commonly observed, and pseudo-Gaucher cells may be present, representing the ingestion of debris by histiocytic cells from ineffective erythropoiesis. Electron microscopy of late erythroblasts also reveals an excess of endoplasmic reticulum parallel to the cell membrane, giving the appearance of a double cell membrane (Fig. 29.15). A third difference, which is also a pathognomonic finding, is that

colonies with erythroblast multinuclearity. Initially, studies of peripheral blood CDA II RBCs identified a number of chemical abnormalities, including unbalanced globin chain synthesis, increased membrane glycolipids, and altered RBC membrane protein patterns demonstrated by two-dimensional electrophoresis. Furthermore, glycoproteins on CDA II RBCs were found to have an abnormal carbohydrate structure, leading to aberrant reactivity with anti-i sera.

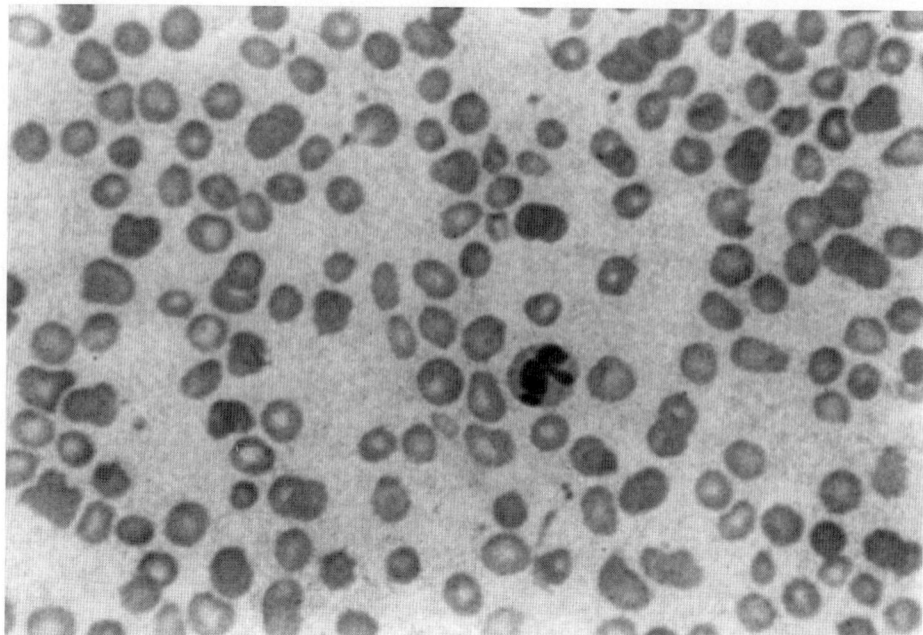

Fig. 29.13 PERIPHERAL BLOOD SMEAR FROM A PATIENT WITH CONGENITAL DYSERYTH-ROPOIETIC ANEMIA TYPE II. Note the marked variation in red blood cell size and shape.

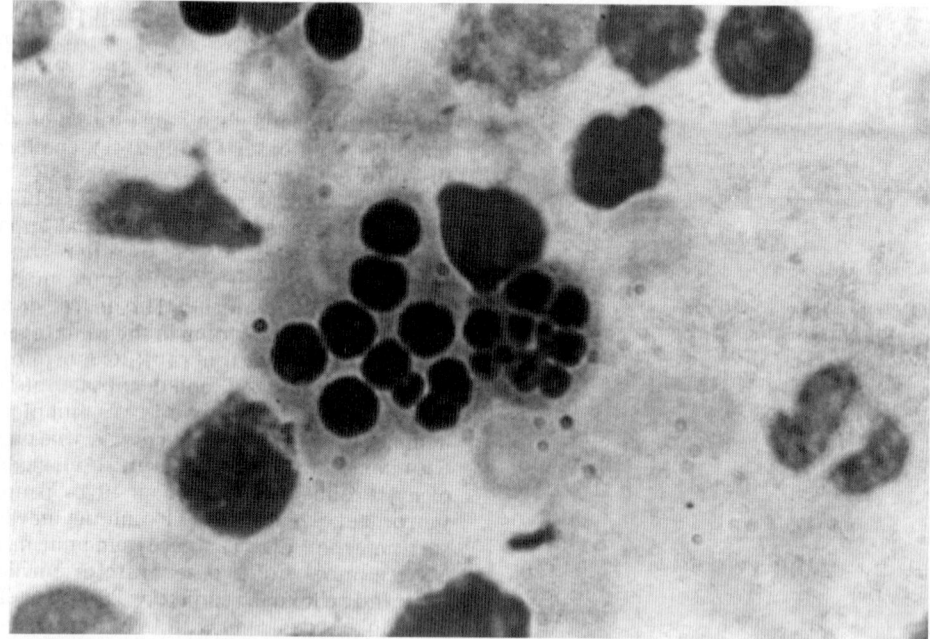

Fig. 29.14 BONE MARROW ASPIRATE FROM A PATIENT WITH HEMPAS (CONGENITAL DYS-ERYTHROPOIETIC ANEMIA TYPE II) SHOWING ERYTHROID HYPERPLASIA AND MULTINU-CLEATED ERYTHROBLASTS. *(Provided by Dr. Jean Shafer, Rochester, NY.)*

CDA II RBCs are lysed by acidified (pH 6.8) sera obtained from approximately 30% to 60% of fresh ABO-compatible sera from normal persons (i.e., a positive Ham test result), but there is no lysis when RBCs are incubated with the patient's own acidified serum. This lysis is a result of a naturally occurring IgM antibody that recognizes an antigen on CDA II cells and binds complement; this antibody can be removed by preincubating normal sera with HEMPAS erythrocytes. However, the specific HEMPAS antigen recognized by this antibody is not known. In contrast to HEMPAS, the erythrocytes of patients with paroxysmal nocturnal hemoglobinuria (PNH) undergo lysis when the acidified serum is from the PNH patient or from normal donors. Another difference is that PNH erythrocytes undergo lysis in isotonic sucrose (sugar water test), but HEMPAS RBCs do not lyse in isotonic sucrose.

The erythrocytes from patients with CDA II also exhibit an increased agglutinability and lysis to anti-i and anti-I sera and manifest increased expression of both antigens. These surface antigens are complex carbohydrate structures found predominantly on fetal and adult RBCs, respectively. Increased expression of i antigen can be demonstrated on all RBCs in CDA II using fluorescent labels. Relatives of patients with CDA II who have normal BM but increased agglutinability to anti-i appear to be heterozygote carriers of this

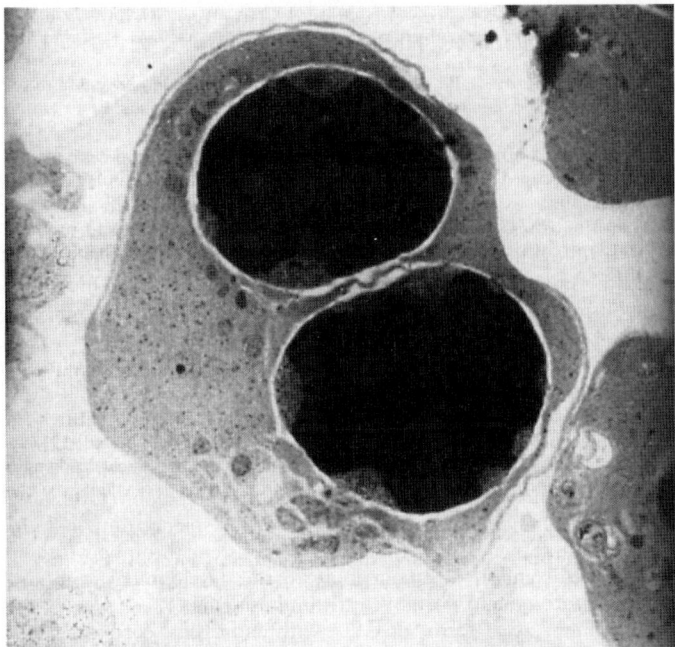

Fig. 29.15 ELECTRON MICROSCOPY OF A BONE MARROW ERYTHROBLAST FROM A PATIENT WITH HEMPAS (CONGENITAL DYSERYTHROPOIETIC ANEMIA TYPE II). Note the appearance of a double cell membrane, reflecting an excess of endoplasmic reticulum. *(Provided by Dr. Raoul Fresco, Maywood, IL.)*

disorder. HEMPAS erythrocytes bind a normal amount of complement (C1), but more antibody and less C4 than normal. This causes binding of an excess of C3 and hemolysis.

The number of erythroid progenitors is probably normal in BM and blood. Although one study found only normal morphology of the erythroblasts produced in culture, subsequent studies reported multinuclearity similar to that seen in the BM. As in CDA I, the defect in CDA II is in the erythroid progenitor cell and is expressed variably in more mature erythroblasts.

Patients with CDA II may develop progressive, lifelong iron overload even in the absence of transfusions, and approximately 20% develop cirrhosis as a consequence. Splenomegaly occurs in the majority of patients with CDA II. A number of other clinical associations with CDA II have been reported such as mental retardation, Sweet syndrome, von Willebrand disease, and Dubin-Johnson syndrome, among others. Rather than true associations, it is likely that the majority represent coincidental occurrences. An adult patient was reported with an extramedullary hematopoietic mass in the posterior mediastinum that was a result of BM expansion associated with ineffective erythropoiesis. In a retrospective study of 41 patients, coinheritance of Gilbert syndrome was associated with a significantly increased risk of hyperbilirubinemia and early-onset gallstone formation.

A large study from Italy and Turkey identified correlation between three genetic groups and clinical phenotype: patients carrying two missense alleles (group 1), patients carrying a missense allele in compound heterozygosity with a nonsense/hypomorphic allele (group 2), and patients carrying either two hypomorphic alleles or a nonsense allele in compound heterozygosity with a hypomorphic allele (group 3). The degree of anemia, hyperferritenemia, and transfusion dependency was most severe in patients who belonged to group 2, followed by the patients in group 1. The patients in group 3 had the mildest phenotype.

CDA Type III

Based on reported CDA cases, type II is the most common CDA, type I is next, and CDA III is the rarest of the three major forms. In contrast to the other two forms, CDA III is inherited as an autosomal dominant disorder. The responsible gene is *KIF23*, which encodes mitotic kinesin-like protein 1 (MKLP1) that localizes to the midbody ring. In vitro studies showed that the mutations in the genes result in cytokinesis failure. It has also been shown that ubiquitination of MKLP1 is required for midbody ring degradation by autophagy; thus abrogation of this process may cause cytokinesis failure and multinuclearity.

In a Swedish family with 31 cases inherited in an autosomal dominant mode, an excess number of cases with a monoclonal gammopathy and myeloma have occurred. Also, an adult patient with CDA III was described with T-cell non-Hodgkin lymphoma. These cases, plus a case of Hodgkin disease occurring in an additional patient, may indicate an increased incidence of lymphoproliferative diseases in CDA III.

Laboratory Abnormalities. In CDA III, splenomegaly is usually minimal or absent. The anemia is usually mild to moderate, but transfusion-dependent patients have been observed. The circulating RBCs can be normal or mildly macrocytic. BM examination shows erythroid hyperplasia. Giant erythroblasts with up to 12 nuclei are the most distinctive feature of CDA III observed on light microscopic examination of the BM. These may appear similar to some of the large multinucleated cells seen in CDA II (see Fig. 29.14). Abnormally large lobulated nuclei and discordance in nuclear maturation are also found. Although they are hallmarks of CDA III, these findings are not pathognomonic and may be seen in erythroleukemia. Electron microscopy demonstrates nuclear clefts and blebs, autolytic areas within the cytoplasm, and iron-filled mitochondria. In some cases of CDA III with presumed autosomal dominant inheritance and in some sporadic cases, electron microscopy reveals that an occasional erythroblast section contains stellate or branching electron-dense intracytoplasmic inclusions. These are morphologically indistinguishable from those in HbH disease and consist of precipitated β-globin chains.

The acidified-serum lysis test result is negative in CDA III. Agglutination and lysis of erythrocytes to anti-i antibody has only been examined in a few cases of CDA III with conflicting findings. Serum thymidine kinase was measured in 20 patients with CDA III and 10 healthy siblings. Elevated thymidine kinase was found in all 20 cases but was normal in the siblings. It is suggested that measuring thymidine kinase levels can allow clinicians to discriminate between affected individuals and healthy siblings without performing a BM aspirate.

CDAs Groups IV to VII

Dozens of cases of CDA have been reported that do not conform to the classification of types I, II, and III. Some of the earlier reports of variants may or may not have been CDAs. In an attempt to sort out some of the better-documented cases, a phenotype-based classification was proposed by Wickramasinghe and Wood that assigns patients to one of four groups (not types), designated groups IV, V, VI, and VII. To qualify for inclusion in this classification, each group contains cases from three or more unrelated families. The features of each are as follows.

CDA Group IV. This group has severe anemia, transfusion dependence from birth, marked erythroid hyperplasia, normoblastic or mild to moderate megaloblastic changes, up to 8% BM erythroblasts with markedly irregular or karyorrhectic nuclei, and an absence of precipitated protein within erythroblasts by electron microscopy. An infant with group IV CDA presented with hydrops fetalis. The spleen is enlarged. The inheritance is not clear.

CDA Group V. Patients have normal or near-normal hemoglobin levels, a normal or slightly elevated MCV, and an increased serum unconjugated bilirubin. The BM shows marked erythroid hyperplasia and normoblastic or mild to moderate megaloblastic changes. The spleen may be palpable. The condition has been previously described as "primary shunt hyperbilirubinemia." Inheritance is variable and appears to be autosomal recessive in some cases but possibly autosomal dominant or X-linked in others. In CDA group V, the BM macrophages engulf morphologically normal but functionally abnormal erythroblasts.

CDA Group VI. This group is characterized by marked macrocytosis (MCV 119–125 fL) with little or no anemia and grossly megaloblastic erythropoiesis. There may be mild jaundice and an increased serum bilirubin. The differential diagnosis includes orotic aciduria and thiamine-responsive anemia. Vitamin B_{12} and RBC folate levels are normal.

CDA Group VII. These patients have severe transfusion-dependent anemia from birth, marked erythroid hyperplasia, normoblastic or nonspecific dysplastic changes, markedly abnormal nuclear shapes in many erythroblasts, and intraerythroblastic inclusions resembling precipitated α-globin chains. The inclusions do not react with monoclonal antibodies against α- and β-globin chains. The diagnosis requires the exclusion of β-thalassemia trait in the parents.

Unclassified CDA Cases

Unclassifiable cases of CDA have been reported with lifelong anemia that was probably inherited. These cases were characterized by marked aniso- and poikilocytosis and occasional teardrop and fragmented erythrocytes in the peripheral blood. Hyperplastic BM showed megaloblastoid features without multinuclearity or ringed sideroblasts, but a case with prominent ringed sideroblasts was also described. Unlike classical CDA, neutropenia or thrombocytopenia has been observed in some of these patients. Cytogenetic studies of BM revealed no clonal chromosomal abnormalities. Reticulocyte response to anemia was absent or inappropriately low in all. Most studies of parents failed to reveal abnormalities, suggesting an autosomal recessive mode of transmission.

Variant CDAs Associated With Specific Gene Mutations

GATA1 is a transcription factor closely linked with erythropoiesis and megakaryopoiesis. The Val205Met mutation in the **GATA1** gene underlies a CDA with dyserythropoiesis and thrombocytopenia.

The **KLF1** gene encodes an erythroid transcription factor. A specific mutation of KLF1 produced a severe form of CDA with basophilic stippling of polychromatic erythroblasts and erythrocytes, marked abnormalities of nuclear shape, and increased expression of embryonic and HbF.

A case of hereditary cryostomatocytosis and dyserythropoiesis was caused by a de novo erythroid anion exchanger **band 3 mutation.** The BM morphology showed dyserythropoiesis characteristic of CDA I and CDA II.

Mutant **MVK** resulted in mevalonate kinase deficiency, dyserythropoietic anemia, and BM findings similar to those in CDA II.

A syndrome of dyserythropoietic anemia, exocrine pancreatic insufficiency, and calvarial hyperostosis was caused by a mutation in **COX412,** a gene highly expressed in BM.

Differential Diagnosis

Marrow erythroblast multinuclearity is seen with other hematologic disorders, but these can be readily distinguished from CDA. The **megaloblastic anemias** have a different clinical presentation and are identified in the laboratory by the presence of hypersegmented neutrophils, decreased RBC folate values, or reduced serum levels of vitamin B_{12}. The **MDS** may manifest as an isolated refractory anemia, but they often present with bi- or trilineage cytopenias that contrast sharply with CDA. The MDS subsets may also show BM granulocytic and megakaryocytic morphologic abnormalities, the presence of myeloblasts, ringed sideroblasts, and clonal cytogenetic changes. **Erythroleukemia** (AML, M6) is another cause of marked dyserythropoiesis, but typically there is pancytopenia, the erythroblasts are avidly positive for the periodic acid–Schiff stain, and the BM cells may show a clonal cytogenetic marker. The **β-thalassemia syndromes**

differ from CDA by the presence of marked microcytosis with elevated levels of hemoglobin A_2, HbF, or both.

Therapy and Prognosis

In general, the CDAs are associated with a favorable long-term prognosis. For example, CDA I can be diagnosed late in life. One reported case was associated with a relatively benign course over a 30-year follow-up. Clinical manifestations of the CDAs may include intermittent jaundice and dark urine caused by increased hemoglobin catabolism or signs and symptoms of anemia. Rarely, hyperbilirubinemia without anemia may be the initial presentation of CDA patients. Cholelithiasis may be present as a consequence of chronic hyperbilirubinemia.

Anemia is typically mild in most cases of CDA and requires no intervention, but in more severe presentations, especially those requiring transfusional support, splenectomy may be beneficial. Most of the experience showing an improvement in hemoglobin levels after splenectomy has been in CDA II; the benefit of splenectomy in CDA I is less clear. Splenectomy may cause a persistent thrombocytosis in CDA types I and II and contribute to the development of Budd-Chiari syndrome and portal vein thrombosis.

Treatment of all forms of CDA with androgens, corticosteroids, vitamin E, vitamin B_{12}, folic acid, pyridoxine, or iron is ineffective in ameliorating the anemia. Iron therapy is also contraindicated because of the underlying propensity for hemosiderosis secondary to ineffective erythropoiesis, transfusional iron overload, increased gut iron absorption, and downregulation of the primary regulator of iron absorption, hepcidin. Even if regular RBC transfusions are not initiated, patients should be routinely monitored for evidence of iron overload. Iron chelation with daily subcutaneous infusions of deferoxamine (Desferal) has been underused in CDA even though deaths have been recorded from hemochromatosis. The value of the oral iron chelator deferasirox (Exjade) has not been defined yet for the CDAs.

Phlebotomy has been carried out to remove iron in selected CDA patients, but this could result in a worsening of the anemia and theoretically enhance gut iron absorption. An additional concern is that CDA patients seem predisposed to hepatic cirrhosis irrespective of body iron burden. The pathogenesis of this is unclear.

Interferon-α-2a or INF-α-2b therapy given two or three times a week or peg-INF-α-2a once a week, increase hemoglobin levels and decrease iron overload in most patients with CDA I who require repeated transfusions for moderately severe anemia. Erythrokinetic studies demonstrate a striking reduction of ineffective erythropoiesis in patients receiving INF, and electron microscopy shows a reduction in nuclear structural abnormalities. INF therapy should also be considered in moderately anemic CDA I patients before treatment of iron overload with phlebotomy. Patients with CDA II do not respond to INF-α.

Hematopoietic stem cell transplantation has been curative in a few severe cases of CDA, including transfusion-dependent CDA type I, CDA type II, Ham test–negative "CDA type II," and an unclassifiable CDA.

Asymptomatic extramedullary hematopoiesis may mimic tumors of the mediastinum, abdomen, and vertebral column. Because of the increased RBC production that occurs, the development of sites of extramedullary hematopoiesis may result in an amelioration of the degree of anemia. Technetium-99m sulfur colloid scintigraphy is useful in delineating the extent of these regions.

Future Directions

Identification of the various mutant genes for the CDA types will facilitate a more precise classification than the phenotype-based system used currently. The wild-type protein product of the CDA genes requires further research to clarify their function in health and their role in producing CDA when mutated. Strategies are required for managing iron overload similar to those for DBA and thalassemia major. In this regard, the therapeutic benefit of oral iron chelators such as Exjade should be explored fully.

INHERITED BONE MARROW FAILURE SYNDROMES WITH PREDOMINANTLY NEUTROPENIA

Kostmann Syndrome and Severe Congenital Neutropenia

Background

Kostmann syndrome (KS) and severe congenital neutropenia (SCN) refer to inherited types of neutropenia with onset in early childhood of profound neutropenia (ANC <200/μL), recurrent life-threatening infections, and a maturation arrest of myeloid precursors at the promyelocyte-myelocyte stage of differentiation. Some experts in the field refer to KS as the autosomal recessive type of severe inherited neutropenia and to SCN to all the other inherited neutropenia with similar phenotype. However, because many IBMFSs are inherited in different modes and because SCN and KS are indistinguishable phenotypically in the majority of the patients, the option to "split" the two disorders is debatable. In this chapter, we will refer to them as Kostmann/severe congenital neutropenia (K/SCN).

The initial description of syndrome made by Dr. Kostmann in 1956 included several neutropenic patients in a large intermarried Swedish kinship. An autosomal recessive mode of inheritance in 24 cases was deduced by inference because of hematologically normal parents with two or more neutropenic children in several families. Recently, homozygous germline *HAX1* mutations have been identified in patients with K/SCN, including some from the original pedigree described by Dr. Kostmann, confirming an autosomal recessive inheritance in these families. Nevertheless, it is now clear that the K/SCN group is genetically heterogeneous despite a shared hematologic phenotype (see Table 29.1). The first identified K/SCN gene was the neutrophil elastase 2 gene (*ELA2* or *ELANE*), which was found mutated on one allele in patients with K/SCN, indicating an autosomal dominant inheritance in many cases.

Epidemiology

K/SCNs are rare. The estimated incidence based on data from CIMFR from 2001–2010 was 4.7 cases per million live births per year. There is equal distribution of the disease between genders. There might be different frequency of specific genetic groups in different countries. For example, *HAX1* mutations in North America was found only in patients who immigrated from certain European countries.

Etiology, Genetics, and Pathophysiology

The discovery of heterozygous mutations in the *ELANE* gene encoding neutrophil elastase in 22 of 25 sporadic and dominantly inherited patients with K/SCN was the entry point for understanding the molecular basis of the disorder in many patients. Among patients with K/SCN enrolled in the North American cohort, the most common mutations are in *ELANE* (about 60%). Mutations in other genes (e.g., in *GFI1* and *GCPC3*) were rare. The rest of the patients did not have identified mutations and no mutations in *HAX1* were found. In Europe *ELANE* mutations are present in 60% of patients, followed by mutations in *HAX1* in 20% to 25% of patients. Mutant *ELANE* also occurs in all cases of classical cyclic neutropenia, but the mutations cluster in exon 4 or 5 on the gene or at the junction of exon 4 with intron 4. Patients with congenital neutropenia have mutations more widely distributed over exons 2, 3, 4, and 5.

Although typical K/SCN patients present early in life with severe neutropenia and life-threatening infections, rare cases with *ELANE*

mutations in phenotypically healthy family members were reported. For example, two siblings with congenital neutropenia inherited the same heterozygous *ELANE* mutation from their hematologically normal father. In another family, a healthy father of a congenital neutropenia patient was mosaic for his daughter's Cys42Arg mutation in peripheral blood hematopoietic cells. The mutation was found in about 50% of his T lymphocytes but only in 10% of his neutrophils. This is congruent with a lack of recurrent infection phenotype in the father. The mutation was evident in myeloid precursors but was selectively lost during myelopoiesis or failed to mature to neutrophils.

The exact mechanism whereby mutant *ELANE* causes neutropenia is unclear. *ELANE* encodes neutrophil elastase, a glycoprotein synthesized in the promyelocyte/myelocyte stages and packed in the azurophilic cytoplasmic granules. It is released in response to infection and inflammation. There are several proposed mechanisms for how mutations in *ELANE* cause neutropenia. The wild-type neutrophil elastase diffusely localizes throughout the cytoplasm. It has been shown that the mutated protein is not reduced, but mistrafficked and is abnormally concentrated in the nucleus and plasma membrane. Interestingly, mutations that disrupt the ATG translation initiation codon or the immediately adjacent Kozak sequence have shown to cause translation from downstream in-frame initiation codons, yielding a protein that lack the amino-terminally domain sequences that are important for ER-localizing. A second theory suggests that the mutant protein leads to accumulation of nonfunctional protein in the endoplasmic reticulum, activation of unfolded protein response, and apoptosis of K/SCN neutrophils. Related to this theory, decreased expression of Bcl-2 was observed in K/SCN myeloid progenitor cells along with constitutive mitochondrial release of cytochrome C and excessive cellular apoptosis. Of note, administration of G-CSF restored Bcl-2 expression and improved survival of myeloid progenitor cells. Another proposed mechanism is downregulation of lymphoid enhancer-binding factor 1 (*LEF-1*) in K/SCN. This leads to reduced transcription of *LEF1*-target genes such as *C/EBP*-α and impaired granulocytic differentiation.

HAX1 was reported to be mutated in 40% of patients with K/SCN in a European study but in only few patients in the CIMFR. HAX1 localizes to the mitochondria. It contains two domains reminiscent of a BH1 and BH2 of the BCL-2 family. It promotes normal potential of the inner mitochondrial membrane and protects myeloid cells from apoptosis. The direct function of HAX1 in promoting survival may explain the accelerated apoptosis reported in K/SCN neutrophils. *HAX1-mutant* K/SCN cells are also characterized by reduced LEF1 levels as in *ELANE-mutant* K/SCN cells.

A constitutively activating mutation in the Wiskott-Aldrich syndrome protein encoded by the *WASP* gene was discovered in five males from a three-generation family. The phenotype was composed of severe neutropenia from birth, bacterial infections, monocytopenia, and shifts of lymphocyte subsets. BM morphology showed a selective maturation arrest at the promyelocyte/myelocyte stage similar to K/SCN. Mutant *WASP* leads to constitutive activation of the WASP protein because of disruption of an autoinhibitory domain in the wild-type protein. This increased WASP protein activity produces marked abnormalities of cytoskeletal structure and dynamics, disruption of mitosis, genomic instability, and apoptosis of neutrophils.

Mutations in the proto-oncogene *GFI1* also cause K/SCN with severe neutropenia and a maturation arrest at the promyelocyte–myelocyte stage. GFI1-deficient mice exhibit severe neutropenia with accumulation of abnormal arrested progenitors and increased HSC/P proliferation. GFI1 is a transcriptional repressor of several transcription programs. The first transcription program is active during the progenitor stage. During this stage, GFI1 downregulates the HoxA9-Pbx1-Meis1 transcription factor complex. Because HOXA9 drives progenitor proliferation, GFI1 deficiency leads to uncontrolled HOXA2 activation and accumulation of arrested-differentiation myeloid progenitors. The second transcription program is activated during terminal granulopoietic differentiation. During this stage, GFI1 represses genes that promote differentiation of nongranulocytic cells such as CSF1. Patient-related mutations also disable the GFI1 repressor activity on *ELANE* expression, which leads to accumulation of neutrophil elastase in all subcellular compartments and might underlie the mechanism for premature apoptosis. Another potential mechanism for neutropenia when GFI1 is deficient might be related to loss of GFI1-mediated regulation of the expression of the microRNAs miR-21 and miR-196b, which regulate myeloid maturation.

A constitutive point mutation was discovered in the extracellular domain of the G-CSF receptor (*GCSFR* or *CSF3R*) in a patient with K/SCN who also had a mutant *ELANE* gene. The receptor mutation affected ligand–receptor complex formation with severe consequences for intracellular signal transduction; the patient was totally unresponsive to G-CSF therapy. As demonstrated in vitro and then clinically, corticosteroids combined with G-CSF produced a corrective action through synergistic activation of STAT5, and the patient responded to G-CSF therapy. Subsequently additional patients with cell-surface *GCSFR* mutations who did not refractory to G-CSF therapy were published, suggesting that this may be a common finding in cases unresponsive to treatment. Importantly, four K/SCN patients from two different families who did not respond to G-CSF treatment were found to have biallelic mutations in *GCSFR*.

Regarding the cellular pathology of K/SCN, many cell culture studies performed in the 1970s and 1980s provided clonogenic data that pointed to intrinsically defective granulocytic progenitors. Further reports confirmed this and excluded other possible pathogenetic factors. To summarize: (1) K/SCN BM myeloid colony growth is defective, (2) K/SCN serum contains normal or increased levels of G-CSF, (3) endogenous K/SCN G-CSF has normal biologic activity, (4) G-CSF receptors are expressed in slightly increased numbers on myeloid cells from K/SCN patients, and (5) the binding constant for G-CSF to its receptor in K/SCN is normal.

Regarding correlation between the mutated gene and phenotype, *ELANE* mutations are associated with severe and early-onset neutropenia with differentiation arrest at the stage of promyelocyte-myelocyte. Typically, the patients do not have physical malformations. The patients have a high risk of MDS/AML but no known risk of solid tumors. Patients with mutations in *HAX1* typically have severe and early-onset neutropenia with differentiation arrest at the stage of promyelocyte–myelocyte. They also have a high risk of MDS/AML but no known risk of solid tumors. About 30% of patients with *HAX1* mutations have neurologic abnormalities such as seizures, learning disabilities, and developmental delay. This is attributable to nonsense mutations (e.g., p.Gln155ProfsX14) that affect the *HAX1* transcript that is expressed in the central nervous system in addition to that expressed in hematopoietic cells. Mutations in *WAS* are associated with moderate to severe neutropenia, reduced phagocyte activity, monocytopenia, lymphopenia, reduced NK cells, reduced lymphocyte proliferation, and recurrent infections (but usually not as frequent as in the classical K/SCN). MDS/monosomy 7 has also been reported. *GFI1* mutations are associated with severe to moderate neutropenia, and monocytosis, reduced B and T cells with normal lymphocytic function. There are no clear data about the BM findings in this type of neutropenia, and the risk of MDS/AML is unknown.

Clinical Features

Approximately half of patients develop clinically significant infections within the first month of life and almost all others develop them by 6 months. Skin abscesses are common, but deep-seated tissue infections and septicemias also occur. Data from the SCNIR illustrate examples of every conceivable form of bacterial and fungal infection in the precytokine era. Especially troublesome in survivors were recurrent episodes of otitis media and pneumonia; advanced gingival stomatitis, sometimes with tooth loss; and in the extreme, gut bacterial flora overgrowth, leading to malabsorption requiring total parenteral nutritional therapy.

In contrast to some of the other IBMFSs, physical malformations are uncommon. Birth weights are generally unremarkable, and physical examination findings are usually normal. There are a small

number of reports of short stature, cataracts, microcephaly, seizures, developmental delay, and mental retardation. As mentioned earlier, neurologic manifestations are part of a small group of patients with *HAX1* mutations. Data from the SCNIR indicate that some patients with K/SCN develop bone demineralization that may be an intrinsic component of the disorder; it has been observed before and during G-CSF therapy. The underlying pathogenesis is unclear, but patients can develop bone pain and unusual fractures. Osteopenia is a common theme with the IBMFSs.

Laboratory Findings

Peripheral Blood and Bone Marrow

Neutropenia is profound and persistent in K/SCN, usually less than 200/μL. A small number of patients have intermittent cycling patterns with regular periodicity that ranges in a low to severely low neutrophil count range. A compensatory two- to fourfold increase in monocytes is seen, sometimes accompanied by eosinophilia. At diagnosis, platelet numbers are normal or increased, and hemoglobin values are usually normal. In survivors in the precytokine era, anemia of chronic disease associated with recurrent infections and inflammation was common. Aside from neutropenia, humoral and cellular immunity is completely normal.

Bone marrow specimens are usually normocellular. The striking classic finding is a maturation arrest at the promyelocyte or myelocyte stage with a paucity of more mature elements. Promyelocytes are abundant and may have atypical nuclei and the cytoplasm may be vacuolated. Neutrophils and bands are usually absent (Fig. 29.16). BM eosinophilia and monocytosis is common. The other hematopoietic lineages are normal, active, and undisturbed.

Predisposition to Leukemia and Myelodysplastic Syndrome

Clearly, K/SCN carries a high risk of leukemia. There were three case reports of patients who developed AML before the use of hematopoietic growth factors and one more recent patient diagnosed with acute leukemia before starting G-CSF. As a rough estimate, in the

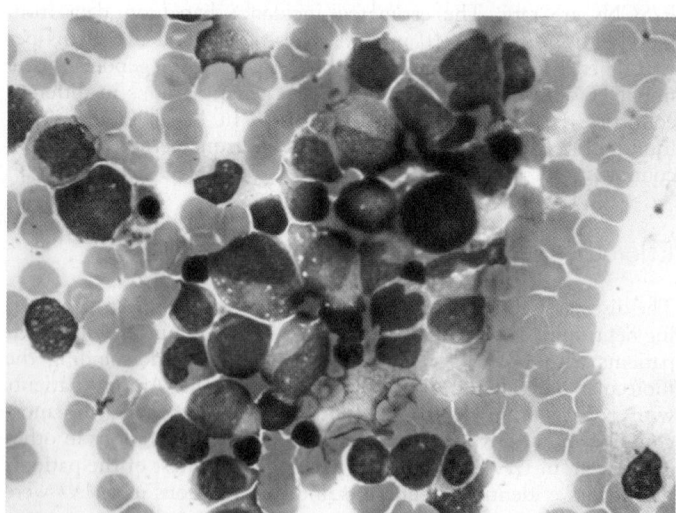

Fig. 29.16 HIGH-POWER VIEW OF A BONE MARROW ASPIRATE FROM A PATIENT WITH KOSTMANN SYNDROME (CONGENITAL NEUTROPENIA) BEFORE GRANULOCYTE COLONY-STIMULATING FACTOR THERAPY. The findings are a "maturation arrest" with recognizable myeloblasts, promyelocytes, myelocytes, and occasional metamyelocytes but total absence of band forms and neutrophils. *(Photomicrograph prepared by Dr. Mohamed Abdelhaleem, Toronto.)*

literature, there were 128 cases of congenital neutropenia reported and three cases of AML up to 1989 (the first year that G-CSF was available for general use), leading to a crude estimated risk of leukemia of 2%. Nevertheless, because most patients with congenital neutropenia died at a young age from bacterial sepsis or pneumonia in the precytokine era, the true risk of patients with congenital neutropenia developing MDS/AML was not clearly defined. Specific mutations (i.e., G214R or C151Y) were associated in one study with a high risk for evolution to AML.

G-CSF therapy completely changed clinical outcomes of K/SCN. Before G-CSF, the median duration of survival was about 3 years; the current median age is more than 40 years. The number of documented cases of MDS/AML has dramatically increased since 1989, which likely reflects the natural history of the disease that is now allowed to manifest by prolonging life. However, whether G-CSF increases this risk or hastens the appearance of leukemia is still debatable.

The risk of MDS/AML is higher in patients requiring higher doses of G-CSF. According to SCNIR data, less responsive patients, defined as those having ANCs of less than 2.1×10^9/L on G-CSF doses greater than 8 µg/kg/day had a cumulative incidence of MDS/AML of 34% after 15 years; more responsive patients, defined as having ANCs of greater than 2.1×10^9/L on G-CSF doses lower than 8 µg/kg/day had a cumulative incidence of 15%. The data were interpreted as indicating that a poor response to G-CSF defines an "at-risk" population and predicts an adverse outcome. The data do not necessarily support a cause-and-effect relationship between development of MDS/AML and G-CSF therapy. The results may only mean that patients requiring higher G-CSF therapy have a more severe clinical and hematologic phenotype. A report from the French Severe Chronic Neutropenia Study Group confirmed that increased exposure to G-CSF with respect to dose and duration in congenital neutropenia patients was associated with a heightened risk of MDS/AML, but they do not speculate on the mechanism.

Conversion to MDS/AML in K/SCN patients is associated with cellular genetic abnormalities that provide insight into the pathobiology of the transformation and may be useful in identifying patients who are at high risk. Several cellular and genetic changes have been found in the BM of patients with K/SCN who received G-CSF. Whether these changes are coupled to G-CSF therapy is unknown. Remarkably, the abnormalities have predictable, similar characteristics in most patients and underscore a fairly specific multistep pathogenesis in the evolution into MDS/AML. At varying time points after starting G-CSF therapy, about half of the congenital neutropenia patients who transform acquire the same activating RAS oncogene mutation, namely a GGT (glycine) to GAT (aspartic acid) substitution at codon 12. More than 90% of patients who transform also show an acquired cytogenetic clonal alteration in BM cells, usually −7 or 7q− but also +21 or +8. Complex cytogenetics (e.g., −7 and +21) have also been identified. More than 80% of patients develop one or more GCSFR point mutations. These GCSFR mutations are nonsense mutations that result in the truncation of the C-terminal cytoplasmic region, a subdomain that is crucial for G-CSF–induced maturation. The acquired mutation is directly operative in the conversion to MDS/AML. In murine models, the mutation results in impaired ligand internalization, defective receptor downmodulation, and enhanced growth signaling that produces an exaggerated hyperproliferative effect in response to G-CSF. This also confers resistance to apoptosis and enhances cell survival that favors clonal expansion in vivo. The detection of GCSFR mutations places patients at high risk for malignant conversion, but the time course from detection of mutations to overt MDS/AML varies considerably and may take years.

Although patients requiring higher doses of G-CSF to attain safe neutrophil levels are at a higher risk of developing MDS/AML, there is no definitive evidence that G-CSF directly causes malignant transformation. G-CSF may simply be an "innocent bystander" that corrects the neutropenia, prolongs patient survival, and allows time for the malignant predisposition to declare itself. Alternatively, G-CSF may accelerate the propensity for MDS/AML in the genetically

altered stem and progenitor cells in congenital neutropenia. G-CSF may rescue malignant clones that would otherwise be destined for apoptosis. The clinical interplay between G-CSF and the receptor mutation was underscored in the report of a patient with congenital neutropenia on G-CSF who developed a receptor mutation and AML. When G-CSF was stopped, the blast count in blood and in BM fell to undetectable levels on two occasions without giving chemotherapy, although the mutant receptor was persistently detectable during the remissions. A similar patient has been observed in Toronto (Y. Dror, unpublished data).

An axiom of oncogenesis is that rapidly dividing cells are more susceptible to mutational events. Because therapeutic G-CSF provides a powerful proliferative signal for BM cells, it is a reasonable hypothesis that congenital neutropenia BM progenitors acquire new mutations. From the evidence cited herein, acquisition of a G-CSF receptor mutation in the face of therapeutic G-CSF in congenital neutropenia can provide the hyperresponsive replicative scenario that can relentlessly evolve into MDS/AML. Is recombinant human G-CSF a carcinogen? This would seem highly unlikely. As a physiologic regulator of hematopoiesis, it would be unexpected for G-CSF to break molecular bonds and cause DNA damage even when used in therapeutic dosages.

In one patient with K/SCN who progressed to MDS/L, clonal evolution was assessed by exome sequencing of whole marrow cells. A pro-proliferative, differentiation-defective GCSFR mutation was found, that persisted and acquired secondary mutations. The frequency of RUNX1 mutations was high in a cohort of K/SCN patients who developed MDS/L. Mutations in RUNX1 and GCSFR cooperate to promote clonal expansion.

Differential Diagnosis

The commonest cause of isolated neutropenia in very young children is **viral-induced BM suppression.** An antecedent history of good health, the occurrence of a viral illness, and the transient nature of the neutropenia distinguish this disorder from K/SCN.

Autoimmune neutropenia of infancy is recognized as a fairly specific syndrome of early childhood. Low neutrophil numbers are often discovered during the course of routine investigation for a benign febrile illness. The illness abates, but the neutropenia persists, sometimes for months and occasionally for years. A BM biopsy is normocellular, and an aspirate shows active granulopoiesis up to the band stage; neutrophils may be normally represented, reduced or absent. The neutropenia is caused by increased peripheral destruction and the diagnosis can be supported by demonstrating specific antigranulocyte antibodies on neutrophils. The prognosis is good, the neutropenia is self-limited albeit protracted, and patients seldom develop serious bacterial infections as a result of it. Other infrequent acquired causes of severe, isolated neutropenia in this age group include BM suppression from a drug or toxin and neutrophil sequestration as part of a hypersplenism syndrome.

Of the IBMFSs, **SDS** can also manifest as isolated neutropenia but can be identified because of growth failure, the malabsorption component caused by pancreatic insufficiency, fatty changes in the pancreas seen on CT scanning or ultrasonography, and characteristic skeletal abnormalities. **Glycogen storage disease type 1b (GSD-1b)** and **Barth syndrome** are also in the differential diagnosis. Neutropenia can also be a prominent part of **antibody deficiency syndromes** and **cellular immunodeficiency disorders** (Table 29.8); investigation of chronic neutropenia of childhood should include an immunoglobulin electrophoresis, T-cell proliferative studies, and quantitation of T-cell subsets and NK cell activity. **Cyclic neutropenia** is distinguished by predictable symptomatology, especially mouth sores about every 3 weeks (19–23 days), often associated with chronic gingivitis. A complete blood count two or three times a week for 4 to 8 weeks demonstrates the diagnostic oscillation pattern with a cyclic nadir. Other **unclassified inherited neutropenia syndromes** with vertical transmission or in siblings have been described. The neutropenia in such cases are typically mild to moderate. When severe

TABLE 29.8	Miscellaneous Inherited Neutropenia Disorders				
Diagnosis	Genetics	Mapping	Mutant Gene	Additional Features
Hyper IgM syndrome, type 1	X-L	Xq26	*CD4OL*	↓ IgG, IgA, IgE, autoimmune cytopenias
Hermansky-Pudlak syndrome, type 2	AR	5q14.1	*AP3B1*	↓ IgG, partial albinism, platelet dysfunction
Griscelli syndrome, type 1	AR	15q21	*MYO5A*	Neurologic dysfunction, partial albinism
Griscelli syndrome, type 2	AR	15q21	*RAB27A*	Same as type 1 plus hemophagocytosis
Chediak-Higashi syndrome	AR	1q42.1-q42.2	*LYST (CHSI)*	Immunodeficiency, partial albinism
Poikiloderma with neutropenia	AR	16q13	*C16ORF57*	Rash, short stature, dystrophic nails
P14 deficiency	AR	1q22	*MAPBPIP*	Immunodeficiency, hypopigmentation
Cohen syndrome	AR	8q22-q23	*VPS13B/COH1*	Retinopathy, retardation, skeletal anomalies
Charcot-Marie-Tooth syndrome, type 2	AD	19p13.2	*DMN2*	Axonal demyelinating neuropathy

AD, Autosomal dominant; AR, autosomal recessive; Ig, immunoglobulin; X-L, X-linked recessive.
Data compiled from Online Mendelian Inheritance in Man (http://ncbi.nlm.nih.gov/omim).

neutropenia is diagnosed in the newborn period, the cause may be passive transfer transplacentally of IgG antineutrophil antibodies from the mother. This can occur if the mother has an autoimmune disorder with neutropenia or by alloimmunization caused by fetomaternal incompatibility for a neutrophil-specific antigen.

Therapy and Prognosis

Before the introduction of G-CSF as a specific therapy of K/SCN, there was limited treatment. Antibiotics were the mainstay of management for active infection and for prophylaxis. Attempts to mobilize neutrophils with lithium had limited application.

Cytokine Therapy

G-CSF has supplanted all other forms of management because more than 90% of K/SCN patients respond. It is recommended to begin G-CSF therapy as front-line treatment when the diagnosis is established. GM-CSF in crossover trials with G-CSF for K/SCN is not as effective and does not induce a neutrophil response consistently. The specific target of ANC when G-CSF is given to K/SCN patients has not been carefully studied. A level of above 1.0×10^9/L is considered as a target by some investigator in the field. However, ANC above 0.75×10^9/L that is not associated with infections might also be acceptable. If the ANC remains below the target after initiation of G-CSF at 5 µg/kg/dose once a day subcutaneously, the dose may be escalated to 10 µg/kg/dose and then by increments of 10 µg/kg/dose at 7- to 14-day intervals until a response is seen. The occurrence of bacterial infection is reduced dramatically with an ANC of 1×10^9/L or above. Patients who are proven to be infection-free with ANC of 0.75 to 1.0 may continue on the same G-CSF doses. The G-CSF dose can be reduced if the ANC increases to 5.0×10^9/L or above to find the lowest dose necessary for maintaining a neutrophil count at 0.75 to 1.0×10^9/L or greater. The SCNIR coinvestigators defined nonresponders as patients who do not respond to G-CSF levels exceeding 120 µg/kg/day. Partial responders show an increase of their ANC to 0.5 to 1.0×10^9/L with the highest dose, but they still experience bacterial infections. In these patients, the dose of G-CSF cannot be increased because of the large volume and frequency of injections required. The only currently available treatment for patients who do not demonstrate sufficient response to G-CSF treatment is HSCT. In one published case of a G-CSF nonresponder, the addition of small dose of prednisone (5 mg/day) to a standard G-CSF dose of about 5 µg/kg resulted in a long-term complete response. HSCT should be considered for patients who require high doses of G-CSF, because of the association with high risk of developing MDS/AML.

All patients on G-CSF therapy should be seen by a physician every 3 to 6 months. Patients requiring more than 8 µg/kg/day are at higher risk for MDS/AML and should be evaluated more often. Blood counts (white blood cells, hemoglobin, platelets, and differential blood counts) should be obtained and a physical examination performed at least every 3 months, including assessment for weight and height in pediatric patients and documentation of intercurrent infections. BM examination for morphology and cytogenetics is recommended once a year to search for acquired cytogenetic abnormalities such as monosomy 7 or trisomy 21 and other early signs of MDS.

From SCNIR data, a sustained hematologic response in patients treated with G-CSF for more than 15 years has been confirmed. With therapy, neutrophil counts rise in more than 90% of K/SCN patients and are maintained at a plateau for protracted periods, resulting in vast clinical benefits. In no instance has there been BM or hematopoietic lineage "exhaustion" or depletion with G-CSF therapy.

Hematopoietic Stem Cell Transplantation

The SCNIR transplant data was reported in 2000. Of 29 who were transplanted, 18 had transformed to MDS, AML, or both, and the dual goal was to cure the malignancy and the neutropenia. Only three of the 18 were successful. The causes for failure included mismatched transplants, progressive refractory AML, serious illness at the time of the procedure, and transplants performed in desperation. The other 11 patients underwent HSCT for reasons other than malignant transformation, mostly because of no response or only partial response to G-CSF. Eight patients received stem cells from an HLA-matched sibling after conditioning mainly with busulfan–cyclophosphamide alone or with additional immunosuppression. In sharp contrast to the MDS/AML group, 9 of the 11 were cured with resolution of neutropenia.

A summary of 18 K/SCN cases transplanted between 1989 and 2005 in Japan for lack of or a partial response to treatment with G-CSF but without MDS/AML was published in 2010. Nine patients received stem cells from an HLA-identical sibling donor and nine from an alternative donor. Twelve received myeloablative regimens, and six patients received varying nonmyeloablative conditioning regimens. Sixteen of the patients were reported alive and in complete remission at a median follow-up of 6.5 years.

A multicenter retrospective analysis of umbilical cord transplants for IBMFs in Europe published in 2011 included 16 patients with K/SCN. The conditioning regimens were myeloablative in nature. One patient received a related cord blood graft, and the other 15 received unrelated grafts. Three patients were transplanted for leukemia or MDS using unrelated cord blood; two died. The other 13 patients were transplanted because of a lack of response to G-CSF. At a median follow-up of 41 months, 11 of the 13 were alive; one received an untreated graft, and 10 received unrelated grafts.

In the English literature, seven patients received nonmyeloaplastive regimens. However, the small number of patients, the different regimens, and the different indications (refractoriness to G-CSF or MDS/AML) do not allow meaningful conclusions.

In general, the best scenario for a curative HSCT is when the procedure is performed before developing MDS/AML using a matched-related donor and when the patient is in good physical condition. In a small series of six transplanted patients for MDS or AML, two with MDS who underwent the procedure without being given induction chemotherapy survived, but four with AML given induction chemotherapy had significantly more morbidity and died posttransplant, raising questions about conditioning strategies for these patients. Two other cases with AML from Japan were published in 2013. In both cases HSCT without prior AML-type chemotherapy was successfully applied.

The discovery of an isolated BM clonal cytogenetic abnormality without other evidence of MDS or AML in patients with congenital neutropenia raises management issues. One option is to perform HSCT if there is a matched donor as soon as feasible. This has generally been recommended for patients with −7, 7q−, or +21. The a priori argument is that the chance for cure is higher when the patient is well and has a low burden of malignant cells. The problem with this decision centers on not knowing the tempo of progression from cytogenetic evolution to clear-cut MDS or AML. Thus there may not be a need to rush to transplant in all patients. Instead, one recommendation is to lower the G-CSF to the lowest dose that maintains neutrophil counts greater than 0.5×10^9/L and to monitor the patient regularly with blood counts and by serial BM testing.

Opinions also vary about the best way to manage patients with other genetic changes such as *G-CSF-R* or *RAS* mutations but without clonal BM cytogenetic abnormalities or morphologic evidence of transformation. In one patient with an isolated G-CSF receptor mutation, an HSCT was performed to eliminate the risk of leukemic conversion. Debate about this approach continues, and watchful waiting is an acceptable option.

Therapeutic options for newly diagnosed patients with K/SCN must be constantly reevaluated. It is largely accepted that G-CSF induces robust neutrophilic responses and eliminates infections almost completely in more than 90% of K/SCN patients. Therefore it should be the first treatment choice. HSCT has been regarded as "salvage" therapy for patients who either acquire evidence of malignant myeloid transformation or fail to respond to G-CSF altogether. For KS patients transplanted with a fully matched donor before transforming to MDS/AML and in stable health, the chance for cure is at least 85%, possibly higher. The SCNIR data support this estimate. Not only is the neutropenia fully corrected by HSCT, but the risk of MDS/AML is also eliminated. The onerous burden of daily subcutaneous injections is removed, the financial expense is relieved, and the side effects of G-CSF are prevented. Clearly, an 85% cure rate stacks up favorably against the high cumulative incidence of incurable MDS/AML over time, particularly in patients who require large doses of G-CSF. HSCT is a reasonable option as front-line therapy for selected higher risk patients instead of G-CSF, and the option should be discussed fairly and sensibly with newly diagnosed patients and families.

Bisphosphonates for Osteoporosis

In 50% of K/SCN patients on G-CSF, bone density measurements show varying degrees of osteopenia and osteoporosis. It is unclear whether the osteopenia in SCN is caused by G-CSF or the underlying disease or a combination of both. Most of the cases with osteopenia are subclinical and asymptomatic, but some patients complain of bone pain and have fractures. Evidence shows that bisphosphonates are an effective treatment for the majority of these cases.

Future Directions

The list of K/SCN genes is by no means complete, and further studies are necessary to discover novel genes. It is also not clear if there is an association between specific mutations and the risk of evolution to MDS and acute leukemia, but studies are ongoing to try to answer this clinical question. At present, diagnosis of cyclic and congenital neutropenia still depends primarily on observations of serial blood cell counts, but it is expected that mutational analysis of the *ELANE* gene will become a routine part of making the diagnosis and the

establishment of a prognosis for these patients in the years ahead. Because apoptosis is a central mechanism of neutropenia in these patients, future studies will determine whether the term *maturation arrest* should be replaced by *accelerated apoptosis* as a descriptive term for the BM findings. It appears that cellular models involving transfection of the mutant genes into human myeloid cell lines provide evidence of how neutropenia occurs. Potentially, these models can also be used to examine new approaches to preventing apoptosis and serve to provide clues to new and more effective therapies. Considerable data now confirm the effectiveness of G-CSF in the treatment of various forms of K/SCN. However, the inconvenient administration, potential long-term effects, and lack of response in 10% of patients require the development of alternative therapies. Gene therapy is still to be developed.

Cyclic Neutropenia

Cyclic neutropenia is an autosomal dominant disorder characterized by a regular, repetitive reduction in peripheral blood neutrophils for 3 to 4 days every 19 to 23 days. Between nadirs, the patients have normal or nearly normal neutrophil counts. Patients usually present in infancy or childhood and have a less severe infectious course compared with those with K/SCN. However, life-threatening infections have been reported. A proportion of patients need treatment. Daily administration of G-CSF typically improves symptoms in most patients.

Cyclic neutropenia is caused by heterozygous mutations in the *ELANE (ELA2)* gene that encodes neutrophil elastase. The mutations usually occur at the active site of neutrophil elastase without disrupting the enzymatic substrate cleavage by the active site. The mutations seem to disturb a predicted transmembrane domain, leading to excessive granular accumulation of elastase and defective membrane localization of the enzyme. The myeloid precursors are characterized by cyclic increases in apoptosis. However, the precise molecular mechanism for the cycling hematopoiesis has not been defined. It is also not clear why the same mutations in *ELANE* are associated with both cyclic and K/SCN phenotypes.

Myelokathexis and WHIM Syndrome

Myelokathexis is a rare autosomal dominant disorder with recurrent bacterial infections caused by a reduced number and function of neutrophils. Neutropenia is typically moderate to severe. Degenerative changes in the granulocytes are characteristic and include pyknotic nuclear lobes, fine chromatin filaments, and hypersegmentation. The BM is usually hypercellular with granulocytic hyperplasia. The pathophysiology of myelokathexis has been attributed to a defective release of BM cells into the peripheral blood. Neutrophil precursors are characterized by decreased expression of BCL-X and accelerated apoptosis. G-CSF ameliorates the neutropenia and leads to clinical improvement during episodes of bacterial infection.

WHIM syndrome refers to the association of myelokathexis with other features (**w**arts, **h**ypogammaglobulinemia, **i**nfections, and **m**yelokathexis). Most cases are caused by mutations in the chemokine receptor gene *CXCR4* but dysfunction of GRK3, a negative regulator of CXCR4, has also been implicated. The mutations result in enhanced chemotactic response of neutrophils in response to the CXCR4 ligand CXCL12 (stroma-derived factor 1) and pathologic retention of neutrophils in the BM. Patients with wild type *CXCR4* might have other genetic defects that lead to an enhanced interaction between CXCR4 and CXCL12 and an enhanced chemotactic response, such as reduced inhibition of CXCL12-promoted internalization, and desensitization of CXCR4 by G protein–coupled receptor (GPCR) kinase-3 caused by decreased transcription of the GPCR kinase-3. G-CSF induces a prompt increase in neutrophil numbers and gamma globulin levels may also increase. Twice-daily injections of plerixafor (CXCR4 antagonist) in three patients were associated with an increase in neutrophil counts, fewer infections and improvement of warts in combination with imiquimod. Immunoglobulin levels and specific antibody response were not fully corrected.

G6PC3-Associated SCN (Dursun Syndrome)

This syndrome is an autosomal recessive form of SCN caused by biallelic mutant *G6PC3*. Wild-type *G6PC3* encodes glucose-6-phosphatase catalytic subunit 3, which, when mutated, confers an increased susceptibility of neutrophils to apoptosis. BM samples morphology varied among the reported patients, but included mild to moderate decrease in mature neutrophils, normal appearing BM or promyelocyte-myelocyte maturation arrest. Neutropenia is usually severe, rendering patients susceptible to severe bacterial infections. Lymphopenia and thrombocytopenia may occur. Structural heart defects, urogenital abnormalities, venous angiectasia on the trunk and extremities, intellectual disability, inflammatory bowel disease, and a broad range of other physical abnormalities are additional features. One reported patient developed MDS and subsequently AML.

Barth Syndrome

Barth syndrome is a rare multisystem metabolic disorder inherited in an X-linked recessive mode. It is the first human disease in which the primary causative factor is an alteration of cardiolipin remodeling. Cardiolipin is a component of the inner mitochondrial membrane necessary for proper functioning of the electron transport chain.

The findings in typical cases are mild to severe neutropenia, dilated or hypertrophic cardiomyopathy, underdeveloped skeletal musculature and muscle weakness, exercise intolerance, growth delay, cardiolipin abnormalities, and 3-methylglutaconic aciduria. ANCs are variable, but total agranulocytosis has been reported. BM morphology includes a maturation arrest at the myelocyte stage. On electron microscopy, mitochondria show concentric, tightly packed cristae and occasional inclusion bodies in various tissues, including granulocyte precursors. Clinically, the cardiomyopathy dominates the clinical picture, but gingivitis, oral problems, and bacterial sepsis from neutropenia can be problematic. Most patients do not need treatment with G-CSF. Anecdotal reports and the authors' experience (Y. Dror, unpublished data) suggest that G-CSF is highly effective in correcting the neutropenia and preventing infections. The myriad clinical problems requires a multidisciplinary approach. Female carriers are healthy and hematologically normal, likely because of extreme skewing of X-inactivation. The initial impression that Barth syndrome was a lethal infantile disease has been modified; age distribution in 54 living patients ranges from 0 to 49 years and peaks around puberty.

The Barth syndrome gene was mapped to Xq28, which led to the cloning of the *TAZ* gene and the various mutations that account for the phenotype. *TAZ* produces several different mRNAs with resultant proteins called tafazzins. Mutations in *TAZ* result in a decrease in tetralinoleoyl species of cardiolipin and an accumulation of monolysocardiolipin within cells. A murine model of Barth syndrome has been developed. Knocked-down cellular models and patient BM cells are characterized by accelerated cell death. However, a recently proposed mechanism for the neutropenia involves exposure of cell surface phosphatidylserine because of ROS, and consequently increased clearance of neutrophils by tissue macrophages.

Glycogen Storage Disease Type 1b

Glycogen storage disease type 1b is caused by a deficiency in glucose-6-phosphate translocase (transporter) because of mutant *G6PT1 (SLC37A4)*. GSD-1b patients experience disturbed glucose homeostasis and quantitative or qualitative neutrophil abnormalities.

The translocase transports glucose-6-phosphate into the lumen of the endoplasmic reticulum, where it is hydrolyzed into glucose and inorganic phosphate. Absence of translocase results in an inability to liberate glucose from glucose-6-phosphate. Consequently, patients with GSD-1b are susceptible to fasting hypoglycemia, lactic acidosis, hepatomegaly, poor linear growth, delayed pubertal development, and other systemic complications.

Most patients have neutropenia, which ranges from mild to severe. A strict correlation between genotype and the degree of neutropenia has not been established. Some studies reported hypocellular BM; however, BM testing on nine patients from the City of Hope National Medical Center in 2001 before G-CSF therapy revealed normal to hypercellularity in all patients. Maturation arrest at the myelocyte stage or later is a feature. Neutrophil apoptosis appears to be a central mechanism leading to granulopoietic failure. Neutrophil dysfunction with defective chemotaxis and an impaired respiratory burst is an additional feature. Patients are consequently susceptible to recurrent infections and to inflammatory bowel disease. Infections most commonly involve the skin, perirectal area, ears, and urinary tract, but septicemia, pneumonia, and meningitis may also occur. The most frequently isolated organisms include *Staphylococcus aureus*, group A streptococci, *Streptococcus pneumoniae, Escherichia coli*, and *Pseudomonas*.

G-CSF therapy is extremely effective in almost all GSD-1b patients. BM cellularity increases, the ANCs increase exuberantly, and impaired oxygen radical formation is corrected. AML while on G-CSF is a rare event. Prospective data on GSD-1b patients receiving G-CSF therapy from the SCNIR identified 40% with splenomegaly before starting G-CSF, 81% with splenomegaly by the first year of treatment, and 100% with splenomegaly by 3 years. Hypersplenism can occur but can be overcome by reducing the G-CSF dosage or by splenectomy. Histology of the surgically excised spleens shows extramedullary hematopoiesis.

Other Inherited Neutropenias

Other inherited neutropenia disorders are associated with specific mutant genes, but they do not necessarily have the K/SCN BM phenotype, nor is their pathophysiology necessarily similar (see Table 29.8). Immune deficiency appears to be an important component of these syndromes. These miscellaneous forms tend to have distinguishing physical abnormalities such as partial albinism and are not predisposed to MDS/AML.

INHERITED BONE MARROW FAILURE SYNDROMES WITH PREDOMINANTLY THROMBOCYTOPENIA

Thrombocytopenia With Absent Radii Syndrome

Background

Thrombocytopenia absent radii syndrome has two essential features, hypomegakaryocytic thrombocytopenia and bilateral radial aplasia with thumbs present. It is one of a group of IBMFSs that includes FA, DBA, and radioulnar synostosis with radial ray anomalies. The manifestations of the phenotype vary widely, and patients can present with abnormalities involving skeletal, skin, gastrointestinal, brain, renal, and cardiac systems. The identification of biallelic mutations in *RBM8A* in patients with TAR syndrome determined the autosomal recessive inheritance of this disorder. Almost always, parents of patients with TAR are phenotypically normal. Women with TAR syndrome can conceive and give birth to hematologically and phenotypically normal offspring. Three cases of AML and one case of acute lymphoid *(lymphoidic)* leukemia in TAR syndrome patients have been reported. Using a denominator of about 300 published cases of TAR, four leukemic episodes (1–2% crude rate) suggests a predisposition to the development of hematologic malignancies.

Etiology and Pathophysiology

Thrombocytopenia in TAR syndrome is the result of a defect in megakaryocytopoiesis and thrombocytopoiesis. It was previously shown that patients with TAR have submicroscopic deletions at 1q21.1 in one allele of *RBMA8* in 100% of cases. The allele carries one of two low-frequency SNPs in the regulatory regions of *RBM8A*. *RBM8A* encodes the Y14 subunit of exon-junction complex, which processes mRNA. The mutations caused reduced expression of the protein in platelets from affected individuals.

Thrombopoietin levels in plasma or serum are consistently elevated in TAR syndrome, thereby excluding a cytokine production defect as a cause for thrombocytopenia in this disorder. BM CFU-MK progenitors are either absent or are present in low to normal frequencies but produce small colonies in vitro with abnormal morphology. CFU-GM and BFU-E colony growth is often increased.

In a detailed study of CD34+ cells, the thrombocytopenia of TAR syndrome was associated with a dysmegakaryocytopoiesis characterized by cells remaining at an early stage of differentiation. Cells expressing CD41 without CD42 accumulated behind the block, and there was a decrease in c-mpl transcripts and mpl protein. The response of platelets to adenosine diphosphate or to the thrombin receptor agonist peptide SFLLRN (TRAP) is normal in patients with TAR. However, in contrast to control participants, platelets from patients with TAR do not undergo activation in vitro in response to recombinant thrombopoietin as measured by testing thrombopoietin synergism to adenosine diphosphate and TRAP. Thrombopoietin-induced tyrosine phosphorylation of platelet proteins in this setting is completely absent or markedly decreased. The results indicate that there is a lack of response to thrombopoietin downstream the c-mpl signal transduction pathway.

No recurrent chromosomal changes are seen in TAR syndrome. Some karyotypic abnormalities found in a few patients are of unclear significance. Clastogenic induced chromosomal breakage analysis in TAR syndrome is normal.

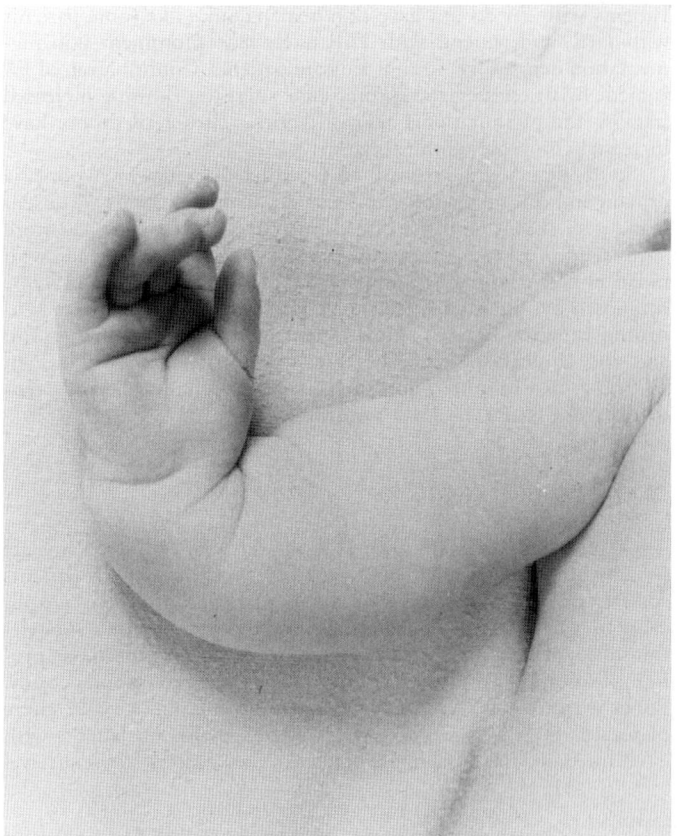

Fig. 29.17 RADIAL APLASIA WITH PRESERVATION OF THE THUMB IN A NEWBORN WITH THROMBOCYTOPENIA WITH ABSENT RADII SYNDROME.

Clinical Features

History and Physical Examination

The diagnosis is made during the newborn period because of the absent radii, and about half of patients develop a petechial rash and overt hemorrhage such as bloody diarrhea. Patients have bilateral radial aplasia (Fig. 29.17) with preservation of the thumbs and fingers on both sides. Additional upper extremity deformities include radial club hands; hypoplastic carpals and phalanges; and hypoplastic ulnae, humeri, and shoulder girdles. Syndactyly and clinodactyly of the toes and fingers are also seen. Characteristic findings include a selective hypoplasia of the middle phalanx of the fifth finger and altered palmar contours. Upper extremity involvement ranges from isolated absent radii to true, often asymmetric, phocomelia. The lower extremities are involved in about half of cases. Malformations include hip dislocation, coxa valga, femoral torsion, tibial torsion, abnormal tibiofibular joints, small feet, and valgus and varus foot deformities. Abnormal toe placement is commonly seen, especially the fifth toe overlapping the fourth. Similar to upper limb involvement, lower extremity deformities range from minimal involvement to complete phocomelia. An asymmetric first rib, a cervical rib, cervical spina bifida, and a fused cervical spine can occur, but trunk involvement is usually minimal. Micrognathia has been associated with the TAR syndrome in up to 65% of cases.

Cardiac abnormalities occur in 15% of patients, including atrial septal defect, tetralogy of Fallot, and ventricular septal defect. Capillary hemangiomas are common (24%) as well as redundant nuchal folds. Genitourinary tract malformations are detected in 23% of cases. About 95% of patients have short stature, 76% have macrocephaly, and 53% show facial dysmorphism. Structural brain abnormalities may be present. Additional findings are dorsal pedal edema, hyperhidrosis, and gastrointestinal disturbances such as diarrhea and feeding intolerance; almost 50% of patients are intolerant of cow's milk.

Prenatal diagnosis can be made by genetic testing, by ultrasound imaging of absent radii with thumbs present, and by measuring platelet numbers obtained by fetoscopy or cordocentesis. A published case describes a prenatal diagnosis of TAR followed by an in utero platelet transfusion to facilitate safe delivery.

Laboratory Findings

Thrombocytopenia as a result of BM underproduction is a consistent finding. BM specimens show normal to increased cellularity with decreased to absent megakaryocytes. The erythroid and myeloid lineages are normally represented. When a few megakaryocytes can be identified in biopsies, they are small, contain few nuclear segments, and show immature nongranular cytoplasm. If platelet counts increase spontaneously in patients after the first year of life, megakaryocytes increase in parallel and appear more mature morphologically. At diagnosis, leukocytosis is seen in the majority of patients and is sometimes extreme, to greater than 100,000/μL with a "left shift" to immature myeloid forms. The cause of this leukemoid reaction is unclear, but it is usually transient and subsides spontaneously. If anemia is present, it is likely attributable to blood loss caused by thrombocytopenia. When platelet numbers are adequate for study, their size is generally normal, and routine testing of function is unremarkable, although some patients may show abnormal platelet aggregation and storage pool defects. Compared with other IBMFSs, RBC size and HbF levels are normal.

Differential Diagnosis

Important clinical differences distinguish TAR syndrome from **FA**. In FA, when radii are absent, the thumbs are hypoplastic or absent.

Patients with FA do not have skin hemangiomas like some patients with TAR, and patients with TAR rarely have prominent skin pigmentation defects like 40% of Fanconi patients. Confirmation of FA is made by the clastogenic chromosome stress test showing increased fragility and by mutational analysis. Patients with TAR do not have increased chromosomal breakage.

Some infants with **trisomy 18** (+18) have absence or hypoplasia of radii and thrombocytopenia. However, in +18, thumbs are absent if radii are absent, and the disorder can also be distinguished from TAR syndrome cytogenetically. There are several syndromes with radial abnormalities but with *normal* platelet counts that can be diagnosed by mutational gene analysis. These include **Roberts syndrome** (mutant *ESC02*); **Holt-Oram syndrome** (mutant *TBX5*); and the clinical spectrum of three disorders caused by mutant *RECQL4:* **Rothmund-Thomson syndrome, Baller-Gerold syndrome,** and **RAPADILINO syndrome.**

Therapy and Prognosis

The risk of hemorrhage is greatest in the first year of life. Deaths are usually caused by intracranial or gastrointestinal bleeding. If patients survive the first year, platelet counts spontaneously increase inexplicably to levels that are hemostatically safe and do not require platelet transfusional support. A minority of patients have sustained, profound thrombocytopenia that does not improve spontaneously. Published cases of TAR syndrome show an actuarial survival curve plateau of 80% by age 1 to 2 years. Many reports of patients with TAR antedated the modern use of platelet transfusions, so the survival is likely much better currently. Patients with TAR do not evolve into having pancytopenia, but may develop acute leukemia in 1% to 2% of cases.

Platelet Transfusions

As in other IBMFSs associated with thrombocytopenia, platelet transfusions should be used judiciously. Bleeding and prophylaxis for orthopedic surgical procedures are appropriate indications. Persistent platelet counts below 10,000/μL may require preventive platelet transfusions on a regular basis, especially in the first year of life when the expectation is that a spontaneous improvement in platelet number will ensue with time in most infants. Single-donor platelets are preferred to multiple random donor platelets to minimize the risk of alloimmunization. HLA-partially matched or fully matched donors for platelets may be required if patients become refractory to transfusions.

Other Therapies

Supportive management is the mainstay, but in exceptional situations, profound, persistent life-threatening thrombocytopenia can be successfully treated by HSCT. Thrombopoietin receptor agonists, such as romiplostim and eltrombopag, have not been studied in TAR syndrome. Elevated serum thrombopoietin levels at baseline in patients with TAR may predict a poor response to these products. IL-11, another thrombopoietic cytokine, has not been studied in clinical trials either; however, endogenous IL-11 serum levels in patients with TAR are also elevated. Androgens, corticosteroids, and splenectomy are ineffective therapies for TAR syndrome.

Inherited Bone Marrow Failure Syndromes (IBMFSs) and Malignant Leukemic Transformation

Historically, the IBMFSs were classified as "benign" hematology to contrast sharply with hematologic cancer. Patients with IBMFSs often died early in life from complications of cytopenias. However, in the current era of advanced supportive care and availability of recombinant cytokines and other effective therapeutics, patients with these conditions usually survive the early years of life and beyond. With the extended lifespan of patients, the natural history of these disorders has dramatically changed. One of the most sobering observations is that the many IBMFSs confer an inordinately high predisposition to developing MDS and AML. These include conditions such as K/SCN, SDS, FA, DC, CAMT, DBA, and TAR syndrome, among others. Thus the distinction between "benign" and "malignant" hematology in the context of the IBMFSs has become blurred, and a new clinical and hematologic continuum is evident. Clearly, these disorders are leukemia-predisposition syndromes and several of them (e.g., FA, DC, and DBA) are broader cancer-predisposition syndromes.

Carcinogenesis occurs as a multistep sequence of events that is driven by genetic damage and by epigenetic factors. In the traditional view, the initiation of cancer starts in a normal cell through mutations from exposure to carcinogens. In the proliferative phase that follows, the genetically altered, initiated cell undergoes selective clonal expansion that enhances the probability of additional genetic damage from endogenous mutations or DNA-damaging agents. Activation of proto-oncogenes, inactivation of tumor-suppressor genes, or inactivation of genomic stability genes may be central in this process. Finally, during malignant conversion and cancer progression, malignant cells show phenotypic changes, gene amplification, chromosomal alterations, and altered gene expression.

With respect to the leukemia-predisposition IBMFSs, there is reason to believe that leukemogenesis is also a multistep process. The first genetic "hit" or leukemia-initiating step may be the syndrome-specific inherited genetic abnormality itself, which initially manifests as the single- or multiple-lineage marrow failure state. The "predisposed" progenitor, already initiated, could conceptually develop decreased responsiveness to the signals that regulate homeostatic growth, terminal cell differentiation, or programmed cell death. Leukemic promotion and progression with clonal expansion heading to MDS or AML could then ensue readily. Because many of the mutant genes that produce the inherited BM failure syndromes have been discovered, the nature of the leukemogenic-initiating events in these conditions should become evident.

Three of the syndromes illustrate the point. The best example is the multistep evolution of leukemic transformation over time in patients with K/SCN. The acquisition of activating *RAS* oncogene mutations, cytogenetic abnormalities involving primarily +7, 7q− and +21, and G-CSF receptor mutation occurs in the majority of patients who transform. In one patient with K/SCN who progressed to MDS/L, clonal evolution was assessed by exome sequencing of marrow cells. A pro-proliferative, differentiation-defective *GCSFR* mutation was found, that persisted and acquired secondary mutations. The frequency of *RUNX1* mutations was high in a cohort of K/SCN patients, who developed MDS/L. Mutations in *RUNX1* and *GCSFR* cooperate to promote clonal expansion.

Other than clonal cytogenetic changes, we know little about the timeline or sequence of events that characterize the malignant phenotype of SDS. It is striking, though, that the syndrome from early age already shares many of the findings of de novo adult MDS, including abnormal hematopoietic colony growth, abnormally short leukocyte telomeres, elevated apoptotic index mediated by FAS/FAS ligand, an abnormal immune system, an aberrant marrow microenvironment that shows impaired support of normal hematopoiesis, increased microvessel density, and impaired mitotic spindle stabilization. Many, if not all, of these findings may evolve in utero.

Finally, FA has a "short-cut" mechanism to leukemic conversion. Biallelic mutant genes from conception result in genomic instability, compromised DNA repair, and chromosome breakage. In a study from France, the investigators used SNP arrays to analyze marrow cells of patients with FA with MDS/leukemia. They identified a relatively high frequency of somatic *RUNX1* gene disruption compared with what is typically seen in patients with de novo MDS/leukemia. The opportunities for blood cancers in this setting are infinite. Actuarial data from the IFAR showed that the risk of acquiring clonal cytogenetic abnormalities was 67% by 30 years of age in patients with BM failure. The actuarial risk of MDS or AML was 52% by 40 years of age. This steady tempo of leukemic evolution implies a stepwise acquisition over time of additional, critical genetic "hits" before overt MDS/AML.

SUGGESTED READINGS

General

Cada M, Segbefia CI, Klaassen R, et al: The impact of category, cytopathology and cytogenetics on development and progression of clonal and malignant myeloid transformation in inherited bone marrow failure syndromes. *Haematologica* 100:633–642, 2015.

Chirnomas SD, Kupfer GM: The inherited bone marrow failure syndromes. *Pediatr Clin North Am* 60:1291–1310, 2013.

Tsangaris E, Klaassen R, Fernandez CV, et al: Genetic analysis of inherited bone marrow failure syndromes from one prospective, comprehensive and population-based cohort and identification of novel mutations. *J Med Genet* 48:618, 2011.

Fanconi Anemia

Auerbach AD: Fanconi anemia and its diagnosis. *Mutat Res* 668:4, 2009.

Longerich S, Li J, Xiong Y, et al: Stress and DNA repair biology of the Fanconi anemia pathway. *Blood* 124(18):2812–2819, 2014.

Quentin S, Cuccuini W, Ceccaldi R, et al: Myelodysplasia and leukemia of Fanconi anemia are associated with a specific pattern of genomic abnormalities that includes cryptic RUNX1/AML1 lesions. *Blood* 117:e161–e170, 2011.

Shwachman-Diamond Syndrome

Donadieu J, Fenneteau O, Beaupain B, et al: Classification of and risk factors for hematologic complications in a French national cohort of 102 patients with Shwachman-Diamond syndrome. *Haematologica* 97(9):1312–1319, 2012.

Finch AJ, Hilcenko C, Basse N, et al: Uncoupling of GTP hydrolysis from eIF6 release on the ribosome causes Shwachman-Diamond syndrome. *Genes Dev* 25:917, 2011.

Hashmi SK, Allen C, Klaassen R, et al: Comparative analysis of Shwachman-Diamond syndrome to other inherited marrow failure syndromes. *Clin Genet* 79:448, 2011.

Sen S, Wang H, Nghiem CL, et al: The ribosome-related protein, SBDS, is critical for normal erythropoiesis. *Blood* 118:6407, 2011.

Dyskeratosis Congenita

Alter BP, Giri N, Savage SA, et al: Cancer in dyskeratosis congenita. *Blood* 113:6549, 2009.

Ballew BJ, Savage SA: Updates on the biology and management of dyskeratosis congenita and related telomere biology disorders. *Expert Rev Hematol* 6(3):327–337, 2013.

Congenital Amegakaryocytic Thrombocytopenia

Ballmaier M, Germeshausen M: Congenital amegakaryocytic thrombocytopenia: clinical presentation, diagnosis, and treatment. *Semin Thromb Hemost* 37(6):673–681, 2011.

Diamond-Blackfan Anemia

Ellis SR, Gleizes PE: Diamond Blackfan anemia: ribosomal proteins going rogue. *Semin Hematol* 48:89, 2011.

Horos R, von Lindern M: Molecular mechanisms of pathology and treatment in Diamond Blackfan anaemia. *Br J Haematol* 159:514–527, 2012.

Vlachos A, Blanc L, Lipton JM: Diamond Blackfan anemia: a model for the translational approach to understanding human disease. *Expert Rev Hematol* 7:359–372, 2014.

Congenital Dyserythropoietic Anemias

Iolascon A, Heimpel H, Wahlin A, et al: Congenital dyserythropoietic anemias: molecular insights and diagnostic approach. *Blood* 122:2162–2166, 2013.

Wickramasinghe SN, Wood WG: Advances in the understanding of the congenital dyserythropoietic anaemias. *Br J Haematol* 131:431, 2005.

Kostmann/Severe Congenital Neutropenia

Dale DC, Welte K: Cyclic and chronic neutropenia. *Cancer Treat Res* 157:97, 2011.

Grenda DS, Murakami M, Ghatak J, et al: Mutations of the *ELANE* gene found in patients with severe congenital neutropenia induce the unfolded protein response and cellular apoptosis. *Blood* 110:4179, 2007.

Hauck F, Klein C: Pathogenic mechanisms and clinical implications of congenital neutropenia syndromes. *Curr Opin Allergy Clin Immunol* 13(6):596–606, 2013.

Makaryan V, Zeidler C, Bolyard AA, et al: The diversity of mutations and clinical outcomes for ELANE-associated neutropenia. *Curr Opin Hematol* 22(1):3–11, 2015.

Rosenberg PS, Zeidler C, Bolyard AA, et al: Stable long-term risk of leukaemia in patients with severe congenital neutropenia maintained on G-CSF therapy. *Br J Haematol* 150:196, 2010.

Skokowa J, Fobiwe JP, Dan L, et al: Neutrophil elastase is severely downregulated in severe congenital neutropenia independent of *ELANE* or HAX1 mutations but dependent on LEF-1. *Blood* 114:3044, 2009.

Skokowa J, Steinemann D, Katsman-Kuipers JE, et al: Cooperativity of RUNX1 and CSF3R mutations in severe congenital neutropenia: a unique pathway in myeloid leukemogenesis. *Blood* 123:2229–2237, 2014.

CHAPTER 30

APLASTIC ANEMIA

Neal S. Young and Jaroslaw P. Maciejewski

Aplastic anemia (AA), the paradigm of the bone marrow (BM) failure syndromes, is most simply defined as peripheral blood pancytopenia and a hypocellular BM (Fig. 30.1). From epidemiologic and clinical features, pathophysiologic studies, and response to therapy, AA is a distinctive disease. However, the diagnosis of AA requires excluding other causes of pancytopenia (Table 30.1). AA can occur as a primary hematologic disorder, most often idiopathic, or apparently result from various proximate causes, including obvious physical and chemical toxins but also drugs and viruses that can act indirectly. Although AA is usually characterized by a severe diminution in BM function that affects all the hematopoietic lineages, granulocyte, platelet, and red blood cell (RBC) levels may not be depressed uniformly, and less severe degrees of BM hypoplasia and odd combinations of bicytopenias and monocytopenias can occur. AA can be especially difficult to distinguish from hypocellular myelodysplasia, a diagnostic dilemma that can rest on real biologic similarities. Even typical AA can vary in its clinical course, from a fulminant illness marked by hemorrhage and infections to an indolent process manageable by transfusions. The reader is referred to previous editions of this textbook for references, as well as to the authors' recent reviews[1]

HISTORY

The study of BM failure dates to 1888, when Paul Ehrlich described a young woman who died after an explosive short illness marked by severe anemia, bleeding, and high fever. As a pathologist, Ehrlich was struck by the absence of nucleated RBCs and the fatty quality of the femoral BM. Vaquez and Aubertin, in a 1904 case report of "pernicious anemia with yellow BM," named the disease and emphasized a pathophysiology of *anhematopoiesis*. The etymologic root of the term *aplastique* is the Greek verb *pl¿Jw*, to create and give shape to (*¿plaztká*, the adjective, unformed).

CLASSIFICATION

AA is a major sequela of irradiation and exposure to cytotoxic chemotherapy. It has been associated with the use of chemicals and drugs, viral infections, and other diseases (Table 30.2). Most patients have an idiopathic form of the disease. Historical associations of environmental exposures and causation are interesting but should be considered with some skepticism because of biases of observation and reporting, and lack of direct evidence in most cases.

EPIDEMIOLOGY

Incidence, Geographic and Age Distribution

The International AA and Agranulocytosis Study (IAAAS) was conducted in Europe and Israel from 1980–1984.[2] This study was performed prospectively and applied strict case definition to pathologically confirmed cases. Using stringent criteria, the overall annual incidence of AA was 2 cases per 1 million people. In Asia, similar methodology was applied by Thai investigators to determine a higher annual incidence, 4.0 cases per 1 million people in Bangkok and 5.6 cases per 1 million people in the northeastern province of Khonkaen.[3] In general, from published, hospital-based series,

personal communications, and first-hand observations, AA appears more prevalent in less developed regions of the world. There are no major sex or racial differences in the occurrence of AA.

AA is a disease of the young (Fig. 30.2). Most patients present between 15 and 25 years of age or older than 60 years of age.

Epidemiologic Clues to Causality

Population-based studies have investigated possible causal associations. Drugs are implicated in only approximately 25% of cases of AA in the West; in Thailand, AA was attributed to drug exposure in only approximately 15% of cases.[3] There are associations with chemical exposures, exposures to viruses, hepatitis, and occupation. There is evidence that geographic variation in AA might result from environmental causes and also genetic predispositions.

Genetic Aspects

In children and young adults, acquired AA should be distinguished from the main inherited forms of BM failure, Fanconi anemia (FA) and dyskeratosis congenita (DKC) (Chapter 29). Identification of constitutional AA has important therapeutic implications. Patients with FA and DKC can lack typical physical anomalies, and the pancytopenia can develop long after childhood, mimicking acquired disease. The distinction between inherited and acquired AA has been blurred with the identification of mutations in the telomerase genes that appear to be risk factors rather than determinants of clinical BM failure (see later). Genomic approaches to the study of AA are likely to uncover other genetic contributions to susceptibility to BM failure.[4,5]

A few histocompatibility types have also been associated with AA, most consistently human leukocyte antigen (HLA)-DR2. HLA-DR subtypes predicted response to immunosuppressive therapy in a large cohort of US AA patients, in which HLA-DR15 was associated with the presence of a paroxysmal nocturnal hemoglobinuria (PNH) clone and responsiveness to immunosuppression. Genetic predisposition may be responsible for some idiosyncratic reactions to drugs and chemicals leading to the development of AA. Polymorphisms in cytokine genes, associated with an increased immune response, are also more prevalent in AA. Genome-wide transcriptional analysis of T and natural killer cells from AA patients has implicated pathologic expression of components of innate immunity, including Toll-like receptors.

ETIOLOGY AND PATHOGENESIS

Hematopoiesis in Bone Marrow Failure

Stem Cells

A consistent laboratory finding for patients with AA is a very low number of hematopoietic progenitor cells. Deficient colony formation by BM cells of AA patients is observed, even in the presence of high levels of hematopoietic growth factors. The total number of progenitors in a BM sample is reduced, and the number of colony progenitor cells assayed from a purified CD34+ cell population is low.

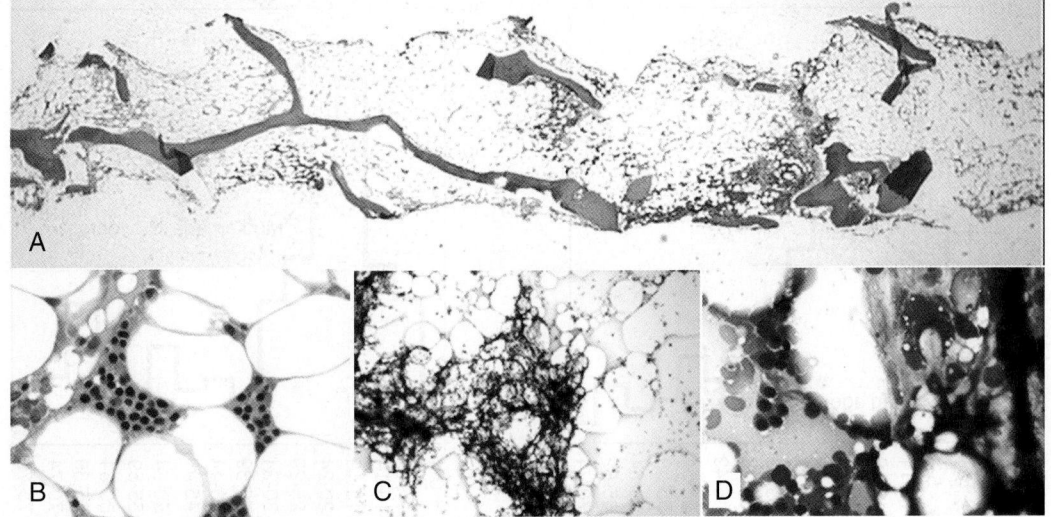

Fig. 30.1 BONE MARROW MORPHOLOGY IN SEVERE APLASTIC ANEMIA. Bone marrow biopsy specimen, of sufficient length (A) shows severe hypocellularity. The corresponding aspirate (B, D) shows empty marrow spicules and residual stoma including lymphoid cells, plasma cells, histiocytes and mast cells.

TABLE 30.1	**Differential Diagnosis of Pancytopenia**

Pancytopenia With Hypocellular Bone Marrow

Acquired aplastic anemia
Inherited aplastic anemia (Fanconi anemia and others)
Some myelodysplasia syndromes
Rare aleukemic leukemia (acute myelogenous leukemia)
Some acute lymphoblastic leukemias
Some lymphomas of bone marrow

Pancytopenia With Cellular Bone Marrow

Primary bone marrow diseases
Myelodysplasia syndromes
Paroxysmal nocturnal hemoglobinuria
Myelofibrosis
Some aleukemic leukemias
Myelophthisis
Bone marrow lymphoma
Hairy cell leukemia
Secondary to systemic diseases
Systemic lupus erythematosus, Sjögren syndrome
Hypersplenism
Vitamin B_{12}, folate deficiency (familial defect)
Overwhelming infection
Alcohol
Brucellosis
Ehrlichiosis
Sarcoidosis
Tuberculosis and atypical mycobacteria

Hypocellular Bone Marrow ± Cytopenia

Q fever
Legionnaires disease
Mycobacteria
Tuberculosis[a]
Anorexia nervosa, starvation
Hypothyroidism

[a]Pancytopenia in tuberculosis only rarely is associated with a hypocellular bone marrow at biopsy or autopsy. Marrow failure in the setting of tuberculosis is almost always fatal; exceptional patients probably had underlying myelodysplasia or acute leukemia.

TABLE 30.2	**A Classification of Aplastic Anemia**

Acquired Aplastic Anemia

Secondary aplastic anemia
Irradiation
Drugs and chemicals
Regular effects
Cytotoxic agents
Benzene
Idiosyncratic reactions
Chloramphenicol
Nonsteroidal antiinflammatory drugs
Antiepileptics
Gold
Other drugs and chemicals
Viruses
Epstein-Barr virus (infectious mononucleosis)
Hepatitis virus (non-A, non-B, non-C, non-G hepatitis)
Parvovirus (transient aplastic crisis, some pure red cell aplasia)
Human immunodeficiency virus (acquired immunodeficiency syndrome)
Immune diseases
Eosinophilic fasciitis
Hyperimmunoglobulinemia
Thymoma and thymic carcinoma
Graft-versus-host disease in immunodeficiency
Paroxysmal nocturnal hemoglobinuria
Pregnancy
Idiopathic aplastic anemia

Inherited Aplastic Anemia

Fanconi anemia
Dyskeratosis congenita
Shwachman-Diamond syndrome
Reticular dysgenesis
Amegakaryocytic thrombocytopenia
Familial aplastic anemias
Preleukemia (e.g., monosomy 7)
Nonhematologic syndromes (e.g., Down, Dubowitz, Seckel)

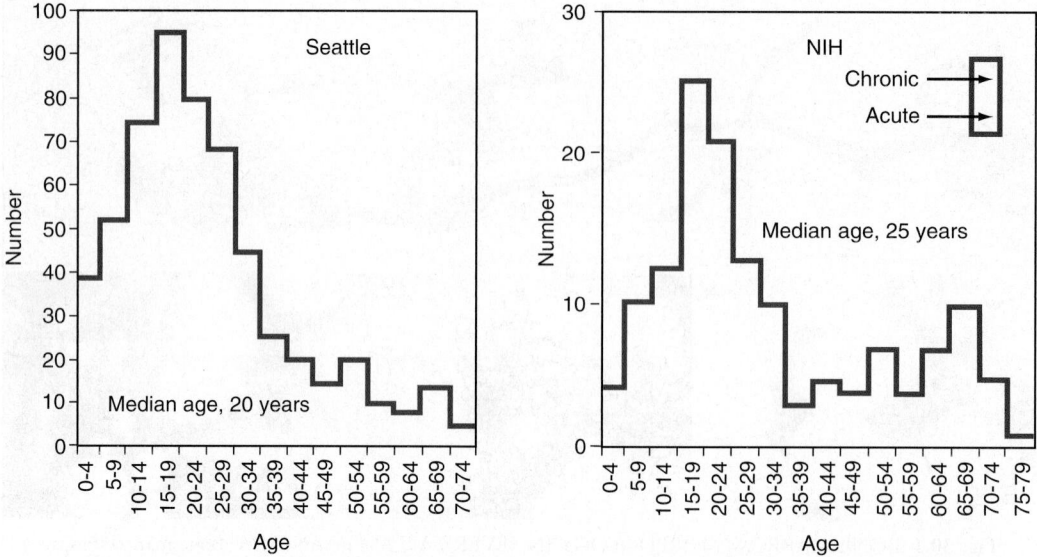

Fig. 30.2 DISTRIBUTION OF APLASTIC ANEMIA BY AGE. For patients at the University of Washington, a major transplantation center, the age given is at the time of first treatment. For the patients at the NIH, where immunosuppressive therapy is offered, the age given is at the time of diagnostic bone marrow biopsy. Acute disease is defined as less than 3 months between diagnosis and presentation at NIH, and chronic disease is defined as more than 3 months. *NIH*, National Institutes of Health. *(Seattle statistics are courtesy of Rainer Storb, University of Washington.)*

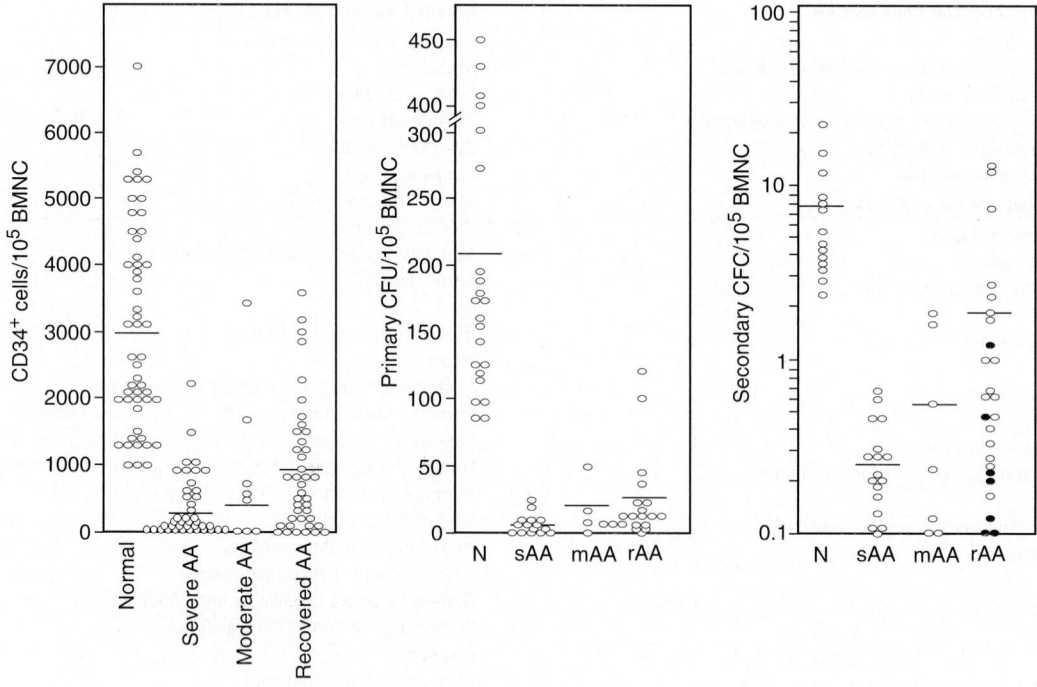

Fig. 30.3 The numbers of CD34 cells, primary CFC, and LTC-ICs were measured in the bone marrow of AA patients. Each dot represents an individual patient's sample studied. sAA includes patients at presentation, cases refractory to immunosuppressive therapy, and patients who relapsed after a period of recovery. Primary CFC were measured in short-term methylcellulose cultures. Secondary CFC after long-term bone marrow cultures reflect LTC-IC numbers. *AA,* Aplastic anemia; *BMNC,* blood mononuclear cell; *CFC,* colony-forming cell; *CFU,* colony-forming unit; *LTC-IC,* long-term culture-initiating cell; *mAA,* moderate aplastic anemia; *N,* normal; *rAA,* recovered from aplastic anemia; *sAA,* severe aplastic anemia.

Long-term culture-initiating cells (LTC-ICs), stem-cell surrogates are also profoundly deficient of stem cells in all patients with severe AA. At clinical presentation, the number of LTC-ICs is usually less than 10% of normal; combined with a reduction in total BM cellularity to 10% or less, the stem-cell number is estimated to be reduced to 1% or less than normal in patients with AA (Fig. 30.3).[6]

Telomeres and Bone Marrow Failure

One peculiar feature of white blood cells in some cases of AA is short telomeres. The discovery by linkage analysis in large pedigrees that the X-linked form of DKC was caused by mutations in *DKC1* and subsequently purposeful identification of mutations in *TERC* in some autosomal dominant patients with this constitutional BM failure syndrome provided a genetic basis for DKC. Central to the repair machinery is an RNA template, encoded by *TERC,* on which telomerase, a reverse transcriptase encoded by *TERT,* elongates the nucleotide repeat structure; other proteins, including the *DKC1* gene product dyskenin, are associated with the telomere repair complex. Systematic surveys of DNA disclosed first *TERC* and later *TERT* mutations in some patients with apparently acquired AA, including older adults.[4] Family members who share the mutation, despite normal or near-normal blood counts, have hypocellular marrows, reduced CD34[+] cell counts and poor hematopoietic colony formation, increased hematopoietic growth factor levels, and of course short telomeres. However, clinical presentation is much later than in typical DKC, and physical anomalies are often absent. Chromosomes are also protected by several proteins that bind directly to telomeres. Mutations in the gene for shelterin, one such protein, produce very severe DKC. Some inherited sequence variants/polymorphism in genes that repair or protect telomeres appear to be genetic risk factors in acquired AA, probably because they confer a quantitatively reduced hematopoietic stem cell compartment that may also be qualitatively inadequate to sustain immune-mediated damage. Accelerated telomere attrition in AA not currently explained by mutations may be caused by subtle or obscure genetic lesions or follow from the pathophysiology of BM stress and excessive stem cell turnover.

Stromal and Hematopoietic Growth Factors

Stromal cell function is usually not defective in cases of AA. Adherent cells from patients support hematopoiesis by normal CD34[+] cells, whereas no hematopoietic colonies develop when patients' CD34[+] cells are cultured in the presence of normal stroma (Fig. 30.4). Stromal cells cultured from patients' BM generally produce normal quantities of hematopoietic growth factors. Serum levels of erythropoietin, thrombopoietin, granulocyte colony-stimulating factor (G-CSF), and granulocyte-macrophage colony-stimulating factor (GM-CSF) are almost always normal or elevated. Adequate stromal function is implicit in the success of BM transplantation in AA because important stromal elements remain of host origin.

PATHOPHYSIOLOGIC PATHWAYS LEADING TO APLASTIC ANEMIA

Direct Hematopoietic Injury

The most common form of AA is iatrogenic; transient BM failure routinely follows treatment with cytotoxic chemotherapeutic drugs or irradiation (Fig. 30.5). Certain chemical or physical agents directly injure proliferating and quiescent hematopoietic cells. However, patients with community-acquired AA rarely have a history of exposure to such physicochemical agents. Even benzene, which can act as a particularly inefficient cytotoxic chemical, is an infrequent cause of AA in developed countries. Medical drugs are associated with acquired AA, and in some instances, they can directly cause BM damage. However, compared with chemotherapeutic agents, which are delivered in high doses, relatively low total quantities of ingested drug apparently cause idiosyncratic hematologic reactions. In addition to their direct toxic effects, chemicals and viruses may induce complex and not well-understood immune reactions leading to BM failure in persons with AA (see Fig. 30.5).

Immune-Mediated Bone Marrow Failure

In the 1970s, Mathé and colleagues observed unexpected improvement of pancytopenia after failed BM transplantation. They speculated that the immunosuppressive conditioning regimen, intended to allow engraftment of the donor BM, might instead have promoted the recovery of host BM function. The effectiveness of diverse treatments that reduce lymphocyte number or block T-cell function and the superior results obtained when agents are combined strongly suggest that such therapeutic success is caused by the immunosuppressive effects of the drugs used. AA shares clinical and pathophysiologic features with other autoimmune or immune-mediated human diseases that are also characterized by T-cell–mediated, tissue-specific organ destruction (inflammatory bowel disease, type 1 diabetes, multiple sclerosis, uveitis, and others).

Immune system destruction of BM occurs in animal models of graft-versus-host disease (GVHD) and in humans with transfusion-associated GVHD, in which AA is the cause of death. Very small numbers of effector cells, which have been conveyed by residual lymphocytes contained within the transfusion product or with solid organ transplants, are sufficient to mediate GVHD under these conditions. AA is associated with rheumatologic syndromes, such as eosinophilic fasciitis, and with systemic lupus erythematosus. AA occasionally occurs in individuals with hypogammaglobulinemia or congenital immunodeficiency syndrome, thymoma, thymic hyperplasia, and thymic carcinoma.

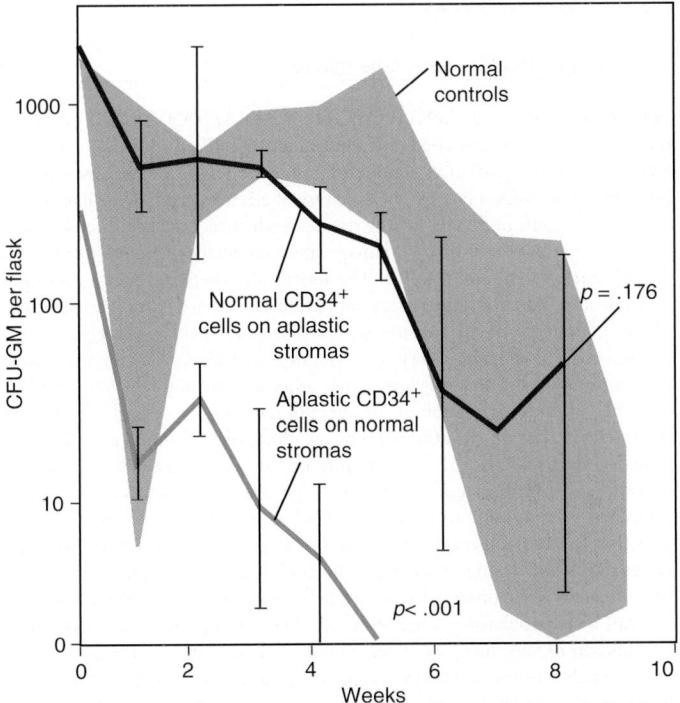

Fig. 30.4 NORMAL STROMAL CELL FUNCTION IN LONG-TERM CULTURE OF APLASTIC ANEMIA BONE MARROW. *CFU-GM,* *(Courtesy Dr. Judith Marsh, St. George's Hospital Medical School, London.)*

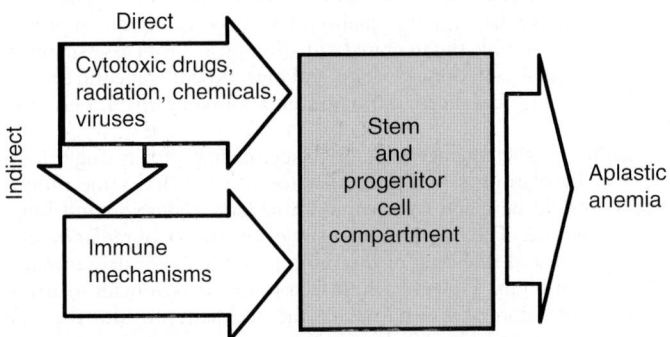

Fig. 30.5 POSSIBLE CAUSES OF DIRECT AND INDIRECT BONE MARROW FAILURE IN PATIENTS WITH APLASTIC ANEMIA.

Laboratory support for the immune hypothesis first came from coculture experiments in which mononuclear cells from AA patients' blood or BM were shown to suppress in vitro colony formation by hematopoietic progenitor cells. T-cell depletion sometimes improved colony formation in vitro. Patients' blood and BM cells were shown to produce a soluble factor that inhibited hematopoiesis, ultimately identified as interferon (IFN)-γ. Patients' T cells overproduce IFN-γ and tumor necrosis factor (TNF), two cytokines that inhibit hematopoietic proliferation. Tbet, a transcriptional regulator that is critical to Th1 polarization, is constitutively expressed in a majority of AA patients. AA blood and BM also contains elevated numbers of activated cytotoxic lymphocytes, and activity and levels of these cytotoxic cells are decreased with antithymocyte globulin (ATG) therapy. T regulatory cells, as in other human immune-mediated diseases, are decreased in AA. IFN-γ and TNF negative effects on the proliferation of early and late hematopoietic progenitor and stem cells is far more potent when these cytokines are secreted into the BM microenvironment than when they were simply added to the cultures. IFN-γ and TNF can suppress hematopoiesis by inhibiting cell proliferation, inducing Fas-mediated apoptosis, and blocking hematopoietic growth factor intracellular signals. The early immune system events that must precede the global destruction of hematopoietic cells are not clear. Involvement of CD4 lymphocytes has been suggested based on the overrepresentation of HLA-DR15 among patients with immune-mediated AA. Clones of HLA-DR–restricted T cells derived from a few patients have been shown to proliferate in response to BM cells.

Many features of human AA can be reproduced in mouse models of GVHD in which the donor inoculum lacks stem cells. Major and minor histocompatibility mismatch demonstrates the potency and specificity of small numbers of T cells, the role of cytokines, efficacy of immunosuppressive therapies, an "innocent bystander effect," and roles for specific lymphocyte regulatory and effector T cell subsets.[7]

Radiation

BM aplasia is a major acute toxic effect of radiation (Fig. 30.6); the dose-related occurrence of pancytopenia 2–4 weeks after exposure to radiation. Mortality from hematologic toxicity is a function of the ability of BM to tolerate damage to stem cells. The capacity for recovery of hematopoietic function after even massive single irradiation exposures is considerable, reflecting the resistance of the quiescent stem cell to damage and their enormous BM repopulating potential. At intermediate radiation doses around the median lethal dose (LD$_{50}$), at which BM toxicity limits survival, supportive efforts can drastically alter outcome. Autopsies of atomic bomb victims in Japan showed acellular BM in the first weeks of the explosion, but later regenerating BM was frequently present. The histologic picture of radiation-mediated aplasia includes necrosis, nuclear pyknosis and karyorrhexis, nuclear lysis, and ultimately cytolysis; the associated phagocytosis, marked congestion, and hemorrhage are rapidly followed by fatty replacement. BM hypoplasia occurs with radiation doses higher than 1.5–2 Gy to the whole body. Precise LD$_{50}$ figures for humans do not exist, and estimates are based on the limited direct human data and extrapolation from animal experiments. The LD$_{50}$ is highly dependent on the quality of medical care, and improved support may double the tolerated radiation dose. From assessment of the outcome of radiation accidents and high-dose therapeutic irradiation, the LD$_{50}$ has been estimated at approximately 4.5 Gy (see Fig. 30.6).

Although the management of pancytopenia after a single large dose of irradiation is similar to that for treating AA, some unique points should be made concerning immediate evaluation and long-term prognosis. The type and intensity of the source of radiation and the distance and shielding of the subject are the major determinants of radiation injury. However, these factors are often difficult to assess. Early recognition of the nature of the accident provides the best opportunity for dosimetry by accident reconstruction and use of blocking, displacement, or chelation agents. Exposure correlates well with the degree of pancytopenia. Because lymphocytes are particularly

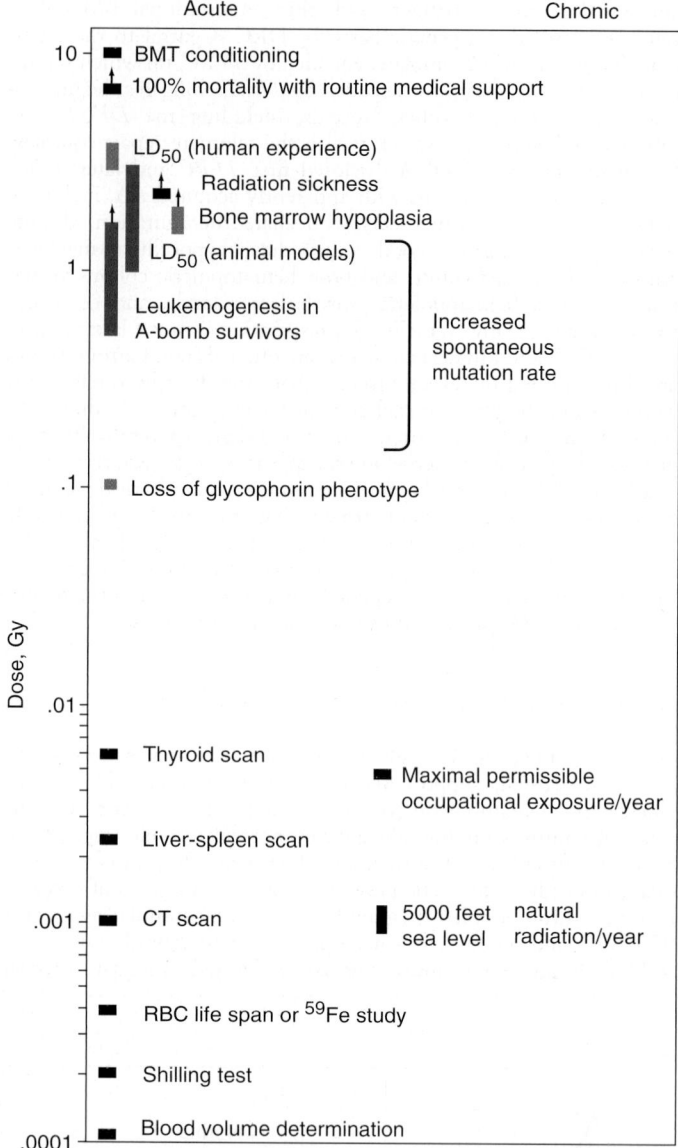

Fig. 30.6 SCALE OF WHOLE-BODY RADIATION DOSES. A Gray (Gy) is a measure of absorbed dose equivalent to 1 J/kg unit mass, and 1 Gy equals 100 rads. Radiation represents radiant energy. When absorbed by biologic tissue, radiant energy causes release of electrons and molecular ionization, which result in further energy release. Radiant energy can directly break chemical bonds and indirectly damage macromolecules through generation of high-energy free radical forms. The relationship between increased mutation rate and radiation dose is very approximate *(hatched bars)*. Measurement of the phenotype of an autosomal recessive gene such as for glycophorin would be expected to be a very sensitive indicator. Because malignant transformation is almost certainly a two-step process, increased leukemogenesis is probably an underestimation of the effect of radiation on a single gene. Even the extensive data on the atomic bomb survivors of Hiroshima are subject to statistical errors because of the small number of cases; a linear or exponential curve fit gives various results, and very high doses of radiation may not be associated with as high a risk of leukemia because of stem cell death. Other data that can bear on mutation frequency lie outside the range shown. In a patient with ankylosing spondylitis who underwent irradiation of the spine, leukemogenesis was observed at relatively low doses (doubling of the leukemia rate can be extrapolated to approximately 7 Gy), but such individuals can be predisposed to leukemia. An increased risk of thyroid cancer after irradiation of the mediastinum in childhood occurred at approximately 4 Gy. *BMT,* Bone marrow transplantation; *CT,* computed tomography; *LD$_{50}$,* median lethal dose; *RBC,* red blood cell.

sensitive to radiation, their rate of decline can be used to estimate the dose of total body exposure to a level of approximately 3 Gy. At higher doses, the fall in granulocytes and the severity of thrombocytopenia and reticulocytopenia can be used as gauges. The survival of some patients who received doses higher than 9 Gy suggests that autologous BM reconstitution may occur in most persons who survive the immediate consequences of radiation exposure.

Pancytopenia may be a late consequence of a single radiation dose, but AA is not well documented as a delayed event after radiation exposure. A variety of hematologic abnormalities are associated with chronic low-level radiation exposure, most commonly lymphocytosis, neutropenia, dysmorphic leukocytes, and giant platelets (see Fig. 30.6). Cytogenetic abnormalities accumulate with time after chronic exposure, but they may not be reliably related to dose. Repeated low doses of radiation have been associated with AA, but even in these circumstances, only a small proportion of exposed individuals develop hematologic disease. AA does not appear to be more frequent among nuclear power plant or thorium processing factory workers or among residents living close to the plants. Excessive numbers of deaths from AA were reported after therapeutic irradiation of the spine for ankylosing spondylitis; later analysis has suggested that the risk may have been overestimated. AA has not been found in unexpected numbers in cancer patients who had received therapeutic irradiation or among persons exposed to higher natural background radiation.

Drugs and Chemicals

AA is frequently associated with medical drug use (Table 30.3). At the end of the 19th century, chemicals were linked to BM function through observations of benzene effects on workers. Establishment of a relationship between the analgesic amidopyrine and agranulocytosis in the early 20th century and an apparent epidemic of AA after the introduction of chloramphenicol in the 1960s also supported this concept. Initially suggested by the accumulation of case reports, drug associations have been established in formal case-control population-based epidemiologic studies. In the IAAAS, relative risks were estimated for individual drugs and large classes of pharmaceutical agents, including nonsteroidal antiinflammatory drugs (NSAIDs), drugs affecting thyroid function, certain cardiovascular agents, some psychotropics, and sulfa-based antibiotics (Table 30.4).[2] Approximately 25% of the cases of AA identified in the IAAAS could be attributed to drug use. Drug use as a risk factor was also assessed by similar methods in Thailand, where the incidence of AA is higher than in the West. Surprisingly, chloramphenicol was not shown to be a risk factor; the etiologic fraction of AA was attributed to only 15%.

Associations between drug exposure and AA can be divided into two classes. Drugs used in cancer chemotherapy are selected for their cytotoxicity, and their regular, dose-dependent induction of BM aplasia is an expected effect. Most AA associated with medical drug use in the community is described as idiosyncratic, meaning that its occurrences are unexpectedly rare. Many of the drugs implicated in AA also appear to cause other, milder forms of BM suppression such as neutropenia. Although difficult to prove, some dose relationship probably does exist even for idiosyncratic reactions. In most case reports, patients received normal or high doses of the agent, usually for a period of weeks to months. Drug-induced aplasia cannot be distinguished by history from idiopathic forms of the disease; the clinical course, including the favorable response to immunosuppressive therapy, is the same as in idiopathic disease.

The low probability of developing AA after a course of drugs may be a reflection of the gene variant frequency for metabolic enzymes (for direct chemical effects) or immune response genes. The rarity of idiosyncratic drug reactions could then arise from the infrequent combination of unusual circumstances: exposure, genetic variations in drug metabolism, the physical properties of the agent, enzymatic pathways that chemically alter the drug, and the susceptibility of the host to the action of a toxic compound. Examples of detoxifying enzyme systems directly applicable to BM failure and that also demonstrate genetic variability include arylhydrocarbon hydroxylase

TABLE 30.3	Classification of Drugs and Chemicals Associated With Aplastic Anemia

I. Agents That Regularly Produce Marrow Depression as a Major Toxic Effect When Used in Commonly Used Doses or Normal Exposures

Cytotoxic drugs used in cancer chemotherapy
Alkylating agents (busulfan, melphalan, cyclophosphamide)
Antimetabolites (antifolic compounds, nucleotide analogs) antimitotics (vincristine, vinblastine, colchicine)
Some antibiotics (daunorubicin, doxorubicin [Adriamycin])
Benzene (and less often benzene-containing chemicals: kerosene, carbon tetrachloride, Stoddard solvent, chlorophenols)

II. Agents Probably Associated With Aplastic Anemia but With a Relatively Low Probability Relative to Their Use

Chloramphenicol
Insecticides
Antiprotozoals (quinacrine and chloroquine)
Nonsteroidal antiinflammatory drugs (including phenylbutazone, indomethacin, ibuprofen, sulindac, diclofenac, naproxen, piroxicam, fenoprofen, fenbufen, aspirin)
Anticonvulsants (hydantoins, carbamazepine, phenacemide, ethosuximide)
Gold, arsenic, and other heavy metals such as bismuth and mercury
Sulfonamides as a class
Antithyroid medications (methimazole, methylthiouracil, propylthiouracil)
Antidiabetes drugs (tolbutamide, carbutamide, chlorpropamide)
Carbonic anhydrase inhibitors (acetazolamide, methazolamide, mesalazine)
D-Penicillamine
2-Chlorodeoxyadenosine

III. Agents More Rarely Associated With Aplastic Anemia

Antibiotics (streptomycin, tetracycline, methicillin, ampicillin, mebendazole and albendazole, sulfonamides, flucytosine, mefloquine, dapsone)
Antihistamines (cimetidine, ranitidine, chlorpheniramine)
Sedatives and tranquilizers (chlorpromazine, prochlorperazine, piperacetazine, chlordiazepoxide, meprobamate, methyprylon, remoxipride)
Antiarrhythmics (tocainide, amiodarone)
Allopurinol (can potentiate marrow suppression by cytotoxic drugs)
Ticlopidine
Methyldopa
Quinidine
Lithium
Guanidine
Canthaxanthin
Thiocyanate
Carbimazole
Cyanamide
Deferoxamine
Amphetamines

(e.g., benzene toxicity), epoxide hydrolases (e.g., phenytoin toxicity), S-methylation (e.g., 6-mercaptopurine, 6-thioguanine, azathioprine) and N-acetylation (e.g., sulfa drugs). Genomic approaches have revealed the complex role of genetic variation in metabolic pathways that process arylhydrocarbons and even links to immune function.

Benzene

Benzene exposure is linked to AA. Benzene myelotoxicity can be placed between the predictable effects of chemotherapeutic agents and idiosyncratic drug reactions. Industrial emissions add greatly to the biologic sources of ambient benzene. Significant benzene exposure can also occur outside of industry. Although the concentrations of benzene to which consumers are exposed are orders of magnitude

TABLE 30.4

Drugs Associated With Aplastic Anemia in the International Aplastic Anemia and Agranulocytosis Study[a]

Drug	Stratified Risk Estimate (95% CI)	Multivariate Relative Risk Estimate (95% CI)
Nonsteroidal Analgesics		
Butazones	3.7 (1.9–7.2)	5.1 (2.1–12)
Indomethacin	7.1 (3.4–15)	8.2 (3.3–20)
Piroxicam	9.8 (3.3–29)	7.4 (2.1–26)
Diclofenac	4.6 (2.0–11)	4.2 (1.6–11)
Antibiotics		
Sulfonamides[b]	2.8 (1.1–7.3)	2.2 (0.6–7.4)
Antithyroid drugs	16 (4.8–54)	11 (2.0–56)
Cardiovascular Drugs		
Furosemide	3.3 (1.6–7.0)	3.1 (1.2–8.0)
Psychotropic Drugs		
Phenothiazines	3.0 (1.1–8.2)	1.6
Corticosteroids	5.0 (2.8–8.9)	3.5 (1.6–7.7)
Allopurinol	7.3 (3.0–17)	5.9 (1.8–19)
Gold	29 (9.7–89)	

[a]The multivariate model included the following factors: age, gender, geographic area, date of interview, reliability of the patient, person interviewed, transfer from another hospital, history of blood disorder or tuberculosis, exposure to benzene and related chemicals, and use of other suspected drugs.
[b]Other than trimethoprim-sulfonamide combination.
CI, Confidence interval.
From Kaufman DW, Kelly JP, Levy M, Shapiro S: *The Drug etiology of agranulocytosis and aplastic anemia,* New York, 1991, Oxford University Press.

lower than those observed in industrial workers, the effect of low-dose chronic exposure is uncertain, but genetic variations in metabolizing enzymes may influence susceptibility to BM suppression at these levels. Benzene metabolites are also generated from the diet.

Water-soluble products of benzene metabolism such as phenols, hydroquinones, and catechols mediate the toxicity to the BM. Benzene and its intermediate metabolites covalently and irreversibly bind to BM DNA, inhibit DNA synthesis, and introduce DNA strand breaks. Benzene acts as a "mitotic poison" and as a mutagen. Acutely, the more mature, actively cycling BM precursor cells are preferentially damaged over more primitive progenitors. Intermittent exposure may be more damaging to the stem cell compartment than is continuous exposure. BM stroma can also be damaged by benzene.

The range of hematologic disease attributable to benzene is broad, from relatively frequent mild alterations in blood counts to AA or leukemia. Studies of exposed North American workers earlier in the 20th century suggested that the risk of AA was 3% to 4% in men exposed to concentrations higher than 300 ppm and that 50% of individuals exposed to 100 ppm developed some blood cell count depression. Leukopenia, anemia, thrombocytopenia, and lymphocytopenia are common consequences of benzene; other manifestations include macrocytosis, acquired Pelger-Huet anomaly, eosinophilia, basophilia, and less often, polycythemia, leukocytosis, thrombocytosis, or splenomegaly. The BM is usually normocellular but can show hypocellularity or hypercellularity; a hypercellular phase can precede complete aplasia. In addition to hypocellularity, chronically exposed workers can have BM necrosis, fibrosis, edema, and hemorrhage. BM failure and leukemia in benzene workers can manifest decades after exposure.

Aromatic Hydrocarbons

The common perception that other molecules resembling benzene or containing a benzene ring can also cause BM suppression is not well supported by evidence. Neither the closely related alkylbenzenes nor pure toluene or xylene are established BM toxins. Often, an aromatic hydrocarbon has been implicated as causative by a clinician only for lack of another apparent etiology. For some substances, toxicity might result from the presence of benzene as a contaminant of the synthesis of the molecule or in the petroleum distillates used to dissolve the compound. However, the total number of AA cases reported with aromatic hydrocarbon exposures is small when the large populations exposed to this heterogeneous group of chemicals are considered. For example, the significance of a handful of case reports associated with insecticide exposure in the context of the vast use of these compounds is questionable. However, the very high prevalence of aromatic hydrocarbons in daily life would greatly amplify even a small individual risk. Pesticides and insecticides have been associated with AA for decades, with almost 300 medical case reports appearing in the medical literature. The most frequently cited insecticides are chlordane, lindane, and dichlorodiphenyltrichloroethane. For the miscellaneous aromatic hydrocarbons, case reports also greatly outnumber series of patients, and systematic epidemiologic surveys have shown mixed results.

Chloramphenicol

Structural similarity of chloramphenicol to amidopyrine, a drug known to cause agranulocytosis, led to early prediction of possible hematotoxicity. During the period of its unrestrained use, chloramphenicol was considered the most common cause of AA in the United States, accounting for 20% to 30% of total cases and 50% of drug-associated cases. Estimates of the risk of AA after a course of chloramphenicol ranged from 1 case per 20,000 to 1 case per 800,000 people. Based on these figures, a course of chloramphenicol was estimated to increase the risk of AA 13-fold. Although the introduction of chloramphenicol into the US market was perceived as having increased the total number of cases of AA, this assumption was only weakly supported by epidemiologic data, and the mortality from AA remained essentially constant during the period of chloramphenicol's introduction and extensive use and after the withdrawal of chloramphenicol from the market. Chloramphenicol has not been associated with AA in Thailand, despite its high rate of use there. In Hong Kong, where the use of chloramphenicol is almost 100 times higher than in the West, drug-associated AA occurs infrequently. The early epidemiologic surveys stressed excessive dosage, high blood levels, repeated or intermittent courses, young age, and oral route of administration as particular risks for chloramphenicol BM toxicity.

Nonsteroidal Antiinflammatory Drugs

Compared with chloramphenicol, it took far longer to associate phenylbutazone with AA. Mortality estimates have ranged from 1 case per 100,000 to 1 case per 1 million treatment courses. The use of other NSAIDs is associated with case reports of AA. A large case-control led investigation in Europe confirmed the risk of AA with phenylbutazone use and identified even higher probabilities with other NSAIDs. There was a suggestion of increased risk with drugs taken regularly for a prolonged period at very high doses, and in some cases, hematologic reactions were reproduced on repeat exposure.

Neuroleptics and Psychotropic Drugs

A variety of drugs used to treat disorders of the central nervous system have been associated with AA: the hydantoins and carbamazepine, antidepressants, tranquilizers, and felbamate. The marketing of felbamate was severely affected by the occurrence of AA in more than 30 patients. Monitoring of drug blood levels and peripheral blood counts in patients receiving carbamazepine was recommended despite fewer than two dozen AA cases reported by 1982. Doubt about the validity of many cases reported in the literature, as well as several large series of patients who did not develop hematologic toxicity and an estimated AA case rate of approximately 1 in 200,000 treated patients, have led to questions concerning the relationship between carbamazepine and AA.

Gold and Heavy Metals

Gold salts have an extraordinarily high frequency of fatal adverse reactions, estimated at 1.6 cases per 10,000 prescriptions. Dose-dependent leukopenia is common, but several dozen cases of AA have been reported. In the IAAAS, exposure to gold salts was the most significant drug association for developing AA, with a relative risk of 29 and an excess risk of 23 cases per 1 million users in 1 week. Spontaneous recovery rarely occurs. Patients have been successfully treated with stem-cell transplantation or immunosuppressive therapy; chelation usually has not been helpful.

TYPICAL AND ATYPICAL PRESENTATIONS

Most patients with AA seek medical attention for symptoms that occur as a result of low blood counts (Fig. 30.7 and Table 30.5). Some patients are diagnosed incidentally and often show few symptoms despite severely depressed blood counts. All of the blood elements can be depressed or a single lineage cytopenia can dominate. The differential diagnosis of pancytopenia includes a variety of diseases (see Table 30.1). Most patients do not have systemic symptoms: weight loss, persistent fever, pain, and loss of appetite point to an alternative diagnosis.

Bleeding is the most alarming manifestation of pancytopenia and frequently sends the patient to a doctor. Thrombocytopenia usually does not cause massive bleeding. Instead, the patient reports easy bruisability and the appearance of red spots, especially over dependent surfaces; gum bleeding with tooth brushing and episodic nose bleeds are common. Heavy menstrual flow or irregular vaginal bleeding can occur in younger women. In AA associated with PNH, red or dark urine may be reported that is caused by free hemoglobin, but visible bleeding from the genitourinary and gastrointestinal tracts is rare. Extensive hemorrhage from any organ can occur but usually late in the course of the disease and almost always associated with infections, drug therapy, or invasive procedures.

The ability to adapt to a gradual reduction in hemoglobin concentration is remarkable. The anemic patient might mention fatigue, lassitude, shortness of breath, or ringing in the ears, but some individuals can tolerate astonishingly low hemoglobin levels without complaint. Even abrupt cessation of erythropoiesis leads to only a slow decline in hemoglobin.

Infection is an uncommon presentation in patients with AA. The sore throat of agranulocytosis is not often observed, presumably because other alarming symptoms appear earlier.

Retrospective studies of AA associated with drugs and viruses and the observation of the occasional patient with serially monitored blood counts suggest a latent period of 6–8 weeks between the inciting event and the onset of pancytopenia. The interval can be more prolonged when pancytopenia is well tolerated or moderate.

With identification of genetic risk factor, the family history has assumed great importance in the evaluation of pancytopenia. Leukemia and myelodysplastic syndrome (MDS) can occur in FA and DKC pedigrees. In the telomeropathies secondary to *TERT* and *TERC* mutations, hematologic findings in other family members may be mild, such as modest thrombocytopenia or macrocytosis with or without anemia. These mutations also contribute to the development of cirrhosis and pulmonary fibrosis, which may be present as diagnoses in the pedigree. Early graying of the hair is sometimes prominent in telomere disease pedigrees. Inherited mutations in other genes predispose to BM failure and myeloid neoplasms. Mutations in *GATA2* also lead to susceptibility to specific infections (which may manifest as warts). Germline mutations in *RUNX1*, *ETV-6*, *CEBP1a* and *MPL* cause AA or leukemia, in childhood. Genetic testing for genes that are mutated in constitutional BM failure is commercially available.

Findings on physical examination usually reflect the severity of the pancytopenia (Table 30.6). However, patients with severe disease can look well. The patient can present with subtle variations from normal or with a dramatic, even toxic appearance. Petechiae are often present over the pretibial surface of the lower legs and the dorsal aspects of the forearms and wrists; a few petechiae can be seen in the oropharynx and on the palate. Scattered ecchymoses typically appear in areas exposed to minor trauma. With severe thrombocytopenia, retinal hemorrhages can be observed on funduscopic examination, there can be gingival oozing or blood in the nares, and hemorrhage can be apparent at the uterine cervical os. The stool can contain traces

TABLE 30.5	Presenting Symptoms of Aplastic Anemia
Symptoms	**Number of Patients**
Bleeding	41
Anemia	27
Bleeding and anemia	14
Bleeding and infection	6
Infection	5
Routine examination	8
Total	101

Adapted from Williams DM, Lynch RE, Cartwright GE: Drug induced aplastic anemia. *Semin Hematol* 10:195, 1973.

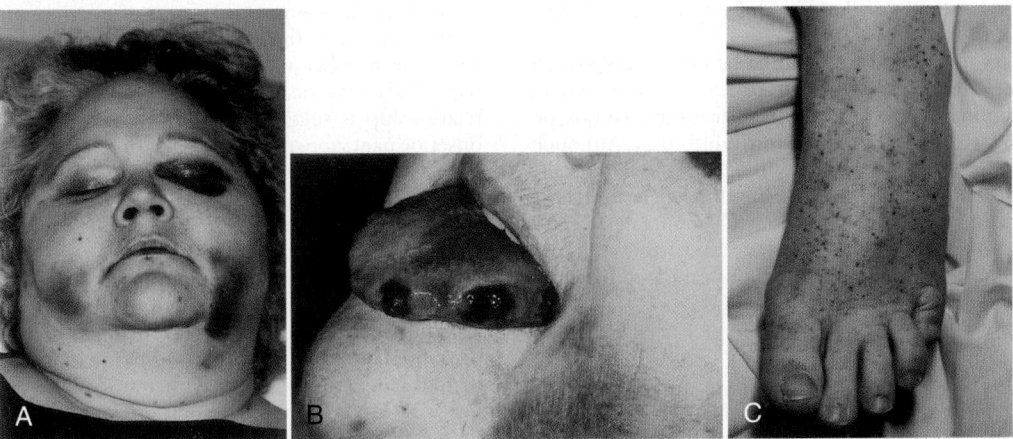

Fig. 30.7 CLINICAL PRESENTATIONS OF APLASTIC ANEMIA. (A) Ecchymosis in pancytopenic women. (B) Submucosal hematomas. (C) Petechial eruptions in a thrombocytopenic patient.

TABLE 30.6	Severity of Aplastic Anemia as Defined by Laboratory Studies

Severe aplastic anemia
Bone marrow cellularity <30%
Two of three peripheral blood criteria:
Absolute neutrophil count <500 cells/mm^3
Platelet count <20,000 cells/mm^3
Reticulocyte count <40,000 cells/mm^3
No other hematologic disease
Moderate aplastic anemia
Patients with pancytopenia who do not fulfill the criteria of severe disease

Diagnostic Algorithm in Aplastic Anemia

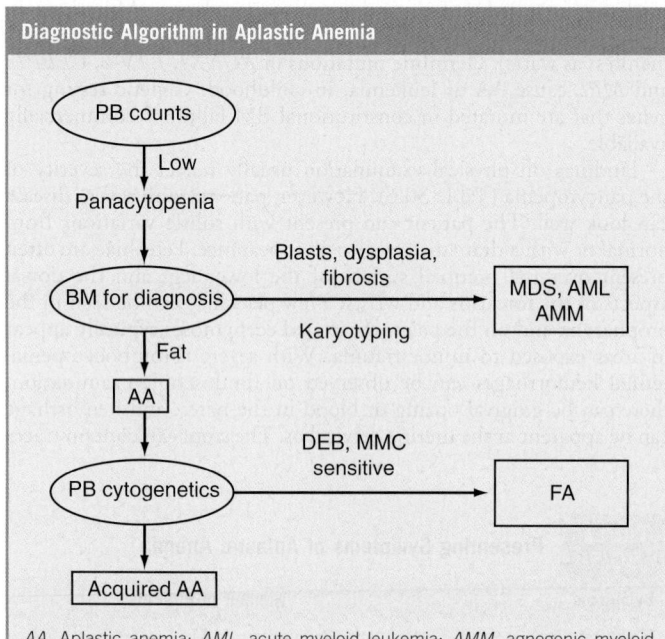

AA, Aplastic anemia; AML, acute myeloid leukemia; AMM, agnogenic myeloid metaplasia; BM, bone marrow; DEB, diepoxybutane; FA, Fanconi anemia; MDS, myelodysplastic syndrome; MMC, mitomycin C; PB, peripheral blood.

TABLE 30.7	Bone Marrow Morphologic Findings That Discriminate Myelodysplasia From Aplastic Anemia

Characteristic[a]	Myelodysplasia	Aplastic Anemia
Cellularity	Usually normal to increased	Decreased
Erythropoiesis		
Megaloblastic	Very common	Common
Dyserythropoietic	Very common	Unusual
Maturation defects	Common	Not found
Ringed sideroblasts	Common	Not found
Myelopoiesis		
Monocyte prominence	Very common	Unusual
Midmyeloid predominance	Very common	Unusual
Increased blasts	Yes	Not found
Megakaryocytes		
Atypical morphology	Very common	Not found

[a]Ringed sideroblasts and myeloblasts are observed by definition, in some of the myelodysplastic syndromes. Dyserythropoietic red blood cell precursors show bizarre forms with multiple or irregular nuclei. Megakaryocytes can show defective nuclear polyploidization and increased internuclear spaces, or they can be small with only a few nuclei and peculiar granulation.
Adapted from Bagby GC: The preleukemic syndrome (hematopoietic dysplasia). In Shahidi NT (ed): *Aplastic anemia and other bone marrow failure syndromes,* New York, 1990, Springer-Verlag, p 199 (provides percentages for myelodysplasia).

Posttransfusion Graft-Versus-Host Disease

Almost uniformly fatal, AA is a constant feature of transfusion-associated GVHD, produced by the transfusion of competent lymphocytes into immunodeficient hosts, including children with congenital syndromes, cancer patients receiving high-dose chemotherapy, and patients with adoptive cellular immunotherapy for leukemia.[8] Rarely, posttransfusion GVHD occurs in an apparently immunocompetent recipient in the special circumstance in which the donor is homozygous for an HLA haplotype also shared by the recipient, as can occur among first-degree family members. Small numbers of lymphocytes are sufficient to produce the syndrome, which is surprisingly resistant to immunosuppressive therapy. Pancytopenia with BM hypoplasia is an almost constant feature of posttransfusion GVHD. Runt disease in animals is a model of this immune-mediated BM failure syndrome.

Pregnancy

Pregnancy is common in the age groups most susceptible to BM failure, and in many cases, its association is probably only coincidental. The true frequency of AA in pregnancy is unknown, but from the number of cases reported, it appears rare, although BM hypoplasia may be relatively common during pregnancy. A causal relationship is suggested by the temporal relationship between the onset of pancytopenia and that of pregnancy and by resolution after delivery and spontaneous or induced abortion; some patients have developed AA that remitted after each delivery. Survival rates for AA in pregnancy have been relatively high for the mother and baby, with most pregnancies successful. Hemorrhage is the most common cause of death from AA during pregnancy. The published data are insufficient to guide management of the pregnant woman with AA, especially because it is clear that AA in some cases is serendipitously diagnosed and can persist beyond parturition. A woman who desires a child can be maintained with transfusions, with the understanding that any clinical deterioration is a criterion for interruption or termination of the pregnancy. The hazard of pregnancy to the woman who has recovered from idiopathic AA is unknown, but most hematologists, recognizing the risk of relapse, advise patients not to

of heme. Pallor is common and is best appreciated on the mucous membranes and palmar surfaces. The newly diagnosed patient can be febrile, but specific or localizing signs of infection are uncommon on presentation. Cachexia, splenomegaly, and lymphadenopathy are not associated with AA, and these findings should strongly suggest another diagnosis. The examiner should look carefully for café-au-lait spots and other physical anomalies of FA and for typical nail changes, leucoplakia, hypopigmentation of the skin and gray hair of telomere disease in children and adults.

Several atypical presentations of AA should be noted. A physician might encounter an elderly patient with pancytopenia in whom subsequent BM examination reveals dysplastic features (see box on Diagnostic Algorithm in Aplastic Anemia and Table 30.7). Although the history of the illness in a newly diagnosed patient is typically short—in the range of months—some patients may recall a long history of bruisability, anemia, and low blood-cell counts reported to them by previous physicians during routine examinations. These patients can have a moderately severe, chronic disease, and pancytopenia from childhood should suggest a constitutional AA.

CLINICAL ASSOCIATIONS

A number of clinical syndromes, usually revealed through a careful history and physical examination, are associated with AA (see box on Diagnostic Algorithm in Aplastic Anemia and Tables 30.2 and 30.3).

become pregnant, especially if thrombocytopenia and a PNH clone are present.

Hepatitis

Hepatitis-associated AA has several distinctive features.[9] Typically, an uneventful episode of apparent viral hepatitis in a young man is followed in 1–2 months, during convalescence from the liver inflammation, by very severe pancytopenia. Depression of blood cell counts during the course of hepatitis is common; leukopenia, atypical lymphocytosis, macrocytosis, and thrombocytopenia mimic in milder forms the hematologic changes of AA. However, posthepatitis AA has a very poor prognosis, with early estimates of mortality of 90% at 1 year, and a history of AA with hepatitis has been considered an indication for early BM transplantation. Patients with posthepatitis AA can successfully undergo BM transplantation without an increased risk of venoocclusive disease. Patients with hepatitis-associated aplasia have markers of immune system activation and respond well to intensive immunosuppressive therapy. Almost all cases have been non-A, non-B, non-C. Posthepatitis AA is linked to fulminant hepatitis of childhood and acute seronegative hepatitis. Acute viral hepatitis that is seronegative differs clinically from hepatitis C disease; parenteral exposure is not a risk factor, liver functions abnormalities are more severe during the acute phase, and late complications are more common. Even next generation sequencing has failed to find evidence of infection in seronegative hepatitis.

Postmononucleosis Aplastic Anemia

Acute infection with Epstein-Barr virus (EBV) causes infectious mononucleosis that is commonly associated with neutropenia and other hematologic abnormalities but, like acute hepatitis, is only rarely complicated by AA. However, EBV may be involved in the cause of AA more frequently than originally appreciated, because a large number of primary EBV infections are unrecognized. Pancytopenia can be first observed during the acute mononucleosis syndrome or shortly thereafter. Some patients have recovered spontaneously, and others after therapy with corticosteroids or ATG. EBV can occasionally be demonstrated in the BM cells of patients with apparently idiopathic AA, in association with serologic evidence of a primary or reactivated viral infection.

Hemophagocytic Syndrome

The BM is hypocellular in approximately one-third of cases with hemophagocytic syndrome. In this disorder, there can be progression from BM hypercellularity to aplasia; myelofibrosis is also common. Pancytopenia occurs in most cases; anemia is a universal finding; thrombocytopenia and neutropenia are also common. In contrast to typical AA, these patients appear systemically ill and have a fulminant course, with fever and constitutional symptoms, and peripheral blood-cell count depression is often associated with abnormalities of other organ systems: hepatosplenomegaly, elevation of transaminases, lymphadenopathy, cutaneous eruptions, and pulmonary infiltrates. The syndrome is associated with a wide variety of diseases. In the infectious category, viral infections are most common and include EBV, cytomegalovirus, herpes simplex, herpes zoster, B19 parvovirus, and HIV-1; bacterial and parasitic infections have also been associated with hemophagocytosis. Hemophagocytosis can be observed on supravital or Wright-Giemsa staining of the BM of patients with idiopathic AA, and it is also a morphologic feature of graft rejection after BM transplantation. In virus-associated hemophagocytosis, there is evidence of immune system activation. The sera of patients have been shown to contain high levels of IFN-γ, TNF-α, interleukin (IL)-6, soluble CD8, and soluble IL-2 receptor, and T cells overproduce IFN-γ in vitro. The clinical response to cyclosporine is consistent with a T cell–mediated pathophysiology of hematopoietic failure. In

younger patients, hereditary forms of the syndrome should be investigated by appropriate testing for germline alterations. The syndrome can be a presentation of lymphomas and seen in the context of hemolysis.

Paroxysmal Nocturnal Hemoglobinuria and Aplastic Anemia

There is a strong association between AA and PNH (see Chapter 31). These diseases are frequently diagnosed concurrently or sequentially in the same individual, and they share similar clinical and pathologic features (i.e., pancytopenia and BM hypocellularity). The presence of an expanded PNH clone is associated with HLA-DR15 and has been reported as a good prognostic marker for responsiveness to immunosuppressive therapy. Clinical BM failure can be present at the onset of PNH or can develop after diagnosis. By flow cytometry of granulocytes for glycosylphosphoinositol-anchored proteins, there is expansion of a PNH clone in 50% or more of AA cases at presentation. Longitudinal studies of patients with de novo PNH or PNH developing from AA indicate a low probability of spontaneous remission; in most patients, the contribution of the PNH clones remains stable for years, but hemolytic disease can develop.

Collagen Vascular Diseases

AA is a component of the collagen vascular syndrome called eosinophilic fasciitis. This severe, scleroderma-like disease is characterized by fibrosis of subcutaneous and fascial tissue, localized skin induration, eosinophilia, hypergammaglobulinemia, and an elevated erythrocyte sedimentation rate. The rheumatologic symptoms of fasciitis respond to corticosteroids, but the associated AA has a very poor prognosis. A few patients have survived after BM transplantation or immunosuppressive therapy. More rarely, AA has complicated systemic lupus erythematosus and rheumatoid arthritis, but in many cases, the role of concomitant drug therapy is confounding. Rarely, AA can accompany Sjögren syndrome, multiple sclerosis, and immune thyroid disease. AA occasionally occurs in individuals with hypogammaglobulinemia or congenital immunodeficiency syndrome, thymoma, or thymic hyperplasia.

LABORATORY EVALUATION

Peripheral Blood

In typical cases of AA, all the blood cell counts are depressed. The blood smear usually shows obvious paucity of platelets and leukocytes but normal RBC morphology; toxic granulations can be present in neutrophils. Automated cell counting shows erythrocyte macrocytosis and a normal RBC distribution of width. Platelet size is normal and not increased as in immune peripheral destruction, but the low number can cause greater heterogeneity of size. Prior transfusions alter platelet numbers, relative reticulocyte counts, and hemoglobin values. Although relative lymphocytosis is common, most patients also have decreased absolute numbers of monocytes and lymphocytes. The severity of AA can be graded based on the peripheral blood cell counts (see Table 30.6 and box on Diagnostic Algorithm in Aplastic Anemia).

DIAGNOSIS OF APLASTIC ANEMIA

Although the ultimate diagnosis of AA rests on the interpretation of an adequate BM biopsy specimen, important clues to the cause of pancytopenia can be obtained from the history, physical examination, and laboratory data. Pancytopenia that is not primarily hematologic in origin but secondary to other disease processes is usually an obvious diagnosis. Patients with severe liver disease and splenomegaly, systemic lupus erythematosus, or overwhelming sepsis can have low blood cell counts, but the clinical presentation is not subtle. Similarly, BM aplasia following cytotoxic drug therapy for cancers and a variety of nonmalignant diseases is anticipated. In the challenging case, obvious medical causes of pancytopenia have usually already been excluded. Pancytopenia almost never results from peripheral blood cell destruction alone. In AA, the blood smear does not show reticulocytes, band forms, or the large platelets typical of increased compensatory BM efforts.

Acquired AA is a disease of the young, as is constitutional aplasia. Patients with FA often, but not always, have physical abnormalities. In the absence of a suggestive family history or the presence of physical anomalies, the distinction between acquired and constitutional disease depends on the results of a clastogenic-stress culture of peripheral lymphocytes (for FA) and telomere length of leukocytes (for DKC and the telomeropathies).

In older patients the major differential diagnosis is between AA and myelodysplasia. There is a gray area between hypocellular myelodysplasia and moderate AA, and even competent hematologists might not agree on the final diagnosis. BM cytogenetics can help in establishing the proper diagnosis.

Myelofibrosis can also produce pancytopenia, but the BM is not aspirable, the spleen is often enlarged, and the peripheral blood smear shows characteristic abnormalities. Acute leukemia in children and the elderly can manifest as BM hypocellularity, requiring a careful search for lymphoblasts or myeloblasts, including phenotypic analysis by flow cytometry. Blood flow cytometry for glycophosphoinositol-anchored proteins should be performed to diagnose PNH (see Chapter 31).

The patient's history can provide clues, such as benzene exposure for myelodysplasia and acute leukemia or a suspicious drug history for AA. Discontinuation of exposure to the incriminated drugs or chemicals is mandatory, and in some instances, patients may then recover. However, given the difficulty of assigning blame with absolute certainty to environmental agents, we treat all patients similarly and do not advocate protracted observation for possible spontaneous recovery. For patients with severe disease (see Table 30.6), suitable and early preparation for BM transplant should be undertaken or immunosuppression begun, whereas for those with moderate disease, the clinical status should be evaluated, and serial blood cell counts are required to assess progression of the disease.

BONE MARROW

The BM must be assessed quantitatively and qualitatively for cellularity and the morphology of residual cells (Fig. 30.8 and see Fig. 30.1). BM aspiration and biopsy should always be performed, and the core

specimen should be at least 1 cm long. There should no hesitation in performing a second procedure if required.

BM cellularity is best estimated from the core biopsy. Point counting under microscopic cross hairs in many parts of a histologic section is the most accurate method of determining cellularity, but hematologists commonly rely on visual estimation only. A crude "eyeball" approximation is almost always adequate in severe aplasia, because the hematopoietic content of the BM specimen is usually close to zero. Estimates of BM cellularity based on examination of the aspirate smear and biopsy specimen are correlated, but dilution of the aspirate by sinusoidal blood often occurs, and the aspirate can be hypocellular when the biopsy specimen is hypercellular or can show focal areas of active hematopoiesis. Normal BM cellularity decreases considerably with age, a variation that is of some importance in assessing the older patient with aplasia or myelodysplasia. In autopsy samples from normal, young children, approximately 80% of the BM space of the iliac crest is cellular. BM cellularity gradually decreases from age 20 to 70 years and more precipitously in the very elderly, to approximately 30% in the eighth decade of life. For practical purposes, the lower limit of normal BM cellularity in adults is accepted at approximately 30%, but the differences at the extremes of life should be recalled when evaluating infants and the elderly. In most patients with AA, total BM cellularity is extremely low, but there can be significant residual lymphocytosis. The increase in BM fat in aplasia is caused by increases in the size and number of individual fat cells. "Hot pockets" of hematopoiesis can be present. The BM tends to contract centripetally with age, and a similar process can be observed in pathologic states, so the sternal BM can be more cellular than iliac crest samples.

Examination of the BM (Fig. 30.9, and see also Figs. 30.1 and 30.8) is basic for the diagnosis of most primary hematologic causes of pancytopenia (see Table 30.1 and box on Diagnostic Algorithm in Aplastic Anemia). A fatty, even watery specimen can usually be aspirated without difficulty from an aplastic patient, whereas a truly dry tap is more typical of a packed or fibrotic BM. The morphology of individual cells is best seen in the Wright-Giemsa–stained aspirate smear, and the architecture of the BM is appreciated in a biopsy section. In acellular specimens, the only cells visible are usually lymphocytes, plasma cells, and stromal elements (fibroblastoid and histiocytic cells). Some degree of dyserythropoiesis is common, usually the megaloblastoid features of macrocytosis and some nuclear-cytoplasmic maturation asynchrony, but sometimes more complex degenerative changes in nuclei and cytoplasm can be observed by light and electron microscopy (see Fig. 30.8). These features are common to AA and myelodysplasia (see Table 30.7), which can be very difficult to distinguish. Hemophagocytosis of RBCs can also be seen in AA. Examination of the cells close to the spicules of a sparse aspirate smear can disclose a distinctive population of leukemic blasts; increased numbers of myeloblasts are not seen in

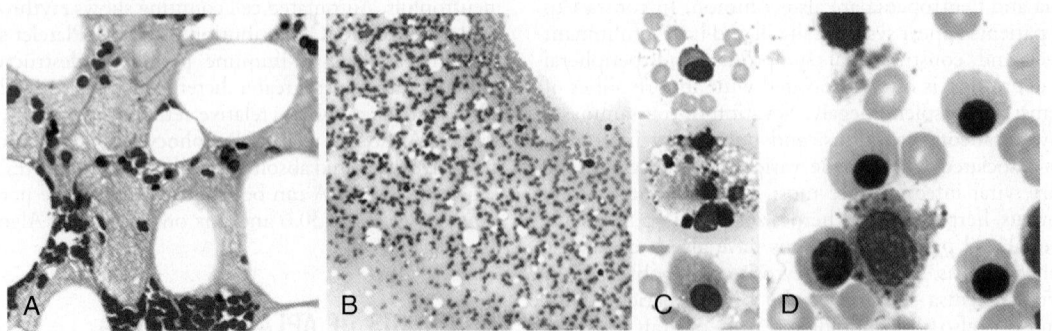

Fig. 30.8 SOME MORPHOLOGIC FEATURES OCCASIONALLY OBSERVED IN PATIENTS WITH APLASTIC ANEMIA. Empty marrow with eosinophilic ground substance consistent with serous atrophy or stromal injury (A), possibly indicative of marrow damage. Scanty marrow aspirate in severe disease (B) showing only rare nucleated elements many of which are from blood. Presence of plasma cells, histiocytes and osteoblasts (C) confirms marrow nature of aspirate. Note: sometimes the histiocytes can show hemophagocytosis. Megaloblastoid erythropoiesis (D) is sometimes seen in aplastic anemia and in recovery.

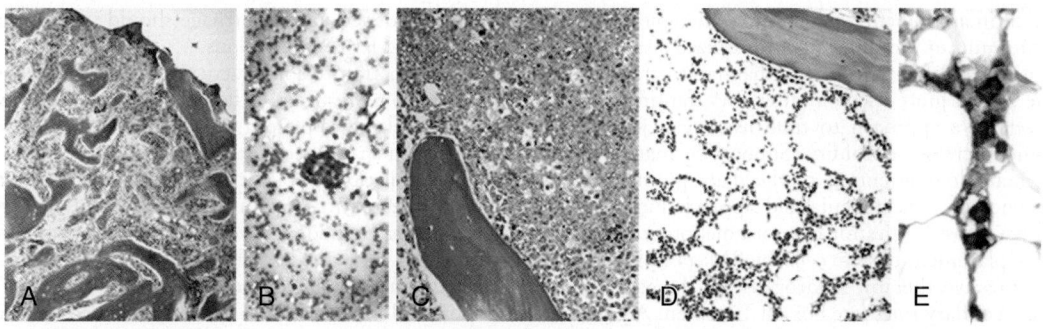

Fig. 30.9 MORPHOLOGY OF OTHER DISEASES THAT MAY MANIFEST WITH PANCYTOPENIA. Bone marrow biopsy from patient with pancytopenia showing myelofibrosis and osteosclerosis associated with metastatic prostate cancer (A). The aspirate was hypocellular but did show occasional tumor clusters (B). Another case where the patient presented with pancytopenia and was found to have a bone marrow packed with lymphoma cells (C). Hairy cell leukemia can present with pancytopenia and with a hypocellular bone marrow (D) difficult to distinguish from aplastic anemia. The diagnosis rests on identifying a B-cell infiltrative process with immunohistochemical stains (E, CD20).

AA and are evidence of aleukemic leukemia or herald the evolution of leukemia. Histochemistry for CD34[+] cells should show staining only of vascular elements in AA, and increased CD34[+] cell numbers is typical of MDS and acute myeloid leukemia (AML).

Karyotyping of BM cells is diagnostically important. Unfortunately, the yield of cells from a hypocellular BM can be inadequate to perform cytogenetic analysis. Chromosome analysis is usually normal in AA but frequently reveals a clonal abnormality in myelodysplasia. Cytogenetic studies, including interphase fluorescent in situ hybridization (FISH) and single nucleotide polymorphisms array–based karyotyping may produce informative results, including detection of cryptic chromosomal abnormalities.[10]

Radiographic Measures of Bone Marrow Function

Magnetic resonance imaging (MRI) with spin-echo sequences can be useful in the study of BM disease. On T1-weighted spin-echo images, fatty BM appears bright and cellular BM exhibits a lower density signal (see Fig. 30.9). The high-fat content of aplastic BM can be readily appreciated on MRI. Magnetic resonance spectroscopy, which detects the type of fat signal, has shown diverse patterns among AA patients.

DIFFERENTIAL DIAGNOSIS OF PANCYTOPENIA

AA is not the most common cause of pancytopenia (see Table 30.1). A rational diagnostic algorithm can be very helpful in establishing a correct diagnosis (see box on Diagnostic Algorithm in Aplastic Anemia). Pancytopenia is unlikely to be the presenting feature of hypersplenism in cirrhosis or of Evans syndrome (autoimmune hemolytic anemia and thrombocytopenia) in systemic lupus erythematosus. Findings on physical examination can point strongly toward another diagnosis. For example, the patient with myelofibrosis usually has splenomegaly, whereas a large spleen is very unusual in AA. Although vitamin B$_{12}$ and folate deficiencies have been reported to be associated with erythroid hypoplasia, this must be an exceedingly rare event. For the practicing hematologist, the most important and difficult choice of diagnoses in patients with pancytopenia is among the primary BM disorders.

In moderate AA, the modest depression of BM cellularity can muddle the single most reliable diagnostic criterion. BM cellularity is imprecisely quantitated at best, and further uncertainty is introduced by large sampling errors. "Hot spots" of hematopoietic activity in an otherwise acellular specimen reflect biologic heterogeneity in the pattern of cell loss. In patients with a syndrome of transient pancytopenia, spontaneous recovery occurs within a few months;

although the blood cell counts can be severely depressed, the BM is much more commonly normo/hypercellular than hypoplastic. In patients with chronic BM failure, serial BM specimens may not be identical because of sampling error or because the original disease was misdiagnosed or has changed its character. Some patients with AA are not pancytopenic; they do not have uniform depressions of RBC, white blood cell (WBC), and platelet production, despite an empty BM, and their clinical course is dominated by failure in two cell lines or a single hematopoietic lineage. Related conditions such as pure red cell aplasia, amegakaryocytic thrombocytopenia, and agranulocytosis, although usually distinctive in their clinical presentation, can evolve into more generalized BM failure. A hypocellular BM often precludes the proper morphologic diagnosis. This problem can be especially evident in the case of a MDS with hypoplastic BM (see Table 30.7).

BM cytogenetics, if positive for chromosome abnormalities, usually leads to a diagnosis of leukemia or MDS (see Chapters 59 and 60). However, some random chromosomal abnormalities may be transient and some believe that typical AA is not incompatible with an abnormal karyotype, in particular when somatic mosaicism is present. Often, an acellular specimen precludes successful culture and generation of metaphase smears. In such cases, single nucleotide polymorphisms arrays–based karyotyping can be performed on interphase cells and may be helpful in detection of clonal abnormalities. Screening for monosomy 7 and trisomy 8 can be also performed using interphase FISH.

Molecular diagnostics has entered the BM failure clinic. To establish the diagnosis of constitutional AA, commercial panels are now available to screen germline DNA for genes responsible for FA, telomeropathy, and Schwachman-Bodian-Diamond syndrome, and implicated genes in other congenital syndromes. Acquired mutations of recurrently mutated genes in MDS/AML can be detected in circulating WBC in about one-third of AA patients. In contrast to MDS and AML, mutations occur in a limited subset of genes, and the clone size, as estimated from variant allele frequency, is also small. Mutations in *DNMT3A* and *ASXL, CBL* and *SETBP1* correlate with patient age but independently predict for a poorer long-term outcome, especially in younger individuals. Only mutations in *PIGA* and *BCOR/BCORL* correlate with responsiveness to immunosuppressive therapy. Detection of unfavorable mutations in a patient who has failed treatment may influence the decision to undertake high risk or alternative stem cell transplantation.[11]

TREATMENT

AA should be considered a medical emergency. Lives are lost, mainly because the grave consequences of severe pancytopenia go unrecognized. The ultimate benefits of definitive therapies such as transplantation or immunosuppression will be unrealized if the patient succumbs to an early clinical catastrophe. A haphazard transfusion policy increases the risk of graft rejection after BM transplantation, but an overly conservative approach to transfusion can jeopardize the patient's life and increase morbidity. Supportive management therefore requires meticulous attention to the daily problems that occur as a consequence of pancytopenia and appreciation of their impact on the ultimate possibilities for cure or amelioration of AA. AA can be cured by replacement of stem cells, by BM transplantation, and by immunosuppressive therapy. Androgens and hematopoietic growth factors have secondary roles (see box on Treatment Algorithm in Aplastic Anemia).

Supportive Management

Bleeding

Bleeding was historically a common symptom in AA, and death from hemorrhage occurred frequently in the premodern era. Platelet transfusions have substantially improved survival in patients with this disease. Measurable correction of the platelet count by transfusion almost always alleviates the minor mucocutaneous bleeding common in thrombocytopenic patients. Major bleeding is usually not caused by thrombocytopenia alone, and other explanations for massive hemorrhage should be sought. The bleeding time improves after erythrocyte transfusion in patients with anemia, and there is a strong inverse correlation between the hematocrit and bleeding. The treatment of serious hemorrhage should include correction of severe anemia and RBC transfusions.

Modern transfusion practice has made platelets readily available and safe to administer. Other than cost and convenience, the major problem related to platelet transfusions is the development of alloimmunization in the recipient. The life span of the transfused platelet in the circulation is dramatically shortened by host antibodies, almost always directed to HLA-A and HLA-B antigens. Alloimmunization is suggested by poor recovery of the 1-hour posttransfusion platelet count and confirmed by finding specific HLA antibodies in serum. Refractoriness can often be overcome by selection of HLA-matched donors. Alloimmunization can be prevented or delayed by the use of single-donor platelets rather than pooled platelets, and by physical leukocyte depletion, by filtration or ultraviolet treatment of blood products. Avoidance of platelet transfusions except when there is active bleeding is another alternative to prevent alloimmunization, but the dose relationship between exposure to different donors' platelets and the probability of developing refractoriness are not clearly established.

Prophylactic transfusion of platelets is not standard but nevertheless frequent in practice. The primary indication for platelet prophylaxis is to prevent intracranial hemorrhage, but the risk of this complication in the chronically thrombocytopenic patient, although real, is low. Prophylactic platelet transfusions have not been shown to alter patient survival. Nevertheless the beneficial effects of avoiding bleeding complications and improving the quality of life justifies their use. Although the 20,000 platelets/μL value has long been used to trigger transfusion, many reports have suggested little difference in the risk of bleeding over a wide range of platelet counts between 5000

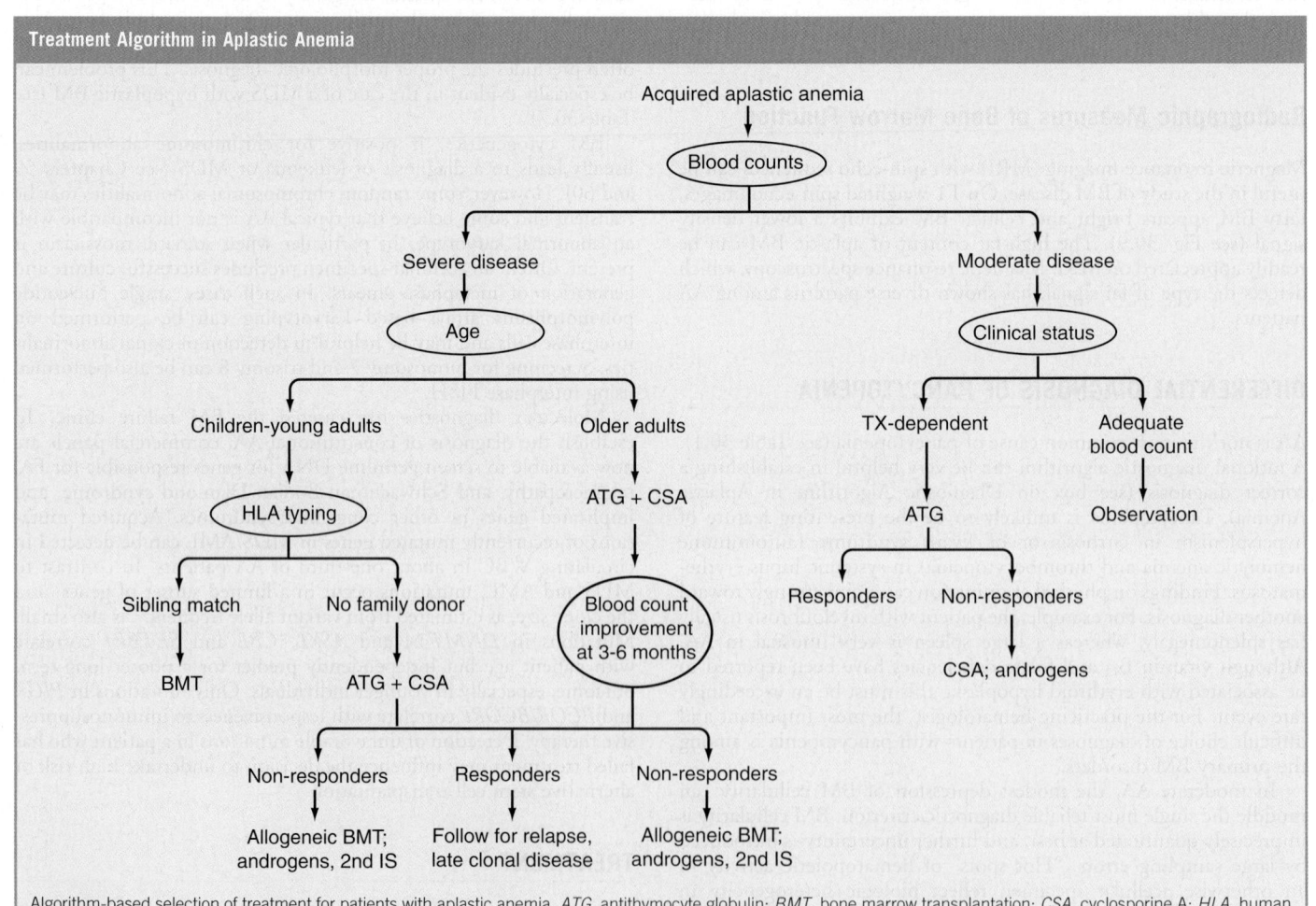

Treatment Algorithm in Aplastic Anemia

Algorithm-based selection of treatment for patients with aplastic anemia. *ATG*, antithymocyte globulin; *BMT*, bone marrow transplantation; *CSA*, cyclosporine A; *HLA*, human leukocyte antigen; *IS*, immunosuppression; *TX*, treatment.

and 100,000 platelets/µL. In a randomized trial of patients with AML, the risk of major bleeding was no different when 10,000 or 20,000 platelets/µL was chosen as the threshold, whereas the lower value led to a 20% reduction in platelet use. Any prophylaxis program must be modified to address the individual patient, but a goal of maintaining platelet counts >10,000 platelets/µL is reasonable. Major surgery can be accomplished in the setting of thrombocytopenia. In one study blood loss and morbidity rates were low even at platelet counts of less than 30,000 platelets/µL.

Anemia

Other than to reduce the risk of graft rejection after receiving an allogeneic stem cell transplant, there is no reason to allow a patient to suffer the symptoms of anemia. After equilibrium is achieved, a constant amount of blood will be required to maintain a given hemoglobin concentration. Physically fit individuals are usually not symptomatic at hemoglobin concentrations higher than 7 g/dL; patients with underlying cardiovascular disease should be maintained at a higher level (≥9 g/dL). Iron chelation should be used in patients with unresponsive chronic anemia who have a reasonable expectation of survival. Chelation may be avoided in the patient who proceeds to transplant soon after diagnosis or who responds in a few months to immunosuppressive therapy. In patients with chronic anemia, institution of a regimen of oral deferasirox (Exjade) or subcutaneous deferoxamine (Desferal) at adequate doses may be initiated as transfusions accumulate and serum ferritin rises.

Alloimmunization because of blood product administration increases the probability of graft rejection and mortality after BM transplantation. Blood products from potential BM donors such as a sibling or a parent (who share histocompatibility antigens) should be avoided. Small numbers of transfusions do not have a major deleterious effect on survival. The 5% risk of graft rejection after transplantation in entirely untransfused patients was increased to 15% with receipt of 1–40 units and to higher than 25% in more heavily transfused patients. Graft rejection would be anticipated to be lower with leucocyte-depletion methods of platelet preparations. Speed in arranging tissue typing and transfer to an appropriate center has a greater impact on the survival of the patient than the judicious transfusion of a few units of RBCs to a severely anemic patient or platelets to a bleeding patient. Transfusions should not be withheld in an older patient in whom immunosuppressive therapy will be the first-line therapy.

Infection

There are very few specific reports of infections and their therapy in patients with AA. The duration of neutropenia is the major difference between the neutropenia of BM failure and that induced by cytotoxic chemotherapy. With longer periods of neutropenia, the probability of serious bacterial or fungal infection increases. A second major difference is that neutropenia is part of a complex of problems associated with malignant disease and its therapy. In AA, the immune system is activated, and with the exception of intravenous catheter placement, the integument is preserved. Studies of cancer patients have usually identified a low-risk category of neutropenia, determined by the relatively brief period of neutropenia; by this criterion, almost all unresponsive patients with AA are at high risk.

In classic studies of leukemic children, neutropenia was shown to increase susceptibility to bacterial infections, and the number of infectious episodes correlated with the degree and duration of neutropenia. Susceptibility to infection is extremely high with an absolute neutrophil count of less than 200/µL, and this value has been used to define a category of very severe AA. As severe granulocytopenia becomes prolonged, infection is inevitable. Recommendations for initiation of empirical antibiotic therapy are similar for AA patients and other patients with neutropenia. The cardinal rule is, if the absolute neutrophil count is less than 500 cells/µL and infection is suspected, broad-spectrum parenteral antibiotic therapy should begin immediately. Any regimen may require modification based on the results of cultures, new symptoms or signs, or a deteriorating clinical course. Bacteremia is present in only 20% of febrile neutropenic episodes, and in only approximately 40% of those can a microbiologic cause or localizing physical findings be identified. Early discontinuation of antibiotics when cultures are unrevealing in persistently neutropenic patients is dangerous. Some experienced practitioners use prophylactic antibiotics to reduce febrile episodes and hospital admissions.

Patients often remain febrile despite antibiotic therapy, or fever reappears. In the absence of additional microbiologic data or clinical clues from the patient's complaints or physical examination, antifungal therapy should be instituted in patients who have remained febrile despite adequate antibacterial therapy. Current infectious disease guidelines recommend introduction of antifungal therapy after 5 days, but earlier addition can be advisable in the AA patient, especially if there are findings on chest tomography and a positive test for galactomannan protein. Fungemia during an initial febrile episode is rare, but fungal infection becomes more likely with repeated courses of antibiotics and ultimately is the major cause of death in AA patients in whom definitive therapy fails. *Candida* and *Aspergillus* species account for almost all fungal diseases in AA. Early aggressive treatment of neutropenic patients can reverse fungal disease. Large randomized trials have shown that newer antifungal agents such as voriconazole and caspofungin are less toxic and as effective or superior compared with amphotericin and liposomal amphotericin for treatment of both persistent neutropenic fever and established *Candida* and *Aspergillus* infection. Improved survival in severe AA is in some part caused by better antifungal drug therapies.[12]

Polymorphonuclear cells have a relatively brief life span in the circulation and their major activity is in infected tissue. There are no simple measures of the therapeutic efficacy of WBC transfusions. The absolute neutrophil count is not measurably increased by standard transfusions. Several controlled trials performed in the 1970s reported improved survival in patients who received granulocyte transfusions; negative studies may have used relatively low numbers of granulocytes transfused (<10^{10}/m²/day). Granulocyte transfusions are expensive and associated with serious toxicity: severe febrile reactions, pulmonary capillary leak syndrome, an increased risk of infection, and inevitable alloimmunization. Administration of G-CSF to normal donors greatly increases the yield of leukapheresis without adverse effects on the volunteers. Excellent results can be obtained from community donors, and the use of allocompatible granulocytes (as determined by lymphocytotoxicity screening assay) can further improve clinical results of granulocyte transfusions. Large numbers of neutrophils can be obtained, allowing dramatic increases in the absolute granulocyte levels in neutropenic recipients, which can improve clinical outcomes; case reports and phase I and II studies have suggested that G-CSF (G-CSF plus dexamethasone)–mobilized granulocyte transfusions can be helpful in the treatment of life-threatening fungal infections in severely neutropenic patients.[13]

Definitive Therapy

Hematopoietic Stem Cell Transplantation

Allogeneic stem cell transplantation from an HLA-matched sibling donor provides curative therapy for AA patients (Fig. 30.10).

Stem cell transplantation in AA is the subject of a large number of reports and reviews.[1,14–16] Cytokine-mobilized peripheral blood has also been used successfully as a stem cell graft but multiple studies favor BM over mobilized peripheral blood stem cell grafts in AA patients because of the lower risk of chronic GVHD.[17] The first studies of allogeneic BM transplants conclusively demonstrated their value compared with conventional supportive therapy. In a controlled trial reported by the International Aplastic Anemia Study Group, patients with severe disease who received transplants early had an actuarial survival rate of more than 60%, compared with

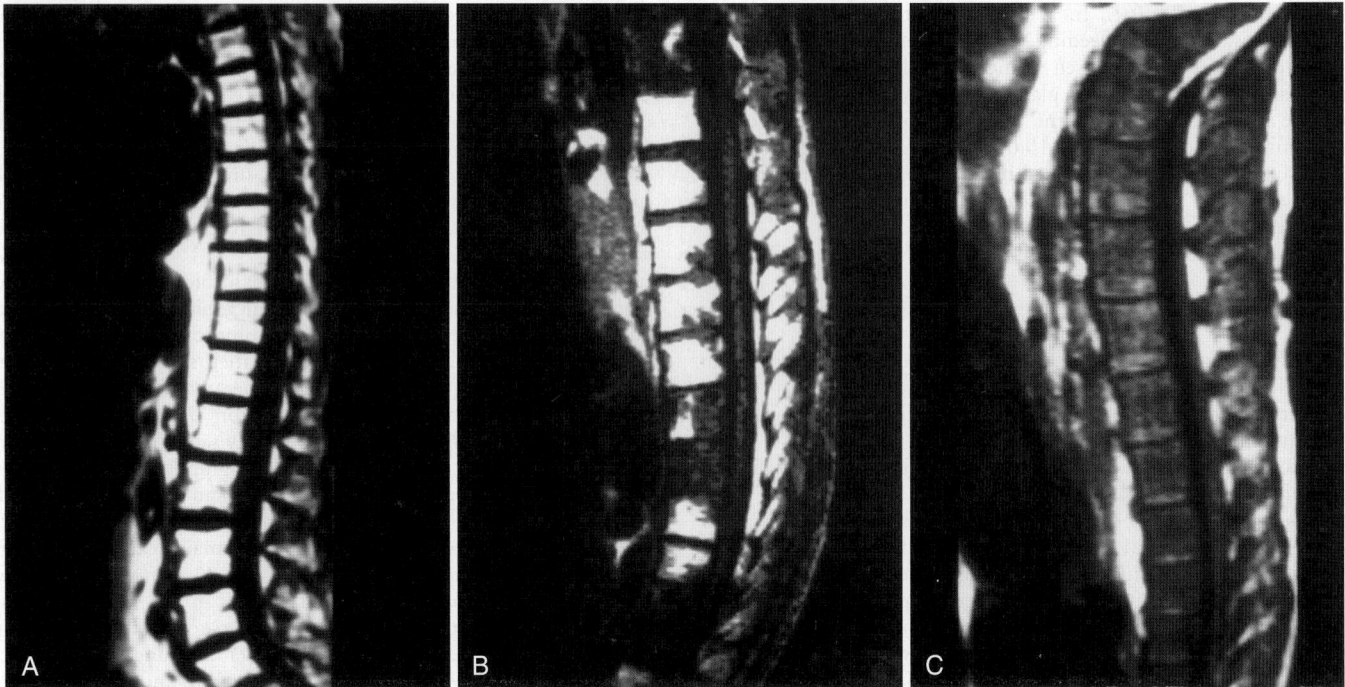

Fig. 30.10 MAGNETIC RESONANCE IMAGING OF BONE MARROW. (A) Bone marrow in a young man with severe aplastic anemia, (B) in a middle-aged woman with severe aplastic anemia, and (C) in a middle-aged woman with myelodysplasia.

approximately 20% in patients who received androgens and blood transfusions only. Results with BM transplantation have improved over time because of a combination of factors: progressive modification of conditioning regimens and lower procedure-related early mortality, improved transfusion support and antibiotic regimens, and the introduction of cyclosporine as prophylactic therapy for GVHD. Some centers report very high rates of survival ranging from 79% to 95%. Registry data indicate lower survival values as the general experience for the same period, with 64% of patients who received transplants during the period of 1985–1991 alive at 5 years after the procedure. Between 1990 and 1994, the European Group for Bone Marrow Transplantation (EGBMT) reported a 72% survival rate at 3.5 years, and 80% at 5 year.[18] In an analysis published in 2015, favorable risk factors were identified and allowed stratification into prognostic categories.[19] When young patients, age less than 20 years, are transplanted within 180 days of diagnosis with BM rather than blood as the stem cell source, and receive ATG in the conditioning regimen, and their cytomegalovirus (CMV) status were combined, low-risk patients had a 90% long-term survival (high-risk patients survival was 67%).

Graft rejection and GVHD are the major complications of allogeneic transplantation in AA. Graft rejection is a strong predictor of posttransplantation survival. The rate of graft rejection decreased with intensification of the immunosuppressive conditioning regimen, from 15% to about 4% in Europe and from 35% to between 10% and 15% in Seattle, and has remained stable in the past decade. Graft rejection may be related to the pathophysiology of AA, a finding supported by the unexpectedly high proportion of failures in unprepared patients receiving syngeneic transplants and even in adequately preconditioned patients receiving syngeneic transplants. In a group of untransfused patients who received allogeneic stem cells, the incidence of graft rejection was 10%, indicating that AA patients may be particularly sensitive to alloimmunization. Nevertheless, the influence of the number of transfusions on graft rejection is relative, and modest numbers of blood donations (40 units in the International Bone Marrow Transplant Registry experience and less than 10 units of erythrocytes or 40 units of platelets in Seattle) did not greatly increase the risk of graft rejection.[20]

Matched Sibling Donor (Hematopoietic Stem Cell Transplantation)

Intensification of immunosuppressive conditioning regimens with the use of total-body or lymphoid irradiation, cyclosporine, or ATG reduces the risk of graft rejection. Such measures, however, have not been shown to influence long-term survival.[21] The effect of the conditioning program on graft rejection probably is achieved through elimination of the recipient's lymphocytes and of subsequent mixed hematologic chimerism, which is associated with rejection. More rapid regeneration of BM grafts has been observed when cyclosporine is used, and second transplantations have been successful when ATG has been added to the conditioning regimen. In a prospective trial, ATG in the conditioning regimen did not significantly improve outcomes, but ATG has appeared advantageous in retrospective analysis of large numbers of patents. Matched sibling transplants should be accomplished without irradiation, and successful nonradiation conditioning regimens have included substitution with ATG, alemtuzumab, or fludarabine, which achieve engraftment and avoid many of irradiation's long-term complications, especially late cancers. With added ATG, sustained engraftment can be achieved by more than 90%, and patients who reject the graft can be still successfully retransplanted. The combination of cyclophosphamide plus fludarabine, with or without ATG, or regimens including alemtuzumab, have also achieved high rates of graft acceptance and survival even in heavily transfused patients who were transplanted with mobilized peripheral blood stem cells, months after proving refractory to immunosuppressive drugs. Overall, reported rejection rates range between 10% and 15%.[22]

Rates of chronic GVHD vary and are related to patient selection and treatment regimens. Age remains the dominant risk factor for the development of chronic GVHD. Chronic GVHD is more frequent and more severe in older patients, and children, including adolescents, have a much lower probability of suffering and dying from chronic GVHD. In an EGBMT analysis, a significant survival difference was observed between those younger than 20 years of age (65%) and those older than 20 years of age (56%), but there was no survival difference between patients 21–30 years old and those 31–55 years old. Young adults have fared better in other series, although morbidity from severe GVHD disease was more prevalent in the young adults than in children (43% versus 10%). Overall, the acute GVHD rate between 1991 and 1997 was approximately 20% for patients younger than 20 years of age and 40% for those over 40 years of age. In general, similar numbers have been cited for chronic GVHD. In more recent reports, the Seattle team's regimen of cyclophosphamide, ATG, cyclosporine, and methotrexate in children produced 100% 5-year survival, with low rates of graft rejection, 7%; high-grade acute GVHD, 3%, and chronic GVHD, 10%; the European collective experience is similar for first-line transplant in very young children (91% long-term survival; 2% rejection, 8% acute GVHD, and 6% chronic GVHD). In contrast, patients over the age of 40 years (who are often transplanted after failing immunosuppressive treatment), have three- to fourfold higher probabilities of developing acute and chronic GVHD.

In summary, excellent survival rates and low morbidity in younger patients make allogeneic BM transplantation the treatment of choice for children and adolescents. Older adults have a higher risk of transplant-related morbidity and mortality. Younger adults have a good opportunity for cure with transplantation but face more complications than do children. In addition to age, a prolonged interval between diagnosis and transplantation, multiple transfusions, and serious infections before transplantation are poor risk factors.

Transplant From Alternative Donors

Haplotype sharing between parents occasionally has allowed identification and successful transplantation between phenotypically matched relatives. Long-term survival after even one-locus-mismatched family donation is inferior to genotypically matched transplants, mainly because of graft rejection and GVHD. In the large European experience, for phenotypically identical family matches, the actuarial survival rate was 45%; for patients with a single-locus mismatch, it was 25%; and for those with two to three loci mismatched, the survival rate was 11%. In a report from Seattle although all patients who received fully HLA-matched transplants survived, those with mismatches at one or more loci had a much poorer outcome, and even with total-body irradiation added to the conditioning regimen, the survival rate was only 50%.

Until recently, most large studies of matched unrelated donor transplants (MUD) have shown inferior long-term survival and higher rates of complications as compared with matched sibling transplants. Even more than in standard sibling transplants, age is a crucial risk factor in unrelated transplants. The degree of match clearly impacts the outcome of the unrelated BM transplantation, and selection of donors based on high resolution typing is a factor in improving outcomes. Different conditioning regimens have been used at various centers, and results are often difficult to compare between institutions because of the large number of variables. Nevertheless, in a recent summary of the large European experience of transplants performed between 2005 and 2009, overall survival was equivalent to matched sibling procedures (76% versus 83%), although with rates of high-grade GVHD (10% versus 5%) and chronic extensive GVHD (11% versus 6%). Factors predictive of a favorable MUD outcome were transplant using BM as a source of stem cells, transplant within 180 days of diagnosis, patient age, use of ATG in the conditioning regimen, and CMV status.[19] MUDs are sufficiently effective in children that they have been tested as first-line therapy in pilot trials, with good outcomes.

Retrospective analysis of 71 AA patients treated with umbilical cord transplantation showed the estimated probability of 3-year overall survival of 38% (median follow-up of 35 months; the cell dose appeared to be the most important factor impacting survival.[23] While umbilical cord transplants have become less frequent, increasingly popular is the use of stem cells from haploidentical family members, who are almost always available. As with MUDs, early experience was poor, but the addition of cyclophosphamide posttransplant, to

eradicate immune cells responsible for GVHD, has apparently been successful, although the literature describing the results is currently sparse; small case series from China and Brazil describe about 70% survival and remarkably low rates of GVHD.

Late Complications of Bone Marrow Transplantation

A study published in 2011 analyzing outcomes of children with AA over the 4 decades indicates that the majority of long-term survivors after transplantation during childhood can have a normal productive life with 30-year survival of 82%.[24]

Very late complications after transplantation include effects on gonadal function, growth and development, avascular necrosis, as well as compromised function of endocrine, neurologic, or other organ systems. About 10% of long-term survivors have significant late effects after matched sibling transplant, and a higher proportion after MUD. A high rate of secondary malignancies has been recorded after transplantation. In a National Cancer Institute retrospective analysis of almost 20,000 transplantations, the risk of late-onset cancer was eightfold higher at 10 years than in the general population and even higher for young patients, for whom the risk of malignancy was increased approximately 40-fold. For AA, multivariate analyses repeatedly implicate radiation as the major risk factor for the development of malignancies, usually solid cancers. For AA, among 320 patients who received transplants in Seattle, four developed cancer, leading to a calculated risk seven times higher than for normal controls. In a recent update, 12% of patients who survived more than 2 years after transplantation developed solid tumors. In a French survey, four of 147 AA patients developed solid tumors, an 8-year cumulative incidence rate of 22%. In an analysis of 700 transplantation patients with AA and FA, the risk of developing a secondary malignancy was 14% at 20 years. The hazard of lymphoid malignancies decreased with the time after transplantation, whereas the risk of solid tumors progressively increased. In general, the rates of secondary malignancies after BM transplantation for AA and other diseases are similar. Immune events such as acute GVHD, treatment with ATG or monoclonal antibodies, in addition to total-body irradiation have been linked to the development of secondary malignancies. Patients with these secondary cancers, except for carcinoma of the skin, have a poor prognosis. The risk of cancer after BM transplantation must be evaluated in the context of other therapeutic options, especially immunosuppression, because a significant risk of late malignancy exists in AA patients independent of transplantation therapy. The risk of malignancy in the large registry of the EGBMT was equivalent for patients who received immunosuppression and for those who underwent transplantation. Compared with the general European population, the relative risk of malignancy was calculated at 5.15 for AA patients treated with immunosuppression (confidence interval [CI]: 3.2–7.9) and at 6.67 (CI: 3–12.6) for patients receiving transplants. Overall, the rate of malignancy after BM transplantation has been calculated to be 3.8-fold higher than in the age-matched population.

Immunosuppression

Antithymocyte Globulins

Immunosuppressive therapy is an effective alternative treatment for patients who are not candidates for BM transplantation (see box on Treatment Algorithm in Aplastic Anemia).[1]

Immunoglobulin preparations made from the sera of horses immunized against human thymocytes are the mainstays of current regimens. Horse ATG is licensed for use in the United States as ATGAM and SAA is an approved indication. Thymoglobulin, a rabbit ATG, is more available worldwide.

The efficacy of antilymphocyte globulin (ALG) in BM failure was discovered serendipitously in the late 1960s, when Mathé observed recovery of autologous hematopoietic function in patients who

Therapy for Aplastic Anemia

After the diagnosis of acquired aplastic anemia (AA) has been established, treatment options must be identified, considered carefully, and chosen with alacrity (see box on Treatment Algorithm in Aplastic Anemia). For patients with moderate disease, an expectant approach can be chosen based on a stable course and adequate blood counts, or for patients dependent on transfusion support, horse antithymocyte globulin (ATG; 40 mg/kg/day for 4 days) can be given. After assessment of the response, patients who improve should be monitored for hematologic signs of relapse, and nonresponders can be offered alternative therapy, such as androgens or cyclosporine. In severe disease for which the prognosis with blood transfusion and antibiotic support alone is poor, bone marrow (BM) transplantation from a histocompatible sibling or immunosuppression are accepted and effective therapies. Although large, retrospective analyses have shown that long-term survival rates from transplantation or immune therapy are equivalent, each has its own advantages and disadvantages. For children, BM transplantation remains the treatment of choice if an appropriate family donor is available, because these patients have a low rate of graft-versus-host disease (GVHD), and the BM disease is cured by stem cell replacement. The risk of therapy-related cancers can be increased, especially in children, after BM transplantation, and is ameliorated by avoiding radiation in the conditioning regimen. Adults with AA also successfully receive transplants, although the risk and severity of chronic GVHD and other treatment-related complications increase with age. BM transplantation has been performed in patients older than 50 years of age, and it is a reasonable approach in a younger adult, less than 40 years old, especially with more severe degrees of neutropenia. Most studies show that transplant early in the course of disease, within 6 months of diagnosis, is desirable.

Most patients with AA do not have a human leukocyte antigen (HLA)–matched sibling donor, and immunosuppression is the treatment of choice in these cases. Patients with severe disease should receive a combination of ATG and cyclosporine. We recommend a regimen consisting of 40 mg/kg/day of horse ATG on days 1–4, followed by cyclosporine for

6 months at a dose of 12 mg/kg. Corticosteroids are added in moderate doses (1 mg/kg of prednisone or methylprednisolone) during the first 2 weeks to ameliorate serum sickness. Improvement should be expected within 6 months. This regimen has produced hematologic responses in approximately 65% of treated patients, who then have an excellent 5-year survival rate.

Although immunosuppressive therapy is generally well tolerated, patients frequently relapse and require further treatment; however, relapse is not associated with a poor prognosis. More serious is the development of late-onset hematologic clonal diseases, paroxysmal nocturnal hemoglobinuria (which may not be clinically significant), myelodysplastic syndrome, and acute myeloid leukemia.

For patients in whom immunosuppressive therapy fails, there are a number of options. For children, alternative donor BM transplantation should be considered early; at the best centers, survival rates now are almost as good as with sibling donors. In children and adults, well matched unrelated donor stem cells provide similar long-term survival as do matched sibling donors, but the rate of chronic and severe chronic GVHD is higher. Patients with AA and telomere disease can respond to androgen therapy. Repeated immunosuppression in a patient in whom a first course of ATG and cyclosporine has failed is successful in about 30% of cases. Eltrombopag is approved for use in patients with refractory AA.

Patients with severe AA should not be subjected to useless early trials of corticosteroids or hematopoietic growth factors as the primary treatment. For the occasional patient who must decide between BM transplantation and immunosuppression, the advice of experts familiar with this disease and careful counseling of the patient are advisable. Age and severity of neutropenia are decisive factors. A limited number of transfusions can be necessary to optimize the patient's condition before definitive therapy and are acceptable. Single-donor platelets should be given and can be obtained from HLA-compatible donors. In severely neutropenic patients, granulocyte colony-stimulating factor therapy can decrease the risk of life-threatening infections. In the absence of overt bleeding, platelet counts as low as 5000 cells/μL appear to be safe.

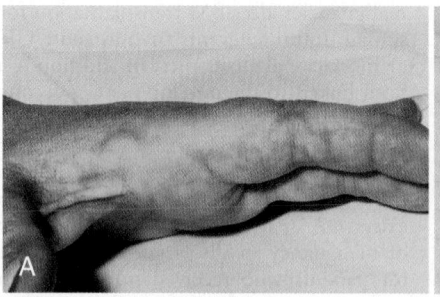
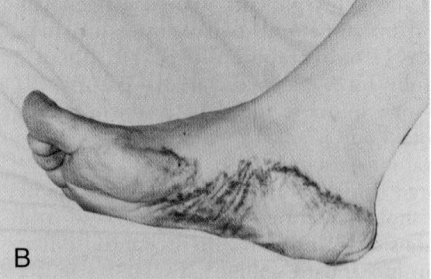

Fig. 30.11 CUTANEOUS ERUPTIONS OF SERUM SICKNESS. (A) On the hand, (B) on the foot.

received antilymphocyte serum as conditioning for BM transplantation. Observations and formal studies in Europe showed that 40% to 70% of patients responded with hematologic improvement and improved survival. Similar results were also obtained in US randomized and multicenter protocols, in which about one-half of patients treated with ATG or ALG showed hematologic improvement, broadly defined as an end to transfusion dependence and an improvement in a neutrophil number to a level protective against infection.

The putative cause of AA is not a factor that predicts response. Virus- and drug-induced aplasia and posthepatitis AA respond similarly compared with idiopathic disease. Cytogenetic abnormalities do not preclude a response because AA with chromosomal abnormalities and some cases of frank myelodysplasia improve after ATG. The response rate to ATG or ALG is not improved by the addition of androgens or very high doses of corticosteroids.

A hematologic response to ATG is usually apparent within a few months of therapy; in some cases, all blood counts rise dramatically, and in others, increases in platelets or RBCs can be delayed (see box on Treatment Algorithm in Aplastic Anemia). The average time to improvement in neutrophil number is 1–2 months; transfusion independence occurs approximately 2–3 months after initiation of

treatment. Continued improvement without further therapy commonly occurs after 3 months; nevertheless, clinical status by 3 months is strongly correlated with long-term survival. Blood counts above the critical values for severity and platelets and reticulocyte counts of more than 50,000 cells/μL are highly prognostic. Reticulocyte count, perhaps reflecting the stem cell reserve, has been the best predictor of response and survival. With new and better tolerated antifungal drugs, survival even of nonresponders has improved and a very low neutrophil count may no longer have prognostic value.

ATG has three major toxic effects: immediate allergic phenomena, serum sickness, and transient blood cell count depression (Fig. 30.11). Fever, rigors, and an urticarial cutaneous eruption are common on the first or second day of ATG therapy, and these symptoms respond to antihistamines and meperidine. Anaphylaxis is rare but can be fatal. Corticosteroids are administered in moderate doses (1 mg/kg of prednisone or methylprednisolone) during the first 2 weeks to ameliorate the symptoms of serum sickness. Doses of ATG and ALG have varied from 5 to 50 mg/kg, and the duration of administration has varied from 4 to 28 days. It is more rational to administer equivalent doses of horse ATG by the schedule originally used in Europe (40 mg/kg/day for 4 days); antiserum will then have reached low levels in the circulation by the time host antibody appears. A short course of therapy is easier to administer, associated with less serum sickness, and equally effective as the same dose given over a more prolonged course. Thymoglobulin, rabbit ATG, has been approved for use in the United States. While rabbit ATG is more potent by weight than horse ATG, a randomized trial (using most commonly applied dosing of thymoglobulin at 3.5 mg/kg × 5 days) showed it markedly inferior to horse ATG in achieving hematologic response, and survival was poorer as well.[25]

ALGs are immunosuppressive. ATGs contain a heterogeneous mix of antibody specificities for lymphocytes. Horse sera fix human complement efficiently, and all preparations are T-cell cytotoxic in vitro, with little difference among ATGs or among lots for lymphocyte killing in vitro. In vitro ALGs efficiently inhibit T-cell proliferation and block IL-2 and IFN-γ production and IL-2 receptor expression. ATG induces Fas-mediated apoptosis of T cells, especially after activation. In patients the administration of ATG results in rapid reduction in the number of circulating lymphocytes, usually to less than 10% of starting values, and lymphopenia persists for several days after discontinuing therapy. Although lymphocyte numbers return to pretreatment values by 3 months, reductions in activated lymphocyte numbers in recovered patients persist. It seems likely that these inhibitory effects on T cells are responsible for the efficacy of ALGs in AA. Nevertheless, the ability of ATG to stimulate lymphocyte function by acting as a mitogen may also have a role in their therapeutic efficacy. Notably, rabbit ATG can stimulate T regulatory cell development in vitro and in patients, although this effect in AA is overwhelmed by rabbit ATG's more potent CD4 cell depletion in comparison to horse ATG.

Cyclosporine

Several groups reported anecdotal success with cyclosporine (CSA) therapy combined with androgens in individual patients with AA, in many of whom other therapies had failed. Some studies suggested efficacy of CSA in patients refractory to ALG or ATG alone, with salvage rates of approximately 50%. The optimal regimen has not been determined. In the United States CSA has usually been used in high doses (12 mg/kg/day for adults and 15 mg/kg/day for children), with adjustment according to plasma drug concentrations and serum creatinine levels. In Europe lower doses (3–7 mg/kg/day) have been reported to be equally efficacious. Hematologic improvement can occur in a few weeks or months. A 6-month trial is warranted. Remissions, when achieved, usually have been durable, but some patients relapse when cyclosporine is discontinued. Most patients who relapse will respond to the reinstitution of CSA; the lowest possible dose should be sought by tapering, but some patients may require long-term maintenance treatment.

CSA has considerable toxicity. Hypertension and azotemia are the most common serious side effects; hirsutism and gingival hypertrophy are also frequent complaints. Increasing serum creatinine levels are an indication for dose reduction. Chronic CSA nephropathy characterized by interstitial fibrosis and tubular atrophy can be irreversible. The risk of nephropathy is increased by high doses and longer duration of therapy and occurs more commonly in older than in younger patients. CSA, especially in combination with corticosteroids, converts patients with AA to a temporary immunodeficiency state and puts them at high risk for opportunistic infections. Monthly aerosolized pentamidine prophylaxis can prevent *Pneumocystis carinii* pneumonia in patients receiving CSA.

Combined or Intensive Immunosuppressive Therapy

The combination for the treatment of AA of an agent that lyses lymphocytes (ATG) with a drug that blocks lymphocyte function is rational. The strategy has resulted in a striking increase in the response rate to immunosuppressive therapy in randomized and multicenter trials, to 60% to 80% at 1-year compared to about 40% with ATG alone, more complete responses, and better 5-year survival rates for responding patients at 80% to 90%. Children do especially well with combined therapy, elderly patients less so, partly because of greater toxicity and poor tolerance of pancytopenia related complications in the presence of comorbidities.

In disease refractory to initial therapy with ATG and CSA, a repeat course of rabbit ATG and CSA or alemtuzumab can be administered as a salvage regimen and can rescue about a third or more of patients.

Cyclophosphamide

Cyclophosphamide in high doses (45–50 mg/kg/day for 4 days) and "moderate" dose (50 mg/kg/day × 2 days) without stem cell rescue can induce hematologic recovery in severe AA, with an overall response rate claimed similar to that achieved with ATG therapy but a higher proportion of complete responses and less relapse and clonal evolution. However, cyclophosphamide severely depresses the neutrophil count, resulting in prolonged hospitalization for suspected or actual infection and a higher risk of invasive fungal infections and death in comparison to ATG and CSA.

Corticosteroids

Methylprednisolone in modest doses (1 mg/kg/day) is administered with ATG to ameliorate the symptoms of serum sickness. Very-high-dose corticosteroids regimens can be effective, especially in recently diagnosed patients. High-dose methylprednisolone has also been added to ATG therapy, with inconsistent results. However, ATG is associated with better response rates and many fewer associated toxic effects than high-dose steroid therapy and is generally preferable as initial therapy. Modest doses of corticosteroids do not have roles in the treatment of AA except in combination with ATG.

Late Complications of Immunosuppressive Therapy

Relapse after immunosuppressive therapy is common. About one-third or more of responding patients may be expected to require reinstitution of immunosuppressive drugs or another course of ATG. Relapse can manifest as a gradual decline in one blood count, need for transfusion after a period of transfusion-independence, or abrupt recurrence of severe pancytopenia. Most relapse responds to retreatment, and there is no clear relationship with inferior survival.

A much more serious complication is the development of late-onset clonal hematologic disorders, especially myelodysplasia and AML. Some of these events likely represent part of the natural history of AA. Before recent improvements in treatment, leukemia was considered an unusual complication but late-onset clonal disorders do not appear to be the result of the introduction of immunosuppressive therapy. In European and National Institutes of Health trials, the overall rate of clonal evolution is 12% to 15% at about a decade. Children appear to be at similar risk for the development of clonal complications as adults, and evolution to MDS can occur in responders and in refractory patients. MDS that develops after AA can transform to AML but can also be surprisingly indolent. Cytogenetic analyses are almost always abnormal in clonal evolution. Monosomy 7 is the most frequent finding and confers a poor prognosis; in contrast to trisomy 8. Clinically monosomy 7 was more likely to occur in primarily refractory patients and had a poor prognosis, whereas patients with trisomy 8 often remain CSA-responsive and have good prospects for survival. Trisomy 6 and 13q– also behave benignly in most cases. A PNH clone can be detected in up to 50% of patients at the time of presentation. Usually the clone size remains stable and it may decrease; over time, only a minority of patients will develop a large clone and the hemolytic or thrombotic form of PNH. Both the presence of somatically mutated clones in the marrow and rapid telomere attrition have been associated as risk factors with the development of MDS and AML after treatment of AA.

Immunosuppression Versus Bone Marrow Transplantation

Immunosuppression and transplantation are both effective therapies for AA (Figs. 30.12 and 30.13). Lack of a matched sibling donor, the

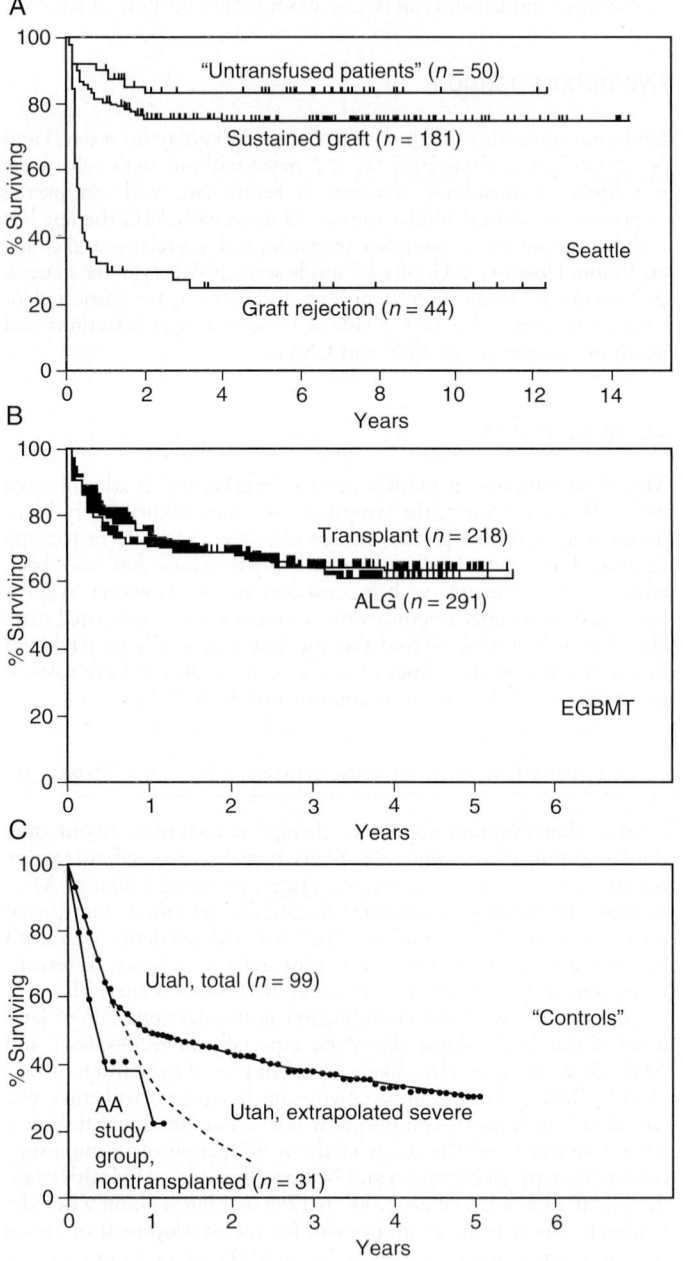

Fig. 30.12 ACTUARIAL SURVIVAL RATES FOR PATIENTS WITH APLASTIC ANEMIA. (A) Data on bone marrow transplantation from the University of Washington. (B) Data from the EGBMT on bone marrow transplantation versus immunosuppression with ALG. (C) Natural history as indicated by survival with supportive and other treatments. Two groups are illustrated. Extrapolated survival curves for patients with severe disease are derived from retrospective reviews from the University of Utah of 101 records collected from the late 1940s to early 1970s. The patients received blood transfusions and, later in this period, also received platelets. Almost all were treated with corticosteroids, and one-half were also treated with androgens. Data for patients who did not receive transplants come from a multicenter study of the efficacy of marrow transplantation performed in the early 1970s; this control group was treated with hendrogens. *AA,* Aplastic anemia; *ALG,* antilymphocyte globulin; *EGBMT,* European Group for Bone Marrow Transplantation.

expense and availability of transplantation, and risk factors such as active infections, advanced age, or a heavy transfusion burden lead most patients to automatically undergo treatment with ATG/CSA. For a few patients with AA, a choice does exist between transplantation and immunosuppressive therapy. BM transplantation offers a permanent cure. Its disadvantages are cost, procedure-related morbidity and mortality (especially GVHD in older patients), and an increased incidence of solid organ malignancies. Immunosuppressive therapy is easier and initially cheaper. However, many patients do not achieve normal blood cell counts and remain at high risk for relapse and the more serious complications of late-onset clonal hematologic disease, especially MDS.

Retrospective analyses of the large number of European patients reported to the EGBMT show consistently improved results with both therapies but have repeatedly failed to demonstrate a survival advantage for transplantation over immunosuppression. Single-center studies are similar. Certain categories of patients, defined by neutrophil number and age, probably benefit from one therapy or the other. In general BM transplantation yields superior results in children, immunosuppression in older adults

Remarkable improvements in results using unrelated donors have made this approach available to many patients who lack a sibling donor. Increasingly, children who have failed a single course of immunosuppression and adults refractory to multiple courses of ATG are offered this procedure, and some transplant groups advocate for early MUD or even haploidentical donor transplant, even before a trial of immunosuppression.

Androgens

Testosterone and synthetic anabolic steroids appeared to be major advances in the treatment of AA when they were introduced in the 1960s. The high response rates in some early series may be retrospectively attributed to the inclusion of patients with moderate acquired and constitutional AA. For severe AA, controlled trials in general have not demonstrated efficacy, as measured by survival rates

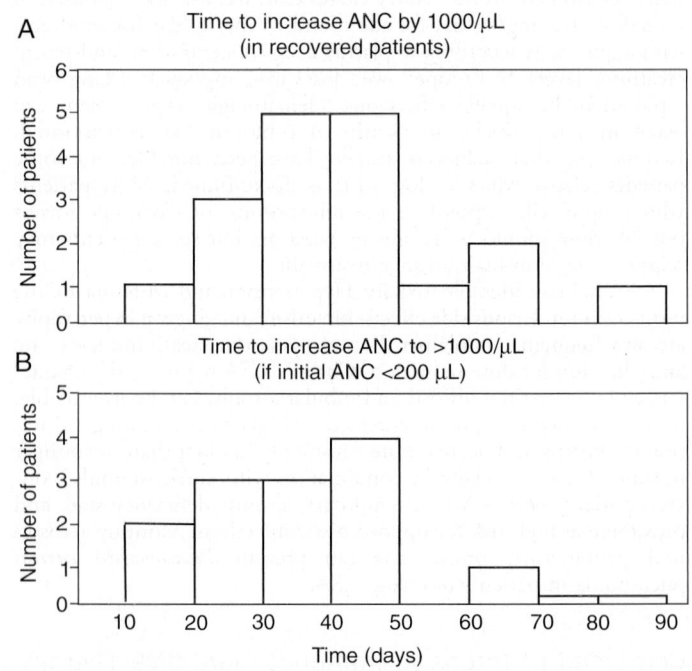

Fig. 30.13 TIME TO RESPONSE AFTER TREATMENT WITH ANTI-LYMPHOCYTE GLOBULIN. (A) Distribution of patients with severe aplastic anemia by time to achieve an increase in the absolute neutrophil count of 1000 cells/mm³. (B) Distribution of patients with an initial absolute neutrophil count of less than 200 cells/mm³ by time to achieve an absolute neutrophil count of 1000 cells/mm³. *ANC,* absolute neutrophil count.

or hematologic improvement. When added to immunosuppressive therapies, androgens failed to result in any increase in response rates.

Androgens continue to be helpful in occasional patients when used as a second-line therapy. Most hematologists have observed patients who appeared to respond or even to develop hormone dependence. Androgen therapy remains popular in developing countries because it is inexpensive, well tolerated, and seemingly effective. Various preparations of androgens at different doses have resulted in similar response rates of 35% to 60% after 6 months of therapy. Sex hormones increase telomerase gene transcription and danazol has been effective in marrow failure due to telomeropathy.[27]

Useful androgens include nandrolone decanoate, oxymetholone, and danazol. The hemoglobin response is frequently more impressive than improvements in granulocyte or platelet levels. An adequate trial is considered to be a full dose given for at least 3 months. Complications occur infrequently, although some are serious and can limit effective therapy, especially in the elderly. The associated liver cholestasis is usually reversible. Hepatotoxicity (e.g., bile duct proliferation, peliosis, atypical hepatocyte hyperplasia, tumors) can occur but is less common with parenteral formulations. Children appear to tolerate high doses of androgens without lasting effects on growth or maturation.

Hematopoietic Growth Factors

Hematopoietic growth factor production is normal or increased in most patients with AA. Nevertheless, many patients are treated with pharmacologic high doses of cytokines, often with uncertain justification. G-CSF and GM-CSF in some cases can increase neutrophil numbers in patients with AA. In general,,neutrophil responses to growth factors are transient, dependent on their continuous administration, and usually restricted to patients with quantitatively less severe forms of AA. Nevertheless, occasional bilineage and trilineage responses have been observed. Children may be more sensitive to the effects of prolonged administration of G-CSF.

A concern has been the possibility that prolonged administration of G-CSF might increase the probability of late clonal disease, especially monosomy 7. In retrospective analyses of Japanese children and adults with severe AA, this syndrome appeared to occur most frequently among patients who had received growth factor; a modest increase in the risk of myelodysplasia and leukemia and monosomy 7 was also seen in European cases. The mechanism of G-CSF's relationship to monosomy 7 may be selection of aneuploid cells bearing an isoform of G-CSF; these cells are less sensitive to G-CSF, but when triggered by the cytokine they proliferate but do not differentiate.

Anemia and pancytopenia in rare patients have responded to prolonged administration of high doses of erythropoietin alone, GM-CSF and erythropoietin, and with IL-3 and G-CSF. In one randomized protocol, the combination of G-CSF and high doses of erythropoietin improved hemoglobin values, mainly in patients with moderate disease.

Growth factors have also been combined with definitive medical therapy to improve neutrophil counts during the early phase of immunosuppression. Neither small pilot trials nor large randomized studies have shown substantial benefit for the routine use of GM-CSF or G-CSF in preventing infection, improving the response rate to immunosuppression, or in survival. A brief therapeutic trial of G-CSF or GM-CSF is often used in severely neutropenic patients who are persistently or seriously infected in the hope of clinical benefit. Growth factors, alone or in combination, are occasionally effective in chronically refractory patients.

New thrombopoietic factors may have utility in AA. An oral c-mpl agonist peptide, eltrombopag, increased not only platelet counts but led to erythrocyte and granulocyte improvement in almost half of 25 patients with chronic refractory severe AA. The mpl receptor is expressed by hematopoietic stem cells, and laboratory and clinical data indicate physiologic stimulation of stem cells by thrombopoietin. This study led to the Food and Drugs Aadministration approval of labeling of eltrombopag as a salvage therapy for AA refractory to immunosuppressive therapy. Whether eltrombopag (and functionally related recombinant c-mpl ligand Nplate) adversely impact the risk of later MDS and AML is not yet established. Ongoing trials combine eltrombopag with immunosuppression as first treatment in SAA and have produced very high response rates and complete response rates, as well as earlier blood count recovery.

PROGNOSIS

The initial blood cell counts of a patient with AA are important indicators of prognosis. The popular "Camitta" criteria used to define severe disease are the presence of two of the following three: neutrophil count of less than 500 cells/μL, platelet count of less than 20,000 cells/μL, and corrected reticulocyte level of less than 1% (<40,000 cells/μL). In the more modern era absolute reticulocytes (>25,000/uL) and absolute lymphocytosis predicted a good response to immunosuppression and survival. The robustness of the platelet and reticulocyte response after immunosuppression also correlates with long-term survival. Clonal evolution, especially −7del(7q), is a poor prognostic factor, and age-adjusted telomere length of leukocytes at diagnosis may predict this serious complication.[26]

The rate of spontaneous recovery is difficult to estimate, but most observers believe it to be low. Untreated severe disease is almost invariably fatal. In contrast, moderate AA has a good prognosis, and some patients with minimal blood cell count depression recover normal blood cell counts with limited or no therapy.

SUGGESTED READINGS

Adkins DR, Goodnough LT, Shenoy S, et al: Effect of leukocyte compatibility on neutrophil increment after transfusion of granulocyte colony-stimulating factor-mobilized prophylactic granulocyte transfusions and on clinical outcomes after stem cell transplantation. *Blood* 95:3605, 2000.

Bacigalupo A. How I treat acquired aplastic anemia. *Blood* 129:1428–1436, 2017.

Chen J, Lipovsky K, Ellison FM, et al: Bystander destruction of hematopoietic progenitor and stem cells in a mouse model of infusion-induced bone marrow failure. *Blood* 104:1671, 2004.

Deeg HJ, Leisenring W, Storb R, et al: Long-term outcome after marrow transplantation for severe aplastic anemia. *Blood* 91:3637, 1998.

Desmond R, Townsley DM, Dumitriu B, et al: Eltrombopag restores trilineage hematopoiesis in refractory severe aplastic anemia that can be sustained on discontinuation of drug. *Blood* 123:1818–1825, 2014.

Dumitriu B, Feng X, Townsley DM, et al: Telomere attrition and candidate gene mutations preceding monosomy 7 in aplastic anemia. *Blood* 125:706–709, 2015.

Heckman KD, Weiner GJ, Davis CS, et al: Randomized study of prophylactic platelet transfusion threshold during induction therapy for adult acute leukemia: 10,000/microL versus 20,000/microL. *J Clin Oncol* 15:1143, 1997.

Herbrecht R, Denning DW, Patterson TF, et al: Voriconazole versus amphotericin B for primary therapy of invasive aspergillosis. *N Engl J Med* 347:408, 2002.

Hughes WT, Armstrong D, Bodey GP, et al: 2002 Guidelines for the use of antimicrobial agents in neutropenic patients with cancer. *Clin Infect Dis* 34:730, 2002.

International Agranulocytosis and Aplastic Anemia Study: Risks of agranulocytosis and aplastic anemia: A first report of their relation to drug use with special reference to analgesics. *JAMA* 256:1749, 1986.

Kojima S, Matsuyama T, Kato S, et al: Outcome of 154 patients with severe aplastic anemia who received transplants from unrelated donors: the Japan Marrow Donor Program. *Blood* 100:799, 2002.

Marsh J, Schrezenmeier H, Marin P, et al: Prospective randomized multicenter study comparing cyclosporin alone versus the combination of antithymocyte globulin and cyclosporin for treatment of patients with nonsevere aplastic anemia: a report from the European Blood and Marrow Transplant (EBMT) Severe Aplastic Anaemia Working Party. *Blood* 93:2191, 1999.

Morgan GJ, Alveres CL: Benzene and the hemopoietic stem cell. *Chem Biol Interact* 30:153, 2005.

Rosenfeld SJ, Follman D, Nunez O, et al: Antithymocyte globulin and cyclosporine for severe aplastic anemia. Association between hematologic response and long-term outcome. *JAMA* 289:1130, 2003.

Socie G, Stone JV, Wingard JR, et al: Long-term survival and late deaths after allogeneic bone marrow transplantation. Late Effects Working Committee of the International Bone Marrow Transplant Registry. *N Engl J Med* 341:14, 1999.

Tichelli A, Socie G, Marsh J, et al: Outcome of pregnancy and disease course among women with aplastic anemia treated with immunosuppression. *Ann Intern Med* 137:164, 2002.

Tisdale JF, Dunn DE, Geller N, et al: High-dose cyclophosphamide in severe aplastic anaemia: A randomised trial. *Lancet* 356:1554, 2000.

Yoshizato T, Dumitriu B, Hosokawa K, et al: Somatic mutations and clonal hematopoiesis in aplastic anemia. *N Engl J Med* 373:35–47, 2015.

Young NS, Calado R, Scheinberg P: Current concepts in the pathophysiology and treatment of aplastic anemia. *Blood* 108:2511, 2006.

REFERENCES

For the complete list of references, log on to www.expertconsult.com.

CHAPTER 31

PAROXYSMAL NOCTURNAL HEMOGLOBINURIA

Robert A. Brodsky

Paroxysmal nocturnal hemoglobinuria (PNH) is a clonal hematopoietic stem cell disorder that has fascinated hematologists for more than a century because of its protean clinical manifestations and captivating pathophysiology (MIM 300818).[1] One of the earliest descriptions of PNH was by Dr. Paul Strübing, who in 1882 described a 29-year-old cartwright who presented with fatigue, abdominal pain, and severe nocturnal paroxysms of hemoglobinuria that were exacerbated by excess alcohol, physical exertion, and iron salts. Strübing deduced that the hemolysis was occurring intravascularly as the patient's plasma turned red following severe attacks of hemoglobinuria. Decades later his prescient deduction was confirmed. Later reports by Marchiafava and Micheli[1a] led to the eponym, Marchiafava-Micheli syndrome, but it was Enneking, in 1925,[1b] who introduced the term *paroxysmal nocturnal hemoglobinuria*.

In 1937, Thomas Ham[1c] found that PNH erythrocytes were hemolyzed when incubated with normal, acidified serum. This seminal discovery resulted in the first diagnostic test for PNH, the acidified serum or Ham test. The cell lysis following acidified serum appeared to be complement dependent because heat inactivation abrogated the reaction; however, it was not until 1954, with the discovery of the alternative pathway of complement activation, that complement was formally proven to cause the hemolysis of PNH red cells. Following the emergence of specific diagnostic tests, additional disease manifestations such as venous thrombosis, bone marrow failure, and development of myelodysplastic syndromes (MDS) and acute leukemia were associated with PNH. These nonerythroid manifestations of the disease foreshadowed the discovery that PNH results from the clonal expansion of a mutated hematopoietic stem cell.

In the 1980s, roughly 100 years after Strübing's initial description of the disease, it was discovered that PNH cells display a global deficiency in a group of proteins affixed to the cell surface by a glycosylphosphatidylinositol (GPI) anchor. Interestingly, several of the missing proteins (e.g., CD55 and CD59) are important complement regulatory proteins. A few years later, the genetic mutation phosphatidylinositol-glycan complementation class A (*PIGA*) responsible for the GPI-anchor protein deficiency was discovered,[2] and most recently, a humanized monoclonal antibody that inhibits terminal complement activation has been shown to ameliorate hemolysis and disease symptoms in PNH patients.[3] Although the pathophysiology of many of PNH's clinical manifestations are now understood, the mechanism of thrombosis, the mechanism of clonal dominance, and the close association with aplastic anemia continue to be areas of intense investigation. PNH is an extremely rare condition; however, the risk for developing PNH in patients with acquired aplastic anemia is 20% to 30%. In addition, more than half of patients with acquired aplastic anemia harbor a small to moderate PNH population at diagnosis.

PATHOPHYSIOLOGY

The Glycosylphosphatidylinositol Anchor

Covalent linkage to GPI is an important means of anchoring many cell-surface glycoproteins to the cell membrane. Alkaline phosphatase was the first GPI-anchor protein recognized after it was discovered that cell surface alkaline phosphatase could be removed by a bacterial enzyme, phosphatidylinositol-specific phospholipase C (PIPLC). PIPLC cleaved the phosphate from phosphatidylinositol and left the enzyme with full activity after its release, suggesting that the protein structure was unperturbed. This fundamental observation led to the discovery of dozens of GPI-anchored proteins.

The GPI anchor consists of a highly conserved glycan core (ethanoloamine-*P*-6Manα1-2Manα1-6Manα1-4GlcN) linked to the 6-position of the D-*myo*-inositol ring of phosphatidylinositol (Fig. 31.1). The anchor is synthesized in the endoplasmic reticulum membrane and involves more than 10 reactions and more than 30 different genes. The first step in GPI anchor biosynthesis is the transfer of *N*-acetylglucosamine (GlcNAc) from uridine diphosphate-GlcNAc to phosphatidylinositol (PI) to yield GlcNAc-PI. This step is catalyzed by GlcNAc-PI α1-6 GlcNAc transferase, an enzyme whose subunits are encoded by seven different genes: *PIGA, PIGC, PIGH, GPI1, PIGY, PIGP,* and *DPM2*. In the second step, GlcNAc-PI is deacetylated by the gene product of *PIGL* to form glucosamine (GlcN)-PI. GPI anchor assembly continues in the endoplasmic reticulum with acylation of the inositol and stepwise addition of mannosyl and phosphoethanolamine residues. The preassembled GPI is linked to nascent proteins that contain a C-terminal GPI-attachment signal peptide, displacing it in a transamidase reaction. The GPI-anchored protein then transits the secretory pathway to reach its final destination at the plasma membrane in compartments known as lipid rafts. If the GPI anchor is not attached to the protein, it is degraded intracellularly, probably in lysosomes.

Given the numerous gene products involved in GPI anchor assembly, it seemed improbable that PNH would be the consequence of a single genetic mutation. However, after intense scrutiny of this pathway, it became apparent that in virtually all PNH cases, the defect can be attributed to mutations in the *PIGA* gene, whose product is essential for the first step of GPI anchor biosynthesis. Later it was determined that the *PIGA* gene is on the X chromosome and that its product is part of a complex that transfers *N*-acetylglucosamine to phosphatidylinositol to form GlcNAc-PI. Thus a single "hit" will generate a PNH phenotype because males have only one X chromosome, and in females one X chromosome is inactivated through lyonization. Conceivably a mutation in any one of the genes in this pathway would cause the disease; however, other genes involved in GPI anchor biosynthesis are located on autosomes. Inactivating mutations in these genes would have to occur on both alleles to produce the PNH phenotype. Rare cases of PNH caused by mutations other than *PIGA* have been described.[4] In one example the disease was caused by a compound heterozygous mutation in the *PIGT* gene. In addition, rare cases of congenital CD59 deficiency have been shown to produce a PNH-like phenotype. These patients have chronic hemolytic anemia and a propensity for thrombosis. In contrast to PNH, patients with germline CD59 deficiency present with a relapsing immune-mediated peripheral neuropathy. Congenital *PIGA* mutations resulting in an absence of GPI-anchored proteins are embryonic lethal; however, germline hypomorphic *PIGA* mutations have now been described.[5,6] The hypomorphic *PIGA* mutations cause a syndrome known as multiple congenital abnormalities-hypotonia-seizure syndrome 2 (MCAHS2; MIM 300868). MCAHS2 patients present with severe intellectual disability, dysmorphic facial features, seizures, and early death. Red cells from these patients tend to have little to no GPI anchor deficiency and hence no hemolysis.

Acetylcholinesterase from erythrocytes and alkaline phosphatase from leukocytes were the first GPI-anchored proteins shown to be missing in PNH. Since then, more than a dozen GPI-anchored proteins with heterogeneous expression on hematopoietic cells have been found to be missing in PNH (Table 31.1). The functions of

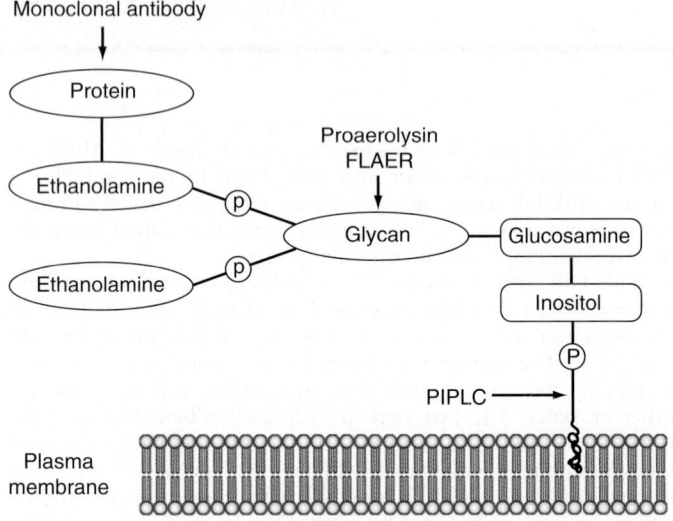

Fig. 31.1 STRUCTURE OF THE GLYCOSYLPHOSPHATIDYLINOSITOL (GPI) ANCHOR. Phosphatidylinositol is inserted into the lipid bilayer of the plasma membrane. The glycan core, which serves as the binding site for aerolysin, proaerolysin, and FLAER, consists of a molecule of *N*-glucosamine, three molecules of mannose, and a molecule of ethanolamine. The representative protein (e.g., CD55, CD59, etc.) is covalently attached through an amide bond to an ethanolamine on the terminal mannose. Individual monoclonal antibodies used for the diagnosis of PNH (e.g., CD55, CD59, etc.) bind to the protein, but not the GPI anchor. Phosphatidylinositol-specific phospholipase C (PIPLC) cleaves the phosphate from phosphatidylinositol and leaves the enzyme with full activity after its release.

these cell surface GPI-anchored proteins are manifold; they can serve as complement regulatory proteins, enzymes, blood group antigens, receptors, and adhesion molecules. Membrane inhibitor of reactive lysis (CD59) and decay accelerating factor (CD55)—both complement regulatory proteins—are the most widely expressed GPI-anchored proteins and can be found on all hematopoietic lineages including $CD34^+CD38^-$ stem/progenitor cells. Certain proteins, CD58 (LFA3) and CD16 (FcγRIII), may exist in both GPI-linked and transmembrane forms.

Phosphatidylinositol-Glycan Complementation Class A Gene

Investigators in Osaka, Japan, first identified the gene that was defective in PNH. The gene was isolated by expression cloning and named *PIGA*. *PIGA* was then cloned into an expression vector and transfected into GPI-deficient cell lines derived from PNH patients; cell surface expression of all the missing GPI-anchored proteins was restored, confirming that *PIGA* mutations are responsible for causing PNH. Since this seminal discovery, somatic mutations of the *PIGA* gene have been found in virtually all PNH patients to date. Little to no GPI anchor is made when the *PIGA* gene is mutated. Consequently, the translated protein (e.g., CD59, CD55, etc.) residing in the cisterna of the endoplasmic reticulum cannot be attached to the GPI anchor and is degraded in situ.

The human *PIGA* gene contains six exons, five introns, and extends over 17 kb (Fig. 31.2); it encodes for a protein that contains 484 amino acids (60 kDa). In humans, there is a single copy of the gene located on the short arm of the X chromosome (Xp22.1), although an intronless pseudogene has been found on chromosome 12q21. A wide range of somatic mutations interspersed throughout the entire coding region of the *PIGA* gene have been described in PNH patients. There are no true mutational "hot spots," although exon 2, which contains almost half of the coding region, is the exon where most mutations occur. Most *PIGA* mutations are small insertions or deletions, usually one or two base pairs, which result in a frameshift in the coding region and consequently a shortened, nonfunctional product. Although *PIGA* function is abolished by these

TABLE 31.1	Cell Surface GPI-Anchored Protein Absent on PNH Blood Cells	
Antigen	**Hematopoietic Lineage**	**Classification**
CD55: decay accelerating factor	All blood cells	Complement regulator
CD59: membrane inhibitor of reactive lysis	All blood cells	Complement regulator
CD58: lymphocyte function associated antigen-3	All blood cells	Adhesion molecule
Acetylcholinesterase	Red blood cells	Enzyme
CD14: monocyte differentiation antigen	Granulocytes, monocytes, macrophages	Endotoxin-binding receptor
CD16: Fcγ receptor III	Granulocytes, NK cells	Receptor
CD66b	Granulocytes	Adhesion
Neutrophil alkaline phosphatase	Granulocytes	Enzyme
CD87: urokinase (plasminogen activator) receptor	Monocytes, granulocytes	Receptor
Leukocyte alkaline phosphatase	Granulocytes	Enzyme
CDw52: Campath-1 antigen	Lymphocytes, monocytes	Unknown
CD24	B lymphocytes, granulocytes	B-cell differentiation
CD48	All leukocytes	Adhesion molecule
CD73: ecto-5′-nucleotidase	Some B and T lymphocytes	Enzyme
Dombrock-Holley/Gregory-bearing protein	Red blood cells	Blood group antigen
Folate receptor	Myeloid and erythroid cells	Receptor
CD109	Activated platelets and T cells	Unknown
CD157	Mature monocytes	Adhesion and transmigration of monocytes

GPI, Glycosylphosphatidylinositol; NK, natural killer; PNH, paroxysmal nocturnal hemoglobinuria.

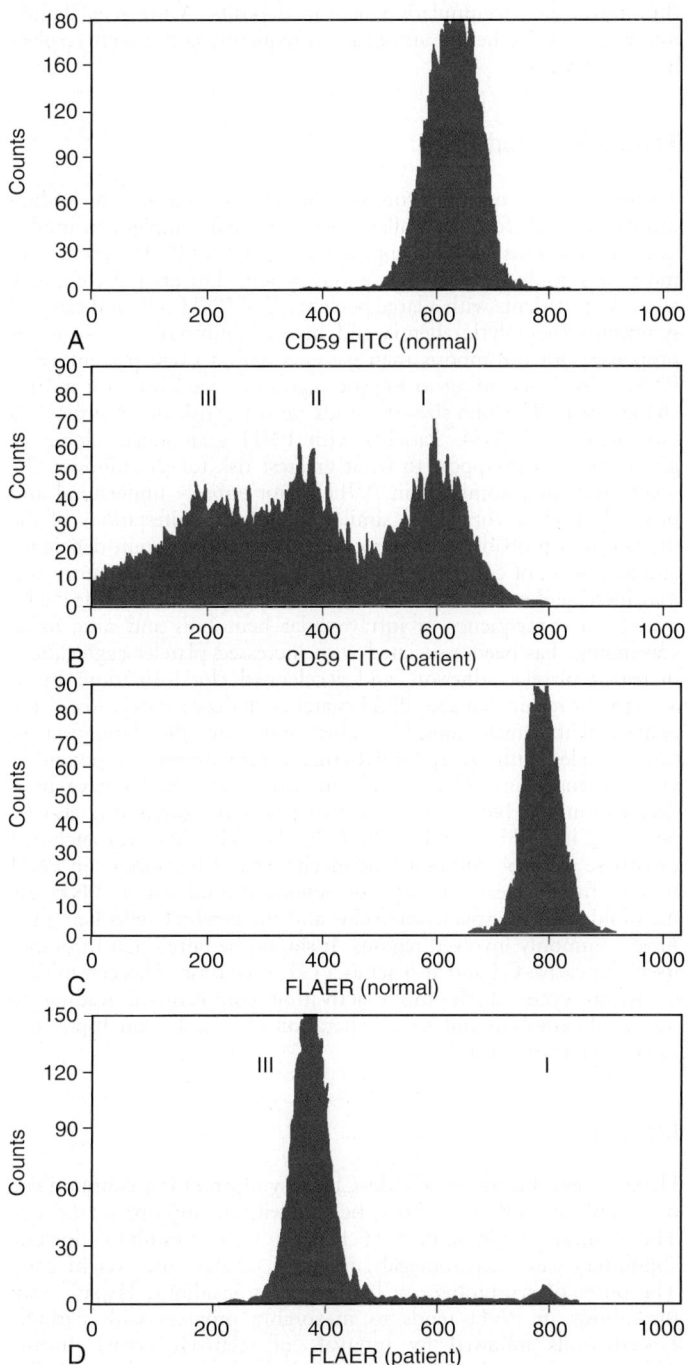

Fig. 31.2 FLOW CYTOMETRIC ANALYSIS OR PERIPHERAL BLOOD CELLS FROM A PAROXYSMAL NOCTURNAL HEMOGLOBINURIA (PNH) PATIENT. (A) Fluorescence intensity of erythrocytes from a healthy control after staining with anti-CD59. (B) Fluorescence intensity of erythrocytes from an untransfused PNH patient after staining with anti-CD59. Type II cells are "blended" between the type I (normal) and type III cells. (C) Fluorescence intensity of granulocytes from a healthy control stained with FLAER. (D) Fluorescence intensity of granulocytes from the same PNH patient as (B) following staining with FLAER. Note that the granulocytes are almost exclusively type III cells. A small population of type I granulocytes is present.

frameshift mutations, missense mutations, where the product of the mutated *PIGA* gene has some residual activity, have also been described. In most patients studied, a single (monoclonal) *PIGA* mutation has been discovered. However, two different mutations (biclonal) and in one case four separate *PIGA* mutations have been found in PNH patients.

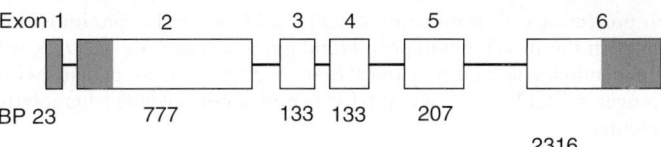

Fig. 31.3 STRUCTURE OF THE HUMAN *PIGA* GENE. Boxes represent exons; intervening lines represent introns. Shaded areas show noncoding regions.

Paroxysmal Nocturnal Hemoglobinuria Stem Cell

PNH is a clonal hematopoietic disorder. The first evidence to support the notion that PNH arises through the mutation of an abnormal multipotent hematopoietic stem cell was derived from glucose 6-phosphate dehydrogenase studies on the red cells of women with PNH.[7] Subsequently, flow cytometric analyses revealed that all hematopoietic lineages—myeloid, erythroid, and lymphoid—were involved. Furthermore, *PIGA* mutations found in granulocytes match those found in other lineages, and CD34$^+$CD38$^-$ stem/progenitor cells have been shown to be missing GPI-anchored proteins in PNH patients. Thus the "hit" in PNH clearly involves a multipotent hematopoietic stem cell. In PNH, both B cells and T cells have been shown to be derived from the malignant clone.

Paroxysmal Nocturnal Hemoglobinuria Red Cells

PNH cells can display one of three phenotypes (Fig. 31.3): cells with normal expression of GPI-anchored proteins (type I cells), cells with intermediate expression of GPI anchor proteins (type II cells), and cells with no expression of GPI anchor proteins (type III cells). These three populations are most easily seen in the erythrocyte and granulocyte populations. Patients with three discreet granulocyte populations (type I, type II, and type III cells) usually have more than one PNH clone. The type II cells are usually the consequence of a missense mutation, whereas the type III cells commonly result from frameshift mutations caused by small base-pair insertions or deletions. However, in many PNH patients the type II cells are not a distinct population, but represent a "spectrum" between the type III and type I cells (see Fig. 31.3).

CLINICAL FEATURES

Hemolytic Anemia and Hemoglobinuria

Hemolysis in PNH results from the increased susceptibility of PNH red cells to complement. Complement consists of a battery of proteins that circulate in the plasma. It is a highly integrative system that is important for host defense, clearance of injured cells, modulation of metabolic and regenerative processes, and regulation of adaptive immunity. Complement can be activated by a variety of pathways (lectin, classical, and alternative) and is tightly regulated. Imbalance between activation and regulation can result in a number of disease states. Normally, membrane proteins regulate the activation of the complement system and protect cells from the deleterious effects of activated complement. PNH red cells are more vulnerable to complement-mediated lysis because of a reduction, or complete absence, of membrane inhibitor of reactive lysis (CD59) and decay accelerating factor (CD55), both of which are GPI-anchored.

CD59 is a 19,000 molecular weight glycoprotein that blocks terminal complement by binding to C8 and C9 in the assembly of the membrane attack complex (MAC); thus interfering with C9 binding, polymerization, and pore formation. CD55, a 68,000 molecular weight glycoprotein, which functions to accelerate the rate of destruction of membrane-bound C3 convertase. Hence CD55 reduces the amount of C3 that is cleaved, and CD59 reduces the number of MAC that is formed. Of the two, CD59 is more important in protecting cells from complement. Red blood cells from individuals with the Inab phenotype, a blood group antigen, lack CD55, yet these individuals have no clinical hemolysis. In contrast, patients with congenital CD59 deficiency have complement-mediated hemolytic anemia.

The classic manifestation from which PNH derives its name—paroxysmal bouts of reddish, brownish, or "cola-colored" urine that strikes predominantly overnight—is described by a minority of PNH patients. Most PNH patients have no noticeable hemoglobinuria or have intermittent episodes of hemoglobinuria with no relation to the time of day. Early speculation that the nocturnal hemoglobinuria was a function of a mild drop in pH that occurs with sleep has not been validated. Patients with a history of hemoglobinuria are more likely to have a large PNH clone and less likely to have a markedly hypocellular bone marrow.

Although hemolysis is often the most conspicuous feature in patients with classical PNH, many patients, particularly those with coexisting bone marrow failure, exhibit mild to barely detectable hemolysis. The hemoglobin concentration can range from normal to severely depressed. The reticulocyte count is often elevated but usually lower than expected for the degree of anemia. Patients with PNH manifest all the usual clinical and laboratory signs of chronic hemolytic anemia: weakness, fatigue, pallor, and dyspnea on exertion. In patients with prominent hemolysis, the magnitude of fatigue can be out of proportion to the degree of anemia. Morphologically, the red cells appear normal, although some cases display mild to moderate poikilocytosis and anisocytosis. The haptoglobin levels are usually low, and the lactate dehydrogenase (LDH) is frequently elevated, sometimes greater than 3000 IU/L, depending on the degree of hemolysis.

Multiple factors influence the degree of hemolysis in PNH, including the size and type of the PNH clone and the degree of complement activation. In general, the percentage of PNH erythrocytes correlates with the degree of hemolysis. However, the type of PNH erythrocytes may also influence the degree of hemolysis. Type III erythrocytes are more readily lysed than type II erythrocytes and almost always constitute a larger percentage of the PNH red cells. Thus patients with a large percentage of type III erythrocytes tend to have more hemolysis than patients with a large percentage of type I or type II cells. Finally, hemolysis is frequently exacerbated by infections (especially gastrointestinal infections), surgery, strenuous exercise, excessive alcohol intake, blood transfusions, and anything else that increases complement activation.

Smooth Muscle Dystonia and Nitric Oxide

Many clinical manifestations of PNH are readily explained by hemoglobin-mediated nitric oxide scavenging.[8] Failure of complement regulation on the PNH erythrocyte membrane leads to intravascular hemolysis resulting in the release of large amounts of free hemoglobin into the plasma. Free plasma hemoglobin leads to increased consumption of nitric oxide resulting in manifestations that include fatigue, abdominal pain, esophageal spasm, erectile dysfunction, and possibly thrombosis. Indeed, hemoglobinuria, thrombosis, erectile dysfunction, and esophageal spasm are more common in patients with large PNH populations (>60% of granulocytes) than in patients with relatively small PNH populations. In a study of 49 PNH patients diagnosed using flow cytometry, Moyo et al.[10] demonstrated that large PNH clones were associated with an increased risk for thrombosis, hemoglobinuria, abdominal pain, esophageal spasm, and male impotence. Thus many of the clinical manifestations of PNH appear to be a direct consequence of intravascular hemolysis, leading to the release of free hemoglobin, scavenging of nitric oxide, and smooth muscle dystonias.

Renal Manifestations

PNH patients have a greater than sixfold increased risk of chronic kidney disease. Renal tubular damage is caused by microvascular thrombosis and accumulation of iron deposits. Acute renal failure following massive hemolysis occurs infrequently and usually resolves in days to weeks.

Thrombosis and PNH

Thrombosis is an ominous complication of PNH and was the leading cause of death before the availability of terminal complement inhibition.[9] Thrombosis occurs in approximately 40% of PNH patients and most commonly involves the venous system, but arterial clots may also occur. Patients with a large percentage of PNH cells and classical symptoms (hemolytic anemia and hemoglobinuria) have a greater propensity for thrombosis than patients with a small percentage of PNH cells.[10] According to logistic regression modeling, for a 10% change in PNH clone size, the odds ratio for risk of thrombosis is estimated to be 1.64. Patients with PNH granulocyte clones of greater than 60% appear to be at greatest risk for thrombosis. The mechanism of thrombosis in PNH is not entirely understood and probably multifactorial, but similar to other manifestations of the disease, it is probably related to the GPI anchor protein deficiency and activation of complement. Indeed, C5a is proinflammatory and may increase the risk for thrombosis. Furthermore, nitric oxide depletion (as a consequence of intravascular hemolysis and nitic oxide scavenging) has been associated with increased platelet aggregation, increased platelet adhesion, and accelerated clot formation. In an attempt to repair damage, PNH platelets undergo exocytosis of the complement attack complex. This results in the formation of microvesicles with phosphatidylserine externalization, a potent in vitro procoagulant. These prothrombotic microvesicles have been detected in the blood of PNH patients. Fibrinolysis can also be perturbed in PNH given that PNH blood cells lack the GPI-anchored urokinase receptor. Although the mechanism of thrombosis in PNH is not entirely clear, the sites of venous thrombosis in PNH are manifold with the splanchnic veins and the cerebral veins being the most commonly involved regions. It should be noted that thrombin itself can cleave C3 and also act as a C5 convertase. This can initiate a viscous cycle of thrombin activating complement, leading to increased hemolysis and more generation of C5a that predisposes to even more thrombosis.

Liver

Hepatic vein thrombosis (Budd-Chiari syndrome) is a common site of thrombosis in PNH and may be fatal without appropriate therapy. The clinical manifestations of hepatic vein thrombosis include abdominal pain, hepatomegaly, jaundice, ascites, and weight gain. The onset of symptoms can be abrupt or insidious. Hepatic vein thrombosis in PNH tends to inexorably progress with periodic exacerbations followed by intervals of relatively stable disease. Although some patients live many years with the condition, it frequently results in death unless complement inhibition or bone marrow transplantation is initiated. The best noninvasive tests to confirm the diagnosis include computed tomography scanning, magnetic resonance imaging, and ultrasonography. Thrombosis can involve the small hepatic veins, large-sized hepatic veins, or both. Thrombolytic therapy has been used successfully to restore venous patency and reverse the hepatic congestion; however, because of the potential danger of this approach, it should be used judiciously. Patients with acute onset disease, preserved platelet counts (>50,000 cells/mm³), and large vessel involvement are the best candidates for thrombolysis. For patients with massive ascites who are not suitable candidates for thrombolytic therapy, transjugular intrahepatic portalsystemic shunting or surgical shunting can successfully palliate some patients. Orthotopic liver transplantation was once considered contraindicated in PNH, but now that the thrombotic risk can be mitigated using complement inhibition, this is no longer true. Long-term survival following liver transplantation and eculizumab administration has been reported.

Portal vein thrombosis is also common in PNH and can occur with or without hepatic vein thrombosis. Patients frequently present with nausea, vomiting, abdominal pain, and liver dysfunction. Management is similar to that of hepatic vein thrombosis.

Other Abdominal Veins

Venous thrombosis in PNH has been described in all abdominal and retroperitoneal venous systems including the splenic veins, mesenteric veins, renal veins, and the inferior vena cava. Thrombosis of minor veins can also occur and can be difficult to diagnose because of the protean manifestations and their relapsing and remitting nature. Often such patients present with recurrent, severe abdominal pain crises sometimes mimicking intestinal obstruction. The consequence of these microthromboses can sometimes be visualized with esophagogastroduodenal endoscopy or colonoscopy. Patients with intestinal thromboses can present with ischemic colitis and can be misdiagnosed as having Crohn disease. Upper gastrointestinal bleeding can be caused by esophageal or gastric varices that develop as a consequence of portal hypertension or splenic vein thrombosis.

Cerebral Veins

Cerebral veins, particularly the sagittal veins and sinuses, are also highly prone to thrombosis in PNH. Patients can present with severe headaches and/or focal neurologic deficits depending on the location of the thrombosis. Similar to hepatic vein thrombosis, cerebral vein thrombosis is an ominous complication that can result in substantial morbidity and mortality. Magnetic resonance imaging to carefully examine the cerebral blood flow is helpful in establishing the diagnosis.

Other Sites

Dermal venous thrombosis can occur virtually anywhere on the body. Patients usually complain of pain, discolorations, and swelling. The lesions can reach several centimeters in diameter and are firm and tender. Necrosis and the formation of a black eschar can occur. Anticoagulation and warm compresses can ameliorate the attacks. Pulmonary emboli and deep venous thrombosis have also been reported in PNH; arterial thrombosis is less common.

CLONALITY AND BONE MARROW FAILURE

PIGA Mutations in Aplastic Anemia and Myelodysplastic Syndrome and Healthy Controls

Small to moderate PNH clones are found in up to 70% of patients with acquired aplastic anemia, demonstrating a pathophysiologic link between these disorders. Typically, less than 20% GPI anchor protein-deficient granulocytes are detected in aplastic anemia patients at diagnosis, but occasional patients can have larger clones. DNA sequencing of the GPI anchor protein-deficient cells from aplastic anemia patients reveals clonal *PIGA* gene mutations that arise from a multipotent hematopoietic stem cell. Moreover, many of these patients exhibit expansion of the *PIGA* mutant clone and progress to clinical PNH. Although it was once thought that PNH evolving from aplastic anemia is more benign than classical PNH, this observation is probably a consequence of lead time bias, as many of these patients eventually develop classical PNH symptoms.

Somatic *PIGA* mutations arising from hematopoietic cells can be found at low frequency (~1 in 50,000 granulocytes) in healthy control subjects. These mutations arise from hematopoietic progenitor cells. Since normal and *PIGA* mutant progenitor cells do not self-renew and only survive for 3 to 4 months, these cells cannot contribute to

disease. PNH granulocytes (0.01–5%) can also be found in up to 25% of patients with MDS; however, unlike acquired aplastic anemia, it is extremely rare for PNH to evolve from MDS patients. These small PNH populations in MDS appear to be clinically irrelevant since the *PIGA* mutations in MDS are transient and also arise from progenitor rather than hematopoietic stem cells.[11] In contrast, *PIGA* mutations in PNH patients and patients with acquired aplastic anemia arise from a multipotent hematopoietic stem cell and are found in all lineages, including T lymphocytes.

Distinguishing hypoplastic MDS from aplastic anemia is often difficult; however, quantitative analysis of bone marrow CD34 positive cells is useful for discriminating between these two entities.

The PNH Stem Cell and Clonal Expansion

To cause PNH, *PIGA* mutations must occur in a self-renewing, hematopoietic stem cell and must achieve clonal dominance. The mechanisms leading to the clonal expansion and dominance of PNH stem cells remain a topic of continued investigation. Any hypothesis must also account for the close pathophysiologic relationship between PNH and acquired aplastic anemia, a T-cell–mediated autoimmune disease characterized by depletion of hematopoietic stem cells. The leading hypothesis is that PNH stem cells have a conditional survival advantage in the setting of an autoimmune attack (e.g., aplastic anemia) that targets the bone marrow. One hypothesis involves natural-killer group 2 member D (NKG2D)-mediated immunity that is activated by the expression of ligands such as major histocompatibility complex class I chain-related peptides A and B (MICA/B) and cytomegalovirus UL-16 binding proteins (ULBPs).[12] MICA/B are transmembrane proteins but the ULBPs are GPI-linked. NKG2D is a common receptor for MICA/B and the ULBPs. It is expressed on natural killer (NK) cells and CD8+ cytotoxic T cells. Engagement of NKG2D with its ligands (MICA/B and ULBPs) promotes cell death of the NKG2D ligand-expressing cells by the NKG2D+ effectors; thus PNH cells would be relatively spared from effector cell-mediated killing because they lack GPI-anchored ULBPs. Recently, it has been proposed that CD1d-restricted, GPI-specific T cells might be responsible for the immune killing in PNH. Under this scenario, PNH cells would be spared immune-mediated killing because CD1d has been shown to associate with GPI. Others have shown that mutations that confer a survival advantage to the PNH clone can contribute to clonal outgrowth.

Clinical observations also provide clues to understanding clonal dominance in PNH and the relationship between aplastic anemia and PNH. Up to 30% of aplastic anemia patients treated with conventional immunosuppressive therapy (antithymocyte globulin and cyclosporine) will develop PNH or MDS, usually several years after therapy. In contrast, allogeneic bone marrow transplantation appears to eliminate the risk for developing PNH in patients with aplastic anemia. These data suggest that secondary clonal disorders (PNH and MDS) are part of the natural history of aplastic anemia. Although immunosuppressive therapy prolongs survival, it does not prevent these late complications.

Clonal Transformation

PNH patients, similar to aplastic anemia and MDS patients, are at increased risk for clonal transformation; however, the incidence of leukemic transformation in PNH is small, probably less than 5%. MDS and acute myeloid leukemia are the most common malignancies to evolve from PNH; the leukemic cells may arise from the GPI anchor-deficient clone in many, but not all cases.

NATURAL HISTORY

The natural history of PNH before the era of anticomplement therapy ranged from indolent to severely debilitating and life-threatening.[13,14] The ability to pharmacologically interfere with terminal complement appears to have altered the natural history of the disease by markedly decreasing the thrombosis rate.[15,16] With appropriate therapy, the natural history of classical PNH is probably no different from age-matched controls. Females and males are equally affected with the median age of diagnosis being 40 years. Without therapy, the median survival from time of diagnosis is 10 to 20 years. Thrombosis, severe pancytopenia, evolution to MDS or leukemia, older age, and thrombocytopenia at diagnosis portend a poor prognosis. Older literature, where patients were diagnosed with PNH based on the Ham test or sucrose hemolysis test, reported the occurrence of spontaneous long-term remissions in up to 10% of PNH cases; however, in patients diagnosed by flow cytometry, the spontaneous remission rate is much less common.

LABORATORY EVALUATION

Blood

Peripheral blood counts in PNH patients vary from severe pancytopenia to nearly normal. Virtually all patients will present with anemia, frequently with mild macrocytosis. Thrombocytopenia and/or neutropenia are also common. A mild to moderate reticulocytosis is usually present in patients with the classical form of the disease; however, in patients with hypoplastic PNH (also referred to as *aplastic anemia/PNH overlap*), the reticulocyte count can be low for the degree of anemia. Similarly, in patients with hypoplastic PNH, the biochemical profile can be normal, but in patients with large PNH clones the indirect bilirubin and LDH are significantly elevated. In patients with vigorous hemolysis, it is not uncommon for the laboratory to report the specimen as "hemolyzed."

Bone Marrow

Bone marrow cellularity can be hypocellular, normocellular, or hypercellular. In patients with classical PNH (not arising from or coinciding with aplastic anemia), the marrow is usually normocellular to hypercellular with erythroid hyperplasia. Mild to moderate dyserythropoiesis is common. Stainable iron is frequently absent because of iron loss associated with the intravascular hemolysis. Cytogenetic abnormalities can be found in a small number of patients.

DIAGNOSIS

Complement-Based Assays

The Ham test and the sucrose hemolysis test (sugar water test) were two of the first assays used to diagnose PNH. Both assays are performed on erythrocytes and discriminate PNH cells from normal cells based on a differential sensitivity to the hemolytic action of complement. In the Ham test, the alternative pathway of complement is activated by acidification of the serum. This results in lysis of PNH erythrocytes but not normal erythrocytes. The Ham test is relatively specific for PNH, but is not very sensitive.

Complement is also activated in a low-ionic-strength sucrose-containing medium. Preferential lysis of PNH erythrocytes through the activation of complement in this sucrose-containing medium forms the basis of the sugar water test. This assay is easier to perform and is more sensitive than the Ham test but not as specific; other hemolytic anemias and even leukemias can produce false positive results. The complement lysis assay in which complement is activated with antibody will also detect PNH erythrocytes. These complement-based red cell assays are important from a historical perspective, but should no longer be used to establish the diagnosis of PNH.

GPI Anchor–Based Assays

Most laboratories use monoclonal antibodies against specific GPI-anchored proteins in conjunction with flow cytometry to diagnose PNH. Anti-CD59 is most commonly used because it is widely expressed and is displayed on all hematopoietic lineages. Anti-CD55, anti-CD14, anti-CD16, anti-CD67, and a variety of other monoclonal antibodies can also be used to establish the diagnosis. Flow cytometry offers several advantages over complement-based assays for diagnosing PNH: it measures the size of the PNH clone in the various cell lineages, it is more sensitive and specific, and it is less affected by blood transfusions. It is noteworthy that rare congenital deficiencies of CD59 and CD55 can lead to a false positive test for PNH if only one monoclonal antibody is used. This, coupled with the variable expression of GPI-anchored proteins on different hematopoietic lineages, accounts for the recommendation that at least two different monoclonal antibodies, directed against two different GPI-anchored proteins, on at least two different cell lineages, should be used to diagnose a patient with PNH. Solely screening patients' red cells for PNH can lead to false negative tests, especially in the setting of a recent hemolytic episode or a recent blood transfusion. Granulocytes and monocytes have a short half-life and are not affected by blood transfusions; the percentage of PNH cells in these lineages best reflects the size of the PNH stem cell pool.

Aerolysin Assays

A fluorescein-labeled proaerolysin variant, FLAER, is commonly used in conjunction with monoclonal antibodies in a flow cytometric assay to diagnose PNH.[17,18] Aerolysin is the principal virulence factor of the bacterium *Aeromonas hydrophila*. It is secreted as an inert protoxin termed proaerolysin, which binds selectively and with high affinity to the GPI anchor. After binding to its receptor (the glycan portion of the GPI anchor), the C-terminal peptide of proaerolysin is cleaved by cell proteases. This activates the toxin and leads to the formation of heptameric channels that insert into the membrane and kill the cell. PNH cells are resistant to aerolysin and proaerolysin because PNH cells lack GPI-anchored proteins. FLAER binds to the GPI anchor without forming channels and gives a more accurate assessment of the GPI-anchor deficit in PNH than anti-CD59. Because the GPI anchor is the major determinant for binding FLAER, it allows for the direct assessment of GPI anchor expression on virtually all cell lineages. Red cells are a notable exception; this may be because both normal and PNH red cells express large amounts of glycophorin, a protein shown to bind aerolysin weakly. Nevertheless, in mononuclear cells FLAER eliminates the need for multiple lineage-specific monoclonal antibodies. These properties make FLAER more reliable for detecting the small PNH populations often found in patients with aplastic anemia.

THERAPY

The major indications for therapy in PNH are thrombosis, transfusion-dependent anemia, severe pancytopenia, disabling fatigue, and debilitating smooth muscle dystonia. The choice of therapy depends on the underlying cause of these manifestations. If the symptoms are from complement-mediated hemolysis or includes thrombosis, terminal complement inhibition with eculizumab is indicated; if the symptoms are mainly from underlying bone marrow dysfunction, immunosuppressive therapy or bone marrow transplant should be considered. Some PNH patients can be managed conservatively with watchful waiting.

Immunosuppressive Therapy

PNH patients with a hypocellular bone marrow, low reticulocyte count, and pancytopenia (hypoplastic PNH) will frequently respond to immunosuppressive therapy. The response rate in this group is more than 50%. In fact, finding a minor population of PNH-like cells in severe aplastic anemia may predict for response to immunosuppressive therapy. The impaired hematopoiesis that occurs in hypoplastic PNH may respond to antithymocyte globulin and/or cyclosporine, but the PNH clone is usually not eradicated. Expansion of the PNH clone ultimately leading to classical PNH may occur several months to years after treatment with immunosuppression; thus patients should be monitored for signs and symptoms of PNH. Immunosuppressive therapy does not benefit patients with classical PNH.

Management of Anemia

The cause of anemia in PNH is often multifactorial. In patients with hypoplastic PNH, bone marrow failure is the major etiologic factor for anemia. Patients with hypoplastic PNH may respond to immunosuppressive therapy. However, in patients with cellular bone marrow, elevated reticulocyte counts, and a high LDH (classical PNH), intravascular hemolysis is the major mechanism of anemia. Terminal complement inhibition is highly effective for decreasing intravascular hemolysis. Iron deficiency caused by intravascular hemolysis can also contribute to the anemia of PNH; thus, in patients with absent iron stores, iron replacement therapy is indicated. Folic acid supplementation is also recommended in PNH because of the high red cell turnover. Erythropoietin is rarely beneficial in PNH. Often red cell transfusions are required to treat severe anemia. PNH patients should receive group-specific blood and blood products. Washing the red cells with saline, once advocated to minimize hemolysis after transfusion in PNH, is unnecessary.

Eculizumab

Eculizumab is a humanized monoclonal antibody against C5 that inhibits terminal complement activation (Fig. 31.4). Because C5 is common to all pathways of complement activation, blockade aborts progression of the cascade regardless of the stimuli. Moreover, prevention of C5 cleavage blocks the generation of the potent proinflammatory and cell lytic molecules C5a and C5b, respectively (see Fig. 31.4). Importantly, C5 blockade preserves the critical immunoprotective and immunoregulatory functions of upstream components that culminate in C3b-mediated opsonization and immune complex clearance. In 2007, the U.S. Food and Drug Administration approved eculizumab for use in PNH based upon its efficacy in two phase III clinical trials.[19,20] Eculizumab is highly effective in reducing intravascular hemolysis in PNH; it does not stop extravascular hemolysis and it does not treat bone marrow failure. Thus eculizumab is most effective in patients with classical PNH. Treatment with eculizumab decreases or eliminates the need for blood transfusions in most patients, improves quality of life, and reduces the risk of thrombosis.[21] Two weeks before starting therapy, all patients should be vaccinated against *Neisseria meningitides* because inhibition of complement at C5 increases the risk for developing infections with encapsulated organisms, particularly *N. meningitides* and *Neisseria gonorrhoeae*. Eculizumab is administered intravenously at a dose of 600 mg weekly for the first 4 weeks. On week 5, the dose is increased to 900 mg IV and thereafter the drug is dosed at 900 mg IV every 14 ± 2 days. Rare patients will break through at this dosage and require a higher dose of eculizumab. Eculizumab is generally safe and well-tolerated, but must be continued indefinitely since it does not treat the underlying cause of the disease. The most common side effect, headache, occurs in roughly 50% of patients, after the first dose or two, but rarely occurs thereafter. Neisserial sepsis is the most serious complication of eculizumab therapy; thus it is imperative to remind patients that they have a 0.5% yearly risk of acquiring neisserial sepsis even after vaccination. Moreover, patients should be revaccinated against *N. meningitides* every 3 to 5 years after starting eculizumab.

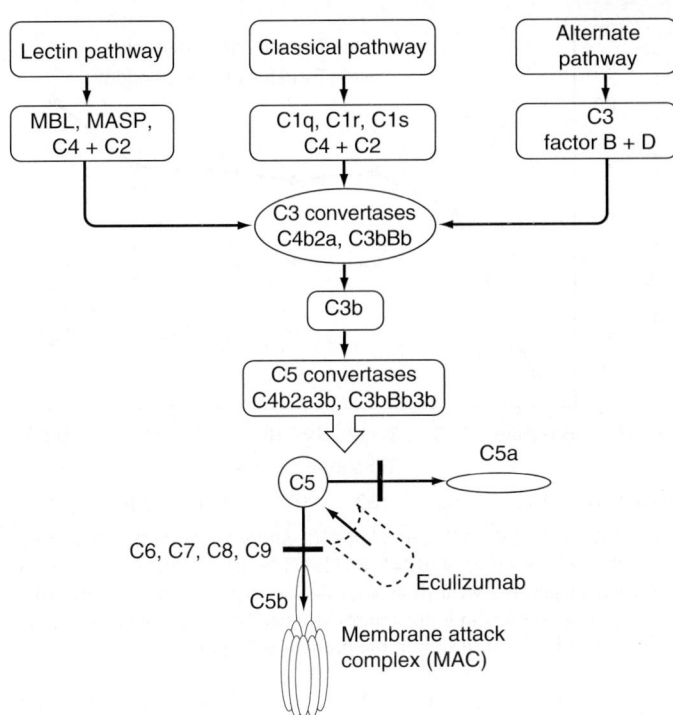

Fig. 31.4 OVERVIEW OF THE COMPLEMENT CASCADE. Classic, alternative, and lectin pathways converge at the point of C3 activation. The lytic pathway is initiated with the formation of C5 convertase and leads to the assembly of the C5, C6, C7, C8, (*n*) C9 MAC. Eculizumab is a monoclonal antibody that binds to C5, thereby preventing the formation of C5a and C5b. C5b is the initiating component of the MAC. *FITC,* Fluorescein isothiocyanate; *MASP,* mannan-binding lectin associated service protease; *MBL,* mannose binding lectin.

Indications for Therapy

Not all patients with a diagnosis of PNH require eculizumab therapy. The best candidates for treatment are those with a large PNH clone associated with disabling fatigue, thromboses, transfusion dependence, frequent pain paroxysms, renal insufficiency, or other end organ complications from disease. Watchful waiting is appropriate for asymptomatic patients or for those with mild symptoms. In patients with hypoplastic PNH, therapy should be directed toward the underlying bone marrow failure with careful monitoring of the PNH clone using flow cytometry. Patients who meet criteria for severe aplastic anemia should be managed with either allogeneic bone marrow transplantation (BMT) or immunosuppressive therapy depending upon the age of the patient and the availability of a suitable donor.

Monitoring Patients on Eculizumab

Most patients notice symptomatic improvement within hours to days after the first dose of eculizumab. Patients should be monitored with a complete blood count, reticulocyte count, LDH and biochemical profile weekly for the first 4 weeks and then monthly thereafter. The LDH usually returns to normal or near normal within days to weeks after starting eculizumab; however, the reticulocyte count usually remains elevated and the hemoglobin response is highly variable. The reticulocyte count often remains elevated because most PNH patients on eculizumab continue to have extravascular hemolysis. Erythrocytes of PNH patients on eculizumab have increased deposition of C3dg caused by CD55 deficiency and these cells are prematurely removed by the reticuloendothelial system. The hemoglobin response is largely dependent

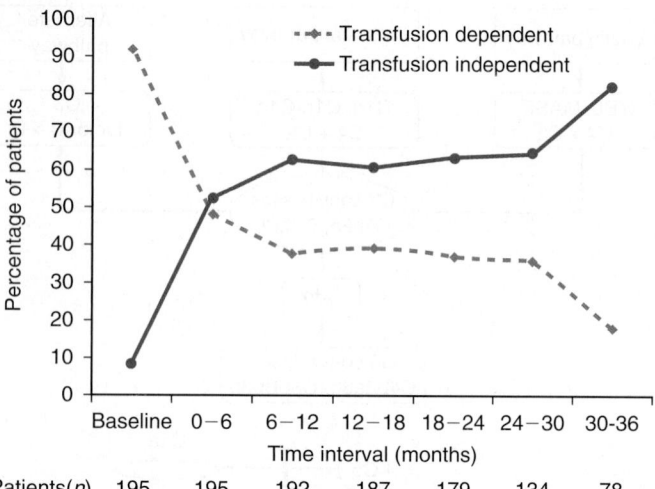

Patients(n) 195 195 192 187 179 134 78

Fig. 31.5 PERCENTAGE OF TRANSFUSION-INDEPENDENT AND TRANSFUSION-DEPENDENT PATIENTS OVER TIME. Transfusion-independent patients were those who did not require a blood transfusion during the previous 6 months; transfusion-dependent patients had received at least one blood transfusion in the previous 6 months.

upon the degree of extravascular hemolysis and the amount of underlying bone marrow failure. In classical PNH patients who are transfusion dependent, a marked decrease in red cell transfusions is observed in virtually all patients, with over 65% achieving transfusion independence (Fig. 31.5). Breakthrough intravascular hemolysis and a return of PNH symptoms occurs in less than 5% of PNH patients treated with eculizumab. This typically occurs a day or two before the next scheduled dose and is accompanied by a spike in the LDH level. If this occurs on a regular basis, the interval between dosing can be shortened to 12 or 13 days or the dose of eculizumab can be increased to 1200 mg every 14 days. It is also important to recognize that increased complement activation that accompanies infections (e.g., influenza or viral gastroenteritis) or trauma can also result in transient breakthrough hemolysis.[22] These single episodes of breakthrough hemolysis do not require a change in dosing. Patients with continued anemia, a normal or near normal LDH, and a robust reticulocyte count are likely to be having substantial extravascular hemolysis. In this setting, a direct antiglobulin test will likely be positive for complement and negative for IgG.

Pharmacogenetics has also been shown to influence response to therapy. Polymorphisms in the complement receptor 1 (*CR1*) gene are associated with response to eculizumab. CR1, through binding C3b and C4b, enhances the decay of the C3 and C5 convertases.[23] The density of CR1 on the surface of red cells modulates binding of C3 fragments to the GPI-negative red cells when C5 is inhibited. PNH patients with polymorphisms in *CR1* that lead to low CR1 levels (L/L genotype) are more likely to be suboptimal responders to eculizumab than patients with intermediate (H/L genotype) or high (H/H genotype) levels of CR1. Missense mutations in C5 (c.2654→A) prevent binding and therefore lead to failure to respond to eculizumab. This rare polymorphism is found in 3.5% of the Japanese population.[24]

Thrombosis

Thrombosis is the most feared complication of PNH and is an indication for eculizumab and anticoagulation.[9] In patients with acute-onset abdominal vein thrombosis, thrombolytic therapy has been successfully used. However, in some patients, thrombolytic therapy and/or anticoagulation is relatively contraindicated because

of severe thrombocytopenia. Terminal complement blockade appears to be the most effective way to prevent further thrombotic events and in many patients may allow for the discontinuation of anticoagulation. Pregnancy, surgery, or the use of oral contraceptives can increase the risk for thrombosis in PNH and should be considered high risk.

Stem Cell Transplantation

Allogeneic stem cell transplantation (ASCT) is the only curative therapy for PNH, but is associated with significant morbidity and mortality.[25] The International Bone Marrow Transplant Registry (IBMTR) reported a two-year survival probability of 56% in 48 recipients of HLA-identical sibling transplants between 1978 and 1995. The median age was 28 years. The majority of the deaths in this study occurred within one year of transplantation. One of seven recipients of alternative donor allogeneic transplants reported to the IBMTR during this period was alive 5 years after transplant. The European Blood and Marrow Transplant group reported a 5-year survival rate of 70% following allogeneic BMT for PNH; however, only 54% met criteria for classical PNH. The median age in the study was 30 years. Graft failure occurred in 6% of patients and acute and chronic graft-versus-host disease (GVHD) occurred in 15% and 20% of patients, respectively.

More recently, the Gruppo Italiano Trapianto Midollo Osseo published a retrospective study of 26 patients (median age, 32 years) who received an ASCT for PNH (4 AA/PNH) in Italy between 1988 and 2006. HLA-matched sibling donors were used as a stem cell source for 22 patients; there was one patient who received stem cells from a matched unrelated donor and three who received stem cells from mismatched donors (2 related and 1 unrelated). A myeloablative conditioning regimen (busulfan + cyclophosphamide) was used for 15 of the patients. The remaining 11 received a variety of different reduced-intensity conditioning regimens, most being cyclophosphamide- or fludarabine-based. GVHD prophylaxis was highly variable, but largely cyclosporine-based. The 10-year probability of survival was 57% for all patients, with a median follow-up of 131 months. There was one primary graft failure in a patient receiving a myeloablative conditioning regimen and secondary graft failure in a patient who received a nonmyeloablative ASCT; both patients eventually died from complications of a second ASCT. Acute GVHD (aGVHD) greater than stage 2 occurred in 3 of the 26 patients; chronic GVHD (cGVHD) occurred in 10 of 20 evaluable patients with four (16%) experiencing extensive cGVHD. The transplant related mortality at one year was 26% in patients receiving a myeloablative conditioning regimen and 63% in the group that received a nonmyeloablative regimen; however, this was likely because of the fact that all three patients in the nonmyeloablative group received an ASCT from a nonidentical donor. There was just one patient in the myeloablative group who received an ASCT from an unrelated or mismatched donor.

In summary, ASCT should not be offered as initial therapy for most patients with classical PNH given the morbidity and mortality. Exceptions are PNH patients in countries where eculizumab is not available or patients who do not have a good response to eculizumab therapy. Patients with hypoplastic PNH and life-threatening cytopenias continue to be reasonable candidates for ASCT. A myeloablative conditioning regimen is not required to eradicate the PNH clone. Allogeneic ASCT following nonmyeloablative conditioning regimen can cure PNH. Whether or not there is an advantage to one approach over the other will require further study; however, nonmyeloablative regimens may be preferable in young patients seeking to maintain fertility or patients with moderate organ dysfunction who may not tolerate a myeloablative regimen. Lastly, since ASCT is the only curative therapy available for PNH, continued use and investigation of this approach in selected patients is reasonable. Recent advances in mitigating GVHD such as posttransplant high-dose cyclophosphamide may particularly be effective in PNH, but further studies are required.[26]

PNH has an estimated incidence of 2 to 5 per million in the United States. This, coupled with its protean manifestations, make diagnosing PNH a challenge for even the most astute diagnostician. However, given the ease and specificity of modern diagnostic assays, the most important attribute a physician can possess in diagnosing PNH is to maintain a high level of suspicion and to be cognizant of the various presentations of the disease. A small sample of peripheral blood sent to an experienced flow cytometric laboratory is usually sufficient to establish or exclude the diagnosis of PNH. These assays are fast, reliable, and inexpensive. If monoclonal antibodies are used to establish the diagnosis, it is imperative that two or more antibodies be used on at least two different lineages. Assaying granulocytes is the most reliable method to diagnose PNH as they are not affected by blood transfusions. I prefer to use FLAER in conjunction with monoclonal antibodies on granulocytes and monocytes because of the improved sensitivity and specificity; anti-CD59 is the most reliable marker on erythrocytes. PNH populations less than 1% are not usually relevant, but if present on multiple lineages in the setting of a hypocellular bone marrow may help to establish an immune-mediated form of aplastic anemia.

Classical PNH is usually more conspicuous than hypoplastic PNH. Patients typically present with a direct antiglobulin negative hemolytic anemia, hemoglobinuria, and mild to moderate cytopenias. Obscure paroxysms of back pain, abdominal pain, fatigue, and/or headaches are often present. The bone marrow is typically normocellular to mildly hypercellular with intense erythroid hyperplasia and mild to moderate dyserythropoiesis. Bone marrow iron stores are frequently, but not always, absent. PNH patients can also present with abrupt, severe abdominal pain and jaundice caused by thrombosis. All patients presenting with unexplained hepatic vein, portal vein, mesenteric vein, or portal vein thrombosis should be screened for PNH.

It is important to distinguish PNH from MDS. Most patients with refractory anemia should be screened for PNH, especially those with moderate to severe cytopenias, an elevated LDH, and a hypocellular bone marrow. In addition, all patients diagnosed with aplastic anemia should be screened for PNH. As few as 3% of PNH erythrocytes may result in an elevated LDH. In rare instances myelofibrosis or autoimmune hemolytic anemias can mimic PNH. Patients with a history of aplastic anemia—especially those managed with immunosuppressive therapy—should be monitored closely for the outgrowth of PNH.

APPROACH TO TREATMENT

It useful to classify PNH patients as either "classical" or "hypoplastic". This can usually be accomplished by ordering a complete blood count, reticulocyte count, LDH, peripheral blood flow cytometry for PNH, and a bone marrow aspirate, biopsy, and cytogenetics. Patients with classical PNH tend to have mild to moderate cytopenias, a normocellular to hypercellular bone marrow, an elevated reticulocyte count, a markedly elevated LDH, and a relatively large PNH granulocyte population (>30%). In contrast, hypoplastic PNH patients present with manifestations similar to that of aplastic anemia or hypoplastic MDS. These patients typically present with moderate to severe cytopenias, a hypocellular bone marrow (<25% cellularity), a decreased corrected reticulocyte count, a normal or mildly elevated LDH, and a relatively small (<20%) PNH granulocyte population. Most, but not all, patients can be readily subdivided into classical versus hypoplastic PNH, a distinction that aids with therapeutic decisions.

Hypoplastic PNH

Because bone marrow failure is the major risk for patients with hypoplastic PNH, therapy is directed towards the pancytopenia. If, in addition to the PNH, the patient fulfills criteria for severe aplastic anemia (see Chapter 30), appropriate therapeutic options include allogeneic bone marrow transplantation, high-dose cyclophosphamide,

or antithymocyte globulin and cyclosporine. Young patients (i.e., <30 years of age) with an HLA-matched sibling should be transplanted; for older patients and for those without an HLA-matched sibling, high-dose cyclophosphamide or antithymocyte and cyclosporine is appropriate. Alternative donor transplants with posttransplant immunosuppression is showing promising results, but more experience with this approach in severe aplastic anemia is needed before this can be recommended as initial therapy. If the patient's cytopenias do not fulfill criteria for severe aplastic anemia, supportive care or a trial of immunosuppressive therapy is appropriate.

Classical PNH

Symptoms in patients with classical PNH vary from mild to severely debilitating to acutely life-threatening. Hence therapy should be directed toward the specific manifestations (e.g., anemia, thrombosis, etc.). Allogeneic stem cell transplantation, preferably from an HLA-matched sibling, is appropriate for patients with debilitating or life-threatening disease. In general, these are patients with recurrent thrombosis or those with clonal evolution to either MDS or acute leukemia. Patients with less severe disease should not be transplanted because of the morbidity and mortality of the procedure. Antithymocyte globulin and cyclosporine or high-dose cyclophosphamide does not appear to benefit patients with classical PNH.

Anemia

All patients with classical PNH should be placed on folic acid (1–2 mg/d). Patients with absent iron stores, usually because of chronic intravascular hemolysis, should be treated with oral iron supplementation. Eculizumab has become the standard-of-care to treat selected patients with classical PNH. It is the only drug demonstrated in a randomized study to benefit PNH patients. Eculizumab has been shown to decrease the need for transfusions, decrease paroxysms, and improve quality of life in patients with classical PNH; however, it has not been shown to benefit patients with hypoplastic PNH. In classical PNH, eculizumab is recommended for patients with disabling fatigue, thromboses, transfusion dependence, frequent pain paroxysms, renal insufficiency, or other end organ complications from disease. Watchful waiting is appropriate for asymptomatic patients or those with mild symptoms.

Thrombosis

Patients who present with acute life-threatening or organ-threatening thrombosis should be considered for thrombolytic therapy followed by long-term anticoagulation. Thrombosis is probably the most compelling reason to start eculizumab in PNH patients. Whether or not anticoagulation can be safely discontinued after eculizumab induction is still unknown, but patients who respond well to eculizumab therapy may not need long-term anticoagulation.

REFERENCES

1. Brodsky RA: Paroxysmal nocturnal hemoglobinuria. *Blood* 124(18):2804–2811, 2014.
1a. Marchiafava E: Anemia emolitica con emosiderninuria perpetua. *Policlinico* [Med] 35:105–117, 1928 (in Italian).
1b. Enneking J: Eine neue form intermittierender haemoglobinurie (Haemoglobinurie paraoxusmalis nocturia). *Klin Wochenschr* 7:2045, 1928.
1c. Ham T: Chronic hemolytic anemia with paroxysmal nocturnal hemoglobinuria. A study of the mechanism of hemolysisin relation to acid-based equilibrium. *N Eng J Med* 217:915–917, 1937.
2. Takeda J, Miyata T, Kawagoe K, et al: Deficiency of the GPI anchor caused by a somatic mutation of the PIG-A gene in paroxysmal nocturnal hemoglobinuria. *Cell* 73:703–711, 1993.

3. Rother RP, Rollins SA, Mojcik CF, et al: Discovery and development of the complement inhibitor eculizumab for the treatment of paroxysmal nocturnal hemoglobinuria. *Nat Biotechnol* 25(11):1256–1264, 2007.

4. Krawitz PM, Hochsmann B, Murakami Y, et al: A case of paroxysmal nocturnal hemoglobinuria caused by a germline mutation and a somatic mutation in PIGT. *Blood* 122(7):1312–1315, 2013.

5. Johnston JJ, Gropman AL, Sapp JC, et al: The phenotype of a germline mutation in PIGA: the gene somatically mutated in paroxysmal nocturnal hemoglobinuria. *Am J Hum Genet* 90(2):295–300, 2012.

6. Belet S, Fieremans N, Yuan X, et al: Early frameshift mutation in PIGA identified in a large XLID family without neonatal lethality. *Hum Mutat* 35(3):350–355, 2014.

7. Oni SB, Osunkoya BO, Luzzatto L: Paroxysmal nocturnal hemoglobinuria: evidence for monoclonal origin of abnormal red cells. *Blood* 36(2):145–152, 1970.

8. Rother RP, Bell L, Hillmen P, et al: The clinical sequelae of intravascular hemolysis and extracellular plasma hemoglobin: a novel mechanism of human disease. *JAMA* 293(13):1653–1662, 2005.

9. Hill A, Kelly RJ, Hillmen P: Thrombosis in paroxysmal nocturnal hemoglobinuria. *Blood* 121(25):4985–4996, quiz 5105, 2013.

10. Moyo VM, Mukhina GL, Garrett ES, et al: Natural history of paroxysmal nocturnal hemoglobinuria using modern diagnostic assays. *Br J Haematol* 126:133–138, 2004.

11. Pu JJ, Hu R, Mukhina GL, et al: The small population of PIG-A mutant cells in myelodysplastic syndromes do not arise from multipotent hematopoietic stem cells. *Haematologica* 97(8):1225–1233, 2012.

12. Hanaoka N, Nakakuma H, Horikawa K, et al: NKG2D-mediated immunity underlying paroxysmal nocturnal haemoglobinuria and related bone marrow failure syndromes. *Br J Haematol* 146(5):538–545, 2009.

13. Hillmen P, Lewis SM, Bessler M, et al: Natural history of paroxysmal nocturnal hemoglobinuria. *N Engl J Med* 333:1253–1258, 1995.

14. de Latour RP, Mary JY, Salanoubat C, et al: Paroxysmal nocturnal hemoglobinuria: natural history of disease subcategories. *Blood* 112(8):3099–3106, 2008.

15. Kelly RJ, Hill A, Arnold LM, et al: Long-term treatment with eculizumab in paroxysmal nocturnal hemoglobinuria: sustained efficacy and improved survival. *Blood* 117(25):6786–6792, 2011.

16. Hillmen P, Muus P, Roth A, et al: Long-term safety and efficacy of sustained eculizumab treatment in patients with paroxysmal nocturnal haemoglobinuria. *Br J Haematol* 162(1):62–73, 2013.

17. Brodsky RA, Mukhina GL, Li S, et al: Improved detection and characterization of paroxysmal nocturnal hemoglobinuria using fluorescent aerolysin. *Am J Clin Pathol* 114(3):459–466, 2000.

18. Borowitz MJ, Craig FE, DiGiuseppe JA, et al: Guidelines for the diagnosis and monitoring of paroxysmal nocturnal hemoglobinuria and related disorders by flow cytometry. *Cytometry B Clin Cytom* 78(4):211–230, 2010.

19. Hillmen P, Young NS, Schubert J, et al: The complement inhibitor eculizumab in paroxysmal nocturnal hemoglobinuria. *N Engl J Med* 355:1233–1243, 2006.

20. Brodsky RA, Young NS, Antonioli E, et al: Multicenter phase III study of the complement inhibitor eculizumab for the treatment of patients with paroxysmal nocturnal hemoglobinuria. *Blood* 111(4):1840–1847, 2008.

21. Hillmen P, Muus P, Duhrsen U, et al: Effect of the complement inhibitor eculizumab on thromboembolism in patients with paroxysmal nocturnal hemoglobinuria. *Blood* 110(12):4123–4128, 2007.

22. DeZern AE, Dorr D, Brodsky RA: Predictors of hemoglobin response to eculizumab therapy in paroxysmal nocturnal hemoglobinuria. *Eur J Haematol* 90:16–24, 2013.

23. Rondelli T, Risitano AM, Peffault de Latour R, et al: Polymorphism of the complement receptor 1 gene correlates with hematological response to eculizumab in patients with paroxysmal nocturnal hemoglobinuria. *Haematologica* 99(2):262–266, 2014.

24. Nishimura J, Yamamoto M, Hayashi S, et al: Genetic variants in C5 and poor response to eculizumab. *N Engl J Med* 370(7):632–639, 2014.

25. Peffault de Latour R, Schrezenmeier H, Bacigalupo A, et al: Allogeneic stem cell transplantation in paroxysmal nocturnal hemoglobinuria. *Haematologica* 97(11):1666–1673, 2012.

26. Brodsky RA, Luznik L, Bolanos-Meade J, et al: Reduced intensity HLA-haploidentical BMT with post transplantation cyclophosphamide in nonmalignant hematologic diseases. *Bone Marrow Transplant* 42:523–527, 2008.

ACQUIRED DISORDERS OF RED CELL, WHITE CELL, AND PLATELET PRODUCTION

Jaroslaw P. Maciejewski and Swapna Thota

ACQUIRED PURE RED CELL APLASIA

Acquired pure red cell aplasia (PRCA) is characterized by the presence of an acquired severe normochromic, most frequently normocytic, anemia associated with a complete disappearance of reticulocytes and erythroid precursors in the marrow and normal production of myeloid cells and platelets. Consequently, it is presumed that the defect lies within erythroid precursors and not within stem cells as seen in aplastic anemia. Initially described *as progressive anemia with exclusive absence of erythroid series in the bone marrow*, PRCA is a rare bone marrow failure disorder without geographic or racial predilection. All ages can be affected, but if present in children, it is called transient erythroblastopenia of childhood (TEC) and may be difficult to distinguish from congenital causes of anemia, mainly Diamond-Blackfan anemia (DBA) (Chapter 29). Former nosology included various terms such as *erythrophthisis, chronic hypoplastic anemia, and pure red cell agenesis.*

ETIOLOGY AND CLASSIFICATION

Acquired forms of PRCA must be distinguished from congenital forms of PRCA, which usually manifest themselves early in life (see Chapter 29). Acquired PRCA occurring in childhood may be difficult to distinguish from DBA. As an acquired disease, PRCA may be a primary disorder or secondary to a variety of systemic diseases, including a number of hematologic malignancies (Table 32.1).

Pathogenesis

The inciting events in the development of PRCA are not known. However, as with idiopathic aplastic anemia, viruses or exposure to chemicals can serve as potential triggers (Fig. 32.1). Theoretically a viral infection could lead to depletion of erythroid precursors. Studies of B19 parvovirus (discussed later) suggest such an etiology. Because hematopoietic stem cells are not affected by B19 parvovirus, myeloid cells and platelets are normally produced, and upon clearance of the virus, normal erythroid production can resume. Similarly, in immune-mediated PRCA, the mechanism of erythroid inhibition may vary and may include (1) antibodies to proteins specific to erythroblasts, (2) direct cytotoxic T lymphocyte (CTL)–mediated killing of erythroid precursors, and (3) production of soluble products by CTLs such as inhibitory or proapoptotic cytokines that directly affect the erythroid series.

Historically, initial studies concentrated on examining the effects of soluble serum inhibitors of erythropoiesis. These investigations revealed a decline in erythroid colony formation in the presence of patient serum or failure to induce erythroid colony formation in the presence of erythropoietin. Such serum inhibitors can be found in 40% of patients with PRCA. In 60% of patients, erythroid colony formation can be induced in vitro with hematopoietic growth factors.

The inhibitory activity is localized to the immunoglobulin (Ig)G fraction and disappears upon remission. The antigenic targets for autoantibodies have not been well characterized, but various stages of erythroid differentiation can be affected (also called PRCA type A), as seen in the reduction of burst-forming unit–erythroid or colony-forming unit–erythroid. In certain cases of antibody-mediated PRCA, the involvement of the complement system is a prerequisite to disease causation. Perhaps the exception and a model for antibody-induced red cell aplasia is the identification of PRCA associated with antierythropoietin antibodies (also called PRCA type B) in rare cases. Consistent with the specificity of the antibodies, myeloid colony formation is not impaired, making it unlikely that a more ubiquitous inhibitory cytokine mediates the specific erythroid inhibition.

Experimental and clinical observations have suggested that PRCA may also be mediated by CTLs, which specifically recognize and kill erythroid precursors similar to CTL-mediated killing of cells in aplastic anemia. Although such a T cell–mediated erythroid response is likely to be polyclonal, rare instances of T-cell large granular lymphocyte (T-LGL) leukemia associated with PRCA or erythroid inhibition may represent an extreme form of the clonal continuum of CTL responses (see T-LGL-associated PRCA). In addition to CTLs expressing α/β T-cell receptors (TCRs), T cells with a γ/δ TCR can mediate PRCA. The antigens/antigenic peptides triggering such a response have not been well described. Similarly, natural killer (NK) cells have also been implicated in mediating cytotoxicity directed against erythroid precursors. NK cells, like γ/γ T lymphocytes and unlike α/β CTLs, do not rely on major histocompatibility complex (MHC)–restricted cytotoxicity, but may use killer-cell immunoglobulin-like receptors (KIRs). KIRs inhibit cytolysis when they encounter a cell bearing human leukocyte antigen (HLA) class I molecules. A lack of appropriate KIRs may predispose cells to increased attack by NK cells or γ/δ CTLs. Physiologic downregulation of KIRs has been implicated in the pathogenesis of PRCA in a patient with concomitant γ/δ T-LGL clonal proliferation. An alternative NK-cell cytotoxic mechanism independent of KIR has been reported in healthy individuals.

Peripheral Th lymphocyte polarization has been implicated in the pathogenesis of PRCA.[56,57] Polarization toward the Th2 functional subtype during disease relapse and normalization of Th1/Th2 ratio after effective treatment has been reported in both monoclonal gammopathy- and thymoma-associated PRCA.

PRIMARY PURE RED CELL APLASIA

Primary PRCA occurs in the absence of any underlying disorder. It may be acute and self-limited or may be a chronic and refractory condition. Acute forms are uncommon. Most cases are protracted and chronic, unlike TEC, which is an acute and self-limited disorder. Most of the cases of classic primary PRCA are autoimmune in origin, but a significant proportion will remain idiopathic in origin in spite of an exhaustive workup.

TABLE 32.1   Classification of Pure Red Cell Aplasia

Congenital (DBA)

Primary	Autoimmune	
	Idiopathic	
Secondary	Thymoma[1–5]	CLL[6,7]
	Hematologic malignancies	T-LGL/chronic NK-LGL leukemia[8–15]
		Myeloma[16]
		NHL[17,18]
		MDS[19]
		ALL[20–22]
	Solid tumors	Renal cell carcinoma[23]
		Thyroid cancer[24]
		Various adenocarcinomas[25,26]
	Infections	Parvovirus B19[27]
		EBV,[28] mumps
		HIV,[29] HTLV-1[12]
		CMV[30]
		Viral hepatitis (hepatitis A,[31–33] hepatitis B[34,35])
		Leishmaniasis[36]
		Gram-positive systemic infections (e.g., staphylococcemia)
		Meningococcemia
	Autoimmune conditions	SLE[37]
		RA[38]
		Sjögren syndrome[39,40]
		Mixed connective tissue disease[41]
		Autoimmune hepatitis[42]
		Anti-EPO antibodies[43,44]
		ABO-incompatible BMT
		Minor incompatibility[45–50]
	Drugs and chemicals	
	Pregnancy[51,52]	
	Severe nutritional deficiencies[53,54]	
	Renal failure[55]	

ALL, Acute lymphoblastic leukemia; *BMT,* bone marrow transplantation; *CLL,* chronic lymphocytic leukemia; *CMV,* cytomegalovirus; *DBA,* Diamond-Blackfan anemia; *EBV,* Epstein-Barr virus; *EPO,* erythropoietin; *HIV,* human immunodeficiency virus; *HTLV-1,* human T-lymphotrophic virus-1; *MDS,* myelodysplastic syndrome; *NHL,* non-Hodgkin lymphoma; *NK-LGL,* natural killer large granular lymphocyte; *RA,* refractory anemia; *SLE,* systemic lupus erythematosus; *T-LGL,* T-cell large granular lymphocyte.

SECONDARY FORMS OF PURE RED CELL APLASIA

Clinical Associations

B-Cell Chronic Lymphocytic Leukemia–Associated PRCA

In B-cell chronic lymphocytic leukemia (CLL), PRCA can be observed in up to 6% of cases. A recent study found 0.5% of their 1750 CLL patients has PRCA. The underlying pathogenetic mechanisms are not clear, and the inhibition of the erythroid series does not appear to be mediated by a soluble factor. The distinction between whether the PRCA is a result of the primary B-cell CLL disease or its therapy becomes difficult in circumstances when PRCA presents as a late event. In most cases, PRCA cannot be attributed simply to infiltration of the marrow by lymphoma cells.

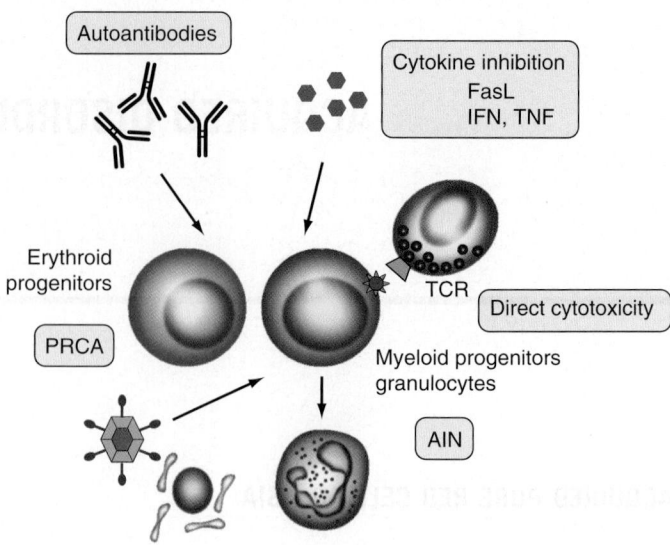

Fig. 32.1 PATHOGENESIS OF PURE RED CELL APLASIA. *AIN,* Autoimmune neutropenia; *FasL,* Fas ligand; *IFN,* interferon; *PRCA,* pure red cell aplasia; *TCR,* T-cell receptor; *TNF,* tumor necrosis factor.

T-Cell Large Granular Lymphocyte–Associated PRCA

Although neutropenia is a typical finding in T-LGL leukemia, PRCA with varying degrees of erythroblastopenia can also be observed in 10% to 15% of patients with T-LGL leukemia. It is found to be commonly associated with signal transducer and activator of transcription (STAT)3 mutant T-LGL leukemia. In such a setting, PRCA is often accompanied by red cells with an increased mean corpuscular volume. It is possible that PRCA associated with T-LGL leukemia represents an extreme form of the T cell–mediated disease that, if polyclonal, might be classified as idiopathic PRCA.

Thymoma-Associated PRCA

Thymoma is associated with PRCA; thus a chest x-ray examination or computed tomographic (CT) scan should be included in the workup for PRCA. Antibodies with direct inhibitory effects against erythroid precursors may be present. T cell–mediated inhibition of erythropoiesis has also been implicated in the pathogenesis of PRCA associated with either benign or malignant thymomas. A late onset immunodeficiency condition; Good syndrome characterized by hypogammaglobulinemia and thymoma is associated with PRCA in 33% of the patients. Thymectomy is the usual initial treatment approach; however, incomplete responders, nonresponders, and patients who relapse are common, necessitating additional therapies in the form of azathioprine, intravenous immunoglobulin (IVIg), and cyclosporine A (CsA).

Pregnancy-Associated PRCA

Pregnancy-associated PRCA is a self-limited syndrome that may occur at any age of gestation. It has a high risk for relapse during subsequent pregnancies and can be safely managed with either blood transfusions or corticosteroids. Patients with other forms of PRCA may also be more prone to relapse during pregnancy.

Parvovirus B19 and Other Viral-Induced PRCAs
Parvovirus B19 is a single-stranded deoxyribonucleic acid (DNA) virus, which in normal individuals causes fifth disease (erythema infectiosum) in children and arthropathy in adults. The cellular

receptor for the virus is the P antigen, a blood group antigen also responsible for the agglutination reaction that occurs in the presence of the virus. Detection of parvovirus B19–specific IgM without antiparvovirus B19 IgG, supports the diagnosis of acute infection, whereas the parvovirus B19–specific IgG suggests immunity. Addition of parvovirus B19 in vitro to cultures of erythroid progenitor cells completely abolishes erythroid colony formation. Primary infection causes lifelong immunity; however, it is possible that a latent virus may persist in a healthy individual for years.

A transient aplastic crisis is a typical complication of a primary parvovirus B19 infection in patients with increased red cell turnover (usually chronic hemolysis, e.g., hemoglobinopathies, and hereditary red blood cell [RBC] membrane disorders, e.g., hereditary spherocytosis). In typical cases, acute reticulocytopenia results in a sudden drop in hemoglobin (Hb)/hematocrit levels as RBC destruction is not supported by a suppressed marrow. Occasionally, characteristic giant pronormoblasts may be seen in marrow aspirates (Fig. 32.2). Aplastic crisis is often self-limiting with the evolution of a protective IgG response. Viral titers in the serum of affected patients may be high.

A more chronic form, parvovirus B19–related PRCA, may develop in immunocompromised patients as, for example, in acquired immunodeficiency syndrome (AIDS). In such cases, IVIg can produce remarkable responses. High doses of IVIg are required (>2 g/kg) because an insufficient dose may not produce the desired effect. DNA dot blot hybridization is the best diagnostic test for the detection of viremia. Parvovirus B19 can also be detected by polymerase chain reaction (PCR), a routinely available test, but this method may provide a high rate of false-positive results. However, if negative, it excludes B19 parvovirus–mediated disease. Improved tests have been developed that allow for the detection of neutralizing antibodies and infectivity of parvovirus B19. Several other viral infections, including viral hepatitis (A and C), Epstein-Barr virus (EBV), cytomegalovirus (CMV), human T-Lymphotropic virus (HTLV)-1, and human immunodeficiency virus (HIV) have been implicated as causative agents of PRCA. Little is known about the exact mechanisms underlying these disorders, but they likely involve T cell–mediated suppression as observed during HTLV-1 infection and EBV or antibody-mediated destruction of RBC precursors, as in hepatitis C–induced PRCA.

Connective Tissue Disease–Associated PRCA

The majority of connective tissue diseases associated with PRCA are autoimmune in nature. Several rheumatologic diseases have been associated with PRCA, including adult-onset Still disease,[58,59] dermatomyositis,[60] mixed connective tissue disease,[41] polymyositis,[61] rheumatoid arthritis,[38,62] Sjögren syndrome,[39,40,63] systemic lupus erythematosus and antiphospholipid syndrome.[37,64,65] The

pathogenesis of the PRCA in this setting may vary and includes autoantibody-mediated erythroid inhibition,[66] autoantibody directed against erythropoietin,[67] and CTL-mediated killing of erythroid precursors.[64]

Drug-Induced PRCA

Various chemical agents and drugs have been associated with PRCA. The mechanisms responsible for erythroid inhibition may be diverse depending on the offending agent (Table 32.2) but may include induction of antibodies targeting the drugs or drugs bound to cellular and plasma proteins. Another possible mechanism involves drug-mediated triggering of T-cell responses, or direct toxicity to the erythroid series as seen with diphenylhydantoin.[68]

Erythropoietin Antibody–Associated PRCA

Recombinant erythropoietin is used in the treatment of anemia of various origins, including anemia of chronic disease, renal disease, and a variety of bone marrow failure syndromes, particularly myelodysplastic syndrome (MDS). Cases of PRCA have developed

TABLE 32.2 Drugs and Chemicals Implicated in Pure Red Cell Aplasia

Alemtuzumab[69]	Isoniazid[92–94]
Allopurino[70,71]	Lamivudine[95]
α-Methyldopa[72]	Linezolid[96]
Aminopyrine[73]	Maloprim[97]
Azathioprine[74,75]	Mycophenolate mofetil[98]
Benzene[76]	Penicillin[99]
Carbamazepine[77]	Phenylbutazone[100]
Cephalothin[78]	Phenytoin[68,101,102]
Chloramphenicol[79]	Procainamide[103–105]
Chlorpropamide[80,81]	Ribavirin[98,106]
Cladribine[82]	Rifampicin[107]
Clopidogrel	Sulfasalazine[108,109]
Cotrimoxazole[83]	Sulfathiozole[110]
D-Penicillinamine[84]	Sulindac[111]
Erythropoietin[43,44]	Tacrolimus[112]
Estrogens[85]	Thiamphenicol[113]
Fludarabine[86]	Ticlopidine[114,115]
FK506[87]	Valproic acid[116,106]
Gold[88]	Zidovudine[117]
Halothane[89]	
Interferon-α [90,91]	

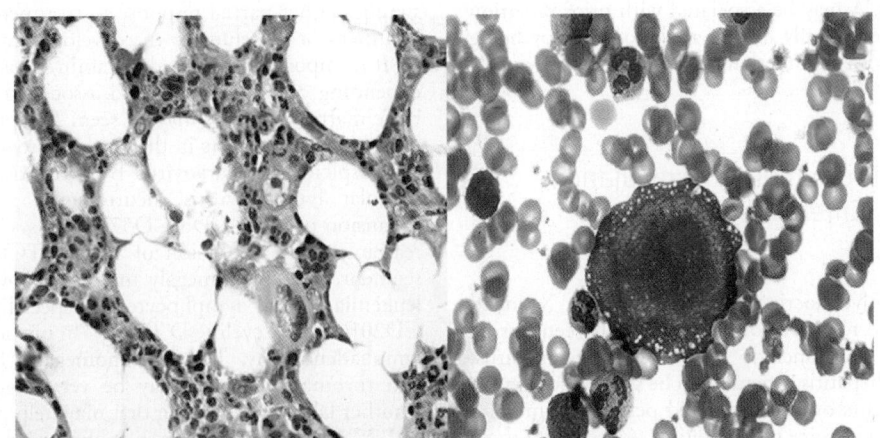

Fig. 32.2 PARVOVIRUS B19–MEDIATED PURE RED CELL APLASIA.

as a consequence of antibody formation against endogenous erythropoietin or while receiving treatment with recombinant erythropoietin. The latter condition has been referred to as *epoetin-induced PRCA* or *EPO-PRCA* with initial cases related to exposure to epoetin alpha (Eprex; 92%) and epoetin beta (NeoRecormon; 8%). There are reports of human erythropoietin (HuEPO) neutralizing antibody PRCA related to the use of biosimilar recombinant HuEPO in Thailand. There are several risk factors to the development of EPO-PRCA, including subcutaneous route of administration, use of epoetin alpha stabilized in a human serum albumin (HSA)–free formulation, use of silicone oil as lubricant in prefilled Eprex syringes, and use in patients with chronic renal disease. This observation has led to modification in the storage, handling, and administration of Eprex favoring IV administration, especially with Eprex stabilized with HSA-free formulation, and avoidance of the subcutaneous (SC) non–HSA stabilized Eprex. Diagnostic criteria have also been proposed incorporating major features (treatment with epoetin for at least 3 weeks, decrease in Hb by 0.1 g/dL/day without transfusions or transfusion requirement of about 1 unit/week to keep Hb level stable, reticulocyte count less than 10×10^9/L, no major drop in other blood lineages), minor features (skin and systemic allergic reactions), and accessory investigations to exclude other causes. The most commonly used tests to detect antibodies are enzyme-linked immunosorbent assay, radioimmunoprecipitation assay, and surface plasmon resonance. Once antibodies are detected, their neutralizing ability is tested using an in vitro bioassay. Following establishment of diagnosis, management should include discontinuation of exogenous erythropoietin, administration of immunosuppressive agents, or, in cases of anemia secondary to renal insufficiency, renal transplantation.

PRCA Following Allogeneic Stem Cell Transplantation

In contrast to HLA matching, ABO blood group incompatibility plays a minor role in the success of allogeneic hematopoietic stem cell transplantation (HSCT). However, PRCA may be associated with major ABO incompatibility between the donor and recipient, leading to inhibition of donor erythroid precursors by residual host isoagglutinins. This complication is more commonly observed following the use of nonmyeloablative conditioning regimens. PRCA may also be resistant to the withdrawal or decrease of immunosuppression, or donor lymphocyte infusions. Responses to rituximab, erythropoietin, plasma exchange and azathioprine have been reported. A case responsive to purified CD34+ cell infusion has also been reported. Resolution of PRCA is generally associated with decrease and subsequent disappearance of host isoagglutinins.

PRCA Postradiation Therapy

In rare circumstances, PRCA may be associated with prior radiation therapy. The cases described usually involve radiation therapy being administered to a patient with an underlying thymoma not previously associated with PRCA.

PRCA Associated With Immune Dysregulation, Polyendocrinopathy, Enteropathy, X-Linked Syndrome

Immune dysregulation, polyendocrinopathy, enteropathy, X-linked syndrome is a rare X-linked recessive condition typically seen during infancy. Clinical features may include type 1 diabetes mellitus, eczema, and autoimmune hepatitis. Anemia can be severe at diagnosis because the fall in Hb occurs over a protracted period of time and patients often exhibit a good degree of adaptation. Arrest of erythropoiesis is obvious with a profound reticulocytopenia.

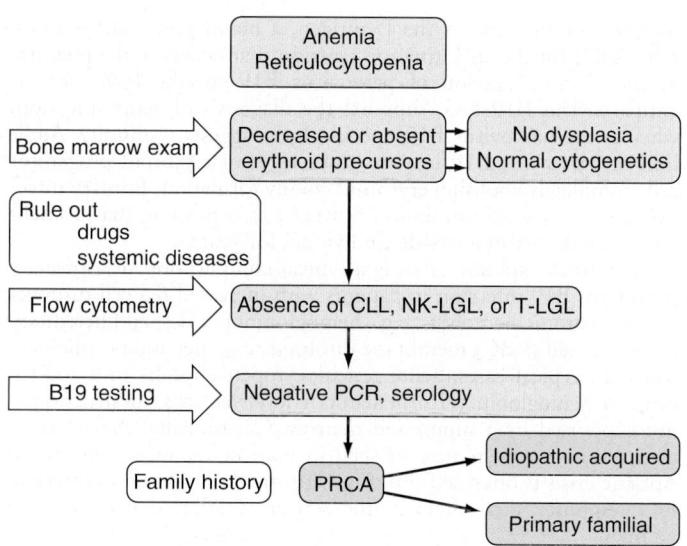

Fig. 32.3 DIAGNOSTIC ALGORITHM IN PURE RED CELL APLASIA. *CLL,* Chronic lymphocytic leukemia; *NK-LGL,* natural killer large granular lymphocyte; *PCR,* polymerase chain reaction; *PRCA,* pure red cell aplasia; *T-LGL,* T-cell large granular lymphocyte.

LABORATORY EVALUATION

A complete blood cell count with differential, peripheral smear review, reticulocyte count, and a bone marrow examination remain the cornerstone in the diagnosis of PRCA. The classic hematologic picture of PRCA includes a normocytic, normochromic anemia (anemia associated with T-LGL leukemia is often macrocytic) with a normal white blood cell and platelet count. The reticulocyte count is significantly reduced to less than 1% (a reticulocyte level greater than 2% is not compatible with the diagnosis of PRCA (Fig. 32.3). The bone marrow examination generally shows absence of cells belonging to the erythroid lineage and the normal appearance of granulocytic and monocytic precursors and megakaryocytes. Erythroid precursors, if present, are usually less than 1%, and only a few residual proerythroblasts or basophilic erythroblasts may be seen. Blast cell numbers and cellularity are within normal limits. There are no dysplastic changes, ringed sideroblasts, or reticulin fibrosis. Cytogenetic evaluation is normal. In some cases, neutropenia, mild thrombocytopenia, eosinophilia, thrombocytosis, leukocytosis, or relative lymphocytosis may be seen. Cytogenetic abnormalities, if present, may indicate concomitant myelodysplasia and is a poor prognostic marker for both response to treatment and propensity to leukemic transformation. During the course of PRCA patients, ineffective erythropoiesis characterized by a maturation arrest at the proerythroblast or basophilic erythroblast stage may be observed and signifies either partial response to treatment or initial recovery from treatment or a prelude to the development of full-blown PRCA.

It is important to exclude vitamin B$_{12}$ and folate deficiencies, and depending on the etiology and associated disease, other blood and bone marrow findings may be seen. The presence of giant and vacuolated pronormoblasts in the bone marrow examination should raise the suspicion for parvovirus B19 infection. The presence of large granular lymphocytosis, neutropenia, and/or thrombocytopenia, expansion of CD3+CD8+CD57+ T cells, clonal cytotoxic TCR gene rearrangement, expansion of specific TCR Vβ region family gene segment, and splenomegaly may point toward concomitant T-LGL leukemia, B-cell lymphocytosis, especially of the CD5+/CD19+/CD20+/CD23+/cyclin D–/SmIg–dim phenotype with concomitant lymphadenopathy, hepatosplenomegaly, hypogammaglobulinemia, and thrombocytopenia may be very suggestive of a B-cell CLL. Another laboratory finding that may help point to a secondary cause of PRCA includes the presence of monoclonal gammopathy. Parvovirus B19 DNA titers (DNA hybridization and amplification techniques) may show high levels of the virus at 10 genome copies per milliliter,[118] but it is important to note that serologic (IgM and IgG) titers are usually absent. Erythropoietin antibodies, antinuclear antibodies, and/or complement consumption may point toward a specific disease mechanism. A radiographic workup may also be useful in the clinical workup because chest x-ray examination or CT scan may show evidence of a thymoma.

DIFFERENTIAL DIAGNOSIS

PRCA can be easily differentiated from aplastic anemia and other types of bone marrow failure syndromes. A distinction between MDS with erythroid hypoplasia and idiopathic PRCA may be more difficult. In childhood, TEC has to be distinguished from DBA, but a history of normal blood counts, late onset of manifestations, and a transient disease course are characteristic of TEC.

THERAPY

The distinction between primary and secondary forms of PRCA is essential because many secondary types have specific and very effective therapies (Table 32.3). All potentially offending drugs should be discontinued, and drug-associated PRCA should remit within 3 to 4 weeks. Nutritional deficiencies (B_{12} and folic acid) should be excluded and treated if present. The therapy of primary and secondary forms of PRCA refractory to the treatment of an underlying disease may be challenging and should include a sequential trial of various immunosuppressive agents until a response is achieved. Spontaneous remissions have been reported.

Surgery or Radiation

In cases associated with thymoma, thymectomy is the usual initial treatment of choice before immunosuppression and may induce remission with return of erythropoiesis in 4 to 8 weeks in about 30% to 40% of patients. Patients who fail to respond to surgery should be treated as patients with idiopathic PRCA. The removal of a thymoma may improve responsiveness to immunosuppressive therapy. Thymectomy in the absence of a thymoma in other forms of PRCA is not recommended. In circumstances where surgical resection of thymoma is contraindicated, radiation therapy with or without chemotherapy may be administered.

Medical

Supportive

Supportive care includes blood transfusions and iron chelation.

Immunosuppression

Prednisone therapy is associated with significant response rates (approximately 40%) and should constitute the initial therapeutic approach. Initial responses are generally observed after 4 to 6 weeks. A slow taper of prednisone is suggested over a period of 3 to 4 months. The disease may relapse, and the minimal maintenance dose of corticosteroids may need to be established to maintain the desired Hb levels. Trials of prednisone therapy without clinical response longer than 8 weeks are not warranted.

Alternative therapies may include cyclosporine, oral cyclophosphamide, azathioprine, antithymocyte globulin (ATG), rituximab, and alemtuzumab (see Table 32.3). Erythropoietin and darbepoietin are usually not effective as a sole agent but may hasten recovery following an adequate trial of cyclophosphamide. No randomized trials exist to favor a particular treatment based on efficacy. The choice of therapy may be influenced by clinical clues. For example, the presence of LGLs may suggest the use of CsA, hypogammaglobulinemia may be corrected with IVIg, whereas detection of hypergammaglobulinemia or monoclonal protein may suggest a choice of rituximab. Most refractory cases may require administration of ATG. The age of the patient may influence the choice of the cytotoxic agent, which may pose a significant risk for the development of secondary leukemias, especially with a prolonged administration.

Danazol is a synthetic attenuated androgen that has been used for many years for the treatment of a variety of hematologic disorders, mainly myelofibrosis.

IVIg is also effective in several types of PRCA. Higher doses of usually 2 g/kg of IVIg for 5 days are necessary for the treatment of parvovirus B19 virus–induced PRCA. In AIDS patients with parvovirus B19 virus–induced PRCA, a regimen consists of induction therapy with 1 g/kg daily for 1–2 days followed by 1 g/kg for 2 days.

Azathioprine is an imidazolyl derivative of mercaptopurine that inhibits DNA synthesis by inhibition of purine metabolism. In PRCA, it may be given at a dose of 2–3 mg/kg/day IV and has been found to be effective in patients nonresponsive to cyclophosphamide.

| TABLE 32.3 | Therapy for Pure Red Cell Aplasia and Its Results |

	Study								
Agent	Chikkappa[119]	Means[120]	Au[121]	Dessypris[122]	Zecca[123]	Lacy[124]	Charles[125]	Sloand[126]	Abkowitz[127]
Steroids				18/41		9/29	9/36	–	
Cytotoxic agents				24/54		14/29	8/27	–	
Antithymocyte globulin				2/6		0/1	8/12		6/6
Cyclosporine A	6/7	6/9		3/4		4/5	2/3		
Splenectomy				4/23		0/1	0/1		
Daclizumab (Zenapax)								6/15	
Rituximab					1/1				
Alemtuzumab (Campath)			2/2						
Methotrexate							2/37		

Oral cyclophosphamide may be started at a dose of 50 mg orally (PO) daily, with a maximal dose of no more than 150 mg daily. Blood counts should be monitored, and the dose may be escalated accordingly. Trials of therapy longer than 3 months without signs of response are not warranted. Monitoring of the reticulocyte count may allow for the early assessment of response. Often, a delayed response may be seen when cyclophosphamide is withdrawn, reflective of balance between immunosuppression and cytotoxicity.

Rituximab given IV infusion weekly for 4 weeks has been found to be efficacious in PRCA. PRCA in a variety of settings, including B-cell CLL, EBV-associated posttransplant lymphoproliferative disease, ABO-incompatible allogeneic HSCT for acute myeloid leukemia, and hairy cell leukemia variant, has been successfully treated with Rituximab. In cases refractory to immunosuppressive agents affecting T-cell function, rituximab or low-dose alemtuzumab constitute a reasonable option. Rituximab is effective in patients with PRCA owing to ABO incompatibility following bone marrow transplantation.

CsA can be administered at a dose of 5–10 mg/kg PO daily in divided doses. CsA can be combined with prednisone at doses of 20–30 mg PO. The trough levels of CsA should be monitored. An adequate trial of therapy is considered 3 months of therapy. The response rates may be as high as 60% to 80%. After a response is achieved, the therapy should be continued for 6 months followed by a slow taper.

Horse ATG may be given to refractory cases at a dose of 40 mg/kg IV daily for 4 days with prednisone at 1 mg/kg. Concomitant prednisone should be administered and then tapered over 2–3 weeks. A therapeutic response should occur within 3 months posttherapy, although responses at or beyond 6 months may be observed.

Daclizumab, an anti–interleukin (IL)-2 receptor antibody (Zenapax, anti-CD25 mAb), may constitute a good alternative to ATG. A dose of 1 mg/kg of body weight IV is administered every 2 weeks. While dacluzimab is not currently on the market other anti–IL-2 are available options.

Methotrexate, an antimetabolite, at low doses (7.5–15 mg/week PO) is useful in treating PRCA, especially in patients with concomitant LGL leukemia. The responses are generally sustained, and therapy is well tolerated. Methotrexate may be given in conjunction with other therapies like CsA.

Alemtuzumab (Campath, anti-CD52 monoclonal antibody) is a recombinant DNA–derived humanized monoclonal antibody directed against the cell surface glycoprotein CD52, which is expressed on the surface of normal and malignant B and T lymphocytes. Currently approved for multiple sclerosis and available on compassionate use for other indication. Former IV dosing has been replaced with SC (initial dose of 3 mg, and subsequent doses at 10 mg once or twice weekly). The usual cumulative dose before response is usually around 50–100 mg. Alemtuzumab has been tested in a variety of lymphoproliferative disorders, including B-cell lymphomas and T-LGL leukemia. Similarly, PRCA occurring in the context of these conditions previously unresponsive to other therapies has been shown to be responsive to this agent.

Hematopoietic Stem Cell Transplantation

Despite advances in immunosuppressive regimens, subsets of patients with PRCA remain refractory and are very difficult to treat. As with other bone marrow failure disorders with autoimmune pathogenesis like aplastic anemia, HSCT is an important treatment option especially for refractory and relapsed PRCA cases. Matched sibling donor allogeneic HSCT results in restoration of normal hematopoiesis in patients with refractory PRCA. In another case, a patient with relapsed PRCA underwent matched sibling donor allogeneic HSCT combined with donor lymphocyte infusions resulting in full donor engraftment and subsequent return of normal hematopoiesis, suggesting a graft-versus-autoimmunity effect as the likely mechanism for response.

PROGNOSIS

The prognosis of secondary PRCA depends upon the underlying disease. Idiopathic PRCA may be very refractory to treatment. Ultimately, remission may be achieved in a significant proportion (approximately 68%) of patients, especially when sequential regimens are used. Spontaneous remissions are observed in 5% to 10% of cases. Relapses are common, especially during the first year postremission but are usually responsive to the same regimen that induced remission. Chronic, low-dose immunosuppressive therapy may be needed in certain cases that have relapsed. In one study, median survival was reported to be 14 years. Unlike a megakaryocytic thrombocytopenic purpura, evolution to aplastic anemia is rare and very few patients (3% to 5%) evolve into acute leukemia.

ACQUIRED WHITE BLOOD CELL PRODUCTION DISORDERS

Neutropenia is a common condition. The majority of cases are secondary to a variety of causes, including systemic or hematologic diseases. We will describe a primary, isolated form of neutropenia in which other hematopoietic lineages are not affected. In such a setting, neutropenia may be the result of peripheral destruction or perhaps less frequently the result of the absence of myeloid progenitors in the marrow. The cutoff value for the diagnosis of neutropenia is an absolute neutrophil count (ANC) of less than 1500 cells/μL. This value is generally accepted as a definition for neutropenia for all ages and ethnic backgrounds except for newborn infants. Clinically, the most concerning consequence of neutropenia is the propensity to develop infections. However, the correlation between ANC and the propensity for infection is variable in different circumstances and determined by marrow neutrophil reserves, duration of neutropenia, and clinical context. This is best illustrated in patients with chronic benign neutropenia of childhood and infancy, where patients may have an ANC as low or less than 250 cells/μL and yet they may be devoid of infections or only have mild infections.

CLASSIFICATION OF ACQUIRED NEUTROPENIAS

Neutropenia as a primary disease should be distinguished from inherited forms of neutropenia, which commonly present during early childhood (see Chapter 29), and secondary forms of neutropenia associated with systemic disorders. In addition, idiopathic neutropenia is distinct from the constitutional or familial benign neutropenia frequently seen in African Americans, Yemenites, and Falasha Jews or black Bedouins. The degree of neutropenia is often mild, and there is no propensity to develop infections. Most cases of neutropenia are secondary to a variety of disorders. Primary autoimmune neutropenia (AIN) and idiopathic neutropenia are less common. We will limit our description to isolated forms of neutropenia (Table 32.4).

Primary Neutropenia

Most cases of neutropenia are secondary to various hematologic and systemic diseases. However, in a small proportion of cases, an inciting cause cannot be identified despite intensive testing. Such idiopathic cases are most likely immune mediated.

Chronic Idiopathic Neutropenia in Adults

Chronic idiopathic neutropenia in adults compared with those in infancy and early childhood has less tendency toward spontaneous remission, although it does generally remain clinically benign. There may be concomitant anemia or thrombocytopenia that may portend a higher incidence of splenomegaly, infectious complications, and antineutrophil antibodies (ANAs) that are complement fixing. A

TABLE 32.4   **Classification of Neutropenia**

Congenital

Primary	Autoimmune neutropenia
	Pure white cell aplasia
	Idiopathic
	Thymoma
	Hematologic malignancies (e.g., T-LGL leukemia)
	Infections/postinfectious
	Viral
	Measles,[128] mumps, roseola,[129,130] rubella,[131] RSV, influenza[132]
	Hepatitis A,[133] B,[133,134] and C[35]
	CMV,[135–137] EBV,[138–140] HIV[141,142]
	Parvovirus[143–145]
	Bacterial
	Tuberculosis[146,147]
	Brucellosis[148–150]
	Tularemia[151]
	Typhoid fever[152]
	Rickettsial
	Rocky Mountain spotted fever[153]
	Ehrlichiosis.[154,155]
	Fungal
	Histoplasmosis[156,157]
	Parasitic
	Malaria,[158] leishmaniasis[36,159]
	Autoimmune conditions, (e.g., SLE,[160,161] RA[162])
	Drugs and chemicals
	Neutropenia associated with immunodeficiency[163,164]
	Severe nutritional deficiencies[165,166]
	Neutropenia caused by increased margination
	Iatrogenic (e.g., hemodialysis[167,168])

CMV, Cytomegalovirus; EBV, Epstein-Barr virus; HIV, human immunodeficiency virus; RA, refractory anemia; RSV, respiratory syncytial virus; SLE, systemic lupus erythematosus; T-LGL, T-cell large granular lymphocyte.

TABLE 32.5   **Human Neutrophil Alloantigens and Autoantigens**

		Nomenclature
Integrin α M chain	CD11b	HNA-4a (MART)
Integrin α L chain	CD11a	HNA-4a (OND)
Gp50-64	CD177	HNA-2a (NB1) PRV-1
Gp70-95		HNA-3a/5b
Integrin β2 chain	CD18	
FcγIII	CD16	
FCGR3B-01		HNA-1a (NA1)
FCGR3B-02		HNA-1b (NA2)
FCGR3B-03		HNA-1c (SH/NA3)

bone marrow biopsy may show evidence of an arrest in myeloid maturation and mild hypercellularity. ANAs may be seen in 36% of patients, suggesting an immunologic pathogenesis. An altered TCR Vβ repertoire, telomere shortening, and activation of Toll-like receptor 4 have been reported to play a role in pathogenesis of chronic idiopathic neutropenia.

Idiopathic neutropenias may be chronic and benign in nature or may be associated with significant morbidity. In certain instances, immune neutropenia may be associated with hemolytic anemia or with immune thrombocytopenia, but these forms likely represent a distinct nosologic entity. Idiopathic neutropenia can occur at any age with a median age at diagnosis being 28.3 years and affects predominantly females (85%). AIN may be associated with moderate and severe depression of neutrophil counts. Monocytosis is frequently present. Some cases present with splenomegaly, which is to be distinguished from cytopenias associated with hypersplenism in Felty syndrome. The frequency of infectious complications rarely correlates with the severity of neutropenia, and patients with severe neutropenia may remain asymptomatic for long periods.

Conceptually, AIN may be caused by peripheral autoimmune destruction of neutrophils caused by lineage-specific inhibition of myeloid precursors, with its extreme form being pure white cell aplasia (PWCA) (see Fig. 32.3). Consequently, increased peripheral destruction is associated with marrow hypercellularity and an increased number of myeloid precursors or, if myeloid progenitors are the targets, decreased myeloid precursors and a myeloid maturation arrest. Autoimmune processes have been implicated in the pathogenesis of AIN and could be mediated by both peripheral destruction of neutrophils and inhibition of myelopoiesis. The antigens involved in these processes include neutrophil antigens NA1, NA2, ND1, ND2, and NB1 (Table 32.5). Both IgG and IgM

antibodies have been implicated. Neutrophil-specific antibodies can be detected using many assays, including specific enzyme-linked immunosorbent assay, opsonization, leukoagglutination, and direct antibody binding. There are several proposed effector mechanisms as to how ANAs can result in neutropenia or affect neutrophil integrity. For example, ANAs may act as opsonins and directly enhance neutrophil destruction. Alternatively, ANAs can indirectly activate, complement, and facilitate opsonization. Immune complexes may also bind to the neutrophil Fc portion, leading to increased neutrophil clearance by the reticuloendothelial system, and finally, ANAs may recognize and damage myeloid precursors. The currently available diagnostic assays used to detect ANAs are generally based on immunofluorescence and agglutination assays. The former allows for the detection of IgM and IgG antibodies from a suspected patient that are attached to normal donor neutrophils detected by flow cytometry performed with the patient's serum and antihuman IgG. The second technique, called agglutination assay, uses serum that leads to agglutination of normal neutrophils into either small or large clumps. These tests suggest an underlying immunologic process but cannot establish the definite cause. If there is a high index of suspicion that ANAs are the causative factor, some authors suggest that a minimum of two methods be used to detect ANAs.

In addition to antibodies, T-cell responses may be associated with neutropenia. The most extreme example of such responses is T-LGL leukemia associated with neutropenia and polarized proliferation of CTLs (see later). In AIN, CTL responses are polyclonal and are often accompanied by the simultaneous presence of antibodies. It is likely that specialized CTL clones are capable of recognizing and killing myeloid precursors, interrupting granulocyte production. Consequently, some cases of AIN may be amenable to therapy with immunosuppressive agents directed against T cells.

Chronic Benign Neutropenia of Infancy and Childhood

Chronic benign neutropenia of infancy and childhood is considered the most common cause of chronic neutropenia in the pediatric age group. The majority of cases are autoimmune in nature and show clinical overlap with childhood idiopathic thrombocytopenic purpura and autoimmune hemolytic anemia. It is therefore considered a type of AIN. This form of neutropenia typically presents in children less than 3 years of age, with a median age of 8–11 months and with a predominance of girls. The ANC is usually less than 250 cells/μL with normal morphologic characteristics and normal Hb and platelet count. Occasionally monocytosis, eosinophilia, and mild thrombocytopenia may be present. In this condition, neutropenia is caused by chronic depletion of mature granulocytes and is accompanied by a compensatory myeloid left shift in the marrow. Most frequent clinical signs and symptoms are oral infections, including bothersome ulcers, but these are often associated with additional functional defects of neutrophils and cellulitis of the labia majora. Of importance is the normal neutrophil count at birth and absence of a history of familial forms of neutropenia. The etiology of this condition is unknown, but the pathogenesis involves ANAs, detectable in the majority of patients. The antibodies are generally directed against similar antigens as seen in adult AIN, especially those involving *NA*, *NB*, and *ND* loci. In about 25% of cases, the antibody is against an allele of neutrophil FcγRIII opsonin receptor called NA1. Immunosuppressive therapy leads frequently to responses supporting the immune pathogenesis of this disease. Although the neutrophil count can be severely depressed, serious infectious complications are uncommon, and therefore treatment to raise the ANC is generally not indicated except if recurrent infections occur. Antibiotics are used to treat infections, and granulocyte colony-stimulating factor (G-CSF) has been shown to be effective in elevating neutrophil counts.

SECONDARY FORMS OF NEUTROPENIAS

Clinical Associations

Drug-Induced Neutropenia/Agranulocytosis

Drug-induced neutropenia is common. The association was first when agranulocytosis was observed in patients taking aminopyrine. The incidence in various studies is 1 to 3.4 cases per million per year. Drugs may induce granulocytopenia by (1) direct toxicity leading to inhibition of myelopoiesis frequently observed in drugs like valproic acid, carbamazepine, and β-lactam antibiotics; (2) immune mediated (either antibody- or complement-mediated) as seen with penicillin and antithyroid drugs or immune complex–mediated (quinidine) destruction of myeloid progenitors and mature neutrophils; and (3) induction of CTL responses to genetic predisposition because of polymorphisms in various genes coding for cytokine and cytokine receptors as demonstrated for clozapine with tumor necrosis factor and HLA polymorphisms as well as variants of genes coding for a variety of metabolizing enzymes.[169,170] Of interest are drugs that directly antagonize important vitamin cofactors necessary in normal bone marrow development. Neutropenia observed in patients treated with trimethoprim-sulfamethoxazole is caused by the inhibitory effects on granulopoiesis by trimethoprim, owing to its antifolate action, which is reversed by folinic acid. A similar finding can be seen with methotrexate owing to its antifolate action.

Most patients present with either asymptomatic neutropenia discovered on routine examination or symptomatic neutropenia with infectious complications, including fever, angular stomatitis, or pneumonia. The reported mortality rates vary from 1% to 25%. Most patients recover with withdrawal of the offending drug without further complications. It has been estimated that drugs account for 72% of cases of agranulocytosis. The usual time to development of overt neutropenia is around 1–2 weeks, and neutropenia resolves upon discontinuation of the offending drug within a 2-week period, although time to recovery may vary. The recovery in neutrophil counts is usually preceded by increases in peripheral blood monocytes and immature granulocytes. The International Agranulocytosis and Aplastic Anemia Study has identified the most commonly associated agents and the relative odds ratios for developing agranulocytosis (Table 32.6).[171] In some instances, the severity of neutropenia is related to the dose and duration of the therapy. The therapy includes discontinuation of the potentially offending agents. In some instances, associated with infections or prolonged recovery, G-CSF may be administered.

Neutropenia as a Manifestation of Systemic Diseases

Postinfectious Neutropenia

Neutropenia is commonly associated with viral infections, particularly in children. Various mechanisms have been implicated in neutropenia associated with systemic viral infections, including inhibition of

TABLE 32.6   Drugs Associated With Agranulocytosis

	Etiologic Fraction	
	Agranulocytosis (%)	Aplastic Anemia (%)
Overall	64	62
IAAAS	12	27
United States	72	17
Thailand	70	2

Drugs associated with agranulocytosis (IAAAS and other drugs of interest)

Acetyldigoxin[172]
ACE inhibitors[173,174]
Allopurinol[175–177]
Amodiaquine[178]
Benzafibrate[179]
β-Blockers[172,180]
β-Lactam antibiotics[181]
Carbamazepine[182]
Cinepazide[183,184]
Corticosteroids[185]
Cotrimoxazole,[186] other sulfonamides
Dipyridamole[172]
Deferasirox (Exjade)[187]
Dypirone[171,188]
Histamine-2 receptor antagonist[189]
Indomethacin[190]
Isoniazid[191,192]
Macrolides[193,194]
Mefloquine[195]
Nifedipine[196]
Phenytoin[197,198]
Procainamide[199,200]
Salicylates[201]
Sulfasalazine[202,203]
Sulfonylureas[204,205]
Tetracyclines[171]
Thenalidine
Thyrostatics[206–208]
Troxerutine[171]

ACE, Angiotensin-converting enzyme; IAAAS, International Agranulocytosis and Aplastic Anemia Study.

hematopoiesis, granulocyte sequestration, margination, and peripheral destruction. Neutropenia generally improves when the viremia resolves. Neutropenia has been associated with hepatitis A, B, and C viruses, EBV, influenza, measles, roseola, CMV, and parvovirus B19 infections. Neutropenia is also frequently encountered in patients with AIDS, with approximately 70% of patients being neutropenic during their illness. The mechanisms vary and may include antibody formation against neutrophils, direct viral inhibition of hematopoietic progenitor cells, abnormal expression of growth factors and other cytokines, and inhibitory effects exerted by HIV-infected accessory cells. The HIV virus not only suppresses hematopoiesis but also increases the risk for acquiring other infections. Furthermore, therapy with antiretroviral agents may dramatically decrease neutrophil counts (see Table 32.4).

Systemic bacterial, fungal, and parasitic infections can be accompanied by neutropenia, including typhoid fever, tularemia, brucellosis, mycobacterial infections, histoplasmosis, malaria, leishmaniasis, and ehrlichiosis. The pathogenesis includes margination and sequestration of leukocytes as observed in malaria, in which there is reduction in the circulating neutrophil pool and enlargement of the marginating granulocytes, primarily in the spleen and lung. Neutropenia can be present during sepsis, especially in newborns or debilitated individuals. In such situations, neutropenia may be caused by inhibition of hematopoiesis by inflammatory cytokines, exhaustion of marrow reserves, or redistribution.

Neutropenia Association With Nutritional Deficiency and Nutritional Excess

Malnutrition, dietary restrictions, malabsorptive states, and concomitant intake of inhibitory drugs are just a few common causes of nutritional deficiencies that may lead to neutropenia. Vitamin B_{12} and folate deficiency, frequently associated with megaloblastic anemia, can also be associated with neutropenia. Lack of these essential vitamin cofactors results in the impairment of normal DNA synthesis, leading to abnormal granulopoiesis. A frequently observed morphologic feature is the presence of hypersegmented neutrophils.

Copper deficiency may also be associated with neutropenia. Possible mechanisms may include arrest in maturation of neutrophil development as shown in studies in mice and increased antineutrophil antibody formation. Most cases have been found in malnourished infants, in patients with zinc intoxication and malabsorption states, and in persons receiving total parenteral nutrition without adequate copper supplementation. Copper deficiency is often accompanied by a normocytic anemia, whereas platelet counts are invariably normal. Other clinical and laboratory manifestations associated with copper deficiency include the presence of ringed sideroblasts in the bone marrow, macrocytic anemia, low ceruloplasmin levels, myeloneuropathy, and skeletal abnormalities. Zinc intoxication in the absence of concomitant copper deficiency has also been associated with neutropenia generally in conjunction with severe anemia.

Neutropenia Associated With Metabolic Disorders

Various acquired or inherited metabolic conditions may be associated with neutropenia. For example, neutropenia has been observed in patients with ketoacidosis and hyperglycemia, orotic aciduria, or methylmalonic aciduria. Similarly, glycogen storage disease type IB is commonly associated with neutropenia responsive to myeloid growth factors.

Acquired Neonatal Neutropenias

Neutropenia has been described in infants of hypertensive mothers. In this syndrome, the ANC can be severely depressed for up to 1 month postpartum. This type of neutropenia is associated with an increased risk for early-onset sepsis in neonates, a prolonged duration of neutropenia, and an increased risk for neonatal nosocomial infections. Granulocyte kinetic investigations suggested that the neutropenia is the result of diminished neutrophil production. An inhibitor released by the placenta and present in cord blood serum has been shown to play a role in this syndrome.

Moderate to severe neutropenia has also been observed secondary to IgG antibodies transferred from mother to infant. This is a condition called *isoimmune neonatal neutropenia* or *neonatal alloimmune neutropenia*. In most cases, antibodies are directed against antigens on neutrophil FcγRIIIb (anti-NA1, anti-NA2, and anti-SH)[209] and NB1,[210,211] but in rare circumstances maternal neutrophil-specific isoantibodies are also produced when there is deficiency of the *FcγRIIIb* gene. The incidence of this condition can be as high as 2:1000 live births. In both neutropenia occurring in hypertensive mothers and isoimmune neonatal neutropenia, differentiation from congenital forms of neutropenia may be difficult. Treatment with G-CSF is usually effective in neutropenia of infants of hypertensive mothers, but higher doses may be needed because preeclampsia-associated inhibitor of rhG-CSF may be present. IVIg and G-CSF are both effective for treatment of isoimmune neonatal neutropenia.

Neutropenia and Hypersplenism

Hypersplenism may be associated with neutropenia, but in most instances other cytopenias will also be present. However, hypersplenism may be a sign of diseases that can result in neutropenia, such as in T-LGL leukemia[212–214] and Felty syndrome. Other than direct sequestration, another potential mechanism leading to neutropenia may be increased neutrophil apoptosis that normalizes after splenectomy.[215] A high incidence of *Helicobacter pylori* infection has also been noted among individuals with neutropenia and splenomegaly. Splenectomy either laparoscopically or through laparotomy may be effective in most cases, although in situations precluding splenectomy, intraoperative splenic artery embolization is also effective.

Pure White Cell Aplasia

PWCA is a rare condition with pathophysiologic overlap with some forms of AIN associated with myeloid suppression. Similar to PRCA, the pathogenesis may vary and includes antibody-mediated suppression of granulopoiesis, T cell–mediated suppression of granulopoiesis, direct myelotoxicity as seen with certain drugs, opsonization of neutrophil precursors in the bone marrow leading to its destruction by macrophages within the bone marrow,[216] and formation of an antibody-complex that may damage myeloid progenitors.[217] A bone marrow examination reveals either a total absence of myeloid precursors or arrest at the promyelocyte stage, with megakaryocytes and the erythroid series remaining quantitatively and qualitatively normal. In many cases, a thymoma is present.[218] PWCA, if associated with thymoma, has a variable clinical outcome. The complete absence of granulocytic precursors portends a poor response to both immunosuppression and thymectomy and is often fatal, whereas the presence of a maturation arrest at the promyelocyte stage may respond to immunosuppressive therapy. PWCA has been described in connection with imipenem-cilastatin, ibuprofen, mesalamine, and chlorpropramide. The discontinuation of the offending drug leads to rapid improvement. PWCA has also been associated with primary biliary cirrhosis.

Therapeutic options may include azathioprine, G-CSF combined with plasmapheresis especially if the disease process is antibody-mediated, methylprednisolone, IV cyclophosphamide combined with plasmapheresis and G-CSF, and thymectomy. Severe depression of counts may require ATG therapy (see later).

Neutropenia Associated With Immunologic Abnormalities

Acquired and inherited defects of the cellular and humoral immune system may be accompanied by secondary neutropenias. In the inherited immunodeficiency syndromes, the initial presentation is neutropenic in children and may be associated with failure to thrive. X-linked agammaglobulinemia is a primary immunodeficiency disorder caused by mutations in the gene for Bruton tyrosine kinase (Btk) expressed in both myeloid and B cells that result in the absence of development of B lymphocytes and hypogammaglobulinemia. Neutropenia is seen in 15% to 26% of patients with X-linked agammaglobulinemia, and most suffer from upper respiratory tract infections. The exact pathogenetic mechanism is not clear but is believed to be related to the crucial role of Btk in myeloid survival under stress. Neutropenia is also seen in 40% to 50% of patients with X-linked hyper-IgM syndrome and has been associated with defects of myelopoiesis. The most common form of hyper IgM syndrome is caused by mutations in the *CD40* gene. This defect also leads to a decrease in IgG and IgA. In addition to chronic anemia, children suffer from various infectious complications. They typically lack ANAs and show an arrest at the promyelocyte-myelocyte stage of neutrophil development. Allogeneic HSCT has been curative in some instances. Common variable immunodeficiency can be associated with neutropenias that can be either chronic or episodic. In addition, hypergammaglobulinemia and hypogammaglobulinemia and T- and NK-cell abnormalities of various causes (both inherited and acquired) can also be associated with neutropenia.

Other Iatrogenic Forms of Neutropenia

Hemodialysis can result in neutropenia. One important mechanism postulated is through activation of the plasma complement pathway by dialyzer cellophane membranes and generation of C5a (desarg) that causes reversible neutrophil aggregation, resulting in transient neutropenia. Similar mechanisms to explain neutropenia have been suggested in other clinical settings, including leukapheresis and cardiopulmonary bypass surgery.

LABORATORY EVALUATION

Laboratory studies aim at the identification of the primary causes of neutropenia, as outlined in Fig. 32.4. Idiopathic and AIN remain, in most instances, diagnoses of exclusion. A careful history, including family history and initial age of first abnormal counts, help to distinguish familial neutropenias (see Chapter 29). Should primary causes such as drugs or systemic diseases be identified, the diagnostic evaluation will concentrate on disease-specific tests. In addition to a complete blood cell count and differential, which will help establish the severity of neutropenia, and tests to diagnose a specific disorder such as T-LGL leukemia, a bone marrow examination is required. Lack of morphologic or cytogenetic signs of primary hematologic diseases (e.g., MDS or aplastic anemia) and peripheral destruction will be supported by the observation of left shift and myeloid predominance. Inhibition of myeloid production is exemplified by an increased erythroid:myeloid ratio.

In some instances, auxiliary tests may help identify the cause of the neutropenia, including vitamin B_{12}, zinc, folate, or copper levels. Determination of immunoglobulin levels may be helpful to establishing the presence of immunodeficiency. Detection of ANAs has a limited significance because most of the currently available tests are not very sensitive and may not be specific. The presence of antibodies, however, may be helpful and supports the diagnosis of autoimmune forms of neutropenia.

DIFFERENTIAL DIAGNOSIS

Differential diagnostic consideration aims to distinguish primary from secondary forms of neutropenia and to exclude familial hematologic diseases. Suspicion of neutropenia secondary to a primary

hematologic disorder requires a bone marrow examination that may be consistent with an early form of aplastic anemia or MDS.

THERAPY

For secondary neutropenias, the therapy is aimed at the primary disease. If potentially offending drugs are present, they should be discontinued. G-CSF may be used for severe cases of both primary and secondary neutropenias. It may help to speed up recovery, but if the primary cause persists, it will have only a temporary effect. Primary or idiopathic neutropenias most often have an autoimmune cause. Prednisone may be used as first-line therapy, but other B cell–targeted agents may be needed, including rituximab. IVIg is effective in certain cases of PWCA. Finally, similar to the treatments applied for T-LGL leukemia, T cell–targeted approaches, such as CsA, can be used. A trial of at least 6 weeks is recommended. Similarly use of ATG has also been effective for cases of PWCA and other idiopathic forms of neutropenia. Weekly oral methotrexate is effective in treating neutropenia related to Felty syndrome and T-LGL leukemia. Of note, is that in many instances, isolated neutropenias may be asymptomatic, and therapy may not be needed. Alemtuzumab has been used with success in treating thymoma-associated PWCA and other cases of neutropenias.

LARGE GRANULAR LYMPHOCYTE LEUKEMIA

LGL leukemia is a chronic clonal lymphoproliferation of cytotoxic T cells (T-LGL) or NK cells (NK-LGL), often associated with cytopenias, including neutropenia, red cell aplasia, and thrombocytopenia. Pancytopenia is less frequently encountered and may be related to splenomegaly. T-LGL leukemia may be an indolent disorder and present with leukopenia or with lymphocytosis. LGLs observed on a peripheral smear are characteristic of T-LGL leukemia, but their frequency can vary.

T-LGL leukemia results from a proliferation of CTLs and often resembles reactive CTL expansion. It is associated with rheumatoid arthritis (11–36%) and B-cell malignancies (5–7%) and to a lesser extent with other autoimmune diseases such as Sjögren syndrome, celiac disease,[219] pulmonary hypertension, hematologic malignancies like MDS and HSCT. Most reactive processes are polyclonal, but immunodominant CTL clones may be present, making a distinction between true T-LGL and a reactive process difficult (Fig. 32.5). A

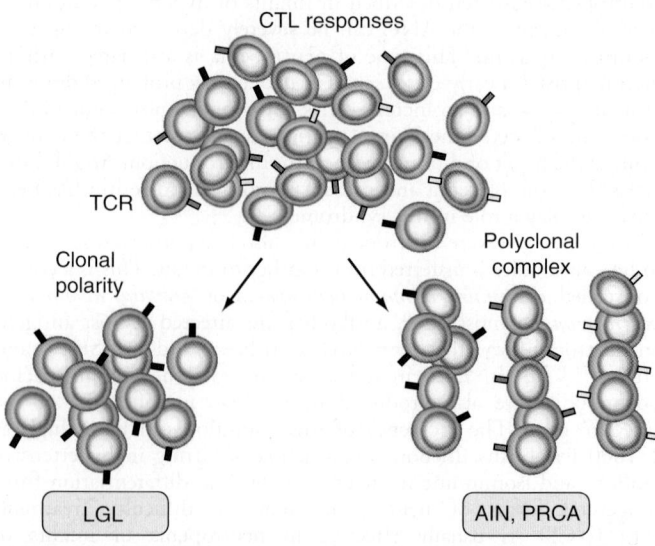

Fig. 32.5 PATHOPHYSIOLOGY OF CYTOTOXIC T-LYMPHOCYTE RESPONSES. *AIN,* Autoimmune neutropenia; *CTL,* cytotoxic T lymphocyte; *LGL,* large granular lymphocyte; *PRCA,* pure red cell aplasia; *TCR,* T-cell receptor.

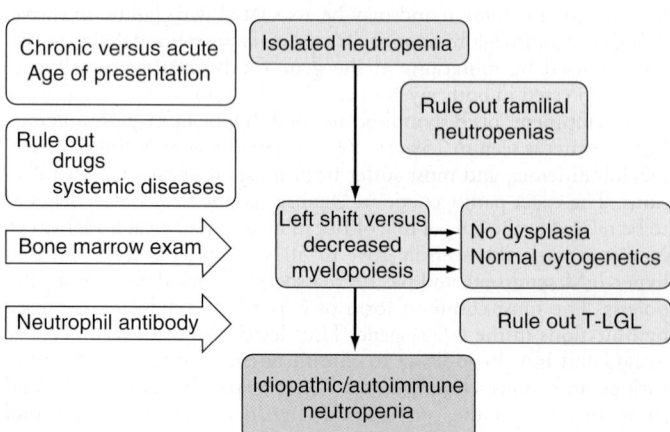

Fig. 32.4 EVALUATION OF PRIMARY AND SECONDARY NEUTROPENIA. *T-LGL,* T-cell large granular lymphocyte.

reduction in the variability of the CTL repertoire can occur in older adults, and clonal or oligoclonal expansion of CTL populations may be more frequent in older individuals. If asymptomatic, this disorder has been termed *monoclonal clonopathy of unclear significance.*

PATHOGENESIS

Inciting Events

T-LGL leukemia frequently arises in the context of a reactive polyclonal CTL expansion undergoing transformation in a manner similar to that proposed for CLL. It is possible also that in T-LGL leukemia one of the effector CTL clones may be initially driven by an inciting antigen, may transform, and consequently the cells fail to undergo apoptosis. The initial or initiating polyclonal response may be a component of the pathophysiologic process associated with infectious agents, rheumatoid arthritis, or other autoimmune disorders.

An initial T cell–mediated process may be responsible for cytopenias in the absence of clonal predominance. In concurrence with this hypothesis, the clinical spectrum of T-LGL is determined by the specificity of the TCR: for example, if myeloid precursors are targets of clonal CTL, neutropenia will be a clinical manifestation. Conversely, if erythroid progenitors are affected, patients will present with anemia (see Fig. 32.1 and Fig. 32.6). However, unlike the cytopenias that resolve following immunosuppression, the CTL clone may persist at a certain level, suggesting that other disease mechanisms involving soluble factors play a role in the development of the cytopenias. Various soluble agents, including (FasL) and perforin, have been implicated in the pathophysiology of the cytopenias in T-LGL leukemia.

Clonal Transformation

Clinically, T-LGL leukemia does not behave like a typical leukemia: excessive accumulation of malignant cells is often absent, and progression to a more malignant phenotype is rare. Instead, the expanded clone in T-LGL leukemia resembles a normal antigen-activated CD8$^+$CD57$^+$ effector cell; both normal and malignant LGL

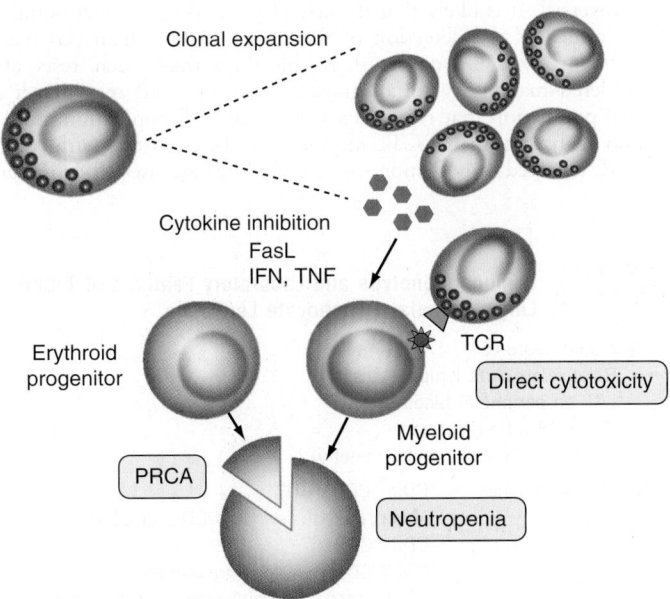

Fig. 32.6 PATHOPHYSIOLOGY OF CYTOPENIAS IN T-CELL LARGE GRANULAR LYMPHOCYTE LEUKEMIA. *FasL,* Fas ligand; *IFN,* interferon; *PRCA,* pure red cell aplasia; *TCR,* T-cell receptor; *TNF,* tumor necrosis factor.

constitutively express perforin and FasL and can suppress neutrophil development in vitro. Typical clonal LGL cells seem to be terminally differentiated and cannot be effectively expanded in vitro by polyclonal mitogens.

It is likely that a polyclonal CTL response predates the outgrowth of the immunodominant T-LGL leukemia clone (see Fig. 32.3). The putative transforming event most likely involves a memory cell that feeds into the mature effector CTL compartment. Under normal physiologic circumstances, activated effector T cells are deleted after antigen-driven expansion by Fas-mediated apoptosis. The failure of an activated memory and/or effector clone to undergo apoptosis may result in its persistent expansion. LGL leukemia cells express high levels of Fas/FasL, yet themselves are resistant to Fas-mediated apoptosis. It is conceivable that persistent LGL leukemia cell expansion may result from this resistance to homeostatic apoptosis. In addition to the high surface expression of Fas/FasL, soluble FasL has been detected in sera from T-LGL leukemia patients and may contribute to the induction of apoptosis of neutrophil precursors in the bone marrow.

An LGL clone persists mostly in the G_0/G_1 phase of cell cycle, and clonal transformation may also be because of a constitutive overexpression of prosurvival and antiapoptotic transcription factors. *STAT3* has been shown to be involved in cellular transformation along with an active Src family kinase and appears to be constitutively activated in T-LGL leukemia cells. In addition, a constitutive activation of an Src family kinase in T-LGL leukemia (likely Lck or Fyn) has been reported that may be related to this increased STAT phosphorylation.[220] It has been proposed that STAT3 activation in T-LGL may inhibit apoptosis downstream of Fas receptor signaling by induction of myeloid cell leukemia-1 (MCL1), a member of the B-cell lymphoma (BCL)2 family of antiapoptotic proteins. This finding is further supported by data showing that blockade of STAT signaling in T-LGL cells leads to the reversal of Fas resistance. Similarly, constitutive activation of the extracellular signal-related kinase mitogen-activated protein kinase pathway seems to play a role in survival of NK- and T-LGL leukemia cells.

Extreme Clonal Expansion and the Nonrandom Nature of the T-LGL

Molecular analysis of the TCR repertoire in T-LGL leukemia has revealed a spectrum of expansion of the T-cell clone in individual patients. In some cases, up to 98% of the CD8$^+$ repertoire consists of only one clone, a surprising finding given the absence of immunodeficiency among T-LGL leukemia patients. In healthy controls, even the most predominant clones, most likely reactive to ubiquitous antigens, represent around 1% of the entire TCR repertoire. It is possible that structurally similar clonotypes present in some patients with T-LGL arise in the context of initial polyclonal CTL response and the initial transformation step is not random (see Fig. 32.3). Once a pathogenic immunodominant clonotype is identified and characterized, its sequence may be used for molecular tracking.

Genetic Alterations in Large Granular Lymphocyte

No recurrent chromosomal aberrations or mutations have been found to be associated with LGL leukemia. Massively parallel second-generation sequencing technology has been used successfully to uncover the genetic background of LGL leukemia. Whole exome sequencing has aided in the discovery of somatic *STAT3* mutation, an oncogene located in chromosome 17 in 40% of the LGL cases. The *STAT3* missense mutations (D661V, D661Y, D661H, Y640F, N647I, and K658N), as well as the insertion mutation (Y657_K658insY), were located in the SH2 domain on the dimerization interface that mediates *STAT3* activation. *STAT3* mutations were detected in one-third cases of NK–LGL unifying T and NK cell lymphoproliferative pathogenesis. Several studies have identified *STAT3* and *STAT5b* mutations specific to LGL at various frequencies.

Of interest, patients with *STAT3* mutations were more likely to have autoimmune conditions and neutropenia and tend to respond to treatment. Sequencing of *STAT3* wildtype cases revealed activating mutations in *STAT5b* in 2% of the cases. *STAT3* and *STAT5b* mutations can be used as molecular markers for LGL leukemia diagnostics, and they present novel therapeutic targets for STAT3 and STAT5b inhibitors. Interestingly not only *STAT* mutations were identified in aplastic anemia and MDS cases with concomitant LGL but they were small clones in 7% of cases without clinical evidence of LGL.

CLINICAL PRESENTATION AND PHYSICAL FEATURES

Patients with T-LGL leukemia present at a median age of about 55 years, with an equal male/female distribution. The clinical course may be indolent and chronic. Patients are asymptomatic in one-third of cases. The most common clinical presentation is neutropenia (observed in approximately 85% of patients) often accompanied by infections or neutropenic fever. However, in contrast to neutropenia associated with other hematologic disorders, LGL leukemia patients may remain surprisingly free of infectious complications for extended periods of time regardless of the depressed ANC. Despite the extreme clonality within the T-cell population (suggesting a decreased antigen recognition spectrum), opportunistic infections are rare. Other single-lineage cytopenias, including PRCA and immune-mediated thrombocytopenia, accompany T-LGL leukemia less frequently than neutropenia. Pancytopenia may be related to splenomegaly reported in 20% to 50% of patients. Hepatomegaly is present in a minority of patients (10–20%). Lymphadenopathy and B symptoms may also occur; however, this is uncommon. It has been reported that pregnancy can improve neutropenia in women with LGL leukemia. Clinical transformation to a more malignant form is rare. The clinical presentation of NK-cell LGL lymphocytosis is very similar to that seen in T-LGL leukemia with regard to lymphocyte counts, associated conditions, treatment responses, and survival.

Clinical Overlap and Associations

In some clinical circumstances, natural or pathologic immune responses can resemble T-LGL expansions. For example, responses to viruses such as CMV or EBV, although of an oligoclonal or polyclonal nature, may display a strong clonal dominance mimicking at times a true clonal process. Consequently, polarized CTL responses in the context of infections have to be distinguished from true LGL leukemia. T-LGL leukemia can occur concomitantly with several autoimmune diseases. Rheumatoid arthritis is likely the most common association, occurring in one-third of patients with T-LGL leukemia, but additional diseases include ulcerative colitis, Sjögren syndrome, systemic lupus erythematosus, multiple sclerosis, and a number of other (auto)immune conditions have been described. Felty syndrome is characterized by neutropenia with rheumatoid arthritis and splenomegaly; 80% of cases express the HLA-DR4 allele, a finding also observed in T-LGL leukemia. This common immunogenetic link and similar patterns of cytotoxic clonal expansion with T-cell infiltration suggest that Felty syndrome and T-LGL leukemia represent components of the same disease process. In addition, PRCA and immune-mediated thrombocytopenia may also be associated with LGL lymphoproliferation. Clonal expansions that characterize T-LGL leukemia can appear similar to oligoclonal CTL responses elicited by strong immunodominant antigens, including certain viruses—thus the distinction between T-LGL leukemia and a reactive lymphoproliferative process. LGL leukemia has also been described after bone marrow and solid organ transplantation, perhaps initiated by an alloantigen or an infectious agent such as EBV.

LGL-like cell expansions may also be present in other hematologic disorders, including MDS, aplastic anemia, and paroxysmal nocturnal hemoglobinuria (PNH), and may coincide with a number of lymphoproliferative disorders as well. In MDS the prognosis is usually determined by the presence of MDS, but the presence of LGL

may provide a rational target for immunosuppressive therapy. In MDS, T-LGL leukemia has been reported to negatively affect the outcome of therapy directed against the CTL clone. LGL leukemia has also been described in conjunction with hemolytic anemia following bone marrow transplantation, perhaps a process initially driven by an alloantigen or infectious agent such as EBV. As with infections, distinction between an LGL leukemia and reactive lymphoproliferation may be blurred. For example, neutropenia may be associated with various degrees of clonality, with an LGL leukemia representing the most extreme form of this process.

LABORATORY DIAGNOSIS

Diagnostic criteria remain a subject of considerable discussion (Table 32.7). Traditionally LGL lymphocytosis (identified by morphologic characteristics and flow cytometry) is a significant diagnostic criterion. However, not all clonal cells display the typical morphologic features, and some patients present with leukopenia. Consequently an LGL count of greater than 2000/μL of blood has been abandoned as a strict diagnostic requirement, and lower numbers such as 0.400/μL of blood have been proposed.[212,221] Most investigators consider the presence of an expanded homogeneous CD3$^+$, TCR-αβ$^+$, CD8$^+$, CD16$^+$, CD28$^-$, CD57$^+$ cell population as diagnostic of T-LGL leukemia and CD2$^+$, sCD3$^-$, CD3ε$^+$, TCR-αβ$^-$, CD4$^-$, CD8$^+$, CD16$^+$, CD56$^+$, CD57$^{(variable)}$ for NK-LGL leukemia. In almost all patients the expanded clone is CD8$^+$ (only very rarely CD4$^+$), and in the majority of cases this population also expresses CD57, but LGL leukemia cases without this marker have been observed. Clinical correlations based on immunophenotypic characteristics have been defined; CD8$^{+(dim)}$/CD57$^+$ LGLs are associated with clonal T-LGL leukemia and neutropenia, CD16 expression with complete or partial loss of CD5 is associated with T-LGL leukemia but not cytopenias, and CD8$^{+(dim)}$/CD57$^+$ with loss of CD5 expression is associated with T-LGL leukemia with severe neutropenia. In addition, clinically aggressive T-LGL leukemia is characterized by expression of CD26. In most cases of LGL leukemia, CD94 is expressed at increased levels, and other receptors for class I MHC molecules are abnormally expressed. Some investigators have suggested that a pool of CD8$^+$ memory cells exists that lack CD57 expression but feed into the mature CD57 effector compartment. The size of the abnormal clone defining T-LGL leukemia remains controversial. It is likely that the size of the leukemic T-cell population influences the detection of the clonal TCR γ-chain (G) rearrangement by PCR or Southern blotting; thus, such tests are considered mandatory for diagnosis. These methods may detect a clonal population that represents 15% of the cell population, but it is also likely that smaller CTL numbers may be consistent with latent T-LGL detected only if more precise methods are used. T-LGL can

TABLE 32.7	Immunophenotype and Laboratory Features of T-Cell Large Granular Lymphocyte Leukemia
Laboratory features	
Relative/absolute lymphocytosis	
LGL on peripheral blood smear	
CD4/CD8 ratio reversed	
Vβ family skewing (flow cytometry)	
Immunophenotype	CD2$^+$, CD5$^+$, CD3$^+$
	Majority CD8$^+$, few CD4$^+$/CD8$^+$ or CD4$^+$
	CD27$^+$CD28$^-$
	CD57$^+$CD16$^+$ perforin/granzyme$^+$
	CD56$^+$ associated with more aggressive forms
TCR rearrangement	TCR-γ PCR
	Southern blot

LGL, Large granular lymphocyte; PCR, polymerase chain reaction; TCR, T-cell receptor.

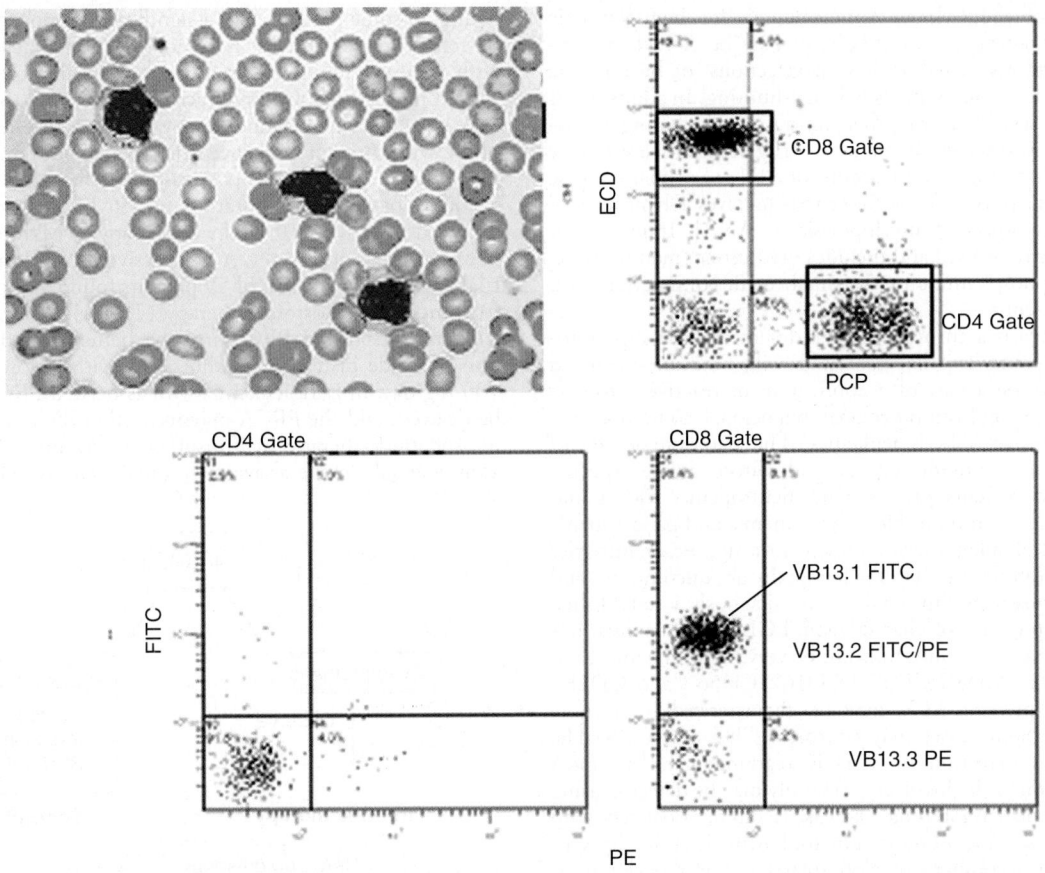

Fig. 32.7 MORPHOLOGIC FEATURES AND FLOW CYTOMETRY OF T-CELL LARGE GRANULAR LYMPHOCYTE. *ECD,* Ethyl cysteinate dimer; *FITC,* fluorescein isothiocyanate; *PCP,* phencyclidine hydrochloride; *PE,* phycoerythrin.

express CD4, but both CD4⁺ as well as double-positive CD4⁺/CD8⁺ cases are rare. Cytogenetic analyses are not useful, although cases with chromosomal aberrations have been described.

Flow cytometric analysis of Vβ utilization pattern with antibodies directed against most of the Vβ-chain types may be helpful in making the diagnosis. The Vβ family expansion by flow cytometry does not prove clonality, but it may help assess the contribution of the T-LGL clone to the CD8⁺ or CD4⁺ population (Fig. 32.7).

Rare immunophenotypic variants of T-LGL exist that coexpress CD4 and CD8, lack both of these markers, or use γ/δ TCR instead of α/β TCR chains. Vβ flow cytometry has been used to assess the size of the LGL clone and its Vβ use; Vβ use can be identified in 80% of patients. The current Vβ antibody panel does not cover 25% to 35% of the Vβ spectrum. In usual cases, T-LGL does not express CD56 antigen; the presence of this marker has been associated with a more aggressive clinical phenotype. A monotypic expression pattern of KIR can be found with monoclonal antibodies to CD157b, CD158a, and CD158e (corresponding to the most prevalent *KIR* genes) in about 50% of patients.

Additional supportive tests include a reticulocyte count, which is low in cases presenting with red cell aplasia. The mean corpuscular volume is usually high. Serologic studies or a DNA titer to detect evidence of an EBV infection is usually not needed but may be helpful to distinguish reactive immunologic responses. The rheumatoid factor is frequently positive. Antinuclear antibodies and ANAs may also at times be positive (see box on Approach to the Diagnosis and Treatment of Acquired PRCA, AIN, and T-LGL).

In cases with thymoma, thymectomy is the usual initial treatment approach; however, incomplete responders, nonresponders, and patients who relapse are common, necessitating the addition of immunosuppressive therapy. In patients with idiopathic PRCA,

---

Approach to the Diagnosis and Treatment of Acquired PRCA, AIN, and T-LGL

Acquired PRCA is characterized by reticulocytopenia, but the diagnosis is based on the morphologic absence of erythroid precursors in the bone marrow. Congenital forms of PRCA, including Diamond-Blackfan anemia, need to be distinguished when presenting in young children. In adults, primary idiopathic disease has to be differentiated from secondary forms of red cell aplasia associated with hematologic diseases such as B-cell chronic lymphocytic leukemia, myeloma, T-LGL leukemia, and parvovirus B19–associated chronic reticulocytopenia or acute transient aplastic crisis. The diagnosis of parvovirus B19 infection can be made on the basis of the presence of parvovirus B19–specific IgM and by DNA hybridization techniques. Parvovirus B19–specific polymerase chain reaction can help rule out an ongoing infection. This diagnosis is important because therapy with IVIg can be curative. The therapy of secondary red cell aplasia includes treatment of the underlying condition. It is also important to distinguish red cell aplasia from myelodysplastic syndromes, which can be associated with erythroid hypoplasia but carry a significantly worse prognosis.

AIN, autoimmune neutropenia; IVIg, intravenous immunoglobulin; PRCA, pure red cell aplasia; T-LGL, T-cell large granular lymphocyte.

---

therapy includes immunosuppressive agents such as prednisone, CsA, or oral cyclophosphamide. Second-line therapies include ATG or rituximab.

Neutropenia may be associated with severe infections, but the risk associated with neutropenia depends on its clinical context, severity, and duration. The management of neutropenia must account for its clinical presentation and the risk for possible life-threatening complications and includes supportive care, clinical monitoring, and implementation of prophylactic antibiotics and/or hematopoietic growth factors. Neutropenia in childhood may be caused by congenital diseases, be associated with viral infections, or be immune mediated. These three causes are usually self-limiting. In adults, most neutropenias are secondary to other conditions, including hematologic or systemic diseases. In general, drug reactions are a very common cause of neutropenia. Idiopathic or AIN as a primary disease is a diagnosis of exclusion. The pathogenesis involves T-lymphocyte/NK–mediated inhibition of myelopoiesis or ANAs. Immunosuppressive therapy may be used and includes prednisone, methotrexate, CsA, IVIg, cyclophosphamide or rituximab or in conjunction with myeloid growth factors.

T-LGL leukemia is a chronic, often indolent clonal lymphoproliferation of cytotoxic T cells associated with immune-mediated cytopenias. It may be a part of a continuum of reactive cytotoxic T-cell responses ranging from polyclonal, oligoclonal, to monoclonal expansions as seen in T-LGL leukemia. The pathophysiology of cytopenias includes cytokine effects and direct antigen-specific cytotoxicity. Most patients present with neutropenia. PRCA and pancytopenia are less common. Hemolytic anemia and pancytopenia may be the result of splenomegaly present in a significant minority of patients. B symptoms and lymphadenopathy are uncommon, and many patients remain asymptomatic. The diagnosis is established according to the presence of characteristic LGL lymphocytosis, but in some patients the LGL count may not be very high. The immunophenotype is $CD3^+$, $CD8^+$, $CD57^+$, $CD16^+$, $CD56^-$, and $CD28^-$. CD56 antigen–expressing LGL may be characterized by a more aggressive course. Some cases may coexpress CD4 and CD8. The diagnosis includes detection of a TCR rearrangement. In most instances, expansion of the involved Vβ family may be detected using Vβ flow cytometric clonotyping. T-LGL is often associated with autoimmune diseases, including rheumatoid arthritis and Felty syndrome. T-LGL can accompany myelodysplasia and, in rare instances, aplastic anemia or PNH. Reactive, often viral infection–associated, CTL proliferation may be difficult to document. Asymptomatic cases are monitored, and development of systemic symptoms or symptomatic cytopenias may prompt therapy. Current treatments include immunosuppressive agents such as prednisone, CsA, oral methotrexate, or cyclophosphamide. Chronic long-term therapy may be more effective than high-dose combination chemotherapy applied in B-cell lymphomas. Second-line treatments may involve alemtuzumab or ATG. The prognosis is generally good, and transformation to a more aggressive lymphoproliferative disorder is rare.

Unless additional hematologic diseases, such as MDS, are suspected, bone marrow examination may not be required. Bone marrow biopsy and aspirate should be obtained in cases of pancytopenia or involvement of several lineages. Morphologic hallmarks of MDS and cytogenetic analysis may help establish a diagnosis of MDS.

DIFFERENTIAL DIAGNOSIS

Differential diagnostic considerations include reactive processes such as viral infections. Occasionally MDS may be present simultaneously or serve as an alternative diagnosis; T-cell oligoclonality may accompany MDS.

THERAPY

A significant proportion of patients will be asymptomatic, and in such cases therapy may be delayed. Lymphocytosis may be significant, but absolute lymphocyte counts more than 40,000/µL is unusual. Symptomatic splenomegaly may be an indication for splenectomy. Pancytopenia may be a result of splenomegaly, and the procedure aids in the treatment of a hemolytic anemia that can be present in some patients.

Patients may tolerate significant degrees of neutropenia for many years. Indications for treatment include neutropenic complications or transfusion dependence (Fig. 32.8). G-CSF therapy will increase

counts in some patients, but a significant proportion of patients will be refractory. Of interest is the observation that high-dose therapy with typical lymphoma regimens may be ineffective and therefore should not be used. Cases refractory to bone marrow transplantation have been described. Monotherapy with prednisone may relieve some of the symptoms and improve neutropenia, but remissions are usually not durable. CsA represents a reasonable first-line therapy; however, a course of sufficient duration has to be given, with a response expected after 8 to 10 weeks of therapy. Weekly oral methotrexate has been used successfully. A prospective phase II multicenter clinical trial analyzing treatment of 59 patients found a response rate of 38% to frontline methotrexate therapy (Table 32.8). Patients with LGL leukemia–associated PRCA may be better treated with oral cyclophosphamide instead of methotrexate with a dose between 50 and 100 mg/day. In LGL leukemia with associated PRCA, responses may be delayed, and the PRCA may recur after discontinuation of cyclophosphamide therapy, or if insufficient treatment (<6–8 weeks) was administered. In the above-mentioned trial, overall response rate to

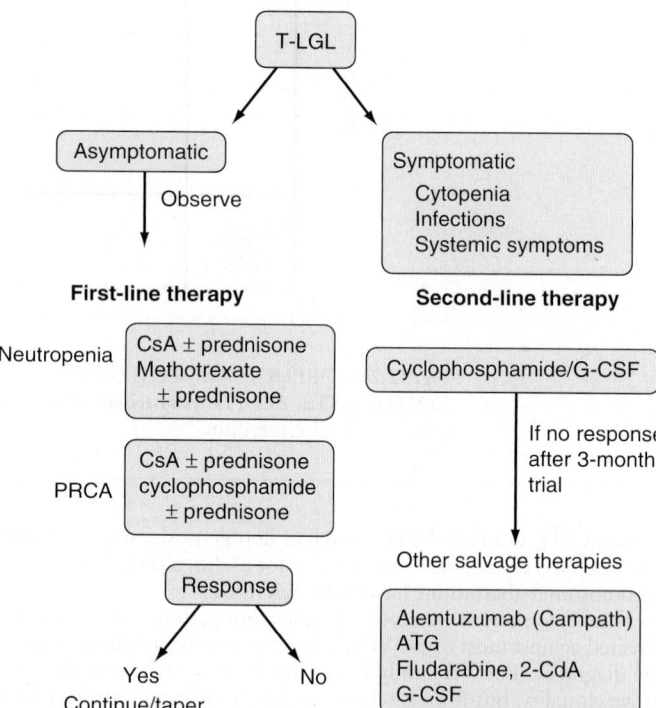

Fig. 32.8 THERAPY OF T-CELL LARGE GRANULAR LYMPHOCYTE LEUKEMIA. *ATG,* Antithymocyte globulin; *2-CdA,* 2-chlorodeoxyadenosine; *CsA,* cyclosporine A; *G-CSF,* granulocyte colony-stimulating factor; *PRCA,* pure red cell aplasia; *T-LGL,* T-cell large granular lymphocyte.

TABLE 32.8	Metaanalyses of Studies for Response to Therapy in Large Granular Lymphocyte Leukemia						
Study	N	MTX (N)	OR (%)	CsA (N)	OR (%)	CPM (N)	OR (%)
French Registry[a]	229	62	34 (55)	24	5 (21)	32	21 (66)
Battiwalla et al[b]	25			25	14 (56)		
Moignet et al[a]	45					45	32 (71)
Osuji et al[a]	29	8	6 (85)	23	18 (78)	4	1 (25)
Dhodapkar[b]	68	2	2 (100)			16	11 (69)
Loughran[c]	59	55	21 (38)			14	9 (64)

[a]Retrospective analysis from multiple centers.
[b]Retrospective analysis in single center.
[c]Multicenter phase 2 trial.
CPM, Cyclophosphamide; CsA, cyclosporine A; MTX, methotrexate; OR, overall response.

cyclophosphamide was 64% following initial methotrexate therapy. Therapy with cyclophosphamide in neutropenic patients may be difficult because of myelosuppression. In most refractory cases, ATG has also been used with success. In recent years, successful therapy with alemtuzumab has been reported. CD52 expression determined by flow cytometry is an important predictive factor for response to alemtuzumab. High response rates with the Janus-activated kinase inhibitor, tofacitinib citrate have been observed (66%) when used as a salvage therapy. Currently such a therapy is approved in cases of LGL with rheumatoid arthritis. Purine analogues like fludarabine given in combination with mitoxantrone and dexamethasone or with dexamethasone alone have been shown to produce impressive responses of 79%, although these were confined to a small group of patients. Allogeneic HSCT has also been used successfully in some cases. Relapses are frequent but are usually responsive to the previously effective therapy. Certain patients may require low-dose maintenance therapy with CsA. In some cases, remarkable improvement of cytopenia can be achieved with splenectomy.

PROGNOSIS

LGL leukemia is a chronic condition and may be indolent. In general, mortality is low. Transformation to more aggressive forms of lymphomas or leukemias is uncommon. In cases of T-LGL leukemia associated with a primary hematologic disease such as MDS, the prognosis is dependent on the therapy of the underlying problem.

ACQUIRED PLATELET PRODUCTION DISORDER

Megakaryocytes, like all formed elements of the peripheral blood, are ultimately derived from undifferentiated hematopoietic stem cells that exist in a developmental continuum (see Chapter 28). Through a series of still incompletely understood events, stem cells undergo an asynchronous division that gives rise to two daughter cells. One daughter cell remains a stem cell, fulfilling the requirement for self-renewal of the stem cell compartment, and the other commits to developing within a given lineage, likely through the induction of specific transcription factors such as GATA1, FOG-1, and Fli-1, in the case of megakaryocytes, and perhaps by downmodulation of other transcription factors, such as c-Myb. Lineage-committed progenitor cells are characterized by a loss of "plasticity" and a remarkable capacity for proliferation. The latter is required because approximately 15 $\times 10^6$ megakaryocytes/kg body weight must be available to produce the roughly 100×10^9 new platelets that are needed daily to maintain a normal platelet count of 150–400 $\times 10^9$/L. As progenitor cell divisional activity proceeds, maturation, as defined by the acquisition of lineage-specific proteins, ensues, largely under the control of the hematopoietic cytokine thrombopoietin. After a variable number of mitoses, proliferative activity eventually declines, giving rise to many daughter cells, which are known as *precursors*. Precursor cells are essentially postmitotic and are capable of one or two additional cell divisions at most. They are often morphologically identifiable as belonging to a given lineage and are primarily engaged in the terminal maturation steps that allow them to function as competent members of their lineage. In the case of megakaryocytes, precursor cells undergo nuclear endoreduplication to increase their ploidy (to a mean of approximately 16 N), a characteristic unique to cells of the megakaryocyte lineage. Nuclear endoreduplication is accompanied by an increase in megakaryocyte cytoplasm and thereby the number of platelets that an individual megakaryocyte can produce.

As discussed in Chapter 28, the process of platelet formation, or thrombopoiesis, occurs during megakaryocyte terminal maturation. It is initiated by the development of the demarcation membrane system in the megakaryocyte's cytoplasm. Among the functions of the demarcation membrane system is delineation of platelet fields. These fields are filled with the granules and proteins that ultimately make up the contents of mature platelets. The latter are shed from pseudopods that mature megakaryocytes extend through endothelial cell junctions into the lumen of marrow capillaries. The pseudopods fracture, because of shear stress in the lumen of these capillaries, and release shards of megakaryocytic cytoplasm, or proplatelets, that are the immediate antecedents of circulating platelets. A fully mature megakaryocyte is estimated to produce approximately 1–1.5 $\times 10^3$ platelets. The molecular regulation of this process is beginning to be better understood. It has been shown, for example, that the apoptosis-stimulating gene *Bax* promotes platelet production. Interestingly, very recent evidence suggests that the life span of circulating platelets is also regulated by the apoptosis proteins. Using the strategy of ethylnitrosourea-inducted mutations, Mason et al[222] have recently demonstrated that mutations in the *Bcl-x_L* gene lead to synthesis of a form of the protein that no longer inhibits *Bax*, and that this in turn leads to accelerated platelet death and a heritable form of thrombocytopenia (Fig. 32.9).

Failure in the process of either megakaryocytopoiesis or thrombopoiesis will result in thrombocytopenia. Under either circumstance, platelet production is characterized as "ineffective," either because there is an absolute decrease in available megakaryocyte cytoplasm (failure of megakaryocytopoiesis) or because cytoplasmic development is defective (failure of thrombopoiesis). Selective impairment of megakaryocytopoiesis may also result from damage to the progenitor cell compartment (the burst-forming units–megakaryocyte or colony-forming units–megakaryocyte [CFU-Mk]; see Chapter 28) or rarely from a compromised ability to synthesize thrombopoietin, the chief cytokine regulator of this compartment (Fig. 32.10). Inherent or acquired defects in megakaryocyte precursor cells may

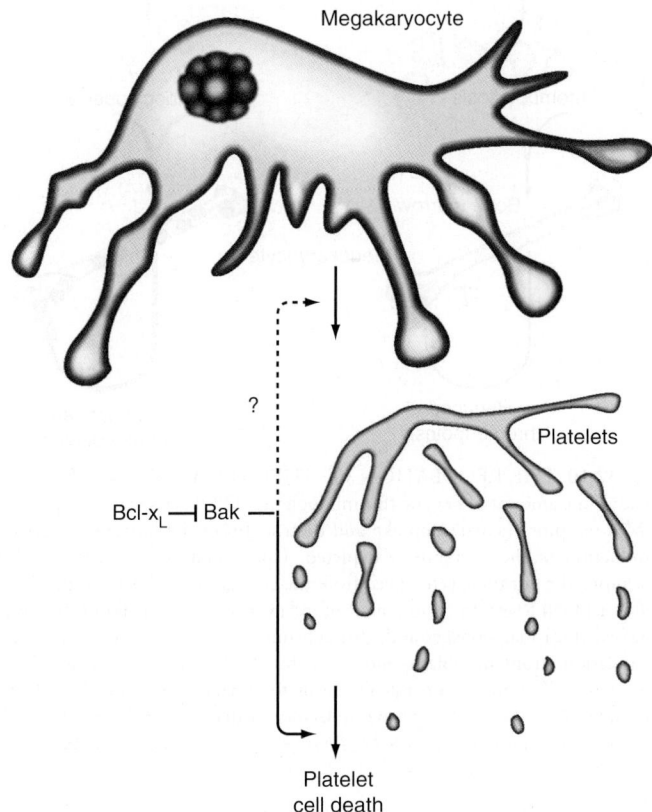

Fig. 32.9 BCL-X_L AND PLATELET LIFE SPAN. Mason et al[222] subjected mice to ethylnitrosourea mutagenesis and screened their first-generation offspring for platelet deficiency. They identified two mutations in the gene encoding the antiapoptotic factor Bcl-x_L that give rise to a dominantly inherited reduction in platelet count. Bcl-x_L appears to promote platelet survival through inhibition of the proapoptotic activity of Bak. Bax promotes production of platelets,[223] and overexpression of antiapoptotic Bcl-x_L impairs the fragmentation of megakayocytes.[224] *(Modified from Qi B, Hardwick JM: A Bcl-x_L timer sets platelet life span. Cell 128:1035, 2007.)*

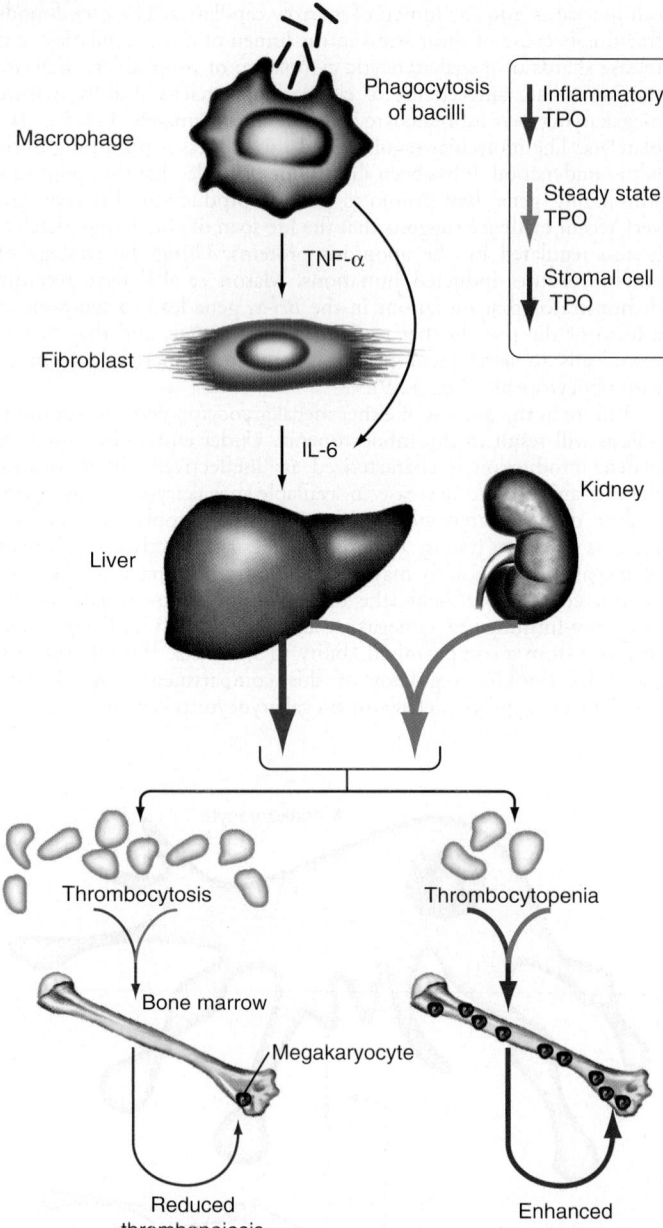

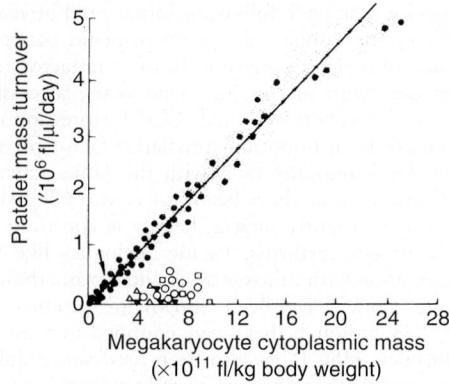

Fig. 32.11 INEFFECTIVE PLATELET PRODUCTION. In thrombocytopenia, the relationship between marrow megakaryocyte cytoplasmic mass and the turnover of platelet mass in the peripheral blood is usually direct. Platelet mass turnover represents the product of the mean megakaryocyte cytoplasmic volume multiplied by the total number of marrow megakaryocytes. The results in normal patients are indicated by the *arrow,* and the *stippled area* represents 95% of confidence limits in thrombocytopenic patients with effective production. Ineffective thrombocytopoiesis is identified as a disparity between available marrow substrate (megakaryocyte cytoplasmic mass) and delivery of platelet mass to the peripheral blood (platelet mass turnover). Results in patients with autosomal dominant thrombocytopenia *(open circles),* Wiskott-Aldrich syndrome *(open triangles),* megaloblastic anemia *(open squares),* and preleukemia *(closed triangles)* are characterized by ineffective platelet production. *(Data from Thompson A, Harker L: Quantitative platelet disorders. In Manual of hemostasis and thrombosis, Philadelphia, 1983, FA Davis, p 65.)*

Fig. 32.10 THE REGULATION OF THROMBOPOIETIN LEVELS. A steady-state amount of hepatic thrombopoietin (TPO) is regulated by platelet c-Mpl receptor–mediated uptake and destruction of the hormone. Hepatic production of the hormone is depicted. Upon binding to platelet c-Mpl receptors, the hormone is removed from the circulation and destroyed, which reduces blood levels. In the presence of inflammation, interleukin-6 (IL-6) is released from macrophages and, through tumor necrosis factor-α (TNF-α) stimulation, from fibroblasts and circulates to the liver to enhance TPO production. Thrombocytopenia also leads to enhanced marrow stromal cell production of TPO, although the molecular mediator(s) of this effect is not yet completely understood. *(Modified from Kaushansky K: The molecular mechanisms that control thrombopoiesis.* J Clin Invest *115:3339, 2005.)*

lead to ineffective thrombopoiesis. The relative effectiveness of platelet production can be calculated by measuring platelet mass turnover, which is defined as the product of the mean megakaryocyte cytoplasmic volume multiplied by the total number of marrow megakaryocytes. A disparity between cytoplasmic mass and platelet delivery to blood (platelet count divided by platelet survival, corrected for splenic pooling) is the hallmark of ineffective platelet production (Fig. 32.11). An examination of the peripheral blood

smear is the first step in the initial assessment of patients who present with thrombocytopenia. The presence of platelet clumps, indicative of pseudothrombocytopenia, or abnormally large, or small, platelets can be very useful in generating a differential diagnosis, as can the presence of inclusion bodies in neutrophils. Nevertheless, the current gold standard for diagnosing thrombocytopenia caused by ineffective platelet production is a bone marrow aspirate and biopsy. At the moment, direct visualization of the marrow and its cellular contents is the only way to judge the quantity and quality of the megakaryocyte population (Fig. 32.12). However, noninvasive methods for making a diagnosis of ineffective platelet production are being developed. For example, the concentration of serum glycocalicin, the soluble fragment of glycoprotein Ib, has been shown to be significantly diminished in patients with platelet production abnormalities when compared with normal control patients.[225] Reticulated platelets, like RBC reticulocytes, contain ribonucleic acid (RNA). It has been suggested that as is true for RBC reticulocytes, the presence of residual RNA in platelets indicates that they have been newly formed. Thus, they may be useful for assessing the dynamics of platelet production under baseline conditions and after marrow insults such as chemotherapy or irradiation. Platelet RNA can be detected by staining with dyes such as thiazole orange, and it has been suggested that assessing the mean thiazole orange staining can be used to construct a reticulated platelet maturation index. Another approach to assessing platelet production is the measurement of serum thrombopoietin levels. Thrombopoietin is synthesized constitutively in the liver and then binds to its receptor c-Mpl on megakaryocytes and platelets. Accordingly, in patients with disorders in which megakaryocytes are reduced in the marrow, thrombopoietin levels rise. However, the wide variation in "normal" thrombopoietin concentrations in serum make this determination somewhat problematic as well. Some of this variability may be attributed to the fact that thrombopoietin synthesis is inducible in marrow stromal cells, perhaps by platelet α-granule proteins. Reports attesting to the increased reliability and precision of measuring several of these parameters at once have appeared, but it remains unclear whether the expense and time involved will prove

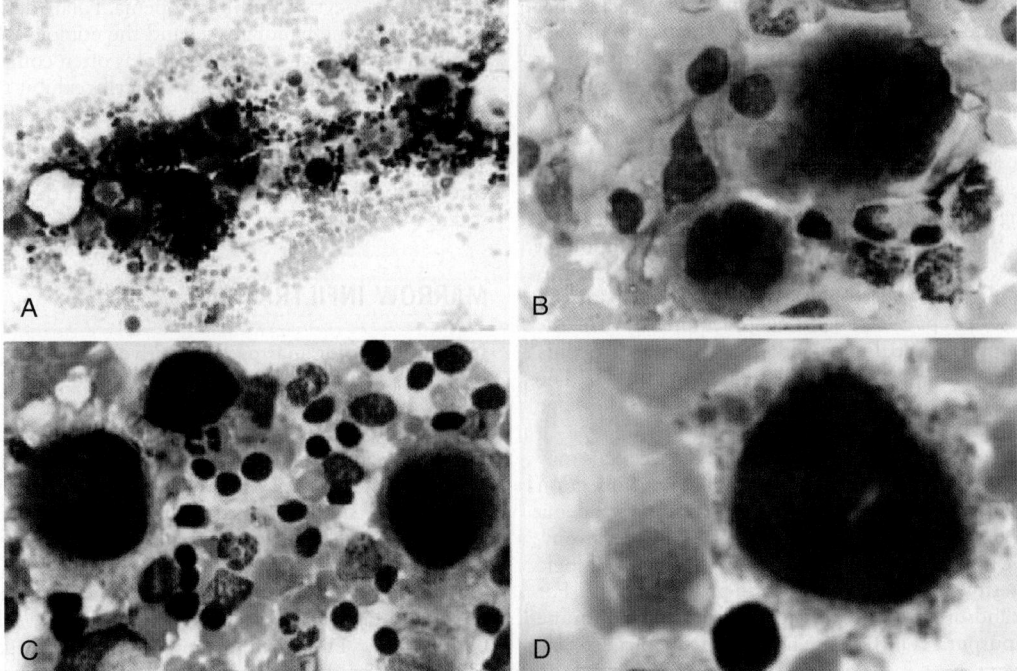

Fig. 32.12 MARROW ASPIRATE OBTAINED FROM A CHILD WITH THROMBOCYTOPENIA AND DYSMEGAKARYOCYTOPOIESIS. The megakaryocytes are small and hypolobular, with diminished cytoplasm. Cells are viewed at magnifications of 250× (A), 1000× (B), 200× (C), and 1600× (D). *(From van den Oudenrijn S, Bruin M, Folman CC, et al: Three parameters: Plasma thrombopoietin levels, plasma glycocalicin levels, and megakaryocyte culture, distinguish between different causes of congenital thrombocytopenia. Br J Haematol 117:390, 2002.)*

cost-effective when compared with the relative simplicity of a bone marrow examination.

As is true for the congenital thrombocytopenias, acquired thrombocytopenia can be caused by a failure of either megakaryocytopoiesis or thrombopoiesis. Of these two possibilities, ineffective thrombopoiesis is the more likely cause, because pure megakaryocyte aplasia or hypoplasia is quite rare. Indeed, thrombocytopenia secondary to decreased marrow megakaryocytes is much more likely to be a prodrome of aplastic anemia, or an early form of MDS. Clues to these conditions can be found in the marrow, where often subtle abnormalities of other hematopoietic lineages, such as macrocytosis or dyserythropoiesis, can be observed.

SELECTIVE MEGAKARYOCYTE APLASIA

Acquired selective amegakaryocytic thrombocytopenia is quite rare. It is almost always because of an autoimmune mechanism, either antibody- or cell-mediated. Autoantibodies reacting with megakaryocytes or their progenitor cells, presumably leading to their destruction, have been described. Antibodies directed to cytokines that regulate megakaryocyte development, in particular thrombopoietin, might also play a role in the biogenesis of such disorders. Cases of cell-mediated suppression of megakaryocytopoiesis leading to a complete selective megakaryocyte aplasia have also been described. In these cases, suppression was shown in one case to be caused by autoreactive T lymphocytes, whereas a macrophage-derived "factor" was implicated in the other.

Patients in whom an autoimmune mechanism is operative may respond to treatment with cyclosporine and ATG, achieving durable remissions. Cytotoxic antibodies directed toward the CFU-Mk may be treated with corticosteroids, plasmapheresis, IVIg, danazol, cyclosporine, or cyclophosphamide. Patients with T cell–mediated inhibition of megakaryocytopoiesis may respond to ATG, cyclosporine, or hematopoietic growth factors. If a particular drug or toxin exposure is believed to be responsible, for example ethanol or a thiazide diuretic, then withdrawal of the offending agent is obviously indicated. If the cause is viral, IVIg or anti-HIV therapies are indicated. Despite the various causes of ineffective thrombopoiesis, immunosuppressive therapy was found to be effective in 8 out of 30 patients.

INFECTION

Many infectious diseases are associated with thrombocytopenia, and it is likely that infection is the greatest noniatrogenic cause of ineffective platelet production. Infectious agents associated with decreased platelet counts include mycoplasma, mycobacteria, ehrlichiosis, and malaria. In these disorders, the cause of the thrombocytopenia is believed to be diminished platelet production although immune-mediated thrombocytopenia has also been described in some patients.

Viral infections are by far the most common infectious agents associated with thrombocytopenia caused by ineffective megakaryocyte or platelet production. Thrombocytopenia has been reported in cases of mumps, rubella, measles, varicella, CMV, infectious mononucleosis, chickenpox, dengue and other hemorrhagic fevers, hepatitis, and parvovirus infections. Live measles virus vaccination can also induce thrombocytopenia arising from decreased production. The mechanism responsible for viral suppression of platelet counts is not completely clear. It is known that megakaryocytes are capable of being infected by a variety of viruses. Infected cells may appear dysplastic, with inclusion bodies, vacuoles, or degenerating nuclei. Naked megakaryocyte nuclei may be seen in particular after HIV infection. That such cytopathic cells might have trouble producing platelets is not difficult to imagine. Recently it has been demonstrated that dengue directly binds to dendritic cell-specific intracellular adhesion molecule-3 on the surface of platelets, and could replicate its viral RNA by usurping the translational machinery of platelets and raising the possibility that other (+)ssRNA viruses may be similarly propagated by these anucleate cytoplasts.

Perhaps the best studied virally induced thrombocytopenia is that associated with HIV infection. Mild to moderate reduction in platelet counts is quite common in patients with this disease. In a large study of HIV-positive patients with hemophilia, the cumulative frequency of thrombocytopenia 6 years after seroconversion was 16% for children and 18% for adults. At 10 years, the frequency increased to 27% in children and 43% in adults. In another study, the frequency of thrombocytopenia was 16% among 103 homosexual men and 37% among 182 IV drug users with a new diagnosis of HIV infection. Thrombocytopenia was also reported to be relatively common in HIV-negative homosexual men (3%) and IV drug users (9%). It was speculated that this might be caused by the high rates of hepatitis in these patient groups. Except for patients who acquire HIV in the background of hemophilia, bleeding secondary to thrombocytopenia is unusual, because the counts are rarely less than 50,000/μL. The principal cause of thrombocytopenia appears to vary with the stage of disease.

Examination of a bone marrow aspirate and biopsy specimens may be required to assess whether infiltration by granulomatous infection or a malignancy is contributing to, or causing, the thrombocytopenia in an HIV patient. Assuming no other obvious cause of the thrombocytopenia, and the presence of typical megakaryocytic morphologic abnormalities, antiretroviral therapy is the principal treatment. For patients with severe and/or symptomatic thrombocytopenia, immune thrombocytopenia purpura (ITP) regimens, including splenectomy, may well be effective.

CHEMOTHERAPY AND IRRADIATION

Chemotherapy and irradiation reliably damage bone marrow in a dose-dependent fashion. Megakaryocytes and their progenitors seem to be particularly sensitive to the effects of these agents. As a result, thrombocytopenia is one of the most frequent adverse effects of total body irradiation and chemotherapy. Allogeneic or autologous marrow transplantation is often complicated by prolonged thrombocytopenia, which may persist long after restoration of neutrophil and RBC counts. Various strategies to ameliorate this problem have been tried, including the use of peripheral blood "stem cells," which may lead to a faster rate of platelet recovery when compared with marrow transplantation. More recently, attempts have been made to expand megakaryocyte progenitor cells, with cMpl agonists including Nplate and Promacta.

Alkylating agents in general produce more prolonged thrombocytopenia than antimetabolites. It has been claimed that some alkylating agents spare megakaryocytes (e.g., cyclophosphamide), but this is a relative phenomenon. Agents such as busulfan, the nitrosoureas, or platinum may cause cumulative damage of the more primitive progenitor cells. Other chemotherapeutic agents, such as the vinca alkaloids, may not decrease the platelet count significantly.

Various potential mechanisms for the relative sparing of platelet production by certain chemotherapeutic regimens have been investigated. For patients who suffer from severe or prolonged thrombocytopenia, reducing the intensity of the chemotherapy is the most appropriate approach to management. It had been anticipated that the use of recombinant thrombopoietin or Promacta might significantly ameliorate this problem.

At the present time, in addition to cMpl-agonists Nplate and Promacta supportive therapy with platelet transfusions and drugs such as ε-aminocaproic acid for patients who have become refractory to platelet transfusions remain the mainstays of therapy.

NUTRITIONAL DEFICIENCIES

Thrombocytopenia of various degrees can be observed in patients with either folate or vitamin B_{12} deficiency. The mechanism of thrombocytopenia is ineffective platelet production. Megakaryocyte numbers are normal or increased in the marrow, and platelet survival is normal or slightly shortened. Vitamin B_{12} deficiency was reported to cause a case

of amegakaryocytic thrombocytopenia. Folate deficiency is frequently associated with ethanol abuse, and the etiology of the thrombocytopenia in patients who abuse ethanol is often complex.

Patients with iron deficiency typically exhibit thrombocytosis, but rare patients may become thrombocytopenic. The extremely rapid increase in platelet counts after initiation of iron therapy suggested an essential role for iron in a late stage of thrombopoiesis. Curiously, thrombocytopenia has been caused by iron therapy in a patient with severe iron deficiency.

MARROW INFILTRATION

It is not rare for marrow infiltrative diseases of any type to cause ineffective hematopoiesis. Blood cell production disorders are commonly observed when the marrow is involved with metastatic cancer, lymphoma, or leukemia. Table 32.3 categorizes the infiltrative processes associated with thrombocytopenia. Physical replacement of marrow is the cause of the thrombocytopenia in many cases; it is also possible that inhibitory factors produced by the infiltrating cells are toxic to the cells of the megakaryocytic lineage or interfere with normal regulatory mechanisms. The diagnosis of infiltrative disease is made by marrow examination, although diagnostic clues are usually provided by history, physical examination, and a leukoerythroblastic blood smear. The marrow shows decreased megakaryocytes, which may be larger than normal because of a compensatory physiologic response to the thrombocytopenia.

ETHANOL-RELATED DISORDERS

Ethanol abuse is very commonly associated with thrombocytopenia, which may result from several different mechanisms. These include, most commonly, increased splenic pooling as a result of portal hypertension and ineffective production related to folate deficiency (which may lead to severe thrombocytopenia). Ethanol itself can be directly toxic to the marrow. In vitro studies have shown that alcohol concentrations achievable in vivo inhibit megakaryocyte maturation but do not inhibit CFU-Mk. Megakaryocyte numbers usually are normal, but markedly decreased megakaryocytes have been observed. Rarely, marrow panhypoplasia has been observed in association with alcohol ingestion. Anemia and macrocytosis accompanied by megaloblastic changes and ringed sideroblasts in the erythroid marrow are typically observed in the marrows of patients who abuse ethanol.

OTHER DRUG-RELATED DISORDERS

A variety of drugs and toxins have been implicated in the etiology of isolated platelet production defects. Estrogen, for example, has been reported to decrease platelet counts through an unknown mechanism. Thrombocytopenia arising from thiazide diuretics has been reported frequently. Although the cause of the thrombocytopenia in most cases is probably increased clearance, decreased marrow megakaryocyte numbers have been noted. Interferon and IL-2 may induce thrombocytopenia. The most likely explanation is inhibition of CFU-Mk. Anagrelide is a very useful drug for lowering platelet counts in patients with myeloproliferative neoplasms and appears to work by reducing megakaryocyte size and ploidy and by disrupting maturation

Paroxysmal Nocturnal Hemoglobinuria

PNH is a clonal disorder resulting from mutations in the X-linked gene PIGA that encodes for an enzyme required in the initial step of biosynthesis of glycosylphosphatidylinositol anchors (PNH is discussed in Chapter 31). Approximately 25% of patients with PNH have significant marrow aplasia. Thrombocytopenia at diagnosis is a poor prognostic indicator. Because platelet survival is usually normal

Compiling a thorough patient history is the first step in a complete workup of a thrombocytopenic patient. Many potential causes will be revealed by a good history, including obtaining a family history of thrombocytopenia, recent infection, medication or substance ingestion, radiation or chemotherapy.

A careful physical examination could also contribute to making a diagnosis. For example, physical findings suggesting any of the inherited disorders described earlier might be discerned, as might findings suggestive of malignancy such as enlarged lymph nodes. Splenomegaly itself is not indicative of a platelet production abnormality but is often found in patients with lymphoma or other processes associated with marrow infiltration and damage that might cause impaired thrombopoiesis.

The peripheral blood smear is next examined, and this is needed to rule out pseudothrombocytopenia. Moreover, the blood smear provides additional clues to both the pathophysiologic mechanism of the thrombocytopenia and the diagnosis. For example, giant platelets suggest a hereditary or myelodysplastic syndrome; oval macrocytosis and hypersegmented neutrophils suggest a folate or vitamin B_{12} deficiency; and a leukoerythroblastic smear points to an infiltrative process.

Examination of the bone marrow is also required to evaluate megakaryocyte number and morphologic features. A biopsy specimen is more reliable than an aspirate to determine whether megakaryocytes are decreased in number. However, an aspirate showing abundant megakaryocytes in the presence of thrombocytopenia is sufficient to suggest platelet destruction or ineffective production. Megakaryocytes are not evenly distributed throughout the marrow, so examination of many fields is required to determine if adequate numbers of cells are present. Megakaryocyte morphologic characteristics are also useful to observe. The normal compensatory response to thrombocytopenia is enlargement of the cells with increased ploidy. Small, microlobulated or hypolobulated megakaryocytes may be seen in myelodysplastic syndromes. Dysmorphic megakaryocytes may also be observed in viral infections, including human immunodeficiency virus. In the future, flow cytometry may provide a more objective analysis of megakaryocytes.

Ultimately a diagnosis of ineffective thrombopoiesis is made by exclusion. The marrow examination reveals quantitatively normal megakaryocytes, and the apparent absence of peripheral platelet destruction together with the appropriate clinical circumstances (e.g., folate or vitamin B_{12} deficiency) often point to this mechanism. Platelet function tests may be helpful in distinguishing ineffective production from platelet destruction. In destructive processes such as immune thrombocytopenia, function is normal, whereas in ineffective platelet production impaired function is not uncommon, as noted earlier. In complex cases, platelet survival studies may be necessary to show that consumption or splenic pooling are not significant contributors to the thrombocytopenia; however, survival studies are rarely required for clinical purposes. In the future, flow cytometric estimation of platelet production rate and measurement of thrombopoietin levels may permit a more facile approach to the differential diagnosis of thrombocytopenia.

---

in cases of PNH, thrombocytopenia is caused by decreased or ineffective platelet production. Megakaryocyte progenitors have a decreased proliferative activity and exhibit increased sensitivity to complement. Treatment with ATG or G-CSF and cyclosporine has ameliorated the thrombocytopenia whereas complement blockade with Eculizumab has little impact on platelet count.

Refractory Thrombocytopenia Caused by Myelodysplasia

MDSs may present as isolated thrombocytopenias rarely. The diagnosis of MDS should be considered when there are clonal chromosome abnormalities. The clinical course of patients with this type of disorder is progressive. Additional cytopenias invariably develop. A significant number of cases will evolve into an acute myeloid leukemia. Some patients with a full-blown MDS associated with marked thrombocytopenia and less than 10% blasts have been reported to experience increases in platelet counts after androgen therapy. Amifostine may be beneficial for some patients. It has been reported that some of these patients have been misdiagnosed as having immune thrombocytopenia purpura. Thrombopoietin agonists like romiplostim have also been used in patients with MDS. In an initial study involving 44 patients, a durable platelet response was achieved in 46% of patients with less bleeding events and transfusions seen in patients who achieved a durable response. Other treatment strategies such as treatment with cytokines and immunomodulating drugs have shown limited activity.

Cyclic Thrombocytopenia

Cyclic oscillations in the platelet count have been reported. The fluctuations in platelet count can be extreme, with thrombocytopenic bleeding occurring in cycles of 20 to 40 days. Women are often affected, and in such patients the cycling occurs in association with the menstrual cycle. The possibility that fluctuating cytokine levels may contribute to the pathogenesis of the disorder has been raised by several studies, although it is difficult to distinguish cause from effect. Cyclic thrombocytopenia may rarely be a presenting manifestation of myelodysplasia. Treatment has been variable; responses to low-dose contraceptives, IV gamma globulin and thrombopoietin mimetics have been reported (see box on Diagnosing Thrombocytopenia Caused by Impaired Thrombopoiesis).[226,227]

SUGGESTED READINGS

Bennett CL, Christie J, Ramsdell F, et al: The immune dysregulation, polyendocrinopathy, enteropathy, X-linked syndrome (IPEX) is caused by mutations of FOXP3. *Nat Genet* 27(1):20, 2001.

Bernard C, Frih H, Pasquet F, et al: Thymoma associated with autoimmune diseases: 85 cases and literature review. *Autoimmun Rev* 15:82–92, 2016.

Bilori B, Thota S, Clemente MJ, et al: Tofacitinib as a novel salvage therapy for refractory T cell large granular lymphocytic leukemia. *Leukemia* 29:2427–2429, 2015.

Caldas CA, de Carvalho JF: Pure red cell aplasia and primary antiphospholipid syndrome: a unique association. *Rheumatol Int* 32:5, 2012.

Dellacasa CM, D'Ardia S, Allione B, et al: Efficacy of plasmapheresis for the treatment of pure red blood cell aplasia after allogeneic stem cell transplantation. *Transfusion* 55:2979, 2015.

Del vecchio L, Locatelli F: An overview on safety issues related to erythropoiesis-stimulating agents for the treatment of anaemia in patients with chronic kidney disease. *Expert Opin Drug Saf* 1–10, 2016.

Frattini F, Crestani S, Vescovi PP, et al: Pure white cell aplasia induced by mesalazine in a patient with ulcerative colitis. *Hematology* 18(3):2013.

Haapaniemi EM, Kaustio M, Rajala HL, et al: Autoimmunity, hypogammaglobulinemia, lymphoproliferation, and mycobacterial disease in patients with activating mutations in STAT3. *Blood* 125:639–648, 2015.

Ishida F, Matsuda K, Sekiguchi N, et al: STAT3 gene mutations and their association with pure red cell aplasia in large granular lymphocyte leukemia. *Cancer Sci* 105:3, 2014.

Jerez A, Clemente MJ, Makishima H, et al: STAT3 mutations indicate the presence of subclinical T-cell clones in a subset of aplastic anemia and myelodysplastic syndrome patients. *Blood* 122(14):2013.

Jerez A, Clemente MJ, Makishima H, et al: STAT3 mutations unify the pathogenesis of chronic lymphoproliferative disorders of NK cells and T-cell large granular lymphocyte leukemia. *Blood* 120(15):2012.

Kerr JR: The role of parvovirus B19 in the pathogenesis of autoimmunity and autoimmune disease. *J Clin Pathol* 69:279–291, 2016.

Koskela HL, Eldfors S, Ellonen P, et al: Somatic STAT3 mutations in large granular lymphocytic leukemia. *N Engl J Med* 366(20):2012.

Landry ML: Parvovirus B19. *Microbiol Spectr* 4:1, 2016.

Lindqvist H, Carlsson G, Moell J, et al: Neutropenia in childhood: a 5-year experience at a tertiary center. *Eur J Pediatr* 2015174:6, 2014.

Loughran TP, Jr, Zickl L, Olson TL, et al: Immunosuppressive therapy of LGL leukemia: prospective multicenter phase II study by the Eastern Cooperative Oncology Group (E5998).

Lown R, Rhodes E, Bosworth J, et al: Acquired amegakaryocytic thrombo-cytopenia: potential role of thrombopoietin receptor agonists. *Clin Adv Hematol Oncol* 8:809–812, 2010.

Malphettes M, Gérard L, Galicier L, et al: Good syndrome: an adult-onset immunodeficiency remarkable for its high incidence of invasive infections and autoimmune complications. *Clin Infect Dis* 15:61, 2015.

Newburger PE, Dale DC: Evaluation and management of patients with isolated neutropenia. *Semin Hematol* 50:198–206, 2013.

Pavlaki KI, Kastrinaki MC, Klontzas M, et al: Abnormal telomere shortening of peripheral blood mononuclear cells and granulocytes in patients with chronic idiopathic neutropenia. *Haematologica* 97:5, 2012.

Rajala HL, Eldfors S, Kuusanmäki H, et al: Discovery of somatic STAT5b mutations in large granular lymphocytic leukemia. *Blood* 121(22):2013.

Rajala HL, Olson T, Clemente MJ, et al: The analysis of clonal diversity and therapy responses using STAT3 mutations as a molecular marker in large granular lymphocytic leukemia. *Haematologica* 100:91–99, 2015.

Sicre de Fontbrune F, Moignet A, Beaupain B, et al: Severe chronic primary neutropenia in adults: report on a series of 108 patients. *Blood* 126:14, 2015.

Spanoudakis M, Koutala H, Ximeri M, et al: T-cell receptor Vβ repertoire analysis in patients with chronic idiopathic neutropenia demonstrates the presence of aberrant T-cell expansions. *Clin Immunol* 137:384, 2010.

Staley EM, Schwartz J, Pham HP: An update on ABO incompatible hema-topoietic progenitor cell transplantation. *Transfus Apher Sci* 54:337–344, 2016.

Steinway SN, Leblanc F, Loughran TP: The pathogenesis and treatment of large granular lymphocyte leukemia. *Blood Rev* 28:87–94, 2014.

Velegraki M, Koutala H, Tsatsanis C, et al: Increased levels of the high mobility group box 1 protein sustain the inflammatory bone marrow microenvironment in patients with chronic idiopathic neutropenia via activation of toll-like receptor 4. *J Clin Immunol* 32:312, 2012.

Visco C, Barcellini W, Maura F, et al: Autoimmune cytopenias in chronic lymphocytic leukemia. *Am J Hematol* 89:1055–1062, 2014.

Worel N: ABO-Mismatched Allogeneic Hematopoietic Stem Cell Transplan-tation. *Transfus Med Hemother* 43:3–12, 2016.

Zelenetz AD: Guidelines for NHL: updates to the management of diffuse large B-cell lymphoma and new guidelines for primary cutaneous CD30+ T-cell lymphoproliferative disorders and T-cell large granular lymphocytic leukemia. *J Natl Compr Canc Netw* 12:797–800, 2014.

Zent CS, Ding W, Reinalda MS, et al: Autoimmune cytopenia in chronic lymphocytic leukemia/small lymphocytic lymphoma: changes in clinical presentation and prognosis. *Leuk Lymphoma* 50:8, 2009.

REFERENCES

For the complete list of references, log on to www.expertconsult.com.

Part **V**

Red Blood Cells

PATHOBIOLOGY OF THE HUMAN ERYTHROCYTE AND ITS HEMOGLOBINS

Martin H. Steinberg, Edward J. Benz, Jr., Adeboye H. Adewoye, and Benjamin L. Ebert

Anemia, polycythemia, and functional derangements of the human erythrocyte together represent a common group of human disorders with a significant impact on public health. Sickle cell disease, hemoglobin E (HbE)–associated disorders, and the thalassemias are humankind's most common single-gene diseases, but the relevance of red blood cell (RBC) disorders to general medicine extends even beyond their individual clinical severities or the number of patients affected. A critical added dimension of erythrocyte disorders is the extraordinarily detailed knowledge available about the basic biochemistry, physiology, and molecular biology of the human RBC and its membrane, metabolism, and major component, Hb. RBCs are especially abundant, relatively simple, and readily accessible for repeated testing in individual patients. These features have facilitated rapid application of the techniques of cellular and molecular biology to studies of the RBC, its component molecules and structures, and syndromes resulting from abnormalities of these entities. Taken as a group, erythrocyte disorders are better understood at the molecular and cellular levels than disorders of any other cell or tissue. It is for this reason that these conditions merit particularly careful scrutiny by students of hematology.

This chapter reviews the concepts about normal RBC homeostasis that form the essential knowledge base for understanding anemias, polycythemias, and functional erythrocyte disorders. The primary focus and the object for detailed discussion within this chapter is Hb, the major component, both quantitatively and qualitatively, of the erythrocyte. Hb molecules dominate the pathophysiology of many RBC disorders and modulate most of the others, in part because of their sheer quantitative predominance in RBC cytoplasm. The other major relevant aspects of human RBCs—the membrane, the enzymes used for intermediary metabolism, differentiation and development, and the process of destruction—are discussed in detail in the introductory portions of other chapters. This chapter surveys these areas only briefly. Detailed descriptions of the RBC membrane can be found in Chapter 45. RBC enzymes and enzymopathies are described in Chapter 44; differentiation and development are described in Chapters 9 and 26; regulation of the RBC mass by erythropoietin is discussed in Chapter 22; and the necessary aspects of RBC destruction are considered in Chapters 43, 46, and 47.

ESSENTIAL FEATURES OF RED BLOOD CELL HOMEOSTASIS

As discussed in Chapter 26, the mature RBC is the product of a complex and orderly set of differentiation and maturation steps beginning with the pluripotent stem cell. By incompletely understood mechanisms involving hierarchic networks of cytokines, a portion of these cells becomes committed to differentiate along the erythroid pathway. Commitment to erythropoiesis provokes a progressively increasing sensitivity to the stimulatory actions of the hormone erythropoietin. As differentiation proceeds, there is preprogramming of certain genes whose expression at high levels will be required during the maturation phase of erythropoiesis. Genes coding for molecules defining the RBC phenotype (e.g., globin) are poised for activation at later maturation steps.

Intermediate progenitor cells arising during differentiation have been characterized experimentally, including the burst-forming unit-erythroid (BFU-E) and the colony-forming unit-erythroid (CFU-E) stages. BFU-Es are progenitor cells that in culture produce bursts or clusters of erythroid colonies, are relatively less sensitive to erythropoietin, and are more plastic with respect to important gene expression parameters, such as the synthesis of adult or fetal Hb (HbF) by their descendants. CFU-Es produce single colonies, exhibit considerably higher sensitivity to erythropoietin, and appear to be more fixed in their potential to express a particular subset of globin genes. CFU-Es appear to give rise to the first morphologically recognizable erythroid cells, the proerythroblasts. At this "primitive" morphologic stage, the program of erythroid cell expression has already been essentially predetermined. The cell is predestined to undergo only a limited additional number of cell divisions, culminating in formation of the enucleate reticulocyte. The terminal maturation stages are morphologically recognizable as erythroblasts exhibiting progressive hemoglobinization of the cytoplasm, condensation and eventual ejection of the nucleus, and remodeling of the plasma membrane. Actual expression of the preprogrammed genes occurs during the 5- to 7-day period of erythroblast maturation.

As discussed in Chapters 9 and 26, the actual reconfiguration of chromatin for activation of the genes and activation itself appear to require the concerted and complex interaction of a diverse but limited group of transcription factors and associated epigenetic regulators. These regulatory proteins recognize a specific array of promoter and enhancer sequences that are embedded as recurrent motifs in and around the appropriate target genes. Even though an enormous amount of information has been gathered about sequences such as the GATA enhancers and their cognate transcription factors (e.g., GATA, FOG, ETS), the precise means by which these sequences and factors cause erythroid differentiation remains mysterious. At this time, this information is of limited clinical relevance to anemias or polycythemias. The orderly 14- to 21-day sequence of differentiation and maturation becomes progressively influenced by the levels of erythropoietin available to the progenitor cells, possibly because of increasing density and affinity of erythropoietin receptors on their cell surfaces. Within 24 hours after enucleation, the reticulocyte traverses the bone marrow–blood barrier membrane and enters the circulation as an immature erythrocyte. These cells retain remnants of nucleated precursors in the form of a relatively small number of polyribosomes actively translating messenger ribonucleic acid (RNA) (>90% of which is globin messenger RNA), a cell membrane that retains some molecules and structures reminiscent of its earlier stages of differentiation, and the complement of enzymes, phospholipids, and cytoskeletal proteins that the cell will possess throughout its remaining life span.

During its first 24 hours in the circulation, the reticulocyte spends considerable amounts of time in the spleen, during which its membrane is "polished." This is a poorly understood remodeling process by which some lipids and proteins, including adhesive molecules such as fibronectin, are removed. The content of polyribosomes and other nucleic acids progressively declines so that stainability with methylene blue is lost by the end of the first day. At this time, the RBC is regarded as a mature erythrocyte, and it circulates largely unchanged for the remainder of its 120-day life span.

Perhaps the most remarkable feature of the human RBC is its durability, given that it is an enucleated cell devoid of organelles that appear to be critical for the survival and function of most other cell types. The RBC has no mitochondria available for efficient oxidative metabolism; no ribosomes for regeneration of lost or damaged proteins; a very limited metabolic repertoire that largely precludes de novo synthesis of lipids; and no nucleus to direct regenerative processes, adaptation to circulatory stresses, or cell division to replenish itself. Given these handicaps, the 120-day survival of these cells is even more striking considering the multiple and often exceedingly hostile environments they must traverse. Mechanical stresses of the circulation include high hydrostatic pressure and turbulence and the shear stresses inherent in a microcirculation networked with many capillaries having diameters only one-third to one-half that of the normal RBC. Biochemical stresses include osmotic and redox fluxes associated with travel through the collecting system of the kidney; the sluggish vascular beds of the spleen, muscle, and bone; and the rapid changes in ambient oxygen pressures occurring in the lungs. All conspire to damage RBCs. Their 4-month survival is truly remarkable.

The ability of the RBC to persist in the circulation depends on its simple but exquisitely adaptive membrane structures; its pathways of intermediary energy metabolism and redox regulation; and its ability to maintain its largest cytoplasmic component, Hb, in a soluble and nonoxidized state. The membrane and enzymes of the RBC appear to be exquisitely crafted to protect the cell from the external ravages of the circulation and the potential internal assaults of the massive amount of iron-rich and potentially oxidizing protein represented by its complement of Hb molecules. For these reasons, a few basic features of these membrane and enzyme systems merit comment before considering the Hb molecule itself.

MAJOR FEATURES OF THE RED BLOOD CELL MEMBRANE

Chapter 45 describes the RBC membrane in considerable detail. Only a few major aspects of that discussion bear repeating for the purposes of this chapter. The RBC membrane and its underlying cytoskeleton have evolved to provide mechanical strength and the necessary pliability and resilience to withstand the mechanical, osmotic, and chemical stresses of the circulation. Because the lipid bilayer membrane essentially has the physical properties of a soap bubble, it would rapidly be emulsified in the circulation. Strength and order are provided to the lipid bilayer by the hexagonal arrays of the highly helical protein spectrin, which forms a latticework underlying the membrane.

The spectrin meshwork is held together by adaptor molecules, such as protein 4.1, adducin, p55, and ankyrin, arrayed at defined points along the highly coiled, rod-like structure of the spectrin oligomers. These protein–protein interactions appear to be critical for holding the latticework together in what has been described as the "horizontal" dimension that permits resistance to shear stress. The involvement of intermediate-length actin fibers and the variability of binding affinities by phosphorylation state appear to provide some flexibility and pliability at these points of interaction. Strength in the "vertical" dimension is provided by additional molecules or additional binding functions of the same molecule, whereby the latticework is attached to the lipid bilayer. For the most part, the physiologically important attachments appear to be indirect. Linkage is mediated through the interaction of the adaptor proteins, such as ankyrin and protein 4.1, with the cytoplasmic domains of abundant transmembrane proteins. These proteins traverse and are embedded in the lipid bilayer, providing a firm anchor. The two most critical of these molecules appear to be band 3 (i.e., the anion transport channel) and a glycophorin, probably glycophorin C/D. A possible additional stabilizing role for the Rh protein complex has been suggested. The construction of these attachments by multiple "hinge" or coupling molecules appears to provide for the flexibility and distensibility of the RBC membrane, a property essential to its ability to flow through small capillaries.

As described in Chapter 46, the complex structure of the membrane is exquisitely sensitive to perturbations impinging on any of its components. In particular, the membrane cytoskeleton and phospholipid structures are each highly susceptible to oxidation, particularly by partially proteolyzed molecules of Hb, which denature to form highly toxic compounds called *hemopyrroles*. This interaction of denatured Hb with the RBC membrane is clinically important, as illustrated by its impact on the pathophysiology of sickle cell anemia (see Chapter 42) or of oxidized and precipitated globin inclusion bodies in thalassemia (Chapter 41). In this chapter, it is sufficient to note that alterations of proteins of the RBC membrane can contribute to shortening the life span of the RBC. Damage can result from direct defects in the cytoskeletal proteins themselves or from susceptibility of these proteins to direct oxidation or attack by oxidized or denatured Hb molecules. Readers are referred to chapters 43 through 47 for detailed descriptions of the relevant phenomena.

ENZYMES OF RED BLOOD CELL INTERMEDIARY

Metabolism

Mammalian erythrocytes possess a highly specialized but remarkably simplified set of metabolic pathways. As discussed in Chapter 44, there are essentially three relevant sets of pathways. The first two are interconnected by the enzyme glucose-6-phosphate dehydrogenase (G6PD). Glucose entering the RBC is metabolized by an anaerobic pathway, the Embden-Meyerhof pathway, which terminates with the enzyme lactic dehydrogenase, forming lactate. Despite its inefficiency (a net of only two adenosine triphosphate [ATP]/glucose molecule), this pathway is the sole source of usable ATP in the cell. Moreover, the pathway generates reduced nicotinamide adenine dinucleotide (NADH), a molecule necessary for driving the reduction of methemoglobin to Hb (see Chapters 44 and 47). A shunt within this pathway, the Rapoport-Luebering shunt, generates the compound 2,3-bisphosphoglycerate (bis[phosphoglyceric acid]) (2,3-BPG), an important cofactor that, when bound to Hb, reduces the affinity of Hb for oxygen (see Hemoglobin Function). The ATP generated is necessary for kinase reactions controlling phosphorylation of membrane and signaling components, for fueling ion pumps and channels, and for maintaining phospholipid levels.

The anaerobic metabolic pathway generates, as one of its intermediates, glucose-6 phosphate, which is the substrate for G6PD. G6PD appears to be the rate-limiting enzyme for a linked pathway called the *oxidative hexose monophosphate shunt*. This pathway involves a cascade of reactions culminating in the reduction of oxidized glutathione to reduced glutathione. Reduced glutathione is used to reverse oxidation of critical structures, including Hb, cytoskeletal proteins, and membrane lipids. Anaerobic glycolysis generates NADH for methemoglobin reduction, 2,3-BPG for modulation of Hb oxygen affinity, and ATP for metabolic energy requirements. Its end product is lactate. The oxidative hexose monophosphate shunt generates NADH phosphate (NADPH) and reduced glutathione for use as the major erythrocyte antioxidant.

During the past decade, most of the enzymes (or at least the erythroid isoforms of these enzymes) involved in RBC intermediary metabolism have been characterized at the molecular level by cloning of their cDNAs, genomic loci, or both. Some of the more relevant information arising from this progress is discussed in Chapter 44. The erythrocyte possesses membrane-based signaling receptors and cytoplasmic signal transduction elements similar, although perhaps less elaborate, than those of nucleated cells. The relevance of these systems to the pathophysiology of RBC disorders is just becoming apparent.

RED BLOOD CELL SENESCENCE AND DESTRUCTION

Erythrocytes, despite their impressive adaptations to circulatory stresses, eventually wear out and are destroyed. RBC survival in humans appears to be remarkably uniform under normal circumstances, spanning approximately 120 days from release of the reticulocyte into circulation to sequestration of the senescent RBC in the reticuloendothelial cells of the liver and spleen. The precise signal, or signals, marking RBCs for destruction remain unknown, as does the underlying pathophysiology within the RBC or on its surface. However, several interrelated theories have emerged; these are discussed only briefly because they are mentioned in other chapters.

RBCs accumulate surface blemishes during their lives in the circulation. These appear to result in part from the accumulation of small amounts of oxygen damage to membrane structures. The altered regions are sensed by the reticuloendothelial cells during passage of the erythrocytes through the liver and spleen. Removal or pitting of these damaged regions from RBC membranes can be documented microscopically; small amounts of normal membrane are also lost during the process.

The biconcave disk shape of the RBC, so important to its distensibility, depends on a high ratio of surface area to volume. This requires redundant membrane surface area. The membrane surface area of the normal biconcave disk is approximately 140 μm^2. To enclose a sphere containing a normal RBC volume (≈ 90 fL), only approximately 95 μm^2 would be needed. Progressive loss of membrane surface by means of the pitting phenomenon should ultimately cause the aging erythrocyte to assume a more rigid spherical shape. A sphere is inevitably far less distensible and far less capable of passing through small apertures than a disk, especially in the sluggish and tortuous circulation of the spleen. This geometric mechanism can lead to the eventual destruction of the RBC.

RBCs progressively lose some of the critical enzymes needed for intermediary metabolism and antioxidant capacity. G6PD levels, for example, progressively decline during the circulating life span, as do levels of several other enzymes. The decline of certain enzymes can be used as a crude means of estimating the relative age of different RBC populations. The biochemical or oxidative mechanism of destruction postulates that aged RBCs are eventually depleted of critical enzymes needed for maintenance of redox status. Oxidation of critical membrane proteins, lipids, and Hb would then ensue, causing distortion and rigidity of the RBC membrane, with accelerated loss as previously described. The end product would be spherocytes incapable of traversing the splenic vascular bed and escaping engulfment by the reticuloendothelial cell.

It has been proposed that an immune-type mechanism can contribute to normal and pathologic RBC senescence. This hypothesis is based on the observation that oxidative damage, regardless of cause, promotes a clustering, or *capping*, of oligomers of band 3 on the RBC surface. Under normal circumstances, band 3 molecules form monomers, dimers, or tetramers. Higher order aggregates appear to be recognized by an endogenous isoantibody possessed by all people. Any RBC accumulating oxidative damage from wear and tear in the circulation, from depletion of enzymes, or from internal pathologic processes such as denaturation of Hb in certain hemoglobinopathies can accumulate these aggregates. The aggregates would then be bound by antibody and be removed by the reticuloendothelial cells as antigen–antibody complexes, using the same means used by reticuloendothelial cells to recognize any immune complex. This mechanism could also provide for the pitting or polishing of damaged RBC membranes. All three of the proposed mechanisms are interrelated by their inception with oxidative damage.

Other membrane-related changes might influence RBC destruction. Bcl-X_L, a suppressor of apoptosis, is present in erythrocyte membranes, and its antagonization may promote cell death. This may be mediated by calcium accumulation and phosphatidylserine exposure. Cholesterol and fatty acids accumulate on the aging RBC membrane and might be targets for oxidation induced by reactive oxygen species. RBCs are removed from the circulation by splenic macrophages, probably by several mechanisms. SHPS-1, a surface glycoprotein and a member of the immunoglobulin superfamily that interacts with RBC membrane CD47, is abundant in macrophages. Studies using mice expressing a mutant SHPS-1 suggested that this molecule might negatively regulate phagocytosis, influencing cell life

span. Increasing phosphatidyl serine exposure and reduced aminophospholipid translocase activity during aging might induce oxidative damage to the cell. It is probable that these mechanisms leading to cell destruction are not mutually exclusive, that no single effect predominates, and that these events occur at different times at different sites of RBC damage.

Regardless of the mechanism(s) fostering eventual senescence and destruction of RBCs, the process itself involves components clinically useful for assessment of anemias associated with accelerated destruction. Chief among these is the generation of indirect or unconjugated bilirubin, the byproduct of heme catabolism occurring within the reticuloendothelial cells. In markedly accelerated states of RBC destruction, hypertrophy of the liver and spleen can also occur, providing a useful physical indicator of hemolytic anemia. These indirect clinical features, coupled with the reticulocyte count, remain more useful for detecting clinical hemolysis than complicated studies of RBC kinetics.

HEMOGLOBIN SYNTHESIS, STRUCTURE, AND FUNCTION

Basic Features

Hbs are the major oxygen-carrying pigments of the body. They are packaged into RBCs in quantities sufficient to carry enough oxygen from the lungs to the tissues to meet the needs of those cells for oxidative metabolism. These quantities are enormous—almost 2 pounds of Hb are present in the body of a reasonably sized human at any given time. Because free Hb in the bloodstream is catabolized and excreted renally in a matter of minutes, packaging in erythrocytes is essential to preserve the newly synthesized molecules for the entire 4-month life span of the RBC. Otherwise, the caloric and biosynthetic resources needed to replace daily losses of Hb would be prohibitive. The RBC's major function is to encase Hb and protect it so it can function as an oxygen transporter for a prolonged period. An additional function of Hb is to modulate vascular tone by its transport of nitric oxide (NO) and possibly nitrous oxide.

The cellular content of blood influences its viscosity; in particular, the hemodynamics are adversely compromised by the presence of too many circulating erythrocytes because blood viscosity correlates especially with hematocrit. To provide for adequate oxygen transport (i.e., enough Hb molecules) in a number of RBCs compatible with tolerable viscosity, each cell must enclose a high concentration of Hb (32–35 g per 100 mL of cytoplasm). This concentration is close to the solubility limit of Hb in physiologic solutions. It follows that even minor perturbations within these molecules (e.g., oxidation) or in the milieu (e.g., changes in pH or ionic strength) can have potentially devastating effects on the solubility of Hb. Because polymerized or precipitated Hbs derange intracellular viscosity, trigger proteolytic reactions that lead to oxidative damage of erythrocytes, and compromise oxygen transport, it is not surprising that the fate of the RBC is inextricably interwoven with the state of its enormous complement of Hb molecules.

Hemoglobin Structure

The Hb tetramer consists of two pairs of unlike globin polypeptide chains, each associated with a heme group. Normal Hb has two α-globin and two non–α-globin chains; the interaction of these chains is responsible for the quaternary structure of the Hb molecule and normal oxygen transport. Functionally, the second exon of each globin gene encodes the major component of the heme-binding pocket, and the α and non-α contacts are regulated by the third exon.

The behavior of Hb is determined by its primary structure, the covalent linking of amino acids to form the polypeptide globin. The higher order structures of Hb depend on the sequence of amino acid residues that make up the globin chain. The α-globin chains contain 141 residues, and the β-globin–like chains are 146 amino acids long (Fig. 33.1). There is considerable homology among these globins,

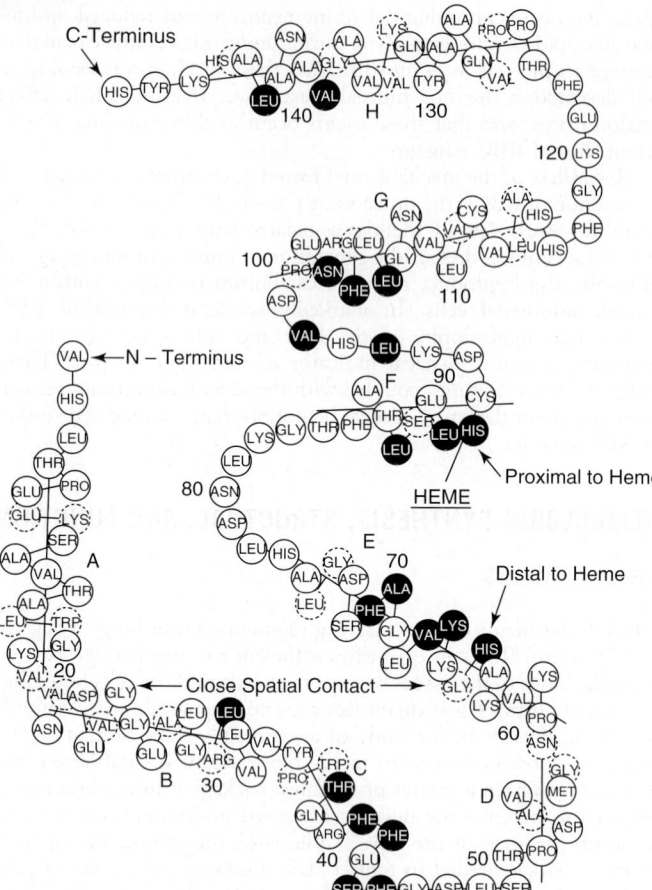

Fig. 33.1 THE β-GLOBIN CHAIN SHOWING HELICAL AND NON-HELICAL SEGMENTS. The helical segments are labeled A through H, and the nonhelical segments are designated *NA* for residues between the N terminus and the A helix, *CD* for residues between the C and D helices, and so forth. *(Reproduced with permission from Huisman THJ, Schroeder WA: New aspects of the structure, function, and synthesis of hemoglobin. Boca Raton, 1971, Fl, CRC Press.)*

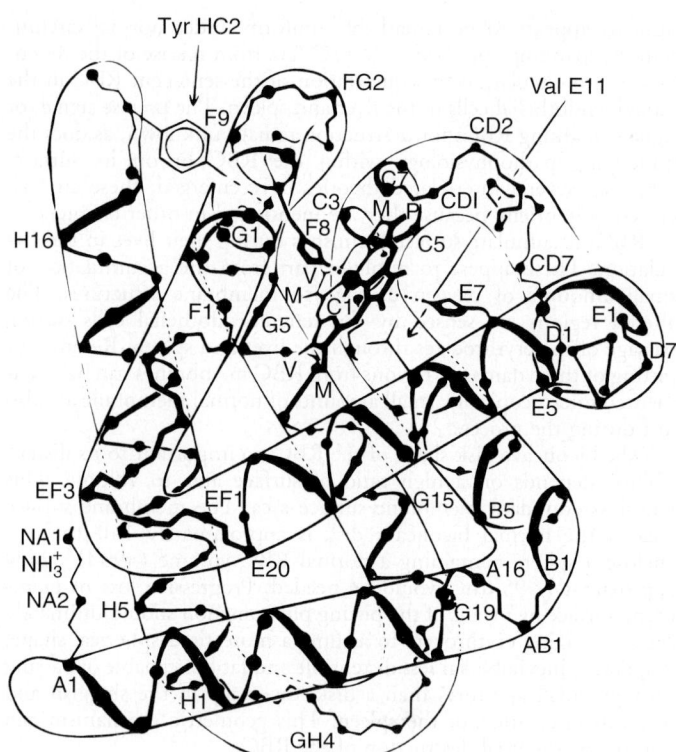

Fig. 33.2 TERTIARY STRUCTURE OF A GLOBIN CHAIN. Globin folds into a tertiary structure such that polar or charged amino acids are located on the exterior of the molecule and the heme ring resides in a hydrophobic niche between the E and F helices. Linked to the heme are the proximal (F8) histidine and the distal (E7) histidine. *(Reproduced with permission from Perutz MF: Molecular anatomy, physiology, and pathology of hemoglobin. In Stamatoyannopoulos G, Neinhuis AW, Leder P, et al, editors: The molecular basis of blood diseases. Philadelphia, 1987, Saunders, p 127.)*

especially among the non–α-globin chains. Whereas the α-globin genes *(HBA2, HBA1)* result from a very ancient gene duplication, the non–α-globin genes *(HBE, HBG2, HBG1, HBD, HBB)* are the result of more recent gene duplications and are more akin to each other than they are to the α-like globin genes. Gene conversion events also ensure the similarity of duplicated genes.

Elements of the secondary structure of globin are shown in Figs. 33.1 and 33.2. Approximately 75% of the globin polypeptide chain forms an α-helix. There are eight helical segments, A through H, separated by short stretches from which the α-helix is absent. These nonhelical segments permit folding of the polypeptide on itself and are often dictated by the presence of prolyl residues, which are generally unable to participate in the formation of α-helices. Although the helical segments of the α-globin and non–α-globin chains do not exactly correspond, it is possible to align amino acid residues in all globin peptides by their helical and nonhelical residue numbers, as indicated in Fig. 33.3. This permits greater appreciation of the homology among globins. Some of the amino acids of globin are invariant, or conserved, in the sense that they are preserved during phylogeny. These residues occur at portions of the molecule that are critical for its stability and function, such as heme binding residues, hydrophobic amino acids of the interior of the molecule, and certain subunit contacts at the α₁–β₂ interface. The introduction of prolyl residues into α-helical segments by mutation leads to interruption of the α-helix and instability of the resulting Hb molecule.

The poorly understood laws that govern the folding of proteins are responsible for the tertiary structure of globin, shown in Fig. 33.3. This folding pattern places polar residues exteriorly and provides a hydrophobic niche for the heme ring between the E and F helices. Numerous noncovalent bonds are formed between the heme and surrounding amino acid residues of globin. An iron atom in the center of the porphyrin ring forms an important bond with the F8 or proximal histidine and through the linked oxygen with the E7 or distal histidine residue. Oxygenation and deoxygenation of Hb occur at the heme iron. Folding of globin and association of chains into dimers and tetramers was once thought to occur spontaneously. However, it is now clear that these processes are assisted by chaperone proteins, which are described in Chapters 5 and 6.

Two α-globin chains and two non–α-globin chains fit together specifically to form a Hb tetramer with a molecular mass of approximately 64,000 daltons and with the quaternary structure shown in Fig. 33.4. The motion of individual globin chains, as well as the movement of globin chains relative to each other during oxygenation and deoxygenation, gives Hb its unique usefulness as a respiratory protein.

Hemoglobin Function

Evolution has honed the Hb tetramer into a molecule ideally suited for its tasks. Because human Hb must behave differently than that of altitude dwelling species or species inhabiting hypoxic locales, many different variants of the same basic molecular design have evolved. Because of the exigencies of molecular evolution, we find in the genome of all animals, including humans, attempts by nature to propagate a variety of different globin genes. The crystallographic

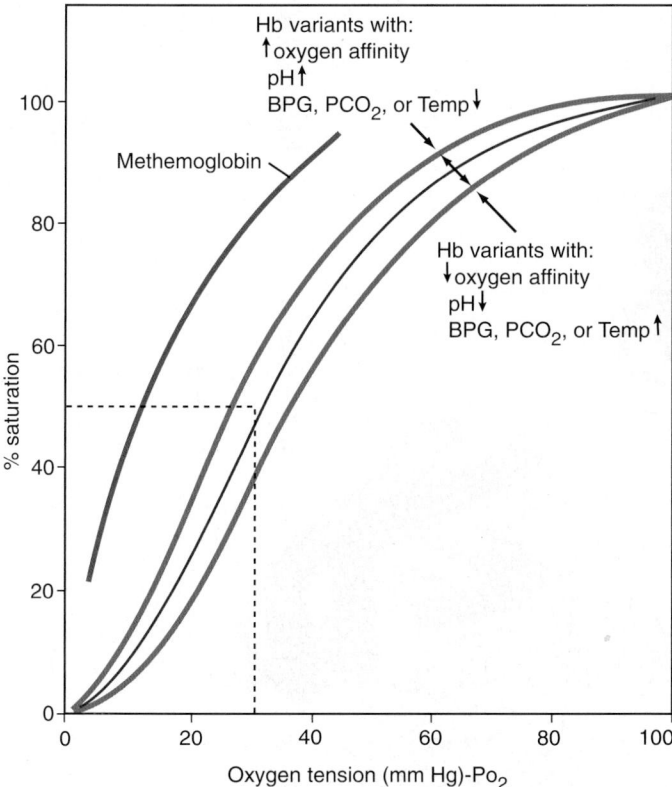

Fig. 33.3 OXYGEN DISSOCIATION CURVE OF HEMOGLOBIN. The percent saturation of hemoglobin (Hb) with oxygen at different oxygen tensions is depicted by the *red sigmoidal curve*. The P_{50} (i.e., oxygen tension at which the hemoglobin molecule is one-half saturated) is approximately 27 mm Hg in normal erythrocytes *(dotted lines)*. Heterotopic modifiers of Hb function can shift the curve leftward by increasing or rightward by decreasing its oxygen affinity. *BPG,* Bisphosphoglycerate *PCO_2,* partial pressure of carbon dioxide; *Po_2,* partial pressure of oxygen. *(Reproduced with permission from Benz EJ, Jr: Synthesis, structure, and function of hemoglobin. In Kelly WN, DeVita VT, editors: Textbook of internal medicine, vol 1. Philadelphia, 1989, JB Lippincott, p 236.)*

studies of Perutz et al defined the oxygenated and deoxygenated structures of Hb at Ångström-unit resolution and provided an exquisitely detailed picture of how the globin chains and individual amino acid residues respond to the loading and unloading of oxygen. All of these, however, share the properties of highly reversible oxygen binding and high solubility in cytoplasm. We know more about the function of Hb than about virtually any other protein, and the knowledge of this mechanism provides a beautiful and intellectually satisfying culmination to decades of study by many investigators.

The oxygen dissociation curve of Hb, shown in Fig. 33.3, describes the percent saturation of Hb with oxygen at different oxygen tensions. The sigmoidal shape of this curve is a result of interaction among the subunits of Hb. Communication within the tetramer is called heme–heme interaction or cooperativity. This implies that the four heme groups do not undergo simultaneous oxygenation or deoxygenation but rather that the state of each heme unit with regard to the presence or absence of bound oxygen influences the binding of oxygen to other heme groups. Myoglobin, a heme-containing protein with virtually the same tertiary structure as globin, exists in muscle as a monomer. The oxygen equilibrium curve of myoglobin is a rectangular hyperbola; in physiologic terms, it rapidly becomes fully saturated at low oxygen tensions and remains saturated as the oxygen tension plateaus. The difference in the oxygen equilibrium curves of myoglobin and Hb lies in the tetrameric nature of the Hb molecule and the cooperativity permitted by the association of similar but unlike subunits. Compared with Hb, myoglobin has a very low P_{50} (i.e., oxygen partial pressure at which the molecule is one-half

saturated). It therefore has an extremely high oxygen affinity and would not be useful for delivering oxygen to tissues. The oxygen in myoglobin is passed on to the mitochondria, where oxidative metabolism occurs. The sigmoidal shape of the oxygen dissociation curve of Hb indicates that the totally deoxygenated Hb tetramer is slow to become oxygenated, but as oxygenation proceeds, the reaction of heme with oxygen accelerates. Perutz has drawn an analogy in which the "appetite" of heme for oxygen grows with the "eating," and conversely, loss of oxygen by heme lowers the oxygen affinity of the remaining heme groups. The Hill coefficient, *n,* which can be calculated from plots of oxygen equilibrium curves, is a description of heme–heme interaction or cooperativity that explains in part the oxygen-binding properties of Hb and myoglobin. The Hill coefficient for myoglobin is 1, indicating no cooperativity; *n* is approximately 3 for the normal human HbA molecule.

The oxygen affinity of Hb within the erythrocyte does not depend solely on the intrinsic properties of the tetramer. The position of the Hb oxygen dissociation curve, and therefore the P_{50}, can be influenced by a number of heterotropic modifiers, including temperature, pH, and small organic phosphate molecules in the cell. The effects of these modifiers on P_{50} are shown in Fig. 33.3.

Hb is the prototype of an allosteric protein; its structure and function are influenced by other molecules. The major intracellular modulator of Hb–oxygen affinity in human erythrocytes is 2,3-BPG, an intermediate product of glycolysis that is present within the erythrocyte at concentrations equimolar to Hb. The synthesis of 2,3-BPG is enzymatically regulated, and its levels can change depending on the conditions extant. 2,3-BPG is able to bind stereospecifically within the central cavity of the Hb tetramer. Hb prepared in the absence of 2,3-BPG has a very high oxygen affinity, but as 2,3-BPG is added to a Hb solution, the oxygen affinity progressively decreases. 2,3-BPG is a polyanion that binds strongly to the deoxygenated form of Hb but poorly to its oxygenated or other liganded forms. Specific amino acids are involved in the binding of 2,3-BPG; these β-chain residues include the N-terminal valines, the H21 histidine (position 143), and the EF6 lysine (position 82). In oxyhemoglobin, the H helices of the β-chains are insufficiently spread to permit firm binding of 2,3-BPG; this, along with other conformational changes, favors the binding of this anion to the deoxygenated rather than the oxygenated form of Hb. The binding of 2,3-BPG stabilizes the tense (T) structure of the deoxygenated form at the expense of the relaxed (R) structure of the oxyhemoglobin tetramer.

Transition from the deoxy (T) to the oxy (R) form of Hb is accompanied by rotation of the αβ dimers along the α_1–β_2 contact region (Fig. 33.5). The T structure is stabilized by salt bridges, which are broken as the molecule switches into the R structure. Some abnormal Hbs with an intrinsically high oxygen affinity, or low P_{50}, occur as a result of an amino acid substitution that leads to loss of bonds that stabilize the tetramer in the T conformation. Hydrogen ions, chloride ions, and carbon dioxide all decrease the affinity of Hb for oxygen by strengthening the salt bridges that lock the molecule into its T conformation. The corollary of the lowering of Hb oxygen affinity by protons is the combination of Hb with protons on deoxygenation. This is known as the Bohr effect and is responsible for carbon dioxide transport in blood, another critical function of the Hb molecule. Deoxyhemoglobin binds the hydrogen ion liberated by the reaction of carbon dioxide with water, increasing the concentration of bicarbonate. Within the lungs, hydrogen ions are lost as Hb binds oxygen; therefore, carbon dioxide leaves solution and is excreted from the body through the lungs. Deoxyhemoglobin can also directly bind carbon dioxide; however, this process involves the minority of carbon dioxide exchanged by the RBCs.

RBCs containing high levels of Hb F have high oxygen affinity because it binds 2,3-BPG poorly. Physiologically, this predicts that the Hb of fetuses should be oxygenated at the expense of the maternal HbA. The high oxygen affinity of HbF is accounted for by a single change in its primary structure, the presence of a serine residue at helical position H21 in place of the histidine found in the β-globin chain. This weakens the binding of 2,3-BPG and leads to stabilization of the molecule in its R state.

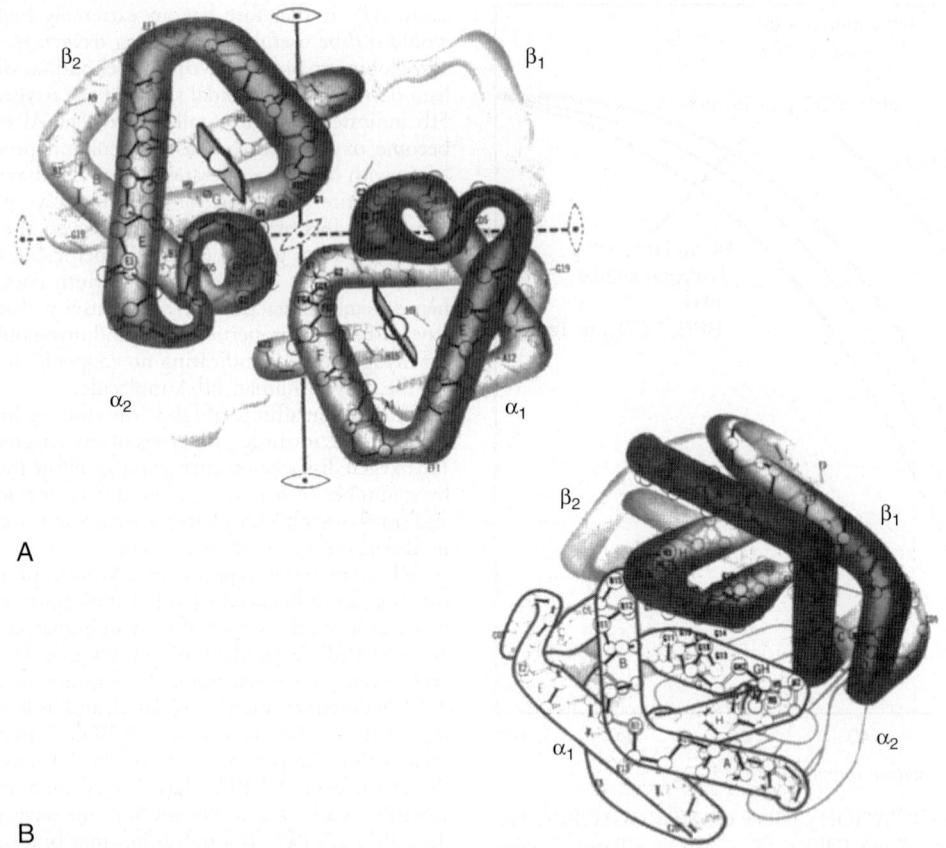

A

B

Fig. 33.4 QUATERNARY STRUCTURE OF HEMOGLOBIN. The contacts between subunits are shown as circled amino acids. In the front view (A), $\alpha_1\beta_2$ contacts are shown, and in the side view (B), α_1-β-β_1 contacts are depicted. *(Reproduced with permission from Dickerson RE, Geis I:* Hemoglobin: Structure, function, and evolution pathology. *Menlo Park, CA, 1983, Benjamin-Cummings.)*

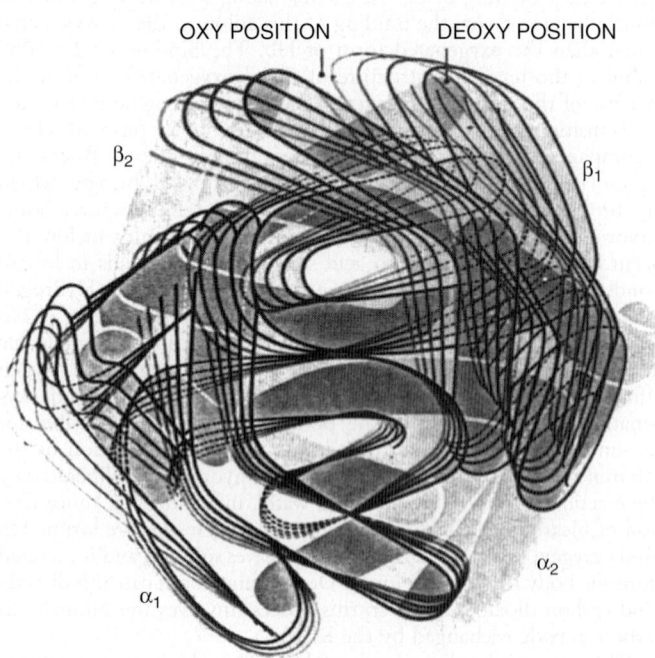

Fig. 33.5 SUBUNIT MOTION IN THE HEMOGLOBIN TETRAMER. The relative motion of hemoglobin subunits on oxygenation and deoxygenation is shown. The $\alpha_1\beta_1$ dimer *(black)* is moving relative to the $\alpha_2\beta_2$ dimer *(shaded)*. The oxyhemoglobin tetramer (R state) is more compact than the deoxyhemoglobin configuration (T state). *(Reproduced with permission from Dickerson RE, Geis I:* Hemoglobin: Structure, function, and evolution pathology. *Menlo Park, CA, 1983, Benjamin-Cummings.)*

Interactions of Hb with NO have been a recent focus of investigation. NO, generated from L-arginine by NO synthases, activates soluble guanylate cyclase to produce the second messenger cyclic guanosine monophosphate. As a potent vasodilator, NO is an important regulator of vascular tone. The reaction of free NO with erythrocytes is diffusion limited. Normally, the primary NO–Hb adduct is nitrosyl (heme) Hb (HbFe[II]NO). Within the erythrocyte, $\beta93$ cysteine is reduced and seems incapable of NO storage and delivery by *S*-nitrosohemoglobin as originally proposed. NO was thought to form *S*-nitrosylhemoglobin in the lungs, where Hb is in its R or oxygenated state, and liberate NO in the microcirculation, where the transition of the R to T conformation induced by deoxygenation released NO from Hb. However, studies suggest that NO binding to heme groups is physiologically a rapidly reversible process. This view supports a model of Hb delivery of NO distinct from its dissociation from the $\beta93$ cysteine residues. Small nitrosothiol molecules could also be involved in NO transfer. The thiol groups of Hb can exchange NO with small nitrosothiols derived from free cysteine and glutathione. Accordingly, the thiol groups of Hb could bind and transfer NO or exchange NO with small shuttle molecules, increasing perfusion of hypoxic tissues. It has been suggested that cytoskeletal and other erythrocyte proteins slow NO influx into the cell and, coupled with NO heme binding, preserve NO bioactivity. NO–Hb interactions, whether through *S*-nitrosohemoglobin formation at the $\beta93$ cysteine or the formation of nitroso intermediates, are likely to be physiologically important. Hb liberated from the intravascularly hemolyzed RBCs rapidly inactivates NO. As the RBC lyses, arginase is also released and destroys the substrate for NO synthases, L-arginine. Together, this leads to a reduction in biologically active NO. With hemolysis as in sickle cell disease or thalassemia, reduced NO bioavailability is associated with disease complications such as pulmonary hypertension, leg ulcers, priapism, and perhaps increased risk of

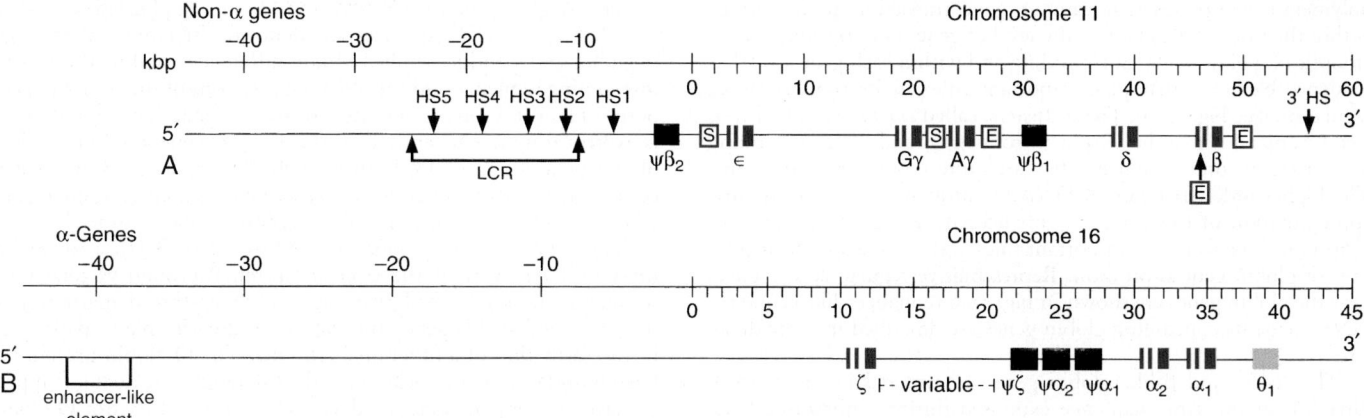

Fig. 33.6 Maps of the β-like and α-like globin gene clusters located on chromosome 11 (A) and chromosome 16 (B). Within each gene cluster are pseudogenes, which are remnants of previously expressed globin genes that have become inactivated as a result of mutation. Active genes are shown in *red boxes* filled with clear introns; inactive or pseudogenes genes are shown in *black boxes,* and the θ-globin gene is shown as a *pink box.* Although this gene is transcribed, it is not clear whether it is represented in a cellular protein. The distance between the functional ζ-globin and pseudo-ζ-globin gene is variable because of the presence of repeated elements. *E,* Enhancer; *HS,* DNase hypersensitive site; *S,* silencer.

stroke. Lactic dehydrogenase also released from the RBC in hemolytic anemia is an excellent marker of these complications.

In summary, the primary amino acid structure of α-globin and non–α-globin chains dictates the inevitable quaternary structure in which resides the ability of Hb to serve as a respiratory protein. Cooperativity ensures rapid binding of oxygen in the lungs and unloading in tissues. Similarly, carbon dioxide is transported from tissues to lungs. The function of Hb may be influenced by mutation and by heterotropic effectors such as protons and 2,3-BPG. The molecule itself changes shape as it provides oxygen for metabolism; it is a lung in miniature, breathing as it allows the body to respire.

Globin Gene Clusters

The amounts and types of human Hb produced at any given age are determined primarily by the selective expression of the individual genes encoding each globin chain. The globin genes of humans are located in two clusters (Fig. 33.6): α-like genes in approximately 30 kb of DNA on the short arm of chromosome 16 between band p13.2 and the telomere and β-like genes in approximately 70 kb of DNA on the terminal portion of the short arm of chromosome 11 (p15). Each gene shares certain basic organizational features. Each contains three exons separated by two introns. Both introns of the α-gene are small (100–300 bp); non–α-genes have one small and one large (1000–1200 bp) intron. The second exon of each globin gene encodes the major components of the heme-binding pocket, and the third encodes the α and non-α contact points.

Flanking each gene at the 5′ and 3′ ends are groups of conserved nucleotides. In conjunction with protein factors, these influence the promotion of gene transcription, ensure the fidelity of the transcript and its translatability, specify sites for the initiation and termination of translation, and improve the stability of the newly synthesized mRNA (Fig. 33.7). Also encoded within the genes are signals that permit the enzymatic machinery within the nucleus to excise precisely the introns from the mRNA precursor and splice together the exons to form a contiguous "mature" mRNA. The spliced mRNA is transported to the cytoplasm and translated into protein. These conserved signals lie at the junction of the exon and intron and within the introns themselves. They are recognized by small nuclear ribonucleoprotein particles, which participate in the formation of a spliceosome, or splicing complex. Their preservation is critical for the splicing process to occur. When mutations occur within splice signal sites, globin synthesis is often impaired. The 5′ end of the mRNA contains

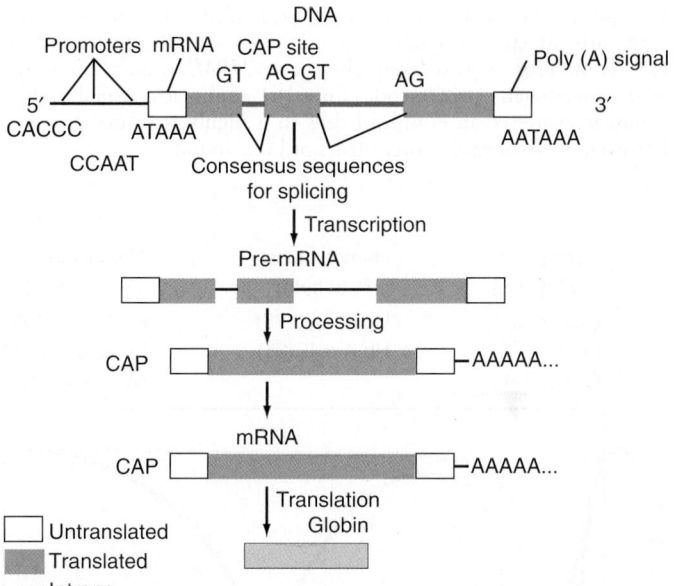

Fig. 33.7 PATHWAY OF GLOBIN BIOSYNTHESIS. Transcription of the globin gene results in a large pre-mRNA molecule containing intervening sequences. During intranuclear processing of this molecule, the intervening sequences are excised and the coding sequences ligated to form a contiguous stretch of RNA, which codes for the globin protein. The message is further processed by the addition of a CAP and a poly(A) tail. The mature message is transported from the nucleus to cytoplasm, where it is translated on polyribosomes by the addition of activated amino acids to a growing polypeptide chain. Globin acquires heme and α: non-α dimers are formed and a hemoglobin tetramer is assembled. *(Reproduced with permission from Steinberg, MH: Hemoglobinopathies and thalassemias. In Stein JH, editor:* Internal medicine, *ed 4, St. Louis, 1994, Mosby-Year Book, p 852.)*

a cap structure, and the 3′ end contains a poly(A) tail, as described in Chapter 1.

Conserved nucleotide clusters 5′ to the coding portion of each globin gene in aggregate act as promoters (see Fig. 33.7). Globin promoters are modular. Some modules are located relatively close to the initiation site of mRNA translation, and some are more distally placed. Promoters ultimately form the binding sites for the RNA polymerase complexes that catalyze gene transcription. Mutations within the promoter can affect the level of gene transcription and the amount of globin made. Surrounding and within each gene are other sequence elements that play important roles in its transcriptional regulation (see Fig. 33.6). These clusters, called *enhancers* and *silencers* (see Chapter 1), may lie within introns or 5' and 3' to the coding sequences; in some instances, they are quite remote from the gene. The higher order structure of DNA in chromatin may permit close approximation of these remote enhancers to the gene during transcription. Enhancers play important roles in the tissue-specific regulation of globin gene expression. Representative regulatory sequences near the globin genes are shown in Fig. 33.6 (enhancer-like element). DNA elements controlling globin genes are described in more detail later.

The α-like and β-like globin genes are ordered in the 5' to 3' direction in the same sequence expressed during embryonic, fetal, and adult development (Fig. 33.8). The functional significance of this arrangement is unclear. However, evidence suggests that the ordering of the ε, γ, δ, and β genes could be an important factor influencing the ability of each locus to interact with distant control elements at different developmental stages.

The α-like and β-like gene clusters probably are the result of an ancient duplication of a primordial globin gene that existed early in the history of vertebrates, approximately 500 million years ago. Each gene cluster probably developed from the duplication of ancestral genes and subsequent divergence through eons of evolution. Within the α-like gene cluster, the ζ-globin gene (*HBZ*) is expressed only very early in embryogenesis and participates in the formation of embryonic Hbs. A μ, α-like globin gene *(HBM)*, originally considered a pseudogene (ψα2), codes for a 141 amino acid α-globin–like chain, is expressed in erythroid cells in a highly regulated fashion; however, an associated protein has not been found.

The α-globin genes (*HBA2, HBA1*) are duplicated and their encoded amino acid sequences are identical; therefore, only a single α-globin polypeptide results. Minor differences within the second intervening sequence and the 3' flanking regions of the α-globin gene permit identification of transcripts from each gene. The 5' or α2-gene is expressed more efficiently than the 3' or α1-gene, so abnormalities of this gene are more likely to be clinically apparent. Both clusters contain genes that are actively transcribed, as well as pseudogenes whose defective structures prohibit expression at any time.

The gene 3' to the α1-gene is the Θ-gene (*HBQ1*), a somewhat mysterious element of the α-gene cluster. Although Θ-gene transcripts are found in fetal tissue and adult erythroid marrow, it is unclear whether this gene's translation product is able to participate in the formation of a functional tetramer. The Θ-globin protein has been found in vivo, but deletion of the Θ-globin gene does not appear to have any implications for developing fetuses. In vitro, Θ-globin mRNA is correctly spliced, and Θ-globin cDNA can direct synthesis of a translatable mRNA and a Θ-globin protein.

The β-like–globin gene cluster consists of the embryonic ε-gene (*HBE*), transcribed only during the first 6–11 weeks of life; the duplicated γ-globin genes (*HBG2, HBG1*) that code for the dominant non–α-globin of fetal life; and the δ- (*HBD*) and β-globin (*HBB*) genes that code for the Hbs of adults. The coding sequences of the two γ-globin genes are identical, except at codon 136, where the 5' or Gγ-gene codes for glutamic acid; the 3' or Aγ-gene encodes an alanine residue. These genes are unequally expressed during fetal development. A switch in their relative rates of expression leads to a similar disparity between the amounts of Gγ and Aγ chains in adults. Although the Gγ/Aγ switch is interesting from the standpoint of the control of gene expression, it is of little clinical importance. HbF in fetuses and adults contains a mixture of Gγ and Aγ chains; the functional qualities of these Hbs are identical.

The δ- and β-globin genes are probably the result of a duplication event that occurred more than 40 million years ago. The β-globin gene has become the predominant gene, coding for most non–α-globin chains of adults. The δ-globin gene has undergone mutation in several critical areas, and its expression is greatly curtailed. Its product, a minor fraction of adult Hb (HbA2), has become functionally insignificant by virtue of its very low level in the erythrocyte. It is likely that the δ-globin gene is a "pseudogene in evolution." HbA2 is clinically useful, however, for characterizing hemoglobinopathies such as β-thalassemia. expression may be totally abolished as it acquires an inactivating mutation. The pseudogenes dispersed within both globin gene clusters provide interesting glimpses into the evolutionary history of globin genes. Pseudogenes are inactive remnants of previously expressed genes. As a result of relaxed selection, their mutation rates are higher than those of surrounding active genes. Because of this, the expression of the δ-globin gene might be totally abolished as it acquires an inactivating mutation.

The expression of the human globin genes is highly regulated. Globin is synthesized in only one tissue—erythroid cells—and only during a narrowly defined stage of erythroid progenitor cell differentiation—the 5–7 days that commence with the proerythroblast stage and end when the enucleated reticulocyte loses the last traces of its RNA. Within the confines of these strict tissue-specific and differentiation stage-specific boundaries, the globin genes are extraordinarily active. By the late normoblast and reticulocyte stages, 90% to 95% of all protein synthesis in these cells is globin synthesis.

Individual globin genes are expressed at different levels in developing erythroblasts of human embryos, fetuses, and "adults" (i.e., 37–38 weeks of gestation and beyond). Different subsets of α-genes and non–α-genes are expressed and silenced at each developmental stage. Moreover, the overall balance of non–α-globin, α-globin, and heme production is maintained throughout each of these complex switching events. The complex mechanisms ensuring the proper tissue-specific, differentiation stage-specific, and ontologic stage-specific expression are incompletely defined. Much information about relevant DNA control elements and transcription factors is emerging. These topics are discussed after a review of the ontogeny of Hb.

Hemoglobins (embryonic)	Hemoglobins (% at birth)	Hemoglobins (% in adults)
Gower 1 ζ₂ε₂	Hb F α₂γ₂ (75)	Hb A α₂γ₂ (97)
Portland 1 ζ₂γ₂	Hb A α₂β₂ (25)	Hb A₂ α₂δ₂ (2.5)
Gower 2 α₂ε₂		Hb F α₂γ₂ (<1)

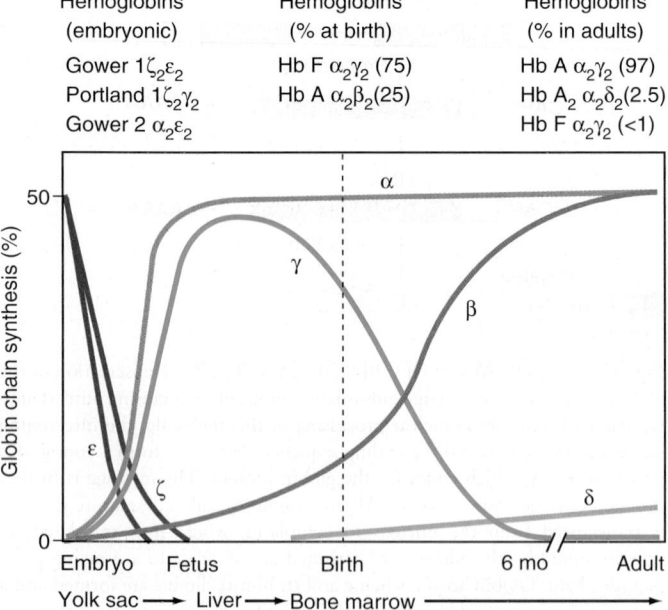

Fig. 33.8 HEMOGLOBIN (Hb) SWITCHING DURING EMBRYONIC, FETAL, AND ADULT DEVELOPMENT. The ζ and ε genes are transcribed during embryonic development and are soon replaced by the fetal γ-globin and adult α-globin gene. At birth, HbF forms approximately 75%, and HbA forms 25% of the total. Transcription of the γ gene begins to decrease before birth, and by 6 months of age, this gene is expressed only at very low levels. Expression of the δ-globin gene begins near birth. In adults, HbA makes up approximately 97%, HbA2 approximately 2.5%, and HbF less than 1% of the total. *(Reproduced with permission from Steinberg MH: Hemoglobinopathies and thalassemias. In Stein JH, editors: Internal medicine, ed 4, St. Louis, 1994, Mosby-Year Book, p 852.)*

Ontogeny of Hemoglobin

The Hb composition of the erythrocyte depends on when in gestation or postnatal development it is measured. This is a result of sequential activation and inactivation (i.e., switching) among genes within the α-globin and non–α-globin gene clusters (see Fig. 33.8). What controls these switches in globin gene transcription is not understood. The two early embryonic Hbs consist of ζ- and ε-globin chains (Hb Gower-1) and α- and ε-globin chains (Hb Gower-2). The ζ-globin gene is akin to the α-globin genes but is expressed only during early embryogenesis. The ε-embryonic globin chain is a β-like element. The combination of ζ- and γ-globin chains forms Hb Portland. These early Hbs are made primarily in yolk-sac erythroblasts and are detectable only during the very earliest stages of embryogenesis except in certain pathologic states, in which they may persist until gestation is complete. The major Hb of intrauterine life is HbF, which consists of two α- and two γ-globin chains. Expression of the γ-globin gene begins early in embryogenesis, peaks during midgestation, and begins a rapid decline just before birth. By 6 months of age in normal infants, only a remnant of prior γ-globin gene expression remains. The level of HbF in the blood declines rapidly thereafter to less than 1% of the total. Expression of the α-globin gene starts early in the first trimester, peaks quickly, and is sustained for life. Expression of the β-globin gene also commences early in gestation and reaches its zenith within a few months after birth. The combination of α-globin with β-globin chains forms HbA the predominant Hb of postnatal life. Adult cells also contain HbA2. The δ-globin gene, which directs synthesis of the non–α-globin chain of HbA2, is very inefficiently expressed. Only low levels of HbA2 are present; defects in the δ-globin gene are of no clinical consequence. In adult blood, HbF is not evenly distributed among erythrocytes and is present in only a very small number of RBCs, called F cells. HbA2 is present in all RBCs, albeit at levels less than 3.5% of the total Hb in adult life.

Hemoglobin Biosynthesis and Its Regulation

Throughout development, genes coding for α-globin, non–α-globin, and heme exhibit coordinated expression. Almost equal amounts of each of the moieties that ultimately constitute the Hb tetramer are made. Excess unpaired globin chains and mutant globins are removed from the cell by ATP-dependent proteases, ensuring a balance between accumulation of α-globin and non–α-globin chains. Balanced chain synthesis and coordination of globin chain production with synthesis of heme are important because Hb tetramers are highly soluble, but the components of Hb (i.e., unpaired chains, protoporphyrin, and iron) are not. Precipitation of any of these is deleterious to cell survival. Erythroblast proteases are not efficient enough to eliminate the substantial excesses of unpaired chains that accumulate when an α-gene or non–α-gene is selectively impaired by severe thalassemia mutations. The mechanisms regulating heme production and some of the interactions between heme and globin synthesis are discussed in Chapter 35.

The proper production of the individual globin chains within erythroid tissues at the appropriate states of differentiation and development is predominantly ensured by regulation at the level of transcription. The onset of phenotypic maturation at the proerythroblast stage is marked by the onset of globin mRNA biosynthesis in dramatically increasing quantities. Expression of α-globin and non–α-globin genes begins at essentially the same time, although some studies suggest a slightly earlier onset for α-globin gene expression. Transcription persists at a high level throughout most of the remainder of erythropoiesis, declines as the nucleus condenses, and is eventually lost in late erythroblasts. Even as the absolute rates of globin gene transcription begin to decrease, however, the relative percentage of total transcriptional activity devoted to globin gene expression continues to increase; this reflects the silencing of transcription of almost every other gene in the erythroblast.

The transcriptional activation of the globin genes is the major event that must be understood to define and manipulate the regulation of Hb biosynthesis and Hb switching. However, posttranscriptional mechanisms contribute to the final distribution of globin and non-globin mRNAs and to the balance of α-globins and non–α-globins within the erythroblasts. When compared with many other mRNAs, such as cytokine mRNAs, globin mRNAs are extraordinarily stable. Their half-lives have been estimated at 30–50 hours. Most other mRNAs have turnover rates, or half-lives, measured within the range of a few minutes to 5 or 6 hours. The increase in the percentage of total mRNA that is globin mRNA is greatly accentuated because the newly transcribed globin mRNAs accumulate and remain quite stable in the cell, but nonglobin mRNAs, which are no longer being produced, are also disappearing at a faster rate. Consequently, the mRNA content of the reticulocytes consists of 90% to 95% globin mRNA.

The transcription rates of the α-globin and non–α-globin genes are not precisely equal. (This phenomenon has been studied in detail only in adult erythroid cells expressing the α- and β-globin genes) A slight, but reproducibly detectable, excess of α-globin mRNA is present in erythroblasts. However, β-globin mRNA is translated somewhat more efficiently than α-globin mRNA. These counterbalancing forces result in almost equal syntheses of α- and β-globin polypeptide chains. There is a very slight excess of α-globin production, resulting in a small pool of free α-globin chains.

Alpha Hb-stabilizing protein (AHSP), a small protein present at high concentrations in RBCs, binds specifically to the α-globin polypeptide, protecting the unstable free α-globin chain by inhibiting heme loss and oxidant-mediated chain precipitation. It remains unclear whether mutations of this protein can modify the phenotype of β-thalassemia by increasing the imbalance in globin chain synthesis. Some α-globin chain variants, because the mutations alter AHSP binding, are associated with mild thalassemia-like features.

Newly synthesized β-globin chains are rapidly and completely incorporated into αβ dimers that spontaneously associate as tetramers. Hb tetramers are remarkably stable throughout the life span of the circulating RBC by virtue of their long half-lives. Only small amounts sustain oxidative or proteolytic damage.

Hb molecules are exposed for prolonged periods to chemically active compounds in the milieu of the bloodstream. They often become nonenzymatically modified by such processes as glycosylation, acetylation, and sulfation. Glycosylation occurs more extensively during periods of hyperglycemia and leads to elevated levels of the glycosylated form of HbA, HbA1c. This phenomenon is the basis of a useful test for control of the blood sugar in diabetes. Other posttranslational modifications are of little clinical importance except as already noted for 2,3-BPG, carbon dioxide, and NO.

Transcriptional Regulation of Globin Gene Expression

Precise regulation of the globin gene clusters involves a complex interplay between trans-acting proteins, such as transcription factors, and cis-acting sequences that act as promoters, enhancers, and silencers of gene activity. DNA-binding proteins interact with sequences in regulatory regions of the globin gene cluster and with other proteins through specific protein–protein interactions, forming DNA–protein complexes that regulate gene transcription. Trans-acting factors mediate the remodeling of chromatin structure, influencing gene expression for the entire globin gene clusters. Mutations in the cis-acting sequences or trans-acting proteins cause dysregulated expression of globin genes, resulting in thalassemia-like syndromes although most thalassemia-causing mutations are in the cognate globin gene clusters. Elucidating the full extent of sequences required for appropriate expression of globin genes will inform the development of constructs for gene therapy.

The nuclei of erythroid cells contain numerous proteins that have been identified as transcription factors, including GATA1, NFE2, LRF, and EKLF. GATA1 is named on the basis of the DNA sequence motif (T/A) GATA (A/G), the GATA motif that it recognizes and binds. It is a zinc finger class DNA-binding protein (see Chapters 22 and 26). Activity of GATA1 requires binding to a zinc finger protein cofactor called FOG1 (named for Friend of GATA1). NFE2 recognizes the DNA sequence motif (T/C) GCT GA (C/G) TCA (T/C). It is a member of the B-zip class of transcriptional activators. GATA1 and NFE2 were originally identified and cloned on the basis of their interactions with their cognate sequences in the globin genes. Erythroid Kruppel-like factor (EKLF, also called KLF1) may be the most specific of the erythroid transcription factors yet discovered. EKLF interacts specifically with the β-globin gene promoter and may influence the γ–β switch. Mice homozygous for disruption of the *Eklf* gene have lethal β-thalassemia. Alone, GATA1, NFE2, EKLF, and FOG1 cannot be the sole determination of tissue specificity of the globin genes. Together, they form a robust transcriptional network that regulates erythroid genes, including the globin genes. Mutations in GATA1 or FOG1 can cause β-thalassemia and thrombocytopenia in patients.

The regions of the globin gene clusters with essential regulatory sequences and erythroid-specific chromatin remodeling extend far beyond the coding sequences of the globin genes. The key regulatory elements for the α-globin gene (HS −48, 40, and 33) lies in erythroid-specific DNase I hypersensitive sites about 40 kb upstream from the α-globin gene. The locus control region (LCR) is critical for high level expression of the β-globin gene cluster, consisting of five sites that are hypersensitive to DNase I (HS 1–5) (see Chapters 1 and 4). Patients with deletion of the HS −40 sites exhibit α-thalassemia, and patients with deletions of the β-globin LCR develop β-thalassemia; however, the thalassemia can be a result of changes in chromatin caused by the large deletion. Similarly, transgenic mice bearing deletions of these critical regulatory regions have severely restricted expressions of the respective globin genes.

The LCRs contain binding sites for the major erythroid transcription factors, including GATA1, EKLF, and NFE2, as well as sites for transcription factors found more widely distributed in many cell types. The LCRs loop to interact directly with the promoters of individual globin genes, resulting in a complex termed the *active chromatin hub*. The resulting structure enables high level expression of globin genes in erythroid cells at the appropriate developmental stages. Additional elements act as insulators, protecting expressed genes from gene silencing through the regulation of chromatin structure.

BCL11A is a transcriptional repressor that decreases HbF expression in adult tissues. Polymorphisms in the *BCL11A* gene are powerfully associated with HbF levels, including in patients with sickle cell disease. Inhibition of *Bcl11a* increases HbF levels and attenuates the phenotype of sickle cell disease in a murine model. The erythroid-specific enhancers of BCL11A have been identified and are an attractive target for genome editing as a therapeutic strategy for the treatment of sickle cell disease and β-thalassemia. The transcription factor LRF or ZBTB7A is also a powerful silencer of HbF gene expression. When this gene and *BCL11A* are knocked out in human erythroid cells, the HbF concentration is more than 90% of the total Hb.

Transcription factors recruit enzymes that remodel chromatin structure. "Open" chromatin, or euchromatin, generally appears cytogenetically uncondensed and is associated with hyperacetylated histones, unmethylated CpG dinucleotides, and active transcription. ATRX is a protein that has been implicated in the modulation of chromatin structure at the α-globin locus. Mutations in the *ATRX* gene, located on the X chromosome, cause a syndrome of α-thalassemia, severe mental retardation, facial dysmorphism, and urogenital abnormalities. ATRX, a member of the SNF2 family of helicase/ATPases, localizes to pericentromeric heterochromatin during interphase and mitosis and contains a plant homeodomain-like domain that is found in chromatin-associated proteins. Cells with a mutated *ATRX* gene have altered patterns of DNA methylation. The ATRX protein therefore exemplifies the connections among DNA methylation, chromatin remodeling, and expression of the α-globin genes.

Chromatin structure can be manipulated pharmacologically through the influence of drugs on methylation and histone acetylation. Cytidine analogs such as 5-azacytidine and its less toxic derivative, decitabine, inactivate DNA methyltransferases, inducing γ-globin gene expression and increasing HbF levels in patients with sickle cell anemia. Histone deacetylase inhibitors are being studied as agents to increase γ-globin expression.

Posttranscriptional, Translational, and Posttranslational Mechanisms

Processed globin mRNA is exported from the nucleus to the cytoplasm by a mechanism that is not clearly defined. mRNA translation occurs in the cytoplasm (see Fig. 33.7). The triplet codons or mRNA are recognized by the anticodons of specific tRNAs that bring activated amino acid residues to the nascent polypeptide chains. The process of translation, in which an mRNA template directs the synthesis of protein, is typically divided into three phases: initiation, elongation, and termination (see Chapters 1 and 4). Each phase is regulated by a variety of protein factors.

The globin mRNA molecule becomes associated with four to six ribosomes, forming the polyribosome. At least 11 eukaryotic translation initiation factors interact with the polyribosome. They mediate stabilization of a preinitiation complex, binding of the initiator methionine tRNA to ribosomal subunits, binding of mRNA to the preinitiation complex, stabilization of mRNA binding, recognition of the cap site at the 5' end of mRNA, and release of initiation factors from the preinitiation complex. Several elongation and termination factors have also been defined. Initiation or an early step in the elongation process is the rate-limiting factor.

The first posttranslational step in tetramer formation is the combination of α-globin and non–α-globin chains to form dimers, an event that appears to depend on the relative charge of each globin subunit. The dimers then form tetrameric Hb. Because of charge differences among non–α-globin chains, there is a hierarchy or affinity of these chains for α-globin chains. The combination of α- and β-globin chains is most favored followed by a combination of α-, γ-, and δ-globin chains. Certain mutant Hbs that have gained or lost a charge may alter this hierarchic arrangement. This may influence the proportion of variant Hb present, especially when the patient also inherits an α-thalassemia syndrome, in which the synthesis of α-globin chains is reduced. The supply of available α-globin chains is then limited, and non–α-globin chains compete with one another to form tetramers with the limiting α-globin chain pool.

Globin chain biosynthesis and heme synthesis are mutually important. Heme plays a role in the regulation of the initiation complex. A deficiency of heme (e.g., in iron deficiency) is associated with the accumulation of a repressor of translation initiation factors. Translation of β-globin mRNA appears to be initiated more efficiently than α-globin mRNA, conferring on the associated anemia some of the features of mild α-thalassemia. This phenomenon occurs because heme deficiency depresses the availability of initiating factors for which the less efficient α-mRNA must compete with the more efficient β-mRNA.

The identification of genetic mutations that cause congenital and acquired forms of anemia provide further insight into the pathways required for the coordinated production of globin and heme. More than half of patients with Diamond-Blackfan anemia, a disorder characterized by a severe macrocytic anemia and a paucity of erythroid progenitor cells, have heterozygous germline mutations in the *RPS19* gene or other genes encoding ribosomal proteins. Similarly, the macrocytic anemia in patients with myelodysplastic syndrome and a deletion of chromosome 5q is caused by heterozygous deletion of another ribosomal protein gene, *RPS14*. Haploinsufficiency for these ribosomal protein genes activates the p53 pathway, leading to cell cycle arrest and apoptosis selectively in the erythroid progenitor cells.

Refractory anemia with ring sideroblasts (RARS) is a subtype of myelodysplastic syndrome characterized by iron-loaded mitochondria evident on Prussian blue staining. In the majority of RARS cases, somatic mutations are present in the *SF3B1* gene, encoding a core member of the RNA splicing machinery. The precise targets of SF3B1 have not been identified.

TABLE 33.1	Classification of Hemoglobinopathies and Thalassemias

Structural hemoglobinopathies—mutations altering the amino acid sequence of a globin chain and altering physical or chemical properties of the hemoglobin tetramer in such a way that function is deranged

Abnormal Hemoglobin Polymerization—Sickle Cell Hemoglobin (HbS); Hemolysis, Vasoocclusion

    Abnormal Hb crystallization (e.g., HbC)
    High oxygen affinity—polycythemia (Hb Zurich)
    Low oxygen affinity—cyanosis (Hb Kansas)
    Hbs that oxidize or precipitate too readily—unstable Hbs (Hb Köln)
    M Hbs—methemoglobinemia, cyanosis (e.g., Hb Milwaukee)

Thalassemia—Defective Production of Globin Chains With Hypochromia, Anemia, Hemolysis, Altered Erythropoiesis

    α-Thalassemia
    β-Thalassemia
    $\delta\beta$-Thalassemias, $\gamma\delta\beta$-thalassemias, $\alpha\beta$-thalassemias

"Thalassemic" Hemoglobinopathies and Dominantly Inherited Thalassemias—Mutations Altering the Synthesis and Structure or Function of the Hemoglobin Gene Products (e.g., HbE, Hb Terre Haute, Hb Lepore, Hb Constant Spring)

    Hereditary persistence of fetal hemoglobin (HbF)—persistence of high levels of HbF into adult life
    Pancellular—high HbF levels in all RBCs
    Nondeletion forms
    Deletion forms
    Hb Kenya
    Heterocellular—inherited increases in the percentage of F cells
    Acquired hemoglobinopathies

Methemoglobinemia Caused by Toxic Exposures

    Sulfhemoglobinemia caused by toxic exposures
    Carboxyhemoglobinemia caused by toxic exposures
    HbH in erythroleukemias
    Acquired elevations in F cells and HbF
    Erythroid stress (e.g., recovery from BM suppression)
    BM dysplasias
    Exposure to agents altering stem cells or gene expression (e.g., hydroxyurea, butyric acid)

BM, Bone marrow; Hb, hemoglobin; RBC, red blood cell.

NOSOLOGY OF HEMOGLOBINOPATHIES

Inherited abnormalities of the Hb molecules that cause morbidity are called hemoglobinopathies and thalassemias. Many of these conditions produce diseases (e.g., sickle cell anemia, thalassemia, unstable Hbs, Hbs with altered oxygen affinity, M Hbs) that are especially important to hematologists. A few acquired conditions lead to modifications of Hb (e.g., carbon monoxide exposure, producing carboxyhemoglobinemia, nitrite exposure causing methemoglobinemia) that produce clinical abnormalities. These situations are summarized by the term acquired hemoglobinopathies or dyshemoglobinemias.

Most of the more than 1200 mutations of the globin gene that have been described produce no disease or only trivial clinical effects. The remainder can be classified according to the hematologic and clinical phenotypes that cause reduced solubility with hemolytic anemia (unstable Hbs and polymerizing Hbs, such as sickle Hb); Hbs with altered oxygen affinity; Hbs predisposing to methemoglobin formation; and the thalassemias involving abnormal synthesis of one or more globin chains with anemia, hemolysis, and alterations of erythropoiesis. Some mutations, such as that responsible for HbE, can alter the structure and synthesis of the molecule. A classification of hemoglobinopathies and thalassemias is provided in Table 33.1. Individual conditions are discussed in the chapters already cross-referenced in earlier sections of this chapter.

SUGGESTED READINGS

Bank A: Regulation of human fetal hemoglobin: new players, new complexities. *Blood* 107:435, 2006.

Boas FE, Forman L, Beutler E: Phosphatidylserine exposure and red cell viability in red cell aging and in hemolytic anemia. *Proc Natl Acad Sci USA* 95:3077, 1998.

Burgess-Beusse B, Farrell C, Gaszner M, et al: The insulation of genes from external enhancers and silencing chromatin. *Proc Natl Acad Sci USA* 99:16433, 2002.

Cantor AB, Orkin SH: Transcriptional regulation of erythropoiesis: an affair involving multiple partners. *Oncogene* 21:3368, 2002.

Chakalova L, Carter D, Debrand E, et al: Developmental regulation of the beta-globin gene locus. *Prog Mol Subcell Biol* 38:183, 2005.

Chiu CH, Schneider H, Slightom JL, et al: Dynamics of regulatory evolution in primate β-globin gene clusters: *cis*-Mediated acquisition of simian gamma fetal expression patterns. *Gene* 205:47, 1997.

Dzierzak E: The emergence of definitive hematopoietic stem cells in the mammal. *Curr Opin Hematol* 12:197, 2005.

Feng L, Zhou S, Gu L, et al: Structure of oxidized alpha-haemoglobin bound to AHSP reveals a protective mechanism for haem. *Nature* 435:697, 2005.

Gibbons RJ, Picketts DJ, Villard L, et al: Mutations in a putative global transcriptional regulator cause X-linked mental retardation with α-thalassemia (ATR-X syndrome). *Cell* 80:837, 1995.

Gladwin MT, Wang X, Reiter CD, et al: S-nitrosohemoglobin is unstable in the reductive erythrocyte environment and lacks O_2/NO-linked allosteric function. *J Biol Chem* 277:27818, 2002.

Gow AJ, Stamler JS: Reactions between nitric oxide and haemoglobin under physiological conditions. *Nature* 391:169, 1998.

Hardison R, Riemer C, Chui DH, et al: Electronic access to sequence alignments, experimental results, and human mutations as an aid to studying globin gene regulation. *Genomics* 47:429, 1998.

Higgs DR, Garrick D, Anguita E, et al: Understanding alpha-globin gene regulation: Aiming to improve the management of thalassemia. *Ann N Y Acad Sci* 1054:92, 2005.

Jenuwein T, Allis CD: Translating the histone code. *Science* 293:1074, 2001.

Kato GJ, McGowan V, Machado RF, et al: Lactate dehydrogenase as a biomarker of hemolysis-associated nitric oxide resistance, priapism, leg ulceration, pulmonary hypertension, and death in patients with sickle cell disease. *Blood* 107:2279, 2006.

Kihm AJ, Kong Y, Hong W, et al: An abundant erythroid protein that stabilizes free alpha-haemoglobin. *Nature* 417:758, 2002.

Li Q, Peterson KR, Fang X, et al: Locus control regions. *Blood* 100:3077, 2002.

Miller IJ, Bieker JJ: A novel erythroid cell-specific murine transcription factor that binds to the CACCC element and is related to the Kruppel family of nuclear proteins. *Mol Cell Biol* 13:2776, 1993.

Rother RP, Bell L, Hillmen P, et al: The clinical sequelae of intravascular hemolysis and extracellular plasma hemoglobin: a novel mechanism of human disease. *JAMA* 293:1653, 2005.

Stamatoyannopoulos G: Control of globin gene expression during development and erythroid differentiation. *Exp Hematol* 33:259, 2005.

Stamler JS, Jia L, Eu JP, et al: Blood flow regulation by S-nitrosohemoglobin in the physiological oxygen gradient. *Science* 276:2034, 1997.

Steinberg MH, Forget BG, Higgs DR, et al: *Disorders of hemoglobin: genetics, pathophysiology, and clinical management*, ed 2, Cambridge, 2009, Cambridge University Press.

Viprakasit V, Tanphaichitr VS, Chinchang W, et al: Evaluation of alpha hemoglobin stabilizing protein (AHSP) as a genetic modifier in patients with beta thalassemia. *Blood* 103:3296, 2004.

Walsh M, Lutz RJ, Cotter TG, et al: Erythrocyte survival is promoted by plasma and suppressed by a Bak-derived BH3 peptide that interacts with membrane-associated Bcl-X(L). *Blood* 99:3439, 2002.

Weatherall DJ, Clegg JB: *The thalassaemia syndromes*, ed 4, Oxford, 2001, Blackwell Science Limited, p 818.

Weiss MJ, Zhou S, Feng L, et al: Role of alpha-hemoglobin-stabilizing protein in normal erythropoiesis and beta-thalassemia. *Ann N Y Acad Sci* 1054:103, 2005.

CHAPTER 34

APPROACH TO ANEMIA IN THE ADULT AND CHILD

Judith C. Lin

Anemia is the clinical state of low red cell mass and one of the most commonly encountered laboratory findings and clinical disorders in hematology. Anemias encompass a broad range of clinical disorders and diseases with a spectrum of subtle to severe clinical impact on health. The approach to anemias can be direct if the cause is a common, singular or monogenic, easily tested and identified one; but in challenging cases, the approach may require a careful, systematic investigation and deduction due to the diverse span of possible pathology and pathogenesis to the red blood cell components, erythropoiesis, and apoptosis. The examination of the patient's blood cell morphology by peripheral smear supports the analysis of anemia and is an integral skill for anemia diagnosis. Epidemiologic studies on the global burden of anemias show that in recent decades iron deficiency accounts for the majority of anemias, with predominance in females and the very young (under 5 years of age) having risen and the anemias of hemoglobinopathies, nutritional deficiency, parasitic infections, and chronic kidney disease significantly impacting quality of life.[1] When analyzing anemia in individuals the approach should be systematic and is often initially categorical, e.g., by relative rates of red cell production, turnover or by characteristic indices and morphologies of red blood cells (RBCs). Additionally, the evaluation of anemia in the adult and child differ primarily in the changing normal ranges for red cells and hemoglobin during childhood as well as the prevalence and onset of congenital hematopoietic diseases and the risks and causes of acquired anemias at different ages in the adult. As population demographics continuously change over time, the evaluation of anemia may also require consideration of the frequent causes of endemic origins.[2]

The evaluation of anemia includes the initial systematic review of laboratory data obtained from the complete blood count (CBC), reticulocyte count, and peripheral blood smear and consideration of the process of RBC production, erythropoiesis.

OVERVIEW OF ERTHROPOIESIS

Erythropoiesis is the regulated process leading to the production of mature RBCs or erythrocytes. Bone marrow (BM) stem cells stimulated by the hormone erythropoietin and other factors, proliferate and differentiate along a pathway of recognizable erythroid precursors that ultimately leads to extrusion of the nucleus to facilitate efficient RBC rheology after the production and accumulation of a high concentration of hemoglobin and RBC enzymes (Fig. 34.1).[1] The early maturing RBCs lose their residual RNA under normal conditions by degradation within a day. Special staining for RNA identifies these cells, termed *reticulocytes* that are useful for both qualitative and quantitative measure of the relative rate of peripheral blood erythropoiesis. Mature RBCs survive in blood circulation 100 to 120 days before being removed from the circulation by macrophages in the spleen and other cells of the reticuloendothelial system.[2] At steady state under physiologic conditions, the production and destruction of erythrocytes is equivalent. This process is driven in large part by the hormone erythropoietin, which is produced in a regulated fashion by periglomerular cells in the kidney (~90%) and constitutively by the liver (~10%).[3] Because preservation of oxygen delivery to tissues is so important, the oxygen-sensing regulatory proteins located in the kidney respond to decreased oxygen tension from any cause such as blood loss, high altitude, or cardiac shunts with the production of erythropoietin (Fig. 34.2). This hormone then travels through the

bloodstream and stimulates RBC production in the BM. Provided that there are adequate nutrients, including folate, vitamin B_{12}, and iron, the precursors in the BM proliferate and mature and are released into the circulation, ultimately expanding the pool of erythrocytes.[4] The increase in oxygen delivery to the kidney then reduces the stimulus for erythropoietin production.

DEFINITION OF ANEMIA

Anemia is defined as a reduction in the RBC mass. Because of a variety of factors, the RBC mass normally changes during the lifespan of an individual and may be different in males and females.[5] Understanding the changes that occur is critical to appropriately identifying what constitutes anemia (Table 34.1). The relatively elevated level of hemoglobin present at birth declines over the first 1 to 2 months of life to levels that are lower than those seen in adulthood. In later childhood, the hemoglobin values are similar and increase modestly over time. Around puberty, girls have reached adult levels of hemoglobin, and androgenic steroids lead to a continued increase in hemoglobin in boys through about age 18 years. This approximately 1.5 g/dL difference between males and females persists through much of adult life until about age 70 years, when the hemoglobin value in men begins to decline. Over the next two decades, the hemoglobin value declines by about 1 g/dL in men while decreasing by only approximately 0.2 g/dL in women.[6] Thus at age 90 years, there is only a modest difference between the mean hemoglobin values observed in men and women (14.1 vs. 13.8 g/dL).

MECHANISMS OF ANEMIA

Although a complete review of all of the mechanisms leading to anemia is beyond the scope of this chapter, an appreciation of some of the mechanisms is useful before approaching the diagnosis of anemia in adults and children. Three broad categories of anemia are blood loss anemia, hypoproliferative anemia, and hemolytic anemia. Blood loss may occur acutely or chronically. When blood is lost acutely through hemorrhage, it may take several hours before a decline in hemoglobin concentration is observed because of the time required for restoration of the plasma volume and equilibration. Several days may elapse before an appropriate reticulocytosis is noted. Chronic blood loss ultimately leads to hypoproliferative anemia because of iron deficiency.

Hypoproliferative Anemia

When used broadly, the term *hypoproliferative anemia* refers to entities that manifest as an inability to produce an adequate number of erythrocytes in response to appropriate signals. Although there are many different causes, the hallmark of hypoproliferative anemia is a low reticulocyte count (Table 34.2). The etiology underlying this class of disorders may relate to the hypoproliferation of precursors within the BM, such as may be seen when there is BM replacement (myelophthisis), or to abnormal maturation of precursors in the BM, such as that which occurs in megaloblastic anemia (folate deficiency, vitamin B_{12} deficiency, myelodysplastic syndromes [MDS], and

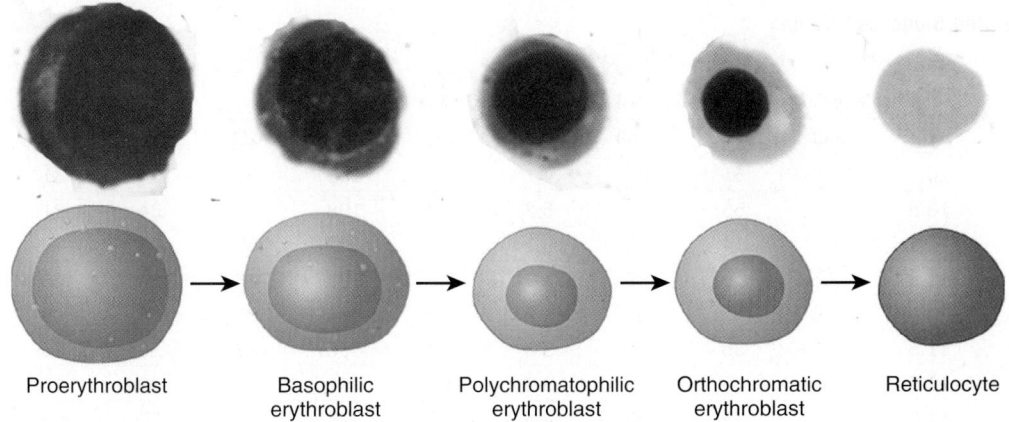

Fig. 34.1 OVERVIEW OF ERYTHROPOIESIS.

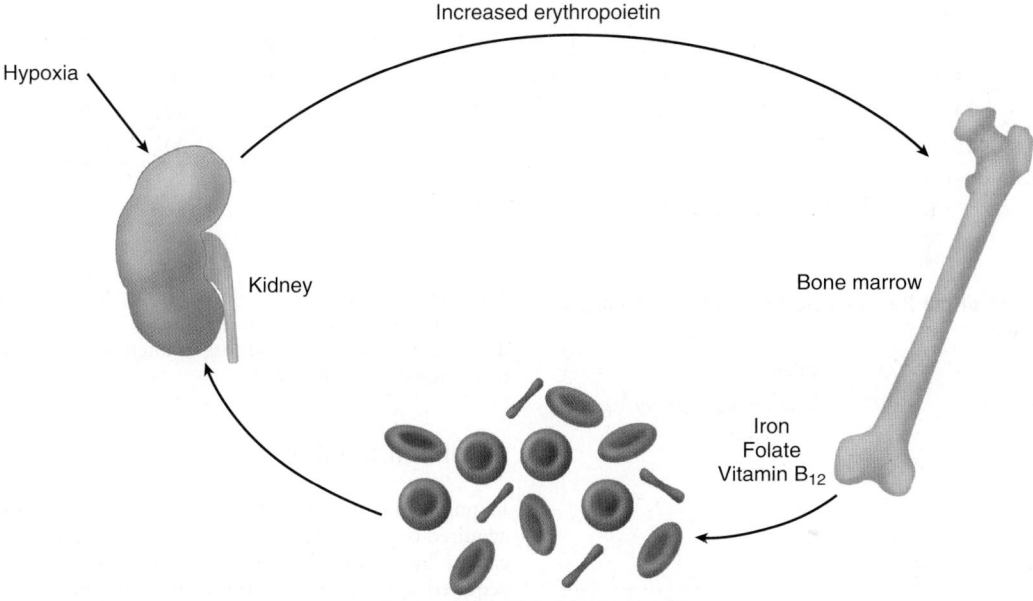

Fig. 34.2 REGULATION OF ERYTHROPOIESIS.

others). In the latter case of megaloblastic anemia, the BM often is packed. However, intramedullary demise of precursors prevents the formation and release of mature RBCs.

By far the most common cause of hypoproliferative anemia globally is iron deficiency.[7] It is estimated that about 2% of infants and children may become iron deficient purely because of inadequate dietary intake, and that 4% of women ages 20 to 49 years of age in the United States have iron-deficiency anemia primarily because of inadequate dietary intake in the setting of menstruation and childbirth. Iron deficiency is also commonly encountered in older individuals as well (~2% of individuals older than age 50 years), and it should provoke a thorough search for its etiology, which in both men and nonmenstruating women frequently is gastrointestinal blood loss. After iron deficiency, acute or chronic inflammation and renal disease are common etiologies of anemia.[8,9] BM failure states and BM replacement caused by hematologic malignancies or solid tumors are less common causes of anemia and are often accompanied by other hematologic manifestations, such as leukopenia and thrombocytopenia.

Hemolytic Anemia

The causes of hemolytic anemia are quite varied and may be congenital or acquired.[10] The hallmark of hemolytic anemia is an elevated reticulocyte count (see Table 34.2). Other features commonly associated with hemolytic anemia include an elevated lactate dehydrogenase (LDH) level, increased unconjugated (indirect) bilirubin level, and decreased haptoglobin level. Hemolytic anemia also may manifest with distinctive changes on the peripheral blood smear. Congenital causes include the hemoglobinopathies, enzymopathies (predominantly glucose-6-phosphate dehydrogenase [G6PD] deficiency), and membrane disorders.[11] Acquired conditions include autoimmune hemolytic anemia, microangiopathic hemolytic anemia, hemolysis related to infections, and acquired membrane disorders such as those caused by liver disease (spur cell of anemia) and paroxysmal nocturnal hemoglobinuria.[12]

COMPARISON OF ETIOLOGIES OF ANEMIA IN ADULTS AND CHILDREN

As already noted, the designation that anemia is present relies on comparison of the patient's hemoglobin or hematocrit with an age- and sex-appropriate normal range (see Table 34.1). Although many types of anemia may occur across the age spectrum, certain types tend to be identified more commonly in either adults or children, and some are primarily identified in neonates. In children, the most common causes of anemia are related to nutritional deficiency or to

TABLE 34.1 Normal Red Blood Cell Values

Age	Hemoglobin (g/dL)		Hematocrit (%)		Red Blood Cell Count (10¹²/L)		MCV (fL)		MCH (pg)		MCHC (g/dL)	
	Mean	−2SD	Mean	−2SD	Mean	−2SD	Mean	−2SD	Mean	−2SD	Mean	−2SD
Birth (cord blood)	16.5	13.5	51	42	4.7	3.9	108	98	34	31	33	30
1–3 days (capillary)	18.5	14.5	56	45	5.2	4.0	108	95	34	31	33	29
1 week	17.5	13.5	54	42	3.1	3.9	107	88	34	28	33	28
2 weeks	16.5	12.5	51	39	4.9	3.6	105	86	34	28	33	28
1 month	14.0	10.0	43	31	4.2	3.0	104	85	34	28	33	29
2 months	11.5	9.0	35	28	3.8	2.7	96	77	30	26	33	29
3–6 months	11.5	9.5	35	29	3.8	3.1	91	74	30	25	33	30
0.5–2 years	12.0	11.0	36	33	4.5	3.7	78	70	27	23	33	30
2–6 years	12.5	11.5	37	34	4.6	3.9	81	75	27	24	34	31
6–12 years	13.5	11.5	40	35	4.6	4.0	86	77	29	25	34	31
12–18 Years												
Female	14.0	12.0	41	36	4.6	4.1	90	78	30	25	34	31
Male 18–49 years	14.5	13.0	43	37	4.9	4.5	88	78	30	25	34	31
Female	14.0	12.0	41	36	4.6	4.0	90	80	30	26	34	31
Male	15.5	13.5	47	41	5.2	4.5	90	80	30	26	34	31

MCH, Mean corpuscular hemoglobin; MCHC, mean corpuscular hemoglobin concentration; MCV, mean corpuscular volume.
From Oski FA: Pallor. In Kaye R, Oski FA, Barness LA, editors: *Core textbook of pediatrics*, ed 3, Philadelphia, 1989, Lippincott, p 62.

TABLE 34.2 Usefulness of the Reticulocyte Count in the Diagnosis of Anemia[a]

Diagnosis	Value
Hypoproliferative Anemias	Absolute Reticulocyte Count <75,000/µL
Anemia of chronic disease	
Anemia of renal disease	
Congenital dyserythropoietic anemias	
Effects of drugs or toxins	
Endocrine anemias	
Iron deficiency	
Bone marrow replacement	
Maturation abnormalities	Absolute reticulocyte count <75,000/µL
Vitamin B₁₂ deficiency	
Folate deficiency	
Sideroblastic anemia	
Appropriate response to blood loss or nutritional supplementation	Absolute reticulocyte count ≥100,000/µL
Hemolytic anemias	Absolute reticulocyte count ≥100,000/µL
Hemoglobinopathies	
Immune hemolytic anemias	
Infectious causes of hemolysis	
Membrane abnormalities	
Metabolic abnormalities	
Mechanical hemolysis	

[a]Note that reticulocyte counts in the range of 75,000 to 100,000/µL can sometimes be associated with appropriate response to blood loss or hemolytic anemia.

a primary hematologic process, either hereditary or acquired. In contrast, the most common causes of anemia in adults are iron deficiency caused by blood loss or anemia caused by systemic illness or malignancy (Table 34.3).

Anemia in Children

Hypoproliferative anemia in children may be associated with either acquired or congenital etiologies. Acquired cases are most commonly caused by nutritional deficiency but also include those caused by acquired aplastic anemia, transient erythroblastopenia of childhood (TEC), the anemia of acute inflammation, and marrow replacement caused by malignancy.[13] Congenital causes include Diamond-Blackfan anemia and other rare syndromes, including refractory sideroblastic anemia and the congenital dyserythropoietic anemias.[14] Iron deficiency may occur in children because of a diet that is rich in cow's milk to the exclusion of other iron-containing foods. This is particularly common during the first 2 years of life. The anemia may be quite severe and may be associated with a mean corpuscular volume (MCV) of 50 to 65 fL. Acquired aplastic anemia, as opposed to pure RBC aplasia, is associated with bicytopenia or pancytopenia. TEC is an acquired disorder that generally occurs during the first 3 years of life in otherwise healthy children, although it can be seen in children from 6 months to 10 years old. It is thought to have a viral or immunologic cause and resolves without specific intervention. The anemia of acute inflammation may be encountered in children who are hospitalized and is generally transient, resolving when the underlying condition has improved. Leukemia may result in BM replacement and is usually associated with abnormalities in other cell lineages in addition to RBCs.

Hemolytic anemia in children is most commonly associated with inherited disorders of hemoglobin or the RBC membrane.[15] However, acquired causes such as autoimmune hemolytic anemia and microangiopathic hemolytic anemia, particularly *Shiga* toxin–associated hemolytic uremic syndrome (HUS), also occur.[16] In older children, many etiologies of hemolytic anemia overlap with those considered in adults, and a similar diagnostic algorithm may be appropriate. However, in newborns, inherited causes of hemolytic anemia must be distinguished from more pronounced cases of the physiologic

<table>
<tr><td>TABLE 34.3</td><td colspan="2">Comparison of the More Common Causes of Anemia in Children and Adult</td></tr>
</table>

Type of Anemia	Children	Adults
Hypoproliferative	• Nutritional deficiency (most commonly iron deficiency) • Acute inflammation • Transient erythroblastopenia of childhood • Acquired aplastic anemia • Marrow replacement caused by malignancy	• Iron deficiency • Anemia of inflammation (anemia of chronic disease) • Anemia of renal disease • Folate or vitamin B_{12} deficiency • Drugs or toxins • Pure RBC aplasia (viral or idiopathic) • MDS
Hemolytic	• Inherited hemoglobinopathies • Inherited membrane disorders • Autoimmune hemolytic anemia • Microangiopathic hemolytic anemia	• Inherited hemoglobinopathies with milder manifestations • Inherited membrane disorders with milder manifestations • G6PD deficiency • Autoimmune hemolytic anemia • Microangiopathic hemolytic anemia (DIC, TTP, HUS, aHUS)

aHUS, Atypical hemolytic uremic syndrome; DIC, disseminated intravascular coagulation; G6PD, glucose-6-phosphate dehydrogenase; HUS, hemolytic uremic syndrome; MDS, myelodysplastic syndrome; RBC, red blood cell; TTP, thrombotic thrombocytopenic purpura.

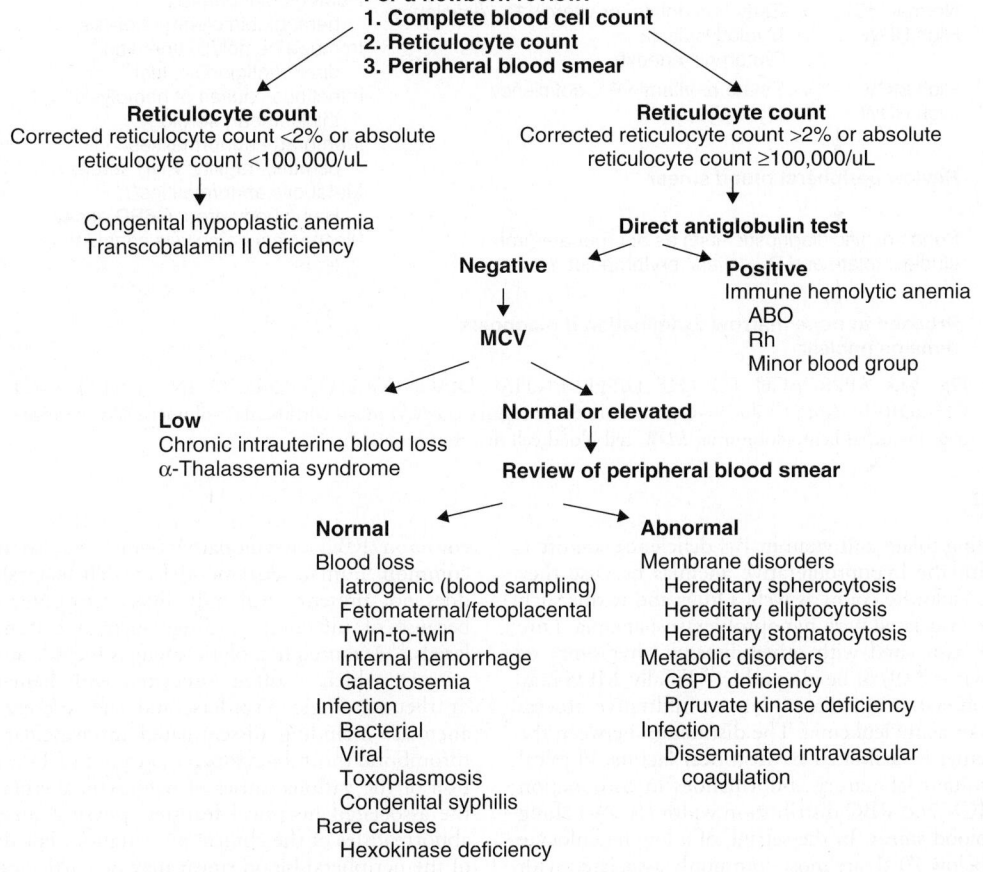

Fig. 34.3 APPROACH TO THE DIFFERENTIAL DIAGNOSIS OF ANEMIA IN A NEWBORN. *G6PD,* Glucose-6-phosphate dehydrogenase; *MCV,* mean corpuscular volume.

hyperbilirubinemia that occurs. After true hemolysis has been identified in an infant, the differential diagnosis is relatively limited (Fig. 34.3). Immune-mediated hemolysis may result from ABO, Rh, or minor blood group incompatibility.[17] Other causes include metabolic disorders and disorders of the RBC membrane. Of note, however, is the fact that hemoglobinopathies, such as sickle cell disease and β-thalassemia, are silent during the newborn period and only become manifest at 4 to 6 months of age when the fetal-to-adult hemoglobin transition has been completed. Newborn screening programs in the United States may provide salient information in this regard on the presence or absence of a hemoglobinopathy.

Alternatively, ethnic background and family history may be helpful in arriving at the appropriate diagnosis.

Anemia in Adults

Hypoproliferative anemia in adults is relatively common. If acute blood loss is excluded, hypoproliferative causes are the most common entities associated with anemia in adults. These are iron deficiency, inflammation (anemia of chronic disease), and renal disease (Fig. 34.4). The megaloblastic anemias that represent maturation

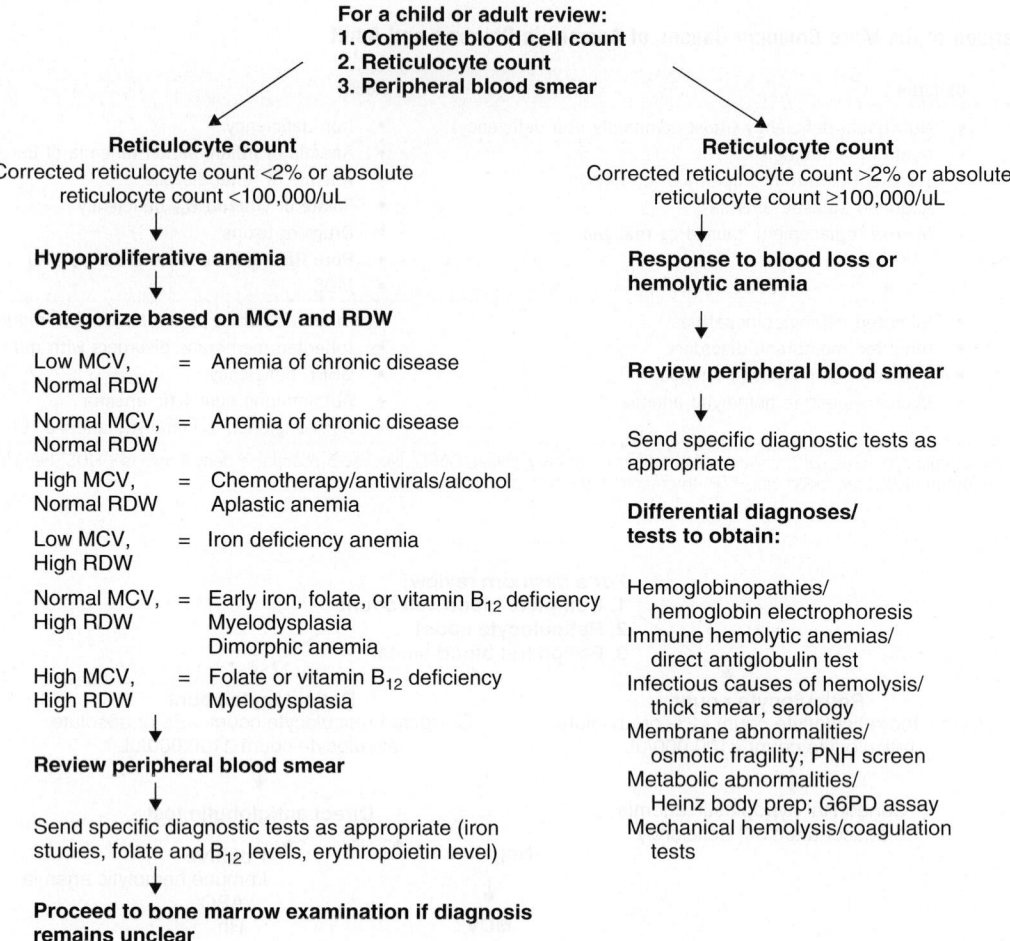

For a child or adult review:
1. Complete blood cell count
2. Reticulocyte count
3. Peripheral blood smear

Reticulocyte count
Corrected reticulocyte count <2% or absolute
reticulocyte count <100,000/uL

↓

Hypoproliferative anemia

↓

Categorize based on MCV and RDW

Low MCV, Normal RDW	=	Anemia of chronic disease
Normal MCV, Normal RDW	=	Anemia of chronic disease
High MCV, Normal RDW	=	Chemotherapy/antivirals/alcohol Aplastic anemia
Low MCV, High RDW	=	Iron deficiency anemia
Normal MCV, High RDW	=	Early iron, folate, or vitamin B$_{12}$ deficiency Myelodysplasia Dimorphic anemia
High MCV, High RDW	=	Folate or vitamin B$_{12}$ deficiency Myelodysplasia

↓

Review peripheral blood smear

↓

Send specific diagnostic tests as appropriate (iron
studies, folate and B$_{12}$ levels, erythropoietin level)

↓

**Proceed to bone marrow examination if diagnosis
remains unclear**

Reticulocyte count
Corrected reticulocyte count >2% or absolute
reticulocyte count ≥100,000/uL

↓

**Response to blood loss or
hemolytic anemia**

↓

Review peripheral blood smear

↓

Send specific diagnostic tests as
appropriate

**Differential diagnoses/
tests to obtain:**

Hemoglobinopathies/
hemoglobin electrophoresis
Immune hemolytic anemias/
direct antiglobulin test
Infectious causes of hemolysis/
thick smear, serology
Membrane abnormalities/
osmotic fragility; PNH screen
Metabolic abnormalities/
Heinz body prep; G6PD assay
Mechanical hemolysis/coagulation
tests

Fig. 34.4 APPROACH TO THE DIFFERENTIAL DIAGNOSES OF ANEMIA IN ADULTS AND CHILDREN. *G6PD,* Glucose-6-phosphate dehydrogenase; *MCV,* mean corpuscular volume; *PNH,* paroxysmal nocturnal hemoglobinuria; *RDW,* red blood cell distribution width.

abnormalities, including folate and vitamin B$_{12}$ deficiency, are often categorized along with the hypoproliferative anemias because they present with a low reticulocyte count as well. Drugs and toxins such as ethanol can also be associated with hypoproliferative anemia. Pure RBC aplasia may be associated with other diseases (thymoma) or viral infection (parvovirus B19) or be idiopathic.[18] Finally, MDS may present with hypoproliferative anemia, as may an infiltrative process such as myelofibrosis or acute leukemia. The distinction between the various causes of anemia is facilitated by historical factors, physical findings, and concomitant laboratory abnormalities in conjunction with review of the MCV and RBC distribution width (RDW) along with the peripheral blood smear. In the setting of a low reticulocyte count, MCV values below 70 fL are most commonly associated with iron-deficiency anemia, and those above 120 fL are most commonly associated with folate or vitamin B$_{12}$ deficiency. The differential diagnosis broadens for MCV values that fall just outside of the normal range. For example, in the setting of a low reticulocyte count, MCV values in the range from 75 to 80 fL may be associated with iron-deficiency anemia, the anemia of inflammation, and endocrine causes of anemia. MCV values between 100 and 110 fL may be associated with folate or vitamin B$_{12}$ deficiency, aplastic anemia, MDS, liver disease, and immune hemolytic anemias.

Hemolytic anemia in adults is less common than hypoproliferative anemia, and the differential diagnosis is broad. Congenital causes associated with mild to moderate hemolysis may be clinically silent until detected later in life.[19] This is particularly the case for milder cases of β-thalassemia intermedia, sickle cell (SC) disease and sickle-β^{+}-thalassemia, and hereditary spherocytosis. Additionally, the most

common RBC enzymopathy (which is also the one of the most common human enzyme defect deficiencies), G6PD deficiency, does not present until individuals encounter oxidant stress either because of infection or drugs such as sulfonamides and antimalarials.[20] Acquired hemolytic anemias include autoimmune hemolytic anemia, which is often associated with hematologic malignancies or rheumatologic disorders, and the microangiopathic hemolytic anemias, including disseminated intravascular coagulation (DIC), thrombotic thrombocytopenic purpura (TTP), and HUS.[21] Distinction of the various causes of hemolytic anemia is also facilitated by the associated historical features, physical findings, and laboratory abnormalities of the clinical presentation. For these disorders, review of the peripheral blood smear may be particularly revealing as to the etiology.

SYSTEMIC APPROACH TO ANEMIA

The correct diagnosis of anemia can often be determined by combining a thorough history and physical examination with review of the CBC, concentrating particularly on the MCV and RDW, along with review of the reticulocyte count and the peripheral blood smear.

History and Physical Examination

Anemia can be a primary disorder or secondary to other systemic processes, thus a careful history and physical examination provide valuable insight into the potential cause. Fatigue often accompanies anemia, but it is very nonspecific and may be related to systemic illness. Nonetheless, determining the concomitant presence of a systemic inflammatory disorder, infection, or malignancy that may be associated with fatigue can be critical in determining the underlying causes of anemia in both adults and children. The medical history may also be quite informative. For example, a history of diabetes mellitus can be associated with significantly impaired renal production of erythropoietin even in the setting of only a mildly elevated creatinine level. Because certain medications may be associated with BM depression or, alternatively, the development of autoimmune hemolytic anemia, all pharmacologic agents, prescribed and over the counter, including alternative medicines, should be reviewed. Occupational history is occasionally relevant, as in the case of individuals, such as welders, who might have been exposed to lead or other potentially BM toxic agents. Social history can be important. A history of intravenous drug use might suggest the possibility of virally transmitted diseases, such as HIV, which may be associated with anemia. Dietary history is also very important, particularly in young and elderly individuals with anemia. The finding of pica in adults (most commonly ice chips or cornstarch) is well known to be associated with iron-deficiency anemia.[22] Ingestion of paint chips may suggest the need to investigate the possibility of toxic lead ingestion. A family history of anemia is highly relevant in the evaluation of children with anemia. However, it is also relevant in adults because certain congenital anemias, such as milder forms of sickle β^+ thalassemia and hereditary spherocytosis, occasionally first become clinically apparent in adulthood.

The significance of pallor on physical examination is in many ways similar to the historic feature of fatigue: it is a common but nonspecific finding. More specific findings may be found in certain types of anemia. For example, angular cheilitis (cracking at the edges of the lips) and koilonychia (spooning of the nails) may accompany iron-deficiency anemia. Splenomegaly may be present in patients with anemia arising from a wide variety of different causes. When present early in life, it is suggestive of a congenital hemolytic anemia, such as thalassemia, sickle cell disease, or hereditary spherocytosis. When found for the first time later in life, splenomegaly may indicate an acquired disorder, such as autoimmune hemolytic anemia, lymphoproliferative disease, or a myeloproliferative disease such as myelofibrosis. Other physical findings can also sometimes provide insight relevant to the investigation of anemia when combined with historical features and laboratory data. Although anemia itself may lead to the presence of systolic cardiac murmurs, the finding of an increased cardiac murmur in an anemic patient with a prosthetic aortic valve and new microangiopathic change on peripheral smear may indicate that investigation into the possibility of perivalvular leak or prosthetic dysfunction is in order.[23] Finally, because neurologic manifestations can accompany or even predate the anemia associated with vitamin B_{12} deficiency, findings such as loss of vibration or position sense in the extremities may be relevant.[24]

Reticulocyte Count

As a marker of RBC production, the reticulocyte count provides essential information in directing the initial investigation of anemia. Modern flow cytometers accurately determine the reticulocyte count using fluorescent probes that bind to the residual ribonucleic acid present in newly released RBCs.[25] These measurements are useful, accurate, and reflect the state of erythropoiesis. However, when significant numbers of nucleated RBCs or nuclear debris are present in the peripheral blood, this diagnostic accuracy declines, and manual counting methods are generally preferable.

When the reticulocyte count is reported as a percentage, it needs to be adjusted for the total number of RBCs present. This correction can be made by multiplying the reticulocyte count by the patient's hematocrit divided by an age- and sex-appropriate normal hematocrit. No such correction is necessary when the reticulocyte count is reported as an absolute number or when it is converted to an absolute number by multiplying the percentage by the RBC number (in RBC/μL).

In the absence of anemia, the normal absolute reticulocyte count is between 25,000 and 75,000/μL. In the presence of anemia, an absolute reticulocyte count of less than 75,000/μL is indicative of a hypoproliferative process, and an absolute reticulocyte count of greater than 100,000/μL is indicative of hemolysis or an appropriate erythropoietic response to blood loss (see Table 34.2). Reticulocyte counts between 75,000 and 100,000/μL require interpretation in the context of other available clinical data, including the severity of anemia present.

Mean Corpuscular Volume and Red Blood Cell Distribution Width From the Complete Blood Count

Automated cell counters provide a wealth of information regarding the size, shape, and hemoglobin content of RBCs. The two parameters most useful in classifying anemia are the MCV and the RDW. MCV is reported in femtoliters (fL) and reflects average cell size. RDW is often reported in percent and represents the standard deviation of RBC volume divided by the mean volume. It reflects the variation in cell size in the population of RBCs.[26] These two parameters are useful because relatively reproducible changes in the MCV and RDW are associated with certain types of anemia (Table 34.4). The MCV and RDW can significantly narrow the

TABLE 34.4	Usefulness of the Mean Corpuscular Value and Red Blood Cell Distribution Width in the Diagnosis of Anemia		
	Low MCV (<80 fL)	**Normal MCV (80–99 fL)**	**High MCV (≥100 fL)**
Normal RDW	Anemia of chronic disease	Acute blood loss	Aplastic anemia
	α- or β-Thalassemia trait	Anemia of chronic disease	Chronic liver disease
	Hemoglobin E trait	Anemia of renal disease	Chemotherapy, antivirals, or alcohol
Elevated RDW	Iron deficiency	Early iron, folate, or vitamin B_{12} deficiency	Folate or vitamin B_{12} deficiency
	Sickle cell-β–thalassemia	Dimorphic anemia (for example, iron + folate deficiency)	Immune hemolytic anemia
		Sickle cell anemia	Cytotoxic chemotherapy
		Sickle cell disease	Chronic liver disease
		Chronic liver disease	Myelodysplasia
		Myelodysplasia	Hereditary spherocytosis, hereditary elliptocytosis, congenital hemoglobinopathies and RBC enzymopathies

MCW, Mean corpuscular value; RDW, red blood cell distribution width.

TABLE 34.5	Combining the Reticulocyte Count and Red Blood Cell Parameters for Diagnosis	
MCV, RDW	Reticulocyte Count <100,000/μL	Reticulocyte Count ≥100,000/μL
Low, normal	Anemia of chronic disease	
Normal, normal	Anemia of chronic disease	
High, normal	Chemotherapy, antivirals, or alcohol Aplastic anemia	Chronic liver disease
Low, high	Iron-deficiency anemia	Sickle cell-β–thalassemia
Normal, high	Early iron, folate, vitamin B₁₂ deficiency Myelodysplasia	Sickle cell anemia, sickle cell disease
High, high	Folate or vitamin B₁₂ deficiency Myelodysplasia	Immune hemolytic anemia Chronic liver disease

MCV, Mean corpuscular volume; RDW, red blood cell distribution width.

differential diagnosis, particularly when combined with the reticulocyte count (Table 34.5).

Examination of the Peripheral Blood Smear

Despite the development and availability of more sophisticated diagnostic testing, review of a well-made peripheral blood smear remains one of the most informative and rewarding diagnostic procedures.[27] It offers the chance to confirm the findings of the automated CBC count, which can be inaccurate in the presence of nucleated RBCs or rouleaux formation. Review of the blood smear also allows for evaluation of other cell lineages, which might suggest a primary BM or infiltrative disease. For example, the finding of hypersegmented neutrophils suggests a megaloblastic process, and this morphologic abnormality can be seen in the blood smear before there are significant changes in the hemoglobin or MCV (see box on Systematic Approach to the Diagnosis of Anemia). Also, only the blood smear reveals the unique morphologic changes occurring with several of the various hemolytic disorders.

Bone Marrow Examination

Bone marrow aspiration and biopsy permit evaluation of cellular morphology and BM architecture, respectively. Special stains, flow cytometry, cytogenetic analysis, fluorescence in situ hybridization (FISH), and molecular testing performed on the BM can provide a wealth of diagnostic information.[28] Because of the discomfort involved in the procedure, however, careful consideration should be given to determining the array of tests required, so that repeated BM aspirates or biopsies need not be performed. If there is any consideration of the possibility of myelodysplasia, leukemia, or lymphoma, an aliquot of anticoagulated aspirate should be set aside at the time of the initial procedure that can be sent, if necessary, for flow cytometry or cytogenetics after review of the aspirate smear. It should be noted that even when properly performed, difficulty obtaining a BM aspirate is commonly observed in certain situations, including myelofibrosis, erythroblastic leukemia (M6), and hairy cell leukemia. In these cases, touch preps of the BM biopsy may help expedite diagnosis.

Diagnostic uncertainty in the setting of hypoproliferative anemia is an indication for BM biopsy. Hematologic disorders such as myelodysplasia, leukemia, lymphoma, or myeloma may be identified. Myelodysplasia in the marrow classically includes megaloblastic

Systematic Approach to the Diagnosis of Anemia

Integration of historic features and physical findings with thoughtful review of the results of the automated complete blood cell count and peripheral smear often significantly narrows down the differential diagnosis of anemia. For example, a patient who has had a gastric bypass eating a normal diet who presents with gradual onset of fatigue accompanied by the more recent onset of distal paresthesias and a finding of decreased vibration sense in the setting of anemia with significantly elevated mean corpuscular volume and red blood cell (RBC) distribution width values and numerous six-lobed polymorphonuclear leukocytes on peripheral blood smear almost certainly has vitamin B₁₂ deficiency. This is suggested even before the return of specific laboratory testing because of the relatively narrow differential diagnosis for megaloblastic anemia and the fact that neurologic abnormalities are not associated with folate deficiency. For the purposes of diagnostic efficiency, the rewards of correlation of historic features and physical findings with a careful review of the peripheral blood smear cannot be overstated.

Special stains of the peripheral blood smear can be helpful in elucidating the cause of anemia. If there is significant nuclear debris present, the reticulocyte count obtained by automated methods can be inaccurate. In such cases, manual counting after staining with new methylene blue, which stains residual RNA in reticulocytes, permits accurate enumeration. If bite cells are detected on peripheral smear, supravital staining with methyl crystal violet can reveal Heinz bodies. These are aggregates of denatured hemoglobin reflecting an oxidative insult, most commonly caused by glucose-6-phosphate dehydrogenase deficiency or, less frequently, by the presence of an unstable hemoglobin (Fig. 34.5H).

Several commonly encountered findings can be seen in RBCs on the peripheral blood smear (Table 34.6 and Fig. 34.5). Whereas microcytic, hypochromic RBCs are suggestive of iron-deficiency anemia or thalassemia (Fig. 34.5F) macrocytic RBCs with ovalocytes (oval RBCs) are suggestive of megaloblastic anemias (Fig. 34.5G). Some findings reflect organ dysfunction, such as echinocytes (burr cells) in uremia (Fig. 34.5R) or acanthocytes (spur cells) in severe liver disease (Fig. 34.5S), although acanthocytes may also be seen in rare conditions such as abetalipoproteinemia. Target cells may be seen in cases of liver disease but may also be present in hemoglobinopathies, including sickle cell disease and thalassemia (Fig. 345W). The presence of schistocytes or RBC fragmentation often reflects systemic disease, such as DIC, TTP, or HUS (Fig. 345P). Finding spherocytes on a smear is suggestive of autoimmune hemolytic anemia or hereditary spherocytosis (Fig. 34.5H). Occasionally, the clue to the correct diagnosis of a systemic illness comes in the form of the observation of intraerythrocytic inclusions, such as malarial (Fig. 34.5O) or babesial forms, and examination of a thick blood smear may be useful for the diagnosis of these disorders when a low parasite burden is suspected.

change and nuclear budding in maturing erythroblasts, as well as morphologic abnormalities in other lineages, such as hypolobated megakaryocytes and hypogranulation of the myeloid lineage.[29] A variety of infiltrative (myelophthisic) processes may be observed.[30] These include malignancies such as small-cell lung, breast, and prostate cancers, which frequently can appear in advanced stages with BM involvement. Alternatively, granulomas may be present, suggesting the possible presence of mycobacterial disease. In children, disseminated neuroblastoma and rhabdomyosarcoma occasionally can appear as a myelophthisic anemia.

FUTURE DIRECTIONS

Anemia may represent a primary hematologic disorder or may represent the manifestation of a systemic process. In children, the former tends to be somewhat more common than the latter, and in adults, the converse is true. However, in both children and adults, a systematic approach to the evaluation of anemia that includes careful review of historic features, the CBC count, and peripheral smear facilitates an efficient diagnosis and minimizes unnecessary testing.

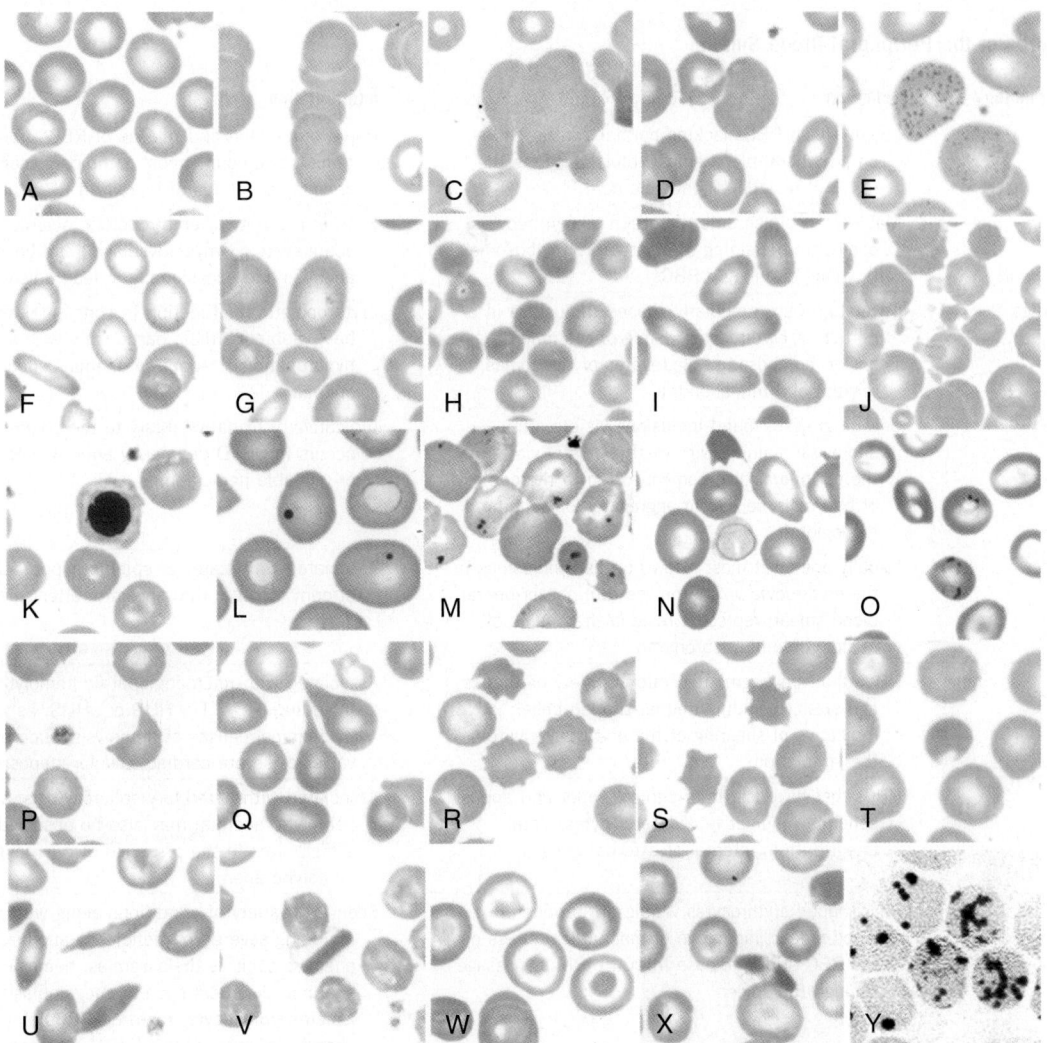

Fig. 34.5 USEFUL PERIPHERAL BLOOD AND RED BLOOD CELL FEATURES IN THE EVALUA-
TION OF ANEMIA. (A) Normal red blood cells (RBCs). Note the central pallor is one-third the diameter
of the entire cell. (B) Rouleaux formation is indicative of increased plasma protein. (C) Agglutination indicates
an antibody-mediated process such as cold agglutinin disease. (D) Polychromatophilic cell. The gray-blue color
is attributable to RNA and the cell is equivalent to a reticulocyte, which must be identified with a reticulocyte
stain. (E) Basophilic stippling. This also is attributable to increased RNA caused either by a left shift in erythroid cells or lead toxicity. (F) Hypochromic microcytic cells typical of iron-deficiency anemia. Note the
widened central pallor and the "pencil" cell in the *lower left*. (G) Macroovalocyte as can be seen in either
megaloblastic anemia or myelodysplastic syndrome. (H) Microspherocytes typical of hereditary spherocytosis.
(I) Elliptocytes (ovalocytes) from a patient with hereditary elliptocytosis. (J) RBC fragments from thermal
injury (burn patient). (K) Nucleated RBC. (L) Howell-Jolly bodies indicative of splenic dysfunction or absence.
(M) Pappenheimer bodies from a patient with sideroblastic anemia. (N) Cabot ring, as can be seen in megaloblastic anemia or MDS. (O) Malarial parasites *(Plasmodium falciparum)*. (P) Schistocyte typical of a
microangiopathic hemolytic anemia. (Q) Tear-drop form indicates marrow fibrosis and extramedullary
hematopoiesis. (R) Echinocyte (Burr cell) with rounded edges. (S) Acanthocyte (spur cell) with more irregular
pointed ends. This was from a patient with neuroacanthocytosis. They can also be seen in patients with liver
disease and lipid abnormalities. (T) "Bite" cell from a patient with glucose-6-phosphate dehydrogenase
(G6PD) deficiency. (U) Sickle cell, from a patient with homozygous sickle cell disease. (V) Hemoglobin C
crystal. (W) Target cells. (X) Hemoglobin C disease. Note that the RBC in center has condensed hemoglobin
at each pole. (Y) Heinz body preparation (supravital stain) from a patient with G6PD deficiency. Note that
the cells to the right have increased precipitated hemoglobin.

TABLE 34.6   Features of the Peripheral Blood Smear

Red Blood Cell Morphology	Definition	Interpretation
Polychromasia	Large, bluish RBCs lacking normal central pallor on peripheral blood smear; bluish stain is the result of residual ribonucleic acid	Rapid production and release of RBCs from BM; elevated reticulocyte count; most commonly seen in any hemolytic anemia and states of increased RBC turnover
Basophilic stippling	Many small bluish dots in portion of erythrocytes; comes from staining of clustered polyribosomes in young circulating RBCs	Seen in a variety of erythropoietic disorders, including acquired (e.g., myelodysplasia) and congenital hemolytic anemias and occasionally in lead poisoning
Pappenheimer bodies	Several grayish, irregularly shaped inclusions in a portion of erythrocytes visible on peripheral smear; composed of aggregates of ribosomes, ferritin, and mitochondria	Erythropoietic malfunction in congenital anemias such as hemoglobinopathies, particularly with splenic hypofunction or acquired anemias such as megaloblastic anemia
Heinz bodies	Several grayish, round inclusions visible after supravital staining with methyl crystal violet of the peripheral blood smear, often in the context of bite cells; represent aggregates of denatured hemoglobin	Indicative of oxidative injury to the erythrocyte, such as occurs in G6PD deficiency and other RBC enzymopathies or unstable hemoglobins
Howell-Jolly bodies	Usually one or at most a few purplish inclusions in the erythrocyte visible on the routine peripheral blood smear; represent residual fragments of nuclei containing chromatin	Associated with states of splenic hypofunction, splenic atrophy, splenic thrombosis or after splenectomy
Schistocytes	RBCs that are fragmented into a variety of shapes and sizes, including helmet-shaped cells; indicative of shearing of the erythrocyte within the circulation	Associated with microangiopathic hemolytic anemias, including DIC, TTP, HUS or aHUS, as well as other mechanical causes of hemolysis, such as prosthetic heart valves or severe cardiac valvular stenosis
Spherocytes	RBCs that have lost their central pallor and appear spherical; indicative of loss of cytoskeletal integrity from internal or external causes	Associated with hereditary spherocytosis, autoimmune hemolytic anemia; may also be observed in addition to schistocytes in the presence of microangiopathic hemolytic anemia
Teardrop cells	Pear-shaped erythrocytes visible on peripheral blood smear; indicative of mechanical stress on the RBC during release from the BM or passage through the spleen	Seen in a variety of conditions along with other poikilocytes including severe iron deficiency anemia, congenital anemias such as thalassemias, hemoglobinopathies, and acquired disorders such as megaloblastic anemia. As isolated poikilocyte, teardrop RBCs may be initial changes of myelophthisis (BM replacement or infiltration), e.g., myelodysplastic syndrome or myelofibrosis.
Burr cells (echinocytes)	RBCs that have smooth undulations present on the surface circumferentially; pathogenesis unknown	Indicative of uremia when present on a properly made peripheral blood smear
Spur cells (acanthocytes)	RBCs that have spiny points present on the surface circumferentially; reflective of abnormal lipid composition of RBC membrane	Most commonly indicative of hemolytic anemia of advanced liver disease when present in significant numbers; also seen in abetalipoproteinemia and in RBCs lacking the Kell blood group antigen

aHUS, Atypical hemolytic uremic syndrome; BM, bone marrow; DIC, disseminated intravascular coagulation; G6PD, glucose-6-phosphate dehydrogenase; HUS, hemolytic uremic syndrome; RBC, red blood cell; TTP, thrombotic thrombocytopenic purpura.

REFERENCES

1. Kassebaum NJ, Jasrasaria R, Naghavi M, et al: A systematic analysis of blobal anemia burden from 1990 to 2010. *Blood* 123:615, 2014.
2. Vichinsky EP: Changing patterns of thalassemia worldwide. *Ann N Y Acad Sci* 1054:18, 2005.
3. Cantor AB, Orkin SH: Transcriptional regulation of erythropoiesis: An affair involving multiple partners. *Oncogene* 13:3368, 2002.
4. Rosse W: The spleen as a filter. *N Engl J Med* 317:704, 1987.
5. Semenza GL: Involvement of oxygen-sensing pathways in physiologic and pathophysiologic erythropoiesis. *Blood* 114:2015, 2009.
6. Hoffbrand AV, Herbert V: Nutritional anemias. *Semin Hematol* 36:13, 1999.
7. Kelly A, Munan L: Haematologic profile of natural populations: Red cell parameters. *Br J Haematol* 35:153, 1977.
8. Nilsson-Ehle H, Jagenburg R, Landahl S, et al: Blood haemoglobin values in the elderly: Implications for reverence intervals from age 70 to 88. *Eur J Haematol* 65:297, 2000.
9. Centers for Disease Control and Prevention: Iron deficiency—United States, 1999–2000. *MMWR Morb Mortal Wkly Rep* 51:897, 2002.
10. Fishbane S: Anemia treatment in chronic renal insufficiency. *Semin Nephrol* 22:474, 2002.
11. Roy CN, Weinstein DA, Andrews NC: 2002 E. Mead Johnnson Award for Research in Pediatrics Lecture: The molecular biology of the anemia of chronic disease: A hypothesis. *Pediatr Res* 53:507, 2003.
12. Tabbara IA: Hemolytic anemias: Diagnosis and management. *Med Clin North Am* 76:649, 1992.
13. Beutler E: Glucose-6-phosphate dehydrogenase deficiency: A historical perspective. *Blood* 111:16, 2008.
14. Gehrs BC, Freidberg RC: Autoimmune hemolytic anemia. *Am J Hematol* 69:258, 2002.

15. Freedman MH, Saunders EF: Transient erythroblastopenia of childhood: Varied pathogenesis. *Am J Hematol* 14:247, 1983.

16. Lipton JM, Ellis SR: Diamond-Blackfan anemia: Diagnosis, treatment, and molecular pathogenesis. *Hematol Oncol Clin North Am* 23:261, 2009.

17. Atweh GF, DeSimone J, Saunthararajah Y, et al: Hemoglobinopathies. *Hematology Am Soc Hematol Educ Program* 14, 2003.

18. Boyce TG, Swerdlow DL, Griffin PM: Escherichia coli O157:H7 and the hemolytic-uremic syndrome. *N Engl J Med* 333:364, 1995.

19. Lee AI, Kaufman RM: Transfusion medicine and the pregnant patient. *Hematol Oncol Clin North Am* 25:393, 2011.

20. Sawada K, Fujishima N, Hirokawa M: Acquired pure red cell aplasia: Updated review of treatment. *Br J Haematol* 142:505, 2008.

21. Tse WT, Lux SE: Red blood cell membrane disorders. *Br J Haematol* 104:2, 1999.

22. Ammus S, Yunis AA: Drug-induced red cell dyscrasias. *Blood Rev* 3:71, 1989.

23. George JN: Evaluation and management of patients with thrombotic thrombocytopenic purpura. *J Intensive Care Med* 22:82, 2007.

24. Moore DF, Jr, Sears DA: Pica, iron deficiency, and the medical history. *Am J Med* 97:390, 1994.

25. Lam BK, Cosgrove DM, Bhudia SK, et al: Hemolysis after mitral valve repair: Mechanisms and treatment. *Ann Thorac Surg* 77:191, 2004.

26. Lindenbaum J, Healton EB, Savage DG: Neuropsychiatric disorders caused by cobalamin deficiency in the absence of anemia or macrocytosis. *N Engl J Med* 318:1720, 1988.

27. Corberand JX: Reticulocyte analysis using flow cytometry. *Hematol Cell Ther* 38:487, 1996.

28. Lombarts AJ, Koevoet AL, Leijnse B: Basic principles and problems of haemocytometry. *Ann Clin Biochem* 23:390, 1986.

29. Bain B: Diagnosis from the blood smear. *N Engl J Med* 353:498, 2005.

30. Hyun BH, Stevenson AJ, Hanau CA: Fundamentals of bone marrow examination. *Hematol Oncol Clin North Am* 8:651, 1994.

CHAPTER 35

PATHOPHYSIOLOGY OF IRON HOMEOSTASIS

Gary M. Brittenham

Each cell in the body needs iron, not too much and not too little. Iron is an essential element required for energy production, oxygen use, and cellular proliferation. Iron, able to act as both an electron donor and an electron acceptor by readily interconverting between ferric (Fe^{3+}) and ferrous (Fe^{2+}) forms, is an irreplaceable component of oxygen transport (hemoglobin); oxygen storage (myoglobin); sensing molecules, cytochromes, iron-sulfur clusters, and heme and nonheme enzymes. The ease with which iron can gain and lose electrons also makes it able to catalyze the formation of highly reactive oxygen species that can damage lipids, proteins, and DNA and injure subcellular organelles, resulting in cellular dysfunction, apoptosis, and necrosis. Consequently, both the total body iron and the amount within each cell are carefully controlled to ensure adequate iron availability but avoid excess iron toxicity. Humans have no regulated means for iron excretion, and obligatory losses are normally minuscule, less than 0.05% of the total body iron each day. As a result, the amount of body iron is determined by control of iron absorption, and human iron homeostasis is distinguished by efficient recycling of iron (Fig. 35.1).

Although all cells require iron, quantitatively most of the iron in the body is found within erythroid cells, and most of the daily movement of iron (approximately 80%) cycles through the erythroid compartment. External exchange of iron through absorption of iron from the gastrointestinal tract and through obligatory losses is very limited. Physiologically, iron is carried into the erythroid marrow and incorporated into hemoglobin, and it enters the circulation within red blood cells (RBCs) dedicated to oxygen transport. At the end of their lifespan, RBCs are phagocytized by a select population of macrophages in the bone marrow, liver, and spleen that then promptly renders up most of the catabolized iron for return to the erythroid marrow. Any surplus is stored within macrophages or hepatocytes. After examining the intricate interrelationship between intracellular and systemic iron homeostasis, this chapter considers in turn each portion of the pathway of iron transport, use, storage, and absorption (see Fig. 35.1). Altogether, iron homeostasis is maintained by effective use of iron for erythropoiesis, efficient recycling of iron from senescent erythrocytes, controlled storage of iron by macrophages and hepatocytes, and careful regulation of intestinal iron absorption.[1-4]

REGULATION OF CELLULAR AND SYSTEMIC IRON HOMEOSTASIS

Each cell in the body needs just enough iron, at just the right time. Iron is required in precise, carefully timed amounts for growth, development, and function. Within the systemic circulation, the varied and varying cellular requirements are met by the transport protein *transferrin*, the physiologic carrier of iron through the plasma and extracellular fluid. Each cell obtains its share of circulating transferrin-bound iron by expressing *transferrin receptor 1*, a glycoprotein on cell membranes that binds the transferrin–iron complex and is internalized in an endocytic vesicle, where iron is released, and then returns to the cell membrane, liberating apotransferrin into the plasma.[1,5] Within the cell, the iron released from the endosome is either used or sequestered with cytosolic *ferritin*, an iron storage protein that holds iron in a nontoxic form ready for prompt mobilization in time of need.[1,6] A prime determinant of the iron supply to

each cell is the number of transferrin receptors expressed on the cell surface. Within each cell, iron self-regulates its intracellular availability, at least in part, through the iron regulatory proteins 1 and 2 that function as sensors of intracellular iron (Fig. 35.2). The iron regulatory proteins recognize and bind to RNA stem–loop structures called iron-responsive elements when iron is absent and dissociate when iron is present.[7] When the iron-responsive elements are within the 3′ untranslated region of a messenger (m) RNA (e.g., transferrin receptor 1 mRNA), binding prevents mRNA degradation, increasing protein expression when iron is lacking. In contrast, when the iron-responsive elements are located in the 5′ untranslated region of an mRNA (e.g., cytosolic ferritin mRNA), binding of the iron regulatory proteins interferes with ribosomal assembly, decreasing protein expression when iron is absent. Accordingly, a *decrease* in intracellular iron availability enhances transferrin receptor 1 protein synthesis, increasing iron import, and reduces cytosolic ferritin protein production and iron storage. Conversely, an *increase* in intracellular iron availability reduces transferrin receptor 1 protein synthesis, inhibiting iron import, and augments cytosolic ferritin protein production and iron storage. In iron-replete cells with sufficient oxygen, F box and leucine-rich repeat protein 5 (FBXL5), a subunit of a ubiquitin ligase complex, monitors cytosolic iron and leads to iron-dependent degradation of iron regulatory protein 2.[8] The presence of two distinct iron regulatory proteins provides for adaptation to cytosolic iron and oxygen over a wide range of concentrations.[7] Altogether, *regulation of intracellular iron homeostasis* is provided principally through iron regulatory proteins 1 and 2 by translational control of the synthesis of transferrin receptor and ferritin and, in specialized cells, of other essential proteins involved in iron homeostasis, including erythroid δ-aminolevulinic acid synthase 2 (eALAS), mitochondrial aconitase, hypoxia-inducible factor 2α (HIF-2α), intestinal divalent metal transporter 1 (DMT1) isoform I, and ferroportin.[7]

Regulation of systemic iron homeostasis is accomplished by control of the entry of iron into plasma for transport by transferrin.[1-4] Circulating transferrin iron is derived from specialized cells that can export iron, primarily reticuloendothelial macrophages that recycle iron from senescent RBCs, hepatocytes that can mobilize iron from stores, and duodenal enterocytes that provide iron absorbed from the diet. To enter plasma, iron in these cells must pass through *ferroportin* (SLC40A1), a multitransmembrane-spanning protein that is the sole known cellular iron export channel.[9] *Hepcidin*, a small 25-amino acid peptide hormone secreted principally by the liver, provides post-translational control of ferroportin expression by binding to and inducing its internalization, ubiquitination, and degradation, thereby inhibiting iron entry into plasma (Fig. 35.3).[2] Hepatic hepcidin synthesis is stimulated by increases in body iron stores, infection, inflammation, or malignancy and inhibited by hypoxemia and increased erythropoietic demand.[3] Increments in plasma hepcidin reduce the amount of ferroportin in cell membranes, causing a prompt fall in plasma iron concentration. Conversely, decrements in plasma hepcidin concentration increase the amount of ferroportin, producing a rise in plasma iron concentration.

MicroRNAs, short (approximately 22 nucleotides), noncoding RNAs that act as antisense regulators of target RNAs, provide a further degree of control of both cellular and systemic iron homeostasis.[10] MicroRNAs help regulate the expression of genes involved in hepcidin expression (HFE, hemojuvelin: miR-122), iron uptake (transferrin receptor 1: miR-320; divalent metal transporter 1:

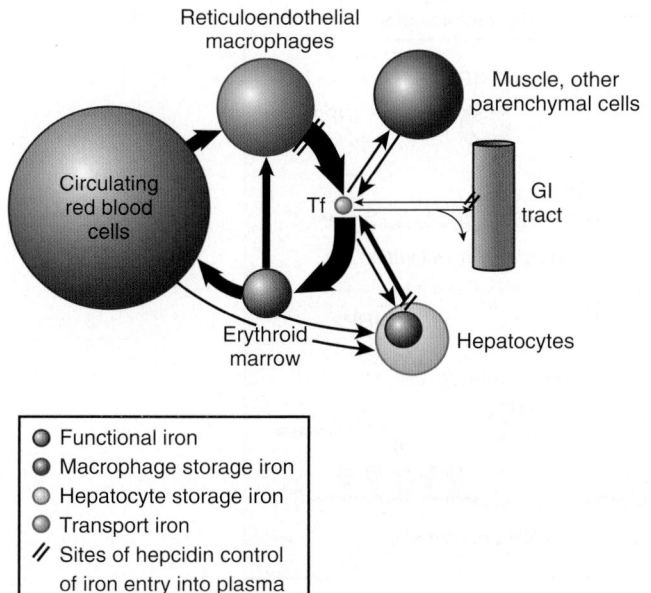

- ● Functional iron
- ● Macrophage storage iron
- ○ Hepatocyte storage iron
- ○ Transport iron
- // Sites of hepcidin control of iron entry into plasma

Fig. 35.1 BODY IRON SUPPLY AND STORAGE. The figure shows a schematic representation of the routes of iron exchange in an adult. The area of each *circle* is proportional to the amount of iron contained in the compartment, and the width of each *arrow* is proportional to the daily flow of iron from one compartment to another. *Double slashes* indicate the sites of hepcidin action, decreasing macrophage release of iron derived from senescent red blood cells (RBCs), diminishing delivery of iron from duodenal enterocytes absorbing dietary iron, and inhibiting release of iron stored in hepatocytes. The concentration of iron in the human body is normally maintained at about 40 mg/kg in women and about 50 mg/kg in men. The major portion of iron is found in the erythron as hemoglobin iron (28 mg/kg in women; 32 mg/kg in men) dedicated to oxygen transport and delivery. Small amounts of erythron iron (<1 mg/kg) are also present in heme and nonheme enzymes in developing RBCs. The remainder of functional iron is found as myoglobin iron (4 mg/kg in women; 5 mg/kg in men) in muscle and as iron-containing and iron-dependent enzymes (1–2 mg/kg) throughout the cells of the body. Most storage iron (5–6 mg/kg in women; 10–12 mg/kg in men) is held in reserve by hepatocytes and macrophages. The small fraction of transport iron (approximately 0.2 mg/kg) in the plasma and extracellular fluid is bound to the protein transferrin (Tf). *GI*, Gastrointestinal.

miR-Let-7d), iron export (ferroportin; miR-485-3p), iron use (iron-sulfur proteins: miR-210), and iron storage (ferritin: miR-200b).[10]

USE OF IRON FOR ERYTHROPOIESIS

The major pathway of iron movement is from plasma transferrin to the erythroid marrow (Fig. 35.4). Each day, almost 200 billion RBCs are produced in a normal adult to replace a similar number reaching the end of their lifespan. Each RBC contains more than 1 billion atoms of iron, four in each tetrameric molecule of hemoglobin, so that more than 200 quintillion (200×10^{18}) atoms of iron are needed daily for erythropoiesis. Transferrin transports iron in a nonreactive, soluble form in the circulation for delivery to erythroid precursors or other iron-requiring cells.[5] Apotransferrin, transferrin without attached iron, is a single-chain glycoprotein with two structurally similar lobes. Binding of a ferric ion to one of these lobes yields monoferric transferrin; binding of ions to both yields diferric transferrin. The transferrin saturation is the proportion of the available iron-binding sites on transferrin that are occupied by iron atoms, expressed as a percentage. In humans, almost all of the circulating plasma apotransferrin is synthesized by the hepatocyte. After delivering iron to cells, apotransferrin is promptly returned to the plasma to again function as an iron transporter, completing 100 to 200 cycles

of iron delivery during its lifetime in the circulation. Apotransferrin is a true carrier that is not lost in delivering iron; the half-life of the protein is about 8 days. In an iron-replete 70-kg man, the amount of transferrin-bound iron in the plasma at any given time is only about 3 mg, but more than 30 mg of iron moves through this transport compartment each day (see Fig. 35.1). Most (approximately 24 mg Fe/d) of this iron is used for erythropoiesis.

Transferrin receptors on the cell surface selectively bind monoferric or diferric transferrin. Two different isoforms of the transferrin receptor exist, encoded by two separate genes. The two glycoproteins have similar extracellular structures but distinct roles in iron homeostasis. Transferrin receptor 1 is ubiquitously expressed and functions as the physiologic transferrin iron importer on all iron-requiring cells. Transferrin receptor 2 is expressed only in hepatocytes, functioning in the control of iron supply by regulating hepcidin expression (see later), and in erythroid precursors, coordinating erythropoiesis with iron availability (see later).[11] Transferrin receptor 1 is a transmembrane glycoprotein dimer composed of two identical subunits linked by a disulfide bond. Each transferrin receptor 1 can bind two molecules of transferrin; if each transferrin is diferric, the dimeric receptor can carry a total of four atoms of transferrin-bound iron. The affinity of transferrin receptor 1 for transferrin depends both on the iron content of transferrin and on the pH. With amounts of iron-bearing transferrin sufficient to saturate receptors at a physiologic pH of 7.4, transferrin receptor 1 has very little affinity for apotransferrin; an intermediate affinity for monoferric transferrin; and the highest affinity for diferric transferrin, estimated at 2×10^{-9} to 7×10^{-9} M. Under such physiologic conditions, the affinity of transferrin receptor 1 for diferric transferrin is more than fourfold greater than that for monoferric transferrin. At a pH of about 5 in the endosome, the affinity of transferrin receptor 1 for apotransferrin increases to that of diferric transferrin.

Iron delivery to an erythroid cell (see Fig. 35.4) begins with the binding of one or two molecules of monoferric or diferric transferrin to transferrin receptor 1.[4,5] The efficiency of iron delivery to the cell depends on the amounts of monoferric and diferric plasma transferrin available. With normal erythropoiesis and a normal transferrin saturation of about 33%, the higher affinity of the receptor for diferric transferrin results in most of the iron supply to cells being derived from this form, providing four atoms of iron with each cycle. At a transferrin saturation of about 19%, equal amounts of iron are provided by monoferric and diferric transferrin; at lower saturations, most of the iron is derived from the monoferric form. Whether monoferric or diferric, the fate of transferrin bound to the transferrin receptor is the same. When bound, the iron-bearing transferrin–receptor complex rapidly clusters with other transferrin–receptor complexes in a clathrin-coated pit. When assembled, the clathrin-coated pit is promptly internalized and detaches from the inner membrane. Within the cytoplasm, the coated vesicle is rapidly stripped of clathrin, and the uncoated vesicles fuse to become multivesicular endosomes. Moving to the interior of the cell, a proton pump lowers the endosome internal pH to about 5.6. In the acidic environment of the endosome, both transferrin and transferrin receptor 1 undergo conformational changes that enhance the rate and completeness of iron release. After release from transferrin within the acidified endosome as ferric iron, the iron is reduced by the ferrireductase six-transmembrane epithelial antigen of the prostate 3 (STEAP3) to the ferrous form and then transported across the endosomal membrane through DMT1 (SLC11A2). Acidification within the endosome increases the affinity of the now iron-free apotransferrin for the transferrin receptor, with the result that the apotransferrin–receptor bond remains intact as the complex is transported back to the cell surface within the endosome. On exposure to the neutral pH of the plasma, the apotransferrin loses its affinity for the transferrin receptor and is released from the membrane, making both the apotransferrin and the transferrin receptor 1 available for reuse (see Fig. 35.4).

Most of the iron transported across the endosomal membrane through divalent metal transporter 1 is then directed to the mitochondria for use in the synthesis of heme and iron-sulfur clusters (Fig. 35.4). Iron can be imported from the cytosol across the

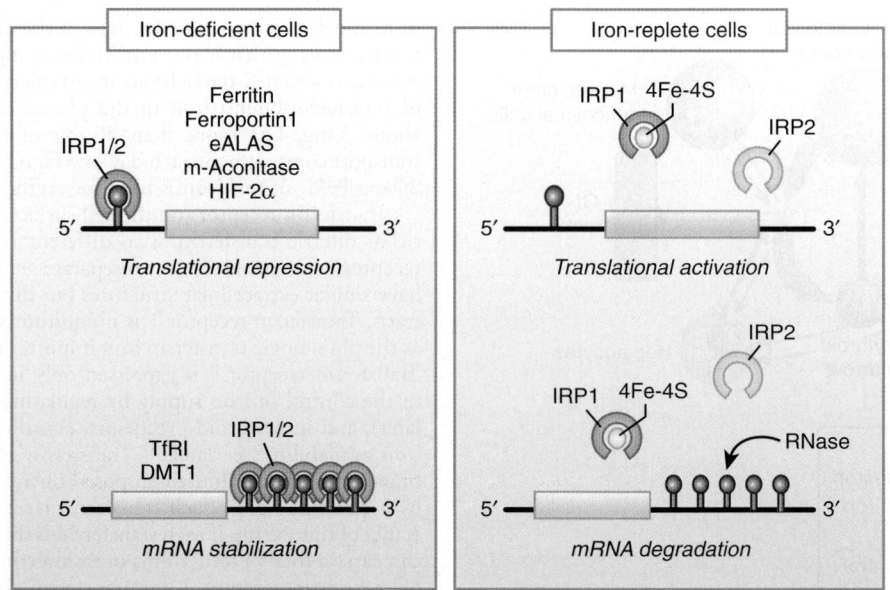

Fig. 35.2 REGULATION OF CELLULAR IRON HOMEOSTASIS BY THE IRON REGULATORY PROTEINS (IRP1 AND IRP2). The iron regulatory proteins recognize and bind to RNA stem-loop structures called iron-responsive elements (IREs) when iron is absent and dissociate when iron is present. Binding IREs within the 3′ untranslated region of mRNA (e.g., transferrin receptor 1 [TfR1]) and some intestinal divalent metal transporter 1 (DMT1) isoforms increases mRNA stability, increasing protein synthesis. In contrast, binding IREs in the 5′ untranslated region of mRNA (e.g., cytosolic ferritin, ferroportin 1, erythroid aminolevulinic acid synthase [eALAS], mitochondrial aconitase [m-aconitase], and hypoxia-inducible factor 2α [HIF-2α]) inhibits protein expression when iron is absent. In iron-replete cells, IRP1 assembles a cubane Fe/S cluster, acquiring aconitase activity while losing the ability to bind to IREs. In iron-replete cells, IRP2 interacts with F box and leucine-rich repeat protein 5 (FBXL5), a subunit of an ubiquitin ligase complex, leading to its ubiquitination and degradation by the proteasome. See text for details. *(Reproduced with permission from Wallander ML, Leibold EA, Eisenstein RS: Molecular control of vertebrate iron homeostasis by iron regulatory proteins. Biochim Biophys Acta 1763:668, 2006.)*

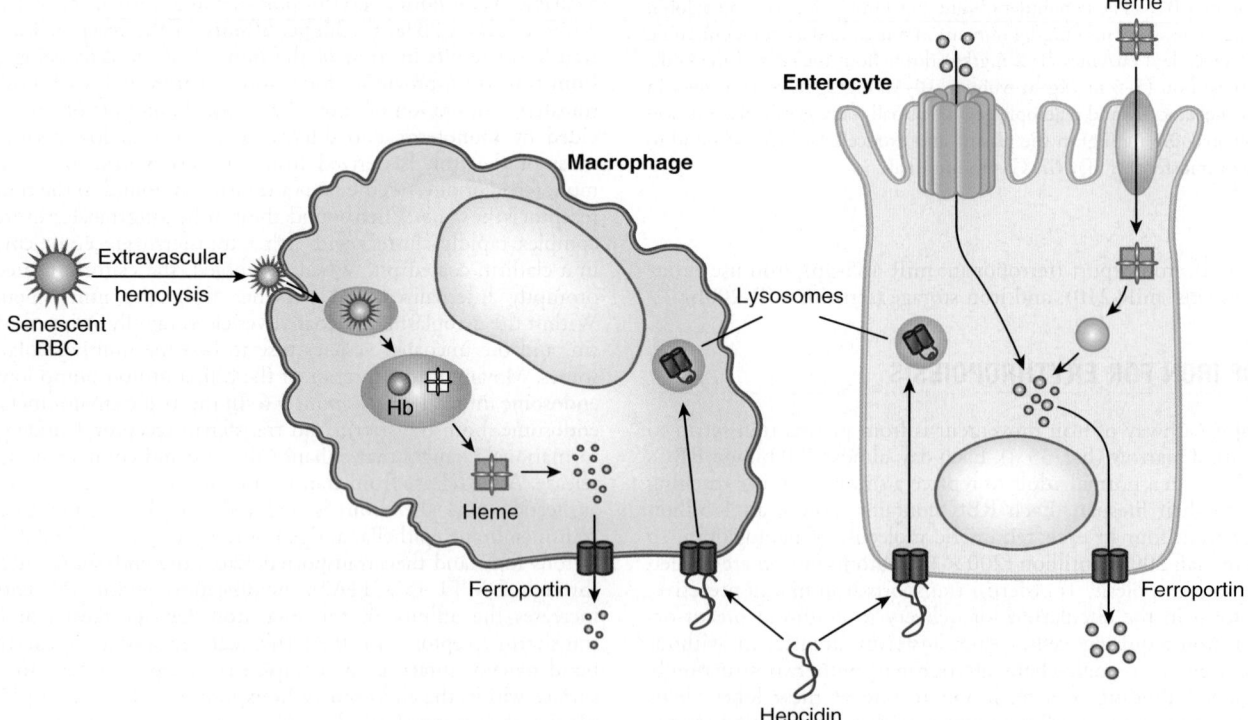

Fig. 35.3 CONTROL OF IRON ENTRY INTO PLASMA BY FERROPORTIN AND HEPCIDIN IN THE REGULATION OF SYSTEMIC IRON HOMEOSTASIS. Ferroportin, a multitransmembrane-spanning protein that is the only known iron exporter in humans, is expressed at high concentrations on the basolateral membrane of duodenal enterocytes, reticuloendothelial macrophages, and hepatocytes (not shown). Plasma hepcidin binds to a specific extracellular domain of ferroportin, inducing the binding and then autophosphorylation of cytosolic Janus kinase 2 (JAK2). JAK2 then phosphorylates ferroportin, leading to ferroportin internalization by clathrin-coated pits and its subsequent degradation in the lysosome. See text for details. *DMT1*, Divalent metal transporter 1.

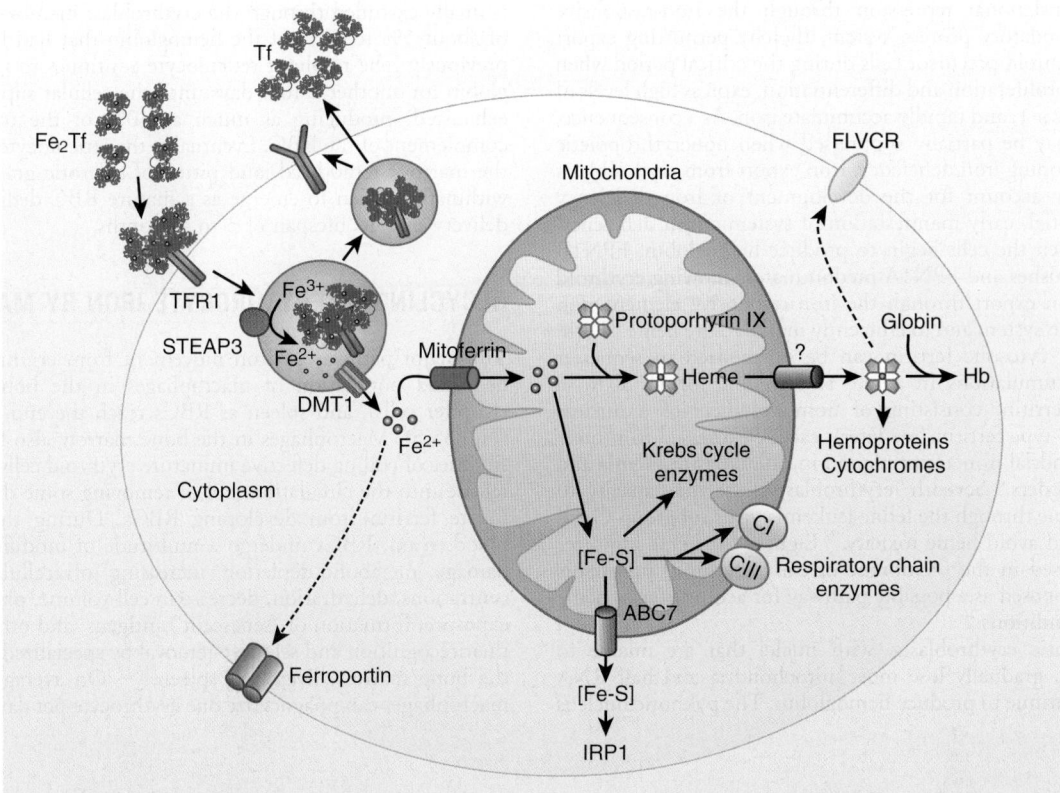

Fig. 35.4 ACQUISITION AND USE OF IRON BY ERYTHROID PRECURSORS. Iron is imported in the transferrin (Tf) cycle and principally used for the synthesis of heme. See text for details. *ABC7*, Adenosine triphosphate–binding cassette, subfamily B (MDR/TAP), member 7; *DMT1*, divalent metal transporter 1; *Fe2Tf*, diferric transferrin; *FLVCR*, feline leukemia virus subgroup C cellular receptor; *Hb*, hemoglobin; *IRP1*, iron regulatory protein 1; *STEAP3*, six-transmembrane epithelial antigen of the prostate 3; *TFR1*, transferrin receptor 1. (*Reproduced with permission from Beaumont C, Delaby C: Recycling iron in normal and pathological states.* Semin Hematol *46:328, 2009.*)

mitochondrial membrane by the transmembrane protein mitoferrin 1 (MFRN1; SLC25A37). Transport of iron from endosomes into mitochondria for heme synthesis by direct contact between the organelles, avoiding the cytosol, also has been proposed.[4] Heme (ferrous protoporphyrin IX), a planar molecule consisting of an atom of ferrous iron in the center of a tetrapyrrole ring, is then synthesized in eight biochemical reactions, with the first and final three reactions catalyzed by mitochondrial enzymes and the four intermediate reactions taking place in the cytoplasm (see Chapter 38). Most heme is then bound to α- or β-globin subunits that combine to form α-β dimers that in turn join to form the functional α_2-β_2-tetramer of hemoglobin (see Fig. 35.4). Small amounts of heme are incorporated into heme enzymes and cytochromes. The fraction of iron not used for heme synthesis can be assembled into iron-sulfur clusters both within mitochondria and in the cytosol[12] (see Fig. 35.4). The cytosolic iron chaperones poly(rC)-binding proteins 1 and 2 (PCBP1, PCBP2) may ferry iron that is in excess of erythroid requirements for heme synthesis to cytosolic ferritin for storage.[13] The same iron chaperones may also carry iron to some cytosolic nonheme enzymes.

Transferrin receptor 2, which binds iron-loaded transferrin with an affinity some 25-fold less than that of transferrin receptor 1, functions as a sensor of iron bound to transferrin and is not involved in cellular iron uptake. In erythroid precursors, transferrin receptor 2 coordinates erythropoiesis with iron availability, a vital mechanism for adaptation to iron deficiency.[11] Transferrin receptor 2, a component of the erythropoietin receptor complex, stabilizes the receptor on the cell surface and modulates the sensitivity of the developing erythroid cells to erythropoietin. By simultaneously sensing the concentration of iron-loaded transferrin in developing erythroid cells

and in hepatocytes (see later), transferrin receptor 2 permits reciprocal adaptation between the extent of erythropoiesis and the level of the iron supply.[11]

Erythroid precursors have a variety of other mechanisms to coordinate erythropoietic activity with iron availability. First, iron regulation of erythroid differentiation helps match the rate of erythropoiesis to iron supply. With iron deficiency, an iron–aconitase–isocitrate pathway also reduces the responsiveness of erythroid progenitors to erythropoietin.[12] With a lack of iron, decreased erythroid use for RBC production helps preserve the supply of iron for vital functions in other tissues. Second, heme synthesis is coordinated with iron availability through an iron regulatory element in the 5′ untranslated region of the mRNA for eALAS, the erythroid-specific initial enzyme in the heme synthetic pathway. If intracellular iron availability is low, binding of an iron regulatory protein will inhibit heme synthesis by preventing translation of the mRNA.[14] Third, if a lack of iron leads to heme deficiency, the heme-regulated translational inhibitor (HRI) is activated and, acting through the α-subunit of eukaryotic initiation factor 2, halts protein synthesis to coordinate the translation of globin mRNAs with the intracellular heme concentration.[15] This action of the HRI is responsible for the physiologic adaptation that produces hypochromic, microcytic erythrocytes in iron deficiency. Fourth, developing erythroblasts synthesize ferroportin to export iron. Their expression of ferroportin is regulated principally by hepcidin, providing another means to coordinate erythroid iron use with systemic iron availability. In erythroid precursors (and in duodenal enterocytes; see later), two ferroportin transcripts are present: the ubiquitously expressed FPN1A, with an iron-responsive element in its 5′ untranslated region, and FPN1B, which lacks the iron-responsive element.[2] During erythroid cell differentiation, FPN1B expression circumvents translational repression through the iron-responsive element, iron regulatory protein system, thereby permitting export of iron from erythroid precursor cells during the critical period when cells commit to proliferation and differentiation, express high levels of transferrin receptor 1, and rapidly accumulate iron. As a consequence, erythropoiesis may be partially suppressed when nonerythropoietic tissues risk developing iron deficiency. Iron export from erythroblasts via FPN1B may account for the development of iron deficiency anemia as an initial, early manifestation of systemic iron deficiency. Nonetheless, when the cells begin to produce hemoglobin, FPN1B expression diminishes and FPN1A predominates, allowing erythroid cells to limit iron export through the iron-responsive element iron regulatory protein system and to efficiently manufacture heme.[2] Fifth, as noted earlier, cytosolic ferritin can be synthesized to sequester surplus iron accumulations in a safe and soluble form.[6] Sixth, a mitochondrial ferritin, consisting of homopolymers of a nuclear gene-encoded H-type ferritin (see later), can be expressed to protect against mitochondrial iron accumulation in sideroblastic anemia and some other disorders.[6] Seventh, erythroblasts have the capacity to export excess heme through the feline leukemia virus subgroup C cellular receptor and avoid heme toxicity.[16] Eighth, the heme importer HRG1 is expressed in the membrane of early erythroid precursors and has been proposed as a possible pathway for acquisition of heme in pathologic conditions.[16]

Orthochromatic erythroblasts, with nuclei that are unable to synthesize DNA, gradually lose most mitochondria and halt RNA synthesis but continue to produce hemoglobin. The pyknotic nucleus is finally extruded through the erythroblast membrane with the loss of about 5% to 10% of the hemoglobin that had been synthesized previously. The resultant reticulocyte continues to synthesize hemoglobin for another 2 to 3 days until the cellular supply of mRNA is exhausted, producing as much as 30% of the total hemoglobin complement of the RBC. Eventually, the reticulocyte is released from the marrow, remodeled, and pitted of siderotic granules and debris within the spleen to emerge as a mature RBC dedicated to oxygen delivery over its lifespan of 3 to 4 months.

RECYCLING OF ERYTHROCYTE IRON BY MACROPHAGES

The major pathway of iron movement from erythroid cells is to a dedicated population of macrophages in the bone marrow, liver (Kupffer cells), and spleen as RBCs reach the end of their lifespan (Fig. 35.5). Macrophages in the bone marrow also have the responsibilities of culling defective immature erythroid cells to prevent their release into the circulation and of removing some deposits of erythrocyte ferritin from developing RBCs. During their time in the bloodstream, RBCs undergo a multitude of modifications (oxidant damage, metabolic depletion, increasing intracellular calcium concentrations, dehydration, decrease in cell volume, phosphatidylserine exposure, formation of "senescent" antigens, and others) that lead to their recognition and selective removal by specialized macrophages in the bone marrow, liver, and spleen.[16,17] On average, each of these macrophages can phagocytize one erythrocyte per day. After ingesting

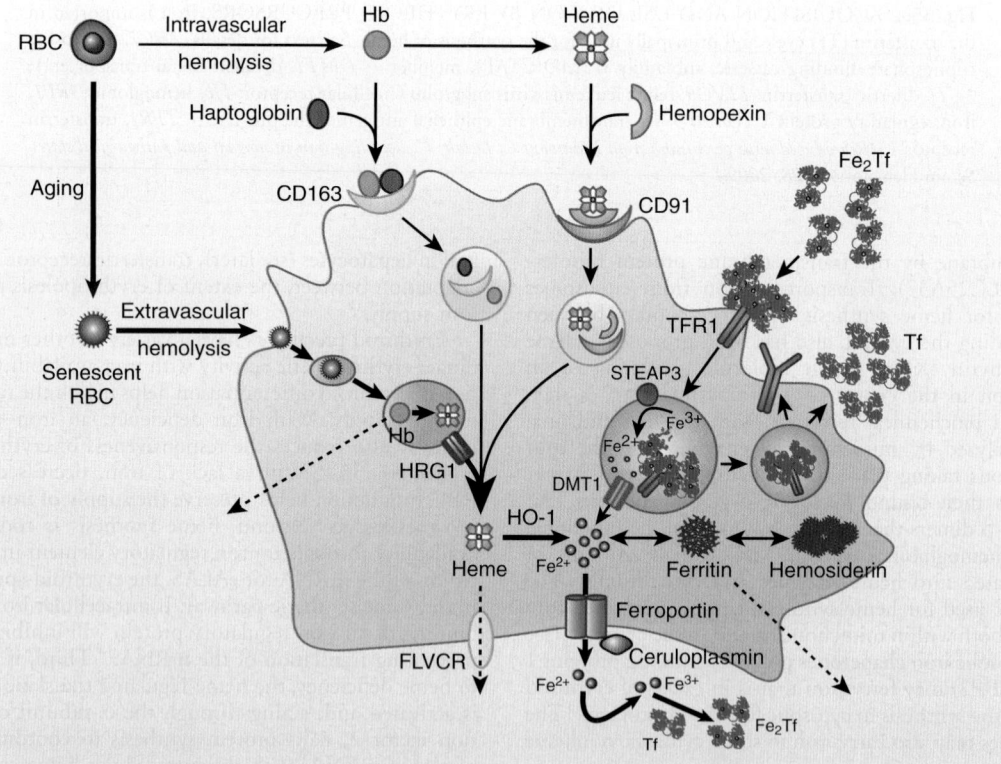

Fig. 35.5 RECYCLING OF ERYTHROCYTE IRON BY MACROPHAGES. Most erythrocyte iron is acquired by erythrophagocytosis of senescent red blood cells (RBCs), but smaller amounts are derived from hemoglobin–haptoglobin and heme–hemopexin complexes. Iron derived from plasma transferrin (Tf) is a minor portion of the total iron flux. Heme is catabolized, and the iron exported through ferroportin and oxidized by ceruloplasmin. In the absence of iron deficiency, a portion of the iron is retained as ferritin and hemosiderin. See text for details. *DMT1,* Divalent metal transporter 1; *Fe₂Tf,* diferric transferrin; *FLVCR,* feline leukemia virus subgroup C cellular receptor; *Hb,* hemoglobin; *HO-1,* heme oxygenase-1; *TFR1,* transferrin receptor 1; *HRG1:* heme importer; *STEAP3,* six-transmembrane epithelial antigen of the prostate 3. *(Reproduced with permission from Beaumont C, Delaby C: Recycling iron in normal and pathological states.* Semin Hematol *46:328, 2009.)*

the erythrocyte in a phagosomal vacuole known as an *erythrophagolysosome*, the erythrocyte membrane is lysed. The hemoglobin within then undergoes oxidative precipitation and rapid catabolism into heme (see Fig. 35.5).[17] Heme is then transported from the erythrophagolysosome into the cytosol via the heme transporter HRG1 (SLC48A1), a heme-transporting permease.[16]

A small proportion of aged or damaged erythrocytes undergo intravascular hemolysis. With normal erythropoiesis, this portion of the total iron flux is minor but can increase substantially in disorders with increased ineffective erythropoiesis or intravascular hemolysis. The hemoglobin released into plasma is then rapidly bound by haptoglobin, a glycoprotein synthesized in the liver.[18] The hemoglobin–haptoglobin complex (M_r 150,000) is too large to be filtered by the kidneys, a feature that helps restrict the renal loss of iron with hemoglobinemia. Macrophages (and hepatocytes; see later) remove the haptoglobin–hemoglobin complex from plasma by binding through the cluster of differentiation 163 (CD163) receptor and after endocytosis digest the complex in lysosomes, liberating heme. In an analogous fashion, any heme released into plasma by intravascular hemolysis complexes with hemopexin and is removed by macrophages (and hepatocytes) expressing the low-density lipoprotein receptor–related protein 1 (LRP1).[18] In macrophages, heme from all these sources is degraded by an enzymatic complex containing nicotinamide adenine dinucleotide phosphate–cytochrome c reductase, the microsomal enzyme heme oxygenase 1, and biliverdin reductase, yielding carbon monoxide (the sole physiologic source in the body), bilirubin, and iron (see Fig. 35.5). Both DMT1 and natural resistance–associated macrophage protein 1 (NRAMP1; SLC11A1), a divalent metal transporter expressed within the late endosomal and phagolysosomal membranes of iron-recycling macrophages,[9] seem to be involved in efficient recycling of this iron.[16,17] Macrophages also can acquire iron from plasma transferrin via the transferrin cycle, but this is a minor portion of their total iron flux.

Ferroportin is the conduit for the outpouring of iron from macrophages in the bone marrow, liver, and spleen to plasma apotransferrin, normally the largest single flux of iron from cells in the body.[19] Ferroportin transcription increases in response to both iron and heme.[19] Ferroportin (FPN1A) levels are also regulated posttranscriptionally through an iron-responsive element in the 5′ untranslated region, with increases in cytosolic iron resulting in increased ferroportin translation. Iron export through ferroportin requires ferroxidase activity, provided by the multicopper oxidase ceruloplasmin in macrophages and by hephaestin in duodenal enterocytes (see later).[19] Ceruloplasmin oxidation may generate a concentration gradient that drives the ferric iron out of the macrophage. In the absence of ceruloplasmin, macrophage ferroportin is rapidly internalized and degraded. Unsaturated transferrin is not required for the release of iron from the macrophages; apotransferrin does not enter the macrophage and accepts iron only after the exit of iron through ferroportin and oxidation by ceruloplasmin.[19] The ferric iron can then be bound by transferrin and transported back to erythroid and other iron-requiring tissues.

Plasma hepcidin regulates iron efflux from macrophages by decreasing the number of ferroportin channels available for iron export.[2] The multimeric composition of ferroportin has not been determined definitively, but a dimeric structure seems most likely, based both on the available evidence and on the autosomal dominant inheritance of ferroportin mutations responsible for iron overload (see Chapter 36).[19] For the most part, ferroportin mutations either interfere with iron export by decreasing the amount of functional ferroportin on the cell surface, resulting in retention and accumulation of macrophage iron, or produce ferroportin resistance to internalization and degradation by hepcidin, resulting in loss of control of macrophage iron export that leads to parenchymal iron loading.[19] Homozygous ferroportin mutations are likely lethal. While the precise pathway of degradation remains uncertain, ferroportin must bind hepcidin for internalization and ubiquitination to occur.[19] Following ubiquitination, ferroportin is degraded after entering the multivesicular body that fuses with lysosomes.

Under normal circumstances, the macrophages in the liver, spleen, and bone marrow that are dedicated to reprocessing hemoglobin iron from senescent erythrocytes maintain an equilibrium between iron storage and release. Synthesis of cytosolic ferritin is induced in response to erythrophagocytosis, and, in the absence of iron deficiency, a portion of the iron derived from the ingested erythrocyte is retained within the macrophage as soluble cytosolic ferritin. With increasing amounts of storage iron within the macrophage, an increasing proportion of iron is stored within amorphous, insoluble masses as hemosiderin. On the basis of studies with heat-damaged erythrocytes labeled with radioactive iron, it is known that the fraction of radioiron sequestered within the macrophage can vary from virtually none in association with iron deficiency to a maximum of almost 80% in the presence of bone marrow aplasia and a fully saturated plasma transferrin.

LIVER REGULATION OF SYSTEMIC IRON HOMEOSTASIS AND IRON STORAGE

The liver (Fig. 35.6) is both the central site for control of systemic iron homeostasis, as the principal source of plasma hepcidin, and a major iron storage organ, sequestering iron in cytosolic ferritin and hemosiderin within hepatocytes and macrophages (Kupffer cells).[3] The dual blood supply of the liver from the portal and systemic circulation is a vital feature, allowing monitoring of both plasma iron in the systemic circulation and newly absorbed iron in the portal circulation. Hepatocytes can acquire iron from plasma transferrin via the transferrin cycle, from hemoglobin–haptoglobin and heme–hemopexin complexes via endocytosis after binding to CD163 and LRP1 receptors, respectively; from lactoferrin, apparently by receptor-mediated endocytosis; and from plasma nontransferrin-bound iron (Fig. 35.6). Plasma non-transferrin-bound iron forms when the rate of iron influx into plasma exceeds the rate of iron acquisition by transferrin.[20] Plasma non-transferrin-bound plasma iron enters specific cells independently of the transferrin mechanism, particularly hepatocytes, pancreatic acinar cells, cardiomyocytes, and anterior pituitary cells, producing toxic accumulations in some forms of iron overload (see Chapter 36). In mice, the ZRT/IRT-like protein 14 (ZIP14; SLC39A14) is reported to be the major route for cellular uptake of plasma non-transferrin-bound iron by hepatocytes and pancreatic acinar cells.[21] In the heart, ZIP14 is not required for uptake of plasma non-transferrin-bound iron and iron loading; L- or T-type Ca^{2+} channels or SLC39A8 are possible alternative transporters.[21]

The liver functions as the central controller of systemic iron homeostasis by being the predominant synthetic source of hepcidin.[3] The biologically active 25-amino acid peptide is produced by proteolytic processing of an 84-amino acid prepropeptide by furin.[2] After secretion, hepcidin circulates in plasma bound to α_2-macroglobulin and is rapidly cleared by the kidneys or degraded after binding to ferroportin.[4] As detailed earlier, hepcidin controls the entry of iron into plasma by decreasing the number of ferroportin channels available for iron export from macrophages, hepatocytes, and duodenal enterocytes. Plasma hepcidin concentrations increase with elevations in iron in plasma and in hepatocytes, and with infection and inflammation, decreasing plasma iron. Plasma hepcidin concentrations decrease with iron deficiency, hypoxia, and increased erythropoietic requirements for iron, increasing plasma iron.[2] The hepatocyte coordinates the congruent or conflicting influences of iron, infection, and erythropoietic demand to determine hepcidin secretion and thereby the systemic supply of iron. Because the amount of plasma iron is small and is replaced every 2 to 3 hours, changes in plasma hepcidin are followed rapidly by changes in plasma iron.

Regulation of hepcidin seems to be entirely transcriptional, integrating signals for induction and inhibition of synthesis both from within and outside the hepatocyte.[22] Intensive investigation has revealed a complex signaling network for transcriptional regulation of hepcidin (summarized graphically in Fig. 35.7) that remains incompletely characterized and with some features that still require

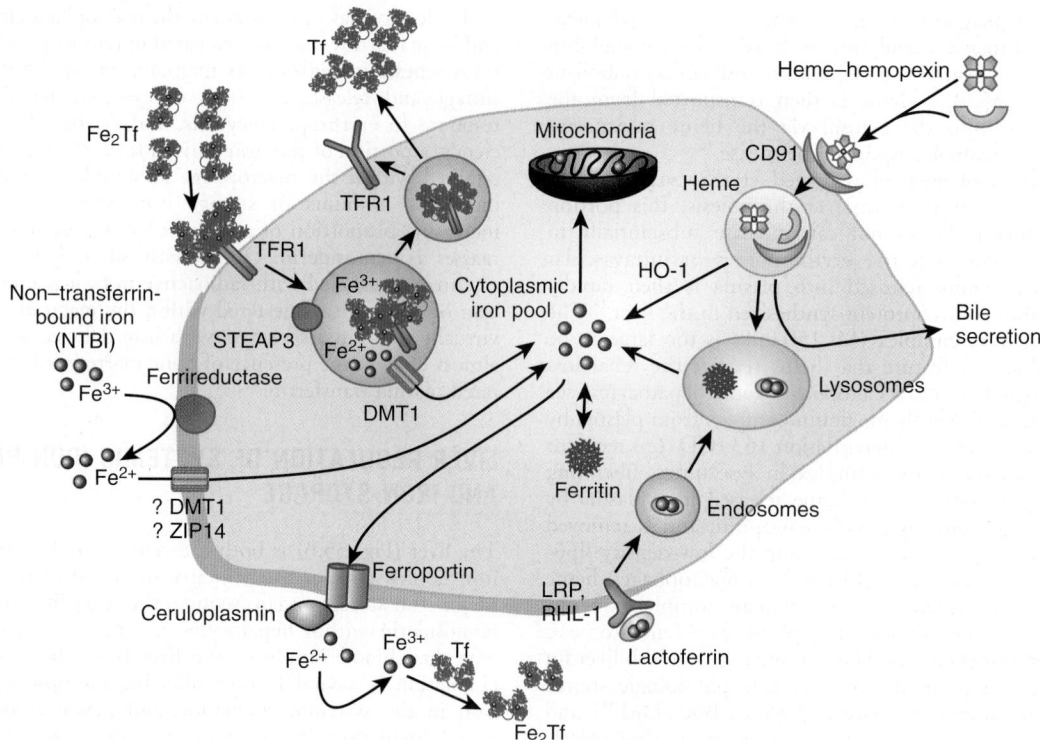

Fig. 35.6 ACQUISITION, USE, STORAGE, AND EXPORT OF IRON BY HEPATOCYTES. Hepatocytes can acquire iron from plasma transferrin (Tf) via the Tf cycle; from heme–hemopexin complexes via endocytosis after binding to CD91 receptors from lactoferrin, apparently by receptor-mediated endocytosis; and from plasma non-Tf-bound iron (NTBI). Iron is used for synthesis of heme and nonheme enzymes, with any excess stored in ferritin and hemosiderin. Iron is exported through ferroportin and oxidized by ceruloplasmin before being taken up by plasma Tf. See text for details. *DMT1,* Divalent metal transporter 1; *Fe₂Tf,* diferric transferrin; *FLVCR,* feline leukemia virus subgroup C cellular receptor; *HO-1,* heme oxygenase-1; *LRP,* low-density lipoprotein receptor-related protein; *RHL-1,* rat hepatic lectin-1 subunit of the asialoglycoprotein receptor; *STEAP3,* six-transmembrane epithelial antigen of the prostate 3; *TFR1,* transferrin receptor 1; *ZIP14,* Zrt- and Irt-like protein 14 (SLC39A14, solute carrier family 39, member 14). *(Reproduced with permission from Graham RM, Chua ACG, Herbison CE, et al: Liver iron transport.* World J Gastroenterol *13:4725, 2007.)*

verification in human studies. The available evidence indicates that major regulators of hepatic hepcidin synthesis include iron (hepatic iron stores, absorbed dietary iron, plasma iron in the systemic circulation), hypoxia, erythropoietic iron requirements, and inflammation and endoplasmic reticulum (ER) stress.[2,4,22] Recent studies have found that the control of hepcidin synthesis is further modulated by a variety of other signal transduction pathways, including nutrient-sensitive mammalian target of rapamycin (mTOR) and proliferative rat sarcoma/rapidly accelerated fibrosarcoma mitogen-activated protein kinase (Ras/RAF MAPK) signaling.[22] The mTOR and Ras/RAF MAPK pathways link hepcidin regulation to nutrient metabolism, cytokines, growth factors, cellular proliferation, and potentially the pathogenesis of hepatocellular carcinoma.[22]

Iron Regulation of Hepcidin Expression

Bone morphogenetic protein 6 (BMP6), a member of the transforming growth factor-β (TGF-β) superfamily, is the key endogenous regulator of hepcidin production (see Fig. 35.7).[2,4] BMP6 seems to be produced primarily (1) by liver nonparenchymal cells in response to hepatocyte iron stores and (2) by duodenal enterocytes in response to dietary iron. BMP6 initiates a signaling cascade by binding to hemojuvelin (HJV), a membrane glycophosphatidlyinositol-linked BMP coreceptor essential for effective induction of hepcidin, and to BMP receptors on the surface of hepatocytes.[2,4] BMP6 binding is followed by phosphorylation of sons of mothers against decapentaplegic (SMAD)1/5/8 and formation of the SMAD1/5/8–SMAD4

complex, which translocates to the nucleus and activates the promoter of the hepcidin gene (*HAMP*).[23] HJV is a critical potentiator of the BMP6-SMAD regulatory pathway.[23] Mutations in *HJV,* the gene for HJV, and in *HAMP* almost abolish synthesis of hepcidin, resulting in juvenile forms of hemochromatosis (types 2A and 2B, respectively; see Chapter 36) with severe iron loading. Neogenin, a deleted in colorectal cancer family member, seems to stabilize HJV, thereby enhancing BMP6 signaling and hepcidin expression.[23] Furin, a proprotein convertase, cleaves membrane-bound HJV to produce a soluble form of HJV that acts as a competitive antagonist of membrane-bound HJV, inhibiting hepcidin activation.[23] TMPRSS6, a transmembrane serine protease, inhibits BMP6 induction of hepcidin synthesis by cleaving HJV from the cell membrane.[24] A variety of inactivating mutations in the *TMPRSS6* gene produce high levels of hepcidin that are responsible for iron-refractory iron-deficiency anemia (see Chapter 36).[24]

Plasma iron, probably as diferric transferrin, is believed to modulate hepcidin synthesis through a distinct pathway that involves HFE, an atypical major histocompatibility complex class I protein that forms a complex with β₂-microglobulin, and transferrin receptor 2 (see Fig. 35.7).[25] Mutations in the genes encoding these proteins, *HFE* (hemochromatosis gene) and *TFR2* (transferrin receptor 2 gene), respectively, are responsible for adult forms of hemochromatosis (types 1 and 3, respectively; see Chapter 36). In these adult forms of hemochromatosis, hepcidin is expressed but fails to be appropriately upregulated as iron stores increase; iron loading is generally less severe than in the juvenile forms. The means whereby these proteins influence hepcidin synthesis are uncertain but may

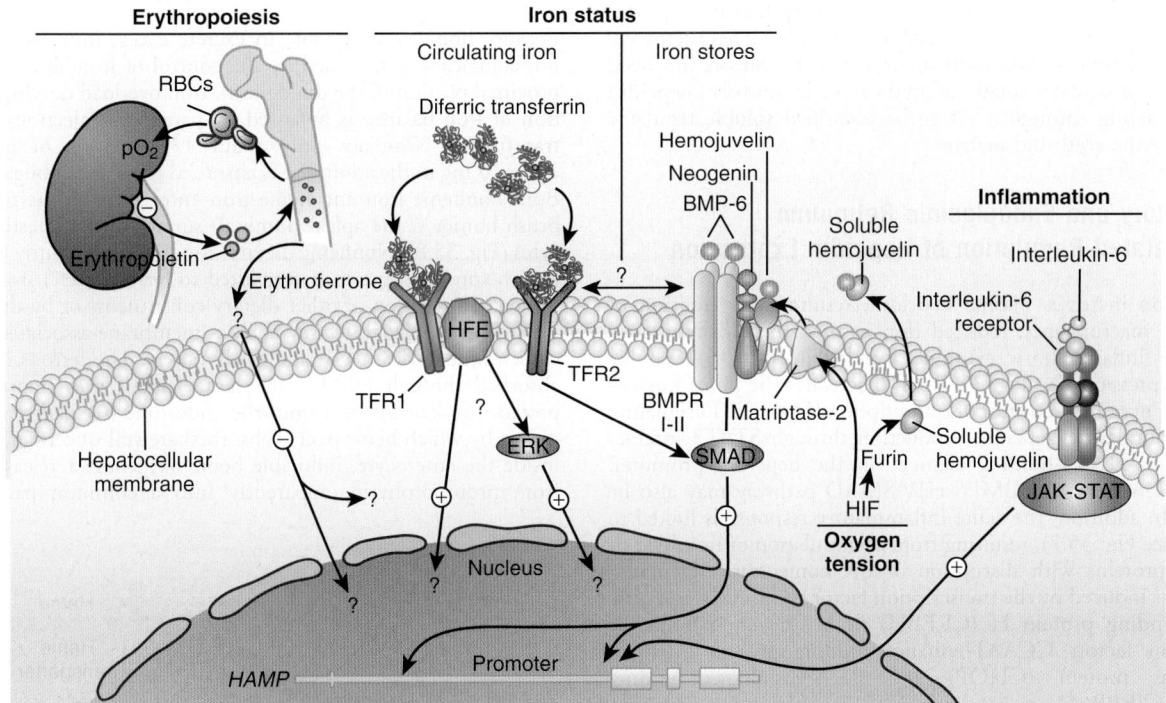

Fig. 35.7 TRANSCRIPTIONAL REGULATION OF HEPCIDIN EXPRESSION IN HEPATOCYTES. Hepatic hepcidin synthesis is regulated by iron, erythropoietic iron requirements, inflammation, and endoplasmic reticulum (ER) stress. Bone morphogenetic protein 6 (BMP6) is the key endogenous regulator of hepcidin synthesis. BMP6 initiates a signaling cascade by binding to the BMP coreceptor hemojuvelin and to two type I and two type II BMP receptors (BMPR I-II) on the surface of hepatocytes. Neogenin may act to stabilize hemojuvelin. BMP6 binding is followed by phosphorylation of sons of mothers against decapentaplegic (SMAD)1/5/8 and formation of the SMAD1/5/8–SMAD4 complex, which translocates to the nucleus and activates the promoter of the hepcidin gene (*HAMP*). The soluble form of hemojuvelin, cleaved by furin, seems to compete for BMP binding with membrane-anchored hemojuvelin. SMAD7, stimulated by iron, interferes with SMAD4 hepcidin activation. TMPRSS6 (transmembrane protease, serine 6; matriptase-2) inhibits BMP6 induction of hepcidin synthesis by cleaving hemojuvelin from the cell membrane. HFE (the hemochromatosis protein) interacts with TfR1 and likely also with TfR2 to modulate hepcidin synthesis through the BMP6-HJV-SMAD pathway and, possibly, through alternative routes involving the extracellular signal–regulated kinase 1 and 2 (ERK1/2), mitogen-activated protein (MAP) kinases, and furin. The erythroid-derived hormone erythroferrone has been identified as a mediator of hepcidin suppression by stress erythropoiesis. The inflammatory cytokine interleukin-6 induces hepcidin expression through a Janus kinase–signal transducer and activator of transcription (JAK-STAT) signaling pathway. Other cytokines and the BMP6-HJV-SMAD pathway may also be involved along with ER stress (not shown), possibly mediated by the transcription factor cyclic AMP response element–binding protein H (CREBH) or by the stress-inducible transcription factors CCAAT/enhancer-binding protein (C/EBP) homologous protein (CHOP) and CCAAT-enhancer-binding protein-α (C/EBPα). See text for details. *HIF,* Hypoxia inducible factor; *RBC,* red blood cell. See text for modulation of hepatic hepcidin synthesis by the nutrient-sensitive mammalian target of rapamycin (mTOR) and proliferative rat sarcoma/rapidly accelerated fibrosarcoma mitogen-activated protein kinase (Ras/RAF MAPK) signaling pathways. *(Modified from Kroot JJ, Tjalsma H, Fleming RE, et al: Hepcidin in human iron disorders: diagnostic implications.* Clin Chem *57:1650, 2011.)*

involve binding of circulating diferric transferrin to transferrin receptor 1, displacing HFE to form a complex with diferric transferrin receptor 2. The complex then acts through the BMP6-HJV-SMAD pathway, alternative routes involving the extracellular signal–regulated kinase 1 and 2, MAPKs, and furin, or some combination of these and other pathways.[4]

Erythropoietic Regulation of Hepcidin Expression

Increased erythropoietic demand for iron reduces hepatic hepcidin synthesis and can override competing influences that induce hepcidin expression, such as iron overload and inflammation (see later). Hemolysis, hemorrhage, and administration of erythropoietin lower

circulating hepcidin concentrations. Patients with marked ineffective erythropoiesis, such as those with β-thalassemia intermedia, have very low or absent plasma hepcidin, increased iron absorption, and high plasma iron despite severe iron overload (see Chapter 36). Neither hypoxia nor erythropoietin decreases hepcidin transcription directly. Studies of earlier candidate mediators, growth differentiation factor 15 (GDF15) and twisted gastrulation protein (TWSG1), have found that neither is involved in the downregulation of hepcidin synthesis after acute blood loss. Erythroferrone, a newly identified hormone produced by erythroblasts in response to erythropoietin, has been established as a physiologic regulator of hepcidin expression that suppresses secretion during stress erythropoiesis.[26] The erythropoietin-regulated pathway of erythroferrone suppression of hepcidin transcription seems to be distinct from and independent of the iron-regulated BMP-SMAD pathway. Still other signal transduction pathways seem likely to be involved in regulating hepatic hepcidin production in response to increased erythropoietic requirements. Transferrin receptor 1 expression on erythroid precursors has been proposed as a proximal mediator of erythropoietic control of hepcidin expression, acting through a yet to be identified soluble regulator produced by the erythroid marrow.[27]

Inflammatory and Endoplasmic Reticulum Stress–Related Regulation of Hepcidin Expression

Inflammation increases plasma hepcidin, resulting in retention of iron within macrophages, reduced iron absorption, and hypoferremia.[28] The inflammatory cytokine interleukin-6 (IL-6) induces hepcidin expression (see Fig. 35.7). IL-6 activates the Janus kinase–signal transducer and activator of transcription (JAK-STAT) signaling pathway, stimulating hepcidin production through STAT3 interactions with a STAT3-binding element in the hepcidin promoter. Other cytokines and the BMP6-HJV-SMAD pathway may also be involved.[4] In addition, the acute inflammatory response is linked to ER stress (see Fig. 35.7), resulting from accumulation of unfolded or misfolded proteins with disruption of ER homeostasis. Hepcidin expression is induced by the transcription factor cyclic AMP response element–binding protein H (CREBH) or by the stress-inducible transcription factors CCAAT/enhancer-binding protein (C/EBP) homologous protein (CHOP) and CCAAT-enhancer-binding protein-α (C/EBPα).[4]

Within hepatocytes and other cells, cytosolic iron is present physiologically in low-molecular-weight forms destined for incorporation into functional compounds or, if present in amounts exceeding cellular requirements, for storage. Recent evidence suggests that protein chaperones and other specialized carriers, membrane transporters, and small molecules provide for distribution of iron within cells. The cytosolic iron chaperone PCBP1, as well as all members of this family of proteins, can deliver excess iron to ferritin, whose structure maintains large amounts of iron in solution in a compact yet bioavailable form, diffusely distributed within the cytosol.[13] Cytosolic ferritin is a heteropolymer consisting of 24 subunits of heavy (H) and light (L) peptides that form a hollow sphere into which as many as 4500 atoms of iron may be deposited in an iron core composed of the hydrous ferric oxide mineral ferrihydrite ($5Fe_2O_3 \cdot 9H_2O$).[6] Iron entry and exit from ferritin seem to be in an equilibrium with the concentration of cytosolic iron. Both uptake and release of iron appear to be intrinsic, autonomous properties of the ferritin molecule. When cytosolic iron is low, iron-containing ferritin particles are randomly dispersed in the cytoplasm. As cytosolic iron increases, concentrations of dispersed ferritin rise, and small clusters of ferritin begin to appear, still soluble and spread throughout the cytosol. With further increases in cytosolic iron, ferritin enters lysosomes by fusion of ferritin clusters with lysosomal membranes, by autophagocytosis, or both, forming siderosomes.[6] Catabolism of ferritin within siderosomes leads to denaturation of ferritin protein subunits and aggregation of the ferritin iron cores, resulting in the formation of amorphous, insoluble masses of hemosiderin.[6] If the extent of iron overload overwhelms the capacity of ferritin to store iron, ferritin iron may act as a prooxidant, contributing to tissue injury. Production of hemosiderin seems to help protect against iron toxicity by sequestering the excess iron away from the cytosol, enclosed within siderosome membranes.[6] As the total amount of tissue iron increases, the proportion stored as hemosiderin rises, from trace amounts in normal individuals to 90% or more with severe iron overload. Depending on the cellular type and iron supply and use, the half-life of cellular ferritin may range from less than 20 hours to 96 hours. Hemosiderin characteristically has a much slower cellular turnover than ferritin. Altogether, for short-term storage of iron, cytosolic iron is in rapid equilibrium with soluble, dispersed ferritin, but for long-term sequestration, the aggregates of iron within hemosiderin undergo slow and limited exchange. Nonetheless, with phlebotomy or iron-chelating therapy, all of the iron within hemosiderin deposits eventually can be mobilized.

INTESTINAL IRON ABSORPTION

Because humans are unable to excrete excess iron, iron balance is physiologically maintained by the control of iron absorption in the proximal portion of the duodenum. Iron overload develops if regulation of iron balance is bypassed by parenteral injections of iron or transfusion. Normally, only about 1 to 1.5 mg of iron of the 10 to 20 mg in the adult diet is absorbed to balance obligatory losses. Both nonheme iron and heme iron enter through the microvillous brush border at the apical (luminal) surface of the intestinal enterocytes (Fig. 35.8). Nonheme dietary iron is predominantly ferric (Fe^{3+}) and, before absorption, is converted to ferrous (Fe^{2+}) iron either by the reducing action of other dietary constituents or by the action of brush border ferrireductases, such as membrane-associated duodenal cytochrome B (DCYTB) and likely others. The ferrous iron is then absorbed through DMT1, the same ferrous iron transporter that provides an exit for iron from the endosome (see earlier). The exact means by which heme iron is absorbed are still uncertain, but, when inside the enterocyte, inducible heme oxygenase 1 releases the iron from protoporphyrin, apparently into a common pathway with

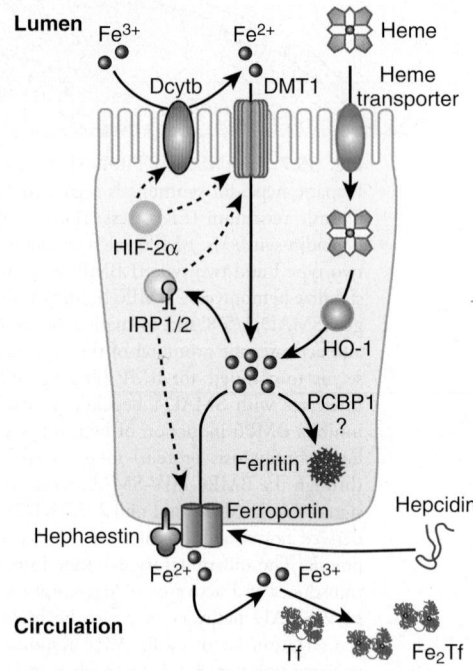

Fig. 35.8 ABSORPTION OF DIETARY IRON BY THE INTESTINAL ENTEROCYTE. In the gastrointestinal lumen, dietary iron is presented to the enterocyte as heme or nonheme iron. Heme iron uptake is not well characterized, and the specific membrane transporter remains uncertain. After absorption, heme oxygenase 1 (HO-1) releases iron from heme into a common cytosolic pool. Nonheme dietary iron is predominantly ferric (Fe^{3+}) and, before absorption, is converted to ferrous (Fe^{2+}) iron either by the reducing action of other dietary constituents or by the action of brush border ferrireductases, such as membrane-associated duodenal cytochrome B (DCYTB) and likely others. Ferrous iron is then transported across the apical membrane by the divalent metal transporter 1 (DMT1) into the common cytosolic iron pool. Iron may be transported into plasma through ferroportin, regulated by hepcidin, with hephaestin or circulating ceruloplasmin acting as ferrioxidases. Cytosolic iron in excess of systemic needs may be carried to ferritin by the cytosolic iron chaperone poly(rC)-binding protein 1 (PCBP1), retained, and then lost when the enterocyte is shed. In addition to regulation by hepcidin, enterocyte iron absorption is modulated by hypoxia inducible factor 2α (HIF-2α), H ferritin, and the iron regulatory proteins (IRP1 and IRP2). The enterocyte also derives iron from plasma transferrin (Tf) via the transferrin cycle (not shown). See text for details. Fe_2Tf, Diferric transferrin. *(Reproduced with permission from Anderson GJ, Frazer DM, McLaren GD: Iron absorption and metabolism. Curr Opin Gastroenterol 25:129, 2009.)*

absorbed dietary nonheme iron. In the enterocyte cytosol, the iron can be (1) retained for cellular requirements or stored in cytosolic ferritin and then lost when the enterocyte is exfoliated or (2) exported through ferroportin on the enterocyte basolateral membrane. Iron export through ferroportin requires oxidation by membrane-bound hephaestin or circulating ceruloplasmin to the ferric form for binding by plasma transferrin. Control of duodenal iron uptake is intricate,[29] depending on both systemic factors (hepcidin control of ferroportin) and local modulation of iron absorption through transcriptional (HIF-2α) and posttranscriptional (by the iron regulatory protein/iron-responsive element system) mechanisms.[29] Expression of FPN1B, which lacks the iron-responsive element in its 5′ untranslated region, allows enterocytes to bypass iron regulatory protein repression of ferroportin iron export even when cells throughout the body are iron-deficient.[29]

FUTURE DIRECTIONS

Remarkable progress has been made in unraveling the molecular mechanisms underlying systemic iron homeostasis, but much remains to be done. Genomic studies are needed to identify additional genes involved in the regulation of iron homeostasis. Little is known about developmental changes in the absorption, use, and storage of iron. Management of iron disposition within the systemic circulation needs further clarification, especially with respect to the basis for the dominant role of erythropoietic iron requirements and to the integration of intracellular and systemic regulatory elements. Control of iron balance needs more elucidation to determine the genetic basis for individual susceptibilities both to iron deficiency and to iron overload. More insight is needed into organ-specific iron handling and into the iron biology of specific disease states. A better understanding is needed of iron homeostasis in the three areas in the body that are outside systemic control: the central nervous system, the testis, and the retina. Nonetheless, a pivotal point has been reached when the advances already made will begin to yield therapeutic benefits from new approaches to biologic therapy using agonists and antagonists to the components of the iron regulatory pathways summarized in this chapter. Clinical trials of hepcidin antagonists have already begun.[30]

REFERENCES

1. Camaschella C: Iron and hepcidin: a story of recycling and balance. *Hematology Am Soc Hematol Educ Program* 2013:1–8, 2013.
2. Ganz T: Systemic iron homeostasis. *Physiol Rev* 93:1721–1741, 2013.
3. Meynard D, Babitt JL, Lin HY: The liver: conductor of systemic iron balance. *Blood* 123:168–176, 2014.
4. Lane DJ, Merlot AM, Huang ML, et al: Cellular iron uptake, trafficking and metabolism: key molecules and mechanisms and their roles in disease. *Biochim Biophys Acta* 1853:1130–1144, 2015.
5. Luck AN, Mason AB: Transferrin-mediated cellular iron delivery. *Curr Top Membr* 69:3–35, 2012.
6. Finazzi D, Arosio P: Biology of ferritin in mammals: an update on iron storage, oxidative damage and neurodegeneration. *Arch Toxicol* 88:1787–1802, 2014.
7. Kühn LC: Iron regulatory proteins and their role in controlling iron metabolism. *Metallomics* 7:232–243, 2015.
8. Ruiz JC, Bruick RK: F-box and leucine-rich repeat protein 5 (FBXL5): sensing intracellular iron and oxygen. *J Inorg Biochem* 133:73–77, 2014.
9. Montalbetti N, Simonin A, Kovacs G, et al: Mammalian iron transporters: families SLC11 and SLC40. *Mol Aspects Med* 34:270–287, 2013.
10. Davis M, Clarke S: Influence of microRNA on the maintenance of human iron metabolism. *Nutrients* 5:2611–2628, 2013.
11. Nai A, Lidonnici MR, Rausa M, et al: The second transferrin receptor regulates red blood cell production in mice. *Blood* 125:1170–1179, 2015.
12. Rouault TA: Mammalian iron-sulphur proteins: novel insights into biogenesis and function. *Nat Rev Mol Cell Biol* 16:45–55, 2015.
13. Leidgens S, Bullough KZ, Shi H, et al: Each member of the poly-r(C)-binding protein 1 (PCBP) family exhibits iron chaperone activity toward ferritin. *J Biol Chem* 288:17791–17802, 2013.
14. Wilkinson N, Pantopoulos K: The IRP/IRE system in vivo: insights from mouse models. *Front Pharmacol* 5:176, 2014.
15. Chen JJ: Translational control by heme-regulated eIF2alpha kinase during erythropoiesis. *Curr Opin Hematol* 21:172–178, 2014.
16. Korolnek T, Hamza I: Macrophages and iron trafficking at the birth and death of red cells. *Blood* 125:2893–2897, 2015.
17. Nairz M, Schroll A, Demetz E, et al: Ride on the ferrous wheel—the cycle of iron in macrophages in health and disease. *Immunobiology* 220:280–294, 2015.
18. Schaer DJ, Vinchi F, Ingoglia G, et al: Haptoglobin, hemopexin, and related defense pathways—basic science, clinical perspectives, and drug development. *Front Physiol* 5:415, 2014.
19. Musci G, Polticelli F, Bonaccorsi di Patti MC: Ceruloplasmin-ferroportin system of iron traffic in vertebrates. *World J Biol Chem* 5:204–215, 2014.
20. Brissot P, Ropert M, Le Lan C, et al: Non-transferrin bound iron: a key role in iron overload and iron toxicity. *Biochim Biophys Acta* 1820:403–410, 2012.
21. Jenkitkasemwong S, Wang CY, Coffey R, et al: SLC39A14 is required for the development of hepatocellular iron overload in murine models of hereditary hemochromatosis. *Cell Metab* 22:138, 2015.
22. Mleczko-Sanecka K, Roche F, da Silva AR, et al: Unbiased RNAi screen for hepcidin regulators links hepcidin suppression to proliferative Ras/RAF and nutrient-dependent mTOR signaling. *Blood* 123:1574–1585, 2014.
23. Zhao N, Zhang AS, Enns CA: Iron regulation by hepcidin. *J Clin Invest* 123:2337–2343, 2013.
24. Heeney MM, Finberg KE: Iron-refractory iron deficiency anemia (IRIDA). *Hematol Oncol Clin North Am* 28:637, 2014.
25. Wu XG, Wang Y, Wu Q, et al: HFE interacts with the BMP type I receptor ALK3 to regulate hepcidin expression. *Blood* 124:1335–1343, 2014.
26. Kautz L, Jung G, Valore EV, et al: Identification of erythroferrone as an erythroid regulator of iron metabolism. *Nat Genet* 46:678–684, 2014.
27. Keel SB, Doty R, Liu L, et al: Evidence that the expression of transferrin receptor 1 on erythroid marrow cells mediates hepcidin suppression in the liver. *Exp Hematol* 43:469–478.e6, 2015.
28. Nemeth E, Ganz T: Anemia of inflammation. *Hematol Oncol Clin North Am* 28:671–681, 2014.
29. Gulec S, Anderson GJ, Collins JF: Mechanistic and regulatory aspects of intestinal iron absorption. *Am J Physiol Gastrointest Liver Physiol* 307:G397–G409, 2014.
30. van Eijk LT, John AS, Schwoebel F, et al: Effect of the antihepcidin Spiegelmer lexaptepid on inflammation-induced decrease in serum iron in humans. *Blood* 124:2643–2646, 2014.

DISORDERS OF IRON HOMEOSTASIS: IRON DEFICIENCY AND OVERLOAD

Gary M. Brittenham

Iron is an essential nutrient required by every cell in the body. Both decreases and increases in the amount of iron may be clinically important. If too little iron is available (iron deficiency), limitations on the synthesis of physiologically active iron-containing compounds can have harmful consequences. If too much iron accumulates (iron overload) and exceeds the body's capacity for safe transport and storage, iron toxicity may produce widespread organ damage and death. The body, with no effective means to excrete excess iron, relies upon control of iron absorption to maintain homeostasis. This chapter focuses on the clinical application of recent remarkable progress in understanding the molecular mechanisms that preserve iron balance.

Iron disorders are principally abnormalities in the amount or distribution of body iron. A fundamental advance has been the recognition that the interaction of hepcidin, the iron regulatory hormone, with ferroportin, the cellular iron export channel, is primarily responsible for the quantity and tissue disposition of body iron. Hepcidin controls iron absorption, use, and storage by binding to and inducing the degradation of ferroportin, decreasing iron entry into plasma from macrophages, hepatocytes, and intestinal enterocytes (see box on Control of Iron Homeostasis by Hepcidin and Ferroportin and Chapter 35). Hepcidin expression is suppressed with iron deficiency, hypoxia, or increased erythropoietic demand but stimulated with iron overload, inflammation, or infection. Genetic and acquired disorders with a deficiency in hepcidin production or with ferroportin resistance to hepcidin action produce iron overload. Hepcidin excess due to genetic causes produces iron-deficiency anemia, but acquired forms, such as those associated with infection, inflammation, or malignancy, result in iron sequestration and anemia.

LABORATORY EVALUATION OF IRON STATUS

Because iron disorders primarily produce quantitative abnormalities in the amount and tissue distribution of iron, laboratory evaluation of iron status relies on indicators of iron supply and storage. The principal routes of iron movement, the amounts and distribution of the major iron pools, and the sites of hepcidin control of iron entry into plasma are shown in Fig. 35.1. The continuum of changes with increased or decreased body iron content is illustrated in Fig. 36.1, which shows schematically the amounts of erythroid iron and storage iron together with the division of iron stores between hepatocyte and reticuloendothelial macrophage deposits and with characteristic values for some clinically available indicators of iron status.

Body iron supply and stores can be evaluated by both direct and indirect means, but no single indicator or combination of indicators is ideal for evaluation of iron status in all clinical circumstances. As body iron content decreases from the iron-replete normal to the amounts found in iron-deficiency anemia or as it increases to the magnitudes found in the various forms of iron overload, each available measure reflects in a different manner the continuum of changes shown in Fig. 36.1. In addition, each indicator may be affected by coexisting conditions that modulate hepcidin expression, such as infection, inflammation, cellular injury, malignancy, ineffective erythropoiesis, hypoxemia, liver disease, and malnutrition (see box

on Control of Iron Homeostasis by Hepcidin and Ferroportin and Chapter 35).

Direct Measures

The direct measures of body iron status yield quantitative, specific, and sensitive determinations of body or tissue iron stores. Quantitative phlebotomy provides a direct measure of total mobilizable storage iron. Quantitative phlebotomy is inapplicable to most anemic disorders but occasionally is useful in the diagnostic evaluation of some forms of iron overload (e.g., in patients with hereditary hemochromatosis who do not undergo liver biopsy). Bone marrow aspiration and biopsy can provide information about (1) macrophage storage iron by semiquantitative grading of marrow hemosiderin stained with Prussian blue (Fig. 36.2) or, if needed, by chemical measurement of nonheme iron; (2) iron supply to erythroid precursors by determining the proportion and morphology of marrow sideroblasts (i.e., normoblasts with visible aggregates of iron in the cytoplasm); and (3) general morphologic features of hematopoiesis. Bone marrow aspiration and biopsy are useful in studies of iron deficiency, but they are of limited applicability in the evaluation of iron overload because no information about the extent of hepatocyte iron deposition is provided. In the evaluation of iron overload, liver biopsy is the best direct test for assessing iron deposition, permitting quantitative measurement of the nonheme iron concentration and histochemical examination of the pattern of iron accumulation in hepatocytes and macrophages (Kupffer cells).

Direct methods for assessing iron status have the disadvantages of being invasive procedures, with their attendant discomfort, lack of acceptability to patients, and, in the case of liver biopsy, risk. A variety of noninvasive means of measuring tissue iron stores has been developed and applied in clinical studies, including determination of hepatic magnetic susceptibility, computed tomography, and magnetic resonance imaging (MRI). MRI, the most widely available method, can provide information about iron deposition in the liver, spleen, pancreas, heart, and brain.[4] When available as appropriately calibrated and validated techniques, these noninvasive methods are helpful in the diagnosis and management of iron overload, but, they lack the accuracy required to detect iron deficiency.

Indirect Measures

Indirect measures of body iron status have the advantages of ease and convenience, but all are subject to extraneous influences and lack specificity, sensitivity, or both. When used to estimate body iron stores, all of the available indirect measures are influenced not only by total body iron stores but also by the effects of acute or chronic changes in plasma hepcidin (see box on Control of Iron Homeostasis by Hepcidin and Ferroportin). Assays for plasma and urinary hepcidin are not yet generally available for clinical use, but they are under development and will likely be helpful in the evaluation of patients with disorders of iron homeostasis.

Measurement of the plasma ferritin concentration provides the most useful indirect estimate of body iron stores. The small amounts

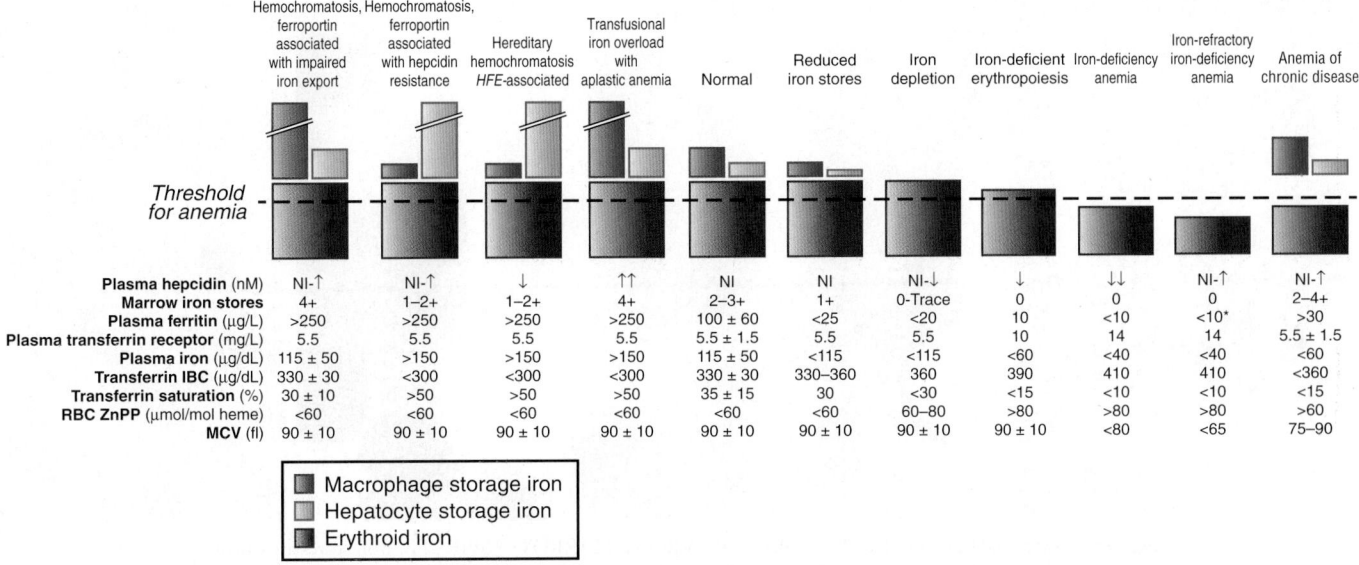

	Hemochromatosis, ferroportin associated with impaired iron export	Hemochromatosis, ferroportin associated with hepcidin resistance	Hereditary hemochromatosis HFE-associated	Transfusional iron overload with aplastic anemia	Normal	Reduced iron stores	Iron depletion	Iron-deficient erythropoiesis	Iron-deficiency anemia	Iron-refractory iron-deficiency anemia	Anemia of chronic disease
Plasma hepcidin (nM)	Nl-↑	Nl-↑	↓	↑↑	Nl	Nl	Nl-↓	↓	↓↓	Nl-↑	Nl-↑
Marrow iron stores	4+	1–2+	1–2+	4+	2–3+	1+	0-Trace	0	0	0	2–4+
Plasma ferritin (µg/L)	>250	>250	>250	>250	100 ± 60	<25	<20	10	<10	<10*	>30
Plasma transferrin receptor (mg/L)	5.5	5.5	5.5	5.5	5.5 ± 1.5	5.5	5.5	10	14	14	5.5 ± 1.5
Plasma iron (µg/dL)	115 ± 50	>150	>150	>150	115 ± 50	<115	<115	<60	<40	<40	<60
Transferrin IBC (µg/dL)	330 ± 30	<300	<300	<300	330 ± 30	330–360	360	390	410	410	<360
Transferrin saturation (%)	30 ± 10	>50	>50	>50	35 ± 15	30	<30	<15	<10	<10	<15
RBC ZnPP (µmol/mol heme)	<60	<60	<60	<60	<60	<60	60–80	>80	>80	>80	>60
MCV (fl)	90 ± 10	90 ± 10	90 ± 10	90 ± 10	90 ± 10	90 ± 10	90 ± 10	90 ± 10	<80	<65	75–90

■ Macrophage storage iron
■ Hepatocyte storage iron
■ Erythroid iron

Fig. 36.1 CONTINUUM OF CHANGES IN THE AMOUNTS OF ERYTHROID IRON AND OF HEPATOCYTE AND RETICULOENDOTHELIAL MACROPHAGE STORAGE IRON IN THE PRESENCE OF INCREASED OR DECREASED BODY IRON CONTENT. Characteristic values for some clinically available indicators of iron status are shown. The *horizontal line* indicates the threshold for anemia. In iron overload, the *diagonal lines* are intended to illustrate increases in excess storage iron from the normal range of 1 g or less to as much as 40 to 50 g. *Plasma ferritin may be normal or increased after administration of parenteral iron. *HFE,* Gene for the hemochromatosis protein, HFE; *IBC,* iron-binding capacity; *MCV,* mean corpuscular volume; *RBC,* red blood cell; *ZnPP,* zinc protoporphyrin.

Control of Iron Homeostasis by Hepcidin and Ferroportin

Hepcidin functions as the chief controller of body iron supply and storage by interacting with ferroportin, a transmembrane protein that is the only known iron exporter in humans (see Chapter 35).[1,2] Hepcidin binds to ferroportin, inducing its internalization and degradation, thereby inhibiting iron efflux from the principal sources of plasma iron-macrophages, duodenal enterocytes, and hepatocytes (see Fig. 35.1). Under physiologic conditions, hepatic hepcidin production coordinates body iron supply with iron need.[1,2] If body iron stores expand, hepatic hepcidin production increases. Increments in plasma hepcidin reduce the amount of ferroportin in cell membranes, causing a prompt fall in plasma iron concentration by decreasing macrophage release of iron derived from senescent red blood cells (RBCs), inhibiting release of iron stored in hepatocytes, and diminishing delivery of iron from enterocytes absorbing dietary iron. Conversely, if body iron stores diminish, hepatic hepcidin production decreases. Decrements in plasma hepcidin concentration increase the amount of ferroportin, producing a rise in plasma iron concentration as a consequence of enhanced delivery from macrophages, mobilization of storage iron from hepatocytes, and increased dietary iron absorption from enterocytes. In addition to the effects of body iron stores, hepcidin production is stimulated by infection, inflammation, cellular injury, or malignancy and inhibited by hypoxemia or increased erythropoietic demand. The influence of infection and inflammation on hepcidin and ferroportin expression link iron sequestration to host defense, and the interaction with erythropoiesis connects iron supply to RBC production.[3] Depending on clinical circumstances, the effects of inflammation or erythropoiesis on hepatic hepcidin synthesis may predominate over those of body iron stores. Liver disease and malnutrition may also impair hepcidin expression. Although hepcidin is the central regulator of iron homeostasis, hypoxia inducible factor 2α and the iron regulatory protein/iron-responsive element system modulate intestinal iron absorption (see Chapter 35).

of ferritin secreted into the circulation can be measured by immunoassay and have a logarithmic relationship to body iron stores in healthy persons. In the absence of complicating factors, plasma ferritin concentrations decrease with depletion of storage iron and increase with storage iron accumulation (see box on Plasma Ferritin

Concentrations). Measurement of the plasma transferrin receptor concentration is helpful in detecting tissue iron deficiency. A majority of plasma transferrin receptors are derived from the erythroid marrow, and their concentration is determined primarily by erythroid marrow activity. While decreased levels of circulating soluble transferrin receptor are found in patients with erythroid hypoplasia (aplastic anemia, chronic renal failure), increased levels are present in patients with erythroid hyperplasia (thalassemia major, sickle cell anemia, anemia with ineffective erythropoiesis, chronic hemolytic anemia). Iron deficiency also increases soluble transferrin receptor concentrations. The plasma transferrin receptor concentration reflects the total body mass of tissue receptor; thus, in the absence of other conditions causing erythroid hyperplasia, an increase in plasma transferrin receptor concentration provides a sensitive, quantitative measure of tissue iron deficiency. In particular, measurement of plasma transferrin receptor concentration may help differentiate between the anemia of iron deficiency and the anemia associated with chronic inflammatory disorders. Although the plasma ferritin concentration may be disproportionately elevated in relation to iron stores in patients with inflammation or liver disease, the plasma transferrin receptor concentration seems to be less affected by these disorders and to provide a more reliable laboratory indicator of iron deficiency.

The erythrocyte zinc protoporphyrin provides an indicator of iron supply to erythroid precursors. In heme biosynthesis, the final reaction is chelation of a ferrous ion by protoporphyrin IX. If no iron is available, zinc is chelated instead to form zinc protoporphyrin. Because zinc protoporphyrin formed during development persists throughout the lifespan of the red blood cell (RBC), the blood concentration changes only as new cells are formed and old cells are destroyed, providing a retrospective view of iron supply over the preceding several weeks. Levels also are increased in many sideroblastic anemias and especially with chronic lead or other heavy metal poisoning. The test is of no value in detecting iron overload.

Measurements of the proportion of hypochromic circulating RBCs (%HRC), the hemoglobin content of reticulocytes (CHr), or the reticulocyte hemoglobin equivalent (Ret He) are possible with some hematology analyzers and offer new means of detecting restriction of the iron supply for erythropoiesis. Measurement of urinary

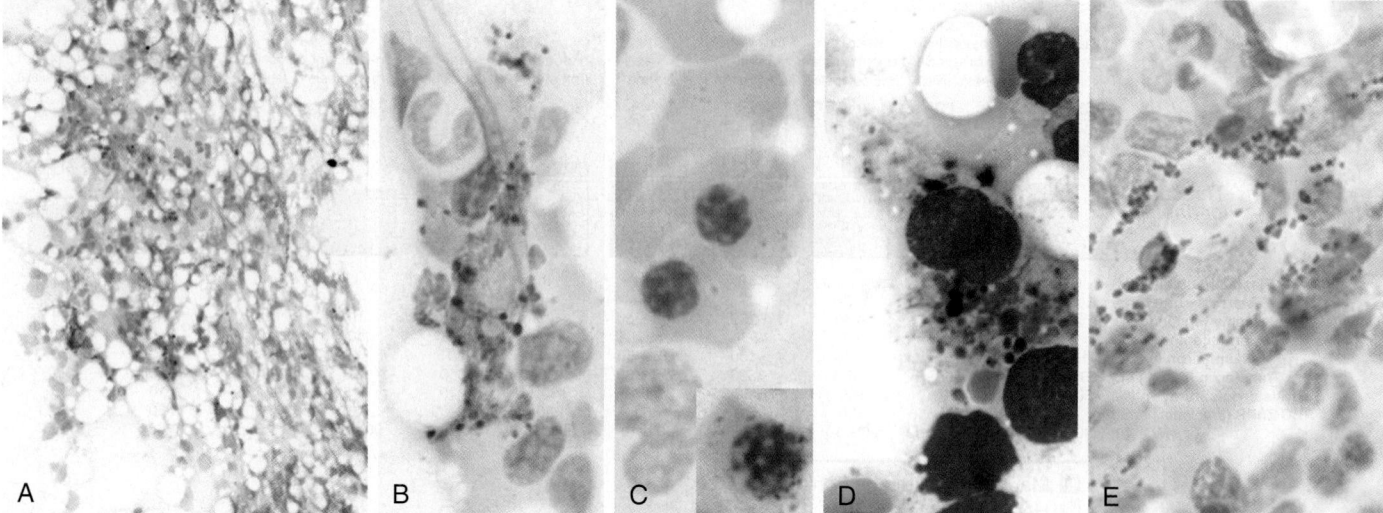

Fig. 36.2 ASSESSMENT OF IRON STORES ON A BONE MARROW ASPIRATE. Iron stores are usually assessed on the aspirate as opposed to the biopsy because the decalcification procedure required for processing the biopsy leaches out the iron and can lead to a false conclusion of absent stores. On the aspirate, a Prussian blue stain is usually used to evaluate iron. This can demonstrate iron stores (blue reaction product), particularly in the cytoplasm of macrophages and histiocytes (A–B). Iron can also be seen in the cytoplasm of some nucleated red blood cells (tiny blue cytoplasmic specks), which would allow these cells to be designated *sideroblasts* (C). These are in contrast to red blood cell precursors with abnormal iron accumulation around the nucleus, or "ring sideroblasts" (C, *inset*). Hemosiderin containing iron can be seen on the Wright-stained aspirate smears as a dark brown or black pigment in histiocytes (D), but generally an iron stain is needed to confirm the presence of iron stores. When parenteral iron therapy is administered, the marrow aspirate can sometimes show coarse iron deposits, frequently in long streaks (E). This is most likely iron in endothelial cells; it does not necessarily indicate marrow iron is present.

Plasma Ferritin Concentrations

Plasma ferritin concentrations are helpful in the detection of both iron deficiency and iron overload. Plasma ferritin concentrations decline with storage iron depletion; a plasma ferritin concentration less than 12 mg/L is virtually diagnostic of absence of iron stores. The only known conditions that may lower the plasma ferritin concentration independently of a decrease in iron stores are hypothyroidism and ascorbate deficiency, but these conditions only rarely cause problems in clinical interpretation. Increased plasma ferritin concentrations may indicate increased storage iron, but a number of disorders may increase the plasma ferritin level independently of the body iron store. Plasma ferritin is an acute-phase reactant. Ferritin synthesis increases as a nonspecific response that is part of the general pattern of the systemic effects of inflammation. Thus fever, acute infections, rheumatoid arthritis, and other chronic inflammatory disorders elevate the plasma ferritin concentration. Both acute and chronic damage to the liver, as well as to other ferritin-rich tissues, may increase plasma ferritin concentration through an inflammatory process or by releasing tissue ferritins from damaged parenchymal cells.

---

iron excretion with chelating agents, usually either deferoxamine or diethylenetriamine pentaacetic acid, offers another means of assessing body iron stores. This test is not helpful for detecting iron deficiency, owing to the overlap between values in persons with normal and those with decreased iron stores; it is used occasionally for the evaluation of iron overload.

Examination of peripheral blood by measurements of hemoglobin concentration, hematocrit, RBC indices, RBC volume distribution, and reticulocyte count and by inspection of erythrocyte morphology reveals abnormalities only after depletion of iron stores restricts the availability of iron for erythropoiesis. The changes are not specific for iron deficiency and may be found in other conditions with defective hemoglobin synthesis, such as thalassemia, infection, inflammation, liver disease, and malignancy. Iron overload does not produce any diagnostic abnormalities in the peripheral blood.

IRON DEFICIENCY

Iron deficiency is a decrease in the amount of body iron resulting from a sustained increase in iron requirements over iron supply. The continuum of decreased body iron is shown in Fig. 36.1. Three successive stages of iron lack can be distinguished. A decrement in storage iron without a decline in the level of functional iron compounds is termed *iron depletion* (see Fig. 36.1). After iron stores are exhausted, lack of iron limits the production of hemoglobin and other metabolically active compounds that require iron as a constituent or cofactor. *Iron-deficient erythropoiesis* (see Fig. 36.1) develops, although the effect on hemoglobin production may be insufficient to be detected by the standards used to differentiate normal from anemic states. Further diminution in the body iron produces frank *iron-deficiency anemia* (see Fig. 36.1). A variety of mechanisms coordinate the rate of erythropoiesis with iron availability (see Chapter 35). Iron deficiency reduces the responsiveness of erythroid progenitors to erythropoietin, helping preserve the supply of iron for vital functions in other tissues by decreasing erythroid use of iron for RBC production.

Epidemiology

Iron deficiency is by far the most common cause of anemia worldwide.[5] In the United States, adequacy of bioavailable iron in the diet, together with food fortification and the widespread use of iron supplements, has reduced the overall prevalence and severity of iron deficiency, but iron nutrition remains a problem in some subpopulations, especially toddlers, adolescent girls, women of childbearing age, and some minority groups. Without iron supplementation, most women will become iron-deficient during pregnancy. Globally, half or more of the populations in many developing countries are iron-deficient, with the highest prevalence among individuals who have diets low in bioavailable iron, who have chronic gastrointestinal blood loss as a result of helminthic infection, or both.[5]

TABLE 36.1	Causes of Iron Deficiency

Increased Iron Requirements

Blood loss
    Gastrointestinal tract
    Genitourinary tract
    Respiratory tract
    Blood donation
Growth
Pregnancy and lactation

Inadequate Iron Supply

Dietary insufficiency of bioavailable iron
Impaired absorption of iron
    Intestinal malabsorption
    Gastric surgery
    Iron-refractory iron-deficiency anemia

Etiology and Pathogenesis

The foremost task in the evaluation of patients with iron deficiency is identifying and treating the underlying cause of the imbalance between iron requirements and supply that is responsible for the lack of iron (Table 36.1). Overall, the iron requirement for an individual includes not only the iron needed to replenish physiologic losses and meet the demands of growth and pregnancy but also any additional amounts needed to replace pathologic losses. Physiologic iron losses generally are restricted to the small amounts of iron contained in the urine, bile, and sweat; shedding of iron-containing cells from the intestine, urinary tract, and skin; occult gastrointestinal blood loss; and, in women, uterine losses during menstruation and pregnancy. In normal men, the daily basal iron loss is slightly less than 1.0 mg/d. In normal menstruating women, the daily basal iron loss is approximately 1.5 mg/d. The median total iron loss with pregnancy is approximately 600 mg, or almost 2 mg/d over the 280 days of gestation.

The most common pathologic cause of increased iron requirements leading to iron deficiency is blood loss.[6] In men and postmenopausal women, iron deficiency almost inevitably signifies gastrointestinal blood loss. Within the gastrointestinal tract, any hemorrhagic lesion may result in blood loss, and the responsible lesion may be asymptomatic. Iron deficiency often is the first sign of an occult gastrointestinal malignancy or other unrecognized conditions such as coeliac disease, or autoimmune, atrophic, or *Helicobacter pylori* gastritis. Chronic ingestion of drugs such as alcohol, salicylates, steroids, and nonsteroidal antiinflammatory drugs may cause or contribute to blood loss. Worldwide, the most frequent cause of gastrointestinal blood loss is hookworm infection,[6] but other helminthic infections, such as *Schistosoma mansoni* and *Schistosoma japonicum,* and severe *Trichuris trichiura* infection also may be responsible.

In women of childbearing age, genitourinary blood loss with menstruation adds to iron requirements.[6] Other, less frequent causes of genitourinary bleeding may be involved, including chronic hemoglobinuria and hemosiderinuria resulting from paroxysmal nocturnal hemoglobinuria or from chronic intravascular hemolysis. Uncommonly, respiratory tract blood loss resulting from chronic recurrent hemoptysis of any cause produces iron deficiency.

In infants, children, and adolescents, the need for iron for growth may exceed the supply available from diet and stores.[7] Premature infants, who have a lower birth weight and a more rapid postnatal rate of growth, are at high risk for iron deficiency unless given iron supplements. With rapid growth during the first year of life, the body weights of term infants normally triple, and iron requirements are at high levels. Iron requirements decline as growth slows during the second year of life and into childhood but rise again with the adolescent growth spurt.

Without supplemental iron, pregnancy entails the net loss of the equivalent of 1200 to 1500 mL of blood. After delivery, resumption

of menstruation usually is delayed for months. If the infant is breast-fed, lactation necessitates an intake of about 0.5 to 1.0 mg of iron daily.

In some instances, an insufficient supply of iron may contribute to the development of iron deficiency.[6] In infants or in women who have experienced heavy menstrual losses or multiple pregnancies, the risk of iron deficiency may be further increased by diets with insufficient amounts of bioavailable iron, such as those with little or no heme iron and with small amounts of enhancers or large amounts of inhibitors of nonheme iron absorption. For older children, men, and postmenopausal women, the restricted availability of dietary iron is almost never the sole explanation for iron deficiency, and other causes, especially blood loss, must be considered.

Impaired absorption of iron in itself infrequently is the sole source of iron deficiency. Nonetheless, in patients in whom evaluation fails to identify a source of blood loss, as well as in those unresponsive to oral iron therapy, celiac disease, autoimmune, atrophic, or *H. pylori* gastritis may be responsible.[6] Iron deficiency frequently complicates gastric surgery, such as partial or total gastric resection, gastroenterostomy for bypass of the duodenum, and bariatric surgery.

Increased iron requirements and an inadequate supply of iron often work in concert to produce iron deficiency. Infants fed cow's milk receive a diet that not only contains small amounts of iron of low bioavailability but also increases iron losses by causing gastrointestinal bleeding.[7] Patients with ulcer disease and increased gastrointestinal blood loss may habitually take antacids or proton pump inhibitors, which diminish dietary iron absorption.

An uncommon heritable cause of iron deficiency is iron-refractory iron-deficiency anemia (IRIDA), an autosomal recessive disorder with severe iron-deficiency anemia and increased concentrations of plasma hepcidin. The anemia is unresponsive to orally administered iron and incompletely responsive to parenteral iron.[8] Mutations in *TMPRSS6,* a gene that normally inhibits hepcidin production, are responsible (see Chapter 35).

Clinical Presentation

Patients with iron deficiency may present with (1) no signs or symptoms, coming to medical attention only because of abnormalities noted on laboratory tests; (2) features of the underlying disorder responsible for the development of iron deficiency; (3) manifestations common to all anemias; or (4) one or more of the few signs and symptoms considered highly specific for iron deficiency, namely, pagophagia, koilonychia, and blue sclerae.[6] In addition, a high prevalence of iron deficiency with or without anemia has been reported among patients with restless legs syndrome, a neurologic disorder characterized by a distressing need or urge to move the legs (akathisia).

An uncomplicated depletion of storage iron generally is not associated with signs or symptoms, although patients without iron reserves will not respond as rapidly to an increased need for iron resulting from blood loss, growth, or pregnancy. Iron-deficiency anemia produces the signs and symptoms common to all anemias, which are pallor, palpitations, tinnitus, headache, irritability, weakness, dizziness, easy fatigability, and other vague and nonspecific complaints. The prominence of these signs depends on the degree and rate of development of the anemia. With greater severity, anemia becomes increasingly debilitating as work capacity and tolerance of physical exertion are restricted and eventually can produce cardiorespiratory failure and even death.

Iron deficiency may produce clinical manifestations independent of anemia. Epithelial tissues have high iron requirements because of rapid rates of growth and turnover and thus are affected in many patients with chronic iron deficiency. Glossitis, angular stomatitis, postcricoid esophageal stricture or web (which may become malignant), and gastric atrophy may develop. Pagophagia, a variant of pica in which ice is the substance obsessively consumed, is a behavioral abnormality that is considered to be a highly specific symptom of iron deficiency, resolving within a few days to 2 weeks after beginning iron therapy. Iron deficiency has other nonhematologic consequences, including impaired immunity and resistance to infection, diminished exercise tolerance and work performance, and a variety of behavioral and neuropsychologic abnormalities. In patients with iron deficiency and heart failure, clinical trials have provided evidence that treatment with intravenous iron improves outcomes.

Laboratory Evaluation

A characteristic sequence of changes in the clinically useful indications of iron status occurs as body iron decreases from the iron-replete normal to the levels found in iron-deficiency anemia.[6] This sequence is illustrated in Fig. 36.1. The patterns shown develop in the absence of complicating factors that increase plasma hepcidin, such as infection, inflammation, liver disease, malignancy, or other disorders (see box on Iron Deficiency and Coexisting Disorders). Initially, as a result of any of the causes listed in Table 36.1, iron requirements exceed the available supply of iron. Iron is mobilized from body stores, and iron absorption is increased. If the amounts of iron available from body reserves and absorption are inadequate, storage iron depletion follows. Exhaustion of iron reserves then results in an inadequate supply of iron to the developing erythroid cell, and iron-deficient erythropoiesis commences. As hemoglobin production becomes

restricted, frank iron-deficiency anemia develops (see box on Plasma Iron Concentration and Transferrin Saturation).

Chronic, long-standing iron-deficiency anemia may produce severe microcytosis and hypochromia, with very pale, distorted RBCs and dramatic reductions in the mean corpuscular volume and mean corpuscular hemoglobin (Fig. 36.3). In contrast, some patients with mild iron-deficiency anemia may have erythrocyte morphology and indices indistinguishable from values found in normal, iron-replete individuals. Nonetheless, laboratory evaluation of uncomplicated iron deficiency in otherwise healthy persons usually is not difficult, and the characteristic patterns of indicators of body iron status shown in Fig. 36.1 typically are diagnostic. In the clinical evaluation of anemia, early or mild iron deficiency must be considered in the workup of normocytic as well as microcytic anemia.

Differential Diagnosis

Iron deficiency is the only microcytic hypochromic disorder in which mobilizable iron stores are absent; in all other disorders, storage iron

---

Iron Deficiency and Coexisting Disorders

Detection of iron deficiency in the presence of chronic infectious, inflammatory, or malignant disorders that increase plasma hepcidin is more problematic than in the absence of such conditions. Even if lack of iron contributes to the anemia of chronic disorders, the increase in plasma hepcidin will lead to a fall in the transferrin concentration (or total iron-binding capacity) and an increase in the plasma ferritin concentration. Because the serum transferrin receptor concentration is less affected by inflammation, its measurement usually can determine whether iron stores are absent. If uncertainty remains, bone marrow examination is definitive. If iron deficiency is present, iron stores are absent; if the anemia of chronic disorders alone is responsible, iron stores are present and typically increased (see Fig. 36.1).

Plasma Iron Concentration and Transferrin Saturation

Plasma iron concentration and transferrin saturation, which equals the ratio of plasma iron to total iron-binding capacity, provide a measure of current iron supply to tissues. After storage iron is depleted, the serum iron concentration falls; a transferrin saturation less than 16% often is used as the criterion for iron-deficient erythropoiesis. In contrast, plasma iron concentration and transferrin saturation are not reliably elevated with increased iron stores within macrophages, as occurs initially with transfusional iron overload, although the transferrin saturation may increase with parenchymal iron loading. Interpretation of the transferrin saturation is complicated by substantial circadian fluctuations in plasma iron concentration with day-to-day variations of 30% or greater. Furthermore, the plasma iron concentration is lowered by ascorbate deficiency and by conditions that increase plasma hepcidin, such as infection, inflammation, cellular injury, and malignancy. Plasma iron is raised by iron ingestion and by conditions that decrease plasma hepcidin, such as hypoxemia, erythroid hyperplasia with ineffective erythropoiesis, and liver disease.

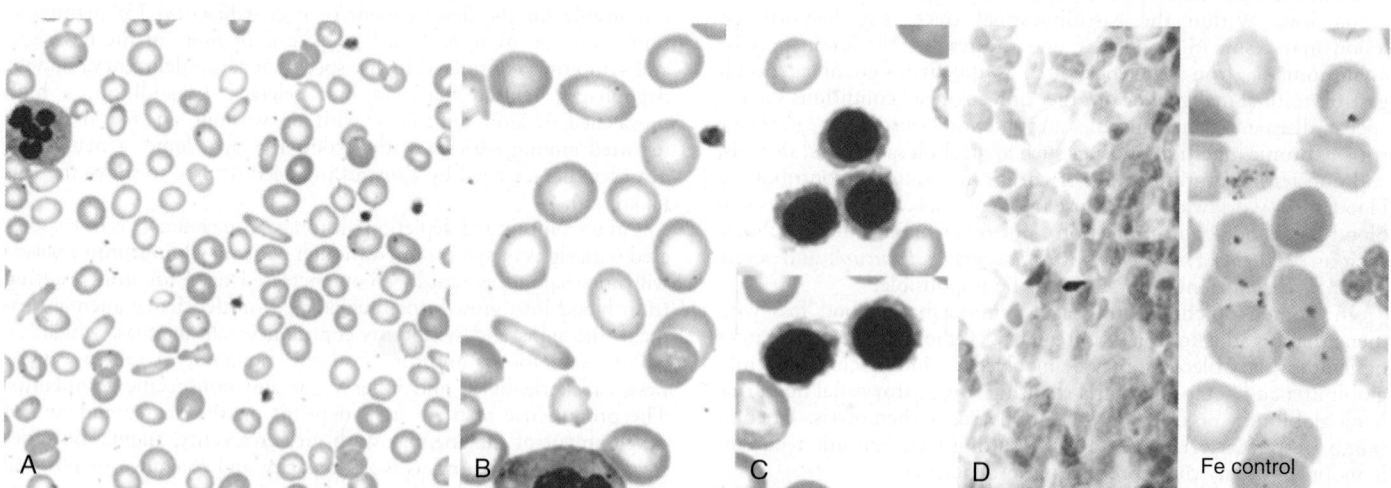

Fig. 36.3 IRON-DEFICIENCY ANEMIA. Peripheral blood smear (A–B), bone marrow (BM) aspirate (C), and Prussian blue stain of BM aspirate (D) with control from a 16-year-old girl with hemoglobin 6.7 g/dL, hematocrit 22.6%, and mean corpuscular volume 59.2 fL. Peripheral smear shows hypochromic microcytic red blood cells (A), with widening of the central pallor and "pencil" cells (B). Polychromatophilic erythroid precursors in the aspirated specimen have scanty cytoplasm that is irregular and vacuolated (C). The Prussian blue-stained aspirate shows no iron stores in multiple spicules (D). Care must be taken not to overinterpret positive staining debris on top of cells *(center)*. Lack of staining on the BM biopsy sample can be misleading because the decalcification process is known to "leach out" iron. An appropriate control should be similar to the patient material. Peripheral blood smears made from a patient with increased iron-containing Pappenheimer bodies and fixed with 100% methanol can serve as an easily accessible control.

TABLE 36.2	Differential Diagnosis of Microcytic Hypochromic Anemia

Decreased Body Iron Stores

Iron-deficiency anemia

Normal or Increased Body Iron Stores

Anemia of chronic disease

Defective absorption, transport, or use of iron

Iron-refractory iron-deficiency anemia after parenteral iron

Atransferrinemia

Aceruloplasminemia

Divalent metal transporter 1 (DMT1 or SLC11A2) deficiency

Ferroportin-associated hemochromatosis with impaired iron export (type 4A)

Heme oxygenase 1 deficiency

Disorders of globin synthesis

    Thalassemia

    Other microcytic hemoglobinopathies

Disorders of heme synthesis: sideroblastic anemias

    Hereditary

    Acquired

Therapeutic Trial of Iron

The diagnosis of iron deficiency often is confirmed by the outcome of a therapeutic trial of iron. A specific orderly response to, and only to, treatment with iron constitutes the final definitive proof that a lack of iron is the cause of anemia. The unequivocal diagnostic response consists of (1) a reticulocytosis, which begins approximately 3–5 days after adequate iron therapy is instituted, reaches a maximum on days 8–10, and then declines; and (2) a significant increase in hemoglobin concentration, which should begin shortly after the reticulocyte peak, is invariably present by 3 weeks after iron therapy is begun, and persists until the hemoglobin concentration is restored to normal. The result of a therapeutic trial of iron must be evaluated for possible confounding factors, such as poor compliance with iron therapy; malabsorption of therapeutic iron; continuing blood loss; and the effects of coexisting conditions, especially infectious, inflammatory, or malignant disorders. The therapeutic trial merely aids in establishing the presence of iron deficiency. The search for underlying causes of iron deficiency must continue despite a positive response to iron therapy.

---

is normal or increased (Table 36.2).[9] In patients with the genetic disorder of IRIDA, iron stores may be normal or increased after treatment with parenteral iron.[8] Difficulties in the evaluation of microcytic hypochromic disorders usually arise when direct assessment of bone marrow iron is unavailable and the diagnosis depends on indirect indicators of iron status (see boxes on Iron Deficiency and Coexisting Disorders and Therapeutic Trial of Iron).

Specific entities to be considered in the differential diagnosis of hypochromic microcytic disorders are listed in Table 36.2; in all of these disorders, body iron stores are normal or increased. The anemia of chronic disease (see Chapter 37) is the most common cause of anemia in hospitalized patients and generally is mild to moderate, typically developing over several weeks in patients with chronic infectious, inflammatory, or malignant disorders. In patients treated with erythropoiesis-stimulating agents for the anemia of chronic renal disease or other disorders, the increased iron requirements of the erythroid marrow cannot be met by iron mobilization from replete stores, resulting in iron-restricted erythropoiesis. This state, sometimes labeled *functional iron deficiency* despite the presence of storage iron, is a form of iron-restricted erythropoiesis resulting from stimulated erythropoietic demand for iron. Uncommonly, a similar pattern can result from endogenous increases in erythropoietin owing to anemia, hypoxemia, and other conditions. The %HRC, CHr, or Ret He may be the earliest indicators that stimulated erythropoietic demand for iron exceeds the available

---

Oral Iron Therapy

Oral iron therapy should begin with a ferrous iron salt taken separately from meals in three or four divided doses and supplying a daily total of 100–200 mg of elemental iron in adults or 3 mg of iron per kilogram of body weight in children.[6] Simple ferrous preparations are the best absorbed and least expensive. Ferrous sulfate is the most widely used, either as tablets containing 60–70 mg of iron for adults or as a liquid preparation for children. Administration between meals maximizes absorption. In patients with a hemoglobin concentration less than 10 g/dL, this regimen initially provides approximately 40–60 mg of iron daily for erythropoiesis, permitting RBC production to increase to two to four times the normal level and the hemoglobin concentration to rise by approximately 0.2 g/dL per day. An increase in the hemoglobin concentration of at least 2 g/dL after 3 weeks of therapy generally is used as the criterion for an adequate therapeutic response. For milder anemia, a single daily dose of approximately 60 mg of iron per day may be adequate. After the anemia has been fully corrected, oral iron should be continued to replace storage iron,[6] either empirically for an additional 4–6 months or until the plasma ferritin concentration exceeds approximately 50 μg/L.

---

supply.[10] Measurement of red cell zinc protoporphyrin concentration also provides a sensitive index of functional iron deficiency, but it is less sensitive than reticulocyte measures to acute changes in iron availability.[10]

Microcytic hypochromic anemias resulting from disorders of heme synthesis (sideroblastic anemias, congenital and acquired) and disorders of globin synthesis (thalassemias, microcytic hemoglobinopathies) are discussed in Chapters 38 and 40, respectively. Other rare congenital or acquired defects with microcytic hypochromic anemia include atransferrinemia,[9] aceruloplasminemia, divalent metal transporter 1 (DMT1 or SLC11A2) deficiency, some forms of ferroportin disease, heme oxygenase 1 deficiency (mutations in *HMOX1*, encoding heme oxygenase 1), several inherited sideroblastic anemias, and a variety of other uncommon disorders.

Therapy

The goal of therapy for iron-deficiency anemia is to supply sufficient iron to repair the hemoglobin deficit and replenish storage iron.[6] Generally, iron therapy for iron deficiency can be deferred until the underlying cause of the lack of iron has been identified. Oral iron is the treatment of choice for most patients because of its effectiveness, safety, and economy and should always be given preference over parenteral iron for initial treatment (see box on Oral Iron Therapy). The risk of local and systemic adverse reactions restricts the use of parenteral iron to patients who are unable to absorb or tolerate adequate amounts of oral iron.[11] Rarely, RBC transfusions are needed to prevent cardiac or cerebral ischemia in patients with severe anemia or to support patients whose chronic rate of iron loss exceeds the rate of replacement possible with parenteral therapy.

Most patients are able to tolerate oral iron therapy without difficulty, but 10% to 20% may have symptoms attributable to iron. The most common side effects are gastrointestinal. Decreasing the amount of iron in each dose usually is effective in controlling side effects, but if symptoms persist, a reduction in frequency to a single daily dose may be helpful. Costly iron preparations with other additives, polysaccharide–iron complexes, or enteric coatings or in sustained-release forms do not appear to offer any advantages that cannot be achieved by simply reducing the dose of plain ferrous salts. Administering iron with food and decreasing the dose will diminish the amount of iron absorbed daily and thereby prolong the period of treatment, but haste in the correction of iron deficiency is rarely needed.

Parenteral iron therapy (see box on Parenteral Iron Therapy), with the risk of adverse reactions, should be reserved for the exceptional patient who (1) remains intolerant of oral iron despite repeated modifications in dosage regimen; (2) has iron needs that cannot be

---

Parenteral Iron Therapy

Parenteral iron preparations that are approved for use in the United States include low-molecular-weight iron dextran, ferric gluconate, iron sucrose, ferumoxytol, and ferric carboxymaltose; iron isomaltoside is approved for use only in Europe.[12] Each preparation has been widely used, often in hemodialysis patients receiving recombinant human erythropoietin, but neither prospective, randomized controlled comparisons among these intravenous agents nor long-term safety studies have been done. Although infrequent, immediate life-threatening anaphylactic reactions constitute the most serious risk associated with use of either intramuscular or intravenous iron preparations, may have a fatal outcome, and can occur with all intravenous iron preparations.[11] Delayed but severe serum sickness-like reactions may also develop, with fever, urticaria, adenopathy, myalgias, and arthralgias.

---

met by oral therapy because of either chronic uncontrollable bleeding or other sources of blood loss, such as hemodialysis, or a coexisting chronic inflammatory state; (3) malabsorbs iron; or (4) has IRIDA.[6,8]

Prognosis

The prognosis for iron deficiency itself is excellent, and the response to either oral or parenteral iron also is excellent.[6] Frequently, both clinical and subjective indications of constitutional improvement are seen within the first few days of treatment, with the patient reporting an enhanced sense of well-being and increased vigor and appetite. Pica may resolve, and soreness and burning of the mouth may abate. Mild reticulocytosis begins within 3 to 5 days, is maximal by days 8 to 10, and then declines. The hemoglobin concentration begins to increase after the first week and usually returns to normal within 6 weeks. Complete recovery from microcytosis may take up to 4 months. With oral iron dosage totaling 200 mg/d or less, the plasma ferritin concentration usually remains less than 12 μg/dL until the anemia is corrected and then gradually rises as storage iron is replaced over the next several months. Although epithelial abnormalities begin to improve promptly with treatment, resolution of glossitis and koilonychia may take several months. The overall prognosis depends on the underlying disorder responsible for the iron deficiency.

Failure to obtain a complete and characteristic response to iron therapy necessitates a review of findings and reevaluation of the patient. A common problem is an incorrect diagnosis, with the anemia of chronic disease (see Chapter 37) mistaken for the anemia of iron deficiency. Coexisting conditions may impede recovery, such as other nutritional deficiencies; hepatic or renal disease; or infectious, inflammatory, or malignant disorders. Occult blood loss may be responsible for an incomplete response. With oral iron therapy, the adequacy of the form and dose of iron used should be reconsidered; compliance with the treatment regimen reviewed; and, finally, the possibilities of malabsorption and of the genetic disorder IRIDA considered.[8]

IRON OVERLOAD

Iron overload is an increase in the amount of body iron resulting from a sustained expansion of iron supply beyond iron requirements. Because requirements are limited and humans lack a physiologic means of excreting excess iron, any persistent increase in iron influx may eventually result in iron overload. The continuum of increased body iron is shown in Fig. 36.1. Whatever the source and the sites of excess iron deposition, when the accumulation overwhelms the cellular capacity for safe storage, potentially lethal tissue damage is the result. The toxic manifestations of iron overload vary with the precise pathogenic defect responsible but are dependent on the amount of excess iron, rate of iron accumulation, cellular pattern of deposition, and presence of complicating factors such as hepatitis or drug or alcohol use.

Epidemiology

The most common form of iron overload in the United States is a genetically determined disorder, the homozygous state for *HFE* hemochromatosis, which occurs in approximately 4 to 5 of every 1000 persons of northern European descent.[13–15] In the United States, other forms of iron overload are less frequent but affect thousands of patients with iron-loading or chronically transfused anemias, such as thalassemia major, sickle cell disease, myelodysplasia, and other acquired refractory anemias.[16] Globally, *HFE* hemochromatosis is the most common genetic disorder in populations of northern European ancestry.[13–15] Thalassemia major and other forms of iron-loading anemia are important public health problems in countries bordering the Mediterranean and in an area extending from Southwest Asia and the Indian subcontinent to Southeast Asia.[17] Dietary iron overload resulting from intake of iron in brewed beverages is a common problem affecting many populations in sub-Saharan Africa and may have a genetic component. Other inherited types of systemic iron overload, the various forms of perinatal iron overload, and the syndromes associated with focal sequestration of iron are uncommon or rare disorders.

Genetic Aspects

The varieties of iron overload known to be genetically determined are listed in Table 36.3, and their cardinal features are summarized in Table 36.4. The known forms of hereditary iron overload all involve defects in the interaction between hepcidin and ferroportin (see box on Control of Iron Homeostasis by Hepcidin and Ferroportin and Chapter 35).[13–15] The autosomal recessive disorders have in common an inappropriately low hepatic hepcidin production that leads to parenchymal iron overload. *HFE* and transferrin receptor 2-associated hemochromatosis and hemojuvelin- and hepcidin-associated juvenile hemochromatosis are the consequence, respectively, of mutations in regulatory genes controlling hepcidin expression *(HFE, TFR2, HJV)* and in the structural gene for hepcidin *(HAMP)*. Hepcidin production is also suppressed in three other rare autosomal recessive disorders with distinctive syndromes of iron overload: DMT1-associated hemochromatosis, atransferrinemia, and aceruloplasminemia.[18] The autosomal dominant disorders have in common mutations in the gene for ferroportin *(FPN)*.[18] In general, these mutations either (1) interfere with iron export, resulting in reticuloendothelial macrophage iron accumulations with only minor clinical manifestations; or (2) produce resistance to the action of hepcidin, resulting in parenchymal iron loading resembling that in the autosomal recessive forms of hereditary iron overload.

Several of the acquired forms of iron overload involve disorders with a genetic origin or component. The genetically determined iron-loading anemias include the inherited sideroblastic anemias (see Chapter 38),[19] some of the hereditary disorders of globin synthesis (see Chapter 40), and some chronic hemolytic anemias (see Chapters 41–47). Similarly, some forms of chronic liver disease and porphyria cutanea tarda (see Chapter 38) are inherited disorders. African dietary iron overload and, possibly, susceptibility to iron accumulation with prolonged medicinal iron ingestion may have genetic components. Many of the disorders requiring chronic RBC transfusion are hereditary, including thalassemia major (see Chapter 40), sickle cell disease (see Chapters 41 and 42), and other chronic refractory anemias. Although the exact etiology of some of these conditions is unknown, subsets of the disorders leading to perinatal iron overload or focal sequestration of iron have an established genetic basis.[20]

Etiology and Pathogenesis

Iron overload is caused by conditions that alter or bypass the normal control of body iron content by regulation of intestinal iron absorption. The known forms of hereditary iron overload (see Table 36.3) have a common pathogenic origin in genetically determined

TABLE 36.3	Causes of Iron Overload

Hereditary Iron Overload

Autosomal recessive hemochromatosis
  Hereditary hemochromatosis
    HFE-associated (type 1)
    Non-HFE-associated: transferrin receptor 2-associated (type 3)
  Juvenile hemochromatosis (type 2)
    Hemojuvelin-associated (type 2A)
    Hepcidin-associated (type 2B)
  DMT1-associated hemochromatosis
  Atransferrinemia
  Aceruloplasminemia
Autosomal dominant hemochromatosis
  Ferroportin-associated with impaired iron export (type 4A)
  Ferroportin-associated with hepcidin resistance (type 4B)

Acquired Iron Overload

From increased iron absorption
  Iron-loading anemia (refractory anemia with hypercellular erythroid marrow)
  Chronic liver disease
  Porphyria cutanea tarda
  African dietary iron overload*
  Medicinal iron ingestion*
From parenteral iron
  Transfusional iron overload
  Inadvertent iron overload from therapeutic injections

Perinatal Iron Overload

Gestational alloimmune liver disease with neonatal hemochromatosis
Trichohepatoenteric syndrome
Cerebrohepatorenal (Zellweger) syndrome
GRACILE (Fellman) syndrome

Focal Sequestration of Iron

Idiopathic pulmonary hemosiderosis
Renal hemosiderosis
Associated with neurologic abnormalities
  Pantothenate kinase-associated neurodegeneration
  Neuroferritinopathy
  Friedreich ataxia

*May have a genetic component.
DMT1, Divalent metal transporter 1; GRACILE, growth retardation, aminoaciduria, cholestasis, iron overload, lactic acidosis, and early death.

abnormalities in the interaction of hepcidin and ferroportin that lead to excessive intestinal iron absorption, resulting in body iron accumulation. The rate, distribution, and harmful effects of tissue iron loading depend on the specific abnormality in the interaction between hepcidin and ferroportin produced by each mutation.

In general, cellular iron loading in the autosomal recessive disorders begins with formation of plasma nontransferrin-bound iron that then enters cells through pathways other than the carefully regulated transferrin–transferrin receptor route.[21] The mechanisms of toxicity in vulnerable iron-loaded cells seem to involve expansion of the pool of cytosolic iron followed by iron-induced generation of reactive oxygen species; damage to lipids, proteins, and DNA; and injury to subcellular organelles, including lysosomes and mitochondria, with cellular dysfunction, apoptosis, and necrosis.[22] The pattern of the organs affected, the timing of the onset of toxic manifestations, and the severity of tissue damage are known to be influenced by a variety of factors in both hereditary and acquired varieties of systemic iron overload. Within the systemic circulation, these factors include (1) the specific underlying genetic or acquired abnormality; (2) the magnitude of iron excess; (3) the rate of iron loading; (4) the distribution of iron load among more innocuous storage deposits in reticuloendothelial macrophages and potentially injurious accumulations in parenchymal cells of the liver, pancreas, heart, and other organs; and (5) the extent of internal redistribution of iron between reticuloendothelial macrophage and parenchymal sites. Genetic studies suggest that genes other than those leading to iron loading have substantial effects on iron accumulation and toxicity.[23] In other forms of iron overload, another level of complexity is introduced because the central nervous system, the testes, and the fetus are functionally separate from the systemic circulation and cannot acquire iron directly from plasma transferrin. Instead, iron must be taken up from the systemic circulation by barrier cells and then exported across the blood–brain and blood–cerebrospinal fluid barriers into the brain interstitial and cerebrospinal fluids, across the blood–testis barrier, and across the placenta to the fetus.[24] As a consequence, disorders affecting the proteins responsible for iron supply to these compartments have distinctive manifestations.

Hereditary Iron Overload

Within the systemic circulation, the specific patterns of iron deposition and damage found in the hereditary disorders of iron overload can be characterized by reference to the pathways of internal iron exchange shown in Fig. 35.1 and the classification given in Table 36.4.

In HFE hemochromatosis, an autosomal recessive disorder, the underlying genetic defect in the regulation of hepcidin production results in an inappropriately elevated iron absorption at any level of body iron, resulting in a chronic progressive increase in body iron stores along with enhanced release of iron from reticuloendothelial macrophages. HFE regulates hepcidin expression through the hepatic bone morphogenetic protein/sons of mothers against decapentaplegic (BMP/SMAD) pathway by binding to the BMP type I receptor Alk3 and preventing its ubiquitination and proteasomal degradation (see Chapter 35).[25] The C282Y and H63D mutant forms of HFE fail to stabilize Alk3 expression and cell surface accumulation, impairing activation of the BMP/SMAD pathway to suppress hepcidin production.[25] Patients are unable to effectively upregulate hepcidin expression as iron stores increase. Intestinal iron absorption, although inappropriately high in hereditary HFE-associated hemochromatosis, is still regulated by body iron levels. As the body iron level rises as a consequence of increased absorption, circulating transferrin becomes saturated and plasma non-transferrin-bound iron is formed.[21] Iron is deposited initially predominantly within hepatocytes (Fig. 36.4), but subsequently the iron accumulates in the pancreas, heart, and other organs.[21] By the time symptoms of organ damage develop, usually in the 4th or 5th decade of life, body iron stores typically have increased from the normal range of 1 g or less to 15 to 20 g or more. Further increments in body iron stores may be fatal, although some patients are able to tolerate a total iron accumulation of as much as 40 to 50 g. Patients with autosomal recessive non-HFE hemochromatosis caused by mutations in the gene for transferrin receptor 2 seem to be clinically similar to those with the HFE-associated form.[14,18] Patients with autosomal recessive juvenile hemochromatosis have a similar pattern of tissue iron deposition found in HFE hemochromatosis but develop severe iron overload much earlier, with hypogonadism and cardiac disease manifesting in the 2nd decade of life.[14,18] The rate of iron accumulation is increased substantially and is estimated to be three to four times greater than that in HFE-associated disease.

Patients with DMT1-associated hemochromatosis have in common a severe microcytic anemia with low hepcidin, high transferrin saturation, and marked hepatic iron deposition but normal to moderately elevated serum ferritin concentration.[14,18] Congenital atransferrinemia (hypotransferrinemia) is a rare disorder of autosomal recessive inheritance in which plasma transferrin is nearly absent and hepcidin is decreased.[14,18] Patients have a severe hypochromic microcytic anemia and die without transferrin infusion or blood transfusions. Hereditary aceruloplasminemia (hypoceruloplasminemia) is a rare disorder of iron homeostasis inherited as an autosomal recessive trait, resulting from absence or severe deficiency of ceruloplasmin occurring as a consequence of mutations in the ceruloplasmin gene.[24] Patients with aceruloplasminemia typically present in the fourth or

TABLE 36.4   Hereditary Iron Overload Disorders

Disorder	Gene, Chromosome Location	Inheritance	Plasma Transferrin Saturation	Plasma Ferritin	Iron Deposition Sites	Clinical Manifestations
Hereditary hemochromatosis, *HFE*-associated (type 1; OMIM 235200)	*HFE*, 6p21	Autosomal recessive	Early increase; >45%	Later increase after 3rd decade of life	Parenchymal iron overload affecting hepatocytes, heart, pancreas, other organs	Liver and heart disease, diabetes, gonadal failure, arthritis, skin pigmentation
Hereditary hemochromatosis, TfR2-associated (type 3; OMIM 604250)	*TFR2*, 7q22	Autosomal recessive	Early increase; >45%	Later increase after 3rd decade of life	Parenchymal iron overload affecting hepatocytes, heart, pancreas, other organs	Liver and heart disease, diabetes, gonadal failure, arthritis, skin pigmentation
Juvenile hemochromatosis, hemojuvelin-associated (type 2A; OMIM 602390)	*HJV*, 1q21	Autosomal recessive	Early increase; >45%	Increased by 2nd decade of life	Parenchymal iron overload affecting hepatocytes, heart, pancreas, other organs	As for hereditary hemochromatosis, but liver involvement less prominent
Juvenile hemochromatosis, hepcidin-associated (type 2B; OMIM 613313)	*HAMP*, 19q13	Autosomal recessive	Early increase; >45%	Increased by 2nd decade of life	Parenchymal iron overload affecting hepatocytes, heart, pancreas, other organs	As for hereditary hemochromatosis, but liver involvement less prominent
Hemochromatosis, DMT1-associated (OMIM 206100)	*SCL11A2*, 12q13	Autosomal recessive	Early increase; >45%	Normal to moderately elevated	Hepatic iron overload, predominantly in hepatocytes	Severe microcytic anemia, liver dysfunction
Atransferrinemia (OMIM 209300)	*TF*, 3q22	Autosomal recessive	No plasma transferrin	Increased	Parenchymal iron overload affecting hepatocytes, heart, pancreas; no iron stores in bone marrow or spleen	Transfusion-dependent iron-deficiency anemia, growth retardation, poor survival
Aceruloplasminemia (OMIM 604290)	*CP*, 3q24-q25	Autosomal recessive	Decreased	Increased	Marked iron accumulation in basal ganglia, liver, pancreas	Diabetes, progressive neurologic disease, retinal degeneration
Hemochromatosis, ferroportin-associated, with impaired iron export (type 4A; OMIM 606069)	*SLC40A1*, 2q32	Autosomal dominant	Remains normal or low	Early increase	Predominantly macrophage iron deposition	None
Hemochromatosis, ferroportin-associated, with hepcidin resistance (type 4B; OMIM 606069)	*SLC40A1*, 2q32	Autosomal dominant	Early increase; >45%	Early increase	Parenchymal iron overload affecting hepatocytes, heart, pancreas, other organs	Similar to *HFE*-associated hemochromatosis

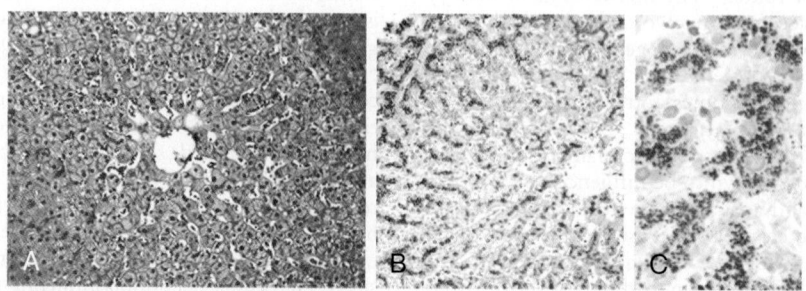

Fig. 36.4 *HFE* HEMOCHROMATOSIS. Liver biopsy sample from a 46-year-old man with homozygous *HFE* hemochromatosis. Hematoxylin and eosin stain of the liver (A) shows intact hepatic architecture. Iron stain (B–C) shows marked diffuse iron deposits in the hepatocytes throughout the lobules. A normal liver would show essentially no iron in the hepatocytes.

5th decade of life with a triad of diabetes mellitus, progressive neurologic disease (dementia, dysarthria, and dystonia), and retinal degeneration.

Patients with autosomal dominant hemochromatosis resulting from mutations in the ferroportin gene that compromise iron export, such as those resulting in ferroportins that are unable to reach the cell surface to interact with hepcidin, have iron deposition predominantly in macrophages, are almost devoid of clinical manifestations, and apparently do not require treatment.[18] Patients with mutations that result in ferroportins that reach the cell surface but do not respond to hepcidin develop a parenchymal pattern of iron overload that resembles that found in patients with the autosomal recessive forms of hemochromatosis.[18]

Acquired Iron Overload

Iron-loading anemias may be associated with excessive absorption of dietary iron that can produce severe iron overload. Iron absorption increases dramatically when accelerated erythropoiesis exceeds the ability of transferrin to provide sufficient iron for hemoglobin production (see Chapter 35).[16,26] The iron-loading anemias are characterized by the combination of erythroid hyperplasia with marked ineffective erythropoiesis and elevated concentrations of erythropoietin. Hepcidin synthesis may be suppressed by erythroferrone, a recently characterized hormone produced by erythroblasts in response to erythropoietin.[27] The decreased concentrations of hepcidin result in increased iron absorption and progressive iron loading. These refractory disorders include thalassemia major and intermedia, hemoglobin E/β-thalassemia, congenital dyserythropoietic anemia, pyruvate kinase deficiency, a variety of sideroblastic anemias, and other anemias associated with blocks in the incorporation of iron into hemoglobin.[16,26] The rate of iron loading is related not to the severity of the anemia but rather to the extent of ineffective erythropoiesis. Patients with nearly normal hemoglobin concentrations may develop massive iron overload; any RBC transfusions will add to the iron burden. Clinical manifestations include liver disease, diabetes mellitus, endocrine disorders, and cardiac dysfunction.

Chronic liver disease with increased absorption of dietary iron may produce mild iron overload in some patients, including individuals with nonalcoholic fatty liver disease (NAFLD), chronic hepatitis C infection, alcohol-related liver disease, or portacaval shunts.[14] In porphyria cutanea tarda (see Chapter 38), the most common type of human porphyria, mild hepatic iron overload is found in most patients, and iron depletion by phlebotomy produces clinical and biochemical remission of the disease. African dietary iron overload occurs in sub-Saharan Africa in association with greatly increased dietary iron intake from a traditional fermented beverage with high iron content, but a genetic component not linked to *HFE* may also be involved. Medicinal iron ingestion can add to the body iron burden of patients with iron-loading disorders, especially iron-loading anemias. In persons without abnormalities affecting iron homeostasis, the extent to which orally administered iron can increase the body iron stores is uncertain.

Parenteral iron overload usually is the result of repeated RBC transfusions in patients with chronic refractory anemia, but occasionally it is unintentionally produced by repeated injections of intravenous iron preparations in patients with anemia unresponsive to iron therapy alone, such as patients undergoing chronic hemodialysis.

Transfusional iron overload progressively develops in patients with chronic refractory anemia who require RBC support (Fig. 36.5).[16,26] In patients with severe congenital anemias such as thalassemia major (Cooley anemia) or Blackfan-Diamond syndrome, transfusional iron loading begins in infancy. Severe iron loading may develop in transfusion-dependent anemias that appear later in life, namely, aplastic anemia, pure RBC aplasia, hypoplastic or myelodysplastic disorders, and the anemia of chronic renal failure. Patients with sickle cell anemia or sickle cell/β-thalassemia are also at risk for iron overload if chronically given transfusions for prevention of recurrent complications such as stroke, severe infections, and incapacitating

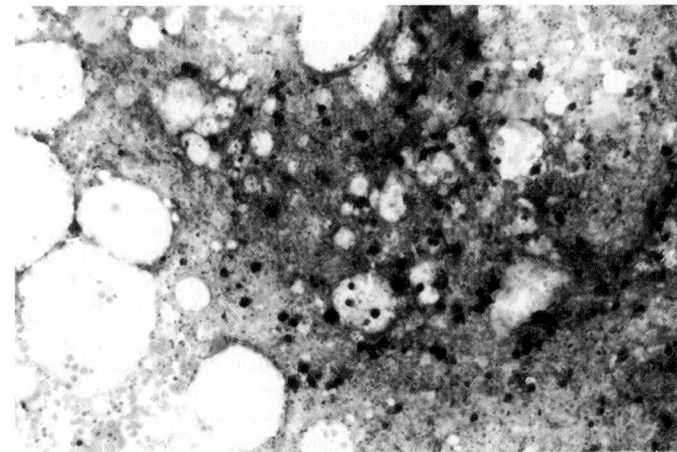

Fig. 36.5 ACQUIRED IRON OVERLOAD. Prussian blue–stained bone marrow (BM) aspirate showing excessive iron stores in acquired iron overload. This occurs in a number of instances as discussed in the text, including transfusional iron overload as illustrated here, in the BM of a patient with a myelodysplastic syndrome.

painful crises. If ineffective erythropoiesis and erythroid hyperplasia complicate the underlying anemia, increased absorption may contribute to the iron burden. The greater the extent of ineffective erythropoiesis, the greater the suppression of hepcidin synthesis and the greater the magnitude of the increase in iron absorption.[27]

Perinatal iron overload (see Table 36.3) develops in some rare or uncommon metabolic disorders of newborns. An important advance has been the recognition that almost all neonatal hemochromatosis is the result of fetal liver injury caused by gestational alloimmune liver disease, with specific maternal anti-fetal liver immunoglobulin G antibodies directed against a fetal liver antigen.[28] The injured fetal liver is unable to produce sufficient hepcidin to regulate placental iron flux, accounting for neonatal iron overload not only in gestational alloimmune liver disease but also in other rare forms of fetal liver disease that result in neonatal hemochromatosis. Treatment with a combination of double-volume exchange transfusion to remove existing reactive antibody and administration of high-dose intravenous immunoglobulin to block antibody action has been much more successful than the previously used regimen of an iron chelator with antioxidants.[28] Focal sequestration of iron in other rare disorders produces various patterns of localized iron deposition, in the lung in idiopathic pulmonary hemosiderosis, and in the kidney in renal hemosiderosis. Finally, remarkable progress is being made in elucidating the molecular bases for disorders with specific patterns of brain iron deposition in association with neurologic abnormalities, including Friedreich ataxia, Alzheimer disease, Parkinson disease, neuroferritinopathy, pantothenate kinase-associated neurodegeneration (formerly called Hallervorden-Spatz syndrome), and other forms of neurodegeneration with brain iron accumulation.[20,24]

Clinical Presentation

Clinical manifestations of iron toxicity generally develop only in patients with forms of systemic parenchymal iron overload in which the magnitude of iron accumulation is sufficient to produce tissue and organ damage.[14,18] Individuals at risk include homozygotes for the types of *HFE* and juvenile hemochromatosis listed in Table 36.3; those with some forms of ferroportin-associated hemochromatosis; those with aceruloplasminemia; and patients with iron-loading anemias, African dietary iron overload, and transfusional iron overload. Patients with forms of iron overload restricted to reticuloendothelial macrophages do not seem to develop clinical complications.[14,18] Specific patterns of neurologic signs and symptoms occur in patients with aceruloplasminemia, pantothenate kinase-associated neurodegeneration, Friedreich ataxia, and neuroferritinopathy that reflect the brain distribution of the excess iron.[20,24]

In patients with systemic parenchymal iron loading, similar clinical features eventually develop with sufficient iron accumulation to produce organ dysfunction and damage.[13-15] At earlier stages, with lower body iron burdens, no distinctive signs or symptoms may be present, and patients may come to attention only because of abnormal laboratory test results. Symptomatic patients may present with any of the characteristic manifestations of parenchymal iron deposition, including liver disease, diabetes mellitus, gonadal insufficiency and other endocrine disorders, cardiac dysfunction, arthropathy, and increased skin pigmentation. Liver disease is the most common complication of systemic iron overload. In all varieties of systemic parenchymal iron overload, the development and severity of liver damage are closely correlated with the magnitude of hepatic iron deposition. Whether derived from increased absorption of dietary iron or from transfused RBCs, progressive parenchymal iron accumulation eventually produces hepatomegaly, functional abnormalities, fibrosis, and finally cirrhosis.[13-15] Hepatocellular carcinoma seems to be the ultimate complication of cirrhosis in iron overload. The development of cirrhosis increases the risk of hepatoma by more than 200-fold.

Diabetes mellitus is another common complication of all forms of systemic parenchymal iron overload. Virtually all of the secondary manifestations of diabetes may develop, including retinopathy, nephropathy, neuropathy, and vascular disease. Gonadal insufficiency and other endocrine abnormalities occur. During the 2nd decade of life, both growth and sexual maturation usually are retarded in untreated patients with transfusional iron overload.

Iron-induced cardiac disease, occurring as a cardiomyopathy with heart failure, arrhythmias, or both, may be a fatal complication of all varieties of systemic parenchymal iron overload. Heart disease is the most frequent cause of death in patients with thalassemia major.[16,26] Severe cardiac disease in particular may be the presenting manifestation in young patients with juvenile hemochromatosis.[18]

Increased skin pigmentation, with a bronze hue in some patients and a slate-gray coloration in others, often accompanies iron overload. Chondrocalcinosis and other forms of arthropathy are common complications of hereditary hemochromatosis and may occur in other forms of systemic parenchymal iron overload. An increased susceptibility to infectious disease may be found in patients with transfusional and other forms of iron overload, especially to infections with certain organisms, including *Vibrio vulnificus, Listeria monocytogenes, Yersinia enterocolitica, Escherichia coli, Candida* spp., and *Mycobacterium tuberculosis*.[13,14,26]

Laboratory Evaluation

The typical sequences of changes in clinically useful indicators of iron status as body iron increases from the iron-replete normal to the amounts found in hereditary hemochromatosis and transfusional iron overload are shown in Fig. 36.1. Characteristic changes in laboratory measures of iron status in the disorders of hereditary iron overload are listed in Table 36.4.

Screening for iron overload can use phenotypical methods, genotypical methods, or both.[13,15] Phenotypical screening can provide biochemical evidence of iron overload in patients with hereditary or juvenile hemochromatosis but does not identify all persons genetically at risk for iron loading. In populations of northern European ancestry, genotypical screening for the C282Y and H63D mutations in *HFE* can identify most persons at risk for developing *HFE* hemochromatosis, but it gives no information about the presence or magnitude of iron overload. In most clinical circumstances, a combination of phenotypical and genotypical methods is the best strategy for screening.[13,15]

In individuals of northern European ancestry, measurement of the serum transferrin saturation usually is the best method for initial phenotypical screening for systemic parenchymal iron overload.[13,15] A persistent value of 45% or greater often is recommended as a threshold

value for further investigation. In the absence of complicating factors, elevated concentrations of serum ferritin provide biochemical evidence of iron overload. Genetic testing then should be considered in persons with abnormal transferrin saturation, serum ferritin concentration, or both. Liver biopsy may be indicated for prognostic purposes to detect cirrhosis if the serum ferritin concentration is greater than 1000 μg/L and may be contemplated in the presence of hepatomegaly or abnormalities on liver function testing, or in patients older than 40 years. Currently, cascade screening of families with affected individuals is recommended, but population screening for *HFE* hemochromatosis is not advised.[15] Individuals who are simply heterozygous for either the C282Y or the H63D mutation in the *HFE* gene do not develop iron overload.[29] Persons with phenotypical evidence of iron overload who are neither C282Y/C282Y homozygotes nor C282Y/H63D heterozygotes can be considered for further genetic testing for less common *HFE* mutations and for non-*HFE* mutations associated with iron loading,[18] for noninvasive assessment of the liver iron concentration, or for diagnostic liver biopsy.

Liver biopsy can establish a definitive diagnosis of hereditary and juvenile hemochromatosis regardless of genotype and can demonstrate the histologic pattern of iron loading found with ferroportin mutations or with chronic liver diseases NAFLD, chronic hepatitis C infection, and alcohol-related liver disease (see box on Testing for Iron Overload). A quantitative determination of the nonheme iron concentration in the liver sample should be made, the pattern of iron deposition examined histochemically, and the extent of tissue injury assessed histopathologically. In patients found to have an increased body iron load, additional clinical and laboratory studies should seek evidence of complications of iron overload. Further investigation may include liver function testing; testing for diabetes mellitus; evaluation of hormonal function; cardiac examination; joint and bone radiography examination; and, especially if cirrhosis is present, screening for hepatocellular carcinoma.[13-15]

Atransferrinemia or hypotransferrinemia is readily demonstrable by measurement of the plasma transferrin concentration. Similarly, aceruloplasminemia or hypoceruloplasminemia can be diagnosed by measurement of the plasma ceruloplasmin concentration.[24] For detection and diagnosis of iron-loading anemia, measurement of the plasma transferrin receptor and examination of the bone marrow may be helpful in demonstrating ineffective erythropoiesis in combination with the erythroid hyperplasia characteristic of these disorders.

Differential Diagnosis

Detection and diagnosis of iron overload are most problematic in the hereditary forms of iron overload (see Table 36.4). A combination of

Testing for Iron Overload

A direct measure of body iron avoids the uncertainties inherent in the interpretation of indirect indicators of iron status. Liver biopsy is the definitive direct test for assessing iron deposition and tissue damage in iron overload, permitting measurement of the nonheme iron concentration, histochemical determination of the cellular distribution of iron between hepatocytes and Kupffer cells, and pathologic examination of the extent of tissue injury.[15] When available as appropriately calibrated and validated techniques, new noninvasive methods using hepatic magnetic susceptibility and magnetic resonance imaging (MRI) may replace liver biopsy when only determination of the liver iron concentration is needed. MRI studies of the heart are particularly useful in patients at risk for cardiac iron deposition.[26] In patients with *HFE* or other forms of hemochromatosis undergoing therapeutic venesection, quantitative phlebotomy provides an accurate retrospective determination of the amount of storage iron that can be mobilized for hemoglobin formation. When liver biopsy is contraindicated in a patient, quantitative phlebotomy is occasionally useful in establishing the diagnosis of *HFE* or other forms of hemochromatosis. Bone marrow aspiration and biopsy provide no information about the extent of parenchymal iron loading and are of limited value in the evaluation of iron overload. Iron overload produces no diagnostic abnormalities in the peripheral blood.

phenotypical and genotypical screening should lead to a definitive diagnosis in most patients. Aceruloplasminemia is a rare disorder, but distinguishing this form of iron overload from hereditary hemochromatosis is important in guiding effective iron-chelating therapy that can prevent or arrest neurologic damage.[24] In patients with iron-loading anemia who are not transfusion-dependent, the severity of anemia provides no indication of the risk of iron loading due to increased dietary iron absorption. Patients with only minor degrees of anemia may accumulate major iron loads. The differential diagnosis directed at the remaining causes of iron overload listed in Table 36.3 poses few problems. Porphyria cutanea tarda is discussed more fully in Chapter 38 and is readily diagnosed by the measurement of urinary porphyrins. The source of iron overload in patients with parenteral iron loading is evident, whether from transfusion or from repeated injections of therapeutic iron. The various causes of perinatal iron overload are clearly distinguished by clinical and pathologic findings. The diagnosis of idiopathic pulmonary hemosiderosis should be considered whenever iron-deficiency anemia develops with coexisting pulmonary abnormalities. Previously, the demonstration of iron deposits in the brain of patients with Friedreich ataxia, pantothenate kinase-associated neurodegeneration, and neuroferritinopathy was possible only at autopsy, but MRI now provides a means for detecting localized brain iron deposits during life.[20,24]

Patients with hyperferritinemia but neither clinical manifestations nor an elevated transferrin saturation may have mutations in the ferroportin gene (see Table 36.4) or in the gene for the iron-responsive element in L-ferritin messenger RNA.[30] The latter mutations are responsible for hereditary hyperferritinemia with cataract, a disorder of autosomal dominant inheritance in which affected family members present with early-onset bilateral nuclear cataracts and moderately elevated plasma ferritin concentrations caused by increased concentrations of L-ferritin.[30] Serum iron concentration and transferrin saturation are normal or low, body iron level as evaluated by phlebotomy is not increased, and no hematologic or biochemical abnormalities are evident in affected persons. Molecular studies have identified mutations in the iron-responsive element of the L-ferritin messenger RNA as responsible.[30] The only consequence of the mutation seems to be an accumulation of L-type ferritin in the lens, resulting in cataract formation.[30] Hyperferritinemia is frequently encountered in disorders *without* iron overload, including malignancy, rheumatologic diseases (such as systemic juvenile idiopathic arthritis, adult-onset Still disease, and hemophagocytic lymphohistiocytosis/macrophage activation syndrome), and chronic infection.

Therapy

The goal of therapy for iron overload is reduction and maintenance of body iron at normal or near-normal levels. If possible, phlebotomy is the treatment of choice for hemochromatosis, iron-loading anemia (if the hemoglobin concentration is high enough to permit venesection), porphyria cutanea tarda, and African dietary iron overload.[14,15] After the diagnosis of iron overload has been established, phlebotomy therapy should begin promptly because any delay extends exposure to potentially toxic iron accumulations.

For most patients, phlebotomy should remove 500 mL of blood, containing 200 to 250 mg of iron, once weekly, until storage iron is depleted.[14,15] The regimen should be individualized. For patients with iron-loading anemia, smaller amounts of blood will need to be withdrawn weekly, but for heavily iron-loaded patients with hereditary hemochromatosis, an even more vigorous program of twice-weekly phlebotomy can be used. The hematocrit or hemoglobin concentration should be measured before each phlebotomy procedure. The progress of iron removal can be followed by periodic measurements of plasma ferritin and iron concentrations and transferrin saturation. The plasma ferritin concentration declines progressively as iron is removed, but the plasma iron concentration and transferrin saturation remain elevated until iron stores near depletion. In a patient with porphyria cutanea tarda, a few weeks of phlebotomy

Timing of Chelation Therapy

In all forms of transfusional iron overload, the most effective means of avoiding complications is to prevent excessive iron accumulation with early iron-chelating therapy.[16,26] In patients who are transfusion-dependent from early infancy (i.e., those with thalassemia major or other congenital refractory anemias), chelation therapy is best started after 10–20 transfusions, usually at approximately 3 years of age. In older patients with acquired refractory anemias who become transfusion-dependent, it seems advisable to begin chelation early after transfusion of 10–20 units of blood. In patients with iron-loading anemia and those with sickle cell disease who are chronically transfused for prevention of complications, early therapy also seems prudent.[16,26] In each of these disorders, delay in beginning chelation therapy only exposes the patient to a greater risk of iron toxicity.

will suffice, but in a patient with hereditary hemochromatosis and an initial body iron burden of 25 g, removal of the iron burden may require 2 years or more of phlebotomy. After complete removal of the iron load, lifelong maintenance therapy is needed, usually necessitating phlebotomy of 500 mL every 3 to 4 months or, in some patients, even less frequently.

For patients with transfusion-dependent refractory anemia, most patients with iron-loading anemia, and rare patients with hemochromatosis for whom phlebotomy is impossible, treatment with an iron chelator is the only means of preventing or removing toxic accumulations of iron (see box on Timing of Chelation Therapy). In patients with hemochromatosis and cardiac failure, a combination of phlebotomy and chelation therapy has been recommended. In the United States, two iron-chelating agents are available for initial treatment of transfusional iron overload: deferoxamine, given parenterally, and deferasirox, administered orally.[16] A third iron chelator—oral deferiprone—is approved in the United States, the European Union, and other countries for patients with thalassemia major when deferoxamine is contraindicated or inadequate.

Over the past 4 decades, clinical experience with deferoxamine, a hexadentate bacterial siderophore purified from *Streptomyces pilosus,* has established the efficacy and safety of this agent in preventing organ dysfunction and prolonging survival in patients with transfusional iron overload.[16,26] Unfortunately, deferoxamine given orally is poorly absorbed. To be effective, the drug must be administered by prolonged subcutaneous or intravenous infusion with a small portable syringe pump, ideally each day, making compliance a demanding task. In patients with modest iron loads and no evidence of iron toxicity, slow subcutaneous infusion of deferoxamine for 9 to 12 hours daily usually provides adequate therapy. In severely iron-loaded patients and in patients with evidence of iron toxicity, particularly those with cardiac complications, chronic slow intravenous infusions given through an indwelling central venous catheter may permit more rapid reduction of the body iron burden. Deferoxamine is a generally safe and nontoxic drug for iron-loaded patients, but systemic complications have been reported, including allergic anaphylactoid reactions, infectious complications, visual abnormalities, auditory dysfunction, and growth retardation.[16,26] The risk of many of these complications may be minimized by adjusting the deferoxamine dose to the magnitude of the body iron load. Adequate deferoxamine therapy should produce a progressive decrease in the body storage iron of almost any patient with iron overload. If no decline is observed, blood and deferoxamine use, compliance, ascorbate status, and other features of the therapeutic regimen should be thoroughly reassessed.

Deferasirox, a synthetic, orally active tridentate iron chelator, was approved for use by the U.S. Food and Drug Administration in 2005 for treatment of transfusional iron overload in adults and in children older than 2 years of age. Deferasirox has a long plasma half-life, making possible once-daily dosing.[16,26] Extensive systematic clinical trials in patients with thalassemia major, sickle cell disease, and other transfusion-dependent anemias have provided evidence that the effectiveness of deferasirox in the management of iron overload is comparable to that of deferoxamine.[16,26] The most common adverse events have been rash, gastrointestinal disturbances, and abnormalities in renal function. Additional clinical studies examining the long-term safety and efficacy of deferasirox are in progress, but the initial experience with this drug suggests that this orally active, iron-chelating agent is a well-tolerated, once-daily treatment for control of transfusional iron overload. Most patients now opt for deferasirox because of the ease of oral administration.

Prognosis

The prognosis for patients with iron overload is influenced by many factors, including the magnitude, rate, and route of iron loading; distribution of iron deposition between reticuloendothelial macrophage and parenchymal sites; amount and duration of exposure to circulating nontransferrin-bound iron; ascorbate status; and coexisting disorders, especially alcoholism.[14,15] The magnitude of iron accumulation seems to be a critical determinant of the risk of cirrhosis of the liver and, in turn, of hepatocellular carcinoma, now the two major causes of death in *HFE* hemochromatosis. If the disease is diagnosed before tissue injury occurs, phlebotomy therapy to remove the excess iron can prevent all of the complications of hemochromatosis, including cirrhosis, and return the patient's life expectancy to normal.[14,15] Even if organ damage is present, phlebotomy prevents further progression, and amelioration of some features of the disease is possible. Skin pigmentation diminishes; hepatic function may improve while fibrosis is arrested or sometimes regresses; and cardiac abnormalities, including even cardiac failure, may resolve. Diabetes and other endocrine abnormalities usually are ameliorated only slightly, if at all, although reversal of hypogonadism has occurred. Arthropathy usually does not subside and may even continue to progress despite phlebotomy.

In patients with iron overload who cannot be treated by phlebotomy, chelation therapy is effective in reducing the body iron burden and improving the prognosis.[16,26] Orally administered deferasirox or chronic infusion of parenteral deferoxamine decreases the hepatic iron concentration, improves hepatic function, promotes growth and sexual maturation, and helps protect against cardiac disease and early death. In all forms of iron overload, the most effective means of preventing complications is prevention of iron accumulation, either by early identification and phlebotomy treatment of hereditary hemochromatosis or by early institution of chelation therapy in patients with iron-loading or transfusion-dependent anemia.

REFERENCES

1. Ganz T: Systemic iron homeostasis. *Physiol Rev* 93:1721–1741, 2013.
2. Lane DJ, Merlot AM, Huang ML, et al: Cellular iron uptake, trafficking and metabolism: key molecules and mechanisms and their roles in disease. *Biochim Biophys Acta* 1853:1130–1144, 2015.
3. Kautz L, Jung G, Valore EV, et al: Identification of erythroferrone as an erythroid regulator of iron metabolism. *Nat Genet* 46:678–684, 2014.
4. St Pierre TG, El-Beshlawy A, Elalfy M, et al: Multicenter validation of spin-density projection-assisted R2-MRI for the noninvasive measurement of liver iron concentration. *Magn Reson Med* 71:2215–2223, 2014.
5. Kassebaum NJ, Jasrasaria R, Naghavi M, et al: A systematic analysis of global anemia burden from 1990 to 2010. *Blood* 123:615–624, 2014.
6. Camaschella C: Iron-deficiency anemia. *N Engl J Med* 372:1832–1843, 2015.
7. Powers JM, Buchanan GR: Diagnosis and management of iron deficiency anemia. *Hematol Oncol Clin North Am* 28:729–745, vi, 2014.
8. Heeney MM, Finberg KE: Iron-refractory iron deficiency anemia (IRIDA). *Hematol Oncol Clin North Am* 28:637–652, v, 2014.
9. DeLoughery TG: Microcytic anemia. *N Engl J Med* 371:1324–1331, 2014.
10. Thomas DW, Hinchliffe RF, Briggs C, et al: Guideline for the laboratory diagnosis of functional iron deficiency. *Br J Haematol* 161:639–648, 2013.
11. Bailie GR, Verhoef JJ: Differences in the reporting rates of serious allergic adverse events from intravenous iron by country and population. *Clin Adv Hematol Oncol* 10:101–108, 2012.
12. Camaschella C: Treating iron overload. *N Engl J Med* 368:2325–2327, 2013.
13. Bardou-Jacquet E, Brissot P: Diagnostic evaluation of hereditary hemochromatosis (HFE and non-HFE). *Hematol Oncol Clin North Am* 28:625, 2014.
14. Barton JC: Hemochromatosis and iron overload: from bench to clinic. *Am J Med Sci* 346:403–412, 2013.
15. Ekanayake D, Roddick C, Powell LW: Recent advances in hemochromatosis: a 2015 update: a summary of proceedings of the 2014 conference held under the auspices of Hemochromatosis Australia. *Hepatol Int* 9:174–182, 2015.
16. Brittenham GM: Iron-chelating therapy for transfusional iron overload. *N Engl J Med* 364:146–156, 2011.
17. McDonald CJ, Wallace DF, Crawford DH, et al: Iron storage disease in Asia-Pacific populations: the importance of non-HFE mutations. *J Gastroenterol Hepatol* 28:1087–1094, 2013.
18. Bardou-Jacquet E, Ben Ali Z, Beaumont-Epinette MP, et al: Non-HFE hemochromatosis: pathophysiological and diagnostic aspects. *Clin Res Hepatol Gastroenterol* 38:143–154, 2014.
19. Bottomley SS, Fleming MD: Sideroblastic anemia: diagnosis and management. *Hematol Oncol Clin North Am* 28:653, 2014.
20. Meyer E, Kurian MA, Hayflick SJ: Neurodegeneration with brain iron accumulation: genetic diversity and pathophysiological mechanisms. *Annu Rev Genomics Hum Genet* 16:257, 2015.
21. Jenkitkasemwong S, Wang CY, Coffey R, et al: SLC39A14 is required for the development of hepatocellular iron overload in murine models of hereditary hemochromatosis. *Cell Metab* 22:138, 2015.
22. Brissot P, Ropert M, Le Lan C, et al: Non-transferrin bound iron: a key role in iron overload and iron toxicity. *Biochim Biophys Acta* 1820:403–410, 2012.
23. McLaren CE, Emond MJ, Subramaniam VN, et al: Exome sequencing in *HFE* C282Y homozygous men with extreme phenotypes identifies a *GNPAT* variant associated with severe iron overload. *Hepatology* 62:429, 2015.
24. Rouault TA: Iron metabolism in the CNS: implications for neurodegenerative diseases. *Nat Rev Neurosci* 14:551–564, 2013.
25. Wu XG, Wang Y, Wu Q, et al: HFE interacts with the BMP type I receptor ALK3 to regulate hepcidin expression. *Blood* 124:1335–1343, 2014.
26. Coates TD: Physiology and pathophysiology of iron in hemoglobin-associated diseases. *Free Radic Biol Med* 72:23–40, 2014.
27. Kautz L, Jung G, Nemeth E, et al: Erythroferrone contributes to recovery from anemia of inflammation. *Blood* 124:2569–2574, 2014.
28. Whitington PF: Gestational alloimmune liver disease and neonatal hemochromatosis. *Semin Liver Dis* 32:325–332, 2012.
29. Zaloumis SG, Allen KJ, Bertalli NA, et al: Natural history of HFE simple heterozygosity for C282Y and H63D: a prospective 12-year study. *J Gastroenterol Hepatol* 30:719–725, 2015.
30. Bowes O, Baxter K, Elsey T, et al: Hereditary hyperferritinaemia cataract syndrome. *Lancet* 383:1520, 2014.

CHAPTER 37

ANEMIA OF CHRONIC DISEASES

Lalitha Nayak, Lawrence B. Gardner, and Jane A. Little

Anemia of chronic disease (ACD) is frequently also called "anemia of inflammation" since it is associated with a variety of diseases including inflammatory conditions, infections, and malignancy.[1] The cause of ACD is multifactorial and includes both inhibition of red blood cell (RBC) production and mildly decreased RBC life span (Table 37.1). Teleologically, ACD may serve to decrease infectious virulence by organisms such as malaria and schistosomiasis in a nutrient-depleted host.[2] Malignancies may also be potentiated in an iron-rich environment in humans. Once described as a "bag of unsolved questions," ACD has become a much smaller bag since the identification of the antimicrobial molecule hepcidin.[3] Hepcidin, a mediator of both innate immunity and iron regulation, plays a major role in the pathogenesis of ACD.

DESCRIPTION AND EPIDEMIOLOGY

ACD is a normocytic and normochromic anemia of underproduction that usually is mild–moderate, with hemoglobin levels in the 8 to 9.5 gm/L range. The anemia can, however, be severe and the mean corpuscular volume may be reduced, sometimes dramatically, in up to one-third of patients with ACD. ACD is the second most common cause of anemia, after iron deficiency anemia,[4] and is the most frequent anemia in hospitalized patients. Over a 2-month period of observation, 52% of hospitalized patients with unexplained anemia met laboratory criteria for ACD. Patients older than 60 years of age had a 24% 3-year incidence of ACD. Anemia is also extremely common in cancer; 39% of cancer patients were found to be anemic. Chemotherapy with or without radiation therapy increases the incidence of anemia to 63% and 42% respectively. Human immunodeficiency virus (HIV) infection is often associated with anemia with a prevalence as high as 55.8%, directly proportional to the burden of symptoms. Rheumatoid arthritis (RA) is associated with mild anemia, with a prevalence from 33% to 60%. The degree of anemia is associated with elevations in markers and/or mediators of inflammation, such as erythrocyte sedimentation rate (ESR), C-reactive protein (CRP), or interleukin-6 (IL-6) level.

Diverse diseases not conventionally considered "inflammatory," such as congestive heart failure, obesity, renal failure, and diabetes, have been associated both with an ACD-type anemia and with cytokine abnormalities more typically associated with inflammatory conditions (e.g., elevated IL-6 and CRP in kidney disease or CRP and fibrinogen in myocardial infarction). Because of the absence of definitive diagnostic criteria or laboratory tests, however, epidemiologic studies in ACD are at the least confounded by this underlying heterogeneity.

ETIOLOGY AND PATHOGENESIS

ACD is a heterogeneous disorder marked by a low serum iron and by disturbances in iron homeostasis. Unlike true dietary iron deficiency, iron is present in the macrophages and total body iron may be normal or elevated. Research over the last decade suggests that synthesis of the iron regulatory antimicrobial peptide hepcidin is induced by inflammatory cytokines during acute and chronic disorders, leading to a state of functional iron deficiency.[5] In addition, other factors such as blunted erythropoietin (EPO) production and reduced RBC life

span also contribute to anemia that cannot be explained by hepcidin alone. Hence the pathogenesis of ACD is multifactorial and complex (Fig. 37.1).

Although Cartwright and Wintrobe describe a modest decrease in the life span of the RBC in ACD, RBCs from patients with ACD have a normal life span when infused into normal subjects, suggesting an abnormality in the surrounding milieu rather than an intrinsic RBC defect. However, the decrease in life span of red cells is insufficient to explain the degree of anemia. Patients with RA have elevated levels of inflammatory cytokines that could theoretically enhance erythrophagocytosis and anemia. Similarly, mice with elevated interferon-γ (IFN-γ) levels (transgenically or exogenously administered) have reduced RBC survival because of RBC removal by cytokine-stimulated macrophages.

Macrophages play a central role in iron homeostasis and participate in the reutilization of iron from senescent red cells, which supplies more than 95% of the daily iron requirements for normal physiologic processes including erythropoiesis. During inflammation, there is iron retention in the macrophage-phagocytic system and decreased delivery of iron for erythropoiesis.[6] Studies using labeled iron show normal iron incorporation into RBCs. This is consistent with the concept that under inflammatory conditions iron release, but not utilization, is primarily impaired. Activation of immune cells during infections, autoimmune processes, and cancer also leads to the production of numerous cytokines that induce hepcidin production in the liver. Hepcidin binds to the iron export protein ferroportin and interferes with cellular iron export through internalization and degradation of ferroportin.[3] When ferroportin is lost in the jejunum, absorption of dietary iron is reduced and serum iron levels are depressed. The same mechanism also inhibits iron export from macrophages, aggravating the low serum iron levels[3] and enhancing iron retention in the macrophage.[7]

Hepcidin-independent mechanisms also contribute to altered iron homeostasis and are mainly orchestrated by cytokines. Tumor necrosis factor-alpha (TNF-α), interleukin-1 (IL-1), IL-6, and IFN-γ all increase uptake of transferrin and nontransferrin bound iron by altering the expression of transferrin-receptor-1 (Tfr1) and divalent metal transporter-1 (DMT1) respectively. In addition, many of these cytokines, including IL-4, IL-10, and IL-13, contribute to increased iron storage within the monocytes/macrophages by increasing the expression of ferritin both transcriptionally and posttranscriptionally. Transcription of ferroportin is also inhibited by IFN-γ and lipopolysaccharide (LPS) thereby contributing to iron sequestration in macrophages.

In addition to effects on iron, a direct inhibition of erythropoiesis and relative deficiency of EPO are seen in ACD. EPO inhibition has been attributed to inflammatory cytokines. In vitro removal of bone marrow-adherent cells (mostly macrophages and monocytes) from patients with ACD leads to increased erythroid colony formation. This effect is lost after coculture with ACD-adherent cells, but not by coculture with control bone marrow-derived adherent cells. Patients with RA have decreased erythroid burst-forming units (BFU-E) that are inversely proportional to circulating TNF levels. In parallel, culture with serum from patients with RA and anemia inhibits BFU-E proliferation, while serum from nonanemic RA patients does not.

In addition, data from clinical studies have documented a relative deficiency of EPO in many chronic diseases associated with anemia.

TABLE 37.1	Suspected Causes of Anemia of Chronic Disease
Shortened erythrocyte survival	
Block in reuse of iron by erythrocyte	
Direct inhibition of erythropoiesis	
Relative deficiency of erythropoietin	

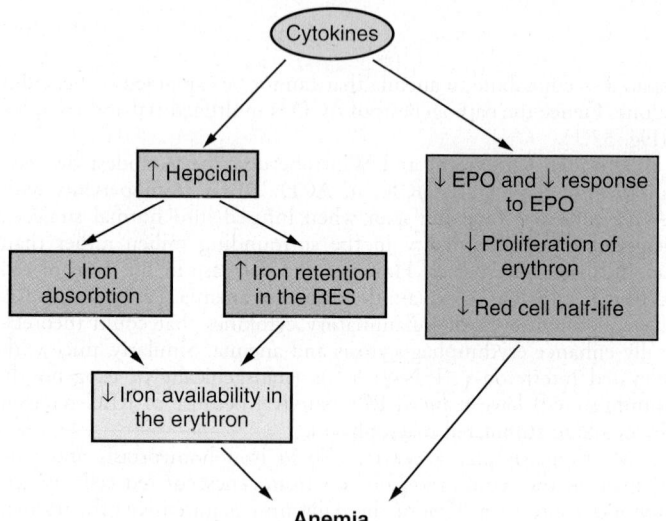

Fig. 37.1 PATHOPHYSIOLOGIC FACTORS ASSOCIATED WITH THE DEVELOPMENT OF ACD. *EPO,* Erythropoietin; *RES,* reticuloendothelial system,.

In a study of 81 patients with solid tumors and clinical ACD and who did not have bone marrow involvement by tumor, EPO levels were higher than in controls without anemia but half that of control subjects with iron deficiency anemia. During inflammation, EPO expression is decreased or inappropriately low for the degree of anemia, which is in part because of cytokine-mediated alterations in binding affinities of EPO-inducing transcription factors and to damage of EPO-producing cells. For example, LPS injections are associated with decreased renal EPO mRNA expression in animal models. Similarly, serum EPO levels are inappropriately low in HIV-positive patients with normochromic, normocytic anemia and in lung transplant recipients.

Finally, EPO may not function optimally in the presence of inflammatory cytokines. EPO-resistant subjects with end-stage renal disease (ESRD) are more likely to have elevations in inflammatory cytokines, and peripheral blood mononuclear cells isolated from EPO-refractory ESRD subjects are more likely to produce inflammatory cytokines than are those from non-EPO-refractory ESRD subjects.

BIOLOGY AND MOLECULAR ASPECTS

The role of inflammatory cytokines in many of the underlying diseases associated with ACD has suggested a mechanistic link for much of the pathophysiology of this anemia, including decreased erythrocyte survival, decreased access to available iron through upregulation of hepcidin, direct inhibition of erythroid progenitor growth, and inadequate EPO response to anemia.

Increased serum levels of cytokines, particularly IL-1, IL-6, IL-10, TNF, IFN-α, IFN-β, and IFN-γ, have been observed in many inflammatory processes, including infections, autoimmune disorders, and solid and hematologic malignancies.[8] Often in these disorders, cytokine levels frequently inversely correlate with the anemia, so as to suggest an association. Serum TNF levels correlate with both disease activity and the degree of anemia in RA. Bone marrows from patients

with RA show increased levels of IL-6 and TNF-α. Experimentally, transgenic mice with endogenous elevations in IFN-γ show increased expression of the proleukocyte, anti-RBC transcription factor PU.1 in hematopoietic precursors and diminished BFU-E. Causality is also suggested by the multiple trials of cytokine antagonists in inflammatory diseases that have shown a decrease in anemia. In patients with Crohn disease, treatment with anti-TNF-α therapy was associated with improvement in disease activity and in anemia. In vitro, anti-TNF-α therapy increased the growth of erythroid progenitor cells obtained from the peripheral blood of patients with active disease.

Cytokine-Induced Decreases in Red Blood Cell Survival

The underlying mechanism for the reduction in RBC life span in ACD is not fully elucidated, but studies support the absence of an intrinsic red cell defect. Alterations in RBC rheology (deformability and aggregation) are seen in intensive care unit patients, especially those with sepsis. In vivo and in vitro experiments suggest that fever itself can induce rheologic changes in RBCs, leading to increased destruction and up to a 15% decline in RBC mass. Rats treated with chronic sublethal doses of TNF had a 25% decline in total RBC mass. The study also demonstrated a simultaneous decrease in RBC survival. This effect may be secondary to increased cytokines e.g., IL-1 in RA patients, that enhance the RBC-phagocytic ability of macrophages.

Cytokine-Induced Abnormalities in Iron Metabolism

Monocytes/macrophages form the major cellular system responsible for an adequate supply of iron for erythropoiesis and they recycle iron from senescent RBCs during the process of erythrophagocytosis.[8-10] Under inflammatory conditions, monocytes/macrophages divert and sequester iron, thus contributing to the generation of anemia.[1,10,11] Proinflammatory cytokines, such as TNF and IL-1, lead to increased iron content in the monocyte/macrophage with induced ferritin expression. The net result is serum hypoferremia and hyperferritinemia. Rats injected with IL-1 or TNF experienced a 40% drop in serum iron levels; further, TNF also caused a significant decrease in iron incorporation into erythrocytes. Animals injected with IL-6 have increased hepcidin levels and develop hypoferremia within 24 hours, but systemic LPS injection (which leads to IL-6 induction) was not associated with hypoferremia in IL-6 knockout mice. Finally, TNF has also been shown to increase radiolabeled iron uptake by peritoneal macrophages without an increase in iron release, suggesting that macrophage sequestration of iron is cytokine-induced. All these studies highlight the importance of cytokines in altering iron metabolism in inflammatory situations.

Molecular evidence implicates both a direct and indirect cytokine effect on iron metabolism. Proinflammatory cytokines IL-1 and IL-6 translationally regulate the expression of ferritin via a 5′ untranslated region within the ferritin mRNA. This mechanism is distinct from the iron-responsive element but similar to a 38-nucleotide consensus sequence found in other IL-sensitive acute-phase reactants. Since the increase in ferritin occurs with concomitant downregulation of transferrin receptor expression, the mode of cellular iron sequestration is not entirely clear. Hepcidin is a 25-amino acid hepatically derived peptide. Fleming and Sly first suggested a link between hepcidin and abnormalities in iron metabolism with inflammation.[12] Recent data show that numerous inflammatory cytokines upregulate hepcidin; however, experimentally IL-6 and the bone morphogenetic proteins (BMPs) are most centrally involved in its synthesis. Hepcidin causes the degradation of ferroportin in duodenal enterocytes and macrophages, leading to the decreased gut iron absorption and increased macrophage iron retention that is classically noted with ACD.

The induction of hepcidin expression by inflammation is mediated through the transcription factors STAT3[13] and SMAD4, both of which are upregulated by cytokines via the BMP type I receptors.

Hence liver specific Smad4$^{-/-}$ mice show an attenuated response to IL-6–mediated hepcidin transcription, and inhibitors of BMP also inhibit IL-6–mediated transcription of hepcidin. In humans, injection with LPS dramatically increases IL-6 levels by hour 3, followed by an increase in urinary hepcidin by hour 6. Direct administration of IL-6 to humans also leads to increased prohepcidin and decreased serum iron. In patients with ACD, increased prohepcidin serum concentrations are associated with decreased expression of ferroportin along with increased ferritin accumulation in circulating monocytes.

Finally, the functional iron depletion mediated by hepcidin may itself augment direct cytokine inhibition of erythropoiesis through the aconitase/iron response protein (IRP) axis.[14] A central contribution to net inhibited erythropoiesis in an inflammatory and functionally iron-depleted state is mediated through an iron-sensing switch. With normal iron levels, heme synthesis and EPO responsiveness are maintained, in part, through a functioning aconitase enzyme bound to an iron-sulfur molecule. However in an iron-depleted state, aconitase ceases to function as an enzyme and becomes an RNA-binding IRP, thereby modulating transcription and translation of iron-regulated proteins.[15] Experimentally, anemia develops following inhibition of aconitase activity, with impaired erythroid progenitor differentiation and viability via a protein kinase C dependent pathway.[15] This anemia can be abrogated experimentally through repletion of the downstream metabolic intermediate isocitrate.[14] Strikingly, in these models, iron depletion uniquely sensitizes erythroid cells to suppression by inflammatory cytokines, and this, too, was mitigated by treatment with isocitrate.

Cytokines Leading to Direct Inhibition of Erythropoiesis

Proliferation and differentiation of erythroid precursors is impaired in patients with ACD. Studies support a role for TNF-α, IL-1, and perhaps IL-6 in this inhibition. There is good evidence that IFN directly inhibits erythropoiesis, such as highly purified CFU-E from murine spleens in a dose-dependent manner. In vitro studies show that IFN-γ modulates cytokine responses and expression of genes that are involved in the proliferation of hematopoietic stem cells, thus affecting self-renewal. IFN-γ can also decrease responsiveness of erythroid progenitors to EPO. In vivo and in vitro studies show that IFN-γ treatment of erythroid progenitors increases the expression of the transcription factor PU.1. Since PU.1 directly interacts with the major erythroid transcription factor GATA-1, it is postulated that IFN-γ treatment affects erythroid progenitors by a PU.1 dependent mechanism.[16]

Serum levels of TNF correlate inversely with the hemoglobin levels and, in RA, with the number of erythroid burst-forming units. Treatment with anti-TNF improves proliferation and decreases apoptosis of erythroid progenitor cells. However, the effect of TNF on erythropoiesis is likely indirect, mediated by the local release of other cytokines including IFN from accessory cells, since the inhibitory effect of TNF on CFU-E was completely abrogated by neutralizing antibodies against IFN-β but not by antibodies to IFN-γ or IL-1. Similarly, the effects of IL-1 also appear to be indirect since growth of purified CFU-E is inhibited by IL-1 only in the presence of adherent T lymphocytes. This inhibition can be reversed by antibodies to IFN-γ, suggesting that IL-1 leads to lymphocyte secretion of IFN.

Cytokines Leading to Decreased Erythropoietin Secretion

EPO is the essential hormone that induces erythropoiesis. Inflammatory conditions are associated with insufficient EPO levels relative to the degree of anemia. Mice injected with LPS have decreased expression of EPO mRNA in kidneys and decreased circulating levels of EPO. In tissue culture, IL-1α, IL-1β, and TNF-α significantly lowered EPO production. IL-1β also inhibited EPO production in perfused rat kidneys. In addition, animal models have suggested that vascular endothelial growth factor, which is commonly elevated

in cancer, wounds, and ischemia, may be a negative regulator of EPO synthesis. Further, autoantibodies to EPO associated with low circulating EPO levels have been detected in subjects with systemic lupus erythematosus.

Perhaps the strongest argument for a causative role of EPO in ACD is that exogenous EPO can partially reverse ACD. Evidence suggests that exogenous administration of EPO may result in decreased levels of hepcidin, via a recently recognized EPO-driven suppressor of hepcidin, erythroferrone, thus leading to improvement in anemia and iron sequestration.[17,18] In rats, low-dose EPO normalized endothelial function, vascular inflammation, and oxidative stress suggesting that EPO may also decrease inflammation. Inhibition by IFN-γ can be reversed by EPO. Moreover, the capacity of patient-derived monocytes from patients with inflammatory bowel disease to secrete TNF predicts the therapeutic response to exogenous EPO.

DIAGNOSIS

Because ACD is both common and multifactorial, an unequivocal diagnosis may be challenging. Further, it is not uncommon that primary hematologic defects are accompanied by inflammation, or vice versa, so other factors that also result in anemia, such as nutritional deficiency, blood loss, hemolysis, renal failure, and primary bone marrow disorders need to be considered. Chronic inflammatory bowel diseases are frequently associated with both chronic gastrointestinal bleeding secondary to the underlying disease and its treatment (with nonsteroidal antiinflammatory drugs [NSAIDs] and glucocorticoids). Iron deficiency can also be secondary to decreased iron absorption, as in autoimmune gastritis and celiac disease. Up to 70% of the anemia associated with RA may be multifactorial. Of the 184 patients admitted to intensive care units, most patients with anemia were found to have EPO levels and iron study results consistent with ACD; however, 13% also had nutritional causes of anemia (iron, folate, or vitamin B12 deficiency). Finally, the contribution of frequent phlebotomy in the hospitalized patients with anemia should not be underestimated (see box on Diagnosis of Anemia of Chronic Diseases).

Contributing causes of anemia, including hemolysis, nutritional deficiency, or sequestration should be evaluated. Iron deficiency plus ACD should be strongly considered in patients with systemic inflammation and a low or "normal" serum ferritin concentration. While some investigators argue that a ferritin level greater than 50 ng/mL excludes any component of iron deficiency even in inflammatory states, a meta-analysis of iron studies in clinical reports from 1842 subjects with serum ferritin levels above 45 ng/mL showed a prevalence of iron deficiency of 6.7%; 3.5% of 1368 subjects with a serum ferritin level of greater than 100 ng/mL had iron deficiency.

Diagnosis of Anemia of Chronic Diseases (Fig. 37.2)

The diagnosis of ACD is primarily one of exclusion and is often difficult. Various laboratory tests have been suggested, but few have proven value in the general population because ACD occurs in too large a variety of acute and chronic illnesses. The best way to diagnose ACD, at least provisionally, is to document an anemia of underproduction (i.e., low reticulocyte index) with low serum iron and low transferrin levels and normal to elevated serum ferritin level in the setting of a systemic, usually inflammatory, illness. A thorough search may be necessary to document the precise underlying illness.

Other causes of anemia, such as hemolysis, nutritional deficiency, or sequestration, should be ruled out, and a component of iron deficiency should be strongly considered in a patient with systemic inflammation and a low or "normal" serum ferritin concentration. These other causes of anemia often accompany ACD. Bone marrow examination is usually not essential for the diagnosis but may be necessary to rule out other diagnoses, including malignancy (e.g., myelodysplastic syndrome), infection, or iron deficiency.

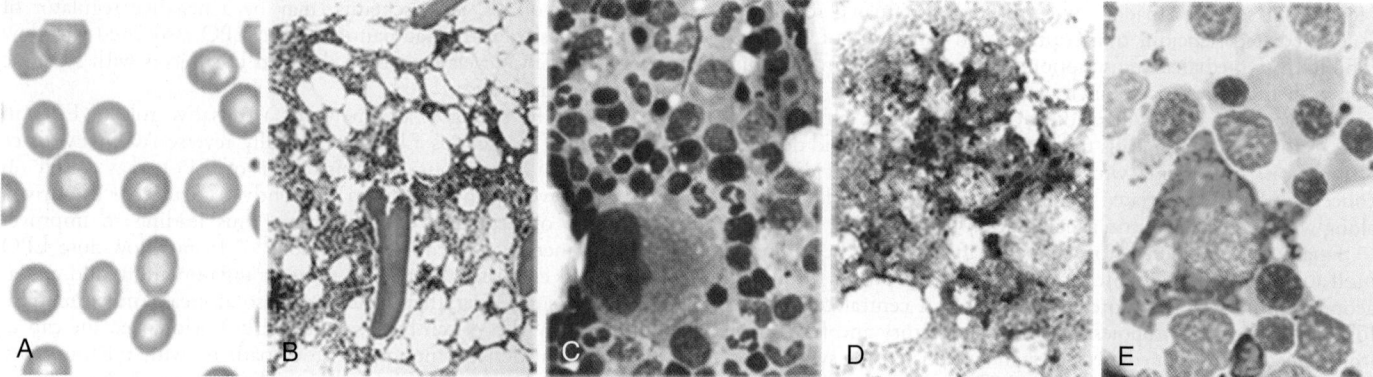

Fig. 37.2 ANEMIA OF CHRONIC DISEASE. (A) Peripheral blood typically exhibits a normochromic, normocytic anemia. (B, C) Bone marrow examination is sometimes performed to rule out other causes of anemia. Typically, the bone marrow is morphologically normal. (D, E) Prussian blue iron stain shows increased iron stores with increased histiocytic iron but decreased sideroblastic iron.

Other researchers have shown that, in acute inflammation, serum ferritin levels greater than 3500 ng/mL can coexist with absent bone marrow iron stores tested by aspirate. In ACD, ferritin levels can be normal or elevated, reflecting increased iron retention in the reticuloendothelial system (RES). Although normograms corrected for the degree of inflammation present have been published, most investigators maintain that serum iron studies cannot predictably rule out iron deficiency. Additional functional tests of iron status have been developed, including soluble transferrin receptors (sTFRs),[19] hemoglobin concentration in reticulocytes (CHr), percent of hypochromic RBCs (%HYPO), and serum hepcidin levels, in an attempt to differentiate ACD alone from ACD complicated with iron deficiency. sTFR levels are elevated in iron deficiency anemia. Several studies show that the numbers of sTFRs on erythroblasts are lower, occasionally dramatically so, in RA patients with ACD than in patients with iron deficiency anemia. The sTFR to the log of serum ferritin ratio may be useful in identifying iron deficiency in the presence of ACD, but is not widely available. While a low ratio index (<1) suggests ACD, an index >2 is indicative of a combination of ACD with iron deficiency.[20] An algorithm that incorporates hepcidin levels has been developed to increase specificity for iron deficiency in ACD, but still requires prospective validation. Hemoglobin concentration in reticulocytes (CHr), distinct from indices of mature RBCs, can reflect the recent status of iron stores in normal or EPO-induced erythropoiesis.[21] sTFR-, CHr-, and hepcidin-based algorithms for iron-replete and iron-deficient ACD are being developed, and a combination of these is likely to be useful in diagnosing and differentiating ACD from ACD with iron deficiency. However, none are fully characterized or yet widely incorporated into clinical practice, and the diagnosis of ACD remains a clinical one.

In a study of mostly older patients with an idiopathic anemia (10 ± 0.6 g/dL), a bone marrow aspirate with biopsy was found to add little to physical examination and serology. However, a bone marrow examination may be necessary to rule out other diagnoses, including iron deficiency, malignancy (e.g., myelodysplastic syndrome), or infection (see Fig. 37.1). Although the clinical setting in which anemia is found helps with the diagnosis of ACD, in 30% of cases no chronic illness can be identified.

ACD may also be undiagnosed in complicated medical patients. Although anemia of renal failure is associated with absolute EPO deficiency, it is also considered an inflammatory condition with associated elevations in cytokine levels. In addition, patients on hemodialysis may have occult infections (e.g., of nonfunctioning arteriovenous grafts) with associated markers of inflammation and EPO resistance; removal of these grafts may correct the anemia. Patients with congestive heart failure and anemia have elevated TNF levels, proportional to the severity of anemia, with EPO levels inadequate to the degree of anemia, all of which are consistent with ACD.

Treatment of Anemia of Chronic Diseases

Treating ACD is unnecessary if the patient is asymptomatic. However, if the anemia is symptomatic or severe, treatment of the anemia itself may be indicated. Epidemiologic studies, such as those in patients with heart failure, HIV, cancer, or kidney disease, suggest physiologic and subjective improvement in signs and symptoms after treatment for anemia. However, treatments need to be individualized because the risks of erythropoiesis-stimulating agents or iron therapy in noniron deficient subjects are theoretically real and practically unknowable given the variety of underlying conditions that are incorporated under the rubric of chronic disease.

The first priority in ACD should be to correct any reversible contributors to the anemia. Because the extent of ACD mirrors the activity of the underlying disease, all efforts should be made to treat the underlying disease. Furthermore, efforts to correct anemia should be modulated by the recognition that the "optimal" target hemoglobin for subjects with ACD is not known. Observations from profoundly anemic subjects without inflammation but religiously opposed to transfusions have suggested a physiologic cutoff for hemoglobin of 5 g/dL, below which increased mortality is seen. In addition, acutely ill patients have not been shown to benefit, in randomized, controlled studies, from transfusion "triggers" above 7 g/dL. Nonetheless, symptomatic improvement is seen in subjects with a range of chronic diseases who are treated for anemia of a more modest degree.

Transfusion therapy may be the most common form of treatment of symptomatic ACD. Newer targeted therapies are emerging in ACD, but are not yet standard-of-care.

TREATMENT

The anemia associated with chronic illness is often mild. In RA, the annual incidence of anemia (<10 g/dL), proportionate with markers of inflammation, was only 1.5%, with a lifetime prevalence of 13.7%. Similarly, in cancer subjects referred for radiation therapy, only 16% had hemoglobin levels of less than 10 g/dL. Although over time the anemia can become more severe, the correction of ACD per se may be unnecessary, especially if the primary disorder contributing to the anemia can be treated and reversed.

There may also be teleologic benefits in the pathophysiologic processes that contribute to ACD. Although fever associated with infections inhibits bacterial growth, decreased iron concentrations (as seen in ACD) synergize with pyrexia to inhibit bacterial growth. This "nutritional immunity" is postulated to be an adaptive factor that contributes to ACD. Further, elevations in serum iron have been associated with an increase in cancer risk. However, iron sequestration is not devoid of risks and ACD can occasionally be severe and warrant immediate attention.

Treatments of anemia in symptomatic patients will need to be individualized, as there are risks with erythropoiesis-stimulating agents as well as iron therapy. The optimal hemoglobin level in ACD patients is not known. Observations of anemia in non-ACD subjects religiously opposed to transfusions have suggested a physiologic cutoff for anemia of 5 g/dL, below which increased mortality is seen.[22] In severe anemia, blood transfusions may be warranted, albeit with recognition of long-term iron overload and human leukocyte antigen–sensitization risks. However, randomized controlled studies indicate that acutely ill patients do not benefit from transfusion triggers >7 g/dL. EPO has improved hemoglobin levels in patients with ACD, with reduction in the necessity for transfusion support; iron supplementation, IV if needed, can be considered in those patients that are unresponsive to EPO supplementation. In anemic AIDS patients, recombinant EPO treatment significantly decreased transfusion requirements, especially with endogenous EPO levels of <500 IU/L; however, all of these patients also received zidovudine, a potential bone marrow suppressant. Recombinant EPO raised the hemoglobin level in patients with a variety of nonhematologic malignancies (with or without chemotherapy), including squamous cell cancer, breast cancer, and colon cancer. However, despite the benefits of decreasing transfusion requirements and improved quality of life, EPO supplementation (both short- or long-acting forms) in patients with cancer and kidney disease increases the risk of stroke and thromboembolic events.[23] Studies have also indicated that critically ill patients and those with cancer undergoing chemotherapy may have an increased rate of thrombosis and overall death when treated with EPO, particularly if target hemoglobins are >10–11 g/dL. Increasing the hematocrit to 42% in a large number of hemodialysis patients with cardiac disease led to an increased number of deaths, and the number of cardiac events was increased in patients with chronic renal disease treated with EPO with a goal of complete normalization of hemoglobin (12.0–15.0 g/dL) as opposed to partial normalization (10.5–11.5 g/dL). Although pretreatment hemoglobin levels have been demonstrated repeatedly to be a predictor of good response to chemotherapy and radiation, studies have demonstrated that patients with breast cancer or head and neck cancer treated with EPO have increased disease progression and worse survival than placebo-treated patients. Based on these and other studies, the U.S. Food and Drug Administration has warned that EPO should be given only in the lowest possible doses necessary to avoid blood transfusions. More recently, consensus has arisen that, for patients with cancer, erythropoiesis-stimulating agents should be used only in those receiving chemotherapy for palliative, rather than curative, intent. EPO should be used sparingly, if at all, with active malignancy.

In the appropriate nonmalignant setting of symptomatic ACD, a starting dose of 20,000 units of EPO given subcutaneously each week can be initiated. If a hemoglobin response is seen, the dose can be decreased and the interval prolonged to titrate the hemoglobin to an asymptomatic level. Follow-up and dose titration are essential to minimize expense, injections, and potential deleterious effects from high hematocrit or exogenous EPO levels. The EPO response may take 4 to 8 weeks and should be monitored for objective symptomatic improvement (e.g., exercise tolerance). About 35% to 40% of patients show primary resistance. Predictors of resistance to EPO include iron or vitamin deficiency, recent need for transfusion therapy, and higher endogenous EPO levels (>100–150 mU/ml) before initiation of therapy. If, after 2 weeks of treatment, the serum EPO level is >100 mU/mL and the hemoglobin concentration has not increased by ≥0.5 g/dL, or if the serum ferritin level remains >400 ng/mL, a response is unlikely.[24] In a multivariate analysis of 80 patients with chronic anemia of cancer, only the absolute hemoglobin value and serum EPO and ferritin levels, but not disease status, bone marrow involvement, or treatment status, were independent predictors of response to EPO.

An important factor limiting response to EPO is functional iron deficiency. Correction of functional iron deficiency with intravenous (IV) iron supplementation can improve the effect of EPO and also decrease the required dosage. IV iron improves EPO responses and

is cost-effective in dialysis patients, even those with elevated ferritin levels; however, the widespread applicability of this approach, and its long-term effects, are not known.

Newer Therapeutic Strategies That Target the Hepcidin-Ferroportin Axis

Treatments to directly address the pathophysiology of ACD via the hepcidin-ferroportin axis,[5] i.e., to decrease hepcidin levels and increase ferroportin activity, are in development, and include direct hepcidin antagonists, RNA interference and gene silencing of hepcidin expression with antisense oligonucleotides,[25] and hepcidin-binding proteins and spigelmers.[5] Strategies targeting upstream regulators of hepcidin production include inhibitors of the BMP6-HJV-SMAD,[5] IL-6, and JAK-STAT pathways.[26] Ferroportin agonists or stabilizers prevent hepcidin-ferroportin interaction and subsequent internalization and degradation of ferroportin.[5] Isocitrate supplementation, which bypasses aconitase in erythroid precursors, may emerge as an adjunct to hepcidin-directed therapies. Of note, the recently identified physiologic repressor of hepcidin, erythroferrone, may play a role in the diagnosis and management of ACD, because of its central role in suppression of hepcidin and in physiologic recovery from experimentally induced anemia of inflammation.[18] These promising approaches, however, are still under investigation and await confirmation in the clinical setting.

SUMMARY AND FUTURE DIRECTIONS

Anemia is a common consequence of many chronic inflammatory, infectious, and malignant conditions; these are characterized by disturbances in iron metabolism, but are often multifactorial. Inflammatory cytokines are thought to be the most important causative factors in ACD. ACD is difficult to diagnose but can usually be strongly suspected based on clinical findings, elimination of other causes of anemia, low serum iron and transferrin levels, and elevated ferritin level. Cytokines such as IFN and TNF have wide-ranging effects, including both direct and indirect inhibition of erythropoiesis and of red cell survival. Direct inhibition of erythropoiesis is mediated by both a relative decrease in EPO as well as a decrease in iron available for hemoglobin synthesis. Many of the abnormalities of iron metabolism in ACD are caused by cytokine-induced increases in hepcidin, and appreciation of the role of hepcidin in ACD may aid in the diagnosis and treatment. Anemia, iron deficiency, and hepcidin may have independent antimicrobial and antitumor roles, and this needs further study. The treatment of patients with ACD should be focused on correcting the underlying disease. Increasing hemoglobin with exogenous EPO can be quite effective, but the potential deleterious results of this strategy, in malignancy, infection, and inflammation, must be considered. Development of new agents that might exclusively target erythropoiesis but not cancer and identification of risk factors for deleterious EPO effects are needed. Since hepcidin overproduction is a key pathogenic feature of ACD, strategies targeting hepcidin, ferroportin, and iron depletion pathways (such as isocitrate) are being studied and could be used in situations where the primary condition is not reversible and the anemia is severe enough to warrant intervention.

REFERENCES

1. Weiss G, Goodnough LT: Anemia of chronic disease. *New Engl J Med* 352:1011–1023, 2005.
2. Nairz M, Haschka D, Demetz E, et al: Iron at the interface of immunity and infection. *Front Pharmacol* 5:152, 2014.
3. Nemeth E, Tuttle MS, Powelson J, et al: Hepcidin regulates cellular iron efflux by binding to ferroportin and inducing its internalization. *Science* 306:2090–2093, 2004.

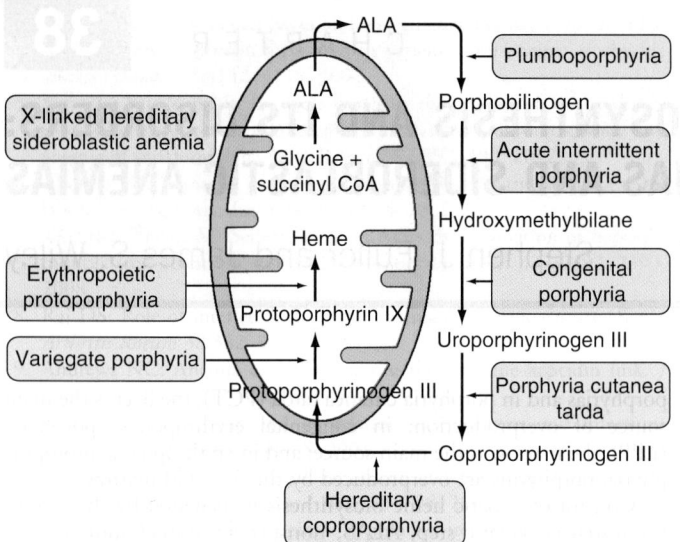

Fig. 38.1 PATHWAY OF HEME BIOSYNTHESIS IN MAMMALIAN CELLS. The first step in the pathway is catalyzed by aminolevulinate synthase (ALAS) and occurs within the mitochondrion using pyridoxal 5′-phosphate as a cofactor. 5-Aminolevulinate (ALA) then leaves the mitochondrion and is converted by ALA dehydratase to give a monopyrrole, porphobilinogen. Four molecules of this compound are converted by porphobilinogen deaminase to a linear tetrapyrrole, hydroxymethylbilane. This molecule is then cyclized by uroporphyrinogen III synthase to uroporphyrinogen III, which is decarboxylated to coproporphyrinogen III. This molecule enters the mitochondrion and is oxidized in succession by coproporphyrinogen III oxidase and protoporphyrinogen III oxidase. The product is protoporphyrin IX, a substrate for ferrochelatase, which catalyzes the insertion of Fe^{2+} to form heme. A mitochondrial heme exporter has been identified as feline leukemia virus subgroup C receptor 1b.[6] The defective steps associated with specific porphyrias and X-linked hereditary sideroblastic anemias are shown.

which is under the control of erythroid-specific promoters such as GATA1, a globin transcription factor. Whether heme inhibits import of pre-ALAS2 into the mitochondrial matrix remains to be unequivocally established. Heme may possibly also prevent the accumulation of intracellular iron by controlling the acquisition of iron from transferrin (see Fig. 38.2B). In addition to transport of iron from plasma to the cytosol by the transferrin receptor, a second transport step is required for mitochondrial uptake of iron. This step is fulfilled by mitoferrin,[22] a member of the solute carrier 25 family of proteins located in the inner mitochondrial membrane, which, to import iron into the mitochondrion, must interact both with ferrochelatase and with the adenosine triphosphate (ATP)-binding cassette transporter ABCB10.[23] Levels of intracellular iron regulate the translation of ALAS2 mRNA. Cellular iron homeostasis is maintained through a posttranscriptional regulatory mechanism, which is mediated by iron regulatory proteins that bind to iron-responsive elements in mRNA of target genes to either increase or decrease translation.[24,25] The RNA binding activity of iron-responsive proteins (IRP) is regulated by mitochondrial iron-sulfur cluster synthesis and cytosolic iron levels.[26–28] When iron is available for heme synthesis, translation of ALAS2 is allowed to proceed as a result of decreased IRP binding to the 5′ UTR iron-responsive elements (IRE) of ALAS2 mRNA. In contrast, under iron-depleted conditions increased IRP binding to ALAS2 mRNA blocks translation and ensures that ALAS2 and protoporphyrin levels are not produced in excess of available iron. Furthermore, to prevent the cell from becoming iron deficient, increased translation of mRNA from genes that increase cellular iron, such as the transferrin 1 gene, results from stabilization of mRNA by binding of IRPs to mRNA (see Chapter 35). This effect ensures that protoporphyrin synthesis is coupled to iron availability.

A second rate-limiting step in the overall heme synthetic pathway lies at the level of porphobilinogen deaminase (PBGD), which has a low endogenous activity and is inhibited by protoporphyrinogen and coproporphyrinogen. There are also two forms of PBGD. The PBGD gene (hydroxymethylbilane synthase; HMBS) encodes two enzymes, which arise from alternative splicing of PBGD mRNA. One isoform

TABLE 38.1	Porphyrias: Clinical Involvement, Enzymatic Etiology, and Chromosomal Location		
Porphyria (Synonym)	**Acute Attack, Skin and Organ Involvement**	**Enzyme of Heme Biosynthesis Affected**	**Chromosome Location**
—	—	Hepatic, 5-aminolevulinate synthase, nonspecific, mitochondrial (ALAS1)	3p21
X-linked sideroblastic anemia	Bone marrow	5-Aminolevulinate synthase, erythroid-specific, mitochondrial (ALAS2)	Xp11.21
X-linked dominant protoporphyria	Skin, red cells, liver	5-Aminolevulinate synthase, erythroid-specific, mitochondrial (ALAS2)	Xp11.21
ALA dehydratase deficiency porphyria (plumboporphyria)	Acute liver	ALA dehydratase (porphobilinogen synthase)	9q33.1
Acute intermittent porphyria (intermittent acute porphyria)	Acute liver	Porphobilinogen deaminase (hydroxymethylbilane synthase)	11q23.3
Congenital erythropoietic porphyria (Günther disease)	Skin, red cells, bone marrow	Uroporphyrinogen III synthase	10q25.2–q26.3
Porphyria cutanea tarda (symptomatic porphyria, cutaneous hepatic porphyria)	Skin, liver	Uroporphyrinogen decarboxylase	1p34
Hereditary coproporphyria	Acute skin, liver	Coproporphyrinogen oxidase	3q12
Variegate porphyria (porphyria variegata)	Acute skin, liver	Protoporphyrinogen oxidase	1q22
Erythropoietic protoporphyria (erythrohepatic protoporphyria)	Skin red cells, liver	Ferrochelatase (heme synthase)	18q21.3

ALA, 5-Aminolevulinate.

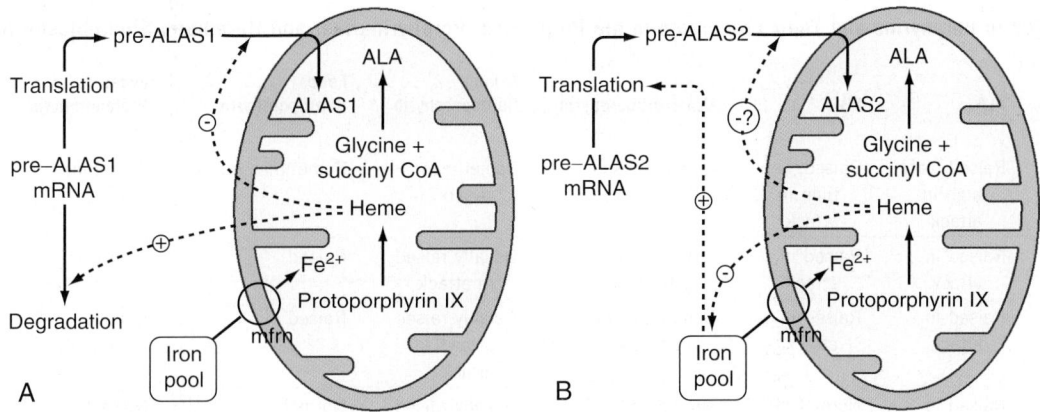

Fig. 38.2 (A) Control of heme synthesis in hepatic and other tissues. The rate of heme synthesis depends on the first and rate-limiting enzymatic step catalyzed by 5-aminolevulinate synthase, nonspecific, mitochondrial (ALAS1). Heme represses transcription of the ALAS1 gene, increases the rate of degradation of its messenger ribonucleic acid (mRNA), and blocks the translocation of the ALAS1 isoenzyme into the mitochondrion. (B) Control of heme synthesis in erythroblasts. Cytosolic iron enhances the translation of mRNA of the pre-ALAS2 by inhibiting the interaction of a repressor protein with an iron-responsive element in the mRNA. The product of the last step, heme inhibits the uptake of iron from transferrin into the cytosol. Heme also may inhibit translocation of ALAS2 into the mitochondrion. The overall result is that the rate of heme synthesis is tightly linked to the availability of iron for the ferrochelatase reaction. Mitoferrin (mfrn) transports Fe^{2+} into the mitochondrial matrix. *ALA,* 5-Aminolevulinate.

TABLE 38.2	Classification of Porphyrias		
Classification	**Disease**	**Biochemistry**	**Clinical Features**
Acute porphyria	Acute intermittent porphyria	Increased ALA and PBG	Acute attack
	Variegate porphyria	Increased ALA and PBG; increased porphyrin	Acute attack; photosensitivity
	Hereditary coproporphyria	Increased ALA and PBG; increased porphyrin	Acute attack; photosensitivity
	ALA dehydratase deficiency porphyria	Increased ALA; increased porphyrin	Acute and chronic neuropathy
Nonacute porphyria	Porphyria cutanea tarda	Increased porphyrin	Photosensitivity
	Erythropoietic protoporphyria	Increased porphyrin	Photosensitivity
	Congenital erythropoietic porphyria	Increased porphyrin	Photosensitivity
	X-linked dominant protoporphyria	Increased porphyrin	Photosensitivity
Porphyrinurias	Lead, alcohol, iron deficiency anemia, liver disease	Various biochemical manifestations	Various clinical presentations

ALA, 5-Aminolevulinate; PBG, porphobilinogen.

is expressed in all cells, whereas a second is restricted to red cells.[29] Erythroid PBGD is stimulated by erythropoiesis in vitro and may play a regulatory role in heme biosynthesis during differentiation.[30]

HMBS, the human PBGD gene, has attracted extensive investigation because of the practical importance of detecting carriers of the gene for acute intermittent porphyria (AIP).[31] Studies of the genetic locus of PBGD on chromosome 11 show great molecular heterogeneity, with 158 nonsense/missense mutations resulting either in single amino acid substitutions or premature chain termination listed in the Human Gene Mutation Database (HGMD Professional 2015.1, www.hgmd.org). Most human mutations have been described in exons 10 and 12,[32] which is consistent with alteration of the binding sites for the dipyrromethane cofactor for the enzyme. The three-dimensional structure of PBGD has been defined by x-ray crystallography, which has allowed study of the structural and functional implications of mutations.[33]

PORPHYRIAS

Biologic and Molecular Aspects

The porphyrias are classified as acute or nonacute (cutaneous) according to their clinical and biochemical features (Table 38.2).

Each of the different types of porphyria is linked to a reduced activity or deficiency of a specific enzyme in the heme biosynthetic pathway, with the exception of the recently described X-linked dominant erythropoietic protoporphyria, which results from inheritance of a gain-of-function mutation in the ALAS2 gene[34] (see Fig. 38.1). When porphyria is caused by a loss-of-function mutation, the resulting enzyme deficiency impairs the production of the end-product heme, and there is overproduction and increased excretion of the heme precursors formed by the steps before the enzyme defect. There is also a compensatory increase in activity of the initial and rate-controlling enzyme ALAS. In the acute porphyrias, there is overproduction of all the porphyrins and porphyrin precursors (e.g., ALA, PBG) formed proximal to the enzyme defect. The increased excretion of porphyrin precursors in the acute porphyrias is caused by decreased activity of PBGD in these conditions. The decrease can be caused by genetic mutation of the enzyme (in AIP) or by inhibition of PBGD by protoporphyrinogen and coproporphyrinogen in variegate porphyria and hereditary coproporphyria, respectively.[35]

In the nonacute porphyrias, there is overproduction of all porphyrins formed before the enzyme defect but no overproduction of porphyrin precursors. The cause of this lack of overproduction of porphyrin precursors in the nonacute porphyrias is unclear, but it may result from a compensatory increase in the activity of the enzyme PBGD in addition to increased activity of ALAS and

TABLE 38.3   Changes in Porphyrins and Their Precursors in the Porphyrias, Porphyrinurias, and Hereditary Sideroblastic Anemia

Porphyrias and Other Conditions	ALA	PBG	Urine Uroporphyrin	Urine Coproporphyrin	Feces Coproporphyrin	Feces Protoporphyrin	Erythrocyte Protoporphyrin
Acute Porphyrias							
Acute intermittent porphyria	Raised, very high in attack	Raised, very high in attack	Usually raised[a]	Sometimes raised	Sometimes raised	Sometimes raised	Normal
Variegate porphyria	Raised in attack	Raised in attack	Usually raised in attack	Usually raised in attack	Raised	Raised	Normal
Hereditary coproporphyria	Raised in attack	Raised in attack	Sometimes raised in attack	Usually raised, always in attack	Raised	Usually normal	Normal
ALA dehydratase–deficiency porphyria	Raised in attack	Normal	Normal	Usually raised in attack	Normal	Normal	Occasionally raised
Nonacute Porphyrias							
Porphyria cutanea tarda	Normal	Normal	Raised (7-/8-carboxylate porphyrin levels very high in attack)	Slightly raised	Isocoproporphyrin raised in remission	Raised in remission	Normal
Erythropoietic protoporphyria	Normal	Normal	Normal	Normal	Normal	Usually raised	Raised, usually very high
Congenital erythropoietic porphyria	Usually normal	Usually normal	Raised, isomer I	Raised, isomer I	Normal	Usually raised	Usually raised
X-linked dominant protoporphyria	Normal	Normal	Normal	Normal	Normal	Usually raised	Raised, usually very high
Other Conditions							
Hereditary sideroblastic anemia	Normal	Normal	Normal	Normal	Normal	Normal	Occasionally raised
Lead poisoning	Raised	Normal	Normal	Sometimes raised	Normal	Normal	Raised when blood lead level >2 μM
Hereditary tyrosinemia	Raised	Normal	Normal	Normal	Normal	Normal	Normal
Iron deficiency anemia	Normal	Normal	Normal	Normal	Normal	Normal	Raised

[a]PBG may cyclize to uroporphyrin nonenzymatically.
ALA, 5-Aminolevulinate; PBG, porphobilinogen.

site-specific heme synthesis.[36] The pattern of overproduction and excretion of porphyrins and porphyrin precursors in the various porphyrias is shown in Table 38.3. A consequence is that each of the different porphyrias is characterized by a different excretion pattern. Quantitative studies of the different porphyrins and precursors in the urine and feces usually identify the particular type of porphyria. The porphyrin precursors ALA and PBG and the more water-soluble porphyrins (with multiple carboxyl groups) are excreted mainly in the urine. Other porphyrins are mainly excreted in the feces by way of the bile (see box on Measurement of Porphyrins and Precursors).

The clinical manifestations of an acute attack of porphyria can be explained by dysfunction of the central, peripheral, and autonomic nervous systems. The mechanism by which altered heme synthesis results in dysfunction is unknown.

Perhaps the most likely hypothesis is that the neurologic and muscular manifestations of acute porphyria arise as a result of heme deficiency within the nerve cells, which causes dysfunction of the energy-dependent Na+/K+ ATPase. The proposal that axonal dysfunction results from impaired energy metabolism is supported by the

findings of axonal membrane depolarization during acute attacks of porphyric neuropathy and reduction in inward rectification between episodes.[37] However, this does not exclude the possibility that ALA may also act as a pharmacologic agent in these diseases, compounding the effects of heme deficiency.[38] ALA has a pro-oxidant effect on rat brain tissues and generates free radical species during its auto-oxidation, and this oxidant stress has been proposed to directly damage myelination by Schwann cells.[39,40] The concept of auto-oxidation or oxidative stress is supported by the hypothesis that manganese excess could contribute to induction of superoxide dismutase[41] and increased indicators of such stress in lead exposure.[42] There is evidence that ALA enters cells by a pathway common to it and γ-aminobutyric acid (GABA).[43]

Genetic Aspects

The enzymatic links and genetic loci in each of the hereditary porphyrias are shown in Table 38.1. Nearly all are inherited as autosomal dominant traits. The Chester porphyria family pedigree (Fig. 38.3)

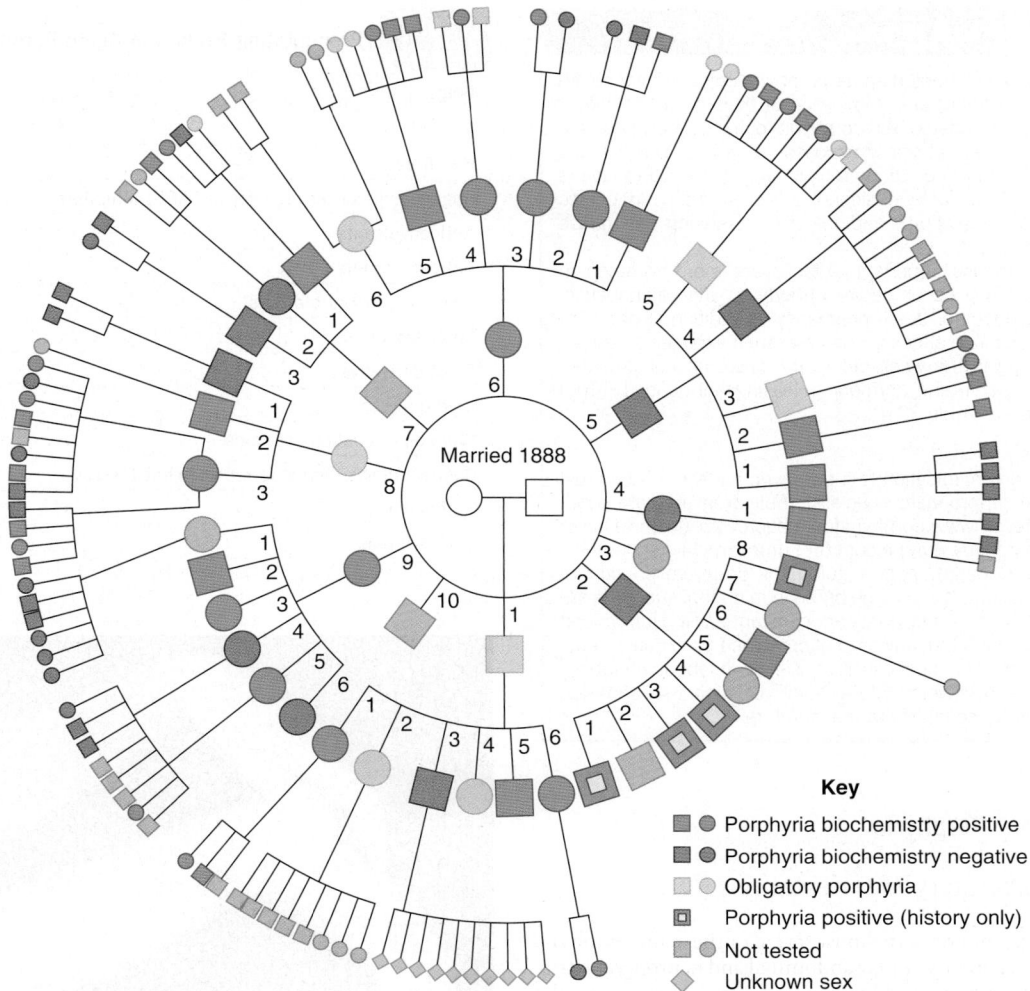

Key
- ■ ● Porphyria biochemistry positive
- ■ ● Porphyria biochemistry negative
- ■ ○ Obligatory porphyria
- ☐ Porphyria positive (history only)
- ■ ● Not tested
- ◆ Unknown sex

Fig. 38.3 THE CHESTER FAMILY PEDIGREE. The propositus, Peter Dobson, was a salmon fisherman from a close-knit community living on the bank of the River Dee, which runs through the city of Chester, UK. Most of the 330 descendants of his marriage in 1888 still live in the city. Many suffered disabling illnesses and psychiatric upsets, which often went unrecognized as porphyria. The family called their illness *Dobson's complaint*. Chester porphyria has recently been confirmed as a variant of acute intermittent porphyria. *Squares* represent male subjects; circles represent females. *(Courtesy Giles R. Youngs.)*

Measurement of Porphyrins and Precursors

Fluorescence of urine under ultraviolet (UV) light is recommended as the initial screening test for the acute porphyrias,[7] whereas plasma fluorescent spectroscopy is the best initial test for diagnosis of cutaneous porphyrias.[44] Diverse techniques such as high-pressure liquid chromatography,[45] quantitative extraction, and various forms of fluorometry are used to measure porphyrins and precursors.[46] The International Federation of Clinical Chemistry and Laboratory Medicine presents diagnostic information on its website (www.ifcc.org).

shows autosomal dominant inheritance of acute porphyria with attacks of neurovisceral dysfunction without cutaneous hypersensitivity. This was originally reported as a dual porphyria[47]; however, identification of a heterozygous truncating mutation in the HMBS gene and no mutations in other heme biosynthesis enzymes in affected individuals has confirmed that Chester porphyria is a variant of classic AIP.[48] HMBS is transcribed from two promoters to produce ubiquitous and erythroid specific isoforms. In classic AIP both isoforms are deficient; however, in the rare, nonerythroid variant only the ubiquitous HMBS variant is defective. The rare congenital EPP

shows autosomal recessive inheritance. The mutations producing each of the acute porphyrias are heterogeneous at the molecular level and include complete or partial gene deletions, alterations of splicing or stability of mRNA, and missense mutations. An exception is variegate porphyria in South Africa, in which the founder effect ensures a predominance of the Arg59Tryp mutation in protoporphyrinogen oxidase.[49,50] Homozygotic or compound heterozygotic inheritance has been found in a number of the porphyrias, as has concurrent inheritance of more than one defect. This may present as two types of porphyria in one family[51] or as two types in one patient.[52,53] Dual porphyrias most commonly arise from a combined deficiency of uroporphyrinogen decarboxylase with PBGD, coproporphyrinogen oxidase, or protoporphyrinogen oxidase.[54]

The prevalence of the different forms varies widely. For example, in northern Europe and North America, approximately 1 of 10,000 individuals carries the gene for AIP, although only about 10% of the affected persons will present with clinical features. It has been suggested that spontaneous mutation accounts for 3% of AIP cases.[55] Variegate porphyria occurs in 1 of 400 white South Africans. There is a reduction in gene frequency in variegate porphyria from generation to generation that suggests that the allele associated with it is selectively deleterious.[56] The same is probably true of the other porphyrias.

TABLE 38.4	Precipitating Factors in Acute Porphyria	
Drugs		**Other Stimuli**
Alcohol		Fasting or dieting
Barbiturates		Hormones, stress
Angiotensin-converting enzyme (ACE) inhibitors		Smoking
Anticonvulsants		
Antidepressants		
Calcium channel blockers		
Cephalosporins		
Ergot derivatives		
Erythromycin		
Steroids or anabolic steroids		
Contraceptives, hormone replacement therapy		
Sulfonamides		
Sulfonylureas		

Acute Intermittent Porphyria

Clinical and Laboratory Manifestations

Acute intermittent porphyria is the most severe of the acute porphyrias. During an attack, patients display abdominal and neuropsychiatric or neurovisceral disturbances. Onset occurs in puberty; female patients exhibit a fourfold greater incidence of attacks than males. Attacks occur mainly in young adults and become less frequent after menopause. It is uncommon to see attacks in children.[57] Crises may vary in duration from several days to months. They are most commonly followed by complete remission, although deaths are still reported, especially with AIP[58] (see box on Precipitating Factors in Acute Porphyria). Late complications of AIP include renal impairment, hypertension, and hepatocellular carcinoma, and patients should be monitored for these complications.[59]

Gastrointestinal symptoms occur in 95% of cases; most patients present with acute colicky central abdominal pain. Examination reveals tenderness but little rigidity, and patients may also experience limb pain or generalized muscular aches. Severe vomiting may occur, and constipation is usual. Hyponatremia occurs in severe attacks.

Motor neuropathy complicates two-thirds of porphyric attacks and may be the presenting feature. Motor involvement is most common, but paresthesias may also occur. Paralysis usually starts peripherally and then spreads proximally; however, in some patients, shoulder girdle involvement may be the first manifestation. The neuropathy may progress rapidly, resulting in respiratory insufficiency. Weakness, usually symmetric, involves proximal and distal limb muscles more often than those of the trunk. Upper limbs and proximal muscles are often affected. Involvement of the wrists, ankles, and small muscles of the hand may lead to a permanent deformity (Fig. 38.4), and trunk muscle weakness can lead to respiratory embarrassment. Death is usually caused by respiratory paralysis. Progressive weakening of the voice may suggest this; treatment requires tracheotomy and intermittent positive pressure ventilation. Paresthesias, numbness, and objective evidence of sensory impairment may occur with loss of pinprick sensation, which is most marked around the shoulder and hip areas; generalized tonic-clonic seizures occasionally occur.

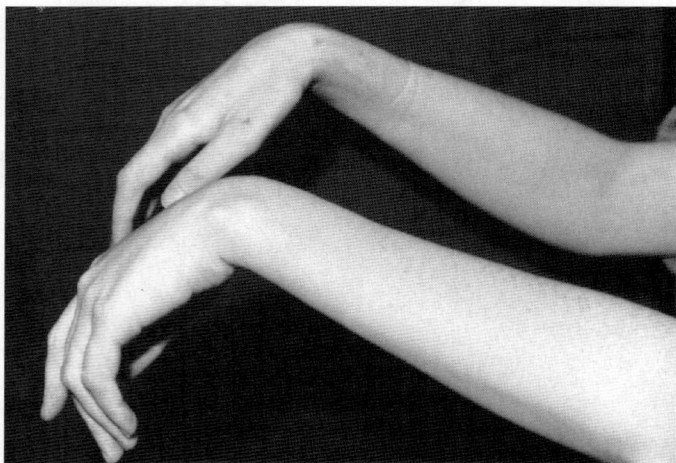

Fig. 38.4 BILATERAL WRISTDROP CAUSED BY PERIPHERAL NEUROPATHY IN A PATIENT WITH ACUTE INTERMITTENT PORPHYRIA.

Severe anxiety, depression, and frank psychosis are the main psychiatric manifestations of porphyric attacks. These psychiatric manifestations may result in a patient being misdiagnosed as suffering from a primary psychiatric disorder. Agitation, mania, depression, hallucinations, and schizophrenic-like behavior may occur. Psychiatric manifestations may persist between attacks.[63] Quality of life is severely affected in those suffering from repeated attacks of acute porphyria.[64]

The cardiovascular system is involved in approximately 70% of attacks. Sinus tachycardia (to 160 beats/min) and hypertension can occur; these elevations usually revert to normal after an attack. There is evidence that hypertension may occasionally be permanent, even in latent cases of AIP (see box on Differential Diagnosis of Acute Intermittent Porphyria).

Other Acute Porphyrias

Hereditary Coproporphyria

Hereditary coproporphyria combines the clinical features of acute porphyria with photosensitive skin manifestations. It results from various mutations in the gene encoding coproporphyrinogen oxidase,

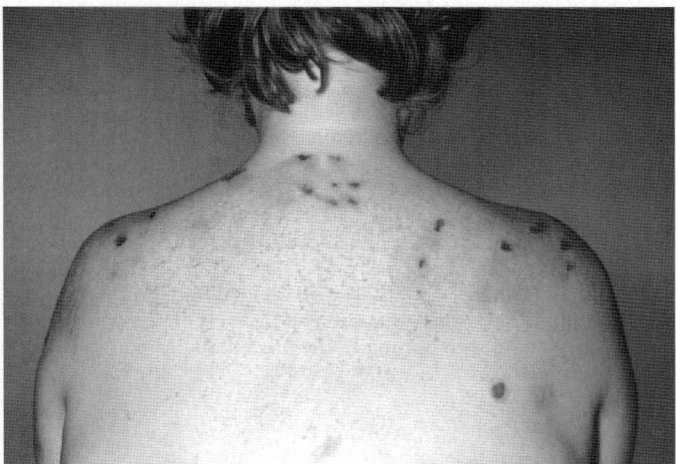

Fig. 38.5 CUTANEOUS LESIONS AND SCARRING IN A PATIENT WITH VARIEGATE PORPHYRIA.

the activity of which is decreased,[67,68] leading to overproduction of coproporphyrin.[69] A clinically distinct variant of hereditary coproporphyria, harderoporphyria, is associated with severe jaundice and hemolysis and is caused by specific mutations that lead to accumulation of harderoporphyrins.[70]

The porphyrin precursors ALA and PBG and the more water-soluble porphyrins (with multiple carboxyl groups) are excreted mainly in the urine. Other porphyrins are mainly excreted in the feces by way of bile.

Variegate Porphyria

Variegate porphyria is similar to hereditary coproporphyria, except that there are more severe skin lesions, sometimes with scarring (Fig. 38.5). Protoporphyrinogen oxidase is the affected enzyme, and protoporphyrin is the major circulating porphyrin. Conventionally, variegate porphyria is most readily diagnosed by measurement of fecal porphyrin concentrations. However, it has been reported[71] that biliary porphyrin levels may provide a better discriminator from normal patients in the asymptomatic phase. As in erythropoietic protoporphyria, there is a tendency toward cholelithiasis. The mechanism by which gallstones form is not certain, but some studies have suggested that porphyrins are cholestatic.[72] In hereditary coproporphyria and variegate porphyria, the pathway intermediates produced in excess, coproporphyrinogen and protoporphyrinogen, respectively, are inhibitors of the secondary rate-controlling enzyme PBGD.[35,73] Numerous mutations in the protoporphyrinogen oxidase gene have

been described leading to 50% reduction in enzyme activity. The functional consequences of many of these mutations have been predicted based on the crystal structure of the enzyme.[74] In a few cases, homozygosity or compound heterozygosity has been described.[49,75]

Acute Hepatic Porphyria

In this porphyria (also known as ALA dehydratase deficiency porphyria or plumboporphyria), the ALA dehydratase activity is depressed, such as seen with a low-function variant of the enzyme in a subject exposed to lead. The clinical picture resembles AIP, but very few cases have been described, and the disease only manifests in homozygous cases when there is a precipitating factor.[76,77]

Concurrent Porphyrias

The concurrent porphyrias are a rare group of conditions in which there is concurrent inheritance of two different defects within the heme biosynthetic pathway, although this requires confirmation from molecular evidence.[78] Previous descriptions[52–54] have shown the presence of concurrent porphyria within a family, and toxicologically there is good evidence that exposure to poisons such as lead can induce multiple changes within the pathway.[79] The first reported example of concurrent porphyria in a family combined the clinical features of acute and cutaneous porphyria, and biochemical analysis confirmed the segregation of variegate porphyria and PCT as independent inherited traits.[80] In another patient, dual genetic defects involving ALA dehydratase and coproporphyrinogen oxidase have been described[52] (see box on Management of Acute Porphyria).

Nonacute or Cutaneous Porphyrias

In all cutaneous porphyrias, porphyrins (which are photosensitizing) are deposited in the upper layers of the skin, and they are responsible for the characteristic skin lesions.[87] In the development of these lesions, reactive oxygen species and other radicals are formed and probably induce oxidative membrane damage, particularly to mast cells, which enables complement activation as one part of the inflammatory reaction[88] (see box on Management of Nonacute Porphyria).

Porphyria Cutanea Tarda or Cutaneous Hepatic Porphyria

Biologic and Molecular Aspects

PCT exists in inherited and acquired/sporadic forms. Type I, or sporadic PCT, comprises 70% to 80% of cases and is associated with 50% level of uroporphyrinogen decarboxylase activity. PCT type II or familial PCT results from heterozygous mutations in uroporphyrinogen decarboxylase, whereas a more severe form, hepatoerythropoietic porphyria (HEP), results from homozygous or compound heterozygous mutations.[99] Mutations in the uroporphyrinogen decarboxylase are found in around one-third of patients with PCT. In inherited and acquired forms, there is diminution in the activity of hepatic uroporphyrinogen decarboxylase, which converts uroporphyrinogen to coproporphyrinogen by the stepwise decarboxylation of the acetyl groups to methyl groups. The mechanism of enzyme inhibition has recently been elucidated, whereby iron-dependent oxidation of uroporphyrinogen generates uroporphomethene, a competitive inhibitor of uroporphyrinogen decarboxylase.[100] Most carriers of mutant uroporphyrinogen decarboxylase are not clinically evident unless precipitating factors are present. Iron alone or chlorinated hydrocarbons can diminish activity of uroporphyrinogen decarboxylase, and this effect is greatly potentiated when both are given together.[101,102] In a murine model, precipitation of uroporphyria by chlorinated hydrocarbons is dependent on hepatic cytochrome P450 Cyp 1A2 oxidase activity, and inherited variations in enzyme function may modulate susceptibility to PCT in humans.[101]

In sporadic (type I) PCT, there is no evident genetic basis for the condition and low uroporphyrinogen decarboxylase activity is restricted to the liver. Patients may have clinical and biochemical evidence of liver disease. Hepatic siderosis invariably occurs, and iron is one of the causative agents in acquired PCT. An association of PCT with hereditary hemochromatosis has been documented, with about 20% of PCT patients being homozygous for the Cys282Tyr mutation in the HFE ("High Fe") gene, a defect that characterizes hereditary hemochromatosis.[103–105] These results strongly implicate the HFE gene as a genetic susceptibility factor in acquired PCT. An association between PCT and hepatitis C infection is well documented, and in countries with high prevalence rates, hepatitis C virus may be the dominant risk factor.[106] An apparent association has emerged between human immunodeficiency virus (HIV) infection and PCT.[107] It is possible that therapy for HIV with zidovudine precipitates the disease, but it is more likely that the association is merely coincidental or that the viral infection unmasks the preexisting uroporphyrinogen decarboxylase defect.[108]

Genetics

Whereas familial PCT is inherited in an autosomal-dominant mode, HEP is inherited in an autosomal-recessive pattern.[109] As in the other genetic lesions in the porphyrias, there is heterogeneity in the mutations causing PCT and HEP phenotypes.[110,111] In the inherited form, more than 120 different mutations (HGMD Professional 2015.1, www.hgmd.org) have been identified in uroporphyrinogen decarboxylase, many of which lie near the dimer interface, resulting in an unstable protein and reduced enzyme activity.[112] In different population groups, it is difficult to find the relative numbers of acquired and familial disease. In one analysis in Hungary, 77.5% of patients were found to suffer from the acquired form, and of the patients with the familial disease, females were affected more than males, suggesting that inheritance may predispose patients to estrogen-precipitated disease.[113]

Clinical Features

The most striking clinical feature of both forms of PCT is a bullous dermatosis on light-exposed areas. This starts as erythema and progresses to vesicles that become confluent to form bullae (Fig. 38.6), which may hemorrhage and leave scars; pruritus is often troublesome. Milia are common and may precede or follow vesicle formation. Facial hypertrichosis is common and may serve as a diagnostic clue. In less severe cases, increased fragility of the skin may be the only clinical sign. In severe cases, photomutilation can result, usually because of infection of slowly healing lesions.

The thickening and scarring with calcification has been described as pseudoscleroderma. Hyperpigmentation is common, and women often complain of hirsutism. Neurologic change is not observed. Patients may have clinical and biochemical evidence of chronic liver

---

Management of Nonacute Porphyria

Patients should avoid exposure to sunlight and use sunblock (to filter Soret band light) and physical barriers such as cotton gloves.

Porphyria Cutanea Tarda

The clinical features are reversed by removing any precipitating agent such as alcohol, halogenated hydrocarbons, and drugs. The patient should be screened for hepatic neoplasm and hepatitis C infection. The mainstay of treatment is to remove liver iron by venesection of 500 mL of blood weekly until clinical remission occurs or until the hemoglobin level falls below 12 g/dL. Chloroquine, at low doses of 125 mg twice per week for several months, has also been helpful because it enhances urinary clearance of porphyrin. When this is not possible, oral cimetidine has been used.[89] When venesection is difficult, parenteral and orally active iron chelators can be used to reduce liver iron stores. It is of value to screen the patient and first-degree relatives for hereditary hemochromatosis.

Erythropoietic Protoporphyria

Oral β-carotene offers effective protection in erythropoietic porphyria (EPP) against solar sensitivity. It does so by quenching the radical formation that is a feature of the skin damage. Yellowing of the skin (i.e., carotenemia) is one side effect. Afamelanotide, an alpha-melanocyte-stimulating hormone, is effective for decreasing photosensitivity in EPP by increasing melanin production, and has shown efficacy and tolerability for the long-term treatment of EPP.[90,91] Interruption of the enterohepatic protoporphyrin circulation by bile salt–sequestering agents such as cholestyramine reduces plasma protoporphyrin levels and may retard the development of the liver disease. Liver transplantation has been reported to be an effective measure in preventing the progression of this disease.[92,93]

Congenital Erythropoietic Porphyria

The severity of hematologic manifestations are predictors of a poor prognosis, and patients with hemolytic anemia or thrombocytopenia should be considered for allogeneic hematopoietic stem cell transplantation (HSCT). The majority of patients treated with allogeneic HSCT have achieved long-term symptomatic cures.[94,95] Erythropoiesis should be reduced by means of erythrocyte hypertransfusion and by hematin or heme arginate infusion.[96] However, care should be taken when prescribing heme arginate, as overdosing may cause acute hepatic failure.[83] Splenectomy and chloroquine therapy (125 mg twice weekly) have an ameliorating effect, as does hypertransfusion, but life expectancy is usually severely shortened. Therapeutic potential has been shown with the use of clinically approved proteasome inhibitors, such as bortezomib, which prevent enzymatically active uroporphyrinogen III synthase (UROS) mutants from early degradation in a murine model, and gene therapy using induced pluripotent stem cells.[97,98]

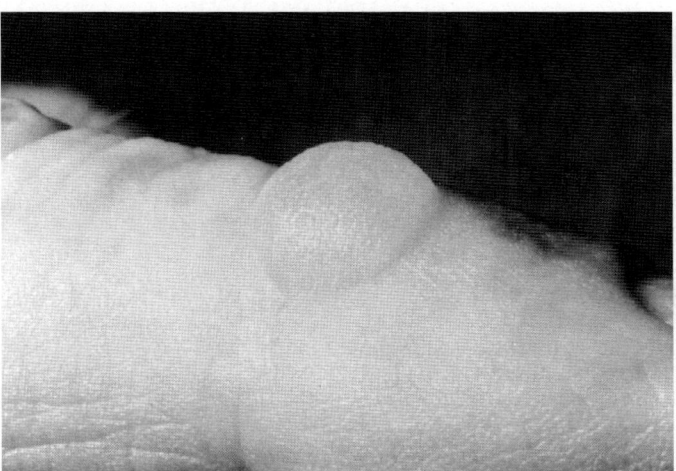

Fig. 38.6 A BULLOUS SKIN LESION OF PORPHYRIA CUTANEA TARDA.

disease, sometimes with cirrhosis. There is an association with hepatocellular carcinoma. Hepatomegaly is particularly common when alcohol intake is excessive.

Precipitating Factors

Many patients with PCT have multiple precipitating factors, including mutations of the HFE gene, hepatitis C infection, or exposure to estrogen.[104,105] Excessive alcohol intake is an important precipitating agent, perhaps because of increased hepatic iron deposition in alcoholics. However, certain halogenated hydrocarbons are sometimes implicated. PCT may also develop in people treated with hemodialysis for kidney failure. An outbreak of cutaneous hepatic porphyria in southeast Turkey in 1956 was traced to seed wheat dressed with the fungicide hexachlorobenzene. A neoplastic subgroup has been identified in which PCT is associated with benign or malignant liver tumors.

Differential Diagnosis

Other causes of bullous or vesicular skin lesions should be excluded, such as a drug reaction (see box on Pseudoporphyria and Renal Dialysis) or chronic renal failure. The distinction between PCT, variegate porphyria, and hereditary coproporphyria rests on biochemical testing of urine and feces, with the highest levels of urinary uroporphyrin found during attacks of PCT (see Table 38.3).

Erythropoietic Protoporphyria

Biologic and Molecular Aspects

Although not described until 1961, this form of EPP, also known as erythrohepatic protoporphyria, is much more common than congenital EPP. Ferrochelatase activity is reduced in peripheral blood, liver, bone marrow, and skin, and protoporphyrin is synthesized in excess.[117] The erythroid progenitor cells (i.e., burst-forming units-erythroid [BFU-E]) in EPP patients show intense fluorescence when viewed under 405-nm light. The gene mutation in EPP shows heterogeneity as in other porphyrias.[118] The last enzyme of the biosynthetic pathway, ferrochelatase, is important because its endogenous activity is relatively low, and it could act as a control point in the pathway. Ferrochelatase ligates iron bound to three cysteine residues in an iron-sulfur cluster,[119] the mutation of which leads to decreased enzyme activity.[120] An oligomeric complex of ferrochelatase, ABCB10 and mitoferrin in the mitochondrial membrane would allow for

channeling of iron from the cytoplasm to the mitochondrial matrix.[121] Immunologic studies on human protoporphyria show that immunologically reactive ferrochelatase is present, but that enzyme activity in three subjects was on average only 17% of normal.[122] Gain-of-function mutations in the ALAS2 gene have recently been described that result in increased erythrocyte protoporphyrin despite normal ferrochelatase activity. This newly described, X-linked dominant erythropoietic protoporphyria, leads to accumulation of protoporphyrin in amounts sufficient to cause photosensitivity and hepatic damage.[34]

Genetics

EPP inheritance resembles an autosomal dominant disorder with incomplete penetrance; however, the disease usually results from inheritance of a FECH null allele together with a low-expression mutation.[123] Haplotype segregation analysis has shown intronic nucleotide polymorphisms in the ferrochelatase gene (FECH) that produces aberrant splicing of mRNA to a form that degrades more rapidly, resulting in enzyme deficiency.[123] Although these disease-associated polymorphisms are common,[124,125] there is heterogeneity of the molecular defect, including aberrant splicing and loss of function of the mitoferrin protein.[19,117,121,126,127] The erythroid-specific ALAS gene resides on the X chromosome, and mutations in exon 11 have been described in X-linked dominant erythropoietic protoporphyria. Recombinant mutants have been shown to increase enzyme activity by two- to threefold, which leads to protoporphyrin overproduction.[128]

Clinical Features

The clinical features are mainly cutaneous on exposure to sunlight and can occur at any age, including infancy and childhood.[129] They include pruritic urticarial swelling and redness of the skin on exposure to sunlight. The most distressing symptom is an unbearable burning sensation on the affected parts. Remarkably, such features are ameliorated during pregnancy, which has been linked to lowered protoporphyrin levels.[130] Hepatic involvement, which occurs in later life, involves deposition of hepatotoxic protoporphyrin in the liver and can lead to fatal liver failure from an active chronic hepatitis with cirrhosis.[131] Such protoporphyrin deposition may also cause cholelithiasis; the gallstones contain high concentrations of protoporphyrin. The liver disease of EPP seems to correlate with erythrocyte protoporphyrin concentrations.[132] Mild microcytic anemia has been reported,[133,134] as well as mitochondrial iron accumulation and ring

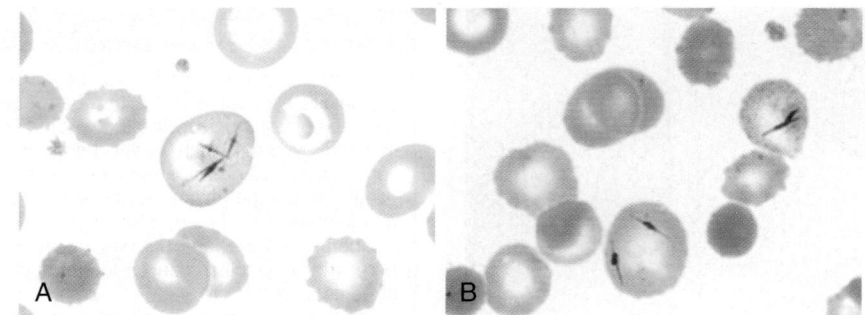

Fig. 38.7 NEEDLE-LIKE INCLUSIONS OF PORPHYRIN IN THE CIRCULATING RED CELLS OF A PATIENT WITH CONGENITAL ERYTHROPOIETIC PORPHYRIA AFTER SPLENECTOMY. *(From Merino A, To-Figueras J, Herrero C: Atypical red cell inclusions in congenital erythropoietic porphyria. Br J Haematol 132:124, 2006.)*

sideroblasts, in about 30% of patients.[135] Late onset of EPP has been reported in patients with myelodysplastic syndrome or overlap myelodysplasia/myeloproliferation. In one patient, EPP has been acquired as a result of expansion of hemopoietic cells containing only one allele of the FECH gene.[136] Inactivation of one allele by deletion involving chromosome 18 thus appears to be sufficient for overproduction of protoporphyrin.[135,137]

Differential Diagnosis

EPP should be distinguished from other causes of a photosensitive rash. The distinction can be made by demonstrating fluorescence in a proportion of red cells (i.e., fluorocytes) in the peripheral blood and confirmed by measurement of greatly increased erythrocyte and fecal protoporphyrin. Patients with EPP have a relatively high incidence of ring sideroblasts in the marrow.[135] This can lead to diagnostic difficulty because some patients with idiopathic sideroblastic anemia have increased levels of erythrocyte protoporphyrin.[138-141] However, EPP can be distinguished by the autosomal dominant inheritance pattern, dermal photosensitivity, normal or low serum levels of iron, and levels of protoporphyrin in red blood cells and feces.

Congenital Erythropoietic Porphyria (Günther Disease)

Biologic and Molecular Aspects

Congenital EPP, or Günther disease, although extremely rare, was the first porphyria to be described in 1874.[142] Unlike the other porphyrias, it is inherited in a mendelian autosomal recessive pattern causing reduced activity of uroporphyrinogen III synthase. The onset of solar photosensitivity results from gross overproduction of porphyrins, caused by deficiency of uroporphyrinogen III synthase. Like other porphyrias, the defective enzyme results mainly from point mutations at multiple sites within the gene.[143] Other enzymes are largely normal, although there is an increase in ALAS activity,[144] which in some cases has been shown to result from gain-of-function mutations in the ALAS2 gene.[145] Excess porphyrins, particularly uroporphyrin-1, accumulate in the normoblasts of the bone marrow and are excreted in the urine and feces. They are also deposited in bones and in the teeth, resulting in a pink-brown discoloration that fluoresces bright red in light of wavelengths around 400 nm. Dental restoration has been used to correct the esthetic appearance of the teeth. There are frequently profound changes in bone structure in patients with congenital EPP. This has been linked to vitamin D deficiency because of light avoidance.[146] However, bone changes can be seen when vitamin D levels are adequate, and it is reasonable to speculate that the porphyrins deposited in bone are cytotoxic because similar bone changes are features of homozygous variegate porphyria and HEP.[147]

Clinical Features

Typically the onset of congenital EPP is from birth, but occasionally late-onset cases have been reported.[96] The skin reaction is severe and can be devastating, and the teeth become brownish pink because of their high porphyrin content. Severe cutaneous photosensitivity is manifested by blistering of light-exposed areas and fragility of the epidermis. Skin thickening occurs, and there is extensive scarring and hypertrichosis. The recurrent damage associated with scarring on the hand may produce a claw-shaped deformity and loss of digits. Dystrophic nails may curl up and drop off. Lenticular scarring may lead to blindness. Hemolytic anemia often occurs and is associated with increased erythrocyte fragility and splenomegaly. Dyserythropoiesis may contribute to the anemia.[148] One patient who underwent splenectomy at 5 years of age has been described with needle-like inclusions of porphyrin in the circulating red cells (Fig. 38.7).[149]

Differential Diagnosis

The most characteristic feature of congenital EPP is the excess production of series 1 porphyrins rather than series 3 isomer produced in the other porphyrias. Red blood cells fluoresce in ultraviolet light, as do the brown-stained teeth, because of high porphyrin content (see box on Pseudoporphyria and Renal Dialysis).

SIDEROBLASTIC ANEMIAS

Sideroblastic anemias are a heterogeneous group of disorders characterized by anemia of varying severity and diagnosed by finding ring sideroblasts in the bone marrow aspirate. The peripheral blood shows hypochromic red cells, which are microcytic in the hereditary forms (Fig. 38.8A) but are often macrocytic in the acquired forms of the disease. The red blood cell parameters from automated cell counting may show bimodal volume distribution curves or widened range of cell sizes (see Fig. 38.8B); however, this dimorphic size distribution is not always present. Tiny inclusions may be visible in the red blood cells; these can be confirmed as iron-containing Pappenheimer bodies by Prussian blue staining of the blood smear (see Fig. 38.8C). The diagnostic test is bone marrow examination together with Prussian blue staining of the bone marrow smears.

The presence of ring sideroblasts (see Fig. 38.8D) is defined as erythroblasts containing five or more iron-positive (siderotic) granules arranged in a perinuclear collar distribution around one-third or more of the nucleus. Electron microscopic examination has shown that these siderotic granules are mitochondria containing amorphous deposits of ferric phosphate and ferric hydroxide. Iron is also bound to mitochondrial ferritin, a molecular form of ferritin that can be distinguished from cytoplasmic ferritin and that accumulates in

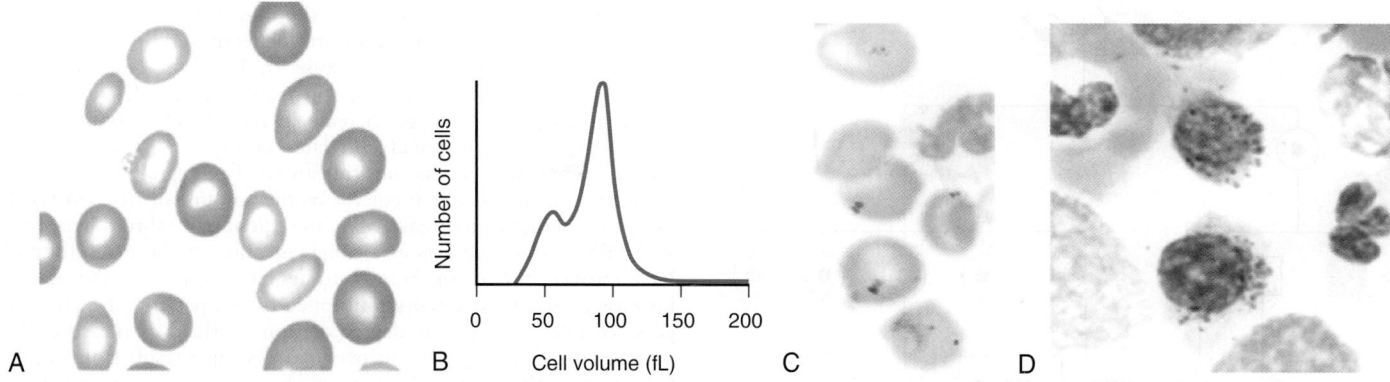

Fig. 38.8 (A) Peripheral blood smear from a patient with hereditary sideroblastic anemia shows a population of hypochromic and microcytic erythrocytes. (B) Erythrocyte volume distribution curve of a patient with hereditary sideroblastic anemia. A dimorphic size distribution is evident. (C) Peripheral blood showing Pappenheimer bodies (Prussian blue stain). (D) The bone marrow smear stained with Prussian blue shows ring sideroblasts.

large amounts in the erythroblasts of subjects with impaired heme synthesis.[150,151]

Iron overload is a common clinical feature of refractory sideroblastic anemia and, in severe cases, may lead to complications that characterize secondary hemosiderosis (e.g., diabetes, cardiac failure). Marrow examination shows prominent erythroid hyperplasia, which is a sign of the ineffective erythropoiesis and is responsible for increased iron absorption. The sideroblastic anemias have diverse causes but have in common an impaired biosynthesis of heme in the erythroid cells of the marrow. Most sideroblastic anemias are acquired as a clonal disorder of erythropoiesis, with various degrees of myelodysplastic features (Table 38.5). The inherited forms are uncommon and occur predominantly in males with an X-linked pattern of inheritance. A number of drugs have been associated with reversible sideroblastic anemia, and ring sideroblasts may be found in patients who abuse alcohol (see Table 38.5). The first descriptions of ring sideroblasts in association with chronic refractory anemias appeared in the late 1950s,[152,153] after an earlier description of familial X-linked hypochromic microcytic anemia.[154]

Hereditary Sideroblastic Anemia

X-Linked Sideroblastic Anemia

Biologic and Molecular Aspects

Approaching 40% of congenital sideroblastic anemias are molecularly unexplained.[155] Erythroid cells from patients with X-linked forms of hereditary sideroblastic anemia generally exhibit low activity of ALAS2[30,156]; however, for a minority of ALAS2 mutations this effect may be difficult to detect in vitro.[155] A defect in this enzyme is firmly established in patients whose anemia responds to pyridoxine therapy, because pyridoxal phosphate is an essential cofactor for ALAS. However, even affected female patients with moderate anemia unresponsive to pyridoxine have been documented to have low levels of ALAS in bone marrow lysates. In some male patients with X-linked pyridoxine-responsive sideroblastic anemia, the low ALAS activity in bone marrow increased to levels above the normal range when the patient took pyridoxine supplements and recovered from the anemia.[157] There are several possible explanations for this enhancement of ALAS activity by dietary pyridoxine supplements. The most likely is that pyridoxine (or its phosphate) may stabilize the ALAS during folding of the mutant enzyme after its synthesis.[156] The gene for the ALAS2 isoenzyme has been localized to the X chromosome, and this gene is known to be the site of most mutations giving rise to X-linked pyridoxine-responsive sideroblastic anemia.[158–160] Approximately 90 different mutations have been identified in individuals

TABLE 38.5	Classification of Sideroblastic Anemias

Hereditary (Nonsyndromic)
X-linked
Autosomal dominant or recessive

Acquired
Idiopathic acquired[a] (refractory anemia with ring sideroblasts)
Associated with previous chemotherapy, irradiation, or in transition myelodysplasia or myeloproliferative diseases

Drugs
Alcohol
Isoniazid
Chloramphenicol
Other drugs

Rare Causes
Erythropoietic protoporphyria
Copper deficiency or zinc overload
Hypothermia

Hereditary (Syndromic)
X-linked sideroblastic anemia with ring sideroblasts and cerebellar ataxia
Myopathy, lactic acidosis, and sideroblastic anemia
Pearson syndrome
Thiamine-responsive megaloblastic anemia
Sideroblastic anemia with immunodeficiency, fevers, and developmental delay

[a]Trial of pyridoxine indicated.

or families with hereditary sideroblastic anemia, and nearly all have resulted from single base alterations in DNA.[161–163] A frequent mutation affects arginine at residue 452 of ALAS2, which occurs in a quarter of all pedigrees but does not affect enzyme activity measured in vitro.[164] All known mutations lie between exons 5 and 11 of ALAS2, the region that codes for the catalytic domain, with most lying within exon 9, which contains the lysine at which binding of pyridoxal 5′-phosphate occurs.[165] A mutation, Asp190Val, has been described in a pyridoxine-refractory patient and appears to affect the proteolytic processing of the ALAS2 during or after import into the mitochondrion.[166] The variety of different mutations in the erythroid ALAS2 gene responsible for X-linked sideroblastic anemia and their pyridoxine responsiveness were reviewed in 2002 and 2010.[159,167]

Genetic Aspects

In most families with hereditary sideroblastic anemia, males are affected with an X-linked pattern of inheritance (Fig. 38.9). However,

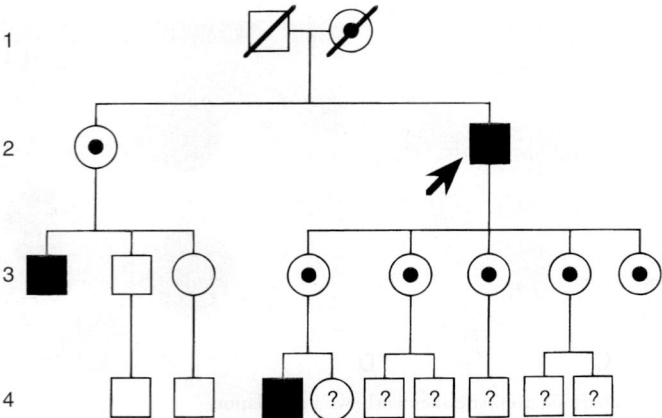

Fig. 38.9 PEDIGREE OF A FAMILY WITH PYRIDOXINE-RESPONSIVE SIDEROBLASTIC ANEMIA SHOWING X-LINKED RECESSIVE INHERITANCE. Affected *(filled box)*, carrier *(filled circle within open circle)*, and unknown status *(question mark within circle or box)* are indicated. Diagonal lines indicate deceased members. This pedigree[47] has been abbreviated to show only the affected branches of the family. The *arrow* indicates the proband.

female carriers, although usually normal, can develop erythrocyte dimorphism or varying degrees of anemia. The assignment of the gene for erythroid ALAS2 to the X chromosome[158] and the many mutations documented in erythroid ALAS2 provide the genetic basis for this X-linked disease. In several families, coinheritance of other X-linked traits (e.g., glucose-6-phosphate dehydrogenase [G6PD] deficiency, ataxia with sideroblastic anemia) has been described.[168,169] Sporadic and familial cases have been described that affect only females, which has been shown to represent skewed X-chromosome inactivation ("unfortunate skewing") affecting the normal allele for the ALAS2 gene.[170] The absence of affected male members in these pedigrees suggests that the ALAS2 defects identified are lethal in hemizygous males.

Clinical and Laboratory Evaluation

Typically the anemia of X-linked sideroblastic anemia manifests in infancy or childhood, but the milder forms of anemia may not be found until midlife. Even elderly patients have been diagnosed with this anemia.[171] Some cases may be discovered only during family surveys, which should always be undertaken when hereditary sideroblastic anemia is diagnosed. Still other patients may present with features of iron overload, such as diabetes or cardiac failure. Iron overload occurs commonly even with mild anemia and may occasionally be seen with female carriers. Enlargement of the liver and spleen may occur with mild abnormalities of liver function tests.

Anemia is extremely variable, but even when little or no anemia is present, the mean corpuscular volume (MCV) is low, and the red cell volume distribution width may be increased. When anemia is severe, the MCV may be as low as 50 fL (50 μm³). The blood smear shows a population of cells with hypochromic, microcytic morphology (see Fig. 38.8), which contrasts with the other normochromic, normocytic cells (i.e., dimorphism). Anisocytosis, poikilocytosis, elongated cells, and siderocytes may also be seen. The characteristic erythrocyte dimorphism is most prominent in patients with milder anemia, in female carriers, and in patients in whom pyridoxine has corrected the anemia but not restored the MCV to normal. In some pedigrees with only affected females, macrocytosis may be present, which contrasts with the typical microcytosis of male hemizygotes.[141,170] Leukocyte values are normal, whereas the platelet count is normal or increased.

Serum iron concentration is increased, and transferrin shows an increased percentage of saturation with iron. Serum ferritin levels are invariably increased. Ineffective erythropoiesis can be confirmed by ferrokinetic measurements showing that plasma iron clearance is

rapid, with subnormal retention of the iron isotope in erythrocytes after 10 to 14 days. Other features of ineffective erythropoiesis may be variably present: a mild increase in bilirubin concentration, decrease in haptoglobin levels, mild increase in lactate dehydrogenase levels, and normal or slight increase in reticulocyte numbers. The magnitude of iron overload correlates poorly with the degree of anemia in patients who are not transfused. The degree of ineffective erythropoiesis is a better predictor of the amount of iron overload. When ferrokinetics are unavailable, the extent of erythroid hyperplasia relative to normal acts as a rough measure of the magnitude of ineffective erythropoiesis. Several studies have shown that the relative increase in erythroid activity multiplied by the patient's age shows a good correlation with the degree of iron overload as measured by plasma ferritin.[172,173] The iron overload does not result from mutations in the HFE gene[174] (see box on Therapy for Hereditary Sideroblastic Anemia).

Differential Diagnosis

Hereditary sideroblastic anemia should be distinguished from idiopathic hemochromatosis, because both have biochemical evidence of iron overload and a similar tissue pattern of iron deposition. Careful hematologic assessment of patient and family members should make the distinction, because the hemoglobin level and MCV are normal in idiopathic hemochromatosis.

Other Nonsyndromic and Syndromic Hereditary Sideroblastic Anemias

X-linked sideroblastic anemia is considered the most common inherited sideroblastic anemia; however, a number of rare forms have recently been identified. These consist of two nonsyndromic sideroblastic anemias, which have a similar phenotype to X-linked sideroblastic anemia, and five syndromic forms where heme synthesis is affected in a variety of other tissues in addition to red cells.

Of the nonsyndromic forms, inherited mutations in both the SLC25A38 and GLRX5 genes have been identified to cause an autosomal recessive pyridoxine-refractory sideroblastic anemia.[178,179] SLC25A38 is located on chromosome 3p22.1 and encodes a mitochondrial carrier protein that may function to import glycine into the mitochondrion or exchange glycine for 5-aminolevulinate.[179] Homozygous or compound heterozygote mutations in SLC25A38 result in a similar phenotype to that seen in X-linked sideroblastic anemia, with onset in infancy of a severe microcytic anemia that is refractory to treatment with pyridoxine and folic acid.[161] GLRX5 encodes a mitochondrial protein, glutaredoxin 5, which when deleted in the zebrafish mutant shiraz results in defective iron-sulfur cluster assembly and blocked synthesis of heme.[180] A late-onset pyridoxine-refractory sideroblastic anemia caused by homozygous mutation in GLRX5 has been described in a patient who in middle age developed symptoms of a microcytic hypochromic anemia, type 2 diabetes, cirrhosis, and liver iron overload.[178]

In addition to genetically defined forms of hereditary sideroblastic anemia, five syndromic types have been described, which present with anemia in combination with either muscle, neurologic, or pancreatic tissue involvement. The first of these disorders to be defined by molecular genetics, the Pearson syndrome, is a rare entity that manifests in early infancy with anemia and exocrine pancreatic dysfunction.[181] The anemia is normocytic or macrocytic, reticulocyte counts are low, and variable degrees of neutropenia and thrombocytopenia are present. The bone marrow shows striking vacuolation and ringed sideroblasts.[182] Although usually fatal, milder forms of the anemia are consistent with survival into adult life. The syndrome, which is related to the Kearns-Sayre syndrome, results from deletions, mutations, or duplications of mitochondrial DNA, variably affecting multiple tissues of the body.[183,184]

A second syndromic congenital sideroblastic anemia, X-linked sideroblastic anemia with cerebellar ataxia (XLSA/A), is a rare mitochondrial disease caused by loss-of-function mutations in the ATP-binding cassette transporter ABCB7.[185–188] ABCB7 is localized to the

Therapy for Hereditary Sideroblastic Anemia

A trial of pyridoxine (100–200 mg/day taken orally) is indicated for 3 months for all patients with hereditary sideroblastic anemia. Response is variable and ranges from complete correction of hemoglobin levels to no effect. Even when pyridoxine completely corrects the anemia (Fig. 38.10), the increase in mean corpuscular volume (MCV) may not reach normal values, and a population of hypochromic, microcytic cells remains.

About 25–50% of patients with hereditary sideroblastic anemia show a full or partial response to pyridoxine, and this vitamin should be continued on a lifelong basis in the responders. A lower maintenance dose should be determined for each responding patient by progressive dose reduction, because long-term therapy with pyridoxine at 100–200 mg/day has been associated with peripheral neuropathy.[175] The adult nutritional requirement for pyridoxine is 1–2 mg/day; some patients have been maintained on as little as 4 mg/day as a supplement.[157] The anemia of thiamine-responsive megaloblastic anemia usually improves with thiamine 25–75 mg/day.[176] Folic acid supplements should also be administered because the erythroid hyperplasia increases demand for this vitamin.

There is one report of successful allogeneic peripheral blood stem cell transplantation in a 19-year-old man with transfusion-dependent hereditary sideroblastic anemia.[177] Transfusions are the mainstay of treatment for severe anemia unresponsive to pyridoxine. Regular administration of packed red cells using white blood cell filters are given to relieve symptoms and permit normal childhood development. Iron overload and secondary hemosiderosis rapidly progress after transfusions begin; chelation therapy with desferrioxamine or oral deferasirox should be initiated from the onset.

Iron removal may be of great benefit for patients who have mild or moderate anemia and evidence of iron overload.[172,173] These patients can often tolerate intermittent phlebotomy, which is preferable to chelation therapy for iron removal, and should be continued to reduce ferritin levels to less than 300 ng/mL. All patients with iron overload should avoid ingestion of ascorbic acid supplements, which enhance iron absorption and increase the tissue toxicity of elemental iron. Alcohol should also be avoided. Splenectomy is contraindicated in this disease.

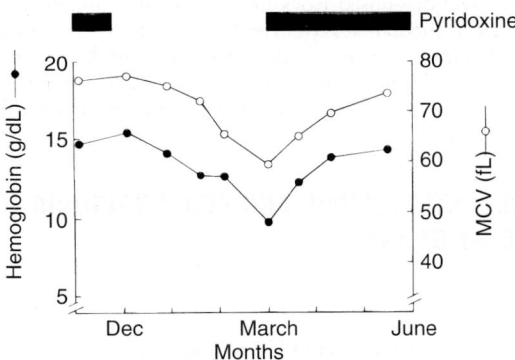

Fig. 38.10 RESPONSE OF THE HEMOGLOBIN CONCENTRATION AND MEAN CORPUSCULAR VOLUME (MCV) TO WITHDRAWAL AND REINSTITUTION OF PYRIDOXINE IN A PATIENT WITH RESPONSIVE HEREDITARY SIDEROBLASTIC ANEMIA.

inner mitochondrial membrane and has been proposed to function as an exporter of mitochondrial iron-sulfur clusters to the cytoplasm[189]; however, a direct role in heme synthesis may arise through an interaction with ferrochelatase.[190] Males affected with XLSA/A usually present in infancy with nonprogressive or slowly progressive ataxia and incoordination, which is accompanied by a mild to moderate hypochromic microcytic anemia and the presence of ring sideroblasts on bone marrow examination.

Mutations in the high-affinity thiamine transporter gene SLC19A2, located at 1q24.2, cause the thiamine-responsive megaloblastic anemia (TRMA) syndrome.[191] TRMA has the unusual bone marrow feature of megaloblastic erythroid maturation with ring sideroblasts. TRMA presents with early-onset megaloblastic anemia, diabetes mellitus, and sensorineural deafness, which respond variably to thiamine treatment.

Missense and nonsense mutations in the PUS1 gene coding for pseudouridine synthase-1 cause the rare autosomal recessive disease, myopathy, lactic acidosis, and sideroblastic anemia (MLASA).[192–195] Mitochondrial and cytoplasmic transfer RNAs (tRNAs) from affected patients lack tRNA pseudouridylation at sites normally modified by PUS1; however, the mechanism by which this affects oxidative phosphorylation and iron metabolism in skeletal muscle and bone marrow are yet to be elucidated.[193] MLASA displays genetic heterogeneity such that an identical phenotype is caused by a homozygous mutation in the mitochondrial tyrosyl-tRNA synthetase gene, YARS2.[194] The homozygous mutation in YARS2, identified in three patients from two consanguineous Lebanese families, causes defective mitochondrial synthesis and, similar to mutations in PUS1, results in defective oxidative phosphorylation.[194] MLASA1 and MLASA2 usually present with progressive exercise intolerance commencing in childhood followed by later development of sideroblastic anemia, basal lactic acidemia, and mitochondrial myopathy.

Over a dozen mutations in the TRNT1 gene, which encodes an essential enzyme that transfers the CCA nucleotide repeat to tRNA molecules, result in sideroblastic anemia with B-cell immunodeficiency, periodic fevers, and developmental delay (SIFD).[196,197] This autosomal recessive syndromic disorder manifests as a severe sideroblastic anemia in infancy, recurrent periodic fevers, B-cell lymphopenia, and hypogammaglobulinemia.

Acquired Sideroblastic Anemia

Acquired sideroblastic anemia is categorized within the myelodysplastic syndromes and may appear de novo or occur after chemotherapy or irradiation (see Table 38.5). The clonal nature of hemopoiesis in this condition was first suggested by Dacie et al.[153] Nearly all cases show evidence of dyserythropoiesis in the marrow, and there may also be dysplastic changes in the myeloid precursors or megakaryocytes, or both. Acquired idiopathic sideroblastic anemia falls within the diagnostic category of refractory anemia with ring sideroblasts as defined by the French-American-British group and World Health Organization classification.[198,199] Acquired sideroblastic anemia is found in myeloproliferative disorders such as idiopathic myelofibrosis or essential thrombocythemia, and distinguishing between idiopathic myelofibrosis and myelodysplasia is sometimes difficult.[199–201] Many patients with refractory anemia with ring sideroblasts and thrombocytosis have a point mutation in the Janus kinase 2 gene (changing valine-617 to phenylalanine), which is a feature usually associated with the myeloproliferative disorders.[202] This latter group have a clinical phenotype that includes normal MCV, marrow fibrosis, and splenomegaly (see Chapter 60).[202] Thus the WHO 2008 classification describes three acquired sideroblastic anemia variants: refractory anemia with ring sideroblasts (RARS); RARS with thrombocytosis (RARS-T), which is included in the myelodysplastic/myeloproliferative neoplasm, unclassifiable category; and, within the refractory cytopenia with multilineage dysplasia (RCMD) category, RCMD and ring sideroblasts (RCMD-RS).

Biologic and Molecular Aspects

Clonal hematopoiesis has been demonstrated in acquired idiopathic sideroblastic anemia and in the related myelodysplastic syndromes. Specific evidence was first provided by finding a single G6PD isoenzyme in erythrocytes, granulocytes, platelets, and B lymphocytes in a woman who was heterozygous for G6PD and carried two isoenzymes in her skin and T lymphocytes.[203] This technique is applicable only to the few women who have G6PD heterozygosity, but restriction fragment length polymorphism analysis can be applied to most women using probes directed at other X-chromosome genes such as that for phosphoglycerate kinase or to an X-linked, variable-copy-number tandem repeat sequence.[204] The results show uniform monoclonality of hematopoiesis in acquired sideroblastic anemia with or without associated myelodysplastic features. Some indirect evidence exists for a primary mitochondrial lesion, perhaps in the mitochondrial respiratory chain, which impairs the reduction of Fe^{3+} because Fe^{2+} is essential for heme synthesis.[205–208] Recurrent mutations in the SF3B1 gene have recently been described in acquired sideroblastic anemia and are found in up to 85% of patients with RARS, RARS-T, and RCMD-RS.[209,210] The product of SF3B1 is associated with mRNA splicing, and mutations in this gene may influence a number of mitochondrial gene networks, including changes in the expression of the iron transporter ABCB7, resulting in iron-laden mitochondria during erythroid development.[211]

Etiology

Clonal chromosomal changes are found in bone marrow cells in approximately 60% of patients with acquired sideroblastic anemia. Characteristic changes are monosomy 7; trisomy 8; deletions involving chromosomes 5, 7, 11, or 20; and a number of balanced translocations.[212] When sideroblastic anemia is acquired after chemotherapy or irradiation, chromosomal changes are usually found and tend to be multiple.[212] Among these changes, the loss of an entire chromosome (5 or 7, or both), deletion of a long arm [del(5), del(7), or del(13)], and an unbalanced translocation are typical.[213,214] When karyotype shows loss of material from chromosomes 5 or 7, or both, a detailed occupational history may show exposure to potentially mutagenic chemical agents in a proportion of patients.[215] However, the development of visible chromosomal changes is probably a late event in acquired sideroblastic anemia and may be preceded by the expansion of a clone of genetically unstable stem cells. This concept is in accord with the view that multiple genetic events underlie the pathogenesis of other myelodysplastic syndromes and acute myeloid leukemia[203,216] (see box on Clinical and Laboratory Evaluation of Sideroblastic Anemia).

Clinical and Laboratory Evaluation of Sideroblastic Anemia

Typically, sideroblastic anemia develops insidiously in a middle-aged or elderly patient with normal or increased mean corpuscular volume (MCV) and a blood smear showing a population of hypochromic red cells. Hepatosplenomegaly may be present. Leukocyte and platelet counts are usually normal, and the presence of a thrombocytosis should prompt investigating for the presence of the JAK2 V617F mutation and RARS-T.[202] If leukopenia or thrombocytopenia is present, a careful search should be made for myelodysplastic features, which lead to the more descriptive term of *refractory cytopenia with multilineage dysplasia* for the condition.[217,218] An iron stain of the bone marrow aspirate shows ring sideroblasts, which should total more than 15% of all erythroblasts to make the diagnosis of acquired sideroblastic anemia.[198,219–221] Iron cannot be assessed in the marrow trephine biopsy core because it may leach out during decalcification.

The bone marrow also shows erythroid hyperplasia. Although mild dyserythropoiesis (e.g., multinuclearity, nuclear budding) and megaloblastoid changes are present, myelopoiesis and megakaryopoiesis are usually normal. When changes are confined to dyserythropoiesis, the condition has been called *refractory anemia with ring sideroblasts*.[220,222] However, dysplasia of myelopoietic and megakaryopoietic elements may be present (i.e., refractory cytopenia with multilineage dysplasia) with the following features: Pelger-Huët–like anomaly, hypersegmentation or hypogranularity of neutrophils, micromegakaryocytes, large mononuclear megakaryocytes, and megakaryocytes with multiple small nuclei (see Chapter 60).[218] Dysmegakaryopoiesis is more easily detected in trephine biopsies than in marrow smears, although the trephine may also show unsuspected islands of myeloblasts characteristic of myelodysplasia.[223] The overall blast count in marrow smears is, by definition, less than 5%, and the peripheral blood monocyte count is less than 1.0×10^9/L. Cytogenetic analysis of marrow aspirates provides important information, because a normal karyotype predicts long survival in any type of acquired sideroblastic anemia.[224]

Differential Diagnosis

Ring sideroblasts are not limited to acquired sideroblastic anemia; they also occur in other myelodysplastic conditions, such as refractory anemia with excess blasts, in which the blast count is higher than 5%.[225] Careful examination of peripheral blood and bone marrow can distinguish acquired idiopathic sideroblastic anemia from these related myelodysplastic conditions. Family surveys are very useful in distinguishing acquired from hereditary forms of sideroblastic anemia, because the latter may present in late adult life.

Prognosis

Acquired idiopathic sideroblastic anemia and the related entity of refractory anemia have the most favorable outlook among the myelodysplastic syndromes, with a median survival of 42 to 76 months and 3% to 12% incidence of leukemic progression in different series.[212,226,227] The prognosis can be correlated with three factors. First is the severity of the anemia, because repeated transfusions markedly increase iron overload and invariably lead to the organ dysfunction characteristic of secondary hemosiderosis (e.g., heart and liver failure, diabetes), and whether neutropenia and thrombocytopenia are associated with the anemia. These cytopenias form the basis of a simple prognostic scoring system in which two or more of the following place the patient in a poor prognostic category: hemoglobin level less than 10 g/dL, neutrophil count less than 1.8×10^9/L, platelet count less than 100×10^9/L.[226,227] Secondly, marrow blasts more than 5% of total nucleated cells predict a poor outcome. Thirdly, karyotypic analysis of marrow aspirates provides valuable information, because a normal karyotype carries a more favorable prognosis. Conversely, chromosome 7 abnormalities impart a high probability of transformation to acute myeloid leukemia. Multiple chromosomal abnormalities and del(20q) are also associated with an increased risk for progression to leukemia; in contrast, trisomy 8 has no adverse prognostic significance.[212] The bone marrow blast percentage, karyotypic analysis, and the presence of peripheral blood cytopenias can be used to group newly diagnosed cases into one of five prognostic groups, which range in median survival from more than 8 years to less than 1 year.[228] Evolution of acquired idiopathic sideroblastic anemia to other myelodysplastic conditions, such as refractory anemia with excess blasts, has been described[229] (see box on Therapy for Acquired Sideroblastic Anemia).

SIDEROBLASTIC ANEMIA AND PORPHYRINURIA CAUSED BY DRUGS

Alcohol

Ring sideroblasts may be found in the bone marrow of malnourished anemic alcoholics, usually in the presence of associated folate

---

Therapy for Acquired Sideroblastic Anemia

Transfusions are indicated for relief of symptomatic anemia. A trial of pyridoxine at 100–200 mg/day for 3 months is worthwhile in patients who have anemia but who do not display neutropenia or thrombocytopenia. However, few patients with acquired idiopathic sideroblastic anemia respond to this vitamin. If any response is achieved, maintenance therapy with pyridoxine at lower dosage is indicated. Cyclosporin (5–6 mg/kg/day) has been reported to benefit the anemia of the closely related myelodysplastic condition of refractory anemia, although the response appeared limited to those with hypoplastic bone marrows.[230] A number of agents, including erythropoietin, 5-azacytidine, decitabine, and lenalidomide, have been studied in therapeutic trials for myelodysplastic syndrome, which have included acquired sideroblastic anemia cases; however, overall outcomes have been poor.[231] It is unclear if iron chelation therapy with the oral iron-chelator, deferasirox is of benefit; however, this question may be answered by ongoing clinical trials.[232,233]

deficiency.[234-236] In contrast, binge drinking or chronic alcohol ingestion in subjects with good nutrition is not associated with sideroblastic abnormality. Sideroblastic change is never the sole cause for the anemia of alcoholism. Alcohol has a direct toxic effect on hematopoiesis.[237] An increased or high-normal MCV and vacuolation of red blood cell precursors is often seen in addition to the ring sideroblast abnormality. Red blood cells show dimorphic morphology; evidence in the marrow of folate deficiency is present in half of cases.[237] Transferrin saturation and marrow iron stores tend to be increased but may be low if gastrointestinal bleeding is present. The ring sideroblasts gradually disappear over 4 to 12 days when alcohol is withdrawn[234]; during this period, there may be a rebound erythroid hyperplasia, reticulocytosis, and thrombocytosis. Folic acid should be given for the associated megaloblastic changes after blood is taken for vitamin B_{12} and folate assays.

Alcohol consumption lowers the plasma concentration of pyridoxal phosphate, a cofactor for ALAS, needed in the first step in heme synthesis.[238] Conversion of ethanol to acetaldehyde is necessary for this effect, and acetaldehyde acts by accelerating the degradation of intracellular pyridoxal phosphate in the liver, lowering plasma levels of this coenzyme.[239]

Chronic alcoholics have an altered heme metabolism with increased urinary excretion of coproporphyrin, mainly isomer III, but normal urinary excretion of uroporphyrin, ALA, and porphobilinogen. Acute and chronic ethanol ingestion markedly depresses the activity of ALA dehydratase in peripheral blood. Ethanol administration to normal subjects results in increased activity of leukocyte ALAS and erythrocyte PBGD, the two rate-controlling enzymes of the pathway. The activities of each of the other four enzymes are depressed. Ferrochelatase, the enzyme that inserts iron into protoporphyrin to form heme, shows the most marked depression, and in alcoholism there is prolonged depression of uroporphyrinogen decarboxylase, which provides a rationale for the role of ethanol in the etiology of PCT.[240,241] As earlier, ethanol is a major precipitating factor in acute porphyria.[242]

Isoniazid

Administration of the antituberculous drug isoniazid has occasionally been associated with development of a sideroblastic anemia after 1 to 10 months of therapy. The anemia is hypochromic and microcytic, with a dimorphic blood smear and ring sideroblasts in the marrow. This complication is thought to occur only in slow acetylators of isoniazid, allowing this drug to react nonenzymatically with pyridoxal and to form a hydrazone that is rapidly excreted in the urine. The anemia can be fully reversed by coadministration of pyridoxine (25-50 mg/day) with isoniazid or by withdrawing isoniazid.[243] Another antituberculous drug, pyrazinamide, may also cause a sideroblastic anemia, which is caused by inhibition of ALAS2 and responds to pyridoxine therapy.[244]

Chloramphenicol

Chloramphenicol is an antibiotic that produces a reversible suppression of erythropoiesis after several days of therapy (plasma levels of 10-15 μg/mL). This effect is predictable and separate from the rare idiosyncratic side effect of aplastic anemia in approximately 1 of 20,000 exposed persons. Nearly all patients given chloramphenicol (>2 g/day) develop vacuolation of the erythroid precursors and ring sideroblasts. These effects are thought to arise from suppression of mitochondrial respiration. Chloramphenicol inhibits mitochondrial protein synthesis and reduces cytochrome a, a_3, and b levels.[245] Serum iron concentrations are increased, and reticulocyte numbers are subnormal; these changes revert on stopping the antibiotic.

Other Drugs

A reversible acquired sideroblastic anemia has been described with penicillamine, linezolid, and with the use of triethylene tetramine

hydrochloride, a copper-chelating agent used in the treatment of Wilson disease.[246,247] Acquired sideroblastic anemia has also been precipitated by progesterone given to a patient on two separate occasions 15 years apart, and this anemia promptly reversed on withdrawal of the drug.[248]

PRESENTATIONS ASSOCIATED WITH SIDEROBLASTIC ANEMIA OR PORPHYRINURIA

Copper Deficiency or Zinc Overload

The copper content of a Western diet averages 0.9 to 1.6 mg each day, which is only a few times greater than the amount needed to maintain homeostasis of this essential element.[249] Copper deficiency has been described in malnourished premature infants,[250] in patients receiving long-term parenteral or enteral hyperalimentation,[251] after gastrectomy,[252] with copper-chelating agents,[246] or on an idiopathic basis.[253] The syndrome of copper deficiency consists of sideroblastic anemia with hypochromic cells in the blood smear, accompanied by ring sideroblasts and vacuolated erythroid and myeloid precursors in the marrow, and of neutropenia with an absence of late myeloid forms in the marrow (Fig. 38.11). In some reports, patients present with neurologic symptoms such as paresthesias, weakness, or ataxia; and demyelination is seen on the magnetic resonance image of the brain.[253] In infants, additional features may be seen, such as osteoporosis and long bone changes, depigmentation of skin and hair, and central nervous system abnormalities. The platelet counts remain normal. Serum copper and ceruloplasmin levels are low, whereas serum iron and transferrin saturation levels are normal. The serum zinc concentration may be increased.[253] Prompt reversal of the hematologic changes follows therapy with 2 to 5 mg/day of copper sulfate taken orally or 100 to 500 μg/day of copper supplement to the intravenous alimentation formula.

Large quantities of ingested zinc interfere with copper absorption and produce the neutropenia and sideroblastic anemia characteristic of copper deficiency.[254] Zinc sulfate is freely available from health food stores, and as little as 450 mg/day for 2 years is sufficient for this effect. Sideroblastic anemia has also been ascribed to zinc toxicity arising from the ingestion of coins over a period of many years.[255] Serum zinc levels are high, whereas serum copper and ceruloplasmin levels are low. Zinc must be discontinued for 9 to 12 weeks for full reversal of the anemia and neutropenia.

Iron Deficiency Anemia

In iron deficiency anemia, there is an accumulation of protoporphyrin in erythrocytes that rarely reaches the level found in EPP. The zinc complex of protoporphyrin is produced because ferrochelatase uses Zn^{2+} during iron-deficient erythropoiesis.[256] Erythrocyte protoporphyrin may be raised before changes appear in peripheral blood and may be helpful in diagnosing iron deficiency when serum iron and ferritin levels are rising as a result of patients having started iron therapy. In iron-deficient erythropoiesis, erythroid ALAS activity is reduced below normal.[257]

Hypothermia

Thrombocytopenia, erythroid hypoplasia, and ring sideroblasts have been described in patients with hypothermia associated with neurologic disease.[258] These changes reverse slowly as body temperature returns to normal.

Other Conditions

In hereditary tyrosinemia, excess urinary ALA is excreted because ALA dehydratase is inhibited by succinyl acetone. Like acute

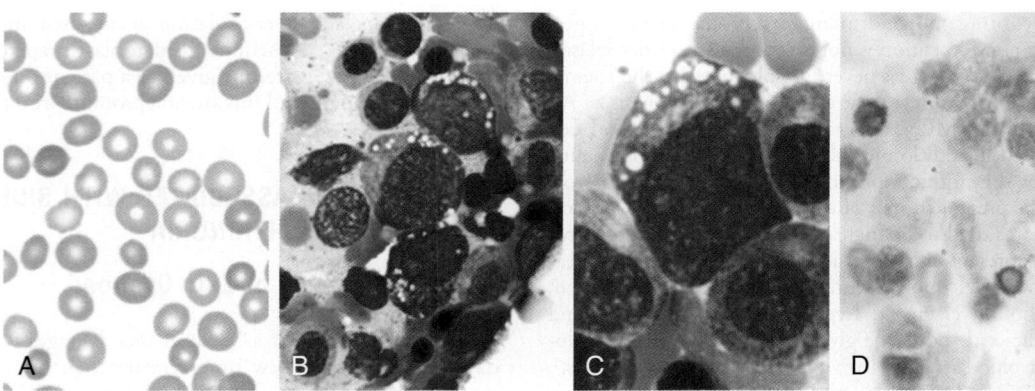

Fig. 38.11 This 70-year-old man was being treated with zinc supplementation and was found to have anemia and neutropenia (hemoglobin, 8.3 g/dL; hematocrit, 23.9%; and white blood cell count, 1200/µL). His peripheral smear (A) showed a biphasic erythroid population with some small slightly hypochromic cells and increased anisocytosis (red blood cell distribution width [RDW], 23.9%). The bone marrow aspirate showed a left shift in granulopoiesis with vacuolization of immature granulocytic and erythroid precursors (B, C). A Prussian blue–stained aspirate revealed ring sideroblasts (D). The patient's copper level was less than 0.1 µg/mL (normal reference range, 0.75–1.45 µg/mL).

Lead Poisoning

It has been known for some time that patients suffering from lead poisoning have an accumulation of protoporphyrin in erythrocytes and increased urinary excretion of ALA and coproporphyrin.[262] There are sex-related differences in the porphyrin synthetic response to lead, with females showing a more profound coproporphyrinuria than men.[263] The elevated protoporphyrin chelated by zinc is retained in the erythrocyte, which may explain the absence of photosensitivity. This accumulation of porphyrins and precursors is caused by the inhibition by lead of the heme biosynthetic enzymes: 5-aminolevulinate (ALA) dehydratase, coproporphyrinogen oxidase, and ferrochelatase. An increase in the activity of the rate-controlling enzyme ALA synthase (ALAS) results.

Many of the clinical manifestations of lead poisoning may be the result of altered heme biosynthesis.[79] A mild to moderate anemia that can be hypochromic and microcytic occurs in a minority of patients, whereas basophilic stippling is prominent because of inhibition of pyrimidine 5'-nucleotidase in the maturing reticulocyte. Ring sideroblasts have not been reported. The abdominal pain, constipation, and peripheral neuropathy that occur in lead poisoning are also seen in acute attacks of hepatic porphyria. Neuropathy, seen in lead poisoning, may also be the result of disorders of heme biosynthesis, as in the porphyrias.[262] Alterations in porphyrin metabolism have provided a useful means of detecting and assessing the severity of lead exposure and poisoning. The diminution in activity of erythrocyte ALA dehydratase and elevated erythrocyte protoporphyrin levels are the most sensitive measures.

may represent mild chronic cases of porphyria or other acquired abnormalities in heme synthesis. However, evidence for this concept is lacking.[263,264]

SUGGESTED READINGS

Aivado M, Gattermann N, Rong A, et al: X-linked sideroblastic anemia associated with a novel ALAS2 mutation and unfortunate skewed X-chromosome inactivation patterns. *Blood Cells Mol Dis* 37:40, 2006.

Ajioka RS, Phillips JD, Weiss RB, et al: Down-regulation of hepcidin in porphyria cutanea tarda. *Blood* 112:4723, 2008.

Anderson KE, Bloomer JR, Bonkovsky HL, et al: Recommendations for the diagnosis and treatment of the acute porphyrias. *Ann Intern Med* 142:439, 2005.

Bergmann AK, Campagna DR, McLoughlin EM, et al: Systematic molecular genetic analysis of congenital sideroblastic anemia: evidence for genetic heterogeneity and identification of novel mutations. *Pediatr Blood Cancer* 54:273, 2010.

Bishop DF, Tchaikovskii V, Nazarenko I, et al: Molecular expression and characterization of erythroid-specific 5-aminolevulinate synthase gain-of-function mutations causing X-linked protoporphyria. *Mol Med* 19:18, 2013.

Bottomley SS, Fleming MD: Sideroblastic anemia: diagnosis and management. *Hematol Oncol Clin North Am* 28:653–670, 2014.

Campagna DR, de Bie CI, Schmitz-Abe K, et al: X-linked sideroblastic anemia due to ALAS2 intron 1 enhancer element GATA-binding site mutations. *Am J Hematol* 89(3):315–319, 2014.

Chakraborty PK, Schmitz-Abe K, Kennedy EK, et al: Mutations in TRNT1 cause congenital sideroblastic anemia with immunodeficiency, fevers, and developmental delay (SIFD). *Blood* 124:2867, 2014.

Chen W, Dailey HA, Paw BH: Ferrochelatase forms an oligomeric complex with mitoferrin-1 and Abcb10 for erythroid heme biosynthesis. *Blood* 116:628, 2010.

Ducamp S, Kannengiesser C, Touati M, et al: Sideroblastic anemia: molecular analysis of the ALAS2 gene in a series of 29 probands and functional studies of 10 missense mutations. *Hum Mutat* 32:590, 2011.

Donker AE, Raymakers RA, Nieuwenhuis HK, et al: Practice guidelines for the diagnosis and management of microcytic anemias due to genetic disorders of iron metabolism or heme synthesis. *Blood* 123:3873, 2014.

Furuyama K, Harigae H, Heller T, et al: Arg-452 substitution of the erythroid-specific 5-aminolaevulinate synthase, a hot spot mutation in X-linked sideroblastic anaemia, does not itself affect enzyme activity. *Eur J Haematol* 76:33, 2006.

Goodwin RG, Kell J, Laidler P, et al: Photosensitivity and acute liver injury in myeloproliferative disorder secondary to late-onset protoporphyria

porphyria and lead poisoning, this disease is associated with neurobehavioral disturbance (see box on Lead Poisoning). In liver disease, there may be increased urinary excretion of coproporphyrin, predominantly isomer I. In the Dubin-Johnson syndrome, which is caused by mutations in the ABCC2 gene, the ratio of coproporphyrin isomer I to isomer III is markedly increased in the urine (>80%), possibly as a result of deficiency of hepatic uroporphyrinogen III cosynthase and increased activity of PBGD.[259] In Rotor syndrome, total urinary excretion of coproporphyrin is markedly increased and consists predominantly of coproporphyrin isomer I.[260] In the unconjugated hyperbilirubinemia of Gilbert syndrome, depressed activity of protoporphyrinogen oxidase and increased activity of ALAS has been found in peripheral leukocytes.[261]

Environmental Intolerances

It has been hypothesized that several otherwise-unexplained chemical-associated illnesses, such as multiple chemical sensitivity syndrome,

caused by deletion of a ferrochelatase gene in hematopoietic cells. *Blood* 107:60, 2006.

Guernsey DL, Jiang H, Campagna DR, et al: Mutations in mitochondrial carrier family gene SLC25A38 cause nonsyndromic autosomal recessive congenital sideroblastic anemia. *Nat Genet* 41:651, 2009.

Harigae H, Furuyama K: Hereditary sideroblastic anemia: pathophysiology and gene mutations. *Int J Hematol* 92(3):425–431, 2010.

Katugampola RP, Anstey AV, Finlay AY, et al: A management algorithm for congenital erythropoietic porphyria derived from a study of 29 cases. *Br J Dermatol* 167(4):888–900, 2012.

Lin CS, Krishnan AV, Lee MJ, et al: Nerve function and dysfunction in acute intermittent porphyria. *Brain* 131:2510, 2008.

Malcovati L, Cazzola M: Refractory anemia with ring sideroblasts. *Best Pract Res Clin Haematol* 26:377, 2013.

Phillips JD, Bergonia HA, Reilly CA, et al: A porphomethene inhibitor of uroporphyrinogen decarboxylase causes porphyria cutanea tarda. *Proc Natl Acad Sci USA* 104:5079, 2007.

Pondarre C, Campagna DR, Antioches B, et al: Abcb7, the gene responsible for X-linked sideroblastic anemia with ataxia, is essential for hematopoiesis. *Blood* 109:3567, 2007.

Puy H, Gouya L, Deybach JC: Porphyrias. *Lancet* 375:924, 2010.

Rand EB, Bunin N, Cochran W, et al: Sequential liver and bone marrow transplantation for treatment of erythropoietic protoporphyria. *Pediatrics* 118:1896, 2006.

Richardson DR, Lane DJ, Becker EM, et al: Mitochondrial iron trafficking and the integration of iron metabolism between the mitochondrion and cytosol. *Proc Natl Acad Sci USA* 107:10775, 2010.

Schultz IJ, Chen C, Paw BH, et al: Iron and porphyrin trafficking in heme biogenesis. *J Biol Chem* 285:26753, 2010.

Szpurka H, Tiu R, Murugesan G, et al: Refractory anemia with ringed sideroblasts associated with marked thrombocytosis (RARS-T), another myeloproliferative condition characterized by JAK2 V617F mutation. *Blood* 108:2173, 2006.

Thunell S, Pomp E, Brun A: Guide to drug porphyrogenicity prediction and drug prescription in the acute porphyrias. *Br J Clin Pharmacol* 64:668, 2007.

Ye H, Jeong SY, Ghosh MC, et al: Glutaredoxin 5 deficiency causes sideroblastic anemia by specifically impairing heme biosynthesis and depleting cytosolic iron in human erythroblasts. *J Clin Invest* 120:1749, 2010.

REFERENCES

For the complete list of references, log on to www.expertconsult.com.

The term *megaloblastic anemia* is used to describe a group of disorders characterized by a distinct morphologic pattern in hematopoietic cells. A common feature is a defect in deoxyribonucleic acid (DNA) synthesis, with lesser alterations in ribonucleic acid (RNA) and protein synthesis, leading to a state of unbalanced cell growth and impaired cell division. Most megaloblastic cells are not resting but vainly engaged in attempting to double their DNA, with frequent arrest in the S phase and lesser degrees of arrest in other phases of the cell cycle. An increased percentage of these cells have DNA values between 2 N (N is the amount of DNA in the haploid genome) and 4 N because of delayed cell division. This increased DNA content in megaloblastic cells is morphologically expressed as larger-than-normal "immature" nuclei with finely particulate chromatin, whereas the relatively unimpaired RNA and protein synthesis results in large cells with greater "mature" cytoplasm and cell volume. The net result of megaloblastosis is a cell whose nuclear maturation is arrested (immature) while its cytoplasmic maturation proceeds normally independently of the nuclear events. The microscopic appearance of this nuclear-cytoplasmic asynchrony (or dissociation) is morphologically described as megaloblastic. Each cell lineage has a limited but unique repertoire of expression of defective DNA synthesis. This is significantly influenced by the normal patterns of maturation of the affected cell line. Additional variables that affect RNA and protein synthesis can lead to the attenuation or modification of megaloblastic expression (see Masked Megaloblastosis).

Megaloblastic hematopoiesis commonly manifests as anemia, but this feature is only a manifestation of a more global defect in DNA synthesis that affects all proliferating cells. The peripheral blood picture is characteristic and reflective of megaloblastic hematopoiesis within the bone marrow. The diagnosis is therefore usually straightforward, but because any condition that specifically perturbs DNA synthesis may lead to megaloblastosis, determination of the precise cause is necessary before institution of therapy. Inappropriate therapy can lead to disastrous consequences for the patient. The biochemical basis for megaloblastosis needs to be understood within the context of evaluation of potential and real variables affecting DNA, RNA, and protein synthesis in a given patient. The most common causes of megaloblastosis are true cellular deficiencies of vitamin B_{12} (cobalamin) or folate, vitamins that are essential for DNA synthesis.

Because of the imperative for conservation of cobalamin within the body, there is a finely tuned mechanism in place to ensure a sequential handover of this precious cargo from one protein to another—from the point of its entry into the mouth through the gut, across the enterocyte, into the circulation with specialized uptake into cells, passage through lysosomes into cytoplasm, and even into mitochondria. Throughout this odyssey, cobalamin is accompanied by several chaperones that sequentially bind, sequester, and thereby ensure that cobalamin does not participate in side reactions. This ensures its fitness for service for critical enzymes.

Despite the greater abundance of folate in the diet relative to cobalamin, there are also specialized means to ensure that the natural folates in food are first chopped and diced before being ushered across the enterocyte through specialized pathways. After passage from the portal blood into the general circulation, folate is extracted by cell surface folate receptors, undergoes endocytosis, and is then shunted together with a proton across another channel into the cytoplasm. It is then received by an overabundance of high-affinity multifunctional enzymes that channel the folate across set pathways to support critical synthesis of thymidine for DNA.

Indeed, the care with which cobalamin and folate are handled is analogous to the swarm of Secret Service agents escorting a president as he walks by a crowd of well-wishers, their sole aim being to prevent him from getting too close to the public—to shake hands, or hug and kiss a baby, and the like, which could also expose him to potential harm by an ill-wisher—and detract him from doing his primary job as chief executive.

A general principle is that the preexisting store of these vitamins will dictate the speed with which overt deficiency develops; this is particularly relevant to pregnant women and children in developing countries with preexisting borderline stores of folate and cobalamin.

The pathophysiology of cellular cobalamin and folate deficiency is most readily discerned by the clinician who approaches megaloblastosis with a clear understanding of the physiology of these vitamins. A detailed discussion of cobalamin and folate therefore follows.

COBALAMIN

The term *cobalamin* refers to a family of compounds with the structure shown in Fig. 39.1. Details of the chemistry, nomenclature, and in vivo substitutions of cobalamin are shown in Figs. 39.1 through 39.3, and excellent reviews are available on the colorful history, chemistry, and biology of cobalamin.[1-4]

Nutrition

Cobalamin is produced in nature only by microorganisms, and humans receive cobalamin solely from the diet.[5,6] Cobalamin is synthesized and used by some microorganisms (e.g., bacteria, fungi). Some strains (such as *Pseudomonas denitrificans*) produce cobalamin during fermentation, making them excellent and cheap commercial sources for cobalamin used in therapy. Herbivores obtain their dietary quota of cobalamin from plants contaminated with cobalamin-producing soil bacteria (rhizobia) that grow in roots and nodules of legumes. Because rhizobia-related organisms are also found in the large intestine of animals (and humans), volitional or inadvertent coprophagy can lead to intake of cobalamin by herbivores; however, cobalamin from manure that contaminates plants is not likely to be a significant source for humans.[5] Nevertheless, colonic cobalamin-producing bacteria—like *Klebsiella pneumoniae* that are related to rhizobia—can be found in the small intestine of some individuals from which cobalamin can be absorbed. For all practical purposes, there is *no* unfortified plant food, including fermented soy products, tempeh/*tempe*, seaweed (which are actually multicellular algae, such as nori [red algae], chlorella [green algae], spirulina [blue-green algae]), or other organic produce that can consistently provide a sufficient amount of active cobalamin to support daily requirements.

Animal protein is the major dietary cobalamin source for nonvegetarians. Meats from parenchymal organs are richest in cobalamin (over 10 μg/100 g wet weight); fish and muscle meats, milk products, and egg yolk have 1 to 10 μg/100 g of wet weight. An average nonvegetarian Western diet contains 5 to 7 μg/day of cobalamin, which adequately sustains normal cobalamin equilibrium.

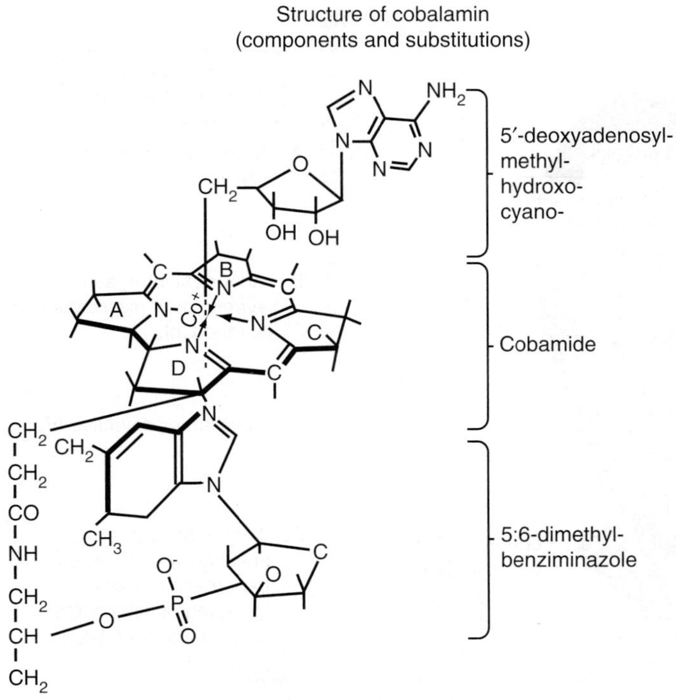

Structure of cobalamin
(components and substitutions)

Fig. 39.1 COBALAMIN (VITAMIN B$_{12}$) CHEMISTRY AND NOMEN-CLATURE. The central cobalt atom of cobalamin forms the focal point of this large complex organometallic molecule (approximately 1300 to 1500 Da). There are up to six ligands that can bind to this cobalt; of these, four involve nitrogen atoms of the planar corrin ring that surround the cobalt atom. The lower α-axial ligand, extending perpendicular below the corrin ring, links to nitrogen of a 5,6-dimethylbenzimidazole phosphoribosyl moiety that is also attached back to the corrin ring through one of its propionamide side chains (this is analogous to the hand guard on the handle on a sabre that covers the knuckles of the hand). The upper or β-axial ligand varies and can exist in the fully oxidized Co^{3+} state, which is referred to as cob(III)alamin; in the Co^{2+} state, called cob(II)alamin (which can be used for the synthesis of methylcobalamin or adenosylcobalamin); or the fully reduced Co$^+$ state (cob[I]alamin). These upper axial ligands include cyano- (cyanocobalamin), hydroxyl- (hydroxocobalamin), methyl- (methylcobalamin), or 5′-deoxyadenosyl- (adenosylcobalamin) and confer a distinct identity to cobalamin for participation in one-carbon metabolism. All these forms with substituted upper axial ligands are cob(III)alamins, which adopt a configuration in which the 5,6-dimethylbenzimidazole nitrogen base is coordinated to the cobalt in the lower axial position. This is referred to as the "base-on" position. However, when cobalamin is bound to the enzymes methionine synthase and methylmalonyl-CoA mutase, another conformational change results in the replacement of the 5,6-dimethylbenzimidazole by a histidine donated by the enzyme; this is the "His-on" position. Thus shifts from "base-on/His-off" conformation to an alternative "base-off/His-on" conformation have an important bearing on the catalytic activity of these enzymes. Conversion of cyanocobalamin to its active cofactor forms requires a decyanation step. *(From Chanarin I: The megaloblastic anemias, Oxford, UK, 1979, Blackwell Scientific Publications.)*

A vegetarian diet supplies between 0.25 and 0.5 μg/day of cobalamin, so all vegetarians *do not* receive adequate dietary cobalamin and are at risk for cobalamin deficiency.[7,8] Even a Mediterranean diet with modest intake of animal-source proteins places mothers and babies at risk for cobalamin deficiency.[9] The current recommended daily allowance is 2.4 μg for men and nonpregnant women, 2.6 μg for pregnant women, 2.8 μg for lactating women, and 1.5 to 2 μg for children 9 to 18 years old.[10] However, reevaluation of cobalamin requirements within a university community (aged 18–50 years) from the USA suggests that a higher intake of 4 to 7 micrograms of cobalamin each day is optimum for adequate cobalamin status.[11] This is in line with earlier studies from the USA and Europe.[12–14]

Food cobalamin is stable to high-temperature cooking but is readily converted to inactive cobalamin analogues by ascorbic acid. Cobalamin is exceptionally well stored in tissues in its coenzyme forms. Of the total-body content of 2 to 5 mg in adults, about 1 mg is in the liver. There is an obligatory loss of 0.1% per day (1.3 μg) regardless of total-body cobalamin content. It takes about 3 to 4 years to deplete cobalamin stores when dietary cobalamin is abruptly malabsorbed, but it may take longer to develop nutritional cobalamin deficiency, because of an efficient enterohepatic circulation, which accounts for turnover of 5 to 10 μg/day of cobalamin.[15]

Absorption

Cobalamin in food is usually in coenzyme form (5′-deoxyadenosyl-cobalamin [adenosylcobalamin] and methylcobalamin), nonspecifically bound to proteins (see Fig. 39.2). In the stomach, peptic digestion at low pH is a prerequisite for cobalamin release from food protein.[15] Once released by proteolysis, cobalamin preferentially binds a high-affinity, 150-kDa, cobalamin-binding protein called *R protein* (a haptocorrin) from gastric juice and saliva that has higher affinity for cobalamin than gastric intrinsic factor (IF). The cobalamin–R protein (holo-R protein) complex, along with excess unbound (apo)-R protein and IF, pass through into the second part of the duodenum, where pancreatic proteases degrade holo-R and apo-R proteins (but not IF). This results in the transfer of cobalamin to IF, a 45-kDa glycoprotein with high-affinity binding (K$_a$ = 1.5 × 10^{10} M^{-1}), 1:1 molar stoichiometry, stability, and resistance to proteolysis over a pH range of 3 to 9.[15] Failure to degrade holo-R proteins by pancreatic protease precludes the involvement of IF in cobalamin absorption because the downstream ileal IF-cobalamin receptors only interact with IF-bound cobalamin.[15] Although R proteins bind cobalamin and most cobalamin analogues with comparably high affinity, IF only binds cobalamin.

IF is produced in parietal (oxyntic) cells in the fundus and cardia of the stomach.[15] IF has two binding sites: one for cobalamin and another for the ileal IF-cobalamin receptor. IF is produced in far greater excess than is actually required for absorption, and the IF in only 2 to 4 mL of normal gastric juice can reverse cobalamin deficiency in adults who lack IF.[15] In the absence of IF, less than 2% of ingested cobalamin is absorbed, whereas in its presence, approximately 70% is absorbed.

IF is secreted in response to food in the stomach in a manner analogous to secretion of acid (i.e., by vagal and hormonal stimulation). IF binds biliary cobalamin and newly ingested cobalamin following its transfer from R protein.[15] Because biliary cobalamin analogues are not transferred from R protein to IF, this is an efficient method for fecal excretion of cobalamin analogues while allowing for reabsorption of biliary cobalamin. The stable IF-cobalamin complex passes through the jejunum to the ileum, where specific membrane-associated IF-cobalamin receptors for IF-cobalamin are located on microvilli of ileal mucosal cells.[15]

The functional IF-cobalamin receptors are composed of a complex of two proteins collectively known as cubam, composed of *cubi*lin[16] and *amn*ionless,[17] that is essential to complete transport of the IF-cobalamin complex from the intestinal lumen into the enterocyte. Cubilin is a large (400-kDa) peripheral membrane protein, which requires the smaller transmembrane protein, amnionless, for its expression at the brush border, and vice versa. Dysfunction of cubam because of mutation in either cubilin or amnionless is the basis for Imerslund-Gräsbeck syndrome. These IF-cobalamin receptors (cubam) require Ca^{2+} for binding at pH above 5.4; they do not bind free IF, cobalamin, or R protein–bound cobalamin; so these receptors are highly specific and have a high affinity for IF-cobalamin (K$_a$ = 1 × 10^9 M^{-1}). The human ileum contains enough cubam receptors to bind up to 1 mg of IF-bound cobalamin; this is the rate-limiting factor in cobalamin absorption.[15]

After the cobalamin-IF complex is internalized by cubam receptor for subsequent processing, cubam is recycled to the cell surface, whereas cobalamin enters the cytoplasm. Subsequent physiologic

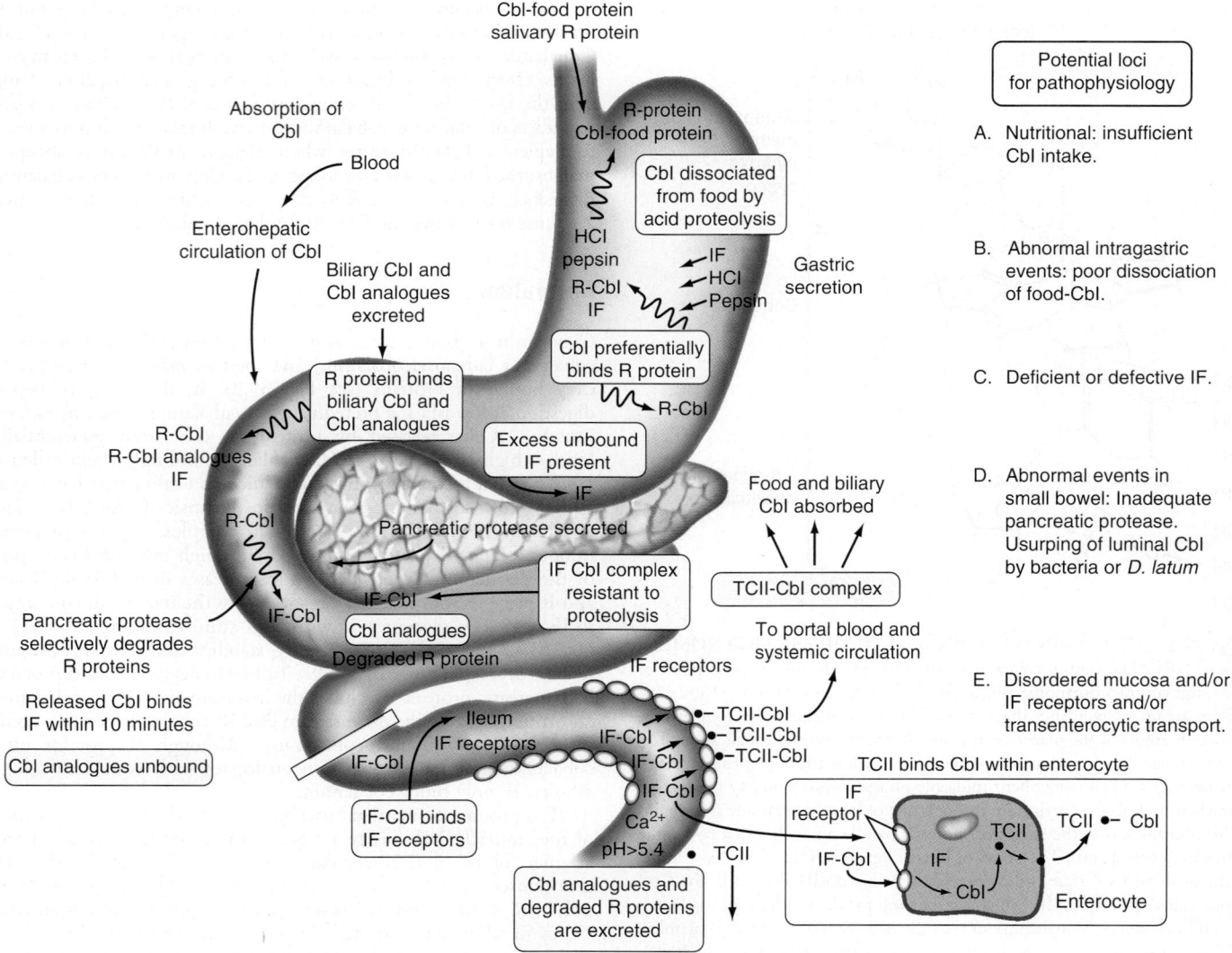

Fig. 39.2 COMPONENTS AND MECHANISM OF COBALAMIN ABSORPTION. *Cbl,* Cobalamin; *D. latum, Diphyllobothrium latum; HCl,* hydrochloric acid; *IF,* intrinsic factor; *R-Cbl,* R-protein bound cobalamin; *TCII,* transcobalamin II.

events are unclear. The multidrug resistance–associated protein (MRP) 1 mediates the cellular export of cobalamin across the basolateral membrane of intestinal epithelium.[18,19] Then cobalamin apparently binds transcobalamin II (TCII) within or at the basal surface of the ileal enterocyte.[15] TCII, which is abundant in the microvascular endothelium, is also available to bind cobalamin. After 3 to 5 hours, cobalamin appears in portal blood largely (over 90%) bound to TCII and reaches peak levels in about 8 hours.[15]

Cobalamin in large doses can also passively diffuse through buccal, gastric, and jejunal mucosa so that less than 1% of a large dose of oral cobalamin appears in the circulation in minutes. This property is used to advantage in individuals with cobalamin malabsorption in lieu of parenteral replacement (discussed later).[15]

Transport

More than 90% of recently absorbed or injected cobalamin is bound to TCII, which is the specific transport protein for delivery of cobalamin to tissues. TCII, a 38-kDa polypeptide synthesized in many tissues, preferentially binds cobalamin with 1:1 molar stoichiometry and high affinity ($K_a = 1 \times 10^{11}$ M^{-1}).[15] The TCII-cobalamin complex is rapidly cleared from the circulation in less

than an hour. TCII-bound cobalamin binds to specific cell surface 58-kDa TCII-cobalamin receptors (encoded by the *CD320* gene) present on several cells.[20,21] High-affinity TCII-cobalamin binding to TCII-cobalamin receptors is specific only for holo- and apo-TCII ($K_a = \sim 5 \times 10^{10}$ M^{-1}). However, because some cobalamin analogues can bind TCII with high affinity, these also have the same potential for cellular uptake as cobalamin.[15]

Circulating cobalamin, which is predominantly in the form of methylcobalamin, is not found free in plasma. Binding to TCII accounts for only 10% to 30% of the total serum cobalamin, with the majority (approximately 75%) of remaining cobalamin being bound to another protein, transcobalamin I (TCI). TCI (another haptocorrin) binds biologically active cobalamins as well as biologically inactive cobalamin derivatives. Because TCI is not a transport protein, it is best viewed as a plasma-storage form of cobalamin; indeed, cobalamin-bound TCI has a slow clearance rate (half-life of 9 to 12 days).[22] A third transport protein, transcobalamin III (TCIII), is closely related to TCI but has a half-life in minutes because it is an asialoglycoprotein. TCIII binds a wide spectrum of cobalamin analogues with high affinity and delivers them via hepatic asialoglycoprotein receptors to hepatic cells, and thence into bile for fecal excretion. Between 0.5 and 9 μg of cobalamin taken up by hepatic TCII receptors is secreted into bile, of which approximately 75% is

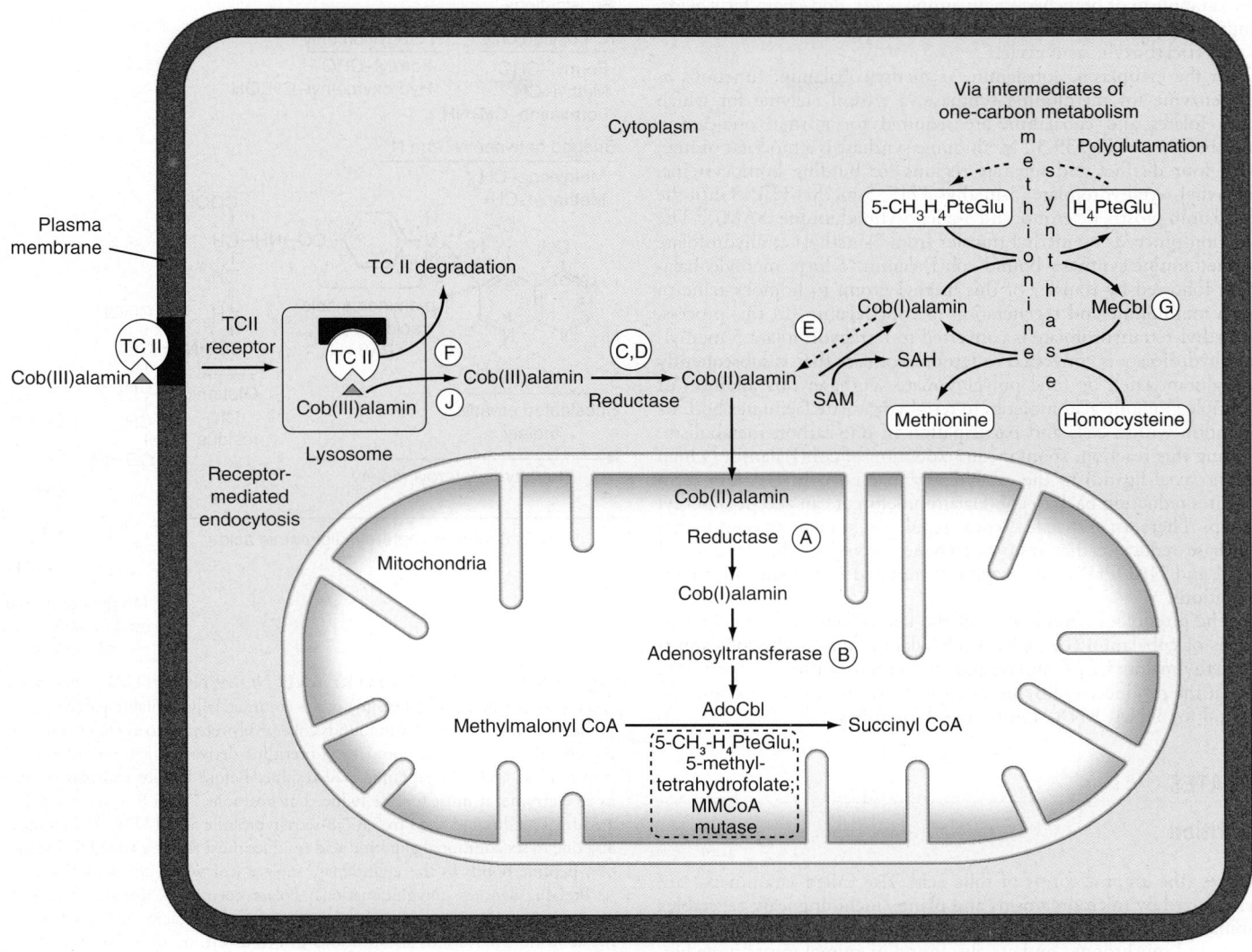

Fig. 39.3 CELLULAR UPTAKE AND INTRACELLULAR REACTIONS INVOLVING COBALAMIN. A large family of natural and synthetic cobalamins can be generated when the cyanide (CN) moiety (upper axial ligand in cyanocobalamin) is replaced. On exposure to light, CN is gradually lost from cyanocobalamin, with the production of hydroxocobalamin. In vivo substitutions include the replacement of hydroxocobalamin or cyanocobalamin by a 5′-deoxyadenosyl group attached by a covalent bond, giving rise to adenosylcobalamin (AdoCbl). Methylcobalamin (MeCbl) is the main form in plasma. In vivo, 5-methyltetrahydrofolate readily donates its methyl group to cob(I)alamin in a reaction involving methionine synthase to form methylcobalamin. Transport of cobalamin across lysosomes requires two distinct membrane proteins, LMBRD1 and ABCD4, which act synergistically and, when lacking, give rise to cblF and cblJ complementation groups, respectively. The approximate loci for defects in cobalamin mutants, cblA to cblJ, are shown. See text for details. *MMCoA mutase,* Methylmalonyl-CoA mutase; *SAH,* S-adenosylhomocysteine; *SAM,* S-adenosylmethionine.

reabsorbed, analogous to food cobalamin,[15] reflecting an efficient enterohepatic circulation of cobalamin.

Cellular Processing

Once bound to TCII receptors, the TCII-cobalamin complex is internalized by conventional receptor-mediated endocytosis (see Fig. 39.3).[15] At the low pH extant in lysosomes, TCII dissociates from cobalamin and is degraded, whereas transport of cobalamin across lysosomes into the cytosol requires two distinct membrane proteins, LMBRD1 and ABCD4, which act synergistically[19] (see Fig. 39.3). Cob(III)alamin, the most "oxidized" form of cobalamin, must be converted to cob(II)alamin and cob(I)alamin by two sequential reductase steps (see Fig. 39.3). Once in the cytoplasm, cobalamin is

bound to CblC, an enzyme that catalyzes removal of the cyano or methyl or adenosyl groups that are bound to cobalt in the cobalamin molecule.[19,23] From here, cobalamin is moved to target enzymes in the mitochondria or the cytoplasm.

Over 95% of intracellular cobalamin is bound to two intracellular enzymes, methylmalonyl-CoA mutase and methionine synthase.[15] When cobalamin interacts with its target enzymes, it exists in a "base-off/His-on" conformation, which reflects a very close relationship with these enzymes (see legend for Fig. 39.1).

In mitochondria, cob(I)alamin is converted to its coenzyme form, adenosylcobalamin, which acts as a coenzyme with methylmalonyl-CoA mutase to mediate the intramolecular exchange of a hydrogen atom attached to one carbon atom with a group attached to an adjacent carbon atom; in this way, methylmalonyl-CoA is converted to succinyl-CoA (methylmalonyl-CoA is normally generated during the catabolism of branched-chain amino acids, odd-chain fatty acids, and cholesterol). When formed, succinyl-CoA can then enter the Krebs tricarboxylic acid cycle.

In the cytoplasm, cobalamin, as methylcobalamin, functions as a coenzyme for methionine synthase, a critical enzyme for which both folates and cobalamin are required for normal one-carbon metabolism (see Fig. 39.3). Methionine synthase is a modular protein with four distinct and separate regions for binding homocysteine, 5-methyl-tetrahydrofolate (5-methyl-THF; 5-methyl-H_4PteGlu), the cobalamin prosthetic group, and S-adenosylmethionine (SAM).[22] The reaction proceeds by methyl transfer from 5-methyl-tetrahydrofolate to methionine synthase–bound cob(I)alamin to form methylcobalamin, followed by transfer of this methyl group to homocysteine to form methionine and regeneration of cob(I)alamin. In this process, 5-methyl-tetrahydrofolate is converted to tetrahydrofolate 5-methyl-tetrahydrofolate is converted to tetrahydrofolate that is subsequently polyglutamylated by folyl polyglutamate synthase; this addition of multiple glutamic acid moieties to tetrahydrofolate facilitates both its retention within cells and participation in one-carbon metabolism. During this reaction, spontaneous oxidation of cob(I)alamin (which has no axial ligand) to the catalytically inactive cob(II)alamin form requires reduction back to cob(I)alamin before it can accept a methyl group. There is a specific redox regulator known as methionine synthase reductase that restores enzyme activity in the presence of SAM and NADPH[24]; this enzyme is mutated in patients with cblE mutations.

The physiologic importance of the key cofactor roles of the two forms of cobalamin (i.e., adenosylcobalamin and methylcobalamin) in methylmalonyl-CoA mutase and methionine synthase, respectively, is that the products and by-products of these enzymatic reactions are critical for DNA, RNA, and protein biosynthesis.

FOLATES

Nutrition

Folates (the anionic forms of folic acid, also called vitamin B_9) are synthesized by microorganisms and plants, including leafy vegetables (spinach, lettuce, broccoli), beans, fruits (bananas, melons, lemons), yeast, and mushrooms, and are also found in animal meats[15]; see Fig. 39.4 for chemistry and nomenclature.

Among natural folates, which are predominantly in polyglutamylated form, only one-half are bioavailable; by contrast, 85% of folic acid that is added to food or ingested as a supplement is bioavailable. Several factors can influence the bioavailability of folates. These include: (1) The stability of the food folate. Natural reduced folates are labile and susceptible to oxidative cleavage by nitrates or light exposure, but folic acid is much more stable. Prolonged boiling or cooking over 30 minutes reduces natural folates by 50% to 80%, whereas ascorbate increases bioavailability, and refrigeration of leafy foods exposed to fluorescent light in supermarkets can double the folate content.[26] (2) Pureed foods allow easier access to the glutamate carboxypeptidase II (also known as folate-polyglutamate hydrolase), which converts folate polyglutamates to simpler folate monoglutamates before absorption[27]; any perturbation of this enzyme by organic acids (orange juice), sulfasalazine, or ethanol can preclude absorption; conversely, folate-binding proteins in human or cow's milk can increase folate absorption for infants and women.[28] (3) Interference with folate absorption across the proximal jejunum from intestinal diseases will affect the bioavailability of food folate. (4) Drugs that interfere with the proton-coupled folate transporter (PCFT) will compromise folate absorption.

The recommended daily allowance of folate is as follows: adult men and nonpregnant women, 400 μg; pregnant women, 600 μg; lactating women, 500 μg; children 9 to 18 years, between 300 and 400 μg.[10] A balanced Western diet contains adequate amounts of folate, but the net dietary intake of folate in many developing countries is often insufficient to sustain folate balance.[15,29–31]

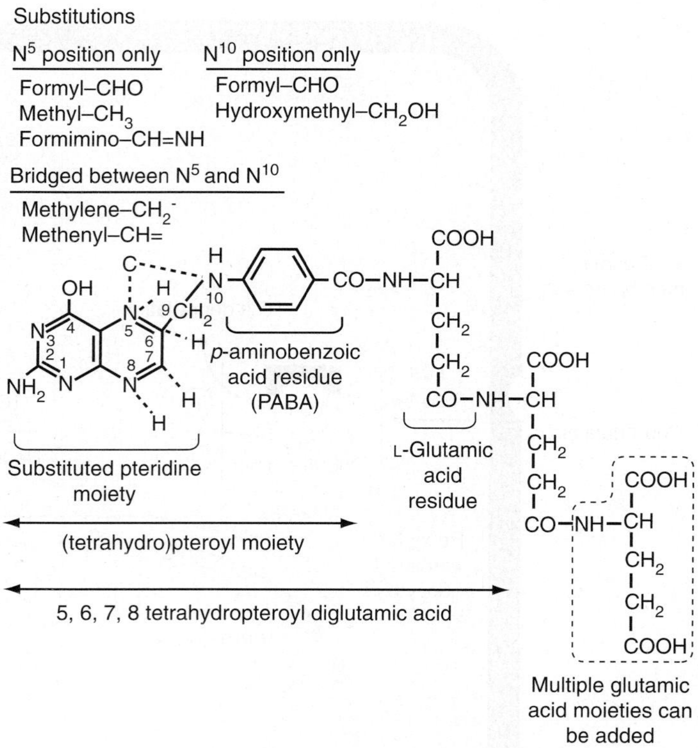

Fig. 39.4 FOLATE CHEMISTRY AND NOMENCLATURE. Folic acid (pteroylmonoglutamate [PteGlu]) is the commercially available parent compound for more than 100 compounds collectively referred to as *folates*. PteGlu consists of three basic components: a pteridine derivative, a *p*-aminobenzoic acid residue, and an L-glutamic acid residue. Before PteGlu can play a role as a coenzyme, it must first be reduced at positions 7 and 8 to dihydrofolic acid (H_2PteGlu) and then to 5,6,7,8-tetrahydrofolic acid (THF; H_4PteGlu), and one to six additional glutamic acid residues must then be added by means of γ-peptide bonds to the L-glutamate moiety (for which the subscripted *n* in PteGlu$_n$ denotes polyglutamation). Folate coenzymes donate or accept one-carbon units in numerous reactions in amino acid and nucleotide metabolism. The various substitutions in H_4PteGlu$_n$ occur at positions 5 or 10, or both; position 5 can be substituted by methyl (CH_3), formyl (CHO), or formimino (CHNH), and position 10 can be substituted by formyl or hydroxymethyl (CH_2OH). Positions 5 and 10 can be bridged by methylene (–CH_2–) or methenyl (–CH=). For an engaging account of the history of folic acid, see the article by Hoffbrand and Weir.[25]

Absorption

After dietary folate polyglutamates are converted to folate monoglutamates at the enterocyte brush border, they are transported through the duodenal and jejunal brush border by physiologically relevant, high-affinity membrane-associated, luminal surface–facing PCFT, which are most efficient in an acidic milieu. At pH 5.5, there is equivalent affinity for transport of physiologic reduced folates and folic acid, but at pH 6.5, reduced 5-methyl-tetrahydrofolate is transported more efficiently.[32] PCFT is a folate-hydrogen symporter, so with each folate molecule transported, there is a net translocation of positive charge. Loss-of-function mutations in PCFT in the enterocyte and choroid plexus result in (congenital) hereditary folate malabsorption,[33,34] a condition associated with an inability to transport folate across the intestine and the choroid plexus. The expression of PCFT is increased in folate-deficient mice, suggesting a physiologic regulatory mechanism. Proton pump inhibitors can reduce expression, and blocking the function of PCFT by sulfasalazine and pyrimethamine can lead to acquired folate malabsorption.[34,35] Within the enterocyte, folates are reduced to tetrahydrofolate and methylated before release into plasma as 5-methyl-tetrahydrofolate. Most of the folic acid taken up by the PCFT in the proximal small intestine is also converted within the enterocyte to 5-methyl-tetrahydrofolate. Folate production by bacteria in the small intestine can also enter the circulation.[36]

The flux of folate from the basolateral membrane of the enterocyte to the portal blood is mediated through MRP3.[34] MRP proteins have low affinity but high capacity and are best visualized as cellular "sump pumps" that eject excess folates (and antifolates) out of cells. Together with MRP2, which mediates folate transport into the bile,[37] these MRPs maintain an efficient enterohepatic circulation, which helps retain folate.[34]

Some bacterially produced folate, especially those produced by probiotic bacteria (genus *Bifidobacterium*), can be absorbed across the large intestine,[38] sufficient to raise the serum folate levels,[39] but normally this accounts for no more than about 5% of the average folate requirement.

Passive diffusion of folic acid (pteroylmonoglutamate [PteGlu]) is probably the primary mechanism of intestinal mucosal folate absorption at high pharmacologic concentrations.[15] The small intestine has a large capacity to absorb folate, with peak folate levels in plasma achieved 1 to 2 hours after oral administration.

Plasma Transport and Enterohepatic Circulation

The normal serum folate level is maintained by dietary folate and a substantial enterohepatic circulation that amounts to about 90 μg/day of folate.[15] Biliary drainage results in a dramatic fall in serum folate (to about 30% of basal levels in 6 hours), whereas abrupt interruption of dietary folate leads to a fall in serum folate levels in about 3 weeks. In the plasma, one-third of the folate is free, two-thirds are nonspecifically bound to serum proteins, and a small fraction binds soluble folate receptors. However, in contrast to cobalamin uptake, there is no specific *serum* transport protein that enhances cellular folate uptake.

Cellular Folate Uptake

Folate Receptors

Plasma 5-methyl-tetrahydrofolate and folic acid are rapidly transported into proliferating cells by specialized, high-affinity, glycosyl-phosphatidylinositol-anchored (membrane) folate receptor-α, which takes up these folates at physiologic concentrations found in serum.[40,41] The plasma membrane containing the folate–folate receptor complex then invaginates and forms an endosomal vesicle that moves into the cytoplasm along microtubules.[42] The perinuclear endosomal compartment then gets acidified to pH 6, which dissociates folate from folate receptors. The released folate then passes across the acidified endosome into the cytoplasm by a transendosomal pH gradient, which is mediated by either the PCFT or related moiety[33,43] (Fig. 39.5).

Folate receptor-α is critical to mediating the cellular uptake of folates in proliferating malignant and normal cells and in transport of folate across the placenta to the fetus,[41,44] into the brain,[45–47] and in renal conservation of folates.[43,48] Folate receptor-α is expressed in several types of cancer cells, whereas folate receptor-β is expressed most in monocytes and macrophages[49–51]; hence these two forms of folate receptors are under intense scrutiny for potential clinical use in detecting (and treating) occult malignancy and inflammation.[49–53]

The physiologic role of the reduced-folate carrier is less clear; it is a "low-affinity" but "high-capacity" system that can also mediate the uptake of 5-methyl-tetrahydrofolate and pharmacologic folates (like methotrexate and folinic acid well, but folic acid poorly) into a variety of cells at physiologic pH.[33,43]

Folate Receptor Regulation and Cellular Folate Homeostasis

Cell surface folate receptor-α is upregulated in response to low extracellular and intracellular folate concentrations through transcriptional, translational, and posttranslational mechanisms.[54–59] Poised in this location facing the external milieu of cells, upregulated folate receptor-α can bind all available folate and thereby help to restore cellular folate homeostasis.

The answer to the more fundamental question—how do cells sense the existence of folate deficiency in the first place so that folate homeostasis can be subsequently restored by upregulating folate receptors?—has finally been discovered.[59] It so happens that the accumulation of intracellular homocysteine during cellular folate deficiency leads to the covalent binding (by homocysteine) of a protein known as heterogeneous nuclear ribonucleoprotein-E1 (hnRNP-E1), which is already known to mediate the translational upregulation of folate receptor-α.[56,60] Homocysteinylation of hnRNP-E1 at specific cysteine–cysteine disulfide bonds leads to the unmasking of an underlying messenger RNA (mRNA)-binding pocket for which folate receptor-α mRNA has a high affinity. This RNA-protein interaction then triggers the biosynthesis of folate receptors, which soon results in a net increase of cell surface folate receptors that are able to bind more available folate and thereby normalize cellular folate levels. In this context, hnRNP-E1 fulfills criteria as a cellular sensor of physiologic folate deficiency (Fig. 39.6) because this protein is able to sense folate deficiency (by interacting with homocysteine) and respond by increasing RNA-protein interaction that triggers the biosynthesis and upregulation of folate receptors.

The broader significance of this mechanism is that *homocysteinylated hnRNP-E1 actually orchestrates a nutrition-sensitive posttranscriptional RNA operon during folate deficiency.* Thus during folate deficiency, the mRNA-binding pocket within homocysteinylated-hnRNP-E1 is actually highly promiscuous, in that it allows the binding of a variety of very diverse mRNAs (perhaps over 100), all of which have a common password composed of short RNA sequences; these RNA-protein interactions can, in turn, trigger the modulation up or down of a variety of several otherwise entirely unrelated proteins that contribute to the biologic features of reduced cell proliferation, differentiation, and apoptosis, which are a hallmark of folate deficiency.[59] In the nucleus, folate receptors also function as a transcription factor by binding to cis-regulatory elements at promoter regions of *Fgfr4* and *Hes1* to regulate their expression.[62]

Folate Receptors and Placental Folate Transport

Placental folate receptors[63,64] that are abundant and polarized to the maternal-facing microvillous membrane of the syncytiotrophoblast (but not on the basement membrane)[65] are critical to transplacental maternal-to-fetal folate transport.[44] Physiologic transplacental folate transport relies on the continued provision of adequate dietary folate intake by the mother. Following capture of maternal folate by placental folate receptors,[66,67] the displacement of this pool by incoming dietary folates, results in an intervillous blood concentration that is three times that of maternal blood. This allows for subsequent transfer of the folate to the fetal circulation along a downhill concentration gradient[44] and ensures continued unidirectional transplacental folate transport. Thus a suboptimum intake of folate by the mother can reduce maternal-to-fetal folate transfer and predispose the embryo/fetus to serious developmental defects.[68–70]

Because PCFT colocalizes with folate receptor-α, this suggests that following binding and internalization of folate into low-pH endosomes, the folate dissociates from folate receptors and presumably passes via PCFT into the cytoplasm. However, because both PCFT and reduced-folate carriers are uniformly distributed in microvillous membrane, cytoplasm, and the fetal-facing basal plasma membrane,[65] the following are all still unclear: the precise handover of folate following endocytosis into the cytoplasm, the potential role of transcytosis of vesicles containing folate, the transport of folate across the syncytiotrophoblast basement membrane into the fetal vasculature, and the role of MRPs in net transplacental folate transport to the fetus.

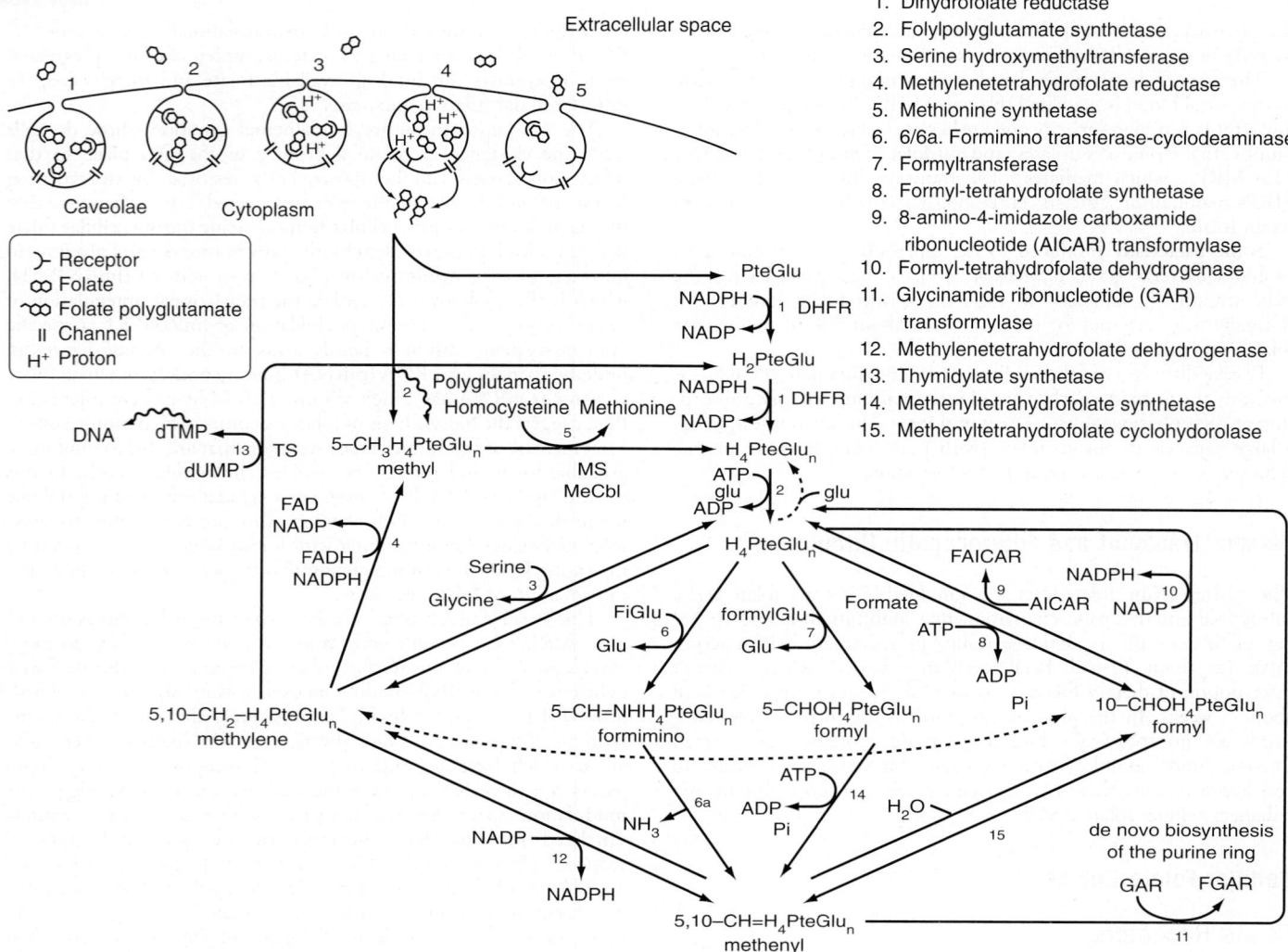

Fig. 39.5 FOLATE RECEPTOR–COUPLED FOLATE UPTAKE AND INTRACELLULAR ONE-CARBON METABOLISM INVOLVING FOLATES. See text for details. The channel within the caveolae/endocytotic vesicle is related to the proton-coupled folate transporter (PCFT). The contribution of the reduced folate carrier–mediated transport and passive diffusion of folate into cells is not shown. *ADP,* Adenosine diphosphate; *ATP,* adenosine triphosphate; *DHFR,* dihydrofolate reductase; *DNA,* deoxyribonucleic acid; *dTMP,* deoxythymidine monophosphate; *dUMP,* deoxyuridine monophosphate; *FAD,* flavin adenine dinucleotide; *FADH,* the reduced form of flavin adenine dinucleotide; *FiGlu,* formimino glutamic acid; *Glu,* glutamic acid; *NADP,* nicotinamide adenine dinucleotide phosphate; *NADPH,* the reduced form of nicotinamide adenine dinucleotide phosphate. *(Modified from Shane B, Stokstad EL: Vitamin B$_{12}$-folate interrelationships. Annu Rev Nutr 5:115, 1985; and Rothberg KG, Ying Y, Kolhouse JF, et al: The glycophospholipid-linked FR internalizes folate without entering the clathrin-coated pit endocytic pathway. J Cell Biol 110:637, 1990.)*

Folate Receptors in Embryonic and Fetal Development

Folate receptor-α is among the earliest genes activated in embryonic stem cells[71] when there is the need for increased folate requirements to support DNA synthesis during spectacular bursts of intense cell proliferation, ranging as short as 2 to 3 hours during brief windows within the proliferative zone in the epiblast.[69,72] Maternal folate deficiency compromises embryonic and fetal development—and probably accounts for an as-yet-uncharacterized number of early miscarriages, as suggested by experimental studies in mice.[57]

Both early-stage neural tube cells and neural crest cells abundantly express folate receptor-α. Experimental perturbation of folate receptor-α can lead to profound abnormalities in neural tube closure and in heart, facial, and eye development.[57,68,70,73–75] Such studies are consistent with a physiologic role for folate receptor-α and the importance of its functioning normally to prevent the development of neural tube defects (NTDs) and neurocristopathies (the latter involve abnormal proliferation and/or migration and/or differentiation of neural crest cells that can result in cleft lip or cleft palate, endocardial cushion defects, and other midline defects).[68–70] Indeed, as predicted,[69] brief experimental perturbation of folate receptor-α expression in these neural crest cells within a short window during embryonic development can impair the mitosis and the migration of these cells into the pharyngeal arches, leading to abnormal development of the pharyngeal arch arteries as well as the outflow tract, predisposing to abnormal heart development.[75] Thus congenital heart defects, which occur at a rate of approximately 1% of live births, and NTDs, among the most common congenital neurologic birth defects, are both dependent on the fidelity of folate receptor-α expression, precisely at the right time and in the right cells during early cardiac and neurologic development. The finding of a significant increase in blocking autoantibodies against placental folate receptor-α in women

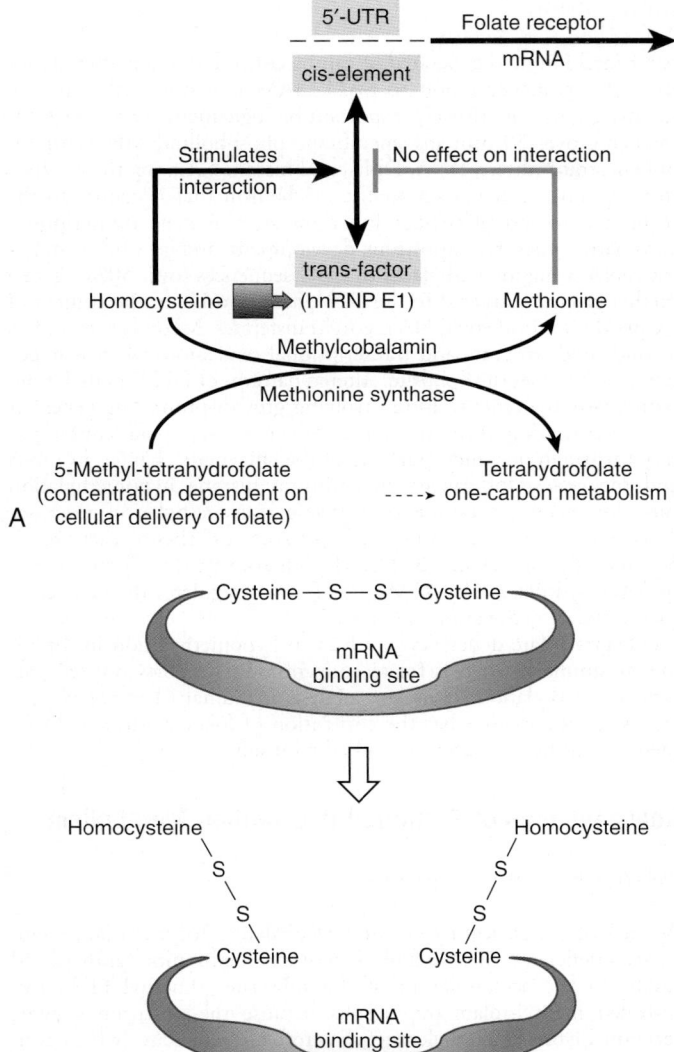

A

B

Fig. 39.6 MODEL FOR HOW THE CELL SENSES FOLATE DEFICIENCY AND RESPONDS BY UPREGULATING FOLATE RECEPTORS. Note how this model links perturbed folate metabolism, ribonucleic acid (RNA)–protein interaction, and coordinated translational regulation of folate receptor to optimize cellular folate uptake and restore folate homeostasis. The prominent *red arrow* highlights the critical role of heterogeneous nuclear ribonucleoprotein E1 (hnRNP-E1) as a candidate sensor of cellular folate deficiency. (A) Reduced folate availability results in inactivation of methionine synthase and intracellular homocysteine buildup, which induces a direct posttranslational homocysteinylation of hnRNP-E1 via targeted homocysteine-*S-S*-cysteine mixed disulfide bonds; this results in the unmasking of a high-affinity folate receptor messenger RNA (mRNA) cis-element binding site and leads to increased translation of folate receptor-α. The net effect is a homeostatic response that aims to restore intracellular folate concentrations to normal by upregulating cell surface folate receptor. Folate repletion reactivates methionine synthase, which converts homocysteine to methionine. Methionine has no effect on the RNA-protein interaction that leads to reduced folate receptor-α synthesis and its downregulation.[56] (Note: other metabolic pathways involving homocysteine[61] are not included.) (B) A proposed mechanism for the unmasking of a cryptic mRNA binding site in hnRNP-E1 following the covalent binding of L-homocysteine, through the replacement of one (of many potential) cysteine disulfide bonds by protein-cysteine-*S-S*-homocysteine mixed disulfide bonds. *5′-UTR, 5′* Untranslated region. *(From Tang YS, Khan RA, Zhang Y, et al: Incrimination of heterogeneous nuclear ribonucleoprotein E1 (hnRNP-E1) as a candidate sensor of physiological folate deficiency. J Biol Chem 286:39100, 2011.)*

with pregnancy complicated by neural tube defects[76] is a striking human correlate of experimental studies in mice using antibodies.[74] Folate receptor-α also provides folate during neuronal regeneration and repair after injury where DNA methylation is also involved.[77]

Folate Receptors and PCFT in Cerebral Folate Transport Across the Choroid Plexus

A new pathway of folate receptor-α dependent basolateral-to-apical transcytosis within vesicles across the choroid plexus cells followed by exosome-mediated folate delivery across the cerebrospinal fluid (CSF) into the brain parenchyma has been discovered.[45] Briefly, 5-methyl-THF is bound by glycosyl-phosphatidyl inositol (GPI)-anchored folate receptor-α on the basolateral surface of choroid plexus cells. Following endocytosis there is sequential transfer of folate receptor-α-bound folate from an early- to a later-endosomal compartment called multivesicular bodies. The inward budding of the limiting membrane of multivesicular bodies leads to formation of several intraluminal vesicles that now contain outward-facing folate receptor-α. Following transcytosis of multivesicular bodies (containing their cargo of intraluminal vesicles) and eventual fusion with the apical membrane, there is discharge of these intraluminal vesicles as 40 to 100 nm exosomes into the cerebrospinal fluid. These exosomes (containing outward oriented folate receptor-α-bound folates) then cross the ependymal cell layer and enter the brain parenchyma.[45]

Some of the endocytosed folate receptor-α-bound folate is transported out of acidified endosomal compartments via proton-coupled folate transporters (PCFT) into the choroid plexus cell cytoplasm.[45] However, more information on the cooperative function of folate receptor-α and PCFT in folate transport to the brain is required, because loss of PCFT-mediated function in hereditary folate malabsorption profoundly compromises choroid plexus transport of folates.[33,78]

Renal Retention of Folates (and Cobalamin)

After glomerular filtration, luminal folate binds folate receptor-α in the brush border membranes of proximal renal tubular cells and is internalized rapidly by folate receptor-α–mediated endocytosis; in the low pH of endocytotic vesicles, there is dissociation of folates and slow transport across basolateral membranes into the blood, with recycling of apo-folate receptor-α back to the luminal brush border membrane.[41,42,48] A large 550-kDa membrane protein called megalin, which interacts with cubilin and is found in renal proximal epithelial cells, functions as a multiligand receptor for a variety of macromolecules.[79,80] Megalin also specifically binds to and mediates endocytosis of TCII-cobalamin complexes as well as filtered folate bound to soluble folate-binding proteins in kidney proximal tubules.[81]

INTRACELLULAR ONE-CARBON METABOLISM AND COBALAMIN–FOLATE RELATIONSHIPS

Cellular Folate Retention and One-Carbon Metabolism

Polyglutamylation of folate by the enzyme folylpolyglutamate synthase catalyzes the addition of multiple glutamate equivalents to their γ-carboxyl residue (see Figs. 39.4 and 39.5). In most eukaryotic cells, the pentaglutamate and hexaglutamate forms predominate. Polyglutamylation is needed to retain folates (and antifolates) within cells; in addition, polyglutamylated folates are more efficient substrates for folate-dependent enzymes. In human erythrocytes (red blood cells [RBCs]), folate is accumulated at earlier stages within the marrow by folate receptors[82,83]; on maturation, more than 90% of $H_4PteGlu_{(n)}$ molecules interact with hemoglobin, which, because of its high capacity, assists in intracellular folate retention.[15] Folate turnover and catabolism in the cytoplasm can be experimentally accelerated by heavy chain ferritin,[84] but the clinical significance is still unclear.

Compartmentalization and Channeling of Folate Metabolism

In an elegant example of conservation of resources, metabolic pathways involving folate are compartmentalized within cells as multienzyme complexes that shuttle one-carbon units along set paths toward key reactions leading to pyrimidine and purine biosynthesis. The major form of folate transported into the cell is 5-methyl-tetrahydrofolate (5-methyl-THF; 5-methy-H$_4$PteGlu) (see Fig. 39.5); folic acid, which is formally called pteroylmonoglutamate (PteGlu), requires reduction to tetrahydrofolate by dihydrofolate reductase in a two-step reaction (PteGlu to *dihydro*pteroylglutamate [H$_2$PteGlu] to *tetrahydro*pteroyl-glutamate [H$_4$PteGlu, or THF]). After cellular uptake, 5-methyl-THF must first be converted to THF via methionine synthase (in the methylation cycle). This is a key reaction because THF is the preferred physiologic substrate for folylpolyglutamate synthase, which adds multiple glutamate moieties to THF (see Fig. 39.4). Only then can the polyglutamylated form of THF participate in one-carbon metabolism where it can be converted to either 10-formyl-THF—used in de novo biosynthesis of purines, or to 5,10-methylene-THF—used for synthesis of thymidylate. Moreover, 5,10-methylene-THF and 10-formyl-THF can be interconverted by intermediates (see Fig. 39.5).

Folate metabolism and folate-dependent enzymes are compartmentalized: approximately 40% are in the mitochondrial matrix, 50% in the cytoplasm, and 10% in the nucleus.[85] The methylation reaction occurs in the cytosol whereas thymidylate synthesis occurs in the nucleus. The mitochondrial compartment *not* shown in Fig. 39.5 contains its complement of folate cofactors, and homologues of the major cytosolic enzymes. For example, cytoplasmic 5-methyl-THF and 5-formyl-THF can enter mitochondria by a mitochondria-specific reduced-folate carrier,[86] whereas SAM, which is also required for mitochondrial methylation reactions, enters mitochondria by a specific transporter.[87] Other one-carbon donors like serine, glycine, dimethylglycine, and sarcosine also enter mitochondria and ultimately generate formate that crosses back into the cytoplasm. In the cytoplasm, C1-THF synthase, a trifunctional enzyme, uses this mitochondria-derived formate with THF to form 10-formyl-THF, which is required for the de novo synthesis of purines (see Fig. 39.5); this enzyme can also catalyze the interconversion of THF, 10-formyl-THF, 5,10-methenyl-THF, and 5,10-methylene-THF. In this way, the continued delivery of mitochondrial formate helps perpetuate cytoplasmic one-carbon metabolism.[85] Another major entry point of one-carbon units into cytoplasmic folate metabolism is through the formation of 5,10-methylene-THF from serine (which is derived from glycolytic intermediates); here the enzyme serine hydroxymethyltransferase catalyzes the addition of carbon 3 from serine to THF to give rise to the key intermediate coenzyme 5,10-methylene-THF.[85] After 5,10-methylene-THF is converted to 5-methyl-THF by the enzyme methylenetetrahydrofolate reductase, it can be used in the methylation cycle that involves methylation of homocysteine via methionine synthase to form methionine and tetrahydrofolate. After 5,10-methylene-THF is converted (via intermediates) to 10-formyl-THF, it can be used for purine nucleotide biosynthesis involving de novo synthesis of purine nucleotides for DNA and RNA. 5,10-Methylene-THF can also be used in the thymidylate cycle via the enzyme thymidylate synthase, which generates thymidylate (by converting deoxyuridine monophosphate [dUMP] to deoxythymidine monophosphate [dTMP]) for DNA synthesis (see Fig. 39.5). Parenthetically, this nuclear one-carbon metabolism compartment is activated during S phase of the cell cycle, following a posttranslational modification of folate-dependent enzymes like thymidylate synthase, serine-hydroxymethyltransferase, and dihydrofolate reductase by specialized small ubiquitin-like modifier (or SUMO) proteins; this modification allows the entry and enrichment of these sumoylated enzymes into the nucleus[88] to provide a buffer against the stress of imminent folate deficiency.[89]

Methylation

After methionine is generated, it can be converted to a methyl donor through its adenosylation to SAM. SAM is a universal donor of methyl groups for critically important biologic methylation reactions involving over 80 proteins, membrane phospholipids, the synthesis of neurotransmitters, RNA, DNA, and histones. Among these, DNA methylation is a major epigenetic mechanism that is central to the regulation of several cellular functions such as gene transcription, chromatin structure, imprinting, development, and genomic instability. DNA is highly methylated in CpG sequences (over 50%); here a methyl group is targeted to the DNA base cytosine in the context of a CpG dinucleotide by DNA methyltransferases. Methylation confers a condensed structure and transcriptional repression, whereas hypomethylation does the opposite. Altered patterns of DNA methylation, particularly hypomethylation involving growth-promoting genes, or hypermethylation of tumor suppressor genes, are popular contemporary themes in our understanding of the epigenetic changes in DNA and the genesis of cancer. In addition, histone hypomethylation can alter gene expression. After these transmethylation reactions that use SAM, the immediate product of these reactions is S-adenosylhomocysteine (SAH), which is converted to homocysteine by SAH hydrolase. The SAM to SAH ratio regulates the balance of such cellular methylation reactions.

Dietary folate deficiency can lead to hypomethylation in experimental animals, whereas folate consumption supports normal patterns of methylation. However, analysis in humans has not yielded consistent results, nor has the correlation of folate status and DNA methylation been rigorously studied clinically.

Consequences of Perturbed One-Carbon Metabolism

Methyl-Folate Trapping

Because of the critical role of methylcobalamin for methionine synthase, a deficiency of cobalamin inactivates methionine synthase and results in the accumulation of the substrate 5-methyl-THF; this so-called methyl-folate trap results because the upstream enzyme reaction involving methylenetetrahydrofolate reductase (which converts 5,10-methylene THF to 5-methyl-THF in preparation for the methionine synthase reaction) is irreversible. Because 5-methyl-THF accumulates and cannot be converted to THF, it leaks out of the cell. (This explains why patients with cobalamin deficiency can have normal to high serum folate values). The ensuing intracellular THF deficiency compromises one-carbon metabolism and initiates the pathophysiologic cascade leading to perturbed DNA synthesis and megaloblastosis.

Hyperhomocysteinemia

Similarly, when methionine synthase is inhibited during either cobalamin or folate deficiency, there is a buildup of the thiol amino acid, homocysteine, which can also leak out of the cell and have multiple deleterious effects on the body through a variety of molecular and biochemical pathways. Indeed, measurement of serum homocysteine is a sensitive measure of clinical folate and cobalamin deficiency in nutritional anemia. The clinical significance of hyperhomocysteinemia is discussed later.

Thymidylate Deficiency and Perturbed DNA Synthesis

With either cobalamin or folate deficiency, there will be a net decrease in 5,10-methylene-THF that interrupts the thymidylate synthase–mediated conversion of dUMP to dTMP. (Although salvage pathways for purine synthesis can compensate for reduced generation of purines through one-carbon metabolism, salvage pathways cannot compensate for reduced thymidine). This results in a high dUMP/dTMP ratio and an increase in deoxyuridine triphosphate (dUTP), which can get misincorporated into DNA. At this juncture, an editorial enzyme recognizes this faulty misincorporation and excises dUTP. However, with a continued inadequate supply of deoxythymidine triphosphate (dTTP), there is a continued cycle of uracil misincorporation into DNA in folate deficiency,[90-92] its removal by uracil-DNA glycosylase,[22] and refilling of the missing base by DNA polymerase β.[93] However, with repetition over several cycles, multiple single-strand nicks are introduced into DNA; this predisposes to chromosome breaks[94] that can contribute to an increased risk of cancer associated with folate deficiency.[91,95,96] In addition, folate deficiency can also lead to double-strand breaks in DNA, which are difficult to repair when the two nicks are close to one another (within 12 bp of each other) on opposite strands.[97] Collectively, such double-strand DNA breaks in folate-deficient cells predispose to the development of acentric chromosomes, DNA fragments, and micronuclei.[94,98] This can even render folate-deficient tissues more permissive to the integration of HPV16 DNA, and trigger (experimental) carcinogenesis.[99]

Chromosome and Cell Cycle Defects

Defective DNA synthesis caused by folate deficiency is reflected by numerous chromosomal abnormalities, including abnormalities in telomeres, which correlate with biomarkers of chromosomal instability and mitotic dysfunction.[100] There is excessive chromosomal elongation with despiralization associated with random breaks and exaggerated centromere constriction, expression of folate-sensitive fragile sites in hematopoietic cells, and reduced biosynthesis, acetylation, and methylation of arginine-rich histone.[22] All this leads to perturbation of the cell cycle with an increased proportion of cells in prophase of the mitotic cycle and G_2 that leads to apoptosis of erythroid precursors and anemia.[22]

MORPHOLOGIC EXPRESSION OF MEGALOBLASTOSIS

There is widening disparity in nuclear-cytoplasmic asynchrony as a cobalamin- or folate-deficient cell divides, until the more mature generations of daughter cells die in the marrow or are arrested (as megaloblastic cells) at various stages of the cell cycle.[15] The plethora of bone marrow morphologic changes can lead an untrained observer to the diagnosis of erythroleukemia. All proliferating cells exhibit megaloblastosis, including the luminal epithelial mucosal cells of the entire gastrointestinal tract, cervix, vagina, and uterus.[15] However, megaloblastic changes are most striking in the blood and bone marrow. Ineffective hematopoiesis extends into long bones, and the bone marrow aspirate (which is superior to the biopsy for observing megaloblastosis) exhibits trilineal hypercellularity, especially of the erythroid series. The appearance of exuberant cell proliferation with numerous mitotic figures is misleading because these cells are actually proliferating very slowly (see box on Morphology in Megaloblastosis from Cobalamin and Folate Deficiency Is the Same).

Erythroid hyperplasia reduces the myeloid-to-erythroid ratio from 3:1 to 1:1. Proerythroblasts are not as obviously abnormal as later forms; they may simply be larger (promegaloblasts). Megaloblastic changes are most strikingly displayed in intermediate and orthochromatic stages, which are larger than their normoblastic counterparts. In contrast to the normally dense chromatin of comparable normoblasts, megaloblastic erythroid precursors have an open, finely stippled, reticular, sieve-like pattern (Fig. 39.7). The orthochromatic megaloblast, with its hemoglobinized cytoplasm, continues to retain its large sieve-like immature nucleus, in sharp contrast to the clumped chromatin of orthochromatic normoblasts. The nucleus is often eccentrically placed in these large oval or oblong cells, and lobulation or indentation of nuclei with bizarre karyorrhexis is often seen. In cells destined for the circulation as macro-ovalocytes, the nucleus may occasionally not be completely extruded. Of the potential progeny of

> **Morphology in Megaloblastosis from Cobalamin and Folate Deficiency Is the Same**
>
> **Peripheral Smear**
> - Increased mean corpuscular volume (MCV) with macro-ovalocytes (up to 14 μm), which is variously associated with anisocytosis and poikilocytosis
> - Nuclear hypersegmentation of polymorphonuclear neutrophils (PMNs) (one PMN with six lobes or 5% with five lobes)
> - Thrombocytopenia (mild to moderate)
> - Leukoerythroblastic morphology (from extramedullary hematopoiesis)
>
> **Bone Marrow Aspirate**
> - General increase in cellularity of all three major hematopoietic elements
> - Abnormal erythropoiesis—orthochromatic megaloblasts
> - Abnormal leukopoiesis—giant metamyelocytes and "band" forms (pathognomonic), hypersegmented PMNs
> - Abnormal megakaryocytopoiesis—pseudo hyperdiploidy

proerythroblasts that develop into later megaloblastic forms, 80% to 90% die in the bone marrow. Marrow macrophages effectively scavenge dead or partially disintegrated megaloblasts. This is the basis for ineffective erythropoiesis (intramedullary hemolysis).

Leukopoiesis is also abnormal. There is an absolute increase in these cells, which are large and have similar sieve-like chromatin. Spectacular giant (20 to 30 μm) metamyelocytes and "band" forms that are often seen are pathognomonic for megaloblastosis (see Fig. 39.7). There may be bizarre nucleoli with small cytoplasmic vacuoles. It is probable that giant metamyelocytes cannot easily traverse marrow sinuses, and their maturation into circulating hypersegmented polymorphonuclear neutrophils (PMNs) is unlikely. Granulation of the cytoplasm remains unaffected.

Megakaryocytes may be normal or increased in numbers and may exhibit additional complexities in megaloblastic expression (see Fig. 39.7). Complex hypersegmentation (i.e., pseudohyperdiploidy) is associated with liberation of fragments of cytoplasm and giant platelets into the circulation. The net output of platelets is decreased in severe megaloblastosis, and abnormal but reversible platelet dysfunction has been documented.[22]

In early cobalamin or folate deficiency, normoblasts may dominate the marrow with only a few megaloblasts seen. Complete transformation to megaloblastic hematopoiesis is observed in florid cases and is reflected by various degrees of pancytopenia.

The earliest manifestation of megaloblastosis is an increase in mean corpuscular volume (MCV) with macro-ovalocytes (up to 14 μm) (see Fig. 39.7). Because these cells have adequate hemoglobin, the central pallor, which normally occupies about one-third of the cell, is decreased. By contrast, thin macrocytes have larger than normal central pallor (Table 39.1). In severe anemia, poikilocytosis and anisocytosis are evident. Cells containing remnants of DNA (i.e., Howell-Jolly bodies), arginine-rich histone, and nonhemoglobin iron (i.e., Cabot rings) may be observed. Extramedullary megaloblastic hematopoiesis may also result in a leukoerythroblastic picture.

Nuclear hypersegmentation of DNA in PMNs strongly suggests megaloblastosis when associated with macro-ovalocytosis (see Fig. 39.7). Normally fewer than 5% of PMNs have more than five lobes, and no cells have more than six lobes in the peripheral blood. If megaloblastosis is suspected (greater than 5% PMNs with more than five lobes or a single PMN with more than six lobes), a formal lobe count/PMN (i.e., lobe index) above 3.5 may be obtained.

Ineffective use of iron results in an increased percentage of saturation of transferrin and increased iron stores. If there is associated iron deficiency, the MCV may be normal, and only iron therapy can unmask the megaloblastic manifestations in the peripheral blood. In thalassemia, the entire erythrocyte morphology normally expected in megaloblastosis is masked[15]; however, megaloblastic leukopoiesis is still observed. Significant intramedullary hemolysis (ineffective

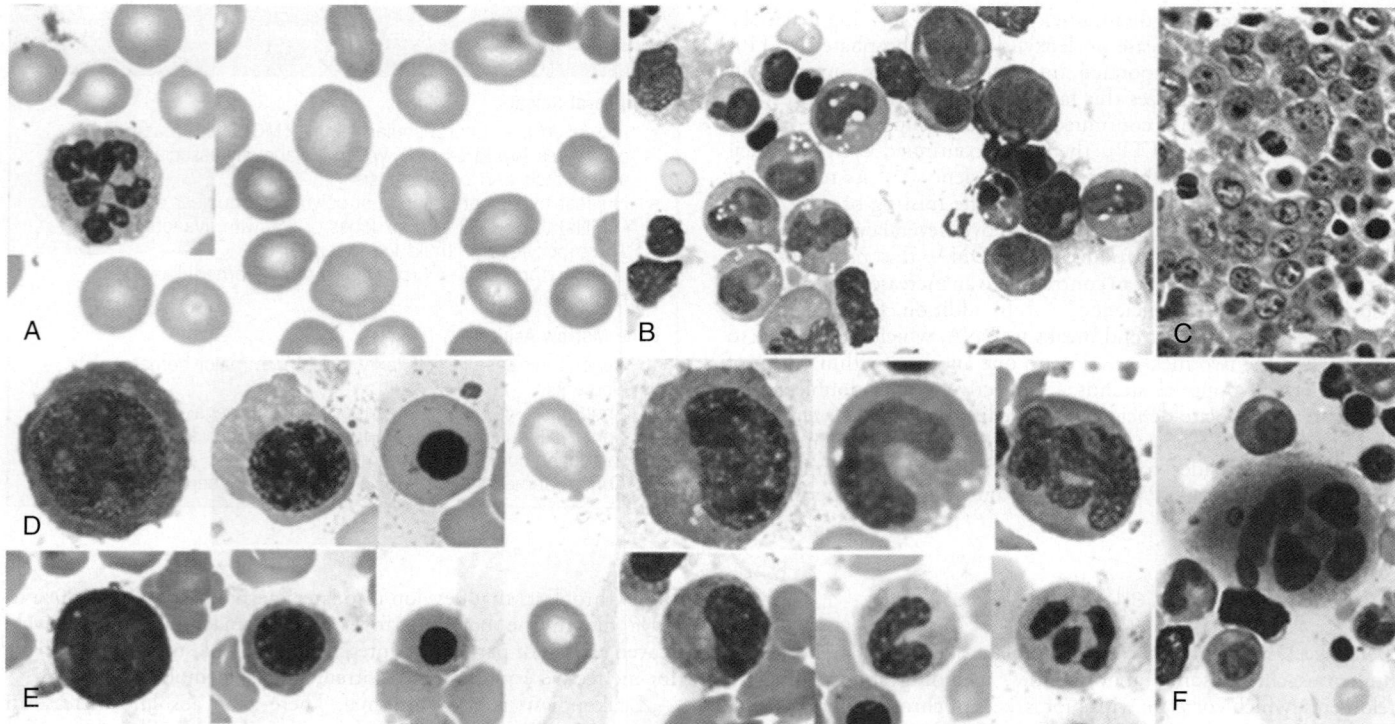

Fig. 39.7 MEGALOBLASTIC ANEMIA. The peripheral smear (A) exhibits macro-ovalocytosis and hypersegmented polys (inset). The bone marrow aspirate (B) shows megaloblastic changes in both granulopoiesis and erythropoiesis. The biopsy (C) is hypercellular and shows sheets of immature erythroid precursors with the appearance of a high mitotic rate. These can mimic acute erythroleukemia or even metastatic tumor cells. Details from the cells in the aspirate (D) compared with normal hematopoiesis at same magnification (E). Note the giant metamyelocyte and band form. In megaloblastic anemia, megakaryocytes also have nuclear atypica, including abnormal nuclear segmentation (F).

TABLE 39.1	Clinical Conditions Not to Be Confused with Megaloblastosis

Macrocytosis[a] Without Megaloblastosis[b]

Reticulocytosis

Liver disease

Aplastic anemia

Myelodysplastic syndromes (especially 5q-)

Multiple myeloma

Hypoxemia

Smokers

Spurious Increases in MCV Without Macro-Ovalocytosis[c]

Cold agglutinin disease

Marked hyperglycemia

Leukocytosis

Older individuals

[a]The central pallor that normally occupies about one-third of the normal red blood cell is decreased in macro-ovalocytes. This contrasts with the finding of thin macrocytes, in which the central pallor is increased.

[b]Although megaloblastosis implies that a bone marrow test has been performed, with the addition of highly sensitive tests for the specific diagnosis of cobalamin and folate deficiency, the need for a bone marrow test is often dictated by the urgency to make the diagnosis.

[c]When the Coulter counter readings of a high MCV are not confirmed by looking at the peripheral smear.

MCV, Mean corpuscular volume.

erythropoiesis) involving more than 90% of megaloblastic precursors is reflected by a lowered absolute reticulocyte count, increased bilirubin (up to 2 mg/dL), decreased haptoglobin, and increased lactate dehydrogenase (LDH) often above 1000 units/mL. There is also a modest decrease in the circulating RBC life span.

Megaloblastosis in rapidly proliferating cells of the gastrointestinal tract leads to a variable degree of morphologic changes and atrophy of luminal epithelial cells. This leads to functional defects, which can include malabsorption of cobalamin and folate in some patients. A vicious cycle whereby megaloblastosis begets more megaloblastosis is established that can be interrupted only by specific therapy with cobalamin or folate.

NEUROLOGIC DYSFUNCTION WITH COBALAMIN DEFICIENCY

Because megaloblastosis caused by folate or cobalamin deficiency leads to a functional folate coenzyme deficiency, the morphologic manifestations of both deficiencies are understandably indistinguishable. However, only cobalamin deficiency results in a patchy demyelination process, which is expressed clinically as cerebral abnormalities and subacute combined degeneration of the spinal cord.[15] The precise role of cobalamin in maintaining the integrity of the central nervous system has not been completely defined (see box on Clues for Distinguishing Cobalamin and Folate Deficiencies).

A series of Japanese patients with apparent folate deficiency–associated neuropathy who exhibited a slowly progressive and sensory-dominant pattern has been reported.[101] While this warrants confirmation, other laboratory and preclinical information provide plausible reasons for the development of abnormal neurophysiology during folate deficiency.[57,59] For example, folate deficiency induces the homocysteinylation and activation of the mRNA-binding protein, hnRNP-E1, which can either activate diverse mRNAs such as tyrosine hydroxylase (which can raise levels of neurotransmitters like dopamine and epinephrine), or neurofilament-M (which can perturb the structure and function of neurons).

The demyelinating process involves patchy swelling of the myelin sheath followed by its breakdown (demyelination), leading to axonal degeneration. Microscopic foci coalesce with one another, giving the

Clues for Distinguishing Cobalamin and Folate Deficiencies

Although the megaloblastic manifestations of cobalamin and folate deficiencies are clinically indistinguishable, certain distinct patterns in mode of presentation provide clues to the type and cause of deficiency. In general, the cause of folate deficiency can be found in the patient's recent past (within 6 months), primarily discerned from the history and physical examination. In contrast, the cause of cobalamin deficiency can remain obscure until specific tests to define the cause are carried out. In the past, by the time anemia was symptomatic, more than 80% of patients had neurologic manifestations, and in 50% this led to some incapacity. Perhaps as a result of widespread use of multivitamins containing folic acid among patients and even in the food given livestock in the West, the hematologic expression of cobalamin deficiency is often substantially attenuated, leading to pure neurologic presentations. Studies highlight the apparent inverse correlation between hematologic and neurologic presentations such that in a third of patients with cobalamin deficiency, the earliest signs are often purely neurologic, and symptoms related to paresthesias and diminished proprioception may cause the patient to see the physician. Based on the multiple potential causes (see box on Etiopathophysiologic Classification of Cobalamin Deficiency or box on Etiopathophysiologic Classification of Folate Deficiency), the warning that "what the mind does not know, the eyes do not see" is a caveat that cannot be taken lightly; failure to recognize cobalamin deficiency as the cause of neurologic disease and treatment of cobalamin deficiency with folate, or misdiagnosis of megaloblastosis as erythroleukemia represent significant extremes of deviation from the dictum *primum non nocere*. Areas of overlap in the symptoms of cobalamin or folate deficiency are related to megaloblastosis (i.e., common cardiopulmonary and some gastrointestinal manifestations). Although pure folate deficiency in the alcoholic with thiamine deficiency (i.e., Wernicke encephalopathy) and peripheral neuropathy is almost indistinguishable from and may mimic cobalamin deficiency, the remaining neurologic manifestations are uniquely characteristic of cobalamin deficiency. Folate deficiency in adults has not been unequivocally shown to give rise to neurologic findings. Coexistence of folate deficiency with neurologic disease should prompt investigations to rule out cobalamin and other nutrient deficiencies arising from dietary insufficiency or malabsorption.

Etiopathophysiologic Classification of Cobalamin Deficiency

I. Nutritional cobalamin deficiency (insufficient cobalamin intake)—vegetarians, poverty-imposed near-vegetarians, breastfed infants of mothers with pernicious anemia
II. Abnormal intragastric events (inadequate proteolysis of food cobalamin)—atrophic gastritis, hypochlorhydria, proton pump inhibitors, H_2 blockers
III. Loss/atrophy of gastric oxyntic mucosa (deficient intrinsic factor [IF] molecules)—total or partial gastrectomy, adult and juvenile pernicious anemia, caustic destruction (lye)
IV. Abnormal events in the small bowel lumen
  A. Inadequate pancreatic protease (R factor–cobalamin not degraded, cobalamin not transferred to IF)
    1. Insufficient pancreatic protease—pancreatic insufficiency
    2. Inactivation of pancreatic protease—Zollinger-Ellison syndrome
  B. Usurping of luminal cobalamin (inadequate binding of cobalamin to IF)
    1. By bacteria-stasis syndromes (blind loops, pouches of diverticulosis, strictures, fistulas, anastomosis), impaired bowel motility (scleroderma), hypogammaglobulinemia
    2. By *Diphyllobothrium latum* (fish tapeworm)
V. Disorders of ileal mucosa/IF-cobalamin receptors (IF-cobalamin not bound to IF-cobalamin receptors [cubam receptors])
  A. Diminished or absent cubam receptors—ileal bypass/resection/fistula
  B. Abnormal mucosal architecture/function—tropical/nontropical sprue, Crohn disease, tuberculous ileitis, amyloidosis
  C. Cubam receptor defects—Imerslund-Gräsbeck syndrome
  D. Drug-effects—metformin, cholestyramine, colchicine, neomycin
VI. Disorders of plasma cobalamin transport (transcobalamin [TCII]-cobalamin not delivered to TCII receptors)—congenital TCII deficiency, defective binding of TCII-cobalamin to TCII receptors (rare)
VII. Metabolic disorders (cobalamin not used by cell)
  A. Inborn enzyme errors—cblA to cblJ disorders (rare)
  B. Acquired disorders (cobalamin inactivated by irreversible oxidation)—nitrous oxide

surface of the spinal cord (on cross section) a spongy appearance; later there is secondary Wallerian degeneration of long tracts. Patchy demyelination usually begins in the dorsal columns in the thoracic segments of the spinal cord (Fig. 39.8) and then spreads contiguously to involve corticospinal tracts. These lesions spread throughout the length of the cord and ultimately involve spinothalamic and spinocerebellar tracts. There is also degeneration of the dorsal root ganglia, celiac ganglia, the Meissner plexus, and the Auerbach plexus. Although demyelination may also extend to the white matter of the brain, it is unclear whether the peripheral neuropathy is caused by a distinct lesion or results from spinal cord disease; the clinical manifestations may be extremely varied.[15]

Vegetarians with cobalamin neuropathy in India[102] had cognitive impairment in nearly one-half of 36 patients; it was mostly global with impaired recall and "serial sevens" (which are useful bedside tests of attention); impaired naming was found among one-quarter of the patients. Nearly one-half had abnormal evoked potential (using the oddball auditory paradigm), which revealed P300 latency that was reversible in 3 months of cobalamin replacement; in one-fifth P300 was unrecordable. Objective tests to document cobalamin neuropathy[102] include nerve conduction studies and motor- and sensory-evoked potentials,[103,104] visual pathway abnormalities,[105] and magnetic resonance imaging that shows T2 hyperintensity and atrophy.

Among another cohort of patients with cobalamin neuropathy from the United States, 65% had mild, about 25% had moderate, and about 10% had severe neurologic deficits.[22] Paresthesias or ataxia were most commonly the first symptoms, and diminished vibratory sensation and proprioception in the lower extremities were the most common objective early signs. Although multiple neurologic syndromes were often seen in the same patient, the spectrum of objective signs could include loss of fine or coarse touch, decreased or increased

Etiopathophysiologic Classification of Folate Deficiency

I. Nutritional causes
  A. Decreased dietary intake—poverty and famine, institutionalized individuals (psychiatric/nursing homes)/chronic debilitating disease, prolonged feeding of infants with goat's milk, special slimming diets or food fads (folate-rich foods not consumed), cultural/ethnic cooking techniques (food folate destroyed)
  B. Decreased diet and increased requirements
    1. Physiologic—pregnancy and lactation, prematurity, hyperemesis gravidarum, infancy
    2. Pathologic
      a. Intrinsic hematologic diseases involving hemolysis with compensatory erythropoiesis, abnormal hematopoiesis, or bone marrow infiltration with malignant disease
      b. Dermatologic disease—psoriasis
II. Folate malabsorption
  A. With normal intestinal mucosa
    1. Drugs—sulfasalazine, pyrimethamine, proton pump inhibitors (via inhibition of proton-coupled folate transporter [PCFT])
    2. Hereditary folate malabsorption (mutations in PCFTs) (rare)
  B. With mucosal abnormalities—tropical and nontropical sprue, regional enteritis
III. Defective folate transport across the choroid plexus into the cerebrospinal fluid—cerebral folate deficiency (mutation or autoantibodies to folate receptors) (rare)
IV. Inadequate cellular utilization
  A. Folate antagonists (methotrexate)
  B. Hereditary enzyme deficiencies involving folate
V. Drugs (multiple effects on folate metabolism)—alcohol, sulfasalazine, triamterene, pyrimethamine, trimethoprim-sulfamethoxazole, diphenylhydantoin, barbiturates

deep tendon reflexes with spasticity or muscle weakness, urinary or fecal incontinence, orthostatic hypotension, amaurosis, dementia, psychosis, or mood disturbances.[22] Overall, although the neurologic deficits were mild in most cases, the severity was judged related to the duration of symptoms before diagnosis; not unexpectedly, those with the shorter duration of symptoms responded most to appropriate replacement.

OTHER EFFECTS OF COBALAMIN AND FOLATE DEFICIENCY

Cobalamin deficiency more often than folate deficiency can also result in sterility from the effects on the gonads. An unexplained finding is generalized melanin pigmentation that is reversible by specific nutrient replenishment. Cobalamin deficiency negatively affects bone development and maintenance,[106] which explains the reduced bone mineral density in those with cobalamin deficiency[107,108] including pernicious anemia.[109,110] Folate is also important for maintenance of regulatory T cells[111]; this may explain the

findings of combined immunodeficiency in hereditary folate malabsorption.[112]

SPECTRUM OF CLINICAL PRESENTATIONS WITH COBALAMIN DEFICIENCY

The age-specific presentations with cobalamin deficiency are discussed in Nutritional Cobalamin Deficiency. Classic presentations of nutritional cobalamin deficiency in developing countries are often accompanied by iron deficiency, and among malnourished populations, many will also have folate deficiency. Among vegetarians in developing countries, cases with nutritional cobalamin deficiency may present in the second and third decades with pancytopenia, mild hepatosplenomegaly, fever, and occasionally thrombocytopenic bleeding.[22] Alternatively, a neurologic and psychiatric syndrome may develop with or independent of anemia. Because neuropsychiatric presentations may dominate the clinical picture and the patient may not have anemia, careful review of the peripheral smear may reveal macrocytosis.[22] In over a quarter of patients with cobalamin neuropathy in the United States, there was no reduction in the hematocrit despite neurologic disease, and only a minority of patients had combined hematologic and neurologic disease. Indeed, the higher the hematocrit, the more severe the neurologic disorder! Conversely, anemic patients may have no neurologic deficits, and the level of cobalamin may have no correlation with the existence or severity of neurologic disease.

BIOCHEMICAL INDICATORS OF EVOLVING DEFICIENCY

Early manifestations of negative cobalamin balance are increased serum methylmalonic acid (MMA) and total homocysteine levels (Table 39.2).[22] This can occur when the total cobalamin in serum is still in the low-normal range. Continued negative cobalamin balance leads to an absolute decrease in serum cobalamin level. Normal levels of MMA and homocysteine rule out clinically significant cobalamin deficiency with virtually 100% certainty.[22]

Likewise, metabolic evidence for folate deficiency (i.e., increased serum total homocysteine level) can be found when serum folates are still in the low-normal range.

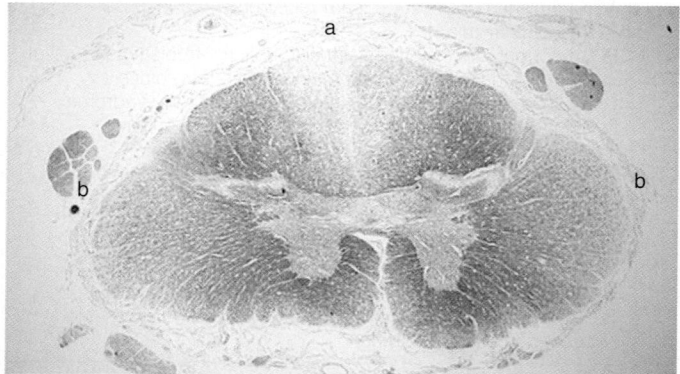

Fig. 39.8 SPINAL CORD IN COBALAMIN DEFICIENCY. The cross section of the spinal cord stained with Luxol blue shows demyelination of the dorsal columns (*a*) and early demyelination of the lateral columns (*b*).

TABLE 39.2	Stepwise Approach to the Diagnosis of Cobalamin and Folate Deficiency

Megaloblastic Anemia or Neurologic-Psychiatric Manifestations Consistent with Cobalamin Deficiency *Plus* Test Results on Serum Cobalamin and Serum Folate

Cobalamin[a] (pg/mL)	Folate[b] (ng/mL)	Provisional Diagnosis	Proceed with Metabolites?[c]
>300	>4	Cobalamin or folate deficiency is unlikely	No
<200	>4	Consistent with cobalamin deficiency	No
200–300	>4	Rule out cobalamin deficiency	Yes
>300	<2	Consistent with folate deficiency	No
<200	<2	Consistent with (1) combined cobalamin plus folate deficiency or (2) isolated folate deficiency	Yes
>300	2–4	Consistent with (1) folate deficiency or (2) an anemia unrelated to vitamin deficiency	Yes

Test Results on Metabolites: Serum Methylmalonic Acid and Total Homocysteine

Methylmalonic Acid (Normal, 70–270 nM)	Total Homocysteine (Normal, 5–14 μM)	Diagnosis
Increased	Increased	Cobalamin deficiency confirmed; folate deficiency still possible (i.e., combined cobalamin plus folate deficiency possible)
Normal	Increased	Folate deficiency is likely
Normal	Normal	Cobalamin and folate deficiency is excluded

[a]Serum cobalamin levels: abnormally low, less than 200 pg/mL; clinically relevant low-normal range, 200 to 300 pg/mL.
[b]Serum folate levels: abnormally low, less than 2 ng/mL; clinically relevant low-normal range, 2 to 4 ng/mL.
[c]Any frozen-over sample from serum folate/cobalamin determination can be subjected to metabolite tests.

Modified Therapeutic Trials

The traditional therapeutic trial using physiologic doses of vitamins (100 µg of folate or 1 µg of cobalamin given daily while monitoring the reticulocyte response)[15] has given way to a modified therapeutic trial. Rather than making the diagnosis of a deficiency, *the intention is often to confirm the clinical suspicion that the patient does not have deficiency.* This can be demonstrated by lack of response to full replacement doses of both vitamins (1 mg of folic acid orally for 10 days and 1 mg of cobalamin intramuscularly or subcutaneously daily for 10 days). Clinical scenarios in which such trials may be applicable (after drawing blood for serum cobalamin and folate levels) are as follows:

1. There is a clinical suspicion that the underlying disease is not caused by a vitamin deficiency, but this idea is not supported by results of clinical, morphologic, and biochemical evaluations. Such conditions include anemia with a megaloblastic bone marrow that may be secondary to chemotherapy, myelodysplastic syndromes, or acute leukemia; when time is of the essence in making the diagnosis; when the levels of cobalamin are likely to be falsely abnormal because of these diseases; or when there is underlying dehydration or renal dysfunction that predictably gives falsely high levels of metabolites.

2. In other situations, (i.e., pregnancy, acquired immunodeficiency syndrome [AIDS], or alcoholism) with a multifactorial basis for anemia, the response or lack thereof to full replacement doses can eliminate cobalamin or folate deficiency and thereby narrow the (often extensive) differential diagnosis.

3. In instances when severe anemia with megaloblastosis is clinically obvious and so serious that the physician cannot wait for the results of specific tests for deficiency. Full doses of both vitamins are administered, and if there is a response manifested by brisk reticulocytosis by days 5 to 7, retrospective assignment of the deficiency is based on the results of blood samples drawn before beginning the trial.

In all therapeutic trials, if there is no evidence of response within 10 days, bone marrow aspiration is indicated to identify another primary hematologic disease.

Serum Homocysteine and Methylmalonic Acid Levels in Cobalamin and Folate Deficiencies

The combined use of homocysteine and methylmalonic acid (MMA) levels can differentiate cobalamin from folate deficiency, because most patients with folate deficiency have normal MMA levels, and the remainder have only mild elevations.[22] These two tests are useful diagnostically. The abnormally high levels of metabolites return to normal only when the patient receives replacement with the appropriate (deficient) vitamin. A positive response to cobalamin, documented by falling levels of homocysteine and MMA, is evidence of cobalamin deficiency. Conversely, therapy with folate results in a decrease in the isolated homocysteine level if folate deficiency is present.[22] Indeed, because several variables that are not related to vitamin deficiency (such as age, mild renal dysfunction) can falsely elevate serum homocysteine and MMA levels, if there is ambiguity, proof of vitamin deficiency would require clear-cut demonstration of a reduction in metabolite levels after specific vitamin supplementation.[22,114]

Laboratory tests are more likely to be accurate when there is a high pretest probability of a particular disease. This can, however, be more vexing in the case of diagnosis of early cobalamin deficiency when symptoms are subtle, nonspecific, or not yet fully manifest. If there is macrocytosis and cobalamin levels are borderline or just below the normal, unequivocal elevation of MMA will support the diagnosis. However, in elderly patients with anemia, there may be several other causes for anemia, and depending on the population studied, cobalamin deficiency may be only one among several possible causes in the differential diagnosis. This is when a modified therapeutic trial—in which a patient is treated with full doses of both cobalamin and folate for 10 days—and the lack of objective response to cobalamin would effectively rule out cobalamin deficiency as a cause (see box on Modified Therapeutic Trials). Alternatively, attribution of the cause of anemia to cobalamin deficiency would be reasonably confirmed retrospectively if there was evidence for resolution of anemia following such therapy with cobalamin. Although reductions from high serum MMA and homocysteine values to baseline following therapy would also be confirmatory, this is impractical because of the expense of multiple testing.

BIOCHEMICAL EVALUATION OF COBALAMIN AND FOLATE DEFICIENCIES

Total Serum Homocysteine and Methylmalonic Acid Levels

Cellular nutrient *deficiency* of cobalamin or folate is reflected by decreased intracellular concentrations. Cobalamin deficiency perturbs methionine synthase activity; this results in substrate (homocysteine) buildup and elevated serum levels of homocysteine, which can be measured by a sensitive assay.[22] In addition, cobalamin deficiency perturbs the activity of methylmalonyl-CoA mutase, which leads to elevated serum MMA levels. Thus homocysteine and MMA are sensitive tests for cobalamin deficiency (see Table 39.2).

Folate deficiency also results in elevated levels of homocysteine because of reduced activity of the methionine synthase–catalyzed reaction.[22] Total homocysteine concentration, which comprises the sum of all homocysteine species in plasma/serum, including free and protein-bound forms, can be measured in plasma or serum.[22,113] In general, plasma levels are slightly lower. Thus an elevation of both homocysteine and MMA, while consistent with cobalamin deficiency, cannot rule out a combined cobalamin and folate deficiency (see Table 39.2); see box on Serum Homocysteine and Methylmalonic Acid Levels in Cobalamin and Folate Deficiencies.

Both homocysteine and MMA levels are elevated in patients with dehydration and renal failure; propionic acid derived from anaerobic fecal bacterial metabolism can also substantially contribute to methylmalonate production.[115] In this setting, the fraction of gut flora contribution to MMA can be reduced by treatment with metronidazole.

The normal value for serum homocysteine is 5.1 to 13.9 µM and serum MMA is 70 to 270 nM, and in general the higher the values, the more severe the clinical abnormalities.[22] However, there is a fairly wide range of "normalcy" in homocysteine values because of age-, creatinine-, gender-, diet-, and race-dependent variables.[113] Basal levels of MMA are usually less than 500 nM, and in renal failure, it rarely increases by more than 1000 nM.[22] If unseparated blood stands at room temperature, homocysteine levels will *increase* over 4 to 24 hours. Frozen serum (from measurements of serum folate or cobalamin) can be used for serum MMA and homocysteine determinations.

Serum MMA levels are elevated in more than 95% of patients with clinically confirmed cobalamin deficiency (with median values of 3500 nM). Serum homocysteine concentrations are elevated in both cobalamin deficiency (median values of 70 µM) and folate deficiency (median values of 50 µM).

Serum Cobalamin Levels

For the most part, a low serum cobalamin level is an established biochemical indicator of cobalamin deficiency. In general, in patients with clinical cobalamin deficiency and megaloblastic anemia or neurologic disease consistent with cobalamin deficiency, the sensitivity of cobalamin concentration less than 200 pg/mL (or less than 148 pmol/L) exceeds 95%[116] when the pretest probability is high. However, up to 10% of adults with true cobalamin deficiency have cobalamin values in the low-normal (200 to 300 pg/mL) range and only metabolite testing with homocysteine and MMA will reveal the deficiency (see Table 39.2).

TABLE 39.3	Serum Cobalamin: False-Positive and False-Negative Test Results

Falsely Low Serum Cobalamin in the Absence of True Cobalamin Deficiency

Folate deficiency (one-third of patients)

Multiple myeloma

TCI deficiency

Megadose vitamin C therapy

Falsely Raised Cobalamin Levels in the Presence of a True Deficiency[a]

Cobalamin binders (TCI and II) increased (e.g., myeloproliferative states, hepatomas, and fibrolamellar hepatic tumors)

TCII-producing macrophages are activated (e.g., autoimmune diseases, monoblastic leukemias and lymphomas)

Release of cobalamin from hepatocytes (e.g., active liver disease)

High serum anti-IF antibody titer

[a]Although a low serum cobalamin level is not synonymous with cobalamin deficiency, 5% of patients with true cobalamin deficiency have low-normal cobalamin levels, a potentially serious problem because the patient's underlying cobalamin deficiency will progress if uncorrected.

IF, Intrinsic factor; *TC*, transcobalamin.

Diagnosing Folate Deficiency

When combined with a clinical picture of megaloblastic anemia and additional results of cobalamin levels, the serum folate concentration is the cheapest and most useful initial biochemical test to diagnose folate deficiency[22] (see Table 39.2). The serum folate level is highly sensitive to folate intake, and a single hospital meal may normalize it in a patient with true folate deficiency. Rapidly developing nutritional folate deficiency first leads to a decline in the serum folate level below normal (less than 2 ng/mL) in about 3 weeks; it is a sensitive indicator of negative folate balance.[15] However, isolated reduction of serum folate level in the absence of megaloblastosis (i.e., false-positive result) occurs in one-third of hospitalized patients with anorexia, after acute alcohol consumption, during normal pregnancy, and in patients on anticonvulsants[22]; unfortunately, these are the very groups at high risk for folate deficiency and the people who exhibit low serum folate levels when they become folate deficient.[15] Conversely, in 25% to 50% of cases (predominantly alcoholics) with folate-deficient megaloblastosis, the serum folate levels may be below normal or borderline (2 to 4 ng/mL).[22] The serum folate level alone should never dictate therapy. It is important to consider the clinical picture, peripheral smear, and bone marrow morphology and also to rule out underlying cobalamin deficiency.

Thus a serum cobalamin concentration is less than 300 pg/mL in 99% of patients with clinical hematologic or neurologic manifestations of cobalamin deficiency,[22] and a cobalamin level of more than 300 pg/mL predicts folate deficiency or another hematologic or neurologic disease (see Table 39.2). However, a low serum cobalamin concentration is not synonymous with cobalamin deficiency, and several associated diseases and conditions can falsely raise or lower cobalamin levels (Table 39.3). Studies have also identified patients with true cobalamin deficiency who have cobalamin levels in the low-normal range. Among 173 unambiguously cobalamin-deficient patients[22] about 5% had normal cobalamin levels.

If the serum cobalamin test is broadly used as a screening test without clinical context, by virtue of the way normalcy is defined, 2.5% of nondeficient individuals will have low levels, which reflects our definition of the lower limit of normal for this test.[22] However, the finding that the same blood sample can give different cobalamin results (one below normal versus one above normal) using different commercial assays is of significant concern.[116] The more recent assays have periodically had such problems, apparently arising from a lack of transparency related to these tests, poor validation using low-cobalamin sera, and poor track record of continuous proficiency testing and tracking of assay performance.[116] It is a particularly serious issue when chemiluminescent tests for serum cobalamin give spuriously elevated levels and fail to detect clinically significant severe pernicious anemia. Such a false negative test result has been attributed to the in vitro binding of anti-IF antibodies (that are found in the serum of a patient with pernicious anemia) to the intrinsic factor found in the manufacturer's reagent.[117,118] However, a recent reevaluation of five different (currently used) automated cobalamin assays found that they are accurate and do not suffer from earlier problems.[119] Nevertheless, the principle that *"a clinical presentation which strongly suggests cobalamin deficiency should always lead to a therapeutic trial (with cobalamin replacement) even if the laboratory assay is nonconcordant"* must be upheld against future vagaries that can lead to dangerous false negative errors in laboratory tests.

So in the absence of availability of metabolite tests, if there are hematologic or neurologic findings that are consistent with clinical cobalamin deficiency, and the serum cobalamin level is normal or borderline low, it is entirely appropriate to treat as for a cobalamin deficiency. If there is no improvement in hematologic parameters within a couple of months, provided there are no other conditions that limit a full response to cobalamin (e.g., iron deficiency or underlying thalassemia trait, hypothyroidism, renal disease, infection, alcoholism, or intrinsic hematologic disease in the bone marrow), cobalamin deficiency would be unlikely.

Cobalamin deficiency can falsely raise serum folate by 20% to 30% via methyl-folate trapping. This will seriously underestimate the

prevalence of an associated folate deficiency among populations (mostly in developing countries, worldwide) where the dietary intake of both vitamins is consistently low. Folate deficiency can also reduce serum cobalamin, but the mechanism is unclear.

Serum Folate Levels

The serum folate level is clinically relevant and widely used. Microbiologic assays for folate, which measure all biologically active forms equally, have been replaced in the West by competitive folate-binding protein assays (from various commercial sources) that are indirect immunoassays, which rely on chemiluminescence methods. These tests are notorious for considerable lack of agreement with one another (see box on Diagnosing Folate Deficiency). Alignment with a new higher-order precision isotope-dilution liquid chromatography–tandem mass spectrometry assay, which demonstrates excellent agreement with the traditional *Lactobacillus casei* method,[120] will allow better standardization of the current competitive folate-binding protein assays.[121]

When negative folate balance continues, hepatic folate stores are depleted in about 4 months.[15] This leads to tissue folate deficiency, which clinically correlates with a decrease in RBC folate (less than 150 ng/mL) by the microbiologic assay.[15] However, current RBC folate tests using different commercial kits have major limitations in sensitivity and specificity and are notoriously unreliable in alcoholics and in pregnancy; furthermore, a reduction of RBC folate also occurs in about 60% of patients with cobalamin deficiency.

The use of red-cell folates as a measure of long-term folate status is valid during clinical trials in which a single kit is used for a cohort of patients; however, it is *not* valuable for routine clinical diagnosis because of the significant variability of performance between different commercial kits and lack of clinical validation.[122] For these reasons, the serum folate level, although labile, is a good initial choice.[15,123–126]

However, there are important caveats to measuring serum folate levels in certain clinical settings (see Caveats Related to the Use of Laboratory Tests in Developing Countries). First, the serum folate level can be artificially raised in a patient with either pure cobalamin deficiency or *combined* cobalamin- and folate- deficiency (Table 39.4). This is because cessation of the cobalamin-dependent methionine synthase reaction leads to a failure in utilization of intracellular folate for one-carbon metabolism. As a result, folate leaks out of cells into the plasma, thereby raising the patient's serum folate level; indeed, replacement of cobalamin alone will return the serum folate level

Summary of the Clinical Usefulness of Tests for Cobalamin and Folate Deficiencies

Within the clinical context of hematologic or neurologic features that suggest the diagnosis of cobalamin deficiency, if the cobalamin levels are suggestive but not definitive, then the MMA and homocysteine tests are an excellent gold standard test to confirm a clinical diagnosis. *Patients with clinical cobalamin deficiency usually have MMA values over 1000 nM and homocysteine values over 25 µM.* The MMA and homocysteine test results are much more sensitive than cobalamin levels and progressively increase much earlier than the drop in cobalamin levels; one or both metabolites was increased in 99.8% of more than 400 patients with proven cobalamin deficiency.[22]

Based on the lower costs of serum cobalamin and folate compared with serum MMA and homocysteine levels, it is recommended (see Table 39.2) to first use the cheaper tests that can assist in the diagnosis of cobalamin and folate deficiency.[22] Clinicians should also restrict use of serum MMA and homocysteine to patients with borderline cobalamin and folate levels; to patients with existing conditions associated with difficulties in the interpretation of test results; to situations in which cobalamin and folate levels are low, when a high MMA level is useful in confirming cobalamin deficiency (rather than attributing the condition to folate deficiency alone); and to patients with clearly low serum levels but for whom there is an alternative explanation for the findings that caused an unusual serum cobalamin level to be obtained (e.g., a diabetic or alcoholic with peripheral neuropathy, an alcoholic with a high MCV and a low serum cobalamin without anemia). In these cases, serum levels of metabolites can assist in the diagnosis of vitamin deficiency.

Diagnostic algorithms consistently stress the value of clinical data to improve the pretest probability of serum cobalamin and serum folate tests.[22] Without detailed clinical information, the combined test results for serum cobalamin, folate, and metabolite (homocysteine and MMA) are not sufficiently unambiguous to diagnose and distinguish cobalamin deficiency from combined cobalamin-plus-folate deficiency. In combined cobalamin-plus-folate deficiency, both vitamins would be needed to restore baseline values, particularly of homocysteine.[22]

to baseline.[127–132] Thus associated nutritional cobalamin deficiency has the potential to consistently mask the coexistence of mild- to moderate folate deficiency if the unwary clinician uses the serum folate level as a gold standard for diagnosing folate deficiency in this clinical setting. Second, such patients (with combined nutritional folate *and* cobalamin deficiency) often reside in malarious regions where there may be ongoing hemolysis from malaria *per se* as well as intrinsic hemolysis from associated hemoglobinopathies that are common in these regions (e.g., thalassemia, sickle cell disease, glucose-6-phosphate dehydrogenase deficiency). In a patient with malaria during hemolysis of *Plasmodium falciparum* infected erythroid precursors, reticulocytes, and mature erythrocytes, there will be substantial release of the 30-fold more folate-rich intraerythrocyte contents *into* serum, thereby artificially raising the baseline serum folate level. Moreover, red cells normally contain substantial amounts of *various forms of folate*, i.e., 5-methyltetrahydrofolate (monoglutamates) and folate-polyglutamates of different glutamate chain lengths[69]; whereas clearance of such released folate monoglutamates would be hindered with associated cobalamin deficiency,[127–132] we also know that the released folate polyglutamates are also inefficiently transported back into cells relative to monoglutamates,[34] thereby also resulting in poor clearance. In this clinical context, the current assays for serum folate (which are primarily designed to measure physiologic serum 5-methyltetrahydrofolate monoglutamate) may not consistently discriminate among these forms of folates. The net result is that a *high* serum folate could be reported in all such individuals with malaria, *even when the patient's tissue folates are significantly depleted.* This predictable masking of tissue folate depletion *argues against* the use of serum tests for folate deficiency in this clinical setting, where assessing the intake of folate-rich foods in the diet is a better method to assess folate status. (See Masking of Nutritional Folate Deficiency by Associated Cobalamin Deficiency and/or Malaria and Table 39.4.)

TABLE 39.4 Serum Folates Are Misleadingly Elevated in Cobalamin (Vitamin B_{12}) Deficiency and/or Malaria Which Are Both Common in Resource-Limited Settings[a],* (From Antony, 2015[133])

	Serum Folates	Erythrocyte Folates	Serum Cobalamin
Pure folate deficiency	Low	Low	Normal/Low*
Pure cobalamin deficiency	Normal/High*,[b]	Low*,[b]	Low
Folate *plus* cobalamin deficiency	Normal*	Low	Low
Pure malaria	Normal*/High*,[c]	High*,[d,e]	Normal
Malaria *plus* folate deficiency	Normal*	Normal*/High*/Low	Normal
Malaria *plus* cobalamin deficiency	Normal*/High*,[c]	Normal*/High*,[e]	Low
Malaria *plus* folate *plus* cobalamin deficiency	Normal*/High*,[c]	Low/Normal*,[e,f]	Low

*The *asterisk* indicates misleading values in the clinical settings shown on the left. The information presented in this table has been synthesized from several sources (see text and references).

[a]Both cobalamin deficiency and clinical malaria and other hemolytic states can complicate the diagnosis of folate deficiency using tests for serum- or erythrocyte-folate concentration.[134]

[b]Cobalamin deficiency is accompanied by inability to use folates for one-carbon metabolism, so folates leak out of erythroid precursors into serum.

[c]Release of the 30-fold excess folate from infected erythroid precursors, reticulocytes, and mature erythrocytes during hemolysis raises serum folate levels. (An as-yet-unknown quantity of folate is released into serum when folate-rich hepatocytes are destroyed during the exoerythrocytic hepatic phase of malaria.)

[d]Hemolysis induces a compensatory reticulocytosis; these reticulocytes are richer in folate than mature erythrocytes.[82,83,127]

[e]*Plasmodium falciparum* can also synthesize folates in erythrocyte cultures in vitro[135] and raises erythrocyte folates in animal models with high levels of parasitemia.[136]

[f]Reticulocytopenia in severe *Plasmodium falciparum* malaria, caused by either combined cobalamin deficiency *plus* folate deficiency, which can trigger a reticulocytopenic (megaloblastic) crisis, or cytokine-induced inhibition of hematopoiesis, will negate an expected rise in erythrocyte folates.

Reused with permission from Antony AC. Megaloblastic anemias. In: Goldman L, Schafer A, eds. *Cecil Medicine*, 25th Edition. Philadelphia, 2015, Elsevier-Saunders: Volume 1, Chapter 164, pp. 1104–1114.

Other Tests

The clinical use of low holo-transcobalamin II (holo-TCII) levels, to provide information on the extent of saturation of serum TCII as an early marker of cobalamin homeostasis[137] or to diagnose cobalamin deficiency in lieu of serum cobalamin values, is still unclear. This test has not yet been sufficiently clinically validated[116,138] to define sensitivity, specificity, and other clinical confounders that can alter the results.

PATHOGENESIS OF COBALAMIN DEFICIENCY

Nutritional Cobalamin Deficiency

Vegetarian diets can be classified as lactovegetarian, ovovegetarian, lacto-ovovegetarian, or vegan, respectively, if they include dairy products, eggs, dairy products and eggs, or no animal products at all.[7] However, all these vegetarian diets contain insufficient amounts of cobalamin. Therefore *all* vegetarians are in various stages of progressive cobalamin depletion and moving inexorably toward cobalamin deficiency.[8] This warrants early supplementation with cobalamin.

In addition, the vast majority of those living in developing countries subsist on a monotonous diet that is intrinsically low in animal-source foods (which are more expensive than plant-based diets). Although they are not strictly considered vegetarians, these individuals are better classified as "near-vegetarians"[7,8] and should also be supplemented with cobalamin. Thus cobalamin deficiency has been widely reported among 45% of Northern Chinese women,[139] and up to 85% of adolescents[140] and 65% of newborns[141] in India. In one series from Pakistan,[142] among those with megaloblastic anemia (hemoglobin <8 g/dL), nearly 80% had cobalamin deficiency. Koreans also do not consume sufficient animal-source proteins.[143] Surprisingly, even those consuming Mediterranean diets that are rich in fruits and vegetables but low in animal-source protein are at risk for cobalamin deficiency; among 180 pregnant women, cobalamin deficiency was found in 72% of mothers and 41% of babies.[144]

The fetus is dependent on the mother's cobalamin stores for a sufficient quota of cobalamin at birth; a close correlation exists between low maternal serum and breast milk cobalamin concentrations and cobalamin insufficiency in the infant.[145] Therefore when mothers do not consume sufficient amounts of animal-source foods, they themselves are at risk for nutritional cobalamin deficiency, and their infants will have smaller stores of the vitamin at birth.[146,147] Although the dictum is that infants should be exclusively breastfed for the first 6 months of life, a large percentage of mothers in developing countries had evidence of cobalamin deficiency.[7,148,149] For example, three-quarters of a cross section of 366 pregnant urban women in South India had cobalamin deficiency.[150] So there is an imperative to raise these values in women and in babies. An important series of studies has shown that treatment of the mother during pregnancy[151] or even the infant shortly after delivery will promptly reverse preexisting cobalamin deficiency.[152]

Cobalamin-deficient infants can present with a spectrum of clinical findings, ranging from feeding difficulties and refusal of both breast milk and complementary food by regurgitation (which results in failure to thrive) to motor and social retardation, reflecting a developmental delay. The child is persistently drowsy and rarely sits up or makes eye contact.[7] There may be lemon-tint jaundice with hypotonia, insufficient head control, and delayed spontaneous turning. There can be brownish-black areas of hyperpigmentation in the dorsal fingers and toes as well as over the medial thighs, arms, and axillae (which usually resolve within 3 months of therapy). Evidence of megaloblastic anemia may be masked with superimposed iron deficiency. If left untreated, there is growth retardation with reduced height and weight, and reduced head circumference with cranial magnetic resonance imaging (MRI) showing delayed myelination and frontoparietal cortical atrophy in affected infants[153]; these can also be reversed within 3 months of cobalamin replacement. Treatment results in a dramatic increase in alertness and responsiveness of the child, who is now miraculously transformed into a normal child who, within a few days, rolls over spontaneously, makes eye contact with its mother, and is much more interested in the surroundings. Any previous abnormal movements (tremors, chorea, or myoclonus) may regress but transiently return within a few days to affect the face or tongue; however, these will resolve in 2 to 3 months.[154] Cobalamin deficiency often resurfaces during wartime, which invariably leaves women and their infants malnourished.[155]

Infants in the West fed a macrobiotic diet (vegan-like with occasional servings of fish) must be rapidly replenished with cobalamin before switching to a cobalamin-rich diet. Otherwise, up to 20% continue to have low cobalamin status, which can lead to impaired psychomotor functioning well into youth and later adolescence with compromise in faculties related to reasoning, abstract thinking, and learning ability.[156]

When children in resource-limited settings grow up on the same monotonous diet as their parents, they are at risk for combined cobalamin, folate (and iron) deficiency.[7,114,157–159] *This problem of vertical intergenerational transfer of a deficient "bank balance" of minerals and micronutrients from one generation to another has been documented in all developing countries.* These affected children with preexisting depleted stores of cobalamin, folate (and iron), and imminent deficiency, who are the unwitting victims of circumstance, limp on through life with cognitive dysfunction and lower intelligence quotient and emotional intelligence (when compared with their better nourished counterparts in developed countries). When they move on into adolescence and (often premature) young motherhood, they pass on their deficient "bank balances" vertically to the next generation and so the cycle continues *ad infinitum*. The number of such affected individuals worldwide is probably in the hundreds of millions.

Recent longitudinal studies from the West among women who apparently consume a balanced nonvegetarian diet confirm that pregnancy places an additional stress on the mother's cobalamin stores and can lead to metabolic evidence of cobalamin deficiency.[160–162] This can negatively affect their breastfed infants' cobalamin status at 6 weeks; indeed, over two-thirds of Norwegian infants of otherwise healthy mothers had a metabolic profile consistent with cobalamin deficiency, which reverted to normal after cobalamin replenishment.[161,162] Among infants with only minor developmental delays and feeding difficulties (regurgitation) and biochemical evidence of cobalamin deficiency, those who were treated with cobalamin responded with significant clinical benefit, a fact that underscores the importance of cobalamin in postnatal neurodevelopment.[163] Thus it is likely that many more breastfed infants in the West probably need cobalamin supplements early in life, as do their mothers in preparation for pregnancy.[11]

Intragastric Events Leading to Cobalamin Malabsorption

Inadequate Dissociation of Cobalamin from Food Protein

Dietary cobalamin is bioavailable only after proteolytic digestion of food by gastric acid and pepsin. Failure to release cobalamin from food protein can lead to food-cobalamin malabsorption and frank cobalamin deficiency despite the presence of IF.[22]

Congenital Intrinsic Factor Deficiency

Congenital IF deficiency arising from mutations in gastric IF,[164] resulting in complete loss of IF, can be transmitted as an autosomal recessive trait and expressed in homozygotes by the age of 2 years as severe megaloblastic anemia (less than 100 cases reported).[165] Dysfunctional IF may lead to only a mild abnormality in binding to cobalamin and result in a delayed presentation into the second decade.

Loss or Atrophy of Gastric Oxyntic Mucosa

IF deficiency, which arises from atrophy of gastric parietal (oxyntic) mucosal cells, can be caused by total or partial gastrectomy; by autoimmune destruction, as observed in adult Addisonian pernicious anemia or, rarely, in a similar disease in children (juvenile pernicious anemia); and after destruction of gastric mucosa by caustic (lye) ingestion.

Total gastrectomy invariably leads to cobalamin deficiency in about 5 years (range, 2 to 10 years); indeed, longitudinal follow-up revealed that all 176 patients developed cobalamin deficiency within 4 years, with earlier clinical presentations occurring in those with lower cobalamin status preoperatively.[143] This condition is often associated with iron deficiency,[15] warranting routine cobalamin and iron replacement prophylactically.

Cobalamin deficiency eventually develops in 10% to 20% of patients 8 years after partial gastrectomy; a minority (about 5%) develops frank clinical manifestations of cobalamin deficiency with megaloblastic anemia. The cause is multifactorial, and contributing factors include decreased IF secretion, hypochlorhydria, intestinal bacterial overgrowth of cobalamin-consuming organisms, and associated iron deficiency. The degree of cobalamin deficiency depends on the size of the remaining gastric remnant. It is more common in Bilroth II than in Bilroth I surgery, and in subtotal than in partial gastrectomy. Morbidly obese patients treated surgically with gastric bypass also have more food-cobalamin malabsorption than patients treated with vertical banded gastroplasty.[22] Even after laparoscopic Roux-en-Y gastric bypass, and despite multivitamin supplementation, iron deficiency was seen in one-half of patients and cobalamin deficiency seen in one-quarter at 3 years[166]; therefore these patients probably need higher oral cobalamin (or addition of parenteral) therapy.

Absent Intrinsic Factor Secretion and Pernicious Anemia

A common cause of cobalamin malabsorption is pernicious anemia, an autoimmune disease in which the fundamental defect is atrophy of the gastric (parietal cell) oxyntic mucosa that eventually leads to the complete absence of IF and hydrochloric acid secretion (Fig. 39.9). The autoimmune gastritis (leading to chronic atrophic gastritis) associated with pernicious anemia involves the fundus and body of the stomach, and the histologic appearance of the gastric mucosa (infiltration with plasma cells and lymphocytes) is strongly reminiscent of the autoimmune type of lesions.[6,167,168] Because cobalamin is absorbed only by binding to IF and uptake by ileal IF-cobalamin receptors, the net consequence is severe cobalamin malabsorption leading to cobalamin deficiency.

The annual incidence of pernicious anemia is approximately 25 new cases per 100,000 persons older than 40 years. Although the average age of onset is about 60 years, pernicious anemia is no respecter of age, race, or ethnic origin. The predisposition to developing pernicious anemia may have a genetic basis, but neither the mode of inheritance nor the initiating events or primary mechanism is precisely understood. There is a positive family history for about 30% of patients, among whom the risk for familial pernicious anemia is 20 times as high as in the general population; about 20% of siblings of patients are projected to develop pernicious anemia by the age of 90 years, and pernicious anemia has developed concordantly in identical twins.

There is a significant association of pernicious anemia with other autoimmune diseases,[15] including Graves disease (30%), Hashimoto thyroiditis (11%), vitiligo (8%), Addison disease, idiopathic hypoparathyroidism, primary ovarian failure, myasthenia gravis, type 1 diabetes mellitus, and adult hypogammaglobulinemia.[15,22]

Autoimmune gastritis progresses over decades to atrophic body gastritis and pernicious anemia. Serum anti-IF antibodies are highly specific (100%) for pernicious anemia, but the sensitivity is only about 50%. Earlier, the clinical use of antiparietal cell antibodies was limited because of low specificity. This necessitated use of additional surrogate markers (high serum gastrin and low pepsinogen I levels) that reflected loss of acid- and IF-secreting parietal (oxyntic) cells. However, newer enzyme-linked immunosorbent assays (ELISA) for antiparietal cell antibodies, which are directed against gastric H^+/K^+ ATPase, are 30% more sensitive than previous (immunofluorescence) assays. A reanalysis of the clinical utility of combining anti-IF and newer antiparietal cell antibody tests to noninvasively diagnose pernicious anemia points to this approach as very promising.[169] Thus among 81 patients with biopsy-proven atrophic body gastritis and pernicious anemia, combining anti-IF antibodies (37% sensitivity; 100% specificity) with newer antiparietal cell antibodies (sensitivity 91%; specificity 90%) significantly increased their diagnostic performance for pernicious anemia, yielding overall 73% sensitivity while maintaining 100% specificity.[169]

Juvenile pernicious anemia can manifest in the second decade with severe cobalamin deficiency in conjunction with many of the associated endocrinopathies and autoantibodies observed in adults.[15]

Undiagnosed pernicious anemia is common among free-living elderly persons (over 60 years of age) who have only minimal clinical manifestations of cobalamin deficiency (i.e., 1.9% of a Southern California survey population had unrecognized and untreated pernicious anemia).[170] The prevalence was 2.7% in women and 1.4% in men, but 4.3% of the African American women and 4.0% of the white women had pernicious anemia.

Abnormal Events in the Small Bowel Lumen

Insufficient Pancreatic Protease

About 30% of patients with severe pancreatic insufficiency fail to degrade R proteins, which will lead to impaired transfer of cobalamin from R protein to IF. Pancreatic extract will normalize cobalamin malabsorption.[15]

Inactivation of Pancreatic Protease

Pancreatic protease can be inactivated by massive gastric hypersecretion arising from a gastrinoma in Zollinger-Ellison syndrome.[15] The

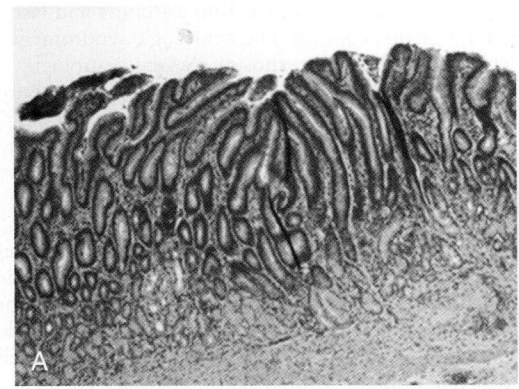
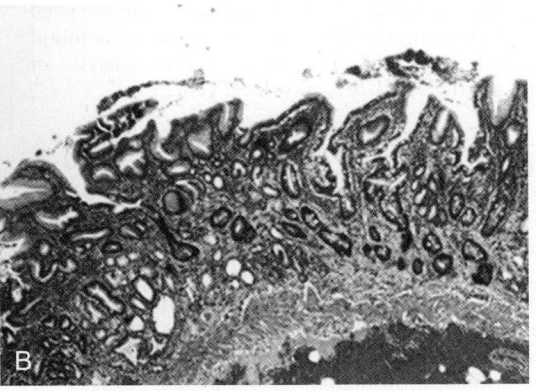

Fig. 39.9 HISTOLOGIC FEATURES OF STOMACH IN PERNICIOUS ANEMIA COMPARED TO NORMAL. The normal gastric mucosa (A) is contrasted to that seen in pernicious anemia (B), in which there is atrophy of gastric glands, intestinal metaplasia with goblet cells, and loss of parietal cells (not visible at this magnification).

continued low pH of the luminal contents reaching the ileum may also perturb interaction of the IF-cobalamin complex with IF-cobalamin receptors (which requires a pH above 5.4).

Usurpation of Luminal Cobalamin

The near-sterile condition of the small bowel is maintained by a combination of the mechanical cleansing action of peristalsis and the chemical action of gastric acid. Disorders conducive to relative stasis, impaired motility, and hypogammaglobulinemia are predisposing factors that favor colonization by bacteria. Many of these bacteria can take up free cobalamin, but not IF-bound cobalamin. However, if colonization extends proximally to the locus at which IF and cobalamin interact, significant cobalamin may be usurped before it can bind to IF.[15] This cobalamin malabsorption can be corrected to some extent by a 7- to 10-day course of antibiotic therapy.

Approximately 3% of individuals infested with the fish tapeworm *Diphyllobothrium latum,* which avidly usurps cobalamin for growth[15] can develop frank cobalamin deficiency. Humans become infected when they eat partially cooked or raw fish containing plerocercoids, which develop into adult worms in the jejunum in about 6 weeks, growing to a length of 10 m, with up to 4000 proglottids[15]; when these worms lay eggs, the life cycle is repeated. After ova have been identified in the stools, expulsion of the worms by praziquantel (10 to 20 mg/kg as a single dose taken orally) and cobalamin replenishment is curative.

Disorders of Ileal Intrinsic Factor–Cobalamin Receptors or Mucosa

Absence of Intrinsic Factor–Cobalamin Receptors

The distal ileum has the greatest density of IF-cobalamin receptors. Disease or removal of only 1 to 2 feet of terminal ileum by resection or bypass reduces ileal IF-cobalamin receptor numbers for interaction with IF-cobalamin, resulting in cobalamin malabsorption.[15,22]

Defective Intrinsic Factor–Cobalamin Receptors or Post-Intrinsic Factor–Cobalamin Receptor Defects

Imerslund-Gräsbeck syndrome is a term used collectively for a heterogeneous group of congenital (autosomal recessive) disorders in children arising from biallelic mutations (in 80% of cases) involving either the *cubilin* (*CUBN*) or *amnionless* (*AMN*) genes that constitute the functional IF-cobalamin receptor (i.e., cubam).[171] This results in selective cobalamin malabsorption. Children present between 3 and 10 years of age with megaloblastic anemia and neurologic presentations with low serum cobalamin levels associated with mild, persistent, benign proteinuria (in 90% of cases). Because cubam also participates in the renal tubular absorption of albumin, this is the basis for proteinuria found in Imerslund-Gräsbeck syndrome. Diagnosis requires analysis of mutational status of gastric IF, *CUBN*, and *AMN* genes.[164,171]

Drug-Induced Defects

Long-term use of H_2 antagonists and/or proton pump inhibitors may interfere with the handover of food-cobalamin to IF, especially in those with preexisting borderline cobalamin stores. Long-term treatment with metformin can interfere with IF-cobalamin binding to ileal cubam receptors[172] and progressively increases the risk for cobalamin deficiency over time.[173] Therefore, screening for cobalamin deficiency and additional confirmation of metabolic evidence of cobalamin deficiency (elevated MMA) can be reason to trigger replacement therapy with cobalamin. Other drugs (e.g., cholestyramine, colchicine, neomycin) probably also impair transepithelial transport of cobalamin.[15]

Disorders of Plasma Cobalamin Transport

Polymorphism or absence of TCI can be associated with low cobalamin levels, but the MMA and homocysteine levels are normal. By contrast, either deficiency or defective TCII can present with megaloblastic anemia in infancy; this can be associated with normal cobalamin levels (because TCI, which binds over 75% of serum cobalamin is normal). However, there will be metabolic evidence of cobalamin deficiency that can be reversed by daily or biweekly injections of 1 mg of cobalamin, which ensures passive cobalamin delivery into cells. Mutations in the gene for the TCII receptor (*CD320*) have also been identified.[174]

Disorders of Intracellular Cobalamin Use

Congenital Metabolic Defects of Cobalamin Metabolism: Cobalamin Mutants A to J

Given the multitude of chaperones or transporters involved in escorting cobalamin intracellularly to their destination to function as coenzymes for methionine synthase and methylmalonyl-CoA mutase, it is not difficult to envision that there would invariably be inborn errors of cobalamin metabolism where one of these escorts or transporters is missing. The combination of megaloblastic anemia with increased levels of homocysteine or MMA, or both, in serum and urine despite normal cobalamin and folate levels should suggest an inborn error of cobalamin metabolism.[175] The inherited defects of cobalamin use (see Fig. 39.3) are heterogeneous and are empirically defined as cobalamin mutations A to J (cblA to cblJ).[175]

These infants must be differentiated from those with nutritional cobalamin deficiency who could have similar clinical features. Patients suspected of having an inborn error of metabolism should be evaluated by specialized laboratories, such as the McGill University laboratory of Prof David Rosenblatt—a premier diagnostic center.[176]

Functional Cobalamin Deficiency After Nitrous Oxide Exposure

Nitrous oxide (N_2O) inactivates coenzyme forms of cobalamin by oxidizing the fully reduced cob(I)alamin to cob(III)alamin; this results in a state of functional intracellular cobalamin deficiency. This syndrome was first identified in patients with tetanus given nitrous oxide for up to 6 days.[15] Subsequently, persons exposed to nitrous oxide for open heart surgery and through chronic (surreptitious, accidental, or occupational) exposure have been recognized as being at high risk for developing megaloblastosis and cobalamin-deficient neuromyelopathy.[15] The slang word for recreational use of nitrous oxide is *nanging;* capsules that are used for making whipped cream are a cheap and easy source of nitrous oxide in the community. Megaloblastosis develops within 24 hours and lasts less than 1 week after a single exposure. The neurologic syndrome is usually seen with chronic intermittent exposure. Severe neurologic deficits have been reported after prolonged intraoperative exposure to nitrous oxide in patients with unsuspected cobalamin deficiency.[22]

Subclinical Cobalamin Deficiency

The entity of subclinical cobalamin deficiency is defined when there is biochemical evidence for cobalamin deficiency, reflected by a low cobalamin value (and increased MMA and homocysteine) but without overt clinical manifestations. Although dependent on the population studied, the frequency of (silent) subclinical cobalamin deficiency in the United States is suspected to be 10 times higher than classic (overt) cobalamin deficiency that is found in 1% to 2% of the population. Nevertheless, the issue of subclinical cobalamin deficiency has been a vexing problem and a semantic dilemma. Many elderly persons may have various symptoms consistent with aging (including fatigue, cognitive changes, lower quality-of-life measures, and subtle symptoms of neuropathy) that cannot be directly attributed to cobalamin deficiency, despite the fact that these very symptoms are often seen in symptomatic cobalamin deficiency; often this triggers testing with a serum cobalamin test, and a borderline result that spontaneously reverts to normal, or minimally fluctuates above or below the cutoff value, or remains stable without change over many years generates a new set of problems, including the need to label this entity and thereby make clinical decisions.

Although some experts do not feel obliged to treat, preferring to wait for overt symptoms, others feel ethically bound to treat even without overt clinical manifestations; indeed, such clinical manifestations can be very subtle and are detected only by sophisticated neurophysiologic or imaging studies that are expensive and impractical for routine clinical practice. In support of earlier therapy in this clinical setting, there is compelling clinical evidence that combined B-vitamin supplementation to reduce homocysteine can reduce brain atrophy[177] and both cognitive and clinical decline[178] (see section on Homocysteine and Mild Cognitive Impairment).

After replenishing potentially depleted cobalamin stores with parenteral cobalamin therapy, oral supplementation for 4 to 6 months on and 4 to 6 months off may afford an adequate cobalamin status in most patients[179] as an alternative to continuous therapy. A key factor is the cost of cobalamin (and the lack of side effects associated with cobalamin therapy); for example, parenteral cobalamin, which can be purchased on the Internet for $15 for each 10 mg/10 mL vial, would last a year after replenishing stores. The additional purchase of 30-gauge $\frac{1}{2}$-inch insulin U100 syringes for monthly subcutaneous injection could be less costly than even generic tablets of 1 mg taken daily.

PATHOGENESIS OF FOLATE DEFICIENCY

Folate deficiency is usually recognized in the course of certain clinical presentations that predispose to negative folate balance and subsequent deficiency. It is instructive therefore to conceptualize cellular folate deficiency as arising from etiologic categories of decreased supply (i.e., reduced intake, absorption, transport, or use) or increased requirement (i.e., metabolic consumption, destruction, or excretion). However, in the same patient more than one mechanism may result in net folate deficiency. The precise contribution of one mechanism over the other is often not obvious, and specific tests to define each mechanism are not routinely available for clinical use. Thus the clinical context is especially important. Megaloblastic manifestations of folate deficiency are discussed within the context of the history and physical examination (discussed later). Cases of neuropathy in adults attributed to folate deficiency are rarely encountered; when they are, the possibility of alcoholism with thiamine deficiency must be considered. In any case, every patient with neuropathy, myelopathy, or psychiatric manifestations associated with megaloblastosis must be investigated in detail to rule out cobalamin deficiency. Gastrointestinal megaloblastosis begets further folate malabsorption, which propagates a vicious cycle of folate deficiency in the short term and cobalamin deficiency in the long term. With the exception of drug-induced defects or inborn errors of folate metabolism that result in decreased use of intracellular folates, all causes, irrespective of mechanism, result in reduced net delivery of folates to normal proliferating cells.

Nutritional Causes of Folate Deficiency

The body stores of folate are adequate for only about 4 months[15] although those with higher folate stores could take longer to become frankly deficient.[180] Individuals who are chronically in negative folate balance may only require a brief "nudge"—from superimposition of an associated illness that leads to hemolysis, anorexia, or folate malabsorption—to "tip" them into frank folate deficiency. The incidence of folate deficiency varies from country to country and even within regions in the same country. This is highly influenced by the

economic status and ethnic diet where cooking and choice of foods vary from region to region. For example, in Benin, central Africa, the prevalence of folate deficiency anemia was 20%, and in Zimbabwe, 30% had low folate levels, whereas in Sudan it was nearly 60%.[181] In Sri Lanka, one-half of schoolchildren had low-folate status, but less than 1% had folate deficiency in Thailand, which likely relates to the abundant consumption of greens and meats by Thais. Even in the United States, before folate fortification of food, about 20% of the population had low-folate status, and in Venezuela, 30% had low-folate status before such fortification. Decreased availability of folate-rich foods (in winter, after natural disasters, or during the wet season in central Africa), poverty, various cultural or ethnic diets (consisting of maize, rice, or well-cooked beans and vegetables), and cooking techniques that destroy food folate, coupled with the anorexia that accompanies chronic illnesses, are just a few of the reasons for rapid development of folate deficiency.[15,22]

In Western countries, food faddism, alcoholism, or unbalanced slimming diets usually lead to decreased folate intake in young to middle-aged individuals.[15] Edentulous or infirm persons or neglected older adults who are too ill to prepare their meals, as well as psychiatric patients, are particularly at risk for nutritional folate deficiency[15] (see box on Etiopathophysiologic Classification of Folate Deficiency).

Folate fortification of foods in the West has led to widespread elimination of folate deficiency and related anemia,[182,183] leading to questions of whether testing for folate deficiency is even justified.[184,185] Vigilance must nevertheless be exercised among the elderly who are still at risk for both folate and cobalamin deficiency.[186-188]

Pregnancy and Infancy

Pregnancy and lactation are associated with significantly higher folate requirements (over 400 µg/day) for growth of the fetus, placenta, breast, and other maternal tissues.[189] Folate requirement increases throughout pregnancy and is maximal near term. There is also increased urinary loss of folate in pregnancy (about 14 µg/day versus approximately 4.2 µg/day in nonpregnant women) because of a lower renal threshold. Poor preparation for pregnancy, with a poorly balanced diet and preexisting multifactorial nutritional anemia that remains unaddressed, is a major factor accounting for serious pregnancy complications and adverse birth outcomes. Therefore additional folate during pregnancy is required to prevent both pregnancy complications (preeclampsia, placental abruption or infarctions, recurrent miscarriage) and poor pregnancy outcomes (preterm delivery, neural-tube defects [NTDs], congenital heart defects, and intrauterine growth retardation). Low-folate status associated with short interpregnancy intervals or twin pregnancies also predisposes to preterm births.[190] All this demand for folate must somehow be met by increased folate intake.

However, the vast majority (over 90%) of pregnant women in resource-poor countries consume less than the estimated average requirement of folate[191]; in addition, a substantial number also consume less than optimum amounts of several other minerals, such as iron, and micronutrients, including cobalamin, as noted earlier. For example, studies on women from groups with low socioeconomic status from North India[29,30] have estimated that the daily intake of folic acid ranged between 75 µg and 167 µg, which is far lower than the 400 µg/day required to prevent birth defects.[64] This is simple to remedy. When given daily or even twice weekly, the combination of iron (100 mg elemental iron) and folic acid (0.5 mg) has been shown to significantly improve several cognitive abilities of schoolgirls in India,[192] which renders them better prepared for pregnancy in the future. This is all the more important because of results from experimental studies designed to define the influence of gestational folate deficiency on the fetus (discussed later). Thus pregnancy with poor folate intake is the most common cause of megaloblastic anemia in the world.

As noted earlier, the placenta has a large number of folate receptors,[64] which facilitate binding and transport of folates to the developing fetus. Preferential delivery of folate to the fetus can cause or aggravate folate deficiency in the mother.[15] This is observed clinically when a mother with severe folate deficiency gives birth to a baby who has normal folate stores.[63]

The rapidly proliferating tissues in children also have an absolute requirement for exogenously supplied folate. Although human milk can maintain folate balance in breastfed infants, the breast milk content of folate is low when the mother's folate status is poor.

Before the advent of routine folate supplementation during pregnancy, the incidence of megaloblastic marrows in the United States, Canada, and the United Kingdom during late pregnancy was about 25%, but in South India, it was about 55%.[15] Folate deficiency is eight times as high in twin pregnancies. Multiparity (multiple frequent pregnancies with a prolonged state of negative folate balance) and hyperemesis gravidarum commonly lead to folate deficiency. Because the anemia of pregnancy is most frequently caused by iron deficiency, combined iron and folate deficiency (dimorphic anemia) is the more frequent clinical presentation. Increased use of folates by the newborn leads to a drop in serum folate levels by about 6 weeks of age. This drop is exaggerated in premature infants (who have feeding difficulties, infection, or hemolytic disease leading to pure folate deficiency); hence supplementation is routine for them.[15]

Folates and Neurodevelopment

All inborn errors of folate metabolism, which result in reduced folate availability to the developing brain, give rise to mental retardation and related mental health problems. The fetal brain is dependent on sufficient provision of maternal folate during embryogenesis. Thus it can been predicted that, under conditions where maternal folate deficiency can compromise the delivery of folate to the developing fetal brain, and depending on the degree of deficiency, there could be a spectrum of neurologic abnormalities; this could range from full-blown NTDs to more subtle changes that manifest in childhood as behavioral abnormalities.[57,69,193] Because routine folate supplementation is now the norm for women, we must rely on experimental studies in animals to clarify the pathologic effects of folate deficiency in pregnancy. Such studies[57] indicate that folate deficiency will significantly compromise early pregnancy outcomes (including the rates of pregnancy, rate of implantation, and effects on the number of live births). Even lesser degrees of folate deficiency to only one-third of optimum dietary folate for 2 months before and throughout gestation in dams, which coincidentally mimics the extent of insufficient dietary folate availability among women in vast areas of Northern India,[64] also resulted in subtle histologic aberrations and defects during murine fetal development.[57] These included increased apoptotic cell loss involving nearly every organ and fine architectural anomalies, as well as adverse influences on fetal brain development and unexpectedly profound abnormalities in the white matter, reflecting perturbed neuronal development.[57] Surprisingly, despite postnatal folate replenishment, these mice exhibited an anxiety phenotype in adulthood.[194] The latter studies indicate a new paradigm for the developmental origin of neuropsychiatric disease that points to poor maternal folate nutrition during pregnancy. These data also suggest the existence of a sensitive window during fetal neurodevelopment when folate deficiency dysregulates the expression of certain genes and/or proteins, which leads to the imprinting of abnormal neural circuits in utero that predispose to anxiety in adulthood. In concordance with these studies in mice, a prospective cohort human study has reported that lower maternal folate status in early pregnancy was associated with childhood hyperactivity/inattention and peer problems in early childhood.[195] The associations between low maternal folate and head circumference at birth[195] are similar to murine studies in which a net reduction in the number of cells (by approximately 20%) in the brains of murine fetuses that experienced gestational folate deficiency[57,193] was observed; this increased brain cell loss was because of apoptosis arising from megaloblastosis of folate-deficient cells during development. Folate is also critical during the early postnatal period and deficiency (in rodents) results in apoptosis of

cochlear cells leading to severe hearing loss[196] and learning and memory deficits.[197]

There is additional clinical support for a relationship between suboptimal folate delivery to the developing fetal brain and abnormal behavior. For example, 18-month-old children of mothers who took folate supplements had less "internalizing" patterns of behavior (emotionally reactive, anxious/depressed, somatic complaints, withdrawn) and less "externalizing" syndromes involving attention problems and aggressive behavior compared to offspring of women who did not take folate supplements.[198] There is a link between periconceptional folic acid supplements for women and a lower risk of autistic disorder (the most severe of the autism spectrum disorders) in their young children.[199] These findings are consistent with other recent studies from Asia, Europe, and North America, suggesting that children of mothers with higher blood folate concentrations or mothers receiving folic acid supplements had improved neurodevelopmental outcomes.[200–203] Conversely, low maternal folate status during early pregnancy is associated with a higher risk of emotional problems in the offspring.[204] Thus it appears that we are likely peering through the mist into a new field whereby nutritional folate insufficiency during fetal neurodevelopment predisposes to neuropsychiatric illness!

The long-lasting benefit to the offspring of women who take iron and folic acid during the early stages of pregnancy appears to be a consistent theme; in Nepalese women, such supplementation provided significant benefits to the proper neurodevelopment of their babies in utero.[200] Children of these women exhibited improved brain function, manifest by improvement in both general intellectual ability and some aspects of executive functions as well as fine motor skills when tested at ages 7 to 9 years. Although this clinical study was unable to assign whether iron or folic acid was the more important, there is sufficient supporting experimental evidence in the literature for both being critically important. Indeed, these human parallels to murine studies are consistent with the Barker hypothesis on the developmental origins of disease. Finally, there is also evidence to suggest that suboptimal folate intake that leads to low-folate status during adolescence can affect cognition and academic achievement, independent of socioeconomic status.[205] And another recent large observational study has also identified that maternal use of folic acid supplements in early pregnancy was associated with a reduced risk for severe language delay in children at age 3 years.[201] Collectively these clinical and experimental studies strongly support the importance of folate during neurodevelopment.

The new finding that homocysteinylated-hnRNP-E1 orchestrates a nutrition-sensitive posttranscriptional RNA operon that includes mRNAs that are important for the integrity of myelin and neuronal intermediate neurofilament-middle molecular mass proteins, as well as tyrosine hydroxylase, which generates dopamine and norepinephrine, provides insight into how folate and cobalamin deficiency during pregnancy can influence neurodevelopment.[57,59,194] Indeed, the activation of multiple members of the hnRNP family by high intracellular homocysteine, via folate or cobalamin deficiency in pregnancy, may in fact activate several such nutrition-sensitive posttranscriptional RNA operons, which, acting together in concert as a higher-order nutrition-sensitive (homocysteine-responsive) posttranscriptional RNA regulon, would lead to the modulation of several diverse mRNAs that exert a profound effect on fetal neurodevelopment.[59]

Folate-Responsive Neural Tube Defects and Neurocristopathies

NTDs are the most common major congenital malformation of the central nervous system. They arise from disturbances in neurulation that involve incomplete closure of neural tissues, leading to major midline defects. The neural tube, which begins as a tiny ribbon of tissue, normally folds inward to form a tube by the 28th day after conception. Thus NTDs originate in the first month of pregnancy (before many women know they are pregnant). The expression of folate receptors on embryonic neural tube and neural crest cells as well as the critical bursts of proliferative activity and the need for folate to support cell proliferation have been discussed earlier. Thus it is critical for a woman to have enough folate in her body before conception (periconceptionally) to ensure sufficient availability for the embryo. Anencephaly and spina bifida, the commonest NTDs, are important factors in fetal mortality (Fig. 39.10). Worldwide, the risk in the general population ranges from less than 1 to 9 cases per 1000 births; for example, the only population-based study in the least-developed area in India identified that the incidence of NTDs was up to 8.21 per 1000 live births, which is among the highest worldwide.[206] Landmark studies have established the preventive role of periconceptional folates in both the *recurrence* of NTD (using folic acid 4000 µg/day) and the *first occurrence* of NTD (using folic acid 400 µg/day). Of significance, the greatest protection by folates occurs in those regions with the highest rates of NTDs. Conversely, the use of folic acid antagonists (trimethoprim, triamterene, carbamazepine, phenytoin, phenobarbital, and primidone) during pregnancy increases the risk for these birth defects by twofold.[207]

Because 50% of pregnancies in the United States and elsewhere are unplanned and compliance with taking folic supplements to prevent NTD is only at about 50%, a consensus developed that fortification of food with folic acid in the United States was the best way to improve overall folate status in women at risk for NTD occurrence. By January 1998, fortification of foods (i.e., rice, flour, pasta, macaroni, breads, and cake with folic acid at 140 µg/100 g of food) was part of American law. This level was chosen to ensure that women of childbearing age would have an increase in folic acid intake of at least 100 µg a day, which is about 25% of the recommended daily intake. Subsequent evaluation has clearly demonstrated that fortification of food with folic acid has had multiple salutary effects during human development and that major congenital abnormalities can be prevented.[189] Table 39.5 shows several documented collateral benefits identified through population-based studies.

There remain questions about the effectiveness of the folic acid fortification program for women in the 15- to 35-year-old age-group in preventing NTDs. Because of an incomplete knowledge base among some women[22,226] and their tendency to consume low-carbohydrate foods (which are the very foods that are fortified), there is continued concern that this group is still not getting adequate amounts of dietary folate. This is the basis for recommendations to continue to educate women of childbearing age to take folic acid supplements at 400 µg/day (beyond what they are already receiving through folate fortification of food). Although regulations for mandatory fortification of wheat flour with folic acid are in place (in 53 countries by 2010), they have not been uniformly implemented.[227]

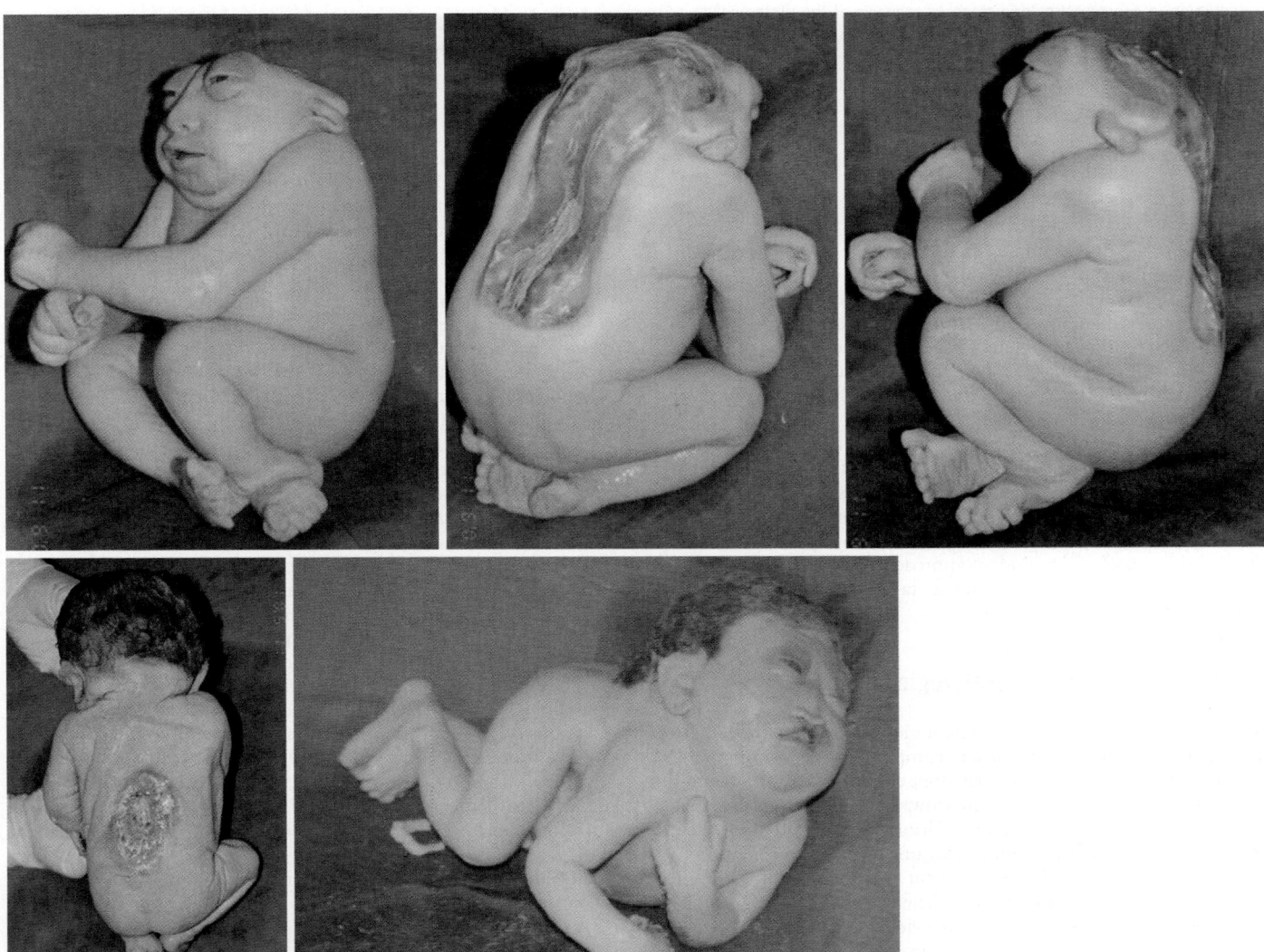

Fig. 39.10 FOLATE-RESPONSIVE NEURAL TUBE DEFECTS. Anencephaly with complete rachischisis *(top panel),* open infected meningomyelocele *(bottom left),* and iniencephaly with cleft lip *(bottom right). (Courtesy Prof. Molly Paul, Anatomy Department Museum, Christian Medical College and Brown Memorial Hospital, Ludhiana, Punjab, India.)*

TABLE
39.5
Beneficial Effects of Homocysteine-Lowering Therapy on Nonhematopoietic Systems

Using Folic Acid, Cobalamin, Pyridoxine Supplementation (Grade A Studies)

Reduction in hip fracture[208,a]

Reduction in the progression of carotid intima media thickness[209,a] (a surrogate marker of early subclinical arteriosclerosis)

Reduction in age-related macular degeneration[210,a]

Reduction in rate of brain atrophy[177,a]

Improvement in cognitive function[178,211,212,a]

Using Folic Acid Supplementation (Grade A Studies)

Reduction in stroke[213,a]

Reduction in the rate of cognitive decline among healthy older adults[211,a]

Reduction in age-related (sensorineural) hearing loss[214,a]

Reduction in first occurrence of NTDs[215,216,a]

Reduction in recurrence of NTDs[217,a]

Reduction in phenytoin-induced gingival hyperplasia[218,a]

Beneficial Effects of Folic Acid Fortification of Food (Population-Based Studies)

Reduction in NTDs[219–221] (anencephaly, spina bifida, encephalocele, meningocele, iniencephaly)

Reduction in cleft lip with or without cleft palate[222]

Reduction in severe congenital heart disease[222,223] (endocardial cushion defects, conotruncal defects)

Reduction in congenital pyloric stenosis, stenosis of the ureteropelvic junction, limb reduction defects[222]

Reduction in stroke mortality[224]

Decreased risk for preterm births,[225] low birth weight, and small-for-gestational-age babies

[a]Paper with randomized controlled trial data; grade A studies.
NTD, Neural tube defect.

Moreover, folate-fortified foods do not reach all women of reproductive age adequately, particularly the most needy women in the lowest socioeconomic bracket.[228,229] So the ideal of folate fortification has not been achieved and over 90% of pregnant women worldwide still do not receive sufficient folate,[191] and over one-half of the world's population still does not have easy access to folate-fortified foods.

Contrary to the assertion in the American Dietetic Association's position paper on vegetarianism,[230] there is an insufficient body of evidence to confidently assert that women in the United States of childbearing age who consume a balanced vegetarian diet with abundant green leafy vegetables will obtain sufficient folate and therefore not be at risk for giving birth to babies with NTDs. Until robust evidence from clinical trials is available to support this association's position paper,[230] a prudent approach is to recommend that all women who are vegetarians must take cobalamin and folate supplements.

Folates and Intrinsic Hematologic Disease

Because folate is necessary for hematopoiesis, folate requirements are increased when there is significant compensatory erythropoiesis in response to peripheral RBC destruction, abnormal hematopoiesis, or infiltration by abnormal cells in marrow. The recognition that folate deficiency developing in hemolytic disorders can lead to an acute aplastic crisis has led to recommendations favoring routine prophylactic administration of folate. A recent metaanalysis of 19 studies have put to rest the concern of iron-folate and malarial progression[231] and a Cochrane analysis identified *no* evidence that this is a problem when combined with antimalarial drugs and insecticide-treated bed nets.[232] Sadly however, this dictum is not followed for the vast majority of children living in malarial regions. An unexpected increase in transfusional requirement or a fall in platelets can also suggest folate deficiency.[15] The case of a patient with sickle cell disease on long-term folate who developed pernicious anemia and presented with

neuropsychiatric dysfunction[233] is a valuable reminder that those on folate prophylaxis need periodic follow-up for symptoms and signs of supervening cobalamin deficiency.

Folate Malabsorption With Normal Intestinal Mucosa

Hereditary Folate Malabsorption

Hereditary folate malabsorption, which is caused by loss of function mutations in the PCFT gene, has been detected in 19 different families; in the USA, those of Puerto Rican descent share a common mutated allele.[234] Loss of PCFT is associated with inability to transport folate across the intestine and into the brain, resulting in low serum and cerebrospinal fluid folate values with megaloblastic anemia, chronic diarrhea, and neurodevelopmental defects with seizures and mental retardation; this syndrome responds to high-dose parenteral folinic acid that bypasses and overcomes the transport defects. Affected patients can also present with a syndrome of reversible subacute combined immunodeficiency syndrome with hypogammaglobulinemia and recurrent infections.[235] If diagnosed early in infancy, hereditary folate malabsorption responds well to parenteral 5-formyltetrahydofolate and can allow normal development into adulthood.[236]

Folate Malabsorption With Intestinal Mucosal Abnormalities

Tropical Sprue

Residents of, and visitors to, endemic areas in the tropics can acquire a disorder characterized by small intestinal malabsorption.[15] Generalized, nonspecific small bowel malabsorption leads to a wide spectrum of clinical manifestations arising from defective absorption of fat, carbohydrate, albumin, calcium, folate, and in later stages, cobalamin.[15] There is abrupt onset of explosive, intermittent, or continuous diarrhea, abdominal distention, and pain, associated with anorexia, vomiting, and extreme fatigue. Stools are fluid or semisolid and frequently contain mucus and blood. This stage is followed weeks to months later by nutrient deficiency. Later, as steatorrhea continues, megaloblastosis dominates the clinical picture. In the short term, malabsorption leads to folate deficiency, but later in the chronic (longer than 3 years) phase of the disease, cobalamin malabsorption contributes additional clinical manifestations of cobalamin neuropathy.[15] There is some degree of villous atrophy and loss of intestinal functional surface. Although less severe than in nontropical sprue, it is more extensive, involving the entire small intestine.

After investigations for associated iron, cobalamin, and folate deficiencies, therapy with folate and a broad-spectrum antibiotic (e.g., tetracycline) is indicated together with symptomatic treatment of diarrhea and vomiting; fluid, mineral, and electrolyte imbalance; and other associated nutritional deficiencies.[15]

The endemic nature of this disorder in the tropics (and in certain households)[15] and the beneficial response to antibiotics all suggest an infectious origin. However, the dramatic response to folate, which is curative in the first year in about 60% of cases (this cure is cited to be almost diagnostic of the disease), has not been explained.[15] It is unlikely that pure folate deficiency is the primary cause, because nutritional folate deficiency does not result in tropical sprue; the clinical response to antibiotics suggests a close interplay among a pathogenic infectious agent, endogenous flora, and the folate status of the enterocyte.

Nontropical Sprue

Nontropical sprue (i.e., celiac disease, gluten-induced enteropathy) is the most common cause of intestinal malabsorption in temperate zones. It results from a possibly inherited sensitivity to gluten (a glutamine-rich protein found in wheat, barley, rye, and other grains) and a related substance, gliadin.[15] The intestinal lesion (i.e., villous atrophy with hypertrophied crypts and lymphocytic and plasma cell infiltrate of the lamina propria) is more florid than that seen in tropical sprue but occurs to a greater extent in the proximal small intestine with relative ileal sparing; as a result, cobalamin malabsorption is less common. The consequences of malabsorption are otherwise the same. Patients present between the ages of 30 and 50 years with intermittent or persistent diarrhea (abrupt in 20%), weight loss, abdominal distention with discomfort, glossitis, and megaloblastic anemia. Iron deficiency may also be prominent. Diagnosis is established by documenting the presence of sensitive and specific serum antiendomysial antibodies IgA type or anti–tissue transglutaminase antibodies, malabsorption, and jejunal biopsy. The megaloblastosis responds well to folate therapy.[15]

Regional Enteritis and Other Small Intestinal Disorders

The distal small intestine is involved in 80% of individuals with Crohn disease, so extensive ileal involvement or ileal bypass can result in malabsorption of cobalamin. Moreover, a poor diet or extensive mucosal disease can increase requirements for folate[237] whereas sulfasalazine can inhibit the absorption of folates via interference with PCFT function.[238]

Cerebral Folate Deficiency

Cerebral folate deficiency is a broad syndrome whereby several diseases can be accompanied by neurologic findings and low CSF folates but with normal serum folate levels.[239,240] The GPI-anchored folate receptor-α on the basolateral surface of choroid plexus cells is critical to the transport of folate from the blood across the CSF into the brain. Predictably, therefore, mutation of folate receptor-α, or the generation of antibodies to folate binding proteins found in cow's milk that cross react with choroid plexus folate receptor-α, can perturb folate transport into the brain and lead to cerebral folate deficiency. Indeed, among a group of 14 children with extremely low (≤ 5 nmol/l) levels of 5-methyl-THF in the CSF, mutations in folate receptor-α, which led to a failure in expression of functional folate receptors, were identified in 10 of them (71%).[46,47] These patients presented at <3 years with symptoms of developmental delay, movement disturbances, ataxia, myoclonic seizures, infantile spasms, and leukodystrophy that was reversed by folinic acid.[46,241] The finding of two older patients (aged 13 and 15 years) with severe polyneuropathy raises the possibility of other patients who may also have such defects that can present in young adulthood with unexplained neurologic disorders.

Acquired infantile-onset cerebral folate deficiency, which is associated with autoantibodies to folate receptor-α,[242,243] usually develops 4 to 6 months after birth and is characterized by agitation, insomnia, delayed development with deceleration of head growth, psychomotor retardation, cerebellar ataxia, pyramidal tract signs in the legs, dyskinesias (such as choreoathetosis and ballismus), a severe polyneuropathy, and in some cases, seizures. Untreated, central visual disturbances can become manifest and lead to optic atrophy and blindness by the third year. The folate receptor autoantibody titer decreases with restriction of bovine milk intake but promptly increases upon rechallenge. Cerebral folate deficiency responds to high doses of folinic acid and a cow's milk–free diet.[244]

Among 93 patients with autism spectrum disorders, 75% had autoantibodies to folate receptor in the serum; treatment with high dose leucovorin led to improvement in one-third of those treated.[245] Of added significance, an adult-onset presentation of cerebral folate deficiency with progressive memory loss and myoclonus caused by perturbation of folate receptor function by autoantibodies has also been described.[246] Finally, although antifolate receptor antibodies are also associated with neural tube defects,[76] infertility,[247] and orofacial clefts,[248] more information is required to confidently assign causality with these conditions.

Polymorphisms and Inborn Errors of Folate Metabolism

Several genetic polymorphisms involve genes that participate in one-carbon metabolism. These genetic polymorphisms merely reflect variants that are more frequent than the expected 1% allelic variation that could be found in any population. Whereas some polymorphisms impinge on normal physiology of folate and explain abnormal laboratory levels of folate, cobalamin, or metabolites, others may redistribute folate toward thymidylate synthesis and be "DNA protective." Predictably, two or more polymorphisms in the same individual (a combined heterozygote) can be associated with an increased risk for certain congenital diseases in offspring such as Down syndrome[249] or other birth defects. However, because disease association is not equivalent to disease causation, much more study is required to strengthen such relationships. A listing of the spectrum of these polymorphisms can be found in specialized texts.[250] Excellent reviews of inborn errors of folate metabolism are available.[165]

MEGALOBLASTIC ANEMIA NOT CAUSED BY FOLATE OR COBALAMIN DEFICIENCY

Several chemotherapeutic agents (e.g., antimetabolites, alkylating agents) kill malignant cells primarily by interfering with DNA synthesis; megaloblastosis is therefore an expected side effect. (See box on Miscellaneous Megaloblastic Anemias Not Caused by Cobalamin or Folate Deficiency.)

Miscellaneous Megaloblastic Anemias Not Caused by Cobalamin or Folate Deficiency

I. Congenital disorders of deoxyribonucleic acid (DNA) synthesis (rare)
   A. Orotic aciduria
   B. Lesch-Nyhan syndrome
   C. Congenital dyserythropoietic anemia
II. Acquired disorders of DNA synthesis
   A. Deficiency—thiamine-responsive megaloblastic anemia (thiamine transporter 1 mutation)
   B. Erythroleukemia, refractory sideroblastic anemias
   C. Drugs—all antineoplastic drugs that inhibit DNA synthesis (including antinucleosides used against human immunodeficiency virus [HIV] and other viruses), alcohol

---

CLINICAL PRESENTATIONS AND EVALUATION FOR FOLATE AND COBALAMIN DEFICIENCY

Clinical presentations and evaluations for folate and cobalamin deficiency are shown in Table 39.6.

The Interview

The patient's general demeanor and answers to questions may reveal a blunted affect with evidence of depression, irritability, forgetfulness, and sleep deprivation (common in pure folate deficiency). Alternatively, cobalamin deficiency may present with paranoid ideation, dementia, cognitive dysfunction, delusions, or lack of energy manifested by slowed responses. Hallucinations or even obtundation may preclude obtaining an adequate history. The family may indicate the progressive evolution of a marked personality change and may be able to help trace the evolution of symptoms and deviations from the time when the patient was last well. Intermittent therapy with

TABLE 39.6	Similarities of Clinical Manifestations and Megaloblastic Sequelae of Folate and Cobalamin Deficiency[a]	
System	**Manifestations**
Hematologic	Pancytopenia with megaloblastic marrow
Cardiopulmonary	Congestive heart failure
Gastrointestinal	Beefy-red tongue and added stigmata of broad-spectrum malabsorption in folate deficiency[b]
Dermatologic	Melanin pigmentation and premature graying
Genital	Cervical or uterine dysplasia
Reproductive	Infertility or sterility
Psychiatric	Depressed affect and cognitive dysfunction
Neuropsychiatric[c]	Unique to cobalamin deficiency with cerebral, myelopathic, or peripheral neuropathic disturbances, including optic and autonomic nerve dysfunction

[a]However, the neurologic spectrum of dysfunction in cobalamin deficiency is distinct. Inadequate hemoglobinization (from inadequate iron stores or globin synthesis) can mask the expected erythroid megaloblastic morphologic findings in the bone marrow and peripheral smear, and only specific therapy (i.e., iron) can unmask classic megaloblastic manifestations (i.e., masked megaloblastosis). Megaloblastic leukopoiesis is unchanged.

[b]If folate deficiency is uncorrected for 2 to 3 years, cobalamin deficiency will supervene.

[c]Dorsal tract involvement is earliest manifestation in more than 70% of patients with cobalamin deficiency. Neuropsychiatric manifestations are not associated with megaloblastosis in up to 30% of patients.

multivitamins, liver pills, or injections (often given by a well-meaning family member or unregistered practitioner) is a common quick fix in many cultures. Family members are a good source for details on the patient's dietary habits (food faddism, vegetarianism, alcohol intake) and family history of medical problems (blood diseases, gluten sensitivity, autoimmune diseases).

A medical history of epilepsy or alcoholism with seizure disorder (anticonvulsant therapy) is important. Rarely, patients with auto-immune hemolytic anemias may be lost to follow-up and return with acute aplastic crises when they run out of folate. A surgical history of total or partial gastrectomy, anastomosis, fistula, or bowel resection can reveal the potential for perturbation of physiologic absorption (loss of IF, bypassing or loss of absorptive surface, blind loop syndromes). Surreptitious or accidental inhalation of nitrous oxide in an occupational setting (dental or anesthesiology professionals) and deliberate inhalation of nitrous oxide (nanging) using cartridges attached to whipped cream dispensers or visits to "houses of laughter," where nitrous oxide can be inhaled for a small fee can be revealed only on direct questioning. Visits to tropical countries and the development of intermittent episodic diarrhea may give a clue to tropical sprue; prolonged (over 3 years) chronic gastrointestinal symptoms followed by insidious development of neurologic problems predicts a combined (folate followed by cobalamin) deficiency (see box on Drugs That Perturb Folate Metabolism).

Systemic review of symptoms may range from none (i.e., incidental increased MCV or PMN hypersegmentation) to severe (i.e., unstable angina from severe anemia). With slow development of anemia, the patient often does not develop cardiopulmonary symptoms until there is a 50% reduction in hemoglobin concentration, which leads to dyspnea on exertion, palpitation, and generalized fatigue or lethargy. Only when the hemoglobin concentration is below 5 g/dL does the patient develop dyspnea at rest and angina on modest exertion or even at rest. Congestive heart failure is heralded by pedal edema, nocturia, orthopnea, and tender hepatomegaly.

Upper gastrointestinal symptoms with anorexia associated with intrinsic gastrointestinal disease or anemia with heart failure must be distinguished from symptoms arising from glossitis. The latter may lead to inability to wear dentures, or tolerate hot drinks or spicy foods

Drugs That Perturb Folate Metabolism

Ethanol. Although beer has higher folate content than other alcoholic beverages, alcoholism may lead to neglect of healthy dietary practices in favor of alcohol. Patients who have one nutritious meal each day tend to stave off the eventual development of folate deficiency. Alcohol consumption leads to a relatively rapid (2- to 4-day) fall in serum folate levels. Excess alcohol consumption is possibly the most common cause of folate deficiency in the United States.[15]

Trimethoprim and *pyrimethamine* bind to bacterial and parasitic dihydrofolate reductase with much greater affinity than to human dihydrofolate reductase, but patients with underlying folate deficiency appear to be more susceptible to the effects of these drugs. The megaloblastosis can be reversed by folinic acid (5-formyl-tetrahydrofolate [5-formyl-THF]; leucovorin).

Methotrexate binds with high affinity to human dihydrofolate reductase and leads to trapping of folate as a metabolically inert form (dihydrofolate). This leads to a true depletion of THF within hours and consequently to functional deficiency of 5,10-methylene-THF and reduced thymidylate synthesis. Although megaloblastosis can develop rapidly, the toxic effects of methotrexate can be avoided by rescue with 5-formyl-THF (leucovorin).

Sulfasalazine produces megaloblastosis in up to two-thirds of patients taking full doses (over 2 g/day) by decreasing absorption of folates and induction of Heinz body hemolytic anemia (i.e., increased requirements).

Anticonvulsants can induce neural tube defects (NTD), and consensus guidelines have stressed the importance of ensuring that pregnant women[22] and children[251,252] with epilepsy be prescribed folates together with anticonvulsants. Whereas folates protect against spontaneous abortion,[253] folic acid supplementation of women receiving antiepileptic drugs, which are known to interfere with folate absorption, also led to a significant reduction of spontaneous abortion.[254] Now there are new clinical data on phenytoin-induced gingival hyperplasia, which is a cosmetically undesirable side effect that affects a large percentage of patients, usually between 2 and 6 months of initiating therapy. A recent randomized controlled trial among children 6 to 15 years of age who were initiated on phenytoin has provided incontrovertible evidence that taking folic acid 0.5 mg daily can largely prevent phenytoin-induced gingival hyperplasia[218]; whereas 88% in the placebo group developed gingival hyperplasia, only 21% in the folic acid group developed this side effect. The data from this paper provide more "ammunition" to encourage young women on antiepileptic drugs to keep taking folic acid to prevent them from getting cosmetically unsightly gingival hyperplasia (particularly if reducing the risk for having a baby with NTD is too nebulous a concept for them). The only caveat is that before initiating long-term folic acid supplements, the cobalamin status must be normalized.

Although *antineoplastics* and *antiretroviral antinucleosides* such as azidothymidine lead to megaloblastosis, the temporal sequence and investigations to rule out cobalamin or folate deficiency should easily lead to a correct causal assignment.

because of burning, and even odynophagia, which may compromise further food intake (seen in cobalamin and folate deficiencies). The patient may volunteer that glossitis is relieved by multivitamin ingestion. Weight loss in cobalamin deficiency is not as severe as in folate deficiency arising from intrinsic gastrointestinal disease. Episodic or chronic diarrhea with steatorrhea is commonly caused by tropical sprue, although it may be brought on by gluten-containing foods. Although these symptoms may be accompanied by abdominal pain, pain in the absence of diarrhea could be caused by tabetic crisis (vomiting, abdominal rigidity, absence of leukocytosis, or fever) accompanying spinothalamic involvement in cobalamin-deficient myelopathy.

The patient with pernicious anemia may have two or three semisolid bowel movements per day; although this may be construed as a normal pattern, it may represent a change since the last time the patient was well. Constipation may be related to obstipation arising from involvement of the Meissner plexus and the Auerbach plexus within the gastrointestinal tract. Similarly, incipient loss of bladder or bowel control caused by cobalamin myelopathy may present with urgency or nocturia.

In contrast to musculoskeletal symptoms (arthralgia or frank arthritis) of autoimmune diseases, nocturnal cramps or pain in upper and lower extremities may indicate spinothalamic tract involvement. Hypoparathyroidism or systemic lupus erythematosus, alone or associated with pernicious anemia, leads to significant overlap of cerebral, musculoskeletal, and neurologic presentations.

Review of skin symptoms may elicit a history of increased diffuse or blotchy generalized brownish skin pigmentation, especially of nail beds and skin creases. This is common in cobalamin and folate deficiency; associated vitiligo suggests autoimmune disease.

Although symptoms related to neurologic dysfunction may be volunteered, a complete detailed questionnaire should be formulated during the interview. Questions should be directed to perversions in taste or smell, decreased visual acuity, changes in color vision, and eye pain (neuritis), tinnitus, or headache. Dizziness with orthostatic hypotension and "blacking out" may be related to severe anemia or cobalamin-deficient autonomic dysfunction, which can also be associated with night sweats.[255] Vertigo or difficulty in walking in the dark (loss of proprioception and position sense), difficulty in ambulation (which may feel like "walking on cotton wool"), stiffness of extremities (corticospinal tracts), or ataxia (spinocerebellar tracts) may be indicative of a serious cobalamin myelopathy. Early symptoms are symmetrical tingling ("pins and needles"), extending from the tips of the toes, to a glove and stocking distribution in later stages. "Burning feet" syndrome, or more commonly, complaints of difficulty in performing simple tasks such as buttoning clothes, may also be a presenting symptom. When loss of bladder and bowel control brings the patient to the physician, advanced neurologic dysfunction is invariably present.

Genitourinary symptoms such as impotence or recurrent cystitis from bladder dysfunction can suggest cobalamin neuropathy. Multiple pregnancies with short intervals between delivery and conception predispose to a high risk for overt folate deficiency and contribute to fetal growth restriction in babies (cobalamin deficiency is more often associated with infertility).

The Physical Examination

Physical examination may reveal different features in well-nourished patients (cobalamin-deficient vegetarians or pernicious anemia) and poorly nourished (folate-deficient) individuals. The latter show evidence of significant weight loss or other stigmata of multiple deficiencies because of either poor diet (malnutrition) or "broad-spectrum" malabsorption. Associated deficiency of vitamins A, D, and K and protein-calorie malnutrition may give rise to angular cheilosis, bleeding mucous membranes, dermatitis, osteomalacia, and chronic infections. Various degrees of pallor with lemon-tint icterus (i.e., a combination of pallor and icterus best observed in fair-skinned individuals) are common features of megaloblastosis.

When anemia is severe, the patient may have a low-grade fever. The skin may reveal a diffuse, brownish pigmentation or abnormal blotchy tanning.[256] A macular hyperpigmentation with follicular accentuation may be observed in the axilla and groin; hyperpigmentation can also involve the dorsal acral distal interphalangeal joints and a reticular pigmentation in the mid–upper back can develop slowly over a year (but resolves within 2 months of cobalamin replacement).[256] Special emphasis should be given to pigmentation of skin creases and nail beds and both palmar and dorsal aspects of hands and feet.[257] (Mucous membrane pigmentation is usually not observed, in contrast to Addison disease.) Premature graying, observed in light- and dark-haired individuals, is reversible within 6 months of cobalamin therapy.

A blunted masklike facies is extremely common in folate deficiency. Alternatively, there may be evidence of classic hyperthyroid or hypothyroid facies (associated with pernicious anemia). Special attention should be given to the eyes and eyebrows for the well-known signs of thyroid dysfunction.

Examination of the mouth may reveal glossitis with a smooth (depapillated), beefy red tongue with occasional ulceration of the lateral surface or gingival hyperplasia (antiepileptics). The neck may reveal thyromegaly (diffuse or with nodules) if there is associated disease. Increased jugular venous distention should alert the examiner to cardiovascular failure, with its attendant gallop, cardiomegaly (with or without pericardial effusions), pulmonary basal crepitations, pleural effusion, tender hepatomegaly, and pedal edema. Nontender hepatomegaly, but more often mild splenomegaly, may rarely be caused by extramedullary hematopoiesis in severe anemia, but a midepigastrium mass raises the ominous possibility of gastric carcinoma, which is up to seven times more likely[258] in patients with pernicious anemia.

An inverse correlation has been identified between the extent of anemia and neurologic dysfunction. Patients with normal complete blood count values often have neurologic signs and symptoms. In prolonged cobalamin deficiency, the neurologic examination reveals clear-cut evidence of involvement of posterior and pyramidal, spinocerebellar, and spinothalamic tracts. Among the earliest signs of posterior column dysfunction are loss of position sense in the index toes (before great toe involvement), which is elicited by passive movement, and loss of the ability to discern vibration of a high-pitched (256 cycles/s) tuning fork. This is a very early elicitable, objective sign, which invariably precedes by many months the loss of ability to sense the vibration of a lower-pitched (128 cycles/s) tuning fork. Usually the patient loses vibration sense to 256 cycles/s from toe to hip before loss of 128 cycles/s vibration sense even begins. Because of the slow coalescence of contiguous spinal cord lesions, a constellation of elicitable signs may be obtained. Upper motor neuron disease is indicated by weakness and progressive spasticity with increased muscle tone, exaggerated deep tendon reflexes with clonus, extensor plantar response, and incoordinate or scissor gait, which may progress to spastic paraplegia. The involvement of peripheral nerves may markedly modify these signs to include flaccidity and the absence of deep tendon reflexes. A positive Romberg sign is not uncommon, and a positive Lhermitte sign may be elicited. Loss of sphincter and bowel control, altered cranial nerve dysfunction with altered taste, smell, and visual acuity or color perception, and optic neuritis (unexplained predominance in males) may be other physical signs indicating cobalamin deficiency. Inability to carry out serial subtraction of 7 from 100 is a valuable test to document reduced cerebral function (the electroencephalogram often reveals slow wave frequency) in pernicious anemia, which can progress over time to presentation with catatonia[259] or delirium.[260]

Diagnostic Issues: Information from the Peripheral Smear and Bone Marrow Aspirate

Although not specific for megaloblastic anemia, macro-ovalocytes are the hallmark of megaloblastosis (see Fig. 39.7). However, only one-half with MCV values greater than 105 fL may have vitamin deficiency. In almost one-half of all cases, macrocytosis per se is not associated with megaloblastosis, and additional tests are necessary for complete diagnosis.

The frequency of hypersegmented PMNs (5% with five lobes or 1% with six-lobed PMNs) in patients with megaloblastic hematopoiesis is 98%. The sensitivity decreases to 78% in alcoholics, although the specificity of this finding is approximately 95%. With a combination of hypersegmented PMNs and macro-ovalocytosis, the specificity is 96% to 98%, and the positive predictive value of folate or cobalamin deficiency is about 94%.[22] Hypersegmentation of PMNs is insufficiently sensitive, when compared with metabolite levels, to be used as a clinical tool in the diagnosis of mild cobalamin deficiency[22] (see box on Diagnostic Bone Marrow Aspiration).

Masked Megaloblastosis

The term *masked megaloblastosis* is reserved for conditions in which true cobalamin or folate deficiency with anemia is not accompanied by classic findings of megaloblastosis in the peripheral blood and

---

Diagnostic Bone Marrow Aspiration

Is bone marrow aspiration always necessary to diagnose cobalamin- or folate-deficient megaloblastosis? With the addition of highly sensitive serum tests for the specific diagnosis of cobalamin and folate deficiency, the need for a bone marrow test is often dictated by the urgency to diagnose megaloblastosis (with results available in an hour). For example, in the case of florid hematologic disease with or without neurologic disease suggestive of cobalamin or folate deficiency, bone marrow aspiration carried out as soon as possible is invaluable in assisting the rapid diagnosis of megaloblastosis. However, in the outpatient setting, when the patient has a characteristic peripheral smear, or for a patient with a primary neuropsychiatric presentation, a case can be made to initiate the sequence of diagnostic tests without bone marrow aspiration by proceeding with measurement of serum levels of vitamins or metabolites (see Table 39.2). In a pregnant patient with pancytopenia with macro-ovalocytes, hypersegmented polymorphonuclear neutrophils, and reticulocytopenia with a history of noncompliance with prenatal supplements (and no neurologic findings suggestive of cobalamin deficiency), bone marrow aspiration may not be necessary to initiate therapy for a strong presumptive diagnosis of folate deficiency. If there is no evidence of response within 10 days, bone marrow aspiration is indicated.

---

bone marrow. This occurs when there is a coexisting condition that neutralizes the tendency to generate megaloblastic cells (usually involving reduction in RBC hemoglobinization, as in iron deficiency or thalassemia).[22] A wide RBC distribution width (RDW) on the Coulter counter readout in the presence of a "normal" mean corpuscular hemoglobin or MCV may reflect megaloblastic anemia[22] or dimorphic anemia (macro-ovalocytes plus microcytic hypochromic RBCs). Because megaloblastic white blood cells and precursors are unaffected by deficient hemoglobinization, these pathognomonic findings (giant myelocytes and metamyelocytes, and hypersegmented PMNs) remain; the latter may persist for up to 2 weeks after replacement with cobalamin or folate.[15] The recognition of masked megaloblastosis should initiate investigations to rule out iron deficiency, anemia of chronic disease, or hemoglobinopathies. Appropriate replacement with cobalamin or folate elicits a maximal therapeutic benefit only when iron deficiency is corrected. Conversely, if combined iron and cobalamin deficiency (total gastrectomy or pernicious anemia) or iron and folate deficiency (pregnancy) is treated with iron alone, megaloblastosis will be unmasked.

APPROACH TO DIAGNOSIS AND THERAPY OF MEGALOBLASTOSIS

In general, there are three stages in approaching a patient: *recognizing* that megaloblastic anemia is present; *distinguishing* whether folate, cobalamin, or combined folate and cobalamin deficiencies have led to the anemia; and diagnosing the *underlying disease* and *mechanism* causing the deficiency. Establishing that the patient does have megaloblastosis is, in theory, straightforward. This is easily done by first evaluating the complete blood count, the MCV, and the peripheral smear, followed by a bone marrow aspiration. Clues to whether cobalamin or folate deficiency is responsible for megaloblastosis can be obtained by serum cobalamin and serum folate levels; if these levels are borderline, additional testing of serum MMA and serum homocysteine can define the true nature of the deficiency.[22] However, this ideal and orderly workup is not always feasible in clinical practice, because the patient may present for the first time with megaloblastosis with or without associated neurologic disease; may be referred after a variable workup has already been initiated for possible megaloblastosis; may present with symptoms primarily attributed to a disease predisposing to cobalamin or folate deficiency; may present with a disease associated with hyperhomocysteinemia (discussed later), in which case anemia or neurologic dysfunction may only be a minor symptom; may present with isolated neurologic disease in the absence of anemia; or may be referred after empirical therapy has been given

for presumed cobalamin or folate deficiency. The immediate question therefore pertains to the overall status of the patient.

If the patient is decompensated or decompensation is imminent, obtain serum folate and cobalamin levels and bone marrow aspiration to confirm megaloblastosis and proceed with transfusion of 1 unit of packed RBCs *slowly,* with vigorous diuretic therapy to obviate further congestive heart failure from fluid overload; this mandates close monitoring and correction of fluid and electrolyte imbalance. Cobalamin and folate should be administered simultaneously in full doses. Transfusion does not alter serum folate or cobalamin levels.

If the patient is moderately symptomatic (but not in heart failure), the strong likelihood of a dramatic response (in the sense of well-being and relief of sore tongue) within 2 to 3 days even before hematologic improvement argues against immediate blood transfusion.[22] Therefore (and provided the patient is unlikely to decompensate in the short-term) proceed with appropriate diagnostic workup as for the well-compensated patient.

If the patient is well compensated and in the outpatient setting, the physician has time to develop an orderly sequence of diagnostic tests. First, check the peripheral smear and rule out other macrocytic anemias (thin macrocytes with a normoblastic marrow in contrast to macro-ovalocytes) (see Fig. 39.7). Draw blood for cobalamin and folate levels (*before* the patient's first hospital meal) to sort out whether the problem is caused by a deficiency of folate or cobalamin, or both, or some other deficiency (see Table 39.2). Assuming that there is no urgency to make the diagnosis, the physician can elect to wait for the results of these tests before proceeding with the next test in the diagnostic workup. If making the diagnosis is urgent, a cost-effective test is the bone marrow aspirate; results indicating megaloblastosis (or not) can be available within an hour. If bone marrow aspiration is performed, samples are sent for special stains and flow cytometry (megaloblastic erythropoiesis can resemble erythroleukemia) and cytogenetic analysis (myelodysplastic syndromes can exhibit some megaloblastic changes in the erythroid series, but megaloblastic granulopoiesis is not seen). If the marrow is not obviously megaloblastic but the iron stain reveals absent stores, review the morphologic evaluation again with special emphasis on granulocytic precursors and promegaloblasts, and look for more subtle megaloblastic changes.

If the serum cobalamin and folate levels are equivocal (i.e., in the low-normal range), and the patient elects to delay or refuses a bone marrow aspiration, a strong case can be made to test for serum homocysteine and MMA. Serum MMA and homocysteine levels are ordered together (the same sample remaining from the serum sent for cobalamin and folate levels may be used if it was frozen). Integrating the results for serum MMA and homocysteine levels (which will be available after a week or more) with those for serum cobalamin and folate levels can help distinguish cobalamin and folate deficiencies (see Table 39.2). A normal MMA and homocysteine level eliminates cobalamin deficiency with 100% confidence, and normal homocysteine levels suggest that megaloblastic anemia is not caused by folate deficiency. These tests are particularly useful if the patient has pure neurologic disease or if there are associated conditions such as iron deficiency or thalassemia that can mask megaloblastosis. Administration of folate or cobalamin will reduce elevated serum homocysteine and MMA levels to basal values by 1 week, so there is only a narrow window to clinch the diagnosis using metabolite tests.[22] In the rare situation when a defect in cobalamin or folate metabolism is suspected, early consultation with experts who have published in this area is advised.*

A reticulocyte count is useful to follow the patient's response to appropriate replacement therapy. Additional supporting studies to document increased serum LDH, haptoglobin, and bilirubin (evidence for intramedullary hemolysis) may be performed.

When the megaloblastic state is established, try to determine the underlying mechanism of cobalamin or folate deficiency. The cause of folate deficiency is usually sorted out by this time from the history, physical examination, and the clinical setting. If pure folate deficiency

---

*References 18,19,46,164,165,175,176,234,261,262.

has been prolonged, expect associated cobalamin deficiency to ensue (special emphasis should be given to identifying subtle manifestations of neurologic disease). If cobalamin deficiency is suspected, test for both serum anti-IF antibodies and the newer more sensitive antiparietal cell antibodies (see section on Pernicious Anemia.) Also see box on Practicing Classic Medicine Without the (Classic) Schilling Test.

THERAPY

Routinely, treatment with full doses of parenteral cobalamin (1 mg/day) and oral folate (folic acid) (1 to 5 mg) before knowledge of the type of vitamin deficiency is established should be reserved for the severely ill patient. An appropriate regimen for conditions in which cobalamin replenishment can correct cellular cobalamin deficiency (but not correct the underlying problem that led to the deficiency, such as pernicious anemia) is 1 mg of intramuscular or subcutaneous cyanocobalamin per day (week 1), 1 mg twice weekly (week 2), 1 mg/week for 4 weeks, and then 1 mg per month for life (about 15%, or 150 µg, is retained 48 hours after each 1-mg cobalamin injection). *Ideally, this protocol for rapid correction of cobalamin deficiency and complete replenishment of cobalamin stores should be used in the beginning for all patients with cobalamin deficiency, regardless of the etiology* (see box on Modified Therapeutic Trials).

Parenteral hydroxocobalamin should be reserved for all inborn errors of cobalamin metabolism. There is no major advantage of other preparations over generic cyanocobalamin. There is equivalence between oral 2-mg cobalamin tablets consumed daily (where cobalamin is passively absorbed at high doses) and traditional monthly parenteral treatment with 1 mg of intramuscular/subcutaneous cobalamin among those requiring long-term cobalamin. So for patients who refuse monthly parenteral therapy, or prefer daily oral therapy, or in those with disorders of hemostasis, cobalamin (1 to 2 mg/day as tablets) can be recommended for all those patients with

cobalamin malabsorption.[15,22] The physician must ensure that the patient is compliant and demonstrates adequate cobalamin levels as well as resolution of hematologic and neurologic abnormalities on follow-up. For nutritional cobalamin deficiency (e.g., vegetarians) when the entire circuitry in cobalamin absorption is intact, daily oral cobalamin of 5 to 10 µg (found in conventional multivitamin tablets in the United States) taken for a lifetime of vegetarianism will suffice. However, if malabsorption of food-bound cobalamin is suspected (especially in the elderly with achlorhydria), higher doses of daily oral cobalamin (equal to or greater than 1000 µg/day) is required.[263]

The bioavailability of oral cobalamin can be reduced by about 40% when it is taken with a meal; taking cobalamin on an empty stomach will lower losses in the stool. More than 98% of all the cobalamin in feces is in the form of cobalamin analogues, and about 80% of the ingested cobalamin is converted to analogues by microorganisms in the gut.[264]

Oral folate (folic acid) at doses of 1 to 5 mg/day results in adequate absorption (even where intestinal malabsorption of physiologic food folate is present). Therapy should be continued until complete hematologic recovery is documented. If the underlying cause leading to folate deficiency is not corrected, folate may be continued. Folinic acid (i.e., 5-formyl-THF [leucovorin]) should be reserved *only* for rescue protocols involving antifolates (methotrexate or trimethoprim-sulfamethoxazole), for 5-fluorouracil modulation protocols, after nitrous oxide toxicity, or in pediatric cases involving cerebral folate deficiency or inborn errors of folate metabolism. It is too expensive for conventional repletion in folate-deficient states in adults.

Response to Replenishment

The response of the patient to appropriate replacement is reversion of megaloblastic hematopoiesis to normal hematopoiesis within the first 12 hours; by 48 hours, normal hematopoiesis is reestablished, and the only evidence for a prior megaloblastic state may be the persistence of a few giant metamyelocytes. Because megaloblastosis caused by cobalamin or folate deficiency can be reversed in 24 hours by administration of folate (i.e., a nutritious hospital meal), delay of a diagnostic bone marrow aspirate should be avoided. Clinically the first 36 to 48 hours are often highlighted by the awakening of an occasional semistuporous individual whose "chief complaint" is amazement at the remarkably improved sense of well-being experienced, with increased alertness and appetite and reduced soreness of the tongue. The elevated serum MMA and homocysteine levels will return to normal by the end of the first week.

Accelerated turnover of normal DNA in erythroid precursors is associated with an increase in serum urate level, which usually peaks by the fourth day, and with increased cellular phosphate uptake for nucleotide synthesis. This may precipitate an attack of gout if the patient has a "gouty predisposition." The reticulocyte count increases by the second to third days and peaks by the fifth to eighth days (the peak reticulocyte count is directly proportional to the degree of preexisting anemia). This is followed by a rise in RBC count, hemoglobin, and hematocrit by the end of the first week, which normalizes in approximately 2 months, regardless of the initial degree of anemia. By the end of the third week, the RBC count should be above $3 \times 10^6/mm^3$; if it is not, additional causes of underlying iron deficiency, hemoglobinopathy, chronic disease, or hypothyroidism should be considered (Table 39.7).

Hypersegmented PMNs continue to remain in the blood for 10 to 14 days; however, the number of normal PMNs and platelets rises and normalizes within the first week. During this process, there may be a transient left shift to include myeloid precursors. The reduced intramedullary hemolysis (as a result of normalized hematopoiesis) leads to a gradual reduction in the serum bilirubin level by the end of the first week, and LDH levels will drop concomitantly.

In response to cobalamin, progression of neurologic damage and dysfunction is inhibited. In general, the degree of functional recovery is inversely related to the extent of disease and duration of signs and symptoms. As a rough estimate, signs and symptoms that have been

TABLE 39.7	Causes of Megaloblastosis Not Responding to Therapy With Cobalamin or Folate

Wrong Diagnosis

Combined folate and cobalamin deficiencies being treated with only one vitamin

Associated iron deficiency

Associated hemoglobinopathy (e.g., sickle cell disease, thalassemia)

Associated anemia of chronic disease

Associated hypothyroidism

TABLE 39.8	Indications for Prophylaxis With Cobalamin or Folate

Prophylaxis With Cobalamin

Infants on specialized diets[a]

Premature infants

Infants of mothers with pernicious anemia[a]

Infants and children of mothers with nutritional cobalamin deficiency

Vegetarianism and poverty-imposed near-vegetarianism[a]

Total gastrectomy[b]

Prophylaxis With Folic Acid[c]

All women contemplating pregnancy (at least 400 µg/day)[d]

Pregnancy and lactation, premature infants

Mothers at risk for delivery of infants with neural tube defects[e,f]

Hemolytic anemias/hyperproliferative hematologic states

Patients with rheumatoid arthritis or psoriasis on therapy with methotrexate[g]

Patients on antiepileptic drugs

Patients with ulcerative colitis

[a]For vegetarians, prophylaxis with cobalamin (5- to 10-µg tablet/day) orally should suffice. In all other conditions involving any abnormality of cobalamin absorption, cobalamin tablets of 1000 µg/day should be administered orally to ensure that cobalamin transport by passive diffusion across the intestine is sufficient to meet daily needs.
[b]Consider late development of cobalamin deficiency and iron malabsorption (prophylaxis with oral cobalamin and iron).
[c]Ensure that the patient does not have a cobalamin deficiency before initiating long-term folate prophylaxis.
[d]For prevention of first occurrence of neural tube defects.
[e]Previous delivery of a child with neural tube defects (e.g., anencephaly, spina bifida, meningocele) imparts a 10-fold greater risk for subsequent delivery of infant with neural tube defects.
[f]Folic acid (4 mg/day) administered periconceptionally and throughout the first trimester.
[g]To reduce toxicity of the antifolate.

present for less than 3 months are usually completely reversible; with longer duration, there is invariable residual neurologic dysfunction. The reversibility of neurologic damage is slow (a maximal response may take 6 months). Substantial increments (in recovery) are unlikely to be gained after the first 12 months of appropriate therapy. However, most neurologic abnormalities have improved in up to 90% of patients with documented subacute combined degeneration.

Follow-up

Patients with neurologic dysfunction from cobalamin deficiency have traditionally been given more frequent doses of cobalamin (biweekly rather than monthly therapy for the first 6 months), despite the lack of evidence that this form of therapy is more beneficial. This approach nevertheless serves a purpose in that improvement in neurologic status can be carefully documented. Once maximal responses have been established, most patients can be treated with life-long cobalamin with a dose that is appropriate for the underlying cause of cobalamin deficiency. Follow-up outpatient visits every 6 months should be instituted to ensure adequate maintenance of hematopoiesis, as well as early diagnosis of other diseases commonly associated with the cobalamin- or folate-deficient state. Patients with pernicious anemia are prone to developing iron deficiency that arises from poor iron absorption from achlorhydria.[22] Therefore when iron deficiency is established, total dose replacement using parenteral iron, such as 1 gram of low-molecular-weight iron-dextran (INFeD) administered over an hour, is indicated.[265]

Patients with pernicious anemia have a twofold increase in proximal femur and vertebral fractures and a threefold increase in distal forearm fractures. The associated antral enterochromaffin cell hyperplasia (driven by hypergastrinemia that accompanies atrophic body gastritis) can be associated with dysplasia, a risk factor for development of neoplasia.[168] In addition, the loss of oxyntic glands and replacement by metaplastic pyloric or intestinal glands is a risk factor for gastric cancer.[168] Finally, three studies (from Sweden, the United States, and Denmark) on a total of nearly 15,000 patients with pernicious anemia have identified an excess risk for gastric cancers within the first few years of diagnosis[266]; so it is prudent to recommend upper endoscopy for these patients despite the lack of prospective data favoring this approach.

ROUTINE SUPPLEMENTATION OF COBALAMIN AND FOLATE

Routine periconceptional supplementation of folate for normal women[22] and in 10 times higher doses for women at risk for delivery of subsequent babies with NTDs,[22] provides effective prophylaxis against the development of NTDs (Table 39.8); this also appears to reduce the risk for congenital heart disease,[223] and isolated cleft lip (with or without cleft palate) by about one-third.[267] Food fortification with folic acid (140 µg/100 g flour) has nearly eliminated folate deficiency[268]—the prevalence of low serum folate level decreased from 18.4% to 0.8% with a small (0.3 g/dL) increase in hemoglobin[269]; it has consistently reduced NTDs[215,270]; and it is a cost-effective intervention.[228,271] Food fortification was intended to provide only

one-quarter of the recommended dietary allowance of folate. A very brief focused interaction involving physician advice combined with a booster phone call and starter bottle of folic acid tablets can markedly increase a woman's regular intake of folic acid (increase by 68% versus 20% in the control group).[272] Although regulations for mandatory fortification of wheat flour with folic acid are in place in 53 countries (by 2010), in many cases, these regulations have not been implemented.[227] Moreover, folate-fortified foods do not reach all women of reproductive age adequately, particularly the most needy women in the lowest socioeconomic bracket.[228,229] As a result, the ideal of folate fortification has not been achieved in developing countries where over 90% of the world's pregnant women still fail to receive optimum folate,[191] and well over one-half of the world's population still does not have easy access to folate-fortified foods. In addition, awareness of the need for folate before pregnancy remains low in the developing world (in Nepal it is a dismal 5%).[273]

The administration of folate and cobalamin in addition to parenteral erythropoietin and parenteral erythropoietin and iron to premature infants significantly improved hemoglobin values[274]; so this should be the standard of care.

Supplementation with folate during pregnancy also helps to prevent premature delivery of low-birth-weight infants,[15] and routine supplementation for premature infants and lactating mothers is also recommended.

In addition to hematologic diseases leading to increased folate requirements (e.g., autoimmune hemolytic anemia, β-thalassemia), folic acid supplements reduce the hepatotoxicity and gastrointestinal intolerance of methotrexate in psoriasis[22,275] and rheumatoid arthritis[276] without impairing the efficacy of methotrexate.

Supplementation with folic acid protects against the development of colorectal neoplasia in high-risk patients with ulcerative colitis.[22]

For schoolchildren in developing countries, simple community-level interventions, such as micronutrient fortification (using a premix added to school lunches), that build upon the infrastructure of an existing program have proven to be contextually acceptable and efficacious in improving folate and cobalamin (in addition to vitamin A and iron) status in Himalayan villages of India.[277] Such programs are critically important to the health of both women and their children (discussed later). Table 39.8 summarizes conditions that warrant routine folate or cobalamin supplementation.

Following food fortification, the total folate intake of most U.S. children 1 to 13 years of age does meet the estimated average requirement,[278] but children given supplements are at risk for exceeding the tolerable upper intake level; this remains a concern because the long-term effects are unknown. Whereas folic acid supplements consumed in excess of 1 mg/day can mask hematologic symptoms of cobalamin deficiency, it has been found that 94% of U.S. adults who do not consume supplements, or who consume less than 400 µg of folic acid per day from supplements, do not exceed the upper limit in intake for folic acid.[279] There is also no evidence that taking high-folate supplements or consuming large amounts of folate-fortified foods places individuals at risk for exacerbating any underlying cobalamin deficiency.[280]

Is there a role for cobalamin fortification of foods? A strong case can be made to consider the fortification of flour (or other contextually relevant food vehicle in developing countries) with small amounts of cobalamin to serve the majority of the population whose dietary intake of animal-source foods is poor. However, this type of fortified food will not benefit those (in developed countries) with food-cobalamin malabsorption; these individuals usually need the equivalent of 1 mg of oral cobalamin daily, an amount that could not possibly be achieved by the small amount of cobalamin added to fortify foods. Other issues related to cobalamin analogue formation upon exposure to light or mixing with other food ingredients and other stability issues during storage have not been resolved; hence this topic remains a work in progress.

Immigrants from developing countries often continue to consume their native diet (which is usually low in animal-source foods) after resettling in the United States; this was earlier documented among Indian physician trainees in New York.[281] Recently, when two-thirds of Bhutanese refugees were diagnosed to have cobalamin deficiency, this prompted the Centers for Disease Control & Prevention to recommend supplemental cobalamin together with nutrition advice.[282]

Although *Plasmodium falciparum* possesses two folate transporter proteins that can facilitate membrane transport of folic acid, folinic acid, the folate precursor *p*-amino benzoic acid (pABA), and the human folate catabolite pABAG$_n$, rescue experiments on parasites in vitro show that pABA was the only effective salvage substrate at physiologic levels.[283] Recently, the safety of using low-dose folic acid (1 mg/day) in 467 pregnant women with malaria was affirmed[284]; however, high-dose folic acid (5 mg/day) will allow for resistance, with potential adverse outcomes in children.[285–287]

HYPERHOMOCYSTEINEMIA

Normally homocysteine is metabolized by the methylation reaction (discussed earlier) and by a second trans-sulfuration pathway, which essentially eliminates homocysteine as a potential source of methionine. In the trans-sulfuration pathway, cystathionine β-synthase catalyzes the condensation of homocysteine with serine in the presence of pyridoxyl phosphate (vitamin B$_6$) to form cystathionine, which is further cleaved by a vitamin B$_6$–dependent γ-cystathionase to form cysteine and α-ketobutyrate. The cysteine that is formed can be used for synthesis of the antioxidant glutathione, a key component that defends against oxidative stress within cells. In some tissues like liver, homocysteine can also be remethylated to methionine by the transfer of a one-carbon moiety from betaine by the enzyme, homocysteine methyltransferase, which is restricted to the liver and kidney. Thus the level of plasma homocysteine depends on genetically regulated levels of essential enzymes in one-carbon metabolism, the intake of folic acid or food folates, vitamin B$_6$, cobalamin, and other acquired conditions (dehydration, renal dysfunction, antifolates, and nitrous oxide).

Caveats Related to the Use of Laboratory Tests in Developing Countries (see Table 39.4)

Masking of Nutritional Folate Deficiency by Associated Cobalamin Deficiency and/or Malaria

In developing countries, the majority of the population is either vegetarian or near-vegetarian; these diets are monotonous, low in fresh vegetables, fruits, and in animal-source foods. Such a diet predisposes to a combination of nutritional cobalamin and folate (and iron) deficiencies, particularly among women and children. With cobalamin deficiency, the failure in utilization of intracellular folate for one-carbon metabolism, results in folate leaking out of cells, thereby raising the serum folate.[125-130] What this means is that the presence of cobalamin deficiency will consistently mask the coexistence of folate deficiency whenever there is (undue) over-reliance by the clinician in using the biomarker of the serum folate level as a gold standard to diagnose folate deficiency. This is a surprisingly common error in the contemporary literature—a fact that inadvertently downplays (with disastrous consequences) the seriousness of folate deficiency among millions of these particularly vulnerable women and children. Added to this is the fact that in many such regions, there is also the scourge of endemic malaria with its propensity for hemolysis (and release of the 30-fold higher red cell folate into plasma). Once again, in such settings, the serum folate concentration will yield normal-to-high values, predictably underestimate the tissue folate status, and serve to mask the diagnosis of mild-to-moderate folate deficiency in these patients who desperately require folate to support compensatory hematopoiesis and for growth and development (See Table 39.4 and Summary of the Clinical Usefulness of Tests for Cobalamin and Folate Deficiencies).

The only solution to correctly identifying whether these patients are at risk for nutritional folate deficiency is to obtain a good dietary history and identify those at risk for nutritional insufficiency.[150] (Other formal assessment includes use of 24-h food recall, estimated/weighed record, or locally validated food-frequency questionnaires to evaluate the quality and quantity of nutrients consumed.)[150] Indeed, knowledge of dietary folate and cobalamin intake should always trump the results of conventional blood tests for folate deficiency, which are flawed in this clinical setting. From the practical standpoint, all individuals at risk for nutritional anemia caused by deficiency of iron, folate, and cobalamin (including both adults[150] and children[288]) should be given prophylactic oral cobalamin, folate (and iron) replacement; and in malarious zones, these should be combined with antimalarial drugs and insecticide-treated bed nets.

Overreliance on Laboratory Data at the Expense of Clinical Information—A Case Study

The majority of women and children in developing countries suffer from combined nutritional iron, cobalamin, and folate deficiency—the three key causes of nutritional anemia. There are often additional congenital or acquired causes for hemolytic anemia in a single individual, such as malaria, bacteremia, hemoglobinopathy, or glucose-6-phosphate dehydrogenase deficiency. There is therefore potential for a clinician to make several critical interrelated errors: First, despite dire poverty and near-famine conditions, mere inattention and failure to obtain a good dietary assessment of (deficient) iron, cobalamin, and folate intake in these vulnerable patients will lead to an underestimation of the extent of deficiency of these nutrients. Second, this can be coupled with a lack of appreciation of the potential for one deficient micronutrient to have on the blood test result of another. For example, cobalamin deficiency or hemolysis will invariably raise the serum folate level and lead to an underestimation (and misdiagnosis) of the fact of *tissue* folate deficiency. Third, a failure to replace all three deficient nutrients in a given individual will invariably lead to a failure in restoring hemoglobin values to optimum; but then again, replacing one or even two out of three key missing nutrients cannot possibly be expected to secure a complete resolution of anemia.

Chronic hyperhomocysteinemia is established as a major risk factor in occlusive vascular diseases. These include myocardial infarctions from coronary atherosclerosis, extracranial carotid artery stenosis, vascular disease in end-stage renal failure, thromboangiitis obliterans, aortic atherosclerosis, venous thromboembolism, placental abruption or infarction, and recurrent stillbirths. Hyperhomocysteinemia is also associated with reduced bone mineral density and increased incidence of fractures,[289] increased small-vessel cerebrovascular disease–related strokes,[290,291] dementia, and Alzheimer disease.[292]

Raised maternal plasma levels of homocysteine primarily from cobalamin and folate deficiency are associated with various pregnancy complications. These include preeclampsia and spontaneous pregnancy loss,[253,293–296] placental abruption,[293,295,297] recurrent pregnancy loss,[293,295,298] fetal growth restriction,[294,295] preterm birth,[299] and stillbirth.[294] The adverse outcomes for the baby include NTDs and congenital malformations.[294,295] Normalization of maternal homocysteine level with cobalamin and folate and improvement of these pregnancy outcomes for some complications[295,298] indicate that some of these risks can be reduced with good nutrition.

Homocysteine-Lowering Trials and Primary Versus Secondary Prevention

Most homocysteine-lowering intervention trials have been underpowered; they have looked at populations in which the serum homocysteine level has been borderline elevated rather than being elevated to the higher level (over 20 μM); and they have only had a follow-up of less than 5 years. Moreover, many of the intervention trials have been compromised by the advent of food fortification with folate or by enrolled patients who were consuming multivitamins containing folic acid. A recent review of this "homocysteine controversy"[300] has noted that the duration of follow-up in most studies has been too short (and likely dictated by the dramatic results from the use of antihypertensives and statins, which required only short follow-up to demonstrate positive effects). The point made is that such expectations are unrealistic for atherosclerosis because the atherosclerotic plaque commonly takes 30 to 40 years to develop into a full-blown clinical event. Moreover, there is a distinct difference between primary prevention of the earliest stages of a disease process and attempts to intervene after demonstrated vascular damage (secondary prevention). (Indeed, it was only longer follow-up for 10 to 15 years that established the primacy of blood glucose control in management of patients with diabetes.)

Despite the failure of homocysteine-lowering therapy in several trials related to secondary prevention of atherosclerotic disease, this has not eliminated the possibility of a beneficial role of lowering homocysteine in primary prevention of diseases. Indeed, clinical trials that used folates have suggested that folate also has a role in reduction in strokes,[213] reduction in the rate of cognitive decline among healthy older adults,[211] and a reduction in age-related (sensorineural) hearing loss.[214] There is also Grade A evidence from randomized controlled trials for a role of folate in combination with cobalamin for reduction of hip fractures,[208] subclinical atherosclerosis,[209] and stroke prevention.[213] In addition, the value of a triple combination of folate, pyridoxine, and cobalamin to reduce age-related macular degeneration in women was shown by a relatively small study[210] (see Table 39.5). Despite support by an observational epidemiology study,[301] larger studies are required.[302]

By inference, in addition to clinical presentation with nutritional anemia, patients can also present with any of these additional clinical conditions, as well as a variety of pregnancy complications with or without poor pregnancy outcomes (affecting the newborn), when they have long-standing untreated hyperhomocysteinemia.

Homocysteine and Mild Cognitive Impairment

All inherited diseases involving a severe elevation of homocysteine are associated with cognitive deficit and poorer neurocognitive performance. Accelerated brain atrophy is often a characteristic among those with mild cognitive impairment who then go on to develop Alzheimer disease. Now a randomized controlled trial from the United Kingdom, where folate fortification of food is not mandatory, among elderly patients with mild cognitive impairment has identified that lowering of homocysteine level by B vitamins over 2 years did slow the rate of brain atrophy by almost 30%.[177] There was also

improvement in cognition by such therapy among those with mild cognitive impairment.[178] This is consistent with another randomized controlled trial (in a region without folate fortification of food) that demonstrated beneficial effects of folates on cognition over 3 years.[211] A randomized controlled trial of oral folic acid and cobalamin supplementation to prevent cognitive decline in community-dwelling older adults with depressive symptoms concluded that long-term supplementation of daily oral 400 μg folic acid plus 100 μg cobalamin promotes improvement in cognitive functioning after 24 months, particularly in immediate and delayed memory performance.[212] While awaiting larger confirmatory trials, these studies suggest that homocysteine-lowering therapy can slow down the accelerated rate of brain atrophy that is found with mild cognitive impairment.

Homocysteine Lowering and the Progression of Diabetic Nephropathy

Even though patients with diabetic nephropathy have elevated levels of homocysteine, attempts to use a combination of high doses of oral B vitamins (folic acid, pyridoxine, cobalamin) to reduce homocysteine concentrations have now been shown to *worsen* their kidney disease and place them at greater risk for dying from serious vascular events.[303] Hence there is *no* justification for using high-dose B vitamins in this setting or outside the framework of properly conducted clinical research.

FOLATE FORTIFICATION OF FOOD AND THE RISK FOR CANCER

Three large prospective studies[304–306] suggest that long-term folate intake actually *decreases the risk* for initiation or early development of colorectal cancer[306]; in addition, there appears to be a diminished to nonexistent influence on (precancerous) adenomas. A recent meta-analysis of 13 randomized trials that compared the incidence of cancer of all types in ~50,000 individuals led to the conclusion that folic acid supplementation does not significantly increase or decrease the risk of cancer over a 5-year treatment period.[307] Collectively, these papers provide reassurance that the fortification of food to prevent NTDs in women of childbearing age has not led to harm among the remaining "nontargeted" population of adults. There also could be long-term benefits in primary prevention (see Table 39.5).

FUTURE DIRECTIONS

In this age of spiraling costs for health care delivery, and the ongoing debate on ways to reduce these costs, few instances in internal medicine and hematology yield more satisfying dividends than diagnosing and treating cobalamin and folate deficiency using generic vitamins that are "dirt-cheap"—costing only a few cents a day. These conditions are devastating when undiagnosed or misdiagnosed or when cobalamin deficiency is treated with folate alone. Recognition of various populations at risk and the clinical scenarios in which folate and cobalamin deficiency are likely to be present, and the availability of sensitive and specific tests, should reduce uncertainty in diagnosis. The studies on folate supplementation during pregnancy that identified new folate-responsive NTDs and neurocristopathies are a paradigm for identification of hitherto unrecognized roles for other nutrients in human development. The significant impact of supplemental folates in relieving human suffering consonant with reducing costs for intensive and long-term care of infants with prematurity or NTDs is a major achievement and an outstanding example of cost-effective preventive medicine. Other recent advances from randomized controlled studies indicate beneficial effects of supplemental folate and cobalamin in the prevention of diverse diseases. The structural characterization of folate receptors offers unprecedented potential to develop a new generation of antifolates that can occupy the receptor-binding pocket and thereby starve cancer cells that primarily depend on folate receptor-mediated uptake of folates.[308,309] Whereas folate receptor-α is overexpressed in many tumors, folate receptor-β is unique to macrophages found at sites of inflammation. To this end, folate receptor-α and -β targeting using monoclonal antibodies or various folate-tagged fluorescent probes,[310] newer radionuclides,[311] drugs, as well as ^{18}F-based folate radiotracers for positron emission tomography (PET) imaging,[312] are under intense scrutiny in the clinic. The influence of folates and cobalamin during development in utero—especially on behavioral neuroscience—allows us to peer into a new field where groundbreaking discoveries will be made in the coming decade. A molecular link between folate deficiency, homocysteinylated-hnRNP-E1, and its role in perturbing the human papillomavirus (type 16) life cycle and in HPV16-induced cancer has been discovered.[99] Because this virus is the most common cause of cervical cancer worldwide (and also responsible for a significant number of vulvar, vaginal, penile, anal, and oropharyngeal cancers), such studies open the door to new investigations into the potential role of these vitamins in the field of preventive oncology. Finally, folate receptor-4 (renamed Juno after the Goddess of Fertility), which is found on the surface of eggs, is what the sperm protein, Izumo1 (named after a Japanese marriage shrine), recognizes and binds to gain entry and fuse to form a single diploid cell.[313] This pair of proteins is essential for reproduction and raises the potential for identifying fertility problems and opens the door to new contraceptives.[314]

SUGGESTED READINGS

Antony AC: Vegetarianism and vitamin-B12 (cobalamin) deficiency. *Am J Clin Nutr* 78:3, 2003.

Antony AC: In utero physiology: role of folic acid in nutrient delivery and fetal development. *Am J Clin Nutr* 85:598S, 2007.

Bjorke-Monsen AL, Ueland PM: Cobalamin status in children. *J Inherit Metab Dis* 34:111, 2010.

Carmel R: Biomarkers of cobalamin (vitamin B-12) status in the epidemiologic setting: a critical overview of context, applications, and performance characteristics of cobalamin, methylmalonic acid, and holotranscobalamin II. *Am J Clin Nutr* 94:348S, 2011.

de Jager CA, Oulhaj A, Jacoby R, et al: Cognitive and clinical outcomes of homocysteine-lowering B-vitamin treatment in mild cognitive impairment: a randomized controlled trial. *Int J Geriatr Psychiatry* 27:592–600, 2012.

Duggan C, Srinivasan K, Thomas T, et al: Vitamin B-12 supplementation during pregnancy and early lactation increases maternal, breast milk, and infant measures of vitamin B-12 status. *J Nutr* 144:758–764, 2014.

Durga J, van Boxtel MP, Schouten EG, et al: Effect of 3-year folic acid supplementation on cognitive function in older adults in the FACIT trial: a randomised, double blind, controlled trial. *Lancet* 369:208, 2007.

Gherasim C, Lofgren M, Banerjee R: Navigating the B(12) road: assimilation, delivery, and disorders of cobalamin. *J Biol Chem* 288:13186–13193, 2013.

Gordon N: Cerebral folate deficiency. *Dev Med Child Neurol* 51:180, 2009.

Grapp M, Just IA, Linnankivi T, et al: Molecular characterization of folate receptor 1 mutations delineates cerebral folate transport deficiency. *Brain* 135:2022–2031, 2012.

Grapp M, Wrede A, Schweizer M, et al: Choroid plexus transcytosis and exosome shuttling deliver folate into brain parenchyma. *Nat Commun* 4:2123, 2013.

Hodis HN, Mack WJ, Dustin L, et al: High-dose B vitamin supplementation and progression of subclinical atherosclerosis: a randomized controlled trial. *Stroke* 40:730, 2009.

Lahner E, Norman GL, Severi C, et al: Reassessment of intrinsic factor and parietal cell autoantibodies in atrophic gastritis with respect to cobalamin deficiency. *Am J Gastroenterol* 104:2071–2079, 2009.

Lee JE, Chan AT: Fruit, vegetables, and folate: cultivating the evidence for cancer prevention. *Gastroenterology* 141:16, 2011.

McFarland R: Cerebral folate deficiency—mishaps and misdirection. *Brain* 135:2002–2003, 2012.

Quadros EV: Advances in the understanding of cobalamin assimilation and metabolism. *Br J Haematol* 148:195, 2010.

Smith AD, Smith SM, de Jager CA, et al: Homocysteine-lowering by B vitamins slows the rate of accelerated brain atrophy in mild cognitive impairment: a randomized controlled trial. *PLoS ONE* 5:e12244, 2010.

Smulders YM, Blom HJ: The homocysteine controversy. *J Inherit Metab Dis* 34:93, 2011.

Stabler SP: Clinical practice. Vitamin B12 deficiency. *N Engl J Med* 368:149–160, 2013.

Toh BH: Diagnosis and classification of autoimmune gastritis. *Autoimmun Rev* 13:459–462, 2014.

Torheim LE, Ferguson EL, Penrose K, et al: Women in resource-poor settings are at risk of inadequate intakes of multiple micronutrients. *J Nutr* 140:2051S–2058S, 2010.

Torsvik I, Ueland PM, Markestad T, et al: Cobalamin supplementation improves motor development and regurgitations in infants: results from a randomized intervention study. *Am J Clin Nutr* 98:1233–1240, 2013.

Visentin M, Diop-Bove N, Zhao R, et al: The intestinal absorption of folates. *Annu Rev Physiol* 76:251–274, 2014.

Wang X, Qin X, Demirtas H, et al: Efficacy of folic acid supplementation in stroke prevention: a meta-analysis. *Lancet* 369:1876, 2007.

Watkins D, Rosenblatt DS: Inborn errors of cobalamin absorption and metabolism. *Am J Med Genet C Semin Med Genet* 157C:33–44, 2011.

Xiao S, Tang YS, Khan RA, et al: Influence of physiologic folate deficiency on human papillomavirus type 16 (HPV16)-harboring human keratinocytes in vitro and in vivo. *J Biol Chem* 287:12559, 2012.

Yang Q, Botto LD, Erickson JD, et al: Improvement in stroke mortality in Canada and the United States, 1990 to 2002. *Circulation* 113:1335, 2006.

Zhao R, Matherly LH, Goldman ID: Membrane transporters and folate homeostasis: intestinal absorption and transport into systemic compartments and tissues. *Expert Rev Mol Med* 11:e4, 2009.

REFERENCES

For the complete list of references, log on to www.expertconsult.com.

THALASSEMIA SYNDROMES

John Chapin and Patricia J. Giardina

The thalassemia syndromes are a heterogeneous group of inherited anemias characterized by defects in the synthesis of one or more of the globin chain subunits of the hemoglobin (Hb) tetramer. The clinical syndromes associated with thalassemia arise from the combined consequences of inadequate Hb production and imbalanced accumulation of globin subunits. The former causes hypochromia and microcytosis; the latter leads to ineffective erythropoiesis (IE) and hemolytic anemia. Clinical manifestations are diverse, ranging from asymptomatic hypochromia and microcytosis to profound anemia, which can be fatal in utero or in early childhood if untreated. This heterogeneity arises from the variable severities of the primary biosynthetic defects and coinherited modifying factors, such as increased synthesis of fetal globin subunits or diminished or increased synthesis of α-globin subunits. Palliative treatment of the severe forms by blood transfusion is eventually compromised by the concomitant problems of iron overload, alloimmunization, and bloodborne infections.

As a group, the thalassemias represent the most common single genetic disorder known. In many parts of the world, they constitute major public health problems. Laboratory analysis of these disorders has been one of the most productive and enlightening endeavors of biomedical research. Study of the molecular defects underlying the thalassemia syndromes has led to fundamental advances in our understanding of eukaryotic gene structure and function. For each of these reasons, a thorough understanding of thalassemia and its related disorders is essential to hematologists. This chapter reviews the major features of these syndromes. Readers wanting more detailed information than can be included here are referred to more comprehensive monographs elsewhere.[1,2]

The classification, genetic basis, and pathophysiology of the thalassemia syndromes are based on a thorough understanding of the human Hbs, their biosynthesis, their encoding *globin* gene families, and their roles as soluble oxygen-carrying molecules. Therefore, readers of this chapter should first familiarize themselves with the material presented in Chapter 31. The material presented in this chapter is also substantially clarified by prior reading of Chapters 33 and 34 because the principles underlying the pathophysiology of and therapy for thalassemia draw heavily on knowledge of iron metabolism.

DEFINITIONS AND NOMENCLATURE

The term *thalassemia* is derived from a Greek term that roughly means "the sea" (Mediterranean) in the blood.[1] It was first applied to the anemias frequently encountered in people from the Italian and Greek coasts and nearby islands.[3–5] The term is now used to refer to inherited defects in globin-chain biosynthesis. Individual syndromes are named according to the globin chain whose synthesis is adversely affected. Thus, α-globin chains are absent or reduced in patients with α-thalassemia, β-globin chains in patients with β-thalassemia, δ-globin and β-globin chains in patients $\delta\beta$-thalassemia, and so forth. In some contexts, it is also useful to subclassify the syndromes according to whether synthesis of the affected globin chain is totally absent (e.g., β°-thalassemia) or only partially reduced (e.g., β^+-thalassemia).

The most common forms of thalassemia arise from total absence of structurally normal globin chains or a partial reduction in their synthesis. In contrast to the "structural" hemoglobinopathies (e.g.,

sickle cell anemia), which are characterized by the production of normal amounts of mutant globin chains having deranged physical or chemical properties, the thalassemias are quantitative disorders: the primary lesion lies in the amount of globin produced. However, some rare forms of thalassemia are characterized by the production of structurally abnormal globin chains in reduced amounts, which are described in more detail in this chapter. These thalassemic hemoglobinopathies share features of thalassemia as well as those of structural hemoglobinopathies.[6]

Some mutations alter the patterns of fetal to adult Hb switching. These conditions, called *hereditary persistence of fetal Hemoglobin,* are not generally associated with clinical symptoms; nonetheless, they merit consideration in this chapter. Their importance lies in their role as modulating factors when coinherited with other hemoglobinopathies. They are also useful models for investigating the molecular basis for *globin* gene regulation during human development and as paradigms for rational therapy for the major β-chain hemoglobinopathies, namely, sickle cell anemia and β-thalassemia.

ETIOLOGY, EPIDEMIOLOGY, AND PATHOPHYSIOLOGY

Thalassemias have been encountered in virtually every ethnic group and geographic location. Thalassemia carriers affect 1.5% of the world population. They are most common in the Mediterranean basin and tropical or subtropical regions of Asia and Africa. The "thalassemia belt" extends along the shores of the Mediterranean and throughout the Arabian peninsula, Turkey, Iran, India, southeastern Asia, especially Thailand, Cambodia, and southern China.[7–10] The prevalence of carriers of thalassemia in these regions is in the range of 2.5% to 15%. Similar to sickle cell anemia, thalassemia is most common in areas historically affected by endemic malaria. Malaria seems to have conferred selective survival advantage to thalassemia heterozygotes in which infection with the malarial parasite is believed to result in milder disease and less impact on reproductive fitness.[1,2,11] Therefore, the gene frequency for thalassemia has become fixed and high in populations exposed to malaria over many centuries.

PATHOPHYSIOLOGY: GENERAL PRINCIPLES

The primary lesion in all forms of thalassemia is reduced or absent production of one or more globin chains. For all practical purposes, the major impact on clinical well-being occurs only when these lesions affect the α- or β-globin chains necessary for the synthesis of adult hemoglobin (Hb A), with a normal structure of $\alpha_2\beta_2$. Severe impairment of γ-, ε-, or ζ-globin production is presumably lethal in utero, and has not been observed in human biology. One consequence of reduced globin-chain production is immediately apparent: reduced production of functioning Hb tetramers. As a result, hypochromia and microcytosis are characteristic of virtually all patients with thalassemia. In the milder forms of the disease, this phenomenon may be barely detectable.

The second consequence of impaired globin biosynthesis is unbalanced synthesis of the individual α- and β-subunits. Hb tetramers are highly soluble and have reversible oxygen-carrying properties exquisitely adapted for oxygen transport and delivery under physiologic conditions. Free or "unpaired" α-, β-, and γ-globin chains are either highly insoluble or form homotetramers (Hb H and Hb Bart) that are incapable of releasing oxygen normally, and because they are relatively unstable, will precipitate as the cell ages. For poorly understood reasons, no compensatory regulatory mechanism exists whereby impaired synthesis of one globin subunit leads to a compensatory downward adjustment in the production of the other (partner) globin chain of the Hb tetramer. Thus, whereas useless excess α-globin chains continue to accumulate and precipitate in β-thalassemia, excess β-globin chains form Hb H in α-thalassemia. The abnormal solubility or oxygen-carrying properties of these chains lead to a variety of physiologic derangements. Indeed, in the severe forms of thalassemia, it is the behavior of the unpaired globin chains accumulating in relative excess that dominates the pathophysiology of the syndrome rather than the mere underproduction of functioning Hb tetramers. The precise complications of this pathophysiologic phenomenon are diverse and depend on the amount and the identity of the globin chain accumulating in excess. The fundamental principle that must be appreciated is that thalassemias cause symptoms by underproduction of Hb and by accumulation of unpaired globin subunits. The unpaired subunits are usually the major sources of morbidity and mortality.

The predominant circulating Hb at the moment of birth is fetal hemoglobin (Hb $F^{\alpha 2 \gamma 2}$) (see Chapter 33). Although the switch from γ- to β-globin biosynthesis begins before birth, the composition of Hb in the peripheral blood changes much later because of the long-life span of normal circulating red blood cells (RBCs) (approximately 120 days). Hb F is thus slowly replaced by Hb A so that infants do not depend heavily on normal amounts and function of Hb A until they are between 4 and 6 months old. The pathophysiologic consequences of these considerations are that whereas α-chain hemoglobinopathies tend to be symptomatic in utero and at birth, individuals with β-chain abnormalities are asymptomatic until 4 to 6 months of age. These differences in the onset of phenotypic expression arise because α-chains are needed to form Hb F and Hb A, but β-chains are required only for Hb A.

β-THALASSEMIA SYNDROMES

Nomenclature

Many different mutations cause β-thalassemia and its related disorders, such as δβ-thalassemia and the silent carrier state. They are inherited in a multitude of genetic combinations responsible for a heterogeneous group of clinical syndromes. β-Thalassemia major, also known as Cooley anemia or homozygous β-thalassemia, is a clinically severe disorder that results from the inheritance of two

β-thalassemia alleles, one on each copy of chromosome 11. As a consequence of diminished Hb A synthesis, the circulating RBCs are very hypochromic, abnormal in shape, and they contain markedly reduced amounts of Hb. Accumulation of free α-globin chains leads to the deposition of precipitated aggregates of these chains to the detriment of the erythrocyte and its precursor cells in the bone marrow (BM). The anemia of thalassemia major is so severe that long-term blood transfusions are usually required for survival.

The term *β-thalassemia intermedia* is applied to a less severe clinical phenotype in which significant anemia occurs but chronic transfusion therapy is not absolutely required. It usually results from the inheritance of two β-thalassemia mutations, one mild and one severe; the inheritance of two mild mutations; or, occasionally, the inheritance of complex combinations, such as a single β-thalassemia defect and an excess of normal α-*globin* genes, or two β-thalassemia mutations coinherited with heterozygous α-thalassemia (in this last form, known as αβ-thalassemia, the α-thalassemia allele reduces the burden of unpaired α-chains).[12–14] Simple heterozygosity for certain forms of β-thalassemic hemoglobinopathies can also be associated with a thalassemia intermedia phenotype, sometimes called *dominant β-thalassemia.*[15,16]

Thalassemia minor, also known as β-thalassemia trait or heterozygous β-thalassemia, is caused by the presence of a single β-thalassemia mutation and a normal *β-globin* gene on the other chromosome. It is characterized by profound microcytosis with hypochromia but mild or minimal anemia. In general, thalassemia minor has no associated symptoms, although cholelithiasis has been reported from the accumulation of pigmented gallstones as a result of hemolysis in this population.[17]

Molecular Pathology

Forms of β-thalassemia arise from mutations that affect every step in the pathway of globin gene expression: transcription, processing of the messenger ribonucleic acid (mRNA) precursor, translation of mature mRNA, and posttranslational integrity of the β-polypeptide chain (Fig. 40.1 and Table 40.1).[18–20] Large deletions removing two or more non–α-genes are found in rare cases, as are smaller partial or total deletions of the β-gene alone (see Fig. 40.1). Most types of β-thalassemia are caused by point mutations affecting one or a few bases.[18–25] Of the more than 200 mutations causing β-thalassemia, approximately 15 account for the vast majority of affected patients, with the remainder responsible for the disorder in only relatively few patients. It has been determined that five or six mutations usually account for more than 90% of the cases of β-thalassemia in a given ethnic group or geographic area (see Table 40.1).[22]

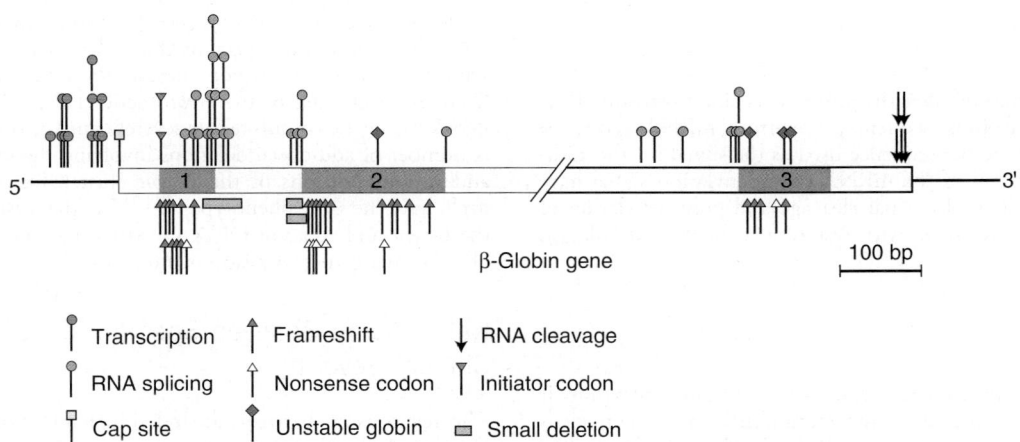

Fig. 40.1 MODEL OF THE HUMAN β-GLOBIN GENE SHOWING SITES AND TYPES OF VARIOUS MUTATIONS CAUSING β-THALASSEMIA. *(Adapted from Kazazian HH Jr: The thalassemia syndromes: molecular basis and prenatal diagnosis in 1990.* Semin Hematol *27:209, 1990.)*

TABLE 40.1	Common β-Thalassemia Mutations in Different Racial Groups
Racial Group	**Description**
Mediterranean	IVS-1, position 110 (G → A)
	Codon 39, nonsense (CAG → TAG)
	IVS-1, position 1 (G → A)
	IVS-2, position 745 (C → G)
	IVS-1, position 6 (T → C)
	IVS-2, position 1 (G → A)
African	–34 (A → G)
	–88 (C → T)
	Poly(A), (AATAAA → AACAAA)
Southeast Asian	Codons 41/42, frameshift (-CTTT)
	IVS-2, position 654 (C → T)
	–28 (A → T)
Asian Indian	IVS-1, position 5 (G → C)
	619-bp deletion
	Codons 8/9, frameshift (++G)
	Codons 41/42, frameshift (–CTTT)
	IVS-1, position 1 (G → T)

Data from Kazazian HH Jr, Boehm CD: Molecular basis and prenatal diagnosis of beta-thalassemia. *Blood* 72(4):1107, 1988; and Kazazian HH Jr, Boehm CD: personal communication, 1993.

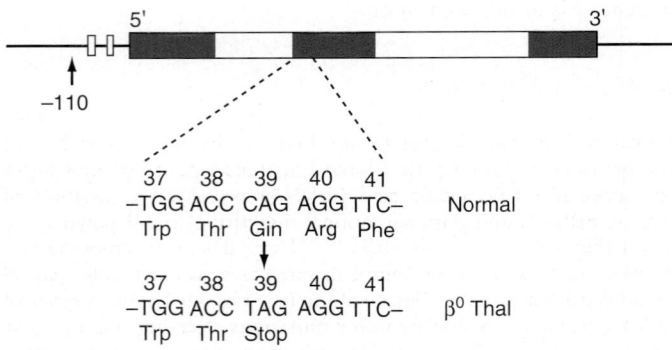

Fig. 40.3 β°-THALASSEMIA ARISING FROM A MUTATION CHANGING AN AMINO ACID CODON TO A TERMINATION CODON (NONSENSE MUTATION). *(Adapted from Takeshita K, Forget BG, Scarpa A, Benz EJ Jr: Intranuclear defects in β-globin mRNA accumulation due to a premature translation termination codon. Blood 64:13, 1984.)*

Transcription

Whereas several mutations alter the promoter region upstream of the β-globin mRNA-encoding sequence, impairing mRNA synthesis, mutations that derange the sequence used as the signal for the addition of the poly-(A) tail of the mRNA polyadenylation signal have been shown to result in abnormal cleavage and polyadenylation of the nascent mRNA precursor, with resulting reduced accumulation of mature mRNA.[19–21]

Processing

Many forms of β-thalassemia are caused by mutations that impair splicing of the mRNA precursor into mature mRNA in the nucleus or that prevent translation of the mRNA in the cytoplasm. The molecular pathology of splicing mutations is complex (Fig. 40.2). Some base substitutions ablate the donor (GT) or acceptor (AG) dinucleotides, which are absolutely required at the intron–exon

boundaries for normal splicing and thereby completely block production of mature functional messenger RNA. Thus, no β-globin can be synthesized (β°-thalassemia). Other mutations alter the consensus sequences that surround the GT- and AG-invariant dinucleotides and decrease the efficiency of normal splicing signals by 70% to 95%, resulting in β⁺-thalassemia; some consensus mutations even abolish splicing completely, causing β°-thalassemia. A third type of splicing aberration results from mutations that are not in the immediate vicinity of a normal splice site. These alter regions within the gene, called *cryptic splice sites,* which resemble consensus splicing sites but do not normally sustain splicing (see Fig. 40.2). The mutations activate the site by supplying a critical GT or AG nucleotide or by creating a sufficiently strong consensus signal to stimulate splicing at that site 60% to 100% of the time. The activated cryptic sites generate an abnormally spliced, untranslatable mRNA species. Only 10% to 40% of the mRNA precursors are thus spliced at the normal sites, which causes β⁺-thalassemia of variable severity. The mutation responsible for the most common form of β-thalassemia among Greeks and Cypriots (Fig. 40.3) activates a cryptic splice site near the 3′ end of the first intron (position 110).[26,27] The determinants that dictate the degree to which each mutation alters splice site use remain largely unknown.

Translation

Mutations that abolish translation occur at several locations along the mature mRNA and are very common causes of β-thalassemia (see Fig. 40.1 and Table 40.1). The most common form of β°-thalassemia in Sardinians results from a base substitution in the gene that changes the codon encoding the 39th amino acid of the β-globin chain from CAG, which encodes glutamine to TAG, whose equivalent (UAG) in mRNA specifies termination of translation (see Fig. 40.3).[28,29] A premature termination codon totally abrogates the ability of the mRNA to be translated into normal β-globin. Premature translation termination also results indirectly from frameshift mutations (i.e., small insertions or deletions of a few bases, other than multiples of three, that alter the phase or frame in which the nucleotide sequence is read during translation).[29] An in-phase premature termination codon is usually encountered within the next 50 bases downstream from a frameshift.

Other Sites

Rare mutations that affect gene function by intriguing mechanisms have been described. An extremely large deletion of the *β-globin* gene cluster has been described that removes the *ε-*, *γ-*, and *δ-*genes.[30] The patient has a severe β-thalassemia phenotype, but the *β-globin* gene and 500 bases of adjacent 5′ and 3′ DNA have an entirely normal nucleotide sequence. The *β-gene* functions normally in surrogate cells. The important aspect of this deletion is that it removes the critical locus control region located thousands of bases upstream from the beginning of the *globin* gene cluster at the 5′ end of the *ε-globin* gene; loss of this region severely impairs *β-gene* expression.[18,31] A number of additional deletions involving the locus control region and various portions of the *β-gene* cluster, but sparing the *β-gene* itself, have the same phenotype.[1,2,19–21] In other cases of β-thalassemia, the *β-gene* and adjacent DNA are structurally normal, and the basis of abnormal gene expression is unknown.[22]

Relationship Between Specific Mutations and Clinical Severity

The relationship between an individual mutation and the clinical severity of the β-thalassemia phenotype associated with that particular mutation is complex.[22] For example, the A to G mutation at position 34 of the *β-gene* promoter commonly encountered in patients of African origin is associated with a different clinical

A

Normal splicing

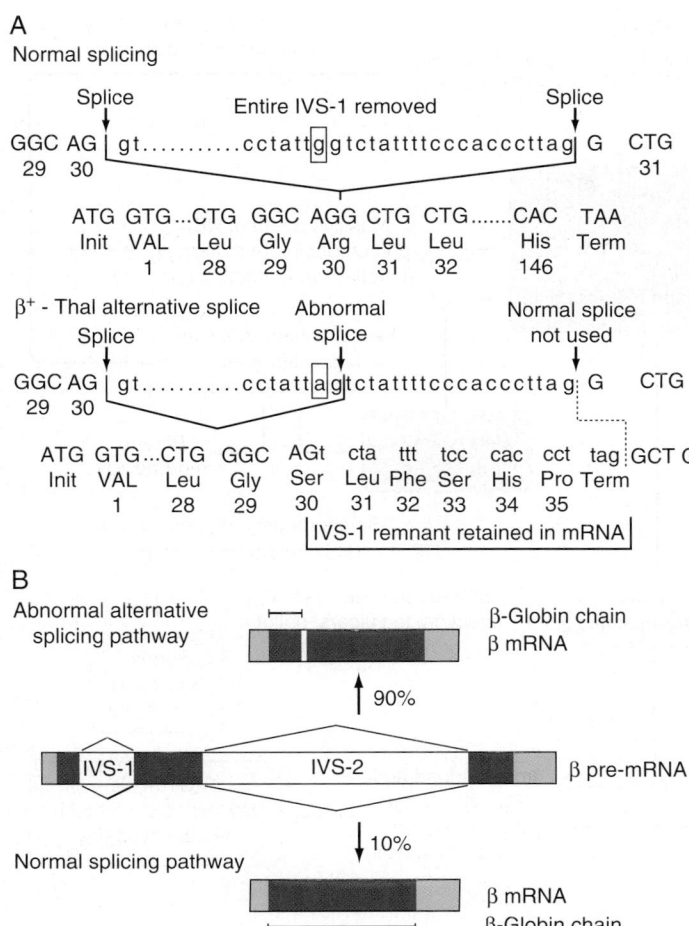

Fig. 40.2 β⁺-THALASSEMIA ARISING FROM ALTERNATIVE MRNA SPLICING CAUSED BY A MUTATION ACTIVATING A CRYPTIC SPLICING SITE. (A) The G→A mutation is shown enclosed in *squares* located near the 3′ end of intron 1 (IVS-1); it creates a sequence motif closely mimicking a pre-mRNA acceptor splice site. The product of the alternative splicing event is also shown. Note that use of the activated cryptic site generates a mature mRNA that contains an in-frame termination codon and therefore does not encode a functional β-globin chain. *(From Benz EJ Jr: The hemoglobinopathies. In Kelly WN, DeVita VT, editors:* Textbook of Internal Medicine, *Philadelphia, 1988, JB Lippincott, p 1423.)* (B) Diagram of the means by which use of the cryptic splice site 90% of the time results in only 10% of the mRNA precursor molecules to be spliced normally into translatable mature mRNA, thus causing β⁺-thalassemia. *mRNA,* Messenger ribonucleic acid. *(Adapted from Bunn HF, Forget BG:* Hemoglobin: molecular, genetic and clinical aspects. *Philadelphia, WB Saunders, 1986.)*

severity than that found in Chinese patients inheriting the same mutation.[32] Clearly, the genetic "context" of the mutation is different in the two populations. The mutant *β-globin* gene in the two different racial groups probably arose in different chromosome backgrounds that have different potentials for γ-gene expression. Multiple forms, or haplotypes, of normal non–*α-globin* gene clusters exist in various human populations. These are defined by the patterns of restriction fragment length polymorphisms detected when DNA is digested with restriction endonucleases and analyzed by Southern gene blotting for the fragments bearing the non–*α-globin* genes.[28] Haplotypes differ according to whether each restriction site is present or absent along the gene cluster. More than 12 haplotypes have been defined by examination of several restriction sites located along the cluster that are present or absent in a polymorphic manner in normal individuals.[28] The clinical variability encountered in two different groups bearing identical primary mutations correlates best with the haplotype or chromosome background on which the

mutation is inherited. The differences in physiologically important functions among haplotypes that modulate severity remain unknown, but a possible explanation lies in the variable abilities of the *γ-globin* genes on different chromosomes to respond to severe erythroid stress by increased expression during postnatal life. The *β-globin* genes carried on some haplotypes differ in the degree to which they can respond in this manner.[33] Because Hb F synthesis reduces the severity of β-chain hemoglobinopathies,[1] the level of γ-gene expression from a given chromosome can play an important modulating role.

Pathophysiology

The biochemical hallmark of β-thalassemia is reduced biosynthesis of the β-globin subunit of Hb A ($\alpha_2\beta_2$). In β-thalassemia heterozygotes, β-globin synthesis is about half-normal, as described by the synthetic ratio of β- to α-chain mRNA (β/α ratio) of 0.5–0.7 (normal = 1.0). This ratio has a direct correlation with clinical severity in β-thalassemia patients.[34] In homozygotes for β°-thalassemia, who account for approximately one-third of patients, β-globin synthesis is absent. β-globin synthesis is reduced to 5% to 30% of normal levels in β⁺-thalassemia homozygotes or β⁺/β°-thalassemia compound heterozygotes, who together account for approximately two-thirds of cases.[1] Alpha hemoglobin stabilizing protein is a chaperone-like protein that assists in binding free α-globin chains, higher levels of alpha hemoglobin stabilizing protein result in a more severe clinical phenotype.[34]

Because the synthesis of Hb A ($\alpha_2\beta_2$) is markedly reduced or absent, the RBCs are hypochromic and microcytic. γ-Chain synthesis is partially reactivated so that the Hb of the patient contains a relatively large proportion of Hb F.[1] However, these γ-chains are quantitatively insufficient to replace β-chain production.

Individuals inheriting two β-thalassemic alleles experience a more profound deficit of β-chain production. Little or no Hb A is produced, and importantly, the imbalance of α- and β-globin production is far more severe (Fig. 40.4). The limited capacity of RBCs to proteolyze the excess α-globin chains, a capacity that probably exerts a protective effect in heterozygous β-thalassemia, is overwhelmed in homozygotes. Free α-globin accumulates, and unpaired α-chains aggregate and precipitate to form inclusion bodies, which cause oxidative membrane damage within the RBC[35] leading to apoptosis and destruction of immature developing erythroblasts within the BM IE.[36,37] Consequently, relatively few of the erythroid precursors undergoing erythroid maturation in the BM survive long enough to be released into the bloodstream as erythrocytes. The occasional erythrocytes that are formed during erythropoiesis bear a burden of inclusion bodies. The reticuloendothelial cells in the spleen, liver, and BM remove these abnormal cells prematurely, which reduces RBC survival as a consequence of this hemolytic anemia.

Defective β-globin synthesis exerts at least three distinct yet interrelated effects on the generation of oxygen-carrying capacity for the peripheral blood (see Fig. 40.4): (1) IE, which impairs production of new RBCs; (2) hemolytic anemia, which shortens the survival of the few RBCs produced; and (3) hypochromia with microcytosis, which reduces the oxygen-carrying capacity of the few RBCs that do survive. The profound deficit in the oxygen-carrying capacity of the blood stimulates production of high levels of erythropoietin (EPO) in an attempt to promote compensatory erythroid hyperplasia. Unfortunately, the ability of the BM to respond is markedly impaired by IE. Massive BM expansion does occur, but very few erythrocytes are actually supplied to the circulation. The BM becomes packed with immature erythroid precursors, which die from their burden of precipitated α-globin chains before they reach the reticulocyte stage. Profound anemia persists, driving erythroid hyperplasia to still higher levels. In some cases, erythropoiesis is so exuberant that masses of extramedullary erythropoietic tissue form in the chest, abdomen, or pelvis.

As described in the following section, massive BM expansion exerts numerous adverse effects on the growth, development, and

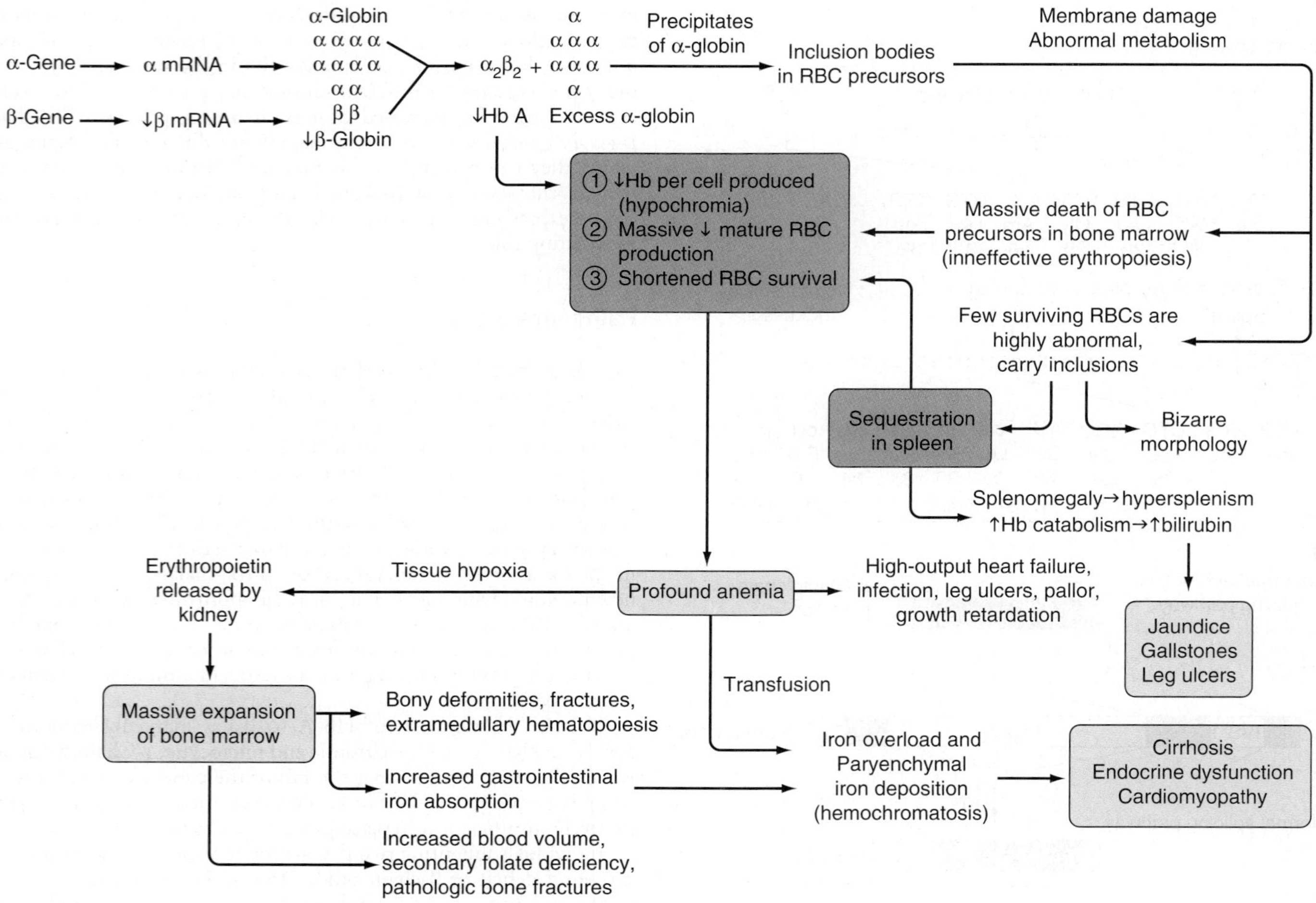

α-Gene ⟶ α mRNA ⟶ α-Globin
                    α α α α
                    α α α α   α
                    α α   α α α
                                  α₂β₂ + α α α   Precipitates   Membrane damage
                                          α   of α-globin   Abnormal metabolism
β-Gene ⟶ ↓β mRNA ⟶ β β   ↓Hb A Excess α-globin   Inclusion bodies
                    ↓β-Globin   in RBC precursors

① ↓Hb per cell produced (hypochromia)
② Massive ↓ mature RBC production
③ Shortened RBC survival

Massive death of RBC precursors in bone marrow (inneffective erythropoiesis)

Few surviving RBCs are highly abnormal, carry inclusions

Sequestration in spleen

Bizarre morphology

Splenomegaly→hypersplenism
↑Hb catabolism→↑bilirubin

Erythropoietin released by kidney

Tissue hypoxia

Profound anemia

High-output heart failure, infection, leg ulcers, pallor, growth retardation

Jaundice
Gallstones
Leg ulcers

Massive expansion of bone marrow

Bony deformities, fractures, extramedullary hematopoiesis

Transfusion

Increased gastrointestinal iron absorption

Iron overload and Paryenchymal iron deposition (hemochromatosis)

Cirrhosis
Endocrine dysfunction
Cardiomyopathy

Increased blood volume, secondary folate deficiency, pathologic bone fractures

Fig. 40.4 PATHOPHYSIOLOGY OF SEVERE FORMS OF β-THALASSEMIA. The diagram outlines the pathogenesis of clinical abnormalities resulting from the primary defect in β-globin chain synthesis. *Hb*, hemoglobin; *RBC*, Red blood cell.

function of critical organ systems and creates the characteristic facies caused by maxillary BM hyperplasia and frontal bossing (Fig. 40.5). Hemolytic anemia results in massive splenomegaly and high-output congestive heart failure. In untreated cases, death occurs during the first 2 decades of life. Treatment with RBC transfusions sufficient to maintain Hb levels above 9.0–10.0 g/dL improves oxygen delivery, suppresses the excessive IE, and prolongs life. Unfortunately, as discussed in more detail later, complications of chronic transfusion therapy, including iron overload, can be fatal before 30 years of age. The addition of iron chelation therapy to regular transfusion therapy now prolongs survival and improves the quality of life.

PATHOPHYSIOLOGY: RECENT FINDINGS

IE is the hallmark of β-thalassemia, triggering a cascade of compensatory mechanisms and resulting in clinical sequelae such as erythroid BM expansion, extramedullary hematopoiesis, splenomegaly, and increased gastrointestinal iron absorption. Several studies demonstrate that erythropoietic iron demand influences hepcidin expression to a greater degree than anemia or nonhematopoietic iron stores.[38,39] In particular, studies in β-thalassemia demonstrate that hepcidin expression is disproportionally low relative to the degree of iron overload.[40–42] (see Chapter 35). Recent studies in mice have begun to shed light on the complex molecular mechanisms underlying IE and the associated compensatory pathways; this new understanding may lead to the development of novel therapies. Increased or excessive

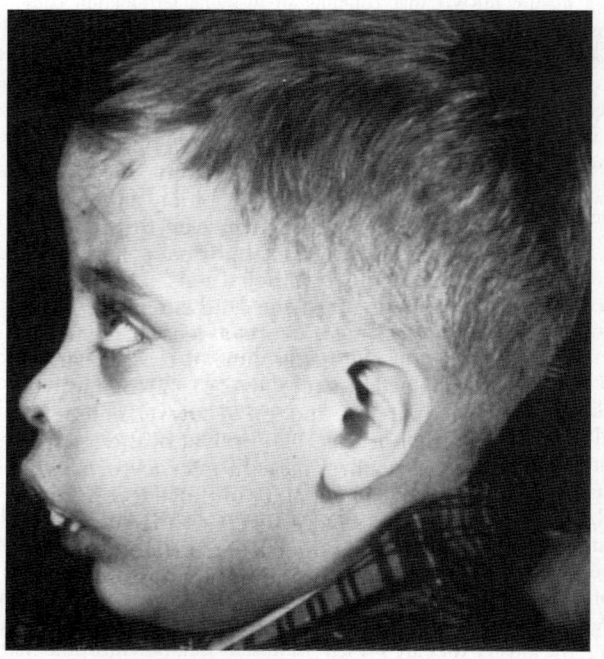

Fig. 40.5 THALASSEMIC FACIES. See text for description. *(From Jurkiewicz MJ, Pearson HA, Furlow LT Jr: Reconstruction of the maxilla in thalassemia. Ann N Y Acad Sci 165:437, 1969.)*

activation of the Janus kinase 2 (JAK2)–STAT5 (signal transducers and activators of transcription 5) pathway promotes unnecessary disproportionate proliferation of erythroid progenitors, but other factors suppress serum hepcidin levels leading to dysregulation of iron metabolism. Preclinical studies suggest that JAK2 inhibitors, hepcidin agonists, and exogenous transferrin may help to restore normal erythropoiesis and iron metabolism and reduce splenomegaly.[43-53]

JAK2

In murine models and patients with β-thalassemia, erythroid precursors express elevated levels of the phosphorylated active form of JAK2 (pJAK2) and other downstream signaling molecules that promote proliferation and inhibit differentiation of erythroid progenitor cells.[54,55] A recent study showed that JAK2 activation upregulated the transcription factor ID1[56]; high levels of ID1 have been found to inhibit cellular differentiation.[55] JAK2 signaling also activates the phosphoinositol-3-kinase (PI3K)–AKT pathway, which plays an important role in regulating cell survival and the activity of the transcription factor forkhead box O3 (FOXO3), which modulates oxidative stress during erythropoiesis.[55] Taken together, findings from these studies suggest a model in which persistent phosphorylation of JAK2 as a consequence of high EPO levels induces erythroid hyperplasia and massive extramedullary hematopoiesis and the early erythroid progenitors that fail to differentiate colonize and proliferate predominantly in the spleen and liver,[54] thus contributing to hepatosplenomegaly. Given the central role of JAK2 in the pathophysiology of IE, it has been hypothesized that JAK2 inhibitors may be effective in modulating some of these compensatory mechanisms that lead to the severe clinical complications associated with β-thalassemia.

The activation of the EPO–EPO-Receptor–JAK2 pathway is not likely the only cause of the limited erythroid differentiation observed in β-thalassemia. It is possible that other factors or abnormal physiologic conditions present in β-thalassemia come into play, interfering with erythroid cell differentiation. Among the possible factors acting together with JAK2, iron overload, reactive oxygen species (ROS), or the unbalanced synthesis of globin chains or heme can be also considered.[57] Iron is essential for all cells but is toxic in excess. It is possible to speculate that thalassemic erythroid cells accumulate an excess of toxic heme associated with free α-chains, leading to the formation of ROS, which has been involved with cell RBC hemolysis and altered differentiation.[58,59]

Serum iron is bound to transferrin and enters erythroid cells primarily via receptor-mediated endocytosis of the transferrin receptor (TfR1). TfR1 is essential for developing erythrocytes, and reduced TfR1 expression is associated with anemia. STAT5-null mice are severely anemic and die perinatally. Two studies associated STAT5 to iron homeostasis showing that ablation of STAT5 leads to a dramatic reduction in the iron regulatory protein 2 and *Tfr1* mRNA and protein.[60,61] Both genes were demonstrated to be direct transcriptional targets of STAT5, establishing a clear link between EPO-R–JAK2–STAT signaling and iron metabolism. Therefore, it is possible that activation of JAK2 might increase erythroid iron intake and that this might be detrimental in thalassemic cells, in which part of the iron ends up in toxic hemichromes (α-chain/heme aggregates), triggering ROS formation.

The persistent phosphorylation of JAK2 leads to an increased number of surviving erythroid precursors, contributing to the IE. Therefore, suppression of JAK2 activity may modulate IE. Based on this hypothesis, a JAK2 inhibitor was used for 10 days in mice affected by thalassemia intermedia (Hbbth3/+) and demonstrated a reduction in splenomegaly ("nonsurgical splenectomy").[54] This study also demonstrated that JAK2 inhibitors decreased the number of cells expressing cell cycle–related genes and partially reversed the IE, ameliorating the ratio between erythroid precursors and enucleated RBCs.[54,62] Thus, although a complete understanding of how JAK2 inhibitors achieve this effect is unavailable, modulation of cell cycle and differentiation are likely involved. Clinical trials of JAK2 inhibitors are currently underway in thalassemia major, and will add clarity to the role of JAK2 in this disease.

Hepcidin

The role of hepcidin in iron regulation is reviewed elsewhere (Chapters 35 and 36).

Several studies demonstrate that erythropoietic iron demand influences hepcidin expression to a greater degree than anemia or nonhematopoietic iron stores.[38,39] In particular, studies in β-thalassemia demonstrate that hepcidin expression is disproportionally low relative to the degree of iron overload.[40-42] These and previous studies proposed that an "erythroid factor" suppresses hepcidin synthesis.[63] Part of this regulation is related to erythroferrone, a hormone produced by erythroblasts in response to EPO and suppresses hepcidin. Mice that are deficient in erythroferrone fail to suppress hepcidin production during erythropoietic stress like experimental hemorrhage. Furthermore, thalassemia intermedia mice (Hbbth3/+) have high levels of erythroferrone expression that contributes to hepcidin suppression.[64]

Other factors are also important in hepcidin regulation. Twisted gastrulation-1 (TWSG1) has been isolated from immature erythroid precursors in β-thalassemic mice.[65] As a small secreted cysteine-rich protein able to influence bone morphogenetic proteins signaling, the expression of TWSG1 is increased in β-thalassemic mice and represses hepcidin in vitro.[65,66] However, whether this factor is present in other conditions and how efficiently TWSG1 represses hepcidin in physiologic conditions are still unclear. Growth differentiation factor-15 (GDF15) has been isolated from the sera of β-thalassemic patients and in other individuals exhibiting features of IE, such as myelodysplastic syndrome (MDS) and congenital dyserythropoietic anemia type I and II and an inverse correlation with hepcidin levels has been demonstrated.[67-69] GDF15 is a member of the transforming growth factor (TGFβ) superfamily of proteins, which are known to control cell proliferation, differentiation, and apoptosis in numerous cell types. However, it is possible that in conditions such as β-thalassemia, multiple "erythroid factors" suppress hepcidin expression.[70,71] The mechanisms of action of GDF15 and TWSG1 in repressing hepcidin expression remain undefined but are likely to alter the function of proteins that modulate hepcidin production.

The TGFβ superfamily of cytokines is important in RBC development. Activin also plays a role in erythropoiesis and red cell differentiation. Recent studies in mice suggest that using an activin receptor IIA ligand trap (sotatercept) may block activin, decreasing deleterious effects of GDF15, and limiting IE. This class of drugs may also improve bone mineral density in thalassemia patients. Clinical trials are currently under way.[72]

Mice affected by thalassemia intermedia (Hbbth3/+) avoid iron overload when placed on a low-iron diet or are engineered to overexpress a moderate level of hepcidin.[73] Reversal of iron overload results in reduced erythroid iron intake, limiting the synthesis of heme and the formation of hemichromes and ROS.[73] Because hemichromes and ROS cause IE in β-thalassemia, iron restriction and decreased erythroid iron intake result in more effective erythropoiesis, normalize RBC morphology and lifespan, increase circulating Hb, and reverse splenomegaly.[62,73] Thus, the use of hepcidin agonists or drugs that increase hepcidin expression, decreases iron uptake from the diet, reduces iron overload, and improves erythropoiesis in TI.[73] In TM, repeated blood transfusions are the principal cause of iron overload. Despite iron overload, hepcidin concentrations are low; transfusion also suppresses endogenous erythropoiesis and, as a consequence, results in a transient increase in hepcidin.[40,74,75] Although intestinal iron absorption contributes part of the total iron load in these patients, hepcidin therapy may be effective in conjunction with transfusion to prevent intestinal iron uptake when endogenous hepcidin falls.

Transferrin

TfR1 takes up iron from duodenal enterocytes where iron is absorbed and from macrophages when iron is recycled from senescent RBCs and delivers it to cells by binding TfR1. Tf saturation is the main player in determining the rate of erythroid iron intake, modulating erythropoiesis. In turn, erythropoiesis influences hepcidin expression in the liver. Therefore, reducing the saturation levels of Tf might have beneficial effects in β-thalassemia, decreasing formation of hemichromes in the RBCs as well as the florid erythropoiesis that suppresses hepcidin expression in the liver. In fact, chronic treatment with apo-Tf injections in *Hbbth1/th1* mice (another murine model of thalassemia intermedia) results in increased Hb production, decreased reticulocytosis and serum EPO levels, reverses splenomegaly, and elevates hepcidin expression.[76] Apo-Tf injections reduce hemichrome formation and change the proportion of erythroid precursors to more mature relative to immature precursors, lower the rates of apoptosis in mature erythroid precursors, and reduce the amount of extramedullary erythropoiesis in the liver and spleen in *Hbbth1/th1* mice. Theses injections also resulted in iron unloading in tissues, normalization of anemia, transferrin saturation, and suppression nontransferrin bound iron levels in plasma. The addition of exogenous apo-Tf results in decreased Tf saturation and likely a shift toward more monoferric-Tf molecules with more Tf molecules available to deliver smaller amounts of iron to more erythroid precursors, resulting in further decreased mean corpuscular hemoglobin (MCH) and fewer hemichromes. Apo-Tf injections also appear to alter erythroferrone expression, HAMP, plasma hepcidin, and ferroportin.[77] Future studies of apo-Tf will be important in understanding iron regulation in vivo.

Clinical Manifestations

Clinical Findings at Diagnosis

Protected by prenatal Hb F production, infants with β-thalassemia major are born free of significant anemia. Nevertheless, deficient β-chain synthesis can be demonstrated at birth. Clinical manifestations usually emerge during the second 6 months of life as the consequences of defective β-globin synthesis on overall Hb production become more pronounced. The diagnosis is almost always evident by 2 years of age.[78] Pallor, irritability, growth retardation, abdominal swelling caused by enlargement of the liver and spleen, and jaundice are the usual presenting features.[79] Facial and skeletal changes caused by BM expansion develop later.

Clinical Findings in Untreated or Undertreated Patients

Untreated patients die in late infancy or early childhood as a consequence of severe anemia. In a retrospective review from Italy, the average survival of children with untreated thalassemia major was less than 4 years; approximately 80% died in the first 5 years of life.[80] Patients who receive transfusions sporadically may live somewhat longer than untransfused patients, but their quality of life is extremely poor as a result of both the chronic anemia and the IE. The low Hb level and massive organomegaly are usually disabling, and the changes in the facial bones are disfiguring. After 10 to 20 years of weakness, stunted growth, and impaired activity, the undertransfused patients usually succumb to congestive heart failure.

This disastrous symptom constellation, so prevalent in the past, is now rare in North America and most industrialized countries. Nonetheless, the clinical manifestations and complications of untreated or undertreated β-thalassemia major illustrate the principles of the pathophysiology. Furthermore, these descriptions accurately characterize the disease that is still prevalent in many parts of the world.

Initial Laboratory Findings

The anemia of thalassemia major is characterized by severe hypochromia and microcytosis. The Hb level decreases progressively during

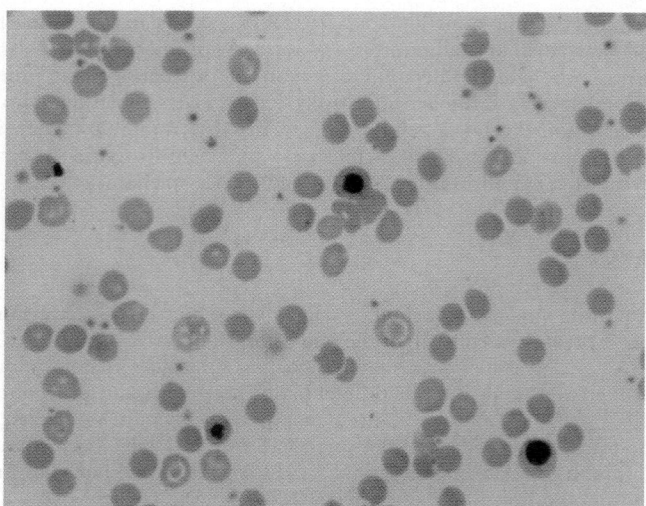

Fig. 40.6 MORPHOLOGIC APPEARANCE OF THE PERIPHERAL BLOOD FILM IN A CASE OF SEVERE β-THALASSEMIA. Note the bizarre cells, the hypochromia, nucleated red blood cells, target cells, and polychromasia.

the first months of life. When the child becomes symptomatic, the Hb level may be as low as 3–4 g/dL. RBC morphology is strikingly abnormal, with many microcytes, bizarre poikilocytes, teardrop cells, and target cells (Fig. 40.6). A characteristic finding is the presence of extraordinarily hypochromic, often wrinkled and folded cells (leptocytes) containing irregular inclusion bodies of precipitated α-globin chains.

Clinical Heterogeneity of Thalassemia

The severity of β-thalassemia is remarkable for its variability in different patients. Two siblings inheriting identical thalassemia mutations sometimes exhibit markedly different degrees of anemia and erythroid hyperplasia. Many factors contribute to this clinical heterogeneity. Individual alleles vary with respect to severity of the biosynthetic lesion. Other modifying factors ameliorate the burden of unpaired α-globin. High levels of Hb F expression persist to widely various degrees in β-thalassemia. Because γ-globin can substitute for β-globin, simultaneously generating more functional Hbs and reducing the α-globin inclusion burden, this is a powerful modulating factor. Theoretically, patients may also vary in their ability to solubilize unpaired globin chains by proteolysis. Occasional heterozygous patients have had more severe anemia than expected, possibly because of defects in these proteolytic systems or because of the type of thalassemic mutation. Inheritance of more than the usual complement of *α-globin* genes may also increase with severity of β-thalassemia because of additional production of unpaired α-globin chains. All of these factors emphasize the essential role of α-globin inclusions in the pathophysiology of β-thalassemia.

Nucleated RBCs are frequently present in peripheral circulation. The reticulocyte count is 2% to 8% lower than would be expected in view of the extreme erythroid hyperplasia and hemolysis. The low count reflects the severity of intramedullary erythroblast destruction. The white blood cell count is elevated. A moderate polymorphonuclear leukocytosis and normal platelet count are typical unless hypersplenism has developed. The BM exhibits marked hypercellularity caused by erythroid hyperplasia. The RBC precursors show defective hemoglobinization and reduced amounts of cytoplasm.

The osmotic fragility is strikingly abnormal. The RBCs are so markedly resistant to hemolysis in hypotonic sodium chloride solution that some are not entirely hemolyzed even in distilled water. Before transfusion therapy is initiated, the serum iron and transferrin saturation are already increased as a result of increased iron absorption.[81]

The Hb profile reveals predominantly Hb F. In patients with homozygous β°-thalassemia, no Hb A is found throughout life. Hb A may be undetectable in the newborn with β+-thalassemia and is present in reduced amounts in later life. The levels of Hb A_2 in thalassemia major are variable, probably because of increased numbers of F cells that have a decreased Hb A_2 content.[1] Other biochemical abnormalities of the RBC in cases of thalassemia major include a postnatal persistence of the i antigen and a decrease of RBC carbonic anhydrase; these findings are probably also caused by the elevated levels of circulating F cells.

The intraerythrocytic inclusions in the peripheral blood cells of patients with thalassemia, first described by Fessas,[82] are especially prominent after splenectomy. These inclusions, best seen by staining with supravital staining (Brilliant Cresyl Blue) or by phase microscopy, are aggregates of precipitated, denatured α-chains.[83] They are also found in large numbers within erythroid precursors in the BM.

The patient is icteric; unconjugated bilirubin levels are in the range of 2.0–4.0 mg/dL at the time of diagnosis but may rise substantially as the anemia worsens in the absence of transfusion. RBC survival in cases of thalassemia major is variable but usually markedly decreased. The ^{53}Cr half-life ranges between 6.5 and 19.5 days compared with the normal half-life of 25–35 days.[36] Increased plasma iron turnover and poor use of radiolabeled iron indicate IE.[36] Serum aspartate aminotransferase levels are frequently increased at diagnosis because of hemolysis. Alanine aminotransferase levels are usually normal before transfusion therapy but may rise subsequently because of iron-induced hepatic damage or viral hepatitis. Lactate dehydrogenase levels are markedly elevated as a consequence of IE. Haptoglobin and hemopexin are reduced or absent.[84]

Later Laboratory Findings

Serum zinc levels may fall to abnormally low levels. A relationship between this finding and growth failure has been postulated but not established.[85,86] Low levels of plasma and leukocyte ascorbic acid are common in thalassemic patients because of increased metabolism of the vitamin to oxalic acid in the presence of iron overload.[87,88] Biochemical evidence of folic acid deficiency may occur as a result of excessive consumption secondary to increased requirements.[89,90] The serum levels of α-tocopherol are often reduced to less than 0.5 mg/dL, and increased RBC membrane lipid peroxidation has been described.[91–93]

Coagulation abnormalities consistent with liver disease (i.e., lowered levels of factors II, V, VII, IX, and X) may occur in older patients with hepatitis or iron-induced hepatic injury.[94] Only rarely are the abnormalities sufficient to require specific therapy. However, the combination of mild thrombocytopenia from hypersplenism and low coagulation factors and platelet dysfunction from liver disease may cause or aggravate bleeding.[95]

Numerous laboratory abnormalities reflect the accumulation of excessive iron and the consequences of iron-induced organ damage, and they are described in the following sections.

Treatment

The advent of modern therapy has had a major impact on the clinical and laboratory features of thalassemia major. Transfusion and chelation therapy, described subsequently in detail, have ameliorated many of the most striking manifestations of the disease. Bone marrow transplantation (BMT) has allowed for the cure in some patients. However, these therapies have created their own complications; therefore, this section addresses the treatment of the complications of thalassemia and its therapy. Current clinical management and associated clinical manifestations and complications have been reviewed in a number of publications.[96–101]

Transfusion Therapy

Transfusion therapy for thalassemia was once sparingly administered as a palliative measure when patients became symptomatic. These periodic transfusion regimens were unsatisfactory even for those limited purposes; symptoms of anemia and the cosmetic and other consequences of overgrowth of erythropoietic tissue rendered life unpleasant and uncomfortable for patients. Consequently, several centers initiated transfusion programs in which patients received regular transfusions to keep their Hb levels high enough to ameliorate these symptoms,[102,103] but the median survival time of patients transfused to maintain Hb levels of 7–8 g/dL in the United States in the 1960s was only 17 years of age.[103,104] So called "hypertransfusion" programs were designed initially to maintain Hb levels above 8 g/dL. In the more modern application of hypertransfusion therapy, Hb levels are usually maintained above 9–10.5 g/dL.

The clinical benefits of hypertransfusion programs are dramatic. The growth of younger children follows normal percentiles for height and weight.[105] Erythropoiesis is significantly suppressed as evidenced by decreased numbers of reticulocytes and normoblasts and TfR1 levels.[106,107] Hypertransfusion reduces or prevents the enlargement of the liver and spleen. Abnormal facies and bone fractures occur less frequently. The overall sense of well-being allows normal age-appropriate activities[108,109] (see box on Guidelines for Transfusion Therapy).

A more vigorous transfusion program (supertransfusion) aimed at keeping Hb levels above 12.0 g/dL is no longer recommended.[110] This approach rested on the assumption that the benefits of further suppression of erythropoiesis and gastrointestinal iron absorption will offset the increased need for RBCs. However, several studies have demonstrated that transfusion requirements (and therefore the rates of transfusional iron loading) increase as the Hb level is raised in both splenectomized and nonsplenectomized patients (Fig. 40.7).[105,111,112] As a result, the consistent maintenance of Hb levels above 11 or 12 g/dL results in excessive iron accumulation without proportional clinical benefit, and supertransfusion protocols should be reserved for patients with poor tolerance of lower Hb levels because of cardiac disease or other reasons.

Alternative approaches to conventional transfusion therapy have been proposed to reduce the rate of transfusion iron loading. These approaches have generally relied on the concept that younger RBCs (neocytes) will circulate longer in the recipient than older RBCs. Preclinical experiments based on the difference in density between younger and older RBCs established the validity of this approach.[113,114] However, in prospective clinical trials, blood requirements were reduced only by 13% to 20%.[115–117] This reduction in iron loading did not outweigh the disadvantages of neocyte transfusions that included increased cost, wastage of 50% of the donor RBCs, and increased donor exposures. The use of automated exchange transfusion has been proposed as another approach to reducing iron loading in patients with thalassemia.[118] With this method, RBCs are removed from the patient at the

---

Guidelines for Transfusion Therapy

Although some of the details of a transfusion program for patients with thalassemia major vary from center to center, the following guidelines are important for achieving the benefits while controlling the risks of a transfusion program. The rationales for these guidelines are discussed in the text.

1. Obtain a complete RBC antigen profile before the first transfusion.
2. Administer 10–15 mL/kg of RBCs every 2–4 weeks to maintain the pretransfusion hemoglobin level above 9–10.5 g/dL.
3. Use packed leukoreduced RBCs that have been stored for less than 7–10 days.
4. Avoid the use of first-degree relatives as blood donors.
5. For patients who come to a new center after receiving transfusions elsewhere, contact the previous blood bank for information about alloantibodies and transfusion reactions.

RBC, red blood cell.

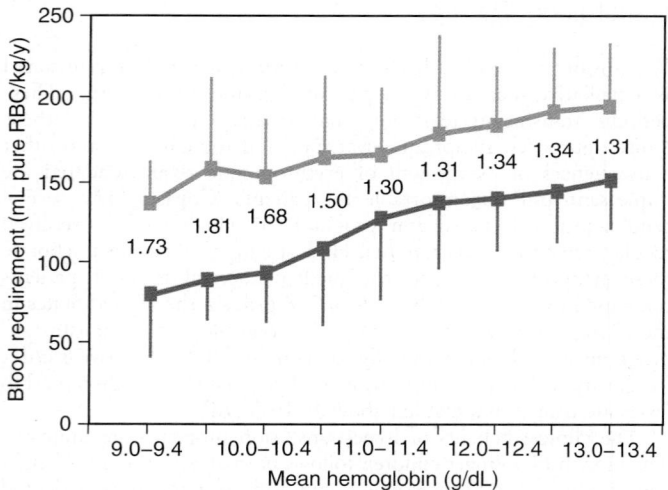

Fig. 40.7 Relationship between transfusion requirements and mean hemoglobin level maintained by patients with thalassemia major. *Blue* = splenectomized patients, *yellow* = nonsplenectomized patients. *RBC,* Red blood cell. *(Adapted from Rebulla P, Modell B: Transfusion requirements and effects in patients with thalassemia major.* Lancet *337:277, 1991.)*

The decision to initiate regular RBC transfusions is one of the most important—and sometimes most difficult—steps in the management of patients with thalassemia. Regular RBC transfusions not only distinguish thalassemia major from thalassemia intermedia but also commit the patient to long-term chelation therapy to control the transfusional iron loading. The decision should include consideration of both clinical and laboratory findings. Children who are growing poorly and developing disfiguring bone changes will benefit from regular transfusions even if their hemoglobin levels are 8–9 g/dL. On the other hand, children who are asymptomatic at hemoglobin levels of 7–8 g/dL may have little to gain from transfusions. Hemoglobin levels below 7 g/dL are usually associated with problems related to both the anemia and the compensatory erythropoiesis. When the hemoglobin level is consistently less than 7 g/dL, there is usually little to be gained from delaying transfusion.

Before the first blood transfusion is given to a child with thalassemia major, a complete RBC antigen profile should be obtained. This information is valuable for identifying minor blood group incompatibility if alloimmunization develops later and helps to distinguish alloantibodies from autoantibodies. The value of extended matching of donor RBCs has not been established in cases of thalassemia, but experience with sickle cell disease suggests that matching for the full Rh system as well as the Kell antigen may reduce the rate of alloimmunization.

In practice, the goal of maintaining the hemoglobin level above 9–10.5 g/dL is usually achieved by administration of approximately 15 mL/kg/mo or 1 to 2 units of donor RBCs every 2 to 5 weeks. Patients with heart disease may need smaller aliquots of RBCs at more frequent intervals to prevent problems related to volume overload. In general, patients can receive the entire unit of donor packed RBCs. However, fractional units are appropriate for infants, small patients, and older patients with heart disease. With the use of current additive solutions, the duration of storage of donor RBCs has only a small effect on the 24-hour recovery and the survival of the RBCs in each transfused unit. However, for patients with thalassemia major who undergo transfusion every 2 to 5 weeks, these small differences may have a significant impact on the annual consumption of blood. Consequently, the use of donor RBCs that have been stored for less than 7 to 10 days strikes a reasonable balance between the potential reduction in transfusion iron loading and the efficient use of the blood bank inventory. The use of volunteer blood donors remains the standard for patients with thalassemia. Although some families of children with thalassemia prefer directed donations, this approach has not reduced the rate of transfusion-transmitted infections among blood recipients in general and has not been shown to reduce the rate of alloimmunization in thalassemia. If directed donations are used, close relatives should be avoided because stem cell transplantation may be a later therapeutic option.

RBC, red blood cell.

same time that new donor RBCs are transfused. This approach has been applied successfully to transfusion therapy for sickle cell disease. However, the goal of transfusion therapy in sickle cell disease is the replacement of Hb S–containing RBCs with Hb A–containing RBCs irrespective of the total Hb level. In contrast, the goal of transfusion therapy in patients with thalassemia is to maintain a specific total Hb level. Despite these different goals, studies of automated exchange transfusion in patients with thalassemia have demonstrated a reduction in net RBC requirements of 30% to 50%, either by reducing the amount of blood administered at the usual transfusion interval or by prolonging the interval between transfusions.[118,119] The benefits of this approach are probably attributable to the removal of previously transfused RBCs from the patients and replacement with younger, recently donated RBCs, reducing the overall age of the circulating RBC population. Further clinical trials of automated exchange transfusion in thalassemia are currently underway.

The decision to initiate transfusion therapy should take into account the overall clinical condition of the patient as well as the Hb level. Patients with severe and persistent anemia (Hb <6–7 g/dL) usually also have failure to thrive, decreased activity level, and irritability. For these patients, transfusion therapy should begin after confirmation of the diagnosis of thalassemia and after demonstration that acute factors such as a febrile illness or folic acid deficiency are not confounding the assessment of the severity of anemia. For patients with higher Hb levels, the decision to begin transfusion depends on the careful assessment of the child's clinical findings. For example, some children with thalassemia have early and pronounced facial bone deformities caused by BM expansion despite a Hb level of 8 g/dL or higher. For such children, the benefits of transfusion therapy may outweigh the risks. In contrast, some patients with thalassemia have little or no clinical difficulty despite a persistent Hb level of 7–8 g/dL, and the benefits of transfusion therapy may be small. Determination of genotype may provide some guidance by distinguishing patients with more severe defects in β-globin production from those with less severe defects, but the overlap between genotype and phenotype in thalassemia still requires reliance on clinical assessment (see box on Deciding to Begin Transfusion Therapy in Patients With Thalassemia).

Chelation Therapy

Each unit of packed RBCs contains approximately 200–250 mg of iron. Based on usual blood requirements in patients with thalassemia

major, the rate of transfusional iron accumulation is approximately 0.30–0.60 mg/kg/d. The massive IE associated with the intermedia and major thalassemias leads to excessive gastrointestinal iron absorption that adds to the transfusional iron burden, although absorption is reduced when a Hb level above 9 g/dL is maintained.[120,121] Humans have no physiologic mechanism to induce significant excretion of excess iron. Phlebotomy, the most efficient method of removing iron in other situations, is precluded in severely anemic patients with thalassemia owing to transfusion dependence.

A pharmacologic approach using specific iron-chelating agents remains the only strategy for removing excess iron in transfusion-dependent patients. Several drugs with chelating properties have been synthesized or recovered from microorganisms. Many lack iron specificity or are inefficient; others cause significant toxicity. To chelate iron, the chelating agent must complex with all of the iron atom's six available coordination sites. Three general classes of iron chelators occur or have been synthesized: hexadentate (deferoxamine), bidentate (deferiprone), and tridentate (deferasirox). Only one hexadentate molecule is necessary to bind one atom of iron, but three molecules of a bidentate iron chelator bind one iron atom and two molecules of a tridentate chelator are required to bind one atom of iron. Chelatable iron is thought to be derived from the intracellular "labile iron pool"[122,123] and from nontransferrin-bound plasma iron.[124,125]

Assessment of Iron Stores

Because excess transfusional iron cannot be actively excreted, it is deposited in the macrophages of the reticuloendothelial system (RES). When the RES is overwhelmed, iron spills over into parenchymal tissue, generating free radical damage with cellular membrane lipid peroxidation and leading to end-organ dysfunction, especially of the liver, endocrine system, and myocardium.

Chelation therapy is initiated after approximately 10 to 25 units of blood have been transfused, serum ferritin levels are above 1000 mg/mL, and liver iron concentration (LIC) is greater than 3 mg Fe/g dry weight.

Measurement of LIC by biopsy provides a direct assessment of tissue iron loading and reflects total body iron stores but liver biopsy requires a skilled technician, at least 1 mg of tissue at least 2.5 cm in length with five portal tracts, and has the risk of hemorrhage and sampling error. The use of magnetic resonance imaging (MRI) to estimate hepatic and cardiac iron in patients with transfusional siderosis has largely replaced liver biopsy for LIC quantification. MRI with proton transverse relaxation rates (R2) with spin-echo imaging, signal intensity ratios, and gradient-echo T2* is currently the preferred method to assess LIC.[126-130] Direct comparisons with hepatic tissue samples demonstrate significant correlations ($r = 0.97$) with biopsy-measured LICs.[127,129-133]. Values between 3 and 7 mg Fe/g dry weight appear to be associated with minimal toxicity, while LIC levels greater than 15 mg Fe/g dry weight are associated with a greater risk of iron-induced heart disease.[134] Experience with cardiac MRI suggests that changes in T2* reflect levels of iron in the heart and may predict adverse changes in cardiac function. Cardiac T2* values are predictive of arrhythmias and cardiac value over 1 year.[135] Cardiac MRI T2*-directed treatment results in improved chelation and iron stores.[136] MRI assessment of iron overload cannot be used in patients with pacemakers or those who are claustrophobic. Future MRI use may involve the quantification of iron concentration of endocrine glands to predict or monitor dysfunction.[137-139]

Measurements of LIC by magnetic susceptometry using a superconducting quantum interference device (SQUID) also correlate well with biochemical measurements of tissue iron.[140,141] At present, measurement of tissue iron by SQUID is limited to the liver, and the instruments are available in only a few sites in the United States of America and Europe. Importantly, the SQUID is not an enclosed space, so claustrophobia is not an issue.

Serum ferritin levels are safe, inexpensive, and readily available, and serial measurements are predictive both of critical complications such as iron-induced heart disease and of adverse effects of chelation therapy such as impairment of vision and hearing. However, single ferritin levels may correlate poorly with LIC because it is an acute phase reactant and may be influenced by inflammation, vitamin C deficiency, hepatitis, and other infectious states. Transferrin saturation is not very useful in evaluating the severity of iron overload in patients with thalassemia because the massive IE usually results in a transferrin saturation greater than 60% even in the absence of iron overload.[142]

Deferoxamine

Deferoxamine mesylate is a naturally occurring hexadentate siderophore isolated from cultures of *Streptomyces pilosus* introduced in 1960. Deferoxamine has a high molecular weight of approximately 600 g/mol, is poorly absorbed by the gastrointestinal tract, and is rapidly removed from the plasma. It has a relatively short half-life of 8 to 10 minutes, which necessitates intravenous or subcutaneous administration. It is highly specific for iron and is associated with relatively low toxicity.[143] Deferoxamine enters cells, chelates iron, and appears in the serum and bile as the iron chelate product, ferroxamine.[144] Deferoxamine chelates iron released by the RES after the catabolism of senescent RBCs and is excreted in the urine.[145] Unbound deferoxamine is absorbed by the hepatic parenchymal cells and chelates iron from the intracellular pool which is excreted in bile. Approximately one-half to two-thirds of the iron excreted in response to deferoxamine is in the stool, with the remainder in the urine.[146] These proportions vary from patient to patient and at different levels of iron overload, dose of deferoxamine, and endogenous erythropoietic activity.[147]

Iron excretion after the administration of deferoxamine is proportional to body iron stores. To achieve negative iron balance, the chelating agent must cause the daily excretion of 0.3–0.6 mg/kg of iron. In the 1960s, deferoxamine was initially administered by daily intramuscular injections of 0.5 g, which led to reduced rates of hepatic iron accumulation and hepatic fibrosis in patients with thalassemia.[148,149] However, intramuscular injections proved to be too painful and were insufficient to achieve negative iron balance. In the mid-1970s, it was demonstrated that iron excretion with deferoxamine at 20–60 mg/kg/d was markedly enhanced and negative iron balance was attained by continuous, prolonged 24-hour intravenous or 8- to 12-hour subcutaneous infusions administered via a lightweight battery-operated or balloon-driven pump.[150,151] In addition, maintaining normal ascorbic acid levels optimizes iron excretion because it increases tissue iron turnover in the plasma.

A pump infuses an aqueous solution of deferoxamine through a small 27-gauge butterfly needle placed under the skin of the abdomen, thigh, or extremities. Most patients use the pump during sleep.[152] Bolus subcutaneous injections of deferoxamine used twice daily induce levels of urinary iron excretion comparable with subcutaneous infusions and may prove helpful as a respite from overnight infusions in some patients not adherent to prolonged infusions.[153,154] In patients who are poorly compliant with subcutaneous therapy, administration of deferoxamine in normal or higher doses can be accomplished intravenously by means of a deep line indwelling catheter, externalized venous catheter, or subcutaneous port. Continuous intravenous administration of deferoxamine is particularly useful for rapidly lowering the total iron burden and is used for reversal of cardiac morbidity (e.g., cardiac arrhythmias or left ventricular dysfunction). Complications of indwelling catheters, including infection and thrombosis rates, have been reported at 1.2 and 0.5 per 1000 catheter days, respectively, in patients treated over 1 to 5 years.

The optimal age for beginning parenteral or oral iron chelation therapy in patients with thalassemia has not been established with certainty. The surprisingly high LICs that have been found in some patients with thalassemia within the first 2 to 3 years of transfusion therapy, occasionally accompanied by histologic finding of fibrosis, provided the rationale for the early initiation of deferoxamine iron chelation.[155,156] Regular deferoxamine chelation therapy begun after the age of 3 to 5 years seems capable of removing previously stored iron and preventing iron-induced liver disease.[104] Data show that deferoxamine started by the age of 2 to 4 years forestalls significant iron overload; however, it also promotes elimination of excess iron in patients if started after significant transfusional iron burden has already developed.[134,157-166] Moreover, deferoxamine may adversely affect bone development and growth in some young patients and the effect of newer oral chelators on growth has yet to be addressed.[167-169] The most common side effect of subcutaneous deferoxamine therapy is inflammation and induration at the site of infusion. Painful lumps may occur despite rotation of infusion sites, appropriate dilution of the drug, and proper placement of the needle. Some investigators have recommended the addition of small amounts of hydrocortisone to the infusion to prevent local reactions. Patients receiving aggressive chelation therapy with lower iron burdens may be more susceptible to toxicity. Neurosensory toxicity of deferoxamine is dose related and inversely correlated with body iron burden. Impairments of visual and auditory acuity are associated with high doses of deferoxamine relative to the iron load.[170] The ototoxicity is characterized by bilateral high-frequency hearing loss. The retinal toxicity is characterized by the loss of night and color vision, retinal atrophy, and cataract formation.[171] Patients receiving deferoxamine should undergo baseline and annual audiograms and ophthalmologic examinations. Deferoxamine should be discontinued if such abnormalities arise, with cautious reinitiation at lower doses when abnormalities improve or resolve. The risk of visual and auditory side effects can be minimized by adjusting the daily deferoxamine dose to the patients' serum ferritin level.[170] Impaired growth associated with growth plate deformities or metaphyseal rickets-like changes in the long bones and histologic evidence of cartilage dysplasia may occur in young children receiving deferoxamine.[167-169] Regular monitoring with plain radiographs of the extremities and vertebral column allows early detection of this complication and reduction in the dose of deferoxamine or temporary interruption of chelation therapy.

Other, less common complications of deferoxamine include anaphylaxis, hypotension, allergic reactions, acute pulmonary disease, impairment of renal function, and infection.[172-178] Severe allergic reactions are rare, and desensitization has been achieved successfully in some patients.[174,175] Acute pulmonary disease and renal failure have occurred in a few patients receiving unusually high doses of deferoxamine by intravenous infusion.[176] The mechanism of this toxicity is unclear. One of the most serious complications of deferoxamine is an increased risk of infection with *Yersinia* and mucormycosis, which uses the deferoxamine iron chelate as a siderophore. Deferoxamine can enhance the growth and virulence of these organisms, leading to colitis, abdominal abscesses, or sepsis.[177,178] The safety of deferoxamine during pregnancy has been inferred from case reports rather than formal studies. A summary of these case reports identified 11 women who received deferoxamine beginning in the first trimester and 33 women who used the chelator beginning in the second or third trimester.[178] None of the infants showed evidence of drug-related toxicity.[179]

Regular chelation with deferoxamine has proven remarkably effective in reducing the transfusional iron burden of thalassemia patients. Increasing evidence indicates that endocrine dysfunction is improved and cardiac disease is delayed or prevented with standard deferoxamine regimens.[180] Cardiac arrhythmias and congestive heart failure have reversed in some patients with standard or aggressive deferoxamine regimens, and life expectancy is significantly prolonged.[181-183] Intense 24-hour intravenous deferoxamine regimens of no more than 15 mg/kg/h have been reported to reverse early cardiac hemosiderosis, but even more conventional doses of 50 mg/kg/d have improved left ventricular ejection fractions and prevented death in some patients.[184,185]

Before subcutaneous deferoxamine therapy, estimated survival was approximately 16 to 17 years of age, with rare patients surviving into their mid-20s.[104,182,186,187] Since regular subcutaneous deferoxamine regimens have been in use, life expectancy has extended into the fourth decade of life.[188-190] The increasing widespread use of deferoxamine has steadily increased survival probabilities worldwide.[189,190] However, long-term European studies have demonstrated that improved survival times are clearly related to the degree of compliance with chelation regimens and are associated with lower serum ferritin levels (<1000 mg/mL).[191] Deferoxamine chelation regimens are clearly cumbersome, inconvenient, and costly. More tolerable approaches are required, and investigations for alternative oral iron-chelating agents have been ongoing and recently more successful.

Although the prevalence of endocrine disturbances, for example, glucose intolerance and diabetes have reduced since the regular use of subcutaneous deferoxamine,[97,100,180] they persist, especially in those in whom deferoxamine was initiated late in their first decade of life.[161] Growth hormone deficiency, hypothyroidism, hypoparathyroidism, vitamin D deficiency, diabetes, and osteoporosis are still observed, and there is little evidence that deferoxamine can reverse established endocrine dysfunctions. The North American Thalassemia Clinical Research Network Registry reported that 96% of thalassemia patients with a median age of 20 years were free of hypoparathyroidism, 91% were free of thyroid disease, 90% were free of diabetes mellitus, and overall 62% were free of any endocrinopathy.[192]

It remains to be determined if starting chelation at a very young age or more easily administered use of oral iron chelation will diminish the endocrine morbidities and further prolong survival associated with iron overload. Direct and indirect measures of iron stores reflect the progress of chelation therapy and help determine appropriate changes in the dose or frequency of chelator use. The serum ferritin level generally declines during regular chelation therapy and may decline rapidly in the first year of treatment in patients with very large iron stores.[193,194] Serum ferritin levels measured over time with use of deferoxamine have predicted the risk of iron-induced heart disease in patients with thalassemia major, and the ratio of the dose of deferoxamine to the ferritin level has identified patients at risk for auditory and visual complications of chelation therapy.[170,183] Although easy to obtain and relatively inexpensive, the serum ferritin level may be increased in the presence of inflammation and may be decreased when iron overload is accompanied by vitamin C deficiency.[195] For these and other reasons, serum ferritin levels frequently correlate poorly with LICs, and clinicians and patients may have a false sense of security when the ferritin level is below 2000 mcg/L. Some studies using deferoxamine suggest ferritin levels lower than 1000 mcg/L are associated with better survival times and less cardiac disease as well as hepatic histology and pathology.[191,196,197]

A relationship between iron overload and ascorbic acid depletion, first suggested by the epidemiology of scurvy among the Bantu, exists in thalassemia major.[87,195] For thalassemia patients with low levels of ascorbic acid, daily supplementation with 100–200 mg of this vitamin increases urinary iron excretion in response to deferoxamine by approximately twofold.[88,198] Ascorbic acid may retard the conversion of ferritin to hemosiderin and therefore allow more iron to remain in the chelatable form.[199,200] However, it can also enhance iron-mediated peroxidation of membrane lipids[201,202] as well as membrane damage in cultured myocardial cells.[203] Cardiac toxicity manifested as arrhythmias and decreased ventricular contractility has been attributed to vitamin C therapy.[204] Ascorbic acid should be used only while deferoxamine is being administered and only in patients who are ascorbate depleted.

Chelation therapy with deferoxamine is expensive and cumbersome because of the need for daily or nightly subcutaneous infusions. Regular infusions require a great deal of dedication and persistence from the patient and family. Noncompliance is common, particularly in the teenage and young adult years, and failure to follow prescribed treatment regimens is the major cause of mortality in patients with thalassemia major.[191] The cost and complexity of deferoxamine administration prevents its availability worldwide, especially in developing countries. The search for a less expensive iron chelator that can be more easily orally administered led to the identification of compounds such as deferiprone and deferasirox.

Deferiprone

One such oral agent is 1,2-dimethyl-3-hydroxypyrid-4-one (L1, deferiprone), a synthetic compound with a low molecular weight of approximately 200 g/mol. It is an orally active bidentate iron chelator that requires three molecules to bind one iron atom. Deferiprone is absorbed by the gastrointestinal tract and has a plasma half-life of approximately 90 minutes (2–3 hours). Chelated iron is excreted predominantly in the urine (90%) and far less in the stool (10%). It was synthesized in the late 1980s and was first tested in uncontrolled clinical trials at the Royal Free Hospital in London, hence the eponym L1.[205,206] A large observational study demonstrated improvement in cardiac iron deposition with deferiprone treatment.[207] At doses of 75 mg/kg/d, deferiprone administered in three divided doses with meals reduces or maintains iron stores, thereby achieving negative iron balance or iron balance in many regularly transfused patients for the most part, particularly those with more severe transfusional iron overload.[208–216] However, some patients remain in positive iron balance and continue to accumulate iron during long-term therapy with this dose of deferiprone.[209,212,217] Regimens using higher doses up to 100 mg/kg/d of deferiprone may be more effective.[218] Combination regimens with deferoxamine also reduce iron stores or prove effective in restoring negative iron balance in some of these patients.[219–221] Enhanced urine and stool iron excretion in thalassemia patients using both deferoxamine and deferiprone have suggested an additive effect postulated by the shuttle hypothesis, that is, deferiprone may chelate intracellular labile iron and shuttle it to deferoxamine.[222] Some studies have also suggested that deferiprone alone or in combination with deferoxamine may be more effective than deferoxamine in removing iron from the heart, improving cardiac function, and preventing iron-induced cardiac disease.[133,216,223–226] Schedules for combination therapy vary but have usually included 5 to 7 days of deferiprone and 2 days of subcutaneous deferoxamine weekly. Intensive combined chelation therapy has been reported to reverse both cardiac and endocrine complications of thalassemia major.[227]

Agranulocytosis occurs in 1% of patients and, although rare, remains the principal concern for patients receiving deferiprone. Milder neutropenia (absolute neutrophil count <1500 but >500) is more common and occurs in approximately 6% to 8% of patients. Severely depressed neutrophil counts represent a significant risk of sepsis and hospitalizations, and in some cases, administration of granulocyte colony-stimulating factor is required. Some reported deaths have been related to deferiprone-induced agranulocytosis or neutropenia. Regular weekly monitoring of blood counts during deferiprone therapy is recommended to detect the rare but important deferiprone-induced complications of neutropenia and agranulocytosis.[212–214,228] In cases where mild neutropenia develops, it may be safe to continue deferiprone therapy with more frequent monitoring of blood counts and clinical symptoms.[229]

Other side effects of deferiprone include gastrointestinal complaints, mostly nausea and some vomiting that occur in approximately 33% of patients and usually resolve without specific intervention. Arthropathy with arthralgias and some joint effusions occur in approximately 15% of patients. The incidence of joint symptoms varies widely among various studies but may be severe enough to require reduction or interruption of chelation therapy. Abnormal liver function tests may occur gradually or suddenly and in the absence of other causes of hepatic dysfunction. These elevations may return to baseline values with the interruption of deferiprone followed by reinitiation beginning with lower doses and close monitoring of liver function tests. Progressive liver disease attributed to deferiprone has not been reported, and concerns about drug-induced hepatic fibrosis have not been substantiated by subsequent studies.[209,211,230,231] However, in vitro evidence shows that deferiprone may potentiate oxidative deoxyribonucleic acid (DNA) damage in iron-loaded liver cells that could occur when the concentration of iron is low relative to the iron chelator (Fig. 40.8).[232] A prospective randomized study comparing the combination of deferiprone at 75 mg/kg/d and deferoxamine at 40–50 mg/kg/d with deferoxamine alone demonstrated that the combination therapy more rapidly reduced hepatic and cardiac iron stores than deferoxamine alone.[233] Further prospective studies are warranted, especially with the combination of deferiprone with deferoxamine. Deferiprone may play a role in shuttling iron

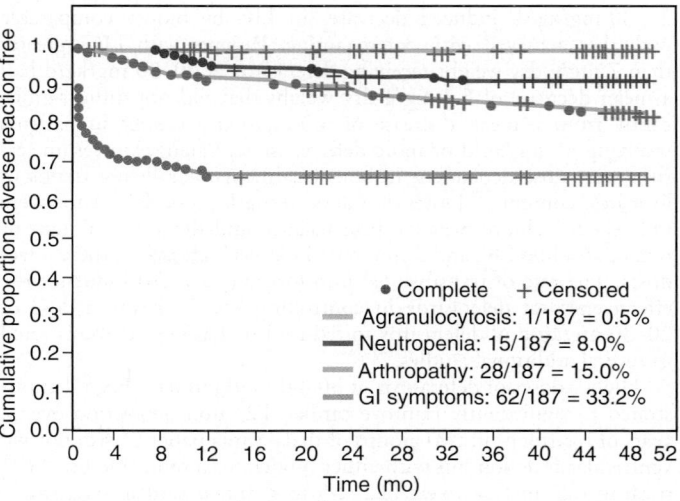

Fig. 40.8 KAPLAN-MEIER CURVES SHOWING THE TIME TO FIRST OCCURRENCE OF IMPORTANT ADVERSE EVENTS IN PATIENTS TREATED WITH DEFERIPRONE. The only case of agranulocytosis occurred in the first year, and gastrointestinal complaints were very uncommon after the first year. Neutropenia and joint problems occurred throughout the 4-year study period but were more common in the first year than in each of the subsequent years. *GI:* gastrointestinal. (*Adapted from Cohen AR, Galanello R, Piga A, et al: Safety and effectiveness of long-term therapy with the oral iron chelator deferiprone.* Blood *102:1583, 2003.*)

from within intracellular pools and enhance the available iron pool to bind with deferoxamine.[211,234–236] Deferiprone continues to be tested in clinical trials alone and in combination with deferoxamine to address its impact on cardiac function.[226] The safety profile of deferiprone has been largely defined by single-center studies, multicenter trials, and postmarketing surveillance largely in European and Asian continents. Deferiprone is currently licensed in both Europe and the United States of America as of 2011 as alternative iron chelation therapy for those who are unable to be successfully treated with other therapies. A liquid formulation of deferiprone is also available, and is particularly advantageous in pediatric patients.

Deferasirox

Deferasirox (ICL670, ExJade) is an orally active iron chelator that was identified by computer technology at Novartis Pharmaceuticals in the 1990s. It is a tridentate compound known as 4-(3,5-bis[2-hydroxyphenyl]-1H-1,2,4-triazol-1-yl)-benzoic acid,[237] wherein two molecules of deferasirox are required to bind one atom of iron. It has a high affinity for iron and a much lower affinity for copper and zinc. Deferasirox is orally bioavailable with a low molecular weight of 373 g/mol and is absorbed by the gastrointestinal tract. It has a dose-dependent plasma half-life of 12 to 18 hours that allows for once-daily oral administration after fasting on an empty stomach.[238] Deferasirox is given as a suspension in water or apple or orange juice.[239] Iron excretion in response to deferasirox is largely in the stool (90%) and far less in the urine (10%).[239] The pharmacodynamic effects of deferasirox tested in a phase I clinical iron balance metabolic study measuring stool and urine iron excretion demonstrated increasing iron excretion at doses of 10, 20, and 40 mg/kg/d, which induced a mean net iron excretion (0.119, 0.329, and 0.445 mg Fe/kg/d, respectively) within the clinically relevant range of the rate of transfusion iron loading for most patients.

The phase III worldwide multicenter open-label randomized active comparator control study of deferasirox compared with deferoxamine was conducted in 65 sites with 586 regularly transfused patients 2 years or more of age with β-thalassemia. Results indicated that chronic daily use of deferasirox, via a single oral dose of

20–30 mg/kg/d, induced decreases in LIC by biopsy comparable with that achieved with deferoxamine. Patients with LICs greater than 7 mg/g dry weight receiving deferasirox at 20–30 mg/kg/d had a mean decrease of 5.3 mg/g dry weight that did not differ significantly from a mean decrease of 4.3 mg/g dry weight in patients receiving 35 mg/kg/d or more deferoxamine. Changes in serum ferritin were dose dependent in both treatments, paralleling trends in liver iron content.[240] Doses of 5 and 10 mg/kg/d of deferasirox were unlikely to achieve negative iron balance and did not maintain or reduce absolute LIC and serum ferritin levels increased at these lower doses. The rate of transfusional iron loading may also influence the effectiveness of deferasirox in controlling LIC.[241] Using a dose of 20–30 mg/kg/d of deferasirox to reduce LIC has been demonstrated in several additional studies.[241–243]

Higher doses of deferasirox at 30–50 mg/kg/d have been demonstrated to significantly improve cardiac T2* iron deposition over 2 years of treatment in two groups of thalassemia patients with normal ventricular function but with either moderate to mild siderosis (T2* = 10 to <20 ms) or severe (T2* >5 to <10 ms) cardiac siderosis.[244] These benefits appear progressive over 5 years with continuing improvement of cardiac T2* and LIC.[245] Furthermore, in the CORDELIA trial, deferasirox appears efficacious and tolerable over time when compared with deferoxamine at reducing LIC and cardiac siderosis.[246] Failure of T2* cardiac siderosis to respond to deferasirox has been predicted by higher baseline LICs and ferritin levels.[247] Deferasirox has also been shown to prevent cardiac iron accumulation in thalassemia patients without evidence of cardiac siderosis as well as improvement in left ventricular function.[248] Deferasirox in combination with deferiprone, an all-oral combination, was as safe as deferoxamine-deferiprone at reducing iron in severely overloaded young β-thalassemia major patients, and superior in patient satisfaction.[249]

Deferasirox was generally well tolerated in these clinical trials. Mild gastrointestinal complaints and skin rashes were the most common adverse events. Discontinuation of deferasirox was rarely required, but abdominal discomfort occurred in 14% of patients, 12% with diarrhea, 10% nausea, and 9% vomiting. Mild increases in serum creatinine occurred in 38% of patients, and a small number exceeded the upper limits of normal; intermittent proteinuria was also observed in 19% of patients. Duplicate serum creatinine level should be assessed before initiating therapy. Close monthly monitoring of serum creatinine needs to be maintained because of nephropathy in animal studies and cases of acute renal failure that were reported after postmarketing use of deferasirox. Severe renal complications may occur in patients with preexisting renal disease. Dose reduction, interruption, or discontinuation should be considered for elevations in serum creatinine. More recent trial data suggests that deferasirox-induced changes in creatinine and renal hemodynamics are usually mild and reversible for up to 2 years of treatment without progression over time.[250] Elevations in serum transaminases also occurred in a small number of patients (6%). Rare reports of fulminant hepatic liver failure have resulted in the recommendation to obtain liver function tests every 2 weeks for 1 month after starting therapy and then monthly thereafter with interruptions or discontinuations of deferasirox if unexplained or progressive transaminase increases occur. Skin rashes also occurred in 15% of patients usually within the first 2 weeks of treatment. The maculopapular eruptions often resolved spontaneously, but severe rashes may require interruption of deferasirox with antihistamine support and possible steroid administration after which deferasirox may be reintroduced at a lower dose with gradual dose escalation. Reports of pancytopenia have occurred in postmarketing reports, but mostly in patients with preexisting hematologic disorders such as MDSs that are frequently associated with BM failure.

A new oral tablet formulation of deferasirox (JadeNu) has recently been approved that does not require dispersion in liquid and can be taken once daily. Dosing is slightly different on a mg/kg dose, based on increased absorption of the new formulation, (e.g., patients on 20 mg/kg/d of the older Exjade formulation would take 14 mg/kg/d of JadeNu). Accordingly, this new formulation may have fewer gastrointestinal side effects. Postmarketing safety studies are currently under way.

Specific Complications and Their Management

Skeletal Changes

Low Bone Mass

With improved survival in patients with thalassemia major, the problem of osteoporosis has assumed greater importance. Approximately 50% to 80% thalassemia patients have an osteoporosis–osteopenia syndrome.[251,252] Vertebral fractures are associated with osteoporosis and cause significant morbidity in this population. Poor bone health begins in childhood and progresses in young adulthood. Lumbar and thoracic vertebrae fractures are present in over 30% of thalassemia patients over the age of 30 years.[253,254] The widespread prevalence of osteoporosis in patients with thalassemia major was first observed across all ages in 1995.[255] Subsequently, others reported a high frequency of abnormal Z scores in pediatric, adolescent, and adult patients. Abnormal bone mineral density has been reported in pediatric and adolescent patients with thalassemia major.[256–258] The Thalassemia Clinical Research Network has identified the overall fracture prevalence of 12% in a contemporary sample of 702 patients with α- and β-thalassemia. The fractures occurred more frequently in thalassemia major (17%) and intermedia (12%) compared with β-E (7%) and α-thalassemia (2%). Facture prevalence increased with age and with sex hormone replacement therapy.[259] More recently an observational study by the Thalassemia Clinical Research Network has demonstrated a high prevalence of low bone mass across all the thalassemia syndromes, including β-thalassemia major, intermedia, β-E, Hb H, H-Constant Spring, and homozygous α-thalassemia, which progresses with aging. In addition, increased serum and urine markers of bone turnover have been described in thalassemia patients with osteoporosis, which correlate with low dual-energy X-ray absorptiometry scores and improve with bisphosphonate therapy.[260] It remains unclear if different chelation therapies and transfusions can alter the progression of osteoporosis.[261] Zinc supplementation may also improve bone density in younger patients with thalassemia.[262]

Skeletal abnormalities (Fig. 40.9) are less common in patients receiving regular RBC transfusions but may still occur as a result of partially unchecked IE and expansion of the erythroid BM.[263] These cause widening of the BM space and thinning of the cortex, with consequent osteoporosis.[255,264] Changes in the skull and facial bones, including expansion of the frontal bone with prominent frontal bossing, may occur before the initiation of transfusion therapy. Radiographs reveal the diploic spaces to be widened. At first, the skull has a granular appearance, but later perpendicular bony trabeculae appear, giving the classic "hair on end" or "crewcut" appearance. Marked overgrowth of the maxilla results in severe malocclusion, jumbling of the upper incisors, and prominence of the molar eminences.[265] These bone changes produce the classic thalassemic facies. Additional skeletal changes are observed in the metacarpals, metatarsals, and phalanges, where expanded medullary cavities produce a rectangular and then a convex shape (see Fig. 40.9). Irregular fusion of the epiphyses of the proximal humerus results in characteristic shortening of the upper arms.[266,267] Marked osteoporosis and cortical thinning may predispose to pathologic fractures of the extremities and compression fractures of the vertebrae (Fig. 40.10).

Several abnormalities in the ribs may occur, including notching and osteolytic lesions.[263,268] The ribs become very wide, especially at the points of their attachment to the vertebral column. BM masses may extrude from these sites, creating the appearance of paravertebral masses and compressing the spinal cord.[269] Although bone deformities and extramedullary hematopoiesis are uncommon in properly transfused patients with β-thalassemia major, it is frequently observed in patients with thalassemia intermedia whose BM is not suppressed by regular transfusions (see the section Thalassemia Intermedia).

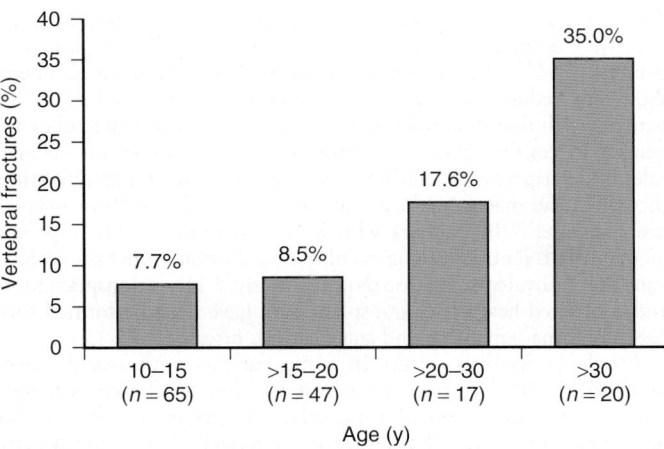

Fig. 40.9 FRACTURE RISK IN THALASSEMIA BY AGE GROUP. Thalassemia patients have increased risk of vertebral fractures by age group. *(Adapted from Pontipa Engkakul, Pat Mahachoklertwattana, Suphaneewan Jaovisidha, Ampaiwan Chuansumrit, Preamrudee Poomthavorn, MD, Niyata Chitrapazt, MD, and Suporn Chuncharunee, MD: Unrecognized vertebral fractures in adolescents and young adults with thalassemia syndromes. J Pediatr Hematol Oncol 35:212–217, 2013.)*

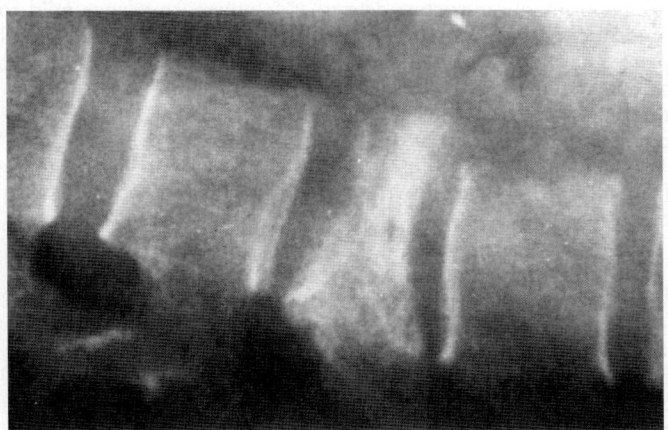

Fig. 40.10 COMPRESSION FRACTURE OF L2 VERTEBRA IN A PATIENT WITH SEVERE β-THALASSEMIA. *(From Pearson HA, Benz EJ Jr: Thalassemia syndromes. In Miller DR, Baehner RL, McMillan CW, editors: Smith's blood diseases of infancy and childhood, ed 5, St. Louis, 1984, CV Mosby, p 439.)*

Growth and Endocrine Status

Growth retardation, including skeletal and dental deformities,[270] was common even in young children until the use of hypertransfusion regimens restored relatively normal growth during the first decade. Without iron chelation therapy, the adolescent growth spurt is often delayed or absent; most patients, even those well maintained by transfusion, may not attain normal stature, partly because of iron-induced damage to the hypothalamic–pituitary axis.[78,271,272] Menarche is frequently delayed. Breast development may be poor, and many female patients have primary or secondary amenorrhea. Boys are frequently immature, with sparse facial and body hair. Although spermatogenesis may be normal, libido is often decreased. A multi-center study of 250 adolescent patients in northern Italy showed that despite hypertransfusion and 7 to 10 years of deferoxamine iron chelation therapy, two-thirds of male patients and one-third of female patients older than 14 years of age were 2 standard deviations or more below the mean for height.[273] Many adolescents between 12 and 18 years of age lacked any secondary sexual changes of puberty. However,

the mean serum ferritin level in the entire group was 3500 ng/mL, indicating persistence of a high level of excess iron burden in most of this group.

Regular chelation therapy started early in the first decade of life frequently allows a normal onset of puberty and development of secondary sexual changes.[274] Administration of recombinant human growth hormone in conventional doses increases height velocity in patients with growth hormone deficiency.[275,276] Normal or higher doses of recombinant human growth hormone increase growth velocity in patients with normal growth hormone reserve but low levels of insulin-like growth factor I.[277,278] For patients with a functional hypothalamic–pituitary axis, treatment with gonadotropin-releasing hormone may induce pubertal changes.[279] In others, administration of sex steroids is necessary to induce secondary sexual characteristics.

Diabetes Mellitus

Abnormal carbohydrate metabolism is common in older patients with thalassemia major. Prepubertal children usually have normal glucose metabolism, but pubertal patients exhibit impaired responses to glucose load. Higher than normal insulin levels despite normal glucose levels are also encountered during puberty.[280] The defect in these patients appears to be related to insulin resistance, with insulin deficiency developing later in the progression to diabetes. Rates of diabetes are reported close to 6% to 8%.[190] Diabetes occurs more frequently in patients with hepatitis C and hepatic dysfunction.[281–283] Oral hypoglycemic agents have been used to regulate hyperglycemia and may reduce the rate of further deterioration of glucose metabolism.[284]

Laboratory findings of hypothyroidism and hypoparathyroidism are present in approximately 14% of patients with thalassemia major.[285–289] Clinical findings associated with these deficiencies are uncommon.[290]

Liver and Gallbladder

Hepatomegaly occurring before the initiation of transfusion therapy in severely affected patients is primarily a consequence of extramedullary hematopoiesis. With the amelioration of the anemia, the liver diminishes in size. However, as transfusion therapy continues, iron accumulation provides a new reason for hepatomegaly and resultant liver injury. Iron deposition, first present in the Kupffer cells, ultimately engorges the parenchymal cells, resulting in an appearance that is indistinguishable from that of idiopathic hemochromatosis.[291–293] The hepatocellular injury of iron overload may be attributable to the liberation of hydrolases resulting from initiation by the ferrous form of iron and peroxidative damage of lysosomal membrane lipids.[294] Fibrosis is usually followed by cirrhosis and an increased risk of hepatocellular carcinoma. The risk of liver damage and the rate of progression may be increased by the concomitant presence of excessive iron with viral hepatitis.

Regular chelation therapy is the key to maintaining normal or near-normal hepatic iron concentrations and preventing iron-induced hepatic fibrosis and cirrhosis. Treatment with deferoxamine slows or prevents iron-induced liver damage and may reduce the severity of preexisting fibrosis in some cases.[148,161,295] Results of treatment of hepatitis C in patients with thalassemia major are similar to those found in other patients. Sustained viral responses occur in 28% to 40% of patients treated with interferon alone and, in two smaller series, 46% to 72% of patients treated with interferon and ribavirin.[296–300] Transfusion requirements increase by 30% to 40% in patients treated with ribavirin as a result of drug-induced hemolysis.[297,299,300] Lower levels of viral RNA and non-1 genotypes are associated with better responses. Higher iron levels adversely affect the response to antiviral therapy in some studies but not in others.[296,298,301] The Thalassemia Clinical Research Network studied the use of pegylated interferon and ribavirin in 16 thalassemia patients. Fifty percent of genotype 1 patients had sustained viral response as well as 25% of genotype 2 and 3 patients; median transfusion requirements increased by 44% after 24 weeks of treatment, and LIC increase of more than 5 mg/g dry weight occurred in 29% of patients, but overall LIC remained stable over the course of the study. In addition, neutropenia occurred in 52% of patients.[300] New oral therapies that do not contain ribavirin or interferon are available to treat hepatitis C, although there is minimal experience in thalassemia to date.

Pigmentary gallstones caused by high levels of bilirubin production are found in an increasing number of patients older than 4-years of age. Two-thirds of patients have multiple calcified bilirubinate calculi after the age of 15 years.[302] Gallbladder surgery is not usually indicated unless biliary colic or obstructive jaundice has occurred.

Heart

Cardiac abnormalities are important causes of morbidity and mortality in patients with thalassemia major. Cardiac enlargement secondary to anemia is almost always present in untransfused children. Before the availability of chelation therapy, myocardial hemosiderosis and serious iron-induced cardiac diseases were inevitable during the second decade. These problems still occur often in older patients with thalassemia who are poorly compliant with chelation therapy, and heart disease, usually in the form of cardiac failure or serious arrhythmias, remains the most common cause of death in patients with thalassemia major.[189,191]

Left-sided heart failure predominates in patients with thalassemia major and is characterized by dyspnea and orthopnea.[303] Right-sided heart failure is less common but may be the presenting cardiac finding in older patients with more severe iron overload. Symptoms include hepatic pain, abdominal discomfort, and peripheral edema. Acute myocarditis, which occurs in approximately 5% of patients with thalassemia, is frequently followed by acute or chronic heart failure.[304]

Early electrocardiographic abnormalities include a prolonged P–R interval, first-degree heart block, and premature atrial contractions. Later, ST-segment depression and ventricular ectopic beats constitute ominous indicators of myocardial damage. Periodic evaluation of cardiac function is essential to detect iron-induced heart disease and to identify patients who will benefit from more intensive chelation therapy (see later discussion). Unfortunately, by the time cardiac results of studies such as echocardiography and 24-hour rhythm monitoring become abnormal, clinical heart disease is imminent. Whether assessment of cardiac iron by MRI using T2* or other measures can better anticipate the development of clinical heart disease is currently under investigation.

In the absence of intensified chelation therapy, ventricular dysfunction progresses rapidly to chronic refractory congestive heart failure, and arrhythmias become increasingly difficult to control. In the past, death usually occurred within 1 year of onset of heart failure. More recent data demonstrate a survival rate of 48% at 5 years.[303] Survival is notably poorer in patients with heart failure after myocarditis or with heart failure accompanied by arrhythmias.[304]

In addition to standard therapy for heart failure and arrhythmias, including angiotensin-converting enzyme inhibitors, β-blockers, diuretics, and antiarrhythmic agents, the pretransfusion Hb level should be maintained between 10 and 12 g/dL. The volume of transfused RBCs should be reduced as needed to prevent acute fluid overload. Because the iron-overloaded myocardium has little capacity to improve its performance unless excess iron is removed, intensive chelation therapy is a critical part of the management of heart disease in patients with thalassemia. Several studies have shown that heart failure can be reversed in many patients with the use of continuous treatment with deferoxamine.[181,305,306] The benefits of this approach may derive from the reduction in cardiac iron stores, the prevention of acute toxicity from nontransferrin-bound iron, or a combination of these two mechanisms. Recent data suggest that deferiprone may be more effective than deferoxamine in reducing the cardiac iron load and treating iron-induced cardiac disease, perhaps because of deferiprone's ability to enter cardiac cells more rapidly than

deferoxamine.[133,223] Deferiprone seems to remove iron from the heart effectively despite its relative inefficiency in controlling hepatic iron content.[133,223,307] Deferasirox treatment for 1 to 2 years has also been shown to reduce cardiac iron and improve cardiac MRI T2* in patients with transfusional iron overload.[308,309] Additional studies are needed to confirm these observations and to establish the relative roles of deferiprone, deferasirox, and deferoxamine or a combination thereof in the management of patients with established iron-related heart disease.[310] In patients who have undergone BMT, improvements in left ventricular contractility and diastolic function accompany the removal of excess iron by phlebotomy.[311] Heart transplantation and combined heart–liver transplantation have been performed successfully in patients with end-stage cardiac disease.[312–314]

Sterile pericarditis occurs in some patients with massive iron overload.[315] Although pericarditis is most often attributed to hemosiderosis, an association with β-hemolytic streptococcal infection and other infectious agents has also been suggested.[316] Therapy usually consists of bed rest, treatment of infection, management of superimposed congestive heart failure, and the use of salicylates or corticosteroids. Occasionally, pericardectomy may be indicated.

Lungs

Mild abnormalities of pulmonary function are common in patients with thalassemia but rarely cause clinical problems. Some patients exhibit primarily restrictive defects[317,318]; others experience mild to moderate small airway obstruction and hyperinflation.[319–321] Most patients have a decreased maximal oxygen uptake and anaerobic threshold; these do not normalize after transfusion.[322] Postsplenectomy thrombocytosis and other prothrombotic changes can predispose to pulmonary vascular occlusion and pulmonary hypertension.[323–326] Treatment with high doses of the iron chelator deferoxamine may also be associated with acute deterioration of pulmonary function.[176,177]

Kidneys

The kidneys are frequently enlarged, partly because of extramedullary hematopoiesis and partly because of marked dilation of the renal tubules.[327] The urine is often dark brown, reflecting the excretion of products of heme catabolism.[328] The urine also contains large amounts of urates and uric acid.

The Thalassemia Clinical Research Network studied the prevalence of renal abnormalities in patients with thalassemia major and thalassemia intermedia receiving deferoxamine chelation. One-third of thalassemia patients who were not regularly transfused had abnormally high creatinine clearance. Regular transfusions were associated with a decrease in clearance ($p = .004$). Almost one-third of patients with thalassemia had hypercalciuria, and regular transfusions were associated with an increase in the frequency and degree of hypercalciuria ($p < .0001$). Albuminuria was found in more than half of patients but was not consistently associated with transfusion therapy. In summary, renal hyperfiltration, hypercalciuria, and albuminuria are common in patients with thalassemia. Higher transfusion intensity is associated with lower creatinine clearance but more frequent hypercalciuria.[329]

Spleen and Splenectomy

Massive splenomegaly is unusual in regularly transfused patients, but even mild or moderate splenomegaly may be associated with findings of hypersplenism, including thrombocytopenia, neutropenia, and increasing anemia. The usual indication for splenectomy is a progressive increase in transfusion requirements caused by hypersplenism. The transfusion requirements, and therefore the rates of iron loading, of splenectomized patients are often considerably less than those of patients whose spleens are intact.[247,307,330,331] A transfusion requirement of more than 180–200 mL/kg/y of packed RBCs usually represents excessive RBC requirements.[330,331] For such patients, a 25% to 60% reduction in transfusion requirements after splenectomy is generally predictable. Before attributing increased transfusion requirements to hypersplenism, it is important to look for other causes, such as RBC alloimmunization or a change in the hematocrit of the units of donor blood. RBC survival studies using ^{52}Cr-labeling are not usually of value for predicting response to splenectomy. Because of the greater risk of postsplenectomy sepsis in younger patients, surgery should be deferred until after 5 years of age whenever possible, so the humoral immune system has developed. For well-transfused and well-chelated patients, splenectomy may have little benefit, and some centers have noted a significant decline in the number of patients undergoing splenectomy in recent years.

Laparoscopic splenectomy has proved safe for patients with thalassemia and has dramatically shortened the recovery time compared with open procedures.[332] Partial splenectomy and partial dearterialization of the spleen have been suggested as alternative approaches to reducing blood requirements without incurring the risk of sepsis.[333-335] The long-term benefits of this approach remain uncertain. Therapeutic embolization of the spleen avoids the need for surgery,[336-338] but this approach is frequently associated with postprocedure pain and fever and does not permit the removal of accessory spleens.

After splenectomy, striking thrombocytosis may occur, which may require thrombosis prophylaxis or platelet deaggregating agents.[339] Increased numbers of nucleated RBCs appear in the blood, and the presence of many RBCs containing inclusion bodies composed of precipitated α-globin chains can be demonstrated by staining with supravital staining.

Patients with thalassemia major are at significant risk for the development of overwhelming, often fatal, infection after splenectomy (postsplenectomy sepsis syndrome).[340] The problem is most common in young children. *Streptococcus pneumoniae* causes two-thirds of cases; *Hemophilus influenzae* type B and *Neisseria meningitidis* account for most of the remaining infections. Typically, there is a fulminant clinical course, proceeding from mild fever and headache to hyperpyrexia, prostration, shock, and death within 6 to 12 hours. Immunization against the most common pathogens before splenectomy, prophylaxis with antibiotics, and early assessment of fever after splenectomy have dramatically reduced the incidence of fatal postsplenectomy sepsis.

Splenectomy should generally be reserved for patients with excessive transfusion requirements from hypersplenism and difficulty controlling iron overload. A large spleen alone does not usually cause significant clinical problems and should rarely, if ever, be the sole reason for splenectomy. Before splenectomy, polyvalent pneumococcal, meningococcal, and *H. influenzae* vaccines should be administered if they have not been given earlier in life.[341,342] Oral penicillin therapy, 250 mg twice daily, is generally used as prophylaxis against postsplenectomy infection in patients with thalassemia. However, the optimal duration of penicillin prophylaxis remains unknown, and compliance is frequently inadequate.[343] Although the risk of postsplenectomy sepsis decreases with age, it does not disappear, and fatal pneumococcal sepsis has occurred many years after removal of the spleen.[344]

Survival in Patients With Thalassemia Major

Improved transfusion therapy and the consistent use of iron chelation therapy have extended the life span of patients with thalassemia major.[103,189,191,345] In a multicenter study of 1079 patients in Italy, the probability of survival to age 20 years was 96% for patients born between 1975 and 1979, the time at which chelation therapy became a regular part of the overall management of thalassemia major (Table 40.2).[189] In contrast, the probabilities of survival at 20 years of age were only 61% and 69% for those born in the periods of 1960 through 1964 and 1965 through 1969, respectively. Other investigators have shown that survival or prevention of life-threatening complications is strongly related to good chelation therapy, assessed either by compliance or by control of iron stores (Fig. 40.11).[134,183,191] The

Patient Age (Years)	Cohort (%)		
	1970–1974	1975–1979	1980–1984
10	98 (96–99)	98 (96–99)	99 (95–100)
15	95 (92–97)	97 (94–98)	98 (93–100)
20	89 (85–92)	96 (93–98)	
25	82 (77–86)		

TABLE 40.2   Survival by Birth Cohort at Different Ages of Patients With Transfusion-Dependent Thalassemia

Data from Borgna Pignatti C, Rugolotto S, De Stefano X, et al: Survival and disease complications in thalassemia major. *Ann N Y Acad Sci* 850:227, 1998.

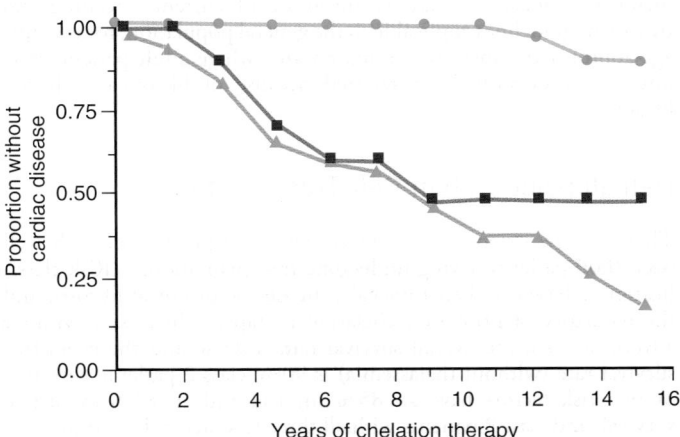

Fig. 40.11 SURVIVAL WITHOUT CARDIAC DISEASE IN PATIENTS WITH THALASSEMIA MAJOR TREATED WITH DEFEROXAMINE ACCORDING TO THE PROPORTION OF SERUM FERRITIN MEASUREMENTS GREATER THAN 2500 NG/ML. The *circles* show cardiac disease-free survival among patients in whom less than 33% of ferritin measurements exceeded 2500 ng/mL; *squares* show survival among patients in whom 33% to 67% of ferritin measurements exceeded 2500 ng/mL; and *triangles* show survival among patients in whom more than 67% of ferritin measurements exceeded 2500 ng/mL. (*Adapted from Olivieri NF, Nathan DG, MacMillan JH, et al: Survival in medically treated patients with homozygous beta-thalassemia. N Engl J Med 331:574, 1994.*)

importance of good compliance with chelation therapy is further demonstrated by data from the United Kingdom showing that the probability of survival for the 1975 through 1984 birth cohort is to date not substantially different than the probability of survival for the 1965 through 1974 birth cohort.[345] The researchers attribute this poorer than expected survival rate, despite the availability of deferoxamine, to a lack of adherence to the recommended schedule of treatment with this chelator.

Chronic Care of the Adult Patient With Thalassemia

Adults with transfusion-dependent thalassemia syndromes are living longer into adulthood, with some approaching their seventh decade of life. It is likely in the coming decades that these patients will have improved life expectancies related to safer transfusion practices, improved screening of the blood supply, and better iron chelation medications. Therefore, the thalassemia patient born in the current era may expect to spend the majority of their life as an adult.

There is currently limited expertise among adult hematologists in the management of adult thalassemia patients. Transition plans are essential for all pediatric patients as they enter adulthood, so that they may receive age-appropriate care. Transition is especially important in thalassemia, as they require the regular uninterrupted schedule of

deferiprone, and deferasirox have all proved to be safe and effective in thalassemia intermedia.[426-428]

Thromboembolic events represent a major complication of thalassemia intermedia, occurring in 10% to 34% of patients.[326,429] These events include stroke, pulmonary embolism, portal vein thrombosis, and deep vein thrombosis of the legs. A hypercoagulable state may also contribute to the pulmonary hypertension that commonly occurs in patients with thalassemia intermedia and is the primary cause of congestive heart failure.[430] Splenectomy is a risk factor for thromboembolic events in patients with thalassemia intermedia, resulting in thrombocytosis and allowing the prolonged circulation of damaged RBCs that generate increased amounts of thrombin.[326] Some investigators consider the risk of thromboembolic events after splenectomy for thalassemia intermedia to be sufficiently high to warrant short-term anticoagulation in the perioperative period and during pregnancy.[326] Oral contraceptives should be used with extreme caution, if at all. Interestingly, known genetic thrombophilias in other populations like factor V Leiden, the prothrombin gene mutation 20210, and MTHFR C677T mutations have not been associated with thrombotic risk in this population.[431]

Extension of hematopoietic tissue beyond the confines of the bones occurs in patients with thalassemia intermedia as a result of the intense erythropoiesis. This complication occurs less frequently in patients with thalassemia major because of the partial suppression of erythropoiesis by regular transfusions. Masses of extramedullary hematopoietic tissue develop in the spinal epidural space, thorax, cranium, pelvis, and elsewhere.[367,432-442] These masses may be detected as incidental findings on imaging studies of the chest or abdomen.[433-439] In other instances, the masses produce symptoms by compressing neighboring structures. For example, patients with extramedullary hematopoietic masses may develop paraplegia from spinal cord compression or loss of visual acuity or visual fields caused by optic nerve compression.[432,435,441,442] Additional clinical presentations of hematopoietic masses include pleural effusions and upper airway obstruction.[437,438,440] Initiation of regular transfusions for patients with thalassemia intermedia or intensification of the ongoing transfusion program for patients with thalassemia major reduces the size of extramedullary hematopoietic masses and helps to prevent recurrences. (Tables 40.4 and 40.5).

β-Thalassemia Minor (Thalassemia Trait)

Inheritance of a single β-thalassemia allele usually results in a mild hypochromic microcytic anemia. The Hb level averages 1 or 2 g/dL lower than that seen in normal persons of the same age and gender. Hb F levels decline more slowly than usual in the first year of life, and the diagnostic elevated Hb A_2 levels are established by approximately 6 months of age.[443-445] Strong intrafamilial correlations of both Hb A_2 and mean corpuscular volume (MCV) are noted.[446,447] Osmotic fragility is decreased; indeed, a one-tube osmotic fragility test has been used in the past for mass screening.[444] The RBC count is increased or normal. The RBCs are characteristically hypochromic (MCH <26 pg) and microcytic (MCV <75 fL). The smear shows varying numbers of target cells, poikilocytes, ovalocytes, and basophilic stippling (Fig. 40.13). The reticulocyte count is normal or slightly elevated. RBC survival is normal, iron utilization is decreased, and slight IE is present.[445] During pregnancy, the anemia of thalassemia trait often becomes more severe, but transfusions are rarely necessary. Increased folic acid supplementation may improve Hb during this period. Because iron deficiency may occur during pregnancy, iron supplementation has been advised to avoid compounding the causes of anemia.[448,449] In general, thalassemia trait carries no direct clinical symptoms or pathologic consequences for the patient. Studies have suggested there may be an increased tendency for gallstones and cholecystitis, but otherwise this condition should be largely asymptomatic.[17] The diagnosis of thalassemia trait assumes particular importance in women who are pregnant or considering pregnancy because of the potential for having a child with thalassemia major.

α-THALASSEMIA SYNDROMES

The α-thalassemias are more difficult to diagnose because characteristic elevations in Hb A_2 or Hb F, seen in many cases of β-thalassemia, do not occur, making Hb electrophoresis difficult to use for diagnostic testing. However, the gene deletions responsible for the most common varieties are readily detectable by molecular biology methods.[450]

TABLE 40.4	Nontransfusion-Dependent Thalassemia Screening Recommendations	
Test Name	**Measurement**	**Frequency**
MRI with T2* liver iron content	Liver iron	every 1–2 years
MRI with T2* cardiac iron content[a]	Cardiac iron	every 1–2 years
Ferritin	Total body iron	every 3 months
History and physical exam	General health, medication compliance	every 3–4 months
Echocardiogram	Pulmonary hypertension TRV	every 1–2 years
Liver function panel	Liver failure, hepatitis	every 3 months
liver ultrasound (if LIC >5/ferritin >800)	Cirrhosis	annually
AFP (if >40 or presence of clinical cirrhosis)	Hepatocellular carcinoma	annually
Hepatitis B, C serologies (if receiving blood transfusions)	Hepatitis B and C viral infection/exposure	annually
Tanner stage/Sexual development evaluation	Sexual development	annually
standing and sitting height	Growth and development	every 6 months
Free T4, TSH	Thyroid function	annually
Calcium, phosphate, vitamin D	Parathyroid function	annually
Fasting blood sugar/oral glucose tolerance test	Diabetes mellitus screening	annually
ACTH test	Adrenal insufficiency	annually
DEXA	Bone mineral density	annually

[a]Cannot be widely recommended because no correlation with LIC
ACTH, Adrenocorticotropic hormone; AFP, α-fetoprotein; DEXA, dual-energy x-ray absorptiometry; LIC, liver iron concentration; MRI, magnetic resonance imaging; TRV, tricuspid regurgitant velocity; TSH, thyroid stimulating hormone.

TABLE 40.5 Transfusion-Dependent Thalassemia Screening Recommendations

MRI with T2* liver iron content	Liver iron	every 1–2 years
MRI with T2* cardiac iron content	Cardiac iron	every 1–2 years
Ferritin	Total body iron	every 3 months
History and physical exam	General health, medication compliance	every 3–4 months
Echocardiogram	Pulmonary hypertension TRV	every 1–2 years
Liver function panel	Liver failure, hepatitis	every 3 months
Liver ultrasound (if LIC>5/ferritin >800)	Cirrhosis screening	annually
AFP (if >40 or presence of clinical cirrhosis)	Hepatocellular carcinoma screening	annually
Hepatitis B, C serologies (if receiving blood transfusions)	Hepatitis B and C viral infection/exposure	annually
Tanner stage/Sexual development evaluation	Sexual development	annually
Standing and sitting height	Growth and development	every 6 months
Free T4, TSH	Thyroid function	annually
Calcium, phosphate, vitamin D	Parathyroid function	annually
Fasting blood sugar/oral glucose tolerance test	Diabetes mellitus screening	annually
ACTH test	Adrenal insufficiency screening	annually
DEXA	Bone mineral density	annually
NTX, CTX, AP	Bone mineral density	annually
Dental evaluation	Maxillofacial disease, periodontal disease, caries	6–12 months

ACTH, Adrenocorticotropic hormone; AFP, α-fetoprotein; AP, alkaline phosphatase; CTX, collagen type 1 cross-linked C-telopeptide; DEXA, dual-energy x-ray absorptiometry; LIC, liver iron concentration; MRI, magnetic resonance imaging; NTX, N-terminal telopeptide; TRV, tricuspic regurgitant velocity; TSH, thyroid stimulating hormone.

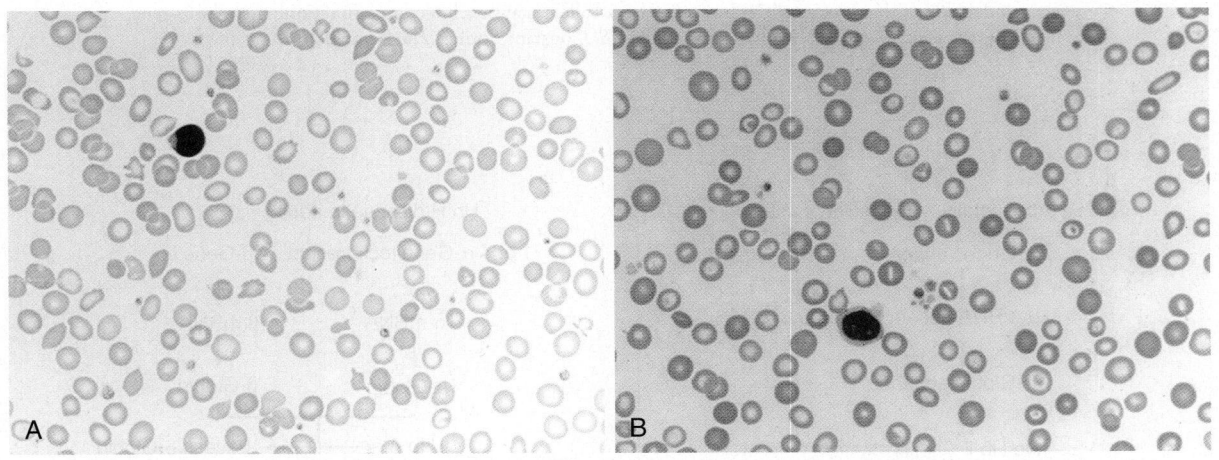

Fig. 40.13 MORPHOLOGY OF THE PERIPHERAL BLOOD FILM IN A PATIENT WITH HETEROZYGOUS β-THALASSEMIA (A) AND A PATIENT WITH HETEROZYGOUS α-THALASSEMIA (B). Note the profound hypochromia and microcytosis and the many target cells. *(From Pearson HA, Benz EJ Jr. Thalassemia syndromes. In Miller DR, Baehner RL, McMillan CW, editors: Smith's blood diseases of infancy and childhood, ed 5, St. Louis, 1984, CV Mosby, p 439.)*

Molecular Pathology and Pathophysiology

The four classic α-thalassemia syndromes are α+-thalassemia trait, in which one of the four *α-globin* genes fails to function; α°-thalassemia trait, with two dysfunctional genes; Hb H disease, with three affected genes; and hydrops fetalis with Hb Bart, in which all four genes are defective. In general, partial deletions are more deleterious and create a more severe phenotype than complete deletions.[451] In the older literature, α°- and α++-thalassemia are referred to as α-thalassemia-1 and α-thalassemia-2, respectively. These syndromes are usually caused by deletion of one, two, three, or all four of the α-globin genes, respectively (Fig. 40.14). Nondeletional forms of α-thalassemia, which account for 15% to 20% of patients, arise from mutations similar to those described for β-thalassemia.[452,453] Fig. 40.15 illustrates the different α-thalassemia mutations and phenotypes. Structurally abnormal Hbs have also been associated with α-thalassemia. The Quong Sze α-globin chain (α125Leu→Pro) is exceedingly labile and is destroyed so rapidly after its synthesis that no Hb tetramers containing the mutant α chain can be formed.[454] α+-thalassemias also exhibit epistasis with haptoglobin variants that alters patterns in malaria protection.[455]

α+-Thalassemia trait is very common in patients of African ancestry, having a genetic frequency of 20% to 30% in some populations. However, the *cis* α°-thalassemia deletion is rare in black patients. Thus, even though α+-thalassemia trait and the *trans* deletion form of α°-thalassemia are very common, Hb H disease is rarely encountered, and hydrops fetalis has not yet been reported in black patients.[456,457]

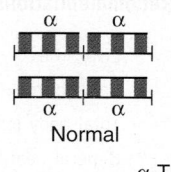

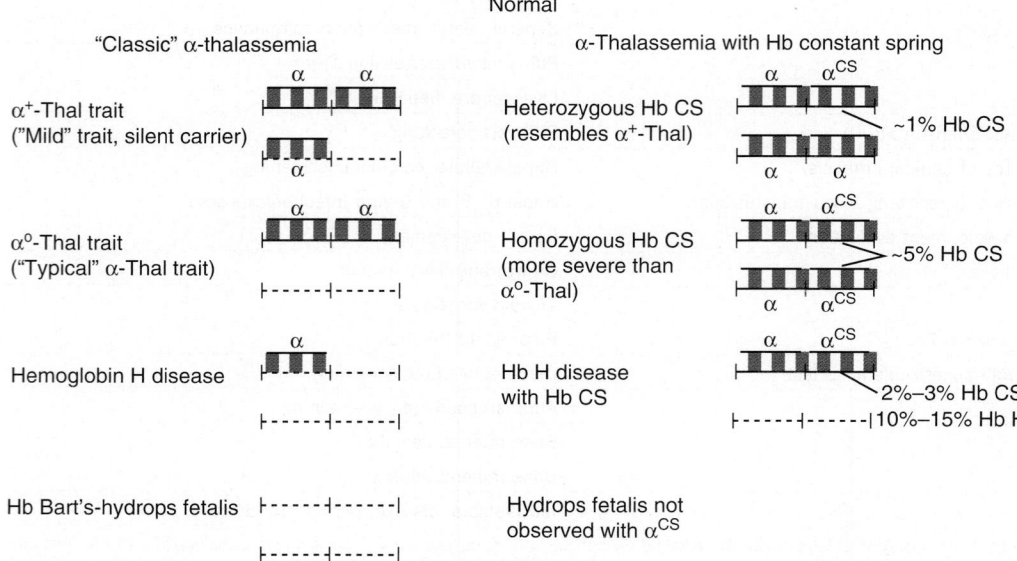

Fig. 40.14 GENETIC ORIGINS OF THE "CLASSIC" α-THALASSEMIA SYNDROMES CAUSED BY GENE DELETIONS IN THE α-GLOBIN GENE CLUSTER. Hemoglobin Constant Spring is an α-globin chain variant synthesized in such small amounts (1–2% of normal) that it has the phenotypic impact of a severe nondeletion α-thalassemia allele; however, the α^{cs} allele is always linked to a functioning *α-globin* gene, so it has never been associated with hydrops fetalis. *CS*, Constant Spring; *Hb*, hemoglobin.

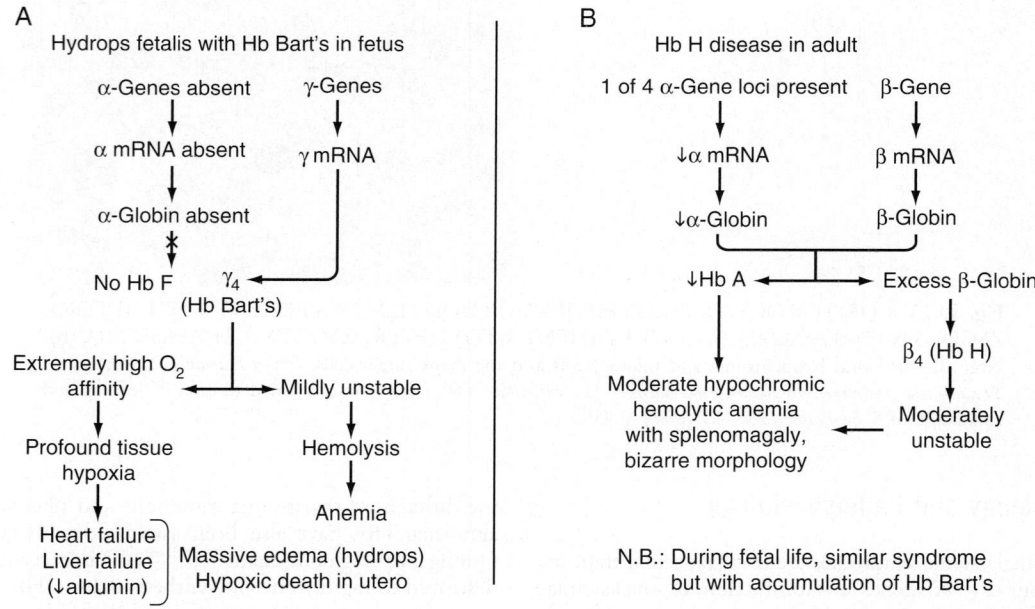

Fig. 40.15 PATHOPHYSIOLOGY OF HEMOGLOBIN H DISEASE AND HYDROPS FETALIS WITH HB BART. *Hb*, Hemoglobin; *mRNA*, messenger ribonucleic acid. *(Adapted from Benz EJ Jr: The hemoglobinopathies. In Kelly WN, DeVita VT, editors: Textbook of internal medicine, Philadelphia, 1988, JB Lippincott, p 1423.)*

Clinical Manifestations

Silent Carrier (α⁺-Thalassemia Trait)

α^+-Thalassemia trait has no consistent hematologic manifestations. The RBCs are not microcytic, and Hb A_2 and Hb F are normal. During the newborn period, small amounts ($\leq$3%) of Hb Bart (γ_4) can be seen by electrophoresis or other techniques. This condition is most often recognized when an apparently normal individual becomes the parent of a child with Hb H disease after mating with a person with α°-thalassemia trait. The mild excess of β-globin chains is probably removed in erythroblasts by proteolysis.[458] α^+-Thalassemia is particularly common in Melanesia, as well as in Southeast Asia and in African Americans, reaching a prevalence of more than 80% in North coastal Papua New Guinea. At the molecular level, α^+-thalassemia has been found to be associated with two common gene deletions resulting from different nonhomologous crossing-over events between the two linked α-globin genes: a 3.7-kb rightward deletion ($-\alpha^{3.7}$) resulting in a fused $\alpha2\alpha1$-globin gene and a 4.2-kb leftward deletion ($-\alpha^{4.2}$) resulting in loss of the 5' (α2) gene.[452,453,459] The level of α-globin gene expression differs in the two conditions, as discussed in the following section.

α-Thalassemia Trait (α-Thalassemia Trait)

Levels of Hb A_2 in the low to low normal range (1.5–2.5%) and β/α synthetic ratios averaging 1.4:1 characterize α°-thalassemia trait. During the perinatal period, elevated amounts of Hb Bart are noted (3–8%). Microcytosis is present in cord blood erythrocytes.

Studies of newborns from the archipelago of Vanuatu in the Southwest Pacific and from Papua New Guinea indicate that homozygotes for the rightward $-\alpha^{3.7III}$ deletion (where only a fused $\alpha2\alpha1$-globin gene, mostly of the α2 type, remains) have lower Hb Bart levels (3.5% ± 0.8%) than those of infants homozygous for the leftward $-\alpha^{4.2}$ deletion (in whom only the $\alpha1$-globin gene remains) (6.0% ± 1.4%). These results suggest that the 5' $\alpha2$-globin gene has a higher output than the 3' $\alpha1$-globin gene, a conclusion supported by direct measurement of α2/α1 mRNA ratios.[460,461]

Hb H is not detected in hemolysates of peripheral RBCs, probably because of rapid proteolysis of Hb H or free β-globin chains. However, approximately 1% of erythroblasts and BM reticulocytes have inclusions. When an α-thalassemia gene occurs in persons who are also heterozygous for α-globin chain variant Hbs, such as Hb S, Hb C, or Hb E, the proportion of the abnormal Hb is lower than that seen in simple heterozygotes.[462] The lower level of the abnormal Hb is attributable to posttranslational control because of higher affinity of β^A chains for a limited pool of α-globin chains coupled with proteolysis of the uncombined $\beta^{variant}$ chains.[463]

Hemoglobin H Disease

Hb H disease is associated with a moderately severe but variable anemia resembling thalassemia intermedia, with osseous changes and splenomegaly.[464] However, the clinical phenotype may be considerably milder in some patients and severe enough to cause hydrops fetalis in others.[465,466] It occurs predominantly in Asians and occasionally in whites (Mediterranean) but is rare in persons of African ancestry. Exacerbations of anemia during febrile illnesses are common and are usually characterized by increasing fatigue and jaundice. Adults with Hb H develop some of the same complications as β-thalassemia including osteoporosis, cholelithiasis, and iron overload.[467]

Because Hb H is unstable and precipitates within the circulating RBCs, hemolysis occurs. Hb H can be demonstrated by incubation of blood with supravital oxidizing stains such as 1% brilliant cresyl blue. Multiple small inclusions form in the RBCs (see Fig. 40.15). Electrophoresis of a freshly prepared hemolysate at alkaline or neutral pH demonstrates a fast-moving component amounting to 3% to 30% of the total Hb. Concomitant iron deficiency may reduce the amount of Hb H in the patient's RBCs.[468] A syndrome of Hb H disease associated with mental retardation, other congenital anomalies, and large deletions on chromosome 16 has been noted in several white families.[469,470]

The degree of deletions in Hb H is also relevant to clinical presentation. Deletional HbH occurs when three deletional alpha (0) mutations occur. Non-deletional HbH occurs when two deletional alpha(0) mutations occur with an alpha (+) mutation (e.g. Constant Spring). Nondeletional Hb H genotypes are more likely to have higher percentage Hb H, more splenomegaly, and more advanced disease.[455]

Hydrops Fetalis With Hb Bart

Hydrops fetalis with Hb Bart occurs almost exclusively in Asians, especially Chinese, Cambodians, Thais, and Filipinos. Affected fetuses are usually born prematurely and are either stillborn or die shortly after birth.[1-4] Marked anasarca and enlargement of the liver and spleen are present. Severe anemia is usually present, with Hb levels of 3–10 g/dL. The RBCs are markedly microcytic and hypochromic and include target cells and large numbers of circulating nucleated RBCs. These morphologic abnormalities and a negative Coombs test result exclude hemolytic diseases caused by blood group incompatibility. Hb electrophoresis reveals predominantly Hb Bart, with a smaller amount of Hb H. A minor component identified as Hb Portland ($\zeta_2\gamma_2$) migrating in the position of Hb A is also seen. Normal Hb A and Hb F are totally absent.[471]

Hydropic infants have massive hepatosplenomegaly. Extreme extramedullary erythropoiesis occurs in response to the profound hypoxia and hemolytic anemia characteristic of this disease. The universal edema characteristic of the hydrops fetalis syndrome is a reflection of severe congestive heart failure and hypoalbuminemia in utero. This is partly a consequence of anemia, but the strikingly abnormal oxygen affinity of the tetrameric Hb Bart is probably the most important determinant of the severe tissue hypoxia. The oxygen dissociation curve of Hb Bart lacks the normal sigmoid form because of noncooperativity during oxygen loading and unloading and is markedly shifted to the left. The shift is so great that little oxygen is released under conditions of low oxygen concentration in the tissues.

Infants with this syndrome do not die in an earlier trimester of pregnancy because of the presence of Hb Portland ($\zeta_2\gamma_2$). This Hb does display cooperativity in a manner similar to that of Hb F and therefore has a much more favorable oxygen dissociation pattern than that of Hb Bart. A high incidence of toxemia of pregnancy has been described in women carrying severely affected infants, providing an increased rationale for prenatal diagnosis of this condition.

Prenatal Diagnosis of α-Thalassemia

Using molecular hybridization technology, Dozy and associates[472] detected the complete absence of α-globin genes in fetal fibroblasts obtained by amniocentesis in a pregnancy at risk of homozygous α-thalassemia and the hydrops fetalis syndrome. A quantitative polymerase chain reaction (PCR) method provides similar information rapidly and accurately.[473] The presence of hydrops can also be detected by ultrasonography. DNA studies or globin synthesis evaluation may be used to confirm the diagnosis in utero. PCR-based assays are available for the detection of the common α-thalassemia deletions.[473-476]

Therapy

Fetuses with homozygous α°-thalassemia usually die in utero because of severe hydrops fetalis and are stillborn. However, some infants have had successful blood exchange transfusion immediately after birth.[477–481] It is also possible to salvage affected fetuses by in utero blood transfusions.[482,483] Limb and urogenital defects are present in a substantial portion of infants with homozygous $\alpha°$-thalassemia who are rescued by these measures, and some infants have developmental delay or other neurologic abnormalities. Management after the perinatal period is similar to the management of patients with thalassemia major and includes transfusion and chelation therapy as well as the possibility of BMT.[484]

Many patients with Hb H disease do not require RBC transfusions. For patients with more severe disease, characterized by lower Hb levels or frequent exacerbations of the anemia, splenectomy can be helpful. Oxidant drugs can accelerate precipitation of Hb H and exacerbate hemolysis; they should therefore be avoided. Exchange transfusion can be used to decrease deleterious levels of Hb H. Infants with heterozygous $\alpha°$-thalassemia trait lose their Hb Bart during the first few months of life and are left with the hematologic findings of α-thalassemia trait, a mild hypochromic microcytosis that persists throughout life.[1] The degree of morphologic abnormality varies greatly among different individuals. That α-thalassemia can be easily diagnosed by Hb electrophoresis at birth gives some impetus to cord blood screening studies. Confusion between heterozygous $\alpha°$-thalassemia trait and iron deficiency may lead to unnecessary evaluations for possible blood loss or unnecessary supplementation with iron unless the overlap in hematologic findings is recognized and more specific diagnostic studies are performed.

De Novo and Acquired Forms of α-Thalassemia

Two distinct α-thalassemia syndromes have been described that are attributable to acquired or de novo mutations: (1) α-thalassemia associated with mental retardation and (2) Hb H disease associated with MDS.

α-Thalassemia Associated With Mental Retardation

α-Thalassemia or Hb H disease can occur as a de novo abnormality in a rare disorder called the α-thalassemia with mental retardation syndrome (ATR).[469,470] In this disorder, affected patients have mental retardation and a number of other developmental abnormalities in association with α-thalassemia trait or Hb H disease that is inherited in a nontraditional manner. Two distinct types of the ATR syndrome have been identified. In some cases, there is the de novo appearance of large (2000 kb or so) deletions involving the entire α-globin gene cluster and adjacent DNA at the tip of chromosome 16, the so-called ATR-16 syndrome. In some of these patients, the deletion produces detectable cytogenetic abnormalities of chromosome 16, indicating that a very large segment of the chromosome is deleted, sometimes because of unbalanced chromosomal translocations involving the telomeres of the affected chromosomes. In some cases, one parent is heterozygous for α^+-thalassemia by various criteria and the other parent is completely normal; in such cases, the child has Hb H disease (- -/- α). In other cases, both parents are normal and the affected child has the hematologic phenotype of heterozygous $\alpha°$-thalassemia (- -/- α) without Hb H disease. In this form of ATR, the clinical findings, such as the degree of mental retardation and associated congenital abnormalities, are variable.

The second type of ATR syndrome is not associated with detectable deletions of the α-globin gene complex. The molecular basis of the disorder consists of mutations of a gene on the X chromosome, and the condition has been called the ATR-X syndrome.[485] In contrast to patients with the ATR-16 syndrome who have a varied phenotype of developmental abnormalities, patients with the ATR-X syndrome have a more uniform or consistent phenotype, particularly severe mental retardation (with IQs of 50–70) and a characteristic dysmorphic facial appearance.[470]

The affected gene in this syndrome encodes a trans-acting factor, called ATRX, that is thought to influence the expression of the α-globin genes as well as that of other genes.[486,487] The structure of this large (280 kDa) DNA-binding protein is complex and contains two major functional domains: an N-terminal cysteine-rich zinc finger–containing domain, called the ADD domain, that has structural features similar to those of DNA methyl transferases, and a C-terminal helicase/ATPase domain. The majority of the mutations associated with the ATR-X syndrome are located in the ADD domain or the helicase domain. The ATRX protein is widely expressed in many different tissues and its intracellular localization is within three different nuclear subcompartments: heterochromatin, ribosomal DNA arrays, and PML bodies. It has been shown to interact with other proteins such as the heterochromatin-associated protein HP1 and Daxx, one of the proteins localized in PML bodies. The prevailing opinion is that the ATRX protein is part of a large chromatin-remodeling complex of the SWI2/SNF2 family. It also has ATPase activity and has translocase activity, that is, it can move along DNA as a "molecular motor." The precise mechanism(s) by which ATRX influences the expression of α-globin (and other) genes remains unknown.

Acquired Hb H Disease Associated With Myelodysplastic Syndrome

Hb H disease has occasionally been observed to develop during the course of different types of MDS and more rarely in patients with other hematologic malignancies.[488] The disorder usually affects elderly men older than the age of 60 years. The degree of imbalance of globin chain synthesis and of α-globin mRNA deficiency in erythroid cells of affected patients is greater than that observed in the hereditary type of Hb H disease. It is conceivable that erythroid cells of the abnormal clone synthesize no α-globin chains at all and that the expression of all four α-globin genes is suppressed or silenced,[489] but this phenomenon is difficult to document in total blood as long as some normal erythroid cells are being produced.

Until recently, the molecular basis of this fascinating disorder remained unknown. Cytogenetic, gene mapping, gene sequencing, and gene or chromosome transfer studies failed to detect any deletion or mutation in the α-globin gene cluster or functional abnormality of α-globin gene of affected patients. The results of all of these prior studies suggested that the defect responsible for this disorder probably involved the abnormal expression or function of a trans-acting factor capable of influencing α-globin gene expression and, indeed, such a factor was recently identified. The discovery of the factor responsible for Hb H disease in MDS results from cDNA microarray analysis of RNA isolated from granulocytes of an affected patient. One of the genes that was found to be markedly underexpressed, compared with results obtained with RNA of normal granulocytes, was the ATRX gene,[490] the same gene that is mutated in the α-thalassemia with mental retardation syndrome of the ATR-X type. Sequence analysis of the ATRX gene in the DNA of blood cells of affected individuals has identified a number of different mutations. It is noteworthy that the mutations of the ATRX gene associated with acquired Hb H disease associated with MDS (ATMDS) occur in the same regions of the gene as the mutations associated with the ATR-X syndrome, that is, in the ADD or helicase domains. In fact, some of the ATRX gene mutations identified in ATMDS are identical or similar in expected functional consequences to various mutations found in the ATR-X syndrome.

The hematologic features in the syndrome are characterized by the presence on blood smear of a dimorphic RBC population, one of which is hypochromic, microcytic, and poikilocytic. Incubation of the blood with the supravital stain brilliant cresyl blue results in the detection of typical Hb H inclusions. Hb electrophoresis or high pressure liquid chromatography detects the presence of Hb H, usually in greater quantities than that typically observed in inherited Hb H disease. In typical MDS, the MCV of the erythrocytes is normal or elevated, frequently higher than 100 fL. However, in ATMDS, the MCV and MCH are low: MCV usually less than 80 fL and MCH usually less than 26 pg.[488] The amount of Hb H usually remains stable but may actually decrease during the course of the disease and no longer persists after transformation of MDS to acute leukemia. This finding suggests that the Hb H–producing clone does not have a selective survival or growth advantage.

The hematologic phenotype, as reflected by the amount of Hb H present in blood, of ATMDS is much more severe than that of the ATR-X syndrome.[486] Some of this difference in severity may be because of the nature of the ATMDS mutations, some of which are null mutations that are likely to be lethal when present in germline DNA of ATR-X embryos. However, the difference in severity is also observed in the case of mutations found in both syndromes that are identical or similar in expected functional consequences. This finding suggests that additional abnormalities in gene expression in ATMDS contribute to the severity of the deficit in *α-globin* gene expression observed in this syndrome. Perhaps the responsible defective cofactor(s) is one or more of the proteins that interact with the ATRX protein to produce a fully functional macromolecular complex that can act as a transcriptional cofactor or that can influence the epigenetic control of *α-globin* gene expression.

THALASSEMIC STRUCTURAL VARIANTS

Certain structural Hb variants are characterized by the presence of a biosynthetic defect as well as abnormal structure.[6] Thalassemic hemoglobinopathies are unusual forms of thalassemia caused by such structural variants.

Hemoglobin Lepore

Hb Lepore ($\alpha 2\beta\delta$) is the prototype of a group of hemoglobinopathies characterized by fused globin chains.[1-4] The chains begin with a normal δ-chain sequence at their N-terminus and end with the normal β-chain sequence at their C-terminus. These hemoglobinopathies arise by unequal or nonhomologous crossover or recombination events that fuse the proximal end of one gene with the distal end of a closely linked structurally homologous gene (Fig. 40.16). During meiosis, mispairing and crossover of the highly homologous δ- and β-globin genes can occur, resulting in a Lepore chromosome, which contains (in addition to *γ-globin* genes) only the fused *δβ gene*, and an anti-Lepore chromosome, which contains the reciprocal fusion product ($\delta\beta$), as well as intact δ- and *β-globin* genes.[1]

Lepore globin is synthesized in low amounts, presumably because it is under the control of the *δ-globin* gene promoter, which normally sustains transcription at only 2.5% the level of the *β-globin* gene.[491] Patients with Hb Lepore have the phenotype of β-thalassemia, distinguished by the added presence of 5% to 15% Hb Lepore. In contrast, the anti-Lepore globin (Miyada) is not associated with a β-thalassemia phenotype because of the presence of an intact and functionally normal *β-globin* gene on the same chromosome.

An analogous but rare variant, Hb Kenya [$\alpha 2(A\gamma\beta)2$], arises from nonhomologous crossing over between the $^A\gamma$ and *β-globin* genes[492] and is associated with the phenotype of Gγ hereditary persistence of fetal Hb. A DNA sequence approximately 600 bases downstream from the *β-globin* gene acts as a strong enhancer, promoting the erythroid-specific expression of the *β-globin* genes in adult cells.[3,4,21] The fused $^A\gamma\beta$ gene as well as the linked upstream $^G\gamma$ gene are believed to come under the influence of the enhancer because of its abnormal proximity and thus are expressed at high levels in adult life.

Hb E

Hb E ($\alpha_2\beta_2^{26Glu\rightarrow Lys}$) is a common variant (15–30% of the population) in Cambodia, Thailand, parts of China, and Vietnam. Hb E is very mildly unstable, but this instability does not significantly alter the life span of RBCs. Hb E trait resembles very mild β-thalassemia trait. Homozygotes exhibit more microcytosis but are still asymptomatic.[493] Compound heterozygotes for Hb E and a β-thalassemia gene (Hb E-β-thalassemia) resemble patients with β-thalassemia intermedia or

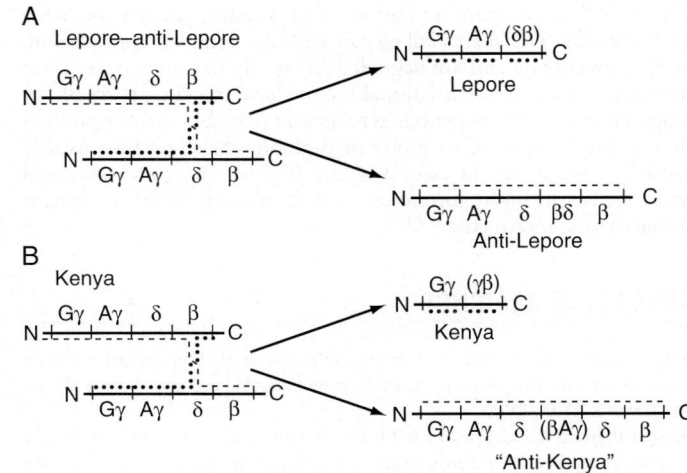

Fig. 40.16 GENETIC ORIGINS OF HEMOGLOBIN (HB) LEPORE, ANTI-LEPORE HB, AND HB KENYA. *(Adapted from Benz EJ Jr: The hemoglobinopathies. In Kelly WN, DeVita VT, editors: Textbook of internal medicine, Philadelphia, 1988, JB Lippincott, p 1423.)*

β-thalassemia major. However, some problems such as infection and pulmonary hypertension may occur more commonly in Hb E-β-thalassemia than in homozygous β-thalassemia.[494]

The only nucleotide sequence abnormality found in the β^E-gene is a base change in codon 26 that causes the amino acid substitution. This mutation, which occurs in a potential cryptic RNA splice region, alters the consensus sequence surrounding a potential GT donor splice site and thus activates the cryptic site. Alternative splicing at this position occurs approximately 40% to 50% of the time, generating a structurally abnormal globin mRNA that cannot be translated appropriately.[495] The other mRNA precursors are spliced at the normal site, generating functionally normal mRNA, which is translated into β^E-globin because the mature mRNA retains the base change that encodes lysine at codon 26.

Hb Constant Spring

Hb Constant Spring (see Fig. 40.14) is an elongated α-globin variant resulting from a mutation that alters the normal translation termination codon.[496] Polyribosomes read through the usual translation stop site and incorporate an additional 31 amino acids until another in-phase termination codon is reached within the 3′ untranslated sequence. The amount of α^{cs} mRNA is markedly reduced, and α^{cs}-globin is synthesized in only minute amounts.[459,497] Six possible mutations of the normal translation termination codon (UAA) in α-globin mRNA could result in the generation of a "sense" codon.[498] Of these, five variants have been identified, each having a markedly underproduced abnormal variant, indicating that disruption of normal translation termination is in some way associated with abnormal mRNA accumulation, presumably because of instability of the mRNA.[459] The output of α-globin from the α^{cs} allele is only approximately 1% of normal, and the gene is thus rendered α-thalassemic. The α^{cs} allele has been identified only on chromosomes containing a *cis*-linked functionally normal *α-globin* gene.[1-4] Thus, α^+-thalassemia trait and Hb H disease–(- /$\alpha^{cs}\alpha$) associated with Hb Constant Spring are common, but hydrops fetalis caused by four abnormal *α-globin* genes cannot occur in association with this variant. Homozygosity for the variant is associated with a relatively mild form of Hb H disease.[1]

EXTRAORDINARILY UNSTABLE HEMOGLOBINS

Rare cases of α-thalassemia (e.g., Hb Quong Sze)454 and β-thalassemia (e.g., Hb Indianapolis, recently renamed Hb Terre

Haute)[499,500] arise from mutations that produce extremely labile globin chains. The chains fail to pair with the complementary chain, or they precipitate and are degraded so rapidly that they never form tetramers. These posttranslational lesions have the same pathophysiologic effects on Hb biogenesis as reduction of globin mRNA production or function. Another group of β-globin chain variants, usually caused by mutations in exon 3 of the *β-globin* gene, are associated with inclusion body formation and a phenotype of dominant β-thalassemia intermedia.[15,16,501]

SUGGESTED READINGS

Angelopoulos NG, Goula A, Rombopoulos G, et al: Hypoparathyroidism in transfusion-dependent patients with beta-thalassemia. *J Bone Miner Metab* 24:138, 2006.

Borgna-Pignatti C, Cappellini MD, De Stefano P, et al: Cardiac morbidity and mortality in deferoxamine- or deferiprone-treated patients with thalassemia major. *Blood* 107:3733, 2006.

Boulad F: Hematopoietic stem cell transplantation for the treatment of beta thalassemia. In Kline R, editor: *Pediatric hematopoietic stem cell transplantation*, New York, 2006, Informa Healthcare, p 383.

Cappellini MD, Cohen A, Piga A, et al: A phase 3 study of deferasirox (ICL670), a once-daily oral iron chelator, in patients with beta-thalassemia. *Blood* 107:3455, 2006.

Cohen A, Glimm E, Porter JB: Effect of transfusional iron intake on response to chelation therapy in β-thalassemia major. *Blood* 111:583, 2008.

Dodd RY: Current safety of the blood supply in the United States. *Int J Hematol* 80:301, 2004.

Gilfillan CP, Strauss BJ, Rodda CP, et al: A randomized, double-blind, placebo-controlled trial of intravenous zoledronic acid in the treatment of thalassemia-associated osteopenia. *Calcif Tissue Int* 79:138, 2006.

Harmatz P, Grady R, Dragsten P, et al: Phase Ib clinical trial of starch-conjugated deferoxamine (40SD02): a novel long-acting iron chelator. *Br J Haematol* 138:374, 2007.

Harmatz P, Olivieri N, Kwiatkowski J, et al: Safety and efficacy of peginterferon alfa-2a and ribavirin for hepatitis C in thalassemia. *Blood* 108:558, 2006.

Hongeng S, Pakakasama S, Chuansumrit A, et al: Outcomes of transplantation with related- and unrelated-donor stem cells in children with severe thalassemia. *Biol Blood Marrow Transplant* 12:683, 2006.

Kattamis A, Ladis V, Berdousi H, et al: Iron chelation treatment with combined therapy with deferiprone and deferoxamine: a 12-month trial. *Blood Cells Mol Dis* 36:21, 2006.

Kolnagou A, Economides C, Eracleous E, et al: Low serum ferritin levels are misleading for detecting cardiac iron overload and increase the risk of cardiomyopathy in thalassemia patients: the importance of cardiac iron overload monitoring using magnetic resonance imaging T2 and T2*. *Hemoglobin* 30:219, 2006.

Kolnagou A, Kontoghiorghes GJ: Effective combination therapy of deferiprone and deferoxamine for the rapid clearance of excess cardiac iron and the prevention of heart disease in thalassemia. The Protocol of the International Committee on Oral Chelators. *Hemoglobin* 30:239, 2006.

Neufeld EJ: Oral chelators deferasirox and deferiprone for transfusional iron overload in thalassemia major: new data, new questions. *Blood* 107:3436, 2006.

Pennell DJ, Berdoukas V, Karagiorga M, et al: Randomized controlled trial of deferiprone or deferoxamine in beta-thalassemia major patients with asymptomatic myocardial siderosis. *Blood* 107:3738, 2006.

Rachmilewitz EA, Giardina PJ: How I treat Thalassemia. *Blood* 118:3479, 2011.

Tanner M, Galanello R, Dessi C, et al: A randomized placebo controlled double blind trial of the effect of combination therapy with deferoxamine and deferiprone on myocardial iron in thalassemia major using cardiovascular magnetic resonance. *Blood* 106:1017A, 2006.

Vogiatzi MG, Macklin EA, Fung EB, et al: Prevalence of fractures among the Thalassemia syndromes in North America. *Bone* 38:571, 2006.

Voskaridou E, Anagnostopoulos A, Konstantopoulos K, et al: Zoledronic acid for the treatment of osteoporosis in patients with beta-thalassemia: results from a single-center, randomized, placebo-controlled trial. *Haematologica* 91:1193, 2006.

Wood JC, Otto-Duessel M, Gonzalez I, et al: Deferasirox and deferiprone remove cardiac iron in the iron-overloaded gerbil. *Transl Res* 148:272, 2006.

REFERENCES

For the complete list of references, log on to www.expertconsult.com.

CHAPTER 41

PATHOBIOLOGY OF SICKLE CELL DISEASE

Robert P. Hebbel and Gregory M. Vercellotti

Since it was recognized as the "first molecular disease," sickle cell anemia caused by homozygosity for the mutant sickle beta globin gene has provided the classic paradigm for single-gene disorders. Predominant clinical features include hemolytic anemia, episodic painful events, chronic organ deterioration, disparate acute and chronic complications, and a foreshortened life span. The genesis of clinical sickle cell disease is complicated, and an understanding of its pathophysiology integrates concepts from multiple disciplines, includes contributions from the red blood cell (RBC) membrane and the vascular wall endothelium, and recognizes the likely participation of multiple genetic influences. This chapter addresses the pathophysiology that underlies the sickle cell disease syndromes described in Chapter 42.

EARLY YEARS OF SICKLE CELL DISEASE RESEARCH

Sickle disease syndromes were known in folk medicine for centuries in parts of Africa, but the eponymous RBC was first reported in the medical literature in 1910 when Herrick described a young Grenadian man with recurrent pain, anemia, and sickle-shaped red corpuscles in the blood (Fig. 41.1). In 1940, Ham and Castle postulated that sickle disease pathophysiology resulted from a "vicious cycle" involving mutually promotive erythrostasis and RBC sickling with adverse viscosity changes. In 1949, Neel validated the Mendelian autosomal dominant inheritance of sickle cell anemia, and Pauling demonstrated presence of an abnormal hemoglobin (Hb) in patients and carriers. This was followed by observation of the poor solubility of deoxygenated sickle Hb (HbS) and the reversible sol-gel transformation of HbS solutions. In 1957, Ingram identified the underlying amino acid substitution. Thereafter, increasingly detailed investigations began to reveal the striking complexities of sickle cell disease pathobiology.

GENETIC CONSIDERATIONS

Molecular Context

The sickle mutation in the *HBB* gene is a GAG→GTG conversion that creates a $\beta^{6Glu\rightarrow Val}$ substitution and thereby forms β^S globin chains. Genes for other β-globin variants are allelic to the β^S gene and have a codominant impact. Examples include genes for the normal β chain (β^A), β mutants (e.g., β^C, β^0 or β^+ thalassemia), and deletional hereditary persistence of fetal Hb (HPFH). Compound heterozygosity for β^S and each one of these results in well-defined clinical syndromes, such as HbAS (i.e., sickle trait), HbSC disease, HbS–β-thalassemia, and HbS-HPFH. Eight percent of African Americans have a β^S gene, 3% have β^C, 1.5% have β-thalassemia, and 0.1% have HPFH. Among African Americans, about 1 in 600 births results in the homozygous state, sickle cell anemia (HbSS), and about 1 in 400 results in some form of sickle cell disease, which additionally includes the compound heterozygous variants other than sickle trait. Worldwide, about 75% of sickle cell anemia births now occur in sub-Saharan Africa, 15% in India, 5% in the Americas, 4% in the Eastern Mediterranean, 1% in Europe.

The *HBB* gene resides in a cluster of β-like genes within which are various nonexonic polymorphic sites. Different combinations of these define discrete β-locus background haplotypes, referred to as the Senegal, Benin, Bantu, Cameroon, and Arab–India haplotypes (Fig. 41.2). Each designation refers to an ethnographic region in which the sickle mutation achieved high gene frequency (typically peaking at 0.10 to 0.15). In most cases, the sickle gene resides on one of these five major haplotypes.

Origin, Selection, and Dispersion of the Sickle Gene

The residence of both β^A and β^S alleles on the distinct regional β cluster haplotypes suggests that the sickle mutation arose independently in the five regions. The β^C mutation arose only once. Historical and biologic data argue that frequency of the β^S gene greatly expanded in Africa about 3000 years ago and in South Asia about 4000 years ago, following the introduction of iron tools. That led to adoption of an agricultural system that promoted both increased human habitation density and favorable breeding conditions for the mosquito vector, *Anopheles,* which in turn enabled development of endemic *Plasmodium falciparum.* In this context, high fixed β^S gene frequencies were reached because of a balanced polymorphism, such that heterozygotes (HbAS) have an adaptive advantage over either homozygote. Thus the Old World geographic distributions of the sickle gene and historical endemic malaria are notably concordant (see Fig. 41.2), suggesting that the sickle gene represents "a biologic solution to a cultural problem."

In hyperendemic areas, *falciparum* malaria uniformly infects the young and is the primary cause of death for children with sickle cell anemia. However, those with sickle trait are less likely to develop high-level parasitemia or to have severe malaria, an effect largely exerted early in childhood. At the level of the RBC, this protection reflects steps after initial parasite invasion. One proposed mechanism links protection to the instability of HbS, immune status, and splenic function. Infection of sickle trait RBCs with *P. falciparum* leads sequentially to augmented Hb denaturation, clustering of membrane protein band 3, attraction of band 3 autoantibody, complement binding, and enhanced erythrophagocytosis, even of the early ring forms. Thereby, an accelerated clearance of parasitized RBC by the spleen could protect those with sickle trait, while HbS homozygotes would lose this protection because of acquiring functional asplenia. In synergy with this scenario, presence of HbS (via a different mechanism) impairs microvascular endothelial cytoadherence of infected RBC, thereby diminishing cerebral symptoms and impeding the sequestration that protects parasitized RBC from splenic exposure. The protective benefit of HbAS is lost if there is concurrent alpha thalassemia (which lowers proportion of HbS). Yet, the blunted malarial susceptibility in sickle trait reflects a complex interrelationship among the sickle gene, host biology, and environmental factors. Malarial severity is affected by polymorphisms in nonglobin genes such as *CR1* (complement receptor 1), *CD36*, *TGFB1* (transforming growth factor β), and *HMOX1* (heme oxygenase 1); a polymorphism in *TLR4* (toll-like receptor 4) prevalent in sub-Saharan Africa exerts a protective effect. Both carbon monoxide (CO) and nitric oxide (NO) blunt severity of experimental malaria. And certain microRNA, enriched in HbS-containing RBC, can inhibit *P. falciparum* growth.

Eventually, the sickle gene spread geographically by means of commerce, migration, and the slave trade. This dispersion has been tracked by analyses of regional β haplotypes, a biologic marker that

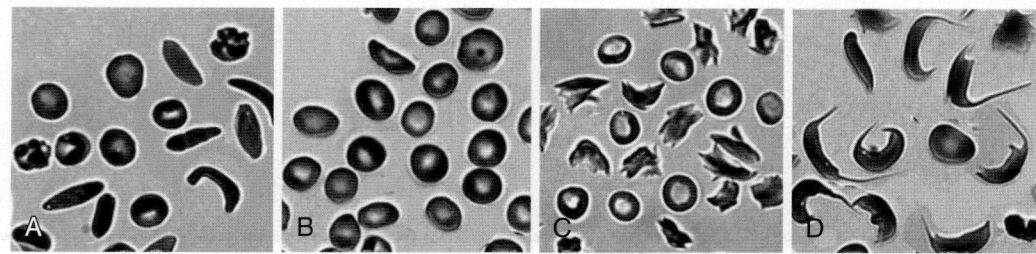

Fig. 41.1 SICKLE RED BLOOD CELL (RBC) MORPHOLOGIES. Blood smears prepared under differing conditions, using antecubital blood from the same sickle cell anemia patient. (A) Venous blood at a P_{O_2} ~40 mm Hg was fixed immediately to document RBC shapes occurring in vivo. Several RBC morphologies are evident, including two granular (raisin-like) cells, five somewhat elongated cells, and two highly elongated and curved cells. (B) Unfixed blood was fully oxygenated. Most cells resumed normal shape, but one elongated, irreversibly sickled cell remains present. (C) The oxygenated cells from (B) were then partially deoxygenated, upon which they assumed classic holly-leaf forms typical of rapid deoxygenation. (D) The partially deoxygenated cells from (C) were then fully deoxygenated (P_{O_2} ~ 0 mm Hg) and display the more elongated shape having fewer spikes that is assumed by sickle RBC that have deoxygenated more slowly. The physical–chemical basis for these shapes is presented in Fig. 41.5. *(Reproduced with permission from Obata K, Mattiello J, Asakura K, et al: Exposure of blood from patients with sickle cell disease to air changes the morphological, oxygen-binding, and sickling properties of sickled erythrocytes. Am J Hematol 81:26, 2006).*

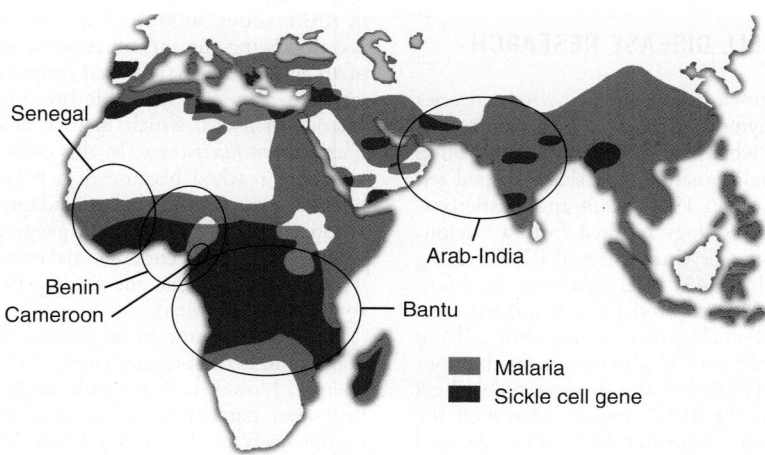

Fig. 41.2 SICKLE GENE AND MALARIA. The five regions in which the sickle gene achieved high allelic frequency are superimposed on shading that identifies the Old World distribution of the sickle gene and of historic, endemic malaria. *(Reproduced with permission from Friedman MJ, Trager W: The biochemistry of resistance to malaria. Sci Am 244:154, 1981; and from Nagel RL, Steinberg MH: Genetics of the β^S gene: origins, epidemiology, and epistasis in sickle cell anemia. In Steinberg MH: Forget BG, Higgs DR, Nagel RL, editors: Disorders of hemoglobin: Genetics, pathophysiology, and clinical management, Cambridge, 2001, Cambridge University Press, p 711.)*

largely corroborates predictions of gene flow derived from historical records. As a generalization, it spread on the Benin haplotype to North Africa and then across the Mediterranean. All three major African haplotypes are present in the western Arabian Peninsula; but on the eastern side, the sickle gene tends to be on the Arab-India haplotype. This is also true in India, although sub-Saharan haplotypes are represented as well. In the Americas, the β^S gene is mostly found on the Benin, Senegal, and Bantu haplotypes.

ABNORMAL MOLECULAR BEHAVIORS OF SICKLE HEMOGLOBIN

Because the $\beta^{6Glu \to Val}$ substitution entails a loss of negative charge and gain in hydrophobicity, HbS exhibits three abnormal molecular behaviors of direct relevance to pathophysiology.

Relationship of HbS Molecular Behaviors to Disease Features
Altered dimer assembly → RBC Hb composition
Hb phenotype and diagnosis
Polymerization risk
HbS instability → Membrane defects
RBC dehydration
Hemolysis
Malaria resistance
HbS polymerization → Sickling
Vasoocclusion
Hemolysis

Hemoglobin S Charge and Tetramer Assembly

Formation of Hb tetramers requires proximate assembly of stable dimers from unlike monomers (e.g., $\alpha + \beta \rightarrow \alpha\beta$), an event governed by electrostatic attraction. The normal α and β chains are positively and negatively charged, respectively. In heterozygous states for β-globin mutants, β-chain competition for dimer assembly is a determinant of the relative proportions of the Hb variants.[1] Mutant β chains with lowered negative charge form $\alpha\beta$ dimers more slowly; the relative rates for dimer association are $\alpha\beta^A > \alpha\beta^S > \alpha\beta^C$, with $\alpha\beta^A$ dimers formed about twice as rapidly as $\alpha\beta^S$ dimers. This explains why those with sickle trait typically have only 40% HbS and why the proportion of HbS exceeds this in HbSC disease. It also explains the effect of concurrent α-thalassemia on the proportion of HbS in sickle trait; as availability of α chains becomes limiting, the percentage of HbS typically drops from 40% to 35% (one α deletion), 30% (two α deletions), or less than 25% (three α deletions).

Hemoglobin S Stability and Oxidant Formation

HbS is modestly unstable, observed in vitro as instability to various applied stresses. Two stresses that are most clearly physiologic involve Hb oxidation.[2] HbS has an abnormal redox potential compared with HbA that may underlie its only modestly (~40%) increased autooxidation rate. Yet, HbS exhibits markedly (~340%) augmented instability and oxidation upon interaction with aminophospholipids characteristic of the membrane's inner leaflet. Its behavior once it enters the plasma environment (caused by intravascular hemolysis) is unknown. Although the physical–chemical mechanism of the destabilizing role of the β^6 valine in HbS is not known, this instability leads to accumulation of various Hb and iron forms at the cytosol–membrane interface.[2] The resulting occurrence of abnormal, oxidative biochemistry promotes a number of prominent defects of the sickle RBC membrane.

Hemoglobin S Solubility and Hemoglobin S Polymerization

Oxy-HbS, oxy-HbA, and deoxy-HbA have very high solubilities, but deoxy-HbS aggregates into densely packed polymers, a process that is fully reversible with reoxygenation.[3,4] This abnormal property causes the eponymous RBC shape change from polymer-mediated distortion, the fundamental basis for disease promotion in sickling disorders.

Polymer Structure

Deoxygenation transforms soluble HbS into a highly viscous and semisolid gel that behaves thermodynamically similar to a crystal in equilibrium with a solution of individual tetrameric Hb molecules. Even complete deoxygenation does not convert all deoxy-HbS to polymer. The insoluble phase is a collection of domains of aligned polymers, the basic unit of which is a double strand in which two strings of deoxy-Hb tetramers make multiple contacts with each other (Fig. 41.3).

Each HbS tetramer has two β^S chains, the β_1 and β_2. Deoxy-HbS undergoes a slight structural shift so that the A helix β^{6Val} "donor" site of the β_2 chain in one tetramer can contact an EF helix "acceptor" site (formed mainly by β^{85Phe}, β^{88Leu}, and β^{70Ala}) in the β_1 chain of a tetramer in the neighboring single string. This critical, lateral association can be made only when HbS is in its deoxy conformation; the EF helix hydrophobic pocket is not a favorable acceptor site for the charged β^{6Glu} of the β^A in HbA. In HbS, the β^{6Val} in the β_1 subunit is located so it cannot participate in such contacts. However, the β_2 chain of the second single string can form chemically similar β^{6Val}-dependent contacts with the β_1 chain of the first single string. There are multiple additional axial and lateral contacts, but these are largely the same for deoxy-HbA and deoxy-HbS and are not themselves sufficient to stabilize a polymeric structure.

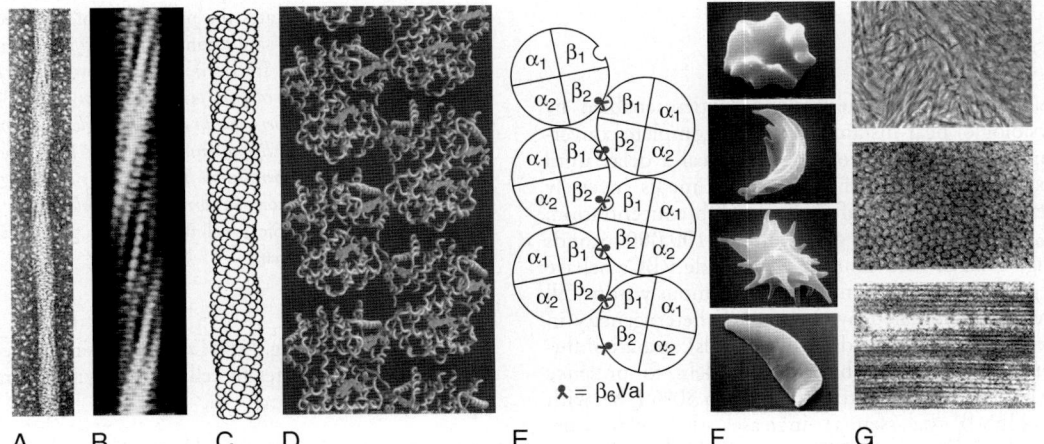

Fig. 41.3 DEOXYGENATED HEMOGLOBIN S (HbS) POLYMER. (A) Electron micrograph of a fiber of polymerized HbS obtained from a sickled red blood cell. (B) Electron density surface map, modeled from authentic HbS fibers, shows pairings that create double strands plus a helical twist. (C) Model of the HbS fiber, with Hb tetramers rendered as solid spheres. (D) Protein backbone shows tetramer staggering in the HbS crystal. (E) Schematic representation of a double strand, emphasizing that only one of the two β^6 valine residues in each HbS tetramer participates in critical lateral contacts. (F) Sickled red blood cells, showing various morphologies *(top to bottom):* granular, holly leaf shaped, classically sickled, and smoother and irreversibly sickled. (G) Electron microscopy of sickled RBC cytoplasm reveals highly ordered polymer domains, as seen from the side *(bottom)* and on end *(middle),* or highly disorganized domains *(top).* (A and C, *Reproduced with permission from Dykes G, Crepeau RH, Edelstein SJ: Three-dimensional reconstruction of the fibres of sickle cell hemoglobin.* Nature *272:506,1978; B, reproduced with permission from Carragher B, Bluemke DA, Becker M, et al: Structural analysis of polymers of sickle cell hemoglobin.* J Mol Biol *199:315,1988; D, reproduced with permission from Harrington DJ, Adachi K, Royer WE, Jr: The high resolution crystal structure of deoxyhemoglobin S.* J Mol Biol *272:398, 1997; F and G, courtesy Dr. James G. White and reproduced with permission from White JG: Ultrastructural features of erythrocyte and hemoglobin sickling.* Arch Intern Med *133:545, 1974.)*

In the physiologic form of the polymer, the component strings of Hb molecules in a double strand are half-staggered and have a slight twist, creating a fiber that is approximately 21 nM in diameter and is composed of one central and six peripheral double strands. The crystal formed in vitro lacks the twist, but its molecular structure is known in great detail.

Role of Hemoglobin S Solubility

The RBC's hydration state dominates the physical-chemical behavior of HbS. The solubility of deoxy-HbS (approximately 16 g/dL, measured under laboratory conditions) is much lower than the RBC mean cell Hb concentration (MCHC). So, even partial cellular deoxygenation can raise deoxy-HbS concentration above its solubility limit, allowing polymerization to occur. The biophysical effect of macromolecular crowding (boosting a protein's activity far above that predicted from concentration alone) confers nonideal behavior upon cytoplasmic constituents, augmenting likelihood for polymerization at any given degree of deoxygenation.

In vitro studies carried out under (nonphysiologic) equilibrium conditions of stable oxygen tension and long-time scale corroborate crystallographic identification of critical amino acids involved in atomic contacts by revealing the influence of other Hbs on HbS solubility (Fig. 41.4).[3] When different Hbs are mixed together, the tetramers dissociate into dimers that intermix and randomly assemble in a binomial distribution to reform tetramers. This clarifies the impact of naturally occurring, intracellular Hb mixtures. In mixtures of HbS and HbA, overall solubility is improved because the hybrid $\alpha\beta^S/\alpha\beta^A$ tetramer integrates into polymer only one half as well as the $\alpha\beta^S/\alpha\beta^S$ tetramer (Fig. 41.4A). Addition of HbF to HbS has a greater sparing effect because neither the $\alpha\gamma/\alpha\gamma$ nor the hybrid $\alpha\beta^S/\alpha\gamma$ tetramer can be incorporated into polymer. In this regard, HbC has the same effect as HbA, and HbA_2 has the same effect as HbF (see Fig. 41.4A). This sparing effect of HbA is such that much lower Hb oxygen saturation is required for polymer to form in HbAS than in HbSS RBCs (Fig. 41.4B).

Kinetics of Polymerization

Laboratory measurements of polymerization kinetics, enabled by inducing (nonphysiologic) near-instantaneous and complete conversion of HbS from R (oxy) to T (deoxy) state, reveal a delay until polymer forms explosively.[4] This inherent delay time is inversely related to an extremely high power of the initial Hb concentration; it is approximately 10 ms at Hb of 40 g/dL, but it is 100,000 seconds at Hb 20 g/dL (Fig. 41.5A). HbS solutions and sickle RBCs behave similarly in this regard. Delay times must vary enormously from cell to cell because they are dominated by the marked heterogeneity in MCHC (i.e., shorter delay for more dehydrated cells) and are influenced by the presence of any non-S Hb (i.e., longer delay for presence of HbA, C, or F) (Fig. 41.5E). Admixture of 20% to 30% HbA with HbS (simulating HbS-β⁺-thalassemia) increases the delay time 10 to 100 fold, and admixture of 20% to 30% HbF with HbS increases it by 10^3- to 10^4-fold.

The mechanism of such polymer formation is hypothesized to proceed by a two-step, double-nucleation process (Fig. 41.5F). Accordingly, the initial homogeneous nucleation takes place in bulk solution, during which small numbers of tetramers associate, with accumulation not favored until a critical nucleus size develops (estimated to be 30 to 50 tetramers). Only then can new tetramers be added lengthwise to form a large polymer. After this occurs, heterogeneous nucleation causes explosive, autocatalytic polymer formation as new fibers form and extend on the surface of the preexisting polymer. It is the time until this explosive formation occurs that laboratory experiments detect as the inherent delay time. It is believed that the striking irreproducibility of long delay times (Fig. 41.5B) reflects stochastic formation of a single (or at least very few) homogeneous nucleation event(s) in cells that slowly polymerize and that

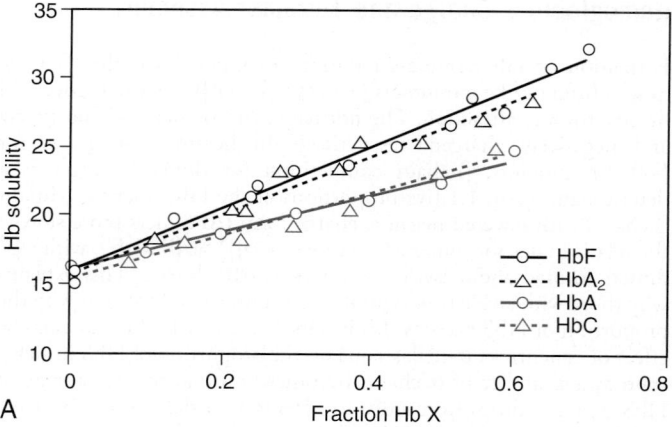

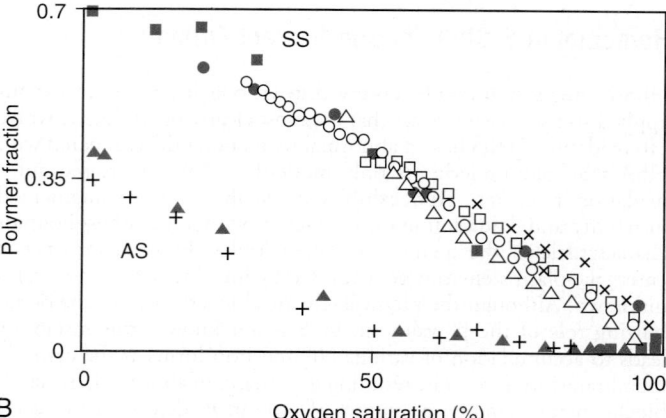

Fig. 41.4 DEOXYHEMOGLOBIN S SOLUBILITY, DEFINED BY STUDIES UNDER EQUILIBRIUM CONDITIONS. (A) Admixture of other hemoglobins with hemoglobin S raises overall solubility in absence of oxygen. The x-axis indicates the proportion of admixed nonsickle Hb. (B) The hemoglobin oxygen saturation required to initiate intracellular polymer formation (i.e., polymer fraction) is much lower for HbAS RBC than for HbSS RBC. (*A, Reproduced with permission from Poillon WN, Kim BC, Rodgers GP, et al: Sparing effect of hemoglobin F and hemoglobin A₂ on the polymerization of hemoglobin S at physiologic ligand saturations.* Proc Natl Acad Sci U S A *90:5039, 1993; B, reproduced with permission from Schechter AN, Noguchi CT: Sickle hemoglobin polymer: Structure-function correlates. In Embury SH, Hebbel RP, Mohandas N, Steinberg MH, editors:* Sickle cell disease: Basic principles and clinical practice, *New York, 1994, Raven Press.*)

short delay times (Fig. 41.5D) reflect simultaneous formation of multiple nucleation sites in cells that polymerize rapidly.

Polymerization Under (Patho)physiologic Conditions

In physiology, sickle RBCs are neither at equilibrium with constant oxygen tension nor undergoing instantaneous or complete deoxygenation. Rather, irrespective of the inherent delay time, the rate of deoxy-HbS polymer growth in vivo is limited by the rate at which RBC deoxygenation develops during microvascular passage. Since this transit time is on the order of ~1 second, it probably effectively renders irrelevant any inherent delay times of less than ~1 second (Fig. 41.5G).[4] Thus kinetic considerations argue that most RBCs in patients with sickle cell anemia are unlikely to sickle during their passage through the microcirculation unless something, such as RBC–endothelial adhesion, slows their transit.

Predictability is complicated by the marked heterogeneity among sickle RBCs in MCHC and HbF content, as well as the natural biologic variability in capillary transit times. A good qualitative

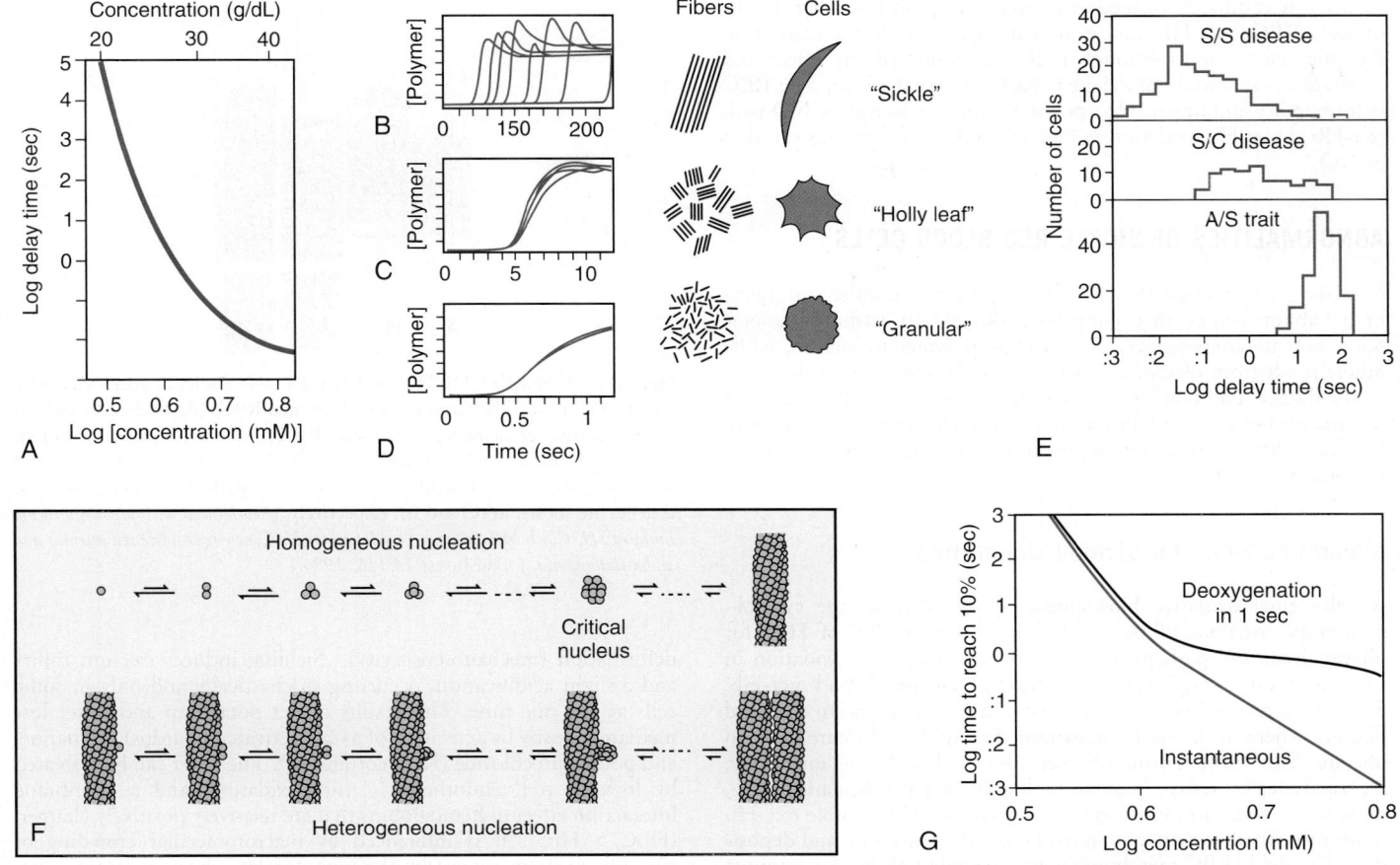

Fig. 41.5 KINETICS OF HEMOGLOBIN S POLYMERIZATION AFTER NEAR-INSTANTANEOUS AND COMPLETE DEOXYGENATION. (A) Extreme dependence of delay time on hemoglobin concentration. (B–D) Kinetic progress curves for polymer formation show that long delay times are highly variable (B), but very short delay times are highly reproducible (D). *To the right* is a representation of domains and corresponding RBC morphology postulated to result from these different scales of polymerization rate (see Fig. 41.1B–E; and Fig. 41.3F). (E) Delay times for individual RBCs are influenced by substituent hemoglobins. (F) A double nucleation process underlies polymer formation, with unfavored homogeneous nucleation (*top*) followed by explosive heterologous nucleation (*bottom*). (G) Physiologically, the finite rate of deoxygenation effectively caps the polymer growth rate and eliminates the relevance of delay times that are short relative to deoxygenation rate (<1 second). *(A–E, Reproduced with permission from Eaton WA, Hofrichter J: Hemoglobin S gelation and sickle cell disease.* Blood *70:1245, 1987; F, reproduced with permission from Ferrone FA, Hofrichter J, Eaton WA: Kinetics of sickle hemoglobin polymerization II. A double nucleation mechanism.* J Mol Biol *183:611, 1985; G, reproduced with permission from Ferrone FA: Oxygen transits and transports. In Embury S, Hebbel RP, Mohandas N, Steinberg MH, editors:* Sickle Cell Disease: Basic Principles and Clinical Practice, *New York, 1994, Raven Press.)*

correspondence between polymerization in solution and within RBCs argues that the fundamental polymerization mechanism (Fig. 41.5F) is not altered by membranes. Yet, emerging evidence indicates that the abnormal sickle RBC membrane can accelerate nucleation, in essence eliminating the inherent delay time. A similar effect would be exerted by any preexisting polymer not completely melted during prior pulmonary transit (expected for fewer than 1% of RBCs). However, neither of these effects would alter the physiologic constraint that bulk polymer growth rate can only parallel RBC deoxygenation rate.

In vitro, sickle RBC can become classically sickled or assume holly leaf or granular forms, depending on deoxygenation rate (slow to rapid, respectively), which determines the number of nucleation domains created (Fig. 41.5B–D; and see Fig. 41.1B–E). In the microcirculation, granular forms are most likely to occur; in contrast, frankly sickled forms are most likely to develop during venous return to the heart. The RBC shape per se is not a determinant of RBC deformability, but rigidification caused by polymer can impede microvascular passage. This would develop dynamically during microvascular transit.

HbF and Its Protective Effect

In sickle cell anemia, HbF in RBC lysates averages ~5% to 8% (range 1% to 25%). However, this HbF is not distributed evenly amongst RBCs.[5] Rather, its heterocellular expression is evident in the presence of F cells (RBC particularly enriched in HbF) that comprise anywhere between 2% and 80% of all RBCs. For most patients, only the small proportion of their F cells that contain at least ~10 pg HbF (roughly one-third of RBC Hb content) are expected to be protected from polymerization under physiologic conditions.[5] Nonetheless, on average, F cells remain better hydrated and exhibit better survival.

Alternative Ligands: Carbon Monoxide and Nitric Oxide

Patients with sickle cell anemia can have nontrivial elevations of CO-Hb levels (reportedly as high as 7.6% in children) because of hemolysis. Hb that is partially liganded with CO is shifted to the R state conformation but has lost a portion of its oxygen carrying capacity. It is difficult to predict whether this produces a net benefit or loss. RBC and Hb appear to participate in NO transport to the microcirculation, although both magnitude of the effect and mechanisms involved are debated. NO is asserted to improve RBC deformability and impair HbS polymerization. Reaction of NO with oxy-Hb causes Hb oxidation to met-Hb and reciprocal consumption of NO.[6]

ABNORMALITIES OF SICKLE RED BLOOD CELLS

Even oxygenated sickle RBCs exhibit a variety of cellular and membrane abnormalities that contribute directly to pathophysiology. Some are the consequence of proximate polymer formation, while others result from oxidative biochemistry. An overarching theme in sickle disease pathobiology is that individual sickle RBC exhibit remarkable heterogeneity in various cellular characteristics. The striking variability in hydration status and HbF content is particularly important.

Membrane Iron and Oxidant Generation

An abnormal oxidative biochemistry takes place at the cytosol–membrane interface of the sickle RBC.[2] The avidity of HbS for bilayer lipid, and perhaps its modestly enhanced auto-oxidation in solution, result in augmented formation of superoxide and met-Hb. This, in turn, can become denatured and lose its heme to the lipid bilayer, where it is easily destroyed by lipid hydroperoxides to liberate "free" iron. Forms of iron associated with the membrane are catalytically active, generating highly reactive oxidants. Also, membrane "free" iron can form a redox couple with soluble oxy-Hb to promote further hemoglobin oxidation, denaturation, and deposition. The sickle RBC membrane thereby acquires abnormal amounts of various iron forms: Hb, denatured hemichrome, free heme, and nonheme iron.[2] A large portion of sickle RBC oxidant generation and stress is from enhanced nicotinamide adenine dinucleotide phosphate (NADPH)-oxidase activity, probably in reticulocytes and exhibiting a responsiveness to certain plasma substances, e.g., endothelin-1.

Of equal importance to excessive oxidant generation, the membrane location of catalytic iron establishes in sickle RBC a unique oxidant risk (not present in normal RBC) because it effectively targets oxidative damage to membrane components. Further, the juxtaposition of iron with bilayer lipid allows reinitiation of peroxidative chain reactions, effectively bypassing protection by vitamin E. Deficient levels of antioxidants (e.g., vitamin E, glutathione, ascorbic acid) in sickle RBC, caused by oxidative consumption and dietary insufficiencies, contribute. The result is abnormal oxidation of membrane protein thiols and peroxidation of membrane lipids. Among the many sickle membrane defects, evidence for an oxidative origin or contribution is strongest for Band 3 clustering, abnormal membrane stiffness, formation of irreversibly sickled cells (ISCs), aberrant cation homeostasis, tendency toward microvesiculation, abnormal mechanosensitivity, and erythrophagocytosis.[2]

Cation Homeostasis and Dehydrated Cells

For normal RBCs, MCHC averages ~32 g/dL and varies from 27 to 38 g/dL, with fewer than 1% of cells having MCHC greater than 38 g/dL. In contrast, the MCHC of sickle RBCs averages ~34 g/dL and ranges from 23 to 50 g/dL, with up to 40% of cells having MCHC greater than 38 g/dL. This extreme density heterogeneity results from reticulocytosis (low-density, low-MCHC cells) and dehydrating mechanisms (higher density, high-MCHC cells) (Fig. 41.6).

The most dramatic ion-handling abnormality of the sickle RBC is sickling-induced permeabilization of the RBC membrane to cations (Na⁺, K⁺, Ca²⁺). Since this depends on cell deformation, it probably partly reflects the sickle RBC's exaggerated leak susceptibility to

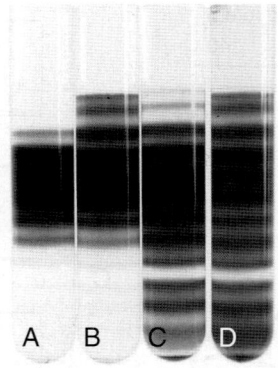

Fig. 41.6 MARKED HETEROGENEITY IN SICKLE RED BLOOD CELL HYDRATION. Compared with normal RBCs (A) studied by discontinuous density-gradient centrifugation, RBCs from a sickle patient with four α genes (D) include cells of unusually low density (mostly reticulocytes) and abnormally high density (dehydrated cells). Sickle patients with three and two α genes are shown in (C and B), respectively. *(Reproduced with permission from Embury SH, Clark MR, Monroy G, Mohandas N: Concurrent sickle cell anemia and alpha-thalassemia.* J Clin Invest *73:116, 1984.)*

deformation (mechanosensitivity).[7] Sickling induces calcium influx and a slight acidification, occurring stochastically and only in some cells at any one time. This results in net potassium and water loss mediated mostly by activation of a Ca²⁺ activated (Gardos) K⁺ channel and potassium chloride (KCl) cotransport. The latter can be activated by lowered pH, endothelin-1, thiol oxidation, and a membrane interaction effect of hemoglobins that are relatively positively charged (HbC > HbS). It is influenced by macromolecular crowding of cytosolic proteins caused by the high MCHC. Even at steady state, sickle RBCs contain increased Ca²⁺ because it is sequestered in cytoplasmic inside-out membrane vesicles, providing evidence of prior cytosolic Ca²⁺ transients.

These aberrancies lead to decrements in RBC hydration and deformability.[7] However, hyperdense RBCs—mostly ISCs—are not necessarily older cells with longer histories of sickling and unsickling. Rather, they can develop via a rapid reticulocyte-to-ISC transformation, with those RBC having lower HbF levels being particularly susceptible. It is unclear whether this rapid induction of cation loss or the gradualism of classic interpretations is the dominant mechanism underlying sickle RBC dehydration. Dehydrated RBCs have diminished deformability and increased propensity for polymerization, the mutually promotive effects of dehydration and sickling comprising a vicious cycle. RBC dehydration is particularly likely to be exaggerated by the renal medullary environment and possibly by nocturnal arterial desaturation accompanying disordered sleep.

Deformability, Fragility, and Vesiculation

Even oxygenated sickle RBCs are poorly deformable.[7] The dominant cause of this is the abnormally high cytoplasmic viscosity of dehydrated cells. Additional factors include abnormal stiffness of the RBC membrane caused, in part, by thiol oxidation and, in part, by a poorly understood direct effect of hemoglobin upon the membrane. Upon RBC deoxygenation in vitro, there is a temporal correspondence between appearance of polymer-induced shape change and deterioration of deformability, as measured by micropipette and laser diffractometer. On the other hand, filtration studies found decreased deformability before morphologic change, and viscometry reveals a large deterioration in bulk viscosity caused by deoxygenated dense discocytes that show little shape change.

Sickle RBCs are somewhat mechanically fragile, which may be a consequence of dehydration and a weakening of critical skeletal associations caused by oxidative protein damage. The tendency of sickled RBCs to lose membrane microvesicles reflects separation of

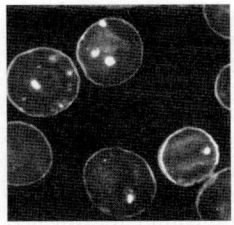
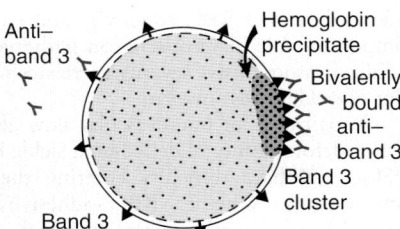

Fig. 41.7 BAND 3 AND IMMUNOGLOBULIN COCLUSTERING. Denatured Hb on the RBC membrane, is associated with clumping of Band 3, and opsonization by naturally occurring anti-Band 3 antibody. Clusters of band 3 are colocalized with immunoglobulin on the membranes of sickle red blood cells (*left*). The drawing shows the colocalization scheme (*right*). (*Reproduced with permission from Schluter K, Drenckhahn D: Co-clustering of denatured hemoglobin with band 3: Its role in binding of autoantibodies against band 3 to abnormal and aged erythrocytes.* Proc Natl Acad Sci U S A *83:6137, 1986.*)

Major Sickle RBC Membrane Defects

Membrane iron deposits →
  Band 3 clumping → Ig attraction → erythrophagocytosis
  Oxidative reactions targeted at membrane →
    Thiol oxidation →
      ISC formation
      ↓ Deformability and ↑ fragility
      PS externalization
      Cation leak
      Microvesiculation
    Lipid peroxidation →
      Mechanosensitivity
      Erythrophagocytosis
Abnormal cation homeostasis →
  RBC dehydration → ↓ deformability
Abnormal microrheology →
  ↓ Deformability
PS externalization →
  Coagulation acceleration
  Erythrophagocytosis
Adhesion to endothelium, monocytes, and macrophages
Enhanced mechanosensitivity → ↑ responsiveness to deformation

the bilayer from the underlying skeleton due to spicules of polymerized hemoglobin, with enhanced susceptibility caused by protein thiol oxidation.

Membrane Proteins and Lipids

Sickle RBC membrane protein function is adversely affected by thiol oxidation and possibly other oxidative protein modifications.[2] Ankyrin interactions with spectrin and Band 3 are abnormal, glycophorin and Band 3 exhibit decreased mobility, and thiol-oxidized β-actin displays abnormal associations in the spectrin–actin-4.1 complex. Band 3 is abnormally clumped from binding of denatured HbS, which enables attraction of naturally occurring anti-Band 3 immunoglobulin (Fig. 41.7).

Normal enforcement of bilayer phospholipid asymmetry is impaired in sickle RBCs. A scramblase that moves phosphatidylserine (PS) outward is activated by calcium transits, and a translocase that restores PS inwardly can be inhibited by thiol oxidation. RBC sickling promotes PS externalization, especially in ISCs, but also in some reticulocytes. Other changes include presence of peroxidation byproducts such as malondialdehyde (MDA) that can cross-link proteins. Notably, the increased presence of bilayer lipid hydroperoxides appears to account for the sickle RBC membrane's abnormal mechanosensitivity, evident in its enhanced cation leak response to deforming stress. Presumably, this deformation susceptibility

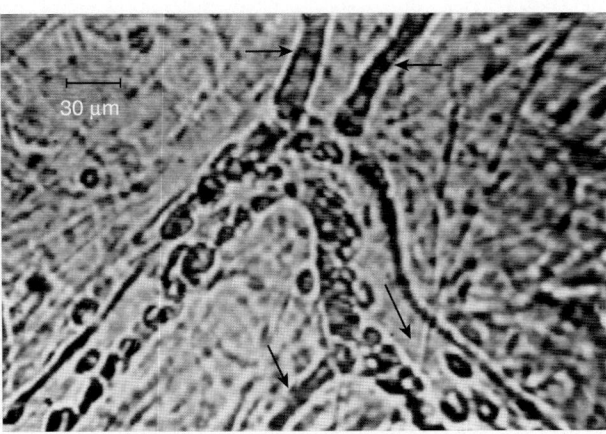

Fig. 41.8 RBC ADHESION TO ENDOTHELIUM. RBCs adhere to the vascular wall endothelium under flow conditions in the microcirculation of a rat infused with human cells. Immobile RBCs are on walls of the postcapillary venule, and the smaller feeder microvessels (*small arrows*) have no flow because of the logjam of RBC. (*Reproduced with permission from Kaul DK, Fabry ME, Nagel RL: Microvascular sites and characteristics of sickle cell adhesion to vascular endothelium in shear flow conditions: Pathophysiological implications.* Proc Natl Acad Sci U S A *86:3356, 1989.*)

contributes to various sickling-induced RBC responses, e.g., microvesiculation.

Irreversibly Sickled Cells

The sickled RBCs seen on a typically-obtained blood smear are mostly ISCs (see Fig. 41.1). Their permanent shape abnormality is caused not by retained polymer but rather by membrane retention of an elongated shape, explained by thiol oxidation of β-actin such that the spectrin–actin-4.1 complex exhibits abnormally slow dissociation. Otherwise, ISCs are similar to other equally dense RBC in having high MCHC, poor deformability, externalized PS, and low HbF content. ISC counts on average are higher in male patients, perhaps reflecting their average lower levels of HbF. The fundamental requirements for ISC formation seem to be RBC dehydration, prolonged deoxygenation, and assumption of a fixed membrane shape. Perhaps there is a prior "conditioning" residence in the microcirculation.

The clinical importance of ISCs lies in their ability to prompt diagnosis of a sickling disorder when seen on blood smear and in their short life span that contributes to overall hemolytic rate. They would contribute to the RBC logjam involved in occlusion, but it is unclear whether ISC count correlates with vasoocclusive manifestations. Although still adhesive to endothelium, ISCs are less so than other sickle subpopulations, but they exhibit greater adherence to macrophages.

Endothelial Adhesivity

Oxygenated sickle RBCs are abnormally adhesive to vascular endothelial cells (Fig. 41.8). About 20 candidate mechanisms have been implicated, most involving adhesion molecules on endothelium, adhesive structures restricted to reticulocytes or present on all RBCs, and with or without bridging by adhesogenic plasma proteins.[8] Some mechanisms require RBC signaling responses to plasma factors for activation. Involvement of mixed cell interactions with endothelium has been proposed. Most described candidate mechanisms involve adhesive reticulocytes and are high affinity, identified using flowing conditions. Yet, in the biologic context microcirculatory blood flow can be intermittent and occurs within vessels of constraining diameters enabling greater potential contact surface area. It seems probable that low-affinity adhesive mechanisms would gain relevance in that situation. Indeed, an unanswered question is whether or not RBC adhesion occurs via a single, dominant mechanism in vivo. To date, only RBC/endothelial adhesion mediated by $\alpha_v\beta_3$ and P-selectin have been verified in vivo in the sickle mouse, in which blockade of P-selectin inhibits adhesion of both RBCs and white blood cells (WBCs) to endothelium and effects improvement in blood flow.

Participation of sickle RBC adhesion in pathophysiology is governed, in part, by endothelial activation state. For example, adhesion events mediated by endothelial vascular cell adhesion molecule 1 (VCAM-1), $\alpha_v\beta_3$, and P-selectin are activated, respectively, by tumor necrosis factor (TNF), platelet activating factor, and thrombin. Each of these endothelial stimulants is elevated in sickle blood. However, there is a multitude of biologic modifiers in the sickle context that can influence endothelial surface features (see Box on Complex Sickle Milieu). Additional influencing factors would include: the reticulocyte count; flow and shear rates; vessel diameter, geometry and vasomotion; marginated WBCs; mixed blood cell interactions with endothelium; concurrent processes (e.g., degree of platelet activation or dehydration); and possibly even environmental exposure to endothelial toxins such as tobacco smoke.

Macrophage Interaction

Sickle RBCs are readily phagocytosed by macrophages because of RBC membrane modifications by malondialdehyde, PS externalization, and opsonization by immunoglobulin. The latter process is triggered by abnormal clustering of membrane protein Band 3 (see Fig. 41.7) and possibly by modification induced by malondialdehyde. The most dense cells have the most surface immunoglobulin and higher PS externalization, and they exhibit the greatest interaction with macrophages and potential for erythrophagocytosis.

THE ROLE OF RED BLOOD CELLS IN DISEASE PATHOGENESIS

Vascular Occlusion

Notwithstanding the conceptual simplicity of the sickling phenomenon, when acute microvascular occlusion occurs, causing an acute painful episode, it is a complex and evolving process. It seems probable that similar events, but of less severe degree and remaining at a subclinical level, are a recurrent or even near-constant feature of sickle vascular pathobiology. The current understanding of microvascular vasoocclusion in sickle cell anemia does carry lingering enigmas.[9]

Insofar as sickling is responsible, risk factors would include anything that would increase RBC dehydration and MCHC (e.g., insufficient clinical hydration, injudicious use of diuretics), foster arterial oxygen desaturation (e.g., lung disease, sleep-disordered breathing), prolong microvascular transit time (e.g., inflammatory milieu), increase blood viscosity (e.g., transfusion, clinical dehydration), right shift the oxygen binding curve (e.g., acidosis), or disturb vascular dynamics (e.g., cold, aberrant neurochemical responses, vasomotive rhythms). The extraordinary heterogeneity amongst sickle RBC undoubtedly confers enormous variability in behavior of individual RBC as they lose oxygen while traversing the microcirculation single-file. Although such behavioral heterogeneity is perhaps the dominant feature of sickle disease pathobiology, it currently is immeasurable at the level of microcirculatory physiology. At the sensitivity of epidemiology, HbF level is inversely related to frequency of vasoocclusive painful crises.[10]

Enabling vasoocclusion, adhesion of sickle RBC to endothelium allows greater deoxygenation by slowing microvascular flow. Indeed, in transgenic sickle mice, vascular occlusion is a two-step process.[11] This model holds that adhesion of less dense (reticulocyte-enriched) sickle RBCs to endothelium in the postcapillary venule initiates vasoocclusion, after which logjamming by dense, poorly deformable, and sickling cells creates retrograde propagation (Fig. 41.8). Thus,

determinants of RBC adhesivity and endothelial activation play an important role in vasoocclusion pathobiology. Consistent with this, clinical vasoocclusive severity correlates with the endothelial adhesivity of sickle RBCs in vitro.

Impairment of microvascular flow also derives from the diminished deformability of dehydrated sickle RBC. Dense cells (especially ISCs) can have difficulty entering the microvasculature, e.g., at bifurcations. Whether RBC adhesivity and poor deformability perhaps exert combined or synergistic effects within the smallest vessels has not been studied, nor has any role for dynamic change of rigidity as deoxygenation progresses during microvascular transit. Clinical vasoocclusive severity in humans correlates with *preservation* of RBC deformability rather than with impairment thereof,[7] perhaps because more dense cells tend to be misshapen and less able to make close adhesive contacts with endothelium.

Hemolytic Anemia

RBC life span in sickle cell anemia averages about 15 days but with marked interindividual variability (from ~7 to ~30 days); in HbSC disease, the average is about 30 days.[12] All four fundamental mechanisms that can underlie RBC removal in hematologic disease—erythrophagocytosis, fragmentation, trapping, and osmotic lysis—probably contribute (Fig. 41.9, bottom). These are consequences of the proximate aberrancies of the sickle RBC discussed earlier (Fig. 41.9, middle) that result from the specific molecular behaviors of the mutant HbS (Fig. 41.9, top). Although speculative, the illustrated, integrated synthesis of extant research data presents a plausible mechanistic blueprint.[12]

Although complex, the routes to accelerated RBC removal seemingly resolve into two contributory mechanistic cascades: one from polymer formation that underlies three terminal processes (trapping, fragmentation, osmotic lysis) that cause intravascular hemolysis; and one from HbS instability that leads to erythrophagocytosis and extravascular hemolysis. Notably, intravascular hemolysis seems to account for only one-third of overall hemolysis, while two-thirds seemingly is explained by extravascular hemolysis. The influence of the instability-based cascade is most evident in enhanced erythrophagocytosis of sickle RBC, promoted by denatured Hb causing Band 3 clumping causing attraction of immunoglobulin.

The shortest survival is exhibited by the sickle RBCs that are most dehydrated and that have the lowest amounts of HbF,[13] consistent with the polymerization-based abnormalities (see Fig. 41.9, left side). Yet, it is not known whether these two RBC features fully explain the very wide range of hemolytic rates. Presumably, the sickle RBCs' fragility is related, and sickled RBCs do lose Hb via microvesiculation when sickling is reversed. Improved RBC hydration caused by concurrent α-globin gene deletion improves RBC survival.[14] Sickle RBC survival drops substantially during acute painful episodes, but whether this precedes or follows vasoocclusion onset is not known. The only biomarkers so far documented to correlate strongly and quantitatively with *measured* RBC lifespan in sickle cell anemia are the (uncorrected) reticulocyte percentage and HbF level.[12]

Consequences of Hemolysis

Hemolysis exerts complex effects. Some are indirect, stemming from expanded erythropoiesis, such as enhanced production of highly adhesive reticulocytes and augmented elaboration of placental growth factor. This growth factor activates blood monocytes and promotes augmented production of endothelin-1 (ET-1) that can exert multiple effects relevant to sickle pathobiology: induce vasoconstriction, cause nociceptive hypersensitization, activate RBC NADPH oxidase activity, and prompt release of inflammatory mediators. Other hemolysis effects derive directly from RBC components released into the blood. Arginase diminishes plasma arginine, possibly impeding endothelial nitric oxide synthase (eNOS). A robust elaboration of PS-positive RBC microparticles exerts a signaling impact upon endothelial cells,

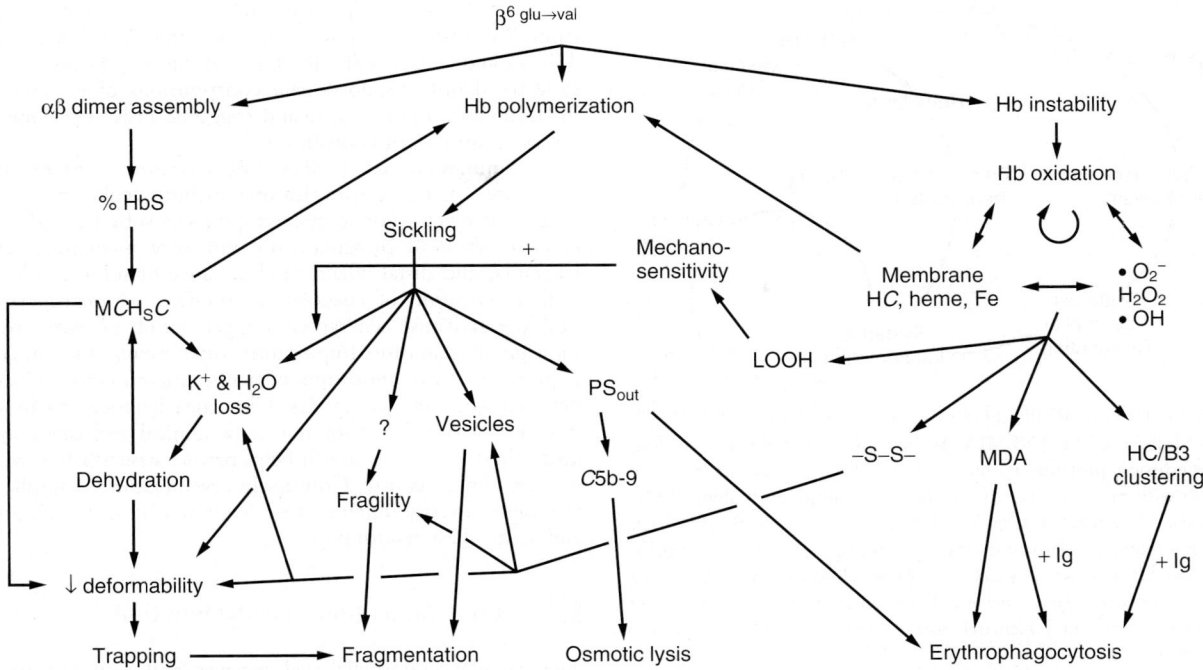

Fig. 41.9 MECHANISMS LEADING TO HEMOLYSIS IN SICKLE CELL DISEASE. This integrated synthesis proposes how the molecular behaviors of hemoglobin S (HbS) *(top)* cause development of multiple RBC abnormalities *(middle)* that lead to the four mechanisms of accelerated RBC destruction *(bottom).* *(Reproduced with permission from Hebbel RP: Reconstructing sickle cell disease: A data-based analysis of the "hyperhemolysis paradigm" for pulmonary hypertension from the perspective of evidence-based medicine. Am J Hematol 86:123–154, 2011.)*

accelerates thrombin generation, promotes pulmonary sequestration of WBCs, and protects disgorged cell-free Hb from scavenging proteins. The oxy-Hb liberated from lysing sickle RBCs can consume NO,[6,15] thus augmenting the diminished NO bioavailability primarily caused by endothelial dysfunction. It has been argued that this phenomenon is the specific cause of multiple specific complications of sickle disease, based upon correlations between them and indirect hemolytic biomarkers.[16] However, this assumption is belied by the extreme complexity associated with hemolysis. It is very likely that biodeficiency of NO in sickle disease contributes to sickle disease complications, but it is improbable that it is a sole causal factor.[12] Deficiency of NO does restrain its normal braking effect on platelet activation and inflammation, as well as its vasodilatory and superoxide buffering functions.

Once HbS in plasma oxidizes to met-HbS, it is abnormally likely to lose its heme[2] and thereby: oxidize blood lipids, induce endothelial activation, stimulate blood monocytes and endothelial cells to produce TNF-α and express tissue factor, and trigger disgorgement of neutrophil extracellular traps, among other effects. Some cell responses to heme are mediated by its binding to TLR4; e.g., in sickle mice this causes enhanced endothelial surface expression of P-selectin and triggers vascular stasis.[17] In the sickle context any potential effects of liberated cell-free Hb would be augmented because of the greatly limited levels of scavenging proteins, haptoglobin and hemopexin.

UNIQUE SYSTEMS BIOLOGY OF SICKLE CELL ANEMIA

Sickle cell anemia is unique amongst human diseases because of the extraordinary complexity arising from concurrent disturbance of multiple biologic processes, such that blood cells and the vessel wall are exposed to a broad spectrum of abnormal inputs (see Box on The Complex Sickle Milieu). Remarkably, this complexity derives from only two proximate events, vasoocclusion and hemolysis. Although it is not possible to identify the proportionate contributions and importance of the resulting disparate aberrancies, two themes emerge.

The Complex Sickle Milieu

Anemia (altered wall shear stress, tissue hypoxia, HIF-1 signaling)
RBC abnormalities (rigidity, sickling, abnormal adhesivity)
Hemolysis (plasma Hb and heme, RBC microparticles, arginase)
Blood cell activation (signaling and adhesive interactions with endothelium)
Systemic inflammation:
    Mediators (TNF, IL-1β, MCP-1, prostaglandins, leukotrienes, others)
    Endothelial glycocalyx degradation
    Activated monocytes, granulocytes, and lymphocyte subsets
    Microparticles (endothelial, monocyte, platelet)
    Mast cell activation (neuroinflammatory mediators)
    NETs
Oxidant stress (activated WBC, xanthine oxidase, NADPH oxidase, mitochondrial, others)
Growth factors (VEGF, PIGF, erythropoietin, others)
Dehydration (vasopressin)
Hemostatic system abnormalities:
    Coagulation activation (thrombin, others)
    Fibrinolysis (D dimer, others)
    Platelet activation (platelet microparticles, plasma TSP, others)
Vasoactive agents (hypoxia, ET-1, thromboxane, vasopressin, prostaglandins, adrenergic agonists, peroxides, CO, NO, others)
Adhesogenic proteins in plasma
Ischemia/reperfusion physiology
Endothelial cell activation and dysfunction
Endothelial cell injury (from occlusion, oxidants, oxidized plasma lipid, mechanic forces)
Inadvertent effects of therapies (iron overload, opioid angiogenesis signaling)

CO, Carbon monoxide; *ET,* endothelin; *Hb,* hemoglobin; *HIF,* hypoxia inducible factor; *IL,* interleukin; *MCIP,* monocyte chemotactic protein; *NETs,* neutrophil extracellular traps; *NO,* nitric oxide; *PIGF,* placenta growth factor; *RBC,* red blood cell; *TNF,* tumor necrosis factor; *TSP,* thrombospondin; *VEGF,* vascular endothelial growth factor; *WBC,* white blood cell.

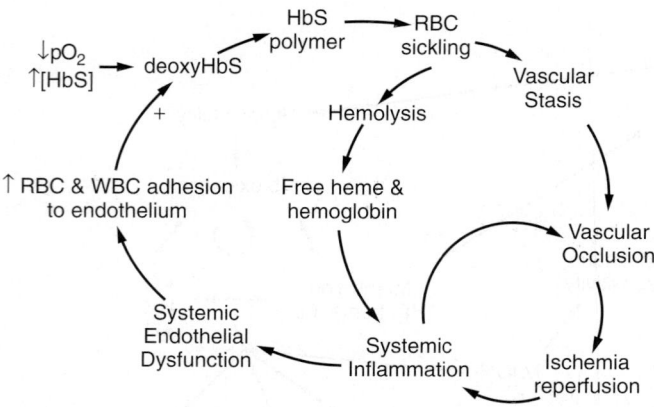

Fig. 41.10 ISCHEMIA/REPERFUSION AS THE CORE DRIVING FORCE IN SICKLE CELL ANEMIA. As the consequence of vasoocclusion, ischemia–reperfusion provides an incessant driving force causing systemic inflammation with microvascular dysfunction. The adhesion biology resulting from activated/dysfunctional endothelial cells creates a positive feedback loop that slows microvascular transit and enables polymer formation. *(Modified from Hebbel RP: Reconstructing sickle cell disease: A data-based analysis of the "hyperhemolysis paradigm" for pulmonary hypertension from the perspective of evidence-based medicine. Am J Hematol 86:123, 2011.)* Hb, Hemoglobin; PS, phosphatidylserine.

First, vasoocclusion and hemolysis are interrelated and mutually promotive. Second, there is an apparent unifying explanation for emergence of this panoply of biologic mediators.

Ischemia-Reperfusion Physiology

The abnormal adhesion of sickle RBC to endothelium creates a positive feedback loop that slows microvascular transit and thereby enables deoxygenation, polymerization, sickling, and occlusion. Experimental studies in transgenic sickle mice indicate that the enabling, proximate instigation of endothelial activation derives from ischemia-reperfusion (I/R) injury physiology, a process that would comprise an incessant driving force for systemic inflammation (Fig. 41.10).[18] This combination of inflammation and endothelial dysfunction can provide a unifying explanation for the multitude of vascular biologic abnormalities in sickle cell anemia, and it establishes a contextual and generative explanation for several of the specific clinical complications.

The complicated biology of I/R injury occurs when a proximate vascular occlusion causing ischemia is followed by reperfusion that reintroduces oxygen to the formerly ischemic area. In the unique sickle context, the initiating occlusive event(s) would be microvascular and multifocal, and they would happen recurrently. As revealed by studies of sickle transgenic mice, this triggers the classic, reperfusion-dependent, early I/R events of localized and rapid onset of oxygen radical generation, nuclear factor kappa-B (NFκB) activation, TNF-α production, and WBC activation. Research on I/R generally illustrates that its pathobiology thereafter explosively arborizes to become vastly complex. Its hallmark, however, is conversion of this localized process into a sterile inflammatory response that is robust and systemic. It initiates widespread microvascular dysfunction and organ accumulations of inflammatory cells by infiltration from blood plus activation of tissue resident macrophages and mast cells. This can lead to disease remote from the initiating occlusion, and it can explain emergence of macrovascular disease from inciting microvascular events.

INFLAMMATION

Many agents comprising the exceedingly complex sickle milieu (see Pink Box) exert proinflammatory effects; a number interact with each other in ways that alter the nature or complexity or magnitude of responses. As one example, the growth factor angiopoietin-2, released from Weibel-Palade bodies, sensitizes the endothelial cell toward TNF-α and consequent adhesion molecule expression. It is not possible to identify proportionate contributions of the many specific inflammatory inputs, but ligand-triggered TLR4 signaling is emerging as an important contributor.[17]

In summation, sickle cell anemia is a chronic, systemic inflammatory state.[19] Characteristic features include: leukocytosis; activation of granulocytes, monocytes, lymphocyte subsets, and mast cells; elevated levels of proximate inflammatory mediators, acute-phase reactants, and distal effectors; abundance of soluble adhesion molecules; activation of coagulation; presence of microparticles from multiple activated cell types; and generation of excess oxidant via multiple mechanisms. Importantly, this systemic inflammatory state is perpetual, with footprints of active inflammation apparent even between acute clinical events. Clinically, leukocytosis in sickle cell disease is a risk factor for mortality, clinical and silent stroke, and acute chest syndrome, and it helps predict which babies will develop a severe clinical course. Conversely, several clinical complications are themselves overtly inflammatory, in particular acute painful episodes and acute chest syndrome.

Endothelial Activation and Dysfunction

The vascular endothelial cell receives and responds to disparate inputs, both sensing and modifying its environment. Although normally adaptive, the endothelial response can become maladaptive. In the sickle context, the extreme complexity of the sickle milieu (see Box on The Complex Sickle Milieu) molds endothelial cell function, leading to a harmful state. The core inflammatory and oxidative input causes a high level of endothelial activation with adverse consequences such as coagulation activation, degradation of the endothelial glycocalyx (a critical determinant of endothelial cell homeostasis), and endothelial dysfunction. An often-overlooked principle predicts that endothelial dysfunction in the sickle context creates unique risk (see Mortality and Sudden Death, later).

Aberrant Vasoregulation

Sickle cell anemia involves deficient endothelial-dependent, flow-mediated conduit artery dilation.[20] Beyond the dominant role of I/R and inflammation-induced endothelial dysfunction, there are several additional contributing processes: TNF-α induction of endothelial L-arginase, limiting L-arginine availability to eNOS; NO consumption by excess superoxide and cell-free oxyHb; elevated asymmetric dimethylarginine; plus other aberrancies (e.g., microparticles, abnormal wall shear stress, elevated phospholipase A2).[12] The proportionate contributions of these processes is unknown. NO bioavailability seems to be higher for females than males, who exhibit substantial non-NO regulation of flow.

Perfusion patterns are complex in sickle cell anemia but can generally be described as impaired microvascular flow and augmented macrovascular flow.[21] Aberrancy of both endothelial-dependent and endothelial-independent vasoregulation is apparent, and the milieu is replete with a multitude of vasoactive substances. A state of vascular instability may derive from tonic upregulation of both vasoconstrictive and vasodilatory systems, in addition to exaggerated α₁-adrenergic vessel wall responsiveness. Sickle humans reveal disruption of autonomic regulation (e.g., with augmented risk for hypoxia-induced perfusion decrements).[22] Systemic blood pressure in patients with sickle cell anemia is lower than in nonanemic controls, yet is higher than in comparably anemic β-thalassemics.

Coagulation Activation

The interplay between inflammation and coagulation often seen in biomedicine is generally highly evident in sickle cell anemia, with chronic activation of coagulation, fibrinolysis, and platelets.[23] This is accompanied by increased whole blood tissue factor (TF) and its increased expression on endothelial cells and blood monocytes. Such abnormalities can follow signaling via heme/TLR4 or TNF or various other perturbing factors. Presence of PS on released microparticles and on some sickle RBC promotes accelerated thrombin generation. Oxidation appears to create resistance to cleavage of ultra-large forms of von Willebrand factor by ADAMTS13. There is excessive consumption of antithrombotic proteins. The extant biodeficiency of NO would contribute to TF expression and augmented platelet activation because it normally inhibits these. Products of platelet and coagulation activation undoubtedly exert signaling and perturbing effects on endothelium.

Genesis of Clinical Disease

For the individual patient, evident clinical disease may not parallel or accurately predict the extent of underlying overall disease burden. It has been argued that some clinical complications (pulmonary hypertension, leg ulcers, priapism, stroke) are caused by hemolysis, while others (acute chest syndrome, acute painful episodes) are caused by vasoocclusion.[17] That different processes underlie different clinical complications is entirely possible, but evidence for there being such dramatic dichotomy of phenotype pathogenesis is very indirect.[12] It is important to recall that effects of the proximate inputs (hemolysis and vasoocclusion) are undoubtedly modulated by the complex sickle milieu, and that multiple biologic systems are concurrently activated. Also, the vessel wall is exposed lifelong to the great variety of stressors and perturbing substances of the complex sickle milieu. Few data in the research literature, whether from general medicine or study of sickle disease, can be extrapolated with any confidence whatsoever to chronicity of this magnitude and complexity.

Pain Syndromes

In adults, a higher frequency of acute painful episodes is associated with increased mortality,[10] presumably reflecting derivation of both from severity of underlying disease activity. The immense further disturbance of multiple biologic processes during such episodes augments risk for complications like acute chest syndrome and sudden death. Pain frequency is higher in association with higher hematocrit and lower HbF level, consistent with the concept that acute painful episodes involve ischemic pain from vasoocclusion. However, pain in sickle disease appears to be multimodal and complex. There probably is a substantial inflammatory contribution to both acute and chronic sickle pain, involving many factors including inflammatory neuropeptides and mast cells.[24] It probably involves a state of nociceptive hypersensitization. The chronic, daily pain affecting many patients seems to be both inflammatory and neuropathic in origin.

Chronic Vasculopathy

The macrovascular component of sickle vascular disease is a chronic inflammatory vasculopathy. Histopathology from the large and medium vessels at the circle of Willis, where some sickle children develop occlusive disease, is characterized by intimal hyperplasia, fibrotic and proliferative changes, and damage to internal elastic lamina. Pathology of arterial lesions at other sites is described similarly. This typical arterial wall response to inflammation occurs, in the sickle case, without the fatty streak and foam cells of atherosclerosis, probably reflecting the absence of hyperlipidemia plus the different spectrum of proximate inflammatory inputs. It is quite possible that the specific generative stressors for vasculopathy could vary somewhat from organ to organ, but it seems likely that universal contributors include inflammation, endothelial dysfunction, growth factor excess, and aberrant wall shear stress.

Thrombosis

The hypercoagulable state suggested by blood biochemistries is accompanied by a thrombotic diathesis.[23] Arterial thrombosis occurs in areas of vasculopathy in the circle of Willis in association with childhood ischemic stroke, and in lungs exhibiting pulmonary hypertension. Incidence of venous thromboembolism is increased, and sickle cell anemia is a complicating condition for pregnancy. Downstream consequences of the coagulation system activation may play a greater role than is currently appreciated.

Stroke and Cerebrovascular Disease

Several stroke syndromes occur in sickle disease and may have differing pathogeneses. Ischemic stroke with clinical deficit develops in 5% to 10% of children with sickle cell anemia, with arterial wall changes that narrow vascular luminal diameter within the circle of Willis being the strongest risk factor and presumptive cause. Completion of the actual stroke tends to involve thrombosis at the site of vessel wall disease. Despite this, most clinical research has focused upon stroke events per se rather than upon separate risks for the apparent fundamental underlying processes, arterial wall disease and thrombotic diathesis. Concurrent α-thalassemia or HbSC disease lowers the risk of this stroke type, and HbF level is not protective. It can be suspected that elevated growth factors are participants in arterial wall disease and the sometimes-associated Moyamoya. In a seemingly separate syndrome, "silent" strokes (but associated with time-dependent degradation of neuropsychologic function) accumulate throughout childhood and are believed to derive from inadequate microvascular blood flow eventuating in multifocal microinfarcts. Yet another syndrome, hemorrhagic stroke, can complicate the vessel fragility of Moyamoya and sometimes aneurysm; otherwise, risk factors and root causes of hemorrhagic stroke are unknown.

Pulmonary Disease

The spectrum of sickle pulmonary complications includes chronic restrictive lung disease, pulmonary hypertension, asthma, infection, in situ and embolic thrombosis, and acute chest syndrome (ACS).

The acute inflammatory syndrome of ACS is associated especially with infection in children and fat embolism (probably from marrow infarction) in adults, but other presumptive triggers are similarly implicated. Risk factors include leukocytosis, lower levels of hemoglobin and HbF, and a history of asthma. The nature of ACS and its occurrence and timing during acute vasoocclusive episodes raise the question whether it might be an event of remote organ injury complicating I/R physiology.[18] Regardless of specific proximate trigger, in this syndrome it is likely that inflammation, adhesion biology, NO deficiency, and endothelial permeability conspire to augment the deleterious effects of hypoxia on the lung. Mast cell activation, another consequence of I/R, may contribute to pulmonary susceptibility generally and to pathobiology of ACS and asthma specifically.

Pulmonary hypertension occurs in about 6% of adults with sickle cell anemia,[25] in half from pulmonary venous disease, in half from pulmonary arterial disease. Genesis is almost certainly multifactorial, as the sickle context involves multiple features associated with pulmonary hypertension in the general population: absence of splenic function and presence of activated platelets, an inflammatory state, and endothelial dysfunction. It is difficult, however, to distinguish between causes and consequences of this pathobiology. Further, the pulmonary arterial wall in sickle cell anemia is awash with suspect mediators, and the biodeficiency of NO emasculates a normal braking mechanism on inflammation, proliferation, and vasoconstriction. Notably, both children and adults with sickle cell anemia not infrequently exhibit sleep-disordered breathing with nocturnal hypoxia, the major pulmonary vasoconstrictor. This justifies suspicion that long-term, repeated exposure to this major stressor plays a role in development of pulmonary hypertension in sickle disease. There may be a substantial problem in sickle cell anemia of transient elevations of pulmonary pressure unrelated to histopathologic pulmonary hypertension, as discussed later under "Mortality and Sudden Death".

Kidney Disease

In sickle cell anemia renal hyposthenuria is a nearly universal problem arising from medullary hypoperfusion resulting from the harsh renal medullary environment; its hypoxia, acidosis, and hyperosmolarity all would promote HbS polymerization and adverse changes in blood viscosity. Indeed, this even occurs in sickle trait as well. The renal cortex, on the other hand, exhibits hyperperfusion, believed to underlie glomerular dysfunction with albuminuria.[21] Patients can also develop acute renal injury, papillary necrosis and chronic renal disease, the latter being a significant contributor to mortality. Hematuria from papillary damage is very common.

Mortality and Sudden Death

Mortality rate is increased in sickle cell anemia patients having higher rates of acute painful episodes,[26] with notable risk indicators including low HbF, high WBC count, chronic renal failure, and elevated tricuspid regurgitant jet velocity. Among apparent causes of death at autopsy, cardiopulmonary disease is most prominent.[27] In 1994, a large study from the United States identified a median survival of 42 years for men and 48 years for women with sickle cell anemia; the comparable ages were 60 years and 68 years, respectively, for HbSC disease.[26] This reflected large past improvement after introduction of prophylactic penicillin for children, revealing the earlier dominance of pneumococcal sepsis in disease natural history. Further improvement has derived from chronic use of hydroxyurea, an agent that boosts HbF level, lowers WBC count, improves RBC hydration and survival, and blunts inflammatory biology and RBC adhesivity. Unfortunately, survival is much worse in parts of the world with less access to medical care and greater abundance of comorbidities (e.g., malaria, diarrheal disease).

Sickle cell anemia entails risk for sudden death, tending to occur during painful episodes or other acute events. Although unexplained, this suggests acute cardiac catastrophe. A candidate mechanism may be occurrence of transient, explosively abrupt elevations of pulmonary artery pressure, even in absence of histopathologic pulmonary hypertension.[12] This derives from an important principle: the underlying, preexisting endothelial dysfunction of sickle disease enables and predicts exaggerated vasoconstrictive responses to unrelated potential vasoconstrictors such as hypoxia, augmented NO consumption and inflammatory signaling. Each can fluctuate in short time scale, e.g., during acute painful episodes, and thereby might create risk for sudden death from rapidly elevated right heart pressure.

Sickle Trait

Sickle trait typically is associated with renal hyposthenuria. More seriously, it comprises risk for exertional sudden death, probably precipitated by effects of dehydration on RBC and blood viscosity. At an epidemiologic level, trait also involves heightened risk for venous thromboembolism, chronic renal disease, and thromboembolism complicating pregnancy. It may predispose toward ischemic stroke.

BASIS OF PHENOTYPIC DIVERSITY

Factors aside from the beta globin contribute to the remarkable interindividual diversity of clinical phenotype and severity in sickle cell anemia. Both can be significantly influenced by environment, nutrition, socioeconomic status, endemic infectious agents, and availability of medical care. Therefore, phenotypic variability is most evident in countries where greater survival and stability derives from accessible medical care, lower infant mortality, and lesser childhood infection burden. The innumerable questions regarding phenotypic diversity are of great importance. In sickle cell anemia, why do some children, but not others, develop stroke? Why do only a small fraction of adults develop pulmonary hypertension, even though all have ongoing hemolysis? Why does pain severity vary so widely irrespective of globin genotype? And so on.

Level of Hemoglobin F

HbF level varies amongst individuals as a quantitative trait and is determined approximately 80% by genetics.[5] After its decline over the first 6 months of life, most of the antisickling protection from its high level at birth is lost, but its level still varies among sickle adults over a 20-fold range. HbF level reflects the number of F cells, the amount of HbF per F cell, and the preferential survival of F cells.[13] Known determinants account for perhaps one-half of its variance: a polymorphic *XmnI* site (11p) upstream of the Gγ gene; the *HBSIL-MYB* intergenic region (6q23); SNPs in *TOX* (8q12.1); and polymorphisms in *BCL11A* (2p16), a transcriptional silencer of the *HBG* gene.[5] HbF is somewhat higher levels in females, hinting at a contributing locus on the X chromosome. Polymorphisms in trans-acting enhancers of *BCL11A* account for some, but not all, of the regional variations in HbF level. Among the African autochthonous haplotypes, the Benin haplotype is associated with higher HbF level; however, it is twice again as high among those with the Arab-India haplotype.

α-Thalassemia

The normal genotype is αα/αα, but about 30% of African Americans have a single α deletion (–α/α), so concordance with sickle cell disease is common; and homozygosity for the allele is seen (–α/–α). Its prevalence elsewhere varies regionally. An α-gene deletion has minimal effect on the HbF level but results in improved RBC hydration (see Fig. 41.6), a lower ISC count, improved RBC survival, and less severe anemia.[14] Perhaps loss of one α gene nudges α/β chain balance toward normal, given the mild instability of βˢ globin.[2] Yet there is no amelioration of pain severity, and some complications (osteonecrosis, retinopathy) increase, possibly because of the increased blood viscosity.

β-Globin Alleles

Compound heterozygosity for the sickle gene and another β allele can affect clinical phenotype, with amelioration to, e.g., in the direction of amelioration by admixing βᴬ or γ chains with βˢ. However, HbSC disease presents a unique case caused by the lesser electronegativity of HbC compared with HbS.[28] Rather than simulating sickle trait (see Fig. 41.5A), presence of HbC stimulates of KCl cotransport, causing RBC dehydration and increasing concentration of HbS. Combined with a concurrent augmentation of HbS proportion (~50% versus ~40% in HbAS), this creates a sickling disorder only somewhat less severe than sickle cell anemia. Although pain and anemia are lessened a bit, there is an increased propensity for retinopathy and osteonecrosis. It has been assumed that this derives from the somewhat higher blood viscosity when anemia is less severe. Other less common β gene alleles can likewise interact with HbS and affect clinical phenotype via impact on polymerization.

Unexplained Phenotypic Diversity

Beyond these well-defined influences, there is still enormous unexplained variability in the clinical phenotype of sickle cell anemia. The disparate biologic processes that participate in vasoocclusion, macrovascular vasculopathy, hemolysis, and specific complications highlight the certainty that phenotypic heterogeneity will be influenced by underlying genetic variations affecting adhesion biology, cation homeostasis, inflammatory signaling, vasoregulation, and so on. Indeed, the spectrum of potential foci at which genetic variation might exert effects and be relevant to sickle disease phenotypic diversity is as vast and complex as human biology itself.

The single-nucleotide polymorphisms (SNPs) that have been detected in association with specific clinical complications are far too numerous to describe here.[29] Of course, much work is still needed to discern whether such associations are actually informative vis à vis pathogenic specifics. Several SNPs seem particularly interesting. A TNF (-308) promoter polymorphism is associated with large vessel stroke in children. Polymorphisms affecting the HO-1 promoter create heterogeneity in GT repeat lengths (the shorter of which enable greater HO-1 responsiveness, e.g., to heme) are described as being associated with lower hospitalization rate for ACS in children. Interestingly, a TLR4 polymorphism prevalent only in sub-Saharan Africa leads to a greater inflammatory TNF-α responsiveness to TLR4 ligands that is protective in malaria, and could well impact sickle biology. A wholly different approach to this general problem was provided by examination of gene expression by, and inflammatory response of, endothelial cells derived from sickle children.[30] Those from children with circle of Willis disease exhibited suggestive inflammatory gene expression, plus an actual exaggerated NFκB response to stimulation with inflammatory mediators. Certainly, the contribution of various nonglobin genetic influences will continue to be identified as modern and creative approaches are being applied to the problem of phenotypic diversity in sickle cell anemia.

REFERENCES

1. Bunn HF: Subunit assembly of hemoglobin: an important determinant of hematologic phenotype. *Blood* 69:1, 1987.
2. Browne P, Shalev O, Hebbel RP: The molecular pathobiology of cell membrane iron: the sickle red cell as a model. *Free Radic Biol Med* 24:1040, 1998.
3. Noguchi CT, Schechter AN: The intracellular polymerization of sickle hemoglobin and its relevance to sickle cell disease. *Blood* 58:1057, 1981.
4. Ferrone FA: Polymerization and sickle cell disease: a molecular view. *Microcirculation* 11:115, 2004.
5. Steinberg MH, Chui DHK, Dover GJ, et al: Fetal hemoglobin in sickle cell anemia: a glass half full? *Blood* 123:481, 2014.
6. Eich RF, Li T, Doherty DH, et al: Mechanism of NO-induced oxidation of myoglobin and hemoglobin. *Biochem* 35:6976, 1996.
7. Ballas SK, Mohandas N: Sickle red cell microrheology and sickle blood rheology. *Microcirculation* 11:209, 2004.
8. Kaul DK, Finnegan E, Barabino GA: Sickle red cell-endothelium interactions. *Microcirculation* 16:97, 2009.
9. Embury SH: The not-so-simple process of sickle cell vasoocclusion. *Microcirculation* 11:101, 2004.
10. Platt OS, Thorington BD, Brambilla DJ, et al: Pain in sickle cell disease. Rates and risk factors. *N Engl J Med* 325:11, 1991.
11. Kaul DK, Fabry ME: *In vivo* studies of sickle red blood cells. Sickle red cell-endothelium interactions. *Microcirculation* 11:153, 2004.
12. Hebbel RP: Reconstructing sickle cell disease: a data-based analysis of the "hyperhemolysis paradigm" for pulmonary hypertension from the perspective of evidence-based medicine. *Am J Hematol* 86:123, 2011.
13. Franco RS, Yasin Z, Palascak MB, et al: The effect of fetal hemoglobin on the survival characteristics of sickle cells. *Blood* 108:1073, 2006.
14. Embury SH, Clark MR, Monroy G, et al: Concurrent sickle cell anemia and alpha-thalassemia. Effect on pathological properties of sickle erythrocytes. *J Clin Invest* 73:116, 1984.
15. Reiter CD, Wang X, Tanus-Santos JE, et al: Cell-free hemoglobin limits nitric oxide bioavailability in sickle-cell disease. *Nat Med* 8:1383, 2002.
16. Taylor JG, 6th, Nolan VG, Mendelsohn L, et al: Chronic hyper-hemolysis in sickle cell anemia: association of vascular complications and mortality with less frequent vasoocclusive pain. *PLoS ONE* 3:e2095, 2008.
17. Belcher JD, Chen C, Nguyen J, et al: Heme triggers TLR4 signaling leading to endothelial cell activation and vasoocclusion in murine sickle cell disease. *Blood* 123:377, 2014.
18. Hebbel RP: Ischemia-reperfusion injury in sickle cell anemia: relationship to acute chest syndrome, endothelial dysfunction, arterial vasculopathy, and inflammatory pain. *Hematol Oncol Clin North Am* 28:181, 2014.
19. Kaul DK, Hebbel RP: Hypoxia/reoxygenation causes inflammatory response in transgenic sickle mice but not normal mice. *J Clin Invest* 106:411, 2000.
20. Gladwin MT, Schechter AN, Ognibene FP, et al: Divergent nitric oxide bioavailability in men and women with sickle cell disease. *Circulation* 107:271, 2003.
21. Nath KA, Katusic ZS, Gladwin MT: The perfusion paradox and vascular instability in sickle cell disease. *Microcirculation* 11:117, 2004.
22. Sangkatumvong S, Khoo MC, Kato R, et al: Peripheral vasoconstriction and abnormal parasympathetic response to sighs and transient hypoxia in sickle cell disease. *Am J Respir Crit Care Med* 184:474, 2011.
23. Sparkenbaugh E, Pawlinski R: Interplay between coagulation and vascular inflammation in sickle cell disease. *Brit J Haematol* 162:3, 2013.
24. Vincent L, Vang D, Nguyen J, et al: Mast cell activation contributes to sickle cell pathobiology and pain in mice. *Blood* 122:1853, 2013.
25. Parent F, Bachir D, Inamo J, et al: A hemodynamic study of pulmonary hypertension in sickle cell disease. *N Engl J Med* 365:4, 2011.
26. Platt OS, Brambilla DJ, Rosse WF, et al: Mortality in sickle cell disease. Life expectancy and risk factors for early death. *N Engl J Med* 330:1639, 1994.
27. Fitzhugh CD, Lauder N, Jonassaint JC, et al: Cardiopulmonary complications leading to premature deaths in adult patients with sickle cell disease. *Am J Hematol* 85:36, 2010.
28. Bunn HF, Noguchi CT, Hofrichter J, et al: Molecular and cellular pathogenesis of hemoglobin SC disease. *Proc Natl Acad Sci USA* 79:7527, 1982.
29. Fertrin KY, Costa FF: Genomic polymorphisms in sickle cell disease: implications for clinical diversity and treatment. *Expert Rev Hematol* 3:443, 2010.
30. Milbauer LC, Wei P, Enenstein J, et al: Genetic endothelial systems biology of sickle stroke risk. *Blood* 111:3872, 2008.

SICKLE CELL DISEASE: CLINICAL FEATURES AND MANAGEMENT

Yogen Saunthararajah and Elliott P. Vichinsky

Hemoglobinopathies are the most common genetic diseases in humans. In sickle cell disease (SCD), a mutated β-globin gene produces sickle hemoglobin (Hb S). This mutation has been positively selected during human evolution because one copy of the sickle gene and one normal *β-globin* gene (sickle cell trait) confers a survival advantage in malaria-endemic regions. With two copies of the sickle gene (Hb SS or sickle cell anemia) or the sickle mutation and another mutated *β-globin* gene, for example, sickle cell–β°-thalassemia (Hb S–β thal) or Hb SC disease (Hb SC) (mixed hemoglobinopathies), the less soluble Hb S can polymerize in deoxygenated regions of the circulation, resulting in red blood cell (RBC) rigidity, RBC adhesion to endothelium, and hemolysis. In addition to hemolytic anemia, these events activate inflammation and coagulation pathways and cause vasoocclusion.[1] Thus the clinical manifestations are chronic hemolytic anemia, recurrent painful episodes, and chronic organ damage from vasoocclusion. This chapter presents the diagnosis and natural history, and describes overall clinical management as well as specific management by organ complications. Clinical interventions are founded on an understanding of underlying pathophysiologic processes. The exigency of living with a painful, life-threatening chronic disease in an ethnically diverse society adds complexity to the psychosocial aspects of this illness. A comprehensive management approach directed at preventing pain crises, chronic organ damage, and early mortality while effectively managing acute complications is recommended. For a full discussion of the fascinating history and molecular pathology of this disease, please see Chapter 42. Normal Hb synthesis, structure, and function are described in Chapter 33, and the thalassemias are considered in Chapter 40.

PREVALENCE

The distribution and frequency of the sickle cell gene in different areas of the world have been influenced by natural selection and gene transmission via trade routes including the slave trade.[2] Among African Americans,[3] the prevalence of sickle cell trait is 8% to 10% among newborns,[4] and in this population, the frequencies of the sickle cell (0.045), Hb C (0.015), and β-thalassemia (0.004) genes[4] indicate that there are 4000–5000 pregnancies a year at risk for SCD. The burden of this disease in the United States is dwarfed by that in the rest of the world, as evidenced by a prevalence of the sickle cell gene as high as 25% to 30% in western Africa and an estimated annual birth of 120,000 babies with SCD in Africa.[5]

DIAGNOSIS

The diagnosis of a sickle cell syndrome is suggested by characteristic findings on the complete blood count (CBC) and peripheral smear that prompt Hb electrophoresis. If a diagnosis of SCD is confirmed, evaluation of the various organ systems at risk is required. These evaluations are discussed in the section on clinical management.

Complete Blood Count and Peripheral Blood Smear

The chronic hemolytic anemia of SCD presents with mild to moderately low hematocrit and Hb levels and a reticulocytosis of approximately 3% to 15%. Additional laboratory features of hemolysis are unconjugated hyperbilirubinemia, elevated lactate dehydrogenase (LDH), and low haptoglobin levels. The reticulocytosis accounts for high or high-normal mean corpuscular volume (MCV). If the age-adjusted MCV is not elevated, the possibility of sickle cell–β-thalassemia, coincident α-thalassemia, or iron deficiency must be considered.

In the peripheral smear (Fig. 42.1), there may be sickled forms, target cells, polychromasia indicative of reticulocytosis, and Howell-Jolly bodies demonstrating hyposplenia. The RBCs are normochromic unless there is coexistent thalassemia or iron deficiency. Sickled forms (irreversibly sickled cells [ISCs]) occur in the peripheral smear only in the SCDs and not in sickle cell trait. In Hb SS disease, ISCs predominate, and target cells may be few; in sickle cell–β-thalassemia, ISCs, target cells, and hypochromic microcytic discocytes are prominent; in Hb SC disease, target cells predominate, and ISCs are rare.

White blood cell (WBC) counts are higher than normal in Hb SS disease, particularly in patients under age 10 years. Mean WBC counts tend not to be elevated in Hb SC disease or sickle cell–β⁺-thalassemia. Mean platelet counts are elevated in Hb SS disease, particularly in patients younger than age 18 years, but are usually normal in those with Hb SC disease and sickle cell–β⁺-thalassemia.

Solubility Tests and Hemoglobin Electrophoresis

Solubility test results (e.g., Sickledex) are positive in both SCD and sickle cell trait. All patients require definitive diagnosis with Hb electrophoresis (which separates Hb species according to amino acid composition) (Fig. 42.2) or high performance liquid chromatography (HPLC).[6] Cellulose acetate electrophoresis at a pH of 8.4 is a standard method of separating Hb S from other variants. However, Hb S, G, and D have the same electrophoretic mobility with this method. Using citrate agar electrophoresis at pH 6.2, Hb S has a different mobility than Hb D and G, which comigrate with Hb A in this system.

Results from electrophoresis or thin-layer isoelectric focusing are similar in Hb SS disease and sickle cell–β°-thalassemia: nearly all of the Hb consists of Hb S. Although differences in the fetal hemoglobin (Hb F) (see Variant Sickle Cell Syndromes) and Hb A₂ levels may be useful in distinguishing these syndromes, the presence of microcytosis or of one parent without sickle cell trait is a more useful indicator of sickle cell–β°-thalassemia. The diagnosis of Hb SC disease is straightforward; nearly equal amounts of Hb S and Hb C are detected. Sickle cell–β⁺-thalassemia and sickle cell trait both have substantial amounts of Hb A and Hb S. This superficial electrophoretic similarity does not provide an obstacle to diagnosis: whereas sickle cell trait is associated with neither anemia nor microcytosis and has an Hb A fraction more than 50%,[7] sickle cell–β⁺-thalassemia is associated with anemia, microcytosis, and an Hb A fraction that ranges from 5% to 30%.

The Hb F level is usually slightly to moderately elevated; the degree varies among patients. The amount of Hb F present is a function of the number of reticulocytes that contain Hb F, the extent of selective survival of Hb F–containing reticulocytes that become mature Hb F–containing erythrocytes (F cells), and the amount of Hb F per F cell.[8] The Arab–Indian and Senegal haplotypes are associated with higher levels of Hb F than the others.[9]

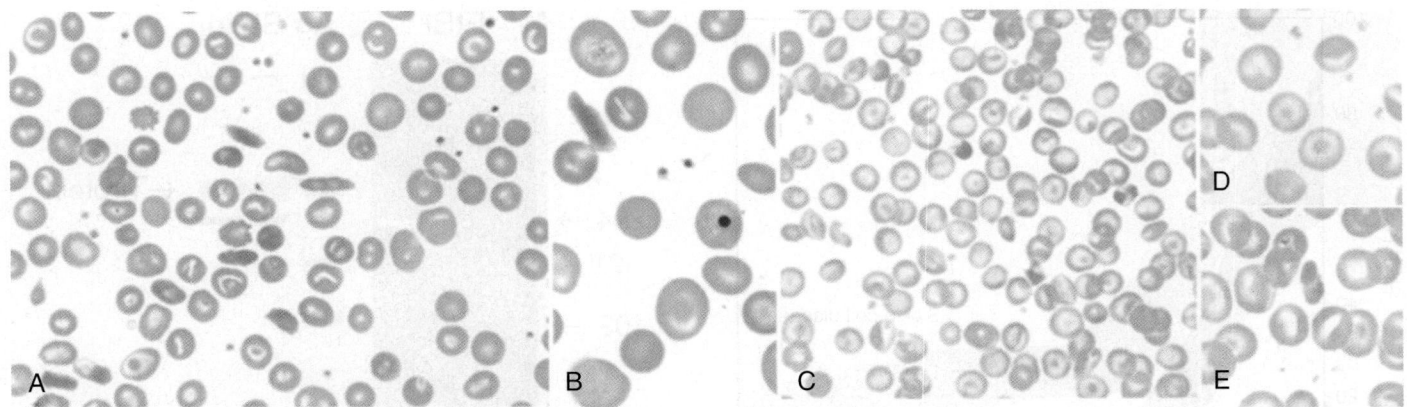

Fig. 42.1 SICKLE CELL DISEASE AND HEMOGLOBIN SC PERIPHERAL BLOOD SMEARS. The peripheral smear in sickle cell disease (A) shows sickle cells that are mostly irreversibly sickled and sometimes referred to as "cigar forms." Higher power detail (B) shows a sickle cell *(upper left)*, red blood cell containing a Howell-Jolly body *(middle right)*, and polychromatophilic cell *(lower center)*. These indicate sickle cell anemia and splenic dysfunction but marrow response with reticulocytosis, respectively. A peripheral smear of a patient with Hgb SC (C) shows no sickled cell, but there are target forms (D) and occasional cells (E) with hemoglobin condensed at each pole of the cell.

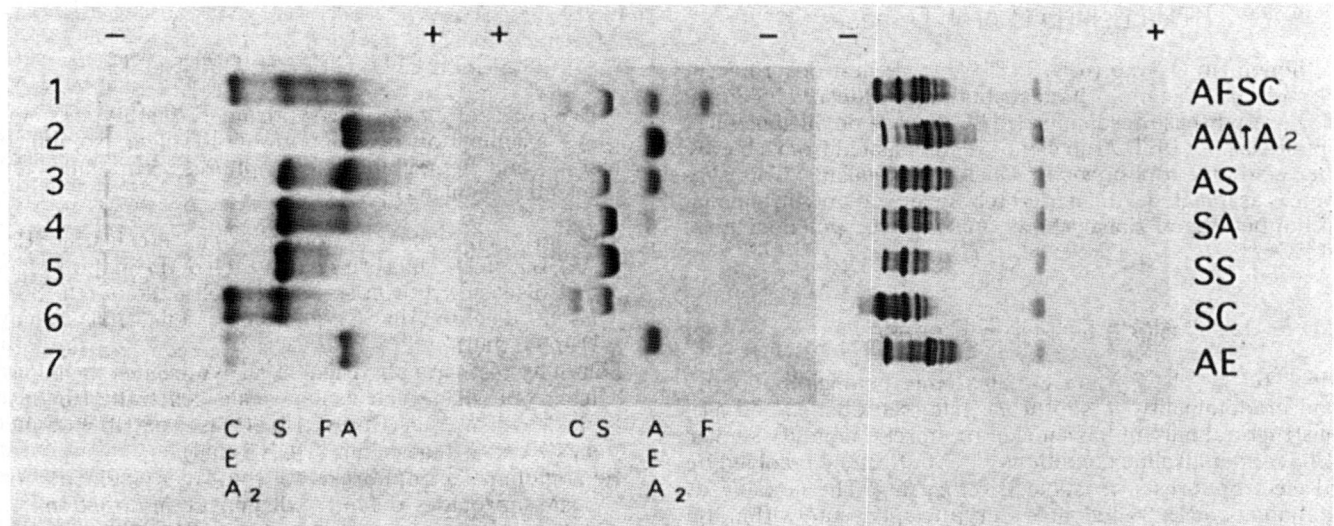

Fig. 42.2 COMPARATIVE ANALYSES OF SEVERAL MUTANT HEMOGLOBINS USING ALKALINE ELECTROPHORESIS, ACID ELECTROPHORESIS, AND THIN-LAYER ISOELECTRIC FOCUSING. On the *right* are shown the components of the standard *(top)* and the phenotypes of the other six samples. Their analyses are shown by alkaline hemoglobin electrophoresis in the *left panel*, acid electrophoresis in the *center panel*, and thin-layer isoelectric focusing in the *right panel*. Locations of the various hemoglobin bands are shown *below the left and center panels*. *A,* Hemoglobin A; *A2,* hemoglobin A2; *C,* hemoglobin C; *E,* hemoglobin E; *F,* hemoglobin F; *S,* hemoglobin S. *(Courtesy M.H. Steinberg.)*

Newborn Screening

The use of prophylactic penicillin[10] and the provision of comprehensive medical care during the first 5 years of life have reduced the mortality rate from approximately 25% to less than 3%, thereby underlining the importance of early identification of infants with SCD. Based on its economy and superiority of detection, universal screening of all newborns is preferred over ethnically targeted approaches.[11,12] Blood samples for testing are obtained by heel stick and spotted onto filter paper for stable transport and subsequent HPLC (solubility testing is unreliable because of the large amount of Hb F present.)

As Hb S increases and Hb F declines in the first months of life (Fig. 42.3), the clinical manifestations of SCD, including anemia, emerge.[13] ISCs can be seen on the peripheral blood smear (Fig. 42.4) of children with sickle cell anemia at 3 months of age,

and by 4 months of age, moderately severe hemolytic anemia is evident.

Tests used in newborn screening must be capable of distinguishing between Hb F, S, A, and C. The Hb distribution pattern is described in descending order according to the quantities detected. Therefore a newborn with sickle cell anemia who has predominantly Hb F with a small amount of Hb S and no Hb A is described as having an FS pattern. An FS pattern is obtained also in newborns who have sickle cell–β°-thalassemia, sickle cell–hereditary persistence of Hb F (HPFH), and sickle cell–Hb D or sickle cell–Hb G (i.e., Hb D and E have the same electrophoretic mobility as Hb S). A newborn with sickle cell trait will have Hb F, Hb A, and Hb S (FAS pattern). The quantity of Hb A is greater than that of Hb S. If the quantity of Hb S exceeds that of Hb A, the presumptive diagnosis is sickle cell–β+-thalassemia (FSA pattern). It may not be possible to distinguish FAS and FSA patterns in newborns, so DNA-based testing or repeat Hb testing at age 3–6 months is recommended.

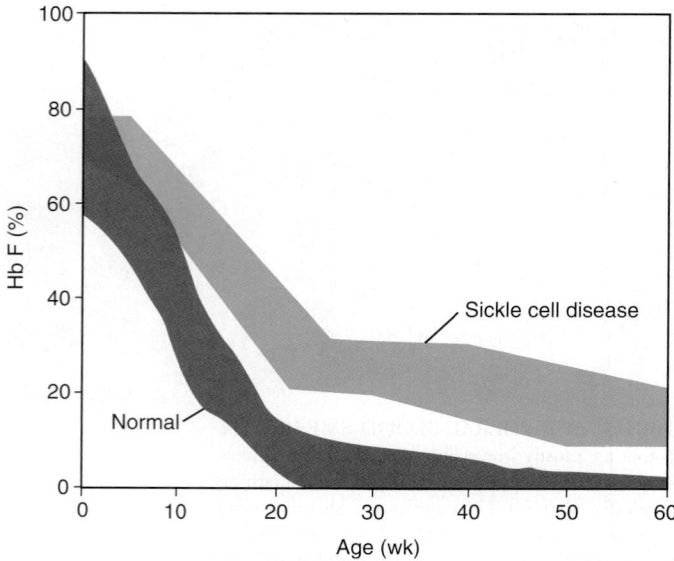

Fig. 42.3 FETAL HEMOGLOBIN (HB F) DECLINE IN CHILDREN WITH HEMOGLOBINS AA AND SS. *HB F*, fetal hemoglobin. *(Data from O'Brien, Mclatosh S, Aspnes AT, et al: Prospective study of sickle cell anemia in infancy. J Pediatr 89:205, 1976.)*

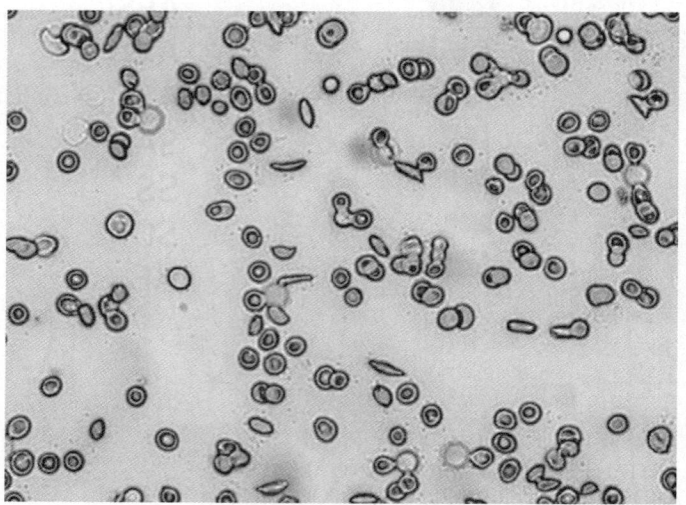

Fig. 42.4 The peculiar elongated shapes of the erythrocytes is what Herrick's intern Ernest E. Irons noted, and together with a report from the German literature of *sichel formen* blood cells, inspired the name by which this condition is now known.

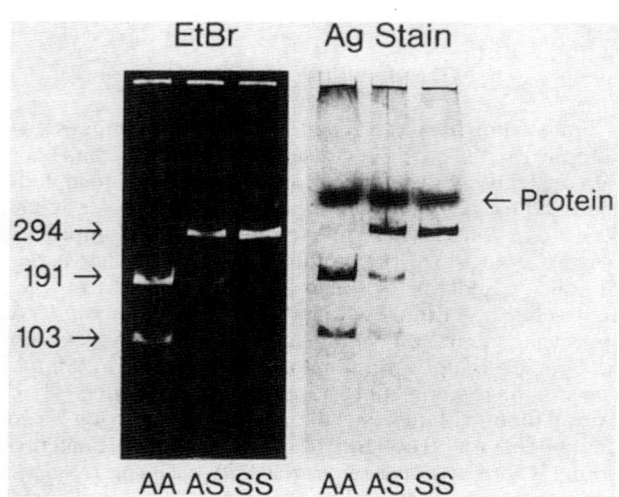

Fig. 42.5 POLYMERASE CHAIN REACTION (PCR)–BASED RESTRICTION ANALYSIS FOR THE SICKLE CELL GENE. The genotypes of the DNA samples tested are shown *below.* The size in base pairs for the undigested PCR product and the products resulting from Oxa Nl are shown at the *left* in base pairs. The fragments from normal β-globin DNA (AA) shows complete Oxa Nl cleavage, from sickle cell trait DNA (AS) shows partial cleavage, and from sickle cell anemia (SS) shows no cleavage. *Ag stain,* Silver stain; *EtBr*, ethidium bromide.

reverse dot-blot methodology to screen the many African American β-thalassemia mutations, as well as the Hb S and Hb C mutations, in a single hybridization reaction.

CLINICAL PRESENTATION AND MANAGEMENT

The cardinal clinical manifestations of SCD are chronic hemolytic anemia; recurrent painful episodes; and chronic organ damage, particularly of the spleen, bones, brain, kidneys, lungs, skin, and heart. The pattern of disease manifestation varies among the major genotypes of Hb SS, Hb SC, and Hb S–β-thalassemia but also within the same genotype. Some of this variability results from coinherited genotypes, for example, α-thalassemia or HPFH (discussed at the end of this chapter).

Typically, patients are anemic but lead a relatively normal life punctuated by painful episodes. However, it is important to realize that chronic organ damage and decreased survival occur even in patients who do not have recurrent pain. This section begins with a brief overview of natural history and survival followed by a discussion of basic management that aims to improve this natural history (disease modification) and then a discussion of management of organ-specific complications.

Prenatal Diagnosis

One large survey found that parents at risk for having a child with SCD were interested in prenatal diagnosis and would consider termination of pregnancy for an affected fetus.[14] Community acceptance of reproductive genetic services depends on the effectiveness of education and counseling. One major ethical issue pertains to our diagnostic skills' having outstripped our ability to predict the severity of diagnosable conditions.

Fetal DNA samples are obtained by chorionic villus sampling at 8–10 weeks' gestation. Polymerase chain reaction (PCR)–based methods for detecting the sickle gene include restriction analysis (Fig. 42.5), allele-specific hybridization, reverse dot blotting, and allele-specific fluorescence PCR. PCR-based diagnosis for Hb SC disease is possible using specific molecular methods for detecting the *Hb C* gene, and the diagnosis of sickle cell–β-thalassemia can be made using

Natural History and Life Expectancy

The manifestations of disease begin after the first few months of life as Hb F levels decline and Hb S levels increase. Certain complications predominate in particular age groups. Between the ages of 1 and 3 years, affected individuals have splenomegaly and splenic sequestration (Fig. 42.6), pneumonia, and meningitis from *Streptococcus pneumoniae* and other encapsulated organisms (because of functional hyposplenism), and hand–foot syndrome; in early childhood, they have stroke, acute chest syndrome, and osteonecrosis; in mid childhood, they have pain crises, osteonecrosis, and acute chest syndrome; between ages 12 and 20 years, they have strokes, priapism, and pain crises; between ages 20 and 30 years, they have renal insufficiency, pulmonary hypertension, disabling osteonecrosis, retinopathy, leg ulcers, and pain crises; and at age older than 30 years, they have renal failure, congestive heart failure, and pain crises.

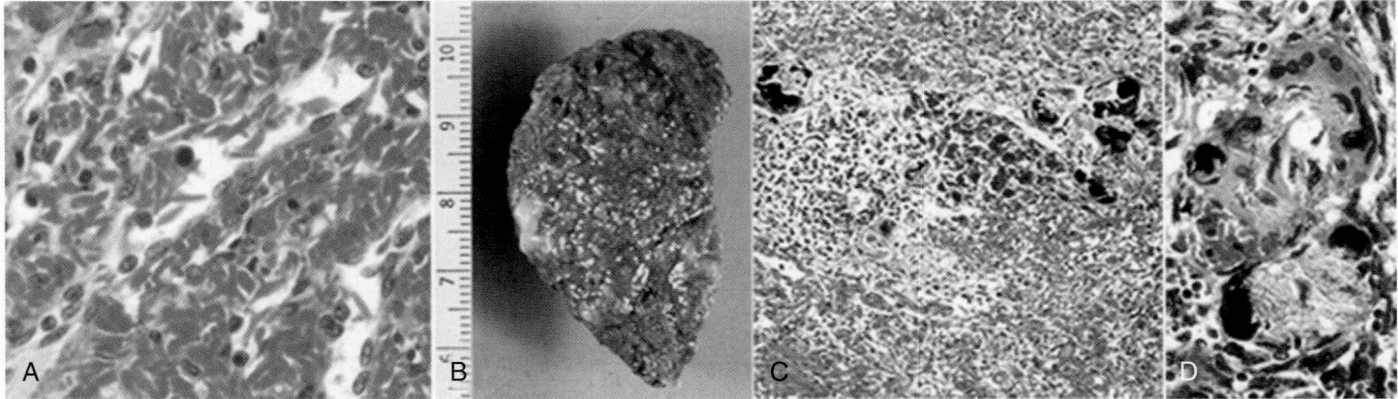

Fig. 42.6 THE SPLEEN IN SICKLE CELL DISEASE. Histologic section (A) of the splenic red pulp shows engorgement of the splenic cords with sickled cells. In infants, excessive pooling in cords can lead to a splenic sequestration crisis. Later in life, the spleen undergoes autoinfarction. The gross pathology (B) shows a tiny 4.5-cm spleen with rough external surface caused by scarring from repeated infarcts. Histologic section reveals classic Gamna-Gandy bodies (C and D) also caused by repeated infarction. These are composed of hemosiderin-laden macrophages, calcium deposits, and foreign body giant cells.

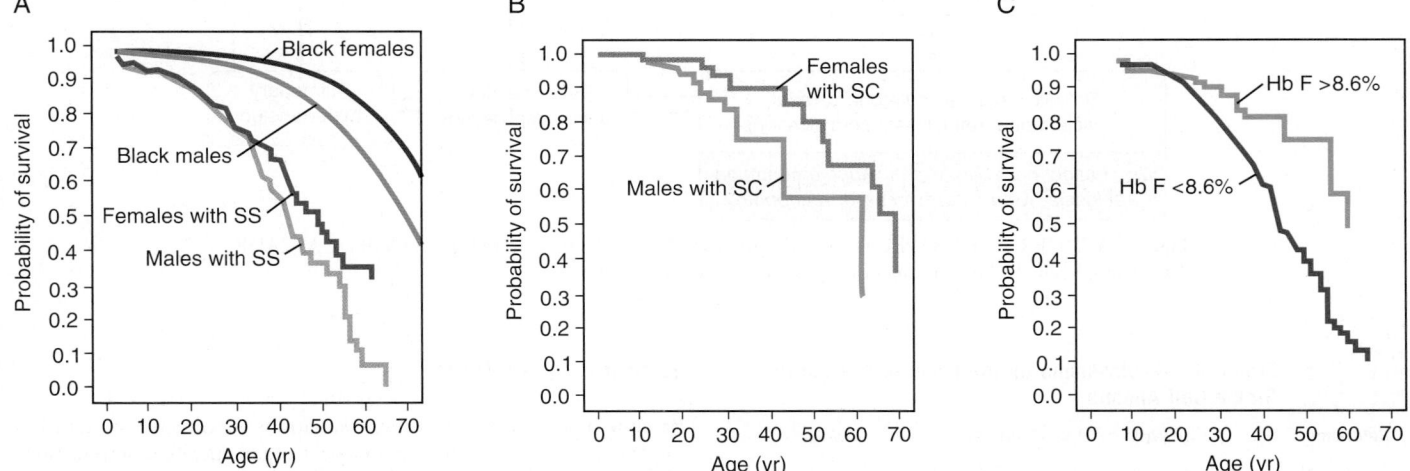

Fig. 42.7 Life expectancy in patients with sickle cell disease for patients with Hb SS disease (A), Hb SC disease (B), and with different levels of fetal hemoglobin (Hb F) (C). *(From Platt OS, Brambilla DJ, Rosse WF, et al: Mortality in sickle cell disease. Life expectancy and risk factors for early death. N Engl J Med 330:1639, 1994.)*

Life expectancy is decreased, although in the past 30 years, this has dramatically improved for patients in the West: in 1973, Diggs[15] reported that the mean survival was 14.3 years; in 1994, Platt et al[16] reported that life expectancy was 42 years for men and 48 years for women with sickle cell anemia (Fig. 42.7). This improvement in survival is most likely the result of improved general medical care, including prophylactic penicillin therapy and vaccination against *S. pneumoniae*.[9] These survival profiles are likely to be relevant even today, although a cohort of patients followed since 1975 show improvement in the probability of survival to age 20 years compared with patients born before 1975 (89% versus 79%).[17] The poor survival and litany of chronic organ damage in survivors emphasize the need for disease-modifying interventions to prevent vasculopathy.[17] There are some indications that disease-modifying agents such as hydroxyurea (HU) can improve survival.[18,19]

Predictors of Disease Severity

The ability to predict clinical course would allow more rational tailoring of therapy to individual patients (e.g., selection of patients for high-risk but effective options such as stem cell transplant). Higher Hb F levels and the coinheritance of an α-thalassemia trait have been identified as favorable disease modifiers in multiple studies (Table 42.1).[20–22] The level of chronic anemia (which is influenced by the presence of an α-thalassemia trait and by Hb F levels) is of considerable predictive value. Patients with more severe anemia are more likely to develop infarctive and hemorrhagic stroke,[23] to have glomerular dysfunction,[24,25] and perhaps to give birth to low-birthweight babies.[26,27] Conversely, they have fewer episodes of acute chest syndrome[28] and (after age 20 years) a lower mortality rate.[28] Progressive anemia from renal endocrine deficiency or a decrease in bone marrow function from vasoocclusion is associated with early death.[18,19]

A number of other genetic polymorphisms may be relevant to disease severity, for example, with regards to the risk of stroke. However, most of these markers are not widely used to guide decision making.[21]

Principles of Management

The twin pillars of therapy are disease modification (prevention of crises, complications, chronic organ damage, and early mortality)

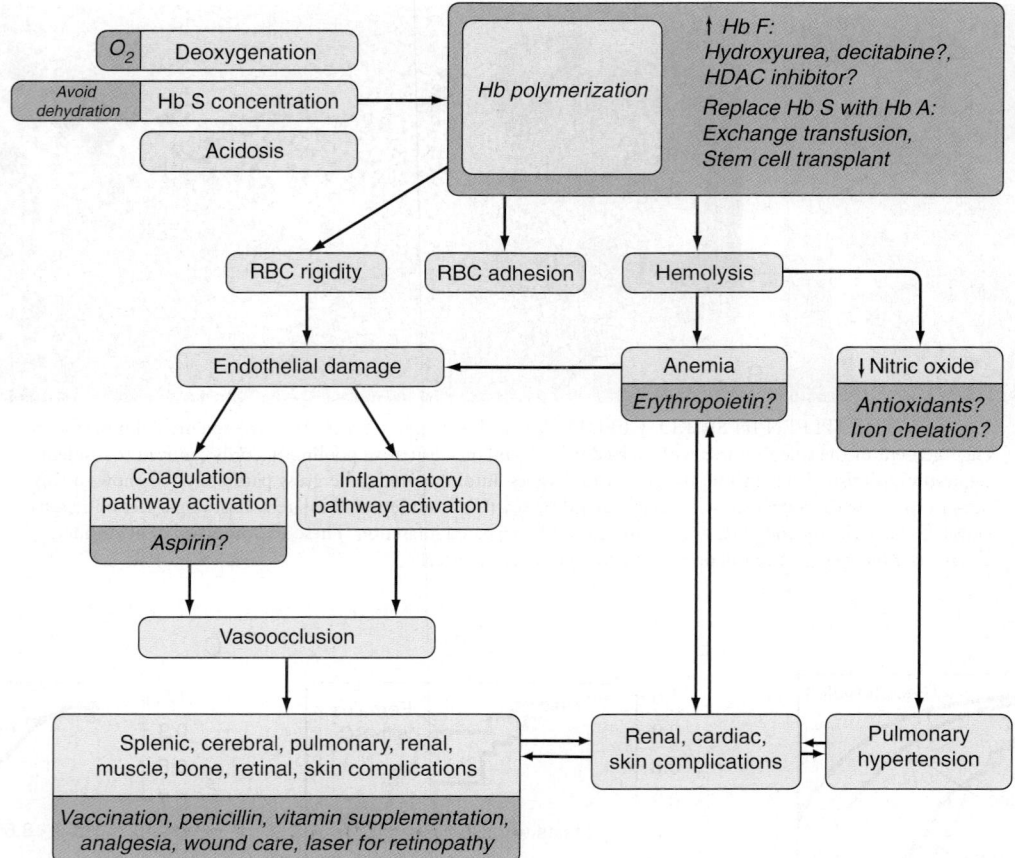

Fig. 42.8 WHERE THERAPEUTICS INTERVENE IN THE PATHOPHYSIOLOGIC CASCADE. *Hb,* Hemoglobin; *HDAC,* histone deacetylase; *RBC,* red blood cell.

TABLE 42.1	Effect of α-Thalassemia on the Level of Anemia in Sickle Cell Anemia		
Reference	**αα/αα[a]**	**–α/αα**	**–α/–α**
Embury et al[29]	7.8[b] (*n* = 25)[c]	9.7 (*n* = 18)	9.2 (*n* = 4)
Higgs et al[30]	7.8 (*n* = 88)	8.1 (*n* = 44)	8.8 (*n* = 44)
Steinberg et al[31]	8.0 (*n* = 73)	9.0 (*n* = 39)	9.5 (*n* = 13)
Felice et al; age 5 years[32]	8.6 (*n* = 88)	8.4 (*n* = 52)	8.3 (*n* = 50)
Felice et al; age 11 years[32]	7.9 (*n* = 40)	8.5 (*n* = 34)	9.6 (*n* = 2)

[a]The different α-globin genotypes indicate the presence of four (αα/αα), three (–α/αα), or two (–α/–α) α-globin genes.
[b]The mean hemoglobin level (g/dL) for each group is shown.
[c]The number of subjects in each group is denoted by *n*.

and compassionate, prompt, effective, and safe relief of acute crises, including pain episodes. Therefore outpatient clinic management is mostly directed at initiating measures to prevent pain crises, prevent organ complications, and improve survival. This effort should include identification of existing organ complications and initiation of measures to prevent further deterioration. Outpatient management can thus be divided into baseline evaluations, basic treatment or disease modification, and additional treatment dictated by the organ complications that are identified. The suggested treatments are based on current understanding of SCD pathophysiology. As shown in Fig. 42.8, some treatments address only one aspect of pathophysiology, but others may have a broader impact. Inpatient management is directed at effective and safe relief of acute crises.

Baseline Evaluations

Baseline blood, urine, and other evaluations are directed at quantifying the chronic hemolytic anemia and organ-specific complications (Table 42.2). They also provide baseline parameters that can be followed to assess response to therapeutic interventions.

In pediatric patients, at least annual assessment of cerebral blood flow in the internal carotid artery and the middle or anterior cerebral artery using transcranial Doppler ultrasonography (TCD) is recommended. This evaluation is a validated predictor of stroke risk. Primary prevention with chronic transfusion is effective in such patients.[33] In adults, magnetic resonance imaging (MRI) or magnetic resonance angiography (MRA) of the brain can be used instead of TCD[34] to assess thrombotic or hemorrhagic stroke risk, especially in those with a history of stroke or seizure. The recognition of cardiopulmonary complications as a cause of early mortality in SCD warrants evaluation for this condition with either echocardiogram or brain natriuretic peptide (BNP) levels. Retinal evaluation is begun at school age and continued on an annual basis. More frequent retinal evaluations are necessary if retinopathy is noted.

Basic Management and Disease Modification

Sufficient evidence suggests that a number of treatments should be considered in all patients. These treatments have been demonstrated to decrease symptoms and complications, increase survival, or both (Table 42.3) (disease modification). There are other treatments for which there are sufficient scientific grounds or clinical data to suggest a potential impact on disease natural history. However, there is presently insufficient clinical data to make firm recommendations (see Fig. 42.8 and Table 42.3). Although treatments such as vaccination

TABLE 42.2	Baseline Evaluations to Consider
Tests	
Blood tests	CBC with differential
	Reticulocyte count
	Hemoglobin HPLC or electrophoresis
	LDH
	Renal function tests
	Liver function tests
	Mineral panel
	Serum iron, ferritin, TIBC
	Vitamin D level
	Hepatitis B sAg
	Hepatitis C antibody
	RBC alloantibody screen
	RBC typing
	D-dimer[a]
	C-reactive protein[a]
	Brain natriuretic peptide
Urine and kidney tests	Urinalysis
	Renal ultrasonography[b]
Radiology	MRI or MRA brain (adults)[c] or transcranial Doppler ultrasonography starting at age 2 years (children)
	Chest radiography[d]
	Hip or shoulder radiograph or MRI (or both)[c]
	Bone density in teenagers and adults
Cardiology and pulmonary	Echocardiogram
Neurocognitive	Neurocognitive testing[d]

[a]Consider following as surrogate markers after initiation of disease-modifying intervention.
[b]If hematuria with red blood cells in urine.
[c]As clinically indicated.
[d]If the patient has poor school performance, an abnormal memory, or abnormal MRI findings.
CBC, Complete blood count; HPLC, high performance liquid chromatography; LDH, lactate dehydrogenase; MRA, magnetic resonance angiography; MRI, magnetic resonance imaging; RBC, red blood cell; sAg, surface antigen; TIBC, total iron-binding capacity.

TABLE 42.3	Disease-Modifying Treatments to Consider[a]
Robust clinical data	Penicillin prophylaxis
	Streptococcus pneumoniae vaccination
	Hydroxyurea
	Chronic exchange transfusion
	Iron chelation for chronic iron overload[b]
Limited clinical data	Daily multivitamin without iron or Folate supplementation AND vitamin D replacement[c]
	Haemophilus influenzae vaccination
	Influenza vaccination
	Erythropoietin
	Phlebotomy
Experimental	Hb F reactivation with decitabine, histone deacetylase inhibitors, or imids
	Erythropoietin for chronic relative reticulocytopenia
	Nutritional supplements and antioxidants (e.g., glutamine, zinc, multivitamins)
	N-acetylcysteine

[a]See text for specific indications and limitations.
[b]Best data from thalassemia patient experience.
[c]Risks minimal therefore, it is generally done.
Hb F, Fetal hemoglobin.

and penicillin prophylaxis do not directly affect the sickling process or vasculopathy, they have had an impact on survival and therefore are included under the umbrella of disease-modifying therapies.

Therapeutic options are further discussed in the sections describing organ-specific complications.

Vaccination and Penicillin Prophylaxis

Children should be immunized against *S. pneumoniae, Haemophilus influenzae,* hepatitis B, and influenza.[35] Vaccination and penicillin prophylaxis can reduce the risk of serious pneumococcal infections.[9,36] Vaccination schedules recommend inoculation with heptavalent pneumococcal conjugated vaccine at 2 months followed by two more doses 6–8 weeks apart (primary series) and a booster at 12 months. This is followed by Pneumovax at age 2 and 5 years. In adults, the Pneumovax should be readministered every 5 years (http://www.cdc.gov/vaccines/pubs/vis/default.htm).

For children younger than age 5 years, prophylactic penicillin recommendations are 125 mg penicillin V orally twice daily until age 2–3 years and 250 mg thereafter.[35] Penicillin prophylaxis begins at 2 months. Randomized, double-blind, placebo-controlled studies of prophylactic penicillin beginning in infancy, including the prophylactic penicillin or placebo study (PROPS), have found that this therapy reduced the incidence of *S. pneumoniae* bacteremia by 84% in children younger than 3 years.[9,36] A randomized, double-blind, placebo-controlled study, the PROPS II study concluded that it is safe to stop prophylactic penicillin therapy at age 5 years in children who have not had prior severe pneumococcal infection or splenectomy and are receiving regular follow-up care.[37] However, the power of the study was restricted by the limited number of *S. pneumoniae* systemic infection events. In an analysis of a patient population receiving penicillin prophylaxis and the Pneumovax, the rate of severe *S. pneumoniae* infections was 2.4 per 100 patient-years. This was favorable compared with the historic prepenicillin prophylaxis rate of 3.2–6.9 per 100 patient-years.[38] These measures reduce risk but do not remove it. The risk of recurrent *S. pneumoniae* sepsis and death in patients who have had previous sepsis is much increased; all patients having a history of pneumococcal sepsis should remain on penicillin prophylaxis indefinitely and are not candidates for outpatient management of febrile episodes.[39] Parents must be aggressively counseled to seek medical attention for all febrile events.

Hydroxyurea and Fetal Hemoglobin Reactivation

The level of Hb F in erythrocytes plays a critical role in determining patient outcomes. Individuals who have SCD and another condition called HPFH have 70% Hb S in their RBCs but are neither anemic nor symptomatic.[40] The uniform distribution of Hb F among their RBCs interferes with Hb S polymerization, increases its solubility, and prevents RBC sickling.[41,42] Even at lower levels of Hb F seen in patients without HPFH, crisis rate and mortality are inversely proportional to Hb F level.[19–22] These findings prompted the idea that pharmacologic reactivation of Hb F production might be of benefit to patients.

HU is an inhibitor of ribonucleotide reductase and a cytotoxic agent that can elevate Hb F levels via an unknown pathway. A double-blind, placebo-controlled, intention-to-treat multicenter study of HU as treatment of pain crisis in SCD found that HU produced definite hematologic changes. HU was started at 0.15 mg/kg/day and escalated to 0.30 mg/kg/day as tolerated and to maintain an absolute neutrophil count no lower than 2000×10^9 L^{-1}. There were significant increases in the levels of Hb, Hb F, F cells, F reticulocytes, packed cell volume (PCV), and MCV and declines in the mean level of leukocytes, polymorphonuclear leukocytes, reticulocytes, and dense sickle cells (Table 42.4).[43] The significant clinical changes were decreased rate of acute painful episodes, longer interval to first and second acute painful episode, fewer episodes of acute chest

TABLE 42.4   Hematologic Effects of Hydroxyurea Therapy

Variable	Hydroxyurea	Placebo	p
Leukocytes (103 cells/μL)	9.9	12.2	.0001
PMNs (103 cells/μL)	4.9	6.4	.0001
Reticulocytes (103 cells/μL)	231	300	.0001
Hemoglobin (g/dL)	9.1	8.5	.0009
PCV (%)	27.0	25.1	.0007
MCV (fl)	103	93	.0001
Hb F (%)	8.6	4.7	.0001
F cells (%)	48	35	.0001
(10^3 cells/μL)	17	15	.0036
Dense sickle cells (%)	11	13	.004

Shown are mean values after 2 years of study. Baseline values, which were not significantly different, are not shown.
Hb F, Fetal hemoglobin; MCV, mean corpuscular volume; PCV, packed cell volume; PMN, polymorphonuclear leukocyte.
Adapted from Charache S, Terrin ML, Moore RD, et al: Effect of hydroxyurea on the frequency of painful crises in sickle cell anemia. Investigators of the Multicenter Study of Hydroxyurea in Sickle Cell Anemia. *N Engl J Med* 332:1317, 1995, with permission.

TABLE 42.5   Clinical Effects of Hydroxyurea Therapy

Variable	Hydroxyurea	Placebo	p
Acute pain crisis rate	2.5/yr	4.5/yr	<.001
Hospitalization rate for acute pain crisis	1.0/yr	2.4/yr	<.001
Interval to first pain crisis	3.0 mo	1.5 mo	<.001
Interval to second pain crisis	8.8 mo	4.6 mo	<.001
Acute chest syndrome	25	51	<.001
Subjects transfused	48	73	.001
Blood units transfused	336	586	.004

Adapted from data in Charache S, Barton FB, Moore RD, et al: Hydroxyurea and sickle cell anemia. Clinical utility of a myelosuppressive "switching" agent. The Multicenter Study of Hydroxyurea in Sickle Cell Anemia. *Medicine (Baltimore)* 75:300, 1996.

syndrome, and diminished number of subjects and units transfused (Table 42.5).[44] In follow-up analysis, higher pre- or posttreatment Hb F levels were associated with a reduction in mortality rate (although no significant changes were observed in the incidence of stroke, hepatic sequestration, or death in the initial study).[18] No short-term toxicity caused by HU was observed. One child born to a patient taking HU and two born to partners of patients taking HU were normal at birth. Although the follow-up analyses suggest the importance of Hb F to better outcomes, it is possible that some HU-induced changes in sickle cell erythrocytes, such as increased water content and decreased Hb S concentration,[45] may be independent of Hb F.

In the original study, only patients with two or more pain crises per year requiring hospitalization were eligible. However, other at-risk patients should be considered for HU therapy. These include patients with evidence of chronic organ damage, patients with severe anemia (unless the reticulocyte count is <250,000 μL^{-1}, in which case consider erythropoietin [EPO] deficiency from renal damage or bone marrow suppression that may require alternative treatment), and patients with indications for chronic transfusion but who have alloantibodies. After obtaining the baseline evaluations per Table 42.2, HU is usually started at 500–1000 mg/day with monitoring of the CBC every 4–8 weeks to ensure that neutropenia (absolute neutrophil count $<2 \times 10^9$ L^{-1}) is not produced. Lower doses may be required

in patients with renal insufficiency and/or relative reticulocytopenia. The dose is increased to a stable maximum Hb F response or neutropenia, but most patients receive between 500 and 2000 mg/day. Response is defined by clinical symptoms, by a persistent and significant (>0.5 g/dL) increase in total Hb or Hb F, and a decrease in LDH. These improvements in symptomatology and hematologic indices may require at least 3–4 months of therapy but can be seen as soon as week 6.

In studies of HU as a therapy for children with SCD, the drug was well tolerated and produced favorable hematologic changes similar to those seen in the adult population.[46] In approximately 10% of the children treated, the increase in Hb F was less than 2%. Baseline Hb F levels, baseline total Hb levels, and compliance were associated with the final Hb F level.[47] Other studies in children have documented a decrease in the number of days of hospitalization and suggest a decreased incidence of vasoocclusive crises.[48] The favorable changes in hematologic indices suggest that HU therapy might be an alternative to blood transfusions for the prevention of recurrent stroke in children with SCD.[49,50] HU therapy appears to lower transcranial Doppler velocities in children with SCD.[51] Studies in the United States and in Belgium support the potential role of HU in the prevention of cerebrovascular accidents (CVAs).[50,52,53] HU was found to improve, but not correct, the abnormal cerebral oxygen saturation associated with SCD.[54]

A persistent concern pertaining to the use of HU in SCD is its putative leukemogenic effect. This concern derives from reports on HU treatment of myeloproliferative diseases, conditions associated with an inherent propensity for leukemic conversion. Although the use of HU combined with ^{36}P or alkylating agents is associated with increased leukemic conversion in patients with myeloproliferative disease,[55] reports claiming a leukemogenic effect for HU alone in polycythemia vera either lacked control subjects[56] or were not designed to assess this issue.[57] In children with the nonmalignant underlying condition of erythrocytosis secondary to inoperable cyanotic congenital heart disease, no leukemic conversion was observed.[58]

Vitamin or Nutritional Supplementation

Chronic hemolysis results in increased utilization of folic acid stores. Megaloblastic crises from folic acid deficiency have been reported.[59,60] Pediatric patients with SCD had higher homocysteine levels than age-matched control African American patients.[61] Folic acid, 1 mg/day orally, is administered as a standard of care.[62] Vitamin B_{12} deficiency can also be seen in patients with SCD. Folate replacement can mask and possibly exacerbate vitamin B_{12} deficiency.[63]

A growing body of research indicates that sickle cell patients have widespread mineral and vitamin deficiencies, including zinc, vitamin C, vitamin E, acetylcysteine, calcium, vitamin D, vitamin A, and others.[64] Fifty percent of children with SCD have evidence of osteoporosis or osteopenia that is associated with inadequate calcium and vitamin D intake.[65–67] Recently, zinc supplementation in a prospective trial documented significant improvement in linear growth and weight gain in children with SCD.[68] Therefore daily supplementation with a multivitamin without iron may be of value, and in individuals with vitamin D deficiency (which is often severe[69]), additional vitamin D replacement therapy should be considered.

Despite increased intestinal absorption of iron in SCD, the combination of nutritional deficiency and urinary iron losses results in iron deficiency in 20% of children with SCD.[70] The diagnosis of iron deficiency may be obscured by the elevated serum iron levels associated with chronic hemolysis, necessitating the detection of a low serum ferritin level or an elevated serum transferrin level for the diagnosis.

Transfusion Therapy

The two main approaches to transfusion in SCD are simple transfusion and exchange transfusion. These transfusions can be administered in an episodic fashion or in a chronic fashion. Therefore transfusion therapy in SCD is of the following types: episodic simple, episodic partial exchange, or chronic partial exchange. In both simple and exchange transfusion, the target Hb level is 10–11 g/dL (hematocrit, 30%).[71,72] Transfusing to a higher Hb or hematocrit level is avoided because a hematocrit level greater than 30% is associated with hyperviscosity if there is a substantial proportion of Hb S in the blood. In exchange transfusion, an additional objective is to achieve an Hb S percentage of less than 30% (or sometimes <50%). In partial-exchange transfusion, a proportion of the patient's diseased RBCs are removed before transfusion of normal donor RBCs; this can be done manually through phlebotomy followed by transfusion or concurrently using an automated device. In patients who need chronic transfusions, partial exchange is recommended because of the reduced iron burden of this approach. Partial exchange is also indicated if the baseline Hb level is more than 10 g/dL. Simple transfusion in this instance risks exacerbating the clinical condition through increased viscosity. For critical illness, exchange transfusion is also preferred. Although the target Hb S level should be less than 30% in exchange transfusion, decreasing Hb S levels to less than 50% may suffice depending on the severity of the complication being treated.

The volumes required for simple and exchange transfusions (Table 42.6) are particularly important for transfusing children. For normal-size adults, the general rule is that each unit of RBCs infused increases the Hb level approximately 1 g/dL.[73]

Episodic simple transfusion should be considered for blood volume replacement in aplastic crisis and splenic sequestration crises and for protection when there is a more than 20% decrease in Hb from baseline from severe illness such as septicemia or severe vasoocclusive crisis or hyperhemolysis or Hb levels of less than 5 g/dL. Episodic simple or exchange transfusion should be considered for acute chest syndrome, priapism, and preoperatively. The choice of simple versus exchange transfusion is determined by the pretransfusion total Hb level and the severity of the illness.

In the preoperative setting, there is good randomized data to support the use of preoperative transfusion to decrease the risk of complications, including severe complications such as acute chest syndrome.[74,75] Preoperative transfusions can be categorized as follows. (1) Top-up transfusions to a target Hb level of 10 g/dL. This is an appropriate intervention for patients with baseline Hb between 6.5–9 g/dL undergoing low or medium risk surgeries (e.g., cholecystectomy, joint replacement). (2) Partial exchange transfusion to achieve a target Hb level of 10 g/dL with an estimated Hb S percentage of <60%. This is an appropriate intervention for patients with baseline Hb levels of >9.5 g/dL undergoing low- or medium-risk surgeries as per above. (3) Exchange transfusion to achieve a target Hb level of 10 g/dL with an estimated Hb S percentage of <30%. This procedure should be considered for patients with SCD undergoing high-risk surgeries (e.g., cardiothoracic surgery). In short, surgery, even low- or medium-risk surgery, is a substantial physiologic stressor for patients with SCD, even those who do not have high risk characteristics at the time of surgery, and preoperative transfusion should be considered. A caveat is that extended phenotyping of transfused red cells, should be performed, as discussed further subsequently.

Chronic partial-exchange transfusion is indicated in primary and secondary prevention of cerebral thrombosis as discussed in the section on neurologic complications.

Transfusion complications include alloimmunization, delayed hemolytic transfusion reactions (discussed in Exacerbations of Anemia), iron overload, and transmission of viral illness. The incidence of alloimmunization is between 19% and 30% and usually occurs with fewer than 15 transfusions.[76] Some patients seem to tolerate multiple transfusions without developing alloantibodies, but others are readily allosensitized. The high rate of alloimmunization in transfused sickle cell patients is partly attributable to minor blood group incompatibilities between the recipient and donor pool, which often differ in ethnicity.[76,77] Antibodies against the C and E antigens of the Rh group, Kell (K) and Lewis, Duffy (Fya, Fyb), and Kidd (Jk) are common.[76] In the Stroke Prevention Trial in Sickle Cell Anemia, the routine use of WBC-reduced RBCs matched for E, C, and Kell decreased the allosensitization rate compared with historical data from 3% to 0.5% per unit transfused and decreased the rate of hemolytic transfusion reactions by 90%.[78] Therefore the recommended approach to preventing alloimmunization is to reduce leukocytes and perform limited phenotype matching for all patients (ABO, C, D, E, and Kell) and extended phenotype matching for patients with alloantibodies.[72] The management of a delayed hemolytic transfusion reaction and transfusional iron overload are discussed under Exacerbations of Anemia, later.

Transmission of human immunodeficiency virus, hepatitis B and C, and human T-cell leukemia/lymphoma virus-1 has diminished with improved screening of banked units but remains an issue. In addition to better screening programs, the use of leukocyte-depleted RBC transfusions can reduce this hazard.[79]

Stem Cell Transplantation

At this time, allogeneic stem cell transplantation remains the only curative option for SCD, and improvements in conditioning approaches suggest both pediatric and adult populations are eligible. The largest series to date has been in a pediatric population with severely symptomatic SCD failing to respond to HU. Using myeloablative conditioning and human leukocyte antigen (HLA)–matched or one-mismatch (two cases) sibling donors, with bone marrow as the source of stem cells in the majority, there was a 10% mortality rate with 90% overall survival and 82% event-free survival at a median follow-up of 54 months.[80] Similar results were obtained when related, HLA-matched umbilical cord blood was used as the source of stem cells.[81] According to these results, stem cell transplant is a therapeutic option for the severely symptomatic child with an HLA-matched sibling donor.

In adults, incorporation of rapamycin (to induce immunologic tolerance) into nonmyeloablative stem cell transplant protocols has enabled stable mixed hematopoietic chimerism with associated full-donor erythroid engraftment and normalization of blood counts. The attainment of tolerance may allow extension of this potentially curative approach to alternative donor sources, an active area of research.[82,83] The issue of the cost-effectiveness of bone marrow transplantation (BMT) gains perspective from the comparative costs in the United States of $150,000 to $200,000 for an uncomplicated BMT versus up to $112,000 annually for conventional medical care of a chronically transfused, iron-overloaded patient.[84]

Education

Education regarding the nature of the disease, genetic counseling, and psychosocial assessments of patients and their families are best

---

TABLE 42.6	Transfusion Formulas

Dilutional effects of transfusion on Hb S: PRBC volume (PRBCV) (mL) = $(Hct_d − Hct_i) × TBV × Hct_{rp}B$

Manual partial-exchange transfusion:[a] Hb Sf = $1 − \dfrac{(PRBCV × Hct_{rp})}{(TBV × Hct_i) + (PRBCV × Hct_{rp})} × Hb\ S_iC$

Automated exchange transfusion: Exchange volume (mL) = $(Hct_d − Hct_i) × TBVHct_{rp} − (Hct_i + Hct_d)2D$

RBC volume (mL) = $Hct_i × TBV$

[a]In these formulas, Hct and Hb S are fractions (e.g., 40% = 0.4). Hct_d, desired hematocrit; Hct_i, initial hematocrit; Hct_{rp}, hematocrit of replacement cells (usually 0.75); Hb S_i, initial Hb S; Hb S_f, final Hb S; PRBC, packed red blood cells; TBV, estimated total blood volume in milliliters (children, 80 mL/kg; adults, 65 mL/kg; nomograms are available). (From Linderkamp et al, with permission. Copyright 1977, Springer-Verlag.) From Nieburg and Stockman, with permission. Copyright 1977, American Medical Association.

accomplished during routine visits. Parents of small children are instructed regarding early detection of infection and palpating enlarging spleens.

Phlebotomy

As mentioned, an Hb level of more than 10–11 g/dL (hematocrit 30%) in the presence of substantial amounts of Hb S (>30%) is associated with hyperviscosity. Some data indicate that phlebotomy to reduce the hematocrit and viscosity (and which may also address iron-overload) can decrease the frequency of crises in Hb SC or Hb S–β+ disease.[85] In Hb SS disease, phlebotomy has successfully been used in combination with HU (which increases the Hb level) in secondary stroke prevention in patients previously treated with chronic transfusion.[86] Phlebotomy alone has also been used in Hb SS disease with baseline Hb levels of more than 9.5 g/dL with favorable results on the frequency and duration of pain crises. This benefit may have resulted from decreased hematocrit and viscosity and from a decrease in intracellular Hb concentration from iron deficiency.[87] One approach to phlebotomy is to remove approximately 10 mL/kg of blood over 20–30 minutes followed by infusion of an equal volume of normal saline. This is repeated every 2 weeks until the target Hb level of 9–9.5 g/dL is achieved.

Erythropoietin or Darbepoetin

The chronic hemolytic anemia of SCD is partially compensated by vigorous reticulocytosis. A decrease in compensatory reticulocytosis will exacerbate already existent anemia and can be expected to increase clinical risk. Accordingly, chronic relative reticulocytopenia (defined as Hb <9 g/dL and absolute reticulocyte count <250,000 × 10^9 L^{-1}) was identified as a significant risk factor for early mortality in a prospective cohort study of patients with SCD.[88]

In the general population, evaluation of EPO levels is usually prompted by the combination of anemia and abnormal serum creatinine level. EPO levels are then interpreted in relationship to the Hb level to assess for the possibility of EPO deficiency. In patients with SCD, this approach to diagnosis has pitfalls. Patients with SCD are already anemic; therefore, gradual anemia exacerbation is easily missed, and clinicians must weigh many possible causes in the context of complex, multisystem SCD pathology. Furthermore, patients with SCD have low serum creatinine levels at baseline. Therefore a substantial increase in serum creatinine from baseline may nonetheless remain below the threshold defined as abnormal for the general population, potentially disguising the presence of renal damage that is sufficient to decrease renal endocrine function. Furthermore, EPO levels are not readily interpreted in the individual patient with SCD: EPO levels in SCD are generally low for the level of Hb.[89] One contributing factor could be increased uptake by the massive compensatory reticulocytosis. However, EPO levels are lower in SCD adults than in children,[89] and EPO levels are inappropriately lower in patients with chronic relative reticulocytopenia.[19] Hence, EPO deficiency should be considered as a possible cause of progressive anemia in patients with absolute reticulocyte counts below 250,000 × 10^9 L^{-1} even if their serum creatinine levels are in the normal range. The cumulative published experience of EPO use in SCD is limited (52 patients).[90] Although EPO by itself has been reported to increase Hb F levels, the most important role for EPO may be as replacement therapy for EPO deficiency that causes relative reticulocytopenia and progressive anemia. EPO replacement can also facilitate enhanced HU dosing and Hb F augmentation.[90] In using recombinant human EPO, caution must be exercised not to elevate the hematocrit to levels that result in hyperviscosity. Also, the reticulocyte fraction is the most adhesive, and it is possible that EPO could exacerbate or trigger sickle cell crises.[90] Patients with SCD may be relatively resistant to EPO and require doses higher than those used in other patients with chronic renal failure. The reasons for EPO resistance are unclear but

may include increased inflammation-mediated suppression of erythropoiesis.[91]

EPO therapy is probably not indicated in patients receiving chronic transfusion therapy in whom encouraging endogenous Hb S containing erythropoiesis may be counterproductive.

Iron Chelation

Early death is well described in association with iron overload from β-thalassemia and hereditary hemochromatosis.[92,93] Similarly, iron overload is likely to be a problem in chronically transfused patients with SCD, although the clinical significance may critically depend on the degree and duration of overload. Chelation guidelines for patients with SCD are similar to those for other chronically transfused, iron-overloaded patients; iron chelation is indicated when the total body iron level is elevated (ferritin >2000 μg/L, quantitative liver iron of 2000 μg/g dry weight, transfusion history >1 year of monthly transfusions).[94] Notably, the serum ferritin level may underestimate clinically significant iron overload.[95,96] Iron chelation options in the United States are deferoxamine (via continuous intravenous or subcutaneous infusion), deferasirox (orally), and deferiprone. There is some data to support greater effectiveness of the oral agents, in particular deferiprone, in cardiac iron unloading, and together with the oral route of administration and toxicity profile, deferasirox or deferiprone are favored over deferoxamine.[97–99]

Newer US Food and Drug Administration (FDA)–approved methods of quantitating iron burden by Ferriscan of the liver[100] can avoid the need for liver biopsies. T2-weighted MRI of the heart indicates hemosiderosis of cardiac tissue, and when the results are abnormal, aggressive chelation is mandated.[101]

Alternatives to Hydroxyurea for Hb F Induction

Alternatives to HU for pharmacologic induction of Hb F that are being studied in clinical trials include the methyltransferase inhibitor 5-aza-2′-deoxycytidine (decitabine) and histone deacetylase inhibitors.[102] These classes of agents act on chromatin processes that regulate gene transcription.

The methyltransferase inhibitors 5-azacytidine and 5-aza-2′-deoxycytidine have produced the largest increases in Hb F of any of the pharmacologic reactivators of Hb F that have been tested.[103,104] Responding patients include those who did not respond to HU, consistent with a different mechanism of action. Although improvements in a number of surrogate clinical endpoints have been demonstrated, larger studies to confirm safety and clinical effectiveness with chronic use are required. In the United States, 5-azacytidine and decitabine have been approved by the FDA for the treatment of myelodysplastic syndrome. The efficacy of the class of agents known as histone deacetylase inhibitors in Hb F reactivation has been reviewed.[104–106] As per the methyltransferase inhibitors, further clinical trials are needed. Other classes of drugs being evaluated for potential Hb F reactivation are the "imid" class of drugs (analogues of thalidomide such as pomalidomide) and inhibitors of lysine demethylase (LSD1/KDM1A).[107]

Preventing Red Blood Cell Dehydration With Ion Channel Inhibitors

Polymerization of Hb S is related to the Hb S concentration within the cell. Therefore a therapeutic strategy could be to reduce the intracellular Hb S concentration. It is possible to reduce the Hb concentration by reducing the Hb content with iron deficiency. It has been observed that spontaneous or induced iron deficiency (see Phlebotomy, earlier) sufficient to reduce the serum ferritin, MCV, and mean cell Hb concentration (MCHC) resulted in variably improved Hb S polymerization, RBC survival, level of anemia, and clinical status.[108]

Anticoagulation or Antiplatelet Therapy

Although there is clear evidence of activation of the coagulation system in SCD, the role of thrombogenesis in vasoocclusive crisis remains unclear.[109] Similarly, there have been no thorough evaluations of the role of antiplatelet or antithrombotic agents for the treatment of SCD. D-dimer levels (a degradation product of cross-linked fibrin) increase during acute vasoocclusive crisis.[110]

Minidose heparin, 5000 to 7500 units every 12 hours, administered to four patients for 2–6 years reduced hospitalization and emergency department time by 75%, and pretreatment pain frequency recurred after heparin was discontinued.[111] Larger clinical studies will be required to better understand the risks and benefits of heparin therapy for acute vasoocclusive crisis in SCD. Heparin has not been studied for acute arterial stroke in patients with SCD but has a role in SCD-associated dural venous sinus thrombosis.[112] The management of stroke is fully discussed under Specific Complications and Their Management.

Acenocoumarol was administered in low doses that achieved a mean international normalized ratio (INR) of 1.64 and reduced the elevated levels of prothrombin activation fragment (fragment 1+2) to 50% of pretreatment levels.[113] Clinical endpoints were not measured. In a crossover study, 29 patients were treated with acenocoumarol to target an INR of 1.6–2.0. No effect on crisis frequency was noted, although again, there were significant reductions in markers of coagulation system activation.[114] In 37 acutely ill sickle cell patients with elevated D-dimers, the effect of low-dose warfarin therapy (1 mg without a target INR) in 12 of them was examined. In multivariate analysis, low-dose warfarin was the only variable associated with a significant decrease in D-dimer levels, suggesting a warfarin-induced decrease in thrombin activity.[110] Therefore oral anticoagulation, even at low doses, is associated with a decrease in laboratory markers of coagulation pathway activation in SCD; however, further clinical trials are required to understand the clinical risks and benefits.

Aspirin was compared with placebo in 49 pediatric patients with SCD in a double-blind crossover study. The frequency and severity of crises were not affected by aspirin therapy.[115] Cerebral thrombosis, which accounts for 70% to 80% of all CVAs in SCD, results from large-vessel occlusion (Fig. 42.9) rather than the more typical microvascular occlusion of SCD. In the United States, there is an ongoing clinical trial testing the safety and efficacy of aspirin in diminishing the incidence and progression of cognitive defects and overt or silent stroke in pediatric patients.

The management of stroke risk and stroke is fully discussed under Specific Complications and Their Management.

Experimental Therapies

Experimental approaches in early stages of clinical evaluation include glutamine supplementation, gene correction using zinc finger nucleases or "CRISPR" that exploit physiologic homology-directed DNA repair, agents that inhibit sickle erythrocyte adhesion to endothelium (recombinant P-selectin glycoprotein ligand-1–immunoglobulin G conjugate), agents that increase the production of nitric oxide (NO) [glutamine], and herbal extracts with unknown mechanisms of action (Niprisan).[116–118]

Specific Complications and Their Management

Pain Crisis

Acute Pain Episode or Crisis

Acute pain is the first symptom of disease in more than 25% of patients and is the most frequent symptom after age 2 years.[119] Pain is the complication for which patients with SCD most commonly seek medical attention.[120] An episode of acute pain was originally

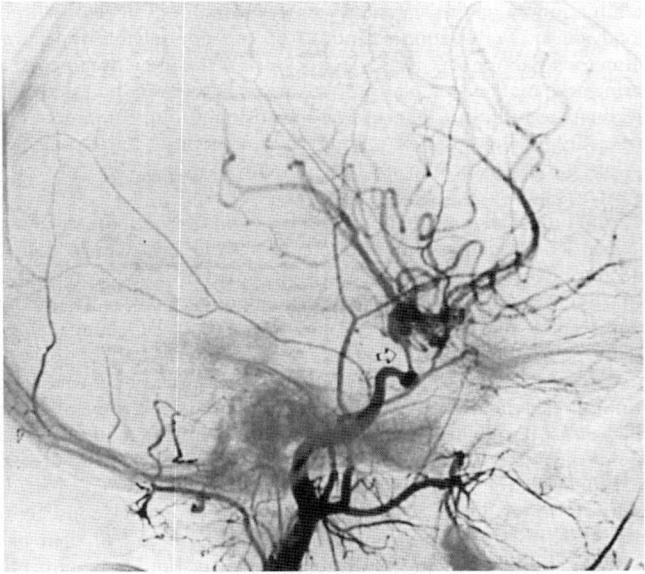

Fig. 42.9 Right common carotid arteriogram taken in anteroposterior projection demonstrating complete occlusion of the origin of the right anterior cerebral artery *(arrowhead). (From Stockman JA, Nigro MA, Mishkin MM, Oski FA: Occlusion of large cerebral vessels in sickle-cell anemia.* N Engl J Med *287:846, 1972.)*

called a "sickle cell crisis" by Diggs, who used the expression "crisis" to refer to any new rapidly developing syndrome in the life of a patient with SCD.[121] The basic mechanism is believed to be vasoocclusion of the bone marrow vasculature causing bone infarction, which in turn causes release of inflammatory mediators that activate afferent nociceptors.[122]

Although a general correlation of vasoocclusive severity and genotype has been posited,[123] there is tremendous variability within genotypes and in the same patient over time. In one large study of patients with Hb SS disease, one-third rarely had pain, one-third were hospitalized for pain approximately two to six times per year, and one-third had more than six pain-related hospitalizations per year.[124] Over a 5-year period in the National Cooperative Study of SCD, 40% of patients had no painful episodes, and 5% of patients accounted for one-third of the emergency department visits. Pain is more frequent with the Hb SS genotype, low levels of Hb F, higher Hb levels,[28] and sleep apnea.[125] The frequency of pain peaks between ages 19 and 39 years. After the age of 19 years, more frequent pain correlates with a higher mortality rate.[28] Medical personnel who see patients only in the emergency department gain a biased view of SCD skewed by a frequently affected minority with severe disease.[126,127]

Pain may be precipitated by events such as cold, dehydration, infection, stress, menses, and alcohol consumption. Any underlying cause should be searched for and corrected, but the majority of painful episodes have no identifiable cause. Pain can affect any area of the body, most commonly the back, chest, extremities, and abdomen; may vary from trivial to excruciating; and is usually endured at home without a visit to the emergency department. There may be premonitory symptoms.[127] The duration averages a few days, with hospital admissions typically lasting between 4 and 10 days. Painful episodes are biopsychosocial events caused by vasoocclusion in an area of the body having nociceptors and nerves.[122] Pain is an effect and, as such, consists of sensory, perceptual, cognitive, and emotional components. Frequent pain generates feelings of despair, depression, and apathy that interfere with everyday life and promote an existence that revolves around pain. This scenario may lead to a chronic debilitating pain syndrome; fortunately, this is rare.

There is no specific clinical or laboratory finding pathognomonic of pain crisis. The diagnosis is established by history and physical examination. Changes in steady-state Hb values, sickled cells on blood smear, WBC counts, and so on are not reliable indicators. Numerous laboratory tests, leukocytosis, D-dimer fragments of fibrin, and markers of platelet activation have been found to lack specificity as indicators of acute vasoocclusion. Often patients can tell if they are having a typical pain crisis or something more sinister. It is thus good practice to ask the patient if it feels like the usual pain-crisis pain.

Initial medical assessment should focus on detection of triggers or medical complications requiring specific therapy, which include infection, dehydration, acute chest syndrome (fever, tachypnea, chest pain, hypoxia, and chest signs), severe anemia, cholecystitis, splenic enlargement, neurologic events, and priapism.[128] Pain management should be aggressive to make the pain tolerable and enable patients to attain maximum functional ability. To make the patient pain free is an unrealistic goal and risks oversedation and hypoventilation, which must be avoided. A pain chart should be started and analgesia titrated against the patient's reported pain together with medical assessment of the patient's overall clinical status, paying particular attention to avoiding oversedation. When clinicians consistently observe a disparity between patients' verbal self-report of their pain and their ability to function, further assessment should be performed to ascertain the reason for disparity. Patients are often undertreated for pain because many physicians and other health care providers are overly concerned with the potential for addiction. Undertreatment of pain is no more desirable than overtreatment and oversedation; undertreatment can prolong the duration of a painful episode and can poison the relationship between the patient and the health care system. In assessing patient responses to conventional doses of

analgesia, it must be remembered that individuals with SCD metabolize narcotics rapidly.[129]

The pain pathway should be targeted at different points with different agents, avoiding toxicity with any one class (Table 42.7). The mainstays are nonsteroidal antiinflammatory drugs (NSAIDs), acetaminophen, and opioids. NSAIDs can be used to control mild to moderate pain and may have an additive role in combination with opioids for severe pain. The most potent NSAID is ketorolac. NSAIDs should be used with caution in those with a history of peptic ulcer, renal insufficiency, asthma, or bleeding tendencies. Within limits, use the agents that the patients know work for them and avoid meperidine (Demerol), which should only be used under very exceptional circumstances. Sedatives and anxiolytics alone should not be used to manage pain because they can mask the behavioral response to pain without providing analgesia.

Treatment of persistent or moderate to severe pain should be based on increasing the opioid strength or dose.[128] One approach is to administer morphine 0.1 mg/kg intravenously or subcutaneously every 20 minutes until pain is controlled. The patient should be checked at 20-minute intervals for pain; respiratory rate, depth, and quality; and sedation until the patient is stable with adequate pain control. Subsequently, the patient should receive a maintenance dose of 0.05–0.15 mg/kg intravenously or subcutaneously every 2–4 hours. A rescue dose of 50% of the maintenance dose can be considered on an as-needed basis every 30 minutes for breakthrough pain.

During maintenance with opioids, pain control; respiratory rate, depth, and quality; and oxygen saturation should be monitored approximately every 2 hours. If respiratory depression is noted, omit the maintenance dose of morphine. For severe respiratory depression

TABLE 42.7   Recommended Dose and Interval of Analgesics Necessary to Obtain Adequate Pain Control in Patients With Sickle Cell Disease

	Dose/Rate	Comments
Severe to Moderate Pain		
Morphine	Parenteral: 0.1–0.15 mg/kg every 3–4 h Recommended maximum single dose, 10 mg PO: 0.3–0.6 mg/kg every 4 h	Drug of choice for pain; lower doses in elderly adults and infants and in patients with liver failure or impaired ventilation
Meperidine	Parenteral: 0.75–1.5 mg/kg every 2–4 h Recommended maximum dose, 100 mg PO: 1.5 mg/kg every 4 h	Increased incidence of seizures; avoid in patients with renal or neurologic disease and those who receive MAOIs
Hydromorphone	Parenteral: 0.01–0.02 mg/kg every 3–4 h PO: 0.04–0.06 mg/kg every 4 h	
Oxycodone	PO: 0.15 mg/kg/dose every 4 h	
Ketorolac	IM: Adults: 30 or 60 mg initial dose followed by 15–30 mg; children: 1 mg/kg load followed by 0.5 mg/kg every 6 h	Equal efficacy to 6 mg MS; helps narcotic-sparing effect; not to exceed 5 days; maximum, 150 mg first day, 120 mg maximum on subsequent days; may cause gastric irritation
Butorphanol	Parenteral: Adults: 2 mg every 3–4 h	Agonist–antagonist; can precipitate withdrawal if given to patients who are being treated with agonists
Mild Pain		
Codeine	PO: 0.5–1 mg/kg every 4 h Maximum dose, 60 mg	Mild to moderate pain not relieved by aspirin or acetaminophen; can cause nausea and vomiting
Aspirin	PO: Adults: 0.3–6 mg every 4–6 h; children: 10 mg/kg every 4 h	Often given with a narcotic to enhance analgesia; can cause gastric irritation; avoid in febrile children
Acetaminophen	PO: Adults: 0.3–0.6 g every 4 h; children: 10 mg/kg	Often given with a narcotic to enhance analgesia
Ibuprofen	PO: Adults: 300–400 mg every 4 h; children: 5–10 mg/kg every 6–8 h	Can cause gastric irritation
Naproxen	PO: Adults: 500 mg/dose initially and then 250 every 8–12 h; children: 10 mg/kg/day (5 mg/kg every 12 h)	Long duration of action; can cause gastric irritation
Indomethacin	PO: Adults: 25 mg every 8 h; children: 1–3 mg/kg/day given 3 or 4 times	Contraindicated in psychiatric, neurologic, renal diseases; high incidence of gastric irritation; useful in gout

IM, Intramuscular; MAOI, monoamine oxidase inhibitor; MS, morphine sulphate; PO, oral.
Adapted from Charache S, Terrin ML, Moore RD, et al. Effect of hydroxyurea on the frequency of painful crises in sickle cell anemia. Investigators of the Multicenter Study of Hydroxyurea in Sickle Cell Anemia. *N Engl J Med* 332:1317, 1995.

or oxygen desaturation, administer naloxone. Incentive spirometry and mandatory time out of bed are helpful in patients with chest pain to decrease the risk for hypoventilation. Adjuvant medications to consider include NSAIDs, acetaminophen, antiemetics, and antihistamines. Laxatives or stool softeners should be prescribed in keeping with close monitoring for constipation.

After 2–3 days, consider decreasing the dose and switching from parenteral to oral administration of opioids. For adult patients whose pain requires several or many days to resolve, a sustained-release opioid preparation is appropriate and provides a more consistent analgesia.

Hydration is a critical part of management. However, cardiac function may be significantly impaired, especially in adult patients, and standard discipline must be followed with intravenous fluid management to avoid iatrogenic fluid overload. Patients with SCD cannot concentrate their urine and are at risk for dehydration when not taking adequate fluids (60 mL/kg/24 h in adults). Intravenous hydration is indicated when the patient is not taking oral fluids adequately. Ideally, the urine specific gravity should be kept under 1.010 by daily testing when in the hospital. Hb may decrease by 1–2 g/dL in an uncomplicated pain crisis; blood transfusion is not routinely indicated for an uncomplicated pain crisis.

Equianalgesic doses of oral opioids should be prescribed for home use when necessary to maintain the relief achieved in the emergency department or hospital ward. Care should be taken to appropriately taper opioids in patients who have received daily opioids over many days. In these patients, there may be physical opiate dependence, which is characterized by the onset of acute withdrawal symptoms upon cessation of opioid administration. For patients at risk for physical dependence, opiates should be titrated downward by 15% to 20% per day to zero. Physical dependence is a physiologic problem, but addiction is a psychologic problem characterized by craving—behavior that is overwhelmingly directed at obtaining the drug; use of the drug for purposes other than pain control; and use of the drug despite negative physical, social, legal, or psychologic consequences.

If the patient is not taking a disease-modifying agent such as HU, consideration should be given to initiating such therapy either as an inpatient or during follow up in the outpatient setting.

Chronic Pain

Chronic pain in SCD usually (but not always) has an identifiable basis such as vertebral fractures, femoral head necrosis, early degenerative changes or osteoarthritis, or chronic skin ulcers. Most patients without such identifiable complications do not require chronic pain medications similar to those used for terminal cancer because the pain from a typical vasoocclusive crisis is episodic. Inappropriately maintaining patients without chronic musculoskeletal degeneration on long-acting opiates can impair their overall psychosocial functioning. On the other hand, adequate analgesia with long-acting opiates (e.g., long-acting morphine preparations similar to those used in cancer patients) is important to maintain the psychosocial functioning of patients who do have complications that cause chronic pain. Also, consider agents such as amitriptyline or antiseizure medications[130] that can address neuropathic components and help decrease the sleep impairment and depression that can occur with chronic pain. If the patient is not taking a disease-modifying agent such as HU, consideration should be given to initiating such therapy.

Chronic Anemia

Chronic hemolytic anemia is one of the hallmarks of SCD. Sickle erythrocytes are destroyed randomly, with a mean life span of 17 days.[131] The overall hemolytic rate reflects the number of ISCs.[132] The degree of anemia is most severe in sickle cell anemia, and Hb S–β°-thalassemia, milder in Hb S–β⁺-thalassemia and Hb SC disease,[133] and, among patients with sickle cell anemia, less severe in those who have coexistent α-thalassemia (Table 42.8 and see Table 42.1).[134]

As already noted, EPO deficiency from otherwise subclinical chronic renal damage may also contribute to a decline in Hb levels below baseline. The level of chronic anemia is a significant prognostic marker.[19]

The treatment options for the chronic anemia of SCD have already been mentioned. These strategies attempt to decrease hemolysis by increasing Hb F (HU and the experimental approaches with EPO, decitabine, and histone deacetylase inhibitors) or decreasing

TABLE 42.8	Bacteria and Viruses That Most Frequently Cause Serious Infection in Patients With Sickle Cell Disease		
Microorganism	**Type of Infection**	**Comments**	
Streptococcus pneumoniae	Septicemia	Common despite prophylactic penicillin and pneumococcal vaccine	
	Meningitis	Less frequent than in years past	
	Pneumonia	Rarely documented except in infants and young children	
	Septic arthritis	Uncommon	
Haemophilus influenzae type b	Septicemia		
Meningitis			
Pneumonia	Much less common in recent years because of immunization with conjugate vaccine		
Salmonella species	Osteomyelitis		
Septicemia	Most common cause of bone and joint infection		
Escherichia coli and other gram-negative enteric pathogens	Septicemia		
Urinary tract infection			
Osteomyelitis	Focus sometimes not apparent		
Staphylococcus aureus	Osteomyelitis	Uncommon	
Mycoplasma pneumoniae	Pneumonia	Pleural effusions; multilobe involvement	
Chlamydia pneumoniae	Pneumonia		
Parvovirus B19	Bone marrow suppression (aplastic crisis)	High fever common; rash and other organ involvement infrequent	
Hepatitis viruses (A, B, and C)	Hepatitis	Marked hyperbilirubinemia	

Data from Buchanan GR, Glader BE: Benign course of extreme hyperbilirubinemia in sickle cell anemia: Analysis of six cases. *J Pediatr* 91:21, 1977.

the intracellular Hb S concentration by preventing RBC dehydration (Gardos channel inhibitors).

Exacerbations of Anemia

The rather constant level of hemolytic anemia may be exacerbated by additional events such as aplastic crises, acute splenic sequestration, acute hepatic sequestration, chronic renal disease, or renal endocrine deficiency that may be present without overt renal failure, bone marrow necrosis, deficiency of folic acid or iron, delayed hemolytic transfusion reactions, autoimmune hemolytic anemia, or hyperhemolysis (hemolytic exacerbations) of unknown etiology. Laboratory evaluations that are very useful in the evaluation of a patient with anemia exacerbation are the reticulocyte count, LDH, alloantibody screening, the direct antiglobulin (Coombs) test, and EPO level.

Aplastic Crises

Aplastic crises are transient arrests of erythropoiesis characterized by abrupt falls in Hb levels, reticulocyte number, and RBC precursors in the bone marrow without necessarily an increase in the LDH. Although these episodes typically last only a few days, the level of anemia may be severe because the hemolysis continues unabated in the absence of RBC production. Although the mechanisms that impair erythropoiesis in inflammation are operative in infections of all types (see Chapter 37), human parvovirus B19 specifically invades proliferating erythroid progenitors, which accounts for its importance in SCD (see Chapters 30 and 32).[135] Parvovirus B19 (Fig. 42.10) accounts for 68% of aplastic crises in children with SCD,[136] but the high incidence of protective antibodies in adults makes parvovirus a less frequent cause of aplasia in this age group (see also Infections, later in this chapter). Other reported causes of transient aplasia are infections by *S. pneumoniae,* salmonella, streptococci, and Epstein-Barr virus. Bone marrow necrosis, which also may be the result of parvovirus infection, characterized by fever, bone pain, reticulocytopenia, and a leukoerythroblastic response, also causes aplastic crisis.[137,138]

Inhaled oxygen therapy also causes transient RBC hypoproduction; supraphysiologic oxygen tensions curtail EPO production promptly and suppress reticulocytosis within 2 days.[139]

The mainstay of treating aplastic crises is RBC transfusion. When transfusion is necessitated by the degree of anemia or cardiorespiratory symptoms, a single transfusion usually will suffice because reticulocytosis resumes spontaneously within a few days. Transfusion may be avoided by keeping severely anemic patients on bed rest to prevent symptoms and by avoiding supraphysiologic oxygen tensions. A useful guideline for transfusion in the context of an aplastic crisis is the reticulocyte count. A patient having an aplastic crisis with a reticulocyte count that is recovering is less likely to require urgent transfusion than one with a normal or low absolute reticulocyte count.

Sequestration Crisis (Spleen or Liver)

Acute splenic sequestration of blood is characterized by acute exacerbation of anemia; persistent reticulocytosis; a tender, enlarging spleen; and sometimes hypovolemia.[140] The LDH level may remain stable or increase. Patients susceptible to this complication are those whose spleens have not undergone fibrosis—young patients with sickle cell anemia and adults with Hb SC disease or sickle cell–β+-thalassemia. Sequestration may occur as early as a few weeks of age and may cause death before SCD is diagnosed. In one study, 30% of children had splenic sequestration over a 10-year period and 15% of the attacks were fatal.[141]

The basis of therapy is to restore blood volume and RBC mass. Because splenic sequestration recurs in 50% of cases, splenectomy is recommended after the event has abated. Alternatively, chronic transfusion therapy is used in young children to delay splenectomy until it can be tolerated safely. Because recurrence is possible during transfusion therapy, parents should be trained to detect a rapidly enlarging spleen and to seek immediate medical attention in this event. Less common sites of acute sequestration include the liver and possibly the lung.[142,143]

Delayed Hemolytic Transfusion Reaction and Autoimmune Hemolytic Anemia

Approximately 30% of patients are predisposed to develop alloantibodies, in part because of minor blood group incompatibilities in racially mismatched blood.[77,78] The corollary is that the other patients can receive multiple transfusions without demonstrating alloantibodies. After alloimmunization, there is a subsequent decrease in antibody titer that can fall below serologically detectable levels. Therefore antigen-positive RBCs appear compatible in cross-matching and are transfused. This can result in a delayed hemolytic transfusion reaction produced by the amnestic response of the immune system (as opposed to the immediate hemolytic reaction that occurs with preformed antibody). The delayed hemolytic transfusion reaction consists of an unexplained fall in Hb, elevated LDH level, elevated bilirubin above baseline, and hemoglobinuria, all occurring between 4 and 10 days after the RBC transfusion. Delayed hemolytic reactions and hyperhemolysis have been shown to occur in 11% of pediatric patients with SCD and a history of alloantibodies.[144] In SCD the delayed hemolytic transfusion reaction can be particularly devastating because it can be accompanied by reticulocytopenia, which together with a

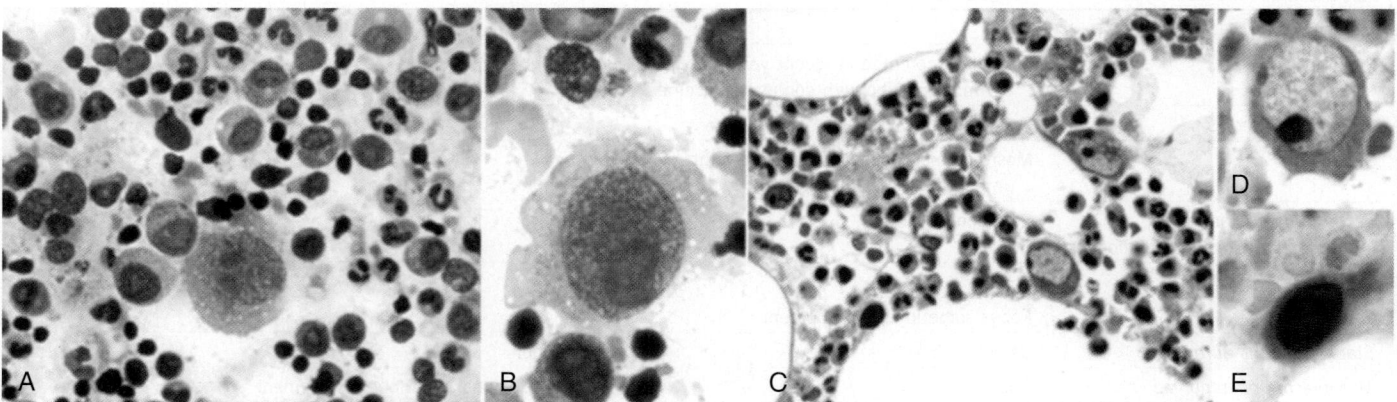

Fig. 42.10 PARVOVIRUS. Bone marrow aspirate in a patient with sickle cell disease and aplastic crisis (A). Note the absence of red blood cell precursors except for the single, large degenerating pronormoblast *(lower center)*. Such pronormoblasts contain large nuclear inclusions (B) as a result of replication of parvovirus B19. The same can be seen in the tissue sections of a bone core biopsy (C and D). The parvovirus can now be recognized immunohistochemically with an immunostain (E).

bystander effect of destruction of recipient blood (not just donor blood) can result in unanticipated worsening of anemia to levels below that seen before transfusion.[145] In addition to the manifestations of a delayed hemolytic transfusion reaction as listed, patients may develop acute congestive heart failure, acute renal failure, or acute chest syndrome (accompanied by vasoocclusive pain crisis). Subsequent transfusions may further exacerbate the anemia.

Resolution of severe anemia may only occur after withholding further transfusions with subsequent reticulocyte count recovery. Corticosteroids at high doses (e.g., intravenous methylprednisolone 500 mg/day for 2–3 days) should be considered if the anemia is life threatening or if further transfusion is deemed necessary to save the patient's life. Intravenous immunoglobulin can also be considered, with proper attention paid to avoiding iatrogenic fluid overload. Approaches to minimizing this complication include transfusing extended-matched (see Basic Management and Disease Modification), phenotypically compatible blood.[76–78] This syndrome may or may not recur with further transfusions after a recovery period.[146]

Hyperhemolytic Crisis

Hyperhemolytic crisis is the sudden exacerbation of anemia with increased reticulocytosis and bilirubin level. If suspected, the approach to management should first be to look for an underlying etiology, which may be one of the events listed earlier: aplastic crisis (during the recovery phase when the reticulocyte count may not be decreased), sequestration crisis, delayed hemolytic transfusion reaction, or autoimmune hemolysis. Another possible cause is glucose-6-phosphate dehydrogenase deficiency.[147]

Erythropoietin Deficiency

This entity is discussed under Basic Management and Disease Modification.

Nutritional Deficiencies: Folate, Iron, or Vitamin B_{12} Deficiency

This entity is discussed under Basic Management and Disease Modification.

Hypothyroidism

Iron overload in SCD can result in hypothyroidism.[148] Therefore hypothyroidism is another etiology to consider in a patient with SCD with an otherwise unexplained decrease in Hb below baseline.

Infections

Immune Deficit

The propensity of children with SCD to contract *S. pneumoniae* infection is related to impaired splenic function[149] and diminished serum opsonizing activity. Even before the anatomic autoinfarction of the spleen in patients with sickle cell anemia, defective splenic function is demonstrable by Howell-Jolly bodies on the peripheral blood smear, visible "pits" on the surface of RBCs, and abnormal results of radionuclide spleen scanning.[150] Specific syndromes exhibiting greater rates of hemolysis cause loss of splenic function at earlier ages—sickle cell anemia earlier than Hb SC disease earlier than sickle cell–β⁺-thalassemia.

Infectious complications of SCD are a major cause of morbidity and mortality[151] even with current vaccination and prophylactic antibiotic regimens. The infections caused by particular organisms are shown in Table 42.8, and the specific organisms affecting different target organs are shown in Table 42.9. By 5 years of age, almost all patients are functionally asplenic, contributing to infectious susceptibility. Historically, pneumococcal sepsis has been the predominant cause of death in those younger than 20 years of age.[152]

Evaluation

The most critical aspect of infectious illness in SCD is the evaluation and treatment of febrile children. Routine evaluation includes a physical examination, a CBC, blood and urine cultures, a lumbar puncture if meningitis is suspected, and chest radiography to evaluate for pneumonia. Results of the CBC are compared with baseline values. A left shift in the differential count suggests bacterial infection.

Penicillin Prophylaxis and Pneumonia Vaccination

Data and recommendations regarding penicillin prophylaxis and pneumonia vaccination are discussed under Basic Management and Disease Modification.

Streptococcus Pneumoniae, Haemophilus Influenzae, Atypical Mycobacteria, and Acute Febrile Illness

Streptococcus pneumoniae bacteremia is accompanied by leukocytosis, a left shift, aplastic crisis, sometimes disseminated intravascular coagulation, and a 20% to 50% mortality rate.[151] Although concerns about *S. pneumoniae* sepsis are largely for young children, this complication also occurs in adults, often with devastating results.[153] *S. pneumoniae* is the major cause of meningitis in infants and young children with SCD, and it occurs in the setting of bacteremia.

The second most common organism responsible for bacteremia in these children, *H. influenzae* type b, accounts for 10% to 25% of episodes. *H. influenzae* bacteremia affects older children and is less fulminant than *S. pneumoniae* bacteremia, but it may be fatal.[151] Conjugated *H. influenzae* type b vaccines produce excellent antibody responses in children with SCD and are now administered in early infancy (http://www.cdc.gov/vaccines/recs/schedules/child-schedule.htm).

Owing to the high mortality rate of bacteremia, hospitalization, blood and cerebrospinal fluid cultures, and parenteral antibiotics have

TABLE 42.9	Organ-Related Infection in Sickle Cell Disease				
Primary Sites of Infection	**Most Common Pathogen(s)**	**Other Pathogens**	**Pathophysiology**	**Prevention**	**Management**
Septicemia	*Streptococcus pneumonia*	*Haemophilus influenza* type b *Escherichia coli* *Salmonella* spp.	Defective splenic function; deficiency of opsonic antibody	Vaccines[a] Prophylactic penicillin	Empiric intravenous antibiotics for fever
Meningitis	*S. pneumoniae*			Same as for septicemia	
Osteomyelitis and septic arthritis	*Salmonella* spp. *S. pneumonia*	*E. coli* *Proteus* spp. *Staphylococcus aureus*		–	Surgical drainage, intravenous antibiotics
Pneumonia	*Mycoplasma pneumoniae* Respiratory viruses	*Chlamydia pneumoniae* *S. pneumoniae*		Vaccines[a]	See pulmonary and therapy sections for management of acute chest syndrome.

[a]Against *Streptococcus pneumoniae* and *Haemophilus influenzae* type b.
Data from Buchanan GR, Glader BE: Benign course of extreme hyperbilirubinemia in sickle cell anemia: Analysis of six cases. *J Pediatr* 91:21, 1977.

been the standard of care for children with fevers higher than 38.5°C. Prompt attention to fever can reduce the risk of severe pneumococcal sepsis. Rapid administration of antibiotics has resulted in a lower incidence of meningitis among patients with bacteremia than 20 years ago when the incidence was 50%.[154] The efficacy of ceftriaxone therapy for *S. pneumoniae* and *H. influenzae* infection[155] has led to new treatment algorithms that recommend outpatient therapy for most patients. However, resistant *S. pneumoniae* have emerged, necessitating a thorough knowledge of local resistance patterns to guide the choice of alternate antibiotics (particularly vancomycin, to which resistance has not been observed).

Please see Pulmonary Complications for further discussions regarding pneumonia and acute chest syndrome.

Meningitis

Meningitis therapy should cover *S. pneumoniae* and probably *H. influenzae* type b and should be continued for at least 2 weeks.

Salmonella and Osteomyelitis

In this patient population, osteomyelitis is commonly caused by *Salmonella* spp.[156] *Staphylococcus aureus*, the most common etiology in patients without SCD, accounts for less than 25% of SCD cases. Infection usually affects long bones, often at multiple sites.

The diagnosis is confirmed by culture of blood or infected bone. Parenteral antibiotics that cover *Salmonella* spp. and *S. aureus* are given, and antibiotic therapy is based on culture results. Parenteral antibiotics are continued for 2–6 weeks.[156] Surgical drainage or sequestrectomy may be required. Most patients are cured by this approach, but there may be recurrences.[156]

Articular infection is less common and is often caused by *S. pneumoniae*.[156]

Parvovirus B19

The specificity of the parvovirus B19 (see also Aplastic Crisis) for erythroid precursor cells, coupled with the accelerated erythropoiesis in hemolytic anemias, leaves sickle cell patients vulnerable to infection by this agent.[157] In SCD, parvovirus infection is a common cause of aplastic crisis, especially in children. It has been reported to cause bone marrow necrosis, acute chest syndrome, pulmonary fat embolism, hepatic sequestration, and glomerulonephritis.[135–138]

Urinary Tract Infections

Patients with SCD are at a higher risk for urinary tract infections and pyelonephritis than the general population. *Escherichia coli* is the most common uropathogen and can cause septicemia in these patients. Persistent urinary tract infections may be secondary to renal papillary necrosis. All urinary tract infections in this patient population should be considered complicated, requiring 10–21 days of appropriate antibiotic therapy.

Neurologic Complications

Neurologic complications occur in 25% or more of patients with SCD.[158] Neurologic complications include CVAs (consisting of transient ischemic attacks [TIAs], overt and silent cerebral infarction, cerebral hemorrhage), seizures (which can be a presenting feature of CVA), unexplained coma, spinal cord infarction or compression, central nervous system infections, vestibular dysfunction, and sensory hearing loss.[159]

Cerebrovascular Accidents, Pathophysiology, Incidence, Risk Factors, and Presentation[160]

Histopathologic evaluation of large-vessel involvement in SCD shows a pattern of smooth muscle proliferation with overlying endothelial damage and fibrosis. Smaller arterioles and capillaries demonstrate distension, thrombosis, and vessel-wall necrosis.[161,162] Aneurysmal dilation associated with hemorrhagic stroke occurs at regions of intimal hyperplasia.[163] The vessel wall changes are likely multifactorial in origin related to endothelial injury from high and turbulent

flow, RBC adherence, and hypoxia; but in addition, it has been speculated that depletion of NO by the free Hb released through intravascular hemolysis may also play a role.[163] The age-specific pattern of stroke risk in SCD may be related to the higher cerebral flow rates in early childhood.[163] Cerebral thrombosis, which accounts for 70% to 80% of all CVAs in patients with SCD, results from large-vessel occlusion (see Fig. 42.9) rather than the more typical microvascular occlusion of SCD.[164] Silent infarcts are thought to result from microvascular vasoocclusion or thrombosis or chronic hypoxia in the periphery stemming from large-vessel disease.[165] In 30% of patients with SCD, major vessel stenosis results in the formation of friable collateral vessels that appear as puffs of smoke (*moyamoya* in Japanese) on angiography.[166] Moyamoya disease predisposes to thrombotic and hemorrhagic strokes, seizures, and cognitive disability.[167]

The relative risk for stroke is 200–400 times higher in children with SCD compared with the children without SCD. The prevalence of clinically overt stroke is 11%. Clinically silent infarction detectable by MRI affects 17% to 20% of patients by age 20 years.[168] Silent infarcts are associated with cognitive impairment. Even in patients without silent or overt cerebral infarction, cognitive functioning can be impaired.[169] Almost 50% of the children with "silent" infarcts eventually require lifelong support or custodial care because of neuropsychologic deficits.[170] Whereas infarctive strokes were common in children and those older than 30 years of age, hemorrhagic stroke was most common between ages 20 and 30 years.[23]

Sickle cell–specific risk factors for CVA include increased cerebral blood flow velocity[171] (discussed further under Primary Prevention of Cerebrovascular Accidents), a history of overt or silent cerebral infarction,[172] nocturnal hypoxia,[173] more severe anemia, higher reticulocyte counts, lower Hb F levels, higher WBC counts, the Hb SS genotype (rather than Hb SC disease or sickle cell–β-thalassemia), nocturnal hypoxemia or sleep apnea, migraines, elevated homocysteine levels, "relative" systolic hypertension (i.e., those at the high end of the lower-than-normal range characteristic of SCD).[23,174] Genetic markers of increased risk are the Central African Republic (CAR) haplotype and the absence of α-thalassemia.[163,175] Both small- and large-vessel thrombosis can occur. Specific HLA alleles separately correlate with small- versus large-vessel stroke risk, suggesting that different pathologic processes may be involved.[163]

In addition to these sickle cell–specific predictors of stroke, one must also consider the well-documented modifiable risk factors for stroke that are operational in the general population; these are hypertension, exposure to cigarette smoke (active smoking or passive exposure), diabetes, atrial fibrillation, dyslipidemia, carotid artery stenosis, postmenopausal hormone therapy, poor diet, physical inactivity, obesity, and fat distribution. Less well-documented but potentially modifiable risk factors include alcohol or drug use, oral contraceptive use, and sleep-disordered breathing.[168]

CVAs are heralded by focal seizures in 10% to 33% of cases and by TIAs in 10%. CVAs are fatal in approximately 20% of initial cases, recur within 3 years in nearly 70%, and are the cause of motor and cognitive impairment in the majority. Intracranial hemorrhage results in the same signs as thrombosis, but in addition, neck stiffness, photophobia, severe headache, vomiting, and altered consciousness may occur. Coma suggests hemorrhage rather than thrombosis. A typical presentation is coma and seizures without hemiparesis. Although the mortality rate may be as high as 50%, the morbidity of survivors is low. Hemorrhage may be subarachnoid, intraparenchymal, or intraventricular, which can be differentiated by angiography. The favorable neurosurgical outcome in subarachnoid hemorrhage caused by ruptured aneurysm justifies an aggressive approach to diagnosis, transfusion, vasodilatory therapy, and surgery.

Primary Prevention of Cerebrovascular Accidents

The overall risk of stroke in pediatric patients with SCD is 1% per year; however, in the subset of patients with transcranial Doppler, evidence of a high (>200 cm/s) cerebral blood flow velocity in the internal carotid artery or middle cerebral artery, the stroke risk is in excess of 10% per year (although this is still much lower than the risk of recurrent stroke in a sickle cell patient after a first event, which is approximately 70%). In the Stroke Prevention Trial in Sickle Cell Disease (STOP), 130 children diagnosed as having clinically silent cerebral artery stenosis on the basis of high cerebral flow rates were randomized to receive chronic transfusion therapy or not. Over a period of more than 2 years, the risk of stroke was reduced to less than 1% per year in the transfused group[171] (a risk reduction of >90%). The ability of transfusion to curtail progression of large-vessel stenosis has also been proven with angiography.[176]

Because of the risks of iron overload and allosensitization with chronic transfusion, a randomized controlled trial of withdrawal of transfusion was conducted (STOP 2). This trial evaluated discontinuation of transfusion after at least 30 months in children who had not had an overt stroke and in whom the cerebral flow rates decreased to low risk (<170 cm/s) with transfusion. This study was terminated early because of a high rate of reversion to high-risk TCD flow rates (34%) and stroke (5%) in the patients taken off transfusion compared with the group who continued transfusion.[177]

In children, MRI can also be used to assess stroke risk: 8.1% of children with an asymptomatic MRI lesion versus 0.5% of those with a normal MRI had a stroke during the ensuing 5 years.[172] A randomized trial of MRI-guided prophylactic transfusion is in progress (Silent Infarct Treatment Trial). In adults, MRI or MRA of the brain should be used[34] to assess thrombotic or hemorrhagic stroke risk.

Chronic transfusion is associated with a significant complication rate. Therefore there is a need for alternatives, especially because some patients and physicians believe that the 10% annual stroke risk does not warrant the risks and burdens of chronic transfusion.[160] The role of aspirin in ischemic stroke prevention in SCD is being evaluated (see Basic Management and Disease Modification). HU significantly lowered the TCD velocity values in a group of 24 children with Hb SS disease compared with an age-matched control group.[51] The role of HU is being formally evaluated in secondary stroke prevention (see Secondary Prevention). Stem cell transplantation has resulted in stabilization of cerebral vasculopathy[178] but there is a mortality risk with this procedure of between 6% and 10%.

Other modifiable risk factors for stroke (see Cerebrovascular Accidents, Pathophysiology, Incidence, Risk Factors, and Presentation) should be identified and treated. Notably, in the general population, hypertension is particularly associated with a risk for hemorrhagic stroke, and effective treatment of hypertension can produce a relative risk reduction of 26% for ischemic stroke and 49% for hemorrhagic stroke.[179] In patients with SCD followed through the Cooperative Study of Sickle Cell Disease, both diastolic and systolic blood pressures were noted to be lower than for matched control participants. Patients with systolic pressures in the higher range for the sickle cell group, even with systolic pressures less than 140 mmHg, had an increased risk of first ischemic stroke (there were insufficient events to make firm conclusions regarding hemorrhagic stroke).[23] Therefore at a minimum, it seems reasonable to follow population-wide recommendations for blood pressure control in patients with SCD.

Evaluation and Management of Acute Cerebrovascular Accidents

Patients with symptoms and signs of CVA should be evaluated immediately using computed tomography (CT) scanning or MRI to distinguish among TIA, cerebral thrombosis, and hemorrhage. In those with hemorrhage, angiography or MRA is indicated after partial-exchange transfusion is performed to avoid complications associated with the injected contrast material. In both thrombosis and hemorrhage, prompt partial-exchange transfusion is performed, and chronic direct transfusion to maintain the Hb S level below 30% is instituted to prevent recurrent events (see also Basic Management and Disease Modification) and promote resolution of arterial stenoses.[176]

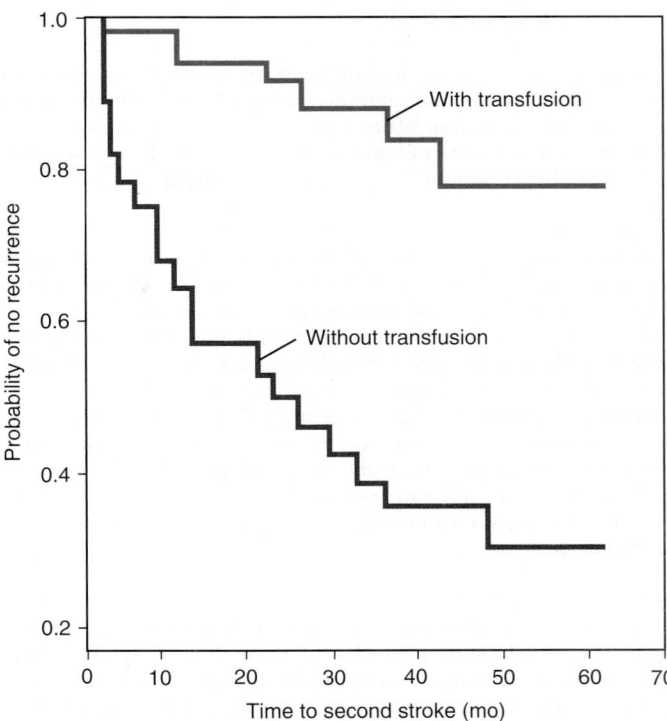

Fig. 42.11 COMPARISON OF STROKE RECURRENCE OVER 62 MONTHS IN A TRANSFUSED GROUP AND IN UNTRANSFUSED HISTORICAL CONTROL GROUPS. *(Adapted with permission from Pegelow CH, Adams RJ, McKie V, et al: Risk of recurrent stroke in patients with sickle cell disease treated with erythrocyte transfusions.* J Pediatr *126:896, 1995.)*

Secondary Prevention of Cerebrovascular Accidents

The risk of recurrent stroke is approximately 70%, a risk that is reduced to around 13% with chronic transfusion.[180] Although recurrent CVAs during chronic transfusion have been reported, this therapeutic modality provides the best means of preventing recurrence (Fig. 42.11). This treatment also provides incidental protection against pain crises, bacterial infections, acute chest syndrome, and hospitalization.

Based on the data from STOP 2 (see Primary Prevention of Cerebrovascular Accidents), chronic transfusion is continued indefinitely. This may not be feasible for administrative reasons or because of allosensitization or iron overload for which the patient is unable or unwilling to undergo treatment. Therefore clinical trials to determine if disease modifiers such as HU or decitabine can reduce stroke risk are indicated. In patients with a history of CVA transitioned from chronic transfusion to HU, the recurrent stroke rate remained stable and in the range seen with continued transfusion.[86]

Per primary prevention, all other identified modifiable risk factors for stroke should be identified and treated.

In patients with moyamoya disease, surgical approaches to therapy, such as extracranial–intracranial bypass, have been useful in improving the perfusion of affected regions of the brain.

Stem cell transplantation has resulted in stabilization of cerebral vasculopathy,[178] but the risk of a second neurologic event is higher in the peritransplant period, and the mortality rate with this procedure is between 6% and 10%.[178]

Seizures

Seizures occur more commonly among patients with SCD. In one study, 21 of 152 patients in a pediatric clinic had seizures, four of which were related to meperidine therapy. Most had nonfocal CT and MRI studies but focal electroencephalographic changes.[181] CVAs are heralded by focal seizures in 10% to 33% of cases. Therefore seizures in SCD ultimately may be related to the underlying vasculopathy.

Pulmonary Complications

Pulmonary disease is the leading cause of death in patients with SCD.[16] Both acute and chronic pulmonary complications are common. The common acute complications are pneumonia and acute chest syndrome, and the common chronic complication is pulmonary hypertension.

Pneumonia

Pneumonia is defined as chest infiltrates on chest radiography or chest CT scan associated with fever and an identified infectious etiology. The risk for and increased frequency of *S. pneumoniae* infections is discussed under Infections earlier. In addition, *Mycoplasma pneumoniae*, *Chlamydia pneumoniae*, and *Legionella* spp. are also relatively common causes of pneumonia in patients with SCD. Antibiotic therapy for pneumonia or acute chest syndrome should cover these agents in addition to pneumococcus and *H. influenzae*. When antibiotics are used to treat the acute chest syndrome, they should cover *S. pneumoniae*, *H. influenzae* type b, *M. pneumoniae*, and *C. pneumoniae*. The combination of cefuroxime and erythromycin is recommended.

Acute Chest Syndrome

Acute chest syndrome occurs in approximately 30% of patients.[182] Acute chest syndrome is defined as a new infiltrate on chest radiography or chest CT scan associated with one or more new symptoms, which include fever, chest pain, cough, sputum production, dyspnea, and hypoxia. This entity is included in discussions of SCD because processes other than infection, such as vasoocclusion, could also lead to pulmonary symptoms, signs, and chest radiographic changes. However, it should be borne in mind that the usual etiology might be both vasoocclusion and infection simultaneously, and in almost all cases of acute chest syndrome, antibiotics should be administered. Many episodes in which common pathogens are not cultured are caused by "atypical" agents (*Mycoplasma*, *Legionella*, and *Chlamydia* spp.), suggesting that antibiotic therapy include agents directed at atypical agents. Pulmonary fat embolus, evidenced by stainable fat in pulmonary macrophages obtained by bronchoalveolar lavage or sputum induction, is found in 44% to 60% of cases of acute chest syndrome.[183] Acute chest syndrome caused by pulmonary fat embolus is associated with more severe hematologic and clinical abnormalities. In adults, the mortality rate is four times higher than in children.[3,184]

Acute chest syndrome is often preceded by febrile episodes in children and by vasoocclusive pain crisis in adults (Fig. 42.12).[184] Elevation of serum phospholipase A2 was detected in patients admitted with vasoocclusive pain crisis 24–48 hours before acute chest syndrome was clinically diagnosed.[185] Pulmonary fat embolus is often preceded by an acute painful episode. Some patients have a rapidly progressive course associated with a precipitous decrease in arterial oxygen tension; they may require intensive care treatment. If there are clinical signs of respiratory distress or when arterial oxygen tension cannot be maintained above 70 mmHg with inhaled oxygen, partial-exchange transfusion is indicated. Artificial ventilation may be required.

In patients with pneumonia or chest syndrome, antibiotics should cover *S. pneumoniae*, *M. pneumoniae*, *Chlamydia pneumoniae*, *H. influenzae*, and *Legionella* spp.

Pulmonary Hypertension

Chronic complications such as pulmonary hypertension occur in as many as 60% of patients.[186-188] There does not appear to be an association with the occurrence of acute chest syndrome,[187] emphasizing that the pathophysiology of these two conditions may differ in some key features. The pathophysiology may involve thrombi in large and small arteries,[189,190] cardiac decompensation from progressive anemia, and potentially reversible increases in vascular tone from NO depletion and medial and intimal hypertrophy.[190] The recognition that pulmonary hypertension is a feature of hemolytic syndromes other than sickle cell and that markers of hemolysis correlate with the risk of pulmonary hypertension supports the idea that depletion

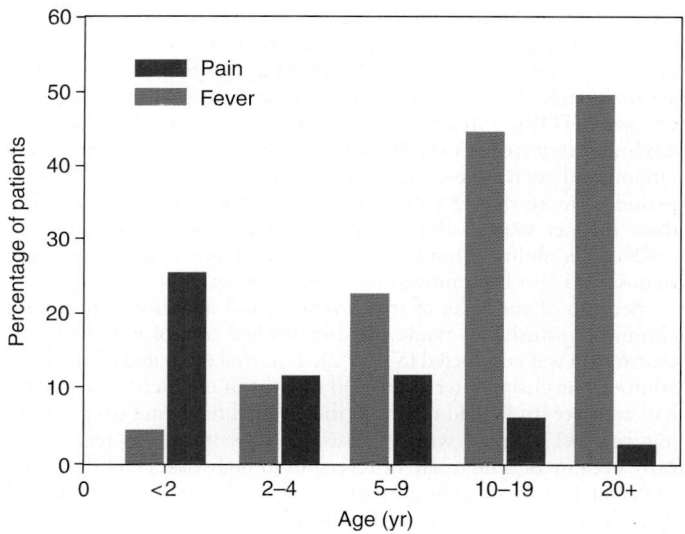

Fig. 42.12 AGE-SPECIFIC ASSOCIATED EVENTS WITHIN 2 WEEKS PRECEDING ACUTE CHEST SYNDROME. *(Adapted with permission from Vichinsky EP, Styles LA, Colangelo LH, et al: Acute chest syndrome in sickle cell disease: Clinical presentation and course. Cooperative Study of Sickle Cell Disease.* Blood *89:1787, 1997.)*

of NO through scavenging by free Hb may have an important role in the pathophysiology of this disease.[187,191] Pulmonary hypertension usually occurs in adults and carries a poor prognosis.[192]

The association with early death and the emerging availability of candidate treatments suggest that efforts should be made to diagnose this condition in all patients with SCD.[187,191] The feasibility of an echocardiogram-determined tricuspid regurgitant jet (TR-jet) velocity measurement of 2.5 m/s to make the diagnosis was suggested by selective cardiac catheterization in a cohort of 195 patients;[186] however, the sensitivity and specificity of this test may have limitations.[191] Elevations in BNP levels correlate with an increased TR-jet and risk of early death.

In a 16-week, double-blind, placebo-controlled trial of sildenafil to treat patients with SCD with increased TR-jet velocity and a low exercise capacity, sildenafil increased hospitalization rates for pain without evidence of improvement in TR-jet velocity or BNP levels.[193] If such patients have chronic relative reticulocytopenia, measures to increase total Hb could be a consideration requiring evaluation in clinical trials (see Basic Management and Disease Modification).

Other Pulmonary Complications

Other findings include restrictive and obstructive lung disease and hypoxemia.[194] High-resolution, thin-section CT scanning of the lungs may show chronic interstitial fibrosis. Airway hyperreactivity occurs in nearly two-thirds of children with SCD not diagnosed as having asthma. Thirty-six percent of 53 children with SCD were found to have sleep-related upper airway obstruction, 16% had hypoxemia, and all 15 who underwent adenotonsillectomy improved symptomatically and had improved hypoxemia.[195] Sleep apnea may be associated with surgically reversible exacerbations of painful episodes and strokes. Blood gas and pulmonary function measurements should be obtained as baseline data for all patients.

Hepatobiliary Complications

Hepatobiliary complications in patients with SCD include cholelithiasis, cholecystitis, acute hepatic cell crisis, acute hepatic sequestration crisis, and sickle cell intrahepatic cholestasis.[196] Chronic transfusion also places patients at risk for infection with hepatitis viruses and for transfusional hemosiderosis. Nontransfusion-related hepatic hemosiderosis can also be seen.

The serum bilirubin level is higher in sickle cell anemia (Hb SS) than in Hb SC disease or sickle cell–β⁺-thalassemia as a result of a greater hemolytic rate. The level rises after the first decade, possibly as a result of chronic hepatobiliary dysfunction. The aspartate aminotransferase (AST) and alanine aminotransferase (ALT) levels are often elevated, particularly in adult patients with sickle cell anemia, but mean levels are normal. Alkaline phosphatase levels are elevated in all genotypes until puberty, which occurred later in males and in those with sickle cell anemia. Percutaneous liver biopsy is associated with a high risk of severe complications and death in patients with SCD with acute hepatic syndromes.[197]

Cholelithiasis and Cholecystitis

The prevalence of pigmented gallstones in SCD is directly related to the rate of hemolysis.[198] In sickle cell anemia, gallstones occur in children as young as 3–4 years of age and are eventually found in approximately 70% of patients. Some have recommended the surgical removal of asymptomatic gallstones to avoid subsequent difficulty in distinguishing gallbladder pain from acute painful episodes. This approach has become more feasible with the availability of laparoscopic cholecystectomy.[199]

Acute Hepatic Cell Crisis

Acute hepatic cell crisis presents with tender hepatomegaly, worsening jaundice, and fever.[196] The likely etiology is hepatocellular cell ischemia. The AST and bilirubin are elevated, but rarely above 300 IU/L and 255 µM, respectively. This syndrome usually resolves within 3–14 days with supportive care alone but can progress to liver failure and fatal outcome, therefore patients should be monitored closely and exchange transfusion initiated if they show signs of progressive liver dysfunction (e.g., increasing AST).

Acute Hepatic Sequestration Crisis

Acute hepatic sequestration crisis presents with acute hepatic enlargement and a dramatic fall in Hb concentration, the most likely mechanism being sequestration of sickled erythrocytes in the liver. Management is with supportive care and transfusions.

Intrahepatic Cholestasis

Sickle cell intrahepatic cholestasis results in severe, asymptomatic hyperbilirubinemia without fever, pain, leukocytosis, hepatic failure, or death.[200] Asymptomatic hyperbilirubinemia without signs of progressive liver dysfunction (e.g., increasing AST) does not require specific therapy. Evidence of progressive liver dysfunction should prompt consideration of acute hepatic cell crisis and exchange transfusion.

Hepatitis C Infection

Chronic hepatitis C infection in SCD occurs with a prevalence that is related to the number of transfusions received; it may be a leading cause of cirrhosis. Liver transplantation has been used successfully as therapy for this complication.[201] If indicated, interferon-ribavirin can be used to treat hepatitis C in patients with SCD.[202]

Obstetric and Gynecologic Issues

Gynecologic complications (delayed menarche, dysmenorrhea, ovarian cysts, pelvic infection, and fibrocystic disease of the breast) are more common in women with SCD. Pregnancy entails increased risks to the mother and child compared with the general population.

Pregnancy

Pregnancy in patients with SCD is associated with increased risks to both the mother and fetus, although these risks are not so great as to prohibit continuation of pregnancy.[203,204] The fetal complications of pregnancy, most of which are related to compromised placental blood flow, are the increased incidence of spontaneous early abortion, intrauterine growth retardation, low birthweight, and fetal death.

Maternal complications include increased rates of painful episodes, severe anemia caused by iron or folate deficiencies, exaggeration of the physiologic "anemia of pregnancy," increased infections (urinary tract infections, pneumonias, endometritis), preeclampsia, and death.[204] It is controversial whether the degree of anemia predicts the birth of babies with low birthweight. The occurrence of a perinatal death in a previous pregnancy and the presence of twins in the present pregnancy are two major risk factors for an unfavorable outcome. The course of pregnancy is more benign in Hb SC disease than in sickle cell anemia.

Better fetal and maternal outcomes in recent years are largely attributable to generally improved antenatal and obstetric care. Patients should be followed in a high-risk obstetric clinic in addition to the hematology clinic and receive the usual vitamin, mineral, and folate supplements. A high-calorie, high-protein diet can be considered. There is no specific therapeutic or preventive treatment for intrauterine growth retardation. Some experts recommend prophylactic transfusion, but a large controlled study showed no improvement in fetal outcome from this management option, although maternal symptoms are reduced. In addition to the usual indications for transfusion therapy in SCD, transfusion therapy is indicated for patients with cardiac or respiratory compromise, in preparation for cesarean section, preeclampsia, twin pregnancy, acute chest syndrome, Hb levels more than 20% below steady state or less than 5 g/dL, and previous history of perinatal mortality. If the Hb is between 8 and 10 g/dL and transfusion is indicated for any of the reasons above, partial exchange should be performed (e.g., phlebotomy of 400–500 mL and transfusion of 2 units of packed RBCs).[203] The type of delivery does not appear to represent a problem, and both spontaneous delivery and cesarean section are well tolerated.

Some experts advise that hypertonic saline injections are contraindicated for elective termination of pregnancy because of the risk of sickling-induced vasoocclusion. However, most methods of abortion are well tolerated. There are anecdotal reports of a higher incidence of acute painful episodes after therapeutic abortion; inpatient intravenous hydration before and for the 24 hours after the procedure is recommended.

Birth Control

Modern nonestrogen-containing intrauterine devices should be considered. Although depot injections of medroxyprogesterone (Depo-Provera) given every 3 months may be safe with regards to stroke risk,[205] there is a risk of bone loss, a consideration in patients with SCD and their propensity to skeletal complications. Oral contraceptives containing low doses of estrogen can be considered with no clear evidence of increased stroke demonstrated to date, although the patients' overall stroke risk should probably still be taken into consideration until there is more phase IV follow-up on the clinical experience. Another caution with low-dose estrogen oral contraception is the risk of contraceptive failure with less than excellent compliance. There may be risks to contraception, but against this must be weighed the risks of unintended pregnancy. Sexually active women should have routine pelvic examinations and birth control instructions.

Renal Complications

Hypertension, proteinuria, hematuria, increasing anemia, and nephrotic syndrome reliably predict progression to renal failure, which are clinical indices to pay attention to because the serum creatinine may be misleading. Patients with sickle cell anemia exhibit an increased proximal tubular secretion of creatinine. Thus patients may have a significant decline in renal function before it is detectable by measuring creatinine clearance.[206] The mean age at presentation with end-stage renal disease is 41 years.[207] Serum creatinine levels are low in all genotypes until age 18 years, when young men experience a rise, apparently related to increasing muscle mass. Creatinine levels increase with age in all genotypes, presumably because of declining renal function (see also organ-specific complications, kidney in Clinical Presentation and Management, later).

Other risk factors for the development of chronic renal failure include use of NSAIDs[208] and a genetic predisposition associated with the CAR β-globin haplotype; the latter has been suggested as an indication for BMT to prevent this outcome.[209] Acute renal failure from infarction may result from hypovolemia, sepsis, hepatorenal syndrome, cardiac failure, renal vein thrombosis, and rhabdomyolysis. These patients typically survive and recover their renal function with no increased risk of developing chronic renal failure.

There are seven well-described nephropathies that affect patients with either sickle cell trait or disease. These are gross hematuria, papillary necrosis, nephrotic syndrome, renal infarction, inability to concentrate urine, pyelonephritis, and renal medullary carcinoma.[206]

Renal transplantation is recommended for patients with sickle cell and end-stage renal diseases.

Renal Endocrine (Erythropoietin) Deficiency

This is discussed under Basic Management and Disease Modification.

Gross Hematuria

Hematuria may result from microthrombi formation in the peritubular capillaries of the renal medulla or from frank papillary necrosis. Significant hematuria may resolve with high urinary flow through oral hydration and bed rest. Hematuria that lasts longer than 1–2 weeks or the need for transfusion may require maintenance of a high urinary flow using a combination of hypotonic fluids and loop diuretics and urinary alkalinization using sodium bicarbonate and acetazolamide. These therapies are aimed at changing the acidic, hypertonic environment of the renal medulla that favors erythrocyte dehydration, increased Hb S concentrations, and Hb S polymerization. If bleeding persists for 72 hours despite these measures, then alternative treatment should be considered. These may include oral urea,[210] ε-aminocaproic acid, and vasopressin. Embolization or nephrectomy should be reserved for prolonged, life-threatening cases of hematuria that require multiple transfusions.

Increased hematuria can also be seen as a consequence of delayed hemolytic transfusion reactions (discussed in Exacerbations of Anemia).

Papillary Necrosis

Papillary necrosis is most often detected incidentally by imaging or microscopic examination of urine in asymptomatic patients. Sloughed papilla may cause ureteral obstruction and urinary tract infection. In addition to broad-spectrum antibiotics, this occurrence requires emergent relief of the obstruction with a retrograde ureteral stent or placement of a percutaneous nephrostomy tube. NSAIDs should be avoided in patients with papillary necrosis. Otherwise treatment is as for hematuria.

Proteinuria

Proteinuria has been found in 20% to 30% of patients with SCD. Increasing age and low Hb levels correlate with proteinuria. Proteinuria can progress to nephrotic syndrome characterized by proteinuria, hypoalbuminemia, edema, and hyperlipidemia. Angiotensin-converting enzyme (ACE) inhibitors produce a significant reduction in sickle proteinuria, although it is unclear if ACE inhibitors might slow or halt the progression of proteinuria to nephrotic syndrome and renal failure.[211,212] Angiotensin II inhibitors are being studied for a potential role in decreasing sickle cell–related proteinuria and renal function deterioration.

Hyposthenuria and Other Abnormalities of Tubular Function

The inability to maximally concentrate urine (hyposthenuria) in response to water deprivation is an early finding of sickle cell nephropathy. Both sickle cell trait and SCD patients may be affected. Hyposthenuria is the cumulative result of recurrent microinfarcts in

the vasa recta caused by sickling (Fig. 42.13). When water deprived, these patients cannot maximally concentrate their urine and develop hypovolemia and dehydration.

Other abnormalities of renal tubular dysfunction found in sickle cell anemia include an incomplete form of distal renal tubular acidosis with hyperchloremic metabolic acidosis and hyperkalemia.[213] The hyperkalemia may respond to oral sodium bicarbonate.

Urinary Tract Infections

Urinary tract infections and pyelonephritis are discussed under infectious complications.

Renal Medullary Carcinoma

Sickle cell trait has been reported to be associated with renal medullary carcinoma.[214] Presentation is with gross hematuria, abdominal or flank pain, or significant weight loss. The disease may be metastatic at diagnosis, and the prognosis is poor. There is a weak association of renal medullary carcinoma with Hb SC disease but no identified association with sickle cell anemia. The reason for these patterns of disease is unknown.

Priapism

Priapism is a condition that is characterized by a sustained erection that does not result from sexual desire and is not relieved by sexual activity. Stuttering priapism is a separate entity that is characterized by multiple, brief episodes of sustained unwanted erection. It has been reported to affect 6.4% to 42% of boys and men with SCD[215] and can also occur in sickle cell trait. Its peak frequencies are between ages 5 and 13 years and 21 and 29 years. Priapism is most likely to develop in patients with lower Hb F levels and reticulocyte counts, increased platelet counts, and the Hb SS genotype. Priapism caused by SCD is usually ischemic, or low-flow, priapism. (High-flow priapism is caused by unregulated arterial flow and can be distinguished from low-flow priapism by a blood gas obtained from the corpora.) Most likely, priapism begins with a physiologic erection. The relative stasis of blood within the corpora leads to a decrease in oxygen tension and development of acidosis, predisposing to Hb S polymerization in the corporal sinusoids, venous occlusion, and low-flow priapism. Pain develops as the corpora become increasingly ischemic after approximately 4 hours of erection. In a minority of patients, usually postpubertal, the engorgement also affects the corpus spongiosum and glans. The mild acidosis that accompanies hypoventilation during sleep may also contribute to the pathophysiology. Impotence is the primary complication of priapism, although some patients with a history of multiple episodes of priapism and significant corporeal fibrosis may report adequate erections and maintain active sex lives. Corporeal ischemia during priapism may induce local inflammation, causing the fibrosis responsible for impotence.

The goal of treatment is to relieve priapism and maintain potency. Patients should be educated to seek medical attention for unrelenting erection of more than 2 hours' duration. Detumescence within 12 hours is optimal to retain potency. After 72 hours, impotence is more likely. The strategy is prompt initiation of supportive medical therapy with intravenous hydration and analgesia and involvement by a urology consultant if the priapism persists for more than 4 hours; aspiration of blood from the corpora with or without irrigation, and injection of an α-adrenergic agonist should be considered (Guidelines of the American Urological Association, https://www.auanet.org/education/guidelines/priapism.cfm). If priapism persists 12 hours, options include partial-exchange transfusion to reduce the Hb S level to less than 30% with a total Hb of less than 10 g/dL or irrigation as outlined earlier. The latter procedure is less effective after 36 hours of priapism. Irrigation should be performed using penile anesthesia (dorsal nerve block; circumferential penile block; or subcutaneous, local, penile shaft block). All irrigation in boys should be performed under conscious sedation. There is anecdotal evidence for the use of hydralazine to treat acute priapism.[216]

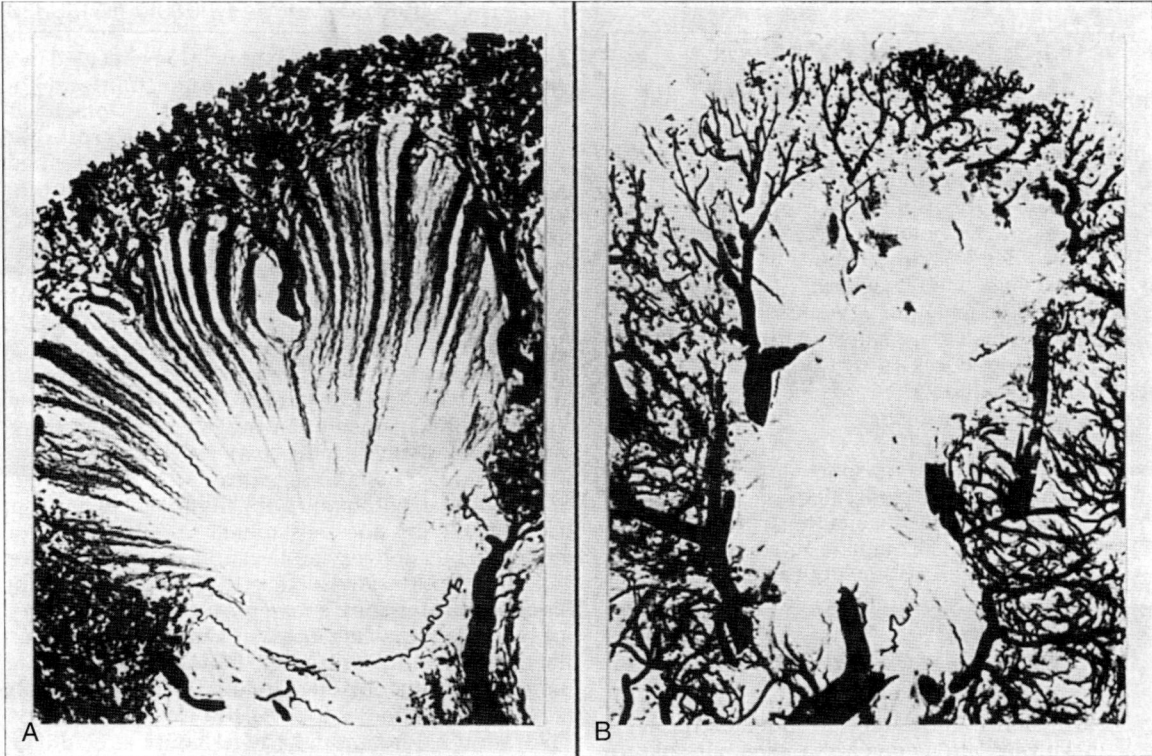

Fig. 42.13 Postmortem microangiographic studies of the vasa recta in a normal individual (A) and a patient with sickle cell anemia (B). *(Reproduced with permission from Elsevier. From LW Statius van Eps et al., Nature of concentrating defect in sickle-cell nephropathy. Microradioangiographic studies, The Lancet, 1970, 295, 450-452.)*

Preventing recurrent priapism is an important component of management. Strategies include HU administration; chronic transfusion; the antiandrogen bicalutamide;[217] self-administration of the α-adrenergic agent etilefrine orally and for episodes lasting over 1 hour, by intracavernous injection; and monthly administration of intramuscular gonadotropin-releasing hormone analogue.[218,219] Prophylactic pseudoepinephrine (Sudafed) appears beneficial in preventing recurrent mild episodes.

Surgical creation of shunts is reserved for severe cases resistant to the above interventions. As many as 45% of patients who have priapism develop some degree of impotence.[220] When impotence persists for 12 months, a semirigid penile prosthesis may be implanted.

Ocular Complications[221]

The retina is particularly vulnerable to vasoocclusion, and annual retinal examination is part of routine health care maintenance for patients with SCD. Superficial retinal hemorrhages have a pink "salmon patch" appearance. Deeper retinal hemorrhages have a "black sunburst" appearance. Other manifestations of sickle cell retinopathy include iridescent spots, retinal neovascularization, and retinal detachment. More subtle signs of sickle cell retinopathy are optic nerve head vascular changes, vascular tortuosity, macular changes (e.g., microaneurysms and vascular loops), and peripheral arteriovenous anastomoses. Other ophthalmologic complications are anterior chamber ischemia, tortuosity of conjunctival vessels, retinal artery occlusion, and angioid streaks. Sickle cell retinopathy is best seen by fluorescein angiography (Fig. 42.14). The earlier onset and greater frequency of proliferative retinopathy in Hb SC disease and sickle cell-β⁺-thalassemia compared with sickle cell anemia and sickle cell-β°-thalassemia suggest that retinal vessels are more susceptible to occlusion by more viscous blood than by more rigid individual cells. Peripheral sickle retinopathy may require vision-saving therapy with laser photocoagulation. Orbital compression syndrome caused by vasoocclusion of the periorbital marrow

space and subperiosteal hemorrhage has been observed to result in headache, fever, and palpebral edema. In this situation, culture, CT scan, and MRI should be used to rule out infectious, neoplastic, and other hemorrhagic etiologies. Conservative therapy, including local measures, analgesia, fluids, transfusion, and careful ophthalmologic surveillance, is recommended unless compression of the optic nerve ensues, in which case surgical decompression should be considered.

Bone Complications

Chronic tower skull, bossing of the forehead, and fish-mouth deformity of the vertebrae are the result of extended hematopoietic bone marrow, causing widening of the medullary space, thinning of the trabeculae and cortices, and osteoporosis. Osteonecrosis may cause a steplike depression of the vertebrae, selected shortening of the cuboidal bones of the hands and feet, and acute aseptic or avascular necrosis. The excruciating pain of bone infarction in the "hand–foot syndrome" that occurs around 2 years of age is often the first symptom of SCD (Fig. 42.15).[222] This dactylitis resolves spontaneously and is treated with hydration and analgesia. Bone infarcts are demonstrable using nuclear medicine scintigraphy or MRI. Serial scans specific for bone osteoclasts, bone marrow macrophages, and inflammatory cells may be useful adjuncts for distinguishing bone marrow infarction from osteomyelitis, but it is essential to obtain cultures directly from the affected tissue before starting antibiotics. Treatment of osteomyelitis is addressed in the Infection sections.

Bone necrosis occurs with equal frequency in the femoral and humeral heads, but the femoral heads more commonly undergo progressive joint destruction as a result of chronic weight bearing. The process is associated with increased intraosseous pressure and is most sensitively detected by MRI. Aggressive physical therapy appears to prevent progression in mild cases and should be considered in the therapy of avascular necrosis. Core decompression surgery to relieve increased intraosseous pressure can be used in early-stage

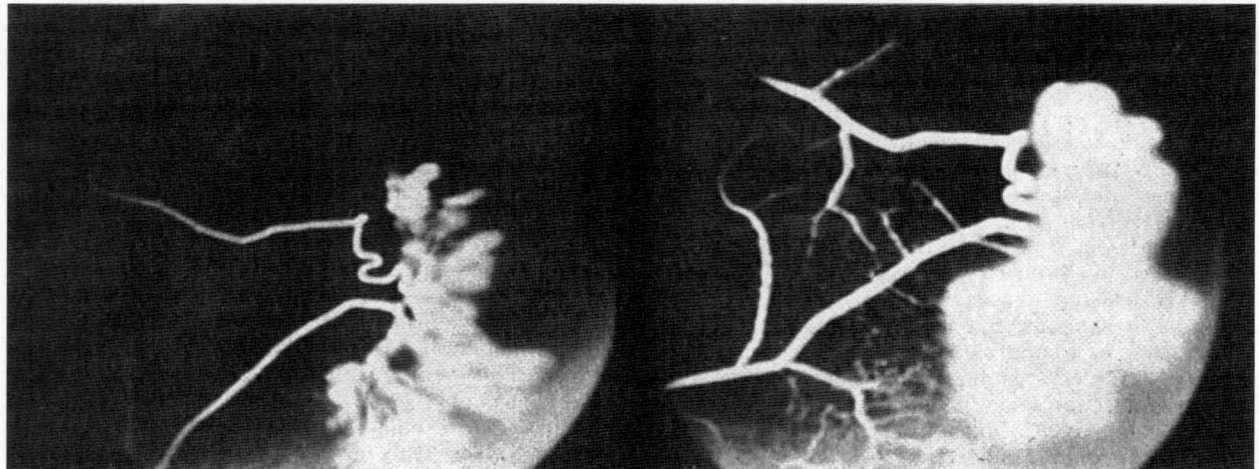

Fig. 42.14 FLUORESCEIN ANGIOGRAPHY DEMONSTRATING A "SEA FAN" APPEARANCE OF SICKLE PROLIFERATIVE RETINOPATHY. *(Courtesy W.C. Mentzer.)*

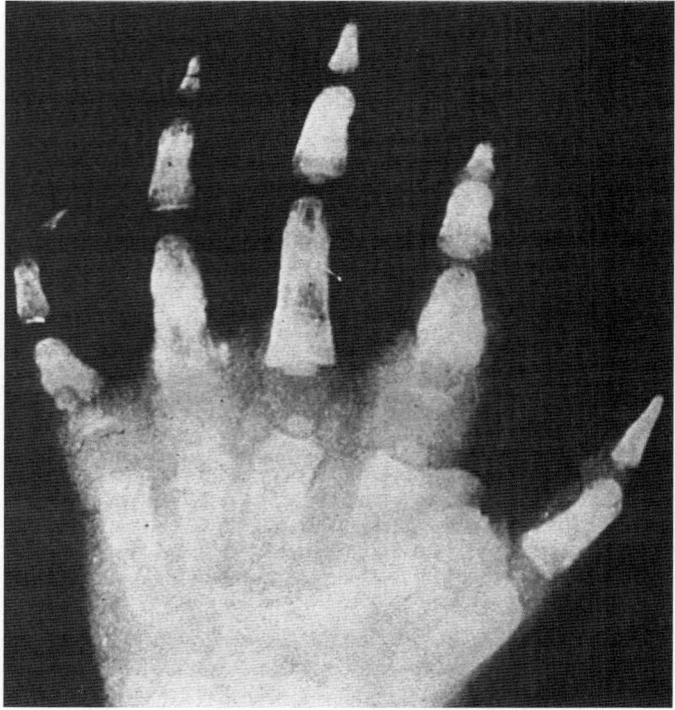

Fig. 42.15 RADIOGRAM SHOWING THE BONE INFARCTIONS IN THE HANDS OF A CHILD WITH THE "HAND–FOOT SYNDROME" DACTYLITIS. *(Courtesy W.C. Mentzer.)*

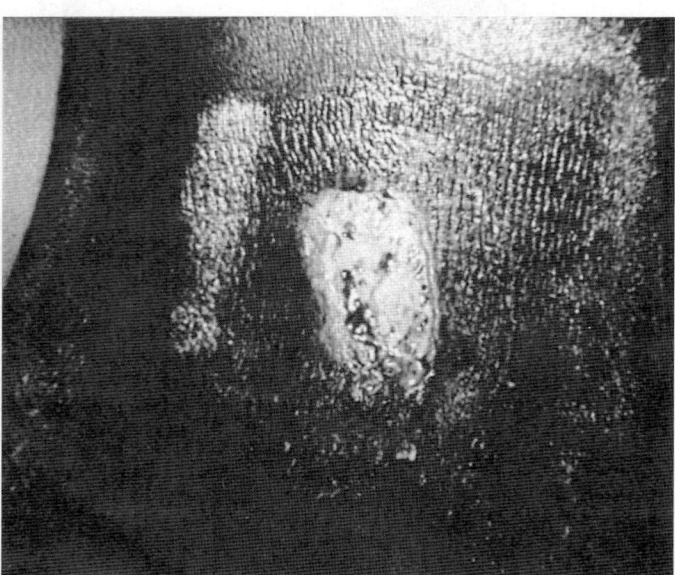

Fig. 42.16 CHRONIC LEG ULCER NEAR THE MEDIAL MALLEO-LUS. *(Courtesy W.C. Mentzer.)*

osteonecrosis (i.e., no radiographic evidence of bone collapse) to prevent disease progression. In more advanced disease, joint replacement can be considered. There is a 30% likelihood that a second hip revision will be required within 4–5 years of prosthetic hip placement in patients with SCD.[223]

Arthritic pain, swelling, and effusion may be related to periarticular infarction or gouty arthritis.

Bone marrow infarction causes reticulocytopenia, exacerbation of anemia, a leukoerythroblastic picture, and sometimes pancytopenia.[137,138] Pulmonary fat embolism is a rare complication of bone marrow infarction.[224] It is associated with fat globules in the sputum and refractile bodies visible in the optic fundi. It is a life-threatening event that may require prompt exchange transfusion and perhaps the use of heparin and corticosteroids.[224]

Dermatologic Complications

Leg ulcers are major causes of morbidity in SCD as a result of their frequency, chronicity, and resistance to therapy. Most occur near the medial or lateral malleolus (Fig. 42.16), may be associated with venous hypertension[225] and hemolytic rate,[226] and are frequently bilateral.[227] They may begin spontaneously or as a result of trauma and may become infected, most commonly by *S. aureus, Pseudomonas* spp., streptococci, or *Bacteroides* spp. Systemic infection, osteomyelitis, and tetanus are rare complications. Ulcers are resistant to healing and tend to be recurrent in well over half of cases. Their incidence has been reported to vary from 25% to 75%.[228] Ulcers rarely occur in patients younger than age 10 years and are most common in sickle cell anemia, less common in sickle cell–β°-thalassemia, and nonexistent in Hb SC disease and sickle cell–β+-thalassemia.[227] The incidence in sickle cell anemia patients declines substantially in those who have coexistent α-thalassemia.[227] Low steady-state Hb levels and low Hb F levels are associated with an increased risk of leg ulceration.[229] Males have a threefold greater risk for developing leg ulcers than females. Treatment of leg ulcers requires persistence and patience; healing usually takes weeks. Therapy[230] begins with gentle debridement to remove nonviable, superficial tissue from more vital areas. Wet-to-dry dressings and DuoDerm hydrocolloid dressings facilitate devitalization. When debridement is complete, zinc oxide–impregnated Unna boots are used to promote healing. Bed rest speeds healing,[231] and topical antibiotics may be required. It may be necessary to use elastic wraps or leg elevation to control edema. Rapid healing of leg ulcers has been reported in patients treated with intravenous arginine butyrate.[232] Oral zinc, local hyperbaric oxygen, chronic transfusion, recombinant EPO, propionyl-L-carnitine, skin grafts, pentoxifylline, and becaplermin (platelet-derived growth factor) may have therapeutic roles and should be considered in individual cases but have not been formally tested for their effectiveness in accelerating resolution of sickle cell–associated leg ulcers.

Myofascial syndromes consist of soft tissue swelling in subcutaneous edema that may have a *peau d'orange* appearance. These may be large or discrete lesions a few centimeters in diameter. These lesions are probably the result of dermal or subdermal vasoocclusion. Treatment is symptomatic.

Cardiac Complications

The chronic anemia of SCD is compensated by high cardiac output, which results in chronic chamber enlargement and cardiomegaly, and mild to moderate mitral and tricuspid regurgitation even in young children. The electrocardiogram shows evidence of left ventricular hypertrophy and less often first-degree block and nonspecific ST-T wave changes. Left ventricular dilation correlates with age and inversely correlates with total Hb.[233] An age-dependent loss of cardiac reserve may predispose to heart failure in adult patients stressed by fluid overload, transfusion, exacerbation of anemia, hypoxia, or hypertension. Cardiac function can be improved by transfusion.[234] Acute myocardial infarction in the absence of coronary disease has been reported, and in one autopsy series, 9.7% of 72 consecutive patients with SCD had myocardial infarction.[235] It appears that myocardial infarction may occur with normal coronary arteries as a result of increased oxygen demand exceeding limited oxygen-carrying capacity or as a result of microcirculatory impairment. As mentioned earlier, pulmonary hypertension (>30 mm Hg) is a relatively common finding in patients with SCD and can be associated with right ventricular hypertrophy. It has been suggested that the increased rate of sudden death observed in SCD may be related to cardiac autonomic dysfunction, as detected by abnormal heart rate variability in response to selected postural maneuvers.[236]

Multiorgan Failure

This disastrous acute event involves multiple organ systems, including the lungs, brain, kidneys, liver, hematologic system, and heart, and usually leads to death.[237] It may be precipitated by infection, vasoocclusion, or fat embolus and consists of a constellation of life-threatening processes, including hypoxemia, acidosis, inflammation, vascular permeability, severe anemia, disseminated intravascular coagulation, renal failure, and hepatic failure. In addition to therapy specific for these processes, exchange transfusion, plasma infusion or exchange, and corticosteroids should be considered.

Psychosocial Issues

Modern insights into the psychosocial adjustment of patients with SCD have provided a level of understanding that allows interventional therapy. Although most patients with SCD are generally well adjusted,[238] there are risks of depression, low self-esteem, social isolation, poor family relationships, and withdrawal from normal daily living.[238] Particular stressors are recurrent and unpredictable pain and the response to it, curtailed activity because of pain, misinterpretation of the meaning of pain, and depression leading to learned helplessness. Although some patients with SCD become addicted to narcotics, this is uncommon and usually is the result of social influences rather than pain therapy. Well-adjusted patients have active coping strategies, family support, and support from the extended family unit common in African American society. Interventional approaches should emphasize recognizing and reinforcing individual strengths; confronting pathologic behavior; and establishing coping skills through reinterpreting pain, diverting attention from pain, and using support systems.[239] Attention to psychosocial concerns is vital to the psychosocial well-being and integration into society of patients with SCD (see Chapter 90).

Growth and Development

By age 2 years, children with SCD have detectable growth retardation that affects weight more than height and has no clear gender difference.[240] By adulthood, normal height is achieved, but weight remains lower than that of control participants. More severe growth delay is noted in children with sickle cell anemia and sickle cell–β°-thalassemia; Hb SC disease is associated with a less severe growth delay. Girls with SCD have retarded sexual maturation that is greater in those with sickle cell anemia and sickle cell–β°-thalassemia than those with Hb SC disease and sickle cell–β+-thalassemia[240]; it is associated with elevated gonadotropin levels for the stage of sexual development and delayed menarche. Boys also have delayed sexual maturation, which is more severe in those with sickle cell anemia than those with Hb SC disease.[240] Retarded sexual maturation in boys can be attributable to primary hypogonadism, hypopituitarism, or hypothalamic insufficiency. The etiology of these multiple endocrine deficiencies may relate to underlying sickle cell pathophysiology or iron overload and emphasizes the importance of a comprehensive basic management and disease modification approach as outlined earlier in this chapter. Improved growth has been reported with HU,[241] transfusion,[241] folic acid supplementation, zinc supplementation,[242] and nutritional supplementation.[243] When children have both SCD and hypersplenism, splenectomy may result in improved protein turnover, metabolic rate, and growth parameters.[244]

VARIANT SICKLE CELL SYNDROMES

The sickle cell syndromes that result from inheritance of the sickle cell gene in simple heterozygosity or in compound heterozygosity with other mutant *β-globin* genes are sickle cell trait, Hb SC disease, and sickle cell–β-thalassemia. These and other less common compound heterozygosity syndromes are reviewed.

Sickle Cell Trait

The prevalence of sickle cell trait is approximately 8% to 10% in African Americans and as high as 25% to 30% in certain areas of western Africa.[4] Approximately 2.5 million people in the United States and 30 million in the world are heterozygous for the sickle cell gene. Sickle cell trait is largely a benign carrier condition with no obvious laboratory hematologic manifestations under basal conditions: RBC morphology, RBC indices, and the reticulocyte count are normal, and ISCs are not seen on the peripheral blood smear. The usual partition of Hb A and Hb S in sickle cell trait is 60:40 owing to a greater posttranslational affinity of α chains for β^A than for β^S chains.[6] When α-thalassemia is coinherited with sickle cell trait, the preferential affinity results in a decreased percentage of Hb S relative to the number of *α-globin* genes deleted (i.e., αα/αα 40% Hb S; −α/αα 35% Hb S; −α/−α 29% Hb S; ——/−α 21% Hb S).[133]

There are a few clinical complications of sickle cell trait; splenic infarction occurs at high altitude.[245] It is a cause of hematuria and hyposthenuria.[246] The frequency of urinary tract infection may be increased. There is an association with renal medullary carcinoma.[214]

There is an increased risk for venous thrombosis with an approximately twofold increase in risk and sickle trait explaining 7% of thrombotic episodes in African Americans.[29] Armed forces recruits in basic training with the sickle cell trait have a substantially increased, age-dependent risk of exercise-related sudden death.[30]

Despite the known complications, past experiences with discrimination in the employment market and health insurance industry provide reminders that the rare clinical events in sickle cell trait provide no real justification for regarding it as anything but a benign carrier condition.[31] Newborn screening programs detect a large number of infants with sickle cell trait; for these parents, genetic counseling is essential. Parents should understand that their child has a benign hereditary condition with some risks as above but that there is a risk for a subsequent child to be born with SCD.

In individuals who appear to have sickle cell trait but are symptomatic, the laboratory diagnosis must be verified. Hemoglobins other than S that polymerize may account for reports of "sickle cell trait" associated with clinical problems. Examples are heterozygous Hb S Antilles and Hb Quebec-CHORI. In the latter case, the Hb variant was distinguished from Hb A using mass spectroscopy.

Hb SC Disease

The gene for Hb C ($\alpha_2\beta_2$ ^{6}Glu→Lys) is approximately one-fourth as frequent among African Americans as the sickle cell gene.[8] Although oxygenated Hb C forms crystals, Hb C does not participate in polymerization with deoxy-Hb S. However, Hb C sustains potassium chloride cotransport and RBC dehydration, raising the intraerythrocytic concentration of Hb S to levels that support polymerization, sickling, and clinical symptoms. As a result of a longer circulatory survival of Hb SC RBCs compared with Hb SS cells (i.e., 27 versus 17 days),[130] the degree of anemia and reticulocytosis is frequently mild: 75% of the patients have a milder level of anemia (hematocrit level >28%) than is usually seen in sickle cell anemia. The predominant RBC abnormality on the peripheral smear is an abundance of target cells; folded ("pita bread") cells, ISCs, "billiard ball" cells, and crystal-containing cells may also be seen.

Splenomegaly may be the only physical finding, and the frequency of acute painful episodes is approximately half that in Hb SS disease, with a life expectancy two decades longer.[16] Nonetheless, significant morbidity can occur. The incidence of fatal bacterial infection is less than in sickle cell anemia, but there is still an increased risk of *S. pneumoniae* and *H. influenzae* infection. Osteonecrosis occurs in approximately 15% of patients.[32] There is a higher incidence of peripheral retinopathy in Hb SC disease than in sickle cell anemia. Coexistent α-thalassemia reduces risk of chronic organ complications.[32] There is an association between renal medullary carcinoma and Hb SC disease.

Sickle Cell–β-Thalassemia

The gene frequency of β-thalassemia among African Americans is 0.004, one-tenth that of the sickle cell gene,[8] and hence there is one-tenth the prevalence of compound heterozygous sickle cell–β-thalassemia in this population. Sickle cell–β-thalassemia is divided into sickle cell–β^+-thalassemia and sickle cell–β°-thalassemia, which have, respectively, reduced or no amounts of Hb A present. Most β-thalassemia mutations among African Americans result in β^+-thalassemia. Sickle cell–β^+-thalassemia is subclassified according to the percentage of Hb A present: type I has 3% to 5%, type II has 8% to 14%, and type III has 18% to 25%. Eighty percent of African American α-thalassemia mutations are attributable to the promoter region mutations (−88 [C to T] and −29[A to G]) that result in a type III phenotype. Compound heterozygous sickle cell–β°-thalassemia occurs infrequently.

In sickle cell–β-thalassemia, the RBCs are hypochromic and microcytic. The ISCs present on the peripheral blood smear are more numerous in sickle cell–β°-thalassemia than in sickle cell–β^+-thalassemia. The hematologic and clinical severity is a function of the amount of Hb A inherited (Table 42.10).

Additional mitigating influences in sickle cell–β-thalassemia are elevated levels of Hb A_2 and, in sickle cell–β^+-thalassemia, levels of Hb A up to 30%. These affect both the solubility and polymerization of Hb S. Hb F is a more active inhibitor of polymerization than Hb A, as shown by Hb S solutions with 15% to 30% Hb A (resembling sickle cell–β^+-thalassemia) having delay times 10–100 times longer than pure Hb S solutions, and Hb S solutions with 20% to 30% Hb F (resembling Hb S–HPFH) having delay times 1000–1,000,000 times longer. A further influence mitigating the polymerization, sickling, and clinical aspects of sickle cell–β-thalassemia is the reduced MCHC, which retards Hb S polymerization. Hematologic values for sickle cell anemia, the sickle cell–β-thalassemias, and Hb S–HPFH are found in Table 42.10.

Sickle Cell–Hb Lepore Diseaseβ

The Hb Lepore gene is a crossover fusion product of the δ- and β-*globin* genes, the product of which, in the case of Hb Lepore Boston, has the same alkaline electrophoretic mobility as Hb S. Therefore patients with the Hb Lepore trait can appear to have sickle cell trait but with only 12% Hb S from thalassemic expression of the abnormal fusion gene. Again, because of the electrophoretic similarity with Hb S, compound heterozygous Hb S–Hb Lepore Boston resembles sickle cell anemia or sickle cell–β°-thalassemia electrophoretically but clinically have less severe anemia, resembling that of sickle cell–β^+-thalassemia. The diagnosis is also suggested by the low to low-normal Hb A_2 levels that result from the incapacitation of one

TABLE 42.10	**Hematologic Variables Associated With Sickle Cell Anemia and the Different Sickle Cell–β-Thalassemia Syndromes**						
Genotype	Hb[a]	%Hb A[b]	%Hb F[b]	%Hb A_2[a]	MCV[a]	Reticulocytes[a]	*n*
Hb SS[c]	7.83	0	4.56	2.87	85.9	10.18	≈123
Hb S–β°-thalassemia[c]	8.85	0	5.86	5.02	69.3	7.2	≈41
Hb S–β^+-thalassemia, type I[d]	8.37	3-5	6.8	4.90	63.7	9.7	3
Hb S–β^+-thalassemia, type II[d]	10.28	8-14	5.2	4.68	70.0	6.6	14
Hb S–β^+-thalassemia, type III[e]	11.55	18-25	5.1	4.66	73.3	1.27	76
Hb S-HPFH[f]	14.6	0	25.8	1.95	81.7	2.4	4

[a]The mean data for each variable are shown. Units of measure are grams per deciliter for Hb, percentage of total hemoglobin for Hb F and A2, fl for MCV, and percentage of total red blood cells for reticulocytes.
[b]Percentage Hb A that defines the Hb S-β$^+$-thalassemia type.[247]
[c]Data from Serjeant et al.[249]
[d]Data from Christakis et al.[248]
[e]Data from Serjeant et al.[250]
[f]Data from Friedman et al.[251]
Hb, Hemoglobin; HPFH, persistence of fetal hemoglobin; MCV, mean corpuscular volume.

δ-globin gene by the crossover. Hb F levels vary. The peripheral smear shows microcytosis, hypochromia, and ISCs. Vasoocclusive complications occur, and splenomegaly is common.

Sickle Cell–Hb D Disease[247]

Because Hb D Punjab or Hb D Los Angeles ($\alpha_2\beta_2^{127}$Glu→Gln) has a similar electrophoretic mobility to Hb S under alkali conditions, Hb SD disease was first reported as an unusual case of sickle cell anemia. Hb D can be distinguished from Hb S by acid electrophoresis or isoelectric focusing. There is moderately severe hemolytic anemia, and the peripheral smear shows marked anisocytosis and poikilocytosis, target cells, and ISCs. The clinical manifestations of this syndrome are similar to those of sickle cell anemia.

Sickle Cell–Hb O Arab Disease[248]

Although Hb O Arab ($\alpha_2\beta_2^{127}$Glu→Lys) was first described in an Israeli Arab family, its distribution is widespread. Sickle cell–O Arab disease resembles Hb SC disease on alkaline electrophoresis, but Hb O Arab can be distinguished from Hb C by acid electrophoresis or isoelectric focusing. This syndrome is associated with moderately severe hemolytic anemia, and the peripheral smear shows anisocytosis, poikilocytosis, and ISCs.

Sickle Cell–Hb E Disease[249]

Hb E ($\alpha_2\beta_2^{26}$Glu→Lys) is a β-thalassemic hemoglobinopathy found predominantly in southeast Asia (see Chapter 40). The structural mutant has an electrophoretic mobility similar to Hb C under alkaline conditions but can be resolved by acid electrophoresis or isoelectric focusing. The GAG→AAG mutation in codon 26 activates a cryptic splice site within the first intron of the β^E gene, causing alternate splicing and decreased expression of the structural mutant. As a result, Hb E makes up only 30% of the total Hb in compound heterozygosity for the sickle cell and Hb E genes. Hb SE disease is essentially benign in at least 50% and possibly most patients, with only mild hemolysis, no vasoocclusive complications, and no remarkable abnormality of RBC morphology. However, vasoocclusive complications and manifestations of chronic hemolytic anemia such as pain crisis, splenic infarction, recurrent pneumonia, and frontal bossing have been reported.

Coinherited Hemoglobin Abnormalities That Interact With Sickle Cell Disease: Hereditary Persistence of Fetal Hemoglobin and α-Thalassemia Trait

Sickle Cell–Hereditary Persistence of Fetal Hemoglobin

Adult Hb (or in the case of sickle cell anemia Hb S) replaces Hb F as a result of the switch from γ- to β-globin synthesis that occurs in fetuses. Because of the inhibitory effect of Hb F on Hb S polymerization and cellular sickling (see Chapter 41), the high fraction of Hb F at birth masks the expression of SCD until Hb S levels increase to 75% at approximately 6 months of age (see Fig. 42.3). Conditions that preserve elevated levels of Hb F into adulthood similarly modulate the course of SCD. The compound heterozygous conditions sickle–HPFH (Hb SS–HPFH) and sickle cell–β°-thalassemia–HPFH both have higher Hb F levels and milder clinical courses than are characteristic of sickle cell anemia.[123]

Hereditary persistence of Hb F results from one of several large deletions of the *δ-* and *β-globin* genes that retard the switch from

the production of Hb F to adult Hb. A more recently discovered variety of HPFH is not caused by a deletion but by one of many point mutations that upregulate the expression of the *γ-globin* gene. The clinical expression of deletional and nondeletional HPFH differs in that the 15% to 35% Hb F in the former is distributed in a pancellular fashion, the 1% to 5% Hb F in the latter is distributed in a heterocellular fashion, and certain mild types of nondeletional HPFH express high Hb F levels not in simple heterozygosity but only in conditions of erythropoietic stress, such as compound heterozygosity with the sickle cell gene. It is likely that many cases of apparent sickle cell anemia with unexplained elevations of Hb F are the result of a nondeletion HPFH mutation.

The gene frequency of the deletional HPFH locus is 0.0005 among African Americans, resulting in a calculated incidence for compound heterozygous sickle cell–deletional HPFH of 1/100 that of sickle cell anemia. Sickle cell–deletional HPFH provided the first evidence that Hb F was a potent inhibitor of Hb S polymerization: individuals with pancellular distribution of 25% Hb F were generally neither anemic nor affected with vasoocclusive manifestations (see Table 42.10).[250] Hb electrophoresis revealed only Hb S, F, and A_2, which resembles sickle cell anemia, sickle cell–β°-thalassemia, and sickle cell–δβ°-thalassemia. Notable differences, however, are the pancellular distribution of 15% to 35% Hb F, Hb A_2 levels less than 2.5%, and the absence of anemia.[251] The generally benign course of sickle cell–deletional HPFH is uncommonly associated with vasoocclusive complication.

Sickle Cell Anemia With Coexistent α-Thalassemia

Prevalences of the silent carrier of α-thalassemia syndrome (genotype −α/αα) and α-thalassemia trait (genotype −α/−α) among African Americans are approximately 30% and 2%, respectively.[252] The peripheral blood smear contains less polychromasia and fewer sickle forms and more hypochromia and microcytosis, commensurate with the numbers of *α-globin* genes deleted. Increased Hb A_2 levels are associated with increasing *α-globin* gene deletions; the Hb F levels are not consistently affected.

Clinically, the impact of *α-globin* gene deletions on sickle cell is not as consistent as that of high Hb F.[21] Because of the powerful effect of Hb S concentration on the kinetics and extent of Hb S polymerization (see Chapter 41), the lower MCHC from *α-globin* gene deletions decreases the hemolytic rate, and anemia is milder in subjects with both α-thalassemia syndrome (genotype −α/αα) and trait (genotype −α/−α) (see Table 42.1). There is a decreased incidence of leg ulcers but an increased incidence of osteonecrosis. The frequency of retinal vessel closure is higher but not the incidence of retinopathy. Complications related to hemolysis (e.g., leg ulcers, chronic renal damage) may be decreased, but the heterogeneity of the patients in previous studies and mixed results make conclusions difficult. Similarly, the influence of α-gene deletions on survival in patients with SCD is not well understood.[21]

SUGGESTED READINGS

Strasser BJ: Perspectives: molecular medicine. "Sickle cell anemia, a molecular disease". *Science* 286:1488, 1999.

Wong TE, Brandow AM, Lim W, et al: Update on the use of hydroxyurea therapy in sickle cell disease. *Blood* 124:3850, 2014.

Yawn BP, Buchanan GR, Afenyi-Annan AN, et al: Management of sickle cell disease: summary of the 2014 evidence-based report by expert panel members. *JAMA* 312:1033, 2014.

REFERENCES

For the complete list of references, log on to www.expertconsult.com.

CHAPTER 43

HEMOGLOBIN VARIANTS ASSOCIATED WITH HEMOLYTIC ANEMIA, ALTERED OXYGEN AFFINITY, AND METHEMOGLOBINEMIAS

Edward J. Benz, Jr. and Benjamin L. Ebert

Hemoglobinopathies are inherited diseases caused primarily by mutations affecting the globin genes. Nearly 1000 mutations are known to alter the structure, expression, or developmental regulation of individual globin genes and the hemoglobins that they encode. Of these, only a few produce clinical disease. Many are highly instructive for students, of gene structure, function, and regulation, but further consideration of most is not warranted in a clinically oriented textbook. The gene mutations that cause sickle cell anemia and the thalassemia syndromes are by far the most important mutations that cause clinical morbidity, in terms of both the complexity of the clinical syndromes they cause and the number of patients affected. These conditions are considered in detail in other chapters (see Chapters 40, 41 and 42). This chapter reviews other abnormalities of the hemoglobin molecule that produce clinical syndromes. Even though each variant is uncommon, these hemoglobinopathies represent, in the aggregate, important problems for hematologists, because they must be considered as possible causes for conditions about which hematologists are often consulted: hemolytic anemia, cyanosis, polycythemia, jaundice, rubor, splenomegaly, and reticulocytosis. In some patients, secondary hematologic complications such as hypercoagulable states are also encountered.

The major inherited hemoglobinopathies producing clinical symptoms (other than sickle cell anemia and thalassemias) can be classified as those hemoglobins exhibiting altered solubility (unstable hemoglobins), hemoglobins with increased oxygen affinity, hemoglobins with decreased oxygen affinity, and methemoglobins (Table 43.1). A few acquired conditions in which toxic modifications of the hemoglobin molecule are important (e.g., carbon monoxide poisoning) also merit consideration.

The sections that follow emphasize hemoglobinopathies that produce the most severe or dramatic alterations in clinical phenotype and those in which a single clinical abnormality (e.g., hemoglobin precipitation) predominates. It is important to emphasize at the outset, however, that although more than 100 mutations affect solubility or affinity, only a few are clinically important. The abnormal functional properties of most mutant hemoglobins can be readily detected in sophisticated research laboratories, but only a few mutant hemoglobins produce laboratory or clinical abnormalities relevant to clinical practice. Moreover, many mutations are pleiotropic, affecting several functional properties of the hemoglobin molecule. Thus a single mutation can increase oxygen affinity and reduce solubility, or produce methemoglobinemia and reduce solubility.

Table 43.2 summarizes the major forms of structurally abnormal hemoglobin, with examples. This table serves as a point of reference for the remaining sections of the chapter.

UNSTABLE HEMOGLOBINS

Unstable hemoglobins are hemoglobins exhibiting reduced solubility or higher susceptibility to oxidation of amino acid residues within the individual globin chains. More than 100 unique unstable hemoglobin mutants have been documented. Most exhibit only mild instability in in vitro laboratory tests and are associated with minimal clinical manifestations. Both α- and β-globin variants can cause this condition. Approximately 75% of the mutations described, however, are β-globin variants. This probably reflects the potential for α-globin variants to exert pathologic effects in utero. Clinical symptoms of unstable hemoglobins also depend, in part, on the quantitative proportion of the abnormal hemoglobin. Because the α-globin genes are duplicated, mutations in an individual locus generally produce only 25% to 35% abnormal globin. By contrast, a simple heterozygote at the single β-globin locus usually produces approximately 50% of the abnormal variant.

The mutations that impair hemoglobin solubility usually disrupt hydrogen bonding or the hydrophobic interactions that either retain the heme moiety within the heme-binding pockets or hold the tetramer together (Fig. 43.1). Some alter the helical segments (e.g., hemoglobin [Hb] Geneva [$\beta^{28Leu \rightarrow Pro}$]), others weaken contact points between the α and β subunits (e.g., Hb Philadelphia [$\beta^{35Tyr \rightarrow Phe}$]), and still others derange interactions of the hydrophobic pockets of the globin subunits with heme (e.g., Hb Köln [$\beta^{98Val \rightarrow Met}$]). The common pathway to reduced solubility invariably involves weakening of the binding of heme to globin. Actual loss of heme groups can occur, for example, in Hb Gun Hill, in which five amino acids, including the F8 histidine, are deleted. In other cases, mutations that introduce prolines into helical segments disrupt the helices and interfere with normal folding of the polypeptide around the heme group. Another feature of these mutations is disruption of the integrity of the tetrameric structure of globin chains. Only the intact hemoglobin tetramer can remain dissolved at the high concentrations that must be achieved within the circulating red blood cell (see Chapters 30 and 40).

Pathophysiology of Unstable Hemoglobin Disorders

The mechanisms by which unstable hemoglobin mutations produce hemoglobin precipitation remain incompletely understood; however, the major outlines of the process have been described (Fig. 43.2). The fundamental step in pathogenesis appears to be derangement of the normal linkages between heme and globin. Loss of appropriate globin chain folding and interaction may ultimately destabilize the heme-globin linkage or lead to partial proteolysis of the chain, thereby releasing heme from that linkage. Once freed from its cleft, heme probably binds nonspecifically to other regions of the globin molecule, forming precipitated hemichromes, which leads to further denaturation and aggregation of the globin subunits. These form a precipitate containing α- and β-globin chains, globin fragments, and heme, called the *Heinz body*.

Heinz bodies interact with delicate red blood cell membrane components (see Chapters 43 and 45), thereby reducing red blood cell deformability. These rigid cells tend to be detained in the splenic microcirculation and "pitted," reflecting attempts by the splenic macrophages to remove the Heinz bodies. Red blood cell damage can be aggravated by the release of free heme into the red blood cell. Several biochemical perturbations correlate with the presence of free heme, such as generation of reactive oxidants (i.e., hydrogen peroxide, superoxide, and hydroxyl radicals). The end result of this process is

TABLE 43.1   Classification of Hemoglobinopathies

Structural hemoglobinopathies: hemoglobins with altered amino acid sequences that result in deranged function or altered physical or chemical properties

Abnormal Hemoglobin Polymerization: HbS
Altered Oxygen Affinity

High affinity: polycythemia
Low affinity: cyanosis, pseudoanemia

Hemoglobins That Oxidize Readily

Unstable hemoglobins, hemolytic anemia, jaundice
M hemoglobins: methemoglobinemia, cyanosis

Thalassemias: Defective Production of Globin Chains

α-Thalassemias
β-Thalassemias
δβ-, γδβ-, αβ-Thalassemias
Structural hemoglobinopathies: structurally abnormal Hb associated
    with coinherited thalassemia phenotype
HbE
Hb Constant Spring
Hb Lepore

Hereditary Persistence of Fetal Hemoglobin: Persistence of High Levels of HbF Into Adult Life

Pancellular: all red blood cells contain elevated HbF levels
Nondeletion forms
Deletion forms
Hb Kenya
Heterocellular: only specific subpopulation of red blood cells contain
    elevated levels of HbF

"Acquired Hemoglobinopathies"

Methemoglobin due to toxic exposures
Sulfhemoglobin due to toxic exposures
Carboxyhemoglobin
HbH in erythroleukemia
Elevated HbF in states of erythroid stress and bone marrow dysplasia,
    usually heterocellular

Hb, Hemoglobin.

TABLE 43.2   Mutations Producing Abnormal Hemoglobin Molecules[a]

Residue	Mutation	Common Name(s)	Molecular Pathology
Abnormal Solubility			
β6	Glu→Val	S	Polymerization
β6	Glu→Lys	C	Crystallization
β121	Glu→Gln	D-Los Angeles, D-Punjab	Increases polymer in S/D heterozygote
β121	Glu→Lys	O-Arab	Increases polymer in S/O heterozygote
Increased Oxygen Affinity			
α92	Arg→Gln	J-Capetown	Stabilizes R state
α141	Arg→His	Suresnes	Eliminates bond to Asn 126 in T state
β89	Ser→Asn	Creteil	Weakens bonds in T state
β99	Asp→Asn	Kempsey	Breaks T state intersubunit bonds
Decreased Oxygen Affinity			
α94	Asp→Asn	Titusville	Alters R state intersubunit bonds
β102	Asn→Thr	Kansas	Breaks R state intersubunit bonds
β102	Asn→Ser	Beth Israel	Breaks R state intersubunit bonds
Methemoglobin			
α58	His→Tyr	M-Boston, M-Osaka	Heme liganded to Tyr not His
α87	His→Tyr	M-Iwate	Heme liganded to both His and Tyr
β28	Leu→Gln	St Louis	Opens heme pocket
β63	His→Tyr	M-Saskatoon	Tyr ligand stabilizes ferriheme
β67	Val→Glu	M-Milwaukee-I	Negative charge stabilizes ferriheme
β92	His→Tyr	M-Hyde Park	Bond of His to heme disrupted
Unstable			
α43	Phe→Val	Torino	Loss of heme contact
v94	Asp→Tyr	Setif	Alters subunit contacts
β28	Leu→Gln	St Louis	Polar group in heme pocket
β35	Tyr→Phe	Philadelphia	Loss of dimer bond favors precipitation
β42	Phe→Ser	Hammersmith	Loss of heme
β63	His→Arg	Zurich	Opens heme pocket
β88	Leu→Pro	Santa Ana	Disrupts helix
β91	Leu→Pro	Sabine	Disrupts helix
β91-95	Deletion	Gun Hill	Shortens F helix
β98	Val→Met	Köln	Alters heme contact

[a]Partial list includes some of the most widely studied hemoglobin structural mutations.
Modified from Dickerson RE, Geis I: *Hemoglobin: Structure, function, evolution, and pathology.* Menlo Park, CA, 1983, Benjamin-Cummings. Copyright Irving Geis.

premature destruction of the red blood cell, producing hemolytic anemia.

Individual unstable hemoglobins vary in their propensity to generate Heinz bodies and hemolysis. For example, Hb Zurich exhibits relatively mild insolubility. Hemolysis is minimal in nonstressed patients with this variant and becomes clinically apparent only in the presence of additional oxidant stresses, such as infection, fever, or the ingestion of oxidant agents. Because of the propensity of unstable hemoglobins to be hypersensitive to oxidation, some patients with unstable hemoglobins can exhibit episodic hemolysis in response to many of the same oxidative stressors as those exacerbating the clinical phenotype of glucose-6-phosphate dehydrogenase (G6PD)–deficient patients (see Chapters 44 and 47).

Patterns of Inheritance and Clinical Manifestations

Unstable hemoglobins are usually inherited as autosomal dominant disorders. However, the rate of spontaneous mutation appears to be high, so the absence of affected parents or siblings does not rule out the presence of an unstable hemoglobin in an individual family. Nonetheless, the presence of a positive family history can be a useful adjunct to diagnosis and should provoke consideration of an unstable hemoglobin as the cause of the familial hemolytic diathesis.

The clinical syndrome associated with unstable hemoglobin disorders is often called *congenital Heinz body hemolytic anemia*. This term derives from the fact that only the most severe cases were detected before the widespread availability of sophisticated methods for detecting and characterizing abnormal hemoglobins. Clinical manifestations are highly variable, ranging from a virtually asymptomatic state in the absence of environmental stressors, to severe hemolytic anemia manifesting at birth. Patients with chronic hemolysis present with variable degrees of typical symptoms, including

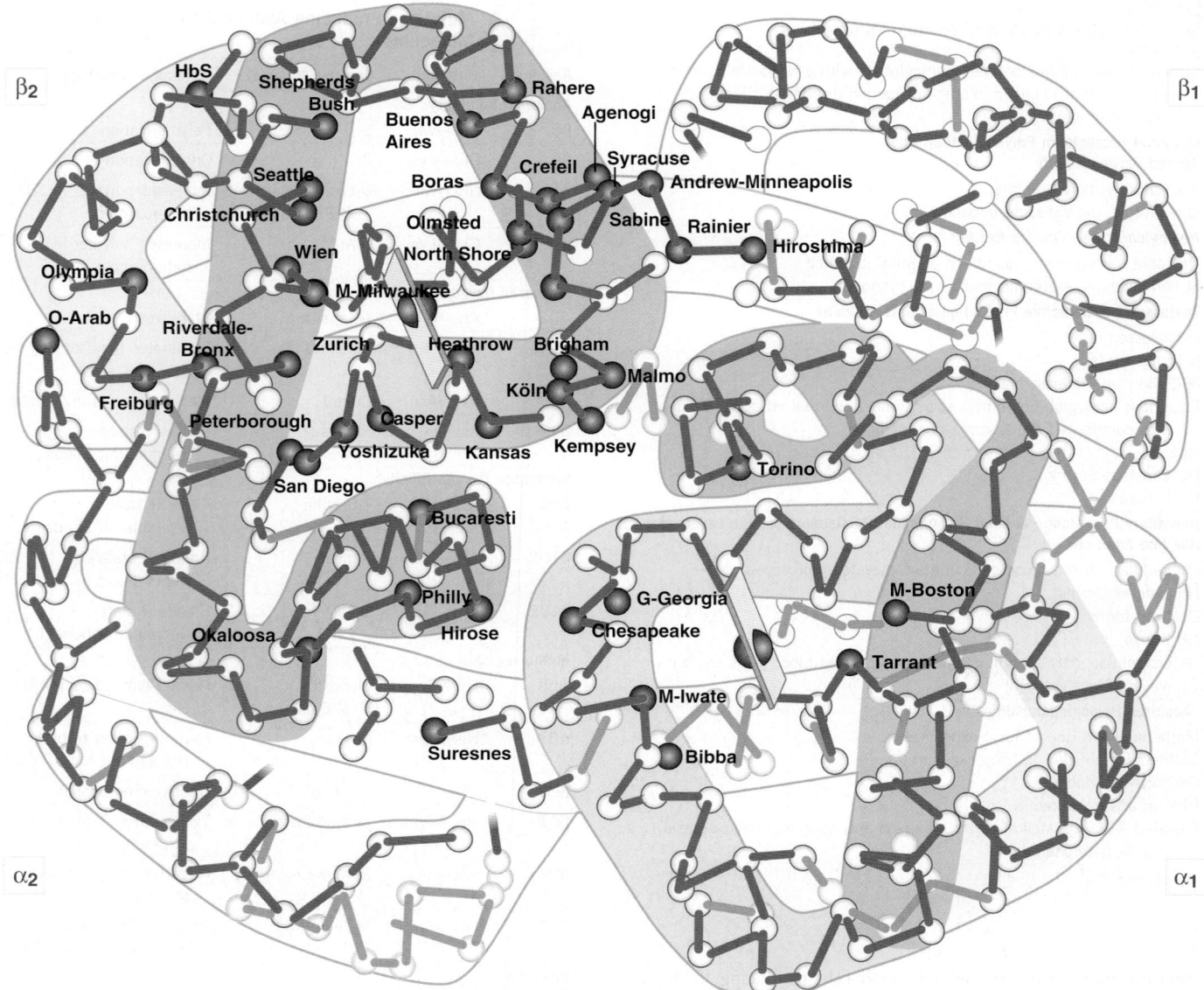

Fig. 43.1 HEMOGLOBIN TETRAMER SHOWING THE POSITION OF THE MORE COMMON, CLINICALLY SIGNIFICANT HEMOGLOBIN MUTANTS. Most of those that have been described occur on the β-chain at invariant residue sites, near critical intermolecular contacts, or in proximity to the prosthetic heme-binding site. *(Modified from Dickerson RE, Geis I: Hemoglobin: Structure, function, evolution, and pathology, Menlo Park, CA, 1983, Benjamin-Cummings. Copyright Irving Geis.)*

anemia, reticulocytosis, hepatosplenomegaly, jaundice, leg ulcers, and a propensity toward premature biliary tract disease.

For hemoglobin variants with a given degree of reduced solubility, the degree of anemia may fluctuate because some of these variants also exhibit altered oxygen affinity. Thus Hb Köln has increased oxygen affinity, resulting in relatively higher levels of tissue hypoxia and erythropoietin stimulation at any given level of hematocrit (see Diagnosis); therefore patients with Hb Köln tend to have higher hematocrit levels than expected on the basis of hemolytic severity because of increased erythropoietin stimulation. By contrast, Hb Hammersmith exhibits decreased oxygen affinity, improving oxygen delivery and allowing patients to function at a lower hematocrit level. Hb Zurich possesses, for complex molecular reasons, a higher-than-normal affinity for carbon monoxide. A high hemoglobin carbon monoxide level develops in patients with Hb Zurich who also smoke. Binding of carbon monoxide protects Hb Zurich from denaturation, thus reducing hemolysis, so these people tend to exhibit lesser degrees of hemolytic anemia than do nonsmoking relatives.

Diagnosis

The presence of an unstable hemoglobin should be suspected in patients with one or more stigmata of accelerated red blood cell destruction: chronic or intermittent hemolytic anemia or jaundice, premature development of bilirubin gallstones or biliary tract disease (as a result of accelerated red blood cell turnover), unexplained reticulocytosis, or bouts of intermittent symptoms that can be related to exposure to oxidant drugs or infections. Other suggestive symptoms include dark urine, transient jaundice, and leg ulcers.

Laboratory diagnosis depends on identification of a mutant hemoglobin that precipitates more easily than normal hemoglobin. The peripheral blood smear may or may not show evidence of hemolysis (i.e., poikilocytosis, polychromasia, or shift cells; Fig. 43.3A). The morphologic evidence for precipitated hemoglobin is the Heinz body, the intraerythrocytic inclusion body detected by staining the peripheral blood smear with a supravital dye, such as brilliant cresyl blue or new methylene blue (see Fig. 43.3B–C). The spleen removes Heinz bodies efficiently, especially if hemolysis is not particularly acute or brisk. Thus Heinz bodies may not be demonstrable at all times. Two provocative laboratory maneuvers are used to aid detection, both of which unmask the tendency of unstable hemoglobins to precipitate: the heat instability test (heating of a hemoglobin solution to 50°C) or the isopropanol instability test (insolubility in 17% isopropanol).

Hemoglobin electrophoresis should be performed but *should not be relied on as the major diagnostic criterion for ruling in or ruling out a hemoglobinopathy.* Many amino acid substitutions that have a profound effect on solubility do not change the overall charge on the hemoglobin molecule. For example, Hb Köln, the most common of the unstable hemoglobin mutations, arises from a mutation changing the valine at position 98 to a methionine. This mutation is electrically neutral; it does not alter electrophoretic mobility. Therefore these variants do not form an abnormal band on an electrophoresis gel. Demonstration of an abnormal band would clearly add

strong evidence in support of the diagnosis. A normal electrophoretogram, however, should never be regarded as strong evidence against the presence of a mutant hemoglobin, especially if the clinical picture or family history otherwise supports the diagnosis. Mass spectrometry analysis of hemoglobin and direct globin gene sequencing are supplanting electrophoresis as diagnostic strategies. They usually provide unambiguous identification of a sequence abnormality. However, electrophoresis is still in use in many clinical settings. Thus the aforementioned precautions in interpretation are still worth noting.

Additional sophisticated analyses of hemoglobin can be obtained from reference laboratories if detailed characterization seems warranted. For example, abnormal hemoglobin or globin bands migrating to novel positions on an isoelectric focusing gel can result from hemoglobin or globin moieties lacking heme in groups. When heme is added to the sample and the proteins are reanalyzed, these bands disappear. This behavior is nearly diagnostic of an unstable variant.

Detection of unstable hemoglobins is occasionally compromised by the selective precipitation of the unstable variant into Heinz bodies. Because most patients are heterozygotes, this phenomenon greatly reduces the apparent percentage of the variant in soluble form. Thus even a variant possessing altered electrophoretic mobility may be very difficult to detect. Indeed, some unstable hemoglobins, such as Hb Geneva or Hb Terre Haute, are so unstable that no mutant gene product can be detected in the steady state. These abnormal hemoglobins actually produce a thalassemic phenotype. They are detectable only by isotope labeling studies or direct analysis of the globin genes.

The amino acid sequence predicted from genetic sequencing may rarely be inaccurate because of posttranslational conversion into an unstable hemoglobin. For example, in the first reported case of congenital Heinz body hemolytic anemia due to Hb Bristol, the DNA sequence predicts a valine-to-methionine substitution at β67. Through posttranslational modification, the methionine is altered to aspartate, a hydrophilic residue that disrupts the heme pocket.

The differential diagnosis of unstable hemoglobin variants is usually straightforward if this general category of hemolytic disorders is suspected. The most common form of G6PD deficiency can also manifest with bouts of intermittent or chronic hemolysis exacerbated by oxidant drugs or infection (see Chapter 44). This diagnosis should be considered, as should other causes of chronic or intermittent hemolytic anemia, including red blood cell membrane disorders (e.g., hereditary spherocytosis) or immune hemolytic anemias. Spherocytes are relatively rare in patients with unstable hemoglobin disorders; this is sometimes a useful discriminant.

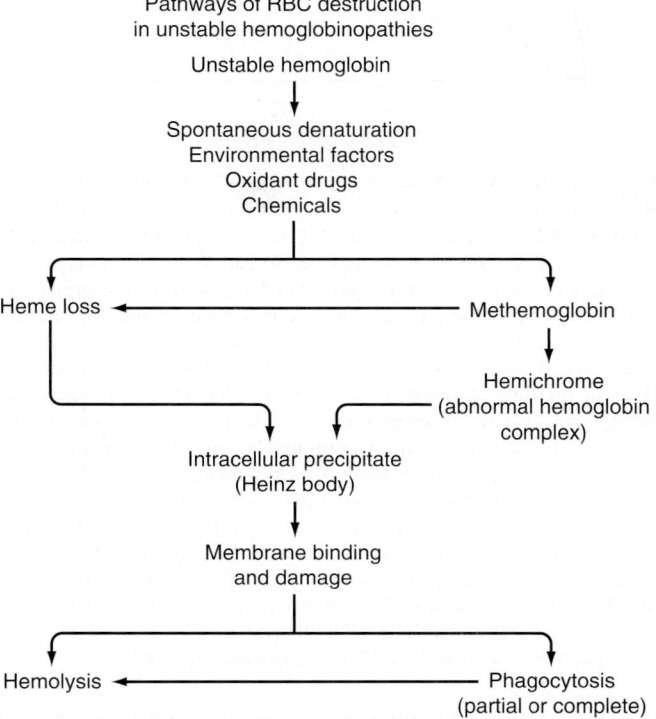

Pathways of RBC destruction in unstable hemoglobinopathies

Fig. 43.2 PRESUMED MECHANISMS BY WHICH DENATURATION OF HEMOGLOBIN LEADS TO ERYTHROCYTE DESTRUCTION. The rate of travel through the various pathways probably differs for the different hemoglobin variants and for a variety of stresses to which the protein is subjected. *RBC,* Red blood cell. *(From Wynngaarden JB, Smith LH Jr, Bennett JC, editors:* Cecil textbook of medicine, *Philadelphia, 1992, WB Saunders.)*

Management

The severity of the clinical complications of unstable hemoglobins varies enormously. Many patients can be managed adequately by observation and education to avoid agents that provoke hemolysis.

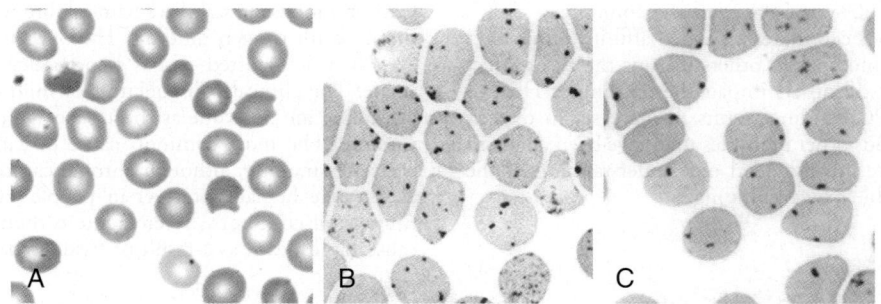

Fig. 43.3 UNSTABLE HEMOGLOBINS; PERIPHERAL BLOOD SMEAR AND HEINZ BODY PREPARATION. The peripheral smear (A) shows "bite" cells with pitted-out semicircular areas of the red blood cell membrane as a result of removal of Heinz bodies by macrophages in the spleen. The Heinz body preparation (B) shows increased Heinz bodies in the same specimen, when compared to a control (C).

Some patients require transfusions during bouts of severe acute hemolytic anemia. Patients who have significant morbidity because of chronic anemia or repeated episodes of severe hemolysis should be considered candidates for splenectomy, especially if hypersplenism has developed. Children with severe hemolysis may require transfusion support until they are old enough (at least 3 or 4 years of age) to undergo splenectomy without unacceptable immunologic compromise. Splenectomy is usually effective for abolition or reduction of anemia. However, splenectomy should be used only as a last resort because of the long-term risks of overwhelming sepsis and thrombosis. Infection often exacerbates hemolysis. Fever should therefore prompt close monitoring of patients for evidence of hemolysis or infection. Postsplenectomy patients with a hemolytic diathesis are also afflicted by a hypercoagulable state, probably due to the deranged membrane architecture resulting from oxidative damage. They thus require monitoring for thrombotic events and may need intermittent or long-term anticoagulant therapy.

HEMOGLOBINS WITH INCREASED OXYGEN AFFINITY

Efficient oxygen delivery by hemoglobin depends on the sigmoid shape of the hemoglobin-oxygen affinity curve. During the transition from the fully deoxygenated to the fully oxygenated state, the initial oxygenation steps occur with difficulty. In fact, the act of binding the first oxygen molecule increases the affinity of the molecule for subsequent oxygen-binding events, thus creating the sigmoid shape of the curve. The necessary intramolecular reorganization occurs only when the precise arrangement of hydrogen bonds, hydrophobic interactions, and salt bridges is broken and formed in the proper sequence.

Mutant hemoglobins exhibiting altered oxygen affinity arise from amino acid substitutions at the interface between α- and β-chains or in regions affecting the hydrogen bonds, hydrophobic interactions, or salt bridges that influence the interaction of heme with oxygen. A second major class of mutations alters binding to 2,3-diphosphoglycerate (2,3-DPG), which in turn alters oxygen affinity when bound to hemoglobin.

Pathogenesis and Pathophysiology

High-affinity hemoglobins exhibit higher avidity for oxygen, causing the oxygen dissociation curve to shift to the left; an example is Hb Kempsey ($\beta^{99Asp \to Asn}$) (Fig. 43.4). These hemoglobins bind oxygen more readily than normal and retain more oxygen at lower partial pressure of oxygen (PO_2) levels. They thus deliver less oxygen to tissues at normal capillary oxygen pressures. The PO_2 in the normal lung (90 to 100 mmHg) is well above that needed to saturate hemoglobin fully with oxygen (60 mmHg). These variant hemoglobins cannot acquire any additional oxygen in the lung despite their higher affinity. At capillary PO_2 (35–45 mmHg), however, high-affinity hemoglobins deliver *less* oxygen. At normal hematocrit levels, a mild tissue hypoxia results, triggering increased production of erythropoietin and red blood cells, thus resulting in polycythemia. In extreme cases, hematocrit levels of 60% to 65% can be encountered.

Many types of mutations can increase oxygen affinity. Some alter interactions within the heme pocket, others disrupt the Bohr effect or the salt-bond site, and still others impair the binding of HbA to 2,3-DPG. Loss of 2,3-DPG binding results in increases in oxygen affinity. These and numerous other examples that have been analyzed at the molecular level have greatly aided our understanding of the molecular basis for reversible oxygen binding.

Diagnosis

High-affinity hemoglobins are a cause of familial unexplained erythrocytosis (see Chapters 63 and 68). Functional testing of the hemoglobin is the key to diagnosis. Oxygen affinity is usually measured as P_{50}, the PO_2 at which hemoglobin is 50% saturated with oxygen (see

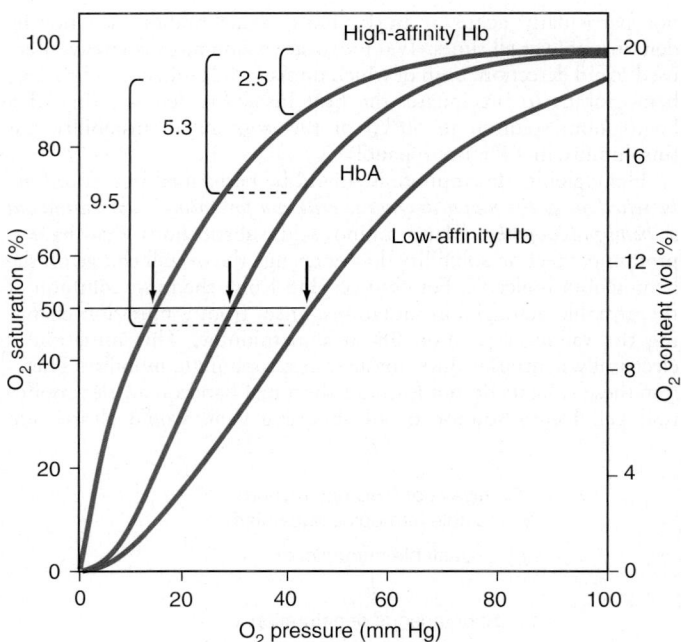

Fig. 43.4 HEMOGLOBIN-OXYGEN DISSOCIATION CURVES ARE ILLUSTRATED FOR NORMAL HEMOGLOBIN (HbA) AND FOR MODEL ABNORMAL HEMOGLOBINS WITH HIGH AND LOW OXYGEN AFFINITIES. On the abscissa, the partial pressure of oxygen (PO_2) is indicated in millimeters of mercury. On the left ordinate, the saturation of hemoglobin with oxygen is indicated as a percentage; on the right ordinate, the oxygen content of the hemoglobin is expressed as volume percent. The three inverted arrows show the PO_2 at which the hemoglobin is 50% saturated (P_{50}) for the three hemoglobins. This value is lowest for the high-affinity hemoglobin. As the PO_2 drops from 100 (arterial) to 40 (tissues) mmHg, hemoglobin desaturates, giving up a portion of its bound oxygen; the numbers on the brackets indicate the amount of oxygen unloaded by the three hemoglobin types expressed as volume percent. Note that the high-affinity hemoglobin delivers less than one-half the oxygen that HbA gives to the tissues, resulting in tissue anoxia, increased erythropoietin secretion, and erythrocytosis. Conversely, the low-affinity hemoglobin is even more efficient than HbA in supplying tissues with oxygen, resulting in diminished erythropoietin production and anemia. *(From Wynngaarden JB, Smith LH Jr, Bennett JC, editors: Cecil textbook of medicine, Philadelphia, 1992, WB Saunders.)*

Fig. 43.4). The hemoglobin preparation is exposed to increasing oxygen pressures, and the relative percentages of oxyhemoglobin and deoxyhemoglobin are determined. The values are plotted on a curve, and the 50% saturation point is determined. A shift to the left means that the hemoglobin reaches 50% saturation at a lower PO_2. High-affinity variants are thus associated with a lower-than-normal P_{50} value. Hemoglobin electrophoresis can, but may not, reveal an abnormal band.

The most common cause of a low P_{50} value is carbon monoxide. Carbon monoxide stabilizes hemoglobin in the R "oxy" state without the need for oxygen binding. The oxygen affinity curve is therefore extremely left-shifted and is hyperbolic, rather than sigmoidal, in shape. The clinical consequences of mild chronic carbon monoxide poisoning are the same as those seen with high-affinity hemoglobin variants. The most common cause of carbon monoxide toxicity is cigarette smoking, although chronic carbon monoxide exposure can elevate the hematocrit level in people such as caisson workers or tunnel toll collectors. Severe acute carbon monoxide poisoning can cause rapid death as a result of tissue hypoxia.

Management

Most patients with high-affinity hemoglobins have mild erythrocytosis; they do not require intervention. Very rarely, the hematocrit level is very high (>55% to 60%). The blood viscosity is then sufficiently elevated to require therapeutic phlebotomy. Carbon monoxide poisoning is treated with supplemental oxygen. When a patient breathes room air, the half-life of carboxyhemoglobin is 4 to 6 hours, but the half-life is 40 to 80 minutes with the use of normobaric oxygen and 15 to 30 minutes with the use of hyperbaric oxygen. Carbon monoxide detectors, designed to detect occult carbon monoxide poisoning, are now required in many municipalities and are predicted to prevent numerous fatalities from occult carbon monoxide poisoning.

HEMOGLOBINS WITH DECREASED OXYGEN AFFINITY

Pathogenesis

Low-affinity hemoglobin variants, such as Hb Kansas ($\beta^{102Asn \to Thr}$), arise from mutations that impair hemoglobin-oxygen binding or reduce cooperativity. In cases of Hb Kansas, the threonine position, β^{102}, cannot form a hydrogen bond with aspartic acid at position α^{94}. Because this aspartate residue stabilizes the R (oxy) state, Hb Kansas binds oxygen less well and exhibits a right-shifted P_{50} value (see Fig. 43.4).

Most low-affinity variants possess enough oxygen affinity to become fully saturated in the normal lung. At the low capillary Po_2 in other tissues, these hemoglobins deliver *higher* than normal amounts of oxygen. They become more desaturated than normal hemoglobins. Two abnormalities result from this high level of oxygen delivery. First, because tissue oxygen delivery is so "overly" efficient, normal oxygen requirements can be met by lower-than-normal hematocrit levels. This situation produces a state of "pseudoanemia," in which the low hematocrit level is deceiving because both oxygen delivery and the patients are completely normal. Second, the amount of desaturated hemoglobin circulating in capillaries and veins can be greater than 5 g/dL. Cyanosis may thus be associated with these variants. This usually ominous finding is entirely misleading in these individuals, because it reflects no morbidity.

Diagnosis

Patients with unexplained anemia or cyanosis who appear to be entirely well in all other respects should be evaluated, especially if there is a positive family history. Testing for the abnormal variant follows the same reasoning as that just described for high-affinity variants. The oxygen dissociation curve will be shifted to the right, and the numeric value of the P_{50} will be higher than normal.

Management

Patients with low-affinity hemoglobins are usually asymptomatic. No treatment is required. It is important to document that a low-affinity hemoglobin is the cause of an apparent anemia or cyanosis to preempt inappropriate workups and provide reassurance to the patient. Cyanosis in some patients can pose a cosmetic problem, but correction with transfusions is rarely justified.

Methemoglobinemias

Methemoglobin results from oxidation of the iron moieties in hemoglobin from the ferrous (Fe^{2+}) to the ferric (Fe^{3+}) state. Normal oxygenation of hemoglobin causes a partial transfer of an electron from the iron to the bound oxygen. Iron in this state thus resembles ferric iron and the oxygen resembles superoxide (O_2^-). Deoxygenation returns the electron to the iron, with release of oxygen. Methemoglobin forms if the electron is not returned. Methemoglobin constitutes 3% or less of the total hemoglobin in normal humans. Under normal circumstances, these levels in humans are maintained at 1% or less

TABLE 43.3	Types of Methemoglobinemia
Congenital	
Defective enzymatic reduction of Fe^{3+}-hemoglobin to Fe^{2+}-hemoglobin	
NADH-methemoglobin reductase (cytochrome-b_5 reductase) deficiency	
Cytochrome b_3 deficiency	
Abnormal hemoglobins resistant to enzymatic reduction (M hemoglobins)	
Acquired	
Excessive (toxic) oxidation of Fe^{2+}-hemoglobin	
Environmental chemicals	
Drugs	

NADH, Reduced form of nicotinamide adenine dinucleotide.

by the methemoglobin reductase enzyme system (the reduced form of nicotinamide adenine dinucleotide [NADH]–dehydratase, [NADH]-diaphorase, erythrocyte cytochrome b_5).

Pathogenesis and Clinical Manifestations

Methemoglobinemias of clinical interest arise by one of three distinct mechanisms: (1) globin chain mutations that result in increased formation of methemoglobin, (2) deficiencies of methemoglobin reductase, and (3) "toxic" methemoglobinemia, in which normal red blood cells are exposed to substances that oxidize hemoglobin iron to such a degree that normal reducing mechanisms are subverted or overwhelmed (see Chapter 44; Table 43.3).

Abnormal hemoglobins producing methemoglobinemia (M hemoglobins) arise from mutations that stabilize the heme iron in the ferric state. Classically a histidine in the vicinity of the heme pocket is replaced by a tyrosine (e.g., Hb M-Iwate, β87 (F8) His $\to$ Tyr); the hydroxyl group of the tyrosine forms a complex that stabilizes the iron in the ferric state (Fig. 43.5). The oxidized heme iron is relatively resistant to reduction by the methemoglobin reductase system.

Methemoglobin has a brownish to blue color that does not revert to red on exposure to oxygen. Patients with methemoglobinemia thus appear to be cyanotic. In contrast to truly cyanotic people, however, arterial partial pressure of oxygen (PaO_2) values are usually normal. Patients with these hemoglobins are otherwise asymptomatic because methemoglobin is usually less than 30% to 50%, the levels at which symptoms become apparent.

Hereditary methemoglobinemia resulting from methemoglobin reductase deficiency (cytochrome-b_5 reductase deficiency) is very rare. Mutations in the b_5 reductase gene cause two distinct phenotypes. In cases of type I methemoglobin reductase deficiency, patients suffer solely from cyanosis; in cases of type II disease, patients manifest both cyanosis and severe mental retardation. One isoform of the b_5 reductase gene is expressed in diverse tissues for participation in a variety of cellular processes. A second isoform, produced by alternative splicing, is expressed in erythrocytes, producing a soluble protein that reduces methemoglobin. Mutations causing type I methemoglobin reductase deficiency occur throughout the gene and result in an unstable protein. Such mutations are primarily significant in erythrocytes that, without nuclei, cannot replace the degraded protein. Mutations causing type II disease occur in the critical NADH or flavin adenine dinucleotide (FAD)–binding domains, causing inactivation of the protein in all tissues and the more severe clinical phenotype.

Like patients with M hemoglobins, patients with methemoglobin reductase deficiency exhibit slate-gray "pseudocyanosis." Even homozygotes, however, rarely accumulate more than 25% methemoglobin, a level compatible with minimal symptoms. Heterozygotes can have normal methemoglobin levels but are especially sensitive to agents causing methemoglobinemia.

A third toxic form of methemoglobinemia is caused by exposure to certain chemical agents and drugs that accelerate the oxidation of

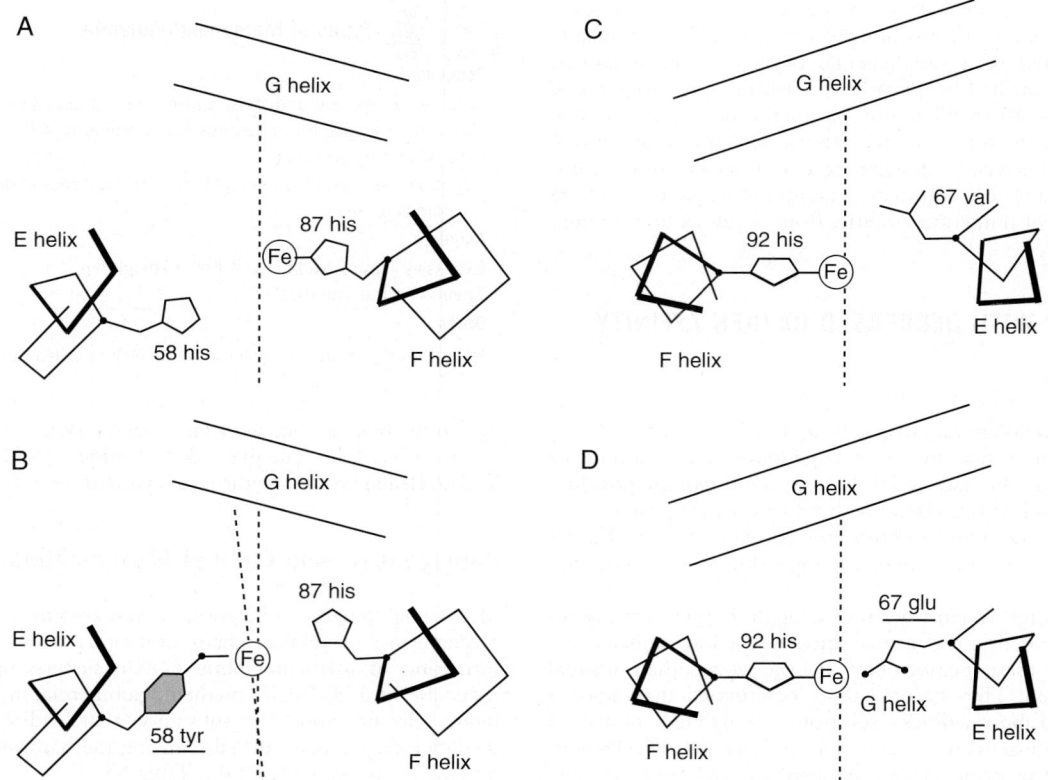

Fig. 43.5 MODIFICATIONS OF THE HEME AND ITS ENVIRONMENT THAT ACCOUNT FOR TWO COMMON M HEMOGLOBINS. (A) Hemoglobin A has a His residue at the α58(E7) position. (B) In hemoglobin M-Boston, the histidine is replaced by a tyrosine, the phenolic side chain of which is capable of covalently binding to the heme iron, resulting in stabilization in the oxidized form. (C) HbA has a Val residue at position β67(E11). (D) Hb M-Milwaukee has a glutamic acid substitution for the β67 valine. The carboxylic side chain of the Glu forms a bond with iron, shifting the equilibrium toward the ferric state. *(Modified from Dickerson RE, Geis I: Hemoglobin: Structure, function, evolution, and pathology, Menlo Park, CA, 1983, Benjamin-Cummings. Copyright Irving Geis.)*

hemoglobin to methemoglobin (Table 43.4). Some compounds directly oxidize hemoglobin, whereas other compounds produce reactive oxygen intermediates that oxidize hemoglobin. Nitrite compounds are especially notorious and common. Some of these compounds also have a propensity to exacerbate G6PD deficiency and the precipitation of unstable hemoglobins.

Nitrates are a frequent environmental cause of toxic methemoglobinemia. Nitrates do not directly interact with either hemoglobin or the reductase pathway but are converted to nitrites in the gut. Well water is a frequently encountered source of excessive nitrates. In general, substantial intake of these agents is required before significant amounts of methemoglobin are generated. Very young infants have lower levels of methemoglobin reductase in erythrocytes and are therefore more susceptible to these agents than are adults. However, all age groups are at risk, given sufficient exposure. Systemic acidosis, particularly in young infants suffering from diarrhea and dehydration, can also cause clinically-significant methemoglobinemia.

Acquired methemoglobinemia is virtually the only situation in which life-threatening amounts of methemoglobin accumulate. In general the only symptom produced when methemoglobin constitutes less than 30% of total hemoglobin is the cosmetic effect of cyanosis. As levels of methemoglobin rise to greater than 30%, however, patients begin to exhibit symptoms of oxygen deprivation, such as malaise, giddiness, and other alterations of mental status. The symptoms reflect a true lack of oxygen availability at the tissue level. Methemoglobin is a markedly left-shifted hemoglobin that delivers little oxygen to the tissues. When methemoglobin accounts for more than 50% of total hemoglobin, loss of consciousness, coma, and death can rapidly ensue. At this level the blood is chocolate brown.

TABLE 43.4 Drugs and Chemicals Having Toxic Effects on Hemoglobin Molecule

Agent	Observed Hemoglobin Derivative	
	Methemoglobin	**Sulfhemoglobin**
Acetanilid, phenacetin	+	+
Nitrites (ferric, amyl, sodium, potassium, nitroglycerin)	+	+
Trinitrotoluene, nitrobenzene	+	+
Aniline, hydroxylamine dimethylamine	+	+
Sulfanilamide	+	+
p-Aminosalicylic acid	+	
Dapsone	+	
Primaquine, chloroquine	+	
Prilocaine, benzocaine, lidocaine	+	
Menadione, naphthoquinone	+	
Naphthalene	+	
Resorcinol	+	
Phenylhydrazine	+	+

Diagnosis

Methemoglobinemia should be suspected in patients with unexplained cyanosis. It is obviously a medical emergency when any patient has cyanosis and altered mental status; a PaO_2 more normal than expected on the basis of the O_2 saturation should trigger a consideration of methemoglobinemia. The ingestion of nitrites as a suicidal gesture, especially in people knowledgeable with respect to chemistry, medicine, or pharmacology, should be considered. Exposure to nitrate-containing therapeutic compounds, e.g., in the setting of the intensive care unit, should also raise suspicion. Methemoglobinemia can be suspected from the brownish color of blood when it is drawn. Laboratory detection is simple; methemoglobin exhibits characteristic peaks of absorption at 630 and 502 nm, rendering it easily distinguishable from normal hemoglobin. Pulse oximetry, using a ratio of absorption at 660 nm and 940 nm, gives an inaccurate reading of 85% oxygen saturation for blood with 100% methemoglobin. The inherited M hemoglobin mutants are frequently detectable by altered electrophoretic mobility, especially if ferricyanide treatment in vitro is used to convert all the hemoglobin solution to methemoglobin.

In the case of toxic methemoglobinemia, recognition of exposure to an appropriate agent provides the most important historical clue. Acute poisoning can represent a life-threatening emergency; therefore laboratory evaluation for methemoglobin should be requested for any person displaying atypical cyanosis or cyanosis occurring along with more normal than anticipated blood gas values. Methemoglobin due to deficiencies of the reductase system can be further evaluated in reference laboratories by direct analysis of these enzymes.

Management

Patients with M hemoglobins are usually asymptomatic and require no management. The secondary cyanosis can present a cosmetic problem. The cyanosis is not reversible because ascorbic acid and methylene blue are usually ineffective.

Patients with deficiency of the reductase system usually do not require treatment. Cyanosis in these cases can be improved by treatment with oral methylene blue, 100 to 300 mg/day, or 500 mg/day of oral ascorbic acid. Riboflavin (20 mg/day) has also been reported to be effective and may be the preferred agent, because methylene blue produces discolored (blue) urine, and ascorbic acid can cause sodium oxalate stones.

Emergency treatment of high levels of toxic methemoglobinemia begins with 1 to 2 mg/kg of intravenous methylene blue as a 1% solution in saline. It is usually infused rapidly (over 3 to 5 minutes);

the dose can be repeated at 1 mg/kg after 30 minutes if necessary. This treatment is usually effective. Methylene blue acts through the reduced form of nicotinamide adenine dinucleotide (NADPH) reductase system, which in turn requires G6PD activity. The method is therefore ineffective in patients who also have G6PD deficiency. These patients, or patients who are severely affected, may require exchange transfusion or hyperbaric oxygen therapy. Oral ascorbic acid is not useful for emergency situations because it acts too slowly. Follow-up maintenance management, however, can be accomplished with either ascorbic acid or oral methylene blue.

Mild cases of methemoglobin intoxication do not require treatment. The patient can be monitored for 1 to 3 days, during which time methemoglobin levels gradually return to normal if the offending agent is eliminated. The most important follow-up therapy for patients with toxic methemoglobinemia involves a thorough search for the offending agent and its removal from the environment.

SUGGESTED READINGS

Bunn HF: Sickle hemoglobin and other hemoglobin mutants. In Stamatoyannopoulos G, Nienhuis AW, Majerus PO, et al, editors: *The molecular basis of blood disease*, ed 2, Philadelphia, 1993, WB Saunders.

Bunn HF, Forget BG: *Hemoglobin: Molecular, cellular and clinical aspects*, Philadelphia, 1985, WB Saunders.

Dickerson RE, Geis I: *Hemoglobin: Structure, function, evolution, and pathology*, Menlo Park, CA, 1983, Benjamin-Cummings.

Ernst A, Zibrak J: Carbon monoxide poisoning. *N Engl J Med* 339:1603, 1998.

Fermi G, Perutz MF: *Atlas of molecular structures in biology. Vol. 2: hemoglobin and myoglobin*, Oxford, 1981, Oxford University Press.

Ho C, editor: *Hemoglobin and oxygen binding*, New York, 1982, Elsevier Biomedical.

Park CM, Nagel RL: Sulfhemoglobinemia: Clinical and molecular aspects. *N Engl J Med* 310:1579, 1984.

Perutz MF: Molecular anatomy, physiology, and pathology of hemoglobin. In Stamatoyannopoulos G, Nienhuis AW, Leder P, et al, editors: *The molecular basis of blood diseases*, Philadelphia, 1987, WB Saunders, p 127.

Smith RP, Olson MV: Drug-induced methemoglobinemia. *Semin Hematol* 10:253, 1973.

Wishner BC, Ward KB, Lattman EE, et al: Crystal structure of sickle-cell deoxyhemoglobin at 5Å resolution. *J Mol Biol* 98:179, 1975.

Wright RO, Lewander WJ, Woolf AD: Methemoglobinemia: Etiology, pharmacology, and clinical management. *Ann Emerg Med* 34:646, 1999.

Wynngaarden JB, Smith LH, Jr, Bennett JC, editors: *Cecil textbook of medicine*, Philadelphia, 1992, WB Saunders.

CHAPTER 44

RED BLOOD CELL ENZYMOPATHIES

Xylina T. Gregg and Josef T. Prchal

Reticulocytes are already enucleated when released from the bone marrow and in the process of maturation into red blood cells (RBCs) they also lose their mitochondria and ribosomes. Unable to carry out oxidative phosphorylation and protein synthesis, RBCs still have to sustain an active metabolism to maintain viability and to preserve hemoglobin in its functional form to ensure adequate oxygen delivery to tissues.

RBC enzymes allow RBCs to accomplish these tasks by supporting glycolysis and the pentose shunt and by providing protection against oxidants by maintaining a high ratio of reduced glutathione (GSH) to oxidized glutathione (GSSG). Other RBC enzymes participate in nucleotide degradation and salvage to remove toxic nucleotides from erythrocytes. Glycolytic enzymes also have diverse, nonenzymatic functions, including stimulation of cell movement, control of apoptosis and modulation of oncogene regulation. These other roles of glycolytic enzymes may explain some of the nonerythroid effects of mutations of the glycolytic enzyme genes. In addition, RBCs contain enzymes, such as glutamine-oxaloacetic transaminase, with no obvious physiologic function; these may be remnants of its nucleated past.

The activities of some RBC enzymes rapidly decrease with aging, but the activities of others decrease slowly or not at all. Clinically significant abnormalities of RBC enzymes cause various hematologic phenotypes, principally acute and chronic hemolytic anemia, polycythemia, and methemoglobinemia. Disorders of some RBC enzymes have no RBC phenotype but their dysfunction in nonerythroid tissues causes systemic disorders such as galactosemia and glycogen storage disorders. Thus the presence of these enzymes in easily accessible RBCs serves as a convenient approach for the diagnosis of these disorders. Deficiencies or abnormalities of other RBC enzymes, such as erythrocyte lactate dehydrogenase (LDH), have no apparent disease phenotype.

METABOLIC PATHWAYS

Glucose is used in two different pathways: glycolysis (Fig. 44.1), which provides two molecules of adenosine triphosphate (ATP), and the pentose shunt (see Fig. 44.1), which generates five and seven carbon carbohydrates and reduces nicotinamide adenine dinucleotide phosphate (NADP to NADPH), the sole source of NADPH in red cells. Under physiologic conditions, approximately 90% of glucose is consumed in the glycolytic pathway and about 10% is used in the pentose shunt. In conditions of increased oxidant stress, however, the contribution of the pentose shunt may be significantly increased. In the glycolytic pathway, the generation of one molecule of ATP could be bypassed by the Rapoport-Luebering shunt (see Fig. 44.1), which generates an important glycolytic intermediate, 2,3 biphosphoglycerate (BPG), that facilitates hemoglobin oxygen delivery.

In addition, RBCs have an active glutathione metabolism comprised of its synthesis and reduction (Fig. 44.2). Maintaining a high ratio of GSH to its oxidized form (GSSG) is the principal antioxidant protective mechanism for RBCs. The release of oxygen from hemoglobin generates reactive oxygen species (ROS). Another source of endogenous ROS in RBCs is NADPH oxidase and, in reticulocytes, mitochondrial derived ROS. Excessive ROS is detrimental to RBCs by affecting membrane deformability and hemoglobin solubility, and thus these immense oxidative stresses must be countered by antioxidant enzymes and other antioxidant protective mechanisms such as the active efflux of oxidized glutathione for the RBC to survive.

ENZYMOPATHIES ASSOCIATED WITH HEMOLYTIC ANEMIA

Deficiencies in three enzymes account for most of cases of hemolytic anemia. The most common is glucose-6-phosphate dehydrogenase (G6PD), which is an enzyme essential for glutathione metabolism, followed by an enzyme defect in the glycolytic pathway, pyruvate kinase, (PK) and lastly pyrimidine 5′ nucleotidase-1 (P5′N1), which is essential for removal of toxic nucleotide precursors. Deficiencies of other enzymes are rarer and have highly variable clinical phenotypes that appear to be specific for each enzymatic defect.

Enzyme disorders affecting glutathione metabolism can cause either chronic or acute intermittent hemolysis and Heinz bodies (precipitated denatured hemoglobin) may be seen in RBCs during an acute hemolytic episode. The glycolytic enzyme deficiencies result in chronic hemolysis by a poorly understood mechanism. These patients are not subject to hemolytic crises after exposure to oxidants and their RBCs do not have any characteristic morphologic abnormalities. The chronic hemolytic anemia that occurs in enzyme deficiencies is termed hereditary nonspherocytic hemolytic anemia.

Glucose-6-Phosphate Dehydrogenase Deficiency

Introduction

G6PD deficiency was the first described and is the most common and best-studied RBC enzyme deficiency. G6PD deficiency is more common where *Plasmodium falciparum* malaria is or has been endemic. It was discovered in the 1950s as a result of investigations into a self-limited hemolysis that occurred after administration of the antimalarial drug primaquine, most commonly in individuals of African or Mediterranean ethnic origin. These early studies also determined that G6PD deficiency is X-linked and subsequent studies in carrier females led to the discovery of X-inactivation, a phenomenon that has been exploited to study the hierarchy of hematopoiesis and the clonality of malignant neoplasms.

Epidemiology

G6PD deficiency is the most prevalent human enzyme deficiency in the world, affecting an estimated 500 million people, although the vast majority of affected individuals are not symptomatic. Although most prevalent in individuals of African, Mediterranean, and Asian ethnic origins, it has been found in almost every population. The highest prevalence is in the tropical belt of sub-Saharan Africa (>32%) and the Arabian Peninsula. In other populations, its prevalence ranges from less than 1 in 1000 among northern European populations to 50% of the males in Kurdish Jews. The distribution across Asia is heterogeneous. Nearly 20% of males in Thailand are affected by one of the five prevalent variants. It is common in southern China (~5% in Hong Kong) and rare in other parts of China, while in India the

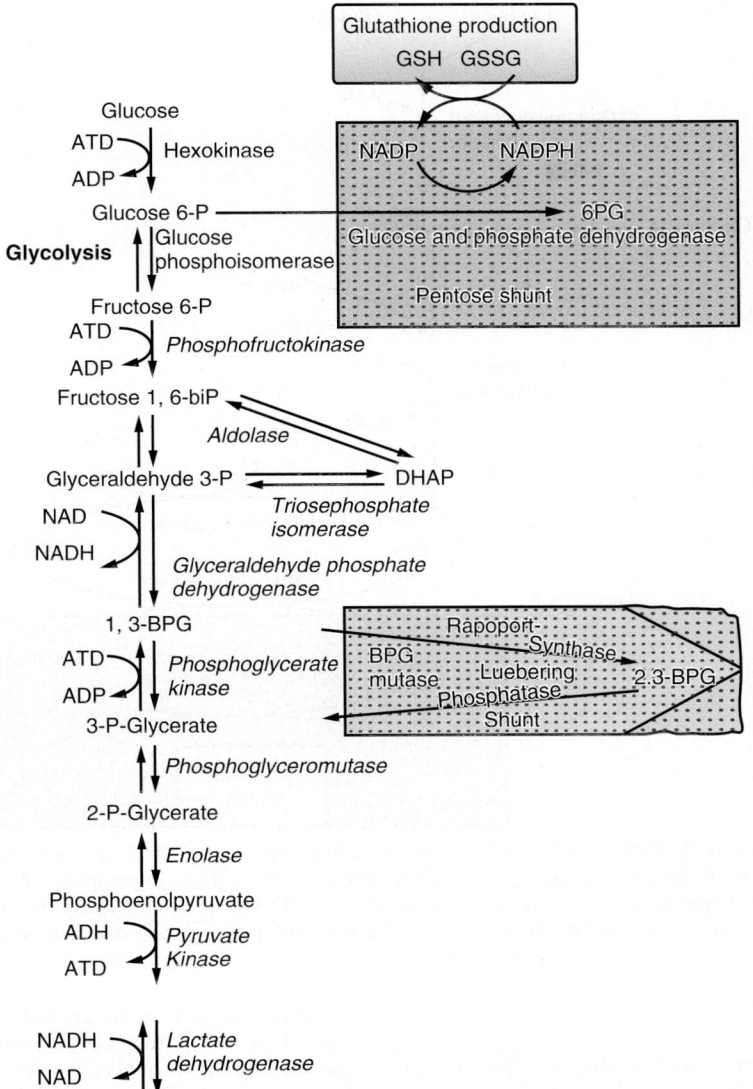

Fig. 44.1 PRINCIPAL COMPONENTS OF THE ERYTHROCYTE METABOLISM WITH CLINICAL RELEVANCE. Glycolysis, Pentose Shunt (*shaded area*), and Rapoport-Luebering shunt (*shaded area*). *ADP,* adenosine diphosphate; *ATP,* adenosine triphosphate; *1,3-BPG,* 1,3- bisphosphoglycerate; *2,3-BPG,* 2,3-bisphosphoglycerate; *DHAP,* dihydroxyacetone phosphate; *GAPD,* glyceraldehyde phosphate dehydrogenase; *GSH,* reduced glutathione; *GSSG,* oxidized glutathione; *NAD+,* nicotinamide adenine dinucleotide; *NADP+,* oxidized form of nicotinamide adenine dinucleotide phosphate; *NADPH,* reduced form of nicotinamide adenine dinucleotide phosphate; *6PG,* 6-phosphogluconate.

prevalence varies from 0% to 27% in different caste, ethnic and linguistic groups. In the United States, G6PD deficiency affects about 10% of African American males. G6PD deficiency is virtually non-existent among indigenous peoples of the Americas and Asian highlanders.

The variable geographic distribution of G6PD deficiency implies that it confers a selective advantage and, as it coincides with the geographic distribution of endemic malaria, suggests protection from lethal malaria, although the exact mechanism has not been fully elucidated. The wild type enzyme is designated G6PD B. The most common G6PD low activity allelic variants are G6PD A- and G6PD Mediterranean. G6PD A- accounts for approximately 90% of G6PD deficient variants in Africa but is also prevalent in North and South America, the West Indies, Italy, the Canary Islands, Spain, Portugal, and the Middle East. The *G6PD A-* mutation (G202A) arose on a *G6PD A+* chromosome (A376G). G6PD A+ has no obvious hematologic phenotype and has a gene frequency similar to that of G6PD A- among African Americans. G6PD Mediterranean is found in the southern part of Italy, Greece, Spain, and Corsica, as well as the Middle East, Iran, and the Arabian Peninsula, India, and Indonesia. G6PD Mediterranean is not homogeneous, but is composed of several distinct mutations, of which *G6PD* Mediterranean[C563T] predominates. Several G6PD variants are pandemic in Asia; there are more than 100 different mutations in various Asian populations.

The high frequency of the most common *G6PD* variants and the diversity of the variants suggest selection of the variants, presumably because of protection from malaria. However, data on which genotype confers protection from malaria has been conflicting. The majority of studies conclude that G6PD deficiency in hemizygous males, and probably also in heterozygous females, confers significant protection against malarial infection. The nature of protection from the mosaic state of G6PD deficiency in heterozygous females remains to be established. However, deficient cells infested with malaria parasites appear be phagocytized more efficiently than normal cells and the host RBCs' impaired ability to restore intracellular NADPH to maintain a high GSH/GSSG ratio may also mean that malarial parasites in G6PD-deficient RBCs are more vulnerable to ROS.

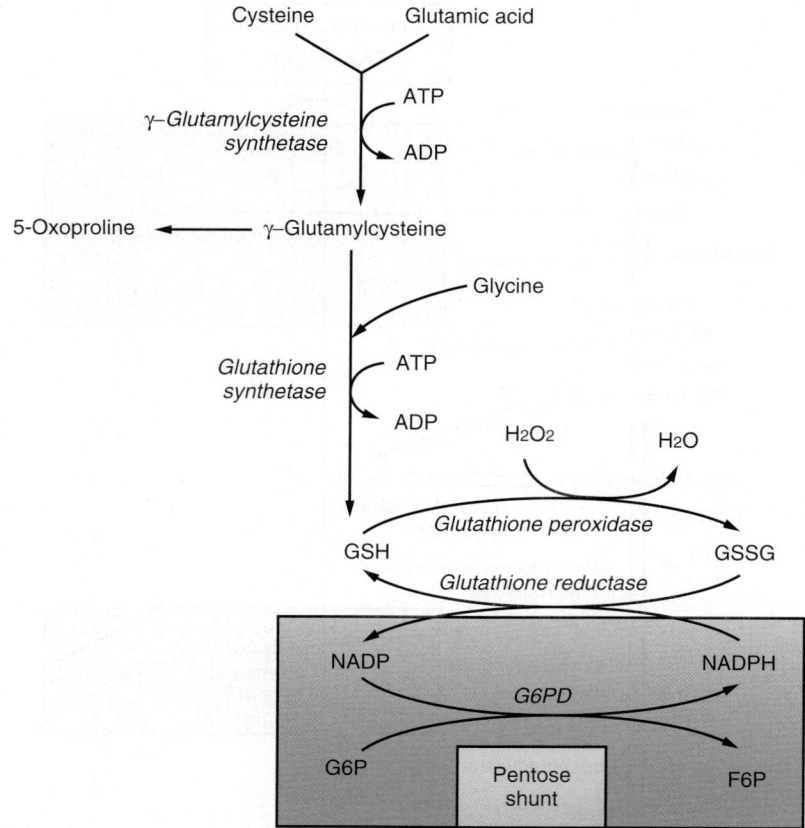

Fig. 44.2 GLUTATHIONE PATHWAY. *ADP,* adenosine diphosphate; *ATP,* adenosine triphosphate; *F6P,* fructose 6-phosphate; *G6P,* glucose 6-phosphate; *G6PD,* glucose-6-phosphate dehydrogenase; *GSH,* reduced glutathione; *GSSG,* oxidized glutathione; *NADP+,* oxidized form of nicotinamide adenine dinucleotide phosphate; *NADPH,* reduced form of nicotinamide adenine dinucleotide phosphate.

Pathobiology

G6PD is a housekeeping enzyme that in the first reaction of pentose shunt catalyzes the oxidation of glucose-6-phosphate to 6-phosphogluconolactone, which reduces NADP$^+$ to NADPH (see Figs. 44.1 and 44.2). In RBCs, the pentose shunt is the only source of NADPH, which is crucial in maintaining high cellular levels of GSH to protect the cell from oxidative stress-induced damage. Within the RBCs, oxidant injury leads to the oxidation of sulfhydryl (SH) groups on the hemoglobin molecule, resulting in the formation of disulfide bridges (-S-S-), which in turn leads to decreased hemoglobin solubility and ultimately the irreversible precipitation of oxidized hemoglobin (Heinz bodies). Under normal conditions these oxidized -S-S- groups of hemoglobin are reduced by GSH to SH-groups by glutathione peroxidase, which in turn is oxidized to GSSG but is restored back to GSH by glutathione reductase in a reaction requiring NADPH. NADPH levels are maintained by G6PD; thus, in G6PD-deficient RBCs, GSH is not restored to adequate levels under oxidative stress, leading to a buildup of free radicals and insoluble hemoglobin within the cell. Precipitated hemoglobin is disruptive to the structure and function of the RBC membrane and leads to increased membrane permeability, osmotic fragility, and cell rigidity. The compromised integrity of the RBC membrane results in both intravascular hemolysis and the rapid removal of these cells within the splenic pulp.

The *G6PD* gene localizes to Xq28, spans 18 kb, and contains 13 exons; the G6PD peptide exists as a tetramer or dimer. Stability of the quaternary structure is crucial for optimal G6PD activity. G6PD activity decreases significantly as erythrocytes age, with a half-life of about 60 days. Reticulocytes have five times higher enzyme activity than the oldest RBC subpopulation. The decrease in G6PD activity with aging is particularly pronounced in some mutant variants such as the African G6PD A-.

G6PD variants can be divided into three categories based on the type of hemolysis they cause: acute intermittent (most common), chronic (rare), or none. The less frequently used World Health Organization classifies the different G6PD variants according to the degree of enzyme deficiency and severity of hemolysis. Class I deficiencies are the most severe and cause chronic hemolysis. Less severe G6PD Mediterranean is a class II deficiency and the even less deficient G6PD A- is a class III deficiency. Classes IV and V do not cause hemolysis and are of no clinical significance.

Over 400 variants of the G6PD enzyme have been identified by biochemical methods, 100 of which reach polymorphic levels. Mutations associated with chronic hemolysis tend to cluster in the vicinity of the NADP-binding domain of the *G6PD* gene and cause more severe deficiency, whereas those associated with acute intermittent hemolysis or no hemolysis are scattered throughout the gene. Most variants are caused by point or missense mutations. Unlike disease-causing mutations of other genes, deletions and insertions causing frameshift and stop codon mutations are not observed; these events would be expected to be fatal, since *G6PD* is a housekeeping gene essential for basic cellular functions.

Clinical Manifestations

Acute Hemolysis

Individuals with the most common forms of G6PD deficiency have no anemia or other clinical manifestations unless they are exposed to triggers of acute hemolysis, such as oxidant drugs, infection, or ingestion of fava beans. Exposure of red cells to certain drugs results in the formation of low levels of hydrogen peroxide as the drug interacts with hemoglobin; other drugs may form free radicals that oxidize GSH without the formation of peroxide as an intermediate. Hemolysis begins in hours to 1–3 days after exposure to the offending drug. However, many drugs implicated in acute hemolysis in G6PD deficiency may not be true culprits, as infection and other stressors can also provoke hemolysis in these people.

The mechanism of hemolysis induced by infection is not well understood, but the generation of hydrogen peroxide by phagocytizing leukocytes or the diffusion of oxidants from neutrophils undergoing oxidative bursts leading to the formation of disulfide bridges of hemoglobin may be factors.

Depending on the G6PD variant, hemolysis can be self-limited or protracted. The RBCs of G6PD A- contain only 5% to 15% of the normal amount of enzyme activity and the age-dependent decline of the activity renders old RBCs severely deficient and susceptible to hemolysis. As this subpopulation is eliminated, younger RBCs and reticulocytes produced in response to hemolysis have higher G6PD activity and are typically not hemolyzed. Thus, the hemolytic process is self-limited, even when the offending agent is continued. In contrast, in G6PD Mediterranean the enzyme activity of the young RBCs is lower compared with G6PD A- and hemolysis continues longer, even days after discontinuation of the culprit drug.

Favism

Fava beans are a staple food in many parts of the world where G6PD deficiency is found at a high gene frequency. The hemolysis precipitated by fava bean ingestion, favism, occurs only in people who are G6PD deficient. It is most frequently associated with the more severe G6PD Mediterranean and G6PD Cairo variants, but rarely has been seen with G6PD A-. Not all individuals with G6PD Mediterranean are susceptible to favism and a tendency toward familial occurrence suggests that additional genetic factors may be important. Favism is more common in children than adults. Hemolysis usually occurs one to several days after fava bean consumption, but onset within the first hours after exposure has been reported.

Chronic Hemolysis

The rare G6PD variants causing chronic hemolytic anemia occur sporadically. The severity of the hemolysis ranges from mild to transfusion dependent. Exposure to the oxidants that cause hemolysis in the acute hemolytic G6PD variants may further exacerbate hemolysis.

Neonatal Jaundice

Neonatal jaundice, which may result in kernicterus, is the most common and often the most serious consequence of G6PD deficiency. The icterus is not only caused by hemolysis but also to inadequate processing of bilirubin by the immature liver of the G6PD deficient infant. Thus, the coinheritance of polymorphic *UGT1A1* promoter alleles (Gilbert syndrome) exacerbates the icterus. Neonatal screening for G6PD deficiency and early phototherapy treatment in endemic areas has been associated with a decreased incidence of kernicterus.

Nonerythroid Effect of G6PD Deficiency

Although patients with the common endemic G6PD variants are not at increased risk for infections, neutrophil dysfunction has been described in some patients with rare severely deficient G6PD variants. Occasionally, cataracts have been observed in patients with some rare variants of G6PD that produce chronic hemolytic anemia. Small studies from the Middle East suggest that decreased G6PD activity may predispose to the development of diabetes. Splenomegaly is generally not seen in G6PD deficient individuals.

Laboratory Manifestations

Under normal conditions, most G6PD-deficient individuals are not anemic and have no laboratory evidence of hemolysis. In the setting of oxidative stress, laboratory findings indicative of acute hemolysis including anemia and reticulocytosis are seen. As the hemolysis is mainly extravascular with a variable intravascular component, variable degrees of hyperbilirubinemia, increased LDH, and decreased

haptoglobin occur. Heinz bodies (denatured precipitated hemoglobin) may be visible in the erythrocytes during an acute hemolytic episode, but not under normal circumstances. "Bite cells" have been described, but this is not specific for G6PD deficiency and these cells are usually not present in acute hemolytic states of patients with common G6PD variants or in G6PD-deficient patients with chronic hemolysis.

Individuals with the chronic hemolytic G6PD variants have varying degrees of anemia and reticulocytosis.

Diagnosis

A biochemical diagnosis of G6PD deficiency can be made using quantitative spectrophotometric analysis to measure the generation of NADPH from NADP in RBC hemolysates. A more convenient rapid fluorescent screening test can be used to test at-risk populations. False-negative results are not unusual, however, especially if enzymatic analysis is performed shortly after resolution of acute hemolytic episodes or in heterozygous females. After acute hemolysis, reticulocytes and young RBCs, which have much higher enzymatic activity, predominate. These false-negative test results are more likely to occur when a screening test rather than a quantitative spectrophotometric analysis of the enzyme activity is used. Females heterozygous for G6PD are particularly difficult to diagnose because of their mosaicism for X-chromosome enzymes and may have total RBC enzymatic activity ranging anywhere from hemizygote to normal; however these females have a variable mixture of deficient and nondeficient RBCs and their deficient RBCs are subject to hemolytic crises. Since the nucleotide substitutions of many G6PD-deficient isoenzymes have been identified, molecular diagnostic methods are more reliable for the accurate diagnosis of females who are heterozygous for G6PD deficiency.

Severe sporadic variants causing chronic hemolytic anemia may be considered for prenatal diagnosis in some circumstances.

Prognosis

Most patients with G6PD deficiency have normal life spans with no clinical sequelae. Neonatal icterus with resultant kernicterus and mental retardation have the gravest consequences.

Therapy

Treatment of an acute hemolytic crisis includes withdrawing any offending agent and supportive care, which in severe cases includes RBC transfusions. Folic acid supplementation is recommended for patients with chronic hemolysis. Rarely, chronic hemolytic anemia is severe enough to require chronic transfusions. Neonatal icterus associated with G6PD deficiency is treated in the same manner as neonatal icterus arising from other causes; G6PD deficiency should be considered in any neonate with hyperbilirubinemia, especially those of high-risk ethnic descent.

Future Directions

In certain areas of the world where G6PD deficiency reaches epidemic proportions and ingestion of fava beans is staple, screening for endemic G6PD-deficient variants would be expected to reduce hospitalizations, RBC transfusions and even mortality (from kernicterus).

Pyruvate Kinase Deficiency

Introduction

PK deficiency is the most common enzyme deficiency causing hemolysis. Although this disorder is far less common than G6PD deficiency, the vast majority of patients with G6PD deficiency never suffer a hemolytic episode, while PK deficiency exhibits a high penetrance of the hemolytic phenotype.

Epidemiology

PK deficiency is distributed worldwide but is more common among people of northern European extraction. The population prevalence of PK deficiency among whites is approximately 50 cases per 1 million. PK deficiency is an autosomal recessive disease, and affected patients are typically double heterozygotes, or, less commonly, homozygous for the same mutation. Homozygous mutations are usually seen in groups with marked consanguinity, and homozygous PK deficiency has been well described in the Amish populations of Pennsylvania and Ohio. Common mutations have well-defined geographic associations. Mutation 1529A is the most common mutation in the United States, northern and central Europe, 1456T in southern Europe, and 1468T in Asia.

PK deficiency does not localize to geographic areas of malarial endemicity. However, there is in vitro evidence that PK deficiency provides protection against infection and replication of *Plasmodium falciparum* in human RBCs, an effect possibly mediated by reduced ATP levels in PK-deficient RBCs. PK deficiency was also shown to be protective in a mouse model of infection with *Plasmodium chabaudi*.

Pathobiology

PK catalyzes the irreversible transfer of phosphate from phosphoenolpyruvate to adenosine diphosphate (ADP) yielding one molecule of pyruvate and one molecule of ATP (see Fig. 44.1). Two genes encode four PK isoenzymes with different tissue expression. PK-R (unique to RBCs) and PK-L (in liver) are products transcribed from two different, tissue-specific promoters of the *PKLR* gene on chromosome 1q21. Other undefined regulatory elements are also involved in *PKLR* gene expression. PK-M1 (in skeletal muscle) and PK-M2 (in leukocytes, kidney, adipose tissue, lungs and fetal RBCs) are formed from the *PKM2* gene by alternative splicing. PK-M2 in fetal erythropoiesis is replaced by the PK-R isoform after birth. PK-R is a heterotetramer whose enzymatic activity is allosterically augmented by fructose 1,6-diphosphate.

More than 230 mutations in the *PKLR* gene have been identified, most of which are missense mutations. Mutations affecting the active site or protein stability are associated with more severe hemolytic anemia. However, the phenotypic expression of identical mutations can be strikingly different. Since most PK-deficient patients are compound heterozygous for two different mutations, rather than homozygous for one, several different tetrameric forms of PK may be present, each with distinct structural and kinetic properties. This complicates genotype-to-phenotype correlations in these individuals, as it is difficult to infer which mutation is primarily responsible for deficient enzyme function and the clinical phenotype. There are even cases in which the activity of PK as measured in vitro is higher than normal, but a kinetically abnormal enzyme is responsible for the hemolytic anemia.

PK deficiency may be also caused by mutations not directly involving *PKLR* gene. Combined heterozygosity for the common 1529A PK mutation and a unique promoter mutation on the other allele that markedly reduced its allelic transcription resulted in a severe hemolytic variant. Mutations in the key erythroid transcription factor KLF1 caused severe congenital hemolytic anemia because of a deficiency of PK.

The mechanism of hemolysis in PK deficiency is not clear. The defect in ATP generation is unlikely to be the cause as ATP deficiency is difficult to demonstrate in many patients and other disorders with more severe ATP deficiency are not associated with significant hemolysis. Increased apoptosis and ineffective erythropoiesis may also be a feature of PK deficiency, although this has only been studied in

splenic erythroid progenitors. Following splenectomy, despite decreased hemolysis and improved anemia, patients paradoxically have a higher number of reticulocytes; this phenomenon is as yet unexplained.

Tolerance of Anemia

The anemia of PK deficiency is better tolerated than a comparable level of anemia seen in patients with hexokinase deficiency, since the block in glycolysis occurs after the Rapoport-Leubering shunt (see Fig. 44.1); (see section on 2,3-BPG deficiency). The resultant accumulation of 2,3-BPG shifts the oxyhemoglobin dissociation curve to the right, leading to better oxygen delivery to the tissue and improved tolerance of anemia.

Clinical and Laboratory Manifestations

The severity of hemolysis in PK-deficient patients is highly variable, ranging from a mild, fully compensated chronic hemolytic process without anemia, to life-threatening transfusion-requiring hemolytic anemia present at birth, to rare hydrops fetalis because of homozygosity for PK null mutations. The disease severity is typically similar among siblings of a given family. In most cases the degree of hemolysis declines after infancy, by a not fully understood pathophysiologic mechanism. Splenomegaly is often but not invariably present. Patients with severe hemolysis may be chronically jaundiced and may develop the clinical complications of chronic hemolytic states, including gallstones, transient aplastic anemia crises (caused by parvovirus infection), folate deficiency, extramedullary hematopoiesis and infrequently, skin ulcers. Pregnancy may precipitate hemolysis. Iron overload has been reported in both nontransfused and transfusion-dependent patients and may be severe; in some cases iron overload has been attributed to coinheritance of mutations in *HFE*, the gene associated with hereditary hemochromatosis. Neonatal icterus may occur and is augmented by coincidental heterozygosity or homozygosity for the *UGT1A1* polymorphism.

Hemolysis is mainly extravascular with a variable intravascular component; thus, increased LDH, hyperbilirubinemia and low haptoglobin levels may be present. The reticulocyte count invariably increases after splenectomy.

Diagnosis

There are no characteristic RBC morphologic findings in PK deficiency. A screening test using crude hemolysate with a single concentration substrate has been used for the detection of pyruvate deficiency but occasionally misses some PK variants. Specialized laboratories can perform quantitative PK enzyme analysis and further analyze the mutant enzyme by comprehensive kinetic studies. In these assays, leukocytes and platelets must be carefully removed as their presence can obscure a deficiency in the red cells. Molecular studies for prenatal diagnosis can be used if the mutation is known.

Therapy

Many patients do not require therapy. Some require RBC transfusions only in transient settings of increased stress, such as the perioperative period, coexistent infections, or pregnancies. However, others require chronic transfusions. Iron chelation may be required in chronic transfusion programs and also in some patients who have never been transfused.

Splenectomy has documented benefit in severe cases; the degree of hemolysis and anemia is ameliorated and the transfusion requirement is generally abolished or markedly decreased. The increase in hemoglobin concentration in nontransfusion requiring patients after splenectomy ranges from 1–3 g/dL. It is recommended to delay splenectomy if possible until after the age of 3 years when the risk of infections with encapsulated organisms declines and because in most cases the degree of hemolysis declines after infancy, by a not fully understood pathophysiologic mechanism. One PK-deficient boy with severe hemolysis was apparently cured by an allogeneic marrow transplant.

A small molecule AG-348 (Agios Pharmaceuticals Inc.) can increase the activity of many PK mutants perhaps by increasing the stability of the PK enzyme. This oral compound is currently in clinical trials and may be able to restore glycolytic pathway activity and normalize ATP and 2,3 BPG levels in PK deficiency.

Prognosis

The clinical course is highly variable ranging from fatal hydrops fetalis, transfusion dependency from birth, and a high risk of kernicterus to normal childhood development with no or rare transfusions, or to compensated hemolysis without anemia. However, hemolysis that is fully compensated because of excessive erythropoiesis may be deceptively benign. In addition to the usual complications of chronic hemolysis such as gallstones and parvovirus-induced aplastic crisis, the excessive number of erythroblasts in these patients produces erythroferrone, which mediates low hepcidin and may result in typical hemochromatosis induced cardiac and hepatic dysfunction.

Future Directions

Small molecular activators of PK are promising, but are being validated in ongoing trials.

New gene therapeutic techniques are also being evaluated in severe PK deficiency. These include the zinc finger nucleases and *CRISPR/Cas9* technology (clustered regularly interspaced short palindromic repeats) that uses noncoding RNAs to guide the Cas9 nuclease to induce site-specific DNA cleavage. The resultant DNA damage is repaired by cellular DNA repair mechanisms that may correct the PK mutation. These technologies hold early promise that will need to be validated by future clinical trials.

Pyrimidine 5′ Nucleotidase-1 Deficiency

Introduction

P5′N1 deficiency is the third most common cause of hemolytic anemia caused by a red cell enzymopathy, after G6PD and PK deficiency. It is inherited in an autosomal recessive manner.

Pathobiology

As the reticulocyte matures, ribosomes and RNA are degraded. P5′N1 assists in the process by catalyzing the dephosphorylation of pyrimidine nucleoside monophosphates into cytidine and uridine, which can diffuse across the cell membrane. P5′N1 activity is specific for pyrimidines and is much higher in reticulocytes than mature red cells; P5′N1 activity rapidly declines during the first few days of red cell maturation. P5′N1 requires Mg^{2+} for its activity and is inhibited by a number of heavy metals, including Pb^{2+}. P5′N1 also has phosphotransferase properties, suggesting an additional role of this enzyme in nucleotide metabolism. Thus far, 27 different mutations have been reported in P5′N1 deficiency. Most patients are homozygous.

P5′N2 is another nucleotidase present in RBCs. Although the activity of this enzyme is generally measured together with that of P5′N1, it is encoded by a separate gene, is not strictly pyrimidine-specific, and is unable to compensate for deficient function of P5′N1. Only P5′N1 deficiency is associated with hemolytic anemia.

The accumulation of pyrimidines in the RBCs because of a deficiency of P5′N1 is presumed to be toxic although the exact mechanism by which P5′N1 causes hemolysis is unknown. The ribosomal aggregates are visible as the characteristic coarse basophilic stippling seen on the peripheral smear. However, deficiency of P5′N1 is at least partly compensated in vivo by other nucleosidases or other nucleotide metabolic pathways. Acquired P5′N1 deficiency occurs in acute lead toxicity because of Pb^{2+} outcompeting the essential cofactor Mg^{2+}.

Clinical and Laboratory Features

P5′N1 deficiency causes chronic hemolytic anemia, with severity ranging from compensated hemolysis without anemia to transfusion dependent anemia. Marked basophilic stippling of RBCs is a laboratory hallmark and thus morphologic examination of the peripheral blood smear provides simple and inexpensive screening. However basophilic stippling is not a specific finding, as it is also found in hemolytic anemia caused by acute lead toxicity and sideroblastic anemia. Confirmation of the diagnosis requires demonstration of decreased P5′N1 activity, normal blood lead levels and, if available, high concentrations of pyrimidine nucleotides in red cells.

Therapy

Chronic transfusion support may be necessary for severe cases. Milder cases may require transfusion only periodically, during pregnancy, infection or other stressors. Iron overload may occur, as in any chronic hemolytic condition, and iron chelation may be needed. Splenectomy was reported to be beneficial in several cases.

OTHER ENZYMOPATHIES OF THE GLUTATHIONE PATHWAY

γ-Glutamylcysteine Synthase Deficiency

γ-glutamylcysteine synthase (GCL) catalyzes the first metabolic step of glutathione synthesis. Deficiency of this enzyme is rare and only a few cases, usually in consanguineous families, have been reported. All patients had hemolytic anemia and approximately half also had neurologic defects, including spinocerebellar degeneration, peripheral neuropathy, and mental retardation. Some patients have been characterized at the molecular level and in all these cases the causative mutation affected the catalytic domain of GCL.

Glutathione Synthetase Deficiency

Glutathione synthetase (GS) deficiency is a slightly more common enzymopathy of glutathione metabolism than GCL deficiency. The clinical severity is variable, but approximately 25% of the patients die in childhood. Mild GS deficiency can manifest as only mild chronic hemolysis. Moderately affected individuals present in the neonatal period with both hemolytic anemia and severe metabolic acidosis caused by the accumulation of the γ-glutamylcysteine metabolite 5-oxoproline, which results from decreased feedback inhibition of GCL by the decreased levels of GSH. Severely affected patients have progressive neurologic defects and animal experiments suggest that 5-oxoproline has a direct neurotoxic effect. The different clinical manifestations are likely compounded by environmental factors as phenotypic variability among siblings with the same mutation has been encountered.

High levels of 5-oxyproline in the urine (found in all severely and moderately affected but in only some of the mildly affected patients) suggest the diagnosis, which is confirmed by documenting deficiency of the enzyme or by demonstrating mutations in the GS gene. Correction of the metabolic acidosis and early supplementation with antioxidants such as vitamins C and E was reported to improve survival and long-term outcome in some but not all affected patients.

Patients with glutathione synthetase deficiency should avoid the same agents known to precipitate acute hemolysis in patients with G6PD deficiency.

Glutathione Reductase Deficiency

Glutathione reductase (GR) restores intracellular GSH by reducing GSSG in the presence of NADPH and flavine adenine dinucleotide (FAD), a derivative of the water-soluble vitamin riboflavin. Hereditary GR deficiency has only been reported in two Dutch families. In one consanguineous family, acute hemolytic anemia after ingestion of fava beans occurred; GR deficiency was caused by a large homozygous deletion. The second family had a compound heterozygous mutation and a clinical phenotype of neonatal jaundice.

Riboflavin is a cofactor of GR. Mild acquired GR deficiency is common and occurs in malnourished individuals because of riboflavin deficiency but has no hematologic phenotype.

Glutathione Peroxidase Deficiency

Glutathione peroxidase is a selenium-containing enzyme that reduces hydrogen peroxide to water. Although a polymorphism affecting the activity of glutathione peroxidase and acquired decreased activity because of selenium deficiency have been described, neither circumstance was associated with a clinical phenotype.

OTHER ENZYMOPATHIES OF THE GLYCOLYTIC PATHWAY

Glucose Phosphoisomerase Deficiency

Glucose phosphoisomerase (GPI) deficiency is one of the three most common RBC enzyme defects causing chronic hereditary nonspherocytic hemolytic anemia (the other two are PK and P5′N1), with approximately 100 affected families described. GPI deficiency is an autosomal recessive disorder, with most patients compound heterozygous for mutations that partially inactivate the enzyme. The severity of the hemolysis is variable. Splenectomy can improve the anemia, eliminating transfusion requirements. Neonatal jaundice is common and hydrops fetalis has been reported. Rarely, severe neuromuscular symptoms, mental retardation and granulocyte dysfunction occur. These symptoms may be caused by nonerythroid functions of GPI, including its actions as a neuroleukin, an autocrine motility factor, a nerve growth factor, and a differentiation and maturation mediator. It has also been suggested that disturbed glycerolipid biosynthesis in GPI deficiency may have significant effects on membrane formation, membrane function, and axonal migration.

Hexokinase Deficiency

Hexokinase (HK), the red cell enzyme with the lowest activity in the glycolytic pathway, catalyzes the initial step in the utilization of glucose and thus is required for both glycolysis and the pentose shunt and produces glucose 6-phosphate. The two HK isoenzymes, HK1 and HKR, are the product of a single gene *HK-1* by use of an alternate translation initiation site. A single nucleotide polymorphism in *HK-1* was strongly associated with reduced hemoglobin and hematocrit levels in a European population. HK deficiency is a rare cause of hereditary chronic nonspherocytic hemolytic anemia with only few dozen cases in 19 families reported. Most patients are of northern European extraction, although one case was reported in a Chinese individual. The molecular defect has been characterized in only four patients; two were homozygous. HK is proximal to the generation of 2,3-BPG and thus decreased levels of 2,3-BPG in HK

deficiency lead to a left-shifted hemoglobin-oxygen dissociation curve and a more symptomatic anemia than comparable levels of anemia seen in patients with other RBC disorders. Splenectomy may be beneficial. A mouse model of HK deficiency demonstrates severe hemolytic anemia with extensive tissue iron deposition and marked reticulocytosis.

Phosphofructokinase Deficiency

Phosphofructokinase (PFK) catalyzes the rate-limiting phosphorylation of fructose-6-phosphate by ATP to fructose-1,6-diphosphate. Red cells contain both M and L subunits of PFK. PFK deficiency is an autosomal recessive disorder with approximately 100 cases and 23 mutant *PFKM* alleles reported. These mutations lead to an almost complete loss of PFK activity in muscle, but only partial loss of activity in erythrocytes. Two common mutations are present in Ashkenazi Jews. The most common manifestation of PFK deficiency is type VII glycogen storage disease (Tarui disease), which causes muscle weakness and exercise intolerance, although a mild chronic hemolytic anemia may also be present. In some patients, hemolysis is present without muscle manifestations.

PFK deficiency in dogs is characterized by hemolytic crises with strenuous exercise. *Pfkm* null mice show exercise intolerance, reduced lifespan and progressive cardiac hypertrophy.

Aldolase Deficiency

Aldolase reversibly cleaves fructose-1,6-diphosphate into glyceraldehyde 3-phosphate and dihydroxyacetone phosphate. Aldolase deficiency is a very rare cause of chronic nonspherocytic hemolytic anemia; myopathy and mental retardation may also occur.

Phosphoglycerokinase Deficiency

Phosphoglycerokinase catalyzes the reversible conversion of 1,3-bisphosphoglycerate to 3-phosphoglycerate, forming ATP in the process. This reaction can be bypassed by the Rappaport-Luebering shunt. Deficiency of this X-chromosome encoded enzyme is variably associated with hemolytic anemia, mental retardation, and myoglobinuria.

Triosephosphate Isomerase Deficiency

Triosephosphate isomerase (TPI) catalyzes the reversible interconversion of the triose phosphate isomers, dihydroxyacetone phosphate and glyceraldehyde 3-phosphate. TPI deficiency is a rare autosomal recessive disorder characterized by chronic hemolytic anemia, increased susceptibility to bacterial infections, cardiomyopathy and progressive neuromuscular disease. Neonatal jaundice may also occur. The neuromuscular disease is likely caused by the formation of toxic protein aggregates of glycated proteins formed by elevated byproducts of dihydroxyacetone phosphate.

Approximately 40 patients with several different mutations have been reported; however, most patients have the same mutation and are descendants from a common British/French ancestor about 1000 years ago. There is no effective therapy and most patients die in childhood, although there are rare exceptions.

OTHER ENZYMOPATHIES

Transaldolase Deficiency

Transaldolase catalyzes the conversion of seduhepulose-7-phosphate and glyceraldehyde-3-phosphate into erythrose-4-phosphate and fructose-6-phosphate. Transaldolase deficiency has been described in

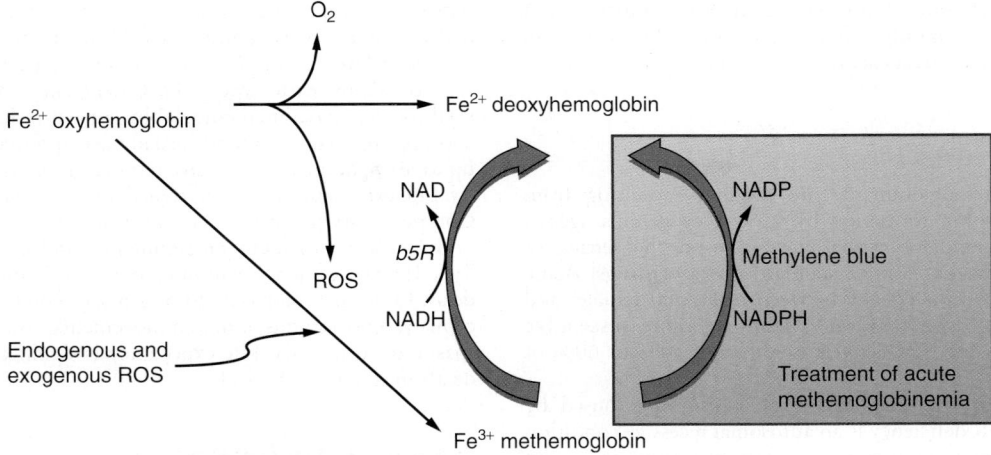

Fig. 44.3 METHEMOGLOBINEMIA. Formation of methemoglobin and it physiologic (*open space*) and therapeutic reduction (*shaded space*). Iron is in the ferrous state (Fe^{2+}) in oxygenated and deoxy-hemoglobin (deoxyHb). When oxygen is released, a small proportion of oxygen bound hemoglobin iron is then converted to ROS converting to the ferric state (Fe^{3+}); i.e., methemoglobin. The NADH, generated in glycolysis is a cofactor for methemoglobin reduction mediated by cytochrome b5 reductase (b5R) depicted in the *open space*, keeping methemoglobin at low levels (<1%). When this physiologic reduction of NADH-dependent methemoglobin reduction is either insufficient because of excessive ROS or decreased b5R activity, methemoglobin reduction can be achieved therapeutically. Exogenously administered methylene blue utilizing NADPH produced by G6PD in pentose shunt can nonenzymatically convert methemoglobin to Fe^{2+} hemoglobin (*shaded space*). *b5R*, cytochrome b5 reductase; *NAD*, nicotinamide adenine dinucleotide phosphate; *NADH*, the reduced form of NAD; *NADP*, oxidized form of nicotinamide adenine dinucleotide phosphate; *NADPH*, reduced form of NADP; *ROS*, reactive oxygen species.

23 patients from 13 families. Transaldolase deficiency presents in the neonatal period and clinical manifestations include dysmorphic features, hepatosplenomegaly, cirrhosis, cardiac and renal abnormalities, skin manifestations, and thrombocytopenia, although the phenotype is highly variable.

Adenosine Deaminase Hyperactivity

Adenosine deaminase (ADA) helps regulate the concentration of adenosine ribonucleotides in the red cell by irreversibly deaminating them to inosine. Hyperactivity of ADA is a rare cause of hereditary nonspherocytic hemolytic anemia and is the only red cell enzyme disorder that is inherited in an autosomal dominant disorder, but the molecular mechanism of this disorder has not been identified. Deficiency of ADA is associated with severe combined immunodeficiency (see Chapter 19).

ENZYMOPATHIES ASSOCIATED WITH POLYCYTHEMIA

Bisphosphoglycerate mutase (BPGM) regulates the concentration of 2,3-BPG (also known as 2,3-DPG) of erythrocytes. 2,3-BPG is an important modifier of RBC oxygen delivery. 2,3-BPG binds to the hemoglobin tetramer and allosterically converts hemoglobin to a low oxygen affinity state, resulting in a rightward shift of the oxygen dissociation curve. BPGM is a multifunctional enzyme with both synthase and phosphatase activity. The synthase activity of BPGM converts 1,3-bisphosphoglycerate to 2,3-BPG, which is then metabolized to 3-phosphoglycerate (3-PGA), an intermediate of the glycolytic pathway, by BPGM-phosphatase (see Fig. 44.1). Deficiency of BPGM results in decreased levels of 2,3-BPG. The consequent left shift of the oxygen dissociation curve increases hemoglobin affinity for oxygen, thus resulting in decreased delivery of oxygen into the peripheral tissues and compensatory polycythemia.

BPGM deficiency is rare and only two families have been comprehensively studied. In a family in France, four siblings were compound heterozygotes for two different BPGM mutations and had polycythemia, markedly decreased 2,3-BPG levels and undetectable BPGM activity. Some of their heterozygote relatives had a milder decrease of 2,3-BPG levels and a mild polycythemia.

ENZYMOPATHIES ASSOCIATED WITH METHEMOGLOBINEMIA

Introduction

Methemoglobinemia occurs when an imbalance arising from either increased methemoglobin production or decreased methemoglobin reduction is present. Methemoglobin is a derivative of hemoglobin in which the ferrous (Fe^{2+}) irons are oxidized to the ferric (Fe^{3+}) state. Methemoglobin is formed spontaneously at a slow rate by the autoxidation of hemoglobin. In the release of oxygen from Fe^{2+}-oxyhemoglobin, one electron is partially transferred to a small portion of released oxygen, generating superoxide and eventually forming other ROS, which convert the iron to the ferric state and form Fe^{3+}-hemoglobin, i.e., methemoglobin (Fig. 44.3). Methemoglobin may also be formed from the oxidation of hemoglobin in other reactions with endogenous and exogenous compounds. The ferric hemes of methemoglobin are unable to bind oxygen and, additionally, if a ferriheme subunit is part of a hemoglobin tetramer, the oxygen affinity of the accompanying ferrous hemes in the hemoglobin tetramer is increased. As a result, the oxygen dissociation curve is left-shifted and oxygen delivery is impaired. Methemoglobin is formed continuously, but reducing mechanisms keep the methemoglobin level at about 1% of the total hemoglobin. The only physiologically important mechanism is the NADH-dependent cytochrome *b5* reductase (b5R). b5R contains a prosthetic FAD group that acts as an electron acceptor. NADH reduces FAD to FADH2, which then reduces the heme protein cytochrome *b5*. Electrons from the reduced cytochrome *b5* are in turn transferred to methemoglobin, reducing iron back to the ferrous state (see Fig. 44.3)

An alternative pathway mediated by NADPH-diaphorase uses NADPH generated by G6PD as a source of electrons to reduce redox dyes, such as methylene blue, and flavin. Reduced methylene blue then reduces methemoglobin. Since these electron acceptors are not physiologic, this pathway is only of importance as it is the mechanism by which methylene blue treats acute toxic methemoglobinemia.

Epidemiology

Most cases of methemoglobinemia are acquired, resulting from increased methemoglobin formation by various exogenous agents. Acute or toxic methemoglobinemia may occur in the setting of overdose or poisoning, but also at standard doses of drugs. Acute methemoglobinemia occurs equally between males and females and over a wide range of ages; however, infants are more susceptible because their erythrocyte b5R activity is normally 50% to 60% of adult activity.

Hereditary methemoglobinemia is most commonly caused by deficiency of b5R. b5R deficiency is an autosomal recessive condition and occurs in all racial and ethnic groups, but is endemic in certain populations, including Navajo and Athabasca Native Americans and natives of Yakutsk, Siberia. Other causes of hereditary methemoglobinemia are the autosomal dominant inheritance of an abnormal hemoglobin in hemoglobin M disease (see Chapter 43) and, very rarely, deficiency of cytochrome b_5.

Pathobiology

Acute Methemoglobinemia

Many drugs and toxins have been implicated in acute methemoglobinemia. More common culprits include dapsone, local anesthetics (benzocaine, lidocaine, prilocaine), and derivatives of the anesthetic phenacetin. Exposure to nitrates and nitrites, widely used as food preservatives and found in well water can also cause methemoglobinemia. Nitrates do not oxidize hemoglobin directly but are converted to nitrites by intestinal bacteria. Infants less than 6 months of age may have increased susceptibility to methemoglobinemia at least in part because of their lower b5R activity. Homemade baby food purees of high-nitrate-containing vegetables, well water contaminated by nitrites and diarrheal illness may all cause acute toxic methemoglobinemia in infants.

B5R Deficiency

In erythrocytes, b5R transfers electrons to methemoglobin to reduce it to hemoglobin. In other cells, b5R transfers electrons from cytochrome b_5 to stearyl-CoA in the endoplasmic reticulum, a reaction that has an important role in cholesterol biosynthesis, fatty acid elongation and desaturation, and drug metabolism. There are two types of b5R deficiency. The more common type I b5R deficiency is usually caused by missense mutations leading to decreased stability of the enzyme. Thus, although b5R is abnormal in all cells, only mature RBCs, which cannot synthesize proteins and replace the enzyme, are significantly affected in patients with type I b5R deficiency. Type II b5R mutations affect the catalytic site or lead to marked structural changes and all cells have decreased b5R activity.

Clinical Manifestations

Methemoglobinemia causes clinically discernible cyanosis when the absolute level of methemoglobin exceeds 1.5 gm%; this correlates with approximately 10% to 15% methemoglobin. Methemoglobinemia should be clinically suspected when "cyanosis" occurs in the presence of a normal PaO_2. Symptoms develop secondary to impaired tissue oxygenation and the onset may be abrupt. Early symptoms include headache, fatigue, dyspnea, and lethargy. At higher levels, respiratory depression, altered consciousness, shock, seizures, and death may occur. As methemoglobin levels rise above 20% to 30%,

patients can experience progressive respiratory compromise, myocardial ischemia, seizures, and coma. Death typically ensues at methemoglobin levels above 70% but can occur at lower levels.

Individuals with type I b5R deficiency, which is limited to erythrocytes, have methemoglobin concentrations of 10% to 35% and appear cyanotic but are usually asymptomatic, even with levels up to 40%. Some patients have reported headache and easy fatigability. Life expectancy is not shortened and pregnancies occur normally. Compensatory polycythemia is at times observed.

In addition to methemoglobinemia and cyanosis, patients with Type II b5R deficiency exhibit mental retardation and developmental delay. Other neurologic symptoms may be present, including microcephaly, opisthotonus, athetoid movements, strabismus, seizures, and spastic quadriparesis. Life expectancy is significantly shortened, and death in infancy is typical.

Laboratory Manifestations

The laboratory diagnosis of methemoglobinemia is based on analysis of its absorption spectra. A fresh specimen should always be obtained because methemoglobin levels tend to increase with storage. Traditional pulse oximetry is unreliable in the presence of methemoglobinemia because of its light absorbance properties; however, co-oximetry can determine the methemoglobin fraction along with all other substances with the optical density at 630 nm.

Methemoglobin detected by co-oximeter should be confirmed by the specific Evelyn-Malloy method if available. This method involves direct spectrophotometric analysis and should be used when methemoglobinemia is suspected. In the Evelyn-Malloy method, blood is lysed in a slightly acid buffer and the optical density is measured at 630 nm before and after adding a small amount of neutralized cyanide Absorption of methemoglobin at this wavelength disappears when it is converted to cyanmethemoglobin. This method remains the most accurate technique for the estimation of methemoglobin concentration.

An eight-wavelength pulse oximeter, Masimo Rad-57 (the Rainbow-SET Rad-57 Pulse CO-Oximeter, Masimo Inc, Irvine, CA, USA), has been approved by the US Food and Drug Administration and appears to be accurate for the measurement of both carboxyhemoglobin and methemoglobin.

Distinguishing the hereditary forms of congenital methemoglobinemia requires interpretation of family pedigrees as well as biochemical analyses. Cyanosis in successive generations suggests autosomal dominant hemoglobin (Hb) M disease, whereas normal parents but possibly affected siblings implies autosomal recessive b5R deficiency. Incubation of blood with methylene blue distinguishes b5R deficiency from Hb M disease, because this treatment results in the rapid reduction of methemoglobin through the NADPH-flavin reductase pathway in cases of b5R deficiency but not in cases of Hb M disease. Types I and II b5R deficiency are distinguished by their clinical phenotype and by analysis of enzymatic activity in erythroid and nonerythroid cells. Because the enzyme defect is found in fibroblasts, analysis of b5R activity in cultured amniotic cells for prenatal diagnosis is possible.

Differential Diagnosis

Sulfhemoglobin in concentrations greater than 0.5 gm% also causes "cyanosis" with a normal PaO_2 and may be erroneously measured as methemoglobin. Other pigments, including methylene blue, may also produce false positive results when methemoglobin is measured by co-oximetry.

Prognosis

Acute methemoglobinemia generally resolves promptly with treatment providing the offending cause is discontinued. Patients with type I b5R deficiency have cyanosis but a normal life expectancy, whereas the pan-deficient type II b5R patients usually succumb in childhood.

Therapy

Offending agents in cases of acquired methemoglobinemia should be discontinued. No other therapy may be required in an asymptomatic patient. However, if the patient is symptomatic or if methemoglobin levels are greater than 20%, specific therapy is indicated. Methylene blue, 1–2 mg/kg intravenously over 5 minutes, is an effective treatment for patients with methemoglobinemia because NADPH formed in the pentose shunt can rapidly reduce this dye to leukomethylene blue in a reaction catalyzed by NADPH diaphorase. Leukomethylene blue, in turn, nonenzymatically reduces methemoglobin to hemoglobin. An exception to the efficacy of this treatment exists in those patients who are G6PD deficient. In these patients, methylene blue would not only fail to give the desired effect on methemoglobin levels but might compound the situation by inducing an acute hemolytic episode. If methylene blue is contraindicated, ascorbic acid can be given. Patients with G6PD deficiency and acute methemoglobinemia have been successfully treated with exchange transfusion. Hyperbaric oxygen has also been used in severe cases of methemoglobinemia.

The cyanosis in hereditary b5R deficiency is of cosmetic significance only but can be treated with methylene blue or ascorbic acid, both of which facilitate the reduction of methemoglobin through alternate pathways. However, this therapy has no effect on the neurologic and other systemic defects seen in type II b5R deficiency.

SUGGESTED READINGS

1. Balasubramaniam S, Duley JA, Christodoulou J: Inborn errors of purine metabolism: clinical update and therapies. *J Inherit Metab Dis* 37:687–698, 2014.
   Purine metabolism reviewed with implications for erythrocyte toxicity.
2. Beutler E: *Red cell metabolism: a manual of biochemical methods*, ed 3, 1984, Grune & Stratton.
   Manual of assays for red cell enzymes and red cell metabolic intermediates.
3. Borron SW, Bebarta VS: Asphyxiants. *Emerg Med Clin North Am* 33:89–115, 2015.
   Review of methemoglobinemia and other conditions impairing oxygen delivery.
4. Cortazzo JA, Lichtman AD: Methemoglobinemia: a review and recommendations for management. *J Cardiothorac Vasc Anesth* 28:1055–1059, 2014.
   Critical review of common causes and management of acute toxic methemoglobinemia.
5. Grace RF, Zanella A, Neufeld EJ, et al: Erythrocyte pyruvate kinase deficiency: 2015 status report. *Am J Hematol* 90:825–830, 2015.
   A summary of current understanding and management of clinical and metabolic features of pyruvate kinase deficiency.
6. Ho HY, Cheng ML, Chiu DT: Glucose-6-phosphate dehydrogenase—beyond the realm of red cell biology. *Free Radic Res* 43:1028–1048, 2014.
   Focus on basic science of glucose-6-phosphate dehydrogenase.
7. Koralkova P, van Solinge WW, van Wijk R: Rare hereditary red blood cell enzymopathies associated with hemolytic anemia—pathophysiology, clinical aspects, and laboratory diagnosis. *Int J Lab Hematol* 36:388–397, 2014.
   A critical review of rarer red cell enzymes.
8. Luzzatto L, Seneca E: G6PD deficiency: a classic example of pharmacogenetics with on-going clinical implications. *Br J Haematol* 164:133–201, 2014.
   Critical review of G6PD deficiency.
9. Prchal JT, Gregg XT: Red cell enzymes. *Hematology Am Soc Hematol Educ Program* 19–23, 2005.
   Summary of red cell enzyme defects in descending order of their clinical importance.
10. van Wijk R, van Solinge WW: The energy-less red blood cell is lost: erythrocyte enzyme abnormalities of glycolysis. *Blood* 106:4034–4042, 2005.
    This review focuses on the impact of energy metabolism of erythrocyte and its pathophysiology.
11. van Zwieten R, Verhoeven AJ, Roos D: Inborn defects in the antioxidant systems of human red blood cells. *Free Radic Biol Med* 67:377–386, 2014.
    A critical review of defects in the antioxidant system of red cells.
12. Viprakasit V, Ekwattanakit S, Riolueang S, et al: Mutations in Kruppel-like factor 1 cause transfusion-dependent hemolytic anemia and persistence of embryonic globin gene expression. *Blood* 123:1586–1595, 2014.
    An unusual cause of pyruvate kinase deficiency.
13. van Solinge WW, van Wijk R: Erythrocyte enzyme disorders. In Kaushansky K, Lichtman MA, Prchal JT, editors: *Williams manual of hematology*, ed 9, New York, 2015, McGraw Hill, pp 689–724.
    Review of red cell enzymes with extensive bibliography of original and recent articles.

CHAPTER 45

RED BLOOD CELL MEMBRANE DISORDERS

Patrick G. Gallagher

Characterization of the structure and function of red blood cell (RBC) membrane proteins and their genes (Fig. 45.1) has led to considerable advances in our understanding of the molecular pathology of membrane-associated disorders, including the definition and characterization of mutations of membrane proteins as a well-defined cause of hereditary hemolytic disease. Likewise, knowledge of the molecular mechanisms underlying changes in RBC deformability, structural integrity, and shape has advanced. RBC shape abnormalities often provide a clue to the pathobiology and diagnosis of the underlying disorder. This chapter categorizes RBC membrane disorders according to the following morphologic and clinical phenotypes: (1) hereditary spherocytosis (HS); (2) hereditary elliptocytosis (HE), hereditary pyropoikilocytosis (HPP), and related disorders; (3) Southeast Asian ovalocytosis (SAO); (4) hereditary and acquired acanthocytosis; and (5) hereditary and acquired stomatocytosis (Tables 45.1 and 45.2).

VERTICAL AND HORIZONTAL INTERACTIONS OF MEMBRANE PROTEINS AND DISORDERS OF RED BLOOD CELL SHAPE

For better understanding of the pathobiology of membrane disorders, membrane protein-protein and protein-lipid interactions are classified in two categories, vertical and horizontal interactions. Vertical interactions, which are perpendicular to the plane of the membrane, stabilize the lipid bilayer. These interactions include spectrin-ankyrin–band 3 interactions, spectrin-protein 4.1R–junctional complex proteins linkage, spectrin-ankyrin–Rh multiprotein complex linkage, and the weak interactions between the skeletal proteins and the negatively charged lipids of the inner half of the membrane lipid bilayer. Horizontal interactions, which are parallel to the plane of the membrane, support the structural integrity of erythrocytes after their exposure to shear stress. Horizontal interactions involve the spectrin heterodimer association site, where spectrin heterodimers assemble into tetramers, the principal building blocks of the membrane skeleton, and the contacts of the distal ends of spectrin heterodimers with actin and protein 4.1R within the junctional complex. Although interactions between proteins of the erythrocyte membrane are significantly more complex than can be classified by horizontal and vertical interactions, the model serves as a useful starting place for understanding erythrocyte membrane protein interactions, particularly in reference to membrane-related disorders.

According to the vertical/horizontal model, HS is considered a disorder of vertical interactions. Although the primary molecular defects in HS are heterogeneous (including deficiencies or dysfunctions of α- and β-spectrin, ankyrin, band 3, and protein 4.2), one common feature of HS RBCs is a weakening of the vertical contacts between the skeleton and the overlying lipid bilayer membrane together with its integral proteins. Consequently, the lipid bilayer membrane is destabilized, leading to release of bilayer lipids from the cells in the form of skeleton-free lipid vesicles. This lipid loss, in turn, results in membrane surface area deficiency and spherocytosis.

In most patients with HE and the related disorder HPP (see Hereditary Elliptocytosis and Related Disorders), the principal lesion involves horizontal membrane-protein associations, primarily spectrin dimer-dimer interactions. In a subset of HE patients with a deficiency or a dysfunction of protein 4.1R or glycophorin C (GPC), the

horizontal defect resides in the junctional complex, where the distal ends of spectrin tetramers connect to actin, in conjunction with protein 4.1R. In patients with severely dysfunctional spectrin mutations, the weakened spectrin dimer-dimer self-association disrupts the skeletal lattice, leading to a marked skeletal instability and cell fragments. In patients with mildly dysfunctional spectrins, RBC shape is that of biconcave elliptocytes. It is speculated that elliptocytes are permanently deformed cells because the weakened horizontal interactions facilitate a shear stress-induced rearrangement of skeletal proteins, precluding recovery of the normal biconcave shape. This hypothesis is not applicable to all forms of elliptocytosis. For example, in SAO, the elliptocytic/ovalocytic cells containing mutant band 3 protein are rigid and "hyperstable" rather than unstable.

Acanthocytosis, Stomatocytosis, and the Bilayer Couple Hypothesis

The mechanism of acanthocytosis and stomatocytosis associated with defects of membrane proteins is much less clear. Most forms of acanthocytosis are associated with either acquired or inherited abnormalities of membrane lipids (e.g., acanthocytosis in end-stage liver disease or abetalipoproteinemia). In rare cases with acanthocytosis, membrane protein abnormalities have been detected, but the associated mechanisms leading to acanthocyte formation are unknown. These abnormalities occur in the McLeod phenotype, the chorea-acanthocytosis syndrome, and other rare disorders. In acanthocytosis erythrocytes, agents that interact with the lipids of the inner lipid bilayer leaflet normalize the shape. These studies suggest that the shape abnormalities reflect an asymmetry in the distribution of membrane lipids between the two halves of the RBC lipid bilayer as predicted by the bilayer couple hypothesis. According to the bilayer hypothesis, the shape of the RBC reflects the ratio of the surface areas of the two hemileaflets of the bilayer. The preferential expansion of the outer leaflet leads to RBC crenation (echinocytosis or acanthocytosis), whereas expansion of the inner lipid bilayer produces a cup shape (stomatocytosis) and surface invaginations.

Hereditary Spherocytosis

Introduction and Epidemiology

The typical features of HS include a dominantly inherited hemolytic anemia of mild to moderate severity, spherocytosis on the peripheral blood film, and a favorable response to splenectomy. The clinical spectrum of HS is variable and includes both mild and asymptomatic forms, as well as severe forms that appear in infancy. The previously reported HS prevalence in Western populations of 1 in 4000 persons is an underestimation, because milder forms of HS might be asymptomatic, suggesting a prevalence of 1 in 2000 individuals. HS has been reported worldwide, particularly in Japanese and African populations, but its prevalence in other ethnic groups is unknown.

Pathobiology

Two major factors are involved in HS pathophysiology: (1) an intrinsic RBC defect and (2) an intact spleen that selectively retains

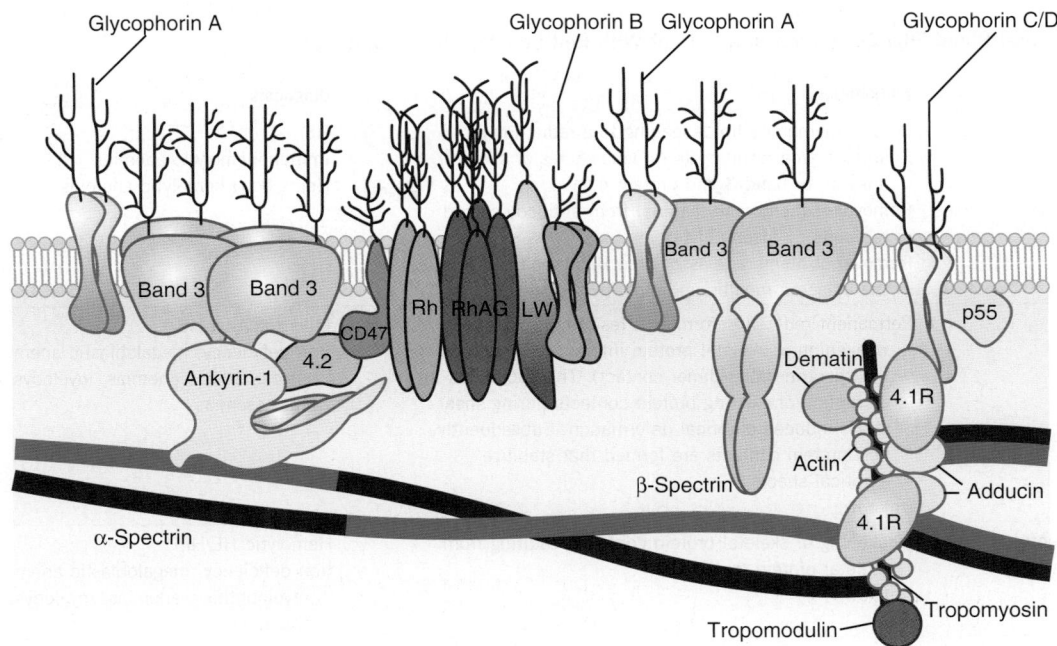

Fig. 45.1 A SIMPLIFIED CROSS-SECTION OF THE ERYTHROCYTE MEMBRANE. The lipid bilayer forms the equator of the cross-section with its polar heads *(small circles)* turned outward. *4.1R,* Protein 4.1R; *4.2,* protein 4.2; *Rh,* Rhesus polypeptide; *RhAG,* Rh-associated glycoprotein; *LW,* Landsteiner-Wiener glycoprotein. *(Reproduced with permission from Perrotta S, Gallagher PG, Mohandas N: Hereditary spherocytosis.* Lancet *372:1411, 2008.)*

TABLE 45.1	Erythrocyte Membrane Abnormalities in Hereditary Spherocytosis, Hereditary Elliptocytosis, and Related Disorders	
Gene	**Disorder**	**Comment**
α-Spectrin	HS, HE, HPP, NIHF	Location of mutation determines clinical phenotype. α-Spectrin mutations are most common cause of typical HE.
Ankyrin	HS	Most common cause of typical dominant HS.
Band 3	HS, SAO, NIHF	In HS "pincer-like" spherocytes on smear presplenectomy. SAO erythrocytes have transverse ridge or longitudinal slit.
β-Spectrin	HS, HE, HPP, NIHF	Location of mutation determines clinical phenotype. In HS, acanthrocytic spherocytes on smear presplenectomy.
Protein 4.2	HS	Common in Japanese HS.
Protein 4.1	HE	
GPC	HE	Concomitant protein 4.1 deficiency is basis of HE in GPC defects.

GPC, Glycophorin C; HE, hereditary elliptocytosis; HPP, hereditary pyropoikilocytosis; HS, hereditary spherocytosis; NIHF, nonimmune hydrops fetalis, SAO, Southeast Asian ovalocytosis.

and damages abnormal HS erythrocytes. An inherited deficiency or dysfunction of proteins of the erythrocyte membrane leads to a multistep process of accelerated HS RBC destruction. Destabilization of the lipid bilayer facilitates a release of lipids from the membrane, leading to surface area deficiency and formation of poorly deformable spherocytes that are selectively retained and damaged in the spleen.

Molecular Pathology

The molecular basis of HS is heterogeneous. Based on densitometric quantitation of membrane proteins separated by polyacrylamide gel electrophoresis, HS can be divided into the following subsets: (1) isolated deficiency of spectrin, (2) combined deficiencies of spectrin and ankyrin, (3) deficiency of band 3 protein, (4) deficiency of protein 4.2, and (5) no abnormality identified.

Isolated Spectrin Deficiency

The reported mutations of isolated spectrin deficiency include defects of both α- and β-spectrin. Mutations of the β-spectrin gene have been identified in a number of patients with dominantly inherited HS associated with spectrin deficiency. A few cases have been associated with de novo β-spectrin gene mutations. With a few exceptions, these mutations are private and may be associated with decreased β-spectrin messenger ribonucleic acid (mRNA) accumulation. Mutations in the highly conserved region of β-spectrin involved in the interaction with protein 4.1R likely lead to dysfunctional binding to protein 4.1R and thereby the linkage of spectrin to actin.

In nondominantly inherited HS associated with isolated spectrin deficiency, the defect involves α-spectrin. In normal erythroid cells, α-spectrin is synthesized in large excess of β-spectrin. Thus patients with one normal and one defective α-spectrin allele are asymptomatic, because α-spectrin production remains in excess of β-spectrin synthesis, allowing normal amounts of spectrin heterodimers to be assembled on the membrane. Patients who are homozygotes or compound heterozygotes for α-spectrin defects suffer from moderate to severe HS.

Combined Deficiency of Spectrin and Ankyrin

The biochemical phenotype of combined spectrin and ankyrin deficiency is the most common abnormality found in the erythrocytes of HS patients. Ankyrin represents the principal binding site for

TABLE 45.2   Peripheral Blood Film Evaluation in a Patient With Red Cell Membrane Disorder

Shape	Pathobiology	Diagnosis
Microspherocytes	Loss of membrane lipids leading to a reduction of surface area resulting from deficiencies of spectrin, ankyrin, or band 3 and protein 4.2 Removal of membrane material from antibody-coated red cells by macrophages Removal of membrane-associated Heinz bodies, with the adjacent membrane lipids, by the spleen	HS Immunohemolytic anemias Heinz body hemolytic anemias
Elliptocytes	Permanent red cell deformation resulting from a weakening of skeletal protein interactions (such as the spectrin dimer-dimer contact). This facilitates disruption of existing protein contacts during shear stress-induced elliptical deformation. Subsequently, new protein contacts are formed that stabilize elliptical shape Unknown	Mild common HE Iron deficiency, megaloblastic anemias, myelofibrosis, myelophthisic anemias, myelodysplastic syndrome, thalassemias
Poikilocytes/fragments	Weakening of skeletal protein contacts resulting from skeletal protein mutations Unknown	Hemolytic HE/HPP Iron deficiency, megaloblastic anemias, myelofibrosis, myelophthisic anemias, myelodysplastic syndrome, thalassemias
Schistocytes, fragmented red cells	Red cells "torn" by mechanic trauma (fibrin strands, turbulent flow)	"Microangiopathic" hemolytic anemia associated with disseminated intravascular coagulation, thrombotic thrombocytopenic purpura, vasculitis, heart valve prostheses
Acanthocytes	Uptake of cholesterol and its preferential accumulation in the outer leaflet of the lipid bilayer Selective accumulation of sphingomyelin in the outer lipid leaflet Unknown	Spur cell hemolytic anemia in severe liver disease Abetalipoproteinemia Chorea-acanthocytosis syndrome, malnutrition, hypothyroidism, McLeod phenotype
Echinocytes	Expansion of the surface area of the outer hemileaflet of lipid bilayer relative to the inner hemileaflet Unknown	Hemolytic anemia associated with hypomagnesemia and hypophosphatemia in malnourished patients, pyruvate kinase deficiency; in vitro artifact of low blood storage (ATP depletion), contact with glass or elevated pH Hemolysis in long-distance runners, renal failure
Stomatocytes	Expansion of the surface area of the inner hemileaflet of the bilayer relative to the outer leaflet Unknown	Exposure of red cells to cationic anesthetics in vitro; in vivo the drug concentrations may not be sufficient to produce similar effect Alcoholism, inherited disorders of membrane permeability (hereditary stomatocytosis)
Target cells	Absolute excess of membrane lipids (both cholesterol and phospholipids: "symmetric" lipid gain), followed by an increase of cell surface area Relative excess of surface area because of a decrease in cell volume	Obstructive jaundice, liver disease with intrahepatic cholestasis Thalassemias and some hemoglobinopathies (C, D, E)

ATP, Adenosine triphosphate; HE, hereditary elliptocytosis; HPP, hereditary pyropoikilocytosis; HS, hereditary spherocytosis.

spectrin on the membrane; thus it is not surprising that ankyrin deficiency is accompanied by a proportional decrease in spectrin assembly on the membrane despite normal spectrin synthesis. Similar to HS associated with β-spectrin mutations, most ankyrin defects are private point mutations associated with decreased mRNA accumulation. In some cases, mutations of the ankyrin promoter leading to decreased ankyrin expression have been found. Approximately 15% to 20% of ankyrin gene mutations reported are de novo mutations.

A number of patients with atypical HS associated with karyotypic abnormalities involving deletions or translocations of the ankyrin gene locus on chromosome 8p have been described. Ankyrin deletions may be part of a contiguous gene syndrome with manifestations of spherocytosis, mental retardation, typical facies, and hypogonadism.

Deficiency of Band 3 Protein

Deficiency of band 3 protein is found in a subset of HS patients who present with a phenotype of a mild to moderate dominantly inherited HS. Most, if not all, of these patients also have concomitant protein 4.2 deficiency. Numerous band 3 mutations associated with HS have been reported, spread throughout both the cytoplasmic and the membrane-spanning domains.

A number of band 3 mutations clustered in the membrane-spanning domain that replace highly conserved arginines have been described. These arginines, which are all located at the cytoplasmic end of a predicted transmembrane helix, exhibit defective cellular trafficking from the endoplasmic reticulum to the plasma membrane.

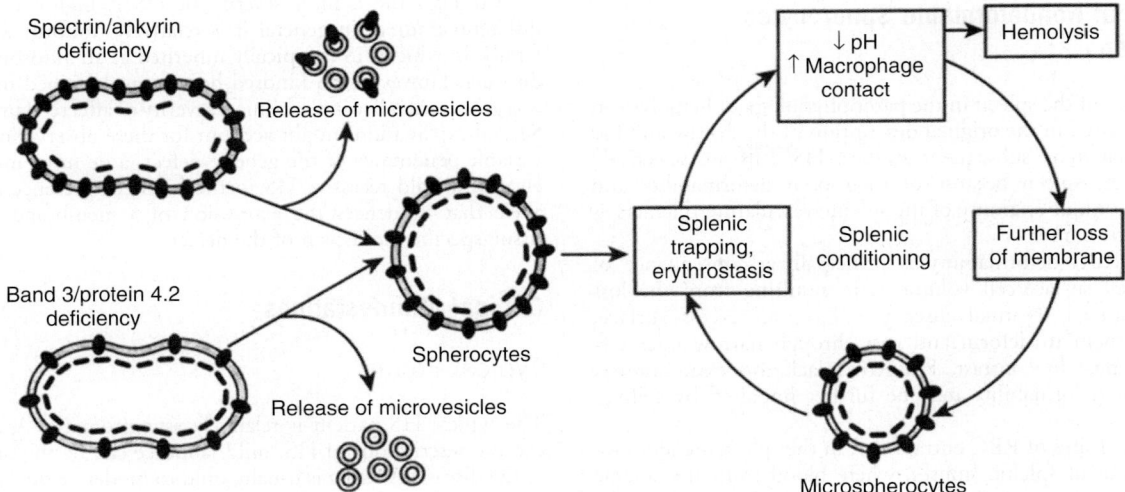

Fig. 45.2 PATHOPHYSIOLOGY OF HEREDITARY SPHEROCYTOSIS. The primary defect in hereditary spherocytosis is a deficiency of membrane surface area. Decreased surface area may be produced by two different mechanisms: (1) Defects of spectrin, ankyrin, or protein 4.2 lead to reduced density of the membrane skeleton, destabilizing the overlying lipid bilayer and releasing band 3-containing microvesicles. (2) Defects of band 3 lead to band 3 deficiency and loss of its lipid-stabilizing effect. This results in the loss of band 3-free microvesicles. Both pathways result in membrane loss, decreased surface area, and formation of spherocytes with decreased deformability. These deformed erythrocytes become trapped in the hostile environment of the spleen where splenic conditioning inflicts further membrane damage, amplifying the cycle of red cell membrane injury.

Alleles have been identified that influence band 3 expression and that, when inherited in trans to a band 3 mutation, aggravate band 3 deficiency and worsen the clinical severity of the disease.

Deficiency of Protein 4.2

Recessively inherited HS caused by mutations in protein 4.2 is relatively common in Japan. In these cases, an almost total absence of protein 4.2 from the erythrocyte membranes of homozygous patients is detected. Protein 4.2–deficient erythrocytes can also have a decreased content of ankyrin and band 3. Protein 4.2 deficiency also occurs in association with band 3 mutations, probably as a result of abnormal binding of protein 4.2 to the cytoplasmic domain of band 3.

Detailed listing of HS mutations is available in mutation databases maintained by the National Human Genome Research Institute and Yale University (http://research.nhgri.nih.gov/RBCmembrane/) and the Human Gene Mutation Database (HGMD®, http://www.hgmd.org).

Molecular Basis of Surface Area Deficiency

Hereditary spherocytes are intrinsically unstable, releasing lipids under a variety of in vitro conditions, including adenosine triphosphate (ATP) depletion or exposure of cells to shear stress. The loss of membrane material occurs through the release of vesicles containing integral proteins devoid of spectrin. During in vitro incubation, the loss of membrane material is sufficient to augment the surface area deficiency, as evidenced by increased osmotic fragility of the cells after incubation. It is assumed but not proved that a similar process takes place in vivo.

The molecular basis of HS is heterogeneous; thus it is likely that surface area deficiency is a consequence of several distinct molecular mechanisms whose common denominator is either a weakening of the vertical connections between the skeleton and the lipid bilayer membrane or a weakening of the stabilizing effect of transmembrane proteins on adjacent lipid molecules of the plasma membrane. Hypothetic pathways that can lead to surface area deficiency are depicted in Fig. 45.2. In patients with isolated spectrin deficiency or a combined deficiency of spectrin and ankyrin, the loss of RBC surface may be caused by an uncoupling of the lipid bilayer membrane from the underlying skeleton. In normal RBCs, the skeleton forms a nearly monomolecular submembrane layer occupying more than one-half of the inner surface of the membrane. Consequently, spectrin deficiency leads to a decreased density of this network. As a result, areas of the lipid bilayer membrane that are not directly supported by the skeleton are susceptible to release from the cells in the form of microvesicles.

In HS associated with a deficiency of band 3 protein, two hypothetic pathways may lead to a loss of surface area. One mechanism may involve a loss of band 3 protein from the cells. Because band 3 protein spans the lipid bilayer membrane many times, it is likely that a substantial amount of "boundary" lipids are released together with the band 3 protein, thus leading to surface area deficiency. Another possible mechanism may involve a formation of band 3-free domains in the membrane, followed by the formation of membrane blebs, which are subsequently released from the cells as microvesicles. Such a hypothesis is based on the observation that aggregation of intramembrane particles (composed principally of band 3) in ghosts leads to the formation of particle-depleted domains from which membrane lipids bleb off as microvesicles. Additional evidence supporting the latter model comes from the band 3 knock-out mouse model and from human, cow, and zebrafish cases of complete band 3 deficiency. Erythrocytes lacking band 3 spontaneously shed membrane vesicles, leading to spherocytosis and hemolysis.

Alterations in Cation Content and Permeability

HS RBCs, particularly those collected from the spleen, are somewhat dehydrated and abnormally permeable to monovalent cations, presumably as a consequence of the underlying membrane defect. The cellular dehydration may be caused by activation of pathways causing a selective loss of potassium and water or a hyperactive Na^+/K^+ pump.

Entrapment of Nondeformable Spherocytes in the Spleen

The importance of the spleen in the pathophysiology of hemolysis in HS was appreciated in the original description of the disease and has been substantiated by subsequent studies. HS cells are selectively destroyed in the spleen because of their poor deformability and because of the unique anatomy of the splenic vasculature that acts as a microcirculation filter.

The poor RBC deformability is principally a consequence of a decreased cell surface/cell volume ratio resulting from the loss of surface material. Normal discocytes have an excess surface, which allows them to deform and pass through narrow microcirculation openings. In contrast, HS RBCs lack this extra surface, and their poor deformability may be further impaired by cellular dehydration.

The principal sites of RBC entrapment in the spleen are fenestrations in the wall of splenic sinuses, where blood from the splenic cords of the red pulp enters the venous circulation. In rat spleen, the length and width of these fenestrations, 2 to 3 μm and 0.2 to 0.5 μm, respectively, are approximately half the RBC diameter. Electron micrographs show that very few HS RBCs traverse these slits. Consequently, the nondeformable spherocytes accumulate in the red pulp, which becomes grossly engorged.

Splenic Conditioning and Destruction

Once trapped in the spleen, HS erythrocytes undergo additional damage or conditioning with further loss of surface area and an increase in cell density, as is evident in cells removed from the spleen at splenectomy. Some of these conditioned RBCs reenter the systemic circulation, as revealed by the "tail" of the osmotic fragility curve, indicating the presence of a subpopulation of cells with a markedly reduced surface area. After splenectomy, this RBC population disappears.

Contributions to conditioning may include a relatively low pH in the spleen as well as in the sequestered RBCs that may further compromise the poor HS RBC deformability, and contact of RBCs with macrophages that may inflict additional damage on the RBC membrane. The conditioning effect of the spleen appears to represent a cumulative injury. The average residence time of HS RBCs in the splenic cords is between 10 and 100 minutes compared with 30 to 40 seconds for normal RBCs, and only 1% to 10% of blood entering the spleen is temporarily sequestered in the congested cords, whereas the remaining 90% of blood flow is rapidly shunted into the venous circulation.

Inheritance

The HS genes are assigned to several chromosomes, including chromosome 1 (α-spectrin), chromosome 8 (ankyrin), chromosome 14 (β-spectrin), chromosome 15 (protein 4.2), and chromosome 17 (band 3). In approximately two-thirds of HS patients, inheritance is autosomal dominant. In the remaining patients, inheritance is nondominant. In many of these patients, HS is caused by a de novo mutation, which is inherited in an autosomal recessive fashion in subsequent generations. Recessively inherited HS cases manifesting with severe hemolytic anemia have been reported. The majority of the affected patients were found to be severely deficient in RBC spectrin, associated with α-spectrin defects. The remaining cases characterized by a recessive inheritance pattern are caused by a defect in protein 4.2, a deficiency that is associated with relatively mild hemolysis.

Only a few cases of homozygous HS have been reported. These patients have a severe hemolytic anemia, whereas their mostly consanguineous parents have a mild to moderate form of the disease or are asymptomatic.

Although the clinical severity of HS is highly variable among different kindred, in general it is relatively uniform within a given family, in which HS is typically inherited as an autosomal dominant disorder. However, HS kindred have been described in which there was great variability in the clinical severity of affected family members. Several explanations might account for these observations, including variable penetrance of the genetic defect, a de novo mutation, presence of a mild recessive HS in the kindred, presence of a modifier allele that influences the expression of a membrane protein, or a tissue-specific mosaicism of the defect.

Clinical Manifestations

Typical Forms

The typical HS patient is relatively asymptomatic. As noted in the earliest descriptions of HS, mild jaundice can be the only symptom of the disease. Anemia is usually mild to moderate but may be absent because of compensatory bone marrow hyperplasia manifest by reticulocytosis. Splenomegaly gradually develops in most patients, with the spleen occasionally reaching large dimensions.

Mild Forms and Carrier State

In some families, anemia is absent, the reticulocyte count is normal or only minimally elevated, laboratory evidence of hemolysis is minimal or absent, and the changes in RBC shape can be mild, escaping detection on the peripheral blood film. The presence of HS is detected only by laboratory testing or during evaluation of a relative with a more symptomatic form of the disease. Some patients are first diagnosed during transient viral infections such as infectious mononucleosis or parvovirus infection, during pregnancy, or even in the 7th to 9th decades of life as the bone marrow's ability to compensate for hemolysis wanes.

Severe and Atypical Forms

The relatively uncommon patients with nondominant forms of HS can present with a severe life-threatening hemolysis early in life. Some patients can be transfusion dependent during early infancy and childhood. The underlying molecular defects include severe spectrin or band 3 deficiency.

Hereditary Spherocytosis and Nonerythroid Manifestations

In most HS cases, the clinical manifestations are confined to the erythroid lineage, probably because many of the nonerythroid counterparts of the RBC membrane proteins (e.g., spectrin and ankyrin) are encoded by separate genes or because some proteins (e.g., protein 4.1R, β-spectrin, ankyrin) are subject to tissue-specific alternative splicing. However, several HS kindred have been reported with a cosegregating neurologic or muscular abnormality, such as a degenerative disorder of the spinal cord, cardiomyopathy, or mental retardation. The observation that both erythrocyte ankyrin and β-spectrin are also expressed in muscles and the brain, particularly the cerebellum, and spinal cord raises the possibility that these HS patients may have a defect in one of these proteins. This hypothesis is further supported by studies of nb/nb mice, a mouse model of HS caused by an ankyrin mutation. These mice develop a neurologic syndrome with a progression that coincides with the loss of ankyrin from the Purkinje cells of the cerebellum.

Mutations of band 3 without HS have been described in patients with distal renal tubular acidosis. With a few rare exceptions, most patients with heterozygous mutations of band 3 and HS have normal renal acidification.

Laboratory Manifestations

Most HS patients have mild to moderate anemia or no anemia at all, reflecting the fact that the hemolytic rate can be very mild and that the hemolysis is fully compensated for by increased RBC production, as evidenced by reticulocytosis. Some patients, however, particularly those with nondominantly inherited HS, are severely anemic, with hemoglobin concentrations as low as 4 to 6 g/dL.

Despite the increased percentage of reticulocytes with a larger volume than mature RBCs, the mean corpuscular volume (MCV) of HS RBCs is often low normal or even slightly decreased, and the mean corpuscular hemoglobin concentration (MCHC) is usually increased (>35 g/dL), together reflecting mild cellular dehydration.

The finding of an MCHC greater than 35.4 g/dL combined with an RBC distribution width (RDW) <14% has been found to be an excellent screening test for HS. Another screening method measures MCV by light scattering and provides a histogram of hyperdense erythrocytes (MCHC >40 g/dL) claimed to identify nearly all HS patients. These hyperdense erythrocytes can be detected with newer laser-based blood counters or using aperture impedance analysis available in many clinical laboratories.

Evidence of accelerated RBC destruction, as indicated by increased lactate dehydrogenase and unconjugated bilirubin levels and by decreased haptoglobin, as well as by reticulocytosis, is present in typical HS patients. However, these abnormalities can be absent in individuals with a mild form of the disease.

Blood Film

In a typical case of HS, spherocytes are readily identified by their characteristic shape on the peripheral blood film (Fig. 45.3). They lack central pallor, their mean cell diameter is decreased, and they appear more intensely hemoglobinized, which reflects both altered RBC geometry and increased cell density. In a three-dimensional view, some spherocytes have a spherostomatocytic shape that is occasionally appreciated on the peripheral blood film. In mild forms of the disease, the peripheral blood smear can appear normal because the loss of surface area can be too small to be appreciated by blood smear evaluation; the cells appear as "fat" disks rather than as true spherocytes.

Additional morphologic features have been described in some HS patients (see Fig. 45.3). A subset of HS patients whose RBCs are deficient in band 3 protein have some pincer-like RBCs on the peripheral blood film, a finding that is both sensitive and specific for this HS subset. These pincer-like cells disappear after splenectomy. Surface spiculations or acanthocytic spherocytes have been described in cases of HS associated with defects in β-spectrin. Frequent sphero-ovalocytes and stomatocytes have been reported in Japanese patients with protein 4.2 deficiency.

Osmotic Fragility and Eosin-5'-Maleimide Binding

Both osmotic fragility (OF) testing and eosin-5'-maleimide (EMA) binding are used in evaluating HS patients.

The osmotic fragility test (Fig. 45.4) measures the in vitro lysis of RBCs suspended in solutions of decreasing osmolarity. The normal RBC membrane is unstretchable and is virtually freely permeable to water. Thus the cell behaves as a nearly perfect osmometer in that it increases its volume in hypotonic solutions progressively until a "critical hemolytic volume" is reached. At this point, the RBC membrane ruptures, and hemoglobin escapes into the supernatant solution. As a result of the loss of membrane and the ensuing surface area deficiency, the critical hemolytic volume of spherocytes is considerably lower than that of normal RBCs. Consequently, these cells hemolyze more than normal RBCs when suspended in hypotonic sodium chloride solutions. However, a finding of increased osmotic fragility is not unique to HS and is also present in other conditions associated with spherocytosis on the peripheral blood film, such as autoimmune hemolytic anemia.

The osmotic fragility curve often reveals uniformly increased osmotic fragility. A "tail" of the osmotic fragility curve can be present in nonsplenectomized HS patients, indicating a subpopulation of particularly fragile RBCs conditioned by splenic stasis. This subpopulation of cells disappears after splenectomy. In patients with mild HS, osmotic fragility can be normal and abnormalities can be found only after incubation that further augments the loss of surface area;

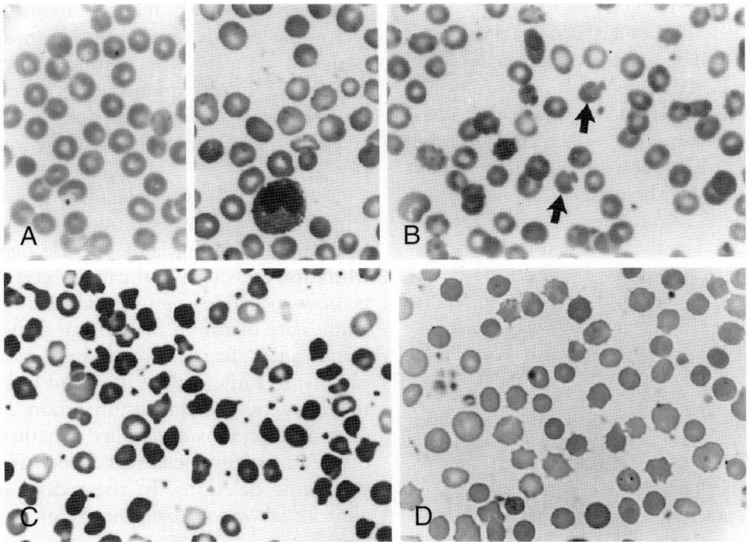

Fig. 45.3 BLOOD FILMS FROM PATIENTS WITH HEREDITARY SPHEROCYTOSIS (HS) OF VARYING SEVERITY. (A) Two blood films of typical moderately severe HS with a mild deficiency of RBC spectrin and ankyrin. Although many cells have a spheroidal shape, some retain a central concavity. (B) HS with pincer-like RBCs *(arrows)*, as typically seen in HS associated with band 3 deficiency. Occasional spiculated RBCs are also present. (C) Severe atypical HS caused by a severe combined spectrin and ankyrin deficiency. In addition to spherocytes, many cells have irregular contour. (D) HS with isolated spectrin deficiency caused by a β-spectrin mutation. Some of the spherocytes have prominent surface projections resembling sphero-acanthocytes.

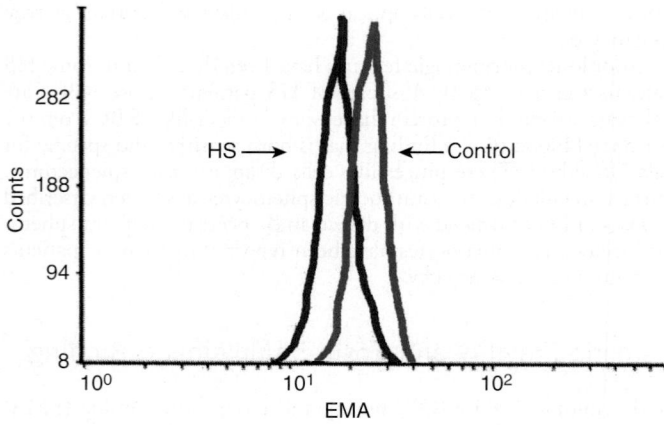

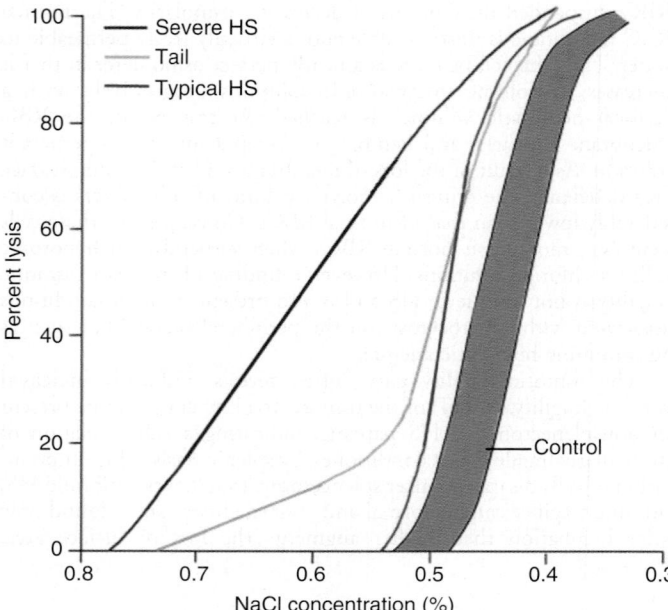

Fig. 45.4 TESTING IN HEREDITARY SPHEROCYTOSIS (HS). *(Top)* Eosin-5-maleimide (EMA) binding. EMA binding, a flow cytometric test that measures the fluorescence intensity of intact RBCs labeled with the dye eosin-5'-maleimide that reacts with membrane band 3 protein, has been shown to be useful as a first-line test for the diagnosis of hereditary spherocytosis. Histogram of fluorescence of EMA-labeled erythrocytes from normal controls *(red)* and a patient with typical hereditary spherocytosis *(blue)*. Decreased fluorescence is observed from HS erythrocytes. *(Bottom)* Osmotic fragility curves in hereditary spherocytosis. The shaded region is the normal range. Results representative of both typical and severe spherocytosis are shown. A tail, representing fragile erythrocytes conditioned by the spleen, is common in spherocytosis patients before splenectomy. *(Reproduced with permission from Gallagher PG: Abnormalities of the erythrocyte membrane. Ped Clin N Am 60:1349, 2013.)*

however, the sensitivity of the incubated osmotic fragility test can be outweighed by a loss of its specificity. The relative contributions of cell dehydration and surface area deficiency can be accurately determined by osmotic gradient ektacytometry, available in specialized laboratories.

OF testing is unreliable in patients who have small numbers of spherocytes, including those who have been recently transfused, and it is abnormal in other conditions where spherocytes are present.

The binding of EMA to band 3 and Rh-related proteins with a 1:1 stoichiometry in the erythrocyte membrane is the basis for the EMA binding test. After binding of fluorescently labeled EMA to erythrocyte membranes, the relative amount of fluorescence, reflect-

ing the amount of EMA binding, is analyzed by flow cytometry. The intensity of EMA binding is decreased in HS erythrocytes (Fig. 45.4). Although defects of band 3 protein are only found in ~25% of typical HS patients, decreased EMA fluorescence is also observed in HS erythrocytes with primary defects in ankyrin and spectrin, thought to be caused by transmission of long range effects of varying protein defects across the membrane, influencing EMA binding. EMA binding has high sensitivity and specificity. In laboratories with the ability to perform fluorescence-activated cell sorting-based studies, it is simple and rapidly performed, even on samples after shipment or storage.

Like osmotic fragility, EMA binding struggles in the diagnosis of mild HS where results may be normal or indeterminate. Other erythrocyte abnormalities such as defects of erythrocyte hydration and variants of dyserythropoietic anemia can also yield abnormal results.

Autohemolysis and Other Tests

RBC autohemolysis, the spontaneous hemolysis of RBCs incubated under sterile conditions without glucose, was previously advocated as a sensitive test for the detection of HS. This test is being used less frequently and is probably no more sensitive than the incubated osmotic fragility test. Other tests described in the literature such as the glycerol lysis test, the pink test, hypertonic cryohemolysis, and the skeleton gelation test are infrequently performed in diagnostic laboratories in the United States. The former two tests, which use glycerol to retard the osmotic swelling of RBCs, are preferred by some laboratories because they are easy to perform and can be adapted to microsamples. Cryohemolysis testing in particular remains popular in Europe.

Detection of the Underlying Molecular Defect

Because the most common finding in erythrocytes of patients with HS is a deficiency of one or more of the membrane proteins, molecular studies often include sodium dodecyl sulfate-polyacrylamide gel electrophoresis (SDS-PAGE) solubilized RBC membrane proteins followed by densitometric quantitation. The results are expressed as ratios of individual red cell membrane proteins to band 3. This technique reveals abnormalities in approximately 70% to 80% of patients, defining the distinct biochemical phenotypes discussed previously. Direct quantitation of membrane proteins by radioimmunoassay is superior to densitometric quantitation and permits accurate measurement of the copy number of the individual proteins per RBC.

Application of molecular genetic analyses including DNA sequencing and other molecular studies complement clinical and laboratory screening and provide definitive diagnosis in most cases. Mutation detection in the major erythrocyte membrane protein genes is now available commercially in the United States. Gene-based studies are of use in diagnosing difficult cases and in cases in which a molecular diagnosis is desired. Molecular analyses have potential pitfalls. In some cases, variants of unknown significance are detected, making genetic diagnosis uncertain. Mutations not detected by study of coding regions and splice junctions may be causative, such as in distant regulatory elements, deep intronic splicing mutations, and intragenic deletions. In these cases, diagnosis is assigned based on clinical, laboratory, and biochemical findings.

Complications

Gallstones

Bilirubin stones are found in approximately 50% of patients with HS, often even in those with a very mild form of the disease. Gallstones have occasionally been detected during infancy, but they are most likely to occur in older children and young adults. The coinheritance of Gilbert syndrome increases the risk for gallstones in HS patients. Because of the high incidence of gallstones, HS patients should be periodically examined by ultrasonography for the presence of gallstones, beginning in childhood.

Crises

True hemolytic crises are relatively rare and only occasionally reported in association with infections. Aplastic crises during viral infections are largely attributable to infection by parvovirus B19. This infection (erythema infectiosum, fifth disease) manifests with fever, chills, lethargy, malaise, nausea, vomiting, abdominal pain with occasional diarrhea, respiratory symptoms, muscle and joint pains, and a maculopapular rash on the face (slapped cheek appearance), trunk, and extremities. The virus selectively infects erythroid precursors and inhibits their growth. The ensuing anemia, often profound, can be the first manifestation of HS. Multiple family members with undiagnosed HS who are infected with parvovirus have developed aplastic crises at the same time. Infection with parvovirus is a particular danger to susceptible pregnant women because it can infect the fetus, leading to fetal anemia, hydrops fetalis, and fetal demise.

Rarely, at least in developed countries, patients present with megaloblastic crises caused by folate deficiency. This typically occurs in patients with increased folate demands, such as those recovering from an aplastic crisis, pregnant women, and older adults. Megaloblastic crisis in pregnancy has been reported as the first manifestation of HS. Folate supplementation is recommended for patients with moderate to severe HS.

Other Complications

In patients with more severe forms of HS, other complications include gout, leg ulcers, or chronic dermatitis of the legs that heal after splenectomy. Symptoms of expanded erythroid space, including paravertebral or renal pelvic masses of extramedullary hematopoiesis, which can mimic an underlying neoplasm, may occur. Several cases of hemochromatosis in HS patients have been reported. In some, iron overload resulted from repeated transfusions; in others, the patients had two genetic defects, one involving HS and the other involving a hemochromatosis carrier state. Other rare complications include thrombosis, pulmonary hypertension, spinocerebellar degenerative syndromes, movement disorders, myopathy, and hypertrophic cardiomyopathy.

More than a dozen cases of HS and hematologic malignancy, including myeloproliferative disorders, multiple myeloma, and leukemia, have been reported. It is unknown if long-standing hematopoietic stress predisposes to the development of these secondary disorders or if they occurred randomly.

DIFFERENTIAL DIAGNOSIS

Because of the relatively asymptomatic presentation of HS, this diagnosis should be considered during an evaluation for unexplained splenomegaly, unconjugated hyperbilirubinemia of unknown cause, gallstones at a young age, severe anemia during pregnancy, or transient anemia during acute infections. The diagnosis of HS can be missed in mild forms of the disease, because spherocytosis might not be apparent on the peripheral blood film. Autoimmune hemolytic anemia should be ruled out by negative results of a Coombs test.

More typical forms of HS, characterized by relatively uniform spherocytosis with increased MCHC, are usually easily distinguished from other disorders manifesting with spherocytosis, such as immune hemolytic anemias and unstable hemoglobins. In some patients, the spherostomatocytes in the rare Rh-null syndrome and the intermediate syndromes of hereditary stomatocytosis can be confused with HS RBCs.

Spherocytosis is transiently improved, and both the osmotic fragility and hemolysis are normalized in patients with obstructive jaundice. This is because of an expansion of RBC surface area that follows an increased uptake of phospholipids and cholesterol from the abnormal plasma lipoproteins. In normal RBCs, this leads to target cell formation; in HS, spherocytes are transformed to discocytes. Spherocytosis and the increased osmotic fragility of HS red cells are likewise improved by iron deficiency, but the RBC life span remains shortened. In addition, coexistence of β-thalassemia trait and HS partially corrects the HS phenotype.

THERAPY AND PROGNOSIS

Splenectomy

Splenectomy is curative in almost all patients with typical forms of HS, because RBC survival is normalized, and anemia and hyperbilirubinemia are corrected. Spherocytosis and the increase in osmotic fragility persist, but the tail of the osmotic fragility curve, indicating the presence of a subpopulation of cells conditioned by the spleen, disappears. In patients with severe, nondominantly inherited HS, splenectomy produces a dramatic clinical improvement, but hemolysis is only partially corrected.

Several weeks to months before splenectomy, patients should be immunized with polyvalent vaccine against pneumococcus as well as vaccines against *Haemophilus influenzae* type b and meningococcus.

Indications for Splenectomy

Risks and benefits should be considered carefully in HS patients before splenectomy is performed (see box on Splenectomy for Hereditary Spherocytosis). A multitude of factors influence the decision for splenectomy in HS patients, including the risk for overwhelming postsplenectomy sepsis, the emergence of penicillin-resistant pneumococci, and the potentially increased risk for cardiovascular disease and pulmonary hypertension later in life. Indications for splenectomy include growth retardation, skeletal changes, symptomatic hemolytic disease, anemia-induced compromise of vital organs, the development of leg ulcers, or the appearance of extramedullary hematopoietic tumors. Whether to perform splenectomy in patients with moderate HS without any of these factors remains controversial.

Because of an increased frequency of postsplenectomy infection in young children, most practitioners avoid splenectomy in infancy and early childhood.

Operative Considerations

When splenectomy is warranted, laparoscopic splenectomy has become the procedure of choice in many centers. Laparoscopic splenectomy has been associated with less postoperative discomfort, a quicker return to preoperative diet and activities, a shorter hospitalization time, decreased costs, and smaller scars. Early complications of splenectomy include local infection, bleeding, and pancreatitis. In general, the morbidity rate of splenectomy is lower in patients with HS than with other hematologic diseases. However, the benefits of surgery must be weighed against possible complications, such as postsplenectomy infections. Although these complications are rare and their frequency is likely to diminish further with appropriate vaccinations, the indiscriminate performance of splenectomy in all HS patients with splenomegaly is unwarranted.

Subtotal (Partial) Splenectomy

Partial splenectomy was developed for infants and young children with severe HS, anemia, and poor growth with the goals of palliating anemia and decreasing transfusion requirements while preserving splenic function. More recently, some have advocated expanding the procedure to all patients being splenectomized for HS. The goal of the operation is to decrease hemolysis while maintaining splenic phagocytic function. In initial cohorts of patients treated with partial splenectomy, stable increases in hemoglobin levels with decreased reticulocyte counts have been observed. The volume of splenic tissue left behind ranges from 10 mL to 30 mL. Although initial data are promising, it is not clear whether the remaining splenic tissue will effectively prevent postsplenectomy sepsis. In addition, regrowth of the splenic remnant has been reported in many patients, which can eventually lead to recurrence of HS and another operative procedure.

There are no specific data to support the use of prophylactic antibiotics postsplenectomy. Some practitioners avoid the prescription of prophylactic antibiotics, others recommend prophylactic antibiotics for at least 5 years postsplenectomy, and others recommend their use for life.

Postsplenectomy Failures
Postsplenectomy failures are caused either by the presence of an accessory spleen missed during surgery (accessory spleens were found in 17% to 39% of all patients) or by the presence of another superimposed RBC disorder such as pyruvate kinase deficiency. The recurrence of hemolytic anemia several years after splenectomy should raise the suspicion of development of splenunculi, resulting from autotransplantation of splenic tissue during surgery. The presence of an accessory spleen or splenunculus is suggested by the absence of both Howell-Jolly bodies and the "pitted" cells with crater-like surface indentations readily seen by interference contrast microscopy. A definitive confirmation of splenosis is made by a radiocolloid liver-spleen scan or by a scan using chromium (Cr)-labeled heated RBCs, which are taken up by the ectopic splenic tissue.

Genetic Counseling

After a patient is diagnosed with HS, family members should be examined for the presence of HS. A history, physical examination for splenomegaly, complete blood count with indices, reticulocyte count, examination of the peripheral blood smear for spherocytes, and biochemical evaluation including bilirubin and haptoglobin levels should be obtained for available close relatives.

Future Directions

Advances in high throughput DNA sequencing methodology have greatly facilitated the precise genetic diagnosis in many cases of suspected inherited membrane-associated disorders. Both targeted gene capture and whole exome sequencing have rapidly developed into effective tools for the identification of disease-causing variants in genetic disease, particularly monogenic disorders. Because they can be applied to disorders with recessive or dominant inheritance or de novo occurrence, like HS, they obviate the need for cumbersome biochemical assays and for linkage analysis in large numbers of individuals. As more patients are studied, it is likely that new HS-associated loci will be discovered. Identification of novel mutations will provide insight into the structure and function of associated membrane protein genes, and our understanding of genotype-phenotype relationships, particularly those with variable influence on disease severity, will be extended.

HEREDITARY ELLIPTOCYTOSIS AND RELATED DISORDERS

Introduction and Epidemiology

Hereditary elliptocytosis designates a group of inherited disorders that have in common the presence of elliptical RBCs on peripheral blood films. Elliptocytosis was first described by Dresbach in 1904, and its heritability was firmly established by Hunter. Subsequent reports have revealed a considerable heterogeneity of clinical expression and have defined several distinct syndromes, including HPP and SAO.

Hereditary elliptocytosis is common in people of African and Mediterranean ancestries. In the U.S. population, the prevalence of HE is approximately 3 to 5 per 10,000. The true incidence of HE is unknown because its clinical severity is heterogeneous and most patients are asymptomatic without anemia. HE is considerably more frequent in areas of endemic malaria. In equatorial Africa, the prevalence of common HE has been estimated at between 0.6% and 1.6%. Worldwide, HE appears to be more common among people of African origin. In Southeast Asian populations, the prevalence of SAO, a variant of HE, is as high as 30%.

The molecular basis of HE remained obscure until a defect of membrane skeletal proteins was suggested. Subsequently defects in the erythrocyte membrane proteins α-spectrin, β-spectrin, protein 4.1R, GPC, and band 3 were described.

On the basis of RBC morphologic characteristics, HE can be divided into three major groups. Common HE, a dominantly inherited condition, is morphologically characterized by biconcave elliptocytes and, in some patients, rod-shaped cells. The clinical severity of common HE is highly variable, ranging from an asymptomatic condition to a severe recessively inherited hemolytic anemia, including hemolytic HE and HPP, in which the blood film reveals numerous RBC fragments, microspherocytes, and poikilocytes. Spherocytic HE, also called hemolytic ovalocytosis, is a much less common condition in which both round "fat" ovalocytes and spherocytes are present on the blood film. SAO, a disorder highly prevalent in the malaria belt of Southeast Asia and the Pacific, is characterized by rigid, spoon-shaped cells that have either a longitudinal slit or a transverse ridge.

Pathobiology of Common Hereditary Elliptocytosis

The possibility that the primary lesion of HE and HPP erythrocytes resides in the proteins of the RBC membrane skeleton was first raised by the findings of thermal instability of HPP spectrin, retention of the elliptical shape in HE membrane skeletons, disintegration of membrane skeletons after exposure to shear stress, defective self-association of spectrin dimers to tetramers, altered susceptibility of spectrin to tryptic digestion, and a deficiency of the membrane skeleton proteins spectrin and protein 4.1R. Gene cloning and determination of the primary structure of these proteins was soon followed by reports of mutations in the genes encoding erythrocyte membrane proteins.

Spectrin Mutations

The most common defects in HE, found in approximately two-thirds to three-quarters of all patients, are mutations of α- or β-spectrin. Both α- and β-spectrin are elongated flexible molecules consisting of triple-helical repeats connected by nonhelical segments. These polypeptides are associated side to side in an antiparallel position, forming a flexible, rod-like αβ heterodimer in which the NH$_2$-terminal of α-spectrin and the COOH-terminal of β-spectrin form the head region of the heterodimer. Spectrin heterodimers associate head to head to form spectrin tetramers, the major structural subunits of the membrane skeleton. Spectrin tetramers in turn are interconnected into a highly ordered two-dimensional lattice through binding, at their distal ends, to actin oligomers with the aid of protein 4.1R.

The contact site between the α- and β-spectrin chains of the opposed heterodimers is a combined "atypical" triple-helical repetitive segment in which the first two helices are contributed by the COOH-terminal of β-spectrin, whereas helix 3 is the first helical segment of α-spectrin. Spectrin dimer-tetramer interconversion is governed by a simple thermodynamic equilibrium that under physiologic conditions strongly favors spectrin tetramers. Most α-spectrin defects are at or near the NH$_2$-terminal of α-spectrin, which is involved in the heterodimer contact (the αI domain defined by limited tryptic peptide mapping; see the discussion under Laboratory Manifestations), and impair the self-association of spectrin into tetramers. Most α-spectrin mutations are point mutations. These mutations create abnormal proteolytic cleavage sites that typically reside in the third helix of a repetitive segment and give rise to abnormal tryptic peptides on two-dimensional tryptic peptide maps of spectrin.

Elliptocytogenic β-spectrin mutations are COOH-terminal point mutations or truncations that disrupt the formation of the combined β triple-helical repetitive segment and consequently the self-association of spectrin heterodimers to tetramers. All of these mutations open a proteolytic cleavage site residing in the third helix of the combined repetitive segment, which gives rise to a 74-kDa αI peptide.

Although most spectrin mutations reside in the vicinity of the αβ-spectrin self-association site, a few mutations remote from the self-association site have been described. These mutations are asymptomatic in the simple heterozygous state but cause hemolytic anemia, which can be severe, in homozygous patients. Unlike mutations located in the self-association contact site, which are predicted to disrupt the conformation of the local protein structure, mutations outside this region are predicted to perturb long-range protein-protein interactions, disrupting the positively coupled, cooperative interactions of αβ spectrin self-association, spectrin-ankyrin interactions, and ankyrin–band 3 interactions. One HE-associated mutation in a linker region remote from the self-association contact site disrupted the stability propagated from one spectrin repeat to the next.

Protein 4.1R Mutations

Another group of elliptocytogenic mutations, although much less common than spectrin mutations, are quantitative or qualitative defects of protein 4.1R. Protein 4.1R is a multifunctional protein that contains several important sites of protein interactions, including the spectrin-binding domain, where 4.1R binds to the distal end of the spectrin αβ heterodimer, markedly increasing the binding of spectrin to oligomeric actin, and the basic NH$_2$-terminal domain, where 4.1R interacts with GPC, phosphatidylinositol, and phosphatidylserine, facilitating the attachment of the distal end of spectrin to the membrane.

Studies of 4.1R mRNA from normal RBCs revealed 4.1R isoforms resulting from complex tissue- and developmental stage-specific patterns of alternate mRNA splicing. Alternate translation initiation sites are present in the protein 4.1R mRNA. When an upstream initiator methionine is used, isoforms greater than 80 kDa are synthesized. During erythropoiesis, this upstream initiator methionine is spliced out and a downstream initiator methionine is used, leading to the production of the 80-kDa mature erythroid protein 4.1R isoform. On SDS-PAGE, protein 4.1R is resolved into two bands of different sizes: 4.1a and 4.1b. The larger band, 4.1a, is typically found in normal RBCs, whereas the shorter one, 4.1b, represents the major isoform of reticulocytes. The 4.1b isoform is converted into the 4.1a isoform by deamidation of Asn 502.

A partial deficiency of protein 4.1R is associated with mild, dominantly inherited HE, whereas a complete deficiency (a homozygous state) leads to a severe hemolytic disease. Homozygous protein 4.1R(–) erythrocytes fragment more rapidly than normal at moderate shear stresses, an indication of their intrinsic instability. Membrane mechanic stability can be restored by reconstituting the deficient RBCs with protein 4.1R or the protein 4.1R/spectrin/actin-binding site. Homozygous protein 4.1R(–) erythrocytes also lack p55 and have only 30% of the normal content of GPC. These homozygous protein 4.1R(–) erythrocytes, as well as GPC-deficient Leach erythrocytes, demonstrate decreased invasion and growth of *Plasmodium falciparum* in vitro.

Mutations associated with protein 4.1R deficiency have included deletions that include the exon encoding the erythroid transcription start size and mutations of the transcription initiation codon. Qualitative defects of protein 4.1R protein include deletions and duplications of the exons encoding the spectrin-binding domain, leading either to truncated or elongated forms of protein 4.1R. Electron microscopic studies of homozygous protein 4.1R(–) erythrocyte membranes revealed a markedly disrupted skeletal network with disruption of the intramembrane particles, suggesting that protein 4.1R plays an important role in maintenance not only of the skeletal network but also of the integral proteins of the membrane structure.

Glycophorin C Deficiency

GPC has been found absent because of a variety of molecular defects. In contrast to other forms of HE, which are dominantly inherited, heterozygous carriers are asymptomatic, with normal RBC morphology, and homozygous patients have no anemia and only mild elliptocytosis apparent on the peripheral blood film.

GPC deficiency with elliptocytosis, the so-called Leach phenotype, caused by reduced expression of GPC, should be distinguished from the immunochemically defined phenotypes Gerbich and Yus, in which abnormal glycoproteins are formed that can functionally substitute for normal GPC and preserve the normal RBC shape. The Leach phenotype is usually caused by a large deletion of genomic DNA (~7 kb) that removes exons 3 and 4 from the GPC/glycophorin D locus. In one patient, the Leach phenotype was caused by a frameshift mutation.

GPC-deficient patients are also partially deficient in protein 4.1R and lack p55, presumably because these proteins form a complex and recruit or stabilize each other on the membrane. It has been speculated that the protein 4.1R deficiency in Leach erythrocytes is the cause of the elliptocytic shape. In contrast, patients deficient in glycophorin A, the major transmembrane glycoprotein, are asymptomatic.

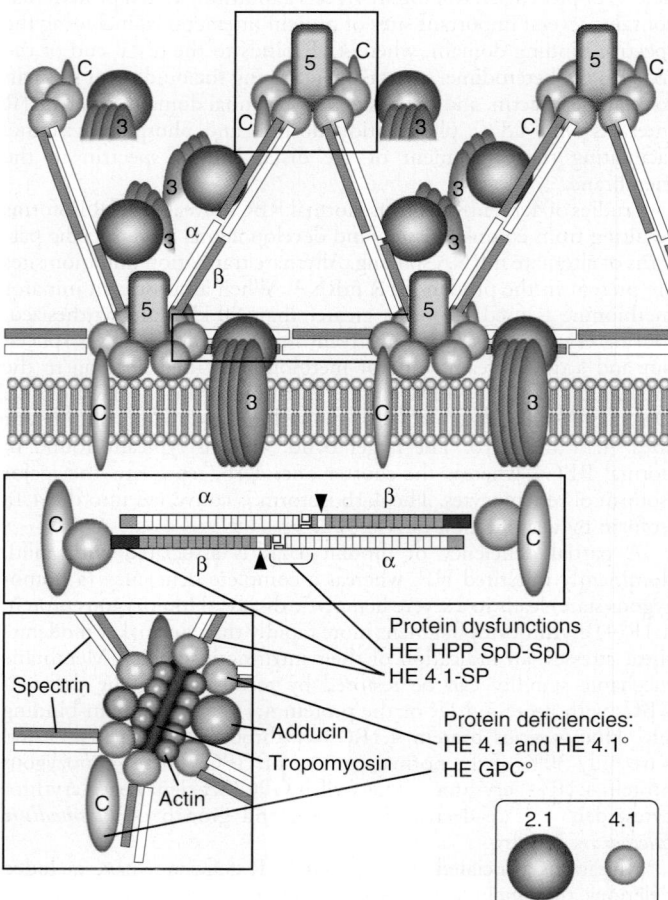

Fig. 45.5 SCHEMATIC REPRESENTATION OF THE MOLECULAR ASSEMBLY OF THE MEMBRANE SKELETON AND THE MOLECULAR DEFECTS IN HEREDITARY ELLIPTOCYTOSIS (HE) AND HEREDITARY PYROPOIKILOCYTOSIS (HPP). Spectrin is composed of α- and β-spectrin heterodimers (SpD) that associate in their head regions into tetramers. At their distal ends, SpD bind to the junctional complexes of oligomeric actin (band 5 *[5]*) and protein 4.1. Additional proteins found in the junctional complex, such as adducin and tropomyosin, are shown in the lower enlarged area. The membrane skeleton is attached to transmembrane proteins by interactions of β-spectrin with ankyrin (protein 2.1; *[black arrowhead]* designates the ankyrin-binding site in β-spectrin), which in turn binds to the cytoplasmic domain of band 3 *(3),* and by linkage of protein 4.1 to glycophorin C (GPC). The known protein dysfunctions in HE and HPP include (1) defects of the SpD head region because of a mutation of either α- or β-spectrin, causing impaired assembly of SpD into tetramers, and (2) defects of proteins of the junctional complex such as a qualitative or quantitative defect of protein 4.1R or GPC. *SP,* Spectrin.

Membrane Effects

Most of the elliptocytogenic mutations of spectrin reside within, or in the vicinity of, the spectrin heterodimer self-association site, disrupting this region and consequently disrupting the two-dimensional integrity of the membrane skeleton (Fig. 45.5). These defects are detected by ultrastructural examination of the membrane skeleton, which reveals disruption of a normally uniform hexagonal lattice. Consequently, membrane skeletons are mechanically unstable, as are whole cell membranes and the cells. In patients with severely dysfunctional spectrin mutations or patients homozygous or doubly heterozygous for spectrin mutations, the membrane instability is

sufficient to cause RBC fragmentation with hemolytic anemia under conditions of normal circulatory shear stress.

The pathobiology of the elliptocytic shape is less clear. RBC precursors in common HE are round and the cells become progressively more elliptical as they age in vivo. RBCs subjected to shear stress in vitro, or RBCs flowing through microcirculation in vivo, have an elliptical or parachute-like shape, respectively. It is possible that elliptocytes and poikilocytes are permanently stabilized in their abnormal shape because the weakened spectrin heterodimer contacts facilitate skeletal reorganization, which follows axial deformation of cells resulting from application of a prolonged or excessive shear stress. This reorganization is likely to involve breakage of the unidirectionally stretched protein connections followed by the formation of new protein contacts that preclude the recovery of a normal biconcave shape. This process has been shown to account for permanent deformation of irreversibly sickled cells.

In HPP, the recessively inherited form of HE characterized by severe hemolysis, RBCs have two abnormalities. They contain a mutant spectrin that characteristically disrupts spectrin heterodimer self-association, and they are also partially deficient in spectrin, as evidenced by a decreased spectrin/band 3 ratio. In some HPP cases, this biochemical phenotype is a consequence of a double heterozygous state for an elliptocytogenic α-spectrin mutation and a defect involving reduced α-spectrin synthesis. Such synthetic defect of α-spectrin is fully asymptomatic in the heterozygous carrier, because under normal conditions, the synthesis of α-spectrin is approximately three to four times greater than that of β-spectrin.

When present in conjunction with an elliptocytogenic mutation of α-spectrin, such a synthetic defect augments the expression of the mutant spectrin. Because the elliptocytogenic α-spectrin mutants are often unstable, the combination of the two defects leads to spectrin deficiency in the cells. Other HPP patients are homozygous or doubly heterozygous for one or two elliptocytogenic spectrin mutations, respectively. In such cases, the spectrin deficiency may be a consequence of spectrin instability that reduces the amount of spectrin available for membrane assembly. Furthermore, in RBCs containing a high fraction of unassembled dimeric spectrin, the spectrin deficiency may in part be related to the stoichiometric ratio of one ankyrin copy per one spectrin tetramer (i.e., two spectrin heterodimers). Consequently, only approximately one-half of spectrin heterodimers succeed in attaching to the ankyrin-binding sites. The phenotype of HPP, characterized by the presence of fragments and elliptocytes, together with evidence of RBC surface area deficiency (as reflected by the presence of microspherocytes on the peripheral blood film), suggests that the membrane dysfunction involves both vertical interactions (a consequence of spectrin deficiency) and horizontal interactions involving the elliptocytogenic spectrin mutation.

The RBC lesion in protein 4.1R deficiency shows similarities in regard to cell shape and membrane stability to the elliptocytogenic mutations of spectrin, suggesting that the deficiency principally affects the spectrin-actin contact (see Fig. 45.5) rather than the skeleton attachment to GPC via protein 4.1R (a vertical interaction).

The molecular basis of elliptocytosis and the mechanical instability of GPC-deficient RBCs are not fully understood. However, recent studies suggest that the deficiency of GPC is not directly responsible for the altered mechanical properties. Instead, the mechanical instability appears to be related to a concomitant partial deficiency of protein 4.1R, as evidenced by a full correction of membrane instability by introduction into the cells of protein 4.1R or its spectrin-binding peptide, which facilitates the contact of β-spectrin to actin. The superimposed deficiency of protein 4.1R is likely to be related to the fact that GPC serves as an attachment site for protein 4.1R to the membrane, recruiting protein 4.1R to the RBC membrane. The effects of these defects on the mechanical stability of GPC-deficient cells appear to be relatively minor, because GPC-deficient patients have no detectable hemolytic anemia and the mechanical properties of the RBCs are normal when tested by micropipette aspiration.

Inheritance

In most patients, HE is inherited as an autosomal dominant disorder. The clinical severity is highly variable among different kindred (reflecting heterogeneous molecular lesions) and, to a lesser extent, within a given kindred, presumably because of other genetic or acquired defects that modify disease expression. Occasionally HE is inherited as an autosomal recessive condition from an asymptomatic parent who carries the same molecular defect of spectrin as the HE offspring. In one kindred with a submicroscopic chromosome X deletion, inheritance was X-linked.

The inheritance of the related disorder HPP is autosomal recessive: one of the parents carries the α-spectrin mutation and either is asymptomatic or has mild HE, whereas the other parent is fully asymptomatic and has no abnormalities detectable by current biochemical approaches. However, several HPP patients have recently been studied who were doubly heterozygous for two α-spectrin mutations; in the heterozygous parents, these mutations were either silent or expressed as mild HE.

Clinical Manifestations

In view of the striking molecular heterogeneity of common HE, it is not surprising that the clinical spectrum of this disorder is variable, ranging from an asymptomatic trait without hemolysis to a life-threatening hemolytic anemia.

Mild Hereditary Elliptocytosis and Asymptomatic Carrier State

In most of these patients, HE is found accidentally during evaluation of the peripheral blood film. Although some HE patients have a mild compensated hemolytic anemia, others do not have any evidence of hemolysis, their RBC survival is normal, and the peripheral blood film may reveal only modest (≥15%) elliptocytosis. The molecular basis of mild HE is heterogeneous, and the reported molecular defects include both α- and β-spectrin mutations, partial deficiency of the 4.1R protein, and the absence of GPC. Some individuals carrying the spectrin mutation are completely asymptomatic, including normal RBC morphologic features; this is often the case in one of the parents of a patient with HPP.

Hereditary Elliptocytosis With Sporadic Hemolysis

Worsening of hemolysis together with the appearance of poikilocytes on the peripheral blood film has been reported in patients with hypersplenism, infections, or vitamin B_{12} deficiency, as well as in those with microangiopathic hemolysis such as disseminated intravascular coagulation or thrombotic thrombocytopenic purpura. In the latter two conditions, worsening hemolysis can be caused by microcirculatory damage superimposed on the underlying mechanical instability of the RBCs.

Hereditary Elliptocytosis With Neonatal Poikilocytosis

Neonatal offspring of parents with mild HE present with symptomatic hemolytic anemia and a marked poikilocytosis. During the first year of life, the hemolysis and poikilocytosis abate, and the clinical picture transforms into that of mild HE. Such patients typically carry one mutant α-spectrin allele. The severity of the molecular defect, in terms of the percentage of spectrin dimers and the amount of mutant spectrin in the cells, is the same in the neonatal period as it is later in life. The worsening of hemolysis in the neonatal period has been attributed to the presence of fetal hemoglobin, which binds poorly to 2,3-diphosphoglycerate (2,3-DPG). The ensuing elevation of free

2,3-DPG levels has a marked destabilizing effect on the spectrin–protein 4.1R–actin interaction, thereby further destabilizing the membrane skeleton.

Hereditary Elliptocytosis With Chronic Hemolysis

Patients with HE with chronic hemolysis present with moderate to severe hemolytic anemia with elliptocytes and poikilocytes on peripheral blood film; some require splenectomy. In some of the kindred, the hemolytic HE has been transmitted through several generations. In some kindred, not all of the HE patients have chronic hemolysis; some have a mild hemolysis only, presumably because of another genetic factor modifying the disease expression.

Homozygous and Compound Heterozygous Hereditary Elliptocytosis

Several HE individuals have been described who were apparent homozygotes for the HE gene. These individuals were found to be either homozygotes or compound (double) heterozygotes for one or two α- or β-spectrin mutations. The clinical severity is variable, from a relatively mild hemolytic anemia to a severe, life-threatening disease, depending on the severity of the underlying molecular defect, and in some cases is indistinguishable from HPP.

Hereditary Pyropoikilocytosis

It is now established that HPP represents a subtype of common HE, as evidenced by the coexistence of both HE and HPP in the same family and by the presence of the same molecular defect of spectrin. Unlike HE patients carrying the spectrin mutation, the RBCs of HPP patients are also partially deficient in spectrin. Typically, one parent of the HPP offspring carries an α-spectrin mutation, whereas the other parent is fully asymptomatic and has no detectable biochemical abnormality. In many such patients the asymptomatic parent carries a silent "thalassemia-like" defect of spectrin synthesis, enhancing the relative expression of the spectrin mutant and leading to a superimposed spectrin deficiency in the HPP offspring. Subsequent studies of the original HPP kindred revealed that defective spectrin synthesis from the null allele was caused by a splicing mutation of the α-spectrin gene. Some HPP patients inherited two α-spectrin mutations; either their parents were hematologically normal or one had mild HE. In these HPP patients, spectrin deficiency may be related to instability of the mutant spectrin. The thermal instability of spectrin originally reported as diagnostic of HPP is not unique for this disorder; it is also found in HE patients carrying this α-spectrin mutation, in the homozygous and in the heterozygous states. HPP is seen predominantly in black patients, but it has also been diagnosed in Arabs and whites.

Molecular Determinants of Clinical Severity

The severity of hemolysis in common HE often varies not only among different kindred but within a given family as well. The two principal determinants of severity of hemolysis are the spectrin content of the cells and the percentage of dimeric spectrin in the crude spectrin extract. The fraction of dimeric spectrin in such extracts in turn depends on several factors. The first of them is the degree of dysfunction of the mutant spectrin. Typically, mutations that are either within or near the combined αβ triple-helical repetitive segment representing the spectrin heterodimer self-association site produce a more severe clinical phenotype and a more severe defect of spectrin function than those seen with point mutations in the more distant triple-helical repeats. Second, the percentage of the dimeric spectrin depends on the fraction of the mutant spectrin in the cells, which in turn is determined by the gene dose (e.g., simple heterozygote versus homozygote or double heterozygote) or the presence of other genetic defects such as the presence, in trans, of a defect leading to a reduced α-spectrin synthesis in some patients with HPP.

The low-expression α-spectrin allele $α^{LELY}$ is the best-characterized abnormality affecting spectrin content and clinical severity. Initially a polymorphism of the αV domain, $α^{V/41}$, was identified in HE patients who, when they inherited $α^{V/41}$ in trans, had more severe HE than expected. Subsequently an amino acid substitution of exon 46, Leu1857Val, and partial skipping of exon 46, linked to the $α^{V/41}$ polymorphism, were identified as the characteristics of the $α^{LELY}$ allele. These abnormalities are located within the site at which spectrin monomers assemble into heterodimers (the spectrin heterodimer nucleation site). In vitro studies suggest that the inability of α-spectrin chains to assemble into the mature membrane skeleton is because of a combination of decreased αβ dimer-binding affinity and increased proteolytic cleavage of the mutant α-spectrin chains. The presence of $α^{LELY}$ in trans diminishes the propensity of the otherwise normal allele to associate with the corresponding β-chain, favoring the attachment of the elliptocytogenic α-spectrin allele. Conversely, coexistence of the α-spectrin mutation in cis and the mutation involving the α-spectrin nucleation site diminishes the propensity of the mutant allele to be incorporated into the spectrin heterodimer, thereby ameliorating the clinical severity of this mutation. The $α^{LELY}$ allele is clinically silent by itself, even when inherited in the homozygous state, probably because α-spectrin is normally synthesized in threefold to fourfold excess.

Laboratory Manifestations

Blood Film and Laboratory Evidence of Hemolysis

A careful blood smear evaluation is essential for the diagnosis of HE and for the classification of the disorder into the three major subtypes outlined previously. In patients in whom elliptocytosis is the only morphologic abnormality, hemolysis is characteristically minimal or absent, with the exception of spherocytic elliptocytosis, in which the presence of round "fat" ovalocytes is associated with accelerated RBC destruction. In patients with hemolytic forms of common HE, poikilocytosis is characteristically found on the blood film. In severe forms of HE, particularly in homozygous HE, many RBCs circulate as cell fragments, producing a marked decrease in MCV. The finding of RBC fragments together with a striking microspherocytosis and often only occasional elliptocytes is characteristic of HPP (Fig. 45.6).

Osmotic and Thermal Fragility

Osmotic fragility is increased in HPP, in spherocytic elliptocytosis, and in HE patients with poikilocytosis apparent on the peripheral blood film. In patients with a mild common HE without poikilocytosis on the peripheral blood film, osmotic fragility is normal.

Thermal instability of RBCs was originally reported as a characteristic feature of HPP. It reflects thermal instability of the mutant

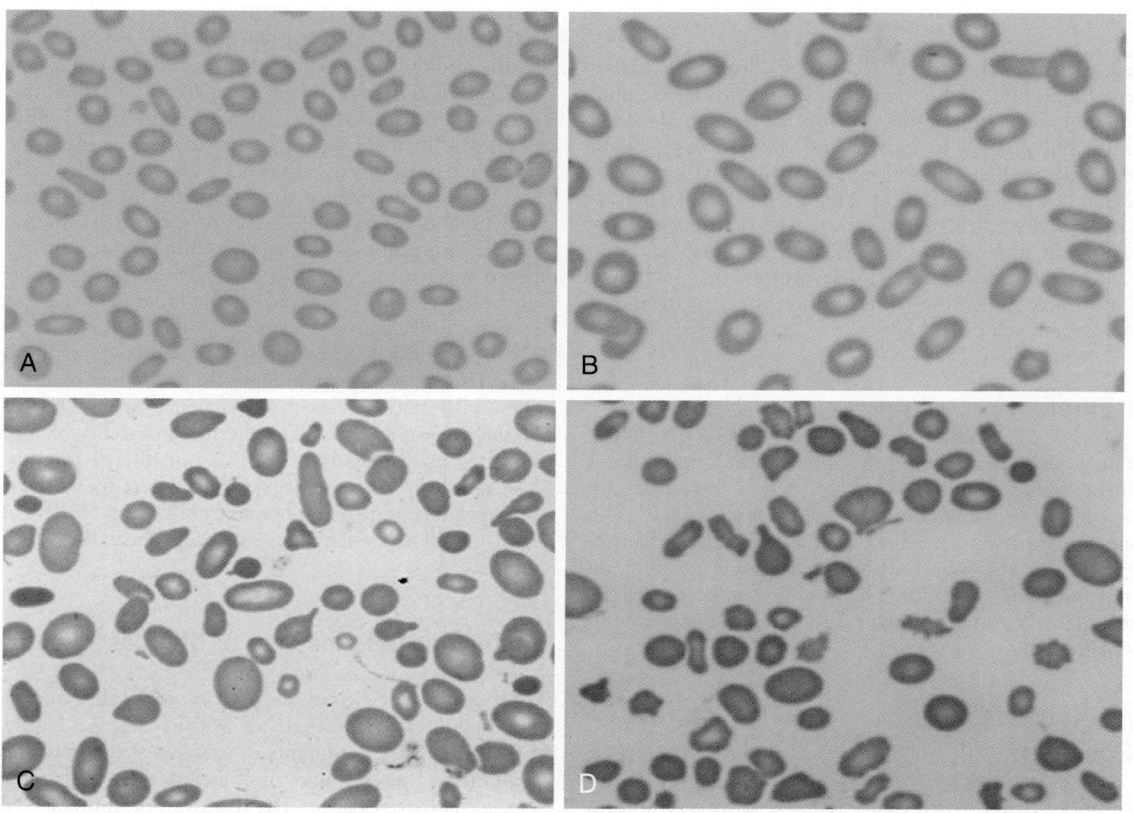

Fig. 45.6 BLOOD FILMS OF PATIENTS WITH VARIOUS FORMS OF HEREDITARY ELLIPTOCYTOSIS (HE). (A) Simple heterozygote with mild common HE. Note the predominant elliptocytosis with some rod-shaped cells *(arrow)* and virtual absence of poikilocytes. (B) Simple heterozygote with severe common hemolytic elliptocytosis. Note the numerous small fragments and poikilocytes. (C) "Homozygous" common HE because of doubly heterozygous state for two mutant α-spectrins. Both parents have mild HE. Note the many elliptocytes, spherocytes, as well as numerous fragments and poikilocytes. (D) Hereditary pyropoikilocytosis. The patient is a double heterozygote for a structural α-spectrin mutant and a presumed α-spectrin synthetic defect. Note the prominent microspherocytosis, micropoikilocytosis, and fragmentation. Only few elliptocytes are present. Some poikilocytes are in the process of budding.

spectrin: In normal RBCs, spectrin is denatured and RBCs fragment at 50°C. HPP RBCs fragment and their spectrin denatures at 41°C. However, the diagnostic value of this test is limited, because thermal instability of RBCs is also noted in HE RBCs containing mutant spectrin. In contrast, an occasional patient with otherwise typical HPP may have normal thermal stability of RBCs and spectrin. RBCs in common HE have unstable membranes and membrane skeletons when subjected to shear stress.

Electrophoretic Separation of Solubilized Membrane Proteins

In HE and HPP, SDS-PAGE can reveal proteins of abnormal mobility, the origin of which can be subsequently identified by Western blotting (e.g., truncated α- or β-spectrins in HE and HPP, or elongated or truncated forms of the 4.1R protein, and a partial or, rarely, complete deficiency of the 4.1R protein in HE). In HPP, SDS-PAGE reveals a partial deficiency of spectrin, as indicated by a decreased spectrin/band 3 ratio. Spectrin deficiency, in conjunction with an elliptocytogenic spectrin mutation affecting the spectrin heterodimer contact, is invariably found in cases of HPP.

Nondenaturing Gel Electrophoresis of Low-Ionic-Strength Spectrin Extract

Analysis of the ratio of tetrameric and dimeric spectrin in the low-ionic-strength extracts reveals the most common functional abnormality in HE (i.e., weakened self-association of spectrin heterodimers into tetramers). Because the spectrin dimer-tetramer interconversion has a high activation energy, it is kinetically immobilized at near 0°C. Consequently, the percentage of spectrin dimers and tetramers in the 0°C crude spectrin extract reflects the relative distribution of these species in the RBC membrane in situ. Mutations of α- or α-spectrin residing within or near the αβ-spectrin heterodimer self-association site invariably lead to an increase in the fraction of dimeric spectrin in the crude 0°C spectrin extract.

Tryptic Peptide Mapping of Spectrin and the Detection of the Underlying DNA Defect

Tryptic digestion of spectrin followed by electrophoretic separation gives rise to highly reproducible tryptic peptide patterns. Among these peptides, the 80-kDa αI domain peptide representing the self-association site of the normal α-spectrin is among the most prominent. Nearly all α- or β-spectrin mutations reported are associated with a formation of tryptic peptides of abnormal size and mobility that are generated from the normal 80-kDa αI domain peptide. The cleavage sites of the most common abnormal tryptic peptides are found in the third helix of a given triple-helical repetitive segment. The reported mutations reside in the vicinity of these cleavage sites either in the same helix or, less commonly, in helix 1 or 2 of a given repetitive segment. Consequently, tryptic peptide mapping remains a powerful tool with which to map the site of the underlying spectrin mutation, which can be subsequently defined by polymerase chain reaction amplification and sequencing of the respective region of the genomic DNA or complementary DNA (cDNA).

Differential Diagnosis

Various acquired and inherited conditions can be associated with elliptocytosis and poikilocytosis, including iron deficiency, thalassemias, megaloblastic anemias, myelofibrosis, myelophthisic anemias, myelodysplastic syndromes, and pyruvate kinase deficiency. The percentage of elliptocytes in these conditions is seldom greater than 60%. However, this is not diagnostically useful, because some HE patients can have a relatively low percentage of elliptocytes. In normal patients the percentage of elliptocytes is not greater than 5%, although in earlier reports it was listed as high as 15%. Previous diagnostic criteria of HE, based on the percentage of elliptocytes, such as 25%, 33%, or 40%, and their axial ratio, do not appear useful. The most reliable differentiation of HE from the other conditions mentioned is based on a positive family history rather than on the percentage of elliptocytes.

Therapy and Prognosis

As in the case of HS, RBCs from patients with more severe forms of HE are retained by the spleen, producing a marked engorgement of splenic pulp. Consequently, patients with symptomatic hemolysis benefit from splenectomy. This procedure is virtually never indicated in heterozygotes with autosomal dominant HE because most do not have clinically significant hemolytic anemia. If hemolysis is still active after splenectomy, folate should be administered daily. Recommendations for antibiotic prophylaxis, immunizations, and monitoring for intercurrent illnesses are similar to those noted earlier for HS patients before and after splenectomy. Serial interval ultrasonographic investigations to detect gallstones should be performed in patients with significant hemolysis.

Spherocytic Elliptocytosis

Spherocytic elliptocytosis, which shares features of HS and HE, has been designated spherocytic HE, HE with spherocytosis, or hereditary hemolytic ovalocytosis. The diagnosis is based on the simultaneous presence of elliptical RBCs and spherocytes or "fat," round sphero-ovalocytes in the peripheral blood film. In contrast to common HE, cells of other shapes, such as rod-shaped cells, poikilocytes, and fragments, are absent. Importantly, hemolysis, despite relatively mild alterations in RBC morphologic features, and increased osmotic fragility are the main diagnostic features distinguishing this disorder from common HE.

The molecular basis of spherocytic HE is unknown. However, patients with mutations, particularly truncations at the C-terminal of β-spectrin, have many of the clinical features of spherocytic HE and probably represent an example of this disorder. Patients who lack GPC have rounded, smooth elliptocytes and could be classified as having a mild, recessively inherited variant of spherocytic HE. Finally, some patients with recessively inherited defects of protein 4.2 can display some features of spherocytic HE, particularly mild ovalostomatocytosis.

Southeast Asian Ovalocytosis

SAO is characterized by the presence of oval RBCs, many containing one or two transverse ridges or a longitudinal slit. The condition is widespread in certain ethnic groups of Malaysia, Papua New Guinea, the Philippines, and Indonesia. Numerous functional abnormalities of ovalocytes have been reported, including increased RBC rigidity, decreased osmotic fragility, increased thermal stability, resistance to shape change by echinocytogenic agents, and a reduced expression of many RBC antigens. A remarkable feature of ovalocytes is their resistance to in vitro invasion by several strains of malaria parasites, including *P. falciparum* and *Plasmodium knowlesi*. In areas of endemic malaria, SAO individuals have reduced numbers of intracellular parasites in vivo, with decreased prevalence and disease severity of malaria in SAO patients compared with controls.

SAO individuals are heterozygotes for two band 3 gene mutations in cis: the deletion of nine codons encoding amino acids 400 through 408 from the boundary of the cytoplasmic and membrane domains of band 3, and the 56 Lys to Glu substitution. The 56 Lys to Glu substitution represents an asymptomatic polymorphism known as band 3 Memphis. The SAO phenotype is associated with a tighter binding of band 3 to ankyrin, increased tyrosine phosphorylation of the band 3 protein, inability to transport sulfate anions, and a markedly restricted lateral and rotational mobility of band 3 protein in the membrane.

Laboratory Manifestations

The finding of 30% or greater of oval RBCs on the peripheral blood film, some containing a central slit or a transverse ridge, in the context of a notable absence of clinical and laboratory evidence of hemolysis in a patient from the ethnic groups noted earlier is highly suggestive of the diagnosis. A useful screening test is the demonstration of the resistance of ovalocytes or their ghosts to changes in shape produced by treatments that produce spiculation in normal cells, such as metabolic depletion or exposure of ghosts to salt solutions. In contrast to normal RBCs, which form spicules in response to such stimuli, SAO RBCs or ghosts do not change shape after these treatments. The mechanism of this resistance to changes in shape is not clear, and it may reflect the high rigidity of the RBC membrane.

Because the underlying cause of SAO is the deletion of 27 bases from the band 3 gene, isolation of genomic DNA or reticulocyte cDNA with subsequent amplification of the deletion-containing region appears to be the most specific test for establishing the diagnosis of SAO. A single, severely affected homozygous SAO individual who was transfusion dependent has been described.

Molecular Basis of Southeast Asian Ovalocytosis Membrane Rigidity and Malaria Resistance

The RBCs of SAO are unique among axially deformed cells in that they are rigid and hyperstable rather than unstable. The SAO mutation is the first example of a defect of an integral membrane protein leading to RBC membrane rigidity, an observation previously attributed to properties of the membrane skeleton. The basis of the increased rigidity is unclear.

The molecular basis of malaria resistance of SAO RBCs is likely related to altered properties of the band 3 protein, which serves as one of the malaria receptors, as evidenced by the inhibition of in vitro invasion by band 3-containing liposomes. In normal RBCs, the invasion process is associated with a marked membrane remodeling that involves redistribution of intramembrane particles that contain band 3 protein. Such particles cluster at the site of parasite invasion, forming a ring around the orifice through which the parasite enters the cell. The invaginated RBC membrane, which surrounds the invading parasite, is free of intramembrane particles. The reduced lateral mobility of band 3 protein in SAO RBCs may preclude band 3 receptor clustering, thereby preventing the attachment of the parasites to the cells. Decreased exchange of anions across the RBC membrane has also been proposed to contribute to the resistance of ovalocytes to malaria invasion. In addition, SAO RBCs consume ATP at a higher rate than normal cells, and the partial depletion of ATP levels in ovalocytes has been suggested to account, at least in part, for the resistance of these cells to malaria invasion in vitro.

Acanthocytosis and Related Disorders

Acanthocytes (from the Greek *acantha*, "thorn") or spur cells are RBCs with prominent thorn-like surface protrusions that vary in width, length, and surface distribution. Spur cells must be distinguished from echinocytes (Greek *echinos*, "sea urchin") or burr cells, characterized by multiple small projections that are uniformly distributed throughout the cell surface (Fig. 45.7). Acanthocytes should also

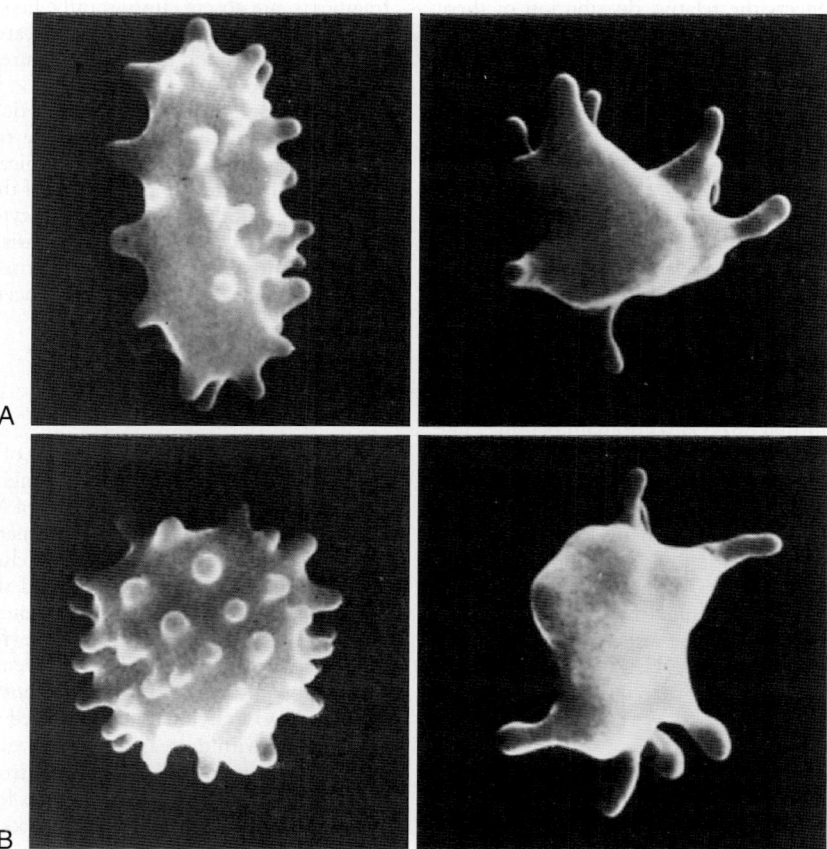

Fig. 45.7 MORPHOLOGIC DIFFERENCES BETWEEN ACANTHOCYTES (A) AND ECHINO-CYTES (B) AS DEMONSTRATED BY SCANNING ELECTRON MICROSCOPY. *(Modified from Bessis M: Red cell shapes: An illustrated classification and its rationale. In Bessis M, Weed RI, Leblond PF, eds: Red Cell Shape Physiology, Pathology, Ultrastructure, New York, 1973, Springer-Verlag.)*

be distinguished from keratocytes ("horn" red cells) that have few massive protuberances.

Acanthocytosis was first described in cases of abetalipoproteinemia and subsequently in severe liver disease, the chorea-acanthocytosis syndrome, the McLeod blood group phenotype, and other conditions. The molecular mechanisms leading to acanthocytosis in abetalipoproteinemia and severe liver disease have been extensively studied and have been attributed to changes in composition of membrane lipids and their altered distribution between the two hemileaflets of the lipid bilayer.

Spur Cell Hemolytic Anemia of Severe Liver Disease

Spur cell hemolytic anemia is an uncommon ominous complication of severe liver disease that is manifested by rapidly progressive hemolytic anemia and acanthocytes on the peripheral blood smear.

Pathobiology

The human RBC membrane contains nearly equal amounts of free (unesterified) cholesterol and phospholipids. The free cholesterol in the plasma readily equilibrates with the RBC membrane cholesterol pool. This is in contrast to esterified cholesterol, which cannot be transferred from plasma into the RBC membrane. The plasma of patients with severe liver disease contains abnormal lipoproteins that have a high free cholesterol/phospholipid ratio. The excess free cholesterol readily partitions into the RBC membrane, leading to a marked increase in free cholesterol in the cells. Consequently, normal cells can develop a spur cell shape after their transfusion into a patient with severe liver disease or after incubation with the liver disease patient's plasma or cholesterol-enriched liposomes.

Spur cell formation involves two steps. The first step is evident in RBCs of splenectomized patients with spur cell hemolytic anemia: RBCs have an expanded surface area with irregular contour and targeting, reflecting accumulation of free cholesterol in the membrane (Fig. 45.8). This extracholesterol accumulates preferentially in the outer bilayer leaflet, as suggested by findings of increased accessibility of cholesterol to cholesterol oxidase and a selective decrease in lipid fluidity of the outer hemileaflet of the lipid bilayer.

The second step in acanthocyte formation involves RBC remodeling by the spleen. As a result, RBCs become spheroidal, and the surface projections are considerably longer and more irregular. The end result of these processes is poorly deformable RBCs with long bizarre projections that are readily trapped in the spleen, which is often markedly enlarged because of passive congestion as a result of underlying portal hypertension. Cholesterol also alters membrane permeability and interacts with several membrane skeletal proteins, but the role of these changes in spur cell lesions is unclear.

Clinical Manifestations

Most patients with chronic liver disease have a mild to moderate anemia related to gastrointestinal blood loss, iron and folic acid deficiencies, or hemodilution or as a direct effect of alcohol on RBC precursors. Peripheral blood smears from these patients often reveal target cells that are particularly prominent in obstructive jaundice.

In some patients, particularly those with end-stage liver disease, anemia rapidly worsens and spur cells appear in high percentage in the peripheral blood. This is accompanied by worsening jaundice, rapid deterioration of liver function, hepatic encephalopathy, and hemorrhagic diatheses. A similar clinical syndrome has been described in patients with advanced metastatic liver disease, cardiac cirrhosis, Wilson disease, fulminant hepatitis, and infantile cholestatic liver disease. The development of spur cell hemolytic anemia is an ominous sign in most patients, predicting a survival seldom exceeding weeks to months. In theory, splenectomy could provide a marked improvement, because the spleen is the major sequestration site of nondeformable acanthocytes; in reality, splenectomy is seldom considered because of severity of the underlying liver disease.

Abetalipoproteinemia

Bassen and Kornzweig first described an association of acanthocytosis with atypical retinitis pigmentosa, progressive ataxic neurologic disease, and a "celiac disease" later attributed to fat malabsorption. Subsequently several investigators reported a congenital absence of β-lipoprotein, accounting for the diverse manifestations of the disorder.

Pathobiology

Abetalipoproteinemia is an autosomal recessive disorder found in people of diverse ethnic backgrounds. The primary molecular defect involves a congenital absence of β-apolipoprotein in plasma. The B apoproteins (B100 and B48) are generated by alternate transcription of a single gene residing on the short arm of chromosome 2. Their deficiency is secondary to defective cellular secretion of the apoprotein

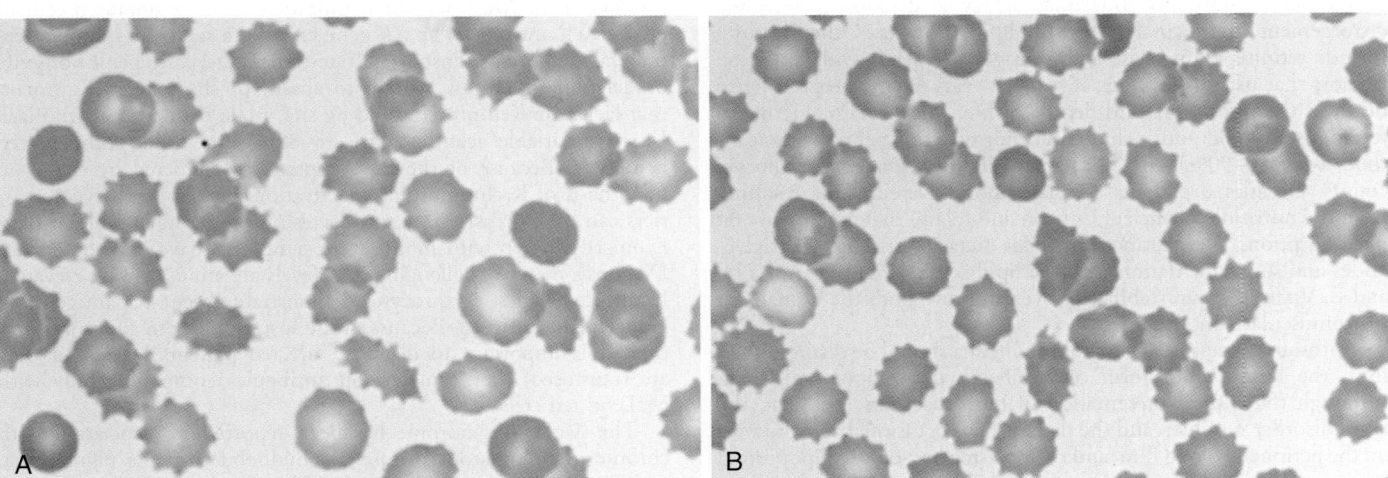

Fig. 45.8 BLOOD FILM OF A PATIENT WITH LIVER CIRRHOSIS AND SPUR CELL ANEMIA. Erythrocytes have an expanded surface area with irregular contour and targeting, reflecting accumulation of free cholesterol in the membrane, preferentially in the outer bilayer leaflet. Splenic remodeling leads to increasing spheroidicity with longer and more irregular surface projections.

by liver cells, caused either by aberrant posttranslational processing or by defective aposecretion. In some patients this is because of qualitative or quantitative defects in the microsomal triglyceride transfer protein, which catalyzes the transport of triglyceride, cholesterol ester, and phospholipid from phospholipid surfaces. Microsomal triglyceride transfer protein is the only tissue-specific component, other than apolipoprotein B, required for secretion of apolipoprotein B-containing lipoproteins. As a result, apoprotein B is absent in plasma, as are the individual lipoprotein fractions that contain this apoprotein. These lipoprotein fractions include chylomicrons and very-low-density lipoproteins that transport triglycerides, as well as the low-density lipoproteins that are products of very-low-density lipoproteins and transport cholesterol. Consequently, preformed triglycerides are not transported from the intestinal mucosa, and they are nearly absent in the plasma. Plasma cholesterol and phospholipids are markedly reduced, with a relative increase in sphingomyelin at the expense of lecithin.

As is the case in acanthocytosis of liver disease, the acanthocytic lesion is acquired from the plasma. Erythrocyte precursors are of normal shape, and the acanthocytic lesion develops as the cells mature and age in the circulation. Normal cells acquire this shape when transfused into the recipient.

The most striking abnormality of RBC membrane lipids involves a net increase in sphingomyelin. Because plasma lipids readily exchange with the lipids of the RBC membrane, it is likely that this change simply mirrors the alterations in plasma lipid composition. In contrast to RBCs in spur cell anemia of severe liver disease, the content of membrane cholesterol is normal or only slightly increased.

The role of membrane lipids in the acanthocyte shape transformation was first established by findings of restoration of biconcave shape after extraction of lipids from the cell membrane by detergents. The molecular basis of the acanthocytic shape is unknown, but several indirect observations suggest that it is related to an increase of the surface area of the outer hemileaflet of the lipid bilayer relative to the inner leaflet. Several other abnormalities have been noted in abetalipoproteinemia, including a decrease in plasma lecithin cholesterol transferase activity and an increased susceptibility of membrane and plasma lipids to oxidation as a result of malabsorption-induced deficiency of vitamin E. The contributions of these abnormalities to the acanthocyte red cell lesions are unknown.

Clinical Manifestations

This autosomal recessive disease can become evident in the first few months of life, manifested by fat malabsorption with normal absorption of other nutrients. Intestinal biopsy is diagnostic, revealing engorgement of mucosal cells with lipid droplets. Other features include retinitis pigmentosa and a progressive ataxia with intention tremors that usually develops at 5 to 10 years of age, progressing to death in the second or third decade of life. The hematologic manifestations are mild and include mild normocytic anemia with acanthocytosis (50–90%) and normal or slightly elevated reticulocyte counts. Occasional patients can have more severe anemia resulting from the nutritional deficiencies (iron and folate) that accompany fat malabsorption. The treatment includes dietary restriction of triglycerides and supplementation with the lipid-soluble vitamins A, K, D, and E. Vitamin E can stabilize or even improve both the retinal and neuromuscular abnormalities.

Autosomal recessive abetalipoproteinemia should be distinguished from the homozygous form of familial hypobetalipoproteinemia. Although the clinical presentation of both disorders is similar, the latter disorder is milder, and the parents have occasional acanthocytes on the peripheral blood film, and their plasma low-density lipoprotein levels are decreased. The molecular lesions in familial hypobetalipoproteinemia involve a variety of apoprotein B gene mutations, leading to aberrant apoprotein B gene transcription or translation.

Varying degrees of acanthocytosis without anemia have also been described with isolated deficiency of apoprotein B100.

Neuroacanthocytosis Syndromes

The neuroacanthocytosis syndromes are a group of degenerative neurologic disorders with phenotypic and genetic heterogeneity that share the feature of acanthocytes on peripheral blood smear. These disorders include chorea-acanthocytosis, the X-linked McLeod syndrome (see McLeod Phenotype), and several other neurodegenerative diseases, including Huntington disease-like 2 caused by mutations in junctophilin-3 and pantothenate kinase-associated neurodegeneration (formerly known as Hallervorden-Spatz syndrome and its allelic variant syndrome—hypobetalipoproteinemia, acanthocytosis, retinitis pigmentosa, pallidal degeneration [HARP]) caused by mutations in pantothenate kinase 2.

Chorea-acanthocytosis syndrome is an autosomal recessive syndrome of adult onset that is manifest by multiple neurologic abnormalities, including limb chorea, progressive orofacial dyskinesia with tics, tongue-biting neurogenic muscle hypotonia, and atrophy. The hematologic manifestations are minimal and include a variable percentage of acanthocytes on the peripheral blood film without anemia and normal or only slightly decreased RBC survival. The mechanism of acanthocytosis in this syndrome is unknown. Studies of plasma and RBC membrane lipids have revealed a high content of unsaturated fatty acids, presumably accounting for reduced RBC membrane fluidity. Additional abnormalities of uncertain significance include an uneven distribution of intramembrane particles, impaired phosphorylation of the erythrocyte actin-bundling protein dematin, abnormal accumulation of transglutaminase products, and altered function and structure of band 3.

Mutations have been identified in the chorein gene (also known as *CHAC* or *VPS13A*—vacuolar protein sorting 13 homolog A) in many affected patients. Chorein does not belong to any known human gene family, and computer searches have not identified any known structural motifs or domains. The function of the chorein gene product remains unknown in either erythrocytes or the brain. In yeast, a chorein homologue is involved in protein sorting and transport and in regulation of levels of phosphatidylinositol-4-phosphate in cell membranes.

McLeod Phenotype

The McLeod syndrome is characterized by a mild compensated hemolytic anemia with a variable percentage of acanthocytes on the peripheral blood film and, in some patients, late-onset myopathy or chorea. The McLeod blood group phenotype is an X-linked anomaly of the Kell blood group system in which RBCs, white blood cells, or both react poorly with Kell antisera. The affected cells lack Kx, the product of the *XK* gene, which appears to be a membrane precursor of the Kell antigens. The *XK* gene encodes a novel 444-amino acid integral membrane transporter. In most patients, pathogenic nonsense or deletion mutations leading to absent or shortened XK protein that lacks the Kell protein binding site. Male hemizygotes who lack Kx have variable acanthocytosis (8–85%) and mild, compensated hemolysis. Because of the RBC mosaicism predicted by the Lyon hypothesis of X chromosome inactivation, female heterozygote carriers can have occasional acanthocytes on the peripheral blood film. Lyonized women with more severe symptoms have been described. Diagnosis may be challenging. CK levels are almost always elevated. In affected males, erythrocytes demonstrate absent Kx antigen and reduced Kell antigens. Because of the susceptibility to alloimmunization, it is important to diagnose affected patients because if they are transfused, they can develop antibodies compatible only with McLeod red cells.

The McLeod syndrome has been reported in association with chronic granulomatous disease of childhood, retinitis pigmentosa, and Duchenne muscular dystrophy. This association is caused by the close proximity of the genetic loci for these disorders in the p21 region of the X chromosome (Xp21), suggesting the occurrence of various manifestations because of contiguous gene syndromes. This may explain the occasional findings of either echinocytes or stomatocytes in Duchenne dystrophy, or a choreiform disorder in some patients with the McLeod phenotype.

The Kell antigen consists of two protein components: a 37-kDa protein that carries the Kx antigen, a precursor molecule necessary for the Kell antigen expression, and a 93-kDa protein that carries the Kell blood group antigen. RBCs with the McLeod phenotype have no detectable Kx antigen, and they have a marked deficiency of the 93-kDa protein that carries the Kell antigen. McLeod RBCs should be distinguished from Kell null (K_0) RBCs, which have a normal shape. In K_0 cells, only the Kell antigen carrying the 93-kDa glycoprotein is absent, whereas these cells have twice the amount of the Kx antigen. As in the other acanthocytic disorders, the surface projections of acanthocytes may be related to asymmetry of the surface area of the two lipid bilayer hemileaflets, as indicated by correction of the acanthocytosis by agents that expand the inner lipid layer, as well as the finding of an increased rate of exchange of phosphatidylcholine (localized preferentially in the outer lipid hemileaflet) with an exogenous source.

Acanthocytosis in Other Conditions

Acanthocytes have also been noted in malnourished patients, including those with anorexia nervosa and cystic fibrosis. In these patients, RBC shape normalizes after restoration of the nutritional status. Likewise, a small number of cells with long spicules resembling acanthocytes are found in patients with hypothyroidism, after splenectomy, and with myelodysplasia.

Differentiation of Acanthocytes From Other Spiculated Red Blood Cells

Echinocytes (Burr Cells)

In contrast to acanthocytes, echinocytes, also called burr cells, have rather uniform surface projections. Although early echinocytic forms have a regularly scalloped cell contour, advanced forms of echinocytes have a spheroidal shape and the surface projections appear as short, narrow spikes (see Fig. 45.8). Although the finding of echinocytes on a peripheral blood film is often an artifact related to blood storage, contact with glass, or an elevated pH, several hemolytic anemias have been reported in association with echinocytosis on peripheral blood films. These conditions include mild hemolytic anemia in long-distance runners and in patients with hypomagnesemia and hypophosphatemia (presumably because of decreased intracellular ATP stores), uremia because of an unknown plasma factor, and pyruvate kinase deficiency.

Inspection of wet blood preparations (but not dried blood films) reveals echinocytosis in most patients with liver disease. In contrast to spur cells in patients with severe liver disease, these echinocytes have a normal cholesterol content, and the molecular abnormality may be related to the binding of abnormal echinocytogenic high-density lipoproteins to the RBC surface.

The mechanisms of echinocytosis in these diverse disorders are likely to be heterogeneous, as suggested by findings that many diverse factors, such as exposure of RBCs to certain drugs, calcium loading, or ATP depletion, can induce the transformation of discocytes to echinocytes in vitro. However, in vitro studies of the discocyte-echinocyte-stomatocyte equilibrium have suggested a possible common denominator. As discussed earlier, the lipid bilayer of normal RBCs is asymmetric in lipid composition: The outer half of the lipid bilayer is relatively enriched in sphingomyelin and phosphatidylcholine, whereas the inner half is preferentially enriched in the negatively charged phosphatidylserine and phosphatidylethanolamine. Agents that preferentially bind to one or another class of these phospholipids dramatically influence RBC shape. Consequently, agents that preferentially accumulate in the outer half of the RBC lipid bilayer, expanding this lipid bilayer, produce an echinocytic shape, presumably by creating an asymmetry between the two surface areas of the two halves of the lipid bilayer. Conversely, agents that asymmetrically expand the inner half of the lipid bilayer, such as chlorpromazine, lead to stomatocytic shape transformation. In the case of echinocytes produced by ATP depletion or calcium loading, the altered phospholipid distribution between the two bilayer hemileaflets may be a consequence of calcium-induced phospholipid scrambling or a decrease in the activity of aminophospholipid translocase, an ATP-dependent enzyme that actively translocates aminophospholipids from the outer leaflet to the inner hemileaflet.

Keratocytes, Bizarre Poikilocytes, and Schistocytes

Mechanical trauma of circulating RBCs has occasionally produced bizarre shapes resembling acanthocytes, such as cells with horny projections (keratocytes). Some acanthocyte-like cells are also seen in splenectomized HE and HS patients. Similar shape changes are seen in heated RBCs, in which spectrin has been damaged by thermal denaturation, suggesting that these cells are bizarre poikilocytes rather than true acanthocytes.

RED BLOOD CELL MEMBRANE DISORDERS MANIFESTED BY TARGET CELL FORMATION

The common feature of target cells is an increase in the ratio of the cell surface area to cell volume. In microcytic RBCs of patients with various forms of thalassemia and hemoglobinopathies, the increased surface to volume ratio, and consequently the target cell shape, reflect at least in part the relative abundance of cell surface area. In liver disease and other disorders discussed subsequently, the target cell formation reflects an absolute expansion of the cell surface area because of a net accumulation of membrane phospholipids and cholesterol.

Liver Disease

The presence of target cells in association with either normal or slightly increased cell volume is characteristically found in patients with obstructive jaundice, including various forms of liver disease associated with intrahepatic cholestasis. These target cells have a normal survival in the peripheral circulation and do not typically account for the anemias often encountered in patients with liver disease.

In these patients, target cell formation is a consequence of a net uptake of both free cholesterol and phospholipids into the RBC membrane from the plasma because of abnormalities in the cholesterol/phospholipid/protein ratios of low-density lipoproteins. Target cells have a decreased osmotic fragility, because the excess of membrane surface area leads to an increase in the critical hemolytic volume.

Lecithin-Cholesterol Acyltransferase Deficiency

The lecithin-cholesterol acyltransferase (LCAT) enzyme catalyzes the formation of cholesterol esters in lipoproteins. It circulates in plasma as a complex with components of high-density lipoproteins. LCAT deficiency, caused by mutations in the *LCAT* gene, is a rare autosomal dominant disorder manifested by hyperlipidemia, premature atherosclerosis, corneal opacities, chronic nephritis, proteinuria, mild anemia, and the presence of target cells on the blood film. The anemia is caused by mild hemolysis together with a diminished compensatory erythropoiesis. As in obstructive jaundice, the target cells in LCAT deficiency have a marked increase in both cholesterol and phospholipids. In addition, the membrane phosphatidylcholine is increased at the expense of sphingomyelin and phosphatidylethanolamine. Bone marrow aspiration and biopsy reveal the presence of sea-blue histiocytes. Analysis of plasma lipoproteins reveals multiple abnormalities secondary to the underlying enzyme deficiency. Inherited

LCAT deficiency should be distinguished from an acquired deficiency of this enzyme, which is found in patients with severe liver disease.

Stomatocytosis and Related Disorders

Stomatocytes were first described in a girl with dominantly inherited hemolytic anemia. On blood films, her RBCs contained a wide transverse slit or stoma (Fig. 45.9). In a three-dimensional view, these cells have a shape of a cup or a bowl. The slit-like appearance is an artifact that results from folding of the cells during blood smear preparation.

Stomatocytes are seen in a variety of acquired and inherited disorders. The latter are often associated with abnormalities in RBC cation permeability that lead to changes in RBC volume, which can be either increased (hence the designation hydrocytosis or overhydrated stomatocytosis) or decreased (xerocytosis or desiccytosis [dessicate]), or in some cases near normal.

There is no unifying theory to explain this morphologic abnormality. In vitro, stomatocytes can be produced by drugs that

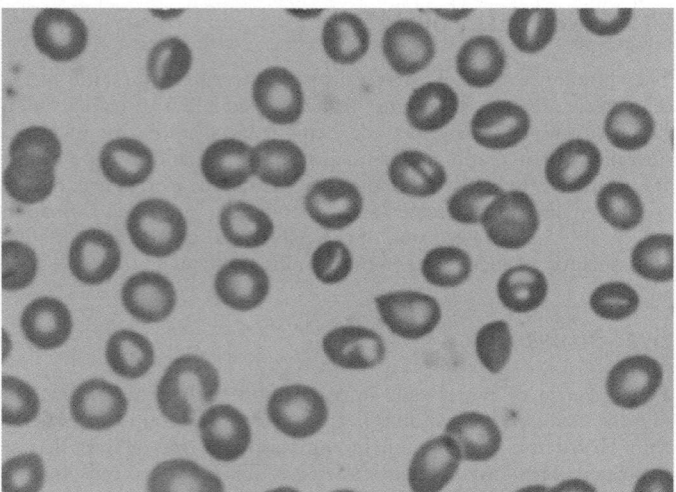

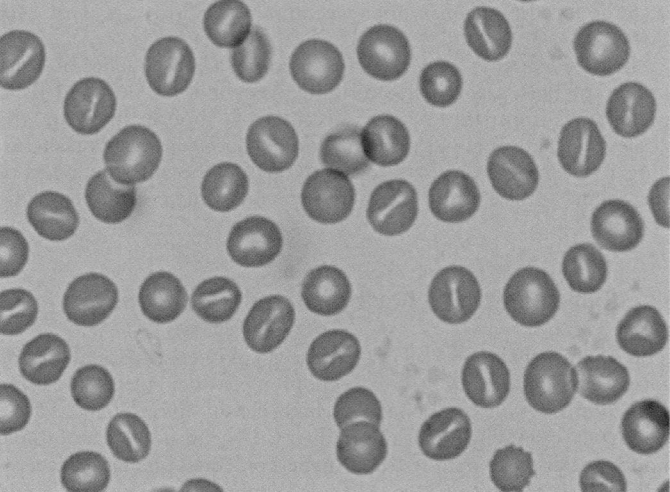

Fig. 45.9 PERIPHERAL BLOOD SMEARS FROM PATIENTS WITH HEREDITARY XEROCYTOSIS (DESICCYTOSIS) (*TOP*) AND STOMATOCYTOSIS (HYDROCYTOSIS) (*BOTTOM*). (*Top*) A Wright-stained peripheral blood smear from a patient with hereditary xerocytosis caused by a PIEZO1 mutation showing rare stomatocytes, occasional dessicytes—dense, abnormal erythrocyte forms where hemoglobin appears puddled at the periphery, and rare target cells. (*Bottom*) A Wright-stained peripheral blood smear from a patient with hereditary hydrocytosis is shown. Numerous stomatocytes, erythrocytes with a central mouth-like "stoma" are seen.

preferentially intercalate into the inner half of the asymmetric lipid bilayer, expanding its surface area relative to that of the outer half of the bilayer.

Hereditary Stomatocytosis-Hydrocytosis

Hereditary hydrocytosis designates a heterogeneous group of hereditary hemolytic anemias that are transmitted in an autosomal dominant manner. The disorder is characterized by a moderate to severe hemolytic anemia with 10% to 30% stomatocytes (see Fig. 45.9), an elevated MCV, and a reduced MCHC. Osmotic fragility of RBCs is markedly increased, as some of the swollen RBCs approach their critical hemolytic volume. For unexplained reasons, RBC membrane lipids and consequently membrane surface area are also increased, but this increase in surface area is insufficient to correct the osmotic fragility of the RBCs. RBC deformability is decreased.

The principal cellular lesion involves a marked increase in intracellular sodium and water content with a mild decrease in intracellular potassium as a result of a marked sodium influx into the RBCs. Despite a marked compensatory increase in active transport of sodium (Na) and potassium by the Na$^+$/K$^+$-ATPase (which normally maintains the low sodium and high potassium concentrations in the cells) and an ensuing increase in glycolysis, the pump hyperactivity is unable to compensate for the vastly increased sodium leak. Stomatin (also known as band 7.2b), an integral membrane protein, is decreased or absent from the erythrocyte membranes of most affected patients. This deficiency appears to be a maturational loss in the bone marrow and in the circulation, perhaps because of a defect in cellular trafficking. Stomatin gene mutations have not been found in unrelated stomatocytosis patients deficient in this protein.

In some patients with hereditary hydrocytosis, missense mutations in RhAG, I61R, or F65S, have been found. In oocytes these mutations induce a monovalent cation leak, possibly opening the pore of an ammonium transporter. Additional studies suggest that the F65S mutation exhibits a gain-of-function phenotype with increased cation conductance/permeability.

Splenectomy can improve, but not fully correct, the hemolysis. In some patients, splenectomy can be deleterious or even contraindicated (see later), perhaps because of altered endothelial cell adherence and membrane phospholipid asymmetry.

Hereditary Xerocytosis and the Intermediate Syndromes

Hereditary xerocytosis or desiccytosis describes an autosomal dominant hemolytic anemia characterized by RBC dehydration and decreased osmotic fragility. Affected individuals have characteristically moderate to severe hemolysis with an increased MCHC, reflecting cellular dehydration. Hydrops fetalis with fetal anemia or fetal ascites or the presence of pseudohyperkalemia have been reported in a number of xerocytosis kindred. Frequently the MCV is mildly increased. In Coulter-type electronic counters, the conversion of pulse height (from the resistance of a cell passing through an electric field) to a cellular volume is dependent on cell shape. Xerocytes do not deform to the same degree as normal cells, which causes the MCV to be approximately 10% too high. The peripheral blood film (see Fig. 45.9) does not always reveal stomatocytes (which are more prominent on wet films), but frequently target cells, dessicytes (dessicate), and spiculated cells are seen. In some of the cells, hemoglobin is concentrated ("puddled") in discrete areas on the cell periphery.

The mechanism of cellular dehydration is unclear and complex, involving a net potassium loss from the cells that is not accompanied by a proportional gain of sodium. Consequently, the net intracellular cation content and cell water are decreased. In some reports a decrease in RBC 2,3-DPG has also been noted.

Most HX patients have heterozygous missense mutations in PIEZO1. *In vitro* studies of HX-associated PIEZO1 mutations demonstrate a gain-of-function phenotype, with many mutants demonstrating delayed channel inactivation, indicating increased cation permeability may lead to dehydration of HX erythrocytes. Piezo proteins are putative ion channels mediating mechanosensory transduction in mammalian cells. Animal models suggest mechanically activated Piezo1 plays a critical role in erythrocyte volume homeostasis. In a small subset of HX patients, defects of the Gardos channel encoded by the *KCNN4* gene have been described.

Some of the reported cases of hereditary stomatocytosis share features of both hereditary stomatocytosis and xerocytosis categorized as "intermediate" syndromes. These patients characteristically have both stomatocytes and some target cells on the peripheral blood smear. Osmotic fragility is either normal or slightly increased. Sodium and potassium permeability is somewhat increased, but the intracellular cation concentration and the RBC volume are either normal or slightly reduced. These cells were reported to have subnormal glutathione content. In some patients, RBCs undergo in vitro hemolysis at 5°C, hence the designation *cryohydrocytosis*. A similar susceptibility to cold-induced cation permeability in which potassium and water loss predominates and xerocytes instead of hydrocytes are present, has also been described.

A study of stomatocytosis, spherocytosis, and spherostomatocytosis patients whose erythrocytes demonstrated significant cation leaks at 0°C and in some cases, band 3–deficient membranes, revealed a series of missense mutations located in an intramembrane domain of band 3. In vitro studies suggest that these mutations convert band 3 from an anion exchanger to a nonselective cation leak channel.

Several investigators have also reported a dominantly inherited hemolytic anemia with stomatocytosis, occasional target cells, spherocytes, and a decreased osmotic fragility in which the main RBC membrane abnormality involved a nearly 50% increase in phosphatidylcholine and a corresponding decrease in phosphatidylethanolamine. Because abnormalities in membrane phospholipid composition have not been systematically investigated, it is uncertain whether the disorder represents a distinct disease entity.

The results of splenectomy in this group of disorders are variable. In some patients, the hemolytic anemia is improved, although often not fully corrected, by splenectomy, whereas in others, the severity of the hemolysis is unchanged. Splenectomy should be carefully considered in patients with hereditary stomatocytosis. Several patients with stomatocytosis (both hydrocytosis and xerocytosis) have developed hypercoagulability after splenectomy, leading to catastrophic thrombotic episodes or chronic pulmonary hypertension. Fortunately, the majority of persons with hereditary stomatocytosis are able to maintain an adequate hemoglobin level, so that splenectomy is not required.

Rh Deficiency Syndrome

Rh deficiency syndrome designates rare individuals who have either absent (Rh$_{null}$) or markedly reduced (Rh$_{mod}$) Rh antigen expression, mild to moderate hemolytic anemia associated with the presence of stomatocytes, and occasional spherocytes on the peripheral blood film. Hemolytic anemia is improved by splenectomy.

The Rh antigens are present in ~20,000 to 30,000 copies per cell and reside on minor transmembrane proteins with an electrophoretic mobility of 28 to 33 kDa on SDS-PAGE. The Rh gene locus encodes two closely linked genes, one encoding the D polypeptide and the other encoding the CcEe proteins, the antigenic expression of which is a consequence of alternate splicing of their pre-mRNA.

Rh proteins are part of a multiprotein complex that includes two Rh proteins and two Rh-associated glycoproteins (RhAG). Other proteins that associate with this complex include CD47, LW, glycophorin B, and protein 4.2. The Rh-RhAG complex interacts with ankyrin to link the membrane skeleton to the lipid bilayer. The Rh proteins share sequence homology to the Mep/Amt family of ammonium transporters in lower organisms and may participate in ammonium transport.

Rh$_{null}$ erythrocytes have no Rh antigen and have reduced or absent LW, Fy5, Ss, U, and Duclos antigens. Rh, RhAG, LW, glycophorin B, CD47, and protein 4.2 are also reduced or absent. Rh$_{null}$ erythrocytes have increased osmotic fragility, reflecting a marked reduction in membrane surface area. These cells are also dehydrated, as indicated by decreased cell cation and water content and increased cell density. The potassium transport and the Na$^+$/K$^+$ pump activity are increased, possibly because of reticulocytosis. Phospholipid asymmetry is also altered.

Although the clinical syndromes are the same, the genetic basis of the Rh deficiency syndrome is heterogeneous, and at least two groups have been defined. The amorph type is caused by defects involving the RH30 locus encoding the RhD and RhE polypeptides. The regulatory type of Rh$_{null}$ and Rh$_{mod}$ phenotypes results from suppressor or modifier mutations at the RH50 locus. When one chain of the Rh-RhAG complex is absent, the complex either is not transported to or is assembled at the membrane.

Familial Deficiency of High-Density Lipoproteins

Familial deficiency or absence of high-density lipoproteins (Tangier disease) because of mutations in ABCA1, a protein involved in cellular export of cholesterol, leads to accumulation of cholesterol esters in many tissues. Clinical manifestations include large orange tonsils, hepatosplenomegaly, lymphadenopathy, cloudy corneas, and peripheral neuropathy. Reported hematologic manifestations include a moderately severe hemolytic anemia with stomatocytosis and thrombocytopenia. Erythrocyte membrane lipid analyses reveal a low free cholesterol content, leading to a decreased cholesterol/phospholipid ratio and a relative increase in phosphatidylcholine at the expense of sphingomyelin.

Sitosterolemia

Sitosterolemia or phytosterolemia is a recessive disorder associated with elevated plasma levels of plant sterols. Affected patients exhibit xanthomatosis and early-onset premature cardiovascular disease. Reported hematologic manifestations include hemolytic anemia with stomatocytosis and macrothrombocytopenia. Mutations in the transporters ABCG5 or ABCG8 lead to gastrointestinal hyperabsorption and decreased biliary elimination of plant sterols as well as altered cholesterol metabolism. Plant sterols are not synthesized endogenously in humans but are passively absorbed in the intestine. ABCG5 and ABCG8 actively pump plant sterols out of the intestinal cells back into the intestine and out of liver cells into bile ducts. It has been hypothesized that the stomatocytic phenotype is caused by intercalation of plant sterols into the inner leaflet of the lipid bilayer.

Acquired Stomatocytosis

Stomatocytes have been noted in diverse acquired conditions, including neoplasms, cardiovascular and hepatobiliary disease, alcoholism, and therapy with drugs, some of which are known to be stomatocytogenic in vitro. In some of these conditions, the percentage of stomatocytes on the peripheral blood smear can approach 100%. However, the clinical significance of this observation is unclear because stomatocytes are absent in most patients with the conditions listed. Furthermore, some stomatocytes can be found in normal individuals (3–5%). The most consistent association is that of stomatocytosis and heavy alcohol consumption.

RED CELL MEMBRANE VARIANTS AND INFECTIOUS DISEASE

Viral, bacterial, and parasitic infection can all cause anemia. Multiple mechanisms leading to hemolysis have been described. As mentioned earlier in this chapter, parvovirus B19 selectively infects erythroblasts through interaction with globoside, which encodes the P blood group antigen and temporarily shuts down erythropoiesis. Although this infection is tolerated well by healthy patients, it can lead to severe, at times life-threatening, aplastic crises in patients with anemias because of premature erythrocyte destruction. As one might predict, parvovirus cannot invade erythroblasts of the rare P-negative individuals.

Most infections cause hemolytic anemias triggered by several distinct, and at times overlapping, mechanisms. *Plasmodium, Babesia,* and *Bartonella* species directly attack the membrane and lyse the red cells. Some bacteria, such as *Clostridium perfringens,* elaborate hemolytic toxins or phospholipases that damage the membrane. Other infectious agents trigger occasional production of autoantibodies against red cell membrane components, which in turn leads to autoimmune hemolytic anemia. Finally, many sepsis syndromes are associated with anemia because of disseminated intravascular coagulation.

Malaria and the Erythrocyte Membrane

The red cell membrane defects described earlier in this chapter cause mild to severe hemolytic anemias. At the same time, many red cell membrane alterations have developed as a defense against microorganisms and parasites invading and lysing red cells. This is especially true for malarial parasites. Although four different species of the malaria parasite *Plasmodium,* including *P. falciparum, P. ovale, P. vivax,* and *P. malariae,* infect humans, almost all of the 1.5 to 2 million annual deaths caused by malaria are attributable to *P. falciparum.*

Because malaria coexisted with humans over the course of human evolution, it comes as no surprise that multiple erythroid genotypes were selected that confer some level of resistance to infection or mitigate disease severity. The ensuing heritable phenotypes include, among others, resistance to red cell adhesion and/or invasion, slower intraerythrocytic growth, decreased or increased adhesion of infected red cells to vascular endothelium, and increased phagocytosis of parasitized red cells.

Malaria and other infections causing hemolytic anemias are described in more detail in Chapter 158, which also discusses hemoglobinopathies and red cell enzyme variants that reduce invasion and/ or retard parasite growth. Consequently, we focus here on the heritable erythrocyte membrane alterations that developed as a defense against malaria.

Erythrocyte Preference

Two parasites, *P. vivax* and *P. ovale,* selectively infect reticulocytes, whereas *P. malariae* infects older erythrocytes. In contrast, *P. falciparum* infects red cells of all ages. This fact and the tendency of *P. falciparum*-infected erythrocytes to sequester in circulation explain the markedly higher severity of *P. falciparum* malaria.

Attachment and Invasion

Duffy Antigen
The *P. vivax* merozoite is completely dependent on attachment to the Duffy blood group antigen (also known as the *Duffy antigen receptor for chemokines [DARC]*) for erythrocyte invasion, and consequently it cannot invade Duffy-negative RBCs. It has been hypothesized that this is why the Duffy-negative phenotype is common in large areas of Africa. The Duffy-negative phenotype is caused by mutation in a *GATA1* motif in the Duffy antigen gene promoter, preventing its expression in erythroid cells, leaving its expression in other tissues intact. Elucidation of this mutation explained a long-standing conundrum of transfusion medicine: why individuals with the Duffy-negative phenotype never develop antibodies against the Duffy antigen.

Glycophorins
All major erythrocyte glycophorins, A, B, and C/D, are involved in attachment of *P. falciparum* to the RBC membrane. Consequently,

invasion of *P. falciparum* into red cells from patients lacking glycophorin A (En[a−]), glycophorin B (S-s-U−), or glycophorins C and D (Gerbich negative, Ge−) is diminished. As noted earlier, the Gerbich-negative phenotype is associated with mild, asymptomatic ovalocytosis.

Protein 4.1R and Spectrin
Deficiency of protein 4.1R or self-association defects of spectrin are associated with elliptocytosis of varying severity. Both phenotypes appear to reduce the burden of RBC invasion.

Band 3 and Southeast Asian Ovalocytosis
Conflicting explanations of the basis of the protective phenotype of SAO (described earlier) from malaria have been described. Initial reports suggested that SAO erythrocytes were resistant to malarial invasion. These results were repeatedly questioned until recent studies demonstrated SAO cells to be resistant to invasion by the more virulent *P. falciparum* strains. This may explain the apparent contradiction with the reports of comparable parasitemias in SAO carriers and patients with a normal red cell phenotype from Papua New Guinea.

The protection from cerebral malaria afforded by SAO erythrocytes is likely because of reduced cytoadherence of SAO red cells to the cerebral vasculature. Under conditions of flow, *P. falciparum*-infected ovalocytes adhere more strongly than normal infected red cells to the endothelial receptor CD36. Because this receptor is not expressed in the brain, this raises a possibility that ovalocytosis protects from cerebral malaria by diminishing the number of parasitized red cells available for adhesion to the cerebral vasculature via alternative receptors. Moreover, ovalocytes appeared resistant to invasion by parasite strains that tend to bind to intracellular adhesion molecule I (ICAM1), the likely receptor for cytoadherence in the brain, but the exact mechanism is not yet known.

Knops Blood Group System
Severe malaria, particularly cerebral malaria, has been associated with the formation of rosettes, clumps of cells formed by the adhesion of malaria-infected erythrocytes to complement receptor 1 (CR1) on uninfected erythrocytes. Identification of the Knops blood group antigens on CR1, followed by observations that frequencies of various Knops antigens varied significantly in whites and individuals of African ancestry, led to the hypothesis that some Knops group antigens might be protective from rosetting and severe malaria. Case control studies with genotyping and/or flow cytometry have yielded conflicting results, but several have linked low-expression CR1 alleles with malaria resistance. Further studies have shown that the expression of CR1 and other complement proteins increases with age. Together these data suggest that genetic and age-related differences in complement protein expression contribute to the variability observed in individuals with severe malaria.

Although these erythrocyte membrane polymorphisms offer fascinating insight into natural defenses against one of the most serious diseases affecting humans, the mechanism of resistance to malaria has not been fully elucidated for any of them. Malaria has clearly had a profound impact on the genetic makeup of populations living in endemic areas and provided us with multiple clues about the host-parasite relationship. Better understanding of these natural defenses might eventually be converted into effective therapeutic interventions.

SUGGESTED READINGS

Bagriantsev SN, Gracheva EO, Gallagher PG: Piezo proteins: regulators of mechanosensation and other cellular processes. *J Biol Chem* 289:31673–31681, 2014.

Barcellini W, Bianchi P, Fermo E, et al: Hereditary red cell membrane defects: diagnostic and clinical aspects. *Blood Transfus* 9:274–277, 2011.

Basu A, Chakrabarti A: Defects in erythrocyte membrane skeletal architecture. *Adv Exp Med Biol* 842:41–59, 2015.

Bianchi P, Fermo E, Vercellati C, et al: Diagnostic power of laboratory tests for hereditary spherocytosis: a comparison study in 150 patients grouped according to molecular and clinical characteristics. *Haematologica* 97:516–523, 2012.

Bolton-Maggs PH, Langer JC, Iolascon A, et al: Guidelines for the diagnosis and management of hereditary spherocytosis—2011 update. *Br J Haematol* 156:37–49, 2012.

Brugnara C, Mohandas N: Red cell indices in classification and treatment of anemias: from M.M. Wintrobes's original 1934 classification to the third millennium. *Curr Opin Hematol* 20:222–230, 2013.

Buesing KL, Tracy ET, Kiernan C, et al: Partial splenectomy for hereditary spherocytosis: a multi-institutional review. *J Pediatr Surg* 46:178–183, 2011.

Christensen RD, Yaish HM, Gallagher PG: A pediatrician's practical guide to diagnosing and treating hereditary spherocytosis in neonates. *Pediatrics* 135:1107–1114, 2015.

Cluitmans JC, Tomelleri C, Yapici Z, et al: Abnormal red cell structure and function in neuroacanthocytosis. *PLoS ONE* 10:e0125580, 2015.

Colin Y, Le Van Kim C, El Nemer W: Red cell adhesion in human diseases. *Curr Opin Hematol* 21:186–192, 2014.

Cordat E, Reithmeier RA: Structure, function, and trafficking of SLC4 and SLC26 anion transporters. *Curr Top Membr* 73:1–67, 2014.

Da Costa L, Galimand J, Fenneteau O, et al: Hereditary spherocytosis, elliptocytosis, and other red cell membrane disorders. *Blood Rev* 27:167–178, 2013.

Das A, Bansal D, Ahluwalia J, et al: Risk factors for thromboembolism and pulmonary artery hypertension following splenectomy in children with hereditary spherocytosis. *Pediatr Blood Cancer* 61:29–33, 2014.

De Franceschi L, Bosman GJ, Mohandas N: Abnormal red cell features associated with hereditary neurodegenerative disorders: the neuroacanthocytosis syndromes. *Curr Opin Hematol* 21:201–209, 2014.

Gallagher PG: Abnormalities of the erythrocyte membrane. *Pediatr Clin North Am* 60:1349–1362, 2013.

Gallagher PG: Disorders of red cell volume regulation. *Curr Opin Hematol* 20:201–207, 2013.

Garnett C, Bain BJ: South-East Asian ovalocytosis. *Am J Hematol* 88:328, 2013.

Glogowska E, Gallagher PG: Disorders of erythrocyte volume homeostasis. *Int J Lab Hematol* 37(S1):85–91, 2015.

Glogowska E, Lezon-Geyda K, Maksimova Y, et al: Mutations in the Gardos channel (KCNN4) are associated with hereditary xerocytosis. *Blood* 126:1281–1284, 2015.

King MJ, Garcon L, Hoyer JD, et al: ICSH guidelines for the laboratory diagnosis of nonimmune hereditary red cell membrane disorders. *Int J Lab Hematol* 37:304–325, 2015.

Mayeur-Rousse C, Gentil M, Botton J, et al: Testing for hereditary spherocytosis: a French experience. *Haematologica* 97:e48–e49, author reply e52, 2012.

Rapetti-Mauss R, Lacoste C, Picard V, et al: A mutation in the Gardos channel is associated with hereditary xerocytosis. *Blood* 126:1273–1280, 2015.

Rice HE, Englum BR, Rothman J, et al: Clinical outcomes of splenectomy in children: report of the splenectomy in congenital hemolytic anemia registry. *Am J Hematol* 90:187–192, 2015.

Sakamoto TM, Canalli AA, Traina F, et al: Altered red cell and platelet adhesion in hemolytic diseases: hereditary spherocytosis, paroxysmal nocturnal hemoglobinuria and sickle cell disease. *Clin Biochem* 46:1798–1803, 2013.

Seims AD, Breckler FD, Hardacker KD, et al: Partial versus total splenectomy in children with hereditary spherocytosis. *Surgery* 154:849–853, discussion 53-55, 2013.

Walker RH, Schulz VP, Tikhonova IR, et al: Genetic diagnosis of neuroacanthocytosis disorders using exome sequencing. *Mov Disord* 27:539–543, 2012.

CHAPTER 46

AUTOIMMUNE HEMOLYTIC ANEMIA

Marc Michel and Ulrich Jäger

Autoimmune hemolytic anemia (AIHA) is caused by autoimmune-mediated destruction of red blood cells (RBCs) by autoantibodies with various properties and target specificities. Exact laboratory diagnosis is often difficult; therefore, experienced diagnostic reference centers play an important role. The disease can be primary (idiopathic) or caused by an underlying condition (secondary), including autoimmune diseases, infections, drugs, or neoplasms. The clinical course of the disease as well as treatment decisions are influenced by the type of antibody involved. Success in treatment and the evaluation of therapies have lagged behind the achievements in laboratory diagnosis but will hopefully improve with the introduction of new effective drugs. Currently, almost all treatments in AIHA are based on experience and opinion but not on evidence. There are no established guidelines. Thus, management of the disease requires general hematologic skills and critical evaluation of treatment recommendations.

HISTORY

The history of diagnostic and therapeutic progress in AIHA has been described by Dacie,[1] one of the great pioneers in this field. Milestones were the discovery of the first RBC autoantibody (Donath–Landsteiner antibody) in 1904, the introduction of the Coombs test in 1945, the establishment of splenectomy as effective treatment of AIHA in the 1950s, and the finding that rituximab is an effective treatment in the past decade. The diagnosis and treatment of patients with AIHA were recently reviewed by several authors.[2-8]

EPIDEMIOLOGY

Because only a low proportion of patients have spontaneous or treatment-induced long-term remissions and the death rate is low, the prevalence of AIHA is relatively high and has been estimated as 17 in 100,000 (in Denmark). The incidence of AIHA in children and teenagers is 0.2–1.0 per million per year.[9] There is some evidence of a familial clustering of AIHA in children, but no hereditary genetic background has been identified.

Primary AIHA and Evans syndrome are slightly more prevalent in women and in children.[10] In secondary AIHA, the female-to-male ratio is very high in systemic lupus erythematosus (SLE), but low in chronic lymphocytic leukemia (CLL)-associated AIHA. The incidence of chronic cold agglutinin disease (CAD) is estimated to be one per million per year, with a female prevalence. Geographical differences have been suggested, with a higher incidence of CAD in Northern climates.

PATHOBIOLOGY

Hemolysis is initiated when an autoantibody binds to the RBC membranes and recruits complement. Destruction of the RBC can occur directly in the circulation (intravascular hemolysis) or by removal of the cell by macrophages in the spleen, liver, or both (extravascular hemolysis) (Fig. 46.1). Several immunoglobulin (Ig) subclasses can fix complement: IgG, IgA, and IgM. Macrophages recognize opsonized erythrocytes via receptors specific for the Fc fragment of IgG and for C3d. RBCs coated with IgG or complement alone are destroyed in the spleen and liver, IgG-coated cells in the spleen, and IgM-coated cells in the liver.[11,12] This has major implications for treatment, particularly for the effect of steroids and splenectomy.

Warm Antibody Hemolytic Anemia

About 70% to 80% of cases of AIHA are caused by WAIHAs. The RBC antibodies in WAIHAs are mostly polyclonal IgG (IgG$_{1-4}$), which have a low capacity to activate the complement system (Table 46.1). The direct antiglobulin test (DAT) in WAIHAs is positive either with IgG (37%) or IgG + C3d (43%). Rarely, the DAT is only positive with C3d (when the amount of IgG on the RBCs is very small). Patients with IgG antibodies may have also IgA antibodies, but IgA antibodies without IgG antibodies are a very rare cause of WAIHAs. WAIHAs are often directed against Rh antigens but also against other blood group antigens (non–Rh-related autoantibodies) such as band 3 protein or glycophorin A. The antibodies fix complement and bind tightly to the RBCs at 37°C. Therefore, there is only a small amount of antibody detectable in the serum. The antibody-coated RBCs are removed from the circulation by splenic (to a lesser degree also by hepatic) macrophages via F$_{c\gamma}$RIII receptors. IgG$_3$ and IgG$_1$ have the highest affinity for the Fc receptors of macrophages. Erythrocytes that are only partially phagocytosed by the macrophages become spherocytes, which are removed in the splenic cords because of their rigid structure. Destruction of RBCs may also be caused by other mechanisms such as antibody-dependent cellular cytotoxicity.[13]

IgM WAIHAs are a very rare cause of AIHA. This type of AIHA can be suspected if RBC autoagglutination occurs at room temperature. The DAT result is positive with C3d alone (65%) or with IgG (24%). Using sensitive methods, IgM on the RBCs can be detected in 71%.[14] Non-Hodgkin lymphoma (NHL) is the underlying disease in some of these cases. This AIHA is severe, often fatal, and refractory to steroids and splenectomy.

Cold Antibody Hemolytic Anemia

CAIHAs in primary or secondary CAIHA are usually monoclonal IgM. The IgM has two binding sites for C1q and fixes complement easily. The targets are polysaccharides (I, I^T, i, or Pr antigens). The "i" antigen is a nonbranched polysaccharide in the cord blood, and the "I" antigen is a similar but branched molecule expressed in the RBCs of adults. The CAIHAs bind to the RBCs at low temperatures and cause their lysis at temperatures above 22°C. The DAT is typically positive with C3d alone. When CAIHAs are present at high titers, they may activate the complement system directly and produce a membrane attack complex and intravascular hemolysis with hemoglobinuria. Usually the complement-coated RBCs are sequestered by liver macrophages.

Paroxysmal cold hemoglobinuria (PCH) is caused by the Donath–Landsteiner (DL) antibody. This is a rare, usually polyclonal IgG cold antibody to P antigen (glycosphingolipid globoside), which binds to the RBCs at 4°C. The cells are lysed at higher temperatures. The DAT is positive with C3d, and the diagnosis is made by the DL test. In this test, normal RBCs and patient and normal serum are

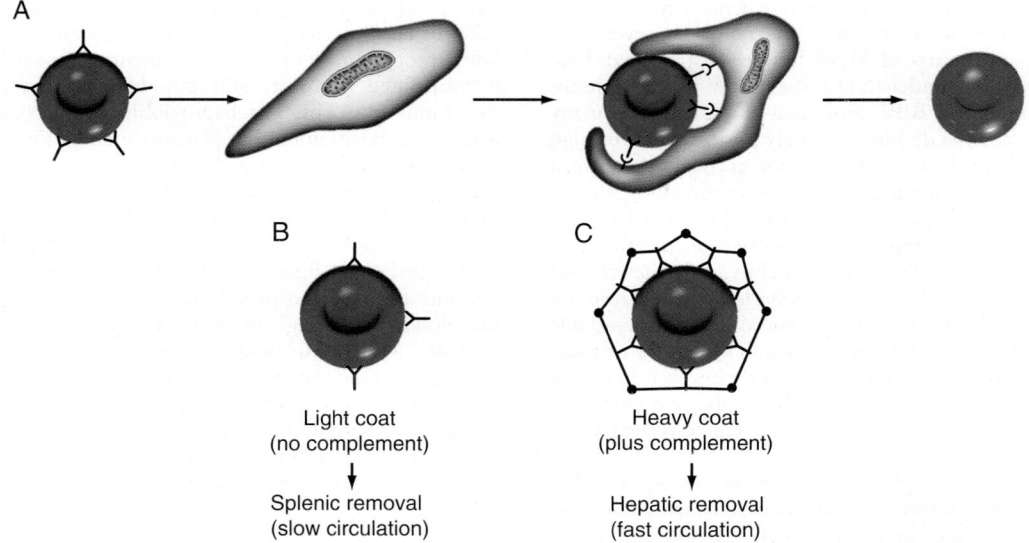

Fig. 46.1 MECHANISM OF EXTRAVASCULAR HEMOLYSIS IN AUTOIMMUNE HEMOLYTIC ANEMIA. (A) Macrophage encounters an IgG-coated erythrocyte and binds to it via its Fc receptors. Thus entrapped, the red blood cell (RBC) loses bits of its membrane as a result of digestion by the macrophage's ectoenzymes. The discoid erythrocyte transforms into a sphere. (B) RBCs lightly coated with IgG (and therefore incapable of activating the complement cascade) are preferentially removed in the sluggish circulation of the spleen. (C) RBCs with a heavy coat of IgG; thus, C3b *(black circles)* can be removed both by the spleen and the liver. *(Courtesy Cunningham MJ, Silberstein LE: Autoimmune hemolytic anemia. In: Hoffman R, Benz EJ Jr, Shattil SJ, et al, eds: Hematology: basic principles and practice, ed 4, Philadelphia, 2005, Elsevier.)*

TABLE 46.1   Properties and Specificities of Red Blood Cell Autoantibodies

	Immunoglobulin (Subclass)	Type of Antibody	Clonality	Specificity	Hemolysis	Site of Removal of Red Blood Cells
WAIHAs	IgG$_{(1-4)}$, IgA	Incomplete	Mostly polyclonal	Rh-antigens and non-Rh-antigens	Extravascular	Spleen (liver)
CAIHAs	IgM	Complete	Mostly clonal	Anti-i, -I^T, -I, -Pr	Intravascular	Liver
Donath–Landsteiner antibody	IgG	—	Polyclonal	P antigen	Intravascular	—

CAIHA, Cold autoimmune hemolytic anemia; Ig, immunoglobulin; WAIHA, warm autoimmune hemolytic anemia.

incubated at 4°C. Agglutination occurs after warming to 37°C. The prominent clinical feature of PCH is a brisk, immediate but sometimes also delayed hemoglobinuria after cold exposure even in patients with low antibody titers. In the past, it has been associated with secondary or tertiary syphilis. Now, two types can be distinguished clinically[15]: (1) an acute, severe form (often associated with hemoglobinuria) but self-limiting AIHA after (respiratory) infections in children, and (2) a rare, chronic AIHA in nonsyphilitic persons with various underlying conditions, including NHL. Patients with chronic PCH respond poorly to steroids and splenectomy.

Mixed Warm and Cold AIHA

A small number of patients have a mixed AIHA with a positive DAT for both IgG and C3d indicating coexistence of warm IgG autoantibodies and high-titer cold agglutinins.[16]

ETIOLOGY AND PATHOPHYSIOLOGY

Our knowledge about the etiology of AIHA is still limited. Factors that may play a role are antigen mimicry; immune deficiency; and, to a lesser extent, probably genetic factors. AIHA, similar to other autoimmune diseases, is a consequence of the loss of immunologic (self-) tolerance against antigens expressed on the erythrocyte surface.

Production of RBC antibodies is a result of the interaction of T and B cells, as well as regulatory factors (e.g., T regulatory cells, cytokines).[17] Disturbances of the Th1/2 T-cell subset balance as well as the occurrence of clonal regulatory T cells specific for a RBC autoantigen have been described. This may be linked to the fact that AIHA does not only occur in immunocompetent individuals but frequently occurs in patients with acquired T-cell defects such as HIV infection or immunosuppressive therapy, particularly after organ transplantation. Polymorphisms or altered expression of negative regulators of T-cell responses such as cytotoxic T lymphocyte antigen 4 (CTLA4) or interleukin-10 may also play a role. Mouse models (New Zealand black mice) have revealed an association of genetic loci with antierythrocyte antibody production or cold agglutinin escape tolerance after *Mycoplasma* infection.

Various target antigens have been described, with Rhesus polypeptides, glycophorin, and erythrocyte band 3 being the most prominent in WAIHA. Cold reactive antibodies frequently target the I or i blood group-specific antigens. Events linked to the development of secondary AIHA by induction of cross-tolerance (molecular mimicry) are infections (*Mycoplasma pneumoniae* [I antigen target], parvovirus, herpes viruses), neoplastic diseases (paraneoplasia), and drugs by various mechanisms. There are important differences in the pathogenesis of WAIHA and CAIHA. The pathogenesis of primary WAIHA is largely unknown. Secondary WAIHA is a complication of several congenital or acquired immune deficiencies. Both moderate (e.g., in CLL) and severe (HIV, posttransplant, congenital severe

T-cell deficiencies) T-cell and humoral immune deficiency predispose to WAIHA, but no correlation between the type and severity of immune deficiency and the risk of AIHA has been established. One phenomenon that is poorly understood is the lack of a clear relationship between the presence of RBC antibodies and anemia. In many instances, there is no anemia despite a strongly positive DAT or high titers of CAIHAs. There is also only a poor correlation between antibody titers and severity of anemia. Another unexplained finding in secondary AIHA is the occurrence of both WAIHAs and CAIHAs in the some condition; for example, in lymphomas or infections.

Antibodies in primary AIHA are frequently polyreactive and polyclonal (no clonal B cells detected by polymerase chain reaction [PCR]). Antibodies in CAD are mostly produced by PCR-detectable oligoclonal or monoclonal B-cell populations. The nature of these antibodies has been extensively studied in CAD. However, in only a few cases has it been established that the RBC antibody is clonal. In most reports, clonality of RBC antibodies was assumed if the patient had a paraproteinemia.

B-cell neoplasms expressing IgMκ antibodies directed against RBC antigens have few somatic mutations, which seem to be fairly restricted to certain Ig heavy and light chain families (VH4-34, VκIV).[18] Moreover, a VH4-34 CLL confounding subclone was shown to arise from a preexisting CAD-producing B-cell population. The restricted clonality of CAD-producing B cells is further corroborated by the detection of clonal Ig rearrangements and recurrent chromosomal aberrations (trisomy 3).[19,20] CLL cells may also drive AIHA by presenting the autoantigen (e.g., erythrocyte protein band 3) to T cells.

SYMPTOMS, CLINICAL FINDINGS, AND RISKS

The symptoms of AIHA depend on the type of antibody, the mode of onset, and the severity of anemia. In patients with WAIHA, the onset is mostly gradual or subacute, and the symptoms (i.e., tiredness, reduction of physical activity, and shortness of breath in elderly patients) are attributable only to anemia. However, patients with postinfectious, drug-induced AIHA, or patients with DL or Pr antibodies often present with acute severe symptoms such as malaise, fever, jaundice, abdominal pain, shortness of breath, and hemoglobulinuria. The course in such patients may be fulminant and even fatal. Patients with chronic CAIHA (CAD) often have an indolent course. Symptoms suggestive of CAIHA are cold sensitivity, cold-dependent acrocyanosis, acral numbness, and rarely livedo reticularis. Anemia worsens after cold exposure or conditions associated with an acute phase reaction.

During clinical examination, a subicterus may be seen. Lymphadenopathy, palpable splenomegaly, or any organomegaly is rare in patients with primary AIHA. Its presence suggests secondary AIHA.

Patients with WAIHA are at an increased risk of venous thromboembolism, sometimes associated with a lupus anticoagulant (LA).[21,22] Older patients with AIHA are at an increased risk of cardiovascular complications, which may also be partly caused by the treatment.

LABORATORY DIAGNOSIS OF AUTOIMMUNE HEMOLYTIC ANEMIA

AIHA is essentially a laboratory diagnosis. The diagnostic pathway of AIHA should proceed in a stepwise fashion answering the following questions:

Step 1: Hemolytic Anemia?

The first step is to establish the diagnosis of hemolytic anemia (see box on Four Important Questions for the Diagnosis and Management of Autoimmune Hemolytic Anemia). This diagnosis is established by the presence of the following pentad of findings: normocytic or macrocytic anemia (male hemoglobin (Hb) <13.0–14.0 g/dL;

female <12.0 g/dL), reticulocytosis (corrected reticulocyte count >2% or absolute reticulocyte count >100,000/μL to 120,000/μL), low haptoglobin, elevated lactate dehydrogenase (LDH), and elevated unconjugated (indirect) bilirubin. Haptoglobin is an α2-globulin that binds Hb. This Hb–haptoglobin complex is degraded in the liver. Hemopexin is another plasma protein with a very high binding affinity to Hb. It scavenges heme released from RBCs and protects the organisms from the adverse effects of circulating Hb. The determination of hemopexin is not essential for the diagnosis of AIHA. Indirect bilirubin is usually not more than 5 mg/dL except in associated liver disease (Epstein-Barr [EBV]-associated AIHA). Additional findings are increased urobilinogen in the urine and spherocytes in the blood smear (Fig. 46.2). Leukoerythroblastosis occurs only in peracute AIHA, but microangiopathic hemolytic anemia should always be suspected in such cases. Bone marrow examination is usually not necessary except in patients in whom secondary AIHA, in particular lymphoma, is suspected. RBC survival is shortened, but its measurement with radioisotopes has no diagnostic value, not even for the prediction of the efficacy of splenectomy.

Four Important Questions for the Diagnosis and Management of Autoimmune Hemolytic Anemia

It is of utmost importance to differentiate between various types of AIHA. A stepwise approach helps in making the right decisions:

Question 1: Hemolytic anemia? The basic features of hemolytic anemia are low haptoglobin levels, elevated indirect bilirubin, and elevated LDH.

Question 2: Autoimmune hemolytic anemia? A DAT is initially performed with a polyspecific antibody to detect IgG or complement C3d bound to RBCs. If the DAT result is positive, the diagnosis of AIHA is established.

Question 3: Warm or Cold Autoimmune Hemolytic Anemia? The DAT is further elaborated with monospecific antibodies to IgG and complement (C3d). If the DAT result is positive with IgG alone or with IgG + C3d, the AIHA is most probably caused by a warm antibody (WAIHA). If the DAT is positive with C3d only, the AIHA is most probably caused by a cold antibody (CAIHA).

Question 4: Primary or secondary AIHA? More than half of AIHAs are secondary to underlying diseases. Secondary AIHA should be suspected in patients with additional findings or who are refractory to initial steroid treatment. In this case, the underlying disease has to be diagnosed (e.g., by serologic tests, computed tomography (CT) scan, or bone marrow biopsy).

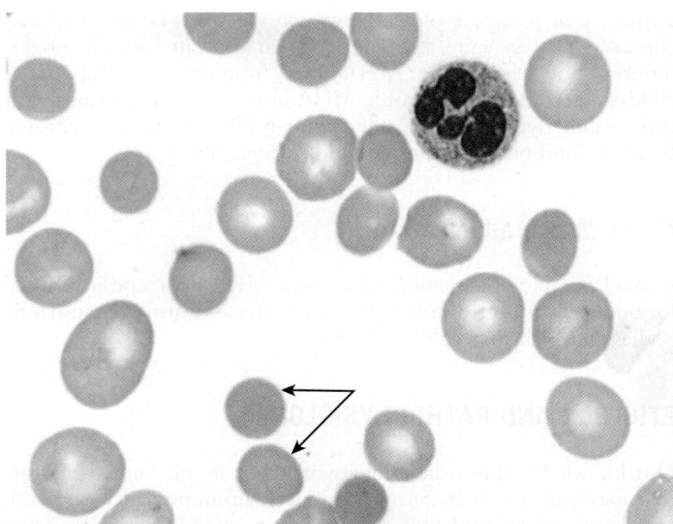

Fig. 46.2 BLOOD SMEAR SHOWING NUMEROUS SPHEROCYTES *(ARROWS).*

Among methodologic diagnostic problems, reticulocyte counting is the biggest, because in many laboratories low-precision microscopic counts are still performed. Automatic flow cytometric methods are more precise, reliable, and convenient. With flow cytometry, the number of highly fluorescent reticulocytes (which are increased in AIHA but are low in hereditary spherocytosis) can also be measured. Falsely very high mean corpuscular volume (MCV) and mean corpuscular Hb concentration occur in some cases of CAIHA because RBC counts are falsely low because of agglutination of RBC at room temperature. If a CAIHA is suspected, blood samples should be sent to the laboratory in warmed containers.

All of the findings of the pentad are not always present. Reticulocytosis is often (in ≈25%) not present at the onset of AIHA. This is mostly because of a delayed initial bone marrow response of erythropoiesis. After 1 week, most of these patients have reticulocytosis. In other patients (particularly in secondary cases), absence of reticulocytosis may be attributable to impairment of erythropoiesis caused by bone marrow infiltration or blunted erythropoiesis caused by an acute-phase reaction. If the reticulocyte count is very low, pure RBC aplasia (PRCA), either immune mediated or induced by a parvovirus (or HHV6) infection, should be suspected. Haptoglobin may be falsely normal or even increased, particularly in patients with malignant or immune diseases, because haptoglobin is an acute-phase protein. Haptoglobin may be falsely low in patients with a haplotype H_0H_0 and in patients with severe liver disease. Both increased bilirubin and elevated LDH have a limited specificity for AIHA.

Step 2: Autoimmune Hemolytic Anemia?

The next step is to find out whether the hemolytic anemia is an AIHA. This is best done by the DAT (Fig. 46.3). In this test, washed RBCs of the patient (obtained from an ethylenediaminetetraacetic acid [EDTA] blood sample) are incubated in a tube with a polyspecific antibody to IgG and complement (C3d). If the RBCs agglutinate, the test result is positive. In many laboratories, the tube test has been replaced by the tube gel test, which is easier to perform, more

reliable, and probably more sensitive (Fig. 46.4). In the indirect antiglobulin test (IAT), patient plasma or serum is incubated with test RBCs, and (after washing) RBC-bound IgG is detected with the DAT. IAT is usually not required for the diagnosis of AIHA except when a drug-dependent antibody is suspected. For the differentiation of drug-dependent antibodies and autoantibodies, an acid eluate of the patient's RBCs should be made and tested in the IAT. If the IAT result is positive, the patient has autoantibodies. The severity of AIHA does not correlate with the strength of the DAT but rather with the immunoglobulin subclass of the antibody (IgG_1 or IgG_3). The result of the DAT is not a reliable marker of treatment success because patients with a complete hematologic remission may remain DAT positive, and DAT positivity or negativity has only limited value to predict the duration of hematologic remission.

Falsely Negative and Positive Direct Antiglobulin Test Results Without Hemolysis or Anemia

If the conventional DAT test result is negative, hemolytic anemia is defined as DAT negative. However, AIHA cannot be definitely excluded because about 5% (2% to 11%) of AIHA patients are DAT negative. If AIHA is suspected for clinical grounds despite a negative DAT result, more sensitive quantitative tests are required to determine the amount of IgG on the RBCs. The threshold of positivity of the conventional DAT is 100–200 IgG molecules per RBC, but in some AIHA patients, the RBC IgG is less than this amount. In about one-third of DAT-negative cases, one of the more sensitive test results (e.g., immunoradiometric tests) will be positive. However, the relationship between the amount of RBC IgG and hemolysis is not clear cut, and there is no "hemolysis threshold."[23] The reasons for these discrepancies between the in vitro and in vivo activity of RBC antibodies are largely unknown. Differences in macrophage activity may be one possible explanation. A search for antibodies in the RBC eluate in which antibodies are more concentrated is also useful. IgA antibodies are rare and sometimes not included in the analysis. Finally, there is the possibility of low-affinity antibodies. Such antibodies are washed out when the washes are made with 37°C saline. A high rate of DAT-negative AIHA has been observed in AIHA induced by nucleoside analogues but also in other secondary AIHA.

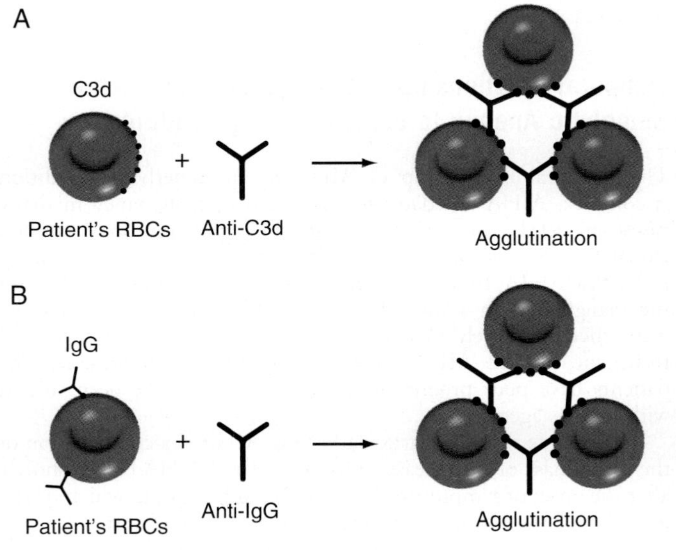

A

C3d

Patient's RBCs   +   Anti-C3d   →   Agglutination

B

IgG

Patient's RBCs   +   Anti-IgG   →   Agglutination

Fig. 46.3 DIRECT ANTIGLOBULIN TEST FOR DETECTION OF (A) ERYTHROCYTE-BOUND C3D OR (B) IGG. Hemagglutination occurs when anti-C3d or anti-IgG can create a lattice structure by bridging sensitized RBCs. *IgG*, Immunoglobulin G; *RBC*, red blood cell. (*Courtesy Cunningham MJ, Silberstein LE: Autoimmune hemolytic anemia. In Hoffman R, Benz EJ Jr, Shattil SJ, et al, eds: Hematology: Basic principles and practice, ed 4, Philadelphia, 2005, Elsevier.*)

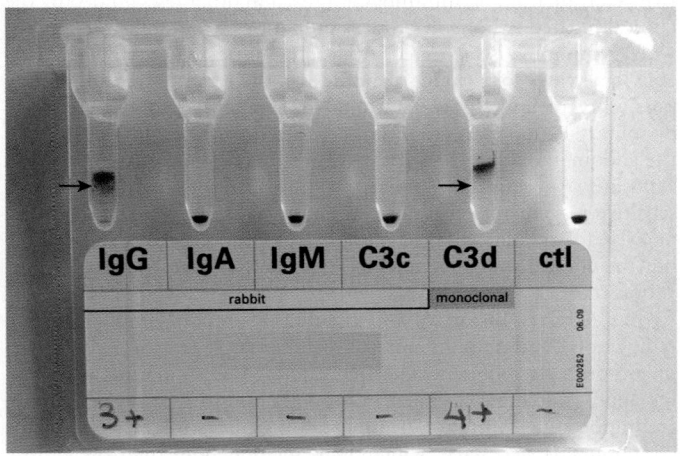

Fig. 46.4 RESULT OF A DIRECT ANTIGLOBULIN TEST PERFOMED ON GEL COLUMNS, WITH A POSITIVE RESULT SHOWN WITH AN ANTI-IGG AND ANTI-C3D. *ctl*, Control; *IgA*, immunoglobulin A; *IgG*, immunoglobulin G; *IgM*, immunoglobulin M.

The DAT result is positive in 1 in 10,000 to 3 in 10,000 normal persons and 10% of hospital patients without anemia or signs of hemolysis.[23a]

Step 3: Warm or Cold Autoimmune Hemolytic Anemia?

In a further step, the DAT is carried out with monospecific antibodies to IgG and complement (C3d) to find out whether a warm or cold antibody is the cause of hemolysis. If the DAT result is positive with IgG alone or with IgG plus C3d, the AIHA is most probably a WAIHA. If the DAT result is positive with only C3d, the AIHA is most probably a CAIHA. The differentiation between WAIHAs and CAIHAs is extremely important for the choice of treatment.

There are some special diagnostic problems in CAIHAs. If CAIHAs are suspected, it must be taken care that the blood that is sent to the laboratory is kept at 37°C to get reliable results. Patients with only RBC C3d may (rarely) have WAIHAs when the amount of RBC IgG is very small. In patients with C3d positivity, the cold agglutinin titer should be determined. If it is greater than 1:512, the diagnosis of a CAD is established. There is no threshold titer that separates normal from abnormal. If the titer is less than 1:512, the thermal amplitude of the antibody must be determined. If the thermal amplitude is above 22°C, the diagnosis is CAD. Mixed type AIHA is rare. The criteria are a positive IgG DAT result and a positive eluate (WAIHAs) result plus a C3d-positive DAT result and the presence of CAIHAs with a thermal amplitude of greater than 30°C (CAIHAs). Many published cases of mixed type antibodies do not fulfill these criteria.[24]

Step 4: Primary or Secondary Autoimmune Hemolytic Anemia?

In the last diagnostic step, it must be determined whether the AIHA is primary or a complication of an underlying disease (secondary). The decision regarding which diagnostic procedures should be used for this purpose depends mainly on the type of AIHA (WAIHAs or CAIHAs) and should include history, physical examination, laboratory tests, and imaging procedures if indicated. In children and younger patients with WAIHA, evidence for an infection should be sought. A list of all recent medication should be made. A history of weight loss, fever, or poor general condition and arthritis points to a malignancy or immune disease as the underlying condition. Palpable lymphadenopathy and splenomegaly do not belong to the clinical picture of primary WAIHA. In this case, lymphoma (particularly splenic marginal zone lymphoma [SMZL]) should be suspected. Laboratory tests should include acute-phase proteins, LDH, quantitative determination of immunoglobulins, and other tests guided by the clinical history. A bone marrow examination is not obligatory except when lymphoma is suspected. Abdominal ultrasonography is reasonable in all cases to exclude splenomegaly, the remote (but important) possibility of an ovarian teratoma (in women), lymphadenopathy, or solitary extranodal lymphomas. Some experts recommend CT of the abdomen or thorax in all cases, but there is concern of radiation exposure. An activated partial thromboplastin time with a lupus-sensitive reagent may reveal a LA. Fluorescence-activated cell sorting or PCR for the detection of monoclonal lymphocytes may be done, but the clinical usefulness of such tests to guide treatment decisions is uncertain.

In CAIHA, a history of a febrile illness should prompt a thoracic radiography, and if results are positive, a serologic test for mycoplasma pneumoniae is required. The quantitative determination of serum Igs and a search for a clonal immunoglobulin by immune fixation are important. If immune fixation findings are positive, a search for lymphoma is necessary, which may include bone marrow biopsy even when there is no lymphadenopathy. In addition to classical CAD, cold agglutinins occurring in association with other cancers, aggressive lymphomas, or infection should be termed *cold agglutinin syndrome*.[25]

Other tests, including blood glucose, Hba_{1c}, renal and hepatic function tests, HIV serology, hepatitis B antigen, and exclusion of latent tuberculosis are necessary to avoid complications of steroids (in WAIHAs) or rituximab (in CAIHAs and WAIHAs).

IMMUNOLOGIC PHENOMENA ASSOCIATED WITH AUTOIMMUNE HEMOLYTIC ANEMIA

Evans syndrome is the combination of WAIHAs with autoimmune thrombocytopenia (ITP), a typical but rare association. Platelet antibodies are usually directed against glycoprotein IIB/IIIA. Neutropenia occurs in 25% of patients. There is no sex predilection; about half of the cases are secondary. Evans syndrome is relatively more common in patients with SLE, antiphospholipid antibodies (APAs), and autoimmune lymphoproliferative syndrome (ALPS).[26] A search for an ALPS is mandatory in younger patients with Evans syndrome. In roughly 50% of the cases, AIHA and ITP occur simultaneously; in 25%, the disease starts with ITP; and in 16%, the disease starts with AIHA. There may be an interval of several years between the onset of AIHA and ITP.[10]

WAIHA, CAIHA, or a positive DAT result without anemia may be associated with PRCA. PRCA may be either immune mediated such as in T-cell neoplasms (particularly T-cell large granulocytic leukemia) or may be caused by an infection with parvovirus. Patients with parvovirus-associated AIHA often present with PRCA.

AIHA is definitely associated with APAs and LA. In one single-center prospective study, LA was found in 30% predominantly idiopathic AIHA. AIHA (4%) and Evans syndrome (10%) are frequent in patients with APAs. It is well established that patients with AIHA have a significantly (2.8-fold to 3.8-fold) elevated risk of venous thromboembolism.[22] It is likely but not proven that patients with AIHA associated with LA are at a higher risk.

In lymphomas, some cases of AIHA are associated with C1-esterase inhibitor deficiency and mixed cryoglobulinemia.

SECONDARY AUTOIMMUNE HEMOLYTIC ANEMIA

About half of cases of AIHA (or probably even more) are secondary. The main causes are immune diseases and malignancies. Other underlying conditions are infections, drugs, transplantation, and congenital defects.

Temporal Relationship of Secondary Autoimmune Hemolytic Anemia to the Underlying Condition

The temporal relationship of AIHA to an underlying condition is complex. AIHA antedates the diagnosis of malignancy in many cases—in NHL, sometimes for years. In population-based studies, clonal B cells have been detected in some patients with seemingly idiopathic AIHA. In most instances, AIHA occurs concurrently with the malignancy. In some other cases, AIHA occurred only at the recurrence and rarely in complete remission (CR) after successful treatment. In CLL, AIHA occurs in a late phase of the disease. The patients have poor prognostic factors and often have been treated with various agents.

In immune diseases, particularly SLE, AIHA is a complication of the early phase of the disease. Infection-related AIHA occurs shortly after the onset of symptoms except in HIV infection, in which AIHA is a complication in the late advanced stage of the disease.

Serologic Type of Autoimmune Hemolytic Anemia in Secondary Autoimmune Hemolytic Anemia

It is an interesting phenomenon that in underlying diseases associated with AIHA, all serologic types of AIHA may occur, but usually one serologic type (WAIHA, CAIHA, or DL antibody) prevails.

The only exception is ovarian teratoma, which is only associated with WAIHA.

Autoimmune Hemolytic Anemia in Immune Diseases

Autoimmune Hemolytic Anemia in Systemic Lupus Erythematosus and Primary Antiphospholipid Syndrome

The prevalence of AIHA in patients with SLE is 7.5% (average of seven studies; range: 5.2% to 12.5%). AIHA may occur at any time during the course of SLE, but two-thirds of cases of AIHA occur at diagnosis or soon thereafter. Almost half of the patients are already taking steroids. Most patients are women and have WAIHA. Evans syndrome is common. Compared with SLE patients without AIHA, those with AIHA are younger; have a higher prevalence of thrombocytopenia, APAs, renal disease, serositis, and central nervous system involvement; and have a higher risk of venous thrombosis.[27]

The prevalence of AIHA in primary antiphospholipid syndrome (PAPS) is about 10%. AIHA precedes PAPS in 25% of cases, but in others occurred after a median time of 4.4 years after the diagnosis of PAPS. Patients with PAPS and AIHA have an increased risk for the development of SLE.[28]

Autoimmune Hemolytic Anemia in Inflammatory Bowel Disease

In the only larger study the prevalence of AIHA in ulcerative colitis was 1.7%.[28a] The mean time from diagnosis of colitis to AIHA was 17 months. Three-quarters of these patients had total colitis. AIHA may also be associated with Crohn disease, but the prevalence is lower than in ulcerative colitis.

Autoimmune Hemolytic Anemia in Other Immune Diseases

A few or single cases of an association of WAIHA with Sjögren syndrome, dermatomyositis, biliary cirrhosis, Graves' disease, Churg-Strauss syndrome, crescentic glomerulonephritis, polymyalgia rheumatica, scleroderma, or autoimmune pancreatitis and of CAIHA with rheumatoid arthritis have been reported. A high prevalence of AIHA was found in small children with giant-cell hepatitis.

Autoimmune Hemolytic Anemia in Transplanted Patients

AIHA is a rare but important and dangerous complication of allogeneic hematopoietic stem cell transplantation (HSCT). Aside from AIHA, causes of hemolytic anemia in transplanted patients may be lymphocyte passenger syndrome and ABO incompatibility. AIHA may be caused by severe immunosuppression by drugs to prevent rejection or graft-versus-host disease (GVHD), viral infections, EBV lymphoproliferative disorder (LPD), or the recurrence of an immune disorder after transplantation (biliary cirrhosis).

The highest rate of AIHA occurred in small children after unrelated cord HSCT for inborn metabolic defects (44%) and in children with severe combined immune deficiency after haploidentical HSCT with T-cell–depleted stem cell grafts.

In adults, the incidence of AIHA ranges from 3.0% to 4.4% after allogeneic HSCT.[29] The median time from HSCT to AIHA is 4–10 months. Most patients have WAIHAs. Risk factors for AIHA are unrelated donor, T-cell depletion, and extensive GVHD. In most cases, AIHA occurred in patients in CR of the underlying disease, but in one study AIHA was associated with a relapse of chronic myeloid leukemia in the majority of patients.

After transplantation of solid organs, the highest risk of AIHA was in patients with pancreatic transplantation. A number of patients with AIHA or CAIHA were observed after liver transplantation but only a small number after cardiac, lung, intestinal, and renal transplantation. The most likely cause of AIHA in these patients is severe drug-induced immunosuppression.

TABLE 46.2	Secondary Autoimmune Hemolytic Anemia in Malignancies		
Malignancy	**Prevalence**	**WAIHAs**	**CAIHAs**
MGUS	Very low	None	All
All NHL	0.23–2.6%		
CLL	4.3–9%	90%	10%
SMZL	10%	2/3	1/3
LPL	3–5%	None	Most
Angioimmunoblastic T-cell lymphoma	13%	One third	Two thirds
Hodgkin lymphoma	0.19–1.7%	All	None
Ovarian teratoma	Very low	All	None
Solid tumors	Very low	Two thirds	One third

CLL, Chronic lymphocytic leukemia; LPL, lymphoplasmacytic lymphoma; MGUS, monoclonal gammopathy with unknown significance; NHL, non-Hodgkin's lymphoma; SMZL, splenic marginal zone lymphoma.

Autoimmune Hemolytic Anemia in Pregnancy and After Blood Transfusion

Very few cases of AIHA and Evans syndrome occurred during pregnancy, all with WAIHAs. In these patients, there seems to be a higher risk for preeclampsia. AIHA responds well to steroids and resolves in most cases after delivery. In two cases, the newborns had mild hemolysis.

Development of RBC autoantibodies is common in multitransfused patients and is associated with the presence of alloantibodies. However, anemia is rare.

Autoimmune Hemolytic Anemia in Malignancies

Autoimmune Hemolytic Anemia in Lymphoproliferative Disorders

AIHA is a typical, relatively common immune-mediated paraneoplastic syndrome in LPD. It occurs in almost all histologic subtypes of NHL, but there is no correlation between the frequency of lymphoma and the risk of AIHA. AIHA is relatively most common in SMZL and angioimmunoblastic T-cell lymphoma (Table 46.2). In most LPD WAIHAs is predominant. Most WAIHAs, particularly in CLL, seem to be polyclonal. The proportion of patients with WAIHAs is highest in CLL and Hodgkin lymphoma; in other malignancies, the ratio of WAIHAs to CAIHAs is 2:1. In lymphoplasmacytic lymphoma (LPL), almost all antibodies are clonal CAIHAs.

Autoimmune Hemolytic Anemia as a Risk Factor for Lymphoproliferative Disorder

In various population-based studies, AIHA emerged as a risk factor for subsequent development of diffuse large B-cell lymphoma, LPL, CLL, monoclonal gammopathy with unknown significance (MGUS), and multiple myeloma. Data regarding the type of AIHA and a possible influence of treatment were not available in these studies. It is uncertain whether autoimmune disorder per se is the causal factor or whether these patients had a clinically silent clonal disorder at the time of AIHA.

Autoimmune Hemolytic Anemia in Chronic Lymphocytic Leukemia

The prevalence of AIHA is highest in CLL, ranging from 4.3% to 9%. The prevalence is highest in poor-risk patients (Binet stage B or C, increased ZAP70 expression, unmutated IgVH status, and CD38 positivity) and patients who had already been treated. However, AIHA may also occur in very early stages of CLL, including B-cell monoclonal lymphocytosis. In a large group of nontreated CLL patients, the prevalence of positive DAT result (with or without anemia) was 14%.[30] Most CLL patients with AIHA are men. The vast majority of patients have (presumably) polyclonal WAIHAs, but in all studies, there is small number of cases with CAIHA (specificity anti-I), often with IgM paraproteinemia.

Autoimmune Hemolytic Anemia in Monoclonal Gammopathy With Unknown Significance and Lymphoplasmacytic Lymphoma

The clinical picture of primary chronic CAD suggests the presence of an "idiopathic" CAIHAs, but in fact, most of these patients have a clonal disease with either only clonal IgM (IgM-MGUS) or LPL with IgM paraproteinemia and bone marrow infiltration (or Waldenström macroglobulinemia). Traditionally, the latter category would be classified as secondary AIHA. More than 90% of patients with "CAD" have a monoclonal IgMκ; 7% had IgG or IgA monoclonal immune globulin with λ chains. The course of CAD is usually indolent. Fewer than half of patients require transfusions, and the risk for progression to highly malignant lymphomas is small.

Autoimmune Hemolytic Anemia in Other Lymphoproliferative Diseases and Myeloma

The prevalence of AIHA is low in NHL, ranging from 0.23% to 2.6%. AIHA has been described in all histologic subtypes of NHL. Based on the prevalence of NHL, the association with AIHA is highest with SMZL, LPL, angioimmunoblastic T-cell lymphoma, and γ heavy chain disease. The antibody may be either a warm (two-thirds) or a cold (one-third) antibody. In NHL, there seems to be a relatively frequent association of AIHA with LA, C1-esterase deficiency, or essential cryoglobulinemia.

A number of predominantly WAIHAs have been described in IgG and IgA myelomas.

Autoimmune Hemolytic Anemia in Myeloid Disorders

Generally, AIHA is rare in patients with myeloid malignancies. A number of cases have been reported in myelodysplastic syndromes, particularly chronic myelomonocytic leukemia. Very few cases were described in acute myelogenous and lymphoblastic leukemia, myelofibrosis, and polycythemia.

Autoimmune Hemolytic Anemia in Solid Tumors

A special, rare, but highly interesting cause of WAIHA is ovarian dermoid cyst. These patients respond very poorly to drug therapies, but the AIHA resolves completely, and the DAT result becomes negative a few weeks after ovariectomy. The same behavior has been described in microcystic adenoma of the pancreas and dermoid cyst of the mesentery associated with AIHA.

AIHA is rarely but definitely associated with solid tumors. It is a very rare complication of lung, renal cell, and ovarian cancer. In some cases of renal cell cancer, AIHA resolved after curative surgery.

Infection-Related Autoimmune Hemolytic Anemia

In immunocompetent patients, AIHA may occur after viral, bacterial, or parasitic infections (Table 46.3). Virus-associated AIHA occurs mostly in newborns and children; bacterial AIHA occurs more often in adults. The onset of AIHA is often shortly after signs of infection but sometimes after a latency time up to weeks. After some specific infections, patients may develop preferentially a warm or a cold antibody (sometimes with specific targets such as I, i, P, or Pr antigen), but in almost all instances beside the dominant antibody (cold or warm), there are a few cases of another antibody (see Table 46.3). Of particular interest is varicella-zoster virus-associated and rubella-associated CAIHAs, because the cold antibody is mostly directed to the Pr antigen and the AIHA is clinically severe. In Mycoplasma-associated AIHA, the antibody target is almost always "I". After Mycoplasma infection, the DAT result is positive in 50% to 60% of cases, but anemia is rare. In some specific infections, the antibody was a DL antibody, but in a large study, most DL antibodies were

TABLE 46.3	Autoimmune Hemolytic Anemia After Infections		
	Infection	WAIHA	CAIHA (Specificities)
Respiratory tract infections (unspecified)	—	—	+ (DL)/PCH
Viral infections (specific)	EBV	+/−	+ (anti-i)
	CMV	+	+/− (anti-i)
	Parvovirus (B19)	+ (often with PRCA)	+/− (DL)
	Varicella	+/−	+ (anti-Pr, anti-I, anti-DL)
	Rubella	—	+ (anti-Pr1) Monotypic IgM
	HIV	+	+ (anti-I, anti-i, anti-Pr)
Bacterial infections (specific)	Mycoplasma	+/−	+ (anti-I, anti-Pr)
	Brucellosis	+/−	+ (anti-I)
	Haemophilus influenzae		+ (DL)
Parasitic infections (specific)	Visceral leishmaniosis	+	—

—, Not reported; +, predominant type of autoimmune hemolytic anemia; +/−, single or few cases reported; CMV, cytomegalovirus; DL, Donath–Landsteiner antibody; EBV, Epstein-Barr virus; PCH, paroxysmal cold hemoglobinuria; PRCA, pure red blood cell aplasia.

found after unspecific respiratory infections.[13] In many cases, the course of AIHA is short, uncomplicated, and self-limited, but some cases with a severe, even fatal, course, particularly in patients with Pr antibodies and in Mycoplasma-associated AIHA, have been reported. In AIHA associated with bacterial infections or in leishmaniasis, treatment of the infection seemed to be beneficial.

AIHA has been described in a few cases of acute hepatitis A, B, C, or E, and in a number of cases of untreated chronic hepatitis C. However, in a large study, an increased prevalence of AIHA has only been found in interferon (IFN)-treated hepatitis C patients.[31]

Anecdotal reports have described patients in whom WAIHAs were associated with measles, Chlamydia pneumoniae, or miliary tuberculosis and CAIHAs with adenovirus, measles, leptospiral pneumonia, Escherichia coli infection (all anti-I), pneumococcal pneumonia (anti-Pr), Haemophilus influenzae (DL), or Bartonella henselae (DAT negative).

Some cases of AIHA have been described after vaccination against hepatitis B, influenza (MF59 adjuvanted), diphtheria–tetanus–pertussis, or rubella. Such associations could not be confirmed in systematic studies.

Drug-Induced Autoimmune Hemolytic Anemia

Historically, methyldopa, an antihypertensive drug, was the first known drug to induce AIHA. The prevalence of methyldopa-induced AIHA is 1% with 10% to 20% DAT-positive patients without anemia, indicating that DAT positivity is not always followed by overt disease. Currently, IFN-α and purine nucleoside analogues are the most common causes of drug-induced AIHA (Table 46.4). The diagnosis of drug-induced AIHA in a patient with AIHA after drug exposure can only be made if the indirect DAT result is positive and the RBC eluate contains a RBC antibody. Such tests have not been performed in all patients in whom drug-induced AIHA was claimed.

The temporal relationship between drug exposure and AIHA is complex. In some instances, AIHA may occur after long-term exposure to a drug (IFN or targeted antibodies). In AIHA caused by

TABLE 46.4	Drug-Induced Autoimmune Hemolytic Anemia				
Drug	**Risk Factors**	**AIHA Onset**	**Type of AIHA**	**Response to Treatment**	**Diseases Treated**
Methyldopa	Not known	Delayed	WAIHA	Resolution after withdrawal	Hypertension
IFN-α	Pretherapeutic positive DAT	Delayed (8–11 months)	WAIHA	Resolution spontaneous or after steroids	Hepatitis C Hematologic malignancies
Efazulimab	Not known	Many months	WAIHA	Resolution after withdrawal	Arthritis (rare)
Etanercept	Not known	Delayed	CAIHA	Resolution after rituximab	Rheumatoid arthritis (rare)
Fludarabine Cladribine Pentostatin	CLL Pretherapeutic positive DAT result	Early (median, 3–4 cycle) or delayed	WAIHA Mixed AIHA	Half of AIHA resolve after steroids	CLL Lymphomas[a] AML[a]
Bendamustin	CLL	No or only very low risk of AIHA			CLL Lymphomas
Chlorambucil	CLL	Delayed onset	WAIHA		CLL
Eculizumab	Patients with incomplete response	After treatment	CAIHA		PNH
Lenalidomide		During treatment	WAIHA	Resolution after withdrawa	One case treated for lymphoma
Checkpoint inhibitors (anti-CTLA4, anti-PD1/PD1L		During treatment	WAIHA		Solid tumors, Hodgkin lymphoma

[a]No or very low risk.
AML, Acute myeloid leukemia; CAIHA, cold autoimmune hemolytic anemia; CLL, chronic lymphocytic leukemia; IFN, interferon; PNH, paroxysmal nocturnal hemoglobinuria; WAIHA, warm autoimmune hemolytic anemia.

purine analogues, AIHA occurs typically after a few cycles of therapy of CLL and is probably dose related (lower incidence and severity at reduced doses of fludarabine). Chlorambucil is said to induce AIHA, particularly after the end of treatment. This has not been found in all studies.

Interferon-induced AIHA has been described in various diseases (particularly hepatitis C and malignant diseases). It is caused by WAIHAs, occurs usually after long exposure to the drug, and disappears spontaneously after cessation of the drug within weeks. AIHA induced by purine analogues (fludarabine, cladribine) occurs mostly during or immediately after the end of drug treatment, but the onset is delayed in some cases. The antibodies are warm or mixed antibodies. This complication occurs predominantly in patients with CLL but seems to be very rare in lymphoma patients treated with these drugs. The incidence of AIHA in patients with CLL after fludarabine or cladribine monotherapy ranges from 2% to 11%. When fludarabine is combined with cyclophosphamide (and rituximab), AIHA is less frequent and probably less severe, but this may be attributable to the lower fludarabine dose in these protocols. Patients with a positive DAT result before treatment have a higher risk of purine analogue-induced AIHA. With steroids alone, about half of the patients achieve a lasting CR. So far no cases of AIHA have been reported after treatment of CLL with bendamustine.

An interesting and as yet unexplained phenomenon is the fact that some patients with CLL-associated AIHA may achieve remissions after fludarabine or cladribine treatment. However, it is general practice to avoid purine analogues in patients with AIHA. Other drugs that have been associated with WAIHAs (in single case reports) were IFN-β, the monoclonal anti-CD11 antibody efalizumab, the recently developed checkpoint inhibitors, namely anti-CTLA4 and anti-PD1/PD-L1 antibodies, and lenalidomide.

A peculiar type of CAIHA has been described in some patients with paroxysmal nocturnal hemoglobinuria who had been treated with the anti-C5 antibody ecuzulimab. These patients had an incomplete response to ecuzulimab. The RBCs of these patients accumulate C3d on their surfaces.

Autoimmune Hemolytic Anemia in Immune Deficiency States

AIHA is one of the classical complications of common variable immune deficiency (CVID). The prevalence of AIHA was 4% to 5.5% in large studies. AIHA preceded the diagnosis of CVID in more than half of the cases (median time from diagnosis of AIHA to CVID: 5.5 years). Evans syndrome is common.

AIHA (often combined with thrombocytopenia) occurs in 23% to 51% of patients with ALPS. The diagnosis of ALPS is made by the demonstration of a high number of circulating TCRαβ+ double-negative (CD4− CD8−) T lymphocytes. The basic defect of ALPS is a disturbance of apoptosis.[26]

AIHA is also common in deficiency of purine nucleoside phosphorylase (a T-cell deficiency with almost normal B cells). At least 15% of patients with Wiskott-Aldrich syndrome have AIHA. AIHA occurs before the age of 5 years and is associated with high serum IgM levels. These patients are candidates for allogeneic stem cell transplantation.

DIFFERENTIAL DIAGNOSIS

In patients with DAT-positive hemolytic anemia, the distinction from drug-dependent immune hemolytic anemia is important. In recipients of ABO- or D-incompatible allografts, anti-RBC antibodies are probably produced by immunocompetent memory B cells from the donor. This so-called *passenger lymphocyte syndrome* (PLS) is frequent in heart and lung transplantation (≤68%). A difficult problem is differential diagnosis of DAT-negative AIHA or Evans syndrome. In younger patients with isolated hemolytic anemia with or without symptoms, hereditary diseases such as hereditary spherocytosis, sickle cell anemia, and thalassemia must be considered. Family history and RBC morphology are most helpful in these cases. In patients with drug-induced hemolytic anemia, nonimmune hemolysis caused by glucose-6-phosphate-dehydrogenase deficiency should be considered. Babesiosis or other infections may cause nonimmune hemolytic anemia. In severely ill patients with hemolytic anemia and thrombocytopenia, idiopathic or cancer-related thrombotic thrombocytopenic purpura, hemolytic uremic syndrome, or disseminated intravascular coagulation should prompt a search for schistocytes in the blood smear.

Paroxysmal nocturnal hemoglobinuria is diagnosed by a deficiency of glycosylphosphatidylinositol anchor proteins on the cell surface caused by a mutation of the *PIG-A* gene. Type II mixed cryoglobulinemia is a condition caused by a monoclonal IgM autoantibody with anti-IgG activity with rheumatoid factor properties frequently associated with hepatitis C. The clinical picture is characterized by a systemic vasculitis syndrome but not by anemia.

TREATMENT

For many years, drugs and procedures routinely used in the treatment of AIHA were not subjected to studies that today are regarded as the gold standard for approval and recommendation. Only a few randomized studies have been performed, and were usually small, and often with a heterogeneous population of patients with a short observation time. Thus, the treatment recommendation in this chapter should be viewed critically.[8]

Goals of Treatment

As in all diseases, the goal of treatment of AIHA is the achievement of a complete clinical and laboratory sustained remission without any residual signs of the disease. Such results can be obtained not only in primary AIHA but also in a substantial number of secondary cases when the underlying disease disappears spontaneously (infection), when the causative drug is withdrawn, or after (curative) treatment (surgery or chemoimmunotherapy) of an underlying malignancy. In most patients with primary WAIHAs, the expectations for success must be tempered. Therefore, a practical goal is the achievement of a good clinical response with freedom from symptoms in the absence of side effects of treatment. Remission of AIHA after treatment is often defined by laboratory values, but there is no consensus on the definition of CR or partial remission (PR) regarding Hb concentration. Formally, one could define CR as absence of transfusion requirement, a normal Hb value (according to the age and sex of the patient), and absence of signs of hemolysis (normal reticulocyte counts, haptoglobin, and LDH; negative DAT result). Such CR is sometimes seen in secondary AIHA. In primary AIHA, CR is often defined as Hb above 11.0 g/dL without sign of hemolysis, but the DAT result may remain positive. A minimal requirement for PR is the absence of transfusion requirement and a satisfactory clinical condition (usually Hb >9–10 g/dL). Thus, in AIHA, the treatment goals must be defined individually and tailored to the patient's needs.

Blood Transfusions

Blood transfusions may be necessary for emergency treatment of AIHA. The problem is to find well-matched RBC concentrates. In critical cases, transfusions should not be avoided or delayed because of uncertainty in matching (see box on Transfusion Therapy in Selected Patients With Severe Autoimmune Hemolytic Anemia). The decision is made on an individual basis depending on the speed of development and severity of anemia, the type and cause of hemolytic anemia (the highest acute death rates were observed in patients with fludarabine-associated AIHA, IgM WAIHAs, and DL antibodies), and the age and clinical condition of the patient. Because the antibody in WAIHAs is directed against blood group antigens, no truly matched blood transfusions are possible, but RBCs can be safely given if alloantibodies are excluded.[3] However, some precautions have to be taken. In patients without a history of previous transfusions or

---

Transfusion Therapy in Selected Patients With Severe Autoimmune Hemolytic Anemia

Immediate blood transfusion should not be withheld from patients with severe anemia. Small amounts of RBCs may be lifesaving in patients with acute cardiac or cerebral dysfunction caused by anemia. However, precautions have to be taken to avoid transfusion reactions. This requires close cooperation between clinicians and the blood bank. The exclusion of alloantibodies is most important. Patients with a low risk for severe reactions caused by an alloantibody are those without a history of previous transfusions or pregnancy. In high-risk patients, extended RBC phenotyping should be performed for selection of compatible RBC concentrates. In all instances, a biologic in vivo compatibility test has to be performed at the beginning of the transfusion.

---

pregnancy the risk of alloantibodies is low, allowing for transfusion of only ABO- and RhD-matched RBCs. In all other patients, extended phenotyping with respect to Rh subgroups (C, c, E, e), Kell, Kidd, and S/s using monoclonal IgM antibodies should be performed for selection of compatible RBC concentrates. Warm autoadsorption or allogeneic adsorption procedures for detection of alloantibodies may be used in exceptional cases. In patients with CAIHAs, transfused blood must be prewarmed using commercial warming coils. In all instances, an important precaution is a biologic in vivo compatibility test, which includes rapid infusion of 20 mL of blood; 20 minutes observation; and, if there is no reaction, further transfusion at usual speed.

Treatment of Primary Warm Antibody Hemolytic Anemia

First-Line Treatment With Steroids

Newly diagnosed severe WAIHAs should be treated immediately with glucocorticoids (steroids) (Fig. 46.5 and Table 46.5; see also box on Initial Steroid Therapy). Therapy starts with an initial dose of 1 mg/kg/day of prednisone orally or an equivalent dose of methylprednisone intravenously. It is recommended to continue with this dose until a hematocrit of greater than 30% or a Hb level of greater than 10 g/dL is achieved. CR or PR is obtained in approximately 80% of patients. Failure to achieve this goal after 3 weeks should result in a switch to second-line therapy. In responding patients, prednisone dose is gradually reduced to 20–30 mg/day within a few weeks. Subsequently, the dose is tapered slowly by 2.5 mg to 5 mg/day per month guided by Hb and reticulocyte counts. If the patient is still in remission after 3–4 months at a dose of 5 mg/day, withdrawal of steroids can be attempted. The exact rate of patients remaining in CR after the end of steroid therapy is not known but is estimated to be around 20% to 40%.[32] Most responders require maintenance steroids to keep the Hb above 9–10g/dL. About 40% to 50% of patients need 15 mg/day or less prednisone (regarded as the highest tolerable dose for long-term treatment). However, 15% to 20% need higher maintenance prednisone doses.

For rituximab, two prospective studies have been reported.[33,34] The first was an open-prospective phase II study testing the efficacy and safety of low-dose rituximab and the second was a randomized phase III open trial that showed the benefit of rituximab in combination with prednisolone over prednisolone alone with an overall response rate (ORR) of 75% at 1 year in the rituximab arm. Combination of rituximab with steroids compared with steroid monotherapy produced an increased response rate (75% vs 36% at 1 year) and a longer relapse-free survival (70% vs 45% at 3 years). Despite these encouraging data, the real value of rituximab in first-line remains to be established.

Therapeutic management of steroid treatment should include blood glucose monitoring, prophylaxis against osteoporosis (commence early), supplementation with folic acid, and heparin treatment in selected cases.

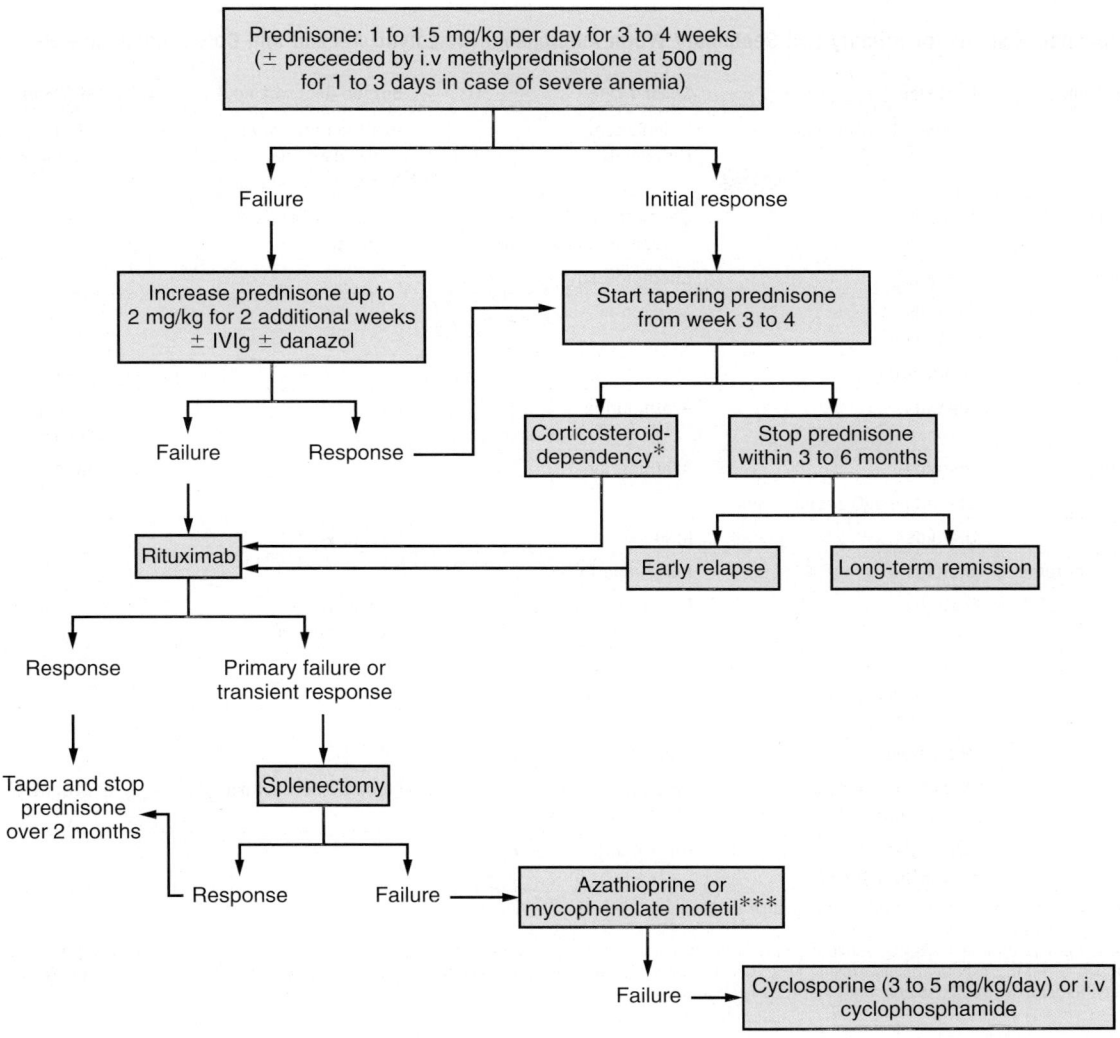

*Dose of prednisone≥10 mg/day to maintain at least a partial response (i.e Hb level >10 g/dL with at least a 2 g increase from baseline without recent transfusion)
**Complete response=normal hemoglobin level without hemolysis.
***The response to each one of these drugs can take as long as 2 to 3 months. They can be considered before splenectomy in case of contra-indication to splenectomy or patient's refusal.

Fig. 46.5 PROPOSED ALGORITHM FOR THE TREATMENT OF PRIMARY WARM ANTIBODY AUTOIMMUNE HEMOLYTIC ANEMIA IN ADULTS. *IV*, intravenous; *IVIg*, intravenous immunoglobulin; *PDN*, prednisone. *(Modified from Lechner K, Jäger U: How I treat autoimmune haemolytic anemias in adults. Blood 116:1831, 2010.)*

Great concerns are osteoporosis, osteonecrosis, and bone fracture, particularly of the lumbar spine. About 30% to 50% of patients on long-term steroid treatment experience fractures. The highest loss of bone density occurs early, even at smaller steroid doses, and the risk of fracture increases by 75% during the first months of treatment.

Thus, patients on steroid therapy should receive bisphosphonates, vitamin D, and calcium from the beginning. Folic acid is also recommended. Steroid-induced diabetes is a major risk factor for treatment-related deaths from infections. Although heparin treatment is not recommended for all patients, the possibility of pulmonary embolism must be considered, particularly in patients with AIHA and LA or recurrent AIHA after splenectomy. Previous studies have also found a beneficial effect of standard heparin in AIHA.

Second-Line Treatment

Second-line treatment is considered in patients (1) refractory to initial steroids as defined earlier, (2) in need of a maintenance dose of more than 15 mg/day of prednisone (absolute indications), or (3) who need between 15 mg/day and 0.1 mg/kg/day (relative indication; Fig. 46.6). Patients with prednisone requirement of 0.1 mg/kg/day or less are potential candidates for long-term, low-dose prednisone. Patients' refractory to steroid treatment should be reevaluated for underlying diseases or warm IgM antibodies.

Currently, there are two major second-line options for primary WAIHAs with proven short- (and long-) term efficacy splenectomy (preferentially laparoscopic) and therapy with the monoclonal anti-CD20 antibody rituximab.[35] From a scientific point of view on the

TABLE 46.5   Treatment Options for Primary and Secondary Warm Autoimmune Hemolytic Anemia and Cold Autoimmune Hemolytic Anemia

Disease or Condition	First Line	Second Line	Beyond Second Line	Last Resort
Primary AIHA	Steroids (+ rituximab)	Splenectomy Rituximab	Azathioprine, MMF, cyclosporine, cyclophosphamide	High-dose cyclophosphamide, alemtuzumab
B- and T-cell NHL	Steroids	Chemotherapy +/− rituximab (splenectomy in SMZL)	Other anti-CD20 antibodies, ibrutinib	
Hodgkin lymphoma	Steroids	Chemotherapy		
Solid tumors	Steroids Surgery			
Ovarian dermoid cyst	Ovariectomy			
SLE	Steroids	Azathioprine	MMF	Rituximab Autologous SCT
Ulcerative colitis	Steroids	Azathioprine		Total colectomy
CVID	Steroids + IgG replacement			
ALPD	Steroids	MMF	Sirolimus	
Wiskott-Aldrich syndrome	Steroids	Allogeneic SCT		
Allogeneic SCT	Steroids	Rituximab[a]	Splenectomy T-cell infusion	
Organ transplantation	Reduction of immunosuppression, steroids			
Drug induced	Withdrawal	Steroids		
Primary CAD	Protection from cold exposure	Rituximab Chlorambucil	Fludarabine + rituximab	Ecuzulimab[b] bortezomid[b]
PCH	Supportive treatment (postinfectious)	Rituximab[a] (chronic)		

[a]Early second-line treatment because of known poor response to steroids.
[b]Off-label use in single cases.
AIHA, Autoimmune hemolytic anemia; ALPD, autoimmune lymphoproliferative disorders; CAD, cold agglutinin disease; CVID, common variable immune deficiency; IgG, immunoglobulin G; MMF, mycophenolate mofetil; NHL, non-Hodgkin's lymphoma; PCH, paroxysmal cold hemoglobinuria; SCT, stem cell transplantation; SLE, systemic lupus erythematosus; SMZL, splenic marginal zone lymphoma.

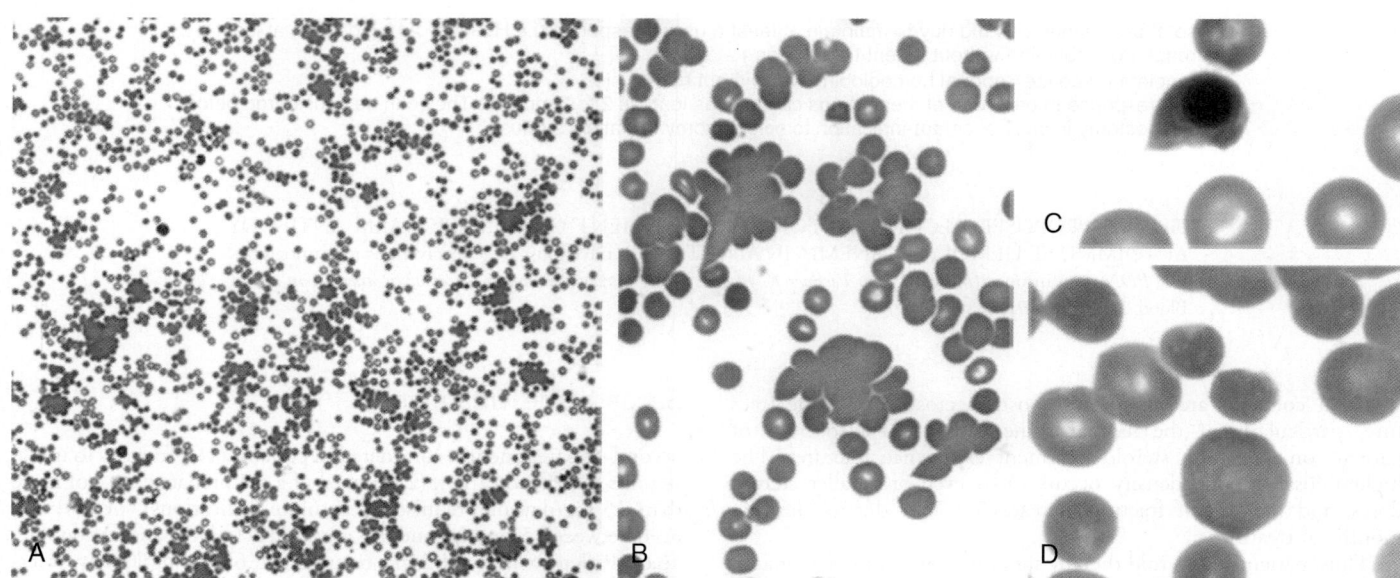

Fig. 46.6 PERIPHERAL SMEAR IN COLD AGGLUTININ DISEASE. Low-power scan shows uneven distribution of red blood cells (RBCs) (A), which at slightly higher power (B) shows the RBCs to be clumped together or agglutinated. This must be distinguished from rouleaux formation. High-power scan shows nucleated RBCs (C), polychromatophilia, and microspherocytes (D).

TABLE 46.6 Second-Line Treatment Options After Steroids

Treatment	Dosing and Application	Side Effects	Precautions
Splenectomy (acute)	Preferentially laparoscopic	Infections, thrombosis	Postoperative thromboprophylaxis
Splenectomy (long term)	—	Infections Venous thrombosis	Vaccination, patient information
Rituximab	375 mg/m² on days 1,8, 15, and 22 IV	Infusional reactions Infections	Premedication with antihistamines (and steroids)
Danazol	200–400/day PO	Hepatotoxicity	None
Cyclophosphamide	PO or IV Dose adjusted to neutrophil count	Neutropenia Mutagenesis	Neutrophil count monitoring, bladder protection after high doses
Azathioprine	2.0–3.mg/kg/day PO Dose adjusted to neutrophil count	Neutropenia	Neutrophil count monitoring; avoid interaction with other drugs (e.g., allopurinol)
MFF	1–2 × 1 g/day PO	Gastrointestinal	
Cyclosporine	PO Dose adjusted to blood levels of CyA Target level, 200–400 ng/mL	Nephrotoxicity Gum hyperplasia	Monitoring of CyA levels and creatinine
Alemtuzumab	SC (variable doses)	Neutropenia	Antiinfectious prophylaxis
Complement inhibition with eculizumab, TNT009		Infections	Vaccination

CyA, Cyclosporine A; IV, intravenous; MMF, mycophenolate mofetil; PO, oral; SC, subcutaneous.

basis of published data, no definite preference for one these treatments is possible because of the insufficient quality of data. For both treatments, there have been no randomized studies comparing these two options. The decision for the preferred treatment in a specific patient has therefore to be made on an individual basis based on judgment of the treating physician, the validity of available data on short- and long-term efficacy, the assumed individual risk of adverse events, and the preference of the patient (Table 46.6).

Splenectomy

For splenectomy, there are more, but older data on the short-term efficacy, few data on long-term efficacy, and good recent data on long-term adverse events. CR or PR is achieved in two-thirds of patients (38% to 82%), depending on the percentage of secondary cases. In addition, there is good evidence that a substantial number of patients will remain in remission without the need for medical intervention for years. In the initial series by Chertkow and Dacie,[36] only 2 out of 28 patients were in remission for more than 5 years, but 6 patients remained in a stable PR for up to 7 years. In 52 splenectomized patients (percentage of primary AIHA unknown), Coon[37] found that 63% had a hematocrit of 30% or greater without steroids after a mean follow-up of 33 months, and 21% had a hematocrit of 30% or greater with a prednisone requirement of 15 mg/day or less after a mean follow-up of 73 months. In a study by Allgood and Chaplin,[38] 44% of patients were in CR after more than 1 year after splenectomy.

Splenectomy can safely be performed laparoscopically in almost all patients with primary AIHA with normal-sized spleens. Withdrawal of steroids after splenectomy should be carried out slowly (as described for primary treatment) to prevent hemolytic crises in case of recurrence. The mortality rate of laparoscopic splenectomy was 0.5% in a large national study. The main short-term risks of splenectomy (in general) are infections, pulmonary embolism, and splenic-portal thrombosis (rare in patients with a normal-sized spleen), but these risks have not been studied specifically in primary WAIHAs.

There is a lifelong increased risk of infections and of venous thrombosis and a very small risk of pulmonary hypertension. The most serious, often fatal, but rare infectious complication is overwhelming pneumococcal septicemia. The risk of infections is highest shortly after splenectomy and decreases after 1 year. In a Scandinavian population-based study, the adjusted relative risk of major infections (requiring hospital contact) in a matched indication comparison 1 year after splenectomy for ITP (with a probably similar risk as AIHA) was 1.4. Although fatal postsplenectomy infections seem to be less common in recent years, it is mandatory to take all measures to reduce this risk. There is good but not definite evidence that preoperative vaccination reduces the risk of severe infections. Vaccination for pneumococci, meningococci, and *Haemophilus influenzae* should be done before splenectomy. Pneumococcal vaccination should be repeated regularly. Long-term antibiotic prophylaxis is probably not required in adults, but patients should be informed about this risk and should take antibiotics immediately in case unexplained fever. Risk in children may be reduced by subtotal splenectomy. The long-term risk of venous thrombosis is moderate. Information for patients about short- and long-term risks is required and may be one of the reasons for the fact that surgical treatment is underused. However, splenectomy is the only therapy so far that may provide freedom from treatment in a substantial number of patients for more than 2 years and possibly cure in about 20%.

Rituximab

Rituximab is currently the best available drug option for second-line treatment. Given at a standard induction dose of 375 mg/m² intravenously on days 1, 8, 15, and 22. In a metaanalysis, the ORR for WAIHAs after rituximab was 70% (67% for primary and 72% for secondary).[39] The CR rate was 42% (32% primary and 46% secondary). The CR rate was highest after 2–4 months. The rituximab schedule and dose are empirically derived from lymphoma treatment, and it is not known whether other schedules including maintenance are equal or better.

There are limited data on short-term and almost no data on long-term efficacy and no data on long-term adverse effects. With regard to short-term efficacy, there seems to be not much difference between rituximab and splenectomy. In one study, almost all patients (10 out of 11) had steroid-refractory primary WAIHAs, but four patients received additional therapies.[40] Eight patients achieved CR and three PR, but six patients still had moderate signs of hemolysis and therefore did not formally fulfill the criteria for a CR. Thus, the true response rates for steroid-refractory WAIHAs seem to be considerably high, but still not completely clear.[39] The efficacy and toxicity of rituximab monotherapy was previously tested in several additional retrospective studies in a mixed population of refractory primary or secondary AIHA. Response usually occurs within 3 weeks. Patients taking steroids before initiation of rituximab should continue on steroids until response to the CD20 antibody. In the D'Arena et al[40] study, at a mean follow-up of 604 days, all patients were still in CR or PR. The longest remission duration was 2884 days. Because of the small patient number, data on long-term efficacy of rituximab should be regarded with caution. Predictors of long-term response are achievement of a CR, conversion to a negative DAT result, and previous splenectomy. Retreatment with rituximab is feasible and may be necessary after 1–3 years. Rituximab has been given to children without apparent safety problems.

The caveats of rituximab therapy are that the drug is not licensed for the indication and that infectious complications are rare but sometimes life threatening, particularly with repeat or maintenance treatment. There is a small long-term risk of progressive multifocal leukoencephalopathy. Nevertheless, rituximab is the preferred option for patients who are not eligible for splenectomy. If one explains the benefits and risks of the two second-line treatments to a patient, he or she usually favors rituximab because it is a noninvasive outpatient treatment, and splenectomy remains an option in case of failure.

Treatment of Patients With Refractory or Recurrent Disease After Splenectomy or Rituximab

In patients failing splenectomy, an accessory spleen should be excluded. Patients who are refractory to splenectomy or with recurrence after splenectomy can be retreated with steroids, assuming that the disease has become more responsive. This may work well in patients with previous requirement of lower steroid doses (≤15 mg/day of prednisone). The other option is to initiate treatment with rituximab immediately.

Patients who are refractory to rituximab should undergo splenectomy, if eligible. There are no data on the influence of initial remission duration on the efficacy of retreatment. In patients relapsing late (>1 year) after rituximab, retreatment with the antibody maybe a good option.

A potentially interesting drug for second-line treatment (which has also been used as first-line treatment along with steroids) is danazol, an attenuated androgen (see Table 46.6).[17] It has established efficacy in C1 esterase deficiency, and efficacy has been claimed in several immune diseases, including WAIHAs. Initial very promising results (ORR: 60% to 70%) in AIHA could not be confirmed in subsequent studies, but it may worthwhile to carry out further studies because the toxicity seems to be relatively low with the exception of a potentially increased risk for hepatocellular carcinoma.

The advantage of high-dose Igs is low toxicity but remission rates are low, and routine use in patients with AIHA is not recommended in a recent guideline.

Treatment Options Beyond Second-Line Therapy in Primary Warm Autoimmune Hemolytic Anemia

Given the nature of the disease, the use of immunosuppressive treatments of all kinds seems logical. Response rates of up to 60% have been reported, but data are frequently based on low patient numbers or anecdotal reports. Cyclophosphamide was very effective in two studies. Other published data of treatment with azathioprine or cyclophosphamide are less favorable, with only about one-third of patients having any response. Evaluation is even more complicated by the fact that patients frequently received concomitant treatment with steroids. Dosing of azathioprine is difficult because of the narrow therapeutic window, hypersensitivity because of genetic defects, and

interaction with other drugs. Cyclophosphamide may have long-term mutagenic effects. Other immunosuppressive drugs such as cyclosporine or mycophenolate mofetil (MMF) have shown high response rates in very small series.

Repeated cycles of high-dose cyclophosphamide (50 mg/kg/day for 4 days) remain an option in selected, highly refractory patients. In a pilot study, six out of nine patients received a CR with a median duration of 15 months or more. Alemtuzumab has also been effective at a dose of 10 mg/day for 10 days. Promising results were recently published for a combination of low-dose rituximab (100 mg on days 1, 8, 15, and 22) with alemtuzumab (10 mg on days 1–3). The results of autologous stem cell transplantation were disappointing, but allogeneic transplantation may be used as a last-resort treatment in patients with Evans syndrome.

In general, second-line treatment should be selected taking into account severity of AIHA, age, comorbidity, and patient preference. Because of the low curative potential of all treatment options, patient safety remains the major concern.

Treatment of Secondary Warm Autoimmune Hemolytic Anemia

In secondary AIHA, the treatment goal depends on the type and severity of the underlying disease. The treatment goal may vary from palliative treatment of AIHA to cure by eradication of the underlying disease. Preferred treatment options are listed in Table 46.6.

Warm Autoimmune Hemolytic Anemia Associated With Systemic Lupus Erythematosus

Steroids used at a similar dosage as in primary WAIHAs induce high response rates. Maintenance treatment with azathioprine, cyclophosphamide, or both may be required. Rituximab is effective against WAIHAs and SLE but may be associated with a higher risk of progressive multifocal leukoencephalopathy in this setting.

Warm Autoimmune Hemolytic Anemia Associated With Chronic Lymphocytic Leukemia

In previously untreated CLL with isolated DAT-positive anemia but no other treatment indication, treatment with prednisone as in primary WAIHAs is the first choice. In case of refractoriness or relapse, rituximab monotherapy is moderately effective but produces response rates of more than 80% in combination with cyclophosphamide and dexamethasone. Cyclosporine also has good activity. In refractory AIHA or in AIHA with advanced or progressive CLL, treatment of the underlying disease with a rituximab-containing regimen according to International Workshop on Chronic Lymphocytic Leukemia guidelines is recommended.[41] In elderly or comorbid patients with active CLL, chlorambucil with prednisone with or without rituximab is a good choice. In general, fludarabine-containing regimens should be used with caution in the presence of a positive DAT result or overt AIHA. In this case, bendamustine with (or without) rituximab is a good alternative. Alemtuzumab has proven activity against CLL and AIHA, and is a good second-line option, particularly in patients with associated PRCA. The tyrosine kinase inhibitor ibrutinib was effective in a patient with WAIHAs and CLL.[42]

Warm Autoimmune Hemolytic Anemia in Other Non-Hodgkin Lymphomas

AIHA in NHLs does not respond well to steroids in general and splenectomy is only effective in SMZLs. Sustained responses in most other lymphoma subtypes have been obtained with lymphoma-specific treatment with or without rituximab.

Drug-Related Warm Autoimmune Hemolytic Anemia

Cessation of the drug may be effective in many cases, and further use of the drug should be avoided. Fludarabine-induced AIHA may be life threatening but responds to steroid therapy.

Treatment of Warm Autoimmune Hemolytic Anemia in Congenital and Acquired Immune Deficiency States and Special Serologic Types

The treatment of WAIHAs in patients with CVID is very similar to that of those with primary WAHA. Additional regular prophylactic treatment with IgG concentrates reduces the risk of recurrence. Splenectomy is effective, but the risk of serious infections is high.

In ALPS, treatment should be started with steroids and then switched to MMF, but sirolimus has the highest efficacy in improving not only AIHA but also lymphadenopathy. AIHA associated with IgM hypergammaglobulinemia in Wiskott-Aldrich syndrome is an indication for allogeneic stem cell transplantation.

Patients with AIHA after allogeneic stem cell transplantation respond poorly to steroids but often do respond to rituximab. An early switch to rituximab may be reasonable in these patients. AIHA in drug-related severely immunosuppressed patients after transplantation of solid organs responds best to reduction of immune suppression. Patients with IgM WAIHAs respond poorly to steroids. These patients are candidates for early rituximab treatment. The same is true for chronic AIHA caused by DL antibodies.

Treatment of Cold Autoimmune Hemolytic Anemia

Primary Chronic Cold Agglutinin Disease

Primary CAD is defined as a CAIHAs in patients with IgM-MGUS or in lymphoma without overt clinical signs but with bone marrow infiltration. All patients should be advised to avoid cold exposure. Drug treatment is required in only half of the patients. Treatment is initiated in symptomatic patients or when Hb levels drop below 9–10 g/dL. Because IgM-coated RBCs are mainly destroyed in the liver, CAIHA does not respond to splenectomy and poorly to steroids. The most effective and best evaluated treatment is rituximab in a standard lymphoma dose. Two studies have provided similar results. In a prospective phase II study, 20 out of 27 patients responded, but most responses ($n = 19$) were partial. The median response duration was 11 months, but most patients responded to retreatment with rituximab. A combination of rituximab and oral fludarabine induced higher ORRs (76%) with a longer duration (median: 66 months).[44] In a metaanalysis, the ORR for rituximab in CAD was 57% with a CR rate of 21%.[39]

Given the role of complement in CAD, it is not surprising that the terminal complement inhibitor ecuzulimab is effective.[45,46] Recent results suggest that inhibition of the complement classical pathway at the level of C1s results in remarkable responses and even CRs (TNT009).[47,48]

Positive results have been obtained with the proteasome inhibitor bortezomib in single rituximab-refractory patients. Preparation of patients with high-titer CAIHAs for surgery by cryofiltration may be required in rare instances.

Secondary Cold Autoimmune Hemolytic Anemia

In CAIHAs associated with lymphomas or solid tumors, treatment of the underlying disease by chemo(immuno)therapy or curative resection results in good responses. Cases of infection-related CAIHAs usually resolve spontaneously, but antibiotic therapy may accelerate the process.

FUTURE DIRECTIONS

Future research should mainly be directed toward generation of better treatment options. The generation of international guidelines is still hampered by the lack of evidence. Every effort should be made to initiate valid comparisons of major treatment options such as steroids, splenectomy, and rituximab, potentially through registries or randomized trials.

Novel therapeutic options may be provided by next-generation anti-CD20 antibodies or antibodies against other targets such as complement factors. Insights into the way T cells drive and control the immune reaction could lead to novels immunotherapeutic approaches. Synthetic peptides modulating Th1 responses via regulatory T cells may be developed into therapeutic tools. Another option would be to target structures on macrophages responsible for RBC destruction (e.g., the CD47–SIRP-α interaction). There is hope that novel targeted therapies will replace splenectomy and even steroid treatment of patients with AIHA.

REFERENCES

For the complete list of references, log on to www.expertconsult.com.

CHAPTER 47

EXTRINSIC NONIMMUNE HEMOLYTIC ANEMIAS

William C. Mentzer and Stanley L. Schrier

By definition, extrinsic causes of hemolysis are abnormalities in the environment in which the red blood cells (RBCs), usually normal themselves, circulate. These abnormalities can be acute or chronic in nature. They can arise from congenital lesions but usually result from acquired lesions. Inherited anomalies of glucose-6-phosphate dehydrogenase (G6PD) deficiency, which reduces the RBCs ability to deal with oxidative insults, can leave RBCs more vulnerable to environmental insults. Determination of hemolysis with various levels of compensation as the cause of an anemia is accomplished using the approaches described in Chapter 34. Signs of extrinsic hemolysis with minimal or no anemia can be valuable clues to diseases of other organ systems. Among the most important forms of extrinsic hemolytic anemia are those caused by immune mechanisms; these are discussed in Chapter 46.

Clinical and morphologic findings suggest the many misfortunes that can befall RBCs in their travels. They can be trapped in an abnormal bone marrow stroma network, sheared by jets in an abnormal heart, cut and fragmented by fibrin strands stretched across damaged areas in the microvasculature, or attacked by parasites. They can undergo stasis and perhaps metabolic depletion in giant hemangiomas or in an enlarged spleen. An abnormally functioning liver or kidney can cause a buildup of substances in plasma that alter RBC shape and metabolism. Drugs can cause oxidation or other metabolic damage. Oxidant injury provokes degradation of hemoglobin with the formation of hemichromes (see Drug-Induced Oxidative Hemolysis later). Degraded hemoglobin and hemichromes bind avidly to the cytoplasmic tail of the major transmembrane protein band 3 (see Chapter 45) and cause clustering of band 3 oligomers. Immunoglobulins (Igs) and complement then bind to the external membrane face over clusters of band 3, promoting immune destruction. Other membrane proteins may be subject to oxidative attack. Toxins, venoms, heat, and mechanical trauma can directly destroy the membrane. These agents may cause an alteration in the asymmetry of the phospholipid bilayer, causing phosphatidylserine to move from the inner leaflet of the membrane bilayer to the outer leaflet, where it can be recognized by macrophages.

In general, only the most devastating damage leads to direct intravascular destruction. Usually, the initial insult leads to an eventual change in the external portion of the RBC membrane, which causes macrophages to retard, hold, remove, or otherwise modify RBCs. Infection or inflammation can activate these macrophages. Some RBC changes are accompanied by a decrease in RBC deformability, which retards flow and thereby facilitates the action of macrophages on the affected RBC. All of these changes lead to extravascular hemolysis.

FRAGMENTATION HEMOLYSIS: MICROANGIOPATHY

Clinical Manifestations

Patients present with various degrees of hemolytic anemia and compensation, with evidence of RBC fragmentation on smear (Fig. 47.1; see box on Differential Diagnosis of Extrinsic Nonimmune Hemolytic Anemias). RBC removal is generally extravascular, with minimal or moderately decreased levels of haptoglobin. If RBC damage is sufficiently severe, signs of intravascular hemolysis may be present. Because of the underlying pathology, some of these syndromes show evidence of platelet removal, leading to thrombocytopenia. Occasionally, the underlying cause produces activation and depletion of procoagulant factors with consequent activation of the fibrinolytic system, consistent with disseminated intravascular coagulation (DIC; see box on Causes of Red Blood Cell Fragmentation Hemolysis).

Pathophysiology

Fragmentation hemolysis occurs when mechanical forces disrupt the physical integrity of the RBC membrane. In vitro shear stresses in excess of 3000 dynes/cm^2 cause RBC fragmentation. In vivo studies in patients with mitral prosthetic regurgitation and hemolysis show high peak shear stresses of 4500 dynes/cm^2, very rapid acceleration or deceleration, or both.

Research suggests alternative mechanisms of producing microangiopathic hemolysis that involve platelets and small vessel thrombi. The platelet-rich, fibrin-poor microvascular thrombi found in many patients with TTP now are thought to be caused by abnormally decreased ADAMTS-13 activity.[1,2] This metalloprotease is responsible for converting the highly thrombogenic ultra large multimers of von Willebrand factor made by platelets and endothelial cells into the smaller forms normally found in circulation. Mutations in or antibodies against ADAMTS-13 result in unusually large multimers of von Willebrand factor attached to endothelial cell surfaces, where platelets may excessively aggregate, leading to formation of microvascular thrombi even in the absence of endothelial damage. In the case of disseminated cancer, the cause of microangiopathy may be microvascular tumor emboli.

Whatever the mechanism of mechanical trauma, the RBC membrane is viscoelastic and has self-sealing properties (see Chapter 45), so that little hemoglobin leaks out as the cell is being cut. However, prolonged distortion of the membrane produces a plastic change; therefore, the smaller RBC fragments usually do not become microspheres or microdisks but continue to display evidence of the shearing event or distortion in the form of typical irregular shapes. These irregular shapes and the rigidity that they reflect subsequently interfere with the ability of RBCs to fold, elongate, and deform sufficiently to pass through 3-μm capillaries and even smaller slits in the walls of the sinusoids of the reticuloendothelial system. This sequence leads to their destruction.

Differential Diagnosis

Generally, the differential diagnosis of fragmentation hemolysis can be deduced from the clinical findings. The presence of a prosthetic heart valve or a regurgitant jet that fragments or accelerates (i.e., Waring blender syndrome) can be readily discerned. The clinical picture of TTP–HUS is generally dramatic and acute (see Chapter 134). Atrioventricular malformations may be associated with DIC and platelet removal; the diagnosis requires a high index of suspicion and imaging studies. The presence of preeclampsia in a pregnant woman with microangiopathic hemolysis usually is obvious, but HELLP syndrome is a serious complication of pregnancy that can occur without other signs of preeclampsia or hypertension. This syndrome can produce hepatic rupture, visual failure, DIC, seizures, and congestive heart failure, and requires treatment by prompt

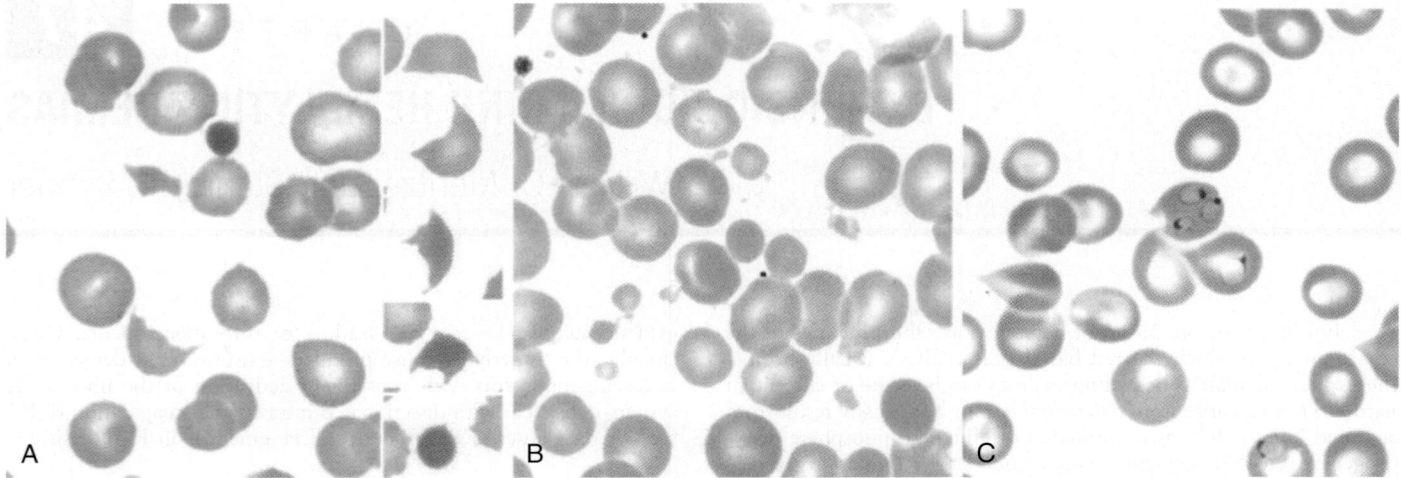

Fig. 47.1 PERIPHERAL BLOOD SMEARS FROM EXAMPLES OF EXTRINSIC NONIMMUNE HEMOLYTIC ANEMIA. (A) Microangiopathic hemolytic anemia. Note the schistocytes, fragmented cells, spherocyte, and polychromasia. More examples of damaged red blood cells (RBCs), including classic "helmet cell" (*top*), are seen to the immediate *right insert*. (B) Thermal injury from a burn. Thermally damaged RBCs form numerous microspherocytes and tiny RBC fragments. (C) Malaria infestation. RBCs containing *Plasmodium falciparum* malaria. Note the high rate of infestation, the presence of only ringed forms, and the multiply infested RBCs (*center*).

Differential Diagnosis of Extrinsic Nonimmune Hemolytic Anemias

There is no simple approach to the differential diagnosis of hemolysis caused by extrinsic nonimmune hemolytic anemia. The physician must pay close attention to the clinical finding. Useful clues come from a determination of whether RBC breakdown is predominantly extravascular or intravascular, but most important in the analysis is the observation of RBC morphology, which can focus the differential diagnosis. Unhelpful terms such as *aniso* and *poik* should be discarded. RBCs are spherocytic, stomatocytic, fragmented, echinocytic, acanthocytic, spurred, or bite cells, or can be mixtures of these types.

Causes of Red Blood Cell Fragmentation Hemolysis

- Damaged microvasculature
- Thrombotic thrombocytopenic purpura–hemolytic uremic syndrome (TTP–HUS)
- Associated with pregnancy: preeclampsia or eclampsia; hemolysis plus elevated liver enzymes plus low platelets (HELLP syndrome)
- Associated with malignancy, with or without mitomycin C treatment
- Vasculitis: polyarteritis, Wegener granulomatosis, acute glomerulonephritis, or *Rickettsia*-like infections
- Systemic lupus erythematosus
- Abnormalities of renal vasculature: malignant hypertension, acute glomerulonephritis, scleroderma, or allograft rejection with or without cyclosporine treatment
- Disseminated intravascular coagulation
- Malignant hypertension
- Catastrophic antiphospholipid antibody syndrome
- Atrioventricular malformations
- Kasabach–Merritt syndrome
- Hemangioendotheliomas
- Atrioventricular shunts for congenital and acquired conditions (e.g., stents, coils, transjugular intrahepatic portosystemic shunt, Levine shunts)
- Cardiac abnormalities
  - Replaced valve, prosthesis, graft, or patch
  - Aortic stenosis or regurgitant jets (e.g., in ruptured sinus of Valsalva)
- Drugs: cyclosporine, mitomycin, ticlopidine, clopidogrel, tacrolimus, or cocaine
- Systemic infection: bacterial endocarditis, brucellosis, cytomegalovirus, HIV, ehrlichiosis, Rocky Mountain spotted fever.

---

delivery of the fetus. Cancer can be an underlying cause of microangiopathy. Vessels supplying malignant tumors are thought to be structurally abnormal. They exhibit the same sort of fibrin stranding that produces fragmentation hemolysis in DIC and TTP–HUS.

Continued use of invasive diagnostic and therapeutic procedures with insertion of foreign bodies into the circulation has been complicated by microangiopathic hemolysis. A transjugular intrahepatic portosystemic shunt can cause the syndrome in approximately 10% of patients. The hemolysis usually disappears after 12–15 weeks. Similarly, use of coil embolization to seal off a patent ductus arteriosus may also cause significant hemolytic anemia. Vasculitis has also been implicated as a cause.

Multiple drugs are associated with microangiopathic hemolysis, most commonly quinine.[3,4] A recent review found that in only 22 of 78 drugs reported to produce drug-induced thrombotic microangiopathy was a definite association found.[4] Cyclosporine, tacrolimus, and mitomycin C have been implicated as causing a HUS picture that typically develops within weeks to months of exposure. Total body irradiation and bone marrow transplantation also are associated with microangiopathic hemolysis. Both chemotherapeutic agents and targeted cancer agents, including immunotoxins, monoclonal antibodies, and tyrosine kinase inhibitors, are associated with thrombotic microangiopathy.[5] The thienopyridines ticlodipine and clopidogrel are both capable of producing a significant thrombotic microangiopathy that differs somewhat in presentation. Ticlodipine-associated TTP typically occurs between 2 and 12 weeks after initiation of therapy and presents with severe thrombocytopenia, microangiopathic hemolytic anemia, highly elevated lactate dehydrogenase, and normal renal function, and is associated with severe deficiency of plasma ADAMTS13 activity.[6] In contrast, clopidogrel-associated TTP usually presents within 2 weeks of drug initiation and is associated with mild thrombocytopenia, microangiopathic hemolytic anemia, mildly elevated lactate dehydrogenase levels, marked renal insufficiency, and near-normal levels of ADAMTS13 activity. Other reported exposures associated with microangiopathic hemolytic anemia include the use of cocaine and the herb Echinacea, The mechanisms of drug-induced thrombotic microangiopathy are not well understood but include immune-mediated causes (as in the case of quinine) and direct toxicity to the endothelium.[4]

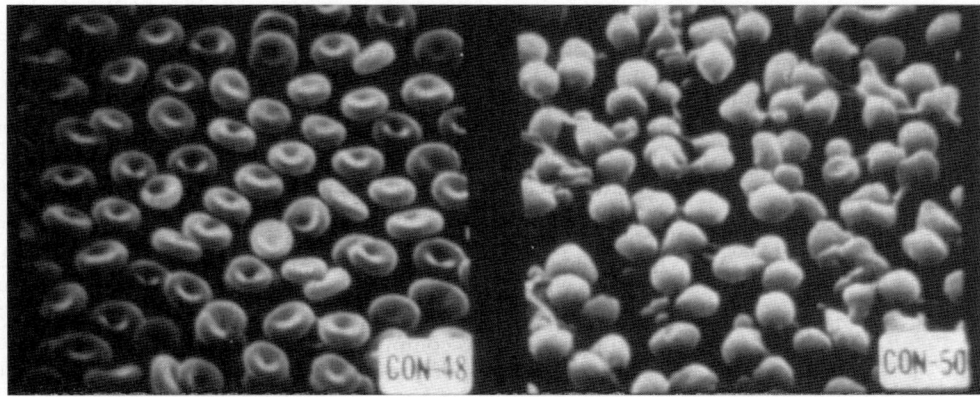

Fig. 47.2 MORPHOLOGIC CHANGES ARE PRODUCED BY HEATING NORMAL RED BLOOD CELLS AT THE INDICATED TEMPERATURES. Budding begins abruptly at 50°C (122°F) and eventually leads to spherocytosis.

Thrombotic microangiopathic hemolytic anemia can also be the presenting feature of severe, systemic infection, including viral (cytomegalovirus [CMV], HIV), fungal, and bacterial infections.[7] Whether infection "triggers" the development of TTP or instead the presentation remains debatable.

In one large series, 10 of 351 (2.8%) patients diagnosed with TTP were subsequently diagnosed with disseminated malignancy.[8] Symptoms suggesting an underlying malignancy include dyspnea, cough, atypical pain, and poor response to plasma exchange. The diagnosis was made by bone marrow biopsy in six of the 10 patients, and all patients died shortly after the diagnosis of malignancy was made.

A current review highlights four hereditary and four acquired disorders that lead to thrombotic microangiopathy.[2] TTP may be hereditary, due to mutations in ADAMTS13, or acquired, due to autoantibody inhibition of ADAMTS13 activity. In addition, complement mutations causing uncontrolled activation of the alternative pathway, mutations in components of cobalamin metabolism, and mutations in a protein kinase C–associated protein, diacylglycerol kinase, are other hereditary causes of thrombotic microangiopathy. Acquired causes in addition to autoantibodies to ADAMTS13 include shiga toxin (hemolytic uremic syndrome), drug mediated on an immune basis (i.e., quinine), drug mediated on a toxic, dose-related basis (i.e., gemcitabine, cyclosporine), and acquired antibodies to complement factor H.

Therapy

Management is primarily directed toward the underlying disease or event. Compensation of RBC production should be optimized by replacing iron or folic acid if the patient is deficient in these nutrients. Occasionally, removal or repair of a damaged native or prosthetic heart valve is necessary when the hemolysis produces a disabling transfusion requirement. Treatment of TTP with plasma exchange has been found to be superior to plasma infusions, with fresh-frozen plasma and cryo-free plasma appearing to have equal efficacy. Thrombotic microangiopathy associated with cyclosporine is often reversible with cessation of cyclosporine.

OTHER FORMS OF MECHANICAL DAMAGE TO RED BLOOD CELLS

Heat Denaturation

Normal RBCs undergo budding and fragmentation when exposed to a temperature of 49°C (120°F) in vitro (Fig. 47.1B). In some of the hereditary hemolytic anemias, this process occurs at temperatures as low as 46°C (115°F; see Chapter 45). Under some clinical circumstances, temperatures sufficient to cause heat denaturation of RBCs have been generated. Occasionally, cell warmers used with transfusions in cold agglutinin disease have malfunctioned and cooked the RBCs about to be transfused. In one case, a patient's mother warmed the RBCs with a hot water bottle, reasoning that such cells would cause less vein irritation to her child. Such transfusion was followed by evidence of intravascular and extravascular hemolysis, and the peripheral smear showed RBC budding and fragmentation (Fig. 47.2). Presumably, similar events can lead to hemolysis in patients who have sustained very extensive burns. In patients with heat stroke, the temperature usually is below 42°C (108°F), a temperature at which little RBC denaturation occurs.

Mechanical Trauma

The classic example of RBC damage caused by mechanical trauma is march hemoglobinuria, which occurs in soldiers after a long march, in joggers after running on a hard road, or in karate or conga drumming enthusiasts after practice. Anemia is rare, and reticulocytosis is uncommon. Evidence of typical intravascular RBC destruction is present and is thought to be caused by direct trauma to RBCs in the vessels of the feet or hands. Switching jogging paths or wearing better footwear often relieves the problem. Some cases show evidence of an underlying RBC membrane abnormality. Strenuous exercise may induce oxidant stress, as evidenced by increased levels of malonyldialdehyde, a marker of lipid peroxidation, in marathon runners after a race. Occasionally, malfunction of the cell savers used during abdominal or thoracic surgery mechanically injures RBCs.

Cardiopulmonary Bypass

Postperfusion syndrome occurs in some patients after cardiopulmonary bypass. The syndrome includes acute intravascular hemolysis and leukopenia as part of a febrile, inflammatory clinical picture. Affected patients may develop pulmonary distress and even adult or acute respiratory distress syndrome. Visible hemoglobinemia occurs, with rising plasma hemoglobin levels, and is associated with an increase in lysed RBC ghosts seen in the whole blood and plasma. These ghosts are coated with the complement complex C5bC9 (see Chapter 24). Presumably, the complement pathway is activated as the blood passes through the oxygenator. The reason why complement activation results in lytic attack on RBCs (and granulocytes) is unknown. Free hemoglobin released into the plasma secondary to intravascular hemolysis may contribute to acute kidney injury after cardiopulmonary bypass. Treatment involves knowledge of the process and requisite support until the situation corrects itself.

Osmotic Attack

Abrupt changes in osmolality can cause hemolysis. Freshwater drowning may be associated with so much water in the lungs that the RBCs swell as they undergo an in vivo osmotic fragility test in the pulmonary vasculature. Conversely, saltwater drowning can cause profound dehydration of RBCs, producing a situation analogous to xerocytosis (see Chapter 45). Rarely, acute hemolysis occurs from mistaken infusion of or exposure to concentrated hypertonic solutions such as those used in hemodialysis. To manage such an event, the physician must recognize its cause, appreciate the shrunken RBCs on a peripheral smear, and restore isotonicity as quickly as possible. In these cases, use of a hemodialysis device, if available, may be helpful.

Hypersplenism

In all organs of the monocyte–macrophage system (i.e., reticuloendothelial system), blood cells leaving the arterial bed are generally unloaded into channels such that the RBCs must pass through the wall of the sinus to reenter the circulation. The sinusoidal wall has slits 2–3 μm long and usually is endothelialized on one side and has a macrophagic lining on the other side. The normal human adult RBC is a discocyte with a surface area 40% larger than a sphere of that volume (see Chapter 33). This excess surface area allows an RBC with a diameter of approximately 8 μm to twist, elongate, and deform sufficiently to squeeze through these 2–3-μm slits. The excess surface area, occasionally referred to as the *ratio of surface area to volume* (SA:V), is critical and is normally approximately 1.4. Any condition that reduces SA:V reduces the ability of RBCs to traverse these sinusoidal slits because plump spheres cannot deform sufficiently.

Factors that interfere with interaction of the cytosol and the membrane also impair the ability of the RBC to deform. Oxidant attack may produce Heinz bodies that come to lie adjacent to the membrane. They interfere with the smooth movement of the membrane over the cytosol, a process called *tank treading*. Such cells are selectively blocked from leaving the splenic cords and entering the sinuses. Inflammation or infection may enhance the ability of splenic macrophages to attack and ingest RBCs. Although not strictly a mechanism of hypersplenism, Kupffer cell erythrophagocytosis is a prominent finding in patients undergoing graft-versus-host hemolysis seen after liver transplantation.

The spleen is more complicated than other reticuloendothelial organs in that the afferent arterioles pass through lymphoid nodules (i.e., white pulp) and then terminate in the cords of Billroth (i.e., red pulp), into which blood cells are discharged. In the slow flow of the cords of Billroth, blood cells are selectively attacked by macrophages and are in direct contact with several classes of lymphocytes. The blood cells must then pass through the cordal walls before they can approach the sinus wall, which they must pass through to reenter the circulation. The spleen provides a double filter, and the blood cells must be remarkably deformable to pass through it. This slow passage permits highly selective action by macrophages, which have receptors that can detect several sorts of alterations in these blood cells. These receptors include the Fc receptor for the appropriate portion of the Ig molecule, receptors for complement components such as C3b, and perhaps receptors that detect alterations in the outer portion of the phospholipid bilayer or in the externally oriented glycopeptides. The macrophage then holds, retards, modifies (i.e., pitting function), or removes (i.e., culling function) the blood cells identified. Normally, the pitting function of the spleen allows it to remove Howell–Jolly bodies and normally occurring endocytic vacuoles (called *pocks* because of their appearance on phase interference or Nomarski microscopy). The normal culling function of the spleen is exemplified by its removal of senescent RBCs.

All the activities of the spleen presumably are markedly accentuated in a large spleen, and if the increased activity is sufficiently extensive, hypersplenism ensues. The size of the spleen, not the portal pressure, is important in determining the degree of RBC sequestration. Other factors that may play a role are the state of activation of

TABLE 47.1	Causes of Splenomegaly
Cause	**Example**
Neoplasia	Lymphoma, hairy cell leukemia
Infection	Bacterial endocarditis, malaria, schistosomiasis, tuberculosis
Portal bed obstruction	Alcoholic cirrhosis, splenic vein thrombosis
Collagen vascular disease	Systemic lupus erythematosus, malignant phase of rheumatoid arthritis
Chronic inflammatory disease	Rheumatoid arthritis
Chronic hereditary or acquired hemolytic anemia	Severe β-thalassemia, autoimmune hemolytic anemia
Lipoidosis	Gaucher disease
Amyloidosis	AL and AA types
Tropical splenomegaly syndrome	Hyperreactive malarial splenomegaly syndrome

the splenic macrophages and the size of the small slits between the splenic cords and sinuses. The macrophages and slits seem to be under a degree of control, as evidenced by variations in splenic removal of RBCs in patients with malaria.

The clinical picture of hypersplenic hemolysis is dominated by the specific cause of the splenomegaly. Although the causes of splenomegaly are legion, there are several general mechanisms (Table 47.1). Usually some degree of anemia is seen, with evidence of a compensatory increase in RBC production. Because stasis and trapping in the spleen are associated with macrophagic attack and remodeling of the RBC surface, the reduction in SA:V leads to spherocytosis. If the RBCs undergo a prolonged period of distortion when traversing the cordal–sinus barrier, tailed RBCs will be present as the RBC membranes undergo a plastic change (see Chapter 45). Because the enlarged spleen can trap and remove platelets and white blood cells, variable thrombocytopenia and leukopenia may occur. The bone marrow may show normal to increased cellularity with erythroid hyperplasia.

Management depends on the cause of splenic enlargement. The anemia or pancytopenia usually is not profound; however, splenectomy may be contemplated if the anemia is severe. Alternatives to splenectomy include splenic embolization and high-intensity focused ultrasound ablation. In most situations, recognition of the possibility of hypersplenism is most important in guiding the approach to diagnosis of an unexplained anemia. Massive splenomegaly is frequently associated with expansion of the plasma compartment, and measurement of hemoglobin, hematocrit, or RBC levels may give a falsely low value of the RBC mass present. In that circumstance, the true RBC mass can be determined by ^{51}Cr assay.

A good example of massive splenomegaly causing plasma volume expansion is tropical splenomegaly syndrome, also known as *hyperreactive malarial splenomegaly syndrome*. Diagnostic criteria include massive splenomegaly more than 10 cm below the costal margin with no other cause identified; immunity to malaria; elevated serum IgM levels; and clinical response to treatment with antimalarial drugs such as chloroquine, proguanil, or pyrimethamine and folic acid. The pathophysiology of the splenomegaly seems to be poorly controlled B-lymphocytic production of antibodies, and IgM stimulation may be a response to malarial antigens or an unidentified mitogen. Malarial parasites are almost never found. The apparent anemia is in large part caused by plasma volume expansion, although RBC survival is reported to be slightly attenuated. Antimalarial therapy for several months reduces spleen size, so splenectomy is unnecessary.

TABLE 47.2	Mechanisms by Which Infection Can Cause Hemolysis	
Mechanism	**Example**
Direct parasitization of red cells	Malaria, babesiosis
Immune mechanisms	Cold agglutinin hemolysis after infectious mononucleosis or mycoplasmal pneumonia (see Chapter 46)
Induction of hypersplenism	Malaria, schistosomiasis
Altered red cell surface topology	*Haemophilus influenzae* infection
Release of toxins and enzymes	Clostridial infection causing thrombotic thrombocytopenic purpura–hemolytic uremic syndrome, *Escherichia coli* 0197, HIV infection

Infection

Infection can cause hemolytic anemia via several pathophysiologic mechanisms (Table 47.2).

Parasite Infections

The classic example of direct parasitization is infection by *Plasmodium falciparum* (Fig. 47.1C), *Plasmodium vivax,* or *Plasmodium malariae.* Infection with malaria, primarily *P. falciparum,* is a major health problem in the developing world, causing an estimated 300–500 million infections and 1–3 million deaths annually.[9] The burden of disease rests most heavily on young children and pregnant women. *Falciparum* malaria can cause a life-threatening anemia, with severe anemia defined as hemoglobin less than 5 g/dL associated with parasitemia and a normocytic blood film.[9] Malaria is primarily a disease of the tropical developing world but is still seen in the United States and its territories, primarily as an import from outside the United States. Of the 1298 cases reported in the United States in 2008, 117 (9%) were classified as severe, two of which were fatal. In each of the malarias, sporozoites injected by the mosquito in its saliva make their way to liver cells. After 1–2 weeks, they become merozoites, which burst out of the liver cells and into the bloodstream. Then, in a remarkable process, the parasite, by means of its apical end and related organelles called *rhoptries,* attaches to a specific receptor on the RBC surface. For *P. vivax,* the Duffy blood group antigen appears to be involved.

P. falciparum binds to sialic acid residues on the RBC surface that are on glycophorin A. After specific attachment, a convulsive movement occurs during which the RBC engulfs the parasite by a process resembling receptor-mediated endocytosis. Upon invasion of the RBC, the malarial parasite starts digesting the hemoglobin, depositing the undigested heme in the form of hemozoin. Knobs appear on the RBC surface, and the RBC becomes a sphere. Many proteins of parasitic origin are inserted into the RBC membrane, and some appear to cluster underneath these knobs. A parasite protein called *mature parasite-infected erythrocyte surface antigen* binds to membrane protein 4.1, and another parasite protein called *ring-infected erythrocyte surface antigen* binds to β spectrin. Both spectrin and protein 4.1 are integral components of the membrane skeleton, and the consequence of the binding of malarial proteins is RBC membrane stabilization. Thus stabilized, the parasitized RBC can continue to survive while the parasite continues to digest its contents.[10]

The parasite recruits the RBC's metabolic machinery, degrades and ingests hemoglobin, and grows, eventually bursting out of the RBC, and the cycle begins again. The RBCs are lysed intravascularly

as a consequence of direct parasitic destruction, extravascularly as a consequence of changes in the splenic microvasculature and in the activation state of the monocyte–macrophage system. Treatment consists of the use of appropriate antimalarials and the support of erythropoiesis, including the use of RBC transfusion or exchange (or both) when indicated.

The anemia of malarial infections also involves mechanisms distinct from lysis of parasitized RBCs. Erythropoiesis is suppressed, leading to suppression of erythroid precursors and inadequate reticulocytosis during acute infection.[11] This inadequate hematopoietic response may be exacerbated by underlying iron deficiency, hemoglobinopathies, or concomitant infection (e.g., HIV), all potential contributors to the severity of anemia. In addition, loss of uninfected erythrocytes plays a major role in the development of anemia, with an 8- to 10-fold greater loss of unparasitized RBCs compared with parasitized cells. Uninfected RBCs have reduced deformability, and the degree of reduced deformability correlates with the severity of infection. Poorly deformable RBCs likely are cleared by the spleen. A recent study in rats indicates that CD8 T-cell–dependent parasite clearance in the spleen is involved in the damage of uninfected RBCs and their subsequent destruction.[12] Evidence of in vivo removal of immature malarial forms prompts the question of whether "uninfected" cells that are lost represent previously infected cells that nevertheless remain abnormal. Insertion of a merozoite rhoptry protein, ring surface protein 2, on RBCs in which infection was aborted has been implicated in the clearance of unparasitized erythrocytes and erythroid progenitors. In addition, uninfected RBCs demonstrate increased binding of Igs that are probably nonspecific immune complexes. Acute malarial infection, particularly with *P. falciparum,* also leads to alteration in splenic function that incites premature destruction of uninfected RBCs.[13]

The lifespan of transfused RBCs is likewise decreased. ^{51}Cr-labeled normal RBCs infused into patients infected with malaria demonstrate a shorter lifespan than in normal control participants; this effect may persist after clearance of the parasitemia. Alternatively, parasites can be removed from RBCs along with the RBC membrane by the process of pitting, producing parasite-free spherocytes. This mechanism potentially explains the observed disparity between anemia and parasitemia.

Other infections that have somewhat similar pathophysiologies include Carrión disease (i.e., bartonellosis), in which a bite from the sandfly injects *Bartonella bacilliformis,* which attaches to the RBC surface of up to 80% of erythrocytes and causes lysis, leading to the massive hemolysis that characterizes acute infection. It appears that invasion of RBCs partly depends on the flagella of *Bartonella* spp. Incubation with antiflagellin antiserum reduces invasion of RBCs. The bacteria also secrete deformin, a factor that leads to deep pitting on the surface of RBCs, presumably providing a portal of entry into the erythrocyte. There also may be a role for splenic clearance of infected cells, and prior splenectomy appeared to protect a patient from hemolysis during acute infection.

Babesia organisms also directly invade RBCs by mechanisms somewhat resembling those seen is malaria,[14] producing fever and hemolytic anemia. The parasite is transmitted by ticks and transfusions of infected blood products,[15] and can be transmitted vertically. Most tick-borne cases occur on the West Coast, particularly in Washington and California, and in the northern portion of the Midwest; cases occurring on the East Coast are concentrated in Massachusetts and Nantucket Island. However, transfusion-associated cases have been reported throughout the United States.[15] In one report of transfusion-associated babesiosis, the median interval from transfusion to onset of clinical manifestations was 37 days. The organisms can be seen invading RBCs on smear examination, somewhat like *P. falciparum* malaria, but these organisms produce no pigment. The highest risk of death from babesiosis occurs in individuals who are older than 50 years or are immunocompromised because of acquired immunodeficiency syndrome (AIDS), drugs, transplantation, or asplenism. Sporadic reports indicate that acquired chronic toxoplasmosis is occasionally associated with hemolytic anemia.

Alteration of the Red Blood Cell Surface by Bacterial Products

Infection can produce hemolysis by altering the RBC surface. An example is the hemolysis caused by *Haemophilus influenzae* type b. Severely affected patients, particularly those with meningitis, have developed hemolytic anemias requiring RBC transfusions. The capsular polysaccharide of the bacterium, composed of polyribosyl ribitol phosphate (PRP), is released during infection and binds to the RBC surface. Infected patients develop antibodies to PRP. When the balance between PRP-coated RBCs and anti-PRP antibodies is correct, an immune-type hemolysis occurs and requires complement. RBC destruction is thought to be both intravascular and extravascular.

Bacterial Products Causing Hemolysis by Direct Damage to Red Blood Cells

The most dramatic example of hemolysis caused by bacterial action is clostridial infection, during which the organism releases enzymes that acutely degrade the phospholipids of the membrane bilayer and the structural membrane proteins. The resulting spherocytes are extremely sensitive to osmotic lysis. The setting can be any infection, but our experience is limited to acute cholecystitis, surgery of the biliary tree, and infections surrounding an obstetric event, including criminal or self-induced abortion, or other infection of the gravid uterus. Patients may also have an underlying gastrointestinal, genitourinary, neuroendocrine, or hematologic malignancy.[16] The signs of infections may be obvious, but fever may be unimpressive. Signs of collapse appear acutely, and the clue is profound intravascular hemolysis, with a spherocytic anemia developing with shocking suddenness. The blood smear characteristically has numerous spherocytes with little evidence of microangiopathy, may be tinged red because of marked hemoglobinemia, and may have ghost cells. A clue to the severity of the process may be the inability of the laboratory to perform chemical determinations or to type and cross-match the blood because the sample is hemolyzed. With even the slightest suspicion of hemolysis caused by bacterial action, the physician immediately starts full doses of penicillin and clindamycin; evaluates the patient for DIC (see Chapter 139); and prepares to support the patient for shock, DIC, acute renal failure, and hemolytic anemia. Whether hysterectomy is lifesaving in the case of septic abortion is unclear.

Hemolysis Caused by Less Well Understood Infections

HIV infection can cause Coombs-positive autoimmune hemolytic anemia, a TTP-like syndrome, and microangiopathic hemolysis. CMV infection has been reported to cause severe Coombs-negative hemolytic anemia in immunocompetent adults.[17] Case reports of autoimmune hemolytic anemia and HUS associated with CMV infection have emerged. The hemolytic anemia in visceral leishmaniasis may be caused in part by generation of oxidative metabolic products. Severe microangiopathic hemolytic anemia has been described in cases of cutaneous anthrax.

Hemolysis Associated With Liver Disease

Hemolysis in liver disease by itself usually is not of overwhelming clinical importance, but it may contribute to the severity of anemia when coupled with defects in RBC production and the type of gastrointestinal blood loss that occurs in several forms of liver disease. Hemolysis in patients with liver disease has several causes. The spleen may be enlarged as a consequence of portal hypertension and produce a hypersplenic picture, a phenomenon seen commonly in hepatic cirrhosis.

Reduction of Dangerous Methemoglobin Levels

Levels of methemoglobin in excess of 20% to 30% can be dangerous, but they can be easily treated with methylene blue (1–2 mg/kg) infused intravenously over 5 minutes as 0.1–0.2 mL/kg of a 1% solution. In the presence of a functioning, intact reduced form of nicotinamide adenine dinucleotide phosphate (NADPH)–methemoglobin reductase system, methylene blue is reduced to leukomethylene blue, which reduces methemoglobin to hemoglobin.

The literature on RBC shape change in liver disease is considerable. The target cell in cirrhosis has an increased SA:V that appears to be a consequence of increased cholesterol and phospholipid content of the membrane bilayer. The cholesterol increase is usually proportionately greater, resulting in an increased cholesterol-to-phospholipid ratio. This increase in lipid probably accounts for the increased RBC surface area, such that more membrane than usual is present in relation to cellular contents. These RBCs probably circulate as bell-shaped RBCs called *codocytes*. However, on dried blood films, they assume the appearance of target cells. Target cells do not have a shortened survival. The RBCs of patients with liver disease frequently are echinocytes when wet preparations are examined, but these echinocytes are not easily apparent on dried blood smears. The echinocytes seem to be produced by a material in the patient's plasma that causes normal RBCs to become echinocytic; this material is an abnormal echinocytogenic high-density lipoprotein. Echinocytes do not necessarily have a shortened survival. Some forms of echinocytic RBCs are normally deformable when studied in the ektacytometer or rheoscope.

A brisk, clinically important hemolysis can occur in some patients with severe liver disease. The peripheral smear in these individuals usually shows acanthocytes (i.e., distorted RBCs). Extreme forms are called *spur cells*, which are probably acanthocytes additionally remodeled by an enlarged spleen (see box on Reduction of Dangerous Methemoglobin Levels) and are considerably enriched in cholesterol. They are rapidly removed in the spleen, which is usually enlarged.

Increased RBC membrane proteolytic activity may be a partial explanation for the differences between acanthocytosis and spur cells, and additional pathophysiologic mechanisms may be involved. Although the adult RBC cannot synthesize phospholipids de novo, it can identify and remove peroxidized fatty acid chains that interfere with normal membrane lipid fluidity. When the fatty acid is removed, a lytic lysoderivative remains; therefore, the missing fatty acid chain must be replaced. A store of acyl groups in the form of acylcarnitine exists in RBC membranes. When needed, the fatty acid (i.e., acyl group) is transferred to acyl-coenzyme A and then inserted into the potentially lytic lysophospholipid by the enzyme lysophosphocholine acyltransferase. Lysophosphocholine acyltransferase is inhibited in spur RBCs, and the same inhibition can be produced by heavily loading RBCs with cholesterol in vitro.

In a case of almost fatal oxidative hemolysis, hydrogen peroxide was injected directly into the Hickman catheter of a patient with AIDS because some persons infected with HIV had circulated a pamphlet suggesting that hydrogen peroxide could be used therapeutically to control HIV infection. We now are seeing AIDS patients with dapsone-induced methemoglobinemia and hemolytic anemia (see Chapter 42). Methemoglobinemia, if severe, is treated as described in the preceding paragraph and in Chapter 24.

In spur cell anemia, the RBCs have an abnormal membrane SA:V ratio, their membrane fluidity is impaired, and they are unable to remove and repair peroxidatively damaged fatty acids. Occasionally, spur cell hemolytic anemia is severe enough to necessitate consideration of splenectomy. Operative morbidity in such cases is considerable because the underlying liver disease usually produces problems with thrombocytopenia and leukopenia, as well as with procoagulants and intolerance to anesthesia. Spur cell anemia is typically associated with alcoholic cirrhosis, but can also be seen in patients with nonalcoholic cirrhosis. The anemia tends to be severe and portends a poor prognosis. Transfusions are of limited efficacy because the membrane abnormalities are acquired by transfused RBCs.[18] In one case, spur cell anemia occurred in a pediatric patient after orthotopic liver transplantation and resolved after retransplantation.[19]

Acute alcoholism can be associated with hypophosphatemia, defined as levels less than 0.2 mg/dL. Such hypophosphatemia presumably interferes with RBC intermediary metabolism (see Chapters 33 and 44), and RBC adenosine triphosphate (ATP) levels fall. Very low ATP levels are associated with RBC rigidity, which leads to fragmentation, loss of surface area, and spheroidicity. The RBCs then are further trapped in the spleen. This hypophosphatemia syndrome can also cause neuromuscular disorders, including weakness, paresthesias, tremors, and seizures. It should be treated aggressively with orally and intravenously administered phosphate supplements. Hypophosphatemia also occurs in patients with cirrhosis, patients receiving total parenteral nutrition whose phosphate intake is not carefully monitored, and patients taking large amounts of phosphate-binding antacids.

Stomatocytosis can occur in severe liver disease and is thought to be a sign of acute alcoholic intoxication. The change in RBC shape can also be seen in acute pancreatitis. The stomatocyte is a cell well on its way to becoming a spherocyte. The reduction in SA:V leads to trapping in the microvasculature of the spleen and other organs of the monocyte–macrophage system, producing various degrees of hemolysis.

Renal Disease

The anemia in renal disease is multifactorial. A major component is impaired RBC production, which can be well controlled with erythropoietin. Renal disease also impairs platelet function, which may lead to occult blood loss. However, hemolysis also can occur and is multifactorial. Disease of the small renal arterioles can produce fragmentation hemolysis of the sort seen in TTP–HUS, preeclampsia, and malignant hypertension (see the box on Causes of Red Blood Cell Fragmentation Hemolysis). Otherwise, whether uremia produces significant shortening of RBC survival is not clear. Patients with chronic renal failure who are undergoing hemodialysis may be particularly susceptible to oxidative damage to their RBCs. RBC glutathione is reduced in some patients, and the activity of the enzymes G6PD and glutathione peroxidase is relatively low. The ability of these RBCs to deal with generation of peroxides probably is impaired.

Venoms, Bites, Stings, and Toxins

The best-known example of toxin-caused hemolysis is discussed in the earlier section, Bacterial Products Causing Hemolysis by Direct Damage to Red Blood Cells.

Insect, Spider, and Snake Bites

Hemolysis occurs after bee and wasp stings, snake bites, and spider bites. Isolated cases of acute intravascular hemolysis after bee and wasp stings have been reported. Two kinds of dangerous spiders live in the United States: the southern black widow and the brown recluse spider. Both sexes of the black widow produce the venom, but only the female has fangs capable of penetrating human skin. Black widow spider bites produce generalized muscle pain and muscular rigidity. Hemolysis is not common. Brown recluse spider bites cause a considerable local reaction, called the *volcano lesion*. DIC and hemolysis may occur after a lag of 24–48 hours. Envenomation results in cleavage of RBC glycophorins, presumably making the RBCs more susceptible.[20] Corticosteroids may be beneficial. The hemolysis appears to be self-limiting, but RBC transfusion support may be needed.

In some parts of the world, cobra bites can cause intravascular hemolysis because the venom contains phospholipases. In the United

States, the two classes of venomous snakes are pit vipers (e.g., rattlesnakes, cottonmouths, moccasins, and copperheads) and coral snakes. Pit viper venom affects hemostasis and may produce DIC with bleeding but rarely hemolysis. Coral snake venom produces severe neurologic impairment. Therapy consists of support and use of the appropriate antivenin and prophylactic antimicrobials, and tetanus injections.

Drugs and Chemicals Exclusive of Those Producing Oxidative Hemolysis

Potassium Chlorate

Potassium chlorate ingestion is listed as a cause of hemolysis, but this compound is no longer available in hospital pharmacies and has no currently recognized medical use. Arsine gas is generated in industrial plants that engage in lead plating, galvanizing, etching, and soldering. Inhalation of a toxic amount produces a severe intravascular hemolysis of unknown pathogenesis and may require urgent RBC and plasma exchange.

Copper

The idea that copper can produce human hemolytic disease is best supported by observations of episodes of severe hemolysis and acute liver failure in patients with Wilson disease. The patient usually is a child, adolescent, or young adult for whom the diagnosis of Wilson disease has not yet been made. The initial clinical presentation is usually dominated by Coombs-negative hemolytic anemia accompanied by weakness and dark urine. Associated findings include coagulopathy, a rapid progression to renal failure, relatively modest rises in serum aminotransferases, and a low alkaline phosphatase level. In addition to the presence of a brisk reticulocytosis, the typical findings of intravascular hemolysis may be present, including elevated lactate dehydrogenase, low haptoglobin, and markedly elevated bilirubin levels. Review of the peripheral smear may not reveal any specific morphologic findings, although both stomatocytosis and blister cells consistent with oxidant injury have been described. In one reported patient with concomitant transfusion-dependent hemoglobin E/β thalassemia, the acute hemolysis led to a severe unexpected drop in the posttransfusion hemoglobin level. Because of the hereditary deficiency in the copper-binding protein ceruloplasmin, urine and serum nonceruloplasmin–bound copper levels in patients with hemolysis are very high.

Free copper can interfere with glucose metabolism by hexokinase inhibition and alternatively can generate oxidative hemolysis, perhaps by acting as a Fenton reagent. It is important to establish the diagnosis promptly. When this condition is suspected, the practitioner should look for Kayser–Fleischer rings on physical examination, and measure serum and urine copper and ceruloplasmin levels. Treatment with penicillamine or trientine plus zinc reduces the serum copper level and stops the hemolysis.[21] In the case of acute liver failure, the treatment is urgent liver transplantation. Plasmapheresis and hemofiltration may be beneficial in reducing the copper level and can serve as a bridge to transplant. In some cases, plasmapheresis in combination with chelation therapy or the use of a fractionated plasma separation and adsorption dialysis system may avert the need for transplant in impending acute liver failure. Other forms of copper poisoning may cause hemolysis in patients who do not have underlying Wilson disease. The amount of copper ingested would have to exceed the copper-binding capacity of normal ceruloplasmin levels.

Lead

There are at least two general forms of lead intoxication. One type is chronic, slow cumulative poisoning (i.e., saturnism). An example is occupational exposure. Symptoms are predominantly neurologic and nephrologic, with variable degrees of anemia, which may be caused by a production defect combined with hemolysis. Relatively acute poisoning occurs when lead inadvertently finds its way into a food source or is consumed as part of an exotic medication. Subacute lead poisoning leads to central nervous system symptoms, hepatitis, nephrotoxicity, hypertension, and abdominal colic along with seizures and severe hemolytic anemia. Physical examination may reveal a lead line on the gums. Peripheral smear shows extensive coarse basophilic stippling and reticulocytosis; however, RBC morphology is not otherwise characteristic. Some researchers state that intravascular destruction occurs, but no proof has been provided. Bilirubin levels are not significantly elevated.

The diagnosis of lead-related hemolysis can be made from the history and findings on physical examination, which include a lead line on the gingiva and coarse basophilic stippling on RBCs, which reflects the pathologic aggregation of ribosomes. The diagnosis is confirmed by measuring blood and urine lead levels. The level of acuity determines the therapy.

The cause of the anemia is complex. Lead interferes with several steps in heme synthesis, particularly those involving heme synthetase and δ-aminolevulinic acid dehydratase (see Chapter 38). The inhibition of heme synthetase probably accounts for the elevation in free erythrocyte protoporphyrin, which provides a useful corroborative diagnostic test for lead toxicity. Inhibition of heme synthesis also probably accounts for the elevated urinary levels of δ-aminolevulinic acid and coproporphyrin. Lead poisoning mimics the basophilic stippling and accumulation of pyrimidines seen in hereditary deficiency of the enzyme pyrimidine 5′-nucleotidase, probably because lead attacks the enzyme (see Chapter 44).

Ribavirin

Current treatment of chronic hepatitis C virus (HCV) infection may consist of combination therapy with pegylated interferon (IFN) and ribavirin, a nucleoside analogue. Ribavirin's activity against HCV includes inhibition of inosine monophosphate dehydrogenase, a key step in de novo guanine synthesis. Treatment with ribavirin may produce dose-dependent hemolytic anemia, which is typically reversible 1–2 months after discontinuing treatment.[22] The hemoglobin drops by an average of 2–3 g/dL and may fall below 11 g/dL in one third or more of patients. The anemia may necessitate a dose reduction of ribavirin or may be treated with recombinant erythropoietin at 40,000 units weekly. A decrease in the total cumulative dose of ribavirin may be associated with decreased sustained virologic response, which would suggest that dose reduction secondary to anemia would have an adverse impact on treatment efficacy. However, in one retrospective study, a drop in hemoglobin of greater than 3 g/dL was instead associated with improved sustained virologic response rate compared with those with a drop in hemoglobin 3 g/dL or less,[23] suggesting conversely that the degree of hemolytic anemia may serve as a biomarker of efficacy. Ribavirin is transported into the erythrocytes and accumulates as ribavirin monophosphates, diphosphates, and triphosphates.[22] The steady-state concentration of ribavirin in erythrocytes is approximately 100-fold higher than that of plasma, and higher erythrocyte ribavirin levels correlate with worsened anemia during therapy. Accumulation of phosphates leads to a decrease in ATP levels compared with control erythrocytes. Because ATP is required to generate the glucose-6-phosphate needed for glycolysis and the hexose monophosphate shunt, reduced levels of ATP may lead to oxidative damage, as evidenced by increased aggregates of band 3, which bind anti-band 3 IgG and complement. The ribavirin prodrug viramidine induces less anemia than ribavirin, although efficacy was decreased when used at fixed doses compared with a ribavirin-containing regimen. Fellay et al[24] have detected two polymorphisms in the inosine triphosphatase (*ITPA*) gene, which encodes a protein that hydrolyzes inosine triphosphate, and were protective against severe anemia in patients treated with HCV. These two polymorphisms were associated with reduced

ITPA activity and accumulation of inosine triphosphate in red blood cells. The mechanism of this protective effect is not yet fully understood. The anemia in patients treated with ribavirin may be exacerbated by concomitant treatment with pegylated IFN, which suppresses hematopoiesis, and may also be associated with autoimmune hemolytic anemia. Anemia may also be exacerbated when ribavirin and IFN are used in combination with the protease inhibitor,[25] a regimen that is efficacious in the treatment of genotype 1 disease.

DRUG-INDUCED OXIDATIVE HEMOLYSIS

General Concepts

The potential for normal RBCs to undergo auto-oxidative destruction is great because the cell is loaded with 20-mM hemoglobin, most of which is bonded to oxygen at the iron(II) atom in heme. The bond that allows the reversible association and dissociation of oxygen from the heme moiety of hemoglobin involves partial transfer of an electron from iron(II) to oxygen. That oxygen then has an extra electron, which makes it a superoxide radical. Ordinarily, when oxygen leaves hemoglobin, it returns the electron. If it does not, a highly reactive superoxide ion is released, leaving behind it an iron(III) moiety called *methemoglobin*.

$$\text{Hb Fe}^{2+}\text{O}_2 \rightarrow \text{Hb Fe}^{3+} + \text{O}_2^{-1}$$

Methemoglobin cannot reversibly bind oxygen. Methemoglobin in itself is not harmful to RBCs, but if the oxidative assault persists, methemoglobin is converted to hemichromes, which are variably denatured hemoglobin intermediates in which the distal histidine unit binds to the oxidized heme. This step is associated with conversion from a high to a low spin state, as measured by electron spin resonance. Continued oxidation leads to irreversibility of hemichrome oxidation, precipitation, and eventually formation of Heinz bodies. Hemichromes and Heinz bodies can destroy membrane function directly or by causing oxidation of membrane proteins and lipids.[26] Approximately 3% of hemoglobin is converted to methemoglobin each day, but the finding that only 1% of hemoglobin normally is in the form of methemoglobin indicates that a mechanism preventing oxidation in RBCs is in effect. These mechanisms are limited because RBCs lack the ability to either efficiently generate ATP or synthesize enzymes. The primary means for preventing or addressing oxidant injury are the generation of the reduced form of nicotinamide adenine dinucleotide (NADH) via the Embden–Meyerhof glycolytic pathway and the generation of NADPH via the hexose monophosphate shunt. NADH is used to reduce methemoglobin by cytochrome b5 reductase, and NADPH is used to reduce glutathione and for catalase activity. Defects in this defense system against oxidation lead to an enhanced tendency to oxidative hemolysis. Examples are G6PD deficiency states.[27] G6PD catalyzes the initial rate-limiting step in the hexose monophosphate shunt. Deficiencies lead to a reduced ability to generate NADPH in response to oxidant stress. Any agent or event that interferes with the smooth offloading of oxygen enhances the generation of O_2^{-1} and methemoglobin, as indicated in the equation. If the reducing power of the RBC is inadequate, hemichromes and Heinz bodies are generated. Many agents appear to cause oxidative hemolysis by interfering with the smooth functioning of the heme cleft.

Pathophysiology

After the oxidative attack has been initiated, the sequence proceeds along a recognizable track. The oxidative attack is directed at hemoglobin and the RBC membrane. However, these structures are not clearly separable because the precipitated hemichrome and Heinz bodies come to lie against the cytosolic face of the membrane. Methemoglobin may be detectably elevated, with levels as

Agents That Cause Oxidative Hemolysis

• Therapeutic agents
  • Nitrofurantoin (Furadantin)
  • Sulfasalazine (Azulfidine)
  • *p*-Aminosalicylic acid
  • Phenazopyridine (Pyridium)
  • Clotrimoxazole
  • Quinolones
  • Phenacetin
  • Rasburicase
  • Dapsone and other sulfones
  • Primaquine
• Recreational drugs
  • Isobutyl nitrate
  • Amyl nitrite
• Miscellaneous agents
  • Naphthalene mothballs
  • Methylene Blue
  • Paraquat
  • Hydrogen peroxide

high as 50% to 60% of total hemoglobin. The hemichromes, by themselves or with their iron portions acting as a Fenton reagent, mediate the generation of hydroxyl free radicals, which add their effect to that of superoxide and hydrogen peroxide. Lipid peroxidation may take place, leading to membrane blebbing and cell lysis, as well as loss of asymmetry of the phospholipid membrane bilayer. Movement of phosphatidylserine and phosphatidylethanolamine to the outer bilayer of the membrane results in increased recognition by macrophages in the reticuloendothelial system. Membrane proteins may be crosslinked, with binding of denatured, oxidized hemoglobin to the membrane cytoskeleton, which may increase splenic macrophage recognition. In addition, the RBCs are rigid and susceptible to trapping in sinusoidal structures, whether or not they have Heinz bodies lying against the membrane. In vitro evidence suggests that oxidized RBCs are increasingly susceptible to phagocytosis by macrophages. These features may account for extravascular destruction. The oxidative lesions can be severe enough to cause intravascular destruction as well, producing hemoglobinemia and hemoglobinuria.

The smear may show bite cells, which look as if a macrophage had taken a bite, removing a Heinz body-containing segment of membrane. RBC rigidity may result in irregularly shaped cells because these undeformable cells are unable to undergo elastic recoil after fighting their way through the sinus wall. Recurrent loss of membrane material may produce spherocytes. Severe hemolysis may produce the kind of circulating ghost or hemighost called a *blister cell* or *bite cell*. These RBCs have an empty veil of membrane on one side and puddled hemoglobin on the other. A Heinz body preparation may be positive. However, the absence of bite cells does not rule out the diagnosis.

The clinical picture is determined by the specific agent used. Screening for G6PD deficiency or a related disorder using an enzyme assay or the ascorbate cyanide test may be useful. Although any defect in the antioxidant defense mechanisms, such as G6PD deficiency, considerably increases the susceptibility to hemolysis, many agents can produce oxidant hemolysis even in persons with normal defense mechanisms (see box on Agents That Cause Oxidative Hemolysis). Paraquat ingestion has occurred inadvertently and in suicide attempts. Profound cyanosis with methemoglobinemia can occur within hours, with levels of 120% or higher. The condition may be succeeded by hemolysis, with Heinz bodies seen in appropriate preparations of RBCs.

Toxic ingestion or inhalation of nitrites may occur in suicide attempts from industrial exposures; via diets high in pickled or smoked foods; through intentional recreational use; or in infants from formulas prepared using well water high in nitrates, which are reduced to nitrites in the infant gut.[28] Nitrites bind to hemoglobin, producing methemoglobinemia, which may be so profound as to produce coma. If methylene blue infusion does not quickly turn the chocolate color of blood back to normal, the physician must consider the possibility that the patient is G6PD deficient and therefore unable to generate adequate amounts of NADPH (discussed earlier in the section Drug-Induced Oxidative Hemolysis: General Concepts). In that case, exchange transfusion may be lifesaving. Benzocaine topical anesthesia in the form of a spray or cream can cause severe methemoglobinemia, with cyanosis and dyspnea requiring methylene blue treatment.

Pyridium (phenazopyridine) can cause oxidative hemolysis even in the absence of renal disease. This agent is commonly used for treatment of bladder irritation. The *Physician's Desk Reference* recommends maximum therapy of 2 days. However, patients not uncommonly are given a prescription for 1–4 weeks of therapy.

It has been recognized for more than 130 years that therapy with dapsone causes oxidative hemolysis. In the past, dapsone was used primarily to treat leprosy and dermatitis herpetiformis, and was not often encountered as a cause of oxidative hemolysis. Dapsone has come into more widespread use in some communities as a very effective prophylactic agent against *Pneumocystis carinii* pneumonia in patients with AIDS. The reduced levels of glutathione reported in patients with AIDS may enhance dapsone toxicity. Dapsone is also used in the treatment of malaria where it regularly causes hemolytic anemia in G6PD-deficient patients.[29] Some clinics screen potential recipients for G6PD deficiency (see Chapter 44) and, if results are negative, proceed with dapsone therapy. However, dapsone can cause oxidative attack on normal RBCs, leading sequentially to methemoglobinemia, Heinz bodies, and hemolysis, all occurring at generally accepted standard doses. Dapsone is metabolized to a hydroxylamine derivative that is directly toxic to RBCs.

MISCELLANEOUS, POORLY CHARACTERIZED CAUSES OF EXTRINSIC HEMOLYTIC ANEMIAS

Interferon-α as a Cause of Hemolytic Anemia

Both microangiopathic and autoimmune hemolysis have been reported with IFN-α use. Zuber et al[30] reported eight patients with chronic myeloid leukemia who developed thrombotic microangiopathy confirmed by renal biopsy. Seven of these patients had identifiable hemolysis, and three had thrombocytopenia. They also reviewed 13 other cases of microangiopathy associated with IFN-α reported in the literature and observed that most cases occurred in the setting of prolonged therapy in chronic myeloid leukemia. Two cases of chronic hepatitis with microangiopathy were notable for having received unusually high doses of IFN for this indication. Cases of autoimmune hemolysis have been reported with IFN-α therapy in the setting of chronic myeloid leukemia or chronic hepatitis C.

Hemolysis With Intravenous Immunoglobulin G

Strictly speaking, hemolysis with intravenous IgG is a form of immune hemolysis. However, preparations of IgG contain anti-A and anti-B antibodies, and rarely cause an alloimmune hemolytic anemia, as described in two young women undergoing treatment for idiopathic thrombocytopenic purpura. If this situation occurs and more intravenous IgG is needed, performing a minor cross-match and choosing a preparation of intravenous IgG that gives no reaction is recommended. In addition to isoantibody production, anemia has been reported with intravenous IgG because of immune complex-mediated complement activation.

For hemolytic anemia with large granular lymphocyte leukemia, see box on Hemolytic Anemia in Chronic Large Granular Lymphocytic Leukemia.

Hemolytic Anemia in Chronic Large Granular Lymphocytic Leukemia

Although large granular lymphocytic leukemia usually manifests as neutropenia and a rheumatoid-like picture, several patients with a severe Coombs-negative hemolytic anemia in the absence of splenomegaly have been described. Large granular lymphocytic leukemia has occurred in a splenectomized patient. The mechanism is unknown, but one report identified direct cytotoxicity against RBCs by the large granular lymphocytic cell lines.

There have been no formal studies on therapy for large granular lymphocytic leukemia-related hemolysis, although immunosuppressive therapy with prednisone or methotrexate has been reported as being partially or wholly successful.

REFERENCES

1. Moake J: Thrombotic microangiopathies: Multimers, metalloprotease, and beyond. *Clin Transl Sci* 2:366, 2009.
2. George JN, Nester CM: Syndromes of thrombotic microangiopathy. *New Engl J Med* 371:654, 2014.
3. George JN: How I treat patients with thrombotic thrombocytopenic purpura: 2010. *Blood* 116:4060, 2010.
4. Al-Nouri ZL, Reese JA, Terrell DR, et al: Drug-induced thrombotic microangiopathy: a systematic review of published reports. *Blood* 125:616, 2015.
5. Blake-Haskins JA, Lechleider RJ, Kreitman RJ: Thrombotic microangiopathy with targeted cancer agents. *Clin Cancer Res* 17:5858, 2011.
6. Zakarija A, Kwaan HC, Moake JL, et al: Ticlopidine- and clopidogrel-associated thrombotic thrombocytopenic purpura (TTP): review of clinical, laboratory, epidemiological, and pharmacovigilance findings (1989-2008). *Kidney Int Suppl* S20, 2009.
7. Booth KK, Terrell DR, Vesely SK, et al: Systemic infections mimicking thrombotic thrombocytopenic purpura. *Am J Hematol* 86:743, 2011.
8. Francis KK, Kalyanam N, Terrell DR, et al: Disseminated malignancy misdiagnosed as thrombotic thrombocytopenic purpura: A report of 10 patients and a systematic review of published cases. *Oncologist* 12:11, 2007.
9. Casals-Pascual C, Roberts DJ: Severe malarial anaemia. *Curr Mol Med* 6:155, 2006.
10. An X, Mohandas N: Red cell membrane and malaria. *Transfus Clin Biol* 17:197, 2010.
11. Chang KH, Tam M, Stevenson MM: Inappropriately low reticulocytosis in severe malarial anemia correlates with suppression in the development of late erythroid precursors. *Blood* 103:3727, 2004.
12. Safeukul I, Gomez ND, Adelani AA, et al: Malaria induces anemia through CD8+ T cell-dependent parasite clearance and erythrocyte removal in the spleen. *MBio* 6:1, 2015.
13. Looareesuwan S, Ho M, Wattanagoon Y, et al: Dynamic alteration in splenic function during acute falciparum malaria. *N Engl J Med* 317:675, 1987.
14. Lobo CA, Rodriguez M, Cursino-Santos JR: Babesia and red cell invasion. *Curr Opin Hematol* 19:170, 2012.
15. Herwaldt BL, Linden JV, Bosserman E, et al: Transfusion-associated babesiosis in the United States: a description of cases. *Ann Intern Med* 155:509, 2011.
16. McArthur HL, Dalal BI, Kollmannsberger C: Intravascular hemolysis as a complication of clostridium perfringens sepsis. *J Clin Oncol* 24:2387, 2006.
17. Veldhuis W, Janssen M, Kortlandt W, et al: Coombs-negative severe haemolytic anaemia in an immunocompetent adult following cytomegalovirus infection. *Eur J Clin Microbiol Infect Dis* 23:844, 2004.
18. Cooper RA, Kimball DB, Durocher JR: Role of the spleen in membrane conditioning and hemolysis of spur cells in liver disease. *N Engl J Med* 290:1279, 1974.
19. Alkhouri N, Alamiry MR, Hupertz V, et al: Spur cell anemia as a cause of unconjugated hyperbilirubinemia after liver transplantation and its resolution after retransplantation. *Liver Transpl* 17:349, 2011.
20. Tambourgi DV, Morgan BP, de Andrade RM, et al: Loxosceles intermedia spider envenomation induces activation of an endogenous metalloproteinase, resulting in cleavage of glycophorins from the erythrocyte surface and facilitating complement-mediated lysis. *Blood* 95:683, 2000.
21. Roberts EA, Schilsky ML: Diagnosis and treatment of Wilson disease: an update. *Hepatology* 47:2089, 2008.
22. McHutchison JG, Manns MP, Longo DL: Definition and management of anemia in patients infected with hepatitis C virus. *Liver Int* 26:389, 2006.
23. Sulkowski MS, Shiffman ML, Afdhal NH, et al: Hepatitis C virus treatment-related anemia is associated with higher sustained virologic response rate. *Gastroenterology* 139:2010, 1602.
24. Fellay J, Thompson AJ, Ge D, et al: ITPA gene variants protect against anaemia in patients treated for chronic hepatitis C. *Nature* 464:405, 2010.
25. Jacobson IM, McHutchison JG, Dusheiko G, et al: Telaprevir for previously untreated chronic hepatitis C virus infection. *N Engl J Med* 364:2405, 2011.
26. Hebbel RP, Eaton JW: Pathobiology of heme interaction with the erythrocyte membrane. *Semin Hematol* 26:136, 1989.
27. Luzzatto L, Seneca E: G6PD deficiency: a classic example of pharmacogenetics with on-going clinical implications. *Brit J Haematol* 164:469, 2014.
28. Greer FR, Shannon M: Infant methemoglobinemia: the role of dietary nitrate in food and water. *Pediatrics* 116:784, 2005.
29. Pamba A, Richardson ND, Carter N, et al: Clinical spectrum and severity of hemolytic anemia in glucose 6-phosphate dehydrogenase-deficient children receiving dapsone. *Blood* 120:4123, 2012.
30. Zuber J, Martinez F, Droz D, et al: Alpha-interferon-associated thrombotic microangiopathy: a clinicopathologic study of 8 patients and review of the literature. *Medicine (Baltimore)* 81:321, 2002.

NON-MALIGNANT LEUKOCYTES

NEUTROPHILIC LEUKOCYTOSIS, NEUTROPENIA, MONOCYTOSIS, AND MONOCYTOPENIA

Lawrence Rice and Moonjung Jung

Abnormalities of leukocyte number are commonly encountered in medical practice. The clinical significance of leukocytosis or leukopenia varies from none at all to being an early clue to a life-threatening process, whether a primary hematologic or secondary reactive process. Potential causes of leukocytosis or leukopenia are myriad. This chapter considers disorders faced by adult practitioners in hospital and outpatient clinics where the predominant hematologic abnormality is neutrophilic leukocytosis, neutropenia, monocytosis, or monocytopenia; other chapters consider lymphocytosis, lymphopenia, eosinophilia, pancytopenia, and hematologic neoplasms.

The normal range for leukocyte count in most laboratories is from about 4500/mm³ to 11,000/mm³. Neutrophils (and band forms) comprise the majority of circulating leukocytes (1800 mm³ to 7700/mm³); monocytes are about 4% of cells (mean absolute count: 300/mm³). The physician must always think in terms of absolute counts of leukocyte subpopulations (total leukocyte count multiplied by the differential percentage). Thus, in a patient presenting with a normal white blood cell (WBC) count of 5000/mm³ and an elevated lymphocyte percentage of 65%, the differential diagnosis to be considered is that of neutropenia, not lymphocytosis, because the absolute neutrophil count (ANC) is decreased but absolute lymphocytes are normal (only relatively increased).

When approaching a patient with abnormal leukocyte number, several factors impact heavily on the differential diagnosis and the vigor with which diagnosis and therapy should be pursued. Diagnostic considerations are vastly different when the abnormality first manifests **in the hospital versus in the outpatient clinic.** Also crucial is the **degree of the abnormality,** providing guidance to its likely cause and consequence. For example, agranulocytosis is a life-threatening disorder in which neutrophils are at or near zero, has a limited spectrum of underlying causes (drug reactions being paramount), and demands immediate interventions. **Duration** has major implications; determining the onset of changes and whether they are stable or progressive informs as to etiology and significance. Whether the abnormality is **symptomatic**—for example, whether a neutropenic or monocytopenic patient has or has had infectious complications—bears on likely etiologies and need for therapy. If there are known or suspected **comorbid conditions,** such as autoimmune or inflammatory disorders, this can crystallize the approach; occasionally, the leukocyte abnormality may be the first sign of a previously unrecognized disorder or may provide important confirmation (e.g., neutropenia in a patient with systemic lupus erythematosus [SLE]). If the leukocyte abnormality is accompanied by **additional hematologic abnormalities** (unexplained abnormalities of red blood cells [RBCs], platelets, or cell morphology), this would point away from disorders considered in this chapter and often toward a primary hematologic disease. Beyond history and physical examination, the peripheral blood smear is key to establish the direction of further evaluation.

NEUTROPHILIC LEUKOCYTOSIS (NEUTROPHILIA)

A high WBC count, particularly a high neutrophil count, is common with any infectious or inflammatory disorder. In the emergency department, leukocytosis is often equated with significant bacterial infection or is at least a sign of illness severe enough to warrant hospital admission rather than outpatient management. Leukocytosis can also be a prominent presenting feature of leukemias and myeloproliferative neoplasms (MPNs). The presence of increased neutrophils assures that acute leukemia is not present. When leukocytosis is extreme, it indicates chronic myeloid leukemia (CML), other MPNs, or a leukemoid reaction.

Leukemoid reaction has been defined as a reactive (nonclonal) neutrophilic leukocytosis with WBC count above 50,000/mm³. This must be differentiated from a neoplastic proliferation.

Leukoerythroblastosis refers to the presence in the peripheral blood of immature myeloid cells (generally myelocytes) and nucleated RBCs, often with giant platelets as well. This is always abnormal. Patients with leukoerythroblastosis do not necessarily have leukocytosis, but they usually do. Most patients (two-thirds) with leukoerythroblastosis have an underlying myelophthisic process, such as primary or secondary myelofibrosis, metastatic tumor, necrosis, or granulomas in the bone marrow (BM). Therefore, BM examination is indicated when leukoerythroblastosis is unexplained. Teardrop poikilocytes and elliptocytes on blood smear would strengthen concerns for myelophthisis. In 20% of patients with leukoerythroblastosis, the cause is hemolytic anemia, and miscellaneous other causes consist mainly of those with shock (septic, hemorrhagic, cardiogenic, anaphylactic) when hypoperfusion of areas of BM disrupt the microenvironment and permit disorderly egress of precursor cells.

Left-shifted neutrophils refer to relative immaturity of circulating cells, often manifest as an increased percentage of band neutrophils. Marked left-shift includes less mature precursor forms, myelocytes and metamyelocytes. Left-shift is nonspecific and may occur with infection or any cause of marked neutrophilia.

Detailed directed history and physical examination are indispensable to the evaluation of neutrophilia (Table 48.1). Fever and chills suggest infection (or inflammation), mandating a search for more specific symptoms that could pinpoint the focus. Examples include a sore throat, pharyngeal erythema, and exudate in pharyngitis; productive cough and abnormal lung auscultation in pneumonia; and dysuria and flank tenderness in urinary tract infection. Medication history mainly explores glucocorticoid use. With mild chronic neutrophilia, smoking habits and obesity become considerations. Recent vigorous exercise, emotional stress, burns, shock, or trauma can increase circulating neutrophils because of catecholamine-induced demargination. A positive family history may suggest hereditary neutrophilia. Often neglected are attempts to delineate the time course of the leukocyte abnormality by seeking prior medical contacts and blood count results at the time. On the physical examination, care should be directed to lymph node palpation because this can be an important clue for infection or malignancy. Palpable splenomegaly may not only direct the evaluation toward hematologic disorders but can be a cardinal sign of a variety of infectious and inflammatory disorders.

Blood smear should always be a part of initial evaluation when there are abnormalities of blood counts. BM aspirate or biopsy morphology may be helpful when pathophysiology and diagnosis are unclear. When appropriate, essential information can be gained by sending BM for microbiologic cultures, cytogenetic or molecular, or other ancillary studies.

1. Hematologic malignancy (CML, CNL, CMML)
2. Infection
3. Inflammation, physiologic stress, hemorrhage, hemolysis
4. Hereditary or congenital neutrophilias
5. Smoking
6. Drugs: colony-stimulating factors, glucocorticoids, epinephrine, lithium
7. Nonhematologic malignancy
8. Asplenia
9. Obesity
10. Recovery from neutropenia

CML, Chronic myeloid leukemia; CMML, chronic myelomonocytic leukemia; CNL, Chronic neutrophilic leukemia.

Leukemoid Reaction Versus Chronic Leukemia

A relatively common reason for hematologic consultation is for very high WBC count. CML is reviewed elsewhere in this text, as are chronic myelomonocytic leukemia (CMML) and the very rare chronic neutrophilic leukemia. Marked neutrophilic leukocytosis or overt leukemoid reaction (WBC count >50,000/mm³) can represent an overly exuberant reaction to any stimulus associated with neutrophilia. In patients with leukemoid reaction, a disproportionate number have infection with *Clostridium difficile*, an organism that elicits a vigorous neutrophil response. Leukemoid reactions may be associated with solid tumors, sometimes due to paraneoplastic production of colony-stimulating factor (e.g., granulocyte colony-stimulating factor (G-CSF) or granulocyte-macrophage colony-stimulating factor [GM-CSF]) or other cytokines (e.g., interleukin [IL]-6 or IL-17), or to particularly aggressive tumors with necrotic areas. The course of neutrophilia usually correlates with the course of solid cancer. It is important to quickly differentiate a reactive neutrophilic leukocytosis from a clonal leukemic proliferation.

The history and clinical context are usually quite different between leukemoid reaction and CML. Most patients with leukemoid reaction are encountered very ill in the hospital with obvious underlying illnesses (e.g., sepsis, organ rejection). Prior WBC counts, which are often available, demonstrate normal WBC counts until the recent onset of acute illness. This contrasts with CML, typically presenting in outpatients with hypermetabolism (weight loss, sweats, low-grade fever), symptoms referable to splenomegaly, or frequently asymptomatic. On physical examination, the spleen is palpable (occasionally massive) in the great majority of patients with CML but splenomegaly is unusual with leukemoid reaction (in the absence of comorbidities such as liver disease).

Laboratory findings reliably differentiate CML from leukemoid reaction. The total leukocyte count is commonly extremely high with CML (median 100,000/mm³ in some series), but counts above 100,000/mm³ are rare and above 150,000/mm³ virtually unheard of with leukemoid reaction. Circulating myelocytes and even a few blasts are more typical of CML, but may be seen in both disorders. Similarly, changes in platelet number and morphology can be seen with both but are more characteristic of CML (especially when changes are extreme). RBC changes do not reliably separate the disorders except in a few cases with prominent teardrops, which point toward MPN. More helpful is the leukocyte differential: patients with CML almost always have some degree of absolute basophilia and eosinophilia, but infection and glucocorticoid excess induce eosinopenia. (When the leukocyte count is 100,000/mm³, realize that 2% to 3% basophils is a substantial absolute increase.)

The leukocyte alkaline phosphatase (LAP) score, high with leukemoid reaction and classically low with CML, has limited utility now that more sensitive and specific tests for CML have emerged. When CML is reasonably considered, testing should be done for the Philadelphia chromosome, t(9;22)(q34;q11.2) by chromosome G-banding,

or *BCR–ABL1* fusion product by fluorescence in situ hybridization or reverse-transcriptase polymerase chain reaction. When other MPNs are judged reasonably possible, *JAK2* V617F mutational status may be informative. In cases with very high suspicion for MPNs but negative *JAK2* V617F mutation, *JAK2* exon 12, *MPL*, and *CALR* mutations can be assessed in a serial manner.

Infection

To protect against the ever-present threats to health and longevity, evolution has armed us with reactant cytokine cascades designed to increase the number of phagocytes and dispatch them to threatened locales. Neutrophilia is classically seen as a response to bacterial infection, responding to such cytokines as IL-6, tumor necrosis factor (TNF), and G-CSF. Neutrophilia is also a frequent response to other types of infections, such as fungal, parasitic, mycobacterial, and sometimes viral.

Changes in neutrophil morphology may be useful in predicting whether bacterial or other infection underlie a neutrophilic response. The authors have confirmed some published reports that prominent neutrophil vacuolization is highly specific and moderately sensitive for serious bacterial infection, as are prominent Dohle bodies (in the absence of a primary hematologic disorder). The authors blindly scored blood smears from 50 patients with serious bacterial infection (half bacteremic), 25 with influenza, 25 with noninfectious fever, and 25 control smears. Toxic granulation of neutrophils, touted as a sign of bacterial infection, was found useless in distinguishing infections from other febrile illnesses.

Inflammation and Stress

Acute or chronic inflammation can cause neutrophilia by mechanisms similar to infection, mediated by the proinflammatory cytokines G-CSF, GM-CSF, TNF, IL-1, IL-6, IL-8, and others. Diseases such as rheumatoid arthritis (RA), vasculitis, inflammatory bowel disease, thyrotoxicosis, eclampsia, and many others are commonly accompanied by neutrophilia. Another rare but notable example is familial Mediterranean fever, in which an inherited *MEFV* mutation leads to dysfunctional pyrin downregulation of neutrophil activation, leading to chronic inflammatory serositis and secondary AA amyloidosis.

Physiologic stresses, including exercise and emotional stress, lead to endogenous catecholamine and glucocorticoid release in addition to inflammatory cytokines. This causes a rapid doubling of circulating neutrophils caused by demargination and by more rapid BM egress of maturing neutrophils. Paulsen found early peaks in M-CSF, growth hormone, and cortisol after exercise followed by increases in G-CSF, IL-6, and monocyte chemoattractant protein 1. Acute hemorrhage and hemolytic anemia are other physiologic stresses. This contributes to increased steady-state neutrophil counts recorded in patients with sickle cell anemia, and the degree of elevation correlates with pain crisis frequency, other complications, and mortality; leukocyte reduction has been postulated to be one mechanism of hydroxyurea's beneficial actions. The stress of acute myocardial infarction is commonly accompanied by mild neutrophilia, and the early magnitude of rise has correlated with poor outcomes.

Hereditary and Congenital Neutrophilias

In newborns, neutrophilia and leukoerythroblastosis are among the hematologic abnormalities associated with trisomy 13, trisomy 18, and trisomy 21 (Down syndrome). A transient clonal MPN can be seen in children with Down syndrome and is usually self-limited, but it does put patients at increased risk for later acute megakaryoblastic leukemia.

Very rare hereditary neutrophilias are sometimes first appreciated in adults. In 1971, Herring reported a mother and three of her four children with lifelong neutrophilia (WBC: 14,000/mm³ to 164,000/

mm³; granulocytes: 9000/mm³ to 62,000/mm³), unusual bleeding, thickened calvariae, and hepatosplenomegaly. They had no increase in infections. The LAP score was high, BM revealed few Gaucher-like histiocytes, karyotype was normal by routine G-banding, but chromatid breaks and gaps were increased. In 2009, French investigators identified a mutation in the *CSF3R* gene in a kindred with hereditary chronic neutrophilia. The point mutation led to constitutive activation of the G-CSF receptor, driving neutrophil proliferation and differentiation. One of 12 affected individuals in this kindred developed overt myelodysplastic syndrome (MDS). The frequency of this and other mutations are unknown with hereditary neutrophilias.

Smoking

Smoking has been well associated with mild neutrophilia in epidemiologic and animal studies. Perry et al found a 27% higher WBC count in smokers. Sunyer et al correlated the degree of leukocytosis and percentage of neutrophils with the number of cigarettes smoked. The effect can persist up to 5 years in those who stop smoking. A suggested mechanism is chronic inflammation because inflammatory markers, including C-reactive protein (CRP) and fibrinogen, are elevated. In a rodent model, cigarette smoke caused overexpression of hematopoietic growth factor genes IL-6, G-CSF, and GM-CSF. Thus, mild neutrophilia without other symptoms in a smoker could be attributed to this practice without further evaluation.

Drugs

Systemic glucocorticoids cause neutrophilia mainly by interfering with neutrophil adhesion to the capillary wall and decreasing neutrophil turnover rate. Maximal neutrophil counts occur 4–6 hours after dexamethasone use in normal volunteers. G-CSF increases circulating neutrophils by increasing BM production and mobilization. Epinephrine increases proinflammatory cytokines and demargination. Suggested mechanisms for lithium-induced neutrophilia are induction of G-CSF and downregulation of CXC-chemokine receptor 4, thus facilitating egress from the BM.

Malignancy

Leukocytosis is frequently associated with solid tumors without direct BM involvement. Some malignant tumors have been reported to produce G-CSF or GM-CSF, occasionally producing leukocytosis in the range of a leukemoid reaction.

Asplenia

Whereas neutrophilia is classically observed early after splenectomy, lymphocytosis predominates in the long run. Nevertheless, chronic mild neutrophilia can also be seen in functionally asplenic individuals. Furthermore, there may be an exaggerated neutrophil response to infections or other stresses. On the blood smear, Howell–Jolly bodies are a very sensitive and specific (when numerous) sign of functional asplenia.

Obesity

Chronic mild neutrophilia has been observed with obesity. Fat tissue can release inflammatory cytokines, creating a state of low-grade inflammation manifest by elevated CRP. Leptin, a hormone released by adipocytes, may act on CD34⁺ cells to promote neutrophil differentiation. More recently, chronically inflamed visceral adipose tissue in obesity was found to simulate BM hematopoietic progenitor cells to proliferate and expand, causing both neutrophilia and monocytosis via IL-1β. In an obese patient with chronic mild neutrophilia

and no obvious other underlying disorder, this can be assumed to be the cause.

NEUTROPENIA (AND AGRANULOCYTOSIS)

The risk of neutropenia-related infection begins to rise at an ANC near 1000/mm³, rising dramatically below 500/mm³ and more so below 100/mm³; thus, an ANC of 500/mm³ to 1000/mm³ is considered moderate neutropenia, and below 500/mm³ is considered severe. This corresponds to National Cancer Institute criteria for medication adverse hematologic event reporting: grade 1 toxicity is 1500/mm³ to lower limit of normal, grade 2 is 1000/mm³–1500/mm³, grade 3 is 500/mm³ to 1000/mm³, and grade 4 is less than 500/mm³. Beyond the ANC, the risk for infection is greatly influenced by the nature of the underlying problem, the BM myeloid reserve, and whether other risk factors for infection are present (e.g., immunoglobulin deficiency or breaks in mucosal barriers). The course with mild and moderate neutropenia is often benign.

The history focuses on the severity and duration of neutropenia, whether infectious complications have occurred (including severe stomatitis or gingivitis), and whether prior blood counts can be obtained. A history of drug exposures and their timing is especially relevant, not only for prescribed medications but also for over-the-counter, herbal, and illicit drugs. Symptoms of systemic inflammatory illness, such as arthritis, skin rash, and photosensitivity, can bear on the etiology and significance of the low WBC count. Fevers, weight loss, and sweats could be clues to many disorders, including malignancy. Liver disorders commonly present with cytopenias, so a history of hepatitis, jaundice, and HIV risk factors should be specifically sought. Symptoms of anemia or bleeding could be clues to more general hematologic disorders. As with most hematologic problems, physical examination should devote extra attention to lymph node areas and the spleen. Oropharynx and skin examination also take on added importance.

Peripheral blood smear review is irreplaceable to direct the workup. MDS does not characteristically present with isolated neutropenia, but this occasionally is the predominant presenting feature in this relatively common syndrome affecting older patients. Specific blood smear findings which could suggest MDS include pseudo-Pelger–Huet neutrophils, hypogranularity, Dohle bodies, and macrocytic and/or dimorphic RBCs with a hypochromic population. Megaloblastic processes, such as vitamin B₁₂ and folic acid deficiency, similarly do not characteristically present with isolated neutropenia, but this occasionally predominates (especially in the presence of acute infection). Hypersegmentation of neutrophils is always present with megaloblastic processes, including those that are drug-induced (e.g., methotrexate, hydroxyurea). Hypersegmented neutrophils are also seen with uremia, as an autosomal dominant benign polymorphism, and in MDS and MPN. In a neutropenic patient, one should always specifically look for large granular lymphocytes (LGLs). A modest increase could indicate a reactive T-cell natural killer (NK) cell process, and a more dramatic increase could alert to clonal T-NK or NK cell proliferations (LGL leukemia). Hairy cells, other morphologic types of circulating lymphoma cells, and blasts are obvious indicators of hematologic malignancy. Morphologic suspicions for such processes could be confirmed by flow cytometry. Reactive lymphocytes may suggest viral infection but also occur with drug reactions and other processes.

Further laboratory testing in patients with neutropenia may often be unnecessary. Especially in mild or moderate cases, the lack of specific diagnostic tests has created some overlap and confusion among what have been called *chronic idiopathic neutropenia, chronic benign neutropenia, ethnic neutropenia,* and *autoimmune neutropenia.* Autoimmune neutropenia is a relatively common cause of both mild and more severe neutropenia, but tests for antineutrophil antibodies are not clinically validated (see later). Serologic tests for antinuclear antibodies and rheumatoid factor can be helpful when autoimmune neutropenia is considered, as positive results may raise suspicion for an undiagnosed collagen vascular disorder or may just support a less specific autoimmune problem. Direct antiglobulin test and antiphospholipid antibodies can also be supportive when there is suspicion for an autoimmune process. Quantitative immunoglobulin levels may reveal an underlying immunodeficiency when there is evidence of autoimmunity or when infectious complications are disproportionate. Serologic tests for some viral infections (HIV, hepatitis, Epstein-Barr virus [EBV]) may sometimes be appropriate. The main utility of flow cytometry occurs when peripheral blood smear suggests an abnormal lymphocyte population (e.g., LGLs or hairy cells). Because LGL leukemia is a relatively common cause of significant neutropenia and because this is a diagnosis frequently initially missed, one should have a low trigger to obtain flow cytometry, assuring that proper markers are analyzed (see later). BM examination may not be helpful or warranted with mild or even moderate isolated neutropenia or in straightforward cases of severe neutropenia (e.g., after drug exposure), but can be essential when the diagnosis is in doubt and especially if other cell lines are compromised.

Severe Congenital Neutropenias

It is beyond the scope of this chapter to review in detail the heterogeneous genetic disorders that manifest in early childhood as severe congenital neutropenia (SCN); nevertheless, consultant hematologists should have some familiarity with this problem both because modern therapy has extended survival for many into adulthood, and because milder forms of these disorders may go undiagnosed until young adulthood. More severe forms of SCN present in infancy with severe stomatitis and recurrent bacterial infections. The molecular bases have been greatly elucidated in recent years, among them being: (1) an autosomal dominant mutation of the neutrophil elastase gene *ELANE* in 50% to 60% of patients, (2) an autosomal recessive mutation of *HAX1*, which is associated with mental retardation and other congenital defects found in Kostmann syndrome, and (3) an autosomal recessive mutation of *SBDS* in Schwachman-Bodian-Diamond syndrome, which presents with variable degree of neutropenia, BM failure, and exocrine pancreatic insufficiency. In young children, the differential diagnosis of SCN includes transient postinfectious neutropenia, alloimmune neutropenia, or hematologic malignancy. BM examination often shows a pattern of maturation arrest. The majority of affected patients are responsive to G-CSF, which has favorably impacted infectious morbidity and mortality. Allogeneic stem cell transplant is another therapeutic option. An intrinsic risk of acute myeloid leukemic transformation, 15% at 20 years, accompanies these disorders, with higher risk in those requiring higher doses and/or responding poorly to G-CSF.

Cyclic neutropenia is a rare autosomal dominant disorder with variable expression, also caused by autosomal dominant mutations of *ELANE* or rarely its transcription regulator. Neutrophil counts vary from mildly to severely low with predictable periodicity, usually about 21 days. The great majority of cases are responsive to G-CSF at low dosage.

Benign Ethnic Neutropenia

Americans of African descent may have chronic mild neutropenia not associated with infectious complications. The 1999–2004 National Health and Nutrition Survey found that black individuals had mean leukocyte counts 900/mm³ lower than white individuals, with ANCs below 1500/mm³ in 4.5% (compared with 0.8% of white individuals). The neutropenia correlates in some individuals with a polymorphism in the Duffy antigen receptor chemokine, a cytokine receptor also responsible for a Duffy-negative RBC phenotype. Some reports find this neutropenia more common in males, but other reports find autosomal dominant inheritance. Marrow granulocyte reserve or release (or both) may be compromised. Benign neutropenia has also been seen in other ethnic populations, including those of Middle Eastern or Japanese descent. Thus, an asymptomatic mildly neutropenic person of appropriate ethnicity without abnormalities on blood smear may require no further diagnostic workup. It may be reassuring to the patient (and the doctor) if prior blood counts can be retrieved to document the chronic, nonprogressive and complication-free course of the neutropenia.

Autoimmune Neutropenia (Primary and Secondary)

Autoimmune neutropenia can be primary or secondary to an autoimmune disorder such as SLE or RA. Neutropenia can be mild or severe. Classically, it is caused by antineutrophil autoantibodies, although autoreactive cytotoxic lymphocytes may also cause this problem. When performed, BM examination often is normocellular or hypercellular, with a late "maturation arrest" picture. Severe cases can display pure WBC aplasia (similar to drug-induced agranulocytosis, which may sometimes also be antibody-mediated). There are several challenges to making the diagnosis. One is that the maturation arrest BM picture is highly nonspecific with regard to mechanism: it could indicate a true stem cell differentiation defect, or the early release of later precursors (as with sepsis or splenic sequestration), or an immune attack aimed at antigens on later myeloid precursors or early recovery from a toxic insult. Another problem is the lack of validated, clinically reliable neutrophil antibody tests. Experimentally, several methods have been used, generally suffering from high false-negative and false-positives rates in detecting antibodies against neutrophil antigens or immune complexes that bind to neutrophil Fc receptors. With no definitive test, diagnosing autoimmune neutropenia rests largely on clinical context and judgment.

Neutropenia caused by antineutrophil antibodies has been seen in infants about 1 year old, usually running a benign clinical course with spontaneous remission in 95% within 2 years. Newborns are at risk of alloimmune neutropenia in the first months of life, but this is not generally accompanied by infectious complications. Secondary autoimmune neutropenias are most common in adults, related to disorders such as SLE, RA, Sjögren syndrome, thymoma, and common variable immunodeficiency. In SLE, neutrophil counts correlate with disease activity and have been related to the induction of TNF–related apoptosis-inducing ligand (TRAIL), a ligand that increases myeloid apoptosis and killing by autologous T cells. Immunosuppressive therapy of the SLE or the use of G-CSF can improve the WBC count.

Felty syndrome was classically described as severe neutropenia and splenomegaly complicating RA, and has been attributed to antineutrophil antibodies, but the distinction between this syndrome and other causes of neutropenia with RA have become blurred. In particular, classic Felty syndrome and LGL syndrome appear to represent points on a disease continuum. About 1% of patients with RA develop Felty syndrome, and it predisposes many to serious infections. Effective therapies have often included methotrexate, gold salts, and rituximab. Because of some risk of exacerbating underlying inflammatory problems, G-CSF should be used with caution.

Large Granular Lymphocyte Syndrome and Natural Killer Cell Proliferations

Proliferations of LGLs (T-NK cells and NK cells) are covered elsewhere, but mention is required here because these are common considerations in adults with neutropenia. These represent heterogeneous disorders, varying from nonclonal reactive processes to indolent clonal proliferations to highly aggressive neoplasms. Both reactive and clonal increases in T-NK cells can be seen with RA, representing a form of Felty syndrome. Reactive LGLs can be seen with other autoimmune disorders, after organ transplantation, with tyrosine kinase inhibitor therapy, or they may be idiopathic. These proliferations are associated with variable degrees of neutropenia, commonly splenomegaly, and increased infectious risks. The diagnosis is suggested on blood smear by large lymphocytes with mature chromatin, excessive cytoplasm, with or sometimes without prominent cytoplasmic granules. Flow cytometry demonstrates increased CD3⁺CD57⁺

lymphocytes with the more common T-NK proliferations or may show CD3⁻ CD56⁺ clones with "pure" NK cell proliferation. Somatic activating mutations in the signal transducer and activator of transcription 3 gene (STAT3) were found in 40 % of patients with LGL leukemia, suggesting aberrant STAT3 signaling pathway is an underlying mechanism of this disease. Somatic activating STAT5b mutations were also found in minority of patients. Variably effective treatments for indolent proliferations are corticosteroids, methotrexate, cyclosporine, cyclophosphamide, and purine nucleoside analogs.

Neutropenia With Infectious Diseases

Leukocytosis is the expected response to most bacterial infections, but leukopenia also occurs and is characteristic of infection by certain organisms. Viral infections often cause transient mild leukopenia, so restraint is wise in the diagnostic approach to a newly recognized moderate leukopenia in a febrile, modestly ill patient. Nonbacterial infections in which neutropenia is frequent or even characteristic include HIV, EBV, cytomegalovirus (CMV), hepatitis A and B, measles, rubella, varicella, rickettsia, and anaplasmosis (ehrlichiosis). Bacterial infections with characteristic leukopenia include typhoid fever and brucellosis, and granulomatous infections (tuberculosis, histoplasmosis) also commonly cause neutropenia, especially when the BM is directly involved. In patients with poor BM reserve (e.g., prior chemotherapy, malnutrition, myelodysplasia) an acute infection very often lowers, rather than raises, the neutrophil count. Profound neutropenia is a known consequence of overwhelming sepsis and has been associated with poor outcomes.

Hypersplenism

Hematologists are frequently consulted for cytopenias, only to find an unappreciated large spleen as the etiology (this most commonly due to liver disease with portal hypertension). Splenic enlargement can lead to sequestration and reduction of circulating WBCs, RBCs, platelets, or any combination of these. The degree of cytopenia is somewhat proportional to the degree of splenic enlargement. Substantial neutropenia out of proportion to the depletion of other cell lines and to the degree of splenomegaly suggests an autoimmune component (which can be seen with hepatitis C or autoimmune hepatitis) or medication effect (e.g., interferon).

Chemotherapy-Induced Neutropenia

The major dose-limiting toxicity of most cancer chemotherapy regimens continues to be neutropenia. This results in hospitalizations, antibiotic costs, reduced quality of life, infectious morbidity, dose reductions and treatment delays that compromise efficacy and outcomes, and result in some deaths: 75% of chemotherapy-related mortality. Febrile neutropenia is defined as an ANC less than 500/mm³ (or expected to decrease to <500/mm³ over the next 48 hours) with fever (>38.3°C or sustained >38°C).

Principles of empiric antibiotic coverage for acute febrile episodes in severely neutropenic patients are covered in detail elsewhere. Basically, there is a high risk of sepsis (even when the source is occult), and a favorable outcome depends on prompt effective antimicrobial coverage, so empiric administration of broad-spectrum antibacterial agents is considered medically emergent. There must be coverage of the traditional aerobic gram-negative rod culprits (particularly *Pseudomonas*), yet vigilance must be maintained for the gram-positive organisms that have emerged as major pathogens. With prolonged or repeated episodes of neutropenia, invasive fungi become common threats to survival, particularly *Aspergillus*, *Candida*, *Mucor*, and *Fusarium* spp. Published guidelines can aid the choice of empiric antimicrobials. Because of difficulty demonstrating favorable impact, enthusiasm for granulocyte transfusions has waned in the past 30 years; clinical studies are readdressing this in the modern era.

TABLE 48.2	Drugs Commonly Associated With Neutropenia

1. Antibiotics: vancomycin, semisynthetic penicillins, chloramphenicol, sulfa, linezolid
2. Antithyroid drugs: methimazole, propylthiouracil
3. Cardiovascular: ticlopidine, procainamide
4. Antipsychotics: clozapine, olanzapine, chlorpromazine
5. Anticonvulsants: phenytoin, carbamazepine, valproic acid
6. Antiinflammatory agents: indomethacin, sulfasalazine, phenylbutazone
7. H2 blockers: cimetidine, ranitidine
8. Analgesics: dipyrone
9. Antineoplastic: rituximab
10. Anthelmintic: levamisole

The utility of prophylactic antibiotics is problematic because of the wide array of potential pathogens and because of concerns of inducing antibiotic resistance. Prophylactic quinolones have had some favorable impact in very high-risk patients after consolidation therapy for acute leukemia or stem cell transplant.

G-CSF is widely used for primary or secondary prevention of neutropenia to decrease morbidity and mortality of febrile neutropenia. Primary prophylaxis is recommended by various guidelines if the risk of developing febrile neutropenia is greater than 20%. This risk is calculated from age, extent of primary cancer, comorbidities, and the known myelotoxicity of the chemotherapy regimen. G-CSF is begun 24–72 hours after the completion of myelotoxic chemotherapy. Pegfilgrastim allows prophylaxis to be given more conveniently (once per cycle).

Drug-Induced Neutropenia

Drug reactions account for a high percentage of acquired neutropenias, both mild but moreover severe cases (agranulocytosis; Table 48.2). Neutropenia often develops abruptly, within 4 weeks of initiation of a causative agent. Pathophysiology may involve immune mechanisms or more direct toxicity such as enhancement of reactive oxygen species made by nicotinamide adenine dinucleotide phosphate oxidase or myeloperoxidase on neutrophil precursors. The diagnosis is generally strongly suspected from an accurate history that plots leukocyte numbers against the time course of drug exposure; confirmation is leukocyte recovery after drug withdrawal. More specific confirmatory testing, such as for drug-dependent antibodies, is mainly an area of research laboratory investigation. BM examination is not usually required but may be helpful when pathophysiology and diagnosis are in doubt, when the course is atypical, and to provide prognostic information (earlier recovery may be anticipated with a picture of "maturation arrest" than one of myeloid aplasia). Treatment demands discontinuation of suspected offending drugs. Although the efficacy of myeloid growth factors (G-CSF) has been questioned, most recommend this therapy because even a modest shortening of severe neutropenia can occasionally be lifesaving. Mortality of drug-induced agranulocytosis is generally reported to be 10%.

The most commonly implicated drugs are listed in Table 48.2. Some merit additional comment. Some drugs have a direct myelotoxic effect rather than induce an idiosyncratic immune-based reaction. Neutropenia will have more gradual onset related to dose and duration, and may be accompanied by suppression of other hematologic cell lines. Linezolid and most instances of chloramphenicol myelosuppression are examples.

Beginning 2007, an epidemic of agranulocytosis was found among intravenous cocaine users. The adulterant levamisole was found in 71% of confiscated cocaine by the Drug Enforcement Agency, with the incidence of agranulocytosis 2.5% to 13% in those exposed. Nadir BM showed severe myeloid hypoplasia. Levamisole had long been linked to agranulocytosis, having been used as an antihelminth and as an immune adjuvant in patients with autoimmune disorders and colorectal cancer.

Severe neutropenia is increasingly recognized in patients treated with rituximab. This neutropenia is unusual for its late onset, generally about 3 months after the last rituximab dose. It occurs with underlying autoimmune disorders, B-cell malignancies, and stem cell transplants—basically in all situations in which rituximab is used—often occurring while the underlying illness is in complete remission. Severe neutropenia has been reported in about 5% of rituximab-treated patients, much higher in some series. Most patients recover quickly, usually after G-CSF therapy, but there have been protracted cases. The authors and others have reported a high risk of relapse (100% in our series) if rituximab is reinitiated. The mechanism is not definitively established, but an intriguing report implicates imbalanced recovery of B-cell clones with a deficiency of stromal-derived factor 1.

MONOCYTOSIS

Monocytosis is extremely nonspecific, usually not requiring investigation per se. Monocytosis has been defined as a sustained absolute increase in monocyte count greater than 800/mm³ to 1000/mm³ (Table 48.3). Transient monocytosis, relative or absolute, is common with recovery from myelosuppression, such as after chemotherapy. Relative or absolute monocytosis may occur in other myelosuppressed states, such as aplastic anemia. This is a favorable factor associated with a lower risk of neutropenic infection, perhaps because some phagocytic capacity is maintained. On the other hand, monocytosis is also very common with hematologic malignancies. In a patient with unexplained cytopenia, monocytosis can be an important clue to an underlying MDS.

Infectious Diseases

Mycobacterial infection is a common cause of monocytosis worldwide, related to its propensity for intracellular infection and tissue granuloma formation. Brucellosis and subacute bacterial endocarditis have also been associated with monocytosis. Certain viral infections, including influenza, varicella-zoster, CMV, and dengue, have been reported to cause monocytosis.

TABLE 48.3   Changes in Monocyte Number

Monocytosis

Infections: tuberculosis, granulomatous infection, brucellosis, subacute bacterial endocarditis
Connective tissue disorder
Recovery from myelosuppression
Hematologic malignancies:
1. MDS, MPD, MDS–MPD overlap, CMML
2. Acute and chronic monocytic leukemia, myelomonocytic leukemia
3. Hodgkin and non-Hodgkin lymphomas
Obesity

Monocytopenia

Hairy cell leukemia
GATA2 deficiency (also known as MonoMAC syndrome, DCML, Emberger syndrome, familial MDS/AML)
Aplastic anemia
Drugs: chemotherapy, IFN-α, glucocorticoids (transient)
Radiation therapy

AML, Acute myeloid leukemia; CMML, chronic myelomonocytic leukemia; DCML, dendritic cell, monocyte and lymphoid deficiency; IFN, interferon; MDS, myelodysplastic syndrome; monoMAC, monocytopenia and mycobacterium avium complex syndrome; MPD, myeloproliferative disorder.

Connective Tissue Disorder

Connective tissue disorders, such as SLE and RA, have been associated with monocytosis in the context of chronic inflammation.

Hematopoietic Malignancies

Monocytosis is common with MDS. CMML is defined as persistent peripheral blood monocytosis greater than 1000/mm³, absent Philadelphia chromosome, and evidence of dysplasia in one or more hematopoietic cell lineages. Juvenile myelomonocytic leukemia, a disease of children that shares pathologic features with CMML, results from defective RAS signaling. Acute myeloid leukemias (AMLs) involving the monocyte line (acute myelomonocytic and acute monoblastic leukemias) may release substantial amounts of lysozyme (muramidase), which is toxic to renal tubules. Serum lysozyme was used to aid in the diagnosis of these leukemias. Monocytosis can result from other myeloid leukemias, MPNs, and lymphomas, particularly Hodgkin disease.

MONOCYTOPENIA

Monocytopenia frequently accompanies granulocytopenia with chemotherapy, aplastic anemia, or other BM-suppressive insults. Isolated or disproportionate monocytopenia is rarely recognized, but observations suggest that this can have serious clinical sequelae when it occurs. In hairy cell leukemia and monoMAC syndrome (GATA2 deficiency), there is a clear association with severe opportunistic infections, particularly those normally engendering a granulomatous response.

Hairy Cell Leukemia

This disorder, considered in detail elsewhere, classically presents with pancytopenia and splenomegaly, often in middle-aged men. The WBC count is sometimes high because of hairy cell proliferation, but monocytes are invariably severely depressed. (Monocytopenia is not seen with "variant hairy cell leukemia.") Neutropenia only partly explains the very high infectious morbidity and mortality. An extraordinary incidence of opportunistic granulomatous infections used to be encountered, including atypical mycobacteria, tuberculosis, histoplasmosis, and other fungi. These are linked to monocytopenia, with impaired granuloma formation. With remission induced by modern therapies (e.g., 2-chloro-deoxyadenosine), monocytopenia and infectious risks have been mitigated.

GATA2 Deficiency

In 2010, investigators at the National Institutes of Health and in the UK simultaneously described an immunodeficiency syndrome characterized by decreased or absent monocytes, NK cells, B cells, and dendritic cells; this clinical syndrome was named *MonoMAC* or *dendritic cell, monocyte and lymphoid deficiency*. This was largely diagnosed in young adults (median age: 33 years). All patients have opportunistic infections, particularly *Mycobacterium avium* complex and other mycobacteria, opportunistic fungi, and viruses, particularly human papillomavirus. Both autosomal dominant and sporadic cases are described, all linked to mutations in the hematopoietic stem cell regulator *GATA2*. Heterozygous haploinsufficiency mutations in *GATA2* are also responsible for Emberger syndrome (primary lymphedema and a predisposition to AML) and familial MDS/AML. BM examination findings are almost always abnormal, usually hypocellular, with increased reticulin fibrosis, multilineage dysplasia with characteristic separated nuclei in megakaryocytes, and absent B and NK precursors. Clonal cytogenetic abnormalities are seen in most patients, particularly monosomy 7 in 16% and trisomy 8 in 24%.

Because leukemic progression with or without death from infection is high, stem cell transplantation is recommended when feasible. When a family member is used as a BM donor, *GATA2* sequencing must be performed to rule out asymptomatic carrier status before donating. When monocytopenia out of proportion to neutropenia is detected in a patient with or without human papillomavirus-associated warts or MAC infection, examination of B- and NK-cell count by flow cytometry will be informative. Detailed family history may reveal additional patients with infectious complications or MDS/AML.

Chronic Mild Neutrophilic Leukocytosis

A 46-year-old man was referred to the hematology clinic for evaluation of neutrophilia that was noted by his primary care physician on a routine blood test. He reported no fevers, chills, or night sweats. He had good energy and was working full time as a lawyer. He denies fatigue, weight loss, or rashes. His past medical history included hypertension and obesity, but was otherwise healthy. He has been an active smoker for 10 years. Family history was negative for blood diseases. Vital signs were normal. Body mass index was 40.5 kg/m^2. Physical examination revealed only an obese abdomen. Laboratory values showed WBC 12,500/mm^3, ANC 8500/mm^3, Hb 14 g/dL, hematocrit (Hct) 42%, platelets 400 K/mm^3. Chemistries were unremarkable. Peripheral blood smear showed only increased neutrophils, with unremarkable RBCs and platelets. A complete blood cell count 2 years ago showed WBC 11,800/mm^3, ANC 8100/mm^3, Hb 14.2 g/dL, platelets 385 K/mm^3. What is the next step in evaluation?

This patient has mild neutrophilia of at least 2 years of duration. Obesity and smoking are common causes of neutrophilia. There is no evidence of chronic infection, inflammation or hematologic malignancy. No further work up is warranted, only follow-up, at the present time.

Acute Severe Neutrophilic Leukocytosis

A 78-year-old woman nursing home resident presented to the emergency department with altered mental status, diarrhea, and abdominal pain. She was recently treated with ciprofloxacin for urinary tract infection. On physical examination, she is difficult to arouse. Vital signs show blood pressure 105/66 mmHg, heart rate 98/min, respiratory rate 18/min, temperature 100.4°F. Abdominal examination reveals distension, active bowel sounds, no organomegaly. Laboratory findings show WBC 88,000/mm^3, Hb 10.5g/dL, platelets 200/mm^3, neutrophils 65%, lymphocytes 5%, monocytes 4%, eosinophils <1%, basophils <1%, bands 25%. Hematology is consulted for the high WBC. Peripheral blood smear shows increased neutrophils, metamyelocytes, and myelocytes. RBCs are normocytic and normochromic. Platelets are unremarkable. Nursing home records show normal blood counts except mild anemia with a Hb of 10.9 g/dL a month ago.

The almost certain cause of the extreme leukocytosis in this patient is leukemoid reaction, perhaps due to urosepsis. *Clostridium difficile* infection is classically associated with severe neutrophilia and the recent antibiotic use with diarrhea and abdominal distention suggests this as another possibility. The absence of splenomegaly, eosinophilia, and basophilia, and near normal blood counts a month ago makes CML or other MPN very unlikely. We would recommend appropriate antibiotics, clinical follow-up, but no molecular testing at this time.

SUGGESTED READINGS

Aapro MS, Bohlius J, Cameron DA, et al: 2010 Update of EORTC guidelines for the use of granulocyte-colony stimulating factor to reduce the incidence of chemotherapy-induced febrile neutropenia in adult patients with lymphoproliferative disorders and solid tumours. *Eur J Cancer* 47:8, 2011.

Akhtari M, Curtis B, Waller E: Autoimmune neutropenia in adults. *Autoimmun Rev* 9:62, 2009.

Aster RH: Adverse drug reactions affecting blood cells. *Handb Exp Pharmacol* 57, 2010.

Bhatt V, Saleem A: Review: drug-induced neutropenia: pathophysiology, clinical features and management. *Ann Clin Lab Sci* 34:131, 2004.

Dale DC, Bolyard AA, Schwinzer BG, et al: The severe chronic neutropenia international registry: 10-Year follow-up report. *Support Cancer Ther* 3:220, 2006.

Dale DC, Link DC: The many causes of severe congenital neutropenia. *N Engl J Med* 360:3, 2009.

Donadien J, Fenneteau O, Beaupain B, et al: Congenital neutropenia: diagnosis, molecular bases and patient management. *Orphanet J Rare Dis* 6:26, 2011.

Freifeld AG, Bow EJ, Sepkowitz KA, et al: Clinical practice guideline for the use of antimicrobial agents in neutropenic patients with cancer: 2010 Update by the Infectious Diseases Society of America. *Clin Infect Dis* 52:e56, 2011.

Gasche C, Reinisch W, Schwarzmeimer JD: Evidence of colony suppressor activity and deficiency of hematopoietic growth factors in hairy cell leukemia. *Hematol Oncol* 11:97, 1993.

Gibson C, Berliner N: How we evaluate and treat neutropenia in adults. *Blood* 124:1251–1258, 2014.

Haas P, Straub R, Beoui S, et al: Peripheral but not central leptin treatment increases numbers of circulating NK cells, granulocytes and specific monocyte subpopulations in non-endotoxaemic lean and obese LEW-rats. *Regul Pept* 51:26, 2008.

Herishanu Y, Rogowski O, Polliack A, et al: Leukocytosis in obese individuals: possible link in patients with unexplained persistent neutrophilia. *Eur J Haematol* 76:516, 2006.

Hsieh MM, Everhart JE, Byrd-Holt DD, et al: Prevalence of neutropenia in the U.S. population: age, sex, smoking status, and ethnic differences. *Ann Intern Med* 146:486, 2007.

Hsieh MM, Tisdale JF, Rodgers GP, et al: Neutrophil count in African Americans: lowering the target cutoff to initiate or resume chemotherapy? *J Clin Oncol* 28:19, 2010.

Koskela HL, Eldfors S, Ellonen P, et al: Somatic STAT3 mutations in large granular lymphocytic leukemia. *N Engl J Med* 366:20, 2012.

Kroft SH: Infectious diseases manifested in the peripheral blood. *Clin Lab Med* 23:253, 2003.

Marchetti M, Falanga A: Leukocytosis, JAK2V617F mutation, and hemostasis in myeloproliferative disorders. *Pathophysiol Haemost Thromb* 36:148, 2008.

Nagareddy PR, Kraakman M, Masters SL, et al: Adipose tissue macrophage promote myelopoiesis and monocytosis in obesity. *Cell Metab* 6:19, 2014.

Neureiter D, Kemmerling R, Ocker M, et al: Differential diagnostic challenge of chronic neutrophilic leukemia in a patient with prolonged leukocytosis. *J Hematop* 1:23, 2008.

Plo I, Zhang Y, Couedic JL, et al: An activating mutation in the CSF3R gene induces a hereditary chronic neutrophilia. *J Exp Med* 206:1701, 2009.

Rajala HL, Eldfors S, Kuusanmäki H, et al: Discovery of somatic STAT5b mutations in large granular lymphocytic leukemia. *Blood* 121:4541, 2013.

Rice L, Harris RL, Lynch EC, et al: Utility of peripheral blood changes in discriminating causes of fever and infection. *Blood* 70:94A, 1987.

Rice L, Shenkenberg T, Wheeler T, et al: Opportunistic granulomatous infections in hairy cell leukemia. *Cancer* 49:1924, 1982.

Seshadri RS, Brown EJ, Zipursky A: Leukemic reticuloendotheliosis. A failure of monocyte production. *N Engl J Med* 295:181, 1977.

Spinner MA, Sanchez LA, Hsu AP, et al: GATA2 deficiency: a protein disorder of hematopoiesis, lymphatics, and immunity. *Blood* 123:6, 2014.

Tesfa D, Keisu M, Palmblad J: Idiosyncratic drug-induced agranulocytosis: possible mechanisms and management. *Am J Hematol* 84:428, 2009.

Weick JK, Hagedorn AB, Linman JW: Leukoerythroblastosis. Diagnostic and prognostic significance. *Mayo Clin Proc* 49:110, 1974.

Wolach O, Bairey O, Lahav M: Late-onset neutropenia after rituximab treatment: case series and comprehensive review of the literature. *Medicine (Baltimore)* 89:308, 2010.

CHAPTER 49

LYMPHOCYTOSIS, LYMPHOCYTOPENIA, HYPERGAMMAGLOBULINEMIA, AND HYPOGAMMAGLOBULINEMIA

Martha P. Mims

Any discussion of quantitative abnormalities of lymphocytes and immunoglobulins is necessarily linked because the B-cell compartment is responsible for immunoglobulin production, and the T-cell compartment helps provide the stimulus. Nevertheless, clinicians are often consulted when a quantitative disorder of one or the other is recognized. Thus, although overlapping, the defects are presented separately.

QUANTITATIVE DISORDERS OF LYMPHOCYTES

The normal number and distribution of lymphocyte subtypes in the peripheral blood varies with age, but no careful study has demonstrated gender or ethnic differences in lymphocyte count. In general, circulating T cells exceed B cells by a ratio of approximately four to one, with that ratio increasing slightly with age (Table 49.1). Natural killer (NK) cells are grouped with lymphocytes but comprise only about 10% of the lymphocyte population. Infants have total lymphocyte counts between 5500/μL and 7000/μL, but this number declines beginning at about 1 year of age to reach 2000/μL to 2400/μL in adults. At birth, the total number of circulating B cells is approximately 1000/μL but decreases over the first 10 years of life to approximately 200/μL to 300/μL by the age of 18 years. A slow decline in circulating B cells continues throughout adulthood and is primarily accounted for by a decline in transitional and naive B cells with a stable or mild increase in circulating memory B-cell numbers with age. Circulating naive B cells represent about two-thirds of the entire naive B-cell pool, and circulating memory B cells represent only about one third of the entire memory B-cell pool.[1]

T cells dominate the circulating lymphocyte population with approximately 3500/μL in infancy, declining to 1500/μL on average in young adults, with even lower numbers (approximately 1200/μL) in elderly adults. In both children and adults, CD4 cells outnumber CD8 cells. Naive CD4 and CD8 T cells decline with age by twofold to fourfold. In one large study, CD4 memory T cells significantly increased with age, but no such trend was seen for CD8 memory T cells.[2]

Against this background, *lymphocytosis* is defined as a lymphocyte count greater than 8000/μL in young children and greater than 4000/μL in teenagers and adults. Lymphocytopenia has been defined as a total lymphocyte count of less than 1000/μL. Given the composition of the circulating lymphocyte pool, it is critically important to define which lymphocyte subsets are over- or underrepresented when there is a quantitative disorder.[2]

Lymphocytosis

As in any clinical disorder, a careful history is critical to defining the origin of lymphocytosis. Inherited causes of lymphocytosis are rare. One recently identified inherited lymphocytosis is BENTA disease (B-cell expansion with nuclear factor kappa-B [NFκB] and T-cell anergy). Germline gain of function mutations in caspase-activating recruitment domain 11 (*CARD11*) drive this disorder, which is characterized by polyclonal lymphocytosis and splenomegaly beginning in infancy. In most cases of lymphocytosis, however, the issue is to determine whether a lymphocyte disorder is clonal/malignant or benign and related to infection, drugs, or physiologic stress. Rarely, neither a malignancy nor an underlying condition can be identified, in which case the lymphocytosis is termed *persistent polyclonal B-cell lymphocytosis*. When an excess of B cells exists, clonality can usually be defined by examining cell surface expression of κ- and λ-light chains using antibody techniques; with T-cell proliferation, it may be important to define clonality by examining T-cell receptor gene rearrangement using molecular procedures. In the case of NK cell disorders, clonality can be quite difficult to determine.

Clonal Disorders

Malignant causes of peripheral blood lymphocytosis are covered in Chapters 76–80, 84, and 86 and include chronic lymphocytic leukemia (CLL), hairy cell leukemia, splenic marginal zone lymphoma, lymphoplasmacytic lymphoma, follicular lymphoma, mantle cell lymphoma, adult T-cell leukemia or lymphoma, and Sézary syndrome. Occasionally, precursor T-cell or precursor B-cell leukemia presents with circulating small cells, which morphologically appear more similar to mature lymphocytes than blasts.

A recently identified clonal disorder causing lymphocytosis is monoclonal B-cell lymphocytosis (MBL), an accumulation of clonal B lymphocytes that does not meet the criteria for CLL (greater than 5000 clonal B cells/μL), but is nevertheless defined by the presence of a clonal population of B cells. Data demonstrate that up to 10% to 15% of patients with lymphocytosis have MBL. Three major subtypes of MBL exist: the CLL immunophenotype (CD5+, CD23+), which is by far the most common; the atypical CLL type (CD5+, CD23−); and non-CLL lymphoproliferative disorder (CD5−). In a systematic study of blood donors more than 45 years of age, 7.1% had detectable MBL. Of these, the majority had the CLL immunophenotype and more than 93% were low-count MBL (B-cell clonal count less than 500 cells/μl). Similar to the relationship between monoclonal gammopathy of uncertain significance and multiple myeloma, only a small proportion of patients with CLL-type MBL (1% to 4% per year) go on to develop progressive disease requiring treatment. Epidemiologic studies of MBL patients have demonstrated strong familial risk for CLL, and the first reports of MBL came from studies of "unaffected" CLL family members. Studies of CLL families suggest that there is an inherited abnormality that increases the risk of developing CLL, and some families exhibit anticipation, with the disease occurring earlier in successive generations. The supposition that MBL is a progenitor lesion for CLL is strengthened by the observation that both low-count and high-count MBL carry the same cytogenetic aberrations observed in good-prognosis CLL. MBL has been identified in up to 30% of individuals infected with hepatitis C virus (HCV), and up to 50% of the HCV-associated cases demonstrate the atypical CLL immunophenotype. The presence of MBL correlates with more advanced liver disease, suggesting that the persistence of viral infection is crucial to development of the B-cell clone. Follow-up for MBL patients is not clearly defined, although it is probably reasonable to evaluate lymphocyte counts with complete blood counts and follow the clone with flow cytometry at periodic

TABLE 49.1	Normal Lymphocyte Subsets With Age[a]				
	Cord Blood	2 Days–11 Months	1–6 Years	7–17 Years	18–70 Years
Total lymphocyte count (×10³ cells/mL)	5.4 (4.2–6)	4.1 (2.7–5.4)	3.6 (2.9–5.1)	2.4 (2.0–2.7)	2.1 (1.6–2.4)
CD4+ T cells (%)	35 (28–42)	41 (38–50)	37 (30–40)	37 (33–41)	42 (38–46)
CD45Ra+ in CD4+ (naive T cells)[b]	91 (82–97)	81 (66–88)	71 (66–77)	61 (55–67)	40 (32–49)
CD8+ T cells (%)	29 (26–33)	21 (18–25)	29 (25–32)	30 (27–35)	35 (31–40)
B cells (%)	20 (14–23)	23 (19–31)	24 (21–28)	16 (12–22)	13 (11–16)
NK cells (%)	20 (14–30)	11 (8–17)	11 (8–15)	12 (9–16)	14 (10–19)

[a]Values are median, with ranges from the 25th to 75th percentiles.
[b]Naive T cells expressed as a percentage of CD4+ T cells.
NK, Natural killer.

intervals depending on the pace of the lymphocyte rise, the clinical scenario, the family history, and the age of the patient.[3]

Infectious Causes

The most common infections causing lymphocytosis are Epstein-Barr virus (EBV) and cytomegalovirus (CMV). In young children, EBV infection frequently presents as an upper respiratory infection, but in adolescents and young adults, it can result in acute glandular fever with pharyngitis, splenomegaly, lymphadenitis, and profound reactive lymphocytosis. Lymphocytosis is less prominent in older adults. Although the B cells are targeted by EBV, the lymphocytosis consists of CD8+ lymphocytes reacting to neoantigens expressed on the surface of infected B cells. The massive T-cell response usually clears the infection in a matter of days to 1 week, and the lymphocytosis resolves. CMV infection can produce a similar lymphocytosis. In the case of CMV, however, the macrophages are the target of infection, and the T-cell lymphocytosis results from a response to the macrophage neoantigen. CMV infection and lymphocytosis are more common in older adults. In both viral infections, lymphocytosis can be profound, with 50% or more of the circulating white blood cells (WBCs) identified as lymphocytes. Examination of the peripheral smear reveals that up to 10% of the circulating lymphocytes are atypical and larger than normal lymphocytes with open chromatin and increased cytoplasm. It is particularly important to recognize lymphocytosis caused by these two viruses in pregnant women because congenital infection can cause fetal death and birth defects. In addition to EBV and CMV, primary infection with human immunodeficiency virus (HIV) can cause lymphocytosis and should be suspected in the presence of a viral syndrome in the appropriate clinical circumstance. In children, infection with Coxsackie A and B6 viruses, echovirus, and adenovirus can cause a brief but profound lymphocytosis. Infections with other viruses, including human herpesvirus 6 (HHV-6) and human herpesvirus 8 (HHV-8) as well as rubella virus, varicella, human T-lymphotropic virus type 1 (HTLV-1), and hepatitis viruses, can cause a lymphocytosis, although much less frequently than CMV and EBV.

Important nonviral infections causing lymphocytosis include *Toxoplasma gondii* and *Bordetella pertussis*. In an immune-competent host, *Toxoplasma* infection is often asymptomatic, but patients can have fever, chills, and lymphadenopathy. Mild lymphocytosis with atypical lymphocytes can be observed. As in the case of EBV and CMV, infections during pregnancy can lead to adverse effects on the fetus. In children and adults, infection with *B. pertussis* can lead to lymphocytosis, with the absolute lymphocyte count frequently greater than 10,000/μL. In more severe cases, lymphocytosis is more pronounced.[4] Unlike viral infections and *Toxoplasma* infection, the lymphocytosis observed in *B. pertussis* infection is caused by increases in all lymphocyte subsets, and it appears that the pertussis toxin blocks migration of the lymphocytes from the bloodstream into lymph nodes.[4] Tuberculosis, rickettsial infection, brucellosis, and shigellosis may also cause lymphocytosis.

Physiologic Stress

Lymphocytosis related to physiologic stress is a poorly studied phenomenon. After strenuous physical exercise, subjects develop lymphocytosis, which returns to preexercise levels within 15 minutes to 1 hour of ceasing the activity. The exercise-induced rise is thought to be attributable to catecholamine and steroid hormones, and their effect on expression of cell adhesion molecules and on cardiac output and shear stress.[5] Exposure to catecholamines increases the expression of β₂-adrenergic receptors on lymphocytes influencing cell trafficking. Reports suggest that a number of other physiologic stresses increase lymphocyte counts, including surgery, trauma, cardiac conditions, sickle cell crises, abdominal pain, and obstetric emergencies. In these cases, all lymphocyte subsets appear to increase, but the increase is most profound for CD4 and CD8 memory T cells. Neutrophil counts also rise in these patients, but in most cases, the lymphocytosis resolves before the peak of the neutrophil count.[6]

Drug Reactions

Drug-induced lymphocytosis can occur as part of a hypersensitivity syndrome. In these cases, the lymphocytosis is usually part of a systemic condition that includes a fever, rash, and lymphadenopathy. Elevation in other WBC counts, including eosinophils and monocytes, is common, and atypical lymphocytes are seen. The time period between drug introduction and the syndrome is usually about 3 weeks with the most common implicated drugs being aromatic anticonvulsants and sulfonamides.[7] Some studies differentiate this syndrome from drug-induced cutaneous pseudolymphomas in which collections of nonclonal lymphocytes appear in the skin after longer periods of drug exposure, but there is no peripheral lymphocytosis.

Polyclonal B-Cell Lymphocytosis

A final entity causing lymphocytosis is persistent polyclonal B-cell lymphocytosis (PPBL). This rare disorder is seen primarily in young to middle-aged women who smoke and results in mild polyclonal lymphocytosis. The lymphocytes are medium sized with abundant cytoplasm and a variable proportion is binucleate. A polyclonal increase in serum immunoglobulin M (IgM) is also observed, and there is an association with the human leukocyte antigen (HLA) antigen D-related 7 (DR7) phenotype. Examination of the B cells reveals that most are CD19+, CD5−, and CD23−, with a normal kappa-to-lambda ratio and a variety of heavy chain rearrangements. Adenopathy, hepatomegaly, or splenomegaly has been observed in some, but not all, patients. Genetic analysis has demonstrated the presence of isochromosome 3q in a proportion of B cells, as well as the presence of multiple B-cell lymphoma immunoglobulin (*BCL2-Ig*) gene rearrangements. Similar gene rearrangements have been identified in family members of PPBL patients along with increases in serum IgM, suggesting that there may be an underlying genetic defect. In vitro studies have shown that PPBL cells proliferate in a CD40-CD154 culture system and secrete both IgM and IgG (isotype switching). This suggests that PPBL may arise from deregulation of the microenvironmment or from a defect in a different B-cell activation pathway resulting in extensive proliferation. Overall, the clinical course of this disorder is benign, and the lymphocytosis is not usually progressive; however, clonal B-cell disorders have been seen in a few patients with the disorder, suggesting that it may represent a preneoplastic state.[8]

Lymphocytopenia

Inherited Disorders

Although there are few inherited causes of lymphocytosis, such is not the case for lymphocytopenia, in which the genetic bases of a number of inherited immunodeficiency disorders have been identified. Chief among these disorders is severe combined immunodeficiency (SCID), which is characterized by the absence of functional T lymphocytes. T lymphocytes, B lymphocytes, and NK cells share progenitors, signaling pathways in development and function, and metabolic pathways; thus B lymphocytes, NK cells, or both are often severely affected in SCID. Moreover, in the absence of functional $CD4^+$ T-helper lymphocytes, B lymphocytes cannot function properly, and hypo- or agammaglobulinemia is observed. In most cases of SCID, the absence of T lymphocytes leads to an extremely low absolute lymphocyte count. As detailed in Chapter 49, SCID can be grouped based on the cellular pathway that is affected. In general, whereas SCID is characterized by complete loss of function of the affected gene, hypomorphic mutations of the same genes lead to quite different phenotypes (Omenn syndrome and atypical SCID). Defects in more than 30 genes are known to lead to SCID. Inheritance is primarily X-linked or autosomal recessive, but in a few cases, such as the DiGeorge anomaly and some cases of Hoyeraal–Hreidarsson syndrome (defects in telomerase), inheritance is autosomal dominant. Until the genetic diagnosis is known, it is useful to characterize SCID syndromes as $T^-B^+NK^+$, $T^-B^-NK^+$, $T^-B^+NK^-$ or $T^-B^-NK^-$ based on the presence or absence of defects affecting B and/or NK cells. SCID can be classified based on the cellular function which is lacking, including deficiency in cytokine-mediated signaling, defects in V(D)J recombination, absent signaling through the T-cell receptor, defects in antigen presentation, and defects in basic cellular processes. Defects in the interleukin-7 receptor alpha chain (IL7RA), actin-regulating protein coronin 1A (CORO1A), CD3 chain components (CD3D, CD3E, CD3Z), and CD45 (PTPRC) lead to $T^-B^+NK^+$ SCID. $T^-B^+NK^-$ SCID defects include deficiencies in cytokine-mediated signaling (IL2RG, JAK3). Defects in V(D)J recombination (RAG1, RAG2) or in nonhomologous end joining for repair of double-strand DNA breaks (DCLRE1C, PRKDC, LIG4, and NHEJ1 mutations) lead to $T^-B^-NK^+$ SCID. Defects that lead to increased lymphocyte apoptosis (AK2, ADA gene mutations) lead to $T^-B^-NK^-$ SCID and are often associated with anomalies outside of the immune system. Defects in thymic embryogenesis and calcium flux, as well as a collection of other abnormalities, including defects in telomerase activity, can also lead to SCID and are usually associated with abnormalities of other organ systems.[9]

In addition to SCID, other inherited disorders can also perturb T- and B-cell numbers. Patients with Wiskott-Aldrich syndrome, caused by mutations in WASP (which encodes a cytoplasmic protein responsible for transducing cell surface signals to the actin cytoskeleton), can present with low T-cell counts early in life and become profoundly lymphopenic over time. Abnormalities in immunoglobulins are also noted in this syndrome, with low levels of IgM and high levels of IgA and IgE.[10] Immunodeficiency affects more than half of all patients with ataxia telangiectasia. Patients with ataxia telangiectasia have homozygous or compound heterozygous mutations in the ataxia-telangiectasia–mutated (ATM) gene, which encodes a protein kinase with functions in the cellular response to DNA damage. Lymphopenia, especially of naive CD4 cells, is observed in about half

of patients with ataxia telangiectasia, with mutations leading to absent expression of ATM kinase activity.[11] Heterozygous germline mutations in GATA2 lead to a spectrum of clinical syndromes characterized by dendritic cell, monocyte, B cell, and NK lymphoid deficiency (DCML deficiency) with elevated 3 ligand (Flt3L). Mononuclear cytopenia appears to evolve in diverse clinical groups of GATA2 mutation including monoMAC syndrome (monocytopenia, B-cell and NK-cell lymphopenia, mycobacterial, fungal, and viral infections and alveolar proteinosis), Emberger syndrome (lymphedema, deafness, and myelodysplastic syndrome [MDS]) and familial (MDS)/acute myeloid leukemia (AML)[12]. GATA2 mutation appears to cause loss of progenitor cells, clonal hematopoiesis and elevation of Flt3L, but the molecular mechanisms of marrow failure and transformation to MDS or AML are as yet unclear.

Infections

A variety of viral and nonviral infections can lead to lymphopenia. HIV is the most common virus associated with lymphopenia. The target of HIV is the CD4 receptor, and the virus selectively targets and infects activated expanding CD4 T cells. Large studies in HIV-infected patients have shown that peripheral blood CD4 T-cell counts fall most rapidly in the year after seroconversion (from approximately 1000/μL before seroconversion to 670/μL at 1 year after infection) and then decline more slowly by about 50/μL per year.[13] In a subset of untreated patients, viremia is absent or well controlled, and lymphocytopenia develops very slowly if at all; particular HLA class I alleles are overrepresented in this group. Lymphopenia is an early and reliable laboratory observation in adult influenza infection and is also detected in infections caused by swine influenza (H1N1) and the highly pathogenic avian influenza (H5N1).[14] Lymphopenia has been reported in patients with severe acute respiratory syndrome (SARS) caused by the SARS-coronavirus. In children, respiratory syncytial virus (RSV) infection is associated with a reduction in lymphocyte count, which is most extreme in the sickest patients; similar effects on lymphocyte counts are seen in measles infections (also a paramyxovirus). In West Nile virus encephalitis, lymphopenia is profound and prolonged, and the initial degree of lymphopenia is predictive of outcome. A variety of other viruses can also cause lymphopenia, including herpes viruses (herpes simplex, HHV-6, HHV-8), parvovirus B19, and Dengue virus. In many viral infections, the degree of lymphopenia is correlated with the severity of the disease.[14]

A variety of nonviral infections cause lymphopenia. Infections with Ehrlichia (a tick-borne obligate intracellular gram-negative bacteria), Salmonella typhi, and Leptospira have all been reported to cause lymphocytopenia during the acute illness. $CD4^+$ T-cell depletion has been described in a subset of HIV-negative patients with tuberculosis and low albumin levels, low body weight, and more extensive disease. Recovery of CD4 count after treatment of tuberculosis suggests that the lymphopenia is caused by the tuberculosis infection.[15] Lymphocytopenia is often observed in sepsis and is thought to occur as a result of cytokine-mediated apoptosis of B cells, CD4 and CD8 T cells, and follicular dendritic cells. In autopsy series, most deaths from sepsis occur during the prolonged hypoimmune state, and the more prolonged the sepsis, the more profound the loss of splenic lymphocytes. In one large retrospective study, severe persistent lymphopenia (defined as an absolute lymphocyte count of less than 600 cells/μL) on the fourth day following a diagnosis of sepsis was predictive of development of secondary infections, as well as short- and long-term survival.[16]

Collagen Vascular Disorders

Autoimmune diseases frequently exhibit decreases in circulating lymphocytes. In systemic lupus erythematosus (SLE), lymphopenia (usually decreases in T cells but occasionally in B cells as well) is not only one of the diagnostic criteria but also a parameter used to assess disease activity. Lymphopenia was observed in more than 60% of patients at diagnosis, with the cumulative incidence over the course of the disease reaching over 90%. Lymphopenia in SLE seems to be more frequent in patients of African descent, and in one study more than half of patients with lymphopenia demonstrated antilymphocyte antibodies. Antigalectin 8 antibodies have been described in patients with SLE, rheumatoid arthritis, and sepsis. In SLE, these autoantibodies are associated with lymphopenia. Apoptosis may also play a role in lymphopenia in SLE, possibly by upregulation of fas antigen on naive peripheral T cells.[17] CD4 T cells may also be decreased in rheumatoid arthritis, and increasing evidence suggests that deficiencies in DNA repair enzymes such as ATM render rheumatoid arthritis T cells sensitive to apoptosis.[18] Apoptotic loss of naive T cells results in lymphopenia-induced proliferation to preserve T-cell homeostasis; this proliferation is now thought to lead to both premature immune aging and an autoimmune-biased T-cell repertoire. In Sjögren syndrome, a minority of patients has been noted to have deficient CD4 counts, and this has been correlated with the presence of anti-CD4 antibodies. Similarly, low lymphocyte counts have been observed in patients with primary vasculitides, type 1 diabetes, and Crohn disease.[17]

Malignancies

Lymphopenia is found in a variety of systemic illnesses; chief among them are cancers. In hematologic malignancies, including Hodgkin lymphoma, diffuse large B-cell lymphoma, and peripheral T-cell lymphoma, patients with lymphopenia have a worse prognosis. Lymphopenia has also been observed in solid tumors, including breast and colon cancer, and soft tissue sarcomas, in which its presence before treatment predicts decreased overall survival. Which specific lymphocyte subsets are involved and the cause(s) of lymphopenia in these tumor types has not been described.

Systemic Disorders

End-stage renal disease (ESRD) has also been associated with lymphopenia, an observation not thought to be exclusively attributable to an effect of dialysis alone. Naive and central memory CD4 and CD8 T cells are significantly reduced in the blood of ESRD patients, apparently because of increased susceptibility of these cells to apoptosis. Lymphopenia occurs in more than 50% of sarcoidosis patients and is associated with chronic disease. Sarcoidosis patients with severe organ system involvement, including neurologic, cardiac, ocular, and advanced pulmonary disease, have lower lymphocyte counts than patients with less severe manifestations (see E-Slide VM03953). Older studies suggest that burn victims have profound decreases in T-cell counts, which may contribute to the infection risk in these patients. Interestingly, lymphopenia is a characteristic of both protein-energy malnutrition and zinc deficiency. Both of these deficiencies perturb the hypothalamic–pituitary–adrenocorticoid axis and increase glucocorticoid levels, which results in increased apoptosis of B and T cells.[19] Intestinal lymphangiectasia, which may be either congenital or secondary to processes that obstruct lymphatic drainage of the gastrointestinal tract, can cause lymphopenia as a result of loss of lymph fluid into the gut along with lymphocytes.

A rare cause of lymphopenia is idiopathic CD4+ lymphocytopenia (ICL), which is defined as a CD4 count less than 300/μL or less than 20% of the T-cell count on two occasions that is not caused by HIV or HTLV infection, drug therapy, or a known immunodeficiency. Patients usually come to clinical notice when they present with opportunistic infections. CD4 T-cell counts typically remain low, but counts do not continue to drop or do not fall rapidly after diagnosis. In one large series, only about 20% of patients recovered from lymphopenia within 3 years of diagnosis. Opportunistic infections plague these patients, and autoimmune diseases occur both before and after the diagnosis of ICL. In ICL, unlike HIV infection, increased activation and turnover are observed in CD4 but not CD8 T lymphocytes.[20]

Drug Effects

A number of drugs are known to cause lymphopenia. Glucocorticoids inhibit production of a number of cytokines and rapidly deplete circulating T cells by enhancing emigration from the circulation, inducing apoptosis, interfering with growth signaling, and inhibiting release from lymphoid tissues. B cells are less affected acutely by glucocorticoid administration, but prolonged administration may result in decreased IgG levels. In clinical trials for multiple sclerosis, delayed release dimethyl fumarate resulted in a decrease in mean lymphocyte count of about 30% in the first year, but about 2% of patients had lymphocyte counts less than 500 cells/μL which persisted for 6 months or longer. Antimetabolite chemotherapeutic agents such as methotrexate, azathioprine, and 6-mercaptopurine lower lymphocyte as well as neutrophil counts, and alkylating agents such as cyclophosphamide have more profound effects on lymphocytes. Purine nucleoside analogs, including cladribine, fludarabine, pentostatin, nelarabine, clofarabine, and others, inhibit DNA synthesis and repair, and cause accumulation of DNA strand breaks. All of these agents are associated with profound lymphoma, which may persist for several years after completion of treatment. In general, T cells are more affected than B cells. Nelarabine in particular is a prodrug of ara-G and is converted to ara-GTP, which accumulates at higher levels in T cells.[21]

Monoclonal and polyclonal antibodies directed against lymphocytes are useful in clinical practice and can induce profound and long-lasting lymphopenia. Whereas antithymocyte globulin and alemtuzumab produce depletion of both T and B cells, the monoclonal antibodies OKT3, daclizumab, and basiliximab produce a more pronounced decrease in T cells. The drugs rituximab and ofatumumab are monoclonal antibodies directed against distinct epitopes on B cells. These drugs deplete peripheral B cells but do not routinely produce lymphopenia.

Finally, radiation exposure commonly results in lymphopenia, which occurs before depression of other cell counts. In fact, lymphopenia can develop within the first 24 hours of exposure if the dose of radiation is great enough, and a drop of 50% or more predicts an increased risk of death. B cells are more sensitive to radiation than T cells and recover more slowly than T-cell numbers.[22]

QUANTITATIVE DISORDERS OF IMMUNOGLOBULINS

In practice, as there are several methods for determining serum immunoglobulin levels it is critical that age-adjusted normal reference ranges are provided by the laboratory when evaluating immunoglobulin level results. Children first achieve adult levels of IgM around 2 years of age, IgG by 6 years of age, and IgA during puberty. Hypogammaglobulinemia is defined as an IgG less than 2 standard deviations from normal, and agammaglobulinemia is usually defined as an IgG level less than 100 mg/dL. Low levels of IgA, IgG, and IgM are characteristic of most forms of SCID.

Hypogammaglobulinemia

Causes of hypogammaglobulinemia can be divided into primary causes related to genetic deficiencies and secondary causes related to malignancies or their treatment, infections, medications, and protein-losing states that deplete antibody.

Secondary Causes

Before embarking on a search for a primary disorder causing hypogammaglobulinemia, it is important to rule out secondary causes. Malnutrition, malabsorption, and any disease state in which large amounts of protein are lost, such as nephrotic range proteinuria, severe burns, lymphangiectasia, or protein-losing enteropathy, can overwhelm the capacity of the B cells to provide adequate immunoglobulin to maintain normal serum levels. Aside from chemotherapeutic agents, a number of medications can produce hypogammaglobulinemia; these include captopril, antiseizure medications (carbamazepine, phenytoin), gold salts, antimalarials, fenoclofenac, penicillamine, and sulfasalazine, as well as glucocorticoids. Infection with HIV and EBV, and congenital infection with rubella, CMV, and *T. gondii* can produce very low immunoglobulin levels and should be ruled out as appropriate. A host of lymphoid malignancies produce hypogammaglobulinemia, but the defect is most profound in CLL, in which up to 85% of patients are said to possess hypogammaglobulinemia even in the absence of treatment.[23]

Primary Immunodeficiencies

The International Union of Immunological Societies has classified the primary immunodeficiency diseases into nine groups, including one class called *predominantly antibody deficiencies.*[9] These disorders present in both adults and children, although some are very rare. Table 49.2 provides a simple grouping of these antibody disorders, some of which are discussed in greater detail in Chapter 49.

The first group is characterized by a severe reduction in all serum immunoglobulin isotypes, with absence or profound reduction in B cells. Patients with these disorders, particularly those with a

well-defined genetic basis, present with severe bacterial infections, most commonly in the respiratory tract (pneumonia, sinusitis, and otitis media), as well as diarrhea caused by bacteria, parasites, and viruses. The prototypic member of this group is X-linked agammaglobulinemia (XLA) caused by a mutation in the Bruton tyrosine kinase *(Btk)* gene, which produces a block in B-cell maturation. Female carriers of a *Btk* mutation are generally asymptomatic, but most boys with XLA come to clinical attention by the age of 1 year. In addition to low-serum immunoglobulins, a clue to the diagnosis is the absence of lymphoid tissue, including tonsils. Autosomal recessive mutations in the μ heavy chain as well as defects in *λ5, Igα, Igβ,* and *BLNK* produce a similar phenotype. Phosphatidylinositol 3-kinase deficiency *(PIK3R1)* and heterozygous mutation of the E47 transcription factor deficiency *(TCF3)* can cause severe reduction in all serum immunoglobulin isotypes. In a small percentage of patients, no clear molecular defect can be identified. Also included in this group are thymoma with immunodeficiency (Good syndrome) and myelodysplasia. Good syndrome is a poorly understood disorder that presents primarily in middle-aged adults. Immunodeficiency can precede or follow the diagnosis of thymoma and does not resolve with thymectomy. In addition to infections, patients experience autoimmune phenomena, including myasthenia gravis, immune thrombocytopenia purpura, pure red blood cell aplasia, and pernicious anemia. Myelodysplastic syndromes can also mimic XLA and

TABLE 49.2	Predominant Antibody Deficiencies		
	Disease	**Mode of Inheritance/Genetic Locus**	**Clinical Features**
Severe reduction in all serum immunoglobulin isotypes with absent B cells	Bruton tyrosine kinase deficiency	XL/Xq21.3–22	Severe bacterial infections (especially of the respiratory tract), absent lymphoid tissue
	μ heavy chain deficiency	AR/14q32.3	Severe bacterial infections
	λ5 deficiency	AR/22q11.21	Severe bacterial infections
	Igα deficiency	AR/19q13.2	Severe bacterial infections
	Igβ deficiency	AR/17q23	Severe bacterial infections
	BLNK deficiency	AR/10q23.2	Severe bacterial infections
	SP110 deficiency	AR/2q37.1	Hepatic veno-occlusive disease, some with frequent infection
	LRRC8A deficiency	AD/9q34.11	Facial anomalies
	PIK3R1	AR/5q13.1	Recurrent bacterial infection
	Thymoma with immunodeficiency (Good syndrome)	None	Recurrent infection with encapsulated bacteria and diarrhea, autoimmune phenomena
	Myelodysplasia	Variable/monosomy 7, trisomy 8, dyskeratosis congenita	Recurrent infections and pancytopenia
Severe reduction in at least two serum immunoglobulin isotypes with low or normal B-cell numbers	Common variable immunodeficiency syndromes	≈10% with family history AR or AD	Recurrent respiratory tract infections leading to chronic sinusitis, hearing loss, bronchiectasis, autoimmune disease, lymphoproliferation, malignancy (especially non-Hodgkin lymphoma and gastric carcinoma)
	TACI alterations	AD and AR/17p11.2	
	BAFFR alterations	AR/22q13	
	MSH5 alterations	Unk/6p22.1-p21.3	
	ICOS deficiency	AR/2q33	Recurrent infections
	CD19 deficiency	AR/16p11.2	Recurrent infections
	X-linked lymphoproliferative disease (mutation in SH2 domain protein 1A)	XL/Xq25–q26	Fulminant infection with EBV, lymphoma, dysgammaglobulinemia
	CD81 deficiency	AR/11p15.5	Recurrent infections
	CD20 deficiency	AR/11q12.2	Recurrent infections
	CD21 deficiency	AR/1q32.2	Recurrent infections
	LRBA deficiency	AR/4q31.3	Recurrent infections, inflammatory bowel disease, EBV infection
	TNSF12 deficiency	AD/17p13.1	Recurrent bacterial infections, thrombocytopenia, neutropenia
	NFKB2 deficiency	AD/10q24.32	Recurrent infections
	CXCR4 activation	AD gain of function/2q22.1	WHIM syndrome

TABLE 49.2	Predominant Antibody Deficiencies—cont'd		
	Disease	**Mode of Inheritance/Genetic Locus**	**Clinical Features**
Severe reduction in serum IgG and IgA with increased IgM and normal B-cell numbers (disorders of immunoglobulin class switching)	CD40 ligand deficiency	XL/Xq26.3-Xq27.1	Recurrent infections with bacteria and opportunistic pathogens, neutropenia, autoimmune disease
	CD40 deficiency	AR/20q11-20q13.2	Recurrent infections with bacteria and opportunistic pathogens, neutropenia, autoimmune disease
	NEMO hypomorphic mutations	XL/Xq28	Recurrent infections with bacteria and opportunistic pathogens, neutropenia, autoimmune disease
	AID deficiency	AR/12p13	Recurrent bacterial infections and diarrhea, marked enlargement of lymphoid organs
	UNG deficiency	AR/12q23–q24.1	Recurrent bacterial infections and diarrhea, marked enlargement of lymphoid organs
Isotype or light-chain deficiencies with normal B-cell numbers	Ig heavy-chain deficiency	AR/14q32	Most patients are healthy
	κ-chain deficiency	AR/2p11.2	Most patients are healthy
	Isolated IgG subclass deficiency	Variable/unknown	Most patients are healthy
	IgA deficiency associated with IgG subclass deficiency	Variable/unknown	Most patients are healthy
	Selective IgA deficiency	Variable/unknown	Most patients asymptomatic, but increased prevalence of infections, autoimmune disease, atopy, and celiac disease
	PRKCδ deficiency	AR/3p21.1	Recurrent infection, autoimmunity, and chronic EBV infection
	Activated PI3K-γ	AD gain of function/1p36.22	Recurrent infection, autoimmunity, chronic EBV, and CMV infection
Specific antibody deficiency with normal immunoglobulin level and B-cell number	Inability to make antibodies to specific antigens	Variable/unknown	Recurrent sinopulmonary infection, bronchiectasis, diarrhea, autoimmune disease
Transient hypogammaglobulinemia of infancy	IgG and IgA deficiency	Variable/unknown	More likely to be male (60%–80%), mild infections and diarrhea, atopy

λ5, Immunoglobulin lambda-like polypeptide (a surrogate light chain subunit that is part of the pre–B-cell receptor); AID, activation-induced cytidine deaminase (thought to be essential for initiation of the DNA cleavage required for class-switch recombination and somatic hypermutation); BAFF-R, B-cell–activating factor receptor; BLNK, B linker (a cytoplasmic linker or adaptor protein that plays a critical role in B-cell development); CMV, cytomegalovirus; CXCR4, CXC-chemokine receptor 4 (mediates migration of resting leukocytes and hematopoietic progenitors in response to its ligand, stromal cell–derived factor 1 [SDF1]); EBV, Epstein–Barr virus; ICOS, inducible T-cell costimulator (belongs to CD28 family of costimulatory surface molecules); Ig, immunoglobulin; Igα, immunoglobulin-associated α (necessary for expression and function of the B-cell antigen receptor); Igβ, immunoglobulin-associated β (necessary for expression and function of the B-cell antigen receptor); LRBA, lipopolysaccharide-responsive, beige-like anchor protein (implicated in regulating endosomal trafficking, particularly endocytosis of ligand-activated receptors); MSH5, mutS homolog 5 (a protein involved with DNA mismatch repair and meiotic recombination); NEMO, NFκB essential modulator; NFκB, nuclear factor kappa-B; PRKCD, member of the protein kinase c family (involved in B-cell receptor-mediated signaling); PI3K-γ, protein kinase C family member (critical for regulation of cell survival, proliferation, and apoptosis); TACI, transmembrane activator and CAML-interactor; TNSF12, tumor necrosis factor ligand superfamily, member 12 (weak inducer of apoptosis); UNG, uracil DNA glycosylase (allows creation of single-stranded breaks essential to class switch recombination and somatic hypermutation); WHIM syndrome, warts, hypogammaglobulinemia, infections, and myelokathexis.

generally present with low B cells and pancytopenia with monosomy 7, trisomy 8, or dyskeratosis congenita.[24]

A second group is characterized by severe reduction of at least two serum immunoglobulin isotypes with normal or low numbers of B cells. Most patients in this group can be categorized as having common variable immune deficiency (CVID), a heterogeneous disorder characterized by recurrent infection and failure to make antibody to vaccine antigens. Both males and females are affected, and patients can have autoimmune and gastrointestinal disease as well as lymphoproliferative disorders. Autoimmune disease can precede the hypogammaglobulinemia. About 10% of patients with a CVID phenotype have a family history of immunodeficiency and can be shown to have mutations in one of five genes expressed in both T and B cells. Homozygous or compound heterozygous mutations in *ICOS* (inducible costimulator), which is expressed on activated T cells and plays a role in activating T-helper cells and providing B-cell help, and *CD19*, a B-cell surface molecule that participates in signaling after antigen binding to the B-cell receptor, have been shown to result in recurrent infections in childhood and hypogammaglobulinemia. Mutations in *TACI* (transmembrane activator and CAML-interactor) and *BAFF-R* (B-cell–activating factor receptor) members of the

tumor necrosis factor (TNF) receptor superfamily, which play roles in B-cell survival and antibody production, and *MSH5*, a mismatch repair gene, are thought to predispose to CVID and IgA deficiency but are not sufficient to independently cause their onset. X-linked lymphoproliferative syndrome caused by mutation in the signaling lymphocyte activation molecular-associated protein SAP (gene, *SH2D1A*) can present atypically or later in life with a CVID phenotype.[25] Single-gene mutations of *TNSF12* (*TWEAK*), *NFKB2*, and *CXCR4* have also been demonstrated to cause low levels of immunoglobulins.

Class-switch recombination defects encompass a third group of antibody deficiencies and result in hyper-IgM syndrome characterized by reductions in serum IgG and IgA with normal or elevated IgM. Mutations in the gene for CD40 ligand make up about 30% of these syndromes. CD40L on the surface of T cells interacts with CD40 on B cells, which is required for immunoglobulin class switching, and CD40 on monocytes, which is required for T-cell response. Patients with *CD40L* mutations and rarer mutations in *CD40* itself and in nuclear factor kappa-B (NFκB) and essential modulator (*NEMO*), required for CD40-induced signaling, have combined antibody and cellular immune deficits, resulting in hypogammaglobulinemia and recurrent bacterial infection, as well as opportunistic infections with organisms similar to those observed in acquired immune deficiency syndrome (AIDS). Defects in the activation-induced cytidine deaminase gene *(AID)* produce hypogammaglobulinemia with recurrent bacterial infections and diarrhea, as well as enlarged lymphoid organs filled with proliferating B cells. A similar clinical picture is produced by homozygous defects in uracil-DNA glycosylase *(UNG)*. AID is thought to deaminate cytosine to uracil, and UNG subsequently deglycosylates and removes the uracil residue, creating an abasic site, which allows for creation of single-stranded DNA breaks. Deficiencies in these enzymes result in defective class switching and somatic hypermutation. Patients with similar phenotypes but without defects in *AID* or *UNG* have been described and probably have mutations in other essential genes involved in class switching.[26]

Additional groups of antibody deficiencies exist in which overall antibody levels are normal, but there are defects in specific isotypes, light chains, or specific antibodies with normal numbers of B cells; the majority of patients with these deficiencies are healthy. The most common member of these groups is selective IgA deficiency, which occurs in about 1 in 500 white individuals. The molecular mechanisms underlying this deficiency are unknown, but there is an association with CVID. Finally, an entity termed *transient hypogammaglobulinemia of infancy* has been described in which the normal decline in immunoglobulins after maternal transfer is prolonged. This entity is poorly understood and usually affects boys, who have mild infections and diarrhea. Recovery usually, but not always, occurs by 3 years of age.[27]

Hypergammaglobulinemia

Hypergammaglobulinemia results from an overproduction of immunoglobulins by plasma cells, either monoclonal and reflective of a plasma cell or lymphoproliferative disorder, or polyclonal and accompanying other disease states. The distinction between polyclonal and monoclonal disorders is made by inspection of the serum protein electrophoretic pattern. Detection of one or several monoclonal bands within a polyclonal background is not unusual, and the literature suggests that small bands frequently disappear and do not become clinically relevant. No data are available to suggest that polyclonal gammopathy drives development of monoclonal gammopathy; however, if a clonal plasmaproliferative disorder is suspected, immunofixation or immunoelectrophoresis should be performed.

Disorders Producing Polyclonal Gammopathy

Polyclonal gammopathy usually reflects one of five major disorders, including liver disease, connective tissue disorders, infections, hematologic disorders, and solid tumors.[28] Interleukin-6 (IL-6) and IL-10 have been implicated in polyclonal gammopathy, as have defects in T cells and chronic antigenic stimulation, but the exact sequence of events leading to polyclonal B-cell activation is not known. In general, treatment is directed at the underlying disease, but there are reports of polyclonal gammopathy leading to symptomatic hyperviscosity. In these cases, plasmapheresis and/or corticosteroids seem to be effective. It should also be noted that polyclonal elevations in serum immunoglobulins can sometimes interfere with the direct Coombs test, possibly via nonspecific antibody binding to red blood cells. The degree of gamma globulin elevation does not seem to be helpful in defining the underlying disease state.

In the largest recent review of polyclonal gammopathy, the majority of patients had liver disease, which covered the spectrum from autoimmune disorders (autoimmune hepatitis, primary biliary cirrhosis, and primary sclerosing cholangitis) to viral hepatitis, and alcoholic liver disease. In fact, elevation of serum gamma globulins is a distinguishing characteristic of autoimmune hepatitis, and the levels usually correlate with activity of disease. The most common etiology for polyclonal gammopathy related to liver disease in the United States is likely infection with HCV, but in any particular clinical setting, the exact distribution likely depends on the population demographic. Other diseases affecting the liver, such as α-1 antitrypsin deficiency and hemochromatosis, are also accompanied by increases in serum immunoglobulins.

Connective tissue diseases, including Sjögren syndrome, SLE, ankylosing spondylitis, and rheumatoid arthritis, are also accompanied by polyclonal gammopathy. In many of these diseases, the degree of gamma globulin elevation may reflect disease activity, although a causative link between the autoimmune phenomena and immunoglobulin levels has not been determined. Several of the periodic fever syndromes, which are sometimes classified with the connective tissue disorders, have elevated immunoglobulin levels as a part of their manifestations. Hyperimmunoglobulinemia D is one such syndrome and is linked to mutations in the mevalonate kinase gene. Patients with this disorder present in the first year of life with febrile attacks, lymphadenopathy, abdominal symptoms, arthritis, and oral and genital ulcers. Most, but not all, patients have elevated levels of polyclonal IgD during and between episodes often accompanied by elevated IgA levels. TNF receptor 1-associated periodic syndrome (TRAPS) results from mutation in the gene *(TNRFRSF1A)* for the TNF receptor 1 and can cause prolonged febrile attacks with abdominal pain, arthralgias, and myalgias. During attacks, polyclonal elevation of immunoglobulins (primarily IgA) is observed.[29]

Infections, usually chronic in nature, are frequently accompanied by polyclonal gammopathy. HIV infection is a common cause, and immunoglobulin levels tend to increase slowly until the diagnosis of AIDS and then decline over the ensuing 6 to 18 months. Polyclonal gammopathy can be a clue to occult infections such as subacute bacterial endocarditis, tuberculosis, perinephric abscess, Lyme disease, and a variety of parasitic infections.

Malignant B- and T-cell disorders can cause polyclonal hypergammaglobulinemia. These diseases include CLL; large granular lymphocytic leukemia; hairy cell leukemia; and angioimmunoblastic T-cell lymphoma (AITL), a rare disease characterized by rash, widespread lymphadenopathy and extranodal involvement, autoimmune phenomena, and polyclonal gammopathy. Interestingly, despite the elevated levels of immunoglobulins observed in AITL, patients exhibit immunodeficiency and a propensity to develop opportunistic infections. Patients with myeloid disorders can also have polyclonal gammopathies; in one large series, nearly 40% of patients with myelodysplastic syndrome had hypergammaglobulinemia, and patients with immunologic abnormalities had inferior survival.[30] The incidence of hypergammaglobulinemia is reported to approach 50% in chronic myelomonocytic leukemia (CMML). Hypergammaglobulinemia has been reported in AML both in adults and children, but it appears to be a rare phenomenon. Among solid tumors, ovarian and hepatocellular cancers are most commonly associated with polyclonal gammopathy. There are case reports of cancers, particularly lung and breast tumors, producing and releasing the secretory component of IgA into the bloodstream with the binding of SC to polyclonal IgA, producing hypergammaglobulinemia of serum sIgA.

A variety of other diseases, including asbestos exposure and several subtypes of hypersensitivity pneumonitis and idiopathic interstitial pneumonia, are associated with polyclonal gammopathy. In general, these disorders represent diffuse activation of B cells.

Disorders Producing Monoclonal Gammopathy

The differential diagnosis of monoclonal gammopathy includes monoclonal gammopathy of undetermined significance (MGUS), multiple myeloma, solitary plasmacytoma of bone or extramedullary plasmacytoma, Waldenström macroglobulinemia, lymphoma, CLL, and primary systemic amyloidosis. These individual disorders are described elsewhere in this text; however, there are a few points to be made about the M protein itself and MGUS. These disorders can produce intact immunoglobulins (IgG, IgM, IgD, or IgE), κ-, or λ-light chains alone or in combination with intact immunoglobulins and rarely heavy chains only. The monoclonal protein is usually detected as a discrete band in the γ or β region in serum or urine

TABLE 49.3 **Diseases Associated With Monoclonal Gammopathy**

Plasma cell and related disorders	MGUS Solitary plasmacytoma: Bone Soft tissue Multiple myeloma Waldenström macroglobulinemia Primary amyloidosis	See Chapters 85–87
Lymphoid disorders	Non-Hodgkin lymphoma	Monoclonal protein observed in CLL (>20% of cases with IgM, ≈50% with IgG, light chains also observed), extranodal marginal zone lymphomas (>30% of cases and correlated with BM involvement), follicular, mantle cell, and diffuse large B-cell lymphomas also reported with serum M proteins as has AITL
	Hodgkin lymphoma	Rare but reported
	Castleman disease	<2% with monoclonal gammopathy
Other hematologic disorders	Acquired von Willebrand disease	IVIG more effective than factor concentrate in increasing factor VIII coagulant and VWF levels
	Gaucher disease	Observed in 25% in one study; M protein declined after splenectomy
	Pernicious anemia, pure RBC aplasia, hereditary spherocytosis, MPD, MDS	
Connective tissue disorders	SLE	IgG, IgM, and IgA have been observed, no difference in disease activity or outcome
	Inclusion body myositis	80% with IgG M protein
	Polymyositis, RA, scleroderma	
Neurologic disorders	POEMS syndrome	Most have M-protein of λ light chain
	Peripheral neuropathy	Most common is IgM followed by IgG and IgA In half, IgM protein binds to myelin-associated glycoprotein Size of M protein not correlated with severity of neuropathy Some benefit from plasma exchange for those with IgG and IgA Fludarabine and rituximab with some benefit for gM
	Myasthenia gravis, ALS, Alzheimer disease	
Dermatologic disorders	Schnitzler syndrome	Neutrophilic urticarial dermatitis, monoclonal IgM protein, and two of: lymphadenopathy, fever, hepatosplenomegaly, joint pain, increased ESR, increased neutrophils, or abnormal bone imaging
	Scleredema	
	Pyoderma gangrenosum	Frequently an IgA protein
Infections	HIV	Both IgG and IgM M proteins observed
	HCV	M protein present in up to 10% of patients
Immunosuppression	Renal transplant	In children CMV infection associated with M protein
	Liver and heart transplant	Most patients with posttransplant lymphoproliferative disorders have M proteins
	BM transplant	Observed in both autologous and allogeneic transplants Appearance of M protein correlated with GVHD

AITL, Angioimmunoblastic T-cell lymphoma; ALS, amyotrophic lateral sclerosis; BM, bone marrow; CLL, chronic lymphocytic leukemia; CMV, cytomegalovirus; ESR, erythrocyte sedimentation rate; GVHD, graft-versus-host disease; HCV, hepatitis C virus; HIV human immunodeficiency virus; Ig, immunoglobulin; IVIG, intravenous immunoglobulin; MGUS, monoclonal gammopathy of uncertain significance; MDS, myelodysplastic syndrome; MPD, myeloproliferative disorder; POEMS, polyneuropathy, organomegaly, endocrinopathy, monoclonal gammopathy, and skin changes; RA, rheumatoid arthritis; RBC, red blood cell; SLE, systemic lupus erythematosus; VWF, von Willebrand factor.

protein electrophoresis (M spike), and then characterized and confirmed by immunofixation electrophoresis (IFE). Monoclonal antibodies have been associated with a wide variety of bacterial antigens as well as various other antigens, including thyroglobulin, von Willebrand factor, and lactate dehydrogenase; however, for most M proteins, the antigen is not recognized. A variety of other disorders are also associated with an M protein (Table 49.3), including connective tissue disorders, neurologic disorders (including POEMS [polyneuropathy, organomegaly, endocrinopathy, monoclonal gammopathy, and skin changes] syndrome), renal disorders, and some infections such as HCV and HIV. Patients undergoing bone marrow and solid-organ transplants in which there is immune suppression are also occasionally observed to have M proteins, but these are usually transient and disappear with recovery of the immune system. Acquired immune disorders such as acquired C1 inhibitor deficiency, type 2 acquired angioedema, and acquired von Willebrand syndrome have also been associated with M proteins.

REFERENCES

1. Morbach H, Eichhorn EM, Liese JG, et al: Reference values for B cell subpopulations from infancy to adulthood. *Clin Exp Immunol* 162(2):271–279, 2010.
2. Erkeller-Yuksel FM, Deneys V, Hulstaert F, et al: Age-related changes in human blood lymphocyte subpopulations. *J Pediatr* 120(2 Pt 1):216–222, 1992.

3. Lanasa MC, Weinberg JB: Immunologic aspects of monoclonal B-cell lymphocytosis. *Immunol Res* 49(1–3):269–280, 2011.

4. Hudnall SD, Molina CP: Marked increase in L-selectin-negative T cells in neonatal pertussis: The lymphocytosis explained? *Am J Clin Pathol* 114(1):35–40, 2000.

5. Walsh NP, Gleeson M, Shephard RJ, et al: Position statement. Part one: Immune function and exercise. *Exerc Immunol Rev* 17:6–63, 2011.

6. Karandikar NJ, Hotchkiss EC, McKenna RW, et al: Transient stress lymphocytosis: an immunophenotypic characterization of the most common cause of newly identified adult lymphocytosis in a tertiary hospital. *Am J Clin Pathol* 117(5):819–825, 2002.

7. Choi TS, Doh KS, Kim SH, et al: Clinicopathological and genotypic aspects of anticonvulsant-induced pseudolymphoma syndrome. *Br J Dermatol* 148(4):730–736, 2003.

8. Cornet E, Lesesve JF, Mossafa H: Long-term follow-up of 111 patients with persistent polyclonal B-cell lymphocytosis with binucleated lymphocytes. *Leukemia* 23(2):419–422, 2009.

9. Al-Herz W, Bousfiha A, Casanova J-L, et al: Primary immunodeficiency diseases: an update on the classification from the International Union of Immunological Societies Expert Committee for Primary Immunodeficiency. *Front Immunol* 5:1–33, 2014.

10. Notarangelo LD, Miao CH, Ochs DH: Wiskott-Aldrich syndrome. *Curr Opin Hematol* 15:30–36, 2008.

11. Staples ER, McDermott EM, Reiman A: Immunodeficiency in ataxia telangiectasia is correlated strongly with the presence of two null mutations in the ataxia telangiectasia mutated gene. *Clin Exp Immunol* 153:214–220, 2008.

12. Dickinson RE, Milne P, Jardine L, et al: The evolution of cellular deficiency in GATA2 mutation. *Blood* 123(6):863–874, 2014.

13. Stein DS, Korvick JA, Vermund SH: CD4⁺ lymphocyte cell enumeration for prediction of clinical course of human immunodeficiency virus disease: a review. *J Infect Dis* 165(2):352–363, 1992.

14. Yuen KY, Chan PK, Peiris M, et al: Clinical features and rapid viral diagnosis of human disease associated with avian influenza A H5N1 virus. *Lancet* 351(9101):467–471, 1998.

15. Turett GS, Telzak EE: Normalization of CD4⁺ T-lymphocyte depletion in patients without HIV infection treated for tuberculosis. *Chest* 105(5):1335–1337, 1994.

16. Drewry AM, Samra N, Skrupky LP, et al: Persistent lymphopenia after diagnosis of sepsis predicts mortality. *Shock* 42(5):383–391, 2014.

17. Fayaz A, Igoe A, Kurien BT, et al: Haematological manifestations of lupus. *Lupus Sci Med* 2(1):e000078, 2015.

18. Shao L, Fujii H, Colmegna I, et al: Deficiency of the DNA repair enzyme ATM in rheumatoid arthritis. *J Exp Med* 206(6):1435–1449, 2009.

19. Prasad AS: Zinc in human health: effect of zinc on immune cells. *Mol Med* 14(5–6):353–357, 2008.

20. Zonios DI, Falloon J, Bennett JE, et al: Idiopathic CD4⁺ lymphocytopenia: natural history and prognostic factors. *Blood* 112(2):287–294, 2008.

21. Robak T, Lech-Maranda E, Korycka A, et al: Purine nucleoside analogs as immunosuppressive and antineoplastic agents: mechanism of action and clinical activity. *Curr Med Chem* 13(26):3165–3189, 2006.

22. Fuks Z, Strober S, Bobrove AM: Long term effects of radiation of T and B lymphocytes in peripheral blood of patients with Hodgkin's disease. *J Clin Invest* 58(4):803–814, 1976.

23. Hamblin AD, Hamblin TJ: The immunodeficiency of chronic lymphocytic leukaemia. *Br Med Bull* 87:49–62, 2008.

24. Conley ME, Dobbs AK, Farmer DM, et al: Primary B cell immunodeficiencies: comparisons and contrasts. *Annu Rev Immunol* 27:199–227, 2009.

25. Jolles S: The variable in common variable immunodeficiency: a disease of complex phenotypes. *J Allergy Clin Immunol Pract* 1(6):545–556, 2013.

26. Qamar N, Fuleihan RL: The hyper IgM syndromes. *Clin Rev Allergy Immunol* 46(2):120–130, 2014.

27. Moschese V, Graziani S, Avanzini MA, et al: A prospective study on children with initial diagnosis of transient hypogammaglobulinemia of infancy: results from the Italian Primary Immunodeficiency Network. *Int J Immunopathol Pharmacol* 21(2):343–352, 2008.

28. Dispensieri A, Gertz M, Therneau T, et al: Retrospective cohort study of 148 patients with polyclonal gammopathy. *Mayo Clin Proc* 76(5):476–487, 2001.

29. Ozen S, Bilginer Y: A clinical guide to autoinflammatory diseases: familial Mediterranean fever and next-of-kin. *Nat Rev Rheumatol* 10(3):135–147, 2014.

30. Mosalpuria K, Bociek RG, Vose JM: Angioimmunoblastic T-cell lymphoma management. *Semin Hematol* 51(1):52–58, 2014.

DISORDERS OF PHAGOCYTE FUNCTION

Mary C. Dinauer and Thomas D. Coates

Phagocytic leukocytes are an essential component of the innate immune system that has evolved to rapidly respond to the presence of invading bacteria, fungi, and parasites. This first line of host defense also includes natural killer (NK) lymphocytes, complement, and other plasma proteins. As reviewed in Chapters 27 and 48, phagocytes are responsible for ingesting, killing, and digesting pathogens. Granulocytic phagocytes (neutrophils and eosinophils) circulate in the bloodstream until they sense chemotactic signals from infected tissues, resulting in adhesion to the vascular endothelium and subsequent migration into the site of infection.[1] Mononuclear phagocytes (macrophages and their circulating precursor, the monocyte), on the other hand, function primarily as resident cells in a variety of tissues such as the lungs, liver, peritoneal cavity, and spleen, where they perform a surveillance role and also interact closely with lymphocytes to promote specific immune responses. Microbial killing is accomplished by two types of mechanisms: (1) de novo synthesis of highly toxic and often unstable derivatives of molecular oxygen by an enzyme known as *respiratory burst oxidase* and (2) preformed polypeptide "antibiotics" and proteases stored within several types of lysosomal granules that are delivered into phagocytic vacuoles containing the ingested microbes.

This chapter reviews the major congenital and acquired disorders of phagocyte function, which from the clinical standpoint largely involve neutrophils. As would be predicted, these disorders manifest clinically by recurrent bacterial and fungal infections, often with atypical pathogens or unusual presentations. Interestingly, the converse of this is only rarely observed. Most patients with recurrent infections do not have any identifiable abnormality in their phagocytes. There are at least two explanations for the clinical rarity of phagocyte disorders. First, given their critical role in host defense, nature may be quite intolerant of major abnormalities in phagocytes. Before the modern antibiotic era, patients with severe disorders probably did not survive into their childbearing years. Second, there is a remarkable redundancy in the antimicrobial machinery of the phagocytes that permits one system to compensate for a defect in another. For example, the host does not rely on a single chemotactic signal or neutrophil membrane receptor to ensure that phagocytes accumulate at sites of infection. Instead, multiple chemotactic signals and receptors are used. A similar phenomenon is seen in the reactions that kill microbes, as both oxidative and nonoxidative systems are used.

This chapter is organized according to the cellular functions outlined above: disorders of the respiratory burst microbicidal pathway, abnormalities of phagocyte adhesion and chemotaxis, and defects in the structure and function of lysosomal granules. This chapter is not meant to be an encyclopedic review of the numerous papers published on phagocyte abnormalities. It is important to note that many of these reports describe marginal in vitro defects, with little evidence that they are responsible for a clinical problem. Comprehensive reviews offering additional information on phagocyte disorders are available.[2,3]

APPROACH TO DIAGNOSIS OF PHAGOCYTE FUNCTION DISORDERS

Inherited and acquired clinical disorders of phagocyte function result from defects in one or more of the major steps leading to microbial killing—adhesion, chemotaxis, ingestion, degranulation, and production of microbicidal oxidants (Fig. 50.1). Patients with inherited disorders typically present in infancy or childhood with recurrent, unusual, or recalcitrant bacterial and fungal infections, and it is usually not difficult to determine that these are outside the range of normal. The presentation of these different inherited disorders can overlap, so that a specific diagnosis cannot be made on clinical grounds alone. Infections commonly seen include those of skin or mucosa, lung, lymph node, deep tissue abscesses, or childhood periodontitis. These can often have an indolent presentation with only low-grade fevers. Bacterial sepsis is an unusual initial symptom and usually reflects dissemination from an infected site. Inherited defects in phagocyte function are rare and represent only about 20% of the primary immunodeficiencies.[2] Thus, children with suspected disorders of host defense should also be screened for defects in humoral, cellular, and complement-mediated immunity. An approach to evaluating the patient with significant recurrent infections is shown in Fig. 50.2. Patients in whom a defect is identified should be referred to a center specialized in care of such patients.

In clinical practice, although nearly all patients with well-characterized phagocyte abnormalities have recurrent or unusual infections, the majority of individuals with histories of persistent or recurrent infections do not have identifiable phagocyte disorders or other immune defects. In some cases, these reflect another underlying medical condition or nonimmunologic problem related to an anatomic or obstructive defect. This chapter focuses largely on disorders in which a good correlation exists between the clinical condition and an identifiable defect in phagocyte function.

DISORDERS OF THE RESPIRATORY BURST PATHWAY

Reactive oxygen species generated by the phagocyte respiratory burst are critical for microbial killing. The enzyme responsible for the initial reaction in this pathway is nicotinamide adenine dinucleotide phosphate (NADPH) oxidase found in plasma and phagolysosomal membranes. Upon activation by inflammatory stimuli, NADPH oxidase catalyzes the transfer of an electron from NADPH to molecular oxygen, thereby forming superoxide (as the O_2^- ion; Fig. 50.3, reaction 1).[3-5] This NADPH oxidase, along with enzymes and reactions that are directly involved in the production or metabolism of O_2^-, constitutes the respiratory burst pathway as depicted in Fig. 50.3. Superoxide is the precursor to numerous microbicidal oxidants, including hydrogen peroxide and hypochlorous acid. Five clinically significant defects have been identified in the respiratory burst, involving the following enzymes: NADPH oxidase (reaction 1), leukocyte glucose-6-phosphate dehydrogenase (G6PD; reaction 8), myeloperoxidase (MPO; reaction 4), glutathione reductase, and glutathione synthetase (reaction 9). These reactions are involved in the production of O_2^- (reactions 8 and 1) in the conversion of O_2^- and hydrogen peroxide to other toxic derivatives (reaction 4) or in the detoxification of excess hydrogen peroxide needed to protect the phagocyte during the respiratory burst (reactions 7 and 9). Of note, NOX homologues to the leukocyte NADPH oxidase are present in the gut, vascular cells, and other tissues, which may generate oxidants for local host defense or for regulation of other cellular functions.[6]

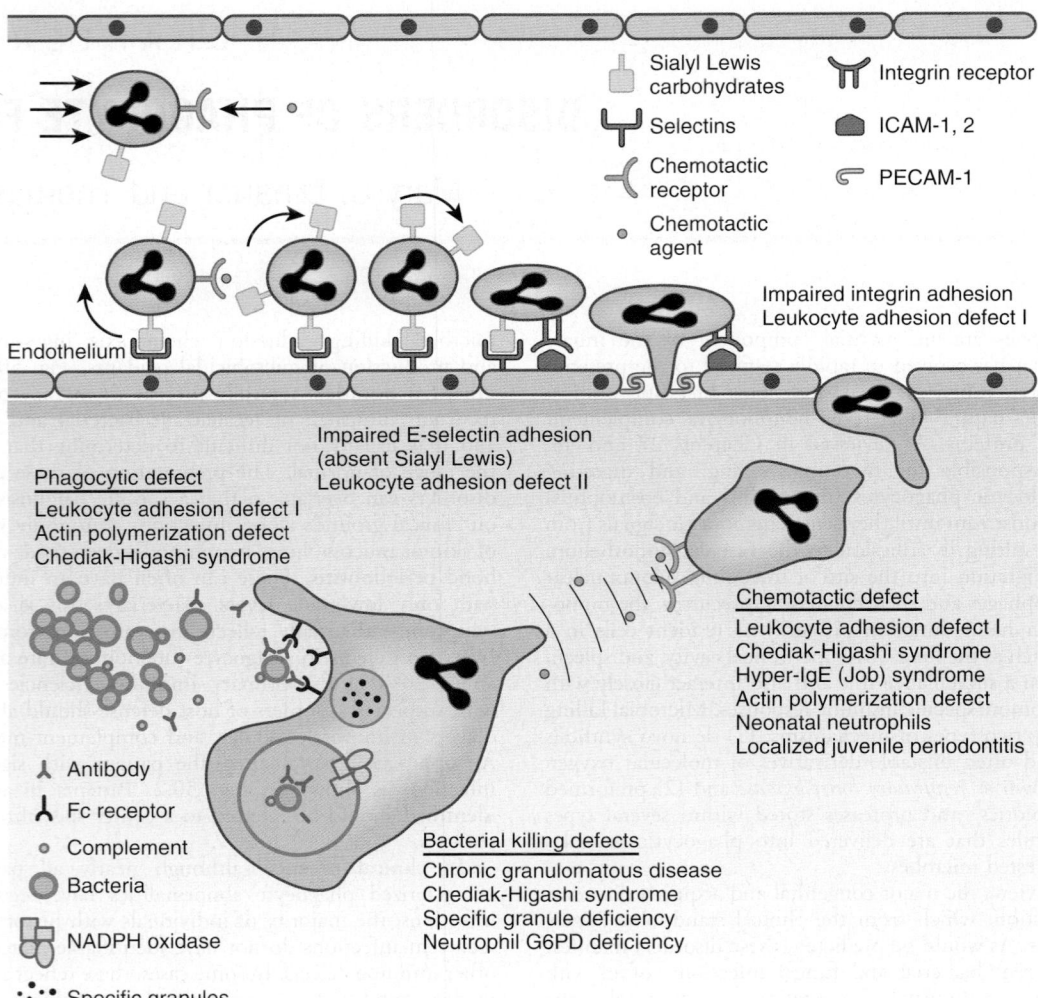

Fig. 50.1 STEPS IN THE RESPONSE OF CIRCULATION NEUTROPHILS TO INFECTION. The adhesion molecule E-selectin is upregulated on endothelial cells in response to inflammatory mediators (interleukin-1 [IL-1], endotoxin, tumor necrosis factor-α), resulting in rolling attachment and margination through interaction with sialyl Lewis carbohydrates on its surface. Chemoattractants such as IL-8 cause upregulation of neutrophil β2 integrins that, in turn, mediate tight adhesion to ICAM-1 and PECAM-1 on endothelial cells. Activated neutrophils can detect as little as a 2% change in the chemoattractant gradient and move to the site of infection. Neutrophils phagocytoze bacteria opsonized by antibody and complement. Both oxidative and nonoxidative antimicrobial mechanisms are then used to kill bacteria. Disorders of phagocyte function associated with each of these steps are noted. *G6PD,* Glucose-6-phosphate dehydrogenase; *ICAM-1,* intercellular adhesion molecule 1; *NADPH,* nicotinamide adenine dinucleotide phosphate; *PECAM-1,* platelet endothelial cell adhesion molecule 1. *(Courtesy Kyoto W, Coates TD: A practical approach to neutrophil disorders.* Pediatr Clin North Am *49:929, 2002, with permission.)*

Chronic Granulomatous Disease

Chronic granulomatous disease (CGD) is a genetically heterogeneous group of defects that share in common the failure of neutrophils, monocytes, macrophages, and eosinophils to undergo a respiratory burst and generate O_2^-.[3,7] CGD is relatively rare, having an estimated incidence of between 1 in 200,000 and 1 in 250,000 live births based on data from the United States CGD Registry,[7] although it is still the most common inherited phagocyte disorder of clinical significance (MPO deficiency is more common, but affected patients are rarely symptomatic). The absence of respiratory burst-derived oxidants results in recurrent, often life-threatening bacterial and fungal infections, and is also associated with formation of inflammatory granulomas.[3,7–9] The disease was first described in 1957 as a syndrome characterized by severe recurrent infections in boys who also had visceral granulomas

containing pigmented histiocytes. The disease was termed *fatal granulomatous disease* owing to this distinguishing histologic feature and the grim clinical course in most patients. It was not until the late 1960s and early 1970s that the defect in oxygen consumption and O_2^- production was identified and a convenient diagnostic assay, the nitroblue tetrazolium (NBT) test, was developed. In the 1980s a combination of biochemical and molecular genetic approaches led to the identification of four critical subunits of NADPH oxidase and the recognition that mutations in the corresponding genes are responsible for four different genetic subgroups of CGD (Fig. 50.4). Recently, a fifth genetic subgroup was identified in a single patient.[10] Databases for the main four genetic subgroups of CGD have been developed that are accessible through the websites http://structure.bmc.lu.se/idbase/ and http://www.hgmd.cf.ac.uk/ac/index.php. Recent publications on disease manifestations and genotypes in large patient registries are also available and support earlier reports.[7,9,11,12]

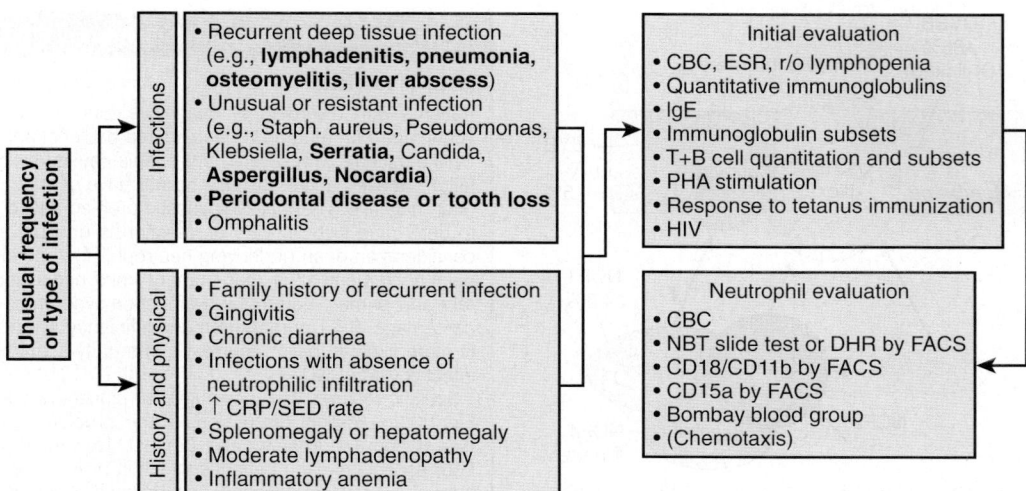

Fig. 50.2 EVALUATION OF PATIENTS WITH RECURRENT BACTERIAL OR FUNGAL INFECTIONS. The history, physical examination, and infections episodes in patients with a possible primary neutrophil dysfunction syndrome are noted. The initial evaluation can be done in most clinical laboratories. A qualified reference laboratory with special expertise in this area should carry out the neutrophil evaluations. Chemotaxis is very difficult to evaluate clinically and should only be attempted in a qualified research laboratory with extensive experience. *CBC*, Complete blood count; *CRP*, C-reactive protein; *DHR*, dihydrorhodamine; *ESR*, erythrocyte sedimentation rate; *FACS*, fluorescence-activated cell sorting; *HIV*, human immunodeficiency virus; *IgE*, immunoglobulin E; *NBT*, nitroblue tetrazolium; *PHA*, phytohemagglutinin; *r/o*, rule out; *SED*, sedimentation.

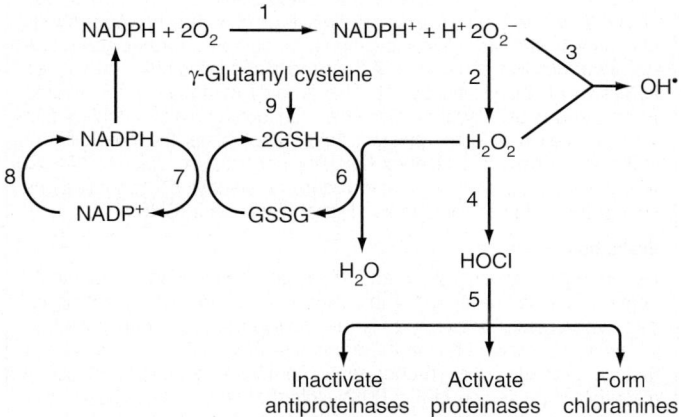

Fig. 50.3 REACTIONS OF RESPIRATORY BURST PATHWAY. *GSH*, Glutathione; *GSSG*, oxidized glutathione; *HOCl*, hypochlorous acid; *NADPH*, nicotinamide adenine dinucleotide phosphate.

Molecular Genetics of Chronic Granulomatous Disease

CGD results from mutations in any of the five genes encoding essential subunits of the NADPH oxidase (Table 50.1).[11,12] In turn, the biochemical and genetic analysis of CGD has been instrumental in characterizing this complex enzyme. The oxidase subunits are referred to by their apparent molecular mass (kDa) and have been given the designation *phox*, for *ph*agocyte *ox*idase. A b-type cytochrome known as flavocytochrome b_{558}, a membrane-bound heterodimer composed of gp91^{phox} and p22^{phox}, is the redox center of the oxidase. Approximately two-thirds of CGD cases result from defects in the X-linked gene encoding the gp91^{phox} subunit of flavocytochrome b_{558}, which contains both the flavoprotein and heme-binding domains responsible for electron transport. A rare autosomal recessive (AR) form of CGD is caused by mutations in the gene encoding p22^{phox}, the smaller subunit of flavocytochrome b_{558}, which provides a critical docking site for p47^{phox}, a regulatory subunit. The remaining cases of AR CGD involve genetic defects in p47^{phox}, p67^{phox}, or p40^{phox}, three regulatory proteins associated with each other in the cytosol of unstimulated cells but which rapidly move to the membrane to activate flavocytochrome b_{558} and superoxide formation when neutrophils are exposed to inflammatory or phagocytic stimuli. The p40^{phox} subunit appears to play a selective role in stimulating high-level superoxide production within phagosomes via membrane-bound phosphatidylinositol-3-phosphate.[10] Formation of the active NADPH oxidase complex also involves the activation of the small guanosine triphosphate (GTP)-binding protein Rac, which then binds to the plasma membrane and p67^{phox}.[3] No cases of CGD have been identified resulting from genetic defects in Rac, although a mutation in the blood cell-specific Rac2 isoform was found in an infant with recurrent infections and abnormal neutrophil adhesion, motility, and partial NADPH oxidase defects.[3]

The gene for gp91^{phox}, termed *CYBB*, spans approximately 30 kb in the Xp21.1 region of the X chromosome. More than 600 distinct mutations have been identified in the gp91^{phox} gene in X-linked CGD (MIM306400), which include deletions, frameshifts, splice site, nonsense, and missense mutations that are distributed throughout the gene (Table 50.2).[11] Approximately 10% to 15% of X-linked CGD is caused by new germline mutations. In most X-linked CGD, gp91^{phox} is completely absent, and there is no measurable flavocytochrome b or superoxide production (the X91° subtype). In about 5% of X-linked cases, gp91^{phox} can be present in normal levels but be nonfunctional (X91$^+$), mutated in such a way that gp91^{phox} is poorly functional (X91$^-$), or expressed in only a small fraction of phagocytes (X91$^+$). The first two "variant" forms of X-linked CGD result from coding sequence mutations, and the latter are caused by mutations in the regulatory portion of the gp91^{phox} gene. Some X-linked CGD patients have large deletions that affect not only the gene encoding gp91^{phox} but also portions of or all the flanking gene loci for McLeod hemolytic anemia syndrome (absence of the Kell erythrocyte antigen, Kx), Duchenne muscular dystrophy, and X-linked retinitis pigmentosa. Rare point mutations in *CYBB* lead to markedly impaired flavocytochrome b expression and activity in macrophages, with much less effect in neutrophils.[13] Affected patients were susceptible to mycobacterial infections but did not have other bacterial and fungal infections characteristic of CGD, highlighting the importance of macrophages for controlling mycobacteria.

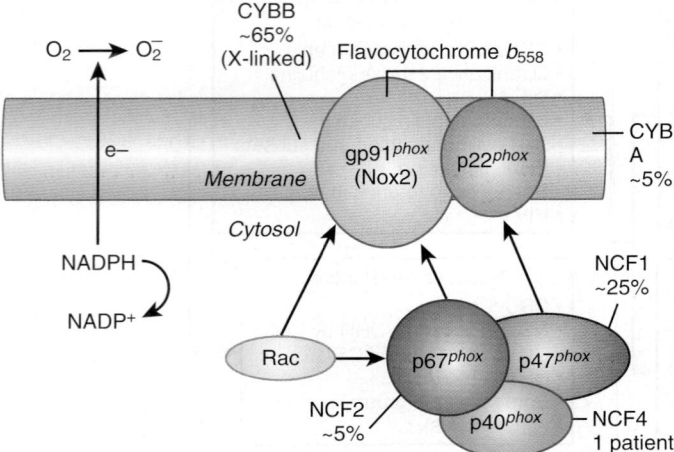

Fig. 50.4 NICOTINAMIDE ADENINE DINUCLEOTIDE PHOS-PHATE OXIDASE AND MOLECULAR GENETICS OF CHRONIC GRANULOMATOUS DISEASE. Shown are the membrane and soluble subunits of NADPH oxidase, indicating how these correspond to the five different genetic subgroups of chronic granulomatous disease (CGD) and their approximate incidence. Flavocytochrome b_{558} is the redox center of the enzyme and is located in plasma, specific granule, and phagolysosomal membranes. This heterodimer is composed of the gp91^{phox} and p22^{phox} subunits of the NADPH oxidase, which are affected in X-linked and an autosomal recessive (AR) form of CGD, respectively. The soluble regulatory proteins p47^{phox}, p67^{phox}, and p40^{phox} are found in the cytosol until phagocyte activation by soluble or particulate inflammatory stimuli, after which they move to the membrane where p47^{phox} and p67^{phox} bind flavocytochrome b558, binds Rac, and p40^{phox} binds phosphatidylinositol 3-phosphate, a phosphoinositide present on phagosome membranes. Mutations in the genes encoding p47^{phox}, p67^{phox} and p40^{phox} account for other AR forms of CGD. Another essential regulatory component of the NADPH oxidase is the small GTPase, Rac, which in its active guanosine triphosphate-bound state, becomes membrane bound, and associates with the oxidase. By a mechanism that is not fully understood, binding of these multiple regulatory subunits activates the flavocytochrome to catalyze the transfer of electrons from cytosolic NADPH across the membrane via the FAD and heme redox centers to molecular oxygen, thereby forming superoxide in the extracellular or intraphagosomal compartment. No cases of CGD have been described owing to mutations in Rac. *FAD,* Flavin adenine dinucleotide; *NADPH,* nicotinamide adenine dinucleotide phosphate

AR CGD involving p22^{phox} (MIM 233690) occurs in approximately 5% of CGD patients and usually involves the complete absence of cytochrome b (A22°), encoded by *CYBA*. Mutations in A22 CGD are heterogeneous and range from large interstitial gene deletions to point mutations associated with missense, frameshift, or RNA splicing defects.[12] Because the full expression of flavocytochrome b in the membrane requires the production of both subunits, a primary deficiency of either component leads to a secondary loss of the other. Thus, neither subunit can be detected on immunoblot analysis in either X91° or A22° CGD. A single patient with A22$^+$ CGD has been described with a missense mutation disrupting the binding site for p47^{phox}.

AR patients with p47^{phox}-deficient CGD (MIM 233700) account for approximately one-fourth of cases in the United States and Europe, but only about 7% of cases in Japan. The p47^{phox} subunit is encoded by the *NCF1* gene. A limited number of mutations have been identified in *NCF1*.[12] Virtually all patients are either homozygotes or compound heterozygotes for a mutant allele with a GT deletion at the beginning of exon 2 that predicts a premature stop codon following the amino acid residue and results in absence of the p47^{phox} protein. The high frequency of the p47^{phox} GT deletion mutation appears to reflect the existence of at least one closely linked highly conserved p47^{phox} pseudogene(s) that contains this GT

deletion. This close physical proximity leads to recombination events between the wild-type gene and pseudogene(s).

A heterogeneous group of mutations in the p67^{phox} gene, *NCF2*, are responsible for A67 CGD, a rare AR form of CGD (MIM233710) accounting for about 5% of cases overall.[12] Almost all mutations identified to date in A67 CGD lead to absent expression of the p67^{phox} protein. However, one A67$^+$ patient has been reported in which a nonfunctional form of p67^{phox} with an amino acid deletion is expressed but is unable to translocate to the membrane or bind to Rac.

Finally, a boy with AR p40^{phox} defects (MIM613960) was recently reported.[10] This patient was a compound heterozygote for two null alleles in *NCF4*. Although NADPH oxidase activity on the plasma membrane was normal, phagosome oxidant production was markedly impaired. The main clinical manifestation in this patient was chronic granulomatous inflammation of the intestinal tract rather than opportunistic infections characteristic of CGD, perhaps related to the more selective role of p40^{phox} in regulating NADPH oxidase activity.

Clinical Approach to Patients With Disorders of Phagocyte Function

Index of Suspicion

Patients with disorders of phagocyte function usually present at a young age with recurrent, deep-seated bacterial and fungal infections. Unlike patients with severe neutropenia caused by bone marrow (BM) failure, these patients usually do not have sepsis. Blood cultures are often negative. The major diagnostic problem faced by the clinician is to determine if the history of infection is unusual enough to warrant consideration of an underlying neutrophil dysfunction defect. The first point to remember is that primary immunodeficiency disorders are rare and primary neutrophil dysfunction syndromes form only a small percentage of all primary immunodeficiency syndromes. The patient is more likely to have recurrent community-acquired *Staphylococcus* infection than CGD.

Specific features that may suggest a phagocytic defect are shown in Fig. 50.2. Excellent discussions of this problem have been published (see Kyono and Coates[2], and Dinauer, Newburger and Borregaard[3]). Four aspects of each patient's infection history should be considered: frequency, severity, location, and responsible pathogen. Patients with unusual features in at least one of these aspects should alert the clinician to a possible underlying phagocyte disorder. When considering frequency, the patient's age and associated medical conditions must be taken into account. For example, recurrent otitis media in a 2-year-old patient is far less worrisome than a similar history in a 40-year-old patient. The more unusual or severe the infections, the less frequently these have to occur before a phagocyte evaluation is indicated. Infections in unexpected anatomic locations, such as hepatic, pulmonary, and rectal abscesses, may indicate an underlying phagocyte defect. Childhood periodontal disease or gingivitis is distinctly uncommon, and in the absence of neutropenic conditions, strongly suggests underlying neutrophil dysfunction. The identification of certain pathogens (e.g., *Serratia marcescens, Klebsiella* spp., *Aspergillus* spp., *Nocardia* spp., *Burkholderia cepacia,* invasive candidiasis) in children and young adults can provide the strongest indications for pursuing further studies. A history of delayed separation of the umbilical cord is often mentioned as a sign of phagocytic defect. This is fairly common as an isolated finding and is usually of no significance. However, this in conjunction with omphalitis or other pyogenic infections raises the possibility of leukocyte adhesion deficiency (LAD) or chemotactic defects. A child with nystagmus, fair skin, and recurrent staphylococcal infections should be evaluated for Chediak-Higashi syndrome (CHS).

Evaluation

Performing a good history and physical examination to eliminate common causes of recurrent infection is important before looking for rare syndromes. For example, is the recurrent pneumonia caused by an aspirated foreign body in the bronchus? In general, patients should first be evaluated for lymphocyte or complement defects. A useful algorithm is presented in Fig. 50.2. Note that testing described in this algorithm is not exhaustive, and patients with truly striking histories of unusual kinds of infections should be referred for further evaluation by specialized research laboratories.

| TABLE 50.1 | Classification of Chronic Granulomatous Disease |

Component Affected	Gene Symbol	Gene Locus	Inheritance	Subtype[a]	NBT Score (% Positive)	O_2^- Production (% Normal)	Flavocytochrome b Spectrum (% Normal)	Defect in Cell-Free NADPH Oxidase Assay	Frequency (% of Cases)[b]
Gp91^{phox}	CYBB	Xp21.1	X	X91°	0	0	0	Membrane	68
				X91$^-$	80–100 (weak)	3–30	Low	Membrane	5
				X91$^-$	5–10	5–10	Low	Membrane	<1
				X91$^+$	0	0	N	Membrane	1
P22^{phox}	CYBA	16p24.3	AR	A22°	0	0	0	Membrane	4
				A22$^+$	0	0	N	Membrane	<1
P47^{phox}	NCF1	7q11.23	AR	A47°	0	0–1	N	Cytosol	17
P67^{phox}	NCF2	1q25.3	AR	A67°	0	0	N	Cytosol	5
p40$^{phox c}$	NCF4	22q13.1	AR	A40$^+$	100	<10 (intracellular)	N	n/a	1

[a]In this nomenclature, the first letter represents the mode of inheritance (X-linked [X] or autosomal recessive [A]), and the number indicates the phox component that is genetically affected. The superscript symbols indicate whether the level of protein of the affected component is undetectable (°), diminished (–), or normal (+) as measured by immunoblot analysis.

[b]Combined data from 209 kindreds evaluated at the Scripps Research Institute/Stanford University CGD Clinic and a cooperative European study representing 57 kindreds and 63 patients. (Courtesy Casimir C, Chetty M, Bohler MC, et al: Identification of the defective NADPH-oxidase component in chronic granulomatous disease: A study of 57 European families. Eur J Clin Invest 22:403, 1992; and Curnutte JT: Chronic granulomatous disease: The solving of a clinical riddle at the molecular level. Clin Immunol Immunopathol 67:S2, 1993.) These frequencies remain similar to those in more recent reports from Europe and the United States.

[c]A single patient reported to date who was a compound heterozygote for a frameshift mutation and a nonfunctional form of p40^{phox} caused by a point mutation. (Matute JD, Arias AA, Wright NA et al: A new genetic subgroup of chronic granulomatous disease with autosomal recessive mutations in p40 phox and selective defects in neutrophil NADPH oxidase activity. Blood 114:3309, 2009.)

AR, Autosomal recessive inheritance; N, normal; NADPH, nicotinamide adenine dinucleotide phosphate; n/a, not applicable; NBT, nitroblue tetrazolium; X, X-linked inheritance.

| TABLE 50.2 | Summary of Mutations in the CYBB Gene Encoding gp91^{phox} in 261 Kindreds With X-linked Chronic Granulomatous Disease |

Type of Mutation	Number of Kindreds	Frequency (%)	Phenotype
Deletions	63	24.2	X91°
Insertions	27	10.3	X91°
Splice-site mutations	42	16.1	X91°
Missense mutations	59	22.6	X91°, X91–, X91+
Nonsense mutations	70	26.8	X91°

Data from Roos D, Curnutte J, Hossle JP, et al: X-CGDbase: A database of X-CGD-causing mutations. Immunol Today 17:517, 1996.

Even though more than 90% of patients with CGD have respiratory burst defects that result in undetectable levels of O_2^- production, there is a surprising heterogeneity in the clinical manifestations of the disease.[7] At one end of the spectrum are patients who begin to have severe bacterial and fungal infections during infancy and who rarely have more than 4 to 12 months between such serious infections. At the other end of the spectrum are patients who are well for many years and then unexpectedly develop a serious infection typical of CGD, such as a staphylococcal hepatic abscess or Aspergillus pneumonia. After their first major infection, some of these patients may be relatively healthy again for another 3 to 10 years before the next severe infection occurs. As a group, patients with X-CGD, A22 CGD, and A67 CGD seem to have a more severe clinical course compared with patients with A47 CGD,[7,9] who have a small amount of detectable oxidant production even in the complete absence of this subunit (Fig. 50.5G). Individuals with partial respiratory burst activity but less than 10% of normal (most X91– patients; see Table 50.1) also tend to have disease of intermediate severity. Polymorphisms in oxygen-independent antimicrobial systems or other components regulating the innate immune response are also likely to play an important role in modifying disease severity.[9] Specific polymorphisms in the MPO, mannose binding lectin, and FcγRIIa genes are associated with a higher risk for granulomatous or autoimmune or

rheumatologic complications.[3,8] Because of this heterogeneity, the diagnosis of CGD should be entertained, not only in young children with recurrent severe infections, but also in adolescents and young adults who experience exceptionally severe or unusual infections.

Clinical Manifestations

In approximately two-thirds of patients, the first symptoms of CGD appear during the first year of life with the onset of recurrent, purulent bacterial, and fungal infections.[7] Table 50.3 summarizes the types of infections and infecting organisms most frequently encountered in CGD. The most common types of infections are those that involve sites in contact with the outside world, which is consistent with the role of neutrophils as a first line of defense against infection. Staphylococcus aureus, enteric gram negatives, Serratia marcescens, B. cepacia, Nocardia spp., and Aspergillus spp. represent the most frequently encountered pathogens in North American patients, but Burkholderia and Nocardia spp. are less frequently seen in Europe.[8] S. aureus is the most frequently isolated organism overall. The most common causes of death have been pneumonia or sepsis caused by B. cepacia and Aspergillus spp., although use of newer azole antifungals has markedly improved the outcome of the latter in recent years.[7,8]

Most CGD pathogens share the property of being catalase negative, and as such inadvertently "lend" H_2O_2 secreted from the pathogen to the peroxide-starved CGD phagocyte, which in turn uses it (after being converted to hypochlorous acid [HOCl] by MPO; see Fig. 50.3) to kill the microbe. It also appears that at least some of the CGD pathogens are resistant to the nonoxidative killing mechanisms of the phagocyte. It is somewhat surprising how often one fails to identify the infecting organism in CGD—perhaps greater than half the time despite aggressive culturing. In this situation, one treats empirically with the antibiotic that should work and if it fails, one then aggressively pursues more invasive diagnostic procedures looking for one (or more) of the less commonly seen microbes such as Nocardia spp., Candida spp., mycobacteria, and a host of other bacteria and fungi (see Table 50.3). Other unusual organisms that cause infection in CGD include other members of the Burkholderia family, including Burkholderia cenocepacia, Burkholderia gladioli, and Burkholderia mallei (the causative agent in melioidosis, a septic illness common in East Asia), and Chromobacterium violaceum, found in

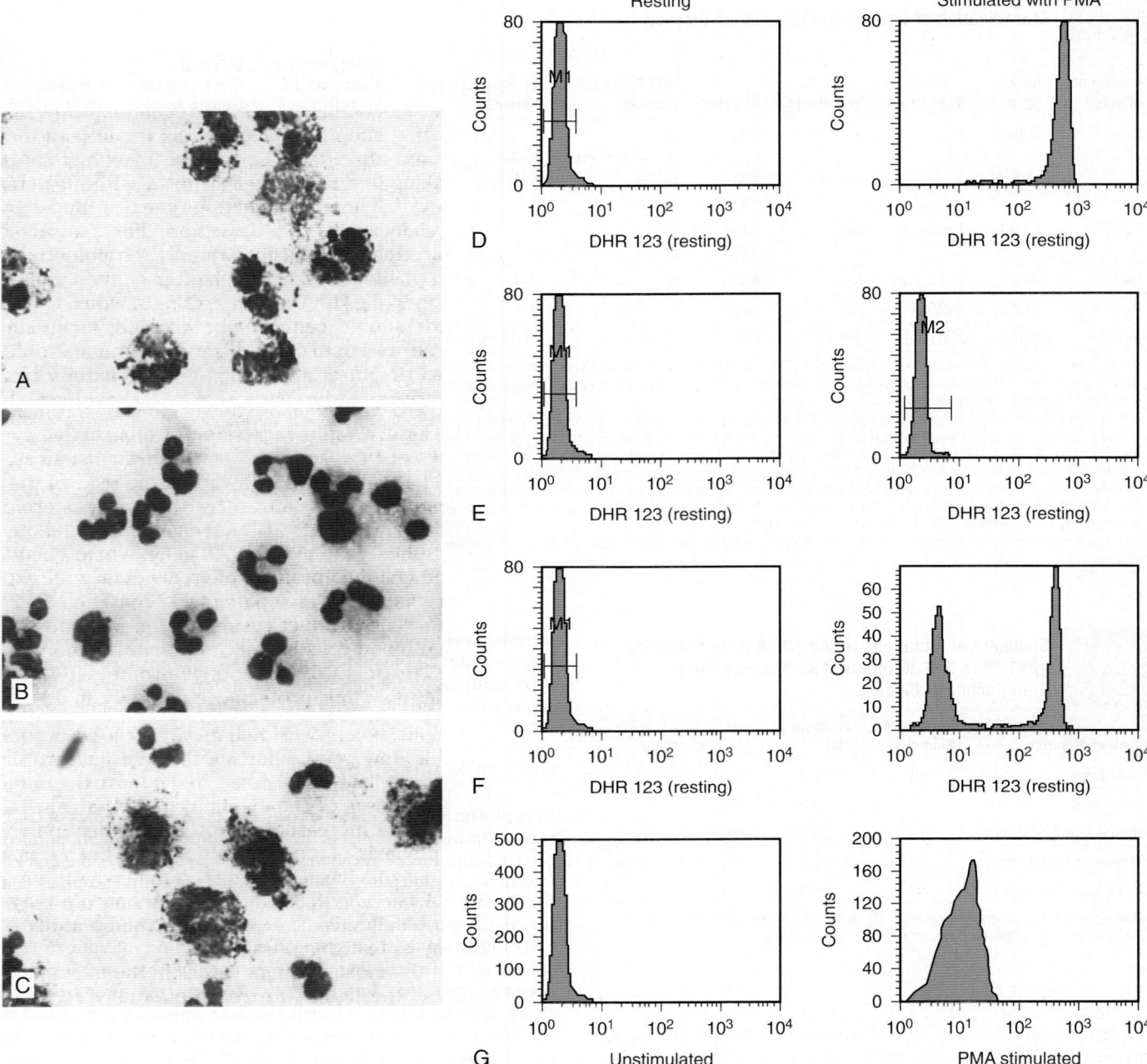

Fig. 50.5 ANALYSIS OF NEUTROPHIL NICOTINAMIDE ADENINE DINUCLEOTIDE PHOS-PHATE OXIDASE ACTIVITY FOR THE DIAGNOSIS OF CHRONIC GRANULOMATOUS DISEASE. (A–C) Nitroblue tetrazolium (NBT) slide test. Peripheral blood neutrophils and monocytes from a drop of fresh whole blood were made adherent to glass slides and stimulated with phorbol myristate acetate. (A) Normal neutrophils and monocytes, all of which are NBT positive. (B) Neutrophils and monocytes from an X-linked chronic granulomatous disease (CGD) patient, which are all NBT negative. (C) A mixture of NBT-positive and NBT-negative neutrophils from the X-linked carrier mother of the patient in (B). (D–G) DHR 123 flow cytometry test. Nonfluorescent DHR 123 is taken up by neutrophils, which become fluorescent after reaction with reactive oxygen species produced in the respiratory burst. (D) Normal neutrophils. (E) Neutrophils from an X-linked CGD patient, which do not fluoresce after stimulation. (F) A mixture of nonfluorescent and fluorescent neutrophils from an X-linked CGD carrier. (G) Neutrophils from a p47^{phox}-deficient patient, which show weak fluorescence after stimulation. *DHR*, Dihydrorhodamine; *PMA*, phorbol myristate acetate.

TABLE 50.3	Infections in Chronic Granulomatous Disease		

Infections	Infections (%)	Infecting Organisms
Pneumonia	70–80	*Aspergillus, Staphylococcus, Burkholderia cepacia, Pseudomonas, Nocardia, Mycobacterium* (including atypical), *Serratia, Candida, Klebsiella, Paecilomyces*
Lymphadenitis	50–60	*Staphylococcus, Serratia, Candida, Klebsiella, Nocardia*
Cutaneous infections/impetigo	50–60	
Hepatic or perihepatic abscesses	20–30	*Staphylococcus, Serratia, Streptococcus viridans, Nocardia, Aspergillus*
Osteomyelitis	20–30	*Serratia, Aspergillus, Paecilomyces, Staphylococcus, B. cepacia, Pseudomonas, Nocardia*
Perirectal abscesses or fistulae	15–30	Enteric gram-negative organisms, *Staphylococcus*
Septicemia	10–20	*B. cepacia, Pseudomonas, Salmonella, Staphylococcus, Serratia, Klebsiella*
Urinary tract infections or pyelonephritis	5–15	Enteric gram-negative organisms
Brain abscesses	<5	*Aspergillus, Staphylococcus*
Meningitis	<5	*Candida lusitaniae, Haemophilus influenzae, B. cepacia*

The relative frequencies of different types of infections in chronic granulomatous disease are estimated from data pooled from several large series of patients in the United States, Europe, and Japan: (1) Mouy R, Fischer A, Vilmer E, et al: Incidence, severity, and prevention of infections in chronic granulomatous disease. *J Pediatr* 114:555, 1989; (2) Bemiller LS, Roberts DH, Starko KM, et al: Safety and effectiveness of long-term interferon gamma therapy in patients with chronic granulomatous disease. *Blood Cells Mol Dis* 21:239, 1995; (3) Forrest CB, Forehand JR, Axtell RA, et al: Clinical features and current management of chronic granulomatous disease. *Hematol Oncol Clin North Am* 2:253, 1988; (4) Hitzig WH, Seger RA: Chronic granulomatous disease, a heterogeneous syndrome. *Hum Genet* 64:207, 1983; (5) Tauber AI, Borregaard N, Simons E, et al: Chronic granulomatous disease: A syndrome of phagocyte oxidase deficiencies. *Medicine (Baltimore)* 62:286, 1983; (6) Cohen MS, Isturiz RE, Malech HL, et al: Fungal infection in chronic granulomatous disease. The importance of the phagocyte in defense against fungi. *Am J Med* 71:59, 1981; (7) Hayakawa H, Kobayashi N, Yata J: Chronic granulomatous disease in Japan: A summary of the clinical features of 84 registered patients. *Acta Paediatr Jpn* 27:501, 1985; and (8) Johnston RB, Newman SL. Chronic granulomatous disease. *Pediatr Clin North Am* 24:365, 1977. These series encompass approximately 550 patients with CGD after accounting for overlap between reports. Unpublished data from the United States CGD Registry encompassing 368 patients was also used to estimate the relative frequencies of infections and the responsible organisms. The infecting organisms are arranged in approximate order of frequency for each type of infection. Note: *B. cepacia* was previously classified as *Pseudomonas cepacia*.

brackish fresh water and which can cause a febrile illness with bacteremia in CGD. A previously unknown gram-negative bacteria, *Granulobacter bethesdensis*, was recently identified in a CGD patient with recurrent fevers associated with chronic necrotizing deep lymphatic infection. This organism is a member of the *Acetobacteraceae* family, which has previously not been linked to invasive human disease.

Pneumonia is the most common type of infection seen in CGD with *S. aureus*, *Aspergillus* spp., *B. cepacia*, and enteric gram-negative organisms as the major pathogens. It is noteworthy that *B. cepacia* has emerged as a particularly lethal organism in CGD. This organism often is not covered with the first line of antibiotics used for *S. aureus* and most gram-negative organisms and can quietly proliferate (with persistent fevers) to the point of quick, explosive collapse caused by endotoxic shock. Intravenous trimethoprim-sulfamethoxazole (TMP-SMX) has been most effective in treating patients if given before widespread dissemination of the infection. Proven or suspected *Aspergillus* infections were treated with amphotericin B therapy, but new azole antifungal agents are now typically used.

Lymphadenitis is the second most common infection and is usually caused by gram-negative organisms, *S. aureus*, or *Serratia marcescens*. Incision and drainage should not be delayed if the lesion fails to respond to parenteral antibiotics. Cutaneous abscesses should be similarly managed. Recurrent perinatal impetigo is almost a signature infection in CGD and often requires months of therapy (mostly oral antibiotics) to clear. Hepatic (and perihepatic) abscesses are also common in CGD and are usually, but not always, caused by *S. aureus*. Most lesions require drainage (needle or surgical) to permit efficient healing to occur. Bone infections, most commonly caused by *Serratia* spp. or *Aspergillus* spp., are particularly problematic in CGD and arise from either hematogenous or contiguous spread (as often is the case with *Aspergillus* infections in the lung invading the ribs, vertebral bodies, or the diaphragm). Perirectal abscesses are difficult to treat, even with months of therapy, and can lead to fistula formations.

Chronic inflammation with granuloma formation is a distinctive hallmark of CGD and contributes to some of its more problematic complications.[8,14] In some cases, this results from imperfectly controlled infections in which stalemates develop between the pathogen

and the patient's leukocytes. These lesions become granulomas as the host uses lymphocytes and activated macrophages to assist in containing the pathogens. However, this complication is not always clearly linked to persistent infection and in these cases, is speculated to involve a dysregulated inflammatory response, inefficient degradation of debris, or both. In the absence of oxidant production, excessive production of cytokines and delayed neutrophil apoptosis at inflammatory sites appear to contribute as underlying mechanisms.

As a result of persistent inflammatory stimulation, CGD patients can have a variety of more chronic complications (Table 50.4). Lymphadenopathy, hepatosplenomegaly, eczematoid dermatitis, and anemia of chronic disease (hemoglobin levels usually 8–10 g/dL) are common manifestations of this process and are most prominent in the first 5 to 10 years of life in those with CGD. Throughout the body, granuloma formation can lead to dysfunction and obstruction in the esophagus, urinary bladder, and kidneys. In the stomach, the gastric antral narrowing can be severe enough in infants and children to resemble pyloric stenosis. Inflammatory involvement of the gastrointestinal tract can be seen in up to one-third of CGD patients, typically in association with the X-linked form. A chronic ileocolitis resembling Crohn disease occurs in about 10% of patients and can range from mild diarrhea to a debilitating syndrome of bloody diarrhea and malabsorption that can necessitate a colectomy. Interestingly, antigliadin antibodies suggesting Crohn disease are positive in more than 50% of CGD patients. Other types of chronic inflammation include gingivitis, chorioretinitis, destructive white matter lesions in the brain, and glomerulonephritis. Discoid lupus has been reported in 10% to 20% of patients, and occasional patients may develop systemic lupus erythematosus, sarcoidosis, or rheumatoid arthritis. The underlying mechanisms are poorly defined, although recent studies suggest that these manifestations may be partly related to subtle defects in the absence of NADPH oxidase in memory B or T cells.

Carriers of CGD, whether the X-linked form or any one of the AR forms, are usually asymptomatic with two important exceptions. First, about one-fourth of X-linked carriers are at risk of developing mild to moderately severe discoid lupus erythematosus characterized by discoid skin lesions and photosensitivity.[3,14] The onset is usually in the second decade of life. The disease does not progress to systemic

TABLE 50.4   Chronic Conditions Associated With Chronic Granulomatous Disease[a]

Condition	Relative Frequency (%)
Lymphadenopathy	98
Hypergammaglobulinemia	60–90
Hepatomegaly	50–90
Splenomegaly	60–80
Anemia of chronic disease	Common[†]
Underweight	70
Chronic diarrhea	20–60
Short stature	50
Gingivitis	50
Dermatitis	35
Hydronephrosis	10–25
Granulomatous ileocolitis	10–15
Gastric antral narrowing	10–15
Ulcerative stomatitis	5–15
Granulomatous cystitis	5–10[b]
Pulmonary fibrosis	<10[b]
Esophagitis	<10[b]
Granulomatous cystitis	<10
Chorioretinitis	<10
Glomerulonephritis	<10
Discoid lupus erythematosus	<10

[a]The relative frequencies of chronic conditions associated with chronic granulomatous disease (CGD) were estimated from the series of reports listed in Table 50.3.
[b]The incidence is estimated from the 50 cases of CGD followed at Scripps Research Institute and Stanford University (unpublished data).

lupus nor does one find serologic evidence of even subclinical disease. Those with severe discoid lupus can be treated with Plaquenil. Recurrent stomatitis, significant gingivitis, or both have also been noted in as many as half of X-CGD carriers. A few also have arthralgias, polyarthritis, and Raynaud phenomenon. The second important complication of the X-linked CGD carrier state is serious infection in women who have an unusually high degree of inactivation of the normal X chromosome in their myeloid cells. If the circulating neutrophil population is skewed to the point that fewer than 10% to 15% of the cells function, then the carrier has an increased risk of bacterial infections that in some cases have been severe.[3]

Diagnosis

The diagnosis of CGD is usually suggested by the unusual clinical histories outlined earlier or by a family history of CGD. The NBT slide test on fresh blood is the classic diagnostic test. A typical result is shown in Fig. 50.5. Fig. 50.5A shows the normal positive staining of a group of seven neutrophils and one monocyte. Fig. 50.5B shows the complete absence of NBT staining in a patient with X91° CGD, the classic X-linked form of the disease. Fig. 50.5C shows the mixed population of NBT-positive and NBT-negative cells observed in that patient's mother, reflecting random X chromosome inactivation. Because nearly 100% of the normal cells in this test are positive, the carrier state in X-linked CGD can be detected when as few as 5% of the cells are NBT negative. This test also permits detection of diffuse populations of weakly positive cells such as those seen in X91⁻ CGD, which are characterized by a partial deficiency of flavocytochrome *b*. Because X-linked CGD can arise by new mutations in the maternal germ line, one does not always see NBT-negative cells in the mother. Flow cytometric assays of oxidase activity, such as those based on the

Diagnosis of Chronic Granulomatous Disease

The diagnosis of CGD is easily established by doing an NBT slide test or flow cytometry of dihydroxyrhodamine (DHR) 123 fluorescence to detect neutrophil NADPH oxidase activity. The NBT slide test is very easy to set up, as is DHR flow cytometry. However, because the probability of getting an abnormal result is very low, there may be confusion in interpretation because of a lack of experience. In the authors' experience, incorrect positive and negative results have been reported for both assays. Thus, if the index of suspicion is high, consultation should be obtained from a center with extensive experience with the test and with the disorder.

Neutrophil respiratory burst activity is preserved in anticoagulated blood maintained at room temperature for several days; thus, DHR testing can be done 1 to 2 days later after shipping to a commercial laboratory. A normal blood sample should always be shipped with the patient specimen as a control for problems in specimen handling during transport.

NBT Slide Test
- No NBT reduction (absence of cells with dark blue formazan deposits) in both X-linked and AR forms of CGD (see Fig. 50.5B).
- Usually no reduction in 50% of cells and normal in 50% for X-linked carrier. The percent positive cells can vary if there is unequal X inactivation and may appear normal or like CGD with extreme lyonization (see Fig. 50.5C).
- False-positive results can occur (i.e., apparent failure to reduce NBT supporting the diagnosis of CGD) if the neutrophils do not adhere to the slide. This happens with greasy slides or with some cases of LAD. Using phorbol myristate acetate to stimulate the cells will avoid this.

DHR Flow Cytometry
- This approach has replaced the NBT slide test in many laboratories. It has the advantage of assessing large numbers of cells and can give quantitation of the amount of oxidant production.
- The change in fluorescence channel number with stimulation is the critical number and not the percent positive cells.
- X-linked CGD patients will not respond at all and show no increase in fluorescence with stimulation (see Fig. 50.5F).
- X-linked carriers will show about 50% of the cells that respond with a normal increase in fluorescence, and the other half will have no response. Degrees of unequal X inactivation are much more accurately quantified by this assay (see Fig. 50.5G).
- AR patients, particularly those with absent p47[phox], have some response to stimulation and show a small increase in fluorescence (see Fig. 50.5H). This level of oxidant production is usually not visible on the NBT test.
- AR carriers have a good response, but the histogram may be broader than normal and may even appear bimodal with a weakly fluorescent peak and a strongly fluorescent peak. This is not distinguishable on the NBT slide test.
- Falsely negative results not supporting the diagnosis of CGD have been reported in specimens that have been run a few days after phlebotomy.
- Falsely abnormal results suggesting CGD can be seen in patients with MPO deficiency because MPO is required to generate strong DHR fluorescence.

Genetic Analysis
- Genetic analysis for X-linked and AR CGD is clinically available and should be performed on at least the proband in each kindred.

Those with fewer than 5% oxidase-positive cells have full-blown CGD.

conversion of dihydroxyrhodamine (DHR) 123 to rhodamine 123, can also provide both quantitative measurements of oxidant generation and the cell-by-cell distribution of activity (see Fig. 50.5D–G). The DHR 123 assay for oxidase activity is now available in many referral centers and through reference laboratories. In addition to X91⁻ CGD neutrophils, weak staining in the NBT test or a small but measurable level of DHR fluorescence can be seen in A47° cells (see Fig. 50.5H) because of a small amount of residual oxidant production. Regardless of diagnostic assay used, is important to have these tests performed on appropriately handled blood samples and by experienced laboratories to avoid inconclusive or false-normal results.

Genetic classification is useful primarily for purposes of genetic counseling and prenatal diagnosis. With the exception of classic X-linked disease in a male whose mother is a carrier, determining the specific oxidase gene affected in a given CGD patient (see Table 50.1) requires additional laboratory studies. Genetic testing for the four most common genetic subgroups is commercially available. Laboratories specializing in neutrophil biochemistry can also perform immunoblot analysis of neutrophil extracts, flavocytochrome b spectroscopy, or functional analysis of membrane and cytosol fractions in the cell-free oxidase assay. In a male with absent flavocytochrome b without clear evidence for a maternal carrier, it is necessary to search for the mutation in both the gp91^{phox} and p22^{phox} genes by DNA sequencing or another method of analysis.

Testing for the McLeod red cell phenotype should be done in all patients diagnosed with X-linked CGD. This causes a mild hemolytic anemia. More importantly, there can be serious problems with development of hemolytic antibodies if these patients are transfused.

Prognosis and Treatment

The cornerstones of therapy in CGD are currently (1) prevention and early treatment of infections, (2) aggressive use of parenteral antibiotics for most infections, (3) use of prophylactic TMP-SMX (5 mg/kg/day of trimethoprim) or dicloxacillin (25–50 mg/kg/day) for sulfa-allergic patients, (4) prophylactic itraconazole (200 mg/day if 13 years of age or older or if weighing at least 50 kg, or 100 mg daily if younger than 13 years of age or weighing less than 50 kg), and (5) use of prophylactic recombinant human interferon-γ (rIFN-γ; 0.05 mg/m^2 or 0.0015 mg/kg if less than 0.5 m^2 three times per week).[3,8] Using these guidelines, the prognosis for patients with CGD has improved dramatically since the disorder was first described in the 1950s, when almost all patients died in childhood. In a large study based on data collected by a CGD registry in the United States in the 1990s, the overall mortality rate was estimated to be 5% per year for X-CGD and 2% per year for AR CGD,[7] and a more recent single-institution study on 76 patients reported an overall mortality rate of 1.5% per year.[8] There is a general consensus that a large majority of newly diagnosed children should survive well into their adult years with aggressive and careful management. As already noted, patients with deficiency of p47^{phox} have a tendency for milder disease compared with those with flavocytochrome-negative CGD. On the other hand, some patients (usually X-linked) prove to have more frequent serious infections or inflammatory complications (or both),

likely because of the effects of modifier genes; these patients may warrant more aggressive treatment such as bone marrow transplantation (BMT; see later).

Several approaches can be used to prevent infections. Patients with CGD should receive all their routine immunizations on schedule (including live virus vaccines), with influenza vaccine administered each year as well. Cuts and skin abrasions should be cleansed promptly with soap and water and a topical antiseptic applied (2% hydrogen peroxide, Betadine ointment, or both). Frequent brushing, flossing, use of antibacterial mouthwash, and professional cleaning of teeth can help prevent gingivitis. Constipation should be avoided because it can lead to rectal or anal fissures and abscesses. Early anal infections can be treated with soaking in soapy water (with or without Betadine). The frequency of pulmonary infections can be reduced by not using commercially available bedside humidifiers; avoiding smoking (cigarettes and marijuana); and refraining from handling decaying plant materials (e.g., hay, mulch, rotting sawdust), which often contain numerous *Aspergillus* spp. Avoidance of construction sites, especially demolition of old buildings that may harbor fungi, is recommended. There have been clear outbreaks of *Aspergillus* pneumonias in immunosuppressed children visiting hospitals undergoing renovation.

There is clear evidence that chronic prophylactic TMP-SMX can decrease the number of bacterial infections in CGD patients by more than half without a concomitant increased risk of fungal infection. In addition, itraconazole is an effective agent for prophylaxis for fungal infections in CGD. Liver function tests should be monitored in patients receiving itraconazole.

Prophylactic rIFN-γ has been another mainstay of current management of CGD.[3,8] The clinical benefit of rIFN-γ is probably related to generally enhanced phagocyte function and killing by nonoxidative mechanisms because its use is not accompanied by any measurable improvement in NADPH oxidase activity in the vast majority of CGD patients. In the original multicenter trial, patients were randomized in a double-blind fashion to receive either placebo or rIFN-γ (0.05 mg/m^2 three times per week). As summarized in Table 50.5, there was a substantial decrease in the number of serious infections in the rIFN-γ arm. Side effects were observed in some of the patients but typically were restricted to mild fever and flu-like symptoms. No additional adverse reactions, including any increased incidence of chronic inflammatory complications, have been noted with more prolonged courses of prophylactic rIFN-γ (more than 10 years), and the patients continued to have a substantial benefit, with fivefold fewer serious infections compared with the placebo group in the phase III study in Table 50.5. On average, this group of patients averaged one serious infection per patient every 4 to 5 years. However, rIFN-γ is used less frequently in Europe as nonrandomized data did not suggest much benefit, and the usage in a cohort followed at the

TABLE 50.5 **Efficacy of Interferon-γ in Preventing Serious Infections in Chronic Granulomatous Disease**

Variable	Clinical Study				
	Phase III Placebo[a]	Phase III IFN-γ[a]	Phase IV (US) IFN-γ[b]	Phase IV (Europe) IFN-γ[c]	Phase IV IFN-γ[d]
Patients (*n*)	65	63	30	28	76
Average duration of therapy on study (years)	0	0.83	1.03	2.4	4.3
Patient-years in study	50.9	52.1	31.10	67.2	328
Serious infections per patient-year	1.1	0.38	0.13	0.4	0.30
Number of hospital days per patient-year	28.2	8.6	2.2	15.0	Not reported

[a]Results from The International Chronic Granulomatous Disease Cooperative Study Group: A controlled trial of interferon gamma to prevent infection in chronic granulomatous disease. *N Engl J Med* 324:509, 1991.
[b]Results from Weening RS, Leitz GJ, Seger RA: Recombinant human interferon-gamma in patients with chronic granulomatous disease—European follow up study. *Eur J Pediatr* 154:295, 1995.
[c]Results from Bemiller LS, Roberts DH, Starko KM, et al: Safety and effectiveness of long-term interferon gamma therapy in patients with chronic granulomatous disease. *Blood Cells Mol Dis* 21:239, 1995.
[d]Results from Marciano BE, Wesley R, De Carlo ES, et al: Long-term interferon-gamma therapy for patients with chronic granulomatous disease. *Clin Infect Dis* 39:692, 2004.
IFN, Interferon.

National Institutes of Health was recently reported to be only 36% because of either lack of access or because of side effects (fever, myalgia); the availability of more potent antifungals and oral antibiotics may be a mitigating factor for reducing serious infectious complications in the absence of prophylactic rIFN-γ.

One of the most frequent errors in the management of CGD patients is the failure to treat potentially serious infections promptly and aggressively with appropriate parenteral antibiotics. Even the best antibiotics can be rendered ineffective if given too late in the course of an infection in CGD. Therefore, early intervention is advisable. Although many of the minor infections and low-grade fevers in CGD patients can be managed on an outpatient basis, episodes of consistently high fever over a 24-hour period or clearly established infections (e.g., pneumonia or lymphadenitis) should be treated with parenteral antibiotics that cover, at least initially, *S. aureus* and enteric gram-negative organisms. Reasonable attempts to define the source of the infection and the responsible microbe should also begin promptly. Monitoring markers of inflammation such as the erythrocyte sedimentation rate (ESR) or C-reactive protein (CRP) can be very useful, both as a clue to the presence of a significant infection as well as following the patient's response to therapy. If the patient fails to respond, then more aggressive diagnostic procedures should be instituted (computed tomography, bone, and gallium scans; open biopsies if indicated) and empirical changes in the antibiotics used to broaden coverage to *Pseudomonas cepacia*. If fungus is identified or strongly suspected, amphotericin B has been the drug of choice in the past, but newer azole antifungal agents such as voriconazole are supplanting its use. Even with appropriate antibiotics, certain types of infections respond slowly and may require many months of therapy. Surgical drainage or resection can sometimes play a key role in accelerating healing of certain types of infection such as lymphadenitis, osteomyelitis, and abscesses of visceral organs such as the liver or lung. Finally, granulocyte transfusions may be of benefit in the treatment of stubborn or life-threatening infections.[3,7,8]

Recurrent fever in CGD always raises the possibility of infection in these patients; however, the macrophage activation syndrome (MAS)–hemophagocytic lymphohistiocytosis (HLH) spectrum of disorders should be considered, especially if the patient has splenomegaly, leukopenia, or thrombocytopenia. As in inflammatory disorders such as rheumatoid arthritis, secondary MAS-HLH has been reported in CGD and is probably often overlooked. Specific treatment may be indicated, especially if the patient has significant cytopenias or evidence of hepatic dysfunction.

Use of corticosteroids should generally be avoided, including extensive topical use, except in cases of severe asthma, esophageal strictures, gastric antral narrowing, granulomatous cystitis, inflammatory bowel disease, or certain cases of pneumonia. Clear evidence shows that corticosteroids are beneficial in these clinical settings because the steroids induce rapid regression of obstructive symptoms at low oral doses (e.g., 1 mg/kg/day of prednisone). Steroids can be lifesaving in young children with airway obstruction because of inflammation. Because of the exaggerated inflammatory reaction seen in CGD, there can be significant swelling in the airway and compression by pulmonary nodes that can block air movement and impede drainage. In these cases, the physician and patient should be aware of the risks of the additional immunosuppression caused by the corticosteroids.

Rare patients with X91° CGD have genomic deletions that span the gp91*phox* gene and the Xk gene, which encodes a membrane protein necessary for expression of the Kell genes.[3] Absence of the Xk gene product results in the McLeod syndrome, in which red blood cells have weak Kell antigens and variable acanthocytosis along with nerve and muscle disorders related to its expression in nonerythroid tissues. Transfusion of patients with McLeod syndrome poses a serious problem because they can develop alloantibodies of wide specificity that can preclude any further transfusions except with Kell-negative blood products. McLeod-matched blood is extremely rare, and patients with this syndrome should have their own blood frozen in case it is needed. Note that use of maternal blood does not solve the problem because only 50% of the mother's blood will match. Because of the difficulty in finding blood, transfusion with non-McLeod blood is likely to occur. Although management is difficult and use of steroids is necessary, the hemolytic anemia can be managed successfully.

Allogeneic BMT can be used to treat CGD, including using matched unrelated donors.[8,15] Because of the risks associated with this procedure, BMT is generally considered only for patients who have a fully human leukocyte antigen-matched sibling and frequent and severe infections despite aggressive medical management. However, reduced-intensity conditioning regimens for allogeneic transplantations have now been successfully used for BMT in CGD, including several cases with ongoing fungal infections.[8,15] Despite improved success rates and decreased complications, which patients with CGD should undergo transplantation remains an individualized decision, particularly for those with residual NADPH oxidase activity and little or no history of serious infection or other complications.[8] Finally, genetic therapies aimed at correcting the defective gene in BM stem cells hold promise for the future if obstacles can be solved to achieve effective and safe gene delivery and their transplantation.[8] Observations on female carriers of X-linked CGD with skewed X-inactivation and preclinical studies in murine CGD models suggest that complete correction of NADPH oxidase activity in 10% of circulating neutrophils will lead to clinically relevant improvements in host defense.

Neutrophil Glucose-6-Phosphate Dehydrogenase Deficiency

NADPH, the primary substrate for the respiratory burst oxidase, is generated by the first two reactions of the hexose monophosphate shunt pathway, which are catalyzed by G6PD (see Fig. 50.3, reaction 8) and 6-phosphogluconate dehydrogenase (6PGD).[16] The leukocyte and erythrocyte G6PD are encoded by the same gene. Thus, a severe deficiency of G6PD in neutrophils can result in a greatly attenuated respiratory burst because of low levels of NADPH. However, the vast majority of individuals with inherited G6PD deficiency do not have problems with a decreased respiratory burst or recurrent infections. A CGD-like syndrome has very rarely been observed in G6PD-deficient patients who have congenital nonspherocytic hemolytic anemia (CNSHA), in whom hemolysis occurs in the absence of redox stress.[3,16] Even in CNSHA, most G6PD mutations cause the enzyme to decay over a period of days and weeks, so that levels in the short-lived neutrophil usually do not become critically low even in some of the most unstable G6PD variants. A few rare and poorly understood G6PD mutations that cause CNSHA are associated with extremely low (<5% of normal) levels of G6PD in the neutrophil, resulting in a deficient respiratory burst and CGD-like symptoms. The combination of chronic, severe hemolytic anemia, recurrent infections, and the laboratory demonstration of extremely low G6PD levels in neutrophils and erythrocytes serves to distinguish this disease from CGD. The treatment for neutrophil G6PD deficiency is the same as for CGD, except that the efficacy of rIFN-γ has not been demonstrated in the former. The chronic hemolytic anemia is treated by supportive means, including transfusions.

Disorders of Glutathione Metabolism

As depicted in Fig. 50.3 (reaction 6), the reduced form of glutathione (GSH) serves to protect the neutrophil from the harmful effects of hydrogen peroxide on NADPH oxidase and other neutrophil proteins. Adequate intracellular levels of GSH are maintained by recycling oxidized glutathione (GSSG) to GSH by glutathione reductase (see Fig. 50.3, reaction 7), as well as by de novo synthesis of glutathione by glutathione synthetase (see Fig. 50.3, reaction 9). Severe deficiencies in either of these enzymes are extremely rare and are apparently inherited in an AR manner.[3] In the case of glutathione reductase deficiency, the respiratory burst terminates prematurely, presumably owing to the toxic effects of accumulating hydrogen peroxide on NADPH oxidase. This brief burst of O_2^-, however, appears to be sufficient for adequate microbial killing because the few patients reported have not had problems with recurrent infections. However, they do have congenital hemolytic anemia during periods of oxidant stress caused by diminished levels of glutathione reductase in erythrocytes. In glutathione synthetase deficiency, the respiratory burst proceeds normally. Patients have severe metabolic acidosis caused by elevated levels of 5-oxoproline, which is the product of the first step in glutathione synthesis and is present in increased levels because of a lack of feedback of GSH on the synthetic pathway. Patients with glutathione synthetase deficiency also have intermittent neutropenia (perhaps caused by the acidosis), as well as oxidant-induced hemolysis. There are mild problems with recurrent infections. Therapy with vitamin E (400 IU/day) has been found to be beneficial in patients with severe glutathione synthetase deficiency with hemolysis and infections.

Myeloperoxidase Deficiency

MPO deficiency is the most common inherited disorder of phagocytes but is almost always asymptomatic.[17] MPO is present in azurophilic granules of neutrophils and monocytes, and catalyzes the production of a potent antimicrobial agent, HOCl from chloride and hydrogen peroxide (see Fig. 50.3, reaction 4).[4,5] HOCl in turn reacts with a variety of primary and secondary amines to form chloramines, some of which can be toxic. Moreover, HOCl is capable of activating latent metalloproteinases (e.g., collagenase) and inactivating antiproteinases.

Complete MPO deficiency is seen in approximately 1 in 4000 individuals, and partial deficiency is even more common (1 in 2000 persons). The key features of MPO deficiency are summarized in Table 50.6. The disorder is inherited in an AR manner. In the few cases reported, several different mutations have been identified, which generally appear to affect the posttranslational processing of a precursor polypeptide for MPO. Acquired forms of MPO deficiency are also seen. The gene that encodes for MPO is located on chromosome 17 at q22–q23 near the breakpoint for the 15-to-17 translocation of promyelocytic leukemia. Subpopulations of MPO-deficient cells can be seen not only in the M3 (promyelocytic) form of acute myeloid leukemia but also in the M2 and M4 forms. MPO-deficient cells are also seen in approximately 25% of patients with chronic myeloid leukemia and myelodysplastic syndromes.

One of the most curious features of MPO deficiency is the remarkable lack of clinical symptoms in affected persons, given the prediction that severe MPO deficiency would cripple important antimicrobial reactions catalyzed by HOCl. In vitro, an impressive defect in killing *Candida albicans* and hyphal forms of *Aspergillus fumigatus* is observed.[17] Bacterial killing in vitro is also abnormal in being somewhat slower than normal, but eventually it is complete. MPO-deficient mice also exhibit abnormalities in host defense against *Candida* and *Klebsiella* spp. Excessive or unusual infections in MPO-deficient patients, however, are uncommon, except for rare individuals who also have diabetes mellitus.[17] In these individuals, disseminated fungal infections (usually candidiasis) are seen.

The discrepancy between the in vitro and in vivo manifestations of MPO deficiency in most patients can be explained in several ways. First, the respiratory burst in MPO-deficient neutrophils is substantially augmented, presumably from the absence of HOCl-mediated toxic effects on the NADPH oxidase. Second, other products of the respiratory burst, together with the oxygen-independent antibacterial proteins, appear to have sufficient potency to compensate for the loss of MPO-dependent reactions. Finally, residual amounts of MPO coupled with the normal levels of eosinophil peroxidase may provide at least some degree of peroxidative activity at the sites of infection.

Treatment is usually not required for MPO deficiency except in those individuals with fungal infections. In these patients, aggressive use of antifungal antibiotics is indicated. The prognosis is excellent in the majority of patients with MPO deficiency.

TABLE 50.6	Summary of Myeloperoxidase Deficiency
Incidence	1 in 2000 (partial deficiency) 1 in 4000 (total deficiency)
Inheritance	Autosomal recessive with variable expression; MPO gene on chromosome 17 at q22–q23
Molecular defect	Defective posttranslational processing of an abnormal MPO precursor polypeptide; eosinophil peroxidase encoded by different gene and levels normal
Pathogenesis	Partial or complete MPO deficiency leads to diminished production of HOCl and HOCl-derived chloramines; MPO products are necessary for rapid killing of microbes (especially *Candida* spp.) but not absolutely required
Clinical manifestations	Usually clinically silent Disseminated candidiasis or fungal disease (rare; usually in conjunction with diabetes mellitus) Acquired deficiency in M2, M3, and M4 AMLs and myelodysplasia
Laboratory evaluation	Deficiency of neutrophil and monocyte peroxidase by histochemical analysis (eosinophil peroxidase normal) Delayed, but eventually normal, killing of bacteria in vitro Failure to kill *Candida albicans* and hyphal forms of *Aspergillus fumigatus* in vitro
Differential diagnosis	Acquired partial MPO deficiency seen in M2, M3, and M4 AML; MDS; and Batten disease
Therapy	None in asymptomatic patients Aggressive treatment of fungal infections when they occur Control of blood glucose levels in diabetics
Prognosis	Usually excellent

AML, Acute myeloid leukemia; *HOCl,* hypochlorous acid; *MDS,* myelodysplastic syndromes; *MPO,* myeloperoxidase.

DISORDERS OF PHAGOCYTE ADHESION AND CHEMOTAXIS

Since 1970, numerous investigators have found in vitro chemotactic abnormalities in neutrophils from patients with a wide variety of clinical disorders associated with increased susceptibility to bacterial and fungal infections.[3] In most circumstances, the chemotactic abnormality identified was only marginal and not always clearly related to the clinical status of the patient. In other instances, clear and major defects were identified in vitro that correlated with the in vivo propensity for infection. Extensive classification systems have been devised to categorize the numerous acquired defects in chemotaxis. The problem in many of these reports is that it is unclear whether the infections were caused by the in vitro chemotactic abnormality or by the medical complications of the underlying disorder (e.g., acidosis, malnutrition, or exposure to nosocomial infections). A further complicating factor is that there are inherent limitations in the in vitro chemotaxis assay, which is subject to laboratory artifacts both as a result of neutrophil purification procedures as well as the assay itself. Furthermore, the extent to which these in vitro chemotactic assay systems faithfully reflect prevailing in vivo conditions is not known. Our understanding of chemotactic disorders has been hampered by the limitations of these assays, just as the elucidation of respiratory burst defects was obscured when the major available assay was in vitro bacterial killing. In this section, the most important and best characterized of the chemotactic disorders, LAD, is discussed in detail. A brief discussion of several other clinically significant chemotactic disorders is also provided.

Leukocyte Adhesion Deficiency Type I

LAD type I (LAD I) is a rare AR disorder of leukocyte adhesion, chemotaxis, and ingestion of C3bi-opsonized microbes as a result of decreased or absent expression of the leukocyte β_2 integrins (Table 50.7).[18,19] The hallmark of LAD I is the occurrence of repeated, often severe bacterial and fungal infections without the accumulation of pus despite persistent granulocytosis (see Table 50.7). The molecular basis for LAD was first suggested by Crowley and colleagues, who found that neutrophils from a patient with this clinical syndrome lacked a high-molecular-weight membrane glycoprotein (see Dinauer,

Newburger, and Borregaard[3]). The patient's neutrophils could not be made to adhere to plastic surfaces or to respond to serum-opsonized particles in terms of ingestion and respiratory burst activity.

The molecular basis of LAD I is now known to result from mutations in the gene for the common CD18 $\beta2$ subunit for these three leukocyte glycoproteins, now termed *$\beta2$ integrins*, that belong to the integrin superfamily of adhesion molecules. Integrins are noncovalently linked heterodimeric glycoproteins consisting of an α and a β subunit. Within each of the eight known integrin subfamilies the β subunit is identical (and defines the subfamily), but the α subunit varies and confers the functional specificity on the integrin. The molecular defect in LAD involves all members of the $\beta2$ integrin subfamily: $\alpha L \beta 2$ (CD11a/CD18), $\alpha m \beta 2$ (CD11b/CD18), and $\alpha x \beta 2$ (CD11c/CD18). CD11a/CD18 is often referred to as *LFA-1* while CD11b/CD18 is also called *Mac-1*, *Mo1*, or *CR3*. LAD I patients have an absent, diminished, or structurally abnormal β 2 subunit (CD18; see later), and as a result, the three types of α chains in the β 2 integrin subfamily cannot assemble into normal α–β heterodimers. Thus, all three β 2 integrins are moderately to severely deficient on all leukocytes in LAD.

The $\beta2$ integrins serve as receptors for the opsonic complement fragment C3bi, the intercellular adhesion molecules 1 and 2 (ICAM-1 and ICAM-2) that are expressed on endothelial cells and leukocytes, and fibrinogen. The diminished or absent expression of $\beta2$ integrins in LAD I leukocytes results in the failure of phagocytes to emigrate from the bloodstream to sites of infection. The early interactions with the endothelium, termed *rolling*, are normal in LAD I because these are mediated by a different family of adhesion molecules known as *selectins*. However, $\beta2$ integrins are responsible for the subsequent tight binding of neutrophils and monocytes to ICAMs on cytokine-activated endothelium, and this step is therefore severely defective in LAD I. Transendothelial migration is also impaired. A second major functional defect in LAD is the failure of phagocytes to bind C3bi-opsonized microbes. Because CD11b/CD18 is the predominant phagocyte receptor for this complement fragment, C3bi-mediated ingestion, degranulation, and respiratory burst activity are severely affected in LAD. Finally, $\beta2$ integrin-dependent signals play a key role in activating neutrophils for enhanced migration, phagocytosis of antibody-opsonized microbes, and degranulation.

Despite in vitro defects in lymphocyte responses dependent on LFA-1 (CD11a/CD18), patients with LAD I rarely have clinical manifestations related to impaired lymphocyte function. It is believed that the role CD11a/CD18 plays in lymphoid cell function can be compensated by other adhesion proteins (CD2, CD4, CD8, and so on).

Molecular Genetics of Leukocyte Adhesion Deficiency Type I

The fact that LAD I involves a deficiency of all leukocyte $\beta2$ integrins focused attention on the common $\beta2$ chain (CD18), and mutations in the corresponding gene, *ITGB2*, have been identified in all LAD I patients who have been analyzed at the molecular level to date.[18,19] Although expression of the leukocyte integrin α subunits is normal in LAD I, these are not transported to the cell surface because the $\beta2$ chain is absent or contains mutations that disrupt its structure or its interaction with the α subunit. Mutations in the α subunits have not been found thus far in patients with LAD I. The CD18 glycoprotein has a large extracellular domain at the N terminus, a single transmembrane domain, and a 46-residue cytoplasmic tail. As with X-linked CGD, CD18 mutations in LAD I are heterogeneous in nature and family specific, and can lead to either undetectable or low (9–20% of normal) levels of α–β dimer expression that correlates with the clinical severity of the disease. More than 50 different mutations have now been characterized in more than 100 families.[18] These include missense mutations, mRNA splicing defects, small deletions, and a premature termination signal. Many patients are compound heterozygotes and have two different mutant alleles for CD18. About half of patients with LAD I in whom the genetic defect

TABLE 50.7	Summary of Leukocyte Adhesion Deficiency Type 1
Incidence	More than 60 patients described in literature
Inheritance	AR
Molecular defect	An absent, diminished, or structurally abnormal β subunit (CD18) caused by one of several types of mutations in the β gene; in the absence of a normal β subunit, the three types of α chains in the β₂ integrin subfamily (CD11a, b, c) cannot assemble into normal α–β heterodimers
Pathogenesis	All three β₂ integrins (CD11a/CD18, CD11b/CD18, and CD11c/CD18) are deficient on all leukocytes, causing multiple abnormalities in cell function: adherence; chemotaxis; and C3bi-mediated ingestion, degranulation, and respiratory burst
Clinical manifestation	Persistent granulocytosis (neutrophil count: 12,000–100,000/mm³) Severe or moderate phenotypes depending on severity of deficiency Recurrent pyogenic infections with absent neutrophil infiltration Delayed umbilical cord separation Severe gingivitis or periodontitis
Laboratory evaluation	Flow cytometric measurement of surface CD11b in stimulated neutrophils with monoclonal anti-CD11b
Differential diagnosis	CGD May be associated with severe neutrophil actin dysfunction
Therapy	Hematopoietic stem cell transplant in clinically severe patients (CD11b <0.3% of normal) Aggressive use of parenteral antibiotics Possible benefit of prophylactic TMP-SMX
Prognosis	Severe: high incidence of death before 2 years of age unless transplantation is performed Moderate: can survive into 20s and 30s but with recurrent infections

AR, Autosomal recessive; CGD, chronic granulomatous disease; TMP-SMX, trimethoprim–sulfamethoxazole.

has been identified have point mutations in a stretch of 250 amino acids in the extracellular domain of CD18. This region is highly conserved among all β subunits and appears to be important for interaction with the α subunit.

Clinical Features

The key features of LAD I are summarized in Table 50.7. The clinical presentation of LAD is heterogeneous and is related to the severity of the deficiency of the β2 integrins. The severe clinical phenotype is associated with less than 0.3% of the normal amount of these glycoproteins on the leukocyte surface; the moderate phenotype has 2.5– 6% of normal levels. In both the severe and moderate forms of the disease, persistent granulocytosis (neutrophil count of 12,000–100,000/mm³) is a constant finding, as are recurrent cutaneous abscesses and aggressive periodontitis and gingivitis. Additional clinical features seen more often in the severe clinical phenotype include delayed umbilical cord separation, omphalitis, perirectal cellulitis, severe ulcerative stomatitis, and bacterial sepsis. A striking finding in LAD I is that abscesses and other sites of infections are devoid of pus despite the marked neutrophilia because neutrophils are unable to emigrate to tissues. *S. aureus* and gram-negative enteric bacteria cause the majority of infections in LAD I. Fungal infections can also occur, particularly from *C. albicans* and *Aspergillus* spp.

Note that infants with delayed separation of the umbilical cord who are healthy and have normal blood counts are very unlikely to have LAD I. Although the mean age of cord separation ranges from 7 to 15 days, 10% of healthy infants can have cord separation at 3 weeks of age or later.

Diagnosis

The diagnosis of LAD I is made by flow cytometric measurement of surface CD11b (Mac1; or the shared CD18 subunit) in unstimulated and stimulated neutrophils using commercially available monoclonal antibodies directed against CD11b or CD18 (see Fig. 50.6). Neutrophils contain an intracellular pool of CD11b/CD18 in their secondary (specific) and tertiary granules, which can be mobilized to the cell surface during stimulation. Therefore, the deficiency of CD11b can be more dramatically demonstrated by using stimulated neutrophils. Carriers of LAD I can be identified by this method because they have been found to express approximately 50% of normal levels of CD11b on the surface of their stimulated neutrophils (see Fig. 50.6).

Prognosis and Treatment

Treatment of LAD I depends on the clinical severity of the disorder. In patients with the moderate clinical phenotype, cutaneous and oral infections can be managed as they occur. The use of prophylactic antibiotics such as TMP-SMX appears to be beneficial, as does aggressive prophylactic treatment of periodontal disease. It is important to note that even patients with the moderate phenotype can die of overwhelming infection. In patients with severe LAD I, aggressive management is indicated because of the high incidence of death before the age of 2 years, and hematopoietic stem cell transplantation is recommended. LAD I should also be amenable to gene-replacement therapy in the future.

Leukocyte Adhesion Deficiency Types II and III

LAD type II is a very rare clinical syndrome closely related to LAD I but caused by a defect in selectin-mediated adhesion events from a deficiency in leukocyte Siayl–Lewis X ligands.[18,19] It was first reported by Etzioni et al in two unrelated boys of Muslim Arab origin and has since described in a total of five individuals (four Arab and one Turkish). The disease is inherited in an AR manner. Patients presented

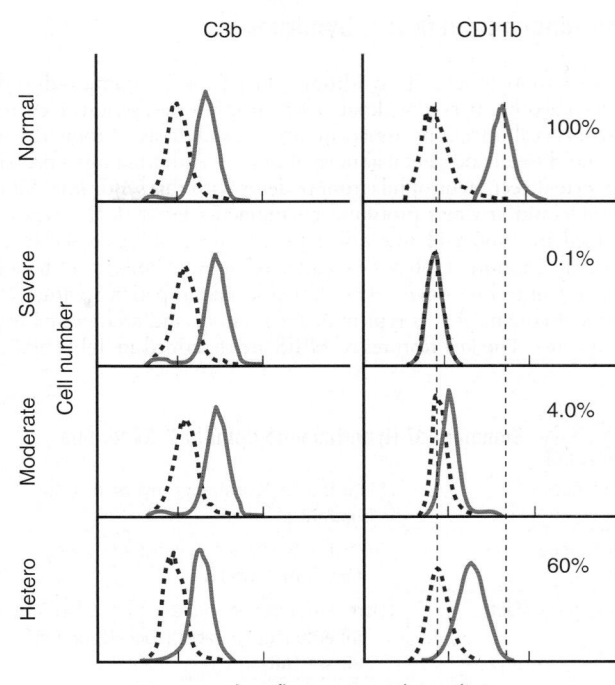

Fig. 50.6 EVALUATION OF ADHESION MOLECULE EXPRESSION FOR DIAGNOSIS OF LEUKOCYTE ADHESION DEFICIENCY. Fluorescence of C3b specific antibody labeled neutrophils (*solid line*) increases compared with a nonspecific control (*dashed line*) after 30-minute exposure to 10-nM fMLP in healthy donors, patients with severe and moderate forms of leukocyte adhesion deficiency(LAD) I, and a heterozygous LAD I carrier. However, the increase in CD11b fluorescence (*solid line*) is markedly diminished in LAD I patients. The respective percent of normal stimulated mean channel number is shown in the *right column*. Note that these results are expressed as percent of normal fluorescence intensity, not as percent of positive cells, as is the case in most flow cytometry assays.

with neutrophilia, recurrent bacterial infections, and periodontitis, similar to LAD I, although these symptoms were generally not as severe. In addition, LAD II is associated with dysmorphic features and psychomotor retardation. LAD II neutrophils express normal levels of CD18. A clue as to the molecular cause of LAD II came from the observation that LAD II red cells were Lewis antigen negative and also had the rare Bombay (hh) erythrocyte phenotype, in which red blood cells express a nonfucosylated variant of the H antigen. These antigenic defects share in common the failure to form certain fucose carbohydrate linkage. The defect in fucose metabolism in LAD II has now been shown to result from mutations in the Golgi guanosine diphosphate–fucose membrane transporter. This leads to a generalized loss of expression of fucosylated glycans on the surface of cells, particularly the sialylated and fucosylated tetrasaccharide, SLeX (CD15a), on the neutrophil surface. As a result, LAD II neutrophils are unable to bind to E- and P-selectin receptors on endothelium and therefore have an impairment in the early steps of rolling and loose binding to blood vessel walls before tight adhesion and emigration into infected tissues. Fucose supplementation has been partially successful in increasing expression of SLeX and decreasing clinical problems.

LAD type III has recently been described in a handful of patients with severe, recurrent infections similar to LAD I, as well as a bleeding tendency similar to Glanzmann thrombasthenia (a β3 integrin-related disorder).[18,19] This disorder results from AR defects in KINDLIN-3, a regulatory protein required for "inside-out" activation of multiple classes of integrins in blood cells. Because the clinical manifestations are typically severe, early BMT may be indicated for patients with LAD III. (see Etzioni[19]).

Hyperimmunoglobulin E Syndrome

Hyperimmunoglobulin E syndrome (HIES) is a complex disorder characterized by markedly elevated serum IgE levels, serious recurrent staphylococcal infections, mucocutaneous candidiasis, chronic dermatitis, and skeletal and dental abnormalities.[20,21] Although not a primary phagocyte defect, neutrophils from patients with this syndrome exhibit a variable and at times profound chemotactic defect. HIES was first described in 1966 and was called *Job syndrome*, in reference to the biblical description of Job as being affected by "sore boils from the soles of his feet unto his crown." The skin abscesses in patients with HIES lack the erythema that is typical of such lesions and are referred to as *cold abscesses*. The key features of HIES are described in Table 50.8.

TABLE 50.8	Summary of Hyperimmunoglobulin E Syndrome
Incidence	More than 200 patients reviewed in the literature
Inheritance	AD with incomplete penetrance; sporadic forms, AR (rare)
Molecular defect	Dominant-negative mutations in STAT3 (AD inheritance; sporadic), Dock8, or Tyk2 kinase (AR)
Clinical manifestations	Staphylococcal pneumonia Pneumatoceles Fungal superinfection of lung cysts "Cold" cutaneous skin abscesses and furuncles Chronic eczematoid dermatitis Mucocutaneous candidiasis Chronic cutaneous viral infections (AR) Severe allergies (AR) Coarse facies, growth retardation (AD) Osteopenia, recurrent fractures (AD) Sinusitis, keratoconjunctivitis Scoliosis (AD) Hyperextensible joints (AD) Delayed shedding of primary teeth (AD) Vascular disease (AD) Malignancy (AR) Stroke/CNS vasculitis (AR)
Laboratory evaluation	Serum IgE >2500 IU/mL Peripheral blood eosinophilia
Differential diagnosis	Atopic dermatitis Wiskott-Aldrich syndrome, DiGeorge syndrome Hypergammaglobulinemia Chronic granulomatous disease
Therapy	Prophylactic anti-*Staphylococcus aureus* antibiotics Aggressive treatment of acute infections with parenteral antibiotics Surgical drainage of deep infections and resection of lung cysts Monitor for scoliosis, fractures, vascular disease
Prognosis	Generally good if managed aggressively Some patients develop lymphoid malignancies; patients with AR HIES have an increased risk and broader spectrum of cancer susceptibility 30% survival by 30 years of age without bone marrow transplant (AR)

AD, Autosomal dominant; AR, autosomal recessive; HIES, hyperimmunoglobulin E syndrome; IgE, immunoglobulin E; STAT3, signal transducer and activator of transcription 3.

Most cases of HIES result from inherited or sporadic autosomal dominant (AD) mutations in signal transducer and activator of transcription 3 (STAT3), a Janus kinase (JAK)-activated transcription factor activated in response to many cytokines and growth factors. These mutations, which are located primarily in regions of the protein that interact with other proteins or with DNA, inhibit the activity of the wild-type STAT3 allele and result in a complex pattern of altered cytokine signaling and impaired T helper type 17 (Th17) cell differentiation. Mutations in *DOCK8*, a guanine nucleotide exchange factor, or *TYK2*, a JAK family member, result in the more rare AR forms of HIES that have more profound impairments in lymphocyte function, leading to a broader risk of infection and other immune dysregulation. Approximately 96% of DOCK8-deficient patients suffered life-threatening infection (58%), malignancy (17% by median age of 12 years) or noninfectious cerebral events (10%) by age 30 years. Only 33% of these patients who were not transplanted survived to 30 years of age.[20]

Insights into how STAT3 signaling defects lead to the clinical syndrome characteristic of AD HIES are now emerging. Defective responses to IL-6 may account for the minimal inflammatory responses characteristic of HIES, and the enhanced IgE production may reflect dysregulated immune responses secondary to impaired signaling by IL-10, a negative regulator. Th17 cells are important for control of mucocutaneous *Candida* infection, which is problematic in many patients. In addition, keratinocytes and bronchial epithelial cells are particularly dependent on Th17 cytokines to produce chemokines and antimicrobial peptides, which may explain the predilection for skin and lung infections. The dental and skeletal abnormalities may be related to defective STAT3 signaling in osteoblasts and osteoclasts.

Diagnosis of Chemotactic Disorders

The direct measurement of neutrophil chemotaxis in a clinical setting is very difficult and requires a specialized research laboratory. Because the assays are biologic assays, the laboratory must run the tests at least monthly to maintain competence and have acceptable normal ranges. Neutrophil chemotaxis is significantly affected by inflammation, complement activation, and medications, making it very difficult, especially in a patient with infection, to determine if the infection is attributable to a chemotactic defect or if the defect is attributable to the infection. This is further complicated by the fact that inflammation activates the neutrophils and affects which populations actually come off of the density gradients required to separate the cells for assay. Unlike the respiratory burst, chemotaxis must be done on fresh cells, so samples cannot be reliably shipped.

The neutrophils from patients with primary chemotactic defects have almost no motility in standard biologic assay systems. Some chemotactic disorders can be diagnosed by assays of other characteristic features.

LAD I

- LAD I has a significant chemotactic defect as well as phagocytic defect, and is characterized by leukocytosis. The diagnosis can be made by flow cytometry of the CD11b complex on the surface.
- Fig. 50.6 indicates surface expression of C3b and CD11b on neutrophils. C3b is used as a positive control and is normal in LAD1. With stimulation, CD11b increases *(top panel)*.
- The results in this assay are expressed as percent of normal stimulated control mean channel number. It is important to note that this is not the percent positive cell, as is the case for most flow cytometry assays.
- Severe LAD1 has no increase with stimulation.
- Moderate LAD1 shows some shift of fluorescence with stimulation.
- Genetic analysis for this disorder is clinically available.

Other chemotactic disorders: Genetic analysis is available for several primary neutrophil defects, and this approach should be pursued before attempting assay of chemotaxis in a clinical setting.

No other primary chemotactic defects are readily diagnosed by a routine clinical laboratory. Measurement of neutrophil chemotaxis itself to look for secondary defects for any kind of clinical decision making is difficult if not impossible to interpret.

Clinical Manifestations

The clinical manifestations of HIES are at times dramatic. Onset is generally in the first 2 months of life and is manifested by chronic dermatitis. By 5 years of age, patients have a history of recurrent skin abscesses, pneumonias, chronic otitis media, and sinusitis. As patients grow older, recurrent staphylococcal pneumonia is a common problem and can be complicated by the formation of pneumatoceles. Septic arthritis, cellulitis, and osteomyelitis are also observed and are usually caused by *S. aureus*, although other bacterial pathogens have also been found. Patients can have chronic mucocutaneous candidiasis and occasionally exhibit keratoconjunctivitis, sometimes complicated by corneal scarring. One feature noted in the majority of patients by the time they reach the teenage years is the presence of coarse facial features (broad nasal bridge, prominent nose). Dental and bone abnormalities are also common features of HIES. Delayed or failure to shed primary teeth occur in the majority. Hyperextensible joints and scoliosis are frequent. Osteopenia of unknown etiology is observed in most patients, and there is an increased risk of fractures to the long bones and vertebral bodies even in the absence of osteopenia. Vascular disease, including aneurysms, tortuosity of middle-sized arteries, and hypertension is also frequently seen.

Patients with the AR form of HIES, the majority of whom have defects of *DOCK8*, which is also referred to as *DOCK8 immunodeficiency syndrome*, also have recurrent sinopulmonary infections, skin abscesses, and dermatitis, with the latter often the first symptom and developing in infancy. Unlike AD HIES, patients with *DOCK8* defects can develop asthma; severe allergies, including to foods, and chronic cutaneous viral infections with human papillomavirus, molluscum contagiosum virus, and herpes family viruses is a distinctive feature seen in approximately 90% of patients. These patients are also at high risk for a variety of malignancies in late childhood to early adulthood, believed to be caused by loss of immune surveillance for tumors.[20] AR HIES patients do not have the nonimmunologic skeletal and dental abnormalities characteristic of AD HIES.

Diagnosis

The diagnosis of HIES should be entertained in any child or young adult who has the above-described clinical picture or simply a history of recurrent infections. The hallmark laboratory finding is a marked elevation of serum immunoglobulin E (IgE), almost always greater than 2500 IU/mL. Levels can be as high as 150,000 IU/mL. Most patients also have peripheral eosinophilia. However, there is no correlation of clinical disease activity with the level of either IgE or peripheral eosinophilia. Atopic dermatitis is the major differential diagnosis because comparably high serum levels of IgE can be seen in patients in this disorder, as well as superficial skin infections. The severe and recurrent nature of the staphylococcal furuncles and pneumonias usually seen in HIES can help distinguish these patients from those with atopic dermatitis. Patients with other primary immunodeficiency syndromes may also manifest elevated IgE levels. Scoring criteria predictive of STAT3 mutations, including recurrent pneumonia, pathologic bone fractures, and lack of Th17 cells, are helpful.[21] DNA testing should be used to make a definitive diagnosis.

Therapy

The therapy for AD HIES is largely supportive.[21] Prophylactic antibiotics (e.g., dicloxacillin or TMP-SMX) can be effective in preventing *S. aureus* infections. Dermatitis can be treated with topical steroids. Bathing in diluted bleach can diminish colonization by *S. aureus*. Prophylactic antifungals can be helpful in patients with chronic mucocutaneous candidiasis. Intravenous antibiotics are used for deep-seated infections or for resistant cutaneous infections. Surgical resection of persistent pneumatoceles is sometimes indicated to prevent superinfection by fungal and gram-negative organisms. Intravenous Ig infusions have shown some success in the management of HIES. Attention should also be paid to blood pressure and other vascular complications. Although a role for hematopoietic stem cell transplantation in AD HIES is unclear, two children with STAT3 mutations who underwent transplantation for non-Hodgkin lymphoma are alive 10 and 14 years later with resolution of all immunologic and nonimmunologic features of HIES.[21] Patients with AR HIES may need prophylaxis for viral infections, and hematopoietic stem cell transplant probably should be considered.[20]

Miscellaneous Chemotactic Disorders

It is extremely rare to have primary defects in neutrophil actin polymerization as a cause of abnormal chemotaxis and recurrent infections.[2,3] In one case, neutrophils had diminished actin polymerization, chemotaxis, and phagocytosis of serum-opsonized particles. Family members had decreased CD11b/CD18 expression and a partial decrease in actin polymerization, which suggested that this disorder might be a variant of LAD I; however, no similar cases have otherwise been described. An apparent AR disorder of actin polymerization has been described in a male infant of Tongan descent who presented with severe skin infections, recurrent pulmonary infiltrates, thrombocytopenia, and invasive *Candida tropicalis* infection. Neutrophil actin polymerization was markedly abnormal and associated with increased expression of an actin-binding protein. Finally, a heterozygous point mutation in β-actin affecting binding to actin-regulatory proteins was discovered in a female patient with recurrent infections, photosensitivity, and mental retardation. Neutrophils had a marked impairment in chemotaxis and in the formyl peptide-induced respiratory burst.

A new syndrome of severe neutrophil dysfunction caused by a dominant-negative mutation in Rac2, a small GTPase expressed in blood cells that acts in many signal transduction pathways, was recently described in an infant boy born to unrelated parents. (see Dinauer and Newburger[3]) This baby presented with rapidly progressive and deep-seated soft tissue infections, along with neutrophilia and poor formation of pus but normal expression of β2 integrins and fucosylated proteins. Neutrophils had marked defects in actin polymerization, chemotaxis, degranulation, and the respiratory burst in response to chemoattractants. Neutrophil responses to other agonists were normal, suggesting that the dominant negative Rac2 mutation produces a selective intracellular signaling defect.

Localized juvenile periodontitis (LJP) is a heterogeneous disorder of unknown etiology characterized by chronic and recurrent periodontal infections and severe alveolar bone loss with onset at the time of puberty.[22] Many patients with LJP have been reported to have defective neutrophil chemotaxis in vitro. At present, it appears that LJP is an acquired disorder in some patients and a genetic disorder in others. It may also be a combination of both in certain patients because they may inherit an unusual sensitivity to the chemotactic inhibitors released by certain periodontal microorganisms. The diagnosis of the disorder is made on the basis of severe periodontal disease and destructive alveolar bone loss involving the first molars and incisors developing during adolescence. It is important to note that many qualitative and quantitative neutrophil disorders are also associated with severe periodontal disease. Therefore, the differential diagnosis should include neutropenia (both chronic and cyclic), LAD, CGD, and Chediak-Higashi syndrome (CHS).

One of the most consistently observed chemotactic abnormalities is seen in neonatal neutrophils.[23] These cells exhibit impaired chemotaxis in vitro in response to a wide variety of chemotactic factors. It appears as though this abnormality is caused, at least in part, by defects in cellular adhesion as a result of diminished mobilization of intracellular adhesion-promoting molecules to the cell surface. Defective neutrophil chemotaxis can be seen in normal neonates between birth and 5 days of age. In severely ill infants, the defect may persist for a longer time.

DEFECTS IN THE STRUCTURE AND FUNCTION OF LYSOSOMAL GRANULES

Two major disorders of neutrophil granules have been described, CHS and specific granule deficiency (SGD). A great deal has been learned about the structural and functional abnormalities of neutrophils from patients with these conditions. Although rare, these disorders are also obligatory components in the differential diagnosis for any patient with recurrent bacterial and fungal infections.

Chediak-Higashi Syndrome

CHS is a rare AR, multisystem disease resulting from widespread defects in granule morphogenesis, with giant lysosomes in leukocytes and other cells throughout the body.[24–26] The disorder is characterized by partial oculocutaneous albinism, frequent (and sometimes fatal) bacterial infections, a mild bleeding diathesis, and peripheral as well as cranial neuropathies associated with defects at the optic chiasm. Those who survive the recurrent infections develop an "accelerated phase" of the disease; one of the hereditary forms of HLH, which, if untreated, is eventually fatal because of a profound pancytopenia that develops.

The most dramatic granule defects are manifested in the various blood cells. Neutrophils contain a highly inhomogeneous population of huge granules derived from coalescence of azurophilic (primary) granules. The giant granules are often more prominent in the BM than in the peripheral blood because many of the abnormal myeloid precursors are apparently destroyed before they leave the BM, resulting in moderate neutropenia with absolute neutrophil counts ranging from 500 to 2000 cells/mm³. Granules are also markedly deficient in antimicrobial granule enzymes such as cathepsin G and elastase, consistent with a defect in granule morphogenesis. Degranulation is delayed and incomplete in Chediak-Higashi neutrophils, resulting in impaired bacterial killing. Chemotaxis is also defective, perhaps related to poor deformability because of the presence of the large granules. Monocytes and macrophages exhibit similar giant cytoplasmic granules, with resultant abnormalities in their phagocytic functions. Giant granules are also seen in lymphocytes and are associated with defects in cytotoxic T-lymphocyte and NK cell function. Eosinophils contain large granules, the functional significance of which is not known. Platelets in this disorder have a storage pool deficiency of adenosine diphosphate and serotonin, presumably caused by the abnormal granule morphogenesis in megakaryocytes, leading to a defect in platelet aggregation.

Abnormal giant granules are also present in other cell types. These include melanocytes, which contain abnormal melanosomes that cannot transfer their contents to adjacent keratinocytes; Schwann cells; astrocytes; and certain cells in the liver, spleen, pancreas, gastric mucosa, kidney, adrenal gland, and pituitary gland.

Molecular Genetics

A gene termed *CHS1* or *LYST* (for its presumed function as a lysosomal trafficking regulatory protein) is affected in the majority of CHS cases and is on the long arm of chromosome 1.[24,25] The encoded protein is very large (3801 amino acids); its specific function is unknown, but recent studies suggest that it may inhibit lysosome fusion with other intracellular membrane vesicles. A variety of frameshift and nonsense mutations that predict synthesis of truncated forms of the protein have been identified in most, but not all, CHS patients studied to date. There is no correlation between the length of the truncated CHS1 protein and the severity of the disease. Disorders similar to human CHS have also been described in many mammalian species, including Aleutian mink, *beige* mice, blue foxes, cats, killer whales, and Hereford cattle. Identification of the human CHS1 gene was aided by positional cloning of the mouse *lyst* homolog affected in *beige* mice.

TABLE 50.9	Summary of Chediak-Higashi Syndrome
Incidence	More than 200 cases described
Inheritance	AR
Molecular defect	A defect in granule morphogenesis in multiple tissues resulting from mutations in the *CHS1* (*LYST*) gene encoding a lysosomal trafficking regulator protein
Pathogenesis	Giant coalesced azurophil granules in neutrophils, resulting in ineffective granulopoiesis and neutropenia, delayed and incomplete degranulation, and defective chemotaxis; abnormal granules in other cells (NK cells, cytotoxic T cells, platelets, melanocytes, neurons)
Clinical manifestations	Partial oculocutaneous albinism Recurrent severe bacterial infections (usually *Staphylococcus aureus*) Cranial and peripheral neuropathies (muscle weakness, ataxia, sensory loss) HLH (accelerated phase)
Laboratory evaluation	Giant granules in peripheral blood granulocytes and in BM myeloid progenitor cells Widespread lymphohistiocytic infiltrates in accelerated phase
Differential diagnosis	Other genetic forms of partial albinism Giant granules can be seen in acute and CMLs
Therapy	Prophylactic TMP-SMX Parenteral antibiotics for acute infections Ascorbic acid (200 mg/day for infants; 6 g/day for adults) HSCT before or at beginning of HLH
Prognosis	Most patients die from infection or complications of HLH during the first or second decade of life unless transplantation is performed

AR, Autosomal recessive; BM, bone marrow; CML, chronic myeloid leukemia; HLH, hemophagocytic lymphohistiocytosis; HSCT, hematopoietic stem cell transplant; NK, natural killer; TMP-SMX, trimethoprim-sulfamethoxazole.

Clinical Manifestations

The key features of CHS are summarized in Table 50.9. The disease usually presents in infancy or early childhood, with infections involving the lungs, skin, and mucous membranes being most commonly encountered. Dental caries and periodontal disease are also common. The most frequent offending organism is *S. aureus*. Gram-negative bacteria, *Aspergillus* spp., and *Candida* spp. also are responsible for many infections. Platelet granule defects result in easy bruising and epistaxis. There is partial oculocutaneous albinism and photosensitivity. Patients may have a white forelock, or an ashen or grayish silver sheen to the hair, which can vary from blond to dark brown. In younger patients, there may be a cartwheel distribution of pigment in the iris and an abnormal red reflex. Neurologic manifestations include peripheral or cranial neuropathies, gait abnormalities, muscle weakness, sensory loss, seizures, or spinocerebellar degeneration. Neurologic symptoms worsen with age.

Approximately 85% of children surviving into the second decade of life develop an accelerated phase of the disease, with fever, lymphadenopathy, and progressive pancytopenia, that is now recognized to be a genetic form of HLH caused by impaired lymphocyte and NK cell function.[26] The development of HLH can sometimes be precipitated by Epstein-Barr virus infection. A reactive-appearing lymphohistiocytic proliferation occurs in the liver, spleen, lymph nodes, and BM, and the prognosis is uniformly fatal unless patients undergo BMT.

Diagnosis

The diagnosis of CHS is made on the basis of the giant peroxidase-positive lysosomal granules in the peripheral blood granulocytes or in BM myeloid cells. Identification of large, acid phosphatase-positive lysosomes in amniocytes and chorionic villus cells has been used to diagnose CHS prenatally. Other clinical features characteristic of CHS can support the diagnosis, including mild oculocutaneous albinism; silvery hair, in which microscopic examination reveals giant melanin granules; and a bleeding diathesis. The development of HLH is characterized by diffuse infiltrates of lymphohistiocytic cells seen on biopsy and by pancytopenia. Occasionally, giant granules that resemble those of CHS can be seen in both acute and chronic myelogenous leukemias.

Therapy

The treatment for the stable phase of CHS is similar to that for other neutrophil disorders. Prophylactic antibiotics such as TMP-SMX appear to be beneficial. Parenteral antibiotics are indicated for acute infections, and responses are often slow. Treatment with high-dose ascorbic acid (200 mg/day for infants; 6 g/day for adults) has been found to improve the clinical status of some patients. Although there is some controversy regarding the efficacy of ascorbic acid, given the safety of this medication, it seems prudent to administer it to all patients. The treatment of HLH (accelerated phase) includes combinations of drugs that suppress the function of activated macrophages and T cells followed by allogeneic hematopoietic stem cell transplantation.[26] Indeed, transplantation is ideally performed before or at the beginning of the accelerated phase. Note that transplantation does not prevent the progressive neuropathy of CHS.

Specific Granule Deficiency

Neutrophil SGD is an extremely rare congenital disorder characterized by recurrent bacterial and fungal infections, primarily involving the skin, ears, and lungs.[3,27] Infections are often indolent and smoldering, and S. aureus, P. aeruginosa, enteric gram-negative bacteria, and C. albicans are the major pathogens. Family studies suggest that it is inherited in an AR manner. Neutrophils from patients with SGD have atypical bilobed nuclei, absent specific granules, and multiple deficiencies of secondary and tertiary granule mRNAs and proteins, including lactoferrin, vitamin B_{12}-binding protein and gelatinase B; although azurophil granules in this disorder are present and contain MPO and lysozyme, they are markedly deficient in defensins. Monocytes display cell surface and functional defects, eosinophils lack eosinophil-specific granule proteins such as eosinophil cationic protein, and platelets have abnormal α granules, suggesting that the underlying defect may be related to regulation of the synthesis of certain granule and membrane proteins. This defect in synthesis is confined to BM-derived cells because lactoferrin secretion is normal in the glandular epithelia of SGD patients despite the severe deficiency in the neutrophils.

The recurrent skin and pulmonary infections characteristic of SGD appear to be caused by two fundamental defects in the neutrophils. One defect is the marked deficiency of at least two important microbicidal granule proteins, lactoferrin and defensins. The other defect is a relatively severe chemotactic abnormality presumably caused by the absence of the intracellular pool of leukocyte adhesion

molecules that normally reside in the specific granules. As discussed earlier, these $\beta2$ integrins play a key role in phagocyte chemotaxis.

The molecular defect responsible for most cases of SGD has recently been shown to involve a myeloid transcription factor known as C/EBPε, which regulates expression of certain genes activated during granulocyte differentiation.[3,27] This came about serendipitously when it was recognized that mice with a targeted deletion in the C/EBPε gene displayed characteristics similar to those of SGD patients, including neutrophils with bilobed nuclei, absent secondary granules, and impaired chemotaxis along with increased susceptibility to bacterial infections. To date, mutations in the C/EBPε gene have been identified in two SGD patients that encode truncated, nonfunctional proteins. However, DNA sequencing of the C/EBPε gene of several other SGD patients has not revealed abnormalities, suggesting that SGD is a genetically heterogeneous disorder.

The diagnosis of SGD can be readily made by microscopic examination. Wright-stained neutrophils are devoid of specific granules but contain normal numbers of azurophilic granules. Electron microscopy reveals small peroxidase-negative vesicles, which presumably represent empty specific granules. The diagnosis of SGD can also be established by demonstrating a severe deficiency in either lactoferrin or vitamin B_{12}-binding protein. An acquired form of SGD can be seen in burn patients or in individuals with various myeloproliferative disorders. The treatment for SGD is similar to that for other neutrophil disorders. If medical management is aggressive, the prognosis appears quite good, with patients surviving into their adult years.

MISCELLANEOUS INHERITED AND ACQUIRED DISORDERS OF PHAGOCYTE FUNCTION

Rare inherited defects in phagocyte production or response to inflammatory cytokines are manifested as recurrent infections.[28,29] HIES also falls into this category (see earlier discussion). A distinctive group of disorders referred to as *Mendelian susceptibility to mycobacterial diseases* (MSMD) involve inherited defects in macrophage IL-12/23–dependent IFN-γ–mediated immunity. Macrophage production of IL-12 and IL-23 after ingestion of mycobacteria triggers IFN-γ production by T and NK lymphocytes, which in turn activates crucial genes in macrophages. MSMD (MIM 20990) can be caused by inherited AR, AD, or X-linked defects leading to impaired T-cell production of IFN-γ, expression of the IFN-γ receptor, or downstream signaling, which results in a spectrum of recurrent and severe atypical mycobacterial infections, as well as susceptibility to *Salmonella* and, in some subgroups, viral infections.[28,29] As mentioned earlier, recessive point mutations in X-linked *CYBB* that selectively impair expression of the NADPH oxidase subunit gp91^{phox} in macrophages but not neutrophils are also considered a subgroup of MSMD.[13] A variety of genetic defects in a scaffolding protein known as *IKK-γ* or *NEMO* that is important for activation of the nuclear factor kappa-B (NFκB) signaling pathway have been reported in patients with anhydrotic ectodermal dysplasia and immunodeficiency; affected children have recurrent pyogenic infections with a minimal systemic inflammatory response and can also develop opportunistic infections with atypical mycobacteria or *Pneumocystis* carinii.[29] Several other kindred have been described with genetic deficiency of another protein, IRAK-4, important for NFκB activation by pyogenic bacteria via the Toll-like receptor/IL-I receptor superfamily. Affected children also had recurrent infections with *S. pneumonia* and *S. aureus*, and a poor inflammatory response but no dysmorphic features or opportunistic infections. Finally, with the increasing use of low-cost gene sequencing, it is likely that new inherited disorders of phagocyte function will be identified in the coming years.

Patients with glycogen storage disease type Ib (GSD-Ib), which results from absence of a glucose-6-phosphate transporter, have impaired neutrophil functions and neutropenia.[30] Neutrophil defects include depressed chemotaxis, phagocytosis, and NADPH oxidase activity. Although neutropenia appears to result from increased neutrophil apoptosis, how impaired glucose homeostasis leads to

Management of Infections

The management of infections in patients with primary neutrophil dysfunction syndromes is quite different than in the normal population, and for the most part different from patients with neutropenias.

- Patients tend to present with relatively low fevers and chronic inflammatory processes associated with marked elevation of ESR and CRP. Unless they have untreated abscesses or inflammatory masses, they tend not to present with frank sepsis and positive blood cultures.
- The frequency of infections decreases somewhat with age in children as their normal T-cell and B-cell–mediated immunity develops.
- Although one should always attempt to obtain culture proof of an infection, more often than not, it is not possible to identify an organism, and it is necessary to treat empirically.
- Because these patients tend to develop deep-seated tissue infections, the ESR can be of great value even though it is quite nonspecific. Elevation in the ESR suggests deep tissue inflammation; CRP is more acute and suggests monocyte activation. Persistent significant elevation of the ESR (>15–20 mm/hour) even in the absence of fever or other symptoms may warrant radiologic search for deep-seated infection.
- The authors advocate an "antibiotic sensitivity by ESR response" approach to empiric therapy in stable patients. One can start at parenteral anti-*Staphylococcus* and gram-negative therapy, and monitor the ESR daily. A monotonic decrease in the ESR within several days that is clear-cut suggests the process is sensitive to the antibiotic selected. Although complete resolution

of inflammatory response may take many weeks, usually there is some clear change in the ESR within 1 week. If there is worsening or no clear response, then an antifungal can be added and the ESR monitored in the same fashion. Return of an elevated ESR can be a sign of development of organism resistance.

- If a patient with CGD is particularly ill appearing or febrile, it is important to make sure that *B. cepacia* complex bacteria are covered.
- There is no fixed duration of therapy for any infections in these patients. If the infections are not completely extinguished, they will return and will contribute to development of chronic pulmonary and hepatic fibrosis. Parenteral antibiotics or antibiotics that can deliver very high tissue levels should be continued significantly past normalization of the ESR and disappearance of any radiographic evidence of deep tissue infection. This can take many months for some pneumonias and liver abscesses.
- Short pulses of steroids (4–6 days) can be lifesaving, particularly for pulmonary infections in young children with CGD. They reduce airway inflammation and promote drainage.
- Young children are susceptible to infections with routine childhood viruses and infections, and tend to do well with standard therapeutic approaches and courses of treatment that are two- to three-times longer than the usual recommended course. Again, monitoring with the ESR can be a guide.

All standard childhood immunizations and influenza vaccinations are strongly recommended. Prophylactic antibiotics may be appropriate (see text).

---

abnormal neutrophil function is uncertain. Interestingly, the BM in the face of neutropenia shows marked hypercellularity with increased mature neutrophils in some patients. The neutrophil count increases within hours of granulocyte colony-stimulating factor (G-CSF) administration, suggesting it is acting in part by releasing neutrophils from the BM. GSD-Ib patients can have infections as well as inflammatory bowel disease. Therefore, in addition to management of the metabolic disruption, these patients are also often treated with G-CSF to improve neutropenia.

There are a variety of noncongenital defects in phagocyte function that can be associated with an increased risk of bacterial or fungal infection.[2,3] Several have already been mentioned, including neonatal neutrophil dysfunction manifested as poor adhesion and chemotaxis. Patients with myelodysplastic syndromes and acute nonlymphoblastic lymphoma can have subpopulations of neutrophils variably defective in adhesion, migration, and production of reactive oxidants, and microbicidal activity that has correlated with an increased risk of infection. Similar defects have been described in diabetes mellitus, Gaucher disease, and renal failure. Severe bacterial infections, surgical trauma, and severe burns can also result in transient depression of a variety of neutrophil functions. The underlying mechanism(s) are incompletely defined and may be related to effects of high levels of inflammatory mediators produced in response to infection or trauma or to products released by bacteria.

REFERENCES

1. Kolaczkowska E, Kubes P: Neutrophil recruitment and function in health and inflammation. *Nat Rev Immunol* 13:159–175, 2013.
2. Kyono W, Coates TD: A practical approach to neutrophil disorders. *Pediatr Clin North Am* 49(929):viii, 2002.
3. Dinauer MC, Newburger PE, Borregaard N: The phagocyte system and disorders of granulopoiesis and granulocyte function. In Nathan DG, Orkin SH, Ginsburg D, et al, editors: *Nathan and Oski's Hematology of infancy and childhood*, ed 8, Philadelphia, 2014, WB Saunders Company, p 773.
4. Klebanoff SJ, Kettle AJ, Rosen H, et al: Myeloperoxidase: a frontline defender against phagocytosed microorganisms. *J Leukoc Biol* 93(2):185–198, 2013.
5. Nauseef WM: How human neutrophils kill and degrade microbes: an integrated view. *Immunol Rev* 219:88, 2007.
6. Al Ghouleh I, Khoo NK, Knaus UG, et al: Oxidases and peroxidases in cardiovascular and lung disease: new concepts in reactive oxygen species signaling. *Free Rad Biol Med* 51:1271, 2011.
7. Winkelstein JA, Marino MC, Johnston RB, Jr, et al: Chronic granulomatous disease. Report on a national registry of 368 patients. *Medicine (Baltimore)* 79:155, 2000.
8. Kang EM, Marciano BE, DeRavin S, et al: Chronic granulomatous disease: overview and hematopoietic stem cell transplantation. *J Allergy Clin Immunol* 127:1319, quiz 27-28, 2011.
9. Kuhns DB, Alvord WG, Heller T, et al: Residual NADPH oxidase and survival in chronic granulomatous disease. *N Engl J Med* 363:2600, 2010.
10. Matute JD, Arias AA, Wright NA, et al: A new genetic subgroup of chronic granulomatous disease with autosomal recessive mutations in p40 phox and selective defects in neutrophil NADPH oxidase activity. *Blood* 114:3309, 2009.
11. Roos D, Kuhns DB, Maddalena A, et al: Hematologically important mutations: X-linked chronic granulomatous disease (third update). *Blood Cells Mol Dis* 45:246, 2010.
12. Roos D, Kuhns DB, Maddalena A, et al: Hematologically important mutations: the autosomal recessive forms of chronic granulomatous disease (second update). *Blood Cells Mol Dis* 44:291, 2010.
13. Bustamante J, Arias AA, Vogt G, et al: Germline CYBB mutations that selectively affect macrophages in kindreds with X-linked predisposition to tuberculous mycobacterial disease. *Nat Immunol* 12:213, 2011.
14. Schappi MG, Jaquet V, Belli DC, et al: Hyperinflammation in chronic granulomatous disease and anti-inflammatory role of the phagocyte NADPH oxidase. *Semin Immunopathol* 30:255, 2008.
15. Güngör T, Teira P, Slatter M, et al: Reduced-intensity conditioning and HLA-matched haemopoietic stem-cell transplantation in patients with chronic granulomatous disease: a prospective multicentre study. *Lancet* 383(9915):436–448, 2014.
16. Beutler E: G6PD deficiency. *Blood* 84:3613, 1994.
17. Lanza F: Clinical manifestation of myeloperoxidase deficiency. *J Mol Med* 76:676, 1998.
18. van de Vijver E, Maddalena A, Sanal O, et al: Hematologically important mutations: Leukocyte adhesion deficiency (first update). *Blood Cells Mol Dis* 48:53, 2012.

19. Etzioni A: Genetic etiologies of leukocyte adhesion defects. *Curr Opin Immunol* 21:481, 2009.

20. Aydin SE, Kilic SS, Aytekin C, et al: DOCK8 Deficiency: Clinical and Immunological Phenotype and Treatment Options—a Review of 136 Patients. *J Clin Immunol* 35(2):189–198, 2015.

21. Sowerwine KJ, Holland SM, Freeman AF: Hyper-IgE syndrome update. *Ann N Y Acad Sci* 1250:25, 2012.

22. Oh TJ, Eber R, Wang HL: Periodontal diseases in the child and adolescent. *J Clin Periodontol* 29:400, 2002.

23. Koenig JM, Yoder MC: Neonatal neutrophils: the good, the bad, and the ugly. *Clin Periodontol* 31:39, 2004.

24. Introne WJ, Westbroek W, Golas GA, et al: Chediak-Higashi syndrome. In Pagon RA, Bird TD, Dolan CR, et al, editors: *GeneReviews*, Seattle (WA), 2010.

25. Kaplan J, De Domenico I, Ward DM: Chediak-Higashi syndrome. *Curr Opin Hematol* 15:22, 2008.

26. Janka GE: Familial and acquired hemophagocytic lymphohistiocytosis. *Ann Rev Med* 63:233, 2012.

27. Gombart AF, Koeffler HP: Neutrophil specific granule deficiency and mutations in the gene encoding transcription factor C/EBP(epsilon). *Curr Opin Hematol* 9:36, 2002.

28. Milner JD, Holland SM: The cup runneth over: lessons from the ever-expanding pool of primary immunodeficiency diseases. *Nat Rev Immunol* 13(9):635–648, 2013.

29. Bustamante J, Boisson-Dupuis S, Abel L, et al: Mendelian susceptibility to mycobacterial disease: genetic, immunological, and clinical features of inborn errors of IFN-γ immunity. *Semin Immunol* 26(6):454–470, 2014.

30. Chou JY, Jun HS, Mansfield BC: Glycogen storage disease type I and G6Pase-beta deficiency: etiology and therapy. *Nat Rev Endocrinol* 6:676, 2010.

CHAPTER 51

CONGENITAL DISORDERS OF LYMPHOCYTE FUNCTION

Sung-Yun Pai and Luigi D. Notarangelo

Over 200 molecular defects that result in primary immune deficiency are known to date. Many of these gene defects have been identified in recent years with the advent of whole-exome and whole-genome sequencing. The study of patients with primary immune deficiencies has unraveled fundamental mechanisms that govern lymphocyte development and function. Importantly, characterization of the molecular basis of these diseases has revealed unanticipated heterogeneity of the clinical and immunological phenotype. This chapter reviews disorders of thymus organogenesis, severe combined immune deficiency (SCID), other combined immunodeficiencies, disorders with immune dysregulation, and defects of humoral immunity.

DEFECTS OF THYMUS ORGANOGENESIS

The thymus is the primary organ where T lymphocytes are generated and educated. Endoderm-derived thymic stem cells derived from the third pharyngeal pouch differentiate into cortical and medullary epithelial cells, which in turn induce the differentiation of hematopoietic precursors into T cells. Thus, defects of thymus organogenesis have important consequences on immune function.

DiGeorge Syndrome

DiGeorge syndrome (DGS) is caused by developmental anomalies of the third and fourth pharyngeal pouches, and is characterized by thymic hypoplasia, hypoparathyroidism, conotruncal heart malformation (especially interrupted aortic arch type B or truncus arteriosus), and facial dysmorphisms (micrognathia, hypertelorism, antimongoloid slant of the eyes, cleft palate, and ear malformations). Hypocalcemic seizures are common. Feeding problems, microcephaly, speech delay, neurobehavioral problems (including bipolar disorders, autistic spectrum disorders, and schizophrenia later in life), and scoliosis are frequently observed.

Between 50% and 90% of patients with DGS carry a hemizygous deletion of chromosome 22q11, which occurs in ~1:3000 newborns, most arising de novo. Fluorescent in situ hybridization readily identifies the 22q11del in most cases. More rarely, DGS is associated with CHARGE syndrome, chromosome 10p deletion, or with mutations of the *TBX1* gene, contained within the 22q11 interval.

Most patients have "partial DGS", manifested by mild T-cell lymphopenia and immunodeficiency. Such patients may be asymptomatic, may have oral thrush and recurrent infections, or may develop autoimmune disease such as juvenile idiopathic arthritis, immune thrombocytopenic purpura, and Raynaud phenomenon. Approximately 1% of DGS patients have "complete DGS", with absence of circulating T cells. Some DGS patients may develop low numbers of oligoclonal T lymphocytes that undergo activation in vivo and infiltrate target tissues, causing skin rash, liver dysfunction, and lymphadenopathy. This condition is known as complete atypical DGS.

Treatment of DGS includes correction of severe heart defects, and supplementation with calcium and vitamin D for hypocalcemia. If a significant immune defect is present, prophylaxis of *Pneumocystis jiroveci* pneumonia with trimethoprim-sulfamethoxazole (TMP-SMZ) is indicated. Live-attenuated vaccines can be safely administered to patients with partial DGS who have good cellular immunity (with $CD8^+$ count >300 cells/μL); however, these vaccines are contraindicated in patients with complete DGS. Use of immunosuppressive drugs is indicated in patients with complete atypical form of the disease.

Ultimately, survival in patients with complete DGS requires immune reconstitution. Bone marrow transplantation from human leukocyte antigen (HLA)-identical donors may allow engraftment of mature T cells contained in the graft. However, because of the absence of thymic tissue, no newly developed T cells are generated, and the patient may remain susceptible to pathogens that are not recognized by donor-derived T cells contained in the graft.

By contrast, thymic transplantation represents the treatment of choice for patients with complete DGS, including the atypical variant. The thymus obtained as discarded tissue from unrelated infants undergoing heart surgery is sliced and cultured in vitro, then implanted in the quadriceps muscles of the infant. Using this approach, 36 out of 50 infants with complete DGS treated by Dr. Markert at Duke University were reported to survive. In most cases, naive T cells appear at around 4–7 months of age; these cells are tolerant to donor thymic cells, display a polyclonal repertoire, and have normal proliferative capacity. Although the number of $CD3^+$ T cells in transplanted patients often remains lower than normal, their diversity and function is sufficient to prevent life-threatening infections.

FOXN1 Deficiency

The transcription factor FOXN1 (whose gene is mutated in the *nude* mouse) plays a critical role in thymus and eccrine glands development. *FOXN1* mutations in humans cause athymia, profound T-cell lymphopenia, alopecia totalis, and nail dystrophy. Similar to DGS, reconstitution of T-cell immunity can be achieved with thymic transplantation.

CHARGE Syndrome

This syndrome is characterized by the association of coloboma, heart anomalies, choanal atresia, mental retardation, genital and ear anomalies, and immunodeficiency. Most cases are sporadic, and represent de novo mutations of the *CHD7* or of the *SEMA3E* genes; less frequently, the disease is inherited as an autosomal dominant trait. The immunodeficiency is secondary to defects of thymic development. There is a variable degree of T-cell lymphopenia, which in some cases is very severe, resembling SCID.

SEVERE COMBINED IMMUNE DEFICIENCY DUE TO EARLY DEFECTS IN T LYMPHOCYTE DEVELOPMENT

SCID, the most severe form of congenital immunodeficiency, is caused by defects that completely abrogate the development of T lymphocytes, and in some cases also that of B and/or natural killer (NK) lymphocytes. Advances in the genes responsible, newborn screening, and gene therapy have had a strong impact on diagnosis and therapy of SCID.

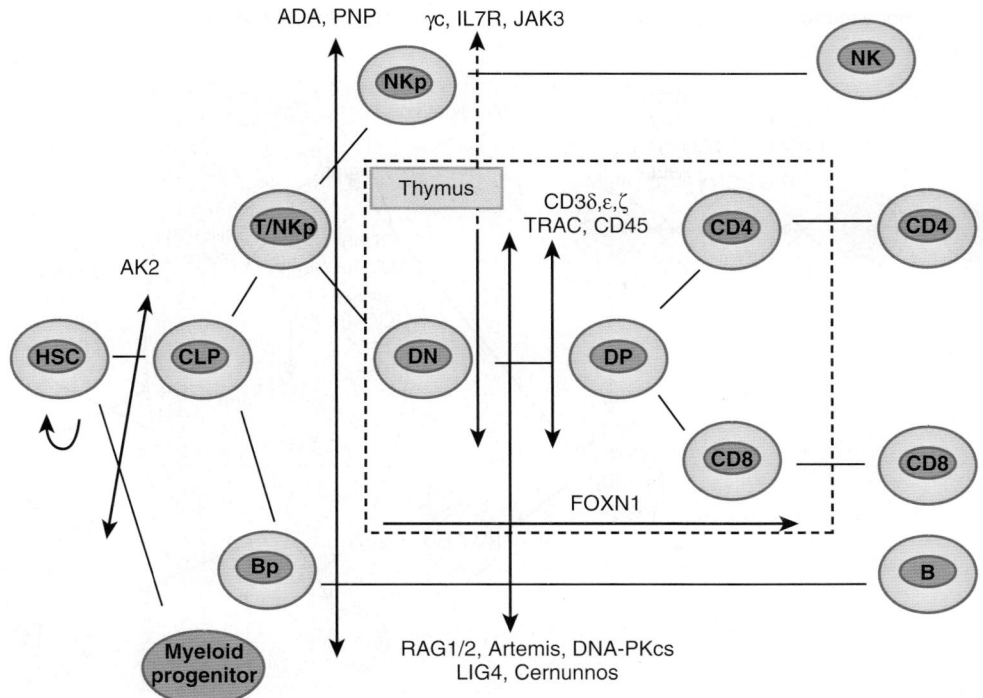

ADA, PNP   γc, IL7R, JAK3

Fig. 51.1 GENETIC DEFECTS ASSOCIATED WITH SEVERE COMBINED IMMUNE DEFICIENCY. Schematic representation of blocks (*arrows*) in lymphoid development associated with genetic defects responsible for SCID. *Dashed line* indicates that the generation of NK lymphocytes is compromised in γc and JAK3 deficiency, but not in IL7R deficiency. *ADA,* Adenosine deaminase; *AK2,* adenylate kinase 2; *B,* B-cell; *Bp,* B-cell progenitor; *CLP,* common lymphoid progenitor; *DN,* double-negative thymocyte; *DNA-PKcs,* DNA protein kinase catalytic subunit; *DP,* double-positive thymocyte; *γc,* common gamma chain; *HSC,* hematopoietic stem cell; *IL7R,* interleukin-7 receptor; *JAK3,* Janus-associated kinase 3; *LIG4,* DNA ligase IV; *NK,* natural killer cell; *NKp,* natural killer cell progenitor cell; *PNP,* purine nucleoside phosphorylase; *RAG,* recombinase activating gene; *T/NKp,* common progenitor of T and natural killer lymphocytes; *TRAC,* T-cell receptor alpha constant chain.

Pathobiology and Genetics

Genetic defects that cause SCID affect various stages in T-cell development (Fig. 51.1), and can be grouped into three major categories: (1) defects in cytokine receptor signaling; (2) defects in lymphocyte survival; and (3) defects of expression and function of the pre–T-cell receptor

Cytokine Receptor Signaling Defects

The most common form of SCID in humans is the X-linked form due to mutations of the *IL2RG* gene, which encodes for the common gamma chain (γc). This protein is shared by receptors for interleukin (IL)-2, IL-4, IL-7, IL-9, IL-15, and IL-21, and signals through the intracellular kinase Janus-activated kinase (JAK)3. Patients with mutations in *IL2RG* or *JAK3* lack both T and NK cells, because development of these subsets depends on IL-7- and IL-15-mediated signaling, respectively. B lymphocytes are present but antibody production is impaired because of the lack of T cells and of defective signaling through IL-21R.

Defects in Lymphocyte Survival

Proliferation and survival of lymphoid progenitor cells are essential to permit generation of a normal number of mature lymphocytes. Some forms of SCID are associated with increased apoptosis. Adenosine deaminase (ADA) converts adenosine to inosine (and deoxyadenosine to deoxyinosine). In patients with ADA deficiency, accumulation of toxic phosphorylated derivatives of deoxyadenosine

causes cell death and results in extreme lymphopenia, with virtual absence of T, B, and NK lymphocytes. Reticular dysgenesis (RD) is a form of SCID characterized by the association of severe lymphopenia, agranulocytosis, and sensorineural deafness. RD is caused by defects in adenylate kinase 2 (AK2), resulting in increased sensitivity to reactive oxygen species and increased apoptosis.

Defects of Expression and Signaling Through the Pre–T-Cell Receptor and the TCR

Rearrangement of the T-cell receptor (TCR) genes by means of VDJ recombination allows expression of the pre-TCR (composed of the pre-Tα and the TCR-β chain), and of mature TCR (either as TCR-αβ or TCR-γδ).

The lymphoid-specific recombinase-activating genes (RAG) 1 and RAG2 proteins initiate VDJ recombination by recognizing recombination-specific sequences that flank the variable (V), diversity (D), and joining (J) elements of the TCR and of immunoglobulin genes, introducing DNA double-strand breaks. These are then repaired through the ubiquitously expressed nonhomologous endjoining (NHEJ) pathway. Mutations of the *RAG1* and *RAG2* genes, and of genes that encode for Artemis, DNA ligase IV, and DNA-protein kinase Cs (PKCs; all components of the NHEJ pathway), result in SCID with a lack of T and B lymphocytes (see Figs. 51.1 and 51.2), but normal numbers of NK lymphocytes. Mutations of Cernunnos/XLF, another component of the NHEJ pathway, severely impair, but do not completely abrogate, T- and B-cell development. Because NHEJ is involved in general mechanisms of DNA repair also in nonlymphoid cells, patients with defects of this pathway also show

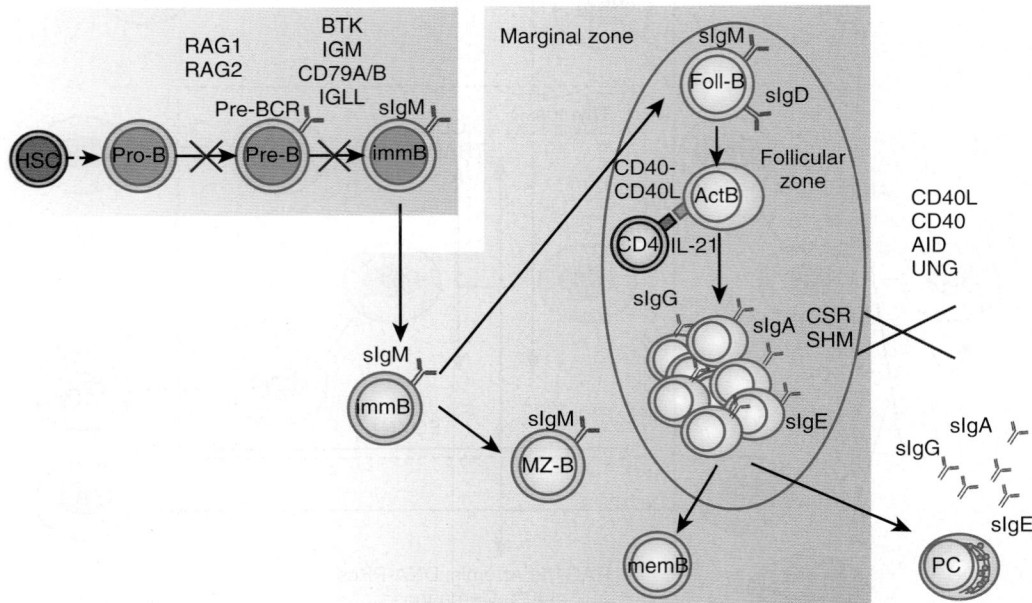

Bone marrow   Spleen/lymph node

Fig. 51.2 GENETIC DEFECTS ASSOCIATED WITH HYPOGAMMAGLOBULINEMIA. Schematic of B-cell development in bone marrow and secondary lymphoid organs, including migration of B cells into the follicular zone where they undergo activation, class-switch recombination (CSR), and somatic hypermutation (SHM). "X" denotes maturation steps at which the genes indicated are required, resulting in a block in differentiation at that stage when the gene is deficient. *ActB*, Activated B cell; *AID*, activation-induced cytidine deaminase; *BTK*, Bruton's tyrosine kinase; *HSC*, hematopoietic stem cell; *IGLL*, immunoglobulin light-like chain; *IL-21*, interleukin-21; *immB*, immature B cell (also termed *transitional B cell*); *memB*, memory B cell; *MZ-B*, marginal zone B cell; *PC*, plasma cell; *Pre-B*, precursor B cell; *Pre-BCR*, pre–B-cell receptor; *Pro-B*, progenitor B cell; *RAG1*, recombination activating gene 1; *RAG2*, recombination-activating gene 2; *sIgA*, surface IgA; *sIgD*, surface IgD; *sIgG*, surface IgG; *sIgM*, surface immunoglobulin M; *UNG*, uracil-DNA glycosylase.

increased cellular radiation sensitivity, are at higher risk of tumors, and may present with neurologic problems.

Signaling through the pre-TCR is essential to promote progression from CD4⁻CD8⁻ double-negative (DN) thymocytes to CD4⁺CD8⁺ double-positive (DP) cells, and is mediated by the CD3 complex. Mutations of the CD3δ (*CD3D*), CD3ε (*CD3E*), and CD3ζ (*CD3Z*) chains interfere with this process and result in SCID. In contrast, mutations of CD3γ (*CD3G*) are more often associated with a milder phenotype that includes autoimmunity. Finally, mutations of the CD45 phosphatase, also involved in cell signaling, cause T⁻ B⁺ SCID.

Clinical and Laboratory Manifestations

Typical clinical features of SCID include early-onset severe infections caused by bacteria, viruses, fungi, and opportunistic pathogens (including *P. jiroveci* pneumonia), protracted diarrhea, candidiasis, and failure to thrive. Engraftment of maternally derived T lymphocytes is common in SCID, occurring in 40% to 56% of infants with the disease. It may be asymptomatic or may manifest similarly to graft-versus-host disease (GVHD): skin rash, elevation of liver enzymes, diarrhea, and cytopenias. Hypomorphic mutations in SCID-causing genes may lead to residual development of T cells that undergo peripheral expansion and infiltrate target organs, causing various symptoms (erythroderma, diarrhea, hepatosplenomegaly, lymphadenopathy, diarrhea). This clinical phenotype is also known as *Omenn syndrome*.

Some forms of SCID may present with additional clinical features (see earlier section on Defects in Thymic Development). In patients with ADA deficiency, accumulation of toxic metabolites may cause

cupping and flaring of the ribs, liver dysfunction, sensorineural deafness and neurobehavioral problems. Microcephaly is typically seen in forms of SCID associated with cellular radiosensitivity and impairment of DNA double-strand break repair. Sensorineural deafness is observed in RD.

Family history (including consanguinity, deaths in infancy, and gender of other affected family members) may be suggestive of X-linked versus autosomal recessive inheritance. Measurement of absolute lymphocyte count (ALC) and the absolute number of CD3⁺ T lymphocytes, CD4⁺ and CD8⁺ T-cell subsets, CD19⁺ B lymphocytes, and NK (CD16⁺/CD56⁺ NK lymphocytes) confirms the diagnosis and may direct the work-up towards specific gene defects. The presence of CD3⁺ cells in a child with clear clinical manifestations of SCID may indicate maternal T-cell engraftment or with hypomorphic mutations that allow residual T-cell development. In both of these situations, the T cells have an activated/memory (CD45RO⁺), whereas T cells in normal infants are predominantly naive (CD45RA⁺). In vitro proliferative response to mitogens is drastically reduced in patients with SCID, but may be partially preserved in infants with Omenn syndrome. Other diagnostic tests that may support the diagnosis of SCID include lack of a thymic shadow at chest x-ray, and low or undetectable serum IgA and IgM. IgG serum levels may be normal early in life, reflecting the transplacental passage of maternally derived antibodies.

Diagnosis by Universal Newborn Screening

SCID can be diagnosed at birth by measuring levels of TCR excision circles (TRECs). TRECs are a byproduct of V(D)J recombination and are present as circularized DNA fragments in newly generated,

Diagnostic Approach to Severe Combined Immune Deficiency

- SCID presents early in life with severe infections of bacterial, viral, or fungal origin.
- Opportunistic infections are common in infants with SCID.
- Respiratory infections, protracted diarrhea, and failure to thrive are typical signs at presentation.
- Lymphopenia is present in 50% to 70% of infants with SCID. Age-specific norms must be used in evaluating the ALC as infants and children have much higher ALCs than adults (3500–13,000 in very young infants versus 1000–2800 in adults).
- T-cell lymphopenia is the hallmark of the disease; abnormalities of the absolute count of B and NK lymphocytes are observed in some forms of SCID. However, T lymphocytes may be present in SCID infants with maternal T-cell engraftment or with hypomorphic mutations in SCID-associated genes that allow residual T-cell development. Thus, a normal ALC does not rule out SCID.
- Maternally engrafted T cells proliferate in the infant with SCID in vivo, but the vast majority do not proliferate in vitro when stimulated with traditionally used mitogens such as concanavalin A and phytohemagglutinin, as measured by thymidine incorporation. Thus, if SCID is suspected, but T cells are detectable, maternal engraftment studies and proliferation to mitogens must be sent.
- Universal newborn screening has now been implemented in the majority of states in the United States. The analyte is detection of TRECs by quantitative PCR. TRECs are high in newly generated T cells and low when T cells are absent or when maternally engrafted T cells are present.
- SCID is genetically heterogeneous. The most common form in Western countries is inherited as an X-linked trait and is T⁻B⁺NK⁻.
- The lack of all lymphocytes (T⁻B⁻NK⁻ SCID) is highly suspicious for the ADA form of SCID, in which toxic metabolites result in death of all lymphocytes. Testing for ADA enzyme level is critical, because if confirmed to be absent, treatment with PEG-ADA can often result in sufficient reconstitution of T-cell immunity to protect the baby from infection.

naive T lymphocytes that express the αβ form of the TCR. Levels of TRECs in circulating lymphocytes are particularly high in newborns and infants, and can be detected by PCR amplification of DNA extracted from the Guthrie card. Newborn screening was recommended for addition to the standard panel in the United States in 2010, and in 2015 >70% of births were screened for SCID. Based on screening of ~3,000,000 infants in the United States, the incidence of SCID is now estimated to be 1 in 58,000 births, higher than with clinical screening alone.

Prognosis, Therapy and Future Directions

Supportive Management

Management of SCID includes observance of strict hygiene measures, prevention of *P. jiroveci* pneumonia with TMP-SMZ, prompt investigation and aggressive treatment of infections, immunoglobulin replacement, and adequate support with enteral or parenteral nutrition. Infections caused by cytomegalovirus (CMV; causing interstitial pneumonia, hepatitis and/or gastroenteritis) and Epstein-Barr virus (EBV; causing lymphoproliferative disease) require active surveillance and preemptive therapy. To prevent transmission of viral infection, blood products from CMV-seronegative donors or leukofiltered products should be used, and must be irradiated to prevent transfusion-associated GVHD. Immunosuppression with steroids and cyclosporine A may be needed to treat GVHD-like manifestations associated with Omenn syndrome or maternal T-cell engraftment. Administration of live vaccines must be avoided in infants with SCID. In spite of these measures, SCID is inevitably fatal within the first few years of life, unless immune reconstitution is achieved with treatment.

Ultimately, infants with SCID should be evaluated for specific gene defects. However, definitive treatment of SCID (typically by hematopoietic cell transplantation; HCT) should not await demonstration of a specific gene defect, as this may take some time. An exception to this general principle is ADA deficiency that can be easily diagnosed by measuring enzyme activity in red blood cells, allowing prompt initiation of enzyme-replacement therapy (ERT), which improves lymphocyte counts. Weekly intramuscular injection of pegylated bovine ADA acts extracellularly to transform adenosine and deoxyadenosine into inosine and deoxyinosine, respectively, thus preventing accumulation of toxic phosphorylated derivatives. Disadvantages of ERT include expense, as it must be continued indefinitely, waning of therapeutic effect over time, and the development in some patients of neutralizing antibodies to PEG-ADA.

General Principles of Hematopoietic Cell Transplantation for SCID

HCT is the standard treatment that promotes long-term immune reconstitution in infants with SCID. HCT for other conditions is generally performed with chemotherapy or radiation conditioning, to prevent graft rejection and eliminate or reduce host hematopoietic stem cells (HSCs), favoring donor hematopoiesis. Because of the lack of T lymphocytes, infants with SCID (especially the NK⁻ forms) are generally considered to have an inherent inability to reject the graft, and may therefore receive HCT from an HLA-identical related donor (sibling) without conditioning. T-cell reconstitution in this case is generally prompt, with initial reconstitution in the first 1–3 months mediated by expansion of mature T cells present in the donor bone marrow, and later reconstitution derived from newly generated T cells that mature in the thymus from donor HSC and progenitors. GVHD prophylaxis is not needed. Unconditioned HCT may also be performed from mismatched related donors (parent), with T-cell depletion of the graft to avoid fatal GVHD. Here the reconstitution is slower, since the generation of T cells is entirely dependent on thymic ontogeny and can take 4–6 months. Engraftment of T cells may not always occur in this setting and up to 25% of patients may require repeat transplantation. GVHD prophylaxis is not needed if the T-cell depletion is sufficiently rigorous. These approaches to HCT without conditioning can lead to sustained T-cell immune reconstitution because of the selective advantage for donor cells differentiating into the T lineage. However, this approach rarely results in significant donor HSC engraftment, which is generally <1%, and thus may fail to correct impairment of humoral immunity.

HCT from matched unrelated adult or cord blood donors has been generally performed with myeloablative conditioning, similar to that used for other nonmalignant disorders. As in the case of sibling donor HCT, memory T cells present in the graft after unrelated adult donor HCT may provide some initial protection against infection (according to their antigen specificity). In contrast, the naive T lymphocytes contained within cord blood provide little antigen-specific immunity early after HCT. Conditioning prior to unrelated donor HCT, or prior to mismatched related HCT, improves the rate of HSC engraftment, but results in short-term and long-term toxicity and increased risk of GVHD. Reduced-intensity conditioning regimens have been proposed with the aim to facilitate stem cell engraftment while reducing the risk of treatment-related toxicity; however, there is no clear evidence that such regimens are associated with better outcome in patients with SCID treated by HCT.

Survival and Long-Term Outcomes After HCT for SCID

While survival after HCT for SCID has improved with time due to advances in early diagnosis and supportive care for infants with SCID, donor type, the presence of infection, and subtype of SCID remain important determinants of outcome. Studies of 10-year survival in 699 infants with SCID in Europe and 5-year survival in 240 infants with SCID in North America confirm excellent survival of 90% and 94%, respectively, after matched sibling donor HCT. Outcomes after mismatched related, unrelated adult volunteer, and umbilical cord blood HCT have improved, although a clear advantage of one alternative donor versus another has not been demonstrated. Mismatched related donor HCT performed without conditioning may be associated with better survival than when conditioning is given.

Respiratory infections and older age at the time of transplant have long been associated with poorer outcome. Infants older than 3.5 months at the time of HCT who have never had infection or had infections that were amenable to treatment prior to HCT interestingly have similar survival to infants younger than 3.5 months at the time of HCT. Among infants who were not actively infected at the time of HCT, survival was very good even for alternative donor recipients. These results suggest that early diagnosis and protection of infection, i.e., through newborn screening, would improve survival significantly. The specific type of SCID also affects outcome: survival after HCT is better in patients with B⁺ than B⁻ SCID.

In infants with SCID, long-term T-cell reconstitution may be achieved in the absence of conditioning and the absence of engraftment of donor-derived stem cells, due to engraftment of committed lymphoid progenitors that seed the thymus. Consistent with this, donor T-cell chimerism and T-cell reconstitution after HCT are achieved in >90% of infants with SCID and the majority have a polyclonal repertoire. The durability of T-cell reconstitution in the absence of conditioning is variable, and some reports have indicated a progressive decline of thymic function after HCT for SCID. Such reports are supported by the finding that survivors after HCT performed with conditioning have higher T-cell counts and higher naive CD4⁺ CD45RA⁺ T-cell counts than those after HCT performed without conditioning. Reconstitution of humoral immunity after HCT for SCID is less uniform; for genetic subtypes that affect B-cell development or function, engraftment of donor B cells is typically required for humoral immune reconstitution. For example, inadequate B-cell function (requiring immunoglobulin-replacement therapy) is often observed in patients with γc and JAK3 deficiency who remain with autologous B cells, due to intrinsic defects in the host B cells' response to γc-dependent cytokines such as IL-4 and IL-21. The number of circulating NK lymphocytes often remains low in patients with γc and JAK3 deficiency, and may contribute to the increased risk of warts.

Rates of acute GVHD (aGVHD) are generally low, ~20%, largely limited to recipients of alternative donor HCT. Patients with poor T-cell reconstitution are at risk for viral and opportunistic infections; autoimmunity (especially cytopenias and hypothyroidism) has been reported in 10% to 20% of these patients, particularly in those with cGVHD. Other long-term complications include nutritional problems, poor growth and development, and neurologic complications (mental retardation, motor dysfunction, sensorineural hearing deficits). Some of these complications are more common in certain subtypes, particularly growth in patients with Artemis-SCID and neurologic problems in patients with ADA deficiency.

Gene Therapy for SCID

Gene therapy, in which the gene of interest is introduced into the patient's own cells, is an attractive therapeutic option for SCID, in particular for infants who do not have an HLA-identical related donor. Expression of the normal copy of the gene in CD34⁺ stem cells confers a selective advantage to the gene-corrected cells during T-cell differentiation. Furthermore, there is no risk of GVHD. Gene therapy has been used successfully to correct SCID in patients with ADA deficiency and with X-linked SCID.

Since the year 2000, more than 70 patients with ADA-deficient SCID have been treated with gene therapy worldwide. Published reports from Milan (Italy), London (United Kingdom) and the United States have collectively described 26 patients who received autologous CD34⁺ progenitor cells transduced with gammaretroviral

> ### Therapeutic Approach to Severe Combined Immune Deficiency
>
> - HSC transplantation is the mainstay of treatment. Optimal survival is achieved when the transplant is performed early in life. This is now possible with newborn screening.
> - Transplantation for SCID can be performed without conditioning, due to the profound absence of T cells and inability to reject. Thus, the bone marrow of a fully HLA-matched sibling can be infused without manipulation and without giving any conditioning to the baby. GVHD prophylaxis is also not necessary. Haploidentical bone marrow from a parent can also be infused without conditioning but must first be T-cell depleted.
> - Such transplants without conditioning can result in T-cell reconstitution that lasts for decades. In the case of a matched sibling graft, initial T-cell reconstitution is rapid, generally within the first 1–3 months, due to proliferation of mature T cells. In the case of a haploidentical graft, mature T cells are removed and thus 4–6 months is required for HSC to develop and emerge from the thymus as mature T cells.
> - Without conditioning, only a low number of donor-derived long-lived HSCs engraft, and this may lead to lack of donor B-cell reconstitution and lack of humoral immunity. With conditioning, donor HSCs are more likely to engraft and give rise to donor B cells. Currently, matched unrelated donor transplants are performed with conditioning.
> - Enzyme replacement may be used in patients with adenosine deaminase deficiency. Gene therapy has offered promising results; however, it is also associated with increased risk of leukemic proliferation due to insertional mutagenesis.

vectors expressing the ADA complementary (c)DNA. All are alive, with sustained production of gene marked T, B and myeloid cells, and the majority of patients have been able to stop ERT. In all trials, engraftment of gene-corrected stem cells has been facilitated by the use of a reduced-intensity chemotherapy regimen with low-dose busulfan.

Twenty patients with X-linked SCID were treated by gene therapy using a gammaretroviral vector in Paris and London at the turn of the century, without chemotherapy conditioning. Eighteen patients are alive, and 17 of them show normalization of T-cell count and function, with sustained thymic output, diversified T-cell repertoire, and ability to mount antigen-specific T-cell responses. In a few cases, improvement of humoral immunity has also been observed. However, leukemic T-cell proliferation due to insertional mutagenesis was observed in 5 out of 20 patients. A modified self-inactivating gammaretroviral vector based on the previously mentioned parent vector has now been reported to be efficacious in nine patients with X-linked SCID in a multicenter trial. Preliminary evidence from this trial suggests that deletion of viral enhancers has decreased expansion of clones bearing insertion sites near lymphoid protooncogenes, suggesting an improved safety profile with regard to leukemogenesis. Self-inactivating lentiviral vectors based on HIV are being developed and/or tested in both ADA and X-linked SCID.

OTHER COMBINED IMMUNODEFICIENCIES

Defects of TCR Signaling

Several forms of combined immune deficiency are caused by genetic defects that affect molecules involved in TCR signaling. In particular, the T lymphocyte-specific protein tyrosine kinase (Lck) associates with CD4 and CD8 molecules and mediates phosphorylation of CD3 chains upon TCR engagement. The Zeta-associated protein of 70 kDa (ZAP-70) tyrosine kinase phosphorylates the CD3 chains, thus promoting downstream TCR signaling. RHOH is an atypical Rho GTPase that participates in receptor-induced signaling in hematopoietic cells. The IL-2-inducible tyrosine kinase (ITK) is a member of the thymic epithelial cell (TEC) family of nonreceptor tyrosine kinases, and modulates the strength of the TCR-induced signal. The serine-threonine protein kinase 4 (STK4) protein induces the transcriptional coactivation of target genes involved in cell proliferation and survival, and is involved in the control of cell death.

At variance with typical forms of SCID, genetic defects of TCR signaling are characterized by residual number and/or function of T cells, consistent with partially preserved thymic architecture and function. Since the thymus of these patients is not empty, the use of chemotherapy is required to facilitate engraftment and T-cell differentiation with donor-derived cells. The immunological phenotype of ZAP-70 deficiency in humans is characterized by a virtual lack of CD8+ lymphocytes; the number of CD4+ cells is preserved, but they are unable to proliferate in response to mitogens and antigens. In contrast, both CD4+ and CD8+ lymphocytes are absent in $Zap7^{-/-}$ mice.

Both RHOH and STK4 deficiencies are characterized by a reduced number of naive T cells, an increased proportion of effector memory T cells (including CD8+ cells with an "exhausted" CD45RA+CCR7− phenotype), and defective lymphocyte proliferation. CD4 lymphopenia and low levels of CD4 and CD8 surface expression have been reported in one patient with LCK deficiency. Progressive CD4 lymphopenia is also commonly seen in patients with ITK deficiency.

All of these forms of impaired TCR signaling are inherited as autosomal recessive traits. Clinically, patients with impaired T-cell signaling present with recurrent, often severe, infections. Cutaneous viral infections are especially common in patients with RHOH and STK4 deficiency. The clinical phenotype of ZAP-70 deficiency is often undistinguishable from SCID; in a few cases, hypomorphic ZAP70 mutations have been associated with Omenn syndrome. Severe lung disease and a high risk of EBV-driven lymphoproliferation are a hallmark of ITK deficiency. Autoimmune manifestations have been observed in several patients with these disorders. Prevention of infections is based on antimicrobial prophylaxis and use of intravenous immunoglobulins; however, ultimate treatment requires HCT.

Coronin-1A Deficiency

Coronin-1A is involved in reorganization of the actin cytoskeleton that allows egress of thymocytes to the periphery. While complete deficiency of coronin-1A in humans is a cause of SCID, hypomorphic mutations have been associated with severe naive T-cell lymphopenia, oligoclonal expansion of activated T cells, and increased risk of EBV-driven lymphoproliferation.

HLA Class II Deficiency

Expression of HLA class II molecules on the surface of thymic epithelial and dendritic cells is essential to promote positive selection of CD4+ lymphocytes. HLA class II deficiency includes a group of autosomal recessive disorders in which mutations in transcription factors (CIITA, RFXAP, RFX5, and RFXANK) that regulate HLA class II gene expression result in profoundly reduced numbers of CD4+ lymphocytes. The clinical phenotype consists of recurrent infections since infancy. Treatment is based on antimicrobial prophylaxis, regular use of immunoglobulins, and HCT. Persistence of CD4 lymphopenia is often observed after HCT, because transplantation of hematopoietic stem cells does not correct defective expression of HLA class II molecules on the surface of TECs, causing defective positive selection of CD4+ lymphocytes.

HLA Class I Deficiency

Presentation of antigens in association with MHC class I molecules is important for thymic development of CD8+ lymphocytes and for the development of antigen-specific cytotoxic T-cell responses. In addition, HLA class I molecules also modulate the function of NK cells that express several HLA class I-binding molecules. HLA class I molecules are assembled and loaded with peptides in the endoplasmic reticulum by transporter associated with antigen presentation (TAP) proteins (TAP1 and TAP2) and the TAP binding or Tapasin protein (TAPBP). Mutations of TAP1, TAP2, or TAPBP cause defective expression of HLA class I molecules, which is associated with a severe reduction in the number of circulating CD8+ TCRαβ+ lymphocytes. NK cells expressing killer inhibitory receptors may not receive HLA class I-dependent inhibitory signals, and hence may mount cytotoxic responses to uninfected cells, causing inflammatory lesions in the lungs and in the skin. There is no definitive treatment for this disease, and management is based on supportive care.

CD40 Ligand and CD40 Deficiencies

CD40 ligand (CD40LG) is expressed by activated CD4+ cells. Interaction of CD40LG-expressing CD4+ cells with B lymphocytes that constitutively express CD40 delivers a signal for B-cell proliferation and class-switch recombination in the presence of appropriate cytokines (see Fig. 51.2). Furthermore, interaction between CD40LG-expressing CD4+ lymphocytes and CD40+ dendritic cells and macrophages promotes secretion of IL-12, and thus enables the development of Th1 responses against intracellular pathogens.

The CD40LG gene is located on the X chromosome (at Xq26). Males with CD40LG mutations suffer from a combined immunodeficiency characterized by recurrent infections, often caused by opportunistic pathogens. P. jiroveci pneumonia classically occurs in the first year of life, but may occur at any age. Cryptosporidium parvum infection may cause chronic watery diarrhea and lead to sclerosing cholangitis. Chronic or intermittent neutropenia has been frequently observed. Patients with CD40LG deficiency are also uniquely prone to tumors of the liver and biliary tract.

Levels of serum IgG and IgA are markedly reduced or undetectable; IgM may be normal or increased, and for this reason the disease is also known as X-linked hyper-IgM syndrome. The number of memory B cells is also markedly reduced.

In vitro activation of T cells with phorbol myristate acetate and ionomycin fails to induce expression of CD40LG on the surface of CD4+ cells, whereas other activation markers (e.g., CD69) are normally expressed.

The prognosis is severe. Death may occur early in life secondary to infections, or during late childhood and young adulthood due to severe liver disease and tumors. Clinical management consists of continuous prophylaxis of Pneumocystis infection with TMP-SMZ, regular use of intravenous immunoglobulins, and hygiene measures to limit the risk of exposure to Cryptosporidium. HCT is the only definitive cure, with survival of ~70% reported in Europe. Preexisting pulmonary disease and Cryptosporidium infection are risk factors for less favorable outcome.

CD40 deficiency is a very rare autosomal recessive disorder, whose clinical and immunological phenotype is indistinguishable from CD40LG deficiency (see Fig. 51.2). The diagnosis is based on the lack of expression of CD40 on the surface of circulating B lymphocytes. Management is as for CD40LG deficiency.

Defects of NF-κB Signaling

The nuclear factor kappa-B (NF-κB) signaling pathway is ubiquitous to all tissues and stages of development, playing critical roles in cell proliferation, oncogenesis, cell survival, and inflammatory responses. Several genetic defects affecting activation of NF-κB have been described that result in combined immune deficiency variably associated with extra-immune manifestations. Hypomorphic mutations in the IKBKG gene, which encodes for the NF-κB essential modulator (NEMO; also known as IKK-γ), the regulatory subunit of the IκB kinase complex, are inherited as an X-linked trait and represent the prototype of disorders of NF-κB signaling. Complete lack of NEMO expression is embryonically lethal in males; females who are heterozygous for null NEMO mutations suffer from incontinentia pigmenti. Typically, males with NEMO deficiency present with ectodermal dysplasia and immunodeficiency (EDA-ID). The phenotypic manifestations of EDA-ID are largely restricted to epithelial tissues and the immune system, with sparse hair, shiny skin, lack of sweat glands and other appendages, and rare conical-shaped teeth. There is often frontal bossing and a characteristic facies. Typical infections are caused by bacteria, including sepsis and meningitis, especially *Streptococcus pneumoniae*, *Staphylococcus*, and *Haemophilus influenzae*; DNA viral infections such as CMV and herpes simplex virus (HSV); and atypical mycobacterial infection. Pneumocystis and other opportunistic infections may also occur. Inflammatory colitis is a frequent manifestation of immune dysregulation. Lymphedema and osteopetrosis have been reported in some patients. Occasionally, manifestations of ectodermal dysplasia may be modest or even absent, thus adding to phenotypic heterogeneity. Immunological abnormalities include variable defects in T-cell proliferation to mitogen and antigens, hypogammaglobulinemia with normal or high IgM, defective antibody production (especially against polysaccharides), and impairment of NK-cell cytotoxicity. Finally, monocytes from patients with NEMO deficiency fail to elaborate inflammatory cytokines such as tumor necrosis factor (TNF)α in response to stimulation by a variety of Toll-like receptor ligands. A similar clinical and immunological phenotype is observed in patients with autosomal dominant EDA-ID caused by gain-of-function mutations of the *IKBA* gene. In these patients, the mutated IKB-α protein cannot be phosphorylated at residues that are critical for its degradation. This prevents release of the cytoplasmic components of NF-κB, which cannot translocate to the nucleus and mediate transcription of target genes.

Aside from supportive therapy with intravenous immunoglobulin replacement, antibiotic prophylaxis and treatment of infections, HCT for these disorders has been used with variable success. Because of the role of NF-κB signaling in nonhematopoietic tissues, certain manifestations of the disease, such as colitis, may not be uniformly ameliorated by HCT.

Mutations of the *IKBKB* gene are responsible for an autosomal recessive disease, characterized by a SCID-like phenotype without ectodermal dystrophy. Patients lack regulatory T cells and TCRγδ+ T cells. The *MAP3K14* gene encodes for NIK, a component of the noncanonical NF-κB signaling pathway. Patients with NIK deficiency suffer from recurrent infections. Immunological abnormalities include reduced T-cell proliferation, hypogammaglobulinemia with reduced number of total and switched memory B cells, and NK deficiency.

The CARD11–BCL10–MALT1 complex regulates NF-κB signaling. Deficiency of any of these proteins causes combined immune deficiency with increased susceptibility to infections. T-cell proliferation is impaired. Defective antibody responses are observed in patients with BCL10 and CARD11 deficiency; the latter condition is also characterized by an increase in the proportion of transitional B cells.

DOCK2 Deficiency

The dedicator of cytokinesis (DOCK) proteins are atypical guanine exchange factors containing a phosphatidylinositol (3,4,5)-triphosphate (PIP3) binding domain and a Rho-family GTPase binding domain with guanine exchange factor activity. DOCK2 is predominantly expressed in various hematopoietic cell lineages (including T, B, NK, and NKT lymphocytes, as well as granulocytes and other myeloid cells), and is activated in response to engagement of the TCR, BCR, and chemokine receptors. DOCK2 activation allows formation of GTP-Rac1, thereby promoting reorganization of the cellular cytoskeleton, and intracellular signaling. DOCK2 deficiency is an autosomal recessive combined immunodeficiency characterized by increased susceptibility to severe infections starting early in life. Severe varicella has been reported in multiple patients. T-cell lymphopenia, with marked reduction of naive T cells and impaired T-cell proliferation, defective antibody responses, reduced NK cell function,

poor migration of T and B lymphocytes in response to chemokines, NKT-cell deficiency, and markedly reduced secretion of interferon-alpha (IFN-α) by plasmacytoid dendritic cells represent the major immunological abnormalities. Low TREC levels at birth have been reported in two patients. The prognosis is very severe, but definitive cure may be achieved with HCT. Use of systemic IFN-α may help in the treatment of severe viral infections.

DOCK8 Deficiency

DOCK8 deficiency is an autosomal recessive combined immunodeficiency characterized by severe and recurrent infections, particularly systemic and cutaneous viral infection (molluscum contagiosium, HSV-1 and HSV-2, human papillomavirus), allergic manifestations (early-onset eczema, food allergies) with elevated serum IgE, impaired humoral immunity (with frequent sinopulmonary infections), and increased risk for squamous cell carcinoma and lymphoma. Large intragenic deletions account for the majority of the mutations. Affected patients have low numbers of naive CD8 T cells, and accumulation of CD8 memory cells with an "exhausted phenotype". A profound impairment in the generation of CD8+ memory T cells in response to influenza or other viral infections has been reported. Humoral immunity is also compromised, with loss of germinal center B cells and defective immunoglobulin affinity maturation. The disease has a severe prognosis, with considerable mortality. HCT represents the only definitive treatment. Use of systemic IFN-α may ameliorate manifestations of severe cutaneous viral infection.

Wiskott-Aldrich Syndrome

Wiskott-Aldrich syndrome (WAS) is an X-linked disorder, characterized by thrombocytopenia with small-sized platelets, eczema, and immunodeficiency. Autoimmune manifestations are common, and there is an increased risk of hematologic malignancies (primarily non-Hodgkin lymphoma, sometimes EBV driven). The estimated incidence is 1 in 100,000 births. The defect is due to mutations in the *WAS* gene, which encodes for an intracytoplasmic protein (WAS protein [WASp]) expressed in hematopoietic cells and involved in cytoskeleton reorganization and immune synapse formation. Deficiency of WASp results in impaired T-cell activation, poor production of antibodies, particularly to carbohydrate antigen, defective NK function, impaired phagocytic cell migration, and defective antigen presentation, thus explaining the immunodeficiency of the disease.

The clinical phenotype may range from typical and severe WAS to isolated thrombocytopenia; milder phenotypes are often associated with residual expression of WASp. Rarely, mutations occurring in the GTPase binding domain of the protein results in a hyperactive form of WASp, resulting in X-linked neutropenia and myelodysplasia without thrombocytopenia, eczema, or immunodeficiency.

Boys with WAS typically present in infancy with bleeding, prompting the discovery of low numbers of platelets with a low mean platelet volume. Bleeding manifestations can range from petechiae and bruising, to severe gastrointestinal and intracranial hemorrhages. Eczema can be mild to severe. Common infections in WAS patients include otitis, sinusitis, pneumonia, and cellulitis. Viral infections (especially from herpesviruses, including CMV, EBV, and HSV-1) and opportunistic infections, such as *P. jiroveci* pneumonia, are also frequent. Approximately 40% of patients with WAS develop autoimmunity, including autoimmune hemolytic anemia, autoimmune thrombocytopenia, thyroiditis, colitis, vasculitis, nephropathy, and arthritis. In addition to thrombocytopenia, typical laboratory findings include inability to mount responses to polysaccharide antigens, low or absent isohemagglutinin titers, high IgE, and poor proliferation of T cells when stimulated with anti-CD3 antibody. Other immune findings are more variable, including progressive T lymphopenia with age, low IgM, and high IgA. Analysis of WASp expression and demonstration of *WAS* gene mutations confirm the diagnosis.

Supportive treatment for WAS consists of monitoring and treatment for bleeding, antimicrobial prophylaxis, immunoglobulin-replacement therapy, and treatment of eczema and autoimmune manifestations with immunosuppressive drugs. Splenectomy can be effective in many to correct thrombocytopenia, but leads to increased risk of sepsis.

Allogeneic HCT (typically with myeloablative regimens) for WAS has become standard at many institutions, and may be indicated early in life, especially in patients with severe mutations that abrogate protein expression.

HCT is usually associated with robust T-cell engraftment, whereas some patients develop mixed chimerism in the B and myeloid lineages, indicating differential requirement for normal WAS protein to promote lineage-specific development or survival. Poor myeloid chimerism is associated with the risk of persistent thrombocytopenia, and mixed chimerism favors autoimmune manifestations.

Survival after HCT for WAS is influenced by donor type and age at transplantation. Optimal results, with approximately 90% survival, are obtained after HCT from an HLA-identical sibling donor. Results of HCT from matched unrelated donors are superior if the transplant is performed at a young age (<5 years), but are good overall even when the transplant is performed later in life. However, mixed chimerism may be associated with increased risk of autoimmunity, and low myeloid chimerism with persistence of thrombocytopenia.

Because outcome after HCT is not uniformly good and many patients lack matched related or unrelated donors, somatic gene therapy is an attractive treatment option for WAS. In a first trial, 10 boys with WAS were treated with gene therapy by transduction of CD34+-selected peripheral blood stem cells using a murine leukemia virus-based gammaretroviral vector after low-dose busulfan conditioning. Immune reconstitution was attained in nine patients; however, seven of these developed leukemia due to insertional mutagenesis. More recently, gene therapy for WAS has been performed using a self-inactivating lentiviral vector. Results show good immune reconstitution and improved safety (with no leukemic events reported); however, the platelet count, although increased, remains abnormally low in most patients.

COMBINED IMMUNODEFICIENCIES WITH OSSEOUS DYSPLASIA

Cartilage hair hypoplasia (CHH) is an autosomal recessive disorder characterized by short-limbed dwarfism, hair abnormalities, increased risk of bone marrow dysplasia, malignancies and Hirschsprung disease, and a variable degree of immunodeficiency. The majority of patients show susceptibility to bacterial and viral infections; however, some may present with SCID, Omenn syndrome, or selective deficiency of CD8+ cells. The disease is more common among certain ethnic groups (the Amish populations and the Finns), and is caused by mutations of the gene encoding for the untranslated RNA component of the ribonuclease mitochondrial RNA processing (RMRP) complex, which is involved in cleavage of ribosomal RNA, processing of mitochondrial RNA, and cell cycle control. Management of the immunologic problems in CHH depends on their severity. HCT may be indicated in cases with severe T lymphocyte defects.

Schimke immunoosseous dysplasia is an autosomal recessive disorder that also combines immunologic and skeletal abnormalities. These children have short stature, skeletal dysplasia, renal dysfunction and T-cell immunodeficiency caused by mutations in the SMARCAL1 gene.

OTHER COMBINED IMMUNODEFICIENCIES

Mutations of ICOS, a molecule expressed by activated T cells, were initially thought to cause a common variable immune deficiency (CVID)-like phenotype, but have more recently been shown to cause combined immune deficiency, with recurrent infections of the respiratory and gastrointestinal tracts, and autoimmunity.

Hepatic venoocclusive disease with immunodeficiency is an autosomal recessive condition caused by mutations of the SP110 gene. In addition to liver disease, patients are highly prone to infections that are often sustained by opportunistic pathogens (CMV, Candida, P. jiroveci). Cerebrospinal leukodystrophy has been observed in several cases. The disease is rapidly fatal, unless treated by HCT.

Autosomal recessive combined immune deficiency with intestinal atresias is caused by mutations in the TTC7A gene, which encodes for a protein involved in maintaining cell polarity in epithelial cells. Variable, but often severe, lymphopenia and panhypogammaglobulinemia are typical immunological abnormalities. The prognosis is generally severe and is determined by the severity of the gastrointestinal involvement and of immune deficiency. Small-bowel transplantation is often necessary. In patients with profound immune deficiency HCT may be required; however, limited data are available on long-term outcome.

The cytidine triphosphate synthase 1 (CTPS1) protein is essential for lymphocyte proliferation. Patients with CTPS1 deficiency have a high risk of recurrent and chronic infections (especially those due to herpesviruses), and of EBV-related lymphoma.

A very high risk of EBV-induced lymphoproliferative disease is also observed in patients with CD27 deficiency, who may also present with signs of hemophagocytic lymphohistiocytosis (HLH). These patients lack memory B cells and often develop hypogammaglobulinemia after EBV infection.

Finally, EBV-associated lymphoma is a common manifestation in patients with magnesium transporter type 1 (MAGT1) deficiency. This condition is inherited as an X-linked trait. The number of naive CD4+ T cells is reduced, and expression of NKG2D, an important activating molecule, on the surface of CD8+ cytotoxic T cells and NK lymphocytes, is markedly decreased. HCT can correct the disease.

IL-21 and IL-21R deficiencies are inherited as autosomal recessive traits. Gastrointestinal manifestations with colitis and Cryptosporidium-associated cholangitis have been reported. A single patient with Kaposi sarcoma and OX40 deficiency has been reported.

DISORDERS WITH T CELL-MEDIATED IMMUNE DYSREGULATION

Along with generation of a diversified repertoire of T and B lymphocytes, purging of self-reactive cells is essential to maintain immune homeostasis and prevent autoimmune diseases. We have already reported how autoimmune manifestations are common in severe forms of immunodeficiency characterized by oligoclonal expansion of T lymphocytes (e.g., Omenn syndrome, complete atypical DGS) and in patients with defects of T-cell signaling. Here, we describe other forms of primary immunodeficiency with faulty control of central or peripheral T-cell tolerance.

Autoimmune Polyendocrinopathy Candidiasis Ectodermal Dystrophy Syndrome

Also known as *autoimmune polyglandular syndrome type 1* (APS1), autoimmune polyendocrinopathy candidiasis ectodermal dystrophy (APECED) is an autosomal recessive disorder characterized by autoimmune endocrine manifestations (hypoparathyroidism, Addison disease), candidiasis, and nail dystrophy. The disease is caused by mutations of the autoimmune regulator (AIRE) gene, which encodes for a transcription factor expressed by medullary TECs (mTECs) where it regulates expression of tissue specific antigens that are presented to nascent T cells, thereby promoting clonal deletion of self-reactive T lymphocytes, or their conversion to natural regulatory T cells (nTreg cells).

In patients with APECED, mucocutaneous candidiasis usually develops first (in infancy or early childhood), followed by autoimmune hypoparathyroidism with hypocalcemia and adrenal failure. Around 15% to 20% of patients may develop insulin-dependent diabetes. Other autoimmune manifestations (hepatitis, ovarian failure) are also common. Hyposplenism has been reported in one study. Candidiasis may reflect elevated levels of antibodies to IL-17 and IL-22, which play an important role in the defense against *Candida* spp.

Management of patients with APECED is based on regular follow-up and search for autoantibodies, which should be repeated every 6 months. Hormone-replacement therapy is indicated for the endocrinopathies. Aggressive management and prevention of candidiasis is important to avoid persistent or recurrent infections that may favor development of squamous cell carcinoma.

Immune Dysregulation Polyendocrinopathy Enteropathy X-Linked Syndrome

Immune dysregulation polyendocrinopathy enteropathy X-linked (IPEX) is an X-linked disorder of systemic autoimmunity. Males with IPEX syndrome present early in life with skin rash, intractable watery diarrhea, insulin-dependent diabetes mellitus, lymphadenopathy, splenomegaly, and failure to thrive. Other autoimmune manifestations include thyroid disease, nephropathy, cytopenias, and vasculitis. In addition, patients with IPEX show elevated levels of IgE.

IPEX is caused by mutations of the *FOXP3* gene, which encodes for a transcription factor that plays a critical role in the development and function of regulatory T (Treg) lymphocytes. These cells have suppressive functions; they have a distinctive phenotype (CD4$^+$ CD25^{hi} FOXP3$^+$) and normally represent 5% to 15% of CD4$^+$ circulating lymphocytes. Most patients with IPEX lack Treg cells; activated self-reactive T lymphocytes infiltrate target tissues and secrete cytokines, causing tissue damage.

IPEX has a severe prognosis. Death often occurs within the first few years of life due to severe malabsorption, failure to thrive, metabolic derangement, or because of severe infections secondary to immune suppression. Use of immunosuppressive drugs (steroids, sirolimus, tacrolimus, rituximab) is necessary to treat the disease. However, the only definitive treatment is allogeneic HCT. Mixed chimerism is sufficient to control the disease; therefore, reduced-intensity conditioning has been used with good results.

CD25 and STAT5B Deficiencies

IL-2 plays an important role in T lymphocyte proliferation and in immune homeostasis. Upon binding to the high-affinity IL-2 receptor, IL-2 promotes phosphorylation and nuclear translocation of the transcription factor signal transducer and activator of transcription (STAT)5, which drives expression of IL-2 target genes, including *FOXP3*. Autosomal recessive mutations of the *IL2RA* (*CD25*) gene, which encodes for the α chain of the IL-2 receptor, cause a disease that is associated with IPEX-like manifestations (lymphadenopathy, hepatosplenomegaly, autoimmune cytopenias, inflammatory bowel disease) and increased susceptibility to severe viral infections. The number of circulating T cells may be normal or slightly reduced, and in vitro proliferative response to mitogens is decreased. The patients' T cells produce reduced amounts of the immunosuppressive cytokine IL-10 upon in vitro activation. HCT represents the only definitive treatment.

Autosomal recessive mutations of the *STAT5B* gene cause a syndrome characterized by autoimmunity (especially cytopenias and autoimmune hepatitis), eczema, severe and/or recurrent infections, lymphocytic interstitial pneumonia, and growth hormone (GH)-insensitive dwarfism. The latter reflects the critical role played by STAT5 in the cellular response to GH. Affected patients have a low number of circulating T and NK lymphocytes and Treg cells, and in vitro proliferative responses to mitogens are reduced. In contrast, IgG levels are often elevated. Aggressive treatment of infections, use of immunosuppressive drugs to treat autoimmune manifestations, and regular monitoring of pulmonary function are the mainstay of treatment.

Cytotoxic T Lymphocyte Antigen 4 Deficiency

Cytotoxic T lymphocyte antigen 4 (CTLA4) is a surface molecule expressed by conventional and regulatory T cells. It competes with CD28 for binding to CD80/CD86 molecules expressed by antigen-presenting cells. However, in contrast to CD28, CTLA4 delivers a suppressive signal that limits T-cell activation. Heterozygous loss-of-function mutations of CTLA4 cause a condition characterized by lymphoid infiltrates in the lung, gastrointestinal tract, and the brain (simulating lymphoma), autoimmune cytopenias, hypogammaglobulinemia, lymphopenia, accumulation of activated T cells, and decreased Treg cell function. The disease is inherited as an autosomal dominant trait with incomplete penetrance. Treatment is based on use of CTLA4-Ig (abatacept) and sirolimus. HCT may be considered in severe cases.

Lipopolysaccharide Responsive Beige-Like Anchor Protein Deficiency

Deficiency of the lipopolysaccharide responsive beige-like anchor protein (LRBA) is inherited as an autosomal recessive trait and causes a combined immunodeficiency with prominent immune dysregulation affecting mostly the gastrointestinal tract (with severe chronic diarrhea and failure to thrive) and the lungs. Autoimmune cytopenias are also common. Typical immunological abnormalities include hypogammaglobulinemia and a variable degree of lymphopenia, with increased proportion of activated T cells. The disease shares some clinical and immunologic manifestation similarities with CTLA4 deficiency. Indeed, LRBA binds to CTLA4 and allows endosomal trafficking of the latter to the cell membrane. In the absence of LRBA, CTLA4 is targeted to the lysosomal compartment where it is degraded. Consistent with this, Treg cells from patients with LRBA deficiency have low levels of expression of CTLA4 and FOXP3, and the actual number and function of Treg lymphocytes are impaired. Treatment with CTLA4-Ig (alone or in combination with sirolimus) may be beneficial.

Defects of Calcium Flux

T lymphocyte activation and homeostasis depend on calcium mobilization. In particular, TCR-induced activation results in release of Ca^{2+} from the endoplasmic reticulum stores, followed by Ca^{2+} entry through the Ca^{2+} release-activated channels (CRAC) located in the cell membrane. Mutations of *STIM1* (which encodes for a sensor of endoplasmic reticulum calcium stores) and of *ORAI1* (which encodes for CRAC) cause severe immunodeficiency in which T-lymphocyte generation in the thymus is not affected, but peripheral T cells are functionally impaired. Autoimmunity and nonprogressive myopathy are distinguishing features of these disorders.

Autoimmune Lymphoproliferative Syndrome

Interaction between Fas (CD95) on activated T and B lymphocytes, and Fas ligand (FASLG) on activated T cells triggers the extrinsic pathway to activation of the caspase cascade, culminating in apoptosis. In addition, cellular stress (including cytokine deprivation) may activate the intrinsic pathway of apoptosis, leading to disruption of mitochondrial membrane permeability, release of cytochrome c, activation of caspase 9 and apoptosis. Defects of Fas- or mitochondrial-dependent apoptosis are responsible for autoimmune lymphoproliferative syndrome (ALPS), characterized by early-onset, chronic (>6 months), nonmalignant lymphoproliferation, autoimmunity, and increased risk of lymphoma.

The majority of patients with ALPS carry heterozygous dominant-negative mutations in the *FAS* (*CD95*, *TNFRSF6*) gene (ALPS-FAS). Somatic mutations of the *FAS* gene are the second most common cause of the disease (ALPS-sFAS). More rarely, ALPS is caused by mutations of the *FASLG* gene (ALPS-FASLG), of caspase 8, caspase 10, Fas-associated death domain (FADD) protein, or by somatic activating mutations of N-RAS or K-RAS. Finally, autosomal recessive deficiency of protein kinase C (PRKCD), which plays an important role in regulating cell survival and apoptosis, also causes an ALPS-like disease with B-cell lymphoproliferative disease.

Lymphoproliferation, manifesting as lymphadenopathy, splenomegaly, or hepatomegaly, is the most common clinical manifestation, with a trend toward progressive remission in adulthood. More than 70% of ALPS patients develop autoimmune disease—most commonly immune cytopenias, less frequently organ-specific autoimmunity. There is an increased risk of malignancies, especially EBV-associated non-Hodgkin lymphoma. Patients with PRKCD deficiency often present SLE-like manifestations, with nephropathy and antiphospholipid antibody syndrome.

An immunologic signature of ALPS is the increased number of DN circulating T lymphocytes that express the αβ form of the TCR, but do not express CD4 or CD8 molecules. There is defective in vitro apoptosis of lymphocytes through the Fas-mediated or intrinsic pathway (depending on the genetic variant). Elevated levels of soluble Fas ligand, vitamin B12, and IL-10, Hypergammaglobulinemia, and anti-phospholipid antibodies are often present in patients with ALPS-FAS. By contrast, patients with PRKCD deficiency have low levels of IgG and an increased proportion of CD5⁺ B cells. Patients with caspase 8 deficiency, FADD deficiency, and PRKCD deficiency have recurrent infections. The number of DN T cells may be normal in patients with *NRAS* or *KRAS* mutations.

Treatment is based on immunosuppression (with steroids, rituximab, mycophenolate mofetil, or sirolimus) and surveillance against lymphoma. Splenectomy may improve cytopenias; however, relapse of autoimmunity has been observed in 50% of the splenectomized patients. Furthermore, severe, invasive bacterial infections have been reported in 30% of splenectomized patients, and the mortality rate for invasive bacterial infection after splenectomy is as high as 13.3%.

Other Conditions With Immune Dysregulation

Gain-of-function mutations of the *STAT1* gene cause a variable clinical phenotype ranging from chronic mucocutaneous candidiasis to increased occurrence of viral, fungal, and bacterial infections, to autoimmunity.

Gain-of-function mutations of the *STAT3* gene cause increased STAT3 signaling and enhanced Th17 differentiation, with lymphoproliferation and solid-organ autoimmunity. The number of Treg cells is reduced.

Deficiency of ITCH, an E3 ubiquitin ligase that regulates activation of phospholipase Cγ1 (PLCγ1), causes multiple autoimmune manifestations (enteropathy, thyroiditis, type 1 diabetes, hepatitis), interstitial lung disease, dysmorphic features, and developmental delay.

Defects of IL-10 and IL-10R are responsible for very early onset inflammatory bowel disease.

Mutations of the tripeptidyl-peptidase II (*TPP2*) gene cause severe autoimmune hemolytic anemia, variable lymphoproliferation, and recurrent infections. Accelerated senescence of lymphoid cells and hypergammaglobulinemia are observed.

DEFECTS OF CELL-MEDIATED CYTOTOXICITY

Mechanisms of immune defense against viral infections are largely dependent on responses mediated by CD8⁺ cytotoxic T lymphocytes (CTLs) and NK lymphocytes. Multimers of perforin, a protein contained in cytolytic granules, form pores through which CTL and NK cells release cytotoxic proteins (granzyme B, granulolysin) into virus-infected target cells, causing activation of caspases and apoptosis. In resting CTLs and NK lymphocytes, cytotoxic proteins are contained in endosomal secretory lytic granules. Following interaction of CTLs or NK cells with the target cell, vesicles containing lytic granules are transported and dock and fuse with the cell membrane, permitting release of cytotoxic proteins into the target cells.

Hemophagocytic Lymphohistiocytosis

Defects in the intracellular transport and release of cytolytic granules are responsible for various forms of familial HLH, including deficiency of Munc13-4 (required to prime vesicles), syntaxin 11 and Munc18-2 (both of which promote vesicle fusion with the cell membrane), and perforin. In these disorders, infections (mostly caused by viruses) trigger an uncontrolled immune response mediated by CD8⁺ T lymphocytes and NK cells that secrete large amounts of IFN-γ, which activates macrophages. Fever, liver, and spleen enlargement, lymphadenopathy, profound cytopenias, hypoalbuminemia, coagulopathy, high levels of ferritin and triglycerides, and immune activation (with increased levels of soluble CD25) characterize these acute episodes, which may lead to multiple-organ failure and death. The diagnosis of these familial forms of HLH is facilitated by flow cytometric analysis of surface expression of CD107a (a protein normally contained in endosomal vesicles) upon in vitro activation of cytotoxic T cells and NK cells. Defective expression of CD107a is observed in patients with Munc13-4, Munc18-2, and syntaxin 11 deficiencies. By contrast, this test is normal in patients with perforin deficiency, in which reduced or absent expression of perforin can be easily demonstrated by flow cytometry.

HLH Associated With Pigmentary Dilution Disorders

Typical features of HLH are also observed in some pigmentary dilution disorders. In particular, Chediak-Higashi syndrome (CHS) is an autosomal recessive disease due to mutations of the *LYST* gene, which encodes for a protein involved in the sorting of proteins to secretory endosomes. This defect affects not only cytotoxic lymphocytes (accounting for FHL-like clinical features), but also melanocytes (that are unable to transfer melanin to keratinocytes and other epithelial cells) and peripheral neurons. Clinical features of CHS include partial albinism (with silvery hair), progressive peripheral neuropathy, recurrent bacterial infections, and mild tendency to bleeding. Neutropenia is often present and may cause bacterial infections. Giant lysosomes can be identified in circulating leukocytes.

Griscelli syndrome type 2 (GS2) is caused by mutations of the *RAB27A* gene, which encodes for a protein involved in docking of secretory granules of cytotoxic lymphocytes and melanocytes to the cell membrane. Accordingly, patients with GS2 present with HLH and hypopigmentation. The diagnosis is facilitated by the demonstration of large clumps of pigment distributed irregularly along the hair shaft, and by reduced expression of CD107a on the surface of CD8⁺ and NK lymphocytes upon in vitro activation.

Hermansky-Pudlak syndrome type 2 is an autosomal recessive disorder caused by mutations of the *AP3B1* gene, which encodes for the β component of the AP-3 complex, involved in sorting of transmembrane proteins to secretory lysosomes. Clinical manifestations include partial albinism, nystagmus, prolonged bleeding, recurrent bacterial and viral infections, and increased risk of HLH. Pigmentary abnormalities, neutropenia, platelet dysfunction (with absence of dense granules and reduced platelet aggregation), and defective cytotoxic activity account for the clinical manifestations of the disease.

Irrespective of the nature of the genetic defect, HLH therapy is based on the prompt and aggressive treatment of underlying infections and immunosuppression to curtail macrophage activation. Administration of humanized anti-IFN-γ monoclonal antibodies may block continuous activation of the immune system and induce remission. Ultimately, definitive treatment is based on allogeneic HCT from a matched related or unrelated donor, and the best results are obtained using reduced-intensity conditioning. Mixed chimerism is sufficient to correct the immunologic abnormalities.

X-Linked Lymphoproliferative Disease

In normal individuals, primary infection with EBV causes infectious mononucleosis, a self-limiting disease. EBV establishes latency in B lymphocytes, salivary glands, and some epithelial cells, and is maintained under control by CD8$^+$ CTLs, and NK lymphocytes. Males with X-linked lymphoproliferative disease type 1 (XLP1) are uniquely susceptible to life-threatening complications of EBV infections. XLP1 is caused by mutations of the *SH2D1A* gene, which encodes for a small adaptor molecule, SLAM-associated protein (SAP). In the absence of SAP, cytotoxic responses to EBV-infected cells are markedly reduced. Persistence of EBV triggers continuous activation of CD8$^+$ CTLs that release high amounts of IFN-γ, ultimately resulting in a macrophage activation syndrome. In addition to HLH, patients with XLP1 are also at high risk of B-cell lymphoma. SAP is also important for the function of follicular helper T cells (T$_{FH}$), which promote maturation of antibody responses. Consistent with this, XLP1 males often develop hypogammaglobulinemia with a lack of memory B lymphocytes. Finally, XLP1 is also associated with impaired development of NK T (NKT) lymphocytes. Flow cytometric analysis of SAP expression and mutation analysis at the *SH2D1A* locus confirms the diagnosis.

A minority of patients with XLP carry defects in another gene (*BIRC4*) that encodes for the X-linked inhibitor of apoptosis (XIAP). Consistent with this, lymphocytes from patients with this disease (XLP2) show increased susceptibility to activation-induced apoptosis. Compared with XLP1, patients with XLP2 have a higher incidence of HLH (with or without EBV infection), but do not show increased risk of lymphoma. Severe inflammatory bowel disease has been reported in several patients. Hypogammaglobulinemia is often present. Flow cytometric analysis of XIAP expression and mutation analysis at the *BIRC4* locus are used to confirm the diagnosis.

Both XLP1 and XLP2 are life-threatening disorders. Administration of immunoglobulins may be beneficial; however, the only curative approach is HCT.

DEFECTS OF B-CELL DEVELOPMENT AND FUNCTION

The previous section covered defects that predominantly affect T lymphocyte development and/or function. This section covers primary immunodeficiencies in which abnormalities of B-cell development and/or function predominate (see Figs. 51.2 and 51.3).

Diagnostic and Therapeutic Approach to Cytotoxicity Defects

- Primary immunodeficiency with defects of cell-mediated cytotoxicity include a heterogeneous group of disorders characterized by increased susceptibility to severe viral infections.
- Typical clinical features include high fever, liver and spleen enlargement, lymphadenopathy, coagulation defects, abnormalities of liver function, and cytopenias after viral infections.
- Two major groups of cell-mediated cytotoxicity defects include familial forms of HLH (fHLH) and X-linked lymphophroliferative disease. In the former, diagnosis is based on demonstration of abnormal cytotoxic function of T and NK lymphocytes. Defective expression of CD107a on activated lymphocytes or reduced expression of perforin may help define the nature of the underlying disorder causing fHLH.
- Prompt recognition and treatment of the underlying infection is essential. Immunosuppression is also required to block exaggerated inflammatory responses. However, the only curative approach to defects of cell-mediated cytotoxicity is represented by hematopoietic cell transplantation. Mixed chimerism is sufficient to allow immune reconstitution. This goal can be achieved with reduced intensity conditioning, with a lower risk of treatment-related toxicity.

X-Linked Agammaglobulinemia

X-linked agammaglobulinemia (XLA), also known as *Bruton's agammaglobulinemia*, is the most common monogenic cause of failure of B-cell development. Males with XLA lack circulating B cells, caused by mutations of the Bruton's tyrosine kinase or *BTK* gene, which encodes for a tyrosine kinase involved in signaling through various receptors, including the pre–B-cell receptor (pre-BCR) and the BCR. Impaired signaling through the pre-BCR causes a severe, but incomplete, block at the pre–B-cell stage in the bone marrow (see Fig. 51.2).

Clinical manifestations of XLA include recurrent sinopulmonary infections (pneumonia, bronchitis, sinusitis, otitis), particularly with encapsulated organisms such as pneumococcus and *Haemophilus influenza*, bacterial skin infections (cellulitis, impetigo, pyoderma gangrenosum, perirectal abscess), and sepsis with *Pseudomonas* or *Staphylococcus*. Symptoms typically begin after 3–6 months of age when maternally derived antibodies disappear. The proportion of circulating B cells is markedly reduced (typically 0.05% to 0.3% of lymphocytes) and there is profound deficiency of all immunoglobulin isotypes. Milder mutations that are permissive for BTK protein expression are associated in vivo with higher levels of serum IgM and later age at diagnosis. Neutropenia, secondary to severe infections, is observed in approximately 10% to 25% of patients; typically, it resolves with antibiotics and immunoglobulin-replacement therapy.

In addition to bacterial infections, patients with XLA are uniquely susceptible to enteroviral infections (including chronic meningoencephalitis) caused by poliovirus, coxsackie virus, and others. However, such complications have become rare after the introduction of optimal doses of immunoglobulin-replacement therapy. Patients with XLA are also at higher risk of infections caused by *Mycoplasma* and *Ureaplasma* species, which affect the joints, prostate, or lungs; and *Giardia lamblia*, causing protracted diarrhea and malabsorption. An increased incidence of lymphoma, colorectal cancer, and gastric adenocarcinoma has been reported in XLA.

Therapy is based on life-long regular administration of immunoglobulins intravenously or subcutaneously, and on prompt and aggressive treatment of infections. With this regimen, survival approaches that of the general population. Antibiotic prophylaxis may be beneficial, but its role has not been firmly established. Patients on immunoglobulin-replacement therapy should be monitored for side effects and adverse reactions, and for liver and renal function.

Autosomal Recessive Agammaglobulinemia

While the majority of agammaglobulinemia cases are caused by the X-linked form, about 15% of cases are presumed to be autosomal recessive (see Fig. 51.2). Mutations of the immunoglobulin μ heavy chain gene (*IGHM*) are the second most common cause of agammaglobulinemia. Other cases are caused by defects in other components of the pre-BCR/BCR complex including the signaling moieties Igα (CD79A) and Igβ (CD79B), and λ5 (IGLL1), the surrogate light chain that pairs with Vpre-B, and the scaffold protein BLNK, which brings BTK into the signaling complex. Finally, congenital agammaglobulinemia may also be caused by mutations of the *PIK3R1* gene, causing complete loss of the p85α subunit of phosphatidylinositol 3-kinase (PI3K), and to heterozygous, dominant-negative mutations of the *TCF3* gene encoding for the transcription factor E47.

Common Variable Immunodeficiency

CVID is the most common primary immunodeficiency severe enough to require treatment, with a prevalence estimated to be 1 in 25,000 to 1 in 30,000 Caucasians, and accounting for approximately 10% to 20% of humoral immunodeficiencies. While a growing number of genetic defects have been found to be associated with a CVID phenotype, these defects account for a minority of cases. The

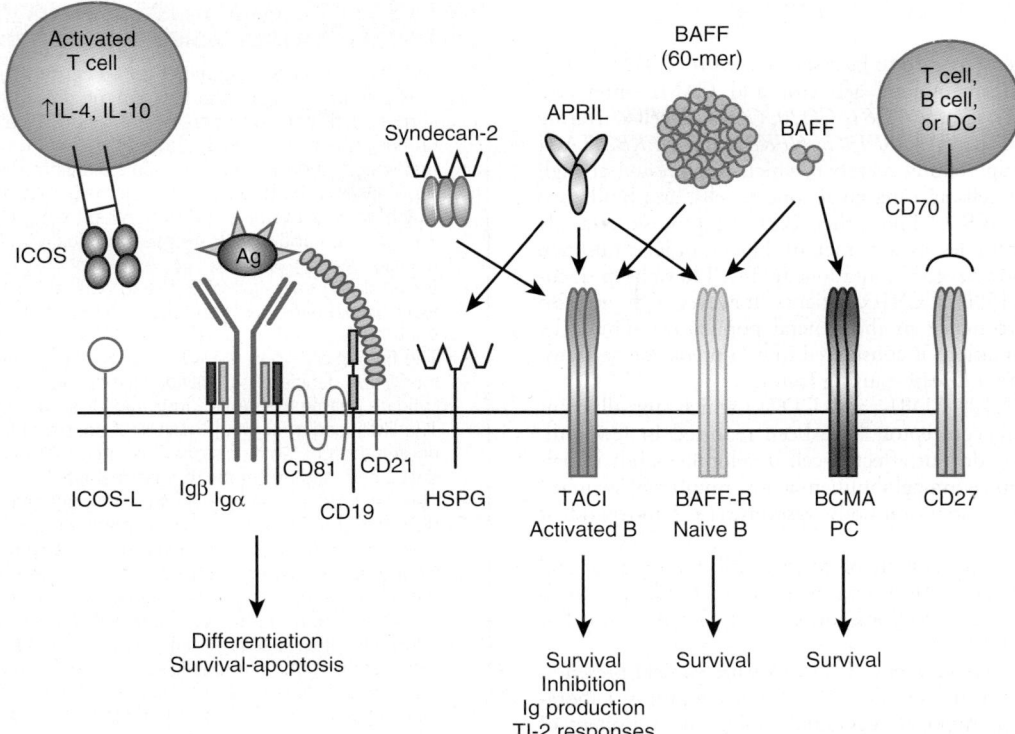

Fig. 51.3 GENETIC DEFECTS ASSOCIATED WITH COMMON VARIABLE IMMUNODEFI-CIENCY. Schematic of cell surface molecules expressed on B cells and their ligands, highlighting those in which defects have been shown to be associated with CVID. *Ag*, Antigen; *APRIL*, a proliferation-inducing ligand; *BAFF*, B-cell–activating factor; *BAFFR*, B-cell–activating factor receptor; *BCMA*, B-cell–maturation antigen; *DC*, dendritic cell; *HSPG*, heparin sulfate proteoglycan; *ICOS*, inducible T-cell costimulator; *ICOS-L*, inducible T-cell costimulator ligand; *Ig*, immunoglobulin; *IL-4*, interleukin 4; *IL-10*, interleukin 10; *PC*, plasma cell; *TACI*, transmembrane activator and calcium modulator and cyclophilin ligand interactor; *TI-2*, T-cell–independent type 2.

"variable" nature of the clinical manifestations of CVID patients could reflect genetic heterogeneity, but also refers to distinct clinical and immunological features that distinguish subgroups of CVID patients. However, the most common genetic variant described to date (mutations in transmembrane activator and calcium modulator and cyclophilin ligand interactor [TACI]) can be found in asymptomatic individuals, and more likely represents a predisposition to CVIDs than primary cause. Thus, the genetic causes of the majority of cases of CVIDs remain obscure and are not clearly monogenic in nature.

Diagnostic criteria for CVIDs were established in 1999 by consensus of European and Pan-American societies, and include the presence of hypogammaglobulinemia (<2 standard deviations below the mean for age of IgG, IgA, and/or IgM) and the lack of specific antibody responses in individuals with onset of symptoms >2 years of age, for whom other causes of humoral immunodeficiency have been ruled out. The number of circulating B cells detected is variable. Specific antibody responses should be assessed for more than one antigen. Because an increasing number of gene defects causing hypogammaglobulinemia early in life have been identified, many experts would recommend limiting the diagnosis of CVID to patients in whom symptoms appeared at >4 years of age.

Consistent with the antibody deficiency, CVID patients have recurrent bacterial infections of the respiratory tract, sepsis with encapsulated organisms, and infections from *Ureaplasma uraelyticum*, *Giardia* species and enteroviruses. However, variable derangement of T-cell numbers and function often results in noninfectious manifestations, including autoimmunity, lymphoid infiltration or proliferation, and malignancy. In one survey only 26% of CVID patients had infections as the only manifestation of disease. Autoimmune cytopenias are quite common (~12%) and may be the presenting feature.

Other autoimmune complications include rheumatoid arthritis, systemic lupus erythematosus, hypothyroidism, vitiligo, psoriasis, diabetes, and autoimmune gastritis with pernicious anemia. Polyclonal lymphocytic granulomatous infiltrates are common and may involve the lungs, liver, or gut (causing enteropathy that is resistant to gluten withdrawal). Finally, both lymphoid (non-Hodgkin lymphoma, chronic lymphocytic leukemia) and nonlymphoid (gastric cancer) malignancies are more frequent in CVID, although the latter may be related to *Helicobacter pylori* infection.

Replacement of immunoglobulins and treatment and prevention of infection remains the mainstay of management of CVID. Immunosuppression may be needed for inflammatory and autoimmune manifestations. Disease manifestations such as autoimmunity, polyclonal lymphocytic infiltrative disease, enteropathy, and malignancy have differential and increasing impact on survival (relative risk of death 2.5, 3.0, 4.0, and 5.5, respectively), while patients with solely infectious manifestations have equivalent survival to the general population. Treatment with HCT has been performed with limited success, and often in the context of consolidative treatment for lymphoproliferation.

Immunophenotyping, genotyping, and recently genome-wide association studies have been performed in an attempt to subcategorize the heterogeneous group of CVIDs into pathobiologically relevant groups. In large part the associations have not been sufficiently robust to direct diagnosis or clinical management, and underscore the genetic heterogeneity of the disease. B-cell subphenotypes most common among CVID patients include a severe reduction in switched memory B cells (CD19⁺CD27⁺IgD⁻); some patients manifest expansion of transitional B cells (CD19⁺CD24ʰⁱCD38ʰⁱ), expansion of CD21ˡᵒʷCD38ˡᵒʷ B cells (the latter thought to play a role in autoimmunity), or reduction in CD4 T-cell number.

Genetic Variants Associated With CVIDs

A few genes have been reported to be associated with CVID (see Fig. 51.3), including transmembrane activator and CAML interactor (TACI; *TNFRSF13B*), *CD19*, *CD81*, *CD20*, *CD21*, B-cell activating factor receptor (BAFF-R; *TNFRSF13C*), *NFKB1*, and *NFKB2*. TACI is a TNF receptor superfamily member, which is expressed at high levels on activated B cells and marginal zone B cells, and binds two ligands, BAFF and APRIL. Like other TNF receptor superfamily members, TACI assembles as a trimer or higher order multimer. Heterozygous and homozygous mutations in TACI have been documented in 10% to 15% of CVID patients; however, they are also found at a lower frequency in the general population. Thus, the presence of TACI mutations is considered to be a predisposing factor to CVID, rather than a disease-causing factor.

Mutations in CD19, CD81, and CD21, which are all components of the B-cell coreceptor, have been reported in few individuals. These defects do not affect B-cell development but impair signaling, causing hypogammaglobulinemia, low number of switched memory B cells, and poor antibody response to T-independent antigens.

CD20 is a surface molecule involved in B-cell development and plasma cell differentiation. Autosomal recessive CD20 deficiency is characterized by recurrent infections, low serum IgG, with normal or elevated IgA and/or IgM.

BAFF-R deficiency is very rare. It has variable clinical presentation, with CVID-like features or even absence of symptoms. Laboratory findings include hypogammaglobulinemia, low numbers of circulating B cells and a defective proportion of memory B cells, and normal antibody response to T-dependent antigen but a defective response to carbohydrate antigens.

A variable clinical phenotype has been also reported in patients with haploinsufficiency of the p50 subunit of NF-κB (encoded by the *NFKB1* gene), causing defective signaling through the canonical NF-κB signaling pathway. In addition to recurrent infections and progressive lung disease, patients often present with autoimmunity (hemolytic anemia, thyroiditis, alopecia) and lymphadenopathy. However, genotypically affected individuals may also remain asymptomatic even through adulthood. Heterozygous mutations of the *NFKB2* gene (affecting mostly the noncanonical NF-κB signaling pathway) cause recurrent infections (especially due to HSV, varicella-zoster virus [VZV], and *Giardia*), central adrenal insufficiency, hypopituitarism, alopecia, trachyonychia, and growth deficiency. Hypogammaglobulinemia, a low number of memory B cells, Treg lymphocytes, T follicular helper (Tfh) cells, and NK lymphocytes have been demonstrated.

B-CELL–INTRINSIC DEFECTS OF CLASS-SWITCH RECOMBINATION

Maturation of the antibody response is marked by class-switch recombination (CSR) and by somatic hypermutation (SHM). With CSR, the μ heavy chain is replaced by other Ig heavy chains. With SHM, mutations are introduced in the Ig V region, allowing affinity maturation. Following CD40LG–CD40 interaction and activation of the NF-κB signaling pathway, expression of activation-induced cytidine deaminase (AID) and of uracil-DNA glycosylase (UNG) occurs in germinal center B lymphocytes (see Fig. 51.3). AID acts on the DNA of Ig heavy chain switch regions and converts cytidine to uridine, which is recognized and removed by UNG. The abasic sites are cleaved by a DNA endonuclease. DNA repair then brings together two different switch regions, allowing CSR.

Mutations in AID and UNG are inherited as autosomal recessive traits. Patients suffer from recurrent bacterial infections. Autoimmune manifestations have been observed in several patients. Circulating B cells are present, but there is a severe reduction of all Ig isotypes with the exception of IgM, which is often elevated. Lymphadenopathy is common and is associated with expansion of germinal centers. Somatic hypermutation is severely compromised in patients with

Diagnostic and Therapeutic Approach to Defects in Humoral Immunity

- Defects in humoral immunity may be caused by intrinsic defects in B-cell development and function, or caused by combined immunodeficiency disorders where lack of T-cell help is the primary cause of B-cell dysfunction.
- Age-specific norms must be used for children. Immunoglobulin (Ig)G levels at birth reflect the maternally transferred antibody, which nadir between 2 and 6 months, then progressively rise with age. IgA and IgM levels rise continually with age until the teenage years.
- Based on enumeration of T, B and natural killer cells, X-linked agammaglobulinemia (XLA; absence of B cells) can be rapidly ruled out.
- The finding of hyper-IgM with low IgG should prompt a work-up for CD40L deficiency, CD40 deficiency, activation-induced cytidine deaminase (AID), and uracil-DNA glycosylase (UNG). The likelihood of each of these is of course different depending on gender and family history. It is important to note that CD40L deficiency may present with a normal IgM.
- The diagnosis of common variable immunodeficiency disorders (CVIDs) should only be made once other causes have been ruled out, and should be made with caution, if at all, in children under 4 years of age. Disorders such as XLA, autosomal recessive agammaglobulinemia, various hyper-IgM syndromes, and XLP should be specifically considered and ruled out. Other diseases that may masquerade as CVID include other combined immunodeficiencies, cystic fibrosis, HIV, and conditions leading to Ig loss such as protein-losing enteropathy. Medications may mimic the symptoms of CVID. Finally, in adults hypogammaglobulinemia may herald the development of thymoma or lymphoid malignancies, and therefore may be secondary to evolving neoplasia.
- Treatment of XLA and the hyper-IgM syndromes other than CD40L deficiency is long-term intravenous Ig replacement, which is very effective.
- Experts disagree on whether CD40L deficiency should be treated with early HSCT, and currently there are no clear predictors to determine who is likely to suffer from opportunistic infections. A patient with CD40L deficiency who has developed cryptosporidium infection and sclerosing cholangitis generally has a much worse outlook with HSCT.
- Treatment of CVID with HSCT is generally reserved for those with an alternate requirement for allogeneic transplant such as lymphoid malignancy or lymphoproliferation, which requires continual immunosuppression.

AID deficiency, and follows an abnormal pattern in patients with UNG deficiency.

Treatment is based on regular administration of Igs, as well as prompt recognition and therapy of infections.

Defects in CSR have also been reported in patients with mutations in *INO80* (encoding for a chromatin remodeling complex) and *MSH6* (involved in the DNA mismatch repair pathway). The latter group of patients is at increased risk of cancer.

Other Immunoglobulin Defects

Gain-of-function mutations of the *PIK3CD* gene (encoding for the p110δ catalytic component of PI3K) cause an immunodeficiency characterized by nodular lymphoid hyperplasia, progressive lung disease with bronchiectasis, chronic or recurrent herpesvirus viremia (CMV, EBV, VZV, HSV), and hepatosplenomegaly. There is an increased risk of lymphomas, which are not necessarily associated with EBV infection. The immunologic phenotype includes CD4 lymphopenia, a reduced proportion of naive T cells, expansion of effector memory and "exhausted" CD8$^+$ T cells, defective T-cell proliferation, variable Ig levels (often with low IgG2), reduced proportion of memory B cells, and poor antibody responses. In these patients, increased PI3K signaling causes hyperactivation of the AKT–mammalian target of rapamycin (mTOR) pathway, shifting the intracellular metabolism of lymphoid cells towards glycolysis and thereby deranging lymphocyte function and differentiation.

A very similar clinical and laboratory phenotype has been observed in patients with heterozygous mutations of the *PIK3R1* gene (encoding for the p85α regulatory subunit of PI3K), which permits expression of a mutated p85α protein lacking the p110δ-interacting domain. Treatment with rapamycin, to reduce mTOR activation, may be beneficial in both conditions. An alternative strategy, currently under investigation, is based on the use of PI3K inhibitors.

SUGGESTED READINGS

Albert MH, Notarangelo LD, Ochs HD: Clinical spectrum, pathophysiology and treatment of the Wiskott-Aldrich syndrome. *Curr Opin Hematol* 18:42–48, 2011.

Alkhairy OK, Abolhassani H, Rezaei N, et al: Spectrum of Phenotypes Associated with Mutations in LRBA. *J Clin Immunol* 36:33–45, 2016.

Bonilla FA, Barlan I, Chapel H, et al: International Consensus Document (ICON): Common Variable Immunodeficiency Disorders. *J Allergy Clin Immunol Pract* 4:38–59, 2016.

Conley ME, Dobbs AK, Farmer DM, et al: Primary B cell immunodeficiencies: comparisons and contrasts. *Annu Rev Immunol* 27:199–227, 2009.

Coulter TI, Chandra A, Bacon CM, et al: Clinical spectrum and features of activated phosphoinositide 3-kinase δ syndrome: A large patient cohort study. *J Allergy Clin Immunol* 2016 Jul 16. [Epub ahead of print].

Ferre EM, Rose SR, Rosenzweig SD, et al: Redefined clinical features and diagnostic criteria in autoimmune polyendocrinopathy-candidiasis-ectodermal dystrophy. *JCI Insight* 2016 Aug 18. [Epub ahead of print].

Feske S: Immunodeficiency due to defects in store-operated calcium entry. *Ann N Y Acad Sci* 1238:74–90, 2011.

Filipovich AH, Chandrakasan S: Pathogenesis of Hemophagocytic Lymphohistiocytosis. *Hematol Oncol Clin North Am* 29:895–902, 2015.

Fischer A, Hacein-Bey Abina S, Touzot F, et al: Gene therapy for primary immunodeficiencies. *Clin Genet* 88:507–515, 2015.

Fischer A, Notarangelo LD, Neven B, et al: Severe combined immunodeficiencies and related disorders. *Nat Rev Dis Primers* 1:15061, 2015.

Hanna S, Etzioni A: MHC class I and II deficiencies. *J Allergy Clin Immunol* 134:269–275, 2014.

Kwan A, Abraham RS, Currier R, et al: Newborn screening for severe combined immunodeficiency in 11 screening programs in the United States. *JAMA* 312:729–738, 2014. Erratum in: *JAMA* 2014;312:2169.

Lo B, Fritz JM, Su HC, et al: CHAI and LATAIE: new genetic diseases of CTLA-4 checkpoint insufficiency. *Blood* 128:1037–1042, 2016.

Notarangelo LD: Combined immunodeficiencies with nonfunctional T lymphocytes. *Adv Immunol* 121:121–190, 2014.

Oliveira JB: The expanding spectrum of the autoimmune lymphoproliferative syndromes. *Curr Opin Pediatr* 25:722–729, 2013.

Orange JS: Natural killer cell deficiency. *J Allergy Clin Immunol* 132:515–525, 2013.

Pai SY, Logan BR, Griffith LM, et al: Transplantation outcomes for severe combined immunodeficiency, 2000-2009. *N Engl J Med* 371:434–446, 2014.

Picard C, Al-Herz W, Bousfiha A, et al: Primary Immunodeficiency Diseases: an Update on the Classification from the International Union of Immunological Societies Expert Committee for Primary Immunodeficiency 2015. *J Clin Immunol* 35:696–726, 2015.

Speckmann C, Doerken S, Aiuti A, et al: etal. A prospective study on the natural history of patients with profound combined immunodeficiency: An interim analysis. *J Allergy Clin Immunol* 2016 Sep 19. [Epub ahead of print].

Su HC, Jing H, Zhang Q: DOCK8 deficiency. *Ann N Y Acad Sci* 1246:26–33, 2011.

Verbsky JW, Chatila TA: Immune dysregulation, polyendocrinopathy, enteropathy, X-linked (IPEX) and IPEX-related disorders: an evolving web of heritable autoimmune diseases. *Curr Opin Pediatr* 25:708–714, 2013.

REFERENCES

For the complete list of references, log on to www.expertconsult.com.

CHAPTER 52

HISTIOCYTIC DISORDERS

Michael B. Jordan and Alexandra Hult Filipovich

The histiocytic disorders comprise a broad grouping of hematologic and immunologic diseases united by the observation that monocyte/macrophages or dendritic cells appear to be prominently involved in disease pathophysiology. The term *histiocyte* refers to phagocytic cells, historically identified on tissue sections but now more precisely defined as cells of the monocyte/macrophage lineage (Fig. 52.1). The ontogeny of these cells continues to be actively studied and debated, and their role(s) in pathogenesis is an active area of investigation. The characteristic cells seen in various histiocytic lesions can, in general, be differentiated by a variety of functional and phenotypic markers. The modern classification of the histiocytoses mirrors this biology (Table 52.1). Although malignant disorders involving monocyte/macrophages or dendritic cells were originally included in this classification, this chapter focuses solely on nonmalignant disorders in this category.

Of the dendritic cell-related histiocytoses, the most clinically common and prominent one is Langerhans cell histiocytosis (LCH). This chapter also briefly discusses other dendritic cell-related histiocytic disorders, including juvenile xanthogranuloma (JXG); Erdheim–Chester disease (ECD); and sinus histiocytosis with massive lymphadenopathy (SHML), also referred to as *Rosai-Dorfman disease* (RDD).

The prominent monocyte/macrophage-related histiocytic disorder, hemophagocytic lymphohistiocytosis (HLH), is discussed in detail later in this chapter. In HLH, activated macrophages, activated T cells, and defective natural killer (NK) cells are the dysfunctional interactive partners.

Table 52.1 lists a currently accepted classification of histiocytic disorders. These disorders are a diverse grouping, ranging from benign skin lesions to rapidly life-threatening systemic disorders. Tables 52.2 and 52.3 list clinical features and commonly used pathologic markers or features that may be used to help distinguish some of these disorders. The clinical diversity of histiocytic disorders is underscored by recent discoveries related to their pathogenesis. Studies dating to the late 1990s have demonstrated that HLH (at least in its familial form) is a unique immune-regulatory disorder. LCH is another disorder, historically considered to be nonmalignant. However, demonstrations of clonality as well as genetic abnormalities of B-Raf now demonstrate that LCH is a benign neoplasm despite its variable clinical phenotype. The pathogeneses of less common dendritic cell- and macrophage-related histiocytic disorders are still unknown.

LANGERHANS CELL HISTIOCYTOSIS

LCH is the most common of the histiocytoses. The central cell of LCH, the Langerhans dendritic cell, was first described in 1868 by 21-year-old Paul Langerhans. Between 1893 and 1920, Hand, Schüller, and Christian described the various nonfatal presentations of LCH, which include bony lesions, skin rash, and diabetes insipidus (DI). Letterer and Siwe (1924 and 1933, respectively) added to the list of clinical presentations by describing cases with liver and spleen involvement in infants and toddlers. These disorders were later grouped under the term *histiocytosis X* (denoting the uncertainty about disease pathogenesis) by Lichtenstein. It was eventually theorized by Nezelof (1973) that histiocytosis X is caused by a proliferation of pathologic Langerhans cells. At present, the term *LCH* has been adopted to refer to all of the varied manifestations of this protean disorder. It is now well recognized that LCH can present at any time in life from the neonatal period to old age. LCH lesions may spontaneously regress or repeatedly "reactivate", contributing to long-term disabilities such as DI or a neurodegenerative disease. Life-threatening forms of LCH, previously referred to as *Letterer–Siwe disease*, typically present in infancy and clearly require intensive therapy and sometimes salvage treatment such as allogeneic bone marrow transplantation (BMT) to cure the children.

Epidemiology

The incidence of LCH has been estimated to be between 5 and 15 cases per million children, per year. The incidence of LCH in adults is believed to be lower than in children but is likely underestimated because of a lack of recognition of LCH in adult medicine. Notably, LCH does not appear to have significant geographic or ethnic predilections. Although families with multiple cases of LCH have been reported, these kindreds are extremely rare. One notable clinical or epidemiologic association reported thus far involves an unexplained coincidence of both LCH and leukemia (of various subtypes) in rare patients.

Pathobiology

The understanding of the pathobiology of LCH is currently undergoing significant evolution, driven by new insights into both normal and disease-associated Langerhans cells. Over the years, LCH has been classified as a neoplasm, a reactive disorder, or an aberrant immune response. LCH cells are pathologic in that they bear heterogeneous characteristics not normally identified in healthy Langerhans cells that are typically resident in the skin. The granulomatous lesions of LCH, which can be found in nearly any organ, represent an accumulation of normal inflammatory cells, including eosinophils, lymphocytes (especially T cells), and macrophages, in addition to the LCH cells. The clinically benign behavior of most cases, including spontaneous remissions and lack of aggressive disease evolution with recurrences, as well as the benign histopathologic appearance of lesions, have suggested a nonmalignant etiology. The failure of many laboratories to culture pathologic Langerhans cells has reinforced this impression. Thus, LCH has been hypothesized to be a reactive or immunologic disorder by many. On the other hand, lesional Langerhans cells have been demonstrated by several investigators to be clonal. This observation, combined with the clinical utility of antineoplastic drugs, has bolstered the opinion that LCH may be a neoplastic disorder.

Several reports in the last 5 years of highly prevalent B-Raf mutations in lesional Langerhans cells have again shifted thinking and strongly support a neoplastic etiology. The mutation in question (*BRAF* V600E) is well described in both malignant melanomas and in benign nevi, among other neoplasms. This mutation leads to activation of the extracellular signal-related kinase (ERK) pathway. More recently, additional mutations associated with the ERK pathway activation have been described in LCH patients. Along with these disease-specific findings, understanding of the biology of normal Langerhans cells has advanced. Cutaneous Langerhans dendritic cells have been shown to arise from in situ precursors,

Bone marrow

Peripheral blood

Tissue compartment

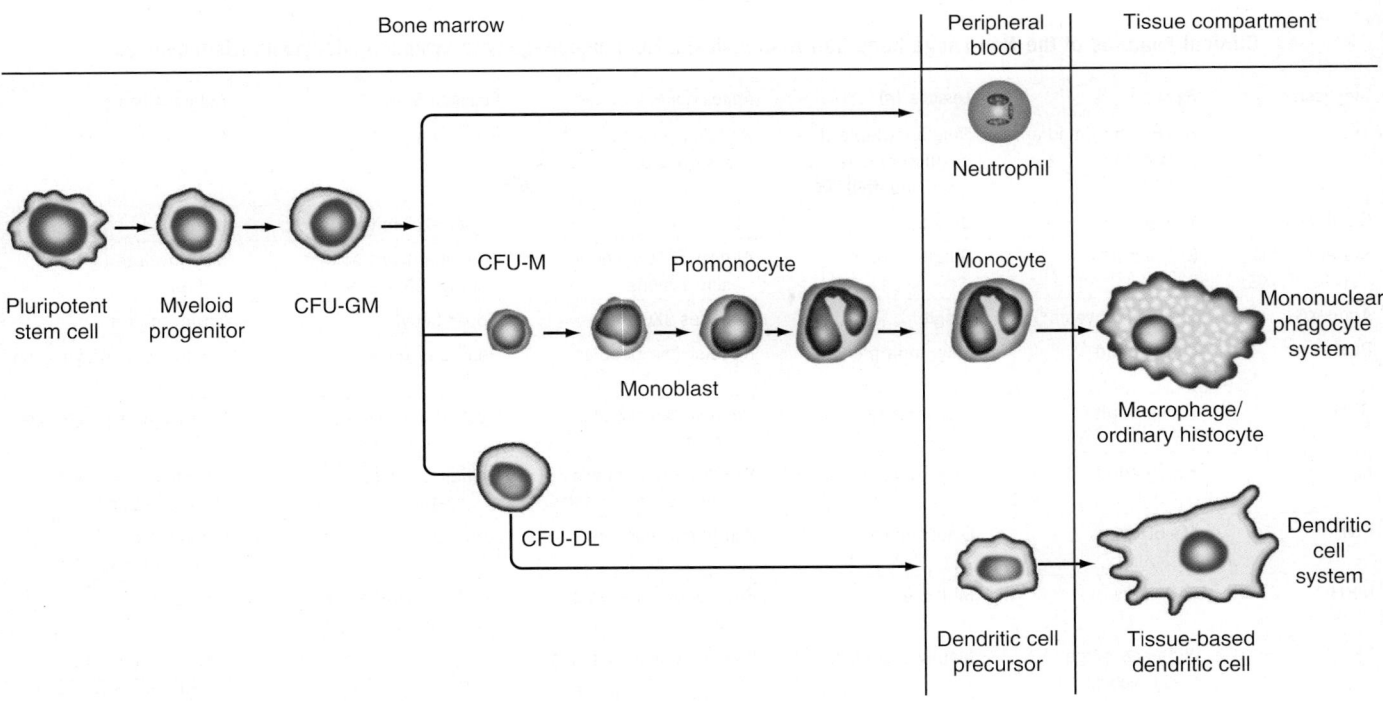

Fig. 52.1 DEVELOPMENT OF CELLS OF THE MONOCYTE/MACROPHAGE LINEAGE. *CFU-DL,* Colony-forming unit–dendritic Langerhans cell; *CFU-GM,* colony-forming unit–granulocyte-macrophage; *CFU-M,* colony-forming unit–macrophage.

TABLE 52.1	Classification of Histiocytic Disorders: Benign Disorders of Varying Biologic Behavior

A. Dendritic cell related
   Langerhans cell histiocytosis
   Juvenile xanthogranuloma and related disorders including:
   • Erdheim–Chester disease
   • Solitary histiocytomas with juvenile xanthogranuloma phenotype
   • Secondary dendritic cell disorders
B. Monocyte/macrophage related
   Hemophagocytic lymphohistiocytosis: familial and sporadic
   Secondary hemophagocytic syndromes
   • Infection associated
   • Malignancy associated
   • Autoimmune associated
   Sinus histiocytosis with massive lymphadenopathy (Rosai–Dorfman disease)
   Solitary histiocytoma of macrophage phenotype

but during inflammation or stress, to arise from circulating myeloid precursors. Therefore, a picture is emerging in which the acquisition of mutation(s), such as *BRAF* V600E, in myeloid precursors may cause a neoplastic proliferation of a terminally differentiated clone that colonizes a distinct anatomic location. Similar to a cutaneous nevus, this neoplasm is a benign one because lesional cells are not fully transformed. Thus, recent findings support the hypothesis that LCH is a benign hematopoietic neoplasm, or a hematopoietic "mole". Thus far, there has been no compelling insight into why LCH has such diverse manifestations, ranging from solitary to widely disseminated disease.

Clinical Manifestations

Clinical involvement with LCH can be highly variable but most often involves bony lesions (present in ≈80% of cases), which may be painful or painless; the latter is common with skull lesions. Skin involvement, typically papulosquamous lesions, often affecting the scalp (and frequently mistaken for cradle cap, seborrhea) is reported in 30% to 60% of patient series. Soft tissue swelling, often in proximity to bony lesions, external ear drainage, enlargement of lymph nodes and thymus, and gum hypertrophy with premature eruption of baby teeth are also well-recognized manifestations. More serious systemic involvement occurs when there is hepatosplenomegaly, liver dysfunction, lung scarring, and hematopoietic failure with or without intestinal involvement. The latter findings are more typical of the widely disseminated form of LCH seen in young infants, which carries a high mortality rate.

Bony Involvement

Solitary or multifocal bony lesions are found predominantly in older children and young adults, usually within the first three decades of life. Such lytic bone lesions are commonly referred to as *eosinophilic granuloma* because of their pathologic appearance. The incidence of bone lesions peaks between 5 and 10 years of age. Solitary or multifocal eosinophilic granuloma (with or without involvement of other organ systems) represents approximately 60% to 80% of all instances of LCH. Patients with systemic involvement frequently have bone lesions in addition to other manifestations of disease. Patients often cannot bear weight and may have tender swelling caused by tissue infiltrates overlying the bone lesions. Radiographically, the lesions are sharply marginated, round, or oval, and usually have a beveled edge on radiography that gives the appearance of depth. Hand–Schüller–Christian disease, referring to the triad of bony involvement, skin lesions, and DI, is most commonly described in younger children aged 2–5 years. It represents 15% to 40% of these patients, although this type of involvement can be observed in patients of all ages. Signs and symptoms include bony defects with exophthalmos, with a tumor mass in the orbital cavity being characteristic. This condition usually occurs owing to involvement of the roof and lateral wall of the orbital bones. In addition, teeth may be lost because of gum infiltration or mandibular involvement (Fig. 52.2).

TABLE 52.2 Clinical Features of the Non-Langerhans Cell Histiocytosis, Nonhemophagocytic Lymphohistiocytosis Histiocytoses

Diagnosis	Ages	Lesions (n)	Appearance	Common Sites	Natural History
JXG	0–18 years (median, 2 years)	Single:multiple 9:1 (disseminated in <6 months)	Reddish progressing to yellow brown	Head and neck	Gradual involution
Giant JXG	Young	Single	>2 cm	Upper extremity or back	Involution
Systemic JXG (4% of JXG)	(3 months*)	Single, multiple	Almost 50% have no skin lesions	Subcutis, liver, spleen, lung, CNS, iris	May involute (4–10% fatal)
Adult XG	18–80 (35 years*)	Single	Same as JXG	Upper body	No involution
BCH	Young child	Few, multiple	Reddish-tan papules	Head and neck	Involution or progression to XG
GEH	Young adult	Disseminated	Reddish-tan papules in crops	Face, trunk, arms	Involution or progression
XD	Young adult	Disseminated	Yellow/reddish-brown plaques and nodules	Eyelids, mucosae, viscerae, CNS	Slow involution or progression
PNH	40–60 years	Disseminated	Xanthoma, nodules	Skin, subcutis	Progression to disfigurement
MRH	>40 years	Multiple	Pink/reddish-brown or yellow	Head, extremities with erosive polyarthritis	Progression
SHML	Wide age range (20 years*)	Mainly systemic	Firm indurated papules	Cervical adenopathy, 80% "B" symptoms, extranodal (43%)	Exacerbations and remissions (5–11% fatal)
ECD	7–84 years (53 years*)	Mainly systemic	Xanthelasma, xanthoma	Long-bone sclerosis, retroperitoneal fibrosis	Highly fatal

*Approximate median age of presentation.
BCH, Benign cephalic histiocytosis; CNS, central nervous system; DI, diabetes insipidus; ECD, Erdheim–Chester disease; GEH, generalized eruptive histiocytosis; JXG, juvenile xanthogranuloma; MRH, multicentric reticulohistiocytosis; PNH, progressive nodular histiocytosis; SHML, sinus histiocytosis with massive lymphadenopathy; XD, xanthoma disseminatum.
Adapted from Weitzman S, Jaffe R: Uncommon histiocytic disorders: The non-Langerhans cell histiocytoses. *Pediatr Blood Cancer* 45:256, 2005.

TABLE 52.3 Biopsy Markers or Features of Various Histiocytic Disorders

Clinical Entity	LCH	JXG Family	HLH	SHML
Cell type involved	LC	DD	M/M	M/M
HLA-DR	++	–	+	+
CD1a	++	–	–	–
CD14	–	++	++	++
CD68	+/–	++	++	++
CD163	–	–	++	++
Factor XIIIa	–	++	–	–
Langerin	++	–	–	–
Fascin	–	++	+/–	+
S100	+	–	+/–	+
Lysozyme	–	–	++	++
Birbeck granules	+	–	–	–
Hemophagocytosis			+/–	
Emperipolesis				+

DD, dermal dendrocyte; HLA-DR, human leukocyte antigen-DR; HLH, hemophagocytic lymphohistiocytosis; JXG, juvenile xanthogranuloma; LC, Langerhans cell; LCH, Langerhans cell histiocytosis; M/M, monocyte/macrophage; SHML, sinus histiocytosis with massive lymphadenopathy.
Adapted from Weitzman, Egeler, eds: *Histiocytic Disorders of Children and Adults*. Cambridge, 2005, Cambridge University Press.

The most frequent sites of skeletal involvement include the flat bones of the skull, ribs, pelvis, and scapula. There may be extensive involvement of the skull, with irregularly shaped, lucent lesions giving rise to the so-called *geographic skull*. Long bones and lumbosacral vertebrae, usually the anterior portion of the vertebral body, are involved less frequently. Involvement of the vertebral bodies may lead to collapse (*vertebra plana*) as the principal or only presenting manifestation. In such cases, the diagnosis may be problematic, although biopsy is typically not advisable unless a soft tissue mass is present. In long bones, growth of lesions in the medullary cavity leads to pressure that may result in erosion through the cortex, stimulating the formation of periosteal new bone accompanied by soft tissue extension. The differential diagnosis includes Ewing and osteogenic sarcoma, bone lymphoma, benign bone tumor and cyst, and infection. Involvement of the wrists, hands, knees, feet, or cervical vertebrae is less common. Orbital involvement may result in vision loss or strabismus caused by optic nerve or orbital muscle involvement, respectively, and may mimic preseptal cellulitis. Oral involvement commonly affects the gums, palate, or both. Erosion of the lamina dura gives rise to the characteristic "floating tooth" seen on dental radiographs. The entire mandible may be involved (see Fig. 52.2), with loss of bone leading to diminished height of the mandibular rami. Erosion of gingival tissue causes premature eruption, decay, and tooth loss. Parents of affected children, particularly infants, frequently report precocious eruption of teeth when, in fact, the gums are receding, leading to exposure of immature dentition. Chronic otitis media caused by involvement of the mastoid and petrous portion of the temporal bone, leading to otitis externa is common.

Cutaneous Involvement

Cutaneous involvement by LCH is both common (occurring in 20–40% of patients) and highly variable. The rash is typically a scaly seborrheic, eczematoid, sometimes purpuric rash involving the scalp, ear canals, abdomen, and intertriginous areas of the neck, face, trunk, and groin (Fig. 52.3). The rash may be maculopapular or nodulo-papular. Ulceration may result, especially in intertriginous areas, and

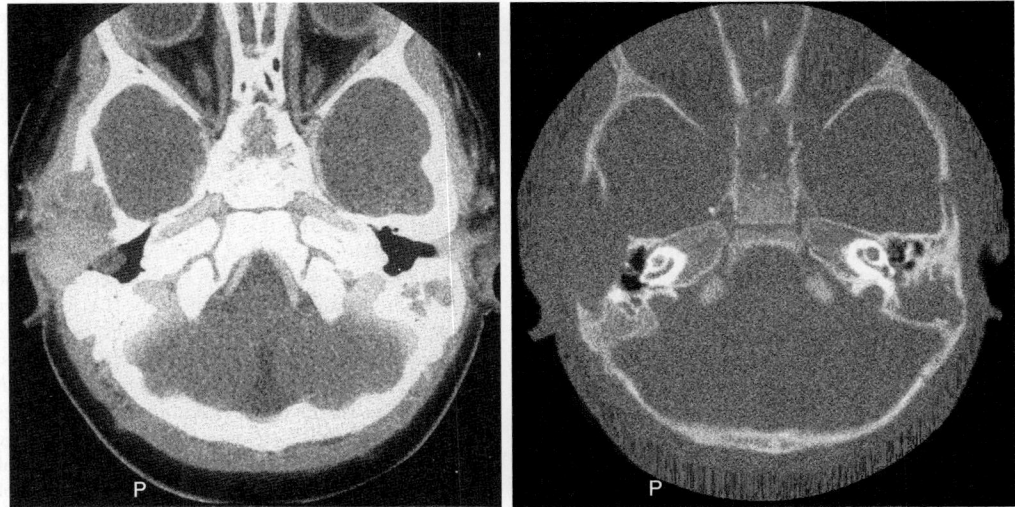

Fig. 52.2 COMPUTED TOMOGRAPHIC SCAN OF A DESTRUCTIVE LANGERHANS CELL HISTIOCYTOSIS ZYGOMATIC LESION IN A CHILD.

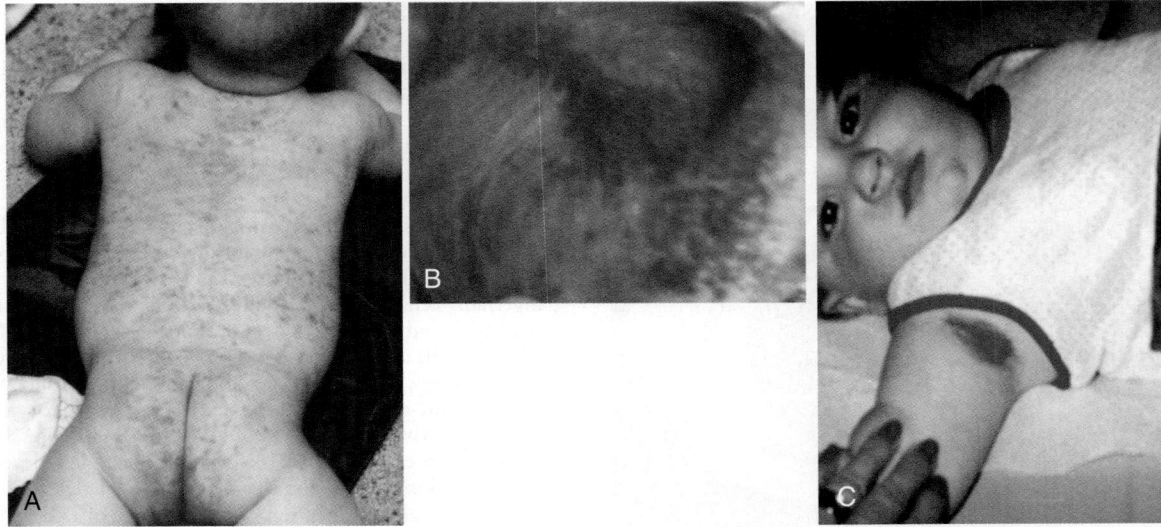

Fig. 52.3 SKIN INVOLVEMENT IN LANGERHANS CELL HISTIOCYTOSIS. (A) Diffuse maculopapular rash. (B) Hemorrhagic scalp rash. (C) Erythematous, "raw" rash typically seen in skin folds such as in the axilla or groin.

may be painful. Mild, isolated cutaneous involvement is relatively common in young infants. Rarely, LCH may present as deep subcutaneous skin nodules only (formerly described as *Hashimoto–Pritzker syndrome*), typically in young infants.

Involvement of Other Organ Systems

A subset of infants and toddlers with LCH have involvement of the spleen, liver, or bone marrow (BM), usually in addition to prominent skin involvement and variable bony disease. This clinical phenotype, previously referred to as *Letterer–Siwe disease*, is the most severe manifestation of LCH and the only form that is likely to be life threatening. Involvement of the BM, usually as evidenced by cytopenias, is an especially poor prognostic factor. Of note, unlike with other tissues, biopsy of the BM in these patients does not typically reveal an obvious infiltrate with CD1a⁺ cells but rather tends to have a dysplastic appearance. Liver involvement may be severe, leading to significant cholestasis, hypoproteinemia, and diminished synthesis of clotting factors.

LCH can have a strictly nodal presentation, not to be confused with SHML, also known as RDD. This presentation is characterized by significant enlargement of multiple lymph node groups with little or no other signs of disease. Thymic involvement is relatively common in children with multisystem involvement. Pancreatic and thyroid involvement has also been reported. Gastrointestinal tract disease has rarely been identified. It is sometimes associated with severe symptoms of diarrhea, malabsorption, and hypoproteinemia.

Isolated pulmonary involvement is usually seen in young adults in their third or fourth decades of life, and occasionally in adolescents. It may follow a severe and often chronic debilitating course; patients may present with pneumothorax. Cigarette smoking has been strongly implicated in primary pulmonary histiocytosis. In contrast, pulmonary involvement in younger patients with systemic disease frequently is mild, although fulminant pulmonary disease may occur. Findings on chest radiographs vary from a diffuse infiltrate consistent with bilateral interstitial pneumonia to a "honeycomb lung" appearance (Fig. 52.4).

Other Clinical Features

DI affects 5% to 40% of patients with LCH, depending on the report. Most instances of DI occur in children who present with systemic disease and involvement of the orbit and skull. Fewer than one-third of children who ultimately develop DI have polydipsia and polyuria as presenting symptoms of LCH. Most cases of DI present within 4 years of diagnosis. DI is caused by infiltration by Langerhans cells and macrophages into the hypothalamus with or without involvement of the posterior pituitary gland (Fig. 52.5). DI may occur at any time during the course of LCH. Patients should be instructed to report signs of DI as soon as they develop because dehydration and electrolyte imbalance may be quite serious. In addition, definitive documentation of DI with measurement of serum and urine electrolytes and osmolality before and after a several-hour water deprivation period should be performed. Vasopressin levels can be measured to document a deficiency. The effectiveness of LCH treatment for reversal of new-onset DI is controversial.

Short stature has been found in up to 40% of children with systemic LCH. Chronic illness and steroid therapy are believed to play an important role in this phenomenon. However, short stature also may be a consequence of anterior pituitary involvement and growth hormone deficiency, which can occur in up to half of patients with initial anterior pituitary dysfunction. Other endocrine manifestations include hyperprolactinemia and hypogonadism caused by hypothalamic infiltration.

A severe complication or manifestation of LCH is the development of a delayed central nervous system (CNS) neurodegenerative syndrome. This CNS involvement is typically seen in children who had classic lytic bony involvement or soft tissue mass lesions in or around the CNS years earlier. Delayed CNS involvement is typically diagnosed after a prolonged, sometimes insidious, decrease in school function. Magnetic resonance imaging (MRI) reveals diffuse or polymorphic lesions involving the white matter of the cerebellum, pons, and cerebral hemispheres. Limited biopsy studies have revealed an inflammatory infiltrate, predominated by CD8+ T cells. Such findings suggest that this form of CNS involvement is analogous to a paraneoplastic syndrome. However, the timing (usually years after disease resolution) and the lack of concurrently active LCH in most patients are unique to this syndrome. Currently, there are no agreed upon diagnostic criteria for CNS LCH, but neurologic involvement (as evidenced by neuropsychiatric testing) with or without MRI findings is essential. Of note, although abnormal MRI findings (with white matter lesions) may precede clinical manifestations, such findings do not always correlate with clinical disease (even in retrospect). Lesions involving the CNS itself or bony lesions of the skull base and facial bones (but not the calvarium or mandible) are thought to confer the greatest risk for subsequent development of this complication.

Laboratory Manifestations

LCH is the most common and prominent of numerous dendritic cell-related histiocytic disorders. Tables 52.2 and 52.3 list the clinical and pathologic features that help to describe and distinguish LCH from other, much rarer, histiocytic disorders (as well as HLH and SHML, discussed in the next section). The typical histologic appearance of LCH varies with the age of the lesion examined (Fig. 52.6). The Langerhans cell is the essential diagnostic feature in the histology of LCH. Early lesions often are locally destructive, with proliferation and accumulation of phenotypically and functionally immature Langerhans cells. Mitoses usually are not present in great numbers, but when found are of no known prognostic significance. Multinucleated giant cells are commonly noted. Other inflammatory cells, such as granulocytes, eosinophils, macrophages, and lymphocytes, are also present. Giant cells and macrophages may be phagocytic and, over time, may accumulate cholesterol. As lesions mature or show signs of regression, fewer Langerhans cells are present, and development of fibrotic reaction is less. The diagnosis of LCH relies on the immunohistochemical identification of the presence of Langerhans cells by cell surface CD1a or by the presence of Birbeck granules by electron microscopy in biopsied lesions. Pathologic criteria for the diagnosis of LCH have been established and were formalized by the Histiocyte Society in 1987. With the availability of antibodies to CD1a for use in routinely processed paraffin-embedded specimens, electron

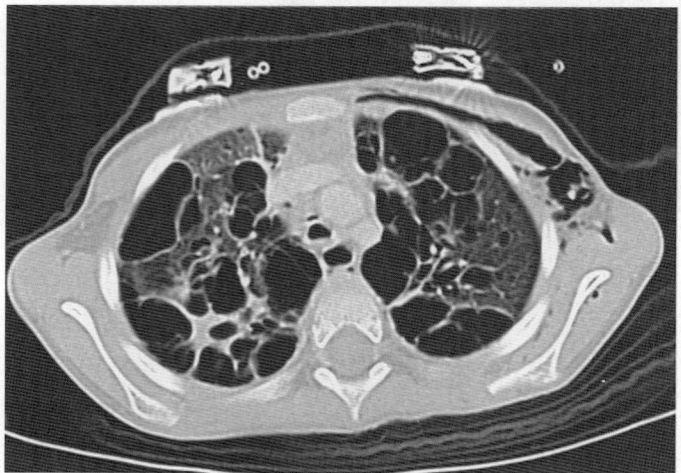

Fig. 52.4 COMPUTED TOMOGRAPHIC SCAN OF THE LUNGS SHOWING CYSTIC CHANGES ASSOCIATED WITH LANGERHANS CELL HISTIOCYTOSIS. *(Courtesy Dr. Melanie Committo.)*

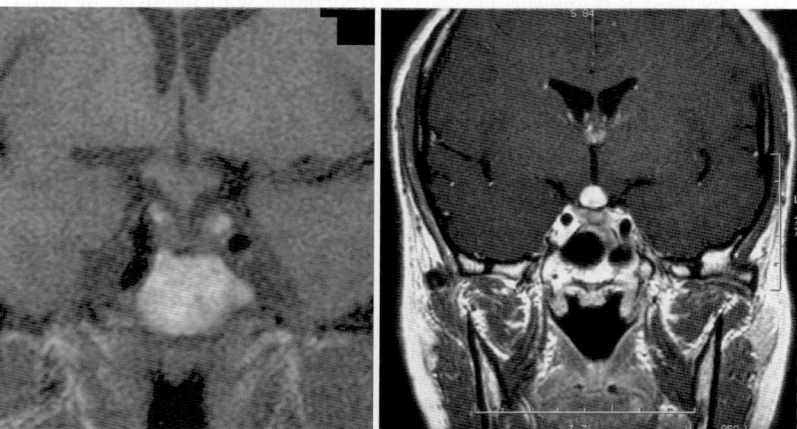

Fig. 52.5 MAGNETIC RESONANCE IMAGING CONTRAST CORONAL VIEWS SHOWING TWO PATIENTS WITH DIABETES INSIPIDUS AND PITUITARY INVOLVEMENT CAUSED BY LANGERHANS CELL HISTIOCYTOSIS.

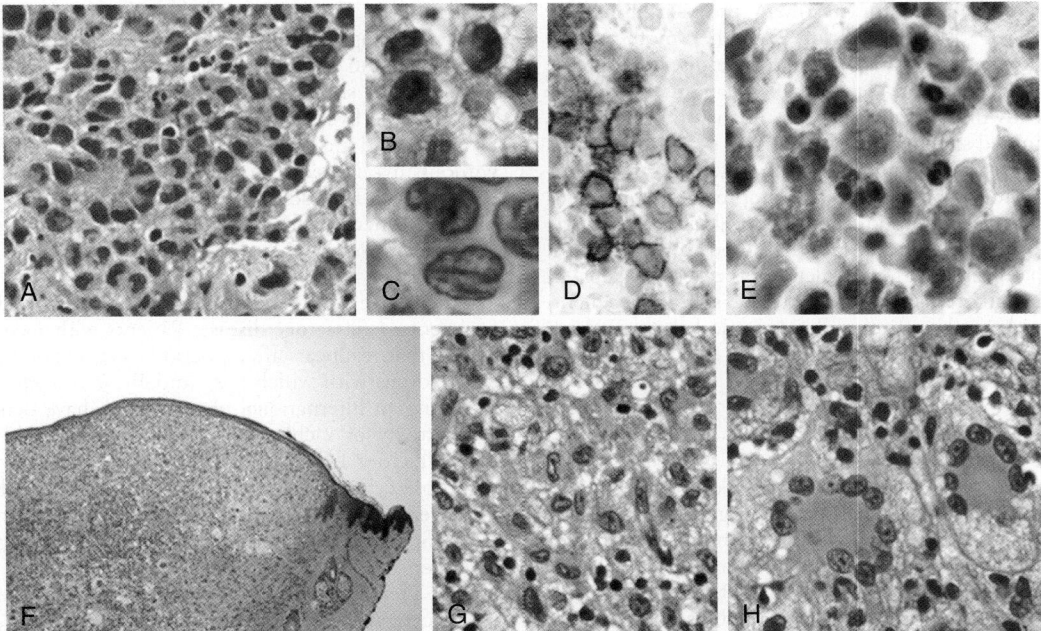

Fig. 52.6 (A–E) Langerhans cell histiocytosis. (A and B) Biopsy sample showing sheets of histiocytes with abundant pink cytoplasm and folded nuclei with prominent nuclear grooves. (C) Cell with a central longitudinal nuclear groove, giving the cell a coffee bean appearance. (D) Immunohistochemical stain for CD1A showing the histiocytic cells are positive. (E) Some cases of Langerhans histiocytosis are associated with prominent eosinophilia. Another term for such cases is *eosinophilic granuloma*. (F–H) Juvenile histiocytosis. Histologic features of juvenile xanthogranuloma vary. (F) In this case, low-power magnification shows a dome-shaped lesion with an attenuated epidermis. (G) At higher power, the bulk of the lesion is composed of a proliferation of histiocytes with abundant pink cytoplasm. Sometimes these histiocytes show more vacuolization or xanthomatization. (H) Scattered Touton-type giant cells are present.

microscopy is rarely needed. Of note, CD1a⁺ Langerhans cells are known to accumulate at the sites of inflammation and may be seen at the margins of malignant lesions. Thus, care should be taken that an adequate biopsy specimen has been obtained to observe the full context of a putative lesion.

Unlike with many malignancies, there are no predictive pathologic features that may define "favorable" or "unfavorable" histology. Although patients are grouped based on their organ system involvement, untreated patients generally do not progress to a different grouping. Within a few months after presentation, it will become apparent that the lesions seen initially are limited to the skeleton or were the "heralding lesion(s)" of diffuse systemic involvement. When cutaneous involvement is the only obvious presenting sign, several months may be required to determine the ultimate extent of disease.

Patients who are suspected to have LCH or who have a new biopsy-proven diagnosis of LCH should have a screening positron emission tomography (or plain radiography and bone scan, although this has been demonstrated to be less sensitive) to help determine the extent of disease involvement. All patients should be evaluated with a complete blood count, chemistries including liver function tests, coagulation workup, and urine osmolality. Dental examination and radiographs should also be considered. The occurrence of cytopenias, particularly thrombocytopenia, in the presence of liver or spleen involvement may be diagnostic of BM involvement.

Differential Diagnosis

The differential diagnosis of LCH depends on the clinical presentation and is typically clarified with a tissue biopsy. Skin involvement frequently mimics seborrheic dermatitis, albeit with a severe or refractory course. Immunodeficiency syndromes or viral infection must be considered as well. The differential diagnosis of bony lesions, although typically quite distinctive, may include bone cyst, lymphoma,

sarcoma, or metastatic solid tumor. Chronically draining ears from temporal bone involvement is often diagnosed as chronic otitis media. Liver and spleen involvement must be distinguished from leukemia and storage diseases.

Prognosis

The prognosis of patients with LCH is largely determined by the nature of their disease presentation and their response to initial therapies. In general, the only patient population with significant mortality rates are those with visceral, or so-called "risk organ", involvement (e.g., liver, spleen, or BM). Furthermore, the international Histiocyte Society conducted a clinical trial (LCH-II) that identified the response after an initial 6 weeks of therapy with weekly vinblastine and daily prednisolone as the single most important factor in predicting mortality in patients with risk organ involvement. Of the approximately 79% of patients who responded to initial therapy, 94% were alive at 5 years, but only 11% of the nonresponders survived. These important data suggest that alternative therapies should be tested early during the course of therapy for patients with poor early responses. Based on early clinical trials, a staging system was developed for the LCH-III trial that is being further modified in the LCH-IV trial.

Therapy

A generally accepted standard for initial treatment of patients with LCH is use of an appropriate amount of the least toxic therapy to treat the disease. In patients with potentially morbid or life-threatening disease at presentation or in those who develop morbid or life-threatening disease during the course of treatment, alternative and sometimes more aggressive treatment should be implemented. This approach emphasizes the need for treatment protocols based on careful prognosis-based risk stratification. Whether more intense upfront therapy in lower risk patients can reduce disease sequelae, such as DI, CNS degeneration, sclerosing cholangitis, or disease recurrence, is currently under evaluation. For the majority of patients with localized or limited systemic disease, the goal of therapy should be minimizing loss of function and preventing cosmetic deformity. Seborrhea-like dermatitis of the scalp may improve with use of a selenium- or phenol-based shampoo. Topical steroids can be effective, but prolonged exposure or use on the face should be avoided. Topical nitrogen mustard has been used for problematic focal skin lesions. In patients with particularly refractory and extensive skin involvement, psoralen ultraviolet A can be effective. These topical therapies have not been studied in clinical trials.

Surgery and Radiotherapy

Patients with disease involving a single bone can usually be managed with local therapy. This most often involves surgical curettage for patients whose lesions are in easily accessible, noncritical locations. Complete "cancer operation" resections are not considered necessary and should be avoided to reduce cosmetic and orthopedic deformities, as well as loss of function. Local soft tissue disease (e.g., scalp, thymus, lymph nodes) generally recurs despite surgery; thus, additional treatment with antiinflammatory or cytoreductive drugs is usually required. Because of concerns about the development of secondary malignancies, systemic therapy is usually favored over radiation. However, local radiotherapy is indicated under certain circumstances; for example, when patients are at risk for visual or hearing loss, skeletal deformity, spinal cord injury, or severe pain when systemic therapy is not rapidly effective.

Chemotherapy

Historically, drugs used in therapy for classic malignant diseases have been used for the systemic or local treatment of LCH. A variety of drugs, including vinblastine, vincristine, cytarabine, nitrogen mustard, cyclophosphamide, procarbazine, chlorambucil, etoposide, methotrexate, corticosteroids, and 6-mercaptopurine (6-MP), have been used, alone or in combination, with variable success. Therapeutic advances for LCH in recent years have largely come from international cooperative trials conducted by the Histiocyte Society. The Histiocyte Society is currently opening the next international trial, LCH-IV, which has strata allowing for the enrollment of all patients with LCH, either as a treatment or as a registry study. For patients not enrolled on LCH-IV, detailed treatment recommendations are available on the Histiocyte Society's website (http://www.histio.org).

A reasonable therapeutic approach to systemic therapy is to observe patients with limited, single-system disease who respond to local (i.e., surgery, radiation) or nonsystemic (i.e., topical steroids) therapy and look for signs of disease resolution. If persistent symptomatic lesions or evidence of progressive disease is seen, systemic treatment should be pursued. Patients with disease that is localized to skin, bone, and lymph nodes (defined as "nonrisk" organs) generally have a good prognosis and may require only minimal treatment. Extensive refractory skin disease may warrant systemic therapy with low-dose oral methotrexate, vinblastine–prednisone, or low-dose cytarabine, or with topical therapy such as nitrogen mustard.

Multisystem disease or multifocal bony disease usually warrants treatment with systemic chemotherapy. The current standard of care is a risk-adapted approach, largely using vinblastine, prednisone, and 6-MP, based on the LCH-III trial. This approach has evolved in a stepwise fashion from previous multicenter trials conducted by international groups (DAL-HX 83/90 protocols [Austria, Germany, Switzerland, The Netherlands], LCH-I, and LCH-II). All of these protocols were risk adapted and were based on different combinations of prednisone, vinblastine, etoposide, methotrexate, and 6-MP. The

Histiocyte Society has stratified patients with LCH into "low-risk" (LR) and "high-risk" (HR) groups based on outcomes related to the extent and location of the LCH lesions. LR patients include patients with skin, bone, lymph node, and pituitary involvement. Patients with liver, spleen, or BM involvement usually have a worse prognosis and are considered higher risk. Children with lung LCH, without involvement of other HR organs, are generally not considered to be HR. Additionally, LR patients believed to have lesions that may increase their future risks of CNS degenerative disease (lesions within the CNS, skull base, or facial bones) are designated as "CNS risk".

Alternative treatment has not been standardized for patients with recurrent or refractory disease. Patients with recurrent disease (i.e., disease that reappears after a period of remission) often respond well to the drugs with which they initially were treated. Several studies, including an international phase II trial, have demonstrated significant activity of 2-chlorodeoxyadenosine (2-CdA) against recurrent and refractory LCH. In addition, the combination of 2-CdA and high-dose cytarabine has been used in refractory, high-risk patients. However, recent reports suggest that clofarabine may be a superior agent for salvage treatment of refractory LCH compared with historical experience (although no direct comparison has been conducted). Finally, a recent report, by Simko et al has demonstrated that upfront use of cytarabine monotherapy is associated with excellent response rates, and may avoid the toxicities of prednisone/vinblastine-based regimens.

Long-Term Follow-up

Retrospective analysis of "CNS risk" patients treated with only surgery, steroid injection, radiation therapy, or a single chemotherapy drug have a 40% incidence of DI. If they receive vinblastine and prednisone for 6 months the incidence of DI is 20%. Complications of developing DI include a significant incidence of anterior pituitary hormone deficiencies or neurodegenerative syndrome. Patients with neurodegenerative syndrome may have ataxia, dysarthria, dysmetria, and learning and behavior difficulties. The diagnosis may be aided by brain MRI, in which T2 hyperintense signals in the cerebellum, basal ganglia, or pons may be present, but such abnormalities do not always correlate with clinical disease or vice versa. Treatment with intravenous immunoglobulin (IVIG) or low-dose cytarabine has anecdotally resulted in stabilization of these symptoms.

A retrospective analysis by Willis et al of 71 patients from a single institution followed for a median of 8.1 years from diagnosis revealed the presence of significant late sequelae in 64% of patients followed for more than 3 years. Skeletal defects were found in 42%, dental problems in 30%, DI in 25%, growth failure in 20%, sex hormone deficiency in 16%, hypothyroidism in 14%, hearing loss in 16%, and CNS dysfunction in 14%. The risk of malignancy in patients with LCH undergoing radiation and chemotherapy is well documented. Thus judicious use of radiotherapy, avoidance of potentially carcinogenic chemotherapeutic agents, and good supportive care are recommended. Leukemia in LCH patients treated with etoposide as a single agent and in combination with other agents has been reported. Because etoposide was not shown to be any more effective than vinblastine in both the LCH-I and LCH-II trials for patients without risk organ involvement, there does not appear to be reason to include this leukemogenic agent in the treatment of these patients with newly diagnosed LCH.

Another serious late effect of LCH is sclerosing cholangitis, which may lead to secondary biliary cirrhosis and liver failure. Sclerosing cholangitis may develop years after successful therapy for LCH and does not typically signify disease recurrence. The only successful treatment of sclerosing cholangitis has been liver transplantation. Other late complications of LCH are pulmonary cyst formation, fibrosis, and chronic pneumothoraces. No effective treatment is available, and progression to cor pulmonale and respiratory failure may occur. Lung transplantation has been used for treatment of such patients. Thus, all patients with LCH require long-term follow up.

In addition to late malignancies, patients should be monitored for signs of long-term disabilities, including cosmetic, orthopedic, and cutaneous deformities that may lead to loss of function and emotional disorders, loss of permanent dentition, endocrinologic disorders and growth failure, hearing impairment, CNS abnormalities and neurocognitive function, sclerosing cholangitis with biliary cirrhosis, and pulmonary fibrosis and cor pulmonale.

Future Directions

The treatment of LCH has undergone significant refinement over the past decade. However, therapy remains empirically defined. With the recent insights into the pathophysiology of LCH, such as B-Raf mutations, new possibilities for more intelligently designed, targeted therapies are conceivable. Trials are ongoing for the assessment of B-Raf and Mek inhibitors in pediatric solid malignancies. It is expected that pilot trials in patients with LCH will commence in the near future. Future clinical trials for such targeted therapies will likely focus on patients with therapy-resistant risk organ involvement because these children have the least satisfactory outcomes.

JUVENILE XANTHOGRANULOMATOUS DISEASE

JXG (or more broadly, the full spectrum of juvenile xanthogranulomatous diseases) is a dendritic cell-related histiocytic disorder. JXG most commonly affects infants and young children, and presents as a solitary or a few "fleshy nodules". These red-yellowish, benign-appearing lesions are sometimes mistaken for molluscum. However, when biopsied, these lesions reveal a distinctive pathology (see Fig. 52.6). Multinucleated, Touton giant cells are usually found, and lesional histiocytes are positive for CD14, CD68, CD163, factor XIIIa, and fascin, suggesting that they are dermal dendrocytes. The cells are usually negative for CD1a, S100, and the plasmacytoid monocyte antigen CD123.

JXG most commonly presents as a single skin lesion in infants and young children. The lesions are nodular and usually yellowish to reddish purple. Lesions may vary significantly in size and number but are often several millimeters to 1 cm in size and solitary. However, in some patients the lesions become widespread and quite disfiguring (Fig. 52.7). Furthermore, JXG may become systemic, involving multiple organs, including the liver, lungs, heart, and CNS. CNS involvement can present with seizures, hemiplegia, and increased intracranial pressure. Patients diagnosed with JXG, particularly multifocal JXG, may benefit from screening computed tomography scans to rule out disseminated involvement, particularly if clinical history suggests this. However, regardless of clinical symptoms, all patients with JXG should have ophthalmologic examination to rule out anterior chamber involvement and prevent potentially blinding complications.

Cutaneous JXG lesions usually resolve over several months and require no treatment. Of note, residual pigmented areas may persist indefinitely even after lesions have regressed. In patients in whom JXG becomes systemic and involves multiple organs, systemic chemotherapy similar to that for patients with LCH has been used. In patients who do not respond to initial treatment with vinblastine and steroids, use of other agents, such as methotrexate, steroids, and 2-CdA, has led to responses, according to anecdotal reports.

ERDHEIM–CHESTER DISEASE

ECD is a rare, non-Langerhans form of histiocytosis first described in 1930 with a wide range of manifestations. The number of new cases has dramatically increased over the past 10 years because of the better recognition of this condition. The natural evolution is variable, but the prognosis in the absence of effective therapy is poor.

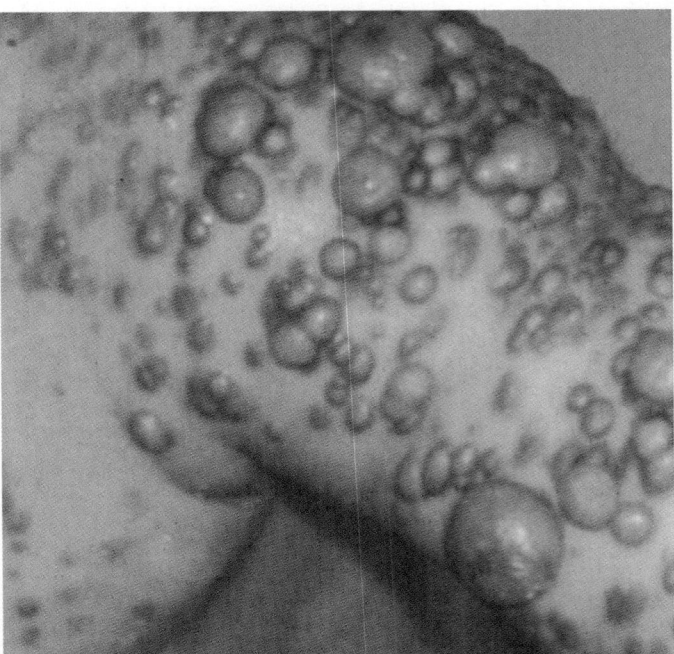

Fig. 52.7 EXTENSIVE JUVENILE XANTHOGRANULOMATOUS DISEASE IN AN INFANT.

ECD is seen most commonly in patients aged 50 years or older. It usually presents with xanthoma-like skin nodules and bilateral lower limb bone pain. Patients with more disseminated disease may have cardiopulmonary insufficiency; renal failure caused by characteristic retroperitoneal and perinephric infiltrative or constrictive changes; and CNS involvement manifested by ataxia, DI, and altered mental status. They may also have periorbital involvement with exophthalmos and impingement on the optic nerves. The disease may be progressive and fatal. The pathophysiology of ECD has been mysterious, although a plasma cytokine profile consisting of elevated interferon-α (IFN-α), interleukin-12 (IL-12), monocyte chemotactic protein-1, IL-4, and IL-7 in these patients suggests a systemic immune perturbation. Recently, mutations in BRAF similar to those in LCH have been identified as the likely initiating event in these patients, although why ECD develops uniquely compared with LCH remains a mystery.

First-line treatment for ECD has consisted of IFN-α. However, a recent report of excellent response to a B-Raf inhibitor may change this standard of care. Other effective treatments have been limited, although responses have been observed with steroids, vinblastine plus steroids, methotrexate, 2-CdA, and bisphosphonates, in addition to IFN-α. Autologous hematopoietic BMT has been reported as a therapeutic modality.

HEMOPHAGOCYTIC LYMPHOHISTIOCYTOSIS

In the broad classification of histiocytic disorders (see Table 52.1), HLH is categorized as a monocyte/macrophage-related histiocytic disorder. HLH derives its name from its sometimes distinctive pathology (hemophagocytosis), in which macrophages appear to be widely infiltrating tissues and engulfing blood and BM cells in a nonspecific fashion. However, HLH is best conceptualized as an immune regulatory disorder, which is characterized by clinical signs and symptoms of extreme inflammation and the development of cytopenias, hepatitis, and CNS dysfunction, which are severe and life threatening. Indeed, it has recently been proposed that the name of this disorder should be changed to "hyperinflammatory lymphohistiocytosis" (also HLH).

HLH was first described as a familial disease by Farquhar and Claireux in 1952, which they named "familial hemophagocytic

TABLE 52.4	Diagnostic Criteria for Hemophagocytic Lymphohistiocytosis, Established for the Conduct of the Hemophagocytic Lymphohistiocytosis-2004 Trial

The diagnosis of HLH may be established by:[a]

A. A molecular diagnosis consistent with HLH: Pathologic mutations of *PRF1*, *UNC13D*, *Munc18-2*, *Rab27a*, *STX11*, *SH2D1A*, or *BIRC4*

or

B. Five of the eight criteria listed below are fulfilled:

1. Fever ≥38.3°C
2. Splenomegaly
3. Cytopenias (affecting at least two of three lineages in the peripheral blood)
4. Hemoglobin <9 g/dL (in infants <4 weeks: hemoglobin <10 g/dL)
   Platelets <100 × 10³/mL
   Neutrophils <1 × 10³/mL
5. Hypertriglyceridemia (fasting ≥265 mg/dL) or hypofibrinogenemia (≤150 mg/dL)
6. Hemophagocytosis in BM, spleen, lymph nodes, or liver
7. Low or absent NK cell activity
8. Ferritin >500 ng/mL
9. Elevated soluble CD25 (soluble IL-2 receptor α)

[a]Additionally, in the case of familial HLH, no evidence of malignancy should be apparent.
BM, Bone marrow; HLH, hemophagocytic lymphohistiocytosis; IL-2, interleukin-2; NK, natural killer.

reticulosis". Through the years, the syndrome of HLH has been recognized as both a sporadic and familial disorder, and in various clinical contexts. Although we prefer to lump each of these clinical variations into a single syndrome (HLH), the medical literature has used a plethora of names: familial erythrophagocytic lymphohistiocytosis, viral-associated hemophagocytic syndrome, and malignancy-associated hemophagocytic syndrome, among others. Furthermore, macrophage activation syndrome (MAS), the systemic inflammatory syndrome observed in association with rheumatologic disorders, is likely a variant of HLH syndrome because both "classic" HLH and MAS have similar clinical phenotypes and appear to share some underlying mechanisms. The International Histiocyte Society formally adopted the name of HLH in 1998 and defined criteria for its diagnosis, which were updated in 2004 (Table 52.4).

Epidemiology

The true incidence and prevalence of HLH are unknown and remain difficult to ascertain accurately. The diagnosis of HLH is challenging because of its variable presentation and the many nonspecific clinical features it shares with other disease processes. HLH is considered to be rare, but increasing awareness and recognition of the syndrome is leading to more frequent diagnoses. Currently, it is estimated that the autosomal recessive forms of familial HLH have a prevalence of 1 in 50,000 live births. A recent report estimated the incidence of HLH in tertiary care pediatric hospitals at 1 case of HLH per 3000 inpatient admissions. Because of the typically autosomal recessive nature of familial HLH, this disorder is reported to occur more frequently in isolated populations or kindreds with consanguinity.

Pathobiology

The immunologic basis of HLH was long suspected because of its inflammatory nature and the finding of cytotoxic deficiencies and other immune abnormalities in patients with HLH. The first confirmation that HLH is an immunodeficiency came in 1999 with the discovery of perforin mutations in affected patients. However, unlike other immunodeficiencies, the principal clinical characteristic of HLH is one of intense, prolonged systemic inflammation rather than unusual or severe infections. Although this inflammation may be triggered by infection or vaccination, the inflammation itself (and not apparently the sometimes benign or transient infection) appears to drive the clinical features of HLH. Thus, familial HLH appears to be a deficiency of immune regulation. Animal studies have begun to detail how this immune regulation functions and how deficiencies may lead to HLH. In brief, cytotoxic lymphocytes kill not only infected cells but also antigen-presenting cells (APCs). These APCs promote T-cell activation during infection. This persistence of activating signals leads to excessive or prolonged acute T-cell activation. Abnormal T-cell activation, in turn, leads to activation of macrophages and the development of disease pathology. In animal models, IFN-γ appears to be the critical nexus between T-cell activation and disease development. In several published series, IFN-γ appears to be elevated in patients with HLH. However, clinical data appear mixed, and it remains uncertain whether IFN-γ is critical for HLH development in all patients. An underlying lesion of immune regulation and the associated pathophysiology is less clear in apparently sporadic cases of HLH, sometimes referred to as *secondary HLH*. However, the traditional dichotomy between primary (familial) HLH and secondary HLH (associated with infections, malignancy, or autoimmunity) is becoming increasingly murky.

HLH may present in a variety of clinical contexts and with a variety of etiologic associations. Patients in the primary HLH category are those with clear familial inheritance or known genetic causes, are usually infants or younger children, and are thought to have fixed defects of cytotoxic function (although this is not always the case). These patients have a clear risk of HLH recurrence and will generally not survive long term without hematopoietic cell transplantation (HCT). Although HLH in these patients can be associated with infections (e.g., cytomegalovirus [CMV] or Epstein–Barr virus [EBV]) or vaccination, the immunologic trigger is often not apparent. The term "secondary HLH" generally refers to older children (or adults) who present without a family history or known genetic cause for their HLH. These patients typically have concurrent infections or medical conditions that appear to trigger their HLH, such as EBV infection, malignancy, or rheumatologic disorders. The list of triggering stimuli for both familial and apparently nonfamilial HLH is extensive. Patients with presumed secondary HLH are sometimes reported as having immune studies, including NK cell function, that normalize with disease resolution, although in the authors' experience this is variable or unclear. Although the mortality rate from HLH may be significant, the risk of recurrence in cases of secondary HLH is poorly defined. Recurrence of HLH in the absence of autoimmune disease or malignancy is generally considered to be good evidence that a patient has primary HLH, regardless of the other clinical features. In the absence of a known genetic defect or family history, it is often not possible to make an initial diagnosis of "primary" or "secondary" HLH. Further obscuring this dichotomy, a recent report by Zhang et al described a large series of adults with HLH who were found to have genetic mutations typically seen in children with familial HLH.

A variety of genetic causes of familial HLH have been identified, all either autosomal recessive or X-linked (Table 52.5). Most of these genetic lesions affect a biologic pathway referred to as *granule-dependent*, or *perforin-dependent*, *cytotoxicity* (Fig. 52.8). This pathway is used by T cells and NK cells to kill target cells, typically those infected by viruses. When triggered, specialized lysosomal granules containing perforin, granzymes, and other proteins are released, leading to apoptotic death of target cells. The first genetic lesions identified in patients with HLH were mutations in *prf1*, the gene encoding the protein perforin. *Prf1* mutations account for about 15% to 20% of HLH in certain geographic areas and are known as familial HLH 2 (FHL2). FHL2 has mild and severe phenotypes that correlate with the degree of mature perforin protein that is produced. Abnormalities of granule formation, mobilization, and extrusion are also identified as causes of HLH. Munc13-4, a protein essential to the exocytotic process, is mutated in FHL3. FHL3 has a worldwide distribution and accounts for 15% to 20% of all heritable HLH.

TABLE 52.5	Hemophagocytic Lymphohistiocytosis-Associated Gene Mutations	
Gene	Location	Disease
PRF1	10q21-22	FHL2
UNC13D	17q25	FHL3
STX11	6q24	FHL4
RAB27A	15q21	Griscelli syndrome
STXBP2	19p13	FHL5
Unknown	9q21.3-22	FHL1
SH2D1A	Xq24-26	XLP1
XIAP	Xq25	XLP2/X-linked HLH

FHL, Familial hemophagocytic lymphohistiocytosis; HLH, hemophagocytic lymphohistiocytosis; XLP, X-linked lymphoproliferative syndrome.

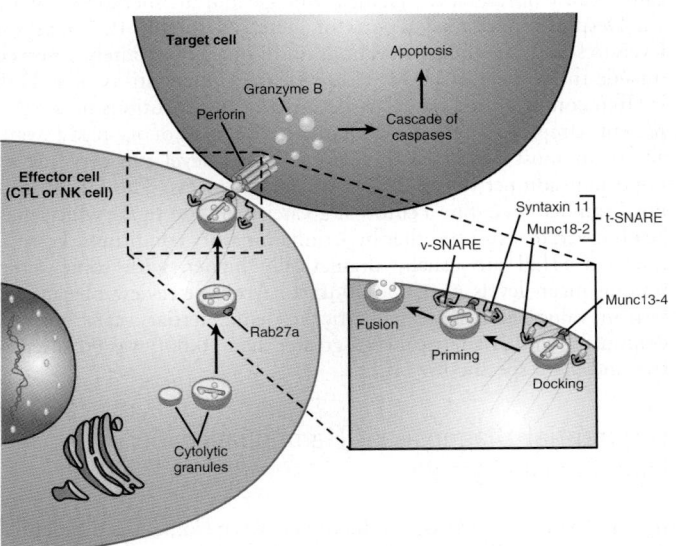

Fig. 52.8 MECHANICS OF CYTOTOXIC FUNCTION REVEALED BY HEMOPHAGOCYTIC LYMPHOHISTIOCYTOSIS-ASSOCIATED GENE MUTATIONS. Hemophagocytic lymphohistiocytosis-associated genetic abnormalities (in the indicated genes) may affect granule-dependent lymphocyte cytotoxicity by impairing trafficking, docking, priming for exocytosis, or membrane fusion of cytolytic granules. The function of this pathway may also be severely impaired by loss of functional perforin, the key delivery molecule for proapoptotic granzymes. Diverse mutations in this pathway all give rise to similar clinical phenotypes (albeit of variable severity). Lyst (the gene affected in Chediak-Higashi syndrome) is not portrayed because its function is not entirely clear, although it appears to play an important role in the maintenance of normally sized (and functional) cytolytic granules. CTL, Cytotoxic T lymphocyte; NK, natural killer, SNARE, soluble N-ethylmaleimide-sensitive fusion attachment receptor protein. (Adapted from Jordan MB, Allen CE, Weitzman S, Filipovich AH, McClain KL: How I treat hemophagocytic lymphohistiocytosis. Blood 118:4041, 2011.)

However, recent discoveries of previously unappreciated intronic mutations in this gene may expand the proportion of patients with FHL3. FHL4 is caused by mutations in the protein syntaxin 11, a member of the soluble N-ethylmaleimide-sensitive fusion attachment receptor protein family of proteins, which is necessary for the fusion of cytotoxic vesicles with the plasma membrane to release their granules. Mutations in the syntaxin-binding protein 2, also important for this process, have been designated FHL5. The genetic defect responsible for FHL1 has not been identified, and no mutations in granzyme proteins have been associated with HLH.

Two X-linked causes of HLH are known. The first, called "X-linked lymphoproliferative syndrome 1" (or XLP1), is caused by

defects in SH2D1A or SAP. This disorder is a complex one characterized by lymphoproliferation, hypogammaglobulinemia, excess risk of lymphoma, and development of HLH. It appears to share some of the pathophysiology with classic familial HLH, although other abnormalities (of B cells and other cells) make this disorder distinctive. The second X-linked cause of HLH, sometimes called "XLP2" (although this is disputed), are abnormalities of a gene/protein called baculoviral inhibitor of apoptosis protein repeat-containing protein 4 (BIRC4)/X-linked inhibitor of apoptosis protein (XIAP). The apparently unique pathophysiology of HLH caused by XIAP deficiency is not understood. Other immunodeficiency syndromes caused by defects in lysosomal trafficking have been linked to life-threatening episodes of HLH. These include Chediak-Higashi syndrome, Griscelli syndrome, and Hermansky-Pudlak syndrome, type II.

Taken together, the nine genetic disorders described above still account for fewer than half of the diagnosed cases of HLH in children, including many familial cases still awaiting molecular definition. Until recently, it was widely believed that symptoms of HLH triggered by genetic causes arose during infancy and early childhood. With the more widespread availability of genetic testing, it is apparent that the first significant episode of HLH can occur throughout life from prenatal presentations through the seventh decade of life. Distinctions between primary (genetically determined) and secondary (acquired) forms of HLH become increasingly blurred together as new genetic causes are identified and patients who develop HLH beyond early childhood or in the contexts of EBV infection or autoimmune disease are being found to share some of the same genetic etiologies.

Clinical Manifestations

The classic presentation of HLH consists of prolonged, hectic fevers (usually present for 1–2 weeks before diagnosis), hepatosplenomegaly, and cytopenias. Neurologic symptoms are common and distinctive features of these patients; these include symptoms of irritability, ataxia, hypotonia or hypertonia, evidence of increased intracranial pressure, meningismus, depressed mental status, cranial nerve palsies, and seizures. Standard diagnostic criteria have been defined by the Histiocyte Society for the conduct of the now closed HLH2004 trial (see Table 52.4). Although imperfect, these criteria are widely accepted for the diagnosis of HLH. However, because HLH is a clinical syndrome, it may present in many forms, including fever of unknown origin (FUO); hepatitis or acute liver failure; and sepsis-like, Kawasaki-like, and primary neurologic abnormalities. Not all of the HLH diagnostic criteria may be present initially, so it is important to follow clinical signs and laboratory markers of pathologic inflammation repeatedly to identify the trends. Typical clinical features seen in patients with HLH, grouped by organ system, are described in the following text.

Prolonged Fever

FUO is a very common diagnosis on general pediatric wards, and differentiating HLH from other causes of FUO may be challenging. In one series, patients ultimately diagnosed with HLH presented with fevers above 102°F for a median of 19 days (range: 4–41 days). In patients with FUO, cytopenias, highly elevated ferritin (>3000 g/dL), or sCD25 significantly above age-adjusted normal ranges generally suggest that a complete HLH diagnostic evaluation should be pursued.

Liver Disease and Coagulopathy

Most patients with HLH have variable evidence of hepatitis at presentation. HLH should be considered in the differential diagnosis of acute liver failure, especially if lymphocytic infiltrates are noted on biopsy. Autopsy evaluation of the liver has shown chronic persistent hepatitis with periportal lymphocytic infiltration in the majority of patients. Neonates with HLH may present with hydrops fetalis and liver failure. Most patients have evidence of disseminated intravascular coagulation (DIC) and are at high risk for acute bleeding. Furthermore, patients with HLH caused by degranulation defects may have intrinsic platelet dysfunction.

Bone Marrow Failure

Anemia and thrombocytopenia occur in more than 80% of patients at the time of presentation with HLH. The cellularity of BM aspirates varies from normocellular to hypocellular or hypercellular. The prevalence of hemophagocytosis in association with HLH diagnosis ranges from 25% to 100%. Although hemophagocytosis in BM is associated with HLH, the morphologic phenomenon may also be induced by more common events, including blood transfusions, infection, autoimmune disease, and other forms of BM failure or causes of red blood cell destruction. Despite the nomenclature of HLH, diagnosis of HLH should never be made or excluded solely on the presence or absence of hemophagocytosis. Infiltration of BM or liver by CD163[+] macrophages, along with global clinical evaluation, may distinguish HLH from other causes of hemophagocytosis.

Skin Manifestations

Patients may have a variety of skin manifestations, including generalized maculopapular erythematous rashes, generalized erythroderma, edema, panniculitis, inflamed papular lesions, petechiae, and purpura. The incidence of skin manifestations ranges from 6% to 65% in published series with highly pleomorphic presentations. Some patients may present with features suggestive of Kawasaki disease, including erythematous rashes, conjunctivitis, red lips, and enlarged cervical lymph nodes. Rashes may correlate with lymphocyte infiltration on skin biopsy, and hemophagocytosis may also be found.

Pulmonary Dysfunction

Patients may develop pulmonary dysfunction that leads to urgent admission to the intensive care unit. In a review of the radiographic abnormalities in 25 patients, 17 had acute respiratory failure with alveolar or interstitial opacities, with fatal outcomes in 88% of those cases.

Brain, Ophthalmic, and Neuromuscular Symptoms

More than one-third of patients present with neurologic symptoms, including seizures, meningismus, decreased level of consciousness, cranial nerve palsy, psychomotor retardation, ataxia, irritability, or hypotonia. The cerebrospinal fluid (CSF) is abnormal in more than 50% of HLH patients with findings of pleocytosis, elevated protein, or hemophagocytosis. MRI findings are highly variable and include discrete lesions, leptomeningeal enhancement, or global edema, and images correlate with neurologic symptoms. Retinal hemorrhages, swelling of the optic nerve, and infiltration of the choroid have been reported in infants with HLH. Diffuse peripheral neuropathy with pain and weakness secondary to myelin destruction by macrophages may also occur.

Laboratory Manifestations

Laboratory manifestations are a critical component of diagnosing HLH. Biochemical abnormalities noted on clinical laboratory assessment include anemia, thrombocytopenia, neutropenia, elevated liver transaminases, hyperbilirubinemia, hypofibrinogenemia, coagulation abnormalities, hypoalbuminemia, hyponatremia, hypertriglyceride-

mia, elevated soluble CD163, elevated soluble CD25 (sCD25; also called "soluble IL-2 receptor"), and hyperferritinemia. Specialized immunologic testing may reveal low or absent NK cell or cytotoxic T lymphocyte function (although this is not always seen), low levels of perforin or other disease-associated proteins (e.g., SAP or XIAP), and decreased degranulation (observed with mutations affecting granule trafficking). Additionally, pathologic examination of BM biopsy, liver biopsy, CSF, spleen or lymph node, or even occasionally peripheral blood may reveal hemophagocytosis and infiltration with CD163[+] macrophages and activated T cells (Fig. 52.9). Examination of CSF reveals pleocytosis, elevated protein, and elevated neopterin levels with CNS involvement. Brain MRI often reveals polymorphic white or grey matter abnormalities in such cases.

Elevations in sCD25 are a particularly useful and notable laboratory feature of HLH. In the authors' experience, this marker is dynamically associated with "active" HLH, and patients with active HLH rarely, if ever, have normal levels of sCD25. Of note, the interpretation of soluble IL-2 receptor levels must be undertaken with care because normal levels change with age and the method of analysis. Despite a few small reports of increased soluble IL-2 receptor levels in sepsis, significant elevations of this marker are rarely observed outside the context of HLH. However, the clinical utility of sCD25 is often compromised by delays because most institutions must send patient samples to referral laboratories. Because of its ready availability in most hospitals, the serum ferritin level can serve as an important adjunct to the decision-making process. The HLH diagnostic guidelines define a cutoff at greater than 500 μg/L, which may be observed in sepsis or other hyperinflammatory conditions. Ferritin levels in HLH are usually dramatically higher, with some series finding mean levels near 45,000 μg/L. A recent review of elevated ferritin values at a large pediatric academic tertiary care hospital demonstrated that a ferritin level greater than 10,000 was 90% sensitive and 96% specific for HLH.

Differential Diagnosis of Hemophagocytic Lymphohistiocytosis

Because HLH presents as an inflammatory syndrome, the differential diagnosis of this disorder is a broad one. Infection must be considered as either a mimic of HLH or as an underlying trigger of the disorder. The list of infections reported as associated with HLH is extensive. If the patient presents with acute multiorgan failure, then sepsis is generally considered first before a diagnosis of HLH is considered. Viral infections, including EBV, CMV, dengue, and severe influenza, should always be considered and treated. Protozoan infections, including malaria, toxoplasmosis, and leishmaniasis, may be a consideration in endemic areas. Visceral leishmaniasis, in particular, may be clinically indistinguishable from primary HLH. In addition to infectious disorders, rheumatologic disorders, including systemic onset juvenile idiopathic arthritis (soJIA) and Kawasaki syndrome, should be considered. Finally, as either a mimic or trigger, malignancy should be considered, particularly lymphoma and leukemia.

Diagnosis

Because of the severe nature of this disorder and the existence of disease-altering therapies, it is crucial to identify patients early in their course. The Histiocyte Society established diagnostic criteria for the HLH-2004 trial, which is widely used for patients not treated in this trial, using both clinical and laboratory findings (see Table 52.4). Laboratory verification of a known genetic defect confirms the diagnosis independent of the presence or absence of any clinical signs or symptoms. However, genetic diagnosis is not usually available in a timely fashion for patients with acute clinical presentations. In the absence of a genetic diagnosis, five of the eight clinical criteria must be met to make a diagnosis. It is important to note that NK cell dysfunction is only present in about 50% of patients with HLH. Additionally, hemophagocytosis may not be present early in the HLH

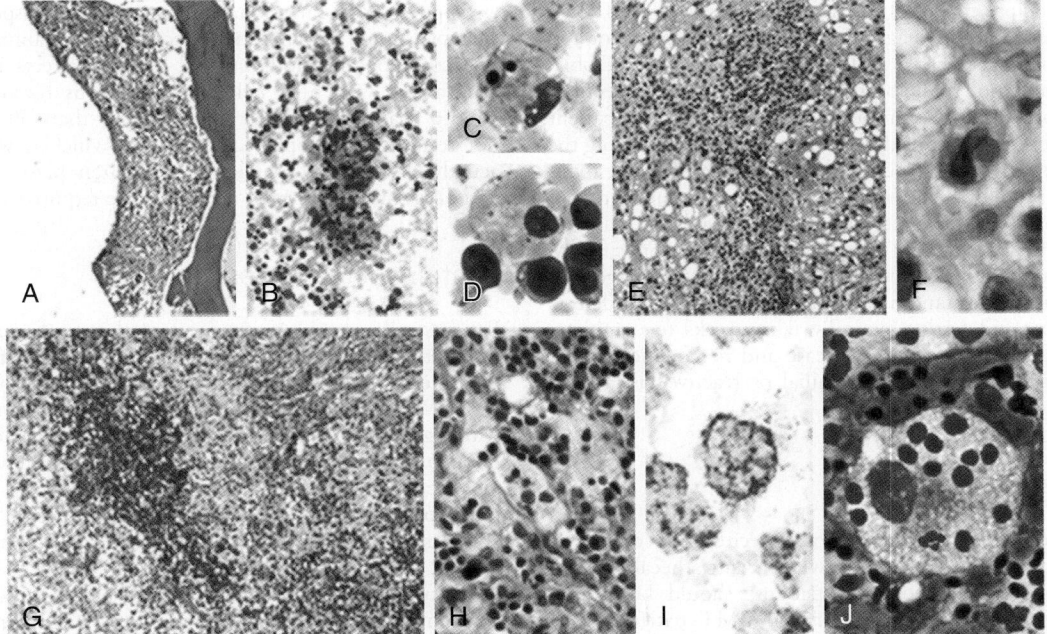

Fig. 52.9 (A–F) Familial hemophagocytic lymphohistiocytosis. Illustrations from a 3-month-old girl who presented with diarrhea, pancytopenia, hepatomegaly, and liver failure. Bone marrow (A and B) showed left-shifted granulopoiesis and increased histiocytes, which at high power (C and D) were undergoing prominent phagocytosis of erythrocytes, platelets, and other cells. Liver biopsy sample (E) showed a lymphohistiocytic infiltrate also associated with hemophagocytosis (F). The patient was shown to harbor a mutation of the perforin gene in exon 2. (G–J) Sinus histiocytosis with massive lymphadenopathy (Rosai–Dorfman disease). Low-power magnification of the biopsy sample (G) shows a mottled appearance of the lesion caused by dark areas containing small lymphocytes and lighter areas containing histiocytes. At higher magnification (H), the histiocytes have abundant pale cytoplasm with scattered cells within. This is emperipolesis, a process of cells traveling through the cytoplasm but not apparently becoming phagocytized or degraded. Note the plasma cells in the background. The emperipolesis can be better visualized with a CD68 stain for histiocytes (I). This process delineates the cell boundary and the cells within the histiocyte cytoplasm. The emperipolesis can also be seen on a Wright-stained touch preparation (J).

disease process; therefore, serial assessments may be required if that diagnostic criterion is to be met.

Therapy

Without therapy, survival of patients with active familial HLH is historically reported to be approximately 2 months. The first international treatment protocol for HLH was organized by the Histiocyte Society in 1994 and led to reported survival of 55%, with a median follow-up of 3.1 years. The HLH-94 protocol, as illustrated in Fig. 52.10, included an 8-week induction therapy with dexamethasone, etoposide, and intrathecal methotrexate. The principal goal of induction therapy is to suppress the life-threatening inflammatory process that underlies HLH. At the end of 8 weeks, patients are either weaned off therapy or transitioned to continuation therapy, which is intended only as a bridge to transplantation.

The Histiocyte Society opened a new trial in 2004, HLH-2004, which is now closed. The major modifications from HLH-94 were to move cyclosporine dosing to the beginning of induction and add hydrocortisone to intrathecal therapy. Results of this trial are not reported at this time. An alternative approach to etoposide-based regimens with comparable survival was published as a single-center retrospective experience over 14 years, in which all patients were treated with corticosteroids and antithymocyte globulin (ATG), followed (rapidly) by HCT. Until this immunotherapy approach can be compared with etoposide–dexamethasone in the setting of a clinical trial and until the results of the HLH-2004 study are published, the standard of care therapy for patients not enrolled in a clinical trial should be based on HLH-94.

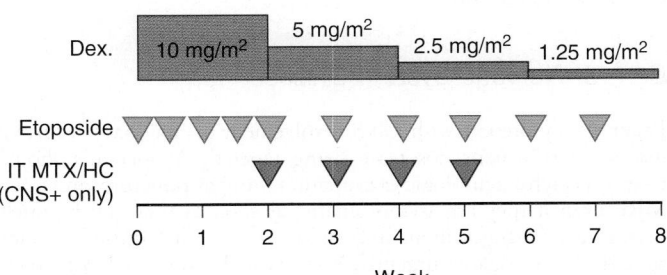

Fig. 52.10 INDUCTION THERAPY FOR HEMOPHAGOCYTIC LYMPHOHISTIOCYTOSIS. Based on the HLH-94 study, this approach should be considered standard of care for all patients not enrolled in clinical trials based on published evidence of efficacy. Etoposide is dosed as 150 mg/m² per dose. Alternatively, for patients weighing less than 10 kg, consideration may be given to dosing etoposide as 5 mg/kg per dose. Dexamethasone (Dex.) is dosed as indicated and may be given orally or intravenously, although the latter is preferred at therapy initiation. IT MTX/HC should be given to patients with evidence of CNS involvement as early as lumbar puncture may be safely performed (which may vary from the diagram) and dosed as follows: age younger than 1 year, 6/8 mg (MTX/HC); age 1–2 years, 8/10 mg; age 2–3 years, 10/12 mg; and age older than 3 years, 12/15 mg. Weekly intrathecal therapy is generally continued until at least 1 week after resolution of CNS involvement (both clinical and cerebrospinal fluid indices). *CNS*, Central nervous system; *IT MTX/HC*, intrathecal methotrexate and hydrocortisone. *(Adapted from Jordan MB, Allen CE, Weitzman S, Filipovich AH, McClain KL: How I treat hemophagocytic lymphohistiocytosis.* Blood *118:4041, 2011.)*

Often, the principal challenge for treating patients with HLH is making a timely and accurate diagnosis. It is critical to search for and treat underlying triggers of HLH and institute specific antimicrobial therapy. Rituximab is often helpful in controlling EBV infection. IVIG is an appropriate adjunct for most viral infections. If the patient is stable and not severely ill, consideration can be given to treating the underlying trigger with disease-specific therapy with or without corticosteroids and close follow-up. However, in most cases, an aggressive therapeutic approach is warranted and may reasonably be initiated before obtaining final results for all diagnostic studies. Specifically, HLH therapy should not be withheld while awaiting results of genetic testing because our understanding of HLH-associated gene defects remains incomplete and testing typically takes weeks to complete. With the exception of autoimmune disease and malignancy, initial therapy for patients with suspected familial or reactive HLH does not differ.

Induction Therapy

The current standard of care consists of a decrescendo course of etoposide and dexamethasone with or without intrathecal therapy (see Fig. 52.10). Ideally, critically ill patients should be treated at facilities familiar with care of cancer and BMT patients. It is important to initiate therapy promptly even in the face of unresolved infections, cytopenias, or organ dysfunction. After starting therapy, patients should be monitored closely for signs of improvement as well as potential complications and toxicities, and therapy may need to be customized. For patients who respond well, with resolution of symptoms and normalization of inflammatory markers, therapy may be weaned per protocol. However, dexamethasone doses and etoposide frequency may need to be increased in response to disease reactivation (see Salvage Therapy section later). Deterioration of liver function and blood counts as well as steady increases in serum ferritin, sCD25, and sCD163 tests may signal relapse of HLH disease activity. If patients do not display at least a partial response within 2 to 3 weeks of therapy initiation, salvage therapy should be considered. Recurrence of fever and increased inflammatory markers after an apparent response should also prompt a careful search for opportunistic infection.

Central Nervous System Disease

Patients may present with CNS involvement or may have recurrent disease as treatment doses are being tapered. All patients should receive a careful neurologic examination, lumbar puncture, and brain MRI, even if they are asymptomatic, as soon as they can be safely performed. Changes in mental status at any time during therapy should be investigated urgently. Patients with proven CNS involvement should be treated with weekly intrathecal methotrexate and hydrocortisone until CSF abnormalities and symptoms normalize. The risk of posterior reversible encephalopathy syndrome (PRES) appears to be significant during induction therapy. Although the etiology of PRES is incompletely understood, it is more frequent in settings of hypertension and is also associated with cyclosporine use. Blood pressure should be aggressively managed during induction. Because CNS involvement suggests a familial etiology and because this disease feature is associated with substantial risks for long-term morbidity, HCT should be considered for patients with this complication.

Supportive Care

Supportive care guidelines for patients on therapy for HLH should be similar to standard practice for patients undergoing HCT, including acute care nursing, *Pneumocystis jiroveci* prophylaxis, fungal prophylaxis, IVIG supplementation, and neutropenic precautions. Any new fever should be evaluated for HLH reactivation, as well

as opportunistic infection, and empiric broad-spectrum antibiotic therapy should be initiated. Because of inflammation, consumptive coagulopathy, and intrinsic platelet defects in some patients, they are at very high risk of spontaneous bleeding. The authors aim to maintain platelet count greater than $50 \times 10^9/L$ and do not recommend prophylactic heparin, which is sometimes used in acutely ill patients. Platelets, fresh-frozen plasma, cryoprecipitate, and occasionally activated factor VII are required for acute bleeding.

Continuation Therapy

Patients who can be weaned off of dexamethasone and etoposide without recurrence, recover normal immune function, and have no identified HLH-associated gene defects may stop therapy after the 8-week induction course. HCT is generally recommended in patients with age younger than 2 years, CNS involvement, recurrent or refractory disease, persistent NK cell dysfunction, or proven familial or genetic disease. Continuation according to HLH-94 consists of pulses of dexamethasone and etoposide (etoposide, 150 mg/m^2 every 2 weeks alternating with dexamethasone 10 mg/m^2/day for 3 days every 2 weeks). Cyclosporine may be added in patients with stable blood pressure and adequate liver and kidney function. Patients on continuation therapy should proceed to HCT as quickly as possible because of the ongoing risks of infection, disease reactivation, or leukemia or myelodysplastic syndrome related to prolonged use of etoposide.

Salvage Therapy

A significant number of patients with HLH either fail to respond adequately to current therapies or relapse before HCT. Approximately 50% of patients treated in the HLH-94 study experienced a complete resolution of HLH, 30% experienced a partial resolution, and approximately 20% died before HCT. Notably, most deaths occurred during the first few weeks of treatment and may reflect either preexisting morbidities or primary refractory disease. Although it is hoped that some patients will fare better with more prompt diagnosis of HLH, others remain unresponsive to standard therapy. Initial treatment with ATG (thymoglobulin, rabbit ATG) has been reported to give higher complete response rates, but partly because of higher relapse rates, long-term outcomes do not appear superior. Although current therapy is effective, there is a need for new treatments for patients with refractory HLH. At present, there are few data regarding potential second-line therapies. Case reports exist describing the use of infliximab, daclizumab, alemtuzumab, anakinra, vincristine, and other agents as salvage therapies for HLH. A recent report found that alemtuzumab has significant activity against refractory HLH in a larger series of patients. Although refractory HLH appears to have a dismal prognosis, approximately 70% of patients in this series survived. Because of its immunoablative qualities, alemtuzumab should be used with caution and by those with experience caring for profoundly immune compromised patients. CMV reactivation and adenoviremia were frequent complications of this therapy. In contrast to refractory patients, those patients who initially respond well to standard therapy but then relapse as treatment is tapered or withdrawn often respond to reintensification of therapy with standard agents. Because of the variability in patient responses, a critical aspect of initial or salvage therapy is close monitoring of the patients for improvement and potential toxicities such as BM suppression or infection.

Hematopoietic Cell Transplantation

Because the time to transplant is a factor in morbidity and mortality from the disease, a donor search should begin at the time of diagnosis even though the precise etiology of HLH (e.g., genetic defect) has not yet been defined. Generally, HCT is recommended in cases of documented familial HLH, recurrent or progressive disease despite intensive therapy, and CNS involvement. Long-term disease-free survival after HCT was approximately 50% to 65% before the year 2000, regardless of whether a matched sibling or closely matched unrelated donor was used. Most patients transplanted during that era succumbed to "transplant-related" complications during the first 100 days after infusion. A significant proportion of fatal complications involved inflammatory conditions termed *acute respiratory distress syndrome, veno-occlusive disease,* and *multisystem organ failure, unspecified.* In rare cases, residual HLH was identified at autopsy despite the use of myeloablative conditioning therapy.

During the past decade, the use of reduced-intensity conditioning (RIC) regimens before HCT has been investigated after encouraging results from an institutional series. Most cases of RIC pretreatment have included alemtuzumab and demonstrated superior early posttransplant survival. In a single-center analysis directly comparing HCT outcomes after myeloablative conditioning versus RIC, a statistically significant improvement was observed after RIC conditioning, with all patients surviving at 6 months after transplant. At present, published data regarding outcome of RIC transplants using umbilical cord blood is not sufficient to draw conclusions regarding safety or efficacy. Donor choice should also take into account the possibility of an occult predisposition to HLH in siblings of patients without identified gene defects. Much remains to be learned and refined regarding the optimal application of alemtuzumab as well as other agents used before HCT. The timing of pretransplant alemtuzumab impacts the probability of graft-versus-host disease, mixed chimerism, and, in rare cases, rejection. Other factors, such as donor source, human leukocyte antigen match, cell dose, and patient condition with regard to HLH disease activity at time of conditioning, may all play roles in determining the likelihood of success after RIC HCT.

Patients with CNS HLH need close posttransplant follow-up. The authors recommend examination of CSF within 100 days of HCT even in asymptomatic patients. Follow-up MRIs are recommended if pretransplant abnormalities were present. In some patients with mixed or full hematopoietic donor chimerism, HLH disease activity in the CSF can be effectively treated with intrathecal therapy during the early posttransplant months. CNS disease is subsequently controlled as donor immune reconstitution progresses.

Prognosis

Significant strides have been made in the treatment of HLH, with survival now generally ranging from 50% to 70%. In children with nonfamilial HLH, overall survival has been reported at 72%, but only 20% of the patients did not require HCT. Survival is increased in children, irrespective of genetic status, who receive HSCT from matched rather than unmatched donors. RIC pretransplant regimens appear to further decrease mortality. The best outcomes in HSCT are seen in children who have a rapid and complete response to pretransplant therapies and who do not exhibit significant neurologic involvement. Prompt initiation of HSCT in familial patients after disease remission is obtained is also likely to increase survival. Patients with significant neurologic involvement may experience severe and permanent sequelae even if they survive.

MACROPHAGE ACTIVATION SYNDROME

MAS is the name commonly given to a severe, potentially fatal inflammatory condition seen in the context of rheumatologic disorders such as soJIA or systemic lupus erythematosus (SLE). The syndrome of MAS shares many similarities with classic HLH, and many investigators view it as a special form of HLH, suggesting that the name may be changed to rheumatologic HLH (or R-HLH). The main manifestations of MAS include fever, hepatosplenomegaly, lymphadenopathy, severe cytopenias, serious liver disease, and coagulopathy consistent with DIC. Hemophagocytosis is often (although not always) seen in the BM of patients with MAS. The true incidence of MAS may be underestimated because relatively mild cases of MAS often remained

unrecognized. Recent evidence suggests that mild subclinical MAS occurs in as many as one-third of patients with active soJIA and may be the first manifestation of soJIA. Infections or change in medications may precede the diagnosis of MAS; in most patients, MAS is triggered by a flare-up of the underlying rheumatologic disease. Published observations suggest that as in HLH, MAS patients have profoundly depressed NK cell function, sometimes associated with abnormal perforin expression, and these abnormalities are associated with specific perforin and Munc13-4 polymorphisms.

Diagnosis and Treatment

There are no validated diagnostic criteria for MAS, and early diagnosis is often difficult. A recent consensus conference has developed expert-based *classification* criteria for MAS, although these have not been validated as *diagnostic* criteria in clinical trials. Thus, in a patient with persistently active underlying rheumatologic disease, a fall in the erythrocyte sedimentation rate (ESR) and platelet count, particularly in combination with persistently high C-reactive protein and increasing levels of ferritin, should raise a suspicion of impending MAS. The diagnosis of MAS is usually confirmed by the demonstration of hemophagocytosis in the BM. Assessment of the levels of sCD25 and sCD163 in serum may help with the timely diagnosis of MAS. Although mild elevation of sCD25 has been reported in many rheumatic diseases, including JIA and SLE, a several-fold increase in the levels of sIL2Rα in these diseases is highly suggestive of MAS. The application of the HLH diagnostic criteria to systemic JIA patients with suspected MAS is problematic. Some of the HLH markers, such as lymphadenopathy, splenomegaly, and hyperferritinemia, are common features of active systemic JIA itself and therefore do not distinguish MAS from a conventional systemic JIA flare. Patients with systemic JIA often have increased white blood cell and platelet counts, as well as serum levels of fibrinogen as a part of the inflammatory response seen in this disease. Therefore, when they develop MAS, they reach the degree of cytopenias and hypofibrinogenemia seen in HLH only at the late stages of the syndrome when medical management becomes challenging. This is even more problematic for the diagnosis of MAS in patients with SLE in whom autoimmune cytopenias are common and difficult to distinguish from those caused by MAS.

Early recognition of this syndrome and immediate therapeutic intervention to produce a rapid response are critical. Prompt administration of more aggressive treatment in these patients may, in fact, prevent development of the full-blown syndrome. To achieve rapid reversal of coagulation abnormalities and cytopenias, most clinicians start with intravenous methylprednisolone pulse therapy (30 mg/kg for 3 consecutive days) followed by 2–3 mg/kg/day divided in four doses. After normalization of hematologic abnormalities and resolution of coagulopathy, steroids are tapered slowly to avoid relapses of MAS. Commonly, however, MAS appears to be corticosteroid resistant, with deaths being reported even among patients treated with massive doses of steroids. Parenteral administration of cyclosporine A has been shown to be highly effective in patients with corticosteroid-resistant MAS. The utility of biologic drugs in MAS treatment remains unclear. Although tumor necrosis factor-inhibiting agents, biologics that neutralize IL-1 and IL-6, have been reported to be effective in occasional MAS patients, other reports describe patients in whom MAS occurred while they were receiving these agents. Based on some success with IVIG administration in virus-associated HLH, this treatment might be effective in MAS triggered by viral infection. If MAS, however, is driven by EBV infection, rituximab, a monoclonal antibody that depletes B lymphocytes (the main type of cells harboring the EBV virus) may be considered.

Future Directions

As an alternative approach to etoposide-based approaches for the treatment of HLH, ATG–prednisone has been used for a number of years in some centers. These two approaches appear to have unique strengths and weaknesses. Although a significant number of patients fail to respond adequately or completely to etoposide-based regimens, ATG-based regimens are complicated by relatively frequent and early relapse (median time to relapse reported by Ouachee-Chardin et al, 5.5 weeks). Thus, a rational combination of these approaches may improve outcomes by increasing initial responses and maintaining them until HCT can be obtained. Currently, a multicenter clinical trial called *hybrid immunotherapy for HLH* (HIT-HLH) is underway in North America, testing the potential of this idea. A sister trial is being conducted in Europe. In this approach, ATG and etoposide are incorporated into one regimen, but the etoposide dose intensity is decreased to minimize potential myelosuppression. No data are available yet regarding the usefulness of this approach. Alternative strategies using anticytokine antibodies for induction therapy are also being developed.

Although HLH appears to be a disease of excessive immune activation, the ideal form of immune suppression and antiinflammatory therapy remains unknown. Although somewhat responsive to corticosteroids and clearly responsive to anti–T-cell serotherapy, such as ATG or alemtuzumab, HLH remains difficult to treat. However, newer, targeted therapies, based on insights from animal models, are on the horizon. A new drug (currently designated NI-0501), a monoclonal antibody targeting IFN-γ, is being tested in a clinical trial in patients with HLH. It is likely that such targeted therapies will eventually supersede current approaches.

SINUS HISTIOCYTOSIS WITH MASSIVE LYMPHADENOPATHY OR ROSAI–DORFMAN DISEASE

First described in 1969, SHML, or RDD, is clinically characterized as a benign, frequently chronic, painless massive lymphadenopathy usually involving cervical lymph nodes and, less frequently, axillary, hilar, peritracheal, and inguinal nodes. Extranodal disease is present in approximately 30% of patients. The upper respiratory mucosa is involved in 20% of patients, bone in 25%, and orbit or eyelid in 10%. Occasionally, there is involvement of the skin, CNS (meninges), lung, liver, and kidney. Ocular manifestations, such as uveitis, have been observed. Although SHML is a histologically reactive and molecularly polyclonal disorder, significant morbidity and death have been associated with massive tissue invasion of the liver, kidney, lung, brain, and other critical structures. In these instances, the disease may have a rapid downhill course.

Eighty percent of patients are diagnosed in the first or second decade of life; however, the disorder also can affect elderly adults. Typically, patients are of African descent; the incidence of SHML is greatest in Africa and the West Indies. Males and females are equally affected.

Laboratory evaluation frequently reveals an elevated ESR, moderate polyclonal hypergammaglobulinemia, anemia, and granulocytosis. Subtle abnormalities of immune indices may also be seen. Involved lymph nodes (see Fig. 52.9) show marked sinusoidal dilation with proliferation of foamy histiocytes within the sinuses (see E-Slide VM03962). Eosinophils are usually low in number, but plasma cells are abundant. A characteristic finding, referred to as *emperipolesis*, demonstrates lymphocytes surrounded by the membranes of histiocytes as observed by electron microscopy. The proliferating histiocytes appear to be macrophages. These large, pale cells show variable expression of S100. They can be distinguished from Langerhans cells found in the lymph nodes of patients with classic LCH by the absence of CD1a or Birbeck granules, the presence of α1-antichymotrypsin, and the absence of CD1a expression.

The etiology of RDD is unknown, but disordered immune regulation has been proposed as a significant contributor. It was originally thought that RDD represented an unusual response to herpesviruses, but this has not been confirmed. Although patients are frequently febrile, infectious agents are not commonly implicated, and the fever is presumed to be a manifestation of systemic disease.

Disease manifestations can subside over several months to years. Of 215 cases in a patient registry, 21% had complete resolution of disease. However, 14 patients died. Five died of "immunologic" causes, such as severe hemolysis; three died of infections; and six probably died as a direct consequence of disease infiltration. As the disease resolves, extranodal disease regresses before nodal disease. Corticosteroids, vinblastine, and low-dose cyclophosphamide are sometimes effective; however, the results with these agents have been inconsistent. A recent report has found that (similar to refractory LCH) clofarabine may be a highly active agent in patients with SHML who require systemic therapy. Attempts at treatment should be reserved for special circumstances, such as tracheal or epidural compression, or invasion of other vital structures, as well as for significant cosmetic disfigurement. Local excision may be useful in selected patients, although the lesions may reappear.

SUGGESTED READINGS

Allen CE, Ladisch S, McClain KL: How I treat Langerhans cell histiocytosis. *Blood* 126(1):26–35, 2015.

Allen CE, Li L, Peters TL, et al: Cell-specific gene expression in Langerhans cell histiocytosis lesions reveals a distinct profile compared with epidermal Langerhans cells. *J Immunol* 184:4557, 2010.

Aricò M, Janka G, Fischer A, et al: Hemophagocytic lymphohistiocytosis. Report of 122 children from the International Registry. FHL Study Group of the Histiocyte Society. *Leukemia* 10:197, 1996.

Arnaud L, Gorochov G, Charlotte F, et al: Systemic perturbation of cytokine and chemokine networks in Erdheim–Chester disease: a single-center series of 37 patients. *Blood* 117:2783, 2011.

Badalian-Very G, Vergilio JA, Degar BA, et al: Recurrent BRAF mutations in Langerhans cell histiocytosis. *Blood* 116:1919, 2010.

Chakraborty R, Hampton OA, Shen X, et al: Mutually exclusive recurrent somatic mutations in MAP2K1 and BRAF support a central role for ERK activation in LCH pathogenesis. *Blood* 124(19):3007–3015, 2014.

Côte M, Ménager MM, Burgess A, et al: Munc18-2 deficiency causes familial hemophagocytic lymphohistiocytosis type 5 and impairs cytotoxic granule exocytosis in patient NK cells. *J Clin Invest* 119:3765, 2009.

Fahrner B, Prosch H, Minkov M, et al: Long-term outcome of hypothalamic pituitary tumors in Langerhans cell histiocytosis. *Pediatr Blood Cancer* 58:606, 2012.

Farquhar JW, Claireaux AE: Familial haemophagocytic reticulosis. *Arch Dis Child* 27:519, 1952.

Feldmann J, Callebaut I, Raposo G, et al: Munc13-4 is essential for cytolytic granules fusion and is mutated in a form of familial hemophagocytic lymphohistiocytosis (FHL3). *Cell* 115:461, 2003.

Gadner H, Grois N, Pötschger U, et al: Improved outcome in multisystem Langerhans cell histiocytosis is associated with therapy intensification. *Blood* 111(5):2556, 2008.

Grom AA, Mellins ED: Macrophage activation syndrome: advances towards understanding pathogenesis. *Curr Opin Rheumatol* 22:561, 2010.

Grom AA, Villanueva J, Lee S, et al: Natural killer cell dysfunction in patients with systemic-onset juvenile rheumatoid arthritis and macrophage activation syndrome. *J Pediatr* 142:292, 2003.

Haroche J, Arnaud L, Amoura Z: Erdheim–Chester disease. *Curr Opin Rheumatol* 24:53, 2012.

Henter JI, Horne A, Aricó M, et al: HLH-2004: Diagnostic and therapeutic guidelines for hemophagocytic lymphohistiocytosis. *Pediatr Blood Cancer* 48:124, 2007.

Jordan MB, Allen CE, Weitzman S, et al: How I treat hemophagocytic lymphohistiocytosis. *Blood* 118:4041, 2011.

Jordan MB, Hildeman D, Kappler J, et al: An animal model of hemophagocytic lymphohistiocytosis (HLH): CD8+ T cells and interferon gamma are essential for the disorder. *Blood* 104:735, 2004.

Marsh RA, Jordan MB, Filipovich AH: Reduced-intensity conditioning haematopoietic cell transplantation for haemophagocytic lymphohistiocytosis: an important step forward. *Br J Haematol* 154:556, 2011.

Marsh RA, Madden L, Kitchen BJ, et al: XIAP deficiency: a unique primary immunodeficiency best classified as X-linked familial hemophagocytic lymphohistiocytosis and not as X-linked lymphoproliferative disease. *Blood* 116:1079, 2010.

Marsh RA, Vaughn G, Kim MO, et al: Reduced-intensity conditioning significantly improves survival of patients with hemophagocytic lympho-histiocytosis undergoing allogeneic hematopoietic cell transplantation. *Blood* 116:5824, 2010.

Minkov M: Multisystem Langerhans cell histiocytosis in children: current treatment and future directions. *Paediatr Drugs* 13:75, 2011.

Minkov M, Steiner M, Pötschger U, et al: International LCH Study Group: reactivations in multisystem Langerhans cell histiocytosis: data of the international LCH registry. *J Pediatr* 153:700, 705, e701-702, 2008.

Nelson DS, Quispel W, Badalian-Very G, et al: Somatic activating ARAF mutations in Langerhans cell histiocytosis. *Blood* 123(20):3152–3155, 2014.

Phillips M, Allen C, Gerson P, et al: Comparison of FDG-PET scans to conventional radiography and bone scans in management of Langerhans cell histiocytosis. *Pediatr Blood Cancer* 52:97, 2009.

Ravelli A, Grom AA, Behrens EM, et al: Macrophage activation syndrome as part of systemic juvenile idiopathic arthritis: diagnosis, genetics, pathophysiology and treatment. *Genes Immun* 13:289, 2012.

Rigaud S, Fondanèche MC, Lambert N, et al: XIAP deficiency in humans causes an X-linked lymphoproliferative syndrome. *Nature* 444:110, 2006.

Risma K, Jordan MB: Hemophagocytic lymphohistiocytosis: updates and evolving concepts. *Curr Opin Pediatr* 24:9, 2012.

Simko SJ, McClain KL, Allen CE: Up-front therapy for LCH: is it time to test an alternative to vinblastine/prednisone? *Br J Haematol* 169(2):299–301, 2015. doi: 10.1111/bjh.13208. [Epub 2014 Nov 16].

Simko SJ, Tran HD, Jones J, et al: Clofarabine salvage therapy in refractory multifocal histiocytic disorders, including Langerhans cell histiocytosis, juvenile xanthogranuloma and Rosai-Dorfman disease. *Pediatr Blood Cancer* 61(3):479–487, 2014. doi: 10.1002/pbc.24772. [Epub 2013 Sep 18].

Stepp SE, Dufourcq-Lagelouse R, Le Deist F, et al: Perforin gene defects in familial hemophagocytic lymphohistiocytosis. *Science* 286:1957, 1999.

Trottestam H, Horne A, Aricò M, et al: Histiocyte Society: Chemoimmuno-therapy for hemophagocytic lymphohistiocytosis: long-term results of the HLH-94 treatment protocol. *Blood* 118:4577, 2011.

Weitzman S, Jaffe R: Uncommon histiocytic disorders: the non-Langerhans cell histiocytoses. *Pediatr Blood Cancer* 45:256, 2005.

Zhang K, Jordan MB, Marsh RA, et al: Hypomorphic mutations in PRF1, MUNC13-4, and STXBP2 are associated with adult-onset familial HLH. *Blood* 118:5794, 2011.

zur Stadt U, Schmidt S, Kasper B, et al: Linkage of familial hemophagocytic lymphohistiocytosis (FHL) type-4 to chromosome 6q24 and identifica-tion of mutations in syntaxin 11. *Hum Mol Genet* 14:827, 2005.

CHAPTER 53

LYSOSOMAL STORAGE DISEASES: PERSPECTIVES AND PRINCIPLES

Edward H. Schuchman and Melissa P. Wasserstein

The lysosomal storage diseases (LSDs) are a diverse group of inherited disorders caused by the defective function of specific lysosomal proteins (Table 53.1). Originally described by de Duve and colleagues,[1] lysosomes are ubiquitous organelles required to metabolize macromolecules. This includes molecules internalized by cells through the process of endocytosis, as well as those produced during the natural turnover of endogenous cell components (autophagocytosis). More than 50 hydrolytic enzymes have been found within the lysosome, as well as several membrane-embedded transport proteins, ion pumps, and other specialized components. Unique to the lysosome is a highly acidic pH, and the enzymes and proteins found within this organelle have evolved to optimally function within this unique environment. Hers[2] was the first to describe enlarged and abnormally shaped lysosomes in a patient with Pompe disease (α-glucosidase deficiency), thus delineating the first LSD. To date, more than 50 disorders have been attributed to defective lysosomal proteins. Most are inherited as autosomal recessive traits, although two are X-linked (Fabry disease and mucopolysaccharidosis [MPS] type II [Hunter disease]). In general, LSDs are categorized according to the type of macromolecule(s) that accumulate (e.g., lipidoses, mucopolysaccharidoses). The pathophysiology of these diseases is directly related to these accumulating material(s), although as the diseases progress many secondary abnormalities also occur. There is also considerable cell and organ specificity among the LSDs that is directly related to the location and function of the specific macromolecules affected.

PATHOBIOLOGY OF LYSOSOMAL STORAGE DISEASES

Biology of the Lysosome and Lysosomal Enzymes: Basic Principles

Lysosomes are formed through the fusion of enzyme-containing vesicles produced in the trans-Golgi network (TGN) with other vesicles such as endosomes or autophagosomes. Central to the formation of a mature lysosome is the establishment of an acidic pH. Mature lysosomes have a pH below 5, which is maintained by proton pumps found within the lysosomal membrane. Acidification of the compartment is required for proper activation of the hydrolytic enzymes and the release of macromolecules from their membrane receptors, providing access to the fully active hydrolytic enzymes. Although lysosomes have been historically considered discrete organelles, it is now known that the lysosomal system is highly dynamic and consists of a series of digestive vesicles with varying pH, hydrolytic enzyme activities, and cellular location.[3]

Lysosomal function requires the coordinated action of acidic hydrolyases, acidification machinery and membrane proteins. It has recently been discovered that the diverse genes/gene products involved in lysosomal function belong to a gene network–the coordinated lysosomal expression and regulation (CLEAR) network–and are transcriptionally regulated by the lysosomal "master gene" TFEB.[4] Transcription factor EB (TFEB) positively regulates the expression of other genes required to form lysosomes, controls the number of lysosomes, and promotes degradation of lysosomal substrates. Key to the formation of the lysosome is the delivery of the hydrolytic enzymes to the acidified vesicles in the TGN. This is accomplished

through a series of specific targeting mechanisms unique to these proteins[5] (see later and box on Lysosomal Protein Biosynthesis and Sorting).

Coincident with the addition of the β-N-acetylglucosamine moiety is the addition of a phosphate group to this sugar by the enzyme N-acetylglucosaminyl-1-phosphotransferase. This modification is essential for targeting of most lysosomal enzymes, and mutations in the gene encoding this enzyme lead to a severe LSD (I-cell disease) characterized by the abnormal targeting and secretion of many lysosomal enzymes.[6] The glucosaminyl residues are subsequently cleaved, exposing terminal mannose-6-phosphate (M6P) residues on the oligosaccharides. Importantly, for any given lysosomal enzyme the oligosaccharide chains may be highly heterogeneous, containing varying amounts of M6P, sialic acid, and glucosaminyl sugars.

In addition to targeting the enzymes to lysosomes, the oligosaccharide side chains also participate in the tertiary structure and folding of the proteins, and are in many cases necessary for their activity. Proteolytic processing within the lysosome also may be required for activity, as well as assembly into macromolecular "scaffolds" that may include protective and/or activator proteins. These events are driven, at least in part, by the low pH of the organelle. Finally, although most lysosomal enzymes use the M6P targeting system, it is also important to recognize that non-M6P targeting systems have been described and may function alone or in combination with M6P.[7] For example, the lysosomal membrane proteins (LIMPs or LAMPs) are sorted to the lysosomal membrane through tyrosine residues located near the carboxyl-terminal end of the proteins.

Pathogenesis of Lysosomal Storage Diseases: General Concepts

The majority of LSDs result from mutations in genes encoding individual lysosomal enzymes, leading to the intralysosomal accumulation of the enzyme's substrate. A small number of the diseases also result from mutations in genes encoding defective transport proteins that reside within the lysosomal membrane, or by the defective function of other nonhydrolytic enzymes required for lysosomal enzyme biosynthesis (e.g., I-cell disease). The type of macromolecules that accumulate distinguishes two main categories of LSDs: i.e., those that accumulate mucopolysaccharides (mucopolysaccharidoses; MPS diseases), and those that accumulate lipids (lipidoses; see Schulze et al[8] and Giugliani et al[9] for reviews). Several carbohydrate storage diseases have also been described.[10] With only a few exceptions (e.g., Wolman disease), the lipid substrates stored in the LSDs share a common structure that includes a ceramide backbone (2-N-acylsphingosine, i.e., the sphingolipids). More than 100 sphingolipids are known with diverse function,[11] and their abnormal accumulation in the LSDs results in a wide range of physiologic, morphologic, and clinical manifestations. For example, progressive lysosomal accumulation of glycosphingolipids in the central nervous system (CNS) leads to neurodegeneration, abnormal neurite sprouting, and synapse deterioration, whereas storage of these lipids in visceral cells can lead to organomegaly, skeletal abnormalities, pulmonary infiltration, and many other manifestations.

TABLE 53.1   Examples of Lysosomal Storage Diseases

Category	Disease	Protein Abnormalities
Lipidoses	Fabry	α-Galactosidase A
	Farber	Acid ceramidase
	Gaucher (types 1, 2, and 3)	β-Glucosidase
	GM₁ gangliosidosis	β-Galactosidase
	GM₂ gangliosidosis	β-Hexosaminidase A and B
	Tay–Sachs	
	Sandhoff	
	Metachromatic leukodystrophy	Arylsulfatase A
	Niemann–Pick	
	Types A and B	Acid sphingomyelinase
	Type C	
	Type 1	NPC1
	Type 2	NPC2/HE1
	Wolman disease (cholesterol ester storage disease)	Acid lipase
Mucopolysaccharidoses	MPS I (Hurler and Scheie)	α-Iduronidase
Other	MPS II (Hunter)	Iduronidase sulfatase
	MPS III (Sanfilippo)	
	Type A	Heparan N-sulfatase
	Type B	N-Acetyl-α-D-glucosaminidase
	Type C	Acetyl-CoA-α-glucosaminide acetyltransferase
	Type D	N-Acetylglucosamine-6-sulfate sulfatase
	MPS IV (Morquio)	
	Type A	Galactosamine-6-sulfatase
	Type B	β-Galactosidase
	MPS VI (Maroteaux-Lamy)	N-Acetylgalactosamine-4-sulfatase (arylsulfatase B)
	MPS VII (Sly)	β-Glucuronidase
	MPS IX	Hyaluronidase
	Aspartylglycosaminuria	Aspartylglycosaminidase
	Cystinosis (Fanconi syndrome)	Cystinosin
	Fucosidosis	Fucosidase
	I-cell (ML-II)	N-acetylglucosamine-1-phosphotransferase
	Pompe	α-Glucosidase
	Mannosidosis	α-Mannosidase
	Schindler	α-Galactosidase B

Lysosomal Protein Biosynthesis and Sorting

All lysosomal enzymes are cotranslationally N-glycosylated in the rough endoplasmic reticulum (ER) through the en block transfer of carbohydrate chains from a lipid intermediate (dolichophosphate). After completion of this process they generally undergo additional proteolytic processing and are assembled into transport vesicles for delivery and further processing in the cis-Golgi apparatus. At this stage, most proteins destined for the lysosomes contain only branched mannosyl oligosaccharide chains that terminate with short-chain α-glucosyl moieites. During transport through the Golgi apparatus they acquire additional, complex oligosaccharide modifications that result in their sorting to lysosomes. A series of glycosyl hydrolases and transferases within specific regions of the cis-, mid-, and trans-Golgi participate in these sequential modifications. For example, in the cis-Golgi, α-glucosidases and α-mannosidases remove terminal glucose and mannose residues, respectively, to produce mannose-terminated core oligosaccharides. Within the mid-Golgi, additional sugars are added, including β-N-acetylglucosamine and β-galactoside. The addition of terminal sialic acid residues occurs in the trans-Golgi.

For the MPS diseases, the mucopolysaccharides (also known as *glycosaminoglycans* [GAGs]) are the primary accumulating macromolecules and are found predominately within connective tissues. The accumulation of these materials results in severe cartilage and bone abnormalities that affect the skeletal system, trachea, and other organs. In some cases the CNS may also be affected, particularly in diseases where the GAG heparan sulfate accumulates.

In general, the storage pattern of a substrate in an LSD patient is dependent on the normal distribution of the molecule in the body, and this tissue-specific storage pattern is responsible for the organ-specific pathology. For example, in Hurler syndrome (MPS type I), two GAGs, dermatan and heparan sulfate, accumulate and result in severe skeletal and neurologic manifestations. In contrast, in Maroteaux–Lamy disease (MPS type VI), only dermatan sulfate accumulates. Because this latter GAG is not normally found in the brain, CNS manifestations do not occur in MPS VI. Similarly, in Tay–Sachs and Sandhoff diseases, the deficiencies of β-hexosaminidase A, or β-hexosaminidases A and B, respectively, results either in primary CNS disease or in combined CNS and visceral disease caused by the different accumulated substrates. Whereas β-hexosaminidase A cleaves the glycosphingolipid (ganglioside) GM2, which is very abundant in the brain, β-hexosaminidase B primarily cleaves sialic acid-containing gangliosides and globosides. Globosides, in particular, are synthesized in visceral tissues, resulting in visceral storage in Sandhoff disease.

Although the primary pathogenic mechanism leading to most LSDs is well understood (i.e., genetic lesions result in primary protein defects and the accumulation of specific substrates), in recent years the complexity of these diseases has been recognized. For example, although GAGs are the primary accumulating macromolecules in the MPS diseases, other compounds, including the neural-specific glycolipids (gangliosides), also accumulate and contribute to disease pathology. In the lipidosis Niemann–Pick disease (NPD) type C, the primary protein defect affects cholesterol transport, although sphingolipids also accumulate and are responsible, in part, for the cellular dysfunction and cell death. In fact, an approved therapy for NPD type C, Miglustat (see later), is based on the principle of reducing ganglioside storage in the brain rather than correcting the primary cholesterol transport defect.[12] Similarly, in NPD types A and B, the sphingolipid sphingomyelin is the primary accumulating substrate, although cholesterol storage also is a major contributory factor.

Indeed, for any individual LSD the pattern of macromolecule accumulation may be extremely heterogeneous and, importantly, also may be tissue and cell specific.[13] Although the mechanism(s) leading to this heterogenous storage pattern is not always known, it presumably relates to a global dysfunction of the lysosomal system, providing a connection between seemingly distinct metabolic pathways.

As the macromolecules accumulate, the lysosomes become distended and destabilized, and may eventually fail to carry out their normal functions related to phagocytosis and autophagocytosis. In turn, this may result in cell dysfunction, senescence, and/or death. In addition, because of the progressive cell and organ disease that occurs in the LSDs, inflammatory pathways are frequently activated in an attempt to repair the damage. However, because the inflammatory cells themselves are dysfunctional, the diseases progress and the inflammatory changes may become chronic. Inflammation is therefore also an important contributory factor to the pathogenesis of LSDs. For example, in the MPS diseases GAG storage is known to activate the Toll-like receptor 4 signaling pathway, leading to the release of tumor necrosis factor-α (TNF-α) and other inflammatory cytokines.[14] TNF-α, in turn, causes elevation of the toxic lipid ceramide within cartilage cells (chondrocytes), contributing to cell death. Treatment of animal models of MPS with anti-TNF-α drugs alone has resulted in the reduction of chondrocyte death and substantial clinical benefits, demonstrating the importance of inflammation in these diseases.[15,16]

GENETICS AND DIAGNOSIS OF LYSOSOMAL STORAGE DISEASES

All LSDs except for two, Fabry disease and MPS type II (Hunter disease), are inherited as autosomal recessive traits. Fabry and Hunter diseases are inherited as X-linked recessive traits. Most mutations causing individual LSDs result in single amino acid changes in the enzyme's polypeptide chain, resulting in absent or defective function. The genes encoding most lysosomal proteins have been cloned, and there is no obvious clustering of these genes within the genome. In some cases, nonfunctional pseudogenes also have been described, which may or may not be transcribed or translated into a nonfunctional protein. Although there is no clustering of the lysosomal genes, most exhibit coordinated transcriptional behavior and are regulated by TFEB.[4,17] In the LSDs TFEB is often translocated from the cytoplasm to the nucleus to "turn on" expression of other lysosomal proteins and enhance lysosomal biogenesis. This is a mechanism by which cells try to compensate for lysosomal dysfunction. However, because the newly formed lysosomes in these diseases will retain the same primary metabolic defect, this may lead to amplification of the disease pathology.

The mutated proteins in LSD patients may be stable and delivered to lysosomes (albeit with reduced catalytic function), or may be unstable with only partial or absent delivery to lysosomes. The effects of the individual mutations may also be cell and tissue specific depending on the normal expression pattern of the enzymes. In general, heterozygous "carriers" of single mutations in a lysosomal gene do not develop clinical symptoms of the disorder, except in the X-linked disorders. For example, in Fabry disease X-inactivation patterns can lead to clusters of cells without enzyme activity, and female individuals carrying one α-galactosidase A mutation may develop disease-related pathology.[18] In addition, one lysosomal gene, SMPD1 encoding acid sphingomyelinase (ASM), is known to be "paternally imprinted" (i.e., preferentially expressed from the maternal chromosome), suggesting that type A and B NPD individuals who inherit "severe" SMPD1 mutations on the maternal chromosome may be more severely affected than those who inherit the same

mutations from the paternal chromosome.[19] This also suggests that some type A and B NPD carrier individuals with maternally derived mutations might exhibit clinical or laboratory manifestations of the disorder, and there is at least one report documenting very low serum high-density lipoprotein levels in such carrier individuals.[20]

Diagnostic assays for patients suspected of having LSDs generally rely on the measurement of specific enzymatic activities in isolated leukocytes, cultured fibroblasts, or transformed lymphoblasts. For some disorders, carrier identification and prenatal diagnosis are available as well. However, because detection of the individual enzyme activities is often complex (e.g., uses nonnatural substrates, detergents, and other specific assay conditions), it is recommended that the enzymatic confirmation of suspected cases be carried out in specialized laboratories experienced in these methods. In addition, because in most LSDs leukocytes and skin fibroblasts are not the clinically relevant cell types, these assay methods are at best indirect measures of the defective lysosomal protein's function at the pathologic sites. For this reason, predicting the clinical outcome from these in vitro measurements is generally not reliable.[21] For example, cells from patients with the infantile, neurologic form of ASM-deficient NPD (type A) and the later-onset, nonneurologic form (type B) often have similar residual enzymatic activities, although their clinical course is markedly different. This likely reflects the function of the individual mutant ASM polypeptides in the brain. Numerous other examples exist for other LSDs as well, posing a unique challenge for predicting phenotypic outcomes in newly diagnosed patients.

As already noted, many genetic abnormalities have been identified for most of the individual LSDs. For most diseases, multiple mutations have been found, and the majority of these are unique (i.e., private) to individual families. However, for some LSDs there are specific populations that may have recurrent mutations caused by founder effects and/or consanguinity, facilitating the use of DNA-based screening methods for the detection of the LSD. This has been most effectively translated into clinical use in the Ashkenazi Jewish population, in which relatively small number(s) of mutations account for several LSDs.[22] This has led to the establishment of a DNA-based "Jewish Genetic Disease" screening panel and the population-based identification of carrier individuals for the same disorder. Such individuals are referred for genetic counseling to assist with family planning and pregnancy outcome choices. The implementation of such screening has led to a dramatic reduction in the incidence of some diseases within this population (e.g., infantile Tay–Sachs disease), and will likely lead to the prevention of other disorders as well. The rapid evolution of cost-effective, high-throughput sequencing methods is also likely to open other populations and disorders to these DNA-based screening approaches.[23] However, it is important to note that the functional consequences of most DNA abnormalities on the protein function have not been confirmed, and thus DNA-based methods alone should not be used to predict clinical outcomes in patients unless the biochemical consequences of these abnormalities are fully established. In general, confirmation of a suspected LSD case should be accomplished by both enzymatic and DNA-based studies, and in only rare cases are these laboratory tests useful to predict clinical outcomes.

THERAPY OF LYSOSOMAL STORAGE DISEASES: AN OVERVIEW

Since the first recognition that LSDs resulted from the defective function of lysosomal proteins, the concept of simply "replacing" the missing protein in individual patients was put forward.[24] This concept was further strengthened in the 1970s by the identification of the M6P-targeting system for lysosomal enzymes and the finding that the secreted forms of many lysosomal enzymes could be rapidly internalized, or "taken up", by cell surface M6P receptors and delivered into the lysosomal system.[25] Today, the principle underlying the treatment of most LSDs remains the replacement of the missing or defective protein. This can be accomplished by stem cell transplantation, protein (enzyme) replacement therapy, or gene therapy. In some cases, treatments have also been developed that are either aimed at slowing the accumulation of undegraded materials (substrate reduction therapy [SRT]) or enhancement of the mutant protein function (chaperone therapy).

The majority of the clinical experience using cell-based therapy in LSDs comes from bone marrow transplantation (BMT).[26] Bone marrow has several advantages as a cell source, including the fact that it contains multiple stem and progenitor cell lineages that can lead to the repopulation of various organs and tissues. However, aggressive immunosuppressive preconditioning is required to achieve effective engraftment in the transplanted patients, leading to high morbidity and, in some cases, mortality. In addition, graft-versus-host disease may occur. These deleterious effects can be severe and may lead to clinical complications in patients that are worse than the disorders themselves. The availability of cord blood repositories and improved transplant methods has reduced these risks, but the possibility of high morbidity remains.

In LSD patients who have successfully undergone BMT and achieved a high level of engraftment, the clinical results have been variable. A number of factors account for this. First, repopulation after BMT is not uniform throughout the body, and depending on the organ systems affected in the patients, clinical improvement may or may not occur. For example, the hematopoietic system is particularly amenable to BMT repopulation, but the skeletal system (cartilage and bone) is not. In the nervous system some transplanted bone marrow-derived cells may cross the blood–brain barrier and repopulate the CNS, but the number of these cells is small and the repopulation efficiency low.[27] A second factor accounting for the variable clinical results after BMT is the age at which the transplant is undertaken. Many of the disease manifestations that occur in LSDs lead to permanent tissue damage (e.g., fibrosis, apoptosis) and are not reversible. Thus, not only must efficient engraftment be achieved after transplantation, but the procedure must also be undertaken before irreversible damage sets in, often in early childhood.

Other than BMT, liver transplantation has been undertaken in several LSDs, also with variable success.[28] Because the liver is a natural secretory organ, the concept underlying liver transplantation is that even partial repopulation of this organ with healthy cells will lead to secretion of these proteins into the circulation and widespread metabolic cross-correction. As with BMT, however, the uptake and distribution of the secreted enzymes will be limited by physiologic barriers (e.g., the blood–brain barrier) and dependent on the vascular supply to the tissue. Unlike BMT, there will no circulating stem cells available for organ engraftment other than in the liver. It is also of interest that early attempts at cell therapy for LSDs used amniotic cells for transplantation. Although the engraftment of these cells was extremely low and the clinical outcomes poor, these studies represented the first embryonic stem cell-based approach for these disorders.

Simultaneous with the development of cell and organ transplantation for LSDs, investigators also began to isolate and study the normal lysosomal proteins involved in the individual LSDs and to explore the idea of protein (enzyme) replacement therapy (ERT). Because this work originated before the development of recombinant DNA technology, it relied on discarded human materials as the enzyme source, usually urine or placentas. "Proof-of-principle" for this approach was first documented by Neufeld and colleagues,[29] who showed in an elegant series of studies that metabolic cross-correction of MPS cells could be achieved by coculture of these cells with normal cells or by replacing the media in MPS cells with "conditioned" media obtained from the normal cells. In addition, at around the same time methods of quantifying the levels or residual enzymatic activities in the LSDs were being developed, and there was also an early recognition that very low levels of functional enzymatic activities in the individual LSDs could have an important impact on the clinical presentation of the individual patients. This suggested that low levels of enzyme uptake were likely required to achieve metabolic cross-correction in vivo.

The first short-term clinical experience with ERT took place in the early 1970s by Brady, Desnick, and others.[30] These early studies revealed (1) that the enzymes were generally well tolerated, (2) that

the half-life of the enzymes in the circulation was short lived, and (3) that the sugar moieties on the enzymes had an important influence on their clearance from the circulation. In general, enzymes with terminal sialic acid residues had longer half-lives in the circulation than those with exposed mannose or M6P residues.

Despite these early successes, the further development of ERT was limited by the inability of the academic-based research laboratories to produce enough of the highly purified enzymes for long-term treatment studies. In addition, due to the very low numbers of diagnosed patients at that time, there was little or no commercial interest in these diseases. In the 1980s, a small biotechnology company (Genzyme, Cambridge, Massachusetts) took on this challenge and began to commercially prepare β-glucocerebrosidase, the enzyme deficient in Gaucher disease, from human placentas. This led to the first long-term experience with ERT in patients with non-neurologic (type 1) Gaucher disease.[31] Importantly, the purified enzyme was chemically modified to expose terminal mannose residues, leading to preferential uptake by macrophages, the primary cellular site of pathology in this disease.

The results of ERT in type 1 Gaucher disease were life changing and included remarkably reduced liver/spleen size and improved hematologic findings. Although the therapy required biweekly intravenous infusions, it led to substantially improved quality of life and was approved by the international regulatory authorities. Based on this remarkable success, over a dozen companies are now involved in the development of ERTs and other therapies for LSDs. In addition, widespread efforts have been undertaken to diagnose patients, including the recent implementation of newborn screening for these disorders. These efforts have revealed that LSDs are more common than originally thought, and it is estimated that they may occur in up to approximately 1 in 7000 live births, and could be even more enriched in some regional, ethnic, and/or disease populations.

By the early 1990s, DNA technologies had evolved to the point where human recombinant β-glucocerebrosidase could be produced in genetically engineered Chinese hamster ovary (CHO) cells, and this eventually replaced the use of placental enzyme. Currently, recombinant LSD enzymes are being produced in various sources, including CHO cells, transformed human cells, plants, and chicken eggs.

Based on the outstanding success in Gaucher disease, ERTs have now been developed for seven other LSDs, including Fabry disease (α-galactosidase), Pompe disease (α-glucosidase), and several of the MPS disorders (MPS I, II, IV and VI). Several others are also under development. With these developments came the recognition that the effects of ERT were disease specific and could be complicated by immune reactions to the infused recombinant proteins. For example, in contrast to the readily accessible hematopoietic system in Gaucher disease, in other LSDs the major cellular targets for ERT (e.g., podocytes in the kidney, myocytes in the muscle, chondrocytes in the cartilage) do not readily take up the intravenously delivered enzymes, either because they do not express the proper cell surface receptors or do not have a sufficient vascular supply. In addition, the costs of these therapies are extremely high, placing a very high burden on reimbursement systems.

These realizations have led researchers to explore other therapies as well, work that has been greatly aided by the development of animal models for most of the LSDs.[32] Considerable early effort was directed towards gene therapies, which have been extensively evaluated in the animal model systems.[33] Numerous clinical and pathologic improvements have been obtained, although the translation of these gene therapy technologies into the clinic has been slow because of safety concerns and issues with large-scale vector production. Recently, the first gene therapy clinical trials for LSDs have been approved in Europe, and over the next decade the evaluation of this approach in several of the individual diseases should be forthcoming.

Other investigators have sought alternative therapeutic approaches for these diseases, focusing on inhibiting the production of substrate in order to reduce accumulation (SRT). For example, Miglustat (OGT 918, N-butyl-deoxynojirimycin; trade name: Zavesca) is a low-molecular-weight compound that inhibits glucosylceramide synthase, the enzyme that catalyzes the first step in the biosynthesis of glucosylceramide and other glycosphingolipids. Miglustat is an orally administered compound that has been shown to effectively decrease organ volume and improve hematologic parameters in patients with type 1 Gaucher disease.[34] However, gastrointestinal side effects are fairly common with oral treatment, so the use of Miglustat has been limited to Gaucher disease patients for whom ERT is not suitable. Miglustat is also used in patients with type C NPD, which causes progressive and severe neurologic disease.[12] Most patients with type C NPD have mutations in an integral membrane protein involved in cholesterol transport (NPC1). However, because NPC1 is a nonsoluble transporter, protein-replacement therapy is not a therapeutic option at the present time. Using animal models, investigators showed that the neurologic pathology in type C NPD was associated with the secondary accumulation of a particular glycolipid, GM_2 ganglioside. Based on this finding, studies were carried out using Miglustat to inhibit glycolipid biosynthesis, resulting in reduction of GM_2 storage and partial neurologic improvements. Clinical trials of Miglustat in type C NPD patients revealed stabilization or improvement of some clinical markers.

Another small-molecule approach under development for the LSDs is based on the use of enzyme-specific inhibitors that can act as "chaperones" of the corresponding mutant proteins, thereby facilitating their delivery to lysosomes and enhancing their residual enzymatic activities. Such "chaperone" therapy is currently being evaluated in clinical trials for several LSDs. Numerous other approaches also have been or are being evaluated in the various LSD animal models, including targeting of inflammatory pathways and stem cell-based therapies, and in the future patients should have access to various therapeutic choices. As with ERT, the effects of these individual therapies are likely to be disease and organ specific, and it is expected that in the future effective treatment of LSD patients will require a combination of these approaches.

HEMATOLOGIC MANIFESTATIONS OF LYSOSOMAL STORAGE DISEASES

Hematologic findings are associated with several LSDs, but in two, Gaucher disease and NPD (types A and B), hematologic abnormalities are among the common presenting features. Hematologic findings should be considered in the differential diagnosis of both disorders, and patients with Gaucher disease or NPD may be seen by hematologists to manage their symptoms. In the next section the hematologic features of these disorders are discussed, as well as several other relevant issues related to hematologic manifestations and LSDs.

Gaucher Disease: β-Glucosidase Deficiency

Cells of the monocyte–macrophage system are the primary sites of pathology in this disorder. In general, these cells are enriched for lysosomes and highly active in phagocytosis. As such, disruption of lysosomes may have a profound effect on their function. An important diagnostic hallmark of Gaucher disease is the presence in a variety of tissues of lipid-filled cells derived from the monocyte–macrophage system, referred to as *Gaucher cells*. These cells are readily evident in the bone marrow, but can also be seen in blood smears and histologically in other tissues, including liver, spleen, lung, and others. As the disease progresses, the deposition of Gaucher cells in these organs increases.

Bleeding is a common presenting symptom of patients with Gaucher disease and is primarily caused by thrombocytopenia. The major sites of bleeding are mucocutaneous, including epistaxis, easy bruising, and gingival hemorrhage. Thrombocytopenia in Gaucher disease is generally thought to be caused by splenic sequestration of platelets. Spleen enlargement is present in all symptomatic patients and is a common presenting sign of the disease. Splenic enlargement in Gaucher disease may be massive, up to 75-fold normal.[35]

Some patients with type 1 Gaucher disease have excessive bleeding that is disproportionate to their platelet counts and coagulation profiles. Abnormal platelet function has been described in patients with type 1 Gaucher disease with abnormal bleeding tendencies.[36] These defects have been attributed to defects in platelet adhesion as well as aggregation. Coagulation deficiencies, particularly low factor levels of factor XI, have also been described.[37] Because both factor XI deficiency and type 1 Gaucher disease are relatively common in the Ashkenazi Jewish population, this finding may reflect concurrence of the two disorders. However, a report describing Egyptian type 1 Gaucher disease patients with deficiencies in factors II, V, VII, VIII, X, XI, and XII supports the concept that the coagulopathy is not limited to Ashkenazi Jewish patients and may have a distinct pathophysiology.[38] In fact, many patients with Gaucher disease have significant deficiencies (less than 50%) of multiple coagulation factors.[37] This is associated with elevations of coagulation activators, suggesting ongoing activation of the coagulation cascade with a resultant consumption of coagulation factors.[38]

Anemia in patients with Gaucher disease is usually mild but occasionally may be severe and can be associated with leukopenia. These findings are also probably attributable to sequestration of cells in the spleen, as well as dysfunctional bone marrow production of cells as the disease progresses. The mainstay of treatment for the hematologic abnormalities in Gaucher disease is ERT. ERT typically produces a remarkable improvement in the platelet count, hemoglobin, and white blood cell count, as well as a reduction in spleen size.[24] ERT may also partially improve the coagulation profile.[38]

In patients with massive splenomegaly, splenectomy is often approached as a treatment option with the expectation that it will improve the platelet count and reduce the risk of splenic rupture. However, the spleen is an important reservoir for storage material, and its removal can displace lipid deposition to other organs, accelerating the rate and severity of disease.

Types A and B Niemann–Pick Disease: Acid Sphingomyelinase Deficiency

The hematologic findings in types A and B NPD are similar to those in Gaucher disease and may include thrombocytopenia and anemia. Splenic enlargement is also a common presenting feature of this disorder, and sequestration of cells in the spleen is thought to be the underlying cause of the low platelets, low hemoglobin, or leukopenia (Fig. 53.1A and B). Some patients with type B NPD have excessive bleeding without significant thrombocytopenia or coagulopathy. Frequent and prolonged epistaxis can be particularly problematic and in some extreme cases may require cauterization, packing, and blood transfusions.

As with Gaucher disease, a primary cellular site of pathology in types A and B NPD is the monocyte-macrophage system, and the characteristic pathological cells are referred to as *Niemann–Pick cells*. These can be distinguished from Gaucher cells by an experienced pathologist, but are frequently misclassified or not recognized, resulting in misdiagnosis. They are also readily evident in blood smears, bone marrow, and other organs, and increase as the disease progresses. As noted above, there is another form of NPD (type C) that is caused by primary defects in cholesterol transport. These patients may also present with mild hematologic findings and an enlarged spleen, although in general the hematologic findings are less severe than in patients with types A and B NPD (see Fig. 53.1C and D)

Fabry Disease: α-Galactosidase Deficiency

Unlike Gaucher and NPD diseases, in Fabry disease the monocyte–macrophage system is not primarily affected. In this disorder, the primary site of accumulation of glycolipids occurs in the vascular endothelial and smooth muscle cells that surround blood vessels. As such, constriction of blood vessels occurs, leading to skin lesions, strokes, and kidney dysfunction. It is noteworthy that several of the

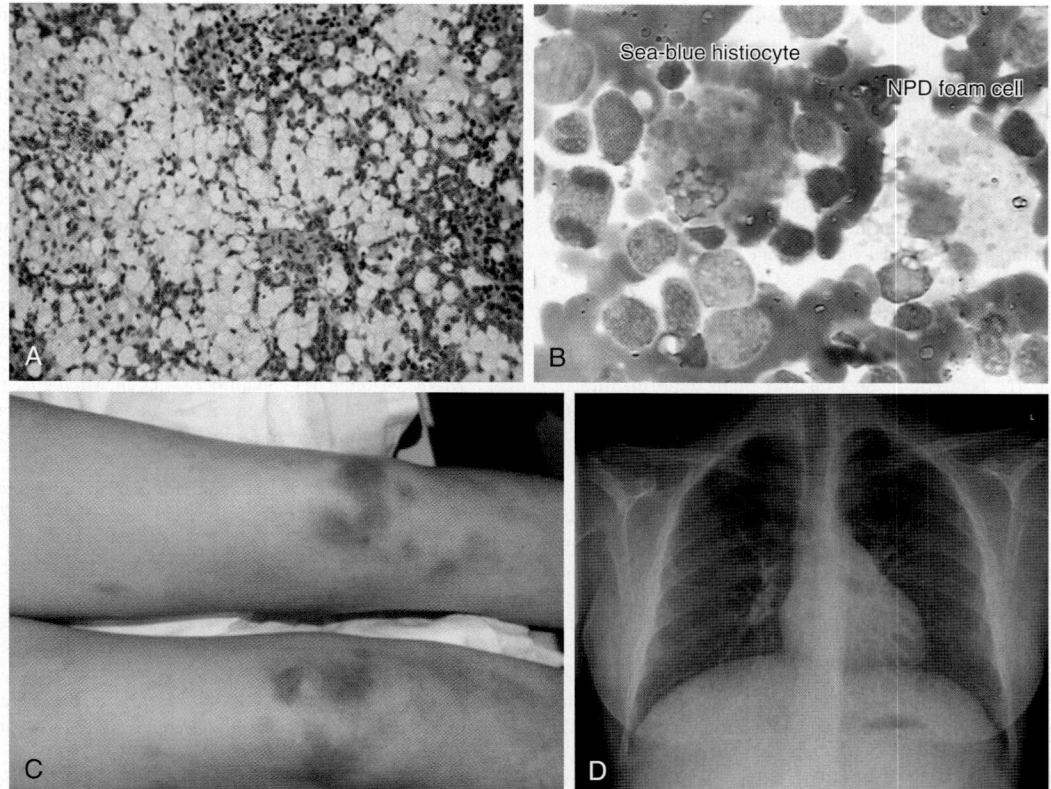

Fig. 53.1 (A) Typical histopathology (hematoxylin and eosin staining) of a liver section from a patient with type B NPD. Note the lipid-filled macrophages (Niemann–Pick cells) that are characteristic of this disorder. (B) Micrograph of the bone marrow from the same patient with type B NPD showing the presence of an NPD cell, as well as a sea-blue histiocyte. Both cells may be characteristically found in the bone marrow of these patients. (C) Bruising that may be seen in type B NPD and is associated with thrombocytopenia. (D) Chest radiograph of a patient with type B NPD showing the diffuse reticulonodular interstitial changes in this disorder. *NPD*, Niemann–Pick disease.

accumulating glycolipids in Fabry disease also are blood group lipids. For example, a number of blood group B glycolipids may contain terminal α-galactosyl moieties, and patients with Fabry disease who have blood groups B and AB will accumulate four glycolipid substrates as opposed to those with A or O blood groups, who will only accumulate two. The clinical consequence of this differential accumulation of blood group lipids in Fabry disease is not clearly understood.

Sea-Blue Histiocytosis and Lysosomal Storage Diseases

Sea-blue histiocytes are lipid-laden macrophages detectable by May–Giemsa staining of the bone marrow, blood cells, or other organs (see Fig. 53.1B). The appearance of these cells may be secondary in many disorders, but for the LSDs they are principally associated with NPD, Gaucher, Fabry, or ceroid storage diseases. For NPD and Gaucher disease specifically, there are several reports in the literature of patients with these disorders being misdiagnosed with primary sea-blue histiocytosis and only later being found to have the primary lysosomal enzyme defect.[34] Thus, the appearance of sea-blue histiocytes should be considered as part of the differential diagnosis of these disorders.

CONCLUSIONS AND FUTURE DIRECTIONS

The LSDs comprise a diverse group of genetic disorders that may present from infancy through adulthood. Most LSDs are caused by single enzyme deficiencies, but these single protein defects can result in a complex array of metabolic abnormalities, leading to a wide range of clinical presentations. The pathophysiology of individual LSDs depends on the specific cells and tissues in which these metabolic abnormalities occur. Phenotypic heterogeneity among patients may be caused by different mutations in the enzyme-encoding genes, resulting in varying levels of residual enzyme activity. Hematologic abnormalities occur in several LSDs, although two diseases, type 1 Gaucher disease and types A and B NPD, primarily affect cells of the monocyte-macrophage system, and hematologic complications can be common and severe in some cases. Several treatment options are available for some of the LSDs, including ERT, and in the case of Gaucher disease ERT is very effective at correcting the hematologic findings. ERT is also under development for type B NPD. Other treatment options, including small molecule and antiinflammatory approaches, also are actively being developed for many LSDs, and in the future most LSD patients are likely to be treated by a combination of these methods. These efforts, together with the development of population-wide enzyme and DNA-based screening for the LSDs, should lead to better medical management and improved quality of life for most patients.

REFERENCES

1. de Duve C: Lysosomes revisited. *Eur J Biochem* 137:391, 1983.
2. Hers HG: Inborn lysosomal diseases. *Gastroenterology* 48:625, 1965.
3. Hasilik A, Wrocklage C, Schroder B: Intracellular trafficking of lysosomal proteins and lysosomes. *Int J Clin Pharmacol Ther* 47:S18, 2009.
4. Sardiello M, Palmieri M, di Ronza A, et al: A gene network regulating lysosomal biogenesis and function. *Science* 325:473, 2009.

5. Kornfeld R, Kornfeld S: Assembly of asparagine-linked oligosaccharides. *Annu Rev Biochem* 54:631, 1985.

6. Reitman ML, Varki A, Kornfeld S: Fibroblasts from patients with I-cell disease and pseudo-Hurler polydystrophy are deficient in uridine 5'-diphosphate-N-acetylglucsamin: Glycoprotein N-acetylglucosaminylphosphotransferase activity. *J Clin Invest* 67:1574, 1981.

7. Bonifacino JS, Traub LM: Signals for sorting of transmembrane proteins to endosomes and lysosomes. *Annu Rev Biochem* 72:395, 2003.

8. Schulze H, Sandhoff K: Lysosomal lipid storage diseases. *Cold Spring Harb Perspect Biol* 1:3, 2011.

9. Giugliani R, Federhen A, Rojas MV, et al: Mucopolysaccharidosis I, II and VI: Brief review and guidelines for treatment. *Genet Mol Biol* 33:589, 2010.

10. Mallat C, Konig JL, Naheedy J: Skeletal and brain abnormalities in fucosidosis, a rare lysosomal storage disorder. *J Radiol Case Rep* 9:30, 2015.

11. Hannun YA, Bell RM: Functions of sphingolipids and sphingolipid breakdown products in cellular regulation. *Science* 243:500, 1989.

12. Patterson MC, Mengel E, Vanier MT, et al: Stable or improved neurological manifestations during miglustat therapy in patients from the international disease registry for Niemann-Pick disease type C: An observational cohort study. *Orphanet J Rare Dis* 10:65, 2015.

13. Walkley SU, Vanier MT: Secondary lipid accumulation in lysosomal disease. *Biochim Biophys Acta* 1793:726, 2009.

14. Simonaro CM, Ge Y, Eliyahu E, et al: Involvement of the Toll-like receptor 4 pathway and the use of TNF-alpha antagonists for treatment of the mucopolysaccharidoses. *Proc Natl Acad Sci USA* 107:222, 2010.

15. Schuchman EH, Ge Y, Lai A, et al: Pentosan polysulfate: a novel therapy for the mucopolysaccharidoses. *PLoS ONE* 8:e54459, 2013.

16. Frohberg M, Ge Y, Meng F, et al: Dose responsive effects of subcutaneous pentosan polysulfate injection in mucopolysaccharidosis type VI rats and comparison to oral treatment. *PLoS ONE* 9:e100882, 2014.

17. Settembre C, Di Malta C, Polito VA, et al: TFEB links autophagy to lysosomal biogenesis. *Science* 332:1429, 2011.

18. Germain DP: General aspects of X-linked disease. In Mehta A, Beck M, Sunder-Plassman G, editors: *Fabry Disease: Perspectives from 5 years of FOS*, Oxford, 2006, Oxford ParmaGenesis, Chapter 7.

19. Simonaro CM, Park JH, Eliyahu E, et al: Imprinting at the SMPD1 locus: Implications for acid sphingomyelinase-deficient Niemann-Pick disease. *Am J Hum Genet* 78:865, 2006.

20. Lee CY, Krimbou L, Vincent J, et al: Compound heterozygosity at the sphingomyelin phosphodiesterase-1 (SMPD1) gene is associated with low HDL cholesterol. *Hum Genet* 112:552, 2003.

21. Balwani M, Grace ME, Desnick RJ: Gaucher disease: when molecular testing and clinical presentation disagree—the novel c. 1226A>G(p. N370S)-RecNcil allele. *J Inherit Metab Dis* 34:789, 2011.

22. Dolgin E: Jewish genetic screening grows despite questions about breadth. *Nat Med* 17:639, 2011.

23. Bell CJ, Dinwiddie DL, Miller NA, et al: Carrier testing for severe childhood recessive diseases by next-generation sequencing. *Sci Transl Med* 3:65ra4, 2011.

24. Brady RO: Enzyme replacement for lysosomal diseases. *Annu Rev Med* 57:283, 2006.

25. Sly WS, Fischer HD, Gonzalez-Moriega A, et al: Role of the 6-phosphomannosyl-enzyme receptor in intracellular transport and adsorptive pinocytosis of lysosomal enzymes. *Methods Cell Biol* 23:191, 1981.

26. Prasad VK, Kurtzberg J: Cord blood and bone marrow transplantation in inherited metabolic diseases: scientific basis, current status and future directions. *Br J Haematol* 148:356, 2010.

27. Krivit W, Sung JH, Shaprio EG, et al: Microglia: the effector cell for reconstitution of the central nervous system following bone marrow transplantation for lysosomal and peroxisomal storage diseases. *Cell Transplant* 4:385, 1995.

28. Ayto RM, Hughs DA, Jeevaratnam P, et al: Long-term outcomes of liver transplantation in type 1 Gaucher disease. *Am J Transplant* 10:1934, 2010.

29. Neufeld EF: The uptake of enzyme into lysosomes: an overview. *Birth Defects Orig Artic Ser* 16:77, 1980.

30. Johnson WG, Desnick RJ, Long DM, et al: Intravenous injection of purified hexosaminidase A into a patient with Tay-Sachs disease. *Birth Defects Orig Artic Ser* 9:120, 1973.

31. Barton NW, Furbish FS, Murray GJ, et al: Therapeutic response to intravenous infusions of glucocerebrosidase in a patient with Gaucher disease. *Proc Natl Acad Sci USA* 87:1913, 1990.

32. Haskins ME: Animal models for mucopolysaccharidosis disorders and their clinical relevance. *Acta Paediatr* 96:56, 2007.

33. Seregin SS, Amalfitano A: Gene therapy for lysosomal storage disorders: Progress, challenges and future prospects. *Curr Pharm Des* 17:2558, 2011.

34. Sharma P, Kar R, Dutta S, et al: Niemann-Pick disease, type B with TRAP-positive storage cells and secondary sea blue histiocytosis. *Eur J Histochem* 23:183, 2009.

35. Sibille A, Eng CM, Kim SJ, et al: Phenotype/genotype correlations in Gaucher disease type I: clinical and therapeutic implications. *Am J Hum Genet* 52:1094, 1993.

36. Gillis S, Hyam E, Abrahamov A, et al: Platelet function abnormalities in Gaucher disease patients. *Am J Hematol* 61:103, 1999.

37. Hollak CE, Levi M, Berends F, et al: Coagulation abnormalities in type 1 Gaucher disease are due to low-grade activation and can be partly restored by enzyme supplementation therapy. *Br J Haematol* 96:470, 1997.

38. Deghady A, Marzouk I, El-Shayeb A, et al: Coagulation abnormalities in type 1 Gaucher disease in children. *Pediatr Hematol Oncol* 23:411, 2006.

INFECTIOUS MONONUCLEOSIS AND OTHER EPSTEIN-BARR VIRUS–ASSOCIATED DISEASES

Carl Allen, Cliona M. Rooney, and Stephen Gottschalk

The initial clinical descriptions of primary Epstein-Barr virus (EBV) infections are credited to Filatov and Pfeiffer at the end of the 19th century. Pfeiffer coined the term *glandular fever,* which described an illness consisting of fever, malaise, sore throat, and lymphadenopathy. In 1920, Sprunt and Evans introduced the term *infectious mononucleosis (IM)* to describe a series of patients with fatigue, fever, lymphadenopathy, and prominent mononuclear lymphocytosis (Fig. 54.1). Serologic diagnosis of IM became available in the 1930s with the heterophile agglutination test developed by Paul and Bunnel and later modified by Davidson.

The identification of EBV as the causative agent of IM was impeded for many years by the inability to transmit the disease to animals or to grow the virus ex vivo. In 1958 Burkitt described a lymphoma in African children and investigators suspected an infectious etiology because the lymphoma's geographic distribution pattern coincided with the African mosquito belt.[1] In 1964 Epstein, Achong, and Barr described herpesvirus-like particles in tumor biopsies from patients with Burkitt lymphoma (BL). Werner and Gertrude Henle developed an indirect immunofluorescent antibody assay to this new virus, now called *Epstein-Barr virus,* and showed that patients with BL, as well as 90% of American adults, had antibodies against EBV. In 1965 the Henles documented seroconversion to EBV of an individual who presented with clinical symptoms of IM. This initial observation was corroborated by larger studies confirming the association of EBV and IM.

Since then, EBV has been linked to a heterogeneous group of diseases (see box on EBV-Associated Clinical Syndromes).[2] EBV was the first human virus implicated in oncogenesis, and the biology of the virus has been studied extensively on a cellular and molecular level.[2] Because primary EBV infection is a self-limiting disease in almost all individuals, therapeutic strategies have focused on the treatment of rare, potentially fatal EBV-associated diseases. Over the last two decades, successful immunotherapeutic approaches have been developed for EBV-associated malignancies, using either monoclonal antibodies or the adoptive transfer of EBV-specific T cells.[3,4]

BIOLOGY OF EPSTEIN-BARR VIRUS

EBV belongs to the family of herpesviruses, which has almost 100 members. Membership is based on the architecture of the virion that is 120 to 300 nm in size and contains (a) a core of linear, double-stranded DNA, (b) an icosadeltahedral capsid with 162 capsomers, (c) an amorphous material between the capsid and envelope designated tegument, and (d) an envelope containing viral glycoproteins. Besides EBV, designated human herpesvirus 4, seven other herpesviruses have been isolated from humans: herpes simplex viruses 1 and 2, cytomegalovirus (CMV), varicella-zoster virus, human herpesvirus 6, human herpesvirus 7, and the Kaposi sarcoma–associated herpesvirus (KSHV, human herpesvirus 8). Herpesviruses are further divided into subfamilies to reflect evolutionary relatedness and similar biologic properties. EBV and KSHV belong to the human gamma herpesvirus subgroup and have a limited tissue tropism to B and T lymphocytes and certain types of epithelial cells. Several variants of EBV have been identified by genomic polymorphisms. Initially, two EBV types were distinguished by sequence changes in EBV nuclear

antigens 2 and 3 (EBNA2 and EBNA3). However, using polymorphisms in the latent membrane protein 1 (LMP1), further subtypes have been described. EBV strains vary by geography and have not been linked to a particular EBV-associated disease.

PRIMARY EPSTEIN-BARR VIRUS INFECTION

Primary EBV infection usually occurs through the oropharynx, where mucosal epithelial cells and/or B cells become productively infected (Fig. 54.2). Infection of B cells by EBV is initiated by binding of the dominant viral glycoprotein gp350/220 to CD21, the C3d complement receptor; subsequent cell entry is mediated by a complex of three viral glycoproteins, gH, gL, and gp42. Gp42 binds to HLA class II, which functions as a coreceptor, and gH is most likely involved in virus-cell fusion. The entry of EBV into epithelial cells may occur through multiple mechanisms because the majority of epithelial cells are CD21 negative. After viral entry, the capsid is dissolved and the EBV genome is transported into the nucleus where it circularizes. Infection of epithelial cells results in lytic or abortive infection, whereas B-cell infection results predominantly in latency, the lytic infection also occurs, resulting in the release of infectious virus into the saliva and other secretions. During primary infection, EBV establishes lifelong latency in B cells and it is estimated that 1 to 50 cells per 1×10^6 B cells in the peripheral circulation are infected with EBV. The number of latently infected B cells within a person remains stable over years; however, intermittent reactivation of EBV in B cells into the lytic cycle at mucosal sites is probably responsible for the observed shedding of infectious virus into the saliva of asymptomatic carriers (Fig. 54.2).

Although EBV can infect any B cell and express the full spectrum of latency proteins, studies suggest that only infection of naive B cells results in persistent infection (Fig. 54.2). EBV infection pushes the naive B cell into a memory state independent of an antigen-dependent germinal center (GC) reaction by upregulation of cytosine deaminase, which induces both class switching and somatic hypermutation. The former also requires the expression of EBV-encoded LMP1, a constitutively activated CD40 molecule, or CD40 ligation, most likely provided by GC T helper (Th)3 cells that can provide T-cell help for B-cell differentiation by provision of CD40 ligand, interleukin (IL)-4, and IL-10 while preventing antigen-dependent effector T-cell–mediated B-cell elimination by expression of transforming growth factor (TGF)-β. This reaction occurs within the lymph node (see E-Slide VM03965) and also involves downregulation of latency proteins and expression of latency type II. On exit from the lymph node, expression of latency proteins is completely inhibited. In this way infected B cells can evade immune elimination. By contrast, primarily infected memory B cells enter and remain in latency type III and are rapidly eliminated by effector T cells and therefore do not contribute to virus persistence.

LATENT EPSTEIN-BARR VIRUS INFECTION

During latent infection, EBV persists episomally in resting memory B cells. Initially, it was thought that EBNA1 and LMP2 were

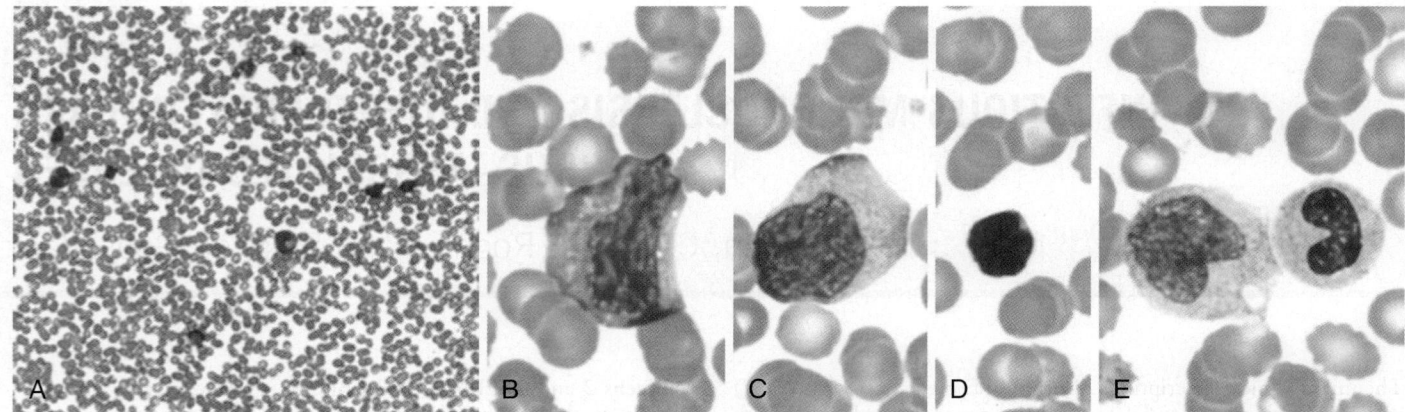

Fig. 54.1 PROMINENT MONONUCLEAR LYMPHOCYTOSIS IN MONONUCLEOSIS. Low power (A) illustrates the leukocytosis, mainly due to activated lymphocytes (B and C), which are contrasted with a normal small lymphocyte (D) and a monocyte and granulocyte (E). The large reactive lymphocytes are frequently confused with monocytes because of their morphologic resemblance and the term *mononucleosis*. Monocytes usually have a finer, lacy chromatin and a gray cytoplasm with small granules and vacuoles when compared with the large activated lymphocytes.

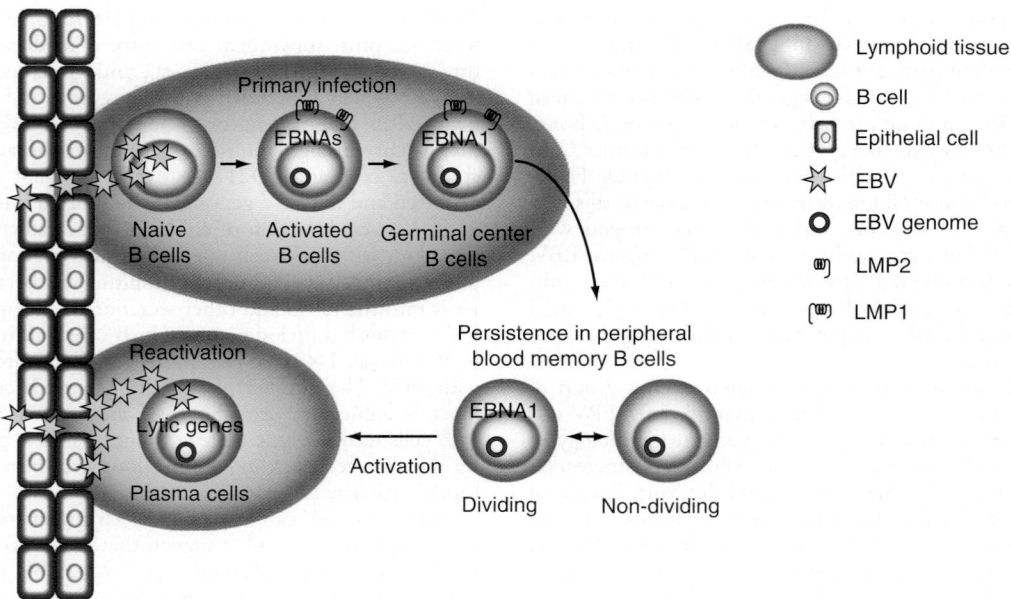

Fig. 54.2 INFECTIOUS LIFE CYCLE OF EPSTEIN-BARR VIRUS. *EBV*, Epstein-Barr virus; *EBNA*, Epstein-Barr nuclear antigen; *LMP*, latent membrane protein.

Epstein-Barr Virus (EBV)–Associated Clinical Syndromes

Infectious mononucleosis
Chronic active EBV infection
Hemophagocytic lymphohistiocytosis
X-linked lymphoproliferative disease
Oral hairy leukoplakia
Multiple sclerosis

expressed in memory B cells; however, more recent studies indicate that the majority of infected cells do not express viral proteins and of the almost 100 viral proteins, only EBNA1 is expressed during memory B-cell division (Fig. 54.2).[2] This extremely limited expression of viral proteins allows EBV to persist long term despite a robust cellular EBV-specific immune response.

Three other distinct types of EBV latency have been characterized in a heterogeneous group of malignancies (Fig. 54.3). Latency type III, which can be readily produced by infecting B cells in vitro with EBV, is expressed in lymphoblastoid cell lines (LCL). These cells express the entire array of nine EBV latency proteins: EBNA1, -2, -3A, -3B, and -3C, EBNA leader protein (LP), and the two viral membrane proteins LMP1 and LMP2. This pattern of EBV gene expression characterizes the EBV-associated lymphoproliferative diseases (EBV-LPD) that occur in individuals severely immunocompromised by solid organ or hematopoietic stem cell transplantation (SOT, HSCT), congenital immunodeficiency, or human immunodeficiency virus (HIV) infection. Latency type II is the hallmark of EBV-positive Hodgkin disease (HD), non-Hodgkin lymphoma (NHL), as well as nasopharyngeal carcinoma (NPC). EBV proteins expressed in these malignancies are EBNA1, LMP1, and LMP2. In addition, BARF1 is expressed in subsets of latency type II associated malignancies. In latency type I, found in EBV-positive BL, only

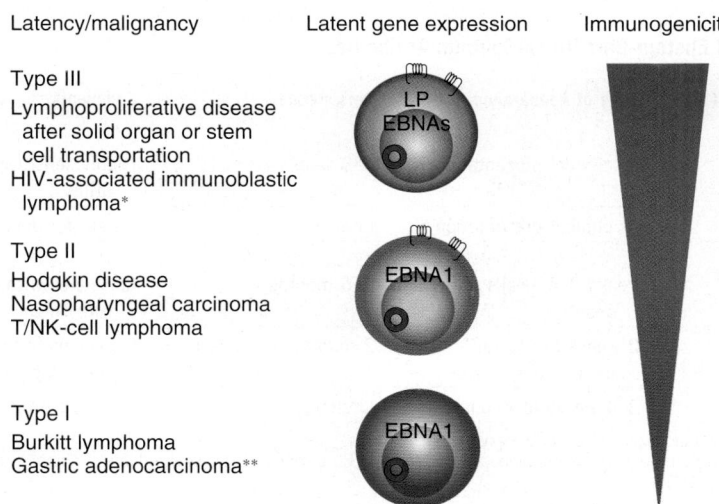

Fig. 54.3 EBV-LATENT GENE EXPRESSION AND IMMUNOGENICITY OF COMMON EBV-ASSOCIATED MALIGNANCIES. *EBV,* Epstein-Barr virus; *EBNA,* Epstein-Barr nuclear antigen; *LP,* leader protein; *NK,* natural killer. For an explanation of symbols, see Fig. 54.2. *Not all lymphomas are latency type III. **Gastric adenocarcinoma can also express latency type II genes.

EBNA1 is expressed. However, variants in which all EBNAs are expressed in the absence of LMP1 have also been described. Latency type I or latency type II is found in EBV-associated gastric adenocarcinoma. While grouping EBV-associated malignancies according to their dominant gene expression profile provided a useful framework for understanding EBV-driven oncogenesis, more recent studies using comprehensive gene expression array profiling have demonstrated expression of lytic cycle genes in BL, or expression of lytic cycle and latency III genes in NPC.[5,6]

The EBV proteins expressed during type III latency are involved in the transformation and growth of EBV-infected B cells. EBNA1 binds to the origin of replication of the latent viral genome and is responsible for the maintenance of the EBV episome in host B cells. EBNA2 upregulates the expression of the viral proteins LMP1 and LMP2 and cellular proteins that contribute to transformation. EBNA3A and EBNA3C are essential for EBV-induced B-cell transformation, and although EBNA3B is not essential for transformation, it is highly conserved and therefore must provide a survival function in vivo. EBNA-LP cooperates with EBNA2 in the induction of viral and cellular genes. LMP1, a viral oncogene, behaves like a constitutively activated CD40 molecule and is essential for EBV-mediated B-cell transformation. LMP2 mimics an activated B-cell receptor (BCR) allowing for long-term B-cell survival in the absence of antigen. In addition, it prevents the reactivation of EBV into the lytic phase of infection.

Besides EBV proteins, small nonpolyadenylated viral RNAs termed *EBERs 1* and *2* and the BamHI-A rightward transcripts (BARTS) are expressed in all forms of latency. In addition, the expression of at least 17 distinct EBV-derived microRNAs has been reported. The EBERs are the most abundant viral RNAs in latently infected cells. They enhance the oncogenic phenotype of EBV-transformed cells but are nonessential for EBV-mediated transformation. The expression pattern of the microRNAs depends on the latency type, and it is therefore likely that they play an important role during the life cycle of the virus.

IMMUNE RESPONSE TO EPSTEIN-BARR VIRUS

Healthy individuals mount vigorous humoral and cellular immune responses to primary EBV infection.[7] Although antibodies to the viral membrane proteins neutralize virus infectivity, the cellular immune response is essential for controlling virus-infected cells during both lytic and latent phases.

Humoral Immune Responses

Heterophile Antibodies

Heterophile antibodies, originally described by Paul and Bunnell, are present in 90% to 95% of EBV infections at some point during the illness. However, in infants and children under the age of 4 years with primary EBV infection, heterophile antibody responses are often not detected. Heterophile antibodies are IgM antibodies, which agglutinate erythrocytes from different species including bovine, camel, horse, goat, and sheep. EBV-induced heterophile antibodies have no reactivity against guinea pig kidney cells in contrast to naturally occurring antibodies (Forssman antibodies) or antibodies present in patients with serum sickness and other conditions.

In addition to heterophile antibodies, cold agglutinins directed preferentially against the anti-I antigen on red cell membranes are frequently detected in the sera of patients with IM; however, hemolytic anemia is rare. Other antibodies (including anti-I, anti-N, Donath-Landsteiner antibodies, platelet antibodies, and anti–smooth muscle antibodies) have been described.

Epstein-Barr Virus-Specific Antibodies

EBV-specific antibody responses are detected with immunofluorescence assays developed in the first decades of EBV research. EBV antibodies are directed against (a) EBNA, (b) early antigen (EA), (c) the membrane antigen (MA) expressed on the surface of cells late in the lytic cycle, and (d) the viral capsid antigen (VCA) expressed within cells late in the lytic cycle. Each antigen is a composite of several distinct viral proteins, and attempts have been made to replace the aforementioned assays with tests using specific viral proteins; however, no single test has attracted widespread use.

VCA-IgM and -IgG antibodies are usually present at the onset of clinical symptoms because of the prolonged viral incubation period (Table 54.1). VCA-IgM antibodies are a good marker for an acute infection because they rapidly disappear within 4 to 8 weeks. VCA-IgG antibodies persist for life and are commonly used to document prior EBV infection. IgG antibodies against EA are present at the onset of the clinical illness in approximately 70% of patients. EA antibodies are divided into methanol-sensitive (anti-D) and methanol-resistant (anti-R) antibodies, and the majority of EA antibodies detected are anti-D antibodies. The presence of anti-D antibodies is

TABLE 54.1   Frequently Determined Epstein-Barr Virus–Specific Antibodies

Antibody Specificity	Positive in IM (%)	Time of Appearance in IM	Persistence	Comments
Viral Capsid Antigen				
VCA-IgM	100	At clinical presentation	4–8 weeks	Highly sensitive and specific; of major diagnostic utility
VCA-IgG	100	At clinical presentation	Lifelong	Useful for documentation of past EBV infection
Early Antigen (EA)				
Anti-D	70	Peaks 3–4 weeks after onset	3–6 months	Correlates with disease severity; seen in patients with NPC
Anti-R	Low	2 weeks to several months after onset	2 months to >3 years	Occasionally seen with unusually severe cases; seen in patients with African Burkitt lymphoma
EBNA	100	3–4 weeks after onset	Lifelong	Presence excludes primary EBV infection

EBV, Epstein-Barr virus; IM, infectious mononucleosis; NPC, nasopharyngeal carcinoma.
Modified from Schooley RT: Epstein-Barr virus (infectious mononucleosis). In Mandell GL, Bennett JE, Dolin R, editors: *Principles and practice of infectious diseases,* Philadelphia, 2000, Churchill Livingstone, p 1599.

consistent with recent infection, because titers disappear after recovery. IgG antibodies to EBNA appear late in the course of almost all cases of EBV infection and persist throughout life; their presence early in a suspected case of primary EBV infection excludes the diagnosis. Aberrations in this pattern of serum reactivity are observed in many EBV-associated diseases and will be discussed under the specific disease sections. For example, the absence of EBNA antibodies despite previous EBV infection is one of the serologic markers suggestive for chronic active EBV infection.

Cellular Immune Responses

In normal individuals, primary EBV infection often results in a massive expansion of activated, antigen-specific T cells. Using tetramer technology to enumerate antigen-specific T cells, it has been documented that the $CD8^+$ T-cell response may be dominated by T cells specific for a limited number of epitopes, as seen with T-cell responses against other herpesviruses. T cells specific for epitopes derived from immediate early and several early EBV proteins of the lytic cycle are dominant during the acute phase of IM, and long-term persistence of EBV-specific, $CD8^+$ T cells has been documented after primary EBV infection. As many as 5.5% of the circulating $CD8^+$ T cells in a healthy virus carrier may be positive for a single EBV epitope, illustrating how persistent EBV infection can influence the composition of the host's T-cell pool. Besides EBV-specific $CD8^+$ T cells, EBV-specific $CD4^+$ T cells play an important role in the control of EBV infections, and EBNA1-specific $CD4^+$ T cells have been implicated in the control of newly infected B cells. As for $CD8^+$ T-cell responses, there is a marked hierarchy of immunodominance, with the majority of $CD4^+$ T cells being specific for EBNA1 and to a lesser extent EBNA3C.

EPSTEIN-BARR VIRUS VACCINE DEVELOPMENT

At present there is only limited experience with human EBV vaccines.[8] Four vaccine studies have been conducted in healthy donors in the prophylactic setting using recombinant vaccinia virus encoding the major viral glycoprotein gp350 (1), recombinant gp350 protein (2), or an EBNA3A peptide. While vaccination with gp350 induced neutralizing antibodies, and in one study prevented the clinical picture of IM, these vaccines did not significantly reduce the incidence of EBV infection. Also no reduction in the incidence of EBV infection was observed with the EBNA3A peptide vaccine. Additionally, a recombinant gp350 protein was evaluated in patients with chronic kidney disease prior to kidney transplantation. Although the vaccine induced transient neutralizing antibodies, it did not reduce the incidence of EBV-LPD posttransplant. Newer vaccines consisting

of gp350-ferritin complexes that induce significantly higher titers of neutralizing antibodies in preclinical models have been developed, but require testing in humans.

Vaccine strategies in the therapeutic setting for the immunotherapy of EBV-associated malignancies should seek to elicit or boost the EBV-specific cellular immune response against EBV latency. Individuals likely to benefit from this approach are EBV-seronegative patients scheduled to undergo SOT or patients who have an EBV-associated malignancy with a low tumor burden or are in remission (see box on EBV-Associated Malignancies). Three vaccine studies have been conducted in patients with EBV-positive NPC. In two studies patients with advanced disease were vaccinated with either dendritic cells (DCs) loaded with peptides derived from LMP2 or DCs transduced with an adenoviral vector encoding full-length LMP2 and an inactive form of LMP1. Administration of DC vaccines was safe, and a transient increase in the frequency of LMP2-specific T cells was observed on the DC/peptide vaccine trial. However, the clinical benefit in both studies was limited. Thus future studies should focus on DC vaccines with greater potency administered to subjects with less tumor burden. In another phase I clinical study, after frontline therapy, patients with NPC were vaccinated with a modified vaccinia virus Ankara encoding the c-terminal portion of EBNA1 and LMP2 (MVA-EL). Induction of $CD4^+$ and $CD8^+$ antigen-specific T-cell responses was observed in the majority of patients after vaccination, and a phase II clinical study is in progress. In addition, a clinical study combining MVA-EL with a PD-L1-specific checkpoint monoclonal antibody (pembrolizumab) is in the planning phase. Lastly, a recombinant adenovirus vaccine encoding LMP2 was evaluated in patients with NPC. While vaccine

---

Epstein-Barr Virus (EBV)–Associated Malignancies

Malignancy	EBV Frequency
Hodgkin disease	~40%
Non-Hodgkin lymphomas	
Burkitt lymphoma	20–95%
Diffuse large B-cell lymphoma and $CD30^+$ $Ki-1^+$ anaplastic large cell lymphoma	10–35%
Lymphomatoid granulomatosis	80–95%
T-cell–rich B-cell lymphoma	20%
Angioimmunoblastic lymphoma	>80%
T-cell, natural killer (NK)-cell, and T/NK-cell lymphomas	30–90%
Nasopharyngeal carcinoma	>95%
Gastric adenocarcinoma	5–10%
Pythorax-associated lymphoma	>95%
Leiomyosarcoma in immunocompromised patients	>95%

administration was safe, no data are available if the vaccine boosted LMP2-specific T-cell responses.

INFECTIOUS MONONUCLEOSIS

Epidemiology

EBV infections occur worldwide and in most populations 90% to 95% of adults have antibodies against EBV. Depending on geographic and socioeconomic factors, there is a wide variation in the age of primary EBV infections. Early, asymptomatic primary EBV infection occurs in individuals from lower socioeconomic groups and in third world countries. In higher socioeconomic groups in industrialized countries, the age of primary infection is often delayed until the second decade of life and clinically apparent IM is more prevalent.

Humans are the only source of EBV. EBV is present in the saliva of patients with IM. A majority of EBV-positive adults shed virus into their saliva, and this percentage is increased in immunocompromised patients such as SOT recipients. EBV is viable outside the body for 2 weeks at 4°C but is susceptible to drying; the virus has not been recovered from environmental sources, suggesting that close contact is needed for viral spread. The incubation period of IM is estimated to be 30 to 50 days.

Clinical Manifestations

Primary EBV infection in infants and young children is either asymptomatic or accompanied by mild, nonspecific symptoms and signs such as fever, upper respiratory tract infection, pharyngitis with or without tonsillitis, and cervical lymphadenopathy. In contrast, approximately 50% of adolescents and young adults present with the clinical picture of IM. Frequently, a prodrome consisting of fatigue, malaise, and low-grade fever is present for 1 to 2 weeks. Prominent pharyngitis with exudative tonsillitis is often the cardinal sign of IM; other signs and symptoms are listed in Table 54.2. The adenopathy in IM most commonly affects the posterior cervical lymph nodes, although diffuse adenopathy can occur. The enlarged lymph nodes are not fixed, may be tender to palpation, and lack overlying skin erythema. Hepatomegaly is uncommon; however, splenomegaly develops in more than 50% of patients and is more prominent in the second to fourth week of the illness. Skin manifestations include a faint, morbilliform rash reminiscent of rubella and less commonly erythema multiforme and erythema nodosum. Most patients with primary EBV infection have symptoms for 2 to 4 weeks and recover without significant complications or sequelae.

Complications of Primary Epstein-Barr Virus Infections

The incidence of complications associated with primary EBV infection is low, although any organ system can be affected.

Hematologic Complications

Patients with IM may present with a wide range of hematologic findings besides the atypical lymphocytosis (Fig. 54.4). These include anemia, neutropenia, thrombocytopenia, and rare cases of aplastic anemia.

Anemia

Autoimmune hemolytic anemia occurs in approximately 3% of patients with IM. It presents in the first 2 weeks of the illness, and

TABLE 54.2 Clinical Manifestations of Infectious Mononucleosis

Manifestation	Percentage (Range)
Symptoms	
Sore throat	82 (70—88)
Malaise	57 (43–76)
Headache	51 (37–55)
Anorexia	21 (10–27)
Myalgias	20 (12–22)
Chills	16 (9–18)
Abdominal discomfort	9 (2–14)
Signs	
Lymphadenopathy	94 (93–100)
Pharyngitis	84 (69–91)
Fever	76 (63–100)
Splenomegaly	52 (50–63)
Hepatomegaly	12 (6–14)
Palatal enanthem	11 (5–13)
Rash	10 (0–15)
Jaundice	9 (4–10)

Modified from Schooley RT: Epstein-Barr virus (infectious mononucleosis). In Mandell GL, Bennett JE, Dolin R, editors: *Principles and practice of infectious diseases*, Philadelphia, 2000, Churchill Livingstone, p 1599.

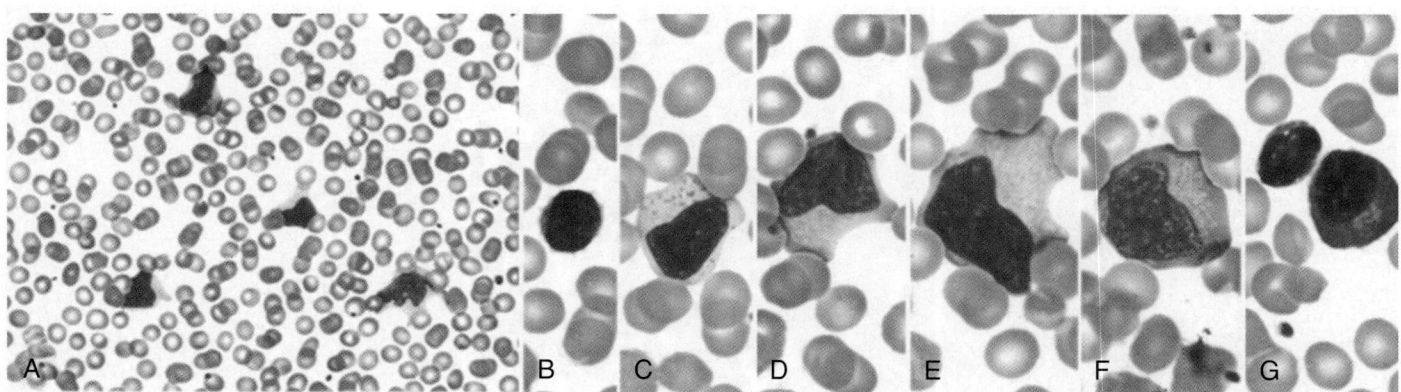

Fig. 54.4 PERIPHERAL BLOOD SMEAR IN INFECTIOUS MONONUCLEOSIS. (A) Low power shows moderately high white blood cell count and high number of reactive, or "atypical" lymphocytes. (B–G) Higher power illustrates spectrum of lymphoid morphology, including small resting lymphocyte (B) for comparison, large granular lymphocyte (C), atypical forms (D–F), also referred to as "reactive" lymphs, and circulating plasma cell (G).

the majority of patients recover within 1 to 2 months. Patients usually have a positive direct Coombs test. Most common anti-I antibodies are present; however, anti-I, anti-N, and Donath-Landsteiner antibodies have also been reported. In addition to hemolysis, IM-associated anemia can be caused by erythroblastopenia.

Neutropenia

Mild, self-limiting neutropenia is a common finding during the first 4 weeks of the disease. However, severe neutropenia associated with fatal bacterial infections has been reported.

Thrombocytopenia

Mild thrombocytopenia (50,000 to 150,000/mm^3) is a common finding in patients with IM. It usually occurs within the first 2 weeks of presentation and resolves within 2 months. Severe thrombocytopenia with overt bleeding is rare; however, death from intracranial hemorrhage has been described. The etiology of the thrombocytopenia is not completely understood, and a variety of explanations have been suggested. Because bone marrow examination shows normal or increased numbers of megakaryocytes, peripheral platelet destruction is most likely due to the presence of antiplatelet antibodies or platelet pooling and destruction within an enlarged spleen.

Splenic Rupture

Splenic rupture occurs predominately in males, with an incidence of 1/1000 to 1/3000 (Fig. 54.5). The incidence of rupture is highest in the second and third week of illness and can be the first sign of IM. Clinical symptoms include abdominal pain or pain referred to either shoulder. Because abdominal pain is an unusual symptom of uncomplicated IM, a splenic rupture should be strongly considered in IM cases when abdominal pain is reported. Although it is a life-threatening complication, with current management the mortality rate is very low.

Neurologic Complications

Neurologic complications develop usually during the first 2 weeks of IM and may be the only manifestation of IM. EBV infection can cause a wide spectrum of neurologic diseases, including encephalitis, meningitis, Guillain-Barré syndrome, acute transverse myelitis, and peripheral neuritis. Patients with neurologic complications have an excellent outcome, with most patients recovering completely.

Other Organ Involvement

Although symptomatic heart disease with IM is uncommon, in one cohort of patients, unspecific ST- and T-wave abnormalities were found in 6% of patients. Renal involvement manifested as microscopic hematuria, and proteinuria is seen in 10% to 15% of patients; however, significant renal dysfunction is rare. Airway compromise due to hypertrophy of the adenoids and tonsils or mucosal inflammation and edema is uncommon but potentially fatal.

Diagnosis

Atypical lymphocytosis is the cardinal hematologic finding in IM (Fig. 54.4). It develops during the first week of the illness and peaks between the second and third week. Atypical lymphocytes represent 60% to 70% of the total white cell count, which ranges between 12,000/mm^3 and 18,000/mm^3. In general, the atypical lymphocytes are large and vary in size. Nuclei are large and eccentrically placed; the cytoplasm is basophilic, and vacuoles are often present. The variable morphologic pattern of atypical lymphocytes in IM distinguishes them from the monotonous appearance of immature leukemic blasts. Atypical lymphocytosis is not pathognomonic for IM and is associated with other diseases such as acute viral hepatitis, CMV infections, mumps, toxoplasmosis, rubella, roseola, and drug reactions.

The diagnosis of EBV infection depends on serologic testing. Tests for heterophile antibodies, including the monospot test and slide agglutination tests, are routinely available. The results of these tests are often negative in children less than 4 years of age, but they identify 90% of cases in older children and adults. Of the available EBV-specific serologic tests, VCA-IgM antibodies are most commonly determined to diagnose primary EBV infection in heterophile-negative IM cases; determining antibodies against EA may also be helpful (Table 54.1). VCA-IgG antibodies are positive during acute infections as well as the convalescent period. The presence of anti-EBNA antibodies excludes an acute infection. Isolation of EBV from throat washings is feasible; however, it is of little diagnostic value because 10% to 20% of healthy adult EBV carriers may shed the virus.

Differential Diagnosis

In the majority of cases, the diagnosis of IM is straightforward. The differential diagnosis includes streptococcal and nonstreptococcal pharyngitis, acute infections with CMV, human herpesvirus 6,

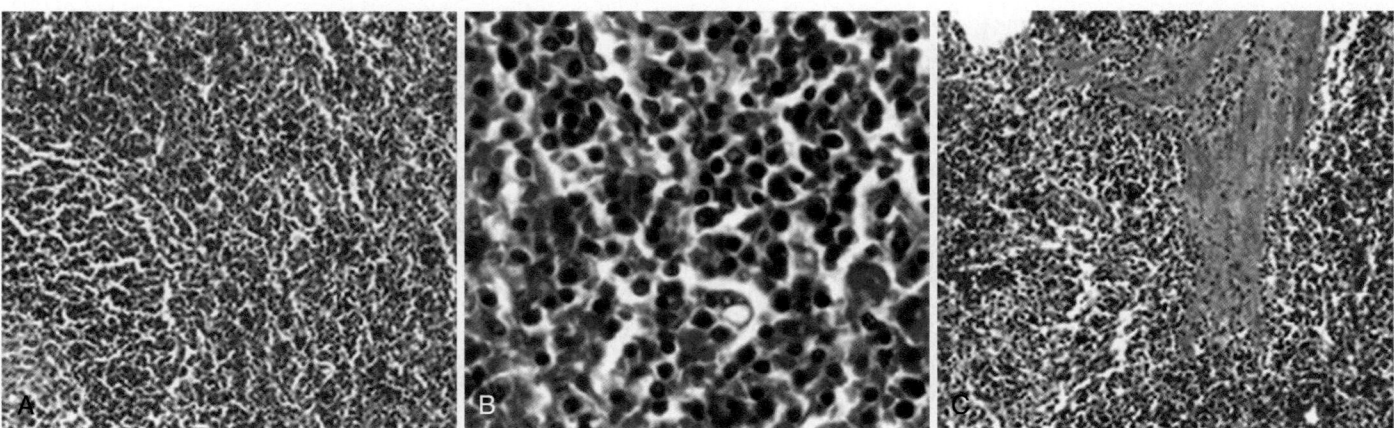

Fig. 54.5 RUPTURED SPLEEN FROM PATIENT WITH INFECTIOUS MONONUCLEOSIS. (A and B) Sections from the spleen show increased white cells in the red pulp. These correspond to the proliferating activated lymphocytes seen in the blood. (C) The lymphocytes can infiltrate into the splenic trabeculae, weakening the integrity of the spleen and making it more prone to rupture.

hepatitis viruses, and toxoplasma. Depending on the presentation, other diseases may be considered such as HIV, rubella, and leukemia or lymphoma.

Treatment

Supportive therapy should include rest and analgesia in the acute stage of IM. Contact sports should be avoided until the patient has fully recovered and the spleen is no longer palpable. The use of corticosteroids is not indicated for uncomplicated IM; however, a trial of corticosteroids is warranted in patients with marked tonsillar inflammation and hypertrophy resulting in impending airway obstruction. Although acyclovir reduces EBV shedding into oral secretions, treatment of IM with acyclovir has resulted in no clinical benefit.

OTHER EPSTEIN-BARR VIRUS ASSOCIATED DISEASES

Most individuals recover from the acute phase of primary EBV infection with no long-term sequelae. However, a minority of patients with intrinsic defects in immune function may respond with potentially lethal uncontrolled pathologic inflammation with fever and multisystem organ failure, meeting diagnostic criteria for hemophagocytic lymphohistiocytosis (HLH). Others may develop chronic active EBV infections (CAEBV) with persistent fever, arthralgia, myalgia, and lymphadenopathy, or develop lymphoproliferative and/or malignant disorders. In addition to primary immunodeficiencies that result in failure to control EBV infection, there is an increasing group of gene defects associated with complex or acquired immune dysfunction (ATM, WAS, PIK3CD, PIK3R1, CTPS1, STK4, GATA2, MCM4, FCGR3A, and CARD11) that predispose not only to complications of EBV infection but also other viruses, bacteria, and/or fungi.[9]

Hemophagocytic Lymphohistiocytosis

HLH is a syndrome characterized by uncontrolled inflammation (see Chapter 52). Diagnostic criteria defined by the Histiocyte Society reflect the clinical features of pathologic immune activation, including persistent fever, splenomegaly, cytopenias, hyperferritinemia, decreased fibrinogen or increased triglycerides, hemophagocytosis (in bone marrow, spleen, or lymph nodes), increased soluble IL-2 receptor α, and decreased or absent natural killer (NK) cell function. The diagnosis of HLH can also be established by a pattern of familial inheritance or proven gene defects. It was first characterized as an inherited disorder in infants in the 1950s, referred to as "familial hemophagocytic reticulosis."

Gene defects resulting in impaired cytotoxic NK- and T-cell function have been associated with autosomal recessive inheritance of HLH, including PRF1 (familial (f)HLH-2), UNC13D (fHLH-3), STX11 (fHLH-4), STXPB2 (fHLH-5), Munc18-2, Rab27a (Griscelli syndrome, type 2), LYST (Chédiak-Higashi syndrome), AP3B1 (Hermansky-Pudlak syndrome, type II), ITK, CD27, and MAGT1 (XMEN syndrome).[10] EBV infection may trigger HLH in patients with any form of familial disease. Gene defects are identified in only 50% of patients with family history consistent with inherited HLH. Therefore, although a diagnosis "primary" or "familial" HLH may be proven, it is impossible to exclude. Familial HLH commonly presents in young children, but there are reports of new onset of HLH in adults as old as 62 years with mutations in HLH-associated genes. Patients with familial HLH typically require prompt treatment with chemotherapy and immune suppression (etoposide/dexamethasone) followed by HSCT.[11] Without therapy, survival of patients with active familial HLH is approximately 2 months. The first international treatment protocol for HLH organized by the Histiocyte Society in 1994 reported long-term survival of over 50%. More recently, survival rates of greater than 90% have been reported with reduced intensity conditioning regimens.[12]

The term secondary HLH generally refers to older children (or adults) who present without a family history or known genetic cause for their HLH. EBV is a common trigger for "secondary HLH," ranging from inflammation that resolves spontaneously to unrelenting disease requiring HSCT. Differentiating infectious mononucleosis from EBV-associated HLH (EBV-HLH) is challenging. Clinical criteria for HLH should be evaluated in patients with persistently high cell-free EBV genome copy numbers in plasma, persistent symptoms of inflammation, or severe symptoms. Patients who initially meet clinical criteria for HLH may occasionally improve spontaneously. Patients with less severe presentations may also respond to corticosteroids, intravenous immunoglobulins or cyclosporine. However, in patients with progressive or severe disease, early initiation (within 4 weeks of onset of symptoms) of etoposide is associated with significant improvement in survival.[13] Because it can eliminate EBV-infected B cells, rituximab may be a beneficial addition to other therapies in patients with progressive EBV-HLH.[14] Some patients with apparently self-resolving HLH after primary EBV infection later develop recurrent HLH requiring immunochemotherapy and HSCT. Therefore it remains important to follow patients beyond resolution of initial symptoms. Alemtuzumab has also been reported to be effective in patients with recurrent or refractory disease.[11] Early clinical data also support the use interferon (IFN)-γ monoclonal antibodies in patients with refractory HLH.

X-Linked Lymphoproliferative Diseases

X-Linked Lymphoproliferative Disease 1

Mutations or deletions in SH2D1A (Src homology 2 domain protein 1A) results in X-linked lymphoproliferative disease (XLP1; Duncan disease), an immunodeficiency characterized by fatal IM meeting the diagnostic criteria for HLH, agammaglobulinemia, or B-cell lymphoma. SH2D1A interacts with SLAM (signaling lymphocyte activation molecule), which plays a central role in the stimulation of B and T cells. SH2D1A controls several distinct key T-cell signaling pathways, and mutant SH2D1A does not bind SLAM, suggesting that it is a natural SLAM inhibitor. SAP association with SLAM receptors is crucial for development of normal NK T cells, formation of normal GCs, and NK- and T-cell killing of EBV-infected B cells. T cells from patients with XLP1 are also resistant to apoptosis by radiation-induced cell death (RICD). Immune hyperactivation induced by primary EBV infection may be due to specific defects in NK+ and CD8+ T-cell cytotoxicity rather than from decreased or absent cytotoxic proteins. Resistance to apoptosis may exacerbate the inflammatory response due to persistence of ineffective activated NK and T cells.

Following infection with EBV, XLP1 patients mount a vigorous, uncontrolled polyclonal expansion of T and B cells. Infiltrating T cells cause extensive tissue destruction of the liver and bone marrow, resulting in death in 50% of XLP1 patients during primary EBV infection. Approximately 30% of patients have acquired hypogammaglobulinemia and 25% of patients develop malignant B-cell lymphomas that are often extranodal, involving the intestinal ileocecal region. It is important to realize that some patients with SH2D1A mutations may only present with hypogammaglobulinemia mimicking common variable immunodeficiency, and a diagnosis of XLP1 should be considered when more than one male patient with hypogammaglobulinemia is encountered in the same family. Patients with fulminant immunologic responses to primary EBV infection may be treated with HLH treatment strategies (steroids and etoposide) and/or rituximab. However, the only curative therapy for XLP1 is HSCT.

X-Linked Lymphoproliferative Disease 2

A second X-linked immune deficiency characterized by recurrent HLH (with or without EBV infection) is XLP2, caused by BIRC4 mutations and XIAP deficiency.[15] Unlike patients with XLP1, those

TABLE 54.3	Classification of Chronic Active Epstein-Barr Virus (EBV) Infection				
		Clinical Symptoms			
EBV-Infected Lymphocyte	**Geography**	**General**	**Skin**	**Clinical Course**	
B cell	Predominant in Western hemisphere	Fever, adenopathy, organomegaly, hepatic, cardiac, or pulmonary dysfunction	None	Chronic	
T cell	Predominant in Asia: Japan, Taiwan, Korea Also in Native Americans: in Mexico, Central and South America		Hydroa vacciniforme	Risk for aggressive lymphoma/leukemia	
NK cell			Hypersensitivity to mosquito bites		

with XLP2 have less pleotropic clinical manifestations. It rarely results in lymphoproliferation or lymphoma and may be more accurately characterized as "X-linked familial HLH." XIAP is a ubiquitously expressed member of a family of proteins defined by baculovirus IAP repeat (BIR) domains that inhibit apoptosis through inhibition of caspases. The mechanism of XIAP-induced HLH remains uncertain. Paradoxically, unlike in cases of XLP1, in which lymphocytes are resistant to apoptosis, XIAP deficiency in XLP2 confers increased sensitivity to RICD. The clinical manifestations of HLH in XLP2 patients with primary EBV infections appear less severe than in patients with XLP1. However, data remain insufficient to make specific therapy recommendations for XLP1 versus XLP2 or other forms of familial HLH.

Chronic Active Epstein-Barr Virus

CAEBV represents a range of clinical manifestations resulting from persistent, uncontrolled infection of B, T, and/or NK cells by EBV (Table 54.3).[16] Inability to control infection is likely due to defects in cytotoxic immune function. CAEBV has considerable pathologic and clinical overlap with HLH, and immune dysfunction is likely due to a variety of causes. Early descriptions of CAEBV primarily reported disease in Asian patients, and almost all cases were due to proliferation of EBV-infected T or NK cells. A recent review of several centers in the United States found a predominance of B cell–associated CAEBV in the Western hemisphere.

To establish the diagnosis of CAEBV, patients must have (a) signs and symptoms for at least 6 months and (b) an abnormal EBV serology with high antibody titers of VCA-IgG and EA-IgG, and little or no antibodies against EBNA. Affected individuals may also have measurable EA-messenger-RNA or EBV-DNA in the peripheral blood, serum, or affected tissues. The life-threatening form of CAEBV is characterized by high fevers, hepatosplenomegaly, and extensive lymphadenopathy, followed by hepatic, cardiac, or pulmonary dysfunction. These patients have very high EBV-VCA titers and EBV-DNA levels in their peripheral blood. Although EBV usually resides in B cells, in severe CAEBV, either T or NK cells are often infected, predisposing the patient to lethal T-cell or NK-cell lymphomas. Severe, often fatal CAEBV is more common in Japan, whereas mild/moderate CAEBV is more common in the Western hemisphere and is predominantly associated with B-cell infection. These patients do not have XLP-associated SH2D1A or BIRC4 mutations, and while the etiology of CAEBV remains poorly understood a recent study demonstrated that GATA2 deficiency is associated with CAEBV and hydroa vacciniforme. Severe allergy to mosquito bites is associated with EBV-infected NK cells, whereas hydroa vacciniforme is associated with EBV-infected T cells. The proposed classification scheme of CAEBV-associated lymphoproliferative disease (LPD) includes three categories: (1) polymorphic LPD without clonal proliferation of EBV-infected cells, (2) polymorphic LPD with clonality, and (3) monomorphic LPD (T- or NK-cell lymphoma/leukemia)

with clonality.[17] In the 2016 WHO Classification of mature lymphoid, histiocytic, and dendritic neoplasms LPDs associated with EBV-infected T cells are classified as systemic EBV-positive T-cell LPDs of childhood; LPDs associated with EBV-infected NK cells, as hydroa vacciniforme-like lymphoproliferative disorder.

Although sporadic clinical improvements of mild/moderate CAEBV have been reported after infusion of IL-2, high-dose immunoglobulin, antiviral drugs, tumor necrosis factor (TNF)-α antibodies, or steroids, the only curative option for severe CAEBV is HSCT. Survival rates vary between 50% and 95%, with better outcomes for patients who (a) are transplanted early after diagnosis, (b) have fewer complications before transplant, and (c) have received a reduced intensity.[18] Besides HSCT, the adoptive transfer of autologous EBV-specific T cells has been explored in five patients with mild or moderate CAEBV. Infusion of EBV-specific T cells resulted in resolution of fatigue, malaise, fever, lymphadenopathy, and splenomegaly lasting for 6 to 36 months. For severe CAEBV in which EBV resides in the T- or NK-cell compartment, the use of EBV-specific T cells has been investigated anecdotally. For example, we have infused donor-derived LMP2-specific T cells with a good partial response as judged by decreasing EBV-DNA load.

Oral Hairy Leukoplakia

Oral hairy leukoplakia (OHL) develops frequently, although not exclusively, in patients who are HIV-positive. It is a nonmalignant hyperplasia of epithelial cells, and most patients present with white, corrugated lesions on the tongue. Besides IM, OHL is the only EBV-associated disease in which active viral replication is apparent, and multiple strains are often present within the same lesion. Inhibiting EBV replication in vivo with antivirals such as valacyclovir results in resolution of OHL. However, after valacyclovir treatment, EBV replication recurs in normal tongue epithelial cells, indicating that productive EBV replication is necessary but not sufficient to induce OHL.

Multiple Sclerosis

Multiple sclerosis (MS) is a rare inflammatory demyelinating disease of the central nervous system. MS is triggered by a combination of genetic as well as environmental factors. The role of EBV in the pathogenesis of MS has been studied for the last 30 years.[19] While the vast majority of EBV-seropositive individuals do not develop MS thereby questioning an association with EBV, the incidence of EBV seropositivity is higher in MS patients than healthy controls. In addition, individuals who have IM as their clinical presentation of primary EBV infection, have a higher incidence of MS. Lastly, increased or decreased cellular immune responses to EBV antigens have been reported in MS patients. If this dysregulation of EBV-specific cellular immune responses contributes to the pathogenesis of MS is the subject of active investigation. Based on findings from these studies, EBV-targeted approaches might be explored in the future.

Epstein-Barr Virus–Associated Malignancies

Over the past decades, EBV has been associated with a heterogeneous group of malignancies.[15] Each year 200,000 cases of EBV-positive malignancies are diagnosed worldwide, with gastric carcinoma being the most common, followed by NPC, and lymphoma. Although there is strong circumstantial evidence linking EBV to these malignancies, the potential causative relationship between EBV and these tumors remains to be firmly established. The following section focuses on EBV-LPD, HD, NHL (including BL), and NPC (Figs. 54.6 and 54.7). All EBV-associated malignancies are associated with viral latency, and spontaneous viral replication occurs at a very low frequency. Because antiviral agents, like acyclovir, only prevent viral replication and do not affect latency, these agents are of limited therapeutic value.

Lymphoproliferative Disease

EBV-LPD develops in patients with congenital or acquired immunodeficiencies, including severe combined immunodeficiency, XLP,

HIV infection, and immunosuppression in SOT recipients (Fig. 54.6, A, B) or HSCT.[20] Besides EBV and a dysfunctional cellular immune system, genetic alterations in B cells have also been implicated in the pathogenesis of posttransplant LPD, especially in SOT recipients, including microsatellite instability, DNA hypermethylation, aberrant somatic hypermutation, and mutations in specific genes such as *MYCC, BCL-6, N-ras,* and *p53.* Most cases of EBV-LPD are lymphomas of B-cell origin, histologic high-grade NHL of the immunoblastic or undifferentiated large cell type that respond poorly to cytotoxic therapy. In the setting of SOT, the reported incidence of EBV-LPD ranges from 1% to 25%, with the highest risk in seronegative recipients, patients receiving intensive immunosuppressive therapy, and patients receiving grafts with a high lymphoid content. After HSCT the incidence of EBV-LPD varies with the transplant regimen and may be as high as 25%. Risk factors for the development of EBV-LPD include the use of stem cells from an HLA-mismatched family member or closely HLA-matched unrelated donor, T-cell depletion of the donor cells, intensive immunosuppression, and an underlying diagnosis of primary immunodeficiency. The incidence is much lower when methods that also deplete B cells are employed. The onset of EBV-LPD seems to be preceded by a large increase in virus load as well as the proliferation of EBV-infected B cells. Frequent monitoring of the EBV-DNA load in peripheral blood is a valuable diagnostic test for early detection of EBV-LPD after HSCT or SOT. However, it remains a subject of debate which is the optimal sample (whole blood, isolated peripheral blood mononuclear cells, plasma)

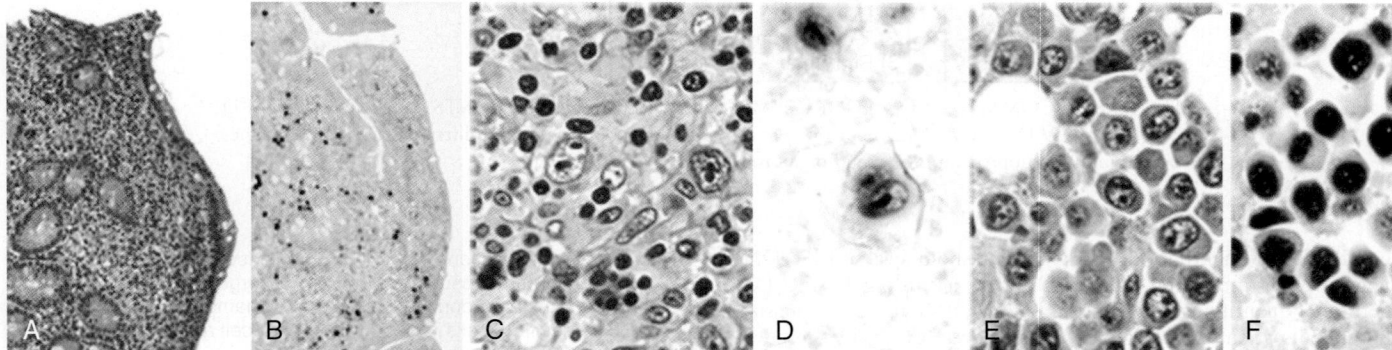

Fig. 54.6 EXAMPLES OF EPSTEIN-BARR VIRUS–POSITIVE LYMPHOID MALIGNANCIES. Posttransplant lymphoproliferative disorder (PTLD), Hodgkin lymphoma, and large B-cell lymphoma. PTLD in the duodenum of a 15-month-old (A) with history of liver transplant. (B) The PTLD was classified as a polymorphic type and was EBV-positive. Hodgkin lymphoma (C) and EBV-positive Reed-Sternberg cells (D). Large B-cell lymphoma (plasmablastic type) in an HIV-positive patient (E), diffusely EBV-positive (F). Note, all EBV studies are in situ hybridizations for EBV mRNA, EBER.

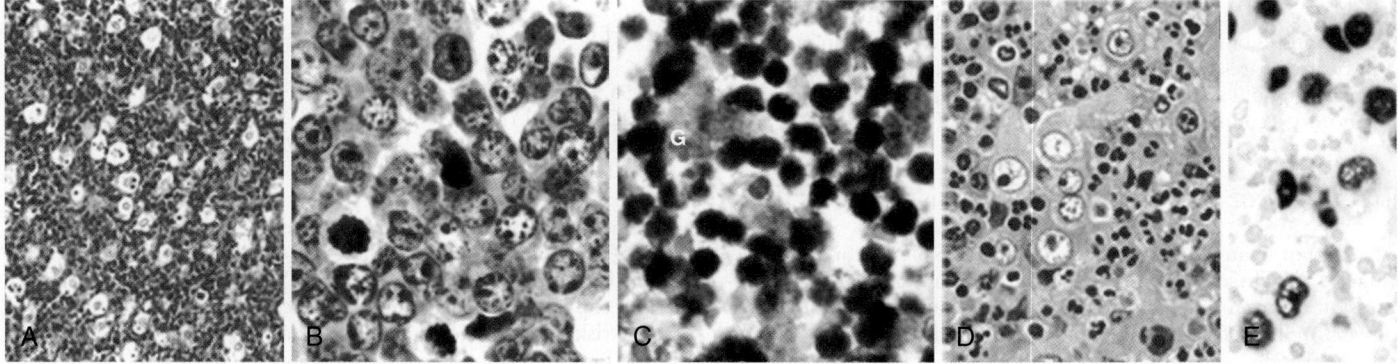

Fig. 54.7 FURTHER EXAMPLES OF EBV-POSITIVE MALIGNANCIES. (A–E) Burkitt lymphoma and nasopharyngeal carcinoma. Low power of Burkitt lymphoma showing the classic "starry sky" appearance (A) and higher power illustrating the highly proliferative lymphoma cells (B), which are uniformly EBV positive (C). Nasopharyngeal carcinoma (D) with EBV-positive cells (E) demonstrated by in situ hybridization for EBV mRNA.

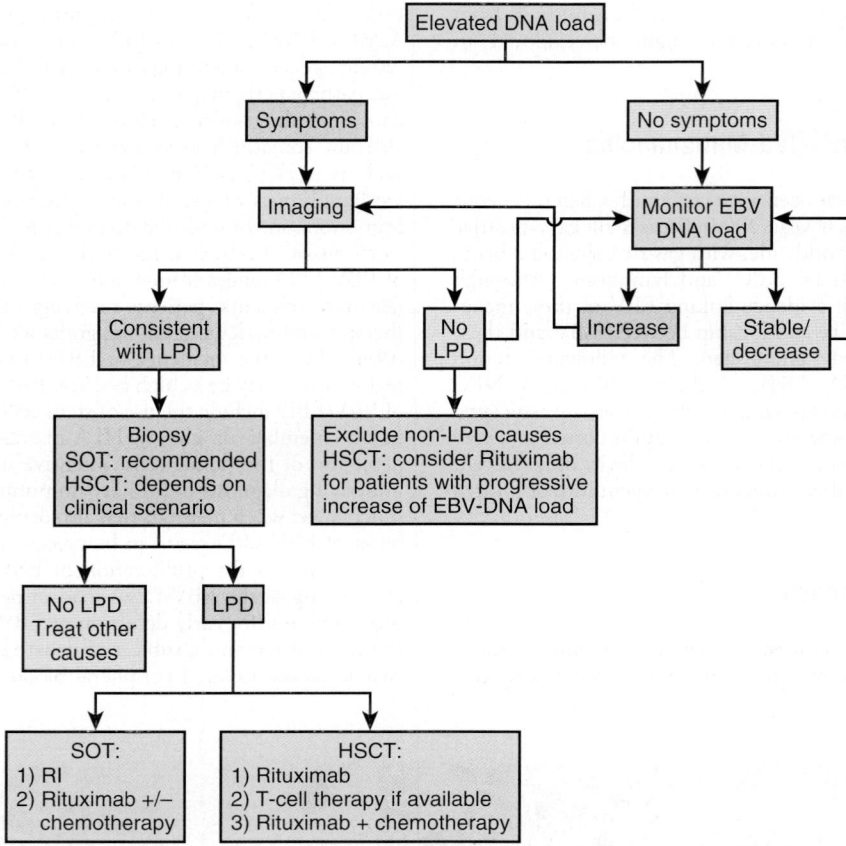

Fig. 54.8 RECOMMENDED ALGORITHM FOR FOLLOWING PATIENTS WITH INCREASED EBV-DNA LOAD. *HSCT,* Hematopoietic stem cell transplant; *LPD,* lymphoproliferative diseases; *RI,* reduction of immunosuppression; *SOT,* solid organ transplant.

for EBV DNA quantitation. Lastly, the threshold level of EBV-DNA suggestive of impending EBV-LPD varies according to the PCR method of quantifying viral DNA. However, it should be emphasized that not all patients with high EBV-DNA levels, especially those with an SOT, develop EBV-LPD. Several distinct patterns of EBV latent gene expression have been identified in the memory B cells of high-load EBV carriers, with type III latency conferring the highest risk for EBV-LPD development. Besides EBV-DNA levels, determining the frequency of EBV-specific T cells or the functionality of T cells in patients with high EBV-DNA load might also assist in identifying patients who are at increased risk for developing EBV-LPD. In addition, host factors such as polymorphisms in the promoter regions of cytokines have been implicated in increasing the risk for developing EBV-LPD. Thus an elevated EBV-DNA load can lead to early diagnosis of EBV-LPD, with consequent reductions in mortality and treatment-related morbidity, although additional results such as clinical signs and symptoms, as well as radiographic findings, must be taken into account before therapy is initiated (Fig. 54.8).[21,22]

Treatment of Lymphoproliferative Disease

A variety of treatment approaches have been explored for EBV-LPD (Fig. 54.9). These include reduction or withdrawal of immunosuppression, conventional chemotherapy, and radiation for localized disease, monoclonal antibodies, adoptive transfer of T cells or EBV-specific T cells, and autologous or allogeneic HSCT for refractory cases. Other potential strategies include eradication of EBV episomes using chemotherapeutic agents like hydroxyurea. Several groups are also developing small molecule inhibitors that block the DNA-binding site of EBNA1, which is critical for EBV episome maintenance.[23] Inducing the lytic cycle of EBV so that the lymphoma cells

Restoring T-cell function
• Reduction of immunosuppression
• Adoptive transfer of donor T cells or EBV-specific T cells

Reduction of B-cell mass
• Surgery, radiation
• Chemotherapy
• B-cell antibodies

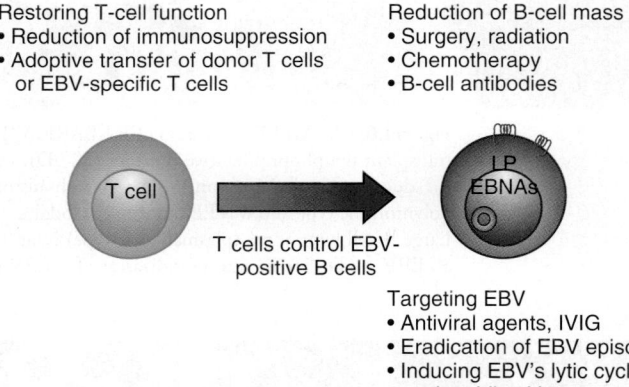

Targeting EBV
• Antiviral agents, IVIG
• Eradication of EBV episome
• Inducing EBV's lytic cycle or thymidine kinase

Fig. 54.9 TREATMENT STRATEGIES FOR EPSTEIN-BARR VIRUS–ASSOCIATED LYMPHOPROLIFERATIVE DISEASES (EBV-LPD). For an explanation of symbols, see Fig. 54.2. *IVIG,* Intravenous immunoglobulin; *LP,* leader protein.

become sensitive to ganciclovir is another therapeutic options. Lastly, in SOT recipients simple withdrawal of immune suppression can result in the regression of localized EBV-LPD by allowing recovery of the suppressed cellular immune system. This approach is limited by the risk for graft rejection, and it is not useful after HSCT because of the profound immunosuppression and the risk for inducing graft-versus-host disease (GVHD).

Monoclonal Antibody Therapy

The CD20 monoclonal antibody rituximab is currently widely used as prophylaxis and as therapy for EBV-LPD. A comprehensive review of the literature that included articles and abstracts published between 1999 and 2008 reported that the use of rituximab as preemptive therapy prevented the development of EBV-LPD in 90% of 341 HSCT recipients, while therapy was associated with a response rate of 63% in 126 HSCT patients.[24] However, response rates varied widely, likely reflecting heterogeneity in patient populations and the fact that early diagnosis and treatment leads to better outcomes. For EBV-LPD after SOT, a recent multicenter analysis of 80 patients reported that rituximab-based therapy had a 3-year progression-free survival of 70% compared with 21% for patients treated without rituximab.[3] Half of the patients treated with rituximab also received chemotherapy, most of them having bulky disease and a high International Prognostic Index. A recent prospective multicenter study suggests that sequential therapy of rituximab followed by chemotherapy results in excellent disease control and overall survival. However, at present it remains unclear for which group of patients rituximab monotherapy is sufficient. Retrospective studies have identified risk factors including extralymphatic disease, high LDH, low albumin, and poor performance status, but these risk factors need to be validated in prospective studies.[25] In summary, rituximab has led to a dramatic improvement in outcome of EBV-LPD. However, rituximab does not restore the cellular immune response to EBV, which may be crucial for the long-term control of EBV-mediated B-cell proliferation. EBV-infected B cells may therefore increase with B-cell recovery, and EBV-LPD may recur. Although rare, the recurrence of CD20-negative lymphomas with the use of rituximab has been reported. Patients who fail to respond to chemoimmunotherapy strategies may respond to high-dose chemotherapy followed by autologous HSCT or adoptive T-cell therapies.

T-Cell Therapies

Donor T-cell infusions have been used successfully to treat EBV-LPD post-HSC transplantation but carry the inherent risk for GVHD. One strategy to prevent GHVD after T-cell infusion is the administration of polyclonal EBV-specific T cells.[26] Initially, donor-derived EBV-specific T cells were generated ex vivo by repeated stimulation with autologous LCLs. Clinical studies in HSCT recipients have shown that these cells are safe, do not cause significant GVHD, reconstitute EBV-specific cellular immunity, and are effective as prophylaxis and therapy for EBV-LPD. In SOT recipients who develop EBV-LPD, donor-derived T cells are of limited value, because the tumor almost always arises in recipient B cells, and donor T cells are unlikely to survive in the recipient's hematopoietic system. Initial studies using autologous EBV-specific T cells for the treatment or prevention of EBV-LPD after SOT have shown promising results but need further investigation.

Although donor-derived EBV-specific T cells have potent clinical activity post-HSCT, their generation using LCLs as antigen presenting cells is a lengthy process, requiring 6 weeks to establish LCLs, then at least 4 weeks for T-cell expansion, followed by 2 weeks for quality control testing. Thus, several groups have developed strategies to rapidly select or generate EBV-specific T cells. Rapid selection strategies rely on the use of HLA-peptide multimers or Streptamers, or so-called interferon (IFN)-γ capture, in which T cells that secrete IFN-γ in response to antigen stimulation are selected. While these selection procedure require no or only limited (>24 hours) ex vivo culture, they require a leukopheresis product. In addition, HLA-peptide multimer or streptamer selection require knowledge of a particular epitope and is restricted to the selection of CD8+ T cells. Our group has therefore focused on rapid expansion protocols in which virus-specific T-cell products are activated and expanded for 10 days with overlapping peptide libraries spanning the viral antigens of interest in the presence of cytokines. Resulting cell lines are polyclonal and contain CD4+ and CD8+ T cells recognizing MHC class I as well as class II restricted viral antigens. EBV-specific T cells were generated as part of multivirus-specific T-cell product, and were effective in five patients with EBV-LPD or EBV viremia. In addition, banked "off the shelf" third-party EBV-specific T cells are actively being explored for the therapy of EBV-LPD as a single or as part of a multivirus-specific T-cell product.[27] Although third-party EBV-specific T cells did not

persist long-term post infusion, they have significant anti EBV-LPD activity, supporting the development of third-party banks for the therapy of EBV-LPD in the transplant setting.

Epstein-Barr Virus-Positive Hodgkin Disease and Non-Hodgkin Lymphomas

EBV is associated with HD as well as NHLs in immunocompetent patients (see Chapters 74, 83). An increased incidence of EBV-positive diffuse large B-cell lymphomas has been seen in older adults.[28] All EBV lymphomas are associated with the virus latent cycle (Fig. 54.3).[2] The majority of immunocompetent patients with EBV-associated lymphomas are latency type II and express EBNA1, LMP1, and LMP2, except for BL, which is latency type I and only expresses EBNA1.

Hodgkin Disease

HD is a malignant neoplasm of lymphoreticular cell origin, and 40% to 50% of cases in immunocompetent individuals are associated with expression of EBV-derived antigens in malignant Hodgkin and Reed-Sternberg (HRS) cells and their variants (Fig. 54.6, B, C). EBV-positive HD is more commonly seen in young children and in less developed countries. EBV association with HD differs by histologic subtype, being highest with the mixed-cellularity subtype. Evidence linking EBV to the pathogenesis of HD includes the findings that (a) every HRS cell in an EBV-positive tumor mass carries the virus, and (b) the EBV genome is clonal, indicating that the malignant HRS cells originated from a single EBV-infected cell. In addition, LMP1, one of the EBV proteins expressed in HRS cells, activates the transcription factor nuclear factor kappa-B (NFκB), which is thought to play an important role in the HD pathogenesis. EBV-positive HD patients also differ in their antibody response to the major EBV-associated antigens in comparison with healthy controls. The overall outcome of EBV-positive and EBV-negative HD is similar; with combination chemotherapy and radiation, the prognosis is excellent for low-stage disease, and overall survival rate for advanced-stage disease is between 65% and 80% (see Chapter 75). Depending on age and histologic subtype, the presence of EBV might be associated with better survival.

Non-Hodgkin Lymphomas

NHLs expressing type II latency include diffuse large B-cell lymphoma (DLBCL), CD30+ Ki-1 anaplastic large cell lymphoma (ALCL) of B-cell type, T-cell–rich B-cell NHLs and lymphomatoid granulomatosis (see Chapter 76). The association of these lymphomas with EBV varies, ranging from 10% to 95%.

EBV-associated NK/T-cell lymphomas include extranodal NK/T-cell lymphoma (nasal type), angioimmunoblastic lymphoma, and large granular lymphocyte (LGL) leukemia/lymphoma (NK- or T-cell type). Between 30% and 100% of these lymphomas are EBV-positive, expressing a type II latency pattern. In addition, CAEBV of NK/T-cell type has been associated with fulminant forms of lymphoma, more than 95% of which are positive for EBV. The overall outcome of EBV-associated NHL depends on histologic subtype and risk factors present at diagnosis, but most are high-grade malignancies with an unfavorable prognosis using current treatment modalities, which are described in detail in Chapters 79 to 85.

Adoptive Immunotherapy for Epstein-Barr Virus-Positive Hodgkin Disease and Non-Hodgkin Lymphomas in Immunocompetent Individuals

In contrast to EBV-LPD only a limited number of EBV-derived antigens (EBNA1, LMP1, and LMP2) are present in EBV-positive HD and NHL. Initial studies with patient-derived, LCL-generated

EBV-specific T cells demonstrated their safety, but infused T cells had limited antitumor activity against HD and NHL in comparison to EBV-LPD. This lack of efficacy could be due in part to immunosuppressive factors secreted by lymphoma cells or may simply be quantitative in that the method used for EBV-specific T-cell generation produces T-cell lines that are dominated by clones reactive to viral proteins not expressed in latency type II lymphoma. To improve T-cell efficacy methods to expand T-cell specific for the EBV proteins LMP1 and LMP2 expressed in latency type II lymphoma and to genetically modify the expanded T cells to render them resistant against inhibitory cytokines have been developed. We conducted two clinical studies with LMP1/2 (LMP)-specific T cells in patients with EBV-positive HD and NHL.[29] The initial trial targeted LMP2 alone and the subsequent LMP1 and LMP2. On both trials combined, 50 patients received LMP-specific T cells. Of 29 patients who received these cells as adjuvant therapy, 28 remained in remission for a median of 3.1 years. Thirteen out of 21 patients infused with active disease had objective clinical responses with 11 patients being complete. While LMP-specific T cells had clinical activity, generation required not only LCLs but also recombinant adenovirus vectors encoding LMP1 and LMP2. After having developed an LMP-specific T-cell production process that is devoid of LCLs and recombinant adenovirus vectors, these cells are currently being tested in clinical studies. To evaluate if rendering LMP-specific T cells resistant to the immunosuppressive lymphoma environment enhances their antitumor activity, we focused on targeting TGF-β, which promotes tumor growth, limits T-cell effector function, and actives inhibitory, regulatory T cells. These detrimental effects of TGF-β can be overcome by modifying T cells to express a dominant negative TGF-β receptor (DNR), which lacks its intracellular signaling domain. DNR expression blocks TGF-β signaling and restores T-cell effector function in the presence of TGF-β. Initial testing in humans indicate that DNR-modified LMP-specific T cells benefit patients who failed therapy with unmodified cells. For a detailed discussion on cell therapy with conventional or genetically modified T cells targeting non-viral antigens for hematologic malignancies see Chapters 98 and 100. In addition to genetically modifying T cells to enhance their antitumor activity, combining the adoptive transfer of T cells with monoclonal antibodies that block immune checkpoints, such as PD-1/PD-L1, hold the promise to enhance their antitumor activity. This approach has not been tested in humans; however, clinical studies are currently being planned.

Epstein-Barr Virus-Associated Non-Hodgkin Lymphoma in HIV Patients

Patients infected with HIV are at high risk to develop NHL. The incidence increases with age, and the male-to-female ratio is approximately 2:1. Depending on certain histologic features, the EBV association ranges from 30% in systemic HIV-related BL (HIV-BL) to 70% to 80% in HIV-related immunoblastic lymphoma (HIV-IBL), and virtually all cases of primary central nervous system lymphoma (PCNSL) are EBV-positive. In biopsies of EBV-associated HIV-NHL, there is considerable variation in the number of EBV-positive cells, and the pattern of EBV latent gene expression varies among tumor types as in immunocompetent individuals (Fig. 54.6, E, F). In HIV-infected patients, the development of EBV-associated HIV-NHL is preceded by a loss of functional EBV-specific T cells, suggesting that strategies to boost the endogenous EBV-specific T-cell response might prevent lymphomas. Restoring CD4+ T-cell counts in patients with HIV with highly active antiretroviral therapy (HAART) has decreased the incidence of PCNSL and HIV-NHL. The clinical experience with T-cell therapy for EBV-associated HIV-NHL is limited.

Burkitt Lymphoma

BL is a high-grade malignant small noncleaved B-cell lymphoma. Histology usually reveals a "starry-sky" pattern resulting from numerous benign macrophages that have ingested apoptotic tumor cells (Fig. 54.7A–C). Although almost all endemic BLs in equatorial Africa are associated with EBV, the virus has been implicated less often in sporadic cases, and in the United States only 20% of BL are EBV positive. In developing countries, an intermediate type of BL has been described, both in its clinical presentation and association with EBV, which varies from 25% to 80%. As with NPC and HD, there is strong circumstantial evidence linking EBV to BL. The EBV genome is clonal as in other EBV-associated malignancies. The majority of BLs carry a translocation between the long arm of chromosome 8, the site of the MYCC oncogene (8q24), and the Ig heavy chain region on chromosome 14, t(8;14). Although the t(8;14) translocation is seen in endemic as well as sporadic BLs, the exact location of the chromosomal breakpoints on chromosome 8 and 14 differ. Other chromosomal translocations seen in BLs are between MYCC and the κ-light chain locus on chromosome 2, t(2;8), or the λ-light chain locus on chromosome 22, t(8;22).

Current treatment strategies rely on intensive chemotherapy, and overall survival depends on extent of disease at presentation, being 90% to 100% for local and 60% to 70% for advanced disease. The prospect for the development of an EBV-specific immunotherapy for BLs is problematic because lymphoma cells evade the immune system by downregulating the expression of EBV latency antigens, cell adhesion molecules, and MHC class I molecules. EBNA1, the only EBV protein expressed in BL, autoregulates its own translation and inhibits HLA class I presentation because of an internal glycine-alanine repeat region. However, the characterization of EBNA1-specific CD4+ T cells, as well as rare CD8+ T cells that can recognize BL through EBNA1, has provided impetus to explore the role of CD4+ T cells in the control and therapy of BL. In addition, EBNA1-specific CD4+ T cells had potent antitumor activity in a murine model of BL. As discussed in the EBV-LPD section, induction of the lytic EBV cycle is another attractive EBV-targeted approach for BL.

Nasopharyngeal Carcinoma

NPC arises from the epithelial cells of the nasopharynx. The WHO classifies NPC into keratinizing squamous cell carcinoma (type 1), nonkeratinizing carcinoma (type 2), and undifferentiated carcinoma (type 3, most common). Type 2 and 3 carcinomas are associated with EBV (Fig. 54.7D, E); however, environmental and genetic factors play an important role in oncogenesis, because the incidence of NPC varies 50- to 100-fold from Southern China to Western countries. EBV was initially linked to NPC by the observation that patients had elevated levels of VCA-IgG, VCA-IgA, and EA-IgG antibodies. Further studies showed that EBV-DNA is present in every tumor cell of type 2 and 3 carcinomas with remarkable consistency. As in HD, the EBV episome in an individual tumor is clonal.

EBV antibody responses have been used to follow tumor burden in patients with NPC; in addition, VCA-IgA antibodies and antibodies against EBV DNase are predictive for NPC in high-risk populations. More recently, detection of EBV-DNA in serum by different PCR methods has shown to be useful for the diagnosis, prognosis, and monitoring of patients with NPC. Most patients with NPC are treated with radiation. Other modalities such as surgery, chemotherapy, and combined approaches may be appropriate in selected circumstances, but a detailed discussion is beyond the scope of this chapter. In NPC, as for EBV-positive lymphomas, only a limited number of EBV latent antigens are expressed. Three therapeutic vaccine studies targeting LMP2, LMP1 and LMP2, or EBNA1 and LMP2 have been conducted, and the results of these trials were discussed in the earlier section EBV Vaccine Development.

The adoptive transfer of autologous EBV-specific T cells is being actively explored. Several groups have reported that the infusion of T cells is safe and has resulted in clinical responses, especially in patients with locoregional disease. In addition, EBV-specific T cells, given as adjuvant after chemotherapy, resulted in a significant increase in 3-year overall survival in comparison to historical controls, who only received chemotherapy.[30] A pivotal, randomized clinical study to validate these findings is in progress.

FUTURE DIRECTIONS

Since its discovery in 1964, EBV has been linked to a heterogeneous group of diseases. EBV was the first human virus implicated in oncogenesis, and the biology of the virus has been studied extensively on a cellular and molecular level. Over the last two decades immunotherapeutic approaches targeting EBV have been developed for EBV-associated malignancies and later phase clinical studies are currently in progress. Although adoptive transfer of T cells so far has been more successful than vaccines, novel, more potent vaccines have been developed that await testing in humans. Combinatorial therapies, for example combining EBV-targeted immunotherapy with antibodies that block immune checkpoints, are starting to be evaluated in clinical studies and hold the promise to improve outcomes. In the next 5 years, rationally designed small molecule inhibitors will be tested for the first time in humans that block the DNA binding site of EBNA-1 with the potential to eradicate EBV. Lastly, whole exome sequencing will continue to identify genes that are associated with life-threatening complications of EBV infections, providing clues into their pathogenesis and novel therapeutic interventions.

REFERENCES

1. Lieberman PM: Epstein-Barr virus turns 50. *Science* 343:1323, 2014.
2. Longnecker RM, Kieff E, Cohen JI: Epstein-Barr virus. In Knipe DM, Howley PM, editors: *Fields virology*, ed 6, Philadelphia, 2013, Lippincott Williams & Wilkins, pp 1898–1959.
3. Evens AM, David KA, Helenowski I, et al: Multicenter analysis of 80 solid organ transplantation recipients with post-transplantation lymphoproliferative disease: outcomes and prognostic factors in the modern era. *J Clin Oncol* 28:1038–1046, 2010.
4. Heslop HE, Slobod KS, Pule MA, et al: Long-term outcome of EBV-specific T-cell infusions to prevent or treat EBV-related lymphoproliferative disease in transplant recipients. *Blood* 115:925–935, 2010.
5. Tierney RJ, Shannon-Lowe CD, Fitzsimmons L, et al: Unexpected patterns of Epstein-Barr virus transcription revealed by a high throughput PCR array for absolute quantification of viral mRNA. *Virology* 474:117–130, 2015.
6. Hu L, Lin Z, Wu Y, et al: Comprehensive profiling of EBV gene expression in nasopharyngeal carcinoma through paired-end transcriptome sequencing. *Front Med* 10:61–75, 2016.
7. Taylor GS, Long HM, Brooks JM, et al: The immunology of Epstein-Barr virus-induced disease. *Annu Rev Immunol* 33:787–821, 2015.
8. Cohen JI: Epstein-barr virus vaccines. *Clin Translat Immunol* 4:e32, 2015.
9. Cohen JI: Primary immunodeficiencies associated with EBV disease. *Curr Top Microbiol Immunol* 390:241–265, 2015.
10. Allen CE, McClain KL: Pathophysiology and epidemiology of hemophagocytic lymphohistiocytosis. *Hematology Am Soc Hematol Educ Program* 2015:177–182, 2015.
11. Jordan MB, Allen CE, Weitzman S, et al: How I treat hemophagocytic lymphohistiocytosis. *Blood* 118:4041–4052, 2011.
12. Marsh RA, Vaughn G, Kim MO, et al: Reduced-intensity conditioning significantly improves survival of patients with hemophagocytic lymphohistiocytosis undergoing allogeneic hematopoietic cell transplantation. *Blood* 116:5824–5831, 2010.
13. Imashuku S: Treatment of Epstein-Barr virus-related hemophagocytic lymphohistiocytosis (EBV-HLH); update 2010. *J Pediatr Hematol Oncol* 33:35–39, 2011.
14. Chellapandian D, Das R, Zelley K, et al: Treatment of Epstein Barr virus-induced haemophagocytic lymphohistiocytosis with rituximab-containing chemo-immunotherapeutic regimens. *Br J Haematol* 162:376–382, 2013.
15. Filipovich AH, Zhang K, Snow AL, et al: X-linked lymphoproliferative syndromes: brothers or distant cousins? *Blood* 116:3398–3408, 2010.
16. Cohen JI, Kimura H, Nakamura S, et al: Epstein-Barr virus-associated lymphoproliferative disease in non-immunocompromised hosts: a status report and summary of an international meeting, 8–9 September 2008. *Ann Oncol* 20:1472–1482, 2009.
17. Ohshima K, Kimura H, Yoshino T, et al: Proposed categorization of pathological states of EBV-associated T/natural killer-cell lymphoproliferative disorder (LPD) in children and young adults: overlap with chronic active EBV infection and infantile fulminant EBV T-LPD. *Pathol Int* 58:209–217, 2008.
18. Kawa K, Sawada A, Sato M, et al: Excellent outcome of allogeneic hematopoietic SCT with reduced-intensity conditioning for the treatment of chronic active EBV infection. *Bone Marrow Transplant* 46:77–83, 2011.
19. Fernandez-Menendez S, Fernandez-Moran M, Fernandez-Vega I, et al: Epstein-Barr virus and multiple sclerosis. From evidence to therapeutic strategies. *J Neurol Sci* 361:213–219, 2016.
20. Gottschalk S, Rooney CM, Heslop HE: Post-transplant lymphoproliferative disorders. *Annu Rev Med* 56:29–44, 2005.
21. Bollard CM, Heslop HE: T cells for viral infections after allogeneic hematopoietic stem cell transplant. *Blood* 127(26):3331–3340, 2016.
22. Weinstock DM, Ambrossi GG, Brennan C, et al: Preemptive diagnosis and treatment of Epstein-Barr virus-associated post transplant lymphoproliferative disorder after hematopoietic stem cell transplant: an approach in development. *Bone Marrow Transplant* 37:539–546, 2006.
23. Gianti E, Messick TE, Lieberman PM, et al: Computational analysis of EBNA1 "druggability" suggests novel insights for Epstein-Barr virus inhibitor design. *J Comput Aided Mol Des* 30:285–303, 2016.
24. Styczynski J, Einsele H, Gil L, et al: Outcome of treatment of Epstein-Barr virus-related post-transplant lymphoproliferative disorder in hematopoietic stem cell recipients: a comprehensive review of reported cases. *Transpl Infect Dis* 11:383–392, 2009.
25. Knight JS, Tsodikov A, Cibrik DM, et al: Lymphoma after solid organ transplantation: risk, response to therapy, and survival at a transplantation center. *J Clin Oncol* 27:3354–3362, 2009.
26. Gottschalk S, Rooney CM: Adoptive T-Cell Immunotherapy. *Curr Top Microbiol Immunol* 391:427–454, 2015.
27. Papadopoulou A, Gerdemann U, Katari UL, et al: Activity of broad-spectrum T cells as treatment for AdV, EBV, CMV, BKV, and HHV6 infections after HSCT. *Sci Transl Med* 6:242ra83, 2014.
28. Dojcinov SD, Venkataraman G, Pittaluga S, et al: Age-related EBV-associated lymphoproliferative disorders in the Western population: a spectrum of reactive lymphoid hyperplasia and lymphoma. *Blood* 117:4726–4735, 2011.
29. Bollard CM, Gottschalk S, Torrano V, et al: Sustained complete responses in patients with lymphoma receiving autologous cytotoxic T lymphocytes targeting Epstein-Barr virus latent membrane proteins. *J Clin Oncol* 32:798–808, 2014.
30. Chia WK, Teo M, Wang WW, et al: Adoptive T-cell transfer and chemotherapy in the first-line treatment of metastatic and/or locally recurrent nasopharyngeal carcinoma. *Mol Ther* 22:132–139, 2014.

PART VII

HEMATOLOGIC MALIGNANCIES

PART

VII

HEMATOLOGIC MALIGNANCIES

PROGRESS IN THE CLASSIFICATION OF HEMATOPOIETIC AND LYMPHOID NEOPLASMS: CLINICAL IMPLICATIONS

Mohamed E. Salama and Ronald Hoffman

Defining and classifying tumors of the hematopoietic and lymphoid tissue accurately is a core requirement for providing optimal treatment to patients with hematologic malignancies. Precise definitions and terminologies are prerequisites for the precise classification of hematologic malignancies. A reproducible classification that is based on consensus definitions and terminologies is fundamentally essential for proper medical practice and the advancement of medical knowledge. Generally, such classifications should be based upon clinically distinct, nonoverlapping disease entities that can be grouped together based on shared distinguishable clinical features, as well as phenotypic and molecular markers which allow for reproducible laboratory testing, clinical outcomes, and responses to therapeutic agents. Traditionally, preliminary attempts at disease classification are initiated by the personal experience of experts, and then evolve after many years or even decades of controversy and exhaustive debate. Subsequently, classification schemes change when new scientific discoveries are validated.

Following many years of controversy, a collaborative project of members of the European Association for Haematopathology and the Society for Hematopathology, along with advice from clinical hematologists and oncologists, resulted in the World Health Organization (WHO) Classification of Tumours of Haematopoietic and Lymphoid Tissues.[1,2] This WHO classification, which is the first true worldwide consensus classification of hematologic malignancies, is based on the principles initially defined in the "Revised European-American Classification of Lymphoid Neoplasms" (REAL) from the International Lymphoma Study Group (ILSG).[3] The most recent WHO classification (4th edition) was formulated in a series of meetings by two clinically advisory committees: one for myeloid neoplasms and other acute leukemias, and one for lymphoid neoplasms.[4] The current WHO classification, which addresses new developments related to disease definitions, nomenclature, grading, and clinical relevance, provides the basis for an approach to hematopoietic and lymphoid neoplasm classification that employs morphology, immune phenotype, genetic features, and clinical features to define diseases.[4] The relative importance of each of these components varies among diseases and is dependent on the current state of knowledge. Morphologic assessment remains a key element of the diagnostic evaluation and classification of hematologic malignancies, as many diseases have characteristic diagnostic features. Morphologic evaluation also remains a decisive step for prioritization of ancillary testing choices that may include phenotyping, as well as molecular or genetic testing. Immunophenotypic studies such as flow cytometry and immunohistochemistry are used routinely to identify the lineage of the benign or malignant process, and often are necessary to reach a definitive diagnosis. In several lymphoid and myeloid neoplasms a specific diagnosis can be facilitated by genetic or molecular abnormalities (e.g., *CCND1* in suspected mantle cell lymphoma [MCL] or *BCR/ABL* for chronic myeloid leukemia [CML]). In addition, some abnormalities can serve as prognostic markers in several diseases (e.g., *TP53*). However, many entities still lack defining genetic or molecular abnormalities.

In some conditions rendering an accurate diagnosis requires knowledge of clinical features such as a patient's age and previous therapy, as well as the anatomic site and/or extent of disease. Although most of the disease entities described in the WHO classification

represent distinct entities, some categories are not as clearly defined and are regarded as provisional entities. In addition, borderline categories have been created for cases that do not clearly fit into one category; thus well-defined categories can remain homogeneous while borderline cases can be further studied and characterized. Furthermore, the WHO classification stratifies hematologic neoplasms according to lineage into three main groups: myeloid, lymphoid, and histiocytic/dendritic cells. In this chapter we provide a summary of neoplasms in these three groups, emphasizing changes that have had an effect on practice guidelines.

PROGRESS IN THE DIAGNOSIS AND CLASSIFICATION OF MYELOID NEOPLASMS

Clinical Implications

The myeloid neoplasms are a heterogeneous group of diseases. In general terms, they are clonal hematopoietic malignancies that can arise in or affect a single myeloid lineage (e.g., monocytic). Alternatively, they can be derived from a pluripotent progenitor cell and can affect multiple or even all myeloid cell types (erythroid, megakaryocytic, monocytic, neutrophilic, basophilic, eosinophilic, and mast cells). The myeloid neoplasms include chronic and acute diseases, along with diseases that evolve from an indolent process to a more aggressive state. As such, they can manifest as proliferative disorders, mostly involving primary mature hematopoietic elements; they can predominately affect immature or blastic cells; or sometimes they can be a combination of these two manifestations. The diseases can result in excess production of blood cells, or they can proliferate in the bone marrow (BM) and exhibit ineffective hematopoiesis, resulting in peripheral cytopenias. Because the diseases range from indolent to acute, they exhibit a wide variation in prognosis. Some disorders are fairly indolent and require only supportive care and transfusional support; others slowly progress but have no successful treatment option. Acute and life-threatening disorders are often curable, even within days or weeks after presentation, if appropriately managed. Accurate, timely diagnosis, and correct classification can have a tremendous impact on outcome.

The diagnosis of the myeloid neoplasms typically requires a multifaceted team approach that relies on cooperation among the clinician, laboratory personnel, and a skilled pathologist. The precise diagnosis requires compiling accurate historical data, clinical information, general laboratory findings, and carefully interpreted observations from the peripheral blood smear, bone core biopsy, and aspirate merged with information from immunophenotyping, cytogenetic analysis, and molecular studies (Table 55.1). Although in some cases a diagnosis can be made with a quick examination of the blood smear, with a single molecular test, or with a simple immunophenotype, in general, careful assessment of the total clinical picture gives the most accurate and clinically relevant diagnosis. Future routine diagnostic modalities may include next-generation sequencing, single-nucleotide polymorphism array karyotyping, gene expression arrays, and genome-wide epigenetic studies.

The myeloid neoplasms are grouped as different categories of diseases. These categories seem to be changing constantly, both in

TABLE 55.1	Components in the Routine Clinical Evaluation of Myeloid Diseases

Current

- Accurate clinical history, including family history and physical examination findings
- General laboratory findings, including CBC, and other specific tests (e.g., EPO) when appropriate
- Evaluation of well-prepared and stained peripheral blood smear with 200 cell differential count
- Review of BM aspirate, including iron stain, and 500 cell differential count
- Evaluation of H&E sections of BM biopsy of sufficient length and reticulin stain
- Phenotyping studies, including cytochemical reactions (nonspecific and specific esterase reactions and myeloperoxidase) and flow cytometric analysis of peripheral blood or BM for phenotype of blasts or other cells when appropriate
- Cytogenetic analysis, including karyotype, and FISH for specific abnormalities when appropriate
- Single-nucleotide polymorphism array karyotyping
- Genetic analysis for particular genetic rearrangements or mutations, including gene sequencing when appropriate
- Next-generation sequencing

Potential Future Clinical Studies

- Gene expression arrays
- Genome-wide epigenetic studies

BM, Bone marrow; CBC, complete blood count; EPO, erythropoietin; FISH, fluorescence in situ hybridization; H&E, hematoxylin and eosin.

TABLE 55.2	WHO Classification of Myeloid Neoplasms

The MPNs, including the myeloid and lymphoid neoplasms with eosinophilia and abnormalities of PDGFRA, PDGFRB, and FGFRA
The AML
The MDS
The MDS/MPN ("overlap") syndromes

AML, Acute myelogenous leukemia; MDS, myelodysplastic syndromes; MPN, myeloproliferative neoplasm.

TABLE 55.3	Tyrosine Kinase Involvement in Myeloproliferative Neoplasms	
Disease	**Tyrosine Kinase Involvement**
Chronic myeloid leukemia, BCR-ABL1+	ABL1 (100%)
Myeloid and lymphoid neoplasms with eosinophilia TK abnormalities	PDGFRA, PDGFRB, or FGFRA
Polycythemia vera	JAK2 V617F (≈95%), JAK exon 12 (≈4%)
Primary myelofibrosis	JAK2 V6174 (≈50%), MPL W515 K/L (5–9%), CALR (35%)
Essential thrombocythemia	JAK2 V617F (≈50%), MPL W515 K/L (≈1%), CALR (35%)
Chronic neutrophilic leukemia	CSF3R (83–90%)
Chronic eosinophilic leukemia, not otherwise specified	—
Mastocytosis	KIT D816V (≈95%)
MPN, unclassified	—

MPN, Myeloproliferative neoplasm; TK, tyrosine kinase.

name and in the components of the disorders. However, refinements have led to an increased understanding of the clinical, pathologic, and genetic basis of the diseases and ultimately serve, or at least strive to, improve diagnosis, treatment and outcome. The current classification of myeloid neoplasms include the categories of myeloproliferative neoplasms (MPNs), acute myeloid leukemias (AMLs), myelodysplastic syndromes (MDS), and MDS/MPNs, which is a category with features that are intermediate between MDS and MPN (Table 55.2). This generally accepted classification system was derived from a number of earlier classification systems,[5] and represents the working system of WHO as of 2008.[4,6] The recent proposal to update the 2008 classification is based on the newer information from molecular testing modalities that further impact the classification and categorization of these neoplasms.[7]

The Myeloproliferative Neoplasms

The MPNs, formerly referred to as *myeloproliferative disorders* (MPDs), are a group of clonal multipotential hematopoietic stem cell disorders that have a proliferative nature, presenting frequently with hypercellular BMs, and an elevation of one or more myeloid cell types in the blood. The MPNs are insidious in onset and chronic in course but have a variable tendency to terminate in BM failure or acute leukemia.[8] The MPNs include CML (Table 55.3), which illustrates how the elucidation of pathways involved in the molecular pathogenesis (i.e., dysregulation of *ABL1* tyrosine kinase [TK] signaling) can

successfully lead to the rational targeted therapy (i.e., imatinib and other TK inhibitors).[9]

The MPNs also include *BCR-ABL1*–negative entities, essential thrombocythemia (ET), polycythemia vera (PV), and primary myelofibrosis (MF) (see Chapters 68–70). These MPNs share common features including multipotential hematopoietic stem cell origin, clonal proliferation, and chronic nature. Although they seem to be distinctive, they can present a diagnostic challenge, and they can have subtle and overlapping presentations. Recent discoveries in the underlying molecular pathology of these entities have demonstrated that, similar to CML and eosinophilic disorders, they too share TK signaling dysregulation, at least to some degree. This is attributable to an associated mutation in the TK, *JAK2* (*JAK2* V617F), which is present in about 50 to 95% of cases of Ph-negative MPNs. Variants of *JAK2* mutations involving exon 12 are also observed in 2% to 3% of PV patients. This association has led to significant revisions in the 2008 WHO criteria for diagnosis, but it also has raised questions as to how a single mutation can be associated with such heterogeneous phenotypic characteristics. Proposed revisions in 2016 WHO classifications for the diagnosis of the Ph-negative MPNs include suggested modifications of lower hemoglobin thresholds for PV. BM biopsy results and the presence of *JAK2* mutations will represent major criteria. A subnormal erythropoietin level will become a minor criterion, and the endogenous erythroid colony assay will no longer be included in the next revision of the WHO diagnostic criteria for MPNs.[10] These changes are intended to capture patients with subtle presentations, such as those with masked PV. Experts also have recommended inclusion of mutations in calreticulin and the thrombopoietin receptor, MPL, which is identified in 20% to 30% of ET and MF cases, and the colony-stimulating factor 3 receptor mutations in the next revision.[10–12]

JAK2 V617F inhibitors are among several agents under investigation for use in patients with MPNs. In 2011 the US Food and Drug Administration (FDA) approved ruxolitinib for the treatment of patients with intermediate or high-risk MF. Subsequently, the FDA also designated ruxolitinib as an orphan product, as it demonstrated potentially significant improvement in safety and efficacy over other available therapies for PV. A number of novel agents that target various pathways are currently being investigated and will be further discussed in detail later (see Chapters 68–70).

Chronic neutrophilic leukemia (CNL) and mast cell disease are currently included in the category of MPNs. CNL is now better defined with the integration of *CSF3R* mutation as a diagnostic tool, and is distinct from atypical CML.[13]

Mast cell disease is yet another disease related to abnormal TK signaling, in this case the *KIT* gene.[14] Its classification system generally considers systemic mastocytosis and cutaneous mastocytosis as main entities but also includes a mast cell proliferation associated with clonal nonmast cell hematopoietic malignancies; this can be another myeloid malignancy or, less commonly, a lymphoid malignancy. With the advances of comprehensive mutational profiling, it is proposed that additional mutations in *SRSF2, ASXL1* and/or *RUNX1* identify a high-risk group of patients with *KIT* D816V⁺ advanced systemic mastocytosis.[15] A more recently improved understanding of the cellular and molecular basis of eosinophilic disorders has translated into more biologically oriented classification schemes that carry therapeutic implications. Thus in 2008 the WHO established a semimolecular classification scheme of separately listed disease subgroups including "myeloid and lymphoid neoplasms with eosinophilia and abnormalities of platelet-derived growth factor receptors (PDGFRA, PDGFRB), or fibroblast growth factor receptor 1(FGFR1)", chronic eosinophilic leukemia (CEL), not otherwise specified (NOS), lymphocyte-variant hypereosinophilia, and idiopathic hypereosinophilic syndrome (see Chapter 71). Although quite uncommon, these are noteworthy because, similar to CML, they have also been found to be caused by dysregulation of TK signaling (caused by mutations in *PDGFRA, PDGFRB*, or *FGFRA*) and at least partially successfully treated with TK inhibitors.[16]

It is important to emphasize that diagnosis of the MPNs does not rest solely with the routine microscopic examination. The diagnostic work-up is more far-reaching and must include reviewing the clinical history and pertinent physical findings, as well as obtaining and assessing laboratory values, including recent complete blood cell counts. Examination of a well-prepared peripheral blood smear and both BM aspirate and biopsy specimens are still crucial. However, ancillary studies, such as cytogenetic and molecular analysis, as well as other more specific laboratory evaluations, are just as important in formulating the correct diagnosis, and in particular, in distinguishing MPNs from reactive myeloid proliferations. This is particularly true, for example, regarding the *JAK2* V617F or other driver mutations, and the impact not only on the diagnosis but also on the prognostication of MPNs.

The Acute Myeloid Leukemias

The historical and emerging classifications systems for AML dramatically illustrate the marked heterogeneity of these diseases. Despite this heterogeneity, however, to date a major breakthrough has not been made in the development of specific initial treatment for AML as an entity apart from acute promyelocytic leukemia. However, to a large extent this concept is changing as newer agents targeting molecularly or genetically defined AML have become available (e.g., FMS-like tyrosine kinase-3 [FLT3] inhibitors for FLT3-mutated cases).[17,18] It is anticipated that the gap between the growing number of unique or genetically defined acute leukemia types and the somewhat limited treatment options may begin to close.

The French–American–British (FAB) classification of AML, introduced in 1976 with its subsequent revision in 1985, provided the first real framework for classifying the AMLs. It also provided fairly reproducible definitions of diseases. The classification was mainly based on morphologic and cytochemical features of the leukemic blasts in the BM. In general, the FAB scheme required that 30% of the BM-nucleated elements be blasts; then it further defined AML subtypes based on the presence of maturation in the granulocytic series, the presence of a monocytic component, and the presence of an erythroid component. Later, as immunophenotyping allowed for improved identification of myeloid precursors, acute megakaryoblastic leukemia and AML with minimal differentiation were added. The types of AML noted in the revised FAB scheme included one with minimal differentiation (MO), one without maturation (M1), one with maturation (M2), and acute promyelocytic leukemia (M3). Also included were a type with combined monocytic and myeloid (neutrophilic) components (M4), a pure monocytic or monoblastic

type (M5A, M5B), a type with a prominent erythroid component (M6), and a megakaryoblastic type (M7) (Table 55.4).

FAB classification provided a framework and defined criteria for different types of acute leukemia. However, leukemia-associated genetic changes, first recognized in the 1980s, seemed to provide more important prognostic information and did not always correlate well with the FAB-defined entities. As the cytogenetic abnormalities became more widely appreciated and their prognostic implications better understood, classification schemes based solely on the "favorable", "intermediate", and "adverse" prognostic cytogenetic findings were introduced and used along with or as an alternative to the FAB scheme (Table 55.4).

The AML WHO classification published in 2001 provided a different strategy from that used by the FAB in two important ways: it redefined AML as requiring only 20% blasts in the BM or blood, and it emphasized the importance of the associated cytogenetic abnormalities. The change in blast percentage came from the recognition that patients with 20% to 30% blasts, who previously were classified as having MDS (refractory anemia with excess of blasts in transformation [RAEB-T] in the FAB MDS classification), often had outcomes similar to those with AML and frequently required treatment as if they had been diagnosed with AML. Furthermore, the inclusion of cytogenetics recognized the important prognostic information associated with these abnormalities, as well as the fact that cytogenetics could point to the underlying molecular pathogenesis. As we learned from our experience with CML, this was critical in developing new drugs and treatment strategies. However, the WHO classification recognized that not all acute leukemias could be defined by cytogenetic abnormalities and that some needed to be defined either clinically or still based on morphologic findings. In this regard, the 2001 classification recognized four major subclasses of AML: AML with recurring cytogenetic abnormalities; therapy-related AML (subclassified further as those with etoposide treatment and those with a history of cytotoxic drug therapy or radiation); AML with multilineage dysplasia; and cases that did not fit into the other subclasses that are referred to as AML not otherwise categorized (Table 55.4).

A 2008 revision of the 2001 classification scheme emphasized risk-based stratification and made a number of changes (Table 55.4).[4] In particular, it expanded the cytogenetic abnormality-associated cases to those with some less common translocations. It added provisional entities defined by mutations often occurring in cytogenetically normal cases, namely those with *NPM1* and *CEBPA* mutations. It combined the different types of therapy-related MDS/AML and renamed this category *therapy-related myeloid neoplasm* (t-MN). It also redefined the dysplasia-associated cases by allowing the cases to be identified by history (of previous MDS), morphology (with multilineage dysplasia), or by cytogenetics (with defined chromosomal changes associated with dysplasia). Additional categories were also added, including AML associated with Down syndrome, acute panmyelosis with MF, granulocytic sarcoma, and blastic plasmacytoid dendritic cell tumor. The 2008 classification eventually defined more than 25 different types of AML. The advent of newer technologies, such as single-nucleotide polymorphism array karyotyping and next-generation sequencing, facilitated the recognition of several relevant driver mutations.[19] Molecular analysis for leukemic driver mutations, particularly in the cytogenetically normal AML subgroup (40% to 50% of AML patients), has been incorporated into routine clinical practice to assess disease progression and prognosis. Important mutations involve *FLT3, NPM1, KIT, CEBPα, TET2, DNMT3A,* and *IDH1.* Although the relevance of many of these mutations to prognosis is defined, some are still debated and their coexisting consequences are yet to be determined.

With the development of more sensitive analysis, the subclassification of AML patients has become more detailed. The proposed revisions to AML classification in 2016 remain largely unchanged for the entities of AML and NOS, with the exception of including the erythroid/myeloid subtype of acute erythroid leukemia with MDS. The 2016 revisions are expected to include recognition of new cytogenetic subgroups such as AML with BCR-ABL and

TABLE 55.4 Classification Schemes for the Acute Myelogenous Leukemias

French–American–British (FAB, 1985)

- **M0:** AML with minimal differentiation
- **M1:** AML without maturation
- **M2:** AML with maturation
- **M3:** APL
- **M3v:** microgranular variant
- **M4:** AMML
- **M4eo:** AMML with abnormal eosinophils
- **M5A:** acute monoblastic leukemia
- **M5B:** acute monocytic Leukemia
- **M6:** erythroleukemia
- **M7:** acute megakaryoblastic leukemia

Cytogenetic

- **Favorable**
  - t(8;21)
  - inv(16)/t(16;16)
  - t(15;17)
- **Intermediate**
  - Normal
  - +8
  - t(v;11q23)
  - del(7q)
  - +21
  - +22
  - Other
- **Adverse**
  - del(5q)
  - −5
  - −7
  - Complex
  - abn (3q)

WHO (2001)

- **Genetic**
  - t(8;21)
  - t(inv16)/t(16;16)
  - t(15;17)
  - t(v;11q23)
- **AML with dysplasia therapy related AML**
  - Etoposide
  - Cytotoxic or radiation
- **Not otherwise specified**
  - With minimal differentiation
  - Without maturation
  - With maturation
  - Myelomonocytic leukemia
  - Monoblastic leukemia
  - Monocytic leukemia
  - Erythroleukemia
  - Erythroid myeloid type
  - Pure erythroid
  - Megakaryoblastic

WHO (2008)

- **With recurrent genetic abnormalities**
  - With t(8;21)(q22;q22)
  - With inv(16)/t(16;16)(p13.1;q22)
  - With t(15;17)(q22;q12)
  - With t(9;11)(p22;q23)
  - With t(6;9)(p23;q34)
  - With inv(3)/t(3;3)(q21;q26.2)
  - With t(1;22)(p13;q13)
  - With mutated NPM1 (provisional)
  - With mutated CEBPA (provisional)
- **With myelodysplasia related changes**
  - Previous history of MDS
  - Multilineage dysplasia
  - MDS-related cytogenetic abnormalities
- **Therapy-related myeloid neoplasms**
  - t-AML/t-MDS (t-MN)
- **Not otherwise specified**
  - With minimal differentiation
  - Without maturation
  - With maturation
  - Myelomonocytic leukemia
  - Monoblastic leukemia
  - Monocytic leukemia
  - Erythroleukemia
  - Erythroid myeloid type
  - Pure erythroid
  - Acute megakaryoblastic leukemia
  - Acute basophilic leukemia
  - Acute panmyelosis with myelofibrosis
- **Myeloid sarcoma**
- **Myeloid leukemia associated with Down syndrome**
- **Blastic plasmacytoid dendritic cell tumor**

WHO (2016)

- **With recurrent genetic abnormalities**
  - AML with t (8;21)(q22;q22.1);RUNX1-RUNX1T1
  - AML with inv(16)(p13.1q22) or t(16;16)(p13.1;q22);CBFB-MYH11
  - APL with PML-RARA
  - AML with t(9;11)(p21.3;q23.3);MLLT3-KMT2A
  - AML with t(6;9)(p23;q34.1);DEK-NUP214
  - AML with inv(3)(q21.3q26.2) or t(3;3)(q21.3;q26.2); GATA2, MECOM
  - AML (megakaryoblastic) with t(1;22)(p13.3;q13.3);RBM15-MKL1
  - Provisional entity: AML with BCR-ABL1
  - AML with mutated NPM1
  - AML with biallelic mutations of CEBPA
  - Provisional entity: AML with mutated RUNX1
- **AML with myelodysplasia-related changes**
- **Therapy-related myeloid neoplasms**
- **AML, NOS**
  - AML with minimal differentiation
  - AML without maturation
  - AML with maturation
  - Acute myelomonocytic leukemia
  - Acute monoblastic/monocytic leukemia
  - Pure erythroid leukemia
  - Acute megakaryoblastic leukemia
  - Acute basophilic leukemia
  - Acute panmyelosis with myelofibrosis
- **Myeloid sarcoma**
- **Myeloid proliferations related to Down syndrome**
  - Transient abnormal myelopoiesis (TAM)
  - Myeloid leukemia associated with Down syndrome

AML, Acute myeloid leukemia; *AMML,* acute myelomonocytic leukemia; *APL,* acute promyelocytic leukemia; *WHO,* World Health Organization.

accompanied cryptic deletions of antigen receptors, particularly immunoglobulin heavy chain (IGH) gene rearrangement; this was recently shown to be specific for de novo disease.[20,21] This update is also anticipated to include new and revised mutations subgroups. For example, AML with *RUNX1* mutations will include only de novo cases. AML with *CEBPα* will be heterozygous/double mutations (Fig. 55.1). In addition, *NPM1* and double mutations in *CEBPα* will trump multilineage dysplasia in de novo disease without MDS-related cytogenetics abnormalities other than del(9q). There will be a greater emphasis on the recognition of familial myeloid neoplasms, with an added classifications section.[19] Overall, the 2016 WHO Classification of AML will have limited changes but will recognize the importance of mutations studies without making the classification overly complex.

The Myelodysplastic Syndromes

The earliest recognition of myelodysplastic disorders as a clinical entity came with the identification of long-standing and treatment-refractory anemia as occasionally representing a preleukemic disorder (see Chapters 60 and 63). MDS patients classically present with pancytopenias and a hypercellular BM with ineffective hematopoiesis and multilineage dysplasia, with or without an increase in blast cell numbers. Although this is fairly typical, it belies the wide pathologic spectrum of MDS, which includes cases that are diagnostically challenging, and which can be difficult to distinguish on one hand from benign causes of cytopenias in older adult patients, and on the other hand from AML and other more aggressive clonal myeloid neoplasms.

The FAB group proposed the first formal classification of MDS in 1982.[5] In this classification scheme, the myelodysplastic disorders were divided into four subtypes based on increasing blast cell numbers or as chronic myelomonocytic leukemia (CMML). The four entities included refractory anemia (RA), refractory anemia with ring sideroblasts (RARS), refractory anemia with excess of blasts (RAEB), and refractory anemia with excess of blasts in transformation (RAEB-T). These entities differed mainly by the percentage of blasts seen in the

BM (Table 55.5). As noted earlier, in the FAB scheme AML was defined by the presence of 30% or more blasts in the blood or BM.

The FAB included CMML in the MDS category, although it was recognized that CMML differed in that it had a proliferative component with increased numbers of circulating monocytes. At times, leukocytosis was a predominant feature of the so-called *myeloproliferative type* of CMML, but this was considered to be a dysplastic form and was classified as a type of MDS when the white blood cell count was less than 13,000/μL.

The 2001 WHO classification of MDS resulted in significant changes to the classification of both MDS (Table 55.5) and AML (as discussed earlier). As mentioned previously, the most notable change was the reduction in the blast percentage required for a diagnosis of AML from 30% to 20%, leading to the elimination of the RAEB-T category. The 2001 classification also included a new subtype of MDS that, despite the lack of increased blasts (less than 5%), had a more aggressive course, probably owing to the presence of more pronounced multilineage dysplasia. This category was called *refractory cytopenia with multilineage dysplasia* (RCMD), and it comprised a substantial proportion of cases previously grouped in the low-grade RA and RARS categories. Although the recognition of RCMD served to deemphasize the importance of the blast percentage for prognosis, these classifications subdivided the RAEB category into two types, with 5% to 9% blasts (RAEB-1) and 10% to 19% blasts (RAEB-2), paradoxically emphasizing the prognostic significance of blast percentage in this category.

An additional significant change in the WHO 2001 MDS classification scheme included the exclusion of CMML from the MDS category, and the development of a separate nosologic group for CMML and other diseases in which there were features of both myelodysplasia and myeloproliferation at the time of diagnosis. These "overlap" disorders are mentioned briefly later.

Further refinements in the WHO classification scheme for MDS were made subsequently in 2008 (Table 55.5). These included expanding low-grade MDS from refractory anemia to refractory cytopenia with unilineage dysplasia (RCUD), thereby recognizing that the megakaryocyte or granulocyte lineage could be equally

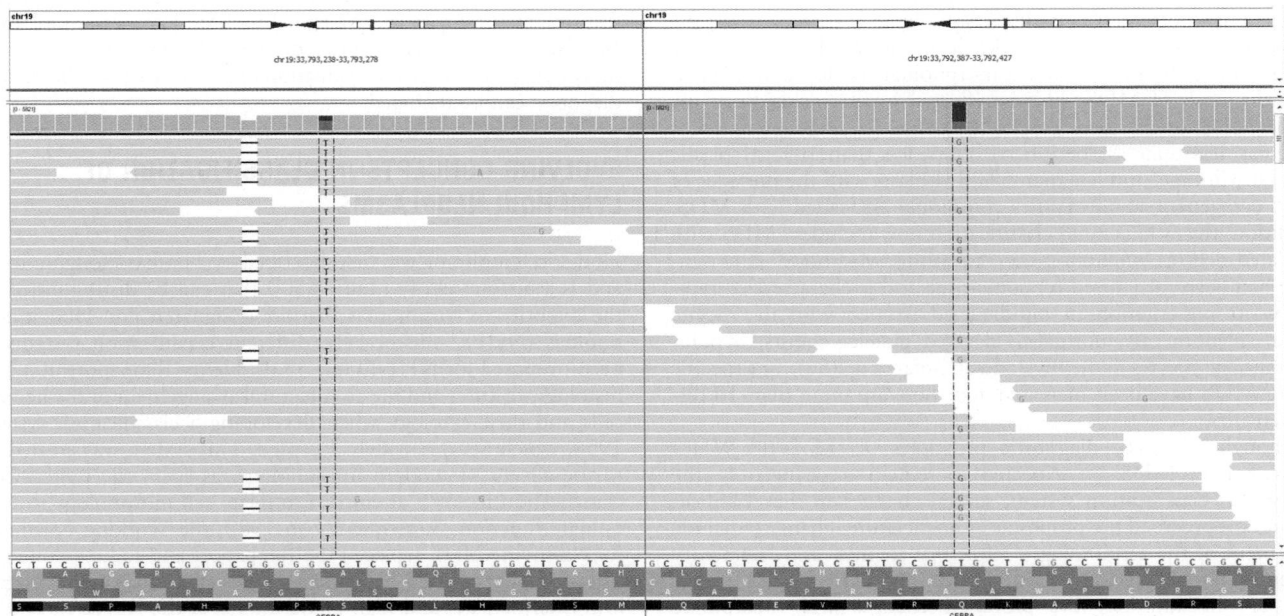

Fig. 55.1 ALIGNMENT DATA OF INTEGRATIVE GENOMICS VIEWER FOR DOUBLE *CEBPA* MUTATIONS IDENTIFIED IN AN AML PATIENT. The *left* side shows c.63_64delinsA, p.Ser21fs, the *right* side shows c.914A>C, p.Gln305Pro. The *CEBPα* N-terminal frame-shift mutation (p.Ser21fs) is predicted to disrupt the normal function of *CEBPα*. The other CEBPA mutation (c.914A>C, p.Gln305Pro) is a C-terminal missense mutation that has been reported in AML patients. Double-*CEBPα* mutations (as seen in this patient) are found in 5% of patients with AML and are associated with a favorable outcome.[44] *CEBPα*-double mutant AML patients also had a significantly better overall survival at 8 years.

TABLE 55.5		Evolving Classifications of the Myelodysplastic Syndromes (MDS)	
FAB 1982	WHO 2001	WHO 2008	WHO 2016
RA	RA	RCUD RA RN RT	MDS with single lineage dysplasia (MDS-SLD)
RARS	RARS	RARS	MDS-RS with single lineage dysplasia (MDS-RS-SLD)
	RCMD RCMD-RS	RCMD (-RS)	MDS with multilineage dysplasia (MDS-MLD) MDS-RS with multilineage dysplasia (MDS-RS-MLD)
RAEB	RAEB-1	RAEB-1	MDS with excess blasts (MDS-EB-1)
	RAEB-2	RAEB-2	MDS with excess blasts (MDS-EB2)
		MDS-U	MDS, unclassifiable (MDS-U)
		MDS with 5q-	MDS with isolated del(5q)
		RCC (provisional)	Refractory cytopenia of childhood
RAEB-T			
CMML			

AML, Acute myeloid leukemia; *AR*, Auer rods; *BM*, bone marrow; *CMML*, chronic myelomonocytic leukemia; *FAB*, French–American–British classification; *MDS-U*, myelodysplastic syndrome, unclassified; *PB*, peripheral blood; *RA*, refractory anemia; *RARS*, refractory anemia with ring sideroblasts; *RAEB*, refractory anemia with excess blasts; *RAEB-T*, refractory anemia with excess blasts in transformation; *RCC*, refractory cytopenia of childhood; *RCMD*, refractory cytopenia with multilineage dysplasia; *RCUD*, refractory cytopenia with unilineage dysplasia; *RS*, ring sideroblasts (% indicates percent RS of total nucleated erythroid precursors); *WHO*, World Health Organization classification.

TABLE 55.6	The Myelodysplastic/Myeloproliferative Neoplasms

- CMML
- "aCML," *BCR-ABL1* negative
- JMML
- RARS-T (provisional)

aCML, "Atypical" chronic myeloid leukemia; *CMML*, chronic myelomonocytic leukemia; *JMML*, juvenile myelomonocytic leukemia; *RARS-T*, refractory anemia with ring sideroblasts and thrombocytosis.

however, its use will not be required in the diagnostic workup of MDS.[22]

The Overlap Myelodysplastic/Myeloproliferative Neoplasms

In 2001 WHO introduced the overlap syndromes—that is, the MDS/MPNs (Table 55.6)—because at the time there was disagreement among committee members as to whether CMML was an MDS, as the FAB suggested, or an MPN, as a number of investigators suggested. This group of diseases was defined to include disorders that share features of the MPNs and of MDS at the time of initial presentation, but that do not fit well into either group. Some of the entities in the MPD/MPN category still are not well understood and may represent a disease in transition from MDS or MPN, although a case should not be placed in this category if initially diagnosed as MDS or MPN. However, without complete knowledge of the historical pathology of each individual patient, it is useful to have this category in order to construct a more reasonable classification. The overlap syndromes include CMML, including the juvenile type and juvenile myelomonocytic leukemia (JMML; see Chapter 63), in addition to "atypical" CML (atypical CML, *BCR-ABL1* negative) and an "unclassifiable" category that includes refractory anemia with ring sideroblasts and thrombocytosis (RARS-T). The MDS/MPNs share proliferative features in some cell lineages but also have dysplastic features, including ineffective hematopoiesis, in others. Similar to the MPNs, the overlap syndromes require a full evaluation of clinical and morphologic findings and evaluation of ancillary studies before a firm diagnosis can be rendered.

EVOLVING CONCEPTS IN CLASSIFICATION OF LYMPHOID NEOPLASMS

Hodgkin lymphoma was first described by Thomas Hodgkin in 1932 and is a distinct entity (Table 55.7) that can be distinguished from the majority of lymphomas that are designated non-Hodgkin lymphomas (NHL).[4] Historically, different classification systems have been proposed for NHL (Table 55.8). Henry Rappaport utilized the histologic features and the architectural arrangement of the neoplastic cells and their cytology when developing a classification system in 1956, which became widely accepted. This system was created prior to the advent of modern immunology; as such, the Lukes–Collins classification in 1975 attempted to relate cell morphology to immunologic function. Subsequently, in 1982, the Working Formulation for classifying NHL replaced the Rappaport and Lukes–Collins classification. This system had three groups based on patient prognosis: low, intermediate, and high grade. In 1994, the REAL classification implemented a new approach for classifying NHL, taking into account immunologic, genetic, and clinical features, and not solely relying on histopathologic characteristics of the tumor cells.[3] In 2001, the WHO classification successfully provided a common language and was adopted as the standard for clinicians and investigators worldwide.[1] The modifications made in the 2008 classification are the result of a successful coordination between pathologists, clinicians, and biologists.[4]

affected. The 2008 WHO classification scheme also emphasized the key role of cytogenetic analysis in the diagnosis of MDS, particularly in cases with otherwise insufficient morphologic evidence to substantiate a diagnosis of MDS. This is reflected in the inclusion of the subtype MDS unclassified (MDS-U), defined by the presence of cytopenias, less than 1% peripheral blasts, less than 10% dysplastic cells in any lineage, and less than 5% BM blasts with the presence of specific cytogenetic abnormalities commonly associated with MDS. In addition, the WHO 2008 classification now includes "MDS with an isolated del(5q)" including the "5q minus syndrome." This syndrome had been recognized for some time and is characterized typically by its presentation in middle-aged women with macrocytic anemia, splenomegaly, normal-to-elevated platelet counts, hypolobated megakaryocytes in the BM, and an isolated del(5q). The specific types of MDS have been increased and there are more than 10 different entities.

Although the basic diagnostic principles of the 2008 WHO classification of MDS are expected to remain unchanged in the 2016 WHO classification system, several changes to the classification are proposed. The proposed nomenclature changes include replacement of the terminology "refractory anemia" and "refractory cytopenia" with "myelodysplastic syndrome with single lineage dysplasia." In addition, the proposed changes will incorporate considerations of the prognostic significance of gene mutations in MDS, revising the diagnostic criteria for MDS entities with ring sideroblasts based on the detection of *SF3B1* mutations, slightly modifying the cytogenetic criteria for MDS with isolated del(5q), reclassifying most cases of the erythroid/myeloid type of acute erythroleukemia, and recognizing the familial link in some cases of MDS.[22] Flow cytometry immunophenotyping will be recognized as a useful ancillary technique in the evaluation of MDS,

<table>
TABLE 55.7 — **Hodgkin Lymphoma**

- **Nodular lymphocyte predominant Hodgkin lymphoma**
- **Classical Hodgkin lymphoma**
  - Nodular sclerosis classical Hodgkin lymphoma
  - Lymphocyte-rich classical Hodgkin lymphoma
  - Mixed cellularity classical Hodgkin lymphoma
  - Lymphocyte-depleted classical Hodgkin lymphoma
</table>

TABLE 55.7 Hodgkin Lymphoma

- **Nodular lymphocyte predominant Hodgkin lymphoma**
- **Classical Hodgkin lymphoma**
  - Nodular sclerosis classical Hodgkin lymphoma
  - Lymphocyte-rich classical Hodgkin lymphoma
  - Mixed cellularity classical Hodgkin lymphoma
  - Lymphocyte-depleted classical Hodgkin lymphoma

TABLE 55.8 Historic Reflection of Lymphoma Classification

1832	Hodgkin	A report of seven lymphoma cases
1966	Rappaport	Rappaport Classification
1974	Lukes–Collins	Lukes–Collins Classification
1978	Lennert	Keil Classification
1982	National Cancer Institute	Working Formulation of Non-Hodgkin Lymphoma
1988	Stansfeld et al	Updated Keil Classification
1994	Harris et al	REAL Classification
2001	Jaffe et al	2001 WHO Classification
2008	Swerdlow et al	2008 WHO Classification

REAL, Revised European-American Classification of Lymphoid Neoplasms; WHO, World Health Organization.

TABLE 55.9 WHO Classification of Mature B-Cell Neoplasms

- Chronic lymphocytic leukemia/small lymphocytic lymphoma
- B-cell prolymphocytic leukemia
- Splenic marginal zone lymphoma
- Hairy cell leukemia
- Splenic lymphoma/leukemia, unclassifiable
- Splenic diffuse red pulp small B-cell lymphoma
- Hairy cell leukemia variant
- Lymphoplasmacytic lymphoma
- Waldenström macroglobulinemia
- Heavy chain diseases
  - μHeavy chain disease
  - γHeavy chain disease
  - αHeavy chain disease
- Plasma cell myeloma
- Solitary plasmacytoma of bone
- Extraosseous plasmacytoma
- Extranodal marginal zone lymphoma of MALT lymphoma
- Nodal marginal zone lymphoma
- Pediatric nodal marginal zone lymphoma
- Follicular lymphoma
- Pediatric follicular lymphoma
- Primary cutaneous follicle centre lymphoma
- Mantle cell lymphoma
- DLBCL, NOS
- T-cell/histiocyte–rich large B-cell lymphoma
- Primary DLBCL of the CNS
- Primary cutaneous DLBCL, leg type
- EBV-positive DLBCL of the elderly
- DLBCL associated with chronic inflammation
- Lymphomatoid granulomatosis
- Primary mediastinal (thymic) large B-cell lymphoma
- Intravascular large B-cell lymphoma
- ALK-positive large B-cell lymphoma
- Plasmablastic lymphoma
- Large B-cell lymphoma arising in HHV8-associated multicentric Castleman disease
- Primary effusion lymphoma
- Burkitt lymphoma
- B-cell lymphoma, unclassifiable, with features intermediate between diffuse large B-cell lymphoma and Burkitt lymphoma
- B-cell lymphoma, unclassifiable, with features intermediate between diffuse large B-cell lymphoma and classical Hodgkin lymphoma

ALK, Anaplastic lymphoma kinase; CNS, central nervous system; DLBCL, NOS, Diffuse large B-cell lymphoma, not otherwise specified; EBV, Epstein-Barr virus; HHV8, human herpesvirus-8; MALT, mucosa-associated lymphoid tissue.

B-cell, T-cell, and NK-cell neoplasms often represent clonal expansion of these cells at certain developmental stages. Although B-cell neoplasms tend to mimic stages of normal B-cell development, some common B-cell neoplasms such as hairy cell leukemia do not conform to a normal B-cell differentiation stage. Additionally, some lymphomas show overt heterogeneity or lineage plasticity; consequently, the normal counterpart of neoplastic cells cannot be used as the sole basis for developing a classification system. The 2008 WHO Classification of Tumors of Hematopoietic and Lymphoid Tissues schema routinely employs a multiple-parameter approach that is based on clinical, morphologic, and biologic features, keeping in mind that a precise separation between entities is not possible in certain cases. Thus, the WHO recognized "gray zones" in which tumor cells may cross boundaries between currently used categories, such as the boundaries between classical Hodgkin lymphoma and primary mediastinal large B-cell lymphoma.[4]

In 2008 WHO expanded the classification of lymphoid neoplasms, with more consideration being given to disease definitions, nomenclature, grading, and clinical relevance. Since then, disease definitions have continued to evolve and expand, with new entities and variants being recognized. Both clinical and laboratory research findings provided new insights that are relevant to these emerging concepts.[23,24] Current areas of development focus on early or in situ lesions, as well as definition of the earlier steps of neoplastic transformation, age as a disease-defining feature (e.g., diffuse large-cell lymphoma of the older adult; Table 55.9), and site-specific impact on disease definition. In addition, there was an emphasis on overlapping or borderline entities, with fuzzy demarcation of morphologic, molecular, and genetic characteristics as areas of diagnostic challenge.[23]

Early Events in Lymphoid Neoplasms

Recent studies have identified additional clonal lymphoid lesions that share genetic and/or phenotypic properties with well-defined neoplasms such as chronic lymphocytic leukemia/small lymphocytic lymphoma (CLL/SLL),[25,26] multiple myeloma (MM), follicular lymphoma (FL) and MCL. However, these entities do not fulfill the diagnostic criteria for these well-defined neoplasms, and many appear to have a limited potential for progression. Monoclonal gammopathy of undetermined significance (MGUS), monoclonal B-cell lymphocytosis (MBL), FL in situ, and MCL in situ are examples of such entities.

MGUS is considered an early form of its malignant counterpart MM, with an age-related increased incidence and a small but definitive risk of progression to MM at an annual rate of 1%. Recent reports have emphasized the significance of genetic profiling in MGUS for risk stratification, and support the view that progression from MGUS to MM results from the selection and expansion of multiple aberrant clones rather than a linear step-wise acquisition of specific genetic abnormalities.[27,28] The International Myeloma Working Group (IMWG) 2010 guidelines recommend a MGUS risk stratification system, with periodic follow-up with serum electrophoresis for low-risk MGUS patients. However, patients with intermediate-risk and high-risk MGUS are suggested to undergo a baseline BM examination including cytogenetics and skeletal survey, and to be followed with serum electrophoresis studies twice in the first year following diagnosis and annually thereafter.[29]

MBL has been diagnosed more frequently than previously reported; this is thought to be related to high sensitivity of flow cytometric analyses. MBL is defined as the presence of a circulating monoclonal B-cell population below 5×10^9/L, persisting for at least 3 months, in otherwise asymptomatic individuals. Based on clonal B-cell counts and clinical significance, MBL is now subdivided into high-count MBL ($0.5-5.0 \times 10^9$/L) and low-count MBL (less than 0.5×10^9/L).[30] High-count MBL progresses to CLL at an annual rate of 1% to 2%, with the clonal B-cell count at presentation being the greatest risk factor. The presence of palpable lymphadenopathy, organomegaly, and/or infiltration of lymphocytes within the BM (greater than 30% of nucleated cells) fulfills the International Workshop on Chronic Lymphocytic Leukemia (IWCLL) criteria for CLL, even in the absence of clonal lymphocytosis, while the WHO diagnosis of CLL/SLL is based upon the presence of extramedullary involvement. Current recommendations for management of CLL-like MBL include yearly monitoring with therapeutic intervention if clinically indicated. Low-count MBL, based on current data, is unlikely to progress to CLL and does not warrant clinical monitoring. MBL with an atypical CLL-like phenotype (CD5+, bright CD20, CD23−) could represent an early leukemic manifestation of MCL, and a thorough staging workup including fluorescence in situ hybridization (FISH) testing for t(11;14) translocation is recommended.

FL in situ was initially described[31] as the localization of atypical B cells that have t(14;18)(IgH-B-cell lymphoma [BCL2]) translocation in the germinal centers of reactive-appearing lymph nodes with strong expression of CD10 and BCL-2. The lymph node architecture is generally intact. The majority of cases of FL in situ do not progress to overt lymphoma, thus the alternate term "follicular lymphoma-like B cells of undetermined significance" was recently proposed. In the 2016 WHO classification revision, alternative term of in situ FL neoplasia is used in order to reflect the uncertain clinical significance of this entity. In situ FL neoplasia must be differentiated from partial involvement by low-grade FL, which usually shows partially effaced nodal architecture with enlarged, crowded follicles, and attenuated mantle zones. This distinction is clinically relevant, as partial involvement by low-grade FL is more likely to be associated with or progress towards overt FL.

Analogous to in situ FL neoplasia, incidental diagnosis of colonization of the mantle cuffs of reactive follicles by cyclin D1-positive B cells has been termed in situ mantle cell neoplasia (MCLIS). In these cases,[32] cyclinD1 highlighted a small subset of B cells within the mantle zone, indicating low-level involvement by lymphoma. This peculiar pattern of cyclinD1 positivity encircling follicles is characteristic of an early or in situ MCL. The in situ variant of MCL is rare and exhibits cyclinD1 positivity within the innermost mantle zone B lymphocytes, and often is reserved for only partial encircling of follicles by MCL cells. In contrast, it has been proposed that full encircling of follicles by cyclinD1-positive cells should be interpreted as an early sign of involvement by MCL. This distinction is important as partial MCL is more likely than MCLIS to progress or coexist with advanced disease. Current management recommendations for MCLIS include whole-body imaging and unilateral BM biopsy (if indicated) to rule out a concomitant overt lymphoma. In the absence of overt disease, no treatment is required and careful follow-up is advised.

Age as a Disease-Defining Feature

The 2008 WHO classification introduced the concept of age as a defining feature in several disease categories.[4] The entities of FL and nodal marginal zone lymphomas (MZLs) that present in the pediatric age group differ from their adult counterparts clinically and biologically. The pediatric variant of FL usually presents with localized disease and is of high histologic grade. These lymphomas lack translocations t(14;18) and do not express BCL2 and have good prognosis, although the optimal management remains to be determined. Nodal MZLs in children also appear to have a low risk of progression. Pediatric nodal MZLs are clonal diseases characterized by marginal zone expansion with fragmentation of germinal centers

and progressive transformation of germinal center-like changes. Presentation with isolated cervical lymphadenopathy is common in pediatric nodal MZL. The WHO classification also recognizes two rare Epstein-Barr virus (EBV)–associated T-cell diseases: systemic EBV+ T-cell lymphoproliferative disease of childhood and hydroa vacciniforme-like lymphoma. These diseases occur almost entirely in children, primarily in those of Asian origin.

On the opposite spectrum of age-related lymphoproliferative disorders is EBV-positive diffuse large B-cell lymphoma (EBV+ DLBCL) of the older adult, which is among the newly included provisional entities in the 2008 WHO classification. The underlying immunologic deficit in this setting is believed to be immunosenescence, which is defined as the natural decay of the immune system as a consequence of aging. This entity also is defined histologically as malignant B-cell lymphoproliferation in people older than 50 years of age, without any known immunodeficiency or prior lymphoma diagnosis, and is associated with an aggressive clinical behavior pattern. Initial studies reported some overlap with classic Hodgkin lymphoma encountered in the older adult.[23] At present, there is a broader understanding than previously appreciated of the wide clinicopathologic spectrum of age-related EBV-positive lymphoproliferative disorder (LPD). This spectrum includes reactive lymphoid hyperplasia, polymorphic extranodal LPD (76% have EBV mucocutaneous ulcer), polymorphic nodal LPD and EBV+ DLBCL. Both polymorphic nodal lesions and EBV+ DLBCL are characterized by poor survival. In this clinicopathologic spectrum, histologic types are highly predictive of outcome; and small-volume disease, particularly in mucosal sites and skin (EBV mucocutaneous ulcer), which are associated with a good prognosis. It is important to keep in mind that although these lymphomas tend to cluster in the very young or the older adult age groups, they are not age restricted. Similarly, EBV+ DLBCL of the older adult can occur in a younger population.[33]

Aggressive B-Cell Lymphoma, Borderline Entities and Site-Specific Categories

The 2008 WHO classification identified several subtypes of DLBCLs (Table 55.9). However, many DLBCLs lack pathologic, clinical, or other defining features that can be used to stratify them. Thus, these are designated DLBCL, NOS in the WHO classification. Stratification according to gene expression profiling as germinal center B-cell (GCB) versus activated B-cell (ABC) types has proven to have prognostic value. The GCB and ABC subtypes are now formally recognized in the 2016 WHO classification, despite the absence of a reproducible routine diagnostic test and the imperfect correlation of immunohistochemical surrogate markers with genomic studies.[34] Digital multiplexed gene expression utilizing formalin-fixed paraffin-embedded–derived RNA at a reasonable cost and turnaround time to classify B-cell lymphomas according to cell of origin is currently being validated as a routine clinical assay.[35,36] The clinical need and utility of this designation is rising, with more studies suggesting that ABC versus GCB lymphomas exhibit differential sensitivity to certain drugs and therapeutic modalities.[34]

In addition to the designation of DLBCL to ABC or GCB subtypes, next-generation sequencing technologies have unveiled the remarkable complexity of DLBCL. More important, it has become increasingly clear that these complexities represent lymphoma subtypes which are driven by very different intracellular oncologic signaling pathways and which can be differentially exploited for therapeutic benefit.[37] Recent studies have demonstrated the high frequency of abnormalities (i.e., noted in greater than 50% of DLBCLs) affecting histone/chromatin-modification enzymes, such as *CREBBP*, *EP300*, *MLL2*, and *EZH2*.[38] The role of therapeutic agents that target the epigenome has been suggested in DLBCL subgroups due to the variability in DNA methylation and its association with outcome.[39,40]

Currently, the role of MYC and BCL2 proteins in DLBCL is an area of an active investigation. It is proposed that cases of DLBCL be evaluated for concurrent MYC and BCL2 dysregulation at diagnosis, in order to determine the presence of translocation/protein overexpression. Patients with dual overexpression of MYC and BCL2 have a significantly poorer outcome compared with patients who express only one or neither protein. In addition, concurrent MYC and BCL2 translocation, known as *double-hit lymphoma*, indicates a subgroup of patients who are refractory to treatment and have a median survival of approximately 8 months.

The 2008 WHO classification emphasizes the importance of integrating morphologic, immunophenotypic, and molecular data to make a final diagnosis. This integration has refined our ability to diagnose several entities such as DLBCL and Burkitt lymphoma (BL). The 2008 WHO classification eliminated the variant category of atypical BL, which had been included in the 2001 WHO classification. Thus, a case with the typical BL phenotype (CD20[+], CD10[+], BCL2[−]) and genotype (so-called *MYC-simple* or *MYC/IG* in the absence of other major cytogenetic anomalies) may be classified as BL even if there is some variability in the morphology of the neoplastic cells. In addition, the 2008 WHO classification recognizes a group of high-grade B-cell lymphomas that are not readily classified as either BL or DLBCL. This provisional category is termed *B-cell lymphoma, unclassifiable*, with features that are intermediate between DLBCL and BL, including double-hit lymphomas.[4] In the 2016 WHO classification DLBCL with MYC and BCL2 and/or BCL6 rearrangements will be included in a single category to be designated high grade B cell lymphoma (HGBL), with MYC and BCL2 and/or BCL6 rearrangements. The category of BCLU will be eliminated. Cases that appear blastoid or cases intermediate between DLBCL and BL, but which lack a MYC and BCL2 and/or BCL6 rearrangement, will be placed in the category of HGBL, NOS. The 2008 WHO classification recognizes another provisional category of B-cell neoplasms with features that are intermediate between DLBCL and classical Hodgkin lymphoma (CHL). These tumors occur predominantly in young men and appear to be more aggressive than either primary mediastinal large B-cell lymphoma or nodular sclerosis CHL. There are other settings in which the distinction between DLBCL and CHL is challenging. For example, some EBV-associated B-cell lymphomas may exhibit features that closely resemble or mimic CHL. The borderline category should be used sparingly but is appropriate when a distinction between CHL and DLBCL is not possible.[4]

Several aggressive B-cell lymphomas have a distinct immunoprofile or resemble a cell-specific stage of differentiation. These include plasmablastic lymphoma, ALK[+] large B-cell lymphoma, human herpesvirus 8-associated malignancies, primary effusion lymphoma, and large B-cell lymphoma associated with multicentric Castleman disease. All of these entities resemble a stage of plasma cell differentiation. Other site-specific categories are primary DLBCL of the central nervous system and primary cutaneous DLBCL, leg type. Both primary central nervous system DLBCL and other DLBCLs arising in privileged sites, such as the testis, may exhibit distinctive biologic features. However, clinical features remain important in clinical management. Interestingly, primary central nervous system DLBCL has a distinctive gene expression signature that may continue to justify it as a separate entity.

Follicular Lymphoma Grading

Revisions to the 2008 WHO classification incorporated changes related to the grading of FL. Both grade 1 and grade 2 were combined in one category and designated "low-grade FL." This revision was the result of questioning the clinical significance of separating grade 1 from grade 2 despite minimal differences in long-term outcome.[4] In addition, several studies identified biologic differences between grades 3A and 3B, with the latter being more closely related to DLBCL. The separation of FL grade 3A from 3B is based on the absence of centrocytes in 3B; however, in routine practice this distinction is difficult. Further studies in this area are needed, as they may be helpful in increasing reproducibility of this distinction. According to the 2008 WHO classification, diffuse areas in grade 3 FL should be designated DLBCL, along with FL, as the bottom-line diagnosis.[4]

Peripheral T-Cell Lymphoma

Peripheral T-cell lymphomas (PTCLs) encompass numerous entities (Table 55.10) that are characterized by a poor prognosis, with the exception of histologic subtype "ALK-positive anaplastic large-cell lymphoma." Most PTCLs lack distinct genetic or biologic features, and the mechanisms underlying the pathogenesis of these lymphomas are not yet fully understood. However, development of genomic high-throughput profiling techniques now allows us to extensively identify the molecular abnormalities present in these entities. The diagnosis of many cases is challenging even for expert hematopathologists, and more than a third of the cases cannot be further classified and consequently are relegated to a "waste basket" category PTCL-NOS. Other frequently encountered entities are angioimmunoblastic T-cell lymphoma (AITL), and anaplastic large cell lymphoma (ALCL). AITL and approximately 20% of PTCL-NOS[4] show phenotypic features of T-cell follicular helper (Tfh) cells; and share a spectrum of genetic abnormalities such as *TET2* and *DNMT3A*, as well as mutations in the motility and adhesion gene *RHOA*.[41]

Despite morphologic and phenotypic similarities ALK[+] ALCL is considered a distinct entity that must be distinguished from the entity of ALK[−] ALCL given the clinical and biologic differences. In the 2016 update to the WHO classification, ALK[−] ALCL are no longer provisional entities and strict criteria are required for the diagnosis of ALK[−] ALCL because CD30 may be expressed in a variety of PTCL subtypes.

Three variants of primary cutaneous PTCL were introduced in the 2008 WHO classification; primary cutaneous gamma-delta T-cell lymphoma, primary cutaneous CD4[+] small/medium T-cell lymphoma as a provisional entity, and primary cutaneous aggressive epidermotropic CD8[+] cytotoxic T-cell lymphoma. Cutaneous gamma-delta T-cell lymphomas have a diverse histologic and clinical spectrum and may display a panniculitis-like pattern. However, this disease has a much poorer prognosis than subcutaneous panniculitis-like T-cell lymphoma, which is defined as a lymphoma exclusively of alpha-beta phenotype in the 2008 WHO classification. Primary cutaneous small/medium CD4[+] T-cell lymphoma is another lymphoma with

TABLE 55.10	WHO Classification of Mature T-Cell and NK-Cell Neoplasms

- T-cell prolymphocytic leukemia
- T-cell large granular lymphocytic leukemia
- Chronic lymphoproliferative disorder of NK cells
- Aggressive NK-cell leukemia
- Systemic EBV-positive T-cell lymphoproliferative disease of childhood
- Hydroa vacciniforme-like lymphoma
- Adult T-cell leukemia/lymphoma
- Extranodal NK/T-cell lymphoma, nasal type
- Enteropathy-associated T-cell lymphoma
- Hepatosplenic T-cell lymphoma
- Subcutaneous panniculitis-like T-cell lymphoma
- Mycosis fungoides
- Sézary syndrome
- Primary cutaneous CD30[−] T-cell lymphoproliferative disorders
- Lymphomatoid papulosis
- Primary cutaneous anaplastic large-cell lymphoma
- Primary cutaneous T-cell lymphoma
- Primary cutaneous aggressive epidermotropic CD8[+] cytotoxic T-cell lymphoma
- Primary cutaneous small/medium CD4[+] T-cell lymphoma
- Peripheral T-cell lymphoma, NOS
- Angioimmunoblastic T-cell lymphoma
- Anaplastic large-cell lymphoma, ALK-positive
- Anaplastic large-cell lymphoma, ALK-negative

ALK, Anaplastic lymphoma kinase; EBV, Epstein-Barr virus; NK, natural killer; NOS, not otherwise specified.

Tfh cell origin that presents commonly as an isolated lesion in the head and neck region.[42] In the 2016 WHO classification a change in the terminology of this entity is proposed—to primary cutaneous small/medium CD4[+] T-cell lymphoproliferative disease instead of lymphoma.

The 2008 WHO classification acknowledged that a variety of PTCLs can present with intestinal disease and that not all of these cases are associated with celiac disease. Intestinal involvement can be seen at presentation, and/or with progression, in extranodal NK/T-cell lymphoma as well as in some gamma-delta T-cell lymphomas. The WHO classification required more stringent criteria to establish a diagnosis known as *enteropathy-associated T-cell lymphoma* Specifically, in order to make the diagnosis of enteropathy-associated T-cell lymphoma, evidence of celiac disease was required either at the genetic level, with the appropriate HLA phenotype, or histologically, in the adjacent uninvolved small bowel mucosa. A new variant, termed the *monomorphic variant of enteropathy-associated T-cell lymphoma*, or *type II*, was introduced into the 2008 WHO classification. Cases exhibiting this variant have some distinctive immunophenotypic and genotypic features. The tumor cells are CD8[+] and CD56[+], and *MYC* amplifications are present in a subset of cases. The monomorphic variant occurs in the setting of celiac disease but also occurs sporadically.[4]

Precursor Lymphoid Neoplasms

The lymphoblastic neoplasms are derived from precursor cells or blasts, most of which are precursor B and T-cell neoplasms that present as leukemia. However, the designation of lymphoblastic lymphoma is used when the neoplasm is confined to a mass lesion without or with only minimal blood or BM involvement. The WHO classification retains the convention that precursor neoplasms are designated *leukemia/lymphoma*. When distinction between leukemia and lymphoma is required for clinical protocol eligibility in presentation with a mass lesion and increased blasts in the BM, a threshold of 25% blasts is used as the defining feature of leukemia.[4]

The 2008 classification recognizes genetic features in the definition of some forms of B-lymphoblastic leukemia (B-ALL). One such example is Philadelphia chromosome-positive (Ph[+]) B-ALL, associated with *BCR-ABL1*, which is more common in adults than in children and is considered very high risk, regardless of other factors. Deletions and other alterations in the *IKZF1* (Ikaros) gene are adverse prognostic indicators in both Ph+ and Ph− patients with B-ALL. Another variant with distinctive clinical features at presentation is B-ALL/lymphoma with t(5;15)(q31;q32) (*IL3-IGH*). These patients present with a marked increase in eosinophils, which may mask a relatively small number of blasts in the BM—a diagnostic pitfall worthy of note. The ongoing and increasing complexity highlights the importance of clinicopathologic correlation and the value of ancillary studies in the classification and workup of patients with B-ALL.[43]

T-lymphoblastic leukemia (T-ALL) is also associated with considerable genetic variability. Routine histopathology, flow cytometry immunophenotyping, conventional cytogenetic analysis, FISH, and/or clonality testing are usually adequate to establish the diagnosis. The most commonly involved genes include the HOX transcription factors. However, genotyping is recommended in the workup of the disease, although at this time it is not used as a criterion to define distinct entities.

DENDRITIC CELL AND HISTIOCYTIC NEOPLASMS: PRINCIPAL CONSIDERATIONS FOR DIAGNOSIS AND TREATMENT

Dendritic and histiocytic neoplasms are hematologic malignancies that have distinct yet variable clinical presentation, and together they make up less than 1% of the neoplastic process of the lymph node or soft tissue.[4] However, the true prevalence of these disorders remains

TABLE 55.11	WHO Classification of Histiocytic and Dendritic Cell Neoplasms

- Histiocytic sarcoma
- Langerhans cell histiocytosis
- Langerhans cell sarcoma
- Interdigitating dendritic cell sarcoma
- Follicular dendritic cell sarcoma
- Fibroblastic reticular cell tumor
- Intermediate dendritic cell tumor
- Disseminated juvenile xanthogranuloma

uncertain because many have been recognized only recently. Several entities are recognized in the 2008 WHO classification of histiocytic and dendritic cell neoplasms (Table 55.11). Traditionally, these tumors are placed into two basic categories based on their derivation from either BM precursors or mesenchymal cells. Histiocytic sarcoma (HS), Langerhans cell histiocytosis (LCH), and interdigitating dendritic cell sarcoma (IDCS) are derived from BM precursors; while follicular dendritic cell sarcoma (FDCS), indeterminate dendritic cell sarcoma, fibroblastic reticular cell tumors, and disseminated juvenile xanthogranuloma are derived from stromal-derived dendritic cells or are mesenchymal in origin. Although divergent differentiation from marrow precursors is the normal histogenesis, hybrid and trans differentiation from lymphoid clones has been proposed in some entities.[39]

Excisional biopsy is the preferred specimen choice from which to render the diagnosis of these disorders. Consultation with an experienced hematopathologist is often required, as morphologic review and an adequate battery of immunohistochemical stains are the most important elements in making an accurate diagnosis of these entities and in differentiating them from other, often-mistaken categories, most commonly NHLs. The rarity of these disorders is the major factor that makes this group of diseases difficult to accurately diagnose and challenging to treat. Advances of immunohistochemistry have contributed to an enhanced understanding of the biology of dendritic and histiocytic neoplasms, and have improved our ability to classify and diagnose these disorders. For example, in contrast to LCH, IDCS are usually positive for S100 but negative for CD1a and langerin (CD207). Unlike FDCS, IDCS do not express follicular dendritic cell markers such as CD21 or CD35.[4]

These entities can involve various organs, although most occur in the lymph nodes and skin, with a unifocal or solitary presentation, and are associated with a good prognosis with surgical resection. On the other hand, cases with disseminated disease have shown a poor outcome, although data on treatment options are limited. Nonetheless, chemotherapy and referral to a tertiary-care center should be considered for patients with these diagnoses. Large pooled analyses or clinical trials will be needed to better understand optimal treatment options of these rare disorders.

REFERENCES

1. Jaffe ES, Harris NL, Stein H: *Pathology and Genetics of Tumours of the Haematopoietic and Lymphoid Tissue*, 2001, IARC Press.
2. Harris NL, Jaffe ES, Diebold J, et al: World Health Organization classification of neoplastic diseases of the hematopoietic and lymphoid tissues: report of the Clinical Advisory Committee meeting-Airlie House, Virginia, November 1997. *J Clin Oncol* 17:3835–3849, 1999.
3. Harris NL, Jaffe ES, Stein H, et al: A revised European-American classification of lymphoid neoplasms: a proposal from the International Lymphoma Study Group. *Blood* 84:1361–1392, 1994.
4. Swerdlow SH, Campo E, Harris NL: *WHO Classification of Tumours of Haematopoietic and Lymphoid Tissues*, Lyon, 2008, IARC Press.
5. Bennett JM, Catovsky D, Daniel MT, et al: Proposals for the classification of the myelodysplastic syndromes. *Br J Haematol* 51:189–199, 1982.

6. Vardiman JW, Thiele J, Arber DA, et al: The 2008 revision of the World Health Organization (WHO) classification of myeloid neoplasms and acute leukemia: rationale and important changes. *Blood* 114:937–951, 2009.

7. Maciejewski JP, Haferlach T: Introduction: molecular pathogenesis of hematologic malignancies. *Semin Oncol* 39:9–12, 2012.

8. Anastasi J: The myeloproliferative and overlap, myeloproliferative/myelodysplastic neoplasms. In Hsi E, editor: *The myeloproliferative and overlap, myeloproliferative/myelodysplastic neoplasms*, St Louis, 2012, Elsevier, p 479.

9. Druker BJ, Talpaz M, Resta DJ, et al: Efficacy and safety of a specific inhibitor of the BCR-ABL tyrosine kinase in chronic myeloid leukemia. *N Engl J Med* 344:1031–1037, 2001.

10. Tefferi A, Thiele J, Vannucchi AM, et al: An overview on CALR and CSF3R mutations and a proposal for revision of WHO diagnostic criteria for myeloproliferative neoplasms. *Leukemia* 28:1407–1413, 2014.

11. Klampfl T, Gisslinger H, Harutyunyan AS, et al: Somatic mutations of calreticulin in myeloproliferative neoplasms. *N Engl J Med* 369:2379–2390, 2013.

12. Nangalia J, Massie CE, Baxter EJ, et al: Somatic CALR mutations in myeloproliferative neoplasms with nonmutated JAK2. *N Engl J Med* 369:2391–2405, 2013.

13. Elliott MA, Tefferi A: Chronic neutrophilic leukemia 2014: Update on diagnosis, molecular genetics, and management. *Am J Hematol* 89:651–658, 2014.

14. Chiu A, Orazi A: Mastocytosis and related disorders. *Semin Diagn Pathol* 29:19–30, 2012.

15. Jawhar M, Schwaab J, Schnittger S, et al: Additional mutations in SRSF2, ASXL1 and/or RUNX1 identify a high-risk group of patients with KIT D816V (+) advanced systemic mastocytosis. *Leukemia* 30:136–143, 2016.

16. Gotlib J: World Health Organization-defined eosinophilic disorders: 2011 update on diagnosis, risk stratification, and management. *Am J Hematol* 86:677–688, 2011.

17. Stone RM, et al: The multi-kinase inhibitor midostaurin (M) prolongs survival compared with placebo (P) in combination with Daunorubicin (D)/Cytarabine (C) induction (ind), high-dose C consolidation (consol), and as maintenance (maint) therapy in newly diagnosed acute Myeloid Leukemia (AML) patients (pts) age 18-60 with FLT3 mutations (muts): an international prospective randomized (rand) P-controlled double-blind Trial (CALGB 10603/RATIFY [Alliance]). *Blood* 16:2015. ahead of print.

18. Pratz K, Levis M: Incorporating FLT3 inhibitors into acute myeloid leukemia treatment regimens. *Leuk Lymphoma* 49:852–863, 2008.

19. West AH, Godley LA, Churpek JE: Familial myelodysplastic syndrome/acute leukemia syndromes: a review and utility for translational investigations. *Ann N Y Acad Sci* 1310:111–118, 2014.

20. Nacheva EP, Grace CD, Brazma D, et al: Does BCR/ABL1 positive acute myeloid leukaemia exist? *Br J Haematol* 161:541–550, 2013.

21. Konoplev S, Yin CC, Kornblau SM, et al: Molecular characterization of de novo Philadelphia chromosome-positive acute myeloid leukemia. *Leuk Lymphoma* 54:138–144, 2013.

22. Arber DA, Hasserjian RP: Reclassifying myelodysplastic syndromes: what's where in the new WHO and why. *Hematology Am Soc Hematol Educ Program* 2015:294–298, 2015.

23. Xie Y, Pittaluga S, Jaffe ES: The histological classification of diffuse large B-cell lymphomas. *Semin Hematol* 52:57–66, 2015.

24. Tirado CA, Chen W, Garcia R, et al: Genomic profiling using array comparative genomic hybridization define distinct subtypes of diffuse large B-cell lymphoma: a review of the literature. *J Hematol Oncol* 5:54, 2012.

25. Henopp T, Quintanilla-Martinez L, Fend F, et al: Prevalence of follicular lymphoma in situ in consecutively analysed reactive lymph nodes. *Histopathology* 59:139–142, 2011.

26. Fend F, Cabecadas J, Gaulard P, et al: Early lesions in lymphoid neoplasia: conclusions based on the Workshop of the XV. Meeting of the European Association of Hematopathology and the Society of Hematopathology, in Uppsala, Sweden. *J Hematop* 5:169–199, 2012.

27. Dhodapkar MV, Sexton R, Waheed S, et al: Clinical, genomic, and imaging predictors of myeloma progression from asymptomatic monoclonal gammopathies (SWOG S0120). *Blood* 123:78–85, 2014.

28. Morgan GJ, Walker BA, Davies FE: The genetic architecture of multiple myeloma. *Nat Rev Cancer* 12:335–348, 2012.

29. Kyle RA, Durie BG, Rajkumar SV, et al: Monoclonal gammopathy of undetermined significance (MGUS) and smoldering (asymptomatic) multiple myeloma: IMWG consensus perspectives risk factors for progression and guidelines for monitoring and management. *Leukemia* 24:1121–1127, 2010.

30. Shim YK, Rachel JM, Ghia P, et al: Monoclonal B-cell lymphocytosis in healthy blood donors: an unexpectedly common finding. *Blood* 123:1319–1326, 2014.

31. Cong P, Raffeld M, Teruya-Feldstein J, et al: In situ localization of follicular lymphoma: description and analysis by laser capture microdissection. *Blood* 99:3376–3382, 2002.

32. Carvajal-Cuenca A, Sua LF, Silva NM, et al: In situ mantle cell lymphoma: clinical implications of an incidental finding with indolent clinical behavior. *Haematologica* 97:270–278, 2012.

33. Beltran BE, Morales D, Quinones P, et al: EBV-positive diffuse large b-cell lymphoma in young immunocompetent individuals. *Clin Lymphoma Myeloma Leuk* 11:512–516, 2011.

34. Sehn LH, Gascoyne RD: Diffuse large B-cell lymphoma: optimizing outcome in the context of clinical and biologic heterogeneity. *Blood* 125:22–32, 2015.

35. Scott DW, Wright GW, Williams PM, et al: Determining cell-of-origin subtypes of diffuse large B-cell lymphoma using gene expression in formalin-fixed paraffin-embedded tissue. *Blood* 123:1214–1217, 2014.

36. Masque-Soler N, Szczepanowski M, Kohler CW, et al: Molecular classification of mature aggressive B-cell lymphoma using digital multiplexed gene expression on formalin-fixed paraffin-embedded biopsy specimens. *Blood* 122:1985–1986, 2013.

37. Zhang J, Grubor V, Love CL, et al: Genetic heterogeneity of diffuse large B-cell lymphoma. *Proc Natl Acad Sci USA* 110:1398–1403, 2013.

38. Pasqualucci L, Dominguez-Sola D, Chiarenza A, et al: Inactivating mutations of acetyltransferase genes in B-cell lymphoma. *Nature* 471:189–195, 2011.

39. Chambwe N, Kormaksson M, Geng H, et al: Variability in DNA methylation defines novel epigenetic subgroups of DLBCL associated with different clinical outcomes. *Blood* 123:1699–1708, 2014.

40. Cerchietti L, Leonard JP: Targeting the epigenome and other new strategies in diffuse large B-cell lymphoma: beyond R-CHOP. *Hematology Am Soc Hematol Educ Program* 2013:591–595, 2013.

41. Ahearne MJ, Allchin RL, Fox CP, et al: Follicular helper T-cells: expanding roles in T-cell lymphoma and targets for treatment. *Br J Haematol* 166:326–335, 2014.

42. Rodriguez Pinilla SM, Roncador G, Rodriguez-Peralto JL, et al: Primary cutaneous CD4+ small/medium-sized pleomorphic T-cell lymphoma expresses follicular T-cell markers. *Am J Surg Pathol* 33:81–90, 2009.

43. Loghavi S, Kutok JL, Jorgensen JL: B-acute lymphoblastic leukemia/lymphoblastic lymphoma. *Am J Clin Pathol* 144:393–410, 2015.

44. Fasan A, Haferlach C, Alpermann T, et al: The role of different genetic subtypes of CEBPA mutated AML. *Leukemia* 28:794–803, 2014.

CONVENTIONAL AND MOLECULAR CYTOGENOMIC BASIS OF HEMATOLOGIC MALIGNANCIES

Vesna Najfeld

Dedicated to the loving memory of Eta Najfeld, MD, a Holocaust survivor and an amazing mother.

Over the past 60 years the cytogenetic analysis of hematologic malignancies has been an area of prolific growth. Chromosome studies and karyotype analysis provide information of both biologic and clinical significance. Refinements in cell culture methods and the application of chromosome banding techniques have advanced our understanding of disease-specific abnormalities, and molecular cytogenetic methods now have made possible the identification of genes involved at translocation breakpoints in specific chromosomal rearrangements. These advances in molecular cytogenetic methods permit mapping of structural rearrangements within a single gene and fundamentally contribute to our knowledge of the biology of leukemia. This evolution in our understanding of cancer genetics has resulted in distinct terminology (Table 56.1). Application of conventional and molecular cytogenetic methods has identified over 600 fusion genes involving over 250 different genes and approximately 1000 recurrent balanced translocations in human cancers. Relevance of these methods has played a pivotal role in the diagnosis, treatment, and prognosis of the hematologic malignancies. This chapter discusses specific cytogenetic events and delineates molecular phenotypes that are important to understand the molecular pathogenesis of hematologic malignancies and provides several genetic testing algorithms. The remarkable hypothesis put forward by Boveri at the turn of the 20th century—namely, that an abnormal chromosome pattern is intimately associated with the malignant phenotype of a tumor cell—has proven correct. Knowledge of the molecular cytogenetic phenotype of hematologic malignancies has led to innovative and specifically tailored treatments. The first example of such gene-targeted therapy has already been successfully applied to chronic myelogenous leukemia (CML).

METHODS

Fig. 56.1 shows the current cytogenomic methods used in detecting clonal chromosomal, gene or other genomic rearrangements and abnormalities in hematologic malignancies.

Cytogenetic Analysis

Cells arrested in metaphase are obtained by exposing marrow cells sequentially to mitotic inhibitors, hypotonic potassium chloride, and fixative. Chromosomes obtained from leukemic marrow are then subjected to the most widely used banding method, trypsin-Giemsa banding (Fig. 56.2). The criteria used to define clonal abnormalities are listed in Table 56.1 and described in the International System for Human Cytogenetic Nomenclature, 2013.

Fluorescence In Situ Hybridization Methods

Fluorescence in situ hybridization (FISH) is a molecular method that allows detection of the number, size, and location of DNA and RNA

segments within individual cells in a tissue sample. It is based on the ability of single-stranded DNA to anneal to complementary DNA. In hematologic disorders, the target DNA is the marrow or peripheral blood DNA present in interphase cells or the DNA of metaphase chromosomes that is fixed on a microscope slide. Other biologic material that may be involved in the leukemic process, such as spleen cells, ascites, and spinal fluid, are particularly useful for FISH studies. In lymphoma, the target DNA is present in lymph nodes, and FISH studies are performed on touch preparations, frozen sections, or paraffin-embedded tissue.

Fig. 56.3 shows four types of FISH probes that are used alone or in combination to determine both numeric and structural rearrangements: (a) centromere enumeration probes, which, as the name implies, are used most frequently in interphase nuclei for detection of numeric chromosome anomalies, (b) whole chromosome painting probes, which are used only on metaphase cells and are very useful in delineating complex rearrangements or the origin of a marker, derivative or ring chromosome, (c) subtelomeric probes, and (d) unique gene loci probes applied to both interphase and metaphase cells in single, dual, triple, or multiple colors to determine specific chromosomal rearrangements, deletions, or amplifications.

The four FISH probe strategies are used in probe design for detection of chromosomal translocations in hematologic malignancies (Fig. 56.4): (a) standard (conventional strategy), (b) extrasensitive strategy, (c) dual-fusion strategy, and (d) "breakapart strategy." The first application of FISH technology for detection of chromosomal translocations in hematologic malignancy was when the *BCR-ABL1* hybrid gene was identified using two-color FISH in interphase cells as well as in metaphase marrow-derived CML cells. In the standard strategy for interphase evaluation of chromosomal translocation, a DNA probe comprising sequences mapped proximal to the breakpoint in one of the chromosomes involved in reciprocal translocations is combined with a differentially labeled DNA probe that includes sequences mapped distal to the breakpoint in the other chromosome. Positive nuclei for the translocation display one dual-color fusion signal, representing one of the derivative chromosomes generated by the translocation, and two single-color signals, one for each of the normal alleles. This standard FISH strategy has been used for detection of translocations in hematologic disorders at diagnosis.

For detection of minimal residual disease, the conventional strategy lacks specificity because cells with random spatial co-localization of normal signals with different colors, found at a frequency from 1% to 10% of scored nuclei, are seen as false positive. To minimize this problem, an extrasensitive method was developed in which a probe for one abnormal chromosome is designed to generate extra, smaller signals in positive nuclei. Hybridization using this strategy results in abnormal cells with co-localization of two signals in dual colors, an additional two signals in one single color and one signal in another single color. Application of the extrasensitive probe has been useful in discriminating between *BCR-ABL1* fusion-positive blast crisis of CML and de novo acute lymphoblastic leukemia (ALL).

A dual-fusion strategy was developed not only to minimize false-positivity but also to detect additional deletions at translocation breakpoints. The dual-color/dual-fusion strategy includes a probe set with DNA sequences that encompasses proximally and distally the translocation breakpoints on both chromosomes involved in the

TABLE 56.1   Glossary of Cytogenetic, Fluorescence in Situ Hybridization and Genomic Terminology

Aneuploidy	Abnormal chromosome number, either gain or loss.
Array CGH	A higher-level CGH technology that provides gene copy information.
Balanced translocation	Exchange of chromosomal material that creates no extra or missing DNA.
Banding	Set of dark and pale segments along the length of chromosomes, resulting from treatment with enzyme before staining. Each chromosome identified by its unique set of bands.
Breakpoint	Specific site on a chromosome containing a break in the DNA that is involved in chromosomal structural rearrangement, such as translocation or deletion.
Centromere	Constriction on the chromosome at the spindle site attachment. During cell mitosis two copies of the DNA in each chromosome are separated by shortening of the spindle fibers attached to opposite sides of the dividing cell. Position of the centromere determines whether the chromosome is metacentric (X-shaped; e.g., 1, 3, 19, 20), submetacentric (centromere positioned more toward the short arms; e.g., 2, 4, 5, 6–12, 16–18, X), or acrocentric (inverted V-shaped; e.g., 13–15, 21, 22, Y).
Centromere enumeration probe (CEP)	Highly repetitive α (or β) satellite DNA, located in the heterochromatin of the centromeric area of chromosomes. CEP targets repetitive α (or β) sequences and produces bright compact signals; particularly useful for detection of numerical loss or gain of chromosomes.
Comparative genomic hybridization (CGH)	Molecular cytogenetic technique that provides a copy-number karyotype at the chromosome and band level. Variety of arrays include disease specialized, chromosome arm specific, and others.
Chromosomal rearrangement	Aberration in which chromosomes are broken and rejoined.
Clonal abnormality	In cytogenetic analysis, two cells showing the same additional or structural abnormality or three cells with loss of the same chromosome. In FISH analysis, any abnormality present after the probe has been validated and normal reference range established, above the normal reference range.
Chromothripsis	A catastrophic DNA damage occurring during a single mitotic division Cytogenomics is the application of molecular biology to determine genomic copy number.
Deletion	Segment of chromosome that is missing (terminal) or segment of chromosome missing between two breakpoints (interstitial).
DNA sequence	Order of nucleotides in a DNA segment, usually displayed from the 5′-triphosphate (5′ end) to the 3′-hydroxyl (3′ end) nucleotides.
Driver mutation	This mutation affects the biology of cell.
Enhancer	DNA sequence that increases the rate of transcription.
Exon	Portion of gene that encodes protein.
Fiber FISH	Application of FISH technology to extended DNA or free DNA fibers.
FISH	Fluorescence in situ hybridization, a method for detection of the number and location of DNA sequences (genes) in tissue section or cell population.
Fluorochrome	Fluorescence molecule that, when conjugated to a molecule, binds to a hapten to facilitate detection of the chromosomal probe. By definition, a fluorochrome is a molecule that will become excited by the light of one wavelength.
Gene construct	Recombinant DNA containing a gene of interest surrounded by sequences engineered to promote a measure of its expression.
Gene map	Order of genes within a chromosome or entire genome.
Genotype	Genetic constitution, usually with reference to particular alleles at a locus.
Haploid	Half of a normal complement (i.e., 23 chromosomes).
Haploinsufficiency	Deletion or inactivation of one allele producing disease caused by inadequate activity of the remaining allele.
Hybrid gene	Fusion of two different genes as a result of a structural chromosomal rearrangement that functions as one transcriptional unit.
Hybridization	Method for rejoining (reannealing) complementary DNA or RNA strands.
Hyperdiploid	Additional chromosomes (e.g., 47 or 48 chromosomes).
Hypermetaphase FISH	Application of FISH to accumulated large number of metaphase cells.
Hypodiploid	Loss of chromosomes (e.g., 45 or 44 chromosomes).
I-FISH	Interphase fluorescence in situ hybridization, application of FISH to nondividing (resting) cells.
Interphase	Stage of mitosis in which the cell is not dividing.
Inversion	Structural chromosomal rearrangement as a result of two breaks occurring in the same chromosome. Paracentric inversion refers to both breaks occurring on the same side of the centromere. Pericentric inversion refers to breaks occurring on the opposite side of the centromere.
Isochromosome	Structural chromosomal rearrangement that consists of doubling of one of the two chromosome arms (connected by the centromere) and loss of the other arm.

Continued

TABLE 56.1 **Glossary of Cytogenetic, Fluorescence in Situ Hybridization and Genomic Terminology—cont'd**

Karyotype	Arrangement of metaphase chromosomes from a particular cell according to size and banding so that the largest chromosome is placed first and the smallest one last (see Fig. 56.2).
kb (kilobase)	Unit of DNA/RNA length = 1000 base pairs of DNA.
Kataegis	Kataegis is a recently discovered phenomenon in which multiple mutations cluster in a few hotspots in a genome. This region is often colocalized with regions of somatic genome rearrangements.
Locus	Unique location of a gene on a chromosome.
Locus (sequence)-specific probe (LSI)	Probe targeted to unique sequence region of the chromosome. Useful for localization of genes on normal chromosomes (gene mapping) and for detection of gene amplification, deletion, inversion, or translocation.
Marker chromosome	Chromosome whose morphology cannot be identified using banding method. Marker chromosomes are frequent in hematologic neoplasms.
M-FISH	Multicolor FISH karyotyping, which allows identification of 24 different human chromosomes (22 autosomes, and the X and Y chromosomes) (see text for details).
NGS	Next generation sequencing.
Nonsilent mutations	Mutations that alter the protein sequences.
Oncogene	Locus that is activated in association with tumor growth. One abnormal allele is sufficient to cause tumor formation or cancer.
SNP	Single nucleotide polymorphism.
Passenger mutation	Is usually a subclone and does not affect the biology of cell.
PCR	Polymerase chain reaction, by which individual gene segments are amplified through sequential cycles of polymerization, heat denaturation, and reannealing.
Pseudodiploid	Diploid number of chromosomes (46) accompanied by structural rearrangement.
Recurrent abnormality	Structural or numerical abnormality observed in multiple patients with the same or similar disease. Recurrent chromosome abnormalities in hematologic neoplasms have prognostic significance.
Telomeric probe	Used to detect repeated DNA sequences present at the end of the chromosome, which is called the telomere. Telomeric DNA contains 10–15 kb of TTAGGG repeats. Adjacent to the telomere is a region called the proximal subtelomeric region, and centromeric to it is a unique chromosome telomeric region. Chromosome-specific telomeric probes are useful for detection of cryptic translocations involving ends of chromosomes.
Translocation	Structural chromosome abnormality resulting from a break in at least two chromosomes with an exchange of material. In reciprocal or balanced translocation, no loss of chromosomal material occurs. In unbalanced translocation, loss of chromosomal DNA occurs.
Tumor suppressor gene	Locus that prevents tumor growth when at least one allele is functional. Loss of both alleles, first through constitutional and then through somatic mutation, is associated with tumor formation or cancer.
Whole chromosome painting probe (WCP)	Spans the entire length of chromosomal DNA sequences and, as the name implies, targets the entire length of DNA sequences. Useful for identification of complex or cryptic structural rearrangements as well as for identification of marker chromosomes.
Nomenclature	
p	= Short arm
q	= Long arm
+	When placed before the chromosome, denotes a gain of a whole chromosome (e.g., +8)
–	When placed before the chromosome, indicates a loss of a whole chromosome (e.g., –7); in rare situations, when placed after the chromosome, as in 5q–, indicates loss of a part of the long arms of chromosome 5
t	translocation
del	deletion
der	derivative
inv	inversion
i	isochromosome
mar	marker chromosome
con	connected
nuc ish	nuclear in situ hybridization
nuc ish 21q22 (D21S65X2)	two copies of D21S65 DNA segment on chromosome 21
nuc ish 9q34 (*ABL1* x2), 22q11.2 (*BCRx2*) (*ABL1* con *BCRx1*)	two *ABL* and two *BCR* loci, but one of each locus is juxtaposed on one chromosome as a result of t(9;22)

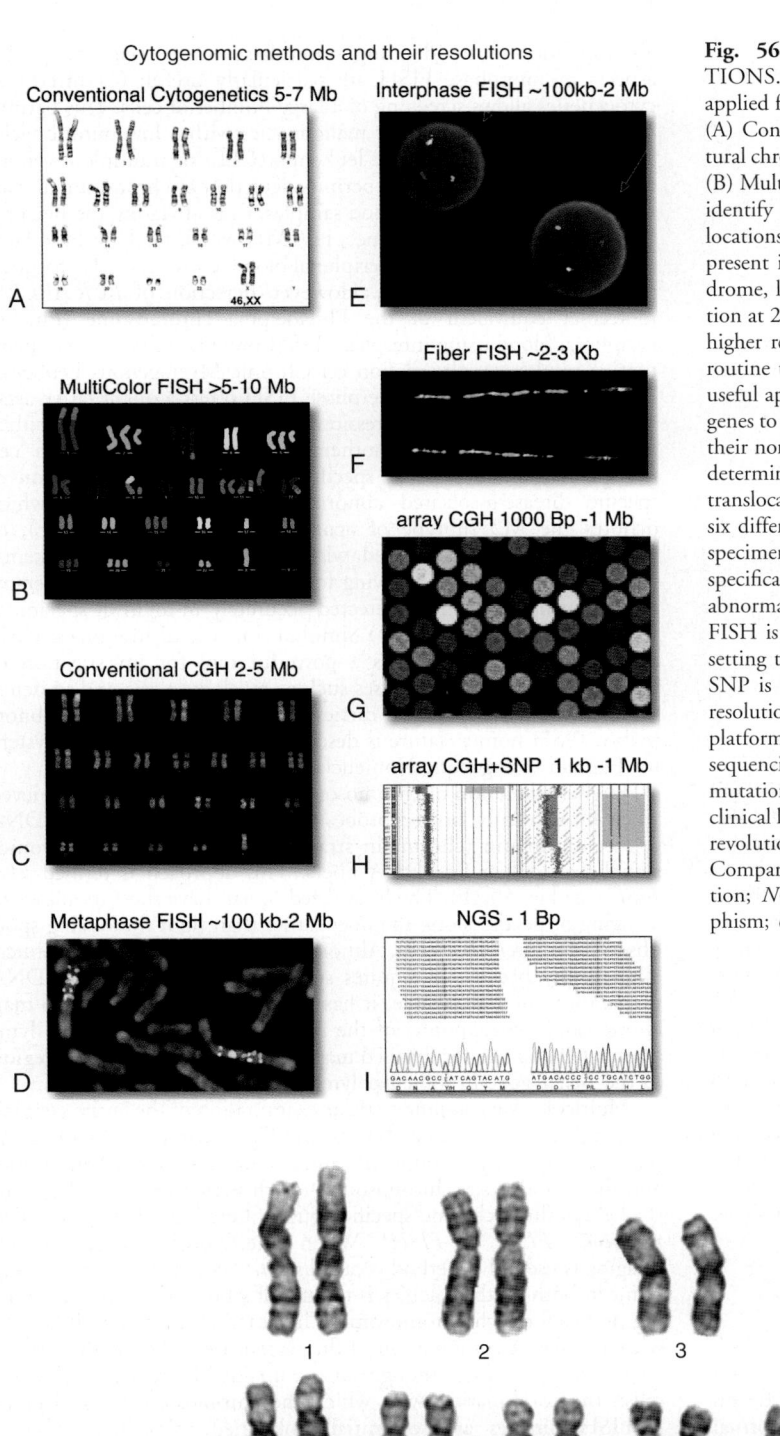

Cytogenomic methods and their resolutions

Conventional Cytogenetics 5-7 Mb

A   46,XX

MultiColor FISH >5-10 Mb

B

Conventional CGH 2-5 Mb

C

Metaphase FISH ~100 kb-2 Mb

D

Interphase FISH ~100kb-2 Mb

E

Fiber FISH ~2-3 Kb

F

array CGH 1000 Bp -1 Mb

G

array CGH+SNP 1 kb -1 Mb

H

NGS - 1 Bp

I

Fig. 56.1 CYTOGENOMIC METHODS AND THEIR RESOLU-TIONS. See text for detailed descriptions of how these methodologies are applied for detection of genomic abnormalities in hematologic malignancies. (A) Conventional cytogenetic methods detects clonal numerical and structural chromosomal abnormalities on a single-cell level, at the level of 5–7 Mb. (B) Multicolor FISH method with 24 different colors is specifically useful to identify the origin of marker chromosomes, complex 3- or more-way translocations, origin of ring chromosomes, and other chromosomal abnormalities present in a complex karyotype such as those seen in myelodysplastic syndrome, lymphoma, and multiple myeloma. (C) Conventional CGH resolution at 2–5 Mb is not used frequently because other technologies have much higher resolution for detection of smaller genomic abnormalities. (D) In a routine tumor cytogenomic laboratory metaphase FISH method has many useful applications. It is the best method for mapping normal and abnormal genes to human chromosomes and therefore localizes genes that have changed their normal positions as a result of multiple chromosomal abnormalities, to determine terminal vs. interstitial deletions as well as to detect cryptic translocations and deletions. (E) As mentioned in the text, there are at least six different reasons to perform interphase FISH on nondividing cells from specimens of patients with hematologic malignancies. Interphase FISH is specifically useful for detection of minimal-residual disease with a diagnostic abnormality has been determined by conventional cytogenetics. (F) Fiber FISH is also used primarily in fine mapping but much more in a research setting than in clinical laboratory. (G and H) Array CGH with or without SNP is the molecular method for detection of small DNA changes at the resolution of a few hundred base pairs to 1 Mb. Addition of SNP array platforms allows for detection of acquired regional UPD. (I) Next generation sequencing is the most powerful method for detection of acquired somatic mutation at the single nucleotide level. Although not yet used routinely in clinical laboratories, the application of NGS to hematologic malignancies has revolutionized the current knowledge of many leukemic entities. *CGH*, Comparative genomic hybridization; *FISH*, fluorescence in situ hybridization; *NGS*, next generation sequencing; *SNP*, single-nucleotide polymorphism; *UPD*, uniparental disomy.

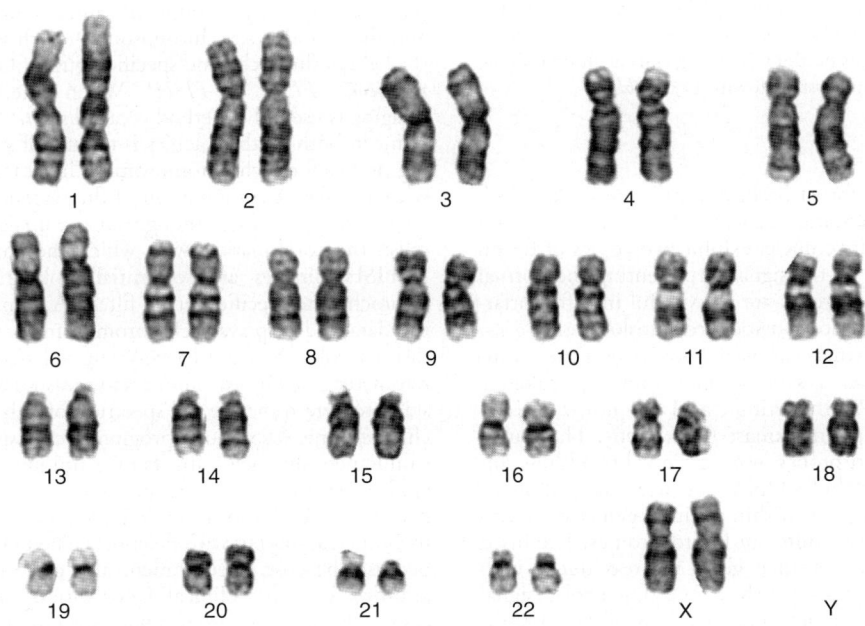

Fig. 56.2 NORMAL ARRANGEMENT OF CHROMOSOMES IN A KARYOTYPE FROM A BONE MARROW METAPHASE SHOWING A SLIGHTLY FUZZY MORPHOLOGY COMPARED WITH A NORMAL KARYOTYPE OBTAINED FROM PHYTOHEMAGGLUTININ-STIMULATED PERIPHERAL BLOOD CELLS.

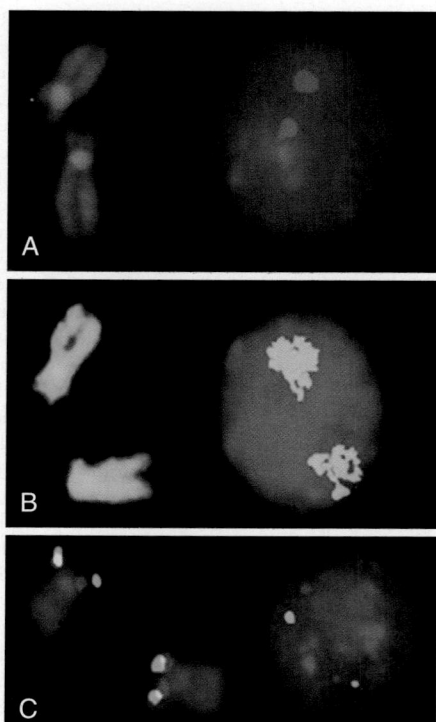

Fig. 56.3 TYPES OF CHROMOSOMAL PROBES (SEE TEXT FOR DETAILS). (A) Pair of chromosome 12 *(left)* and interphase cell *(right)* after fluorescence in situ hybridization (FISH) study with centromere enumeration probe (CEP) showing two hybridization signals *(red)* in the centromeric area of chromosome and two tight signals in interphase cell consistent with disomy (normal copy number). CEP probes are most useful for detection of numerical abnormalities. (B) Hybridization with a whole chromosome 8 painting probe showing the hybridization signal *(green)* along the length of the entire chromosome 8 *(left)* and hybridization domains in interphase cell *(right)*. Whole chromosome painting probes are useful for identifying unknown chromosomes in metaphase cells. (C) Target of locus-specific indicators are specific gene sequences such as P53 seen after hybridization as two small signals *(red)* on chromosome 17, band p13. The main applications of locus-specific indicator (LSI) probes are gene mapping, numerical enumeration in interphase cells, and detection of translocations. Telomeric probe, shown in green for the short arms of chromosome 17, are repetitive probes and are useful for detection of cryptic translocations involving ends of chromosomes. Chromosomes and nuclei are counterstained with DAPI *(blue)*.

translocation. The sequences for each chromosome are labeled with a specific color, and the translocation generates fused signals in both derivative chromosomes. Positive nuclei exhibit two copies of fusion signals and one copy of each of the signals representing the normal alleles. Dual-color/dual-fusion probes are very useful in differentiating various leukemia and lymphoma-associated translocations.

Multiple translocation partners are well known for genes commonly associated with leukemia such as mixed-lineage leukemia (*MLL*) now known as *KMT2A*, the retinoic acid receptor α (*RARA*) gene, and the anaplastic lymphoma kinase (*ALK*) gene. The fourth FISH strategy, with breakapart probes, was developed to address this issue. The breakapart probe includes DNA sequences mapped proximally and distally to the breakpoint within a critical gene (the 3′ end and the 5′ end) labeled with two different fluorochromes. The fused fluorescence signals represent a normal gene, whereas nuclei with rearrangements within the target gene show one single-color signal and one for each derivative chromosome, regardless of which chromosome is the partner in translocation.

One of the most significant advances in diagnostic leukemia cytogenetics has been the application of interphase FISH. Interphase cytogenetics is the term used to describe detection of chromosomal

abnormalities in nondividing, interphase nuclei (Fig. 56.5). Six aspects of interphase FISH are particularly useful: (1) Interphase cytogenetics allows screening of a large number of cells. This permits investigation of hematologic malignancies with a low mitotic yield, such as chronic lymphocytic leukemia (CLL) or multiple myeloma (MM). (2) Interphase FISH permits detection of chromosomal rearrangements in peripheral blood samples, thus obviating the need for marrow aspiration. For instance, in CML, which rarely yields a large number of dividing cells in peripheral blood, conventional cytogenetics usually is uninformative. However, detection of *BCR-ABL1*, a molecular equivalent of the Philadelphia chromosome (Ph), in peripheral blood using interphase FISH provides reliable, fast, quantitative results (see the section on Chronic Myelogenous Leukemia later in this chapter). (3) Interphase FISH offers a quantitative assay for monitoring disease progression or detection of minimal residual disease after ablative chemotherapy or hematopoietic stem cell transplantation. (4) Use of specific probe sets allows detection of specific disease-associated abnormalities such as t(8;21), which denotes the M2 subtype of acute myeloid leukemia (AML), or t(15;17), which is associated with acute promyelocytic leukemia (APL), within 4 hours, allowing for timely and appropriate therapy. (5) Abnormalities can be detected accurately in archival specimens stored for up to 15 years. (6) Simultaneous use of interphase FISH and immunophenotyping is a powerful tool for investigation of lineage involvement in diseases such as myelodysplasia and to determine which cell population carries the specific chromosome abnormality. FISH nomenclature is described in the International System for Human Cytogenetic Nomenclature.

Higher resolution of chromosomal abnormalities can be achieved when fluorescently labeled probes are hybridized to extended DNA or free chromatin (chromatin strands released from their chromosomal scaffold) or free DNA fibers. This approach is termed *fiber FISH* (see Fig. 56.1F). The hybridized signals have the appearance of a "string of pearls" along the fiber rather than tight fluorescing spots observed in interphase cells. Although fiber FISH has limited clinical applicability because it requires special techniques of target DNA preparation on a glass slide, it has been successfully applied to map chromosomal breakpoints of the *cyclin D* gene in mantle cell lymphoma (MCL) and for detailed mapping of the breakpoint site region in the *BCL2* gene in follicular lymphoma (FL).

Multicolor karyotyping permits examination of the entire genome in a single analysis (see Fig. 56.1B, and Fig. 56.6). In 1996 it became possible to identify 24 different human chromosomes (12 autosomes and the X and Y sex chromosomes), each with a unique color, with the help of fluorochrome-specific optical filters. This method is called *multicolor FISH (M-FISH)*. When interferometer-based spectral imaging is used, the method is called *spectral karyotyping*. The starting point in both methodologies is the use of whole chromosome painting probes for each chromosome. Thus each chromosome is labeled with a different combination of fluorescent dyes. The fluorochrome colors are not distinct enough for the unaided human eye to distinguish the combination with which the chromosome is labeled. In M-FISH, images are sequentially obtained using five different fluorochrome-specific optical filters. A computer program combines the data and displays each chromosome as if it were stained with a distinct color. Spectral karyotyping is based on the use of an interferometer (used by astronomers to measure the light spectra of distant stars) to determine the full spectrum of light emitted by each stained chromosome. A computer program then displays all the chromosomes simultaneously, each with its own unique color. These methods are applied with increasing frequency to resolve complex karyotypes, to detect cryptic translocations in patients with a normal karyotype, and to define karyotypes with deletions. Their clinical use may be limited because the cost of equipment and probes is beyond what can be afforded by most clinical laboratories. The M-FISH technology cannot be used to discriminate structural intrachromosomal rearrangements such as duplications, deletions, and inversions.

Although the mBAND technique helps to analyze peri- and paracentric inversions in chromosomes this technique has rarely been used in clinical laboratory practice and it remains a research tool.

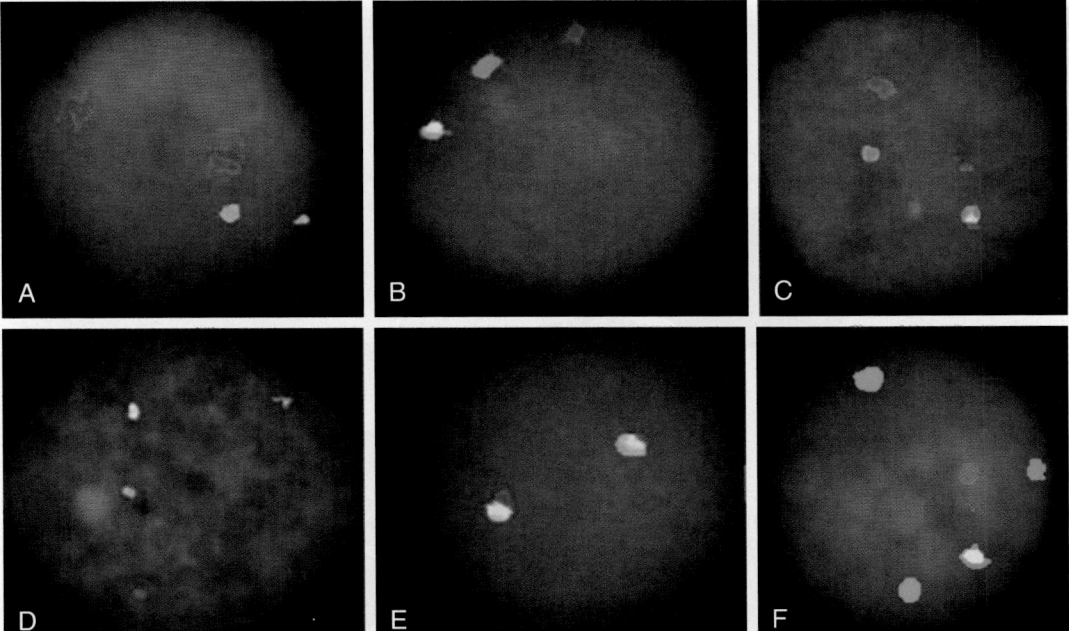

Fig. 56.4 FOUR DIFFERENT PROBE STRATEGIES FOR DETECTION OF CHROMOSOMAL TRANSLOCATIONS (SEE TEXT FOR DETAILS). (A) Normal cell after in situ hybridization with BCR *(green)* and ABL *(red)* showing a normal distribution of two red and two green single signals. (B) Conventional fusion strategy after in situ hybridization shows one fusion *(yellow)* signal representing derivative chromosome generated by the translocation and one single-color signal, red and green, for normal homologues in positive nuclei. (C) An extrasensitive fusion approach generates an extra small *(red)* signal, as well as a fusion signal *(yellow)* and one signal in single color *(green and red)* on normal homologues. (D) Dual-fusion strategy generates two fusion signals *(yellow)* on two derivative chromosomes and one single-color signal on each of two normal chromosomes. (E) Breakapart approach in a normal cell appears as two fusion signals *(yellow).* In this strategy, the 3′ end and the 5′ part of the gene are labeled in two colors. (F) When the rearrangement occurs, the normal chromosome shows co-localization of red and green *(yellow)* as a result of the proximity of the sequences on the chromosome, whereas abnormal derivative chromosomes each have one single red and single green signal, indicating that the rearrangement occurred between the two ends of the gene separating the green and red signals on two different chromosomes. The third-color probe *(blue)* can be used as an internal control (usually centromere enumeration probe) to determine the disomic number of chromosomes.

Comparative Genomic Hybridization and Next Generation Sequencing Methods

Another powerful method used for identifying the location of chromosomal gains, losses, deletions, or amplifications, without prior knowledge of the chromosomal target that may be altered, is comparative genomic hybridization (CGH) (see Fig. 56.1C). Briefly, isolated DNA from leukemic marrow or tumor tissue is labeled with a one-color fluorochrome (e.g., red), whereas DNA isolated from normal control tissue is labeled with a different color (e.g., green). These differently labeled DNAs are hybridized against each other in a competitive hybridization reaction onto normal metaphase spreads. Computer-assisted image analysis detects colors generated after hybridization, which indicate equal hybridization, relative excess, or deficiency of the target DNA (relative to control). The ratio of color intensity provides a "copy number" karyotype. Low resolution CGH, 5–10 Mb, has been successfully applied to study many leukemias, but its clinical use remains limited because it cannot detect balanced translocations, which are the hallmark of many hematologic malignancies. Nevertheless, CGH is an efficient approach to scanning the entire genome for variations in DNA copy number.

A particularly useful investigational approach is a "microchip array" in which labeled DNA or RNA from the sample of interest is hybridized with defined target sequences immobilized on a solid support. The advantage of this method is its ability to screen genes that are gained/amplified or deleted from the genome on a large scale

or, in the case of RNA, to learn whether such genes are expressed at a particular stage of disease. The first example of successful RNA application of the microchip array technique was the differentiation of AML from ALL based solely on gene expression. As shown in Fig. 56.1G, in the array CGH (aCGH) procedure, large-insert genomic clones, oligonucleotides, or single-nucleotide polymorphisms (SNPs) have replaced metaphase chromosomes used in the regular CGH. Array CGH is a higher-resolution CGH technology of approximately 5–50 kb, and provides diagnostic information for diseases associated with DNA dosage. It can also be used to discover previously unexpected sites of altered gene dosage associated with specific hematologic malignancy type. The concept of obtaining gene copy number from multiple genome locations in a single measurement has been used to characterize numerous hematologic malignancies over the last 15 years, and its clinical utility is demonstrated throughout this chapter. Nowadays, SNP arrays are also used that help to genotype few hundred to millions of SNPs to detect rare and common genomic rearrangements (see Fig. 56.1H). These arrays require hybridization of only the test sample onto the array, unlike aCGH, which relies on co-hybridization of test and reference DNA. At this time aCGH + SNP are frequently used together in one study. The most advanced genomic technologies currently known is the next generation sequencing or NGS (see Fig. 56.1I). Also known as massively parallel sequencing, these approaches use a range of techniques that enable sequencing of hundreds of thousands of nucleic acid molecules simultaneously. In order of complexity, these approaches include sequencing of gene panels, exome sequencing (protein-coding genes),

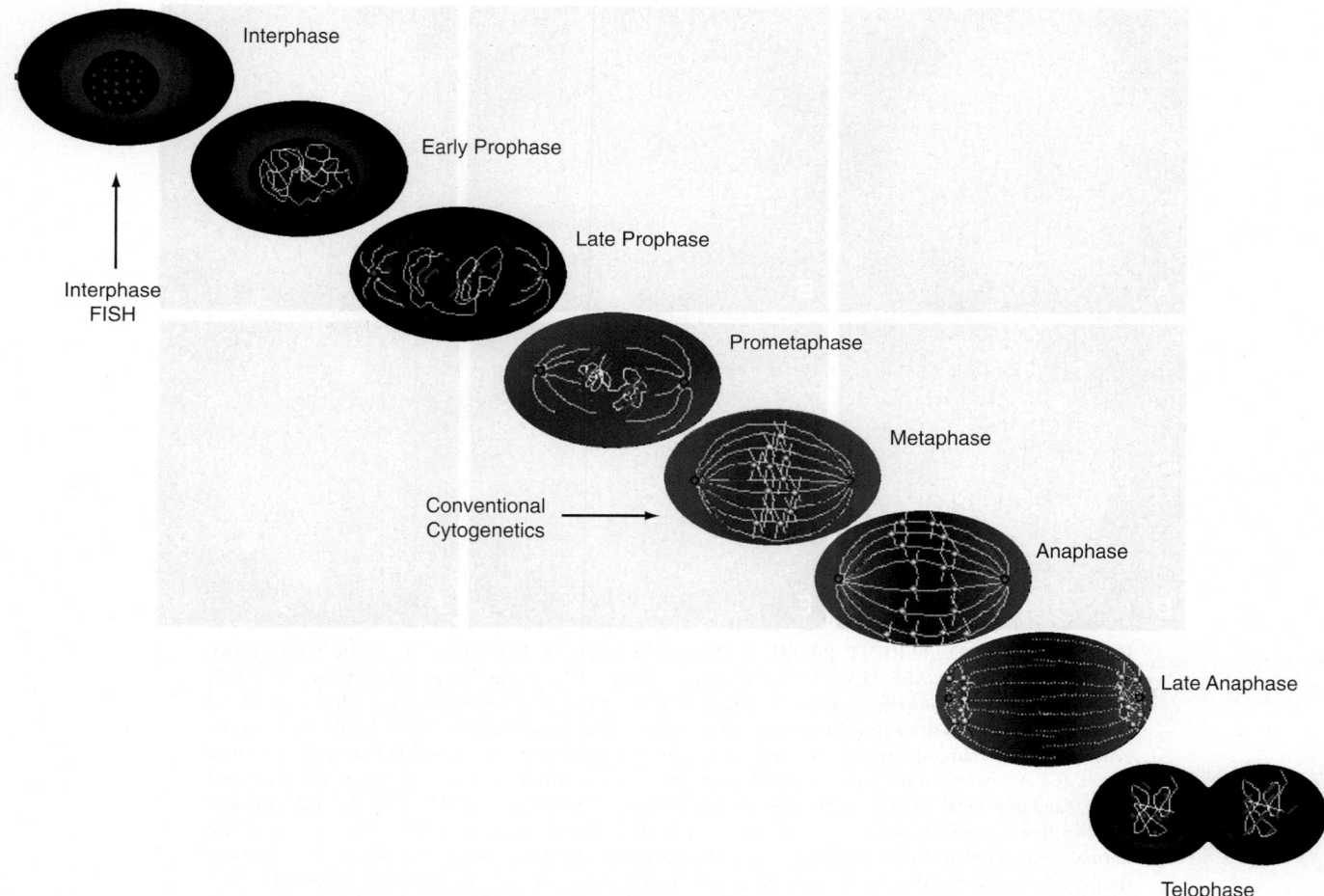

Fig. 56.5 SCHEMATIC REPRESENTATION OF CELL DIVISION. Most clinical FISH studies are performed on nondividing interphase cells, whereas conventional cytogenetics is performed at the metaphase stage of cell division. *(Courtesy Dr. Ari Melnik, Cornell Medical Center, New York.)*

transcriptome (expressed RNA), and sequencing the whole genome (WGS). These techniques have several arrays of several hundred thousand sequencing templates in parallel generating up to several hundred million short reads of DNA sequence per lane. The basic principle of NGS methods involves a process of DNA fragmentation, adapter ligation and immobilization of the fragments via the adapters to create libraries. The libraries then undergo a process of amplification, generating multiple copies of each DNA fragment which are then sequenced in parallel by a fluorescence- or chemiluminescence-based method, yielding billions of short sequence reads. These reads are then aligned to the human reference genome and highly efficient algorithms are used to perform the mapping of these complex genomes. Because of its cost effectiveness and enormous sequencing capacity, NGS is gradually changing the scenario of hematologic malignancy research by discovering disease-causing mutations, identifying novel drug targets, and implementing therapeutic individualization. Exome sequencing is a relatively inexpensive approach to identify protein-coding mutations, but has a major limitation in identifying structural genetic rearrangements, deletions and insertions of DNA, a hallmark of many hematologic malignancies. Exome sequencing is performed at a depth of 100–200-fold coverage of the haploid genome, which enables detection of mutations present in leukemic subclones, which is important in a study of relapse. Transcriptome sequencing involves sequencing of genes actively expressed and can be adjusted to selectively study RNA transcripts that encode proteins (mRNA), transcripts regardless of coding potential (RNA) or a variety of small and noncoding RNA transcripts. RNA sequencing is a highly informative approach and enables identification of

chromosomal rearrangements that result in the expression of chimeric fusion genes and sequence mutation detection. WGS usually involves sequencing leukemic and nonleukemic DNA of an individual. Although it is the most comprehensive modality, WGS may not identify all genetic alterations caused by variation in sequence coverage and difficulties in sequencing complex and GC-rich regions of the genome (including gene promoters).

These modern cytogenomic methods have increased the resolution at which chromosomal and gene rearrangements can be identified. Whereas in conventional cytogenetics the targets are whole chromosomes in metaphase spreads at a resolution of approximately 5 Mb, molecular cytogenetics methods may be used to analyze interphase nuclei at a resolution of 50 kb to 2 Mb or fiber FISH analysis of chromatin strands at a resolution of 5–500 kb. Moreover, the current resolution of aCGH is restricted only by clone size and by the density of clones on the array, some of which may contain resolution at the level of a single nucleotide.

Conventional cytogenetics, FISH, and aCGH along with NGS are complementary. Each has its own advantages and limitations in investigating genomic rearrangements of malignant cells. Although conventional cytogenetics is the comprehensive study of all chromosomes, it requires a large number of dividing cells, which, in some diseases, such as myelofibrosis, is difficult to obtain. Furthermore, many small deletions or structural rearrangements are beyond the microscopic level of detection. FISH is to be used in conjunction with conventional cytogenetics with both interphase and metaphase cells. It is a more sensitive method and detects rearrangements smaller than 1 kb. The main disadvantage of interphase FISH is that it

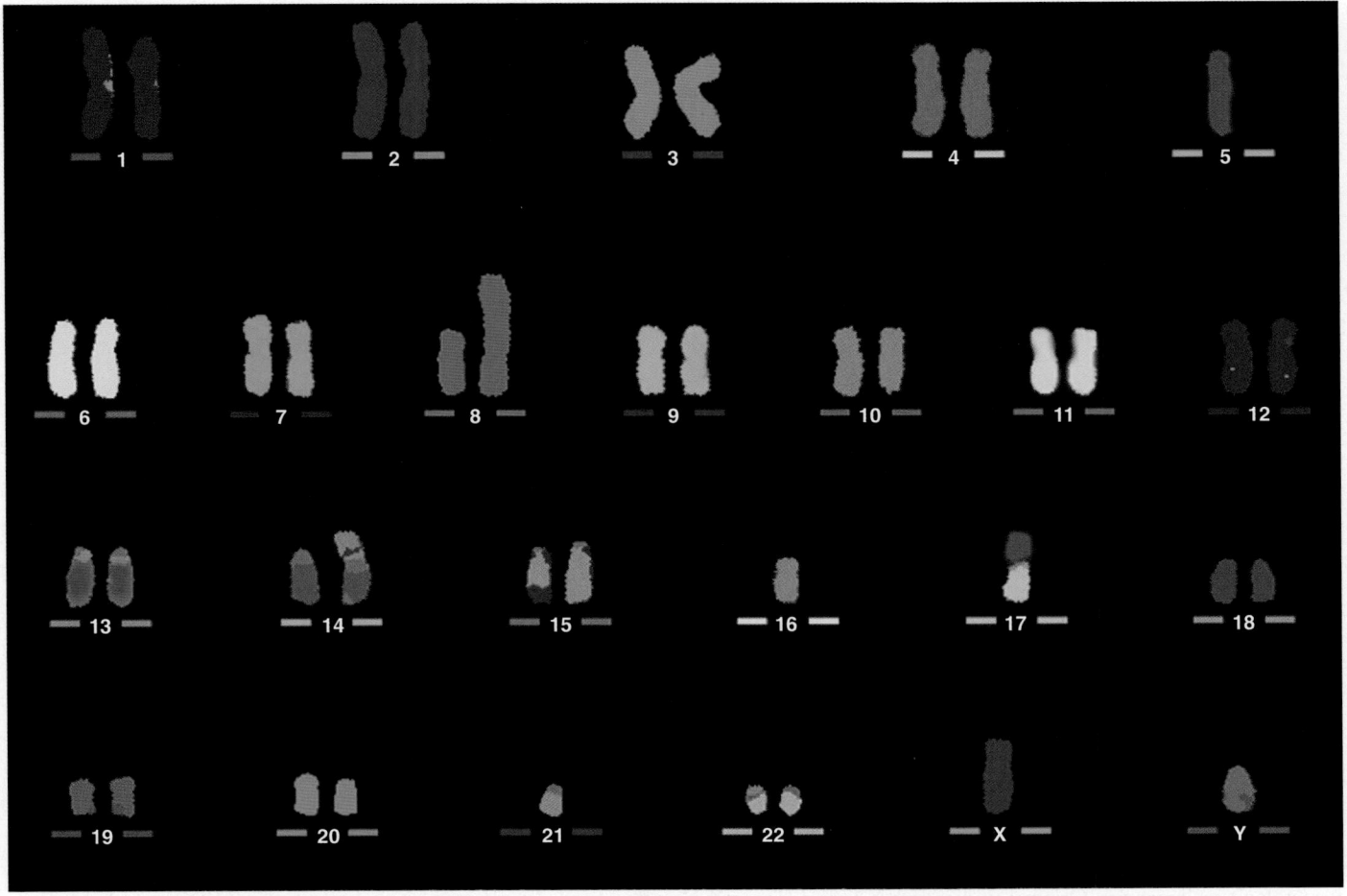

Fig. 56.6 Multicolor metaphase FISH of a bone marrow cell from a patient with myelodysplastic syndrome documenting 43,XY, −5, der(8)t(8;8)(p23;q11.2), der(14;16)(p12;p11.1), inv(15)(q21;q24), der(17)t(5;17) (p13;p13), −21 karyotype. The origin of t(8;8) and der(14;16) could not have been determined by conventional cytogenetic study alone.

cannot be used unless a known abnormality is suspected. When the abnormality is known, interphase FISH identify the clonal aberration at the single-cell level. Because of higher resolution and genome-wide analysis combined aCGH + SNP provides information of genomic changes in patients with a normal karyotype as well as acquired loss of heterozygosity, both important as a prognostic and a predictive tool. With the introduction of high throughput genomic technologies such as NGS, FISH-based chromosome level detection has gradually changed focus to genome-wide detection of single nucleotide and copy number variants that are common in leukemia. It is evident that identification of chromosomal aberrations by molecular cytogenomic techniques is important in detecting novel chromosomal rearrangements and genes involved in leukemogenesis Understanding the basis of these techniques and their application is critical in the accurate diagnosis of hematologic malignancies.

Clonal Origin of Leukemia

The question of whether cell proliferation is monoclonal or polyclonal is fundamental to understanding the underlying etiology of hematologic malignancies. Markers of clonality are used to determine the origin of disease; to differentiate malignant from nonmalignant populations; to establish hematopoietic hierarchy, clonal evolution, and clonal remission; and to delineate steps involved in the multistep pathogenesis of hematologic malignancies.

The clonal origin of leukemias and lymphomas can be assessed by either intrinsic or extrinsic cellular markers. Intrinsic cellular markers

are specific for a cell population, arising either during normal differentiation or as a part of disease process. For instance, cell surface-associated immunoglobulin (Ig) markers such as the λ or κ light chain or idiotypes and T-cell receptors (TCRs) can be useful for evaluating lymphoid diseases. Application of *IgH* markers demonstrated for the first time that MM was of clonal origin. Somatic cytogenetic alterations are useful intrinsic markers for identifying abnormal clones and following disease progression. Thus the observation of identical chromosome anomalies in different cells of the same tumor is evidence of clonality. Since the discovery of the Ph in 1960 it has been well established that nonrandom, recurrent chromosomal abnormalities characterize many hematopoietic malignancies. The finding of the Ph in different CML-derived hematopoietic cell lineages led to the hypothesis that CML originates in a single precursor cell that has a clonal development pattern. Moreover, the presence of additional recurrent chromosomal abnormalities in the Ph-positive clone (such as trisomy 8, duplication of the Ph, or trisomy 19) not only indicates the clinical progression of the disease to accelerated phase or blast crisis, but also demonstrates the subclonal evolution of the Ph-positive clone. Currently, disease-associated somatic genomic mutations, such as rearrangements of *KMT2A (MLL)*, runt-related transcription factor gene (*RUNX1*), *ETV6, PML-RARA*, and many others, can be identified by polymerase chain reaction (PCR)–based assays, FISH assay, and novel aCGH and NGS technologies, and may serve, with or without conventional cytogenetics, as intrinsic markers of disease processes.

On the other hand, extrinsic marker systems use cellular mosaicism that is completely independent of the disease being studied and

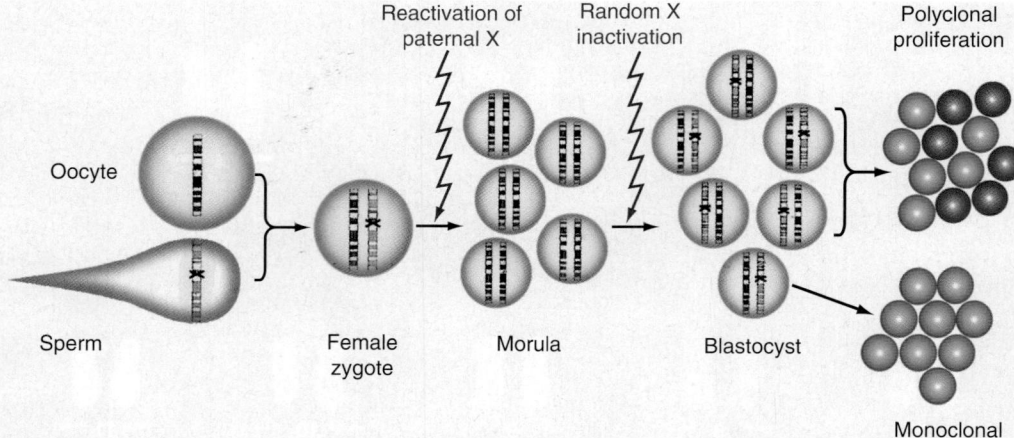

Fig. 56.7 X-CHROMOSOME–LINKED ENZYME GLUCOSE-6-PHOSPHATE DEHYDROGENASE (G6PD) AS A MARKER TO INVESTIGATE CLONAL DEVELOPMENT OF HUMAN HEMATOPOIETIC DISORDERS. Early in embryogenesis, regions of all but one X chromosome are inactivated in each cell containing two or more X chromosomes. The choice of maternal versus paternal X chromosome for inactivation is random. Once the inactivation occurs, it is fixed and is stably transmitted to daughter cells during mitosis (Lyon hypothesis). Females who are heterozygous for the common B type and the less frequent A type, G6PD (localized on Xq27), are mosaic. This cellular mosaicism is used to study monoclonal versus polyclonal cell proliferation and development of malignant hematopoietic diseases. *(Courtesy Dr. W Raskind, University of Washington, Seattle.)*

is not restricted to the cell lineages. Individuals with Turner or Klinefelter syndrome are mosaic for XX or XY and monosomy X cells or XXY and XY cells, respectively. The mosaicism created by X-chromosome inactivation in females is much more widely applicable and has provided fundamental insights into the pathogenesis of hematologic malignancies. Original studies with X-linked glucose-6-phospate dehydrogenase (G6PD) as a marker of clonality were based on the Lyon hypothesis, which asserts that early in embryogenesis, one X chromosome in females is inactivated in somatic cells and the activation status is stably transmitted to daughter cells during mitosis (Fig. 56.7). The choice of maternal versus paternal X-chromosome inactivation is random; however, once it occurs, it is maintained in all daughter cells. Random X inactivation occurs by embryonic day 6.5 around the start of gastrulation and results in a mosaic pattern that characterizes adult females. Therefore an adult female is a mosaic for two-cell populations, one expressing genes from an active X chromosome and the other expressing genes from the inactive X chromosome. Incidentally, mammalian X-chromosome inactivation is a mechanism that equalizes the dosage of X-linked genes between sexes. Although the exact mechanism of X-chromosome inactivation remains to be elucidated, the process of X inactivation starts with methylation of CpG islands. The inactivation process is believed to occur before differentiation of the embryonic stem cell into various cell lineages. Hematopoietic cells do not originate from a single embryonic stem cell but from several progenitors, thereby allowing for gene expression from both X chromosomes.

The observation that human females are heterozygous for the G6PD variant A and A⁻ and that two mosaic cell populations may be distinguishable by electrophoretic mobility was reported in the 1960s. The X-inactivation G6PD mosaic system was then applied to the study of clonality in human tumors (uterine leiomyomas) in 1964 by Gartler and Linden. In females who are heterozygous for the G6PD polymorphism and have malignant hematologic disorders such as CML, the finding of a single G6PD type in marrow or blood cells and both the A and B type G6PD in tissues not involved by the malignant process demonstrated that CML was of clonal origin and provided evidence that the malignant transformation occurred at the level of a stem cell common to most hematopoietic cell lineages. Additional studies with heterozygous G6PD females who had CML demonstrated that some CML-derived B lymphocytes had a single

G6PD type, but these clonal cells were Ph-negative; thus leukemic transformation predates development of the chromosomal abnormality. This observation provided evidence that CML has a multistep pathogenesis. Application of G6PD studies to hematologic malignancies demonstrated the clonal and stem cell origin for AML, ALL, Ph-negative myeloproliferative neoplasm (MPN), myelodysplastic syndrome (MDS), and CLL. G6PD studies were particularly useful in the investigation of red blood cells and platelets in hematologic malignancies because the absence of nuclei in these cells means they cannot be studied by cytogenetics or DNA analysis. Although it is now considered common knowledge that hematologic malignancies are characterized by clonal development, this understanding is greatly owing to what is now known as classic Fialkow's work, whose profound insight contributed much to current concepts and understanding.

Despite the importance of the G6PD approach, it is limited by the rarity of females who are heterozygous for the G6PD isoenzyme. An alternative and more extensive DNA-based X-chromosome clonal assay uses common polymorphic markers that are caused by changes in DNA methylation patterns that accompany inactivation of the X chromosome. These X-linked loci, such as phosphoglycerine kinase, hypoxanthine phosphoribosyltransferase, DXS25 (M27β), and human androgen receptor (HUMARA), have been subsequently extensively used in assessment of clonality, and now it is possible to identify clonal cell populations in virtually all females. DNA-based marker systems rely on a sequence polymorphism that has adjacent differences in methylation on the active and inactive X chromosomes. The inactive X chromosome is more highly methylated than its active homologue, but this is only true for certain regions of genes as 10% to 20% of X-linked genes escape inactivation and can be found both in clusters and in isolation. The most widely used HUMARA assay appears to maintain the stringent methylation differences. The number of CAG tandem repeats differentiates the maternal from the paternal X chromosome.

The DNA-based X-chromosome clonal assay is limited to females younger than 60 years because they usually have 1:1 distribution of two-mosaic–cell population. A ratio greater than 3:1 is found in women older than 60 years, probably as a result of stem cell kinetics influenced by X-linked genetic factors. When the ratio of two cell populations is greater than 3:1, this phenomenon is called a *skewed X-inactivation pattern*. With the HUMARA assay, acquired unequal or skewed X-chromosome inactivation (excessive lyonization) is found in 35% to 40% of women older than 60 years. Thus X-chromosome–based clonality studies must incorporate age-matched controls. Despite the enormous contribution of clonality assays to the understanding of disease processes, they are usually performed in research investigations and are rarely used as diagnostic tools.

More recently acquired somatic mutations are detected using NGS, also known as high-throughput sequencing, the catch-all term used to describe a number of different modern sequencing technologies whereby millions of small fragments of DNA can be sequenced at the same time, creating a massive pool of data. This pool of data can reach gigabites in size, which is the equivalent of 1 billion (1,000,000,000) base pairs of DNA.

Although NGS makes genome sequences handy, the data analysis and biologic explanations are still the bottle-neck in understanding leukemic genomes.

In Utero Mutations and Clonal Origin

The observation that monozygotic twins share identical but nonconstitutive and clone-specific fusion gene sequences (e.g., *ETV6-RUNX1*) in pediatric ALL provided the first unambiguous evidence (in 2003) that genetic lesions, generated by chromosomal translocation, arise in utero. These sophisticated series of studies initiated by Mel Greaves and his colleagues at the Institute for Cancer Research in London, have contributed for the past 13 years to a wealth of knowledge about founder mutations, subclonal development, clonal origin, and the evolution of disease. The initiating lesion and premalignant clone is shared by the twins as a consequence of intraplacental vascular anastomoses and blood cell chimerism. The twin data are endorsed by backtracking of prenatal-initiating genetic lesions in the archived blood spots, or Guthrie cards, of patients with ALL. These data were interpreted to suggest that *ETV6-RUNX1* is likely to be a critical initiating lesion for *ETV6-RUNX1*–positive ALL. However, such fusions are detectable in cord blood from newborn infants at rates approximately 100-fold higher than the incidence of ALL, suggesting an obligatory requirement for additional mutations in leukemia development. Over a period of 10 years these results were confirmed and in utero origin of *MLL*, *BCR-ABL1*, and *RUNX1-RUNXT1* fusion rearrangements were documented, providing direct evidence for a prenatal origin of many childhood leukemias.

Results from genome sequencing of *ETV6-RUNX1* fusion region suggests it arises as a consequence of nonhomologous end-joining in the pro-B cell stage with possible self-renewal capacity to downstream B-cell precursors. Additional evidence was provided by screening for trisomies in stored cord blood and the data indicated that ~6% of enriched CD34$^+$/CD19$^+$ B lineage progenitors carry trisomies frequently seen in hyperdiploid childhood ALL. With novel SNP and other technologies, it has become apparent that ALL has multiple genome copy number variations (CNVs), mostly deletions and these CNVs are distinctive between a pair of twins, indicating a secondary, postnatal origin.[1]

When genotyping sequencing combined with other molecular technologies of five pairs of monozygotic twins with concordant *ETV6-RUNX1*-positive ALL, Greaves and his colleagues demonstrated that all recurrent CNVs (32 in total) were different within twin pairs providing strong evidence that they are probably secondary mutations and postnatal in origin in both twins as well as in nontwins with ALL. Another two twin pairs who shared a monochromaric placenta and had Ph-positive ALL, also studied by Greaves and his colleagues, provided confirmation for the previous observation that *BCR-ABL1* is not sufficient to cause Ph- positive leukemia. Twin A presented with ALL at age 3.8 years and twin B presented at age 4.1 years. Both had an identical *BCR-ABL1* fusion transcript and both received an allogeneic stem cell transplantation from the same human leukocyte antigen (HLA) identical sibling donor but 7 months later twin B died whereas twin A is in good health 8 years following the transplantation. SNP analysis revealed that twin A had a subclone with trisomies for chromosomes 4, 6, 9, 14, 17, and X, tetrasomy 21,

and a gain of 22q11.1–q11.23 region, whereas twin B had deletions of *EBF1* and *IKZ1*. These genotyping results provide direct evidence that rearrangements additional to *BCR-ABL1* are obviously postnatal in origin, they represent a subclonal evolution, and *BCR-ABL1* by itself is not sufficient for development of Ph-positive ALL.

These mutation-driven natural history studies provide evidence for sequential multistep pathogenesis with sequential accumulation of genetic changes, which may be linear through clonal succession as originally proposed by Peter Nowell in 1976, but as Greaves indicated, clonal evolution in most leukemia is rather complex and may represent also a branching structure, as predicted by Darwin.[2]

EARLY MUTATIONS IN LEUKEMOGENESIS AND AGE-RELATED CLONAL HEMATOPOIESIS

As indicated earlier and throughout the chapter, the progress of high-throughput sequencing has provided novel observations in the current understanding of the initial mutations in premalignant stem cells and the clonal development through the accumulation of genetic changes. For example, the evolving concept of the clonal origin of AML involves the mutation in the gene encoding DNA methyltransferase 3A, *DNMT3*.[3] Approximately 22% of patients with AML have a mutation in *DNMT3* gene, localized on the short arms of human chromosome 2, 2p23. However, mutations of this gene are also described in other myeloid malignancies as well as in T cell leukemia/lymphoma. Deep sequencing of patients with AML showed that *DNMT3* mutations are typically found at higher frequencies than other accompanied mutations in AML, such as *NPM1*, *FLT3* or others, suggesting that they were among the first to arise. Two studies demonstrated that patients with AML and *DNMT3* mutations had the same mutation in T and B lymphocytes, indicating that in these patients the mutation had occurred in a primordial cell giving rise to all hematopoietic lineages, which may represent a "founder" clone population from which the AML leukemic population expands. Co-occurrence of *DNMT3* mutations in patients with chromosomal abnormalities such as t(15;17), inv(16), and t(8;21) (see later in the chapter) have not been described. In sharp contrast, approximately 60% of patients with *DNMT3* mutation also carry an *NPM1* mutation whereas only 13% of the patients with the wild type *DNMT3* carry *NPM1* mutations. These patterns imply a temporal acquisition of mutations in AML. Collectively these and other observations indicate that the *DNMT3* mutation is a primary mutation in premalignant stem cell whereas *NPM1* and *FLT3* are common secondary mutations in more differentiated cells that lead to an acute phase of disease, and combined, they may represent a distinct AML entity. It has been further documented that *DNMT3* mutant hematopoietic stem cells and their differentiated progeny persisted in the peripheral blood of these patients even when their AML is in remission following chemotherapy, indicating that at least some of these preleukemic ancestral cells are resistant to treatment. These studies have significant implications for the development of targeted therapies.

Clonal mosaicism for large chromosomal anomalies (duplications, deletions, and uniparental disomy [UPD]) using SNP microarray data from 50,000 subjects in the GENEVA study determined that clonal hematopoiesis is infrequent (<0.5%) from birth until 50 years of age after its frequency rapidly increases to 2% to 3% in the elderly. It has been estimated that individuals with clonal hematopoiesis have 10-fold higher risk of a subsequent hematologic malignancy. These age-related mutations were confirmed by analysis of mutation acquisition in hematopoietic stem cells, over time, through whole-exome sequencing of single hematopoietic stem cell-derived colonies, which showed that the total number of mutations in healthy individual stem cells increases with age. Moreover, sequencing of multiple elderly women provided evidence of clonal hematopoiesis based on X inactivation pattern and recurrent somatic mutation in *TET2* gene. Subsequent analysis of 182 additional elderly women with clonal hematopoiesis determined that more than 5% of these individuals had mutations in *TET2*. Most recent reports by Ebbert and his colleagues in USA on 17,182 persons and by Cross and his colleagues in UK, suggests that peripheral blood of normal individuals showed clonal mutations in 9.5% of individuals between 70 and 79 years of age, 11.7% in individuals between 80 and 89 years of age and in 18.4% of individuals between 90 and 103 years of age. As in previous studies of healthy individuals, the majority of the mutations were in three genes, *DNMT3*, *TET2* and *ASXL1*, all known to occur in myeloid malignancies. The presence of mutations in these three genes is associated with an increase in the risk of hematologic malignancy.[3] However, individuals with clonal hematopoiesis may live for many years and decades without hematologic malignancies though they are at increased risk as compared with those without mutations. These studies may explain the higher frequency of myeloid malignancies in the elderly population.

CHRONIC MYELOPROLIFERATIVE NEOPLASMS

The World Health Organization (WHO) characterizes MPNs as clonal stem cell disorders. CML has a unique place among hematologic malignancies and is described separately from the other Ph-negative MPNs.

Chronic Myelogenous Leukemia (see Chapter 67)

Knowledge of the origins of CML has accumulated over the last 56 years and serves as a classic example of molecular medicine at its best (Table 56.2). The Ph chromosome is the first example of a specific chromosomal abnormality associated with a malignant disease.[4-5] *ABL1* and *BCR* genes are the first oncogenes localized at the site of a chromosomal breakpoint in t(9;22)(q34;q11.2). The *BCR-ABL1* fusion leads to a "hybrid" gene, resulting in the production of a dysregulated tyrosine kinase protein. Finally, imatinib mesylate, a specific tyrosine kinase inhibitor (TKI), was the first rationally designed targeted form of cancer therapy.

The Ph chromosome, named in honor of Philadelphia, the city of its discovery, was described for the first time in 1960. It represents a signature genomic rearrangement occurring in more than 95% of patients with CML. Approximately 3% of all pediatric leukemias are Ph-positive CML. The incidence in children increases with age and it is exceptionally rare in infants. The Ph chromosome results from a balanced translocation t(9;22)(q34;q11.2) (Fig. 56.8A–B). The Ph chromosome arises postzygotically, being found only in hematopoietic tissue. The findings of the Ph chromosome in myeloid cells, erythroid cells, eosinophils, monocytes/macrophages, basophils, and B lymphocytes, along with the absence of the Ph chromosome in cultured marrow fibroblasts, support the concept that the Ph chromosome results from a specific rearrangement in a multipotent hematopoietic stem cell and that it is an acquired rather than an inherited abnormality. Of interest, the Ph chromosome is rarely identified in T cells. T lymphocytes are long-lived cells and may antedate the development of CML. These observations combined with studies exploiting G6PD heterozygosity provide further evidence for the concept that CML is a clonal disease arising in a stem cell capable of differentiation into all hematopoietic cell lineages.

In a review of 1129 Ph-positive patients, the 9;22 translocation was identified in 1036 (92%) cases. Karyotypic analysis of marrow cells in patients with CML is a time-consuming task. However, it

TABLE 56.2	History of Discovery of Philadelphia Chromosome and BCR-ABL1 Fusion
1960	Philadelphia chromosome (Ph) is identified.
1973	Ph is t(9;22)(q34;q11.2).
1983	*ABL1* is translocated from chromosome 9 to chromosome 22.
1984	*BCR* is localized to 22q11.
1987	Ph' is *BCR-ABL1* fusion.

demonstrates not only the presence of the Ph chromosome but also the presence of other chromosomal rearrangements (clonal evolution) of clinical significance.

The reciprocal nature of the Ph-positive translocation was confirmed when studies showed that its molecular consequence is the translocation of the *ABL1* gene from chromosome 9, band region q34, and subsequent fusion to the breakpoint cluster region (*BCR*) gene on chromosome 22, band q11.2 (Fig. 56.9). This creates a hybrid *BCR-ABL1* gene that is transcribed into a chimeric BCR-ABL1 messenger RNA (mRNA) and translated into a specific chimeric protein.

Three major breakpoint locations along the *BCR* gene on chromosome 22 result in three chimeric proteins. They include P210$^{BCR-ABL1}$, P190$^{BCR-ABL1}$, and P230$^{BCR-ABL1}$ and are associated with three distinct types of leukemia. P210$^{BCR-ABL}$ is found in the majority of patients with classic Ph-positive, *BCR-ABL1*-fusion–positive CML and approximately 30% of patients with Ph-positive ALL. Expression of P190$^{BCR-ABL1}$ is seen in 20% to 30% of adults and 80% of children with Ph-positive ALL. Expression of P230$^{BCR-ABL1}$ is associated with a rare indolent chronic neutrophilic leukemia variant and up to 1.6% of CML (approximately 50 patients in the worldwide literature have been described). Approximately 1% to 2% of Ph-positive patients with CML express both P21$^{BCR-ABL1}$ and P190$^{BCR-ABL1}$ and their response to TKI therapy is inferior to patients showing only P210$^{BCR-ABL1}$. The *BCR-ABL1* fusion is present in both standard and variant forms, in cases where chromosome 9 involvement is cytogenetically not detectable, and when a masked Ph is present. In the majority of patients, the fusion of *ABL1* and *BCR* takes place on chromosome 22 (Fig. 56.10 A–B). However, in a small group of patients the *BCR* gene is translocated to chromosome 9, and the fusion of the two genes is localized to 9q34. The prognosis of these patients may be inferior, but the number of reports is too small for a definitive conclusion. The *BCR-ABL1* fusion transcript is present in neutrophils, monocytes, eosinophils, erythrocytes, B cells, rarely in T cells, and in CD34$^+$ cells and is associated with increased proliferation of CD34$^+$ myeloid progenitor cells but not of other more mature myeloid precursors. These observations confirm the hypothesis that CML originates in a multipotent stem cell capable of differentiating to all hematopoietic cell lineages with the exception of T cells. These and other studies provide also evidence for the existence of clonal *BCR-ABL1* fusion-negative stage. The formation of *BCR-ABL1* and the Ph chromosome occurs in an already abnormal and genetically unstable clone of pluripotent hematopoietic cells. Thus it is the preexisting genetic instability that predisposes to formation of *BCR-ABL1* and in Ph[6] chromosome. Once Ph chromosome formation occurs, it confers a further selective growth advantage over normal cells, resulting in overwhelming *BCR-ABL1*–positive, Ph-positive marrow cells at the time of diagnosis of CML.

In the 5% of patients with CML who are Ph-negative by cytogenetic studies, clonal and stem cell origin of these hematologic malignancies can still be demonstrated, and molecular analysis reveals the *BCR-ABL1* fusion in approximately 2% to 3% of these patients (Fig. 56.11). In the majority of Ph-negative patients, an *ABL1* insertion from chromosome 9 to 22q11.2 results in a *BCR-ABL1*–fusion product without reciprocal translocation of sequences from chromosome 22 to chromosome 9. Approximately 2% of patients truly are Ph-negative and *BCR-ABL* fusion-negative. These patients may not have CML but rather another MPN. The concept that the *BCR-ABL1* fusion plays a central role in the pathogenesis of CML is strongly supported by two lines of evidence: (a) retroviral transduction experiments in which P210$^{BCR-ABL1}$ is expressed in murine marrow cells, resulting in a myeloproliferative disorder (MPD) resembling CML, and (b) the fact that imatinib, a TKI, selectively inhibits the BCR-ABL1 fusion protein in mice and specifically inhibits the growth of human Ph-positive cells in vitro and in vivo. Although considered necessary, *BCR-ABL1* may not be initial or sufficient to cause the malignant transformation resulting in CML (see earlier clonal origin section).

Genomic PCR analysis can determine the exact breakpoints of DNA fusion products. Reverse transcriptase PCR (RT-PCR) and

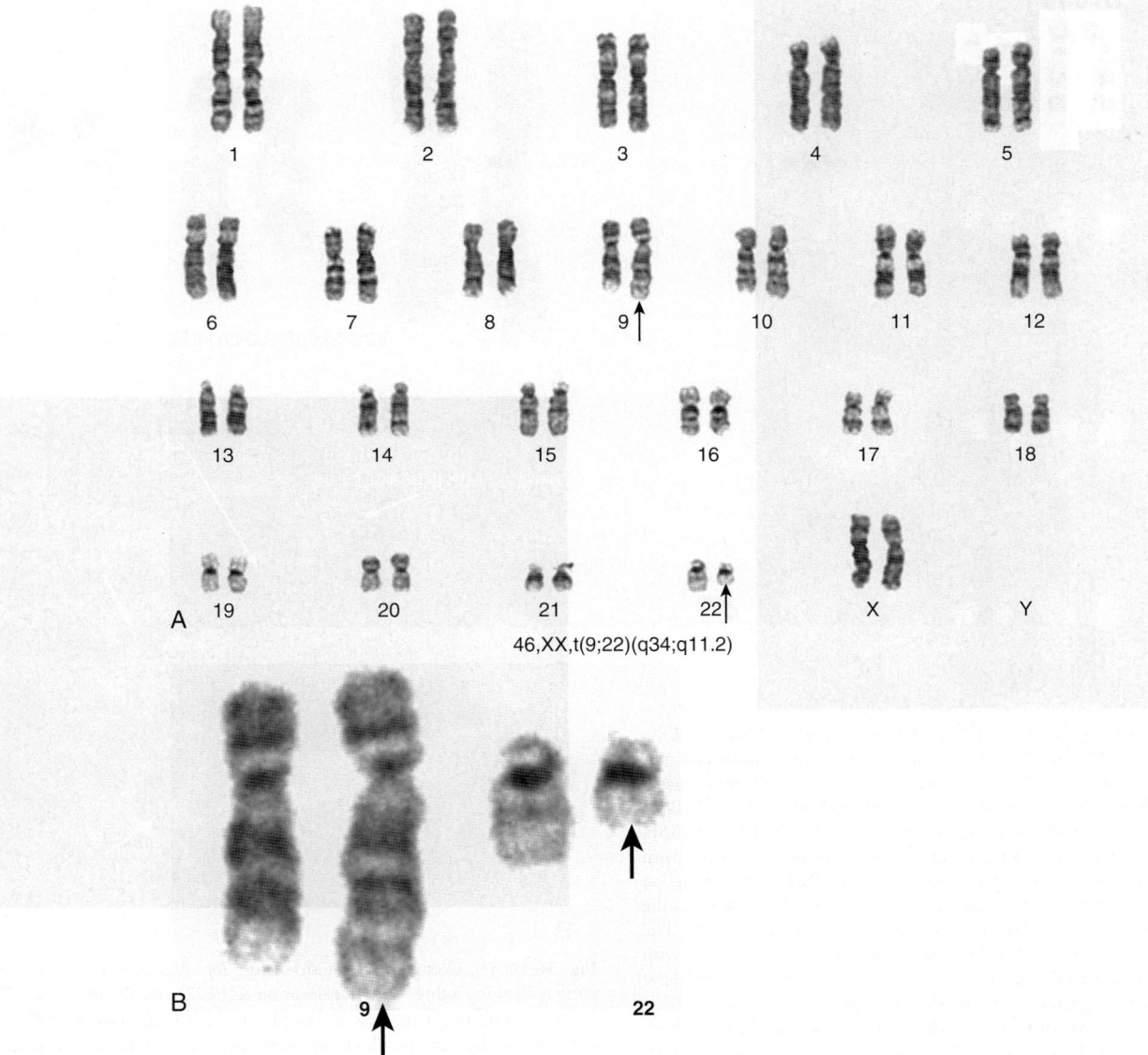

Fig. 56.8 (A) The karyotype of a female patient showing a balanced t(9;22)(q34;q11.2), also known as the Ph chromosome. (B) Isolated t(9;22) showing two-thirds of the long arms of chromosome 22 translocated to one homologue of chromosome 9.

Northern blot analysis allows detection of *BCR-ABL1* transcripts at the RNA level. Current FISH studies for detection of *BCR-ABL1* fusion at diagnosis use a dual-color *BCR-ABL1* ES probe or *BCR-ABL1* dual-fusion probe (Fig. 56.12, see also Fig. 56.6A–B). A triple-color *BCR-ABL1-ASS* probe is used for detection of deletions on both chromosomes 9 and 22 (see Fig. 56.12). Approximately 12% to 15% of patients with CML have large deletions adjacent to the Ph chromosome translocation breakpoint on the derivative 9 chromosome, and initial reports demonstrated inferior survival in these patients. These deletions are heterogeneous and may involve both chromosomes 9 and 22 (majority of cases), only chromosome 9 (8% of patients with deletions), or only chromosome 22 (4% of cases with deletions). Moreover, deletion size is variable, ranging from 0.5 Mb to greater than 10 Mb. A more refined study applying genomic SNP microarrays revealed three common deletion regions: (1) a 162-kb loss at 9q34, (2) a 138-kb deletion at 22q11.2, and (3) a 102-kb deletion at 22q11.2. It appears that the partial deletion of the *ABL1-BCR* fusion on derivative 9 chromosome occurs as a part of the same process as the formation of the *BCR-ABL1* translocation. Before imatinib therapy, these deletions were associated with an adverse prognosis; however, in a study of 521 patients with CML, the cumulative incidence of complete cytogenetic responses and major molecular responses and the overall survival (OS) were comparable after 5-years of follow-up between CML patients with and without the del(9q).

At diagnosis, conventional cytogenetics remains the gold standard because the chromosome analysis will identify not only the t(9;22) but also other chromosomal abnormalities that may indicate accelerated or blast phase of the disease or clonal proliferation of Ph-negative cells.

Imatinib mesylate (Gleevec) has revolutionized therapy for CML and, for most patients, has transformed a deadly disease into a chronic disorder that is compatible with normal life. The standard method for monitoring a patient's response to therapy is conventional cytogenetic analysis of cells obtained from a marrow aspirate. In the phase III International Randomized Interferon and STI-571 (IRIS) study, 89% of patients had Ph-negative marrow aspirates as determined by conventional cytogenetics after 5 years of treatment. However, conventional cytogenetics has limited sensitivity. The degree of tumor load reduction is determined to be an important prognostic factor

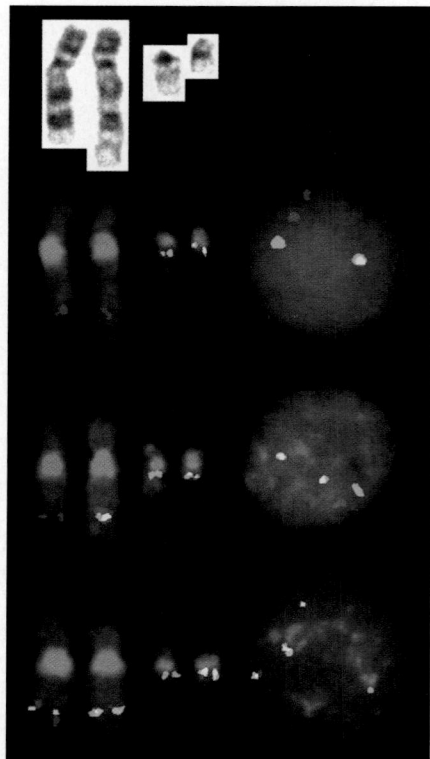

Fig. 56.9 CURRENT FISH PROBE STRATEGIES FOR DETECTING BCR-ABL1 FUSION. Partial karyotype showing the Philadelphia chromosome as a result of t(9;22)(q34;q11.2) *(top row)*. The same chromosomes 9 and 22, as well as a bone marrow nucleus, after hybridization with BCR *(green)* and ABL1 *(red)* using an extrasensitive dual-color, single-fusion FISH strategy *(second row)*. Chromosomes and a nucleus are counterstained with DAPI *(blue)*. In the extrasensitive strategy, a part of ABL1 *(red)* remains on der(9) and is shown in interphase nucleus as a smaller red signal, whereas the normal-size ABL1 hybridization signal is seen on normal homolog 9. The other part of ABL1 is on the Ph chromosome and is seen co-localized with BCR as yellow in interphase nucleus. Therefore interphase nuclei will have one normal-size red signal, one smaller-size red signal, one normal-size BCR signal, and co-localization of BCR and ABL1, producing a yellow signal both in interphase cells and metaphase chromosomes. In the dual-color, dual-fusion strategy *(third row)*, there are two co-localized signals on both der(9) and the Ph chromosome, as well as one red signal of ABL1 on chromosome 9 and one green signal of BCR on normal chromosome 22. In the triple-color, dual-fusion strategy, *ASS* gene *(aqua)* is added. It is used to determine whether sequences from der(9) are deleted at the time of the Ph formation. As shown in the fourth row, ASS is localized centromeric from ABL1 on 9q34, and in patients without deletion, ASS is present as two signals in nucleus and on the chromosome 9.

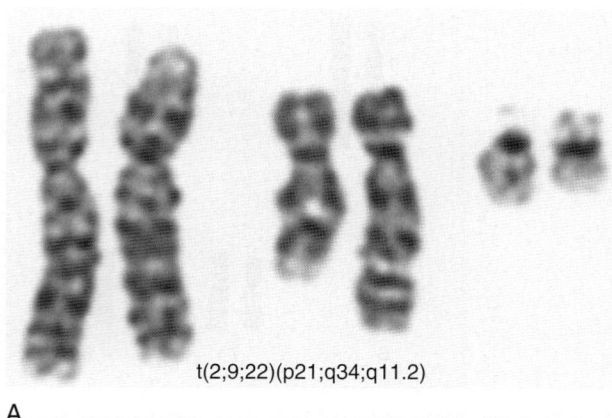

t(2;9;22)(p21;q34;q11.2)

A

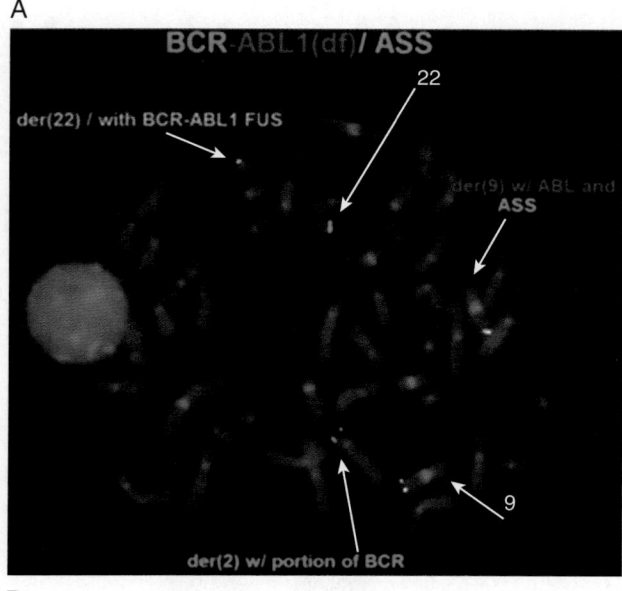

B

Fig. 56.10 (A) Complex Ph translocation. *Top:* A partial karyotype from a patient showing a three-way translocation t(2;9;22) and (B) metaphase FISH *(bottom)* indicating that even in complex karyotype the fusion of *BCR* and *ABL1* takes place on the Ph chromosome or der(22) indicated in *yellow*.

for patients with CML on therapy. Patients with CML without a discernible Ph chromosome detected by conventional cytogenetics analysis may still harbor up to 10^{10} leukemic cells.

Interphase FISH does not depend on the cycling status of cells, and use of double-fusion probes has reduced false-positive results to approximately 1%. However, if peripheral blood cells rather than marrow aspirate cells are used to monitor residual disease, the high percentage of *BCR-ABL1* fusion-negative lymphoid cells may underrepresent the actual residual tumor load. In most direct comparison studies, interphase FISH of peripheral blood compared with conventional cytogenetics of marrow in patients who are treated with imatinib showed good correlations ($r = 0.91–0.97$). Real-time quantitative PCR (RQ-PCR) is by far the most sensitive method. It provides an accurate measure of the total leukemia cell mass and the degree to which *BCR-ABL1* transcripts are reduced by therapy, and it correlates with progression-free survival.

The goal of therapy in CML is to achieve a molecular remission as measured by the reduction or elimination of *BCR-ABL1* transcripts. In the IRIS study, at 5-year follow-up, complete cytogenetic response combined with major molecular response at 12 months was associated with a 97% progression-free survival rate. This compares with an 89% progression-free survival for those with complete cytogenetic response but without a major molecular response. Current international recommendations for optimal molecular monitoring of patients receiving imatinib treatment includes an RQ-PCR assay expressing the *BCR-ABL1* transcript levels on an internationally agreed upon scale. The term *major molecular response* corresponds to ≤0.1% *BCR-ABL1*, whereas the designation *complete molecular response* should be used only for patients with undetectable *BCR-ABL1*, where the limit of detection is confirmed to be at least ≈4.5 log reduction from baseline response. The two major obstacles to successful imatinib-based therapy for patients with Ph-positive, *BCR-ABL1* fusion-positive CML are the persistence of *BCR-ABL1* fusion-positive cells and relapse of the disease because of emergence of resistance to imatinib. Acquired resistance to imatinib treatment is manifested in two ways: amplification of *BCR-ABL1* fusion product (Fig. 56.13) and mutations in the ABL kinase domain. Currently, 100 different ABL1 kinase domain mutations have been described, although only about 15 are common and they account for more than 85% of all mutations detected.

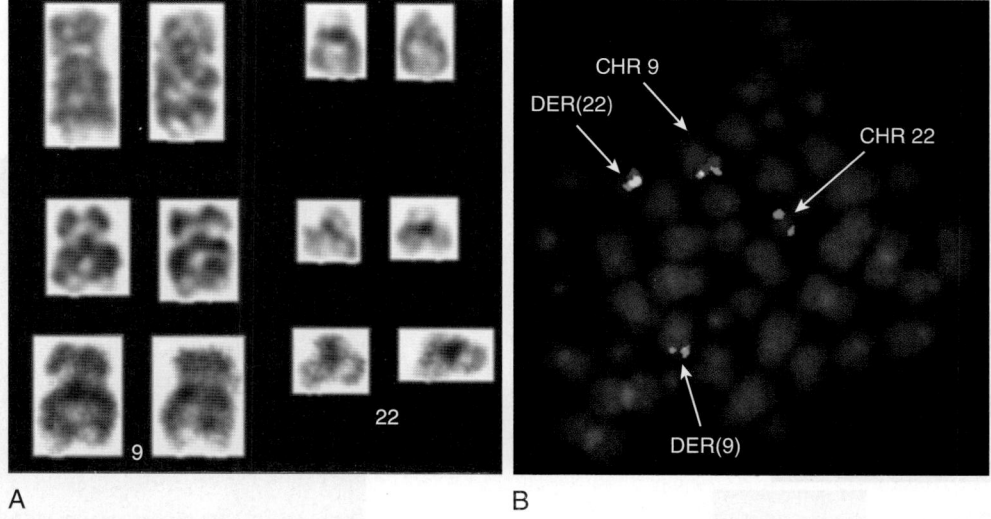

Fig. 56.11. *BCR-ABL1* FUSION IN A PATIENT WITH THE Ph-NEGATIVE, NORMAL KARYOTYPE. *Left panel* shows a partial karyotype from three cells showing normal homologs 9 and 22. The *right panel* shows the *BCR-ABL1* fusion *(yellow)* on der (22) and diminished *ABL (red)* on der(9). The fusion has occurred as a result of *ABL1* insertion into *BCR* without apparent chromosomal translocation. Note an intact ASS *(aqua)* on both chromosomes 9.

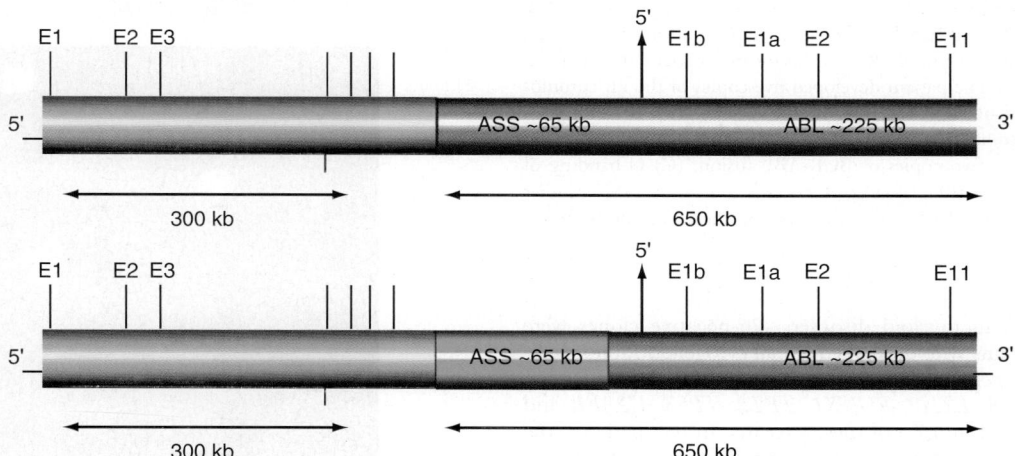

Fig. 56.12 SCHEMATIC REPRESENTATION OF THE MOST FREQUENTLY USED BCR-ABL PROBES. Dual-color/single-fusion extrasensitive probe strategy, as indicated in text, uses a 650-kb probe in which two loci, *ABL* and *ASS,* both are labeled in red. BCR-ABL fusion-positive nuclei show three red signals: one small red signal on der(9), one red signal on normal homologue 9, and a third red signal in fusion with BCR. When a triple-color probe is applied, the *ASS* locus usually is labeled in aqua and the BCR-ABL fusion-positive cells show two aqua signals, unless there is deletion of der(9). The most useful application of triple-color probe is documentation of deletion of derivative chromosome 9.

Patients with CML who cannot tolerate or are resistant to imatinib may benefit from the second and now third generation of TKIs, such as dasatinib, nilotinib, bosutinib, and ponatinib.[7] These agents bind to the ABL kinase domain in a matter distinct from that of imatinib and thereby retain activity against nearly all imatinib-resistant mutations. Recent meta-analysis revealed ABL mutation rates with imatinib 9.7%, dasatinib 1.7%, and nilotinib 3.3%. The most common specific mutations were T315I, E255k, and M315I. T315I mutations constitute 58% of dasatinib-related mutations and 13% of imatinib related mutations. These mutations inhibit the binding of the TKIs, hindering the treatment of patients with CML. The introduction of ponatinib, a new formulation of TKI, has been shown to overcome resistance incurred by the T315I mutation (see Chapter 67).

Between 5% and 8% of patients undergoing treatment with imatinib will develop chromosomal abnormalities such as trisomy 8, monosomy 7, del(20q), and other anomalies in *BCR-ABL1* fusion-negative cells. Imatinib may induce chromosomal abnormalities in *BCR-ABL1⁻* cells. Alternatively, imatinib may uncover chromosomal abnormalities present before therapy after significant reduction of overlying Ph-positive cells (Fig. 56.14). Presence of +8 and other chromosomal anomalies in Ph-negative cells in patients treated with imatinib suggests that CML has a multistep pathogenesis and that clonal Ph-negative cells precede the development of the Ph-positive clone (Fig. 56.15). This important observation about the pathogenesis of CML demonstrates the power of conventional cytogenetics, even in the era of molecular assays, and should be used at least annually while patients are undergoing imatinib treatment. This hypothesis that clonal development occurs in Ph-negative cells before development of the Ph chromosome in the multistep CML pathogenesis was recently confirmed using NGS by targeting 25 genes

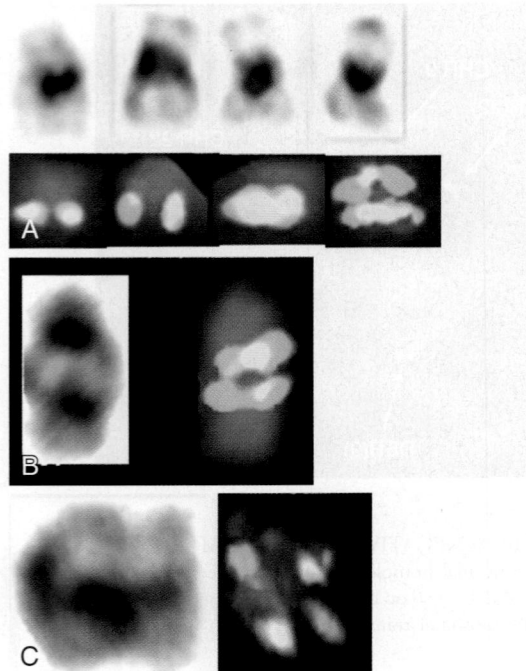

Fig. 56.13 EXAMPLES OF UNUSUAL Ph CHROMOSOME ASSOCI-ATED WITH IMATINIB RESISTANCE AND BLAST CRISIS OF CHRONIC MYELOGENOUS LEUKEMIA. (A) Amplification of the Ph chromosome *(top row)* and the BCR-ABL fusion in a patient treated for 3 months with imatinib. The patient developed five copies of the Ph chromosome and five copies of the BCR-ABL fusion *(yellow)*. (B) G-banding of dicentric Ph chromosome *(left)* dic der(22)t(9;22)(q34;q11.2) and after FISH studies *(right)* showing two copies of BCR-ABL fusion. (C) G-banding of isoderivative Ph, ider(22)t(9;22)(q34;q11.2) *(left)* and after FISH studies showing two copies of BCR-ABL fusion *(yellow)* on the end of both arms.

frequently mutated in myeloid disorders. Ph-negative clones were analyzed in 14 patients who developed clonal cytogenetic abnormalities in Ph-negative cells during TKI treatment. Mutations affecting the genes *DNMT3A, EZH2, RUNX1, TET2, TP53, U2AF1,* and *ZRSR2,* were detected in 43% of these patients. In two patients, the mutations were found also in corresponding Ph-positive diagnostic samples. Moreover, somatic mutations additional to *BCR-ABL1* are found in 33% of patients affecting *ASXL1, DNMT3A, RUNX1,* and *TET2* genes. When individual hematopoietic colonies were analyzed from patients with CML at diagnosis, most mutations were present in the Ph-positive cells. By contrast, deep sequencing of subsequent samples during TKI treatment revealed that one *DNMT3A* mutation occurs in Ph-negative cells that was also present in Ph-positive cells at diagnosis, strongly implying that *DNMT3A* preceded the formation of the *BCR-ABL1* rearrangement and provides support for the initial hypothesis (in 1980) that *BCR-ABL1* and the formation of the Ph chromosome are not initiating events in the pathogenesis of CML. Another example of clonal evolution in MPNs evolving over time is the co-occurrence of the *JAK2V617F* mutation and *BCR-ABL1*. These rare patients usually have a long (10–20 years) history of *JAK2V617F*[+] polycythemia vera (PV) before *BCR-ABL1* and the Ph chromosome were formed. Single cell genotyping revealed both the *JAK2V617F* mutation and *BCR-ABL1* can occur concurrently in hematopoietic stem cells and that *JAK2V617F*[+] mutation occurs before the acquisition of *BCR-ABL1*. The contribution of *BCR-ABL1* to disease progression appears to be greater than that of *JAK2V617F,* because these patients display a clinical phenotype that is consistent with CML rather than PV.

The mechanism of transformation to advanced-phase CML is heterogeneous and poorly understood. In blast crisis of CML, 80% to 85% of patients show karyotypic evolution, that is, new

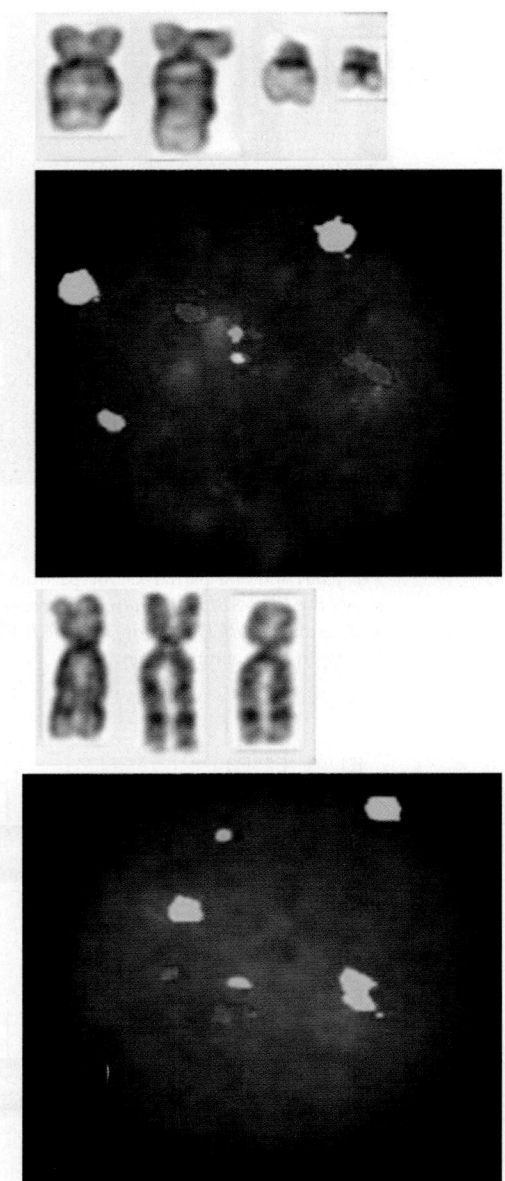

Fig. 56.14 TWO DIFFERENT CELL POPULATIONS FROM A PATIENT TREATED WITH IMATINIB. One population shows t(9;22) *(top row,* partial G-banded karyotype) and the BCR-ABL fusion signal *(yellow, second row)* as well as disomy 8 *(aqua)*. In contrast, the second population shows trisomy 8 *(third row,* partial G-banded karyotype) in the BCR-ABL fusion-negative cells *(fourth row),* showing disomy for the *BCR (green),* ABL *(red)* as well as trisomy for chromosome 8 *(aqua)* (see text for details).

chromosomal abnormalities in very distinct patterns are present in addition to the Ph chromosome. The most common changes include gain of chromosome 8 (33%) or +19 (12%), gain of a second Ph chromosome (30%), i(17q)(20%), alone or in combination, to produce modal chromosome numbers of 47–50 (Fig. 56.16). In males, a loss of Y chromosome is frequently observed. Isochromosome 17q occurs almost exclusively in myeloid blast crisis. Others less frequently observed abnormalities include monosomies of chromosomes 7 and 17, and trisomies of chromosomes 17 and 21. In addition to these common karyotypic evolutions, additional chromosomal aberrations specific for AML—for example, t(8;21) (Fig. 56.17), inv(16), t(3;21)(q26;q22), and most frequently, inv(3q)/t(3;3), resulting in the overexpression of *EVI1*—have been observed. Simultaneous presence of t(9;22) and inv(3) at diagnosis or following TKI therapy appears to be associated with a lack of response to treatment

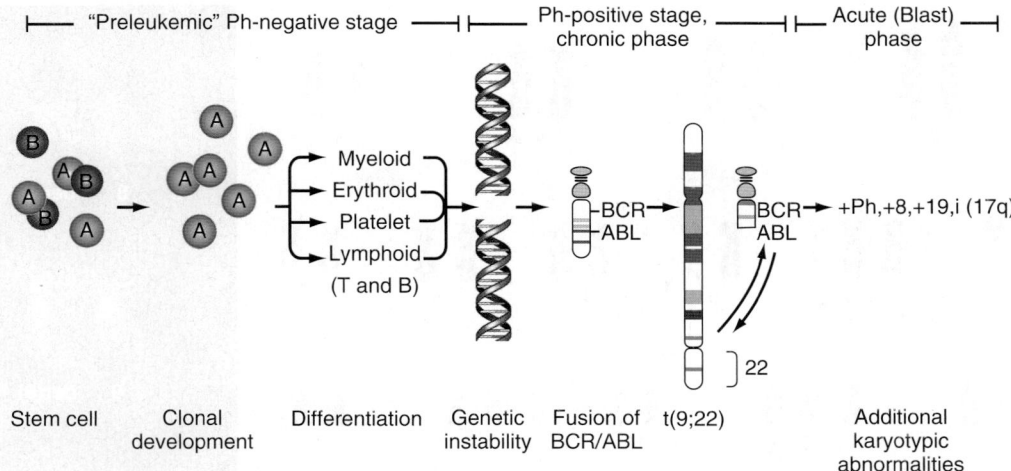

Fig. 56.15 HYPOTHETICAL MODEL OF MULTISTEP PATHOGENESIS OF Ph-POSITIVE CHRONIC MYELOGENOUS LEUKEMIA. The first detectable event is a clonal proliferation of cells that are capable of differentiating to all hematopoietic lineages. These cells are genetically unstable and give rise to BCR-ABL fusion and the Ph chromosome. The blast crisis is characterized by nonrandom abnormalities occurring in a genetically unstable Ph-positive clone. At least six events can be delineated. *(Courtesy Dr. W Raskind, University of Washington, Seattle.)*

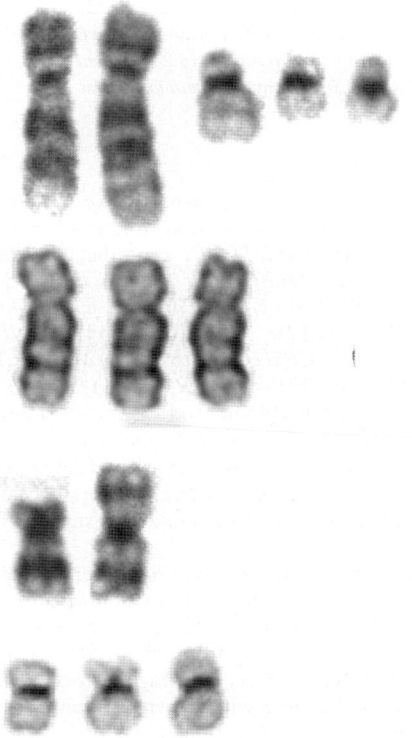

Fig. 56.16 THE FOUR MOST FREQUENT ABNORMALITIES ASSOCIATED WITH THE BLAST CRISIS OF CHRONIC MYELOGENOUS LEUKEMIA. Duplication of the Ph chromosome *(top row)* is identified in about 30% of patients, trisomy 8 *(second row)* is found in 30%, isochromosome of the long arms of chromosome 17 *(third row)* is found in 20%, and gain of chromosome 19 *(fourth row)* is seen in approximately 12% of patients with blast crisis of chronic myelogenous leukemia.

Genetic Testing for Chronic Myelogenous Leukemia (CML)

At diagnosis of CML, perform quantitative cytogenetic analysis using the bone marrow aspirate, which is the sine qua non because peripheral blood cells rarely contain sufficient numbers of mitotic cells at the time of presentation. If the bone marrow aspirate is a "dry tap," perform interphase FISH using a *BCR-ABL1* extrasensitive dual-fusion color probe. To monitor patients with CML during therapy, use FISH to study blood or bone marrow to track changes in the percentage of cells with *BCR-ABL1* fusion at 3-month intervals. Once the patient is in complete cytogenetic and FISH remission, the consensus recommendation is to perform real-time quantitative polymerase chain reaction and to follow the patient at 3-month intervals until molecular remission is achieved. According to ELN 2013 recommendations, a single measurement of rising *BCR-ABL1* transcript numbers is not sufficient to change therapy, whereas two tests at 3 and 6 months, and supplementary tests in between, provide more support for the decision to change treatment. At relapse, perform a chromosome study to assess the karyotype of the malignant clone and to determine whether a new chromosomally abnormal clone has developed or a new subclone in the Philadelphia chromosome–positive clone.

---

extra copy of the Ph chromosome. The second group includes chromosomal abnormalities that are associated with a relatively poor prognosis including i(17q), −7/del(7q) and 3q26.2 rearrangements. The concurrent presence of two or more ACAs conferred an inferior survival and can be categorized into the poor prognostic group. Complete cytogenetic remission for patients in accelerated phase or blast crisis CML treated with imatinib is rarely accompanied by a normal karyotype; however, 6% to 17% of these patients may have some cytogenetic response (see box on Genetic Testing for Chronic Myelogenous Leukemia).

High-resolution cytogenomic studies have demonstrated that in contrast to the chronic phase (which is characterized only by genomic imbalances in or around *BCR* and *ABL1*, specifically deletions), during the blast phase, many additional genomic imbalances occur. Using aCGH, 44 patients in chronic phase of CML as well as in 11 in myeloid and 1 in lymphoid blast crisis were investigated, and a spectrum of recurrent genomic imbalances was associated with disease progression, including losses at 1p36, 5q21, 9p21, and 9q34 and gains at 1q, 8q24, 9q34, 16p, hend 22q11. Moreover, analysis of 78 CML patients in lymphoid blast crisis demonstrated a unique signature of genomic deletions within the Ig heavy-chain and *TCR* genes,

and the clinical course is similar to that of cases with inv(3) without any other chromosomal abnormality. In patients treated with TKI, additional chromosomal abnormalities (ACAs) were classified into two groups based on their impact on survival. ACAs in the good prognostic group include trisomy 8, loss of Y chromosome, and an

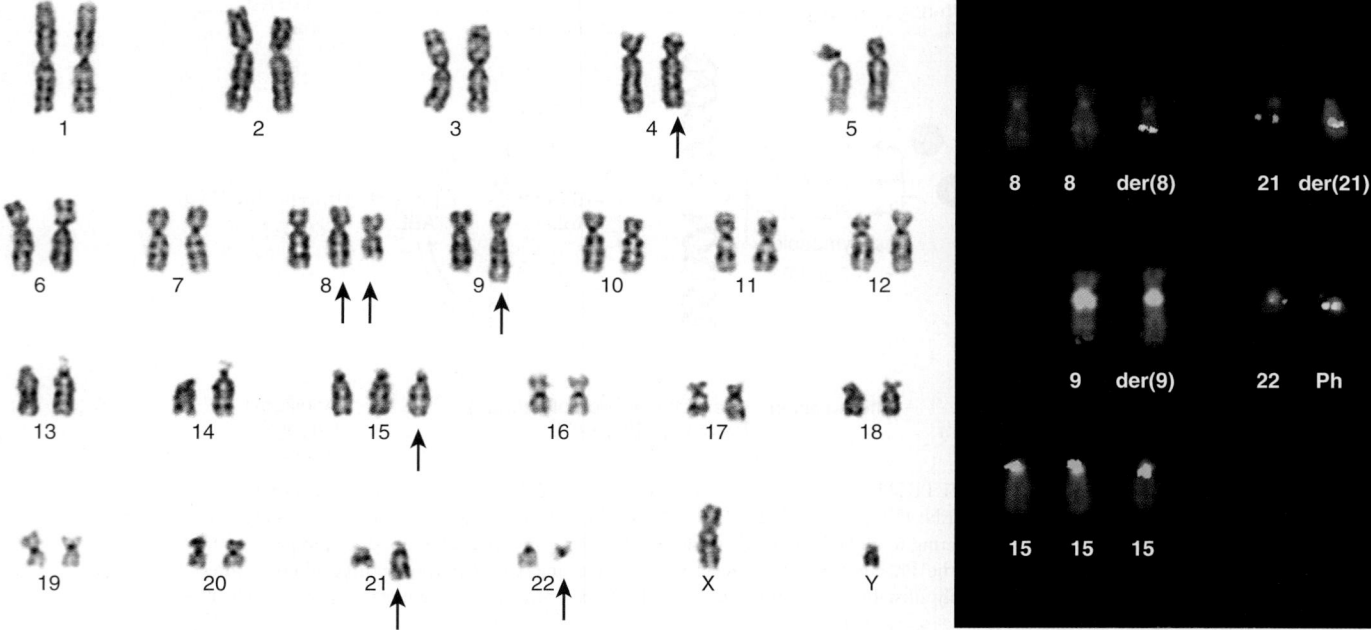

Fig. 56.17 SIMULTANEOUS DETECTION OF t(9;22) AND t(8;21) IN A PATIENT WITH BC-CML: A karyotype *(left)* from a patient with chronic myelogenous leukemia who failed three tyrosine kinase inhibitor treatments and progressed into blast crisis showing 46, XY, del(4)(q31q33), t(8;21)(q22;q22), +8, t(9;22) (q34;q11.2), +15. Metaphase FISH studies *(right panel)* confirmed that in the BCR-ABL1 fusion–positive cells *(middle row, yellow* co-localization), the patient had RUN1-RUNXT1 fusion as a result of t(8;21) [*yellow* signals on der(8) and der(21)] and a gain of chromosome 8 *(top row)* as well as trisomy 15 *(bottom row)* as shown using centromeric FISH probe specific for chromosome 15 *(aqua)*.

indicating that their presence is essential for the development of a malignant clone with the lymphoid phenotype. The most common mutations in myeloid blast phase involve tumor suppressor gene *TP53* (about 25% of cases) and the *RUNX1* in about 40% of cases. In lymphoid blast crisis, 50% of patients have mutation in cycline-dependent kinase inhibitor *CDKN2A*. Recently, mutations in genes frequently found in Ph-negative MPNs such as *CBL, TET2, ASXL11,* and *IDH1/2* were also identified in patients in accelerated/blast phase. Moreover, deletions of *RB1,* gain of function mutations in *GATA-2* and *RAS* are just some of the spectrum of cytogenomic changes characterizing progression of CML. The current thinking is that progression of CML is the result of increased genomic instability combined with defective or insufficient ability to repair DNA.

Ph-Negative Chronic Myeloproliferative Neoplasms

Ph-negative MPNs are disorders arising in a single clone of multipotent precursor cells in which one or all myeloid lineages are abnormally amplified. Classic and more frequently encountered Ph-negative MPDs include PV, primary myelofibrosis, and essential thrombocytopenia (ET). Their cytogenetic and genomic profiles are described in Chapters 68, 70 and 71.

Less frequently encountered MPNs include chronic neutrophilic leukemia, hypereosinophilic syndrome/chronic eosinophilic leukemia, systemic mast cell disorders, atypical CML, and unclassifiable MPNs. Rare recurrent balanced abnormalities in atypical Ph-negative MPN generally involve the *PDGFRB* gene localized at 5q33, *FGFR1* gene on 8p11, and *PDGFRA* gene on 4q12. The best described are t(5;12)(q33;p13), resulting in *ETV6-PDGFRB* fusion protein, and t(8;13)(p11;q12), resulting in the *ZNF198-FGFR1* fusion gene. The disorder known as *8p11 myeloproliferative syndrome* has been recognized and classified by WHO as belonging to the group of myeloid neoplasms associated with multilineage involvement characterized by chronic myelomonocytic leukemia with eosinophilia and an increased incidence (approximately 30%) of T-cell lymphoblastic lymphoma.

This disease is related to fusion genes between *FGFR1* located on 8p11 and various translocations fusing at least 14 different 5′ partner genes to the 3′ part of the *FGFR1* gene that encodes the tyrosine kinase domain (Table 56.3). They include *TPR* (1q25), *LRRFIP1* (2q37), *SQSTM1* (5q35) *FGFR10P* (6q27), *TRIM24* (7q34), *CUX1* (7q22), *PLAG1* (8q12), *CEP110* (9q33), *NUP98* (11p15), *FGFR1OP2* (12p11), *CPSF6* (12q15), *ZMYM2* (13q12), *MYO18A* (17q23), *HERVK* (19q13), and *BCR* (22q11) (Fig. 56.18). The most frequent translocation is t(8;13), and cases with the submicroscopic deletion of the 5′ part of the *FGFR1* gene have also been reported, similar to the formation of t(9;22) with deleted sequences from der(9q) and/or 22q identified in CML. The presence of 8p11 abnormalities in both myeloid and lymphoid cells suggests its origin from a common stem cell.

In patients with chronic eosinophilic leukemia/hypereosinophilic syndrome the most frequent recurrent abnormality is the cryptic deletion on 4q12 as a result of *FIP1L1-PDGFRA* fusion gene reported to occur at frequencies ranging from 3% to 56% (Chapter 71). The disparity in frequencies reflects differing levels of stringency criteria in the diagnosis of disorders with hypereosinophilia as well as different technologies used for detection of *FIP1L1-PDGFRA* fusion. A most recent investigation of 376 patients with persistent unexplained hypereosinophilia revealed an 11% incidence of the *FIP1L1-PDGFRA* fusion gene detected using highly sensitive RQ-PCR. Patients with *FIP1L1-PDGFRA* fusion are characterized by male predominance, marrow fibrosis, increased number of mast cells, elevated serum tryptase levels, and a favorable response to low doses of imatinib. Most of these patients have a normal karyotype because a cryptic deletion of *CHIC2* locus on 4q12 which is only 800 kb in size. This abnormality is detectable using a more sensitive FISH technology and RQ-PCR in the majority of cases. Moreover, the most recent commercially available tricolor FISH probe will detect not only deletion 4q12 as a result of *FIP1L1-PDGFRA* but also a rare *BCR-PDGFRA* fusion resulting from the t(4;22)(q12;q11.2) rearrangement (Fig. 56.19). Serial monitoring with RQ-PCR demonstrates exquisite sensitivity of *FIP1L1-PDGFRA*–positive patients to low-dose

TABLE 56.3   Chromosomal Translocations in Ph-Negative Myeloproliferative Neoplasms

Chromosomal Abnormality	Genes Involved	MPD Entity
t(9;12)(q34;p13)	ETV6-ABL	CML-like, T-ALL
5q32	PDGFRB	**Associated Translocations**
t(1;5)(q25;q32)	TPM3-PDGFRB	Atypical MPN
t(2;5)(p21;q32)	SPTBN1-PDGFRB	Atypical MPN
t(4;5)(q21;q32)	PRKG2-PDGFRB	Atypical MPN
t(5;7)(q32;q11)	HIP1-PDGFRB	CMML-like
t(5;10)(q32;q21)	CCDC6-PDGFRB	Ph-negative MPN
t(5;12)(q32;p13)	ETV6-PDGFRB	CEL, CMML
t(5;12)(q32;p13.3)	ERC1-PDGFRB	Atypical MPN
t(5;14)(q33;q24)	NIN-PDGFRB	Atypical MPN
t(5;14)(q32;q32)	KIA1509-PDGFRB	Atypical MPN
t(5;14)(q32;q32)	TRIP11-PDGFRB	AML
t(5;15)(q23;q15)	TP53BP1-PDGFRB	CEL
t(5;15)(q32;q22)	TPS3BP1-PDGFRB	Atypical MPN
t(5;16)(q32;p13)	NDE1-PDGFRB	Atypical MPN
t(5;17)(q32;p11)	HCMOGT1-PDGFRB	Juvenile CMML
t(5;17)(q32;p11,2)	MYO18A-PDGFRB	Atypical MPN
t(5;17)(q32;p13)	RABEP1-PDGFRB	CMML
t(5;17)(q32;q21)	COL1A1-PDGFRB	Atypical MPN
8p11	FGFR1	**Associated Translocations**
t(2;8)(q37;8p11)	LRRFIP1-FGFR1	MPN syndrome
t(6;8)(q27;p11)	FGFR1OP-FGFR1	Stem cell MPD
t(7;8)(q32;p11)	TRIM24-FGFR1	MPN
t(7;8)(q22;p11)	CUX1-FGFR1	MPN syndrome
t(8;9)(p11;q22)	CEP110-FGFR1	MPN syndrome
t(8;11)(p11;p15)	Nup98-FGFR1	MPN syndrome
t(8;12)(p11;p11)	FGFR1OP-FGFR1	MPN syndrome
t(8;12)(p11;q12)	CPSF6-FGFR1	MPN syndrome
t(8;13)(p11;q12)	ZMYM2-FGFR1	MPN syndrome, leukemia, lymphoma
t(8;17)(p11;q11)	MYO18A-FGFR1	MPN syndrome
t(8;19)(p11;q13)	HERVK-FGFR1	MPN syndrome
t(8;22)(p11;q11.2)	BCR-FGFR1	Lymphoproliferative disorder
4q12	PDGFRA	
del(4)(q12;q12)	FIP1L1-PDGFRA	CEL
t(4;22)(q12;q11.2)	BCR-FGFR1	Atypical CML
4q12	KIT	SM
9p24	JAK2	
t(9;22)(p24;q11.2)	BCR-JAK2	CML-like
t(9;12)(p24;p13)	JAK2-ETV6	CML-like
der(9)t(9;12)(p24;q13)	JAK-NF-E2	MDS
t(8;9)(p22;p24)	PCM1-JAK2	CMPD, AL
der(9;18)t(p13;p11)	Not reported	PV, PV→MF
der(9;18)(p10;q10)	Not reported	PV, PV→MF, ET→AML
der(9)t(1;9)(q12;q12)	Not reported	PV, MF
der(1;7)(q10;p10)	Not reported	ET
t(12)(q21 or q21)	Not reported	MF

AL, Acute leukemia; ALL, acute lymphoblastic leukemia; AML, acute myeloid leukemia; CEL, chronic eosinophilic leukemia; CML, chronic myelogenous leukemia; CMML, chronic myelomonocytic leukemia; CMPD, chronic myeloproliferative disorder; ET, essential thrombocytopenia; MF, myelofibrosis; MPD, myeloproliferative disorder; MPN, myeloproliferative neoplasm; PV, polycythemia vera; SM, systemic mastocytosis.

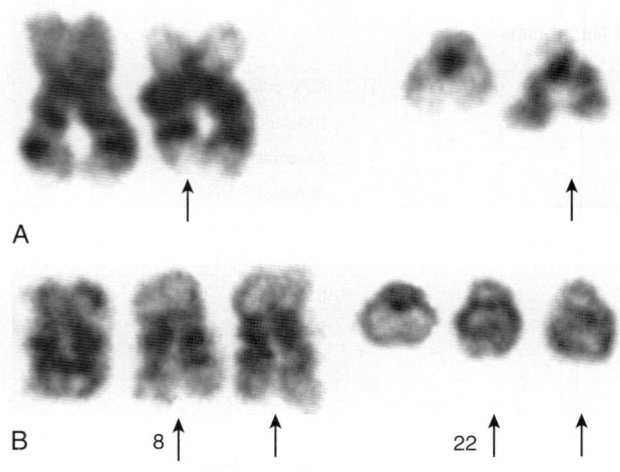

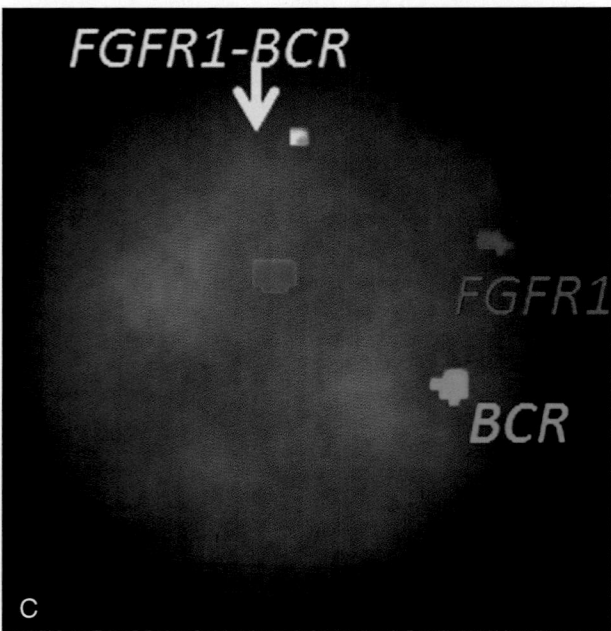

Fig. 56.18 (A) A partial karyotype from a patient diagnosed with Ph-negative myeloproliferative neoplasm showing t(8;22)(p11;q11.2). (B) Six months later the patient developed hyperdiploid karyotype, acute lymphoblastic leukemia, and two copies of t(8;22). (C) Interphase FISH confirmed a FGFR1 *(red)*-BCR *(green)* fusion *(yellow)*.

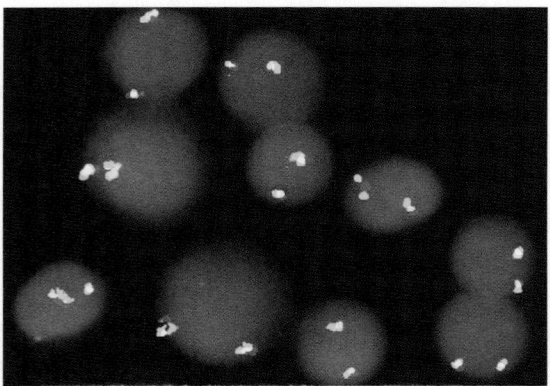

Fig. 56.19 BONE MARROW INTERPHASE NUCLEI AFTER FISH STUDIES USING TRICOLOR PROBE FOR CHROMOSOME 4, BAND REGION q12. The *green* color covers an approximately 750-kb region centromeric from FIP1L1. The *red* probe is telomeric of the FIP1L1 gene. The *aqua* color probe begins between exons 15 and 16 of the *PDGFRA* gene and extends toward the 4q telomere. In normal nuclei, as shown here, the probe appears as two tricolor fusions because of close proximity of probes in interphase DNA. Patients with hypereosinophilic syndrome have fusion of FIP1L1 and PDGFRA genes by interstitial deletion and produce one signal with *green-aqua* fusion and a missing orange signal. If the translocation involves the *PDGFRA* gene with loci on other chromosomes, the expected signal pattern is one *orange–green* fusion and one separate aqua signal.

Genetic Testing for Ph-Negative Myeloproliferative Neoplasms

At diagnosis, perform a real-time alleles-specific polymerase chain reaction for *JAK2*V617F, as well as mutational studies for *CALR* and *MPL*. Cytogenetic analysis of marrow cells is recommended for patients with essential thrombocytopenia and polycythemia vera. Unstimulated peripheral blood can be used instead of marrow aspirate for patients with primary myelofibrosis. Perform FISH studies with *BCR-ABL1* for patients with thrombocythemia to exclude the diagnosis of chronic myelogenous leukemia. FISH studies can be performed when cytogenetics is uninformative for detection of the most frequent abnormalities: +8, +9, +9p, del(13)(q14), and del(20)(q11q13). A panel of five probes includes CEP9, *CDKN2A/B* at 9p21, D8Z2 as a centromeric probe for chromosome 8, *RB1* for deletion 13q, and *D20S108* for deletion of 20q12. For diagnostic purpose and to monitor treatment response in patients with hypereosinophilic syndrome, perform FISH using triplecolor *FIP1L1* probe. For 5q32 rearrangements perform FISH with a *PDGFRB* FISH probe.

---

imatinib treatment. The *FIP1L1-PDGFRA* has been also detected in histopathologically defined cases of systemic mastocytosis with associated eosinophilia, and in cases of AML and T-cell lymphoblastoic lymphoma associated with eosinophilia. In an Italian prospective cohort of 27 patients with *FIP1L1-PDGFRA* who were treated with imatinib, a complete hematologic response was achieved within 1 month and all patients became PCR negative for *FIP1L1-PDGFRA* after a median of 3 months (range 1–10 months). In contrast to CML, very few cases of acquired imatinib resistance have been reported. Those rare reported cases have a mutation in T674I within the ATP-binding domain of PDGFRA, analogous to the T315I mutation in CML.

Although translocations involving *PDGFRB* at 5q32 region have been identified with 22 different fusion partners, they are indeed very rare. Any patient with a 5q31–q33 chromosomal abnormality with or without eosinophilia should be investigated for *PDGFRB* rearrangements by FISH testing.

Once the *PDGFRA*, *PDGFRB*, and *FGFR1* rearrangements are excluded, the only other recurrent secondary abnormalities include

trisomy 8 and trisomy 21 (see box on Genetic Testing for Ph-Negative Myeloproliferative Neoplasms).

In the WHO 2016 classification, *mastocytosis* is no longer listed under Ph-negative MPN. These are rare and heterogeneous diseases characterized by accumulation of clonal mast cells in one or multiple organs. Mastocytosis can affect both children and adults. In most pediatric patients, the disease affects only the skin. In contrast, in most adult patients, the disease is systemic and chronic and almost invariably affects the bone marrow. These cases are called systemic mastocytosis. Over 80% of patients with systemic mastocytosis are characterized by *KIT* mutations, specifically in the activation loop of *KIT*, *KIT* D816V. *KIT* is encoded by a 21-exon-containing gene located on the long arms of chromosome 4, 4q12. Other rare *KIT* mutations have been described in adult and pediatric patients. The knowledge of the type and structure of *KIT* mutation is important because the A-loop mutations D816V/H/Y/N disrupt the structure of the receptor, leading permanently to an active conformation and resistance to imatinib. In patients with advanced systemic mastocytosis other mutations not infrequently include *TET*2 (up to 39%), *SRSF2* (up to 36%), *ASXL1* (up to 21%), and *RUNX1* (23%). At diagnosis testing for *KIT* D816V in peripheral blood leukocytes, using highly sensitive and specific PCR-based assays, is mandatory to determine the *KIT* allelic burden rapidly, which is now used as a gold standard for assessing disease burden.

MYELODYSPLASTIC SYNDROMES

The MDSs (see Chapter 63) are a clinically heterogeneous group of hematologic neoplasms with differing biology and clinical manifestations. They have in common a clonal origin, dysplastic cellular morphology, cytopenias, abnormalities of cellular maturation, and an increased propensity to develop acute leukemia (20%–40%). They predominantly occur in elderly people as a result of multistep pathogenesis. Cytogenetic studies can provide both diagnostic and prognostic information. A chromosomally abnormal clone can be detected in 50% to 60% of patients with de novo MDS and in approximately 90% of patients with therapy-related MDS. There appears to be a correlation between the frequency of chromosomal abnormalities and the severity of disease. Approximately 35% of patients with less aggressive MDS, such as refractory anemia and refractory anemia with ring sideroblasts, have clonal chromosomal rearrangements, whereas approximately 60% to 70% of patients with refractory anemia with excess blasts in transformation have such chromosomal abnormalities. A single or complex chromosomal abnormality may

be present initially, and evolutionary change may occur during the course of the disease. Even at diagnosis, complex genomic lesions involving five or more different chromosomes are not unusual. Despite heterogeneity of chromosomal defects (gain, loss, deletion, amplification, rare balanced translocations, transcriptional silencing via methylation or point mutation), the unifying concept of genetic instability in MDS is hemizygosity of specific genes or chromosomal regions. The most common chromosomal anomalies in MDS involve gain of 1q, del(5q)/−5, del(7q)/−7, trisomy 8, del(11)(q23), del(12p), +13/del(13q), t(11q23), del(12p), del(17p), del(20)(q11q13), +21, and idic(X)(q13).

In 2012 a new cytogenetic classification of MDS was established that includes five different risk groups[8] (Fig. 56.20 and Table 56.4).

The clinical relevance and the power of conventional cytogenetics in MDS were recognized by the WHO, which documented a strong association between del(5)(q13q33) and 5q− syndrome. The 5q− syndrome is a unique subtype of low-risk MDS with a favorable prognosis, lack of other cytogenetic abnormalities, low rate of leukemic transformation, and more common occurrence in older adult females (see Fig. 56.20, *second row*).

Among patients who do not have 5q− syndrome (with or without other chromosomal abnormalities), interstitial deletions of the long arms of chromosome 5 occur in 10% to 15% of patients and are among the most frequent chromosomal abnormalities in MDS (see

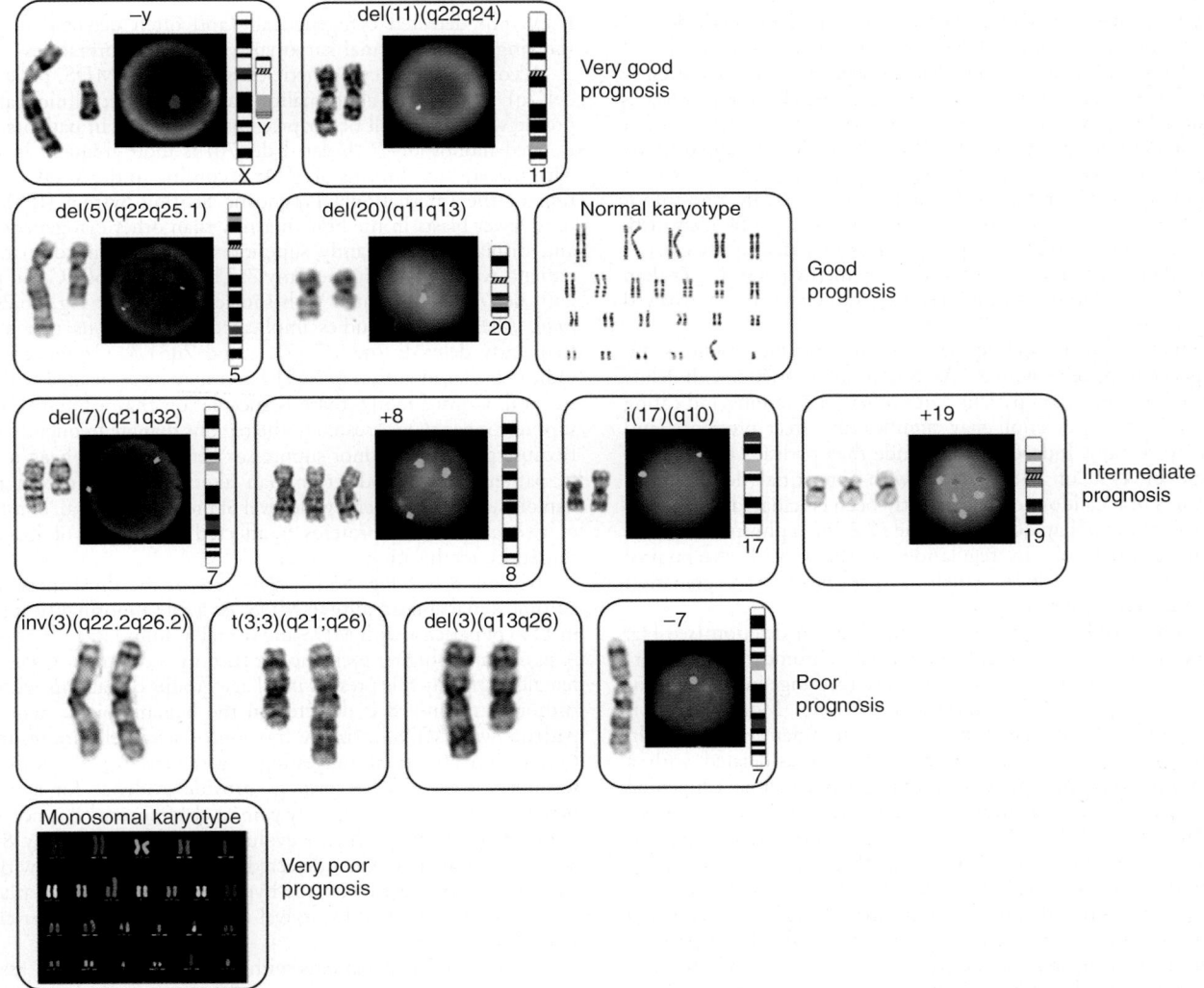

Fig. 56.20 PROGNOSTIC SIGNIFICANCE OF THE RECURRENT CHROMOSOMAL ABNORMALITIES IN MYELODYSPLASTIC SYNDROME, ACCORDING TO THE NEW COMPREHENSIVE CYTOGENETIC SCORING SYSTEM.

TABLE 56.4	Recurrent Chromosomal Abnormalities in Primary Myelodysplastic Syndrome
Abnormality	**Frequency (%)**
−5 or del 5q	10–15
−7 or del 7q	10
trisomy 8	10–17
i(17q) or t(17p)	2–3
del(12p) or t(12p)	1–2
del(11q)	1–2
−13 or del(13q)	1–2
del(9q)	1–2
idic(X)	1
inv(3)(q21q26.2)	1
t(6;9)(p23;q34)	1
t(3;21)(q26.2;q22.1)	<1
t(1;3)(p36.3;q21.2)	<1
t(11;16)(q23;p13.3)	<1
t(2;11) (p21;q23)	<1

Modified from Malcovati et al: *Blood* 122:2943, 2013.

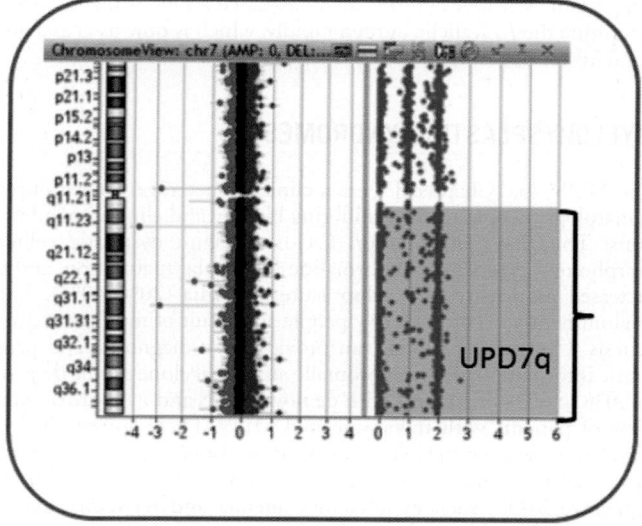

Fig. 56.21 ARRAY COMPARATIVE GENOMIC HYBRIDIZATION PLUS SINGLE-NUCLEOTIDE POLYMORPHISM FROM A PATIENT WITH MYELODYSPLASTIC SYNDROME AND NORMAL CHROMOSOME 7. Note acquired uniparental disomy (UPD) of the long arms of chromosome 7, known to be associated with worse prognosis.

Fig. 56.20, *second row*). The finding of del(5q) in CD34CD38− cells indicates its occurrence in a stem cell capable of differentiating into myeloid and lymphoid cell lineages, which represents an early event in the pathogenesis of MDS. Data on 1432 patients with del(5q) show a significant amount of heterogeneity in breakpoints. FISH studies delineated a commonly deleted segment that is currently estimated to be 1.5 Mb in size, on 5q31.1. The clustering of genes responsible for growth and differentiation of hematopoietic cells at this site and recurrent nature of −5/del(5q) in MDS caused many investigators to speculate that (a) tumor suppressor gene(s) was/were located in the 5q31 or 5q22–23 band region. To date, the tumor suppressor gene responsible for MDS on 5q has yet to be identified. Because the mechanism causing the interstitial del(5q) is elusive, haploinsufficiency or inactivation caused by methylation, rather than a typical tumor suppressor gene, has been speculated to be involved in this process.

Patients with isolated del(5q) have a more favorable prognosis and live longer than patients with ACAs. Specifically, patients with del(5)(q13q31) live longer than patients with other 5q deletions, indicating that the type of 5q deletion may significantly affect prognosis and response to therapy. Indeed, lenalidomide therapy leads to a normal karyotype in 44% of 148 patients with interstitial del(5q). The effectiveness of lenalidomide has recently been elucidated and attributed to inhibition of haplodeficient gene *PP2Acα*, a phosphatase, that plays an essential role in regulation of the G2/M checkpoint. Lenalidomide inhibits *PP2A*, which in turn causes P53 degradation and restores cell-cycle reentry.

In de novo MDS, isolated monosomy 7 or 7q deletion (see Fig. 56.20) occurs in 20% of patients. Frequently, chromosome 7 abnormalities occur with ACA, most commonly rearrangements of 3q or del(12p) (see Fig. 56.20, *third* and *fourth row*). Monosomy 7 is present in all MDS subtypes and is seen predominantly in males. In pediatric patients with constitutional disorders associated with a predisposition to develop AML including Fanconi anemia, congenital neutropenia, neurofibromatosis type 1, Down syndrome, or Kostmann syndrome, −7/del(7q) may be seen as an isolated abnormality. Therefore the question remains to whether these patients have genetic imprinting and preferentially lose chromosome 7. Unequivocal evidence exists that shows that preferential parental origin of the missing chromosome 7 does not occur; approximately half of the patients have loss of either the maternal or paternal homologue, excluding the genomic imprinting hypothesis. Embryonic origin of partial chromosome 7 deletion in monozygotic twins with juvenile chronic myelomonocytic leukemia has been reported. As shown in Fig. 56.21, acquired UPD of 7q is a known recurrent genomic rearrangement in

MDS not detected cytogenetically and often detected in patients showing either a normal karyotype or other abnormalities.

According to the cytogenetic classification of MDS, patients with del(7q) as a single abnormality have a distinct clinicopathologic profile with an overall better prognosis than seen in patients with an isolated monosomy 7. Isolated del(7q) is more frequent in patients with less advanced forms of MDS according to the WHO classification or the International Prognostic Scoring System (IPSS). They have fewer blasts in the bone marrow than other cytogenetic groups and display a significantly superior survival when compared with patients with isolated monosomy 7. The presence of ACA in patients with del(7q) is associated with shortened OS (see Fig. 56.20, *third row*). Allele typing studies implicated three regions that are most frequently deleted: 7q22, 7q31.1, and 7q31.3. Cytogenetic results indicated that retention of 7q31 band may be associated with longer survival. Consequently, there is speculation that a putative myeloid suppressor gene(s) is located in the regions that are frequently deleted. Because prototypic tumor suppressor genes have not been identified in patients with 7q deletions, an alternative explanation may be haploinsufficiency whereby the level of protein is critical, or a complex of two cooperating proteins is affected as a result of inactivation caused by methylation.

Trisomy 8 (see Fig. 56.20, *third row*) is the third most frequent chromosomal abnormality in MDS. As a sole abnormality, it is found in 11% of patients with MDS and overall is found in 17% of patients. A significantly higher incidence of trisomy 8 occurs in males than in females. Trisomy 8 is present in all age groups of patients with MDS. Although trisomy 8 is detected in the hematopoietic stem cells of patients with MDS, a sizable fraction of stem cells are disomic but functionally abnormal, suggesting that the trisomy 8 acquisition is a secondary event. These findings provide evidence for a multistep pathogenesis of MDS, whereby gain of chromosome 8 is not an early event in the stepwise disease evolution. Although trisomy 8 carries an intermediate risk when detected at diagnosis, patients with MDS with trisomy 8 treated with the hypomethylating agent 5-azacitidine have a significantly better survival than patients with other chromosomal abnormalities.

The first series of patients with MDS or MDS/MPN associated with trisomy 11 as a sole abnormality or as a part of noncomplex karyotype was recently reported. This rare recurrent abnormality has an overall frequency of approximately 0.3% and is associated with a significantly inferior survival in patients with IPSS intermediate-risk disease (*p* = .0002) but comparable to the poor-risk group (*p* = .97). Trisomy 11 is associated with clinical aggressiveness and represents a high-risk cytogenetic abnormality.

Deletions of 17p are seen in 3% to 4% of MDS and AML patients. These patients often display several other chromosomal rearrangements, including monosomy 17, isochromosome 17q (see Fig. 56.20, *third row*), and unbalanced translocations between chromosome 17 and another chromosome. Approximately 30% of these deletions are related to therapy. The extent of 17p deletion in all cases involves the *TP53* gene. There appears to be a close correlation between dysgranulopoiesis (e.g., pseudo–Pelger-Huet hypolobulation) and small vacuoles in neutrophils with 17p abnormalities and *TP53* deletion. The median survival of these patients is poor.

An isodicentric X chromosome in Xq13-idic(X) is a rare but recurrent abnormality that has been associated with refractory anemia with ringed sideroblasts. All MDS patients with idic(X)(q13) are females, most likely because the formation of idic(X) would result in nullisomy for Xq13-qter in males. The median age at the time of diagnosis is 73.5 years. The outcome of idic(X)-positive cases is variable; some investigators report aggressive and rapidly fatal disease and others a relatively favorable clinical course with survival for several years. The fact that idic(X) most often occurs as the sole cytogenetic abnormality suggests that it may in itself be sufficient for leukemogenesis. Using a high-resolution SNP array, the breakpoints on idic(X)(q13) were mapped into two distinct breakpoint clusters,

at approximately 70.9 Mb (five cases) and 72.1 Mb (seven cases) on the X chromosome. None of the 11 breakpoints occurred in a gene, strongly indicating that the idic(X)(q13) does not result in a fusion gene. Instead, the functional outcome of the abnormality confers a gene dosage effect because of the concurrent gain of Xpter-q13 and loss of Xq13-qter. This region of the X chromosome is enriched for repeated sequences and most likely, these repeats may facilitate the formation of idic(X). The isodicentric X chromosome was inactive in some patients and active in other patients; hence idic(X) appears to be leukemogenic regardless of X_a or X_i involvement.

Gain of 1q, usually in the form of an unbalanced translocation, is a recurrent abnormality in MDS and appears to be a marker of disease progression. Specifically, the gain of 1q in the form of jumping translocations either at diagnosis or the subsequent acquisition of jumping 1q translocations appears to be associated with imminent transformation to AML in patients after an average of 9 months (Fig. 56.22). Once acquired, the patient's prognosis tended to be dependent on the copy number of 1q, indicating that gain of jumping 1q translocations was associated with both disease progression and poor prognosis. In MDS, the average time to develop jumping 1q was less than 2 years. Treatment (azacitidine, chemotherapy, or stem cell transplant) may temporarily reduce or eradicate the clone, but the responses were not durable. These findings did not provide any common pattern as to the role of the partner chromosomes in unbalanced jumping 1q translocations. However, 81% of recipient

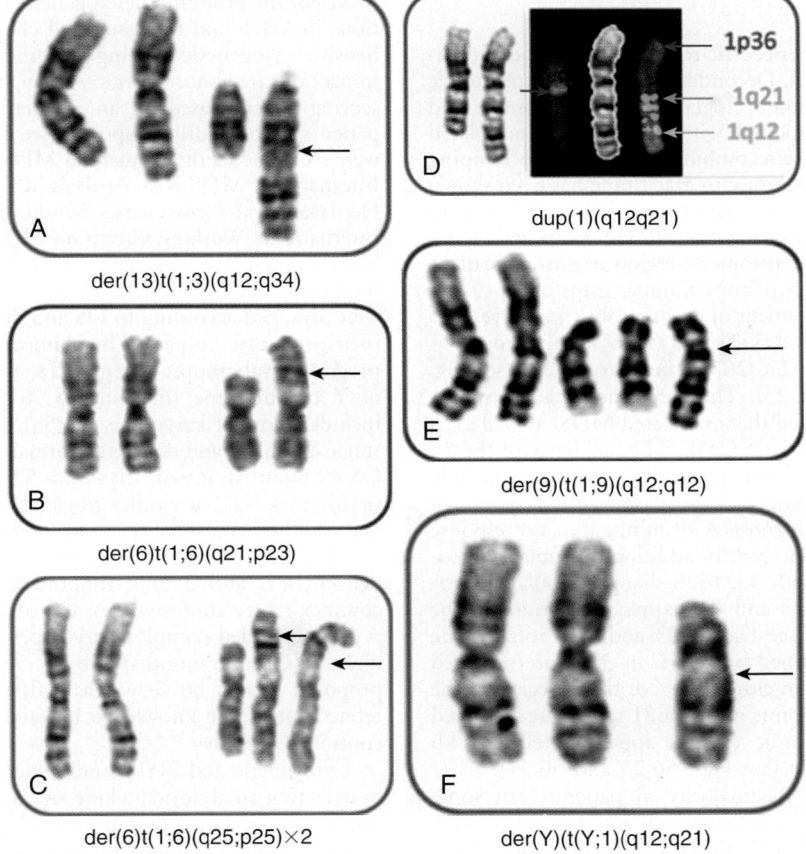

der(13)t(1;3)(q12;q34)

der(6)t(1;6)(q21;p23)

der(6)t(1;6)(q25;p25)×2

dup(1)(q12q21)

der(9)(t(1;9)(q12;q12)

der(Y)(t(Y;1)(q12;q21)

Fig. 56.22 GAIN OF LONG ARMS OF CHROMOSOME 1 IN MYELODYSPLASTIC SYNDROME AND MYELOPROLIFERATIVE NEOPLASM PATIENTS. Partial karyotypes in these six cases represent examples of gain or duplication of 1q. Trisomy 1q in the form of der(13) with an extra 1q is translocated to the terminal portion of the long arms of chromosome 13; (B) Gain of 1q in the form of der(6) whereby the entire long arms of 1 are translocated to the short arms of chromosome 6; (C) Two copies of der(6) resulting in tetrasomy 1q in a patient with an advanced myelodysplastic syndrome; (D) Duplication of region 1q12–q21 in a patient with essential thrombocytopenia; (E) Trisomy 1q translocated to the short arms of chromosome 9 resulting in a gain of 9p and 1q in a patient with polycythemia vera (PV) who transformed to myelofibrosis. This is a PV-specific and recurrent abnormality. (F) Trisomy 1q translocated to the terminal portion of the Y chromosome.

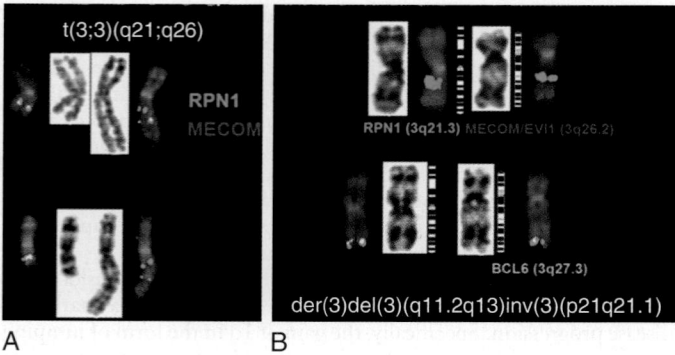

t(3;3)(q21;q26)

RPN1
MECOM

RPN1 (3q21.3)   MECOM/EVI1 (3q26.2)

BCL6 (3q27.3)

A

B

der(3)del(3)(q11.2q13)inv(3)(p21q21.1)

Fig. 56.23 CHROMOSOME 3 ABNORMALITIES IN MYELODYS-PLASTIC SYNDROME (MDS). (A) A partial karyotype from a patient with MDS showing a recurrent t(3;3)(q21;q26). In this rearrangement metaphase FISH showed on the left, *RPN1 (green)* and a part of *MECOM (red)* gene on 3q21 giving an impression of a "yellow" signal because of their proximity on a metaphase chromosome. The right chromosome 3 shows *RPN1 (green)* at 3q21, part of *RPN1 (green)* and *MECOM (red)* on 3q26 as well as unrearranged *MECOM* translocated from the left chromosome 3 homolog. (B) An unusual chromosome 3 rearrangement in MDS showing a deletion of 3q11–q13 region, followed by inversion with two breakpoints at p21 and q21.2. All three genes *RPN1 (green), MECOM (red),* and *BCL6 (yellow)* remained in their normal loci.

breakpoints were localized in pericentric regions whereas the remaining 19% were telomeric fusions. Decondensation of pericentromeric heterochromatin of chromosome 1 together with centromere and repeat DNA sequences interspersed with histones and acetylated sequences may favor illegitimate recombinations leading to jumping 1q translocations. Moreover, exposure to azacitidine has been shown to be associated with alterations of pericentromeric heterochromatin of chromosome 1, as well as an increase in Alu DNA repeats. Hypomenthilation of 1q12–21 pericentromeric region of chromosome 1 appears to be at least one aspect of copy number gains of 1q.

The most frequent rearrangement of chromosome 3 involves two bands on chromosome 3—band 3q21 and 3q26 simultaneously—which produces either t(3;3)(q21;q26) or inv(3)(q21q26) (see Fig. 56.20, *fourth row* and Fig. 56.23). These chromosomal rearrangements are present in de novo and therapy-related MDS, as well as in AML and megakaryoblastic crisis of CML. The incidence of the 3q rearrangements is 2% to 5%. Characteristic clinical features include an elevated platelet count, marked hyperplasia with dysplasia of megakaryocytes, and a poor prognosis with minimal or no response to chemotherapy and a short survival. In addition to similar clinico-pathologic features, patients with 3q21q26 share molecular hetero-geneity in both the breakpoints and the expression pattern of the genes near these breakpoints (see Fig. 56.23 and Fig. 56.24). The chromosomal breakpoints, defined by FISH, in 3q26 are scattered over several hundred kilobases in either the 5′ or the 3′ region of the *EVI1* gene, whereas the breakpoints in the 3q21 region are restricted to two smaller different genomic clusters approximately 100 kb downstream of the *RPN1* gene (see Figs. 56.23 and 56.24). *EVI1* overexpression is observed in the majority of patients, but some patients with the 3q21q26 rearrangement do not have detectable *EVI1* expression, and at least 9% of patients with AML without 3q26 abnormalities overexpress *EVI1*. Therefore the poor prognosis of these patients may be independent of *EVI1* expression, despite the fact that extensive 3q26 breakpoint FISH mapping of both meta-phases and interphase nuclei suggests *EVI1* involvement in numerous novel sporadic and recurrent 3q26 rearrangements. A fusion transcript of *RPN1-EVI1* is rarely observed in patients with 3q21q26 rearrange-ments. Interestingly, functional genomic studies and allelic-specific analysis revealed experimentally that inv(3)/t(3q) results simultane-ously in haploinsufficiency of *GATA2* and upregulation of *EVI1* as a result of rearrangements in noncoding regulatory sequences of these

genes, indicating the importance of mutations residing outside the coding exome.

A monosomal karyotype (MK), a new cytogenetic category, is defined as a karyotype showing two or more distinct autosomal chromosome monosomies or one single autosomal monosomy (excluding isolated loss of X or Y) in the presence of a structural abnormality (see Fig. 56.20, *bottom row*). Initial reports indicated that the MK in MDS, with or without monosomy for chromosomes 5 and 7, was prognostically worse than other complex karyotypes, although later reports could not confirm these results. The reason may be that treatment with azacitidine may have reduced the negative impact of MK in high-risk patients with MDS.

The clinical significance of loss of the Y chromosome, observed in 10% of patients with MDS and approximately 7% of older adult males without MDS, is undefined. Older adult males with MDS and loss of Y chromosome who achieve complete hematologic remission regain the Y chromosome in their marrow cells.

The prognosis of patients with MDS is very heterogeneous. In 1997, based on the cytogenetic abnormalities identified in 816 patients with MDS, as well as percentage of blasts and number of cytopenia, an IPSS was proposed.[9] According to the IPSS, 86% of all cytogenetic findings can be explicitly classified according to their prognostic impact. The system is highly reproducible and very simple to use, but it has certain limitations. Moreover, in the remaining 14% of patients with cytogenetic abnormalities the chromosomal abnor-malities had unknown prognostic significance (Fig. 56.25). This limitation underscores two major cytogenetic classification problems in MDS: the profound heterogeneity of acquired cytogenetic aberra-tions in MDS and the associated challenge of designing a compre-hensive cytogenetic scoring system that predicts the prognostic impact of rare abnormalities. A new and comprehensive cytogenetic scoring system based on an international data collection of 2902 patients was recently proposed (see Fig. 56.20). Patients included were from the German-Austrian MDS Study Group ($n = 1193$), the International MDS Risk Analysis Workshop ($n = 816$), the Spanish Hematological Cytogenetics Working Group ($n = 849$), and the International Working Group on MDS Cytogenetics ($n = 44$) data-bases. In total, 19 cytogenetic categories were defined, providing clear prognostic classification for 91% of all patients. All abnormalities were arranged according to OS and development of AML to classify their prognostic impact. The abnormalities were classified into five prognostic subgroups: very good ($n = 81$) included del(11q) and loss of Y chromosome (median OS, 61 months); good ($n = 1809$) included normal karyotype, del(5q), del(12p), and del(20q) (all as single anomaly) and double abnormalities including del(5q) (median OS 49 months); intermediate ($n = 529$) included del(7q), +8, i(17q) (q10), +19, +21, any other single abnormality, independent clones, and double abnormalities not harboring del(5q) or −7/del(7q) (median OS 26 months); poor ($n = 148$) included inv(3)/t(3q)/del(3q), −7, and double abnormalities including −7/del(7q) and complex (three abnormalities; OS of 16 months); and very poor ($n = 197$) included complex karyotypes with more than three abnor-malities (OS of 6 months) (see Fig. 56.20). This new scoring system proposed should be viewed as a dynamic model, open to further refinement as the knowledge in karyotypic abnormalities of MDS continues to evolve.[10]

Cytogenetic and FISH studies have relatively similar sensitivities in detecting an abnormal clone among patients with MDS. A FISH test for targeted recurrent abnormalities in MDS should use probes to detect numerical and structural anomalies of chromosome regions 1q, 3q, 5q, 7, 7q31, 8, 11q, 12p, 13q, 17p, 20q, and 21. Occasional patients with normal karyotype show an occult neoplastic clone by FISH. On the other hand, using conventional cytogenetic studies, some patients exhibit a neoplastic clone that is not detected by FISH (see box on Genetic Testing for Myelodysplastic Syndrome and Fig. 56.20).

Familial MDS is very rare. However, a recent description of four families with telomerase mutations, both in the RNA component (TERC) and in the reverse transcriptase component (TERT), has raised the awareness of the pathologic role of telomerase mutations

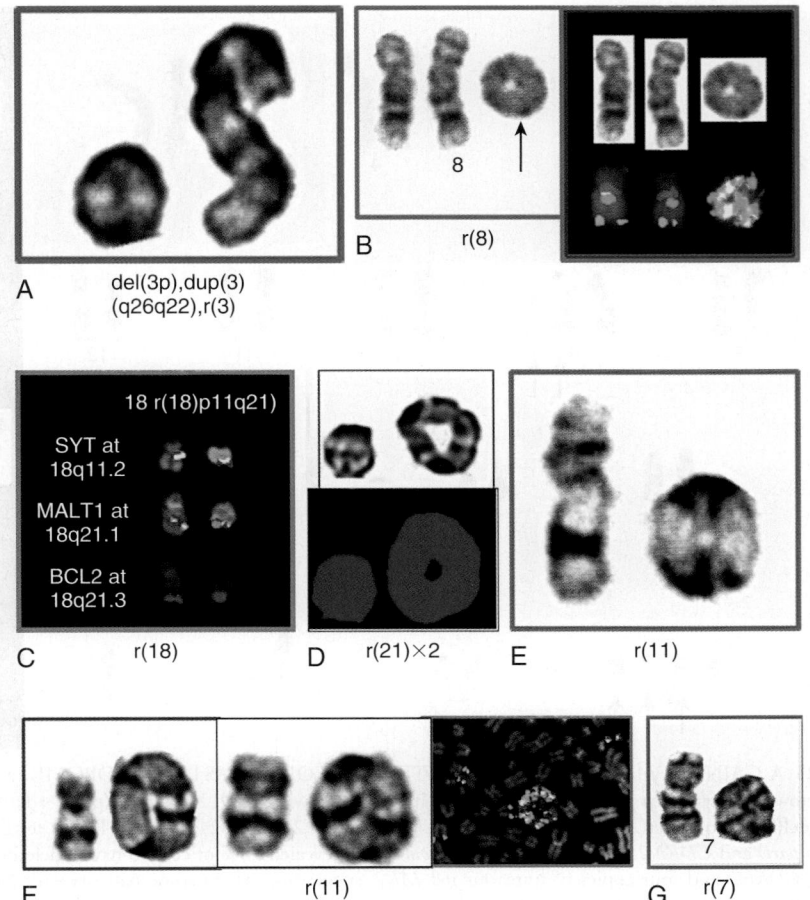

Fig. 56.24 RING CHROMOSOMES IN MYELODYSPLASTIC SYNDROME (MDS) AND OTHER HEMATOLOGIC MALIGNANCIES. (A) Ring 3 of one homolog and deletion 3p and duplication 3q of another homolog 3 in a patient with MDS and a complex karyotype. (B) A gain of ring of chromosome 8 in a patient with acute lymphoblastic leukemia. Metaphase FISH revealed amplification of *FGFR1 (red)* and *D8Z2 (green)* and loss of chromosome 8 region telomeric from 8p12 and below centromere *(green)* resulting in almost total loss of 8p and 8q because *MYC (aqua)* at 8q24 was deleted in r(8). r(18) with breakpoints at p11 and q21 in a patient with acute myeloid leukemia at diagnosis. Metaphase FISH revealed that *SYT*, *MALT1* and *BCL2* were retained in the ring 18. (D) Two different ring 21, as revealed by multicolor FISH in a patient with hairy cell leukemia and a complex karyotype. (E) Ring 11 in a patient with MDS. (F) Two different ring 11 in a patient with multiple myeloma. Metaphase FISH revealed *MLL* amplification *(yellow)* but not amplification of *CCND1 (red)*, *IGH (green)*, or centromere 11 *(aqua)*. (G) ring of chromosome 7 in a patient with T-cell leukemia. *TCRB* and *TCRG* are localized at 7p14 and 7q34, respectively.

in development of MDS/AML. The telomerase activity of the mutations identified in the four of 20 families with familial MDS/AML was between 0% and 11% of the wild-type levels. Patients with telomerase mutations have short telomeres. The recognition of familial MDS/AML arising from constitutional mutations in *TERC* or *TERT* is important because these mutations probably act as disease initiating mutations. Moreover, subsequent generations present with increasingly more severe phenotypes at an earlier age so that each successive generation inherits progressively shorter telomeres, which increasingly promote genomic instability and may lead to earlier development of marrow failure, MDS, or AML. The recommendation is that inherited lesions always be considered in a young patient presenting with MDS, even in the absence of preexisting morphologic or hematologic abnormalities. Another constitutional abnormality that appears to predispose to MDS/AML is a deletion of band region q22.1–q22.2 of chromosome 21 with a complex phenotype (dysmorphic features, organ malformations, growth delay, and mental retardation), germline *RUNX1* deletion, and congenital thrombocytopenia. Three of nine reported patients subsequently developed MDS/AML.

Table 56.5 shows the acquired recurrent somatic mutations observed in patients with MDS. According to the European Leukemia Net report 52% to 74% of patients with a normal karyotype have at least one genomic point mutation or MDS-related copy number change as detected by aCGH + SNP or genomic sequencing. When sequencing and cytogenetics were combined, 78% of MDS patients were found to have acquired genetic lesions. Most recently, Haferlach and colleagues screened MDS patients for known and putative mutations and deletions in 104 genes using targeted NGS and aCGH. They found 90% of patients harbored at least one mutation. Univariate analysis revealed that mutation in 25 genes had an effect on survival.

MDS is a disease of older people with a median age at diagnosis of 65–70; less than 10% of the patients are younger than 50 years. Using SNP array data from 50,000 subjects recruited for genome-wide association studies demonstrated that 0.5% of healthy individuals possessed genomic lesions. In contrast, recent whole-exome sequencing data of DNA from the peripheral blood of 17,182 persons showed clonal mutations leading to clonal outgrowth of hematopoietic cells in 10% of persons over the age of 70 years and in 18.4% among people aged 90–108 years. The most commonly mutated such genes were *DMT3A*, *TET2*, and *ASXL1*, which are frequent mutations in MDS and AML. These elderly people with clonal

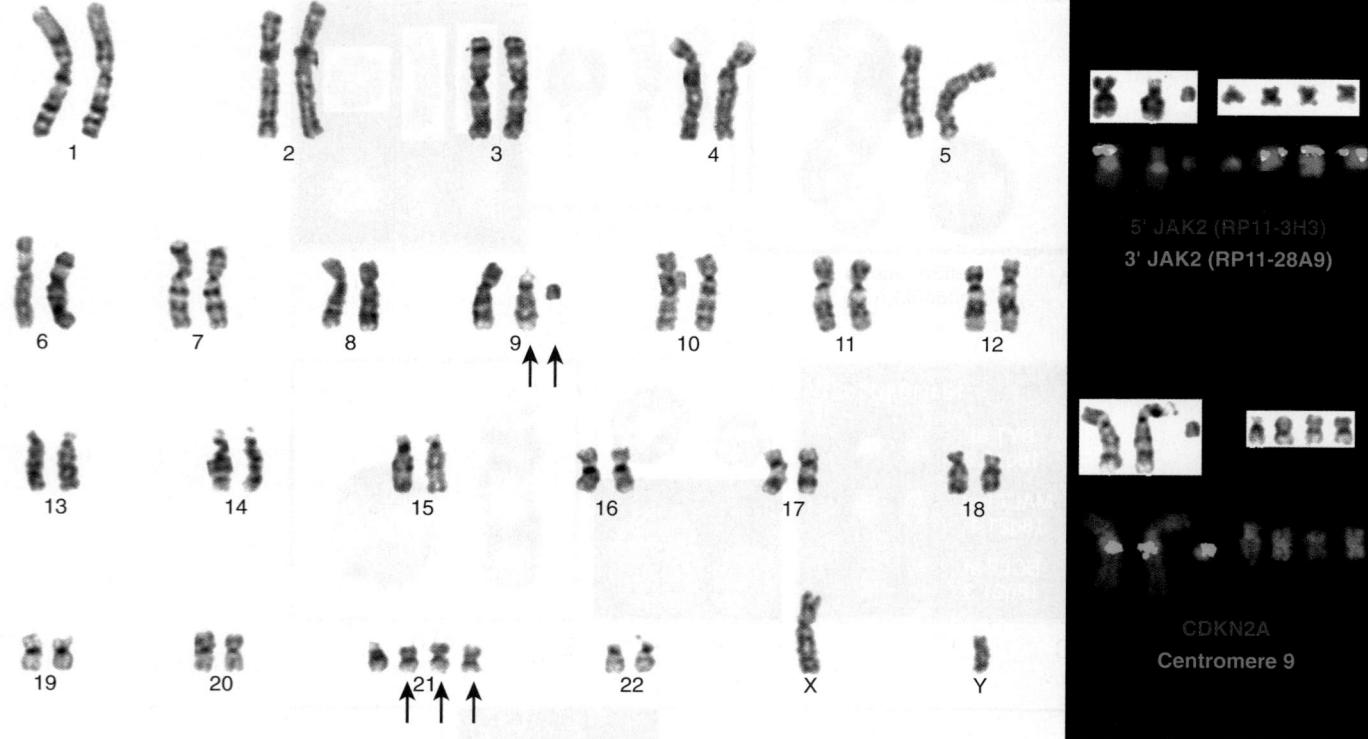

Fig. 56.25 A GAIN OF *JAK2* IN A PATIENT WITH MYELODYSPLASTIC SYNDROME (MDS). A bone marrow karyotype *(left panel)* from a patient with MDS showing a 49, XY, add(9)(p12), +der(9)del(9) (p12p24)del(9)(q12q34)der(21)t(9;21)p21p24;p11), +der(21)t(9;21)(p21p24;p11)×2. FISH testing with *JAK2 (top part)* and *CDKN2* and centromere 9 *(bottom panel)* revealed 70% of cells to have a deletion of 9p, including *CDKN2* and four copies of unrearranged *JAK2*, suggesting that in some patients with MDS the underling mechanism may be a gain of *JAK2*.

TABLE 56.5	Recurrently Mutated Genes in Myelodysplastic Syndrome		
Gene	**Chromosomal Location**	**Frequency (%)**	**Prognosis**
SFRB1	2q33.1	25–30	Favorable?
TET2	4q24	20–25	Neutral
RUNX1	21q22.12	10–20	Unfavorable
ASXL1	20q11.21	10–15	Unfavorable
SRSF2	17q25.1	10–15	Unfavorable
TP53	17p13	5–10	Unfavorable
U2AF1	19q13.42	5–10	Unfavorable
NRAS/KRAS	1p13.2/12p12.1	5–10	Unfavorable
DNMT3A	2p23.3	5	Unfavorable
ZRSR2	Xp22.2	5	Neutral?
EZH2	7q35-36	5	Unfavorable
IDH1/IDH2	2q33.3/15q26.1	2–3	Unfavorable
ETV6	12p13	2	Unfavorable
CBL	11q23.3	1–2	Unfavorable
NPM1	5q35.1	1–2	?
JAK2	9p24	1–2	Unfavorable
SETBP1	18q12.3	1–2	?
SF3A1	22q12.2	1–2	?
SF1	11q13.1	1–2	?
U2AF65	19q13.42	1–2	Unfavorable
PRPF40B	2q23.3	1–2	?

Modified from Malcovati et al: *Blood* 122:2943, 2013.

Genetic Testing for Myelodysplastic Syndrome Disorder

The best genetic test at diagnosis is conventional cytogenetic studies. FISH for targeted loci is useful for some clinical situations, such as marrow samples lacking analyzable metaphases, or to follow the percentage of abnormal cells with known cytogenetic anomalies for patients undergoing treatment (see Fig. 56.20 for selection of appropriate fluorescence in situ hybridization probes). Integrating cytogenetics, FISH and microarray comparative genomic hybridization (CGH), particularly in patients with a normal karyotype, allows greater confidence in detection of genomic change fostering improved patient-specific management.

mutations in their peripheral blood did not have MDS or any other hematologic malignancy, indicating that age-related clonal hematopoiesis is a common premalignant condition and individuals with clonal mutations have an increased risk of developing hematologic malignancy.

ACUTE MYELOID LEUKEMIA

AML refers to a group of heterogeneous diseases with respect to clonality, molecular lesions, chromosomal aberrations, and response to treatment (see Chapter 59). Initially, using G6PD as a marker of clonality, it was determined that AML originates from a single clone and has a multistep pathogenesis. In adults, at the time of diagnosis all hematopoietic cell lineages are clonal. In children younger than 16 years, erythroid cells and platelets often are not part of the leukemic clone.

The application of nucleotide-polymorphism technologies has confirmed the clonal origin of AML and have further revealed that most, if not all, patients with AML evolve through a process of constrained clonal evolution. Multicolor metaphase analysis, FISH, CGH arrays, SNP arrays, PCR arrays, and NGS have all greatly improved detection of subclones and established the concept of a clonal hierarchy in AML. To understand the branching evolution of AML development, each mutation must be placed in the context whether it is a "driver" versus "passenger" and an "initiation" versus "progression" event. Driver mutations directly affect the biology of the cell, whereas passenger mutations do not. Initiation mutations are present within the founding clone and are found in all AML cells. Progression mutations emerge during leukemic evolution, can be found as subclones, and exist in only a fraction of AML cells. Selection pressure, such as chemotherapy, can favor the elimination or outgrowth of different branches within the AML evolutionary hierarchy.

Modern genomic technologies have provided a better understanding of normal and leukemic hematopoiesis. A subset of AML cases evolves from a preceding clinically overt phase such as MDS by subclonal evolution with an increased number of genomic changes. The founder mutations present in preleukemic cells are retained in AML blasts, implicating them as putative initiating events and establishing clonal expansion as the first step in leukemogenesis. However, some recurrent leukemia-associated somatic mutations, such as *TET2,* have been also linked to multilineage clonal hematopoiesis in aging healthy individuals. For the majority of de novo AML without any prior clinical symptoms, the cell of origin, and biologic consequences of initiating mutations and order of subsequent mutations remain poorly understood. Recent evidence revealed that approximately 25% of adult AMLs are associated with *DNMT3A* mutations, which occurs in preleukemic hematopoietic stem cells before acquiring additional mutations such as *NPM1*. These initiating *DNMT3A* mutation–carrying cells persist during remission suggesting that preleukemic hematopoietic stem cells are resistant to induction chemotherapy and may represent a reservoir from which a future relapse develops.

Initial observations by the International Workshop on Chromosomes in Leukemia asserted that cytogenetic findings may serve as the single most important prognostic marker in AML; these observations were subsequently validated through studies conducted by the Medical Research Council (MRC), the Cancer and Leukemia Group B (CALGB), and the Southwest Oncology Group. Finally, in 2008, the WHO incorporated cytogenetic findings along with morphology, immunologic markers, and molecular genetics into their classification system. Cytogenetics is the most powerful independent prognostic factor in AML and provides the framework for risk stratification schemes that have been generally adopted to guide treatment approach. Based on karyotype status, two major groups of AML can be distinguished: (a) those with an abnormal karyotype, which accounts for approximately 52% of patients, and (b) those with a normal karyotype by conventional cytogenetics, which accounts for 48% of patients with AML.

Acute Myeloid Leukemia with a Normal Karyotype

Patients with AML with a normal karyotype who present between the ages of 16 and 60 years carry an intermediate prognosis. However, cytogenetically normal AML is highly heterogeneous at the molecular level, both mutations and overexpression of single genes have been identified, and their complex interactions are frequently refined to provide more accurate risk stratification. Within the normal cytogenetic category, 45% to 62% of patients with AML have nucleophosmin 1 (*NPM1*) mutations, 25% to 35% show *FLT3* mutations, 5% to 10% have *MLL* tandem duplications, and 8% to 15% have *CEBPA* mutations. The prognosis of patients with normal karyotype differs in the presence of each of these mutations (Table 56.6). Patients with *NPM1* mutations alone have a favorable prognosis, with 60% of patients living longer than 11 years. Even in patients age 70 or older, the presence of an *NPM1* mutation is an independent predictor of a more favorable outcome. More than 20 different mutations have been described in the C-terminal portion of the protein that lead to loss

TABLE 56.6	Gene Mutations in Patients with Acute Myeloid Leukemia and a Normal Karyotype		
Gene	Chromosomal Location	Frequency (%) of Patients With Normal Karyotype	Prognosis
NPM1	5q35	45–62	Favorable, increased CR rates and prolonged OS in the absence of FLT3 mutation
FLT3-IDT	13q12	25–35	Unfavorable, specifically when the mutant to WT allelic ratio is high
FLT3-TKD	13q12	7–10	Controversial
CEBPA	19q13.1	15	Favorable
MLL-PTD	11q23	10	Not known
IDH1	2q33.3	15–20	Most likely unfavorable
IDH2	15q26.1	20	Most likely unfavorable
DNMT3A	2p23.2	36	Most likely unfavorable
TET2	4q24	5	Likely unfavorable
ASXL1	20q11.21	9–10	Inferior outcome

CR, Complete remission; OS, overall survival.

of tryptophan residues and generation of a nuclear export signal that acts in concert to cause delocalization of *NPM1* from the nuclei to the cytoplasm. Because the functional integrity of *NPM1* is dependent on its ability to shuttle between the nucleus and cytoplasm, this ability is severely compromised in *NPM1*-mutated AML. *NPM1*-mutated AML is associated with distinctive biologic and clinical features including older age, female predominance, multilineage involvement, extramedullary disease, high blast percentages and increased white blood cell counts, and lack of CD34 expression. As an isolated molecular abnormality, *NPM1*-mutated AML is associated with a highly favorable prognosis, with complete remission (CR) rates between 70% and 80%. The most common mutation (type A, accounting for 75% of all mutations) generates an aberrant extra nuclear export signal. Although *NPM1* mutations are heterozygous, hetero/homodimerization with wild-type *NPM1* results in cytoplasmic mislocalization of both mutant and wild-type protein. This alteration in subcellular location perturbs normal *NPM1* function, including the mislocalization and stabilization of critical proteins such as the TP53 regulator p14ARF, and leads to transformation. This process also generates a distinct transcriptional signature in *NPM1* AML that facilitates the generation of leukemia. *NPM1* mutation is considered to be an early event in the pathogenesis of AML. In childhood AML with normal cytogenetics, *NPM1* mutations are relatively uncommon, occurring at a frequency of 8%.

In contrast, the presence of *FLT3* and *MLL* mutations are associated with an adverse prognosis, and coexistence of *FLT3* and *NPM1* does not improve the prognosis. Internal tandem duplications (ITDs) of the *FLT3* gene confer an increased risk for relapse and death when compared with patients without *FLT3*-ITD. Three types of *FLT3* gene changes are present, ITD of the juxtamembrane domain-coding sequence, a point mutation within the activation loop domain and the copy-neutral loss of heterozygosity. Although both mutations lead to the constitutive activation of the receptor, only presence of *FLT3*-ITD with high allelic ratio has been associated with an inferior outcome. This mutation initially develops as a heterozygous mutation and over time the *FLT3*-IDT blasts acquire copy-neutral loss of heterozygosity resulting in homozygous mutated allele and high *FLT3*-ITD allelic ratio.

Intact functioning of the CCAAT/enhancer binding protein (*CEBPA*) gene is essential for normal granulocytic differentiation. It is a lineage-specific transcription factor that is required for the formation of committed myeloid progenitors from multipotent progenitor cells. *CEBPA* execute this function by coupling the direct transcriptional activation of myeloid-specific genes with the arrest of cell proliferation. *CEBPA* is an intronless gene whose mRNA can be translated into two different AUG codons to give rise to two distinct isoforms, p42 and p30. Only the p42 isoform of *CEBPA* can promote proliferation arrest. *CEBPA* mutations, leading to arrest of differentiation, are seen in 5% to 10% of de novo AML and in up to 15% of normal karyotype AML. Only mutations affecting both alleles, double mutations, confer superior survival as compared to single mutations. Concomitant *GATA1* and *WT1* mutations are seen more often in double mutants while *FLT3*-ITD, *NPM1*, *ASXL1*, and *RUNX1* are mutations more commonly associated with single mutations, possibly contributing to the poorer prognosis.[11]

A rare but specific subset of adult AML can be defined by the cytogenetically cryptic *NUP98-NSD1* fusion gene that involves the nucleoporin gene 98 (*NUP98*) on chromosome11p15, and the nonhomeobox gene *NSD1* present on chromosomal band 5q35. *NUP98* encodes a 98-kDa protein of the nuclear pore complex, and is known to fuse with at least 21 different fusion gene partners in chromosomal rearrangements in various hematologic malignancies. NSD1 is thought to function both as a transcriptional co-activator and a co-repressor. Among 293 pediatric and 808 adult cytogenetically normal cases of AML the *NUP98-NSD1* fusion gene has been described in 16.1% of pediatric and 2.3% of adult AML cases. Apparently *NUP98-NSD1* has been shown to correlate with *FLT3*-ITD, which is associated with increased blast percentages.

TET2 proteins are necessary for the conversion of 5-methylcytosine to 5-hydromethylcytosine and play a role in demethylation processes within the cell. *TET2* mutations have been reported in 10% to 23% of patients with AML with a normal karyotype. The impact of *TET2* mutations on the prognosis and outcome remains poorly defined.

DNMT3A mutations, which affect the DNA methyltransferase enzymes and subsequent epigenetic modulation, have been described in about 27% to 33% of normal karyotype AML and are associated with a worse OS (see earlier sections on Clonal Origin and Early Mutations).[12,13]

Currently, a newly diagnosed patient with AML and a normal karyotype should be checked for more common mutations such as *FLT3*, *NPM1*, *CEBPA*, *RUNX1*, *MLL-PTD*, or *EVI1*, *TET2* and *DNMT3A*, which may have prognostic and possibly therapeutic implications. Patients with overexpression of other single genes should stay, until more data are collected, in a research setting of clinical trials (Table 56.6).

Acute Myeloid Leukemia with an Abnormal Karyotype

Among patients with an abnormal karyotype, 25% have balanced translocations and 27% showed unbalanced abnormalities or a complex karyotype.

The pretreatment karyotype in AML constitutes an independent prognostic determinant for attainment of CR and risk for relapse and survival. Four broad cytogenetic risk categories of AML are useful in clinical practice: favorable, intermediate, unfavorable, and unknown (Figs. 56.26 and 56.27 and Table 56.7). It is important to perform appropriate cytogenetic and FISH studies to establish the correct cytogenetic risk category.[14] Table 56.8 lists 72 of approximately 250 recurrent chromosomal translocations in leukemia, including AML

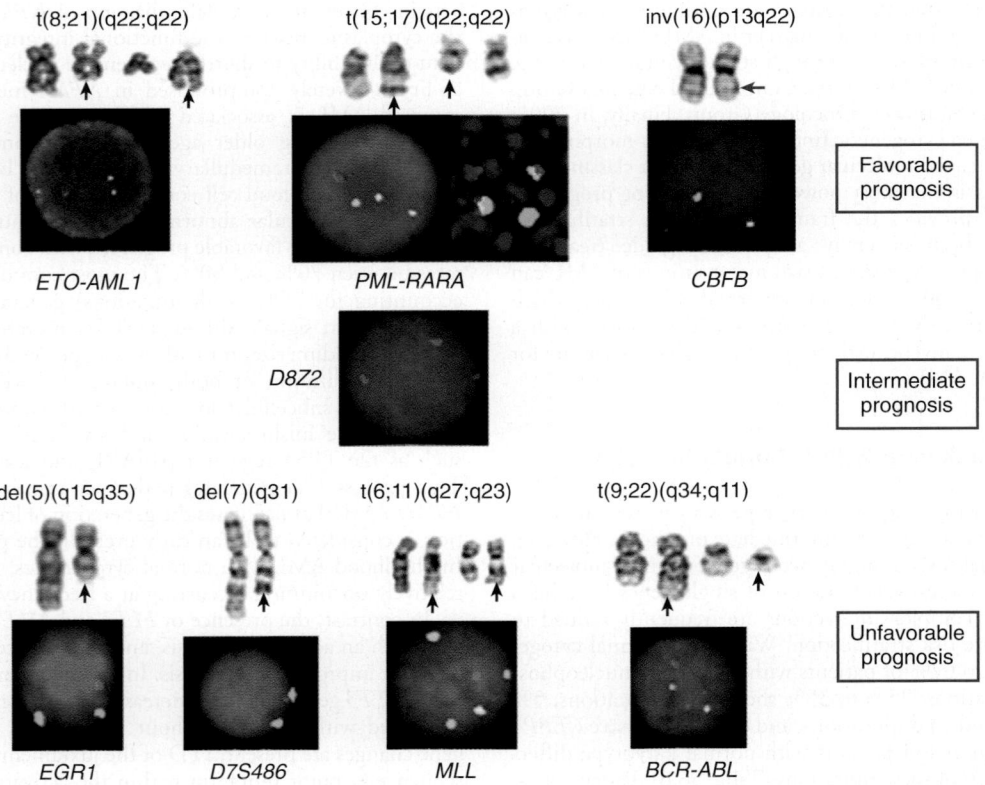

Fig. 56.26 PROGNOSTIC CYTOGENETIC RISK CATEGORIES IN ACUTE MYELOID LEUKEMIA. Favorable prognosis includes t(8;21) and ETO-AML1 fusion, t(15;17) and PML-RARA fusion, and inv(16) and rearrangements of *CBFB* on 16q22. Trisomy 8 is associated with intermediate prognosis. Unfavorable cytogenetic risk categories include monosomy 5/del(5q), −7/del(7q), and translocations of 11q23 and *MLL*, represented here by t(6;11), and the Philadelphia chromosome.

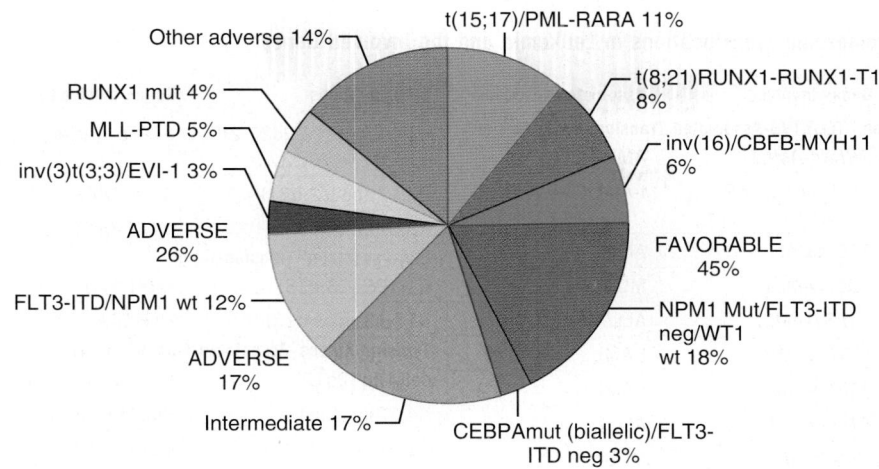

Fig. 56.27 INTEGRATION OF CYTOGENETIC ABNORMALITIES AND MOLECULAR MARKERS TO REFINE RISK GROUPS IN ACUTE MYELOID LEUKEMIA. *(Reprinted from Smith ML, Hills RK, Grimwade D: Independent prognostic variables in acute myeloid leukemia.* Blood Rev *25:39, 2001; with permission.)*

TABLE 56.7   Modification of European Leukemia Net Prognostic System in Acute Myeloid Leukemia

Prognostic Group	Subset	CR rate; relapse with 3+7 without HCT	Comments
Favorable	inv(16)/t(16;16) NK and *NPM1+/FLT3* ITD-NK and *CEBPA* +/+	>80%–90%; 35%–40%	Outcome worse in older patients, with t-AML, KIT mutations, and poor response to initial therapy
Intermediate	Mutated NPM1 and FLIT3-ITD (without adverse-risk genetic lession), t(9;11)(p21.3;q23.3)/MLL-KMT2A	50%–80%; 50%–60%	Outcome worse in older patients, with t-AML, and poor initial response
	Cytogenetic abnormalities Not in favorable or adverse group *FLT3* ITD+		Outcome worse in older patients, with t-AML, and poor initial response
Adverse	−5, −7, 5q abn, 3q, 17p, 11q (other than 9;11), t(6;9), complex, monosomal karyotype, wild type NMP1 and FLT3-ITD, Mutated RUNX1, Mutated ASXL1 and mutated TP53, insufficient metaphases for analysis	<50%; >90%	Outcome worse in older patients, with t-AML, and poor initial response

CR, Complete remission; HCT, hematopoietic cell transplant; NK, normal karyotype; +/+, double mutation.

and excluding *MLL* translocations (see later) (see Fig. 56.26). Because of their specific association with distinct subtypes of leukemia, some AML-specific translocations have been incorporated into the WHO classification as criteria for subclassification of AML, including t(8;21), t(15;17), inv(16), and 11q23 rearrangements, regardless of the morphology or percentage of blast cells.

Two specific cytogenetic types of AML—t(8;21)(q22;q22) and inv(16)(p13q22) or t(16;16)(p13;q22) (see Fig. 56.27)—are called *core-binding factor (CBF)* AMLs and are usually grouped in clinical studies because of similarities between their molecular and prognostic features. However, the morphologic features of these two AML subtypes are very different, suggesting that individual approaches may enhance clinical benefits in future studies. Patients with t(8;21) exhibit large myeloid blasts with abundant basophilic cytoplasm, numerous azurophilic granules, and occasional Auer rods. Patients with 16q22 abnormalities show variable numbers of eosinophils, usually in increased numbers, in all stages of maturation. The immature eosinophilic granules are larger than normal and may contain purple-violet cytoplasmic granules. The t(8;21) subtype may be present alone, although 30% to 35% of patients also display loss of Y chromosomes in males and loss of X chromosome in females (see Fig. 56.26, *top left*). Another 20% of patients with t(8;21) have a deletion of 9q12–23, including a commonly deleted segment that spans 7 to 8 Mb. Trisomies for chromosomes 4 and 8 together with t(8;21) are observed in 6% to 10% of patients. Virtually all patients with t(8;21) achieve CR. Additional cytogenetic abnormalities, irrespective of their nature or complexity, do not have a deleterious effect on rates of remission, relative risk of relapse, and OS. The t(8;21)

interrupts two genes—*RUNX1* (*CBFA2*) on chromosome 21, band q22, in intron 5, and *RUNX1T1* (*ETO* [eight, twenty-one gene], on chromosome 8, band q22—and joins them to form a new chimeric gene on the abnormal der(8) chromosome. *RUNX1* is a gene on chromosome 21, also known as *CBFA2* because it encodes for a DNA-binding component of CBF and binds DNA through a specific sequence called the *runt domain*. The *RUNX1* gene locus on chromosome 21 spans 120 kb; the *RUNX1T1* gene on chromosome 8 is distributed over 87 kb.

The *RUNX1* gene has been identified in more than 39 chromosomal translocations in leukemia and plays a critical role during hematopoiesis (see different *RUNX1* chromosomal partners: *http://atlasgeneticsoncology.org/Genes/AML1ID52.html*). The fusion gene is located on the partner chromosome in the majority of *RUNX1* translocations. Its disruption is associated with the development of myeloid and lymphoid leukemias. Therefore *RUNX1* is viewed as a master regulatory switch that controls development of a definitive hematopoietic lineage. Moreover, the *RUNX1* transcription factor is critical for proliferation and differentiation of hematopoietic stem cells. Haploinsufficiency of *RUNX1* has been linked to a propensity to develop AML, and biallelic nonsense mutations in the *RUNX1* gene have been identified in the primitive AMLs of the French-American-British (FAB) M0 subtype. The RUNX1T1 protein belongs to the ETO family of proteins involved in protein–protein interactions but not in protein–DNA interactions.

In the hybrid RUNX1-RUNXT1 protein, the C-terminus of RUNX1 is replaced by the entire RUNXT1 protein. The main functional characteristic of RUNX1-RUNX1T1 chimeric protein is

TABLE 56.8   Recurring Chromosome Translocations in Leukemia and the Involved Genes

Translocations	Genes Involved	Associated Diseases	Translocations	Genes Involved	Associated Diseases
CBF (AML1/CBFA and CBFB)- and TEL/ETV6-Associated Translocation/Inversion			t(17;17)(q21.2.;q21.2)/ del(17)(q21.2	STATB-RARA	APL
t(X;21)(p22;q22)	PRDX4-AML1	AML	t(X;17)(p11.2;q21)	BCOr-RARA	APL
t(3;21)(q26;q22)	EVI1-MDS1-EAP-AML1	t-AML/CML-ACC/BC	t(3;5)(q25;q35)	MLF1-NPM	AML/MDS
t(8;21)(q22;q22)	ETO-AML1	AML	**E2A-Associated Translocations**		
t(8;21)(q23q22)	FOG2-AML1	MDS	t(1;19)(q23;p13)	PBX1-E2A	B-ALL
t(8;21)(q24q22)	TRPS1-AML1	ALL/AML	t(17;19)(q23;p13)	HLF-E2A	B-ALL
t(16;21)(q24;q22)	MTG16-AML1	t-AML	**Tyrosine Kinase–Associated Translocations**		
t(19;21)(q13;q22)	AMP19-AML1	t-AML	del(4)(q12q12)	FIP1L1-PDGFRA	HES
t(12;21)(p12;22)	ETV6-AML1	ALL	t(4;22)(q12;q11)	PDGFRA-BCR	MPN
t(21;21)(q11;q22)	UPS25-AML1	MDS	t(3;5)(q25;q35)	MLF1-NPM	AML/MDS
inv(16)/t(16;16) (p13;q22)	MYH11-CBFB	AML-M4	t(1;5)(q23;q33)	Myomegalin-PDGFRB	MPD
t(1;12)(p36;p13)	MDS2-ETV6	CML/MDS	t(5;7)(q33;q11.2)	PDGFRB-HIP1	CMML
t(1;12)(q21;p13)	ARNT-ETV6	AML	t(5;10)(q33;q21)	PDGFRB-H4	MPD
t(1;12)(q25;p13)	ARG-ETV6	AML	t(5;12)(q33;p13)	PDGFRB-ETV6	CMML, CEL
t(3;12)(q26;p13)	MDS1-EV1-ETV6	MPD	t(5;14)(q33;q32)	PDGFRB/-AV14	AML
t(4;12)(p11;p13)	BTL-TV6	AML	t(5;14)(q33;q24)	PDGFRB/-IN	MPD
t(5;12)(pq31;p13)	ACS2-ETV6	AML	t(5;15)(q33;q15)	PDGFRB/-P53BP1	MPD
t(5;12)(q33;p13)	PDGFRB-ETV6	CMML	t(5;17)(q33;p13)	PDGFRB-RABEPI	CMML
t(6;12)(q23;p13)	STL-ETV6	ALL	t(5;17)(q33;p11.2)	PDGFRB-HCMOGT	JMML
t(7;12)(q36;p13)	HLXB9-ETV6	AML	t(q;22)(p24;q11.2)	BCR-JAK2	CML-
t(9;12)(p24;p13)	JAK2-ETV6	ALL, aCML	t(9;12)(p24;q13)	JAK2-ETV6	CML-
t(9;12)(q22;p13)	SYK-ETV6	MDS	t(8;9)(p22;p24)	PCMI-JAK2	MPD, AL
t(9;12)(p34;p13)	ABL-ETV6	CMML	**NUP98/NUP214-Associated Translocations**		
t(12;13)(p13;q12)	ETV6-CSX2	AML	t(1;11)(q23;p15)	PMX1/NUP98	AML
t(12;13)(p13;q14)	ETV6-TTL	ALL	t(2;11)(q31;p15)	HOXD13/NUP98	t-AML
t(12;15)(p13;q25)	ETV6-NTRK3	AML	t(4;11)(q21;p15)	RAP1GDS1/NUP98	T-ALL
t(12;17)(p13;p12)	ETV6-PER1	AML	t(5;11)(q35;p15)	NSD/NUP98	AML
t(12;21)(p13;q11)	ETV6-MN1	AML	t(7;11)(p15;p15)	HOXA9/NUP98	AML
t(12;16)(p13;p11)	CHOP-TLS/FUS	AML	t(9;11)(p22;p15)	LEDGF/NUP98	AML
t(16;21)(p11;q22)	TLS-FUS/-RG	AML, MLS	inv(11)(p15q22)	NUP98/DDX10	t-AML
RARA-Associated Translocation			t(11;20)(p23;q34)	NUP98/TOP1	t-MDS
t(15;17)(q22;21)	PML-RARA	APL	t(6;9)(p23;q34)	DEK/NUP214(CAN)	AML
t(5;17)(q32;q21)	NPM-RARA	APL	Normal karyotype	SET/NUP214(CAN)	AML
t(2;17)(q32.3;q21)	NABP1-RARA	APL	**FGFR1-Associated Translocations**		
t(4;17)(q12;q21)	FIP1L1-RARA	APL	t(8;13)(p11;q12)	ZNF198-FGFR1	MPN
t(11;17)(q23;q21)	ZBTB16-RARA	APL	t(7;8)(q32;P11)	TRIM24-FGFR1	MPN
t(11;17)(q13;q21)	NuMA-RARA	APL	t(6;8)(q27;P11)	FGFR1OP-FGFR1	MPN
t(11;17)(q23;q21)	MLL-RARA	APL	ins(12;8)(p11;p11p22)	FGFR1OP2-FGFR1	MPN
			t(8;17)(p11;q11)	MYO18A-FGFR1	MPN
			t(8;22)(p11;q11,2)	BCR-FGFR1	MPN

ACC/BC, Accelerated blast crisis; AL, Acute leukemia; aCML, atypical CML; ALL, acute lymphoblastic leukemia; AML, acute myeloid leukemia; APL, acute promyelocytic leukemia; CBF, core-binding factor; CEL, chronic eosinophilic leukemia; CML, chronic myelogenous leukemia; CMML, chronic myelomonocytic leukemia; HES, hypereosinophilic syndrome; JMML, juvenile myelomonocytic leukemia; MDS, myelodysplastic syndrome; MLS, myelodysplastic syndrome; MPD, myeloproliferative disorder; MPN, myeloproliferative neoplasm; T-ALL, T-cell ALL; t-AML, therapy-related AML; t-MDS, therapy-related MDS.

its ability to bind DNA containing RUNX1 binding sites and thereby exert a dominant negative inhibition of the endogenous RUNX1 protein. The exact role of the RUNX1-RUNX1T1 fusion protein in determining the onset and progression of AML is not fully understood; however, accumulating evidence indicates that even a point mutation in the RUNX1 protein, responsible for assembling and organizing the machinery for hematopoietic gene expression at multiple sites in target genes, results in a block of differentiation of myeloid progenitors to granulocytes. RUNX1 mutations are present in 46% of patients with AML with the M0 subtype and in 80% of patients with AML with trisomy 13. As mentioned earlier, the FLT3 gene is localized on chromosome 13, and quantitation of FLT3 transcript levels is associated with a fivefold increase in patients with RUNX1 mutations and trisomy 13 compared with patients without trisomy 13. The exact relationship between FLT3 and RUNX1 in leukemogenesis remains unknown. Multiple copies of RUNX1/

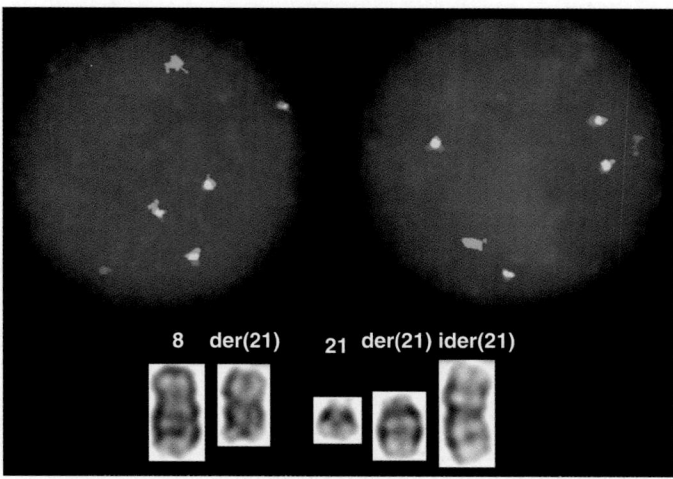

Fig. 56.28 DUPLICATION OF t(8;21). Four copies of ETO-AML1 (RUNX) fusion *(yellow)* shown in two interphase cells *(top)* from a patient with acute myeloid leukemia and t(8;21) *(bottom)* karyotype, as well as ider(21). This formation is equivalent to the Ph duplication in the blast crisis of chronic myelogenous leukemia because of duplication of der(21) without accompanying t(8;21).

RUNXT1 fusion have been demonstrated (Fig. 56.28). The t(8;21) is the most common translocation in pediatric patients with AML (10%–20%). Prenatal origin of t(8;21) was established for approximately 50% of pediatric patients using Guthrie card analysis.

Although 60% to 70% patients with t(8;21) achieve complete and long-term remission, monitoring minimal residual disease using t(8;21) marker is important in identifying patients with a high risk for relapse. Multiparametric approaches, such as flow cytometry, RQ-PCR, and interphase FISH, are complementary methods and provide useful clinical information on relapse kinetics. It should be noted that 18% of healthy individuals have *RUN1-RUNXT1* transcript by PCR and the fusion transcript has been detected in 40% of cord blood samples, suggesting that *RUNX1-RUNXT1* by itself may not have overt leukemic manifestations.

In patients with 16q22 abnormalities such as inv(16)(p13;q22) and t(16;16)(p13;q22), the marrow contains an increased percentage of abnormal eosinophils (Fig. 56.29). Combined May-Grünwald-Giemsa staining with FISH demonstrates that the abnormal eosinophils have inv(16) and are therefore part of the leukemic clone. Trisomy 22 is a frequent accompanying abnormality. Both inv(16) (see Fig. 56.26, *top right*) and t(16;16) (see Fig. 56.29) are abnormalities of the *CBFβ* gene at 16q22 and are associated with M4Eo subtype, according to the FAB classification of AML. Both rearrangements result in fusion of *CBFβ* and *MYH11* (myosin heavy-chain) gene on 16p13. The exact role of the resulting hybrid protein, CBFβ-SMMHC (smooth muscle myosin heavy chain), is unknown, but it probably is involved in impaired hematopoietic differentiation. Both t(8;21) and inv(16) rearrangements result in abnormal repression of CBF target genes. CBF is a heterodimeric transcription factor complex that consists of three distinct DNA-binding CBFα subunits *RUNX1, RUNX2,* and *RUNX3* and a common *CBFβ* subunit, which is non–DNA-binding. The binding affinity of *RUNX1* subunit to the DNA promoter sequences is significantly increased by association with *CBFβ*, which does not directly interact with DNA and protects the *RUNX1* subunit from proteolysis. The breakpoints in t(8;21) affect *RUNX1* exon 5 and *RUNX1T1* exon 2. The breakpoint in *MYH11* involved in inv(16) and t(16;16) is variable and gives rise to at least 10 different fusion variants. In contrast, the breakpoints in *CBFβ* at 16q22 are at intron 5. Both translocations are associated with a favorable prognosis, but they exhibit different leukemic cell morphology.

Approximately 4% of patients with *CBFβ-MYH11* rearrangement do not have a cytogenetically detectable inv(16) or t(16;16).

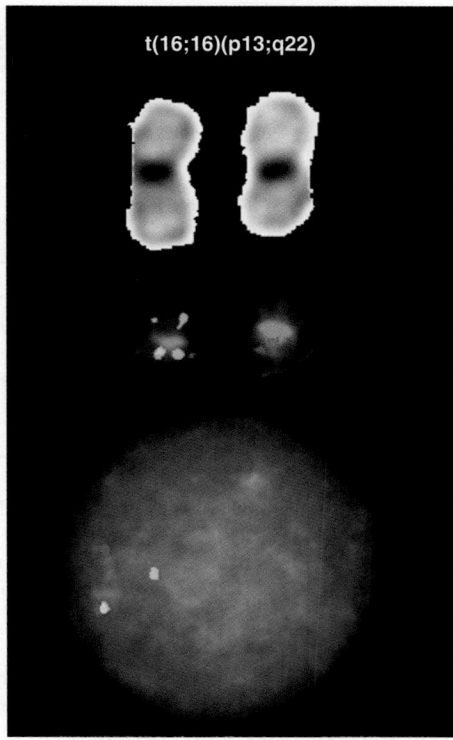

Fig. 56.29 Partial G-banded karyotype from a patient with M4 acute myeloid leukemia showing t(16;16) *(top)*, after FISH study using a breakapart CBFB probe (at 16q22), demonstrating that the 5′ end *(red)* of the gene remains on 16q of one chromosome 16, whereas the 3′ end *(green)* translocated to the short arms of the other chromosome 16. Separation of 5′ and 3′ ends as single signals is indicated in the bone marrow nucleus *(bottom)*.

Cytogenetic detection of inv(16) may be difficult, and interphase FISH with a dual-color *CBFβ* probe at diagnosis is a crucial genetic test. Detection of *CBFβ-MYH11* fusion by either RT-PCR or FISH is found in patients without eosinophilia; therefore *CBFβ* testing should be included in the standard AML testing panel. The presence of additional abnormalities, such as trisomy 8, do not adversely affect clinical outcomes. The *CBFβ-MYH11* chimeric fusion is detected in utero approximately 10 years before development of childhood leukemia. This observation suggests that formation of *CBFβ-MYH11* is not sufficient to cause leukemia and that subsequent genetic events must occur before clinically recognizable leukemia occurs.

Most clinical studies have found that the CBF AML group is associated with a better CR rate, OS, and lower relapse risk than patients with cytogenetically normal AML. However, a recent retrospective analysis of 113 patients with CBF AML demonstrated that at diagnosis, patients with inv(16) were less likely to have any normal metaphases when compared with patients showing t(8;21) karyotype. Moreover, the identification of an increasing number of cells with normal metaphases increased the risk for relapse and negatively affected the survival of patients with inv(16); identifying at least one normal metaphase at diagnosis and 19 with inv(16) had a significant impact on 5-year survival (60% versus 14%, $p = .00005$). These factors, along with age, were the only independent variables associated with refractory disease and higher relapse. Nevertheless, CBF AML has been defined as a favorable genetic group by National Comprehensive Cancer Network (NCCN) guidelines and ELN recommendations.

NCCN guidelines have classified t(8;21) and inv(16) AMLs with c-*KIT* mutations as having intermediate risk disease, whereas the ELN has provided no further recommendations for those with c-*KIT* mutations. Mutations in the *KIT* gene are the most recurrent molecular abnormalities, occurring in 15% to 46% of the cases, and are associated with a higher risk for relapse. The mutation frequency was similar for pediatric and adult patients with t(8;21) whereas pediatric

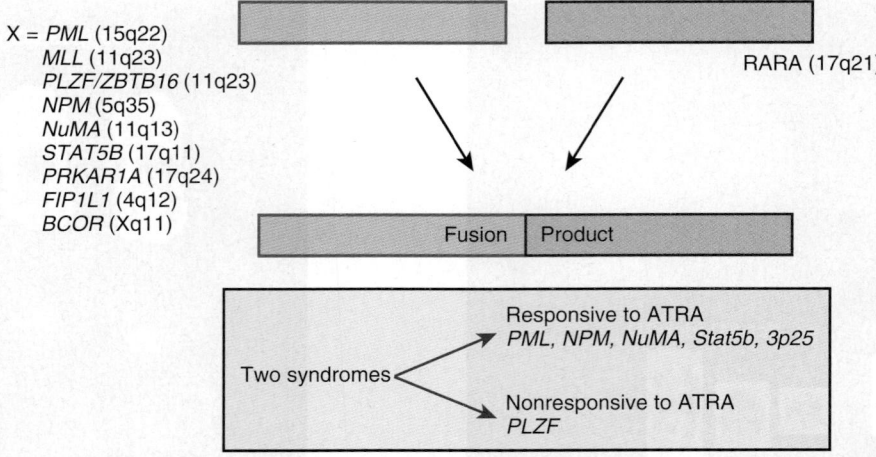

X = *PML* (15q22)
MLL (11q23)
PLZF/ZBTB16 (11q23)
NPM (5q35)
NuMA (11q13)
STAT5B (17q11)
PRKAR1A (17q24)
FIP1L1 (4q12)
BCOR (Xq11)

RARA (17q21)

Fusion Product

Two syndromes

Responsive to ATRA
PML, NPM, NuMA, Stat5b, 3p25

Nonresponsive to ATRA
PLZF

Fig. 56.30 MOLECULAR CYTOGENETIC DEFECTS IN ACUTE PROMYELOCYTIC LEUKEMIA ARE RESPONSIBLE FOR DIFFERENT RESPONSE TO ALL-*TRANS* RETINOIC ACID DIFFEREN-TIATION THERAPY. Patients with t(11;17)(q23(q22) and PLZF(ZBTB16)-RARA fusion do not respond to all-*trans* retinoic acid (ATRA) differentiation therapy, whereas patients with classic t(15;17) and other four cytogenetic variants have exquisite sensitivity to differentiate in response to all-trans retinoic acid.

patients with inv(16) AML tend to have higher frequency of *KIT* mutations than adult patients. The mutations are clustered within exon 17, which encodes the *KIT* activation loop (A-loop) in the kinase domain, and in exon 8, which encodes an evolutionarily highly conserved region in the extracellular portion of the *KIT* receptor. *KIT17* mutations occur almost exclusively at codon D816 in patients with inv(16), and at codons D816 or N8822 in patients with t(8;21). *KIT* mutations represent not only a prognostic indicator but also a potential therapeutic target for TKI therapy. In adults the mutation frequency in exon 17 is significantly higher in t(8;21) than in inv(16) patients with AML (35.6% vs. 6.9%, respectively, *p* < .0001), whereas the mutation frequency in exon 8 is significantly lower in t(8;21) than inv(16) patients with AML (4.4% versus 18.8%, respectively, *p* = .0003). The prognostic value of *KIT* mutations in CBF AML remains debatable. The incidence, characteristics and prognostic effects of *KIT* mutations are different for different subgroups. It appears that mutations in exon 17 have a strong adverse impact on the relapse and survival of adult patients with t(8;21) AML.

Other activated mutations associated with CBF AML include *FLT3*, *CBL*, *NRAS* or *KRAS*, and *ASXL2*. *FLT3* point mutations (most common D835), are frequently associated with inv(16) (6%–24%) and 6% of patients have *CBL* mutations associated with improved OS. *NRAS*- and *KRAS*-activating mutations are preferentially observed in inv(16) and do not impact on prognosis. *ASXL2* mutations (11.5%) are exclusively associated with t(8;21) and were not observed in inv(16) patients. The ASXL2 protein is involved in epigenetic regulation of gene transcription and seemingly confers a worse prognosis but these results need broader validation. *RUNX1* mutations present in about 5% to 15% of patients with M0 AML, are mutually exclusive when t(8;21) and inv(16) are present. Approximately 5% to 10% of CBF AML patients, mostly those with t(8;21), have concurrent systemic mastocytosis with *KIT* mutations and a good prognosis.

As mentioned earlier, there are 39 recurrent abnormalities involving the 21q22 chromosomal site where *RUNX1* is localized. Some of the more frequent rearrangements are discussed here.

The t(16;21)(q24;q22) is a rare but recurrent chromosomal abnormality associated with therapy-related AML. Studies using FISH and RT-PCR methods have demonstrated fusion of *RUNX1* on 21q22 and *CBFA2T3* on chromosome 16, which produces an *RUNX1/CBFA2T3* fusion gene on chromosome 16. The breakpoints of both t(8;21) and t(16;21) occur within the same intron of the *RUNX1* gene. *RUNX1/CBFA2T3* fusion results in the production of a protein that is very similar to the RUNX1/RUNX1T1 protein in t(8;21).

The (16;21)(p11;q22) is a rare chromosomal rearrangement associated with M1-M2 AML. A proportion of these patients may have additional abnormalities. This translocation fuses the *FUS/ERG TLS/FUS* gene on chromosome 16, band p11, to the *ERG* gene on chromosome 22, band q22. The *ERG* gene is a member of the E twenty-six (ETS) family of transcription factors and is a sequence-specific transcriptional activator. The presence of a fusion transcript is detected by RT-PCR, at the time of diagnosis, at relapse, and during remission. These observations are consistent with the impression that patients with t(16;21) have a poor prognosis and may benefit from early detection of this chimeric gene to determine the need for more aggressive therapy.

The t(15;17)(q22;q21) involves the promyelocytic leukemia (*PML*) gene on chromosome 15, band q22, and *RARA* on chromosome 17, band q21. This abnormality constitutes the genetic basis for approximately 95% of all cases of APL (see Fig. 56.26, *middle panels*).[15] The remaining 5% of cases include nine rare variant translocations: t(11;17)(q23;q21)/*ZBTB16-RARA* and *MLL-RARA*, t(11;17)(q23;q21)/*NUMA1-RARA*, t(5;17)(q35;q21)/*NPM1-RARA*, t(2;17)(q32.3;q21)/*NABP1-RARA*, t(17;17)(q21.2;q21.2)/*STATB-RARA* or del(17)(q21.2q21t), t(4;17)(q12;q21) *FIP1L1/RARA*, t(X;17)(p11.2;q21)/*BCOR-RARA*, and cryptic *PRKAR1A-RARA* detected in a patient with a normal karyotype (Fig. 56.30). Therefore APL, which accounts for 10% to 15% of AML cases, is associated with several different genetic rearrangements fusing the *RARA* gene with a different partner gene in each case. Based on these genomic rearrangements, a FISH assay, using a breakapart probe strategy with dual-color *RARA*, can identify two different clinical syndromes: those responsive to all-*trans* retinoic acid (ATRA) (more than 99%) therapy and those carrying a *ZBTB16-RARA* or *STAT5B-RARA* fusion genes, which are not responsive to ATRA and are naturally resistant to arsenic trioxide (AS_2O_3) therapy. Patients with promyelocytes that have exquisite sensitivity to differentiate in response to ATRA treatment have one of the other six RARA fusion rearrangements (see Fig. 56.30). ATRA resistance is heterogeneous and commonly involves mutations in the RARA ligand-biding domain of the fusion protein. FISH studies have also identified patients with cryptic translocations and unusual chromosomal variants (Fig. 56.31). It is important to recognize patients who will or will not respond to ATRA so that appropriate therapy can be administered.

The t(15;17) is often the only chromosomal abnormality present in 70% to 100% of bone marrow metaphase cells. The most frequent additional abnormality is trisomy 8, but this abnormality does not influence the rate of CR. The *RARA* gene is a nuclear hormone receptor, spanning 7.5 kb, and contains nine exons. The breakpoint

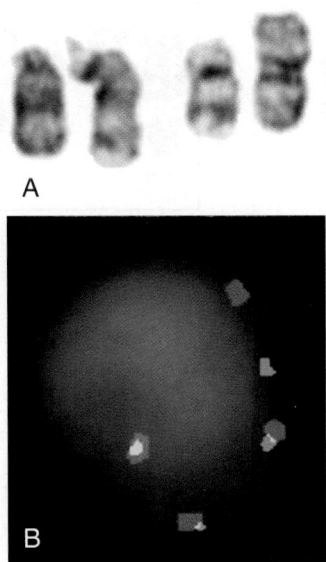

Fig. 56.31 ISOCHROMOSOME 17 IN ACUTE PROMYELOCYTIC LEUKEMIA WITH A GAIN OF PML-RARA FUSION. (A) Partial karyotype from a patient with acute promyelocytic leukemia, showing ider(17) t(15;17)(q22;q21). The karyotype shows isochromosome for the long arms of chromosome 17 and deletion of the short arms. (B) FISH studies revealed three copies of PML-RARA fusion in bone marrow nucleus, confirming that the first event in the pathogenesis was PML-RARA fusion and the subsequent event was a structural rearrangement of isochromosome. *(From Cheng L, Zhang DY, editors: Molecular genetic pathology, Totowa, NJ, 2008, Humana Press, a part of Springer Science.)*

occurs almost exclusively in intron 2 of the *RARA* gene. The *PML* gene locus spans 35 kb and contains nine exons coding for mRNA of 4.6, 3.0 and 2.1 kb. The breakpoints in *PML* occur in three distinct clusters leading to mRNA of different length. The existence of different breakpoint regions in the *PML* gene and the presence of alternative splicing of PML transcripts are responsible for the heterogeneity of *PML RARA* junctions and variants.

APL is a disease characterized by accumulation of blasts blocked at the promyelocytic stage of granulocytic differentiation. APL accounts for only 5% to 8% of pediatric AML, and 95% of children with APL show a classic t(15;17). However, almost 35% of pediatric APL have *FLT3-ITD* mutations. The clinical signs of these mutations on relapse rate and OS is not yet apparent.

Our current understanding of the molecular pathogenesis of APL is that *PML-RARA* behaves as a potent transcriptional repressor and that supraphysiologic doses of retinoic acid can overcome this repression. In the presence of retinoic acid, *PML-RARA* behaves as a transcriptional activator. In patients with variant *ZBTB16-RARA*, an additional co-repressor complex binding site is present, and histone deacetylase inhibitors are used to restore sensitivity to retinoic acid. It appears that *PML-RARA* fusion-induced differentiation arrest of leukemic blasts and increased self-renewal of progenitors are two distinct features of APL and are probably driven by two different gene programs. The *RARA* fusion protein has a dual action, activating transcription of a number of genes and repressing transcription of others. *PML-RARA* and *ZBTB16-RARA* repress several DNA repair genes and activate the Wnt signaling and the NOTCH pathway leading to increased stem cell renewal. Many of the genes targeted by retinoid acid are known to play a key role in regulating myeloid cell proliferation and differentiation. Therefore it is possible that inhibition of their expression by RARA fusion proteins may lead to differentiation blockage.

Accurate identification of the APL-associated genomic lesion at diagnosis is important because APL is a medical emergency that frequently presents with abrupt onset, high risk for early death

(10%–20%), and potential for high cure rate (>80%) if appropriate treatment, based on its genetic profile, is initiated. Initial workup may include conventional karyotyping, FISH studies, RT-PCR, and anti-PML antibodies. Longitudinal monitoring of disease with Q-PCR is currently recommended to provide early intervention if relapse should occur.

Less than 1% of patients with AML have the Ph chromosome (see Fig. 56.26, *bottom left*) and it remains a controversial entity as it is not listed in the WHO 2016 classification as a separate entity. Ph + AML may be cytogenetically distinguished from the myeloid blast crisis of CML by monosomy 7 (also frequently found in Ph + ALL) and inv(16). Moreover, *NPM1* mutations found in 40% to 60% of AML as well as in Ph + AML have not been described in Ph-positive CML. All Ph + AML examined to date showed a unique loss of Ig genes with a specific genomic signature, suggesting a distinct biologic entity. Both P210$^{BCR-ABL1}$ and P190$^{BCR-ABL1}$ were observed, but P190 appears to be prevalent. Before TKI therapy, the median survival of the Ph chromosome +AML was 9 months and has been improved to a median survival of 18 months (range 6–71) with the use of imatinib therapy. In rare patients with AML, late appearance of a Ph chromosome either as a sole abnormality or in a clone showing t(8;21) is taken as evidence that the Ph chromosome in these patients is a secondary event. The late-appearing Ph chromosome in AML is characterized by P190$^{BCR-ABL1}$ protein. The coexistence of the Ph chromosome and inv(16) is a rare but recurrent finding in both CML and AML. In CML the fusion transcript is P210$^{BCR-ABL1}$, whereas in AML the fusion transcript is P190$^{BCR-ABL1}$. The presence of both the Ph chromosome and inv(16) in AML seems to have a favorable prognosis, whereas in CML, the coexistence of *BCR-ABL1* and *CBFB-MYH11* is predictive of rapid transformation to blast crisis.

Using extrasensitive BCR-ABL1 FISH probe Ph-positive AML expressing P190$^{BCR-ABL1}$ protein may be recognized, and distinguished from the Ph-positive CML because it will show a second co-localized "fusion" signal, because the breakpoint on chromosome 22 in AML is more centromeric with two signals closer to each other giving an impression of two fusion signals.

The *KMT2A* [lysine (K)-specific methyltransferase 2A], (*MLL*) gene at 11q23.3 is responsible for 95% of all 11q23 translocations, including those in patients with AML and ALL (Figs. 56.32 and 56.33 and Table 56.9). *MLL* abnormalities are found in approximately 15% of patients with AML and ALL. As of 2013 there were a total of 121 different *MLL* rearrangements of which 79 were characterized at the molecular level.[16] In nearly all direct and reciprocal *MLL* recombinomes, the 3′ portion of the *MLL* gene is retained causing a direct fusion of the 5′ *MLL* gene portion with a gene portion localized telomeric to *MLL*. Of note, an abnormal FISH signal pattern, using dual-color, breakapart FISH, shows an abnormal signal pattern arising from 3′ *MLL* deletions in up to 28% of cases, and very rarely a gain of 3′ *MLL* portion of the gene, usually as a result of an additional derivative partner chromosome.

The seven most frequent rearrangements of the *MLL* gene occur either with a translocation partner gene such as *AFF1/AF4/*t(4;11)(q21;q23), *MLLT3/AF9* /t(9;11)(q21;q23) (Fig. 56.34), *MLLT1/ENL/*t(11;19)(q23;p13.3), *MLLT10/AF10/*t(10;11)(p12;q23), *ELL/*t(11;19)9q23;p13.1), *MLLT4/AF6/*t(6;11)(q27;q23), or derived from *MLL* gene internal duplication *(MLL-PTDs)* of the amino-terminus region of the gene (see Table 56.9 and Fig. 56.32).

The BCR for about 96% of patients is localized between *MLL* exon 9 and *MLL* intron 11. Patients with a breakpoint in *MLL* intron 11 have a worse prognosis compared with those patients with upstream breakpoints. The breakpoint in *MLL* intron 11 causes a *cis to trans* conversion and switches the MLL protein from a transcriptional activator/maintenance factor to a transcriptional repressor.

MLL rearrangements are initiated by DNA damage, which induces DNA repair via the nonhomologous-end-joining DNA repair mechanism. These genetic recombinations produce (1) reciprocal chromosomal translocations which fuse the 5′-*MLL* gene portion with the corresponding gene; (2) partial tandem repeats, frequently in AML; (3) inversions or deletions on 11p and 11q in which inversions lead to reciprocal *MLL* fusions whereas deletions cause fusion of the 5′

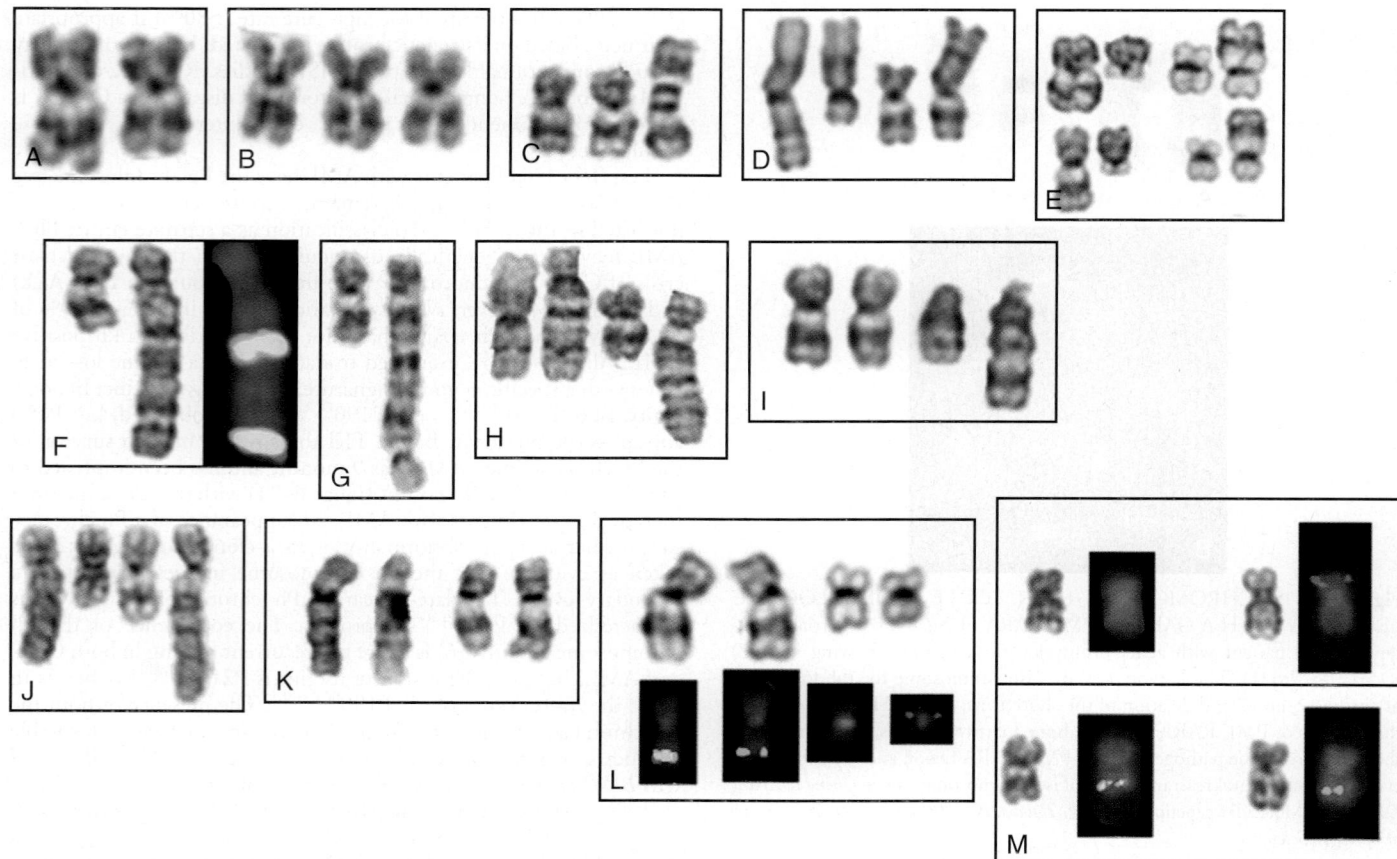

Fig. 56.32 EXAMPLES OF CHROMOSOME 11 ABNORMALITIES. (A) Deletion of chromosome 11 at band q23. (B), Gain (trisomy) of chromosome 11. (C) Gain of isodicentric, idic(q11) in myelodysplastic syndrome (MDS). (D) Balanced t(1;11)(q13;p15) in MDS. (E) t(11;19)(q13;p13) in a pediatric patient with acute myeloid leukemia. (F) Duplication of the long arms of chromosome 11 and FISH image of *MLL* duplication. (G) Duplication (11;22) in the form of dicder(11;22)dup(11)(q13q14)t(11;22)(q23;p11) in a patient with MDS. (H) der(11)dic(1;11)(q12;q23) in a patient with myelofibrosis transforming to acute myeloid leukemia. (I) der(14)t(11;14)(q23;q23), resulting in trisomy for part of the long arms of chromosome 11. (J) t(4;11)(q23;q23) in pediatric acute lymphoblastic leukemia. (K) t(6;11)(q27;q23) in pediatric acute lymphoblastic leukemia. (L) t(11;19)(q23;p13) in pediatric acute lymphoblastic leukemia and after FISH study, showing separation of *MLL* breakapart probe where the 5′ end of the *MLL* (*green*) remains on der(11), and the 3′ end (*red*) is translocated to 19p. (M) t(9;11)(p22;q23) in pediatric acute myeloid leukemia and after metaphase FISH study (*right*), showing that the 3′ end of the *MLL* (*red*) is translocated to 9p but the 5′ end (*green*) remains on der(11).

MLL directly to another gene located further downstream (*ARHGEF12, BCL9L, CBL* and *CEP164*); and (4) complex *MLL* rearrangements involving three- or four-way translocations resulting in more than two fusion alleles (Fig. 56.35) or ring chromosomes (see Fig. 56.25). About 15% of *MLL* recombinations represent in-frame fusions that can be readily expressed into a fusion protein and 85% are out-of-frame fusions and express a 5′ truncated MLL protein.

The t(9;11), which has been associated with a more favorable outcome in adult and pediatric AML, is distinguished as a separate entity in the latest WHO classification (see Fig. 56.34). Other frequent *MLL* translocations are t(6;11)(q27;q23) involving *MLLT4(AF6)* and t(11;19)(q23;p13.3) involving *MLLT1 (ENL)*. A partial tandem duplication of the amino-terminus region of the *MLL* gene is associated in patients with or without trisomy 11 (see Figs. 56.32B, C and F), and *MLL* is an epigenetic regulator that plays a critical role in hematopoiesis, modulating *HOX* gene expression.

The *MLL* gene is encoded by 37 exons. It is recruited to the promoters of select cell-cycle regulatory genes, suggesting its role in cell-cycle control. MLL protein regulates gene expression and cell cycle control via chromatin modification. Translocations of 11q23 cluster within an 8.3-kb region that encompasses exons 8–14 of *MLL*

and fuses the N-terminal portion of *MLL*, which contains the AT hook and methyltransferase domains, to numerous different proteins. In infant and in therapy-related AML, the *MLL* genomic breakpoints cluster at the 3′ end, near exon 12. In childhood and adult de novo AML, the breakpoints usually occur in the 5′ end, between exons 9 and 10. The most frequent MLL rearrangements in pediatric and adult patients as well as in ALL and AML are summarized in Fig. 56.33.

Patients with AML with *MLL* rearrangements have a poor prognosis despite treatment with aggressive multiagent chemotherapy. Identical *MLL* rearrangements have been detected in three pairs of infant monozygotic twins, indicating in utero *MLL* rearrangement that result in clinical manifestations developing some time during the first year of life. The contribution of various *MLL* fusion partners to transformation has been recently clarified. More recently, a retrospective analysis demonstrated that the prognosis of *MLL*-rearranged leukemia may be influenced by the fusion partner. Survival associated with the rare t(1;11)(q21;q23) translocation was favorable, in contrast to very poor outcomes with the more frequent t(4;11), t(10;11), and t(6;11) translocations. Even now novel translocations, such as the one shown in Fig. 56.36, are still being discovered and their prognostic indication is currently unknown.

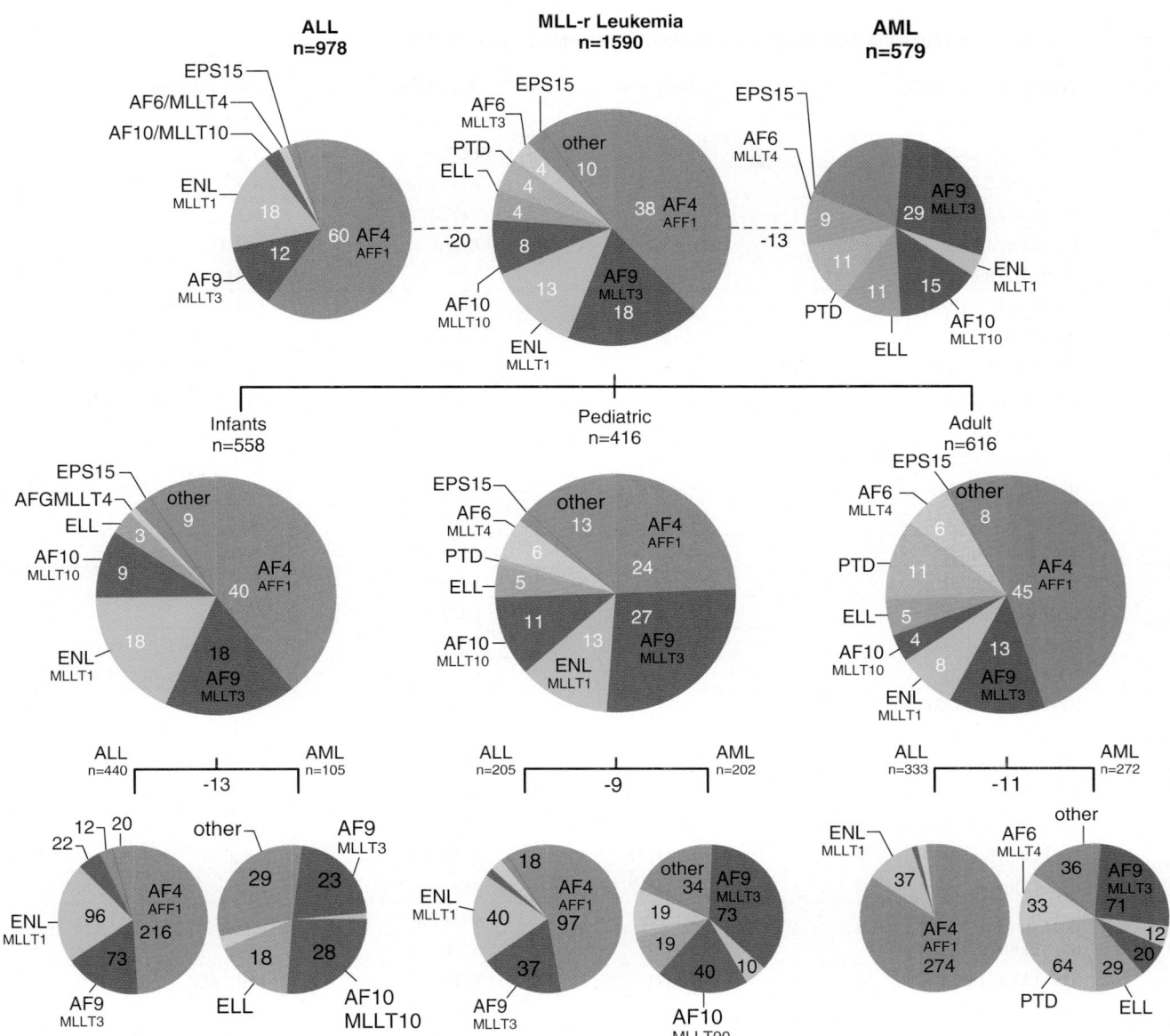

Fig. 56.33. THE *MLL* RECOMBINOME IN ACUTE LEUKEMIA. Classification of patients according to age classes and disease type. (*Top*) Frequency of most frequent translocation partner groups in the investigated patient cohort of *MLL*-rearranged acute leukemia patients (*n* = 1590). This patient cohort was divided into ALL (*left*) and AML patients (*right*). Gene names are written in black, and percentages are indicated as white numbers. Thirty-three patients could not be classified into the ALL or the AML disease types, respectively. (*Middle*) TPG frequencies for the infant, pediatric, and adult patient group. (*Bottom*) Subdivision of all three age groups into ALL and AML patients. Negative numbers refer again to the number of patients who were neither classified to the ALL nor to the AML subgroup. *ALL*, Acute lymphoblastic leukemia; *AML*, acute myeloid leukemia; *TPG*, translocation partner group. (*Reproduced with permission from Meyer et al: Leukemia 27:2165, 2013.*)

TABLE 56.9	**Mixed Lineage Leukemia Translocations and Rearrangements 2015**			
#	Cytogenetic Abnormality	Breakpoint	Hugo Name	Leukemia Type
Characterized on the Molecular Level				
1	t(1;11)(p32;q23)	1p32	*EPS15*	ALL, AML, CML
2	t(1;11)(q21;q23)	1q21	*MLLT11*	AML
3	ins(2;11)(q11.2–q12;q23)	2q11.2–q12	*AFF3*	ALL
4	t(2;11)(q33;q23)	2q33	*ABI2*	AML
5	t(2;11)(q37;q23)	2q37	*SEPT2*	t-AML, AML, t-MDS
6	t(3;11)(p21.3;q23)	3p21.3	*SACM1L*	N/A

Continued

TABLE 56.9	Mixed Lineage Leukemia Translocations and Rearrangements 2015—cont'd			
#	Cytogenetic Abnormality	Breakpoint	Hugo Name	Leukemia Type
7	t(3;11)(p21;q23)	3p21	NCKIPSD	t-AML
8	t(3;11)(p21.1;q23)	3p21.1	DCP1A	ALL
9	t(3;11)(q12~13;q23)	3q13.13	KIAA1524	AML
10	t(3;11)(q21.3;q23)	3q21.3	EEFSEC	ALL
11	t(3;11)(q24;q23)	3q24	GMPS	t-AML
12	t(3;11)(q28;q23)	3q28	LPP	t-AML
13	t(4;11)(p11;q23)	4p11	FRYL	t-ALL, t-AML, t-MDS
14	t(4;11)(p12;q23)	4p14	PDS5A	t-ALL, AML
15	t(4;11)(q21.1;q23)	4q21.1	SEPT11	CML, t-ALL, t-AML
16	t(4;11)(q21;q23)	4q21	AFF1	ALL, t-ALL, BAL, (AML)
17	t(4;11)(q35.1;q23)	4q35.1	SORBS2	AML
18	Complex chromosomal abnormalities	5q12.3	CENPK	AML
19	t(5;11)(q23.3q23)	5q23.3	PRRC1	t-ALL
20	ins(5;11)(q31;q13q23)	5q31	AFF4	ALL
21	t(5;11)(q31;q23)	5q31	ARHGAP26	JMML
22	t(6;11)(q13;q23)	6q13	SMAP1	AML
23	t(6;11)(q15;q23)	6q15	CASP8AP2	AML
24	t(6;11)(q21;q23)	6q21	FOXO3	t-AML, t-ALL
25	t(6;11)(q27;q23)	6q27	MLLT4	AML, t-AML, ALL, T-ALL
26	t(7;11)(p22.1;q23)	7p22.1	TNRC18	ALL
27	t(7;11)(q21;q23)	7q21.12	RUNDC3B	T-ALL
28	t(9;11)(p22;q23)	9p22	MLLT3	AML, t-AML, ALL, BAL
29	t(9;11)(q33.1–q33.3;q23);	9q33.1–q33.3	DAB2IP	AML
30	ins(11;9)(q23;q34)inv(11)(q13)(q23)	9q34	FNBP1	AML
31	t(9;11)(q31–q34;q23)	9q31–34	LAMC3	t-AML
32	t(10;11)(p11.2;q23)	10p11.2	ABI1	AML
33	ins(10;11)(p12;q23q13)	10p12	MLLT10	AML, t-AML, ALL, T-ALL
34	t(10;11)(p12;q23)	10p12	NEBL	AML
35	t(10;11)(q21;q23)	10q21	TET1	AML, ALL
36	inv(11)(p15q23)	11p15.5	AP2A2	AML
37	inv(11)(p15.3q23)	11p15.3	NRIP3	AML
38	INV(11)(q12.1q23)	11q12.1	BTBD18	ALL
39	INV(11)(q12.2q23)	11q12.2	PRPF19	ALL
40	t(11;11)(q13.4;q23)	11q13.4	ARHGEF17	AML
41	inv(11)(q13.4q23)	11q13.4	C2CD3	AML
42	inv(11)(q14q23)	11q14	PICALM	AML, ALL
43	inv(11)(q21q23)	11q21	MAML2	t-T-ALL, t-AML, t-MDS
44	t(11;15)(q23q;q21)inv(11)(q23q23)	11q23	LOC100131626	MDS
45	inv(11)(q23q23)	11q23	BUD13	AML
46	del11q23	11q23.3	CEP164	t-ALL
47	del(11)(q23q23.3)	11q23.3	CBL	AML, t-AML
48	del(11)(q23q23.3)	11q23.3	ARHGEF12	AML, t-AML
49	del(11)(q23q23.3)	11q23.3	BCL9L	ALL
50	del(11)(q23q24.2)	11q24.2	DCPS	AML
51	t(11;12)(q23;q13.2)	12q13.2	SARNP	AML
52	t(11;14)(q23.3;q23.3)	14q23.3	GPHN	AML, t-AML
53	t(11;14)(q32.33;q23.3)	14q32.33	CEP170B	t-AML
54	t(11;15)(q23;q14)	15q14	CASC5	AML, ALL, t-MDS
55	t(11;15)(q23;q14)	15q14	ZFYVE19	AML

TABLE 56.9	Mixed Lineage Leukemia Translocations and Rearrangements 2015—cont'd			
#	Cytogenetic Abnormality	Breakpoint	Hugo Name	Leukemia Type
56	t(11;15)(q23;q21)	15q21	TCF12	t-AML
57	t(11;15)(q23;q24)	15q24–q25	AKAP13	t-AML
58	t(11;17)(q23;p13)	17p12–p11.2	TOP3A	AML
59	t(11;16)(q23;p13.3)	16p13.11	MYH11	AML
60	t(11;16)(q23;p13.3)	16p13.3	CREBBP	t-MDS, t-AML, AML, t-ALL, t-CML
61	t(11;17)(q23;p13.1)	17p13.1	GAS7	t-AML,
62	ins(11;17)(q23;q21)	17q21	ACACA	AML
63	t(11;17)(q23;q21)	17q21	MLLT6	AML
64	t(11;17)(q23;q11–q21.3)	17q11–q21.3	LASP1	AML
65	t(11;17)(q23;q25)	17q25	SEPT9	t-AML, AML, MDS
66	t(11;18)(q23;q21)	18q21	ME2	t-AML,
67	t(11;19)(q23;p13.1)	19p13.1	ELL	AML, t-AML, ALL, BAL
68	t(11;19)(q23;p13)	19p13.3	SH3GL1	AML
69	ins(11;19)(q23;p13.2)	19p13.2	VAV1	AML
70	t(11;19)(q23;p13.3)	19p13.3	MLLT1	ALL, T-ALL, AML, t-AL
71	t(11;19)(q23;p13.3)	19p13.3	ACER1	ALL
72	t(2;11;19)(p23.3;q23;p13.3)	19p13.3	LOC100128568	AML
73	t(11;19)(q23;p13.3–p13.2)	19p13.3–p13.2	MYO1F	AML
74	t(11;19)(q23;q13)	19q13	ACTN4	t-ALL, t-AML
75	t(11;20)(q23;q11)	20q11	MAPRE1	ALL
76	t(11;22)(q23;q11.21)	22q11.21	SEPT5	AML, T-ALL
77	t(11;22)(q23;q13.2)	22q13.2	EP300	t-AML
78	t(X;11)(q13.1;q23)	Xq13.1	FOXO4	ALL, t-ALL, AML
79	ins(X;11)(q24;q23)	Xq24	SEPT6	AML
80	ins(X;11)(q26.3;q23)	Xq26.3	CT45A2	BAL
81	ins(11;X)(q23q28q13.1)	Xq28	FLNA	AML
No Partner Gene Is Directly Fused to the MLL Gene				
1	t(1;11)(p13.1;q23)	1p13.1		
2	t(9;11)(p13.3;q23)	9p13.3		
3	del(11)(q23q23.3)	11q23.3		
4	INV(11)(q23q23.3)	11q23.3		
5	del(11)(q23q23.3)	11q23.3		
6	t(11;21)(q23;q11.21)	21q22		
Not Characterized on the Molecular Level				
1	t(1;11)(p36;q23)			
2	t(1;11)(q31;q23)			
3	t(1;11)(q32;q23)			
4	t(2;11)(p21;q23)			
5	t(2;11)(q37;q23)			
6	t(3;11)(p13;q23)			
7	t(4;11)(p11;q23)			
8	t(6;11)(q13;q23)			
9	t(7;11)(p15;q23)			
10	t(7;11)(q22;q23)			
11	t(7;11)(q32;q23)			
12	t(8;11)(q11;q23)			
13	t(8;11)(q21;q23)			
14	t(8;11)(q24;q23)			
15	t(9;11)(p11;q23)			
16	t(9;11)(q33;q23)			

Continued

TABLE 56.9	Mixed Lineage Leukemia Translocations and Rearrangements 2015—cont'd			
#	Cytogenetic Abnormality	Breakpoint	Hugo Name	Leukemia Type
17	t(10;11)(q25;q23)			
18	t(11;11)(q11;q23)			
19	t(11;11)(q13;q23)			
20	t(11;11)(q21;q23)			
21	t(11;12)(q23;p13)			
22	t(11;12)(q23;q13)			
23	t(11;12)(q23;q24)			
24	t(4;13;11)(q21;q34;q23)			
25	t(11;14)(q23;q11)			
26	t(11;14)(q23;q32)			
27	t(11;15)q23;q15)			
28	t(11;17)(q23;q11)			
29	t(11;17)(q23;q23)			
30	t(11;18)(q23;q12)			
31	t(11;18)(q23;q23)			
32	t(11;20)(q23;q13)			
33	t(11;21)(q23;q11)			
34	t(Y;11)(p11;q23)			
35	t(X;11)(q22;q23)			

AL, Acute leukemia; ALL, acute lymphoblastic leukemia; AML, acute myeloid leukemia; BAL, biphenotypic acute leukemia; CML, chronic myelogenous leukemia; JMML, juvenile myomonocytic leukemia; MDS, myelodysplastic syndrome; t-AL, therapy-related AL; t-ALL, therapy-related ALL; T-ALL, T-cell ALL; t-AML, therapy-related AML; t-CML, therapy-related CML; t-MDS, therapy-related MDS; t-T-ALL, therapy-related T-cell ALL.
Courtesy C. Meyer and Rolf Marschalek, Diagnostic Center of Acute Leukemia (DCAL), Institute for Pharmaceutical Biology, Goethe University, Frankfurt, Germany, February 14, 2015.

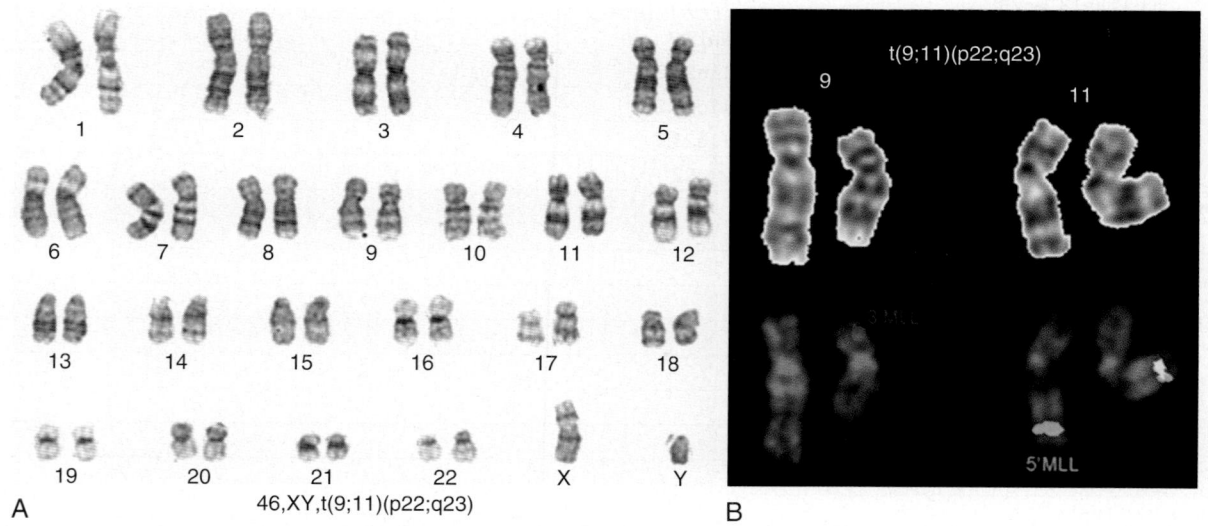

Fig. 56.34 THE MOST FREQUENT *MLL* TRANSLOCATION IS t(9;11)(p22;q23). (A) The G-banded karyotype and (B) a partial karyotype, from another metaphase, after hybridization with dual color "break-apart" MLL probe showing the *5′ MLL (green)* being retained on 11q23 and the *3′ MLL (red)* moved as a result of the translocation to 9p22. This translocation results in a fusion of *MLLT3-AF9*.

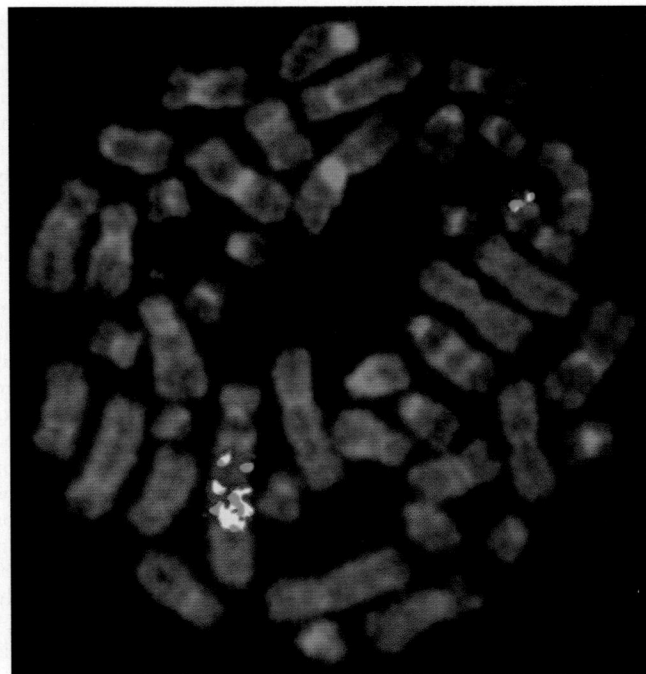

Fig. 56.35 MLL AMPLIFICATION. Metaphase cell from a patient with acute myeloid leukemia after DAPI staining *(blue)* showing *MLL* amplification *(yellow)* along the abnormal chromosome 11. At least 15 copies of *MLL* amplicon were inserted into an abnormal chromosome 11. A normal copy of chromosome 11 with one copy of *MLL* is shown on the right side of the metaphase.

The partner genes in the translocations do not appear to have any common characteristics that would clarify their role in leukemogenesis. However, two observations suggest that *MLL* fusion partners are not randomly chosen. First, a precise localization of genomic *MLL* breakpoints in 414 samples with *MLL* rearrangements, using a long-distance inverse PCR method, showed that the most frequent translocation fusion partners (*AF4, MLLT3, MLLT1, AF10*) belong to the same nuclear protein network involved in histone methylation. Second, several chromatin structural elements, such as topoisomerase II cleavage sites, DNase I hypersensitive sites, and other chromatin sites, are associated with *MLL* rearrangements observed in infant and therapy-related AML. These characteristics of *MLL* suggest that specific chromatin sites are functionally selected in *MLL* rearrangements rather than randomly chosen.

Gene expression studies have demonstrated clear differences between *MLL*-rearranged AML and ALL in expression of lineage-associated genes, but there appears to be a core gene expression profile found in all *MLL*-rearranged leukemias, independent of the lineage markers.

t(8;16)(p11;p13)/MYST3-CREBBP rearrangements are a distinct pediatric subtype of AML with 97% of cases showing FAB subgroup M4 or M5 (Fig. 56.37). This specific association has also been observed in adult AML. Gene expression analysis revealed that t(8;16) cases clustered strongly together with, but separate from, *MLL* rearranged AML.

t(6;9)(p23.3;q34.1) is a rare cytogenetic abnormality, found in approximately 1% of AML cases, and subsequently reported to be associated with AML and marrow basophilia (Fig. 56.38). Basophilic leukemia is now recognized by the WHO classification as a separate entity. In addition to t(6;9), other chromosomal abnormalities such as t(8;21)(q22;q22), del(12)(p11–13), t(X;6),(p11;q23), and t(2;6) (q23;p22) may be associated with basophilic leukemia. As a result of t(6;9), the 3′ end of the *NUP214*, nuclear pore complex protein 214 kDa, gene located on chromosome 9, band q34, is fused to the 5′ end of the *DEK* gene located on chromosome 6, band p23. The resulting *DEK-NUP214* fusion gene is a derivative of chromosome

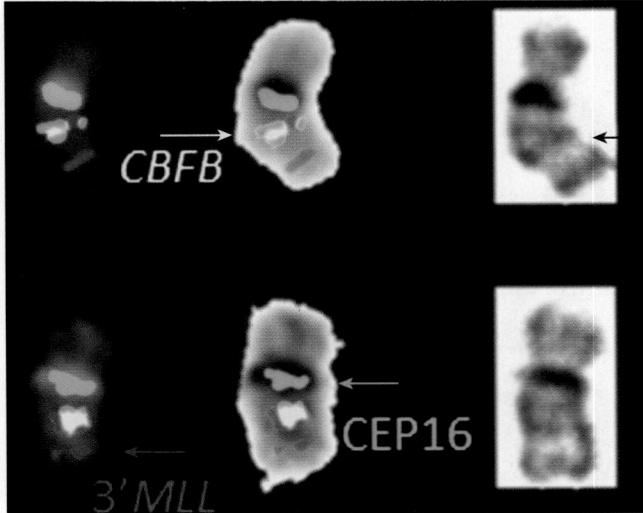

Fig. 56.36 A NOVEL *MLL* PARTNER. A partial karyotype showing an abnormal chromosome 16 from two different metaphase cells from a patient with acute myeloid leukemia showing t(11;16)(q23;q23) karyotype as a sole abnormality. On the *left* is chromosome 16 stained with DAPI *(blue)* after metaphase FISH with three probes: centromere 16 in *aqua*, *CBFB* "break-apart" probe in *yellow*, and 3′ *MLL* in *red*. *Middle panel* is an "inverted" DAPI image and on the *right* is the G-banding of an abnormal chromosome 16. As a result of t(11;16) a part of 11q23 was translocated to 16 and the 3′ *MLL* moved at 16q23.

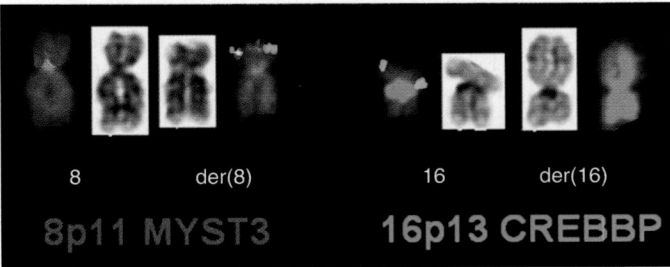

Fig. 56.37 THE t(8;16). A partial karyotype from a patient with acute myeloid leukemia showing a t(8;16)(p11;p13) which results in fusion of *MYST3 (red)* and *CREBBP (green)*.

6. The translocation breakpoints occur in exon 6 in the *NUP214* gene and in exon 2 in the *DEK* gene. As a result, the presence of the *DEK-NUP214* fusion can be identified by PCR methods. Dual-color commercial FISH probes are not available for this translocation. Approximately 70% of patients with *DEK-NUP214* have an *FLT3* tandem duplication.

The nuclear pore complex is a massive structure that extends across the nuclear envelope, forming a gateway that regulates the flow of macromolecules between the nucleus and the cytoplasm. *NUP214* may serve as a docking site in the receptor-mediated import of substrates across the nuclear pore complex and plays a role in nuclear protein import, mRNA export, and cell cycle progression. The role of the DEK-NUP214 protein in leukemogenesis awaits elucidation.

inv(3)(q21q26.2) or t(3;3)(q21;q26.2) (see Fig. 56.23) is a distinct subtype of AML with recurrent chromosome abnormalities and according to 2008 WHO classification, occurring in about 1% to 2.5% of all AML cases. Each rearrangement is associated with the juxtaposition of the *RPN1* (ribophosphorin 1 located on 3q21) gene with the transcription factor *EVI1* (located in the 3q26.2 band). Two alternative forms exist, one generated from *EVI1*, the other *MECOM* (*MDS1* and *EVI1* complex locus) through intergenic splicing with *MDS1*, a gene located 140 kb upstream of *EVI1*. Both rearrangements may present as de novo or secondary AML and are characterized by

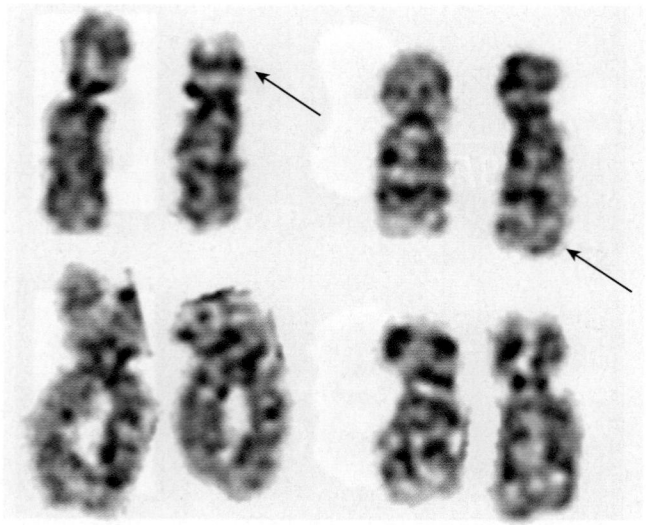

t(6;9)(p23.3;q34.1)

Fig. 56.38 MARROW BASOPHILIA WITH CHARACTERISTIC t(6;9). t(6;9)(p23;q24). Shown as partial karyotype from a patient with acute myeloid leukemia and marrow basophilia. This translocation results in a fusion between *NUP214* gene on 9p34 and *DEK* gene on 6p23.

normal or increased platelet counts and abnormal megakaryopoiesis. They are also observed in MDS, blast crisis of CML, as well as in Ph-negative MPN. De novo AML associated with t(3;3)/inv(3) is an aggressive type of leukemia with minimal response to chemotherapy and poor clinical outcome. Rare patients with an inversion on both chromosome 3 have been described and the second inv(3) appears to be a secondary event that carries an even worse prognosis. Breakpoints in band 3q21 are distributed in a 235-kb region centromeric to and including the *RPN1* locus, whereas those in band 3q26.2 are scattered over a 900-kb region located on each side of and including the *EVI1* locus. There are a few cluster breakpoints within 3q21 region. The first BCR of about 30 kb is located 15 kb centromeric of the *RPN1* gene and the other breakpoints are centromeric to the first one, located up to 60 kb. In contrast to most of the translocations and inversions associated with de novo AML, that lead to the fusion genes, inv(3)/t(3;3) does not generate a chimeric gene, but rather induces gene overexpression. Approximately 68% of reported patients with inv(3)/t(3;3) showed one additional chromosomal abnormality, including −7/del(7q) present in 75% of cases.

Therapy resistance in patients with inv(3)/t(3;3) is linked to the inappropriate activation of the *EVI1* as a consequence of the 3q structural rearrangement. *EVI1* is a hematopoietic stemness factor and transcription factor with chromatin-remodeling activity. *EVI1* is also expressed in approximately 11% of patients with AML in the absence of 3q aberrations and represents an independent adverse prognostic factor. *EVI1* is activated as a consequence of inv(3)/t(3;3) via structural repositioning of a distal *GATA2* enhancer from 3q21 to the *EVI1* locus at 3q26. Relocation of the enhancer additionally confers reduced and monoallelic *GATA2* expression. Besides deregulated expression of *EVI1*, a molecular hallmark of patients with 3q structural rearrangements, 98% of these patients harbor mutations in genes activating RAS/receptor tyrosine kinase signaling pathways including hemizygous mutations in *GATA2*, heterozygous alterations in *RUNX1*, *SF3B1* and genes encoding epigenetic modifiers.

t(3;5)(q25;q35), *NPM1/MLF1*: translocation (3;5)(q25;q35) is present in approximately 0.5% cases of AML and has an intermediate prognosis, it is observed in all age groups, but more commonly in younger patients. These patients have shown to have a 34% survival rate after 10 years. In younger patients, this translocation is usually the sole karyotypic abnormality, whereas older patients may demonstrate a more complex karyotype. This translocation generates an

NPM1/MLF1 chimeric gene, which includes approximately half of the 24-kb *NPM1* gene, localized on 5q35, extending from exons 1–6, juxtaposed to virtually the entire 35-kb *MLF1* gene, localized on 3q25, starting at exon 2. The chimeric NPM1/MLF1 fusion protein totals 426 amino acids with 175 amino acids from *NPM1* fused to 251 amino acids from *MLF1*, which excludes only the initial 16 amino acids from *MLF1* in this chimeric protein. In approximately 88% of patients with t(3;5) the translocation results in *NPM1/MLF1* fusion. In some patients with balanced t(3;5) the fusion is not apparent because of the variant 3;5 translocations that may include multiple genes at 3q21–25 and 5q31–35.

The presence of a hyperdiploid karyotype in acute erythroleukemia occurs in 47% to 56% of patients, along with a loss of genetic material in chromosomes 5, 7, and 18. A monosomal karyotype was identified in 43% of cases in one series. Balanced translocations are rare in erythroleukemia, although rare cases of *MLL* rearrangements have been reported. The frequent occurrence of a complex karyotype with abnormalities of chromosomes 5 and 7 may be one reason for the poor prognosis associated with acute erythroleukemia. Mutations frequently seen in other subgroups of AML (such as *FLT3*, *KIT* or *RAS* mutations) have not been reported in acute erythroleukemia. In pediatric patients, acute erythroleukemia is very rare, present in 2.3% of all patients with AML. Congenital erythroleukemia is exceedingly rare with only six cases reported in the literature.

Pure erythroid leukemia (PEL) is a rare subtype of AML that is often secondary leukemia or therapy related. The uncontrolled proliferation of immature erythroid precursors comprises at least 80% of the marrow. A complex karyotype is present in 83% of cases and the median OS of 2.9 months. Compared with AML with more than 50% erythroblasts, cases of PEL demonstrate a higher incidence of poor-risk chromosomal abnormalities. Within the complex karyotype monosomy 7 appears to be the most frequent abnormality.

The M7 or megakaryocytic subtype of AML is a rare clonal disease, with an estimated frequency of 0.7% among AMLs, arising in a multipotent stem cell capable of differentiating along the megakaryocytic and granulocytic pathway. This acute leukemia subtype has a variety of genetic and morphologic characteristics. The M7 subtype is more frequent in children than in adults. In adults, megakaryocytic leukemia is frequently observed as a secondary leukemia after chemotherapy or leukemic transformation of several chronic MPNs, including CML. Approximately 65% of acute megakaryocytic leukemia is associated with myelofibrosis. No specific chromosomal abnormality is associated with the adult form of megakaryocytic leukemia. After multivariate analysis, the AML megakaryocytic subtype is an independent predictor of increased mortality. Approximately 50% of patients with M7 AML have chromosomal abnormalities at diagnosis. Observed abnormalities include 3q21–3q26 rearrangements, partial or total deletion of chromosomes 5 and 7, gain of chromosomes 8 and 19, and t(9;22). Three manifestations of childhood megakaryocytic leukemia have been observed. First is the t(1;22)(p13;q13) with constitutional trisomy 21 associated with GATA1 mutations. Children with constitutional trisomy 21 have a 10- to 20-fold increased risk of developing leukemia. The incidence of developing M7 leukemia is up to 500 times higher in children with constitutional trisomy 21 than in normal children. However, children with constitutional trisomy 21 and megakaryocytic leukemia have a more favorable prognosis as compared with patients without constitutional trisomy 21. In these patients, somatic mutations of the transcription factor *GATA1* leads to exclusive expression of a truncated form of GATA1. The second form of childhood acute megakaryocytic leukemia involves t(1;22)(p13;q13) encoding the OTT-MAL (RBM15-MKL1) fusion protein in infants without constitutional trisomy 21 (Fig. 56.39). It is a very rare abnormality, described in about 40 cases worldwide (about 5% of infant AML cases), and associated with infantile M7 and with children younger than 3 years of age. Detection of t(1;22) is diagnostic. Adults with t(1;22)(p13;q13) encoding the OTT-MAL fusion protein have not been reported to date. Third, approximately 19% of infants with constitutional trisomy 21 (or mosaic trisomy 21C) and transient MPD subsequently develop M7 leukemia at a mean age of 20

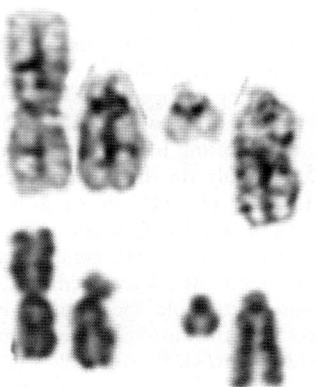

Fig. 56.39 MEGAKARYOCYTIC LEUKEMIA WITH t(1;22). Partial karyotype from two metaphase cells from a 4-week-old baby with M7 megakaryocytic leukemia showing a diagnostic t(1;22)(p13;q13) abnormality.

months. With development of leukemia, these children acquire diverse chromosomal abnormalities, most notably tetrasomy 21 and trisomy 8. The t(1;22) rearrangement has been observed in a set of monozygotic twins, suggesting an in utero origin in some cases. To date there are 16 cases of *GATA1* mutation-related transient MPDs and M7 AML in phenotypically and cytogenetically normal children. Thirteen of the 16 children were diagnosed during the first few months of life and in six cases, the blasts disappeared spontaneously without chemotherapy and the patients did not develop M7 AML. Gene expression profiling (GEP) has provided the first insight into the molecular pathogenesis of M7 leukemia in children with and without constitutional trisomy 21. These patients have distinct molecular phenotypes, with increased expression of chromosome 21 genes in patients with constitutional trisomy 21 as compared with M7 leukemia patients without constitutional trisomy 21. The *RUNX1* gene, localized on chromosome 21 which is essential for normal megakaryopoiesis, is expressed at lower levels in children with constitutional trisomy 21 and M7 leukemia, indicating a mechanism that may contribute to a block in differentiation

Down Syndrome–Associated Acute Myeloid Leukemia

The myeloid leukemia of Down syndrome (DS) was given a special WHO subclassification (ML-DS) because of its unique clinical and biologic features. These erythromegakaryoblastic leukemias are diagnosed before the age of 5 years and often present with thrombocytopenia and/or myelodysplasia. ML-DS is always preceded by the neonatal preleukemic syndrome, transient abnormal myelopoiesis (TAM; also known as transient MPD) that may, or may not, be clinically apparent. Unlike acute megakaryoblastic leukemias in patients without DS, these patients usually respond well to therapy with most patients being cured. Genetically, ML-DS is characterized by an acquired mutation in the *GATA1* gene. The mutation in *GATA1* is necessary but insufficient for development of ML-DS. Virtually all cases of TAM and ML-DS have N-terminal truncating *GATA1* mutations. *GATA1* mutations are present at birth in both neonates with DS with TAM and, through retrospective analysis of neonatal blood spots, also in children with ML-DS without a previous history of TAM. It is not clear at what stage in fetal development *GATA1* mutations arise; the earliest point in gestation at which mutations have been identified is 21 weeks. *GATA1* mutations disappear when TAM (or ML-DS) enters remission, indicating that these are acquired.

Monosomal Karyotype

MK is defined by the presence of at least two separate autosomal monosomies or one monosomy plus one or more structural

abnormalities. The overall frequency of MK in AML varies between 6% and 20%. Although in a study of 1058 patients with AML and abnormal karyotype, 30% had MK (see Fig. 56.27, *bottom row*). AML with MK is frequently associated with other adverse risk cytogenetic abnormalities, such as inv(3), −5 or del(5q), −7 or del(7q), abnormal (12p), −18/del(18q), abnormal (17p), and a complex karyotype. The frequency of these recurrent monosomies are: −7 and −17 in 6%, −18 in 5%, −5 and −21 in 4%, −20 in 3%, −3, −12, and 22 in 2% and loss of chromosomes 2, 4, 9, 13, and 19 in 1%. MK is a strong prognostic predictor of poor outcome compared with a traditionally defined complex karyotype. Patients with MK had a 4-year OS of 4% as compared with 21% in patients with other unfavorable karyotypes but without MK. Responses to induction therapy and OS of patients who have AML with MK are dismal: CR rates of 32% and a 4-year survival of 9%. MKs in a study of 248 patients with AML was found to be associated in more than 50% of patients with deletion of P53, whereas in another study of newly diagnosed 369 patients with AML, MK predicted an adverse treatment outcome and was associated with multidrug-resistance functional activity of leukemic blasts. A low frequency of mutations such as *FLT3* and *NPM1* was found in patients with MK AML.

Gain or Loss of Chromosomes in Acute Myeloid Leukemia

Approximately 15% to 20% of patients with AML have a numerical gain or loss of a single chromosome as the sole primary karyotypic abnormality. Each of the autosomes and sex chromosomes can contribute to the numerical changes. The most common trisomies in decreasing order of frequency are gain of chromosome 8, 22, 13, 21, and 11. The gain of chromosome 8, the most frequent abnormality seen in AML, is found as a sole abnormality in 6.3% of cases and overall occurs in 16% of cases. The incidence of +8 detected by FISH varies between 19% and 25% of AML cases. The prognosis of AML with +8 depends on whether +8 occurs as an isolated abnormality or accompanies other cytogenetic aberrations. In the latter situations, +8 does not appear to adversely affect the favorable outcome of patients with t(15;17), inv(16)t(16;16), and t(8;21). By contrast, patients with +8 and a complex karyotype and/or an unfavorable aberration such as del(5q) or −7 usually have a very poor outcome. Isolated +8 has been considered to be associated with either intermediate or unfavorable prognosis.

Deletion of 17p often results in the loss of tumor suppressor *TP53* gene on band p13.1, which has been reported in 5% to 9% of adult AML patients. The abnormalities of 17p are often associated with other chromosomal aberrations such as del(5q), −5, −7, but is also an independent poor-risk prognostic factor. *TP53* mutations are more common in older patients and those who have received previously alkylating agents. These patients were found to have an increase in the number of CD34+ cells, suggesting that the loss of *TP53* function could cause cell cycle arrest at an immature stage.[17]

Detection of Genomic Abnormalities

Whether PCR-based molecular screening, conventional cytogenetics, or both, should be used at diagnosis of AML is an important question with major consequences for developing a treatment strategy, monitoring therapy, and overall genetic risk assessment. A prospective study demonstrated an approximately 20% discrepancy between results using broad molecular screening with using a multiplex RT-PCR system and cytogenetic testing. This discrepancy has the potential to influence treatment strategies. Cryptic translocations detected as submicroscopic genetic lesions detected by RT-PCR may have no influence on prognosis or treatment strategy. In contrast, cytogenetic results influence treatment decisions by conferring unfavorable risk assignment on patients with negative broad molecular screening. These methodologies provide complementary genetic information for diagnosis, treatment, and follow-up.

Cytogenetic studies are valuable in assessing the effectiveness of therapy (see box on Genetic Testing for Acute Myeloid Leukemia and Fig. 56.26). In most patients with AML, a clonal cell population cannot be detected during remission. However, some mutations, as mentioned earlier, such as *DNMT3A*, have been found during clinical remissions—hence the fourth aspect of AML heterogeneity. When disease relapses, cells with the original chromosome anomalies are observed. If an appropriate FISH or RT-PCR test is available, these are the genetic tests of choice for predicting relapse because these methods are less expensive and more sensitive than chromosomal studies.

Acute Myeloid Leukemia with Complex Karyotype

Any karyotype with at least three chromosomal aberrations, regardless of their type and the individual chromosomes involved, is designated as "complex." Several studies have shown that patients with t(8;21), t(16;16)/inv(16) and t(15;17) constitute a separate biologic and clinical entity even if they contain additional abnormalities, because these additional cytogenetic abnormalities do not adversely affect the clinical outcome. Therefore the category of AML patients with a complex karyotype exclude patients with t(8;21),inv(16)/t(16;16) and t (15;17). Approximately, 10% to 12% of AML patients have three or more chromosome abnormalities whereas 8% to 9% have five or more abnormalities. The incidence of a complex karyotype increases with age. In patients with AML, age 18–60, 6% to 8% have three or more chromosomal abnormalities whereas 17% to 19% of patients older than 60 have a complex karyotype. In three large series of AML patients with a complex karyotype analyzed using multicolor FISH, more than 90% of patients had at least five abnormalities, with a median number of chromosomal aberrations being between 6 and 10. Approximately 80% of all patients with a complex karyotype have deletion 5q, followed by deletions 17p and 7q, occurring in approximately 50% of cases. At least 85% of all patients with AML with a complex karyotype showed one of the three deletions. The prognosis of patients with a complex karyotype is generally very poor. Among patients with AML above the age of 60, which constitute the majority of patients with complex karyotype, only 10% to 44% of those who harbor three or more chromosomal abnormalities achieve a CR, usually after a very short duration (median 6–8 months). CR rates of karyotypically complex patients are slightly higher in younger patients.

The impact of cytogenetics on outcome in a pediatric group of patients with AML (excluding APL) demonstrated about 80% OS for 10 years in patients with CBF AML. In contrast, patients with *MLL* abnormalities had an intermediate prognosis (61% OS at 10 years) with no evidence of heterogeneity according to the translocation partner of *MLL*. Additional abnormalities among the 11q23 leukemia have diverse prognoses; trisomy 8 is an independent favorable, whereas trisomy 19 is considered an adverse prognostic factor in *MLL* rearranged group of pediatric patients.

The striking clinical, cytogenetic, and biologic heterogeneity of AML is only partly explained by the known chromosomal or molecular rearrangements. DNA microarray technology provides a higher resolution and has been demonstrated to detect cryptic copy number alterations (CNA) and UPD. The current clinical implications of aCGH + SNP microarray analyses in AML remains limited. However, in cases with UPD, gene mutations precede mitotic recombination, resulting in loss of the remaining wild-type allele, which can act as a "second hit" mutation. UPD has been shown to be predictive of poor event-free and OS. For example, SNP microarray analysis of patients with AML with a normal karyotype demonstrated UPD of chromosome 13q, leading to duplication of a mutant *FLT3* allele at band 13q12, which was associated with significantly inferior OS. Approximately 20% of patients with AML and a normal karyotype have UPD. The most common chromosomal regions of UPD are 1p, 2p, 2q, 4q (*TET2*), 6p, 7q (*EZH2*), 11p (*WT1*), 11q, 13q (*FLT3*), 14q, 16p, 17p (*TP53*), 19q (*CEBPA*), 21q (*RUNX1*), and Xq. The analysis of genes located within a UPD chromosomal region has shown a copy-neutral loss of heterozygosity with duplication of gene mutations that have been already implicated in AML pathogenesis and a loss of the corresponding normal allele.

Numerous studies using cytogenomics have uncovered a broad range of cryptic CNAs in patients with AML and a normal karyotype, as well as in patients exhibiting balanced translocations or chromosomal imbalances. Not only do these studies reveal a tremendous degree of genetic diversity of AML; they also have shown that the estimated average number of CNAs per genome is 2–2.5. This finding implies either that most AML genomes are relatively stable or that more sensitive methods are required (e.g., complete genome sequences) to capture the whole spectrum of genetic alterations. Genomic imbalances (and their associated target genes) include gains of regions 4q25–26 (*PRDM5*), 8p11.21 (*ZMAT4*), 8q24.21 (*CCDC26*), 13q32 (*ABCC4*), 14q23.1 (*PRKCH*), 16q24.1 (*USP10, CRISPLD2*), and 21q22.3 (*PRMT2*), as well as losses of regions 6q27 (*RPS6KA2*), 7p22.3 (*FAM20C*), 8q24.12 (*TRPS1*), 9p21.2 (*TISCI*), 10q11,21 (*HNRNPF*), 15q21.3 (*RFX7*), Xp11.4 (*BCOR*), and Xp25 (*STAG2*) (Fig. 56.40). The biologic consequences of these small genomic imbalances are not fully understood. In some cases, submegabase-sized CNAs may uncover cryptic rearrangements, as has been shown for *NSD1-NUP98* and *MALT4-MLL* fusion genes. The systemic analysis of CNAs and regions of UPD in AML in the future may fully uncover genomic changes that contribute to AML pathogenesis.

Acute Myeloid Leukemia in the Elderly

The biology of AML changes with age. The spectrum of cytogenetic abnormalities in older adults includes a higher percentage of patients with abnormalities involving −5/del(5q), −7/del(7q), and 17p and a lower incidence of translocations associated with a favorable prognosis and treatment outcome. Older patients with a complex karyotype have an extremely poor prognosis, with only 26% achieving CR owing to high rates of resistant disease. Multidrug resistance is present in 57% of patients over 75 years of age and in 33% of patients with AML younger than 56 years of age. The OS rate in older adult patients with AML is only 2% at 5 years. The biology of AML in the elderly patients may be a consequence of the age of hematopoietic stem cells, shortened telomere length (associated with older cells), presence of fewer normal stem cells to compete with the malignant clones and repopulate marrow following chemotherapy and as mentioned earlier, the increased frequency of age-related somatic mutations present in over 10% of healthy individuals over 70 years of age.

Therapy-Related Acute Myeloid Leukemia and Therapy-Related Myelodysplastic Syndrome

Therapy-related AML and MDS are distinct clinical syndromes occurring as late complications following high-dose chemotherapy, radiation therapy, or autologous stem cell transplantation. A normal karyotype is observed in 8%, and an abnormal karyotype is detected in 92% of the patient population.[18] From the cytogenetic point of view, two different categories of therapy-related AML and MDS can be identified. The first group includes patients who develop AML/MDS following exposure to alkylating agents approximately 5 years after therapy. These leukemias are associated with the presence of monosomy 5/del(5q) or monosomy 7/del(7q) (see Fig. 56.26, *third row*). Many of these patients initially develop myelodysplastic features before transforming into frank AML. Recurrent abnormalities of chromosomes 5, 7, or both account for 70% of all abnormalities observed in therapy-related leukemia. These patients respond poorly to therapy and have a poor OS. A second group of patients develop therapy-related AML without prior MDS. Leukemia cells in these patients often exhibit 11q23 (3%) and 21q22 (3%) balanced rearrangements, attributed to the late effects of topoisomerase II inhibitors combined with alkylating agents and radiation (see Figs. 56.32 and 56.33). AML may develop within a few months to 3 years after

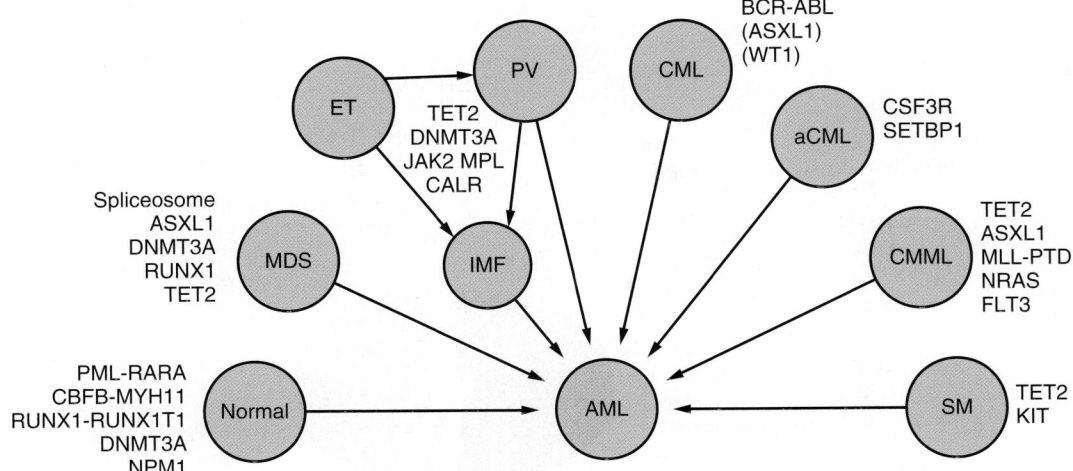

Fig. 56.40 COMMON MUTATIONS IN DE NOVO AND SECONDARY AML. A number of clonal blood disorders with a myeloid phenotype are represented. Each of these disorders is characterized by recurrent mutations in specific genes, some of which are shared between several different phenotypes (e.g., *TET2*). All of these disorders can transform to secondary AML upon acquisition of additional somatic mutations. When AML arises in the absence of an antecedent clonal blood disorder, it is known as primary AML. *aCML,* Atypical CML; *AML,* acute myeloid leukemia; *CML,* chronic myeloid leukemia; *ET,* essential thrombocytopenia; *IMF,* idiopathic myelofibrosis; *PV,* polycythemia vera; *SM,* systemic mastocytosis. *(Reprinted with permission from Grove CS, Vassiliou GS: Acute myeloid leukaemia: a paradigm for the clonal evolution of cancer?* Dis Model Mech *7:941, 2014.)*

therapy. Polysomy (tetrasomy, pentasomy, hexasomy) of chromosome 8 defines a clinicocytogenetic entity associated with therapy-related myeloid malignancies and poor OS (see box on Genetic Testing for Therapy-Related Neoplasms). When the genome of 22 patients with therapy-related AML was sequenced and compared to whole genome sequence data from patients with de novo AML and secondary AML arising from MDS, the mutational burden of therapy-related AML genomes was found to be similar to that of de novo AML indicating that prior chemotherapy does not induce genome-wide DNA damage. However, a distinct subset of mutated genes is present in therapy-related AML/MDS. The whole genome sequence data revealed that *TP53* mutations and mutations in ABC transporter genes (a subset of which have been implicated in chemotherapy resistance) are significantly increased in therapy-related AML/MDS compared with de novo AML/MDS. *TP53* mutations are present in approximately 33% of patients with therapy-related AML/MDS and are associated with poor risk cytogenetics and a worse prognosis. More recent genomic data suggest that cytotoxic therapy does not directly induce *TP53* mutations. Rather, these studies support a model in which rare stem cells carrying age-related *TP53* mutations that are resistant to chemotherapy expand preferentially following treatment.[19]

A novel hierarchical prognostic model of AML solely based on molecular mutations was proposed by a German group in 2012. This model was based on 1000 patients with AML at diagnosis after a median follow-up of 23.7 months. According to Grossman and her colleagues molecular screening for the recurrent balanced rearrangements (*PML-RARA, RUNX1-RUNX1T1, CBFB-MYH11*) and mutations in *CEBPA, NPM1, RUNX1, ASXL1,* and *TP53* as well as for *FLT3-IDT* and *MLL-PTD* can be used to create a prognostic classification system in AML that improves any prognostic model based on cytogenetics alone.[20] Five distinct prognostic subgroups have been identified: (1) very favorable: *PML-RARA* rearrangement or *CEPBA* double mutations with OS at 3 years of 82.9%; (2) favorable: *RUNX1-RUNXT1, CBFB-MYH11* or *NPM1* mutations without *FLT3*-ITD, OS at 3 years of 62.6%; (3) intermediate: none of the mutations leading to assignment into groups 1, 2, 4 or 5; OS at 3 years 44.2%; (4) unfavorable: *MLL*-PTD and/or *RUNX1* mutation and/or *ASXL1* mutation: OS at 3 years 21.9% and (5) unfavorable *TP53* mutation: OS at 3 years 0%. However, using whole-genome or exome sequencing from 71 patients with AML treated with

> **Genetic Testing for Acute Myeloid Leukemia**
>
> At diagnosis, the recommended general practice includes FISH studies using the panel of chromosomal probes for acute myeloid leukemia (AML), including *RUNX1-RUNXT1, PML-RARA, CBFB, BCR-ABL1, MLL,* and *TP53*. Conventional cytogenetic studies must be also performed at diagnosis. Patients with core-binding factor (CBF) AML subtype should be tested for *KIT* exon 17 mutations because these mutations adversely impact the prognosis. These tests are performed at diagnosis to establish a benchmark for the percentage of neoplastic cells and are used in follow-up studies to assess the effectiveness of therapy. In patients with a normal karyotype, mutation studies for the most common genes (*DNMT3, NPM1, FLT3, CEBPA,* and *TET2*) are recommended.

> **Genetic Testing for Therapy-Related Neoplasms**
>
> The best genetic test for therapy-related myelodysplastic syndrome or acute myeloid leukemia is a conventional cytogenetic study. FISH studies with probes for loci on chromosomes 5 and 7, *MLL,* and *RUNX1* should be performed if therapy-related leukemia is suspected. This approach is useful for t(8;21), t(9;22), t(11;var), t(15;17), inv(16), −5/del(5q), −7/del(7q), rearrangements of *ETV6,* and some others.

standard induction therapy demonstrated that for risk stratification the clearance of somatic mutations after chemotherapy is more important than the identification of specific mutations at the time of diagnosis. In this study, the detection of persistent AML-associated mutations in at least 5% of bone marrow cells in day-30 remission samples was associated with significantly increased risk of relapse and reduced OS.

ACUTE LYMPHOBLASTIC LEUKEMIA

ALL accounts for at least 85% of acute leukemias in children and 20% of acute leukemias in adults.[21] The susceptibility to ALL varies with age; the first peak is between 2 and 5 years of age after birth,

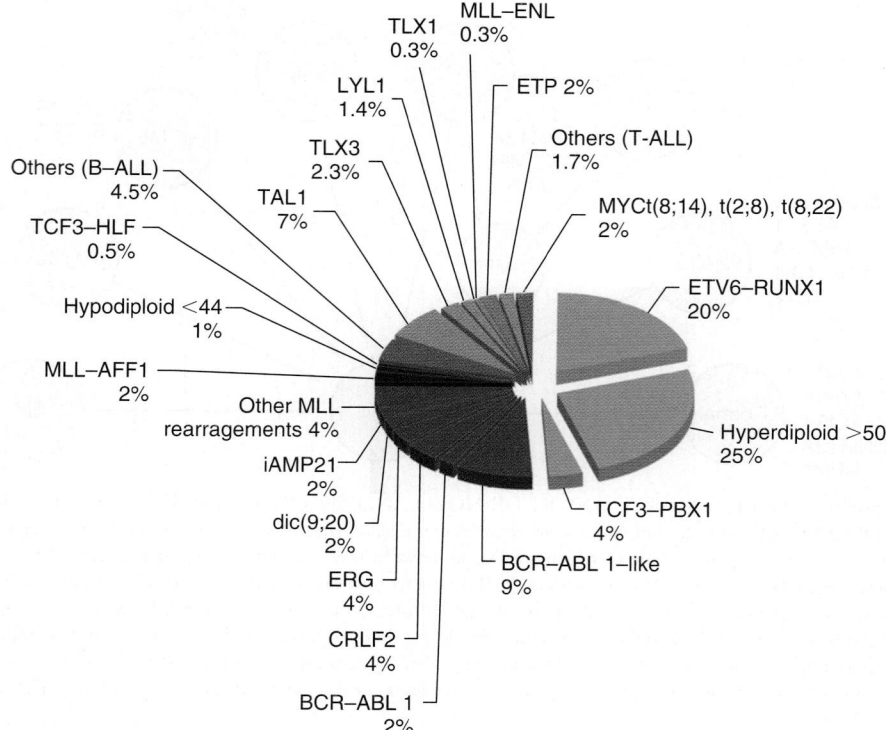

Fig. 56.41 ESTIMATED FREQUENCY OF SPECIFIC GENOTYPES IN CHILDHOOD ACUTE LYMPHOBLASTIC LEUKEMIA (ALL). The genetic lesions that are exclusively seen in cases of T-cell ALL are indicated in *gold* and those commonly associated with precursor B-cell ALL in *blue*. The darker gold or blue color indicates those subtypes generally associated with poor prognosis. *BCR-ABL1*-like cases can be separated into one group with CRLF2 dysregulation and the other with activating cytokine receptor and kinase signaling. *(Reproduced with permission from Pui et al: Pediatric acute lymphoblastic leukemia: where are we going and how do we get there? Blood 120:1165, 2012).*

followed by a gradual decrease during adulthood but an increase in incidence again in individuals older than age 70 years, suggesting that different combinations of environmental and genetic factors contribute to leukemogenesis at different ages. Most published series of patients with acute ALL indicate that 70% to 75% have an abnormal clone by conventional cytogenetic studies (Figs. 56.41 and 56.42). Genomic rearrangements detected with intensive interphase FISH screening have been found in up to 91% of cases. The application of contemporary genome-wide molecular analysis continues to reveal many additional genetic rearrangements that are not detectable with chromosome studies.[22] At least one clonal aberration has been detected in 60% to 79% of adults and 57% to 82% of children with ALL.[15] Today, cytogenetic analyses combined with FISH and/or RT-PCR are mandatory in most ALL clinical trials, and genetic findings play a pivotal role in proper risk stratification and identifying treatment options.[23] Several of the ALL-specific chromosome aberrations and their molecular counterparts have been included in the 2008 WHO classification.

Pretreatment cytogenetics is an independent prognostic factor in children and adults presenting with ALL and is important in determining risk categories.[16]

As shown in Fig. 56.42 and Table 56.10, the risk categories in children include (a) low risk: high hyperdiploidy (trisomies for chromosomes 4, 10, and 17) and t(12;21)/*TEL-RUNX1*; (b) high risk: t(1;19)/*TCF3-PBX1*; and (c) very high risk: t(9;22)/*BCR-ABL1*, *BCR-ABL1*-like, 11q23/*MLL* rearrangements, and iAMP21. In adults the low-risk category includes high hyperdiploidy and del(9p), whereas the high-risk category includes hypodiploidy/near triploidy, t(9;22)(q34;q11), t(4;11)(q21;q23), t(8;14)(q24;q32), and a complex karyotype (five or more chromosomal abnormalities).

Approximately 20% of children and 26% of adults with B-cell ALL are *hyperdiploid*. Two groups are distinguished based on

cytogenetics: (a) those with 51–55 chromosomes whose prognosis is poorer, and (b) those with 56–67 chromosomes whose prognosis is excellent. Both groups have a more favorable prognosis than do children with hypodiploidy or near-haploid ALL. In a study of 1880 children with ALL, patients with 45 chromosomes have an outcome similar to that of pseudodiploid or low hyperdiploid patients with ALL (47–50 chromosomes). Children and adolescents with ALL and hypodiploidy with fewer than 44 chromosomes have a poor outcome. The distribution of specific chromosome gains is not random, with the most often gained chromosomes being 21, X, 14, 6, 18, 4, 17, and 10, each of which is gained in more than 50% of hyperdiploid patients with ALL, followed by gains in chromosomes 8, 5, 11, and 12, that occur more often in patients with 57 or more chromosomes. The prognosis of children with high hyperdiploidy is excellent with a 5-year event-free survival (EFS) rates of between 71% and 83% and a 5-year OS rate of approximately 90%. Pretreatment cytogenetic analyses of more than 5400 children with ALL unequivocally shows that simultaneous trisomies for chromosomes 4, 10, and 17 are associated with a higher long-term EFS (see Fig. 56.42D). By contrast with children who have a favorable prognosis when a hyperdiploid karyotype is present, such a favorable constellation has not been found in patients with adult ALL. The reason for this discrepancy may be that adults often have poor-risk chromosomal translocations, such as the Ph chromosome. Approximately 50% of the high hyperdiploid patients harbor other structural abnormalities, such as gains of 1q, del(6q), which do not appear to influence prognosis, with a possible exception of prognostically adverse isochromosome 17q. Frequently, hyperdiploid leukemic cells fail to proliferate in culture; therefore the use of an ALL panel for FISH is strongly recommended.

Modal chromosome numbers of 45 or less occur in 2% to 3% of cases (specifically, the near-haploid numbers of 24–36)

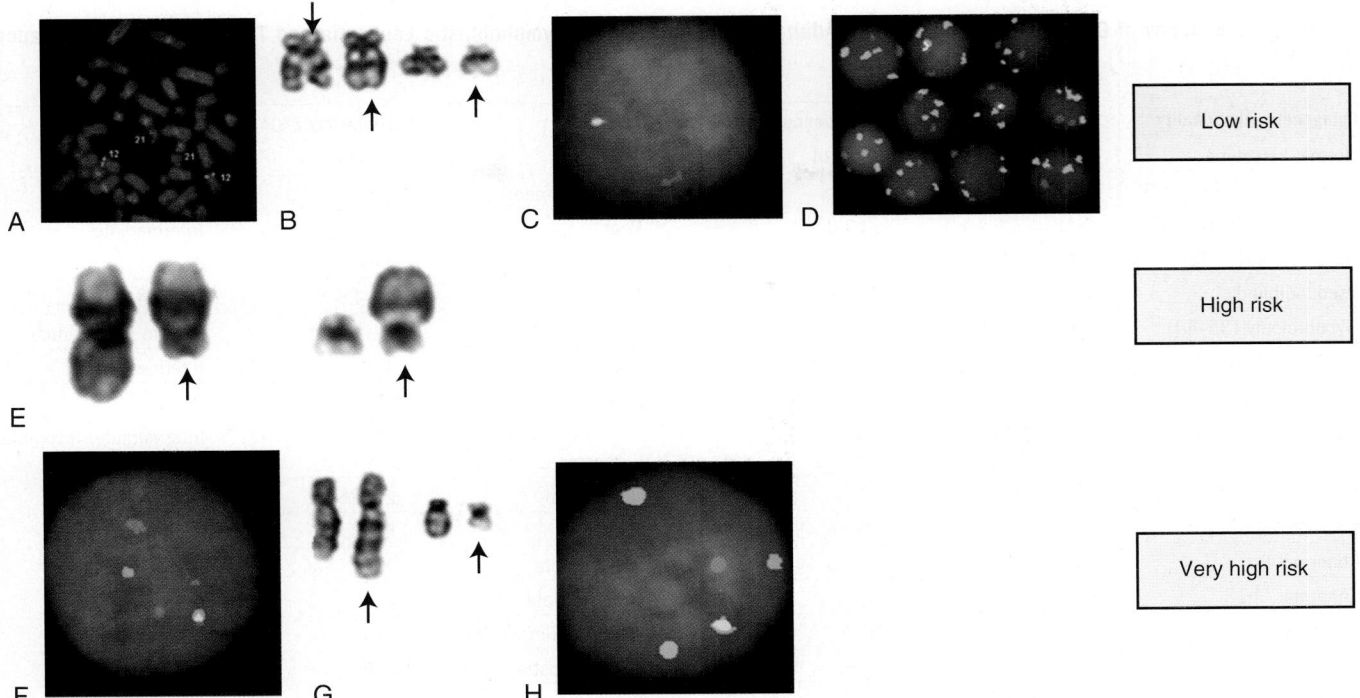

Fig. 56.42 PROGNOSTIC CYTOGENETIC CATEGORIES IN ACUTE LYMPHOBLASTIC LEUKE-MIA. (A) Localization of TEL/ETV6 and AML1 fluorescence probes to chromosomes from a normal bone marrow metaphase cell. TEL/ETV6 is on 12p13 *(green)* and AML1 is on 21q *(red)*. (B) Partial karyotype showing t(12;21)(p13;q22) *(arrows)*. The short arrow at 12p indicates a possible TEL deletion from normal chromosome 12. (C) FISH study showing loss of TEL *(green)* from normal 12 homologue in interphase nucleus, a frequent subclonal evolution in patients with t(12;21). (D) Hyperdiploidy, specifically trisomies for chromosomes 4 *(green)*, 10 *(red)*, and 17 *(aqua)*, is associated with low-risk cytogenetic category (see text for details) and is present in disomy in interphase cells *(top left)*. (E) Partial G-banded karyotype showing t(1;19) (q23;p13.3), which occurs in approximately 6% of patients with B-cell precursor childhood acute lympho-blastic leukemia. (F) FISH hybridization to bone marrow nucleus showing BCR-ABL fusion *(yellow)*. (G) As a consequence of t(9;22), occurring in 5% of children and 20% to 25% of adults with acute lymphoblastic leukemia. (H) Interphase nucleus after FISH study with tricolor probe. Dual-color/breakapart MLL shows separation of the 3′ end and the 5′ end as a result of 11q23 rearrangement. CEP11 *(aqua)* indicates disomy for chromosome 11, used as internal control. MLL rearrangements in acute lymphoblastic leukemia are associ-ated with unfavorable prognosis.

that confer a poor prognosis. Similarly, ALL in adults presenting with low hyperdiploid/near-triploidy have poor outcomes. Loss of chromosome 7 is frequent in adult patients with ALL and the majority of these patients also have t(9;22). Hypodiploid ALL can be further divided into multiple subgroups according to chromosome number. Genomic profiling have shown that near haploid (24–31 chromosomes) and low-hypodiploid (32–39 chromosomes) childhood ALL are distinct subtypes: near-haploid-ALL is associated with a high frequency of *RAS*-activating mutations including focal deletions of *NF*-1 whereas low-hypodiploid ALL has biallelic alterations of the *TP53* locus, deletions of *CDKN2A/B* and/or *Rb1*. *TP53* mutations are also present in nonhematopoietic cells in half of childhood patients with a low-hyperdiploid karyotype, indicating that this disease is a manifestation of Li-Fraumeni syndrome. Diagnosis of low hyperdiploid ALL requires *TP53* testing and genetic counseling.

In childhood ALL, *t(12;21)* was first reported in 1994 as a fortuitous FISH finding. This translocation is difficult to detect by conventional cytogenetics because the translocated portions of 12p13 and 21q22 have virtually identical G-banding patterns. In contrast, the *ETV6-RUNX1* fusion product of t(12;21) is detected using PCR or FISH in 17% to 30% of pediatric patients with ALL (see Fig. 56.42A–C). The *ETV6-RUNX1* fusion, found almost exclusively in children 1–15 years old with B-precursor ALL, represents the most frequent molecular rearrangement in childhood cancer. Children

with the *ETV6-RUNX1* fusion gene have significantly lower rates of relapse than do *ETV6-RUNX1*–negative patients. *ETV6-RUNX1* positive B-precursor ALL is characterized by a prolonged duration of first remission and excellent cure rates. Prospective analyses have demonstrated that the survival rate in t(12;21)-positive patients is significantly better when compared with cases lacking this abnormality; however, this abnormality in multivariate analysis was not found to be an independent predictor of outcome. The *ETV6-RUNX1* fusion is rare in adult ALL. t(12;21)(p13;q22) fuses the helix-loop-helix domain of the *ETV6* gene, located on chromosome 12, band p13, to the DNA-binding and transactivation domain of the *RUNX1* gene, located on 21q22. FISH studies allow visualization of the fusion gene on 21q22. Fusion with *ETV6* converts *RUNX1* from an activator to a repressor of transcription. The *ETV6-RUNX1* fusion is accompanied in 55% to 70% patients by the loss of the other normal nonrearranged *ETV6* allele.[17] This deletion probably represents subclonal evolution. *ETV6-RUNX1* has been detected in utero, probably in a committed B-cell progenitor, and is present in normal cord blood and peripheral blood samples at frequencies 100-fold greater than the risk for corresponding leukemia. The current view of development of *ETV6-RUNX1*–positive leukemia is that these early events are followed by a long "preleukemic" phase followed by loss of the normal *ETV6* homologue, which appears to be an important event in the multistep pathogenesis of this form of leukemia. Currently, of the 397 children with *ETV6-RUNX1*–positive leukemia reported,

TABLE 56.10   Frequency of Cytogenetic Aberrations in Adult and Childhood Acute Lymphoblastic Leukemia and Their Prognostic Relevance

Cytogenetic Abnormality	Genes Involved	Adults Frequency (%)	Adults Prognosis	Children Frequency (%)	Children Prognosis
Normal karyotype	NA	15–34	Good	31–42	Favorable
High hyperdiploidy (>55)	NA	7–8	Good-intermediate	23–30	Good
Low hyperdiploidy (>50)	NA	10–15	Poor	10–11	Intermediate
Near haploidy (<35)	NA	Rare	NA	1–4	Poor
Pseudodiploidy	NA	31–50	Poor	18–26	Intermediate
Hypodiploidy (35–44)	NA	4–9	Poor	6	Poor to intermediate
t(9;22)(q34;q11.2)	BCR-ABL1	11–29	Poor	1–3	Intermediate
t(4;11)(q21;q23)	MLL-AFF1[a]	4–9	Poor	2	Poor
t(1;19)(q23;p13.3)	TCF3-PBX1	1–3	Poor, intermediate favorable	1–6	Intermediate, favorable
t(12;21)(p12;q22)	ETV6 (TEL)-RUNX1	0–3	Not known	22–26	Good
t(8;14)(q24;q32)	MYC-IGH	5–15	Poor	5	Poor
Abnormal 9p	CDKN2A	7–13	Intermediate	7–11	Adverse
Abnormal 9p13	PAX5	2	?Intermediate	2–5	Poor
Abnormal 12p	ETV6	0–3	Favorable/unfavorable	3–9	Not prognostic
del(6q)	Not known	3–6	Not prognostic	6–9	Adverse
del(7p)/del(7q)/–7	Not known	6–11	Not prognostic	1	Adverse
del(5q)	Not known	<2	Not prognostic	2	Not known
Trisomy 8	NA	10–12	Poor	3–4 (17%–22% in T-ALL)	Not prognostic
14q11	TCRα	5–7 (26% in T-ALL)	Excellent	Rare	Poor
t(10;14)(q24;q11)	TRD-TLX1	1–3	Excellent, intermediate		
BCR-ABL1-like	ABL, JAK, EPOR CRLF2, IKZF del	17	High risk	15	High risk
iAMP21	RUNX1	0.5	Poor	2	Poor, unless treated on intense protocol
Monosomal karyotype	NA	9.2	Treated on high risk protocol	12.8	Treated on high risk protocol

[a]See Table 56.8 for all other mixed lineage leukemia rearrangements.
NA, Not applicable; T-ALL, T-cell acute lymphoblastic leukemia.

approximately 60% harbor additional karyotypic abnormalities that contribute to their pseudodiploid or near-diploid karyotypes. The most common secondary change, which occurs in approximately 50% of cases with additional abnormalities, is trisomy 21.

A rare group of patients with B-precursor ALL lack fusion of *TEL* and *RUNX1* but have 3 to 15 copies of the q22 band of chromosome 21, including the *RUNX1* locus. Intrachromosomal amplification of the 21q22 band of chromosome 21 is a clonal marker of the leukemic cells that defines a distinct ALL subgroup (Fig. 56.43A). The British Childhood Leukemia Working Party prospectively screened 1630 patients with childhood ALL and identified 28 children with intrachromosomal amplification of chromosome 21 (iAMP21) (see Fig. 56.43D).[24] Approximately 2% of children and less than 0.5% of adults display iAMP21. Children with iAMP21 have a common or pre–B-cell immunophenotype, a median age of 9 years at presentation, and a significantly inferior event-free and OS at 5 years compared with children exhibiting other cytogenetic subgroups. Even children with Ph-positive ALL have a better 5-year EFS as compared with children with iAMP21. These children have a threefold increased risk for relapse and are twice as likely to die than are their counterparts without iAMP21. The complexity and variability of the iAMP21 includes multiple regions of gains, amplification, inversion, and deletions. In spite of their differences in genomic profiles, the consistent features of patients with ALL and iAMP21 include a common region of highest level amplification spanning 5.1 Mb from 32.8 to 37 Mb,

within which the *RUNX1* gene is located. These observations confirmed that FISH, using probes directed to *RUNX1* locus, to determine the number of copies of the most amplified region, provides a reliable detection method. Thus the finding of three or more extra copies of *RUNX1* on a single abnormal chromosome 21 (a total of five or more *RUNX1* signals per interphase cell) is currently used as the international definition of iAMP21.

Recent genomic, cytogenetic and transcriptional analysis coupled with novel bioinformatic approaches revealed that individuals born with a rare constitutional Robertsonian translocation, t(15;21)(q10;q10)c have an approximately 2700-fold increased risk of developing iAMP21ALL compared with the general population. In these patients, amplification is initiated by a chromothripsis event (a process whereby localized genomic regions are shattered and rearranged in one catastrophic event) that affects both sister chromatids of the Robertsonian chromosome. In sporadic iAMP21, breakage-fusion-bridge (BFB) cycles are typically the initiating event, often followed by chromothripsis. In both sporadic and rob(15;21)c-associated iAMP21, the final stages frequently involve duplications of the entire abnormal chromosome. The end-product is a derivative of chromosome 21 or the rob(15;21)c chromosome with gene dosage optimized for leukemic potential, showing constrained copy number levels over multiple linked genes.

Patients with iAMP21 display a unique spectrum of secondary chromosomal abnormalities and they include gain of X chromosome,

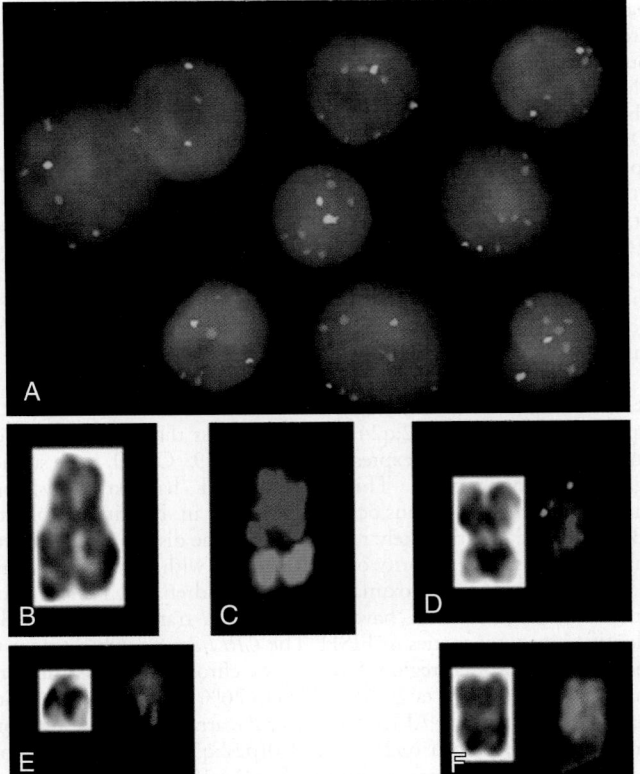

Fig. 56.43 DETECTION OF AML1 AND 21q22 AMPLIFICATION. (A) Intrachromosomal amplification of AML1 *(red)* (TEL *[green]*, present in disomy) in a pediatric patient with pre–B-cell acute lymphoblastic leukemia. This finding is associated with poor prognosis. (B) G-banding of der(18) chromosome and after FISH study (C) with WCP 18 *(green)* and LSI 21q22.13 *(red)*, documenting der(18)t(18;21) and amplification of 21q22 region in a patient with myelodysplastic syndrome/acute myeloid leukemia. (D) Amplification of 21q22 region in myelodysplastic syndrome may be present in another formation: der(21) (G-banding, *left*). FISH study shows amplification of 21q22.13 locus *(red)* and identified der(21) as t(5;21) with 5p15.2 probe *(green)*. (E) Localization of 21q22.13 LSI probe on normal chromosome 21. (F) Homogeneous staining region (hsr)(21), G-banding *(left)*, and after FISH study *(right)* with locus-specific probe for 21q22.13 *(red)* consistent with 21q22.13 band amplification in a patient with myelodysplastic syndrome.

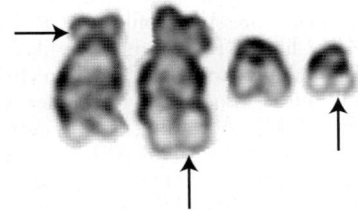

Fig. 56.44 The Ph CHROMOSOME IN ACUTE LYMPHOBLASTIC LEUKEMIA. t(9;22)(q34;q11) *(arrows)* in a patient with acute lymphoblastic leukemia. Note that the first chromosome 9 has deletion of the short arms, a frequent finding in both adult and pediatric patients with acute lymphoblastic leukemia.

10 or 14, or monosomy 7/deletion 7q deletions of 11q, including *ATM* and *MLL* genes, deletions of *ETV6* and *RB1*.

Both the UK and US Children Oncology groups demonstrated that patients with ALL and iAMP21 when stratified as a high-risk group and treated on the most intensive treatment arm have a 5-year EFS (from 29% to 78%), a risk of relapse (reduced from 70% vs. 16%) and OS from 67% versus 89%.

The *ETV6* transcription factor gene, was first identified as a part of a *TEL*–platelet-derived growth factor receptor β fusion [*TEL (ETV6)-PDGFRB*] created by t(5;12)(q33;p13) in chronic myelomonocytic leukemia. It was detected using FISH owing to difficulties in detecting cytogenetic rearrangements at the 12p13 site. As a result of this translocation, the helix-loop-helix domain of *ETV6* is fused in frame to the *PDGFRB* transmembrane and tyrosine kinase domain. Fusion of *ETV6* to a tyrosine kinase also occurs as a result of t(9;12)(q34;p13), leading to the *ABL1-ETV6* fusion that has been observed in patients with ALL, AML, and atypical CML. More than 39 partner genes are known to participate in fusions with *ETV6*, primarily in ALL and less frequently in myeloid malignancies.

Other rearrangements involving 12p include deletions, duplications, and translocations and are observed most often as part of a complex karyotype, frequently associated with chromosome 5 and/or 7 abnormalities. Deletion of 12p13 is much more frequent in children than in adults with ALL and is observed in patients with myeloid disorders, specifically in adults with MDS. Two other genes residing on 12p are also rearranged: *CCND2* is frequently amplified, and *CDKN1B* is often deleted.

Approximately 5% of children and 20% to 25% of adults with ALL have a Ph chromosome, making it the most common structural rearrangement in adult ALL (Fig. 56.44). The breakpoint on the Ph chromosome is more centromeric than in CML (see Chronic Myelogenous Leukemia section, earlier). It includes the 5′ breakpoint on chromosome 22, distal to the first exon (falling between exon e1 and e2) of the *BCR* gene, resulting in the P190$^{BCR-ABL1}$ variant, providing a diagnostic distinction between the lymphoid blast crisis of CML and de novo ALL. Ph-positive ALL is characterized by a smaller BCR-ABL1 (P190) protein, containing less BCR than the P210 and P230 fusion proteins. Among Ph-positive patients with ALL, approximately 58% to 70% of adults and 80% of children have this breakpoint variant. Up to 19% of Ph-positive patients with ALL may express both the P190 and the P210$^{BCR-ABL1}$ proteins. A number of earlier studies indicated that the P190 type of the *BCR-ABL1* breakpoint is associated with a more aggressive form of disease, with greater transforming ability than the P210 protein. Ph-positive ALL has been classified as a stem cell disorder because of the presence of the *BCR-ABL1* transcript in both the myeloid and lymphoid cells.

The *BCR-ABL1* fusion variants are easily detectable by FISH using the extrasensitive probe strategy, and *BCR-ABL1* leukemia can be identified in up to 10% of Ph-negative cases using conventional cytogenetics. Moreover, FISH will identify *ABL* rearrangements in *BCR-ABL1* patients with fusion-negative ALL.

Reactivation of BCR-ABL1 kinase activity is most commonly associated with the emergence of point mutation in the ABL1 kinase domain implicated in imatinib resistance (see Chronic Myelogenous Leukemia section, earlier). Recent studies have indicated that kinase domain mutations are present in 70% of imatinib resistant patients with T315I (37%), E255K (18%) and Y253H (18%) mutations accounting for 75% of these cases. Moreover, 78% of patients resistant to second-generation TKIs were positive for such mutations, and 58% of them had multiple mutations.

More than 60% of adult patients with Ph-positive ALL show additional chromosomal abnormalities in the Ph-positive clone. Most frequent are gain of Ph chromosome, monosomy 7, +8, +X, del(9p), and high triploidy. The additional chromosomal abnormalities have no effect on survival of these patients. High hyperdiploidy is detected in approximately 15% of Ph-positive ALL. According to the WHO classification, 1% of all leukemias are mixed phenotype acute leukemias with t(9;22)(q34;q11.2) and leukemic blast cells expressing B-cell and myeloid phenotypic markers. Occasional T-cell phenotype and trilineage *BCR-ABL1* mixed phenotype leukemia have been rarely reported.

"BCR-ABL1-like" Acute Lymphoblastic Leukemia

Retrospective studies have demonstrated that GEP can be used effectively to classify ALL into prognostically important subtypes.

BCR-ABL1-like ALL is a newly described ALL subtype lacking *BCR-ABL1*, but with a similar expression profile to *BCR-ABL1*+ leukemia. This new "*BCR-ABL1*-like" ("Ph-chromosome-like") ALL includes approximately 15% of all precursor B-cell ALL in children and 17% of adults with ALL and is associated with higher relapse rate and lower EFS (see Fig. 56.41). According to the currently used risk stratification system, 43% of the "BCR-ABL-like" patients are classified as having high-risk disease. Large-scale genomic profiling and sequencing studies of over 1700 childhood and young adult patients with ALL has revealed rearrangements of *ABL*-class genes, rearrangements of *JAK2*, *EPOR*, and *CRLF2*. *ABL*-class rearrangements result in the expression of fusion genes that activate *ABL1*, *ABL2*, *CSFR1*, and *PDGFRB*. In this group of patients *IKZF-1* deletions occur in 40% of pediatric and in 46% of adult patients.[19] *CRLF2* (Xp22.33/p11.3) rearrangements are observed in approximately 50% of patients with BCR-ABL1-like ALL. The gene encodes for cytokine receptor-like factor 2, also known as thymic-stromal–derived lymphopoietin receptor which in combination with the interleukin-7 receptor forms the receptor for the thymic stromal lymphopoietin. *CRLF2*-rearranged leukemic cells have activated JAK-STAT and PI3K signaling pathways.

t(1;19)(q23;p13.3)/*TCF3–PBX1* occurs in 5% to 6% of patients with B-cell precursor childhood and adult ALL. However, among patients with a pre-B (cytoplasmic Ig–positive) t(1;19) is found in approximately 25% of cases (see Fig. 56.32E). Cytogenetically, two forms of t(1;19) have been identified: 25% of cases have a balanced reciprocal t(1;19), whereas 75% have a rearrangement of unbalanced der(19)t(1;19)(q23;p13.3). The unbalanced der(19)t(1;19) arises from the initial trisomy of chromosome 1 followed by the t(1;19) translocation, with subsequent loss of the derivative chromosome 1. More than 95% of t(1;19) are associated with the *TCF3–PBX1* chimeric gene protein product which arrests cell differentiation. The *TCF3* gene (originally identified by the binding of E2A proteins to the kE2DNA sequence motif contained in the Ig κ light-chain enhancer) on chromosome 19, band p13.3, is fused to the *PBX1* (homeobox) gene on chromosome 1, band q23. Approximately 1% of pediatric patients with B-ALL have a variant t(17;19)(q21–q22;p13) translocation resulting in two different genomic rearrangements. The first is the fusion between the *HLF* gene (breakpoint in intron 3) on chromosome 17 and the *TCF3* gene (within intron 13) on chromosome 19, associated with disseminated intravascular coagulopathy. The second is the breakpoint in intron 12 of *TCF3* and intron 3 of *HLF*, which is associated with hypercalcemia. In contrast to *ETV6-RUNX1* rearrangements, which have a prenatal origin, current evidence suggests a postnatal etiology for t(1;19) translocations.

Currently, it is thought that an unbalanced der(19) in pediatric patients with ALL is associated with significantly improved outcome as compared with patients with balanced t(1;19). In adults as the sole abnormality, t(1;19)/der(19)t(1;1.9) is associated with an intermediate prognosis; however, within the context of a hyperdiploid karyotype, it is associated with a poor prognosis. Patients with *TCF3-PBX1* fusion also display *PAX5* (19p13.2) haploinsufficiency, detectable both by conventional and molecular cytogenetics. A variant t(17;19) rearrangement is associated with a poor prognosis. A recent study of adult patients with ALL has suggested that prognosis of patients with t(1;19) can be substantially improved by the treatment with hyper-CVAD regimen. Both t(1;19) and t(17;19) are easily identifiable by conventional cytogenetics, FISH, and RT-PCR, the latter two methodologies are particularly useful in posttreatment specimens that are cytogenetically normal.

In ALL, the most frequent *MLL* (*KMT2A*) translocations include t(4;11) (1%–2% incidence in children and two-thirds of *MLL*-positive adults) (see Fig. 56.33) leading to a *MLL-AFF1* (AF4) fusion and t(11;19)(q23;p13.3) (see Fig. 56.32L) resulting in *MLL-MLLT1* (ENL) fusion. These abnormalities are present in more than 80% of patients with infant leukemia and 10% of childhood and adult *MLL*-positive leukemia. *MLL* rearrangements are associated with a poor outcome in both children and adults (see Acute Myeloid Leukemia, earlier, and T-Cell Lymphoproliferative Diseases, later). One-third of patients with t(4;11) have secondary abnormalities; the most frequent are +X, i(7q), abnormalities of 9p, including i(9q), and +8. The outcomes of patients with t(11;19) is generally poor, especially in children younger than 1 year of age. The most frequent additional abnormalities in patients with t(11;19) are +X, +8, and del(6q). Other less common *MLL* translocations include t(9;11)(p22;q23)/*MLL-MLLT3*, t(10;11)(p13–15;q23)/*MLL-MLLT10* and others. A large multiinstitutional study has determined that secondary aberrations do not affect prognosis of children with ALL and t(4;11),t(11;19) or other *MLL* translocations.

Secondary forms of ALLs are rarely reported but the majority of them are associated with *MLL* rearrangements, the most frequent being t(4;11). Most of these patients have received topoisomerase II inhibitors which are known to cause double-strand DNA breaks.

t(8;14)(q24;q32) is seen in fewer than 5% of all patients with ALL (children and adults) (Fig. 56.45). Variant translocations t(8;22)(q24;q11) and t(2;8)(p12;q24) are seen in less than 1% of children and adults. These cells express CD10, CD19, CD20, and surface IgM immunophenotype. This form of ALL has extremely poor prognosis. The same translocation is found in Burkitt lymphoma (BL), and both entities likely represent the same disease with different manifestations. The majority of adult patients with t(8;14) die within 1 year of diagnosis. Approximately 4% of children and 11% of adult pre–B-cell precursor ALL have recurrent *IGH* translocations usually identified by cytogenetics or FISH. The *CRLF2* gene, which maps to the pseudoautosomal region 1 of the sex chromosomes, is the gene that is most frequently targeted in 20% to 26% of *IGH* translocations in pre–B-cell precursor ALL. *IGH-CRLF2* rearrangements result from the cryptic t(Y;14)(p11;q32) or t(X;14)(p22;q32). The second most frequent *IGH* translocation resulting in t(14;19)(q32;q13), resulting in *IGH-CEBP* chimeric fusion. The third most frequent translocation partner involves *CEBPD* gene (8q11) resulting in t(8;14)(q11;q32) and *IGH-CEBPD* fusion, which is primarily found in children and young adults and is strongly associated with Down syndrome (about 30% of cases). This subgroup frequently have a gain of X chromosome, trisomy 21 as an acquired abnormality, and the Ph chromosome/t(9;22)(;q34;q11). The t(14;19)(q32;q13)/*IGH-EPOR* appears to be causally related to pre–B-cell precursor ALL because it always appears always as the single abnormality. The inv(14) (q11q32)/ins(14;14)(q11;q32) leads to *IGH-TRA/D,* which represent a rearrangement mediated by an interlocus site-specific recombination event between *IGH* and the *TRA* and *TRB* genes. The t(14;20)(q32;q13) results in *IGH-CEBPB*. Collectively, patients with *IGH* translocations may be included in a subgroup of pre–B-cell precursor ALL.

Abnormalities of the short arms of chromosome 9 (p21–22) occur at a frequency of 7% to 13%. In adults the presence of del(9p) appears to be associated with a favorable outcome, whereas in children with ALL, del(9p) is associated with poor outcome. The most frequent abnormalities are co-deletions of two genes, *CDKN2A* and *CDKN2B*, as well as the interferon α and β genes found in many cases. Among the structural rearrangements involving the short arms of chromosome 9, t/dic(9;12)(p11–12;p11–13) is a rare recurrent abnormality associated with L1 morphology (FAB classification), a pre–B-cell phenotype, and an excellent prognosis.

The *IKZF1* gene at 7p12.2 codes for IKAROS, an essential transcription factor in hematopoiesis primarily involved in lymphoid differentiation and is an essential player in the regulation of both T- and B-cell lineage specification.[25] The gene is composed of eight exons, spanning a total of 6.2 kb and coding for a 519-amino acid protein. Deletions of *IKZF1* have been reported in 15% of pediatric and 30% to 50% of adult patients with ALL, and in 75% of Ph-positive B-cell ALL. Both focal and nonfocal *IKZF1* deletions have been shown to be associated with an increased risk of relapse and decreased EFS in both pediatric and adult ALL. Most laboratories use SNP array technique to detect *IKZF1* deletion. Recent genomic studies of patients with ALL have confirmed a higher hazard of relapse in adult ALL with focal *IKZF1* deletions.

Other chromosomal abnormalities detected in nonrandom fashion in adult patients with ALL include deletions, both terminal and interstitial, of the long arm of chromosome 6, and isochromosomes

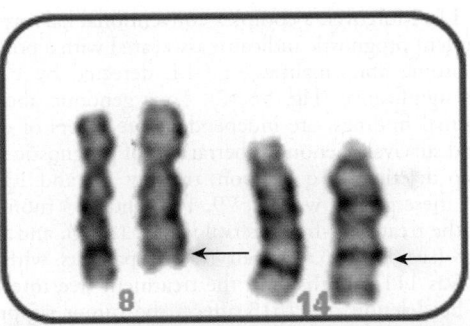

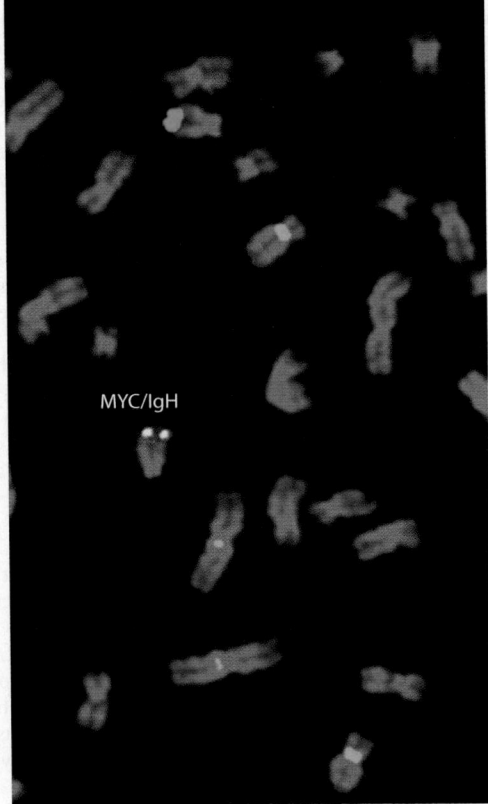

Fig. 56.45 t(8;14)(q24;q32) IN ACUTE LYMPHOBLASTIC LEUKEMIA. *Top panel* shows a partial G-banded karyotype of chromosomes 8 and 14 with *arrows* indicating the breakpoints on each chromosome. The *bottom panel* is a partial metaphase (chromosomes are stained blue with DAPI) after FISH testing using three probes: *IGH* signal *(green)* is seen on normal chromosome 14, *aqua* signals for centromere 8 are observed on both chromosome 8, *MYC* *(red)* is seen on both chromosomes 8 but note a more bold signal on one chromosome 8 when compared to the other. Because *MYC* is broken as a result of t(8;14), the third copy of *MYC* is on chromosome 14 where it is fused to *IGH* and seen as a *yellow* signal.

of 7q, 9q, 17q, and 21q. Adult patients with ALL with t(9;22), t(4;11), t(8;14), −7, +8 chromosomal aberrations have a poorer prognosis and significantly lower probability of long-term CR and survival than do patients with a normal karyotype or patients with other chromosomal rearrangements.

Complex and Monosomal Karyotype

Patients with ALL and a complex karyotype have a poorer outcome in terms of OS and EFS, with most relapses occurring during the first 2 years after diagnosis. More recently a study found that 9.2% of adult patients with ALL had a complex karyotype and 12.8% had a monosomal karyotype. In this study, neither was associated with a

worse prognosis when treated with risk-adapted or subtype oriented protocols. Monosomal karyotype did not have an impact on prognosis in Ph-positive ALL irrespective of imatinib treatment.

The lymphoid leukemias associated with Down syndrome (DS-ALL) are almost exclusively B-precursor ALLs. In a recent large series of DS-ALLs, there were only five cases of T-ALL among 700 patients. Also, in a sharp contrast to the myeloid neoplasms, they almost never occur in infants. Clinically the outcome of DS-ALL is significantly worse than sporadic childhood B-cell precursor ALLs because of intrinsic resistance to therapy and increased treatment-related mortality. Although all known cytogenetic subgroups of childhood B-cell ALLs have been observed, the common abnormalities such as *ETV6/RUNX1* fusion and hyperdiploidy, are less frequent.

Up to 60% of DS-ALLs have aberrant expression of the cytokine receptor *CRLF2* that is often associated with additional mutations activating JAK-STAT signaling. The aberrant expression of this receptor is caused by genomic rearrangements consisting either of a translocation into the *IgH* locus control region or a microdeletion upstream to the *CRLF2* gene, located on the pseudoautosomal component of the sex chromosomes. This deletion fuses *CRLF2* with the promoter of an upstream constitutively expressed *P2RY8* gene. Analysis of the breakpoint sequences suggest that this rearrangement is mediated by *RAG1* or *RAG2* in early B-cell precursors.

Somatic Mutations

The most commonly altered pathways in ALL, involving the transcriptional regulation of lymphoid development, such as *PAX5* (9p13.2), *IKZF1* (7p12.2) and *EBF1* (5q33.3), are frequently mutated. *PAX5* is required for B-lymphoid lineage commitment and maturation. *PAX5* genetic alterations include deletions, sequence mutations, and chimeric genes with at least 16 different chromosomal partners (http://atlasgeneticsoncology.org/Genes/PAX5ID62.html). *IKAROS* is required for the development of all lymphoid lineages and its genetic lesions are implicated in resistance to chemotherapy and TKIs.

Other commonly mutated pathways in ALL include genes involved in tumor suppression and cell cycle regulation (*TP53*, *Rb1*, and *CDKN2A*), cytokine receptor, RAS-signaling, lymphoid signaling and epigenetic modification such as *EZH2*.

Multistep Pathogenesis of Acute Lymphoblastic Leukemia

Epidemiologic and twin studies indicate a multistep pathogenesis of B-cell ALL in infants and children, with an initial leukemogenic event(s) occurring in utero and subsequent genomic changes occurring postnatally. Most of the current thinking of the natural history of childhood ALL was based on the exquisite work of Mel Greaves who studied the clonal origin of leukemia in monozygotic twins. Greaves found that most common chromosomal translocations and their resultant gene fusions can be documented by molecular analysis of neonatal blood spots or Guthrie cards. If a unique gene fusion sequence is present in at least one cell per 30,000 in the peripheral blood, it can be detected by a sensitive PCR assay. The first observations of an in utero origin of an acute leukemia were demonstrated with *MLL* rearrangements in three children with ALL, in monozygotic twins who shared the identical *ETV6-RUNX1* fusion, and in a pair of twins diagnosed at age 3 with B-precursor ALL. Subsequently in utero occurrence of *BCR-ABL1*, and loss of *IKZ1, PAX5*, and biallelic loss of *CDKN2A* have been documented prenatally on Guthrie cards. The concordance rate of twins who share a monochorionic placenta and develop leukemia is nearly 100%, whereas older twins have a discordance rate of 90%, indicating that additional postnatal leukemic events are needed. The frequency of an in utero origin of a B-cell precursor ALL in nontwins as measured by clonal *IGH* rearrangements is reported to be 71%, supporting the notion that in the majority of infants older than 1 year, the development of ALL occurs during fetal development because they share a single placenta resulting in blood cell chimerism. The prenatal mutation occurs commonly, exceeding the actual rate of developing leukemia by some 100-fold, indicating a low rate of reentrance or evolution. The acquisition of the additional genetic lesions, such as copy number alterations of *ETV6*, *PAX5* and *CDKN2* (25%–75% of cases) are recurrent and contribute to leukemogenesis. After testing five pairs of monozygotic twins with concordant *ETV6-RUNX1*–positive ALL, Greaves and his colleagues demonstrated that all recurrent driver mutations detected (32 in total) were different within twin pairs, indicating that they are postnatal in origin in both twins and most likely represent secondary mutations. Further single cell analyses revealed considerable complexity within a tree-like or branching structure of genetically distinct subclones, and as Greaves and colleagues suggested, very reminiscent of Darwin's original 1837 evolutionary divergence diagram (see box on Genetic Testing for Acute Lymphoblastic Leukemia, and earlier section on clonal origin).

B-CELL CHRONIC LYMPHOCYTIC LEUKEMIA

Historically, classic metaphase cytogenetic analyses of CLL were difficult because of the low mitotic yield of neoplastic B cells despite the use of polyclonal B-cell mitogens. FISH analysis of nondividing interphase cells was applied for the first time to hematologic malignancy, for the risk stratification of CLL. Introduced in 2000 by Dohner, the FISH hierarchical prognostic model stratifies patients into good [normal cytogenetics, del(13q)], intermediate with trisomy 12, and poor prognostic groups [del(11q) and del(17p)] and remains the most accepted and validated genomic prognostic model.[26] Moreover, current guidelines still recommend FISH analysis before treatment initiation and also following relapse or lack of response to therapy.

Cytogenetically CLL is characterized by relatively stable genome with a gain or loss of chromosomal regions; balanced translocations, a hallmark of AML, are rare in CLL. With improved detection rate of aberrant karyotypes in CLL using cultivation with CD40 ligand (DSP30) and interleukin 4 and the application of molecular cytogenetics, such as FISH, aCGH, as well as NGS, the detection rate of genomic changes has been raised to 80% to 90%. Analysis of clinically relevant chromosomal loci, combined with immunophenotyping, mutational analyses of the Ig heavy-chain variable region (IgV$_H$), and ZAP-70 overexpression, are of prognostic importance, even though the oncogenic events that lead to the origin of B-CLL remain unknown (Tables 56.11 and 56.12 and Fig. 56.46; see also box on Genetic Testing for B-Cell Chronic Lymphocytic Leukemia). Although microarray and high-density SNP array studies have not identified genes involved in the pathogenesis of CLL, they are helpful in clarifying the heterogeneous nature of CLL, which is a single disease entity with a common genetic phenotype resembling memory B lymphocytes. Genetic testing is strongly recommended for all patients with CLL, particularly in the context of novel therapeutic

trials for CLL. Moreover, a complex conventional karyotype remains an independent prognostic indicator associated with a poor outcome.

Chromosome abnormalities in CLL detected by FISH are of prognostic significance (Fig. 56.47). Four genomic aberrations, as well as normal findings, are independent predictors of disease progression and survival. Genomic aberrations of prognostic significance include 17p deletion, 11q deletion, trisomy 12, and 13q deletion. Survival in these groups was 32, 79, 114, and 133 months, respectively, and the treatment-free interval was 8, 12, 33, and 92 months, respectively (see Fig. 56.46). Survival of patients with a normal karyotype was 111 months, and the treatment-free interval was 49 months. The deletion of 17p13 affects the tumor suppressor gene *TP53*. In 80% to 90% of the cases, a deletion of 17p is associated with mutated *TP53* on the remaining copy. This is one possible reason why p53 pathway–based therapies are not effective in patients with 17p deletion. TP53 mutations have been found in 4% to 15% of patients with early-stage CLL and are associated with poorer outcome. Deletion of 11q and deletion of the *ATM* gene on 11q23.1 are found in 18% of patients with CLL. In about one-third of patients with deleted 11q, a simultaneous mutation of *ATM* has been found. The OS of these patients is shorter.

FISH-detected anomalies are frequent in B-CLL cases with Rai stages 0 to 1 disease, but are more frequent among patients with progressive disease (88%) than in those with stable disease (66%). Two risk groups have been recognized: (a) low risk disease includes patients with a normal karyotype or isolated del(13q); (b) high risk includes patients with del(11q) and del(17p). Patients with +12 are high risk, but in contrast to del(11q) and del(17p), they respond to fludarabine-based therapies (see Fig. 56.46). A comparison of quantitative PCR method with FISH for assessment of the four most frequent aneuploidies revealed a tight correlation in 103 of 110 patients examined, with FISH being more sensitive in detecting subclonal genetic evolution.

The frequency of chromosome 13 abnormalities in CLL detected by conventional cytogenetics is 10% to 15%. However, with the use of FISH, smaller or larger deletions of band q14.3 are detected in up to 60% of patients over time. When multiple DNA probes are used, D13S319 and D13S25 DNA markers are deleted more frequently than is *RB1*. Molecular analyses have detected deletions of 13q in cells that are cytogenetically normal as well as abnormal. These deletions can either be heterozygous (76%) or homozygous (24%). Heterozygous deletions most frequently occur in the early stage of the disease and homozygous deletions occur in the more advanced stages. In a study examining loss of heterozygosity and subchromosomal copy losses of chromosome 13, two types of deletions were defined: type 1 aberrations occurred in 60% of cases and were associated with loss of Rb1 and breaks close to the *miR16/15a* locus; and type 2 aberrations that included Rb1 occurred in 40% of cases. The 13q14.3-deleted segment contains micro-RNA (miRNA) genes. miRNAs are normally made by cells, including B lymphocytes, and they regulate the function of many genes. All patients with homozygous 13q deletion have a dramatic downregulation of miRNA15a, whereas patients with hemizygous 13q deletions are indistinguishable from controls, providing the first molecular clues for pathogenesis of CLL. The percentage of CLL cells with del(13q) is predictive of survival: a high percentage (>80%) of del(13q) cells results in a shorter survival as compared with patients with a lower percentage (<80%) of del(13q) cells. The clinical correlation with del(13q) cells include a higher lymphocyte count, a tendency to exhibit a diffuse pattern of bone marrow infiltration, and splenomegaly. Trisomy 12 or 13q rearrangements are found separately in a substantial proportion of patients with CLL. They co-exist in only 2% to 5% of patients, suggesting that each change may have a distinct pathogenetic route. The presence of del(13q) as the sole abnormality in CLL is associated with the most favorable prognosis, with a median survival of 11 years.

Among the first-degree relatives of patients, population studies have demonstrated a sevenfold increased risk for developing CLL and a twofold increased risk for developing other lymphoproliferative disorders. More than 80 families with CLL affecting multiple family

TABLE 56.11 Most Frequent Clinically Relevant Chromosomal Abnormalities and Copy Number Alterations in Chronic Lymphocytic Leukemia

Chromosomal Abnormality	Frequency %	Likely Gene Target	Clinical Associations and Consequence	miRNAs	Prognosis
amp(2p)	7	REL, XPO1, BCL11A	Unknown		Poor
amp(3q26.32)	6	PIK3CA	Unknown		Poor
del(6q)	~6	Unknown	Associated with prominent lymphocytosis Atypical morphology Splenomegaly Higher rates of CD38 positivity		Poor
del(8p)	5	Unknown	Unknown		Poor
amp(8)(q24.21)	5	MYC			Poor
del(10)(q24)	2	NFkB2	Unknown		Unknown
del(11)(q22.3)	10–20	ATM, BIRC3	Defect in DNA repair Deregulation of P53 Deregulation of cell cycle Extensive lymphadenopathy	↑miR-29b ↑miR-155 miR-29a miR-34b miR-34c	Poor
Trisomy 12	10–23	Unknown	Atypical morphology Aggressive clinical phenotype	↑miR-148a ↑miR-146a	Poor
del(13)(q14)	57–61	miR15a/16 in an intron of DLEU2 Its deletion leads to the release of BCL2	BCL2 expression Resistance to apoptosis	↑miR-155 ↑miR-7–1 ↑miR-154 ↓miR-220 ↓miR-221	Good
del(15)(q15.1)	4	MGA	Unknown		None
del(17)(p13.1)	6–8	TP53	Defect in DNA repair Deregulation of cell cycle Aggressive clinical phenotype	↑miR-151 ↓miR29C ↓miR34a ↓miR148a ↓miR-181	Poor

TABLE 56.12 Genomic Risk Stratification Based on Array CGH[a]

Outcome	Frequency	Gain	Loss
Good[b]	32.5	None	13q14
Intermediate	53.1	1p,7p,12, 18p,18q,19	4p,5p,6q,7p
Adverse	20.6	2p,3q[b],8q[b],17q	7q,8p,11q,17p[b],18p

[a]223 naive patients with chronic lymphocytic leukemia.
[b]Gain of 3q and 8q and loss of 17p are independent unfavorable prognostic biomarkers.

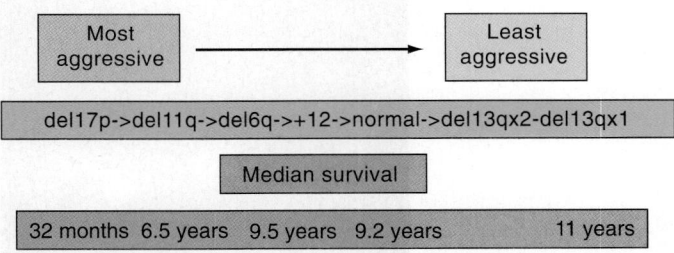

Fig. 56.46 SURVIVAL OF PATIENTS WITH SPECIFIC GENOMIC DEFECTS IN CHRONIC LYMPHOCYTIC LEUKEMIA.

members have been reported. Linkage studies suggest a region of interest in band q22.1 of chromosome 13 (marker D13S156). Fine FISH mapping of six CLL-prone families (63 individuals) reveals deletion of 13q14 in 85% of patients with familial CLL, and four CLL families shared a 3.6-Mb minimal region in 13q21.33–q22.2. This region included 12 candidate genes, but thus far informative candidates have not been identified.

Trisomy 12 was the first recurrent abnormality reported in CLL. It is detected by classic cytogenetics in 7% to 15% of all cases. FISH detects +12 in 15% to 20% of patients with CLL. Trisomy 12 may be present as the sole abnormality or in combination with other chromosomal rearrangements. Because only a proportion of cells are trisomic, normal cells or disomic neoplastic cells may also be present. Follow-up analysis over a 4-year period demonstrates clonal expansion of cells with trisomy 12 as the disease progresses. These observations suggest that trisomy 12 might be relevant in the cell proliferation

process in CLL cells. The observation that trisomy 12 is documented in B cells and is absent from T lymphocytes and CD34 cells in the majority of patients is consistent with the original hypothesis that CLL has a clonal origin and that trisomy 12 arises in a progenitor cell already committed to the B-cell pathway. The exact mechanism by which trisomy 12 contributes to the pathogenesis of CLL remains unknown.

Increased expression of the CLLU1 gene on 12q22 has been observed in CLL samples from patients with or without trisomy 12. Overexpression of CLLU1 in patients with CLL without IgV_H hypermutation combined with restricted and CLL-unique expression pattern suggests that CLLU1 is among the first disease-specific genes identified in CLL. Small duplications have also been reported encompassing the 12q15 region that harbors the MDM2 gene locus.

Recent studies utilizing whole genome sequencing detected NOTCH1 mutations in 42% of patients with trisomy 12. Almost all

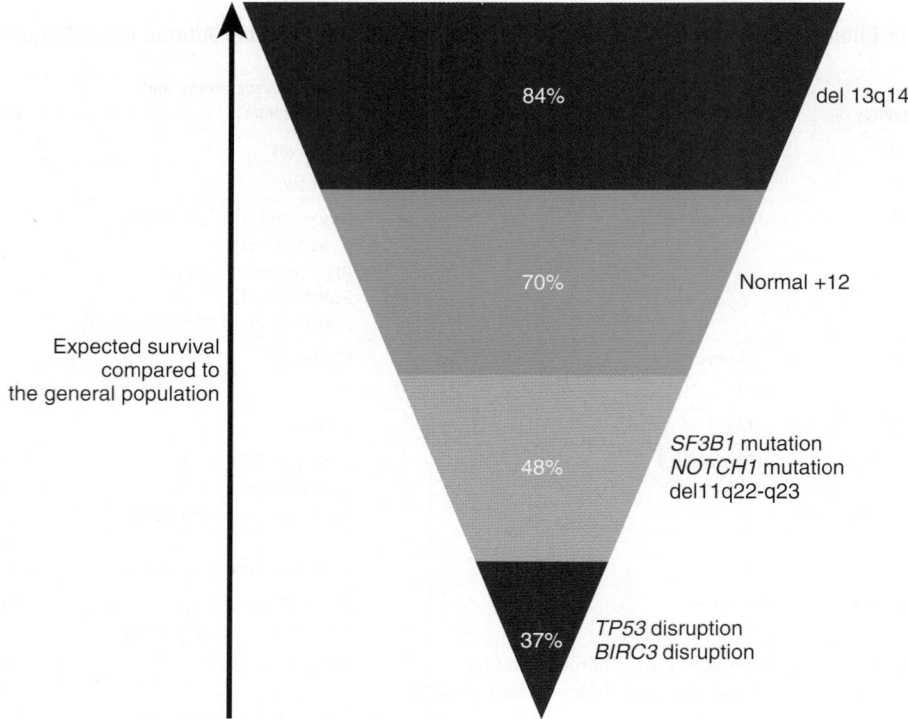

Fig. 56.47 SURVIVAL IN CHRONIC LYMPHOCYTIC LEUKEMIA ACCORDING TO GENETIC DEFECTS. Expected survival of patients with chronic lymphocytic leukemia stratified according to the integrated mutational and cytogenetic model and compared to the matched general population. Expected survival is calculated at 10 years. *(Reprinted with permission from Foa et al: Clinical implications of the molecular genetics of chronic lymphocytic leukemia.* Haematologica *98:675, 2013.)*

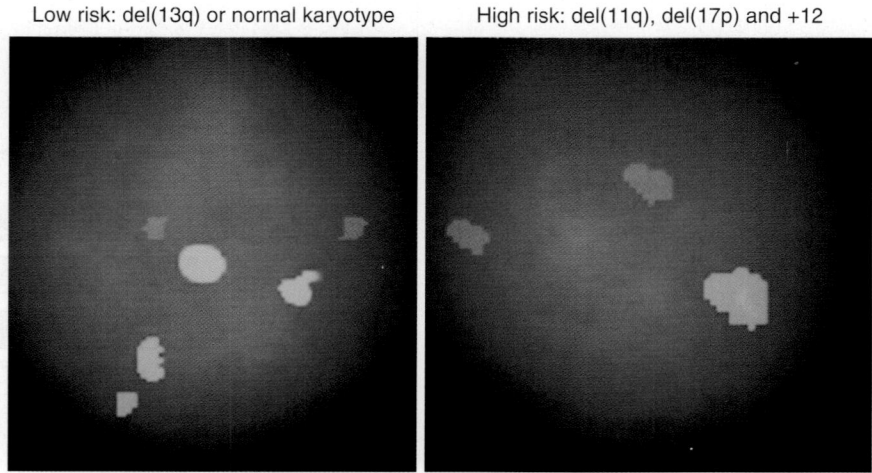

Fig. 56.48 PANEL OF CHROMOSOMAL PROBES USED FOR DETECTION OF GENOMIC DEFECTS IN CHRONIC LYMPHOCYTIC LEUKEMIA. They include 13q14.3 *(red)*, 13q34 *(aqua)*, and CEP12 (all present in disomy; *left*) and 11q22.3 (ATM, *green*) and 17p13.1 (P53; *red, right*). Note there is only one copy of the *ATM* gene *(green, right)* consistent with deletion of sequences from the 11q22.3 band region, which is associated with unfavorable prognosis.

NOTCH1 mutations resulted in a truncated protein, lacking the C-terminal PEST degradation domain, rendering it constitutively active.

Deletions of the long arm of chromosome 11 in CLL as detected by conventional cytogenetics have been reported in 5% to 8% of cases. An interphase FISH study identified deletion of 11q22.3–23.1 in 10% to 20% of cases. FISH characterization of aberrations involved in 11q21–q23 demonstrate a minimal consensus deletion segment of 2–3 Mb, containing a number of genes including *ATM*

at 11q22.3 (Fig. 56.48). Up to 12% of patients have simultaneous deletions of *ATM* and *MLL* at 11q23. Mutations in *ATM* gene are responsible for the ataxia-telangiectasia syndrome. *ATM* functions as a cell-cycle checkpoint regulator. Somatic disruptions of both *ATM* alleles by deletion or point mutation are detected in 25% to 34% of cases. This finding strongly suggests the pathologic role of *ATM* in some patients with B-CLL. A study revealed discontinuous deletions at 11q23.1–q23.3, indicating that genes in this region may have pathogenic significance because they constitute independent targets for amplification or deletion in cases of B-CLL. Most of the patients with del(11q) are relatively young. The appearance of this deletion is clinically associated with lymphadenopathy, rapid disease progression, poor response to treatment and a shorter OS.

Structural aberrations of chromosome 17 are observed in 4% of cytogenetically evaluable B-cell CLL cases. This abnormality frequently affects the short arm of chromosome 17, the site of the *TP53* tumor suppressor gene. Monoallelic deletions of *TP53*, detected by FISH, are present in 7% to 20% of patients and represent the strongest predictor of inferior survival. The median survival of these patients is only 32 months. P53 mutations are associated with aggressive disease and a lack of response to conventional therapy. A novel recurrent dic(8;17)(p11;p11) abnormality also results in loss of *TP53*, and low copy repeats in 17p12 and 8p11 may represent the origin of the translocation by nonallelic homologous recombination on a single chromosome 17. B-CLL in patients with deletion of the *TP53* gene is associated with progressive disease, resistance to treatment, and shortened survival. Patients with 17p deletions or *TP53* mutations are resistant to purine analogs.

Deletion 6q is a relatively rare chromosomal change occurring in approximately 6% of CLL cases and is associated with marked lymphocytosis, abnormal morphology, splenomegaly, overexpression of CD38, and unmutated *IGH* heavy chain variable region.

Because the leukemic phase of certain lymphomas can clinically mimic B-CLL, FISH for translocations using an *IGH* probe is important. Fewer than 7% of patients with CLL/prolymphocytic leukemia patients have t(11;14)(q13;q32), and these conditions usually transform into prolymphocytic leukemia. Moreover, *IGH* testing in CLL is important for detecting patients with recurrent del(14)(q24.1) associated with unmutated IgV$_H$ status (66%) and trisomy 12 (47%). Other rare chromosomal aberrations in CLL include trisomy 3q27 (3%), trisomy 8q24 (5%), gains of 15q15-qter, trisomy 18 and trisomy 19. Other recurrent rearrangements involving loss of 8p21-pter and del(9)(q11) have been reported. A complex karyotype remains a poor prognostic indicator associated with a significantly shorter OS.

Based on the recent CGH results, CLL may be classified into three groups: those with poor outcome (20.6%) exhibit at least one aberration: gain of 2p, 3q, 8q, 17q, and loss of 7q, 8p, 11q, 17p, and 18p; good outcome (32.5%) includes 13q14 loss without any of the other 10 aberrations (gain: 1p, 7p, 12, 18p, 18q 19, loss: 4p, 5p, 6q,7p) and the third, intermediate outcome are all other abnormalities. The three groups are significantly separated with respect to time to first treatment and OS ($p < .001$). Gain of 3q and 8q and 17p loss are independent unfavorable prognostic biomarkers.

Cumulative evidence over the last 20 years of over 20,000 patients with CLL suggests that FISH and Ig heavy chain variable region (*IGHV*) mutation status are standard clinical tests for all patients with newly diagnosed CLL for initial risk stratification.

Gene Mutations as Diagnostic and Prognostic Biomarkers

Approximately 60% to 65% of patients with CLL have somatic mutations in the *IGHV*. The remaining 35% to 40% lack *IGHV* mutations. *IGHV* gene mutations (M-CLL) are markers for a favorable prognosis, whereas an unmutated *IGHV* gene (U-CLL) in CLL is associated with clinically more aggressive disease. The OS rate for U-CLL is 8–9 years whereas that for M-CLL is more than 24 years. The frequency of other somatic mutations is shown in Table 56.13. Mutations in *ATM* may occur in patients with and without a del(11q) in 10% and 25% of patients, respectively. Because del(11q) includes loss of hundreds of other genes, or miRNAs, obviously other genes such as *BIRC3* may play a role in CLL pathogenesis. Thus far the *ATM* mutation remains the most important marker of poor outcome in del(11q) CLL patients. As mentioned earlier, in addition to del(17p) resulting in deletion of *TP53*, 17p may be targeted by acquired copy neutral loss of heterozygosity (cnLOH) which results from somatic recombination event that duplicates a single mutated

TABLE 56.13	Most Frequent Somatic Mutations in Chronic Lymphocytic Leukemia			
Chromosomal Location	Gene	Pathway	Co-Segregation	Frequency
Alterations Associated With M-IGHV				
15q26	CDH2	Chromatin modification		5
3p22	MYD88	Inflammatory pathway	del(13q)	3–5
Alterations Associated With U-IGHV				
11q22.3	ATM	DNA damage response	del(11q)	9–14
11q22	BIRC3	Cell cycle control	del(11q)	1–5
7q31.33	POT1	Cell cycle control	SF3B1	5
17p13.1	TP53	Cell cycle control	del(17p)	5–27
2q33.1	SF3B1	mRNA processing	del(11q)	10–19
9q34.3	NOTCH	NOTCH signaling	Trisomy 12, XPO1, TP53	12–24
4q31.3	FBXW7	NOTCH signaling	Trisomy 12	4
Other Recurrent Mutations				
	NFKB1E			10
	FAT1			10
	EGR2			1–8
	LRP1B			5
	ZMYM3			4
	DDX3X			3
	MAPK1			3
	HIST1H1E			3
	BCOR			3
	RIPK1			3
	SAMHDI			3
	SI			3
	XPO1			2.5
	KLHL6			2
	BRAF			2
	KRAS			2
	MED12			2
	NRAS			1–3
	IRF4			1.5

M-IGHV, Mutated immunoglobulin heavy chain variable; U-IGHV, unmutated *IGHV* gene.

TP53 allele. Sanger sequencing has identified *TP53* mutations without loss or cnLOH of the other *TP53* allele, and these patients exhibit poor survival. Most CLL patients with *TP53* mutations are refractory to chemotherapy. Most *TP53* somatic mutations are missense and located within the DNA binding domain of *TP53* encoded by exons 5–8, and six "hot spots" are mutated in approximately 20% of patients. A subset of patients with CLL exhibit 17p genomic changes, mutated *IGHV* genes and have a stable disease course.

Recently, mutations of *NOTCH1*, *BRAF*, *SF3B1*, *NFKBIE* and *EGR2* have detected in CD34$^+$ cells and CD14$^+$ (myeloid) progenitors in patients with CLL suggests involvement of early immature hematopoietic cells before B-cell differentiation.[21] These observations may indicate that CLL develops from preleukemic multipotent hematopoietic progenitors as a result of deregulation of B-cell receptor intracellular signaling and that CLL develops from a preleukemic phase.

Genome Complexity in Chronic Lymphocytic Leukemia

Most patients with CLL have two chromosomal abnormalities suggesting genomic stability at the microscope level. Solid evidence exists that chromosomal translocations detected by conventional cytogenetics independently predict treatment failure, treatment-free survival, and OS in untreated and treated patients with B-cell CLL. When CLL-derived metaphase cells were obtained following systematic stimulation using B-cell mitogens and activators, balanced and unbalanced translocations were observed in 34% to 42% of patients, respectively. Following multivariate analysis, unbalanced translocations have independently been associated with risk for treatment failure. Because del(13q) usually is cryptic by conventional cytogenetics but easily detected with FISH, both conventional cytogenetics and interphase FISH should be performed at baseline in patients with advanced CLL.

Array CGH and NGS studies have effectively clarified the level of genomic complexity in CLL and revealed that the average number of mutations in CLL cells at diagnosis of CLL lies between 10 and 20, which is one of the lowest among the adult cancers, confirming previous cytogenetic observations. The recent studies also revealed that no single unifying mutation is responsible for CLL. Array-based genomic profiling has extended previous cytogenetic data demonstrating that a subset of patients with CLL have complex genomic profiles pointing to the interplay between chromosomal abnormalities and somatic mutations that are associated with reduced OS. Moreover, telomere dysfunction in CLL and acute telomere attrition results in fusion events that contribute to genomic complexity such as *chromothripsis*, which is a high level of DNA damage that may occur during a single mitotic division. In 2011, using NGS technique, a new phenomenon called chromothripsis (from the Greek *chromos*, meaning "chromosomes," and *thripsis*, meaning "shattering into pieces") was identified in CLL (Fig. 56.49). Chromothripsis describes a process whereby hundreds of genomic rearrangements have been acquired as a result of a single catastrophic event. A chromosomal region or a chromosome or telomere of other chromosomes is shattered into hundreds of pieces, some but not all are stitched together by the DNA repair machinery in a mosaic patchwork of genomic fragments. Cells not only survive this crisis but emerge with a genomic landscape that confers a selective advantage, thereby promoting further malignant evolution. Chromothripsis has been observed in cancer patients with *TP53* mutations. In addition to the clustering of structural variants, multiple base-pair mutations can also be acquired in a single mitotic explosion, called *kataegis*. This process drives cytosine-specific mutagenesis in regions flanking sites of genomic rearrangement, and can result in the rapid occurrence of up to 20 base-pair substitutions. Chromothripsis have been shown to occur in approximately 5% of patients, primarily in patients with unmutated *IGHV* status (74%) and high-risk genomic aberrations (79%). The presence of chromothripsis and kataegis in CLL implies that multiple cancer genes can be disrupted in a single step, providing a "quantum leap" for the malignant potential of the initial CLL clone.

Whole exome sequencing methodologies combined with follow-up studies have revealed that early genomic events include *MYD88*, trisomy 12, and del(13q) and subclonal evolution are followed by late events such as acquisition of mutations of *SF3B1* and *TP53*. Other studies have demonstrated the prognostic value of four driver mutations in *SF3B1*, *NOTCH1*, *BIRC3*, and *TP53*. Patients who have received therapy exhibited a greater degree of clonal evolution and increased heterogeneity, which has been linked to a poor clinical outcome. How treatment affects clonal evolution in CLL remains the subject of investigation. In 18 patients monitored at two time points, two general patterns were observed: clonal equilibrium, in which the

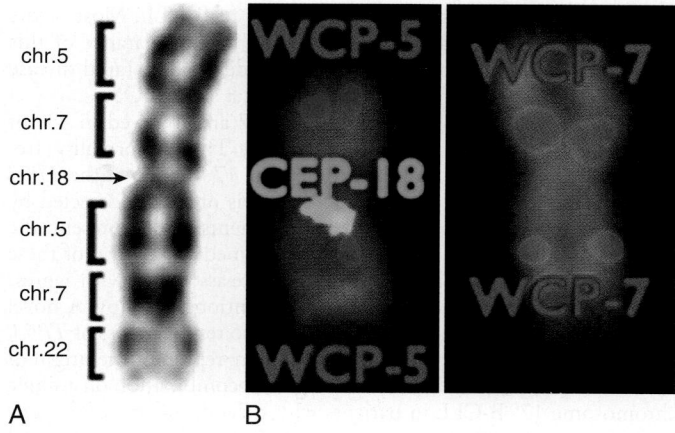

A   B

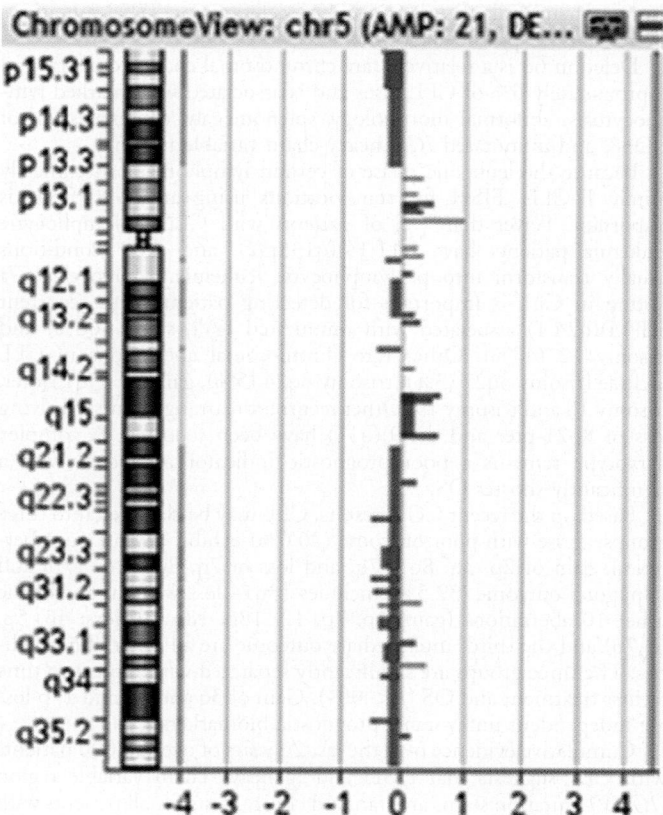

C

Fig. 56.49 CHROMOTHRIPSIS. (A) Conventional G-banded cytogenetic analysis showed a derivative chromosome 18 composed of additional chromosomal segments. (B) Various FISH probes confirmed that the derivative chromosome 18 is composed of segments of chromosome 5, 7, 18, and 22, whereby the fragments of multiple chromosomes are stitched together by paired end joining. (C) Array comparative genomic hybridization (aCGH) of chromosome 5 shows segments within both the p arm and q arm with gains (*blue bars*) and loss (*red bars*) of genomic DNA illustrating that there are frequent copy number changes in a localized region of a chromosome as a result of chromothripsis.

relative size of each subclone has maintained, and clonal evolution, in which some subclones emerge as dominant. More recent studies not only confirmed that molecular lesions in CLL are temporally ordered with del(13q) and +12 occurring initially followed by co-segregation of 11q22–3 deletions and mutations of *SF3B1* observed within the intermediate time point. Therefore two distinct and mutually exclusive evolutionary paths in CLL have been delineated. The first path involves acquisition of trisomy 12 and *NOTCH1* mutations followed by clonal evolution proceeding with *TP53* and *BIRC3* genomic lesions. The second evolutionary pathways involves del(13q) and proceeds towards acquisition of SF3B1 mutations and BIRC3 abnormalities. These molecular events confirmed earlier cytogenetic observations, that trisomy 12 coexists with 13q rearrangements in rare patients. Recent integration of cytogenetic and mutation studies in 637 patients with newly diagnosed CLL consistently showed that patients with TP53 or BIRC3 lesions had a worse prognosis, followed by patients with mutations in *SFRB1* and *NOTCH1* and del(11q). The presence of a minor subclone composed of as little as 2% of the tumor cells within a population in early CLL predated its emergence as a dominant subclone at relapse and the development of a chemoresistant phenotype.

Richter Syndrome

Approximately 15% of patients with CLL transform eventually to Richter syndrome (RS), a highly aggressive phase of CLL, which morphologically mimics diffuse large B-cell lymphoma (DLBCL) and frequently has a dismal outcome. RS is characterized by a complex karyotype, *TP53* disruption (50%–60%), *NOTCH1* activation (30%), and *MYC* abnormalities (30%). The majority of RS cases are derived from the original CLL clone with an average of 20 acquired molecular lesions during the evolution to RS. There appears to be considerable heterogeneity regarding the number and type of genomic abnormalities.

Several clinical and biologic risk factors may predict future RS development. Patients with CLL with an unmutated *IGHV* are four times more likely to develop RS as compared to those with mutated *IGHV*. High ZAP70 expression and CD49d have also been associated with an increased risk of RS in some studies.

Recently, two genetic pathways that lead to transformation of RS from CLL have been delineated. Approximately 50% of patients with RS have cell-cycle deregulation via inactivation of *TP53*, loss of *CDKN2A* (9p21.3), gains or translocations of *MYC*, and loss of 13q14.3 region. These patients had a high cell proliferation rate (Ki-67 >70%) and a worse OS than patients with wild-type *TP53* and *CDKN2A*. The loss of *CDKN2A* function appears to be acquired at the time of transformation, as evidenced by its presence in the RS but not CLL cells. The second group of patients with RS (30%) is characterized almost exclusively by trisomy 12 and *NOTCH1* mutations. The remaining 20% represent a heterogeneous group, and do not exhibit either *TP53/CDKN2A* inactivation or trisomy 12 and individual cases are characterized by del(11q), del(14q), *MYC* activation, *IGH* translocations, and *NOTCH1* mutations. Using paired-sample analysis CLL-specific lesions are almost always present in the RS cells along with RS-specific abnormalities. These observations imply that RS develops through a linear model of clonal evolution from the underlying CLL. Genome-wide DNA analysis confirmed that RS DNA profile remains clearly separate when compared to DLBCL DNA profile.

Newly diagnosed RS is an oncologic emergency requiring assessment of a karyotype and at least FISH detection of *TP53* and *MYC*.

MULTIPLE MYELOMA

MM is a malignancy of terminally differentiated B cells (see Chapter 86). MM plasma cells have a very low proliferation rate, a characteristic that has limited the field of cytogenetic studies. Conventional karyotyping reveals chromosomal abnormalities in 25% to 30% of newly diagnosed patients, especially in cases with an exceptionally high plasma cell proliferative rate. Karyotypes obtained from these cells usually are complex and exhibit more than 20 aberrations in approximately 10% of cases.

When reassessed by FISH, CGH, and multicolor karyotyping using a large panel of centromere-specific and translocation-specific probes, interphase plasma cell nuclei have been shown to be characterized by chromosomal aneuploidy in almost all patients with MM or monoclonal gammopathy of unknown significance (MGUS). Array CGH indicates that 100% of patients with newly diagnosed MM have copy number alterations and frequent homozygous deletions of genes including *TRAF3*, *BIRC1/BIRC2*, *RB1* and *CDKN2C*. Even during CR, after therapy, 12% to 71% of plasma cells still have numerical gain or loss of chromosomes 3, 7, 8, 9, 11, 13, 15, 21, and X.

Table 56.14 lists the most frequent chromosomal rearrangements that occur in patients with MM. Analysis of numerical abnormalities reveals two groups of MM patients: those who are hyperdiploid and those who are not hyperdiploid.

TABLE 56.14	Most Frequent Chromosomal Abnormalities in Multiple Myeloma and Their Frequencies	
Genetic Lesion	**Frequency (%)**	**Oncogenes/Fusion Genes**
Hyperdiploid	~50	Gain of odd-number chromosomes
Nonhyperdiploid		IGH translocations
Translocations		
t(4;14)(p16.3;q32.3)	15	FGFR3, MMSET-IGH
t(11;14)(q13;q32.3)	15–20	CCND1-IGH
t(14;16)(q13;q23)	5–10	MAF-IGH
t(8;14)(q24;q32.3)	<10	MYC-IGH
t(14;20)(q32.3;q11)	5	IGH-MAFB
Gain of Chromosomal Region		**Candidate Oncogenes**
1q21–q22	55	BCL9, IL6R
3q27.1–3q27.2	47	POLR2H, EIF4G1
5p12	44	?
7p11.2	44	?
9q34.11–9q34.3	54	ABL1, ANAPC2
11q13.4–11q14.1	52	SPCS2
15q24.2	44	IMP3
19q13.1	47	PDCD5
21q22.3	37	MCM3AP, HRMT1L1
Loss of Chromosomal Region		**Candidate Tumor Suppressor Gene**
1p13.1–1p12	41	DENND2D
8p23.3–8p21.3	28	DLC1
10q26.2–10q26.3	18	PTPRE
13q34	49	RFP2, micro RNA 15/16
1432.13–13q32.2	33	?
16q11.2–16q12.3	31	CYLD

Modified from Anderson KC, Carrasco RD: Pathogenesis of myeloma. *Ann Rev Pathol* 6:249, 2011.

Genetic Testing for B-Cell Chronic Lymphocytic Leukemia (CLL)

Interphase FISH is used in lieu of karyotype studies because FISH detection of abnormalities in CLL correlates with clinical risk groups and prognosis. FISH studies should be performed on blood for detection of trisomy 12, deletions of 11q22.3, 13q14.3, and the *P53* loci, as well as rearrangement of 14q32.3, *IGH* locus. The FISH test can distinguish between patients with B-cell chronic lymphocytic leukemia and those with the leukemic phase of certain lymphomas, such as mantle cell lymphoma and follicular lymphoma. If FISH for these loci is negative then somatic mutations for *ATM*, *BIRC3*, *NOTCH 1* and *TP53* should be performed.

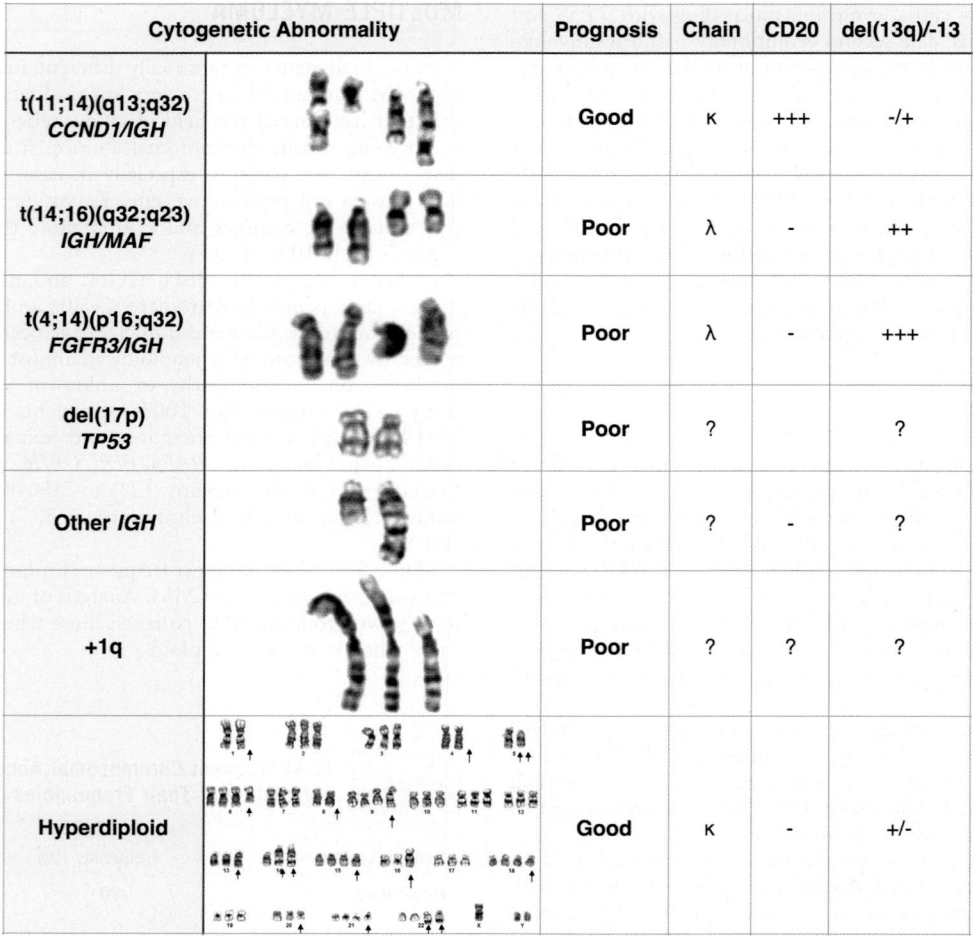

Cytogenetic Abnormality		Prognosis	Chain	CD20	del(13q)/-13
t(11;14)(q13;q32) *CCND1/IGH*		Good	κ	+++	-/+
t(14;16)(q32;q23) *IGH/MAF*		Poor	λ	-	++
t(4;14)(p16;q32) *FGFR3/IGH*		Poor	λ	-	+++
del(17p) *TP53*		Poor	?		?
Other *IGH*		Poor	?	-	?
+1q		Poor	?	?	?
Hyperdiploid		Good	κ	-	+/-

Fig. 56.50 RECURRENT CHROMOSOMAL ABNORMALITIES ASSOCIATED WITH MULTIPLE MYELOMA.

Hyperdiploid Multiple Myeloma

Approximately 55% to 60% of patients with newly diagnosed MM are characterized by a hyperdiploid karyotype with the number of chromosomes ranging from 48 to 74 and trisomies of odd-numbered chromosomes including 3, 5, 7, 9, 11, 15, 19, and 21 and few *IGH* translocations (Fig. 56.50 *bottom row*, and Fig. 56.51). The prognostic relevance of numerical abnormalities using classic cytogenetics is unknown, although the presence of cells with abnormal metaphases cells is an indicator of poor prognosis. However, hyperdiploid MM detected by FISH tend to have a better prognosis than do those with nonhyperdiploid disease. This prognostic benevolence is lost in cases where hyperdiploidy is also associated with other genetic markers of progression or aggressiveness such as gain of 1q21 and deletion of 17p13. A study of 847 patients with MM has demonstrated a median OS of 60.8 months for hyperdiploid patients with MM with no adverse cytogenetic lesions as compared to 33.7 months for those hyperdiploid patients with MM who had one or more of the adverse cytogenetic abnormalities such as t(4;14), t(14;16), t(14;20), del(17p), and +1q (see Figs. 56.50 and 56.51). The exact origins of hyperdiploidy remain unknown, although four processes are proposed: (1) a near-haploid cell doubles all chromosomes; (2) a tetraploid cell experiences subsequent loss of chromosomes; (3) a diploid cell undergoes sequential gains of chromosomes during clonal evolution; and (4) a diploid cell suffers a single mitotic catastrophe resulting in simultaneous gain of additional chromosomes. The data suggest that a single mitotic catastrophe may be the most likely mechanism of acquisition of hyperdiploidy, which may be followed by the secondary gain of extra chromosomes during subclonal evolution.

Nonhyperdiploid Multiple Myeloma

Approximately 45% to 50% patients with MM have nonhyperdiploid MMs that include patients with hypodiploid, near diploid, pseudo-diploid, or near-tetraploid chromosome numbers (fewer than 48 or more than 74 chromosomes), which are characterized by a high frequency of *IGH* translocations (>85%) (see Fig. 56.50 *fifth row*). With the exception of t(11;14)(q13;q32), most of the nonhyperdiploid patients have an aggressive disease course characterized by a short time to relapse and limited survival.

Table 56.15 outlines a lists risk stratification system of patients with MM based upon chromosomal abnormalities.

These patients are at risk of acquiring genetic events such as deletion of chromosomes 13 and 14, chromosome 17 abnormalities, as well as 1q amplification and 1p deletion.

Both hyperdiploidy and nonhyperdiploidy are also present in patients with MGUS, suggesting that such abnormalities occur early in the evolution of disease. More detailed analyses using genome-wide CNAs have revealed numerical aberrations in 98% of MM cases and identified amplification of 1q and deletions of 1p, 12p, 14q, 16q, and 20p to be associated with a poor prognosis, whereas amplification of chromosomes 5, 9, 11, 15, and 19 conferred a superior outcome in patients with MM.

Hypodiploid karyotype (<44 chromosomes) in MM accounts for one-fifth of all patients with MM and represents an aggressive subtype. In these patients, abnormalities such as monosomy of chromosomes 13, 14, and 22 as well as deletions for 1p, 12p, 16q, and 17p are common. These genotypes are associated with a poor outcome and disease progression. Hypodiploid chromosomal status is an independent risk factor for a poor survival.

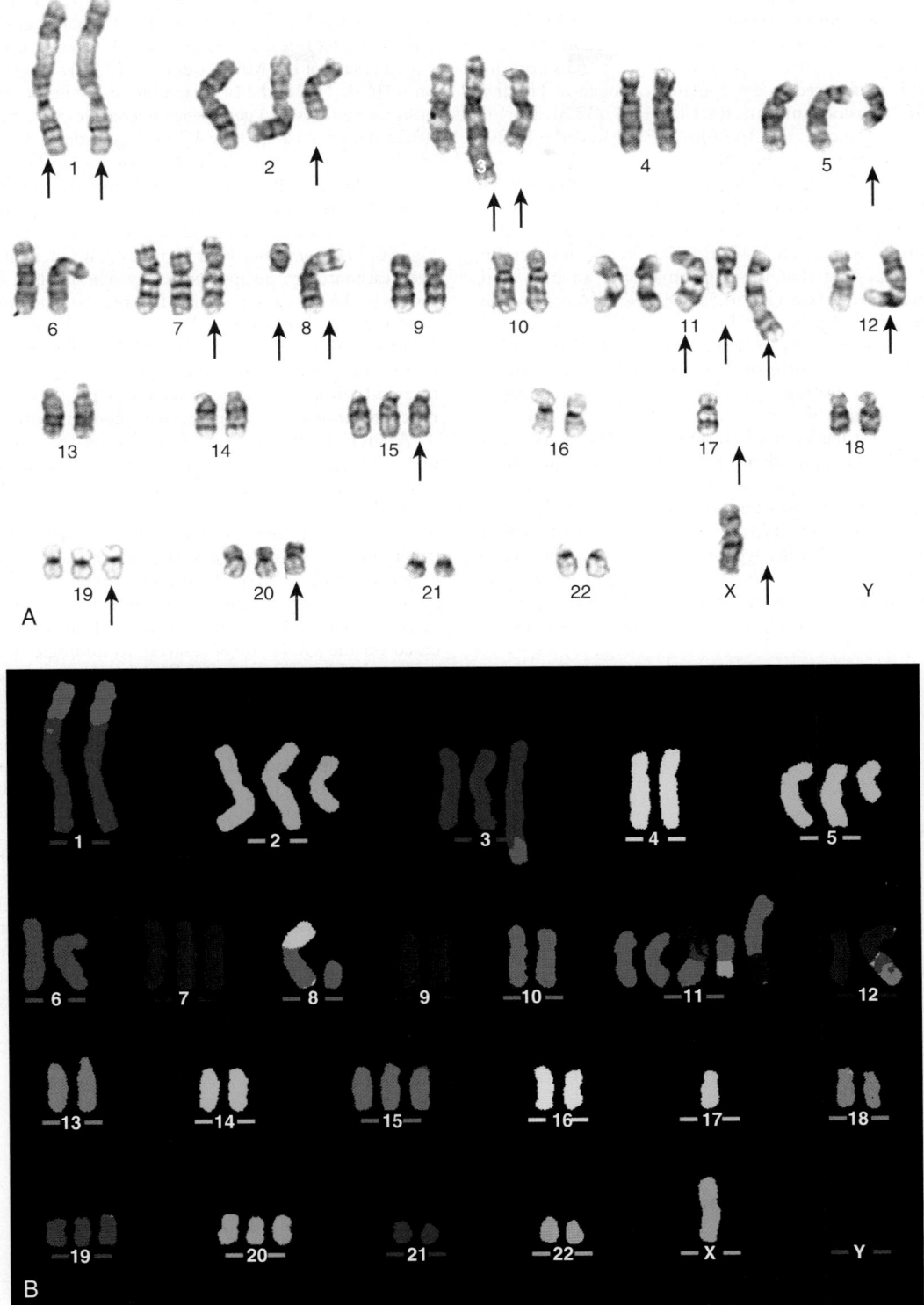

Fig. 56.51 A complex hyperdiploid karyotype from a patient with multiple myeloma (A) and after multicolor FISH (B), which was used to resolve a number of complex derivative chromosomes: 54, X,–X, der(1)t(1;8) (q34;q21q24)×2, der(2)del(2)(p13p25)t(X;2)(p21p22.3;p13), t(3;8)(q27;q22q24), +i(5)(p13p15), +7, der(8;17)(p23;q11.2q25), +der(11)t(1;9;11(?p36;q21q31;p15), t(11;20)(q13;q11.2, der(11)t(9;11) (q13q34;q25), t(12;13)9(p13;q14q34), +15, +19, +20.

Translocations

Primary translocations appear to occur early during the course of MM, whereas secondary translocations occur later on and are involved in tumor progression. Most primary translocations are simple balanced translocations that juxtapose an oncogene and one of the Ig enhancers. An *IGH* rearrangement on 14q32.3 is found in most patients with MM. This rearrangement consists of complex and heterogeneous translocations with the breakpoint involving either the switch region of IGH or the *V, D,* or *J* gene (see Fig. 56.50 *fifth row* and Table 56.10). The primary translocations are caused by somatic hypermutation or errors in the VDJ portion of the switch recombination region. The translocations include a promiscuous array of at least 20 nonrandom chromosomal partners. The characterization of these translocations has led to the identification of critical dysregulated oncogenes (e.g., *BCL2*, cyclin D). In each translocation, a potent enhancer is juxtaposed to dysregulated oncogenes. The five most frequent *IGH* translocations are t(4;14)(p16.3;q32.3), t(6;14) (p21;q32.3), t(11;14)(q13;q32.3), t(14;16)(q32.3;q23), and t(14;20) (q32.3;q12) (see Table 56.12 and Fig. 56.50).

A recurrent *CCND1-IGH* rearrangement is characterized by overexpression of cyclin D1. In contrast to MCL, breakpoints on 11q13 with MM are not clustered but are scattered over a relatively large genomic region. Virtually all MM and MGUS cells have cyclin D dysregulation, suggesting that this abnormality is an early and unifying pathogenetic event (see Fig. 56.50, *first row*). In contrast to other abnormalities involving the *IGH* locus, t(11;14) MM cells tend to be diploid. There appears to be an association of t(11;14) with an oligosecretory or light chain form of MM with CD20 expression, and a lymphoplasmacytic morphology. This chromosomal rearrangement is the most common genetic lesion in MM (15%–20% of patients with MM) but it has been also observed in MGUS, primary plasma cell leukemia, and light chain amyloidosis. Two groups of patients with t(11;14) are recognized: one with a rather indolent course and the other associated with a more aggressive course.

Approximately 15% of patients have a recurrent t(4;14)(p16.3; q32.3) abnormality associated with aggressive disease (see Fig. 56.50 *third row*). This cytogenetic abnormality is associated with IgAλ form of MM with immature plasma cell morphology, and a poor response to therapy. This abnormality is cytogenetically cryptic and is detected

<table>
<tr><td>**TABLE 56.15**</td><td>**Risk Stratification of Myeloma**</td></tr>
</table>

A. Standard Risk
   Trisomies (hyperdiploidy)
   t(11;14)
   t(6;14)
B. Intermediate Risk
   t(4;14)
C. High Risk
   17p deletion
   t(14;16)
   t(14;20)
   High-risk gene expression profiling signature

by FISH. Two genes on chromosome 4p16.3 and the *IGH* switch region on 14q32.3 are involved. The fibroblast growth factor receptor 3 gene (*FGFR3*) is detected on der(14), where it is overexpressed along with a fusion of the MM set domain (*MMSET*) gene, which is located on 4p16.3. This is the first example of a translocation that simultaneously deregulates two genes with oncogenic potential: the *FGFR3* gene detected on der(14) and the *MMSET* gene detected on der(4). *FGFR3* is 50–100 kb telomeric to *MMSET*. Loss of *FGFR3* on der(14) is detected in approximately 20% of cases. A significant number of these patients have del(13q) within the same clone and are hypodiploid.

Translocation (14;16)(q32.3;q23) can only be detected with (see Fig. 56.50 *second row*) FISH studies. The incidence of t(14;16) has been estimated to be approximately 5% of cases. This translocation results in the relocation of the *MAF* proto-oncogene from its position on 16q23 to chromosome 14, band q32.3, and it is overexpressed. Rare variants t(14;20)(q32;q11)/*IGH-MAFB* and t(8;20) are included within this group because they share a similar gene expression signature and clinical outcome. Survival of patients with t(14;16) is significantly shorter as compared with patients without t(14;16).

A large number of *secondary chromosomal aberrations* are found during disease progression. Disease progression is accompanied by four main abnormalities including translocations of *MYC*, the loss or deletion of chromosome 13, deletions of short arms and amplification of long arms of chromosome 1, and the deletion of short arms of chromosome 17. Translocations and/or amplification of *MYC* (8q24) may involve up to 45% of patients with an advanced MM, and then cytogenetic study frequently involves very complex nonreciprocal rearrangements, duplications, and amplifications. More recent data based on the CGH- or SNP-array technologies has revealed homozygous deletions such as *BIRC2/3* on chromosome 11, deletions of *TRAF3* on chromosome 14, and deletions of *CYLD* on chromosome 16. Another recurrent double deletion that has been observed in a limited number of the patients occurs on chromosome 1, targeting the tumor suppressor *CDKN2C* gene at 1q21 chromosomal site.

Deletion of either band q14 or q14.3 (*RB1*, DNA marker D13S319) on chromosome 13 is detected in 10% to 20% of patients using conventional cytogenetics and in 50% using interphase FISH. Microarray CGH data of the critical region on chromosome 13 is consistent with previous findings (Fig. 56.52). Loss of the entire chromosome 13 (82%) is more frequent than is deletion of the long arms of chromosome 13. The most commonly deleted region has not been delineated. The median percentage of plasma cells carrying del(13q), as identified by FISH, ranges from 75% to 90%. Deletion of 13q is associated with specific clinicopathologic features, including

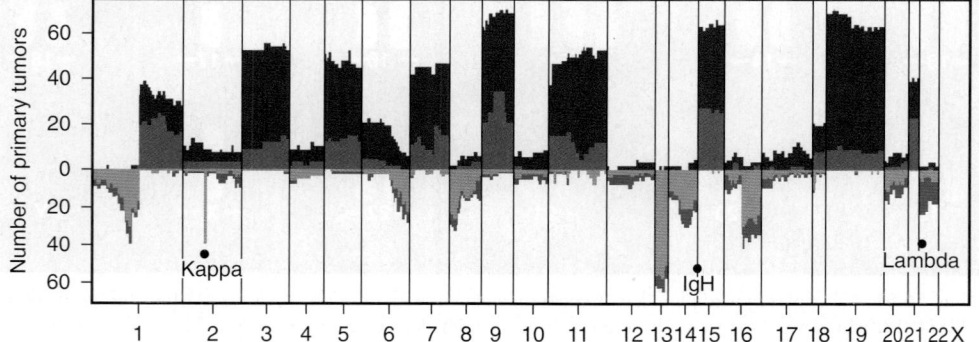

Fig. 56.52 CYTOGENOMIC PROFILES IN MULTIPLE MYELOMA. Summary of genomic profiles and recurrence of chromosomal alterations in primary tumors demonstrated by array comparative genomic hybridization. The recurrence plot mirrors the frequencies of previously reported chromosomal gains and losses, including the deletions of 1p and amplifications of 1q. Integer-value recurrence of copy number aberrations across the samples in segmented data is plotted on the y-axis. The x-axis is in chromosomal order. *Dark red* or *green* bands denote the number of samples with gain or loss of chromosome material, and *bright red* or *green* bars represent the number of samples showing amplification or deletion. *Black dots* show focal deletions of the kappa (2p12), IgH (14q32), and lambda (22q11) loci physiologic in B-cell postgerminal center neoplasms. (*Reprinted with permission from Carasco DR, Tonon G, Huang Y, et al: High resolution genomic profiles define distinct clinic pathogenic subgroups of multiple myeloma patients. Cancer Cell 4:313, 2006.*)

a higher frequency of λ-type MM, high plasma cell-labeling index, female predominance, and inferior survival after standard chemotherapy. Numerous earlier studies have demonstrated that del(13q) represents an adverse prognostic marker in patients with MM treated with conventional chemotherapy. However, more recent studies have demonstrated that del(13q) no longer has adverse prognostic significance in patients treated with bortezomib. Molecular cytogenetics analyses have revealed that del(13q) is present in 90% of patients with t(4;14) or t(14;16); therefore the apparent adverse impact of del(13q) may be related to translocation events.

Deletion of *TP53* at 17p13.1, which occurs in 10% of patients with MM, is a powerful independent predictor of shortened survival and is associated with clonal evolution, drug resistance, and genetic instability (see Fig. 56.50 *fourth row*). This deletion is not found in patients with other high-risk abnormalities such as t(4;14) or t(14;16), and it appears to be mutually exclusive. Patients with P53 deletion have a significantly shorter OS regardless of therapy. The 17p deletion, identified by FISH, is considered the most important molecular cytogenetic factor when determining prognosis.

The gain of 1q21 locus has been identified in 45% of cases of MGUS, 43% of newly diagnosed MM, and 72% of relapsed MM, and represents one of the most frequent recurrent chromosomal abnormalities in MM (see Fig. 56.50 *sixth row* and Fig. 56.53). Gain of 1q is observed cytogenetically as an isochromosome, duplications,

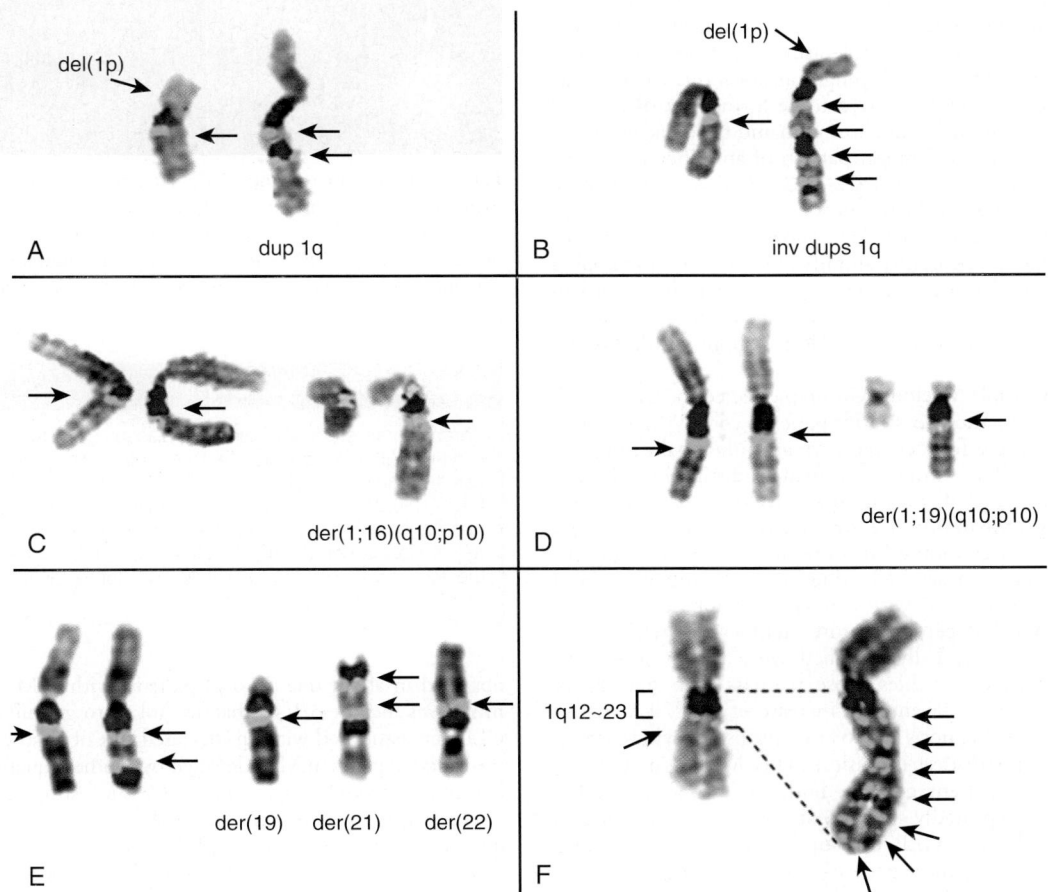

Fig. 56.53 REPRESENTATIVE PARTIAL KARYOTYPES OF METAPHASE CHROMOSOMES DEMONSTRATING THE DIFFERENT TYPES AND DEGREE OF AMPLIFICATION OF CHROMOSOME 1. FISH probes for 1q12 *(red)*, 1q21 *(green)*, and 16q11 *(aqua)* are shown on inverted DAPI images of chromosomes. (A) Interstitial deletion of 1p *(arrow)* in the homolog on the left and a direct dup1q12–q23 on chromosome on the right. (B) Normal homolog 1 on the left and the abnormal homolog on the right, demonstrating both an interstitial deletion of 1p and the amplification of 1q in the same chromosome. Note four copies of 1q21 *(arrows)* in an inverted duplication pattern. (C) Examples of an unbalanced whole-arm translocation of 1q to chromosome 16q. Chromosomes 1 are on the left, and chromosomes 16 are on the right. Aqua probe denotes 16q11 heterochromatin. Note the loss of 16q distal to the aqua probe on the der(1;16)(q10;p10). The entire long arm 1q is translocated to the pericentromeric region of 16q, and a total of three copies of 1q21 *(arrows)* are present. (D) Examples of an unbalanced whole-arm translocation of 1q to 19q. Note that the result of this translocation is the der(1;19)(q10;p10) chromosome, which shows an extra copy of 1q21 *(arrows)* and loss of the entire 19q. (E) Examples of jumping 1q, in which all or a part of 1q is translocated to three copies of 1q *(arrows)* on the three different nonhomologous chromosomes. The whole-arm der(19)(q10;p10) in this case is the same type seen in patient in (D). The der(21) results from the segmental translocation of the inverted dup of 1q to the short arm of 21. The der(22) results from the whole-arm 1q translocated to the short arm of 22. (F) Homologous of chromosome 1 demonstrating amplification of 1q12–q23 by breakage-fusion-bridge cycles. Note multiple copies of 1q21 *(arrows)* on the abnormal homologue on the right. The copies of the 1q12–q23 amplicon occur in an inverted repeated pattern, with a deletion of the 1q distal to the amplified region. Dotted lines between normal homologue 1 *(left)* and abnormal homologue denote the size of expansion of the 1q12–q23 region by break-fusion-bridge cycles. *(Reprinted from Sawyer JR: The prognostic significance of cytogenetics and molecular profiling in multiple myeloma. Cancer Genetics 204:3, 2011; with permission.)*

or jumping translocations and is detected with a 1q21-specific FISH probe. Among 479 patients with newly diagnosed MM, 43% with amp lq21 with either a hypodiploid and hyperdiploid karyotype and del(13q) was associated with poor prognosis as compared with patients lacking amp1q21 (see Fig. 56.53). In a study of 92 patients treated with lenalidomide and dexamethasone, del(17p) and gain of 1q21 was associated with a dismal OS. In the most comprehensive expression profiling survey of patients with MM, reported by the Arkansas Multiple Myeloma Group using GEP70 (gene expression profiling of 70 genes), 30% of these genes were located on chromosome 1, with most of the downregulated genes located on the short arms of chromosome 1 and most of the upregulated genes on 1q. The mechanism for the amplification of 1q is believed to involve 1q12 pericentromeric instability, which most commonly increases the copy number of 1q by a direct and/or inverted duplication. Further instability can result in adding a whole-arm segment of 1q to non-homologous chromosomes by jumping translocations of 1q. The 1q12–q23 amplicon has been reported to be formed by BFB cycles of the 1q12 pericentromeric heterochromatin and the adjacent bands of 1q, resulting in an inverted repeat pattern of amplification of the 1q12–q23 region. Copies of the 1q12–q23 amplicon can become integrated into complex multichromosome translocations during tumor progression. In vitro studies have shown that treatment with hypomethylating agents apparently amplify any 1q region juxtaposed to 1q12 chromosome band producing copy number aberrations in the bone marrow of these patients. Frequent additional deletions detected by conventional cytogenetics include regions within 6q, 8p, 12p, 14q, 16q, or 20p.

The Arkansas Multiple Myeloma Group pioneered the use of GEP as a highly sensitive method to stratify patients with MM in terms of outcome and to more fully characterize an individual's tumor at the molecular level. This group identified a distinctive 70-gene molecular signature (GEP70) for high-risk myeloma that was correlated with a strong probability of early recurrence and shorter OS. These 70 genes have overlapping functions and are involved in cell-cycle regulation, angiogenesis, cell adhesion, cell migration, and proliferation. When compared with standard metaphase and interphase FISH, the GEP70 gene signature significantly reduces the number of patients traditionally classified with a poor prognosis, while at the same time identifies those patients who may be at increased risk for relapse. The marked increase of GEP70 high-risk patients from 13% at diagnosis to 76% at relapse provides strong molecular evidence for disease evolution. This MM signature was validated using many patient cohorts, both in European and US institutions and have repeatedly shown that 15% to 30% of patients identified as high risk using GEP70 is superior to conventional risk stratification in identifying these patients. The GEP 70 gene assay is now commercialized under the name "MyPRS" (Myeloma Prognostic Risk Score) and is currently generated with as little as 15 ng of total RNA from approximately 30,000 CD138⁺ plasma cells.

Although GEP is being widely used for MM classification and survival risk prediction it remains unclear whether GEP-based signatures can predict response to specific therapies. Therefore GEP-based signature in MM has a limited ability to predict the probability of attaining a CR. Gene expression by itself may not delineate eventual cellular behavior and responses to various therapeutic interventions.

Even with the application of GEP, CGH + SNP arrays and other DNA-based approaches such as NGS, MM-specific oncogenes or mutations have not been identified to date. The median number of mutations per MM genome is about 55–60, with a very large range (21–488). Moreover, in contrast to leukemia, "good-risk" cytogenomic abnormalities have not been described. The current data indicate that genetic abnormalities have a major role in determining prognostic value.[27] The current thinking is that development of subclones is a very early event in MM, probably soon after the cell undergoes transformation.

Frequent mutations in MM include *KRAS* (particularly in previously treated patients), *NRAS*, *BRAF*, *FAM46C* (hyperdiploid subgroup), *TP53*, and *DIS3* (in nonhyperdiploid MM with *IGH* rearrangement). Subclonal *KRAS*, *NRAS*, and *BRAF* mutations are

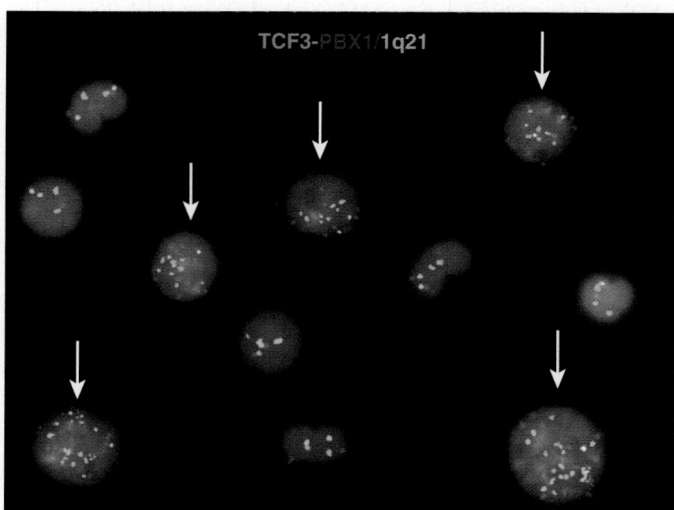

Fig. 56.54 Bone marrow nuclei from a patient with multiple myeloma after hybridization using three probes: 1q21 *(aqua)*, PBX1 *(red)* localized on 1q25, and TCF3 *(green)* localized on 19q13. Note amplification (up to 17 copies) of 1q21 an2 1q25 *(white arrows)*, as well as multiple copies of 19q loci. Amplification of 1q21–q25 is associated with disease progression and very poor prognosis in multiple myeloma despite novel therapies.

Genetic Testing for Multiple Myeloma

Chromosome studies of isolated plasma cells from the marrow are very useful at diagnosis. Perform interphase FISH and molecular genetic studies for detection of *CCND1-IGH* [t(11;14)], del(13)(q14.3)/D13S319, del(17)(p13.1)/P53, *IGH*/14q32.3, and 1q21 locus. If *IGH* rearrangements are detected using a breakapart *IGH* locus and *CCND-IGH* fusion is not identified, refine the translocation partner and use the following set of probes: *MAF-IGH* for detection of t(14;16) and *FGFR3-IGH* for detection of t(4;14).

---

observed in about one-third of patients with MM.[22] Other recurrent mutations include *SP140* that are linked to germline susceptibility to CLL and associated with an increased risk of relapse in MM. Most of the mutated genes in MM detected by exome sequencing have limited, low, or no known biologic significance, suggesting a silent biologic role.

Testing for genetic lesions in MM is an integral part of proper disease management. A simple approach is to identify high-risk genetic subtypes using FISH or genetic expression profiling. If FISH is to be used, preferably after isolation of purified plasma cells, the probes should include, at minimum, t(4;14)(p16;q32), t(14;16) (q32;q23), t(14;20)(q32;q11), gain of 1q and loss of 17p (Fig. 56.54). In our laboratory we also include testing for the t(11;14) and an *IGH* breakapart probe because if the t(11;14) as well as other *IGH* lesions mentioned earlier are not detected, *IGH* translocations without known partners are associated with adverse prognosis. GEP studies require the isolation of purified plasma cells and highly specific dedicated platforms (including very sophisticated bioinformatics), which are not widely available to the majority of physicians. However, the GEP70 analysis and numerous other reports have indicated that gains of 1q12–q44 are an independent marker associated with disease progression and that deletion of TP53 defines a group of patients with ultra high-risk MM (see Figs. 56.50, 56.53 and 56.54). Hence testing with FISH for alterations of 1q21 and/or 1q25 loci, as well as for deletion of the 17p13.1 chromosomal region, will identify patients with unfavorable prognoses (see Fig. 56.54).

LYMPHOMA

Non-Hodgkin lymphoma (NHL) is a heterogeneous group of disorders characterized by a localized proliferation of lymphocytes (see

Chapters 76 through 84). Analogous to other hematopoietic neoplasms, the pathogenesis of NHL is attributable to a multistep process involving progressive and clonal accumulation of genetic lesions. The majority of NHLs are of B-cell origin and involve translocations of Ig loci (see Table 56.10 and Fig. 56.55). *IGH* translocations usually are detected by cytogenetics, often in conjunction with FISH probes that span the *IGH* loci and/or PCR-based technologies. These molecular abnormalities exhibit enormous complexity with multiple and complex translocations, deletions, and amplifications within one clone (Table 56.16). Genetic anomalies represent one of the most reliable criteria for classification of malignant lymphomas. The most common associations between chromosome anomalies and specific lymphomas include t(14;18)(q32;q21) and FL; t(8;14)(q24;q32) and BL; t(11;14)(q13;q32) and MCL; and t(11;18)(q21;q21) and mucosa-associated lymphoid tissue (MALT) lymphoma (see box on Genetic Testing for Non-Hodgkin Lymphoma and Fig. 56.55). However, identification of a specific translocation is not diagnostic of a specific lymphoma subtype (see later). Chromosome studies are difficult and expensive for the study of lymphomas. Thus many investigators use FISH and/or molecular genetic methods to study touch-cell preparations or paraffin-embedded biopsy material to detect genetic anomalies.

Approximately 85% to 90% of patients with FL and some patients with DLBCL exhibit t(14;18)(q32.3;q21.3), resulting in fusion of *BCL2* on 18q21 and *IGH* on 14q32. This translocation is one of the most common chromosomal abnormalities in NHL (see Fig. 56.55D). This somatic rearrangement places *BCL2* gene under the influence of transcriptional enhancers associated with *IGH*, resulting in overexpression of the antiapoptotic BCL2 protein. Translocation 14;18 appears to originate from erroneous *IGH* rearrangement, during B lymphopoiesis in the bone marrow (pre-B cells) and therefore represents a very early genomic event. About 75% of the *BCL2* breakpoints occur within a remarkably narrow region of 15–20 bp at the 3′ end of the *BCL2* gene, whereas the breakpoints in *IGH* fall within the D_H and J_H regions. With regular and fiber FISH methods using *BCL2* breakpoint flanking probes, individual 5′ and 3′ breakpoints can be detected. With disease progression, 100% of patients have BCL2 protein overexpression. Variant translocations, such as t(2;18)(p12;q21) and t(18;22)(q21;q11) involving the *IGK* or *IGL* gene, respectively, rather than *IGH*, are also associated with overexpression of *BCL2*.

Although t(14;18) is most likely an early genetic event in the pathogenesis of FL, it is not sufficient for malignant transformation. It has been known for many years that approximately 50% of healthy individuals harbor low levels of circulating t(14;18) cells but do not develop FL, indicating that ectopic BCL2 expression is necessary but not sufficient for lymphoma progression. Recent studies of 520,000 healthy participants enrolled in the European Prospective Investigation into Cancer and Nutrition study determined that approximately 20% of healthy individuals with t(14;18) will subsequently develop FL up to 20 years later.[23] Progression to FL was significantly associated with elevated t(14;18) burdens in peripheral blood as measured by Q-PCR. They determined that individuals with t(14;18) frequency reaching one in every 10,000 blood cells had a 23-fold greater incidence of progression to FL.

Numerous secondary chromosomal abnormalities have been identified by conventional cytogenetics, and at least five recurrent anomalies, each occurring in at least 20% of FL, may distinguish two subgroups of patients with FL. Patients with t(14;18) and additional trisomy for chromosome 2, 7, or 8 are associated with a more favorable course of disease as compared with patients with del(1p), del(1q), del(6q), der(18), del(22q), or gain of chromosome 12 and X. Interstitial del(6)(q25–q27) is the strongest predictors of a poor prognosis and a shorter survival time. Rearrangements of chromosome 1, such as del(1)(p32–36), +1(p11–q44), and unbalanced translocations of der(1)(1;1)(p36;q11–23) are among the most frequent secondary chromosomal abnormalities in FL. Progression of FL to DLBCL occurs in 60% to 80% of patients and is accompanied by the accumulation of secondary abnormalities, including homozygous del(9p).

TABLE 56.16	Recurrent Chromosomal Translocations in B-Cell Lymphoproliferative Disorders	
Translocations	Genes Involved	Associated Diseases
Immunoglobulin (Ig)-Related Translocations		
t(1;14)(p22;q32)	CNN3-IGH	B-cell ALL, NHL
t(1;14)(q21;q320)	BCL9-IGH	Pre–B-ALL
t(1;14)(q21;q32)	MUC1-IGH	Multiple myeloma
t(1;14)(q24;q32)	LHX4-IGH	
t(2;14)(p13;q32)	BCL11A-IGH	CLL/SLL, ALL, NHL
t(2;8)(p12;q32)	IGK-cMYC	ALL (Burkitt)
t(4;14)(p16.3;q32.3)	FGFR3-IqH	Multiple myeloma
t(5;14)(q31;q32)	IL3-IGH	B-CLL
t(6;14)(p25;q32)	IRF-IGH	Multiple myeloma
t(6;14)(p22;q32)	ID4-IGH	Plasma cell leukemia
t(6;14)(p21;q32)	CCND3-IGH	B-ALL
t(7;14)(q21;q32)	IGH/-CDK6	B-CLL
t(8;14)(q24;q32)	IGH/-cMYC	ALL (Burkitt)
t(8;22)(q24;q11)	IGL-CMYC	ALL (Burkitt)
t(10;14)(q24;q34)	NFKB2-IGH	T-cell ALL, CLL, NHL
t(11;14)(q13;q32.3)	CCND1-IGH	Multiple myeloma
t(11;14)(q23;q32)	DDX6-IGH	
t(11;14)(q23;q32)	PAFAH1B2-IGH	
t(11;14)(q23;q32)	PCSK7-IGH	
t(12;14)(p13;q32)	ETV6-IGH	Pre–B-ALL
t(14;14)((q11;q32)	TCRA-IGH	T-PLL
t(14;16)(q32.3;q23)	IGH-MAF	Multiple myeloma
t(14;19)(q32;p13)	IGH-BCL-3	B-CLL
t(14;20)(q32;q11)	IGH-MAFb	Multiple myeloma
t(14;20)(q32;q13)	IGH-CEPBP B-ALL	
Lymphoma-Associated Translocations		
t(1;14)(p22;q32)	BCL10-IGH	MALT
t(3;14)(q14;q32)	FOXP1-IGH	MALT
t(5;14)(q35;q32)	ODZ2-IGH	MALT
t(11;14)(q13;q32.3)	CCNDI-IGH	Mantle cell
t(14;18)(q32.3;q21)	IGH-BCL2	Follicular
t(3;14)(q27;q32)	BCL6-IGH	Follicular
t(11;18)(q21;q21)	API2-MALTI	MALT
t(14;18)(q32.3;q21)	IGM-MALT	MALT
t(1;14)(p22;q32.3)	BCL10-IGH	MALT
3q27 rearrangements	BCL 6	Diffuse large B cell
t(14;15)(q32.3;q11–13)	IGH-BCL8	Diffuse large B cell
t(3;14)(p14;q32.3)	FOXPIF-IGH	MALT
t(9;14)(p13;q32.3)	PAX5-IGH	LPL

ALL, Acute lymphoblastic leukemia; B-ALL, B-cell ALL; B-CLL, B-cell CLL; CLL, chronic lymphocytic leukemia; LPL, lymphoplasmacytoid lymphoma; MALT, mucosa-associated lymphoid tissue; NHL, non-Hodgkin lymphoma; PLL, prolymphocytic leukemia; SLL, small lymphocytic leukemia; T-PLL, T-cell PLL.

Mutations in the *BCL2* gene are found in 12% of patients with FL at diagnosis and in 53% at the time of progression/transformation. The presence of *BCL2* mutations at the time of diagnosis correlates with increased risk of transformation and an increased risk of death owing to lymphoma (the median survival of patient with *BCL2* mutations is 9.5 years vs. 20.4 years without). Currently it is unknown whether acquired mutations in *BCL2* gene cause FL.

As mentioned earlier, the *IGH-BCL2* fusion is believed to represent a very early event in the pathogenesis of FL. FL-like cells (FLLC)

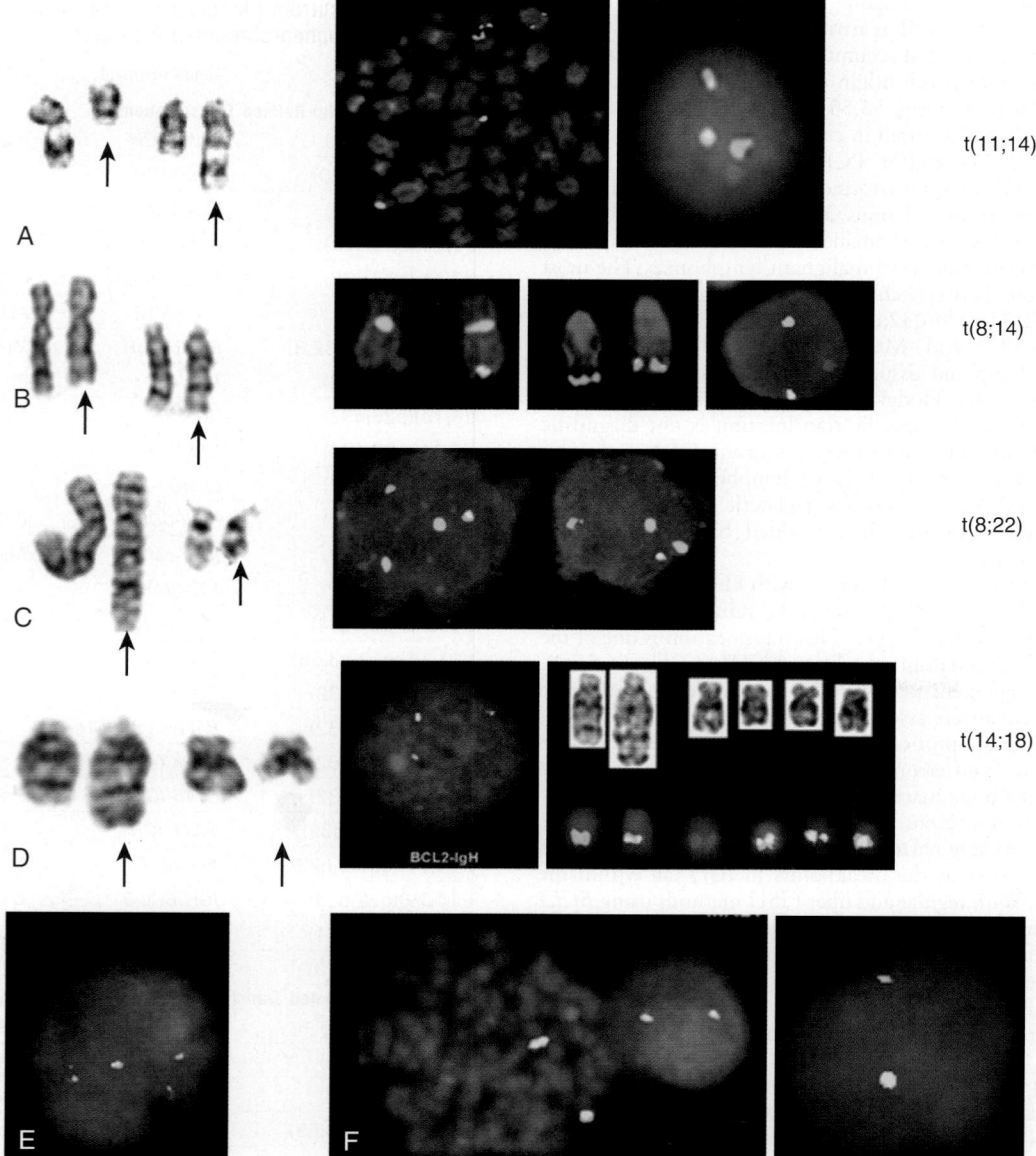

t(11;14)

t(8;14)

t(8;22)

t(14;18)

Fig. 56.55 MOST FREQUENT CHROMOSOMAL ABNORMALITIES IN NON-HODGKIN LYM-PHOMA. (A) Partial G-banded karyotype of t(11;14)(q13;q32.3) *(left),* resulting in CCND1-IGH fusion *(yellow)* on metaphase *(middle)* and in interphase cell *(right)* present in the majority of patients with mantle cell lymphoma. (B) Partial G-banded karyotype of t(8;14)(q24;q32.3) *(left),* resulting in MYC-IGH fusion [*yellow* on der(8) on isolated chromosomes]. Application of *MYC* breakapart probe shows separation of red and green signals consistent with *MYC* rearrangement. Approximately 80% of Burkitt lymphomas are characterized by t(8;14). (C) Partial G-banded karyotype of t(8;22)(q24;q11), a variant of Burkitt lymphoma *(left).* Two interphase lymph node cells after hybridization with MYC breakapart probe and CEP8 *(aqua).* Separation of green and red signals is consistent with MYC relocation from 8q24 to 22q11. (D) Partial G-banded karyotype of t(14;18)(q32.3;q21.3) *(left),* resulting in IGH-BCL fusion (two yellow signals, *middle).* A composite image on the *right* shows both a partial karyotype and FISH study of triplicated der(18)t(14;18) and three copies of *IGH-BCL2* fusion *(yellow),* as well as normal chromosome 14 and 18. Multiple copies of abnormal der(18) chromosome are associated with progressive disease similar to a duplication of the Philadelphia chromosome in the blast crisis of chronic myelogenous leukemia. (E) Lymph node cell from a patient with diffuse large B-cell lymphoma, showing four copies of *BCL6* (breakapart probe). BCL6 is localized at 3q27 and is numerically or structurally rearranged in 35% of diffuse large B-cell lymphoma. (F) Bone marrow metaphase and interphase cell hybridized with breakapart *MALT1* gene at 18q21 *(left)* indicating two fusion *(yellow)* signals when *MALT1* gene is intact. In contrast, rearrangement of the *MALT1* gene in MALT lymphoma usually is the consequence of t(11;18)(q21;q21.1), as shown in the cell *(right)* with clear separation of the 3′ end *(green)* and the 5′ end *(red).*

reside in the germinal center of normal lymph nodes. In a study of 85 reactive lymph nodes of healthy individuals 14% were found to contain high levels of t(14;18) by Q-PCR. These studies provide evidence that FLLCs consistently accumulate within the germinal center, as nonproliferating, early precursor cells that have not acquired other genetic events leading to FL transformation.[28]

GEP has revealed a distinct pattern associated with an indolent form of FL (median survival 11.1 years) and a more aggressive form (median survival 3.9 years), indicating that these different conditions may represent distinct stages in the evolution of FL. Detailed genetic analyses have confirmed that a single mechanism driving the transformation of FL to DLBCL does not exist, rather several discrete mechanisms are operational, including alterations of cell-cycle control (mutations and deletions of cyclin-dependent kinase, *CDKN2A/B*), *MYC* rearrangements and impairment of the DNA damage response (loss of *TP53* and/or *CDKN2A/B*). NGS has shown that each is associated typically with between 20 and 200 small somatic mutations. At least 21 different tumor suppressor genes are altered in FL at frequencies between 2% and 86%, suggesting that FL requires multiple collaborative genomic events acquired over many years.

Three translocations, all affecting the *MYC* gene at 8q24, have been recognized in BL. In 80% of patients a reciprocal translocation t(8;14)(q24; q32) is observed between the *MYC* gene and the *IGH* locus (Figs. 56.56 and 56.57). In the remainder of patients, the reciprocal translocation t(8;22)(q24;q11) or t(2;8)(p12;q24) occurs juxtaposing *MYC* to one of the light-chain loci (κ on 2p12 and λ on 22q11). The t(8;14) translocation was originally described in Epstein-Barr virus (EBV) tumor cells obtained from patients in Africa (see Fig. 56.56B–C). Variant translocations involving *MYC* with a variety of other non-*IG* loci subsequently have been reported. In most patients with sporadic BL, the breakpoints on 8q24.1 are located on 5′ end of the coding region of *MYC* gene. By contrast, in most cases of endemic BL and in non-*IG* translocations, the *MYC* breakpoints are at the 3′ end. As a result of the translocation, control of *MYC* is lost, and the intact protein is constitutively expressed throughout the cell cycle.

Although *MYC-IGH* translocations are sine qua non for the diagnosis of BL, they are not restricted to BL because they also occur in other forms of lymphoma, such as DLBCL (see later), plasma cell myeloma, ALL, MCL, and CLL.

MYC regulates almost 15% of human genes. The *MYC* gene can function as both a transcriptional activator and a transcriptional repressor. MYC forms a heterodimer with MYC associated factor X (MAX). MYC-MAX heterodimer binds to the E-box consensus sequence (CACATG) and serves as a platform for other proteins involved in chromatin remodeling and transcriptional regulation. *MYC* represses genes when it is not bound directly to DNA, but instead is recruited by the *MIZ1* transcription factor, which in turn recruits DNA methyltransferase (*DNMT3*) and histone deacetylase 3 (*HDAC3*) which alter chromatin configuration making it less accessible.

An increased level of constitutive *MYC* syntheses in leukemic disorders is found not only as a result of a translocation but also as a result of mutations and amplification of *MYC* (see Fig. 56.57). Approximately 65% of BL are associated with *MYC* point mutations. As mentioned previously, overexpression of MYC protein is linked to amplification of *MYC* genes reported in plasma cell leukemia, AML, CML, and T-cell lymphoma. *MYC* both directly and indirectly activates *CCND2* and cyclin dependent kinases and downregulates cell cycle inhibitors, promoting the transition from G0 to S phase. MYC has a role in the formation and maintenance of germinal centers.

The most common secondary change associated with t(8;14) in BL is duplication of the long arms of chromosome 1, and these were associated with disease progression. A common duplicated region of 93 kb at 1q21.2 has been defined by FISH studies. A rare complex BL karyotype is shown in Fig. 56.56. Rearrangements of *MYC* can now be detected in nondividing cells as well as in paraffin-embedded lymph node biopsies using a very sensitive interphase FISH assay for t(8;14).

According to the WHO classification, three BL variants are recognized: endemic, sporadic, and immunodeficiency-associated BL. In contrast, many cases of Burkitt-like lymphoma (a separate WHO entity), lack BL translocations but do exhibit increased MYC expression.

High-throughput RNA sequencing has revealed acquired somatic mutations in the *CCND3* gene in 38% of sporadic BL cases. This is an important gene in cell cycle progression and 70% of these patients acquire mutations affecting the transcription factor *TCF3* or its negative regulator *ID3*. In an extended study mutations in the *ID3* gene were detected in 50% of all *IGH-MYC* translocation-positive sporadic BL and these mutations were found to be rare in other *IG-MYC*-positive lymphomas. These findings suggest that disruption of *ID3* function may be a key mechanism in the pathogenesis of BL. Moreover, recurrent mutations in *TP53*, *SMARCCA4* (chromatin modulating complex gene), and *DDX3X* (chromatin modulating complex gene) may contribute to BL evolution.

Approximately 35% of patients with DLBCL and approximately 5% to 10% of patients with FL have rearrangements in the *BCL6* gene which resides at 3q27. Translocation and dysregulation of *BCL6* gene represents a key mechanism of transformation of DLBCL. Chromosomal rearrangements of the *BCL6* locus occur in about 35% to patients with DLBCL, and at least 33 different partners have been described as participating in these rearrangements (http://atlasgeneticsoncology.org/) (see Fig. 56.55E). The most frequent chromosomal band partners are 2p13, 4p13, 6p22, 7p12, 8q24, 13q14, 14q32, 18p11.2, and 22q11. These translocations juxtapose the coding domain of *BCL6* downstream to heterologous promoters derived from different chromosomal partners, leading to dysregulated expression of an intact protein by preventing its downregulation during postgerminal center differentiation. The *BCL6* 5′ sequences are targeted by multiple point mutations in over 70% of cases. Most of the breakpoints in 3q27 occur within a 10-kb region. The fact that the 3q27 region is affected in different lymphomas, irrespective of the translocation partner chromosomes, strongly suggests that alterations of *BCL6*, and not the reciprocal loci, are important in the pathogenesis. The alterations in 3q27 are small so most can be detected with PCR-based assays, or FISH. *BCL6* functions as a transcriptional repressor of genes containing its binding sites; therefore the mechanism responsible for the malignant phenotype is transcriptional deregulation.

Over the past decade NGS has enhanced our understanding of the complex multiple pathways by which DLBCL develops. Approximately 30% of patients with DLBCL harbor mutations and/or deletions inactivating *CREBBP* and more rarely *EP300*, two acetyltransferases that modify lysine residues on both histone and nonhistone nuclear proteins, and therefore modulate the activity of a large number of DNA-binding transcription factors. About one-third of patients with DLBCL harbor mutations in the *MLL2* gene, which broadly affects chromatin structure. Inactivating mutations of both *CREBBP* and *MLL2* have also been observed in FL (49% and about 89%, respectively). Gain-of-function somatic mutations in *MEF2B* transcription factor gene are observed in 10% to 15% of patients with DLBCL. Other genetic lesions include loss-of function/deletions of *FBX011* (4%), which causes *BCL6* dysregulation by impairing proteosomal-mediated degradation of the BCL6 protein. Mutations and deletions of *TP53* remain an important genetic lesion in about 20% of patients with DLBCL, including those resulting from transformation from FL.

t(14;15)(q32;q11–13) occur in 3% to 4% of DLBCL, which results in fusion of the *BCL8* gene on chromosome 15 to the V_H segment of the *IGH* locus. The most common secondary abnormalities are trisomies of chromosomes 3, 5, 7q, 11, 12p, 18q, and Xq, which are observed in greater than 10% of cases. Amplification of *REL*, *MYC*, *BCL2*, *GLI*, *CDK4*, and *MDM2* genes are most frequently associated with advanced-stage disease. The most frequent monosomies include chromosomes 13, 14, and 15. A complex karyotype may have an adverse impact on prognosis.

The use of modern molecular studies identified two major subgroups in DCLBC: activated B cell–like DLBCL (ABC-DCLBC)

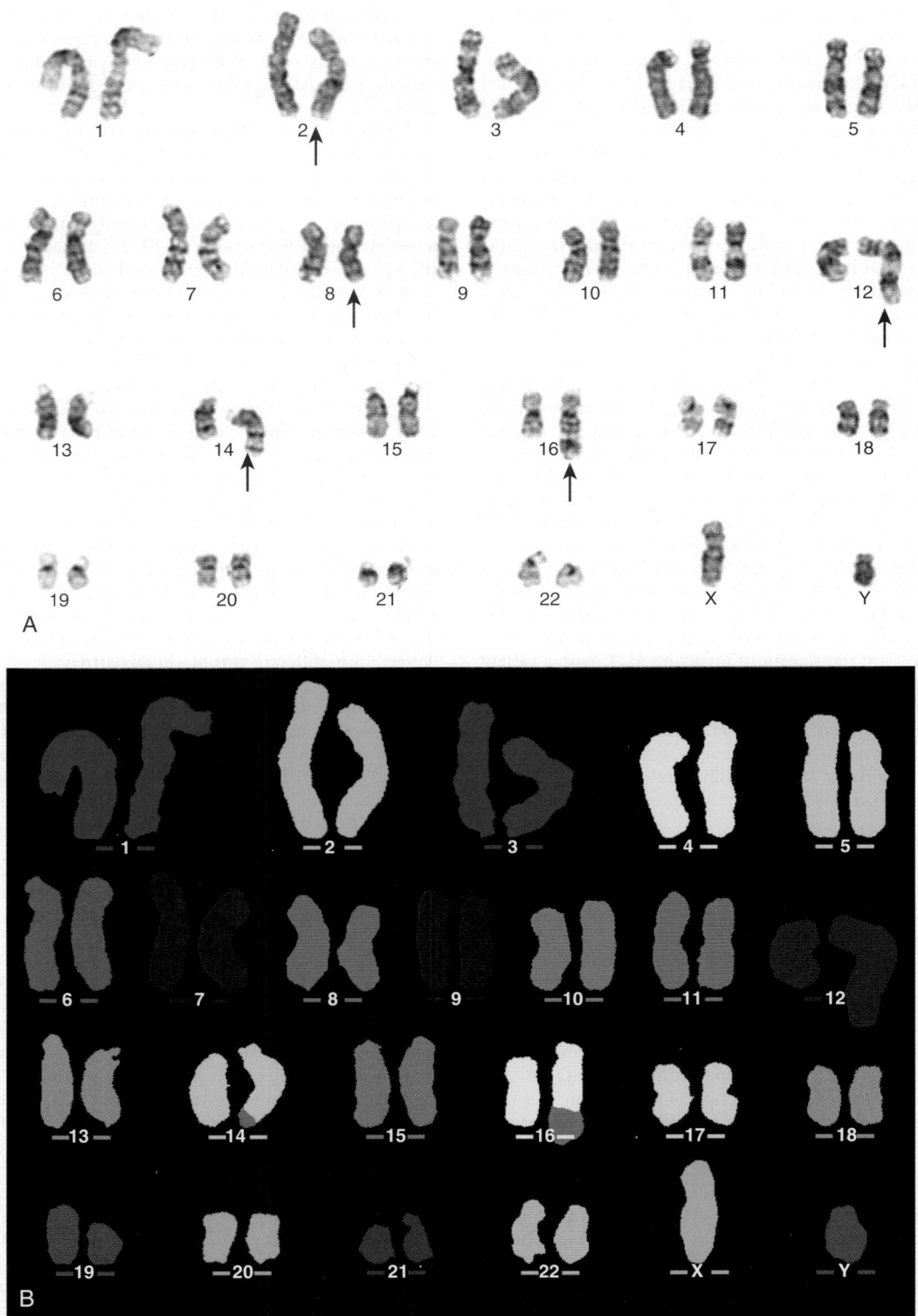

Fig. 56.56 COMPLEX KARYOTYPE OF BURKITT LYMPHOMA. Bone marrow karyotype of a patient diagnosed in an advanced stage of Burkitt lymphoma (A) and after application of the multicolor FISH (B) to resolve complex derivative chromosomes, showing 46, XY, del(2)(p21p23), t(8;14)(q24;q32), dup(12) (q13q24.3), der(16)(t(11;16)(p11.2;q24)) karyotype. *Arrows* indicate abnormal chromosomes. In addition to the classic t(8;14), both duplications of 11q and 12q were identified with multicolor FISH technology.

and germinal center B (GCB)–like DLBCL. According to the WHO 2016 classification, these two subgroups of DLBCL the GCB and ABC subgroups differ in their chromosomal alterations activation of signaling pathways and clinical outcome. Patients with ABC-DCLBC frequently exhibit trisomy of 3, gains of 3q and 18q21–23, and loss of the 6q21–23 region. Patients with GCB DLBCL have frequent gains of the 12q12 chromosomal region. Patients with primary mediastinal lymphoma have gains of 2p14–p16 and 9p21-pter. Apparently, gains in several regions of chromosome 3 are significantly associated with inferior survival. Moreover, genomic gains involving

MYC Amplification

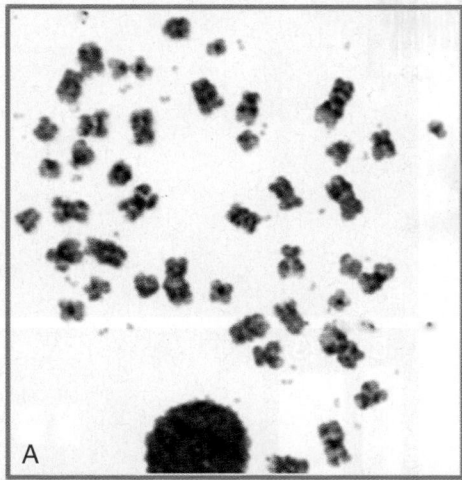

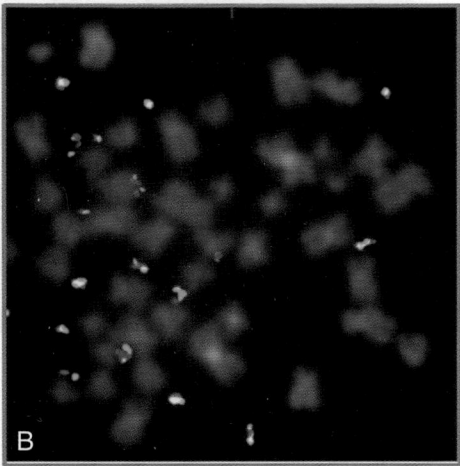

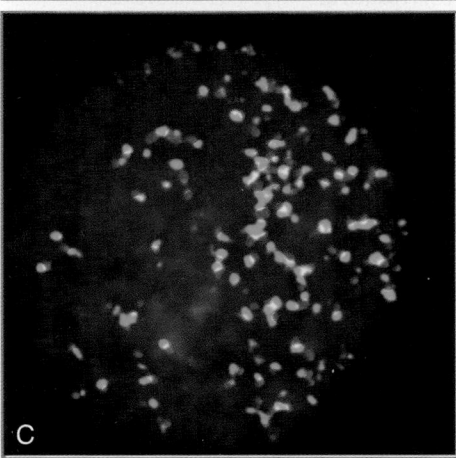

Fig. 56.57 *MYC* AMPLIFICATION. (A) A conventional G-banded bone marrow metaphase from a patient with non-Hodgkin lymphoma. Note very pale doublets of chromatin material all over metaphase cells. They are termed double minutes. (B) All double minutes after hybridization with *MYC* breakapart probe were hybridized to *MYC* consistent with *MYC* amplification. (C) Interphase, nondividing bone marrow cell showing a very high number of *MYC* amplicon. Note that *MYC* gene is not rearranged, only amplified.

the 3p11–p12 region have an independent prognostic power for survival based on previously defined optimal gene expression–based models. Somatic point mutations of the polycomb-group oncogene *EZH2* have been reported in 22% of patients with GCB-DLBCL. The differentiation of GCB B cells into plasma cells requires *PRDM1*,

a sequence-specific transcriptional repressor that is upregulated; 25% of ABC-DLBCL have deletions of *PRDM1* as a result of truncated mutations, or genomic deletions, while an additional fraction of patients lacks the PRDM1 protein as a result of transcriptional repression by a constitutively active translocated *BCL6* gene.

Patients with non-BL may have *MYC* translocations without additional mutation in *BCL2* or *BCL6* and they are described as having single hit lymphomas. Although the most recent studies suggested that patients with *MYC+*, but *BCL2–* and *BCL6–* DLBCL do not have an inferior outcome when compared to those who are *MYC* negative, the clinical relevance of *MYC* rearrangement as sole abnormality in DLBCL is still controversial with some studies indicating an adverse prognosis.

Double hit lymphoma (DHL) refers to B-cell lymphoma with multiple activating oncogenes, one of them being *MYC*. Among DHL, those with alterations in *MYC* and *BCL2* are the most common by far, occurring in 87% of patients, followed by *MYC* and *BCL6* rearrangements, found in 5% of patients. Triple hit lymphoma (THL) involves rearrangements of *MYC, BCL6*, and *BCL2* in a single cell and are observed in about 8% of patients with DLBCL (Fig. 56.58).

DHL can be detected cytogenetically but cryptic gene rearrangements may be missed. FISH therefore should be used for the detection of DHL and THL. FISH studies can be successfully performed using formalin-fixed paraffin embedded tissue sections as well as fresh smears, touch-cell imprints.

Because one of the translocations may be cryptic, a combination of three FISH probes, labeled with three colors, is especially useful in identifying these very complex translocations (see Fig. 56.43). Non-*IG* genes also act as *MYC* translocation partners in 35% to 53% of *MYC* rearranged DLBCL. The t(8;9)(q24;p13), which results in the juxtaposition of *MYC* to *PAX5*, has been frequently reported, accounting for 20% of non-*IG/MYC* rearrangement. Both the DHL and THL have complex karyotypes. Complex karyotypes are not seen in BL, which by definition always have single abnormality.

The detection of increased number of cells expressing *MYC*s correlates well with the presence of gene rearrangements, but the relationship varies. Tumors with more than 70% of *MYC*-positive cells usually are associated with gene rearrangements, but *MYC* translocations can be present in up to 17% of cases with less than 30% *MYC*-positive cells. The variability between the protein expression and gene alterations makes it difficult to recommend the use of MYC immunohistochemistry as a screening method to detect gene rearrangements. The current recommendation is that all patients with DLBCL have FISH for *MYC* rearrangements because combined alterations in *MYC, BCL2*, and *BCL6* confers a more aggressive disease phenotype.

All patients with MCL exhibit t(11;14)(q13;q32) abnormality as detected by FISH (see Fig. 56.55 *top panel*). t(11;14)(q13;q32) is also found in a variety of other B-cell malignancies, including MM, splenic lymphoma with villous lymphocytes, and B-cell prolymphocytic leukemia. Most breakpoints on chromosome 11, band q13, are dispersed over a region of approximately 130 kb centromeric to the cyclin D1 (*CCND1*) gene. At the molecular level, the *BCL1* locus (*CCND1*) on chromosome 11q13 is juxtaposed to an enhancer sequence within the *IGH* gene on 14q32, leading to overexpression of the *cyclin D* gene (involved in cell cycle control), which is not expressed in normal B and T cells or in other malignant lymphomas.

Because the breakpoints within 11q13 are scattered along a 130-kb distance, dual-color FISH has proved to be the most sensitive assay for detection of *IGH-CCND1* fusion in MCL. Furthermore, the *CCND1* fusion rearrangement can also be detected in formalin-fixed, paraffin-embedded samples, making this a rapid and reliable method (see Fig. 56.42A).

Gene expression studies have identified a subset of D1-negative MCL patients, so called because of the lack of cyclin D1 expression and t(11;14). However, both cyclin D1–positive and cyclin D1–negative patients have the same secondary genomic alterations. These secondary chromosomal alterations include gains of 3q, 8q, and 15q

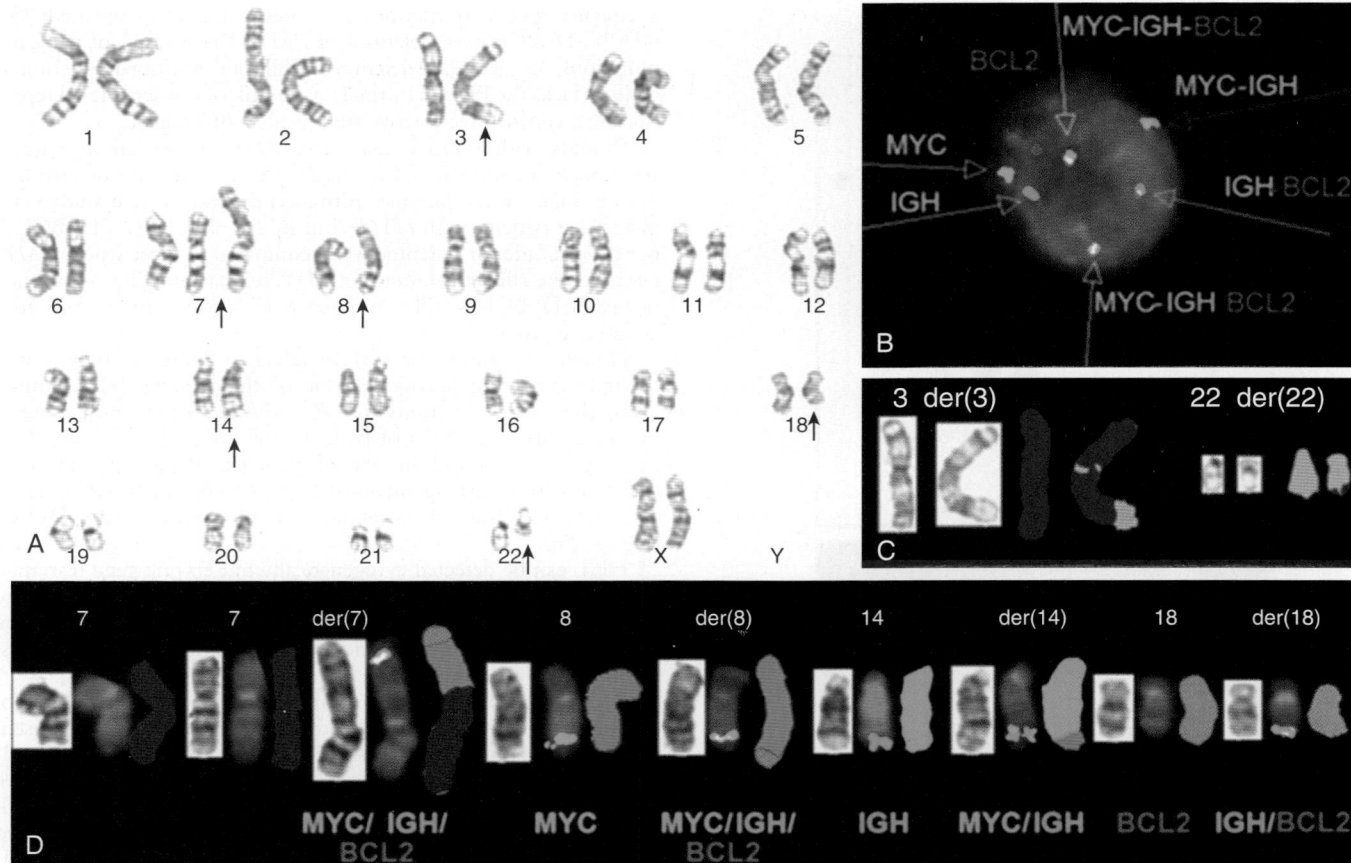

Fig. 56.58. TRIPLE HIT LYMPHOMA (A) A karyotype of patient with triple hit lymphoma with *arrows* pointing the abnormal chromosomes. Note a gain of der(7;8) resulting in three copies of 7q and three copies of rearranged 8q, and the three-way translocation between chromosomes 8, 14, and 18 as well as a translocation (3;22). (B) A bone marrow nucleus showing normal *MYC (aqua), IGH (green)* and *BCL2 (red)* as well as two copies of *MYC-IGH-BCL2* fusion, *MYC-IGH,* and *IGH-BCL2* fusion. (C) A partial karyotype after multicolor metaphase FISH study, using chromosome paining probes, showing a t(3;22) resulting in *BCL6* rearrangement. (D) A partial karyotype of chromosomes 7, 8, 14, and 18. G-banded chromosomes are on the left, DAPI-stained chromosomes with *MYC (aqua), IGH (green)* and *BCL2* are in the middle and multicolor stained chromosomes are on the right. Note der(7) is composed of 7q *(brown),* gain of 8q *(dark green),* and the third copy of *MYC-IGH-BCL2* fusion is on the tip of the 8q. The patients had three copies of *IGH2-BCL2* although cytogenetically this was manifested as a gain of 8q. *(Reprinted with permission from McFarland et al: Two cases of triple hit lymphoma: A call for imperative MYC, BCL2 and BCL6 testing by FISH in aggressive lymphomas. Personalized Medicine in Oncology, April 2015 Vol 4, 16-22. Copyright 2015. Green Hill Healthcare, LLC.)*

and losses of 1p, 8p23-pter, 9p21-pter, 11q21–23, and 13q. Some of the genes residing in these chromosomal regions are dysregulated and are involved in cell proliferation, DNA repair, cellular homeostasis, and apoptosis. In MCL, DNA amplification of several chromosomal regions appears to be associated with a blastoid variant. Loss of 9p21-pter, inactivation of *TP53*, gain of 3q, and high cyclin D expression are biomarkers of a shorter survival and a more aggressive clinical phenotype. The prognostic value of 3q27-qer gains and loss of 9q21–32 region have been determined to be independent of the gene expression–based signature. Extra copies of 3q are prognostic in patients with low proliferation, whereas loss of 9q has improved clinical value in a subgroup of patients with high proliferation. Exome sequencing of patients with MCL has identified genetic heterogeneity underlying MCL with relatively few genes mutated in more than 10% of the cases. Genes most frequently and recurrently showing acquired mutations include *ATM, CCND1, TP53, RB1, WHSC1, POT1, SMARCA4, NOTHCH1,* and *UBR5.*

Extranodal marginal zone lymphoma and MALT lymphoma are considered the third most frequent subtypes of NHL. An etiologic link between low-grade gastric MALT lymphoma and a lymphoid reaction associated with *Helicobacter pylori* infection has been well established. Growing evidence suggests that chronic antigenic stimulation caused by autoimmune diseases, such as Hashimoto thyroiditis, also contributes to an increased risk for developing MALT lymphomas.

The most frequent and specific aberration occurring in MALT lymphomas is t(11;18)(q21;q21.1) (Fig. 56.55F). Although it has been described in other B-cell lymphomas, t(11;18) in MALT lymphoma is usually the sole lesion. It is the only recurrent translocation that does not involve *IG* genes, even though it presents as a B-cell lymphomas. As a consequence of t(11;18), *API2* gene on chromosome 11, band q21, which encodes an inhibitor of apoptosis (also known as IAP2, HIAP1, and MIHC), and a novel gene *MALT1* on chromosome 18, band q21, characterized by several Ig-like C2-type domains, are often rearranged. The resultant chimeric transcript consists of 5′-*API2* and 3′-*MALT* located on der(18). More than 90% of breakpoints in the *API2* locus occur in intron 7, whereas the breakpoints within *MALT1* are variable and occur in four different introns. The *API2-MALT1* fusion is easily identified using a dual-color *API2-MALT1* FISH probe or the breakapart dual-color *MALT1* probe on lymph node biopsy specimens (see Fig. 56.55F). However, detection of deletions and duplications occurring at high frequencies in both the *API2* and *MALT1* genomic sequences require more precise molecular cytogenetic methods.

t(1;14)(p22;q32) and its variant t(1;2)(p22;q12) occur in less than 5% of MALT lymphomas, and are associated with an advanced stage of the disease. This translocation relocates the entire *BCL10* gene from 1p22 to chromosome 14, bringing it under the control of an *IGH* enhancer. Currently, a specific probe for detecting *BCL10-IGH* fusion is not commercially available, but an *IGH* dual-color break-apart FISH probe may determine *IGH* rearrangements without identifying the partner chromosome. The recurrent t(3;14)(p13;q32) abnormality, which results in fusion of the *FOXP1F* gene on chromosome 3 to *IGH*, is a rare rearrangement that causes *FOXP1F* overexpression. Its significance in lymphoma remains unknown. The t(14;18)(q32;q21), which occurs in 2% to 18% of all MALT lymphomas, results in fusion of *IGH-MALT*. The 18q21 breakpoint involving the *MALT1* gene is 5 Mb centromeric from the *BCL2* breakpoint on chromosome 18, which is associated with FL. In contrast to *API2-MALT1* cases, patients with *IGH-MALT1* fusion have disease outside the gastrointestinal tract, usually presenting with ocular, skin, liver, or salivary gland tumors. FISH studies are useful for detecting the *IGH-MALT* fusion in paraffin-embedded lymph node biopsies. Compelling evidence links these translocations to constitutive activation of the NF-κB pathway.

Splenic marginal zone lymphoma (SMZL) lacks recurrent chromosome translocations although approximately 30% of patients have heterozygous 7q deletions. Studies utilizing whole-exome sequencing have identified a novel and recurrent inactivating mutations in Krupel-like factor 2 (*KLF2*) in 42% of patients. These mutations are rarely observed in other B-cell lymphomas. Different *KLF2* mutations compromise the ability of *KLF2* gene to suppress *NF-κB* activation, leading to an altered gene expression pattern favoring B-cell homing to the marginal zone. *KLF2* inactivation alone is insufficient for malignant transformation and requires cooperating genetic events. Other common mutations found in SMZL include *NOTCH2*, *TRAF3*, *TNFAIP3*, and *CARD11*. These mutations with and without *KLF2* mutations indicate that *KLF2* mutation identifies a subset of patients with SMZL with distinct genotype. NGS has demonstrated that 40% of patients with SMZL have mutations in fours genes: *TP53, KLF2, NOTCH2,* and *TRAF3*, of which *TP53* mutations were associated with a shorter survival whereas mutations in *MYB* gene were predictors of a longer OS.

Lymphoplasmacytoid lymphoma (LPL) is a small lymphocytic lymphoma with plasmacytoid differentiation (CD5⁻CD10⁻) characterized by t(9;14)(p13;q32) in approximately 50% of cases. As a result of this translocation, the paired homeobox 5 (*PAX5*) gene on 9p13 moves to the *IGH* locus on der(14), causing dysregulation of *PAX5*. Molecular characterization of t(9;14) has revealed that the coding region of the *PAX5* gene remains intact in some patients. t(9;14) should be considered a regulatory mutation in which the *PAX5* gene is brought under the control of the *IGH* locus. In other cases, molecular studies of t(9;14) reveal that the breakpoint occurs upstream of the *PAX5* promoter, leading to insertion of the *IGH* enhancer upstream of the *PAX5* gene. Recurrent mutations in *MYD88*, specifically L265P mutation, have been identified in over 96% of patients with LPL whereas mutations in chemokine receptor, *CXCR4*, has been observed in about 36% of cases. These mutations identify a subgroup of LPL with aggressive disease.

Waldenström macroglobulinemia (WM) (see Chapter 87) is characterized by a lymphoplasmacytic clonal expansion in the marrow. Historically recurrent chromosomal abnormalities include deletion of the long arms of chromosome 6 in 21% to 55% of cases and trisomy 4 present in approximately 20% of cases. In contrast to other B-cell disorders, abnormalities of *IGH* at 14q32 as detected by FISH are rarely observed. Whole-genome sequencing of WM lymphoplasmacytic cells has led to the identification of a recurring sequence variant at position 38182641 in chromosome 3p22.2. A single-nucleotide change from T to C in the *MYD88* gene resulted in a leucine-to-proline change at amino acid position 265. *MYD88* (3p22 locus) mutations are detected by PCR in the peripheral blood of untreated patients. The *MYB88* L265P mutation is highly specific and is the

most frequent mutation in WM. It is found in over 91% of cases, including those with a gain of chromosome 3 (approximately 12%). This mutation may be considered as the first detectable genetic hit in WM that promotes NF-κB and JAK-STAT signaling pathways. *MYD88* L265P mutation is also seen in SMZL and MALT lymphoma. *MYD88* L265P cannot be used to differentiate between WM and IgM MGUS. Patients with mutated *MYD88* have a shorter survival as compared with patients with unmutated *MYD88*. The *CXCR4* (2q22.1 locus), one of the main regulators of B-cell homing is mutated in almost 30% of patients with WM and 20% of patients with IgM MGUS. Collectively these results indicate that *CXCR4* is an activating mutation in WM and has a critical role in WM pathogenesis.

Little progress has been made in delineating recurrent chromosomal abnormalities in Hodgkin lymphoma (HL) (see Chapter 75). Less than 1% of the cells in HL are Reed-Sternberg cells, of B-cell origin. The most specific chromosomal abnormalities in HL are hyperdiploidy/tetraploidy with tremendous variations in chromosome number, indicating heterogeneity from patient to patient. Even with use of nine different centromeric probes, no specific numerical chromosomal abnormality has been identified. Deletions of 1p, 4q, 6q, and 7q are recurrent, and *JAK2*, located on 9p21, frequently is amplified in patients with HL. Another gene, *REL*, on chromosome 2, band region p14–p15, is amplified in 50% of patients. Of note, *REL* is under the influence of *NF-κB* transcription factor, and constitutive NF-κB activation is a critical prerequisite for Reed-Sternberg cell survival and proliferation.

The genome of Reed-Sternberg cells was largely unexplored because of the technical difficulties in isolating these cells. This difficulty was recently overcome and preliminary results of full-exome deep sequencing of 10 patients revealed inactivating mutations in β2-microglobulin gene (*B2M*, localized at 15q21.1) in 7 of 10 patients. These mutations lead to the loss of major histocompatibility complex class I (MHC1) expression. A lack of *MHC1* expression in Reed-Sternberg cells was previously reported as an independent adverse prognostic factor. Therefore molecular mechanisms leading to MHC1 downregulation in Hodgkin lymphoma is through inactivating mutations in *B2M* gene.

HAIRY CELL LEUKEMIA

No recurrent chromosomal aberrations have been identified in hairy cell leukemia (HCL) although as shown in Fig. 56.59 some patients may have a complex bone marrow karyotype at diagnosis. HCL is a mature B-cell malignancy with the bone marrow, spleen and liver infiltrated by leukemic B cells that have abundant cytoplasm with hairy-looking projections and unique immunophenotyping features. High-density genome-wide SNP genotyping have shown a remarkable balanced genomic profile. In 2011, a *BRAF*-V600E mutation was described for the first time in every one of 47 patients. The *BRAF*-V600E mutation defines HCL, is present in virtually all patients with HCL, and is absent in other B-cell malignancies except a small number of patients with MM.[29] BRAF is a kinase within the RAS-RAF-MEK-ERK pathway that plays a pivotal role in regulating hematopoietic stem cells from patients with HCL. Quantitative

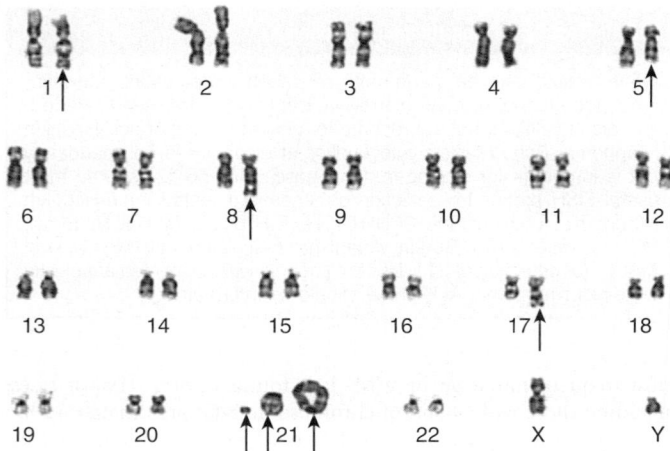

Fig. 56.59 A COMPLEX KARYOTYPE FROM A PATIENT WITH HAIRY CELL LEUKEMIA. In this karyotype there are nine complex structural abnormalities as indicated by *arrows* and the karyotype is 47, XY, del(5)(q15;q31), der(8)t(3;8)(p21p26;q24), der(17)t(1;17) (p36.1;p13) t(17;21)(q25q22.2), −21, +r(21)×2.

sequence analysis revealed a mean *BRAF*-V600E-mutant allele frequency of 4.9% in human hematopoietic stem cells from patients with HCL and functional studies showed that these cells have self-renewal capacity, indicating that this mature B-cell malignancy originates within the hematopoietic stem cell compartment. Detection of the *BRAF*-V600E mutation by PCR is the gold standard for the genetic diagnosis of HCL.

T-CELL LYMPHOPROLIFERATIVE NEOPLASMS

This is a diverse group of hematologic disorders that includes T-cell ALL and T-cell CLL/PML, as well as several indolent T-cell disorders, large granular lymphocyte leukemia, natural killer leukemia/lymphoma, and anaplastic large cell lymphoma (ALCL).

T-cell ALL represents 15% of childhood ALL cases and 25% of adult ALL cases. At diagnosis, approximately 50% of patients have a normal karyotype. Table 56.11 lists recurrent cytogenetic and molecular genomic changes associated with T-cell ALL and Table 56.18 lists the frequency of recurrent chromosomal abnormalities in T-ALL. Immunophenotypic and gene expression analyses are consistent with genetic heterogeneity in T-cell ALL, reflecting, to some degree, distinct stages of T-cell maturation arrest.

One of the common themes in T-lymphoid malignancies is the juxtaposition of the *TCR* gene enhancer element adjacent to a variety of transcription factors located at or near breakpoints on the partner chromosome. The chromosomal bands most frequently involved are 14q11, where *TCRA* and *TCRD* are located (see Fig. 56.60); 7q35, the site of *TCRB*; and 7p15, the site of the *TCRG*. TCR translocations are found in approximately 35% of T-cell ALL cases (Table 56.17). The rearrangements of *TCRB* and *TCRG* are relatively rare, whereas 14q11 rearrangements involving both *TCRA* and *TCRD* are frequent in T-lymphoid neoplasms (see Table 56.13).

In children, the overall frequency of T-cell ALL translocations is 40% to 50%, and several molecular/cytogenetic abnormalities have prognostic relevance (see Table 56.14). *TAL1* rearrangements include t(1;14)(p32;q11), t(1;7)(p32;q35), rare t(1;3)(p32;p21), t(1;5) (p32;q31) and t(14;19)(q11.2;q13.1) (Fig. 56.61). In general, *TAL1* rearrangements are submicroscopic and best identified with FISH. Disruption of *TAL1* is frequently associated with a submicroscopic interstitial deletion (90 kb) between the 5′ untranslated region of the *TAL1* (1p32) and the *SIL* (*STIL*) genes (1p32) in 9% to 26% of cases depending on the different studies. The *SIL-TAL1* fusion product gives rise to inappropriate expression of TAL1 protein. Among 382 children, 16% showed the presence of *SIL-TAL1*, which was more

frequently observed in older children. These 1p32 rearrangements are less frequent in adult ALL. *TAL1*-positive ALL is characterized by an arrest in differentiation at the CD4$^+$CD8$^+$ stage of thymocyte development, when *TAL1* gene is normally silent. *TAL1* gene encodes a transcription factor and several of the core components of the transcription complex include *GATA3*, LIM domain only, and *RUNX1*.

TAL2, residing at 9q32, is detected in rare t(7;9)(q34;q32) rearrangement as a result of juxtaposition of *TAL2* to *TCRB*. *LYL1*, originally described as a fusion partner of *TCRB* in rare (7;19) (q34;p13), and is associated with poor prognosis. Rearrangements of *HOX11L2*, which include cryptic t(5;14)(q35;q32), t(5;7)(q35;q21), and other variants, occur at a frequency of 24% in children and represent a predictor of poor outcome, regardless of treatment strategies. Similarly, the presence of t(10;11)(p13;q14), which results in the *CALM-MLL10* fusion gene and occurs at a frequency of 2% to 5% in children, may be associated with poor outcome. Abnormalities of *HOX11* are more common in adults than in children (31% versus 7%) and are associated with t(10;14)(q34;q24) and t(7;10)(q34;q24). t(10;14) is the most frequent chromosomal translocation in patients with T-cell ALL. It is associated with excellent outcome in both children and adults with t(10;14) and in these patients the homeobox gene *HOX11* is fused with *TCRD*. The coding regions of *HOX11* are not disturbed by the translocation. In the variant translocation t(7;10)(q35;q24), *HOX11* is juxtaposed to *TCRB*, which results in overexpression of normal *HOX11* mRNA by bringing *HOX11* under the influence of *TCR* promoter sequences.

MLL rearrangements are present in 8% of T-cell ALL cases (see Fig. 56.33). The most frequent *MLL* translocation partners in T-cell ALL include *ENL*, which results from t(11;19)(q23;p13.3) and is associated with a better prognosis than T-cell ALL with other fusion partners. GEP has characterized T-cell ALL with *MLL* rearrangements as a distinct molecular subtype. Homeobox genes, regulators of embryonic development, are known targets of *MLL* and are overexpressed in patients with T-cell ALL and *MLL* rearrangements.

Dysregulation of *NOTCH*, tyrosine kinase genes (*ABL1, JAK2*), and LIM domain genes (*LMO1, LMO2*) is also common in T-cell ALL. *NOTCH1* is a fusion partner of *TCRB* in t(7;9)(q34;q34.3). These mutations are present in 56% of T-cell ALL cases. The *NOTCH1* gene is important in lymphoid lineage specification, and resequencing of functional domains of *NOTCH1* have revealed that activating *NOTCH1* mutations are present in most primary pediatric and adolescent molecular cases of T-ALL as well as in adult ALL. Mutations in the heterodimer domain as well as ITD result in constitutive ligand-independent activation of *NOTCH1*.

The LIM family of genes is found at the breakpoint of rare but consistent chromosomal translocations in T-cell ALL. *LMO1*, located at 11p15, is involved in t(11;14)(p15;q11). *LMO2*, located at 11p13, is involved in t(11;14)(p13;q11) and t(7;11)(q35;p13). As an oncogenic transcription regulator, *LMO2* overexpression in erythroid and T cells leads to a differentiation arrest, which is a prerequisite for development of T-cell malignancies.

The *MYB* gene, which is localized on chromosome 6, band q23.3, is rearranged in a rare T-cell ALL subtype observed in young patients (median 2.2 years). Two types of recurrent *MYB* genomic alterations are found in T-cell ALL: (a) a reciprocal t(6;7)(q23;q34) that results in juxtaposition of *MYB* near *TCRB* regulatory sequences on chromosome 7 and (b) a short genomic tandem duplication, identified using genome-wide copy-number analysis. Both rearrangements are cytogenetically cryptic. The breakpoints in t(6;7) are subtelomeric and usually missed. The translocation was discovered using a locus-specific FISH probe for *MYC*.[30] The tandem *MYB* duplication is cryptic using both conventional cytogenetics and locus-specific FISH. It is mapped using high-density oligonucleotide aCGH. Discovery of *MYB* highlights the strength of high-density aCGH in identifying cryptic copy-number abnormalities associated with leukemia.

Although only 1% of Ph-positive ALL have a T-cell phenotype, the *ABL1* gene, is also involved in fusion with *NUP214* (9q34.11), creating the *NUP214-ABL1* chimeric gene/t(9;22)(q34.11–q22.1), which is identified in up to 6% of T-cell ALL. This fusion gene is

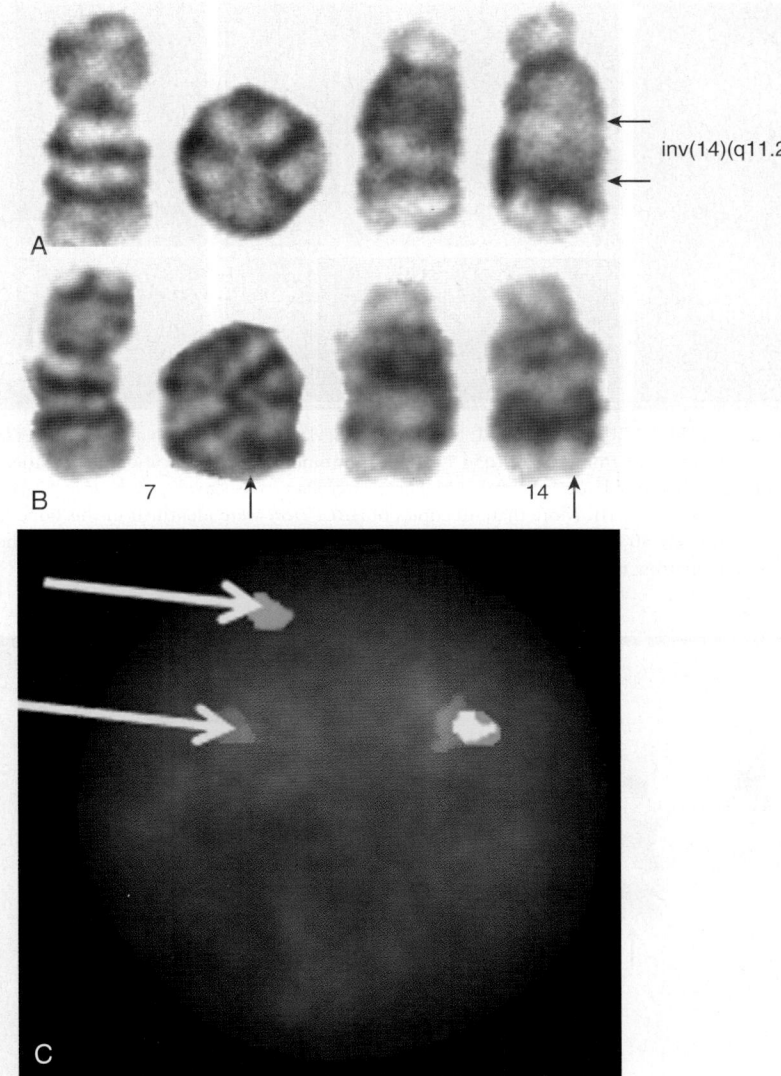

inv(14)(q11.2q32)

Fig. 56.60 REARRANGEMENTS OF T-CELL RECEPTOR (TCR) GENES IN T-CELL MALIGNAN-CIES. A partial karyotype of chromosomes 7 and 14 from a patient with T-cell prolymphocytic leukemia. (A) Ring chromosome 7 and inversion of chromosome 14. *Black arrows* indicate two breakpoints on chromosome 14, q11.2 and q32, where inv(14) have occurred. (B) Different partial karyotype from the same patient showing a dicentric ring 7. (C) An isolated bone marrow nuclei after hybridization with TCRα/δ FISH probe. *Yellow arrows* indicate separation of the 3′ and 5′ of *TCR*, consistent with inv(14). Because of the ring (7) this patient also had rearrangements of TCR β/γ.

<table>
<tr><td rowspan="2">TABLE
56.17</td><td colspan="3">**Frequency of T-Cell Receptor (TCR) Rearrangements
Using Conventional Cytogenetics Versus FISH**</td></tr>
</table>

Locus	Conventional Cytogenetics (%)	FISH (%)	
		Total Karyotype	Abnormal Karyotype
TCRαδ	9.5	17.4	24.7
TCRβ	3.1	19	26.9
TCRγ	0	0	0

found amplified only in T-cell ALL. When identified with FISH using the *ABL1* probe, it appears as an amplified episome between the chromosomes in metaphase cells, usually showing 5–50 copies/cell and very rarely identified by conventional cytogenetics (Fig. 56.62). RT-PCR can also be used for its detection. The most common fusion gene involves the breakpoint in exon 2 of *ABL1* and the

breakpoint in exon 31 of *NUP214*, although variant breakpoints in both genes have been reported. *NUP214-ABL1* is a constitutively activated tyrosine kinase activating similar pathways as *BCR-ABL1* and is sensitive to inhibition with TKIs, especially nilotinib and dasatinib. These patients usually have homozygous or heterozygous deletions of *CDKN2A* at 9p21 chromosomal site as well as trisomy 8, t(7;10)(q35;q24), or t(10;14)(q24;q11), indicating that *NUP214-ABL1* is not a primary genetic event. Patients with *NUP214-ABL1* usually present with high-risk T-cell ALL and their outcome is poor. del(9)(q34.11–q34.13) or rare t(9;9)(q34;q34) results in the formation of a *SET-NUP214* fusion gene frequently observed in T-cell ALL (Fig. 56.63). In rare cases of T-cell ALL, *JAK2* has been identified as a partner chromosome with *ETV6* in t(9;12)(p24;q13), with *PCM1* in t(8;9) and in multiple amplified copies (Figs. 56.64–56.66), two of the three *JAK2* fusion transcripts seen in hematologic malignancies (see Ph-Negative Myeloproliferative Neoplasms, earlier, and Table 56.13).

Adult T-cell ALL is characterized by an aberrant karyotype in almost 70% of cases and by recurrent acquisition of somatic

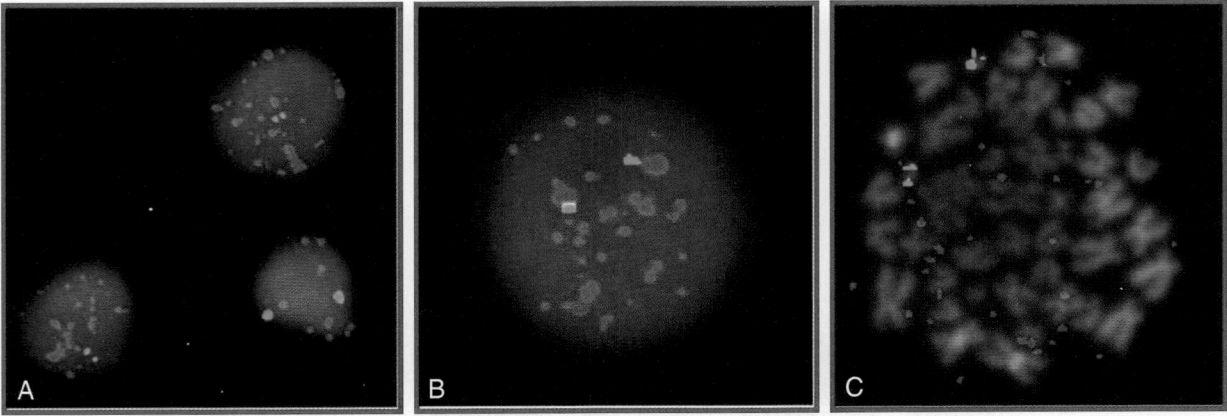

Fig. 56.61 *BL1* AMPLIFICATION IN T-CELL NEOPLASMS. *ABL1* amplification as a result of *NUP214-ABL1* chimeric gene resulting from t(9;22)(q34.11;q22.1) chromosomal translocation in a patient with Ph-positive T-cell acute lymphoblastic leukemia. (A) Three interphase cells showing 2 *BCR* loci *(green)* and numerous copies of *ABL1 (red)*. (B) More than 40 copies of *ABL1 (red)* were identified in this bone marrow nucleus. (C) Approximately 30 copies of *ABL1 (red)* were shown as an amplified episome between the chromosomes in this bone marrow metaphase cell.

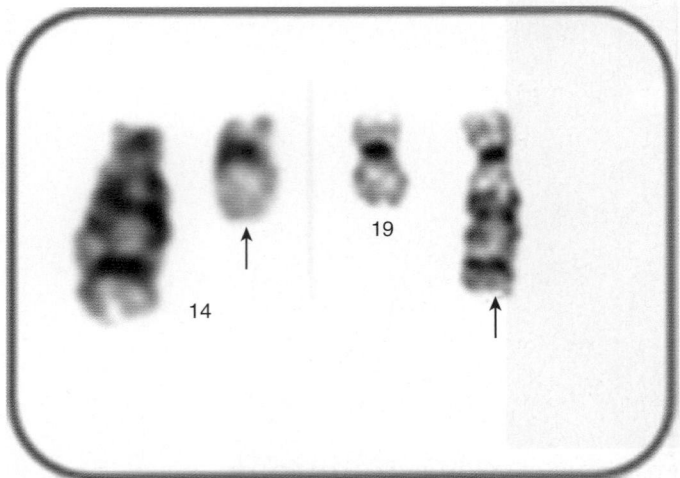

Fig. 56.62 A PARTIAL KARYOTYPE FROM A PATIENT WITH T-CELL LEUKEMIA AND t(14;19)(q11.2;q13.1) KARYOTYPE.

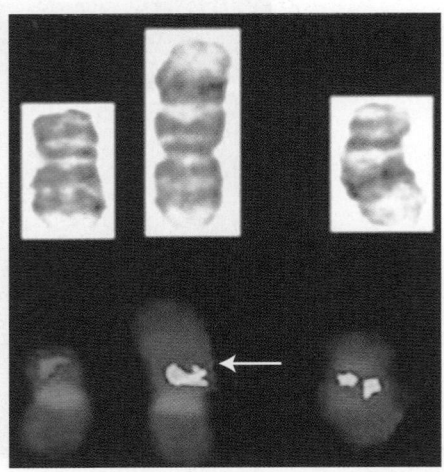

Fig. 56.64 *JAK-TEL* FUSION. Partial karyotype of t(9;12)(p24;q23) *(top)* and after FISH study *(bottom)* with JAK2 *(red)* and TEL/ETV6 *(green)*, showing JAK2-TEL fusion *(yellow)* at 9p24.

T(9;9)(q13;q33)

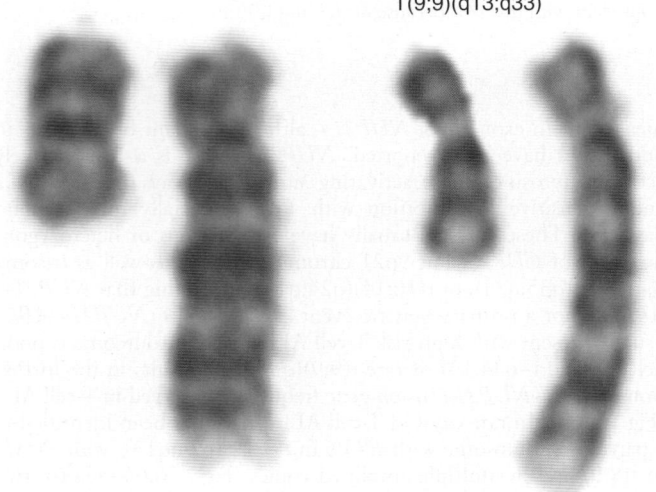

Fig. 56.63 A PARTIAL BONE MARROW CHROMOSOME 9 KARYOTYPE FROM TWO METAPHASE CELLS FROM A PATIENT WITH T-CELL ACUTE LYMPHOBLASTIC LEUKEMIA. The rare variant t(9;9) (q22;q34) also results in *SET-NUP214* fusion gene.

mutations in 93% (Table 56.18). The most frequent recurrent molecular lesions observed in adult T-cell ALL include mutations in the following genes: *NOTCH1* (71%), *PHF6* (39.5%), *FBXW7* (18.9%), *DNMT3A* (17.8%), *RUNX1* (15.5%), *PTEN* (10%), *FLT3-IDT* (2.2%), *FLT3-TKD* (1.1%), and *CDKN2A* (3.3%). Combining these data with frequent *CDKN2A/B* deletions and aberrant *CDKN2B* methylation status, 98.9% of adult T-cell ALL have a minimum of one genetic defect. *DNMT3A* and *RUNX1* mutations are preferentially found in early immature T-cell leukemias and are associated with poor OS.

Early T-cell precursor ALL (ETP) is an aggressive subtype of T-cell ALL that comprises up to 15% of T ALL cases. Whole-genome sequencing of 94 T-ALL cases revealed a mutational spectrum similar to AML and global transcriptional profile is similar to that of normal and myeloid hematopoietic stem cells. ETP ALL is characterized by activating mutations in genes regulating cytokine receptor and RAS signaling (67% of cases: *NRAS*, *KRAS*, *FLT3*, *IL7R*, *JAK3*, *JAK1*, *SH2B3*, and *BRAF*), inactivating lesions disrupting hematopoietic development (58% of cases: *GATA3*, *ETV6*, *RUNX1*, *IKZ1*, and *EP300*) and histone modulating genes (48% of cases: *EZH2*, *EED*, *SUZI2*, *SETD2*, and *EP300*).

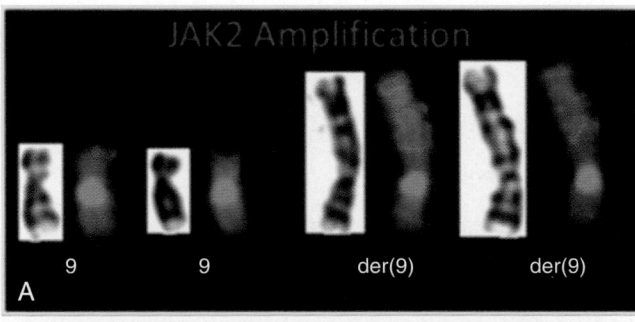

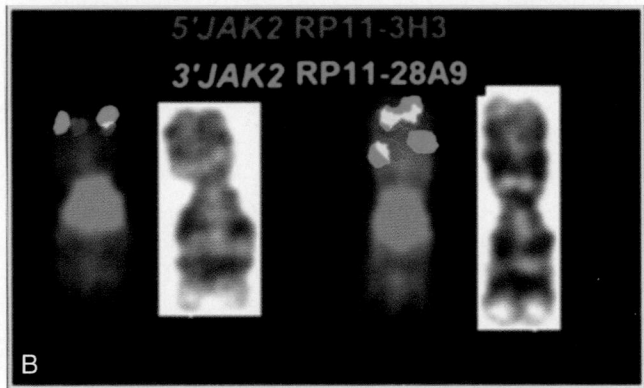

Fig. 56.65 GAIN OF *JAK2* IN ADULT T-CELL LEUKEMIA/
LYMPHOMA. (A) A partial karyotype of der(9) chromosome from a patient
with adult T-cell leukemia/lymphoma showing *JAK2 (red)* amplification.
(B) A partial dup(9)(p24) karyotype showing duplication of JAK2 (*red* is
5′ JAK2, green is *3′ JAK2*).

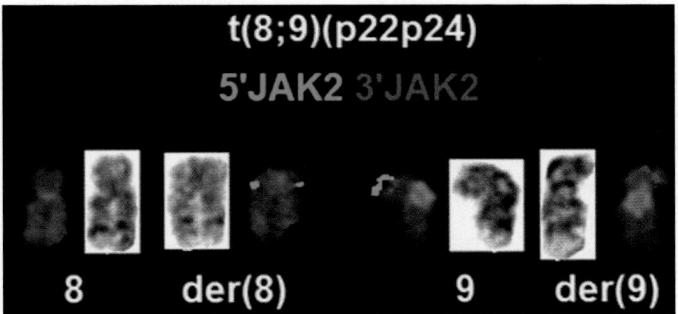

Fig. 56.66 t(8;9)/*PCM1-JAK2* IN T-CELL ACUTE LYMPHOBLASTIC
LEUKEMIA. (T-ALL) A partial karyotype from a patient with T-ALL
showing t(8;9)(p22;p24) resulting in *PCM1-JAK2* fusion also observed in
patients with Ph-negative myeloproliferative neoplasms. In this translocation
5′ JAK2 (*green*) is translocated from 9p24 to 8p22 using JAK2 two-color
breakapart FISH probe.

MYC translocations identify a genetic subtype of T-cell ALL,
which occurs in about 6% of cases within a cohort of 196 patients
with T-cell ALL, including both children and adults. Two types
of translocations were observed: those involving the *TCR* loci and those
with other partners. Specifically, *MYC* translocations were significantly associated with TAL/LMO subtype of T-cell ALL and trisomies
for chromosomes 6 and 7. GEP has revealed that *MYC* translocations
occur as secondary abnormalities present either in subclones at
diagnosis or following disease progression.

In contrast to childhood B-cell ALL, the majority of childhood
T-cell ALL cases develop after birth. In utero origin of this form of
leukemia is rare.

T-cell CLL and prolymphocytic leukemia are characterized by
T-cell leukemia 1 (*TCL1*) gene rearrangements. These include inv(14)
(q11q32.1), t(14;14)(q11;q32.1), and t(7;14)(q35;q32.1) (see Fig.
56.60). In patients showing these karyotypic changes, *TCL1* is found
to be dysregulated.

Adult T-cell leukemia/lymphoma is associated with human T-cell
lymphotropic virus type 1. The most frequent genetic lesions include
altered expression of *CDKN2* (cyclin-dependent kinase inhibitor)
gene on 9p21 (15%–20%) and loss of heterozygosity at 6q15 to q21.
The most frequent chromosomal abnormalities are gain of 3p, 7q,
and 14q and loss of 6q and 13q. Translocations involving 14q32 or
14q11 are frequently observed.

Natural killer lymphoma/leukemia is a group of highly aggressive
lymphoid malignancies of natural killer cell origin. They exhibit
chromosomal rearrangements in greater than 80% of cases by conventional karyotyping. The most frequent abnormalities include
del(6)(q21–23) and gain of the X chromosome. FISH, CGH, and
spectral karyotyping have confirmed the presence of del(6) in
CD3⁻CD56 tumor cells. Other less common but recurrent karyotypic
changes include isochromosome 1q, 6p, and 17q, as well as del(11q),
13q, and 17p, and trisomy 8.

Angioimmunoblastic T-cell lymphoma and unspecified peripheral
T-cell lymphoma are the most frequent nodal T-cell lymphomas.
Losses of 5q/10q/12q, identified by CGH, characterize a subtype of
peripheral T-cell lymphoma associated with a better prognosis. Gain
of 11q13 may represent a primary change in angioimmunoblastic
T-cell lymphoma. In general, chromosomal imbalances are more
common in unspecified peripheral T-cell lymphoma than in angioimmunoblastic T-cell lymphoma. Both disorders may share similar
genomic imbalances.

The molecular basis of ALCL is the result of t(2;5)(p23;q35), which
fuses part of the *NPM* gene on 5q35 with part of the *ALK* receptor
tyrosine kinase gene on 2p23 to produce a chimeric *NPM-ALK* gene.
This encodes a chimeric protein that has activated kinase function.
ALK is thought to play a direct role in the malignant transformation
of lymphoid cells, probably by aberrant phosphorylation of intracytoplasmic substrates. ALCL is a distinct clinical entity, with t(2;5)
detected by cytogenetics in 60% to 85% of patients. The *NPM-ALK*
fusion is identified by FISH (Fig. 56.67) and by RT-PCR assay in
88% of pediatric patients and 60% of adult patients. The other cases
of ALCL have variant translocations with at least 21 different fusion
genes and include rearrangements with *TPM3* (1q24), *EML4* (2p24),
RANBP2 (2q13), *ARIC* (2q35), *TCG* (3q21), *SEC31A* (4q21), *CARS*
(11p15), *CLTC* (17q23), *ALO17* (17q25), *TPM4* (19p13), *CLTC1*
(22q11), *MYH* (22q11.2), and *MSN* (Xq11). Detection of *ALK* rearrangements by FISH corresponds to a cytoplasmic staining pattern
associated with translocations other than t(2;5) in 100% of cases.
Recently two copies of *NPM-ALK* and *TPM3-ALK* fusions were
reported in children with an aggressive form of ALCL.

The prognosis of patients with t(2;5) or variant translocations
is excellent, with 5-year survival rates of 70% to 90%. By contrast,
ALK-negative ALCL is associated with a 5-year survival rates of
40% to 60%. The true nature of ALK-negative ALCL remains
obscure. Most cases have clonally rearranged *TCR* genes. Recurrent rearrangements of the *DUSP22-IRF4* locus on 6p25.3 has
been identified in about 30% of *ALK*-negative ALCLs resulting in
t(6;7)(p25.3.q32.3). Other recurrent rearrangement in *ALK* negative
cases involves inv(3)(q26q26) resulting in *TBL1XR-TP63* fusion.
CGH showed that *ALK⁻* ALCL have more complex copy number
abnormalities than *ALK+ACLC*, specifically gains of 1q41-ter, 5q, 6p,
8q, 12q, and 17q and losses of 6q21 and 13q21–22. The interferon
regulatory factor 4 (*IRF4*), localized at 6p25.3, is highly expressed
in both *ALK+* and *ALK⁻* ALCLs. GEP has revealed that *MYC* is the
primary target of *IRF4* and that *MYC* itself is essential for ALCL
cell survival. Collectively these observations indicate that ALCL is
dependent on *IRF4* and *MYC* signaling. Immunochemical analysis
has revealed that both proteins are co-expressed in 82% of patients
with ALCL.

A variety of genomic rearrangements are seen in the T lymphocytes
of patients with mycosis fungoides and Sézary syndrome. However,
specific cytogenetic abnormalities are not associated with these disorders. Most frequent abnormalities involve loss of chromosome 10,

TABLE 56.18   Genetic Rearrangements in T-ALL

Transcription factor oncogenes

Genetic Lesion	Gene	Frequency %	Outcome
t(1;14)(p32;q11)	TAL1	3	Poor/None
t(1;7)(p32;q34)	TAL1	<1	Poor/None
1p32 deletion	TAL1	25	Poor/None
5'super-enhancer generating mutations	TAL1	5	Unknown
t(7;9)(q34;q32)	TAL2	1	NA
t(19)(q34;p13)	LYL1	1	NA
t(14;21)(q11.2;q22)	BHLHB1	1	NA
t(11;14)(p15;q11)	LMO1	1	NA
t(7;11)(q34;p15)	LMO1		NA
t(11;14)(p13;q11)	LMO2	6	No impact
t(7;11)(q34;p13)	LMO2	<1	No impact
11p13 deletion	LMO2	3	No impact
t(10;14)(q24;q11)	TLX1	5–10 Pediatric T-ALL	No impact
t(7;10)(q35;q24)	TLX1	30 Adult T-ALL	No impact
del(10(q24-q26)	TLX1		No impact
t(5;14)(q35;q32)	TLX3	20–25 Pediatric ALL and 5 Adult T-ALL	Unknown
inv(7)(p15q34)	HOXA	3	
t(7;7)(p15q34)	HOXA	3	
t(10;11)(p13;q14)	PICALM-MLL10	5–10	Poor
t(11;19)(q23;p13)	KMT2A-MLL1	5	Poor
9q34 deletion	SET-NUP214	3	Unknown
inv(14)(q11.2q13)	NKX2-1	5 Pediatric T-ALL	Unknown
inv(14)((q13q32.33)	NKX2-1		
t(7;14)(q34;q13)	NKX2-1		
t(14;20(q11;p11)	NKX2-2	1	Unknown
t(2;14)(q22;q32)	ZEB2	<1	NA
t(6;7)(q23;q34)	MYB	3	NA
t(8;14)(q24;q11)	MYC	1	NA

NOTH1 pathway

t(7;9)(q34;q34.3)	NOTH1	<1	NA
Activating mutations	NOTH1	>60	good
Activating mutations	FBXW7	8–30	poor/none

Cell Cycle

9p21 deletion	CDKN2A	>70	good
t(7;12)(q34;p13)	CCND2	3	NA
13q14.2 deletion	RB1	12 Pediatric T-ALL	No impact
12p13.2 deletion	CDKN1B	12	NA

Transcription factor tumor suppressors

Inactivating mutation or deletion	WT1	10	no imact
Inactivating mutation or deletion	LEF1	10–15	NA
Inactivating mutation or deletion	ETV6	13	No impact
Inactivating mutation or deletion	BCL11B	10	no imact
Inactivating mutation or deletion	RUNX1	10–20	no imact
Inactivating mutation or deletion	GATA3	5	poor

Signal transduction

10q23 deletion	PTEN	10–15	poor
Inactivating mutation	PTEN	10–15	no imact
Episomal 9q34 amplification	NUP214-ABL1	5	poor
t(9;14)(q34;q32)	EML1-ABL1	<1	NA

TABLE 56.18	Genetic Rearrangements in T-ALL—cont'd			
Genetic Lesion	**Gene**	**Frequency %**		**Outcome**
Activating mutation	NRAS	5		no imact
Activating mutation	KRAS	2		NA
Activating mutation	JAK1	4–18		no imact
t(9;12)(p24;p13)	ETV6-JAK2	<1		no imact
Activating mutation	FLT3	5–10		no imact
t(X;7)((q22;q34)	IRS4	<1		NA
t(X;14)(q22;q11.2)	IRS4			
Inactivating mutation	DNM2	15		NA
t(9;22)(q34;q11.2)	BCR-ABL1	1		poor

Modified from Belver and Ferrando Nature 16: 494, 2016.
NA, Not available.

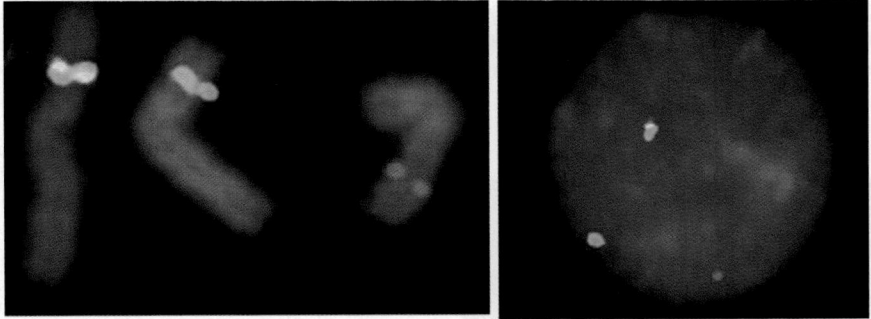

Fig. 56.67 FISH STUDY WITH BREAKAPART *ALK* GENE AT 2p23 IN A PATIENT WITH ANAPLASTIC LARGE CELL LYMPHOMA. *Partial karyotype shows a normal chromosome 2 (left) with yellow signal,* as the 3′ end and the 5′ end of *ALK* gene are in close proximity on chromosome 2. The other chromosome 2 homologue *(middle)* has only a single green signal (5′ end) as a result of t(2;5)(p23;q35), the most frequent translocation in anaplastic large-cell lymphoma. The 3′ end *(red)* of the *ALK* gene is translocated to 5q35. Abnormal *ALK* gene is also shown in interphase cell *(right)*.

deletion of 1p, isochromosome 17q, additions of 17p and 19p, and translocations involving 1p, 10q, and 14q. Both CGH and M-FISH identify chromosome 10, region 10q22–26, as the most frequent abnormality in these disorders.

Posttransplant lymphoproliferative disorder (PTLD) is a morphologically diverse group of lymphoid disorders that occurs in immunosuppressed organ transplant recipients. Chromosomal abnormalities are detected in 51% to 72% of B-cell variant and in almost all T-cell variants, as measured by CGH, FISH, and conventional karyotyping. In general, three groups of nonrandom abnormalities are of importance. The pathogenetic roles of abnormalities known to be involved in lymphomas, such as *MYC*, *TP53*, and 18q21 associated with *BCL2* and *MALT1*, and those associated with large genomic imbalances, such as 2p24–25, 9q22–34, 12q22–24, and 14q32, await elucidation. Trisomy of chromosomes 9 and 11 appears to be associated with EBV PTLD and prolonged survival. In contrast, patients with PTLD showing *MYC* rearrangements (about 50%) are associated with BL, an aggressive clinical course. T-cell PTLD develops late after transplantation. These disorders are EBV⁻ and are associated with a poor outcome and short survival.

ALLOGENEIC HEMATOPOIETIC CELL TRANSPLANTATION

Molecular and cytogenetic analyses can be used to characterize the origin of engrafted cells and the development and evolution of recurrent malignancies after allogeneic hematopoietic cell transplantation (HCT). Hematopoietic cells that emerge after allogeneic HCT may

be of host origin, donor origin, or both. Genetic studies of posttransplant hematopoiesis are termed *chimerism analysis*. Chimerism should be distinguished from mosaicism, which is characterized by two or more different cell populations originating from one zygote. Monitoring chimerism in recipients of allogeneic HCT is essential to identify early engraftment, monitor residual disease, predict relapse, and optimize posttransplantation therapy in case of graft failure.

Historically, karyotype analysis was used to evaluate engraftment after sex-mismatched allogeneic HCT. Polymorphism of chromosomes 1, 9, and 16, as well as satellite polymorphism of chromosomes 13, 14, 15, 21, and 22, were used to differentiate donor from recipient cells in sex-matched allogeneic HCT. Karyotype analysis could identify not only chimerism but also recurrence of the hematologic malignancies. However, this is a time-consuming process and has low sensitivity (5%). In the past two decades, many methods for detection of chimerism have been developed. All follow the basic principle of using the differences in polymorphic genetic markers to distinguish donor from recipient hematopoiesis. These methods include restriction fragment length polymorphism, red cell phenotyping, and interphase FISH, but do not offer the possibility to study all patients. The most widely used technique is PCR for a variable number of tandem repeats/short tandem repeats (VNTR/STR-PCR). This technique has a sensitivity of 3% to 5%, but the quantitation of donor and recipient cells may be cumbersome. The method that allows study of chimerism in all patients involves fluorescence labeling of the primers and resolution of PCR products with capillary electrophoresis. It provides high quantitative accuracy with 1% to 5% sensitivity. Real-time PCR or RQ-PCR for analysis of the *SRY* gene on the Y chromosome allows identification of male cells in the background of 100,000 female cells, providing a high sensitivity for mixed chimerism. However, this approach is limited to the 50% of patients who receive sex-mismatched transplants. Nevertheless, it remains the most sensitive and the fastest method of chimerism analysis, providing reliable quantitative results within 2 hours.

Detection of SNPs by chimerism analysis (SNP-PCR) is highly sensitive. In one study using 11 different SNP loci, SNP-PCR analysis identified independent predictors of relapse after HCT. The two most commonly used methods for detection of chimerism after HCT are fluorescence-based PCR amplification of short tandem repeats (STR-PCR) and interphase FISH. Both methods are accurate and reproducible. The sensitivity of both methods approaches 1%; however, STR-PCR is sex independent and can be applied to all patients. FISH analysis, on the other hand, permits simultaneous evaluation of chimerism and residual disease in the same cell when high sensitivity is not a requirement. FISH analysis for diagnostic genomic abnormalities in conjunction with conventional cytogenetics remains useful and reliable in determining the presence of residual disease (Fig. 56.68).

Leukemia relapse in donor cells after allogeneic HCT is a rare complication occurring in 0.12% to 5% of cases. It was first described in 1971, and more than 90 cases have been reported. Careful genetic analysis of relapse cells is essential. VNTR, restriction fragment length polymorphism, STR analysis, or FISH XY analysis alone may not definitively assign the origin of the leukemic clone because genomic deletions or amplifications of chromosomal segments may occur during transplantation or disease process. The increased use of unrelated cord blood as a source of stem cells for allogeneic HCT raises the concern that hematopoietic progenitors containing preleukemic clonal molecular rearrangements may be inadvertently transplanted. Systematic screening of unselected cord blood samples revealed putative preleukemic rearrangements such as *ETV6-RUNX1* and *RUNX1-RUNXT1*. In a study of 1417 umbilical cord blood samples evidence for the *ETV6* or *RUNX1/RUNXT1* fusions were not found. However, recent reports comparing clinical characteristics of donor-cell derived leukemia (DCL) from the standpoint of the transplant source, with umbilical cord blood and bone marrow, showed in some studies, that AML and MDS were recognized more frequently in DCL after cord blood transplant, but not in other studies, whereas the incidence of AML and ALL was similar after bone marrow transplant. The median duration between the occurrence of DCL following cord blood and bone marrow transplant was 14.5 and 36 months, respectively ($p < .0001$). DCL occurred in a significantly shorter period after cord blood transplant than after marrow transplant. Abnormal karyotypes involving chromosome 7 were observed in 52.4% of cord blood recipients and 17.3% of marrow recipients ($p < .003$). The types of abnormal karyotypes in DCL following marrow transplant were similar to those characteristically observed in adult de novo AML and MDS. Patients with DCL generally have a poor prognosis in both groups. Stem cell transplantation is the best treatment for curing DCL. Therefore DCL appears to have different clinical features according to the transplant source. The reason for an increased risk for leukemia or myelodysplasia in donor cells is not understood and may be a function of the conditioning regimen used or the less stringent HLA matching required for unrelated cord blood stem cell transplantation. Specific mechanisms that result in development of DCL leukemia are unknown. Proposed mechanisms include the following: (a) sustained host-origin antigenic stimulation, (b) impaired hematopoietic microenvironment and defective stromal support system, (c) immune surveillance escape secondary to posttransplant immunosuppressive therapy, (d) similar genetic susceptibility in cases of related donors, (e) viral driven pathogenesis (cytomegalovirus, EBV), (f) delayed effects of conditioning regimen, and (g) transfection of host cell oncogene into donor cells. Most likely, the underlying cause is a combination of these mechanisms operating in individual cases. A very compelling hypothesis for the mechanisms leading to the development of DCL is the "2-hit" hypothesis. A donor HSC that has an inherent susceptibility to malignant transformation (hit 1) is placed within a defective stromal structure creating a microenvironment that elaborates repeated stress signals (hit 2), inducing additional genetic or even epigenetic mutations promoting malignant transformation.

Nevertheless, these patients must be carefully evaluated using an array of molecular methods for determination of leukemia in donor cells (see box on Genetic Testing for Hematopoietic Cell Transplantation). Ideally an examination of every sample before transplantation to determine whether the cord blood cells contain abnormal clones is suggested. In addition, long-term surveillance of stem cell transplant recipients and donors is also required (Fig. 56.69).

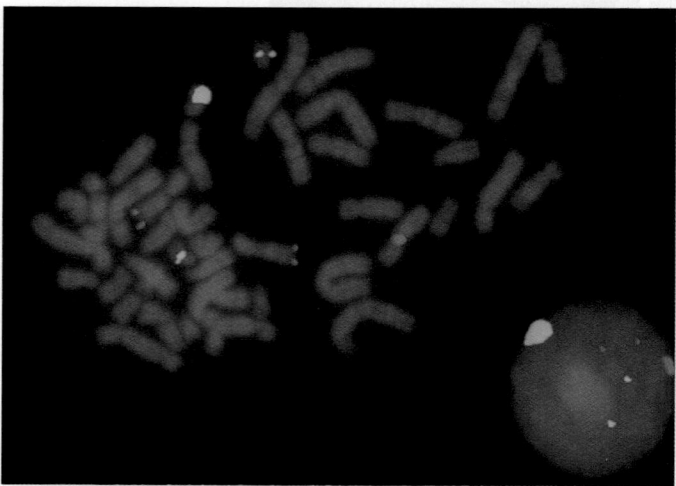
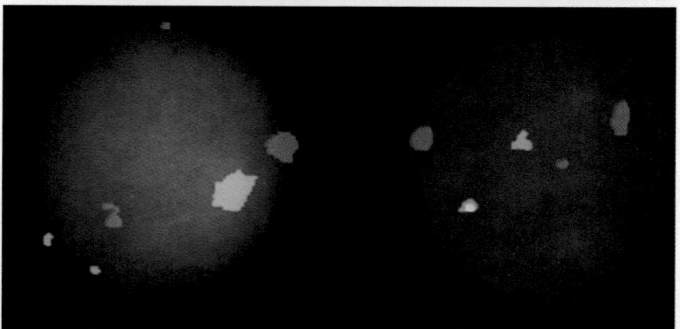

Fig. 56.68 DETECTION OF ENGRAFTMENT AND RESIDUAL DISEASE WITH FISH IN SEX-MISMATCHED HEMATOPOIETIC CELL TRANSPLANTATION. Metaphase and nondividing cell *(blue)* after DAPI counterstaining, hybridized with X *(large red)* and Y *(large green)* for detection of engraftment and with ABL *(small red)* and BCR *(small green)* for detection of residual chronic myelogenous leukemia *(top panel)*. Left nucleus *(bottom panel)* shows a donor male (XY) cell origin and lack of BCR-ABL fusion. In contrast, a host female (XX), BCR-ABL fusion *(yellow)*–positive cell is shown on the *right*. Combination of XY FISH probes with diagnostic genomic markers is a powerful and fast FISH method for simultaneous detection of chimerism and minimal residual disease.

Genetic Testing for Hematopoietic Cell Transplantation

Testing consists of either variable number of tandem repeats/short tandem repeats PCR for detection of engraftment in patients with sex-matched hematopoietic cell transplantation (HCT) or single-nucleotide polymorphism PCR, which has a high sensitivity. In sex-mismatched HCT, both interphase FISH with XY probes and real-time quantitative PCR for analysis of *SRY* gene on the Y chromosome can be used for detection of engraftment. Detection of both engraftment and minimal residual disease is best accomplished by FISH, simultaneously using probes for XY and the explicit probe for diagnostic genetic defect, such as XY and *BCR-ABL1*.

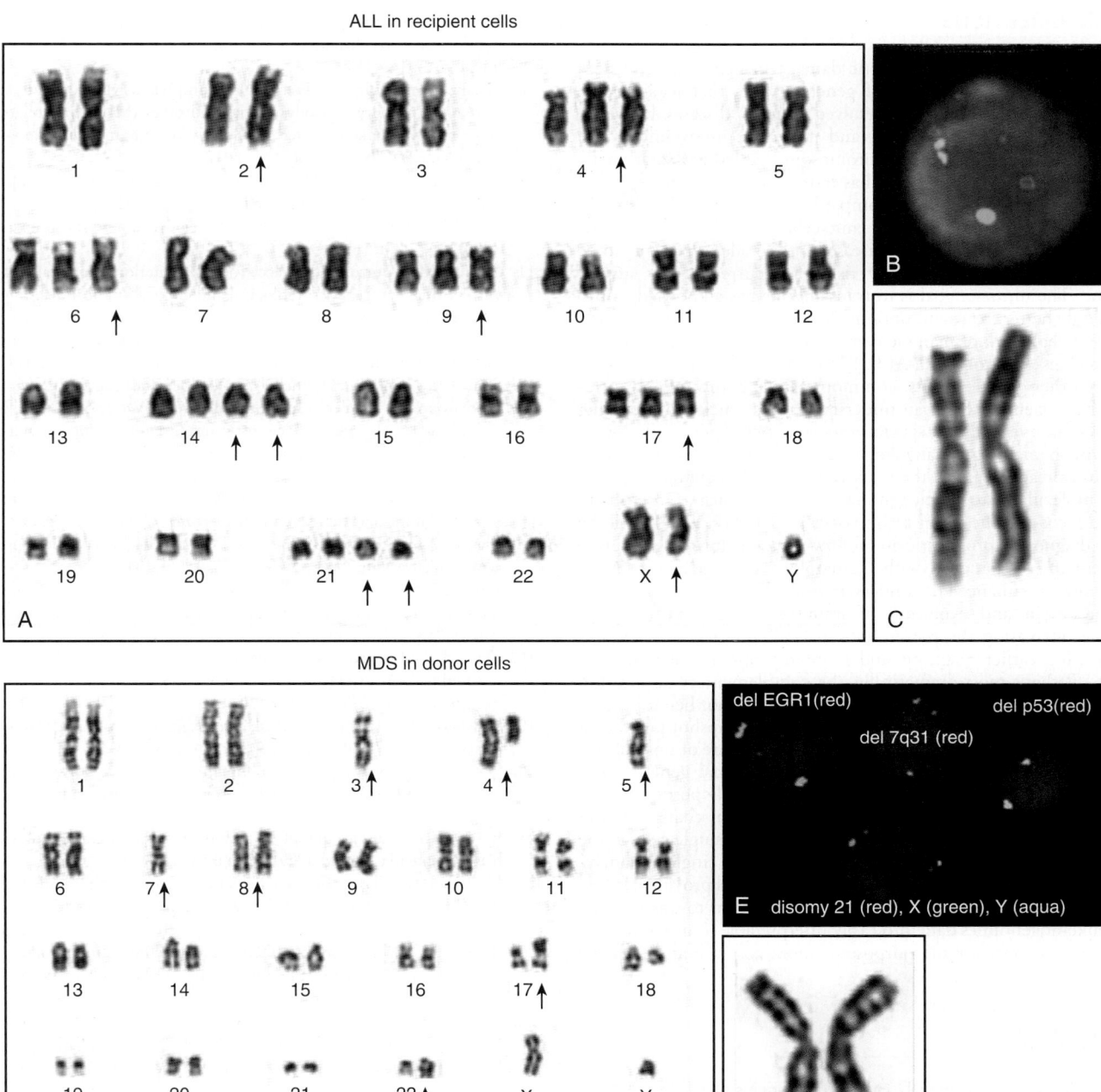

Fig. 56.69 DONOR-DERIVED MYELODYSPLASTIC SYNDROME (MDS) FOLLOWING CORD BLOOD TRANSPLANTATION IN ACUTE LYMPHOBLASTIC LEUKEMIA. (A) At diagnosis of acute lymphoblastic leukemia, in January 2006, cytogenetic analysis of bone marrow revealed a 56, XY, +X, inv(2)(p11.2q13), +4, +6, +9, +14, +14, +17, +18, +21, +21 hyperdiploid karyotype (*arrows* indicate abnormal chromosomes) hyperdiploid karyotype (*arrows* indicate abnormal chromosomes). (B). A bone marrow nucleus from a specimen obtained in January 2007 after FISH showed 5% of cells with tetrasomy 21 *(red signals)*, two copies of X chromosome *(green signals)*, and one copy of Y chromosome *(aqua)*. (C) A partial karyotype of chromosome 2 from the peripheral blood specimen, PHA-stimulated for 72 h, obtained in May 2006, showing a constitutional inversion (2)(p11.2q13). (D) At the time of the diagnosis of MDS in May 2011, bone marrow cytogenetic analysis revealed 65% of cells with a 44, XY, −3,del(4)(q23q33), der(5;17)(p10;q10), −7,t(8;22)(p21;q13), +mar karyotype (*arrows* indicate abnormal chromosomes). (E) Five bone marrow nuclei after FISH studies from the June 2011 specimen showing 75% cells with deletion of *EGR1* at 5q31 chromosomal location *(red)* and deletion of P53 at 17p13.1 chromosomal localization *(red)* as a result of der(5;17); 71% showing a loss of 7q31 locus as a result of monosomy 7, as well as disomy 21 *(red)*, one X *(green)*, and one Y *(aqua)* chromosome. (F) A partial bone marrow karyotype of chromosome 2 from May 2011 specimen showing a normal chromosome 2 from the donor cells and absence of inv(2) observed in the bone marrow and PHA-stimulated PB at the time of diagnosis peripheral blood specimen, PHA stimulated for 72 h, obtained in May 2006, showing a constitutional inversion (2)(p11.2q13). (D) At the time of the diagnosis of MDS in May 2011, bone marrow cytogenetic analysis revealed 65% of cells with a 44, XY, −3,del(4)(q23q33), der(5;17)(p10;q10), −7, t(8;22)(p21;q13), 1mar karyotype (*arrows* indicate abnormal chromosomes). (E) Five bone marrow nuclei after FISH studies from the June 2011 specimen showing 75% cells with deletion of *EGR1* at 5q31 chromosomal location *(red)* and deletion of *P53* at 17p13.1 chromosomal localization *(red)* as a result of der(5;17); 71% showing a loss of 7q31 locus as a result of monosomy 7, as well as disomy 21 *(red)*, one X *(green)*, and one Y *(aqua)* chromosome. (F) A partial bone marrow karyotype of chromosome 2 from May 2011 specimen showing a normal chromosome 2 from the donor cells and absence of inv(2) observed in the bone marrow and PHA-stimulated PB at the time of diagnosis. *(Reproduced with permission from Cotter R et al: Am J Hematol 87:931, 2012.)*

FUTURE DIRECTIONS

The question of how initial genetic damage in hematopoietic stem cell disorders causes a cascade of genetic events that leads to the development of malignancy is unresolved for many diseases. However, major advances have been made, and molecular unraveling of the consequence of the Philadelphia chromosome has led to the rationally designed imatinib treatment that has transformed CML from a fatal disease into a chronic disorder compatible with normal life. Precise molecular characterization of leukemic cells not only provides more insight into the pathogenesis of disease but also allows patients to be stratified as having high or low risk for recurrence and adverse outcome. The ultimate goal is to translate this basic knowledge into increasingly better treatment options. Molecular diversity is currently the genetic hallmark of many leukemias, even within a single disease entity such as AML or T-cell ALL. We are at the threshold of understanding other genetic events, common genetic pathways and intratumor heterogeneity. Such an understanding is crucial to designing molecular interventions for specific abnormalities of genetic pathways underlying hematologic malignancies. It is clear that the genetic revolution has already changed the practice of clinical hematology. In the future, molecular cytogenetics and cytogenomics, such as interphase-directed locus-specific FISH technologies and aCGH + SNP, will be the key diagnostic, prognostic and follow-up tools during the routine management of patients with hematologic malignancies. NGS technology has enhanced the understanding of leukemic pathogenesis and the origin and evolution of mutations and their temporal sequence, increasing the power for subclassifying leukemic entities and allowing earlier diagnosis and more appropriate treatment for patients. Perhaps most dramatically, the complementary application of these genetic methods has demonstrated intratumor heterogeneity. Nonetheless, modern genomic studies provide a snapshot portrait of the total DNA within the tumor along with a mixture of normal and abnormal cells. Systematic interrogation of subclonal genetic complexity and clonal architecture or phylogeny currently poses a technical challenge because three categories of mutational change; fusion genes, CNVs, and SNPs, need to be identified in a single cell. In the future, to construct a clonal evolutionary phylogeny, single cell analysis using genetic profiling at diagnosis and relapse will provide detailed subclonal genetic architecture. The challenge remains to translate the large leukemogenomics data into easily interpretable results accessible to the hematologist for the purpose of more accurate and effective therapies.

REFERENCES

1. Alpar D, Wren D, Ermini L, et al: Clonal origins of ETV6-RUNX1+ acute lymphoblastic leukemia: studies in monozygotic twins. *Leukemia* 29:839, 2015.
2. Greaves M: Darwin and evolutionary tales in leukemia. *Hematology* 3–12, 2009.
3. Yang L, Rau R, Goodell MA, et al: DNMT3A in haematological malignancies. *Nat Rev* 15:152, 2015.
4. Nowell PC, Hungerford DA: A minute chromosome in human chronic granulocytic leukemia. *Science* 132:1497, 1960.
5. Rowley JD: A new consistent chromosomal abnormality in chronic myelogenous leukemia identified by quinicrine fluorescence and Giemsa staining. *Nature* 243:290, 1973.
6. Martin PJ, Najfeld V, Hansen JA, et al: Involvement of the B-lymphoid system in chronic myelogenous leukemia. *Nature* 287:49, 1980.
7. Bhaskar A, Raturi K, Dang S, et al: Current perspectives on the therapeutic aspects of chronic myelogenous leukemia. *Expert Opin Ther Pat* 24:1117, 2014.
8. Schanz J, Tuchler H, Sole F, et al: New comprehensive cytogenetic scoring system for primary myelodysplastic syndromes (MDS) and oligoblastic acute myeloid leukemia after MDS derived from an international database merge. *J Clin Oncol* 30:820, 2012.
9. Jonas B, Greenberg P: MDS prognostic scoring systems – Past, present, and future. *Best Pract Res Clin Haematol* 28:3, 2015.
10. Ades L, Itzykson R, Fenaux P, et al: Myelodysplastic syndromes. *Lancet* 383:2239, 2014.
11. Martelli MP, Sportoletti P, Tiacci T, et al: Mutational landscape of AML with normal cytogenetics: biological and clinical implications. *Blood Rev* 27:13, 2013.
12. Jaiswal S, Fontanillas P, Flannick J, et al: Age-related clonal hematopoiesis associated with adverse outcomes. *N Engl J Med* 371:2488, 2014.
13. Shlush LI, Zandi S, Mitchell A, et al: Identification of pre-leukaemic haematopoietic stem cells in acute leukaemia. *Nature* 506:328, 2014.
14. Grimwade D, Mrózek D: Diagnostic and prognostic value of cytogenetics in acute myeloid leukemia. *Hematol Oncol Clin North Am* 25:1135, 2011.
15. De Braekeler E, Douet-Guilbert N, De Braekeler M: RARA fusion genes in acute promyelocytic leukemia. *Expert Rev Hematol* 7:347, 2014.
16. Meyer C, Hoffmann J, Burmeister T, et al: The MLL recombinome of acute leukemias in 2013. *Leukemia* 27:2165, 2013.
17. Wong TN, Ramsingh G, Young AL, et al: Role of TP53 mutations in the origin and evolution of therapy – related acute myeloid leukaemia. *Nature* 518:552, 2014.
18. Kayser S, Dohner K, Krauter J, et al: The impact of therapy-related acute myeloid leukemia (AML) on outcome in 2853 adult patients with newly diagnosed AML. *Blood* 117:37, 2011.
19. Welch JS, Ley TJ, Link DC, et al: The origin and evolution of mutations in acute myeloid leukemia. *Cell* 150:264, 2012.
20. Grossman G, Schnittger S, Kohlmann A, et al: A novel hierarchical prognostic model of AML solely based on molecular mutations. *Blood* 120:2963, 2012.
21. Bhojwani D, Yang J, Pui CH, et al: Biology of childhood acute lymphoblastic leukemia. *Pediatr Clin N Am* 62:47, 2015.
22. Mulligan CG: The genomic landscape of acute lymphoblastic leukemia in children and young adults. *Hematology Am Soc Hematol Educ Program* 2014:174, 2014.
23. Roberts KG, Mullighan CG: Genomics in acute lymphoblastic leukaemia: insights and treatment implications. *Nat Rev Clin Oncol* 12:344, 2015.
24. Harrison CJ: Blood Spotlight on iAMP21 acute lymphoblastic leukemia (ALL); a high-risk pediatric disease. *Blood* 125:1383, 2015.
25. Olsson L, Johansson B: Ikaros and leukaemia. *Br J Haematol* 169:479, 2015.
26. Dohner H, Stilgenbauer S, Benner A, et al: Genomic aberrations and survival in chronic lymphocytic leukemia. *N Engl J Med* 343:1910, 2000.
27. Bolli N, Avet-Loiseau H, Wedge DC, et al: Heterogeneity of genomic evolution and mutational profiles in multiple myeloma. *Nat Commun* 5:2997, 2014.
28. Correia C, Schneider PA, Dai H, et al: BCL2 mutations are associated with increased risk of transformation and shortened survival in follicular lymphoma. *Blood* 125:658, 2015.
29. Tiacci E, Trifonov V, Schiavoni G, et al: BRAF mutations in hairy-cell leukemia. *N Engl J Med* 364:2305, 2011.
30. Starza RL, Borga C, Barba G, et al: Genetic profile of T-cell acute lymphoblastic leukemias with MYC translocations. *Blood* 124:3577, 2014.

PHARMACOLOGY AND MOLECULAR MECHANISMS OF ANTINEOPLASTIC AGENTS FOR HEMATOLOGIC MALIGNANCIES

Stanton L. Gerson, Paolo F. Caimi, Basem M. William, and Richard J. Creger

The treatment of patients with hematologic malignancies has been revolutionized over the past decades as new therapeutic targets continue to be identified through cellular and molecular studies of these conditions. These investigations have spawned the discovery, clinical evaluation, and US Food and Drug Administration (FDA) approval of new mechanistic-based therapeutic agents. A surprising number of these agents have progressed from the discovery phases to validation, animal modeling, and successful clinical testing. The results have led to a virtual explosion in the therapeutic armamentarium and an increase in the spectrum of drugs including small molecules, monoclonal antibodies, radiolabeled antibodies, drug immunoconjugates, immunotoxins, and complex delivery systems. This chapter provides information on new and existing therapeutic agents available for the treatment of patients with hematologic malignancies. The chapter reviews the "classic" agents as well as the newly developed, target-based agents. Both cytotoxic and growth-inhibitory agents are covered; however, the use of therapeutic antibodies and antibody conjugates is reviewed within the chapters dealing with specific diseases.

TUMOR CELL HETEROGENEITY OF HEMATOLOGIC MALIGNANCIES

Whereas hematologic malignancies are of clonal origin (i.e., they are derived from a single transformed cell), individual neoplastic cells from a patient's malignancy exhibit a great deal of phenotypic diversity and acquire secondary mutations that affect proliferation, drug sensitivity, and resistance. This diversity likely arises from the progeny of clonal populations and subsets of stem cells. In animal models, it has been shown that the clones themselves can give rise to progeny that can transmit the clonal malignancy after transplantation into secondary recipients, suggesting that stem cells are not required to transmit the malignant phenotype.

New evidence indicates that leukemia stem cells are more quiescent, have higher levels of protective proteins such as efflux pumps for drugs, and have higher levels of DNA repair proteins or antiapoptotic proteins than the more abundant cell making up the circulating population of cells. Tumor cell heterogeneity arises as a consequence of spontaneous mutational events, changes in gene promoter methylation, abnormal expression of transcription factors, lymphoid reactivity, and cytokine responsiveness. For example, a mutation or change in expression that renders a hematopoietic cell clone autonomous or growth factor–independent would be expected to render such cells less susceptible to adverse environmental conditions (e.g., growth factor withdrawal). Similarly, one would also predict that a genetic change facilitating cell cycle entry or disruption of cellular maturation would ultimately lead to overgrowth of affected clones. For obvious reasons, mutations that interfere with drug metabolism or the cell death pathway itself would provide a net survival advantage, particularly under the selection pressure of cytotoxic drug treatment.

Malignant myeloid and lymphoid cells have many reasons to have increased mutational rates. Genomic instability can arise from dysregulation of the cell cycle machinery because of a number of events, including perturbations of cyclins leading to MYC overexpression; AKT activation; disruption of replication sequences; loss of DNA repair enzymes such as mismatch repair (MMR) enzymes; loss of proper homologous recombination from a defect in the BRCA–Fanconi pathways; and loss of ATM/ATR kinases, which can give rise to chromosomal recombination, loss, and microsatellite instability, and loss of checkpoint regulation. These events can give rise to intraclonal emergent point mutations, translocations, and intragenic losses that might not only result in malignant transformation, but also lead to disruption of genomic stability and selection in favor of proliferative and apoptosis-resistant subclones. Leukemic clonal evolution favors drug resistance.

Common mechanisms may be involved in events associated with malignant transformation and the development of mutations that result in tumor heterogeneity. For example, the cell cycle checkpoint and tumor suppressor gene, *TP53*, is induced during DNA damage, leading to G_1 arrest and, if the damage is too severe to repair, cell death by apoptosis occurs. The presumed goal of this process is to eliminate cells that develop deleterious mutations as a result of damage to the genome. Loss of *TP53* may not only increase cellular survival by inhibiting the cell death process, but may also promote the transmission of mutations that would otherwise be deleted. In this manner, a defect of the cell death pathway can have multiple consequences, including (1) selection of cells exhibiting a growth advantage over their normal counterparts, (2) development of drug resistance, and (3) promotion of mutations that result in either (1) or (2), as well as neoplastic cell heterogeneity. Age-dependent changes in these processes may explain the more favorable behavior of leukemias and lymphomas in response to chemotherapy in young patients than older patients.

A model of the relationship between tumor growth rate, the occurrence of spontaneous mutations, and the development of drug resistance was first described by Goldie and Coldman and is referred to as the Goldie and Coldman hypothesis. In this model, the size of a tumor depends on a complex interaction between tumor growth rate and cell loss, the latter stemming from the status of the cell death process, exhaustion of available nutrients, and outstripping of the blood supply. As tumors increase in size, the cell death rate tends to increase. The heterogeneous nature of additional mutations makes it likely that multiple mechanisms of resistance will develop as well. From an operational standpoint, this model has clear implications for the rational design of therapeutic strategies and provides a basis for early and intensive combination drug therapy. The successful implementation of this strategy is exemplified by the administration of dose-intensive multidrug regimens (i.e., the BEACOPP [bleomycin, etoposide, Adriamycin, cyclophosphamide, vincristine (Oncovin) procarbazine, and prednisone] regimen in Hodgkin lymphoma, CODOX-M-IVAC [cyclophoshamide, vincristine, doxorubicin, high-dose methotrexate alternating with ifosfamide, etoposide and high-dose cytarabine] in Burkitt lymphoma [non-Hodgkin lymphoma (NHL)]) and combinations of cytotoxic agents with monoclonal antibodies, such as CHOP (cyclophosphamide, hydroxydaunorubicin, vincristine [Oncovin], and prednisone)–rituximab, which are potentially curative when given early in the course of the disease. Other examples include combined use of multitargeted agents such as lenalidomide and bortezomib for myeloma, fludarabine, cyclophosphamide and rituximab for chronic lymphocytic leukemia (CLL), or maneuvers to overcome resistance of pretreated disease outside of cell-based therapies. However, as predicted by the model, administration of these or other intensive regimens in patients with relapsed or late-stage disease generally fails because of a generalized resistance of tumor cells to all classes of chemotherapeutic agents.

DEVELOPMENT OF CHEMOTHERAPEUTIC AGENTS

The quest for anticancer agents for hematologic malignancies began with the nitrogen mustard class of compounds developed from the chemical warfare agent sulfur mustard gas used in World War I. Since that time, the National Cancer Institute (NCI) and the pharmaceutical industry have developed complex approaches to drug development, screening, and evaluation. Initial screening consisted of toxicity assessment against murine tumor cell lines. Currently, screening is directed toward numerous cell targets, including receptor and downstream signaling kinases; inducers of cell death pathways, including those at the cell surface; mitochondrial enzymes; nuclear DNA and DNA replication, processing and repair proteins, including base excision repair, PARP, CHK1, topoisomerases, and telomerase; and inhibitors of histone deacetylase (HDAC) and histone methylation, cell cycle proteins, proteasomes, and the mitosis and spindle machinery. Therapeutic agents targeting microenvironment, angiogenesis, and immune checkpoints round out the spectrum of therapeutic approaches. Whereas killing cells had been the backbone of chemotherapeutic approaches to human malignancies, the field of antineoplastic agent development, which in the first decade of the 21st century was at a tipping point, has now embraced novel targeted and highly effective compounds that block the function of specific kinases with surprising efficacy, even at late stages of disease. Ultimately a balanced approach is likely, with much more precision in drug selection, use of mechanism-based combinations, and attention towards and anticipation of tumor heterogeneity, complex subclonality, and emergence of predictable resistance patterns that dictate proactive drug selection and utilization.

Examples include Bruton tyrosine kinase (Btk) and phosphatidylinositol 3-kinase (PI3K) inhibitors in lymphoid malignancies as well as Janus kinase (JAK) inhibitors for treatment of myelofibrosis and polycythemia vera. A number of differentiating agents, kinase inhibitors, and immunomodulatory and cytostatic agents complete the antineoplastic armamentarium. The field of drug development also has to contend with much more complex assessments of toxicities due to both on- and off-target effects, as well as normal tissue effects. In the sections that follow these toxicities will be noted because they restrict the utility of many drugs and toxicities need to be monitored when using new drug combinations.

Screening for Antitumor Activity Among Chemotherapeutic Agents

Identification of critical targets for therapy in cancer cells and the microenvironment starts with the recognition of a known or novel target that appears critical for cancer development, dormancy, growth, or metastasis. The NCI Division of Cancer Treatment has a well molecularly characterized cell bank of malignancies that are available for new drug screening. A more contemporary cell line resource is the Cancer Cell Line Encyclopedia (CCLE), developed to assist in drug analysis. It is a compilation of gene expression, chromosomal copy number, DNA sequence, and RNA data from 947 human cancer cell lines collected across databases and repositories. Many cell lines have drug sensitivity profiles from more than 20 anticancer drugs. Both academia and pharma utilize high-throughput gene knockdown (shRNA and siRNA) library approaches, drug screening using large compound libraries, and in silico screening based on protein and drug structures for docking analysis. Repurposed drugs that are FDA approved or for which there are extensive data provide a rich resource for lead compound identification. Medicinal chemistry can then be

applied to improve potency and specificity, solubility, kinetic profile, and tissue penetration and residence. For instance, to screen for a kinase inhibitor, cells overexpressing an activated kinase may be used. After an initial in vitro screen, human tumor cell activity is evaluated using a series of athymic mouse xenograft studies targeting tumors from tissues that show promise in vitro assays. More informative data is generated from banks of patient-derived tumor cell lines, often using Rho-associated kinase (ROCK) inhibition, and using patient-specific tumor xenografts for drug screening. These in vivo models consist of primary malignancies grown in immunodeficient mice, typically NSG mice. Some genetically engineer mice to express needed human cytokines that promote leukemic cell growth, or reconstitute mice with a human immune system to evaluate immunomodulatory drugs and cell-based immune responses. Another model system mimics the human disease by establishing mice with specific chromosomal translocations and oncogene mutations found in human cancers. Drug efficacy endpoints are complex, since target effects may produce cell death, senescence, apoptosis, differentiation, polyploidy, inhibition of metastasis, and loss of cancer stem cell populations. Drugs with promising efficacy and novel mechanisms of action then go on to formulation and toxicology testing, and are ultimately developed for phase I clinical testing through academic centers, industry, or the NCI Cancer Therapy Evaluation Program. Effective drug screening includes evidence of target effect specificity and potency, consideration of effects across tumor types, recognition of predictors of sensitivity and resistance that depend on the mechanism of action and known pathways of resistance, characterization of genetic changes associated with resistance and acquired resistance, and pharmacokinetic preclinical analysis. In all instances, animal studies often fail to provide accurate prediction of therapeutic efficacy, pharmacokinetics, emergence of resistance, or even toxicities.

Variants of patient-specific tumor xenograft (PDX) models, which allow for direct passage of human tumors in mice, include orthotopic models that assess the tissue microenvironment for tumor growth and drug efficacy, metastatic models that allow for removal of primary tumor and metastasis to the brain, lungs and bone, and direct implantation and metastasis, for instance into colon, spleen or marrow sites.

Phase I Clinical Trial Design

New anticancer agents are assessed through a series of clinical trials termed *phase I, phase II,* and *phase III* (Table 57.1). The purpose of phase I clinical trials is to establish the safe and optimal biochemically active dose of the compound in question with acceptable toxicity that can be used in disease-targeted phase II testing. During phase I development, pharmacokinetics and pharmacodynamic measures are studied in detail so that appreciable information can be forthcoming from the very first set of patients targeted for treatment and to allow confirmation of these observations in larger phase II disease-focused trials. Dose schedule and route of administration are key

TABLE 57.1	Clinical Trial Design

Phase I

Evaluate safety by dose escalation and multiple dose schedules

Establish maximum tolerated dose and dose-limiting toxicity

Consider use of hematopoietic support if myelosuppression is dose limiting

Phase II

Establish response (complete, partial, objective) in specific diseases

Phase III

Compare new treatment with established regimen for the disease in randomized trials

considerations in early phase I development. Numerous considerations have guided dose-escalation strategies that accompany phase I trial development. The starting dose is typically 10% of the lethal dose in animals adjusted for species dose equivalency. In classic phase I development, a modified Fibonacci dose schedule is used. Groups of three patients are treated at each of the following doses until the maximum tolerated dose is observed: 1N (the starting dose), 2N, 5N, 7N, 9N, 12N, and 16N. Typically, the maximum tolerated dose is defined as the maximum dose not causing irreversible toxicity of any type and causing less than grade 4 toxicity in any organ. Newer agents often have off-target toxicities, and these complicate drug evaluation because the dose-dependent toxicities are replaced by rashes, cardiac effects from prolonged QT intervals, activation or inhibition of other pathways, and unusual side effect profiles such as pleural and pericardial polyserositis. Typically, if one dose-limiting toxicity is observed, the patient cohort is expanded to six patients, and if two patients develop dose-limiting toxicity, typically defined as grade 4 toxicity except as previously noted, then further entry at this dose is not pursued, and the next lower dose level is used to establish the maximum tolerated dose with a total of six patients accrued at that dose level.[1]

Alternative strategies of drug escalation have included the use of toxicity grades to enhance dose escalation in early drug development, allowing that if no toxicity is observed, fewer patients might be accrued to each dose. Using the modified Fibonacci scheme, one patient is entered at each dose level until grade 2 toxicity is observed, at which point cohorts of three patients are entered at each level. Early in drug development, level skipping may take place if no toxicity is observed. The overall impact of this is to reduce the number of patients treated at suboptimal doses of therapy and to increase the number of patients evaluated at biologically active doses.

More importantly, biomarker-driven studies can be used to optimize inhibition of the target rather than treating to toxicity. This can then be extended in phase II to determine whether the drug effects on its biochemical target correspond to efficacy and tolerance.

Phase II Drug Development

Phase II drug development uses the established phase I dose to define therapeutic efficacy, typically in a two-stage design. If an expectant response rate in excess of 20% is deemed clinically significant, 15 patients are accrued, and if two or more responses are seen, accrual is continued to a total of 26 patients to establish the definite response rate. Modifications include phase Ib/II designs in specific diseases with dose escalations and efficacy assessments in a disease-specific manner. Phase II combination therapies optimize therapeutic efficacy, often with dose escalation of one or both agents. For instance, topotecan was found in phase I testing to have efficacy against refractory leukemias, leading to combinations of topotecan with ara-C. When a new agent is combined with an established agent, the new agent undergoes dose escalation. In the past, strategies for combination chemotherapeutic agents have included the use of non–cross-resistant agents with nonoverlapping toxicities. Mechanism-based therapeutic combinations have been more successful. In rare diseases, and now with genomic-driven studies, randomized phase II trials in a specific disease comparing standard to novel therapy can be used as evidence for drug approval, a "registration" trial.

Most phase III trials randomize patients between an established standard therapy and a new therapy that has appeared promising in the phase II setting. These studies are usually multi-institutional and many involve large national (e.g., National Clinical Trials Network) and international cooperative groups. The endpoint of these studies is disease response, time to progression (TTP), survival, and patient tolerance. Phase III trials are important for positive and negative results.[2] All trials must have rigorous objective data collection, safety and quality review, and reporting. All clinical trials should be registered at clinicaltrials.gov and all should have public reporting of results.

TRADITIONAL CYTOTOXIC ANTINEOPLASTIC AGENTS TARGETING THE CELL CYCLE AND DNA

Targeting Tumor Cell Growth Kinetics

Malignant hematopoietic cells proliferate more and differentiate less than their normal counterparts. The cell cycle consists of a series of stages through which normal and neoplastic cells proceed during the course of cellular replication (shown schematically in Fig. 57.1). The cell cycle is divided into G_1 (pre-DNA synthetic phase), S phase (in which DNA replication takes place), G_2 (post-DNA synthetic phase), and mitosis (M), during which chromosomal division and segregation occur. In addition, nonproliferating, resting cells reside in G_0, a phase that may theoretically last for an indefinite period. Such cells remain in G_0 until they are induced to cycle (at G_1) by specific triggers (e.g., hematopoietic growth factors). The growth fraction of a tumor

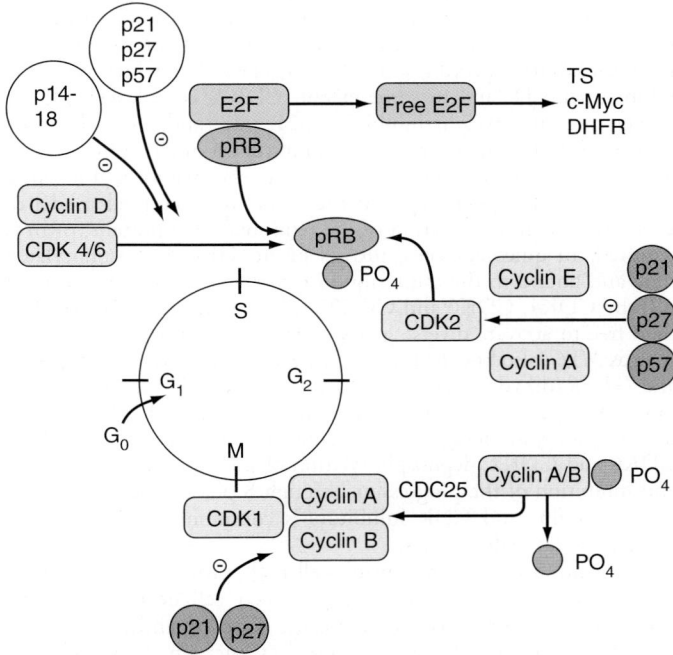

Fig. 57.1 PROGRESSION THROUGH THE CELL CYCLE IS CONTROLLED THROUGH COMPLEX INTERACTIONS AMONG CYCLINS, CYCLIN-DEPENDENT KINASES, AND CYCLIN-DEPENDENT KINASE INHIBITORS. Progression across the G_1S interface and through S phase involves the E2F transcription factor, which activates numerous enzymes (e.g., thymidylate synthase, dihydrofolate reductase) required for DNA replication. The pRb in its dephosphorylated state binds to and inactivates E2F in conjunction with DP proteins, thereby inhibiting S-phase progression. Conversely, phosphorylation of pRb antagonizes binding to E2F, allowing S-phase events to proceed. Phosphorylation of pRb results from activation of (1) CDK2:cyclin A/E and (2) CDK4/6:cyclin D complexes. The former complexes are inhibited by the CDK1s p21, p27 (and p57), and the latter are inhibited by the low-molecular-weight CDK inhibitors (p14–18) but also by p21 and p27. The complex formed by CDK1 (p34^{cdc2}) and cyclins A and B regulates G_2M progression and is inhibited by the "universal" CDK inhibitor, p21. Moreover, its phosphorylation status, which plays a major role in determining activity, is regulated by the phosphatase cdc25. Proteins such as pRb, E2F, p21, and p27 can influence the response of cells to chemotherapeutic agents by controlling cell cycle progression and possibly via cell cycle–unrelated actions. *CDK*, Cyclin-dependent kinase; *CDK2*, cyclin-dependent kinase-2; *DHFR*, dihydrofolate reductase; *pRb*, retinoblastoma protein.

represents the percentage of cycling cells relative to the total cell population. The generation time represents the time required for a cell to proceed through a single cell cycle (generally 24–36 hours for hematopoietic tissues). Surprisingly, in the case of acute myeloid leukemia (AML), the generation time of leukemic blasts is not shorter than that of normal hematopoietic progenitors and may be longer. The proliferative advantage of malignant hematopoietic cells (and of many nonhematopoietic tumors) stems, at least in part, from the fact that a higher percentage of cells are in cycle at any one point in time (i.e., the growth fraction is higher). The doubling time represents the period required for a tumor to double in mass and is, in general, inversely related to the tumor's growth fraction. Tumor-doubling times range from longer than 120 days in the case of some solid tumors (e.g., lung and colon) to less than 2 weeks (in some leukemias and lymphomas). Tumors with high growth fractions and short doubling times tend to be more sensitive to chemotherapy than slowly growing neoplasms with low growth fractions and long doubling times.

Cell cycle progression is governed by a complex network of proteins consisting of cyclins, cyclin-dependent kinases (CDKs), and CDK inhibitors. Progression through S phase is regulated primarily by CDK2 in association with cyclins A and E; progression through G_2M is regulated by CDK1 ($p34^{cdc2}$) and cyclins A and B; and progression through G_1 involves CDKs 4–6 in conjunction with cyclin D. CDK inhibitors fall into two major categories: the low-molecular-weight inhibitors (pINK14, -15, -16, -17, and -18), which primarily inhibit cyclin D (and to some extent, CDK2) complexes, and the higher molecular-weight inhibitors, p21, p27, and p57, which are more universal in their actions and inhibit most or all CDKs. Signals for the progression of cells through G_1S are essential for maintenance of the neoplastic phenotype. In the commonly accepted model of G_1S progression, inactivation of the retinoblastoma protein (pRb) is required. In quiescent cells, pRb is in an active dephosphorylated state and bound to the transcription factor E2F. Phosphorylation of pRb by CDK4, CDK6 and CDK2 leads to release of E2F, which is then free to activate diverse genes essential for S-phase progression, such as *MYC* (also known as c-Myc), *TYMS* (thymidylate synthetase), and *DHFR* (dihydrofolate reductase). Conversely, induction of CDK inhibitors (e.g., by transforming growth factor-β [TGF-β] or differentiation-inducing agents) results in inactivation of CDK4, CDK6 and CDK2, dephosphorylation of pRb, inactivation of E2F, and inhibition of the progression through S phase. Aberrant expression of cyclins and CDK inhibitors is commonly encountered in hematopoietic malignancies.

In addition to growth control, cell cycle proteins are intimately involved in the regulation of programmed cell death (apoptosis) and checkpoint control mechanisms. Consequently, cell cycle regulatory proteins can exert a major influence on the response of neoplastic cells to cytotoxic agents. For example, when cells undergo DNA damage, they may arrest in G_2M or G_1, during which repair occurs, or if the damage is too severe, the cells undergo apoptosis. In particular, the tumor suppressor gene *TP53* and its downstream inducible target p21 have been implicated in the G_1 arrest process after genotoxic insult. Dysregulation of various cell cycle regulatory proteins can have a major impact on the sensitivity of neoplastic cells to chemotherapeutic agents. Loss of the *TP53* gene renders cells resistant to diverse chemotherapeutic agents, presumably by preventing cells from undergoing repair in G_1 and thereby inhibiting the cell death processes and allowing DNA damage to accumulate, culminating in cellular transformation. Conversely, transfection of P53-negative cells with wild-type P53 restores responsiveness to most drugs. Dysregulation of the CDK inhibitors p21 (a downstream target of P53) and p27 increases the sensitivity of neoplastic cells to various cytotoxic agents, possibly by uncoupling S-phase progression and mitosis. After DNA damage, checkpoints block the cell cycle, but loss of the CDK inhibitors p21 or p27 prevents cells from arresting in G_1 and cells die during G_2M. Mutations in the E2F protein have been shown to lengthen S phase and increase the sensitivity of malignant cells to S-phase–specific agents. Furthermore, cells lacking functional pRb have been shown to be

significantly less sensitive to the actions of antimetabolites, including methotrexate.

In vivo the growth of tumors is limited by various factors such as vascular supply, nutritional requirements, and possibly physical restraints. Consequently the rate of tumor growth declines as the number of cells increases. To the extent that tumor-doubling times are inversely correlated with drug responsiveness, large, late-stage tumors are less susceptible to cytotoxic drugs than early-stage tumors, with higher growth fractions. Most chemotherapeutic drugs kill by first-order kinetics. The implication of this phenomenon is that it requires the same drug dose to reduce the number of tumor cells from 10^4 to 10^1 cells as it does to reduce the tumor burden from 10^{10} to 10^7 cells.

Hematopoietic malignancy-initiating or stem cells, such as leukemia stem cells, appear to explain resistance and treatment failure. These cells express high levels of hematopoietic stem cell proteins and markers, and are resistant to cell cycle–specific agents because of an increase in quiescent cell populations. They overlap with normal hematopoiesis stem cells and there appears to be a set of HSCs that contain preleukemic-promoting mutations that both predispose and may be sufficient for conversion to leukemic stem cells. The proteins expressed by these cells have become targets of therapy, including alterations in DNA damage, quiescent cell cycle factors such as the thrombopoietin receptor MPL, stem cell proliferation signals such as NOTCH and WNT protein families, and niche occupancy proteins such as KIT.

Cytotoxic agents may be divided into several categories with respect to their effects on the cell cycle or the cell cycle specificity of their actions, or both.

1. *Noncycle-active drugs* kill both cycling and noncycling cells in all phases of the cell cycle. Examples include steroids and antitumor antibiotics (except bleomycin).
2. *Cycle-active, nonphase-specific drugs* are more active against cycling cells and can kill cells in each phase of the cell cycle. However, such drugs may preferentially kill cells in a particular phase of the cell cycle. Examples include alkylating agents, cisplatin, and 5-fluorouracil (5-FU).
3. *Cycle-active, phase-specific drugs* primarily kill cells in a specific phase of the cell cycle. Examples include most antimetabolites, which are active against cells engaged in DNA synthesis (S-phase cells), and microtubule-active drugs (e.g., vinca alkaloids, taxanes), which kill cells in G_2M.

An example of a cytokinetically rational approach to chemotherapy involves the combination of a noncycle-active agent (e.g., daunorubicin) with a cycle- and a phase-specific agent (e.g., ara-C, fludarabine, decitabine, gemcitabine, clofarabine and nelarabine). From a theoretical standpoint, administration of a noncycle-active agent may reduce tumor mass, leading in turn to an increase in the growth fraction caused by recruitment of cells into cycle. Such cells would then be more susceptible to a cycle- and phase-specific agent, particularly one administered over a prolonged interval. In the case of hematopoietic malignancies, attempts have been made to recruit neoplastic cells into the more susceptible S phase of the cell cycle through the use of hematopoietic growth factors. The success of such a strategy has been limited because of several factors, including the inability of growth factors to increase the S-phase fraction significantly, the lack of selectivity of this strategy, and the theoretical possibility that growth factors may protect neoplastic cells from apoptosis.

Unfortunately, cytokinetic differences between normal and neoplastic tissues have been difficult to exploit. Both normal hematopoietic stem cells and hematologic malignant stem cells have a low proportion of cells in G_1. However, prolonged dosage schedules can provoke these malignant cells into cell cycle and may explain their efficacy. Consequently, rapidly dividing normal tissues such as gastrointestinal epithelium and normal hematopoietic progenitors tend to be very sensitive to most chemotherapeutic agents. As a result, mucositis and myelosuppression represent frequent dose-limiting toxicities for many cytotoxic drugs.

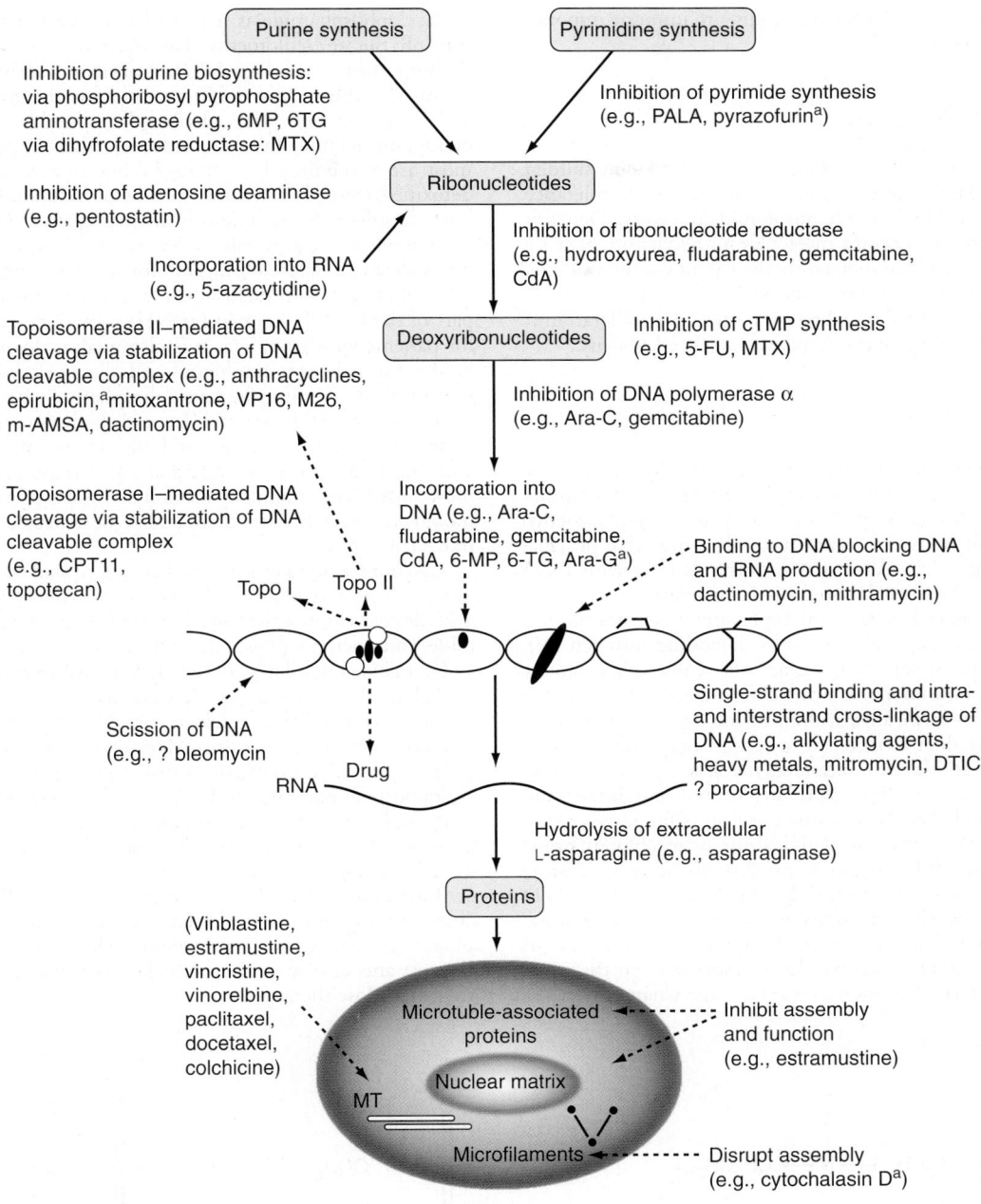

Fig. 57.2 OVERVIEW OF SITES AND MECHANISMS OF ACTION OF THE MOST USEFUL CHEMOTHERAPEUTIC AGENTS. *5-FU,* 5-Fluorouracil; *6-MP,* 6-mercaptopurine; *ara-C,* cytarabine; *ara-G,* 9'-β-D-arabinofuranosylguanine; *DTIC,* dacarbazine; *Topo,* topoisomerase.

Newer agents that target cell cycle proteins are often first utilized in patients with hematologic malignancies. As noted in the section on CDK and CHK1 inhibitors, these agents can have potent cytotoxic effects on dividing cells.

PHARMACOLOGY OF TRADITIONAL CHEMOTHERAPEUTIC AGENTS

Traditional agents are classified by their site of action, and as such all have a targeted mechanism, albeit not that of newer kinase targeted agents. They are divided into alkylating agents, antimicrotubule agents, antimetabolites, topoisomerase I or II inhibitors, platinum analogs, and miscellaneous agents. The pharmacology and cellular mechanisms of action of these agents are schematically presented in Fig. 57.2.

Alkylating Agents

Drug treatment for cancer began with the use of the mustard class of alkylating agents, initially mechlorethamine (nitrogen mustard), which entered into clinical use in the mid-1940s. Alkylating agents are used in many regimens but are rapidly being supplanted by newer classes of agents.

All alkylating agents undergo molecular rearrangements to form covalent bonds to DNA bases. Some form monoadducts, while others form cross-links either with intrastrand or interstrand bases, or with adjacent proteins. All alkylating agents are cytotoxic to tumor cells through interruption of DNA replication, induction of DNA damage repair and stress response, or through checkpoints in the cell cycle that result in apoptosis, senescence, or necrosis. All alkylating agents induce DNA strand breaks directly or through the damage response. Alkylating agents can also cause DNA mutations that can induce a cytotoxic response or can alter proteins, leading to immune responses to novel protein sequences.

Mechanisms of Resistance

Efficient removal of the DNA adducts reduces the lesion burden, while loss of DNA damage recognition can invoke damage tolerance, as in the case of loss of MMR and temozolomide tolerance. Detoxifying enzymes can serve as acceptor molecules for alkylation, alter the agent prior to DNA attack, or metabolize the parent compound. Loss of TP53 results in loss of cell cycle checkpoint induction of DNA repair signals. Increased AKT signaling promotes cell proliferation to compensate for the DNA damage response-associated toxicity.

Nitrogen Mustard

The nitrogen mustard class includes mechlorethamine, cyclophosphamide, 4-hydroperoxy cyclophosphamide, ifosfamide, chlorambucil, and melphalan. These drugs all share a common bischloroethyl group attached to nitrogen and a substituted "R" group that provides drug specificity (Fig. 57.3). All nitrogen mustards react with DNA in an SN_2 reaction, a bimolecular nucleophilic displacement reaction also called a *second-order reaction*. Although numerous sites are targeted for alkylation, nucleophiles in DNA, including nitrogen (N), oxygen (O), and phosphate (P), attract the chloroethyl moiety attached to the R–N backbone, and the chlorine is displaced by the nucleophilic atom to form an aziridinium moiety. The remaining chloroethyl group is then attracted to a second nucleophilic atom, forming a second aziridinium intermediate, leading to a second alkylation, forming a cross-link. Both intrastrand and interstrand cross-links are formed. The N^7 guanine position is the most critical for cytotoxic cross-link formation. Clinical use of mechlorethamine is limited because the MOPP regimen (mechlorethamine, vincristine [Oncovin], procarbazine, prednisone) has been replaced by ABVD (doxorubicin [Adriamycin], bleomycin, vinblastine, dacarbazine [DTIC]) in Hodgkin lymphoma (see Chapter 75). Local use of mechlorethamine occurs in a dermatologic suspension for the treatment of cutaneous T-cell lymphomas (CTCLs; see Chapter 85).

Cyclophosphamide is a nitrogen mustard with a ringed structure off the end-chloroethyl backbone that decreases spontaneous decomposition (see Fig. 57.3). Enzymatic activation is required through multifunction P450 enzymes in the liver. Phenobarbital and corticosteroids may alter activation. The bioavailability of cyclophosphamide orally and intravenously is quite similar, although most use of the drug is by bolus IV injection. Cyclophosphamide is detoxified through oxidation to 4-keto-cyclophosphamide and carboxyphosphamide by aldehyde dehydrogenase. Cyclophosphamide is used in doses as small as 50–100 mg/day orally (PO) and in bolus doses of 400–700 mg/m² for solid tumors and 750 mg/m² in combination with doxorubicin and vincristine and prednisone as part of the CHOP regimen for NHLs, or alone or with bortezomib for patients with myeloma. It is also used at doses of up to 60 mg/kg/day for 4 days in autologous and allogeneic bone marrow (BM) transplantation protocols. Cyclophosphamide is used in numerous treatment protocols for NHLs and high-dose therapy regimens designed to eradicate tumor and BM in patients with lymphomas and leukemias and those undergoing BM transplantation. It is commonly used with granulocyte colony-stimulating factor (G-CSF) for mobilizing hematopoietic stem cells to be collected before autologous transplantation.

Cyclophosphamide is metabolically activated by cytochrome P450 mixed function oxidases in the liver to 4-hydroxycyclophosphamide. 4-Hydroxycyclophosphamide is further converted to aldophosphamide and then to phosphoramide mustard, the alkylated species, and acrolein. High levels of aldehyde dehydrogenase detoxify cyclophosphamide in hematopoietic stem cells and, thus, high doses are not marrow ablative. Acrolein is a highly reactive aldehyde and the cause of hemorrhagic cystitis. Mercaptoethane sulfonate (Mesna) is used to provide prophylaxis against hemorrhagic cystitis caused by cyclophosphamide and ifosfamide, and is now standard for doses of cyclophosphamide and ifosfamide above 1000 mg/m². Mesna is given in divided doses every 4 hours or as a continuous infusion for 18–24 hours in a dose equivalent to either cyclophosphamide or ifosfamide. Other than hemorrhagic cystitis, BM suppression is dose limiting and can be rescued by reinfusion of autologous or allogeneic hematopoietic progenitor cells. Other toxicities include alopecia and cardiac toxicity, which is unusual and most often seen after high-dose therapy.

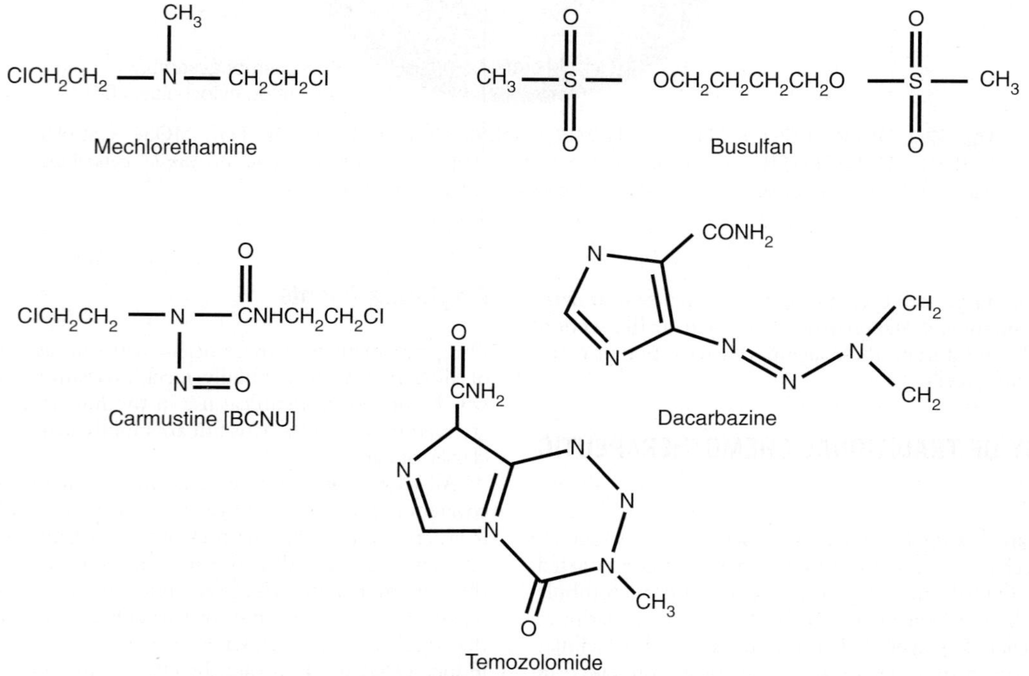

Fig. 57.3 STRUCTURE OF COMMON ALKYLATING AGENTS.

4-Hydroperoxycyclophosphamide, a chemically stable form of the reactive intermediate of cyclophosphamide, 4-hydroxycyclophosphamide, is more toxic to committed hematopoietic progenitors such as colony-forming unit–granulocyte/macrophages (CFU-GM), burst-forming unit–erythroids (BFU-E), and colony-forming unit–erythroids (CFU-E).

Melphalan, or phenylalanine mustard, has an amino acid side chain that alters its cellular uptake and stabilizes its structure, allowing PO administration (see Fig. 57.3). It is available in both PO and IV forms, and has a similar effect on DNA cross-linking as cyclophosphamide and the other nitrogen mustards. Melphalan uptake by cells is by means of a neutral amino acid transporter. Its rate of cross-link formation is much slower than that of mechlorethamine, presumably because of delayed metabolism. Oral melphalan is used predominantly for the standard treatment of multiple myeloma (MM) and IV in high-dose regimens in preparation for stem cell transplantation (see Chapter 86) for MM patients.

Chlorambucil has been used for more than 40 years for the treatment of CLL. Chlorambucil is the phenylbutyric acid derivative of nitrogen mustard and is very stable, entering the cell by diffusion rather than by a specific uptake mechanism. It is typically administered orally on a daily basis or intermittently. It appears to have greater bioavailability than melphalan and a more consistent half-life of approximately 2 hours.

Busulfan is an alkylsulfonate unique among alkylating agents because of two sulfur groups and lack of a chloroethyl moiety (see Fig. 57.3). Busulfan, similar to the nitrogen mustards, reacts predominantly at the N^7 position of guanine and produces an N^7–N^7 biguanyl DNA cross-link, although the precise nature of this cross-link appears different than that of the nitrogen mustards. The pharmacokinetics of busulfan is important for its use in high-dose therapy for ablation of the BM in patients undergoing autologous transplantation for acute leukemia or allogeneic stem cell transplantation (see Chapter 104). Because the incidence of venooclusive disease is lower in patients receiving high-dose busulfan with predosing pharmacokinetics performed, this is now recommended in high-dose regimens, the target being an area under the curve (AUC) of 1125 μmol/L × min (range 900–1350) with every 6 hour dosing. Busulfan is a potent stem cell toxin, killing both early and late hematopoietic progenitor cells and damaging the BM stroma. Other toxicities of busulfan include nausea and vomiting, and pulmonary interstitial and intraalveolar edema leading to fibrosis. The pulmonary fibrosis is distinct from the interstitial pneumonitis, which accompanies allogeneic stem cell transplantation and is not related to cytomegalovirus or other viral infections.

Nitrosoureas

Four chloroethyl nitrosoureas and one methyl nitrosourea are in clinical use. These agents are different from the nitrogen mustards in that they alkylate through an SN^1 reaction, forming a highly reactive intermediate in the presence of N, O, and P nucleophiles in DNA. The commonly used clinical agent is (2-chloroethyl)-N-nitrosourea (BCNU). N-[(4-amino-2-methyl-5-pyrimidinyl) methyl]-N-(2-chloroethyl)-N-nitrosourea (ACNU) is commonly used in Japan. A third agent, N-(2-chloroethyl)-N-cyclohexyl-N-nitrosourea (CCNU), is used predominantly as an PO nitrosourea in children with brain tumors. All of these compounds have high hydrophobicity, actively penetrating the blood–brain barrier.

The DNA alkylation sites include N^7 and O^6 of guanine. Chloroethylation at the O^6 position of guanine appears critical to cytotoxicity. DNA cross-linking by chloroethyl nitrosoureas include at 1-(3-cytosinyl), 2-(1-guanyl) ethane, and 1-2-bis(7-guanyl) ethane. The former is responsible for much of the cytotoxicity observed with the chloroethyl nitrosoureas. It is formed after alkylation at the O^6 position of guanine. This adduct undergoes intramolecular rearrangement to a circular intermediate, N^1. O^6 ethanoguanine is formed, which can then rearrange by attack at the opposite hydrogen-bonded base N^3 of cystine, forming the interstrand cross-link. This is a unique

DNA cross-link and is poorly recognized by DNA repair processes, leading to marked cytotoxic potency of this cross-link.

The pharmacokinetics of the chloroethyl nitrosoureas reveal a very short half-life. BCNU is predominantly used for high-dose treatment of recurrent lymphomas. Regimens including BCNU induce sustained complete remission (CR) rates of approximately 40%–60%. Doses of between 300 and 600 mg/m² have been safely administered. The chloroethyl nitrosoureas cause profound and cumulative BM suppression at conventional doses of 120–150 mg/m², limiting treatment to three to five cycles at 6-week intervals.

Complications of high-dose BCNU therapy include pulmonary toxicity and renal toxicity at doses higher than 600 mg/m². Pulmonary toxicity, as evidenced by a decrease in the DL_{CO} (diffusing capacity of the lung for carbon monoxide), occurs in up to 40% of patients. It can be managed with high-dose oral steroids during the inflammatory phase. Interstitial nephritis with glomerulosclerosis, interstitial fibrosis, and dropout of tubules has been reported with BCNU or CCNU.

Methylating Agents

Four methylating alkylating agents are in clinical use. These include procarbazine, DTIC, streptozotocin, and temozolomide. Procarbazine and DTIC are triazines. Streptozotocin is a monofunctional methyl nitrosourea derivative with an attached sugar moiety, and temozolomide is an imidazotetrazine. All react with DNA by undergoing SN^1 reactions forming a methyldiazonium ion, resulting in methylation of N^7 guanine (67%), O^6 guanine (9%), O^4 and O^2 thymine (2%), and N^3 adenine (3%). None form DNA cross-links. However, all induce high levels of DNA methylation, and their recognition and repair results in both single- and double-strand breaks. N^7 methylguanine is removed through the BER system. Recognition by the N-methylpurine glycosylase results in removal of the adducted base with formation of an abasic site that is recognized by the apurinic (AP) endonuclease, which then cleaves the backbone at the AP site. Subsequently, the free 5′ sugar is released by DNA lyase, with repair initiated by β-polymerase and DNA ligase. BER effectively removes N^7 methylguanine and N^3 methyladenine, and restores DNA to normal. Inhibition of BER by the investigational agent methoxyamine (TRC102) blocks this pathway and increases toxicity.

O^6 methylguanine mispairs with thymine during DNA synthesis, resulting in a lesion recognized by the MMR system. Mispair recognition proteins are MSH6, MSH3, and MSH2. Recognition of the mispair recruits additional proteins to the complex, including MLH1 and PMS1/PMS2. These proteins initiate exonuclease cleavage of a long patch in the newly synthesized strand of DNA. This is then repaired by polymerases-δ and -ε. If unrepaired, a thymine is repeatedly inserted opposite the O^6 methylguanine, resulting in multiple single-strand breaks. Cells expressing high levels of the DNA repair protein for O^6 methylguanine, O^6 methylguanine-DNA methyltransferase (MGMT), are approximately 10-fold more resistant to methylating agents than MGMT-negative cells. Cells lacking MMR are very resistant to methylating agents. Acquisition of MMR defects is associated with acquired resistance to methylating agents and cisplatin, which is also recognized by this protein complex.

Procarbazine was synthesized as a monoamine oxidase inhibitor and has been used since the 1950s for the treatment of Hodgkin lymphoma and NHL, as well as a component of combination therapies for gliomas. DTIC is metabolically activated by cytochrome P450 microsomal oxidoreductases, ultimately leading to formation of the methyldiazonium ion and DNA methylation. DTIC is used in combination with ABVD for treating Hodgkin lymphoma (see Chapter 75) and is also used for patients with metastatic malignant melanoma in combination with BCNU, cisplatin, and tamoxifen. Activation of DTIC requires hydroxylation of one terminal methyl group caused by demethylation forming 5-[3-methyl-triazen-1-yl]-imidazole-4-carboxamide (MTIC), with spontaneous decomposition to the methyldiazonium ion, which alkylates the DNA, as noted earlier. Maximum tolerated doses of DTIC are approximately

1000 mg/m^2, with myelosuppression and gastrointestinal toxicity (including severe watery diarrhea) being the most common side effects.

Temozolomide represents an imidazotetrazinone. It differs from DTIC in that it is chemically degraded to the monomethyl triazine, MTIC, at neutral pH and does not require P450 enzymatic demethylation. Compared with DTIC, temozolomide has much more consistent pharmacokinetic parameters, including peak serum concentrations, volume of distribution and clearance, and conversion to MTIC. Clinical studies documented considerable activity in acute leukemias. The dose-limiting toxicity was thrombocytopenia and, less frequently, neutropenia, with maximum tolerated doses of 1000 mg/m^2 given over 5 days on a daily or twice-daily regimen. Nausea and vomiting were the other common side effects, easily controlled with antiemetics.

Bendamustine

Bendamustine is comprised of a 2-chloroethylamine nitrogen mustard alkylating group, a benzimidazole ring, and a butyric acid side chain. Its mechanism of action is unknown but appears to be different to other alkylating agents, causing DNA damage that is repaired predominantly by the base-excision repair system and has activity against lymphoid cell lines resistant to alkylating agents.[3] Myelosuppression with leukopenia and thrombocytopenia is the most frequent side effect, with mild nonhematologic side effects including nausea, fatigue, constipation and diarrhea. Phase III studies comparing standard treatment with bendamustine and rituximab in front-line treatment of CLL[4] and indolent lymphomas (see Chapter 77) have established this combination as first-line treatment. Bendamustine is also active against MM, and combinations with steroids and bortezomib or the immunomodulatory agents thalidomide and lenalidomide have been reported to result in high response rates in patients with relapsed or refractory disease.

Alkylating Agent–Induced Leukemias

Alkylating agents induce dose-limiting myelosuppression and cause sublethal DNA damage to hematopoietic progenitors, causing mutational events that lead to malignant transformation to preleukemic and leukemic states. A concern exists about the use of hematopoietic growth factors after exposure to alkylating agents (see Chapter 59). There is evidence of increased cytotoxicity to hematopoietic progenitors during simultaneous exposure to these agents and growth factors. Treatment-related AML (T-AML) accounts for approximately 15% of all adult AML. Approximately 50% of T-AML patients have a preleukemic phase compared with only 10% of patients with de novo AML. CRs are achieved in 15%–30% of patients with T-AML and a mean remission duration of 2 months. Chromosomal abnormalities and gene mutations characteristic of T-AML establish this as a distinct disease requiring novel therapeutic approaches. Loss or deletion of all or part of the long arm [q] of chromosomes 5 or 7 is common, as are trisomy 8 and deletions of the short arm of chromosomes 12, 17, and 21.

Historically, patients with Hodgkin lymphoma treated with mechlorethamine and procarbazine in the MOPP regimen or with CCNU were at the highest risk if exposed to radiation as well as an alkylating agent combination. Patients with polycythemia vera treated with chlorambucil were at much higher risk than patients treated with phlebotomy alone, which can contribute to a shift in treatment strategy. Patients with myeloma and ovarian cancer have developed T-AML, especially after prolonged exposure to alkylating agents. Patients treated with alkylating agents for benign diseases such as nephritis, lupus, psoriasis, rheumatoid arthritis, and Wegener granulomatosis also have an increased risk of T-AML. The mean latency between exposure and T-AML from alkylating agents is 4–5 years, in contrast to T-AML from etoposide, which has a latency period as short as 1 year. The cumulative risk of developing T-AML is between 10% and 17% at 4–6 years for myeloma patients treated with melphalan and between 2% and 10% at 7–10 years in patients with Hodgkin lymphoma. Alkylating agent-associated T-AML has also been recognized in patients with breast and colon cancer.

Antimicrotubule Agents

The antimicrotubule drugs include the vinca alkaloids (e.g., vincristine, vinblastine, vinorelbine and vindesine), taxanes (e.g., paclitaxel and docetaxel), and epothilones (ixabepilone).

Molecular Targets

The vinca alkaloids are naturally occurring (vincristine and vinblastine) or semisynthetic (vinorelbine) nitrogenous bases derived from the pink periwinkle plant, *Catharanthus roseus*. Paclitaxel was originally isolated from the bark of the Pacific yew, *Taxus brevifolia*. Paclitaxel can also be isolated from other members of the *Taxus* genus and from a fungal endophyte that grows on the Pacific yew. Docetaxel is derived semisynthetically from 10-deacetyl-baccatin III, which is obtained from the needles of the European yew, *Taxus baccata*.

The vinca alkaloids bind to the protein tubulin at a site distinct from that of the taxanes and, at low concentrations, inhibit microtubule dynamics. At higher concentrations, these vinca alkaloids disrupt microtubules and mitotic spindle, resulting in cell cycle mitotic arrest and apoptosis of cells (see Fig. 57.3). In contrast, after binding to α-tubulin, taxanes kinetically stabilize microtubule dynamics at their plus ends and shift the equilibrium toward tubulin polymerization into microtubule bundles. This also causes mitotic arrest and apoptosis of cells. The mitotic arrest caused by antimicrotubule drugs is associated with phosphorylation of the B-cell lymphoma (BCL2) protein and increased intracellular levels of the BCL2-associated X protein (Bax), which promote apoptosis.

As natural products, overexpression of the efflux pump multidrug resistance gene-1 (MDR-1) and the ABCB-1 transporter mediate resistance. Intracellular resistance to mitotic spindle and microtubule formation is mediated by numerous pathways and proliferative signals including MYC, nuclear factor kappa-B (NFκB) and AKT.

Antimicrotubule agents, particularly the vinca alkaloids, are used in the management of lymphomas and leukemias, and continue to be used in the mainstay of clinical chemotherapeutic regimens. Because of their mechanism of action, they are best used in multiagent combinations, in which potentiation of efficacy with other classes of agents, such as antimetabolites and DNA-damaging agents, provide better therapeutic responses and well-tolerated treatments.

Inhibitors of Nucleotide Synthesis

Within this class are two important agents used for hematologic malignancies, hydroxyurea and methotrexate. They both serve to disrupt nucleotide synthesis, and slow or stop DNA and RNA synthesis.

Hydroxyurea

Hydroxyurea inhibits ribonucleotide diphosphate reductase, blocking de novo synthesis of purines and pyrimidines. S-phase arrest is commonly observed. Given this exquisite cell cycle specificity, resting and quiescent cells are rarely affected and there is virtually no hematopoietic stem cell toxicity. As a consequence of disruption of nucleotide synthesis and direct binding to telomere binding factors, telomere synthesis and function are compromised in leukemic cells. In cells arrested in S phase, apoptosis and senescence are observed.

Hydroxyurea is used in the treatment of myeloproliferative neoplasms including essential thrombocythemia, polycythemia vera and myelofibrosis (Chapters 68–70). It may also be used for acute cytoreduction prior to induction therapy of AML and for management of chronic myelomonocytic leukemia. It is commonly used for extended periods of time to induce fetal hemoglobin and reduce sickle crisis in patients with sickle cell anemia (Chapter 42).

Folic Acid Analogs (e.g., Methotrexate)

Folic acid analogues block the formation of thymidine, resulting in accumulation of UMP, leading to high levels of UTP, which is incorporated into DNA and causes purine nucleotide pool imbalance, slowing DNA synthesis. These agents bind thymidylate synthase and dihydrofolate reductase, and disrupt cell cycle progression and cell division. Methotrexate polyglutamation results in higher affinity binding to DHFR and improved inhibition. Aminopterin, the first antifolate, was used by Sidney Farber (reported in 1948) and became one the first chemotherapeutic agents to be administered with success to children with acute lymphocytic leukemia (ALL). Methotrexate is the agent currently used in hematologic diseases, while the family of agents includes pemetrexed and trimetrexate. Inhibition of folate-dependent methyl transfer enzymes disrupts purine synthesis pathways. Toxicity of methotrexate is reversed by N^5-formyl FH$_4$, or leucovorin, which serves as a direct folate coenzyme. Since it has no tumor selectivity, normal tissues in active cell cycle are affected, including mucosa, bone marrow and hair follicles, resulting in mucositis, pancytopenia and alopecia. Prolonged use is associated with pulmonary and liver fibrosis. High-dose therapy and excessive periods of high blood levels result in interstitial nephritis, sometimes requiring dialysis,

The most common resistance is due to amplification of DHFR expression by upregulation of translation and gene amplification, including the establishment of minichromosomes with the DHFR gene. A second mechanism is decreased affinity of DHFR to methotrexate. A third mechanism is decreased thymidylate synthase, and the fourth mechanism of resistance is impaired methotrexate polyglutamate formation.

While use has diminished in recent years, methotrexate remains part of the regimen for maintenance in children and adults with ALL (Chapter 66). It is also used to depress T-lymphocyte proliferation after allogeneic stem cell transplantation to prevent acute graft-versus-host disease (GVHD). High-dose methotrexate, with careful blood level monitoring to prevent acute renal toxicity and mucositis, and leucovorin rescue, is effective in the management of CNS leukemias, primary CNS lymphoma, and high proliferative fraction (myc positive, bcl6 positive and high KI67) intermediate- and high-grade lymphomas, including Burkitt.

Nucleoside Analogues

The nucleoside analogs exhibit structural similarities to naturally occurring nucleosides and are incorporated into either DNA or RNA with lethal consequences. Alternatively, they block key enzymes in de novo purine or pyrimidine biosynthesis. There are two broad categories:

1. Pyrimidine analogs (e.g., ara-C, 5-azacytidine, gemcitabine)
2. Purine analogs (e.g., 6-thioguanine [6-TG], 6-mercaptopurine, fludarabine, chlorodeoxyadenosine, deoxycoformycin, clofarabine, nelarabine)

These categories are not mutually exclusive; for example, some nucleoside analogs (e.g., ara-C and 6-TG) also inhibit enzymes involved in DNA or deoxyribonucleotide biosynthesis. These agents are predominantly cycle-active agents and in most cases are phase specific, being primarily active against cells in S phase. Because the growth fraction of hematologic malignancies tends to be higher than that of nonhematologic malignancies, nucleoside analogs are particularly useful in the former disorders. In contrast to alkylating agents, nucleoside analogs have limited carcinogenic and leukemogenic potential. The fluorinated pyrimidines (e.g., 5-FU) are generally not used in treating hematologic disorders and are not discussed further.

ara-C has been used in the treatment of acute leukemias—particularly acute nonlymphocytic leukemias, aggressive lymphomas

including Burkett, and CNS lymphomas for over 30 years. It is incorporated into DNA during replication and inhibits polymerase-α, is cell cycle specific, and penetrates the blood–brain barrier. In rapidly replicating cells, it stalls polymerase function, leading to replication fork collapse and strand breaks at the replication fork, signaling apoptosis and differentiation.

Mechanisms of Resistance

Although ara-C remains the backbone of therapy for aggressive hematologic malignancies, resistance has been observed that is both specific to the drug and nonspecific. Specific resistance could be due to nucleotide transport down regulation, uncommon in dividing cells. Inside the cell, ara-C is phosphorylated by deoxycytidine kinase to the active 5′-triphosphate derivative ara-CTP, whereas catabolism of ara-C by cytidine deaminase (CDD) to the nontoxic metabolite arabinoside uridine is a major pathway of detoxification that can be overcome by high-dose therapy. Low penetration into the cerebrospinal fluid is overcome by bolus administration of very high doses: 1–2 g/m^2 over 1 hour. Other resistance mechanisms appear nonspecific and result in leukemia tolerance to cell cycle arrest and induction of apoptosis, tolerance to DNA strand breaks, and rapid cell division after therapy.

Clinical Use

Standard induction therapy for AML includes a 5–7-day continuous infusion of 100–200 mg/m^2 or high-dose ara-C at doses of 1–3 g/m^2 over 1 hour every 12 hours. Many modifications to these schedules have improved tolerance without sacrificing efficacy. For CNS leukemia, a depo form of ara-C has been developed with improved tolerance and sustained cerebrospinal fluid levels (Chapter 60).

Subcutaneous administration has provided responses in older individuals with AML or MDS who do not respond well to more intensive induction therapy.

5-Azacytidine and Decitabine

These agents were initially developed as antimetabolites but are more effective at low doses that inhibit the function of histone demethylation, and are described below.

Gemcitabine

Developed as an agent for the treatment of pancreatic cancer, gemcitabine has gained therapeutic attention for use in patients with Hodgkin lymphoma and NHL, particularly in the relapsed state.

Like other nucleotide analogues, gemcitabine is a prodrug that is phosphorylated by deoxycytidine kinase to gemcitabine diphosphate (FdCDP) and gemcitabine triphosphate (dFdCTP), which, when incorporated into DNA, stalls the polymerase-α, which adds one more deoxynucleotide to the elongating strand. The polymerase replication complex then falls off the DNA, causing replication fork collapse and chain termination. In addition, FdCDP is a potent inhibitor of ribonucleoside reductase, causing depletion of deoxyribonucleotide pools and further encouraging dFdCTP incorporation while disrupting DNA synthesis.

Specific resistance is caused by upregulation of deoxycytidine deaminase, which metabolizes gemcitabine to 2,2′-difluorodeoxyuridine. Nonspecific resistance emerges due to upregulation of membrane transporters, although their role in clinical resistance is less clear.

Numerous studies have identified the utility of adding gemcitabine to cisplatin and other agents for the treatment of both relapsed Hodgkin lymphoma and NHL, and CTCLs. The combination of oxaliplatinum or cisplatin and gemcitabine is effective and well tolerated, and the majority of patients remain eligible for autologous stem cell collection and transplantation.

Fludarabine

Fludarabine was introduced 25 years ago as an agent with potent activity against lymphoid malignancies and remains an active agent in CLL and other low-grade lymphomas. It has since emerged as an agent in combination that is effective in leukemias, and in induction therapy for nonmyeloablative conditioning prior to allogeneic stem cell transplantation. It is recognized for its immunosuppressive function and inducing tolerance to allografts transplantation. Fludarabine phosphate is the 2-fluoro, 5'-monophosphate derivative of vidarabine (9'-β-D-arabinofuranosyladenine [ara-A]) and is converted to the di- and triphosphate by intracellular kinases, as are gemcitabine and ara-C. It has greater potency because it confers resistance to deamination by adenosine deaminase (ADA) and improved solubility. It is incorporated into DNA as a nucleotide and causes chain termination. It is a potent inhibitor of cytosolic 5'-nucleotidase II. It is also a substrate for uracil glycosylase, causing abasic sites as the first stem in BER and has recently been used in combination with TRC102, which binds to these sites and prevents their repair. Like other nucleoside analogues, it causes replication fork collapse, double-strand breaks, and induction of P53, leading to apoptotic signaling. Its efficacy against normal lymphoid T and B cells appears linked to both cytotoxicity against proliferating cells and resting cells; the latter effect is mediated by interference with the normal activity of the nucleotide excision repair pathway.

Fludarabine is a complex agent. Resistance is multifactorial including active transport, decreased cytosolic 5'-nucleotidase II and deoxycytokine kinase, and Ku80 binding to telomerase. Other non-specific mechanisms include mutations in *p53* or loss due to chromosome deletion, which is important in many cases of CLL, and other proliferation-associated genes such as *NOTCH1*, *SF3B1*, and *BIRC3*. Low-level miR-34a is also associated with fludarabine resistance.

Fludarabine, at a standard dose of 25 mg/m² for 5 days and rituximab with or without cyclophosphamide were the mainstay of primary treatment for CLL (Chapter 77). Fludarabine has also been used in refractory leukemias, marginal cell and other low-grade lymphomas. Recognition of the appearance of lymphopenia after treatment led to studies establishing fludarabine as part of the non-myelosuppressive preparative regimens for allogeneic transplantation, used particularly for older individual recipients. This is most often at a dose of 30–35 mg/m² for 5 days and used in combination with radiation, melphalan, or cyclophosphamide. In addition to lymphopenia, multiple cycles are associated with prolonged myelosuppression and a chronic peripheral neuropathy.

Clofarabine

Clofarabine (2-chloro-2'-arabino-flouro-2'-deoxyadenosine) is a purine analog with activity in patients with relapsed acute leukemia. Its activation requires cellular uptake and conversion to the triphosphate nucleotide. It then decreases ribonucleotide reductase; alters nucleotide precursors; inhibits and reduces the function of antiapoptotic proteins such as Bcl-X(L), Mcl-1, and Bax with dephosphorylation of akt; and inhibits DNA synthesis.

It appears more active against B-cell than T-cell lymphomas, but also has activity in AML and myelodysplastic syndromes (MDS). It is well tolerated. Recent studies show its significant efficacy in ara-C–refractory AML. Reversible liver toxicity and myelosuppression can be dose limiting (see Chapter 59).

Nelarabine

Nelarabine (9-β-D-arabinofuranosylguanine) is another FDA-approved purine analog for the treatment of refractory T-cell leukemias and lymphomas (Chapter 85).

As a nucleotide analogue, it preferentially accumulates in T cells and is incorporated into DNA, causing chain termination and inhibiting DNA synthesis. The FDA approved this drug after analyzing the results of two phase II clinical trials, one in pediatric T-cell acute lymphoblastic leukemia (ALL) and the other in adults with T-cell lymphoblastic lymphoma. In both cases, patients had relapsed after at least two induction regimens. Because CRs were seen in 13% of the 39% of pediatric patients and in 18% of the 28 adult patients, the FDA granted approval. Neurologic toxicity is dose limiting. Good response rates, including CRs, have been seen in patients with refractory T-cell leukemias.

Reduced ara-G incorporation into DNA is likely due to both altered nucleotide transport, increased nucleotidase activity, reduced nucleoside kinase activity, and nonspecific resistance mechanisms as described earlier for this class of agent.

Inhibitors of DNA Topoisomerase I and II

Inhibitors of DNA topoisomerases I and II include such drugs as doxorubicin, daunorubicin, mitoxantrone, etoposide, and topotecan. Before describing the specific inhibitors, a brief review of the drug targets (topoisomerase enzymes) will be presented (Table 57.2).

DNA Topoisomerase I

Topoisomerase I is a ubiquitous enzyme whose function in vivo is to relieve the torsional strain in DNA, specifically to remove positive supercoils generated in front of the replication fork and to relieve negative supercoils occurring downstream of RNA polymerase during transcription. Topoisomerase I is catalytically active as a 100-kDa

---

TABLE 57.2   Characteristics of Mammalian DNA Topoisomerases

	Topoisomerase I	Topoisomerase IIα and Topoisomerase IIβ	
Size of monomer (kDa)	100	170	180
mRNA (kb)	4.2	6.2	6.5
Chromosome	20q12–13.2	17q21–22	3p24
DNA cleavage	Single-strand breaks	Double-strand breaks	Double strand
Covalent intermediate	3'PO₄-Tyr⁷²³	5'PO₄-Tyr⁸⁰⁴	5'PO₄-Tyr⁸²¹
ATP requirement	No	Yes	Yes
Nuclear location	Nucleoli, diffuse	Nuclear matrix and scaffold, nucleoli	Nucleoli Nuclear matrix
Cell cycle dependence	None	Yes, maximum in G₂/M	None
Nuclear localization signal	NH₂-end	COOH-end	COOH-end
Phosphorylation	By CK II and PKC (increases activity)	By CK II, PKC, p34ᵒᵈᶜ², MAPK	Increases mass to 190 kDa
Role	In replication, transcription, and recombination	In replication, transcription, chromosome condensation/segregation, and recombination	rRNA transcription
Inhibitors	Camptothecins	(see Table 57.3)	

MAPK, mitogen-activated protein kinase; PKC, protein kinase C.

monomer and is concentrated in nucleoli, although smaller amounts are found in a diffuse nuclear distribution. The gene for this enzyme is located on human chromosome 20q12–13.2. Topoisomerase I does not require ATP for catalytic activity. It binds double-strand DNA over 15–25 bp (with a preference for supercoiled or bent DNA) followed by cleavage of one DNA strand and forming a transient covalent phosphotyrosyl bond at the 3'-end of DNA. DNA torsional strain is then relieved by a "controlled rotation" mechanism (see Fig. 57.1), subsequent to which the cleaved DNA is religated. The three-dimensional crystal structure of human topoisomerase I, both in covalent and noncovalent complexes with DNA, has defined the structural elements of the enzyme that contacts DNA. The association between topoisomerase I and the 3'-end of cleaved DNA has been termed the *cleavable complex*, which is stabilized by topoisomerase I inhibitors.

DNA Topoisomerase II

Two isoforms of human topoisomerase II (α and β) exist. They act as homodimers to cleave double-stranded DNA and require ATP for full activity. Their role in vivo is to relieve torsional strain in DNA, and their cellular distribution is determined by nuclear localization signals contained in the C-terminal domain. These isoforms are distinct in that they have different-size monomers (see Table 57.2), their genes are located on separate chromosomes, their nuclear distribution is different, and only the α-isoform shows cell cycle variations in amount and activity (with maximal activity being in G_2/M). The mechanism of action of topoisomerase II involves several steps (Fig. 57.4): DNA

recognition and binding (curved and supercoiled DNA, as well as DNA crossovers, are preferred), the sequential cleavage of the two strands of DNA with covalent attachment of a monomer to each 5'-end of the cleaved DNA, passage of another DNA duplex through the break site (e.g., to relieve DNA torsional strain or decatenate daughter chromosomes at the end of replication), religation of the cleaved DNA, and ATP hydrolysis-dependent enzyme turnover. The binding of ATP by topoisomerase II is required for the strand passage reaction. Again, the association between topoisomerase II monomers and the 5'-end of the cleaved DNA has been termed the *cleavable complex*, the stabilization of which generally correlates with the cytotoxic activity of specific topoisomerase II inhibitors.

Because topoisomerase I and II inhibitors convert their respective enzymes into DNA-damaging agents, it is usually true that the more enzyme target a cell contains (provided it is in the nucleus), the more cytotoxic is the specific inhibitor. An exception to this generalization is CLL cells, which have abundant topoisomerase I but are not very sensitive to topoisomerase I inhibitors because topoisomerase I inhibitors are S-phase specific and CLL cells have very few cells in S phase. Finally, in addition to topoisomerase I and II, a mammalian DNA topoisomerase III has been described and found to be essential for early embryogenesis in the mouse. In addition to the presumed lethality of a homozygous deletion of the topoisomerase II gene, topoisomerases I and III appear to be essential for cell growth and division in mammals. The specific role of topoisomerase III in humans is unknown at present.

DNA Topoisomerase I Inhibitors

Camptothecin is a plant alkaloid first identified in 1966 from the tree *Camptotheca acuminata*. Early clinical studies with camptothecin were stopped primarily because of hemorrhagic cystitis resulting from conversion of the sodium salt form to the active lactone form owing to its acidic pH in the bladder. Renewed interest in camptothecin occurred in 1985 when topoisomerase I was identified as the target of this drug and as new more water-soluble analogs became available. At present, two topoisomerase I inhibitors have been approved by the FDA as second-line agents for the treatment of ovarian carcinoma and colorectal cancer; these are topotecan and irinotecan (CPT-11; Fig. 57.5). Topotecan has been shown to be active in the treatment of MDS and inactive in the treatment of CLL. Responses to topotecan have also been seen in refractory MM, refractory large-cell lymphoma, and refractory acute leukemia.

The lactone forms of topotecan and SN-38 (the active form of CPT-11 generated in vivo by the action of a carboxylesterase) are as

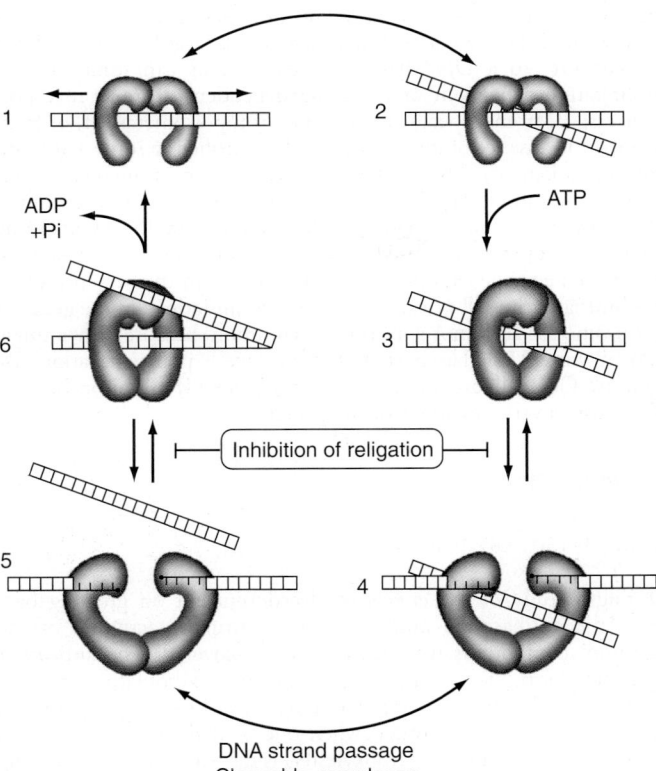

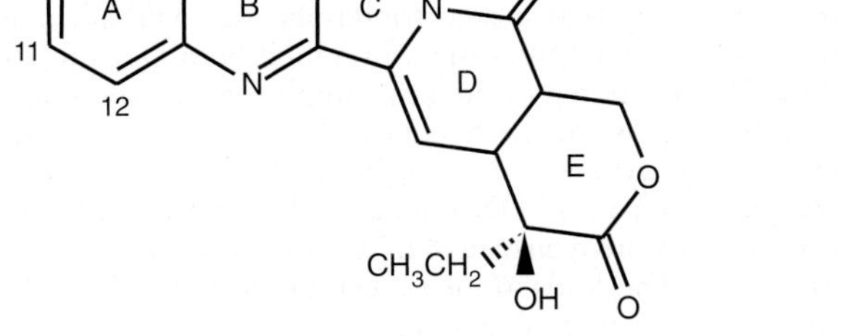

Fig. 57.4 DNA TOPOISOMERASE II CATALYTIC CYCLE. (1) Noncovalent binding of DNA by the topoisomerase II homodimer. (2) DNA recognition and preferential binding to crossovers by topoisomerase II. (3) Binding of ATP promotes the formation of a topologic complex. (4) DNA cleavage with covalent linkage of each topoisomerase II monomer to the 5'-DNA terminus of the break. (5) Poststrand passage cleavable complex. (6) Religation of the cleaved DNA is followed by ATP hydrolysis and enzyme turnover. DNA topoisomerase II inhibitors generally increase cleavable complexes by inhibiting the religation activity.

	C-10	C-9	C-7
Camptothecin	H	H	H
Topotecan	OH	$(CH_3)_2NCH_2$	H
9-Aminocamptothecin	H	NH_2	H
SN-38	OH	H	CH_3CH_2
CPT-11	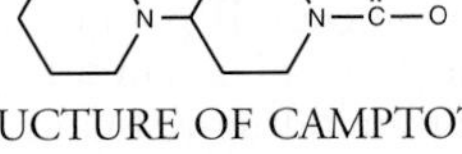	H	CH_3CH_2

Fig. 57.5 STRUCTURE OF CAMPTOTHECIN ANALOGS.

TABLE 57.3	Mechanism(s) of Action of Antineoplastic Agents That Are Primarily Topoisomerase II Inhibitors			
Drug	**Topoisomerase II Inhibition Poison**	**DNA Suppressor**	**Free Radical Intercalation**	**Formation**
Epipodophyllotoxins	+++	–	–	+
VP-16				
VM-26				
Anthracyclines				
Doxorubicin				
Daunorubicin	++	++	++	+
Idarubicin				
Epirubicin				
Anthracenedione				
Mitoxantrone	++	++++	++	+
Acridine				
m-AMSA	+++	+	+	–
Catalytic inhibitors				
Aclarubicin	–	+++	+	–
Others (merbarone, fostriecin, bis-2,6-dioxopiperazines)	–	+++	–	–

m-AMSA, Amsacrine.

much as 1000-fold more active inhibitors of DNA topoisomerase I than are their carboxylate forms. The lactone form predominates at an acidic pH. Topoisomerase I inhibitors stabilize the DNA–enzyme cleavable complex and thus inhibit DNA religation, but the production of DNA double-strand breaks results from a collision of the DNA replication fork with the ternary drug–enzyme–DNA complex, which is the lethal event (see Fig. 57.4). Topoisomerase I inhibitors are considered S-phase–specific agents because they require ongoing DNA synthesis to exert their cytotoxic effect.

DNA Topoisomerase II Inhibitors

Inhibitors of DNA topoisomerase II are commonly used for the treatment of hematologic malignancies. Three general types of topoisomerase II inhibitors exist (Table 57.3). The first are the topoisomerase II poisons, typified by etoposide, which results in the stabilization of cleavable complexes. The second group are the catalytic inhibitors, represented by aclarubicin, merbarone, and the bis-2,6-dioxopiperazine derivatives (ICRF-193, ICRF-159, ICRF-187); these are drugs that, except for aclarubicin, do not bind DNA and do not stabilize cleavable complexes, but rather interfere with some aspect of topoisomerase II catalytic activity (e.g., ICRF-187 inhibits topoisomerase II adenosine triphosphatase [ATPase] activity). The final class includes drugs that can inhibit both DNA topoisomerases I and II, and are represented by intoplicine and saintopin.

DNA topoisomerase II poisons (see Fig. 57.5 for structures) are most likely cytotoxic because they trap DNA topoisomerase II complexes on nascent DNA in the nuclear matrix. The topoisomerase II poison-stabilized enzyme–DNA complex likely acts as a replication fork barrier and leads to the generation of irreversible DNA damage and cell death in proliferating cells. Whereas experiments in yeast show that although DNA synthesis is a major determinant for cell killing by topoisomerase I inhibitors, topoisomerase II poisons are also cytotoxic during other phases of the cell cycle.

Drug Resistance to Topoisomerase Inhibitors

Essentially all of the topoisomerase II poisons (see Tables 57.2 and 57.3) are substrates for the drug efflux pump P-glycoprotein (PGP), and many are substrates for multidrug-resistance protein (MRP) and

lung resistance-related protein. In addition, several point mutations and gene deletions have been defined in the gene for topoisomerase II, resulting in the production of an enzyme with altered catalytic or cleavage activity. The third mechanism of resistance is a decrease in expression of the enzyme such that there is less target for the inhibitor to "convert" to a DNA-damaging agent. This can result from a proliferation-dependent or cell cycle–dependent decrease in topoisomerase II, from a specific attenuation of topoisomerase II, or from an intrinsic absence of topoisomerase II (identified in some acute and chronic leukemias). The fourth resistance mechanism involves alterations in the subcellular distribution of the enzyme. Truncation of the COOH-end of topoisomerase II has resulted in the cytoplasmic distribution of enzyme caused by a loss of nuclear localization signals, so that the enzyme cannot interact with DNA in the presence of an inhibitor and the cell is resistant. However, mutations in the gene for topoisomerase II do not appear to be common, because only a single patient with AML has been found to have a point mutation. By contrast, CLL cells are resistant to topoisomerase II inhibitors because they express very low levels of the protein.

Platinum Analogs

Mechanism of Action

During a study of the effects of electric current on growing bacteria, the antibacterial and, later, the antitumor activities of the platinum compounds were fortuitously discovered. The antitumor agent cisplatin, its *cis*-carboxylester analog, carboplatin, and the diaminocyclohexane-containing oxaliplatin, are heavy-metal platinum complexes. They are activated when one of their ligands (cisplatin; chloride and carboplatin; carboxylester) is displaced by water, leading to the formation of positively charged aquated platinum complexes, allowing platinum to stably bind DNA, RNA, proteins, or other critical biomacromolecules (see Fig. 57.2). With DNA, platinum complexes form covalent links to the N^7 position of guanine and adenine. The N^7 adducts at d(GpG) or d(ApG) result in intrastrand or interstrand DNA cross-links that bend the DNA helix and inhibit DNA synthesis. The cytotoxicity of platinum analogs correlates with the total platinum binding to DNA, as well as with the intrastrand or interstrand cross-links. This results in DNA damage, which triggers apoptosis of sensitive cells.

Clinical Activity

Cisplatin, carboplatin, and oxaliplatin are used in the treatment of refractory lymphomas in a variety of combinations, and as part of high-dose and intensification therapy for lymphomas as definitive treatment including prior to autologous stem cell transplantation.

Miscellaneous Agents

Among the agents included in this category, only plicamycin, bleomycin, procarbazine, L-asparaginase, gallium nitrate, and glucocorticoids are of current interest to hematologists; these are discussed in Appendix 57.6.

PHARMACOLOGY OF TARGETED ANTINEOPLASTIC AGENTS

Since the year 2000, the therapeutic arsenal available for treatment of hematologic malignancies has expanded to include a group of drugs that have collectively been termed as "targeted agents." Traditional chemotherapeutic drugs affect specific targets, many times identified after the cytotoxic and clinical activity of these agents have been demonstrated. Dobbelstein and Moll describe three "waves" or "epochs" in anticancer drug development.[4] The first wave includes traditional chemotherapeutic agents, comprised mostly of drugs that affect DNA replication, repair and cell division; these drugs are nonspecific and can affect normal cells, but take advantage of the increased proliferation of cancer cells to exert their cytotoxic activity. Second-wave drugs target cellular signals, including those mediated by surface receptors and protein kinases. Monoclonal antibodies are included in this second wave. The targets of signaling inhibitors are diverse, and include the products of oncogenes, essential for the development and survival of neoplasms ("oncogene addition"). The prototype of this class of agents is imatinib, targeting the chimeric product of B-cell receptor (BCR)-ABL in CML. Other cellular signaling proteins are not the product of oncogenes, but have an essential role in intracellular processes of malignant cells. This state is known as "nononcogene addiction" and has expanded the number of targets that can be used for cancer treatment with signaling inhibitors. Examples of the latter agent class include inhibitors of mammalian target of rapamycin (mTOR) and BTK. The third wave of anticancer drugs target cellular mechanisms and effector systems distinct from those targeted by drugs of the first two waves, but that are still essential for the survival of cancer cells. The cellular processes targeted by drugs of the third wave are those that contain several types of constitutive stress experienced by cancer cells (separate from replicative stress), including proteotoxic stress leading to abnormal protein folding and increased protein degradation (targeted by heat-shock protein inhibitors and proteasome inhibitors), DNA damage (targeted by PARP inhibitors), DNA modifications (targeted by hypomethylating agents and HDACs), prosurvival balance in organelles governing cell survival (targeted by BCL2 inhibitors), increased need for protein transport (inhibited by nuclear transport inhibitors), as well as transcriptional, ribosomal, metabolic, and oxidative stress, targeted by several other drugs in development. Other agents not easily included in these three waves include immunomodulatory drugs (thalidomide, lenalidomide, and pomalidomide), as well as agents promoting cancer cell differentiation (all-*trans* retinoic acid).

Signaling Inhibitors (Table 57.4)

Imatinib Mesylate and Other BCR-ABL Kinase Inhibitors

Imatinib Mesylate

Imatinib mesylate is a phenylaminopyrimidine developed as an inhibitor of the constitutively active tyrosine kinase (TK) BCR-ABL, expressed in the leukemic cells of most patients with CML. The recognition that the constitutively active TK BCR-ABL played a central role in the pathogenesis of chronic myeloid leukemia led to the search for potential inhibitors. The introduction of the TK inhibitor imatinib for treatment of CML is a major milestone in the development of targeted therapy for hematologic and neoplastic disorders. The role of the BCR-ABL kinase in the pathogenesis of CML and ALL and the use of BRC/ABL inhibitors in the treatment of these disorders are discussed in further detail in Chapter 67.

Imatinib mesylate is the founding agent in the class of TK inhibitors. It causes direct inhibition of the BCR-ABL kinase, but is not absolutely specific for this molecule, as it also inhibits other kinases, including KIT (formerly designated c-KIT), platelet-derived growth factor (PDGF), stem cell factor (SCF), and TEL-ARG.

Radiographic crystallography studies show that imatinib mesylate competitively binds to the ATP-binding site of the ABL kinase and stabilizes it in an inactive conformation. The 50% inhibitory concentration (IC_{50}) of imatinib mesylate for BCR-ABL is in the submicromolar range, and is substantially lower than the supramicromolar levels achievable in the plasma of patients receiving the drug by the oral route.

Despite the success with imatinib mesylate in the treatment of chronic-phase CML and, to a lesser extent, accelerated or blast-phase CML, the preexistence or development of resistance represents a major therapeutic challenge that can occur at any stage of the disease. Primary or secondary resistance can develop through a variety of mechanisms. BCR-ABL–dependent mechanisms correspond to the emergence of mutations in ABL kinase domain, which can be located in the imatinib binding site, the P loop, the catalytic domain, or the activation loop. Many of these mutations are present at the time of diagnosis and resistant clones emerge after exposure to imatinib. Resistance mechanisms independent of BCR-ABL include development of multidrug resistance mechanisms (e.g., PGP related); decreased levels of human organic cation transporter; acquisition of additional genetic abnormalities (clonal evolution) including acquisition of an additional Philadelphia-positive chromosome (Ph+), trisomy 8 and isochromosome 17q, increased expression of the BCR-ABL protein, and SRC kinase overexpression.

Imatinib also has activity in diseases dependent on other kinases, such as PDGF receptor (PDGFR)α, PDGFRβ, or KIT, and is active against myeloproliferative disorders associated with eosinophilia and FIP1L1/PDGFRα or PDGFRβ fusion genes, as well as against systemic mastocytosis without KIT^{D816V} mutation (Chapters 71 and 72).

Common adverse events due to imatinib include fluid overload and edema, and development of heart failure, fatigue, rash, and myelosuppression. Gastrointestinal side effects are common, and nausea and vomiting are frequent reasons for poor compliance.

Dasatinib

Dasatinib is a second-generation ABL kinase inhibitor approved for the treatment of CML. Dasatinib is an oral multikinase inhibitor, affecting BCR-ABL, KIT, PDGFR and src kinases. It binds the ATP binding site of ABL in an opposite direction to imatinib, can inhibit active and inactive forms of the kinase, and requires fewer points of contact. This reduced structural stringency in kinase inhibition allows for inhibition of all kinase mutations, with the exception of the *T315I* mutation.

Compared with imatinib, dasatinib is several hundred times more potent as an inhibitor of ABL. Initial studies demonstrated dasatinib-induced responses in patients who had developed resistance to imatinib treated in the chronic, accelerated, and blast phase of CML.

There is a high response rate in patients with wild-type sequences of *bcr-abl* and also in patients with mutations in the ABL protein conferring resistance to imatinib, with the exception of the *T315I* mutation.

As a multikinase inhibitor, dasatinib has a broader and alternative toxicity profile, with pulmonary edema, pleural effusions, and thrombocytopenia being the more frequent adverse effects. Recently, higher rates of pulmonary hypertension have been observed in patients receiving dasatinib.

TABLE 57.4   Targets and Approvals for Signaling Inhibitors

Agent	Identified Target Molecules	Approved Indications
Imatinib	BCR-ABL, KIT, PDGFRα, PDGFRβ, SCF, RET	CML, KIT-positive GIST, Ph+ ALL, myeloproliferative syndromes with PDGFR gene rearrangements Systemic mastocytosis without C-Kit mutation D816V Chronic eosinophilic leukemia and adult hypereosinophilic syndrome with FIP1L1-PDGFRα fusion or with unknown status of this fusion
Nilotinib	BCR-ABL, Kit, Lck, Ephrins, PDGFRβ, MAPK11, ZAK	CML
Dasatinib	BCR-ABL, Kit, Src, Lck, Yes, Fyn, Ephrins, PDGFRβ, STAT5B	CML Ph+ ALL
Bosutinib	BCR-ABL, Kit, Src, HCK, Lyn, MAPK1-2	CML
Ponatinib	BCR-ABL, Kit, PDGFRα, VEGFR, Src, Lyn, Lck, FGFR1–4, FLT3, TEK	CML with *T315I* mutation ALL with *T315I* mutation
Ibrutinib	BTK	Relapsed CLL, CLL with del(17p), relapsed mantle cell lymphoma, Waldenström's macroglobulinemia
Idelalisib	PI3Kδ	Relapsed CLL, SLL and follicular lymphoma
Ipatasertib	AKT	
Afuresertib	AKT	
Temsirolimus	mTOR	Renal cell carcinoma
Everolimus	mTOR	Renal cell carcinoma Advanced hormone receptor positive, HER2-negative breast cancer
Crizotinib	ALK, HGFR	ALK-positive non-small–cell lung cancer
Sorafenib	BRAF, VEGFR, FLT3, PDGFRβ, Kit, FGFR1, Ret	Hepatocellular carcinoma Renal cell carcinoma Recurrent thyroid cancer
Ruxolitinib	JAK1, JAK2,	Intermediate or high risk myelofibrosis Polycythemia vera refractory to hydroxyurea
Pacritinib	JAK2, FLT3	

ALL, Acute lymphoblastic leukemia; CML, chronic myeloid leukemia; CLL, chronic lymphocytic leukemia; FLT3, fms-like tyrosine kinase 3; HGFR, hepatocyte growth factor receptor; mTOR, mammalian target of rapamycin; PDGFR, platelet-derived growth factor receptor, PI3K, phosphatidylinositol 3-kinase; SCF, stem cell factor; SLL, small lymphocytic lymphoma; STAT5B, signal transducer and activator of transcription 5B; VEGFR, vascular endothelial growth factor receptor.

Nilotinib

Nilotinib is the other second-generation ABL kinase inhibitor approved for treatment of CML. Nilotinib is structurally related to imatinib, but has structural modifications that increase affinity for the ABL kinase site, binding with an improved topological fit to the kinase site in its inactive form. Nilotinib is 10–30 times more potent that imatinib.

In contrast with imatinib and dasatinib, nilotinib is a selective inhibitor of BCR-ABL. Nilotinib is active in chronic- and accelerated-phase CML patients who have developed resistance to imatinib. As with dasatinib, nilotinib was compared with imatinib in a phase III randomized trial as initial therapy for chronic-phase CML patients, with nilotinib achieving higher rates of complete cytogenetic and major molecular responses, and with fewer cases of CML phase progression or clonal evolution in the nilotinib-treated cohorts (PMID21856226). Nilotinib is active against all *BCR-ABL* mutations that confer resistance to imatinib, with the exception of T315I.

Common adverse events with nilotinib include rash, gastrointestinal disturbances (nausea, vomiting, diarrhea), as well as neutropenia and thrombocytopenia. Pleural effusion and peripheral edema are less common than with dasatinib. In addition, QT prolongation and risk of pancreatitis are serious side effects of nilotinib.

Bosutinib

Bosutinib is a dual kinase inhibitor of Src and ABL kinases. Although originally described as a Src-selective TK inhibitor, cell line screening assays allowed discovery of its ABL inhibitory activity. ABL kinase assay studies showed the IC$_{50}$ was 1.4 nM. Cell line and animal studies supported the potential therapeutic activity of bosutinib against CML. Bosutinib has does not inhibit wild-type c-KIT of PDGFR, although recent studies have shown inhibitory activity of other kinases, including CSK, Eph receptors, Trk, Tek, and Axl kinases, as well as some epidermal growth factor receptor and KIT mutants.

Bosutinib docks inside the intermediate conformation of the ATP binding site of ABL (in contrast to imatinib, which binds to the inactive conformation of the site). Binding to the intermediate conformation overcomes the resistance to imatinib conferred by mutations *Y253F*, *E255K*, and *D276G*, but does not confer activity against cells expressing *T315I*. In addition, Bosutinib appears to be a poor substrate of MDR transporters, overcoming this additional mechanism of resistance.

Common adverse events observed with bosutinib include gastrointestinal upset (diarrhea, vomiting, and abdominal pain), whereas the more common serious adverse events include diarrhea, myelosuppression, and elevated serum lipase and transaminases.

Ponatinib

Ponatinib is a third-generation, dual Src-ABL inhibitor. It was developed using computational and structure-based design to have activity against BCR-ABL forms with mutations that convey resistance to other TKIs, in particular *T315I* mutation. Ponatinib binds

ABL in its inactive form as imatinib. Differences in the chemical structure allow ponatinib to maintain interaction with ABL even in the presence of isoleucine in position 315, in cases with a *T315I* mutation. Initial cell- and murine-based studies showed that ponatinib inhibits cells expressing mutant or native *BCR-ABL*. Subsequent human studies demonstrated that ponatinib had activity in CML, including those with *T315I* mutation. Toxicities observed in early clinical trials included pancreatitis and elevation in pancreatic enzymes, fatigue, rash, and elevated aminotransferase levels. Ponatinib received FDA-accelerated approval in 2012 for the treatment of resistant or intolerant CML and Ph+ ALL. However, subsequent trials showed increased arterial thrombosis events in patients randomized to ponatinib arms, leading to limitations in the indications for ponatinib and the requirement for thrombosis prevention strategies in subjects treated with this drug.

Bruton Tyrosine Kinase Inhibitors

Btk is a cytoplasmic TK with a well-defined role in B-cell receptor signaling that is fundamental in B-lymphocyte development, differentiation, and signaling. Btk is a member of the Tec family of kinases (see Chapter 77). Activation of Btk triggers a cascade of signaling events that culminates in the generation of calcium mobilization and fluxes, cytoskeletal rearrangements, and transcriptional regulation of NFκB and nuclear factor of activated T cells.[5] Ibrutinib (PCI-32765) is a first-in-class, selective, irreversible, small-molecule inhibitor of Btk. Ibrutinib binds covalently to a cysteine (Cys 481) in the Btk active site, with potent and irreversible enzymatic activity. Clinical trials demonstrated a favorable toxicity profile with remarkable clinical activity in patients with relapsed CLL, mantle cell lymphoma (MCL), and Waldenström macroglobulinemia, with additional activity observed in activated B-cell–like diffuse large B-cell lymphoma and other lymphoid malignancies.

An early transient phase of lymphocytosis has been associated with response in CLL and MCL patients. Bruising can be observed in up to half of patients treated with ibrutinib. Serious adverse events associated with ibrutinib occurred in approximately 10% of patients, including rash, febrile neutropenia, diarrhea, and life threatening bleeding. The diarrhea follows two patterns: an early diarrhea that usually presents in the first weeks of treatment, which can usually be managed with antidiarrheal agents, and a late diarrhea that has an inflammatory bowel component and that may require more aggressive therapies, including corticosteroids and other antiinflammatory therapies. Atrial fibrillation or flutter has been observed in 6%–9% of patients. The mechanism for increased bleeding risk appears to be related to a platelet function defect secondary to interference of collagen receptor glycoprotein VI signaling.

Dosing for CLL and Waldenström's macroglobulinemia patients is 420 mg PO once daily; MCL patients is 560 mg once daily.

PI3K/AKT/mTOR Inhibitors

The PI3K/AKT/mTOR pathway is involved in the regulation of diverse cellular functions, including cell growth, protein synthesis, cell cycle regulation, glucose metabolism, and motility. PI3K represents a family of enzymes with multiple subunits. These subunits cooperate to transduce upstream signals (from RTKs, G-protein–coupled receptors, and other intracellular stimuli) into the enzymatic conversion of phosphatidylinositol diphosphate (PIP_2), to phosphatidylinositol triphosphate (PIP_3). The dual-specific phosphatase and tensin homolog (PTEN) opposes the actions of PI3K. PTEN is one of the most frequently mutated tumor suppressor genes in human malignancies, with inactivating mutations, genetic losses, and epigenetic silencing leading to PTEN loss. Phosphatidylinositol triphosphate, through phosphoinositoside-dependent kinase-1 (PDK1), leads to the phosphorylation and activation of the serine/threonine kinase AKT.

AKT signals to multiple downstream targets, in particular mTORC1, to promote cell survival and growth. Additional targets of AKT include molecules involved in cell survival and proliferation (e.g., Bad, Bim, procaspase 9, CREB, forkhead transcription factors [FHKR], IB), cell cycle regulators ($p21^{CIP1}$, $p27^{KIP1}$, cyclin D_1), glycogen synthesis (GSK3), and protein synthesis (FRAP1, $p70^{S6K}$).

The mechanistic target of rapamycin (also known as mTOR) operates through two complexes: mTORC1 (mTOR-Raptor) and mTORC2 (mTOR-Rictor). mTORC1 is activated by AKT and mediates its downstream proliferation, growth, and survival signaling, specifically through phosphorylation and inactivation of the repressor of mRNA translation initiation factor 4E-binding protein 1 (4E-BP) and ribosomal protein S6 kinase 1 (S6K1; see Fig. 57.6), resulting in enhanced translation of transcripts relevant to lymphoma pathogenesis, including CCND1, MYC and MCL1. The mTORC1 complex is activated by AKT whereas mTORC2 is capable of activating AKT. The majority of the downstream canonical functions are conduced by mTORC1.

Because of the frequency of PTEN losses or mutations (less common in hematologic malignancies) in transformed cells and the dependence of numerous cancers on an intact PI3K/AKT/mTOR pathway for survival, this cascade has become an attractive therapeutic target.

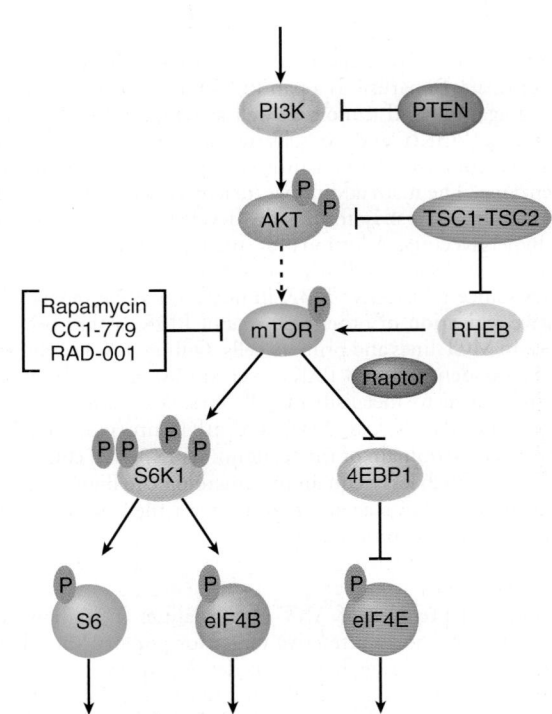

Translation-initiation of mRNA with highly structured 5'UTR
(C-MYC, CYCLIN D1, etc.)

Fig. 57.6 RAPAMYCIN OR ITS ANALOGS INHIBIT MAMMALIAN TARGET OF RAPAMYCIN AND THE DOWNSTREAM PHOSPHORYLATION OF S6K1 AND 4EBP1, THEREBY ATTENUATING THE TRANSLATION INITIATION OF mRNAS WITH HIGHLY STRUCTURED 5'-UTR. Activation of the receptor (FLT-3) or cytosolic tyrosine kinase (e.g., BCR-ABL) can lead to increased activity of PI3K/AKT. Although it can directly phosphorylate mTOR, AKT activity inhibits the TSC1–TSC2 complex, thereby derepressing RHEB and activating mTOR. The phosphorylation and activation of S6K1, and phosphorylation and inactivation of 4E-BP through Raptor, results in the phosphorylation of S6, eIF4B, and eIF4E, which are involved in the cap-dependent translation of mRNAs with highly structured 5'-UTR. *eIF*, Eukaryotic translation initiation factor; *mTOR*, mammalian target of rapamycin; *PI3K*, phosphatidylinositol 3-kinas; *PTEN*, phosphate and tensin homolog; *RHEB*, Ras homolog enriched in brain; *TSC*, tuberous sclerosis; *UTR*, untranslated region.

PI3K Inhibitors

Idelalisib (CAL-101, GS 1101) is a highly selective inhibitor of the p110d isoform of PI3K (PI3Kδ), an isoform of PI3K that is expressed selectively in hematopoietic cells, in particular those of the lymphoid lineage. Idelalisib has in vitro activity against lymphoid cell lines and primary CLL and MCL cells, but does not affect normal B-cell viability (see Chapter 77). Idelalisib inhibits not only the B-cell receptor signaling pathway-induced survival signals but also appears to disrupt the effects of microenvironmental signals on neoplastic cells,[6] affecting chemotaxis of tumor cells, which could explain the transient lymphocytosis observed after treatment of CLL patients with this agent. Clinical trials have shown that idelalisib is active in treating patients with relapsed CLL and other relapsed indolent lymphoid malignancies. Additional trials are investigating the activity of idelalisib in combination with other chemotherapeutic agents for the treatment of aggressive and indolent lymphoid malignancies, as well as its role in the treatment of AML and ALL.

Idelalisib is currently approved as a single agent for relapsed follicular lymphoma and SLL and in combination with rituximab for CLL patients. The approved dosing is 150 mg PO twice daily. Common dose-limiting toxicities include diarrhea, fever, and rash. Elevation of liver function tests is also commonly observed, requiring interruption of idelalisib. Serious adverse events include hepatotoxicity occurring in the first 3 months of treatment, diarrhea and colitis, intestinal perforation, pneumonitis, and neutropenia.

Other PI3K Inhibitors

Several other PI3K inhibitors are currently in various stages of development. Buparlisib is a pan PI3K inhibitor that appears to have activity against solid tumors as well as lymphoid malignancies. Pictilisib is a PI3Kα and -δ selective inhibitor that may overcome resistance conferred by constitutive expression of the α isoform of the enzyme. The main additional toxicity observed with PI3K inhibitors that target the α isoform is the development of insulin resistance and hyperglycemia. Additional agents have specificities that include other isoforms such as PI3Kβ, -δ and -γ.

Resistance to selective PI3K inhibitors may be mediated by constitutive activation of other isoforms of PI3K, as has been observed in certain MCL lines and primary cells. O-linked N-acetylglucosamine transferase, dendrin, and PAK1 overexpression have been associated with resistance to idelalisib in cell lines. Mechanisms of resistance may include PTEN loss, MYC and eIF4e upregulation. Mutations of the catalytic domain of the α subunit (PIK3CA), common in solid tumors, are much less frequent in hematologic malignancies, although treatment with these agents may increase the selective pressure for emergence of this abnormality.

AKT Inhibitors

The frequent presence of AKT abnormalities in human neoplasms makes this enzyme an attractive target for potential novel treatment strategies. Several drugs have been developed using dephosphorylation of the active enzyme, allosteric enzyme inhibition, and ATP competition as strategies for targeting AKT. Allosteric inhibitors bind the lipid-binding domain of AKT, resulting in a change in conformation that prevents localization to the plasma membrane and subsequent activation. The allosteric inhibitor perifosine had modest clinical activity as a single agent in patients with Waldenström macroglobulinemia and in patients with myeloma alone or in combination with bortezomib. Phase III studies failed to demonstrate clinical benefit. MK2206 is another oral allosteric inhibitor with minimal single-agent activity against solid tumors and hematologic malignancies.

Early ATP-competitive AKT inhibitors had significant off-target effects. More recently, ipatasertib (GDC-0068), an oral pan AKT inhibitor, has been observed to have significant selectivity for AKT. Clinical development has focused on solid tumors. Afuresertib (GSK 2110183) is a reversible ATP-competitive AKT inhibitor with in vitro activity against ALL, CLL, lymphoma, and myeloma. A phase I study of single-agent afuresertib showed activity in MM, with a maximum tolerated dose of 125 mg PO once daily. Subsequent studies have demonstrated activity of afuresertib when used in combination with bortezomib and dexamethasone for the treatment of myeloma, and with ofatumumab for the treatment of CLL. Frequent adverse events include gastrointestinal complaints (diarrhea, nausea, dyspepsia, gastrointestinal reflux, and anorexia) and fatigue. Severe adverse events include rash, fatigue, elevations in liver function tests, and thrombocytopenia.

Inhibitors of the Mammalian Target of Rapamycin

The first mTOR inhibitor discovered was the naturally occurring macrolide rapamycin (sirolimus), widely used as an immunosuppressant (see Chapter 108). The importance of the mTOR pathway in cancer suggested this agent would have antineoplastic activity. Improvements in solubility and pharmacokinetic properties led to development of rapamycin analogs (rapalogs), of which everolimus and temsirolimus are available as antineoplastic agents.[7] The mechanism of rapamycin and its analogs is similar: after complexing with the small protein FKBP12, they bind irreversibly to the FKBP12-rapamycin binding site on the mTOR protein. Acute rapamycin treatment only affects mTORC1 because the FKBP12-rapamycin is occluded in mTORC2. Prolonged rapalog exposure may result in decreased mTOR availability and therefore indirectly decreased mTORC2 activity through limited mTORC2 complex formation. It is well recognized that growth factor signaling initiated through the receptor tyrosine kinases (RTKs) or caused by the activity of cytosolic tyrosine kinases (TKs), such as BCR-ABL, results in activation of PI3K/AKT signaling. AKT has been shown to phosphorylate and inactivate tuberous sclerosis (TSC)2 (also known as tuberin), thereby disrupting its interaction with TSC1 (or hamartin; see Fig. 57.6). Inhibition of the TSC1–TSC2 complex derepresses RHEB, which is a small G protein that activates mTOR. When RHEB is in an active GTP-bound state, its localization to the membrane stimulates mTOR-mediated phosphorylation of the downstream eukaryotic initiation 4E-BP and ribosomal protein S6K1 (see Fig. 57.6). However, the association of mTOR with the 150-kDa Raptor (regulatory-associated protein of mTOR) is necessary for the phosphorylation of 4E-BP and S6K1. mTOR-mediated phosphorylation and activation of S6K1 results in the phosphorylation of the ribosomal S6 protein and eIF4B (see Fig. 57.6). AKT has also been shown to directly activate S6K1. S6K1 activity is involved in regulating the translation of a group of mRNAs that have a highly structured 5'-UTR (untranslated region), including mRNAs that have a 5'-TOP (terminal oligopyrimidines; a stretch of 4–14 pyrimidines).[8]

The rapalogs temsirolimus and everolimus have been tested in lymphoid malignancies, and as single agents they have demonstrated activity, although modest, against a variety of lymphomas (see Chapter 82). In the initial phase II study in patients with MCL, temsirolimus was administered at a dose of 250 mg based on a phase II study done in renal cell carcinoma patients. A modest response rate was noted (overall response rate [ORR]: 38%), but the majority of patients required a dose reduction because of myelosuppression, particularly thrombocytopenia. A second trial in relapsed refractory MCL patients was conducted to determine if a lower dose of temsirolimus could be used. In a follow-up phase II study, temsirolimus was given at a dose of 25 mg IV weekly and was found to be as effective as the 250-mg IV dose, with a modest improvement in the toxicity profile and dose reductions. This dose and schedule were also noted to be efficacious in nonmantle cell NHL, with thrombocytopenia being the main dose-limiting toxicity. A recent phase III study in relapsed refractory MCL patients evaluated two different dosing regimens of temsirolimus; 175 mg weekly for 3 weeks followed by 75 mg weekly versus 175 mg weekly for 3 weeks followed by 25 mg weekly versus the investigator's choice.[9] At the conclusion of this study, it was determined that the temsirolimus regimen with 175/75 mg dosing had a significant improvement in progression-free survival (PFS) and objective response rate compared with the investigator's choice. Everolimus, given orally at a daily dose of 10 mg has single-agent activity against Hodgkin lymphoma (PMI, Waldenström macroglobulinemia, diffuse large B-cell lymphoma [DLBCL], CLL, and other relapsed lymphomas).

The most common side effect of rapalogs is myelosuppression; other common side effects include fatigue, oral ulcers, and dermatologic abnormalities. Metabolic abnormalities are common, including hyperglycemia, hypercholesterolemia, and hypertriglyceridemia. An uncommon pulmonary toxicity manifested as interstitial lung disease has also been observed with rapalogs.

Anaplastic Lymphoma Kinase Inhibitors

Anaplastic lymphoma kinase (ALK) encodes for a 210-kDa RTK, a member of the insulin receptor superfamily closely related to leukocyte TK. While ALK has a normal role in nervous system development, translocations involving ALK have been described in a variety of malignancies, including anaplastic large-cell lymphoma (NPM-ALK, TFG-ALK, ATIC-ALK, and CLTC-ALK translocations), DLBCL (NPM-ALK, CLTC-ALK, SQSTM1-ALK, and SEC31A-ALK translocations), as well as non-small-cell lung cancer (NSCLC; EML4-ALK translocation and others). These translocations result in ALK chimeras, with fusion of the intracytoplasmic domain of ALK with partner proteins that provide a dimerization domain that results in ALK-mediated autophosphorylation and constitutive activation. Subsequent signaling promotes cellular proliferation, survival and growth via phospholipase Cγ, RAS/mitogen-activated protein kinase (MAPK), PI3K and c-Src.

Crizotinib

Crizotinib is a dual ALK/c-MET inhibitor with additional inhibitory activity against the kinase ROS1 (c-ros). It inhibits kinase activation through binding to the kinase domain and displacing the kinase activation loop, interfering with ATP and substrate binding. Crizotinib was shown to be 20-fold more selective for ALK and MET than other kinases, and inhibited cell proliferation and induced apoptosis in NPL-ALK–dependent cell lines. The initial clinical studies done in patients with NSCLC showed the maximum tolerated dose was 250 mg PO twice daily. Although initially tested as a c-MET inhibitor in these patients, ALK translocations were reported to be associated with marked responses in patients treated with crizotinib. Subsequent studies in ALK-rearranged NSCLC confirmed the activity of crizotinib in NSCLC with *ALK* translocations. In 2011, the FDA granted approval for crizotinib in this patient population. Subsequent studies conducted in relapsed and refractory ALK-positive anaplastic large-cell lymphoma showed a high rate of response to single-agent crizotinib. Additional trials testing crizotinib for ALK-positive lymphomas are ongoing.

The most common adverse events include gastrointestinal symptoms (nausea, vomiting, diarrhea), visual impairment, asthenia, cough, and myelosuppression (neutropenia, lymphopenia), as well as elevations of hepatic function tests.

Inhibitors of the RAF1/Mek/ERK Pathway

The MAPK pathways consist of three parallel serine-threonine kinase modules that are intimately involved in the control of cell survival, proliferation, and differentiation. Two of these, c-Jun N-terminal kinase (JNK) and p38 MAPK, are activated in response to environmental stresses, including DNA damage and osmotic stress, but p42/44 MAPK (also known as extracellular signal-regulating kinase [ERK]) is primarily induced by growth factors and other mitogenic stimuli. Although exceptions exist, JNK and p38 MAPK primarily exert proapoptotic functions, but ERK activation is generally associated with cell survival. The only well-defined activator of ERK is the serine-threonine kinase mitogen-activated protein kinase 1/2 (MEK1/2), but numerous ERK targets have been identified, including ELK-1, CREB, BCL2, Bad, FRAP1 (also known as mTOR), and caspase 9, among numerous others. The activating effects of MEK1/2 on ERK are opposed by phosphatases that dephosphorylate and inactivate the enzyme (e.g., MAP kinase phosphatase 1/2).

The major activator of MEK1/2 is the serine-threonine kinase RAF, of which three forms exist: RAF1, B-RAF, and A-RAF. RAF can be activated by Ras (discussed earlier), as well as through various RAS-independent pathways, including PKC, KSR, as well as the SRC and JAK family of kinases, among others. The activation of RAF involves several processes, including recruitment to the plasma membrane, phosphorylation on serine and threonine residues, and dimerization. Interference with any of these processes can lead to inhibition of Raf activation as well as downstream targets.

Dysregulation of the RAF/MEK/ERK pathway has been observed in most hematopoietic malignancies, including acute leukemia, CLL, MM, and lymphomas. Consequently, there has been considerable interest in the development of pharmacologic inhibitors of the RAF/MEK/ERK pathway in these disorders. In addition to their potential intrinsic activity against malignant hematopoietic cells, evidence indicates that such agents might also enhance the activity of conventional cytotoxic drugs.

Sorafenib

Initial approaches to RAF inhibition focused on efforts to destabilize the protein. For example, geldanamycin and the related compound 17-AAG act as inhibitors of HSPCA, a chaperone protein necessary for Raf processing and stabilization. Interference with HSPCA results in destabilization and proteasomal degradation of RAF as well as numerous other proteins, including AKT. More recently, however, a Raf kinase inhibitor, sorafenib, which is approved for use in kidney cancer, has been developed and has entered phase I and II clinical trials in humans with leukemia. In preclinical studies, induction of leukemic cell death by sorafenib has been shown to stem from inhibition of translation and downregulation of the short-lived antiapoptotic protein Mcl-1 and induction of endoplasmic reticulum (ER) stress with bim-mediated apoptosis. In the clinical setting, modest response rates of 10% were observed in two studies, suggesting the need to consider combination therapy.

Janus Kinase 2 Inhibitors

JAK2 is a non-RTK that plays a central role in the transduction of differentiation and proliferation signals in hematopoietic progenitor cells. Ligand binding to surface receptors for hematopoietic growth factors leads to phosphorylation of JAK2 with subsequent activation of transcription factors in the JAK/signal transducer and activator of transcription (STAT) pathway, including STAT3 and STAT5 (see Chapters 68–70). Identification of the JAKV617F mutation in patients with myeloproliferative neoplasms, including polycythemia vera, essential thrombocythemia, and primary myelofibrosis, represented a fundamental step in understanding the pathophysiology of these disorders. The genetic abnormality corresponds to a point mutation in nucleotide 1849 of the molecule, where guanine replaces thiamine, resulting in substitution of a valine for phenylalanine in the JH2 pseudokinase autoinhibitory domain of the molecule. The result is either hypersensitivity to cytokine signals or constitutive activation of the kinase. Development of JAK2 inhibitors followed as a rational, targeted therapeutic strategy for these neoplasms (see Chapters 68–70).

Ruxolitinib

Ruxolitinib (INCB018424, Jakafi) is a small-molecule inhibitor of JAK1 and JAK2, and the first-in-class JAK inhibitor to receive FDA approval for treatment of intermediate- and high-risk myelofibrosis[10,11] (see Chapter 70). It exerts its inhibitory activity through competitive inhibition of the kinase's ATP-binding catalytic site. In preclinical studies, JAK1/2 inhibition with ruxolitinib decreased STAT3/5 signaling both in wild-type cells and those carrying *JAKV617F*. In the initial phase I/II study, the maximum tolerated dose was 25 mg when given twice daily and 100 mg on once-daily dosing. After 3 months of therapy, 44% of patients with splenomegaly experienced a reduction of more than 50%. Responses were observed in patients with the *JAKV617F* mutation as well as those with wild-type *JAK2*. Importantly, the majority of patients experienced a decrease in constitutional symptoms and improved exercise tolerance and performance status, as well as weight gain. In larger, randomized trials, while clinical improvement was superior with ruxolitinib treatment, this agent was not effective in reversing histologic, cytogenetic, or molecular abnormalities in peripheral blood or BM, suggesting that ruxolitinib is not curative. Recent studies have also shown ruxolitinib to be effective in controlling symptoms, spleen size and hematocrit in patients with polycythemia vera. Dosing of ruxolitinib in myelofibrosis patients is based on platelet count, ranging from 5 mg twice daily for patients with platelet counts lower than 50,000/μL to 20 mg twice daily if platelet counts are above 200,000/μL; in patients with polycythemia vera the starting dose of ruxolitinib is 10 mg twice daily. Rapid redevelopment of splenomegaly and symptom exacerbation can occur after abrupt interruption or discontinuation of ruxolitinib. Common side effects of ruxolitinib include myelosuppression, primarily anemia, and thrombocytopenia requiring dose modifications; increased risk of infections and herpes zoster; gastrointestinal symptoms (abdominal pain, diarrhea), fatigue and headache.

Other JAK2 Inhibitors

Several other inhibitors with activity against JAK2 are under investigation.

Pacritinib (SB1518) is a JAK2 inhibitor with activity against the wild-type kinase as well as the JAKV617F-mutated kinase; it also inhibits fms-like tyrosine kinase 3 (FLT3). It achieves high rates of reduction in spleen volume. The tested dose is 400 mg daily. Recent studies confirm the activity of pacritinib in the treatment of MF, resulting in improvements in hematologic, radiologic, and clinical symptom endpoints. The main side effects are gastrointestinal, predominantly diarrhea, nausea, vomiting, and abdominal pain, while hematologic adverse events are modest.

Momelotinib (CYT387) is an oral multikinase inhibitor affecting JAK1/2, TYK2, TBK1, PRKD1, ROCK2, PRKCN, MAPK8, and CDK2/cyclin A. Early trials in myelofibrosis patients resulted in decreased splenomegaly and improvement in symptoms in the majority of patients treated. Of note, more than one-third of patients with improved splenomegaly had previously been treated with ruxolitinib. The most common side effects included myelosuppression, primarily thrombocytopenia. Nonhematologic side effects included headache, QTc prolongation, neuropathy, and abnormal liver test results. The maximum tolerated dose has been established at 300 mg/day given continuously in 28-day cycles.

Immunomodulatory Agents

Thalidomide and its related compounds provide effective oral immunomodulatory (see Chapter 86) therapy for patients with hematologic malignancies, in particular plasma cell dyscrasias and lymphoid malignancies. They have complex mechanisms of action. Further details on their therapeutic impact are found in Chapters 86 and 81–82.

Thalidomide

Experimental studies have identified that thalidomide reduces expression of the cellular inhibitor of apoptosis protein and potentiates proapoptotic processes such as TNF-related apoptosis-inducing ligand (TRAIL)/po2L. Thalidomide also reduces NFκB and IκB expression, thereby reducing IL-6 expression. In addition, thalidomide decreases vascular endothelial growth factor (VEGF) and reduces angiogenesis and vessel density in the bone marrow of patients with MM. The lack of a simple mechanism of action has been confusing because it is unclear which, if any, biomarker is an appropriate correlate for clinical success or toxicity. Thalidomide has been in clinical use for more than 50 years and has well-documented and sometimes serious side effects, including severe birth defects, somnolence, axonal length-dependent peripheral neuropathy, orthostatic hypotension, neutropenia, bradycardia and occasional heart block, and increased viral load in HIV-positive patients. The risk of developing thrombotic

events is elevated, giving rise to the recommended use of an anticoagulant regimen such as aspirin, low-molecular-weight heparin or Coumadin. Nonetheless, efficacy is certainly seen clinically and has been validated in SCID models of human myeloma. Data also point to its potential clinical efficacy in patients with solid tumors and MDS. The approved dose of thalidomide for treatment of plasma cell myeloma is 200 mg PO given once daily. Dose reductions should be considered in the presence of hematologic toxicity.

Lenalidomide

Lenalidomide was identified as an analog of thalidomide with more potent immunomodulatory functions but fewer side effects. Lenalidomide also has antiangiogenic properties, blocks IL-6 production, and reduces NFκB and IκB levels. In addition, lenalidomide induces caspase 8-mediated apoptosis and mitochondrial-mediated cell death. T-cell activation and increased natural killer (NK) activity are observed, thus increasing the anticancer immune response. Lenalidomide can cause a similar dose-dependent peripheral neuropathy as thalidomide, and causes more significant myelosuppression, which can be dose limiting. The risk of thrombosis is also increased and the administration of lenalidomide should be accompanied by antithrombotic prophylaxis. Hypersensitivity rash occurs in up to 10% of patients. In trials of CLL and lymphoma, initial treatment with lenalidomide can result in tumor flare, characterized by fever, rash and painful lymphadenopathy; lower initial doses should be considered in patients with high tumor burden and CLL. A variety of dosing schedules provides a flexible therapeutic approach and a high response rate in relapsed myeloma patients, with an ORR of 25% and median overall survival (OS) of 28 months. In 5q- MDS patients, response in over 40% of patients was observed, indicating more based on the achievement of transfusion independence (see Chapter 60). The activity of lenalidomide has been observed in several lymphoid malignancies, with its current approval limited to MCL that has relapsed after two lines of therapy. The approved starting dose of lenalidomide is 25 mg PO once daily (days 1–21 of a 28-day cycle) for plasma cell myeloma and MCL. A dose of 10 mg once daily is used in 5q- MDS patients.

Pomalidomide

Pomalidomide is a third-generation member of the immunomodulatory drugs (IMiDs) class. In addition to its immunomodulatory and antiangiogenic activity, pomalidomide has direct activity against myeloma cells, affecting gene expression, and promoting apoptosis and cell cycle arrest. Pomalidomide upregulates expression of p21^{WAF} and downregulates interferon (IFN) regulatory factor 4. p21^{WAF} inhibits CDK2, which in turn results in phosphorylation of the retinoblastoma (Rb) protein and cell cycle arrest at G1. Apoptosis is also induced via activation of caspase 8. In vitro studies showed that pomalidomide was active in cell lines resistant to thalidomide and lenalidomide.

Phase I studies established that the maximum tolerated dose of pomalidomide was 4 mg given PO on days 1–21 of 28-day cycles, which corresponds to the currently approved starting dose. Results of a phase II study combining pomalidomide with dexamethasone in patients with relapsed myeloma showed an encouraging ORR of 63% (partial response [PR] or better), including 60% of patients who were refractory to bortezomib and 40% of patients who were refractory to lenalidomide. The most common severe adverse events are myelosuppression (anemia, neutropenia, and thrombocytopenia), infections, and fatigue. Venous thromboembolic events were observed in early-phase studies and subsequent trials have required thromboprophylaxis, under which the rate of VTE with pomalidomide is less than 5%.

Proteasome Inhibitors

The 26S proteasome is the central proteolytic machinery of the highly conserved ubiquitin proteasome system. In eukaryotic cells, whereas the lysosomal pathway degrades extracellular proteins imported into the cell through endocytosis or pinocytosis, the proteasome controls the degradation of intracellular proteins. Numerous studies have demonstrated that the ubiquitin–proteasome system controls basic cellular functions such as cell cycle progression, signal transduction, and programmed cell death, hence the interest in therapeutic interventions that manipulate proteasomal activity and potentially restore cellular homeostasis into transformed cells (see Chapter 4).

Ubiquitin is a highly conserved 76-amino–acid polypeptide that is expressed in all eukaryotic cells. Under the sequential action of E1 (ubiquitin-activating enzyme), E2 (ubiquitin-conjugating enzyme), and E3 (ubiquitin ligase), ubiquitin is activated and covalently conjugated to potential proteasome substrates via an isopeptide bond between the C-terminal glycine residue of ubiquitin and the ε-amino group of internal lysine residues in target proteins. The same set of enzymes also catalyzes the formation of the isopeptide bond between G76 and the lysine residue (K48) of previously conjugated ubiquitin, leading to formation of a polyubiquitin chain. Polyubiquitinated substrates are usually targeted for proteasomal degradation.

The 26S proteasome is a large (2000-kDa) threonine protease present in the nucleus and cytoplasm of all eukaryotic cells. This ATP-dependent, multicatalytic protease eliminates damaged or misfolded proteins and regulates cyclins and CDK inhibitor cell cycle regulatory proteins as well as other proteins that govern the transcription factor activation, apoptosis, and cell trafficking. Its structure consists of two parts: the 20S core and the 19S cap regulatory particle (Fig. 57.7). The 19S cap is involved in the recognition, binding, and unfolding of ubiquitinated proteins and in the regulation of the opening of the 20S core. The 20S core is a cylinder composed of four stacked heptameric rings, each containing seven different α or β subunits (α7β7β7α7; Figs. 57.7 and 57.8). Three different active sites are located inside the cylindrical core within the β-subunit rings. Proteasome inhibitors target the 20S subunit of the proteasome. At least three distinct proteolytic activities are associated with the proteasome: chymotryptic, tryptic, and peptidylglutamyl. After release from the substrate, the polyubiquitin chain is hydrolyzed into single ubiquitin moieties, and tagged proteins are degraded to small peptides. Both the assembly of the 26S proteasome and the degradation of protein substrates are ATP dependent. The mechanism leading to cell death after proteasome inhibition are not fully understood, but it is hypothesized that accumulation of incompatible regulatory proteins within the cell, accumulation of mis-folded proteins from the ER ("ER stress") leading to suspension of protein synthesis, and interference with degradation of proteins that inhibit NFκB, leading to inhibition of NFκB, are the major contributors to cell death induced by proteasome inhibitors. Synergism between proteasome inhibition and cytotoxic chemotherapy is an area of active research. The activated B-cell subtype of DLBCL (ABC-DLBCL), which has inferior survival after anthracycline-based chemotherapy, is characterized by constitutive activation of the NFκB pathway, leading to resistance to apoptosis via the mitochondrial pathway through upregulation of NFκB-regulated genes (including bcl-2, bcl-XL, X-linked inhibitor of apoptosis [XIAP], and survivin). This explains the clinical benefit seen with the addition of bortezomib, the first-in-class proteasome inhibitor to anthracycline-based chemotherapy in ABC-DLBCL.

Transformed cells are much more sensitive to blockade of the proteasome than are normal cells; the exact mechanism of this selective susceptibility is not fully understood. Early studies revealed that proteasomes are abnormally highly expressed in rapidly growing metazoan embryonic and human neoplastic cells, but not in their well-differentiated and normal proliferating cells. The selectivity of proteasome inhibitors is not solely dependent on proliferative status since both transformed and normal fibroblasts have similar growth rates, although proteasome inhibitors are selectively toxic to SV-40–transformed cells.

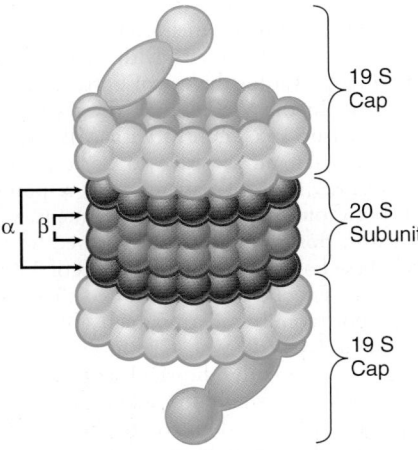

Fig. 57.7 26S PROTEASOME.

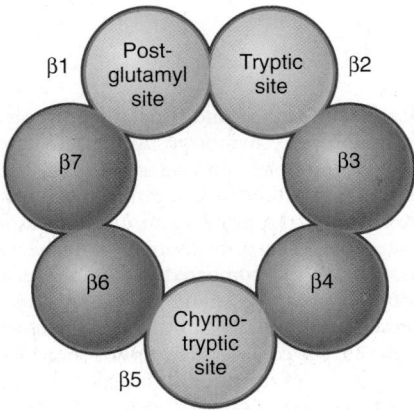

Fig. 57.8 CROSS-SECTION OF THE BETA RING OF THE 20S CORE OF THE 26S PROTEASOME.

Mechanisms of Resistance to Proteasome Inhibitors

Initial studies conducted using bortezomib-resistant cell lines identified mutations that affected the shape of the S1 pocket of the B5 subunit of the proteasome that is responsible for chemotrypsin-like activity. However, the clinical relevance of this finding is less certain, as mutations in the B5 subunit have not been identified in myeloma patients who are resistant to proteasome inhibitors. Upregulation of glutathione/oxidative injury defense systems (such as MUC1) was also demonstrated in bortezomib-resistant cell lines. Other mechanisms of proteasome resistance that have been observed in myeloma cell lines and disease models include upregulation of heat-shock proteins (such as heat-shock protein [HSP]90 and HSP27), which function as ubiquitin chaperones facilitating NFκB signaling and bortezomib efflux from cells through expression of PGP transporter. Gene expression signatures associated with bortezomib sensitivity and resistance have been characterized in cell lines derived from animal models of myeloma, yet the clinical relevance of such signatures awaits confirmation in large clinical trials.

Bortezomib

Bortezomib (pyrazylcarbonyl-Phe-Leu-boronate), the first in this class of agents to enter clinical trials, is a dipeptidyl boronic acid that is a specific and selective inhibitor of the 26S proteasome. The Boron atom interacts reversibly with the catalytic threonine residue of the proteasome, primarily inhibiting its chymotrypsin-like activity. The inhibition of the ubiquitin–proteasome pathway with bortezomib was demonstrated to arrest the growth of malignant cells (breast, colon, prostate tumor cell lines, Burkitt lymphoma, adult T-cell leukemia, Lewis lung carcinoma, CLL, and myeloma cell lines) and sensitize them to chemotherapeutic agents (5-FU, cisplatin, taxol, doxorubicin, CPT-11, and gemcitabine). Bortezomib mediates these effects through multiple mechanisms by regulating the expression of proteins involved in cell cycle progression (P21^{cip1}, P27^{Kip1}), oncogenesis (P53, IκB), apoptosis (BCL2, BIRC2, BIRC3, BIRC4, Bax), and, more recently, DNA repair (DNA-PKcs, ATM). Loss of IκB destabilizes NFκB, reducing expression of a critical plasma cell cytokine stimulatory molecule, interleukin (IL)-6 (see Chapter 86). The process of cell death appears to be p53 independent and to result in mitotic catastrophe, although the classical caspase 8-dependent apoptosis pathway has also been implicated. A recent study found a strong correlation between immunoglobulin production and apoptotic sensitivity to bortezomib, suggesting that the active requirement for protein folding in the ER provides a direct target and explains sensitivity to proteasome inhibition. It also suggests a selective mechanism that could explain the emergence of less differentiated myeloma cells with decreased immunoglobulin production during treatment. These processes also increase oxidative stress and contribute to apoptotic signaling, explaining the sensitivity of myeloma cells to proteasome inhibition.

Preclinical Studies With Bortezomib

Screening of the NCI tumor cell lines revealed that bortezomib is active against a broad range of tumor types. The average growth inhibition of 50% (GI$_{50}$) across the entire NCI cell panel (60 human-derived cell lines) occurred at 7 nM. Among solid tumor cell lines, those of the prostate, breast, colon, and pancreas were exquisitely sensitive to proteasomal inhibition. PC-3 prostate carcinoma cells, treated with bortezomib, underwent growth arrest in G2-M phase with a parallel increase in P21 levels and decreased activity, but not the levels of CDK-4. Bortezomib treatment also led to caspase activation, PARP cleavage, and apoptotic cell death with an IC$_{50}$ of 20 nM. Bortezomib exhibited synergistic effects when combined with SN-38 and radiation against colon tumor cells and in mouse xenografts. Similarly, pancreatic tumor xenografts were sensitive to the cytotoxic effect of bortezomib, particularly when combined with gemcitabine or CPT-11. Cytotoxic activity was reported as well against Lewis lung carcinoma cells and nasopharyngeal squamous cell carcinoma cells. In most of these studies, an increase in the cellular levels of P21WAF1, P27KIP1, P53, and IκB was observed.

In hematologic malignancies, proteasome inhibitors exhibited cytotoxic activity in a wide range of cell lines, including MM, U937 human monocytic leukemia, HL-60 promyelocytic leukemia, Jurkat T-cell leukemia, K562 CML, Ramos Burkitt lymphoma, and primary B-cell CLL. In MM cells, bortezomib induced p53 and MDM2 protein expression, induced phosphorylation (Ser15) of p53 protein, and activated JUN NH$_2$-terminal kinase (JNK), which in turn activated caspase 8 and caspase 3. Bortezomib was also shown to activate the intrinsic (mitochondria–cytochrome C [cyt c]–caspase 9) and extrinsic (JNK–death receptor-activated caspase 8) apoptotic pathways of the myeloma cells. Bortezomib blocked tumor necrosis factor (TNF)-induced NFκB activation through inhibition of IκB degradation. TNF-induced intracellular adhesion molecule (ICAM)–1 expression on RPMI8226 and MM.1S cells was also inhibited. The unfolded protein response not only was increased in plasma cells producing large quantities of immunoglobulin, but also induced a stress apoptosis response. Bortezomib also induced osteoblast activity through the Runx2/Cbfa2 pathway. Furthermore, bortezomib inhibited receptor activator of NFκB ligand -induced osteoclastogenesis through inhibition of P38 kinase. Increased osteoblast activity has the potential to restore the osteoporosis associated with MM when used with or without bisphosphonates. Moreover, it prevented the adherence of myeloma cells to BM stromal cells and the NFκB-dependent production of IL-6. Importantly, bortezomib demonstrated synergistic activity with dexamethasone, thalidomide, melphalan, and doxorubicin and did not appear to be a substrate for multidrug-resistance transporters. However, the NFκB blockade could not account for all of the antimyeloma activity of bortezomib, and other mechanisms clearly contribute to its antineoplastic effects. Finally, an IC$_{50}$ concentration of bortezomib in myeloma cells had no effect on peripheral blood mononuclear cells from healthy volunteers and did not affect cultured BM stromal cells. This did not preclude the observation of myelosuppression during treatment of patients with bortezomib as a single agent.

Pharmacology of Bortezomib

Bortezomib is primarily metabolized through cytochrome P450 (CYP) and not via phase II pathways (e.g., glucuronidation and sulfation). In vitro studies indicated that the primary metabolic pathway was deboronation mediated by CYP3A4. Bortezomib was also metabolized by CYP2D6, but the rate of metabolism was slower than that observed with CYP3A4. The deboronated metabolites have been shown to be inactive in the 20S proteasome assay. Bortezomib rapidly exits the plasma compartment, with more than 90% cleared within 15 minutes of IV administration. In whole-body autoradiography of [^{14}C] bortezomib-treated rats, the CNS, testes, and eyes appeared to be protected from bortezomib. Bortezomib specifically and selectively inhibits proteasome function by binding tightly (dissociation constant [K_i] >0.6 nM) and reversibly to the enzyme's chymotrypsin-like site. In ex vivo 20S proteasome activity bioassays, the proteasome was inhibited within 1 hour of bortezomib administration, and baseline proteasome activity was restored within 48–72 hours. An intermittent but high level of inhibition (>70%) of proteasome activity was better tolerated than sustained inhibition. Thus, a twice-weekly clinical dosing regimen is better tolerated. Nonetheless, this dose schedule is often associated with significant myelosuppression and the onset of peripheral neuropathy. Reducing the dose schedule to a weekly regimen ameliorates these toxicities and appears to increase patient tolerance without jeopardizing clinical efficacy.

Clinical Studies With Bortezomib

Phase II clinical trials (11 years ago) with bortezomib demonstrated the effectiveness of this agent in relapsed/refractory MM were reported. In the SUMMIT study of 202 patients with relapsed MM, 27% of patients achieved a PR or complete response (CR), and median time to progression was 7 months. The FDA approved the drug for use in relapsed/refractory MM in 2003 on the basis of this study. In 2008, the VISTA trial presented evidence demonstrating the superiority of bortezomib plus melphalan and prednisone (VMP) compared to MP alone for patients with newly diagnosed MM, which led to FDA approval for the use of bortezomib combinations as front-line therapy. In the VISTA trial, the median TTP was 24 months for VMP versus 16.6 months with MP. After initial treatment, many patients remain sensitive to bortezomib and can be retreated upon relapse; 63% of patients who responded to initial treatment with bortezomib respond to retreatment, with a median TTP of 9.3 months. Bortezomib is also approved for the treatment of relapsed MCL based on a demonstrated ORR of 33% in the phase II PINNACLE trial. Friedberg et al[11a] showed that the addition of bendamustine to bortezomib and rituximab (BVR) resulted in an ORR of 83% with a 2-year PFS of 47% in patients with relapsed/refractory MCL. More recently, the results of the phase III LYM-3002 trial were published where 487 adults with MCL ineligible for intensive therapy were randomized to R-CHOP vs VR-CAP (replacing vincristine with bortezomib). The VR-CAP arms had a median PFS of 24 months with a relative improvement of 59% over the R-CHOP arm and 4-year OS was also better (64% vs. 54%).

Second-Generation Proteasome Inhibitors

Carfilzomib: Carfilzomib is a second-generation proteasome inhibitor that selectively inhibits the chymotrypsin-like activity of the proteasome and is active in bortezomib-resistant patients. Carfilzomib induces irreversible inhibition (once carfilzomib binds to its active site within the barrel of the proteasome, the proteasome is permanently inactivated and new proteasomes must be synthesized to restore proteasome activity) compared with the reversible effects of bortezomib (duration of proteasome inhibition lasts about 72 h). Carfilzomib was approved in 2012 for the treatment of patients with myeloma who have received at least two prior therapies. As a monotherapy in phase II studies, carfilzomib induced an ORR of 20% in patients refractory to bortezomib. Carfilzomib appears to be less likely to cause peripheral neuropathy, and is safe in patients with renal impairment. Phase III studies of carfilzomib are ongoing. Higher response rates are observed when carfilzomib is used in combination with other agents such as lenalidomide and low-dose dexamethasone. The current FDA-approved dose of carfilzomib is 20 mg/m^2 for cycle 1, and 27 mg/m^2 for cycle 2. Recent data have shown MTD of carfilzomib is higher; therefore, a phase II study is underway to compare the two different doses of carfilzomib in combination with dexamethasone in a randomized fashion to determine if a higher dose can improve the efficacy while maintaining a safe toxicity profile.

Oprozomib (ONX-0912): Oprozomib is a structural analog of carfilzomib that is orally bioavailable. Oprozomib had demonstrated clinical activity in a phase I trial in patients with hematologic malignancies (myeloma and CLL). A once-daily administered oral dose was introduced in a phase Ib/II trial in order to improve gastrointestinal tolerability, and is demonstrating a good safety profile and promising preliminary response data.

Ixazomib (MLN9708): Ixazomib is a boronic acid-containing peptide with chymotrypsin- and caspase-like proteasome inhibitory activity, formulated for oral administration. Clinical trials, as single agent and in combination with HDAC inhibitors (HDIs), are underway to assess its effects in bortezomib-refractory patients. Early indications suggest that ixazomib may be associated with less neuropathy than bortezomib.

Delanzomib (CEP-18770): Delanzomib is a boronic acid-containing peptide formulated for oral administration. Early indications suggest that delanzomib may be associated with less neuropathy than bortezomib but it was noted to cause rash. A phase II trial of this drug has been terminated due to lack of efficacy in relapsed/refractory myeloma patients.

Marizomib (NPI-0052): Marizomib is a novel nonpeptidic, orally active, irreversibly-binding proteasome inhibitor with broad activity at all three catalytic sites of the proteasome. Since it is not peptide based, marizomib is resistant to degradation by endogenous proteases. It is capable of overcoming bortezomib resistance in vitro; clinical trials are underway but are still in early stages. Dose-limiting toxicities in phase I trials have included cognitive changes, transient hallucinations, and loss of balance, which were reversible. The most common drug-related adverse effects included fatigue, gastrointestinal adverse events, dizziness, and headache. There was no evidence of neuropathy or thrombocytopenia. Since marizomib has a different mechanism of action from bortezomib, and a nonoverlapping toxicity profile, combinations of these agents may be evaluated in future studies.

This is a very active area of research; there are over 10 structurally distinct classes of proteasome inhibitors in development, with new agents expected to enter clinical testing in the hopes of finding drugs with optimal potency, reduced toxicity and oral bioavailability. Table 57.2 outlines some of the ongoing clinical trials investigating the combination of second-generation proteasome inhibitors with other agents.

Toxicities of Proteasome Inhibitors

Given their broad application, prolonged exposure, and use in combination with other agents with similar toxicities (especially vinca alkaloids and IMiDs), there has been a considerable effort to characterize and mitigate the side effects of proteasome inhibitors. One of the major motivations for the development of the second-generation agents has been to reduce the occurrence of neuropathy. Unlike IMiDs, proteasome inhibitors, as a class, do not appear to induce chromosomal abnormalities and therefore are not associated with an increased risk for secondary malignancies. Proteasome inhibitors may therefore be safer for long-term use/maintenance therapy than other agents. (see Table 57.2).

Peripheral Neuropathy

The peripheral neuropathy associated with bortezomib is typically a sensory neuropathy affecting the hands and feet in a "stocking and glove" distribution, and is frequently painful. Grade ≥ 3 PN occurs in 5%–15% of patients but is reversible in the most cases (in the phase III VISTA trial, 60% of instances of neuropathy showed complete resolution within a median of 5.7 months). The mechanism by which bortezomib produces peripheral neuropathy is unknown, but is hypothesized to be due to aggresome formation and cytoskeletal collapse in dorsal root ganglion sensory neuron axons, alterations in mitochondrial function, or other off-target effects. It is possible that the boron moiety is implicated in the peripheral neuropathy since carfilzomib (which does not contain a boron atom) is much less likely to cause neuropathy than bortezomib. The incidence of peripheral neuropathy with bortezomib is reduced by subcutaneous (SC) administration and weekly dosing. The lower incidence of neuropathy of SC vs. IV administration of bortezomib has been attributed to IV dosing achieving peak serum levels of bortezomib that exceed the threshold that causes peripheral neuropathy, whereas the slower pharmacokinetics of SC administration deliver an effective antimyeloma dose without exceeding the neuropathy threshold.

Hematologic Toxicity

Hematologic adverse events appear to be a class effect associated with proteasome inhibitors; all agents tested so far are associated with thrombocytopenia, neutropenia, anemia, and lymphopenia. Differences in the tendency of the different agents to cause hematologic toxicity remain to be established as newer agents undergo further testing in clinical trials (there is hope that second-generation drugs may have lower rates of hematologic toxicity). Bortezomib, carfilzomib, and ixazomib cause transient, cyclical thrombocytopenia, with platelet counts dropping and then returning to baseline prior to the next cycle of treatment. The exact mechanism of bortezomib-induced thrombocytopenia remains to be fully elucidated. Bortezomib does not appear to adversely affect stem cell function. One hypothesis is that proteasome inhibition with bortezomib prevents the activation of NFκB, which leads to impairment of platelet budding from megakaryocytes.

Herpes Zoster Reactivation

Bortezomib has been associated with a significantly increased rate of herpes zoster reactivation. In the phase III study of bortezomib plus melphalan and prednisone versus MP alone, zoster reactivation was observed in 13% of patients in the VMP group versus 4% in the MP group. In the subgroup of patients in the VMP group who were receiving antiviral prophylaxis, the rate of zoster reactivation was reduced to 3%. The increased susceptibility to herpes zoster reactivation in patients treated with bortezomib may be due to the effect of bortezomib treatment on the number and function of specific lymphocyte subsets.

Other Toxicities

Infusion reactions (chills, fever, and dyspnea) have been observed with carfilzomib. Therefore, it is recommended that dexamethasone (4 mg PO or IV) be administered prior to each dose during cycle 1 and prior to the first of the higher doses during cycle 2. Carfilzomib has been associated with pulmonary complications, renal toxicity, and cardiac events (including congestive heart failure and cardiac arrest) in 7% of treated patients. Chest pain and acute congestive heart failure may have been related to prehydration with normal saline. Ixazomib may cause transient rash. Marizomib has been reported to cause reversible CNS toxicities (hallucinations, loss of coordination). The toxicities of the newer agents will ultimately be important in determining whether these drugs are suitable for first-line use.

Targeting Apoptosis Signaling in Hematologic Malignancies

The processes of cell division and cell death are tightly coupled so that a net increase in cell numbers does not occur. Alterations in the expression or function of the genes controlling cell division and cell death can upset this delicate balance and are hallmarks of cancer. Although conventional anticancer drugs cause cell cycle perturbation or DNA damage, they do not directly interact with the intracellular machinery involved in apoptosis. Tumor selectivity of conventional agents is largely caused by the increased sensitivity to apoptosis of tumor cells after DNA damage or cell cycle perturbation. Novel therapeutic agents or strategies that target critical regulators or effectors of apoptosis are under development and clinical testing, and these agents or strategies have the potential to exert selective cytotoxicity against cancer cells.

Caspases are the "executioners" for apoptosis. They are proteases that exist as inactive zymogens and are activated by proteolytic cleavage of their proforms in response to a variety of death stimuli. This processing occurs at conserved aspartic acid residues, thus generating the enzymatically active caspases. Caspase activation is organized as a cascade, with an upstream initiator and downstream effector caspase. Upstream initiator caspases contain large prodomains that interact with specific proteins involved in triggering the cascade. The downstream caspases, which function as the ultimate effectors of apoptosis, possess small prodomains and are activated predominantly by proteolytic cleavage by upstream caspases. The irreversible cleavage of specific protein death substrates by the downstream effector caspases directly or indirectly accounts for the biochemical and morphologic changes that are recognized as apoptosis.

At least three pathways of caspase activation leading to apoptosis have been identified (Fig. 57.9): (1) the receptor-initiated apoptosis pathway, where the TNF family of cytokine receptors activate initiator caspases such as caspase 8; (2) the mitochondria-initiated apoptosis pathway, where cyt c and other prodeath effectors are released from mitochondria into the cytosol that results in activation of caspase 9; and (3) a pathway of caspase activation, which involves a serine protease, granzyme B, that directly cleaves and activates several caspases, including procaspase 3.

Proapoptotic Targets of Anticancer Agents

Most cancer cells have active antiapoptotic pathways that prevent cell death in response to growth, checkpoint, DNA damage, and metabolic stimuli. A number of current anticancer agents in development target these pathways and are designed to be effective alone or in combination with other agents that disrupt the cell cycle, DNA synthesis, invoke DNA damage, and so on.

Death Receptor–Initiated Apoptotic Signaling

Several TNF family receptors are known to transduce signals that result in apoptosis. These include TNFRSF1A (also known as CD120a and previously designated tumor necrosis factor receptor-1 [TNFR1]), TNFRSF6 (also known as CD95, APO-1, or FAS), TNFRSF25 (also designated TRAMP and known as DR3 or APO3), TNFRSF10A (also known as DR4 or TRAIL-R1), and TNFRSF10B (also known as DR5 or TRAIL-R2). These receptors, also called *death receptors*, are characterized by the presence of a death domain within their cytoplasmic region, and have been shown to trigger apoptosis upon binding to their cognate ligands or specific agonist antibody. The activating ligands for these death receptors are structurally related molecules that also belong to the TNF gene superfamily such as TNFSF6 (also known as Fas ligand), TNF, and TRAIL.

Ligation of death receptors produces receptor trimerization and formation of a death-inducing signaling complex (DISC). This is composed of TNFRSF6, Fas (TNFRSF6)-associated via death domain (FADD), and procaspase 8, an apical signaling complex that mediates receptor-induced apoptosis. FADD binds directly to FasR, TNFRSF10A, or TNFRSF10B and indirectly to TNFRSF1A via TNFRSF1A-associated via death domain protein (TRADD). FADD is essential for cell death signaling from all three receptors. FADD interacts through its C-terminal death domain to cross-link TNFRSF6, TNFRSF10A, or TNFRSF10B receptors and recruits procaspase 8 and procaspase 10, or TRADD, through its N-terminal death effector domain (DED) to the DISC (see Fig. 57.9). Oligomerization of caspase 8 within the DISC results in a high local concentration of the zymogen. The induced proximity under these crowded conditions generates low levels of intrinsic proteolytic activity of caspase 8, enough to allow the various proenzymatic molecules

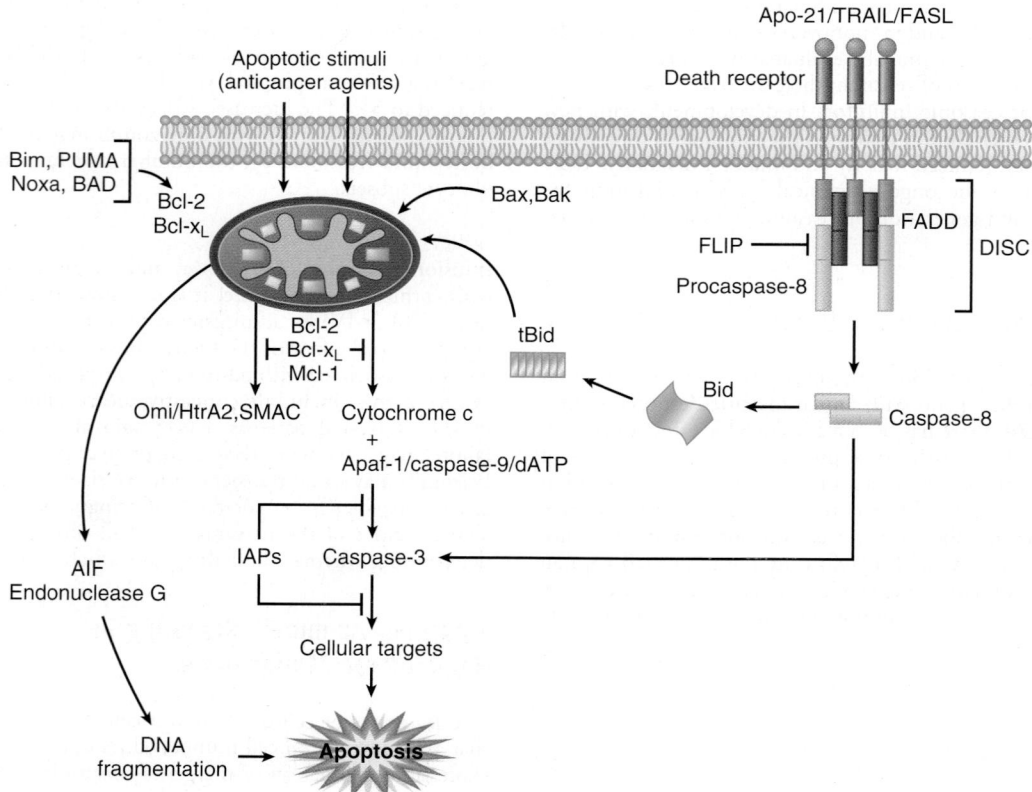

Fig. 57.9 SCHEMATIC REPRESENTATION OF APOPTOTIC PATHWAYS.

to mutually cleave each other. Processing of caspase 8 removes the DED-containing prodomain, thus releasing the activated protease into the cytosol, where it can cleave and activate other downstream procaspases. In certain types of cells (type I), enough caspase 8 is activated by the activation of the death receptor to cause apoptosis. In other cell types, such as hepatocytes (type II), a sufficient level of caspase 8 activation is not achieved and the apoptotic signal is amplified by the mitochondrial pathway. The active caspase 8 cleaves the cytosolic p22 Bid into a BH3-only domain-containing, proapoptotic, truncated p15 tBid fragment, which translocates to the mitochondria and triggers the release of cyt c into the cytosol. Cleavage by caspase 8 has been shown to cause exposure of a glycine residue on p15 Bid that is myristoylated, thereby targeting p15 Bid to the mitochondria. Thus, N-myristoylation acts as an activating switch that enhances tBid-induced release of cyt c and apoptosis. The ability to cleave Bid may not be limited to caspase 8. Other caspases, such as caspase 3, as well other proteases, such as granzyme B and lysosomal proteases, have been shown to activate Bid. This indicates that Bid probably serves to amplify the caspase cascade rather than to initiate it (see Fig. 57.9).

Fas ligation has also been shown to initiate an alternative pathway leading to apoptosis, involving activation of JNK/SAPK. After ligation, Fas recruits an adaptor protein called Daxx that interacts with the apoptosis signal-regulating kinase 1 (ASK1), activating the transcription factors AP-1 and ATF-2. After activation, ASK-1 launches a phosphorylation cascade that culminates in the activation of JNK. Activated JNK phosphorylates substrates such as c-Jun, p53, and a pro-death Bcl-2 member Bim. This, in turn, has been shown to trigger mitochondrial or death receptor-initiated apoptotic signaling.

Mitochondria-Initiated Apoptotic Signaling

Mitochondria sequester a potent cocktail of proapoptotic proteins. These proteins promote apoptosis by activating caspases (e.g., by cyt c), by inducing DNA fragmentation (e.g., by endonuclease G or apoptosis-inducing factor [AIF]), or by neutralizing cytosolic inhibitors of apoptosis (IAPs; e.g., by SMAC or Omi/HtrA2). On induction of apoptosis, unlike other proapoptotic proteins, mitochondrial AIF translocates to the nucleus to induce DNA fragmentation and apoptosis. Cyt c is a well-known component of the mitochondrial electron transfer chain. Cyt c is released from the mitochondria during apoptosis. After release into the cytosol, cyt c binds to apoptosis-activating factor (Apaf-1), a cytosolic adapter protein that contains a caspase recruitment domain (CARD), a nucleotide-binding domain, and multiple WD-40 repeats. Binding of cyt c to Apaf-1 increases its affinity for dATP or ATP by approximately 10-fold. It also triggers the oligomerization of Apaf-1 into a multimeric Apaf-1–cyt c complex, also called the *apoptosome*. This exposes the CARD domain of Apaf-1, which recruits several molecules of procaspase 9, inducing their autoactivation. Only the caspase 9 bound to the apoptosome is able to efficiently cleave and activate a downstream executioner caspase, caspase 3.

SMAC/DIABLO is a 25-kDa mitochondrial protein that is released by mitochondria into the cytosol during apoptosis. SMAC contains a mitochondria-targeting sequence at its N-terminus. This sequence is removed on import into the mitochondria, generating the mature SMAC protein. In the mitochondria-initiated and common effector pathways of apoptosis, the processing and proteolytic activity of caspase 9 followed by caspases 3 and 7 are inhibited by the IAP family of proteins. IAP family members include XIAP, cIAP1, cIAP2, and survivin. All IAPs contain at least one baculovirus repeat (BIR) domain, although some contain three. Another region, the RING domain, has ubiquitin ligase activity and promotes the self-degradation of IAPs through proteasomes in response to some apoptotic stimuli. Furthermore, during Fas death receptor-mediated apoptosis, XIAP is cleaved by activated caspase 3 into the N-terminal BIR1 and 2 and BIR3-RING finger fragments. The BIR3 domain binds and sequesters the monomeric and inactive caspase 9, thereby

inhibiting its activation. Overexpression of XIAP inhibits anticancer drug (including ara-C)–induced caspase activity and apoptosis. In contrast, downregulation of XIAP sensitizes cancer cells to apoptosis induced by chemotherapeutic drugs. The antiapoptotic activity of NFκB has also been shown to be mediated by the induction of IAPs. The first four amino acids of the mature SMAC, Ala-Val-Pro-Ile (AVPI), bind to the BIR domain of IAP proteins. The four amino acids (AVPI) of SMAC that bind to the BIR3 domain of XIAP are similar to the XIAP-binding sequence of active caspase 9. In addition, SMAC has been shown to form a stable complex with the BIR2 domain of XIAP. SMAC binds to the linker-BIR2 domain and presumably disrupts its inhibition of the active caspase 3 and caspase 7 by steric hindrance. On induction of apoptosis, another mitochondrial protein, Omi/HtrA2 (a serine protease), is released from mitochondria and can induce caspase-independent cell death. Additionally, like SMAC, the mature Omi protein contains a conserved IAP-binding motif (AVPS) at its N-terminus. Omi complexes with XIAP at high stoichiometry and promotes apoptosis by neutralizing the caspase-inhibitory effect of XIAP. Recently, Omi has also been shown to process XIAP and promote its proteasomal degradation.

The Bcl-2 family of proteins is divided into three subfamilies. Members of the subfamily that include Bcl-2, Bcl-x_L, and Mcl-1 inhibit apoptosis (see Fig. 57.9). The Bax subfamily members that promote apoptosis, including Bax and Bak, share with Bcl-2 three of the four Bcl-2 homology domains, BH1–BH3. A C-terminus hydrophobic tail is responsible for the localization of these proteins to the outer membranes of the mitochondria and ER. The third BH3-only subfamily of proteins that includes Bid, Bim, and Bad also promotes apoptosis by binding and inactivating prosurvival Bcl-2 family members. The prosurvival Bcl-2 family members, to a variable degree, are bound to the membranes of the mitochondria, the ER, and the nuclear envelope. In the event of an apoptotic stimulus, BH3-only proteins require Bax and Bak to trigger mitochondrial apoptotic signaling. For example, the exposed BH3 domain of tBid oligomerizes with Bak and Bax, causing their mitochondrial membrane insertion and cyt c release. In response to apoptotic stimuli, Bax and Bak undergo conformational change and form membrane-associated homo-oligomers, disrupting the outer membrane of the mitochondria and ER and releasing the pro-death molecules into the cytosol. Besides tBid, Humanin peptide has been shown to activate Bax. Bcl-2 can block these events involving Bax activation by titrating tBid or Bim and/or heterodimerization with Bax and preventing mitochondrial permeabilization.

Induction of P53^wt in cells triggers apoptosis by transcriptional activation of prodeath effectors, including Bax, Noxa, Puma, Apaf-1, and DR5, and by transcriptional repression of Bcl-2 and IAPs. p53-dependent apoptosis has also been shown to occur in the absence of any gene transcription or translation. In response to apoptotic stimulus such as irradiation, p53 translocates to the mitochondria, where it directly induces permeabilization of the outer membrane by forming complexes with the protective Bcl-2, resulting in the release of cyt c into the cytosol. The E2F transcription factor, normally restrained by the Rb tumor suppressor to inhibit cell proliferation, has been shown to induce apoptosis though p53-dependent and p53-independent mechanisms. These mechanisms include transcriptional activation of ARF (the alternate reading frame product of the INK4a/ARF tumor suppressor locus) or p73 (a member of the p53 family), repression of Mcl-1, and inducing the levels of caspase proenzymes.

Selective Antiapoptotic Agents or Strategies

BCL2 Family of Proteins as Targets for Anticancer Drug Design

The antiapoptotic protein BCL2 was originally identified during the process of the discovery of the t(14;18) in human follicular lymphoma. Overexpression of BCL2 has been reported in both hematologic and solid malignancies and to mediate resistance to traditional chemotherapeutic agents, radiation, and other antitumor treatments.

Bcl-2 Antisense

Liposomal antisense Bcl-2 oligonucleotide (Bcl-ASODN) has been created and shown to cause apoptosis of many types of cancer and leukemia cells. Bcl-2-ASODN also sensitized tumor cells in vitro and in vivo to chemotherapeutic drugs. The most promising agent to target Bcl-2 is Genasense (oblimersan sodium; G3139), an 18-mer phosphorothioate oligodeoxynucleotide antisense compound. Clinical studies suggest safety and efficacy in solid and hematologic malignancies. In a phase III trial, 241 patients were randomly assigned to receive oblimersen 3 mg/kg/day as a 7-day continuous infusion in addition to fludarabine–cyclophosphamide versus fludarabine–cyclophosphamide. This study met its primary objective by demonstrating a significantly superior CR or nodular partial remission (CR/nPR; 17% vs. 7%; $p = .025$); however, no significant differences in ORRs as well as TTP were found. However, at 5-year follow-up a significant improvement in survival was noted, with a hazard ratio of 0.6 for those treated with oblimersen. Results of another phase III study were reported in which the addition of oblimersan to high-dose dexamethasone did not improve OS or TTP in myeloma patients.

BH3 Peptide/Mimetics or Bcl-2/Bcl-XL Small-Molecule Antagonists

Another strategy to create Bcl-2 inhibitors has focused on developing small molecules that mimic the action of the endogenous Bcl-2-binding death agonists. Compounds that mimic the BH3-only class of death agonists such as Bad inhibit the survival proteins Bcl-2 and Bcl-x_L but do not appear to have independent proapoptotic activity. Two classes of novel small-molecule cell-permeable inhibitors of the Bcl-x_L-BH3 domain (BH3I) have been identified. Studies have demonstrated that BH3Is induce apoptosis by preventing BH3 domain-mediated interaction between proapoptotic and antiapoptotic members of the Bcl-2 family. Two natural products have been suggested to antagonize the antiapoptotic function of Bcl-2 or Bcl-x_L. Tetrocarin A was reported to inhibit mitochondrial functions of Bcl-2 and suppress its antiapoptotic activity. In another report, Antimycin-A was shown to mimic activity of BH3 peptides and selectively induce apoptosis in cell lines overexpressing Bcl-x_L. Certain green tea catechins and black tea theaflavins were identified as potent inhibitors (K_i in the nanomolar range) of the antiapoptotic Bcl-2 family of proteins. On the basis of the high-resolution three-dimensional structure of the target receptor, small organic molecules that bind to this interface have been designed. ABT-737 is a BH3 mimetic that binds to Bcl-2, Bcl-xL, and Bcl-w with high affinity (K_i <1 nM) but not to Mcl-1. Preclinical data demonstrate cytotoxic activity in B lymphoid tumor cell lines, human follicular lymphoma, myeloma, and CLL cells, as well as synergism with other chemotherapeutic agents. Also, ABT-737 effectively kills AML blast, progenitor, and stem cells without disturbing normal hematopoietic cell development. However, the clinical utility of ABT-737 is limited, as it undergoes rapid metabolism and is not orally bioavailable. Targeted modifications of ABT-737 led to synthesis of navitoclax (ABT-263), an orally bioavailable BH3 mimetic. In the initial phase I trial[12] more than half of patients had a decrease in their lymphocytosis, with 35% achieving partial remission. The main toxicity was dose-dependent thrombocytopenia, which occurred early in the treatment cycle (days 2–5 of a 21-day cycle). Neutropenia occurred at higher dose levels. Other adverse events included gastrointestinal side effects and fatigue. The remarkable activity of this agent in early trials validated Bcl-2 as a target for the treatment of CLL. The clinical development of navitoclax was suspended because of thrombocytopenia; which is an off-target effect due to inhibition of Bcl-XL.

Venetoclax (Abt-199) was subsequently developed to replace navitoclax as a highly selective, orally available small-molecule Bcl-2 family protein inhibitor that binds with high affinity (K_i <0.10 nM) to Bcl-2 and with lower affinity to other Bcl-2 family proteins Bcl-XL and Bcl-w (>480-fold and >2000-fold lower affinity than to Bcl-2, respectively). Thrombocytopenia is less frequent with venetoclax due to its lower affinity to Bcl-XL. Early clinical experience with venetoclax is very promising, with remarkable efficacy in a patient population with relapsed or refractory CLL with high ORR (75%–79%) and impressive CR rates (22%–29%) and clearance of MRD even in the high-risk subsets of patients with the adverse-risk del(17p) chromosomal abnormality associated with p53 mutation/dysfunction, an unmutated immunoglobulin heavy chain gene (IGHV), and those with disease refractory to fludarabine in a phase I trial. The early clinical trials of venetoclax were suspended initially because all patients treated developed tumor lysis syndrome (TLS), which led to two deaths. That led to modification of the clinical protocol with a gradual dose escalation of venetoclax on a 2–3-weekly basis up to the target dose of 400 mg daily with stringent monitoring and aggressive prophylaxis and management of TLS. Although laboratory evidence of TLS remain highly prevalent in patients with CLL treated with venetoclax, no deaths due to TLS have been observed after adoption of these modifications. ORR rates as high as 61% have been reported in a mixed cohort of patients with relapsed NHL in combination with bendamustine and rituximab with no added toxicity. The responses were few in patients with relapsed DLBCL; however, responses (37.5%) were seen in patients with indolent lymphomas. A phase III clinical trial is in progress in patients with relapsed/refractory CLL comparing venetoclax and rituximab to bendamustine and rituximab. Venetoclax has received approval for relapsed/refractory CLL with del(17p) based on impressive clinical activity. However, the risk of TLS may be prohibitive to limit its use to clinicians with expertise in management of hematological malignancies and TLS.

Cyclin-Dependent Kinase Inhibitors

Orderly progression through the cell cycle is regulated by the coordinated expression of a variety of genes and proteins, and effected by the interactions between cyclins, CDKs 1–9 and endogenous CDK inhibitors (e.g., p21^{CIP1}, p27^{KIP1}, and p57^{KIP2}; see Fig. 57.1). CDK1, in association with cyclins A and B, is involved in G_2M progression; CDK2, CDK4, and CDK6, in association with cyclins A, D, and E, are involved in G_1S progression. Activation of CDKs results in phosphorylation of the pRb, which leads to its dissociation from the E2F transcription factor. Once freed, E2F triggers the transcription of diverse genes involved in cell cycle progression (thymidylate synthase and dihydrofolate reductase, among numerous others). Endogenous small-molecule CDK inhibitors such as P21^{CIP1} and P27^{KIP1} bind stoichiometrically to CDKs and inhibit their activity. CDK activity can also be regulated through inhibitory or activating phosphorylation. Interference with the activation of CDKs results in dephosphorylation of pRb, leading in turn to binding and inactivation of E2F and inhibition of cell cycle progression.

Cell cycle dysregulation is a cardinal characteristic of cancer. A classic example of this phenomenon is the association of increased expression of cyclin D_1 in MCL. Regulation of the cell cycle has been found to be closely related to apoptosis, and disruption of normal cell cycle transit has been shown to be a potent cell death stimulus. A corollary of this observation is that agents that interfere with the cell cycle, in addition to blocking cell cycle progression, can be potent inducers of programmed cell death. Cell cycle inhibitors can be subdivided into several categories. For example, they can act directly, as in the case of CDK inhibitors, or indirectly, as in the case of HDIs, compounds that block cell cycle progression by inducing endogenous cell cycle inhibitors such as P21^{CIP1}. The latter agents are discussed later in this chapter. CDK inhibitors can also be classified as specific (i.e., directed against a particular CDK, such as CDK2) or those that nonspecifically inhibit most CDKs (e.g., flavopiridol).

Flavopiridol

Flavopiridol (L86-8275) is a semisynthetic flavonoid derived from the Indian plant *rohitukine*. It was the first CDK inhibitor to enter clinical trials in humans. Flavopiridol binds to the ATP-binding site of CDKs, resulting in reversible, competitive enzyme inhibition at concentrations of less than 100 nM. As noted earlier, flavopiridol is a relatively nonspecific CDK inhibitor and inhibits all CDKs, although it is less effective against CDK7. Flavopiridol induces G_1S or G_2M arrest, presumably a consequence of inhibition of CDK1 and CDK2. Flavopiridol may also act to block cell cycle progression by downregulating cyclin D_1 levels, inhibiting the CDK-activating complex (CDK7), or both.

In addition to blocking cell cycle progression, flavopiridol has been shown to be a potent inducer of apoptosis in malignant hematopoietic cells (e.g., acute and chronic leukemia) at low concentrations (e.g., <100 nM). Moreover, flavopiridol has shown activity against MM cells in vitro.

The proapoptotic actions of flavopiridol have been attributed to its capacity to inhibit the positive transcription elongation factor-β (PTEF-β), cyclin T/CDK9 complex by inhibiting phosphorylation of the C-terminal domain of RNA polymerase II. This leads to downregulation of several antiapoptotic proteins, including BIRC4, $P_{21}{}^{CIP1}$, and, in the case of MM cells, Mcl-1. Flavopiridol has also recently been shown to block the antiapoptotic actions of the IAP family member survivin.

In clinical studies, flavopiridol was initially administered as a 72-hour continuous infusion every 2 weeks, with a maximally tolerated dose of 40 mg/m^2. Steady-state plasma levels in excess of those necessary to inhibit CDKs and induce apoptosis in leukemia cells (e.g., 350 nM) were achieved. Dose-limiting toxicities were fatigue, diarrhea, nausea, and myelosuppression. However, the occurrence of thromboembolic phenomena and the general lack of single-agent activity have limited enthusiasm for administering flavopiridol by this schedule. Flavopiridol has also been administered as a daily IV bolus for 1, 3, or 5 days every 3 weeks with manageable toxicity, and other schedules are being examined, including a hybrid schedule with half the dose administered as an IV bolus and the other half as a more prolonged infusion. When administered as a daily bolus infusion for 3 days every 3 weeks, flavopiridol exhibited modest activity in patients with MCL. A novel pharmacologically directed schedule of flavopiridol has been developed in which half of the dose (e.g., 30 mg/m^2) is administered as a 30-minute bolus-loading infusion and 30 mg/m^2 as a 4-hour infusion. In a phase I study, objective response rates of 45% were obtained with this schedule in patients with progressive CLL, including some with high-risk disease.[13] Because of the rapidity of response, particularly in patients with high white blood cell counts, aggressive measures designed to avoid TLS (e.g., hydration, alkalinization of the urine, administration of rasburicase) are advisable. Efforts are now underway to use this novel flavopiridol schedule in combination with other agents and in other hematologic malignancies.

Because of limited single-agent activity, combination regimens involving flavopiridol are being explored in hematologic malignancies. On the basis of preclinical evidence of synergism with the antimetabolite ara-C, a regimen combining flavopiridol on a daily IV bolus schedule followed by high-dose ara-C has been initiated in patients with AML and has shown some activity. In a phase II study, flavopiridol was administered as a 1-hour bolus infusion of 50 mg/m^2 daily for 3 days before administration of high-dose ara-C (day 6) and mitoxantrone (day 9). CR rates of 67% were obtained in patients with high-risk AML and more than half were durable. More recently, evidence of synergism between flavopiridol and other signal transduction modulators has become the focus of considerable attention. For example, the observation that flavopiridol interacts synergistically with imatinib mesylate against CML cells, including some that are imatinib mesylate resistant, has prompted the initiation of a phase I trial of flavopiridol and imatinib mesylate in patients with progressive BCR-ABL$^+$ hematologic malignancies. Four out of 21 patients responded. Evidence that flavopiridol interacts synergistically with HDAC and proteasome inhibitors in human leukemia cells has appeared, and clinical trials combining flavopiridol with the HDI vorinostat or the proteasome inhibitor bortezomib in patients with refractory AML/MDS and MM/indolent NHL are currently underway.

SNS032

SNS032 is a small-molecule CDK inhibitor discovered through high-throughput screening that is primarily active against CDK2. In preclinical studies, SNS032 has shown potent antiproliferative activity against ovarian and breast cancer cells in vitro. As is the case with other CDK inhibitors, SNS032 induces cell cycle arrest, pRb dephosphorylation, and, under some circumstances, apoptosis in CLL and myeloma cell lines. At least in some tumor cell lines, however, CDK2 may be dispensable for cell cycle progression. In CLL cells, SNS-032 was cytotoxic in vitro in untreated and refractory cell lines. RNA synthesis was suppressed after treatment, with evidence of CDK 2 and 7 inhibition.[14]

Several phase I trials of SNS032 have been initiated. SNS032 has been administered as either a 24-hour or 1-hour infusion every 3 weeks. Dose levels of 4–59 mg/m^2 have proven to be tolerable; the maximum tolerated dose for either of these schedules has not been reached. Toxicities have been mild and include rash, nausea and vomiting, diarrhea, and fatigue. In a clinical trial in patients with CLL (19 patients) and myeloma (18 patients), CDK7 and -9 inhibition was observed, but responses as a single agent were modest.

Hypomethylating Agents

Promoter methylation within CpG islands regulates gene expression in all cells. Disruption of normal gene expression profiles accompanies malignant transformation, giving rise to complex patterns of gene expression. As a consequence, promoters of many genes have an altered pattern of methylation, resulting in either gene activation or gene repression. The link between these concepts and the interest in agents that alter promoter methylation began with the realization that azacitidine, an agent used sparingly for treating myeloid leukemias, had efficacy when given at low doses either IV or SC for extended periods of time, and that in these cases, altered gene expression accompanied responses. Both azacitidine and 5-aza-2′-deoxycytidine (decitabine) act by irreversible inhibition of the DNA methyltransferases responsible for methylation of the cytidine in CpG islands and are thus S-phase–specific agents. Wijermans et al[14a] first described that a related compound, 5-aza-2′-deoxycytidine, was effective when given as a continuous infusion to elderly patients with high-risk MDS, with a 54% response rate. The mechanism of action included both a direct change in promoter methylation and independent changes, with up to 70% genome-wide demethylation, suggesting either that genes with altered expression either up- or downregulated a second set of genes through altered pathways such as induction of WAFp21, p15, and p16, or in a more direct fashion through altered transcription factor expression. More recent studies have identified activity of these agents in both AML and CML. Most often, PRs or short-lived CRs are seen in AML, with CRs more common in MDS. Recent studies also describe a number of extended therapy regimens. Kantarjian et al[14b] reported a comparison of 20 mg/m^2 decitabine IV for 5 days with 20 mg/m^2 SC daily for 5 days and 10 mg/m^2 IV for 10 days. The 5-day IV dose schedule was judged superior on the basis of clinical outcome with 39% CR, a higher proportion of reactivation of p15, and achievement of a hypomethylation state as well as clinical tolerance. Azacitidine has been given after allogeneic stem cell transplantation, at lower doses, as a "maintenance" regimen, to prevent relapse. De Lima et al[14c] established the MTD of azacitidine after transplant as 32 mg/m^2 for 5 days. Posttransplant azacitidine may also augment graft-versus-leukemia effect and attenuate GVHD after transplant through expansion of T-regulatory cells. An oral formulation of azacitidine is currently in clinical development which would permit convenient and prolonged exposure to the drug, which may translate into better outcomes. It was recently shown that pretreatment with azacitidine, followed by R-CHOP chemotherapy, can restore chemosensitivity in DLBCL cells in vitro and in clinical samples from patients with DLBCL. The combination between azacitidine and R-CHOP was feasible, safe, and associated with a higher ORR compared with historic controls treated with R-CHOP alone. Azacitidine "priming" decreased SMAD1 methylation, and increased SMAD1 mRNA, in DLBCL cells obtained from patients. SMAD1 is the major downstream effector of TGF-β. TGF-β exerts an antiproliferative effect in most NHL, and loss of antiproliferative response to TGF-β has been demonstrated in the majority of NHLs. SMAD1 hypomethylation has been associated with an abundance of SMAD1 mRNA and restoration of chemosensitivity in DLBCL cells after azacitidine "priming."

Histone Deacetylase Inhibitors

Histone acetyl transferases (HATs) control gene expression through the modification of chromatin structure through acetylation of chromatin-bound histones. Regulation of acetylation is through histone deacetylation. Without the ability to fine tune histone binding to chromatin regions, gene expression is perturbed. Inhibition of this process by a group of agents termed *histone deacetylation inhibitors* alters gene expression in both normal and malignant cells. Often the result is differentiation of malignant cells or induction of apoptosis. Given the long history of the use of differentiating agents in leukemias, for APL (retinoids), low-dose ara-C and azacytidine, it is not surprising that newer HDIs have undergone extensive evaluation in leukemias.

Posttranslational Histone and Nonhistone Protein Modifications and Gene Transcription

Nucleosomes are regularly repeating, structural units of chromatin, which are essential in packaging eukaryotic DNA. Each unit is composed of 146 base pairs of DNA tightly wrapped around a core histone octamer. Each histone octamer consists of two units each of histones H2A, H2B, H3, and H4, and each nucleosome in turn is connected to its neighbor by a short segment of linker DNA approximately 10–80 base pairs in length. Histone H1 binds and stabilizes linker DNA. Each core histone has an N-terminal tail, which is lysine rich and positively charged. Specific amino acid residues at the N-terminal undergo a variety of enzymatic posttranslational modifications. Modifications can also occur within the globular domain of histones that make extensive contacts with DNA. *Histone code* is the name given to the combination of biochemical modifications affecting different histone residues that specify chromatin function. However, it has been suggested that various postsynthesis histone modifications be considered an epigenomic alphabet. Each modification is a letter, and the combination of modifications at a specified genomic region is a word that may have different functional meanings depending on the context.

HATs and HDACs are two classes of enzymes that mediate the acetylation and deacetylation, respectively, at evolutionarily-conserved N-terminal lysine residues. Acetylated histones are negatively charged and do not bind as tightly to negatively charged DNA, thereby facilitating gene transcription. In contrast, deacetylated histones bind closely to DNA, preventing transcription. Acetylation status of chromatin and hence gene transcription is dictated by balanced activity of HATs and HDACs. Acetylation of core histone bases has also been implicated in chromatin assembly, DNA repair, and replication timing of specific genomic regions. Cross-talk also exists between acetylation and ubiquitination. Thus, HDACs can decrease the half-lives of substrates by exposing the lysine residue for ubiquitination. Other crucial functions affected by the delicate balance between HATs and HDACs include activation of the apoptotic program via interaction between Ku70 and Bax; protein localization (nuclear vs. cytoplasm); and DNA binding of transcription factors such as p53, E2F1, GATA1, RelA, YY1, and hormone receptors. There is a growing list of nonhistone proteins that are modulated by HATs or HDACs. These include hypoxia-inducible factor-1α (HIF-1α), β-catenin, α-tubulin, Ku70, importin-α 7, cortactin, and, most recently, HSP90. HATs and HDACs can be classified into subfamilies according to the presence of highly conserved structural motifs. Please refer to Table 57.5 for details.

Aberrant Histone Acetyl Transferase and Histone Deacetylase Activity in Hematologic Malignancies

Aberrant activity of HATs and HDACs resulting in aberrant gene transcription is a hallmark of many cancers, including many hematologic malignancies. Several chromosomal translocations in leukemia that produce chimeric fusion oncoproteins have been shown to recruit HDACs to promoters and repress genes involved in cell cycle growth inhibition and differentiation. For example, PML-RARα in APL and AML1-ETO generated by t(8;21) translocation in AML recruit HDACs to their target genes, resulting in chromatin modification and repression of genes, leading to blocked differentiation and inhibition of apoptosis. HDACs have also been found in complexes with proteins that regulate cell cycle checkpoints such as Rb and its family members. Resistance to chemotherapy can occur because of increased levels of thioredoxin, a thiol reductase, and decreased levels of thioredoxin-binding protein (TBP-2) in many cancers; HDIs can reverse this phenomenon. These effects create a strong rationale for developing inhibitors of HDAC activity that would correct transcriptional deregulation of genes involved in cell cycle regulation and apoptosis as cancer therapeutic agents.

TABLE 57.5	Human Histone Deacetylases			
Characteristics	**Class I**	**Class IIa**	**Class IIb**	**Class III**
Members	HDAC1, 2, 3, 8, 11	HDAC4, 5, 7, 9	HDAC6, 10	SIRT1, 2, 3, 4, 5, 6, 7
Localization	Nuclear	Nucleocytoplasmic	Nucleocytoplasmic	Nuclear/cytoplasmic/mitochondrial
Substrates	Histones p53 (HDAC1) NFκB (HDAC3)	Histones HSP90	Histone Tubulin HSP90?	Histones Tubulin (SIRT2) p53 (SIRT1) TAF(I)68 (SIRT1)
Binding site inhibitors	Zn²⁺ TSA SAHA/LAQ824 Depsipeptide Trapoxin Butyrate VPA	Zn²⁺ TSA SAHA/LAQ824 Trapoxin Butyrate VPA	Zn²⁺ TSA SAHA/LAQ824 Tubacin	NAD⁺ Nicotinamide

HDAC, Histone deacetylase; NAD, nicotinamide adenine dinucleotide; NFκB, nuclear factor kappa-B; SAHA, suberoylanilide hydroxamic acid; TSA, tricostatin A; VPA, valproic acid.

Mechanisms of Anticancer Activity of Histone Deacetylase Inhibitors

Treatment with HDIs modulates expression of 2%–10% of a selective, but variable, subset of genes in various cell types with as many genes upregulated as are downregulated. Normal cells are more resistant than cancer cells to the effects of HDIs. HDI-induced cell cycle arrest and apoptosis is usually correlated with upregulation of p21, p27, and p16, and attenuation of cyclin A and D levels, leading to decreased activity of CDK4 and CDK2. Induction of GADD45α and -β and upregulation of TGF-β, which inhibits c-Myc, may also contribute to the cell cycle arrest in G1 or G2. Promoter regions of p21 and the telomerase catalytic unit telomerase mutation in the reverse transcriptase (TERT) have been shown to contain SP1 sites that bind HDAC-recruiting transcription complexes. HDIs also activate the mitochondrial apoptotic pathway by transcriptional activation of apoptotic proteins such as TBP-2, Bad, Bim, Bid, BAK, Bax, and caspases 3 and 9, and repression of antiapoptotic proteins such as thioredoxin, bcl-2, XIAP, and Mcl-1. HDIs have also been shown to upregulate Fas and the Apo-2L/TRAIL receptors DR4 and DR5, downregulate c-FLIP, and enhance Apo-2L/TRAIL-induced DISC and apoptosis.

Treatment of leukemias with HDI alone or in combination with other agents such as all-trans retinoic acid has been shown to overcome the inhibition of differentiation caused by chimeric fusion oncoproteins such as PML-RARα, PLZF-RARα, or AML-ETO. HDIs have also been shown to induce the expression of gelsolin, an actin-binding protein involved in morphologic and cytostructural changes associated with differentiation. Several HDIs have been shown to induce acetylation of HSP90 and inhibit its chaperone association with important prosurvival client proteins such as AKT and c-Raf. This directs these client proteins to polyubiquitylation and proteasomal degradation, thus contributing to the lowering of the threshold for apoptosis in cancer cells. Inhibition of HDAC6 results in marked accumulation of ubiquitinated proteins (inhibition of the aggresome), via acetylation of α-tubulin, which in turn results in increased cellular stress and cytotoxicity.

HDIs may also act by exerting antiangiogenic and immune modulatory effects via downregulation of HIF-1α and epidermal growth factor. HDIs also affect cancer cell migration, invasion, and metastasis by altering expression of extracellular matrix proteins and metastasis genes in favor of reduced cell invasion.

Two reports have provided potential insights into biomarkers for response to HDIs. The first demonstrated that enhanced JAK/STAT signaling negatively affected HDI-induced death of CTCL cells, and constitutive accumulation of STAT1 in the nucleus and high levels of phosphorylated STAT3 correlated with a lack of response to vorinostat in clinical trials. The second approach incorporated a sophisticated loss-of-function genetic screen that identified human RAD23 homolog B (HR23B) as important for HDI-induced apoptosis. Subsequent studies showed a correlation between HR23B expression and clinical response to vorinostat, and the interaction between HSP90 and HDAC6 was identified as being the crucial functional effector mechanism delineating relative sensitivity to HDI-induced apoptosis through regulated HR23B expression. Whether there is any functional interplay between JAK/STAT signaling and HR23B remains uncertain. Moreover, as HR23B expression can regulate sensitivity to HDIs that are very weak inhibitors of HDAC6 (e.g., apicidin, romidepsin), it is unlikely that direct effects on the HDAC6/HSP90 functional interaction account for the mechanistic role of HR23B in regulating HDI-induced apoptosis.

How or why tumor cells are more sensitive to HDI-induced apoptosis compared with matched, normal cells remains an intriguing and largely unanswered question. Previous studies indicated that tumor cells treated with HDI preferentially accumulate reactive oxygen species (ROS) compared with treated normal cells, concomitant with enhanced expression of the reducing molecule thioredoxin in normal but not tumor cells. Recently, we utilized donor-matched normal and transformed cells treated with vorinostat to identify a tumor cell-selective, proapoptotic gene expression signature containing effectors of the intrinsic apoptotic pathway that conferred tumor cell-selective apoptosis mediated by vorinostat and romidepsin. It is not clear why matched tumor and normal cells selectively regulate a subset of genes that confer tumor cell-selective, HDI-mediated apoptosis. It is tempting to speculate that the cancer epigenome is altered in such a way as to predispose to altered expression of apoptotic genes in response to the transformation process, but definitive mechanistic evidence remains to be obtained.

Classes of Histone Deacetylase Inhibitors

Several structurally diverse classes of naturally occurring and synthetic compounds have been investigated for their ability to inhibit HDAC activity (Table 57.6). These include short-chain fatty acids (e.g., valproic acid [VPA]), hydroxamic acid derivatives (e.g., vorinostat, panobinostat), synthetic benzamides (e.g., entinostat), and cyclic tetrapeptides (e.g., romidepsin). All of these have undergone clinical evaluation.

Short-Chain Fatty Acid Histone Deacetylase Inhibitors

Sodium butyrate, a well-studied member of this class of compounds, induces in vitro growth arrest and differentiation of human leukemia cells at millimolar concentrations. Its clinical development has been hampered by its short half-life and difficulty in achieving millimolar levels in vivo. Phenylbutyrate, another derivative of butyric acid, is able to induce in vitro growth arrest and differentiation of leukemia cells at clinically achievable submillimolar concentrations. Importantly, at these levels, phenylbutyrate is able to synergize with retinoids in inducing cell cycle arrest, differentiation, and apoptosis of myeloid leukemia cells, and with ara-C in myeloid leukemias. VPA, a well-tolerated antiepileptic, was shown to be as effective as an HDI at levels ranging between 0.5 and 2.5 mM.

Two phase I trials have examined the therapeutic effects of phenylbutyrate in patients with AML and MDS. No responses were noted in either study, with neurotoxicity being the dose-limiting toxicity. Several studies have used VPA as monotherapy or in combination with other agents in hematologic malignancies. As monotherapy in MDS, response rates have been as high as 16% using the IWG criteria. Neurotoxicity has been the major side effect. Other side effects of VPA include thrombocytopenia, weight gain, asthenia, and rarely hepatic failure and pancreatitis. Given the low response rate, emphasis has shifted to newer HDIs.

Vorinostat and Other Hydroxamic Acid Derivative Histone Deacetylase Inhibitors

Members of this class are some of the most potent HDIs. They contain a functional group that interacts with the critical zinc atom at the base of the catalytic pocket of the class I and II HDACs. These HDIs also possess a hydrophobic cap and an aliphatic side chain that interacts with the edge and fits into the hydrophobic catalytic pocket, respectively, of the HDACs. Members of this class inhibit both class I and II HDACs. Vorinostat (SAHA, Zolinza) is a second-generation polar–planar compound that induces in vitro growth arrest, differentiation, or apoptosis of a variety of cancer, leukemia, and MM cells by restoring function of aberrantly silenced genes, among other effects. In phase I studies, vorinostat was administered IV to patients with solid tumors or hematologic malignancies daily × 3 or daily × 5 for up to 3 weeks. The maximum tolerated dose of vorinostat in patients with hematologic malignancies was 300 mg/m² daily × 5 for 3 weeks; thrombocytopenia and leukopenia were the notable toxicities, but induced no significant responses as a single agent in refractory AML. In sequential treatments in vitro, a schedule-dependent synergy was seen with other agents used to treat AML, but in some instances, antagonistic activity was observed. In a phase II study of vorinostat combined with gemtuzumab ozogamicin as induction therapy for elderly AML patients, a CR rate of more than 20% was observed. In a phase I trial of relapsed AML, vorinostat with idarubicin induced a 17% response rate with modification of histone acetylation patterns.

TABLE 57.6	Histone Deacetylase Inhibitors[a]			
Name	**Type of Compound**	**Cell Culture (Activity)**	**Animal Tumor Models**	**Clinical Trial**
Butyrates	Short-chain fatty acids	Yes (µM)	Yes	Phase I/II
Valproic acid	Short-chain fatty acid	Yes	Yes	Phase I/II
Trichostatin A	Hydroxamic acid	Yes (nM)	Yes	–
Pyroxamide	Hydroxamic acid derivative	Yes (nM)	Yes	Phase I
Oxamflatin	Hydroxamic acid derivative	Yes (µM)	Yes	–
SAHA	Hydroxamic acid derivative	Yes (nM)	Yes	Phase I/II
TPX-HA analog (CHAP)	Hydroxamic acid derivative	Yes (nM)	Yes	–
LAQ824	Hydroxamic acid derivative	Yes (nM)	Yes	Phase I
MS-275	Benzamide derivative	Yes (µM)	Yes	–
CI-994 (*N*-acetyl dinaline)	Benzamide derivative	Yes	Yes	Phase I
Depsipeptide (FR901228, FK-228)	Cyclic tetrapeptides	Yes (nM)	Yes	Phase I/II
Trapoxin	Cyclic tetrapeptides	Yes (nM)	–	–
Apicidin	Cyclic tetrapeptides	Yes (nM)	Yes	–

[a]Activity reported as "Yes" indicates that the compound has been shown to inhibit histone deacetylase (HDAC) activity, that is, growth of transformed cells in culture and in vivo tumor growth in animal studies. (–) indicates no data reported. CI-994 is reported to inhibit histone deacetylation but does not directly inhibit HDAC.
SAHA, Suberoylanilide hydroxamic acid.

More impressive responses have been seen in patients with lymphoma. Specifically, treatment of patients with progressive, persistent, or recurrent T-cell cutaneous lymphoma showed strong evidence of significant responses, resulting in rapid FDA approval (see Chapter 85). In the pivotal study, 74 patients with stage IB and higher T-cell cutaneous lymphoma who had failed two systemic therapies were treated with vorinostat at a dose of 400 mg PO once daily. Sixty one patients (82%) had stage IIB or higher CTCL and 30 patients (41%) had Sézary syndrome. The objective response rate was 30% based on a standardized scoring system, and the median time to tumor progression was 202 days. In these studies, the common toxicities were diarrhea (52%), fatigue (52%), nausea (41%), and anorexia (24%). Although the definitive mechanism of action of this high degree of response is not known, a recent review outlines the current hypotheses. Furthermore, highly significant synergy has been observed in preclinical models combining vorinostat with bortezomib.

Progress with other lymphomas has been more complex. Thirty nine patients with advanced hematologic malignancies were enrolled in a trial composed of two cohorts examining IV and PO formulations of vorinostat. Up to 70% of patients had DLBCL. The median numbers of prior treatments were seven and five in the IV and PO cohorts, respectively. A substantial number of patients had undergone a prior stem cell transplant. Most patients tolerated vorinostat well. Responses were seen in about 15% of patients.

In patients with refractory follicular lymphoma, NHL, or MCL, ORRs of 47% were seen, and responses were observed in two of nine patients with marginal zone lymphoma. The duration of response was longer than 1 year. The largest recent study, by the Southwest Oncology Group (SWOG) in NHL, showed a very low response rate as a single agent, which resulted in combination therapy studies. A number of such studies are underway, but none to date has generated significant results showing combined agent clinical synergy.

Belinostat is another hydroxamic acid HDI that was recently FDA approved for the treatment of relapsed and refractory peripheral T-cell lymphoma (PTCL) based on a multicenter, single-arm BELIEF trial of 120 evaluable patients with PTCL that was refractory or had relapsed after prior treatment. Among patients with histologically confirmed PTCL (*n* = 120), the ORR was 25.8%. Similar to other two FDA-approved HDIs, belinostat was also tested in phase I and II clinical trials for both solid and hematological cancers.

Panobinostat is a second-generation hydroxamic acid-based hybrid polar HDI tested both in in vitro and in vivo tumor models, and in clinical trials. Panobinostat induces apoptosis in a dose-dependent manner on human CML blast crisis K562 cells and acute leukemia MV4-11 cells with the activating length mutation of *FLT-3*. Exposure to panobinostat is associated with hyperacetylation of H3, H4, and Hsp90; increase in p21; and induction of cell cycle G1 phase accumulation.

Fifteen patients with a median age of 63 years and refractory AML, ALL, or MDS received IV panobinostat in a phase I trial at the following dose levels (mg/m^2): 4.8, 7.2, 9.0, 11.5, and 14.0. Grade III QTc prolongation was observed in four patients at the 14.0 mg/m^2 level and in one patient at the 11.5 mg/m^2 level. QTc prolongation was asymptomatic and reversible on drug discontinuation. Other toxicities included nausea, diarrhea, vomiting, hypokalemia, and thrombocytopenia. Eight out of 11 patients with peripheral blasts had transient reductions in blast counts, which increased shortly after drug discontinuation. Panobinostat has also been shown to be highly effective in CTCL[15] but not more effective than vorinostat. However, unlike vorinostat, single-agent activity has been seen, with response rates of almost 40% in refractory Hodgkin lymphoma. Even more impressive have been recent results in Hodgkin lymphoma patients relapsing after autologous transplantation, in which overall responses of greater than 70% and objective and durable responses were seen in 27% in a large cohort of 129 patents.[16] Recently, the use of panobinostat has been approved in combination with bortezomib and dexamethasone in patients with relapsed and refractory MM.[17] Many other hydroxamic acid derivative-based HDIs have entered preclinical or clinical studies as anticancer agents with promising results, including abexinostat, pracinostat, resminostat, givinostat, panobinostat, and CUDC-101.

Synthetic Benzamide Derivative Histone Deacetylase Inhibitors

Benzamide-containing HDIs are another class of compounds that showed both in vitro and in vivo anticancer activities. Among them, mocetinostat (MGCD0103) and entinostat (MS-275) are two examples of benzamide derivatives that had been taken to clinical trials. Mocetinostat (MGCD0103), a benzamide derivative HDI, is selective for both Class I and Class IV HDACs. A phase I trial of mocetinostat in patients with leukemia or MDS showed the drug was safe and exhibited antileukemia activity in these patients. Three patients also achieved a complete bone marrow response (blasts ≤5%). A phase II clinical trial in patients with CLL also demonstrated efficacy with a manageable side effects profile. The safety and efficacy of this compound was tested in patients with relapsed classical Hodgkin lymphoma during a phase II clinical trial. Even though the treatment showed promising clinical activity with manageable toxicity in patients with relapsed classical Hodgkin lymphoma, four patients died during the study, of which two may have been treatment-related deaths. As a result, this study has been terminated. Entinostat is another Class I selective HDI and is well tolerated either as a single agent or in combination with other drugs. A phase I trial tested entinostat in patients with refractory solid tumors and lymphomas. Prolonged disease stabilization was seen in some patients, and the drug was well tolerated and demonstrated antitumor activity.

Cyclic Tetrapeptide Histone Deacetylase Inhibitors

The principal members of this class of agents are depsipeptide (romidepsin). Romidepsin has recently been approved by the FDA as an IV agent for the treatment of patients with relapsed or refractory CTCL. It is a potent HDI that exerts in vitro antitumor effects at nanomolar levels against several cancer cell types. It also induces apoptosis of human acute leukemia and CLL cells. It is a natural product derived from *Chromobacterium violaceum*, a bacterium isolated from Japanese soil samples. Additionally, romidepsin was shown to exert antiangiogenic effects by modulating the expression of genes involved in angiogenesis. FDA approval for rhomidepsin in relapsed/refractory CTCL is based on two large phase II studies: a multi-institutional study based at the NCI in the United States (71 patients), and an international study (96 patients). The treatment schedule was identical across both studies and the ORR was 34% in both studies. Romidepsin also induced complete and durable responses in patients with relapsed or refractory PTCL across all major PTCL subtypes, regardless of the number or types of prior therapies, with an objective response rate of 25%, which led to the approval of single-agent romidepsin for the treatment of relapsed or refractory PTCL in the United States. Similarly, a phase II trial enrolling 47 patients with PTCL of various subtypes including PTCL not otherwise specified, angioimmunoblastic, ALK-negative anaplastic large-cell lymphoma, and enteropathy-associated T-cell lymphoma also showed an ORR of 38%. A phase I study of romidepsin in patients with CLL and AML at a dosage of 13 mg/m^2 IV on days 1, 8, and 15 of a 4-week cycle showed antitumor activity in several patients, although no CRs or PRs were observed. Response was greater in patients with CLL than AML. There were no life-threatening toxicities, but constitutional symptoms characteristic of HDAC inhibition were observed in the majority of patients.

Depsipeptide shows substantial activity against CTCL and it has been approved by the FDA for treatment of CTCL patients who have received at least one prior line of systemic therapy at a dose of 14 mg/m^2 IV over 4 hours on days 1, 8, and 15 of a 28-day cycle. Another phase II study of depsipeptide as a single agent has shown an encouraging 38% response rate in PTCL. In relapsed myeloma, no objective responses have been observed.

Toxicity of Histone Deacetylase Inhibitors in Clinical Trials

The most common grade 3 and 4 adverse events observed with the use of HDIs were thrombocytopenia, neutropenia, anemia, fatigue, and diarrhea. In some cases, HDI-induced thrombocytopenia can be rapidly reversible upon withdrawal of the drug. Nausea, vomiting, anorexia, constipation, and dehydration were also seen in patients receiving HDIs. Deaths have been reported in clinical studies involving HDIs. For example, when mocetinostat was tested in patients with relapsed Hodgkin lymphoma four patients died, of which two were treatment-related deaths. Similarly, deaths were also reported in clinical trials involving vorinostat, givinostat, and many other HDIs.

Combinations of Histone Deacetylase Inhibitors With Other Agents

With an increased understanding of the function of HDIs, rational combinations of chemotherapies and HDI inhibitors have been investigated. The acceptable toxicity profile associated with HDI

treatment permits a broad integration into currently approved chemotherapy regimens. A variety of HDIs synergistically enhance the growth inhibition and apoptosis of DNA-damaging agents and irradiation. This occurs, in part, through a HDI-mediated increase in chromatin accessibility and downregulation of DNA repair. A small phase I study examined the MTD of vorinostat with standard-dose CHOP chemotherapy in 14 patients with untreated PTCL. The MTD of vorinostat was 300 mg daily. The combination was tolerated, with diarrhea being the most common toxicity observed, and with a 2-year PFS and OS of 79/70% and 81/75% in the two dosing schedules tested, respectively. Synergy between HDI and proteasome inhibitors has been demonstrated in preclinical and clinical studies in myeloma. The most well-characterized model of synergy between proteasome inhibitors and HDIs are the dual inhibition of the proteasome and aggresome pathways. Targeting both the proteasome with bortezomib and the aggresome with HDAC6 inhibitors in tumor cells induces greater accumulation of polyubiquitinated proteins, resulting in increased cellular stress and apoptosis. More specifically, proteasome inhibition drives the formation of aggresomes, which are dependent on the interaction of HDAC6 with tubulin and dynein complex. Moreover, the proteasome inhibitor (bortezomib) and HDAC6 inhibitors (tubacin or panobinostat) lead to increased hyperacetylation of tubulin and generation of polyubiquitinated proteins, thus increasing cellular stress response (i.e., c-Jun N-terminal protein kinase activation) and leading to apoptosis, which is, in part, dependent on caspase activity. The addition of panobinostat to bortezomib improved PFS by about 3 months in a recent randomized phase III trial of 768 patients with relapsed/refractory myeloma that led to FDA approval. Clinical trials are ongoing to test the combinations of HDI with hypomethylating agents, mTOR inhibitors, and other proteasome inhibitors.

Denileukin Diftitox

Denileukin diftitox (DD) or DAB389IL-2 (Ontak) is a fusion protein in which the receptor binding domain of diphtheria toxin has been exchanged for that of the IL-2 molecule. Because of the specificity of the IL-2 domain, the DT-mediated cytotoxic activity will predominately affect cells that express the IL-2 receptor (IL-2R). The IL-2R is selectively expressed on activated T-lymphocytes, B cells, and NK cells. It has been shown that IL-2 fusion toxin is cytotoxic against in vitro T-cell lines. It has been estimated that approximately 50% of CTCL cases express the IL-2R (CD25), as demonstrated by immunohistochemical staining. DD was approved by the FDA for the treatment of relapsed or persistent, CD25$^+$ CTCL based on demonstrated efficacy in a placebo-controlled multinational dose-ranging study that enrolled 144 patients with CD25$^+$ stages Ia–III CTCL. Patients who had three or fewer prior therapies were randomly assigned to receive an IV infusion of either DD at 0.018 mg/kg or 0.009 mg/kg on days 1–5 of a 21-day cycle (maximum eight cycles) or saline placebo. The ORR for patients receiving the 0.018 mg/kg dose was 46%, with a median response duration of 220 days. The ORR for patients receiving the 0.009 mg/kg dose was 37%, with a median response duration of 277 days. Patients receiving the saline placebo had an ORR of 16% and median response duration of 81 days. Significant improvements of PFS at both doses of DD was noted (hazard ratio: 0.27 comparing 0.018 mg/kg vs. placebo, p = .0002; hazard ratio: 0.42 comparing the 0.009 mg/kg vs. placebo, p = .02). Treatment-emergent adverse events that occurred in at least 20% of patients in the 0.018 mg/kg group, and more frequently than in the placebo arm, were fever, nausea, rigors, fatigue, vomiting, headache, peripheral edema, diarrhea, anorexia, rash, and myalgia. Serious adverse events in patients receiving DD included infusion reactions, capillary leak syndrome, and loss of visual acuity, including loss of color vision. Laboratory abnormalities reported included hypoalbuminemia and hepatic transaminitis. Both bexarotene and alitretinoin were shown to increase the expression of CD25 in the CTCL cell line. Cells that were subsequently exposed to DD showed a 50%–70% decrease in protein synthesis. This observation suggests that increases in expression of components of the IL-2R can be achieved by retinoids and rexinoids, which may enhance the cytotoxicity of DD. A phase I trial investigating the use of bexarotene in conjunction with DD in patients with relapsed or refractory CTCL was undertaken, and eight out of 12 treated patients showed a greater than 50% increase in CD25 expression after treatment with bexarotene. A phase II trial of DD demonstrated an ORR of 48% in relapsed/refractory PTCL (excluding CTCL) with median PFS of 6 months. Higher responses (61%) were seen in CD25$^+$ tumors. In a phase II trial in patients with relapsed/refractory NHL, the ORR was 25%, with similar responses in CD25$^+$ and CD25$^-$ tumors. DD has also demonstrated promising activity in 30 patients with steroid-refractory acute GVHD, with 71% of patients responding with either complete (50%) or partial resolution (21%) of GVHD. Hepatic transaminase elevation was the dose-limiting toxicity.

Heat Shock Protein Inhibitors

Heat shock proteins (HSPs) are molecular chaperones that increase their expression in response to cellular stresses, including heat shock, nutrient deprivation, oxidative stresses, heavy metals, and alcohol exposure. They form multimolecular complexes with cellular proteins (called *clients*), regulating their correct folding, repair, degradation, and function. A number of multigene families of HSPs exist, and their individual products vary in cellular expression, function, and localization; they are classified according to their molecular weight (e.g., HSP90, HSP70, HSP27). Exceptions to this rule are the chaperones identified as glucose-regulated proteins (GRP94 and GRP75).

HSP90 is one such molecular chaperone that regulates the function and stability of more than 200 proteins, many essential for maintaining cell signaling and survival during stress states. The protective actions of HSP90 also allow cancer cells to escape the inherent toxicity of their environment, evade the effects of chemotherapy, and protect themselves from their own genetic instability. In humans, HSP90 consists of four genes, cytosolic HSP90α and HSP90β, GRP94, and HSP75/TNF-associated protein 1 (TRAP1). The monomer HSP90 consists of a conserved 25-kDa N-terminal and a 55-kDa C-terminal domain. The N-terminus contains a highly conserved ATP-binding domain. Dimerization of these nucleotide-binding domains is essential for chaperone actions, ATP binding and hydrolysis. Phosphorylation leads HSP90 to interact with co-chaperones such as HSP70 and p23 to form heteroprotein complexes, which are essential for interaction with protein clients, including protein kinases, transcription factors (e.g., steroid hormone receptor, retinoid receptors, and HIF-1α), and other proteins with various functions (e.g., mutant *p53*, the catalytic subunit of telomerase hTERT, TNFR1, and Rb). HSP90 inhibition leads to misfolded client proteins that are involved in malignancy to be polyubiquitinated and degraded by proteosomes.

The first generation of HSP90 inhibitors, benzoquinone ansamycins (herbamycin A, geldanamycin, and tanespimycin) was observed to have some antineoplastic activity, but their clinical development was limited by difficulties in formulation, hepatotoxicity and unexpected deaths in clinical trials. Newer, nongeldanamycin agents have improved bioavailability and water solubility, and have been observed to have limited single-agent activity against hematologic malignancies. In phase I studies in lymphoid malignancies, the HSP90 inhibitor AUY922 had an overall response of 10%, and was associated with grade 3 fatigue, visual disturbances, and anemia. With data suggesting possible synergy with other antineoplastic agents, it is possible that HSP90 inhibitors may be used in combination strategies.

Protein Translation Inhibitors

The increased proliferation and cell survival of cancer cells imposes a requirement for increased levels of short-lived proteins involved in cell division and survival. As a result, protein translation is markedly upregulated in cancer cells, making ribosomal function and protein synthesis a potential therapeutic target.

Protein translation is divided into three phases: initiation, elongation, and termination. As discussed in earlier sections of this chapter, mTOR inhibitors disrupt the initiation phase by preventing assembly of the eIF4F complex, responsible for ribosomal recruitment. Other agents aimed at impeding translation by directly targeting the function of eIF4F have not yet had successful clinical applications.

Omacetaxine

Omacetaxine mepesuccinate (homoharringtonine, HHT, synribo), is a semisynthetic, highly purified compound derived from a plant alkaloid discovered more than 40 years ago. Omacetaxine prevents peptide elongation by binding the A site in the peptidyl cleft of the large ribosomal subunit, thus blocking correct positioning of the amino-acid side chains of tRNAs. The clinical activity of omacetaxine has been correlated with its capacity to decrease translation of short-lived proteins such as c-Myc, MCL-1, and Cyclin D1. The initial clinical studies of omacetaxine in CML were done with IV administration, before the introduction of BCR-ABL inhibitors, and were focused on patients who had failed IFN-α. Interest decreased after approval of imatinib for CML, but subsequent studies focused on the use of SC omacetaxine in patients who developed resistance to TK inhibitors and those carrying the T315I mutation. The maximum tolerated dose was 1.25 mg/m^2 subcutaneously twice daily. Subsequent studies demonstrated omacetaxine was capable of achieving major cytogenetic response in 23% of chronic-phase CML patients carrying the T315I mutation. Omacetaxine dosing was 1.25 mg/m^2 twice daily for 14 days every 28 days until achievement of a hematologic response, after which maintenance was given at the same dose for 7 days every 28 days. Hematologic toxicity was frequent (neutropenia 44%, anemia 39%, and thrombocytopenia 76%), particularly in the initial stages of treatment, and was managed by reducing the number of days of drug administration. The most common nonhematologic toxicities were infections, diarrhea, nausea, and fever. Severe nonhematologic toxicities included infection (10%), fatigue (5%), and increased alanine aminotransferase (3%). Omacetaxine received FDA approval in 2012 for the treatment of CML patients who have failed two or more TKI treatments.

DRUG RESISTANCE TO CHEMOTHERAPEUTIC AGENTS OR MULTIDRUG RESISTANCE

Although many hematologic malignancies develop resistance to a specific class of chemotherapeutic agents, especially to targeted therapeutics, through the development of kinase region point mutations, emergence of resistance to multiple cytotoxic chemotherapeutic agents is also common among hematologic malignancies. The basis for resistance includes specific drug resistance mechanisms, overexpression of the ATP-binding cassette (ABC) transporters such as MDR-1 for drug efflux, and overexpression of antiapoptotic proteins. The Goldie-Coldman hypothesis predicts that drug-resistant tumor cell clones survive because of a favorable spontaneous mutation, which occurs in approximately one in a million cells. Because 1 g of tumor contains 1×10^9 cells, it becomes obvious that high tumor burden states contain cells with a tremendous number of mutations, which can contribute to drug resistance. This is the rationale for using combination chemotherapy at specific dose intervals to maximize dose intensity.

Drug-resistance mechanisms have been discovered and subsequently defined at the molecular level by investigators working in vitro with tumor cell lines selected in the presence of specific antitumor agents, by analysis of primary samples of untreated and treated hematologic malignancies, and through screening of tumor banks. Classes of resistance include acquired protein deficiency, loss of sensitivity to apoptotic signals, and age-related defects in the cellular pathways that normally lead to apoptosis.

P-Glycoprotein (ABC-B1 Transporter)

Structure and Function

The ABC superfamily of membrane transporters mediates the cross-membrane flux of xenobiotics, naturally occurring toxic compounds, drugs, peptides, and ions. The ABC family has a profound impact on homeostasis and is critically important to proliferation and differentiation signals in normal progenitor cells. It also mediates drug sensitivity. The terminology remains challenging because many earlier works referred to PGP and MRP, but the more recent consensus on the ABC superfamily has created a more simple approach going forward. PGP (ABC-B1 transporter) has been the subject of intense biochemical and clinical studies since it was first discovered in drug-resistant cell lines more than 20 years ago. The biochemistry of PGP has been reviewed in detail by several investigators. This phosphorylated glycoprotein has a molecular mass of approximately 170 kDa and is localized to the plasma membrane, where it functions as a drug efflux pump (Table 57.7). The ATP-dependent extrusion of antineoplastic agents confers a relative level of resistance to the cell that overexpresses PGP. Recently, the family of drug-transporting proteins has been more carefully characterized, leading to the use of the term *ATP-binding cassette transporters*. The observation of double-minute chromosomes and homogeneously staining regions in several MDR cell lines suggested that gene amplification is involved in PGP-mediated MDR. The human *MDR1* gene, which codes for PGP and is involved in antitumor drug resistance, and the human *MDR2* gene (the product of which is expressed by hepatocytes) are located very near each other on human chromosome 7q21.1. The human *MDR1*

gene has 28 exons and codes for a protein of 1280 amino acids. The PGP molecule has two homologous halves, each with a hydrophobic region containing six transmembrane domains and a hydrophilic region containing an ATP-binding site. *N*-linked glycosylation occurs on the extracellular side (Fig. 57.10). PGP is a member of the ABC superfamily, which includes, among more than 100 others, the MRP; the *pfmdr* pump in *Plasmodium falciparum*, which results in chloroquine resistance; STE6, the transporter of the "a" peptide mating factor in yeast; the cystic fibrosis transmembrane conductance regulator (CFTR); and the TAP-1 and TAP-2 proteins that transport antigenic peptides for association with class I molecules and surface antigen presentation. MRP has been demonstrated in several MDR mammalian cell lines and in human tumors (see later), but a recent study in human tumor cell lines has shown TAP overexpression associated with MRP, as well as drug resistance resulting from transfection of the *TAP* genes.

PGP has a broad specificity for hydrophobic compounds and can both reduce the influx of drugs into the cytosol and increase efflux from the cytosol. To accomplish the former, this "hydrophobic vacuum cleaner" must detect drugs and expel them while they are still in the plasma membrane. Drugs are thought to be effluxed from the cytosol through a single barrel of the PGP transporter, although an exact mechanism has been lacking. A recent study has used electron microscopy to generate an initial structure of PGP to 2.5-nm resolution. The structure was further refined by three-dimensional reconstructions from single-particle image analysis of detergent-solubilized PGP and by Fourier projection maps of small crystalline arrays of PGP. This demonstrates that PGP is monomeric, with the shape of a cylinder 10 nm in diameter with a maximum height (in the plane of the membrane) of 8 nm (see Fig. 57.10). Approximately half of

TABLE 57.7	Characteristics of Three Mechanisms of Multidrug Resistance That Result From Overexpression of PGP, Multidrug Resistance-Associated Protein, or Lung Resistance-Related Protein		
	PGP	**MRP**	**LRP**
Gene on chromosome	7q21.1	16p13.1	16p11.2
Protein			
Molecular mass	170 kDa	190 kDa	110 kDa
Cellular location	Plasma membrane	Plasma membrane	Cytoplasm ≫ nuclear membrane
Function	Efflux pump, chloride channel	Drug transporter	Major vault protein (nucleocytoplasmic transport?)
Energy source	ATP	ATP	
Posttranslational modifications	*N*-glycosylation, phosphorylation	*N*-glycosylation, phosphorylation	No *N*- or *O*-glycosylation
Analogs	Member ABC superfamily	Member ABC superfamily; GS-X pump, MOAT, LTC$_4$ transport	
Drug-Resistance Phenotype			
Antitumor agents	Act-D, *m*-AMSA, dauno, dox, epi, ida, mito-C	Act-D, chlor, CDDP-GSH, dauno, dox, epi, mel, tax (low), vbl (low), vcr, VM-26, VP-16	Carbo, CDDP, dox, mel, vcr, VP-16
	(Low), mtz, nav, tax, txtr, tpt (low), vbl, vcr, VM-26, VP-16	As, Cd, colch (low), GSH	
Other drugs	Colch, rhod	Conjugates, GSSG, LT$_4$, Sb	
Reversing agents	CSA, FK506, nifed, PSC833, quin, rap, verap	CSA, gnstn, indo, nicard, prbn, PSC833, verap, VX-710	
Normal hematopoietic tissues with increased expression	NK (CD56$^+$) T cells, suppressor T cells (CD8$^+$), B cells, CD34$^+$ stem cells	PBMNs (especially T cells), red blood cell membranes; liver and spleen low level	Macrophages
Prognostic significance	AML, MM, NHL	AML (inv 16)	AML, ALL

ABC, ATP-binding cassette; act-D, actinomycin D; ALL, acute lymphoblastic leukemia; AML, acute myeloid leukemia; As, arsenicals; ATP, adenosine triphosphate; carbo, carboplatin; Cd, cadmium; CDDP-GSH, cisplatin glutathione conjugate; chlor, chlorambucil; colch, colchicine; CSA, cyclosporin A; dauno, daunomycin; dox, doxorubicin; epi, epirubicin; gnstn, genistein; GS-X, glutathione conjugate; GSSG, oxidized glutathione; ida, idarubicin; indo, indomethacin; LRP, lung resistance-related protein; LTC$_4$, cysteinyl leukotriene; *m*-AMSA, amsacrine; mel, melphalan; mito-C, mitomycin C; MM, multiple myeloma; MRP, multidrug resistance-associated protein; MOAT, multispecific organic anion transporter; mtz, mitoxantrone; nav, navelbine; NHL, non-Hodgkin lymphoma; nicard, nicardipine; NK, natural killer; nifed, nifedipine; PGP, P-glycoprotein; prbn, probenecid; quin, quinidine; rap, rapamycin; rhod, rhodamine; Sb, antimonials; tax, taxol; tpt, topotecan; txtr, taxotere; vbl, vinblastine; vcr, vincristine; verap, verapamil; VM-26, teniposide; VP-16, etoposide.

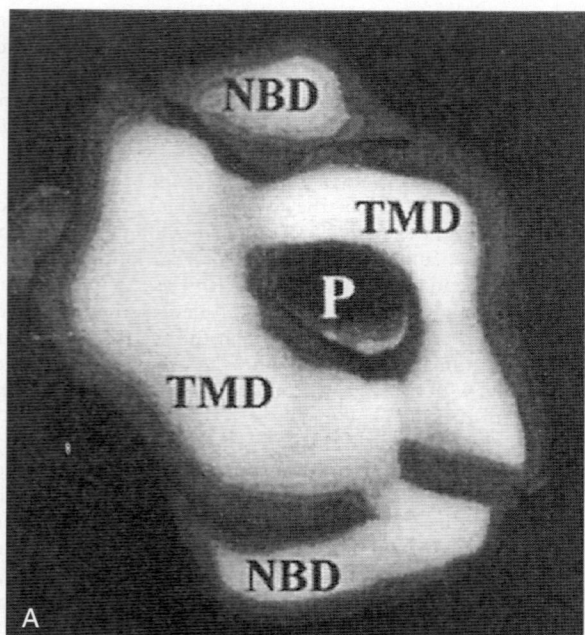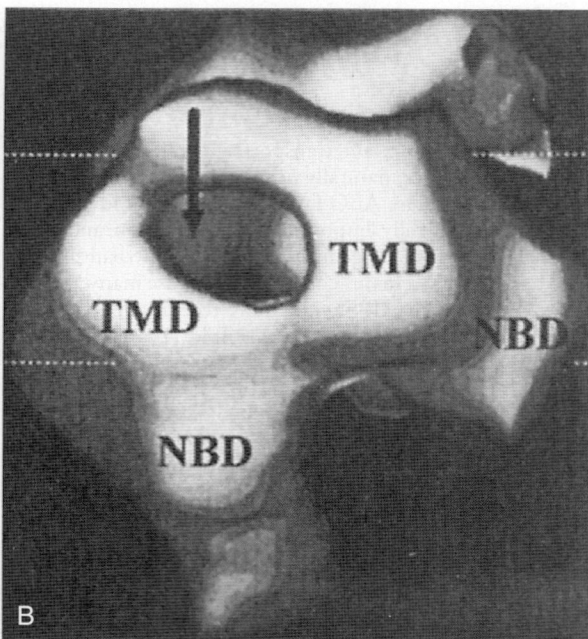

Fig. 57.10 STRUCTURE OF P-GLYCOPROTEIN DETERMINED BY ELECTRON MICROSCOPY. A computer graphic representation of the three-dimensional reconstruction is shown as a shaded surface representation of the structure. The *straight arrow* shows the putative ATP-binding domains. *P* represents the aqueous pore open at the extracellular face of the membrane. *TMD*, two thumbs, each of which probably corresponds to one of the two transmembrane domains. *NBD*, 3-nm lobes projecting from the structure at the cytoplasmic face of the membrane, probably corresponding to the two nucleotide-binding domains. (A) View perpendicular to the extracellular surface of the lipid bilayer; (B) side view of P-glycoprotein in which the approximate position of the lipid bilayer is indicated by the two horizontal *dashed lines. Arrow* indicates asymmetric opening providing access from the lipid phase to the aqueous core of the protein. *(Reproduced with permission from Rosenberg MF, Callaghan R, Ford RC, et al: Structure of the multidrug resistance P-glycoprotein to 2.5 nm resolution determined by electron microscopy and image analysis.* J Biol Chem 272:10685, 1997.)

the PGP molecule is within the membrane because the lipid bilayer is approximately 4 nm in depth. When viewed from the extracellular surface of the membrane, PGP is pteroidal with a large central pore 5 nm in diameter. This large aqueous chamber in the membrane that is open to the extracellular space is closed on the cytoplasmic side, presumably by the two 3-nM intracellular lobes (putative nucleotide-binding domains) and the hydrophilic cytoplasmic loops between the transmembrane domains. Thus, this large pore has a "gate" on the cytoplasmic side of the membrane that can regulate the transport of different-sized substrates.

Substrates of PGP include (see Table 57.7) anthracyclines (doxorubicin, daunorubicin, epirubicin, and idarubicin), anthracenediones (mitoxantrone), aminoacridines (amsacrine), taxanes (taxol and taxotere), epipodophyllotoxins (VP-16 and VM-26), vinca alkaloids (vincristine, vinblastine, and vinorelbine), bortezomib, and actinomycin D. Mitomycin C and one of the topoisomerase I inhibitors (topotecan) are both weak substrates for PGP. Several drugs reverse the resistance mediated by PGP overexpression and sensitize cells to the cytotoxic effects of antineoplastic agents. These drugs compete with antitumor agents for efflux from the cell, effectively increasing the intracellular concentration of the cytotoxic drug, and include immunosuppressants (cyclosporin A [CSA], FK 506, rapamycin, PSC 833), calcium channel blockers (verapamil, nifedipine), antiarrhythmics (quinidine), and other miscellaneous agents. Several of these MDR-modulating agents have been used in clinical trials in an effort to sensitize resistant tumor cells (see later).

Methods of Detection

Several monoclonal antibodies that recognize PGP and are commercially available for routine analyses have been described. Monoclonal antibodies C219 and JSB-1 recognize internal epitopes of PGP,

whereas antibodies MRK16 and UIC2 detect external antigens and are more suited for fluorescence-activated cell sorting analysis.

P-Glycoprotein Expression in Normal Human Tissue

High levels of expression of *MDR1*/PGP have been found in the epithelium of several human tissues with excretory function, suggesting that PGP is normally involved in transporting both exogenous toxic compounds and endogenous metabolites. These tissues include the adrenal cortex, renal proximal tubule epithelium, biliary hepatocytes, small and large intestinal mucosa, pancreas, and endothelial cells of the brain and testis. Normal human hematopoietic tissues with high levels of *MDR1*/PGP include CD34+ progenitor cells, CD56+ (NK) cells, and CD8+ (T-suppressor) cells. Lower levels of expression have also been observed in CD4+ (T-helper) cells, CD19+ B cells, and CD14+ cells (monocytes).

P-Glycoprotein Expression in Human Malignancies

Increased expression of PGP has been observed in several human tumors, especially those malignancies that arise in tissues that normally have high levels of PGP expression. An analysis of 61 human tumor cell lines (from leukemia, CNS tumors, melanoma, breast cancer, ovarian cancer, colon cancer, lung cancer, and kidney cancer) that were not selected for resistance to antitumor agents demonstrated co-expression of two or three of the MDR proteins (PGP, LRP, or MRP) in 64% of the cell lines. PGP and LRP were overexpressed in 3% of the tumors; MRP and LRP in 43%; and PGP, LRP, and MRP in 18%. The cell lines with the highest levels of drug resistance were found to overexpress all three proteins. Whether this is true in primary human tumors awaits further investigations.

Acute Myeloid Leukemia

An earlier meta-analysis of studies that examined the expression of *MDR1*/PGP in blasts of patients with AML found that 40% (105 out of 261 patients) who were PGP positive achieved a CR, but 81% (192 out of 238) of PGP-negative patients obtained a CR. An analysis of 96 untreated patients with AML showed that PGP expression predicted induction failure ($p < .0001$) and decreased OS ($p < .001$), as did unfavorable cytogenetics. PGP expression was not detected in patients with favorable cytogenetic abnormalities [t(15;17), inv(16), t(8;21)], was found in 29% of those samples with a normal karyotype, and was expressed in 62% of patients with an unfavorable cytogenetic abnormality. PGP was also detected in 63% of those with secondary AML compared with 25% of those with de novo disease. PGP analysis with the MRK16 antibody in 211 elderly patients (older than 55 years) with untreated AML again showed that PGP expression is significantly associated with a decreased CR rate and resistant disease. Patients in this report with de novo PGP-negative AML with favorable cytogenetics have a CR rate of 81% compared with 12% for those with secondary AML, which is PGP positive and has unfavorable cytogenetics. Clinical trials using the PGP substrate Valspodar (PSC833) acting as a competitive inhibitor did not show the dramatic benefit expected, especially in older patients with acute leukemias.

Impact of P-Glycoprotein in Other Hematologic Malignancies

The role of PGP in the drug resistance of NHL, myeloma, and ALL is ill defined. CLL is another chronic leukemia in which few PGP-related antineoplastic agents are used. However, a single study has shown a correlation between *MDR1* expression and survival, in which the 10 B-CLL patients who were *MDR1* positive had a median survival of 19 months compared with 46 months for the 17 patients who were *MDR1* negative ($p < .01$). Nonetheless, a recent study identified bortezomib as a substrate for PGP, raising the possibility that myeloma PGP levels affect clinical response. There have not been recent studies of the role of PGP in drug resistance in NHL in the past 5 years. With the newer kinase inhibitors, it has recently been noted that nilotinib and dasatinib are high-affinity substrates of ABCG2. These agents appear to inhibit the function of this transporter, but whether this will translate into clinical impact has not received prospective attention.

Clinical Studies With Modulators of P-Glycoprotein

The clinical trials that have used various modulators of PGP have been reviewed by several investigators. An early study in VAD-refractory MM resulted in short-lived PRs to VAD plus racemic verapamil in five out of 22 patients. Four of the five responders overexpressed PGP; however, cardiac side effects precluded further dose escalation of IV *R,S*-verapamil. Continuous IV infusion of CSA with VAD in VAD-resistant myeloma patients resulted in seven out of 15 responses, which were more common in those who overexpressed PGP. A randomized SWOG phase III study of VAD and PO verapamil in 120 patients with refractory myeloma demonstrated a 41% and 36% response in the VAD and VAD/verapamil arms, respectively, with median survival times of 10 and 13 months, respectively. Continuous-infusion CSA has been dose escalated in combination with daunorubicin and ara-C. Transient hyperbilirubinemia was seen in 62% of the patients; these same patients had increased serum daunorubicin levels and a higher response rate. A CR was seen in 26 out of 42 patients; however, the MDR phenotype was not found to influence the response. A study of PSC833 in patients with acute leukemia treated with cytarabine, daunorubicin, and etoposide showed a modest benefit in patients younger than 45 years of age, raising the potential of developing an effective strategy in patients older than 60 years of age in whom PGP expression in leukemic cells is more common. Zosuquidar, a PGP inhibitor, was tested for efficacy in a phase III trial by ECOG in 449

patients older than the age of 60 years. No benefit in response rate or survival was noted. Likewise, in a CALGB study, in adults with untreated leukemia younger than the age of 60 years, PSC833 also did not improve survival or response rates. Thus, the future role of modulation of PGP in leukemia management remains ill defined.

Multidrug Resistance-Associated Protein (ABC G2 Transporter)

Structure and Function

The MRP was first described in 1992 in the doxorubicin-selected small-cell lung cancer cell line, and its biochemical characteristics and biologic properties have been reviewed.[18] It has now been classified within the larger context of ABC transporters, termed *ABC G2 transporters*. Because much of the literature uses the MRP nomenclature, we refer to this herein except for the studies using the ABC terminology. This *N*-glycosylated plasma membrane phosphoprotein has a molecular mass of 190 kDa (1531 amino acids) and is a member of the ABC transporter superfamily (see Table 57.7 and Fig. 57.11). This transporter has 18 transmembrane domains (12 in the amino end and six in the carboxyl end) and is coded on human chromosome 16p13.1.

The overexpression of MRP has been shown in vitro to result in different levels of drug resistance to several classes of antineoplastic agents, represented by actinomycin D, chlorambucil, melphalan, cisplatin (CDDP), daunomycin, doxorubicin, epirubicin, teniposide (VM-26), etoposide (VP-16), and vincristine. Low levels of resistance have also been reported for taxol, vinblastine, and colchicine. In addition to antitumoral agents, MRPs (and its isoforms) are capable of transporting heavy metals (arsenicals, cadmium, and antimonials) as well as glutathione conjugates and cysteinyl leukotriene. Compounds reported to modulate MRP-mediated drug resistance in vitro include the calcium channel blocker verapamil nocardipine; the

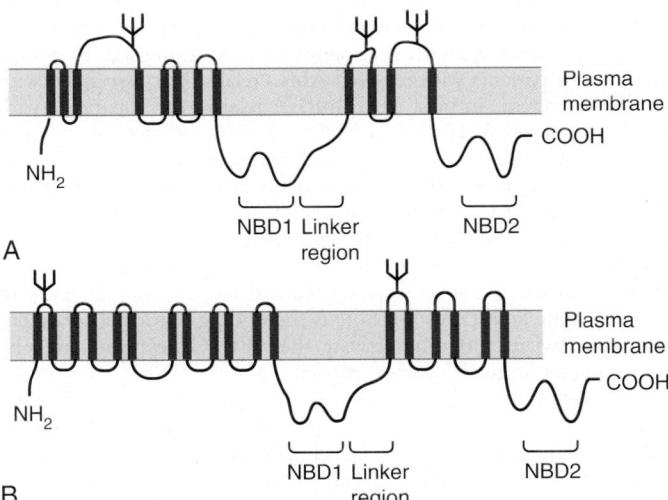

Fig. 57.11 MODELS OF MULTIDRUG-RESISTANCE PROTEIN MEMBRANE TOPOLOGY. Multidrug-resistance protein (MRP) possesses features common to all members of the ATP-binding cassette transporter superfamily in that each half of the protein is predicted to consist of several transmembrane domains followed by a cytosolic nucleotide-binding domain (MBD). The first model (A) is based on computer-assisted hydropathy analyses of the human MRP amino acid sequence and predicts that MRP is composed of 12 transmembrane domains *(solid bars)*, eight of which are within the NH₂-proximal half of the protein. The second model (B), based on a comparison of human and murine MRP with other ATP-binding cassette transporters, suggests that there are up to four additional transmembrane domains in the NH₂-proximal half of the protein. *(Adapted from Loe DW, Deley RG, Cole SPC: Biology of the multidrug resistance-associated protein, MRP. Eur J Cancer 32A:945, 1996.)*

protein kinase C inhibitor GF109203X; the cyclosporin analog PSC833; the TKI genistein; the gyrase-inhibiting antibiotic difloxacin; and amiodarone VX-710. Amiodarone VX-710, a nonmacrocyclic ligand of the FK506-binding protein FKBP12 and a potent modulator of PGP-mediated MDR, has been found to restore sensitivity of MRP-expressing HL60/ADR cells to the cytotoxic action of doxorubicin, VP-16, and vincristine. Other investigational agents include danusertib, a potent pan-aurora and ABL kinase inhibitor being developed for CML. The nonsteroidal antiinflammatory drug indomethacin has also been shown to significantly increase the sensitivity of HL60/ADR cells to doxorubicin and vincristine, and may be a specific inhibitor of MRP.[19]

Multidrug-Resistance Protein Expression in Hematologic Malignancies

The expression of MRP mRNA or the level of MRP protein has been assessed in 148 patients with hematopoietic malignancies. MRP mRNA expression was found to be significantly increased in 84% of patients with CLL and in 30% of those with AML. The vast majority of patients with ALL, CML, MM, hairy cell leukemia, and NHL were found to have low levels of MRP mRNA expression. MRP protein was assayed using the monoclonal antibody MRPr1, and the results were generally similar with increased expression in most patients with CLL. A study of 40 patients with refractory lymphoma and 16 with newly diagnosed lymphoma suggests a limited role for MRP mRNA expression in drug resistance in NHL because 15 paired samples in the refractory group showed no difference in MRP expression pre- and post-EPOCH treatment. In addition, the untreated patients had MRP mRNA levels that were no different from the pre- or post-EPOCH patient levels. A study of 49 patients with AML and 29 with ALL demonstrated significantly higher expression of MRP in ALL ($p < .007$) and in secondary AML ($p < .016$), but not in de novo AML. Combining overexpression of ABC G2 and FLT3-ITD, an Italian group identified that in adult AML patients, overexpression of ABC G2 was detected in 83 (50%) and FLT3-ITD in 47 (28%) patients. Although the response rate was not affected, the duration of remission was much shorter when these proteins were overexpressed. In a small study of 14 patients with relapsed AML, relapse was associated with a twofold increase in blast MRP mRNA relative to 29 patients with newly diagnosed AML ($p < .01$). Paired blast samples (obtained at diagnosis and at relapse) from 13 AML and four ALL patients showed a twofold increase in 80% of the patients at relapse, suggesting that the expression of the MRP transporter at relapse may be involved in drug resistance. Because purine nucleoside antimetabolites may be exported by ABC G2, as noted earlier, it is of note that clofarabine is also a substrate, but its function is mediated inversely by levels of deoxycytidine kinase. Also of note is the finding that drug treatment can demethylate and thus activate the ABC G2 exporter, thereby increasing its protective tumor impact.

The larger family of transporters, the ABC group that includes ABC G2 and ABC B1, are overexpressed in leukemic cells and in many malignant stem cells. In fact, in addition to CD44, high levels of ABC transporters assist in the characterization and isolation of the transplantable subpopulation of malignant stem cells. Brendel and coworkers found that both imatinib and nilotinib used to block the ABL kinase in CML were effectively blocking the ABC transporter in CML cells. This suggested both that these agents might function in part by blocking expression of an important leukemic stem cell protein, and that they would sensitize CML cells to other agents transported by the ABC system.

DNA Repair Pathway Mechanisms of Drug Resistance

O⁶-Alkylguanine-DNA Alkyltransferase

As noted previously, the nitrosoureas and methylating agents are cytotoxic largely because of formation of DNA adducts at the O^6

position of guanine. The most efficient means of protection from the cytotoxicity of adducts at the O^6 position of guanine is rapid repair by the O^6-alkylguanine-DNA alkyltransferase (AGT or MGMT). This protein serves as the stoichiometric acceptor protein for O^6-alkylguanine DNA monoadducts, transferring the alkyl group from DNA to the active site of the protein, inactivating the protein, and restoring DNA to normal. However, the $N^1G–N^3C$ DNA cross-link that follows chloroethylation is not a substrate for AGT. There is a striking correlation between drug resistance and alkyltransferase activity. Of interest, high levels of AGT are found in many leukemias, but low AGT is observed in normal human CD34 cells, perhaps explaining why nitrosoureas are not used in leukemia management and why nitrosoureas are effective myeloablative agents used in high-dose chemotherapy regimens. A novel inhibitor of AGT, O^6-benzylguanine (BG) has been used to sensitize human tumors to BCNU. Studies indicate activity of the combination of BG and BCNU in myeloma and in cutaneous lymphomas. Therapeutic benefit from the methylating and alkylating agent cloretazine appears to be related to lower levels of AGT. Likewise, temozolomide has some therapeutic efficacy in leukemia in a manner inversely related to AGT levels in the tumor cells. A study in five pediatric patients pointed out that response to temozolomide was greater in those with MGMT promoter methylation and no evidence of MMR. This has been tested in a prospective phase II trial of older patients with leukemia. Temozolomide was given in a dosing schedule dependent on MGMT promoter methylation status, with a shorter course of therapy in those with low MGMT expression in the leukemic cells. The ORR in elderly leukemia patients who would otherwise not be candidates for treatment was about 40%, with a median duration of about 29–35 weeks.

Mismatch Repair

The spectrum of drug resistance and sensitivity to methylating agents does not end with AGT. Evidence suggests that methylating agent-induced cell death involves an aborted effort at MMR. Karran and others,[20] in mammalian systems, have shown that the replicative DNA polymerase pauses at O^6-mG and the repair polymerase pauses at O^6-mG and preferentially inserts a thymine (T) at the site. The O^6-mG:T base pair is recognized by the MMR system, which initiates (see later). In human cells, the MMR complex consists of at least six proteins involved in the recognition and repair of mismatch lesions: HMLH1, hMSH2, hMSH3, hPMS1, hPMS2, and GTBP (GT-binding protein, also called *MSH6*), all of which appear to be homologs of MMR proteins found in *Escherichia coli* and in yeast. After binding recognition, an endonuclease removes a patch of approximately 100–1000 bp containing the T mismatch, DNA polymerase-δ or -γ fills in the patch, with reinsertion of a T opposite the O^6-mG, and a DNA ligase closes the strand break. Because the O^6-mG:T is reformed, cytotoxicity ensues as a result of repetitive efforts at DNA repair and induction of chromosomal breakage, rearrangements, energy depletion, and apoptosis. Drug resistance based on mutation or loss of expression of an MMR protein, owing to mutation within one of the gene coding regions, or promoter methylation leading to loss of gene expression, has been noted in solid tumors and in leukemias and lymphomas. The mutator phenotype was originally described in cells with acquired resistance to methylnitrosourea, methylmethanesulfonate, or *N*-methyl-*N*-nitroso-*N*-nitrosoguanidine, which were tolerant to G→A point mutations according to the inability to repair O^6-mG and are cross-resistant to 6-TG used in childhood leukemia maintenance regimens, which form the 6-TG:T mismatch.

Major Molecular Response Mutations and Methylating Agent Resistance

MMR defects in humans were initially described in hereditary nonpolyposis colon cancer, which comprises approximately 15% of all colon cancer, lymphomas, and relapsing acute leukemias. The genetic defect results in a high rate of spontaneous mutations within microsatellite DNA, resulting in the RER phenotype arising as the expansion or contraction of mono-, di-, or tri-nucleotide repeats within the microsatellites. Tumor cells defective in MMR are remarkably resistant to temozolomide regardless of AGT activity or its inhibition by BG, confirming the importance of MMR in sensitivity to methylating agents. Of interest, MMR mutant cells are also two- to threefold resistant to cisplatin, perhaps because the cisplatin DNA adduct is bound by the MMR complex, slowing its recognition and repair by the nucleotide repair pathway and increasing its cytotoxicity. Such MMR-deficient cells also exhibit microsatellite instability, a measure of genomic instability and the propensity to develop further mutations during therapy, leading to subclones of resistant cells. Loss of PMS2 has been identified in a family of childhood lymphomas. Microsatellite instability is seen in acute leukemias and in T-cell leukemias, suggesting both that these malignancies have lost MMR function and that they are more prone to drug resistance and acquisition of additional mutations that give rise to further drug resistance. Evidence of microsatellite instability and loss of MMR is present in some leukemias but is much more common in treatment-related leukemias, again providing a mechanism of drug resistance.

Base Excision Repair

Methylating agents such as procarbazine and temozolomide form large numbers of N^3-A and N^7-G adducts in addition to O^6-mG (with TMZ, the relative amounts are 72 N^7mG:8 O^6mG:5 N^3mA). Thus, under normal circumstances, cells process many more N^7mG and N^3mA lesions than O^6mG lesions, even though the latter appear much more cytotoxic except in MMR-defective cells. Repair of N^3-A and N^7-G adducts through BER is efficient and normally leads to cell survival rather than cell death. Adducts are recognized by the methylpurine glycosylase with removal of the base, generating an abasic (or AP) site. The AP site is then cleaved by the class II hydrolytic endonuclease (or AP endonuclease) generating a single-strand break with a 5′ PO$_4$, which becomes the substrate for DNA polymerase-β, and to a lesser extent, polymerases-δ and -γ, followed by DNA ligase (reviewed by Sancar[21]). Other compounds induce nucleotide pool imbalance, leading to misincorporation of bases that become substrates for BER. These compounds include folate antagonists such as methotrexate, 5-FU, and, to a lesser extent, nucleoside analogs such as fludarabine. Misincorporation of uracil after 5-FU inhibition of thymidilate synthase also leads to BER. Compounds to disrupt BER, such as TRC102, are now being developed and may lead to combination therapy for hematologic malignancies. An initial phase I trial with TRC102 has been completed with pemetrexed, and a second trial with temozolomide continues. A third trial using the combination of fludarabine and TRC102 in patients with CLL has found remarkable efficacy in the first cohorts after relapsing from fludarabine (unpublished).

Drug Resistance to Antimetabolites

Although overlap exists, antimetabolites can be classified into nucleoside analogs that are incorporated into RNA or DNA (or both) and agents that inhibit de novo purine and pyrimidine biosynthetic pathways. Mechanisms of resistance to these agents fall into several broad categories. For example, many antimetabolites are prodrugs in that they must be converted intracellularly into active nucleotide forms to exert their cytotoxic actions. Consequently, events that interfere with cellular accumulation of drug or nucleotide formation will reduce activity. Examples include decreased transport of methotrexate or decreased nucleotide formation of ara-C and 6-TG by reductions in activity of deoxycytidine kinase or hypoxanthine–guanine phosphoribosyltransferase, respectively. Alternatively, enhanced drug catabolism reduces cytotoxicity. Examples include the deamination of ara-C (to inactive ara-U) by CDD or catabolism of 6-TG by thiopurine methyltransferase. A third mechanism of resistance stems from the presence of increased intracellular levels of a competing metabolite (e.g., dCTP in the case of ara-C, or hypoxanthine or guanine in the case of 6-TG). Fourth, alterations in the level of activity of a target enzyme or the presence of a mutant form that is a poor target of inhibition will also confer resistance. Examples include increased

activity or a mutant form of DHFR (in the case of methotrexate), an altered DNA polymerase-α (in the case of ara-C), or increased activity of ribonucleotide reductase (through overexpression of either subunit). Finally, cytokinetic factors represent a common theme in the case of most (but not all) antimetabolites, in that a reduction in the S-phase fraction generally leads to reduced drug sensitivity. Note that these resistance mechanisms are agent specific and are distinct from the more general modes of resistance (e.g., increased expression of BCL2) associated with defects in the distal cell death pathway.

Mechanisms of Resistance to Signaling Inhibitors

The introduction of signaling inhibitors to the therapeutic armamentarium represents a significant advance in the treatment of hematologic malignancies. As discussed in the previous sections, these agents can inhibit with relative selectivity cellular signaling pathways essential for the survival of neoplastic cells. However, development of resistance has been observed in vitro and in clinical practice, and appears to be the rule rather than an exception with these agents. The mechanisms of resistance related to drug influx/efflux also can affect sensitivity to targeted agents. In addition, several other mechanisms have been described for signaling inhibitors, including genetic alterations, changes in protein expression, and activation of alternative pathways.

Genetic Modifications Leading to Resistance to Signaling Inhibitors

Cancer cells treated with kinase inhibitors tend to acquire genetic modifications that overcome the inhibitory effects of these agents.

Point mutations are the most common mechanism of resistance to TK inhibitors. The development of resistance against a specific inhibitor can be the result of a preexisting cancer cell subpopulation carrying the mutation; once exposure to the drug occurs and sensitive cells die, this cell population experiences selective advantage. On the other hand, cell line studies have been able to induce the emergence of resistance to specific signaling inhibitors, suggesting that the genomic instability experienced by neoplastic cells facilitates emergence of new mutations that may affect drug sensitivity.

Mutations that confer resistance to a kinase inhibitor commonly affect the affinity of the drug for the kinase domain without affecting its catalytic activity. Other mutations affect the conformation of the kinase, making it less available to the inhibitor, and others decrease the affinity of the kinase for ATP, affecting the efficacy of ATP-competitive inhibitors.

Genetic amplifications are common in cancer cells. Many signaling inhibitors target pathways that present amplification of one of its components. Further increases in gene amplification can affect the drug–target balance in favor of the latter. Gene amplifications resulting in increases in target may be overcome by increasing the inhibitor dose, as it is done in clinical practice with imatinib; however, this is limited by the higher potential for adverse events.

Genetic modifications that don't involve the target can also result in resistance. This can occur when mutations or amplifications result in increased activity or expression of signaling molecules located downstream or parallel to the point of inhibition. These "escape" mechanisms may be taken into consideration when designing combination strategies for treatment with multiple targeted agents.

FUTURE DIRECTIONS

The treatment of hematologic malignancies has seen significant progress over the last decades. The continuing expansion of the therapeutic armamentarium with the addition of target-based therapies presents clinicians and researchers with several challenges. The first problem is one of choice; with several agents identified as effective for a single malignancy, an evidence-based choice will be more difficult to make in the absence of head-to-head comparison in clinical trials. In addition, a major question remains whether the newer signaling inhibitors, "third-wave" agents, and newer immunotherapies only achieve disease control and potentially prolong survival, without definitive disease eradication and cure. It is possible that the former objective is sufficient for approaching normal lifespan in certain disorders, particularly those of indolent nature affecting patients of more advanced age. However, aggressive disorders that represent a life-threatening condition when relapsed would be better treated with curative intent. Strategies for aggressive, resistant, or relapsed disease will likely require inclusion of multiple agents of different generations and mechanisms of action. Current clinical trials are exploring the use of combinations of signaling inhibitors or anti-apoptotic agents with "traditional" chemotherapeutic agents. These combinations, along with the addition of monoclonal antibody and antibody–drug conjugate-based therapies as well as future strategies may achieve sufficient disease control to achieve disease eradication and cure in a larger number of patients. Researchers and clinicians will need to also take into account the cost of these therapies and their impact on quality of life, particularly as several target-based agents have been demonstrated to have activity as maintenance therapies. The long-term effects of many of these agents are still unknown. Future clinical trial design and planning should include answers to these questions: potential for cure versus disease control, rational use strategies, and identification of the most effective and least toxic therapeutic approaches for each disease.

Certainly future considerations include the incorporation of genetic and genomic information into the clinic, as well as other markers of abnormalities of the "signalome" of a specific hematologic malignancy. Application of these diagnostic strategies to a specific patient will allow for individual tailoring of the treatment strategy, both based on the characteristics of the tumor and the individual capacity to tolerate and metabolize drugs. Extensive validation studies will be necessary to understand the true value of these tests in the management of patients with hematologic malignancies.

REFERENCES

1. LoRusso PM, Boerner SA, Seymour L: An overview of the optimal planning, design, and conduct of phase I studies of new therapeutics. *Clin Cancer Res* 16:1710, 2010. [Epub 2010 Mar 9]. Review. PubMed PMID: 20215546.

2. Seymour L, Ivy SP, Sargent D, et al: The design of phase II clinical trials testing cancer therapeutics: consensus recommendations from the clinical trial design task force of the National Cancer Institute Investigational Drug Steering Committee. *Clin Cancer Res* 16:1764, 2010. [Epub 2010 Mar 9]. PubMed PMID: 20215557; PubMed Central PMCID: PMC2840069.

3. Cheson BD, Rummel MJ: Bendamustine: rebirth of an old drug. *J Clin Oncol* 27:1492, 2009. [Epub 2009 Feb 17].

4. Dobbelstein M, Moll U: Targeting tumour-supportive cellular machineries in anticancer drug development. *Nat Rev Drug Discov* 13:179–196, 2014.

5. Mohamed AJ, Yu L, Bäckesjö CM, et al: Bruton's tyrosine kinase (Btk): function, regulation, and transformation with special emphasis on the PH domain. *Immunol Rev* 228:58, 2009. Review. PubMed PMID: 19290921.

6. So L, Fruman DA: PI3K signalling in B- and T-lymphocytes: new developments and therapeutic advances. *Biochem J* 442:465, 2012. PubMed PMID: 22364281.

7. Zaytseva YY, Valentino JD, Gulhati P, et al: mTOR inhibitors in cancer therapy. *Cancer Lett* 319:1, 2012. [Epub 2012 Jan 17]. Review. PubMed PMID: 22261336.

8. Liu Q, Thoreen C, Wang J, et al: mTOR mediated anti-cancer drug discovery. *Drug Discov Today Ther Strateg* 6:47, 2009. PubMed PMID: 20622997; PubMed Central PMCID: PMC2901551.

9. Hess G, Herbrecht R, Romaguera J, et al: Phase III study to evaluate temsirolimus compared with investigator's choice therapy for the treatment of relapsed or refractory mantle cell lymphoma. *J Clin Oncol* 27:3822, 2009. [Epub 2009 Jul 6]. PubMed PMID: 19581539.

10. Mascarenhas J, Hoffman R: Ruxolitinib: the first FDA approved therapy for the treatment of myelofibrosis. *Clin Cancer Res* 2012. [Epub ahead of print]. PubMed PMID: 22474318.

11. Harrison C, Kiladjian JJ, Al-Ali HK, et al: JAK inhibition with ruxolitinib versus best available therapy for myelofibrosis. *N Engl J Med* 366:787, 2012. PubMed PMID: 22375970.

11a. Friedberg JW, Vose JM, Kelly JL, et al: The combination of bendamustine, bortezomib, and rituximab for patients with relapsed/refractory indolent and mantle cell non-Hodgkin lymphoma. *Blood* 17(10):2807–2812, 2011.

12. Roberts AW, Seymour JF, Brown JR, et al: Substantial susceptibility of chronic lymphocytic leukemia to BCL2 inhibition: results of a phase I study of navitoclax in patients with relapsed or refractory disease. *J Clin Oncol* 30:488, 2012. [Epub 2011 Dec 19]. PubMed PMID: 22184378.

13. Tong WG, Chen R, Plunkett W, et al: Phase I and pharmacologic study of SNS-032, a potent and selective Cdk2, 7, and 9 inhibitor, in patients with advanced chronic lymphocytic leukemia and multiple myeloma. *J Clin Oncol* 28:3015, 2010. [Epub 2010 May 17]. PubMed PMID: 20479412.

14. Chen R, Wierda WG, Chubb S, et al: Mechanism of action of SNS-032, a novel cyclin-dependent kinase inhibitor, in chronic lymphocytic leukemia. *Blood* 113:4637, 2009. [Epub 2009 Feb 20]. PubMed PMID: 19234140; PubMed Central PMCID: PMC2680368.

14a. Wijermans PW, Krulder JW, Huijgens PC, et al: Continuous infusion of low-dose 5-Aza-2′-deoxycytidine in elderly patients with high-risk myelodysplastic syndrome. *Leukemia* 11(Suppl 1):S19–S23, 1997.

14b. Kantarjian H, Oki Y, Garcia-Manero G, et al: Results of a randomized study of 3 schedules of low-dose decitabine in higher-risk myelodysplastic syndrome and chronic myelomonocytic leukemia. *Blood* 109(1):52–57, 2007.

14c. de Lima M, Giralt S, Thall PF, et al: Maintenance therapy with low-dose azacitidine after allogeneic hematopoietic stem cell transplantation for recurrent acute myelogenous leukemia or myelodysplastic syndrome: a dose and schedule finding study. *Cancer* 116(23):5420–5431, 2010.

15. Ellis L, Pan Y, Smyth GK, et al: Histone deacetylase inhibitor panobinostat induces clinical responses with associated alterations in gene expression profiles in cutaneous T-cell lymphoma. *Clin Cancer Res* 14:4500, 2008. PubMed PMID: 18628465.

16. Younes A, Sureda A, Ben-Yehuda D, et al: Panobinostat in patients with relapsed/refractory Hodgkin's lymphoma after autologous stem-cell transplantation: results of a phase II study. *J Clin Oncol* 2012. [Epub ahead of print]. PubMed PMID: 22547596.

17. Richardson PG, Hungria VT, Yoon SS, et al: Panobinostat plus bortezomib and dexamethasone in previously treated multiple myeloma: outcomes by prior treatment. *Blood* 127(6):713–721, 2016.

18. Mo W, Zhang JT: Human ABCG2: structure, function, and its role in multidrug resistance. *Int J Biochem Mol Biol* 3:1, 2012. [Epub 2011 Mar 30]; PubMed PMID: 22509477; PubMed Central PMCID: PMC3325772.

19. Tiwari AK, Sodani K, Wang SR, et al: Nilotinib (AMN107, Tasigna) reverses multidrug resistance by inhibiting the activity of the ABCB1/Pgp and ABCG2/BCRP/MXR transporters. *Biochem Pharmacol* 78:153, 2009. [Epub 2009 Apr 11]. PubMed PMID: 19427995.

20. Karran P, Macpherson P, Ceccotti S, et al: O6-methylguanine residues elicit DNA repair synthesis by human cell extracts. *J Biol Chem* 268(21):15878–15886, 1993. PubMed PMID: 8340413.

21. Sancar A, Lindsey-Boltz LA, Unsal-Kaçmaz K, et al: Molecular mechanisms of mammalian DNA repair and the DNA damage checkpoints. *Annu Rev Biochem* 73:39–85, 2004. Review. PubMed PMID: 15189136.

22. Egorin MJ, Van Echo DA, Tipping SJ, et al: Pharmacokinetics and dosage reduction of cis-diammine(1,1-cyclobutanedicarboxylato)platinum in patients with impaired renal function. *Cancer Res* 44:5432–5438, 1984.

23. Calvert AH, Newell DR, Gumbrell LA, et al: Carboplatin dosage: prospective evaluation of a simple formula based on renal function. *J Clin Oncol* 7:1748–1756, 1989.

CLINICAL PHARMACOLOGY OF ALKYLATING AGENTS

MECHLORETHAMINE (MUSTARGEN)

Chemistry: Mechlorethamine, also called *nitrogen mustard*, is a water-soluble and alcohol-soluble analog of sulfur mustard gas. It is a bifunctional chloroethylating agent that alkylates DNA, RNA, and protein.

Absorption, Fate, and Excretion: The parent compound is highly reactive and has a biologic half-life of approximately 15 minutes. The principal route of degradation is spontaneous hydrolysis, but some enzymatic demethylation also occurs.

Preparation and Administration: Mechlorethamine is supplied in vials of 10 mg with 100 mg of sodium chloride and is reconstituted with 10 mL of sterile water to yield a 1-mg/mL solution, ideally prepared immediately before use. However, the manufacturer considers the drug expired 1 hour after reconstitution. The drug is injected over a few minutes through tubing as a freely running intravenous (IV) infusion. For topical application (e.g., in mycosis fungoides), 10 mg of drug is dissolved in 60 mL of tap water. Alternatively, a 10 mg% ointment has been used by dissolving the drug in 95% ethyl alcohol and petrolatum (Aquaphor). Mechlorethamine is a powerful vesicant. In the event of extravasation, vigorous irrigation followed by 0.25% sodium thiosulfate injection at the site of extravasation should be attempted. Ice packs may be placed for 6–12 hours to minimize the local reaction.

Toxic Effects: Myelosuppression is the dose-limiting systemic side effect. This worsens with each additive cycle. Severe nausea and vomiting, infertility, alopecia, and pain at the site of injection, which can sometimes spread to involve the venous system (tracking), are also common. Occasionally, a macular papular rash is observed, but this does not appear to be allergic in nature and does not contraindicate continuation of therapy. Infertility is common but may be reversible. Infrequent adverse effects include alopecia, anorexia, weakness, and diarrhea. The drug has also been shown to induce chromosomal abnormalities and may contribute to the development of secondary leukemias, as seen in patients treated with this agent as part of the MOPP (mechlorethamine, vincristine [Oncovin], procarbazine, prednisone) regimen.

Potential Drug Interactions: None reported.

Therapeutic Indications in Hematology: Mechlorethamine is incorporated in many chemotherapy combinations used in the treatment of Hodgkin lymphoma (MOPP and MOPP/ABV [Adriamycin, bleomycin, and vinblastine] hybrid) and in some non-Hodgkin lymphomas (NHLs; prednisone, etoposide, methotrexate, doxorubicin [Adriamycin], cyclophosphamide, Leucovorin [PROMACE]/MOPP). However, its use has largely been supplanted by other agents.

Cyclophosphamide (Cytoxan)

Chemistry: Cyclophosphamide is a cyclic phosphamide ester of mechlorethamine. After being metabolically activated, it alkylates DNA, forming cross-links.

Absorption, Fate, and Excretion: The drug is relatively well absorbed orally, with approximately 75% oral bioavailability. The parent compound is not active. The drug is metabolized by the hepatic cytochrome P450 (CYP) system, which ultimately generates at least two active compounds, phosphoramide mustard and acrolein. The latter appears to be responsible for cyclophosphamide's bladder toxicities. The plasma half-life of cyclophosphamide varies from 4 to 6.5 hours. Approximately 15% of the drug is excreted unchanged in the urine. Dose reduction should be considered in patients with severe renal failure.

Preparation and Administration: Cyclophosphamide is supplied as 25- and 50-mg tablets and as a powder for parenteral administration in 100-, 200-, and 500-mg and 1- and 2-g vials. It is dissolved by adding 5 mL of preservative-free sterile water for every 100 mg of drug. Cyclophosphamide is chemically stable for 24 hours at room temperature and for 6 days if refrigerated.

Toxic Effects: Bone marrow suppression is the major side effect. The myeloid series is primarily affected, although thrombocytopenia also occurs at high doses and alopecia is common. Nausea and vomiting can be severe and are usually delayed, occurring 6–8 hours after administration. Hemorrhagic cystitis occurs in 10% of patients receiving nontransplant doses and is apparently caused by the formation of the urotoxin acrolein. Because of this potential side effect, patients should be well hydrated. Mesna disulfide (sodium 2-mercaptoethanesulfonate disulfide) has also been used on a weight-equivalent basis to ameliorate cyclophosphamide-induced bladder toxicity. Other potential toxic effects include stomatitis, skin and nail hyperpigmentation, interstitial pulmonary fibrosis, and the syndrome of inappropriate secretion of antidiuretic hormone. Rare episodes of acute congestive heart failure have been reported. After bone marrow transplant doses, hemorrhagic cystitis is common, and cardiac toxicity (cardiomyopathy) may be seen. Late sequelae include bladder fibrosis (more common with daily [oral] therapy), bladder cancer, leukemogenesis, and infertility.

Potential Drug Interactions: Corticosteroids may increase P450 enzyme–induced metabolism and is often avoided in high-dose therapy. When combined with doxorubicin, it may increase cardiac toxicity. This may be prevented by amifostine. In animal studies, conflicting results were reported when the P450 enzyme inducer phenobarbital was given with cyclophosphamide. Most investigators, however, have observed a reduction in the amounts of active metabolites. Conversely, when cimetidine (but not ranitidine) was administered in leukemia-bearing mice before treatment with cyclophosphamide, a significant prolongation of their survival and higher plasma concentrations of alkylating metabolites were observed. Although one should remain alert for these potential drug interactions, none has been demonstrated in humans. Cyclophosphamide reduces serum pseudocholinesterase levels, which may prolong the neuromuscular blocking effects if given simultaneously. Caution must be exercised when administering high doses of these two drugs to critically ill patients. Life-threatening hyponatremia may develop when used in conjunction with indomethacin, although the precise incidence is unknown.

Therapeutic Indications in Hematology: Cyclophosphamide is a key drug in the treatment of lymphomas and myeloma. It is incorporated in many chemotherapy regimens, including CHOP, MACOP-B, PROMACE/CYTABOM, CVP, and VMCP (see Chapters 81 and 85 for details). In addition, cyclophosphamide is the drug most commonly used in preparatory regimens for bone marrow transplantation. It is also used in solid tumors and as an immunosuppressant in nonmalignant conditions such as glomerulonephritis and systemic lupus erythematosus.

Ifosfamide (Ifex)

Chemistry: Ifosfamide is an oxazaphosphine nitrogen mustard that differs from cyclophosphamide by the placement of chloroethyl groups.

Absorption, Fate, and Excretion: As in the case of cyclophosphamide, the parent compound is inactive and is metabolized by the CYP system in the liver. The metabolism of ifosfamide is influenced by the dose and schedule of administration. When administered as a single bolus, 60% is eliminated into the urine, 53% as unchanged inactive drug. When administered daily for 5 consecutive days, 56% is excreted into the urine, 15% as the inactive parent compound. The half-life is 7 hours when administered daily for 5 consecutive days and 15 hours when given as a single bolus dose. There is poor penetration across the blood–brain barrier. Its longer half-life and slower metabolic activation allow higher doses to be given.

Preparation and Administration: The drug is provided in 1-g vials and should be reconstituted in sterile water or bacteriostatic water to a final concentration of 50 mg/mL. Ifosfamide can be diluted further in 5% dextrose, normal saline, or Ringer solution for injection to achieve concentrations of between 0.6 and 20 mg/mL. The solution should be infused over 30 minutes. To prevent hemorrhagic cystitis, patients must receive Mesna disulfide for protection against urotoxicity and must be kept well hydrated (2 L/day). Mesna is a thiol compound that is rapidly oxidized to dimesna in vivo. Mesna and dimesna are filtered by the glomeruli, reabsorbed in the proximal tubule, and finally secreted back into the tubular lumen of the kidney. In the tubules, approximately one-third of the filtered dimesna is readily converted back to Mesna. The free sulfhydryl group of this compound reacts with the urotoxic metabolite acrolein produced by both ifosfamide and cyclophosphamide (see Fig. 57.7). This reaction creates a nontoxic acrolein–Mesna thioether that is safely eliminated in the urine. Mesna has also been shown to inhibit the degradation of ifosfamide or cyclophosphamide to acrolein.

Mesna has been given in combination with ifosfamide in different doses and schedules. One recommended schedule uses IV bolus injection in a dosage equal to 20% of the ifosfamide dose (on a milligram-to-milligram basis) at the time of ifosfamide administration and 4 and 8 hours after each dose of ifosfamide. Mesna has also been given by continuous infusion with excellent results. The two agents may be mixed together in the same IV solution; however, Mesna is not compatible with cisplatin.

Toxic Effects: With the use of Mesna to protect against urotoxicity, myelosuppression—especially leukopenia and, to a lesser extent, thrombocytopenia—is the dose-limiting side effect. Renal tubular acidosis can occur. CNS effects, observed in approximately 10% of patients treated, include somnolence, confusion, depressive psychosis, and hallucinations. Less commonly, dizziness, disorientation, and cranial nerve dysfunction occur. Nausea and vomiting are common. Low serum albumin and elevated serum creatinine may enhance CNS toxicity. As with cyclophosphamide, such side effects as alopecia, leukemogenesis, and infertility also occur. Cardiac toxicity is rare.

Potential Drug Interactions: Because ifosfamide is also metabolized by the P450 system, physicians should remain alert for the same type of potential drug interactions that have been reported with cyclophosphamide. A recent report advises close monitoring of warfarin anticoagulant control in patients receiving ifosfamide/ Mesna.

Therapeutic Indications in Hematology: Ifosfamide was recently approved for treatment of patients with refractory testicular cancer. In hematologic malignancies, its major indication is in the treatment of refractory lymphomas.

Melphalan (Melphalan)

Chemistry: Melphalan is synthesized from nitrogen mustard and phenylalanine. It is a bifunctional chloroethylating agent that forms DNA cross-links.

Absorption, Fate, and Excretion: The oral bioavailability of melphalan is quite variable, 20%–50% of the drug being excreted in the stool. Some patients show virtually no oral absorption. This fact is particularly pertinent in the treatment of patients with myeloma, in whom a lack of response to melphalan may simply be caused by poor oral absorption. Melphalan has a half-life of approximately 90 minutes. It is extensively metabolized, with only approximately 10%–15% of an administered dose excreted unchanged in the urine.

Preparation and Administration: Melphalan is commercially available in 2-mg tablets and in IV formulation for high-dose therapy.

Toxic Effects: The dose-limiting toxicity is myelosuppression, manifested by leukopenia and thrombocytopenia, and generally occurring 2–3 weeks after therapy. Recovery may take 6 weeks, however, in patients who have been heavily pretreated with chemotherapy drugs, radiotherapy, or both. Nausea, vomiting, and alopecia are uncommon side effects and are usually mild. Occasionally, amenorrhea and azoospermia, pulmonary fibrosis, dermatitis, and secondary malignancies (e.g., leukemia) occur, especially in patients receiving the drug over the long term. At cumulative doses of less than 600 mg, the incidence of second hematologic malignancy is probably less than 2% but may be greater than 15% at higher doses. Higher doses used in transplant patients result in gastrointestinal toxicity that is dose limiting. At these doses, the syndrome of inappropriate secretion of antidiuretic hormone, pneumonitis, and hepatic venoocclusive disease have been observed.

Potential Drug Interactions: Administration of high-dose IV melphalan with cyclosporine increases the risk of cyclosporine nephrotoxicity.

Therapeutic Indications: The major use of melphalan is for the treatment of multiple myeloma (MM), either as a single agent or in combination with other alkylating agents and prednisone (e.g., the MP and VMCP regimens). The IV formulation has been approved for isolated limb perfusion in melanoma. It is used in high-dose protocols for myeloma and solid tumors at doses of 140–200 mg/m^2.

Chlorambucil

Chemistry: Chlorambucil is an aromatic derivative of mechlorethamine.

Absorption, Fate, and Excretion: Chlorambucil is well absorbed after oral administration. It is extensively metabolized in the liver to its major metabolite, phenylacetic acid mustard (PAAM), which also has bifunctional alkylating activity. The half-lives of chlorambucil and PAAM are 1.5 and 2.5 hours, respectively; less than 1% of either chlorambucil or PAAM is excreted in the urine.

Preparation and Administration: Chlorambucil is commercially available as 2-mg tablets.

Toxic Effects: Treatment is usually well tolerated, with myelosuppression the dose-limiting toxic effect. Patients on a daily oral schedule should have biweekly complete blood counts. Nausea and vomiting are uncommon, but mild alopecia and skin rashes occasionally occur. As with the other alkylating agents, azoospermia (especially above a cumulative dose of 400 mg), amenorrhea, and secondary leukemia are potential risks of prolonged therapy. Rare cases of pulmonary fibrosis have also been reported.

Potential Drug Interactions: None reported.

Therapeutic Indications in Hematology: The major uses are in the treatment of Waldenström macroglobulinemia, low-grade lymphomas, chronic lymphocytic leukemia (CLL), and Hodgkin lymphoma. Except for CLL, chlorambucil has been supplanted by newer agents.

Busulfan (Myleran)

Chemistry: Busulfan is an alkylsulfonate bifunctional alkylating agent not chemically related to mechlorethamine. It forms DNA intrastrand and interstrand cross-links.

Absorption, Fate, and Excretion: Busulfan is well absorbed after oral administration. When given by the IV route, greater than 90% is cleared from the plasma after 3 minutes. The drug is extensively metabolized to inactive compounds that are excreted renally. The major metabolite is methane sulfonic acid, although more than 10 other not fully identified metabolites exist. Virtually no intact busulfan is found in the urine. The biologic half-life of busulfan is approximately 2.5 hours.

Preparation and Administration: The drug is commercially available as 2-mg tablets.

Toxic Effects: Although at low doses the major effect of busulfan is on the granulocytic series, at high doses all three hematologic series are affected. Compared with the other alkylating agents, its nadir of myelosuppression may be relatively late, in a range of 11–30 days. Hematologic recovery is also prolonged and may take approximately 54 days. A relatively common side effect is an Addisonian-like syndrome characterized by skin hyperpigmentation and weakness but without abnormalities in adrenal function. Cumulative pulmonary toxicity has been well described and consists of a mixed alveolar and interstitial pneumonitis. As with the other alkylating agents, infertility and leukemogenesis can occur. Nausea and vomiting are rare. At high doses, it is associated with hepatic venoocclusive disease in up to 19% of patients. Seizures may also occur and are controlled by diphenylhydration.

Potential Drug Interactions: A metabolic interaction may take place between busulfan and various anticonvulsant medications; however, further description of the specific effects is awaited.

Therapeutic Indications in Hematology: Busulfan is used mainly in the treatment of chronic myeloid leukemia. More recently, high-dose busulfan has been incorporated into preparatory regimens for bone marrow transplantation. Blood level monitoring with adjustment for higher dose levels improved therapeutic outcome and reduced toxicity.

Carmustine (BCNU)

Chemistry: Carmustine, also called BCNU (1,3[bis]-2-chloroethyl-nitrosourea), decomposes spontaneously into a chloroethyl hydroxide that can alkylate the DNA and into an isocyanide molecule, which may produce carbamylation of proteins. Cytotoxicity is caused by DNA cross-links.

Absorption, Fate, and Excretion: IV-administered carmustine is rapidly metabolized, with a half-life of 70 minutes. Approximately 30%–80% of metabolites are eliminated in the urine within 24 hours. The drug, its metabolites, or both readily cross the blood–brain barrier, resulting in cerebrospinal fluid concentrations within the range of 15%–70% of plasma levels. Peak serum levels vary widely in patients treated at 200–600 mg IMF.

Preparation and Administration: Carmustine is commercially available in 100-mg vials as a white lyophilized powder. The drug is reconstituted with 3 mL of absolute alcohol provided by the manufacturer and 27 mL of sterile water, and can be further diluted with normal saline or 5% dextrose in water. It should be used immediately after reconstitution and can be infused over 1–2 hours.

Carmustine is chemically stable for 3 hours at room temperature and for 24 hours when refrigerated.

Toxic Effects: Myelosuppression is the dose-limiting toxic effect and tends to increase with successive cycles of therapy. Leukopenia and thrombocytopenia are characteristically delayed and reach their maximum between the third and sixth weeks after drug administration. Nausea and vomiting can be severe. Abnormal liver function test results may be found, but the abnormalities are usually mild and reversible. Two rare but serious toxic effects include cumulative pulmonary or interstitial pneumonitis progressing to fibrosis and progressive renal damage, which are dose related. Secondary leukemias can also occur 5–10 years after treatment. Patients who receive greater than 1100 mg/m^2 are at increased risk of pulmonary fibrosis. Carmustine is not a vesicant, but rapid infusion often produces a burning sensation at the injection site.

Potential Drug Interactions: Cimetidine may enhance the myelosuppressive effect of carmustine. Carmustine may decrease the pharmacologic effects of phenytoin. In rats with intracerebrally implanted tumors, pretreatment with phenobarbital eliminated the antitumor activity of carmustine. The reduction in carmustine antitumor activity correlated with increased carmustine metabolism, which is apparently the result of hepatic microsomal enzyme induction.

Therapeutic Indications in Hematology: Carmustine in combination with other cytotoxic agents may be used in the initial treatment of Hodgkin lymphoma (BCVPP regimen) and multiple myeloma (VBAP regimen). In high-dose therapy, it appears in BEP for relapsed lymphomas.

Lomustine (CCNU)

Chemistry: Lomustine, also called CCNU, is a nitrosourea derivative with chloroethyl and cyclohexyl side chains.

Absorption, Fate, and Excretion: The drug is rapidly absorbed from the gastrointestinal tract and is rapidly and completely metabolized. Its active metabolites have prolonged plasma half-lives, within a range of 16–48 hours. Approximately 50% of an administered dose is detectable (as metabolites) in the urine within 24 hours, and 75% is detectable within 4 days. Active metabolites cross the blood–brain barrier and can be detected in significant concentrations in the cerebrospinal fluid.

Preparation and Administration: The drug is commercially available in 10-, 40-, and 100-mg capsules.

Toxic Effects: The toxicity profile of lomustine is similar to that of carmustine. Because lomustine can produce vomiting and the drug is given orally, special attention should be directed to emesis control. If the patient vomits soon after ingestion, the vomitus should be inspected for the presence of intact capsules. The drug should be given again if capsules are identified with certainty. Secondary leukemias are reported 3–10 years after use.

Potential Drug Interactions: These are similar to those of carmustine.

Therapeutic Indications in Hematology: Lomustine is occasionally used as second-line treatment for patients with Hodgkin lymphoma and NHL and for childhood gliomas.

Streptozocin (Zanosar)

Chemistry: Streptozocin is a naturally occurring nitrosourea derived from *Streptomyces acromogenes*. The drug is a glucosamine-1-methyl-nitrosourea, which, unlike the other nitrosoureas, methylates DNA and is cytotoxic owing to induced mismatch repair.

Absorption, Fate, and Excretion: After IV administration, the drug is rapidly metabolized, with no intact drug detectable in the plasma after 3 hours. Its half-life is 40 hours. Within the first 24 hours after administration, approximately 10% of the parent compound is excreted in the urine.

Preparation and Administration: The drug is commercially available in 1-g vials and is reconstituted with either 9.5 mL of normal saline or 5% dextrose in water for injection to form a 100-mg/mL solution. IV infusion of the drug over 30–45 minutes usually prevents discomfort at the injection site. Patients should be kept well hydrated to preclude renal tubular toxicity.

Toxic Effects: Although nausea and vomiting have been considered by some investigators to be the limiting toxic effects, in most phase I trials nephrotoxicity was the principal dose-limiting effect. Nausea and vomiting are severe and require aggressive antiemetic support. Streptozocin may also aggravate duodenal ulcers. Renal toxicity frequently occurs and includes mild proteinuria, glycosuria, hypophosphatemia, renal tubular acidosis, and occasionally irreversible azotemia. Although the myelosuppressive effect of streptozocin is mild, it can potentiate the bone marrow suppression of other cytotoxic drugs. Slight increases in hepatic enzymes can also occur. Occasionally, patients (primarily those with insulinomas) may experience transient alterations in glucose metabolism.

Potential Drug Interactions: Streptozocin can potentiate the hyperglycemic effect of glucocorticosteroids. Phenytoin therapy decreases the cytotoxic effect of streptozocin on the pancreatic β-cells, leading to potential interference with its therapeutic effect in patients with pancreatic islet cell tumors. Streptozocin is a potent renal toxin, and every effort should be made to avoid concomitant administration of other nephrotoxins.

Therapeutic Indications in Hematology: Streptozocin has been used in the initial treatment of Hodgkin lymphoma and, less commonly, in NHLs.

Dacarbazine

Chemistry: Dacarbazine is also called DTIC [5-(3,3-dimethyl-1-triazeno)imidazole-4-carboxamide]. After undergoing metabolic activation by microsomal enzymes in the liver, it acts primarily as an alkylating agent.

Absorption, Fate, and Excretion: After IV administration, the drug is extensively metabolized. Activated DTIC has an elimination half-life of 5–7 hours. Approximately 40%–50% of the parent drug is found in the urine within the first 24 hours after administration.

Preparation and Administration: DTIC is commercially available in 100- and 200-mg vials, which must be protected from light and stored at a temperature of 2–8°C. The drug is reconstituted with normal saline or sterile water to produce a 10-mg/mL solution. It can be administered as a slow IV push or by infusion over 15–30 minutes.

Toxic Effects: Myelosuppression, primarily represented by leukopenia, is the dose-limiting toxic effect. Use of the drug leads to considerable problems with emesis and requires aggressive antiemetic support. A flulike syndrome consisting of fever, malaise, and myalgias may occur. Direct sunlight during the first 2 days after drug administration may result in facial flushing, facial paresthesias, and lightheadedness. Hepatotoxicity and diarrhea have also been reported.

Pain along the injection site can occur if the drug is rapidly infused but can usually be lessened by prolonging the infusion rate. Secondary leukemias are reported between 3 and 10 years after use.

Potential Drug Interactions: DTIC activation may be enhanced by phenytoin or phenobarbital, although the clinical significance of this potential interaction remains uncertain. There may be a potential (as yet poorly characterized) drug interaction with levodopa, whereby the response to levodopa is diminished.

Therapeutic Indications in Hematology: DTIC is used primarily in the treatment of Hodgkin lymphoma as part of the ABVD (doxorubicin [Adriamycin], bleomycin, vinblastine, and DTIC) regimen and for melanoma.

Procarbazine

Chemistry and Mechanism of Action: Procarbazine is a substituted hydrazine derivative with a chemical structure similar to that of the monoamine oxidase inhibitors (MAOIs). Accordingly, procarbazine exhibits weak MAOI effects. Procarbazine itself is inert and must undergo metabolic activation to generate cytotoxic reactants, the mode of action of which is not clear. They may inhibit transmethylation of methyl groups of methionine into tRNA or may also directly damage DNA. Hydrogen peroxide, formed during the autooxidation of procarbazine, may attack protein sulfhydryl groups contained in residual proteins tightly bound to DNA.

Absorption, Fate, and Excretion: Procarbazine is rapidly and completely absorbed by the oral route, with peak plasma levels occurring within 60 minutes. It penetrates well into the cerebrospinal fluid. The drug is readily metabolized in the liver and has a plasma half-life of 10 minutes after IV injection. The major sites of elimination are the kidneys, where approximately 70% of the drug is excreted as *N*-isopropylterephthalamic acid and less than 5% is excreted unchanged.

Preparation and Administration: Procarbazine is commercially available as 50-mg capsules.

Toxic Effects: The usual dose-limiting toxic effect is myelosuppression. Occasionally, nausea and vomiting may be dose limiting, although tolerance to those effects may develop during continued administration. Other less common side effects include paresthesias, headache, dizziness, depression, apprehension, insomnia, nightmares, hallucinations, drowsiness, ataxia, foot drop, decreased reflexes, tremors, coma, confusion, convulsions, skin rash, alopecia, myalgia, and arthralgia. Procarbazine may possibly be leukemogenic.

Potential Drug Interactions: Combination chemotherapy that includes procarbazine may result in a decrease in digoxin plasma levels. Because procarbazine is a weak MAOI, hypertensive reactions could theoretically occur after concurrent ingestion of sympathomimetics, levodopa, tricyclic antidepressants, or foods with high tyramine content (e.g., dark beer, yogurt, cheeses, and red wines). However, such reactions have not been reported. Concomitant use of narcotics or other strong sedatives may result in exaggerated depressant effects, leading to coma and possibly death. Procarbazine also interacts with alcohol, causing a disulfiram-like reaction.

Therapeutic Indications in Hematology: Procarbazine is often used in combination with other cytotoxic agents in the treatment of Hodgkin lymphoma (MOPP and MOPP derivatives) and to a lesser extent in the treatment of NHL (PROMACE-MOPP).

Temozolomide

Chemistry and Mechanism of Action: Temozolomide is not active but undergoes rapid nonenzymatic conversion at physiologic pH to the reactive compound monomethyl 5-triazino imidazole carboxamide (MTIC), which is also the active methyl group–donating metabolite of DTIC. Unlike DTIC, formation of MTIC from temozolomide does not require metabolic activation (liver); thus there is much more consistent conversion from temozolomide to the methyl-donating MTIC. The cytotoxicity of MTIC is thought to be primarily caused by alkylation of DNA. Alkylation (methylation) occurs mainly at the O^6 and N^7 positions of guanine. Cytotoxicity results from processing of these lesions by methylguanine methyltransferase, mismatch repair, and base excision repair.

Absorption, Fate, and Excretion: Temozolomide is rapidly and completely absorbed after oral administration; peak plasma concentrations occur in 1 hour. Food reduces the rate and extent of temozolomide absorption.

Temozolomide exhibits a mean elimination half-life of 1.8 hours and exhibits linear kinetics over the therapeutic dosing range. Temozolomide is spontaneously hydrolyzed at physiologic pH to the active species, MTIC and to temozolomide acid metabolite. MTIC is further hydrolyzed to 5-amino-imidazole-4-carboxamide (AIC), which is known to be an intermediate in purine and nucleic acid biosynthesis and to methylhydrazine, which is believed to be the active alkylating species. Approximately 38% of the administered temozolomide total radioactive dose is recovered over 7 days; 37.7% in urine and 0.8% in feces. The majority of the recovery of radioactivity in urine is as unchanged temozolomide (5.6%), AIC (12%), temozolomide acid metabolite (2.3%), and unidentified polar metabolite(s) (17%). Overall clearance of temozolomide is approximately 5.5 L/hour/m^2.

Preparation and Administration: Temozolomide is given orally with each capsule containing either 5, 20, 100, 140, 180, or 250 mg of temozolomide. The inactive ingredients for TEMODAR capsules are lactose anhydrous, colloidal silicon dioxide, sodium starch glycolate, tartaric acid, and stearic acid.

Toxic Effects: Bone marrow depression, including neutropenia, lymphopenia, anemia, and thrombocytopenia, occurs frequently with temozolomide. Mild transaminase elevations of up to 40% of patients and hyperbilirubinemia of up to 19% are seen. Mild-to-moderate headache is among the most commonly reported adverse effects along with moderate nausea and vomiting, although these may be secondary to the use of antiemetics.

Drug Interactions: None described.

Therapeutic Indications in Hematology: Temozolomide may have some activity in both acute myeloid leukemia (AML) and acute lymphocytic leukemia (ALL), but the correct dose is presently unknown. Temozolomide has no activity in NHL.

Bendamustine

Chemistry and Mechanism of Action: Bendamustine is a bifunctional alkylating agent (mechlorethamine analogue). Its structure is characterized by a nitrogen mustard group linked to a benzimidazole nucleus, which forms covalent bonds with electron-rich nucleophilic moieties, resulting in interstrand DNA cross-links. Bendamustine is active against both quiescent and dividing cells.

Absorption, Fate, and Excretion: Although absorbed well orally, bendamustine is only administered intravenously. It is highly protein bound, averaging approximately 95%. The half-life of bendamustine is approximately 40 minutes. Bendamustine is primarily metabolized in the liver via hydrolysis, and little is excreted in urine unchanged, but the pharmacokinetics in patients with significant renal failure are unknown.

Preparation and Administration: Bendamustine is available for IV use in single-use vials containing either 25 mg or 100 mg of bendamustine HCl. Sterile water for injection is added to each vial to obtain a 5-mg/mL solution. The lyophilized powder should completely dissolve in 5 minutes. After being diluted with either 0.9% sodium chloride injection, US Pharmacopeia (USP), or 2.5% dextrose/0.45% sodium chloride injection, USP, the final admixture is stable for 24 hours when stored refrigerated or for 3 hours when stored at room temperature.

Toxic Effects: Bendamustine frequently causes anemia, severe neutropenia, and thrombocytopenia. Infusion reactions presenting as fever, chills, pruritus, and rash have been seen. Antihistamines, antipyretics, and corticosteroids have been effective in preventing these reactions. Tumor lysis syndrome has been seen with the first dose of bendamustine, so appropriate precautions should be taken. Local reactions are seen with extravasation, and care should be taken when administering the drug in a peripheral site. Headache, nausea, and vomiting, as well as skin reactions including rash, toxic skin reactions, and bullous exanthema, have occurred with bendamustine. AML has been reported in patients after use of bendamustine HCl.

Drug Interactions: Although their clinical significance is unknown, ciprofloxacin, fluvoxamine, and omeprazole may increase bendamustine levels and decrease levels of active minor metabolites.

Therapeutic Indications in Hematology: Bendamustine has been effective in treating chronic lymphoid leukemia, MM, Hodgkin lymphoma, NHL, and indolent B-cell lymphomas.

APPENDIX　57.2

CLINICAL PHARMACOLOGY OF ANTIMICROTUBULE AGENTS

Vincristine (Oncovin) and Vinblastine (Velban)

Chemistry and Mechanism of Action: Both vincristine and vinblastine are asymmetric dimeric compounds that bind to the protein tubulin at a site distinct from that for the taxanes. At low concentrations vincristine and vinblastine inhibit microtubule dynamics. At higher concentrations they disrupt microtubules that constitute the mitotic spindle, resulting in metaphase arrest. They are relatively M-phase specific. Owing to their lipophilicity, vinca alkaloids are rapidly taken into cells and achieve several-hundred-fold higher intracellular than extracellular concentrations. Whereas overexpression of the multidrug resistance transporters P-glycoprotein (PGP) or multidrug resistance protein can reduce the intracellular accumulation, alterations in the α- or β-tubulins can affect drug–target interaction for vinca alkaloids.

Absorption, Fate, and Excretion: After IV injection, both drugs are rapidly distributed to the body tissues, especially the red blood cells and platelets. Their elimination follows a triphasic pattern. The elimination half-lives are as follows α, less than 5 minutes; β, 50–155 minutes; and γ, 20–85 hours. Both vinca alkaloids are primarily eliminated through the liver into the bile and feces, making patients with obstructive liver disease more susceptible to toxic effects. A 50% reduction in the dose is recommended for serum bilirubin concentrations of 1.5–3.5 mg/dL. Dose modification for renal dysfunction is not indicated. After brief IV bolus administration, peak plasma vincristine concentrations of 100–400 mM are achieved, which decline to less than 10 mM in 2–4 hours. Continuous infusion doses of 1.0 mg/m^2/day produce vincristine plasma concentrations ranging from 1 to 10 nM.

Preparation and Administration: Vincristine is commercially available in 1-, 2-, and 5-mg vials. Each milliliter contains 1 mg of vincristine sulfate, 100 mg of mannitol, 1.3 mg of methylparaben, and 0.2 mg of propylparaben. Vincristine is a powerful vesicant that should be administered only IV into a freely running infusion of normal saline or dextrose solution. If the drug is given by continuous infusion, it must be infused through a central IV line. In case of extravasation, infusion should be discontinued and any residual drug aspirated through the line. The manufacturer also recommends infiltrating the area with 1–2 mL of hyaluronidase, 150 U/mL, and then applying warm compresses for 72 hours to facilitate dispersion of the drug. Vinblastine is commercially available as a lyophilized powder and a 1-mg/mL solution in 10-mg vials. The lyophilized drug is reconstituted by adding sodium chloride for injection (which may be preserved with either phenol or benzyl alcohol) to the 10-mg vial. Administration of vinblastine should follow the same guidelines described for vincristine.

Toxic Effects: Vincristine's dose-limiting toxic effect is neurotoxicity, which appears to be related to its relative polarity. Peripheral neurotoxicity usually manifests as sensory impairment, decreased deep-tendon reflexes, and paresthesias. Less commonly, severe painful dysesthesias, ataxia, foot drop, and cranial nerve palsy (e.g., affecting the extraocular and laryngeal muscles) can occur. Autonomic neurotoxicities include constipation, abdominal cramps, and ileus, which may be prevented by use of mild laxatives. Alopecia occurs frequently, but myelosuppressive effects are minimal. Rare side effects include inappropriate secretion of antidiuretic hormone and ischemic cardiac toxicity. Vinblastine's dose-limiting toxic effect is myelosuppression, with leukopenia more pronounced than thrombocytopenia. Anemia is uncommon. Neurotoxicity can also occur but is significantly less common than with vincristine. Vinblastine is also a vesicant.

Potential Drug Interactions: Both vinca alkaloids have been reported to increase the accumulation of methotrexate and etoposide in tumor cells. Acute shortness of breath and bronchospasm can occur when vincristine or vinblastine is given in conjunction with mitomycin C. Because asparaginase may impair the hepatic clearance of vincristine, it is preferable to administer the vincristine 12–24 hours before L-asparaginase. Vincristine may decrease the absorption and plasma levels of orally administered drugs such as digoxin. Dilantin may increase the cytotoxicity of vincristine in multidrug-resistant tumor cells; however, this remains to be demonstrated in the clinic. When concurrently administered, erythromycin may increase the toxicity of vinca alkaloids, especially vinblastine.

Therapeutic Indications in Hematology: The vinca alkaloids are among the most important drugs in the treatment of hematologic malignancies. They have a broad spectrum of activity and are often incorporated into many chemotherapy regimens used in the treatment of ALL, Hodgkin lymphoma, NHL, CLL, and MM.

Vinorelbine (Navelbine)

Chemistry and Mechanism of Action: Vinorelbine is a semisynthetic derivative of vinblastine (5′-nor-hydrovinblastine) with an eight-member catharanthine ring. Similar to other vinca alkaloids, it also binds to tubulin, inhibits microtubule assembly, and produces a mitotic arrest of cells. These occur at concentrations that relatively spare axonal microtubules, which may reduce neurotoxicity.

Absorption, Fate, and Excretion: Short (6–10 minutes) IV infusions of 30 mg/m^2 produce peak plasma concentrations approximately 1.0 μg/mL with a triphase decay. Rapid α (<5 minutes) and β (49–168 minutes) half-lives result in a rapid decline in the plasma concentration in the first hour posttreatment followed by a prolonged terminal half-life of 18–49 hours, reflecting slow efflux from the peripheral compartment. The volume of distribution at steady state is 20–75.6 L/kg. The drug is extensively bound to platelets, lymphocytes, and plasma proteins. The major site of metabolism is the liver, with 33%–80% of the drug excretion in feces and approximately 20% in urine.

Preparation and Administration: Vinorelbine is available for injection in single use as 10 mg/mL in 1- or 5-mL vials without preservatives. The calculated dose is diluted to 1.5–3.5 mg/mL for a slow injection (6–10 minutes) by a syringe with 5% dextrose or 0.9% saline, or between 0.5 or 2.0 mg/mL in an IV bag. Because vinorelbine is a strong vesicant, it should be administered through a freely flowing IV access avoiding all extravasation.

Toxic Effects: Vinorelbine shares many of the principal toxicities of vinblastine. Myelosuppression is dose limiting but not cumulative, with nadirs occurring 7–10 days after administration.

Anemia and thrombocytopenia occur infrequently. Because of lower affinity for axonal versus spindle microtubules, neurotoxicity is less prominent with vinorelbine. Mild-to-moderate peripheral neuropathy and constipation occur in approximately 30% of patients, and the incidence of neuropathy increases with the duration of treatment. Mild-to-moderate nausea and vomiting is seen in 33% of patients. Stomatitis and diarrhea are less frequent. Transient elevations of transaminases have been reported. Among the miscellaneous side effects noted are chest pain with or without electrocardiographic changes (6%, most with underlying cardiac disease), as well as bronchospasm and dyspnea (5%). Alopecia is seen in 10% of patients.

Therapeutic Indications in Hematology: Objective responses have been observed in approximately 33% of patients with Hodgkin lymphoma or NHL.

Paclitaxel (Taxol) and Docetaxel (Taxotere)

Chemistry and Mechanism of Action: Both paclitaxel and docetaxel are complex diterpene alkaloid esters consisting of a taxane system linked to an oxetane ring and a C-13 side chain that is necessary for their cytotoxic effects in mammalian cells. After binding to the N-terminal 31 amino acids of the β-tubulin subunit in the tubulin oligomers or polymers, these taxanes kinetically stabilize microtubule dynamics at plus ends. They also decrease the lag time and shift the equilibrium toward tubulin polymerization into microtubule bundles. The disequilibrium of tubulin–microtubule polymerization results in mitotic arrest and apoptosis of cells. Taxane-induced mitotic arrest is associated with phosphorylation of B-cell lymphoma (BCL2) protein and increased intracellular levels of free BAX protein, which promote apoptosis. Compared with paclitaxel, docetaxel demonstrates 1.9-fold greater affinity for tubulin binding sites and greater potency in mediating BCL2 phosphorylation.

Absorption, Fate, and Excretion: Taxanes generally are administered by IV infusion lasting over 3, 24, or 96 hours (paclitaxel) or 1 hour (docetaxel). Depending on the dose and schedule, peak plasma concentrations of paclitaxel range between 0.05 and 15.0 mM. Its steady-state volume of distribution ranges between 48 and 182 L/m^2, with rapid uptake in almost all tissues except the CNS and 98% plasma protein binding. Plasma decay for paclitaxel is biphasic, with α and β half-lives of 0.34 and 5.8 hours, respectively. Saturable distribution and elimination appear to be responsible for paclitaxel's nonlinear pharmacokinetics. This means that paclitaxel dose escalation in shorter schedules may result in disproportionate increases in area under the concentration–time curve and peak plasma concentration. It is metabolized to 6-hydroxy paclitaxel by the CYP3A isoform of the PU_{50} mixed-function oxidases in the hepatic microsomes. Total fecal and urinary excretion of paclitaxel and its metabolites is approximately 70% and 10%, respectively. Although dose modification is not necessary for renal insufficiency, a 50% reduction in dose is recommended even for moderate hyperbilirubinemia or significant elevations in hepatocellular enzymes. When administered as a 1-hour IV infusion, docetaxel has linear pharmacokinetics that fit a three-compartment model. Similar to paclitaxel, docetaxel also has a high clearance rate (0.36 L/hour), a steady-state volume of distribution (67.3 L/m^2), and a terminal half-life of 12 hours. Docetaxel also has high protein binding (97%) and extensive tissue distribution. The drug or its metabolites also have high fecal (80%) and low urinary elimination (5%). Metabolism of docetaxel also primarily occurs in hepatic microsomal P450 mixed-function oxidases, CYP3A, CYP2B, and CYP1A.

Preparation and Administration: Paclitaxel is available as a 30-mg/5 mL single-dose vial in polyoxyethylated castor oil (Cremophor EL) 50% and dehydrated alcohol, USP 50%. The contents of the vial must be diluted before use. Docetaxel for injection is available as a concentrate in polysorbate 80 in two vial contents (23.6 mg/0.59 mL or 94.4 mg/2.36 mL) along with the appropriate diluent (1.83 or 7.33 mL) in separate vials. Adding diluent that is 13% (w/w) ethanol in water for injection to the concentrate produces a final premix concentration of 10 mg docetaxel/mL. The required amount of premix is transferred by a calibrated syringe into 0.9% saline or 5% dextrose to produce a final concentration of 0.3 or 0.9 mg/mL. The IV infusion is administered over 1 hour.

Toxic Effects: Hypersensitivity reaction (HSR) was noted in up to 30% of patients in the early phase I studies. HSR occurs early in the first or second infusion and may be caused by vehicle Cremophor EL or paclitaxel itself. HSR consists of dyspnea, bronchospasm, urticaria, and hypotension. Most HSRs regress completely after stopping the infusion and treatment with antihistamines, fluids, and vasopressors. Prolonged infusions (>3 hours) and premedication (dexamethasone 20 mg PO, 12 and 6 hours before treatment, diphenhydramine 50 mg, and ranitidine 150 mg IV 30 minutes before treatment) have reduced the incidence of major HSRs to less than 3%. Patients with a history of HSR may be rechallenged with paclitaxel at a markedly slower infusion rate, 20 mg dexamethasone IV every 6 hours for four doses before treatment. Although not formulated in Cremophor EL, HSRs can occur in up to 25% of patients receiving docetaxel. Most HSRs are minor, consisting of flushing, chest tightness, and low back pain. Premedication with dexamethasone 8 mg PO twice daily for 3 days starting 1 day before treatment with docetaxel considerably reduces the incidence of HSRs and fluid retention. Neutropenia is the main toxicity of paclitaxel and docetaxel, but it is not cumulative. With higher doses of paclitaxel (250 mg/m^2 over 24 hours), this can be ameliorated with subsequent administration of granulocyte colony-stimulating factor. Severe thrombocytopenia and anemia are rare. Symmetric, distal, peripheral sensory neuropathy is usually seen with higher doses or multiple doses of paclitaxel. This often limits chronic use of paclitaxel. Diffuse areflexia and neuronopathy are less commonly seen. Higher doses can also cause motor and autonomic neuropathy as well as myalgias, especially in patients with preexisting neuropathy or when paclitaxel is used with cisplatin. Severe peripheral neuropathy or myalgias are less common after repetitive docetaxel at 100 mg/m^2. Cardiac rhythm abnormalities, especially bradyarrhythmias and (rarely) heart blocks, have been reported secondary to paclitaxel treatment. A direct causal link between paclitaxel and myocardial ischemic episodes and tachyarrhythmias has not been established. Although noted, a direct link has also not been established between the occurrence of cardiac conductance abnormalities or ischemia and docetaxel treatment. Nausea, vomiting, diarrhea, and stomatitis are uncommon and generally mild to moderate. Alopecia is universal with both drugs. Skin toxicity is more severe and common with docetaxel. It is characterized by an erythematous pruritic maculopapular rash affecting the forearms and hands. Onychodystrophy with discoloration, ridging, and brittleness of fingernails also occurs. Docetaxel can cause cumulative fluid retention, resulting in peripheral edema, third-space fluid collection, and weight gain, which usually resolves slowly after stopping docetaxel. Concurrent treatment with dexamethasone, as noted earlier, delays the onset and decreases the incidence of these side effects.

Potential Drug Interaction: When paclitaxel infusion (24 hours) is administered after cisplatin, there is a 33% reduction in the clearance rate of paclitaxel. This produces suboptimal antitumor cytotoxicity and more profound neutropenia. Hence, the sequence of paclitaxel followed by cisplatin is commonly recommended. The use of carboplatin after paclitaxel has been reported to cause less thrombocytopenia than carboplatin alone. Mucositis is more pronounced when paclitaxel is used before doxorubicin, a sequence that reduces the clearance of doxorubicin. Hematologic toxicity is more prominent with the sequence of cyclophosphamide followed by paclitaxel compared with the reverse sequence of administration. Anticonvulsants such as phenytoin and phenobarbital induce the metabolism of paclitaxel and docetaxel by the P450 mixed-function oxidases. Conversely, in vitro studies have shown that inhibitors of the P450 system can interfere with the metabolism of both drugs. These inhibitors include erythromycin, testosterone, ketoconazole, and fluconazole.

Therapeutic Indications in Hematology: Both paclitaxel and docetaxel have significant activity against previously treated patients with NHL. Paclitaxel is also very active against HIV-associated Kaposi sarcoma.

APPENDIX   57.3

CLINICAL PHARMACOLOGY OF ANTIMETABOLITES

Cytosine Arabinoside

Chemistry and Mechanism of Action: Cytosine arabinoside (1′-β-D-arabinofuranosylcytosine; ara-C) is a nucleoside analog that differs from its naturally occurring counterpart (2′-deoxycytidine) by virtue of the presence of a hydroxyl group in the 2′-β configuration. The altered reactivity of the resulting arabinosyl sugar moiety confers on ara-C its cytotoxic activity. Ara-C enters the cell by a facilitated nucleoside diffusion mechanism and is converted to its nucleoside monophosphate form, ara-CMP, by the pyrimidine salvage pathway enzyme, deoxycytidine kinase. This represents the rate-limiting step in ara-C metabolism. Ara-C may also be catabolized intracellularly to an inactive form, ara-U, by the enzyme cytidine deaminase (CDD). Ara-C is ultimately converted to its lethal triphosphate derivative, ara-CTP, by a mono- and diphosphate kinase. Ara-CTP is an inhibitor of DNA polymerases α, β, and γ, and is also incorporated into replicating DNA strands, leading to inhibition of chain initiation and elongation and premature chain termination. The extent of incorporation of ara-C into DNA closely correlates with lethality in leukemic cells. Although ara-C is generally thought of as a prototypical S-phase–specific agent, its ability to interfere with DNA repair polymerases (e.g., β and γ) as well as lipid biosynthetic enzymes may account for lethal effects in noncycling cells.

Absorption, Fate, and Excretion: After IV administration, ara-C is rapidly deaminated to an inactive form, ara-U, by CDD. This enzyme is present in the plasma, liver, and kidney but is present at very low levels in the CNS. The initial plasma half-life of ara-C has been estimated to be 10–12 minutes. Approximately 90% of the administered ara-C dose is excreted by the kidneys as ara-U or other inactive metabolites. The terminal half-life of ara-C is approximately 2–3 hours. CNS ara-C levels after a 2-hour infusion approximate 50% of plasma concentrations. Steady-state plasma concentrations after standard-dose therapy (e.g., 100–200 mg/m²/day as a continuous infusion) approximate between 10^{-7} and 10^{-6} M. When ara-C is given as a high-dose bolus infusion (e.g., 1–3 g/m² over 1–3 hours), plasma levels as high as 100 μM can be achieved.

Preparation and Administration: Ara-C is provided as a sterile, lyophilized powder for reconstitution in vials containing 100 mg, 200 mg, 1 g, or 2 g of material. The powder is reconstituted with sterile bacteriostatic water for injection with benzyl alcohol (0.945%) added as a preservative. When reconstituted in this way, solutions are stable for up to 48 hours under controlled temperatures (e.g., between 15°C and 30°C or 60°F and 86°F). Material reconstituted without preservative should be used immediately. For intrathecal injection, ara-C should be reconstituted in a diluent that does not contain preservative (e.g., preservative-free 0.9% sodium chloride, USP) and used immediately.

Toxic Effects: Ara-C is primarily toxic to rapidly dividing tissues; consequently, myelosuppression and gastrointestinal toxicity represent the major side effects of this agent. Patients receiving ara-C regularly experience leukopenia, anemia, and thrombocytopenia, with nadirs appearing 7–14 days after drug administration. Gastrointestinal toxicity includes nausea and vomiting, abdominal pain, mucositis, and a chemical hepatitis characterized by elevation of liver function enzymes. The latter is generally reversible. Patients receiving ara-C as a high-dose infusion (e.g., 1–3 g/m² repeated every 12 hours for a total of 6–12 doses) experience standard toxicities and several unique

ones. These include alopecia, an exfoliative dermatitis, a chemical conjunctivitis (generally ameliorated by the prophylactic administration of a steroid or saline ophthalmic solution), a respiratory distress–like syndrome (characterized by the appearance of rales, abnormal radiography findings, and pulmonary insufficiency), and cerebellar toxicity. The latter, which is characterized by nystagmus, ataxia, and other cerebellar signs, may be irreversible, and its appearance mandates discontinuation of therapy. Intrathecal administration of ara-C has been rarely associated with the toxicities described later for methotrexate.

Potential Drug Interactions: None reported.

Therapeutic Indications in Hematology: Ara-C represents a mainstay in the treatment of AML (e.g., as part of the "7 and 3" regimen, in which it is given in conjunction with daunorubicin). It is also incorporated into some induction regimens for ALL. High-dose ara-C (HIDAC), either alone or in combination with anthracycline antibiotics, is frequently used in the treatment of refractory or relapsed AML or ALL. High-dose ara-C has also been used in some salvage regimens for NHL (e.g., ESHAP). Chronic low-dose ara-C has been used in the treatment of patients with myelodysplastic syndrome (MDS).

Methotrexate

Chemistry and Mechanism of Action: Methotrexate (*N*-[4-[[(2,4-diamino-6-pteridinyl)methyl]methylamino]benzoyl]-L-glutamic acid) represents a member of a class of compounds referred to as *antifolates*. Methotrexate is a potent inhibitor of dihydrofolate reductase, an enzyme responsible for the reduction of dihydrofolates to tetrahydrofolates. The latter are required in 1-carbon transfer reactions involved in de novo purine and pyrimidine biosynthesis, including conversion of deoxyuridylate (dUMP) to thymidylate (dTMP) by thymidylate synthase. As in the case of most antimetabolites, methotrexate is primarily active against S-phase cells. Methotrexate is transported across cell membranes by an energy-dependent, temperature-sensitive concentrative process involving folate-binding proteins, after which it is polyglutamylated by the enzyme folylpolyglutamyl synthetase. Polyglutamylation of methotrexate enhances its intracellular retention and in some studies has been shown to correlate with the sensitivity of leukemic cells to this agent. The mechanism by which methotrexate kills cells may stem from interference with DNA synthesis (leading to a "thymine-less death") secondary to DHFR inhibition, disruption of purine biosynthesis, or a combination of these actions. The lethal actions of methotrexate may be reversed by reduced folates such as 5-formyltetrahydrofolate (leucovorin). The possibility that tumor cells may exhibit impaired transport of such reduced folates serves as the basis for strategies involving administration of high-dose methotrexate in conjunction with leucovorin rescue.

Absorption, Fate, and Excretion: In adults, oral absorption is dose dependent, with mean bioavailability approximating 60% at doses of 30 mg/m² or less. At higher doses (e.g., ≥80 mg/m²), bioavailability is less. Peak plasma concentrations occur 1–2 hours after oral administration. Methotrexate bioavailability approximates 100% for parenteral routes of administration; with these routes, peak plasma methotrexate levels are achieved within 30–60 minutes after administration. For each route, the steady-state volume of distribution ranges from 40% to 80% of body weight. Methotrexate tends to accumulate in third-space fluids (e.g., ascites or pleural effusions) and can result in prolonged release and accompanying toxicity. Consequently, it is generally not advisable for patients with fluid accumulations to receive methotrexate. Methotrexate competes with reduced folates for transport across cell membranes; however, at high doses (e.g., ≥ 100 mg/m^2), passive diffusion is the primary mechanism through which intracellular accumulation occurs. Methotrexate is approximately 50% protein bound and does not penetrate the CNS barrier when administered orally or parenterally at conventional doses. However, when given by the intrathecal route, high CNS levels are achieved. Administration of high-dose methotrexate with leucovorin rescue can also result in therapeutic CNS levels.

The primary route of excretion is renal, with 80%–90% of the drug appearing unchanged in the urine within 24 hours after IV administration. The terminal half-life of methotrexate is 4–10 hours for patients receiving low-dose therapy and 8–15 hours for those receiving high-dose therapy. Because of the primary renal rate of excretion and the possibility of nephrotoxicity, methotrexate should be withheld or administered at reduced doses in patients with impaired renal function. Patients receiving high-dose methotrexate therapy should be hydrated and their urine alkalinized before administration to reduce the risks of toxicity.

Preparation and Administration: Methotrexate is available in multiple formulations: (1) tablets, containing 2.5 mg methotrexate and inactive ingredients (lactose, magnesium stearate, and pregelatinized starch; (2) methotrexate sodium injection, available in vials of 25, 50, and 250 mg, containing benzyl alcohol as a preservative, sodium chloride, and water for injection (preservative-containing solutions should not be used for intrathecal or high-dose administration); (3) methotrexate sodium injection without preservative, which can be used for IV, intraarteriolar, intrathecal, and high-dose administration; and (4) lyophilized powder, which is provided in 20-mg vials and is reconstituted with preservative-free sodium chloride or 5% dextrose in water to a final concentration not exceeding 25 mg/mL.

For intrathecal administration, solutions of 1–1.5 mg/mL should be prepared using preservative-free 0.9% sodium chloride as the diluent. For high-dose therapy, leucovorin rescue is required to prevent significant toxicity. Leucovorin is administered 12–24 hours after methotrexate at a dose of between 15 and 25 mg IV, intramuscularly (IM), or PO every 6 hours until the methotrexate dose declines to levels of less than 5×10^{-7} M.

For patients receiving intermediate or high-dose methotrexate (e.g., ≥ 500 mg/m^2), serum methotrexate and creatinine levels should be monitored at 24-hour intervals. If, after 48 hours serum methotrexate levels are greater than 5×10^{-7} M but less than 1×10^{-6} M, leucovorin is continued at a dose of 25 mg/m^2 every 6 hours for eight doses until methotrexate levels decline to below 5×10^{-7} M. If levels are greater than 1×10^{-6} M but less than 2×10^{-6} M at 48 hours, the dose of leucovorin is increased to 100 mg/m^2 every 6 hours for eight doses. For methotrexate levels $\geq 2 \times 10^{-6}$ M at 48 hours, the dose of leucovorin is 200 mg/m^2 every 6 hours for eight doses.

Toxic Effects: Methotrexate primarily exhibits its toxic effects toward proliferating tissues. Consequently, dose-limiting toxicities include bone marrow suppression (leukopenia, thrombocytopenia, anemia), mucositis, and diarrhea. High-dose therapy is occasionally accompanied by transient elevations in liver function test results, but chronic low-dose therapy is more often associated with hepatic fibrosis. Standard-dose therapy is rarely associated with nephrotoxicity, but acute renal failure can be seen with high-dose therapy secondary deposition of 7-*OH*-methotrexate in the renal tubules. The risk of methotrexate nephrotoxicity is significantly reduced by ensuring adequate hydration and alkalinization of the urine. Other reported toxicities include a maculopapular rash and an idiosyncratic pulmonary toxicity characterized by cough, fever, dyspnea, hypoxia, and interstitial infiltrates.

A necrotizing leukoencephalopathy has been reported in patients receiving methotrexate who have had prior cranial irradiation. Intrathecal methotrexate has been associated with several toxicities, including (1) chemical arachnoiditis; (2) motor paralysis accompanied by cranial nerve dysfunction, seizures, and coma; and (3) chronic demyelinating syndrome. Each of these may be exacerbated by prior craniospinal irradiation.

Potential Drug Interactions: Methotrexate exhibits many potential drug interactions that are related to plasma protein binding. For example, many compounds are known to displace methotrexate from serum albumin, potentially increasing its bioavailability. These agents include sulfonamides, salicylates, tetracyclines, chloramphenicol, and phenytoin. However, the clinical implications of such interactions are not clear. Nonsteroidal antiinflammatory drugs should not be administered in conjunction with methotrexate when the latter is given at intermediate or high doses owing to the potential for elevation and prolongation of methotrexate plasma concentrations. Penicillins can reduce renal clearance of methotrexate and should be used with caution in this setting. Probenecid may also reduce renal transport of methotrexate. Administration of methotrexate can also reduce the clearance of theophyllines, and concomitant use of these agents requires careful monitoring. Increases in methotrexate toxicity have been observed in some patients receiving trimethoprim–sulfamethoxazole, possibly as a consequence of enhanced antifolate effects. Administration of folates in vitamin preparations may reduce the efficacy of methotrexate by bypassing dihydrofolate reductase inhibition. Methotrexate may increase the toxicity (and potentially the activity) of various antineoplastic agents in a schedule-dependent manner (e.g., when given before 5-fluorouracil).

Therapeutic Indications in Hematology: Methotrexate is widely used in the treatment of ALL, particularly in the maintenance phase. Methotrexate is frequently administered intrathecally in patients with CNS leukemia and prophylactically in certain patients with ALL. It also represents a component of various multidrug regimens used in the treatment of NHL (e.g., M-BACOD, PROMACE-CYTABOM).

Hydroxyurea

Chemistry and Mechanism of Action: Hydroxyurea is an inhibitor of the ribonucleotide reductase system that catalyzes the rate-limiting step in the de novo biosynthesis of purine and pyrimidine deoxyribonucleotides, that is, the conversion of ribonucleotide diphosphates to their deoxyribonucleoside diphosphate derivatives. Ribonucleotide reductase consists of two subunits: a binding and allosteric effector component and an iron-binding catalytic component. Hydroxyurea binds to and inactivates the catalytic subunit of the enzyme. Similar to most antimetabolites, hydroxyurea is an S-phase–specific agent and blocks cells in the G_1S phase of the cell cycle. Exposure of cells to hydroxyurea leads to a depletion of deoxyribonucleotide triphosphate (dNTP) pools, the extent of which correlates with DNA synthesis inhibition and cell death. Two consequences of hydroxyurea administration include potentiation of the metabolism or cytotoxicity of nucleoside analogs (e.g., ara-C) as a result of dNTP pool depletion and elimination of amplified genes present extrasomally in double-minute chromosomes.

Absorption, Fate, and Excretion: Hydroxyurea is generally administered PO, although IV regimens are currently being investigated. The drug is readily absorbed from the gastrointestinal tract, with peak plasma levels as high as 2.0 mM occurring approximately 2 hours after oral administration. Serum concentrations decline to undetectable levels after 24 hours. The drug is primarily excreted via the renal route, with 75%–80% of the drug appearing in the urine 12 hours later. The drug penetrates the cerebrospinal fluid, although it has not been established that therapeutic levels are achieved after standard oral administration.

Preparation and Administration: Hydroxyurea is provided as 500-mg capsules. The drug is stored at room temperature in tightly capped containers and protected from heat.

Toxic Effects: The most common adverse reactions include myelosuppression (leukopenia, thrombocytopenia, anemia), gastrointestinal symptoms (e.g., nausea and vomiting, stomatitis, anorexia, appetite disturbances), and dermatologic toxicity (e.g., rashes, skin ulcerations, facial erythema). Rarer toxicities, generally seen at high doses include neurologic disturbances, such as drowsiness, dizziness, headache, and convulsions; altered renal function; and alopecia. The mutagenic potential of hydroxyurea is unknown, and the drug should be avoided when possible in pregnant women.

Potential Drug Interactions: As noted earlier, hydroxyurea may increase the toxicity of certain nucleoside analogs. Hydroxyurea may also serve as a radiosensitizing agent; consequently, patients receiving concurrent radiation therapy may experience enhanced toxicity.

Therapeutic Indications in Hematology: Hydroxyurea has also been successfully used in the treatment of Philadelphia chromosome negative myeloproliferative neoplasms, including myelofibrosis, polycythemia vera, and essential thrombocythema. Its leukemogenic potential is uncertain, however, and it should be used with caution, particularly in younger patients. Hydroxyurea has also been shown to reduce the incidence of painful crises in individuals with sickle cell anemia in a subset of patients, a phenomenon that may result from increases in red blood cell fetal hemoglobin levels.

Fludarabine

Chemistry and Mechanism of Action: Fludarabine phosphate is a fluorinated derivative of the nucleotide analog ara-A, which is resistant to deamination by the degradative enzyme CDD. It is converted intracellularly to its triphosphate derivative, which inhibits ribonucleotide reductase, as well as DNA polymerase-α and DNA primase. Fluoro-ara-ATP is also incorporated into DNA, a process that appears to be essential for the induction of apoptosis in leukemic cells. Fludarabine is toxic to S-phase cells, but its ability to interfere with DNA repair may contribute to lethality in their noncycling counterparts.

Absorption, Fate, and Excretion: After IV injection, fludarabine phosphate is rapidly deaminated (i.e., within minutes) in the plasma to its nucleoside derivative, 2′-fluoro-ara-A, which is then converted intracellularly to its nucleotide form, 2′-fluoro-ara-AMP by the pyrimidine salvage pathway enzyme, deoxycytidine kinase. The half-life of 2′-fluoro-ara-A is approximately 10 hours; the primary mode of elimination is renal, with 25% of the total dose appearing in the urine as unchanged 2′-fluoro-ara-A. Total body clearance of fludarabine is inversely correlated with serum creatinine.

Preparation and Administration: Fludarabine is supplied as a sterile powder in 50-mg vials containing 50 mg of mannitol and sodium hydroxide to adjust the pH to 7.7. Material is reconstituted in 2 mL of sterile water to yield a 25-mg/mL solution for injection. The material may be stored at 4°C (40°F); because the reconstituted solution contains no antimicrobial preservative, the drug should be administered within 8 hours of formulation.

Toxic Effects: The most common dose-limiting toxicity is myelosuppression (neutropenia, thrombocytopenia, and anemia). Other toxicities include fever, chills, infection, nausea, and vomiting. Rarer toxicities include malaise, fatigue, anorexia, and weakness. Patients with CLL receiving fludarabine have experienced serious opportunistic infections and tumor lysis syndrome. The most serious toxicity of fludarabine when administered at high doses (>40 mg/m²/day for 5 days) is irreversible neurotoxicity, including cortical blindness, necrotizing leukoencephalopathy, and death. This phenomenon has

rarely, if ever, been seen in patients receiving conventional doses (e.g., 25 mg/m²/day for 5 days). Rare reports of interstitial pneumonitis have appeared.

Potential Drug Interactions: Fludarabine has been shown to potentiate the intracellular metabolism and activity of ara-C, although the toxicity of this combination may also be enhanced. No other interactions have been reported.

Therapeutic Indications in Hematology: Fludarabine has shown marked activity in both untreated CLL and in disease refractory to standard alkylating agent therapy. Fludarabine has also shown activity as a single agent, and particularly in combination with others (e.g., mitoxantrone, Cytoxan) in indolent NHL.

2′-Chlorodeoxyadenosine

Chemistry and Mechanism of Action: 2′-Chlorodeoxyadenosine (CdA; cladribine) is a derivative of deoxyadenosine that differs from its parent compound by the presence of a chlorine moiety at the 2′-position of the purine ring. It is transported intracellularly by facilitated nucleoside diffusion and phosphorylated by the pyrimidine salvage pathway enzyme deoxycytidine kinase. CdA is relatively resistant to deamination by CDD. CdA is readily converted to its triphosphate derivative, 2′-chlorodeoxyadenosine-5′-triphosphate, particularly in cells of lymphoid origin, and is incorporated into tumor cell DNA by DNA polymerase-α. CdATP is also an effective inhibitor of ribonucleotide reductase, which may contribute to lethal effects. CdA induces cell death (apoptosis) in both cycling and noncycling cells, possibly by promoting DNA fragmentation and by depleting cells of ATP or NAD, or both.

Absorption, Fate, and Excretion: Relatively little pharmacokinetic information concerning CdA is available. The drug is most commonly administered as a 7-day continuous infusion or as a 2-hour infusion over 5 days. The bioavailability of CdA after subcutaneous (SC) administration approximates that of the IV route but is less than that after oral administration. Renal excretion appears to be the major route of elimination. When given as a 2-hour infusion, CdA has a relatively long terminal half-life (e.g., ≈6 hours), and plasma concentrations after such a schedule may approximate those associated with the continuous infusion. Cerebrospinal fluid levels are approximately 25% of plasma concentrations.

Preparation and Administration: For daily infusions, CdA is diluted under sterile conditions in bags containing 500 mL of 0.9% sodium chloride injection, USP. The use of 5% dextrose solutions is not recommended because of enhanced degradation of the drug. For preparation of longer infusions (e.g., 7 days) the use of bacteriostatic sodium chloride injection, USP, is recommended. After being prepared, solutions of CdA should be refrigerated at a temperature between 4°C (40°F) and 8°C (47°F) for no more than 8 hours before administration.

Toxic Effects: The major toxicity of CdA is myelosuppression, which is primarily observed after intermittent rather than continuous infusion. Other toxicities include fever, generally beginning several days after initiation of therapy, and increased susceptibility to opportunistic infections. Rare side effects include nausea and hepatic and renal toxicity.

Potential Drug Interactions: None reported.

Therapeutic Indications in Hematology: CdA has shown significant activity in CLL and hairy cell leukemia. However, response rates in the former disorder appear to be somewhat less than those obtained with fludarabine; moreover, patients who have progressed on fludarabine therapy infrequently respond to CdA. Other diseases in which CdA has shown activity include NHL and Waldenström macroglobulinemia.

2′-Deoxycoformycin

Chemistry and Mechanism of Action: 2′-Deoxycoformycin (pentostatin; DCF) is an adenosine analog that is a highly effective inhibitor of the purine biosynthetic enzyme adenosine deaminase (ADA). It is transported across cell membranes by facilitated nucleoside diffusion, where it binds tightly to ADA. Inhibition of ADA results in accumulation of deoxyadenosine metabolites, most notably dATP. dATP exerts its toxic effects through inhibition of ribonucleotide reductase and induction of global imbalances in dNTP pools. These result in interference with DNA synthesis and repair. 2′-Deoxycoformycin is particularly toxic to certain lymphoid cells with low levels of ADA activity. It is also toxic to both cycling and resting cells; the mechanism underlying its cytotoxicity toward quiescent cells is unknown.

Absorption, Fate, and Excretion: After IV injection of 2′-deoxycoformycin, the plasma clearance follows a biphasic pattern, with a terminal elimination half-life of 3–15 hours. Protein binding is limited. The drug is only partially metabolized, with approximately 60%–80% of the drug appearing unchanged in the urine after 24 hours. The total-body clearance of 2′-deoxycoformycin correlates well with creatinine clearance. Patients with impaired renal function may require reductions in the 2′-deoxycoformycin dose.

Preparation and Administration: 2′-Deoxycoformycin is unstable when reconstituted in solutions of pH less than 5.0. Consequently, it is customarily reconstituted in normal saline. 2′-Deoxycoformycin is provided in vials containing 10 mg of drug, 50 mg of mannitol, and sodium hydroxide to adjust the pH to less than 7.0. It is administered as an IV infusion over 20–30 minutes. Hydration is recommended before and after 2′-deoxycoformycin administration.

Toxic Effects: The major toxicities of 2′-deoxycoformycin include myelosuppression, nausea and vomiting, immunosuppression, acute renal failure, keratoconjunctivitis, fever, and elevations of liver function enzymes. At high doses, neurologic toxicity, including somnolence, seizures, and coma, have been reported, although these are seen infrequently in patients receiving standard dose therapy. When administered at such doses (e.g., 4 mg/m^2 biweekly), side effects are relatively minor.

Potential Drug Interactions: 2′-Deoxycoformycin may augment the toxicity of ara-A as a consequence of inhibition of ADA.

Therapeutic Indications in Hematology: 2′-Deoxycoformycin is primarily used in the treatment of hairy cell leukemia, in which response rates of up to 90% have been reported, even in patients refractory to other therapy, including interferon-α (IFN-α). Activity has also been reported in other lymphoid malignancies, such as T-cell lymphoma, CLL, prolymphocytic leukemia, and Waldenström macroglobulinemia, although its precise role in the treatment of these disorders remains to be fully evaluated.

6-Thioguanine

Chemistry and Mechanism of Action: Thioguanine (6-TG) is a guanine analog in which the 6′-hydroxyl group is replaced by a sulfhydryl group. It interferes with de novo purine biosynthesis at multiple levels. After transport across the cell membrane by facilitated diffusion, 6-TG competes with hypoxanthine and guanine for phosphorylation by hypoxanthine–guanine phosphoribosyltransferase and is converted to its nucleotide form, 6-thioguanylic acid (TGMP), which accumulates within cells. TGMP inhibits several purine biosynthetic enzymes, including glutamine-5-phosphoribosylpyrophosphate aminotransferase and IMP dehydrogenase. 6-TG nucleotides are also incorporated in DNA and RNA, where they function as fraudulent bases. It is presently unknown which of these actions (interference with purine interconversions, blockade of de novo purine biosynthesis, or nucleic acid incorporation) is primarily

responsible for 6-TG cytotoxicity, although DNA incorporation appears to play a significant role. 6-TG is considered to be an S-phase–specific agent.

Absorption, Fate, and Excretion: After oral administration, the bioavailability of 6-TG is variable, ranging from 14% to 46% of the administered dose (mean: 30%). Peak plasma levels are achieved 8 hours after administration and decline slowly thereafter. The average plasma disappearance of 6-TG is approximately 80 minutes, with a range of 25–240 minutes. Relatively little unchanged material appears in the urine; the major excreted product is the methylated derivative 2-amino-6-methyl thiopurine. CNS penetrance after parenteral administration is minimal.

Preparation and Administration: 6-TG is available in tablet form for oral administration. Each tablet contains 40 mg of 6-TG and inactive ingredients, including gum acacia, lactose, magnesium stearate, potato starch, and stearic acid. IV preparations are available only in experimental settings.

Toxic Effects: The major dose-limiting toxicity of 6-TG is myelosuppression. Other less common toxicities include gastrointestinal disturbances (nausea and vomiting, anorexia, diarrhea), jaundice, and elevated liver function test results.

Potential Drug Interactions: In contrast to 6-MP, the metabolism of 6-TG is not modified by allopurinol; consequently, dose adjustments do not have to be made when these agents are administered concurrently.

Therapeutic Indications in Hematology: The primary indication for 6-TG is in the treatment of AML, generally in conjunction with other agents (e.g., daunorubicin and ara-C). However, it has not been firmly established that addition of 6-TG to such regimens improves therapeutic efficacy. 6-TG also has activity in chronic myeloid leukemia, although it has been supplanted by other agents (e.g., hydroxyurea, IFN-α in this disorder).

6-Mercaptopurine

Chemistry and Mechanism of Action: 6-Mercaptopurine (1,7-dihydro-6*H*-purine 6-thione monohydrate; 6-MP; purinethol) is an analog of the purine bases adenine and hypoxanthine. It is both an antineoplastic and immunosuppressive agent. Similar to 6-TG, 6-MP and its metabolites act at multiple levels to interfere with purine biosynthesis and interconversions. It competes with hypoxanthine and guanine for hypoxanthine–guanine phosphoribosyltransferase, and after conversion to thioinosinic acid (TIMP), blocks conversion of IMP to xanthylic acid and IMP to AMP. Both TIMP and another metabolite, 6-methylthioinosinate (MTIMP), inhibit glutamine-5-phosphoribosylpyrophosphate aminotransferase. 6-MP is also incorporated into RNA and DNA, thereby functioning as a fraudulent base. It is unknown which of these actions is primarily responsible for the lethal actions of 6-MP, although available evidence points to DNA incorporation as a prime determinant of cytotoxicity.

Fate, Absorption, and Excretion: After oral administration, the bioavailability of 6-MP is highly variable, presumably because of interpatient differences in gastrointestinal absorption, which averages 50% of the administered dose. Extensive catabolism by hepatic xanthine oxidase also contributes to drug elimination. Approximately 50% of the administered 6-MP or its metabolites are recovered in the urine. The volume of distribution generally exceeds the total body water. After IV administration, the plasma disappearance half-life was 47 minutes in adults. Plasma protein binding is modest (approximately 19%), and CNS penetrance is minimal.

Preparation and Administration: 6-MP is supplied as tablets for oral administration. Each tablet contains 50 mg of 6-MP and the inactive ingredients corn and potato starch, lactose, magnesium stearate, and stearic acid. An IV preparation containing 500 mg of 6-MP per vial is available for investigational use.

Toxic Effects: The major dose-limiting toxicity of 6-MP is myelosuppression. This is dose related and is manifested by leukopenia, thrombocytopenia, and anemia. The hematologic effects of 6-MP may be delayed, so it is important to withdraw the medication temporarily at the first sign of unusual hematologic toxicity. Individuals with an inherited disorder of thiopurine methyltransferase deficiency may be particularly susceptible to 6-MP–mediated hematopoietic suppression. Other toxicities include hepatotoxicity (elevated liver function test results, cholestasis, hepatic necrosis, ascites), nausea, vomiting, mucositis, fever, rash, and diarrhea. The hepatotoxicity, which occurs in 10%–40% of patients, requires close monitoring and discontinuation of therapy until recovery occurs. Patients receiving 6-MP uniformly experience immunosuppression.

Potential Drug Interactions: Allopurinol, an inhibitor of xanthine oxidase, significantly reduces the catabolism of 6-MP when the latter is given orally, leading to major increases in plasma concentrations. Allopurinol does not alter the pharmacokinetics of IV 6-MP, presumably because of the absence of first-pass metabolism of 6-MP when administered by this route. When administered in conjunction with allopurinol, the dose of 6-MP should be reduced by one-third to one-fourth. Increased toxicity has been reported in patients receiving concurrent 6-MP and trimethoprim–sulfamethoxazole. 6-MP may also modify the effects of warfarin.

Therapeutic Indications in Hematology: The major use for 6-MP is in the maintenance phase of treatment for ALL. 6-MP has also been used in the treatment of patients with immune thrombocytopenia purpura or autoimmune hemolytic anemia refractory to all other forms of therapy.

5′-Azacitidine

Chemistry and Mechanism of Action: 5′-Azacitidine is an analog of the nucleoside cytidine, differing from the parent compound by virtue of the presence of nitrogen at the 5′ position of the heterocyclic ring. 5′-Azacytidine is transported across the cell membrane by facilitated nucleoside diffusion and is converted to its nucleotide monophosphate form, 5′-aza-CMP, by the pyrimidine salvage pathway enzyme uridine–cytidine kinase. 5′-Azacytidine is also a substrate for the degradative enzyme CDD. It is ultimately converted to its lethal derivative, 5′-aza-CTP, which is incorporated into RNA, and to a lesser extent, DNA. The lethal actions of 5′-azacytidine are believed to result from its ability to interfere with protein synthesis through disruption of RNA processing. The chemical instability of the 5′-azacitidine ring structure is also believed to contribute to the cytotoxicity of this compound.

Absorption, Fate, and Excretion: The drug distributes into a volume corresponding to the total body water after IV administration and is also well absorbed after SC injection.

It is extensively deaminated in the plasma and liver and displays minimal plasma binding. Peak plasma concentrations after IV injection approximate 1.0 mM. The initial half-life of 5′-azacitidine (or its metabolites) is approximately 4 hours, although the drug is rapidly converted to various derivatives within minutes of administration. There is minimal cerebrospinal fluid penetrance.

Preparation and Administration: Azacitidine is available in 100-mg vials and can be administered both IV and SC. When given SC, it should be reconstituted with 4 mL of sterile water for injection. The diluents should be injected slowly into the vial. Vigorously shake or roll the vial until a uniform suspension is achieved. The suspension will be cloudy. The resulting suspension will contain azacitidine 25 mg/mL. Do not filter the suspension after reconstitution. Doing so could remove the active substance. Azacitidine reconstituted for

SC administration may be stored for up to 1 hour at 25°C (77°F) or for up to 8 hours between 2°C and 8°C (36°F and 46°F). To provide a homogeneous suspension, the contents of the dosing syringe must be resuspended immediately before administration. To resuspend, vigorously roll the syringe between the palms until a uniform, cloudy suspension is achieved. When given IV, reconstitute each vial with 10 mL of sterile water for injection. Vigorously shake or roll the vial until all solids are dissolved. Withdraw the required amount of solution to deliver the desired dose and inject into a 50–100-mL infusion bag of either 0.9% sodium chloride injection or lactated Ringer solution.

Toxic Effects: The major toxicity of 5′-azacitidine has been leukopenia and, to a lesser extent, thrombocytopenia. Nausea and vomiting, which are often refractory to standard antiemetic therapy, have also been encountered, most frequently in patients receiving bolus infusions. Gastrointestinal toxicity is ameliorated by administering 5′-azacitidine as a continuous infusion. Other potential side effects include diarrhea, fever, hepatotoxicity (most frequently in patients with preexisting hepatic disease), neuromuscular toxicity, rash, and hypotension.

Drug Interactions: None reported.

Therapeutic Indications in Hematology: 5′-Azacitidine is primarily used in the treatment of refractory AML, with response rates ranging from 17% to 30% when used as a single agent. 5′-Azacitidine has also yielded clinical responses in a subset of patients with the MDS when administered as a low-dose continuous infusion. In early trials, low-dose 5′-azacytidine increased fetal hemoglobin levels in some patients with sickle cell anemia and thalassemia; however, its mutagenic potential has limited the use of this agent in nonmalignant conditions.

Decitabine

Chemistry and Mechanism of Action: Decitabine is a synthetic nucleoside analog of 2′-deoxycytidine, a cytotoxic S-phase pyrimidine analogue that induces hypomethylation of DNA at concentrations that do not cause major suppression of DNA synthesis. It also causes cellular differentiation or apoptosis. This is accomplished by intracellular phosphorylation of decitabine to its triphosphate form, which is incorporated into DNA and blocks methylation of newly synthesized DNA by binding to DNA methyltransferase. Nonproliferating cells seem relatively insensitive to decitabine.

Absorption, Fate, and Excretion: Decitabine is widely distributed with less than 1% protein binding and is tolerated after SC injection. There is some CNS penetration after subcutaneous injection with cerebrospinal fluid concentrations in patients with meningeal leukemia that were approximately 20% of corresponding steady-state plasma levels. The mean half-life is 0.5–0.6 hours. The route of metabolism appears to be deamination by CDD, principally found in the liver but also in granulocytes, the intestinal epithelium, and whole blood.

Preparation and Administration: Decitabine is available in 50-mg vials, which are reconstituted with 10 mL of sterile water for injection (USP); upon reconstitution, each milliliter contains approximately 5.0 mg of decitabine at a pH of 6.7–7.3. Immediately after reconstitution, the solution should be further diluted with 0.9% sodium chloride injection, 5% dextrose injection, or lactated Ringer solution injection to a final drug concentration of 0.1–1.0 mg/mL. Unless used within 15 minutes of reconstitution, the diluted solution must be prepared using cold (2°–8°C) infusion fluids and stored at 2°–8°C (36°–46°F) for up to a maximum of 7 hours until administration.

Toxic Effects: The major toxicity of decitabine has been bone marrow suppression, including leukopenia, thrombocytopenia, and anemia. Nausea and vomiting are mild. Other potential side effects include diarrhea, fever, and hepatotoxicity, including hyperbilirubinemia, transamination elevations, and electrolyte abnormalities.

Drug Interactions: None reported.

Therapeutic Indications in Hematology: Decitabine is indicated for treatment of patients with MDS, including previously treated and untreated, de novo, and secondary MDS. It has also been used as salvage therapy both alone and in combination for AML, chronic myeloid leukemia, and acute lymphoid leukemia.

Gemcitabine

Chemistry and Mechanism of Action: Gemcitabine (2',2'-difluorocytidine monohydrochloride) is a nucleoside analog that differs from 2'-deoxycytidine by virtue of the presence of fluorine atoms in the 2'α and 2'β positions of the cytidine ring. It is transported across the cell membrane by facilitated nucleoside diffusion, phosphorylated by deoxycytidine kinase, and ultimately converted to its lethal metabolites, dFdCDP and dFdCTP. The diphosphate form (dFdCDP) inhibits ribonucleotide reductase, leading to disruption of dNTP pools and resultant interference with DNA synthesis and repair. The triphosphate form (dFdCTP) competes with dCTP for incorporation into DNA. Reductions in dCTP pools (secondary to ribonucleotide reductase inhibition) result in self-potentiation of gemcitabine action. Incorporation of gemcitabine into DNA in S phase inhibits elongation of the replicating strand, leading to DNA chain termination. The lethal actions of gemcitabine in leukemia cells have been related to the induction of apoptosis and are not restricted to cells actively engaged in DNA synthesis. Gemcitabine has been shown to be considerably more potent in inducing apoptosis in cultured human leukemia cells than ara-C.

Absorption, Fate, and Excretion: In studies involving IV administered labeled gemcitabine, up to 98% of the drug was recovered in the urine after 1 week. The excreted dose was composed of a minor fraction (gemcitabine; <10%) and inactive metabolites (e.g., 2'-deoxy-2',2'-difluorouridine). Plasma protein binding was minimal. In studies involving both short and long gemcitabine infusions, the pharmacokinetics were found to be linear and best described by a two-compartment model. Plasma half-life and clearance are influenced both by age and gender. For short infusions, half-lives varied from 32 to 94 minutes; for longer infusions, half-lives varied from 245 to 638 minutes. The volume of distribution was approximately 50 L/m² for short infusions and 370 L/m² for long infusions.

Preparation and Administration: Vials of gemcitabine contain 200 mg or 1 g of the HCl derivative formulated with mannitol (200 mg or 1 g) and sodium acetate (12.5 mg or 62.5 mg) as a sterile lyophilized powder. HCl or NaOH has been used for pH adjustment.

Toxic Effects: The major dose-limiting toxicity of gemcitabine is myelosuppression, although anemia and thrombocytopenia have also been encountered. Other toxicities include nausea and vomiting, transient elevations in liver function test results, mild hematuria, proteinuria (and in rare cases, hemolytic uremic syndrome), fever, rash, dyspnea, edema, and a flulike syndrome. Other infrequent toxicities included alopecia, paresthesias, and bronchospasm.

Potential Interactions: Gemcitabine may function as a radiosensitizing agent and can increase the toxicity of ionizing radiation. No other interactions are known.

Indications in Hematology: The primary indication for gemcitabine is in the treatment of patients with pancreatic carcinoma. However, as an experimental agent, gemcitabine is being evaluated for the treatment of ALL and CLL.

Nelarabine, Arabinofuranosylguanine (Ara-G)

Chemistry and Mechanism of Action: Nelarabine is a prodrug of the deoxyguanosine analog 9'-β-D-arabinofuranosylguanine, also known as *ara-G*. Accumulation of a metabolite ara-GTP in leukemic blasts allows for incorporation into DNA, leading to inhibition of DNA synthesis and cell death.

Absorption, Fate, and Excretion: Nelarabine is demethylated by ADA to ara-G, then monophosphorylated by deoxyguanosine kinase and deoxycytidine kinase, and subsequently converted to the active 5'-triphosphate, ara-GTP. Nelarabine is only available in an IV formulation. Nelarabine and ara-G are both partially eliminated by the kidneys. Approximately 5%–10% of nelarabine is excreted by the kidneys compared with 20%–30% of ara-G. Nelarabine exhibits a half-life of 30 minutes, and ara-G, the active metabolite, has a half-life of 3 hours.

Preparation and Administration: Nelarabine for injection is supplied as a clear, colorless, sterile solution in glass vials. Each vial contains 250 mg of nelarabine (5 mg of nelarabine/mL) and sodium chloride (4.5 mg/mL) in 50 mL of water for injection, USP. Nelarabine is not diluted before administration. The dose is transferred into polyvinylchloride (PVC) infusion bags or glass containers and administered as a 2-hour infusion in adult patients or as a 1-hour infusion in pediatric patients.

Toxic Effects: Bone marrow suppression encompassing all cell lines causing anemia, leucopenia, thrombocytopenia, and neutropenia occurs in all patients. Neurologic complications of nelarabine include asthenia, altered mental states including severe somnolence, CNS effects including convulsions, and peripheral neuropathy ranging from numbness and paresthesias to motor weakness and paralysis. Demyelinating disease of the CNS may occur when combining nelarabine with other drugs that may have CNS toxicity. Nausea and vomiting are seen and antiemetics are necessary.

Drug Interactions: Pentostatin has been shown to be a strong inhibitor of ADA in vitro. Concurrent administration of nelarabine and pentostatin may result in reduced ADA-dependent conversion of nelarabine to its active moiety, thereby potentially decreasing nelarabine efficacy or altering nelarabine's adverse event profile. Therefore, concomitant administration of nelarabine and pentostatin is not recommended.

Therapeutic Indications in Hematology: Nelarabine is effective in T-cell ALL, T-cell lymphoma, and T-cell lymphoblastic lymphoma. The dosage in adults of nelarabine is 1500 mg/m² administered IV over 2 hours on days 1, 3, and 5 repeated every 21 days. The pediatric dosage of nelarabine is 650 mg/m² administered IV over 1 hour daily for 5 consecutive days repeated every 21 days. The proper number of cycles for adult and pediatric patients has not been determined.

Clofarabine

Chemistry and Mechanism of Action: Clofarabine is a purine nucleoside antimetabolite formulated in unbuffered normal saline with a pH range of 4.5–7.5. It inhibits DNA synthesis by decreasing cellular deoxynucleotide triphosphate pools by inhibiting ribonucleotide reductase, terminating DNA chain elongation, and inhibiting repair through incorporation into the DNA chain by competitive inhibition of DNA polymerases.

Absorption, Fate, and Excretion: Clofarabine is 47% bound to plasma proteins, primarily albumin. Clofarabine is phosphorylated intracellularly to the cytotoxic active form (clofarabine triphosphate) by deoxycytidine kinase. The terminal half-life is estimated to be 5.2 hours with the metabolite clofarabine triphosphate, yielding a half-life greater than 24 hours, and 49%–60% of the dose is excreted in the urine unchanged. Systemic clearance and volume of distribution at steady state were estimated to be 28.8 L/hour/m^2 and 172 L/m^2, respectively.

Preparation and Administration: Clofarabine is supplied in a 20-mL, single-use vial that contains 20 mg of clofarabine in 20 mL of unbuffered normal saline at a concentration of 1 mg/mL. Clofarabine should be filtered through a sterile 0.2-μm syringe filter and diluted with 5% dextrose injection, USP, or 0.9% sodium chloride injection, USP, before IV infusion to a final concentration between 0.15 and 0.4 mg/mL.

Toxic Effects: Bone marrow suppression encompassing all cell lines causing anemia, leucopenia, thrombocytopenia, and neutropenia occurs in all patients. A capillary leak syndrome, also known as *systemic inflammatory response syndrome* (SIRS), thought to be related to cytokine release leading to respiratory distress, hypotension, pleural effusions, pericardial effusions, and multiorgan failure may occur in a small number of patients. Elevations of liver transaminases are seen and are transient (typically, less than 2 weeks' duration) and occurred within 1 week of clofarabine initiation. Elevations in bilirubin may also occur.

Drug Interactions: None described.

Therapeutic Indications in Hematology: Clofarabine is effective in treating ALL. The recommended pediatric dose is 52 mg/m^2 administered by IV infusion over 2 hours daily for 5 consecutive days. Treatment cycles are repeated after recovery or return to baseline organ function, approximately every 2–6 weeks. Clofarabine has been used in adults at a dosage of 40 mg/m^2 administered by IV infusion over 2 hours daily for 5 consecutive days. Clofarabine has also been used in combination with cytarabine. Because this drug is excreted to a major extent by the kidneys, extreme caution should be used in patients with renal dysfunction.

APPENDIX   **57.4**

TOPOISOMERASE I INHIBITORS AND TOPOISOMERASE II INHIBITORS

TOPOISOMERASE II INHIBITORS

Etoposide (Vepesid), Etoposide Phosphate (Etopophos), Teniposide (Vumon)

Chemistry and Mechanism of Action: Etoposide (VP-16), etoposide phosphate, and teniposide (VM-26) are semisynthetic derivatives of epipodophyllotoxin. The mechanism of action of these drugs appears to be related to their ability to stabilize a topoisomerase II–DNA cleavable complex, which acts as a replication fork barrier and leads to the generation of irreversible DNA damage and cell death in proliferating cells.

Absorption, Fate, and Excretion: Etoposide has an oral bioavailability of 25%–75%. Its terminal half-life is 6–8 hours, with approximately 30%–40% excreted in the urine, two-thirds as unchanged drug. There is no accumulation with consecutive daily administration, but cytotoxicity has strict schedule dependency. Clinical studies suggest that in patients with a plasma creatinine level greater than 130 mol/L, the etoposide dose should be reduced by more than 25%.

Etoposide phosphate is rapidly and completely converted in vivo to VP-16 by the activity of phosphatase and has been shown to have the same pharmacokinetics as VP-16. Because of its increased water solubility, etoposide phosphate can be given IV in much less volume. In addition, the metabolic acidosis and hypotension seen with the infusion of VP-16 are not seen with this prodrug.

Teniposide has a multiphasic pattern of clearance from plasma with a terminal half-life of 9.5–21 hours. Unlike those of etoposide, metabolites of teniposide account for greater than 80% of the drug excreted in the urine. Similar to etoposide, there is significant inter-patient and intrapatient variation in clinical pharmacokinetics. There are currently no formal recommendations for dose modification in patients with renal insufficiency.

Preparation and Administration: Etoposide is commercially available as 50-mg capsules and in vials of 50 and 100 mg at a concentration of 20 mg/mL. When the drug is diluted with normal saline or 5% dextrose in water to a concentration of 0.2 or 0.4 mg/mL, it is stable for 96 or 48 hours, respectively. Etoposide must be administered slowly over more than 30 minutes to prevent hypotension.

Etoposide phosphate is available commercially as single-dose vials containing etoposide phosphate equivalent to 100 mg of etoposide. When it is diluted with water, 5% dextrose, or normal saline to a concentration of 10–20 mg/mL, it can be administered without dilution over 5–10 minutes. When reconstituted, etoposide phosphate is stable for 24 hours at room temperature or under refrigeration.

Teniposide is supplied in 50-mg vials for IV use only. The IV solution may be taken orally but is unpalatable. Currently, no oral preparation is available in the market; however, for investigational purposes, each 50-mg vial may be dissolved in 50–100 mL of syrup or juice. To achieve optimal absorption, a single oral dose of 60 mg/m^2, which may be repeated at 6-hour intervals, is advised. As with etoposide, rapid infusion can produce hypotension.

Toxic Side Effects: Myelosuppression, especially leukopenia, is the dose-limiting toxic effect of etoposide and teniposide. Nausea and vomiting are usually mild and easily prevented with antiemetics. Rapid infusion of etoposide (<30 minutes) may cause hypotension. Anaphylactoid reactions (e.g., bronchospasm) occur in fewer than 2% of patients and may be related to the Cremophor vehicle. Alopecia occurs in approximately 20% of patients treated with etoposide. This side effect is more common with teniposide. When the drug is given in bone marrow transplantation doses, mucositis and diarrhea are prominent and may be dose limiting.

Potential Drug Interactions: Theoretically, any drug that increases the S-phase fraction will increase the cytotoxicity of epipodophyllotoxins and other topoisomerase inhibitors. Conversely, drugs that inhibit DNA synthesis antagonize the effect of etoposide and teniposide (e.g., 5-fluoro-2'-deoxyuridine given before etoposide in some human cancer cell lines decreases the cytotoxicity of the latter). More recent in vitro data suggest that synergistic cytotoxic effects are seen when VP-16 is given after a topoisomerase I inhibitor, which appears to upregulate the amount of topoisomerase II enzyme. Antagonistic effects have been reported when a topoisomerase II inhibitor is given before a topoisomerase I inhibitor. In hematology, etoposide and teniposide may inhibit intracellular ara-CTP formation leading to reduced ara-C cytotoxicity. Potentiation of teniposide activity has been seen with methotrexate and dipyridamoles. There is at least a twofold increase in the clearance of teniposide with concomitant administration of phenobarbital or phenytoin. Cyclosporine and other PGP antagonists (PSC 833) potentiate the cytotoxic effects of etoposide.

Therapeutic Indications: Etoposide is used in the treatment of NHL and as a second-line treatment for Hodgkin lymphoma. It is also incorporated in the preparatory regimens for bone marrow transplantation of refractory lymphomas (CBV) and acute leukemia. Teniposide has been approved as a front-line agent with combination chemotherapy for childhood ALL. Combination chemotherapy with teniposide has been used successfully in some cases of refractory adult ALL and acute monocytic leukemia, but the duration of remission is not significantly different from that with other standard salvage regimens. In NHL, teniposide has shown comparable activity to vincristine. Etoposide phosphate has been given in both standard-dose and high-dose (as a single agent) chemotherapy regimens and appears to have the same pharmacokinetics and antitumor activity as VP-16.

Daunorubicin

Chemistry and Mechanism of Action: Daunorubicin is an anthracycline that inhibits DNA topoisomerase II, acting as a poison at lower concentrations and a suppressor of cleavable complex formation at higher doses. Daunorubicin is also a DNA intercalator and generates reactive oxygen intermediates.

Absorption, Fate, and Excretion: After IV injection, daunorubicin undergoes rapid tissue uptake and concentration. It is rapidly metabolized in the liver, where approximately 25% of the drug concentrates and has a half-life of 20–50 hours. The principal metabolite is daunorubicinol, which also displays antineoplastic activity. Biliary excretion accounts for approximately 75% of the drug and metabolite elimination. Patients with significant hepatic dysfunction should receive an attenuated dose of daunorubicin.

Preparation and Administration: Daunorubicin is supplied with 100 mg of mannitol in 20-mg vials, from which it is reconstituted with 4 mL of sterile water for injection. The vial should be protected from sunlight. Daunorubicin is a powerful vesicant that should be administered into the tubing of a freely flowing IV infusion of either 5% dextrose in water or normal saline. In the event of extravasation, as much infiltrated drug as possible should be aspirated from the tissue, and cold compresses should be maintained on the site for several hours. Despite these measures, skin grafting may be necessary. Daunorubicin is not physically compatible with heparin, and the two drugs should not be co-administered in the same IV tubing. The patient should be informed that daunorubicin may impart a red color to the urine for up to 72 hours after administration.

Toxic Effects: Myelosuppression, predominantly leukopenia, is the dose-limiting toxic effect. Mucositis, nausea and vomiting, and alopecia are common. Facial flushing, conjunctivitis, and lacrimation may occur in rare cases. Erythematous streaking near the site of injection occurs as a benign local allergic reaction and should not be confused with extravasation. The drug can produce a severe local reaction (e.g., pneumonitis, esophagitis) in previously irradiated areas, even when both therapies are not administered concomitantly (radiation recall). Cardiac toxicity is a unique characteristic of the anthracycline antibiotics and can be acute or chronic. In the acute form, abnormal ECG changes such as ST-T wave elevation and arrhythmias may be seen. Transient reduction in the ejection fraction can also occur acutely and is often associated with pericarditis (pericarditis-myocarditis syndrome). The chronic form of anthracycline cardiac toxicity is related to the cumulative dose. The dose limit of doxorubicin is generally considered to be 450–500 mg/m^2, where the risk of clinical cardiotoxicity is between 1% and 10%. The corresponding cumulative dose limit for daunorubicin is 900–1000 mg/m^2. The cardiac toxicity is clinically characterized by congestive heart failure, usually refractory to medical therapy. Cardiac irradiation or the administration of cyclophosphamide may increase the risk of cardiotoxicity. The cardiotoxic effects appear to be related to the formation of free radicals and not to the inhibition of DNA topoisomerase II. The cardioprotective agent dexrazoxane (Zinecard) is now available and recommended to be started at a doxorubicin cumulative dose greater than 350 mg/m^2.

Potential Drug Interactions: Daunorubicin is not physically compatible with heparin or dexamethasone. The drug interactions described for doxorubicin (description follows) probably occur with daunorubicin as well.

Therapeutic Indications in Hematology: Daunorubicin is used in combination with other drugs in the treatment of AML and ALL.

Doxorubicin (Adriamycin)

Chemistry and Mechanism of Action: Doxorubicin is also an anthracycline glycoside antibiotic. It differs from daunorubicin at C-8, in which a hydroxyacetyl group replaces an acetyl group. Because of this, doxorubicin is also called *hydroxyl daunorubicin*. Its mechanisms of action also involve stabilizing DNA–topoisomerase II complexes, DNA intercalation, and free radical formation.

Absorption, Fate, and Excretion: Doxorubicin has a triphasic plasma clearance with a half-life of approximately 30 hours. The drug is extensively metabolized in the liver to yield an active metabolite (doxorubicinol) and a number of inactive metabolites (aglycones). Within 7 days, more than 50% of an injected dose is excreted in the bile, but only 5%–10% of the drug is excreted in the urine. Penetration into the cerebrospinal fluid is poor.

Preparation and Administration: Doxorubicin is commercially available in vials of 10, 20, 50, 150, and 200 mg. The lyophilized powder is reconstituted with either normal saline or sterile water for injection to yield a 2-mg/mL solution. The reconstituted solution must be protected from sunlight. The drug should be injected slowly into the tubing of a freely running IV infusion of normal saline or 5% dextrose in water. Erythematous streaking along the vein is often an indication that the administration rate is too rapid. The drug is a powerful vesicant, and in case of extravasation, the measures described for daunorubicin should be followed.

Toxic Effects: The toxic effects are similar to those of daunorubicin. It is important to emphasize that weekly low-dose regimens or administration by continuous infusion can decrease the risk of cardiotoxicity with doxorubicin.

Potential Drug Interactions: When used in combination with other drugs as treatment for leukemia or lymphoma, doxorubicin may decrease the oral bioavailability of digoxin. It is not physically compatible with heparin or 5-fluorouracil. Barbiturates may increase the plasma clearance of doxorubicin and decrease its cytotoxic effect. Doxorubicin is compatible with vincristine, and the two drugs can be administered together in the same IV solution.

Therapeutic Indications in Hematology: Doxorubicin is one of the most important drugs in the treatment of hematologic malignancies. It is used in the treatment of Hodgkin lymphoma (ABVD regimen), NHL (CHOP, MACOP-B), and MM (VBAP, VAD).

Idarubicin (Idamycin)

Chemistry and Mechanism of Action: Idarubicin, also called 4′-demethoxydaunorubicin (4-DMDR), is an analog of daunorubicin in which the methoxy group from the aglycone has been replaced with hydrogen. Idarubicin is also a topoisomerase II inhibitor and generates free radicals.

Absorption, Fate, and Excretion: The elimination half-life of the parent compound is 11.3 hours and that of the primary metabolite, 13-epirubicinol, is 40–60 hours. The major metabolite is as active as idarubicin. The oral bioavailability of this drug is approximately 30%; 80% of the drug is excreted in the urine as 13-epirubicinol.

Preparation and Administration: Idarubicin is supplied in 5- and 10-mg vials from which it is reconstituted with sterile water or normal saline to obtain a 1-mg/mL solution. The drug should be infused for 10–15 minutes through the tubing of a freely running IV infusion. Extravasation precautions should be instituted during administration. The oral formulation remains investigational.

Toxic Effects: The side effects of idarubicin are similar to those of daunorubicin and doxorubicin but are of lesser intensity at equal myelosuppressive doses.

Potential Drug Interactions: None reported.

Therapeutic Indications in Hematology: Idarubicin in combination with ara-C is equivalent, if not superior, to combination chemotherapy with daunorubicin in the treatment of adult AML and MDS. Idarubicin has been approved for use in combination therapy for adult AML.

Mitoxantrone (Novantrone)

Chemistry and Mechanism of Action: Mitoxantrone is a synthetic anthracenedione. Its mechanism of action appears to primarily involve the inhibition of DNA topoisomerase II. Its reduced potential for free radical formation may explain the decreased cardiotoxicity of this drug.

Absorption, Fate, and Excretion: Mitoxantrone is excreted via the renal and hepatobiliary systems, but the hepatobiliary elimination accounts for approximately 30% of active drug elimination and appears to be of greater importance. The half-life is quite variable, with a range of 23–42 hours. Patients with severe hepatic dysfunction have been shown to eliminate the drug more slowly.

Preparation and Administration: Mitoxantrone is commercially available as a 2-mg/mL solution in 10-mL, 12.5-mL, and 15-mL vials (20, 25, and 30 mg per vial, respectively). The drug is further diluted in normal saline or 5% dextrose in water for injection and is administered for approximately 15–30 minutes into the tubing of a freely running IV infusion. As with the anthracyclines, erythema or streaking along the vein of infusion indicates that the drug is being infused too rapidly. Although mitoxantrone is not a vesicant, there have been rare reports of tissue necrosis after extravasation.

Toxic Effects: Myelosuppression, principally leukopenia, is the dose-limiting toxic effect. Thrombocytopenia is relatively mild. Nausea, vomiting, and alopecia are usually mild and occur in fewer than 30% of patients treated. Rarely, mucositis and elevation of liver enzymes occur. The drug imparts a blue color to the urine of patients treated. One of the primary advantages of mitoxantrone, compared with doxorubicin, is its reduced incidence of cardiac toxicity. Occasionally, patients develop congestive heart failure after treatment with mitoxantrone in the absence of prior anthracycline exposure, although the incidence appears to be less than 5%.

Potential Drug Interactions: None reported.

Therapeutic Indications in Hematology: Mitoxantrone is approved for induction therapy of AML in adults.

TOPOISOMERASE I INHIBITORS

Topotecan (Hycamtin)

Chemistry and Mechanism of Action: Topotecan is a semisynthetic derivative of camptothecin that stabilizes a complex between DNA topoisomerase I and DNA. The cytotoxic effect of this drug is believed to result from the collision of DNA replication forks with a ternary complex of topoisomerase I, DNA, and topotecan. The resulting double-strand DNA breaks are lethal. The lactone form of topotecan, which predominates at an acidic pH, is a much more potent inhibitor of DNA topoisomerase I.

Absorption, Fate, and Excretion: At neutral or physiologic pH the carboxylate form of topotecan is favored, and at a pH of less than 7 the lactone form is favored. Topotecan has been given as a bolus or by continuous infusion. In less than 1 hour after infusion, most of the circulating drug in the plasma is in the carboxylate form as a result of the physiologic pH. Whereas the terminal half-life of the lactone form of this S-phase–specific agent is 2.6 hours, the terminal half-life of the total drug is 3.3 hours. In an IV dose, 36% is excreted unchanged in the urine, and there is a 1.5-fold concentration of the drug in bile. Cerebrospinal fluid levels of topotecan lactone reach approximately 32% of plasma levels. Dose adjustment is required for creatinine clearance less than 60 mL/min, but no adjustment is necessary for bilirubin up to 10 mg/dL.

Preparation and Administration: Topotecan is commercially available as 4-mg vials that are reconstituted with 4 mL of sterile water. This solution can be further diluted in normal saline or 5% dextrose in water and should be used immediately.

Toxic Effects: The dose-limiting toxicity for topotecan for all schedules is neutropenia. Thrombocytopenia and anemia are less common, although there is an increase in thrombocytopenia with continuous infusion schedules. Other less common and mild toxicities include nausea, vomiting, diarrhea, fever, fatigue, alopecia, skin rash, and increased liver function tests. Mucositis has been seen with prolonged infusion schedules over 5 days or when topotecan is given in higher doses.

Potential Drug Interactions: In vitro data suggest that there may be some synergism if a topoisomerase I inhibitor is given before a topoisomerase II inhibitor. In vitro data also suggest that synergism may be seen if a topoisomerase I inhibitor (topotecan) is given after an alkylating agent, suggesting that topoisomerase I may be involved in the repair of alkylator-induced DNA damage.

Therapeutic Indications in Hematology: Phase II studies suggest that topotecan has activity in MDS, AML, and MM.

Irinotecan (Camptosar or CPT-11)

Chemistry and Mechanism of Action: Irinotecan (Camptosar or CPT-11) is a prodrug that has a bulky piperidino side chain at C-10 that is cleaved in vivo by a carboxylesterase-converting enzyme to generate SN-38. SN-38 is approximately 1000-fold more potent a topoisomerase I inhibitor than CPT-11. The lactone forms of both SN-38 and CPT-11 are more potent inhibitors of topoisomerase I than the carboxylate forms, which is felt to be the mechanism of action of these drugs as described for topotecan.

Absorption, Fate, and Excretion: The terminal half-life of the lactone form of CPT-11 is 7 hours, and that of the total drug is 10.5 hours. The terminal half-life of SN-38 lactone is 8.7 hours, and that of the total drug is 14.7 hours. Of a dose of irinotecan, 22% is excreted unchanged in the urine. SN-38 is excreted into the bile and can undergo glucuronidation. Whereas the plasma protein binding of CPT-11 is reported to be between 30% and 68%, that of SN-38 is 95%.

Preparation and Administration: Irinotecan is available as a 100-mg single-dose vial with 20 mg/mL of irinotecan. This preparation also contains 45 mg of sorbitol/mL and 0.9 mg of lactic acid/mL with the pH adjusted to 3.5. This solution can be diluted with 5% dextrose in water (preferred) or in normal saline to a final concentration of 0.1–1.2 mg/mL. The solution is stable for up to 24 hours at room temperature or 48 hours when refrigerated. The dose should be modified for severe diarrhea.

Toxic Effects: The major toxic effect of irinotecan is diarrhea. This can be early-onset diarrhea, occurring within hours of administration, or during the infusion, which can be associated with cramping, vomiting, flushing, and diaphoresis. These side effects are attributable to the cholinergic effects of CPT-11 and can be managed with atropine. Severe later onset diarrhea can be treated with high-dose loperamide, which has been found to decrease the incidence of grade 4 diarrhea from 20% to 2%. Diarrhea has been found to be the dose-limiting toxicity when irinotecan is given on a weekly schedule, and neutropenia is the dose-limiting toxicity when the drug is given every 3 weeks. Also seen are alopecia, nausea, vomiting, mucositis, fatigue, increased liver function test results, and rare cases of pulmonary toxicity.

Potential Drug Interactions: As described for topotecan, in vitro data suggest some synergism when topoisomerase I inhibitors precede topoisomerase II inhibitors or follow alkylating agent administration.

Therapeutic Indications in Hematology: Phase I and phase II studies have shown responses in refractory leukemia and lymphoma.

CLINICAL PHARMACOLOGY OF PLATINUM ANALOGS

Cisplatin (Platinol)

Chemistry and Mechanism of Action: Cisplatin [cisdiamined ichloroplatinum(II)] is an inorganic heavy-metal complex. This complex can have *cis*- and *trans*-isomers; the *cis*-isomer is the active antitumor drug. In the relatively higher chloride concentrations of plasma, cisplatin is uncharged in the dichloroform and passes through plasma membranes. Intracellularly, the low chloride concentrations allow the displacement of the chloride ligands by water to form the positively charged aquated complex. This forms covalent cross-links between two nucleophilic atoms of macromolecules such as the N^7 positions of guanine and adenine in DNA. The cytotoxicity of cisplatin correlates closely with total platinum binding to DNA, to interstrand cross-links and to the formation of intrastrand bidentate N^7 adducts at d(GpG) and d(ApG), resulting in intrastrand cross-links that bend the DNA helix and inhibit DNA synthesis. Cisplatin damage to DNA induces apoptosis of sensitive cells.

Absorption, Fate, and Excretion: After IV injection, the drug concentrates in the liver, kidneys, and bowel. Plasma levels of cisplatin decay in a biphasic manner, with an initial half-life of 25–49 minutes and a terminal half-life of 58–73 hours. Although 15% of the administered cisplatin is excreted unchanged in the urine, up to 90% of the administered dose of the drug can be recovered from the urine.

Preparation and Administration: Cisplatin is commercially available as a lyophilized powder, supplied in 10- and 50-mg vials also containing mannitol, sodium chloride, and hydrochloric acid, and as an aqueous solution in 50- and 100-mg vials. Reconstitution of the powder for injection is achieved by adding sterile water to make a 1-mg/mL solution. The reconstituted solution should be further diluted in normal saline (usually 500 mL to 1 L) and administered over 1–3 hours. To prevent nephrotoxic effects, 25–50 g of mannitol is often added to the saline solution, and patients are aggressively hydrated before and after cisplatin infusion. Magnesium sulfate (12–24 mEq) is commonly added to the saline solution to preclude the development of hypomagnesemia.

Toxic Effects: Nephrotoxicity is the dose-limiting toxic effect. Cisplatin produces a dose-dependent impairment of renal tubular function manifested by an increase in serum creatinine as well as potassium and magnesium wasting. The renal dysfunction is usually reversible, but repeated treatments may produce a cumulative and permanent mild-to-moderate impairment of renal function. Administration of other nephrotoxic agents such as aminoglycosides, even between courses, can potentiate its toxicity. Nausea and vomiting are usually severe and require the use of aggressive antiemetic support. When doses greater than 70 mg/m² are used, it is also important to protect against delayed nausea and vomiting by administering antiemetic agents (e.g., prochlorperazine plus dexamethasone) for 3 days after therapy. Myelosuppression is usually mild. High-frequency hearing loss, tinnitus, and frank deafness may occur. Peripheral neurotoxicity, characterized by paresthesias or sensory loss in a glove-and-stocking distribution or as muscular weakness, is relatively common in patients who receive total cumulative doses of greater than 500 mg/m². The peripheral neuropathy may take many months to resolve, if it does at all. Vestibular toxicity and anaphylactic reactions may occur rarely.

Potential Drug Interactions: Aminoglycosides and amphotericin may enhance cisplatin nephrotoxicity. Caution should be exercised when cisplatin is administered with bleomycin and methotrexate because cisplatin-induced renal damage may delay the excretion and thus increase the toxicity of these agents.

Therapeutic Indications in Hematology: Cisplatin is used in the treatment of refractory lymphomas, usually in combination with ara-C and high-dose dexamethasone.

Carboplatin (Paraplatin)

Chemistry and Mechanism of Action: Carboplatin is a second-generation platinum (II) complex. Its mechanism of action is very similar to that of cisplatin. However, the carboxyl ester groups in this platinum complex are less easily displaced and less chemically reactive. The peak levels of DNA cross-linking also occur 6–12 hours later for carboplatin than for cisplatin.

Absorption, Fate, and Excretion: Carboplatin is primarily eliminated through the kidneys. Its elimination is slower than cisplatin with a terminal half-life between 2 and 6 hours. After IV injection, approximately 60% of the total drug is excreted within 24 hours.

Preparation and Administration: Carboplatin is commercially available as a lyophilized powder in 50- and 150-mg vials containing carboplatin and mannitol. It is reconstituted with sterile water to a final concentration of 10 mg/mL. For injection, further dilution with 5% dextrose and water or normal saline to a concentration of 0.5 or 2 mg/mL, in which it is stable for 8 hours at room temperature. Carboplatin is often administered by IV injection over 15–30 minutes. Patients with reduced renal function (creatinine clearance of <60 mL/min) should have the dose of carboplatin decreased according to the formula described by Egorin et al.[22]

For previously untreated patients:

$$\text{Dosage (mg/m}^2) = (0.091)(\text{Creatinine clearance/Body surface area}) \times [\text{Pretreatment platelet count} - \text{Platelet nadir desired/Pretreatment platelet count} \times 100] + 86$$

For heavily pretreated patients:

$$\text{Dosage (mg/m}^2) = (0.091)(\text{Creatinine clearance/Body surface area}) \times [(\text{Pretreatment platelet count} - \text{Platelet nadir desired/Pretreatment platelet count} \times 100) - 17] + 86$$

A formula developed by Calvert and colleagues[23] also takes into account the patient's pretreatment renal function, as follows:

$$\text{Dose (mg)} = \text{Target AUC (mg/mL} \times \text{min) H [GFR (mL/min)} + 25]$$

where the dose in mg (not mg/m² body surface area) equals target AUC (area under the plasma clearance curve) × GFR (glomerular filtration rate) + 25.

In previously untreated adults, the AUC can be estimated at 7 when carboplatin is used alone and 4.5 when used in combination. If AUC is set lower, less toxicity is expected.

Toxic Effects: The dose-limiting toxic effect is myelosuppression, thrombocytopenia being more significant than leukopenia.

Carboplatin leads to less emesis than cisplatin. Although nausea and vomiting are common, they can be easily controlled with antiemetics. At high doses such as those used for bone marrow transplantation, hepatotoxicity, renal dysfunction, and moderate-to-severe cytotoxicity can occur.

Potential Drug Interactions: None reported.

Clinical Indications in Hematology: Carboplatin has been recently approved for the treatment of ovarian cancer. It is also used to treat small-cell lung, testicular, head and neck, and genitourinary cancers. High-dose carboplatin is presently under evaluation in acute leukemias and lymphomas.

HISTONE DEACETYLASE INHIBITORS

Panobinostat

Chemistry and Mechanism of Action: Panobinostat is a histone deacetylase (HDAC) inhibitor that inhibits the enzymatic activity of HDACs at nanomolar concentrations. HDACs catalyze the removal of acetyl groups from the lysine residues of histones and some non-histone proteins. Inhibition of HDAC activity results in increased acetylation of histone proteins, an epigenetic alteration that results in a relaxing of chromatin, leading to transcriptional activation. In vitro panobinostat caused the accumulation of acetylated histones and other proteins, inducing cell cycle arrest and/or apoptosis of some transformed cells. Panobinostat shows more cytotoxicity towards tumor cells compared with normal cells.

Absorption, Fate, and Excretion: The oral bioavailability of panobinostat is approximately 21%, and is 90% bound to human plasma proteins and is independent of concentration. Panobinostat is metabolized in the liver via reduction, hydrolysis, oxidation, and glucuronidation. About 40% of hepatic elimination occurs via CYP3A, while CYP2D6 and CYP2C19 are minor pathways.

Preparation and Administration: Panobinostat is available as a 10-mg size #3 light-green opaque capsule, a 15-mg size #1 orange opaque capsule, and a 20-mg size #1 red opaque capsule.

Toxic Effects: Panobinostat has been associated with severe diarrhea, severe and fatal cardiac ischemic events, severe arrhythmias, serious hemorrhage, myelosuppression, and elevations in aminotransferases and total bilirubin.

Potential Drug Interactions: All drugs undergoing metabolism by the CYP3A and CYP2D6 pathways should be used with caution.

Therapeutic Indications in Hematology: Multiple myeloma.

Romidepsin

Chemistry and Mechanism of Action: Romidepsin is a HDAC inhibitor. HDAC catalyzes the removal of acetyl groups from acetylated lysine residues in histones, resulting in the modulation of gene expression, which induces cell cycle arrest and apoptosis.

Absorption, Fate, and Excretion: Romidepsin undergoes extensive metabolism primarily by CYP3A4, with minor contribution from CYP3A5, CYP1A1, CYP2B6, and CYP2C19. It has a 3-hour half life and is >90% protein bound.

Preparation and Administration: Romidepsin is supplied as a kit including a sterile, lyophilized powder in a single-use vial containing 10 mg of romidepsin and 20 mg of the bulking agent, povidone, USP. In addition, each kit includes one sterile diluent vial containing 2 mL (deliverable volume) of 80% propylene glycol, USP, and 20%

dehydrated alcohol, USP. Romidepsin is administered IV over a 4-hour infusion.

Toxic Effects: Romidepsin is associated with cardiac toxicities including ST-segment changes and T-wave changes, along with QT prolongation, hypotension and ventricular arrhythmia, severe myelosuppression along with gastrointestinal symptoms, and TLS.

Potential Drug Interactions: All drugs undergoing metabolism by the CYP3A and CYP2D6 pathways should be used with caution.

Therapeutic Indications in Hematology: Cutaneous and peripheral T-cell lymphomas.

TYROSINE KINASE INHIBITORS

Bosutinib

Chemistry and Mechanism of Action: Bosutinib is a TK inhibitor, specifically BCR-ABL kinase.

Absorption, Fate, and Excretion: Bosutinib is primarily metabolized by CYP3A4. The major circulating metabolites identified in plasma are oxydechlorinated (M2) bosutinib (19% of parent exposure) and N-demethylated (M5) bosutinib (25% of parent exposure), with bosutinib N-oxide (M6) as a minor circulating metabolite. All the metabolites were deemed inactive. The half life of bosutinib is 22.5 hours and 95% is protein bound. Food increases the absorption of bosutinib. The bosutinib dose should be reduced in patients with severe (creatinine clearance [CLcr] <30 mL/min) or moderate (CLcr 30–50 mL/min) renal impairment.

Preparation and Administration: Bosutinib is available as a 100-mg yellow oval and a 500-mg red oval tablet.

Toxic Effects: Bosutinib is associated with gastrointestinal toxicity including diarrhea, nausea, vomiting, abdominal pain, myelosuppression, and hepatic transaminase elevations. Fluid retention occurs with bosutinib and may manifest as pericardial effusion, pleural effusion, pulmonary edema, and/or peripheral edema.

Potential Drug Interactions: All drugs undergoing metabolism by the CYP3A4 pathway should be used with caution.

Therapeutic Indications in Hematology: Philadelphia chromosome-positive (Ph+) chronic myelogenous leukemia (CML).

Crizotinib

Chemistry and Mechanism of Action: Crizotinib is an inhibitor of RTKs including ALK, hepatocyte growth factor receptor (c-Met), reactive oxygen species 1 (c-ros), and Recepteur d'Origine Nantais (RON). Crizotinib prevents the expression of oncogenic fusion proteins from activating gene expression. This inhibition impairs cell proliferation and survival of these proteins.

Absorption, Fate, and Excretion: Bioavailability ranges from 32% to 66%. Crizotinib is metabolized in the liver by CYP3A4/5. The primary pathways include oxidation of the piperidine ring to crizotinib lactam and O-dealkylation, with subsequent phase 2 conjugation of O-dealkylated metabolite. No starting dose adjustment is needed for patients with mild (CLcr 60–89 mL/min) or moderate (CLcr 30–59 mL/min) renal impairment based on a population pharmacokinetic analysis. Increased exposure to crizotinib occurred in patients with severe renal impairment (CLcr <30 mL/min) not requiring dialysis. Administer XALKORI at a dose of 250 mg PO once daily in patients with severe renal impairment not requiring dialysis.

Preparation and Administration: Crizotinib is provided as a hard, 250-mg gelatin capsule, size 0, and a hard, 200-mg gelatin capsule, size 1.

Toxic Effects: Rare but serious toxicities include hepatotoxicity, interstitial lung disease/pneumonitis, QT prolongation, and bradycardia. Other toxicities seen are vision disorders presenting as visual impairment, photopia, blurred vision, sensory neuropathy, renal cysts, nausea, vomiting and diarrhea, dizziness, and fluid retention.

Potential Drug Interactions: Co-administration of crizotinib with strong CYP3A inhibitors increases crizotinib plasma concentrations. Co-administration of crizotinib with strong CYP3A inducers decreases crizotinib plasma concentrations.

Therapeutic Indications in Hematology: ALK-positive anaplastic large-cell lymphoma.

Sorafenib

Chemistry and Mechanism of Action: Sorafenib blocks Raf kinases, which are serine/threonine protein kinases that are downstream effector molecules of Ras proteins. Theses kinases activate the Raf/MEK/ERK signaling pathway mediating cell proliferation, differentiation, and transformation. Sorafenib also inhibits tumor angiogenesis by VEGF receptor (VEGFR)-2, VEGFR-3, PDGFRβ, Flt3, c-KIT, and p38-α.

Absorption, Fate, and Excretion: Bioavailability ranges from 38% to 49%. Sorafenib is metabolized through oxidative metabolism by CYP3A4 and glucuronidation with a mean elimination half-life of 25–48 hours. No correlation between sorafenib exposure and renal function was observed following administration of a single PO dose of 400 mg to subjects with normal renal function and subjects with mild (CLcr 50–80 mL/min), moderate (CLcr 30 to <50 mL/min), or severe (CLcr <30 mL/min) renal impairment who were not on dialysis. No dose adjustment is necessary for patients with mild, moderate, or severe renal impairment who are not on dialysis.

Preparation and Administration: Tablets containing sorafenib tosylate (274 mg) equivalent to 200 mg of sorafenib.

Toxic Effects: Sorafenib has been associated with cardiac ischemia, infarction hemorrhage, congestive heart failure and hypertension, and QT interval prolongation. Adverse dermatologic effects including hand-foot skin reaction, rash, Stevens-Johnson syndrome and toxic epidermal necrolysis, gastrointestinal perforation, drug-induced hepatitis, and impairment of TSH suppression in DTC have also been reported. Sorafenib also causes leukopenia, lymphopenia, anemia, neutropenia, and thrombocytopenia.

Potential Drug Interactions: Any drug that has an effect on or is metabolized by CYP3A4 has potential interactions.

Therapeutic Indications in Hematology: FLT3-ITD positive AML.

Nilotinib

Chemistry and Mechanism of Action: Nilotinib is a selective TK inhibitor active against BCR-ABL kinase. Nilotinib binds to and stabilizes the inactive conformation of the kinase domain of ABL protein. Nilotinib is 30-fold more potent than imatinib.

Absorption, Fate, and Excretion: Nilotinib is rapidly absorbed and reaches its peak concentration in 3 hours. The AUC of nilotinib increases by 82% when given 30 minutes after a high-fat meal compared with a fasting state. Its elimination half-life is approximately 17 hours. It is metabolized by oxidation and hydroxylation,

as well as undergoing metabolism by CYP3A4. None of the nilotinib metabolites have significant pharmacologic activity.

Preparation and Administration: Nilotinib is available in capsules for oral use, containing a 150- or 200-mg nilotinib base, anhydrous (as hydrochloride, monohydrate) with the following inactive ingredients: colloidal silicon dioxide, crospovidone, lactose monohydrate, magnesium stearate, and polyoxamer 188.

Toxic Effects: Nilotinib may cause anemia, neutropenia, and thrombocytopenia. Prolonged QT interval and sudden death has occurred. Pruritus, rash, and nausea are common. Also seen with nilotinib are arthralgias and myalgias. Cough has also been associated with nilotinib.

Drug Interactions: Nilotinib is a competitive inhibitor of cytochrome P450 (CYP) isoenzymes 3A4, 2C8, 2C9, and 2D6, and has the potential to increase concentrations of drugs metabolized by these enzymes. Nilotinib plasma concentration is increased during concomitant use with potent CYP3A4 inhibitors (e.g., atazanavir, clarithromycin, indinavir, itraconazole, ketoconazole, nefazodone, nelfinavir, ritonavir, saquinavir, telithromycin, voriconazole). Decreased nilotinib plasma concentration occurs during concomitant use with potent CYP3A4 inducers (e.g., dexamethasone, carbamazepine, phenobarbital, phenytoin, rifabutin, rifampin, and St. John's wort). Drugs that increase the pH of the upper gastrointestinal tract may decrease the solubility of nilotinib and reduce its bioavailability. The oral administration of esomeprazole results in a 34% reduction in the AUC of nilotinib.

Therapeutic Indications in Hematology: Nilotinib has demonstrated activity in the case of CML resistance resulting from BCR-ABL kinase mutations from treatment with imatinib. This includes accelerated-phase CML resistant or intolerant to prior therapy. ALL, Ph+, relapsed/refractory. Blastic phase chronic myeloid leukemia, Resistant or intolerant to imatinib. Chronic phase, Ph+, newly diagnosed. Chronic-phase CML, resistant or intolerant to prior therapy.

Ponatinib

Chemistry and Mechanism of Action: Ponatinib is a kinase inhibitor that inhibits the in vitro TK activity of ABL and T315I mutant ABL with IC_{50} concentrations of 0.4 and 2.0 nM, respectively. Ponatinib inhibits the in vitro activity of additional kinases with IC_{50} concentrations between 0.1 and 20 nM, including members of the VEGFR, PDGFR, FGFR, EPH receptors and SRC families of kinases, and KIT, RET, TIE2, and FLT3. The drug also inhibits the in vitro viability of cells expressing native or mutant BCR-ABL, including T315I.

Absorption, Fate, and Excretion: Phase I (oxidative) and phase II (hydrolysis) metabolism are involved in at least 64% of a ponatinib dose. In phase I metabolism, CYP3A4 is primarily involved, with CYP2C8, CYP2D6, and CYP3A5 involved to a lesser extent. Ponatinib is also metabolized by esterases or amidases. Ponatinib has a half-life of 24 hours.

Preparation and Administration: Ponatinib is provided as 15- and 45-mg round white tablets.

Toxic Effects: The use of ponatinib has led to arterial and venous thrombosis and occlusions, including fatal myocardial infarction, stroke, and stenosis of large arterial vessels of the brain, and severe peripheral vascular disease. Fatal and serious heart failure or left ventricular dysfunction has occurred. Hypertension. Other toxicities include peripheral neuropathy pancreatitis, ocular toxicity, serious bleeding events, fluid retention, and myelosuppression.

Potential Drug Interactions: All drugs undergoing metabolism by the CYP3A4 pathway should be used with caution.

Therapeutic Indications in Hematology: Philadelphia chromosome–positive chronic myelogenous leukemia and Philadelphia chromosome–positive acute lymphoblastic leukemia.

JANUS KINASE INHIBITORS

Ruxolitinib

Chemistry and Mechanism of Action: Ruxolitinib is a JAK inhibitor (JAK1 and JAK2) that inhibits dysregulated JAK signaling associated with myelofibrosis. JAK signaling involves recruitment of signal transducers and activators of transcription (STATs) to cytokine receptors, activation, and subsequent localization of STATs to the nucleus, leading to modulation of gene expression.

Absorption, Fate, and Excretion: Ruxolitinib is 95% absorbed and 97 % protein bound. Ruxolitinib is metabolized primarily by CYP3A4, with a half-life of approximately 3 hours. Ruxolitinib is not removed by dialysis, although some active metabolites may be removed; therefore, the drug should be administered after dialysis.

Preparation and Administration: Ruxolitinib is supplied as a 5- and 10-mg round tablet, a 15- and 25-mg oval tablet, as well as a 20-mg capsule. For patients unable to ingest tablets, Jakafi can be administered PO by suspending one tablet in approximately 40 mL of water with stirring for approximately 10 minutes.

Toxic Effects: Ruxolitinib has been shown to cause myelosuppression, progressive multifocal leukoencephalopathy, and infections such as Herpes zoster.

Potential Drug Interactions: All drugs undergoing metabolism by the CYP3A4 pathway should be used with caution,

Therapeutic Indications in Hematology: Myelofibrosis and polycythemia vera,

APPENDIX **57.6**

CLINICAL PHARMACOLOGY OF MISCELLANEOUS AGENTS

Idelalisib

Chemistry and Mechanism of Action: Idelalisib is an inhibitor of PI3Kδ kinase, which is expressed in normal and malignant B cells. Idelalisib induces apoptosis and inhibits proliferation in cell lines derived from malignant B cells and in primary tumor cells. Idelalisib inhibits several cell signaling pathways, including B-cell receptor (BCR) signaling and CXC-chemokine receptor (CXCR)4 and CXCR5 signaling, which are involved in trafficking and homing of B cells to the lymph nodes and bone marrow.

Absorption, Fate, and Excretion: Idelalisib is metabolized via aldehyde oxidase and CYP3A to an inactive metabolite. It is 84% protein bound, with a half-life of 8.2 hours. AUC is increased up to1.7-fold in subjects with ALT or AST, or bilirubin values greater than the upper limit of normal (ULN) compared with subjects with normal AST or ALT or bilirubin values. CLcr has no effect on idelalisib exposure. No dose adjustment is needed for patients with CLcr ≥15 mL/min.

Preparation and Administration: Idelalisib is available as a 100-mg orange oval tablet as well as a 150-mg pink oval tablet.

Toxic Effects: Fatal and/or serious hepatotoxicity occurred in 14% of patients treated with idelalisib. Severe diarrhea or colitis with possible perforation occurred in 14% of patients. Fatal and serious pneumonitis as well as grade ≥3 cutaneous reactions were also seen. 31% of patients treated also had significant neutropenia.

Potential Drug Interactions: All drugs undergoing metabolism by the CYP3A pathway should be used with caution.

Therapeutic Indications in Hematology: Follicular lymphoma, small lymphocytic lymphoma, and CLL.

Oblimersen

Chemistry and Mechanism of Action: Oblimersen is an 18-mer phosphorothioate antisense oligonucleotide that targets human Bcl-2 mRNA and prevents Bcl-2 expression. Oblimersen downregulates Bcl-2 expression, with enhancement of tumor cell apoptosis.

Absorption, Fate, and Excretion: The half-life of oblimersen averages 0.5–2 hours, and it is excreted primarily unchanged in the urine.

Preparation and Administration: Oblimersen is given by continuous IV infusion or subcutaneously.

Toxic Effects: Oblimersen is associated with hyperglycemia, diarrhea, thrombocytopenia, and hepatic toxicity.

Potential Drug Interactions: Unknown.

Therapeutic Indications in Hematology: AML, NHL, and MM.

Thalidomide

Chemistry and Mechanism of Action: The mechanism of action of thalidomide is not fully understood. Thalidomide has immunomodulatory, antiinflammatory, and antiangiogenic properties. The immunologic effects vary substantially under differing conditions but seem to suppress TNF-α production and downmodulate cell surface adhesion molecules. Other antiinflammatory and immunomodulatory properties include suppression of macrophage involvement in prostaglandin synthesis and modulation of IL-10 and IL-12 production by peripheral blood mononuclear cells. Angiogenesis inhibition is described, but the exact mechanism is not yet definitively defined.

Absorption, Fate, and Excretion: Thalidomide absorption is slow after oral administration, and the bioavailability of capsules has not yet been determined, but based on radiolabeled thalidomide, greater than 90% is recovered in urine, suggesting good oral absorption. The mean elimination half-life of thalidomide ranges from 3 to 6.7 hours, but the exact metabolic fate of thalidomide is unknown. Protein binding is 55%–66%.

Preparation and Administration: Thalidomide is available as 50-, 100-, 150-, and 200-mg PO capsules. A 20-mg/mL PO suspension may be prepared with capsules and a 1 : 1 mixture of Ora-Sweet and Ora-Plus by emptying the contents of twelve 100-mg capsules into a glass mortar. Add small portions of the vehicle and mix to a uniform paste; mix while adding the vehicle in incremental proportions to almost 60 mL; transfer to an amber calibrated bottle and add quantity of vehicle sufficient to make 60 mL. Stable for 35 days refrigerated.

Toxic Effects: Thalidomide frequently may cause deep venous thrombosis and pulmonary embolism. Thalidomide causes birth defects in humans. It must not be given during pregnancy. Leucopenia along with thrombocytopenia is observed. Pruritus and rash as well as constipation are seen.

Drug Interactions: Thalidomide increases cyclosporine A metabolism and clearance. An increase in the thrombogenic state in patients with MDS has been observed in patients receiving darbepoetin alfa and thalidomide. The addition of docetaxel to thalidomide increases the risk of venous thromboembolism.

Therapeutic Indications in Hematology: Thalidomide has been used to treat MM and MDS.

Lenalidomide

Chemistry and Mechanism of Action: Lenalidomide, a thalidomide analog, is an immunomodulatory agent with antineoplastic and antiangiogenic activity. Lenalidomide affects ligand-induced responses (angiogenesis, inflammation, cell adhesion, immune response), inhibits production of TNF, increases production of IL-2 and IFN-γ, and increases cytolytic T-cell and NK cell responses. It inhibits trophic signals to angiogenic factors in cells, and inhibits growth of myeloma cells by inducing cell cycle arrest and apoptosis.

Absorption, Fate, and Excretion: Lenalidomide is rapidly absorbed after oral administration. Lenalidomide has a half-life of 3 hours with 67% of the drug excreted unchanged in the urine. Adjustment to the initial dosage is recommended in patients with moderate or severe renal impairment. Compared with patients with normal renal function, those with moderate and severe renal impairment have a 66%–75% decrease in drug clearance, and patients on hemodialysis have an 80% decrease in clearance. Although the drug is 30% protein bound, lenalidomide is partially removed by hemodialysis and should be given after dialysis. Food does not alter the extent of absorption nor the AUC of lenalidomide.

Preparation and Administration: Lenalidomide is available in 2.5-, 5-, 10-, 15-, and 25-mg capsules for PO administration. Each capsule contains lenalidomide as the active ingredient along with lactose anhydrous, microcrystalline cellulose, croscarmellose sodium, and magnesium stearate.

Toxic Effects: Lenalidomide frequently may cause deep venous thrombosis and pulmonary embolism. Severe myelosuppression across all cell lines is common. Pruritus and rash as well as constipation and hypokalemia are seen. Lenalidomide is an analogue of thalidomide and may cause birth defects in humans. It must not be given during pregnancy.

Drug Interactions: Lenalidomide increases digoxin plasma concentrations. Dexamethasone increases the thrombogenic effect of lenalidomide.

Therapeutic Indications in Hematology: Lenalidomide has activity in MM when used in combination with dexamethasone. It also is has activity in chronic lymphoid leukemia as well as MDS with deletion 5q abnormlalities.

Pomalidomide

Chemistry and Mechanism of Action: Pomalidomide is structurally and functionally related to thalidomide. Its mechanism is not fully understood but it has effects on angiogenesis, alters inflammatory and regulatory cytokines, and may affect T cells.

Absorption, Fate, and Excretion: Pomalidomide is administered orally. Pharmacokinetic data are still being elucidated.

Preparation and Administration: Pomalidomide is an investigational agent administered orally.

Toxic Effects: Pomalidomide has extensive bone marrow toxicity affecting all three cell lines, peripheral neuropathy, orthostasis, rashes, pulmonary toxicity, and clotting abnormalities.

Drug Interactions: Data not available.

Therapeutic Indications in Hematology: Pomalidomide has been studied in MM.

Temsirolimus

Chemistry and Mechanism of Action: Temsirolimus is an inhibitor of mammalian target of rapamycin (mTOR) and binds to an intracellular protein (FKBP-12). This protein–drug complex inhibits the activity of mTOR and results in G1 growth arrest. When mTOR is inhibited, its ability to phosphorylate p70S6k and S6 ribosomal protein, which are downstream of mTOR in the PI3K/AKT pathway, was blocked.

Absorption, Fate, and Excretion: Temsirolimus is predominately metabolized in human liver microsomes by cytochrome P450 3A4 (CYP3A4). Temsirolimus is extensively metabolized to sirolimus. Four other metabolites account for less than 10% in the plasma. The mean half-life of temsirolimus is 17.3 hours, and the mean half-life of sirolimus, the active metabolite, is 54.6 hours. Neither the parent drug nor its metabolite is dialyzable. Dosage reduction or discontinuance may be warranted in patients with hepatic impairment to reduce the potential for toxicity.

Preparation and Administration: Temsirolimus is supplied as a kit consisting of two vials: temsirolimus injection (25 mg/mL) and a diluent of 1.8 mL. Temsirolimus is mixed with 1.8 mL of the diluent. The resultant solution contains 10 mg/mL. The concentrate–diluent mixture is stable below 25°C for up to 24 hours. To administer, withdraw the required amount of concentrate–diluent mixture and further dilute into an infusion bag containing 250 mL of 0.9% sodium chloride injection, USP. Patients should receive prophylactic IV diphenhydramine 25 mg before the start of each dose.

Toxic Effects: Temsirolimus causes a decreased lymphocyte count, leucopenia, decreased hemoglobin, and thrombocytopenia. Hyperglycemia, edema, and rash (which may progress to Stevens-Johnson syndrome) have also been seen.

Drug Interactions: The concomitant use of strong CYP3A4 inhibitors (e.g., ketoconazole, itraconazole, clarithromycin, atazanavir, indinavir, nefazodone, nelfinavir, ritonavir, saquinavir, telithromycin, and voriconazole) may increase plasma concentrations of sirolimus (a major metabolite of temsirolimus). The use of concomitant strong CYP3A4 inducers (e.g., dexamethasone, phenytoin, carbamazepine, rifampin, rifabutin, rifampicin, phenobarbital) may decrease plasma concentrations of sirolimus (a major metabolite of temsirolimus).

Therapeutic Indications in Hematology: Temsirolimus has been shown to have activity in MCL.

Everolimus

Chemistry and Mechanism of Action: Everolimus is an analogue of rapamycin (sirolimus) with immunosuppressive and antiproliferative activity. Everolimus is an inhibitor of rapamycin (mTOR), a serine–threonine kinase, downstream of the PI3K/AKT pathway. After binding and forming a complex with the cytoplasmic FK506-binding protein 12 (FKBP-12), the complex binds to and inhibits mTOR and phosphorylates P70 S6 ribosomal protein kinase (a substrate of mTOR). Everolimus reduces the activity of S6 ribosomal protein kinase (S6K1) and eukaryotic elongation factor 4E–binding protein. In addition, everolimus inhibits the expression of hypoxia-inducible factor 1 and reduces the expression of VEGF.

Absorption, Fate, and Excretion: Peak everolimus concentrations are reached 1–2 hours after oral administration with protein binding of 74%. Everolimus is extensively metabolized by the liver, with everolimus being a substrate of CYP3A4 and PGP. Metabolism involves demethylation, hydroxylation, and ring degradation. There are six main metabolites of everolimus, which have approximately 100-times less activity than the parent everolimus compound, including three monohydroxylated metabolites, two hydrolytic ring-opened metabolites, and a phosphatidylcholine conjugate of everolimus. The elimination half-life is 30 hours and is prolonged to a mean of 79 hours in patients with moderate hepatic impairment.

Preparation and Administration: Everolimus is available in 2.5-, 5-, 7.5- and 10-mg nonscored tablets.

Toxic Effects: Everolimus causes bone marrow suppression across all cell lines, hyperglycemia, rash, and mucositis along with pulmonary toxicity.

Drug Interactions: Everolimus concentrations are increased when administered with CYP3A4 or PGP inhibitors such as ketoconazole, itraconazole, clarithromycin, atazanavir, nefazodone, saquinavir, telithromycin, ritonavir, indinavir, nelfinavir, voriconazole, amprenavir, fosamprenavir, aprepitant, erythromycin, fluconazole, verapamil, diltiazem, grapefruit, grapefruit juice, or St. John's wort. Everolimus concentrations are decreased when administered with strong CYP3A4 inducers such as phenytoin, carbamazepine, rifampin, rifabutin, rifapentine, or phenobarbital.

Therapeutic Indications in Hematology: Everolimus has been used in MCL, diffuse large B-cell lymphoma, and Hodgkin lymphoma.

Arsenic Trioxide

Chemistry and Mechanism of Action: The mechanism of action of arsenic trioxide is not completely understood. Arsenic trioxide causes morphologic changes and DNA fragmentation characteristic of apoptosis in NB4 human promyelocytic leukemia cells in vitro, possibly mediated by activation of cysteine proteases (caspases). Arsenic trioxide also causes damage or degradation of the fusion protein PML-RARβ.

Absorption, Fate, and Excretion: The metabolism of arsenic trioxide involves reduction of pentavalent arsenic to trivalent arsenic by arsenate reductase and methylation of trivalent arsenic to monomethylarsinic acid and monomethylarsinic acid to dimethylarsinic acid by methyltransferases. The main site of methylation reactions appears to be the liver. The pharmacokinetics of trivalent arsenic, the active species, have not been characterized.

Preparation and Administration: Arsenic trioxide is available in 10-mL, single-use ampules containing 10 mg of arsenic trioxide. It is formulated as a sterile, nonpyrogenic, clear solution of arsenic trioxide in water for injection using sodium hydroxide and dilute hydrochloric acid to adjust to pH 8. Trisenox should be diluted with 100–250 mL of 5% dextrose injection, USP, or 0.9% sodium chloride injection, USP. Arsenic trioxide should be administered IV over 1–2 hours. The infusion duration may be extended up to 4 hours if acute vasomotor reactions are observed. A central venous catheter is not required.

Toxic Effects: Arsenic trioxide has electrocardiographic abnormalities, including QT interval prolongation, T-wave flattening, and atrioventricular block. Nonspecific edema and weight gain have been reported. Dry skin, pruritus, and rashes have occurred relatively frequently. Anemia, thrombocytopenia, and neutropenia are also observed.

Drug Interactions: Arsenic trioxide can cause QT interval prolongation and complete atrioventricular block. QT prolongation can lead to a torsade de pointes–type ventricular arrhythmia. The risk of torsade de pointes is related to the extent of QT prolongation, and concomitant administration of QT-prolonging drugs may exacerbate this phenomenon.

Therapeutic Indications in Hematology: Arsenic trioxide is effective in newly diagnosed acute promyelocytic leukemia, FAB M3. Moreover, in patients who are refractory to or have relapsed from retinoid and anthracycline chemotherapy, arsenic trioxide has some activity as a single agent for relapsed or refractory MM. Arsenic trioxide produced hematologic improvement in a subset of patients with MDS.

Bortezomib (Velcade)

Molecular Formula: The molecular formula is $C_{19}H_{25}BN_4O$, molecular weight 384.24 g/mol, N-pyrazinecarbonyl-L-phenylalanine-L-leucine boronic acid.

Absorption, Fate, and Excretion: After IV administration of a 1.3-mg/m² dose, the median estimated maximum plasma concentration of bortezomib was 509 ng/mL (range: 109–1300 ng/mL). The mean elimination half-life of bortezomib after the first dose ranged from 9 to 15 hours at doses ranging from 1.45 to 2.00 mg/m² in patients with advanced malignancies. In vitro studies with human liver microsomes and human cDNA-expressed cytochrome P450 isozymes indicate that bortezomib is primarily oxidatively metabolized via cytochrome P450 enzymes 3A4, 2D6, 2C19, 2C9, and 1A2. The major metabolic pathway is deboronation to form two deboronated metabolites that subsequently undergo hydroxylation to several inactive metabolites.

Preparation and Administration: Bortezomib for injection is supplied as a lyophilized powder for reconstitution. Each sterile single-use vial contains 3.5 mg of bortezomib and 35 mg of mannitol, USP. Each vial is reconstituted with 3.5 mL normal (0.9%) saline such that the reconstituted solution contains bortezomib at a concentration of 1 mg/mL. The pH of the reconstituted solution is between 5 and 6. The drug is given without any further dilution as an IV bolus over 3–5 seconds. Intact vials of lyophilized bortezomib for injection are stored in a refrigerator at 2–8°C (35–47°F) and protected from light. Stability studies are ongoing to monitor each clinical lot. Product should be administered immediately after reconstitution. The solution as reconstituted is stable for 43 hours at room temperature. Bortezomib is administered as an IV bolus (over 3–5 seconds) twice weekly for 2 weeks followed by a 1-week rest period.

Toxic Effects: The most commonly reported adverse events are asthenic conditions (including fatigue, malaise, and weakness; 65%), nausea (64%), diarrhea (51%), decreased appetite (including anorexia; 43%), constipation (43%), thrombocytopenia (43%), peripheral neuropathy (including peripheral sensory neuropathy and peripheral neuropathy aggravated; 37%), pyrexia (36%), vomiting (36%), and anemia (32%). Fourteen percent of patients experienced at least one episode of grade 4 toxicity, with the most common being thrombocytopenia (3%) and neutropenia (3%).

Potential Drug Interactions: No formal drug interaction studies have been conducted with bortezomib. In vitro studies with human liver microsomes indicate that bortezomib is a substrate of cytochrome P450 3A4, 2D6, 2C19, 2C9, and 1A2. Bortezomib may inhibit 2C19 activity (IC_{50} = 18 μM, 6.9 μg/mL) and increase exposure to drugs that are substrates for this enzyme. Patients who are concomitantly receiving bortezomib and drugs that are inhibitors or inducers of cytochrome P450 3A4 should be closely monitored for either toxicities or reduced efficacy. Patients on oral antidiabetic agents receiving bortezomib treatment may experience hypo- or hyperglycemia and require close monitoring of their blood glucose levels and adjustment of the dose of their antidiabetic medication. Finally, patients should be cautioned about the use of concomitant medications that may be associated with peripheral neuropathy (e.g., amiodarone, antivirals, isoniazid, nitrofurantoin, or statins), or with a decrease in blood pressure.

Therapeutic Indications in Hematology: Bortezomib is approved by the US Food and Drug Administration (FDA) for the initial treatment of MM patients.

Carfilzomib

Chemistry and Mechanism of Action: Carfilzomib is an epoxomicin derivate that irreversibly binds to and inhibits the chymotrypsin-like activity of the 20S proteasome. Inhibition of proteasome-mediated proteolysis results in an accumulation of polyubiquinated proteins, which may lead to cell cycle arrest, induction of apoptosis, and inhibition of tumor growth.

Absorption, Fate, and Excretion: Carfilzomib is an investigational product. It has rapid clearance with an elimination half-life of less than 30 minutes and a clearance higher than liver blood flow, which suggests there are multiple clearance pathways.

Preparation and Administration: Carfilzomib currently is available investigationally as an IV product.

Toxic Effects: Carfilzomib has been shown to produce mild-to-moderate nausea and diarrhea. Respiratory symptoms occur and include cough, dyspnea, and exertional dyspnea. Neurologic symptoms include hypoesthesia, headache, and paresthesia. Additional adverse events seen are fatigue, pyrexia, and peripheral edema.

Drug Interactions: Data not available.

Therapeutic Indications in Hematology: Carfilzomib has been approved by the FDA for the treatment of MM of patients who have received at least two prior therapies, Hodgkin lymphoma, and NHL.

Ibrutinib

Chemistry and Mechanism of Action: Ibrutinib is a first-in-class oral therapy that is a selective, irreversible inhibitor of Bruton tyrosine kinase (BTK) and inhibits BTK activity, preventing B-cell activation and B-cell–mediated signaling, and inhibiting the growth of malignant B cells that overexpress BTK.

Absorption, Fate, and Excretion: No data available.

Preparation and Administration: Ibrutinib is an approved agent available as an oral dose.

Toxic Effects: Ibrutinib may cause diarrhea, fatigue, nausea, and skin bruising. Also, transient high lymphocyte counts are frequently seen.

Drug Interactions: No data available.

Therapeutic Indications in Hematology: Ibrutinib is used in CLL/small lymphocytic lymphoma, MCL, diffuse large B-cell lymphoma, and MM. It is approved for the treatment of MCL patients who have received two prior therapies and CLL patients with the 17p deletion.

Dasatinib

Chemistry and Mechanism of Action: Dasatinib is an orally active TK inhibitor against BCR-ABL, SRC family, c-KIT, EPH receptor A2, and PDGFRβ. The primary mechanism of resistance to dasatinib is the *T315I* mutant clone.

Absorption, Fate, and Excretion: Dasatinib is orally absorbed and extensively metabolized in human liver microsomes, primarily by cytochrome P450 CYP3A4, to an active metabolite. CYP3A4 is the primary enzyme responsible for the formation of the active metabolite. Flavin-containing monooxygenase 3 and uridine diphosphate-glucuronosyltransferase enzymes are also involved in the formation of dasatinib metabolites. In human liver microsomes, dasatinib was a weak time-dependent inhibitor of CYP3A4. The exposure of the active metabolite, which is equipotent to dasatinib, represents approximately 5% of the dasatinib AUC.

Preparation and Administration: Dasatinab is an oral agent usually taken twice daily without regard to meals.

Toxic Effects: Treatment with dasatinib is associated with severe thrombocytopenia, neutropenia, anemia, and platelet dysfunction. Also seen is fluid retention, including pleural and pericardial effusion, pulmonary edema, severe ascites, and generalized edema. A prolonged QT interval has been observed as well as extensive skin rashes.

Drug Interactions: Dasatinib is a CYP3A4 substrate. Administration with drugs that are CYP3A4 inhibitors may cause increased dasatinib plasma concentrations and subsequent increase in toxicities.

Drugs that induce CYP3A4 activity may decrease dasatinib plasma concentrations and decrease its effectiveness. The solubility of dasatinib is pH dependent. Simultaneous administration of SPRYCEL with antacids should be avoided, and there should be 2 hours' separation in the administration of dasatinib and antacids. Long-term suppression of gastric acid secretion by H_2 blockers or proton pump inhibitors may reduce dasatinib exposure, and antacids are preferred. Dasatinib is a time-dependent inhibitor of CYP3A4; therefore, CYP3A4 substrates may have their plasma concentration altered by dasatinib.

Therapeutic Indications in Hematology: Treatment with dasatinib results in hematologic and cytogenetic responses in patients with lymphoid blast crisis, Ph+ chronic myeloid leukemia, and Ph+ ALL as initial treatment and in disease-resistant or intolerant to imatinib.

Bleomycin

Chemistry and Mechanism of Action: Bleomycin is a glycopeptide. Its antitumor effect correlates with its ability to cause scission of both double- and single-stranded DNA via activated oxygen formed by the iron–bleomycin complex. Bleomycin also affects DNA repair by inhibiting DNA ligase.

Absorption, Fate, and Excretion: Bleomycin is rapidly distributed throughout the body and concentrates in the skin, lungs, kidneys, peritoneum, and lymph nodes. Its plasma half-life is 2–4 hours. Within 24 hours of injection, approximately 50% of an administered dose is excreted unchanged in the urine. Bleomycin elimination correlates well with creatinine clearance; accordingly, patients with renal failure should receive reduced doses. In the tissues, bleomycin is inactivated by bleomycin hydrolase. Tissues lacking this enzyme, such as the lungs and skin, are more susceptible to the drug's toxic effects.

Preparation and Administration: Bleomycin is commercially available in vials containing 15 U (approximately equivalent to 15 mg), from which it is reconstituted for injection with 3–5 mL of sterile water, normal saline, 5% dextrose in water, or bacteriostatic water. For IV infusion, the reconstituted solution can be further diluted with either normal saline or 5% dextrose in water and administered over 5 minutes. Bleomycin can also be administered by the SC, IV, IM, intracavitary, and intraarterial routes. Because patients with lymphomas are at an increased risk of anaphylactoid reactions, which may not occur until 12 hours after administration, the first two doses should be IM "test doses" of 1–2 mg. If no reactions occur, full doses may be given.

Toxic Effects: The most serious toxic effect is interstitial pneumonitis, which is dose related and occurs in approximately 10% of patients treated with cumulative doses of greater than 350–400 U. The interstitial pneumonitis may evolve into life-threatening pulmonary fibrosis. Pulmonary toxicity is more common in patients older than 70 years, in those receiving a total dose of greater than 400 U, and in those who received prior radiotherapy to the lung. It is important to emphasize, however, that the pulmonary toxicity is unpredictable; it has been reported in patients who had none of these risk factors and has occurred in a patient after administration of only 20 U. Some reports suggest that an increased concentration of inspired oxygen acts synergistically with bleomycin to produce pulmonary fibrosis. During critical illness and perioperatively, therefore, an attempt should be made to maintain the inspired oxygen concentration at 21%. The early phases of the pulmonary toxicity are clinically manifested by dyspnea and fine rales. Although corticosteroids are often used in this setting, it is not clear that they are of benefit.

Mucocutaneous toxicity occurs in 50% of patients treated and is manifested by hyperpigmentation, pruritic erythema, mucositis, desquamation of the plantar surface skin of the hands or feet, ridging of the nails, and alopecia. The mucositis can be severe and is the acute dose-limiting toxic effect. Febrile reactions, which occur a few hours after bleomycin administration and may last 4–12 hours, are also common. Fever becomes less frequent with continued use of the drug and can usually be prevented by concurrent administration of gluco-corticosteroids (e.g., 100 mg of hydrocortisone). Bleomycin has virtually no myelosuppressive effect. Anaphylactoid reactions are observed in approximately 1% (up to 8% in some series) of patients with lymphomas treated with bleomycin.

Potential Drug Interaction: Bleomycin, administered with other drugs for the treatment of lymphorrhea, can decrease the oral bio-availability of digoxin and the pharmacologic effect of phenytoin and certain anesthetic drugs.

Therapeutic Indications in Hematology: Bleomycin is often incorporated in the chemotherapy regimens of Hodgkin lymphoma (ABVD and MOPP-ABV hybrid regimens) and NHL (MACOP-B, PROMACE-CYTABOM, M-BACOD, and CHOP-Bleo).

Asparaginase

Chemistry and Mechanism of Action: Asparaginase contains the high-molecular-weight enzyme L-asparaginase amidohydrolase, type EC-2, derived from *Escherichia coli*. Asparaginase hydrolyzes serum asparagine to nonfunctional aspartic acid and ammonia, depriving tumor cells of a required amino acid; thus, tumor cell proliferation is blocked by the interruption of asparagine-dependent protein synthesis. The drug appears to be most active in the G_1 phase.

Absorption, Fate, and Excretion: Asparaginase is not absorbed orally. Its plasma half-life varies from 8 to 30 hours and is not influenced by dosage, age, sex, surface area, or renal or hepatic function.

Preparation and Administration: Asparaginase is commercially available in vials containing 10,000 IU of asparaginase in 80 mg of mannitol. For IV use, the drug should be reconstituted with 5 mL of either sterile water or sodium chloride for injection and injected in the tubing of a freely running infusion of either normal saline or 5% dextrose in water over 30 minutes. For IM or SC use, each vial should be reconstituted with 2 mL of sodium chloride for injection to obtain a 5000-U/mL solution. For dosages that exceed 2 mL, use of two injection sites is recommended. For both IV and IM administration, the drug must be used within 8 hours of reconstitution, and only if it is clear. Because of the possibility of HSRs (particularly in patients with lymphomas), an intradermal skin test is recommended before initial administration of asparaginase or when 1 week has elapsed between doses. For this test, 2 IU should be injected intradermally and observed for a wheal or erythema for 1 hour. A negative skin test result, however, does not preclude possible development of a HSR. It is recommended that oxygen, epinephrine, and corticosteroids be available at the bedside during administration of the drug. For allergic patients, the *E. coli* form of asparaginase should be replaced by the asparaginase derived from *Erwinia carotovora*, provided by the NCI as an investigational group C agent.

Toxic Effects: The toxicity of asparaginase is reported to be greater in adults than in children. Anorexia, nausea, or vomiting occurs in approximately one-third of patients. Most of the other side effects can be divided into two main groups, those related to HSRs to the foreign protein and those resulting from decreased protein synthesis. The HSR is characterized by urticaria, laryngeal edema, broncho-spasm, or hypotension and may occur with the initial dose of the drug even if the skin test result is negative. More commonly, however, allergic phenomena are observed after multiple courses of treatment. Adverse effects related to the inhibition of protein synthesis include hypoalbuminemia and decreases in serum fibrinogen, prothrombin, antithrombin III, and other coagulation factors, which may lead to both clotting and hemorrhagic complications; decreased serum

insulin with hyperglycemia; and decreased serum lipoproteins. In 25% or fewer of patients, cerebral dysfunction, characterized by confusion, stupor, and frank coma, can occur. Although the neuro-toxic effects resemble those of ammonia toxicity, they are apparently caused by low concentrations of either L-asparagine or L-glutamine in the brain. Acute pancreatitis, which may progress to severe hemor-rhagic pancreatitis, may occur in 15% of patients. Elevation of liver enzymes and serum bilirubin is almost universal and is histologically represented by fatty metamorphosis. Liver toxicity, although usually not clinically significant, has resulted in occasional fatalities. Aspara-ginase can occasionally produce renal functional impairment with oliguric renal failure.

Potential Drug Interactions: When asparaginase is administered immediately before or concurrent with methotrexate, it decreases the cytotoxic effect of the latter. When administered to patients with acute leukemia 9–10 days before or shortly after methotrexate, however, asparaginase appears to enhance the cytotoxic effect of methotrexate. Concurrent administration of asparaginase with vin-cristine may increase vincristine's neurotoxic effects, but this effect appears to be less pronounced when asparaginase is given after vin-cristine. The effects of asparaginase on liver function may potentially interfere with the activation or metabolism of other cytotoxic agents.

Therapeutic Indications in Hematology: Asparaginase is used in combination therapy for remission induction of ALL.

Glucocorticoids

Chemistry and Mechanism of Action: Glucocorticoids are synthetic compounds derived from the natural adrenal hormone cortisol. Glucocorticoids mediate their biologic actions predomi-nantly by binding to their cytosolic receptor, which then translocates to the nucleus. There, as a homodimer, it binds to specific DNA sequences located in the regulatory regions of a number of genes. Gene transcription can be upregulated or downregulated by gluco-corticoids. They can also inhibit binding of the AP-1 transcription factor to its DNA consensus sequence site. Lymphocytes treated with glucocorticoids undergo apoptosis mediated by glucocorticoid recep-tors. An early cytostatic phase is marked by growth inhibition and cessation of proliferation caused by inhibition of cellular uptake of glucose, amino acids, and nucleosides, as well as inhibition of mac-romolecular synthesis. This is followed by a cytolytic phase character-ized by chromatin condensation and internucleosomal DNA cleavage.

Absorption, Fate, and Excretion: Many synthetic glucocorti-coids are available, the three most commonly used in hematology being prednisone, dexamethasone, and methylprednisolone. Gluco-corticoids are well absorbed orally and are primarily metabolized in the liver. Unlike the other two glucocorticoids, the activity of pred-nisone depends on hepatic conversion to the 11-hydroxy form (prednisolone). Whereas the biologic half-lives of prednisone and methylprednisolone are approximately 12–36 hours, dexamethasone has a biologic half-life of 36–72 hours. Plasma half-lives for all three drugs are within the range of 3–4 hours. Compared with cortisol, the relative antiinflammatory potencies of dexamethasone, methyl-prednisolone, and prednisone are 25, 5, and 4, respectively, for equivalent doses.

Preparation and Administration: Prednisone is available only for oral administration, but methylprednisolone and dexamethasone are available in oral and parenteral dosage forms.

Toxic Effects: When glucocorticoids are used for less than 14 days, as is often done when they are used in combination with other cytotoxic agents, the most common side effects include euphoria, insomnia, psychosis, hyperglycemia, hypokalemia, increased appetite, metabolic alkalosis, proximal muscular weakness, and fluid retention with edema formation and hypertension. When used on a chronic basis, glucocorticoids also may induce a "Cushingoid" appearance, easy bruisability, peptic ulcers, osteoporosis, subcapsular cataracts, and an increased susceptibility to infections related to impaired cellular immunity. Because of this, H_2 blockers, antifungal agents (e.g., ketoconazole), and sulfamethoxazole–trimethoprim have been used in certain glucocorticoid chemotherapy combinations.

Potential Drug Interactions: Glucocorticoids interact with a variety of drugs, including barbiturates, oral contraceptives, erythromycin, hydantoins, rifampin, isoniazid, and salicylates. Given the wide range of doses of glucocorticoids used, however, these interactions are of no major clinical relevance.

Clinical Indications in Hematology: Glucocorticoids have direct anticancer activity in many hematologic malignancies, including ALL, CLL, Hodgkin lymphoma, NHL, and plasma cell neoplasms. Because of their efficacy and toxic profiles, which do not overlap with the toxic effects of the other cytotoxic agents, glucocorticoids are used in many chemotherapy regimens. In addition, they are useful in the management of hypercalcemia secondary to myeloma and lymphomas, and are of paramount importance in the treatment of autoimmune hematologic disorders.

Flavopiridol

Chemistry and Mechanism of Action: Flavopiridol is a semisynthetic flavone and selective inhibitor of CDKs 1, 2, 4–7, PKC, PKA, and PDGF causing cell cycle arrest. It also may inhibit CDK9/TEFb, which causes downregulation of McI-1, BIRC4, cyclin D1, and p21CIP1.

Absorption, Fate, and Excretion: Flavopiridol is 94% protein bound and is metabolized by the UDP glucuronyltransferase isoenzymes. Its half-life varies with infusion duration and ranges from 3.5 hours (1-hour infusion) to 27 hours (72-hour infusion).

Preparation and Administration: Flavopiridol is supplied as a 10-mg/mL yellow-greenish solution in a 5-mL vial. Contents may be diluted in either 5% dextrose injection or 0.9% sodium chloride injection to achieve a final concentration of 0.09–1 mg/mL. If the drug is administered through peripheral IV access, a concentration of less than 0.5 mg/mL is thought to decrease thrombotic complications. Flavopiridol has been administered as a 1-, 24-, and 72-hour infusion.

Toxic Effects: Grade 4 neutropenia and grade 3 lymphocytopenia occur and are more common with shorter durations of infusion. Thrombocytopenia is seen infrequently. Secretory diarrhea is a dose-limiting toxicity and may last for up to 3 days. Orthostatic hypotension is a frequently seen occurrence. Thrombosis with the 72-hour infusion duration was far more common than in the shorter infusion durations. A fatigue rate approaching 75% has been reported. Other toxicities include pleuritic chest pain, hyperbilirubinemia, and nausea.

Potential Drug Interactions: Paclitaxel in combination with flavopiridol has been associated with severe dose-limiting neutropenia.

Therapeutic Indications in Hematology: Flavopiridol's place in therapy is still being assessed. It has activity and use in hematologic malignancies, including MCL, leukemias, and MM. It may cause potential solid tumors in combination with other agents. The FDA has granted orphan drug status for flavopiridol to treat patients with AML.

Tanespimycin (17-AAG, Geldanamycin, NSC 330507)

Chemistry: Tanespimycin is a water-soluble benzoquinone ansamycin antibiotic that binds to HSP90.

Fate, Absorption, and Excretion: Tanespimycin has a mean terminal half-life of 2.3 hours and is primarily metabolized by liver microsomal enzymes, specifically CYP3A4. One metabolite, 17-AG, is known to be active and has a mean terminal half-life of 4.6 hours. Peak plasma concentrations of 17-AAG and 17-AG occur at 30 and 60 minutes, respectively. 10.6% of 17-AAG and 7.8% of 17-AG is recovered in the urine over a 72-hour period.

Preparation and Administration: Tanespimycin is available as a single-use amber vial containing 50 mg of tanespimycin in 2 mL of dimethylsulfoxide. Before administration, the tanespimycin concentrate must be completely thawed at room temperature (over a period of ≤1 hour). Incomplete thawing affects the concentration of the drug because of changes in volume. Tanespimycin concentrate must be diluted to 1 mg/mL by withdrawing 2 mL and adding it to 48 mL of EPL diluent 2% egg phospholipids with 5% dextrose in water. A clear solution should be obtained with gentle mixing. Shaking should be avoided to prevent foaming. No further dilution is required and the final solution should be dispensed in a glass bottle. A 0.45-μm filter may be used, but is not required. The infusion should be completed within 8 hours of mixing. Intact vials of Tanespimycin should be stored in the freezer (–10° to –20°C). EPL diluent should be stored in the refrigerator (2°–8°C) and not frozen. Administration is by IV infusion.

Toxicity: Anemia, diarrhea, nausea, vomiting, fatigue, transaminitis, and muscle pain.

Drug Interactions: Tanespimycin is metabolized by CYP3A4. Agents that alter CYP3A4 activity may affect drug levels and metabolism, although this has not been shown to affect clinical use.

Therapeutic Uses: Lymphoma and leukemia in clinical trials.

Imatinib (Gleevec)

Chemistry and Mechanism of Action: Imatinib, a phenylaminopyrinadine derivative, is a selective protein TK inhibitor effecting BCR-ABL TK. This enzyme is found commonly in chronic myeloid leukemia and in some clones of ALL. Imatinib also inhibits the kinases for PDGF, SCF, and KIT.

Absorption, Fate, and Excretion: Imatinib is well absorbed and achieves peak levels within 2–4 hours and follows linear pharmacokinetics at the standard doses. Cytochrome P450 is the major route of metabolism, with CYP3A4 being the primary pathway. An *N*-desmethyl piperazine is the main metabolite and is active. Pediatric patients follow the same pharmacokinetics as in adults.

Preparation and Administration: Imatinib is available in a film-coated tablet. In its pure form, it is a white to brownish to yellowish powder and is soluble in aqueous buffers of less than 5.5.

Toxic Effects: Gastrointestinal effects are common and include nausea and diarrhea. Muscle cramps are seen in one-third of patients receiving imatinib. Myelosuppression reflected as thrombocytopenia, anemia, and neutropenia occurs, with thrombocytopenia and neutropenia seen more frequently in patients in accelerated phase or blast crisis. Fluid retention is dose related and is exhibited as edema and weight gain, but pleural and pericardiac effusions are also seen. Fatigue and headache, although low grade, occur in 25% of patients.

Potential Drug Interactions: Drugs that inhibit CYP3A4 may increase imatinib plasma concentrations; these include ketoconazole, itraconazole, erythromycin, and clarithromycin. CY3A4 inducers that may decrease plasma concentration of CY3A4 are dexamethasone, rifampin, phenytoin, and carbamazepine. Imatinib increases concentrations of simvastatin, cyclosporine, and warfarin, along with other medications that are metabolized by CYP3A4.

Therapeutic Indications in Hematology: Imatinib is considered first-line therapy in Ph+ CML and has activity in accelerated or blast-phase CML. Some effect has been shown in ALL as well as hypereosinophilic syndrome and polycythemia vera.

Topotecan (Hycamtin)

Chemistry and Mechanism of Action: Topotecan is a semisynthetic derivative of camptothecin that stabilizes a complex between DNA topoisomerase I and DNA. The cytotoxic effect of this drug is believed to result from the collision of DNA replication forks with a ternary complex of topoisomerase I, DNA, and topotecan. The resulting double-strand DNA breaks are lethal. The lactone form of topotecan, which predominates at an acidic pH, is a much more potent inhibitor of DNA topoisomerase I.

Absorption, Fate, and Excretion: At neutral or physiologic pH, the carboxylate form of topotecan is favored, and at a pH less than 7, the lactone form is favored. Topotecan has been given as a bolus or by continuous infusion. In less than 1 hour after infusion, most of the circulating drug in the plasma is in the carboxylate form because of the physiologic pH. The terminal half-life of the lactone form of this S-phase–specific agent is 2.6 hours, and the terminal half-life of the total drug is 3.3 hours. Thirty six percent of an IV dose is excreted unchanged in the urine, and there is a 1.5-fold concentration of the drug in bile. Cerebrospinal fluid levels of topotecan lactone reach approximately 32% of plasma levels. Dose adjustment is required for a creatinine clearance less than 60 mL/min, but no adjustment is necessary for a bilirubin up to 10 mg/dL.

Preparation and Administration: Topotecan is commercially available as 4-mg vials that are reconstituted with 4 mL of sterile water. This solution can be further diluted in normal saline or 5% dextrose in water and should be used immediately.

Toxic Effects: The dose-limiting toxicity for topotecan for all schedules is neutropenia. Thrombocytopenia and anemia are less common, although there is an increase in thrombocytopenia with continuous infusion schedules. Other less common and mild toxicities include nausea, vomiting, diarrhea, fever, fatigue, alopecia, skin rash, and increased liver function test results. Mucositis has been seen with prolonged infusion schedules over 5 days or when topotecan is given in higher doses.

Potential Drug Interactions: In vitro data suggest that there may be some synergism if a topoisomerase I inhibitor is given before a topoisomerase II inhibitor. In vitro data also suggest that synergism may be seen if a topoisomerase I inhibitor (topotecan) is given after an alkylating agent, suggesting that topoisomerase I may be involved in the repair of alkylator-induced DNA damage.

Therapeutic Indications in Hematology: Topotecan has activity in MDS, AML, chronic myeloid leukemia, and MM.

Vorinostat (Zolinza)

Chemistry and Mechanism of Action: Vorinostat is a HDAC inhibitor. It inhibits HDAC 1, HDAC2, HDAC3, and HDAC6 at nanomolar concentrations. Inhibition prevents removal of the acetyl groups from lysine residues in target histones and transcription factors. Loss of deacetylase function results in persistence of acetyl groups on histones, resulting in larger segments of open chromatin and a general increase in gene expression. Often this promotes differentiation and cell cycle arrest with apoptosis. The number of genes affected continues to grow so that the impact of vorinostat is complex.

Absorption, Fate, and Excretion: Reported pharmacokinetics after a 400-mg oral administration are an AUC of 5.5 micromolar-hours, a C_{max} of 1.2 micromolar, and T_{max} of 2–10 hours. Fatty meals decrease the rate of absorption but increase overall drug levels. There is no recommended dosing relative to meals. Vorinostat is heavily plasma protein absorbed. It undergoes glucuronidation hydrolysis, and later β-oxidation to inactive metabolites. Little is excreted unchanged.

Preparation and Administration: Oral dosing of 400 mg with food is standard. If side effects are noted, reduce the dose to 300 mg. There is no approved pediatric dosing.

Toxic Effects: Many side effects are noted. Common are fatigue, thrombocytopenia, muscle spasms, and anorexia. Serious reported adverse effects in clinical trials included pulmonary embolism in 4.7% and anemia in 2.3%.

Potential Drug Interactions: Vorinostat can prolong the effect of coumadin, raising the international normalized ratio. It can also induce glucose intolerance.

Therapeutic Indications in Hematology: Vorinostat is approved for cutaneous manifestations of CTCL in patients who have become refractory to standard treatments. It is being tested in other disorders such as myeloma and leukemias to determine whether it works through the HDACs or through altered expression of numerous proteins.

CHAPTER 58

PATHOBIOLOGY OF ACUTE MYELOID LEUKEMIA

Andrew M. Brunner and Timothy A. Graubert

Acute myeloid leukemia (AML) is a cancer of hematopoietic stem/progenitor cells, characterized by recurrent genetic and epigenetic alterations. Historically, human leukemias were distinguished according to clinical and histological features, and subsequently by morphology. More recently, analysis of the AML genome at increasing resolution, from the level of whole chromosomal changes to individual base pairs, together with an appreciation of epigenetic changes and interactions within the bone marrow microenvironment, have furthered the understanding of the biology and clinical behavior of this disease.

PHENOTYPE OF ACUTE MYELOID LEUKEMIA

Normal hematopoiesis is characterized by self-renewal and differentiation of long-term hematopoietic stem cells (HSCs) to short-term HSCs, multipotent progenitors, and common lymphoid and myeloid progenitors. These lineage-committed progenitors further differentiate to mature lymphoid or myeloid cells, including erythrocytes, granulocytes, macrophages, and platelets. This process is regulated by lineage-specific transcription factors at key points during normal hematopoiesis. Functional analysis of recurrent chromosomal, molecular, and epigenetic alterations in AML has revealed that many of these lesions cause aberrant activation or derepression of hematopoietic differentiation programs, impacting proliferation, survival, and maturation of myeloid progenitor cells. Consequently, a hallmark of the AML phenotype is an accumulation of immature myeloid precursors. A myeloblast count of 20% or greater distinguishes AML from other myeloid malignancies.

Historically, leukemias were classified according to morphologic criteria using the French–American–British (FAB) classification, first proposed in 1976. This system classifies AML by the extent of maturation and lineage specificity, ranging from M0 (undifferentiated) to M3 (promyelocytic), M4eo (myelomonocytic with eosinophilia), M6 (erythroid), or M7 (megakaryocytic). Certain FAB subtypes were subsequently found to correlate with underlying cytogenetic abnormalities, notably M3 with t(15;17), M4eo with inv(16), and M2 with t(8;21). As greater understanding of recurrent cytogenetic and now molecular and epigenetic aberrations have been identified, it has become clear that morphology alone is inadequate to fully describe the disease spectrum of AML.

ETIOLOGY OF ACUTE MYELOID LEUKEMIA

The majority of patients who develop AML lack any recognized antecedent disease or predisposition, and for these patients their disease is classified as sporadic or de novo. In these cases, AML appears to result from the accumulation of spontaneously acquired somatic mutations in self-renewing hematopoietic cells. In contrast, a diagnosis of secondary AML (sAML) is preceded by a known predisposing condition, including environmental exposure, antecedent hematologic malignancy, or inherited factors.

Toxins and Exposures

A number of environmental, occupational, and iatrogenic exposures have been identified that contribute to sAML via genotoxic damage to hematopoietic cells. Exposure to benzene, an organic component of many commonly used chemicals including plastics, dyes, pesticides, solvents, and petroleum products, has been linked to the subsequent development of AML. This relationship was identified in the 19th century, when bone marrow aplasia and myeloid leukemia were noted among workers exposed to benzene-containing chemicals. Individuals with occupational benzene exposure have an approximately threefold increased relative risk of developing AML. Workplace benzene exposures have decreased significantly since this discovery, but other sources of benzene exposure remain a concern; for example, through cigarette smoking. Although cytopenias can occur within months of benzene exposure, there is a latency of several years between benzene exposure and the development of leukemia.

Two classes of chemotherapy drugs are associated with an increased risk of sAML; cases of AML arising after chemotherapy or radiation have been historically designated as therapy-related AML (tAML). One class of drugs with clear links to tAML are the topoisomerase II inhibitors. The most commonly used topoisomerase II inhibitors are anthracyclines, such as doxorubicin, idarubicin, and daunorubicin, and the epipodophyllotoxin etoposide, which are critical components of many treatment regimens for both solid tumors and hematologic malignancies. Topoisomerase II is an adenosine triphosphate-dependent enzyme that re-ligates DNA at sites of double-strand breaks to manage supercoils; inhibition of this enzyme increases the number of double-strand breaks. Resolution of these double-strand breaks may occur via error-prone nonhomologous end joining, resulting in accumulation of DNA damage or apoptotic cell death. tAML arising after exposure to topoisomerase II inhibitors typically occurs with a latency of 1–3 years, and is often characterized by balanced chromosomal translocations, with the majority involving the Mixed Lineage Leukemia (*MLL*) locus on chromosome 11q23. Typical lesions are reciprocal translocations such as t(9;11)(p21;q23) and t(11;19)(q23;p13); other translocations that do not involve the *MLL* locus have also been described, including the t(15;17), t(8;21), and inv(16) rearrangements. The risk of tAML varies based on the chemotherapy dosing schedule, cumulative dose received, additional cytotoxic agents, and underlying disease characteristics, but generally does not exceed 5% of patients treated with topoisomerase II inhibitors.

Alkylating agents are the second class of chemotherapy drugs with a clear role in the pathogenesis of tAML. The first leukemogenic agents identified in this category were nitrogen mustards. Frequently implicated drugs in contemporary clinical practice include cyclophosphamide, ifosfamide, and melphalan; weaker associations have been described with other alkylating agents such as busulfan, thiotepa, and cisplatin. Alkylating agents create adducts in DNA bases, which are variably mutagenic or cytotoxic. Cytogenetic lesions in alkylator associated tAML are typically unbalanced, including loss of the long arms of chromosomes 5 or 7 [del(5q), del(7q)], or complete loss of these chromosomes (−5, −7). The risk of tAML following alkylator exposure is up to 1% per year, but typically has a longer latency (5–7 years), compared with topoisomerase II-associated tAML. The risk increases with age and cumulative exposure to these agents. Given the long latency period, it is likely that alkylating agents cause genomic instability, which accumulates over time prior to progression to AML. Consistent with this, heterozygous loss of *TP53* appears to be a common event leading to gain of additional somatic mutations and development of tAML. In some cases of tAML, small clonal populations harboring *TP53* mutations antedate chemotherapy exposure. *TP53* deficiency may confer enhanced fitness on these clones, allowing them to expand under the selective pressure of therapy.

Exposure to ionizing radiation also has been identified as a causative mechanism for tAML. This relationship was identified in the context of occupational exposures during the development of radiography, and subsequently in the setting of mass exposures such as the atomic bomb detonations or nuclear power plant disasters, where a time-limited spike in leukemia incidence occurred following the event. Outside of these events, therapeutic radiation therapy represents the most common setting for significant radiation exposure, which is associated with a small but significant increase in tAML risk. Radiation-associated tAML is characterized by an increased frequency of mutations otherwise implicated in de novo AML pathogenesis—for instance, mutations in *RUNX1*, as well as balanced translocations such as *RUNX1-RUNX1T1* and *DEK-NUP214*—suggesting some selectivity in the patterns of DNA damage.

Prior Hematologic Malignancy

Other myeloid malignancies, including myelodysplastic syndromes (MDS) and myeloproliferative neoplasms (MPNs), carry a risk of disease evolution to sAML. The risk varies depending upon the underlying disease, and may be facilitated by certain exposures, including genotoxic chemotherapy.

Patients with MPNs have an approximately 10% risk of evolution to AML over 10 years, which varies according to the underlying disease. The risk is lowest in essential thrombocythemia and as high as 20% for myelofibrosis. There is a clear association between therapies used in treating MPNs, specifically alkylating agents and radioactive phosphorus, and AML evolution; treatment with these agents results in a three to fourfold increase in incident AML. Another mechanism that may contribute to clonal evolution and disease progression may be a chronic inflammatory state related to the underlying MPN. Sequencing of sAML cases developing in the background of an MPN has identified recurrent mutations in *TET2*, *JAK2*, *IDH*, *IKZF1*, and *ASXL1*. Moreover, a number of patients with a *JAK2* mutated MPN may develop *JAK2* wild-type AML, thought to arise either from a common pre-*JAK2* founding clone, or due to parallel expansion of a distinct hematopoietic clone. Post-MPN AML with mutated *JAK2* typically proceeds through an accelerated myelofibrosis phase, while post-MPN AML that no longer harbors a *JAK2* mutation tends to arise from chronic phase disease and may be associated with the use of cytotoxic therapies.

Prior to the introduction of tyrosine kinase inhibitors (TKIs) for CML, patients with CML typically progressed from chronic phase to blast phase within 5 years, at a rate of over 20% per year. Most cases of blast phase CML have a myeloid phenotype, while approximately 30% of patients have a lymphoid phenotype. Additional mutations may occur during transformation of CML, and approximately 80% of patients have additional cytogenetic abnormalities, such as duplication of the Philadelphia chromosome, and other trisomies that are recurrent in de novo AML. Up to one-third of patients with CML in myeloid blast phase harbor mutations in the tumor suppressor genes *P16* or *TP53*. Additionally, *BCR-ABL* signaling upregulates transcription factors implicated in AML pathogenesis, including *HOXA9* and *EVI1*, which may contribute to leukemic transformation. Underscoring the continued requirement for *BCR-ABL1* signaling in CML evolution, the rate of transformation to blast phase CML in the TKI era has decreased markedly to approximately 1% per year.

Approximately one third of patients with MDS progress to sAML, although this varies significantly according to the underlying MDS subtype and disease characteristics, including the percentage of bone marrow blasts, presence of characteristic cytogenetic abnormalities, and cytopenias. Progression to leukemia is associated with acquisition of additional somatic mutations as well as epigenetic alterations within the MDS clone. Mutations in transcription factors and cytokine signaling genes, including *RUNX1*, *NRAS*, and *ETV6*, are more common at progression to sAML, compared with the frequency of these mutations at MDS diagnosis. Mutations in *RUNX1* are enriched in populations with tAML and other forms of sAML.

Epigenetic modifications of the MDS genome appear to also play a significant role in AML progression, particularly through DNA methylation-mediated silencing of tumor suppressor genes.

Congenital Bone Marrow Failure Syndromes

A number of inherited bone marrow failure syndromes are associated with an increased risk of developing advanced myeloid malignancies. This may be due to the proliferative stress imposed by chronic cytopenias or defects in DNA repair that are hallmarks of several of these syndromes.

Fanconi anemia (FA) is the most common inherited bone marrow failure disorder, and is caused by germline mutations in factors involved in DNA repair. These disorders have an autosomal recessive inheritance pattern except for *FANCB*, which is X-linked. To date, 17 genes have been identified as a part of the *FANC* gene family, and together their protein products are responsible for identifying DNA damage and targeting these sites for repair. The FA core complex is recruited to the site of DNA damage after exposure to crosslinking agents. FANCD2 is ubiquitinated by the core complex, and forms the link between the FA and BRCA DNA repair pathways. Phenotypically, patients with FA have short stature, abnormalities of the thumb and radius, skin findings including hyperpigmentation and café au lait spots, microphthalmia, endocrinopathies, and often present with aplastic anemia later in childhood. The cumulative risk of AML or MDS among FA patients is approximately 10% to 15%, with peak incidence during the teenage years.

Dyskeratosis congenita (DKC) is a bone marrow failure syndrome characterized by inherited mutations in the telomere maintenance pathway. DKC can be inherited in an autosomal dominant (Online Mendelian Inheritance in Man [OMIM] 127550), autosomal recessive (OMIM 224230), or X-linked recessive pattern (OMIM 305000). Mutations in *TERT*, *DKC1*, *TERC*, or *TINF2* account for most cases. Typical findings among patients with DKC include the "triad" of skin hyperpigmentation, nail dystrophy, and oral leukoplakia, and these patients will typically develop bone marrow failure by 20–30 years of age. As a result of the underlying mutation, patients have markedly shortened telomeres, which contribute to bone marrow failure, as well as damage to other organs including pulmonary fibrosis and hepatic cirrhosis. Transformation to AML occurs in approximately 10% of patients, and is thought to occur via genomic instability related to shortened telomeres and associated DNA damage, resulting in dysplasia and an increased risk of hematopoietic malignancy.

Shwachman–Diamond syndrome (OMIM 260400) is an autosomal recessive disorder caused by mutations in *SBDS*. Hematopoietic manifestations of Shwachman–Diamond syndrome most often include isolated neutropenia, although many patients will eventually develop pancytopenia, which may progress to aplastic anemia. AML or MDS occurs in up to a third of patients by 30 years of age, and is thought to relate to chromosomal instability and accelerated rates of apoptosis, which may be due to the role of *SBDS* in stabilizing the mitotic spindle during mitosis.

Severe congenital neutropenia or Kostmann syndrome is associated with neutropenia at birth and has been associated with a variety of genetic mutations. The pattern of inheritance can be autosomal dominant (*ELANE* or *GFI1*), autosomal recessive (*HAX1*, *G6PC3*, *VPS45*, or *JAGN1*), or X-linked (*WAS*). The clinical course is marked by bacterial infections from a young age; some patients may be responsive to granulocyte colony-stimulating factor (G-CSF), but the rate of leukemic transformation is high among this group, with nearly a third of patients developing AML or MDS within 10 years. Transformation into AML is frequently characterized by the acquisition of somatic mutations in *CSF3R*, which encodes the G-CSF receptor. The causal relationship to chronic G-CSF therapy remains controversial.

Diamond–Blackfan anemia (DBA) (OMIM 105650) is characterized by red cell aplasia and typically spares the leukocyte and platelet lineages. DBA is typically inherited in an autosomal dominant fashion and is associated with mutations in a number of ribosomal proteins. Defects in ribosome function result in anemia early in life and patients with DBA may have characteristic skeletal anomalies, including craniofacial defects, and at times the classic triphalangeal thumb; this anemia is often steroid responsive but many eventually require chronic transfusional support and hematopoietic cell transplantation. AML can occur in up to 20% of patients and typically occurs after 40 years of age.

Congenital amegakaryocytic thrombocytopenia (CAMT) (OMIM 604498) and thrombocytopenia with absent radii (TAR) (OMIM 274000) syndrome are both characterized by hypoplastic thrombocytopenia. CAMT is inherited in an autosomal recessive manner via mutations in the *MPL* gene, which encodes the receptor for thrombopoietin (TPO). Patients have concomitant elevations in serum TPO levels, and thrombocytopenia from birth, which typically progresses to aplasia. CAMT is associated with an increased incidence of AML, typically in the second decade of life. While CAMT does not have phenotypic manifestations outside of thrombocytopenia, TAR syndrome is also associated with thrombocytopenia at birth, as well as characteristic absence of the radii. TAR syndrome has been associated with mutations in *RBM8A*, which is involved in messenger RNA (mRNA) splicing. The thrombocytopenia in TAR syndrome often improves over time; both acute lymphoblastic leukemia and AML have been reported among patients with this rare disorder.

Down syndrome, caused by trisomy 21, is associated with an approximately 10–20-fold elevated relative risk of AML and MDS compared with the general population, and in particular an increased risk for acute megakaryocytic leukemia, FAB M7. Infants with Down syndrome may experience transient abnormal myelopoiesis (TAM), where circulating peripheral blood blasts are seen and may be accompanied by hepatic dysfunction, effusions, and rash; this occurs in approximately 10% of these patients. The majority of TAM cases harbor somatic mutations in *GATA1*, resulting in altered function of this transcription factor that plays an important role in hematopoietic cell maturation, particularly in the megakaryocyte lineage. Decreased *GATA1* expression results in megakaryocyte proliferation. Indeed, up to 30% of persons with TAM will progress to AML, commonly acute megakaryocytic leukemia. The development of AML in patients with Down syndrome likely relates both to acquired somatic mutations, such as *GATA1*, and also the presence of additional copies of genes on chromosome 21 that facilitate leukemogenesis, such as the oncogenes *RUNX1*, *ERG*, and *ETS2*.

Mendelian Acute Myeloid Leukemia Predisposition Syndromes

A number of genes that are targets of recurrent somatic mutation in AML are also mutated in the germline in families with predisposition to myeloid malignancy without a prodrome of bone marrow failure. These include mutations in *RUNX1*, *CEBPA*, and *GATA2*. Predisposition to AML is also associated with germline variants in *ANKRD26*, *SRP72*, *ETV6*, and *DDX41*. Although these familial syndromes are rare, they are important to recognize, since affected individuals and asymptomatic carriers require specific clinical management.

Familial platelet disorder with predisposition to acute myelogenous leukemia (OMIM 601399) is associated with autosomal dominant inheritance of germline mutations in *RUNX1*. Mutation carriers frequently present with easy bruising/bleeding due to quantitative or qualitative platelet dysfunction and have an approximately 40% lifetime risk of developing AML, typically in the third or fourth decade.

Germline mutations in the *CEBPA* gene are a rare cause of autosomal dominant familial predisposition to AML (OMIM 116897). The germline mutations are typically truncating at the N-terminus of the protein, with acquisition of a C-terminal somatic mutation as a common event in the development of AML among these patients. These cases have a relatively favorable prognosis, similar to de novo AML with somatically-acquired biallelic *CEBPA* mutations.

Inherited mutations in *GATA2* cause a spectrum of disorders with overlapping features, including Emberger syndrome (OMIM 614038) and immunodeficiency 21 (IMD21) (OMIM 614172), also described as monocytopenia with susceptibility to mycobacterial, fungal, and papillomavirus infection and myelodysplasia (MonoMAC syndrome) or dendritic cell, monocyte, B-lymphocyte and natural killer lymphocyte deficiency (DCML). Patients with IMD21 have decreased monocyte counts, natural killer and B-cell deficiency, and are at increased risk of viral and nontuberculous mycobacterial infections. Emberger syndrome patients have a similar presentation, but also have deafness and lymphedema, and often develop pancytopenia. AML or MDS arises in approximately 70% of carriers and is associated with cooperating genetic events, such as mutations in *ASXL1* or hemizygous deletions involving chromosome 7.

GENETIC AND EPIGENETIC ALTERATIONS IN ACUTE MYELOID LEUKEMIA

AML is characterized by a large number of recurrent cytogenetic, molecular, and epigenetic modifications that illustrate the pathophysiologic role of acquired somatic alterations affecting specific gene products. These mutations have been incorporated into strategies for prognostic stratification and risk-adapted treatment, in addition to providing a framework for targeted therapy. The World Health Organization (WHO) classification now recognizes a number of recurrent genetic abnormalities, including balanced translocations and inversions, as defining features of AML.

Early understanding of the pathogenesis of AML suggested a model where AML occurred in the setting of acquired mutations in two pathways: class I mutations, which activate cell proliferation and survival pathways, and class II mutations, which block normal mechanisms of differentiation. This arose out of the identification of mutations that commonly arose together or were both required in mouse models to produce leukemia, such as class I mutations in cytokine signaling pathways, and class II mutations in hematopoietic transcription factors. However, this model does not account for the wide spectrum of more recently described somatic alterations, nor do all patients carry class I and class II mutations.

Chromosomal Abnormalities

The central role of acquired mutations in AML was first recognized through the identification of recurrent nonrandom cytogenetic alterations in the mid-20th century. Recurrent karyotypic lesions are frequent events in AML, present in roughly 50% to 60% of patients at diagnosis, and have distinct prognostic significance that are central to treatment decisions, including the identification of patients for whom hematopoietic cell transplantation should be considered in first remission, as well as patients likely to achieve a favorable outcome with chemotherapy alone (Fig. 58.1). Common chromosomal abnormalities include chromosome translocations or inversions, chromosome deletions, and monosomies or trisomies. Patients can be stratified according to karyotype into favorable, intermediate, and poor-risk categories. Typically, favorable risk includes patients with t(15;17), t(8;21) or inv(16)/t(16;16), and adverse risk includes inv(3q)/t(3;3), t(6;9), monosomy 7, monosomy 5, loss of 5q, 7q, or 17p, and complex (greater than 3) chromosomal abnormalities, as well as most translocations involving the *MLL* locus on chromosome 11q23. In lieu of additional molecular studies, all other karyotypic lesions are generally classified as intermediate risk. This includes patients with a normal karyotype, which comprise approximately 45% of all AML cases.

Retinoic Acid Receptor Rearrangements

A distinct subset of AML, acute promyelocytic leukemia (APL) or FAB M3, comprises approximately 10% of adult AML cases, and is defined by the presence of a translocation involving the retinoic acid

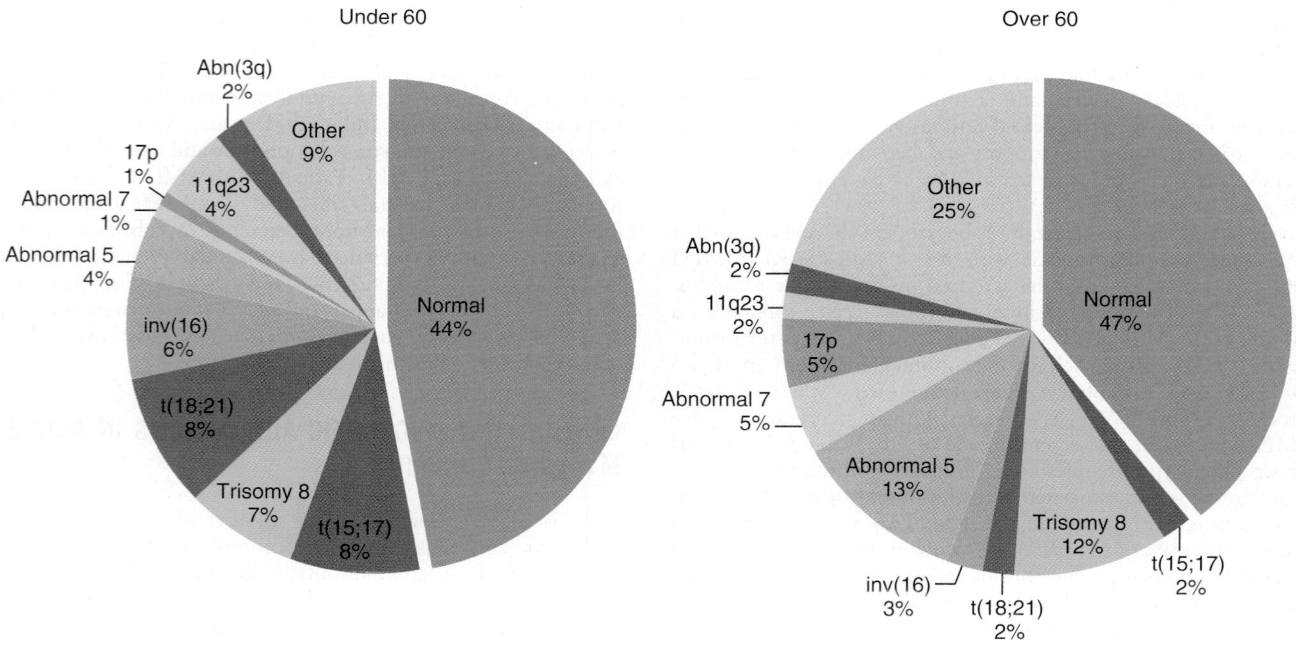

Fig. 58.1 FREQUENCY OF CHARACTERISTIC CYTOGENETIC ABNORMALITIES IN ADULT PATIENTS WITH ACUTE MYELOID LEUKEMIA. The proportion of recurrent cytogenetic abnormalities in patients 15–60 years old and patients greater than 60 years old at diagnosis is shown. *Abn,* Abnormal; *Inv,* inversion; *(Data derived from previously reported cytogenetic studies by CALGB, MRC, SWOG, ECOG, EBMT, and AMLSG.)*

receptor-α *(RARA)* on chromosome 17q21. This results in a distinct phenotype characterized by a maturation arrest at the promyelocyte stage. APL is often accompanied by a coagulopathy that can be immediately life-threatening. RARs heterodimerize with retinoid X receptors (RXRs) to bind DNA at retinoic acid response elements, where they control gene expression during development and differentiation. In the majority of cases, *RARA* is fused with the *PML* gene on chromosome 15q22 as a consequence of t(15;17)(q22;q21). Other rare fusion partners include PML-like zinc finger *(PLZF),* nucleophosmin *(NPM1),* nuclear mitotic apparatus protein *(NUMA1),* and signal transducer and activator of transcription 5B *(STAT5B).* Each of these fusion partners has a self-association domain, similar to RXRs, and the fusion product interferes with expression of retinoic acid transcriptional targets. In mouse models, transgenic expression of *PML-RARA* results in APL after a long myeloproliferative phase; the long latency period prior to leukemia development implies a requirement for acquisition of cooperating mutations for full transformation. Introduction of the *FLT3-ITD* hastens APL onset in mice. Consistent with this finding, over 35% of human patients with APL have *FLT3-ITD* mutations and nearly 20% have *FLT3-TKD* mutations. *PML-RARA* appears to have a dominant negative effect on RARα transcriptional function, as well as a role in DNA and chromatin modification, resulting in impaired myeloid differentiation. Additionally, the fusion protein disrupts the organization of PML nuclear bodies, which are subcellular structures that are involved in a number of cell cycle, metabolic, and apoptotic regulatory pathways.

Core Binding Factor Rearrangements

Rearrangements involving genes encoding components of the core binding factor (CBF) are present in roughly 15% of AML cases. CBF is a heterodimeric transcription factor that is comprised of an alpha subunit (encoded by *RUNX1*) that binds to a consensus DNA sequence, and a beta subunit (encoded by *CBFB*) that increases the affinity for DNA binding. The t(8;21) translocation is found in up to 10% of AML cases and creates an in-frame fusion of *RUNX1* with *RUNX1T1.* This rearrangement is enriched in the FAB M2 subgroup,

and comprises up to 40% of this patient subgroup. This fusion protein alters the CBF transcription factor complex, allowing it to oligomerize and interact with the nuclear corepressors *SMRT* and *N-CoR,* resulting in impaired hematopoietic differentiation. The *RUNX1-RUNX1T1* fusion protein functions as a dominant negative inhibitor of wild-type CBF, and consequently impairs hematopoietic differentiation. The fusion protein also leads to activation of TP53 response genes, which may in part explain the relative chemosensitivity of t(8;21) AML. *RUNX1* is involved in other rare translocations, including t(16;21)(q24;q22) with myeloid translocation gene on chromosome 16 *(MGT16),* and also t(3;21)(q26;q22), with *EVI1.*

Chromosomal alterations involving *CBFB* include inv(16) and t(16;16)(p13;q22), which create an in-frame fusion between *CBFB* and *MYH11,* the gene encoding smooth muscle myosin heavy chain 11. AML with inv(16) or t(16;16) often has the FAB M4eo phenotype. The *CBFB-MYH11* gene product exerts a dominant negative effect on *RUNX1,* and can recruit nuclear corepressors to inhibit transcription of CBF gene targets. Mouse models with a *CBF-MYH11* knock-in mutation require additional mutations to progress to AML, and in humans up to two-thirds of all patients with inv(16) also harbor mutations in *KIT, FLT3,* or *RAS.* Given the clear link between CBF rearrangements, as well as the *PML-RARA* translocation, and the development of AML, the presence of any of these is sufficient for a diagnosis of AML, regardless of the percentage of myeloblasts in the bone marrow or peripheral blood.

Mixed-Lineage Leukemia Gene Rearrangements

Translocations in the mixed-lineage gene *(MLL)* are seen in up to 10% of patients with AML. *MLL* rearrangements are common in tAML leukemia following exposure to topoisomerase II inhibitors, and are enriched in cases with the FAB M5a phenotype. Wild-type MLL binds DNA and methylates histone H3K4 via its C-terminal SET domain, and regulates expression of target genes, including homeobox *(Hox)* genes. Members of the homeobox A cluster, including *HOXA7* and *HOXA9,* play critical roles in the regulation of hematopoiesis, and are normally expressed in early hematopoietic cells. Rearranged MLL retains its N-terminal DNA binding domain, while the C-terminal portion is replaced by a fusion partner. More than 70 unique fusion partners have been identified, including AF4, AF9, AF10, and ENL; these can interact with and recruit the histone methyltransferase disruption of telomeric silencing 1-like (DOT1L), which methylates H3K79, and results in the expression of *HOXA* genes implicated in leukemic transformation. Expression of the *MLL-AF9* fusion in mice generates AML with high penetrance and short latency. Another mechanism by which *MLL* plays a role in leukemia is through an in-frame partial tandem duplication of exons 5–12 (*MLL-PTD*). Mouse knock-in models with *MLL-PTD* develop acute leukemias characterized by overexpression of *Hox* genes and an increase in H3/H4 acetylation with associated H4K4 methylation.

Rare Translocations

Less common cytogenetic abnormalities implicated in the pathogenesis of AML include the t(6;9), which fuses the *DEK* oncogene, which encodes a DNA binding protein involved in transcription regulation and introduction of supercoils, with *Nucleoporin 214* (*NUP214* or *CAN*), which encodes a nuclear envelope pore protein that regulates nuclear/cytoplasmic transport. This rearrangement is found in approximately 1% of patients with AML and is associated with a poor prognosis. It typically occurs as a sole chromosomal rearrangement; however, there is a high frequency of concurrent mutations in *FLT3-ITD*. The fusion retains most of the open reading frame from both proteins, but the molecular consequences of the fusion protein are not well understood. Retroviral transduction of long-term HSCs generates leukemias after transplantation into mice.

t(3;3)(9q21;q26.2) and inv(3)(q21q26.2) are included in the "acute myeloid leukemia with recurrent cytogenetic abnormalities" category in the WHO classification. Collectively, the inv(3)/t(3;3) rearrangements are present in less than 5% of AML cases and are associated with poor survival. These rearrangements juxtapose *EVI1* (*MECOM*) with regulatory elements of the *RPN1* locus. EVI1 interacts directly with DNA methyltransferase 3A (DNMT3A) and DNMT3B, which may account for the distinct DNA hypermethylation signature associated with dysregulated EVI1 expression. Patients with this translocation may have preceding MDS, and often the bone marrow morphology shows multilineage dysplasia with atypical megakaryocytes.

t(8;16)(p11;p13) is a rare translocation that occurs in de novo AML and topoisomerase II-associated tAML. The disease typically has a FAB M4 or M5 phenotype, and patients often present with extramedullary disease, coagulopathy, and hemophagocytosis. This translocation fuses two histone acetyltransferases: KAT6A (also known as MOZ or MYST3) and CREB binding protein. The fusion protein binds to DNA and the colocalized proteins result in upregulation of the *HOX* genes *HOXA9* and *HOXA10*, as well as their cofactor, *MEIS1*.

The t(1;22) involving one twenty two (*OTT*; or RNA-binding motif protein 15 [*RBM15*]) and megakaryocytic acute leukemia (*MAL* or *MKL1*) is a rare translocation found in infant acute megakaryocytic leukemia. MAL functions as a transcriptional coactivator of DNA-bound serum responsive factors (SRFs) and triggers histone modifications, including acetylation of H3K9. The translocation generates the *OTT-MAL* fusion protein, which alters MAL function, resulting in SRF-directed expression of *MYL9* and *MMP-9*, which play a role in megakaryocyte development and migration, and may contribute to the phenotype of t(1;22) megakaryocytic leukemia. Mice engineered to express *OTT-MAL* have altered megakaryocyte development and dysregulated NOTCH signaling. With concurrent activating mutations in *MPL*, these mice develop acute megakaryocytic leukemia.

Amplifications and Deletions

Recurrent cytogenetic abnormalities in AML also include somatically acquired chromosome copy or segment gains, chromosomal monosomies, as well as the accumulation of karyotypic abnormalities, classified

as complex karyotype, which typically has at least three or more distinct chromosomal abnormalities. Common abnormalities include those involving chromosomes 5 and 7, particularly in AML arising out of the background of MDS, and each of which are seen in approximately 5% to 10% of patients with AML. Enhancer of zeste 2 polycomb repressive complex 2 subunit (EZH2) is a histone methyltransferase that may play a role in leukemogenesis via haploinsufficiency in the setting of loss of material from the long arm of chromosome 7. Interstitial deletions on the long arm of chromosome 5 at 5q33.1 are associated with the 5q minus syndrome, which has a low risk of progression to sAML. RPS14 and miR145/146a have been implicated in the pathogenesis of this syndrome. In contrast, deletions involving a more proximal region at 5q31.2 are associated with higher risk of sAML transformation. Most chromosome 5 deletions in high-risk MDS and AML are large, including most of the long arm or the entire chromosome. Many genes have been implicated in diseases associated with these larger deletions, including *APC*, *CTNNA1*, *HSPA9*, *EGR1*, and *NPM1*.

Loss of chromosome 17p, including the *TP53* locus at 17p13, is associated with complex cytogenetics as well as abnormalities in chromosome 5 and 7. Indeed, there appears to be cooperativity between 17p alterations and deletions at chromosome 5q13 at the site of *SSBP4*, another tumor suppressor gene, which may influence the progression to leukemia. Alterations in 17p are enriched in patients with alkylator-associated tAML and sAML rising from an underlying MPN or MDS. In contrast to AML with balanced translocations, leukemias that develop in the context of 17p alterations are characterized by greater genomic instability.

Common trisomies in AML include somatic acquisition of trisomy 8 and trisomy 21, seen in approximately 10% and 3% of patients, respectively. Trisomy 8, the most common chromosomal gain seen in AML, may contribute to leukemogenesis via amplification of *MYC*, which is located at chromosome 8p24 and is implicated in a number of malignancies including AML. Acquired trisomy 21, similar to AML in Down syndrome, appears to progress to AML via the subsequent acquisition of mutations in *RUNX1* or *GATA1*. Unlike Down syndrome, acquired trisomy 21 often occurs in conjunction with other cytogenetic aberrations, in particular with complex cytogenetic rearrangements.

Recurrently Mutated Genes

For many patients, a recurrent chromosomal abnormality cannot be detected by either cytogenetic analysis or fluorescence in situ hybridization, using probes for common rearrangements and copy number alterations. This group of patients with normal cytogenetics accounts for approximately 45% of AML cases and has historically been categorized as having intermediate prognosis with standard treatment. Molecular testing of this group, as well as patients in other cytogenetic risk groups, has identified a number of recurrent genetic alterations that play critical roles in AML pathogenesis, prognosis, and response to therapy. On average, AML genomes contain fewer somatic mutations compared with other adult cancers (fewer than 20 mutations in protein-coding genes per case). Genes that are mutated across multiple AML cases at a frequency higher than expected by chance are more likely to be biologically relevant. AML mutations can be categorized according to the type of gene that is affected and the functional impact of the mutation. Many gene mutations cooperate with other alterations, including the large-scale copy number changes and rearrangements described earlier (Fig. 58.2).

Cytokine Signaling

A number of mutations have been identified that result in altered signal transduction, enhancing leukemic cell proliferation and survival. These include mutations in the fms-related tyrosine kinase 3 (*FLT3*) gene, *RAS* genes, and *KIT*. Mutations in *FLT3* can occur either as an in-frame internal tandem duplication within the juxtamembrane

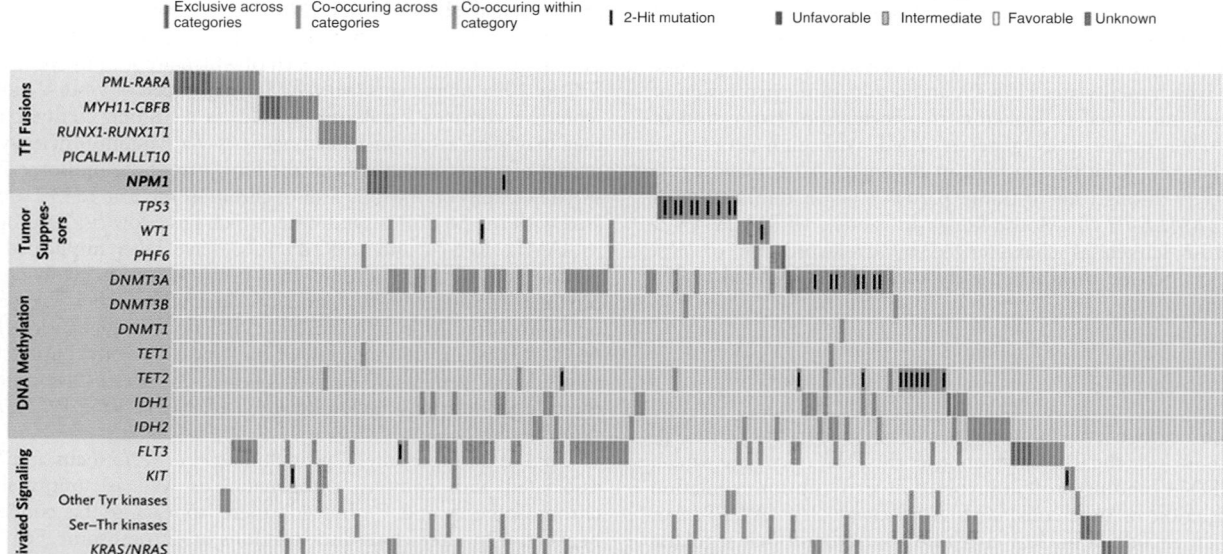

Fig. 58.2 COOCCURENCE AND MUTUAL EXCLUSIVITY OF SOMATIC MUTATIONS AMONG PATIENTS WITH ACUTE MYELOID LEUKEMIA. A combination of exome, genome, and transcriptome sequencing in 200 patients with de novo acute myeloid leukemia identified a number of mutations which cooccur or are mutually exclusive according to nine categories of biological function: transcription factor fusions, cytokine signaling, transcription factor mutations, tumor suppressor genes, regulators of DNA methylation, polycomb complex, spliceosome, cohesin complex, and nucleophosmin. *TF,* Transcription factor. *(From Ley TJ, Miller C, Ding L, et al: The Cancer Genome Atlas Research Network. Genomic and epigenomic landscapes of adult de novo acute myeloid leukemia. N Engl J Med 368:2059, 2013. Copyright © 2013 Massachusetts Medical Society. Reprinted with permission.)*

domain of the receptor (*FLT3-ITD*), found in up to 30% of AML patients, or as a mutation in the tyrosine kinase domain (*FLT3-TKD*), the most common being a point mutation resulting in an aspartate to tyrosine substitution at codon 835, detectable in 5% to 10% of AML cases. Both mutations result in constitutive activation of the receptor. *FLT3* signaling activates the RAS/mitogen-activated protein kinase (MAPK) signaling pathway, and mutated *FLT3-ITD* can also activate the STAT5 pathway, which induces the serine-threonine Pim kinases, and results in enhanced cell growth and survival. Murine models that combine *FLT3-ITD* with other mutations, such as *PML-RARA*, *MLL-ENL*, or *NUP98-HOXD13*, have demonstrated cooperativity between these mutations with respect to latency and penetrance of leukemia, while either mutation on its own has low efficiency for disease initiation. The *FLT3-ITD* alteration in particular appears to be associated with increased rates of relapse and worsened patient outcomes; it is not clear whether *FLT3-TKD* mutations have the same impact on outcomes. The *FLT3-ITD* alteration may be present at the time of diagnosis, and can be acquired or lost at relapse. Moreover, the length of the duplication, position of the mutation, and number of distinct ITDs can vary within a given patient. Together, this suggests that the *FLT3-ITD* alteration may be a later event in the development of AML and illustrates the subclonal heterogeneity of AML.

CD117, encoded by *KIT*, is another example of a protooncogenic receptor tyrosine kinase implicated in a number of malignancies. KIT is the receptor for stem cell factor, and is upregulated in most patients with AML. *KIT* mutations are most frequently seen at codons D816 or N822 in the tyrosine kinase domain, or in the extracellular domain; rare internal tandem duplications have also been identified in AML. Mutations at D816 or N822 occur in the activating loop of the kinase domain, interrupt autoinhibitory feedback, and result in constitutive activation. Mutations in *KIT* occur in less than 10% of patients and are enriched in patients with AML harboring CBF alterations. In mouse models, *KIT* mutations cooperate with *RUNX1-RUNX1T1* and *CBFB-MYH11* to induce AML. *KIT* mutations in patients with CBF AML, particularly with *RUNX1-RUNX1T1*, are associated with increased rates of relapse.

Mutations in the *RAS* proto-oncogenes, most commonly *NRAS* and *KRAS*, are also recurrent events in AML, identified in approximately 10% and 5% of patients, respectively. *RAS* family members are small membrane-associated guanosine triphosphatase signaling proteins that activate the MAPK/extracellular signal-related kinase (ERK) pathway, leading to cell growth and survival. The most common mutations in *NRAS* occur at codons 12, 13, and in *KRAS* at codon 12. These mutations result in a guanosine triphosphate-bound state of the RAS protein, leading to constitutive activation. In murine models, expression of mutant *NRAS* or *KRAS* results in a spectrum of myeloid disease, with variable features of acute leukemia, myeloproliferation, or MDS/MPN overlap. Consistent with this finding, *RAS* is frequently mutated in patients with MPNs and CMML.

Transcription Factors

In addition to their frequent identification in novel fusion proteins, transcription factors are also recurrently mutated in AML. *RUNX1* mutations occur in approximately 5% to 15% of all patients with AML, but are slightly more common in patients with intermediate-risk AML, particularly in association with trisomy 8 or trisomy 13. Approximately 80% of *RUNX1* mutations are located in a DNA-binding domain that is homologous to the *Drosophila runt* protein. C-terminal domains of RUNX1 are involved in nuclear matrix localization and recruitment of transcriptional trans-activating and repressing factors. Overexpression of mutant *RUNX1* in mice causes AML with dysplastic changes, and, in combination with *EVI1* mutations, results in a more rapid AML phenotype.

CEBPA is mutated in almost 10% of AML cases; these mutations are enriched in younger patients and patients with otherwise normal cytogenetics. *CEBPA* encodes the CCAAT/enhancer binding protein-alpha, a basic leucine zipper transcription factor. Patients with *CEBPA* mutations most often have normal cytogenetics; mutations result in loss of function and typically arise in the transactivation domain or in the basic leucine zipper domain. Favorable prognosis is restricted to cases with biallelic *CEBPA* mutations, which is associated with a distinct gene expression signature. When biallelic mutations were engineered in a mouse model, hematopoietic differentiation was impaired, but cooperating mutations were required for AML transformation, such as the addition of *FLT3-ITD*.

Tumor Suppressor Genes

Mutations in tumor suppressor genes facilitate the development of AML. Common examples include the canonical tumor suppressors *TP53* and Wilms tumor 1 (*WT1*). Mutations in *TP53* are found in fewer than 10% of AML cases overall, but are enriched in patients with AML with a complex karyotype, two-thirds of which will also harbor a mutation in *TP53*. TP53 is a transcription factor that regulates multiple signaling pathways in response to cellular stress, with an output that may culminate in cell cycle arrest, senescence, or apoptosis. Mutations occur throughout the *TP53* gene, usually resulting in loss of function; over half of cases have loss of heterozygosity at 17p.

Mutations in *WT1* occur in fewer than 10% of patients with AML, but wild-type *WT1* is frequently overexpressed. WT1 is a zinc finger transcription factor that is required for normal development. Mutations may occur throughout the gene and generally predict loss of function. One mechanism by which loss of WT1 may influence tumorigenesis appears to relate to DNA methylation; mutations in *WT1* result in a DNA methylation pattern similar to that in *TET2* mutated AML, apparently due to a lost interaction between WT1 and wild-type TET2. In addition to loss of function, *WT1* may also have oncogenic effects. In a *RUNX1-RUNX1T1* mouse model of AML, forced overexpression of *WT1* resulted in more rapid progression to AML.

Regulators of DNA Methylation

Methylation of cytosine residues is an important epigenetic mark that contributes to regulation of gene expression. Genes encoding factors directly or indirectly involved in DNA methylation or demethylation, including *TET2*, *DNMT3A*, and isocitrate dehydrogenase-1 (*IDH1*) or *IDH2*, are recurrently mutated in AML.

DNMT3A encodes a de novo methyltransferase that catalyzes cytosine methylation at CpG dinucleotides. These mutations are seen in approximately 20% of patients with de novo AML, but nearly 30% of patients with a normal karyotype. Nearly 50% of the *DNMT3A* mutations are heterozygous missense substitutions at codon R882 (most frequently R882H); the remainder are deletions, frameshifts, and missense substitutions throughout the open reading frame.

Mutations in ten-eleven-translocation 2 (*TET2*), have been identified in 10% to 30% of patients with AML, and are enriched in patients with prior MDS or MPN. Members of the TET gene family include *TET1* and *TET2*; *TET1* is also rearranged in t(10;11)(p12;q23). TET2 converts 5-methylcytosine to 5-hydroxymethylcytosine, an initial step in the reversion to unmethylated cytosine. Hydroxylation of methylated CpG-rich regions by TET2 activates gene programs important for cellular differentiation, including the homeobox A cluster. By contrast, TET2 loss-of-function mutations are associated with impaired differentiation. Mice harboring a *TET2* null allele display enhanced stem cell self-renewal and develop myeloid malignancies with underlying features consistent with CMML or MDS. *TET2* mutations do not have a consistent impact on AML prognosis in multivariate analysis.

Mutations in *IDH1* or *IDH2* are also involved in *TET* deregulation via the oncometabolite 2-hydroxyglutarate (2-HG). IDH1 is primarily cytosolic, while IDH2 localizes to mitochondria. These proteins normally decarboxylate isocitrate to form α-ketoglutarate via the reduced form of NADPH, a key reaction in the Krebs cycle. Mutational hotspots include codon R132 in *IDH1* and codons R140 or R172 in *IDH2*. *IDH1/2* mutations are found in approximately 5% to 10% and 15% to 20% of patients with AML, respectively. The mutations are enriched in cases with a normal karyotype and frequently co-occur with *NPM1* mutations. Mutant IDH1/2 catalyzes the conversion of α-ketoglutarate to 2-HG, which suppresses TET2 due to competitive inhibition at the α-ketoglutarate binding site. Through this mechanism, excess 2-HG results in a DNA hypermethylation pattern similar to that observed in *TET2*-mutated AML; however, this oncometabolite also interferes with other α-ketoglutarate–dependent enzymes, including members of the Jumonji-C domain-containing histone demethylases. Mouse models with *IDH1* mutations in hematopoietic cells develop a disease phenotypically similar to human MDS.

Polycomb Complex

The polycomb complex plays a major role in silencing transcription during development; it functions in conjunction with trithorax group proteins, which activate transcription, to epigenetically modulate genes during embryogenesis. Recurrent mutations in polycomb complex genes or regulators have been identified in several cancers, including AML. Additional Sex Combs-Like 1 (ASXL1) is an enhancer of the trithorax and polycomb genes; it plays a critical role in *HOX* gene expression during embryogenesis. Mutations in *ASXL1* in AML typically occur in exon 12 and result in loss of function. Expression of mutated *ASXL1* in mice results in aberrant *HOX* gene activation, and, when conditionally deleted in hematopoietic cells, results in anemia and leukopenia with multilineage myeloid dysplasia. Acquired somatic mutations in *ASXL1* occur in approximately 10% to 20% of patients with AML and are enriched in those with underlying MDS.

ASXL2 is also involved in regulation of the polycomb repressor complex, and mutations in *ASXL2* are present in over 20% of patients with AML harboring the *RUNX1/RUNX1T1* translocation; they are mutually exclusive with *ASXL1* mutations in this group.

The nuclear receptor binding SET domain protein 1 (*NSD1*) gene encodes a histone methyltransferase, which similarly has a role in normal development; germline mutations result in Sotos syndrome, which is associated with a number of childhood cancers. NSD1 methylates H3K36 and is associated with transcriptional activation. *NSD1* is involved as a fusion partner in the recurrent translocation t(5;11)(q35;p15.5) with *NUP98*, seen in approximately 15% of pediatric AML, but less than 5% of adult AML, and is associated with a poor response to therapy. This fusion protein binds regulatory elements of the polycomb complex and results in *HOX* gene activation.

Spliceosome Complex

The spliceosome complex consists of a number of proteins around a small nuclear ribonucleic acid (snRNA) core, which identifies splicing motifs in pre-mRNA, removing introns and religating exons, to generate a diversity of mRNA isoforms from each coding gene. The splicing machinery is highly conserved, and in addition to five snRNAs, there are numerous associated proteins. Recurrent mutations have been identified in hematologic malignancies in a number of the core splicing components, most often affecting *SF3B1*, *U2AF1*, *SRSF2*, or *ZRSR2*. These mutations are typically heterozygous and tend not to cooccur within patients, suggesting that a second mutation in the pathway confers no additional selective advantage or is not tolerated by hematopoietic cells. Alternative splicing was noted in AML samples prior to the discovery of spliceosome mutations, but the cause and biological consequences were not understood. Collectively, splicing factor mutations are detectable in approximately 15% of patients with AML. These mutations are highly associated with specific subtypes of MDS and MPNs; consequently, AML with splicing factor mutations frequently have a history of these antecedent disorders. *SF3B1* is the most common mutation in the splicing complex; mutations in this gene are tightly associated with the refractory anemia with ringed sideroblasts MDS subtype. *SRSF2* mutations are common in CMML and are retained when these patients progress to sAML.

Cohesin Complex

The cohesin complex is involved in the alignment of sister chromatids throughout replication, from the initial DNA synthesis during S-phase and on through mitosis and segregation during M-phase. The cohesin core complex is comprised of the structural maintenance of chromosomes (SMC) proteins SMC1, SMC3, RAD21 (SCC1), and stromalin antigens STAG1 or STAG2. These core proteins form a ring structure, with a hinge formed by SMC1 and SMC3, and a closed loop formed through the binding of RAD21 with STAG1 and STAG2, which regulates chromosome segregation. Recurrent mutations in the genes for this core complex have been identified in approximately 15% of AML cases. The cohesin complex preferentially localizes at "super enhancers," which regulate gene expression related to cell lineage and self-renewal. Perturbation of this mechanism may be more relevant to the pathogenesis of AML, since cohesin mutations have not been associated with increased risk of aneuploidy in this disease.

Nucleophosmin

Nucleophosmin (*NPM1*) is a molecular chaperone with multiple functions, including ribosomal protein assembly, the prevention of nucleolar protein aggregation, and regulation of the tumor suppressors TP53 and alternative reading frame (ARF). *NPM1* mutations are seen in approximately one third of patients with AML, and are enriched in patients with normal karyotypes. They occur as insertions in exon 12, most frequently of the four base pairs TCTG (type A), causing a frameshift mutation with an added nuclear export signal motif at the carboxy-terminus, and resulting in cytoplasmic localization and loss of function. Less common mutations with similar effect include alternate insertions of CATG (type B) or CCTG (type D), among others; there does not appear to be a clinical impact according to the type of mutation. Murine models incorporating the *NPM1* type A mutation result in increased megakaryocytes, but do not develop AML. Consistent with this, mutations in *NPM1* are thought to represent early events in the development of AML. Rarely, *NPM1* is involved in chromosomal translocations, including t(2;5)(p23;q35) with *ALK*, and t(5;17)(q35;q21) with *RARA*, the latter resulting in an uncommon variant of APL.

Epigenetic Alterations in Acute Myeloid Leukemia

AML is frequently characterized by epigenetic alterations, including covalent modifications to DNA and chromatin factors, dysregulated expression of small and large noncoding RNAs, and changes in long-range DNA interactions resulting in altered gene expression. In many cases (discussed earlier), these epigenetic regulators are targets of somatic mutation or are aberrantly recruited by fusion proteins in AML.

Methylation of cytosine on DNA at CpG sites, which are enriched at gene promoter regions, is a key regulator of gene expression. The AML genome has increased methylation when compared with normal tissues, and certain genetic subtypes of AML, such as AML with *RUNX1-RUNX1T1* or *PML-RARA* rearrangements, have distinct gene methylation patterns. Recurrent missense mutations in the de novo DNA methyltransferase, DNMT3A, likely function in a dominant negative fashion and lead to focal regions of reduced DNA methylation. Oxidation of 5-methylcytosine to 5-hydroxymethylcytosine by the TET enzymes is an intermediate step toward subsequent demethylation. TET2 inhibition, either through an acquired loss-of-function mutation, or via 2-HG produced preferentially in the setting of *IDH1/2* mutations, results in aberrant hydroxymethylation, particularly at key *HOX* sites, which leads to myeloid expansion and a dysplastic phenotype in mouse models. Causal links between mutations in these regulatory enzymes, cytosine modifications, altered gene expression, and leukemogenesis remain elusive, but it is unlikely that global changes in methylation are responsible for the leukemic phenotype.

DNA methylation and histone modification are often coordinately regulated. For example, *EVI1* has DNA methylation activity, but also associates with histone deacetylases and methyltransferases. The polycomb repressive complex 2 (*PRC2*) catalyzes the methylation of histone H3K27, resulting in gene silencing. PRC2 is comprised of a noncatalytic subunit, as well as a SET domain with methyltransferase activity via *EZH1* or *EZH2*. Mutations in *EZH2* found in myeloid malignancies are predicted to be loss of function. In mouse models, EZH2 appears to have either tumor suppressor or oncogene characteristics, depending on the timing of the mutation in relation to the stage of disease, and has a role in inhibiting hematopoietic cell differentiation. Similarly, *ASXL1* interacts with PRC2, resulting in trimethylation at H3K27; loss-of-function mutations may promote leukemia due to relative activation of PRC2-specific genes. Finally, MLL rearrangements bring a diversity of fusion partners to targets normally regulated by MLL. Many of these fusion partners interact with DOT1L, a histone H3K79 methyltransferase, which then methylates critical *MLL*-dependent regulatory genes, such as *HOXA9*.

BIOLOGY OF ACUTE MYELOID LEUKEMIA

Role of the Bone Marrow Microenvironment

AML arises in hematopoietic cells residing in a bone marrow microenvironment known as the *niche*, where the stromal infrastructure helps to promote leukemic cell survival. AML cells in culture have improved survival when in the presence of bone marrow fibroblasts, which increase expression of the antiapoptotic proteins Bcl-2 and Bcl-XL. Moreover, the bone marrow stroma contributes to chemoresistance via the binding of fibronectin on stromal cells to VLA-4 expressed on AML blasts. Bone marrow stromal cells also produce the chemokine SDF-1, or chemokine CXC motif ligand 12 (CXCL12), which binds to CXC-chemokine receptor 4 (CXCR4), a chemokine receptor expressed on hematopoietic progenitors as well as leukemic cells. This signal maintains the normal hematopoietic progenitor niche; it also facilitates proliferation and survival.

A variety of strategies that interfere with the interactions between leukemic and stromal cells have been tested as a means to enhance the efficacy of cytotoxic agents. In addition, there is evidence that AML blasts sustain an immunosuppressive microenvironment via an arginase-dependent mechanism that may be amenable to pharmacologic inhibition.

Clonal Hierarchy of Acute Myeloid Leukemia

The recognition that some mutations may be lost or acquired at relapse (e.g., *FLT3-ITD*), while others are present at diagnosis and remain stable (e.g., *NPM1*, *PML-RARA*, and *CBF* rearrangements) suggests that distinct clonal populations can coexist in an AML sample. Sequencing of serially obtained samples has revealed a clonal hierarchy in AML, beginning with a founding clone that represents the initial population that becomes dominant in the bone marrow. The founding clone spawns subclones that retain founding clone mutations, but gain additional mutations that confer a growth advantage. The clonal architecture evolves over time as a feature of the natural history of the disease, or in response to selective pressure imposed by therapy. Analysis of AML cases that entered morphologic remission after cytotoxic chemotherapy, and later relapse, revealed that the dominant clone at relapse retains founding clone mutations. These observations raise the hypothesis that therapies directed at eradicating drivers of the founding clone may be more effective than therapies targeting subclones.

Somatic mutations accumulate in an age-dependent manner in normal individuals without perturbing hematopoiesis in most cases. However, several large cohort sequencing studies have demonstrated that up to 10% of apparently healthy individuals over 65 years of age have detectable clonal populations that are marked by somatic mutations, often in genes that are recurrently mutated in MDS/AML (particularly in epigenetic regulators, including DNMT3A, TET2, and ASXL1). Although clonally skewed hematopoiesis has been associated with an elevated risk of later developing a hematologic malignancy, the vast majority of these individuals do not progress to MDS or AML. Additional epidemiologic study will be required to determine how often clonal hematopoiesis is a precursor to MDS/AML and whether surveillance and/or early intervention are warranted.

Leukemia Stem Cells

Normal HSCs are characterized by their capacity for self-renewal and multilineage differentiation, properties that can only be assessed in vivo using functional assays such as xenotransplantation into immune deficient mouse models. The pioneering studies of John Dick and colleagues demonstrated that a similar cellular hierarchy exists in AML, in which rare cells with an immunophenotype similar to normal stem/progenitor cells are enriched for the capacity to initiate leukemia in xenotransplantation models. Further work has led to the identification of several cell surface antigens that are preferentially expressed on leukemia-initiating cells compared with normal HSCs, including CD123, CD99, and TIM3.

Interestingly, cells with an HSC immunophenotype that are capable of engraftment in mice and multilineage differentiation in vivo can be recovered from the bone marrow of patients with AML. These "preleukemic stem cells" may harbor the same class of mutations detected in individuals with clonally skewed hematopoiesis (e.g., DNMT3A), but lack the full complement of mutations found in the bulk AML sample, suggesting that they are ancestral. The contribution of these preleukemic stem cells to chemotherapy resistance and relapse remains to be determined.

FUTURE DIRECTIONS

AML comprises a heterogeneous spectrum of disease, which shares a common myeloid phenotype and is characterized by accumulation of abnormal leukemic myeloblasts. The development of AML occurs through serial acquisition of somatic mutations, resulting in clonal expansion and genetic evolution of this disease. As our understanding of the genetic underpinnings has grown, it is clear that there are various pathways to the development of AML (Fig. 58.3). Moreover, some mutations appear to be earlier, founding events, while other mutations are typically acquired during disease progression. The further identification of the sequence of mutation acquisition, as well as cooccurring and mutually exclusive genetic pathways, will help to better distinguish different subsets of this disease.

A broader understanding of the mutational landscape of AML has provided a basis for development and testing of novel targeted therapies and monitoring of disease. The role of residual disease monitoring may occur through cytogenetic, flow cytometric, and now also molecular assessment. The incorporation of these residual disease markers into clinical practice remains under intense investigation; similar to patients with chronic myeloid leukemia, it may eventually inform treatment duration and maintenance therapies.

Molecular Diagnostics in Acute Myeloid Leukemia

The various mutations and dysregulated pathways integral to the pathobiology of acute myeloid leukemia (AML) also yield specific therapeutic targets and offer clear prognostic implications for patients. As such, molecular testing at the time of AML diagnosis has become the standard of care, to assist with subclassification of disease, risk stratification, selection of an induction regimen, and consolidation preferences. Diagnosis of AML requires analysis of a specimen demonstrating excess myeloblasts. For patients with high levels of circulating disease, some studies may be performed with the use of peripheral blood samples; however, assessment of a bone marrow biopsy and aspirate is essential.

Standard Evaluation

The cornerstone of the diagnosis of AML remains morphologic assessment. In the current WHO guidelines, at least 20% of the bone marrow cellularity must be comprised of myeloblasts, except in the presence of the t(8;21), t(16;16)/inv(16), or t(15;17) rearrangements, which are sufficient for an AML diagnosis regardless of blast count. In addition, promonocytes in acute monocytic leukemia, megakaryoblasts in acute megakaryocytic leukemia, and abnormal promyelocytes in acute promyelocytic leukemia are added to the blast percentage. Only in pure erythroleukemia are erythroblasts included in the blast count.

Flow cytometry utilizes multiparametric analysis of single cells to assess cellular granularity and size, cell surface, intracellular antigen expression, and other features. The coexpression of certain cell surface markers may help to confirm myeloid cell origin, identify immature blasts, typically CD34+ and CD117+, and also to distinguish an aberrant phenotype of a leukemic blast population. Flow cytometry can enumerate small populations of leukemic cells, below the limit of detection by morphology. For this reason, flow cytometric analysis has been developed as a platform to monitor minimal residual disease (MRD). The role of MRD assessment by flow cytometry in routine AML care remains under investigation.

A critical element in the initial laboratory assessment of AML is cytogenetic analysis of a bone marrow aspirate specimen. This provides important prognostic data for risk stratification and informs therapeutic strategies. Cells from the aspirate are cultured, mitosis is interrupted, and the paired chromosomes are arranged to identify missing, translocated, or duplicated segments. Fluorescence in situ hybridization utilizes fluorescently labeled DNA probes and can identify gains and losses of chromosomal material, as well as rearrangements that may be cryptic using conventional banding techniques.

Detection of somatic mutations that are known drivers of AML biology can aid in the initial risk classification of patients with AML, particularly those with intermediate-risk cytogenetics. Current National Comprehensive Cancer Network guidelines recommend testing of four genes (*KIT, FLT3, NPM1,* and *CEBPA*) at diagnosis, because their prognostic significance has been validated in large cohorts (level 2A evidence). Testing for mutations in *RUNX1* is recommended for WHO classification. In addition, use of targeted therapies is increasingly dependent on detection of a specific tumor genotype.

Investigational Testing

Given the rapidly expanding number of genes that are recognized targets of recurrent somatic mutation in AML, more comprehensive mutational profiling is beginning to enter routine clinical practice. With increasing numbers of genes to query, next-generation sequencing approaches offer advantages in sensitivity, cost, and efficiency over traditional testing methods (e.g., polymerase chain reaction, Sanger sequencing). Large panels of genes can be tested simultaneously by pre-enriching for the targets of interest (by automated amplicon generation, or hybridization capture). With further improvements in analytical workflow and cost reduction, whole-genome and transcriptome sequencing could displace some existing diagnostic tools, as these platforms can provide simultaneous detection of mutations, gene expression, copy number alteration, and structural variation.

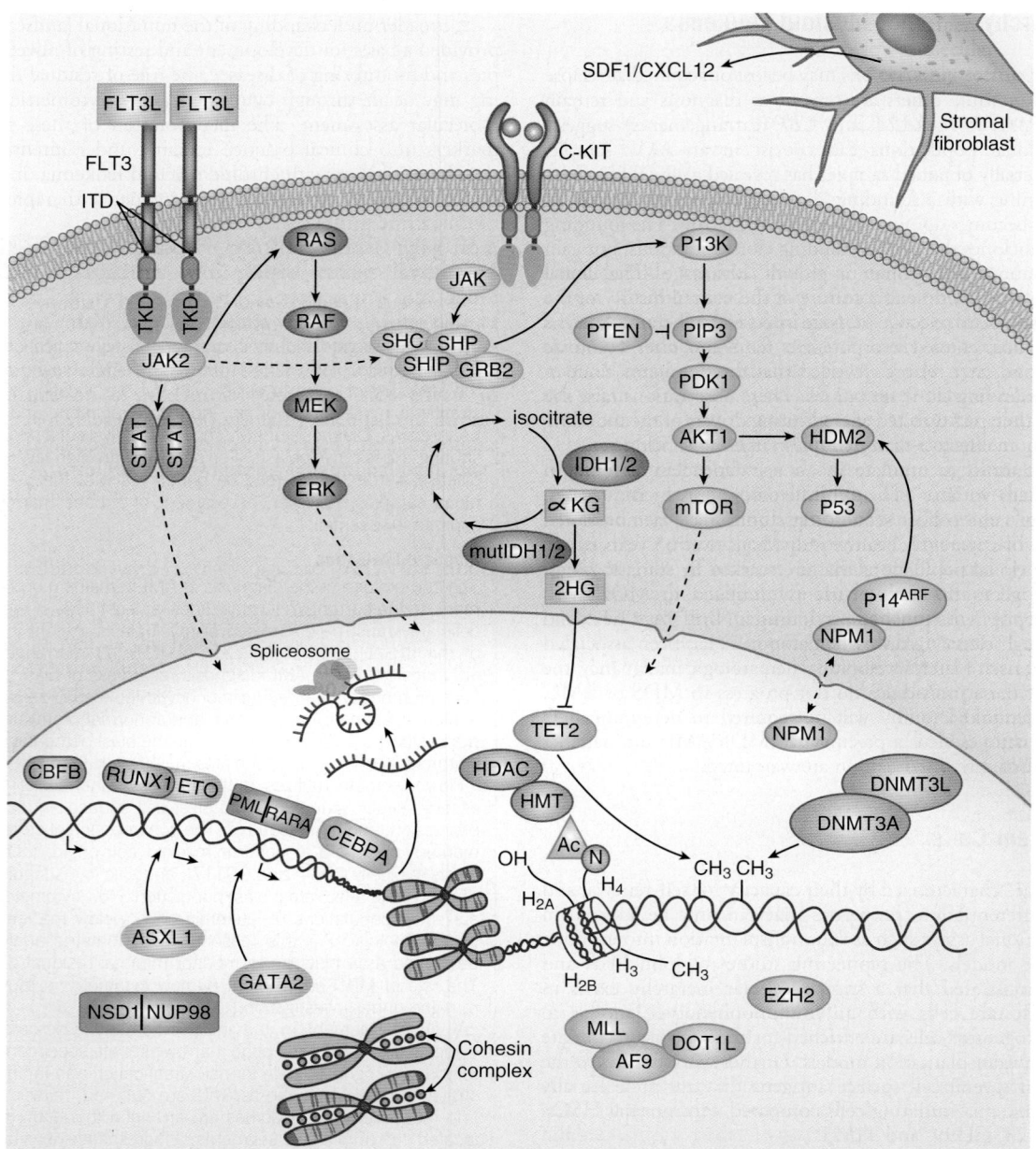

Fig. 58.3 COMMONLY ALTERED CELLULAR PATHWAYS IN ADULT ACUTE MYELOID LEUKE-MIA. Mutations in acute myeloid leukemia commonly affect pathways related to cell signaling, differentiation, secondary modifications of DNA, and tumor suppressor genes. Collectively, these lesions interfere with self-renewal, differentiation, and survival pathways. *Ac*, acetyl; *AF9*, ALL1-fused gene from chromosome 9 protein; *α-KG*, α-ketoglutarate; *ARF*, ADP-ribosylation factor; *AKT1*, AKT serine/threonine kinase 1; *ASXL1*, additional sex Combs-like 1; *CBFB*, core binding factor b; *CEBPA*, CCAAT/enhancer binding protein-alpha; *CH₃*, methyl; *CXCL12*, CXC-chemokine ligand 12; *DNMT3A*, DNA methyltransferase 3A; *DNMT3L*, DNA methyltransferase 3 like; *DOTIL*, disruption of telomeric silencing 1-like; *ERK*, Extracellular signal-related kinase; *ETO*, eight twenty one or RUNX1T1; *EZH2*, Enhancer of zeste homolog 2; *FLT3L*, FMS-like tyrosine kinase-3 ligand; *GATA1*, GATA binding protein 1; *GRB2*, growth factor receptor–bound protein 2; *H*, histone; *HDAC*, histone deacetylase; *HDM2*, human homolog of double minute 2, P53-binding protein; *HMT*, histone methyltransferase; *IDH1/2*, isocitrate dehydrogenase 1/2; *ITD*, internal tandem duplication: *JAK*, Janus-activated kinase; *MEK*, mitogen-activated protein kinase kinase; *MLL*, mixed lineage leukemia; *mTOR*, mammalian target of rapamycin; *N*, nitrogen; *NPMI*, nucleophosmin; *NSD1*, nuclear receptor binding SET domain protein 1; *Nup98*, nucleoporin 98; *OH*, hydroxyl; *P14^{ARF}*, cyclin-dependent kinase inhibitor 2A; *p53*, tumor protein p53; *RARA*, retinoic acid receptor alpha; *PDK1*, phosphoinositide-dependent kinase-1; *PI3K*, phosphatidylinositol 3-kinase; *PIP3*, phosphoinositide-3,4,5-trisphosphate; *PML*, promyelocytic leukemia; *PTEN*, phosphatase and tensin homolog; *RAF*, RAF kinase family; *RAS*, RAS family kinase; *RUNX1*, runt-related transcription factor 1; *SDF-1*, stromal cell–derived factor 1; *SHC*, Src Homology 2 Domain-Containing; *SHIP*, SH₂-containing inositol phosphatase; *SHP*, small heterodimer partner; *STAT*, signal transducer and activator of transcription; *TET2*, TET oncogene family member 2; *TKD*, tyrosine kinase domain.

SUGGESTED READINGS

Alter BP, Giri N, Savage SA, et al: Malignancies and survival patterns in the National Cancer Institute inherited bone marrow failure syndromes cohort study. *Br J Haematol* 150:179–188, 2010.

Bennett JM, Catovsky D, Daniel MT, et al: Proposals for the classification of the acute leukaemias. French-American-British (FAB) co-operative group. *Br J Haematol* 33:451–458, 1976.

Bonnet D, Dick JE: Human acute myeloid leukemia is organized as a hierarchy that originates from a primitive hematopoietic cell. *Nat Med* 3:730–737, 1997.

Byrd JC, Mrózek K, Dodge RK, et al: Pretreatment cytogenetic abnormalities are predictive of induction success, cumulative incidence of relapse, and overall survival in adult patients with de novo acute myeloid leukemia: results from Cancer and Leukemia Group B (CALGB 8461). *Blood* 100:4325–4336, 2002.

Corral J, Lavenir I, Impey H, et al: An Mll–AF9 fusion gene made by homologous recombination causes acute leukemia in chimeric mice: a method to create fusion oncogenes. *Cell* 85:853–861, 1996.

Ding L, Ley TJ, Larson DE, et al: Clonal evolution in relapsed acute myeloid leukaemia revealed by whole-genome sequencing. *Nature* 481:506–510, 2012.

Döhner H, Estey EH, Amadori S, et al: Diagnosis and management of acute myeloid leukemia in adults: recommendations from an international expert panel, on behalf of the European LeukemiaNet. *Blood* 115:453–474, 2010.

Dong F, Brynes RK, Tidow N, et al: Mutations in the gene for the granulocyte colony-stimulating–factor receptor in patients with acute myeloid leukemia preceded by severe congenital neutropenia. *N Engl J Med* 333:487–493, 1995.

Druker BJ, Guilhot F, O'Brien SG, et al: Five-Year follow-up of patients receiving Imatinib for chronic myeloid leukemia. *N Engl J Med* 355:2408–2417, 2006.

Erickson P, Gao J, Chang KS, et al: Identification of breakpoints in t(8;21) acute myelogenous leukemia and isolation of a fusion transcript, *AML1/ETO*, with similarity to *Drosophila* segmentation gene, *runt*. *Blood* 80:1825–1831, 1992.

Ernst T, Chase AJ, Score J, et al: Inactivating mutations of the histone methyltransferase gene *EZH2* in myeloid disorders. *Nat Genet* 42:722–726, 2010.

Falini B, Mecucci C, Tiacci E, et al: Cytoplasmic nucleophosmin in acute myelogenous leukemia with a normal karyotype. *N Engl J Med* 352:254–266, 2005.

Figueroa ME, Abdel-Wahab O, Lu C, et al: Leukemic IDH1 and IDH2 mutations result in a hypermethylation phenotype, disrupt TET2 function, and impair hematopoietic differentiation. *Cancer Cell* 18:553–567, 2010.

Grimwade D, Hills RK, Moorman AV, et al: Refinement of cytogenetic classification in acute myeloid leukemia: determination of prognostic significance of rare recurring chromosomal abnormalities among 5876 younger adult patients treated in the United Kingdom Medical Research Council trials. *Blood* 116:354–365, 2010.

Kakizuka A, Miller WH, Jr, Umesono K, et al: Chromosomal translocation t(15;17) in human acute promyelocytic leukemia fuses RAR alpha with a novel putative transcription factor, PML. *Cell* 66:663–674, 1991.

Ley TJ, Ding L, Walter MJ, et al: DNMT3A mutations in acute myeloid leukemia. *N Engl J Med* 363:2424–2433, 2010.

Ley TJ, Miller C, Ding L, et al: The Cancer Genome Atlas Research Network. Genomic and epigenomic landscapes of adult de novo acute myeloid leukemia. *N Engl J Med* 368:2059–2074, 2013.

Liu P, Tarlé SA, Hajra A, et al: Fusion between transcription factor CBF beta/PEBP2 beta and a myosin heavy chain in acute myeloid leukemia. *Science* 261:1041–1044, 1993.

Lu C, Ward PS, Kapoor GS, et al: IDH mutation impairs histone demethylation and results in a block to cell differentiation. *Nature* 483:474–478, 2012.

Mitchell JR, Wood E, Collins K: A telomerase component is defective in the human disease dyskeratosis congenita. *Nature* 402:551–555, 1999.

Nakao M, Yokota S, Iwai T, et al: Internal tandem duplication of the flt3 gene found in acute myeloid leukemia. *Leukemia* 10:1911–1918, 1996.

Pabst T, Mueller BU, Zhang P, et al: Dominant-negative mutations of CEBPA, encoding CCAAT/enhancer binding protein-alpha (C/EBPalpha), in acute myeloid leukemia. *Nat Genet* 27:263–270, 2001.

Pappaemmanuil E, Gerstung M, Bullinger L, et al: Genomic classification and prognosis in acute myeloid leukemia. *N Engl J Med* 374:2209–2221, 2016.

Paschka P, Marcucci G, Ruppert AS, et al: Adverse prognostic significance of KIT mutations in adult acute myeloid leukemia with inv(16) and t(8;21): a cancer and leukemia group B study. *J Clin Oncol* 24:3904–3911, 2006.

Pedersen-Bjergaard J: Insights into Leukemogenesis from Therapy-Related Leukemia. *N Engl J Med* 352:1591–1594, 2005.

Shigesada K, van de Sluis B, Liu PP: Mechanism of leukemogenesis by the inv(16) chimeric gene CBFB/PEBP2B-MHY11. *Oncogene* 23:4297–4307, 2004.

Shlush LI, Zandi S, Mitchell A, et al: Identification of pre-leukaemic haematopoietic stem cells in acute leukaemia. *Nature* 506:328–333, 2014.

Walter MJ, Shen D, Ding L, et al: Clonal architecture of secondary acute myeloid leukemia. *N Engl J Med* 366:1090–1098, 2012.

Welch JS, Ley TJ, Link DC, et al: The Origin and Evolution of Mutations in Acute Myeloid Leukemia. *Cell* 150:264–278, 2012.

Wong TN, Ramsingh G, Young AL, et al: Role of TP53 mutations in the origin and evolution of therapy-related acute myeloid leukaemia. *Nature* 518:552–555, 2015.

CLINICAL MANIFESTATIONS AND TREATMENT OF ACUTE MYELOID LEUKEMIA

Stefan Faderl and Hagop M. Kantarjian

INTRODUCTION

Acute myeloid leukemia (AML) is a clonal disorder of hematopoietic stem or progenitor cells causing a differentiation block and unregulated proliferation of hematopoietic cells in the marrow, blood, and in some cases extramedullary sites. The consequences of this malignant transformation include marrow failure, profound immune deficiencies, and not infrequently manifestations of a systemic inflammatory response of varying severity. The high malignant potential of AML with rapid progression, universally fatal outcome if left unattended to, and challenging clinical course and management continue to attract a high level of interest.

Knowledge of the pathobiologic aspects of AML as it relates to origin of blast cells, their biologic behavior, sensitivity to therapeutic interventions, and their interactions with and interdependence on the microenvironment is growing. Extensive application of whole-genome sequencing has identified numerous gene mutations and molecular footprints in AML, highlighting the heterogeneity of AML, devising better tools for prognosis, and identifying abnormal cellular and signaling pathways as central to the development of the leukemic phenotype against which novel targeted therapies are increasingly being developed.

Progress in basic, translational, and clinical research is cutting inroads into decade-old management paradigms. Although standard induction therapy for most patients with AML has not changed much in four decades and remains rooted in cytarabine/anthracycline combinations, newer studies are addressing a variety of questions: higher doses of cytarabine and/or anthracyclines during induction therapy, incorporation of novel drugs into existing chemotherapy backbones, separate approaches to core-binding factor (CBF) leukemias, chemotherapy-free treatment of most patients with acute promyelocytic leukemias (APL), alternative ways of treating AML in older patients, the expanding role of epigenetic therapies, and a steadily increasing armamentarium of small-molecule targeted therapies in AML salvage. New drugs allow old concepts such as maintenance therapy to be revisited. More extended application of measurements of minimal residual disease (MRD) may have the same helpful impact in AML as it proved to have in other forms of acute leukemias. A major challenge for the future lies in the ability to effectively incorporate and utilize the vast amount of generated data in the most effective way to extend to patients with AML the benefit of the exploits of research.

EPIDEMIOLOGY

In 2014, 18,860 new cases of patients with AML were diagnosed in the United States and an estimated 10,460 patients with AML died from it.[1] The age-adjusted incidence rate of AML is 3.6/100,000 population. However, with a median age at diagnosis of 66 years, incidence rates are as high as >15/100,000 in the older age group, and about 70% of all diagnoses of AML are in patients over 55 years of age. This is important as older patients have more comorbidities, respond less well to chemotherapy than younger patients, and carry the worst prognosis of any age group. AML is slightly more frequent in men than women (lifetime risk of acquiring AML: 1 in 227 [male] to 1 in 278 [female]). Based on Surveillance, Epidemiology, and End Results (SEER) data from 2005 to 2009, small differences in frequency also exist by race; AML is more common in whites than other ethnic groups (http://seer.cancer.gov). According to one study of 27,525 patients with AML, based on the SEER database from 1999 to 2008, African–Americans and Hispanics had a 12% and 6% increased hazard of death, respectively. This unfavorable hazard rate pertained despite the higher rate in these two ethnic groups of AML with translocations t(8;21) and t(15;17), both associated with a better outcome.

Several studies have suggested associations between leukemia diagnosis and season of the year. One study looking at this association found December and January as the two months with the highest number of new diagnoses, particularly for patients older than 65 years and men. Observations such as these raise interesting questions about the role of infectious agents in the etiology of AML.

PATHOBIOLOGY

Molecular genetic analysis has greatly contributed to a better understanding of the pathobiology that underlies the initiation and evolution of AML. AML is characterized by a relatively well-defined set of a small number of recurrent mutations. A series of transforming events (e.g., mutational processes intrinsic to the particular cell, exposure to external mutagens, genotoxic treatment of unrelated malignancies) leads to the development of preleukemic stem cells. Through the aggregate action of a network of mutated genes, these cells are characterized by impaired self-renewal properties, blocks in differentiation, limited capacity to undergo apoptosis, and altered signaling and metabolic pathways. Frequently, a given type of mutation is not sufficient to elicit the full leukemogenic phenotype and a second set of mutations is necessary for the fully transformed leukemic stem cells to develop. The transformation of immature hematopoietic cells that arises out of genetic changes in hematopoietic stem and more committed progenitor cells is thus considered a stepwise process in which genes of complementary mutation classes act together. This view gave rise to the two-hit model of leukemogenesis. In this model, two separate classes of mutations are operative: mutations that activate signal induction pathways and lead to uninhibited proliferation and survival; and mutations that affect transcription factors or other transcription elements that cause impaired hematopoietic differentiation and aberrant acquisition of self-renewal properties. Whereas mutations between these two groups easily coexist, mutations within one class are typically mutually exclusive. Since the initial publication of this model in 2002, whole-genome sequencing has identified many more gene mutations involved in AML pathobiology. Although most of these more recently described genes do not neatly fit into one or the other mutation classes, the principle of synergistic activity in the process of malignant transformation remains nevertheless valid.

Once compromised by a set of genetic mutations and in the context of propitious interactions with the microenvironment, leukemic cells may quickly accrue additional abnormalities (on a genetic or epigenetic level), and a new level of genomic instability may result in evolution and progression. An interesting aspect of such a dynamic model of acquisition of genetic abnormalities is the possibility that AML therapy itself may induce further genetic changes and become a driving force in selection of some AML clones over others.[2,3]

CLINICAL AND LABORATORY MANIFESTATIONS

Signs and symptoms of AML mostly reflect the effect of cytopenias. Patients typically present with a short history (1–8 weeks) of constitutional complaints (fatigue, lack of energy, malaise, profuse sweats), manifestations of bleeding (such as from gums, bruising in the skin, epistaxis, menorrhagia), or fevers. Fevers should always be presumed to be secondary to infections even in the absence of an identifiable focus and lead to rapid institution of antibiotic therapy. "Tumor fever" remains a diagnosis of exclusion. Extramedullary infiltrations of leukemia cells in the gingiva, skin, lymph nodes, or other organs occur occasionally. Bone pains are infrequent even with excessive leukocytosis and should raise the suspicion of an acute lymphoblastic leukemia (ALL), especially in children. Likewise, signs and symptoms referable to central nervous system (CNS) involvement (cranial nerve defects and other focal neurologic abnormalities, mental status changes, seizure activity) are rare, with the exception of AML with monocytic/monoblastic differentiation or in any AML with considerable leukocytosis (>100,000/μL).

Signs at physical examination are often nonspecific but in their aggregate can lead to a correct diagnosis. It is impossible to distinguish AML from ALL based solely on clinical presentation or examination findings. Patients may demonstrate pallor, ecchymoses or petechiae, enlargement of lymph nodes, or rarely, hepatosplenomegaly. Examination of the lungs may reveal signs of symptoms of an infectious process. Some patients with AML have no abnormal findings on physical examination.

The laboratory evaluation should include blood counts with evaluation of the blood smear, a standard chemistry panel (electrolytes, urea nitrogen, creatinine, total bilirubin, transaminases, uric acid, lactate dehydrogenase [LDH]), and coagulation studies, including prothrombin time (PT), partial thromboplastin time (PTT), and fibrinogen levels. Anemia and thrombocytopenia are universal. The white blood cell (WBC) count can vary from low to high and will range from 5000/μL to 100,000/μL in most patients. The highest degrees of leukocytosis can be seen in AML with myelomonocytic differentiation. Leukocytosis of 100,000/μL or higher is considered an emergency and requires immediate efforts to reduce the disease burden (e.g., leukapheresis, chemotherapy) because (1) leukostasis in some vascular beds may have catastrophic consequences (e.g., lung, brain), and (2) it may elicit a systemic inflammatory response with serious secondary organ damage (e.g., diffuse alveolar injury, hepatic failure). However, there is not always a good correlation between the severity of leukocytosis and immediate adverse clinical effects, and far lower WBC levels may elicit life-threatening symptoms. The WBC must therefore be assessed in the context of the patient's overall physical condition and other clinical and laboratory abnormalities (e.g., LDH, uric acid, coagulation parameters). Disseminated intravascular coagulation (DIC) is often seen in patients with myelomonocytic AML, APL, and any high-WBC AML. PT, PTT, and fibrinogen levels should be carefully followed and coagulation factors be replaced as clinically indicated. Subclinical DIC is common in many forms of AML and can worsen with the institution of therapy. Abnormalities of renal and hepatic values may represent infiltration of these organs, even in the absence of clinical symptoms.

Imaging studies are of little help in diagnosis but allow assessment of complications (pneumonia, cerebral bleed). If patients present with any neurologic deficit, the threshold for computed tomography (CT) scan (noncontrast if bleeding is of concern) or any other imaging modality of the brain should be low. Further evaluations should be based on the clinical assessment of the patients.

DIAGNOSIS AND CLASSIFICATION

The diagnosis of AML relies on morphologic evaluation (cytochemical stains), immunophenotyping by flow cytometry, and assessment of karyotype and molecular studies (Fig. 59.1).

Blast percentage is best determined on a 500-cell differential of the marrow aspirate. Three broad types of myeloblasts are described based on the granular content and nuclear features of the blasts (type 1: agranular basophilic cytoplasm, nucleus with fine chromatin, and two to four distinct nucleoli; type 2: basophilic cytoplasm with 20 or fewer azurophilic granules and similar nuclear features as type 1 blasts; type 3: basophilic cytoplasm with more than 20 azurophilic granules), although the morphologic variety of blasts exceeds the defined categories (Fig. 59.2). Promyelocytes have moderately basophilic cytoplasm with numerous azurophilic granules, and monoblasts and promonocytes usually exhibit folded/convoluted nuclei and may contain prominent acidophilic nucleoli. Promyelocytes, promonocytes, and atypical pronormoblasts are considered blast equivalents in some subgroups (e.g., APL, acute monoblastic leukemia, and acute erythroleukemia, pure erythroid type). Micromegakaryocytes and pronormoblasts are not considered blasts (see Fig. 59.2K and L). Auer rods are rod-like filaments of aggregated primary granules that are found in 30% to 50% of newly diagnosed patients with AML and, if present, are one of the hallmark morphologic features to establish a diagnosis of AML (see Fig. 59.2C). AML marrows are typically hypercellular with decreased or absent megakaryocytes. Exceptions are marrows of older patients or those with therapy-related AML, which may be hypocellular with dysplastic changes of one or several hematopoietic lineages. Prominent dysplasia may suggest a previous diagnosis of myelodysplastic syndrome (MDS) but can also be found in patients with de novo AML, where the prognostic significance of dysplastic changes is less clear. Cases with extensive fibrosis may represent a preceding myeloproliferative neoplasm or acute megakaryocytic leukemia.

Several cytochemical reactions further highlight morphologic characteristics (myeloperoxidase [MPO], periodic acid–Schiff, Sudan black B, naphthol AS-D chloroacetate esterase [specific esterase], α-naphthyl acetate/butyrate esterases [nonspecific esterases], acid phosphatase; Fig. 59.3). MPO is the most specific granulocytic marker, and MPO positivity in at least 3% of the blasts is consistent with a diagnosis of AML. On the other hand, lack of MPO staining does not rule out AML because it is often not present in AML with minimal differentiation, acute monoblastic leukemia, and acute megakaryocytic leukemia. Monoblastic leukemias are stained by nonspecific esterases. Whereas the MPO reaction is relatively uncomplicated and results are available quickly, this is not the case with most of the other cytochemical reactions, and their diagnostic utility is nowadays mostly outdone by immunophenotyping by flow cytometry.

The first systematic attempt of an AML classification goes back to the French–American–British (FAB) group, and was based solely on morphology (blast percentage, degree of differentiation, lineage involvement). Because of its limited scope, the FAB system is now considered inadequate. Rapidly growing insights from genetic mutation analyses, their association with prognosis, and, in some cases, prediction of response to therapy triggered a revision of the old system and led to the changes in the 2008 edition of the World Health Organization (WHO) classification of AML. The focus has shifted to identification of recurrent cytogenetic–molecular abnormalities, information regarding exposure to prior chemotherapy and/or radiation therapy, and morphologic features related to dysplasia-related changes and remnants of the FAB system (Table 59.1). Several categories have been defined:

1) AML with recurrent genetic abnormalities. This includes AML with relatively common cytogenetic changes: AML with t(8;21) (q22;q22), *RUNX1-RUNX1T1* (Fig. 59.4); AML with inv(16) (p13.1q22) or t(16;16)(p13.1;q22), *CBFB-MYH11* (Fig. 59.5); AML with t(15;17)(q22;q12); *PML-RARA* (Fig. 59.6); and AML with t(9;11)(p22;q23), *MLLT3-MLL* (Fig. 59.7). Less common

Text continued on p. 930

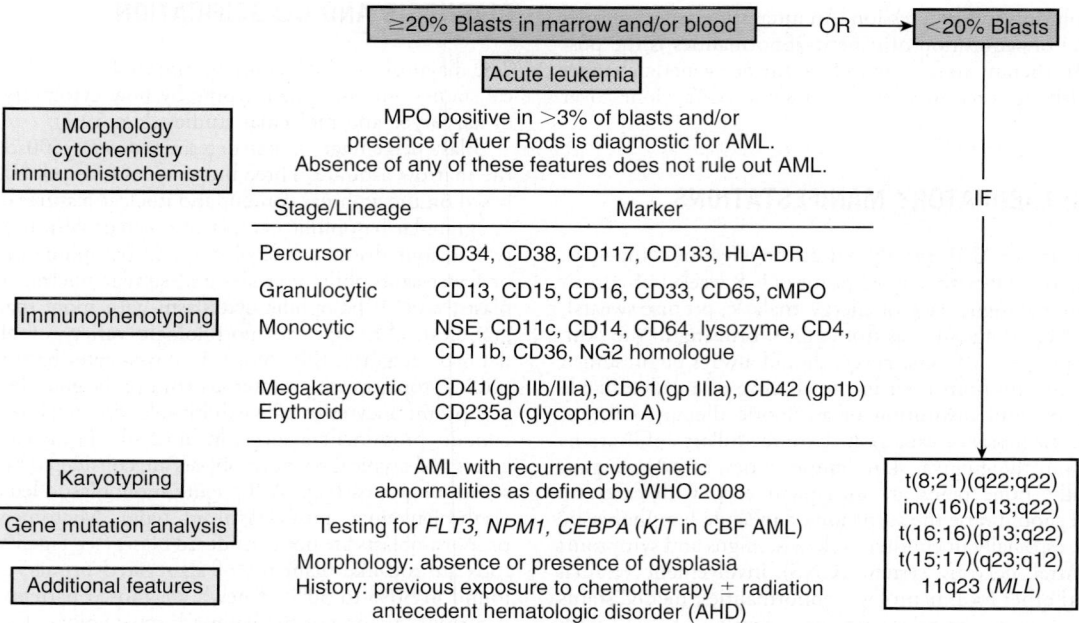

≥20% Blasts in marrow and/or blood — OR → <20% Blasts

Acute leukemia

Morphology cytochemistry immunohistochemistry

MPO positive in >3% of blasts and/or presence of Auer Rods is diagnostic for AML. Absence of any of these features does not rule out AML.

Stage/Lineage	Marker
Percursor	CD34, CD38, CD117, CD133, HLA-DR
Granulocytic	CD13, CD15, CD16, CD33, CD65, cMPO
Monocytic	NSE, CD11c, CD14, CD64, lysozyme, CD4, CD11b, CD36, NG2 homologue
Megakaryocytic	CD41(gp IIb/IIIa), CD61(gp IIIa), CD42 (gp1b)
Erythroid	CD235a (glycophorin A)

Immunophenotyping

IF

Karyotyping

AML with recurrent cytogenetic abnormalities as defined by WHO 2008

Gene mutation analysis

Testing for *FLT3, NPM1, CEBPA* (*KIT* in CBF AML)

Additional features

Morphology: absence or presence of dysplasia
History: previous exposure to chemotherapy ± radiation antecedent hematologic disorder (AHD)

t(8;21)(q22;q22)
inv(16)(p13;q22)
t(16;16)(p13;q22)
t(15;17)(q23;q12)
11q23 (*MLL*)

Fig. 59.1 WORKUP OF ACUTE MYELOID LEUKEMIA. The diagnostic workup consists of a morphologic assessment, immunophenotyping by flow cytometry, assessment of the karyotype, and a panel of gene mutations. Whereas morphologic assessment by itself is often not sufficient to render a diagnosis, flow cytometry will confirm the lineage assignment (myeloid vs. lymphoid) and stage of differentiation in more than 95% of cases. In the remainder, either no lineage-specific antigens are expressed (acute undifferentiated leukemia) or antigens of more than one lineage are present (mixed-phenotype acute leukemia). In the latter scenario, antigens of several lineages can be found on one (biphenotypic) or separate populations of blasts (bilineal). Karyotyping and gene mutation analysis may add diagnostic information in morphologically ambiguous situations but is otherwise of more interest in determining prognosis. Additional information (exposure to previous chemotherapy and/or radiation therapy, history of an antecedent hematologic disorder, dysplasia) forms the basis for the 2008 revision of the WHO classification of AML (see Table 59.1). *AHD*, Antecedent hematologic disorder; *AML*, acute myeloid leukemia; *CBF*, core-binding factor; *MPO*, myeloperoxidase; *WHO*, World Health Organization.

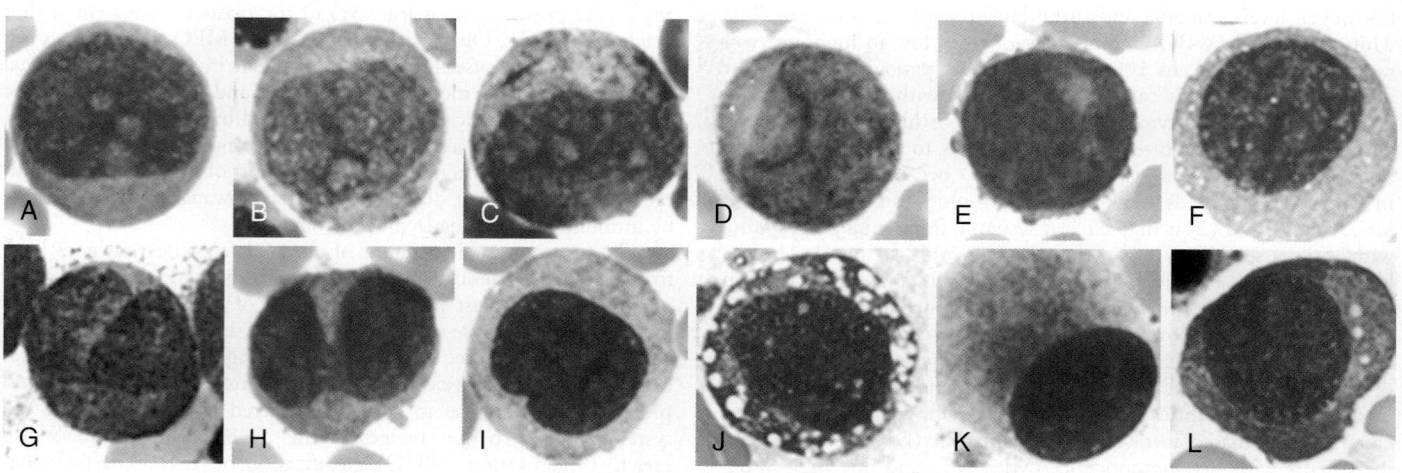

Fig. 59.2 SPECTRUM OF BLASTS, BLAST EQUIVALENTS, AND OTHER CELLS. Blast cells in acute myeloid leukemia (AML) exhibit a wide spectrum of morphologic features. The French–American–British classification described three types of blasts depending on the granule content (A–C). However, blasts with nuclear invagination (frequently associated with *NPM1* and/or *FLT3* mutations) (D); blasts with pseudopods (frequently shown to be megakaryoblasts) (E); and monoblasts (F) are also quite distinctive. Blast equivalents include granular or hypogranular promyelocytes (G and H) for acute promyelocytic leukemia, promonocytes (I) for AML with a monocytic component, and atypical pronormoblasts (frequently with cytoplasmic vacuoles) (J) for acute erythroleukemia of the pure erythroid type. Micromegakaryocytes (K) and pronormoblasts (L) are not considered blasts.

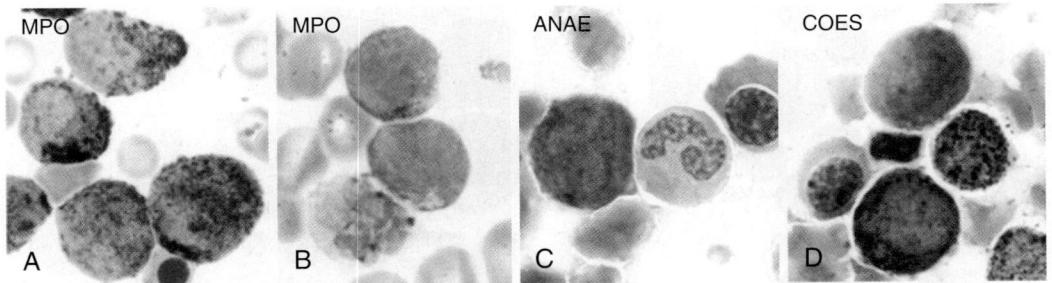

Fig. 59.3 CYTOCHEMISTRY: MYELOPEROXIDASE, α-NAPHTHYL ACETATE ESTERASE, AND COMBINED ESTERASE REACTIONS. The MPO reaction is easily performed, can be done in less than a few minutes, and provides important initial information about the lineage of the blasts, particularly in cases in which morphologic assessment is difficult. In many laboratories it is routinely performed for all new acute leukemias. The MPO reaction should be interpreted in the blast population and expressed as a percentage of blasts that are positive. (A) The positive MPO reaction is strong. (B) The reaction is weak and seen in only some blasts. A counterstain would have obscured the weak reaction product. A weak MPO reaction is not uncommon in cases of acute myeloid leukemia (AML) associated with myelodysplasia (as in [B]). The neutrophils in such cases are also only weakly positive (*bottom cell* [B]). The ANAE reaction is a nonspecific esterase reaction positive in most monocytic cells ([C] *orange-brown* cell on *left* compared to negative neutrophil, and erythroid cell, *middle* and *right*). The ANAE reaction is interpreted as positive in cells as a percentage of nonerythroid elements. A significant monocytic component is usually defined as 20% or greater of the nonerythroid elements and is usually required for making a diagnosis of acute myelomonocytic leukemia. It is notable that in some cases of AML with inv(16) (i.e., AML with abnormal eosinophils), the monocytes are ANAE negative. A COES reaction uses another nonspecific esterase reaction for monocytes, α-naphthyl butyrate esterase, together with the specific esterase, chloroacetate esterase, for granulocytes. The combination allows simultaneous evaluation of granulocytes (blue reaction product) and monocytes (orange-brown reaction product). (D) Acute myelomonocytic leukemia. A monocyte *(top)*, a granulocyte *(right)*, and a myelomonocytic hybrid cell that exhibits both the orange-brown and blue reaction products *(bottom)*. *ANAE,* α-Naphthyl acetate esterase; *COES,* combined esterase; *MPO,* myeloperoxidase.

TABLE 59.1	WHO Classification of Acute Myeloid Leukemia (2008)			
Category	**Subtype/Definition**		**Category**	**Subtype/Definition**
AML with recurrent cytogenetic abnormalities	t(8;21)(q22;q22); *RUNX1-RUNX1T1*[a]		**Myeloid sarcoma**	
	inv(16)(p13.1q22); *CBFB-MYH11*[a]		**Myeloid proliferations related to Down syndrome**	Transient abnormal myelopoiesis
	t(16;16)(p13.1q22); *CBFB-MYH11*[a]			Myeloid leukemia associated with Down syndrome
	t(15;17)(q22;q12); *PML-RARA*[a]			
	t(9;11)(p22;q23); *MLLT3-MLL*			
	t(6;9)(p23;q34); *DEK-NUP214*		**Blastic plasmacytoid dendritic cell neoplasm**	
	inv(3)(q21q26.2); *RPN1-EVI1*			
	t(3;3)(q21;q26.2); *RPN1-EVI1*			
	t(1;22)(p13q13); *RBM15-MKL1*		**Acute leukemia of ambiguous lineage**	Acute undifferentiated leukemia
AML with MDS-related changes	Morphologic features of MDS, or			Mixed phenotype acute leukemia with t(9;22)((q34;q11.2); *BCR-ABL1*
	Prior history of MDS or MDS/MPN, or			t(v;11q23); *MLL* rearranged
	MDS-related karyotype, and			Mixed phenotype acute leukemia, B/myeloid, NOS
	None of the recurrent genetic abnormalities above			Mixed phenotype acute leukemia, T/myeloid, NOS
Therapy-related myeloid neoplasms	Late complications of cytotoxic chemotherapy (alkylating agents, topoisomerase II inhibitors) and/or ionizing radiation therapy[b]		**Provisional entities**	AML with mutated *NPM1*
				AML with mutated *CEBPA*
AML, not otherwise specified	AML with minimal differentiation			NK-cell lymphoblastic leukemia/lymphoma
	AML without maturation			
	AML with maturation			
	Acute myelomonocytic leukemia			
	Acute monoblastic/monocytic leukemia			
	Acute erythroid leukemia			
	Acute megakaryoblastic leukemia			
	Acute basophilic leukemia			
	Acute panmyelosis with myelofibrosis			

[a]Diagnosis of AML regardless of percent blasts
[b]Excluded are patients with AML who have transformed from MPN
AML, Acute myeloid leukemia; MDS, myelodysplastic syndrome; MPN, myeloproliferative neoplasm; NK, natural killer cell; NOS, not otherwise specified.

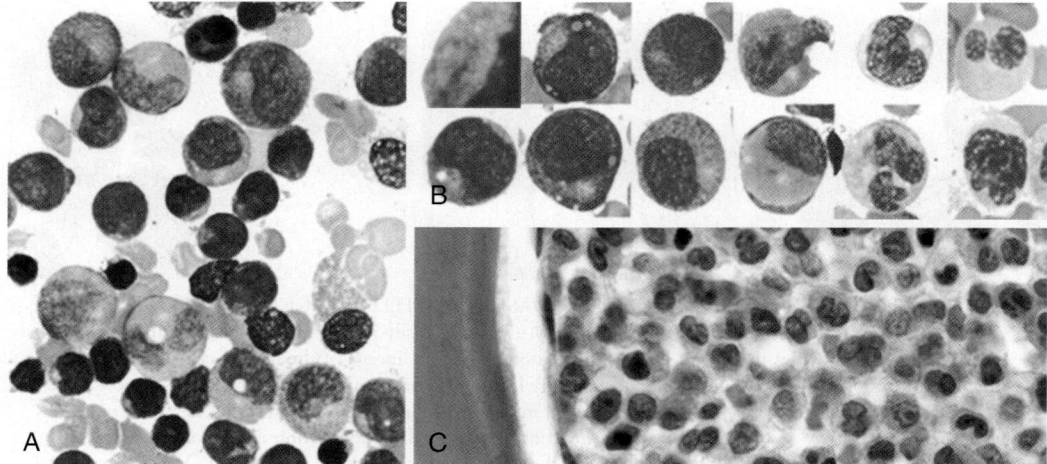

Fig. 59.4 ACUTE MYELOID LEUKEMIA WITH t(8;21)(q22;q22), (*RUNX1-RUNX1T1*). (A) Low-power, Wright-stained bone marrow aspirate smear showing increased blasts associated with differentiating myeloid cells. (B) Details illustrating some of the features associated with this leukemia. They include blasts with long thin Auer rods *(top left)*, immature cells with abnormal eosinophilic globules *(top and bottom, second from left)*, abnormal salmon-colored granulation in the maturing cells, sometimes associated with a basophilic periphery *(top and bottom, fourth from left)*, and slightly abnormal features in the mature neutrophils *(far right)*. Pseudo–Chediak-Higashi granules were not seen in this case. (C) Biopsy specimen illustrates the significant degree of maturation that can sometimes be seen. In fact, in some cases the blast count can be less than 20%, but the diagnosis of acute myeloid leukemia is still made with the cytogenetic finding of t(8;21).

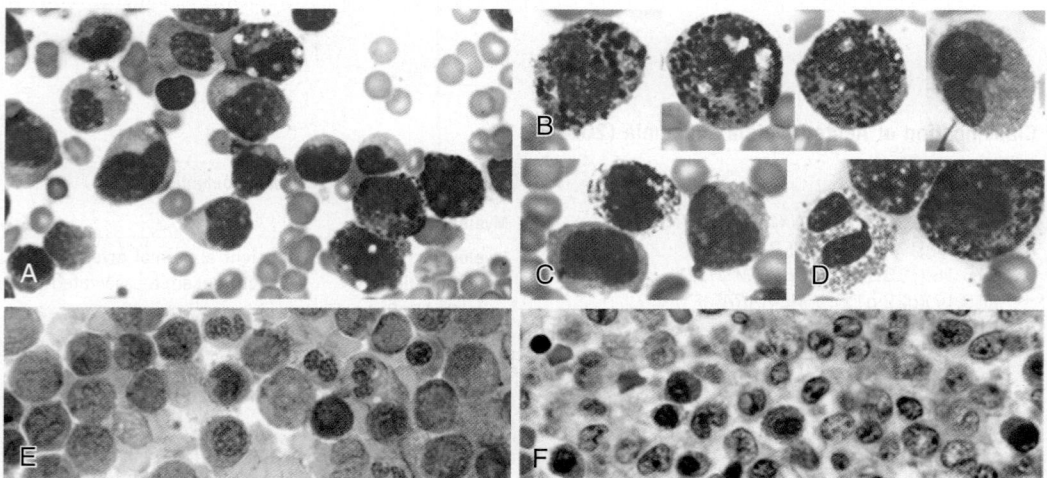

Fig. 59.5 ACUTE MYELOID LEUKEMIA WITH ABNORMAL BONE MARROW EOSINOPHILS AND INV(16)(p13.1;q22) OR t(16;16)(p13.1;q22), (*CBFB-MYH11*). (A) Low-power, Wright-stained bone marrow aspirate showing blasts, monocytic cells, granulocytic cells, and abnormal eosinophils. (B) Features of the abnormal eosinophils in three abnormal eosinophils *(left three cells)*. Note the abnormal basophilic granules in the eosinophilic myelocytes. These granules are large, tend to cluster or coalesce, and are interspersed among the large eosinophilic granules, which are more difficult to see. As the eosinophils mature, the abnormal basophilic granules are less prominent and sometimes disappear *(far right)*. A common misconception is that the basophilic granules are the granules of basophils and that the abnormal eosinophils are "hybrid cells." (C) A basophil in the same case *(top cell)* for comparison. (D) Cells from a case of reactive eosinophilia, also for comparison. Immature eosinophils *(cell to the right)* do have primary blue granules. However, they are usually less prominent and less atypical than the basophilic granules of the abnormal eosinophils. It is notable that the monocytes in cases of AML with inv(16) or t(16;16) are sometimes α-naphthyl acetate esterase (ANAE) reaction negative. (E) Negative ANAE reaction. (F) Abnormal eosinophils cannot be recognized in hematoxylin and eosin-stained sections of the biopsy.

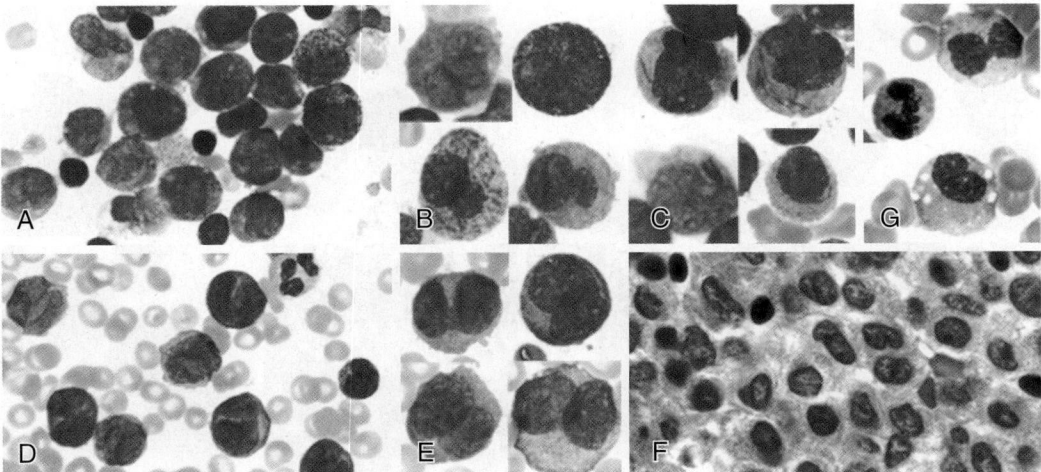

Fig. 59.6 ACUTE PROMYELOCYTIC LEUKEMIA, ACUTE MYELOID LEUKEMIA WITH t(15;17) (q22;q12), (*PML-RARA*). (A–C) Acute promyelocytic leukemia (APL). (D and E) Hypogranular or microgranular subtype. (F) Bone marrow biopsy. (G) APL cells maturing after all-trans retinoic acid (ATRA) therapy. In the typical granular type of APL (A), the abnormal promyelocytes can exhibit variable morphologic features. Even within the same case, the granules can range from coarse, dark, and dense to fine and dust-like (B). The nuclei in the abnormal promyelocytes frequently exhibit a bilobed, dumbbell, or reniform shape. This is a diagnostically important feature, which can sometimes be difficult to recognize beneath the granules (B). Auer rods can be single, multiple, coalesced into Auer bodies, and even present in maturing cells (C). The microgranular type usually presents with an elevated white blood cell count (D). Although granules cannot be readily appreciated at the light microscope (E), granules can be demonstrated by electron microscopy. The abnormal nuclear shapes (bilobed, dumbbell, and reniform) can be easily appreciated (E). Bone core biopsy sample typically shows sheets of cells with abundant granular cytoplasm (F). After ATRA therapy the abnormal promyelocytes mature to abnormal neutrophils ([G] *top and bottom right*, compared with normal neutrophil, *left*). These can be seen for weeks after therapy and do not signify a failed response to the differentiating agent.

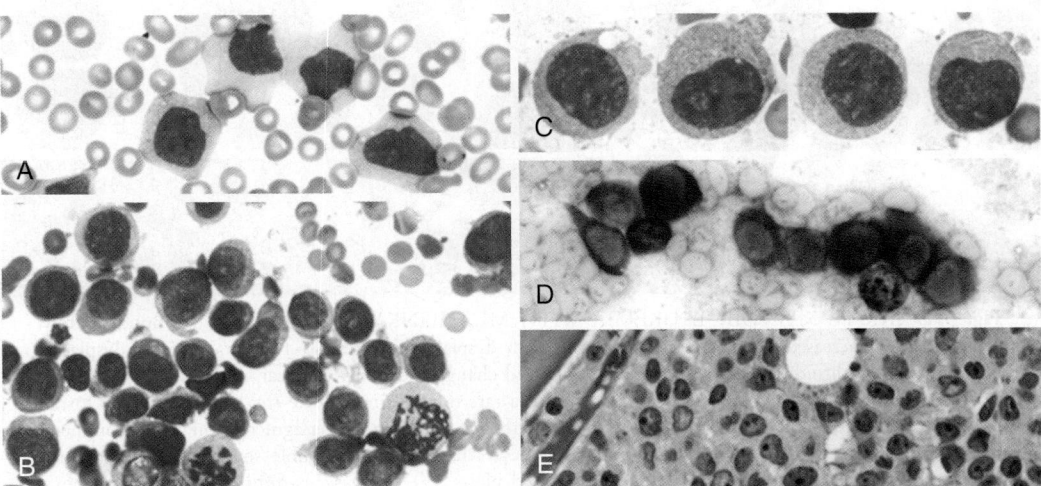

Fig. 59.7 ACUTE MONOBLASTIC LEUKEMIA WITH t(9;11)(p22;q23), (*MLLT3-MLL*). Acute monoblastic leukemia with t(9;11). (A) Such cases typically present with high counts because of circulating monoblasts. (B and C) Bone marrow aspirate is packed with monoblasts and shows few granulocytic elements. (D) Absence of a granulocytic component can be illustrated with the combined esterase reaction, in which most of the cells show the α-naphthyl butyrate reaction product *(orange-brown)*, with only rare granulocytes with the blue reaction product from the chloroacetate esterase reaction. (E) The biopsy sample is usually packed with sheets of monoblasts with fine nuclear chromatin and abundant pink cytoplasm.

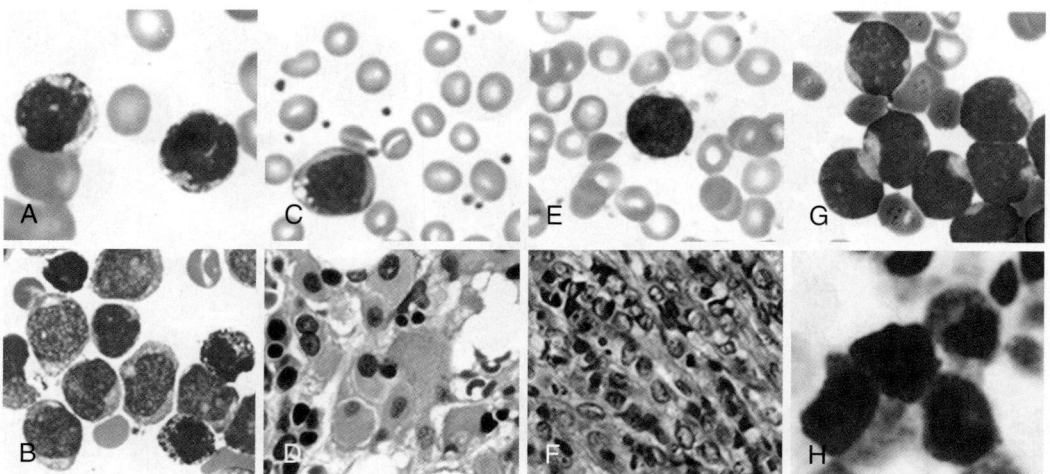

Fig. 59.8 ACUTE MYELOID LEUKEMIA WITH LESS COMMON CYTOGENETIC AND GENETIC CHANGES. (A and B) Acute myeloid leukemia (AML) with t(6;9)(p23;q34). These cases are characterized by marrow dysplasia and basophilia. However, the morphologic characteristics can be quite varied among cases. AML with inv(3)(q21q26.2) or t(3;3)(q21;q26.2) is characterized by normal or high platelet counts, (C) and by a bone marrow with numerous micromegakaryocytes (D). AML with t(1;22)(p13;q13) is uncommon and occurs in infants. The blasts are megakaryoblasts (E) but in the bone marrow can have a sarcomatous appearance (F). AML with *NMP1* or *NPM1* and *FLT3* mutations frequently presents with high peripheral blast counts, and the blasts sometimes have nuclear invaginations (G). *NPM1* mutation is associated with the abnormal cytoplasmic localization of *NPM1* rather than the normal nuclear staining (H).

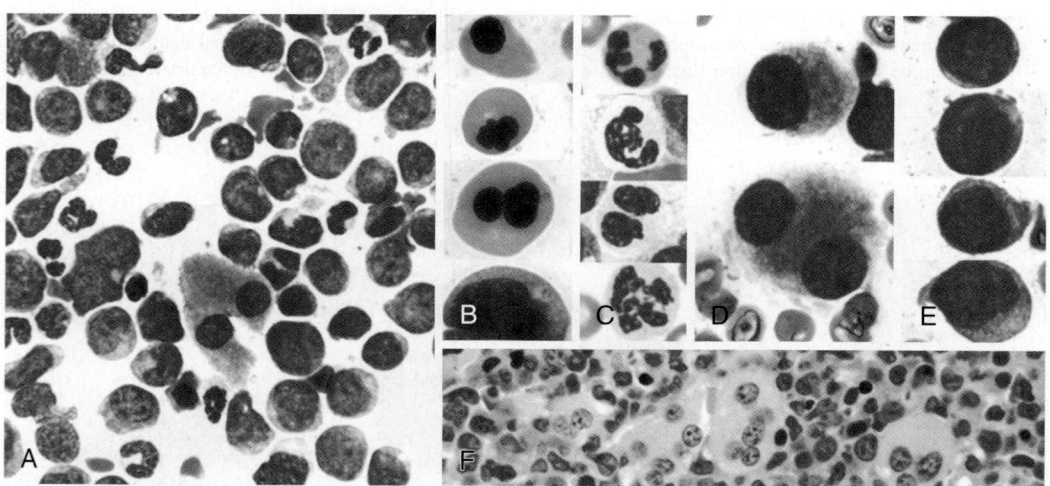

Fig. 59.9 ACUTE MYELOID LEUKEMIA WITH MULTILINEAGE DYSPLASIA. (A) Bone marrow aspirate shows increased blasts and maturing cells with dysplastic features. (B–D) Details of the dysplasia. (B) Maturing erythroid elements exhibit megaloblastoid change and bizarre nuclear abnormalities. (C) Dysplastic granulocytes *(bottom three)* are compared with a rare normal granulocyte *(top)*. The dysplastic forms have pale cytoplasm and abnormal nuclear shapes with hypolobation, hypersegmentation, and prominent nuclear excrescences. (D) Dysplastic micromegakaryocytes have single or double small nuclei but mature cytoplasm with platelet material within. (E) Increased blasts. (F) Dysplasia is difficult to appreciate on a biopsied section. This is true except for the megakaryocytes. Dysplastic megakaryocytes can be recognized on the biopsy specimen by their abnormally small nuclei, which are sometimes multiple and widely spaced.

subtypes are AML with t(6;9)(p23;q34), *DEK-NUP214*; AML with inv(3)(q21q26.2) or t(3;3)(q21;q26.2), *RPN1-EVI1*; and AML with t(1;22) (p13;q13), *RBM15-MKL1* (Fig. 59.8). Diploid AML with mutations of the nucleophosmin gene (*NPM1*; see Fig. 59.8G and H), and *CEBPA* (and in the absence of additional mutations) have been assigned a provisional status. This group of AML is expected to expand with subsequent editions.

2) AML with myelodysplasia-related changes is defined in one of three ways: a) AML in patients with a preceding history of MDS; b) AML with multilineage dysplasia recognized morphologically (Fig. 59.9); and c) AML associated with a myelodysplasia-related cytogenetic abnormality.

3) The category of therapy-related AML was retained from the 2001 WHO classification, although the distinctions between AML associated with alkylating agents or radiation and those with topoisomerase II inhibitors were abandoned. Many patients receive complex therapeutic regimens, making this distinction difficult and impractical.

4) Not otherwise specified subtypes of AML are a "wastebasket" of sorts for AML cases that do not fit the categories already described

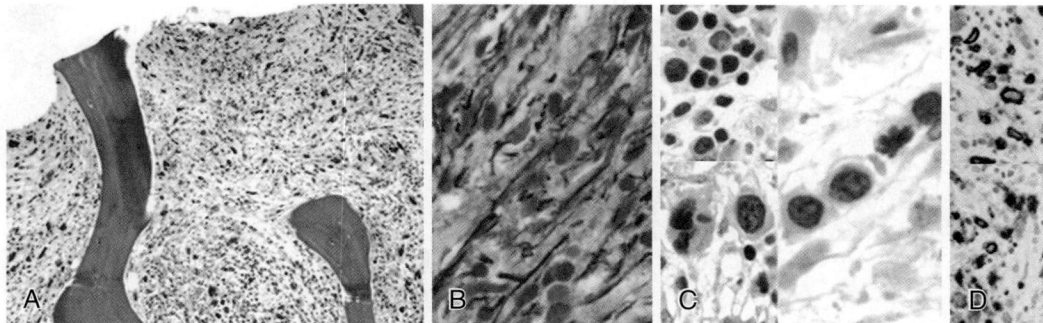

Fig. 59.10 ACUTE PANMYELOSIS WITH MYELOFIBROSIS. (A) Bone marrow biopsy specimen shows a loosely packed marrow with a swirling appearance to the cellular elements due to underlying fibrosis. (B) The latter is illustrated on the reticulin stain. (C) Proliferations of erythroid cells *(top left)*, megakaryocytes *(bottom left)*, and immature cells within the fibrotic areas *(right)*. (D) Immunohistochemical staining shows increased megakaryocytes *(top,* CD61) and increased blasts *(bottom,* CD34).

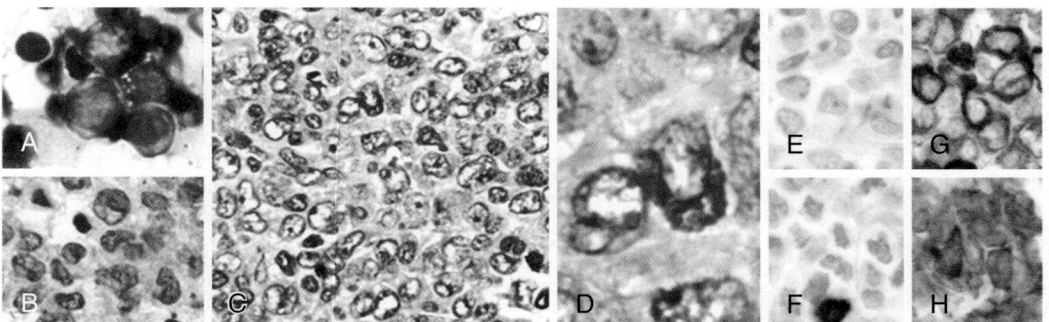

Fig. 59.11 MYELOID SARCOMA. Myeloid sarcomas can sometimes present a diagnostic challenge. In this case the touch imprints (A) and frozen section preparation (B) from a mass lesion in the cecal area from a 44-year-old patient were thought to represent a high-grade lymphoma. However, initial immunohistochemical stains did not support the diagnosis, and on closer inspection of the tumor and with subsequent immunomarkers, a diagnosis could be reached. The tumor (C) is composed of sheets of noncohesive cells. A diagnostic clue to the origin was the presence of eosinophilic myelocytes (D), which indicate that some tumor cells have the capacity to differentiate into eosinophils. The granules of neutrophilic myelocytes cannot be recognized on tissue section. The immunohistochemical stains showed the cell to be CD45+ (not shown), (B) and T marker negative (E and F), but myeloid marker (myeloperoxidase and CD33) positive (G and H). Cytogenetic analysis showed the case was inv(16)(p13.1;q22).

and for the most part are classified using the FAB scheme (AML with minimal differentiation, AML without maturation, acute myelomonocytic leukemia, acute monocytic or monoblastic leukemia, acute erythroleukemia, acute megakaryoblastic leukemia, AML with maturation, acute basophilic leukemia). The AML-like disease of acute panmyelosis with myelofibrosis is included here (Fig. 59.10).

5) Lastly, the classification now includes myeloid sarcoma (Fig. 59.11), myeloid proliferations associated with Down syndrome (see chapter), and the rather rare entity of blastic plasmacytoid dendritic cell neoplasm (Fig. 59.12).

PROGNOSIS

Prognosis in AML is dependent on patient- and disease-related factors. The former determine the likelihood of surviving induction chemotherapy and are strongly influenced by age, performance status, and a basic assessment of organ function (hepatic, renal, cardiac).[4] There is no standardized assessment tool and physicians may variably apply weighted integer prognostic scores or comorbidity scores such as the Charlson comorbidity index and the hematopoietic cell transplantation comorbidity index. Comorbidity indices (ideally as part of a more global geriatric assessment strategy) are particularly useful in older patients where the question of intensive chemotherapy versus

lower intensity interventions assumes more significance. Disease-related factors determine resistance to therapy. They include antecedent hematologic disorders (e.g., MDS), prior exposure to chemotherapy or radiation therapy (therapy-related AML), and biologic features of the blasts. Among the latter, karyotype has historically been considered as the most important prognostic factor dividing patients into those with favorable (CBF leukemias associated with t(8;21) and inv(16) or t(16;16); APL with t(15;17)), unfavorable (complex abnormalities and monosomies, among others), and intermediate prognosis (mainly diploid; Fig. 59.13).[5]

Karyotype is increasingly supplemented by analyses of commonly mutated genes. Whereas prognosis is hardly or not at all augmented by gene mutation testing in cytogenetically favorable and unfavorable groups, the situation is different in the intermediate-risk group, which is characterized by its size and heterogeneity in outcome. It is here where fine tuning of prognostic markers matters most. Early identified commonly mutated genes (FMS-like tyrosine kinase-3 [FLT3], NPM1, CEBPA) have formed the basis of many revised cytogenetic–molecular risk stratifications which led to identification of patients with more favorable outcome (e.g., diploid and $NPM1^{mutated}/FLT3\text{-}ITD^{wild\text{-}type}$ or $CEBPA^{double\ allele\ mutated}/FLT3\text{-}ITD^{wild\text{-}type}$) and others with unfavorable prognosis ($FLT3\text{-}ITD^{mutated}$; $KIT^{mutated}$ in CBF AML). Ongoing efforts at whole-genome sequencing have identified additional repetitively mutated genes that are being considered in risk assessment with partly incongruous results (e.g., KIT,

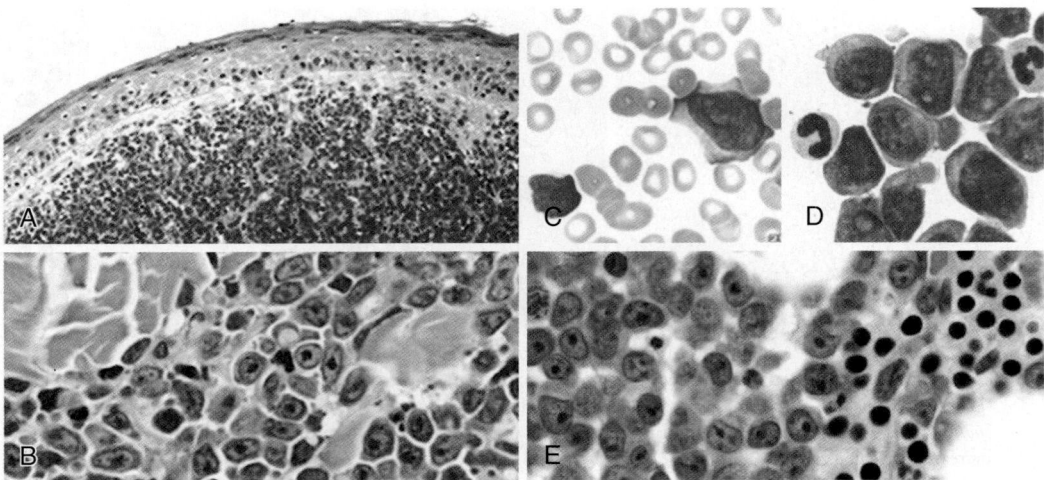

Fig. 59.12 BLASTIC PLASMACYTOID DENDRITIC CELL NEOPLASM. The blastic plasmacytoid dendritic cell tumor is an unusually aggressive malignancy that was previously called *hematodermic* malignancy. It is now classified in the acute myeloid leukemia category of myeloid neoplasms. It frequently presents in the skin with a blastic proliferation of cells in the dermis (A and B), which inevitably spreads to the blood (C) and bone marrow (D and E).

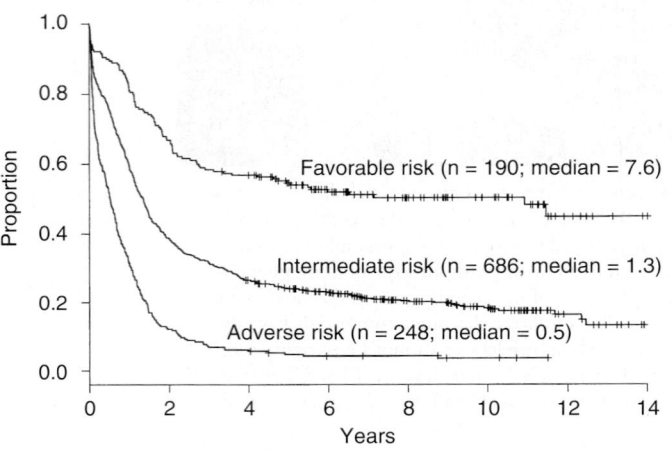

Fig. 59.13 DISEASE-FREE SURVIVAL BY CYTOGENETIC RISK GROUP. *(Data from Byrd JC, Mrózek K, Dodge RK, et al: Pretreatment cytogenetic abnormalities are predictive of induction success, cumulative incidence of relapse, and overall survival in adult patients with de novo acute myeloid leukemia: Results from Cancer and Leukemia Group B [CALGB 8461],* Blood *100:4325, 2002.)*

TABLE 59.2	Risk Groups Based on Cytogenetic-Molecular Features (According to European Leukemia Net)		
Risk Group	**Karyotype**	**Molecular Abnormality**	**Estimated 4-Year Survival (%)**
Favorable	t(15;17)	PML-RARa	60-80+
	t(8;21)	AML-ETO (KIT^wt)	
	inv(16)	CBFB-MYH11 (KIT^wt)	
	t(16;16)	CBFB-MYH11 (KIT^wt)	
		CEBPAdm (CN) (FLT3-ITD^wt)	
		NPM1mut (FLT3-ITD^wt)	
Intermediate-1	t(8;21)	NPM1mut/FLT3-ITD^mut	30-50
	inv(16)	NPM1wt/FLT3-ITD^mut	
	t(16;16)	NPM1wt/FLT3-ITD^wt	
		AML-ETO1 plus KIT^mut	
		CBFB-MYH11 plus KIT^mut	
		CBFB-MYH11 plus KIT^mut	
Intermediate-2	t(9;11)	KMT2A-MLLT3	20-40
	Karyotype neither favorable nor adverse		
Adverse	inv(3)	RPN1-EVI1	< 10-15
	t(3;3)	RPN1-EVI1	
	t(6;9)	DEK-NUP24	
	t(v;11)	KMT2A (formerly MLL) *rearranged*	
	-5; del(5q); -7		
	Abnl 17p	TP53	
	Complex		
	Monosomal		

abnl, Abnormal; *CN,* cytogenetic normal (diploid); *dm,* double allelic mutation; *mut,* mutated; *Wt,* wild type (unmutated).

Data from Döhner H, Estey EH, Amadori S, et al: Diagnosis and management of acute myeloid leukemia in adults: recommendations from an international expert panel, on behalf of the European LeukemiaNet. *Blood* 115:453, 2010.

IDH1 and *IDH2, MLL-PTD, TET2, DNMT3A, ASXL1, RUNX1, PHF6, TP53*).[6] In general practice, testing is recommended for mutations of *NPM1, CEBPA,* and *FLT3* in all patients with a new presentation of AML, and *KIT* in patients with CBF AML. The European Leukemia Net has published a revised risk model based on integration of cytogenetic and gene mutation information (Table 59.2).[7]

Assessment of posttherapy response provides additional valuable information. Traditional criteria such as achievement of complete morphologic remission (CR) after one course of induction therapy retain significance, whereas others (assessment of early blast response based on a midcycle marrow evaluation during standard induction therapy) are of more limited predictability. The most powerful posttreatment prognostic factor is MRD. MRD is defined as disease that remains below the threshold of detection by morphology and immunohistochemical assays. It is estimated that patients in morphologic CR still harbor up to 10^9 leukemic cells, which constitute an important reservoir for later recurrences. Assessing MRD has several advantages: (1) better determination of the quality of response, (2) more timely diagnosis of an impending relapse and improvement of

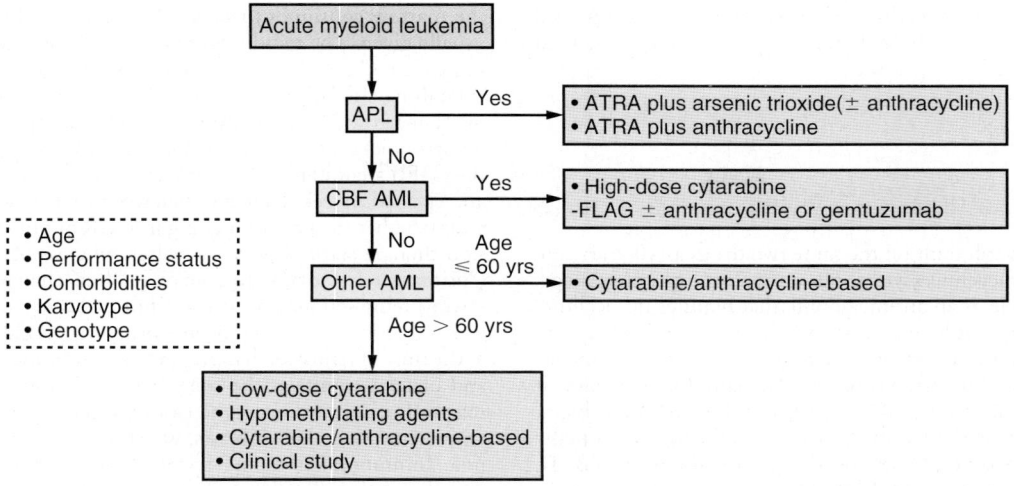

Fig. 59.14 GENERAL APPROACH TO ACUTE MYELOID LEUKEMIA THERAPY. *AML*, Acute myeloid leukemia; *APL*, acute promyelocytic leukemia; *ATRA*, all-trans retinoic acid; *CBF*, core binding factor; *FLAG*, fludarabine, cytarabine (ara-C), and granulocyte colony-stimulating factor.

outcome by early intervention, and (3) support in decision to intensify postremission therapy (transplant) or not. Efficacy of preemptive therapy based on MRD has been established for APL but data in support for other subtypes of AML are still accumulating.

MRD can be detected by reverse-transcriptase polymerase chain reaction (RT-PCR) or multiparameter flow cytometry (MPFC). Both assays have comparable sensitivity. RT-PCR requires a suitable molecular target such as fusion transcripts (e.g., *PML-RARA, RUNX1-RUNX1T1, CBFB-MYH11, DEK-CAN*) or overexpressed (WT1) or mutated genes, and thus applies to a more limited number of patients than MPFC. MPFC is based on the identification of a leukemia-associated immunophenotype, which can be detected in the majority of patients with AML in various ways: a) "different-from-normal" antigen expression in leukemic blasts; b) detection of lineage-foreign markers; c) asynchronous expression of markers; d) altered density of surface antigens; e) detection of surrogate marker profiles (associated with cytogenetic–molecular markers); f) detection of leukemia stem cells.[8] Commonly, a level of 0.1% has been determined to distinguish patients with MRD from those without. This level is a log higher than what defines the threshold for MRD in ALL (<0.01%). MRD levels following induction or early in consolidation have been associated with relapse and survival in all age groups regardless of cytogenetic and mutational status. Even though MRD levels tend to be higher in patients with unfavorable pretreatment characteristics, the prognostic impact of MRD extends to all risk groups and has shown to improve standard risk classification independently of cytogenetic–molecular markers. Evaluation of MRD has led to renewed interest in strategies for its elimination. Besides intensification of therapy by means of hematopoietic stem cell transplantation (HSCT) as a response to persistence of MRD, other approaches have been or are being pursued: maintenance therapy (interleukin-2 [IL-2] based), cellular therapy (dendritic cell vaccination, T-cell manipulations), monoclonal antibodies (e.g., anti-CD123), epigenetic priming, or maintenance.

THERAPY: FRONTLINE

AML therapy is one of the most challenging of oncologic interventions. Treatment often needs to be fast, physicians need to deal with a multitude of complications (disease or treatment related), and from the start a patient's condition can deteriorate rapidly. Given its complexity, treatment of patients with AML requires a multidisciplinary effort including oncologists, pharmacists, a well-educated and committed nursing staff, and various consulting services (e.g., infectious disease, pulmonology, nephrology, cardiology). Supportive care

measures including transfusion services and symptom control have played an important part in improving the outcome of patients with AML over the last decade.

The general approach to AML therapy is summarized in Fig. 59.14. Besides AML subtype (APL, CBF leukemias, other) attention needs to be paid to age and a more global assessment of fitness (performance status, comorbidities, geriatric assessment scores). Treatment of patients "unfit" for standard intensive induction therapy (often equaled to patients older than 60 to 65 years) is frequently approached differently from that of younger patients, and hence this chapter addresses therapy separately for each age group. It should be understood, though, that age alone is increasingly considered inadequate to assess a patient's fitness status.

Treatment of AML consists of induction and postremission therapy. The goal of induction is to produce a CR and that of postremission therapy to maintain it by eliminating residual disease. CR is defined as achievement after chemotherapy of less than 5% marrow blasts, a neutrophil count of greater than 1000/μL, a platelet count of greater than 100,000/μL, independence of red blood cell transfusions, and resolution of all signs and symptoms referable to AML. CR defines a landmark point in time because patients who achieve CR on any given day after beginning therapy have longer survival subsequent to that day than patients who are resistant to therapy on the day in question. Lesser response criteria (CR without platelet recovery, CR with incomplete blood recovery including neutropenia, partial remission, morphologic leukemia-free state) may serve as useful end points in the context of investigational studies (phase I, II, or III), but they do not carry the same significance for survival as does CR. Postremission therapy consists of repeated cycles of chemotherapy or HSCT in its various forms (autologous, allogeneic, haploidentical, cord blood, reduced intensity). The role of HSCT for AML therapy will be the topic of a separate chapter of this book. The debate as to which patients should receive chemotherapy consolidation versus HSCT is most divisive for patients with intermediate-risk disease. In this population, characterization of the genotype has become helpful in guiding that decision.

Leukemia has been at the forefront of the development of "targeted" therapy, mostly small-molecule drugs directed against defined intracellular proteins (e.g., kinases). Given the increasing number of genetic abnormalities and the identification of diverse intracellular pathways of blast cells, the specter of "personalized therapy" looms high in AML therapy. Yet, despite intense research activity, to date no "targeted" drug has been approved for any type of AML (exceptions: gemtuzumab ozogamicin [GO], an anti-CD33 monoclonal antibody–calicheamicin conjugate with activity in some subtypes of AML was approved in 2000, but then withdrawn in the United States in 2010; decitabine, a DNA methyltransferase inhibitor, was approved in 2013 for older patients with AML in Europe, but not in the United States).

Induction Therapy

Patients Less Than 60 Years of Age

Induction therapy is still built on the same two drugs as 40 years ago: cytarabine and anthracycline. Cytarabine, an analogue of a physiologic pyrimidine nucleoside, is an antimetabolite that requires intracellular conversion to its triphosphate compound, ara-CTP, and incorporation into DNA to become active. When given by itself at standard doses of 100–200 mg/m^2 intravenously (IV) daily for 5–7 days, it produces CR rates of around 40%. Anthracyclines (daunorubicin, idarubicin, mitoxantrone, aclarubicin) act by stabilizing the normally occurring complex between DNA and the enzyme topoisomerase II, thereby leading to apoptotic cell death. Daunorubicin, the anthracycline that was first available, achieves similar CR rates as does cytarabine alone. The combination of cytarabine 100–200 mg/m^2 as a continuous IV infusion (its serum half-life is only 15 minutes) daily for 7 days and daunorubicin 45–60 mg/m^2 IV daily for 3 days on days 1–3 has become known as the "3 + 7" regimen and, for more than 40 years, has been the standard induction combination for most patients with AML. Remission rates range from 60% to 80%, and long-term disease-free survival is about 35%.[9]

In clinical practice, patients undergo a repeat marrow study between 14 and 21 days from the start of treatment (Fig. 59.15). If the marrow continues to show blasts and is cellular, a reinduction is usually given. The reinduction may be an attenuated repetition of the induction ("2 + 5") or an intensification with intermediate-dose cytarabine (IDAC) or high-dose cytarabine (HiDAC). If the day 14 or 21 marrow is hypoplastic and hence appropriately chemoablated, hematopoietic growth factors (granulocyte colony-stimulating factor [G-CSF]) are initiated and supportive care continues. Marrow studies are repeated 2 weeks later and then weekly if necessary until it becomes clear whether the patient is going into CR or not. If in CR, postremission therapy starts shortly thereafter, whereas in case of no response ("primary refractory"), treatment is often changed. Remissions following reinductions are usually shorter lasting than remission after one induction cycle. The degree of neutrophil and platelet recovery at the time of remission has prognostic significance. Higher neutrophil and platelet counts at the time of remission are predictive of better relapse-free survival. In some cases a regenerating marrow may have an increased number of blasts, which may look like persistent leukemia. Immunophenotyping by flow cytometry often helps to make that distinction. Further follow-up marrow studies will show reduction in blasts concomitant with a rise of neutrophils and platelets.

Many modifications to the 3 + 7 regimen have been tried over the years. Giving 10 instead of 7 days of cytarabine (3 + 10), increasing the dose of cytarabine from 100 mg/m^2/day to 200 mg/m^2/day, adding a third drug (e.g., etoposide, thioguanine, topotecan, fludarabine) or modulators of drug resistance, and priming leukemic blasts with hematopoietic growth factors (G-CSF and granulocyte-macrophage colony stimulating factor) have not proven superior.

However, in 2012, the Polish Adult Leukemia Group published the outcome of an open-label, randomized study where addition of

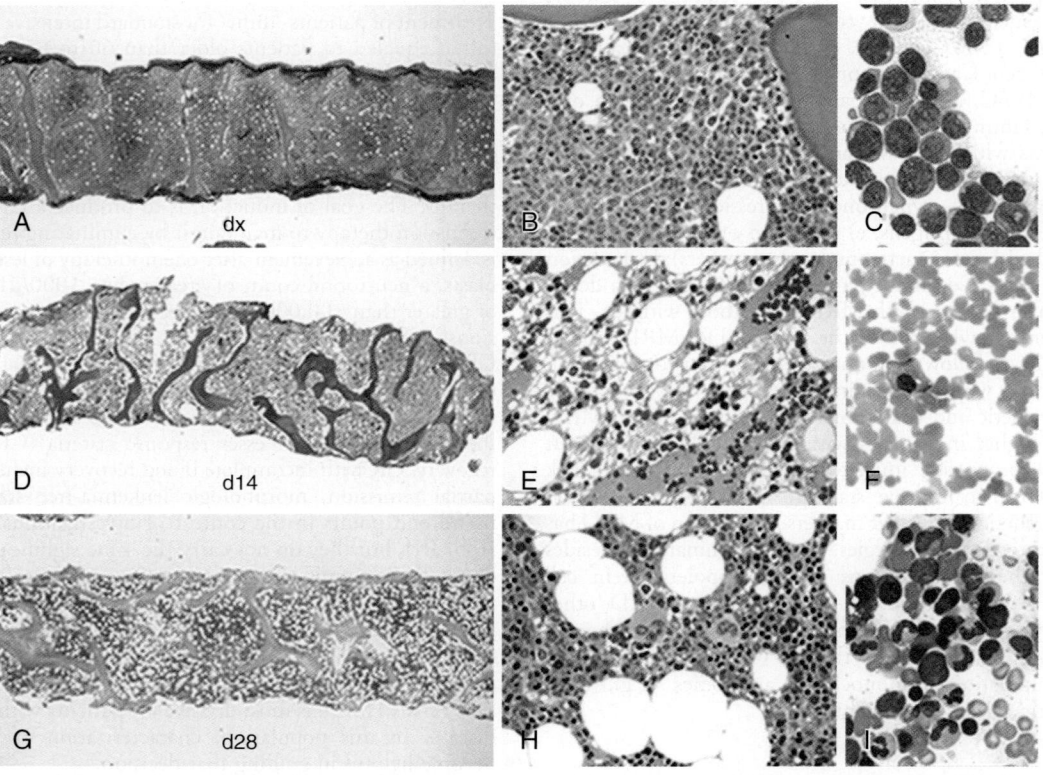

Fig. 59.15 ACUTE MYELOID LEUKEMIA AT DIAGNOSIS AND AT DAY 14 AND DAY 28 FOLLOWING THE START OF STANDARD INDUCTION CHEMOTHERAPY. A 43-year-old man presented with fatigue and was found to have a white blood cell count of 70,300/μL composed of mostly blasts. A bone marrow study (A–C) showed a 90% cellular marrow packed with blasts (80%). The blasts were myeloperoxidase positive and had the following phenotype: CD34$^+$, HLA-DR$^+$, CD117$^+$, CD13$^+$, CD33$^+$ with partial CD15 and CD11b. Cytogenetic analysis demonstrated a normal male karyotype, and molecular studies showed wild-type *FLT3* and *NPM1*. The patient was treated with standard induction chemotherapy, and a day-14 bone marrow study (D–F) showed chemoablation effects with an empty marrow, stromal injury, dilated sinuses, and only scattered stromal cells and plasma cells with no obvious blasts. A bone marrow study performed at day 28 (G–I) showed regenerative changes of trilineage hematopoiesis.

cladribine, but not fludarabine, to a standard daunorubicin/cytarabine backbone resulted in significantly increased rates for remission (68% versus 56%; $p = .01$) and 3-year overall survival (OS; 45% versus 33%; $p = .02$). In a publication in 2013 by the MD Anderson Cancer Center, addition of clofarabine, a second-generation nucleoside analog, to idarubicin and cytarabine (IA) led to significantly better event-free and OS in the three drug combination when compared with a historical IA-treated group, especially in patients younger than 40 years of age. The use of fludarabine, idarubicin, HD-AC versus 3 + 7 in the Medical Research Council (MRC) trials is discussed later.

The choice and dose of anthracyclines has been the subject of debate. Substitution of daunorubicin by doxorubicin produced more toxicity without added benefit. Idarubicin is a 4-demethoxy anthracycline analogue of daunorubicin, which results in increased lipophilicity and better cellular uptake compared with daunorubicin.

A study by the Eastern Cooperative Oncology Group (ECOG 1900) randomized patients between the ages of 17 and 60 years with untreated AML to a 3 + 7 combination with either standard-dose daunorubicin (45 mg/m² daily × 3) or high-dose daunorubicin (90 mg/m² daily × 3).[10] High-dose daunorubicin achieved higher rates of CR (70.6% versus 57.3%, $p < .001$) and improved median OS (23.7 months versus 15.7 months, $p = .003$). This improvement was limited to patients younger than 50 years and with intermediate cytogenetics in the absence of *FLT3* mutations. A more recent follow-up of the study suggested that the benefit extends to all cytogenetic risk groups regardless of age. The study also found a significant association with improved survival between the high-dose daunorubicin arm and presence of *DNMT3A* mutations.[6] The daunorubicin dose of 90 mg/m²/day did not lead to a higher incidence of adverse events (particularly cardiomyopathy and infectious complications). The study can be criticized on the basis that the dose of the comparator arm, daunorubicin 45 mg/m² daily for 3 days, is no longer considered the standard of care in AML, and instead 60 mg/m²/dose should be considered standard. A recent MRC trial compared daunorubicin 60 mg/m² versus 90 mg/m² during induction and showed equivalent results (Burnett ASH 2014). Daunorubicin 90 mg/m² daily × 3 equals 270 mg/m², which may prohibit further anthracyclines therapy (cumulative cardiotoxic dose of daunorubicin 360–450 mg/m²).

A metaanalysis of 29 randomized controlled trials compared the efficacy of different anthracyclines and dosing schedules during AML induction therapy.[11] Idarubicin compared with daunorubicin improved remission rates, although this effect was limited to studies with a daunorubicin/idarubicin ratio of <5. Likewise, higher dose compared with lower dose daunorubicin improved remission rates. Survival estimates suggest that both high-dose daunorubicin (90 mg/m²/dose × 3 days or 50 mg/m²/dose × 5 days) and idarubicin (12 mg/m²/dose × 3) can achieve 5-year survival rates of between 40% and 50%. Rather than the type of anthracycline, what matters most is to use equitoxic doses.

A metaanalysis of trials using HiDAC during induction encompassed 1691 patients and arrived at the following conclusions: there were no differences between HiDAC and standard-dose cytarabine (SDAC) with respect to percent CR and rates of persisting leukemia and early death; 4-year OS and recurrence-free survival, on the other hand, were significantly better with HiDAC but at the cost of more toxicities (infections, nausea/vomiting, CNS).[12] HiDAC benefited mostly patients who already were more likely to achieve CR (i.e., patients with intermediate and favorable karyotype). The major drawback of HiDAC during induction is that it may make further consolidation therapy difficult.

The MRC AML 15 trial randomized 1268 patients to receive fludarabine, high-dose cytarabine (ara-C), G-CSF, and idarubicin (FLAG-Ida; fludarabine 30 mg/m² on days 2–6, cytarabine 2 g/m² on days 2–6, idarubicin 10 mg/m² on days 4–6, and G-CSF on days 1–7) and 1983 to receive cytarabine (ara-C), daunorubicin, and etoposide (ADE; daunorubicin 50 mg/m² on days 1, 3, 5; cytarabine 100 mg/m² on days 1–8; and etoposide 100 mg/m² on days 1–5), the latter representing the SDAC arm.[13] FLAG-Ida resulted in higher

response rates following the first induction and fewer patients on FLAG-Ida relapsed. However, more myelosuppression and deaths in CR offset the survival benefit unless FLAG-Ida treated patients were able to receive four courses (FLAG-ida × 2, HiDAC × 2) where 8-year survival was 63% for patients (versus 47% with 3 + 7) with intermediate risk and 95% for those with favorable risk.

The European Organization for Research and Treatment of Cancer (EORTC)-Italian Group for Haematological Diseases in Adults (GIMEMA) AML-12 trial randomized 1942 newly diagnosed AML patients between 15 and 60 years of age to an induction with SDAC or HiDAC (3 g/m² every 12 hours on days 1, 3, 5, and 7).[14] With 6-year of follow up the study demonstrated significantly higher CR rates in all patients and significantly improved event-free (43.6% versus 35.1%; $p = .003$) and OS (51.9% versus 43.3%; $p = .009$) for patients between 15 and 45 years of age. The impact on survival was particularly evident in younger patients with secondary AML, high-risk cytogenetics, and mutations of *FLT3*, emphasizing that HiDAC may overcome poor-risk features during induction that SDAC cannot.

Patients Aged 60 Years or Older

In an analysis of SEER data spanning the years from 1977 to 2006, the 1- and 2-year OS of patients aged 65–74, 75–84, and >85 years was only 30.3%, 14.8%, 7.8%, and 15.8%, 5% and 1.7%, respectively.[15] Although AML is mostly diagnosed in patients over age 60 years, available AML therapy has had its least impact in this age group and prognosis has not appreciably changed to the better in decades. Older patients do worse for various reasons. Comorbidities are frequent, and they are more likely to have a poor performance status. Hence, tolerance to the myelosuppressive and immunosuppressive consequences of intensive chemotherapy is diminished. There are also differences intrinsic to the blast biology between older and younger patients. Patients over 60 years of age are more likely to have secondary AML (following MDS or another antecedent hematologic disorder), demonstrate unfavorable cytogenetics, have reduced sensitivity to anthracyclines, and more often express multidrug-resistant phenotypes. Assuming that therapy is mostly futile and palliation more appropriate, only about one-third of older patients receive treatment for AML. Yet, patients over age 60 years of age should not be precluded from therapy. In a landmark randomized analysis by the EORTC from 1989 comparing intensive chemotherapy to supportive care, intensive therapy produced a measurable survival advantage. Other studies have also demonstrated the benefits of therapy over supportive care only, with respect to survival and quality of life.

To pursue a middle ground between supportive care and intensive treatment, lower intensity therapies are increasingly used. Although they hold promise for many older patients with AML, a select group of patients may still benefit from more intense interventions. Older patients are not a homogeneous group and several models have been devised to identify variables that predict which patients may do well with conventional therapy versus those who will not (Table 59.3). These models are comprised of patient characteristics, easily accessible clinical variables, and tumor characteristics. Although performance status can be a powerful predictor of the probability to survive intensive therapy, age remains an arbitrary variable and is increasingly understood to be a poor discriminator of outcome. Efforts are therefore underway to capture multiple patient characteristics (physical and cognitive function, nutritional status, comorbidity, psychological state and social support) as part of a comprehensive geriatric assessment and to better distinguish patients into fit, vulnerable, and frail (indicating a significantly increased risk of treatment complications).[16]

Three broad avenues of therapy in older patients with AML are standard intensive chemotherapy, lower intensity therapy (low-dose cytarabine, hypomethylating agent [HMA]), and clinical studies. Intensive chemotherapy follows the outline already discussed in the section on younger patients. Given current data, the benefit of intensive therapy may be restricted to diploid AML with mutated

TABLE 59.3	Prognostic Models in Older Patients With Acute Myeloid Leukemia	
Study	Outcome	Unfavorable Characteristics
Study Alliance Leukemia	Survival Disease-free survival	CD34 expression >10% WBC >20 × 10⁹/L Age >65 years LDH >700 U/L NPM1 status wild-type[a]
UK Medical Research Council	Survival	Adverse cytogenetic group Elevated WBC[b] Poor performance status[b] Older age[b] Secondary AML
Acute Leukemia French Association	Survival	High-risk cytogenetics ± Age ≥75 years Performance status ≥2 WBC ≥50 × 10⁹/L
MD Anderson Cancer Center	Remission rate Induction mortality Survival	Age ≥75 years Secondary AML[c] AHD duration ≥6[c] (12) months Treatment outside LAFR Unfavorable cytogenetics WBC ≥25 × 10⁹/L[c] Hemoglobin ≤8 g/dL[c] Creatinine >1.3 mg/dL Performance status >2 LDH >600 U/L[d]
Hematopoietic Cell Transplantation Comorbidity Index	Early mortality Survival	Dyspnea Coronary artery disease, CHF, MI, or EF <50% Chronic hepatitis, elevation of bilirubin and/or transaminases Cirrhosis Elevations of creatinine, dialysis, renal transplant Secondary AML Depression/anxiety requiring therapy Continued use of antimicrobial therapy after day 0 BMI >35 kg/m²

[a]Favorable and high-risk groups were defined solely by cytogenetic aberrations. Above factors served to further divide the intermediate risk group into good intermediate versus adverse intermediate.
[b]As continuous variables.
[c]Only significant for prediction of remission.
[d]Only significant for prediction of survival.
AHD, Antecedent hematologic disorder; BMI, body mass index; CHF, congestive heart failure; EF, ejection fraction; LAFR, laminar air flow room (isolation floor);LDH, lactate dehydrogenase; MI, myocardial infarction; WBC, white blood cell count;

NPM1 and wild-type FLT3-ITD, and possibly also to patients with CBF AML. Once a choice for standard therapy is made doses should not be attenuated. The optimal dose of cytarabine lies between 100 mg/m² daily × 7 days to up to 1.5 g/m² daily for 3 or 4 days and all anthracyclines are equal (if given attention to dose). Intensive induction chemotherapy is not appropriate for frail or vulnerable patients (simplified as reflected in a poor performance status), for those presenting with an adverse cytogenetic-molecular profile, and rarely for those over age 80 years.

Lower intensity therapy is therefore indicated for patients who are accordingly "unfit" for standard chemotherapy. In the National Cancer Research Institute AML 14 Trial, 217 unfit patients were randomized to low-dose cytarabine 20 mg subcutaneously twice daily for 10 days or hydroxyurea.[17] Both survival and remission rate (18% versus 1%; p < .001) were superior with low-dose cytarabine with the exception of patients with adverse cytogenetics, who did poorly on either treatment arm. Achievement of CR was related strongly to survival, with those patients in CR surviving for a median of 19 months compared to only 2 months in nonresponders. Multiple clinical trials are exploring combinations of low-dose cytarabine with other (mainly investigational) agents to improve response rates and survival over low-dose cytarabine alone. Although many agents have been tried (e.g., clofarabine, sapacitabine, lenalidomide, vosaroxin, volasertib, plerixafor, all-trans retinoic acid [ATRA]), as of the end of 2014 no combination has unequivocally demonstrated superior outcomes over standard therapy alone.

HMAs have found widespread use in the treatment of myeloid disorders including MDS and AML. Their different mechanism of action associated with a manageable toxicity profile, low incidence of mortality, and administration in the outpatient setting make them ideal agents for use in older patients. Azacitidine 75 mg/m² subcutaneously daily for 7 days was compared with conventional care (best supportive care, low-dose cytarabine, or intensive chemotherapy) in a subset of 113 patients (median age: 70 years) entered on a randomized MDS study but with 20% to 29% blasts ("oligoblastic AML").[18] Median OS was 24.5 months in the azacitidine group and 16 months in the conventional care group (p = .005). A more recent study of azacitidine versus conventional care in older patients with AML and more than 30% marrow blasts comes to similar conclusions in favor of azacitidine, with a median survival of 12.7 months versus 6.3 months. The survival difference was maintained when comparing azacitidine with specifically low-dose cytarabine-treated patients among the conventional care group (American Society of Hematology meeting 2014). Decitabine 20 mg/m² IV daily for 5 days every 4 weeks was compared to supportive care or low-dose cytarabine in a large randomized multicenter study across the United States and Europe.[19] The decitabine arm achieved a higher CR rate (17.8% versus 7.8%; p = .001), and in a post hoc sensitivity analysis of the mature data a survival advantage was observed at fixed time points over 2 years. The results of this study led to approval of decitabine for the treatment of AML in older patients in Europe but not in the United States.

Higher response rates have been reported with a 10-day schedule of decitabine, although these results have not yet been validated pending results from a randomized trial comparing it to the more common 5-day schedule. Data from single studies suggesting higher response rates of decitabine in patients expressing higher baseline levels of miR-29b or mutations of DNMT3A or TET2 are awaiting confirmation. In almost all comparisons between intensive induction therapy and HMA-based treatments, patients receiving intensive therapy achieve higher CR rates, yet OS is similar. Besides the lower treatment-related mortality associated with HMAs, the beneficial effect of HMAs on survival appears to extend to patients with lower levels of responses (defined by traditional criteria). In this context it is also noteworthy that HMAs elicit responses in patients with unfavorable karyotypes, an important difference from low-dose cytarabine.

Postremission Therapy

Patients Under 60 Years of Age

In CR, as many as 10⁹ leukemia cells survive as MRD below the threshold of detection by morphologic assessment. Further therapy is therefore necessary to reduce this number and minimize the chances of relapse. In a series of clinical studies in which patients did not receive postremission therapy, relapse was universal, and the median remission duration was about 4 months. Postremission therapy is mainly predicated by pretreatment prognostic factors and can take the form of intensified therapy (HSCT) or continued chemotherapy.

As for the latter, debate continues with regard to dose, number of cycles, and whether or not there is a role for maintenance.

In a landmark study by the CALGB, patients with newly diagnosed AML in CR following a 3 + 7 induction were randomized to SDAC (100 mg/m² continuous IV infusion daily × 7), IDAC (400 mg/m² continuous IV infusion daily × 5), or HiDAC (3 g/m² IV over 3 hours every 12 hours on days 1, 3, and 5) for a total of four cycles.[20] This was followed by an additional four cycles of 2 + 5, a consolidation-maintenance omitted from all subsequent CALGB studies. The probability of remaining in continuous CR after 4 years was 24% for SDAC, 29% for IDAC, and 44% for HiDAC (*p* = .002). Over the ensuing years, studies have shown that there is no benefit by extending consolidation therapy by a fifth cycle and that even three cycles may be equivalent. HiDAC in consolidation holds less benefit for patients older than 60 years and those with intermediate and especially unfavorable karyotypes.

CBF leukemias are characterized by translocation t(8;21), inv(16), or t(16;16) and, at the molecular level, by a disruption of *CBF* transcription genes, which play a crucial role in hematopoietic differentiation. CBF AMLs comprise about 15% to 20% of patients with AML. They stand out in that they are very sensitive to cytarabine-based therapy, which is reflected in high remission rates (80–90%) and more patients achieving long-term OS (about 60% at 5 years). Postremission therapy with HiDAC (e.g., 3 g/m² IV every 12 hours on days 1, 3, and 5) for three to four cycles is most commonly used. Questions remain with regard to the optimal number of cycles, intensification, and addition of further drugs. One cycle (with a cumulative dose of up to 18 g/m² of cytarabine) is worse than three or four cycles (cumulative dose: 54–72 mg/m²). On the other hand, giving two cycles in combination with idarubicin, daunorubicin, or mitoxantrone is comparable to three or four cycles with HiDAC. According to the MRC AML10 trial, one consolidation cycle of IDAC (cumulative dose: 5 g/m²) was equivalent to three or four consolidation cycles as given in the CALGB studies. Addition of GO to cytarabine-based conventional chemotherapy resulted in lower risk or relapse and higher OS, especially in patients with favorable karyotype.[21] Given the excellent responsiveness to chemotherapy vis-à-vis the higher risk for treatment-related mortality and morbidity with stem cell transplant, there is no role for transplant as consolidation in these patients. Less frequently in the United States compared with other regions, autologous transplant is sometimes performed following one or two cytarabine-based consolidations, albeit with comparable results to chemotherapy-only regimens. Subgroups of patients with CBF AML have been identified with worse than expected outcome. Long-established poor prognostic factors include older age, a high WBC at diagnosis, presentation with granulocytic sarcoma in t(8;21), and expression of CD56. Worse survival has also been described in the presence of *KIT* mutations (more frequently of exon 17 than exon 8). These mutations occur in up to one-third of patients with inv(16) and about 20% of those with t(8;21). Although remission rates are similar, CBF AML with mutated *KIT* are more likely to relapse. Screening for *KIT* mutations should therefore be routinely added to cytogenetic analysis. Clinical trials adding tyrosine kinase inhibitors active against KIT (e.g., dasatinib) to chemotherapy are being conducted. Given the worse prognosis, allogeneic stem cell transplant in this situation is also advocated by some.

Patients with diploid karyotype and mutations of *NPM1* or biallelic mutations of *CEBPA* without mutations for *FLT3-ITD* have a similarly favorable outcome to that of patients with *KIT* wild-type CBF AML. They also do not benefit from allogeneic stem cell transplant in first remission and are typically treated with standard consolidation chemotherapy.

Patients in the intermediate-risk group comprise the largest (about 60%) and most heterogeneous AML population (about 60% of AML). The majority demonstrate a diploid karyotype. It is in this group of patients where there is an ongoing debate about the role of chemotherapy versus stem cell transplant in consolidation. It is also in this group where the prognostic impact of gene mutation analysis is most helpful to facilitate this decision, at least in select patients (Table 59.4).

TABLE 59.4	Indications for Postremission Hematopoietic Stem Cell Transplantation Based on Cytogenetic–Molecular Profile	
Prognostic Group	**Subgroups**	**HSCT**
CBF AML	*KIT^wt*	No
	KIT^mut	Possible
Intermediate	*FLT3-ITD^mut*	Yes
	FLT3-D835^mut	Possible
	NPM1^mut [a]	No
	CEBPA^mut [a]	No
Unfavorable	Not relevant	Yes

[a]Without concomitant mutations of *FLT3-ITD*. In the case of *CEBPA*, only if the mutation is biallelic.

AML, Acute myeloid leukemia; CBF, core-binding factor; HiDAC, high-dose cytarabine; HSCT, hematopoietic stem cell transplant; mut, mutated; wt, wild type.

No advantage for HSCT has been observed for patients with cytogenetically normal karyotype and mutations of *NPM1* or biallelic mutations of *CEBPA* without mutations of *FLT3-ITD*. On the other hand, transplant in first CR should be considered for all other patients with intermediate- or high-risk disease. A systematic review and metaanalysis of 24 prospective trials including 6007 patients demonstrated significant relapse-free and OS benefit in these patient groups when compared with nonallogeneic HSCT.[22]

Outcome following standard chemotherapy remains poor for patients with adverse-risk cytogenetics and unfavorable gene mutations, most notably of *FLT3-ITD* (but not the kinase domain mutation of *FLT3* at D835) and *TP53*. There is an ongoing discussion about the significance of allele burden with respect to *FLT3-ITD* mutations in that patients with a low allelic ratio (usually <0.5) have similar outcomes to patients without the mutation. Contrary to earlier reports, however, increasing evidence suggests that the allele burden has little significance and that the detection of the mutation per se is what matters for treatment decisions. Although the same prognostic markers also worsen prognosis following HSCT, the latter still carries a better survival. Patients with high-risk disease are appropriate candidates for clinical trials in lieu of standard chemotherapy and even HSCT.

Patients Aged 60 Years or Older

The value of intensive postremission therapy is a matter of debate for older patients with AML. Unlike in younger patients, HiDAC is less effective and given its higher potential for toxicities, it is less feasible to administer four repetitive cycles. There are conflicting data as to the number of postremission cycles (one cycle has been shown to be as effective as several cycles) and to the required intensity of postremission therapy. It is generally accepted that intensive postremission therapy most benefits patients with mutations of *NPM1* (without *FLT3-ITD* mutations) and possibly leukemias expressing CBF rearrangements.

Reduced-intensity and nonmyeloablative conditioning regimens have opened HSCT to a wide range of especially older patients. Age only retains significance by virtue of its association with other covariates (performance status, comorbidities), but per se is not a predictor for nonrelapse mortality. This notion comes with the caveat that very little data exist for HSCT in patients over 75 years of age. The fact that less than 10% of older patients are receiving an allogeneic HSCT underlines the need for better tools in decision-making between HSCT and chemotherapy. The European LeukemiaNet AML Working Party has proposed an integrated dynamic risk-adapted assessment tool that takes into account disease-specific biological factors, clinical and laboratory characteristics, as well as estimates for relapse and nonrelapse mortality following either intervention.

Molecular markers and MRD serve to distinguish favorable from unfavorable subsets, although it needs to be recognized that ostensibly favorable molecular groups of older patients carry a higher risk of relapse than what would be expected for younger patients.

Maintenance Therapy

Maintenance therapy (i.e., additional therapy following consolidation) aims to improve the quality of remission, eliminate residual disease, and maximize the chances to remain disease free. The concept is effective in some acute leukemias (ALL, APL), but to date has not led to any appreciable improvement in the outcome of patients with AML.

The antileukemic effect of the immune system is displayed in the graft-versus-leukemia effect following allogeneic HSCT (not if T-cell depleted), resulting in decreased relapse rates. Initial studies focused on stimulation by IL-2 of immune effector cells such as tumor-specific cytotoxic lymphocytes and natural killer cells. Although IL-2 has demonstrated antileukemic activity in preclinical models, not one study applying low-dose IL-2 (high doses of IL-2 were not feasible because of drug-related toxicities) showed any improvement of disease-free or OS. Only with the combination of IL-2 plus histamine dihydrochloride could an improvement of leukemia-free survival at 3 years be demonstrated when compared with a randomized observation cohort (40% versus 26%; $p = .01$). The benefit was restricted to patients in CR1 and did not extend to OS. Recent success with chimeric antigen receptor-transfected T cells and the emergence of bispecific T-cell antibodies (although harder to apply in AML than lymphoid malignancies) has revived the specter of cellular therapy in maintenance strategies.

Other concepts have been developed based on lenalidomide and HMAs (azacitidine, decitabine), including following HSCT. Results as to their impact remain inconclusive and maintenance therapy remains investigational.

Therapy: Salvage

Most patients with AML relapse and do so within the first year following achievement of remission. In an analysis of 1069 consecutive AML patients in first CR who were treated and followed at the MD Anderson Cancer Center, the risk for treatment failure was 69%, 38%, 17%, 8%, and 7% in the first to fifth year, respectively. With a 6-year relapse-free survival of 84% for patients who were alive and disease free at 3 years, it is reasonable to consider patients cured once in CR for at least 3 years. For patients over 60 years of age, relapse-free survival was only 56% and therefore a substantial relapse risk persists without any discernible "safe haven".

The prognosis for patients in relapse remains poor, but outcomes are more heterogeneous than first impressions suggest. An important predictor for prognosis is the duration of first remission. In a study of 243 patients with AML in first relapse, the likelihood of CR was 60% if the duration of first remission exceeded 2 years and 19% if it was shorter than 1 year. Treatment was not associated with prognosis. In a multivariate analysis of 667 patients in first relapse, a prognostic score was derived from four clinical parameters (duration of first remission, karyotype at diagnosis, age at relapse, and previous HSCT or not) that identified three risk groups: a) favorable group: CR 85% and 5-year OS 46%; b) intermediate group: CR 60% and 5-year survival 34%; c) poor risk group: CR 18% and 5-year survival 4%. In another prognostic model for relapsed/refractory AML, disease status (relapse <12 months), FLT3-ITD mutation, and high-risk cytogenetics were independent adverse prognostic factors for OS and event-free survival (EFS). Three subgroups with different outcomes at 2 years were identified: a) favorable (no adverse features): OS 58%, EFS 45%; b) intermediate (one adverse factor): OS 37%, EFS 31%; c) poor (≥ two adverse factors): OS 12%, EFS 12%. Prognosis is worse for patients after more than one salvage attempt, but even then 1-year survival probabilities vary between 2% and 24%. Patients who are primary refractory to at least one cycle of HiDAC-based induction therapy do equally poorly, with a subsequent CR rate of 22%, median CR duration of around 9 months, and survival of 3.8 months.

The goal of salvage therapy is to recapture a remission or at least achieve sufficient reduction of disease burden (absence of circulating blasts, marrow blasts <10%) to transition patients to HSCT. Five-year survival expectations following HSCT vary from 30% to 40% (first relapse/second CR) to <10% (refractory relapse), but remain superior to nontransplant therapies across all scenarios.

There is no one standard salvage regimen. An intensive chemotherapy regimen may benefit the few patients with favorable prognostic features at relapse. Commonly used intensive regimens are fludarabine, cytarabine, G-CSF (FLAG), fludarabine, cytarabine, idarubicin (FAI), high-dose cytarabine, mitoxantrone (HAM), mitoxantrone, etoposide, cytarabine (MEC), and cytarabine, daunorubicin, etoposide (ADE). Outcome is similar with any of the combinations. The MEC regimen is not infrequently associated with severe mucositis. Large randomized studies are rare. One international multicenter trial randomized 326 patients ≥55 years of age with relapsed and refractory AML to cytarabine 1 g/m^2 daily for 5 days or cytarabine plus clofarabine. CR rate and EFS were superior in the combination arm but the primary OS endpoint was not met. Another more recent multicenter study randomized 711 patients with first relapse and refractory AML ≥18 years of age to cytarabine 1 g/m^2 daily for 5 days versus the combination of cytarabine with vosaroxin, a first-in-class anticancer quinolone derivative. Without an increase in early mortality, the combination arm achieved significantly higher CR rates (30.1% versus 16.3%, $p = .00001$) and OS benefit (median 7.5 versus 6.1 months; $p = .06$; stratified = 0.02), which was more obvious if patient groups were censored for subsequent allogeneic HSCT (median 6.7 months versus 5.3 months, $p = .02$).[23] Benefit was greatest in patients aged ≥60 years and those with early relapse.

Any of these strategies only rescue a minority of patients with AML relapse. It therefore remains imperative to pursue more effective treatments with investigational agents through clinical trials.

Therapy: Investigational

Anti-CD33–Directed Therapy

CD33 is a cell surface antigen that is present in more than 80% of patients with AML but is absent from pluripotent hematopoietic stem cells. GO is a humanized anti-CD33 monoclonal antibody linked to the DNA-binding cytotoxin calicheamicin. As a single agent in relapsed/refractory patients with AML, it achieved response rates close to 30% and resulted in GO's accelerated approval in the year 2000 by the US Food and Drug Administration (FDA). Subsequent combinations of GO with chemotherapy demonstrated hepatic toxicities (in particular sinusoidal obstruction syndrome), which were not observed before. This problem was largely resolved by reducing GO doses to as low as 3 mg/m^2 in combinations. The expanded spectrum of toxicities plus the observation that GO failed to improve outcome of patients in a large randomized trial by the Southwest Oncology Group (SWOG S0106) led the FDA to revoke the approval in 2010 and GO was voluntarily withdrawn from the market (except for Japan). However, subsequent randomized trials in which GO was combined with standard chemotherapy produced favorable results. A metaanalysis of five randomized trials (including SWOG S0106) with a total of 3325 patients can be summarized as follows: 1) GO does not increase remission rate; 2) although early mortality is higher in GO-treated patients, OS is improved as the reduction in the relapse rate of GO-treated patients far outweighs early mortality; 3) the survival benefit is mostly seen in patients with favorable and intermediate-risk cytogenetics, but not with adverse karyotype; 4) doses of 3 mg/m^2 are as effective as higher doses and were associated with fewer early deaths.[24] In other studies, GO has also been shown to be effective and safe for patients with APL.

Whether GO will return to the United States market is unknown. Yet, interest in anti-CD33–directed therapies persists. SGN–CD33A is an anti-CD33 engineered cysteine antibody conjugated to an average of two molecules of a pyrrolobenzodiazepine dimer, a highly potent DNA crosslinking agent. SGN-CD33A has shown single-agent antileukemia activity, and combinations with standard AML and MDS therapy are underway. AMG 330 is a novel CD33/CD3-directed bispecific T-cell engaging (BiTE) antibody. It is highly active against CD33$^+$ AML cell lines and can potently lyse leukemic blasts from AML patients. Clinical studies are in progress.

CPX-351

CPX-351 is a liposomal formulation of cytarabine and daunorubicin at a fixed 5:1 molar ratio within 100-nm bilamellar liposomes. This formulation allows delivery of a maximally synergistic drug ratio to tumor cells and may enhance treatment efficacy. In a phase II randomized study of CPX-351 versus 3 + 7 in older patients with untreated AML, the investigational combination achieved significantly higher remission rates than standard 3 + 7 and significantly better OS in the subgroup with secondary AML. Final results of a randomized phase III study of CPX-351 versus standard 3 + 7 in patients aged 60 to 75 years with high-risk (secondary) AML confirmed the significant improvement in remission rate and median OS with CPX-351. Pending filing and FDA assessment of this compound, CPX-351 may become a new standard of care for this patient group.

FLT3 Inhibitors

Inhibitors of FLT3 have been in clinical trials for many years. Yet no FLT3 inhibitor has received FDA approval. The clinical activity of single-agent first generation inhibitors (midostaurin, lestaurtinib, sunitinib, sorafenib, semaxanib, tandutinib) has been limited, only demonstrating transient reductions in blood and/or marrow blasts but, for most, without achievement of objective responses. In a randomized study of standard salvage therapy versus addition of lestaurtinib, no benefit with regard to response rate or survival was observed. A randomized study of standard induction therapy in patients 18 to 60 years of age with or without sorafenib (regardless of FLT3 status) demonstrated superior relapse and event free survival for the sorafenib treated group. The CALGB 10603 (RATIFY) study randomized 717 patients between ages 18 and 60 with newly diagnosed FLT3 positive (both ITD and TKD) AML to receive a standard 3 + 7 induction alone or in combination with midostaurin. Ten years after conception the final results were presented in 2016. Although the addition of midostaurin did not improve remission rates, the FLT3 inhibitor group enjoyed a statistically significant event free and overall survival benefit that extended to both ITD and TKD groups and persisted regardless of mutation load. The outcome of this study defines the combination of 3 + 7 and midostaurin (FDA approval pending) as a new standard of care for this patient population.

Higher single-agent activity (including objective remissions) has been observed with the next generation FLT3 inhibitors quizartinib, gilteritinib, and crenolanib. They are being actively evaluated in combination with standard chemotherapy in various clinical trials in frontline and relapsed FLT3 positive patients.

Various factors influence the activity of FLT3 inhibitors. Blasts with a low mutant allelic burden of *FLT3/ITD* may be less dependent on FLT3 signaling. Whether or not there is an association of the size of the ITD fragment with outcome is controversial. Secretion of FLT3 ligand is another resistance mechanism under discussion. The spectrum of activity of most of the FLT3 inhibitors extends to other kinases so that there are differences with regard to specificity between these agents. Next generation FLT3 inhibitors are more specific towards FLT3 compared to other kinases than is observed in the first generation compounds.

IDH Inhibitors

Somatic mutations in the metabolic enzymes IDH1 and IDH2 result in accumulation of the oncometabolite R-2-hydroxyglutarate (2-HG). High levels of 2-HG lead to epigenetic changes and impaired cellular differentiation. Several compounds have been developed that specifically target *IDH1 R132H* and *IDH2 R140Q*. Data from a phase I study of AG-221, an oral, reversible, and selective inhibitor of *IDH2*, showed high levels of clinical activity with objective response rates of 50%.

Inhibitors of Polo-Like Kinases

Polo-like kinases belong to a family of serine/threonine protein kinases that play a key role in mitotic checkpoint regulation and cell division. Volasertib is a low–molecular-weight, ATP-competitive kinase inhibitor that potently inhibits Polo-like kinases and has shown in vivo efficacy in AML xenograft models. A randomized phase II trial of low-dose cytarabine with or without volasertib in patients not suitable for intensive induction therapy (median age 75 years) showed higher rates of CR and significantly better EFS and OS with the addition of volasertib.[25] The volasertib arm was also associated with a higher frequency of adverse events (mainly myelosuppression, neutropenic fever, and gastrointestinal toxicities).

Other Novel Agents

Sapacitabine is an oral cytarabine analog whose cyano structure causes irreparable single-strand DNA breaks. It is active in AML and patients with MDS, including those who have lost response to standard HMAs.

Guadecitabine (SGI-110) is a second-generation dinucleotide of decitabine and deoxyguanosine with prolonged half-life and activity in AML and high-risk AML.

Signaling through the RAS/RAF/MEK pathway is activated in many cancers and has been one of the first targets for small-molecule kinase inhibitors. Inhibitors of MEK1/2 have demonstrated clinical activity in the salvage therapy for AML. Of 39 patients with relapsed or secondary AML, a third responded in the presence of KRAS or NRAS mutations compared with only 8% in the absence of mutations.

Inhibitors of DOT1L have shown activity in patients with *MLL*-rearranged AML.

Other targets are BCL2 and MDM2 and other antiapoptotic proteins; nuclear export proteins; multidrug resistance proteins; the ubiquitin–proteasome pathway; aurora kinases, which play an important role in the formation and organization of the mitotic spindle apparatus; the mammalian target of rapamycin/phosphatidylinositol 3-kinase/AKT pathway; components of the microenvironment (e.g., CXC-chemokine receptor 4 and CXC-chemokine ligand 12 inhibitors). Venetoclax is a recently approved BCLR inhibitor for the treatment of chronic lymphocytic leukemia. Its activity in AML and MDS is being evaluated in clinical studies.

ACUTE PROMYELOCYTIC LEUKEMIA

APL is a rare subtype (approximately 10% of all AML diagnoses) with unique pathophysiologic, clinical, and therapeutic features. The median age at diagnosis of 40 years is younger than for other types of AML; APL occurs more frequently in Hispanics and the obese. If diagnosed promptly and managed appropriately, APL has the most favorable prognosis of all AMLs. On the other hand, catastrophic bleeding events (coagulopathies, thrombocytopenia), differentiation syndrome, or infectious complications can be associated with a high early mortality (in some reports 20–30%). In 80% of the cases, APL cells are hypergranular with many Auer rods. A microgranular variant

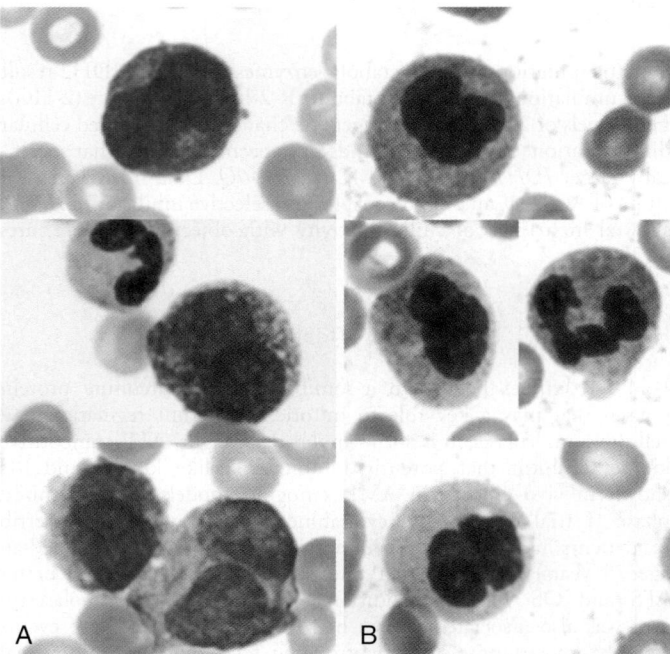

Fig. 59.16 EFFECT OF ALL-TRANS RETINOIC ACID THERAPY ON ACUTE PROMYELOCYTIC LEUKEMIA CELLS. All-trans retinoic acid (ATRA) therapy in acute promyelocytic leukemia (APL)causes the malignant promyelocytes (A) to differentiate, and the effects of differentiation can be seen within days of treatment (B). The differentiated APL cells are still somewhat atypical, frequently with bilobed nuclei (compare with normal neutrophil [B, *inset center right*]).

(M3v) is often associated with leukocytosis. APL cells are strongly positive for MPO staining and lack expression of CD34 and HLA-DR.

APL is almost always the result of translocation t(15;17), which fuses the retinoic acid receptor alpha (*RARA*) gene with the promyelocytic leukemia (*PML*) gene. In very rare cases (<5%) translocation partners other than *PML* result in alternative fusion genes (e.g., *PLZF-RARA*, *NPM-RARA*, *NuMA-RARA*, *STAT5-RARA*), which often convey resistance to ATRA. PML-RARA is an abnormal retinoic acid (RA) receptor that represses transcription of RA-activated target genes by recruiting large protein complexes through the coiled-coil domain of PML, which in turn act as potent transcriptional corepressors. Pharmacologic doses of RA release the corepressors and allow recruitment of coactivators, resulting in the transcription of previously silenced genes. This leads to a sudden arrest in proliferation and a differentiation response that can be seen in vitro and in vivo within a few days following administration of ATRA (Fig. 59.16). APL is the most dramatic example of the success of differentiating therapy, which has proved disappointing in other forms of AML.

The clinical activity of ATRA was first demonstrated in a study from China, where oral ATRA alone when given over 30 to 90 days achieved CR rates of 85%, an observation that was later confirmed by groups in North America and Europe. ATRA has a dramatic effect on the coagulopathy, substantially reducing the risk of serious bleeding events, and should be instituted immediately upon suspicion of a diagnosis of APL even in the absence of confirmatory testing. ATRA therapy has also been associated in 10% to 25% of patients with "retinoic acid syndrome" (more appropriately called *differentiation syndrome* because it is also seen with other differentiating agents such arsenic trioxide [ATO]). It occurs within a few days of the start of therapy and is reminiscent of manifestations of capillary leak and respiratory distress syndrome: fever, dyspnea, hypoxemia, pulmonary infiltrates, weight gain, peripheral edema, renal and hepatic dysfunction, and ascites. Differentiation syndrome carries a high mortality unless recognized and managed promptly. Therapy consists of

immediate administration of steroids (dexamethasone 10 mg twice daily until resolution of signs and symptoms) and interruption of therapy if no response or in the case of life-threatening complications. This intervention will rapidly reverse the manifestations of differentiation syndrome and has substantially reduced mortality to below 5%. Some investigators have proposed prophylactic use of dexamethasone 2.5 mg/m² every 12 hours for the first 15 days in patients with WBC exceeding 5000/µL.

Subsequent clinical studies confirmed significantly better disease-free survival for the combination of ATRA plus chemotherapy. In the French APL 93 trial, concurrent administration of ATRA with chemotherapy achieved identical CR rates of 92% but a lower relapse rate at 2 years (6%) compared with sequential administration (16%, $p = .04$). As standard induction therapy for patients with APL hence emerged the combination of ATRA with an anthracycline (daunorubicin or idarubicin). In two large trials from Italy (GIMEMA) and Spain (PETHEMA), CR rates were 95% and 89%, respectively, and 2-year disease-free survival was 79%.[26] A risk-stratification model was proposed based on WBC and platelet count. High risk was defined as a WBC of greater than 10,000/µL at diagnosis with significant differences in relapse-free survival between patients with high- and those with intermediate-/low-risk disease. The role of cytarabine in APL therapy is controversial. In two randomized studies of ATRA/anthracycline ± cytarabine from the AML MRC15 trial and the European APL Group, rates for CR and induction failure were comparable, but in the European trial (using daunorubicin as opposed to idarubicin in the MRC trial), the risk for relapse was increased when cytarabine was omitted. On the other hand, in the MRC15 trial not only was there no difference in relapse rate, the cytarabine-treated patients experienced a small increase of deaths and higher use of medical resources. In a joint analysis of the European results with those of the PETHEMA group, the benefit of cytarabine was restricted to patients with higher risk disease.

ATO has potent antiapoptotic activity in APL cells. Whereas its precise mechanism of action is not well defined and almost certainly depends on additional mechanisms, it is the most active drug available against APL. Based on previously published data by the MD Anderson Cancer Center, a phase III multicenter trial compared ATRA plus chemotherapy with ATRA plus ATO in low- to intermediate-risk patients.[27] CR rates between the ATRA/ATO and the ATRA/chemotherapy group were similar (100% vs. 95%, $p = .12$). Although designed as a noninferiority trial, EFS and OS at 2 years were superior in the ATRA/ATO-treated patients. The ATRA/ATO arm was also associated with less hematologic toxicity and fewer infections, but higher rates of hepatic toxicity. The combination of ATRA and ATO can therefore be considered a new standard of care for patients with non–high-risk APL.

Single-agent ATO induction may be particularly attractive where medical resources are scarce and access to cheaper therapies is an economic necessity. In two studies, one from India and one from Iran, single-agent ATO achieved CR rates close to 85%, with 3-year survival rates of 86% (India) and 5-year survival rates of 64% (Iran). Patients with higher risk disease responded equally favorably. ATO can cause prolongation of the QTc interval, which may rarely lead to serious cardiac arrhythmias. It is recommended to check an electrocardiogram before each course of therapy and maintain electrolytes such as potassium and magnesium at high-normal levels throughout therapy.

Monitoring response during induction consists of morphologic assessments of marrow smears and measurements of PML/RARA by RT-PCR. As the differentiation response of leukemic blasts may be delayed, repeat marrow studies are not recommended before blood counts recover at around 4 to 6 weeks of therapy. No change of therapy should be undertaken during this time. At the end of induction and by the time a morphologic and cytogenetic remission is achieved, PML/RARA is frequently still detectable, which at this early point in therapy is common and should not be interpreted as a sign of treatment resistance.

Postremission therapy consists of consolidation and maintenance, with the goal to convert a morphologic and cytogenetic remission into a durable molecular (PCR-negative) response and maintain PCR negativity throughout. For patients who are treated with an ATRA/chemotherapy combination, common practice is to give another two or three anthracycline-based cycles. Addition of ATO to a standard consolidation has significantly improved EFS and disease-free survival in a large randomized United States Intergroup study.[28] For ATRA/ATO-treated patients, the combination is continued throughout consolidation. Following consolidation, maintenance therapy for 1 to 2 years with ATRA ± mercaptopurine and methotrexate has been recommended. There is debate as to the benefit of maintenance and it is very likely that the impact of maintenance on overall outcome will change now that ATRA and ATO are a standard treatment for lower risk patients during induction. High-dose ara-C and mercaptopurine-methotrexate maintenance may not add benefit in the context of optimal novel therapies using ATRA-ATO with or without anthracyclines or GO. PCR testing is essential in the follow-up of patients with APL. In no other leukemia, with the possible exception of chronic myeloid leukemia and emerging in CBF leukemias, does molecular testing play such a critical role and influences clinical decision-making processes. Patients who do not achieve a molecular response by the end of the consolidation (usually 3 months into CR) have a poorer prognosis with a higher likelihood of relapse. Furthermore, these patients have a better survival with early intervention at the time of molecular rather than morphologic relapse. Whereas no further monitoring may be necessary for molecular responders with low-risk disease because of the very low relapse likelihood, monitoring should take place every 3 months for 2 years for patients with high-risk disease, those older than 60 years, and patients for whom treatment delays occurred during consolidation. Positive PCR test results should be confirmed by a second PCR test within 1 to 4 weeks. If the repeat test results are negative, no further action is necessary; however, close prospective monitoring should be applied.

ATO is effective therapy for patients with relapsed APL, including those with persistent PCR-positive disease. Morphologic remissions are achieved in up to 90% and molecular remissions in 70% to 80% of patients, respectively. Three-year survival rates are between 50% and 70%. Addition of ATRA to ATO may provide little further benefit if ATRA was already part of the induction/consolidation, which is the case most of the time. HSCT should follow achievement of a second remission. Autologous HSCT is recommended for patients who have again achieved a molecular response. For those whose PCR results remain positive despite ATO-based therapy, allogeneic HSCT is favored. CNS involvement at the time of relapse is rare, so that there is no commonly agreed-upon strategy of CNS prophylaxis. Whereas some groups such as the National Comprehensive Cancer Network advocate prophylactic intrathecal therapy for patients in second morphologic remission, the Spanish PETHEMA group showed that two independent risk factors for CNS disease are a WBC >10,000/μL and occurrence of CNS hemorrhage during induction. Under those circumstances the incidence of CNS involvement has been as high as 5.5%, but it was not higher than 1.2% at 5 years for the remainder of the patients.

ADDITIONAL ISSUES IN ACUTE MYELOID LEUKEMIA

Hyperleukocytosis

Hyperleukocytosis is often understood as a WBC >100,000/μL (Fig. 59.17), although this definition is not always followed very closely in clinical practice. It should be noted that lesser degrees of hyperleukocytosis can have grave consequences dependent on the biologic properties of the blasts. Myeloid blasts are less deformable than normal myeloid cells or even lymphoid blasts, and adhere to vessel walls and extramedullary tissues due to a complex array of adhesion molecules. Hyperleukocytosis is a medical emergency with a high mortality rate, mainly due to pulmonary and CNS complications from bleeding (intravascular sludging, anatomic disruption of the endothelium, DIC, or a combination) and direct tissue infiltration

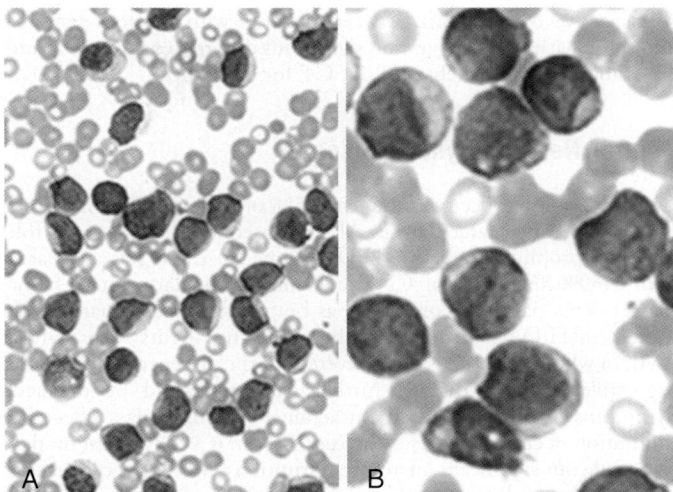

Fig. 59.17 HYPERLEUKOCYTOSIS IN ACUTE MYELOID LEUKEMIA. The patient was a 23-year-old man who presented with several weeks of abdominal pain, weight loss, and fatigue. He was found to have a marked leukocytosis of 165,300/μL composed of mostly blasts ([A] and higher power [B]), which were shown to be myeloblasts by flow immunophenotyping. The patient developed some shortness of breath and hypoxia, and underwent two cycles of leukapheresis and hydroxyurea before induction. Molecular analysis revealed the leukemia to have an *FLT3-ITD* mutation.

triggering inflammatory responses. It is therefore imperative that efforts be undertaken to reduce the blast burden as soon as possible. Because red blood cell transfusions increase the viscosity of blood flow, they should be used judiciously or if possible avoided as long as the WBC remains high. Leukapheresis is a fast and effective method for WBC reduction. Although it has an immediate effect in reducing early mortality, there has been no impact on survival. Leukapheresis does not affect cellular plugs that are already formed in a vascular territory, nor does it abate inflammatory reactions in tissues infiltrated by blasts. Rapid administration of cytotoxic chemotherapy with or without leukapheresis therefore plays an important role. The most effective drug is cytarabine. Hydroxyurea is an oral alternative that is well tolerated and easy to administer. However, hydroxyurea does not effectively infiltrate tissues and thus may not reach extravascular blast infiltrates. Care must be taken to avoid tumor lysis syndrome, using adequate hydration and uricosuric agents, and to meticulously follow electrolyte levels and renal function.

Myeloid Sarcoma

Myeloid sarcoma (granulocytic sarcoma, chloroma) is an extramedullary myeloid tumor composed of myeloid blasts. Myeloid sarcomas can occur in any tissue but most commonly present in the skin (leukemia cutis), lymph nodes, gastrointestinal tract, testes, CNS, soft tissue, and bones. They can easily be confused with lymphomas and soft-tissue sarcomas. Myeloid sarcomas can be isolated, occur together with marrow involvement, or precede it. In a few instances they may be the relapse manifestation of patients who have been treated for AML in the past, particularly following allogeneic stem cell transplantation. In the context of chronic myeloid malignancies (e.g., MDS, myeloproliferative neoplasms, chronic myeloid leukemia, chronic myelomonocytic leukemia), their appearance represents progression to a blast phase. Even when isolated, myeloid sarcoma should be treated systemically with chemotherapy, as for any other AML. Radiation therapy may be of help to optimize local control in challenging anatomic compartments. However, in the absence of systemic therapy, subsequent progression to systemic AML is very likely. There is controversy over whether patients with myeloid sarcoma do better or worse than those with AML. The majority of retrospective comparisons between patients with myeloid sarcoma and those with AML suggest no significant differences in survival and a possible survival benefit with HSCT for all groups.[29]

Central Nervous System Disease

CNS involvement occurs in less than 5% of patients with AML and is therefore much rarer than in ALL. Consequently, there is no role for CNS prophylaxis. Before HiDAC, inv(16) AML was associated with a 30% incidence of CNS leukemia, particularly intracerebral masses. This particular problem has been virtually eliminated with the use of HiDAC but may still be noted in patients with inv(16) AML in whom HiDAC is not delivered. In the presence of symptoms suggestive of CNS disease, further workup should be pursued. Symptoms are due to raised intracranial pressure, mass effect, or infiltration of cranial nerves. Whereas CT scan is a convenient modality to rule out significant anatomic disruptions, it is not very sensitive to detect more subtle signs of leptomeningeal disease, and, if concerns persist, a magnetic resonance image of any CNS structure where disease is suspected should be obtained. Lumbar puncture is a crucial component of the workup. Blasts in the cerebrospinal fluid may range from a few cells to several thousand. Treatment consists of intrathecal therapy with cytarabine and/or methotrexate via lumbar route or Ommaya reservoir. The dose of methotrexate should be reduced by 50% if administered into an Ommaya reservoir. A typical schedule includes twice-weekly intrathecal doses until the cerebrospinal fluid becomes clear. The frequency is then changed to weekly for 2 months, then every other week for 2 months, followed by monthly injections for up to 1 year (various similar schedules are used in practice). Radiation therapy can be a useful alternative, especially in the case of localized lesions such as isolated cranial nerve findings. Although high-dose cytarabine penetrates the blood–brain barrier and may have contributed to a lower rate of CNS involvement over the years, it alone is not sufficient therapy once there is CNS disease. The risk for CNS involvement is higher in AML with any type of monoblastic differentiation and those cases with a high WBC (>100,000/µL) at presentation (high LDH >100 IU/L), and perhaps in FLT3-positive AML. Although some authorities have recommended routine intrathecal therapy once in remission, this is not common practice.

Pregnancy

AML is rarely diagnosed during pregnancy. In a case-control study of 785 women with AML aged 15 to 50 years compared with 1576 age- and sex-matched controls, AML occurred at a rate of 1.3% in the pregnant group and 3.4% in the control group (odds ratio: 0.44 in favor of pregnant women). The response to treatment is not affected by pregnancy. AML therapy during the first trimester is problematic due to the toxic and teratogenic effects of chemotherapy on the fetus. Under those circumstances, termination of pregnancy before institution of induction therapy should be strongly considered. Pregnancy outcome during the second and third trimester is more favorable, and successful treatment of the AML and delivery of normal infants have been reported. Daunorubicin is preferable over idarubicin because the latter is more lipophilic and has higher DNA affinity, raising the question of higher maternal–fetal transfer and toxicity to the fetus. It is not advisable to delay therapy once the diagnosis of AML is made given the high risk for maternal death. In situations where the leukemia behaves indolently and women are close to delivery, a conservative approach can be chosen with supportive care and induction of labor as soon as possible. These decisions are based on clinical judgment and discussion with the patient.[30]

FUTURE DIRECTIONS

Although standard induction therapy has not substantially changed over the previous four decades (unchanged 3 + 7 dose and schedule),

the context in which it is delivered has become more refined. More significance is given to particular subsets of patients: a) patients unfit for standard chemotherapy (often but not always rightfully understood as those over age 60 years) frequently receive lower intensity therapies or are enrolled in clinical studies with novel agents (e.g., volasertib, vosaroxin, guadecitabine, venetoclax, SGN-CD33A); b) more and more particular cytogenetic–molecular abnormalities are amenable to targeted, often single-agent, approaches (e.g., FLT3 inhibitors, IDH1/2 inhibitors, DOT1L inhibitors, multikinase inhibitors); c) addition of the FLT3 inhibitor midostaurin to standard induction therapy improves survival in FLT3 mutated AML; d) CPX-351 improves survival in older patients with secondary AML; e) the studies of immunotherapy may open up new options. Response assessment extends beyond morphologic and cytogenetic remissions and increasingly includes MRD measurements similar to what has been happening in adult ALL. Molecular signatures and cellular pathways that are abnormally activated or regulated in AML blasts are contributing to a more complex picture of the biology of AML and, besides providing prognostic information, offer targets for drug development.

REFERENCES

1. Siegel R, Ma J, Zou Z, et al: Cancer Statistics, 2014. *CA Cancer J Clin* 64:9, 2014.
2. Pandolfi A, Barreyro L, Steidl U: Concise Review: Preleukemic stem cells: molecular biology and clinical implications of the precursors of leukemia stem cells. *Stem Cells Transl Med* 2:143, 2013.
3. Grove CS, Vassiliou GS: Acute myeloid leukaemia: a paradigm for the clonal evolution of cancer? *Dis Model Mech* 7:941, 2014.
4. Walter RB, Othus M, Borthakur G, et al: Prediction of early death after induction therapy for newly diagnosed acute myeloid leukemia with pretreatment risk scores: a novel paradigm for treatment assignment. *J Clin Oncol* 29:4417, 2011.
5. Byrd JC, Mrózek K, Dodge RK, et al: Pretreatment cytogenetic abnormalities are predictive of induction success, cumulative incidence of relapse, and overall survival in adult patients with de novo acute myeloid leukemia: results from Cancer and Leukemia Group B (CALGB 8461). *Blood* 100:4325, 2002.
6. Patel JP, Gönen M, Figueroa ME, et al: Prognostic relevance of integrated genetic profiling in acute myeloid leukemia. *N Engl J Med* 366:1079, 2012.
7. Döhner H, Estey EH, Amadori S, et al: Diagnosis and management of acute myeloid leukemia in adults: recommendations from an international expert panel, on behalf of the European LeukemiaNet. *Blood* 115:453, 2010.
8. Paietta E: Minimal residual disease in acute myeloid leukemia: coming of age. *Hematology Am Soc Hematol Educ Program* 2012:35, 2012.
9. Freireich EJ, Wiernik PH, Steensma DP: The leukemias: a half-century of discovery. *J Clin Oncol* 32:3463, 2014.
10. Fernandez HF, Sun Z, Yao X, et al: Anthracycline dose intensification in acute myeloid leukemia. *N Engl J Med* 361:1249, 2009.
11. Teuffel O, Leibundgut K, Lehrnbecker T, et al: Anthracyclines during induction therapy in acute myeloid leukemia: a systematic review and meta-analysis. *Br J Haematol* 161:192, 2013.
12. Kern W, Estey EH: High-dose cytosine arabinoside in the treatment of acute myeloid leukemia. *Cancer* 107:116, 2006.
13. Burnett AK, Russell NH, Hills RK, et al: Optimization of chemotherapy for younger patients with acute myeloid leukemia: results of the medical research council AML15 trial. *J Clin Oncol* 31:3360, 2013.
14. Willemze R, Suciu S, Meloni G, et al: High-dose cytarabine in induction treatment improves the outcome of adult patients younger than age 46 years with acute myeloid leukemia: results of the EORTC-GIMEMA AML-12 trial. *J Clin Oncol* 32:219, 2014.
15. Thein MS, Ershler WB, Jemal A, et al: Outcome of older patients with acute myeloid leukemia. *Cancer* 119:2720, 2013.
16. Klepin HD, Geiger AM, Tooze JA, et al: Geriatric assessment predicts survival for older adults receiving induction chemotherapy for acute myelogenous leukemia. *Blood* 121:4287, 2013.

17. Burnett AK, Milligan D, Prentice AG, et al: A comparison of low-dose cytarabine and hydroxyurea with or without all-trans retinoic acid for acute myeloid leukemia and high-risk myelodysplastic syndrome in patients not considered fit for intensive treatment. *Cancer* 109:1114, 2007.

18. Fenaux P, Mufti GJ, Hellström-Lindberg E, et al: Azacitidine prolongs overall survival compared with conventional care regimens in elderly patients with low bone marrow blast count acute myeloid leukemia. *J Clin Oncol* 28:562, 2010.

19. Kantarjian HM, Thomas XG, Dmoszynska A, et al: Multicenter, randomized, open-label, phase III trial of decitabine versus patient choice, with physician advice, of either supportive care or low-dose cytarabine for the treatment of older patients with newly diagnosed acute myeloid leukemia. *J Clin Oncol* 30:2670, 2012.

20. Mayer RJ, Davis RB, Schiffer CA, et al: Intensive postremission chemotherapy in adults with acute myeloid leukemia. Cancer and Leukemia Group B. *N Engl J Med* 331:896, 1994.

21. Hills RK, Castaigne S, Appelbaum FR, et al: Addition of gemtuzumab ozogamicin to induction chemotherapy in adult patients with acute myeloid leukaemia: a meta-analysis of individual patient data from randomized controlled trials. *Lancet Oncol* 15:986, 2014.

22. Koreth J, Schlenk R, Kopecky KJ, et al: Allogeneic stem cell transplantation for acute myeloid leukemia in first complete remission: systematic review and meta-analysis of prospective clinical trials. *JAMA* 301:2349, 2009.

23. Ravandi F, Ritchie E, Sayar H, et al: Improved survival in patients with first relapsed or refractory acute myeloid leukemia (AML) treated with vosaroxin plus cytarabine versus placebo plus cytarabine: results of a phase 3 double-blind randomized controlled multinational study (VALOR). *Blood* 124:LBA-6, 2014.

24. Hills RK, Castaigne S, Appelbaum FR, et al: Addition of gemtuzumab ozogamicin to induction chemotherapy in adult patients with acute myeloid leukaemia: a meta-analysis of individual patient data from randomized controlled trials. *Lancet Oncol* 15:986, 2014.

25. Döhner H, Lübbert M, Fiedler W, et al: Randomized, phase 2 trial of low-dose cytarabine with or without volasertib in AML patients not suitable for induction therapy. *Blood* 124:1426, 2014.

26. Sanz MA, Martin G, Rayon C, et al: A modified AIDA protocol with anthracycline-based consolidation results in high antileukemic efficacy and reduced toxicity in newly diagnosed PML/RARalpha-positive acute promyelocytic leukemia. PETHEMA group. *Blood* 94:3015, 1999.

27. Lo-Coco F, Avvisati G, Vignetti M, et al: Retinoic acid and arsenic trioxide for acute promyelocytic leukemia. *N Engl J Med* 369:111, 2013.

28. Powell BL, Moser B, Stock W, et al: Arsenic trioxide improves event-free and overall survival for adults with acute promyelocytic leukemia: North American Leukemia Intergroup Study C9710. *Blood* 116:3751, 2010.

29. Bakst RL, Tallman MS, Douer D, et al: How I treat extramedullary acute myeloid leukemia. *Blood* 118:3785, 2011.

30. Thomas X: Acute myeloid leukemia in the pregnant patient. *Eur J Haematol* 95:124, 2015.

CHAPTER 60

MYELODYSPLASTIC SYNDROMES

Christopher J. Gibson, Benjamin L. Ebert, and David P. Steensma

Myelodysplastic syndromes (MDS) are clonal hematopoietic disorders characterized by ineffective hematopoiesis and peripheral blood cytopenias, abnormal cell morphology on blood and bone marrow examination (Fig. 60.1) and a risk of progression to acute myeloid leukemia (AML). It has a variable clinical course, manifesting in some patients as indolent cytopenias necessitating occasional transfusions and in others as aggressive diseases that rapidly evolve into treatment-refractory leukemias, with a broad spectrum of severity in between.

Despite this phenotypic variability, individual cases of MDS share many pathophysiologic mechanisms at the molecular and cellular levels, and our understanding of these mechanisms has evolved substantially in the last decade. At the same time, although MDS also shares features with AML and other myeloid malignancies, mounting evidence shows that it is appropriately conceived as a distinct class of diseases, and that the older conceptualization of MDS as "preleukemia" is overly simplistic.

While understanding of MDS pathophysiology is improving, the condition remains difficult to treat, and outcomes for patients with MDS have unfortunately not improved substantially since the last edition of this textbook. This chapter describes our current understanding of the classification, pathobiology, clinical features, and treatment approaches for this heterogeneous group of disorders.

HISTORY

Central to an understanding of how MDS is diagnosed and classified is the concept of *morphologic dysplasia*, a pathologic term that was originally introduced as a shortening of the phrase *dysmorphology of neoplasia*. Although specific criteria for diagnosis of MDS as a distinct clinical syndrome exist and are discussed subsequently, the term myelodysplasia refers more generally to an abnormal appearance of hematopoietic precursors during pathologic examination of bone marrow, which may result from many different causes (e.g., drug toxicity, nutritional deficiency, viral infection). The process by which our understanding of MDS has evolved from that of a morphologic oddity to that of a distinct disease process has been a century in the making, propelled forward at several points by paradigmatic shifts in pathologic and molecular characterization of hematologic diseases.[1]

In describing the history of MDS as a distinctly categorized disease entity, it is perhaps most useful to separately describe the history of its major conceptual components. The earliest recognized of these, not surprisingly, was that of dysplasia itself. Although studies of peripheral blood in anemic patients were reported in the 19th century,[2] the first real characterization of actual dysplasia was probably made by Giovanni di Guglielmo in Pavia in 1923, when he described abnormal erythroid forms in the marrows of patients with various types of cytopenias.[3] A second major concept, that of ineffective hematopoiesis, was developed in the 1930s with the description of *refractory anemia* in patients unresponsive to iron pills or liver extract (the precursor to vitamin B_{12} supplementation);[4] in the 1950s, others expanded this to include similarly refractory leukopenia and thrombocytopenia and termed the collective disorder "refractory cytopenias."[5] Importantly, however, ineffective hematopoiesis and marrow dysplasia were initially incompletely linked, and the ineffective hematopoiesis of many early refractory anemia patients was probably rooted in other disorders, such as anemia of inflammation caused by advanced rheumatologic disease or nonmyeloid neoplasia.

The third major component of MDS, and possibly the most prominent, is its temporal positioning as a potential preleukemic state. This was first conceptualized in 1942 as *odo-leukemia* ("odo" from the Greek for edge or threshold) by a group from France led by Paul Chevallier to describe a case of anemia evolving into leukemia,[6] which they attributed to benzene exposure. A similar disorder was termed *preleukaemic anemia* by a British hematologist, J.L. Hamilton-Paterson, in 1949.[7] This term was adopted and expanded by an American group based in Chicago in the early 1950s,[8] providing one of the clearest descriptions of a disorder clinically defined by both cytopenias and a risk of leukemia. Other groups in the 1950s and 1960s published similar descriptions under different terminologies.[9]

The 1970s saw some of the greatest strides toward our modern conceptualization of MDS. In 1970, Dreyfus and colleagues coined the term *refractory anemia with excess blasts* (RAEB, described in French as *les anémies réfractaires avec excès de myéloblasts*)[10] and later attempted to further characterize components of RAEB based on morphology and clinical characteristics.[11] The term *hematopoietic dysplasia* was used in the early 1970s to describe a heterogeneous group of disorders distinct from AML, and the term was later simplified to *myelodysplasia*.

One of the key events in the history of myeloid disease classification was the formation of the French-American-British (FAB) Cooperative Group in 1976, which in that year issued a comprehensive and influential categorization of AML[12] based on the 1975 classification of Galton and Dacie.[13] The FAB classification persisted as the dominant descriptive system for AML until the early 2000s. The original FAB AML formulation from 1976 included two types of "dysmyelopoietic syndromes" that should not be confused with AML: RAEB and chronic myelomonocytic leukemia (CMML), which had first been described in the late 1960s.[14] However, it was not long before MDS was recognized as a separate group of diseases and accorded a distinct classification system, described in more detail later.

CLASSIFICATION

The currently accepted classification scheme for MDS was initially published by the World Health Organization (WHO) in 2001 and most recently revised in 2008 (Table 60.1), with a third revision planned for 2016. Like the classifications of the FAB group, the WHO classification is principally a morphologic system and classifies disease chiefly based on the number of dysplastic lineages and the percentage of marrow blasts, though it also includes one specific cytogenetically defined subtype, MDS with isolated del(5q). The other WHO 2008 subtypes include refractory cytopenia with unilineage dysplasia (RCUD), which is most commonly refractory anemia (RA); refractory cytopenia with multilineage dysplasia (RCMD); refractory anemia with ringed sideroblasts (RARS); RAEB (subdivided into RAEB-1, 5%–9% blasts, and RAEB-2, 10%–19% blasts); and unclassifiable MDS (MDS-U) for those cases that do not clearly fall into any other category. In addition, the WHO system classifies cases with myeloproliferative features separately; this group includes CMML and RARS with thrombocytosis (RARS-T).

The WHO classification was intended to replace the prior FAB classification system, which was initially proposed in 1982 as an MDS correlate to the FAB system for classifying AML.[15] The 1982

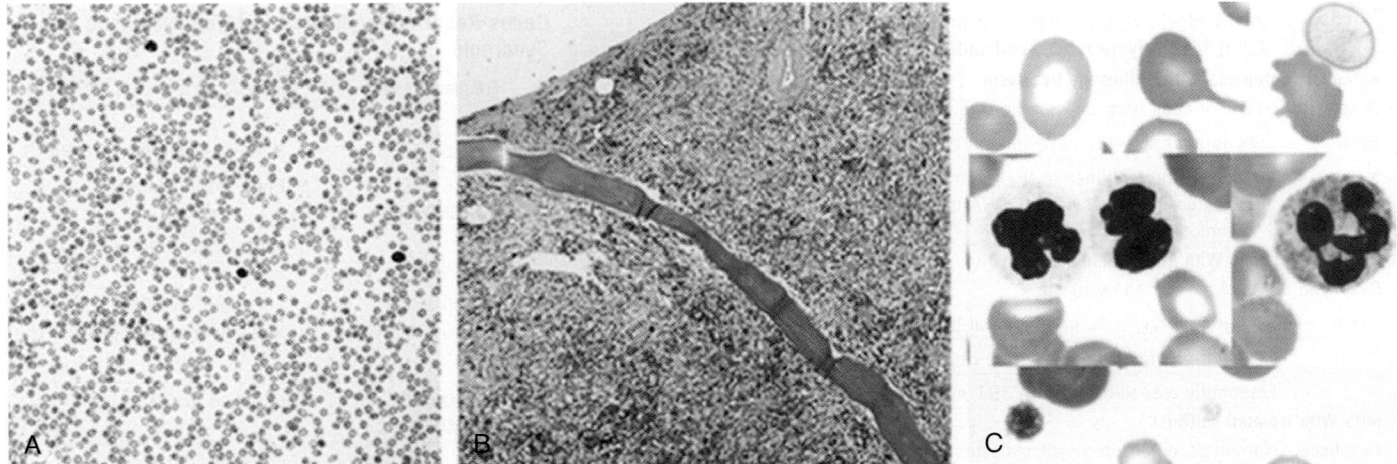

Fig. 60.1 ELEMENTS OF MYELODYSPLASTIC SYNDROME. Myelodysplastic syndromes are generally characterized by cytopenias (A) caused by ineffective hematopoiesis (B), which is related to multilineage dysplasia (C). (A) This patient presented with a white blood cell count of 1500/μL, hemoglobin 8.9 g/dL, and platelet count 47,000/μL. (B) The bone marrow was hypercellular, indicating ineffective hematopoiesis. (C) Evidence of trilineage dysplasia was apparent on the peripheral smear. Anisocytosis with macroovalocytes and poikilocytosis is seen in the red blood cells (C, *top*). The latter included the somewhat uncommon finding of Cabot ring forms *(right)*. A large proportion of the granulocytes were severely hypogranular (C, *middle left*) compared to some normal forms still in the circulation *(right)*. Platelets (C, *bottom*) were decreased in number, and many were severely hypogranular *(middle,* barely visible) compared with residual normal platelets *(left)*.

FAB system distinguished five subtypes of MDS, namely (1) RA, (2) RARS, (3) RAEB (defined as 5%–19% blasts in the marrow), (4) RAEB in transformation (defined as 20%–29% blasts in the marrow), and CMML.

The WHO system thus bears some similarities to the FAB scheme, but there are several notable changes. First, the WHO system recognizes that MDS may present with isolated leukopenia or thrombocytopenia, albeit uncommonly, hence the change from RA to the broader RCUD and the addition of a second distinct class for patients with more than one affected cell line. Second, a mounting body of evidence suggested that MDS with proliferative features is clinically and biologically distinct from MDS without such features and thus warrants separate designation.[16,17] Third, the unique clinical syndrome associated with isolated del(5q), in combination with its particular responsiveness to treatment with lenalidomide, warranted its designation as a specific entity.[18] Finally, the cutoff for diagnosis of AML was changed from 30% to 20% bone marrow blasts or greater, rendering the designation of RAEB in transformation obsolete, although this change was not without its detractors.[19]

The WHO revision improved on certain aspects of the FAB system. In particular, the FAB system required that patients display at least 10% dysplasia in two different cell lineages to achieve even a diagnosis of RA; this excluded patients with mild or unilineage dysplasia, many of whom had natural histories indistinguishable from those who met the diagnostic criteria. While the WHO guidelines eliminated the dual-lineage requirement and allows a diagnosis of MDS in patients with unilineage dysplasia, it nevertheless draws arbitrary lines of distinction between subclasses of a heterogeneous disease, and patients with minimal dysplasia are still typically excluded from the diagnosis.[20] Artificial boundaries such as the 10% dysplasia, 15% ring sideroblasts and 5%/10%/20% blast cutoffs often prove themselves to be of variable relevance, both biologically and clinically, because they fail to capture a number of variables important in MDS, including age, sex, and most cytogenetic and genetic data.

Although some of the FAB and WHO subgroups imply very rough prognostic information—for instance, patients with FAB RAEB or WHO RAEB-2 are at higher risk of progression to AML than subgroups without excess blasts[21]—other systems specifically dedicated to estimating disease risk, such as the International Prognostic Scoring System (IPSS; see later), are better suited to this task.

Future iterations of a classification system may incorporate elements of genetic or clinical data that better group MDS patients based on disease biology, prognosis and natural history, or anticipated responsiveness to treatment modalities.[22] For now, however, this classification scheme remains only one of several descriptive tools applied to patients with MDSs.

EPIDEMIOLOGY AND ETIOLOGY

Most available data suggest that MDS is one of the most common hematologic malignancies, although this claim has been difficult to validate until recently because of confusing terminology and incomplete reporting of cases to registries.[23,24] Cases of MDS were not reported to the National Cancer Institute's Surveillance, Epidemiology, and End Results (SEER) until 2001, and initial reports to the registry suggested an incidence of only about 10,000 new cases per year.[25] Subsequent comparison of these data with Medicare and insurance claims for MDS suggested that a substantial proportion of MDS cases went unreported to SEER, with an estimated age-adjusted incidence of >5.3 per 100,000, compared to the SEER estimate of 3.3.[26]

The reporting difference was especially stark in patients age 65 and older, where it was estimated that the actual incidence of MDS might actually be close to fourfold higher than what was captured in the database (75 versus 20 per 100,000). Some of the underreporting was likely related to specific criteria for entry into the database (for instance, myeloid malignancies could only be counted once, such that patients presenting with a new diagnosis of secondary AML were usually coded as AML, without mention of MDS). Much of the underreporting, however, was likely because of the complexity of diagnosing and classifying MDS, as described earlier. The rate of reporting appears to have recently improved, with annual incidence in the 2007–2011 SEER database estimated at around 20,500 and an age-adjusted incidence of 4.9 per 100,000.[27]

Even the most accurate database, however, would probably underestimate the total global burden of MDS, which is likely present in a substantial percentage of older patients with idiopathic cytopenias who never undergo bone marrow analysis.[28] Although some proportion of this uncaptured population likely has biologically indolent

TABLE 60.1	2008 World Health Organization Classification of the Adult Myelodysplastic Syndromes

Refractory Cytopenia With Unilineage Dysplasia

Dysplasia	≥10% of cells from a single lineage
Blasts	<5% in marrow; <1% in peripheral blood; no Auer rods
Notes	Includes refractory anemia (RA), refractory neutropenia, refractory thrombocytopenia; RA is by far the most common subtype

Refractory Anemia With Ring Sideroblasts

Dysplasia	Isolated erythroid dysplasia
Blasts	<5% in marrow; <1% in peripheral blood; no Auer rods
Notes	≥15% of erythroid precursors are ring sideroblasts
	Frequently associated with SF3B1 mutations

MDS With Isolated del(5q)

Dysplasia	Normal or increased megakaryocytes with hypolobated nuclei
Blasts	<20% (though usually much less)
Notes	del(5q31) must be sole chromosomal abnormality

Refractory Cytopenia With Multilineage Dysplasia

Dysplasia	≥10% of cells from two or more myeloid lineages
Blasts	<5% in marrow; <1% in peripheral blood; no Auer rods
Notes	Peripheral monocyte count must be <1 × 10⁹/L; ring sideroblasts may be present

Refractory Anemia With Excess Blasts

Dysplasia	No specific requirement
Blasts	RAEB-1: 5%–9% in marrow, <5% in peripheral blood, AND no Auer rods
	RAEB-2: 10%–19% in marrow, 5%–19% in peripheral blood, OR Auer rods
Notes	Old designation of RAEB-t (20%–30% blasts) now considered AML

Unclassifiable MDS

Dysplasia	Minimal, or not meeting criteria for another subtype
Blasts	<5% in marrow; <1% in peripheral blood; no Auer rods
Notes	In presence of *clonal cytogenetic finding* considered diagnostic of MDS

Note: excludes refractory cytopenias of childhood. MDS/myeloproliferative neoplasms such as chronic myelomonocytic leukemia and RARS with thrombocytosis are classified separately.
AML, Acute myeloid leukemia; MDS, myelodysplastic syndrome; RAEB, refractory anemia with excess blast.

TABLE 60.2	Genes Recurrently Mutated in Myelodysplastic Syndrome

Gene	Frequency (%)	Notes
Splicing Factors		
SF3B1	20–30	Strong association with RARS
SRSF2	10–15 (MDS) 40 (CMML)	Enriched in CMML
U2AF1	5–12	Association with del(20q)
Epigenetic Modifiers		
TET2	20–30 (MDS) 40–50 (CMML)	Enriched in CMML Mutually exclusive with IDH
DNMT3A	8–13	
ASXL1	10–20 (MDS) 30–40 (CMML)	Enriched in CMML
EZH2	5–10 (MDS) 20–30 (CMML)	Enriched in CMML May be functionally involved in 7q−
IDH1/2	<5	More frequent in AML
ATRX	Rare	Associated with acquired thalassemia
Transcription Factors		
RUNX1	10–15	Can be somatic or germline
GATA2	Rare	Mostly germline
ETV6	<5	Can be somatic or germline
TP53	10–12	Association with complex karyotype, therapy-related disease
Kinases and Receptors		
JAK2	<5	Enriched in RARS-T
NRAS	5–10	Seen in progression to AML
CBL	<5	Enriched in JMML
PTPN11	<5	More common in JMML
BRAF	Rare	Also seen in hairy cell leukemia
Cohesin Complex		
STAG2	5–10	Cohesin class mutations enriched in high-risk MDS and secondary AML.
RAD21	<5	
SMC3	<2	
SMC1A	<2	
GCPR Complex		
GNAS	Rare	Mutations recently described in wide range of hematologic malignancies, including MDS.
GNB1	Rare	

AML, Acute myeloid leukemia; CMML, chronic myelomonocytic leukemia; GCPR, G-coupled protein receptor; IDH, isocitrate dehdryogenase; JMML, juvenile myelomonocytic leukemia; MDS, myelodysplastic syndrome; RARS, refractory anemia with ring sideroblasts; RARS-T, RARS with thrombocytosis.

disease that would never require therapy, more thorough cross-sectional studies, particularly in older patients, would help clarify the distinction between this end of the MDS spectrum and more aggressive biology that brings patients to clinical attention.

As referenced earlier, MDS is by and large a disease of older adults and reflects the inexorable acquisition of genetic mutations by aging hematopoietic progenitor cells (Table 60.2). In the United States, the median age at diagnosis is approximately 71 years,[29] and in the absence of a congenital disorder or exposure to radiation or cytotoxic chemotherapy for another disease, diagnosis before the age of 50 is rare.[30] Recent data suggest that a substantial proportion of older adults, perhaps as many as 10% of those over age 70, harbor hematopoietic clones defined by the presence of mutations recurrently found in MDS and AML, and that this state of "clonal hematopoiesis of indeterminate potential" progresses to MDS at a rate of 0.5% to 1% per year.[31,32] MDS occurs in children much more rarely, at an estimated annual rate of 1 per 1 million.[33] Most cases are classified as oligoblastic myelogenous leukemia (essentially RAEB), and other subtypes are even less common.[34] Several genetic syndromes confer an increased risk of MDS; these include Down syndrome,[35] Fanconi

anemia,[36] dyskeratosis congenita and other telomeropathies, and germline mutations in GATA2,[37] RUNX1,[38] and ETV6.[39] In Fanconi anemia and the telomeropathies,[40] MDS during young adulthood may be the initial presenting sign of the disease.

Most subtypes of MDS appear to be more common in men than women, with the most recent SEER data suggesting respective age-adjusted incidences of 6.7 versus 3.9 per 100,000.[41] The one exception to this is MDS with isolated del(5q), which most series show to be more common in women.[42] The reason for these sex differences is unclear; some have postulated a protective factor encoded on the X chromosome, or a similar protective factor on the Y chromosome (which is clonally lost in some cases of MDS). Others have suggested that the increased incidence in men overall is likely caused by differences in occupational exposures, but this has never been clearly demonstrated. Indeed, the only toxic chemical exposure definitively proven to cause MDS is benzene,[43] which is now significantly less prevalent in industrial workplaces than it had been in the past. Other environmental exposures, including cigarette smoking, have been postulated but never definitively proven to predispose to MDS.[44]

MDS in the United States and Western Europe is epidemiologically similar, but there are differences between these geographic regions and other parts of the world. In Asia[45] and Eastern Europe,[46] for instance, the average age at MDS diagnosis is younger, and the frequency of both severe cytopenias and risk of progression to leukemia may differ.[47] Some of these differences are likely caused by variance in environmental exposures. In Japan, for example, broad population-wide exposure to ionizing radiation from the atomic bombings of Hiroshima and Nagasaki in the 1940s continued to influence MDS incidence well into the 1990s.[48] However, the cause of differences in MDS subtypes, such as the low incidence of RARS in Japan compared with the West, remain unclear.

Indeed, the two exposures most consistently associated with subsequent development of MDS are ionizing radiation and cytotoxic chemotherapy, and MDS arising in these settings, known as therapy-related MDS or t-MDS, is frequently characterized by TP53 mutations,[49] multiple large-scale chromosomal abnormalities including complex karyotypes (most commonly defined as ≥3 clonal chromosomal anomalies),[50] and frequent transformation to treatment-refractory AML.[51] In the United States, radiation is most frequently encountered as treatment for other cancers, and radiation fields that include the hips or pelvis, the most active sites of hematopoiesis in adults, probably pose the greatest risk.[52] Less commonly, exposure to radiation can occur as the result of occupational exposures (e.g., workers at nuclear reactors) or industrial accidents. Among chemotherapeutic agents, there is a substantial difference in the risk of subsequent MDS. In particular, alkylating agents (e.g., cyclophosphamide and melphalan)[53] appear to carry the greatest risk, while the risk with nucleoside analogues is lower. Of particular note, the rapidly progressive AML seen in association with topoisomerase inhibitors (e.g., doxorubicin, etoposide) is not typically preceded by MDS.[54]

PATHOBIOLOGY

The past 10 years have witnessed significant advances in our understanding of the rich and complex pathobiology underlying MDSs. MDS is now recognized to arise from interactions between acquired genetic mutations in hematopoietic precursor cells, alterations in the microenvironment of the bone marrow, and dysregulated immune surveillance. Broadly speaking, the acquisition of sequential mutations in precursor cells drives the development of a malignant clone, and alterations in the microenvironment and the immune response allow that clone's expansion. This section details our current understanding of these concepts.

Myelodysplastic Syndrome Stem Cells

One of the central challenges in understanding the pathogenesis of MDS has been isolating the cell of origin and understanding that cell's mechanisms of self-renewal and propagation, both of which are necessary for the establishment of a malignant clone.[55] In theory, the exact state of hematopoietic differentiation from which a malignant clone arises could vary between cases of MDS, but the capacity for self-renewal implies that the origin cell was either a hematopoietic stem cell (HSC), and thus possessed intrinsic self-renewal capabilities, or it was a more differentiated myeloid progenitor that acquired the ability to self-renew. Clonal expansion then occurs through the acquisition of new mutations or epigenetic alterations that either enhance proliferation or confer resistance to apoptosis. MDS presumably becomes morphologically apparent when the dominant clone acquires a subsequent genetic lesion that leads to dysplasia within one or more hematopoietic compartments; this may or may not coincide with genetic lesions that lead to ineffective hematopoiesis and cytopenias, at which point MDS also becomes clinically evident.[56]

Proving that MDS is a clonal disease was not as straightforward a proposition as it was for AML, in which examination of the bone marrow typically identifies sheets of abnormal, morphologically identical blasts. In contrast, for MDS—particularly low-risk disease in which blasts are rare and the marrow architecture is disorganized and heterogeneous—a clonal origin was not immediately obvious based on morphology alone. Nonetheless, the clonal nature of MDS was established in the 1980s by studies that showed skewed inactivation of glucose-6-phosphate dehydrogenase (G6PD), an X-linked gene, in the hematopoietic cells of female MDS patients heterozygous for G6PD deficiency.[57] More recent studies have used deep sequencing techniques to track the clonal evolution from MDS into AML and have confirmed that in these cases, the preexisting MDS is as highly clonal as the resulting secondary AML.[58]

That MDS is a disorder of stem or early progenitor cells has been more difficult to prove.[59] Some of this difficulty is a reflection of the elusiveness of human HSCs themselves: the ability of different human cell populations to self-propagate after xenotransplantation into immunodeficient mice, considered the functional hallmark of "stemness," varies with the exact degree of immunodeficiency of the mice into which the cells are transplanted.[60] Moreover, xenotransplant experiments using immunophenotypically defined hematopoietic stem and progenitor cells (HSPCs; classically CD34+ CD38− Lin−) from MDS patients have not shown a striking proliferative or self-renewal advantage for the MDS cells compared to normal controls,[61] and the degree to which these experiments accurately depict the clonal dynamics of MDS in humans is unclear. Some have further been troubled by the observation that lymphoid clonal expansion, which should occur with near-equal frequency to myeloid clonal expansion if MDS is indeed a disorder of very early hematopoietic progenitors, is only rarely observed.[62,63] However, more recent studies combining immunophenotypic analysis with deep sequencing of clonal mutations in MDS cells have shown that the mutations appear to originate exclusively in the most primitive, stem-cell-like compartment,[64] and others have shown that differential expansion of specific progenitor compartments may vary between different phenotypes and risk profiles of MDS.[65] This evidence has contributed to the conclusion that MDS is, in fact, a disorder of transformed HSCs.[66]

The conceptualization of MDS as a stem cell disorder explains, in large part, why it is so refractory to most attempts at conventional therapy. Both normal HSCs and leukemia stem cells remain quiescent for much of their lifetimes, and during these periods they are largely impervious to any agents, such as most chemotherapeutic drugs, that exert their effects during active DNA replication.[67] Overcoming the intrinsic resistance to therapy conferred by the existence of quiescent reservoirs of disease is one of the central challenges in developing effective treatments for MDS.[68]

Genetic Alterations

Like other cancers, the core hypothesis underlying MDS pathogenesis is that the originating clone of MDS becomes increasingly abnormal, and ultimately malignant, through the sequential accumulation of acquired genetic or epigenetic abnormalities.[69] Improvement in our understanding of how these abnormalities are acquired, how they interact with each other, and their impact on pathways affecting proliferation, self-renewal, and differentiation, has been one of the major advancements in the study of MDS over the last decade.

Several different classes of genetic abnormalities may be found in MDS. The first to be recognized were cytogenetic abnormalities on standard karyotyping,[70] which are present in about 50% of patients.[71] A second category of cryptic chromosomal aberrations, including microdeletions and copy number-neutral loss of heterozygosity, are too small to be detected by karyotype but may be found with fluorescence in-situ hybridization (FISH)[72] or single nucleotide polymorphism (SNP) arrays.[73] The most common type of abnormality, mutations in single genes, has been increasingly well characterized, and clinical tests for recurrent mutations are becoming increasingly available, though as discussed later, it appears that not all mutations have equal clinical relevance.[74] Finally, epigenomic alterations—global aberrations in histone and chromatin modification—are common in MDS, and are often, though not always, associated with mutations in genes involved in epigenetic regulation.[75]

Somatic Mutations

Of the types of genetic abnormalities found in MDS, acquired mutations in individual genes are the most recently recognized; they are also the most frequent, currently estimated to be present in around 80% of MDS patients.[69] Although certain environmental exposures increase the risk of acquiring potentially deleterious mutations, most are acquired randomly, either spontaneously (e.g., deamination of cytosine to uracil), during DNA replication before cell division, or during DNA repair.

One of the central challenges of understanding the genetics of MDS has been determining which mutations contribute to the pathogenesis of the disease and which do not. Accumulating evidence has shown that HSCs acquire nonsynonymous exonic mutations with translational consequences at a rate of about one mutation per decade.[76] Since the incidence of MDS increases with age, HSPCs from an average MDS patient should typically contain between 5–10 such mutations (though the actual number varies widely between patients), against a background of hundreds of noncoding single nucleotide variations. The vast majority of these mutations, both coding and noncoding, are of no pathogenic consequence and are thus termed *passenger* mutations, while a minority, the so-called driver mutations, actually contribute to the development of the disease.[77]

Distinguishing driver mutations from passenger mutations is not always trivial. Passenger mutations, without conferring clonal advantage, tend not to recur with any significant frequency in cohorts of MDS patients; however, whereas a few driver mutations are relatively common in MDS, many have been found in only a small fraction (<5%) of cases, suggesting novel mechanisms of disease pathogenesis.[78] Similarly, whereas noncoding mutations are unlikely to contribute to pathogenesis and can thus be ignored when analyzing MDS genomes, the majority of coding mutations, even those present within a majority of cells in the malignant clone, are also nonpathogenic and are simply artifacts captured by an aging HSPC. Classifying a mutation as a driver thus involves accumulating evidence that the mutation occurs recurrently in MDS, that its putative function could plausibly contribute to MDS pathogenesis, and, in the best-case scenario, that this function can be recapitulated using in vitro or in vivo models.

Large-scale genomic studies of MDS cohorts have shown that many of the recurrently mutated genes can be segregated into one of a few functional categories,[78–81] and this functional characterization has in turned revealed insights about how an MDS clone develops over time. Genes affecting RNA splicing (*SRSF2, SF3B1, U2AF1*) are the most commonly mutated and tend to be early events in MDS pathogenesis. Genes affecting epigenetic regulation (*TET2, ASXL1, EZH2, DNMT3A*) are the next-most commonly mutated and also tend to occur early. On the other hand, mutations in genes for growth factors (*NRAS, JAK2*) tend to occur late and in subclonal populations.

These observations have contributed to an overarching model of how sequential somatic mutations cooperate to bring about MDS. In this model, early mutations in splicing factors and epigenetic genes do little to affect proliferation or differentiation on their own, but rather create a permissive environment for the acquisition of subsequent mutations in genes that confer proliferative advantages or blocks in differentiation. The latter group of mutations contributes more directly to the clinical features of MDS, but the former is responsible for its tendency towards genomic and epigenomic instability, which in turn may contribute to the disease's poor response to treatment. This section is a brief summary of our current understanding of some of the most important genes and pathways that are recurrently deranged in MDS.[82]

Splicing Factor Mutations

Genes encoding splicing factors, which excise introns to create mature messenger RNA (mRNA) transcripts, are the most commonly mutated class of genes in MDS, with between half and two-thirds of patients harboring such a mutation.[83] As opposed to most of the other classes of mutations discussed here, which occur in other malignancies with significant frequency, splicing factor mutations are rarer in other cancers than MDS, and some have unique associations with specific morphologic phenotypes.[84] Splicing factor mutations tend to be mutually exclusive within MDS clones, and most of the affected genes encode proteins that comprise the E/A splice site recognition complex that acts at the 3′ end of pre-mRNA, suggesting that the mutations converge on a shared biologic pathway.[85] Exactly how splicing factor mutations predispose to the development of MDS, and whether they can help predict aspects of natural history or treatment response, remain areas of active investigation.

SF3B1

SF3B1 encodes the U2 small nuclear riboprotein complex (snRNP) responsible for 3′ branch site recognition and is the most frequently mutated splicing factor gene. *SF3B1* mutations can be found in about 20% to 30% of all MDS patients; there is a particularly strong association with ring sideroblast morphology, with mutations found in 60% to 85% of patients with RARS or RARS-T and substantial percentages of other MDS subtypes in which ring sideroblasts can be found.[86,87] The most common mutations are missense substitutions that change lysine to glutamate at codon 700, with other smaller hotspots in the same vicinity. These mutations all occur within a cluster of 26 nonrepeating HEAT domains that are thought to be involved in binding of *SF3B1* to other members of the U2 snRNP.[88] As with other splicing factor mutations, they tend to be heterozygous and imply a gain of function. How exactly the mutations affect MDS pathogenesis is not completely clear, but they are often acquired early in disease development, tend not to be associated with complex karyotypes, and tend not to be associated with poor-prognosis mutations.[89] *SF3B1* mutations are clinically associated with a distinct phenotype of isolated, transfusion-dependent anemia with preserved white blood cell and platelet counts relative to *SF3B1*-wildtypes, as well as a lower risk of progression to AML.[90] Indeed, in larger studies of MDS cohorts, *SF3B1* mutations appear to confer an improvement in relative survival, making them somewhat unique among MDS-associated mutations.[80]

SRSF2

SRSF2 encodes a member of the serine/arginine (SR)-rich family of pre-mRNA splicing factors that interacts with the U2 and U1 components of the spliceosome. After *SF3B1*, it is the second-most commonly mutated splicing factor, with mutations present in 10% to 15% of MDS[91] and 40% of CMML.[92] The overwhelming majority of mutations are heterozygous missense substitutions for proline at codon 95, implying a gain of function. A small minority of in-frame insertions or deletions affects the same region. *SRSF2* mutations co-occur with several other mutations, many of which are also frequently found in CMML, including *TET2, ASXL1, CUX1, IDH2,* and *STAG2*. In contradistinction to patients with *SF3B1* mutations, patients with *SRSF2* mutations tend to have more dysplasia in the granulocytic lineage and less in the erythroid lineage, and patients consequently tend to have a less prominent transfusion requirement, more enrichment in the RAEB subtypes, and, at least in some studies, a greater risk of progression to AML.[93] This phenotype is more heterogeneous than that associated with *SF3B1*, but most studies have nevertheless shown that *SRSF2* mutations appear to confer an inferior prognosis.[91]

U2AF1

U2AF1 encodes an auxiliary factor in the U2 spliceosome that is responsible for recognizing the AG splice acceptor dinucleotide at the 3′ end of introns. *U2AF1* mutations occur in about 12% of patients with MDS.[94] Similar to other commonly mutated splicing factor genes, the two most common mutations are both heterozygous missense substitutions, again implying a gain of function, and both appear to alter sequence specificity of pre-mRNA binding and splicing.[95] The two mutations are in separate zinc finger DNA binding domains, one at codon 34 toward the N-terminal of the protein, and one at codon 157 toward the C terminal. Some studies have shown an increased tendency of MDS with *U2AF1* mutations to evolve into secondary AML,[96] but given the small numbers of patients in these studies, the strength of this effect is unclear.

Epigenetic Modifier Mutations

Epigenetic changes are biochemical modifications that affect chromatin structure, and thereby gene expression, without actually altering the DNA sequence itself. The two types of epigenetic changes most relevant to MDS are DNA methylation and histone modification.[75] DNA methylation involves the addition of a methyl group to the cytosine residues of cytosine-guanine pairs by members of the DNA methyltransferase (DNMT) family of enzymes. These cytosine-guanine pairs frequently cluster together in "CpG islands," which are typically located just upstream of promoter regions. CpG islands tend to be unmethylated at baseline, but their progressive methylation leads to transcriptional silencing of the downstream genes. Studies have shown that many MDS patients display aberrant methylation patterns compared to healthy controls, with isolated hypermethylation in the promoters of critical tumor suppressors despite global hypomethylation elsewhere. This phenomenon has been hypothesized to play a role in the pathogenesis of MDS, but attempts to glean prognostic or predictive information from specific methylation patterns in MDS patients have been largely unsuccessful, and the success of so-called hypomethylating agents such as 5-azacitidine and decitabine (which may in fact not truly act by reducing global methylation) has been variable.

A second type of epigenetic regulation involves the biochemical modification of histones, the structural protein complexes that form scaffolding for chromatin packaging. The interaction between histones and chromatin represents an additional level of transcriptional control, in which unwinding of chromatin is required for the transcription machinery to physically access DNA. The dynamics of chromatin-histone interactions are largely mediated by complex biochemical modifications of specific histone amino acids. In MDS and other myeloid disorders, these modifications can either be affected directly by mutations in genes coding for histone-modifying enzymes or indirectly by the permutation of biochemical pathways that regulate the balance between open and closed chromatin.

TET2

TET2, which encodes a member of the Ten-Eleven Translocation gene family, is the most commonly mutated epigenetic regulator in MDS.[97] *TET2* mutations occur in 20% to 30% of all MDS and are particularly enriched in CMML, where they can be found in 40% to 50% of cases.[98] The *TET2* protein is a methylcytosine oxygenase responsible for converting 5-methylcytosine (5mC) into 5-hydroxymethylcytosine (5hmC) using iron and α-ketoglutarate (α-KG, produced by *IDH1* and *IDH2*), and for further oxidizing 5hmC to 5-formyl- and 5-carboxycytosine.[99] These reactions are thought to contribute to active demethylation through base excision repair back to unmodified cytosine.[100] Mutations in *TET2* tend to be inactivating frameshift or nonsense mutations or specific missense substitutions predicted to lead to abrogation of protein function, and

many patients are either compound heterozygotes or have uniparental disomy (UPD) at chromosome 4q, leading to effective abrogation of TET2 function.[101] Indeed, patients with *TET2* mutations have been shown to have globally altered methylation profiles.[102] *TET2* mutations often occur early in MDS pathogenesis and are thought to alter HSC homeostasis, a theory supported by the fact that HSCs in *TET2* knockout mice display enhanced self-renewal and repopulation capacity. In humans, however, *TET2* mutations do not appear to themselves confer a specific phenotype;[79] rather, they may create an epigenomic environment permissive to the acquisition of other mutations that are responsible for determining these factors. Recent evidence suggests that *TET2* mutations appear to predict a favorable response to hypomethylating agents, particularly in the setting of wildtype *ASXL1*.[103] *TET2* mutations were not previously felt to confer prognostic information, but newer data suggest that, at least in patients undergoing stem cell transplant, they predict an inferior outcome.[104]

DNMT3A

DNMT3A is a member of the family of DNMTs, which catalyze the addition of methyl groups to cytosine residues of CpG dinucleotides. These dinucleotides tend to cluster in 5′ promoter regions upstream of genes, and increased methylation of these CpG islands is associated with decreased expression of the associated downstream gene.[105] The observation that many cancers often display aberrant methylation relative to healthy tissue has led to the hypothesis that hypermethylation, particularly in the promoters of tumor suppressor genes, plays a role in cancer pathogenesis. This hypothesis has been somewhat supported by the efficacy, albeit imperfect, of so-called hypomethylating agents like decitabine and 5-azacitidine in MDS and AML (see section on Therapy, later).

The *DNMT3A* gene consists of 29 exons and encodes a 908-amino acid protein that, along with DNMT3B, is one of the two enzymes responsible for de novo CpG methylation independent of replication, whereas a third methyltransferase, DNMT1, is responsible for maintenance of baseline hemimethylation during active replication. Only *DNMT3A* mutations, however, have been found to occur recurrently in myeloid malignancies, perhaps suggesting differential expression in hematopoietic cells. Analysis of *DNMT3A* mutations in patients with MDS has shown a preponderance of missense single nucleotide variations predicted to alter protein function, although nonsense mutations, insertions, and deletions (indels) have been observed as well. The mutations occur throughout the gene, although a mutational hotspot at R882H, in the methyltransferase domain, has been described in a minority of MDS patients.[106] In AML, the R882H mutant protein has been shown to inhibit wildtype *DNTM3A*, suggesting a dominant negative mechanism.[107]

In earlier studies, *DNMT3A*-null HSCs transplanted into mice displayed aberrant global methylation patterns, increased self-renewal, and impaired differentiation capacity compared to wildtype HSCs, but the mice themselves did not develop dysplasia or other hematologic malignancies.[108] In more recent studies, however, mice transplanted with *DNMT3A*-null HSCs had shortened overall survival and developed a spectrum of hematopoietic malignancies similar to that seen in humans, including leukemia and MDS.[109] The different outcomes in these two studies is thought to be caused in large part by the fact that mice in the older experiments were serially transplanted at 18 weeks, before they had a chance to develop overt hematologic disease, whereas mice in the later experiments were observed for 6 months. The long latency to development of malignancy in these experiments may speak to the subtlety of the epigenomic abnormalities initially conferred by acquisition of *DNMT3A* mutations.

In humans, the significance of *DNMT3A* mutations in the pathogenesis of MDS is not clear. They occur with somewhat less frequency than the most common recurrent mutations (between 8 and 13% in most studies[80,110] although some studies have quoted much lower frequencies below 5%).[111] On the other hand, clonal

DNMT3A mutations have recently been shown to exist with modest frequency in healthy older adults and are in fact significantly more common than mutations in any other single gene,[31] with an overall frequency that is significantly higher than their aggregate representation among hematologic malignancies. This discrepancy could either reflect the same long latency of *DNMT3A*-mutated hematologic malignancy that was observed in mouse models, or it could suggest that *DNMT3A* mutations have a relatively less potent pathogenic effect than some other genes (e.g., *TET2* mutations, which are less frequent in the general population but more frequent in MDS).

DNTM3A mutations appear to be negatively correlated with mutations in certain other genes, particularly *SRSF2* and *ASXL1*,[80] and in low-risk MDS they seem to have a positive correlation with *SF3B1* mutations.[112] There is evidence that *DNMT3A* mutations confer a poor prognosis in cytogenetically normal AML,[106] but that prognostic significance so far has not been convincingly shown to apply to *DNMT3A*-mutated MDS.

ASXL1

ASXL1 codes for a polycomb chromatin-binding protein and is involved in epigenetic regulation of gene expression. It acts as a co-activator of the retinoic acid receptor and directly interacts with chemical modifiers of histones (e.g., NCOA1, a histone acetyltransferase, and LSD1, a histone demethylase). *ASXL1* mutations occur in about 10% to 29% of total MDS and myeloproliferative neoplasm (MPN),[113] 17% of AML, and 40% of CMML.[114]

The specific mechanisms by which *ASXL1* mutations affect the development of MDS are not clear. The first mice engineered to have constitutive *ASXL1* germline insufficiency survived to adulthood with relatively mild lymphopenia and modest splenomegaly, and did not develop myelodysplasia.[115] Subsequently, *ASXL1* mutations were found to confer global reduction H3K27 trimethylation by disrupting normal recruitment of polycomb recessive complex 2 (PRC2), which places the H3K27 mark in vivo.[116] This was followed by a more physiologic attempt at conditional *ASXL1* knockout in murine hematopoietic cells, which did induce abnormal myeloid differentiation that was compounded by additional loss of *TET2*. In this study, *ASXL1*-deficient cells displayed differential expression of a set of genes largely related to hematopoietic differentiation.[117]

In humans, most MDS-associated *ASXL1* mutations affect the C-terminal portion of the protein, specifically the plant homeo protein interaction domain.[118] This observation has led to speculation that the mutant protein retains DNA-binding activity and thus exerts a dominant-negative effect on wildtype *ASXL1*, which may not have been captured in the mouse experiments. In studies of MDS cohorts, investigators have observed that *ASXL1* mutations co-occur less frequently with certain other recurrent genetic lesions, particularly *DNTM3A* and *JAK2*.[119] On the other hand, *ASXL1* mutations have been found to cooccur with both *RUNX1* and *TET2* abnormalities.[120] The most recent rigorous studies suggest that *ASXL1* mutations have a modestly poor prognosis, but tend to occur in patients with low IPSS scores who would otherwise be felt to have indolent disease, perhaps suggesting a more profound pathogenic effect than might be suspected.[79]

EZH2

EZH2 encodes the catalytic subunit of PRC2, which promotes the di- and trimethylation of lysine 27 on histone 3 (H3K27). Locally, methylated H3K27 results in closed chromatin and transcriptional repression, and global H3K27 trimethylation in particular is associated with reduced pluripotency and cellular senescence, suggesting a role for *EZH2* in regulation of cell fate.[121] Recent studies have shown that α-KG also regulates relative levels of methylation at this locus, suggesting a possible henvergence with the TET2/IDH pathway.[122] *EZH2* resides on the long arm of chromosome 7, and its loss has been hypothesized to be at least part of the reason 7q− is such a

deleterious cytogenetic occurrence in MDS,[123] though not all 7q deletions affect the *EZH2* locus.[124] Mutations in *EZH2* itself are found in 5% to 10% of patients with MDS[80] and 20% to 30% of patients with CMML.[125] Consistent with the model of *EZH2* as a negative regulator of pluripotency and survival, mutations tend either to be inactivating frameshift or nonsense mutations, or missense mutations concentrated in the gene's SET domain, which is critical for DNA binding.[126,127] *EZH2* mutations confer a negative prognosis in MDS that appears to be independent of other prognostic factors, including the IPSS score, in part because they tend not to be associated with specific clinical characteristics that are incorporated into these systems.[79]

IDH Genes

The isoforms of isocitrate dehydrogenase, encoded by *IDH1* and *IDH2*, are responsible for the conversion of isocitrate to α-KG, which as above is used by TET2 in the conversion of 5mC to 5hmC. Mutations in *IDH1* and *IDH2* lead to enzymes with neomorphic activity that convert α-KG to d-2-hydroxyglutarate, which accumulating data suggests is an oncometabolite that can inhibit both TET2 and other epigenetic enzymes, including prolyl hydroxylases and a number of histone demethylases.[128] Mutations in *IDH1/2* and other members of the IDH pathway (including *WT1*) have repeatedly been shown to be important in AML,[129] but *IDH* mutations are relatively infrequent in MDS, occurring in 5% or fewer of patients.[79,80] Both *IDH1* and *IDH2* mutations can cooccur with most other recurrent mutations besides *TET2*, with which they are essentially mutually exclusive.

Transcription Factor Genes

Transcription factors represent a third class of genes commonly mutated in MDS. Similar to epigenetic and splicing genes, mutated transcription factors can have pleiotropic effects on a number of gene targets, and these mutations are indeed also often early events in MDS pathogenesis.

RUNX1

RUNX1 (formerly known as *AML1*) is the transcription factor gene most commonly mutated in MDS, and its biology is complex. It encodes the alpha subunit of the core binding transcription factor and is involved in determining the lineage fate of HSCs.[130] *RUNX1* was initially identified as one of the genes involved in two different common pathogenic translocations: t(8;21), found in AML, and t(12;21), found in acute lymphoblastic leukemia.[131,132] Subsequently, germline point mutations in *RUNX1* were identified in autosomal dominant familial platelet disorder with propensity for AML,[38] and later as somatic events in both sporadic AML and MDS.[133] Reflecting the complexity of *RUNX1* biology, mutations occurring throughout the gene, can be either monoallelic or biallelic, and can be frameshift insertions or deletions or nonsense or missense substitutions.[134] However, most mutations appear to have an inactivating effect on *RUNX1* function, either by affecting the DNA-binding RUNT domain or by disrupting the C-terminal protein interaction domain.[135] Many of the remaining mutations outside these regions appear to affect RUNX1 interactions with epigenetic regulators like MLL, thereby affecting histone methylation.[136] Both clonal and subclonal *RUNX1* mutations appear to confer a poor prognosis in MDS patients, irrespective of other prognostic factors.[78]

ETV6

ETV6 encodes an ets-like transcription factor with mostly repressive activity.[137] It is situated on the short arm of chromosome 12, and its role in hematologic malignancy has been best characterized by its involvement in recurrent translocations, including t(3;12)(q26;p13)[138] and deletions of 12p.[139] In MDS, however, both missense and inactivating frameshift point mutations have been described as well. There is some data that the missense mutations, which mostly cluster in the DNA-binding ETS domain, have a dominant negative effect on the wildtype allele.[140] However, whether malignant transformation requires ETV6 activity below a critical threshold remains unclear, as not all frameshift mutations occur with loss of heterozygosity (and some frameshifts can confer dominant negative function as well). *ETV6* mutations are relatively rare events in MDS, occurring in at most 5% of cases;[79] recently, familial cases of MDS and AML because of inherited *ETV6* mutations have also been described.[39]

GATA2

GATA2 encodes a transcription factor with pleiotropic effects in early hematopoietic progenitor cells.[141] In contrast to most other genes described here, acquired mutations in *GATA2* are quite rare, but there are a number of clinical syndromes associated with germline *GATA2* mutations, several of which involve a risk of developing MDS and AML. These include Emberger syndrome (congenital lymphedema and risk of AML),[142] autosomal dominant monocytopenia and mycobacterial infection syndrome,[143] and dendritic cell, monocyte, B and natural killer (NK) lymphoid deficiency syndrome.[144] In addition, *GATA2* mutations have also been described in kindreds with no accessory phenotype beyond a strong history of early-onset MDS/AML.[37] Several phenotypic components appear to be dependent on the type of mutation. For instance, nearly all patients who develop MDS or AML have mutations in or immediately 5′ to the second zinc finger domain, which tend to be missense substitutions predicted to affect DNA binding.[145] On the other hand, a second group of patients with truncating frameshift mutations in the N-terminal region of the gene tend to present at younger ages with more pronounced immune deficits, but have a lower risk of MDS or AML. Although the mechanism by which these patients develop MDS is not completely clear, the subset of patients with *GATA2* germline mutations who develop MDS or AML has been observed to acquire *ASXL1* mutations with frequency much greater than would be expected to occur by chance.[146]

TP53

TP53 mutations occur in about 10% of patients with MDS, and as in other settings imply a poor prognosis and response to therapy.[79] They are closely associated with a complex karyotype and tend not to cooccur with other recurrent driver mutations.[147,148] They frequently cooccur with del(5q) and may represent a progression pathway for patients with 5q− syndrome.[149] They are also frequently found in t-MDS and AML.[49] Recently, a small series of patients with t-AML showed that TP53 mutations present in the leukemia were detectable in samples collected 3–6 years earlier, which in at least two patients predated their original chemotherapy.[150] This suggests that the expansion of rare preexisting clones harboring TP53 mutations may be the leukemogenic mechanism in at least some patients with therapy-related disease, rather than accumulation of DNA damage induced by the chemotherapy itself.

Tyrosine Kinases and Growth Factor Receptors

Mutations in tyrosine kinase and growth factor receptor genes are typically associated with proproliferative signals and occur in a wide range of myeloid malignancies, including AML (*FLT3*[151]), MPNs (*JAK2*[152] and *MPL*[153]), and mast cell disorders (*KIT*).[154] While they do occur in MDS, they are usually late, subclonal events that often mark progression to secondary AML.[155] A few of these deserve specific mention. Activating mutations in *NRAS* are the most frequent

tyrosine kinase mutations found in MDS,[156] but still only occur in about 5% of cases and as mentioned earlier, tend to begin as subclonal, proproliferative events that frequently drive the transition to AML.[157] Best known for its role in MPNs, *JAK2* is mutated in about 3% to 5% of MDS, particularly RARS-T and CMML.[158] *JAK2* mutations in MDS tend not to be associated with overproduction of mature hematopoietic cells as they are in MPNs, likely as a consequence of concomitant biologic defects contributing to ineffective hematopoiesis.[159]

Cohesin Complex Genes

Genes encoding members of the cohesin complex family, including *RAD21*, *STAG2*, *SMC3*, and *SMC1A*, are each mutated in a small minority of MDS cases, but collectively, cohesin mutations can be found in about 10% of MDS.[160] Their physiologic role is in the maintenance of chromatid structural fidelity, particularly during mitosis. How cohesin complex mutations affect MDS pathogenesis is not completely understood, since they do not appear to directly promote chromosomal instability. Clinical studies, however, have shown that they appear to be disproportionately associated with multilineage dysplasia, and confer inferior survival and an increased risk of progression to AML.[161]

Other Genes

The genes described previously collectively account for the majority of mutations found recurrently in MDS, but this list is certainly not exhaustive. Even very recent, broad surveys of patients with MDS using the most updated panels of gene mutations and high-resolution FISH and karyotyping have shown that between 10% and 20% of patients lack a detectable genetic abnormality.[78–81] There are multiple possible explanations for this observation. For example, some of these patients may have other types of aberrations not captured by sequencing or karyotyping, such as small copy number abnormalities that might be detected by SNP arrays, which are not routinely performed in clinical practice. More likely, however, many of these patients probably have mutations in genes that are less frequently altered in MDS pathogenesis. Some of these mutations are in pathways represented by other, better-known genes; for example, rare mutations have been described in *PTPN11*, a tyrosine phosphatase that acts as a downstream effector in the RAS pathway,[162] and in *BRAF*, better known for its association with melanoma and hairy cell leukemia.[163] Similarly, rare mutations have been described in *EED* and *SUZ12*, other components of the PRC2 that affiliate with EZH2 and collectively interact with ASXL1.[164] Other times, MDS can occur in the setting of mutations in genes better known for being associated with other diseases, such mutations in *CBL*, a gene better known for its association with juvenile myelomonocytic leukemia that encodes an E3 ubiquitin ligase responsible for degrading several tyrosine kinases.[165] Finally, mutations are occasionally described in relatively novel gene classes, including genes encoding the G-protein subunits *GNAS*[166] and *GNB1*[167] and the DNA repair enzymes *hOGG1*, *XRCC3*, and *XPD*.[168] Some patients may have mutations in other genes that have yet to be described. While it is unlikely that a major, frequently mutated pathway remains undiscovered in MDS, study of these low-frequency, "long-tail" mutations may yield valuable further insights into the molecular pathogenesis of the disease.

Karyotypic Abnormalities

Chromosomal abnormalities, larger-scale genetic aberrations that can be detected on either karyotype or FISH, are also common events in MDS.[169] The most common types of abnormalities in MDS are deletions or duplications of very large chromosomal regions; as opposed to some other hematologic cancers, translocations and inversions are less common. Several of the most common karyotypic abnormalities have been shown to have prognostic value, and one, del(5q), has enough unique biologic features to be its own subclassification within the WHO criteria.

del(5q)

Interstitial deletion of the long arm of chromosome 5 [del(5q)] is the most common chromosomal abnormality in MDS,[42] and del(5q) is the only karyotypically-defined subtype recognized by the WHO.[170] Although the specific region affected varies between patients, there are two commonly deleted regions (CDRs), one on 5q31.1 and the other at 5q32-33.3, with most patients having a deletion that includes both CDRs.[171] MDS patients in whom del(5q) is the sole karyotypic abnormality often display the "5q-minus syndrome," which is clinically characterized by anemia, normal or elevated platelet count, female predominance,[172] lower risk of transformation to AML, and a striking response to lenalidomide.[173]

Our understanding of the pathobiology underlying del(5q) MDS has improved substantially over the past several years; a key observation was the lack of recurrent point mutations in genes located on 5q in other patients with MDS, which, coupled with the fact that most patients with del(5q) retain one normal chromosome 5, suggested that the pathobiology could be best explained by haploinsufficiency of deleted genes.[174] Indeed, it now appears that different genes lost in the CDRs are responsible for different aspects of the 5q- phenotype. For instance, haploinsufficiency of *RPS14*, a ribosomal subunit gene located at 5q31.2, leads to p53 activation in erythroid progenitors and is responsible for the dyserythropoiesis seen in the syndrome,[175] and deletion of a key microRNA, miR-145, is responsible for the megakaryocytic component of the phenotype.[176] Separately, haploinsufficiency of *CSNK1A1*, which is located at 5q32 and encodes casein kinase 1-alpha, is responsible for the sensitivity to lenalidomide, which accelerates the ubiquitination and degradation of remaining casein kinase 1-alpha through a cereblon-dependent process.[177] Other studies have suggested that additional genes on 5q, including *EGR1*, *APC*[178], *HSPA9*[179], *NPM1*[180], and others[181] may contribute to features of the disease via a similar mechanism of haploinsufficiency in select cases.

These points apply only to del(5q) as a sole karyotypic abnormality in MDS. When del(5q) is found with other chromosomal abnormalities, especially in the context of a complex karyotype (three or more karyotypic abnormalities, a finding often associated with TP53 mutations or 17p loss), the prognosis is poor and the response to lenalidomide seen in 5q- syndrome usually does not exist.[149] Cooccurrence of del(5q) with TP53 mutation or 17p loss, in fact, occurs more frequently than would be expected by chance, suggesting cooperativity of the two abnormalities. Del(5q) seen in the context of AML, even if the sole karyotypic abnormality, is a universally poor prognostic sign.[182]

Chromosome 7 Abnormalities

Deletion of one entire copy of chromosome 7 (i.e., monosomy 7) is also characteristic of MDS and portends a poor prognosis.[183] The pathogenesis of chromosome 7 abnormalities is incompletely understood. Several genes recurrently mutated in MDS, including *EZH2*,[123] *MLL3*,[124] and *CUX1*,[184] lie on 7q, and it has been hypothesized that loss of some or all of chromosome 7 contributes to MDS pathogenesis via a haploinsufficiency mechanism similar to that seen in del(5q). If such a mechanism exists, however, the evidence supporting it has not yet been produced. Part of the difficulty in proving its existence lies in the fact that unlike del(5q), there is no common deleted region on chromosome 7 in which to focus efforts at driver gene discovery.[185] It is important to note that in the revised IPSS (IPSS-R), del(7q) is considered to be an intermediate-prognosis abnormality distinct from monosomy 7, which is classified as poor prognosis.[186]

Trisomy 8

Trisomy 8 is present in about 5% of MDS patients and can be found in a wide range of other myeloid disorders, including AML, MPNs, and aplastic anemia. In MDS, it can often be seen as a late, subclonal event.[187] Although its contribution to pathogenesis is incompletely understood, MDS patients with trisomy 8 appear to upregulate *WT1*, an oncogene that can be mutated in AML (but very rarely in MDS), which may behave as a neoantigen that stimulates the expansion of oligoclonal CD4+ and CD8+ T cells.[188] Some evidence suggests that these populations may contribute to impairment of hematopoiesis in MDS patients with trisomy 8,[189] which may explain why some patients with isolated trisomy 8 can have substantial responses to immune suppression with antithymocyte globulin (ATG).[190] Trisomy 8 has also been associated with the development of paraneoplastic autoimmune phenomena, such as Behçet disease,[191] again reflective of the immune dysregulation characteristic of this cytogenetic abnormality.

del(20q)

del(20q) is an infrequent chromosomal aberration in MDS, occurring in about 2% of patients.[192] Patients with del(20q) frequently have prominent thrombocytopenia, may have concomitant mutations of *U2AF1*, and appear to have an intermediate prognosis,[193] although 20q loss can also be a late event that indicates clonal progression of disease.[194] The best candidate driver gene lying within the common deleted region is a tumor suppressor gene known as *MYBL2*,[195] but recent studies suggest that in myeloid models, a reduction in *MYBL2* levels below what would be predicted for classic haploinsufficiency is required to drive clonal expansion.[196] Although *ASXL1* resides on 20q, it sits outside the CDR,[197] and most patients with 20q abnormalities do not have concomitant *ASXL1* mutations.

17p Deletions

Chromosome 17 abnormalities occur most often in MDS in association with complex karyotypes, which is most likely related to the fact that *TP53* resides within the common deleted region on 17p.[147] In MDS, many patients with loss of 17p will have an inactivating mutation of their remaining copy of *TP53*, implying that haploinsufficiency is not in and of itself enough to drive pathogenesis.[198] At the same time, patients almost never lose both copies of 17p as part of a larger chromosomal event, suggesting that some other gene or genes in this region may be essential for hematopoietic cell survival. As with *TP53* point mutations, loss of 17p is an exceedingly poor prognostic factor in MDS, is frequently seen in cases of therapy-related disease,[53] and often presages the development of treatment-refractory AML.[199]

Complex and Monosomal Karyotypes

Complex karyotypes, meaning those with three or more cytogenetic abnormalities, are one of the more common abnormalities in MDS.[169] About half are associated with *TP53* mutations; conversely, many, but not all, patients with TP53 mutations have complex karyotypes.[147] As opposed to 17p abnormalities, which are reflective of the *TP53* loss itself, complex karyotypes are instead downstream effects of p53 loss and represent the type of structural DNA damage that would have triggered p53-mediated apoptosis in normal cells. The exceedingly poor prognosis associated with complex karyotypes is in fact probably a proxy for p53 loss; the half of patients with complex karyotypes who have intact p53 function appear to have prognoses similar to patients with normal cytogenetics. Monosomal karyotypes, defined as complete loss of at least two entire chromosomes or one monosomy plus one other abnormality, are also common and also tend to confer a poor prognosis, particularly when associated with monosomy 7 or monosomy 5.[200] When monosomal and complex karyotypes occur together, however, the monosomy does not appear to confer an additional poor prognosis beyond that of the complex karyotype.[201]

Other Karyotypic Abnormalities

A number of other cytogenetic abnormalities have been repeatedly described in MDS, including −Y,[202] del(13q),[203] del(11q),[139] del(12p) or t(12p),[204] del(9q),[192] idic(X)(q13),[192] t(11;16)(q23;p13.3),[205] t(3;21) (q26.2;q22.1),[206] t(1;3)(p36.3;q21),[207] t(2;11)(p21;q23),[205] inv(3) (q21q26.2)[207] and t(6;9)(p23;q34).[208] Most of these do not have specific phenotypes or associated with them, but some do confer prognostic information and are included in the IPSS-R. In particular, −Y and del(11q) are designated "very good" prognosis; del(12p), del(20q), isolated del(5q), and normal karyotypes are considered "good;" trisomy 8, del(7q), isochrome 17(q), trisomy 19, and trisomy 21 are considered "intermediate;" monosomy 7, double deleted (7q), derivative (3q), and complex karyotype with exactly three abnormalities are considered "poor," and complex karyotypes with more than three abnormalities are considered "very poor." In addition, finding any of these in the appropriate clinical context, regardless of whether they are known to carry prognostic information, is typically enough to warrant a diagnosis of MDS, even in the absence of clear morphologic dysplasia.

The Microenvironment in Myelodysplastic Syndrome

The malignant transformation of hematopoietic progenitors in MDS occurs not in isolation, but within the rich microenvironment of the bone marrow stroma, which has come to be known as the "hematopoietic niche."[209] Evidence has shown that under normal circumstances, hematopoiesis is in part regulated by paracrine signals released from nonhematopoietic mesenchymal cells,[210] and evolving data suggest that some of these processes are dysregulated in MDS. Early circumstantial clues came from findings that patients with MDS and other hematologic malignancies have abnormal circulating levels of cytokines known to affect hematopoiesis, including monocyte-colony stimulating factor, interleukin (IL) 1a, and granulocyte-monocyte colony stimulating factor (GM-CSF),[211] and other studies have shown that hematopoietic cells from MDS patients respond abnormally to these cytokines compared to cells from healthy controls.[212] More recent studies have shown that hematopoietic progenitor cells transplanted into older mice display a narrower range of clonal expansion than identical cells transplanted into younger mice, suggesting that an aging niche might exert selective pressure on dominant hematopoietic progenitor cell clones.[213] Furthermore, it has been discovered that conditional deletion of the gene encoding dicer1, a microRNA processing enzyme, in osteoprogenitor cells can induce myelodysplasia and secondary AML in mice;[214] concurrently, other studies have shown altered expression of DICER and DROSHA, another microRNA-processing enzyme, in mesenchymal cells of MDS patients.[215] Even more intriguing, it has recently been shown that introduction of an activating B-catenin mutation in mouse osteoblasts can induce the development of AML through induction of the Notch ligand jagged1, which leads to Notch activation in HSCs.[216] As tantalizing as these findings are, the extent of their pervasiveness across all MDS patients, and how microenvironmental alterations interact with the well-validated recurrent mutations found in hematopoietic cells, has yet to be determined. It is worth noting that HSC transplantation, which involves only the transplantation of hematopoietic elements and not stroma, can be curative for some patients with MDS, implying that at least in these patients, the niche is not sufficient to sustain disease.

Immune Dysregulation

In normal human tissues, both the innate and adaptive immune systems play important roles in identifying, isolating, and destroying early clones with malignant potential before they are able to transform into clinically evident cancers. Perturbation of this immune response presumably allows the persistence and propagation of abnormal clones in MDS, but the extent to which this is pathogenically important is not clear.[217]

Several aspects of innate immunity have been shown to be abnormal in MDS patients.[218] Some toll-like receptors, including TLR4, are overexpressed on MDS progenitor cells,[219] and increased TLR signaling has been associated with higher degrees of apoptosis and the development of cytopenias. In patients with del(5q), loss of miRs 145 and 146a from the common deleted region has been shown to upregulate tumor necrosis factor (TNF) receptor–associated factor 6, a TLR adaptor E3 ubiquitin ligase, as well as Toll IL-1 receptor domain-containing adaptor protein (TIRAP), two important downstream effectors of TLR4.[220] del(5q) may also lead to the upregulation of CD14 on granulocytes via heterozygous loss of mDia1, a scaffolding protein involved in actin polymerization, which appears to confer abnormalities of the innate immune response.[221] More recently, myeloid-derived suppressor cells have been shown to be significantly expanded in some patients with MDS, and increased signaling in these cells via interaction with S100A9, an important inflammatory mediator, has been shown to similarly stimulate inappropriate apoptosis in hematopoietic precursor cells.[222] Coincident with these findings, population-level data have suggested that patients with chronic inflammatory stimulation appear to be at increased risk of developing MDS and AML.[223]

Abnormalities in the adaptive immune system also exist in MDS. These have been particularly well described in hypoplastic variants, which have similarities to aplastic anemia at both the cellular and genetic level, and both can respond to immune suppression.[224] More broadly, oligoclonal T-cell receptor gene rearrangements can be found in MDS patients of all subtypes,[225] and clinically detectable abnormalities of NK-cell, B-cell, and T-cell number and function can be detected in a subset of patients as well.[226–228]

Abnormal Apoptosis

Although MDS is typically characterized by normal or increased marrow cellularity, abnormalities of apoptosis are frequently described, particularly in low-risk variants, where increased apoptosis has been hypothesized to contribute to the development of ineffective hematopoiesis.[229] There are two major mammalian apoptosis pathways. The death receptor pathway, also known as the external pathway, is triggered by ligation of TNF family members, which leads to the recruitment and activation of caspases at the cell surface.[230] There is ample evidence of abnormalities in this pathway in MDS; for instance, TNF-α levels have been shown to be increased in all MDS subtypes,[231] and other proapoptotic cytokines, including IL-8, transforming growth factor β, interferon-γ, and Fas ligand, have been shown to be elevated as well.[232] The other major apoptotic pathway, known as the BCL-2 or intrinsic pathway, involves a complex balance between proapoptotic (BAX, BAK, BAD, PUMA, and others) and antiapoptotic molecules (BCL-2, BCL-XL, MCL-1, and others),[233] and has also been shown to be abnormal in MDS. For example, ratios of proapoptotic (Bax/Bad) to antiapoptotic (Bcl-2/Bcl-XL) molecules are elevated in patients with lower-risk subtypes of MDS (RA and RARS), but the ratio reverses in RAEB and secondary AML, primarily driven by increased BCL-2 expression.[234] Coordinate with this observation, but somewhat paradoxically, inhibition of apoptosis by BCL-2 appears to prevent leukemic transformation in murine models of MDS.[235] Preclinical studies further suggest that inhibition of BCL-2 and other antiapoptotic molecules may delay progression of disease[236] and may sensitize MDS cells to hypomethylating agents such as azacitidine, but clinical trials combining these approaches have not yet been performed.[237]

Transformation to Acute Leukemia

Although MDS and AML are often uttered in the same breath and conceptualized as two facets of a similar disease process, this is an overly simplistic view that ignores the complexity and heterogeneity of each disease on its own.[82] Although MDS can and often does transform into secondary AML, other types of de novo AML are biologically quite distinct from MDS, and conversely, some low-risk forms of MDS are biologically distinct from secondary AML. At the same time, however, there is a continuum between the two diseases that is only now starting to become fully understood. Recently, for instance, it has been shown that cases of AML harboring mutations in any of eight genes (*SF3B1*, *SRSF2*, *U2AF1*, *ZRSR2*, *ASXL1*, *EZH2*, *BCOR*, or *STAG2*) are highly likely to have evolved out of MDS, even when no antecedent stage of MDS was clinically evident.[148] The converse, that AML with driver mutations in other genes must have arisen de novo, is not necessarily true; *NPM1* mutations appear to be restricted to de novo AML, but mutations in *DNMT3A*, *TET2*, and *IDH1/2* can occur in both secondary and de novo AML and thus do not appear to be ontogeny-specific. In this study, *TP53*-mutated AML comprised its own category and was associated with prior chemotherapy and complex karyotypes, consistent with prior studies.

Understanding this shared genetic basis of MDS and secondary AML has also shed light on the transition from one to the other. Although the eight genes defining secondary ontogeny (i.e., disease arising from antecedent MDS) have different functions, they all tend to have broad, pleiotropic effects and for the most part have in mouse models been shown to be insufficient for leukemogenesis when they occur in isolation. The fact that they occur infrequently in de novo AML may imply that they have effects strong enough to commit cells to an MDS phenotype, with increased self-renewal and inhibitory effects on differentiation and hematopoiesis, whereas *TET2* and *DNMT3A* mutations may have more subtle effects that increase self-renewal but do not in and of themselves predispose to a specific phenotype in the absence of specific secondary mutations.

In most cases, progression of MDS to AML involves the acquisition of proproliferative mutations, which tend to be late, subclonal events.[238] These mutations frequently occur in tyrosine kinase genes like *FLT3*,[155] *NRAS*,[239] or *KIT*,[240] or in certain transcription factor genes such as *CEBPA*,[241] and lead to constitutively activated growth and proliferative pathways. As discussed elsewhere, patients who develop secondary AML from an antecedent MDS tend to have a poorer prognosis, with both a lower rate of complete remission and a poorer overall survival, independent of remission, than patients with de novo AML.[242] In unselected populations, some of this difference in outcome can be explained by proximate characteristics of the secondary AML cohorts, which tend to be older and have more comorbidities, mirroring the demographics of the MDS population. However, patients with secondary AML have inferior outcomes even compared to age-matched controls with de novo AML,[235] which has remained the case when redefining ontogeny based on the genetic stratification outlined earlier.[243] This inferior outcome has been presumed to reflect the intrinsic refractory nature of the antecedent MDS, and this presumption is now being proven true by sequencing bone marrow samples from secondary AML patients who morphologically appear to be in remission—in fact, the proliferative mutations are often eliminated but the preexisting driver mutations remain, suggesting that chemotherapy simply reverted the marrow to the preexisting clonal state.[58,148] Overcoming the intrinsic resistance to therapy that appears to be common to most patients with MDS remains one of the central challenges of treating the disease.

Integrating the Pathobiology of Myelodysplastic Syndrome

With the continuous, deepening accumulation of data describing the pathogenesis underlying MDS, one of the central future challenges will be integrating these data into coherent models that correctly reflect fundamental aspects of the disease. The need for integration is twofold. First, there is a need to integrate disparate components of the biology itself, including somatic mutations, changes in gene expression, epigenetic disruption, and cell-cell interactions within the marrow microenvironment and beyond. Second, it will also be necessary to integrate these biologic storylines with clinical information, in the hope that a fuller understanding of MDS biology may uncover new treatment approaches and better predictive and prognostic models than do single biologic features alone. Such work is already beginning; for instance, a recent report suggested that an algorithm integrating sequencing for common driver mutations with principal component analysis of gene expression better predicts some clinical features of MDS than sequencing or expression data considered in isolation, and the algorithm outperformed the IPSS in predicting overall survival (76% versus 64% accuracy).[244] Thus far, however, these types of integrative studies remain in relative infancy. Making significant gains in this type of deep understanding will be a substantial undertaking, requiring large, well-coordinated clinical trials with rigorous banking of serial blood and marrow samples, careful annotation of clinical features and outcomes, and intensive collaboration between academics, industry, and clinicians in devising strategies for rationally targeting key elements of MDS biology.

CLINICAL FEATURES OF MYELODYSPLASTIC SYNDROME

Compared to other hematologic disorders, the clinical features of MDS are often underemphasized relative to laboratory aspects of the disease. This is in part because of the fact that the major common physiologic defect, ineffective hematopoiesis, usually leads to somewhat vague signs or symptoms. Nevertheless, it is important to understand these features within the context of the disease's pathogenesis and management. Some patients with MDS have distinct clinical phenotypes that are largely related to genetics or specific pathologic features. MDS can also coexist with other hematologic malignancies, including multiple myeloma (even in previously untreated patients)[245], hairy cell leukemia,[246] chronic lymphocytic leukemia (CLL),[247] non-Hodgkin lymphoma,[248] and large granular lymphocyte leukemia (LGL).[249] Parsing the components of presentation that could be caused by a coexisting process (e.g., in a patient with both MDS and CLL, which is the primary contributor to the patient's cytopenias?) is an important task for clinicians and pathologists.

Differential Diagnosis

In the absence of clonal markers or excess blasts, MDS is a diagnosis of exclusion, requiring that other potential contributors to cytopenias and myelodysplastic morphology be ruled out to the greatest extent possible.[250] Since cytopenias are the most common presenting clinical feature, the differential diagnosis is in theory broad and includes numerous other entities covered in more detail elsewhere in this book. In practice, however, all patients suspected of having MDS should undergo a bone marrow aspirate and biopsy, since the diagnostic criteria are almost entirely pathologic and marrow findings are critical for risk stratification and treatment planning.

Several nutritional deficiencies can cause cytopenias and morphology similar to MDS. Folate deficiency can cause macrocytosis and, in extreme cases, megaloblastic morphology in the marrow.[251] Vitamin B_{12} (cobalamin) deficiency is a more classic cause of megaloblastic changes, and patients with severe B_{12} deficiency can have bizarre morphology with an abundance of early forms that can occasionally be confused with evolving AML, especially erythroleukemia.[252] Since the hematologic changes of B_{12} deficiency can occur in the absence of classic neurologic symptoms, B_{12} and folate levels should be checked on all patients in whom a potential diagnosis of MDS is being entertained, and methylmalonic acid and homocysteine levels may help clarify whether deficiency is truly present in cases with borderline levels.[253]

Copper deficiency is less common than B_{12}/folate deficiency, but can also be mistaken for MDS. It classically arises in patients who have had gastrectomies or certain forms of gastric bypass surgery, particularly biliopancreatic diversion,[254] and can also develop in patients taking high doses of zinc, which competes with copper for absorption in the small bowel[255] (it is important to note that newer forms of gastric bypass, including gastric sleeve procedures and newer iterations of the roux-en-y, maintain small bowel absorption such that patients do not typically develop copper deficiency). Clinically, patients with copper deficiency develop an anemia that can be normocytic or macrocytic and can occasionally be profound. Mild neutropenia can also be seen, while clinically significant thrombocytopenia is rare.[256] Such patients can also develop neurologic symptoms similar to those seen in vitamin B[12] deficiency, including peripheral neuropathy, myelopathy, demyelination, and rarely optic neuritis.[257] In the marrow, copper deficiency is classically associated with ring sideroblasts and erythroid and neutrophil vacuolization.[258] In the right clinical setting, negative testing for somatic *SF3B1* mutations in the presence of definite ring sideroblasts should elevate the degree of suspicion.

Alcohol is a common cause of hematologic abnormalities, especially macrocytic anemia, even in the absence of folate or vitamin B[12] deficiency.[259] Bone marrow examination often reveals sideroblastic changes, and sometimes megaloblastic morphology, but frank dysplasia is uncommon.[260] Patients with borderline marrow findings who are suspected of significant alcohol intake should be advised to completely abstain from drinking (such advice is occasionally heeded), with a repeat marrow examination in 2–3 months.

Other drugs and toxins have also been associated with dysplastic changes in the marrow. Well-described offenders include valproic acid,[261] mycophenolate mofetil,[262] ganciclovir,[263] alemtuzumab,[264] nucleoside analogues such as fludarabine[265] and cytarabine, and the antimetabolites mercaptopurine and methotrexate.[266] These tend to cause macrocytic anemias and can also cause neutropenia and thrombocytopenia. On the other hand, isoniazid[267] and chloramphenicol,[268] and to a lesser extent cycloserine[269] and pyrazinamide,[270] have been associated with modest sideroblastic anemia. The anemia associated with isoniazid, in particular, can often be reversed with high doses of vitamin B[6] (pyridoxine).[271] Chloramphenicol can separately cause an idiosyncratic pancytopenia that is particularly distinguished by prominent vacuolization of erythroid precursors.[272]

Among infectious agents, HIV infection has specifically been associated with dysplastic changes in the marrow. Patients typically have hypercellular marrows with evidence of trilineage dysplasia most predominant in the erythroid line.[273] The erythroid hematopoiesis almost always is megaloblastic, and reticulated fibrosis is often seen in bone marrow biopsies. The marrows also often have polyclonal plasma cell expansion, lymphoid aggregates, and granulomas are often seen. The differential diagnosis of erythrodysplasia in patients with HIV infection includes the influence of medications, opportunistic infections, or a direct effect of HIV on the hematopoietic progenitor cells.[274] Since the US Preventive Services Task Force now recommends a one-time HIV test for all adults,[275] essentially all patients in whom MDS is being considered should be tested to rule out HIV.

Other primary hematologic disorders are also on the differential diagnosis with MDS. Hypoplastic MDS, for example, can be difficult to distinguish from aplastic anemia and in the absence of characteristic cytogenetic or genetic abnormalities.[276] Similarly, some patients with MDS may have a significant degree of co-existing fibrosis, which can complicate the distinction from a myeloproliferative disorder.[277] Again, genetic analysis may help make this distinction clearer.[278]

Signs and Symptoms

Signs and symptoms of MDS are typically vague. Although some patients profess to being asymptomatic, fatigue is extremely common, as is a sense of general malaise.[279] Rarely, patients may complain of diffuse arthralgias that can lead to suspicion for an underlying rheumatologic disorder like systemic lupus erythematosus.

Smaller proportions of patients may present with severe or recurrent infections as a result of immune defects,[280] most commonly neutropenia. Bleeding or easy bruising as a result of thrombocytopenia or qualitative platelet defects also bring some patients with MDS

to medical attention.[281] When present, fever is most commonly a sign of infection, though a small number of patients may run low-grade fevers in the absence of a discernible infection. Splenomegaly or hepatomegaly are rare and should prompt consideration of either an alternate diagnosis or an MDS/MPN overlap syndrome.

Dermatologic Manifestations

Although dermatologic manifestations of MDS are uncommon,[282] a few deserve specific mention. Neutrophilic dermatosis (Sweet syndrome) is characterized by painful plaques on the face, neck, or extremities, often in association with fever and diffuse arthralgias.[283] While neutrophilic dermatosis can be seen in any subclass of MDS, it is classically associated with an impending transformation to AML. It frequently responds to steroids or dapsone therapy, but may recur as steroids are tapered.[284] Recently, Sweet syndrome in MDS patients has been associated with heterozygous mutations in *MEFV*, a gene linked to Mediterranean fever.[285]

Pyoderma gangrenosum (PG) is an ulcerative, necrotic lesion that most frequently develops on the extremities.[286] Histologically it is also characterized by neutrophilic infiltrates; clinically, it may be associated with pathergy and frequently develops at the site of recent minor trauma, such as intravenous (IV) catheter insertion sites. PG can be associated with a wide range of underlying conditions other than MDS. A high index of suspicion is necessary to distinguish it from necrotizing infections, since treatment of PG involves systemic steroids, and surgical debridement is contraindicated.

Other dermatologic manifestations of MDS include monocytic infiltrates, classically of the gingiva and other mucosal surfaces, a process most frequently seen in CMML;[287] the development of a chloroma or granulocytic sarcoma, which by definition implies progression to AML; and petechial lesions, which most frequently develop on the lower extremities and imply severe thrombocytopenia.

Autoimmune Manifestations

A percentage of patients with MDS may have overlapping immunologic or rheumatologic features to their disease, which may in part arise from the immune dysregulation that occurs during disease pathogenesis.[288] In a few patients, these may be the presenting complaint. Such manifestations can include episodes of seronegative oligoarthritis or polyarthritis,[289] cutaneous vasculitis,[290] polymyositis,[291] or autoimmune peripheral neuropathies. Rare patients can present with a lupus-like syndrome that can include fever, polyarthralgias, polychondritis, pleuritis, pericarditis, and cytopenias (including hemolytic anemias). Other autoimmune phenomena have also been reported, including mucocutaneous ulcerations, iritis, polymyositis, inflammatory bowel disease, and erythrocyte aplasia. Many of these, which are essentially paraneoplastic syndromes, respond to the initiation of immunosuppressive agents such as corticosteroids.[292]

Some reports have additionally documented cases of patients who were diagnosed with rheumatologic conditions only weeks or months before they were found to have MDS, including relapsing polychondritis,[293] polymyalgia rheumatica or temporal arteritis,[294] Raynaud phenomenon, Sjögren syndrome, and autoimmune glomerulonephritis.[295] However, since some of these conditions are relatively common themselves, particularly in older populations, whether they represent a true association with MDS or are merely coincidental occurrences is not entirely clear.

Objective Findings: Erythroid Lineage

The majority of patients with MDS present with some degree of anemia, which contributes significantly to fatigue and lethargy, the most common presenting complaint.[296,297] The anemia is often macrocytic, and the peripheral blood smears of MDS patients

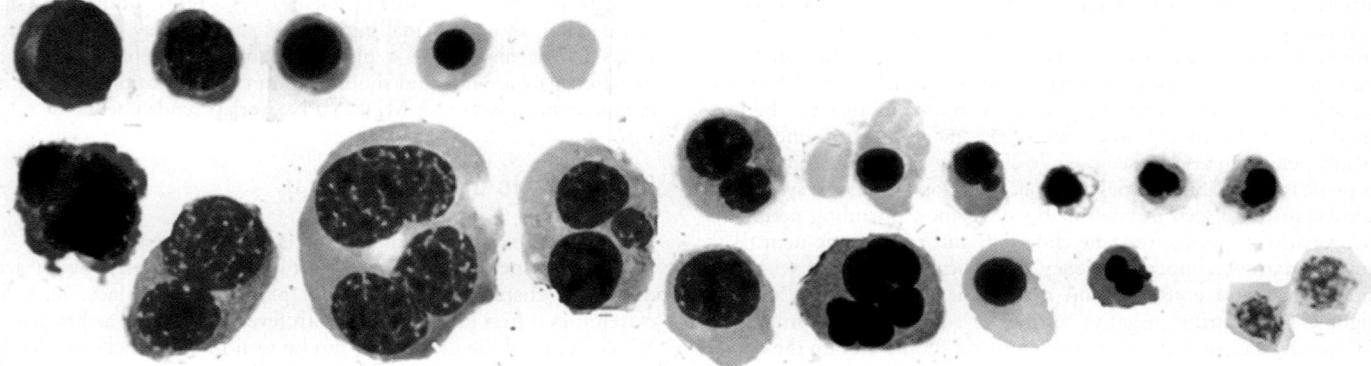

Fig. 60.2 ERYTHROID DYSPLASIA. Examples of dysplastic erythroid precursors *(bottom)* compared to those with normal morphology in the sequence of erythroid maturation *(top)*. The dysplastic forms include *(left* to *right)* abnormal immature forms with multinucleation; maturing forms with multinucleation and nuclear-to-cytoplasmic dyssynchrony; and more mature forms with megaloblastoid change, nuclear budding, cloverleaf forms, cytoplasmic vacuolization, and cytoplasmic stippling. Ringed sideroblasts *(far right)* also are evidence of erythroid dysplasia. Photomicrographs are from patients with refractory cytopenia with multilineage dysplasia and ringed sideroblasts.

frequently show a variety of abnormal forms, including oval macrocytes, and less commonly dacrocytes, elliptocytes, or acanthocytes.

Anemia in MDS is usually caused by ineffective hematopoiesis. Consequently, the erythropoietin (EPO) level is typically normal or modestly elevated, though in many elderly patients it is still lower than would be expected for the degree of anemia, in some cases because of subclinical renal insufficiency.[298] The ineffective hematopoiesis causes abnormal iron utilization in a substantial number of patients, many of whom have evidence of iron overload based on ferritin or transferrin saturation.[299] Studies have shown other abnormalities of erythrocytes as well, including increased levels of fetal hemoglobin,[300] aberrant surface antigens,[301] increased osmotic fragility, and low levels of pyruvate kinase,[302] although none of these are routinely checked in clinical practice. Hemolysis is not routinely observed in MDS patients, but may occur in those with some of these latter abnormalities or with concomitant autoimmune disorders.

Morphologic changes in the erythroid lineage on bone marrow examination can vary widely from patient to patient. Many patients have megaloblastoid erythroid precursors that contain multiple nuclei or asynchronous maturation of the nucleus and cytoplasm (Fig. 60.2). It is this asynchrony, with continued membrane synthesis in the absence of normal nuclear maturation, which is thought to give rise to the macrocytosis displayed by most patients. Ring sideroblasts, erythroid precursors containing iron-laden mitochondria, are another relatively common finding.[303] They are defined by the presence of at least five granules that are positive with the Prussian blue reaction and line at least one-third of the circumference of the cell nucleus. Ring sideroblasts are not in and of themselves diagnostic of MDS and can be seen in a number of other disorders (including congenital sideroblastic anemias and nutritional deficiencies), but their presence in association with other dysplastic changes is highly specific for MDS and, as described earlier, is tightly linked to acquired *SF3B1* mutations.[88] Ring sideroblasts may be seen in all subtypes of MDS; the specific designation of RARS is made when ring sideroblasts comprise at least 15% of the cellularity, blasts are not increased, and dysplasia in other lineages is minimal.

In a normal bone marrow, myeloid precursors typically outnumber erythroid precursors by a ratio of 2–4 to 1. A special case arises in cases of MDS in which this normal ratio is significantly skewed towards the erythroid lineage, that is, 50% or more of the total cellularity is erythroid. If in this case 30% or more of the remaining cellularity is comprised of myeloblasts, the case may be diagnosed as erythroleukemia (WHO AML, not otherwise specified, subtype acute erythroid leukemia, erythroid/myeloid type; formerly FAB-M6A).[15,170]

Acquired hemoglobin H disease is a rare but well-described development in MDS that has been associated with acquired mutations of *ATRX*,[304] a gene encoding a chromatin-remodeling protein; when mutated in the germline, *ATRX* has been associated with X-linked alpha thalassemia/mental retardation (ATR-X) syndrome. The pathogenesis of the syndrome is related to severe reduction in synthesis of alpha globin chains, and indeed, patients with acquired *ATRX* mutations have clinical features resembling alpha thalassemia, including microcytosis, anisocytosis, poikilocytosis, target cells, schistocytes, dacrocytes, and beta-chain tetramers on crystal violet staining.[305] As opposed to the macrocytosis seen in most MDS patients, those with acquired *ATRX* mutations are typically profoundly microcytic, again similar to thalassemia.

Myeloid Lineage

About one-half of patients with MDS are neutropenic at the time of diagnosis.[306] Many also have defective neutrophil function irrespective of the absolute neutrophil count (ANC), and patients with MDS have been shown to have inadequate inflammatory responses to infections. Many have diminished production of hematopoietic growth factors like granulocyte colony-stimulating factor (G-CSF) and GM-CSF, and their neutrophils often have reduced phagocytic, chemotactic, or bactericidal capabilities.[307–309] In place of neutrophils, the proportion of monocytes is often elevated, which can sometimes be shown to have been the case for months or even years before diagnosis. Such a history can be observed patients with pure MDS, not just those with MDS/MPN overlaps like CMML.

The granulocytes of MDS patients also display frequent morphologic abnormalities (Fig. 60.3). In the marrow, either myeloid hyperplasia or hypoplasia can occur, and there is often a prominent left shift towards immature forms. Myeloid precursors often display asynchronous maturation of the nucleus and cytoplasm. In promyelocytes this can manifest as an early hypergranulation coupled with reticulated nuclei and a prominent Golgi apparatus, but more mature myeloid forms are usually hypogranulated and hypolobated. The myeloid series may also be abnormally localized: rather than differentiating in an organized fashion inwards from the endosteum, immature cells often cluster centrally in a morphologic process known as abnormal localization of immature precursors (ALIP).

Morphologic characterization of the myeloid series is particularly important with regard to the blast count, since ≥20% myeloblasts is characterized as AML using the WHO classification, and ≥5% qualifies as RAEB. Even patients with lower blast percentages, however,

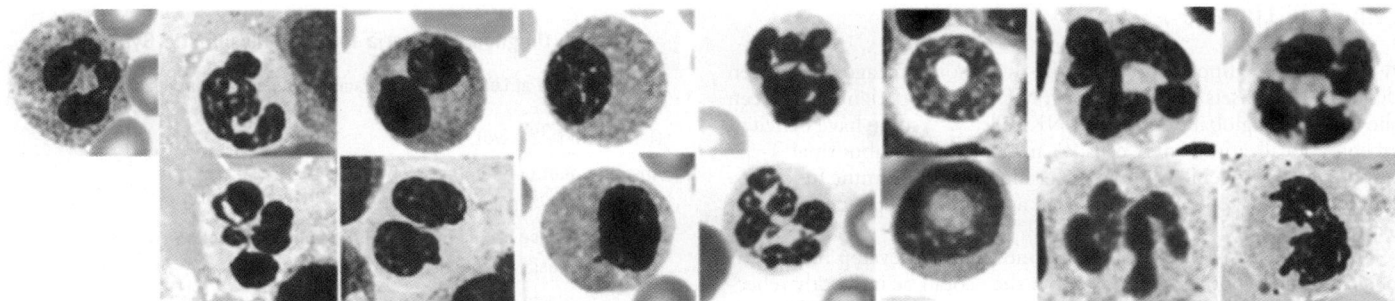

Fig. 60.3 GRANULOCYTIC DYSPLASIA. Granulocytic dysplasia is most evident in mature neutrophils and can be contrasted to features of normal forms *(far left, top),* which are usually still present as a subpopulation of the total cells in most cases. Granulocytic dysplasia is characterized by *(left to right, starting at second column)* reduced cytoplasmic granulation, nuclear hypolobation (resulting in the binuclear or single-lobed pseudo–Pelger-Huët forms), hypersegmentation, ringed forms ("rodent cells"), cells with nuclear twinning, and cells with excessive nuclear excrescences. Photomicrographs are from a number of cases of refractory cytopenia with multilineage dysplasia and refractory anemia with excess blasts.

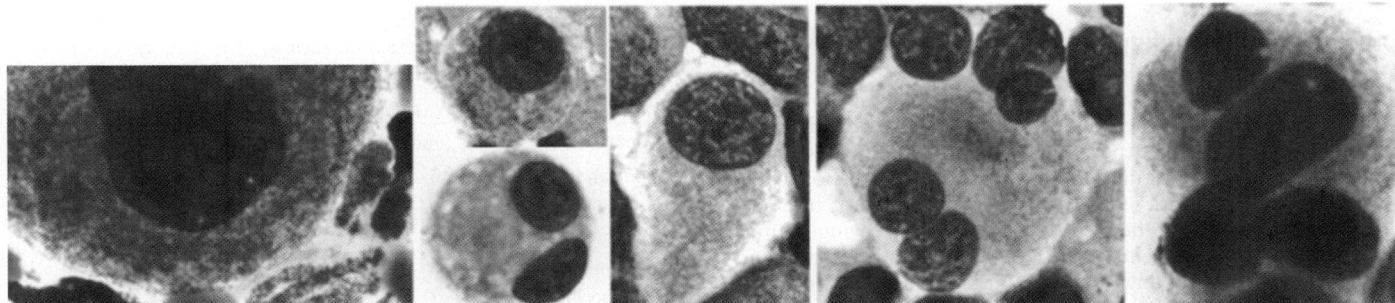

Fig. 60.4 MEGAKARYOCYTIC DYSPLASIA. Dysmegakaryopoiesis is most obvious with the presence of micromegakaryocytes and abnormal larger forms *(panels 2–5).* These are compared with a normal megakaryocyte at same magnification *(panel 1, far left).* Micromegakaryocytes have single, two, or four small nuclei, which indicate a low-ploidy level. Normal low-ploidy megakaryocytes can be seen in the bone marrow, but these are immature forms and do not have mature granular cytoplasm with platelet material, as do the micromegakaryocytes. Larger dysplastic megakaryocytes have multiple, small, widely spaced nuclei. Photomicrographs are from a number of cases of refractory anemia with excess blasts and refractory cytopenia with multilineage dysplasia.

still have an increased risk of developing AML, and some have proposed designating any MDS patient with more than 2% marrow blasts as having "oligoblastic leukemia."[310] ALIP has been shown to occur in most cases of RAEB and in about a third of cases in which the blast percentage is less than 5%.[311] In these latter cases ALIP has been shown to be an independent risk factor for subsequent development of AML.[312]

In the peripheral blood, visible morphologic abnormalities include so-called pseudo Pelger-Huët cells, which have condensed chromatin and bilobed nuclei resembling an old-fashioned pince-nez (true Pelger-Huët cells are a benign congenital abnormality seen in children). Granulocytes may display other nuclear abnormalities as well, including hypersegmentation reminiscent of vitamin B_{12} deficiency, and aberrant ring shapes. The hypogranulation visible in the marrow typically persists in the peripheral blood, and the left shift typical of MDS marrows is often, though not always, present to some degree in the blood as well.

Despite these quantitative and qualitative defects in leukocytes, only a minority of MDS patients have problems with recurrent infections.[313] When infections do occur, they tend to be bacterial and often arise from the lower respiratory tract, skin, and mucous membranes. Patients without absolute neutropenia may still develop recurrent infections as a consequence of abnormal neutrophil function. Even though only some patients have recurrent infections, an infection is the most common cause of MDS-associated death.

Megakaryocytic Lineage

Thrombocytopenia is present in 25% to 50% of MDS patients at the time of presentation,[296,306] and some patients with normal platelet counts can have functional platelet defects.[314] Laboratory abnormalities include prolonged bleeding times, defective granulation, and abnormal platelet aggregation indices mediated by hypofunctional platelet glycoprotein IIb/IIIa, leading to what is known as a *Glanzmann-type defect.*[315,316] These defects can occasionally manifest as spontaneous bleeding, or can be unmasked after trauma or surgery.

Thrombocytosis, by contrast, is relatively unusual in patients with MDS, except in those with MDS/MPN overlap syndromes, 5q-syndrome, or RARS-T.[317] *JAK2* mutations, in particular, are associated with thrombocytosis. Thrombocytosis can occasionally be subtle, especially in patients with advanced disease, in whom a normal platelet count may in fact represent a relative thrombocytosis counteracted by dwindling megakaryocytic reserves.

In the marrow, megakaryocytes are most commonly present in normal or increased numbers. A number of morphologic abnormalities can be observed, including abnormally small forms (micromegakaryocytes), hypersegmentation, and nuclear hypolobation (Fig. 60.4).[318,319] Megakaryocytes may also be abnormally distributed in clusters scattered throughout the marrow in MDS, rather than their normal parasinusoidal positioning.

Lymphoid Lineage

A number of abnormalities in the lymphoid lineage have been described in subsets of patients with MDS. Some patients have been shown to have global decreases in NK cells,[226,320] some have deficient receptor localization on B cells,[228] and some have abnormal T-cell responses to mitogenic stimuli.[227] Certain types of immune functions, however, appear to be preserved, such as antibody-dependent cellular cytotoxicity.[321]

The mechanism by which these abnormalities develop in MDS is unclear. One hypothesis proposes that they could be indirectly reflective of shared somatic defects in a multipotent progenitor. Although this has not been directly proven, it is theoretically possible given data showing that most driver mutations in MDS patients are present in the long-term hematopoietic stem cells (LT-HSC) compartment and could therefore be passed both to myeloid and lymphoid cells.[64] Alternatively, a number of immune functions, including both B-cell and T-cell diversity, diminish as a function of normal aging,[322,323] and in this context, deficiencies of immune function could develop as a consequence of lymphoid cells arising from and interacting with an abnormally aged hematopoietic niche.

Other Objective Findings

Patients with MDS may have a variety of other laboratory abnormalities as a consequence of their disease. Ineffective erythropoiesis may lead to inappropriate iron deposition, resulting in abnormally elevated ferritin and transferrin saturation.[324] Nonspecific markers of cellular turnover, such as elevations in lactate dehydrogenase,[325] uric acid, and phosphate, may also be seen. Reflective of underlying immune dysregulation, some patients may have abnormalities of immunoglobulins (Igs), including hypogammaglobulinemia, polyclonal hypergammaglobulinemia, and even monoclonal gammopathies.[326,327] Whether this latter phenomenon is directly related to MDS or to an unrelated, early plasma cell dyscrasia has not been definitively established, and the answer may indeed be different in different patients.

DIAGNOSTIC SYSTEMS AND CLINICAL SYNDROMES

As discussed throughout this chapter, MDS is heterogeneous in both morphology and clinical course, a characteristic that requires diagnostic criteria sufficiently broad to capture the entire spectrum of disease, and diagnostic criteria are typically left purposefully vague to allow for inclusion of patients in whom a high suspicion of MDS exists but who do not specifically meet these formal criteria (Table 60.3). Patients with MDS typically have at least one persistent, otherwise unexplained cytopenia (hemoglobin less than 11 g/dL, ANC <1,500/mm³, or platelet count less than 100,000/mm³), plus one of the following: (1) ≥5% blasts in the bone marrow, (2) any of several chromosomal abnormalities that are found recurrently in MDS; (3) a meaningful degree of dysplasia, usually 10% or more, detectable in at least one cell lineage on bone marrow examination, or (4) other evidence of clonal hematopoiesis.[170] In the past this latter category has usually comprised either karyotype or FISH results demonstrating chromosomal abnormalities missed by conventional karyotype, but evidence of clonal hematopoiesis based on detection of recurrent somatic mutations may need to be considered as well. However, given that at least 10% of the population aged 70 or older harbor point mutations in genes associated with myeloid malignancies,[31,32] detection of such a mutation in the absence of other diagnostic criteria cannot be considered equivalent to MDS.

As described elsewhere, the 2008 WHO criteria divide adult MDS into six general categories: RCUD (including RA, RARS, refractory neutropenia, and refractory thrombocytopenia), RCMD, RAEB-1, RAEB-2, MDS with isolated del(5q), and MDS-U. Despite the detail of the criteria, they still have a number of limitations, a fact that is probably inescapable when attempting to categorize a disease with so many disparate manifestations. The most obvious limitation is the

TABLE 60.3	Diagnostic Criteria for Myelodysplastic Syndrome

A. Presence of at Least One Unexplained Cytopenia for at Least 6 Months[a]

Hemoglobin <11 g/dL, *or*
Absolute neutrophil count <1.5 × 10⁹/L, *or*
Platelet count <100 × 10⁹/L

***plus* B. Presence of One or More MDS-Qualifying Criteria:**

>10% dysplasia in one or more hematopoietic lineage, *or*
5%–19% blasts in bone marrow, *or*

MDS-defining cytogenetic abnormality, such as:

t(1;3)(p36.3;q21.1)	t(2;11)(p21;q23)	inv(3)(q21;q26.2)
t(3;21)(q26.2;q22.1)	−5 or del(5q)	t(6;9)(p23;q34)
−7 or del(7q)		del(9q)
del(11q)	t(11;16)(q23;p13.3)	del(12p) or t(12p)
−13 or del(13q)	i(17q) or del(17p)	idic(X)(q13)

***plus* C. Exclusion of Alternative Diagnoses**

AML (i.e., <20% blasts, and no t(8;21), inv(16), t(16;16), t(15;17), or erythroleukemia) or *ALL*

Other hematologic diseases (aplastic anemia, PNH, LGL, lymphoma, myelofibrosis and other MPN)

Viral infections (HIV, EBV, parvovirus)

Nutritional deficiencies (iron, copper, B₁₂, folate)

Medications (methotrexate, azathioprine, isoniazid, cytotoxic chemotherapy)

Alcohol or other toxins

Autoimmune diseases (SLE, Felty syndrome, ITP, autoimmune hemolytic anemia)

Congenital disorders (Diamond-Blackfan anemia, Shwachman-Diamond syndrome, Fanconi anemia, and others)

[a]Diagnosis can be made earlier than 6 months if no other cause is apparent for cytopenias, or there are excess blasts or an MDS-defining cytogenetic abnormality
ALL, Acute lymphoblastic leukemia; *AML,* acute myeloid leukemia; *EBV,* Epstein-Barr virus; *HIV,* human immunodeficiency virus; *ITP,* immune thrombocytopenic purpura; *LGL,* large granular lymphocyte leukemia; *MDS,* myelodysplastic syndrome; *MPN,* myeloproliferative neoplasm; *PNH,* paroxysmal nocturnal hemoglobinuria; *SLE,* systemic lupus erythematosus.

complexity of the criteria themselves, which can make them cumbersome for clinicians to use. Second, as described previously, there are a number of conditions that can mimic aspects of MDS, and the diagnostic criteria assume these diagnostic possibilities have been eliminated. Third, morphologic criteria are still based around strict, arbitrary percentages of dysplasia and blasts, which can be interpreted differently by different pathologists or may be vulnerable to sampling variations.[328,329] Finally, although WHO criteria incorporate cytogenetics to a limited extent, the criteria have not yet been updated to include types of newer genetic results that have been shown to have diagnostic value, and it is likely that incorporating some of these features will improve diagnostic clarity. A 2016 revision of the WHO criteria eliminated the term "refractory anemia" so that, for example, RAEB-1 is now known as "MDS with excess blasts" (MDS-EB). This revision also noted that MDS with ring sideroblasts (MDS-RS) can be diagnosed with 5% to 14% ring sideroblasts if a somatic SF3B1 mutation is present; if SF3B1 is wild-type, at least 15% ring sideroblasts are needed.

IPSS and IPSS-R

Although the WHO classification system (and the FAB system before it) is the accepted standard for diagnosing MDS, it does not confer

TABLE 60.4 1997 International Prognostic Scoring System for Myelodysplastic Syndromes (IPSS)

Variable	Score			
	0	0.5	1	1.5
Marrow blasts (%)	<5	5–10	–	11–20
Karyotype	Good	Intermediate	Poor	–
Cytopenias	0–1	2–3	–	–

TABLE 60.5 Survival Based on International Prognostic Scoring System for Myelodysplastic Syndromes (Percent)

IPSS Risk Group	# Patients	2 Years	5 Years	10 Years	15 Years
Low	267 (33%)	85	55	28	20
Intermediate-1	314 (38%	70	35	17	12
Intermediate-2	179 (22%)	30	8	0	–
High	56 (7%)	5	0	–	–

TABLE 60.6 2012 Revised International Prognostic Scoring System for Myelodysplastic Syndrome (IPSS-R)

Cytogenetic Risk	Included Karyotypic Abnormalities
Very good	del(11q), −Y
Good	Normal, del(20q), del(5q) alone or +1 other abnormality, del(12p)
Intermediate	+8, del(7q), i(17q), +19, +21 Any other single or double abnormality Two or more independent clones
Poor	der(3q), −7, double with del(7q), complex with exactly 3 abnormalities
Very poor	Complex with >3 abnormalities

Scoring Table Parameter	Category/Score				
Cytogenetic risk	Very good 0	Good 1	Intermediate 2	Poor 3	Very poor 4
Marrow blasts (%)	≤2 0	3–4 1	5–10 2	>10 3	
Hemoglobin (g/dL)	≥10 0	8–9.9 1	<8 1.5		
Platelet count (× 10^9/L)	≥100 0	50–99 0.5	<50 1		
Neutrophil count (× 10^9/L)	≥0.8 0	<0.8 0.5			

IPSS-R Risk Group	Total Score	% of Patients	Median Survival (Years)	25% With AML (Years)
Very low	≤1.5	19	8.8	NR
Low	2–3	38	5.3	10.8
Intermediate	3.5–4.5	20	3	3.2
High	5–6	13	1.6	1.4
Very high	>6	10	0.8	0.73

AML, *Acute myeloid leukemia*; NR, *not reached*.

much specific prognostic information, and other systems have been developed expressly for this purpose. The most widely used has been the IPSS[330] and its newer revised iteration, the IPSS-R.[331] The original IPSS was first published in 1997 and was derived by analyzing baseline characteristics in over 800 newly diagnosed MDS patients from all diagnostic categories. Patients were scored based on three characteristics: the percentage of blasts in the marrow, the presence of specific cytogenetic abnormalities, and the number of cytopenias in the blood. They were then stratified based on total score into four risk groups (low, intermediate-1, intermediate-2, and high) that were shown to have prognostic value, both in estimating the chance of progressing to AML and in estimating the duration of overall survival. This is shown in Table 60.4 and Table 60.5. The original IPSS excluded patients with t-MDS, patients with proliferative CMML, and patients who ultimately underwent allogeneic stem cell transplantation or other disease-modifying therapy.

The original IPSS had several limitations that ultimately necessitated its revision. First, it was formulated 4 years before the adoption of the first iteration of WHO classification criteria, and some of changes in those criteria (for instance, changing the cutoff for AML from 30% blasts to 20% blasts) effectively invalidated certain aspects of the IPSS. Furthermore, broad application of the criteria to larger populations of MDS patients began to reveal that the original IPSS gave insufficient weight to some important clinical features, particularly the presence of severe cytopenias. The IPSS was only validated in de novo disease, not t-MDS, and only in patients treated with supportive care alone. In response to some of these evident limitations, several alternative prognostic systems have been proposed over the last decade, but none of them have been widely adopted.[332–334]

The IPSS-R (Table 60.6), which was introduced in 2012, revised the MDS blast cutoff to 20% and assigned a point for each individual cytopenia present at the time of diagnosis, stratifying on the basis of severity. Furthermore, it incorporated a broader range of cytogenetic abnormalities than the original IPSS, and stratified patients into five risk categories instead of four. The resulting system thus incorporates more informative biology and offers better refinement of prognosis than its predecessor.[335,336]

The median survival times estimated by the IPSS and IPSS-R are largely reflective of natural history since they were originally derived in patients who did not receive any therapy for their MDS (Table 60.5). However, IPSS-R stratifications have been shown to retain relevance when applied to treated populations, including risk stratification of patients receiving hypomethylating agents[337] and those who undergo allogeneic stem cell transplantation.[338]

Nevertheless, the IPSS-R still has prognostic limitations. It does not incorporate laboratory findings, such as lactate dehydrogenase

and the serum ferritin, that have been shown to have independent prognostic value in dedicated studies. It does not capture the kinetics of disease or comorbid conditions. In addition, similar to the WHO classification criteria, IPSS-R does not include any molecular data other than cytogenetics.

Other Risk Stratification Systems

The limitations of the IPSS prompted attempts at more refined risk stratification using alternative models. Few of these have gained much traction in clinical practice but retain value for use in clinical trials and retrospective studies. For instance, a need for better stratification of lower-risk patients (i.e., IPSS-low or Int-1) led to the creation of the Lower-Risk Prognostic Scoring System (LR-PSS) by the MD Anderson group.[332] The LR-PSS uses criteria similar to the IPSS but sets lower thresholds for point assignment (e.g., 2 points for a platelet count <50 × 10^9/L and 1 point for bone marrow blasts ≥4%). Subsequent studies have confirmed the ability of LR-PSS to risk-stratify patients, with those in the highest risk group having the greatest risk of developing AML, and the poorest overall survival,[339] and addition of genetic sequencing has shown that in these low-risk patients, EZH2 mutations, though rare, portend a poor prognosis.[112] Other attempts to improve prognostic systems have included attempts to incorporate formal measures of comorbidity into the IPSS,[340] and an attempt to combine the WHO classification system with the IPSS that has been dubbed the WPSS.[341] This latter system was formulated before the introduction of the IPSS-R, but subsequent studies have suggested that the WPSS and the IPSS-R are about equal in their accuracy of predicting prognosis.[342]

Specific Clinical Syndromes

Although MDS is a heterogeneous disorder, it contains a number of specific entities, either defined by cytogenetics, pathologic findings, or clinical features, which possess distinctive clinical features or biologic behaviors. Some of these are discussed in more detail later.

The 5q– Syndrome

Patients with isolated loss of the long arm of chromosome 5 [so-called del(5q) or 5q minus syndrome] are a unique group whose biology is described in more detail earlier. Clinically, 5q– syndrome is characterized by a predominant anemia with preservation or even elevation of platelet counts, striking pathologic feature is the presence of mononuclear micromegakaryocytes identified in the bone marrow biopsy (Fig. 60.5A–C) and an indolent course with progression to AML in fewer than 25% of cases.[343,344] For unclear reasons, it is more common in women, who comprise 60% to 70% of cases. The anemia in lower risk del5q MDS is usually very responsive to the initiation of lenalidomide,[173] which is discussed in more detail in the subsequent section on Treatment. Those patients who become refractory to lenalidomide

typically remain transfusion dependent, and management of iron overload then becomes increasingly important.

The designation of 5q– syndrome applies only to patients in whom loss of 5q is the only cytogenetic abnormality. Patients in whom 5q– is only one of several cytogenetic aberrations in fact tend to have a worse prognosis than average, with a more rapid progression to AML. As referenced previously, loss of 5q often occurs in tandem with *TP53* mutations (or loss of 17p), another poor-prognosis combination.[149]

Hypocellular Syndromes

Most patients with MDS have hypercellular or normocellular marrows. Hypocellular marrows, in contrast, are found in fewer than 15% of patients, and delineate the entity of hypoplastic MDS (Fig. 60.5D–E).[224] These patients have substantial overlap, both morphologically and clinically, with other hypoplastic syndromes, including aplastic anemia,[345] paroxysmal nocturnal hemoglobinuria (PNH),[346] and T-cell LGL.[249,347] In fact, distinction between these entities can sometimes be difficult, as patients with MDS may occasionally have PNH or LGL clones detectable by flow cytometry, though these are usual small and transient. Some of the resemblance may in fact reflect a shared pathogenesis; for instance, studies have shown that a sizable minority of aplastic anemia cases harbor clonal somatic mutations in genes recurrently mutated in MDS, including *ASXL1* and *DNMT3A*,[348] and that these patients have an inferior

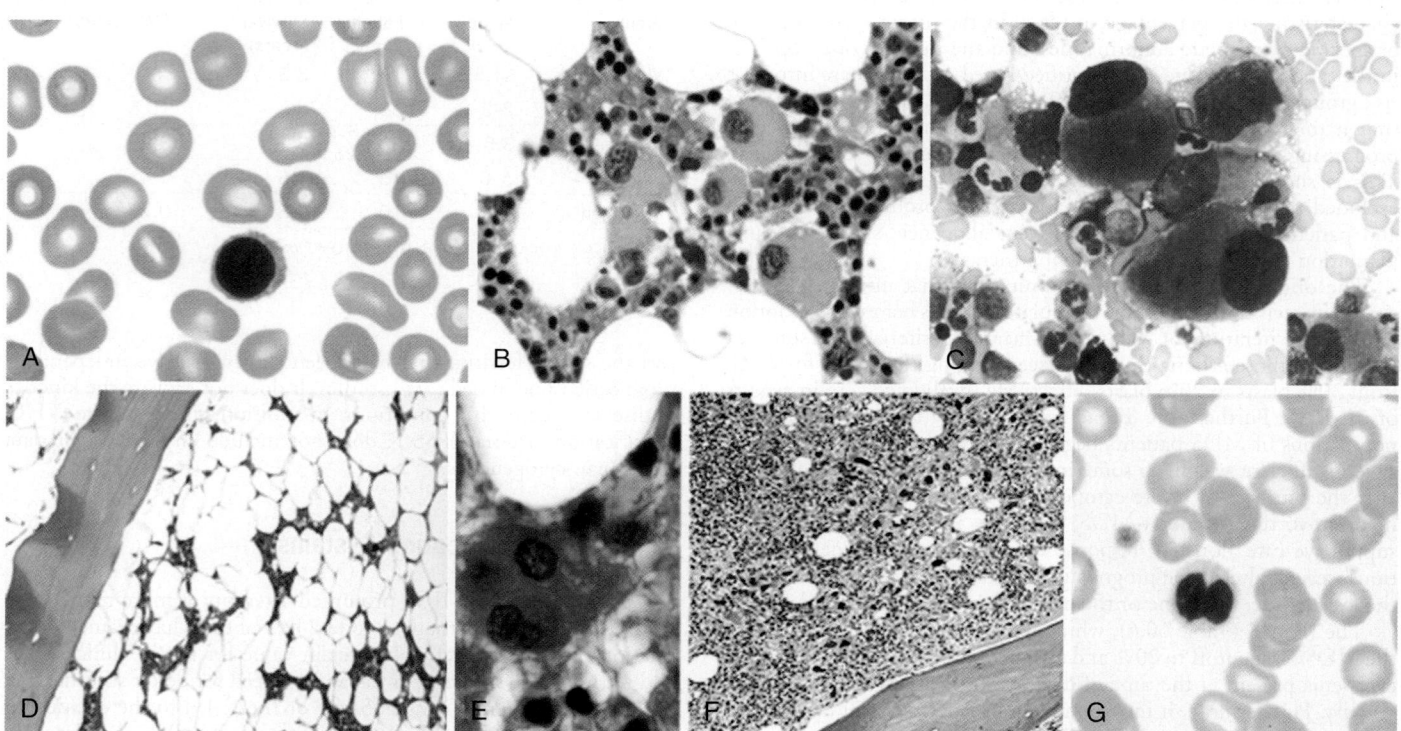

Fig. 60.5 SPECIFIC MYELODYSPLASTIC SYNDROMES. The 5q– syndrome (A–C); hypocellular myelodysplastic syndrome (D and E), and myelodysplastic syndrome with fibrosis (F and G). The 5q– syndrome has specific morphologic correlates. There is a macrocytic anemia (A) and a cellular bone marrow characterized by increased small monolobated megakaryocytes (B and C). The megakaryocyte nuclei have little segmentation and are fairly round. Although some true micromegakaryocytes may be present (C, *inset*, same magnification), the typical monolobated forms are not as tiny as the micromegakaryocytes. Hypocellular myelodysplastic syndrome (D and E) can present a diagnostic problem and can be difficult to differentiate from aplastic anemia. Dysplasia may be difficult to evaluate if the smears are paucicellular. The finding of dysplastic megakaryocytes (note small widely separated nuclei, E) on the biopsy sample can be helpful. Myelodysplastic syndrome with fibrosis (F) can be difficult to differentiate from myeloproliferative neoplasms (MPNs). However, the lack of large megakaryocytes, which typically are see in the MPNs along with presence of dysplasia in the circulating neutrophils (G) are useful clues to the correct diagnosis.

prognosis compared to patients with mutations in *PIGA* and *BCOR*.[349] It is therefore possible that these studies are defining distinct disease processes within a homogeneous-appearing morphology, with *ASXL1* and *DNMT3A* mutations defining disease more similar to MDS, and *BCOR* and *PIGA* mutations defining disease more akin to true, immune-mediated aplasia. At the same time, finding somatic mutations characteristic of the alternative diagnoses (for instance, members of the telomerase family in aplastic anemia,[40] or *STAT3* mutations in LGL[350]) may clarify the picture as well.

Myelodysplastic Syndrome/Myeloproliferative Neoplasm Overlap Syndromes

Although previously included as a subtype of MDS, disorders with overlapping features of both MDS and MPN are no longer included in the WHO classification system and are now considered an entity unto themselves; they are discussed in more detail elsewhere.

Myelodysplastic Syndrome With Fibrosis

Marked fibrosis rarely occurs in cases of MDS (Fig. 60.5F–G) without myeloproliferative features, but when it does occur, it can be difficult to distinguish these cases from MPN.[351] Evaluation for somatic mutations may be helpful, since finding a *JAK2*, *CALR*, or *MPL* mutations is more common in pure MPNs than in MDS,[352] while certain other mutations, including *TET2* and *SRSF2*, are somewhat enriched in MDS-MPN overlap syndromes.[101,353] On the other hand, extensive dysplasia is more suggestive of MDS. In addition, a few genetic lesions appear to be more specific for pure MDS syndromes, including *SF3B1* mutations and complex cytogenetics.

Patients with overlapping MDS and fibrosis often have severe, progressive cytopenias with evidence of myelophthisis on peripheral smear, but the splenomegaly associated with myelofibrosis in an MPN background is less common. Nevertheless, the prognosis for these patients appears to be relatively poor.

Therapy-Related Myelodysplastic Syndrome

t-MDS is a well-recognized and feared consequence of cytotoxic chemotherapy for other cancers, but the overall incidence is difficult to estimate.[243,354] This is partly because of the fact that it is not usually reported as a distinct entity, and in part because it can be difficult to establish causality in all patients who develop MDS following treatment for a prior cancer. t-MDS has been best characterized in patients with a prior history of breast cancer,[52,355,356] lymphoma,[357,358] and myeloma,[359] where the overall incidence is usually reported at around 1%. On the other hand, t-MDS is rare following treatment for other types of tumors, such as gastrointestinal and genitourinary cancers. This difference is largely attributed to differences in the types and intensities of chemotherapeutic agents used to treat different tumor types. In particular, high doses of alkylating agents, such as cyclophosphamide, ifosfamide, melphalan, and busulfan, have been associated with classic t-MDS,[360] as has extensive radiation therapy.[361] A distinct, well-characterized class of therapy-related myeloid malignancies occur after treatment with topoisomerase inhibitors but largely consists of AML without an antecedent MDS phase.[54,205,362]

t-MDS has a relatively distinct clinical behavior. It is typically characterized by a latency of years and recurrent large-scale chromosomal abnormalities, especially of chromosomes 5 and 7 or 11q23. Complex karyotypes are also common.[363] These karyotypic abnormalities, which occur in only about 10% to 15% of patients with de novo MDS, have a frequency of around 50% to 70% in t-MDS. They tend to have a more aggressive clinical course than patients with de novo disease, with more frequent progression to acute leukemia. They also tend to respond poorly to all classes of treatment, and even for those patients who undergo allogeneic stem cell transplantation, relapse is not infrequent.[364]

As discussed elsewhere in this chapter, the mechanism of pathogenesis for t-MDS has long been thought to involve the acquisition of severe, large-scale chromosomal damage, a theory that is circumstantially supported by the mechanism of alkylators (which induce double-stranded DNA breaks) and the fact that many patients with t-MDS have complex karyotypes. On the other hand, it has previously been observed that some patients with t-MDS have point mutations in *TP53*, which would not be expected to directly arise from alkylator-induced damage,[360] but which can lead to the acquisition of chromosomal rearrangements even in the absence of chemotherapy. Recent deep studies of a small group of patients with therapy-related AML harboring *TP53* mutations have shown that clones harboring the mutations preceded the development of leukemia by years, and in some cases could be detected before the original initiation of chemotherapy.[150] This recapitulates older data showing that cytogenetic abnormalities present in the bone marrow of patients who developed therapy-related leukemia after autologous transplant for lymphoma could be found in the stimulated autologous specimens, which had been banked years before the development of t-AML.[365] These findings suggest an alternate method of t-MDS pathogenesis, in which rare clones harbor preexisting mutations that either confer a selective growth advantage during marrow reconstitution, tolerance of DNA damage that would otherwise trigger apoptosis, or both, thus promoting clonal selection and expansion upon exposure to chemotherapy.

Refractory Anemia With Ringed Sideroblasts and Thrombocytosis

Although thrombocytopenia is the most common platelet abnormality in MDS, rare patients present with marked thrombocytosis.[317] This most frequently occurs in the setting of RARS, and in the second iteration of the WHO criteria, these patients are classified as having RARS-T.[366] On bone marrow examination, there are often features of both MDS, such as frequent ringed sideroblasts, and MPNs, such as megakaryocytic hyperplasia. Molecularly, patients often have concomitant *SF3B1* mutations, which drive the ring sideroblast morphology,[366] and *JAK2* mutations, which drive the thrombocytosis and are otherwise uncommon in MDS.[367] Patients meeting criteria for RARS-T are relatively uncommon and prognostic information is thus limited, but one small series of patients had better 5-year survival than matched patients with RARS, perhaps because the proliferative drive of the JAK2 mutation helps preserve blood cell counts.[368]

TREATMENT OF PATIENTS WITH MYELODYSPLASTIC SYNDROMES

Treating patients with MDS presents a number of challenges. First, MDS patients are often elderly and thus frequently have serious comorbid conditions and poor performance status. Second, the protean nature of MDS, which is particularly heterogeneous even compared with other cancers, means that treatments appropriate for some patients may be unhelpful for others. Third, a number of biologic factors, most importantly the disease's origin in a quiescent stem cell, make MDS highly refractory to most conventional treatments like intensive cytotoxic chemotherapy (which many MDS patients are not healthy enough to receive anyway).

In addition, although the biology of MDS is increasingly well understood, most of the common derangements, like mutations in splicing factors and epigenetic regulators, have wide-ranging, pleiotropic effects that render narrowly targeted therapies infeasible. While some agents like hypomethylators and histone deacetylase inhibitors are matched to biologic processes that are frequently deranged in MDS, their usual clinical impact is modest at best. Allogeneic stem cell transplantation remains the only curative therapy for MDS, but is unavailable to many because of age and comorbidities, and even for those who undergo it, relapse is not uncommon.

Despite these challenges, all patients with MDS should be offered some form of therapy. For elderly patients or those with serious comorbid conditions who are too unwell to undergo active treatment, this may consist primarily of supportive care and possibly hospice or palliative care service referral. Other patients with lower-risk disease may benefit from a period of observation, or judicious use of transfusion and growth factor support, balanced in carefully selected cases with chelation therapy to prevent or relieve iron overload. Patients with higher-risk disease may derive benefit from treatment with hypomethylating agents or other conventional therapies, and those patients with high-risk disease who meet other selection criteria should be referred for consideration of hematopoietic stem cell transplantation (HSCT). Finally, patients should whenever possible be encouraged to participate in clinical trials to the extent that this remains consistent with their personal goals of care.

Once the decision to pursue active treatment has been made, there are at least three major points to consider. One is the choice of initial treatment modality, which is guided in large part by risk stratification. This should typically start by computation of the IPSS-R, but IPSS-R score should not be the sole consideration in choosing therapy; for instance, a very young patient with otherwise lower-risk MDS that has evolved quickly may still warrant consideration of a stem cell transplant, and an elderly patient with very high risk disease may nevertheless opt not to pursue treatment with a hypomethylating agent after a thorough discussion of the risks and potential benefits. Second, there are a number of special cases for which there is no clear consensus about the single best treatment strategy; these include patients with lower-risk disease who have a dominant cytopenia other than anemia, anemic patients with lower-risk disease who lack del(5q) but also have an elevated serum EPO, and patients with high-risk disease who have progressed on a hypomethylating agent but are not candidates for transplant.

Finally, since therapies other than allogeneic HSCT are rarely if ever curative, defining what constitutes a meaningful response can be a nontrivial endeavor. Objective criteria for response were proposed by an International Working Group (IWG) in 2000 and revised in 2006, and include hemoglobin, number of metaphases with abnormal karyotypes, and percentage of the marrow involved by blasts.[369] However, improvements in these objective variables may not always coincide with the ways patients perceive changes in their quality of life[370,371] or MDS-related symptoms,[279] and these perceptions may be more likely to impact patients' decisions to continue or discontinue active therapy for their disease.

Lower-Risk Disease

Many patients with lower-risk MDS do not require active treatment directed at the underlying disease process, but this does not mean they require no treatment at all. In fact, providing appropriate supportive care is an important undertaking that can at times be complex and time-consuming, and requires a detailed understanding of the evidence behind the available supportive measures.[372]

Management of Anemia

Because most MDS patients become anemic at some point during their disease, appropriate management of their anemia is of critical importance.[373] Management can be broken down into two main components: transfusion support and use of erythropoiesis-stimulating agents (ESAs).

Transfusion Support

Many, if not most, patients with MDS will require packed red blood cell (PRBC) transfusion during the course of their disease. To minimize the risks associated with repetitive transfusion, it is usually appropriate to reserve transfusion until the hemoglobin is below 8–9 mg/dL or the patient has symptoms referable to anemia. More restrictive transfusion strategies, such as those suggested by studies in inpatient or critical care settings,[374,375] may be appropriate in younger, healthy patients, while some older patients, particularly those with significant comorbid cardiac disease, may benefit from more liberal strategies targeting a hemoglobin of 9–10 mg/dL.[376,377] Unless the patient is an HSCT candidate (in which case irradiated blood is essential), there is no consensus about leukocyte depletion or irradiation of the product.[378] Since many patients with MDS will receive hundreds of units of PRBCs over the course of their disease, prevention and appropriate management of iron overload is also of substantial importance.[379,380]

Erythropoiesis-Stimulating Agents

Transfusion dependency is a negative predictor of outcome in MDS.[381] While transfusion requirement may to some extent may be a marker of more severe hematopoietic insufficiency and worse disease not captured by other prognostic markers, the poor outcomes may also be a reflection of the adverse effects of repetitive transfusion, including accumulation of toxic iron species, immune modulation, and a risk of infection.[382] Given these facts, the administration of ESAs has been heavily investigated in MDS in an attempt to spare patients from unnecessary transfusions.

More than 20 studies of ESAs have been conducted in MDS, and 20% to 50% of patients experience meaningful, sustained improvements in their hemoglobin level in response to ESA supplementation.[383–388] Predictors of response include lower pretreatment serum EPO levels (<500 U/L, but especially <100 U/L),[389] lower IPSS scores,[390] normal blast counts, normal or low-risk cytogenetics,[391] and lower serum and marrow levels of inflammatory cytokines.[392] The serum EPO level should be evaluated in the context of the degree of anemia; a trial of an ESA is usually reasonable in patients with EPO levels up to 200–300 U/L, which, while technically elevated on most laboratory reference scales, is still lower than would be predicted for most MDS patients' degree of anemia. Patients with EPO levels over 500 U/L, on the other hand, are unlikely to respond to any dose or duration of ESA.

There are two major formulations of ESA available in the United States. Epoetin alfa, the shorter-acting of the two, can either be given at a dose of 150–300 U/kg three times weekly, or in a fixed dose of 40,000 to 60,000 units once weekly.[388] Higher doses above 60,000 U/weekly have not proven to be more effective.[393] Darbepoetin alfa is longer acting and is typically given in doses of 500 μg once every 3 weeks.[394] Retrospective comparisons of the two agents have not shown a significant difference in efficacy.[395] Other ESA formulations are available outside the Unites States, such as epoetin zeta and bioequivalent ESAs. Although there is some increase in response with longer duration of therapy,[396] in practical terms, a trial of 12 weeks is reasonable. Before starting therapy, other causes of anemia should be ruled out. In particular, response can be suboptimal if patients are absolutely or even relatively iron deficient, and oral or parenteral iron supplementation may be reasonable in patients with ferritin levels at the lower end of the normal range.

One limitation of the numerous studies of ESAs in MDS patients is the lack of a consistent definition of response, since most studies predated uniform IWG criteria. Some studies define this based on a hemoglobin increase (usually improvement by 1–2 g/dL),[397,398] while others have defined response by transfusion reduction or quality of life metrics.[399] In practice, any of these improvements could be a reasonable criterion for continuation of therapy. Of particular interest, supplementation with ESA has not been shown to increase the rate of progression to acute leukemia, and one comparative trial showed a nonsignificant trend toward a decreased risk of leukemia, although the biologic basis for this is not clear.[400] In addition, several studies have shown an improvement in response in patients supplemented with a combination of ESA and G-CSF, especially in RARS, likely caused by pleiotropic effects of both growth factors on hematopoietic progenitors.[399,401]

ESAs are no longer routinely used for management of anemia in solid tumor patients, where studies have shown them to be associated with an increased risk of poor outcomes.[402] Similar findings have also been noted in patients without cancer receiving ESAs for anemia associated with renal failure.[403] Such a risk has not consistently been shown in MDS, although most studies published to date have not had long follow-up periods. The risk of thromboembolism has largely been correlated with the degree of improvement in hemoglobin, with patients targeted to hemoglobins over 12 mg/dL at greatest risk. Given this, the consensus recommendation in MDS is to initiate an ESA at hemoglobin <10 g/dL and target a level between 11–12 g/dL.[404]

Management of Neutropenia and Infections

As referenced previously, patients with MDS often become neutropenic but also appear to have other qualitative immune defects that are not accurately represented by the ANC,[392,393] and infection is the leading cause of death in MDS.[280] Despite this, supplementation with either G-CSF (filgrastim, tbo-filgrastim and others) or GM-CSF (sargramostim) has not consistently been shown to improve outcomes in MDS patients.[405–407] Nevertheless, it is reasonable to consider a trial of growth factor (usually G-CSF, because of less frequent adverse effects) in lower-risk IPSS patients with significant neutropenia, typically defined as an ANC <1000/mm³. Supplementation in higher-risk patients, particularly those with any degree of excess blasts, is not usually recommended in the absence of chemotherapy, because of lingering concerns about promoting expansion of leukemic clones.[408] Other therapeutic strategies for immune supplementation, including granulocyte transfusion and cytokine administration, have not been shown to be helpful.[409]

A thorough understanding of appropriate antibiotic use is an important component in the care of MDS patients. Patients should be counseled to seek medical attention for any fever greater than 100.4°F/38.4°C, and those who are neutropenic should be hospitalized and started on antibiotics while an appropriate search for infection is undertaken. A thorough discussion of treating febrile neutropenia can be found elsewhere in the text, but should begin with an antibiotic that covers a broad spectrum of gram-negative organisms including *Pseudomonas* species.[410] Although prophylactic antibiotics should not be started routinely, they may be appropriate for selected patients who demonstrate a pattern of recurrent infections.[411,412] There is less consensus about prophylactic antivirals or antifungal medications, and the efficacy of the latter depends on local microbiologic isolates and epidemiologic patterns.

Management of Thrombocytopenia and Bleeding

Modest thrombocytopenia is common across many subtypes of MDS, while severe depression of platelet counts is more frequently seen in patients with higher-risk IPSS scores or those undergoing active treatment with hypomethylating agents or chemotherapy. Overall, bleeding is the second most common cause of nonleukemic death in MDS patients.[413] Conventional wisdom and observational studies indicate that the risk of bleeding with trauma begins to increase at a platelet count near 50×10^9 cells/L and that of spontaneous hemorrhage does not increase significantly until the count is below 10–20 $\times 10^9$ cells/L. However, these cutoffs may underestimate the bleeding risk in MDS patients, many of whom have qualitative defects in platelet function that are not captured by the platelet count. A number of retrospective studies have evaluated the significance of thrombocytopenia in MDS, all of which have found that thrombocytopenia confers a poor prognosis caused by both the risk of bleeding and, in some cases, an elevated risk of transformation to AML.[330,413–415]

As with red blood cells, management of thrombocytopenia can either involve transfusions or use of growth factors. Many institutions use a standard transfusion threshold of 10×10^9 cells/L,[416] but as discussed earlier, a higher goal may be appropriate in selected patients

who show a predilection for bleeding. In general, patients should be transfused prophylactically rather than waiting for bleeding to occur. Although there are few large studies comparing transfusion strategies specifically for MDS patients, a recent study of patients with other hematologic malignancies showed that for most patients (including those with AML), a prophylactic strategy using a trigger of 10×10^9 cells/L led to fewer significant hemorrhages than a therapeutic strategy in which patients were transfused only when bleeding.[417]

Thrombopoietin (TPO) analogs, which are standard therapeutic options for refractory chronic idiopathic thrombocytopenia purpura (ITP),[418] are not yet approved by any regulatory agencies for use in MDS. The two major formulations approved in ITP are romiplostim, a "peptibody" consisting of 14 amino acid peptides that bind the extracytoplasmic domain of the TPO receptor fused to an IgG1 heavy chain, and eltrombopag, a small molecule without TPO homology that nevertheless binds and activates the TPO receptor.[419] Romiplostim is administered as intermittent subcutaneous injections, whereas eltrombopag is an oral formulation that is taken daily.

Both agents have shown efficacy in terms of reducing platelet transfusions and clinically significant bleeding events and increasing platelet counts in early-phase trials in MDS.[420–424] In patients with IPSS low or intermediate-1 risk MDS who had platelet counts less than 50×10^9/L, romiplostim consistently led to significant improvements in platelet count, which were durable in about half of patients.[421] A similarly designed phase I/II trial of eltrombopag is ongoing.

However, concerns have been raised about the safety of TPO agonists in patients with MDS. First, a number of studies in ITP have shown an increase in marrow reticulin fibrosis in subsets of patients.[425] While the absolute risk of fibrosis has not been determined, and fibrosis has been moderate in most patients, some have speculated that the process could be accelerated within the abnormal marrow microenvironment of MDS patients.[426] Second, there is concern about increased blast proliferation in the presence of TPO agonists, since some blasts have functional TPO receptors. A randomized controlled trial of romiplostim versus placebo (the only phase III study of either agent in MDS to date) was stopped early by the study's safety monitoring committee because of interim analysis suggesting a higher rate of progression to AML in the romiplostim arm.[427] At the time the study was stopped, 10 of 167 patients in the romiplostim group had progressed to AML, compared to two of 83 in the placebo group. Since the study was far from completion of accrual at the time it was stopped, the risk of disease progression could not be definitively assessed and the AML progression rate eventually nearly equalized; nevertheless, the manufacturer has now added a warning of risk of MDS progression to romiplostim's label. Until there is more conclusive evidence evaluating the link between TPO analogs and the risk of disease progression, neither romiplostim or eltrombopag can be recommended for routine treatment of MDS-associated thrombocytopenia outside a clinical trial, although patients with refractory bleeding who fail to respond to platelet transfusions could consider trying one of these agents palliatively.

Management of Iron Overload (Transfusional Hemosiderosis)

Although it is clear that MDS patients who undergo repeated blood transfusions carry an increased risk of developing iron overload,[381] the importance of this relative to other disease-related risks, and how to assess and respond to it, remains a matter of some debate.[382] MDS is distinct from pediatric illnesses associated with iron overload, in which the benefit of chelation has been well established,[428] in that many MDS patients will not live long enough for the clinical impact of end-organ iron deposition to be realized. Registry data suggest that patients with higher transfusion requirements have a greater risk of complications,[429,430] but registry data cannot prove the direction of the relationship—that is, whether the transfusions lead to complications or whether the need for transfusion is simply a marker of more severe disease or underlying comorbidities. Other retrospective studies have provided circumstantial evidence for deleterious effects of iron overload. For instance, one study has shown a higher rate of death from heart failure among MDS patients,[431] and another has shown increased rates of heart and liver failure among MDS patients with high lifetime numbers of transfusions,[432] but these observations again cannot prove causality.

There are two major formulations of chelating agent available in the United States, deferoxamine and deferasirox (a third agent, deferiprone/L1, is available only for thalassemia patients via a restricted distribution program). Deferoxamine is administered as a continuous subcutaneous or IV infusion, a cumbersome mechanism that has limited its applicability in widespread practice. Deferasirox, an oral formulation, is more convenient so is much more widely used, but is quite costly.

Deferasirox is typically started at 20 mg/kg (14 mg/kg for the new tablet form of deferasirox FDA approved in 2015) once daily and escalated to 30–40 mg/kg/day (28 mg/kg for the new tablet form of deferasirox FDA approved in 2015), depending on iron kinetics and patient tolerance. Although deferasirox has been shown to rapidly mobilize stored iron and reduce labile plasma iron species, it is frequently discontinued either as a result of disease progression or caused by side effects, which include gastrointestinal distress, renal impairment, and rash.

To date, there have been no randomized controlled trials to definitively evaluate the impact of iron chelation on outcomes in MDS. The largest prospective trial to date, a single-arm cohort study of 1744 patients treated with deferasirox, included a prespecified MDS subgroup of 341 patients. Over the study's single year, median ferritin levels decreased significantly compared to baseline regardless of whether patients were chelation naive or not, as did the median alanine aminotransferase, which was tracked as a marker of hepatic toxicity from iron overload. On the other hand, 48.7% of the MDS patients discontinued treatment because of side effects. Since there was no control arm and the study period was short, no conclusions could be drawn about the impact of chelation on more meaningful clinical outcomes. Other studies have shown improvements in hematopoiesis in patients started on chelation therapy,[433,434] but these observations were not tied to longer-term outcomes either.

There are data from retrospective studies showing better outcomes for patients who undergo iron chelation, but all of these are subject to patient selection bias. In one, a Canadian study of 178 patients, only 18 received chelation therapy, suggesting that these patients were carefully selected and destined to have a better outcome anyway.[435] In another, a French study of 97 patients in whom 46% received chelation, the regimen and duration of chelation therapy varied considerably, and no baseline assessment of iron stores was performed.[436] A recent metaanalysis of iron chelation studies in MDS found that use of chelation therapy was associated with an increase in length of survival (overall 61.2 months longer for patients receiving chelation),[437] but since the analysis included only retrospective studies, it is very possible that these numbers are again largely reflective of selection bias, with healthier or younger patients more likely to receive chelation therapy than those who were older or sicker.

Despite the limitations of the available data, there are several published consensus opinion guidelines regarding the use of chelation therapy in MDS.[324,438] Although they differ with respect to their specific recommendations, most operate on similar principles that the patients best suited to iron chelation therapy are either those with lower-risk disease and significant anemia who presumably face a long period of transfusion dependency, or those who could potentially be eligible for stem cell transplantation, since in the transplant setting numerous studies have shown that a high ferritin is associated with inferior outcomes.[439] A third category of patients comprises those with suspected end-organ damage as a result of iron overload.

Some of the guidelines recommend waiting to start chelation therapy until the ferritin is greater than 1000 μg/L or the patient has had more than 20–30 lifetime transfusions, but they also note that neither of these criteria is supported by high-level evidence. Serum ferritin is problematic since it is subject to variability based on

inflammatory state, and is an imperfect marker of total body iron burden. For quantitative assessment of hepatic iron overload, T2*-weighted magnetic resonance imaging of the liver has supplanted biopsy as the preferred method of validation.[440]

Other Therapies for Lower-Risk Disease

The literature is replete with attempts to treat lower-risk MDS with a variety of different drugs, especially so-called differentiating agents such as retinoic acid or arsenic trioxide (ATO). With the exception of lenalidomide for 5q− syndrome, most of these have been inconsistently effective at best.

Lenalidomide

As described previously, lenalidomide is a derivative of thalidomide that is uniquely effective in reversing the severe anemia associated with isolated del(5q). This was previously thought to be related to poorly characterized immunomodulatory effects (as implied by "Imid," the name given to the class of thalidomide derivatives).[441] However, more recent work has shown that lenalidomide actually exerts its effect in 5q− syndrome by mediating the binding of the E3 ubiquitin ligase cereblon to casein kinase 1α, thus triggering casein kinase's proteasomal degradation.[442] Casein kinase 1α is an essential kinase whose gene, CSNK1A1, lies within the minimally deleted region on 5q.[177] In normal cells, treatment with lenalidomide is insufficient to deplete casein kinase 1α to lethal levels, but the haploinsufficiency of CSNK1A1 induced by loss of 5q renders 5q− cells sensitive to the drug through a p53-dependent mechanism and allows for repopulation of the marrow by wildtype hematopoietic progenitors. This activity appears to be unique to lenalidomide and is not shared, for instance, by thalidomide. Unfortunately, the effect is not permanent and resistance eventually develops in most cases, often through inactivating mutations in TP53.[443] Hopefully, however, these new insights will enable further studies of how these resistance mechanisms arise.

Lenalidomide's efficacy was first observed in MDS-001, a phase I study of 32 patients with symptomatic anemia who had not responded to ESAs.[444] Twenty of the 32 patients became independent of transfusion for some period of time, including 10 of 12 patents with del(5q). Of the responders, those with del(5q) had a significantly longer duration of response. This prompted further study of lenalidomide specifically in del(5q) patients in MDS-003, a phase II study in which 76% of 148 enrolled patients had an improvement in anemia and 67% achieved transfusion independence, with a median improvement in hemoglobin near 5 mg/dL. A second phase II trial, MDS-002, showed that lenalidomide was also effective in a substantially smaller subset of patients without del(5q), with an overall response rate of 43% and a transfusion independence rate of 26%. The factors that determine lenalidomide responsiveness in non-del(5q) MDS have not been determined.

The most conclusive evidence of lenalidomide's efficacy in del(5q) comes from the phase III MDS-004 trial,[173] a randomized, double-blinded study in which patients were randomized 1:1:1 to receive lenalidomide 10 mg/day on days 1–21 of a 28-day-cycle, lenalidomide 5 mg/day on days 1–28, or placebo on days 1–28. Those without an erythroid response at 16 weeks were unblinded and became eligible for open-label treatment. At the conclusion of the study, significantly more patients in both lenalidomide groups had achieved transfusion independence for at least 26 weeks than those in the placebo group (56% in the 10-mg group versus 43% in the 5-mg group versus 5.9% in the placebo group), with those in the 10-mg group having a longer median duration of response (82.9 weeks) than those in the 5-mg group (41.3 weeks). Intriguingly, treatment with lenalidomide also appeared to lower the risk of transformation to AML; at a median follow up of around 3 years, 36.4% of patients who had received placebo only and 30.4% who had started with placebo and crossed over to lenalidomide had developed AML, compared to 23.2% in the 5-mg group and 21.7% in the 10-mg group, though the crossover model prevented an assessment of statistical significance.

Given recent progress in understanding of lenalidomide's mechanism of action, it is perhaps unsurprising that it demonstrates considerably lower efficacy in MDS patients who do not have del(5q). In these patients, studies have consistently shown an overall response rate of about 25%, which on average lasts less than a year.[445,446] It is not known whether the patients who respond have abnormalities of casein kinase 1α, or whether their sensitivity to lenalidomide occurs via a different mechanism.

Lenalidomide is generally well tolerated, especially compared to thalidomide. The most common side effects are neutropenia and thrombocytopenia, which are most common in the first month of treatment and which have some correlation to treatment response.[447] Pretreatment thrombocytopenia, a feature atypical of pure del(5q), appears to negatively correlate with response and perhaps serves as a phenotypic proxy for cooperating genetic events that blunt the molecular sensitivity to the drug.[149] Significant thromboembolism has been observed in studies of patients with myeloma who receive lenalidomide, an effect that largely seems to be confined to co-administration of lenalidomide and dexamethasone;[448] the manufacturer thus recommends thromboprophylaxis in del(5q) patients as well, though it is not clear that the thrombotic risk is the same in these populations, and thrombocytopenia may limit the safety of this approach.

Low-Dose Cytarabine

Cytarabine, also known as cytosine arabinoside or Ara-c, is a pyrimidine analog that is widely used in the treatment of a number of hematologic malignancies. In MDS, its use dates to the 1980s.[449,450] The typical dosing schedule is 5–20 mg/m^2 per day via subcutaneous injection (daily or twice daily) or continuous IV infusion. Although 10% to 20% of patients with MDS have some degree of pathologic response during Ara-c therapy, these tend to last only a few months, and treatment has not been shown to improve survival or reduce the rate of transformation to AML.

One of the drawbacks to treatment with cytarabine or any other conventional chemotherapeutic agent is that they cause cytopenias as a primary side effect, and since cytopenias are a central problem in most MDS patients, the agents rapidly become limited in utility.[451] The worsening of cytopenias is likely one of the primary reasons for the lack of survival benefit for cytarabine in MDS.

Antitumor Necrosis Factor Therapy

The observation that MDS patients often have elevated levels of inflammatory cytokines and increased rates of apoptosis led to the postulate that blockade of these pathways might ameliorate the ineffective hematopoiesis found in many patients with MDS. Etanercept, a soluble TNF-α inhibitor, has been analyzed in two small pilot studies of MDS patients, with mixed results: cytopenias improved in one trial,[452] whereas no effect was seen in the other.[453] The drug has also been combined with both ATG[454] and azacitidine,[454] but in neither case was it clear that the addition made a difference. A separate case report described sustained erythroid responses in two patients treated with infliximab, a monoclonal anti-TNF antibody.[455] TNF-α and other inflammatory mediators may play a greater role in some subsets of MDS than others,[456] and better delineation of these groups may make future study of anti-TNF therapy reasonable in selected patients.

Immunosuppressive Therapy

Corticosteroid therapy was once a mainstay of treatment for MDS, but despite reported response rates in the range of 10% to 20%,[457]

the complications of long-term steroid use in this population came to outweigh the benefits. Nevertheless, immunosuppressive therapy may be reasonable for certain subsets of MDS patients in whom autoreactive T-lymphocytes contribute to the inhibition of effective hematopoiesis. Patients with hypoplastic MDS, in particular, have been shown to have similarities to aplastic anemia, and may respond to treatment with ATG.[458] Other studies have shown that patients with underlying PNH clones, which can be assessed by flow cytometry for PIG-anchored glycoproteins CD55 and CD59, may also respond to ATG, as may patients with a human leukocyte antigen (HLA) DR15 phenotype.[459]

Retrospective analysis of data from the International Myelodysplasia Risk Assessment Workshop showed that treatment with immunosuppression was associated with an improvement in overall survival (8.1 vs. 5.2 years, $p < .001$) and a lower risk of leukemic transformation, but these results could have been subject to selection bias since fewer patients with higher-risk disease are treated upfront with immunosuppression.[460] On the other hand, a randomized study comparing ATG plus cyclosporine to best supportive care suggested a slight improvement in hematologic response in the ATG + cyclosporine A group, but there was no difference in disease-free or overall survival.[461] Subgroup analysis suggested that patients with hypocellular marrows were more likely to respond to immunosuppression, again hinting at biologic similarities to aplastic anemia. In studies making careful distinction between MDS and aplastic anemia, however, mortality with ATG treatment was higher in MDS than in aplastic anemia.[345]

Alemtuzumab, a monoclonal antibody against anti-CD52, has activity in highly selected subsets of MDS patients. In particular, one small phase I/II study of patients yielded a 77% overall response rate among patients with IPSS intermediate-1 disease.[462] Some patients with cytogenetic abnormalities normalized their karyotype, and the rate of complete response appeared to increase with time in those patients who were not lost to follow up. However, alemtuzumab is severely immunosuppressive and the study was hampered by a high rate of attrition and careful selection of patients, and the results have not yet been repeated. The biologic basis for the high response rate in this single study remains unclear.

Manipulating the Microenvironment: Vascular Endothelial Growth Factor and Other Targets

Observations of increased microvessel density in the bone marrow of MDS[463] patients have led to some enthusiasm for targeting vascular growth factors and other molecules associated with the marrow microenvironment, but results so far have been somewhat disappointing. For instance, a phase II trial of bevacizumab, a monoclonal antibody directed against vascular endothelial growth factor (VEGF), showed a decrease in VEGF levels and a significant reduction in microvascular density, but only one of 21 patients had any type of hematologic response.[464] Similarly, a phase II study of vatalanib, an oral VEGF receptor inhibitor, showed hematologic responses in only 5% of patients, though many patients had to withdraw from the study because of side effects.[465]

Other therapies directed at the microenvironment have similarly shown responses in only a minority of patients. For instance, the combination of pentoxifylline, a phosphodiesterase inhibitor, with dexamethasone and ciprofloxacin (PCD) has been shown to induce hematologic responses in some patients, but most of these are transient and probably represent neutrophil demargination from the corticosteroid.[231] A more recent study combining PCD with amifostine, an antiangiogenic agent usually used as a chemoprotectant, showed a hematologic response rate of 66%, but long-term results have not been reported.[466] Lenalidomide and thalidomide were both previously thought to act via effects on the microenvironment,[467] but with the discovery of lenalidomide's role as a catalyst for cereblon-mediated ubiquitination, as described earlier, the extent to which it also affects the microenvironment is unclear.

Signal Transduction Inhibitors

Activating mutations in receptor tyrosine kinases like *NRAS* and *FLT3* are relatively uncommon in MDS, not because they never occur in this population, but because they usually act as catalysts for progression to secondary AML.[238] The consideration for use of FLT3 inhibitors in MDS is similar to those in s-AML, and data are limited. A more thorough discussion of these agents may be found in Chapter 59 (AML).

Other Agents

A number of other agents have been used in MDS and reported either in anecdotes or small, nonrandomized series of patients. Historically, many patients with RARS were started on vitamin B₆ because of its efficacy in familial sideroblastic anemia, but it has shown little efficacy in adults.[468] Other dietary supplements, include retinoids (vitamin A analogues), vitamin D,[469] and vitamin K2,[470] have all been tried because of favorable effects on differentiation in vitro, but have not been effective in humans. A number of other drugs have also been trialed in humans based on similar observations of prodifferentiation effects in preclinical experiments, all without comparable efficacy in human patients. These include amifostine as a single agent,[471] the solvent hexamethyl bisacetamide,[472] and alpha and gamma interferon. Interferon, in particular, has recently been shown to cause normal HSCs to exit quiescence in mouse models,[473,474] but whether it can be used for similar purposes to "prime" MDS stem cells for subsequent treatment with cytotoxic therapy has not yet been explored.

Given their efficacy in promyelocytic leukemia, both all-*trans* retinoic acid (ATRA) and ATO have been trialed in small numbers of MDS patients in a similar attempt to induce differentiation. ATO has shown responses in up to 20% of MDS patients in several small series,[475–478] but the molecular basis for this action and how to predict who will respond are unclear. ATRA by itself has largely been ineffective, likely caused by the absence of the PML-RARA fusion protein that is the basis for its efficacy in acute promyelocytic leukemia (APML).[479,480] In vitro data suggest that in some AML models, downstream targets of the retinoic acid receptor may be epigenetically silenced by abnormal induction of histone demethylases such as LSD1, which can be inhibited by tranylcypromine, a monoamine oxidase inhibitor (MAOI) approved in Europe to treat depression.[481] In vitro, the combination of ATRA with tranylcypromine in non-APML leukemia derepresses targets of the retinoic acid receptor and significantly impairs the ability of leukemia stem cells to engraft in immunodeficient mice. Whether this pathway can be similarly reactivated in MDS, and whether this is a viable therapeutic combination in patients, also remain as yet unexplored.

A number of other novel agents remain in clinical trials for lower-risk MDS at the time of this writing.[482] These include inhibitors of the transforming growth factor-beta receptor,[483] inhibitors of toll-like receptors, chimeric antibodies to activin, mitochondrial modulators, RAS pathway inhibitors, and anti-CD33 molecules. In addition, there are ongoing trials evaluating combinations of existing therapies, including hypomethylating agents, histone deacetylase (HDAC) inhibitors, lenalidomide, and hematopoietic growth factors. While some of these trials may identify novel therapies or combinations with efficacy for subsets of MDS patients, whether any of them will have substantial impact on the treatment landscape for low-risk MDS remains to be seen.

Higher-Risk Disease

Hypomethylating Agents

MDS genomes frequently display aberrant methylation patterns relative to normal hematopoietic cells. This observation was initially made in the 1990s, when investigators noted hypermethylation in the promoters of numerous tumor suppressor genes, including *CDKN2A, CDKN2B*,[484] *FHIT*,[485] *SOCS1*,[486] *CTNNA1*,[487] and others. Later, with the advent of genome-wide methylation profiling, it was further observed that this aberrant methylation is often a global phenomenon in MDS and that global hypermethylation, in particular, appears to confer a poor prognosis.[488]

This characterization of aberrant methylation in MDS soon led to the identification of hypomethylating agents (HMA) as a candidate class of MDS drugs. The prototypical hypomethylator, 5-azacytidine (azacitidine), was synthesized in the 1960s and its hypomethylating activity first clearly characterized in 1980.[489] It is an azo-substituted pyrimidine analogue that incorporates into RNA and is from there converted to a deoxynucleotide and incorporated into DNA, where it binds and irreversibly inhibits DNMT1. The in vitro result is a global decrease in cytosine methylation, which leads to differentiation in some leukemia cell lines. Of note, azacitidine also appears to have nonepigenetic mechanisms of action, including some degree of direct cytotoxicity and immune stimulation.[490] Both azacitidine and the related compound decitabine (5-aza-2'-deoxycytidine) are now frequently administered in both MDS and AML.

Standard dosing of azacitidine is 75 mg/m² administered subcutaneously once per day for 7 consecutive days each month.[491] This was the dosing schedule used in the first major study of hypomethylating agents in MDS, CALGB 9221, in which azacitidine was found to be superior to best supportive care both in terms of quality of life and risk of progression to AML.[492] In this study, about 60% of patients had some degree of response to azacitidine, although consensus response criteria were not used. Most of these responses were minor hematologic improvement, but about 15% of patients had a pathologic complete response. Most of those who responded did so within 6 months. There was a nonsignificant trend toward an improvement in overall survival with azacitidine, and side effects tended to be mild, including nausea and vomiting and transient myelosuppression.

Based on these data and a large increase in requests for compassionate use of the drug after CALGB 9221 was first presented in 2002, the Food and Drugs Administration (FDA) granted approval to azacitidine for MDS in 2004. A subsequent study, AZA-001, comparing azacitidine 1:1 to the patient and doctor choice of either standard induction, low-dose cytarabine, and best supportive care in 358 patients with higher-risk MDS or CMML showed a median 9-month improvement in overall survival for those treated with azacitidine (24 versus 15 months).[493] This represents the only major study to date in which a survival benefit has been shown for a drug in MDS. Other studies have shown that a more convenient 5-day azacitidine dosing schedule appears to be effective, but this has not been directly compared to the 7-day schedule, which remains the standard. One recent study suggested an improvement in response from prolonged administration of azacitidine, though all patients in this study had higher rates of hematologic normalization compared to historical controls, for unclear reasons.[494]

The other major hypomethylating agent, decitabine (5-aza-2'-deoxycytidine), is also FDA-approved for treatment in all subclasses of MDS. Although structurally similar to azacitidine, decitabine has a deoxyribose backbone that permits it to be directly incorporated into DNA. At higher doses it introduces DNA cross-linking and cell-cycle arrest, a mechanism more akin to a cytotoxic agent, but at lower doses it appears to primarily act as a hypomethylating agent.[495]

Similar to azacitidine, decitabine has been shown to improve outcomes for patients with MDS, including a reduced transfusion requirement and slower transformation to AML. It may induce responses more quickly than azacitidine; for instance, in the multicenter ADOPT (alternative dosing of decitabine for outpatient therapy) study, 90% of patients responded after four cycles, rather than the six cycles seen in the largest azacitidine trials.[496] In contrast to azacitidine, however, decitabine has never been shown to confer an overall survival benefit. Some of the difference in outcomes may be explained by difficulties establishing the optimal dose and schedule; in the earliest trials it was administered at a dose of 15 mg/m² given IV every 8 hours for 3 days,[497] but subsequent studies showed better hypomethylation and an improved overall response rate when it was given at a dose of 20 mg/m^2 once daily for 5 consecutive days,[498] the dosing strategy used in ADOPT. Some recent small studies have suggested an even different dosing strategy, using frequent administration of low doses of decitabine (0.1–0.2 mg/kg/day) in an attempt to minimize the cytotoxic effects of the drug while catching more cells in S phase, when the demethylating activity of the drug would be most effective.[499]

Despite the widespread use of hypomethylating agents in MDS, a number of key questions persist. Although studies have shown that each can demethylate the promoters of specific tumor suppressors (e.g., *P15INK4B*[500] for decitabine and *PLCB1*[501] for azacitidine), it is not clear that this is the dominant in vivo mechanism. Some studies have shown increased demethylation in patients who respond to hypomethylating agents,[502] but this has not been a universal observation, and neither pretreatment methylation levels (either global or at specific promoters) nor the net change in methylation with treatment have been consistently predictive of treatment responsiveness.[488,503] Recent studies have also interrogated the impact of somatic mutations on hypomethylating agent sensitivity, and *TET2* mutations in particular have been shown to increase the likelihood of HMA response,[103] but the overall impact of these findings in the long term remains unclear.

"Histone" Deacetylase Inhibitors

The observation that MDS frequently involves epigenomic abnormalities has provoked interest in other modalities beyond the hypomethylating agents. To date, the next most-studied class of agent is the histone deacetylase inhibitors, which as their name implies block the deacetylation of histone residues as well as deacetylation of other cellular protein. In vitro, application of these drugs leads to large-scale epigenetic modifications, but in vivo, the drugs have so far not proven as effective as hypomethylating agents, at least when used alone.[504] Several agents, however, remain in trials, including valproic acid,[505] vorinostat,[506] panobinostat,[507] and belinostat.[508] Many of these trials combine the HDAC inhibitor with some other therapy. One cooperative trial of azacitidine with or without entinostat, E1905, showed no improvement in hematologic response in the entinostat arm, which in fact displayed less demethylation than azacitidine alone, perhaps suggesting some degree of pharmacologic antagonism.[494] However, in vitro data have also shown significant pharmacologic differences between the different HDAC inhibitors, suggesting that results for one drug may not be generalizable to the class as a whole. Similar negative results were recently reported in the U.S./Canadian Intergroup S1117, a large three-arm trial comparing azacitidine alone to azacitidine plus vorinostat to azacitidine plus lenalidomide, as well as a study of azacitidine with or without pracinostat.[509]

Induction Chemotherapy

AML-like induction regimens (e.g., cytarabine plus an anthracycline) are not effective for most patients with MDS, with available studies suggesting a remission rate of less than 20%. Hematologic recovery is often incomplete, and in many cases the chemotherapy mainly serves to select for the malignant clone. In fact, a randomized trial comparing azacitidine to daunorubicin plus cytarabine in elderly patients with higher-risk MDS showed that the patients treated with azacitidine had better outcomes, although only small numbers of patients were treated with induction.[493]

Induction chemotherapy, however, may be reasonable in selected younger patients; some studies have suggested remission rates of up to 50% in patients younger than 60, though these may have contained some patients with de novo AML,[510] and the studies were performed before the widespread availability of deep sequencing techniques that might have shown persistence of clonal mutations even in the ablated marrows.[148] Adding other agents, such as liposomal doxorubicin,[511] topotecan,[512] and thalidomide, do not seem to improve the rates of

remission. Conventional chemotherapy alone is rarely curative in MDS, and even those younger patients who achieve a complete remission will need further consolidation, usually with an allogeneic stem cell transplant.

Allogeneic Stem Cell Transplantation

Allogeneic HSCT is the only known curative therapy for MDS.[513] This is thought to arise from the fact that MDS progenitor cells, being transformed stem cells, are mostly quiescent and are thus relatively resistant to most chemotherapy. Allogeneic HSCT, on the other hand, leverages both the chemotherapy of the conditioning regimen and the antitumor effect of the newly transplanted stem cells to eliminate all vestiges of the prior hematopoietic system. This is, of course, a simplified description of the best-case outcome for HSCT. The reality for most MDS patients is significantly more complicated, although outcomes have steadily improved in recent years as centers have gained more experience in transplanting older patients using unrelated and even unmatched donors.[514]

An exhaustive review of stem cell transplantation is beyond the scope of this chapter, but a few points specific to MDS bear mention. Identification of patients for whom transplant might be a reasonable option is an important first step. This group typically includes patients younger than 60 years, who are often in otherwise good health and would otherwise be predicted to have a long life expectancy. Older patients who are in otherwise excellent health may be considered for transplantation as well, usually with a reduced-intensity conditioning regimen. Although there is no official upper age limit to eligibility, most centers are hesitant to transplant patients older than 75.[515]

The stage of disease is also important: in older patients, transplant is usually reserved for those with excess blasts or other forms of higher-risk disease, but it is important to proceed to transplant before the disease has evolved into acute leukemia. On the other hand, some centers occasionally offer transplantation to younger patients with lower-risk categories of disease given that they have a longer latency period in which their disease could progress or evolve into leukemia. This decision, however, is not completely uniform, and some data suggest that delayed stem cell transplantation is associated with better overall survival in patients with low and intermediate-1 IPSS scores regardless of age.[516]

Once a decision has been made to proceed to transplant, other decisions must follow. The first involves the source of the stem cells. If a healthy, HLA-matched sibling is available, this is often preferable;[517] however, reflective of the average age of MDS patients, most siblings are older and often have comorbidities, such as cancer or other illnesses, that preclude them from consideration as donors. If a related donor is unavailable, the next best option is a search of the national donor registry for an HLA-matched unrelated donor.[518] Compared to related donors, transplant from unrelated donors carries a higher rate of graft-versus-host disease as a consequence of minor antigen mismatch. If a matched unrelated donor cannot be found, options then include an unrelated donor transplant mismatched at one (or occasionally more) HLA loci, or an "alternative donor source," which includes umbilical cord blood[519] and haploidentical donors.[520] In the case of MDS patients, this latter type of transplant is often obtained from one of the patient's children.

The specific choice of conditioning regimen is likely less important in MDS than in other hematologic diseases given the disease's intrinsic chemoresistance, as described earlier. Options include fludarabine plus busulfan, fludarabine plus melphalan, busulfan plus cyclophosphamide, or cyclophosphamide plus irradiation. Many older patients with MDS are unlikely to tolerate myeloablative doses of conditioning agents and are instead given reduced doses of conditioning agents. These "reduced intensity conditioning" transplants rely more heavily on the graft-versus-tumor effect of the transplant to eliminate the malignant clone.[521,522] Given the intrinsic chemoresistance of MDS stem cells, however, this is usually a reasonable tradeoff. Following transplant, patients must remain on immunosuppressive medications to prevent the emergence of graft-versus-host disease. A full discussion of posttransplant considerations is outside the scope of this chapter, but most aspects of this area are less specific to MDS than those discussed previously.

As mentioned, despite being potentially curative therapy, transplant in MDS is associated with significant morbidity and mortality. One study has suggested that 50% to 60% of lower-risk patients and 20% to 40% with higher-risk disease can expect long-term disease-free survival following transplant,[523] but the alternative view of these data is that a substantial proportion of patients (40%–50% of low risk and 60%–80% of high risk) either relapse or die of nonrelapse complications of transplant.

Numerous studies have attempted to dissect patient and disease attributes that may predict outcomes following transplant. Poor-risk cytogenetics, including monosomy 7 and complex karyotypes,[524] have been shown to predict a high rate of relapse, and recent data suggest that pathogenic *TP53*, *DNMT3A*, and *TET2* mutations are predictors of poor outcomes following transplantation as well.[104] So far, no cytogenetic or genetic profiles have been clearly associated with a favorable response to transplant. Preexisting neutropenia has been shown to predict an increased risk of serious infections in the posttransplant setting.[525] On the other hand, a low blast count (fewer than 5%) is associated with better outcomes, and other data show that patients who achieved a remission or significant response to pretransplant chemotherapy have better outcomes as well.[526]

Other Therapies for Higher-Risk Disease

Autologous Stem Cell Infusion

Though rarely used in current practice, infusion of autologous stem cells has been attempted in the past, primarily for patients with oligoblastic disease.[527,528] There are a number of reasons why this approach is suboptimal for MDS patients. The most obvious drawback is that MDS is by definition a disorder of stem cells, such that any autologous infusion will ultimately lead to repopulation of the marrow with the original malignant clone, but without the graft-versus-leukemia effect imparted by an allogeneic transplant. Moreover, autologous stem cell infusion is really meant to serve as a rescue after high-dose chemotherapy, and is thus most successful when given for a chemotherapy-sensitive disease, which MDS is not. Finally, given the ineffective hematopoiesis many patients experience before treatment, hematopoietic recovery following high-dose chemotherapy is often poor. Since most patients who would be candidates for autologous stem cell rescue would also be eligible for other, more effective modalities of therapy, there are usually few reasons to pursue this avenue.

Other Drugs

Most drugs known to have activity in AML have been tried for MDS as well, usually with suboptimal results. These include etoposide,[529] irinotecan, gemcitabine,[530] low-dose melphalan,[531] idarubicin,[510] and clofarabine.[532] Both hydroxyurea and low-dose oral etoposide can be used to control proliferation in patients with excess blasts, but they do not target the underlying disease. Clofarabine is sometimes effective as a bridge to transplant therapy in patients with excess blasts despite hypomethylating agent therapy, but renal and hepatic toxicity and severe skin rash are limiting.[533]

As with lower-risk disease, there are a number of ongoing trials for patients with high-risk MDS as of this writing. Reflective of the poorer prognosis of these patients compared to those with lower-risk disease, many of these trials either examine different combinations of high-dose chemotherapy or modification of protocols for allogeneic stem cell transplant, and are often open to both MDS and AML patients. However, there are a number of novel or repurposed agents in trials as well, including immunotherapies (ipilimumab,[534] adoptive T-cell transfer,[535] and NK cell therapy[536]), small molecules

(PIM kinase inhibitors, B-catenin degraders[537]), and radioisotope-conjugated monoclonal antibodies. As mentioned earlier, whether any of these drugs will significantly change the landscape of MDS therapy is unclear.

FUTURE DIRECTIONS

While the last ten years have witnessed substantial improvements in our understanding of the molecular pathophysiology underlying MDS, similar strides have not been made in its treatment: at the time of this writing, it has been almost 10 years since the FDA last approved a new drug for treatment of MDS (decitabine in 2006). There are few therapies in clinical trials that offer hope of broad or deep efficacy, and much of the ongoing clinical effort is directed at incremental changes to current practice, such as adjusting dosing schedules of currently approved therapies or using modestly effective drugs in combination. The lack of progress is to a great extent caused by unfortunate facts of MDS biology, including its origin in quiescent stem cells, a paucity of targetable activating mutations, and enrichment for poorly targetable mutations with much more subtle effects on growth and differentiation. Efforts are further complicated by the heterogeneity of biology both between and within individual patients, as well as the advanced age and poor overall health of many patients with MDS.

Despite these significant challenges, there is nevertheless great opportunity for improvements in care. Advances in stem cell transplant techniques, including the availability of alternative donor sources, refinements of posttransplant immunosuppression, and augmentation of the graft-versus-tumor effect, should continue to improve the outcomes for MDS patients able to undergo transplant. An equally difficult challenge lies in treatment of those patients ineligible for transplant, and it is in these patients that effective unification of our improving biologic understanding of MDS with clinical care is most essential.

SUGGESTED READINGS

Abel GA, Klaassen R, Lee SJ, et al: Patient-reported outcomes for the myelodysplastic syndromes: a new MDS-specific measure of quality of life. *Blood* 123(3):451–452, 2014.

Bejar R, Stevenson K, Abdel-Wahab O, et al: Clinical effect of point mutations in myelodysplastic syndromes. *N Engl J Med* 364(26):2496–2506, 2011.

Bejar R, Stevenson KE, Caughey B, et al: Somatic mutations predict poor outcome in patients with myelodysplastic syndrome after hematopoietic stem-cell transplantation. *J Clin Oncol* 32(25):2691–2698, 2014.

Bejar R, Stevenson KE, Caughey BA, et al: Validation of a prognostic model and the impact of mutations in patients with lower-risk myelodysplastic syndromes. *J Clin Oncol* 30(27):3376–3382, 2012.

Cogle CR, Iannacone MR, Yu D, et al: High rate of uncaptured myelodysplastic syndrome cases and an improved method of case ascertainment. *Leuk Res* 38(1):71–75, 2014.

Damm F, Fontenay M, Bernard OA: Point mutations in myelodysplastic syndromes. *N Engl J Med* 365(12):1154–1155, author reply 155, 2011.

Della Porta MG, Tuechler H, Malcovati L, et al: Validation of WHO classification-based Prognostic Scoring System (WPSS) for myelodysplastic syndromes and comparison with the revised International Prognostic Scoring System (IPSS-R). A study of the International Working Group for Prognosis in Myelodysplasia (IWG-PM). *Leukemia* 2015.

Genovese G, Kähler AK, Handsaker RE, et al: Clonal hematopoiesis and blood-cancer risk inferred from blood DNA sequence. *N Engl J Med* 371(26):2477–2487, 2014.

Gerds AT, Gooley TA, Estey EH, et al: Pretransplantation therapy with azacitidine vs induction chemotherapy and posttransplantation outcome in patients with MDS. *Biol Blood Marrow Transplant* 18(8):1211–1218, 2012.

Greenberg PL, Tuechler H, Schanz J, et al: Revised international prognostic scoring system for myelodysplastic syndromes. *Blood* 120(12):2454–2465, 2012.

Haferlach T, Nagata Y, Grossmann V, et al: Landscape of genetic lesions in 944 patients with myelodysplastic syndromes. *Leukemia* 28(2):241–247, 2014.

Hahn CN, Chong C-E, Carmichael CL, et al: Heritable GATA2 mutations associated with familial myelodysplastic syndrome and acute myeloid leukemia. *Nat Genet* 43(10):1012–1017, 2011.

Hahn T, McCarthy PL, Hassebroek A, et al: Significant improvement in survival after allogeneic hematopoietic cell transplantation during a period of significantly increased use, older recipient age, and use of unrelated donors. *J Clin Oncol* 31(19):2437–2449, 2013.

Jaiswal S, Fontanillas P, Flannick J, et al: Age-related clonal hematopoiesis associated with adverse outcomes. *N Engl J Med* 371(26):2488–2498, 2014.

Kon A, Shih L-Y, Minamino M, et al: Recurrent mutations in multiple components of the cohesin complex in myeloid neoplasms. *Nat Genet* 45(10):1232–1237, 2013.

Kuter DJ, Begley CG: Recombinant human thrombopoietin: basic biology and evaluation of clinical studies. *Blood* 100(10):3457–3469, 2002.

List A, Kurtin S, Roe DJ, et al: Efficacy of lenalidomide in myelodysplastic syndromes. *N Engl J Med* 352(6):549–557, 2005.

Lyons RM, Marek BJ, Paley C, et al: Comparison of 24-month outcomes in chelated and non-chelated lower-risk patients with myelodysplastic syndromes in a prospective registry. *Leuk Res* 38(2):149–154, 2014.

Nikoloski G, Langemeijer SMC, Kuiper RP, et al: Somatic mutations of the histone methyltransferase gene EZH2 in myelodysplastic syndromes. *Nat Genet* 42(8):665–667, 2010.

Papaemmanuil E, Cazzola M, Boultwood J, et al: Somatic SF3B1 mutation in myelodysplasia with ring sideroblasts. *N Engl J Med* 365(15):1384–1395, 2011.

Papaemmanuil E, Gerstung M, Malcovati L, et al: Clinical and biological implications of driver mutations in myelodysplastic syndromes. *Blood* 122(22):3616–3627, quiz 3699, 2013.

Pascal L, Beyne-Rauzy O, Brechignac S, et al: Cardiac iron overload assessed by T2* magnetic resonance imaging and cardiac function in regularly transfused myelodysplastic syndrome patients. *Br J Haematol* 162(3):413–415, 2013.

Saunthararajah Y, Sekeres M, Advani A, et al: Evaluation of noncytotoxic DNMT1-depleting therapy in patients with myelodysplastic syndromes. *J Clin Invest* 2015.

Schanz J, Tüchler H, Solé F, et al: New comprehensive cytogenetic scoring system for primary myelodysplastic syndromes (MDS) and oligoblastic acute myeloid leukemia after MDS derived from an international database merge. *J Clin Oncol* 30(8):820–829, 2012.

Schneider RK, Ademà V, Heckl D, et al: Role of casein kinase 1A1 in the biology and targeted therapy of del(5q) MDS. *Cancer Cell* 26(4):509–520, 2014.

Steensma DP: Dysplasia has A differential diagnosis: distinguishing genuine myelodysplastic syndromes (MDS) from mimics, imitators, copycats and impostors. *Curr Hematol Malig Rep* 7(4):310–320, 2012.

Steensma DP: Historical perspectives on myelodysplastic syndromes. *Leuk Res* 36:1441, 2012.

Walter MJ, Shen D, Ding L, et al: Clonal architecture of secondary acute myeloid leukemia. *N Engl J Med* 366(12):1090–1098, 2012.

Yoshida K, Sanada M, Shiraishi Y, et al: Frequent pathway mutations of splicing machinery in myelodysplasia. *Nature* 478(7367):64–69, 2011.

Yoshizato T, Dumitriu B, Hosokawa K, et al: Somatic mutations and clonal hematopoiesis in aplastic anemia. *N Engl J Med* 373(1):35–47, 2015.

REFERENCES

For the complete list of references, log on to www.expertconsult.com.

61

ALLOGENEIC HEMATOPOIETIC STEM CELL TRANSPLANTATION FOR ACUTE MYELOID LEUKEMIA AND MYELODYSPLASTIC SYNDROME IN ADULTS

John Koreth, Joseph H. Antin, and Corey Cutler

Recent advances in molecular diagnostics are shedding considerable light on genetic underpinnings of myelodysplastic syndrome (MDS) and acute myeloid leukemia (AML). However, with notable exceptions both diseases remain therapeutic challenges. Fortunately our ability to provide more precise prognostic information has corresponded with advances in transplantation technology. We are increasingly able to apply transplantation to older people and those with comorbidities and to use alternative donors in patients without matched family members. By applying molecular prognostic criteria we can provide transplantation to patients with poor outcomes on conventional therapy, and we can avoid transplant-related toxicity in those patients who are likely to do well with supportive care or nontransplant therapy.

Allogeneic hematopoietic stem cell transplantation (HSCT) is curative in MDS and AML because of a combination of the cytotoxicity of the preparative conditioning regimen and the donor-mediated immunologic graft-versus-leukemia (GVL) effect. Regimen intensity ranges from high-dose myeloablative conditioning (MAC) that induces profound and prolonged pancytopenia to reduced-intensity conditioning (RIC) that induces milder cytopenias and is more appropriate for older patients and those with comorbidities in whom MAC may be intolerable. The risk-benefit ratio of conditioning regimen intensity varies with factors like patient age, comorbidities, and relapse risk. In general, more intense regimens cause more treatment-related morbidity and mortality but are associated with a lower relapse rate. Conversely, there are more relapses in RIC HSCT, but the procedure is more tolerable.[1]

ACUTE MYELOID LEUKEMIA

AML displays clinical heterogeneity with markedly variable survival, traditionally defined by prognostic factors of patient age, white blood cell count, prior MDS or cytotoxic therapy, remission status, and karyotype, but increasingly further refined by its molecular heterogeneity. In addition to new prognostic indicators, there are now novel AML therapeutic agents in clinical trials, which also constitute an alternative to conventional cytotoxic chemotherapy and are potentially intercalatable with HSCT.

However, AML also constitutes the leading indication for HSCT worldwide, and accounts for 20,905 of 61,825 allogeneic transplants (34%) in the United States and reported to the Center for International Blood and Marrow Transplant Research (CIBMTR) in the decade 2003–13 (M. Pasquini, personal communication). Moreover, the use of molecular tissue typing in conjunction with better control of treatment-related complications has increased the use of alternative donors. Data from the CIBMTR indicate that 1286 of 1778 allogeneic HSCT (72%) undertaken for AML in 1998 involved related donors, compared with 1223 of 2557 allogeneic HSCT (48%) in 2008. In contrast, the number of unrelated donor HSCT for adult AML increased from 297 in 1998 to 1017 in 2008, while the number of umbilical cord blood (UCB) transplantations increased from 11 to 130 over the same time period.[2] As shown in a recent

analysis from the European Society for Blood and Marrow Transplantation, the ability to use donors that are not histocompatible will further increase the pool of patients in whom HSCT is an effective therapy.[3,4]

Matched Related Donor HSCT for Adult Acute Myeloid Leukemia in First Complete Remission

Currently cytogenetics remains the most powerful prognostic indicator in AML, both at the time of diagnosis and at relapse, and can also direct choice of curative postremission therapy, especially for adult patients less than 60 years of age.[5,6] Adult AML patients can be stratified into good-risk, intermediate-risk, and poor-risk groups on the basis of numeric and/or structural chromosomal abnormalities and the presence of specific mutations (see Chapter 58). Increasingly molecular genotyping supplements, and may ultimately supplant, karyotype-based AML prognostication. For instance, current European LeukemiaNet consensus incorporates molecular mutations to derive AML prognostic risk groups (Table 61.1).[7]

Numerous groups have evaluated prospectively the relative benefits of allogeneic HSCT versus nonallogeneic therapies (consolidation chemotherapy or autologous HSCT) in adult AML patients 18 to 60 years of age in first complete remission (CR1). Treatment allocation was by biologic assignment as a surrogate for true randomization, with allogeneic HSCT for patients with available human leukocyte antigen (HLA)–matched sibling donors (donor group) and nonallogeneic consolidation for those lacking matched sibling donors (no-donor group). Some studies further stratified postremission outcomes by cytogenetic risk. Individual studies, when analyzed on an intent-to-treat (ITT) donor versus no-donor basis, typically demonstrated that allogeneic HSCT was effective at improving disease-free survival, but overall survival benefit was hard to document because of graft-versus-host disease (GVHD) and other treatment-related mortality. Moreover, transplantation in CR2 salvages some of the patients who relapsed, thus making overall survival (OS) similar with the two approaches.

A meta-analysis of over 6000 patients in 24 biologic treatment assignment trials, however, confirmed that OS was in fact better in allogeneic matched related donor transplantation in AML-CR1, with a hazard ratio (HR) of death at 0.90 (95% confidence interval [CI], 0.82 to 0.97).[7] Importantly, when stratified by cytogenetic risk, there was an OS benefit of allogeneic transplantation (Table 61.2) for both intermediate-risk (HR, 0.83; 95% CI, 0.74 to 0.93) and poor-risk (HR, 0.73; 95% CI, 0.59 to 0.90) cytogenetic groups, but not for good-risk AML-CR1 (HR, 1.07; 95% CI, 0.83 to 1.38) (Fig. 61.1). These findings were particularly relevant for patients with normal cytogenetic AML, who constitute the largest subgroup and for whom no consensus regarding optimal postremission treatment was previously available. These studies did not, however, have the benefit of prognostic assignment based on FLT3, NPM1, or other molecular markers.

TABLE 61.1	European LeukemiaNet AML Risk Classification[10]
Genetic Group	**Subsets**
Favorable	t(8;21)(q22;q22); *RUNX1-RUNX1T1*
	inv(16)(p13.1q22) or t(16;16)(p13.1;q22); *CBFB-MYH11*
	Mutated *NPM1* without *FLT3*-ITD (normal karyotype)
	Mutated *CEBPA* (normal karyotype)
Intermediate-I[a]	Mutated *NPM1* and *FLT3*-ITD (normal karyotype)
	Wild-type *NPM1* and *FLT3*-ITD (normal karyotype)
	Wild-type *NPM1* without *FLT3*-ITD (normal karyotype)
Intermediate-II	t(9;11)(p22;q23); *MLLT3-MLL*
	Cytogenetic abnormalities not classified as favorable or adverse[b]
Adverse	inv(3)(q21q26.2) or t(3;3)(q21;q26.2); *RPN1-EVI1*
	t(6;9)(p23;q34); *DEK-NUP214*
	t(v;11)(v;q23); *MLL* rearranged
	−5 or del(5q); −7; abnl(17p); complex karyotype[c]

[a]Includes all AMLs with normal karyotype except for those included in the favorable subgroup; most of these cases are associated with poor prognosis.
[b]For most abnormalities, adequate numbers have not been studied to draw firm conclusions regarding their prognostic significance.
[c]Three or more chromosome abnormalities in the absence of one of the WHO designated recurring translocations or inversions, that is, t(15;17), t(8;21), inv(16) or t(16;16), t(9;11), t(v;11)(v;q23), t(6;9), inv(3) or t(3;3)

Prognostic Factors for Acute Myeloid Leukemia in First Complete Remission

Good-Risk Acute Myeloid Leukemia

In general, the 15% to 20% of AML patients with core binding factor (CBF) leukemia—t(8;21) (q22;q22) and inv(16)(p13.q22)—are considered to have good-risk disease, with a long-term disease-free survival of approximately 50–60% after consolidation chemotherapy, and allogeneic HSCT is not routinely recommended for patients achieving CR1. However, retrospective studies have identified activating mutations in C-KIT *(mKIT)*—a member of the type III receptor tyrosine kinase family—at exon 17 *(mKIT 17)* or exon 8 *(mKIT 8)* in approximately 30% of CBF AMLs that are associated with increased relapse incidence and likely poorer survival, though results from individual studies vary.[8,9] For instance, in an analysis of 61 patients with inv(16), *mKIT* was associated with 5-year relapse rate of 56% compared with 29% ($p = .05$) without *mKIT* mutations. This effect is especially prominent with mKIT17, where 80% relapsed compared with 29% without the mutation ($p = .002$). Similarly, in 49 patients with t(8;21), the 5-year relapse rate was 70% in the presence of *mKIT* mutations compared with 36% with wild-type *mKIT* ($p = .017$). These relapse rates are similar to that of poor-risk AML, suggesting a potential benefit of allogeneic HSCT in this subset. Importantly, relative mutant level (mutant/wild-type allelic ratio [AR]) may also be relevant, with a retrospective analysis of prospective AML trials suggesting the negative prognostic impact of *mKIT* in CBF AML is restricted to cases with AR ≥0.25.[10]

Intermediate-Risk Acute Myeloid Leukemia

The intermediate-risk cytogenetic group is heterogeneous and includes cytogenetically normal disease as well as those with karyotypic abnormalities not meeting criteria for good- or poor-risk AML.

It constitutes the largest risk category, accounting for approximately 40–50% of adult AML patients less than 60 years of age. Long-term disease-free survival of approximately 40–45% is anticipated after consolidation chemotherapy. However, identification of mutations with prognostic importance such as mutant FLT3 internal tandem duplication *(FLT3-ITD)*, nucleophosmin 1 *(NPM1)*, and *CEBPA* (CCAAT/enhancer binding protein-α) can help further individualize the decision regarding allogeneic transplantation.

Patients with *FLT3-ITD* have inferior survivals compared with those without *FLT3-ITD*.[10,11] The negative impact of *FLT3-ITD* appeared abrogated by allogeneic transplantation in CR1 when assessed on an ITT donor versus no-donor basis, although in this analysis the patients were not preferentially assigned transplantation on this basis. In an updated analysis, the *FLT3-ITD* mutant level appeared relevant to AML prognosis and HSCT benefit, with high levels (AR ≥0.51) associated with lower CR rates and poor survival. Importantly, these patients benefit from allogeneic HSCT, while those with low *FLT3-ITD* mutant levels clinically behave similarly to those without *FLT3-ITD*.[12] The *NPM1* and *CEBPA* mutations are associated with good outcomes independent of HSCT, and most investigators do not offer HSCT in first remission.[10,12–14] The favorable impact of *NPM1* mutations appears to persist even in older patients, although this belief is in evolution, and allogeneic HSCT may be a consideration in older AML.[15–17] There is a growing list of additional prognostic markers undergoing evaluation in AML. These include mutation analysis of *RAS, WT1, RUNX1, MLL, TET2, IDH1/2, TP53*; expression levels of individual genes like *EVI1, ERG, MN1*, and *BAALC*; and gene expression and microribonucleic acid (miRNA) profiling.[6,10,16] In a large analysis to develop a prognostic model for AML based solely on molecular markers, Grossmann et al documented five distinct AML prognostic subtypes: (1) very favorable: *PML-RARA* rearrangements or *CEBPA* double mutations (3-year OS: 82.9%); (2) favorable: *RUNX1-RUNX1T1, CBFB-MYH11*, or *NPM1* mutation without *FLT3-ITD* (3-year OS 62.6%); (3) intermediate: none of the mutations leading to assignment in the other groups (3-year OS: 44.2%); (4) unfavorable: *MLL-PTD* and/or *RUNX1* mutation and/or *ASXL1* mutation (3-year OS: 21.9%); and (5) very unfavorable: *TP53* mutation (3-year OS: 0%).[18] If validated, such analyses highlight the ability of molecular markers to further delineate prognosis within AML, especially within intermediate-risk AML. This suggests that this category of risk will gradually disappear as prognostic precision improves. Although the better-prognosis subgroup within intermediate-risk AML may not benefit from early allogeneic transplantation, HSCT appears to be the preferred postremission therapy for intermediate-risk AML patients at higher risk for relapse, including those lacking favorable gene mutations like *NPM1* without *FLT3-ITD*, or double mutant *CEBPA*. With the advent of mutation analysis an interesting question will be whether patients in remission but with detectable clonal hematopoiesis are better served going to HSCT despite the good-risk cytogenetics.

Poor-Risk Acute Myeloid Leukemia

In poor-risk AML relapse rates are high and survival rates are anticipated to be 15% or lower with conventional therapy. Allogeneic HSCT with a matched sibling or unrelated donor results in long-term survival of 30–40% and is considered the treatment of choice for adults less than 60 years of age with poor-risk AML. There is, however, a subgroup of poor-risk AML that may have particularly adverse prognosis, for whom additional novel therapeutic strategies may be necessary.

The monosomal karyotype (MK) is defined by the presence of a single autosomal monosomy, in association with at least one additional monosomy or non–good-risk structural chromosomal abnormality (i.e., excluding CBF mutation AML).[17] In the original report, MK-positive AML patients had a long-term survival of only 3–4%, and these generally dismal chemotherapeutic outcomes have been confirmed by other investigators.[18] Allogeneic transplantation

TABLE 61.2	Allogeneic Transplantation Guidelines for Adult Acute Myeloid Leukemia Based on Commonly Assessed Cytogenetic and Molecular Markers			
AML Category	**Prognostic Impact**	**Allogeneic Transplantation**		**Notes**
AML-CR1: Younger Adults				
Good-risk disease				
APL	Favorable	No		APL is treatable by chemotherapy
CBF-AML *without mKIT*	Favorable	No		t(8;21) AML with high WBC count at diagnosis may have worse prognosis
CBF-AML *with mKIT*	Intermediate	Possible: MRD, MUD Uncertain: MMUD, UCB, haplo		
Intermediate-Risk Disease				
CN-AML *with CEBPA*	Favorable	No		Benefit likely restricted to *DM-CEBPA*
CN-AML *with mutant NPM1 but not FLT-3-ITD*	Favorable	Possible: MRD		Emerging data suggests allogeneic HSCT benefit for this category, with reduced relapse and improved DFS in patients >40 years.
CN-AML *with FLT-3-ITD*	Unfavorable[a]	Yes: MRD, MUD Possible[b]: MMUD, UCB, haplo		Unfavorable risk may be restricted to AML *with FLT-3-ITD allelic ratio >0.51*
Other intermediate-risk disease	Intermediate or Unfavorable	Yes: MRD Likely acceptable[a]: MUD Possible[b]: MMUD, UCB, haplo		Likely considerable underlying clinical heterogeneity. Molecular risk profiling may further delineate risk in this category.
Poor-Risk Disease				
Monosomal karyotype *absent*	Unfavorable	Yes: MRD, MUD Likely acceptable[b]: MMUD, UCB, haplo		
Monosomal karyotype *present*	Very unfavorable	Yes: MRD, MUD. Acceptable[b]: MMUD, UCB, haplo		
Abnormal 17(p)	Very unfavorable	Yes: MRD, MUD Acceptable[b]: MMUD, UCB, haplo		
AML-CR1: older adults	Unfavorable	Yes: MRD, MUD Likely acceptable[b]: MMUD, UCB, haplo		
AML-CR1: t-AML, AML/MDS	Unfavorable	Yes: MRD, MUD Acceptable[b]: MMUD, UCB, haplo		Molecular risk profiling may supersede clinical classification of secondary AML, especially in older patients
AML-CR2	Very unfavorable	Yes: MRD, MUD Acceptable[b]: MMUD, UCB, haplo		
AML not in remission	Very unfavorable	Yes: MRD, MUD Uncertain: MMUD, UCB, haplo		For selected patients: good performance status, little comorbidity, lower leukemic burden; CIBMTR risk score may be useful

[a]If no sibling donor available.
[b]If no timely matched donor available.
AML, Acute myeloid leukemia; APL, acute promyelocytic leukemia; CBF, core binding factor; CIBMTR, Center for International Blood and Marrow Transplant Research; CN, cytogenetically normal; CR1, first complete remission; CR2, second complete remission; haplo, haploidentical; MDS, myelodysplastic syndrome; MMUD, mismatched unrelated donor; MRD, matched related donor; MUD, matched unrelated donor; t-AML, therapy-related AML; UCB, umbilical cord blood; WBC, white blood cell.

appears to only partly ameliorate the impact of MK-positive karyotype, which remained an adverse prognostic factor after HSCT, and was associated with a relapse risk of 62% and poor survival of 15% at 4 years.[19]

Importantly, some if not all of the negative impact of MK and complex karyotype (CK) AML is its association with deletions of chromosome 5 (−5/5q−) and especially with abnormal 17p (site of TP53 gene). In a retrospective analysis of 236 high-risk AML-CR1 patients of whom nearly half (49%) received reduced-intensity allogeneic HSCT, patients with abn(17p) had a 2-year event-free survival (EFS) of 11%, those with −5/5q− but no abn(17p) had a 2-year EFS of 29%, and those with high-risk AML (including MK or CK) without either abn(17p) or −5/5q− had a 2-year EFS of 49%.[20] Further, in updated analyses, the negative impact of abnl(17p) appears minimally improved after allogeneic HSCT.[21,22] Improving HSCT outcomes in TP53 mutant AML must be a high priority for the future.

Transplantation Regimen Intensity

Myeloablative HSCT remains the standard of care for younger adults with AML. However, treatment-related mortality after MAC remains appreciable. Lower-intensity regimens offering less treatment-related toxicity are increasing in popularity. One report retrospectively compared RIC transplantation with chemotherapy in high-risk AML on a donor versus no-donor basis. They identified a leukemia-free survival benefit in the donor group (54% versus 30%, $p = .01$).[23] Several groups have compared MAC versus RIC transplantation, documenting similar overall and leukemia-free survival, with some reporting lower treatment-related mortality offset by increased relapse risk, especially for patients not in complete remission at time of HSCT. A CIBMTR study compared 3731 MAC, 1041 RIC, and 407 nonmyeloablative (NMA) transplantations, reporting adjusted 5-year OSs of 34%, 33%, and 26%, respectively.[24] The authors concluded that, although NMA transplantation increased relapse and

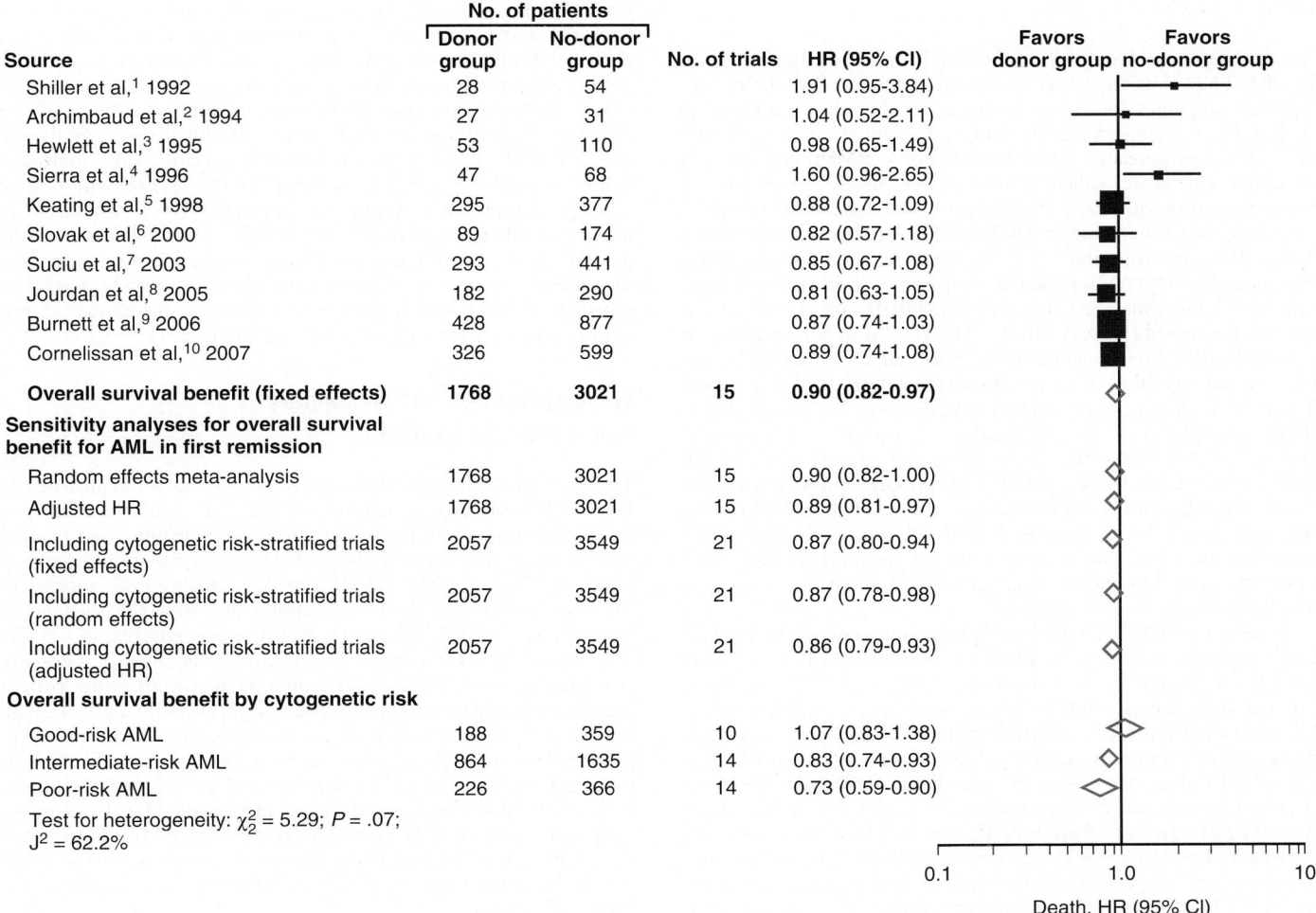

Source	No. of patients		No. of trials	HR (95% CI)	Favors donor group	Favors no-donor group
	Donor group	No-donor group				
Shiller et al,[1] 1992	28	54		1.91 (0.95-3.84)		
Archimbaud et al,[2] 1994	27	31		1.04 (0.52-2.11)		
Hewlett et al,[3] 1995	53	110		0.98 (0.65-1.49)		
Sierra et al,[4] 1996	47	68		1.60 (0.96-2.65)		
Keating et al,[5] 1998	295	377		0.88 (0.72-1.09)		
Slovak et al,[6] 2000	89	174		0.82 (0.57-1.18)		
Suciu et al,[7] 2003	293	441		0.85 (0.67-1.08)		
Jourdan et al,[8] 2005	182	290		0.81 (0.63-1.05)		
Burnett et al,[9] 2006	428	877		0.87 (0.74-1.03)		
Cornelissan et al,[10] 2007	326	599		0.89 (0.74-1.08)		
Overall survival benefit (fixed effects)	**1768**	**3021**	**15**	**0.90 (0.82-0.97)**		
Sensitivity analyses for overall survival benefit for AML in first remission						
Random effects meta-analysis	1768	3021	15	0.90 (0.82-1.00)		
Adjusted HR	1768	3021	15	0.89 (0.81-0.97)		
Including cytogenetic risk-stratified trials (fixed effects)	2057	3549	21	0.87 (0.80-0.94)		
Including cytogenetic risk-stratified trials (random effects)	2057	3549	21	0.87 (0.78-0.98)		
Including cytogenetic risk-stratified trials (adjusted HR)	2057	3549	21	0.86 (0.79-0.93)		
Overall survival benefit by cytogenetic risk						
Good-risk AML	188	359	10	1.07 (0.83-1.38)		
Intermediate-risk AML	864	1635	14	0.83 (0.74-0.93)		
Poor-risk AML	226	366	14	0.73 (0.59-0.90)		

Test for heterogeneity: $\chi^2_2 = 5.29$; $P = .07$; $J^2 = 62.2\%$

Death, HR (95% CI)

Fig. 61.1 META-ANALYSIS OF OVERALL SURVIVAL BENEFIT IN FIRST COMPLETE REMISSION OF ACUTE MYELOID LEUKEMIA FOR YOUNGER ADULTS. *AML*, Acute myeloid leukemia; *CI*, confidence interval; *HR*, hazard ratio. *(Redrawn from Koreth J, Schlenk R, Kopecky KJ, et al: Allogeneic stem cell transplantation for acute myeloid leukemia in first complete remission: Systematic review and meta-analysis of prospective clinical trials, JAMA 301:2349, 2009. Sources cited within Fig. 61.1 can be found following the reference list online at expertconsult.com.)*

impaired survival, RIC and MAC regimens had similar overall and leukemia-free survival. Although a small randomized trial documented similar outcomes of MAC versus RIC transplantation in AML-CR1,[25] a larger prospective randomized trial of MAC versus RIC transplantation in AML or MDS patients (Blood and Marrow Transplantation Clinical Trials Network protocol 0901) closed after accrual of 272 of planned 356 patients because of an increased relapse risk in the RIC arm (http://www.nlm.nih.gov/databases/alerts/2014_nhlbi_bmt_ctn.html). RIC transplantation does, however, offer the option of curative allogeneic HSCT in older or sicker patients with AML-CR for whom the toxicity of MAC transplantation might be prejudicial. Conversely, patients with good performance status but high AML relapse risk might be preferentially selected for MAC.

Alternative Donor Transplantation

HSCT from an HLA-matched sibling donor has been the standard of care for prospective biologic treatment assignment studies evaluating postremission therapies. Patients lacking sibling donors could be considered for alternative donors: unrelated adult donors, UCB, or haploidentical donor transplantation.

Unrelated Adult Donors

Given the very poor outcomes after nonallogeneic therapy in poor-risk AML, and the documented benefit of HLA-matched sibling donor HSCT, clinical practice has been to undertake HLA-matched unrelated donor transplantation for younger adults with poor-risk AML in CR1 who lack sibling donors. A retrospective analysis of HLA-matched sibling compared with unrelated donor HSCT in poor-risk AML-CR1 documented comparable outcomes with HLA-matched siblings and HLA well-matched unrelated donors with 3-year OS of 45% compared with 53% ($p = .63$).[26] Outcomes were not as good for partially HLA-mismatched unrelated donors (one-locus HLA mismatch), with 3-year OS of 31% ($p = .026$). Smaller prospective studies have also shown equivalent results, confirming the suitability of well-matched unrelated donor HSCT in poor-risk AML.[27,28]

There is limited data comparing HLA-matched sibling with unrelated donors in intermediate-risk AML, although at least one study documented similar outcomes with either donor type.[29] Current practice is to offer HLA-matched unrelated donor HSCT to intermediate-risk AML patients in first remission, especially if there are adverse molecular lesions.

Umbilical Cord Blood

Another important issue is the use of UCB transplantation for AML in CR1. These data are harder to interpret because most studies have reported outcomes for "acute leukemia," rather than restricted to AML-CR1. A European registry study documented similar outcomes of UCB versus unrelated donor bone marrow (BM) transplantation in adults with acute leukemia, whereas a CIBMTR study showed better outcomes with HLA-matched unrelated donor BM transplantation but similar outcomes of UCB and HLA-mismatched unrelated donor BM transplantation.[30,31] A large analysis of adult acute leukemia (including 880 AML patients) compared the outcomes of single-unit 4–6/6 HLA-matched (HLA-A, -B, -DRB1) UCB with 8/8 or 7/8 HLA-matched (HLA-A, -B, -C, -DRB1) BM or peripheral blood stem cell (PBSC) transplantation and documented similar leukemia-free survival regardless of stem cell source or degree of HLA match. There was higher treatment-related mortality after UCB transplantation.[32] Transplantation in CR1 resulted in similar 2-year leukemia-free survivals of 44%, 50%, 52%, 39%, and 41% with UCB, 8/8 PBSC, 8/8 BM, 7/8 PBSC, and 7/8 BM transplantation, respectively. In contrast, a Japanese study evaluated outcomes of 484 AML patients receiving 4–6/6 UCB compared with 8/8 unrelated donor BM transplantation and documented a similar relapse risk with UCB transplantation, but higher treatment-related mortality and worse overall and leukemia-free survival.[33]

Double-unit UCB (DUCB) transplantation is commonly used for larger patients. Indeed, since 2005 the number of adults receiving DUCB has exceeded those receiving single-unit UCB products. Limited data suggest similar outcomes of myeloablative DUCB, HLA-matched unrelated, and sibling donor HSCT in hematologic malignancies.[34] However, only a subset of patients had AML. The role of DUCB in AML remains to be better delineated. Reducing treatment toxicity will be important to advance UCB transplantation. A recent phase trial of 79 adult AML cord recipients (60% DUCB), identified a low 2-year NRM incidence of 20%, suggestive of progress in this metric.[35] In general however, current clinical practice envisages use of UCB transplantation in younger adults with high-risk AML in CR1 who lack suitable HLA-matched donors.

Haploidentical Donors

There is insufficient data on haploidentical transplantation to allow a precise recommendation for patients with AML. Several strategies have been used in high-risk patients, and the outcomes are encouraging.[3,36–38] Haploidentical transplantation is particularly interesting given the potential enhancement of GVL activity by natural killer cells and allogeneic T cells responding to the HLA disparity. Regimens incorporating posttransplantation cyclophosphamide for the prevention of GVHD after haploidentical transplantation have gained increasing prominence, with low rates of treatment-related mortality and GVHD.[39–41] For AML/MDS, a retrospective analysis found no significant differences between outcomes of matched unrelated ($n = 108$) and haploidentical ($n = 32$) donor HSCT with posttransplantation cyclophosphamide.[42]

Relapsed, Refractory, and Induction-Failure Acute Myeloid Leukemia

Outcomes are typically poor for AML patients not in remission at the time of allogeneic HSCT, although the literature in this regard is limited, heterogeneous, and likely subject to patient selection and publication bias. A large analysis of MAC HSCT for acute leukemia in relapse or in primary induction failure (including 1673 AML patients) documented a 3-year OS of 19% in AML.[43] On multivariable analysis, risk factors at time of HSCT of poor-risk cytogenetic AML, CR1 duration of less than 6 months, circulating AML blasts, performance score of less than 90%, and lack of an HLA-matched

sibling donor predicted for 3-year survival ranging between 42% (zero risk factors) and 6% (three or more risk factors). The major cause of death remains AML relapse, and innovative strategies to reduce leukemic burden before transplantation and enhance GVL effect after transplantation are required to improve survival of this extremely high-risk patient population.[44] In this patient population, the ability of novel agents for targeting specific AML molecular lesions or pathways (e.g., *FLT3-ITD, IDH 1/2, mTOR*) with limited off-target toxicity, as a bridge to allogeneic HSCT, would be an important albeit putative clinical benefit. The ability to rapidly proceed to allogeneic transplantation may also be important given the dismal outcome of chemotherapy alone, suggesting a role for expeditious UCB and haploidentical BM transplantation in this setting, especially for patients achieving a remission.

Therapy-Related and Secondary Acute Myeloid Leukemia

Therapy-related AML (t-AML) currently accounts for approximately 10% to 20% of newly diagnosed AML, and its incidence is likely to rise in the future given increasing cancer survivorship. Postremission therapy using conventional chemotherapy is usually not curative in secondary AML (s-AML: t-AML and AML arising from antecedent MDS or MPD) with the rare exception of CBF-AML, specifically inv(16) and t(15;17). Allogeneic HSCT is less effective in s-AML. The poorer survival appears multifactorial, because of poor-risk cytogenetics, lower likelihood of entering remission, older patient age, and impaired organ function from prior cancer therapy; although some reports documented similar posttransplantation survival compared with de-novo AML when adjusted for risk factors like disease status and cytogenetics.[2,45] An observational analysis of 545 patients with t-AML identified four risk factors influencing HSCT outcomes: age greater than 35 years, poor-risk cytogenetics, AML not in remission, and lack of well-matched donors. A prognostic score could stratify outcomes from 5-year OSs of 50% (zero risk factors) to 4% (four risk factors).[46]

Molecular genotyping offers insights into the clinical heterogeneity of s-AML. In a seminal analysis, Lindsley et al identified eight genes specifically mutated in s-AML (*SRSF2, SF3B1, U2AF1, ZRSR2, SXL1, EZH2, BCOR, STAG2*) that also identify worse prognosis in "de-novo" elderly patients with AML, likely indicating undiagnosed antecedent MDS. They also identified a molecular signature of "de-novo" type AML. Finally, they confirmed that patients with *TP53* mutations comprised a distinct set of AML with the worst outcomes. Molecular risk stratification offers the potential to redefine the clinical diagnosis of s-AML, refine AML risk prognostication, and potentially, better select remission-inducing and postremission therapy.[47]

Acute Myeloid Leukemia in Older Adults

AML incidence rises with age, with a median age at diagnosis of 67 years (Surveillance, Epidemiology and End Results data: http://seer.cancer.gov/). For AML patients older than 60 years, consolidation chemotherapy is unlikely to be curative (Fig. 61.2). Even after adjusting for increased incidence of poor prognosis features like adverse cytogenetic and molecular markers, secondary AML, comorbidities, and poorer performance status, older age remains an independent predictor of poor survival with conventional chemotherapy. A priori, age-related clonal hematopoiesis may be a relevant variable for impaired survival, though this remains to be confirmed.[48,49] Although allogeneic HSCT is a curative therapy in the older age-group, there is considerable reluctance to refer these patients for transplantation, in contrast to younger adults with AML, in part because of outdated assumptions regarding the tolerability of allogeneic transplantation, but also because of lack of comparative data regarding outcomes.

Several reports have documented the feasibility of RIC transplantation with acceptable toxicity and reasonable survival in patients

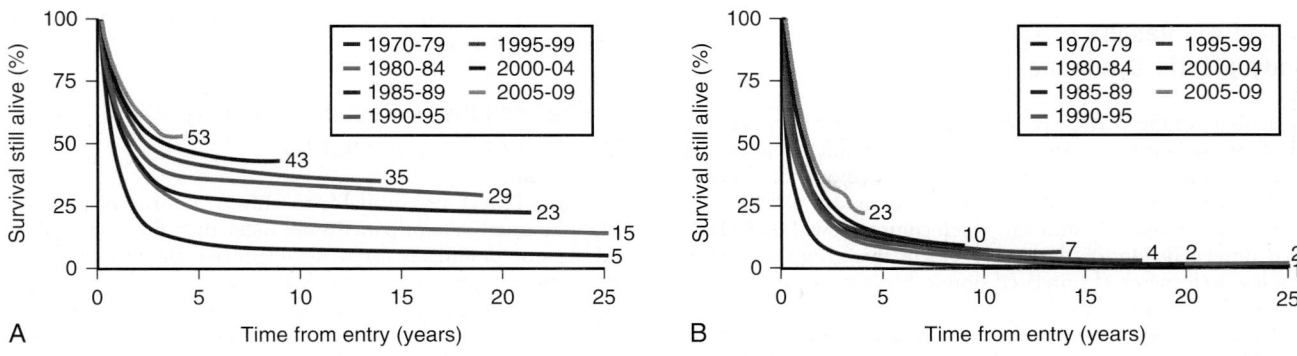

Fig. 61.2 CHANGE IN ACUTE MYELOID LEUKEMIA OVERALL SURVIVAL WITH TIME. (A) Age 15 to 59 years. (B) Age 60 years or greater. (*Data from Burnett A, Wetzler M, Lowenberg B: Therapeutic advances in acute myeloid leukemia, J Clin Oncol 29:487, 2011.*)

60 years of age and above, including those with AML. Indeed, chronologic age alone does not appear to be a prognostic factor in RIC allogeneic transplantation for AML.[50,51] In a case-control study comparing RIC transplantation with chemotherapy for AML patients 60 to 70 years of age, allogeneic HSCT was associated with lower relapse risk (32% versus 81%, *p* < .001), greater treatment-related mortality (36% versus 4%; *p* < .001), and longer 3-year leukemia-free survival (32% versus 15%, *p* = .001), with a borderline 3-year OS benefit (37% versus 25%, *p* = .08).[52]

Overall, for physically fit older patients with AML, especially those between 60 and 70 years of age, a donor search should be undertaken promptly at diagnosis, disease control with intensive induction chemotherapy is beneficial, and they should be considered for potentially curative allogeneic transplantation upon entering complete remission. Broadly speaking, molecular and karyotypic AML risk prognostication also applies to older patients being considered for RIC HSCT, with several caveats. First, favorable risk (e.g., CBF-AML) disease retains a relatively favorable impact in older patients, though it is unknown if data indicating equivalent outcomes of nontransplantation and allogeneic HSCT treatment can be extrapolated to the older patient. Emerging data suggests that allogeneic HSCT offers additional benefit in the older patient with favorable risk disease. For instance, in the UK National Cancer Research Institute (NCRI) AML trial of 16 patients with median age >65 years, *NPM1* mutant *FLT3-ITD* negative AML treated patients with intensive chemotherapy had a 3-year OS of only 26%, with a relapse incidence of 73%.[53] Additionally, in a combined SWOG/NCRI cohort, patients with *NPM1* mutant *FLT3-ITD* negative AML who were aged 55–65 years had a significantly improved 2-year OS of 70% versus 27% for those aged >65 years (*p* < .001). The survival benefit of *NPM1* mutant *FLT3-ITD* negative AML was absent in patients aged >65 years.[54] Importantly, in a separate donor versus no-donor analysis, *NPM1* mutant AML patients with an allogeneic donor had significantly lower 3-year relapse rates (14% versus 46%) and improved relapse-free survival (71% versus 47%), indicating a beneficial antileukemic effect of allogeneic HSCT in this AML subgroup.[55] Secondly, MK and *TP53* mutant AML have an extremely poor prognosis,[21,22,56] and the adequacy of RIC HSCT is questionable in this AML subgroup. Such patients should be appropriately counseled prior to proceeding with allogeneic HSCT, with consideration to conditioning intensity escalation if possible. Novel clinical trials are a priority for this AML subgroup.

Relapse After Transplantation

AML relapse after allogeneic transplantation is common, has a very poor prognosis, and remains a leading cause of death in this disease. Early identification of HSCT recipients at risk of disease relapse is therefore of considerable importance. While falling donor chimerism after HSCT can identify cohorts at higher relapse risk,[57,58] more

specific detection of minimal residual disease in the HSCT context has included multi-parameter flow cytometry and molecular markers (e.g., AML-specific translocations or mutations).[59,60]

Importantly, the identification of patients at high risk of relapse after allogeneic HSCT offers the opportunity for targeted early intervention. For instance, early phase trials of hypomethylating agents for MDS/AML (e.g., azacytidine), and targeting of *FLT3-ITD* AML (e.g., sorafenib) have been reported, with early evidence indicating safety and possible efficacy.[61,62] Future prospective trials focused on those at high relapse risk (e.g., MRD or chimerism-based selection) offers an informative population for evaluation of intervention efficacy, and is a high priority for improving AML outcomes.

The treatment options for patients with disease relapse after HSCT include withdrawal of immune suppression, donor lymphocyte infusion (DLI), chemotherapy (including novel agents), second allogeneic transplantation, or supportive care.[63] Tapering of immune suppression and DLI are used especially in patients without GVHD to enhance antileukemic graft versus leukemia (GVL) effect. DLI has limited efficacy, in the range of 15% to 30%, for patients with relapsed AML, and many responses are incomplete or temporary. Outcomes are better in patients who relapsed beyond 6 months after HSCT, those with lower leukemic burden (less than 35% BM blasts), patients with good-risk cytogenetics, and those who achieved remission before DLI.[64] Novel options to enhance curative GVL effect include infusion of donor lymphocyte subpopulations (e.g., CD25-depleted DLI, enriched for T effector cells), and immune checkpoint inhibitors (e.g., *CTLA-4* blockade).[65,66] A second allogeneic HSCT has demonstrable but limited efficacy, and duration of remission of more than a year after initial HSCT is the major predictor of survival.[67]

TRANSPLANTATION FOR MYELODYSPLASTIC SYNDROME

The MDSs comprise a heterogeneous group of clonal hematologic stem cell disorders characterized by varying degrees of cytopenias and risk for transformation into acute leukemia[68] (see Chapter 60). The incidence and prevalence of MDS has increased significantly over the last 20 years as a result of increasing longevity of the population and increasing physician awareness.[69–71] New therapeutic options such as hypomethylating agents, immunomodulatory drugs, and differentiation induction agents may improve hematologic parameters and reduce transfusion requirements,[72] and even prolong survival,[73] but allogeneic HSCT is the only known curative therapeutic option.

MDS is currently the third most common indication for allogeneic HSCT as reported to the CIBMTR. MDS is a disease predominantly of older individuals, and with the increased use and acceptance of RIC into the eighth decade of life, it is anticipated that transplantation volume for MDS will continue to increase in the coming years.

Contemporary Results of Transplantation for Myelodysplastic Syndrome

Recent analyses of the CIBMTR have suggested improving outcomes for MDS transplantation. An analysis of 701 adult subjects that received a transplant between 2002 and 2006 demonstrated nearly 50% OS when a matched sibling donor was used.[74] While these results were not statistically different when compared with 8/8 HLA-matched unrelated donors, the 3-year OS in this group was 38%. Using a less well matched unrelated donor, however, was associated with poorer long term survival.

It is becoming increasingly evident that allogeneic transplantation offers a survival advantage over conventional therapies in MDS. One prospective trial that assigned subjects in a donor vs. no donor analysis demonstrated a survival advantage in the donor arm over those without a donor. Importantly, in this analysis, there did not appear to be a decrement in early survival in the donor arm, suggesting that early transplant-related mortality after transplantation is comparable to mortality associated with nontransplant therapies in a high-risk subject cohort. To confirm these findings, two additional large prospective biologic assignment trials have been initiated in Europe and North America.

Clinical Results in Myeloablative Transplantation

There are few reports of transplantation uniquely for patients with the myelodysplastic disorders, because most reports include both patients with AML and those with MDS. Those few analyses that do exist unfortunately often present biased results, because there is inherent patient selection in the reported studies. The bias in these analyses, although recognized by physicians and patients alike, is often overlooked, because patients who choose early HSCT often identify with those included in the analysis to justify their decision.

One of the largest reports of MAC HSCT for MDS is from the Seattle group. Using a targeted busulfan strategy in patients undergoing related or unrelated donor HSCT, results were stratified by pretransplant International Prognostic Scoring System (IPSS; see Chapter 60) risk score.[75,76] Patients were prospectively enrolled in the targeted busulfan treatment program; however, the decision to undergo transplantation was based upon physician and patient preference. Results in this study were correlated with IPSS stage, suggesting that outcomes were improved with HSCT at an earlier disease stage. This would be expected because patients with earlier-stage disease have received less treatment (thus less comorbidity) and may also have more indolent disease biology. Among the patients in the lowest IPSS score group there were no relapses, whereas the relapse rate was 42% for patients in the highest IPSS category. As a consequence, 3-year survival was 80% in the lowest IPSS risk group but was under 30% for patients in the high IPSS category. Mutation analysis will need to be incorporated into prognostic systems as we go forward.

Similarly, de Witte et al[77] examined outcomes of HSCT for patients with earlier-stage MDS (refractory anemia or refractory anemia and ringed sideroblasts). This analysis studied 374 patients who underwent HSCT from either matched, sibling, or unrelated donors. Both standard MAC and RIC regimens were used. IPSS score could be calculated in fewer than half of the patients, and HSCTs were performed over a decade-long period, such that inherent differences in transplantation technology resulted in improved overall survival over time. Although factors such as conditioning intensity, stem cell source, and donor status did not affect outcome, recipient age and duration of identified MDS diagnosis were important predictors of overall survival. Earlier transplantation was associated with an absolute increase in overall survival of 10% at 4 years (57% versus 47%, $p = .02$) and was associated with improved relapse-free survival in multivariable analysis. Despite the finding of improved outcome with earlier HSCT, this should not be interpreted as a recommendation for early HSCT in individuals with low-risk MDS, because the authors did not compare outcomes to a cohort of patients treated with supportive care alone.

Clinical Results in Reduced-Intensity Conditioning Transplantation

Previously HSCT was available to only a minority of patients with MDS, because 75% of patients are older than 60 years at diagnosis and are not candidates for MAC regimens. Because older patients have a poorer prognosis than their younger counterparts, there is a great impetus to develop strategies for older individuals. Within the RIC literature, there is great variability in the reported conditioning intensity; however, the commonality of these regimens is that they can be safely offered to patients previously deemed too old or to have too much comorbidity for high-dose therapy. It appears that late relapses after MAC HSCT are not common,[78] but high-intensity regimens are associated with higher treatment-related mortality.[79] This further justified the shift towards reduced intensity conditioning.

The City of Hope group reported on their outcomes using a RIC regimen of fludarabine and melphalan in 43 patients with MDS or AML. OS was 53% at 2 years, with a 16% relapse rate.[80] Treating over 90 patients with AML ($n = 74$) or AML ($n = 22$) using a targeted busulfan and fludarabine regimen, de Lima et al[81] reported 1-year treatment-related mortality of only 3%, without a compromise in antitumor activity. Using the more commonly applied RIC regimen of fludarabine with busulfan, albeit with different intensities (and including some patients with AML), other groups have demonstrated similar outcomes, with treatment-related mortality of 13–27%, relapse rates of 23–32%, disease-free survival of 38–68%, and OS of 39–79%.[82–85]

Comparative Results: Myeloablative and Reduced-Intensity Regimens in Myelodysplastic Syndrome

Several analyses have compared RIC with conventional MAC transplantation, and the majority of them suggest similar outcomes. The premise behind all of these comparisons is that RIC should be associated with a reduction in early treatment-related mortality, whereas MAC approaches should be associated with a reduction in disease relapse. The net effect of these two opposing risks is no difference in outcomes. For example, at the Dana-Farber Cancer Institute, the outcomes of 136 patients with advanced MDS or acute myelogenous leukemia who underwent transplantation were compared when stratified by conditioning regimen intensity.[1] OS at 2 years was the same following RIC as for MAC transplantation (28% versus 34%, $p = .89$); however, the causes of treatment failure were significantly different, with more relapse in the RIC group (61% versus 38%, $p = .02$), but higher treatment-related mortality in the MAC group (32% versus 15% at 100 days) as anticipated. Overall treatment-related mortality, however, was no different ($p = .28$). In this report, patients were treated according to patient and physician preference, whereas in a similar single-center analysis reported by Martino et al,[86] patients were prospectively assigned to RIC or CD34+ selected MAC transplantation based on patient age. In this analysis, nonrelapse mortality and OS were no different between groups.

Similar to single-center studies, large retrospective database studies comparing RIC and high-intensity HSCT have been performed. A CIBMTR review of the outcomes of 550 patients 50 years of age or older who underwent matched sibling donor HSCT showed no difference in MAC and RIC outcomes. In an even larger CIBMTR analysis that included both patients with MDS and those with AML, patients were stratified into MAC, RIC, and truly NMA subgroups. Although results for MDS alone are not available, overall outcomes indicated less-favorable long-term results for NMA regimens when compared with higher-intensity regimens.[24] In an analysis by the European Group for Blood and Marrow Transplantation (EBMT) of over 800 patients with MDS, the 3-year relapse rate was significantly

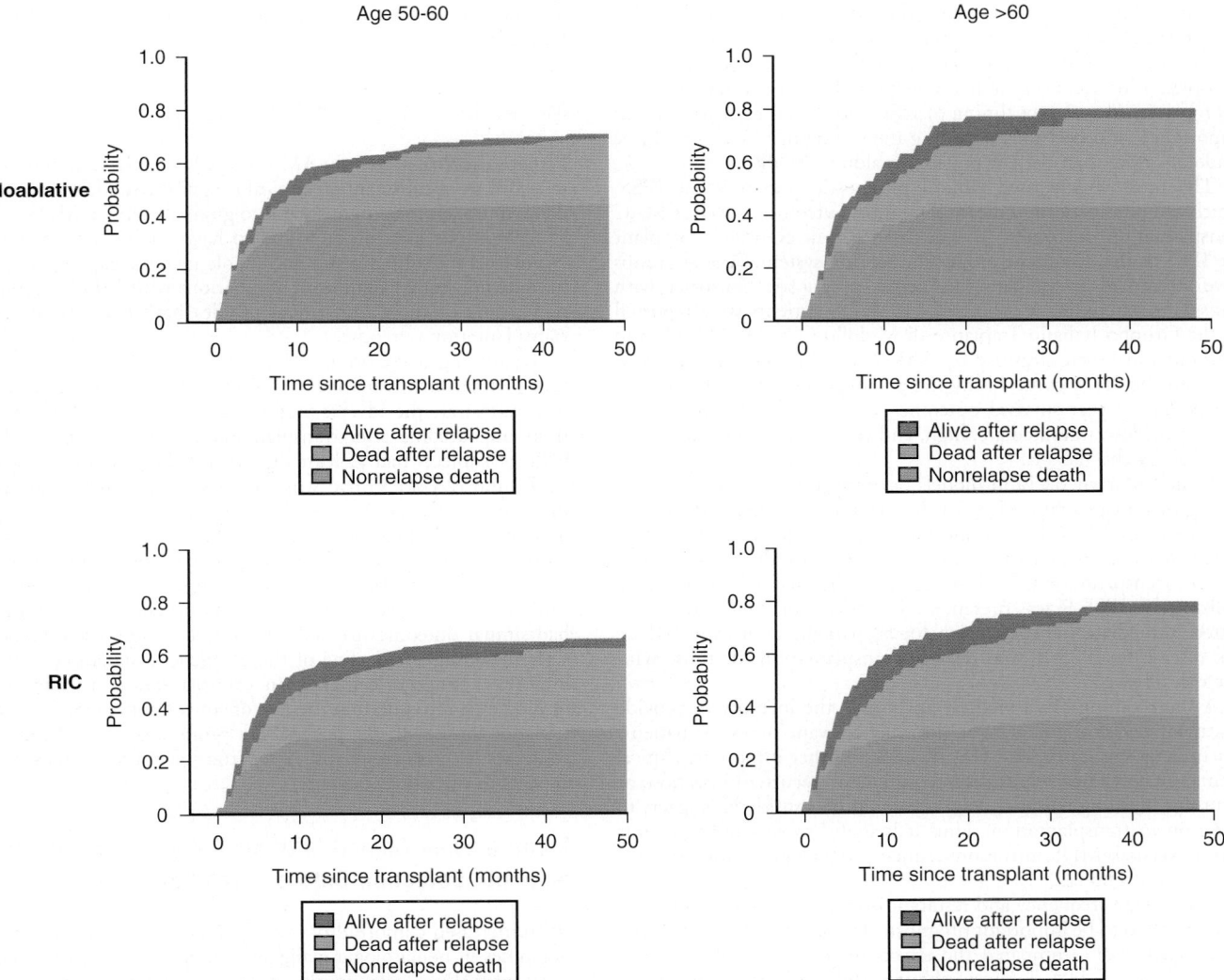

Fig. 61.3 COMPETING RISK CUMULATIVE INCIDENCES FOR RELAPSE AND NONRELAPSE MORTALITY AMONG INDIVIDUALS ABOVE AGE 50 YEARS. *RIC,* Reduced-intensity conditioning. *(Data from Lim Z, Brand R, Martino R, et al: Allogeneic hematopoietic stem-cell transplantation for patients 50 years or older with myelodysplastic syndromes or secondary acute myeloid leukemia,* J Clin Oncol *28:405, 2010.)*

higher after RIC (HR, 1.64; $p = .001$), but with less treatment-related mortality (HR, 0.61; $p = .015$), leading to similar 3-year OS (45% versus 41%, $p = .8$). When limited to individuals above 50 years of age, no difference in outcome stratified by conditioning intensity (32% versus 30%, $p = .73$) was noted.[87] Competing risk cumulative incidences for relapse and nonrelapse mortality are shown in Fig. 61.3.

It is important to consider that none of these retrospective studies adjusted for comorbidity, and it is almost certain that if reanalyzed, the RIC cohorts would contain a higher proportion of patients with more comorbid conditions. Because only a minority of studies suggested that regimen intensity is important for long-term outcomes, some patients, including those without significant comorbidity, have now opted for earlier RIC transplantation, because treatment-related morbidity and mortality after this procedure is lower than after traditional MAC transplantation. In order to compare outcomes prospectively among patients eligible to undergo both MAC and RIC transplantation, the Bone Marrow Transplant Clinical Trials Network initiated a randomized, controlled trial in patients 18 to 65 years of age. This trial was closed prior to completion of accrual because of better outcomes in the myeloablative cohort; however, the results for patients with MDS have not been released at the time of this publication.

A second prospective randomized trial was recently reported by the EBMT. The RIC-MAC trial randomized 129 subjects up to age 65 (60 with an unrelated donor) to either an ablative or reduced-intensity busulfan regimen. There were no statistical differences in nonrelapse mortality, relapse or disease-free survival, but in multivariable regression modeling, there was a survival advantage for subjects who received reduced-intensity conditioning.[88]

Using Prognostic Models to Define the Role and Timing of Transplantation

Clinical, Laboratory, and Cytogenetic Prognostic Factors

Comparative registry analyses have documented the benefit of HSCT over conventional supportive and disease-modifying agents in MDS[89]; however, this should not be interpreted as an indication for HSCT in all patients. Despite the curative potential of HSCT, transplantation carries substantial risk for early morbidity and mortality, and careful consideration must be made regarding the appropriateness of each potential recipient and the timing at which transplantation is offered. Despite this, all patients who are potential candidates for HSCT should be referred to a transplantation center early in their disease course so that a discussion regarding the appropriateness of transplantation can occur and a donor search can be initiated, where appropriate. The correct timing of HSCT is therefore of paramount importance, and decisions regarding the timing of HSCT should be made on more than patient preference alone.

The most widely used clinical prognostic system is the IPSS, which can predict both nontransplantation outcomes as well as MAC transplantation outcomes.[90,91] The IPSS-R will eventually supplant the IPSS as the dominant prognostic scoring system. Several groups have attempted to validate this newer prognostic construct with transplant outcomes. A cohort of 519 MDS patients were reported by the Gruppo Italiano Trapianto di Midollo Osseo (GITMO) and their outcomes were stratified by IPSS-R. In addition to the IPSS-R, MK and the HCT comorbidity index independently predicted outcomes. The 5-year survival outcomes were 71%, 58%, 39%, and 23% in the low, intermediate, high, and very high risk patients when classified by the IPSS-R.[92]

Several Markov decision models have suggested that the optimal timing of transplantation is with the diagnosis of Intermediate-2 or higher disease,[90,93] although one more heterogeneous analyses suggested that even patients with Intermediate-1 risk disease should be offered transplantation.[94] Most recently, the first decision model utilizing the IPSS-R was presented. The results of this analysis suggested immediate transplantation for all patients with Intermediate risk disease by IPSS-R, and delayed transplantation for those with low risk disease.[95]

A shortcoming of all of these analyses is the inability to provide treatment decision guidance at clinically relevant times for patients not undergoing immediate HSCT, because other important clinical events, such as a new transfusion requirement, recurrent infection, or recurrent bleeding episodes certainly could be considered triggers to move on to transplantation. Thus it is useful to subdivide patients with lower-risk MDS into more-refined prognostic groups that may benefit from HSCT.

Transfusion frequency and resultant iron overload have both been demonstrated to be important prognostic factors in HSCT outcomes. Platzbecker et al[66] compared the effects of transfusion dependency at the time of HSCT. Even though the transfusion-dependent group had more low-risk features, OS was inferior, with a 3-year OS of 49% compared with 60% in the transfusion-independent group ($p = 0.1$). The Pavia group examined a cohort of patients stratified by IPSS to determine the relevance of the newer World Health Organization (WHO) histologic classification scheme and to determine if transfusion requirement influenced outcomes among different IPSS groups. For patients with low- and intermediate-1 risk IPSS scores, the WHO histologic classification scheme significantly differentiated survival among the different histologic subtypes within each IPSS range.[67] More importantly, the authors demonstrated a significant effect on survival based on the requirement for transfusion support. As would be expected, outcomes in patients with higher-grade myelodysplasia were affected less by transfusion requirement than were patients with less-advanced WHO histologic classifications. As a result, the impact of transfusion requirement was then incorporated into the WHO Prognostic Scoring System (WPSS).[96] In this system, the effect of regular transfusion requirement (defined as requiring at least one transfusion every 8 weeks in a 4-month period) was given the same regression weight as progressing between cytogenetic risk groups. In contrast to the initial IPSS publication, which carries prognostic information only at the time of initial MDS diagnosis, this model was time dependent, such that patients could be continually reevaluated by the scoring model and updated prognostic information could be generated at any time in the patient's treatment course. As such, the development of new cytogenetic changes or the development of a transfusion need adds useful information that helps guide treatment decisions, including the decision to proceed to HSCT as well as estimating transplantation outcomes.[97] Determining at which WPSS stage transplantation outcomes are superior to nontransplantation therapy has yet to be determined, although this prognostic scoring system is used less frequently.

Molecular Prognostic Factors

Perhaps even more than in AML, mutation analysis undoubtedly led to a shift from rudimentary clinical prognostic models to molecularly defined models for prognosis and to guide therapy in MDS. As many as 75% of patients can be found to have one or more mutations.[98] Numerous individual genes and whole genome expression profiling have demonstrated significant associations with MDS outcome, and now, some of these mutational profiles have been associated with transplantation outcome.

Examining a cohort of 87 patients who underwent allogeneic transplantation at Dana-Farber Cancer Institute, Bejar et al were able to demonstrate the adverse prognostic impact of three specific mutations on outcome after transplantation.[99] In this cohort, although 92% of subjects had at least one identifiable mutation, those with *TET2* and *DNMT3A* had worse prognoses that those without these mutations, whereas those with mutations in *TP53* had the worst outcomes, with no subjects surviving beyond 2 years after transplantation. Mutations in *TP53* were extremely powerful predictors of relapse, and were better prognosticators than cytogenetic status; subjects with complex karyotypes in the absence of *TP53* mutations had similar outcomes to subjects without complex karyotypes, possibly heralding the decline of the cytogenetic signature as the most important prognostic marker in transplantation. In addition, this finding calls into question the role of conventional HSCT off clinical trials for those with the poorest risk profiles, since in the absence of strategies to reduce relapse after transplantation, transplantation appears to offer little benefit.

Incorporating Comorbidity for Patient and Conditioning Intensity Selection Before Transplantation

With increased comorbidity comes an increase in the rate of adverse outcomes in hematologic malignancies, and, in particular, the treatment of MDS.[100] Previously, it was demonstrated that age alone cannot be used as a surrogate for comorbidity, as demonstrated by an analysis of over 500 individuals with MDS who underwent a first RIC transplantation.[101] Several comorbidity scores have been developed to help provide prognostic information in myeloid malignancies. In MDS, the Hematopoietic Cell Transplantation Comorbidity Index, developed by Sorror and colleagues,[102,103] has been shown to carry prognostic value, even in patients with MDS not undergoing transplantation.[104] The consideration of comorbidity before HSCT is even more relevant now that RIC has been shown to be effective in the treatment of MDS, and patients can elect to undergo RIC transplantation. Patients were divided into four separate groups, with each group being defined on the basis of comorbidity and malignant disease risk. Within each of the four risk groups, patients who underwent MAC and RIC were compared with each other. As expected in each of the four groups, the RIC arm experienced higher relapse rates but lower treatment-related mortality rates when compared with the MAC arm. As a result, disease-free and overall survival was similar between conditioning arms in all four groups.[103] More recently, an enhanced index that incorporates both age and clinical comorbidity was developed and demonstrated even more prognostic power than either of the components alone. In this scoring system those with the highest age-adjusted comorbidity scores have nonrelapse mortality that might exceed 50% at 5 years, with concomitant survival that is less than 20%.[105] Transplantation for this group of individuals should be seriously considered outside the spectrum of routine practice.

The effects of elevated ferritin levels on HSCT until recently have been largely limited to patients undergoing MAC transplantation.[5] We previously reported that an elevated pre-HSCT serum ferritin level was strongly associated with lower overall and disease-free survival in patients with AML and MDS after transplantation, and this was largely attributable to increased treatment-related mortality.[5] Similarly, a prospective single-institution study of 190 adult patients undergoing MAC HSCT demonstrated that elevated pretransplantation serum ferritin level was associated with increased risk for 100-day mortality, acute GVHD, and bloodstream infections or death as a composite endpoint.[106] It has now been recognized that elevated ferritin level can predict inferior outcomes even after RIC transplantation.[87] As a laboratory prognostic factor, ferritin should be considered a marker of comorbidity, because ferritin is a marker of inflammation. As such, ferritin levels could influence the decision to pursue high-intensity or reduced-intensity HSCT. Optimally, if high-intensity HSCT is planned, proceeding before the accumulation of a critical amount of iron should be pursued, or, alternatively, chelation therapy before HSCT can be considered, although this latter approach has not yet been demonstrated to be effective in prospective clinical trials.

Pretransplantation Therapy

The role of cytoreductive chemotherapy before HSCT for MDS remains controversial. Many analyses have demonstrated that outcomes are improved with lower disease burden at the time of HSCT,[107] but previously only conventional chemotherapy was offered. The analyses that compare chemotherapy to no chemotherapy before HSCT are inherently biased, because patients who do poorly or expire with chemotherapy are not included in HSCT outcome data and might have had favorable outcomes if not exposed to cytotoxic agents. On the other hand, responsiveness to chemotherapy may indicate more favorable disease biology and this has been correlated with improved outcomes after HSCT.[108]

With the advent of DNA hypomethylating therapy, the use of conventional chemotherapy has diminished for MDS patients. The effect of DNA hypomethylating therapy on HSCT outcomes has recently been studied by several groups.[94-96] Compared retrospectively, it does not appear that pretransplantation hypomethylating therapy offers a survival advantage,[109] but these agents continue to be used widely to prevent disease progression and to reduce transfusion needs while donor selection is performed in patients destined to undergo transplantation. Two recent analyses have compared the use of traditional chemotherapy with hypomethylating therapy prior to transplantation. In the smaller of the two analyses, there was no advantage to hypomethylating therapy over conventional chemotherapy,[110] while in the larger of the two, the use of both chemotherapy and hypomethylating therapy prior to transplantation was associated with adverse outcomes, presumably on the basis of identifying subjects with more aggressive disease biology.[111] Only a prospective randomized trial with survival measured from the time of randomization to pretransplant therapy can rationally answer the question as to the most appropriate pretransplant therapy.

There may be some advantage to the use of these agents before HSCT, because DNA hypomethylating therapy has been shown to upregulate the expression of cancer-testis antigens,[112,113] killer immunoglobulin-like receptor (KIR) ligands,[114] HLA molecules,[115] and other minor antigens on tumor cells,[116] all of which may enhance graft-versus-MDS effects. Hypomethylating agents have been used after transplantation to reduce the risk for relapse,[62] but more studies will need to be undertaken before this type of therapy can be routinely recommended.

FUTURE DIRECTIONS

Despite the progress that has been made in conventional therapy for both AML and MDS, allogeneic HSCT has the best track record for curing the disease. Although HSCT has limitations, reductions in toxicity, improvements in donor availability, and new strategies to enhance GVL while limiting GVHD promise to further improve survival. Advances in mutation analysis provide insights into the pathophysiology of MDS and AML and suggest routes for targeted therapy. However, in many circumstances targeted therapy may not be feasible, and thus the utility of molecular prognostic indicators is to identify patients who will benefit from early transplantation.

REFERENCES

For the complete list of references, log on to www.expertconsult.com.

SUGGESTED READINGS

Alessandrino EP, Della Porta MG, Bacigalupo A, et al: WHO classification and WPSS predict posttransplantation outcome in patients with myelodysplastic syndrome: a study from the Gruppo Italiano Trapianto di Midollo Osseo (GITMO). *Blood* 112:895, 2008.

Bornhauser M, Kienast J, Trenschel R, et al: Reduced-intensity conditioning versus standard conditioning before allogeneic haemopoietic cell transplantation in patients with acute myeloid leukaemia in first complete remission: a prospective, open-label randomised phase 3 trial. *Lancet Oncol* 13:1035, 2012.

Brunstein CG, Fuchs EJ, Carter SL, et al: Alternative donor transplantation: results of parallel phase II trials using HLA-mismatched related bone marrow or unrelated umbilical cord blood grafts. *Blood* 118:282, 2011.

Burnett A, Wetzler M, Lowenberg B: Therapeutic advances in acute myeloid leukemia. *J Clin Oncol* 29:487, 2011.

Cutler CS, Lee SJ, Greenberg P, et al: A decision analysis of allogeneic bone marrow transplantation for the myelodysplastic syndromes: delayed transplantation for low-risk myelodysplasia is associated with improved outcome. *Blood* 104:579, 2004.

Dohner H, Estey EH, Amadori S, et al: Diagnosis and management of acute myeloid leukemia in adults: recommendations from an international expert panel, on behalf of the European LeukemiaNet. *Blood* 115:453, 2010.

Eapen M, Rocha V, Sanz G, et al: Effect of graft source on unrelated donor haemopoietic stem-cell transplantation in adults with acute leukaemia: a retrospective analysis. *Lancet Oncol* 11:653, 2010.

Farag SS, Maharry K, Zhang MJ, et al: Comparison of reduced-intensity hematopoietic cell transplantation with chemotherapy in patients aged 60-70 years with acute myelogenous leukemia in first remission. *Biol Blood Marrow Transplant* 2011.

Fenaux P, Mufti GJ, Hellstrom-Lindberg E, et al: Efficacy of azacitidine compared with that of conventional care regimens in the treatment of higher-risk myelodysplastic syndromes: a randomised, open-label, phase III study. *Lancet Oncol* 10:223, 2009.

Greenberg P, Cox C, LeBeau MM, et al: International scoring system for evaluating prognosis in myelodysplastic syndromes. *Blood* 89:2079, 1997.

Gupta V, Tallman MS, He W, et al: Comparable survival after HLA-well-matched unrelated or matched sibling donor transplantation for acute myeloid leukemia in first remission with unfavorable cytogenetics at diagnosis. *Blood* 116:1839, 2010.

Gupta V, Tallman MS, Weisdorf DJ: Allogeneic hematopoietic cell transplantation for adults with acute myeloid leukemia: myths, controversies, and unknowns. *Blood* 117:2307, 2011.

Koreth J, Schlenk R, Kopecky KJ, et al: Allogeneic stem cell transplantation for acute myeloid leukemia in first complete remission: systematic review and meta-analysis of prospective clinical trials. *JAMA* 301:2349, 2009.

Lee JH, Lim SN, Kim DY, et al: Allogeneic hematopoietic cell transplantation for myelodysplastic syndrome: prognostic significance of pre-transplant IPSS score and comorbidity. *Bone Marrow Transplant* 45:450, 2010.

Lim Z, Brand R, Martino R, et al: Allogeneic hematopoietic stem-cell transplantation for patients 50 years or older with myelodysplastic syndromes or secondary acute myeloid leukemia. *J Clin Oncol* 28:405, 2010.

Litzow MR, Tarima S, Perez WS, et al: Allogeneic transplantation for therapy-related myelodysplastic syndrome and acute myeloid leukemia. *Blood* 115:1850, 2010.

Luger SM, Ringden O, Zhang MJ, et al: Similar outcomes using myeloablative vs reduced-intensity allogeneic transplant preparative regimens for AML or MDS. *Bone Marrow Transplant* 47:203, 2012.

Malcovati L, Germing U, Kuendgen A, et al: Time-dependent prognostic scoring system for predicting survival and leukemic evolution in myelodysplastic syndromes. *J Clin Oncol* 25:3503, 2007.

Malcovati L, Porta MG, Pascutto C, et al: Prognostic factors and life expectancy in myelodysplastic syndromes classified according to WHO criteria: a basis for clinical decision making. *J Clin Oncol* 23:7594, 2005.

McClune BL, Weisdorf DJ, Pedersen TL, et al: Effect of age on outcome of reduced-intensity hematopoietic cell transplantation for older patients with acute myeloid leukemia in first complete remission or with myelodysplastic syndrome. *J Clin Oncol* 28:1878, 2010.

Rockova V, Abbas S, Wouters BJ, et al: Risk stratification of intermediate-risk acute myeloid leukemia: integrative analysis of a multitude of gene mutation and gene expression markers. *Blood* 118:1069, 2011.

Schanz J, Steidl C, Fonatsch C, et al: Coalesced multicentric analysis of 2,351 patients with myelodysplastic syndromes indicates an underestimation of poor-risk cytogenetics of myelodysplastic syndromes in the international prognostic scoring system. *J Clin Oncol* 29:1963, 2011.

Schlenk RF, Dohner K, Krauter J, et al: Mutations and treatment outcome in cytogenetically normal acute myeloid leukemia. *N Engl J Med* 358:1909, 2008.

Walter RB, Pagel JM, Gooley TA, et al: Comparison of matched unrelated and matched related donor myeloablative hematopoietic cell transplantation for adults with acute myeloid leukemia in first remission. *Leukemia* 24:1276, 2010.

SOURCES CITED IN FIG. 61.1

1. Schiller GJ, Nimer SD, Territo MC, et al: Bone marrow transplantation versus high-dose cytarabine based consolidation chemotherapy for acute myelogenous leukemia in first remission. *J Clin Oncol* 10:41, 1992.

2. Archimbaud E, Thomas X, Michallet M, et al: Prospective genetically randomized comparison between intensive postinduction chemotherapy and bone marrow transplantation in adults with newly diagnosed acute myeloid leukemia. *J Clin Oncol* 12:262, 1994.

3. Hewlett J, Kopecky KJ, Head D, et al: A prospective evaluation of the roles of allogeneic marrow transplantation and low-dose monthly maintenance chemotherapy in the treatment of adult acute myelogenous leukemia (AML): a Southwest Oncology Group study. *Leukemia* 9:562, 1995.

4. Sierra J, Brunet S, Granena A, et al: Catalan Group for Bone Marrow Transplantation: feasibility and results of bone marrow transplantation after remission induction and intensification chemotherapy in de novo acute myeloid leukemia. *J Clin Oncol* 14:1353, 1996.

5. Keating S, de Witte T, Suciu S, et al: European Organization for Research and Treatment of Cancer, Gruppo Italiano Malattie Ematologiche Maligne dell'Adulto: the influence of HLA-matched sibling donor availability on treatment outcome for patients with AML: an analysis of the AML 8A study of the EORTC Leukaemia Cooperative Group and GIMEMA. *Br J Haematol* 102:1344, 1998.

6. Slovak ML, Kopecky KJ, Cassileth PA, et al: Karyotypic analysis predicts outcome of preremission and postremission therapy in adult acute myeloid leukemia: a Southwest Oncology Group/Eastern Cooperative Oncology Group Study. *Blood* 96:4075, 2000.

7. Suciu S, Mandelli F, de Witte T, et al, EORTC and GIMEMA Leukemia Groups: Allogeneic compared with autologous stem cell transplantation in the treatment of patients younger than 46 years with acute myeloid leukemia (AML) in first complete remission (CR1): an intention-to-treat analysis of the EORTC/GIMEMAAML-10 trial. *Blood* 102:1232, 2003.

8. Jourdan E, Boiron JM, Dastugue N, et al: Early allogeneic stem-cell transplantation for young adults with acute myeloblastic leukemia in first complete remission: an intent-to-treat long-term analysis of the BGMT experience. *J Clin Oncol* 23:7676, 2005.

9. Burnett AK, Wheatley K, Goldstone AH, et al: Longterm results of the MRC AML10 trial. *Clin Adv Hematol Oncol* 4:445, 2006.

10. Cornelissen JJ, van Putten WL, Verdonck LF, et al: Results of a HOVON/SAKK donor versus no-donor analysis of myeloablative HLA-identical sibling stem cell transplantation in first remission acute myeloid leukemia in young and middle-aged adults: benefits for whom? *Blood* 109:3658, 2007.

CHAPTER 62

ACUTE MYELOID LEUKEMIA IN CHILDREN

Tanja A. Gruber and Jeffrey E. Rubnitz

Acute myeloid leukemia (AML) is a complex and heterogeneous group of malignancies in which genetic and epigenetic alterations lead to the transformation of myeloid cell precursors. The tremendous diversity of abnormalities across subtypes of AML suggests that we must strive to develop therapies that target specific subgroups. Nevertheless, intensification of broadly active chemotherapy, the selective use of hematopoietic stem cell transplantation (HSCT; Box 62.1), improvements in supportive care and risk stratification, and the use of minimal residual disease (MRD) to monitor response to therapy, have contributed significantly to improvements in the treatment outcome for children with this disease. Survival rates for children with AML who are treated on contemporary clinical trials are now greater than 60%. A subset of patients, including those with acute promyelocytic leukemia (APL), Down syndrome and acute megakaryoblastic leukemia (AMKL), and core-binding factor (CBF) leukemia, have excellent outcomes, with survival rates that approach 90%. However, the cure rates for other subtypes of AML are unacceptably low and cannot be improved simply by further intensification of standard chemotherapy. Genomic and biologic insights into the mechanisms of leukemogenesis have provided opportunities to develop targeted and less toxic therapies for the treatment of AML. Their ability to improve outcomes, however, will be dependent on the requirement of the biologic targets for the survival of the leukemic cell. Thus, a comprehensive understanding of compensatory processes and mechanisms of resistance are critical for the ultimate success of these agents.

EPIDEMIOLOGY

AML accounts for approximately 20% of cases of acute leukemia in children and adolescents younger than 20 years of age. The incidence rates have remained constant over the past 40 years, are similar between boys and girls and, in general, are highest during the first 2 years of life. However, the age distribution may vary between subtypes. For example, APL and CBF leukemia are rare in children younger than 3 years of age, whereas the incidence of AMKL is highest in this young age group and rare among teenagers. The distribution of AML subtypes may also vary among ethnic groups, with some studies suggesting a higher incidence of APL among Hispanic populations.

Although we have learned much about the biology and genetics of AML, the causes remain elusive. The majority of cases are believed to result from interactions among genetic factors that may be inherited or acquired and environmental factors. Constitutional syndromes that are associated with an increased predisposition to AML include Down syndrome, Fanconi anemia, Bloom syndrome, neurofibromatosis, Noonan syndrome, congenital neutropenia, and germline haploinsufficiency of the *RUNX1* gene. Exposure to ionizing radiation, alkylating agents, topoisomerase II inhibitors, and benzene are among the few environmental factors proven to increase the risk of AML. In the majority of cases of childhood AML, neither a genetic nor environmental cause can be identified.

PATHOBIOLOGY

The morphologic and histochemical features of the leukemic cells served as the initial way to subdivide AML into distinct clinical entities, with the French-American-British (FAB) classification being the prototype of this approach. This classification scheme, however, was limited in biologic, prognostic, and therapeutic significance. The identification of specific cytogenetic alterations and submicroscopic molecular genetic lesions led to newer classification schemes, with the most recent widely used approach being the World Health Organization classification of AML (Table 62.1). With the development of genome-wide gene expression profiling, array-based comparative genomic hybridization methodologies, and next-generation sequencing, newer insights have been gained into the heterogeneity within AML. These studies have helped to validate the distinct nature of some of the previously described genetic subtypes, including AMKL, APL, the CBF leukemias, and AML with translocations involving the mixed lineage leukemia (*MLL*) gene. In addition, these approaches have identified new genetic subtypes as well as lesions that are enriched within leukemias that have normal karyotypes or miscellaneous chromosomal alterations (Fig. 62.1). Some of these lesions provide prognostic information and may serve as therapeutic targets for directed therapies.

AML-associated chromosomal translocations are genetic drivers that are believed to be initiating lesions, but are generally insufficient on their own to induce a full leukemic phenotype. Thus, like all cancers, multiple genetic and epigenetic alterations are necessary to convert a normal lineage-restricted stem or progenitor cell into a fully transformed leukemia cell. Although the exact number of mutations necessary to generate a leukemia is likely to differ between specific subtypes of AML, it has been useful to conceptualize the mutations as falling into two broad classes: class I mutations confer a proliferative or survival advantage; and class II mutations block differentiation and result in enhanced self-renewal (Fig. 62.2). It appears that it takes at least one mutation in each class to transform a normal cell into a leukemic one. Interestingly, many of the class II mutations arise from translocation events that lead to chimeric transcription factors with oncogenic properties. The recent efforts to more deeply explore the molecular lesions that underlie AML have significantly expanded the list of genes whose alterations contribute to leukemogenesis. One of the most surprising findings from these studies was the identification of a very limited number of somatic mutations in AML compared with the much larger numbers seen in other malignancies, such as breast cancer, pancreatic cancer, small-cell lung carcinoma, and melanoma. The number of mutations in pediatric AML is also significantly lower than the number of mutations seen in pediatric acute lymphoblastic leukemia (ALL), with one study finding an average of only 2.38 somatic copy-number alterations (CNAs; e.g., deletions and/or amplifications) in AML compared with an average of 6.46 CNAs in pediatric ALL. Even more striking was the lack of any CNAs in 34% of patients.

One of the early dogmas of cancer biology purports that tumors are clonal and arise from single cells. In support of this are cytogenetic studies demonstrating that leukemia cells within a patient are uniform in their abnormalities. As our ability to detect mutations has increased with the advent of next-generation sequencing, it has become apparent that while there is typically a founding clone that carries a subset of mutations present in all tumor cells, there is also significant tumor heterogeneity at diagnosis when taking into account the full complement of lesions. This is perhaps not surprising, given that cells can acquire new mutations with each cellular division. Furthermore, this heterogeneity provides an advantage to the tumor cells in that

Although the use of allogeneic hematopoietic stem cell transplantation (HSCT) in first remission is controversial, we recommend it for high-risk patients, including those with -7, t(6;11)(q27;q23), t(10;11)(p12;q23), t(10;11)(p11.2;q23), t(5;11)(q35;p15.5), t(6;9)(p23;q34), t(8;16) (p11;p13), inv(16)(p13.3q24.3), and t(16;21)(q24;q22). Until the impact of FLT3 inhibitors on the outcome of patients with *FLT3* internal tandem duplication (ITD) has been determined, we recommend HSCT for patients with *FLT3*-ITD and high allelic ratios or poor response to therapy. Patients who do not have high-risk genetic features but who have high (>1% after the first course of therapy) or persistent (>0.1% after two courses of therapy) levels of minimal residual disease (MRD) are also at high risk of relapse and are therefore candidates for HSCT in first remission. Because recent studies have demonstrated that outcomes after HSCT are similar regardless of donor type, we believe that the decision to perform HSCT in first remission should be based on the factors described above, rather than on the availability of a matched donor. Thus, patients who are classified as high-risk acute myeloid leukemia based on genetic features or MRD should undergo HSCT using a matched sibling donor, matched unrelated donor, haploidentical donor, or cord blood in first remission. Prior to transplant, reasonable efforts should be made to reduce the level of MRD as much as possible without causing organ toxicity or infectious complications that may increase transplant-related morbidity or mortality.

TABLE 62.1   2016 World Health Organization Classification of Acute Myeloid Leukemia and Related Neoplasms

Acute myeloid leukemia with recurrent genetic abnormalities
  AML with t(8;21)(q22;q22); RUNX1-RUNX1T1
  AML with inv(16)(p13.1q22) or t(16;16)(p13.1;q22); CBFB-MYH11
  APL with t(15;17)(q22;q12); PML-RARA
  AML with t(9;11)(p22;q23); MLL-MLLT3
  AML with t(6;9)(p23;q34); DEK-NUP214
  AML with inv(3)(q21q26.2) or t(3;3)(q21;q26.2); RPN1-EVI1
  AML (megakaryoblastic) with t(1;22)(p13;q13); RBM15-MKL1
  AML with mutated NPM1
  AML with mutated CEBPA
  Provisional entity: AML with BCR-ABL1
  Provisional entity: AML with mutated RUNX1
Acute myeloid leukemia with myelodysplasia-related changes
Therapy-related myeloid neoplasms
Acute myeloid leukemia, not otherwise specified
  AML with minimal differentiation
  AML without maturation
  AML with maturation
  Acute myelomonocytic leukemia
  Acute monoblastic/monocytic leukemia
  Pure erythroid leukemia
  Acute megakaryoblastic leukemia
  Acute basophilic leukemia
  Acute panmyelosis with myelofibrosis
Myeloid sarcoma
Myeloid proliferations related to Down syndrome
  Transient abnormal myelopoiesis
  Myeloid leukemia associated with Down syndrome

AML, Acute myeloid leukemia.
Modified from Arber DA, Orazi A, Hasserjian R, et al: The 2016 revision to the World Health Organization classification of myeloid neoplasms and acute leukemia, Blood 127:2391, 2016.

different subclones may have different growth characteristics and drug sensitivities depending on the complement of mutations present. However, the most robust AML clones in the laboratory, as determined by engraftment hento immunodeficient mice, do not necessarily equate to the dominant clone at diagnosis nor the clone that leads to relapse. It is thus clear that we still have an incomplete understanding of the molecular pathology of pediatric AML. Ongoing DNA sequencing efforts and studies on the epigenetic state of leukemia cells, coupled with biologic studies to understand the role of individual mutations as well as the spectrum of mutations within a given patient, will likely produce a much deeper understanding of the disease and mechanisms of drug resistance over the next several years. In this chapter we discuss the major subtypes of AML and our current understanding of the biologic processes that mediate disease.

The Core-Binding Factor Leukemias

The CBF transcription complex is a heterodimeric complex composed of an alpha DNA-binding subunit (RUNX1, RUNX2, or RUNX3), and a non-DNA-binding beta subunit (CBFβ). The complex functions as a master regulator that controls the birth of the definitive hematopoietic stem cell (HSC) during embryogenesis and plays important roles in normal hematopoietic cells, both in the control of their differentiation state as well as their effector functions. *RUNX1* was the first identified mammalian CBF gene and was isolated as part of the AML-associated translocation t(8;21)(q22;q22.3). Following the discovery of *RUNX1*, the inv(16) and the less common t(16;16)(p13;q22), which are found in the majority of acute monoblastic leukemias with eosinophilia (FAB-M4Eo), were cloned and shown to result in a fusion between *CBFβ* and *MYH11*, the gene that encodes smooth muscle myosin heavy chain (SMMHC). Subsequently, rare somatic mutations of *RUNX1* were detected in de novo AML, with the highest frequency (40%) seen in the FAB-M0 subtype. These mutations lead to impairment in DNA binding or decreased transcriptional activity. Collectively, these data reveal that mutations in the genes encoding the RUNX1/CBFβ transcription factor complex are one of the most common lesions seen in de novo AML, occurring in approximately 25% of cases.

The most frequently observed rearrangement in AML is the t(8;21), which fuses the 5′ portion of *RUNX1* to almost the entire coding region of *RUNX1T1*. The *RUNX1-RUNX1T1* fusion product functions primarily as a transcriptional repressor, inhibiting the expression of lineage-specific genes that are normally activated by the RUNX1-CBFβ complex to promote myeloid differentiation. In human and murine systems, expression of *RUNX1-RUNX1T1* is insufficient to induce leukemia, but does establish a preleukemic population that has enhanced self-renewal properties and can acquire additional mutations over time to lead to overt leukemia. Consistent with this hypothesis, in bone marrow samples from patients that have achieved a clinical remission, rare progenitors expressing *RUNX1-RUNX1T1* are present and can persist for years without expanding. These cells also retain the ability to differentiate into multiple lineages, so arguably they are not fully leukemic in nature. Cooperating mutations that promote full transformation identified in patients with CBF alterations include *FLT3*, *c-KIT*, and *RAS* among others, many of which confer a proliferative advantage.

The inv(16)/t(16;16)-encoded CBFβ-MYH11 fusion protein retains the RUNX1 binding domain and therefore its ability to interact with wild-type RUNX1. This chimeric protein functions in a dominant manner to inhibit normal RUNX transcriptional activity. Interestingly, 90% of *CBFβ-MYH11* conditional knock-in mice spontaneously developed AML with a latency of 5 months, implying that fewer cooperating mutations are necessary for this chimeric oncogene than *RUNX1-RUNX1T1*. These results may be explained by increasing evidence that CBFβ-MYH11 has functions independent of RUNX1 repression. Knock-in mice expressing a mutant Cbfβ-MYH11 allele that has low binding affinity for Runx1 demonstrate decreased repression of Runx1, but this did not correlate with reduced leukemogenesis. In fact, the mice developed leukemia faster, suggesting that there are Runx1-independent mechanisms of transformation by the chimeric protein. An analogous setting occurs in patients as well, whereby a small percentage of inv(16) AML patients produce a fusion protein that lacks the high-affinity binding domain responsible for enhanced binding to RUNX1. The clinical course and characteristics of these cases do not differ from cases in which the

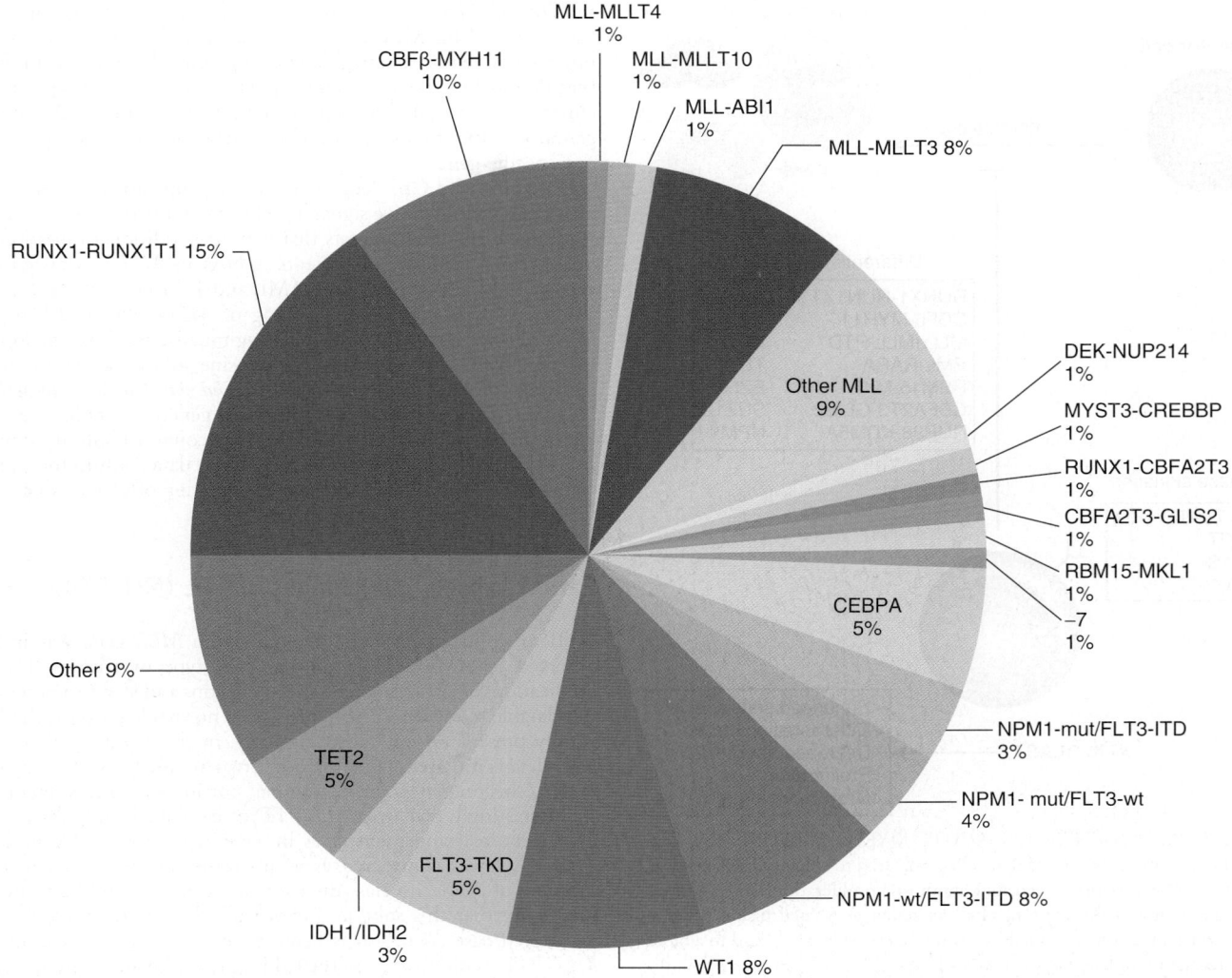

Fig. 62.1 FREQUENCIES OF RECURRENT GENETIC LESIONS IN CHILDHOOD ACUTE MYELOID LEUKEMIA. *MLL*, Mixed lineage leukemia.

fusion protein retains the high-affinity binding domain, further suggesting that dominant repression of RUNX1 is not the only mechanism through which the fusion gene contributes to leukemogenesis. The targets of the RUNX1-independent mechanism are unknown, as are the relative importance of the dependent and independent activities.

MLL Gene Rearrangements

The *MLL* gene, located on chromosome 11 band q23, is a mammalian homologue of the *Drosophila* trithorax (Trx) protein. The trithorax protein in *Drosophila* positively regulates homeodomain (*HOX*) genes, a set of transcription factors that specify cell identity along the anteroposterior axis of segmented animals during embryonic development. Their positive regulation is countered by Polycomb-group (PcG) proteins, such as BMI1, which act as transcriptional repressors of the *HOX* genes.

MLL encodes a protein of approximately 500 kDa with multiple domains that form part of a multiprotein complex involving transcription regulators including TFIID, SWI/SNF, NuRD, hSNFsH, and SIN3A. This complex is responsible for chromatin remodeling, including acetylation, deacetylation, and methylation of nucleosome-attached histones. MLL is thought to play a role in the recruitment of proteins, assembly of the complex, and is required for transcriptional elongation of its target genes. Experiments evaluating the

contribution of MLL-deficient embryonic stem cells in chimeric animals found an absence of lymphoid and myeloid populations derived from the MLL-deficient stem cells, demonstrating a requirement for MLL in either the specification or expansion of HSCs during development. Conditional knockout of the *Mll* gene in adult mice leads to bone marrow failure within 3 weeks, providing evidence that MLL is not only required for definitive hematopoiesis, but is also required for maintenance of HSCs in postnatal hematopoiesis.

Chromosomal translocations involving the *MLL* gene are associated with both AML and ALL leukemias, with more than 50 different translocation partners identified. *MLL* rearrangements are found in 60%–70% of infants with leukemia, regardless of immunophenotype, but are less common in older children and adults. The distribution of translocation partners varies depending on the age of the patient and the immunophenotype of leukemia, with *MLLT3*, *MLLT10*, *MLLT4*, and *ELL* being more frequent in pediatric AML. With the exception of internal partial tandem duplications (PTD) of *MLL* (*MLL*-PTD), the majority of *MLL* rearrangements contain the N-terminus of MLL and the C-terminus of the fusion partner gene. Some of the partner genes are nuclear proteins with transcription modulation activity that lead to activation of MLL target loci, while others are either cytoplasmic or membrane bound with diverse functions but share in common the presence of dimerization/oligomerization domains. Oligomerization promotes enhanced recruitment of transcription cofactors as well as stabilization of the large multiprotein transcriptional complex.

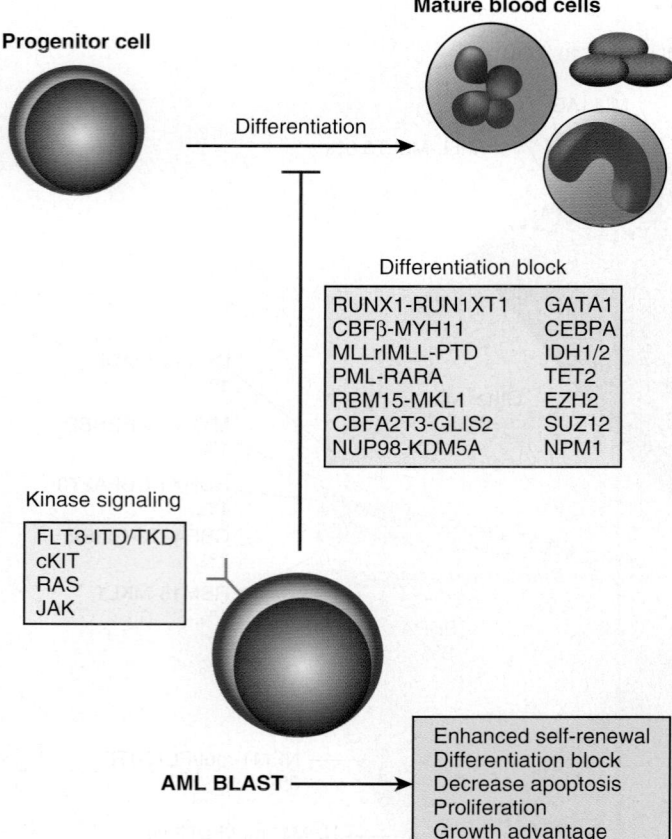

Mature blood cells

Progenitor cell

Differentiation

Differentiation block

RUNX1-RUN1XT1	GATA1
CBFβ-MYH11	CEBPA
MLLrIMLL-PTD	IDH1/2
PML-RARA	TET2
RBM15-MKL1	EZH2
CBFA2T3-GLIS2	SUZ12
NUP98-KDM5A	NPM1

Kinase signaling

FLT3-ITD/TKD
cKIT
RAS
JAK

AML BLAST ⟶

Enhanced self-renewal
Differentiation block
Decrease apoptosis
Proliferation
Growth advantage

Fig. 62.2 PATHOGENESIS OF ACUTE MYELOID LEUKEMIA. Leukemic blasts contain mutations that collectively lead to enhanced self-renewal, a block in differentiation, decreased apoptosis, proliferation, and a growth advantage. Many of the acute myeloid leukemia–associated fusion genes as well as point mutations and small insertion/deletions in genes lead to a block in differentiation of hematopoietic progenitor cells, resulting in an immature phenotype. Cooperating mutations in genes that activate kinase signaling pathways are often present that enhance proliferation and lead to robust cytokine-independent growth, providing a survival advantage. Examples of mutations conferring these characteristics are shown.

In addition to the recruitment of transcriptional transactivators by these fusion proteins, several have been shown to recruit hDOT1L, a histone methyltransferase that methylates H3 lysine residues (H3K79). hDOT1L recruitment is ubiquitously coupled with active transcription and is responsible for H3K79 methylation in the proximal part of a given gene. A global loss of H3K79 methylation significantly affects heterochromatin formation; therefore the aberrant recruitment of hDOT1L by MLL fusions and the resulting H3K79 methylation are thought to affect gene expression by altering chromatin accessibility.

Leukemias with *MLL* translocations show increased expression of multiple *HOX* genes, including *HOXA4, HOXA5, HOXA9*, and *HOXA10* regardless of their immunophenotype. *HOX* genes encode transcription factors whose deregulated expression is identified in multiple cancers, although the mechanisms by which they contribute to carcinogenesis are extremely varied. All hematopoietic progenitors express a characteristic pattern of *HOX* genes dependent on their lineage and stage of differentiation. Overexpression of individual *HOX* genes results in disturbance of stem cell pools and differentiation patterns, some of which lead to myeloproliferation and even overt AML in mice. HOXA9, in particular, leads to increased self-renewal of hematopoietic progenitors and overexpression in AML patients has been frequently described, specifically in patients with *MLL* gene rearrangements. In multiple models, HOXA9 is required for MLL-mediated leukemogenesis, although this does not hold true

in *MLL-MLLT3* transgenic mice. Although HOXA9 was not specifically required for MLL-MLLT3-mediated leukemogenesis, multiple other *HOX* genes are upregulated in this model and it was proposed that due to functional redundancy within members of a given Hox cluster, a "Hox code," as defined by upregulation of multiple *HOX* genes, is sufficient for the development of leukemia as opposed to one specific gene.

In contrast to CBF leukemias, where cooperating genetic lesions providing a proliferative signal have been described, analysis of *MLL*-rearranged leukemia suggests that very few additional mutations are present in this subset of patients. CNAs in *MLL*-rearranged cases average only 1.33 for pediatric AML and 1 for pediatric ALL in two studies. Next-generation sequencing of *MLL*-rearranged leukemias has confirmed a paucity of cooperating mutations, although approximately 50% carry an activating tyrosine kinase mutation in this pathway, providing the so-called *second hit* for leukemogenesis. However, cases exist that lack additional genetic alterations, and the kinase mutations for those samples that contain them are typically subclonal and often absent at relapse. These data confirm the strength of the *MLL* fusion genes and suggest targeting of cooperating mutations will not result in a therapeutic benefit.

Partial Tandem Duplications of MLL (MLL-PTD)

Tandem duplication of the 5′ end of the *MLL* gene was initially observed in AML with a normal karyotype or trisomy 11. The duplications are in-frame repetitions of exons and lead to a potentially translatable sequence. In patients with a normal karyotype, the PTD is only present on one allele; similarly, in trisomy 11 patients only one allele is mutated while the other two are unchanged. In contrast to *MLL* fusion genes, the C-terminal portion of MLL is retained.

Interestingly, pediatric *MLL*-PTD cases failed to cluster with other *MLL* gene rearrangement cases in gene expression profiling. When *MLL*-PTD was considered as a subgroup and compared to other subtypes of AML, no class-discriminating genes could be identified, suggesting that this subtype is not only distinct from other *MLL*-rearranged cases, but also is heterogeneous. In addition, unique to *MLL*-PTD is the absence of the wild-type *MLL* gene transcript. AML cases with the *MLL-MLLT3* translocation retain expression of the normal *MLL* allele, and this coexpression is required for leukemogenesis in murine hematopoietic cells. The wild-type *MLL* transcript is absent in *MLL*-PTD; however, antisense oligodeoxynucleotides against *MLL*-PTD result in reexpression of the wild-type transcript, suggesting MLL-PTD is silencing transcription at the wild-type locus. In addition to antisense oligodeoxynucleotides, the silencing could also be reversed by DNA methyltransferase and histone deacetylase inhibitors. Reexpression of the wild-type allele was associated with increased cell death and reduced proliferation, indicating that the repression of wild-type *MLL* contributes to transformation.

Despite expression array data suggesting *MLL*-PTD is a distinct biologic entity, experiments have shown that the mechanism of *MLL*-PTD–mediated leukemogenesis shares many similarities with other MLL fusion proteins. MLL-PTD is able to induce strong transactivation in a *MYC*-luciferase reporter assay similar to a dimerized *MLL* fusion gene construct. The duplication of the N-terminal domains may therefore allow dimerization, leading to altered gene expression and malignant transformation. A mouse knock-in model in which exons 5–11 of murine *Mll* were targeted to intron 4 of the endogenous locus resulted in upregulated *HoxA9* gene expression, increased CFU replating capacity, and enhanced proliferation, similar to MLL fusion proteins.

Acute Promyelocytic Leukemia

APL is morphologically identified as AML-M3 by the FAB classification and is characterized by a balanced reciprocal translocation between chromosomes 15q22 and 17q1221. In the late 1970s, it was discovered that leukemia cells could be forced to differentiate in vitro when exposed to retinoic acid. Based on this observation, Zhen-Yi Wang treated a 5-year-old girl with refractory APL who was in a critical condition with all-*trans*-retinoic acid (ATRA). With single-agent ATRA, she achieved a complete remission (CR) and remains disease free to this day. Wang and colleagues subsequently treated 24 patients with APL and were able to improve the CR rate to 96% with ATRA alone. In addition to high CR rates, ATRA has improved long-term outcomes, with 5-year EFS rates as high as 85% in adults and 91% in children. This remarkable response rate to ATRA was specific for APL, leading researchers to explore the retinoic acid receptor (RAR) in this population. In the early 1990s, several groups simultaneously demonstrated that the translocation that characterizes this malignancy encodes a chimeric protein fusing the *PML* gene with the RAR (*RARA*) gene. In contrast to the expected paradigm, whereby molecular biology leads to the development of a targeted agent, ATRA was found to be effective prior to the understanding of the mechanism. In studying the response of APL to this agent, much of the biology of APL has come to light, demonstrating the constant interplay that exists between science and medicine.

Greater than 98% of patients with APL carry t(15;17)(q22q1221), which fuses the *PML* gene with the *RARA* gene to create the chimeric oncogene *PML-RARA*. Retinoid signaling is relayed by two families of nuclear receptors, the RARs and the retinoid X receptor, that together form heterodimers. In the absence of retinoic acid, these heterodimers bind to target gene promoters and repress transcription through the recruitment of NCoR, SMRT), and HDAC corepressors. When retinoic acid binds, a conformational change allows the recruitment of coactivators and histone acetyltransferases, resulting in activation of transcription. *RARA* is highly expressed in myeloid cells, and activation of its transcriptional targets promotes granulopoiesis. *PML-RARA* expression impairs normal responses to retinoic acid as the fusion protein binds to transcriptional corepressors and histone deacetylases with a higher affinity than wild-type RARA.

In addition to the effects on transcription, the fusion gene alters localization of PML. In wild-type cells, PML is localized in discrete nuclear subdomains, called *nuclear bodies*, which likely play a role in senescence, growth control, telomere lengthening, and DNA repair. These nuclear bodies are disrupted by PML-RARA in a manner that is reversible by treatment, suggesting that they are important in apoptosis and growth control. PML is in fact a p53 target gene, and regulates p53 stability by sequestering Mdm2, a negative regulator of p53, to the nucleolus, thus providing a mechanism for this phenotype. PML contains a sumoylation site that is present on the PML-RARA chimeric protein and is required for leukemic transformation.

The mechanism whereby retinoic acid induces differentiation of APL cells carrying *PML-RARA* was delineated following the demonstration of its clinical efficacy. Retinoic acid binds to the hormone-binding site of PML-RARA, inducing a conformational change that triggers co-repressor release and co-activator recruitment, opening up the chromatin structure and relieving the transcriptional repression. Global transcription and protein alterations following treatment with retinoic acid are significant for a large number of genes involved in granulocyte differentiation, such as CEBPs, cytokines, cytokine receptors, and molecules downstream of cytokine signaling. Another effect of ATRA is to induce proteasome degradation of the chimeric oncogene.

ATRA is not the only targeted agent for APL. Ai-ling 1, a Chinese remedy historically used to treat a variety of illnesses, was tested by a group from Harbin Medical University in the 1970s in more than 1000 patients with different cancers and was found to induce remissions in approximately two-thirds of patients with APL. Zhu Chen, a scientist in Shanghai, collaborated with the Harbin team in 1994 to demonstrate that the effective component of this remedy was arsenic (III) trioxide. Importantly, arsenic was able to induce remissions in patients who had failed ATRA and conventional chemotherapy. Subsequently, many groups confirmed these findings and the mechanism of action has been under study ever since. At high concentrations, arsenic induces apoptosis of APL, while low doses promote maturation and differentiation. Arsenic treatment causes

PML to be localized to the nuclear matrix where it becomes sumoylated and subsequently degraded by proteasomes. When global transcription and protein patterns affected by arsenic were compared to those altered by ATRA, it was found that while arsenic regulated a significant number of genes also regulated by ATRA, the total number of affected genes was much less. Arsenic altered a more significant change in protein patterns than ATRA, suggesting that its main mechanism was through protein alterations as opposed to gene expression modulation.

Acute Megakaryocytic Leukemia

AMKL is a subtype of AML characterized by abnormal megakaryoblasts that express platelet-specific surface glycoprotein. Bone marrow biopsy frequently demonstrates extensive myelofibrosis, often making aspiration in these patients difficult. AMKL is rare in adults, occurring in only 1% of AML patients, but comprises between 4% and 15% of childhood AML cases. In pediatrics, the disease is divided into two major subgroups: AMKL in patients with Down syndrome (DS-AMKL) and AMKL in patients without Down syndrome (non-DS-AMKL). AMKL is the most frequent type of AML in children with Down syndrome, and the incidence in these patients is 500-fold higher than in the general population. Somatic mutations in *GATA1* are found in almost all cases of DS-AMKL and precede the development of leukemia, as indicated by their presence in patients with transient myeloproliferative disease (TMD) in the neonatal period. Pediatric non-DS-AMKL is a heterogeneous group of patients, a significant proportion of which carry chimeric oncogenes including *RBM15-MKL1*, *CBFA2T3-GLIS2*, *NUP98-KDM5A*, and *MLL* gene rearrangements.

DS-AMKL is associated with a hematologic disorder in infancy, termed TMD. In this disorder, a clonal population of megakaryoblasts accumulates in the peripheral blood. These blasts are phenotypically indistinguishable from AMKL leukemic blasts, and in the majority of cases remission is spontaneous within 3 months in the absence of treatment. In approximately 20% of TMD cases patients will develop MDS or AMKL. TMD is felt to originate in utero, as mutations in *GATA1*, the genetic lesion associated with TMD, have been found to be present at birth in patients that suffered from TMD. Exome sequencing of TMD has revealed that nonsilent mutations in these blasts are primarily limited to the *GATA1* gene. In contrast, AMKL blasts carry a higher burden of mutations, with additional lesions in epigenetic and kinase-signaling genes leading to progression of the disease. Collectively, these findings support a model whereby TMD blasts arise secondary to *GATA1* mutations, acquiring this so-called *first hit* and persist in the bone marrow. Additional lesions can then occur, providing the cooperating events that are necessary for full blown leukemia to develop.

The GATA proteins are transcription factors, three of which are expressed principally in hematopoietic cells (*GATA1*, *GATA2*, and *GATA3*). GATA1 is required for the development of erythrocytes, megakaryocytes, eosinophils, and mast cells. Mutations detected in DS patients with AMKL consist of short deletions, insertions, and point mutations within exon 2 that introduce a premature stop codon. This shorter mutant protein retains the ability to bind DNA and interact with its cofactor, but lacks the transcriptional activation domain and hence has reduced transactivation potential. GATA1 is able to activate lineage specific genes and repress progenitor maintenance genes depending on the cofactors present. Deregulation of these targets contributes to the differentiation arrest seen with the truncated GATA1 that is no longer able to transactivate transcription of lineage-specific genes. Given that only 20% of TMD progresses to leukemia, what then are the subsequent events or alterations that promote the preleukemic state to that of a fully transformed malignancy? Exome and targeted sequencing of 46 genes has provided insight to this question, identifying recurrently mutated genes in three major categories: cohesin, epigenetic regulators, and signaling molecules. These include the cohesin complex genes *STAG2*, *RAD21*, *SMC3*, *SMC1A*, *NIPBL* and *CTCF*; PRC2 complex genes *EZH2* and

SUZ12; as well as kinases such as *JAK1, JAK2, JAK3, MPL, KRAS,* and *NRAS*.

t(1;22), which is seen exclusively in infants with AMKL, fuses *RBM15* and *MKL1. MKL1* is a transcriptional coactivator for serum response factor (SRF), a transcription factor that regulates the expression of genes involved in cell growth, proliferation, and differentiation, as well as genes that control the actin cytoskeleton. In unstimulated cells MKL1 associates with G-actin monomers and is retained in the cytoplasm. Following stimulation and Rho-mediated actin polymerization, G-actin pools are depleted and MKL1 translocates to the nucleus, associating with SRF to activate gene transcription. RBM15 encodes a protein containing three N-terminal RNA recognition motifs that bind to nucleic acids and a Spen paralogue and orthologue C-terminal (SPOC) domain that is thought to interact with the SMRT and NCoR corepressor complexes, as well as RBPJ, a transcription factor downstream of Notch signaling. The fusion of MKL1 to RBM15 deregulates the normal intracellular localization of MKL1 such that it is becomes constitutively localized to the nucleus, resulting in SRF activation even in the absence of stimuli. In addition to the SRF transcriptional program, the fusion also aberrantly activates RBPJ transcriptional targets. While both transcription programs have been shown to be deregulated by the fusion gene, the degree to which they contribute to transformation is still unclear.

Until recently, with the exception of the *RBM15-MKL1* fusion, the genetic etiology of non-DS-AMKL had remained elusive. Transcriptome sequencing of a small cohort identified a cryptic inversion on chromosome 16 [inv(16)(p13.3q24.3)] in half of the patients that resulted in the joining of *CBFA2T3*, a member of the ETO family of nuclear corepressors, to *GLIS2*, a member of the GLI family of transcription factors. The gene expression profile of *CBFA2T3-GLIS2* AMKL was distinct from that of AMKL cells lacking this chimeric transcript, and from other genetic subtypes of pediatric AML. Furthermore, the *CBFA2T3-GLIS2* fusion gene conferred a poor prognosis, a finding that has since been confirmed. Expression of *CBFA2T3-GLIS2* in *Drosophila* and murine hematopoietic cells induces bone morphogenic protein (BMP) signaling, a pathway not previously implicated in AML, and results in a marked increase in the self-renewal capacity of hematopoietic progenitors. *CBFA2T3-GLIS2*-expressing cells remained growth factor dependent in vitro and fail to induce leukemia in mice, consistent with a requirement for cooperative mutations. Overall, the total burden of somatic mutations in *CBFA2T3-GLIS2*-expressing cases is low; however, several have been found to carry lesions in either a Janus kinase(JAK) gene and/or a somatic amplification of the Down syndrome critical region on chromosome 21.

In addition to *CBFA2T3-GLIS2*, approximately 8% of pediatric non–DS-AMKL cases carry the *NUP98-KDM5A* fusion. *NUP98*, a nucleoporin family member with transactivation activity, fused to *KDM5A*, an H3K4me3-binding PHD finger, was initially described in adult AML. When introduced into murine bone marrow, this fusion oncogene induces a myeloid differentiation arrest and mice develop AML with an average latency of 69 days. Wang and colleagues demonstrated this fusion to be bound to H3K4me3 mononucleosomes, showing the PHD finger plays a role in targeting the fusion to the genome. Interestingly, microarray analysis identified several polycomb proteins carrying H3K4me3 marks to be transcriptionally upregulated in response to the fusion, while housekeeping genes with constitutive H3K4me3 marks remained unchanged. Affected polycomb targets confirmed by chromatin immunoprecipitation include genes upregulated in *MLL*-rearranged leukemia such as HOXA5, HOXA7, HOXA9, HOXA10, MEIS1, and PBX1. Furthermore, the authors demonstrate a block in PRC2 binding, the complex that antagonizes polycomb proteins through transcriptional repression of target genes. Therefore, the *NUP98-KDM5A* fusion is able to prevent silencing of critical transcription factors that play a role in maintaining hematopoietic progenitor status, similar to *MLL* gene rearrangements. It is perhaps not surprising then, that *MLL-AF9* and *MLL-AF10* fusion events have also been detected in non-DS-AMKL. As these lesions are also found in other subtypes of AML,

there are likely additional factors contributing to the development of megakaryoblastic disease. Cooperating mutations, the target cell, and the microenvironment all have the potential to direct lineage during the process of transformation.

Cytogenetically Normal AML

Approximately 20%–25% of pediatric AML cases lack chromosomal aberrations and are prognostically defined as intermediate risk. To understand the underlying lesions driving this form of AML and to use this information to further refine risk stratification of these patients, efforts have been made by a number of groups to identifying the genetic lesions within this AML subtype. Identified genetic lesions have included mutations within the genes *FLT3, NPM1, IDH, RAS,* and *CEBPA*. More recent whole-genome sequencing analysis of cytogenetically normal adult AML has identified these previously described mutations, as well as the mutation of a number of other genes including DNMT3A, which are thought to contribute to tumorigenesis. Below we discuss the most frequent somatic mutations identified within pediatric AMLs with a normal karyotype.

Nucleophosmin
Nucleophosmin (*NPM*) is often mutated in cytogenetically normal AML and is unique in that it has both oncogenic and tumor suppressor functions. The protein shuttles between the nucleus and cytoplasm, taking part in many cellular processes including regulation of ribosomal RNA transcription/processing, transport of preribosomal particles to the cytoplasm, DNA-histone and nucleosome assembly, as well as regulating the activity and stability of tumor suppressors such as p53 and ARF. Alterations of *NPM* in cancer include its overexpression in a variety of epithelial cancers; involvement in chromosomal translocation in several hematological malignancies including the t(2;5)[NPM-ALK] in anaplastic large-cell lymphoma (ALCL), t(3;5)[NPM-MLF1] in myelodysplastic syndrome and AML and t(5;17)[NPM-RARA] in variant APL; and point mutations that alter its C-terminus resulting in the creation of a new nuclear export signal. Each of these genetic alterations result in alteration of the normal shuttling of NPM between the cytoplasm and nucleus, resulting in constitutive cytoplasmic localization. Mutations in *NPM* are found in 35% of cytogenetically normal adult AMLs but only between 2% and 12% of pediatric AMLs with normal cytogenetics.

The tumor suppressor function of NPM in hematologic malignancies is attributed to its role in maintenance of genomic stability and in the regulation of the ARF-p53 tumor suppressor pathway. Wild-type NPM forms a complex with ARF and HDM2, which stabilizes ARF and prevents HDM2-mediated p53 degradation. More recently, it has also been shown that in the absence of NPM or in the presence of an NPM mutant, cells express increased protein levels of the MYC proto-oncogene due to a loss of degradation by the NPM-stabilized ubiquitin ligase, FBW7G. Given that mutations in NPM are able to suppress the ARF-p53 tumor suppressor pathway and enhance the oncogenic MYC pathway, it is perhaps not surprising that the mutation occurs in the context of cytogenetically normal AML with a minimal number of secondary lesions.

Isocitrate Dehydrogenase and TET2
Isocitrate dehydrogenase 1 (*IDH1*) was initially identified as a target of cancer-associated mutations in a study that performed whole-exome sequencing on glioblastoma multiforme (GBM). Subsequent analyses revealed *IDH1* or *IDH2* mutations in up to 16% of adult and about 7% of pediatric AMLs with normal cytogenetics. The mutations in both GBM and AML have been heterozygous and restricted to arginine 132 in exon 4 of *IDH1*, or to either the homologous residue in IDH2, R172, or to a second arginine, R140, also located in its substrate binding pocket. Although the distribution of specific *IDH1/IDH2* mutations varies between GBM and AML, each results in a loss of the enzyme's ability to catalyze the oxidative carboxylation of isocitrate to α-ketoglutarate (α-KG), coupled with a

gain of function to catalyze the NADPH-dependent reduction of α-KG to 2-hydroxyglutarate (2-HG). The altered activity of the enzyme leads to an increase in the level of 2-HG, which has pleotropic effects including the inhibition of the enzymatic activity of the α-KG-dependent enzyme TET oncogene family member 2 (TET2), responsible for catalyzing the conversion of 5-methylcytosine to 5-hydrozymethylcytosine. Loss-of-function mutations of *TET2* have also been identified in a variety of hematopoietic malignancies including MDS, myeloproliferative neoplasms and AML. Interestingly, mutations in *IDH1/2* and *TET2* appear to be mutually exclusive, confirming a common downstream effect of these lesions. Alterations of the enzymatic activity of TET2, either through direct mutations or mutation of *IDH1/2*, lead to enhanced self-renewal of hematopoietic progenitors and an expansion of the stem cell and progenitor cell compartment, and thereby directly contribute to leukemogenesis.

FMS-like Tyrosine Kinase 3

FMS-like tyrosine kinase 3 (FLT3, FLK2) is a class III receptor tyrosine kinase that is normally expressed in early hematopoietic progenitors that are $CD34^+/c\text{-}Kit^+$. When bound by its ligand (FLT3 ligand or FL) the receptor dimerizes, leading to activation of the receptor's intrinsic tyrosine kinase activity. The activated kinase signals through a variety of pathways including the phosphatidylinositol 3-kinase (PI3K) and RAS signal-transduction cascades through phosphorylation of cytoplasmic substrates. Two major classes of FLT3-activating mutations have been identified in AML, internal tandem duplication (ITD) in the juxtamembrane domain and point mutations in the tyrosine kinase domain (TKD). Both classes of mutations result in ligand-independent constitutive activation of the receptor's kinase activity and induce factor-independent growth of the murine pro-B–cell line Ba/F3. *FLT3* mutations are frequent cooperating lesions, being found not only in cytogenetically normal AML, but in APL, CBF AML, and *MLL*-rearranged leukemia as well.

The *FLT3*-ITD mutation results from a fragment of the juxtamembrane-domain coding sequence that is duplicated and inserted, the length of which varies from 3 to 400 bp. The juxtamembrane domain is a negative regulator of the kinase activity and the ITD leads to a disruption of this autoinhibitory activity. As a result of the disruption of this domain, the mutant *FLT3*-ITD undergoes ligand-independent dimerization and tyrosine autophosphorylation, and this constitutively active tyrosine kinase activates the downstream targets that are normally regulated by the native receptor. Transplantation of bone marrow cells transduced with *FLT3*-ITD into mice leads to a myeloproliferative disorder but not leukemia, underscoring the importance of cooperative mutations in *FLT3*-ITD–positive malignancy. In a study of 144 cases of newly diagnosed adult AML, 24 out of 28 *FLT3*-ITD–positive cases had second mutations/alterations, the most frequent of which were mutations of *NPM1*, *MLL*-PTD, *CEBPA*, and *PML-RARA*.

FLT3-TKD mutations occur in the activation loop of the kinase domain, leading to constitutive activation. In a wild-type setting, ligand-induced activation of FLT3 causes an active configuration to form, allowing kinase activity. The TKD mutations interfere with the inhibitory loop and thus are similar to ITD in disrupting the regulation of signaling, but differ in that they do not require dimerization for constitutive activation. While both mutations lead to constitutive activation of AKT and extracellular signal-related kinase (ERK)1/2 from the PI3K and RAS signaling cascades, respectively, data suggest that strong signal transducer and activator of transcription (STAT5) activation is only observed in *FLT3*-ITD cells.

RAS

RAS proteins couple receptor activation with downstream effector pathways, altering proliferation, differentiation, and apoptosis. Overall, approximately 30% of cancers express a mutant or so-called *oncogenic* RAS. Three RAS genes are encoded in the human genome: *HRAS*, *KRAS*, and *NRAS*, and the frequency of mutations for these genes vary significantly between cancer types. In myeloid leukemia, *NRAS* mutations predominate, followed in frequency by *KRAS*, while *HRAS* mutations have not been reported. RAS proteins cycle between an inactive GDP-bound state and an active GTP-bound state. Somatic mutations occur at amino acid residues, which impair their intrinsic GTPase activity and also confer resistance to GTPase-activating proteins leading to persistence of a GTP-bound (and therefore active) state. Active RAS mediates effects through a multitude of downstream effector pathways including RAC, PI3K, RAF, RAL, and PKC, all of which confer abnormal functional properties in cancer cells. These pathways affect cell cycle progression, promote survival, and stimulate actin reorganization and vesicle trafficking, all of which have been shown in various model systems to contribute to RAS-induced tumorigenesis. In AML, cooperating lesions found in *NRAS* mutant cases include *NPM1*, *C/EBPA*, *PML-RARA*, *MLL* rearrangements, *RUNX1-ETO*, and *CBFB-MYH11*. In a pediatric cohort of 111 AML cases, activating mutations in *NRAS* were found in 45%, 44%, and 24% of *RUNX1-ETO*, *CBFB-MYH11*, and *MLL* rearranged cases, respectively.

CCAAT Enhancer-Binding Protein Alpha

CCAAT enhancer-binding protein alpha (C/EBPα) is a transcription factor that contains two N-terminal transcriptional activation domains (TAD1 and TAD2) and a C-terminal DNA-binding basic region followed by a leucine zipper domain that mediates homo- and hetero-dimerization with other CEBP family members. DNA binding requires dimerization and is critically dependent on the distance between the leucine zipper domain and the DNA-binding basic region. *CEBPA* encodes an mRNA that contains alternative translation initiation sites resulting in two major protein isoforms: the fully translated C/EBPα (p42), and an N-terminally truncated protein (p30) lacking the N-terminal transactivation domain TAD1. In the hematopoietic system, *CEBPA* is expressed in myeloid progenitors and granulocytes but not macrophages, and has been shown to regulate the expression of many myeloid genes. Conditional knockout of *Cebpa* in adult mice blocks the transition from common myeloid progenitors to the more differentiated granulocyte monocyte progenitor, leading to an accumulation of myeloid blasts.

Mutations that reduce the transcriptional activity of C/EBPα occur in between 5% and 14% of AML patients, and are primarily seen in FAB-M1/2 AMLs with a normal karyotype. Two classes of *CEBPA* mutations have been defined: mutations that occur within the first 300 bp of the *CEBPA* gene and result in frameshifts or stop codons that eliminate expression of the p42 isoform but have no effect on the translation of p30; and mutations in the 3′ end of the gene that result in in-frame insertions or deletions that disrupt the relationship of the basic and leucine zipper domains and alter DNA-binding activity. The most frequent pattern seen in patients is a combination of the two types of mutations, one on each allele. Knock-in mice that eliminate p42 translation while allowing expression of p30 have been generated, and these mice uniformly die of AML by 60 weeks of age, providing direct evidence that *Cebpa* mutations contribute to the process of leukemogenesis.

CLINICAL AND LABORATORY MANIFESTATIONS AND DIAGNOSIS

Most children with AML have signs and symptoms of bone marrow failure, including pallor, fatigue, bleeding, bruising, and infection. Hepatosplenomegaly, lymphadenopathy, and bone pain are common, but usually less prominent than in children with ALL. Because of the acute nature of the process, weight loss and other signs of chronic disease are rare. In some cases, the predominant clinical signs result not from bone marrow disease, but from extramedullary myeloid tumors, referred to as *chloromas* or *granulocytic sarcomas*, which most often arise in the orbital or spinal regions. Other clinical manifestations include gingival hypertrophy, commonly seen in AML cases with a monocytic component, and skin or subcutaneous nodules. Cutaneous lesions may be single or multiple violaceous papules or nodules, are most common in infants, and may be mistaken for the blueberry muffin lesions that are associated with congenital infection. Skin nodules sometimes develop before bone marrow involvement and may regress spontaneously. Patients with elevated leukocyte counts (hyperleukocytosis) may also present with central nervous system (CNS) symptoms (seizure or stroke) or pulmonary symptoms related to hyperviscosity.

Among children with AML, the median leukocyte count at diagnosis is approximately $20 \times 10^9/L$, with a median hemoglobin concentration of approximately 9 g/dL and a median platelet count of $60 \times 10^9/L$. Although about 10% of children with AML do not have morphologically detectable circulating blasts, careful examination of the peripheral blood smear will reveal leukemic cells in most cases. Prolonged prothrombin, thrombin, and partial thromboplastin times, as well as decreased fibrinogen levels, are seen in the majority of patients with APL and about 5% of other AML cases. Abnormalities of serum chemistries may include hyperuricemia, although this is less common and less severe than hyperuricemia associated with ALL. The presence of hypokalemia, a rare finding in patients with ALL, suggests a diagnosis of monoblastic leukemia.

Among patients who present with circulating blasts, the differential diagnosis is generally limited to various types of leukemia, including AML, ALL, and juvenile myelomonocytic leukemia (JMML). For patients who do not have blasts in their blood at the time of presentation, the differential diagnosis is determined by signs and symptoms and may include aplastic anemia, autoimmune or inflammatory disease, infection, and solid malignancies. In most cases, the diagnosis of AML is made by bone marrow examination. A bone marrow aspiration should be performed for morphologic examination, immunophenotyping, genetic, and molecular studies, whereas a bone marrow biopsy is used to assess cellularity. A diagnosis of AML is confirmed when 20% or more of nucleated bone marrow cells are blasts of myeloid origin or when the blasts contain AML-specific genetic lesions, regardless of blast percentage. When a diagnosis of AML is confirmed, most investigators classify each case according to the World Health Organization criteria (Table 62.1). Since AML may involve the CNS, examination of the cerebrospinal fluid (CSF) should also be performed as part of the workup of all patients. Although CNS leukemia is traditionally defined as the presence of at least five leukocytes/μL of CSF with leukemic blast cells present, the significance of lower levels of CNS involvement is not known. The diagnosis of CNS involvement may also be based on the presence of cranial nerve palsies or radiologic evidence of leukemic infiltration.

Prognostic Factors

Genetic features, some of which can be identified by conventional karyotyping and others that require molecular techniques, are strongly associated with outcome (Table 62.2). An equally important predictor of outcome is response to therapy, which can be assessed by morphologic, immunophenotypic, or molecular examination of the bone marrow before and after each course of chemotherapy.

Investigators from almost all study groups consider children whose leukemic blasts contain the t(8;21)(q22;q22)/*RUNX1-RUNX1T1*, inv(16)(p13.1;q22)/*CBFβ-MYH11*, or t(16;16)(p13.1;q22)/*CBFβ-MYH11* (collectively referred as *CBF leukemia*) to have low-risk AML. In contemporary clinical trials, the overall survival (OS) rates are approximately 90% for this group of patients. Although *KIT* mutations confer an inferior prognosis in adults with CBF leukemia, their prognostic significance in children is not clear. Thus, most clinical trials classify children with CBF leukemia as having low-risk disease, regardless of other genetic abnormalities.

Mutations of the *NPM1* gene are seen primarily in AML cases with normal karyotypes, with or without internal tandem duplications of the *FLT3* gene (*FLT3*-ITD). Children whose blasts contain *NPM1* mutations, normal karyotypes, and wild-type *FLT3* appear to have an excellent prognosis, although the data to support their classification as low-risk patients are not as strong as that for children with CBF leukemia. Similarly, biallelic mutations of *CEBPA* are

TABLE 62.2	Prognostically Important Genetic Abnormalities in Pediatric Acute Myeloid Leukemia
Favorable	
t(8;21)(q22;q22)/*RUNX1-RUNX1T1*	
inv(16)(p13.1;q22)/*CBFβ-MYH11*	
t(16;16)(p13.1;q22)/*CBFβ-MYH11*	
t(1;11)(q21;q23)/*MLL-MLLT11*	
NPM1/wt-*FLT3*	
CEBPA	
t(15;17)(q22;q12)/*PML-RARα*	
Unfavorable	
t(6;11)(q27;q23)/*MLL-MLLT4*	
t(10;11)(p12;q23)/*MLL-MLLT10*	
t(10;11)(p11.2;q23)/*MLL-ABI1*	
t(6;9)(p23;q34)/*DEK-NUP214*	
t(8;16)(p11;p13)/*MYST3-CREBBP*	
t(16;21)(q24;q22)/*RUNX1-CBFA2T3*	
t(5;11)(q35;p15.5)/*NUP98-NSD1*	
inv(16)(p13.3q24.3)/*CBFA2T3-GLIS2*	
FLT3-ITD	
Monosomy 7	
Likely Unfavorable	
IDH1, IDH2	
RUNX1	
TET2	
DNMT3A	
Intermediate or Unknown	
t(9;11)(p12;q23)/*MLL-MLLT3*	
Other *MLL*	
t(1;22)(p13;q13)/*RBM15-MKL1*	

associated with normal karyotypes and a favorable outcome in adults with AML, but occur in less than 5% of childhood AML cases. Nevertheless, they are likely to be associated with a favorable outcome and are included as a low-risk feature in many treatment protocols.

Genetic abnormalities, for which there is strong evidence of an association with a high risk of relapse, include monosomy 7 and *FLT3*-ITD. The outcome of patients with *FLT3*-ITD is especially poor in cases with high ratios of *FLT3*-ITD to wild-type *FLT3*. Translocations that create chimeric fusion genes and likely confer a poor prognosis include the t(6;11)(q27;q23)/*MLL-MLLT4*, t(10;11)(p12;q23)/*MLL-MLLT10*, t(10;11)(p11.2;q23)/*MLL-ABI1*, t(5;11)(q35;p15.5)/*NUP98-NSD1*, t(6;9)(p23;q34)/*DEK-NUP214*, t(8;16)(p11;p13)/*MYST3-CREBBP*, t(16;21)(q24;q22)/*RUNX1-CBFA2T3*, and inv(16)(p13.3q24.3)/*CBFA2T3-GLIS2*. The prognostic impact of other lesions, such as mutations of *WT1, IDH1, IDH2, RUNX1, TET2*, or *DNMT3A*, is not known. However, because they are associated with a high risk of relapse among adults with AML, it is likely that they also confer a poor outcome in children.

Response to therapy reflects features specific to the leukemia (genetic alterations and inherent sensitivity to chemotherapy), characteristics of the patient (pharmacogenomics and drug metabolism), as well as the intensity and components of therapy, and is therefore a key predictor of outcome. However, morphologic examination of the bone marrow, especially during periods of brisk hematopoietic recovery after intensive chemotherapy, is subjective and lacks the sensitivity and specificity required to accurately assess response. Methods that rely on leukemia-specific features that distinguish residual leukemia cells from normal hematopoietic precursors can provide more precise estimates of MRD. Techniques applicable to AML include RNA-based PCR analysis of leukemia-specific gene fusions, quantitative analysis of *WT1* expression, deep sequencing to detect leukemia-specific mutations, and flow cytometric detection of aberrant immunophenotypes. Although PCR detection of fusion transcripts is sensitive to a level of 0.01%–0.001%, it can be applied to only about 50% of cases. In addition, the significance of persistence

TABLE 62.3	Results of Recent Clinical Trials for Pediatric Acute Myeloid Leukemia						
Study	Years of Enrollment	Eligible Age (Years)	Number of Patients	CR (%)	EFS (%)	OS (%)
AIEOP AML 2002/01	2002–2011	≤18	482	87	55	68
AML-BFM 2004	2004–2010	<18	611	89	All: 55 L-DNR: 59 Ida: 53	All: 74 L-DNR: 76 Ida: 75
COG AAML0531	2006–2010	≤29	1022	87	GO: 53 No GO: 47	GO: 69 No GO: 65
JCACSG AML99	2000–2002	≤18	240	95	62	76
MRC AML12	1995–2002	<16	529	92	54	64
NOPHO AML 2004	2004–2009	≤18	151	92	57	69
SJCRH AML02	2002–2008	≤21	216	94	63	71

AIEOP, Associazione Italiana di Ematologia e Oncologia Pediatrica; BFM, Berlin-Frankfurt-Münster Study Group; COG, Children's Oncology Group; CR, complete remission; EFS, event-free survival; GO, gemtuzumab ozogamicin; Ida, idarubicin; JCACSG, Japanese Childhood AML Cooperative Study Group; L-DNR, liposomal daunorubicin; MRC, Medical Research Council; NOPHO, Nordic Society of Paediatric Haematology and Oncology; OS, overall survival; SJCRH, St Jude Children's Research Hospital.

of fusion transcript expression is not consistent across subtypes of AML. For example, persistent expression of *PML-RARA* is associated with a high risk of relapse among patients with APL, whereas the *RUNX1-RUNX1T1* and *CBFβ-MYH11* transcripts can be detected in patients with CBF leukemia who are in long-term remission. In contrast, the sensitivity of flow-based MRD assays is only 0.1%–0.01%, but this technique can be applied to more than 90% of cases and has been used successfully by investigators from the Children's Oncology Group (COG), the Berlin-Frankfurt-Münster (BFM) study group, St. Jude Children's Research Hospital (SJCRH), and the Dutch Childhood Oncology Group (DCOG). For example, among children with AML who were treated in the St. Jude AML02 trial, the 3-year cumulative incidence of relapse was 17% for patients without detectable MRD, 39% for those with >0.1% MRD, and 49% for patients with MRD levels >1%. It is clear, however, that better methods are needed to identify patients who are MRD negative by current techniques, but who still suffer relapse of their disease.

THERAPY

CR and OS rates are now greater than 90% and 60%, respectively, for children with AML (Table 62.3). Most induction regimens are based on the combination of cytarabine and daunorubicin, first developed in the 1970s. Attempts to improve remission induction rates have included the addition of other nucleoside analogues (cladribine or fludarabine), dose-intensification of cytarabine, the replacement of daunorubicin with idarubicin, mitoxantrone, or liposomal daunorubicin, and the addition of gemtuzumab ozogamicin (GO). Although all these interventions were found to be safe, randomized clinical trials demonstrated similar remission rates regardless of the dose of cytarabine, the addition of other nucleoside analogues, the substitution of daunorubicin with another anthracycline, or the addition of GO. It is likely that the increases in CR rates are largely due to improvements in supportive care, rather than to the development of better chemotherapy.

Clinical trials conducted during the 1980s and 1990s demonstrated that intensive postremission therapy, administered as intensive chemotherapy or HSCT, significantly improves outcome and is an essential component of therapy for all children with AML. By contrast, low-dose maintenance therapy may actually lower the survival rates. Trials performed during the past 20 years (Table 62.3) have sought to determine the optimal duration of postremission therapy, the benefit of new agents, the value of MRD monitoring, and the role of HSCT. However, like the interventions used to improve

remission induction rates, many of the postremission interventions have had only modest effects on survival.

Examples of large, well-designed randomized trials that have produced excellent results despite the lack of major differences between treatment arms include the AML-BFM 2004 and the COG AAML0531 trials. In the BFM trial, 521 children with AML were randomly assigned to receive liposomal daunorubicin (80 mg/m²/day for 3 days) or idarubicin (12 mg/m²/day for 3 days) in combination with cytarabine and etoposide during induction therapy. Results were similar between the liposomal daunorubicin and idarubicin treatment arms: OS, 76% versus 75%; EFS, 59% versus 53%, and cumulative incidence of relapse, 29% versus vs 31%. Subgroup analyses suggested that patients with t(8;21) may benefit from the use of liposomal daunorubicin. In the COG trial, 1022 patients were randomly assigned to receive standard chemotherapy with or without the addition of three doses of GO. Although the incorporation of GO was associated with a better EFS (53% vs. 47%), there was no difference in OS between arms (69% vs. 65%). In this trial, GO had the greatest impact among patients with favorable karyotypes and had no effect on the outcome of high-risk patients. These trials illustrate the difficulties encountered when performing randomized studies of nonspecific agents in a heterogeneous disease with small subgroups.

Attempts to improve the results obtained with chemotherapy have included the use of autologous and allogeneic HSCT. Although autologous transplantation is rarely recommended for patients with AML, allogeneic HSCT is a reasonable option, as many studies have demonstrated that HSCT is associated with lower rates of relapse compared with chemotherapy. However, because HSCT is accompanied by higher rates of treatment-related mortality and morbidity than chemotherapy, the indications for performing HSCT in first remission remain controversial

In general, study groups in the United States recommend HSCT in first remission for a larger proportion of patients than do European investigators, who often reserve the use of HSCT for patients who are in second remission. However, improvements in supportive care, more comprehensive HLA typing, and the selection of killer inhibitory receptor (KIR)-mismatched donors, have led to fewer short- and long-term side effects and greater benefits. In recent trials the outcomes are similar regardless of donor type. For example, among children with high-risk AML who were treated in the St. Jude AML02 trial and underwent HSCT at our institution, the 5-year OS rates were 68%, 74%, and 77% for patients who received matched sibling donor, matched unrelated donor, and haploidentical donor transplants in first remission, respectively. In addition, the 5-year OS estimate was 67% for patients who had detectable disease (0.01%–5%)

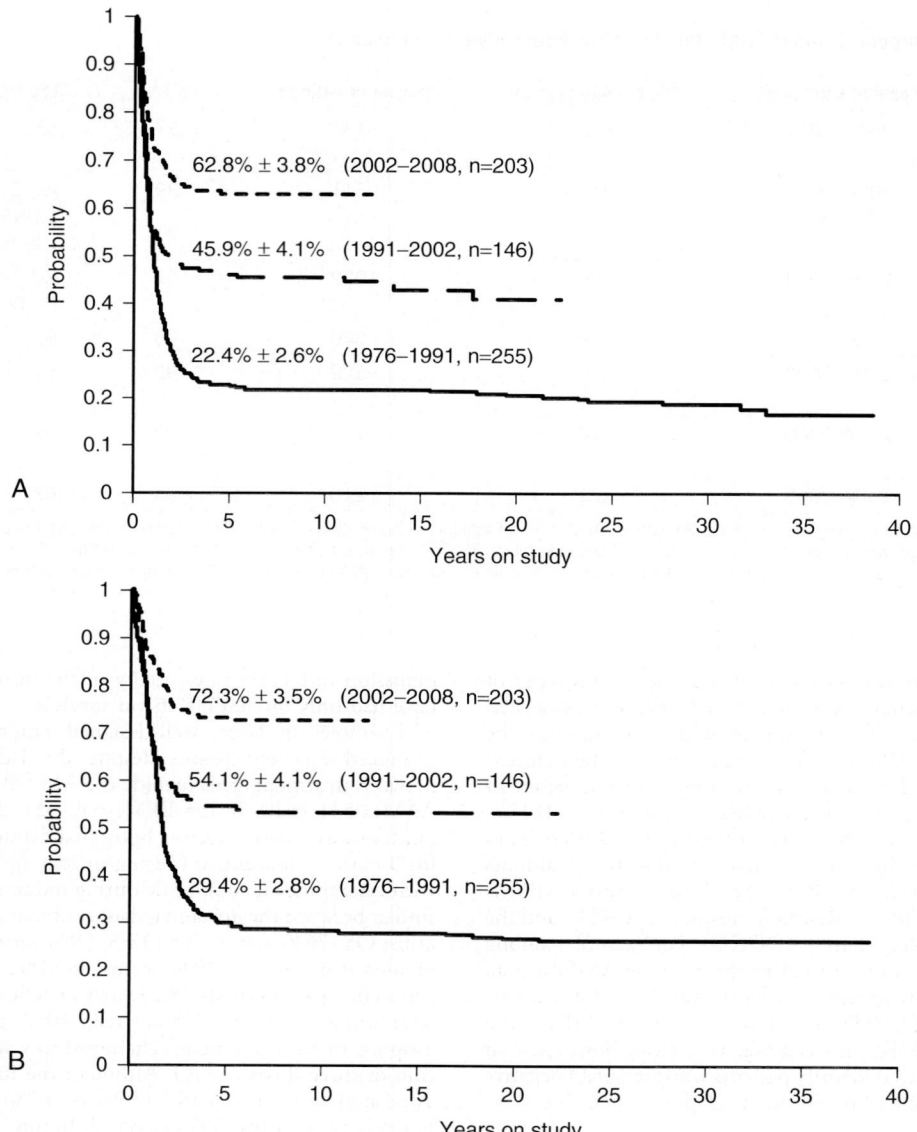

Fig. 62.3 EVENT-FREE SURVIVAL (A) AND OVERALL SURVIVAL (B) FOR PATIENTS WITH ACUTE MYELOID LEUKEMIA TREATED ON ST. JUDE TRIALS.

at the time of transplant, indicating that even though MRD is an important predictor of posttransplant outcome, it is not a contraindication to HSCT (Fig. 62.3).

Children with Down syndrome and AML have a favorable prognosis, with OS rates greater than 90%, and should be treated in cooperative group trials that are designed to minimize toxicity while maintaining high cure rates. The excellent outcome has been at least partly attributed to increased levels of cystathionine-β-synthetase, a high frequency of cystathionine-β-synthetase polymorphisms, and decreased levels of cytidine deaminase in the blasts of patients with Down syndrome, all of which result in altered metabolism of cytarabine. Approaches to the diagnosis, supportive care measures, and treatment of childhood APL are similar to those in adults with APL, including the immediate initiation of all-*trans* retinoic acid (ATRA) followed by the continued use of ATRA and arsenic trioxide, with or without the addition of conventional chemotherapy.

SUPPORTIVE CARE

Supportive care is an essential component of the management of children with AML. Initial leukocyte counts greater than 100,000/μL

are associated with risks of intracranial hemorrhage and respiratory insufficiency secondary to leukostasis. Therefore, all patients with hyperleukocytosis, as well as those with symptoms of leukostasis regardless of leukocyte count, should immediately receive interventions to reduce the leukemic burden, such as leukapheresis, exchange transfusion, hydroxyurea, or low-dose cytarabine (100–200 mg/m^2/day).

Infectious complications are a major cause of morbidity and mortality in children with AML. In fact, the cumulative incidence of documented infection is greater than 60% among AML patients who do not receive prophylactic antibiotics. Randomized, controlled trials conducted in adults with AML demonstrated that prophylactic antibiotics, such as oral levofloxacin, are effective at reducing the incidence of bacterial infection, but similar studies have not yet been completed in children. However, nonrandomized trials performed in pediatric patients with AML have shown that the use of prophylactic antibiotics, such as cefepime alone or the combination of vancomycin and ciprofloxacin, dramatically reduce the incidence of bacterial infection and decrease the length of hospital stay compared with historical controls. Although the emergence of drug-resistant bacteria is a concern, we believe that the benefits of prophylactic antibiotics outweigh this potential risk (Box 62.2).

As a result of prolonged periods of neutropenia secondary to myelosuppressive therapy, patients with acute myeloid leukemia (AML) are at high risk of bacterial and fungal infections. Prior to our implementation of prophylactic antibiotics 10 years ago, we observed documented bacterial infections, most commonly caused by viridans group streptococci, in approximately two-thirds of AML patients. We subsequently demonstrated that the use of prophylactic antibiotics, such as cefepime alone or the combination of vancomycin and ciprofloxacin, dramatically reduced the incidence of bacterial infection, decreased length of hospital stays, and could be safely administered by caregivers in the outpatient setting. Although the emergence of drug-resistant bacteria is a concern, we believe that the benefits of prophylactic antibiotics outweigh this potential risk. To further address the risks and benefits of prophylactic antibiotics, the Children's Oncology Group is currently evaluating prophylactic levofloxacin in children with leukemia who are at high risk of infection. Because disseminated fungal infections are also common in children with AML, we recommend that all patients receive antifungal prophylaxis with micafungin, caspofungin, voriconazole, or posaconazole. Micafungin and caspofungin provide excellent coverage for infections caused by *Candida* species, but are less active than voriconazole and posaconazole against *Aspergillus* species. Our use of prophylactic voriconazole has been associated with a decrease in the incidence of *Aspergillus* infections, but we have seen the emergence of other molds, such as *Fusarium*, *Mucor*, and *Rhizopus*. Although we have successfully treated these infections with posaconazole, we must be wary of the development of posaconazole resistance.

Disseminated fungal infections, most commonly caused by *Candida* and *Aspergillus* species, are also frequently seen in children with AML. Because several randomized, controlled trials demonstrated the benefits of prophylactic antifungal therapy in adults with cancer, many pediatric oncologists recommend antifungal prophylaxis for children with AML. Available agents include fluconazole, itraconazole, voriconazole, posaconazole, micafungin, and caspofungin. Among the azoles, fluconazole and itraconazole are not ideal because they are less active against *Aspergillus* species than voriconazole and posaconazole. Although the latter agents are both active against *Aspergillus* species, posaconazole has greater activity against other molds, such as *Fusarium*, *Mucor*, and *Rhizopus*. Micafungin and caspofungin are not as broadly active as voriconazole and posaconazole, but their ease of administration (daily intravenous infusion), compatibility with other drugs, and less variable pharmacokinetic properties suggest that they are reasonable choices as well.

FUTURE DIRECTIONS

Tyrosine Kinase Inhibitors

AML cells commonly possess aberrant receptor tyrosine kinase activity as a result of genetic alterations, such as *FLT3*-ITD. These alterations are seen in approximately 15% of pediatric and 30% of adult AML cases, and are associated with a poor outcome, particularly in cases with high ratios of *FLT3*-ITD to wild-type *FLT3*. Evidence that *FLT3* mutations are driver lesions suggests that they are rational targets to which inhibitors should be tested. Recent studies have demonstrated that sorafenib, sunitinib, and other FLT3 inhibitors are highly active in patients with *FLT3* mutations, but that prolonged use of these agents is associated with the development of resistance, most commonly caused by the acquisition of point mutations in the kinase domain. Crenolanib, a novel tyrosine kinase inhibitor, is active in sorafenib-resistant AML mouse models that contain the *FLT3* D835 or F691 mutations, suggesting that this agent may extend clinical benefit. Further studies are needed to determine the optimal dose, schedule, and combination of inhibitors that are required to improve the long-term outcome of patients with *FLT3* mutations. Although tyrosine kinase inhibitors represent a distinct approach to

AML therapy, target validation is slow and new therapeutic strategies are needed.

Epigenetic Agents

Abnormal regulation of epigenetic modification, such as histone acetylation and DNA methylation, is likely a key factor in the pathogenesis of AML. A central role for epigenetic dysfunction in AML is supported by the observation of mutations and translocations in genes involved in these processes, such as *TET2*, *DNMT3*, *IDH1*, *IDH2*, and *MLL*. These findings suggest that histone deacetylase inhibitors and demethylating agents may be active, either alone or in combination with chemotherapy, in AML. The histone deacetylase inhibitor vorinostat as well as the DNA hypomethylating agents decitabine and 5-azacytidine have shown promising activity and are currently being tested in combination with chemotherapy. A related epigenetic target in childhood AML is the DOT1L histone methyltransferase, which is required for transformation by MLL fusion proteins. A DOT1L inhibitor (EPZ-5676) is now in phase I trials for adults and children with relapsed *MLL*-rearranged leukemia. Recently, the bromodomain and extraterminal (BET) family of proteins (BRD2, BRD3, BRD4, and BRDT), which bind acetylated lysines in histone tails and regulate gene expression by recruiting multiprotein complexes such as MLL to super enhancer regions, have also been explored as drug targets in AML. Preclinical models show that BET inhibitors are active against a variety of malignancies, including AML, and at least four such inhibitors are in early clinical trials.

Antibody-Based Therapies

Most antibody-directed therapies for AML have focused on CD33, which is expressed on the surface of leukemia blasts in greater than 90% of cases. GO, a humanized anti-CD33 antibody conjugated to calicheamicin, was approved by the United States Food and Drug Administration in 2000, but was later withdrawn from the market because of concerns of toxicity. However, the results of randomized trials that were completed after the withdrawal of GO suggest that the addition of GO to conventional chemotherapy reduces the risk of relapse and improves event-free survival. Metaanalyses demonstrate that the benefit of GO was greatest among low-risk patients, with only modest benefits seen in intermediate-risk patients and no benefits in patients with high-risk disease. Recently, a novel anti-CD33 conjugate (SGN-CD33A), in which calicheamicin is replaced with a synthetic pyrrolobenzodiazepine, was shown to be more potent than GO at inducing apoptosis in AML in preclinical models, and is now being evaluated in Phase I clinical trials.

An alternative approach to enhancing the efficacy of CD33-directed therapy is through the development of CD33/CD3-directed bispecific T-cell engager (BiTE) antibodies. By bridging CD33 with T-cell receptors (TCRs), BiTE antibodies can direct T-cell effector functions to AML cells. In preclinical models, the CD33/CD3 BiTE AMG 330 was able to recruit T cells, resulting in potent CD33-dependent cytotoxicity. Analogous to BiTE antibodies, bispecific killer cell engagers (BiKE) target CD16 on natural killer (NK) cells and tumor-specific antigens, such as CD33. A CD33/CD16 BiKE has recently been shown to induce NK cell function and eliminate CD33$^+$ AML cells in preclinical models. It is likely that BiTE and BiKE antibodies will soon be tested in clinical trials for patients with relapsed AML (Box 62.3).

Natural Killer Cell Therapy

The beneficial effects of KIR-mismatched donor NK cells in the setting of allogeneic HSCT for AML has led to interest in the use of allogeneic NK cells in the non-HSCT setting. We performed a pilot study that demonstrated that infusions of haploidentical NK cells in patients with AML were well tolerated and associated with transient engraftment, expansion of donor NK cells, minimal toxicity, and no graft-versus-host disease. Although these results suggest that treatment with haploidentical mismatched NK cells is a safe and potentially valuable approach to reduce the risk of relapse in patients with AML, clinical trials are required to investigate its benefits. In addition, it is likely that enhancement of NK cell activity will be required to provide optimal antileukemic effects. Potential methods to increase NK cell activity include the expansion of activated NK cells, the addition of lineage-specific antibodies, the use of anti-KIR antibodies to block inhibitory KIRs, and the depletion of host regulatory T cells, which may inhibit the proliferation of donor NK cells.

Chimeric Antigen Receptor-Modified T Cells

T cells can be redirected to target cells of interest through the use of chimeric antigen receptors (CARs), which link a target cell ligand-recognition domain to signaling regions from the TCR. First-generation CARs typically incorporated the TCRζ cytoplasmic domain, but it was later demonstrated that tandem signaling domains incorporating the TCR along with costimulatory or coreceptor signals provided more robust stimulation and enhanced the survival, expansion, and activity of CAR-modified T cells. The clinical effectiveness of CAR-modified T cells was first established in B-cell malignancies using a CD19-41BB–ζ CAR, originally developed by Imai and Campana at St. Jude.

A major challenge to extending the success achieved with CD19-specific CARs to AML is identifying the proper recognition domain, because effective therapy will require eradication of the leukemic initiating cells as well as their more mature descendants. The widespread expression of CD33 on leukemic cells and the absence of downmodulation after GO treatment indicate that it is a robust target. Preclinical studies performed in NOD-SCID mouse models suggest that CD33 CAR-modified T cells should be investigated. However, the potential depletion of normal hematopoietic precursors or committed myeloid progenitor cells may cause unacceptable long-term neutropenia. In addition, the absence of CD33 expression on leukemic stem cells in some cases may limit the efficacy of such therapy. Future clinical trials and additional modifications of CD33 CARs will address these important issues.

CONCLUSION

Recent studies of the genetics and biology of AML have identified new therapeutics targets and have led to the development of novel therapies, many of which are now in early-phase clinical trials. We hope that these efforts will lead to the development of more effective and less toxic treatments in the near future. However, the evaluation of these treatment strategies will require collaboration between cooperative groups to ensure that adequate numbers of patients to which each therapy is directed can be studied.

SUGGESTED READINGS

Andersson A, Ma J, Wang J, et al: The landscape of somatic mutations in infant MLL rearranged acute lymphoblastic leukemias. *Nat Genet* 47:330, 2015.

Creutzig U, Zimmermann M, Bourquin JP, et al: Randomized trial comparing liposomal daunorubicin with idarubicin in induction for pediatric acute myeloid leukemia: results from Study AML-BFM 2004. *Blood* 122:37–43, 2013.

Fujisaki H, Kakuda H, Shimasaki N, et al: Expansion of highly cytotoxic human natural killer cells for cancer cell therapy. *Cancer Res* 69:4010–4017, 2009.

Gamis AS, Alonzo TA, Meshinchi S, et al: Gemtuzumab ozogamicin in children and adolescents with De Novo acute myeloid leukemia improves event-free survival by reducing relapse risk: results from the randomized phase III Children's Oncology Group trial AAML0531. *J Clin Oncol* 32:3021–3032, 2014.

Gibson BE, Webb DK, Howman AJ, et al: Results of a randomized trial in children with Acute Myeloid Leukaemia: medical research council AML12 trial. *Br J Haematol* 155:366–376, 2011.

Grisendi S, Mecucci C, Falini B, et al: Nucleophosmin and cancer. *Nat Rev Cancer* 6:493–505, 2006.

Gruber TA, Larson GA, Zhang J, et al: An Inv(16)(p13.3q24.3)-Encoded CBFA2T3-GLIS2 Fusion Protein Defines an Aggressive Subtype of Pediatric Acute Megakaryoblastic Leukemia. *Cancer Cell* 22:683–697, 2012.

Hitzler JK, Zipursky A: Origins of leukaemia in children with Down syndrome. *Nat Rev Cancer* 5:11–20, 2005.

Inaba H, Coustan-Smith E, Cao X, et al: Comparative analysis of different approaches to measure treatment response in acute myeloid leukemia. *J Clin Oncol* 30:3625–3632, 2012.

Inaba H, Gaur AH, Cao X, et al: Feasibility, efficacy, and adverse effects of outpatient antibacterial prophylaxis in children with acute myeloid leukemia. *Cancer* 120:1985–1992, 2014.

Inaba H, Rubnitz JE, Coustan-Smith E, et al: Phase I pharmacokinetic and pharmacodynamic study of the multikinase inhibitor sorafenib in combination with clofarabine and cytarabine in pediatric relapsed/refractory leukemia. *J Clin Oncol* 29:3293–3300, 2011.

Kaspers GJ, Zimmermann M, Reinhardt D, et al: Improved outcome in pediatric relapsed acute myeloid leukemia: results of a randomized trial on liposomal daunorubicin by the International BFM Study Group. *J Clin Oncol* 31:599–607, 2013.

Klco JM, Spencer DH, Miller CA, et al: Functional heterogeneity of genetically defined subclones in acute myeloid leukemia. *Cancer Cell* 25:379–392, 2014.

Krivtsov AV, Armstrong SA: MLL translocations, histone modifications and leukaemia stem-cell development. *Nat Rev Cancer* 7:823–833, 2007.

Kung Sutherland MS, Walter RB, Jeffrey SC, et al: SGN-CD33A: a novel CD33-targeting antibody-drug conjugate using a pyrrolobenzodiazepine dimer is active in models of drug-resistant AML. *Blood* 122:1455–1463, 2013.

Laszlo GS, Gudgeon CJ, Harrington KH, et al: Cellular determinants for preclinical activity of a novel CD33/CD3 bispecific T-cell engager (BiTE) antibody, AMG 330, against human AML. *Blood* 123:554–561, 2014.

Leung W, Campana D, Yang J, et al: High success rate of hematopoietic cell transplantation regardless of donor source in children with very high-risk leukemia. *Blood* 118:223–230, 2011.

Leung W, Pui CH, Coustan-Smith E, et al: Detectable minimal residual disease before hematopoietic cell transplantation is prognostic but does not preclude cure for children with very-high-risk leukemia. *Blood* 120:468–472, 2012.

Ley TJ, Mardis ER, Ding L, et al: DNA sequencing of a cytogenetically normal acute myeloid leukaemia genome. *Nature* 456:66–72, 2008.

Loken MR, Alonzo TA, Pardo L, et al: Residual disease detected by multidimensional flow cytometry signifies high relapse risk in patients with de novo acute myeloid leukemia: a report from Children's Oncology Group. *Blood* 120:1581–1588, 2012.

Meshinchi S, Alonzo TA, Stirewalt DL, et al: Clinical implications of FLT3 mutations in pediatric AML. *Blood* 108:3654–3661, 2006.

Miyamoto T, Nagafuji K, Akashi K, et al: Persistence of multipotent progenitors expressing AML1/ETO transcripts in long-term remission patients with t(8;21) acute myelogenous leukemia. *Blood* 87:4789–4796, 1996.

O'Hear C, Heiber JF, Schubert I, et al: Anti-CD33 chimeric antigen receptor targeting of acute myeloid leukemia. *Haematologica* 100:336–344, 2015.

Radtke I, Mullighan CG, Ishii M, et al: Genomic analysis reveals few genetic alterations in pediatric acute myeloid leukemia. *Proc Natl Acad Sci USA* 106:12944–12949, 2009.

Renneville A, Roumier C, Biggio V, et al: Cooperating gene mutations in acute myeloid leukemia: a review of the literature. *Leukemia* 22:915–931, 2008.

Rubnitz JE, Inaba H, Dahl G, et al: Minimal residual disease-directed therapy for childhood acute myeloid leukaemia: results of the AML02 multicentre trial. *Lancet Oncol* 11:543–552, 2010.

Rubnitz JE, Inaba H, Ribeiro RC, et al: NKAML: a pilot study to determine the safety and feasibility of haploidentical natural killer cell transplantation in childhood acute myeloid leukemia. *J Clin Oncol* 28:955–959, 2010.

Rujkijyanont P, Chan WK, Eldridge PW, et al: Ex vivo activation of CD56(+) immune cells that eradicate neuroblastoma. *Cancer Res* 73:2608–2618, 2013.

Schubbert S, Shannon K, Bollag G: Hyperactive Ras in developmental disorders and cancer. *Nat Rev Cancer* 7:295–308, 2007.

Schuettengruber B, Chourrout D, Vervoort M, et al: Genome regulation by polycomb and trithorax proteins. *Cell* 128:735–745, 2007.

Sung L, Aplenc R, Alonzo TA, et al: Effectiveness of supportive care measures to reduce infections in pediatric AML: a report from the Children's Oncology Group. *Blood* 121:3573–3577, 2013.

Tasian SK, Pollard JA, Aplenc R: Molecular therapeutic approaches for pediatric acute myeloid leukemia. *Front Oncol* 4:1–11, 2014.

Tsukimoto I, Tawa A, Horibe K, et al: Risk-stratified therapy and the intensive use of cytarabine improves the outcome in childhood acute myeloid leukemia: the AML99 trial from the Japanese Childhood AML Cooperative Study Group. *J Clin Oncol* 27:4007–4013, 2009.

Wang ZY, Chen Z: Acute promyelocytic leukemia: from highly fatal to highly curable. *Blood* 111:2505–2515, 2008.

Zimmerman EI, Turner DC, Buaboonnam J, et al: Crenolanib is active against models of drug-resistant FLT3-ITD-positive acute myeloid leukemia. *Blood* 122:3607–3615, 2013.

MYELODYSPLASTIC SYNDROMES AND MYELOPROLIFERATIVE NEOPLASMS IN CHILDREN

Franklin O. Smith, Christopher C. Dvorak, and Benjamin S. Braun

The myelodysplastic syndromes (MDS) and myeloproliferative neoplasms (MPN) are a heterogeneous group of clonal stem cell disorders that result in ineffective hematopoiesis and an increased risk of developing acute myeloid leukemia (AML). In children, MDS and MPN are now classified into three main groups: MDS, juvenile myelomonocytic leukemia (JMML), and transient abnormal myelopoiesis (TAM) in children with Down syndrome. Whereas in MDS, ineffective hematopoiesis results in progressive cytopenias, in MPN, at least initially, ineffective hematopoiesis leads to excessive proliferation frequently characterized by increased peripheral blood counts. MDS and MPN are rare in children. Chronic myeloid leukemia (CML), characterized by the Philadelphia chromosome (*BCR/ABL* positive) is seen in both children and adults, but other forms of MPN (polycythemia vera [PV], essential thrombocythemia [ET], primary myelofibrosis, chronic neutrophilic leukemia, chronic eosinophilic leukemia, chronic basophilic leukemia, chronic myelomonocytic leukemia, systemic mastocytosis [SM], and stem cell leukemia–lymphoma syndrome) are exceedingly rare in children. Readers interested in CML and disorders that are predominantly found in adults are referred to in Chapters 67–70. In contrast, two MPNs are uniquely pediatric: JMML and Down syndrome–associated TAM.

MYELODYSPLASTIC SYNDROMES

The MDS are a heterogeneous group of clonal disorders characterized by ineffective hematopoiesis, impaired maturation of hematopoietic cells, progressive cytopenias, and dysplastic changes in the bone marrow (BM).

Epidemiology

MDS is a common malignancy of adults with an incidence of 50 cases per million in people older than the age of 60 years.[1] In contrast, MDS accounts for only 3%–7% of all hematologic malignancies in children, with an unknown true incidence, owing in part to the inclusion of children with Down syndrome in some estimates. Several population-based studies have been performed with reported incidences of 4.0 cases per million in Denmark,[2] 3.1 per million in British Columbia (Canada),[3] and 1.35 per million in the United Kingdom.[4] The median age of presentation is 6.8 years with an equal sex distribution.[4–6] However, in a study of children with advanced or high-risk MDS, the median age of presentation was older at 10.7 years with a 2:1 male to female ratio.[7]

Pathobiology

As in adults, MDS in children can be considered as primary (de novo) or secondary. In adults, two predominant patterns of primary, de novo MDS have been observed. In the first of these patterns, the disease is indolent in nature and is characterized by prolonged survival, little accumulated genetic damage, and a low probability of progression to AML. This group of diseases is best exemplified by the 5q– syndrome, an entity not seen in children. Far more common in adults is a disease characterized by the accumulation of genetic damage, progression to BM failure, and a high probability of developing AML. This form of the disease is characterized as a mutator phenotype.[8] The primary MDS seen in children appear to share this mutator phenotype.

As in adults, secondary MDS in children can also arise as sequelae from exposure to chemotherapy and radiation, and from genetic conditions including monosomy 7 syndrome, Down syndrome, paroxysmal nocturnal hemoglobinuria (PNH), neurofibromatosis, Bloom syndrome, and Li-Fraumeni syndrome. However, MDS in children may often result from inherited constitutional BM failure syndromes including Fanconi anemia (FA), severe congenital neutropenia, Shwachman-Diamond syndrome, congenital amegakaryocytic thrombocytopenia, dyskeratosis congenital, Diamond-Blackfan anemia, and MonoMAC syndrome. Unlike de novo MDS in the elderly, the true incidence of de novo MDS in children may become less frequently diagnosed as genetics and inherited constitutional BM failure syndromes (IBMFS) causes of secondary MDS are increasingly identified in children.

Ongoing studies are now defining the molecular pathogenesis and interrelationships among MDS, MPN, and AML.[9–11] Accumulating data suggest that aberrant signal transduction resulting from acquired somatic mutations encoding proteins leading to hyperactivation of the Ras pathway may stimulate proliferation without concomitant differentiation.[10] This has been clearly demonstrated in CML (*BCR-ABL*).[12,13] A number of other putative pathogenetic mutations have been identified in other myeloproliferative disorders, including *JAK2* V617F mutations in PV, ET, and primary myelofibrosis[14]; *KIT* D816V mutations in SM[15]; *FIPL1-PDGFRA* in chronic eosinophilic leukemia-SM[16]; *ZNF198-FG4FR1* mutations in stem cell leukemia–lymphoma syndrome[17]; *RAS/NF1/PTPN11* mutations in JMML[18–20] (Fig. 63.1); and *GATA1* mutations in TAM.[21]

AML is the result of cooperating mutations in genes that confer a proliferative and survival advantage (e.g., activating mutations in receptor tyrosine kinases [FLT3, c-kit]) and genes that impair differentiation and apoptosis (e.g., loss-of-function mutations in transcription factors [CBF, AML/ETO]) (Fig. 63.2). This multistep model for the pathogenesis of AML is supported by murine models,[22,23] the analysis of leukemia in twins,[24–27] and the analysis of patients with familial platelet disorder with a propensity to develop AML (FDP/AML syndrome).[28]

Recent advances in sequencing techniques and a rapidly evolving understanding of the biology of epigenetics (global methylation and histone modification) and mRNA slicing machinery have transformed our understanding of oncogenic driver mutations in adult MDS.[29–32] In adults with MDS, approximately 50% of patients have recurrent mutations in a slicing factor (*SF3B1, U2AF1, SRSF2, ZRSR2*), a novel class of cancer-associated genes that was only recently recognized to be important in MDS. Similarly, the same percent of adult patients have at least one mutated epigenetic regulator (*TET2, ASXL1, DNMT3A, EZH2, IDH1,* and *IDH2*), whereas approximately 25% of adults will have mutations in both splicing factors and epigenetic regulators. Karyotypic abnormalities (5/5q–, 7/7q–, 3q, 20q) alone occur in approximately 5% of adults. Approximately 15% of adult patients have mutations in other genes (without associated mutations

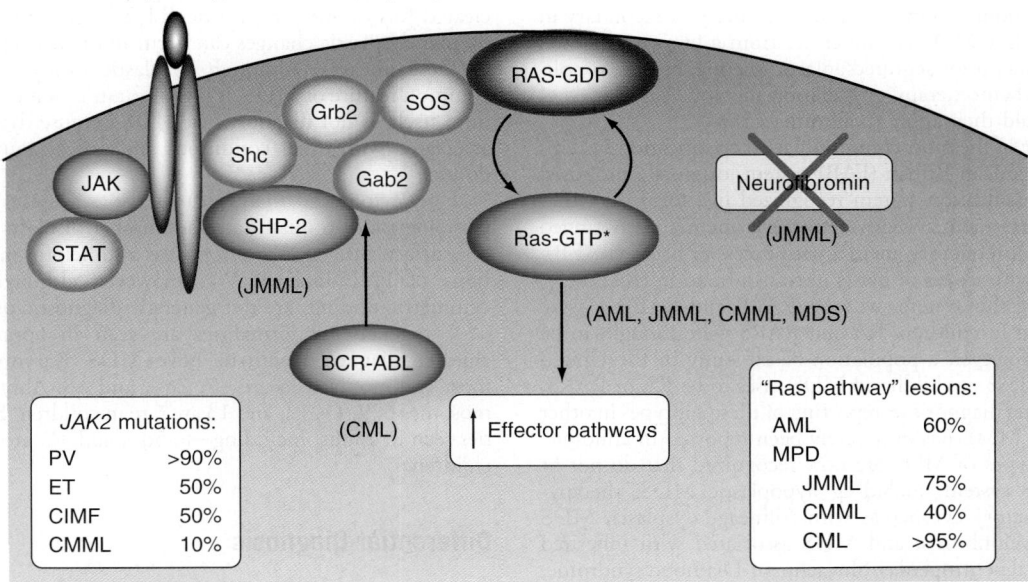

Fig. 63.1 OVERVIEW OF RAS SIGNALING WITH MOLECULES HARBORING MUTATIONS IN PATIENTS WITH MYELOID MALIGNANCIES. *AML*, Acute myeloid leukemia; *CML*, chronic myeloid leukemia; *CMML*, chronic myelomonocytic leukemia; *ET*, essential thrombocythema; *GDP*, guanosine diphosphate; *GTP*, guanosine triphosphate; *JAK*, Janus-activated kinase; *JMML*, juvenile myelomonocytic leukemia; *MDS*, myelodysplastic syndromes; *MPD*, myeloproliferative disorder; *PV*, polycythemia vera.

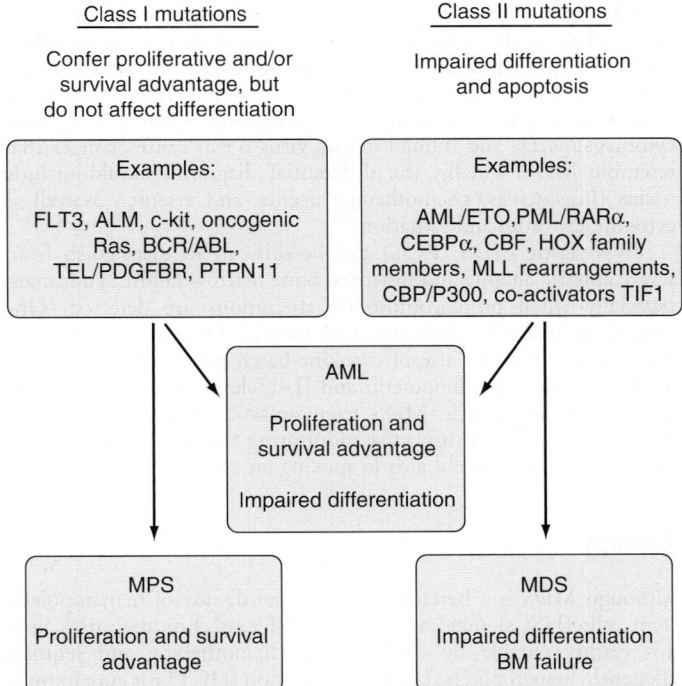

Fig. 63.2 COOPERATING MUTATIONS IN ACUTE MYELOID LEUKEMIA, MYELOPROLIFERATIVE SYNDROMES, AND MYELO-DYSPLASTIC SYNDROMES. *AML*, acute myeloid leukemia; *BM*, Bone marrow; *MDS*, myelodysplastic syndromes; *MPS*, myeloproliferative syndromes.

in mRNA spicing genes or DNA methylation genes) including transcription factors (*RUNX1*, *ETV6*, *PHF6*, *GATA2*), kinase signaling genes (*NRAS*, *KRAS*, *JAK2*, *CBL*), and cohesion genes (*STAG2*, *SMC3*, *RAD21*). Finally, approximately 10% of adult patients have no mutations detectable.[32] This remarkable improvement in the understanding of the genetic events underlying adult MDS is leading to improved methods of risk-group stratification and prognosis (e.g., *TP53* mutations are associated with adverse disease features and outcomes).[33–35]

The patterns of genetic and karyotypic abnormalities in children with MDS are increasingly distinctive from that of adults. Although a few karyotypic abnormalities are shared (e.g., 7/7q–), many that are common in adults are only rarely found in children (e.g., 5q–). Importantly, mutations in mRNA spicing genes and other genes are only rarely found in children with de novo and secondary MDS.[36–39] Mutations in epigenetic genes that control DNA methylation and histone function are also only rarely identified in children, making their role in MDS uncertain. For example, although mutations in *TET2* are identified in 20%–25% of adults with MDS, only one out of 19 children with refractory cytopenia of childhood (RCC) had a mutation in *TET2*.[40] Instead, the genetic abnormalities in children with MDS are most often those associated with inherited BM failure syndromes and other genetic disorders (*FANC* member genes, *DKC*, *TERT*, *TREC*, *WAS*, *GATA-2*, *SBDS*, etc.).

Finally, three exceedingly rare familial forms of MDS/AML are associated with mutations in *RUNX1/AML1* (familial platelet disorder with a predisposition to AML), *CEBPα* (familial AML), and *GATA-2*.[39,41–43]

Classification

Until recently, MDS in children was poorly defined, characterized, classified, and reported. In fact, MDS was not included in the International Classification of Childhood Cancer until 2005.[44] Also contributing to this lack of information was the use of classification and prognostic systems designed for adults that have had limited applicability to children. A number of classification systems for children and adults have now been proposed. Taken together, it may be useful to think about childhood MDS as primary or secondary in nature, with secondary MDS arising either from a known inherited BM failure syndrome, prior acquired aplastic anemia, or as a complication from prior chemotherapy or radiation therapy. A diagnosis of primary MDS would then apply to all other cases.

Historically, one of the most commonly used classification systems was the French-American-British (FAB) system, originally proposed in 1982.[45] This classification system recognized five forms of MDS in adults: refractory anemia (RA), refractory anemia with ringed sideroblasts (RARS), refractory anemia with excess of blasts (RAEB), refractory anemia with excess of blasts in transformation (RAEB-T), and CMML. Using this system, whereas RAEB and RAEB-T were commonly reported in children, RA and RARS were thought to be rare in children. However, a population-based study in the United Kingdom showed 25% of childhood MDS cases to be RA or RARS, suggesting inaccurate diagnosis or reporting of these subtypes in other pediatric studies. CMML has only rarely been reported in children.

Additional subtypes of MDS are now recognized that do not fit well into the FAB system, including hypoplastic MDS, therapy-related MDS, refractory cytopenias with trilineage dysplasia, MDS associated with myelofibrosis, and MDS associated with inherited disorders (congenital neutropenias, Shwachman-Diamond syndrome, FA), Down syndrome, neurofibromatosis type 1, and mitochondrial cytopathies.[46,47] Therefore the World Health Organization (WHO) proposed changes to the FAB criteria to account for many of these subtypes.[48,49] Importantly, whereas adults commonly present with RA without cytopenias in the myeloid or platelet lineages, this is very rare in children since they more often have cytopenias in more than one cell line. Therefore children with low-grade MDS are classified as having refractory cytopenia as opposed to RA. Thus in 2008 the WHO classification of pediatric MDS included the provisional category of RCC based on persistent cytopenia with less than 5% blasts in the bone marrow and less than 2% blasts in the peripheral blood.[50] Under this classification, it is recommended that children with refractory cytopenia with multilineage dysplasia (RCMD) be classified as RCC until it is clarified whether the number of lineages involved is an important prognostic discriminator in childhood MDS. Under the 2016 revision of the WHO classification of myeloid and neoplasms and acute leukemia, RCC remains a provisional entry.[51]

Clinical Manifestations

Signs and symptoms of MDS are nonspecific and are usually attributable to pancytopenia (fever, infections, pallor, fatigue, bruising, and petechiae). Lymphadenopathy, hepatomegaly, and splenomegaly are uncommon presenting signs in children with MDS.

Laboratory Manifestations

Commonly accepted minimal diagnostic criteria for pediatric MDS include the absence of common de novo AML karyotypic abnormalities and at least two of the following: (1) sustained, unexplained anemia; neutropenia or thrombocytopenia; dysplastic morphology in the erythroid; granulocytic or megakaryocytic lineages (at least bilineage), and (2) an acquired, sustained clonal cytogenetic abnormality and 5% or more blasts in the BM.[8,52] Almost half of all children with MDS in one series presented with refractory cytopenia, most notably neutropenia and thrombocytopenia.[53]

Morphologically, the BM may be hypocellular, normocellular, or hypercellular. A diagnosis of MDS is made based on the presence of dysplastic changes in at least two cell lineages. The dysplastic changes in the granulocytes (hypogranulation, nuclear hyposegmentation, megaloblastoid maturation, and a left shift with an increased number of myeloblasts), megakaryocytes (micromegakaryocytes, abnormal megakaryocyte nuclei), monocytes (increase in BM monocytes, abnormal granulation with persistence of azurophilic granules,

hemophagocytosis, abnormal nuclei, and giant forms), or erythroid lineages (megaloblastoid maturation, nuclear budding and multinucleated forms, and ringed sideroblasts) can be multiple and varied. Similar dysplastic changes can occur in the peripheral blood for each of these lineages. Although dysplastic changes in the BM are a common feature of MDS, it is important to remember that dysplasia, unto itself, is not diagnostic of MDS because dysplastic features are associated with other conditions and can be found in normal BM donors.[54]

Flow cytometric analysis can serve as a useful addition to histopathology and to quantitate the number of blasts based on aberrant cell surface antigen expression. It is also helpful in detecting populations of PNH-like cells[55,56]. However, although beneficial, flow cytometric findings are not generally diagnostic of MDS.

Cytogenetic abnormalities are seen in approximately half of children diagnosed with de novo MDS. Karyotypic abnormalities most commonly seen are −7, 7q−, and +8. Abnormalities in chromosomes 6, 9, 11, 12, and 13 are rare in children. Specific abnormalities seen in adults, including −5, 5q−, and −Y, are very rarely seen in children.

Differential Diagnosis

Although the history, physical examination, evaluation of the BM and peripheral blood, and cytogenetic analysis often make the diagnosis of MDS, other diseases should be considered. Congenital disorders such as Down syndrome, FA, Shwachman-Diamond syndrome, Diamond-Blackfan anemia, congenital dyserythropoietic anemias, and hereditary sideroblastic anemia should be considered. The differential should also include AML with a low blast count, mitochondrial cytopathies such as Pearson syndrome, rheumatic diseases including juvenile idiopathic arthritis, and myeloproliferative disorders. Specifically, PNH, although rare in children, should be considered. Deficiencies of vitamin B_{12} and folate can cause megaloblastic changes that resemble the dysplastic changes seen in MDS. Other nutritional deficiencies, including copper, iron, thiamine, riboflavin, and pyridoxine, should be considered. Infections caused by human immunodeficiency virus, parvovirus, Epstein-Barr virus, cytomegalovirus, and human herpes virus 6 can cause changes that resemble MDS. Finally, the differential diagnosis should include toxins (insecticides, chemotherapy agents, and arsenic), as well as cytokine exposure and radiation.

Hypoplastic MDS (RCC) can be difficult to distinguish from severe aplastic anemia and inherited bone marrow failure syndromes, especially when no chromosomal aberrations are detected. One interesting area of research that may help in differentiating between these diagnoses is the use of cytokine-based programs. In one preliminary study, thrombopoietin and IL-17 levels were useful in differentiating hypoplastic MDS from aplastic anemia.[57] When the diagnosis is unclear, prospective monitoring and serial BM examinations may serve as useful aids in making an accurate diagnosis.

Therapy

Although MDS is a heterogeneous, clonal disease of hematopoietic stem cells (HSCs) that can manifest different clinical courses, it is not readily curable by conventional chemotherapy and requires allogeneic hematopoietic cell transplantation (HCT) for cure in most cases. Some children with RCC and RCMD who do not have life-threatening neutropenia and who do not require transfusions may only require close observation (see box on Treatment Overview for Children With MDS). Although children with this disease may eventually develop progressive disease requiring HCT, they may have long periods when minimal treatment is required.[53] The use of AML-like chemotherapy for patients with RCMD with excess blasts (RCMD-EB) is controversial but may serve to "debulk" patients with a high percentage of blasts before HCT.[6,58,59] However, this potential benefit may be offset by toxicities associated with AML-like

Treatment Overview for Children With MDS

A multitude of agents have been studied for the treatment of myelodysplastic syndromes (MDS) in adults, but only rarely in children. These include low-dose chemotherapy (cytosine arabinoside, melphalan, hydroxyurea, etoposide, topotecan, 6-mercaptopurine, and busulfan), hormones (glucocorticoids and androgens), differentiating agents (13-*cis*-retinoic acid, all-*trans* retinoic acid), hematopoietic growth factors (granulocyte-macrophage colony-forming factor, granulocyte colony-forming factor, and erythropoietin), demethylating agents (decitabine, 5-azacytidine), proteosome inhibitors, antiangiogenic agents, and arsenic.[60–75] This has resulted in three drugs (lenalidomide, azacitidine, and decitabine) that are now approved by the US Food and Drug Administration for the treatment of MDS in adults. However, as there are currently no safety or efficacy data to support the use of these agents in children with MDS, these drugs are not approved for MDS in children.

In addition, a large number of agents are being tested in clinical trials in the broad categories of kinase inhibitors, deacetylase inhibitors and DNA methyltransferase inhibitors, altered cell metabolism, cytotoxics, cell cycle inhibitors, immunomodulators and immunosuppressive agents, apoptosis modulators, and others.[76]

The difficulty in assessing the safety and efficacy of new agents in children with MDS is illustrated by the Children's Oncology Group's recent prospective study of amifostine.[77] This prospective Phase II cooperative group study was unable to be completed because of lack of accrual. As a result, the safety and efficacy of amifostine in children with MDS remains uncertain. Despite a lack of successful prospective clinical trials in children with MDS, there are limited retrospective data on the use of the hypomethylating agent azacytidine in children with newly diagnosed MDS, and in the palliative setting, children with relapsed MDS. These children had RCC, advanced and secondary MDS,[78] and prior to allogeneic hematopoietic cell transplantation (HCT).[79] These retrospective reviews suggest that azacytidine is tolerable and responses are possible, although the safety and efficacy in these various clinical settings have not been demonstrated in prospective clinical trials in children.

Most children with MDS require allogeneic HCT for curative therapy. Although children have been included in published HCT studies for MDS that are largely focused on adult patients, several studies focus specifically on children.[80–85] Taken together, these studies suggest a probability of disease-free survival in about 50% of patients undergoing human leukocyte antigen–matched related donor HCT. The Center for International Blood and Marrow Transplant recently published results for 118 children with MDS who underwent unrelated donor HCT.[84] Forty-six children had refractory cytopenia, 55 with RAEB and 17 with RAEB-T. Relapse of disease was most likely in children with RAEB and RAEB-T, with transplant-related mortality highest in recipients of human leukocyte antigen–mismatched grafts. The 8-year probabilities of disease-free survival for children with refractory cytopenia, RAEB, and RAEB-T were 51%, 35%, and 29%, respectively (Fig. 63.3).

HCT has also been reported in children and young adults with secondary MDS and secondary AML after aplastic anemia,[86] and as a salvage, second transplant procedure after relapse or graft failure.[87] Current areas of investigation include the predictive value of Wilms tumor 1 expression prior to HCT,[88] monosomal karyotype at the time of diagnosis or time of HCT[89] and hematopoietic chimerism after transplantation.[90]

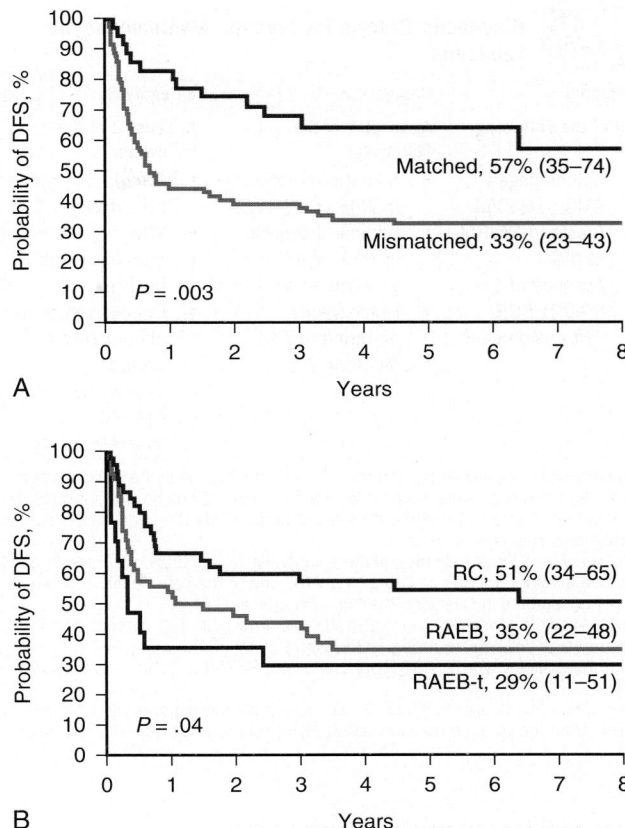

Fig. 63.3 (A) The 8-year probabilities of DFS after bone marrow transplantation (BMT): 57% for patients who received matched BMT (matched at human leukocyte antigen A, B, C, DRB1) and 33% for patients who received mismatched BMT. (B) The 8-year probabilities of disease-free survival after BMT: 51% when transplantation was performed for RC, 35% when transplantation was performed for RAEB, and 29% when transplantation was performed for RAEB-T. *DFS*, Disease-free survival; *RAEB*, refractory anemia with excess of blasts; *RAEB-T*, refractory anemia with excess of blasts in transformation; *RC*, refractory cytopenia. (*Reproduced with permission from Woodard P, Carpenter PA, Davies SM, et al: Unrelated donor bone marrow transplantation for myelodysplastic syndrome in children.* Bio Blood Marrow Transplant 17: 723, 2011.)

chemotherapy. Finally, patients with advanced MDS (RAEB-T or t-MDS) should be treated like those with AML.

Prognosis

Although a number of methods have been developed to predict the outcome of adults with MDS, the systems now most commonly used in adults are the International Prognostic Scoring System[91] that uses percentage bone marrow blasts, karyotype, and number of cytopenias to assign a score that is then used to predict outcome, and the WHO classification-based prognostic scoring system (WPSS) that includes more recently identified prognostic factors (e.g., transfusion dependency and multilineage dysplasia).[92] A recent study demonstrated

that both systems "well represent" the prognostic risk for patients whose MDS is defined by the WHO classification criteria.[93] Although these are effective tools for adults, their value for children is very limited.[94]

Secondary Myelodysplastic Syndrome

Secondary MDS can develop in both children and adults after exposure to chemotherapy and radiation. Alkylating agents used to treat Hodgkin disease, non-Hodgkin lymphoma, and Ewing sarcoma are particularly concerning in children.[95–107] Interestingly, there is also evidence to suggest that the cardioprotectant dexrazoxane, a topoisomerase II inhibitor with a mechanism of action that is different from etoposide and doxorubicin, may have increased the incidence of secondary MDS and AML in children treated for Hodgkin disease.[108]

Treatment options for children with secondary MDS are limited. Although AML-like chemotherapy can induce a period of remission and reduction in BM blasts, it is not curative. Allogeneic HCT has curative potential, but outcomes remain poor, with only 20%–30% of children surviving in reported series.[106,109,110] However, as noted earlier, recent data from the Center for International Blood and Marrow Transplant demonstrate that treatment failure with unrelated donor HCT is not higher compared with primary MDS.[84]

TABLE 63.1	Diagnostic Criteria for Juvenile Myelomonocytic Leukemia		
Category 1	**Category 2**	**Category 3**	
All of the Following:	**At Least 1 of the Following:**	**At Least 2 of the Following:**	
• Splenomegaly[a]	• Somatic mutation in RAS or PTPN11	• Circulating myeloid precursors	
• AMC >1000/µL	• Clinical diagnosis of NF1 or NF1 gene mutation	• WBC >10,000/µL	
• Blasts in PB/BM <20%		• Increased Hgb F for age	
• Absence of the t(9;22) BCR/ABL fusion gene	• Homozygous mutation in CBL	• Clonal cytogenetic abnormality excluding monosomy 7	
	• Monosomy 7	• GM-CSF hypersensitivity	

The diagnosis of juvenile myelomonocytic leukemia is made if a patient meets all of the Category 1 criteria and one of the Category 2 criteria without needing to meet the Category 3 criteria. If there are no Category 2 criteria met, then the Category 3 criteria must be met.

[a]For the 7%–10% of patients without splenomegaly, the diagnostic criteria must include all other features in Category 1 AND one of the parameters in Category 2 OR no features in Category 2 but two features in Category 3.

AMC, Absolute monocyte count; BM, bone marrow; GM-CSF, granulocyte-macrophage colony-stimulating factor; Hgb F, fetal hemoglobin; NF1, neurofibromatosis type 1; PB, peripheral blood; PTPN11,; WBC, white blood cell.

From Chan RJ, Cooper T, Kratz CP, et al: Juvenile myelomonocytic leukemia: A report from the 2nd International JMML Symposium. *Leuk Res* 33:355, 2009.

MYELOPROLIFERATIVE NEOPLASMS

Juvenile Myelomonocytic Leukemia

JMML is classified by the WHO as an overlap of MDS and MPN. It is an aggressive myeloid malignancy of young children with poor outcomes to conventional therapies. The diagnostic criteria are complex (Table 63.1), but recent advances in elucidating the molecular genetics of the disorder demonstrate that approximately 85% of children will harbor an alteration in one of five genes. Thus there is now international agreement on the diagnostic criteria[111] (see Table 63.1), with an emphasis on incorporating these molecular genetic criteria, as well as a recent definition of common response criteria.[112]

Epidemiology

The incidence of JMML in the United States has been estimated as 0.69–1.2 per million.[4,113] There is a male predominance with a median age of diagnosis of 1.8 years. The apparent incidence and demographic distribution may change in coming years because of refinement of diagnostic techniques such as molecular testing. In particular, mutation analysis may identify patients with less aggressive disease or at a younger age.

Pathogenesis

Early clonality studies suggested that JMML arose at the level of at least an immature myeloid precursor cell.[111,114–118] More recent data suggest that JMML may arise in a pluripotent stem cell with involvement of the myeloid, erythroid, and megakaryocyte lineages, as well as B lymphocytes and T lymphocytes.[111,119–122] This is supported by finding pathogenic mutations in immature hematopoietic cells identified by flow cytometry.[123]

Somatic mutations that augment signaling through the Ras pathway occur in approximately 85% of JMML patients. These include biallelic inactivation of NF1 (15%),[124] activating mutations

in NRAS or KRAS (25%),[125–127] mutations in the PTPN11 gene (see Fig. 63.1) (35%), and mutations in CBL (10%–15%).[128–131] This synopsis reflects decades of research, beginning with the seminal observation that JMML is associated with neurofibromitosis type 1 (NF1). A rough comparison of incidence rates suggests that NF1 carries a 500-fold increased risk of acquiring JMML. At a molecular level, these children inherit a defective allele of the NF1 gene, which encodes a negative regulator of Ras named *neurofibromin*. In JMML, the normal allele is lost as a somatic event in the initiating cell, most often by loss of heterozygosity in which the overall copy number remains unchanged (uniparental isodisomy). This completely ablates neurofibromin and thereby increases Ras activity.

Such interplay of inherited and somatic mutations is also relevant to the other JMML genes. Germline mutations in PTPN11 cause Noonan syndrome (NS), a common genetic condition that overlaps phenotypically with NF1 and sometimes includes a mild JMML-like myeloproliferative syndrome. This finding led directly to the discovery of somatic PTPN11 mutations in sporadic JMML, a lesion now recognized as the most common pathogenic mutation in this disease. Furthermore, rare germline mutations in KRAS have also been associated with related genetic syndromes including NS and cardiofaciocutaneous syndrome.[132–137] The PTPN11 and KRAS mutations present in the germline generally have less severe biochemical consequences than those in sporadic cases. This suggests that strong signal activation is not tolerated during development. Accordingly, the most common NS-associated PTPN11 alleles have relatively weak effects on signal transduction, and the myeloproliferative syndrome in these patients is usually transient.[138–140] However, a more recent and comprehensive analysis has suggested that a cohort of NS patients may inherit more deleterious mutations and develop fatal neonatal JMML.[141] Thus cytoreductive therapy or HCT may be considered for select NS patients with severe disease.

Similar to NF1, mutations in CBL are heterozygous in the germline, with subsequent reduction to homozygosity in hematopoietic cells. This contrasts with the lesions described in adults.[130] The heterozygous germline mutations appear to cause a genetic syndrome with features that can overlap with NS, termed *CBL syndrome* or *Noonan syndrome-like disorder with or without juvenile myelomonocytic leukemia*. The phenotypic manifestations of NSLL are variable and incompletely penetrant, and they include cryptorchidism, hearing loss, and skeletal abnormalities. Importantly, major vascular abnormalities have been described in patients with CBL-mutant JMML, and this could also reflect an NSLL phenotype. As expected for a heterozygous mutation, transmission is autosomal dominant, although 50% of cases arise spontaneously.[129,131,142–145] In contrast to the loss of function mutations in NF1, the mutations in CBL selectively inactivate the ubiquitin ligase activity of the Cbl protein while leaving the molecule otherwise intact. When homozygous, this alteration eliminates the negative regulatory activity of Cbl while sparing positive signaling functions.[130]

It has been speculated that the 15% of patients without mutations in the five major JMML genes have heretofore undetected mutations that also activate Ras signaling. In recent genomic studies, rare mutations in SH2B3, RRAS, RRAS2, RAC2, or JAK3 seem to be consistent with this idea.[146–148] Collectively, these data support the idea that hyperactive Ras is essential for initiation of JMML, but suggest that initiating mutations beyond the five major genes will be diverse and infrequent.

These so-called *Ras pathway* or *driver* mutations are largely mutually exclusive, supporting the idea that each provides a similar function in JMML. However, patients with two such lesions or duplication of the mutant allele have been reported, typically co-occurring in the same cells.[146,147] This likely reflects clonal evolution and positive selection for increased Ras signaling even beyond that provided by the initiating mutation. Growing evidence demonstrates that negative feedback prevents the Ras pathway from being fully activated by a single lesion, leading to a dosage effect of mutant alleles on signaling outputs.[149] Consistent with predictions from model systems, cases with multiple Ras pathway mutations have a more aggressive clinical course.[147]

Genomic studies have also begun to address the question of whether mutations outside the Ras pathway contribute to the pathogenesis of JMML.[123,146–148] A wide variety of so-called secondary mutations have now been recognized. They are primarily associated with relapse of JMML after HCT, or with transformation to AML. However, they often can be detected at a low level in the blood or bone marrow when JMML is first diagnosed. This suggests that clonal evolution selects for chemotherapy resistance and eventually leukemic transformation. This is supported by the striking observation that secondary mutations of any kind have a major prognostic impact, even when they are present in a very small proportion of hematopoietic cells at diagnosis.

In the few JMML cases in which clonal history has be inferred, mutations appear to be acquired sequentially, beginning with a Ras pathway lesion. This linear evolutionary path contrasts with the highly branched patterns typical of high-grade neoplasms. Thus despite the discovery of a variety of secondary mutations in JMML, it remains a disease with much less genetic complexity than most cancers. This may have important implications for therapy, as any individual patient is likely to harbor a relatively small number of distinct subclones that need to be eradicated to achieve cure.

The cellular function of cooperating mutations in JMML is under active investigation. Most can be categorized into three groups. Some amplify signaling beyond the level provided by the initial Ras pathway mutation. As described earlier, some second mutations directly alter core Ras pathway genes. Janus-activated kinase (JAK)/signal transducer and activator of transcription (STAT) signaling is enhanced by activating mutations in *JAK3* or loss-of-function mutations in *SH2B3*, which encodes the negative regulatory adaptor protein LNK. Mutations in *RRAS*, *RRAS2*, and *RAC2* represent a novel signaling complex in JMML that is implicated in regulating the PI3K/Akt pathway.[147] Dominant point mutations in *SETBP1* remain somewhat unexplored, but may augment signal transduction by inhibiting the phosphatase PP2A or regulate gene transcription and strengthen self-renewal programs. Other secondary lesions have broad effects on gene expression, through inactivation of the PRC2 polycomb repressor complex or alteration of spliceosome components. Many of these genes and cellular functions are also implicated in the pathogenesis of other myeloid neoplasms such as CMML or AML.

Model Systems

Genetically engineered mouse models of JMML have been based on directed mutation of *Nf1*, *Kras*, *Nras*, *Ptptn11*, and *c-Cbl*. These are reviewed in detail elsewhere.[150,151] In general terms, these mice reproduce many key features of JMML, but penetrance and severity of disease vary across these models. In an alternative approach, induced pluripotent stem cells have recently been generated from germline and neoplastic cells from JMML patients.[152] These can be differentiated into myeloid progenitors that also recapitulate signal transduction and cell biology phenotypes characteristic of JMML. Together, these systems provide a robust set of tools for investigating the biology of JMML and also enable preclinical testing of novel therapeutic strategies.

Cell Biology of JMML

Hematopoiesis in JMML is altered in a distinctive way that is much more subtle than in acute leukemias, although nonetheless usually fatal if not corrected. A consensus has emerged that the disease initiates with a somatic Ras pathway mutation, presumably in a single HSC. This implies that the mutation imparts a competitive advantage over normal stem cells. This is supported by evidence from multiple mouse models.[153–156] Interestingly, however, *Nf1*[−/−] HSCs fail to cause an overt disease when mixed with wild-type cells, suggesting a limit to the advantage imparted by *Nf1* loss. Furthermore, there is also evidence that excessive signaling in Ras or phosphatidylinositol 3-kinase (PI3K) induces substantial stress in HSCs.[153,157–162]

More overt effects are seen in myeloid and erythroid progenitor cells, as manifested clinically by the circulation of immature erythroid and myeloid forms in the peripheral blood. In normal hematopoiesis, proliferative myeloid precursors are only present in the bone marrow and are strictly dependent on exogenous cytokines. By contrast, myeloid colonies arise from cultures of either blood or bone marrow from JMML patients, and they often do not require additional cytokines.[163] Importantly, they uniformly demonstrate a hypersensitive dose-response curve to the cytokine granulocyte-macrophage colony-forming factor (GM-CSF). Finally, aberrant differentiation generates excessive monocytes and insufficient mature erythrocytes. Although the mechanisms underlying abnormal hematopoiesis in JMML remain under investigation, both cell-intrinsic and cell-extrinsic mechanisms are likely to contribute.

Similarly, the precise biochemical signaling events responsible for the MDS/MPN phenotype are poorly understood. Ras proteins potentially signal through a wide variety of effector proteins,[164] but cancer is most closely linked to the Raf/MEK/ERK and PI3K/Akt pathways. Evidence from model systems suggests that each of these plays an important role in directing the abnormal growth and differentiation that defines JMML. Inhibitors of MEK cause substantial improvements in MDS/MPN in *Kras* or *Nf1* mutant mice.[165,166] Similarly, attenuation of PI3K signaling counteracts the effects of mutant *Ptpn11* and *Kras* alleles in mice.[167–169] The relevant downstream targets of these signaling networks in JMML are poorly characterized, but several studies have implicated specific hematopoietic transcription factors that integrate aberrant upstream signals to alter hematopoietic cell fate decisions.[170,171]

JAK/STAT signaling is also implicated in JMML. The GM-CSF receptor requires the nonreceptor tyrosine kinase Jak2 to initiate signaling. Therefore JAK2 is upstream of Ras as well as STAT5 in this context. STAT5 phosphorylation in myeloid progenitors from JMML patients is hypersensitive to GM-CSF, mirroring the abnormal colony forming activity of these cells.[172] The acquisition of *JAK3* or *SH2B3* mutations in advanced JMML also implies involvement of this pathway in JMML pathogenesis.

Clinical Manifestations

Children with JMML typically present with signs and symptoms attributable to a heavy burden of organ-infiltrating cells that results in hepatosplenomegaly, lymphadenopathy, and skin rash. As a result of the association with neurofibromatosis, patients may also have café-au-lait spots or juvenile xanthogranulomas. Death is usually the result of organ dysfunction caused by infiltrating cells, infection, or bleeding. Approximately 10%–20% of children progress to a blast-like phase consistent with AML.

Laboratory Manifestations

Laboratory abnormalities may include an elevated white blood cell count with absolute monocytosis, anemia, and thrombocytopenia (Figs. 63.4 and 63.5). Monocytes, either circulating in the peripheral blood or in the BM, frequently appear dysplastic. The peripheral smear shows leukoerythroblastic changes, and there are often circulating nucleated red blood cells. Fifty percent of patients may also present with elevated fetal hemoglobin levels and hypergammaglobulinemia, which is of interest given that there are patients recently described with autoimmune lymphoproliferative syndromes who also harbor *RAS* mutations (see later). International criteria mandate that the BM have fewer than 20% blast cells at diagnosis. Other findings typical in the BM may include micromegakaryocytes.

Differential Diagnosis

Traditionally, establishing a diagnosis of JMML was not easy because its clinical and laboratory presenting features can also be associated

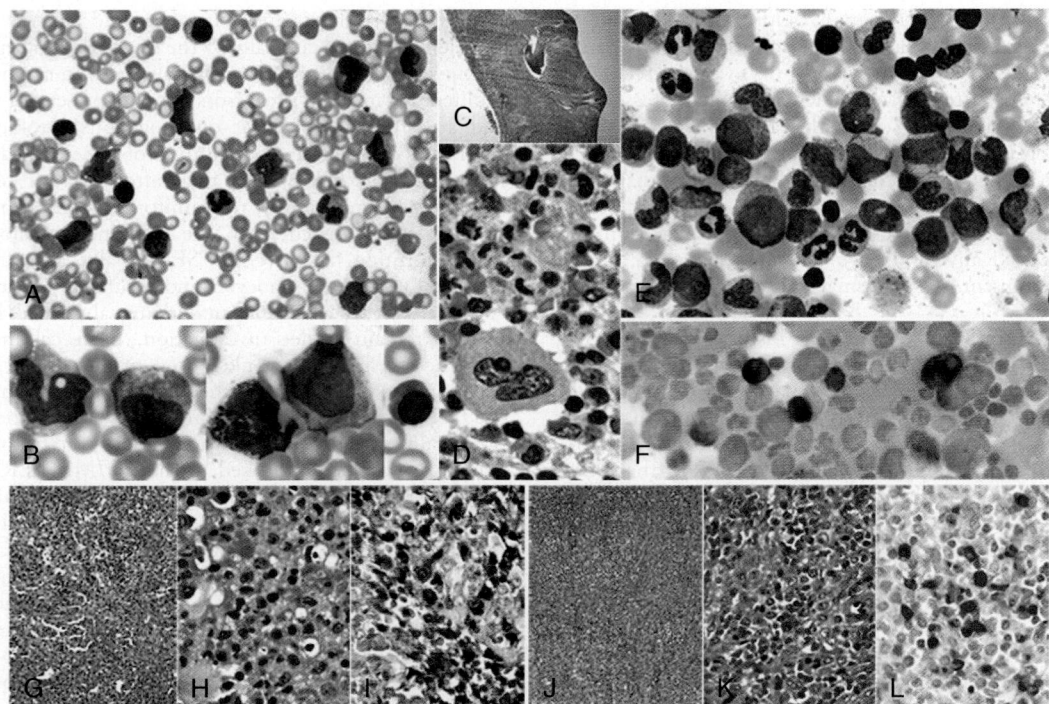

Fig. 63.4 JUVENILE MYELOMONOCYTIC LEUKEMIA: BLOOD, BONE MARROW, LUNG, AND SPLEEN. The illustrations are from the case of a 3-year-old boy who was diagnosed with neurofibromatosis at birth. At 1 year of age, he presented with leukocytosis (58 K/μL). The peripheral blood (A and B) showed left-shifted granulocytes and increased monocytes (16%). A bone marrow biopsy (C and D) was hypercellular as a result of increased granulocytic and monocytic cells that could also be appreciated on the aspirate (E). Blasts accounted for only 4% of the bone marrow elements. A combined esterase reaction (F) illustrated the increased monocytes (α-naphthol butyrate esterase reaction positive; *orange/brown*) in the background of granulocytes (chloroacetate esterase reaction positive; *blue*). Cytogenetic analysis revealed monosomy 7. At age 2 years, the patient presented with respiratory distress, and a lung biopsy (G and H) demonstrated a monocyte infiltrate (lysozyme stain, I) consistent with involvement by juvenile myelomonocytic leukemia. This is not uncommon in such patients. At age 3 years, his blast count began to rise, and he underwent a splenectomy (which showed a marked infiltrate of immature and mature monocytes and granulocytic cells [J and K; lysozyme stain, L]). After the splenectomy the patient underwent a successful stem cell transplant.

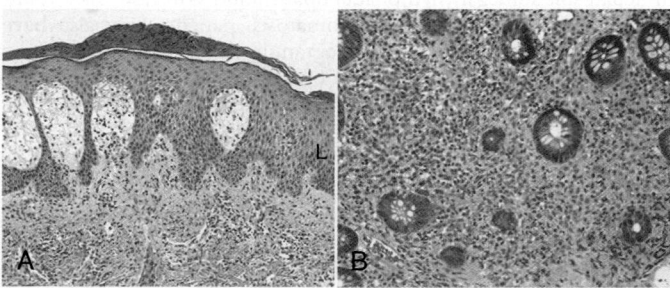

Fig. 63.5 JUVENILE MYELOMONOCYTIC LEUKEMIA: SKIN AND GASTROINTESTINAL TRACT. Patients with juvenile myelomonocytic leukemia sometimes present with or develop skin nodules, which on biopsy show a myelomonocytic infiltrate in the upper and lower dermis (A). Involvement can also be seen in the gastrointestinal tract (B). *(The case was kindly provided by Dr. Elizabeth Hyjek, University of Chicago.)*

with other disorders, including Wiskott-Aldrich syndrome,[173] infantile osteopetrosis,[174] infections (Epstein-Barr virus, cytomegalovirus, human herpesvirus 6, histoplasmosis, mycobacterium, and toxoplasmosis), class I Langerhans cell histiocytosis, hemophagocytic lymphohistiocytosis, FA, Kostmann syndrome, Shwachman syndrome, and Down syndrome. However, with a positive molecular mutation, patients who exhibit the category 1 features are now more easily diagnosed.

Recently, the term "Ras associated lymphoproliferative disorder (RALD)" has been coined to describe patients with autoimmunity and lymphoid proliferation with activating *RAS* mutations in the blood.[175] These mutations were initially thought to be in the germline but later were established to be somatically acquired in the bone marrow. These patients also exhibit splenomegaly and monocytosis, and they tend to meet clinical diagnostic criteria for JMML. At this time, there is no accepted method for distinguishing JMML from RALD, except to note that patients diagnosed with RALD have less fulminant myeloid disease and relatively more prominent immune dysregulation. Further study is needed to determine whether these diagnoses represent distinct clinicopathologic entities or rather represent the spectrum of hematologic phenotypes specified by Ras pathway mutations. Along with reports of rare JMML patients who survive without chemotherapy despite persistent Ras pathway mutations, this idea has raised the controversial question as to whether select patients can be monitored without definitive therapy. However, given the difficulty of prospectively diagnosing RALD, its extremely low incidence, and the strong tendency of JMML to become more aggressive over time, most patients meeting JMML criteria should be treated as such.

Therapy

Children with JMML can have a variable course, with rare patients having a spontaneous remission and long-term survival without treatment but others having a rapidly fatal course despite aggressive treatment.[176,177] The patients likely to do well without HCT are those with somatic NRASG212S or KRASG12V mutations, or germline mutations in CBL.[178-180] Older age, lower platelet count, and elevated hemoglobin F levels have been used to predict a more aggressive clinical course for patients.[181-185] Currently, the most adverse prognostic factor for outcome is the presence of >20% blasts or an AML-like gene expression profile,[181,184] which have survival rates of <10% even with allogeneic HCT.

A wide variety of agents have been used to treat children with JMML, including AML-like chemotherapy,[59,186-191] low-dose chemotherapy,[192,193] interferon-α (IFN-α),[194] and 13-cis-retinoic acid. Tipifarnib, a farnesyl transferase inhibitor, was tested in a Phase II window by the Children's Oncology Group (COG) where it produced some responses, but did not appear to impact long-term survival.[195] Perhaps because the evaluation of these treatment regimens has been complicated by small patient numbers, a prior lack of consistent response criteria, and until recently, lack of assays to measure the burden of clonogenic JMML stem cells, the utility of chemotherapy prior to HCT is unclear. One report showed no difference in univariate post-HCT outcomes in patients who did or did not receive AML-like chemotherapy, but this was limited by the inclusion of patients with AML and the lack of multivariate analysis.[181] Several newer reports show trends towards better post-HCT outcomes in patients who either received AML-like chemotherapy (without mention of response)[182] or who had normalization of WBC count and organomegaly prior to HCT.[195] With the advent of uniform response criteria[112] and the ability to follow molecular disease burden in patients with mutations in PTPN11, NRAS, and KRAS,[196] more definitive data on the role of pre-HCT chemotherapy may soon be forthcoming. For most children with JMML, allogeneic HCT offers the only known potential for cure, with about half of transplanted children surviving disease free.[182,197,198] Rapid withdrawal of immunosuppression appears to be important in this disease, as mounting evidence supports a graft-versus-leukemia effect.[199,200] A number of issues related to HCT for JMML remain uncertain. Among these are the value of pretransplant splenectomy and the optimal conditioning regimen and graft-versus-host disease prophylaxis. Splenectomy, a procedure not without long-term risks, had a trend towards improved outcomes in patients undergoing umbilical cord blood transplant,[182] but no benefit in those getting transplants from other donors.[181,195] Radiation-containing preparative regimens, which have significant long-term risks in small children, have not shown benefit when compared with other published reports,[195] although they did decrease the risk of rejection in patients undergoing cord blood transplant.[182] The most common cause of death after HCT is recurrent disease, but a second HCT can be lifesaving for some children.[181,201,202] Donor leukocyte infusions have variable response rates.[200,203]

Down Syndrome–Associated Transient Abnormal Myelopoiesis

Epidemiology

Down syndrome is one of the most common congenital disorders, affecting approximately one in every 800–1000 live births. It has been demonstrated in a recent population-based study that children with Down syndrome have a 10–20-fold overall increased risk of developing leukemia,[204] a 150-fold increased risk of developing AML, and a 500-fold increased risk of acute megakaryocytic leukemia. The median age of diagnosis of myeloid leukemia of Down syndrome (ML-DS), as defined by the WHO classification system, in children with Down syndrome is 2 years.[205] TAM, also known as transient myeloproliferative disorder (TMD) and transient leukemia, is thought to occur in at least 10% of children with trisomy 21 Down syndrome, although 7%–16% of TAM cases have mosaic trisomy 21. It has also been suggested that when cases of TAM that develop and resolve in utero or result in death before delivery are taken into account, the incidence may be as high as 20%.[206] Currently, it is estimated that approximately 20%–30% of children with TAM subsequently develop AML, usually by 3 years of age. This estimate was validated in a recent prospective study conducted by the COG.[207] In this study, AML developed in 16% of Down syndrome children who had TAM at a median of 441 days (118–1085 days).

Pathobiology

The molecular pathogenesis of TAM and ML-DS in children with Down syndrome is now providing valuable insights into myeloid leukemogenesis.[21] Current research suggests that the development of TAM and subsequent progression to ML-DS are the result of a three-step process: perturbation of fetal hematopoiesis by trisomy 21; an acquired GATA1 mutation; and the acquisition of additional oncogenic mutations.[208,209]

It is increasingly clear that trisomy 21 results in genome-wide changes in gene expression that affect, directly or indirectly, most chromosomes.[210] This results in perturbed hematopoiesis with increased numbers and clonality of HSCs, increased frequency of megakaryocyte and erythroid progenitors, and reduced numbers of granulocyte- and macrophage-committed progenitor cells.[211,212]

Recent studies have shown that virtually all patients with TAM and most patients with ML-DS harbor mutations in exon 2 and occasionally in exon 3 of the hematopoietic transcription factor GATA1.[213-217] GATA1 is a double–zinc finger DNA-binding transcription factor expressed primarily in hematopoietic cells. It is required for the development of red blood cells, megakaryocytes, mast cells, and eosinophils. A number of different mutations in GATA1 have been identified, including insertions, deletions, missense mutations, nonsense mutations, and slice site mutations. All of these mutations lead to a block in the expression of the full-length 50-kd isoform of GATA1 but allow for the expression of a smaller, 40-kd isoform (GATA1s).[218] This smaller isoform lacks the N-terminal transactivation domain but retains both zinc fingers involved in DNA binding as well as interactions with its cofactor, friend of GATA1 (FOG1).[213] Recent studies have shown that mutations that alter GATA1-FOG1 binding in the N-terminal zinc finger or result in the expression of the GATA1s isoform uncouple megakaryocyte growth and differentiation.[219-221] Similar studies in cell lines derived from children with ML-DS have demonstrated that expression of GATA1 led to erythroid differentiation whereas expression of GATA1s did not alter the characteristics of the cell line.[217] Taken together, current data suggest that the loss of GATA1 and expression of GATA1s directly contribute to leukemogenesis.

Although mutations in GATA1 may be sufficient to cause TAM, these mutations are not sufficient for the development of ML-DS, as evidenced by the latency period between resolution of TAM and the development of ML-DS, as well as the observation that not all children with TAM and GATA1 mutations will ultimately develop ML-DS. Therefore a multistep pathogenesis model is proposed in patients with Down syndrome in whom ML-DS develops in clones with GATA1 mutations and additional cooperating mutations. A large number of potential target genes have been proposed and are the subject of ongoing investigation.[222] Among this long list of candidate targets are mutations in the gene for JAK3, a member of the JAK family of nonreceptor tyrosine kinases. Several gain-of-function mutations[223,224] and loss-of-function mutations in JAK3[225] have been identified in both TAM and ML-DS patient samples. Although mutations in JAK3 might indeed represent an additional "hit" in this three-step model, the finding of mutations in TAM patients who have not progressed to ML-DS may argue against JAK3 as a cooperating mutation.

Another particularly important area of investigation is the interaction between GATA1 and chromosome 21. Identification of critical interactions between GATA1 and relevant genes on chromosome 21 will serve to further inform us about the pathogenesis of leukemia in children with Down syndrome.

Clinical Manifestations

Patients with Down syndrome typically present with TAM within 3 months after birth, although TAM can be manifest at birth. Some of these children present with hydrops fetalis secondary to anemia and cardiac dysfunction. Although some patients may be asymptomatic, others can have myeloblast infiltration of the heart, liver, and spleen that can result in hepatosplenomegaly; hepatic fibrosis; pleural, pericardial, and peritoneal effusions; and disseminated intravascular coagulopathy. In some cases, organ dysfunction can be severe, with failure of the liver, heart, kidneys, and lungs. In the COG's recently published prospective study, death occurred in 21% of patients, although only 10% died as a result of TAM-associated problems.[207]

Laboratory Manifestations

The complete blood count in infants with TAM typically demonstrates an elevated white blood cell count with myeloblasts present (see Fig. 63.6). The percentage of circulating myeloblasts exceeds the percentage of BM myeloblasts. Rarely, a neonate without stigmata of Down syndrome will present with similar features—in these cases, workup for either trisomy 21 mosaicism or a *PTPN11* mutation should be pursued. Flow cytometric analysis of the myeloblasts from TAM patients and ML-DS associated with Down syndrome show many similarities between these disorders as well as patterns of cell surface antigen expression that is distinct from other types of AML in children.[226] Specifically, all TAM and ML-DS blasts express CD45, CD38, and CD33, but the majority of cases express CD36 and CD34. CD41 and CD61 also are expressed, consistent with megakaryocyte differentiation. CD14 and CD64 are usually negative. Most cases have aberrant expression of CD7, a T-lineage antigen.

Therapy

The treatment of infants with TAM is generally supportive. Patients without significant organ dysfunction can be followed closely without medical intervention. In the COG's prospective study, peripheral blood blasts and TAM-associated symptoms resolved in 36 and 49 days, respectively, for observation patients.[207] In infants with significant organ impairment, a number of therapeutic approaches aimed at reducing the burden of myeloblasts are routinely used, including exchange transfusion, leukophoresis, and chemotherapy. According to reports using cytosine arabinoside in children with Down syndrome and ML-DS,[227,228] cytosine arabinoside is the chemotherapeutic agent now most commonly used in infants with TAM. The efficacy of very low doses of cytosine arabinoside is being tested in prospective clinical trials. Several additional questions related to the treatment of infants with TAM are also the subject of ongoing clinical trials. Among these is the identification of high-, intermediate-, and low-risk populations, with treatment stratified on the basis of risk group and a determination of whether treatment with very low-dose cytosine arabinoside will prevent progression of TAM to ML-DS and hepatic fibrosis.

Prognosis

Recent data from the COG reporting the results of the POG-9481 prospective clinical trial offer insights into the natural history of TAM and the identification of prognostic factors.[229] This study followed 48 children with TAM. Eighty-nine percent of infants achieved a spontaneous remission, 74% had a normalization of peripheral blood counts, and 64% maintained a clinical remission. Seventeen percent of infants had an early death. Factors associated with early death included a high white blood cell count ($p < .001$), increased bilirubin and liver function test values ($p < .005$), and a failure to normalize blood counts ($p < .001$). Nineteen percent of patients had a progression to ML-DS at a median of 20 months. The greatest risk factor for progression to leukemia was the presence of karyotypic abnormalities in addition to trisomy 21 in blasts cells.

The COG's more recent A2971 study identified three groups of children with different outcomes based on the presence or absence of hepatomegaly and life-threatening symptoms.[207] Children with neither hepatomegaly nor life-threatening symptoms were at low risk of death (overall survival [OS], 92%); children with hepatomegaly alone had an intermediate risk of death (OS, 77%), and children with both hepatomegaly and life-threatening symptoms were at high risk of death (OS, 51%).

OTHER MYELOPROLIFERATIVE NEOPLASMS

Essential Thrombocythemia

ET has an estimated incidence of 1–1.25 cases per million in adults but is even rarer in children, with an estimated incidence of 0.09 cases per million.[230–234] ET is a genetically heterogeneous disease. Mutations in *JAK2* have been reported in adults with *BCR-ABL*–negative MPNs, including ET, PV, and idiopathic myelofibrosis (IM). It has been proposed that ET consists of several subtypes, with some children and adults having monoclonal disease but others having polyclonal disease. Further investigation into the mutational status of *JAK2* V617F also demonstrates mutation-positive (roughly 55%) and mutation-negative patients.[231,235] Another cause of ET was recently demonstrated to be mutations in CALR (calreticulin).[236] Studies suggest that a similar proportion of children and adults with somatic ET display polycythemia rubra vera-1 (PRV-1) RNA overexpression, *JAK2* V617F mutations, and monoclonal disease.[237] Rare cases of familial ET have been shown to be caused by dominant activating mutations in both c-*MPL*[237] and in *JAK2*.[238]

Patients with ET have thrombocythemia with an increased number of megakaryocytes in the BM. Platelet clumps on peripheral blood smears are common. Some patients have a concomitant increase in the number of peripheral blood granulocytes. The differential diagnosis includes familial ET, other forms of MPS, and increased platelets as a reactive process.

Although the clinical course can be uncomplicated, patients can develop thromboembolic complications, including deep venous thrombosis, and arterial thrombosis such as transient cerebral ischemia and peripheral vascular ischemia. The clinical course for children is typically less aggressive than in adults, with fewer thrombotic episodes.[237,239] Adult patients have a median survival of at least 10 years, with most deaths caused by thrombosis.[240,241] Progression to AML has been reported in adult patients, usually those with a prior exposure to chemotherapy agents.

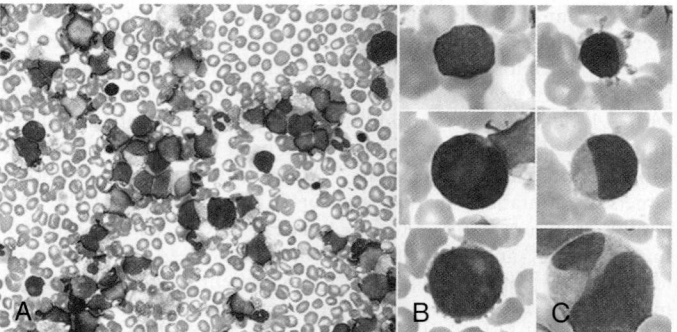

Fig. 63.6 TRANSIENT ABNORMAL MYELOPOIESIS AND TRANSIENT LEUKEMIA OF DOWN SYNDROME. The patient was a premature newborn girl with trisomy 21 and a white blood cell count of 195,000/μL with 67% blasts (A). The blasts were CD34+, CD33+, and CD117+, and a portion exhibited CD41, a megakaryocyte marker. Morphologically, some of the blasts appeared to be megakaryoblasts (B), sometimes with slight differentiation toward megakaryocytes (C).

Asymptomatic children do not require treatment. There is no clear association with platelet count and thrombotic events. As such, there is not a clear role for treatment with aspirin, which can increase the risk of paradoxical bleeding episodes.[242] Risk factors for thrombosis include leukocytosis and presence of a *JAK2* V617F mutation.[243] A number of treatment approaches aimed at controlling thrombocytosis have been attempted for symptomatic patients, including hydroxyurea, IFN-α, and anagrelide.[244-246] The JAK inhibitor ruxolitinib may benefit some patients with ET, especially those with *JAK2* V617F mutations, although pediatric-specific data with this agent are lacking. The successful use of allogeneic HCT has been reported for a number of adult patients with ET, especially after transformation to myelofibrosis or AML.[247-249] Younger patients, and those with matched related donors, did especially well, suggesting that allogeneic transplant should be considered in pediatric patients with ET.

Idiopathic Myelofibrosis

IM is very rarely diagnosed in children[250] and should be differentiated from acute megakaryocytic leukemia; metastatic neoplasms; and connective tissue, metabolic, and bone diseases. It is characterized by BM fibrosis, megakaryocytes with bizarre morphology, splenomegaly, anemia, and extramedullary hematopoiesis. IM is a clonal disorder, with approximately half of adult patients having mutations in *JAK2* V617F.[251] Recent studies have suggested that angiogenic cytokines produced by megakaryocytes and monocytes and their receptors (platelet-derived growth factor receptors, vascular endothelial growth factor receptor-2, and fibroblast growth factor receptor) may be involved in the pathogenesis of the myelofibrosis.[252]

Numerous treatment approaches have been attempted with variable degrees of success. These include splenectomy, splenic radiation, transfusions, androgens, corticosteroids, hydroxyurea, and IFN-α.[253-255] More recently, based on preliminary studies about the potential role of angiogenic cytokines and their receptors, newer approaches have been tested, including the tyrosine kinase inhibitor imatinib[256,257] and the antiangiogenic agent thalidomide.[258,259] Selective JAK inhibitors have been successfully used in patients with IM with a dramatic improvement in the quality of life but without generalized reduction of the *JAK2* V617F burden allele.[260] In 2011, the United States Food and Drug Administration granted approval to the first of these agents, ruxolitinib, for adults with IM. However, the safety and efficacy of ruxolitinib in children is still unknown. Further trials are investigating the combination of JAK inhibition in combination with other therapeutic modalities, such as PI3K inhibition, mammalian target of rapamycin inhibition, histone deacetylase inhibition, and antifibrotic agents.[261] Finally, allogeneic transplantation is the only potentially curative option for IM, with resolution of BM fibrosis in donor-engrafted patients but high rates of transplant-related complications.[248,262-265] The survival in children is unknown, with a median survival in adults of 4 years.

Polycythemia Vera

PV has an incidence of three cases per 100,000 in adults but is very rarely seen in children, with fewer than 0.1% of PV patients diagnosed before 20 years of age.[265] PV in children is far more often the result of congenital or acquired causes of an increased red blood cell mass. These include primary familial polycythemia (characterized by specific mutations in the erythropoietic receptor gene)[266] and secondary polycythemias caused by abnormal hemoglobins, cardiac and pulmonary disease, excessive erythropoietin, and a relative polycythemia that is the result of decreased plasma volume.

PV in children and adults is associated with clonal hematopoiesis,[267] *JAK2* V617F mutations (in 95% of patients; with mutations in *JAK2* exon 12 representing 2%–4%),[237,268-273] overexpression of PVR-1 RNA,[274,275] and endogenous erythroid colony growth.[276,277] In contrast to adults, children with PV may be less likely to have *JAK2*

V617F mutations and endogenous erythroid colony growth,[237,278] such that the proposed revision to WHO's diagnostic criteria,[279] may be less helpful in the diagnosis of PV in children, although other reports suggest that the proposed WHO criteria are equally applicable to children.[280] The proposed criteria include: (1) a hemoglobin >16.5 g/dL in men or >16.0 g/dL in women; (2) a BM biopsy showing trilineage myeloproliferation and pleomorphic megakaryocytes; and (3) either a *JAK2* mutation or a serum erythropoietin level below the normal reference range.[281] Although the pathogenesis is currently unclear, patients also have abnormalities in tissue factor, endogenous anticoagulants mechanisms, hyperhomocysteinemia, and acquired von Willebrand syndrome.

Children with PV may present with signs and symptoms associated with an increased red blood cell mass such as headache, dizziness, fatigue, pruritus, night sweats, and a ruddy complexion. Mild splenomegaly may be present, but massive hepatosplenomegaly is rare. As a result of hyperviscosity of the blood, elevated platelet counts, and coagulation abnormalities, patients can develop thromboses and CNS ischemia, although the incidence of thrombotic events may be lower than that reported in adults.[237,278]

Many different agents have been used to treat patients with PV, including chlorambucil,[282] melphalan,[283] 6-thioguanine,[284] uracil mustard,[285] busulfan,[286] carboquone,[287] anagrelide,[288] imatinib,[289] hydroxyurea,[290] radioactive phosphorous,[291] and IFN.[292] Despite these efforts, the best approach to patients with PV remains unclear. Therefore the British Committee for Standards in Haematology formulated recommendations for the initial management of PV.[293] Recommendations include phlebotomy to maintain a hematocrit level less than 45%;[294] low-dose aspirin unless contraindicated; and cytoreduction if there is poor tolerance to phlebotomy, symptomatic or progressive splenomegaly, evidence of disease progression, or thrombocytosis. For patients younger than 40 years of age, pegylated IFN was the recommendation for first-line cytoreduction, with hydroxyurea as second line. However, the JAK inhibitor ruxolitinib was recently found to have excellent results in controlling the hematocrit and splenomegaly with minimal side-effects in an open-label phase III trial.[295] This may eventually supplant IFN and hydroxyurea as front-line therapy once pediatric-specific dosing is available. Finally, allogeneic transplantation has been successfully used to treat some adult patients,[247-249] especially those with progression to myelofibrosis or AML. Younger patients, and those with matched related donors, did especially well, suggesting that allogeneic transplant should be considered in pediatric patients with PV.

FUTURE DIRECTIONS

Although a clearer understanding of the biologic mechanisms underlying MDS in children is slow in coming, dramatic progress has been made in our understanding of the genetic and biologic mechanisms contributing to TMD, JMML, PV, ET, and IM. There exists a potential for targeted therapeutics for many of these disorders, with the first targeted agents now receiving approval for use in adults. However, the use of these approved agents in children remains investigational.

Progress for both MDS and MPN in children will require international cooperation. The rarity of these disorders and limitations in resources for pediatric cooperative cancer groups make clinical trials within each individual cooperative group increasingly difficult.

SUGGESTED READINGS

Arber DA, Orazi A, Hasserjian R: The 2016 revision to the World Health Organization classification of myeloid neoplasms and acute leukemia. *Blood* 127:2391, 2016.

Bhatia S, Krailo MD, Chen Z, et al: Therapy-related myelodysplasia and acute myeloid leukemia after Ewing sarcoma and primitive neuroectodermal tumor of bone: a report from the Children's Oncology Group. *Blood* 109:46, 2007.

Crispino JD: GATA1 mutations in Down syndrome: implications for biology and diagnosis of children with transient myeloproliferative disorder and acute megakaryoblastic leukemia. *Pediatr Blood Cancer* 44:40, 2005.

Gamis AS, Alonzo TA, Gerbing RB, et al: Natural history of transient myeloproliferative disorder clinically diagnosed in Down syndrome neonates: a report from the Children's Oncology Group Study A2971. *Blood* 118:6752, 2011.

Gamis AS, Smith FO: Transient myeloproliferative disorder in children with Down syndrome: clarity to this enigmatic disorder. *Br J Haematol* 159:277, 2012.

Glaubach T, Robinson LJ, Corey SJ: Pediatric myelodysplastic syndromes: they do exist! *J Pediatr Hematol Oncol* 36:1, 2014.

Hasle H, Niemeyer CM: Advances in the prognostication and management of advanced MDS in children. *Br J Haematol* 154:185, 2011.

Hasle H, Niemeyer CM, Chessells JM, et al: A pediatric approach to the WHO classification of myelodysplastic and myeloproliferative diseases. *Leukemia* 17:277, 2003.

Loh ML: Recent advances in the pathogenesis and treatment of juvenile myeolomonocytic leukemia. *Br J Haematol* 152:677, 2011.

Maloney KW, Taub JW, Ravindranath Y, et al: Down syndrome preluekemia and leukemia. *Pediatr Clin North Am* 62:121, 2015.

Niemeyer C, Kang M, Shin D, et al: Germline CBL mutations cause developmental abnormalities and predispose to juvenile myelomonocytic leukemia. *Nat Genet* 42:794, 2010.

Strahm B, Nollke P, Zecca M, et al: Hematopoietic stem cell transplantation for advanced myelodysplastic syndrome in children: results of the EWOG-MDS 98 study. *Leukemia* 25:455, 2011.

Tefferi A, Gilliland DG: Oncogenes in myeloproliferative disorders. *Cell Cycle* 6:550, 2007.

Tefferi A, Thiele J, Orazi A, et al: Proposals and rationale for revision of the World Health Organization diagnostic criteria for polycythemia vera, essential thrombocythemia, and primary myelofibrosis: recommendations from an ad hoc international expert panel. *Blood* 110:1092, 2007.

Tefferi A, Vainchanker W: Myeloproliferative neoplasms: molecular pathophysiology, essential clinical understanding and treatment strategies. *J Clin Oncol* 29:573, 2011.

Webb DK, Passmore SJ, Hann IM, et al: Results of treatment of children with refractory anaemia with excess blasts (RAEB) and RAEB in transformation (RAEBt) in Great Britain 1990-99. *Br J Haematol* 117:33, 2002.

Wlodarski MW, Hirabayashi S, Pastor V, et al: Prevalence, clinical characterisitcs and prognosis of GATA2-related myelodysplastic syndromes in children and adolescents. *Blood* 127:1387, 2016.

Woodard P, Carpentaer PA, Davies SM, et al: Unrelated donor bone marrow transplantation for myelodysplastic syndrome in children. *Biol Blood Marrow Transplant* 17:723, 2011.

Woods WG, Barnard DR, Alonzo TA, et al: Prospective study of 90 children requiring treatment for juvenile myelomonocytic leukemia or myelodysplastic syndrome: a report from the Children's Cancer Group. *J Clin Oncol* 20:434, 2002.

Yoshida K, Toki T, Okuno Y, et al: The landscape of somatic mutations in Down syndrome-related disorders. *Nat Genet* 45:1293, 2013.

REFERENCES

For the complete list of references, log on to www.expertconsult.com.

CHAPTER 64

PATHOBIOLOGY OF ACUTE LYMPHOBLASTIC LEUKEMIA

Melissa Burns, Scott A. Armstrong, and Alejandro Gutierrez

Normal lymphoid precursors undergo somatic recombination at their immunoglobulin (Ig) or T- cell receptor (TCR) gene loci,[1] and the successful completion of V(D)J recombination, with the resultant formation of a functional Ig or TCR, is required for the survival of lymphocyte precursors. Positive and negative selection steps ensure that only lymphocytes with Ig or TCRs that function appropriately within the context of an individual's immune microenvironment are allowed to proceed through the proliferation and differentiation steps required for the development of mature lymphocytes. This developmental process generates a repertoire of mature lymphocytes with unique variations in the antigen-recognition portions of the Ig or TCR genes; together these form the foundation of the adaptive immune system that can recognize a countless variety of foreign antigens. The acquisition of mutations of oncogenes or tumor suppressors during this developmental process, which can be mediated by off-target activity of the V(D)J recombination machinery,[2,3] can lead to the dysregulated proliferation and differentiation arrest that are characteristic of acute lymphoblastic leukemia (ALL). Many of these genetic alterations have prognostic significance and are used in modern ALL treatment protocols to adjust the intensity of therapy. Although the incidence of specific genetic alterations in ALL varies according to patient age (Fig. 64.1), evidence suggests that the pathogenesis underlying malignant transformation in molecularly defined subsets of ALL is similar across age groups.[4,5]

CLONAL ORIGIN OF LEUKEMIC LYMPHOID CELLS

The clonal origin of leukemia was first suggested by the identification of the Philadelphia (Ph) chromosome in chronic myeloid leukemia (CML).[6] Subsequently, numerous lines of evidence have provided additional support for this theory, which is now generally accepted. Uniform structural and numerical chromosomal abnormalities are frequently demonstrated in all leukemic lymphoblasts from an individual patient. Identical rearrangements of Ig or TCR genes, which are somatic in origin, have been demonstrated in ALL cell populations.[7,8] Additionally, identical patterns of X-chromosome inactivation have been demonstrated within all cells of individual patients with ALL by allelic analysis of the glucose-6-phosphate dehydrogenase gene on the X chromosome.[9] Moreover, the methylation patterns of restriction fragment length polymorphisms in X-linked genes, as detected by Southern blot analysis, have been used to show that even rare ALL cases with two completely different cytogenetic clones probably arise by clonal evolution from a single transformed progenitor.[10]

LINEAGE-SPECIFIC FEATURES OF LEUKEMIC LYMPHOBLASTS

Malignant lymphoblasts share many of the features of normal lymphoid progenitors.[11,12] Thus, ALL cells rearrange their Ig and TCR genes and express components of antigen receptor molecules and other differentiation-linked cell-surface glycoproteins in ways that correspond to features of developing normal B and T lymphocytes. In many cases, leukemic cells appear to represent the clonal expansion of a lymphoid progenitor that has arrested its development at an early stage of B- or T-cell differentiation.[13] However, in many cases of ALL,

the blast cell phenotypes differ from those of normal lymphocyte progenitors, which is likely a result of aberrant regulation of gene expression. Still the general concept that leukemic cells should be classified according to their "normal" developmental stage remains an important one, providing a basis for the study of immunophenotype-specific genetic changes.

Mature B-Cell Acute Lymphoblastic Leukemia

The diagnosis of mature B-cell ALL, also termed *Burkitt leukemia*, is based on the detection of surface Ig on leukemic blasts. This rare phenotype accounts for only 2%–3% of ALL cases, and the lymphoblasts generally have distinctive morphology, with deeply basophilic cytoplasm containing prominent vacuoles; this morphologic pattern is designated L3 in the French-American-British (FAB) system.[14–16] Mature B-cell ALL is a disseminated form of Burkitt lymphoma, as these conditions share common cytogenetic, molecular, phenotypic, and clinical features.[17] Mature B-cell ALL does not respond well to chemotherapy traditionally used for childhood ALL. However, good outcomes have been obtained with treatments designed for Burkitt lymphoma, which involve relatively brief but intensive regimens that emphasize cyclophosphamide and the rapid rotation of antimetabolites in high dosages.[18–22] Thus, mature B-cell leukemia was the first form of ALL to be recognized as a distinct clinical entity based on immunophenotypic and cytogenetic features, and the first to be treated by separate protocols designed specifically for the leukemia's unique features.

Precursor B-Cell Acute Lymphoblastic Leukemia

Approximately 80% of ALL patients have lymphoblasts with phenotypes corresponding to those of B-cell progenitors.[16,23] These cases can be identified on the basis of cell surface expression of CD19 and at least one other recognized B lineage-associated antigen: CD20, CD24, CD22, CD21, or CD79.[16,23] The most common subtype of precursor B-cell ALL, termed *common precursor B-cell ALL*, also expresses CD10. These lymphoblasts may also express nuclear terminal deoxynucleotidyl transferase (TdT) or CD34. About one-fourth of precursor B-cell ALL cases express cytoplasmic Ig μ heavy-chain proteins and are designated *pre-B ALL*.

DNA rearrangement of Ig genes occurs before heavy-chain gene expression in B-cell development, providing a genetic marker of B-lymphocyte ontogeny. Korsmeyer and coworkers pioneered the use of heavy- and light-chain gene rearrangements to support an early B-lineage origin of most ALL blasts.[24,25] However, Ig heavy-chain gene rearrangements have also been documented in about 15% of T-cell ALL cases and in a similar percentage of acute myeloid leukemia (AML) cases.[26–28] Thus, caution must be exercised when assigning cell lineage on the basis of studies of Ig gene rearrangement.

The identification of specific immunophenotypic, genetic, and clinical features that predict response to therapy in patients with B-lineage ALL, and the incorporation of these predictors into clinical decision making, are now widespread in modern ALL treatment protocols. This ability to predict outcome has been closely tied to the remarkable improvements in therapy for children with this disease, which 50 years ago was universally fatal. However, many subgroups

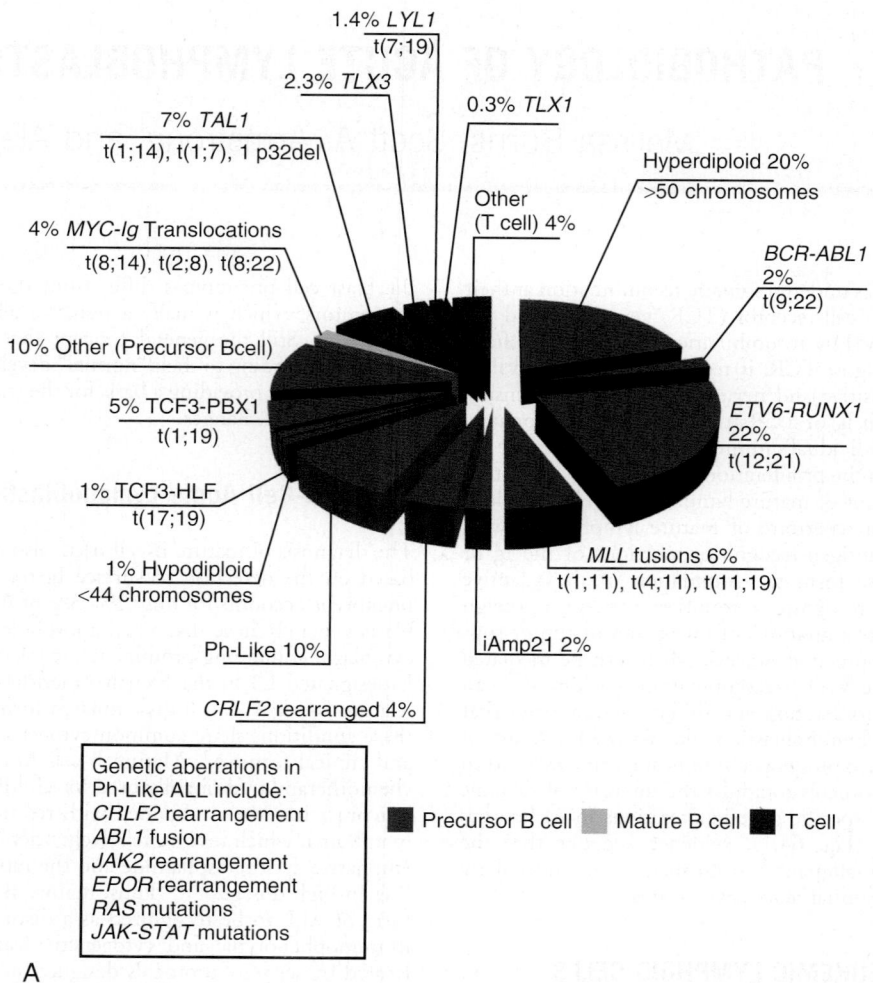

Pediatric acute lymphoblastic leukemia

1.4% *LYL1*
t(7;19)

2.3% *TLX3*

0.3% *TLX1*

7% *TAL1*
t(1;14), t(1;7), 1 p32del

Other
(T cell) 4%

Hyperdiploid 20%
>50 chromosomes

4% *MYC-Ig* Translocations
t(8;14), t(2;8), t(8;22)

BCR-ABL1
2%
t(9;22)

10% Other (Precursor Bcell)

ETV6-RUNX1
22%
t(12;21)

5% TCF3-PBX1
t(1;19)

1% TCF3-HLF
t(17;19)

MLL fusions 6%
t(1;11), t(4;11), t(11;19)

1% Hypodiploid
<44 chromosomes

iAmp21 2%

Ph-Like 10%

CRLF2 rearranged 4%

Genetic aberrations in
Ph-Like ALL include:
CRLF2 rearrangement
ABL1 fusion
JAK2 rearrangement
EPOR rearrangement
RAS mutations
JAK-STAT mutations

■ Precursor B cell   ■ Mature B cell   ■ T cell

A

Fig. 64.1 FREQUENCY OF THE MAJOR CYTOGENETIC ABERRATIONS IN PEDIATRIC (A) AND ADULT (B) ACUTE LYMPHOBLASTIC LEUKEMIA. The Ph-like (also known as BCR-ABL1-like) acute lymphoblastic leukemia subtype comprises a number of chromosomal translocations and mutations in oncogenic kinase and cytokine receptor pathways, which are shown in the *insert*.

of pediatric and adult patients face a much poorer prognosis, and much progress remains to be made.

T-Cell Acute Lymphoblastic Leukemia

Lymphoblasts with a T-cell phenotype comprise approximately 15% of cases of ALL. These cases can be classified according to the sequence of expression of T-cell–associated surface antigens during normal thymocyte ontogeny.[29,30] Numerous investigators, using a battery of monoclonal antibodies specific for T-cell surface glycoproteins, have confirmed the close relationship between the recognizable patterns of surface antigen expression on leukemic T cells and the normal stages of thymocyte development.[31–34] T-cell ALL is often associated with distinctive clinical features that include high circulating leukocyte counts, a male predominance, CNS involvement, and a radiographically evident thymic mass in many cases at presentation. Historically, patients with T-cell ALL had an adverse prognosis compared with patients with B-lineage ALL, but this gap has narrowed with the intensification of therapy for these patients.[35,36] In marked contrast to precursor B-cell ALL, in which the availability

of a wide range of clinical and genetic prognostic markers has allowed the development of treatment protocols tailored to an individual patient's risk of relapse, robust pretreatment prognostic markers had been lacking in T-cell ALL[37] until the recent identification of biomarkers of differentiation arrest at the earliest stages of T-cell development.[38,39]

Recent work has identified a subset of T-cell ALL cases at particularly high risk of treatment failure, which are characterized by differentiation arrest at the earliest identifiable stages of T-cell development. These cases are defined either by absence of biallelic TCRγ deletion (ABD), indicating differentiation arrest prior to the completion of T-cell receptor (TCR) gene rearrangement, or by expression of a characteristic "early T-cell precursor" (ETP) phenotype.[38,39] In addition to harboring oncogenic lesions typical of T-cell ALL, ETP cases also harbor gene mutations that are characteristic of AML or myelodysplastic syndrome, including *DNMT3A*, *IDH1/2*, and *EZH2*,[40,41] suggesting that the cell of origin of ABD/ETP T-cell ALL may be a multipotent hematopoietic stem or progenitor cell rather than a committed T-cell progenitor. ETP appears to comprise 8%–15% of pediatric T-cell ALL but may account for a much higher fraction of T-cell ALL in adults,[41] thus providing one possible

Adult acute lymphoblastic leukemia

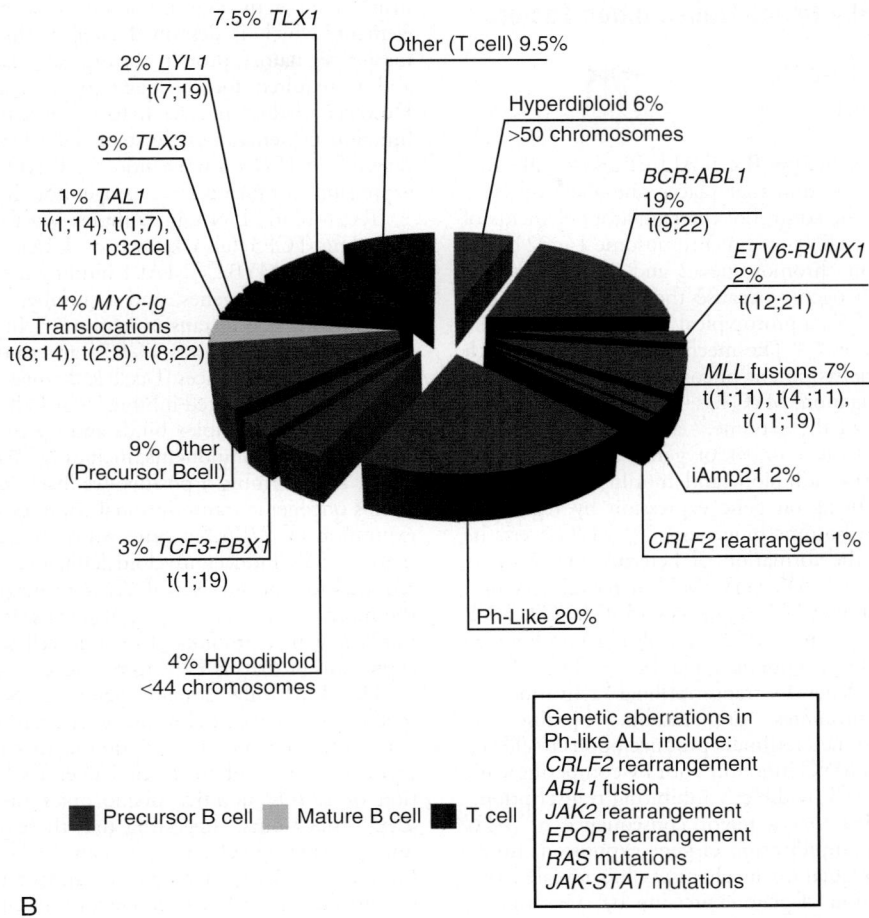

B

Fig. 64.1, cont'd

explanation for the significantly inferior outcomes of adults versus children with T-cell ALL.

Mixed-Lineage Leukemia

Acute mixed-lineage leukemia (MLL) is defined by blast cells that coexpress markers of both the lymphoid and myeloid lineages. Two distinct forms of these leukemias are recognized: biphenotypic leukemia, which accounts for the majority of MLLs and can be the result of cells with lymphoid morphology coexpressing myeloid-associated antigen,[42,43] or those with myeloid morphology and reactivity to myeloperoxidase staining that coexpress cell-surface antigens normally restricted to lymphoid cells, and bilineal leukemia, in which there are two distinct population of cells (generally one lymphoid and one myeloid). The origin of MLLs has not been established. One possibility is malignant transformation of pluripotent hematopoietic stem or progenitor cells that retain the ability to differentiate in both the myeloid and lymphoid lineages; another is immortalization of rare progenitor cells that normally coexpress features of both lineages; and a third is aberrant gene expression caused by specific genetic alterations.[44] Despite initial controversy, coexpression of myeloid antigens in ALL, or of lymphoid markers in AML, does not appear to have significant prognostic value in the setting of contemporary treatment regimens.[45–47]

GENETIC BASIS OF ACUTE LYMPHOBLASTIC LEUKEMIA

An in-depth analysis of the genetics of ALL is beyond the scope of this chapter, but we present here an overview of select genetic lesions that have provided key insights into the mechanisms of leukemogenesis. Mutations are classified based on their predominant cellular consequences, which is an imperfect classification scheme because some mutations can induce more than one type of cellular aberration. Nevertheless, we believe this provides a useful conceptual framework for understanding the molecular pathogenesis of ALL.

Aberrant Activation of Oncogenic Transcriptional Programs

Dysregulated activation of oncogenic transcriptional programs is a central theme in the pathogenesis of ALL. Many of the proto-oncogenes recurrently activated by genetic lesions are transcription factors that regulate proliferation and differentiation during the development of various embryonic tissues. Thus, co-option of normal developmental pathways plays a central role in human leukemogenesis. Transcription factors are commonly activated by chromosomal translocations in ALL, but the consequences of translocations tend to vary according to the ALL subtype. In mature B-cell ALL and in T-cell ALL, these genetic lesions often lead to the aberrant expression of structurally intact genes. By contrast, the chromosomal transloca-tions that often occur in precursor B-cell ALL generally lead to the expression of chimeric fusion proteins.

Activation of Structurally Intact Transcription Factors

MYC in Mature B-Cell Acute Lymphoblastic Leukemia

The vast majority of cases of mature B-cell ALL (Burkitt leukemia) are characterized by a translocation that places one allele of *MYC* from chromosome 8 under the control of the regulatory elements of an *Ig* gene, either the heavy-chain gene on chromosome 14q32 or the κ or λ light-chain genes on chromosomes 2 and 22, respectively. These translocations are oncogenic because they result in lineage-specific overexpression of *MYC*, a prototypical basic helix-loop-helix oncogenic transcription factor.[48–56] The mechanisms through which the MYC oncoprotein exerts its potent oncogenic effects have been the subject of intense investigation. MYC has been estimated to regu-late the expression of 15% of the genome,[57] and leads to the tran-scriptional activation of a large number of genes involved in cell division, growth, metabolism, adhesion, and motility.[58] MYC also exerts posttranscriptional effects on gene expression by regulating microRNA expression and ribosome biogenesis.[59–62] MYC exerts its transcriptional activity via the formation of heterodimers with its DNA-binding partner protein MAX. MYC-MAX heterodimers bind to canonical hexameric E-box DNA sequences (5′-CACGTG-3′), where they activate transcription.[63] MAX can also heterodimerize with other basic helix-loop-helix proteins, including MAD,[64] MXI-1 (MAD2),[65] and MNT.[66] Whereas transcriptional activation by MYC-MAX complexes promotes proliferation, binding by MAD-MAX and other MAX heterodimers produce opposite effects. For example, MAD inhibits MYC function both by competing with MYC for binding to MAX and by directly inhibiting transcription.

Recent work has revealed that a major consequence of *MYC* overexpression is the global amplification of gene expression. Inves-tigation of transcriptional regulation mechanisms has revealed two distinct steps in the regulation of gene expression by transcription factors. First, RNA polymerase II and its associated transcriptional apparatus are loaded onto a gene promoter by one set of transcription factors,[67,68] but RNA polymerase is often initially "paused" near the proximal promoter.[69–71] Subsequent release from transcriptional pause is a distinct and highly regulated step in the control of gene expres-sion. Unexpectedly, recent studies have revealed that a major conse-quence of *MYC* overexpression is the release of transcriptional pause at genes that were already loaded with RNA polymerase, rather than the recruitment of RNA polymerase to new target genes.[72–74] These findings support a model in which *MYC* overexpression functions to amplify the expression of genes that are already being transcribed, thus "locking in" a cell's existing transcriptional program. The acqui-sition of a *MYC*-activating lesion in a cell with a highly proliferative gene expression program that is normally transient, such as an immature B-cell progenitor, can lock this cell in this highly prolifera-tive state, thus providing one mechanism to explain *MYC*-driven oncogenesis.

TAL1 and LMO Genes in T-Cell Acute Lymphoblastic Leukemia

In leukemia with a T-cell phenotype, the breakpoints of recurrent chromosomal translocations consistently juxtapose TCR gene regula-tory elements, which are highly active in committed T-cell progeni-tors, to the protein-coding sequence of oncogenic transcription factors, which then become aberrantly overexpressed as a result of these translocations. The best characterized of the oncogenic tran-scription factors involved is TAL1 (; also known as SCL). *TAL1* is overexpressed as a result of the recurrent t(1;14) translocation or intrachromosomal deletions in approximately one-fourth of

childhood T-cell ALL cases.[75–80] However, *TAL1* is aberrantly expressed in the leukemic cells of 60% of children and 45% of adults with T-cell ALL, implicating additional pathogenic mechanisms leading to *TAL1* overexpression. One such recently described mecha-nism is an activating mutation of a noncoding gene-regulatory element, which is described later in this chapter. TAL1 acts as a master regulatory protein during early hematopoietic development and is required for the generation of all blood cell lineages.[81,82] However, it does not seem to be required for the generation and function of hematopoietic stem cells (HSCs) during adult hemato-poiesis.[83] *TAL1* is a bona fide T-cell ALL oncogene, as its aberrant expression in murine T-cell progenitors induces T-cell ALL.[84,85]

TAL1 binds DNA in complex with other transcription factors including TCF3 (also known as E2A), HEB, LMO1/2, GATA3, RUNX1 and MYB.[86–88] TAL1 binding can activate or repress expres-sion of its target genes, and a number of these targets have been implicated in T-cell transformation.[89,90] In murine T-cell progenitors, *TAL1* expression inhibits TCF3 transcriptional activity,[91] and loss of TCF3 function induces T-cell leukemias in mice,[92,93] supporting a role for TAL1-mediated inhibition of TCF3 function in leukemogen-esis. The TAL1 complex binds and upregulates expression of several of its own core components, including TAL1, GATA3, RUNX1, and MYB, thus forming a positive-feedback loop that reinforces activity of this oncogenic transcriptional complex.[88,90] TAL1 also upregulates expression of *TRIB2*, a gene whose overexpression in mouse bone marrow cells induces myeloid leukemia,[94] and whose expression is required for the survival of *TAL1*-overexpressing T-cell ALL.[90] Fur-thermore, TAL1 also upregulates expression of the microRNA mir223, which promotes leukemic cell survival by downregulating expression of the FBXW7 tumor suppressor.[95]

The LIM-only domain genes, *LMO1* and *LMO2*, are also involved in recurrent chromosomal translocations in T-cell ALL.[96–98] These genes encode transcription factors that interact with *TAL1* in erythroid cells and in T-cell leukemias.[99–101] Homozygous disrup-tion of *LMO2* in mice phenocopies the hematopoietic defect of *TAL1* knock-outs, suggesting that these proteins function together during hematopoietic development.[102,103,104,105] In addition, overex-pression of *LMO1* or *LMO2* in murine thymocytes leads to T-cell transformation[106–110] and accelerates the onset of leukemias in *TAL1* transgenic mice.[101]

Homeobox Genes

The homeobox gene *TLX1* (also known as *HOX11*) is the found-ing member of a family of homeobox genes that includes *TLX2* (*HOX11L1*) and *TLX3* (*HOX11L2*), each of which plays key roles in embryonic development.[111–114] *TLX1* was originally isolated from the recurrent t(10;14) translocation in T-cell ALL,[27,115–117] and is aber-rantly expressed in 5% of pediatric and approximately 25% of adult T-cell ALL cases.[118–120] *TLX3* is also involved in a recurrent t(5;14) (q35;q32) translocation,[121] and is overexpressed in approximately 25% of pediatric but only 5% of adult T-cell ALL.[118,120,122–124] *TLX1* and *TLX3* encode very similar proteins, suggesting they have similar oncogenic mechanisms. Overexpression of *TLX1* or *TLX3* induces differentiation arrest at a cortical stage of T-cell development, an effect that is mediated by *TLX*-induced transcriptional repression of the pre–T-cell receptor alpha, whose expression is required for pro-gression beyond this stage in normal T-cell development.[125,126] *TLX1* expression in murine T-cell progenitors induces T-cell ALL, and these tumor cells have a defective mitotic checkpoint due to transcriptional repression of the checkpoint kinase *CHEK1*.[127] These findings, together with the previous observation that TLX1 binds the catalytic subunits of the phosphatases, PP2A and PP1, and disrupts the G2/M check-point,[128] thus provide a mechanistic explanation for the association of *TLX1/TLX3* overexpression with aneuploidy, which is otherwise rare in human T-cell ALL.[127] *RUNX1*, which is directly bound and repressed by TLX1 and TLX3, has been implicated as a downstream mediator of the oncogenic function of these transcription factors in T-cell ALL.[129]

The cluster of *HOXA* genes on chromosome 7 is affected by a recurrent chromosomal inversion that places it in the vicinity of TCR beta gene regulatory elements, leading to aberrant expression of the entire *HOXA* cluster in approximately 5% of cases of T-cell ALL.[130,131] Many of these cases also carry cooperating oncogenic lesions consisting of *NOTCH1* gene mutations and deletions of 9p21.[132] This new translocation that directly activates *HOXA* gene expression provides additional evidence for the role of aberrant *HOXA* activation in leukemogenesis and in the pathogenesis of *MLL*- and *CALM-AF10*–rearranged leukemias, as reviewed in more detail later.

Chimeric Transcription Factor Oncogenes

Chromosomal translocations resulting in the formation of chimeric proteins represents a second mechanism for aberrant transcription factor activation, which is more prevalent in precursor B-cell ALL. These translocations juxtapose exons that encode the DNA-binding and protein-binding domains of different genes, resulting in expression of a chimeric fusion protein. The generation of such fusions is facilitated by the modular structure of transcription factor genes, in which discrete exons encode particular functional domains. This feature of gene structure facilitates organismal evolution, but is commonly co-opted during oncogenesis.

TCF3-PBX1 Fusion Genes in Precursor B-Cell Acute Lymphoblastic Leukemia

A well-known example of an oncogenic chimeric transcription factor is the *TCF3-PBX1* (also known as *E2A-PBX1*) rearrangement, which results from the t(1;19)(q23;p13) chromosomal translocation present in about 5% of all B-lineage ALLs and in 25% of cases with a pre-B (cytoplasmic Ig-positive) phenotype.[133,134] This translocation fuses the two N-terminal transactivation domains of the *TCF3* transcription factor on chromosome 19 to the DNA-binding domain of the homeobox gene *PBX1*, leading to the expression of hybrid TCF3-PBX1 oncoproteins.[135–140] The transforming potential of TCF3-PBX1 was first demonstrated by the rapid induction of AML in lethally irradiated mice repopulated with hematopoietic progenitors transduced with *TCF3-PBX1* genes.[141] This fusion has also been shown to transform NIH-3T3 fibroblasts and induce T-cell lymphomas in transgenic mice.[142,143] Additional studies have shown that deletion of one of the TCF3 activation domains diminishes its transforming activity, but deletion of the *PBX1* homeodomain has no effect.[143,144] The presence of the *TCF3-PBX1* translocation was originally associated with a poor prognosis.[145] However, this translocation no longer imparts an adverse prognosis in the setting of modern risk-adjusted protocols for childhood ALL.[134,146–148]

TCF3-HLF Fusion Genes in Early Pre-B Acute Lymphoblastic Leukemia

The t(17;19) is a rare recurrent chromosomal translocation that fuses the N-terminal transactivation domains of *TCF3* to the C-terminal DNA-binding and dimerization domains of *HLF*,[149,150] a basic leucine zipper domain transcription factor. Although the TCF3-HLF fusion protein can bind DNA either as a homodimer or as a heterodimer with HLF and related proteins, no other PAR proteins are expressed in hematopoietic cells, and the TCF3-HLF fusion binds DNA as a homodimer in cells harboring the t(17;19). Similar to *TCF3-PBX1*, *TCF3-HLF* can transform NIH-3T3 fibroblasts, a process that requires the HLF leucine zipper domain and the TCF3 transactivation domains.[151] *TCF3-HLF* can also induce lymphoid tumors in transgenic mice.[152,153] A major consequence of *TCF3-HLF* expression in lymphoid precursors is inhibition of apoptotic cell death. In normal pro-B lymphocytes, expression of *TCF3-HLF* blocks apoptosis induction by either interleukin (IL)-3

or p53.[154] In *TCF3-HLF*–expressing human ALL cells, inhibition of TCF3-HLF function by expression of a dominant-negative form of TCF3-HLF results in apoptosis induction.[154] HLF is the mammalian homologue of the worm protein ces-2, a transcription factor that is necessary for the death of two specific nerve cells during *Caenorhabditis elegans* development.[154–156] This pathway, which is evolutionarily conserved, is inhibited by the TCF3-HLF fusion. Thus, in contrast to the proapoptotic role of the wild-type HLF homolog (ces-2) in worms, TCF3-HLF blocks apoptosis by inducing the expression of SLUG, a transcription factor that blocks DNA damage-induced apoptosis in hematopoietic cells.[157–160] The t(17;19) is seen in less than 1% of ALL cases, but is associated with characteristic clinical features including adolescent age, disseminated intravascular coagulation and hypercalcemia at diagnosis.

CALM-AF10 Fusion Gene in T-Cell Acute Lymphoblastic Leukemia

The t(10;11)(p13;q14) is detected in approximately 3%–10% of T-cell ALL cases and in occasional AML cases. This translocation results in the fusion of *CALM* (also known as *PICALM*), encoding a protein with high homology to the murine clathrin assembly protein ap3, with *AF10*, a gene identified as an *MLL* partner in the *MLL-AF10* fusion resulting from the t(10;11)(p13;q23).[161] Expression of the *CALM-AF10* fusion transcript has been associated with early arrest in T-cell development and to differentiation into the gamma-delta lineage in T-cell ALL.[162] Additionally, aberrant upregulation of *HOX* gene expression appears to be involved in *CALM-AF10*–mediated leukemogenesis, at least in AML cells that carry this translocation.[163] Interestingly, analysis of a mouse model of *CALM-AF10*–induced AML suggests that the leukemic stem cell in this model has lymphoid characteristics, and cells from human patients with AML can be identified that have similar characteristics to the disease-propagating cell in this animal model.[164] More recent evidence has demonstrated a dependence of *CALM-AF10*–mediated leukemogenesis on the H3K79 methyltransferase DOT1L, thus implicating targeted therapy with DOT1L inhibitors in this ALL subtype.[165,166]

ETV6-RUNX1 (*TEL-AML1*) Fusions in Precursor B-Cell Acute Lymphoblastic Leukemia

Although most t(12;21) translocations are not detectable by standard cytogenetic analysis, this translocation is detectable by molecular techniques in approximately 25% of childhood B-lineage ALL, which makes this the most common translocation in pediatric ALL (see Fig. 64.1). The *ETV6-RUNX1* translocation often arises prenatally and is likely to be the initiating mutation in at least a subset of ALL, as evidenced by the identification of identical *ETV6-RUNX1* translocations in identical twins with concordant ALL, and in retrospectively analyzed neonatal blood specimens of children who were diagnosed with ALL many years later.[167,168] However, *ETV6-RUNX1* alone is not sufficient for leukemogenesis because the incidence of detectable *ETV6-RUNX1* fusions in the blood of normal newborns is about 100-fold greater than the incidence of leukemia.[169]

The molecular mechanisms mediating *ETV6-RUNX1*–induced leukemogenesis remain poorly understood. This fusion gene encodes a chimeric protein that contains the helix–loop–helix (HLH) domain of *ETV6* fused to nearly all of *RUNX1* (also known as *AML1* or *CBFA2*), including both the transactivation domain and the DNA- and protein-binding Runt homology domains. Both of these genes are found in other leukemia-related translocations, and both are essential for normal hematopoiesis. *ETV6* was first identified in the t(5;12) in chronic myelomonocytic leukemia, where it is fused to the platelet-derived growth factor receptor gene (*PDGFRB*), and is also fused to *ABL*, *MN1*, and *EVI1* in AML and to *JAK2* in T-cell ALL.[170] *ETV6* is required for fetal hematopoiesis in the mouse. Interestingly, the inactivation of *Etv6* in adult mice leads to the selective loss of

HSCs from adult bone marrow, but hematopoiesis is sustained by committed precursors.[171] Most *ETV6-RUNX1* leukemias show loss of the normal *ETV6* allele, suggesting that the leukemogenic effect of *ETV6-RUNX1* may be mediated in part by loss of wild-type *ETV6* function.[172–175] Interestingly, germline loss-of-function *ETV6* mutations have been recently identified in patients with familial thrombocytopenia and a predisposition to hematologic malignancies including ALL,[176,177] further implicating wild-type *ETV6* as an ALL tumor suppressor.

RUNX1 is the DNA-binding component of the RUNX1-CBFβ transcription factor complex disrupted by the t(8;21), t(3;21), and inv(16) in AML. RUNX1 is a transcription factor that is required for the expression of several hematopoietic genes involved in myeloid and lymphoid development, including *PU.1* and *IL-3*, although it can also act as a transcriptional repressor in some settings.[178] Homozygous disruption of the murine *Runx1* or *CBFB* genes results in the lack of definitive hematopoiesis, indicating that genes regulated by RUNX1 are essential for normal hematopoietic development.[179,180] Additionally, rare familial mutations in the *RUNX1* DNA-binding domain lead to familial platelet disorder and predisposition to both myeloid and lymphoid malignancies.[177,181]

The presence of the *ETV6-RUNX1* translocation is associated with an excellent prognosis, with event-free survival rates of approximately 90% in a variety of studies.[182–184] However, *ETV6-RUNX1* may not represent an independent predictor of prognosis when age and white blood cell count at the time of diagnosis are taken into account in multivariate analysis.[184] Nevertheless, this translocation identifies a large subset of children with precursor B-cell ALL who appear to represent good candidates for less intensive therapy.

Activating Point Mutations of Oncogenic Transcription Factors

NOTCH1 in T-Cell Acute Lymphoblastic Leukemia

The *NOTCH1* gene was originally discovered as a partner gene in an exceedingly rare t(7;9) chromosomal translocation in T-cell ALL, in which *NOTCH1* is truncated and placed under the control of the *TCRβ* locus.[185] Despite the rarity of *NOTCH1* translocations, a search for point mutations within the *NOTCH1* gene revealed activating mutations in more than 50% of cases of T-cell ALL.[186] *NOTCH1* plays several critical roles during T-cell development,[30,187–189] and its overexpression in murine hematopoietic cells potently drives T-cell ALL.[190] NOTCH1 is a transmembrane protein that is proteolytically processed during its transit to the cell surface, where it exists as a heterodimer consisting of extracellular and transmembrane subunits (Fig. 64.2). Upon ligand binding, the transmembrane subunit undergoes additional proteolytic cleavage within the plasma membrane, which leads to the release of its intracellular domain, known as ICN1 (intracellular domain of NOTCH1), into the cytosol. ICN1 subsequently translocates into the nucleus, where it is active as a transcription factor. Activating *NOTCH1* mutations in T-cell ALL can occur as either missense mutations in the heterodimerization domain, which allow constitutive proteolytic activation of the ICN1 domain,[186,191] or as frameshift or stop codon mutations that lead to truncation of the PEST domain. The PEST domain regulates proteasomal degradation of the protein, and these PEST-inactivating mutations result in aberrant stabilization of ICN1 protein.[186,192] Mutations in both regions are often found on the same allele in cases of T-cell ALL, and are synergistic in increasing *NOTCH1* transcriptional output.[186] Additionally, the NOTCH1 oncoprotein can also be stabilized by inactivating mutations of tumor suppressor genes involved in its proteasomal degradation, including *FBXW7* and *Cyclin C*, as discussed later in this chapter.[193,194] *MYC* is an important transcriptional target of *NOTCH1*, and it mediates many of the leukemogenic properties of *NOTCH1* in human T-cell ALL cells.[195–198] However, *NOTCH1* also has *MYC*-independent oncogenic activity, as evidenced by its ability to induce T-cell ALL in zebrafish, where *NOTCH1* does not upregulate *MYC* expression.[199]

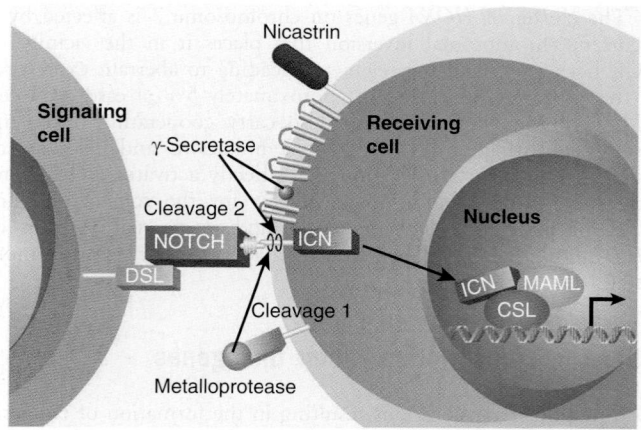

Fig. 64.2 THE NOTCH1 ONCOGENIC SIGNALING PATHWAY. Binding of the NOTCH1 cell surface receptor with δ serrate ligand (DSL) stimulates proteolytic cleavage of NOTCH by metalloproteases and γ-secretase. This leads to the release of the intracellular domain of NOTCH1 (ICN), which translocates to the nucleus, where it acts as a transcription factor to regulate gene expression. *(Adapted from Armstrong SA, Look AT: Molecular genetics of acute lymphoblastic leukemia. J Clin Oncol 23:6306, 2005, with permission.)*

Additional *NOTCH1* targets implicated in T-cell ALL pathogenesis include the *IL7R* interleukin receptor,[200] and the long noncoding RNA *LUNAR1*, which is upregulated by *NOTCH1* and functions to upregulate expression of the insulin-like growth factor 1 receptor (*IGF1R*).[201]

Small-molecule inhibitors of γ-secretase impair the proteolytic activation of NOTCH1 (see Fig. 64.2), and these drugs were previously developed due to the role of this enzyme in Alzheimer's disease. More recently, SERCA calcium channel inhibitors have also emerged as an alternative approach to target oncogenic NOTCH1 signaling. Small-molecule SERCA inhibitors induce endoplasmic reticulum (ER) stress, impair NOTCH1 maturation in the ER, and effectively inhibit NOTCH1 signaling with a preference for mutant rather than wild-type alleles.[202] SERCA inhibition also has activity in human T-cell ALL xenograft models.[202]

The clinical experience with NOTCH1 inhibitors to date has been limited to γ-secretase inhibitors. Although these drugs have activity in vitro in a subset of T-cell ALL cell lines,[186] early clinical trial results have been disappointing.[203,204] In part, this reflects the fact that prolonged systemic NOTCH inhibition is intolerable due to development of severe secretory diarrhea. This is an on-target toxicity of NOTCH inhibition, which drives intestinal epithelial cells to a secretory goblet cell fate.[205,206] Interestingly, dexamethasone has been shown to mitigate the intestinal toxicity of γ-secretase inhibitors, and this is an especially appealing therapeutic combination because NOTCH1 inhibition can simultaneously reverse resistance to dexamethasone.[207] In vivo preclinical data support the utility of this combination,[208] which awaits testing in human clinical trials.

Investigation of mechanisms of resistance to NOTCH1 inhibition has revealed several potential strategies for therapeutic intervention. Activation of the phosphatidylinositol 3-kinase (PI3K)-AKT pathway, which commonly results from loss of its negative regulator *PTEN* in T-cell ALL,[209] provides one mechanism for resistance to NOTCH1 inhibition.[210] The PTEN-PI3K-AKT pathway also mediates resistance to MYC inhibition in this disease.[211] However, work in a murine model of Kras-induced T-ALL, where leukemias commonly acquire activating *NOTCH1* mutations and are sensitive to PI3K inhibitors, revealed that the development of resistance to PI3K inhibition was unexpectedly associated with loss of oncogenic NOTCH1 signaling.[212] This finding thus raises the possibility that dual PI3K-NOTCH1 inhibition may actually promote the emergence of drug resistance. Additional studies are needed to define the optimal strategy for clinical application of NOTCH1 and PI3K inhibition in patients with T-cell ALL.

Recent work has also revealed that some T-cell ALL cases in which the bulk cell population is sensitive to NOTCH1 inhibition harbor minor populations of so-called "persister" cells that are resistant to NOTCH1 inhibitors. This "persister" state is not driven by genetic mutations, but is instead a reversible cellular state characterized by chromatin compaction.[213] These NOTCH1 inhibitor-resistant cells maintain expression of *MYC*, a crucial downstream target of *NOTCH1*, despite effective inhibition of NOTCH1 activity.[213,214] However, the survival of these cells is specifically dependent on BRD4,[213,214] a transcriptional regulator whose ability to bind acetylated chromatin can be specifically inhibited using small molecules.[215] Combination therapy with inhibitors of both BRD4 and NOTCH1 can block emergence of this resistance mechanism, and this approach has promising in vivo activity in preclinical models.[213,214]

MYC Mutations in Mature B-Cell Lymphoblastic Leukemia

As reviewed previously in this chapter, mature B-cell ALL is characterized by chromosomal translocations that place the *MYC* coding sequence under the control of *Ig* gene-regulatory elements. Although the *MYC* coding region is not structurally altered by these translocations in most cases, point mutations of *MYC* commonly arise in these tumors at codons 58 or 62.[216–218] These codons encode phosphorylation sites that regulate the activity and proteasomal degradation of MYC.[219] These mutations lead not only to the aberrant stabilization of MYC protein,[220–222] but also inhibit the ability of MYC to activate apoptosis, while its ability to stimulate proliferation remains intact.[223]

Mutations of Histone-Modifying Enzymes

DNA exists in cells in complex with histone proteins and other molecules in a complex known as chromatin. Posttranslational modifications of histone proteins play prominent roles in the regulation of chromatin structure. Chromatin structure at individual loci can be broadly categorized as euchromatin, or "open" chromatin, where transcription factor binding sites in DNA are readily accessible to the transcriptional machinery, or heterochromatin, where chromatin is compacted and DNA is generally not accessible to the transcriptional machinery. Alternations in chromatin structure can have profound effects on the gene expression program activated by transcription factors. Several enzymes that catalyze covalent histone modifications are recurrently mutated in ALL, highlighting a central role for dysregulation of chromatin structure in human leukemogenesis.

MLL Fusion Genes

Translocations involving the *MLL* gene (also known as *KMT2A*) on chromosome 11q23 occur in approximately 80% of infant ALL cases, 5% of AML cases, and 85% of secondary AML cases that occur in patients treated with topoisomerase II inhibitors.[182] *MLL* is the human ortholog of the *Drosophila* trithorax gene.[224–227] Trithorax proteins are positive regulators of homeobox gene expression and act antagonistically to polycomb proteins.[228] Wild-type *MLL* positively regulates *HOX* gene expression and is required for both primitive and definitive hematopoiesis.[229–231] Wild-type *MLL* is a member of a large transcriptional regulatory complex, together with histone deacetylases and members of the SWI/SNF chromatin-remodeling complex.[232]

The MLL protein undergoes proteolytic processing by Taspase1, a specialized protease that cleaves the MLL protein into N-terminal (MLL^N) and C-terminal (MLL^C) fragments that remain associated through intramolecular protein–protein interaction domains.[233–235] MLL^N contains several DNA-binding domains, including AT-hook domains that nonspecifically bind the minor groove of DNA, a methyltransferase homology region (CxxC domain) that specifically

binds unmethylated DNA, four plant homeodomain zinc fingers with an embedded bromodomain, and a transcriptional repression domain.[228] The C-terminal fragment MLL^C contains a transcriptional activation domain that recruits the histone acetyltransferase cAMP response element-binding protein (CBP) and a SET domain that is responsible for its histone 3 lysine 4 (H3K4) methyltransferase activity.[235]

Wild-type *MLL* encodes a H3K4 lysine methyltransferase, and H3K4 methylation is associated with transcriptional activation. Strikingly, the H3K4 methyltransferase domain is invariably lost in MLL fusion oncoproteins. *MLL* fusion oncogenes result from translocations whose breakpoints cluster between exons 5 and 11 of *MLL*, and the resultant fusion proteins retain the N-terminal region of MLL, including the AT-hook and CxxC domains that bind DNA in a sequence-nonspecific manner.[236] By contrast, the C-terminal domains that mediate the association of wild-type *MLL* with its endogenous chromatin remodeling complex and its H3K4 methyltransferase activity are invariably lost from oncogenic MLL fusion proteins. Instead, the C-terminus of MLL fusion proteins is provided by one of more than 60 different translocation partners, with common translocations such as the t(4;11), t(9;11), and t(11;19)(q23;p13.3) resulting in the in-frame fusion of *MLL* to AF4, AF9, and ENL, respectively. The unrelated t(11;19)(q23;p13.1) translocation results in fusion of *MLL* to ELL, the RNA polymerase II elongation factor.[237,238]

Formal proof that *MLL* fusions play a critical role in the development of leukemias has come from the generation of murine models of *MLL*-induced leukemias. Chimeric mice harboring a *MLL-AF9* fusion gene generated by homologous recombination developed leukemias with a latency of 4–12 months.[239] Retroviral transduction of *MLL-ENL*, *MLL-ELL*, and *MLL-CBP* fusion genes in hematopoietic precursors induces transformation upon transplantation into recipient mice.[240–242] Similar results were obtained with a model in which chromosomal translocations involving the *MLL* locus are induced by directed interchromosomal recombination in mice, a strategy that experimentally reproduces the initiating events in the pathogenesis of *MLL*-rearranged leukemias.[243] Interestingly, the introduction of *MLL-AF9* into committed granulocyte-macrophage progenitors in the mouse leads to the reactivation of a subset of genes normally expressed only in HSCs, and transforms these committed precursors into AML leukemic stem cells by imparting the properties of self-renewal,[244] suggesting that the leukemogenic lesion in *MLL*-rearranged leukemia might occur in a committed progenitor rather than in a pluripotent HSC.

MLL-rearranged B-lineage leukemias have a characteristic gene-expression signature that includes the upregulation of several *HOX* genes and the expression of numerous myeloid markers.[245–247] Both early B- and T-cell ALLs with MLL rearrangements showed a characteristic upregulation of specific *HOX* genes, including *HOXA9*, *HOXA10*, and *HOXC6*, and the *HOX* gene regulator *MEIS1*.[245–247] These results, together with the demonstration that *HOXA9* plays important roles in the transformation of hematopoietic precursors by *MLL* fusion oncogenes in murine leukemia models,[248,249] emphasize the central role of *HOX* gene dysregulation in the pathogenesis of *MLL*-rearranged leukemias. Additionally, as discussed later in this chapter, overexpression or activating mutations of the *FLT3* receptor tyrosine kinase are frequent in *MLL*-rearranged leukemias.[245,246,250,251]

Until recently, the precise mechanisms mediating the oncogenic activity of MLL fusion proteins were unclear, because *MLL* translocation partners have no sequence similarity. However, recent work has shown that several distinct *MLL* translocation partners are functionally linked through their association in protein complexes that regulate transcriptional elongation (Fig. 64.3).[252] Oncogenic MLL fusion proteins have been implicated in the DOT1L, SEC, and PAFc transcriptional complexes. The DOT1L complex consists of DOT1L, a H3K79 methyltransferase, and multiple MLL fusion partners, including AF9, ENL, and AF10.[253–258] The SEC (also known as p-TEFb or AEP) complex consists of a CDK9 and cyclin T heterodimer (known as p-TEFb) that phosphorylates RNA polymerase II,

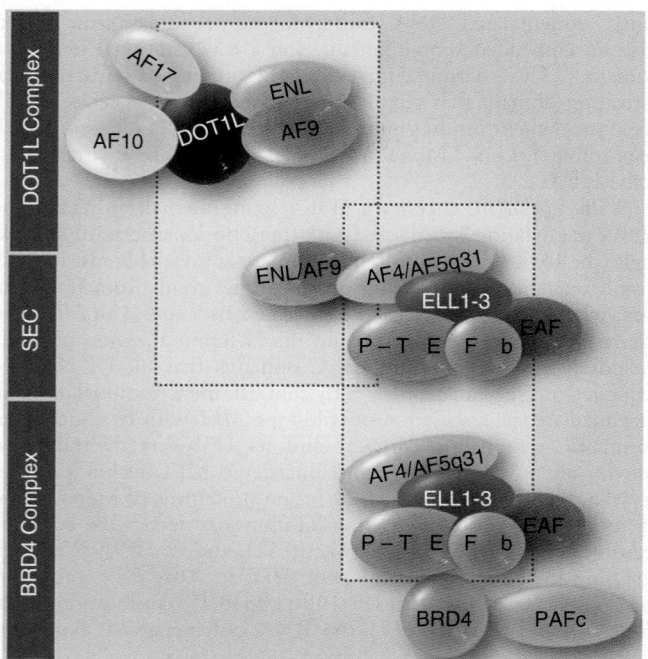

Fig. 64.3 TRANSCRIPTIONAL ACTIVATION COMPLEXES IN MIXED-LINEAGE LEUKEMIA-REARRANGED ACUTE LYMPHO-BLASTIC LEUKEMIA. Mixed-lineage leukemia (MLL) can be fused to several distinct translocation partners with little sequence similarity, but many of the MLL translocation partners have been found to be functionally related via roles in multimeric protein complexes that regulate transcriptional elongation and activation, some of which are shown here. The DOT1-like histone lysine methyltransferase (DOT1L) complex has drawn particular interest given the requirement for this enzyme for leukemogenesis driven by MLL fusions. Small molecule DOT1L inhibitors have promising activity in preclinical models of *MLL*-rearranged leukemia. SEC, Super elongation complex; PAFc, polymerase-associated factor complex; P-TEFb, positive transcription elongation factor complex. *(Adapted from Deshpande, AJ, Bradner J, Armstrong SA: Chromatin modifications as therapeutic targets in MLL-rearranged leukemia. Trends Immunol 33:563, 2012, with permission.)*

interacts with several MLL fusion partners, including ENL, ELL, AF4, and AF5, and copurifies with several MLL fusion proteins.[259,260] PAFc regulates RNA polymerase II and associates with the N-terminus of both wild-type MLL and MLL fusions.[261]

The observation that DOT1L interacts with multiple MLL translocation partners suggests that MLL fusion proteins may drive ectopic gene expression through recruiting excessive DOT1L activity to their target loci, implicating the DOT1L complex as a potential therapeutic target. DOT1L encodes a histone H3K79 methyltransferase, and many of the target genes directly upregulated by oncogenic MLL fusions are characterized by aberrant histone H3 lysine 27 (H3K27) methylation, including the 5′ *HOXA* cluster genes and *MEIS1*.[262–264] Interestingly, the DOT1L methyltransferase is required for transformation of murine bone marrow progenitors by MLL fusion oncoproteins, but it plays a less prominent role in normal hematopoiesis, thus suggesting a therapeutic window for therapeutic targeting of DOT1L in *MLL*-driven leukemias.[166,257,265–269] Indeed, small-molecule inhibitors of DOT1L have recently been developed and demonstrate promising activity against *MLL*-rearranged leukemia cells in vitro and in vivo, with little toxicity in murine models.[270–273] The antileukemic activity of DOTL1 inhibition is mediated, at least in part, by the recruitment of SIRT1, a histone deacetylase that induces chromatin compaction and silences gene expression. Moreover, the combination of DOT1L inhibitor with a pharmacologic SIRT1 activator demonstrates significantly better therapeutic activity than DOT1L inhibition alone.[274]

The oncogenic activity of MLL fusions also requires their physical interaction with Menin, the tumor suppressor protein encoded by the multiple endocrine neoplasia 1 (*MEN1*) gene. Menin binds an N-terminal domain of *MLL* that is conserved in all MLL fusion proteins.[275,276] Moreover, abrogating the interaction of Menin with MLL, either by deleting Menin or by mutating the Menin-binding domain of *MLL*, impairs both transcriptional and oncogenic functions of MLL fusions.[275,277] These findings spurred the development of small-molecule inhibitors of the MLL–Menin interaction, and one such inhibitor has demonstrated promising activity in preclinical models, both in vitro and in vivo.[278]

The presence of *MLL* rearrangements is associated with dismal outcomes despite aggressive chemotherapy in most cases of B-precursor ALL.[16,279–281] Although bone marrow transplantation (BMT) in first remission does not appear to improve outcomes for all infants with *MLL*-rearranged ALL,[281,282] a recent comprehensive study revealed significantly improved outcomes with BMT in infants with *MLL*-rearranged ALL who have particularly high-risk features.[283] Recent data demonstrating the therapeutic utility of small-molecule inhibitors of DOT1L and of the MLL–Menin interaction have generated considerable enthusiasm for the application of these novel therapeutic strategies for patients with *MLL*-rearranged leukemias.

PRC2 Mutations in T-Cell ALL

The polycomb repressive complex 2 (PRC2) is a transcriptional repressor complex best known as a "writer" of H3K27 methylation, a chromatin mark associated with transcriptional repression. Up to 25% of T-cell ALL cases harbor inactivating mutations of core components of the PRC2, including *EZH2*, *SUZ12*, and *EED*.[40,284,285] EZH2 deficiency is sufficient to initiate T-cell leukemogenesis in murine models,[285] implicating PRC2 as a tumor suppressor in this disease. Genome-wide analysis of NOTCH1 occupancy and histone methylation patterns have revealed that NOTCH1 binding is associated with loss of the repressive histone mark placed by the PRC2 complex, H3K27 trimethylation.[284] Recent work has revealed that the H3K27 "eraser" demethylase JMJD3 (also known as *KDM6B*) is a component of the NOTCH1 transcriptional complex.[286] These data thus support a model in which NOTCH1 recruits the H3K27 "eraser" demethylase JMJD3 to its target genes, where it antagonizes the activity of the H3K27 "writer" PRC2. Thus, one pathogenic consequence of PRC2 inactivation in T-cell ALL may be the release of inhibition of oncogenic NOTCH1 signaling. Interestingly, a small-molecule inhibitor whose effects include inhibition of JMJD3 function has therapeutic activity in T-cell ALL,[286] thus suggesting the need to investigate JMJD3 inhibition as a potential therapeutic strategy for patients with PRC2-mutant T-cell ALL.

Focal Activating Mutations of Non-coding Gene Regulatory Elements

Activating mutations of *cis*-acting gene-regulatory elements are common events in ALL pathobiology. This mechanism was first revealed through investigation of recurrent translocations that juxtapose the protein-coding sequences of *MYC* with *Ig* enhancer elements in mature B-cell ALL (Burkitt leukemia), as discussed earlier in this chapter. However, monoallelic oncogene overexpression often occurs in the absence of identifiable chromosomal translocations, suggesting the existence of unrecognized mutations of *cis*-acting gene regulatory elements. However, our ability to identify pathogenic mutations of nonprotein-coding elements has been hampered by the difficulty of distinguishing pathogenic "driver" mutations from nonspecific "passenger" events that represent nonspecific consequences of genetic instability, which are much more common in cancer genomes. Two recent studies provide experimental paradigms for the identification of such pathogenic mutations of gene-regulatory elements, based on colocalization of genetic lesions with markers of active gene-regulatory elements.

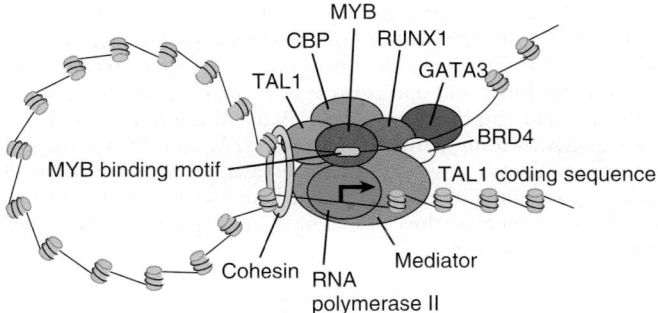

Fig. 64.4 ONCOGENIC SUPERENHANCER IN T-CELL ACUTE LYMPHOBLASTIC LEUKEMIA. Noncoding insertion mutations upstream of *TAL1* create binding sites for the myeloblastosis (MYB) transcription factor, which then recruits it's H3K27 acetylase binding partner CBP (CREB-binding protein) leading to the recruitment of core components of a major leukemogenic transcriptional complex containing *RUNX1, GATA3,* and *TAL1,* and to the formation of a de novo superenhancer that drives expression of the *TAL1* oncogene in a subset of T-cell ALL. *(Adapted from Hnisz D, Abraham BJ, Lee TI, et al: Super-enhancers in the control of cell identity and disease. Cell 155:934, 2013.)*[287]

TAL1 Super-Enhancer Mutations in T-Cell ALL

Advances in the ability to map transcription factor occupancy and chromatin modifications genome-wide have revealed the presence of unusually dense clusters of enhancer elements at select genomic locations. These elements have been termed *super-enhancers* (also stretch enhancers or locus control regions), and are characterized by dense and broad occupancy by core components of the transcriptional machinery, such as Mediator, as well as histone marks associated with active enhancer elements, including H3K27 acetylation. Super-enhancers have been implicated in the expression of genes responsible for cellular identity in normal and malignant cells.[287–291]

Recent work has revealed the presence of focal mutations affecting a specific hotspot in a noncoding locus 23 kb upstream of the *TAL1* oncogene in 5% of T-cell ALL cases.[292] These mutations uniformly introduce a binding motif for the MYB transcription factor, and this occurs at a locus that already harbors binding motifs for core components of the TAL1 complex, including TAL1 itself, RUNX1 and GATA3. These mutations lead to the discovery that the *MYB* oncogene is a core component of the TAL1 complex. Indeed, the introduction of this novel MYB binding site is sufficient to recruit the entire TAL1 transcriptional complex to this locus (Fig. 64.4), which leads to the generation of an aberrant super-enhancer that drives aberrant overexpression of *TAL1* specifically from the mutated allele.[88]

Duplications of the *NOTCH1*-Driven Enhancer of *MYC* in T-Cell ALL

Aberrant NOTCH1 activation is pathogenic, at least in part, due to NOTCH1-driven overexpression of *MYC*, as reviewed earlier in this chapter. Recent work has revealed an enhancer element downstream of *MYC* that is highly bound by NOTCH1, and is affected by recurrent somatic duplications in 3% of human T-cell ALL.[293] This enhancer forms a looping interaction with the *MYC* proximal promoter, and it drives NOTCH1-dependent overexpression of *MYC*. Mice in which this enhancer element has been deleted have a defect in T-cell development that specifically mimics that seen in mice with T-cell–specific *MYC* inactivation. Moreover, murine bone marrow cells lacking this enhancer element are completely resistant to leukemic transformation by NOTCH1. Finally, duplication of this enhancer element drives increased gene expression in a reporter assay, suggesting that this enhancer duplication is pathogenic because it potentiates signaling though the oncogenic *NOTCH1-MYC* axis.[293,294]

Aberrant Growth Factor Signaling

BCR-ABL1 in B-Cell Acute Lymphoblastic Leukemia

The Ph chromosome, which arises from the t(9;22)(q34;q11), was originally identified in patients with CML; however, it is also found in about 2% of childhood cases and 20% of adult cases of ALL, which are almost always of the precursor B-cell subtype.[182] The t(9;22) generates a *BCR-ABL1* fusion gene, consisting of 5′ (upstream) sequences from *BCR* and 3′ (downstream) sequences of *ABL1*. The t(9;22) breakpoints on the distal tip of the long arm of chromosome 9 are scattered over a distance of nearly 200 kb within the first intron of the *ABL1* proto-oncogene, upstream of the tyrosine kinase domain.[295–297] The breakpoints in the *BCR* gene on chromosome 22 cluster in two separate regions of that gene, known as the *major breakpoint cluster region (M-BCR)* or *minor breakpoint cluster region (m-BCR)*. In two-thirds of cases of Ph-positive ALL, the breakpoint in the *BCR* gene occurs in the minor breakpoint cluster region (*m-BCR*), but in all cases of CML and about one third of cases of ALL, the breaks occur in the major breakpoint cluster region (*M-BCR*).[298] The fusion transcript more commonly present in ALL (*m-BCR*) encodes a 190-kd protein (p190), whereas the transcript found in CML and in some cases of ALL (*M-BCR*) encodes a 210-kd hybrid protein (p210).[299–302] Both types of fusions generate chimeric oncoproteins that are activated as a tyrosine-specific protein kinase, similar to the v-abl protein.[303–305]

The ABL1 tyrosine kinase is localized both in the nucleus and in the cytoplasm of proliferating cells. It is normally activated by DNA damage downstream of *ATM* and appears to promote p53-mediated growth arrest.[306–309] Mice deficient in *Abl1* develop a wasting syndrome and die soon after birth.[310,311] In contrast to the nuclear and cytoplasmic distribution of normal ABL1, the BCR-ABL1 fusion oncoprotein has a cytoplasmic location and shows increased tyrosine kinase activity.[312,313] When expressed in murine hematopoietic precursors, both p190 and p210 transform hematopoietic cells in vitro and induce a syndrome similar to CML in mice.[314–317] Transformation by the BCR-ABL1 oncoprotein involves activation of the RAS- mitogen-activated protein kinase (MAPK) pathway, PI3K and JUN kinase, c-CBL and CRKL, JAK-STAT, nuclear factor kappa-B (NFκB), SRC, and cyclin D1.[318–325] The BCR–ABL1 oncoprotein affects multiple aspects of cell homeostasis, including apoptosis, differentiation, and cell adhesion. An important cellular effect of BCR-ABL1 is the induction of cellular resistance to DNA damage agents such as cytostatic drugs and irradiation. After DNA damage, BCR-ABL1 extends the duration of the G2/M cell cycle checkpoint and facilitates DNA repair. It also upregulates the antiapoptotic *BCLXL* gene, contributing to the suppression of apoptotic cell death.[326]

The presence of the Ph chromosome has historically been associated with an extremely poor prognosis in ALL patients despite treatment with intensified chemotherapeutic regimens.[327–329] These patients have been shown to have particularly good responses to allogeneic BMT in first remission, whether from matched sibling or from unrelated donors.[330–334] However, the development of imatinib mesylate, a pharmacologic tyrosine kinase inhibitor targeting the BCR-ABL1 oncoprotein, opened novel therapeutic opportunities for the management of Ph-positive ALL. The utility of imatinib as a single agent for Ph-positive ALL is limited by the rapid development of drug resistance.[335,336] However, the combination of BCR-ABL kinase inhibitors with conventional chemotherapy has led to remarkable improvements in outcome for patients with Ph-positive ALL.[337–341]

Despite its activity, imatinib resistance remains a barrier to further therapeutic improvements in Ph-positive ALL. Resistance most commonly emerges because of point mutations in the kinase domain of *BCR-ABL1*. As a result, a series of novel BCR-ABL1 kinase inhibitors have been developed that retain activity against many of these mutant oncoproteins.[342–344] Although not all *BCR-ABL1* mutations that confer resistance can be overcome with newer agents, the potential of these newer BCR-ABL inhibitors with broader specificity to further improve outcomes is actively being investigated. Additionally, a novel pathway mediating resistance to BCR-ABL1 inhibition has been uncovered in Ph-positive ALL. Upon BCR-ABL1 inhibition, these cells markedly upregulate expression of the *BCL6* transcription factor, a well-known oncogene that is often translocated in diffuse large B-cell lymphomas.[345] BCL6 then blocks activation of the p53 pathway via transcriptional repression of ARF and thus blocks the therapeutic efficacy of monotherapy with imatinib in Ph-positive ALL cells. Importantly, inhibition of BCL6 activity genetically or using a peptide inhibitor of BCL6 has demonstrated marked activity in patient-derived BCR-ABL1 xenografts grown in immunodeficient mice, highlighting the therapeutic relevance of these findings.[346]

BCR-ABL1–Like Acute Lymphoblastic Leukemia

Analysis of the gene expression signatures of patients with ALL has led to the identification of a new subtype of precursor B-cell ALL, termed *BCR-ABL1–like* or *Ph chromosome-like (Ph-like) ALL*. These cases were identified because they lack *BCR-ABL1* translocations, yet are characterized by a gene expression signature nearly identical to that of BCR-ABL1-positive ALL. These patients are at very high risk of treatment failure, mirroring the poor prognosis of BCR-ABL1 ALL.[347,348] One common genetic feature common to both BCR-ABL and BCR-ABL–like ALL is the deletion of the Ikaros tumor suppressor.[348] However, in-depth genomic investigation of BCR-ABL1–like ALL has also revealed that most of these cases harbor chromosomal translocations or point mutations leading to dysregulated activation of growth factor signaling pathways. These include activating translocations of the *ABL1* kinase to "noncanonical" fusion partners, of the cytokine receptor *CRLF2* or the erythropoietin receptor *EPOR*, or activating mutations of the RAS or JAK-STAT pathways.[349–351] These findings have important clinical implications, as many of these mutated genes are targetable with clinically relevant inhibitors, and clinical trials testing specific targeted agents in genetically defined subsets of the disease are underway.

NUP214-ABL1 in T-Cell Acute Lymphoblastic Leukemia

Although the BCR-ABL1 translocation is rare in T-cell ALL, amplified episomes containing *NUP214-ABL1* fusion genes have recently been described in approximately 6% of children and adults with T-cell ALL.[352] These episomes appear to arise via a mechanism in which the genomic region of chromosome 9q34, which contains both the *NUP214* and *ABL1* genes, is circularized in a manner that leads to the fusion of these two genes. The breakpoint in the *ABL1* gene in all of these cases occurs in intron 1, which is the same breakpoint observed in Ph-positive CML and precursor B-cell ALL, but the *NUP214* breakpoints are variable. The wild-type NUP214 protein is a component of the nuclear pore complex and may contribute oligomerization motifs to the *NUP214-ABL1* fusion oncogene. The NUP214-ABL1 fusion protein has constitutively activated ABL1 tyrosine kinase activity, which is inhibited by the BCR-ABL kinase inhibitor imatinib.[352] The therapeutic potential of imatinib or second-generation tyrosine kinase inhibitors for NUP214-ABL1–positive T-cell ALL is of considerable interest.

B-Cell Receptor Signaling in Acute Lymphoblastic Leukemia

Despite its importance in the molecular pathogenesis of mature B-cell lymphomas, the role of B-cell receptor signaling in ALL was poorly understood. However, a recent study has revealed that 10%–15% of cases of ALL are characterized by active signaling through the B-cell receptor.[353] Such B-cell receptor-positive cases were identifiable by expression of the Ig μ heavy chain or of BCL6 protein on flow

cytometry, and were strongly associated with the presence of the *TCF3-PBX1* rearrangement or 6q21 deletion, but rare in other ALL subsets.[353,354] Interestingly, the oncogenic *TCF3-PBX1* translocation itself directly binds and upregulates genes encoding key components of the B-cell receptor in these cases.[353] Active B-cell receptor signaling leads to downstream activation of *SRC*, *SYK*, and *PI3K* oncogenic signaling pathways. Importantly, these cases are sensitive to small-molecule inhibitors of kinases that mediate B-cell receptor signaling in preclinical models, thus providing a novel potential therapeutic strategy for these patients.[353,354]

RAS Gene Mutations

Pioneering studies into the molecular etiology of cancer led to the identification of activated homologs of either *HRAS* or *KRAS* in human tumor DNA.[355,356] These proto-oncogenes were originally identified on the basis of their homology with viral oncogenes. Gene-transfer methods identified an additional member of the *RAS* gene family, called *NRAS*,[357,358] that had not been observed as a component of a transforming retrovirus. Proto-oncogenes of the *RAS* family (*HRAS*, *KRAS*, and *NRAS*) encode 21-kDa proteins that are associated with the inner surface of the cytoplasmic membrane and are involved in growth factor receptor signaling.[359] RAS proteins are guanosine nucleotide-binding proteins (G proteins) that are GTP-bound in their active form and GDP-bound in their inactive form. The *RAS* proto-oncogenes are converted to the status of transforming oncogenes by somatic mutations that most commonly alter the amino acids specified by codons 12, 13, or 61. Mutated *RAS* genes lose their intrinsic GTPase activity, thus accumulating in their active, GTP-bound conformation, even in the absence of growth factor binding to surface receptors. Aberrant RAS-mediated signaling contributes to transformation through activation of the *PI3K* and *MAPK* pathways.[359]

In ALL, mutations of codons 12, 13, or 61 of *NRAS* have been found in approximately 10% of patients, while *KRAS* mutations have been identified in 5%–10% of patients.[360,361] *RAS* mutations are considerably more common in specific molecular subsets of ALL. Up to 50% of cases of *MLL*-rearranged ALL harbor mutations of *NRAS* or *KRAS*,[361,362,363] although these mutations can be subclonal and lost at relapse.[363] *RAS* mutations have also been identified in approximately 30% of Down syndrome-associated precursor B-cell ALL and appear to be mutually exclusive of *JAK2* mutations in this setting.[364] *RAS* mutations appear to be more frequently found in the setting of relapsed ALL and are associated with a poor prognosis in this setting.[365] The development of an effective pharmacologic approach for direct inhibition of RAS has been elusive.[366] However, recent studies in preclinical models of *RAS*-driven ALL have revealed the therapeutic potential of inhibitors of key downstream effectors of RAS signaling in ALL, including MEK and PI3K, thus providing a rationale for clinical trials testing such an approach for *RAS*-mutant ALL.[365,367,368]

PTEN-PI3K-AKT Mutations in T-Cell Acute Lymphoblastic Leukemia

The PI3K-AKT signal transduction pathway, which is negatively regulated by the PTEN tumor suppressor, induces cellular growth and proliferation while inhibiting apoptosis and is aberrantly activated in a range of human cancers.[369–371] In T-cell ALL, recent work has identified a very high frequency of mutational activation of oncogenic signaling through this pathway, most often via deletions or truncating mutations of *PTEN,* but activating mutations of *PI3K* and *AKT* genes also occur.[209,210,372,373] Moreover, deletions of *PTEN* have been found to predict treatment resistance in clinical specimens.[40,209] Studies in zebrafish and patient-derived xenograft mouse models have identified that acquisition of the PI3K-AKT pathway during clonal evolution of leukemic blasts leads to primary glucocorticoid resistance, an effect mediated by direct phosphorylation of the glucocorticoid receptor by AKT.[374,375] In addition, both MYC and the PI3K-AKT pathway have been identified as key suppressors of the proapoptotic factor BIM, which is required for mitochondrial apoptosis in normal T-cell development.[210,211,376,377] Taken together, these findings thus suggest the potential clinical utility of PI3K-AKT pathway inhibitors in high-risk T-cell ALL, many of which are currently in human clinical trials.[378]

FLT3 in MLL-Rearranged Acute Lymphoblastic Leukemia

FLT3 encodes a receptor tyrosine kinase that is highly expressed in early hematopoietic precursors, where it plays important functional roles.[379,380] Multiple studies have shown that activating mutations of *FLT3*, which lead to constitutive receptor tyrosine kinase activity even in the absence of ligand, are common in leukemic myeloblasts in patients with AML but are rare in adults with ALL.[381–383] However, gene expression studies demonstrated high expression of *FLT3* in most cases of ALL that involve *MLL* gene rearrangements or hyperdiploidy.[245,246,250] Additionally, activating mutations were identified in 18% of infants with *MLL*-rearranged ALL,[251] in 21%–24% of hyperdiploid ALL cases,[251,384] and in all three cases of the prothymic CD117/KIT+ subtype of T-cell ALL in adults examined.[385]

In the absence of FLT3 ligand, wild-type FLT3 receptors are inactive because of autoinhibition mediated by the juxtamembrane domain of the receptor. Upon binding of FLT3 ligand, normal FLT3 receptors homodimerize, become activated by phosphorylation, and lead to the activation of signal-transduction pathways that promote proliferation and cell survival.[386] Activating mutations of *FLT3* found in leukemias occur in two separate regions of the gene. In-frame tandem duplications in the juxtamembrane domain lead to loss of the autoinhibition mediated by this domain, with subsequent dimerization and receptor activation in the absence of FLT3 ligand.[387] Alternatively, point mutations or insertions in the second tyrosine kinase domain of the FLT3 receptor lead to autophosphorylation and activation of downstream signaling in the absence of FLT3 ligand.[383,388,389] Small-molecule inhibitors of the FLT3 kinase lead to apoptosis in AML cell lines in vitro. A phase I study of the FLT3 inhibitor, quizartinib, demonstrated an acceptable toxicity profile and is currently being investigated in phase II trials, both as monotherapy and in combination with chemotherapy or BMT in adults with AML and MDS.[390,391] These small-molecule inhibitors are also active against *MLL*-rearranged ALL cell lines,[250,392] and hold promise as targeted therapies for cases of ALL that rely on aberrant activation of FLT3.

CRLF2 and JAK2 Mutations in Precursor B-Cell Acute Lymphoblastic Leukemia

The CRLF2 cytokine receptor binds its ligand, thymic stromal lymphopoietin (TSLP), as a heterodimeric complex with the IL-7 receptor subunit (IL-7R). TSLP-CRLF signaling plays physiologic roles during normal B-cell development and in inflammation. Genomic analyses of precursor B-cell ALL patient samples revealed recurrent deletions within the pseudoautosomal region of Xp22.3/Yp11.3 that result in overexpression of the entire coding region of *CRLF2* under the control of gene regulatory elements of P2RY8, a purinergic receptor that is expressed at high levels in ALL cells.[393–395] In some cases, such rearrangements are also accompanied by a Phe-232Cys point mutation in *CRLF2* that promotes constitutive dimerization and cytokine-independent growth.[394,395] Interestingly, aberrant *CRLF2* expression very frequently co-occurs with *JAK2*-activating mutations, and these two genetic lesions collaborate to induce ligand-independent activation of downstream signal transduction pathways, suggesting that *CRLF2* may act as a scaffold that is required for activation of oncogenic JAK-STAT signaling by *JAK2* mutations in precursor B-cell ALL.[393–395] Overall, *CRLF2* rearrangements occur with especially high frequency in patients with Down

syndrome[323–325] and have been found to portend a poor prognosis in adults[324]; however, more recent studies in the pediatric population suggest that *CRLF2* may not be as poor a prognostic indicator as originally thought, suggesting that in the absence of a Ph-like ALL expression profile, *CRLF2* mutations are not an independent poor prognostic indicator.[396,397]

A number of JAK2 inhibitors have been developed for the treatment of myeloproliferative syndromes,[398] which generated considerable excitement for the application of such inhibitors to *CRLF2/JAK2*-mutant precursor B-cell ALL. However, one problem with first-generation ("type 1") JAK2 inhibitors that stabilize JAK2 in its active conformation is that these drugs induce paradoxical hyperactivation of JAK2, and these drugs have little therapeutic activity in *JAK2*-mutant ALL.[399] Paradoxical JAK2 phosphorylation following treatment with type 1 JAK2 inhibitors is mediated by heterodimerization and trans-phosphorylation of JAK2 by other JAK family kinases, including JAK1 or TYK2.[400] One promising approach to overcome this obstacle is to target the chaperone protein HSP90, which binds and stabilizes both wild-type and mutant JAK2 proteins. Indeed, treatment with small-molecule HSP90 inhibitors, which are in human clinical trials, triggers JAK2 degradation and has promising activity in preclinical models.[399,401] An additional approach has been the development of second-generation ("type 2") JAK2 inhibitors that stabilize JAK2 in its inactive conformation. One such type 2 JAK2 inhibitor has been shown to have significant activity as a single agent, and to synergize with dexamethasone, both in vitro and in vivo in preclinical models of ALL.[402] These findings support the need for human clinical trials testing this approach in patients with *CRLF2*-rearranged or *JAK2*-mutant precursor B-cell ALL.

Interleukin-7 Receptor Mutations in T-Cell Acute Lymphoblastic Leukemia

IL7R is required for normal T-cell development, with loss-of-function *IL7R* mutations leading to severe combined immunodeficiency.[327] The IL-7R protein can heterodimerize with either IL2Rγ, resulting in the receptor for IL-7, or with CRLF2 to form the receptor for TSLP.[403,404] Recently, point mutations in the *IL-7R* have been described in approximately 10% of T-cell ALL cases.[40,405,406] These point mutations typically introduce a novel cysteine residue in the transmembrane domain of the protein that permits formation of a neomorphic disulfide bond between mutant IL-7R homodimers. This leads to ligand-independent receptor dimerization and activation of downstream oncogenic signal transduction pathways, including JAK–STAT and PI3K–AKT. A potential therapeutic strategy to target oncogenic activation of mutant IL-7R proteins is the reduction of the neomorphic disulfide bond. Indeed, *N*-acetylcysteine, a reducing agent developed clinically for the treatment of acetaminophen overdose, has been shown to reduce the extracellular cysteine bond and inhibit signaling by mutant IL-7R proteins.[407] Clinical trials testing this approach are under development.

Tumor Suppressor Gene Inactivation

Much attention has been focused on tumor suppressors, whose loss of function via deletion or mutational inactivation leads to malignant transformation. Knudson first proposed that inactivation of both alleles of a single locus is needed to initiate the development of retinoblastoma, basing his hypothesis on the observed frequencies of hereditary and sporadic forms of this disease.[408] Allelic loss of defined regions of many different chromosomes has been linked to specific types of human tumors. By analogy with the findings in retinoblastoma, a reasonable hypothesis is that each of these regions harbors a tumor suppressor gene whose product is uniquely involved in the inhibition of cell cycle progression and promotion of terminal differentiation of the normal cells that give rise to these different types of tumors.

p53 and CDKN2A mutations

p53 (also known as TP53) is a classic tumor suppressor gene whose activation induces apoptosis, cell cycle arrest, or senescence in response to distinct stimuli, including DNA damage or aberrant oncogene activation.[409–411] p53 is mutated or deleted in a wide variety of human tumors,[412] and occurs as a heritable cause of cancer in families with Li-Fraumeni syndrome.[413–416] p53 is inactivated in a variety of hematopoietic malignancies, including mature B-cell ALL, but is mutated or deleted in fewer than 3% of pediatric precursor B-cell or T-cell ALL cases at diagnosis.[417–419] However, p53 mutations are seen in approximately 25% of relapsed T-cell ALL cases, as well as in association with early treatment failure, suggesting a role for p53 inactivation in the development of resistant disease.[417,418]

Despite the rarity of p53 mutations in ALL specimens at the time of diagnosis, the p53 pathway is commonly inactivated by loss-of-function mutations of the CDKN2A locus in ALL.[420–423] CDKN2A encodes two distinct tumor suppressor proteins, ARF (also known as p14ARF in humans and p19ARF in mice) and p16INK4a. ARF is induced by oncogene stress, such as acute MYC overexpression, and it binds and sequesters mouse double-minute 2 homolog MDM2, leading to p53 activation. p16INK4a is a cyclin-dependent kinase inhibitor, a family of proteins that also include p15INK4B, p18INK4C, p19INK4D, p21, p27, and p57. These constitute a family of tumor suppressors that negatively regulate the cell cycle by inhibiting CDK phosphorylation of pRB.[424] In particular, human leukemia and lymphoma show a high frequency of 9p21 deletions involving both the p16INK4A/p14ARF and the p15INK4B loci. Epigenetic silencing of these tumor suppressor genes through hypermethylation of their promoter sequences represents an alternative mechanism of gene inactivation. Although p16INK4A/p14ARF and p15INK4B are homozygously deleted in 20%–30% of precursor B-cell ALL cases and in 70%–80% of T-cell ALL cases, epigenetic silencing of the p15INK4B promoter has been observed in 44% of primary B-lineage ALLs.[382,420–422,425–433]

FBXW7 and Cyclin C in T-Cell Acute Lymphoblastic Leukemia

FBXW7 (also known as FBW7) is an E3 ubiquitin ligase that targets the transcriptionally active intracellular form of NOTCH1 (ICN), MYC, and cyclin E for degradation, and this gene is inactivated by mutation or deletion in approximately 10% of T-cell ALL cases.[193] In T-cell ALL cell lines, FBXW7 mutation or homozygous deletion leads to resistance of NOTCH1 pathway inhibition by γ-secretase inhibitor therapy, presumably because intracellular NOTCH1 protein levels remain high in the absence of FBXW7-mediated degradation despite inhibition of γ-secretase activity. Additionally, tumor-derived FBXW7 mutations maintain their ability to bind MYC but do not lead to its degradation, and may act as dominant-negative mutants that protect MYC from degradation.[193] FBXW7 also targets the antiapoptotic protein MCL1 for proteasomal degradation in T-cell ALL, providing an additional oncogenic consequence resulting from inactivation of the FBXW7 tumor suppressor.[434]

Recent work has implicated cyclin C as a key component of the FBXW7-dependent pathway that mediates degradation of NOTCH1.[194] Cyclin C, which was originally identified as a growth-promoting cyclin, is involved in recurrent heterozygous deletions in human T-cell ALL. In a murine model, loss of one cyclin C allele accelerates the onset of NOTCH1-induced T-cell ALL, implicating this gene as a tumor suppressor. Mechanistically, cyclin C binds and activates the cyclin-dependent kinases CDK18, CDK8, and CDK3 to phosphorylate the intracellular domain of NOTCH1, and promote its FBXW7-mediated proteasomal degradation. Thus, cyclin C deficiency and FBXW7 are both key components of a degradation pathway heat controls physiologic NOTCH1 activity. The model that emerges from these findings is that impaired function of either of these tumor suppressors promotes T-cell oncogenesis by inducing aberrant nuclear accumulation of transcriptionally active NOTCH1.[194]

PAX5 and Other B-Cell Developmental Gene Alterations in Precursor B-Cell Acute Lymphoblastic Leukemia

A high-resolution genome-wide analysis of precursor B-cell ALL cases using single-nucleotide polymorphism arrays identified copy number alterations in a number of genes that play important roles in B-cell development.[435] Genes involved in B-cell development were found to be altered by deletion, amplification, mutation, or rearrangement in 40% of cases of precursor B-cell ALL. The most common abnormalities identified were deletions of PAX5. Upon further analysis of other cases, other mechanisms that led to inactivation of PAX5 were identified. These included a number of translocations that led to fusion proteins that maintained the ability to bind to PAX5 transcriptional targets but lost regulatory ability, thus having dominant-negative activity, and inactivating point mutations that altered the transcriptional activity of PAX5. More recently, a recurrent germline PAX5 mutation affecting Gly183 in the octapeptide domain of the gene has been identified in two unrelated kindreds, thus implicating PAX5 in an autosomal dominant leukemia predisposition syndrome.[436] Deletions were also detected in the TCF3, EBF1, LEF1, IKZF1, and IKZF3 genes, all of which play important roles in B-cell development.

Ikaros Mutations in High-Risk Precursor B-Cell Acute Lymphoblastic Leukemia

Ikaros is a DNA-binding transcription factor that is required for the development of all lymphoid lineages, and expression of a dominant-negative Ikaros mutation in mice was shown to lead to T-cell lymphomas.[437,438] However, the role of Ikaros in human leukemias was not appreciated until genomic analyses of precursor B-cell ALL patient samples revealed Ikaros (IKZF1) deletions in 29% of pediatric samples.[435] Ikaros deletions are strongly associated with BCR-ABL–positive ALL, and are characteristically acquired at transformation of CML to ALL (lymphoid blast crisis), as well as with Ph-like ALL.[423] Ikaros deletions predict a very high risk of treatment failure that appears to be independent of BCR-ABL1, with patients with Ikaros-deleted, BCR-ABL1–negative ALL faring as poor as those with BCR-ABL1–positive ALL.[348] Interestingly, recent work has implicated mutational activation of a variety of kinases or cytokine receptors in Ikaros-deleted, BCR-ABL1–negative ALL,[349,351,439] as reviewed earlier in this chapter. Given the remarkable clinical activity of imatinib in high-risk BCR-ABL1 ALL, these findings strongly support the need for clinical trials testing specific targeted inhibitors for patients with such targetable oncogenic alterations.

Inactivation of LEF1 in T-Cell Acute Lymphoblastic Leukemia

The LEF1 transcription factor, a member of the lymphoid enhancer binding factor/T-cell specific transcription factor (LEF/TCF) family of DNA-binding transcription factors, is best known for its role as a positive mediator of β-catenin transcriptional activity, a well-established oncogene.[440] Recent genomic analyses have identified mono- and biallelic deletions and truncating mutations of LEF1 in 18% of primary T-cell ALL patient samples, unexpectedly implicating LEF1 as a T-cell ALL tumor suppressor.[87] LEF1 inactivation is associated with a very young age at diagnosis, T-cell differentiation arrest at an early cortical stage of T-cell development, and activating NOTCH1 mutations. Moreover, T-cell ALL cases with LEF1 inactivation are characterized by very high expression of MYC mRNA, a surprising finding given that LEF/TCF transcription factors transactivate MYC expression when bound to β-catenin.[441,442] In addition to their well-established functions as transcriptional activators, *LEF/TCF* transcription factors can also act as transcriptional repressors when bound to Groucho/TLE family members in the absence of β-catenin activation.[443] Although the precise mechanisms responsible for the pathogenic effect of *LEF1* inactivation in T-cell ALL have not yet been established, one potential explanation is that *LEF1* may actively repress *MYC* in T-cell ALL cells lacking β-catenin activation, and that *LEF1* inactivation in this context may promote maximal *MYC* overexpression downstream of other oncogenic lesions that drive *MYC* overexpression, such as *NOTCH1* mutations.

BCL11B Inactivation in T-Cell Acute Lymphoblastic Leukemia

The *BCL11B* transcription factor is required for normal T-cell development. In murine T-cell progenitors, inactivation of *BCL11B* leads to developmental arrest at double-negative stages, acquisition of natural killer-like features, and aberrant self-renewal activity.[444-447] Monoallelic *BCL11B* deletions or point mutations have recently been identified in 9%–16% of primary T-cell ALL patient samples.[127,448] The point mutations identified typically occur within the DNA-binding domains of *BCL11B* and are predicted to disrupt their ability to bind DNA. Moreover, previous work in murine models has shown that *BCL11B* suppresses T-lymphoblastic malignancies induced by *p53* haploinsufficiency, radiation, or the *BCR-ABL1* oncogene,[449,450] and *BCL11B* inactivation is a particularly common cooperating lesion in murine T-cell ALL induced by the *TLX1* oncogene or by *ATM* deficiency.[127,451] In human T-cell ALL, recurrent cryptic t(5;14)(q35;q32) translocations juxtaposing *BCL11B* and *TLX3* have been described, which result in *BCL11B* gene regulatory elements driving overexpression of *TLX3*.[121,452,453] These translocations were long thought to be pathogenic because of the resultant overexpression of the *TLX3* oncogene. However, these recent findings indicate that both *BCL11B* inactivation and *TLX* oncogene overexpression are important pathogenic consequences of this translocation, thus representing two oncogenic events from a single genomic lesion. *BCL11B* has recently been implicated as a core component of the SWI/SNF chromatin remodeling complex, a key tumor suppressor in diverse human malignancies. Thus, SWI/SNF complex inactivation provides one potential mechanism to explain the pathogenic consequences of *BCL11B* in T-cell ALL.[454]

PHF6 Mutations in T-Cell Acute Lymphoblastic Leukemia

T-cell ALL has a conspicuous male predominance, suggesting the potential involvement of tumor suppressors on the X-chromosome. Targeted mutational analysis of the X chromosome revealed one such candidate tumor suppressor, PHF6, which is a nucleolus ribosomal RNA (rRNA) promoter-associated protein that directly interacts with upstream binding factor through its PHD1 domain and suppresses rRNA. Germline mutations of *PHF6* were first described in association with Borjeson-Forssman-Lehmann syndrome (OMIM 301900), which is associated with severe mental retardation and facial dysmorphisms but until recently had not been associated with T-cell ALL. Ferrando and colleagues identified somatic nonsense and frameshift mutations leading to loss of *PHF6* expression in 16% of pediatric and in 38% of adult T-cell ALL patient samples, and which were associated with overexpression of the *TLX1* or *TLX3* oncogenic transcription factors.[455] The pathogenic consequences of *PHF6* inactivation in T-cell ALL are not fully understand and remain an area of ongoing investigation. However, recent work has suggested that *PHF6* plays a role in cell proliferation, and that loss of *PHF6* leads to arrest at the G_2/M checkpoint and increased DNA damage at the ribosomal locus. Thus, it is postulated that *PHF6* acts as a tumor suppressor with a regulatory role in rRNA synthesis and genome maintenance.[456]

Ribosomal Protein Gene Mutations in T-Cell Acute Lymphoblastic Leukemia

Mutations in ribosomal proteins that lead to impaired ribosome biogenesis and function are well characterized in disorders of normal hematopoiesis, such as Diamond-Blackfan anemia and in 5q- myelodysplastic syndrome; however, until recently they were not known to be associated with the development of ALL. Using whole-exome sequencing, recurrent mutations in *RPL5* and *RPL10* have been identified in pediatric T-cell ALL.[457] Moreover, gene expression analysis of pediatric T-cell ALL samples has identified monoalleleic focal deletions of *RPL22*, a ribosomal gene that is required for the development of normal T-cell progenitors.[458] While functional studies investigating ribosomal proteins in T-cell ALL have revealed a role transformation and cell proliferation, the exact mechanism through which this may provide an advantage to the lymphoblasts remains unknown.[457,458]

Abnormalities of Leukemia Cell Ploidy

Abnormalities of chromosome number, which generally occur in the absence of specific chromosomal translocations, have important prognostic and biologic implications in childhood ALL.

Hyperdiploidy

Found in 25%–30% of childhood ALL cases, high hyperdiploidy, defined as the presence of 51–65 chromosomes in the leukemic clone, is a powerful favorable prognostic indicator in childhood ALL.[183] Trisomies of chromosomes 4, 10, and 17 impart a particularly good prognosis, while high hyperdiploidy in the absence of these trisomies is less of a favorable prognostic factor.[459] Near triploid (68–80 chromosomes) and near tetraploid ALL (>80 chromosomes) appear to be biologically distinct entities with less prognostic significance. Patients with high hyperdiploidy can expect favorable long-term outcomes, and typically present with favorable prognostic indicators, such as age between 2 and 10 years, a low white blood cell count, and precursor B-cell immunophenotype.[460-462] The mechanisms accounting for the favorable outcome of patients with hyperdiploid ALL remain elusive but may reflect an increased sensitivity to antimetabolite therapy[463] and a greater propensity to undergo apoptosis.[152]

Hypodiploidy

In marked contrast to the favorable outcomes associated with hyperdiploidy, the occurrence of hypodiploidy (<45 chromosomes) carries an extremely poor prognosis.[183,464] A recent large-scale genomic study has revealed that hypodiploid ALL comprises two molecularly distinct biologic entities.[465] Near-haploid ALL (24–31 chromosomes) commonly harbors activating mutations in the *RAS* pathway, with activating mutations of *RAS* genes or loss-of-function mutations of its negative regulator *NF1* being particularly common. By contrast, low hypodiploid ALL (32–39 chromosomes) has an exceptionally high frequency of *p53* mutations, which are otherwise very rare in ALL. Strikingly, nearly half of these cases had *p53* mutations identified in remission DNA, strongly suggesting these patients have germline *p53* mutations. Despite the differences in underlying genetic alterations, both near haploid and low hypodiploid ALL are associated with activation of RAS and PI3K signaling pathways, and preclinical data support the potential therapeutic utility of PI3K pathway inhibitors for these patients.[465]

Polysomy 21

Gains of additional copies of chromosome 21 are the most common somatic aneuploidy in precursor B-cell ALL, and patients with germline trisomy 21 (Down syndrome) are at increased risk of this disease.[466,467] Additionally, chromosome 21 is never lost in ALL cases with hypodiploidy,[465] highlighting the role of additional copies of chromosome 21 in ALL pathobiology.

In addition to whole-chromosome 21 gains, 1%–2% of precursor B-cell ALL cases are characterized by amplification of material from an approximately 5-Mbp region of chromosome 21 that includes *RUNX1*, the so-called *intra-chromosomal amplification of chromosome 21* (iAMP21).[468,469] Interestingly, iAMP21 is 2700-fold more common in individuals with a germline Robertsonian translocation involving chromosomes 15 and 21. These translocations result in the fusion of the long arms of chromosomes 15 and 21 into a single chromosome. Both of these chromosomes are acrocentric with little genetic material on their short arms, thus little genetic material is lost and heterozygous carriers are phenotypically normal. Whole-genome sequencing analysis of ALL cases with iAMP21 has revealed highly complex structural and copy number rearrangements within the amplified region.[470] Interestingly, reconstruction of the evolution of this lesion strongly suggests that the initiating event for this lesion is chromothripsis, or the shattering of a chromosome in a single catastrophic event,[471] followed by additional amplification via breakage-fusion-bridge cycles.[470] These data strongly suggest that the abnormal structure of the Robertsonian chromosome predisposes it to focal genomic instability involving chromosome 21, possibly because it is prone to mitotic segregation errors,[472,473] thus providing a potential mechanism linking germline chromosome 21 Robertsonian translocations and iAMP21. Children with iAmp21 ALL are often older at presentation with a mean age of 9 years and have a low white blood cell count. Several studies have demonstrated increased risk of relapse and overall worse outcomes with this chromosomal aberration; however, more recent studies have shown improved outcomes with intensification of therapy for patients with iAMP21.[474]

Until recently, the molecular mechanisms linking trisomy 21 to B-cell leukemogenesis were unknown. Recent work with a murine model harboring triplication of 31 genes that are orthologous to a segment of chromosome 21q22[475] revealed that chromosome 21q22 triplication leads to aberrant self-renewal and differentiation arrest of B-cell progenitors.[476] Moreover, chromosome 21q22 triplication accelerates the onset of B-ALL induced by either *BCR-ABL1* or the combination of *CRLF2* and activated *JAK2*. Polysomy 21 was found to induce loss of the repressive histone mark H3K27 trimethylation, indicating suppression of activity of the PRC2. This effect was mediated, at least in part, by overexpression of the histone remodeling gene *HMGN1*, a gene encoded on the triplicated region of chromosome 21q22.[476] These findings thus formally prove that polysomy 21 is oncogenic in the B-cell lineage, and provide a molecular mechanism linking this chromosomal lesion to B-cell pathobiology.

CHEMOTHERAPY RESISTANCE MECHANISMS AND NOVEL THERAPEUTIC TARGETS

Apoptosis Resistance and Mitochondrial Apoptosis

Despite the clinical application of conventional cytotoxic chemotherapy for more than 50 years, the molecular determinants of chemotherapy response have received relatively little attention. Recent work has implicated a major role for resistance to cell death through the mitochondrial pathway. The mitochondrial pathway of apoptosis is regulated by the relative activity of pro- and antiapoptotic BCL2 family members, which converge at the mitochondrial outer membrane. When survival signals predominate, the BAX and BAK1 effector proteins are in an inactive conformation. However, induction of mitochondrial apoptosis culminates in the activation of BAX and BAK1, which oligomerize to form pores in the mitochondrial outer membrane.[477] This step triggers mitochondrial depolarization, cytochrome c release, and subsequent caspase activation, and is generally considered the point of irreversible commitment to cell death. Recent work using an assay to measure the ability of a fixed proapoptotic stimulus to trigger mitochondrial depolarization has

revealed that a tumor cell's sensitivity to mitochondrial apoptosis is a major determinant of chemotherapy response. Indeed, resistance to mitochondrial apoptosis can predict clinical outcome for patients with a wide range of tumors, including ALL.[478] Investigation of the dependence of ALL cells on specific antiapoptotic factors revealed that most cases of precursor B-cell ALL and of ETP ALL are dependent on the antiapoptotic BCL2 protein, whereas "typical" T-cell ALL cases are most often dependent on a distinct antiapoptotic protein, BCL-XL. Small-molecule inhibitors of both of these proteins are under preclinical development and demonstrate promising activity in preclinical models.[479] There is considerable interest in the clinical application of these antiapoptotic inhibitors for the treatment of ALL.

NT5C2 Nucleosidase Gene Mutations in Acute Lymphoblastic Leukemia

Genomic analyses of relapsed ALL clinical specimens have revealed activating point mutations in the cytosolic 5′-nucleotidase II gene (*NT5C2*), occurring in approximately 20% of relapsed T-cell ALL cases and in 3% of relapsed precursor B-cell ALL.[480,481] *NT5C2* encodes a 5′-nucleotidase enzyme that metabolizes and inactivates nucleoside analog chemotherapeutics, including 6-mercaptopurine and 6-thioguanine. Point mutations within *NT5C2* lead to increased enzyme activity in vitro, and their expression is sufficient to induce resistance to 6-mercaptopurine and 6-thioguanine in ALL cells. Patients with *NT5C2* mutations presented with early relapse, defined as within 36 months of achieving remission, and had a uniformly poor prognosis.[480,481] These findings highlight the need for alternative therapeutic strategies for these patients.

Pharmacologic *PP2A* Activation in T-Cell Acute Lymphoblastic Leukemia

A small-molecule screen in a zebrafish model of MYC-induced T-cell ALL revealed that perphenazine has activity against zebrafish and human T-cell ALL.[482] Perphenazine is a US Food and Drug Administration-approved antipsychotic best known as an inhibitor of dopaminergic signaling, but its antileukemic activity could not be explained by any of its known molecular targets. Using a mass spectrometry-based approach, PP2A was identified as a novel target of perphenazine. Perphenazine was found to bind and activate the phosphatase activity of PP2A, leading to dephosphorylation and inactivation of several oncoproteins with well-known roles in leukemogenesis, including MYC and AKT.[482] Despite its key role as a tumor suppressor, *PP2A*-inactivating mutations have not been described as a recurrent event in T-cell pathobiology. This is likely because each subunit of PP2A is encoded by multiple redundant genes, making it easier for a tumor cell to inactivate PP2A function by overexpression of a negative regulator, such as the *TLX1* oncogene.[128] Although the dopaminergic neurotoxicity of perphenazine is an obstacle to immediate clinical translation of these findings, the development of more potent and specific PP2A activators could have important therapeutic applications for patients with T-cell ALL and other cancers driven by hyperphosphorylated PP2A substrates.

FUTURE DIRECTIONS

The immediate applications of the emerging molecular information include a redefinition of risk-classification schemes to emphasize the roles of somatically acquired genetic abnormalities that carry a defined prognosis and likelihood of therapeutic failure. Currently, patients are assigned to treatment according to their initial clinical features and, increasingly, the genetic and biologic properties of their leukemic cells. We are now in a position to view ALL as a group of heterogeneous diseases defined by discrete molecular lesions. As these lesions have been systematically analyzed in larger numbers of patients, it has been possible to devise new classification schemes for ALL that reflect prognosis with precision. The development of new drugs based on the molecular biology of ALL, whose promise is highlighted by the early success of imatinib in BCR-ABL1–positive ALL, is clearly a priority for the future and will likely take the form of compounds developed to specifically interfere with oncoprotein function and other prosurvival mechanisms specific to each patient's leukemic blasts. Additionally, the discovery that enzymes such as kinases and histone methyltransferases play important roles in ALL pathogenesis has provided new opportunities for targeted drug development. The opportunity is now at hand to improve therapy through randomized trials coordinated on a nationwide or even worldwide scale that focus on key subsets of patients with acute leukemia whose lymphoblasts harbor specific genetic abnormalities.

SUGGESTED READINGS

COMPREHENSIVE REVIEWS

Armstrong SA, Look AT: Molecular genetics of acute lymphoblastic leukemia. *J Clin Oncol* 23(26):6306–6315, 2005.

Roberts KG, Mulligan CG: Genomics in acute lymphoblastic leukaemia: insights and treatment implications. *Nat Rev Clin Oncol* 12(6):344–357, 2015.

Roti G, Stegmaier K: New Approaches to Target T-cell ALL. *Front Oncol* 4:170, 2014.

Van Vlierberghe P, Ferrando A: The molecular basis of T cell acute lymphoblastic leukemia. *J Clin Invest* 122(10):3398–3406, 2014.

SPECIFIC GENETIC LESIONS IN ACUTE LYMPHOBLASTIC LEUKEMIA

Andersson AK, Ma J, Wang J, et al: The landscape of somatic mutations in infant MLL-rearranged acute lymphoblastic leukemias. *Nat Genet* 47(4):330–337, 2015.

Holmfeldt L, Wei L, Diaz-Flores E, et al: The genomic landscape of hypodiploid acute lymphoblastic leukemia. *Nat Genet* 45(3):242–252, 2013.

Lane AA, Chapuy B, Lin CY, et al: Triplication of a 21q22 region contributes to B cell transformation through HMGN1 overexpression and loss of histone H3 Lys27 trimethylation. *Nat Genet* 46(6):618–623, 2014.

Li N, Fassl A, Chick J, et al: Cyclin C is a haploinsufficient tumour suppressor. *Nat Cell Biol* 16(11):1080–1091, 2014.

Li Y, Schwab C, Ryan SL, et al: Constitutional and somatic rearrangement of chromosome 21 in acute lymphoblastic leukaemia. *Nature* 508(7494):98–102, 2014.

Mansour MR, Abraham BJ, Anders L, et al: An oncogenic super-enhancer formed through somatic mutation of a noncoding intergenic element. *Science* 346(6215):1373–1377, 2014.

Ntziachristos P, Tsirigos A, Van Vlierberghe P, et al: Genetic inactivation of the polycomb repressive complex 2 in T cell acute lymphoblastic leukemia. *Nat Med* 18(2):298–301, 2012.

Ntziachristo P, Tsirigos A, Weltead GG, et al: Contrasting roles of histone 3 lysine 27 demethylases in acute lymphoblastic leukaemia. *Nature* 514(7523):513–517, 2014.

Perez-Andreu V, Roberts KG, Harvey RC, et al: Inherited GATA3 variants are associated with Ph-like childhood acute lymphoblastic leukemia and risk of relapse. *Nat Genet* 45(12):1494–1498, 2013.

Roberts KG, Morin RD, Zhang J, et al: Genetic alterations activating kinase and cytokine receptor signaling in high-risk acute lymphoblastic leukemia. *Cancer Cell* 22(2):153–166, 2012.

Weng AP, Ferrando AA, Lee W, et al: Activating mutations of NOTCH1 in human T cell acute lymphoblastic leukemia. *Science* 306(5694):269–271, 2004.

Yoda A, Yoda Y, Chiaretti S, et al: Functional screening identifies CRLF2 in precursor B-cell acute lymphoblastic leukemia. *Proc Natl Acad Sci USA* 107(1):252–257, 2010.

Zhang J, Ding L, Holmfeldt L, et al: The genetic basis of early T-cell precursor acute lymphoblastic leukaemia. *Nature* 481(7380):157–163, 2012.

CLINICAL IMPLICATIONS AND NOVEL THERAPEUTIC STRATEGIES

Bernt KM, Zhu N, Sinha AU, et al: MLL-rearranged leukemia is dependent on aberrant H3K79 methylation by DOT1L. *Cancer Cell* 1:66–78, 2011.

Chen L, Deshpande AJ, Banka D, et al: Abrogation of MLL-AF10 and CALM-AF10-mediated transformation through genetic inactivation or pharmacological inhibition of the H3K79. *Leukemia* 27(4):813–822, 2013.

Coustan-Smith E, Mulligan CG, Onciu M, et al: Early T-cell precursor leukaemia: A subtype of very high-risk acute lymphoblastic leukaemia. *Lancet Oncol* 10(2):147–156, 2009.

Den Boer ML, van Slegtenhorst M, De Menezes RX, et al: A subtype of childhood acute lymphoblastic leukaemia with poor treatment outcome: a genome-wide classification study. *Lancet Oncol* 10(2):125–134, 2009.

Gutierrez A, Pan L, Groen RW, et al: Phenothiazines induce PP2A-mediated apoptosis in T cell acute lymphoblastic leukemia. *J Clin Invest* 124(2):644–655, 2014.

Knoechel B, Roderick J, Williamson KE, et al: An epigenetic mechanism of resistance to targeted therapy in T cell acute lymphoblastic leukemia. *Nat Genet* 46(4):364–370, 2014.

Piovan E, Yu J, Tosello V, et al: Direct reversal of glucocorticoid resistance by AKT inhibition in acute lymphoblastic leukemia. *Cancer Cell* 24(6):766–776, 2013.

Schultz KR, Bowman WP, Aledo A, et al: Improved early event-free survival with imatinib in Philadelphia chromosome-positive acute lymphoblastic leukemia: A children's oncology group study. *J Clin Oncol* 27(31):5175–5181, 2009.

van der Veer A, Waanders E, Pieters R, et al: Independent prognostic value of BCR-ABL1-like signature and IKZF1 deletion, but not high CRLF2 expression, in children with B-cell precursor ALL. *Blood* 122(15):2622–2629, 2013.

REFERENCES

For the complete list of references, log on to www.expertconsult.com.

CHAPTER 65

CLINICAL MANIFESTATIONS AND TREATMENT OF CHILDHOOD ACUTE LYMPHOBLASTIC LEUKEMIA

Sima Jeha and Ching-Hon Pui

INTRODUCTION

Serial risk-directed clinical trials have optimized the combination of chemotherapeutic agents and, along with advances in supportive care, have led to current cure rates of childhood acute lymphoblastic leukemia (ALL) exceeding 85% compared with those of less than 10% in the 1960s.[1] However, because ALL is the most common cancer in children, relapsed ALL remains a leading cause of death from a disease in this age group. Over the last decade, minimal residual disease (MRD) has become the most important determinant in risk stratification. Prophylactic cranial irradiation has been successfully omitted from virtually all patients in several frontline protocols, and the Abelson (ABL) tyrosine kinase inhibitors imatinib and dasatinib have revolutionized the treatment of patients with Philadelphia chromosome (Ph)-positive ALL. Significant advances in biotechnology, such as next generation sequencing (NGS), have led to a deeper understanding of the molecular pathways involved in ALL, which in turn helped identify new ALL subtypes and their driver mutations.[2] Precision medicine ALL strategies based on inherited and leukemia-specific genomic features, host pharmacogenomics, and targeted molecular and immunologic treatment approaches are increasingly implemented to improve cure rates and reduce toxicity.

EPIDEMIOLOGY

ALL accounts for approximately 75% of all cases of childhood leukemia, and is the most common pediatric cancer, representing 23% of cancer diagnoses among children younger than 15 years of age. About 3600 children and adolescents are diagnosed with ALL each year in the United States, with an annual rate of 30 to 40 per million. The peak incidence of ALL occurs around 3 to 5 years of age. This young age peak historically has been associated with major periods of industrialization in many countries, suggesting a causative role for environmental changes. Recent studies disclosed that hyperdiploid (>50 chromosomes) and ETV6-RUNX1 (also known as TEL-AML1) ALL account for more than half of the cases in this peak age group, and are associated with specific germline genetic polymorphisms. In fact, the differences in the prevalence of specific germline genetic polymorphisms can largely explain the racial or ethnic differences in the incidence and proportion of genetic subtypes of ALL. ALL, especially T-cell subtype, occurs more frequently in boys than in girls.[3]

Certain inherited genetic and acquired factors are associated with the development of ALL, but most patients have no recognized risk factors. Children with constitutional trisomy 21 (Down syndrome) are up to 15 times more likely to develop leukemia than children without Down syndrome. Genetic instability and DNA repair disorders (e.g., Bloom syndrome, ataxia-telangiectasia, Fanconi anemia) are also associated with an increased risk of developing ALL.[4] Among identical twins, if one is diagnosed with ALL during the first year of life, the risk that the other twin will develop ALL is over 70%, approaching 100% in twins with a single monochorionic placenta. The extraordinarily high concordance rate in monozygotic infant twins compared with dizygotic infant twins or nontwinned siblings results from the metastasis of leukemic cells from one twin to the other through shared placental circulation. Highest in infancy, this risk diminishes with increasing age. If the first twin develops ALL by 5 to 7 years of age, the risk to the second twin is approximately twice that in the general population, regardless of zygosity.[5] After the age of 7 years, the risk to the unaffected twin is similar to that for persons in the general population. The majority of infants with ALL have a chromosome translocation that results in the fusion of the MLL gene at 11q23 with a variety of partner genes, the most common of which is AF4. Identical twin infant pairs with concordant ALL share the same acquired MLL gene rearrangements.

The most common chromosome translocation in childhood ALL, t(12;21), results in ETV6-RUNX fusion. In contrast to MLL-rearranged ALL, ETV6-RUNX1 leukemias present after infancy and have a concordance rate of only 10% in identical twins. ETV6-RUNX1 fusion can be found in as many as 1% of cord blood samples of normal newborn babies, a frequency 100 times higher than the prevalence of this subtype of leukemia, suggesting that additional postnatal mutations are necessary for malignant transformation. Analysis of Guthrie cards of 2- to 6-year-old children with ALL showed that most did have detectable, clonotypic ETV6-RUNX1 sequences at birth. In addition, identical ETV6 and RUNX1 breakpoints were present in each of the twin pairs with a very asynchronous diagnosis supporting the requirement for one or more additional postnatal events following in utero initiation. This interpretation suggests that ETV6-RUNX1 initiates leukemogenesis but is insufficient for overt disease, and further genetic alterations are required. ETV6 deletions on chromosome 12p, the most frequent additional genetic abnormalities described in cases of ALL with ETV6-RUNX1, appear to be subclonal in fluorescence in situ hybridization (FISH) analysis of leukemic cells from nontwin patients. These findings indicate that ETV6 deletion is a secondary or later event in leukemogenesis, and suggest that leukemia might be initiated in utero but requires at least an essential second postnatal event (two hits).[6] Indeed, recent next generation studies show that virtually all cases of ALL, with the exception of MLL-AF4–positive ALL, have 8 to 12 cooperative mutations.

Several genetic, dietary, and environmental factors have been proposed to modify the risk of leukemia initiation. Children with various congenital immunodeficiency diseases, including Wiskott-Aldrich syndrome, congenital hypogammaglobulinemia, and ataxia-telangiectasia, have an increased risk of developing lymphoid malignancies, as do patients undergoing chronic treatment with immunosuppressive drugs. The loss of cellular immune surveillance capability for tumor antigens and the inability to self-regulate lymphoproliferative processes may contribute to malignant transformation in these patients. Absence of exposure to common infections in the first year of life is associated with a higher risk of developing ETV6-RUNX1–positive or hyperdiploid ALL (>50 chromosomes) in older children. A possible explanation is that in the absence of infection-driven modulation of the naive immune network in infants, subsequent infectious exposures could result in a highly dysregulated response to infections in older children contributing to leukemogenesis. Exposure to ionizing radiation and certain toxic chemicals could also facilitate the development of acute leukemia. The high incidence of leukemia among survivors of atomic bomb explosions in Japan during World War II is well documented. Among survivors of the atomic bomb, there was no increase in the incidence of leukemia in children exposed to radiation in utero. This experience contrasts with other reports of an increased incidence of ALL in children exposed to medical diagnostic radiation both in utero and in childhood. Other evidence linking most environmental exposures to risk of childhood ALL has largely been inconsistent. Causation pathways are likely to be multifactorial and it is probable that the risk of ALL from environmental exposure is influenced by germline genetic variations through the co-inheritance of multiple low-risk variants.

PATHOBIOLOGY

Acute leukemias comprise a group of clonal disorders of maturation at an early phase of hematopoietic differentiation. ALL subtypes are a heterogeneous group of malignancies with distinctive immunophenotype and molecular pathogenesis that result in varying clinical characteristics and response to therapy. Accurate pathobiologic diagnosis is not only important for prognostic stratification, but can also help define patient-specific therapeutic approaches.[7]

Lymphoblastic leukemias can arise from either B- or T-cell mutant hematopoietic progenitor cells capable of indefinite self-renewal. T-cell ALL can be classified into several distinct genetic subgroups that correspond to specific T-cell development stages, and is frequently associated with translocations of T-cell receptor genes on chromosome 14q11 or 7q34 with other gene partners. Early T-cell precursor (ETP) ALL comprises 12% to 15% of T-ALL and is characterized by immature genetic and immunophenotypic features (CD1a-negative, CD8-negative, and CD5-weak and the coexpression of stem-cell or myeloid markers), and gene expression reminiscent of double-negative 1 thymocyte that retains the ability to differentiate into both T-cell and myeloid, but not B-cell lineages. The discovery of its mutational spectrum recapitulated that of acute myeloid leukemia (AML) by whole genome sequencing and global transcription profile similar to that of normal hematopoietic stem cells, and granulocyte macrophage precursors suggest that this subtype of leukemia is a stem-cell leukemia. The prevalence of mutations in genes regulating cytokine receptor and RAS signaling, and histone modification further suggests that the addition of targeted therapy might improve the outcome of this subtype.[8] Most B-lineage leukemias are early precursor B cells, expressing CD19 and CD10 (or cALLa, the common acute leukemia antigen) but lacking surface or cytoplasmic immunoglobulin. The mature B-cell ALL, or Burkitt cell leukemia, are stratified separately and not included in this chapter.

Recent advances in global genome analysis have enabled the identification of recurring alterations in genes and pathways with key roles in cell growth and tumorigenesis. Several observations suggest that multiple lesions are acquired subsequent to founding translocations to induce leukemogenesis. A single nucleotide polymorphism (SNP) array demonstrated substantial differences in the frequency of copy number abnormality (CNA) among various ALL subtypes. MLL-rearranged cases had less than one CNA per case, suggesting that MLL is a potent oncogene that requires very few cooperating lesions to induce leukemia transformation, especially in infants, while other subtypes such as ETV6-RUNX1 and BCR-ABL1 leukemias have over eight lesions per case.

Deletion or sequence mutation of the IKZF1, a gene that encodes the early lymphoid transcription factor IKAROS, is present in over 80% of Ph-positive (BCR-ABL1–positive) ALL and is common in Ph-like ALL that has a gene expression profile similar to that of Ph-positive ALL but lacks BCR-ABL1 fusion. The Ph-like ALL constitutes around 10% of B-ALL in children, its prevalence increases among young adults, and it is more common in patients with Hispanic ethnicity and Native American genetic ancestry with germline GATA3 polymorphism.[9] Approximately half of the Ph-like cases have rearrangements of the cytokine receptor–like factor 2 gene CRLF2, with concomitant Janus kinase (JAK) mutations in one-third of the CRLF2-rearranged cases. This genotype is associated with increased risk of relapse. Remarkably, CRLF2 alterations occur in approximately 50% of the cases with Down syndrome. JAK inhibitors have not yet been studied in patients with Down syndrome ALL, and could

be of therapeutic interest given the increased toxicity with standard chemotherapy in this patient population. Genome sequencing of other Ph-like cases identified structural alterations and mutations activating kinase and cytokine receptor signaling, including EBF1-PDGFRB, NUP214-ABL1, RANBP2-ABL1, BCR-JAK2, STRN3-JAK2, and activating mutations of IL7R or FLT3. Importantly, preclinical studies showed that primary leukemic cells harboring PDGFRB or ABL1 fusion responded to ABL1 tyrosine kinase inhibitors, and those harboring BCR-JAK2 or mutated IL7R responded to JAK2 inhibitor, suggesting that these patients would benefit from the targeted therapy.[10]

Historically, association studies of ALL based on the candidate gene approach have implicated a few genes involved in the metabolism of carcinogens, folate metabolism, protection of DNA from carcinogen-induced damage, and cell-cycle regulation in the development of ALL. However, none of these genes can be confirmed by the recent genome-wide association studies that instead have identified polymorphic variants in several other genes (including ARID5B, CEBPE, GATA3, CDKN2A, BMI1-PIP4K2A, and IKZF1) that are associated with an increased risk of ALL or specific ALL subtypes.[11] Rare germline mutations in PAX5 and ETV6 are linked to familial ALL.[12] In addition to identifying common, low-penetrance susceptibility alleles, these data provide insights into disease causation by identifying risk variants annotating genes involved in transcriptional regulation and differentiation of B-cell progenitors.

CLINICAL MANIFESTATIONS

Children with ALL present with nonspecific symptoms and signs reflecting the degree of disruption in bone marrow (BM) function and the extent of extramedullary infiltration. The most common presenting symptoms are fever, fatigue, pallor, petechiae, bruising, bleeding from mucosal surfaces, and pain. Patients, especially young children, may present with bone pain, arthralgia, or refusal to walk due to leukemic infiltration of the bone or joint, or to expansion of the marrow cavity by leukemic cells (Table 65.1). The evolution of

TABLE 65.1	Clinical Presentation of ALL	
Symptoms/Signs	**Etiology**	**Management**
Fever	Disease or infection	Always conduct fever work up and provide broad antimicrobial coverage until infectious etiology is ruled out
Fatigue, pallor	Anemia (ALL infiltrating bone marrow)	Packed red blood cell transfusion (slow if anemia is severe, avoid in hyperleukocytosis)
Petechiae, bruising, bleeding	Thrombocytopenia (ALL infiltrating bone marrow)	Transfuse with platelets
Pain	Leukemia infiltrating bones/joints, or expanding marrow cavity	Establish diagnosis and start chemotherapy
Respiratory distress/ superior vena cava syndrome	Mediastinal mass	Avoid sedation in presence of tracheal compression. Establish diagnosis as soon as possible and start chemotherapy

ALL, Acute lymphoblastic leukemia.

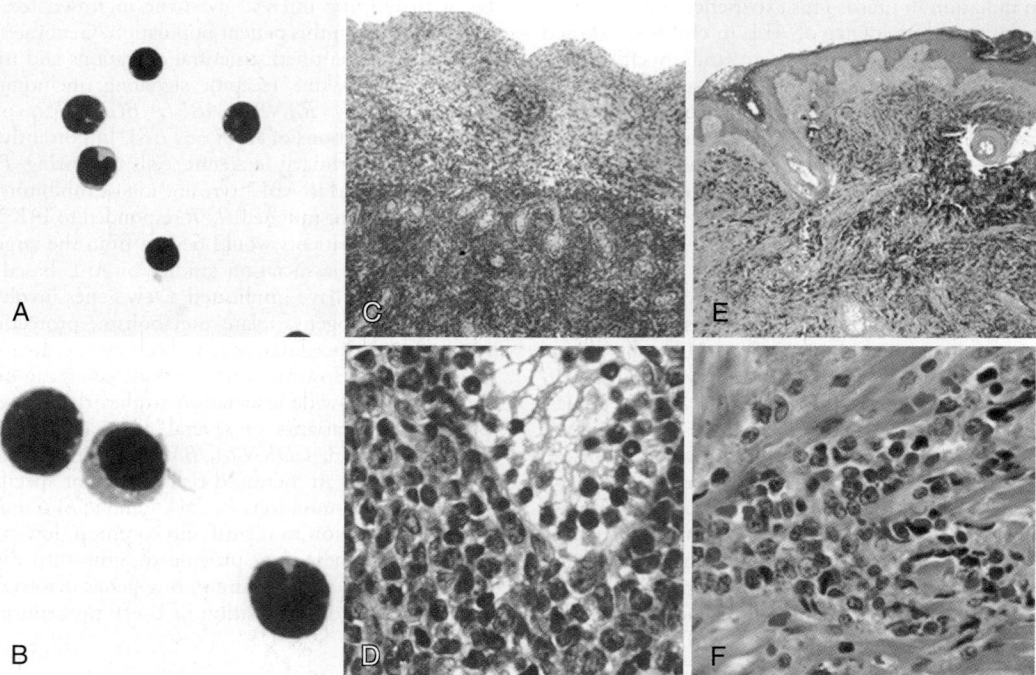

Fig. 65.1 CENTRAL NERVOUS SYSTEM (CNS), TESTICULAR, AND SUBCUTANEOUS INVOLVEMENT IN CHILDHOOD ACUTE LYMPHOBLASTIC LEUKEMIA (ALL). CNS disease identified in the cerebrospinal fluid (CSF) by screening lumbar puncture at the time of diagnosis in a 12-year-old boy with high-risk precursor B-cell ALL. The total count of the CSF specimen was 6131/μL with 6076 white blood cells/μL and 98% blasts. (A, B) The cytospin preparation shows mostly blasts, slightly altered morphologically by the preparation. In (B), there is a small lymphocyte *(middle)* for comparison with the blasts. (C, D) Testicular disease noted at relapse in a 13-year-old boy with precursor B-cell ALL. Note the infiltrate of blasts in the parenchyma of the testes, surrounding the seminiferous tubules. Immunostaining (not shown) demonstrated that the blasts were CD19+, CD10+, and TdT+. (E, F) Cutaneous disease at diagnosis. The patient was an 8-year-old boy with a scalp lesion for 2 months that was initially treated with antibiotics. (F) On biopsy there was much crush artifact, but deep in the specimen there was an infiltrate of blasts separating fibers shown to be B-cell lineage. Interestingly, the patient had a normal complete blood count, but bone marrow was packed with blasts that had a precursor B-cell phenotype and a hyperdiploid karyotype.

symptoms may proceed over a few days, weeks, or months. Less common presenting symptoms include headache, visual complaints, vomiting, respiratory distress, oliguria, and anuria. Occasionally, patients present with life-threatening infection or bleeding.

On physical examination, fever, pallor, petechiae, and ecchymoses may be present. The lymphoproliferative nature of the disease may be manifested as lymphadenopathy, splenomegaly, or hepatomegaly. Overt central nervous system (CNS) involvement is uncommon at presentation, but leukemic cells can be detected by screening lumbar puncture (Fig. 65.1A,B) in as many as 20% of children with ALL, especially those with high-risk disease who are asymptomatic at the time of the puncture. Papilledema, retinal hemorrhages, and cranial nerve palsies may be present. CNS involvement usually is restricted to leptomeninges, and parenchymal mass lesions are uncommon. Epidural spinal cord compression is a rare but serious presenting finding and requires immediate chemotherapy including high-dose glucocorticoid therapy. Laminectomy or radiotherapy is generally not necessary because leukemias are very sensitive to chemotherapy at diagnosis. Overt testicular involvement occurs in only 2% of boys and usually presents as painless, asymmetric enlargement that can be distinguished from hydrocele by ultrasonography (Fig. 65.1C,D). Less common presenting features include ocular involvement, subcutaneous nodules (leukemia cutis) (Fig. 65.1E,F) and enlarged salivary glands (Mikulicz syndrome). Approximately 55% of T-cell cases present with an anterior mediastinal mass. A bulky mediastinal mass can compress the great vessels and trachea, resulting in superior vena cava syndrome and respiratory distress. Patients with large mediastinal mass generally present with cough, dyspnea, orthopnea, dysphagia,

stridor, cyanosis, facial edema, increased intracranial pressure, and sometimes syncope. When significant tracheal compression is present, general anesthesia should be avoided and procedures should be performed under local anesthesia. Immediate diagnosis and initiation of steroids and chemotherapy is essential to prevent respiratory failure. Lumbar puncture and intrathecal therapy can be delayed for a few days, allowing the relief of airway compression and decrease in circulating blasts, without compromising ultimate clinical outcome.

Clinical laboratory data often reveal a broad spectrum of abnormal findings. Various degrees of anemia and thrombocytopenia are usually present at diagnosis. The presenting leukocyte counts range widely from 0.1 to 1500×10^9/L. Leukemic blasts may not be appreciated morphologically in the peripheral blood smear in 10% of the patients. Approximately 45% of children have leukocyte counts less than 10×10^9/L, and 15% present with hyperleukocytosis (>100×10^9/L). Patients with hyperleukocytosis are at increased risk of CNS disease, tumor lysis syndrome, and leukostasis. Leukostasis may manifest as dyspnea, chest pain, alteration in mental status, cranial nerve palsies, or priapism. The majority of childhood ALL cases are B cell in derivation with approximately 12% to 15% of children with ALL having a T-cell immunophenotype. T-cell ALL usually occurs in patients older than 9 years of age with elevated leukocyte count, and is associated with CNS involvement. Coagulopathy, usually mild, can occur in T-cell ALL and is only rarely associated with severe bleeding. Elevated serum uric acid and lactate dehydrogenase levels are common in patients with a large leukemic cell burden. Patients with massive renal involvement can have increased levels of creatinine, urea nitrogen, uric acid, and phosphorus; intrathecal methotrexate should be delayed for a few days to avoid undue delay in methotrexate clearance resulting in systemic toxicity in these patients. Approximately 0.5% of patients have hypercalcemia at diagnosis, attributable to the release of parathyroid hormone–like protein from lymphoblasts and leukemic infiltration of bone; these patients tend to be in the older age group and present with low blast cell count; and this complication generally resolves rapidly with hydration and chemotherapy. The chromosomal rearrangement t(17;19), observed in less than 1% of precursor B-ALL, has been associated with hypercalcemia, coagulopathy, and dismal outcome. Liver dysfunction due to leukemic infiltration occurs in 10% to 20% of patients, is usually mild, and has no prognostic consequences Because vincristine and daunorubicin are metabolized primarily through biliary excretion, modifications of the dosage of these agents are recommended if direct bilirubin level is elevated.

Abnormalities of the bone, such as metaphyseal banding, periosteal reactions, osteolysis, osteosclerosis, or osteopenia, can be demonstrated by radiographic studies in one-half of the patients, especially those with low presenting leukocyte counts. Routine bone surveillance is not necessary because these findings have no clinical or prognostic implication. Vertebral compression fracture that can be found in 2% of the cases in routine chest x-ray to detect mediastinal mass, is usually associated with low leukocyte count and hyperdiploidy (>50 chromosomes), and is not associated with adverse prognosis.

DIFFERENTIAL DIAGNOSIS

Children with ALL present with a variety of nonspecific symptoms that may mimic other conditions. Pancytopenia and fever are also presenting symptoms for aplastic anemia. Failure of a single cell line, as in transient erythroblastic anemia, idiopathic thrombocytopenic purpura, and congenital or acquired neutropenia, sometimes produces a clinical picture that is difficult to distinguish from ALL. Routine BM aspiration is not necessary for patients with severe thrombocytopenia and no other hematologic or physical evidence of leukemia. However, BM aspiration should be performed to exclude leukemia in patients who require glucocorticoid treatment. Children with infectious mononucleosis or other acute viral illnesses may present with fever, adenopathy, splenomegaly, lymphocytosis, or pancytopenia. Fever, arthralgia, or a limp may frequently be confused with juvenile rheumatoid arthritis, which can also be associated with anemia, leukocytosis, and mild splenomegaly. Children with prominent bone pain frequently have nearly normal blood counts, a finding that can contribute to a delay in diagnosis. Immunostains and molecular studies help differentiate ALL from AML and other small blue cell malignancies that invade the BM including neuroblastoma, rhabdomyosarcoma, Ewing sarcoma, and retinoblastoma. Infants may present with subcutaneous nodules (leukemia cutis) that look clinically like Langerhans cell histiocytosis.

PROGNOSIS

Contemporary regimens have abolished the prognostic impact of many clinical and biologic features, demonstrating that the single most important prognostic factor in childhood ALL is appropriate risk-directed therapy (Table 65.2). Accurate assessment of relapse hazard is an integral part of ALL therapy, so that only high-risk patients are treated aggressively, with less toxic therapy reserved for cases at lower risk of failure.

To facilitate comparison of treatment results among different clinical trials, participants in a 1993 workshop sponsored by the United States National Cancer Institute adopted a uniform risk classification based on age and leukocyte. Two-thirds of the patients who were 1 to 9 years old with precursor B-cell ALL and a leukocyte count less than $50 \times 10^9/L$ were considered to be at standard risk of relapse, while the other third were classified as high risk. This classification proved to be of limited prognostic value because up to a third of

patients designated as standard-risk may relapse, and this criterion cannot be applied to T-cell ALL. Moreover, the prognostic impact of age and, to a lesser extent, leukocyte count is largely due to their association with specific genetic abnormalities. For example, the overall poor prognosis of infants less than 12 months of age can be explained by the very high frequency of *MLL* rearrangements (70% to 80%) in this age group, and the overall favorable outcome of patients aged 1 to 9 years is related to the preponderance of cases (70%) with hyperdiploidy (>50 chromosomes) or *ETV6-RUNX1* fusion, both favorable genetic features. Thus a more reasonable strategy would be to develop clinical prognostic risk categories based on their major immunophenotypic features and genetic characteristics. As discussed below, the most important prognostic factor is the early response to remission induction treatment, as determined by MRD level.

B-ALL, lacking immunoglobulin synthesis, is the most common form of acute leukemia in children, and can be further divided into several subtypes based on the stage of differentiation. The high-risk features previously ascribed to pre-B ALL (presence of cytoplasmic IgM) are closely associated with the presence of the t(1;19) translocation with *E2A* (*TCF3*)-*PBX1* fusion. Prognostic distinctions among ALL immunophenotypes, including the negative prognostic impact once associated with T-cell ALL and pre-B ALL with *E2A-PBX1* fusion, have been abolished by recent improvements in risk-directed treatment. Aberrant expression of myeloid-associated antigens has been observed with certain genetic subtypes. CD15, CD33, and CD65 are expressed in ALL cases with a rearranged *MLL* gene, and CD13 and CD33 are expressed in cases with the *ETV6-RUNX1* fusion. Once associated with a poor outcome in some studies, myeloid-associated antigen expression has no prognostic impact in contemporary risk-directed treatment programs.

ALL can be classified according to modal chromosomal number (ploidy) and specific genetic abnormalities of the leukemia stem line. Hyperdiploidy (>50 chromosomes per cell) occurs in 25% to 30% of children with pre-B ALL and is associated with an age of 1 to 10 years, a lower median leukocyte count, increased sensitivity to antimetabolite agents, and a favorable prognosis. In contrast, a hypodiploid karyotype (<44 chromosomes per cell) occurs in 2% to 3% of children with pre-B ALL and predicts a poor outcome among those who respond poorly to remission induction. Low hypodiploidy (30 to 39 chromosomes) is associated with the presence of *TP53* mutations that are frequently inherited, and is a manifestation of the Li-Fraumeni syndrome.[13] Molecular analysis can identify prognostically and therapeutically relevant subgroups that cannot be identified by karyotyping. *ETV6-RUNX1*, the most common specific genetic rearrangement in childhood ALL, has been associated with the most favorable prognosis. With the exception of T-cell ALL with the t(11;19), 11q23/*MLL* rearrangements are generally associated with higher risk of relapse.

Genetic features do not entirely account for treatment outcome and their prognostic impact also depends on the treatment efficacy. As many as 15% of patients with hyperdiploidy >50 or *ETV6-RUNX1* fusion and poor response to induction may suffer recurrences of their leukemia. On the other hand, 70% or more of the patients with the t(9;22) and *BCR-ABL1* fusion, once associated with dismal prognosis, can be cured with chemotherapy and ABL tyrosine kinase inhibitor without the need of allogeneic hematopoietic cell transplantation if they can achieve a solid remission with no detectable MRD.[14,15] Among patients with *MLL-AF4* fusion, infants and adults have a worse prognosis than children. Interindividual variability in the pharmacokinetics and pharmacodynamics of many antileukemic agents also contributes to the heterogeneity in treatment response among patients with specific genetic abnormalities.

The degree of reduction of the leukemic cell clone early during remission induction therapy is determined by leukemic cell genetics, microenvironment, and host pharmacogenetics and pharmacodynamics, and has shown greater prognostic strength than any other individual biologic or host-related feature.[16] Measurements of MRD, by flow-cytometric detection of aberrant immunophenotypes or by polymerase chain reaction (PCR) of clonal antigen-receptor gene

TABLE 65.2	Prognostic Factors in ALL		
Factor	**Prognosis**		**Clinical Application**
Age			
<1 year	MLL⁺ (70–80% infants) poor outcome; MLL⁻ same outcome as older children		MLL⁻ do well on standard ALL therapy. Potential role for FLT3 inhibitors, proteasome inhibitors, histone deacetylase inhibitors, and hypomethylating agents for MLL⁺
1–9 years	Lower (standard) risk		ALL biology may change risk
>9 years	Higher risk		ALL biology may change risk
WBC			
<50 × 10⁹/L	Lower (standard) risk		ALL biology may change risk
≥50 × 10⁹/L	Higher risk		ALL biology may change risk
CNS			
CNS3	Higher risk of CNS and bone marrow relapse		Therapy intensification
CNS2 Traumatic lumbar puncture with blasts	Higher risk of CNS relapse		CNS directed therapy intensification
Testicular	Higher risk		Therapy intensification
Immunophenotype			
T cell	Higher risk		Poor outcome abolished with current therapy
pre-B (cIgM+)	Standard risk		Poor outcome abolished with current therapy
Early pre-B	Standard risk		Genetics may change risk
Early T-cell precursor	Adverse prognosis		Ongoing studies exploring targeted therapies
Ploidy			
>50 (DI > 1.16)	Low risk		Good response to antimetabolites
<44	Higher risk		Therapy intensification
Genetic Alterations			
t(9;22)/BCR-ABL1	Higher risk		ABL TKI
t(4;11)/MLL-AF4	Higher risk		Potential role for FLT3 inhibitors, proteasome inhibitors, histone deacetylase inhibitors, and hypomethylating agents
t(1;19)/E2A-PBX1	Higher risk of CNS relapse		Improved outcome with current therapy
t(12;21)/ETV6-RUNX1	Low risk		
IKZF1	Poor prognosis. Present in 80% Ph+ and also in Ph-like ALL		Potential role for tyrosine kinase, JAK inhibitors
NUP214-ABL1	High risk		Potential benefits from TKI
CRLF2	In half of Ph-like cases, associated with Hispanic/Latino, poor outcome		Potential role for JAK inhibitors
CREBBP	Associated with drug resistance and relapse		Potential benefit from histone deacetylase inhibitors
MRD			
Day 15 <0.01%	Excellent outcome		No benefit from 2nd delayed intensification
Slow early responders	Higher MRD = higher risk of relapse		Benefit from augmented delayed intensification
End of induction >1%	Dismal prognosis		Transplantation in first CR
4 months after diagnosis >0.01%	Dismal outcome		Transplantation in first CR

ALL, Acute lymphoblastic leukemia; CNS, central nervous system; CR, complete remission; DI, DNA index; JAK, Janus kinase; MRD, minimal residual disease; TKI, tyrosine kinase inhibitor; WBC, white blood cell.

rearrangements and more recently by next generation deep sequencing, provides a level of sensitivity and specificity that cannot be attained by traditional morphologic assessment of early treatment response. Patients who achieve an immunologic or molecular remission, defined as leukemic involvement of less than 10^{-4} nucleated BM cells on completion of remission induction, have a much more favorable prognosis than do those who do not achieve this status. Patients who are in morphologic remission but have a postinduction MRD level of 1% or more, fare as poorly as those who do not achieve clinical remission by conventional criteria (≥5% blasts). About half of all patients show a disease reduction to 10^{-4} or lower after only 2 weeks of remission induction, and they appear to have an exceptionally good treatment outcome.[16] The persistence of MRD (≥0.01%)

beyond 4 months from diagnosis was associated with an estimated 70% cumulative risk of relapse. Patients with 0.1% MRD or more at 4 months had an especially dismal outcome. Most contemporary clinical trials have incorporated MRD detection into the risk-classification system. Although MRD positivity is strongly associated with known presenting risk features, it has independent prognostic strength, and is increasingly used in risk stratification of ALL in contemporary regimens.

Currently, pediatric patients with ALL are typically classified into three risk groups: low-, intermediate-, and high-risk (also referred to as standard-, high-, and very high-risk) categories based on age, leukocyte count at diagnosis, blast cell immunophenotype and genotype, as well as early treatment response. More recently, genome-wide

Minimal Residual Disease	Consolidation Therapy
The rapidity of response to induction therapy is an important independent predictor of outcome. There is strong concordance between the assessment of MRD by flow cytometry and by PCR methods. We monitor MRD primarily using the flow cytometry method because it is simple and rapid, and we reserve the PCR method for the few patients (less than 5%) whose leukemic cells lack a suitable immunophenotype. About half of all patients show a disease reduction to 10^{-4} or lower after only 2 weeks of remission induction, and these patients appear to have an exceptionally good treatment outcome. Persistence of MRD of 10^{-4} or more at 4 months from diagnosis is associated with an especially dismal outcome. The adverse prognosis of high-risk slow early responders can be improved with intensification of induction and consolidation. Low-risk cases may be spared the increased risk of early morbidity and mortality from intensive induction provided that they receive postinduction intensification therapy. Novel approaches at measuring MRD using deep sequencing are being evaluated.	The importance of a consolidation phase following remission induction is undisputed, but the treatment regimen and duration varies in the different childhood ALL studies. Commonly used strategies include high-dose methotrexate plus mercaptopurine, frequent pulses of vincristine and corticosteroid plus high-dose asparaginase for 20 to 30 weeks, and re-induction treatment with the same agents given during initial remission induction. Re-induction treatment has become an integral component of contemporary protocols. In one randomized study, double re-induction further improved treatment outcome in patients with intermediate-risk ALL, while additional pulses of vincristine and prednisone after a single re-induction course was not beneficial, suggesting that the increased dose intensity of other drugs, such as asparaginase, was responsible for the observed improvement. An "augmented" regimen including additional doses of vincristine and asparaginase during periods of myelosuppression, improved outcome of patients with a slow early response to therapy.

analyses with SNP array and especially NGS have discovered many nonrandom genetic abnormalities, several of which have already been found to have prognostic and therapeutic implications.

THERAPY, INCLUDING STEM CELL TRANSPLANTATION

In contrast to Burkitt leukemia, which is treated with short-term intensive chemotherapy, therapy for B-ALL or T-ALL is administered over 2 to 3 years. Treatment starts with a 4- to 6-week remission-induction phase aiming at eradicating the initial leukemic cell burden and restoring normal hematopoiesis. The induction phase typically includes the administration of a glucocorticoid (prednisone or dexamethasone), vincristine, and at least a third drug (asparaginase or anthracycline, or both). A three-drug induction regimen appears sufficient for most low-risk cases, provided they receive intensified postremission therapy. The benefit in long-term survival of using four or more drugs during induction is widely accepted in higher risk patients but less clear in lower risk patients. With this approach, 98% to 99% of patients can attain remission, as defined by <5% blasts in the marrow and a return of neutrophil and platelet counts to near normal levels. Intrathecal chemotherapy is usually initiated at the start of treatment but may be delayed in selected patients, as mentioned earlier.

Following remission induction, consolidation (or intensification) is given to eradicate drug-resistant residual leukemic cells. Therapy is tailored to the leukemia subtype and risk group. All patients benefit from a delayed intensification (or delayed re-induction), consisting of using drugs similar to those used in remission induction therapy after a 3-month period of a less intensive, interim maintenance chemotherapy. Double-delayed intensification with a second re-induction at week 32 of treatment improves outcome in patients with intermediate-risk leukemia but does not benefit patients with rapid early response. An augmented intensification regimen consisting of the administration of additional doses of vincristine and asparaginase during the myelosuppression period following delayed intensification has improved the outcome of intermediate- and high-risk patients.

After completion of induction and consolidation, patients receive a 2- to 2.5-year continuation (or maintenance) phase consisting of low intensity metronomic chemotherapy designed to eradicate any residual leukemic cell burden. Weekly low-dose methotrexate and daily oral mercaptopurine form the backbone of most continuation regimens. Many groups add regular pulses of vincristine and corticosteroids to this regimen, although the benefit of these pulses and their optimal duration and frequency of administration in the context of contemporary therapy have not been established.[17] Adjusting chemotherapy doses to maintain white cell count between 2 and 3×10^9/L and neutrophil counts between 0.5 and 1.5×10^9/L has been associated with a better clinical outcome. Overzealous use of mercaptopurine, to

the extent that neutropenia necessitates chemotherapy interruption, reduces overall dose intensity and is counterproductive. The optimal duration of therapy remains unknown. Attempts to shorten therapy duration from 24 months to 12 or 18 months have resulted in a significant increase in relapses. Several studies showed no advantage to prolonging treatment beyond 3 years. A small number of patients with particularly poor prognostic features may undergo allogeneic hematopoietic cell transplantation during first remission.

Radiation therapy was the first modality successfully used to prevent CNS relapse. The effectiveness of cranial radiation as preventive therapy was offset by substantial late effects in long-term survivors, including learning disabilities, multiple endocrinopathies, and an increased risk of second malignancies. Subsequent trials demonstrated that, in the context of optimal systemic and intrathecal therapy, cranial irradiation can be omitted in all patients but reserved for a few patients who developed subsequent CNS relapse.[18] A recent collaborative group study showed that prophylactic cranial irradiation failed to improve outcome of any high-risk subgroups and in fact was associated with poor survival in several subgroups. Patients with high-risk genetic features, T-lineage ALL, and leukemic cells in the cerebrospinal fluid (CSF) even from iatrogenic introduction from a traumatic lumbar puncture at diagnosis, require more intensive CNS-directed therapy to reduce CNS relapse.[18] Studies have successfully used early triple intrathecal therapy with methotrexate, hydrocortisone, and cytarabine or intrathecal methotrexate alone. Systematically administered agents including high-dose methotrexate, dexamethasone, and asparaginase also contribute to prevention of extramedullary relapse.

Based on reports of more potent in-vitro antileukemic activity and better CNS penetration, dexamethasone has replaced prednisone in many continuation regimens. Prednisone remains the preferred glucocorticoid during induction because of the relative increased toxicity associated with dexamethasone use.[19] Polyethylene glycol–conjugated asparaginase, a long-acting and less allergenic form, is progressively replacing the native *Escherichia coli* asparaginase, and is being increasingly administered intravenously instead of intramuscularly. Asparaginase derived from *Erwinia chrysanthemi* has a short half-life and its use is currently limited to patients who are allergic to the *E. coli* formulations.[20] The dose schedule for asparaginase should take into account the variability in the pharmacokinetic profile and potency among the different preparations. Intensifying asparaginase therapy during the early phase of treatment benefits high-risk patients, particularly those with T-cell disease. Significant improvement was also reported in the outcome of patients receiving early intensification consisting of intermediate- or high-dose antimetabolite therapy.[21] The optimal dose of methotrexate depends on the leukemic cell genotype and phenotype, as well as host pharmacogenetic and pharmacokinetic parameters. Methotrexate at 2.5 g/m^2 is adequate for most patients with standard-risk B-ALL, but a higher dose (5 g/m^2) may benefit those with T-cell or high-risk B-ALL. This observation is consistent with the finding that T-lineage blast cells accumulate methotrexate polyglutamates less avidly than do B-lineage blast cells. The increased ability of hyperdiploid ALL blasts cells to accumulate methotrexate polyglutamate could partially explain the excellent outcome of children with hyperdiploid >50 ALL treated on regimens based on low-intensity antimetabolites. Leucovorin rescue is necessary after treatment with high-dose methotrexate; however, overzealous rescue might counteract the antileukemic activity of methotrexate. While the intensive asparaginase and high-dose methotrexate treatment has significantly improved the outcome for patients with T-cell ALL, the emergence of specific therapy like the purine nucleoside analog nelarabine will likely increase the tendency to assign patients with T-cell ALL to a specific treatment protocol or stratum.

About 10% of the population inherit one wild-type gene encoding thiopurine methyltransferase (TPMT) and one nonfunctional variant allele, resulting in intermediate enzyme activity, while 1 in 300 people inherit two nonfunctional variant alleles and are completely deficient of this enzyme that catalyzes the S-methylation of mercaptopurine to its inactive metabolite. Patients with heterozygous and especially homozygous deficiency of TPMT are at high risk of severe myelosuppression. Patients with poor tolerance to antimetabolite treatment should be tested for TPMT genotype or activity for selective dose reduction of mercaptopurine. Recently, *NUDT15* polymorphism was found to account for the poor tolerance of Asian and to a lesser degree Hispanic populations to mercaptopurine. Substituting thioguanine for mercaptopurine during continuation therapy was associated with a high incidence of profound thrombocytopenia and hepatic venoocclusive disease. Thioguanine use has therefore been limited to short pulses administered during consolidation therapy in some trials, and some patients who develop mercaptopurine-induced pancreatitis.

As optimizing the administration of existing therapies is reaching its limit, further improvements in outcome will require the development of therapeutic approaches directed against rational therapeutic targets. The expanded understanding of the biologic, immunologic, and genetic heterogeneity of ALL has enabled development of several novel therapeutic strategies. Various monoclonal antibodies, bispecific T-cell engager antibody (blinatumomab), and autologous CD19 chimeric antigen receptor (CAR) T cells are showing promise in early clinical trials and may be incorporated into ALL regimens in the future.[22]

Autologous transplantation has failed to improve the outcome in ALL. Comparisons between allogeneic hematopoietic cell transplantation and intensive chemotherapy for high-risk patients have yielded inconsistent results due to the small number of patients studied and differences in case selection criteria. It is generally accepted that allogeneic transplantation is a treatment modality for patients with ALL who are predicted to respond poorly to intensive chemotherapy.[23] At present, patients with refractory leukemia (failure to enter morphologic remission after 4 to 6 weeks of induction therapy), high level of MRD (>1%) after remission induction, persistent MRD after consolidation treatment, and early hematologic relapse are candidates for allogeneic transplantation. It is crucial to reduce residual disease to, or close to, undetectable levels as the outcome is superior if MRD

is undetectable prior to transplantation, and worsens with increasing MRD levels at time of transplant. Whether CAR T-cell therapy can replace transplantation in selected patients will need to be tested in prospective clinical trials.

Treatment approaches for adolescents and young adults with ALL have evolved considerably with the widespread adoption of pediatric-based protocols that appears to have significantly improved survival and decreased the need for transplantation in this age group. The benefit of allogeneic transplantation in infants with t(4;11) ALL remains controversial, and should be evaluated in the context of emerging molecular therapies such as FLT3, DNA methyltransferase, proteasome, and histone deacetylase inhibitors. Patients with the recently identified ETP ALL and Ph-like ALL may benefit from molecularly targeted therapy that will improve their outcome without relying on transplantation. Matched unrelated-donor or cord blood transplantation has yielded outcomes comparable to those obtained with matched related-donor transplantation, and should be considered reasonable alternatives if a matched donor is not available. Many advances have been made in stem cell transplantation, such as prevention of graft-versus-host disease, expansion of the pool of suitable unrelated or related donors, donor selection and tissue typing, acceleration of engraftment, enhancement of the graft-versus-leukemia effect, and supportive care. Because improvements in transplantation tend to parallel those in chemotherapy, the indications for transplantation in newly diagnosed and relapsed patients should be re-evaluated periodically. For example, the presence of the Philadelphia chromosome is no longer a clear indication for transplantation with the advent of ABL tyrosine kinase inhibitors.

ACUTE LYMPHOBLASTIC LEUKEMIA RELAPSE

Most relapses occur during treatment or within the first 2 years after its completion, although relapses have been reported as late as 10 years after initial ALL diagnosis. The most common site of relapse is the BM.[24] Relapse in extramedullary sites, such as the CNS and testes, has decreased to less than 3% and 1%, respectively. Leukemia relapse occasionally occurs at other sites, including the eye, ovary, uterus, bone, muscle, tonsil, kidney, mediastinum, pleura, and paranasal sinus. Extramedullary relapse in children with ALL frequently presents as an isolated clinical finding. However, in studies that included the MRD assay, many extramedullary recurrences were associated with MRD in the BM. A small fraction of patients experience a recurrence of acute leukemia with an immunophenotype different from that determined at diagnosis. Some of the cases represent relapse of original leukemic clones with a shift in immunophenotype, but others are secondary malignancies caused by the mutagenic effects of leukemia treatment, especially from epipodophyllotoxin. Patients with isolated BM relapse generally fare worse than those with isolated extramedullary relapse or combined BM and extramedullary relapse.[25] Factors indicating an especially poor prognosis are short initial remission and T-cell immunophenotype. The presence of MRD at the end of second remission induction is also a strong adverse prognostic indicator. While chemotherapy may secure a prolonged second remission in children with ALL who experience late relapse (defined as more than 6 months after cessation of therapy), allogeneic transplantation is the treatment of choice for patients who experience

---

Dose Schedule

The biologically equivalent doses among the different formulations of corticosteroids, thiopurines, and asparaginase are not clear. Trials comparing such agents should be cautiously interpreted taking into account the dose schedule and route of administration, and the effect of variability in the pharmacokinetic profile and potency among the agents involved. Simple modification of dose, schedule, or route of administration may result in significant differences in efficacy and toxicity. Also, when comparing regimens containing high-dose intravenous methotrexate, the dose schedule of leucovorin rescue should not be ignored as it plays a crucial role in modulating the activity and toxicity of methotrexate.

Therapeutic Innovations Being Incorporated Into Contemporary Personalized ALL Therapy

1. Targeting genetic alterations that drive high-risk Ph-like ALL with ABL tyrosine kinase inhibitors and JAK inhibitors
2. Immunotherapeutic approaches with bispecific T-cell engager antibodies and chimeric antigen receptor (CAR) T cells
3. Proteasome inhibitors
4. Histone deacetylase inhibitors

hematologic relapse during therapy or shortly thereafter and for those with T-cell ALL. Patients with late-onset isolated CNS relapse who had not received cranial irradiation as initial CNS-directed therapy have a very high remission retrieval rate, with long-term prognosis approaching that of newly diagnosed patients.

Genome-wide studies using paired diagnosis and relapse samples from the same patients are exploring the genetic basis of relapse. Although 90% of the cases exhibit differential gaining or losing genetic lesions from diagnosis to relapse, most relapse samples are clonally related to diagnosis samples. Relapse clones could be present as minor populations at diagnosis and selected during treatment to emerge in the predominant clone at relapse, displaying alterations of genes that have been implicated in treatment resistance. Almost 20% of relapsed cases have sequence or deletion mutations of *CREBBP*, which impair histone acetylation and transcriptional regulation of CREBBP targets, suggesting that the mutations may confer drug resistance and raising the possibility of using drugs to reverse the aberrant epigenetic programs, such as histone deacetylase inhibitors.[26] The next generation of deep sequencing technologies promises to unravel many more, if not the full repertoire of genetic alterations in leukemia.

SUPPORTIVE CARE

Stringent supportive care significantly contributes to a favorable ALL outcome, and should be initiated at diagnosis as remission induction is associated with an increased risk from cardiovascular, metabolic, and infectious complications. All febrile patients with or without documented infection should be given broad-spectrum intravenous antibiotics until an infectious disease can be excluded. Rapid turnover of leukemia cells before and immediately after the initiation of chemotherapy leads to metabolic disturbances including hyperkalemia, hyperuricemia, hyperphosphatemia, and secondary hypocalcemia. Patients with high levels of uric acid are at risk for the development of acute kidney injury secondary to uric acid deposition in the kidneys. All patients require intravenous hydration to prevent or treat hyperuricemia and hyperphosphatemia. Allopurinol, a xanthine oxidase inhibitor, can prevent uric acid formation. Rasburicase, a recombinant urate oxidase that breaks down uric acid to allantoin (a readily excretable metabolite with 5- to 10-fold higher solubility than uric acid), is more effective than allopurinol but is associated with methemoglobinemia or hemolytic anemia in patients with glucose-6-phosphate dehydrogenase deficiency because hydrogen peroxide is a byproduct of the uric acid breakdown.[27] Phosphate binders should also be used to prevent or treat hyperphosphatemia. Transfusions should be administered slowly in patients with severe anemia to prevent congestive heart failure. In patients with extreme hyperleukocytosis, prompt diagnosis can be established on peripheral blood, and chemotherapy should be urgently initiated (usually steroids with gradual introduction of other agents to achieve adequate response while avoiding massive tumor lysis). Packed red blood cell transfusion should be delayed until after the leukocyte count is decreased to prevent complications of leukostasis, but platelet transfusion should be administered to prevent bleeding. All blood products should be irradiated in patients who are receiving immunosuppressive therapy to prevent graft-versus-host disease. Patients should avoid foods that may be contaminated with pathogens and reduce salt intake, which could induce hypertension and resultant seizure in patients receiving glucocorticoids during induction. Adolescents, obese individuals, and patients with Down syndrome are at increased risk of hyperglycemia and other complications. Prophylactic use of trimethoprim-sulfamethoxazole (or pentamidine or atovaquone in patients with poor tolerance to trimethoprim-sulfamethoxazole) successfully prevents *Pneumocystis jiroveci* (formerly *carinii*) pneumonia. Dental evaluation at diagnosis and meticulous oral hygiene during chemotherapy minimizes the oral complications of leukemia and its treatment. It is important to distinguish between herpes simplex viral infection and chemotherapy-induced oral mucositis. Occasionally, patients have nausea and substantial pain on swallowing because

of esophageal herpes simplex viral infection, candidiasis, or both. Oral candidiasis occurs frequently, especially in young children. Azole compounds (e.g., fluconazole, itraconazole, ketaconazole) are frequently used to treat fungal infections. It should be recognized that they can inhibit cytochrome P450 enzymes and increase the toxicities of various antileukemic agents, especially vincristine. On the other hand, concomitant administration of anticonvulsants that induce cytochrome P450 enzymes (e.g., phenytoin, phenobarbital, carbamazepine) increases the systemic clearance of several antileukemic agents and may adversely affect treatment outcome. Anticonvulsants that are less likely to induce the activity of cytochrome P450 enzymes (e.g., levetiracetam [Keppra]) are recommended in patients receiving chemotherapy. Photosensitive skin rash can occur during antimetabolite therapy. The rashes are erythematous, maculopapular, similar to atopic eczema, and most prominent on the face. Topical administration of simple emollients or a weak steroid preparation, and avoidance of external exposure to sunlight, should improve the skin condition. Patients with Down syndrome tolerate methotrexate poorly, and appropriate dose adjustment is indicated in them. During each clinic visit, a thorough review of all drugs should be undertaken because of potential adverse interactions among them. In fact, chemotherapy can also interact with various food (e.g., grapefruit) and supplements (e.g., St. John's wort, folic acid).[28]

LATE EFFECTS OF TREATMENT

The most problematic late effects of contemporary ALL therapy include neuropsychologic impairments, bone morbidity, and obesity.[29] While neuropsychologic deficits are well-recognized side effects of cranial irradiation, intrathecal and systemic chemotherapy (especially methotrexate) can also cause brain atrophy and spinal cord dysfunction and contribute to the development of neurocognitive toxicities. Severe CNS toxicity has been attributed to cranial irradiation at doses of 2400 cGy or higher, but lower doses have also been associated with long-term neuropsychologic impairments, especially in younger children. Obesity, most prevalent among female survivors of childhood ALL, may be related to metabolic syndrome caused by treatment with cranial radiation and corticosteroids. Osteopenia, fractures, and osteonecrosis have been observed in up to 30% of survivors of childhood ALL. Osteonecrosis, which can lead to significant pain, loss of function, and total joint replacement, has been reported in approximately 8% of children with ALL, with the highest frequency observed in those diagnosed in adolescence. Testicular function (in boys treated with less than 6 g/m[2] cumulative dose of cyclophosphamide) and especially ovarian function are relatively unaffected by antileukemic therapy. Offspring of patients successfully treated for childhood ALL are generally expected to be as normal as the general population. However, recent studies showed that about 5% of patients with ALL inherit major cancer predisposing genes, some of which (such as TP53) have important clinical implication to the immediate family members.[30] Second malignant neoplasms, including malignant gliomas, meningiomas, and myeloid malignancies, occur with increased frequency in patients treated with regimens that included irradiation, epipodophyllotoxins, or alkylating agents.[31]

FUTURE DIRECTIONS

As the cure rate approaches 90%, treatment response assessed by MRD measurements of submicroscopic leukemia has emerged as a powerful and independent prognostic indicator for gauging the intensity of ALL therapy. Children at high risk of relapse may now benefit from early intensification of therapy. The next goal is to reduce the intensity of therapy in children at very low risk of relapse, hence avoiding undue toxicity. The successful elimination of preventive cranial irradiation indicates that treatment reduction is feasible if done with caution and appropriate substitution with less toxic alternatives. Global genome analysis, in addition to refining leukemia classification, is helping identify potential molecular targets for therapy. Expanding the application of pharmacogenomics, a science that aims to define the genetic determinants of drug effects, will allow further personalized therapy in the future.

REFERENCES

1. Pui CH, Yang JJ, Hunger SP, et al: Childhood acute lymphoblastic leukemia: progress through collaboration. *J Clin Oncol* 33:2938–2948, 2015.
2. Hunger SP, Mullighan CG: Acute lymphoblastic leukemia in children. *N Engl J Med* 373(16):1541–1552, 2015.
3. Pui CH, Robison LL, Look AT: Acute lymphoblastic leukaemia. *Lancet* 371(9617):1030–1043, 2008.
4. Bienemann K, Burkhardt B, Modlich S, et al: Promising therapy results for lymphoid malignancies in children with chromosomal breakage syndromes (Ataxia teleangiectasia or Nijmegen-breakage syndrome): a retrospective survey. *Br J Haematol* 155(4):468–476, 2011.
5. Schmiegelow K, Lausten Thomsen U, Baruchel A, et al: High concordance of subtypes of childhood acute lymphoblastic leukemia within families: lessons from sibships with multiple cases of leukemia. *Leukemia* 26(4):675–681, 2012.
6. Zelent A, Greaves M, Enver T: Role of the TEL-AML1 fusion gene in the molecular pathogenesis of childhood acute lymphoblastic leukaemia. *Oncogene* 23(24):4275–4283, 2004.
7. Pui CH, Carroll WL, Meshinchi S, et al: Biology, risk stratification, and therapy of pediatric acute leukemias: an update. *J Clin Oncol* 29(5):551–565, 2011.
8. Zhang J, Ding L, Holmfeldt L, et al: The genetic basis of early T-cell precursor acute lymphoblastic leukaemia. *Nature* 481(7380):157–163, 2012.
9. Harvey RC, Mullighan CG, Chen IM, et al: Rearrangement of CRLF2 is associated with mutation of JAK kinases, alteration of IKZF1, Hispanic/Latino ethnicity, and a poor outcome in pediatric B-progenitor acute lymphoblastic leukemia. *Blood* 115(26):5312–5321, 2010.
10. Roberts KG, Li Y, Payne-Turner D, et al: Targetable kinase-activating lesions in Ph-like acute lymphoblastic leukemia. *N Engl J Med* 371(11):1005–1015, 2014.
11. Trevino LR, Yang W, French D, et al: Germline genomic variants associated with childhood acute lymphoblastic leukemia. *Nat Genet* 41(9):1001–1005, 2009.
12. Shah S, Schrade KA, Waanders E, et al: A recurrent germline PAX5 mutation confers susceptibility to pre-B cell acute lymphoblastic leukemia. *Nat Genet* 45(10):1226–1231, 2013.
13. Holmfeldt L, Wei L, Diaz-Flores E, et al: The genomic landscape of hypodiploid acute lymphoblastic leukemia. *Nat Genet* 45(3):242–252, 2013.
14. Arico M, Schrappe M, Hunger SP, et al: Clinical outcome of children with newly diagnosed Philadelphia chromosome-positive acute lymphoblastic leukemia treated between 1995 and 2005. *J Clin Oncol* 28(31):4755–4761, 2010.
15. Schultz KR, Carroll A, Heerema NA, et al: Long-term follow-up of imatinib in pediatric Philadelphia chromosome-positive acute lymphoblastic leukemia: Children's Oncology Group study AALL0031. *Leukemia* 28(7):1467–1471, 2014.
16. Pui CH, Pei D, Coustan-Smith E, et al: Clinical utility of sequential minimal residual disease measurements in the context of risk-based therapy in childhood acute lymphoblastic leukaemia: a prospective study. *Lancet Oncol* 16(4):465–474, 2015.
17. Eden T, Pieters R, Richards S, et al: Systematic review of the addition of vincristine plus steroid pulses in maintenance treatment for childhood acute lymphoblastic leukaemia—an individual patient data meta-analysis involving 5,659 children. *Br J Haematol* 149(5):722–733, 2010.
18. Pui CH, Campana D, Pei D, et al: Treating childhood acute lymphoblastic leukemia without cranial irradiation. *N Engl J Med* 360(26):2730–2741, 2009.
19. Teuffel O, Kuster SP, Hunger SP, et al: Dexamethasone versus prednisone for induction therapy in childhood acute lymphoblastic leukemia: a systematic review and meta-analysis. *Leukemia* 25(8):1232–1238, 2011.
20. van den Berg H: Asparaginase revisited. *Leuk Lymphoma* 52(2):168–178, 2011.
21. Matloub Y, Bostrom BC, Hunger SP, et al: Escalating intravenous methotrexate improves event-free survival in children with standard-risk acute lymphoblastic leukemia: a report from the Children's Oncology Group. *Blood* 118(2):243–251, 2011.
22. Bhojwani D, Pui CH: Relapsed childhood acute lymphoblastic leukemia. *Lancet Oncol* 14(6):e205–e217, 2013.
23. Pulsipher MA, Peters C, Pui CH: High-risk pediatric acute lymphoblastic leukemia: to transplant or not to transplant? *Biol Blood Marrow Transplant* 17(1 Suppl):S137–S148, 2011.
24. Bailey LC, Lange BJ, Rheingold SR, et al: Bone-marrow relapse in paediatric acute lymphoblastic leukaemia. *Lancet Oncol* 9(9):873–883, 2008.
25. Gaynon PS, Qu RP, Chappell RJ, et al: Survival after relapse in childhood acute lymphoblastic leukemia: impact of site and time to first relapse—the Children's Cancer Group Experience. *Cancer* 82(7):1387–1395, 1998.
26. Mullighan CG, Zhang J, Kasper LH, et al: CREBBP mutations in relapsed acute lymphoblastic leukemia. *Nature* 471(7337):235–239, 2011.
27. Howard SC, Jones DP, Pui CH: The tumor lysis syndrome. *N Engl J Med* 364(19):1844–1854, 2011.
28. Haidar C, Jeha S: Drug interactions in childhood cancer. *Lancet Oncol* 12(1):92–99, 2011.
29. Essig S, Li Q, Chen Y, et al: Risk of late effects of treatment in children newly diagnosed with standard-risk acute lymphoblastic leukaemia: a report from the Childhood Cancer Survivor Study cohort. *Lancet Oncol* 15(8):841–851, 2014.
30. Zhang J, Nichols KE, Downing JR: Germline mutations in predisposition genes in pediatric cancer. *N Engl J Med* 374(14):1391, 2016.
31. Walter AW, Hancock ML, Pui CH, et al: Secondary brain tumors in children treated for acute lymphoblastic leukemia at St Jude Children's Research Hospital. *J Clin Oncol* 16(12):3761–3767, 1998.

CHAPTER 66

ACUTE LYMPHOBLASTIC LEUKEMIA IN ADULTS

Shira Dinner, Sandeep Gurbuxani, Nitin Jain, and Wendy Stock

Acute lymphoblastic leukemia (ALL) is a heterogeneous group of diseases characterized by clonal proliferation of lymphoid progenitors (lymphoblasts). Improved diagnostic tools permit accurate and prompt diagnosis, and aid in evaluation of minimal residual disease (MRD). There have been significant advances in the past decade toward understanding disease pathogenesis, refinement of prognostic groups, and the development of exciting new therapies directed towards specific disease subsets. These molecular targeted and immunotherapeutic approaches are transforming the treatment strategies for adults with ALL and are beginning to result in significant improvements in survival.

EPIDEMIOLOGY

It is estimated that in the year 2015, approximately 6250 new cases of ALL will be diagnosed and 1440 deaths will occur due to the disease in the United States. ALL is primarily a cancer of childhood; the peak incidence (7.7 in 100,000) occurs between the ages of 1 and 4 years, and approximately 60% of the patients are diagnosed before the age of 20 years. The incidence of ALL begins to decline with increasing age after the first decade of life. A second upward trend starts to emerge in the sixth decade of life, and a much smaller peak is seen in patients older than 85 years of age (1.8 in 100,000). Men have a slightly higher incidence of ALL than women (male-to-female ratio, 1.4 : 1). The overall age-adjusted rate of ALL has increased from 0.93 in 100,000 in the year 1975 to 1.47 in 100,000 in the year 2008. Similar increases in the incidence of ALL have also been reported in Scandinavia, the United Kingdom, and Italy. Although most investigators agree that this increase in the incidence is beyond what might be expected from better reporting, the actual cause(s) of this increased incidence remains largely speculative.

ETIOLOGY

A small minority of ALL cases (<5%) are associated with predisposing inherited syndromes such as Down syndrome, Bloom syndrome, ataxia telangiectasia, and Nijmegen breakage syndrome. However, the underlying etiology is not known in most cases. Although parental tobacco or alcohol use, exposure to pesticides or solvents, and cigarette smoking have all been implicated, only ionizing radiation has been significantly linked to increased risk of developing ALL. The vast majority of literature that attempts to identify causative agents for ALL is at best correlative; most of it borders on pure speculation and conjecture. Only recently has it been appreciated that the interaction between genetic predisposition and environmental factors involved in leukemogenesis is complex and may be different for different subtypes of ALL. Epidemiologic studies designed to identify environmental agents involved in leukemogenesis will therefore have to take into account the biologic subsets defined by morphology, immunophenotype, karyotype, and the molecular abnormalities, and consider the possibility that for each of these subtypes the causative agent may well be different. To adequately investigate these issues, future studies will require collaborative efforts studying large patient populations.

Despite the limitations described, it is relevant to review some of the recent advances in our understanding of the etiology of ALL.

Greaves and colleagues have used DNA obtained from neonatal blood spots to demonstrate that ALL-associated chromosomal translocations (and hence a preleukemic clone) can be demonstrated in neonatal blood spots that are acquired in utero. Furthermore, these are present at 100-fold higher rate than the incidence of leukemia. These investigators hypothesize that overt leukemia evolves as a consequence of an abnormal lymphoid proliferation that occurs in response to exposure to an as yet unidentified infectious agent(s). Supporting this hypothesis are data that suggest that day care attendance associated with early exposure to common infectious agents is associated with a lower incidence of ALL. Similarly, industrialization associated with improved socioeconomic status and exposure to common infectious agents later in life has been postulated to result in abnormal and excessive lymphoid proliferation and leukemic transformation. Finally, an infectious etiology can also be evoked to explain leukemic clusters that occur when a previously unexposed community is exposed to infectious agents brought into the community by a large influx of residents, as happens during urbanization of rural communities. However, it needs to be reiterated that all of these studies are at best correlative and not supported by direct experimental evidence. Furthermore, the infectious or environmental agent(s) responsible for this abnormal lymphoid proliferation remains elusive.

CLINICAL MANIFESTATIONS

The clinical presentation of ALL encompasses a wide spectrum of symptoms that correlate with the degree of bone marrow (BM) involvement and the resultant cytopenias, as well as the leukemic cell burden. Typical symptoms include fatigue, anorexia, night sweats, pallor, shortness of breath, bone pain, fever, and bleeding diathesis. Involvement of extramedullary sites may present with lymphadenopathy, hepatomegaly, or splenomegaly. Less commonly, ALL can involve the central nervous system (CNS), leading to headache, vomiting, lethargy, and cranial nerve palsies. Other extramedullary sites of involvement include the testis, tonsils, adenoids, breast, and gastrointestinal tract. Precursor T-cell ALL often presents with a large mediastinal mass with associated respiratory distress or possible signs of superior vena cava syndrome. Burkitt leukemia/lymphoma is frequently associated with CNS involvement and bulky adenopathy.

CLINICAL AND LABORATORY EVALUATION

The initial workup for patients with suspected ALL is detailed in Table 66.1. All patients should undergo a detailed history and physical examination. Family history should be ascertained. Laboratory evaluation should include complete blood count (CBC) with differential; comprehensive metabolic panel, including liver function tests, lactate dehydrogenase (LDH), and uric acid. Coagulation profile should also be obtained, although coagulation parameters are frequently normal at diagnosis. Human leukocyte antigen (HLA) testing should be obtained for patients who are potential candidates for allogeneic stem cell transplantation (aSCT).

All patients should undergo BM aspiration and biopsy for confirmation of diagnosis, and for cytogenetic and molecular genetic evaluation. It is particularly important to send an aspirate (or peripheral

TABLE 66.1	Initial Evaluation of a Patient With Acute Lymphoblastic Leukemia

- Complete history (including family history)
- Physical examination
- CBC with differential
- Comprehensive metabolic profile, including LFTs
- LDH, uric acid
- Coagulation profile
- BM aspiration and biopsy (morphology, immunohistochemistry, flow cytometry, molecular and cytogenetic analysis)
- HLA typing of the patient (if a potential aSCT candidate)
- Lumbar puncture
- Chest radiography or CT imaging of the chest

aSCT, Allogeneic stem cell transplantation; BM, bone marrow; CBC, complete blood count; CT, computed tomography; HLA, human leukocyte antigen; LDH, lactate dehydrogenase; LFT, liver function test.

blood if lymphoblasts are present) to the molecular oncology diagnostic laboratory to evaluate for the presence of the *BCR-ABL* fusion transcript using reverse-transcriptase polymerase chain reaction because these patients will receive frontline therapy that includes a tyrosine kinase inhibitor (TKI).

A lumbar puncture should be performed at diagnosis to determine CNS involvement. In the event of increased risk of bleeding caused by severe thrombocytopenia or risk of cerebrospinal fluid contamination caused by high peripheral blood blasts, the lumbar puncture should be performed by an experienced operator. It is prudent to administer intrathecal chemotherapy at the time of the diagnostic lumbar puncture after obtaining the necessary samples.

APPROACH TO DIAGNOSIS

While evaluation of morphology and immunophenotype are sufficient for making the diagnosis, current risk stratification relies on additional cytogenetic and molecular genetic information. Data from these tests is therefore an important adjunct to the initial diagnostic work up.

Initial laboratory evaluation starts with a CBC and morphologic evaluation of a Giemsa-stained peripheral blood smear. An abnormality of at least one of the CBC parameters is detected in more than 90% of ALL patients at the time of diagnosis. Anemia and thrombocytopenia are common. The anemia is usually a normochromic, normocytic anemia accompanied by reticulocytopenia. The hemoglobin levels range from 30–174 g/L, and almost 50% of the patients have hemoglobin levels below 100 g/L. The median platelet count at presentation is approximately 55–60 × 10^9/L, and almost 60% to 70% of patients have platelet counts below 100 × 10^9/L. Although the total white blood cell (WBC) count may be low, normal or elevated, neutropenia is commonly present. In a Cancer and Leukemia Group B (CALGB) study, the median WBC count at presentation was 19.3 × 10^9/L. Almost one-third of the patients are likely to present with WBC count greater than 30 × 10^9/L. Blasts account for a variable proportion of the circulating WBCs, and the percent blast population can range from 0% to 100%. A leukoerythroblastic picture can sometimes be seen. In an extreme form, immature myeloid precursors and myeloblasts constitute the vast majority of cells in the peripheral blood. This should be kept in mind when attempting to make a diagnosis exclusively from peripheral blood. Eosinophilia as a presentation of ALL is extremely uncommon and is seen in association with specific chromosomal abnormalities, including t(5;14)(q31;q32) or, even less frequently, with 8p11-associated ALL. Eosinophilia associated with t(5;14) is reactive and due to overexpression of interleukin-3 on chromosome 5 driven by the immunoglobulin H (IgH) promoter on chromosome 14. The eosinophilia can be extremely pronounced and mask the blast population in this subset of patients.

Several metabolic abnormalities are present at the time of diagnosis and frequently reflect tumor burden. For example, LDH levels are frequently elevated, and almost 50% of the patients have levels between 300 and 1000 U/L. Elevated serum levels of calcium, potassium, and phosphorous have been noted. More importantly, elevated serum uric acid levels are frequently present and reflect tumor burden. Hyperuricemia needs to be carefully monitored and aggressively corrected to avoid renal failure, especially at the time of starting induction therapy.

MORPHOLOGY

Romanowsky-based stains such as Wright Giemsa and Giemsa provide the greatest cytoplasmic detail for evaluation of cytomorphology of the cells in the peripheral blood smear, BM aspirate smear, and touch imprints (Fig. 66.1). Most frequently, lymphoblasts are small to intermediate in size and have scant, agranular cytoplasm. B lymphoblasts are morphologically indistinguishable from T lymphoblasts, and this distinction relies on immunophenotyping. The nuclei are usually round, with uniformly dispersed "smudgy" chromatin and inconspicuous nucleoli (see Fig. 66.1C). However, variations in morphology are common, and larger cells with abundant bluish gray cytoplasm, larger, somewhat irregular nuclei, and variably prominent nucleoli can be frequently seen (see Fig. 66.1D). Even though the nuclear chromatin of these cells can be fine, it is never as finely dispersed as in a myeloblast. At the other end of the morphologic spectrum are smaller cells with uniformly condensed, mature lymphocyte-like chromatin (see Fig. 66.1E), and distinction from mature B-cell malignancies relies on immunophenotyping. Coarse azurophilic granules (see Fig. 66.1F) can be seen in a subset of blasts in 5% to 8% of childhood ALLs and even more frequently in adult ALL patients. These have been reported in association with Philadelphia chromosome-positive (Ph+) ALL and in ALL in Down syndrome patients. The granules are coarser than the granules seen in myeloblasts and are invariably myeloperoxidase negative (see later discussion of cytochemistry). Morphologic distinction between the L1 and L2 category recommended in the French–American–British (FAB) classification has proven to be poorly reproducible and of little prognostic value. It has been abandoned in the current World Health Organization (WHO) classification.

Cytoplasmic vacuolation (see Fig. 66.1H) can be seen in as many as 28% of childhood ALL patients. These lymphoblasts can be distinguished from leukemic presentation of BL (see later discussion) based on other morphologic features such as a smaller cell size, lack of deep blue cytoplasm, and less coarse chromatin. However, when morphology is confounding, the distinction relies on immunophenotyping of the malignant cells. In contrast to BL cells, ALL blasts are precursor B cells that express terminal deoxynucleotidyl transferase (TdT) and lack surface immunoglobulin (Ig) expression (see later discussion).

The trephine biopsy sections show hypercellular BM (Fig. 66.2). The sections are evaluated after staining with hematoxylin and eosin. The BM is usually packed with a relatively uniform population of small round blasts with round to oval nuclei. Less frequently, the blasts can be more pleomorphic, with indented, convoluted, and variably sized nuclei. The chromatin is described as being finely dispersed or stippled and the nucleoli are usually not conspicuous. Brisk mitotic activity is almost always present. The effacement of the BM space is almost complete and uniform at the time of initial presentation. Minimal residual hematopoiesis is present; in most instances this is represented by a few megakaryocytes and some erythropoiesis. Normocellular or even hypocellular BMs at presentation have been described but are uncommon. Rarely, the initial presentation of ALL can be with an aplastic or markedly hypocellular BM. Making the diagnosis in this hypocellular context can be particularly challenging because of a paucity of material available for supporting studies such as cytogenetics and immunophenotyping.

BM biopsy can show partial or complete necrosis (see Fig. 66.2C). When extensive necrosis is present, making a diagnosis can be

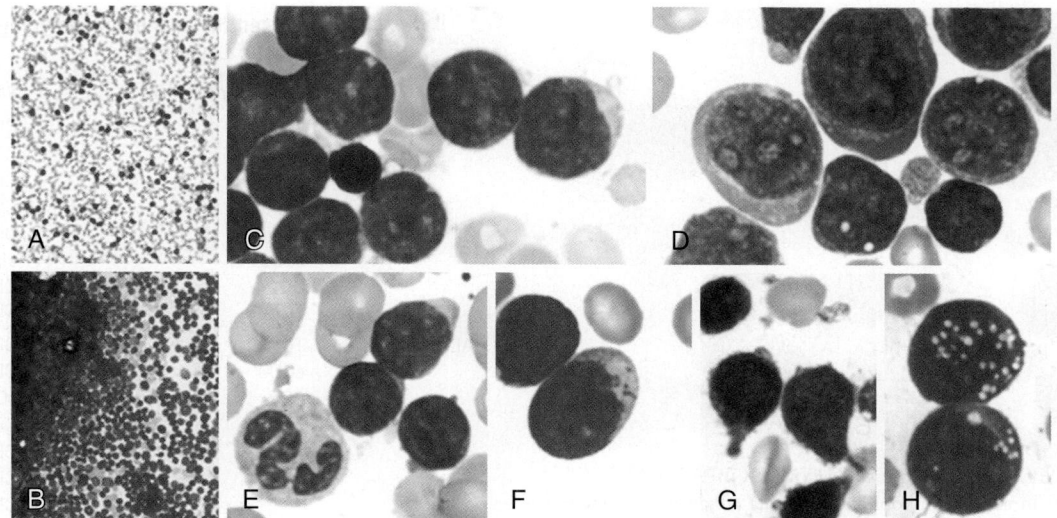

Fig. 66.1 MORPHOLOGIC FEATURES OF ACUTE LYMPHOBLASTIC LEUKEMIA IN THE BLOOD AND BONE MARROW ASPIRATE. (A) In acute lymphoblastic leukemia (ALL), the peripheral blood count can be low, normal or high, although frequently it is high and composed of mostly blasts. (B) A similar range in cellularity is true regarding the bone marrow. Typically, lymphoblasts are small to intermediate in size and have round nuclei with dispersed chromatin and indistinct nucleoli. (C) They have scant pale blue cytoplasm. A small lymphocyte (C, *middle, left*) is useful for comparison. (D) In many cases, the lymphoblasts are monotonous, but in some cases, the lymphoblast morphology is varied with some large cells, some cells with abundant cytoplasm, and other cells with prominent nucleoli. In the older French–American–British classification, these two patterns were referred to as ALL-L1 and ALL-L2, respectively, although they have been shown not to have any clinical significance. Other cytologic variants of lymphoblasts are shown in (E–H). These include (E) lymphocyte-like blasts, (F) blasts with azurophilic granules, (G) blasts with "hand-mirror" morphology, and (H) blasts with vacuoles. The small lymphocyte-like blasts can be difficult to distinguish from chronic lymphocytic leukemia cells in the blood, making flow immunophenotyping important in the distinction. Lymphoblasts with granules can be misleading as they can be mistaken for myeloblast or monoblasts. The hand-mirror cells appear to be an artifact because they can be seen only focally on a smear. Vacuoles in the blasts can make the blasts difficult to distinguish from Burkitt cells (see also Fig. 66.7). However, flow cytometry can easily distinguish the immature ALL blasts from the mature B cells seen in a leukemic presentation of Burkitt lymphoma.

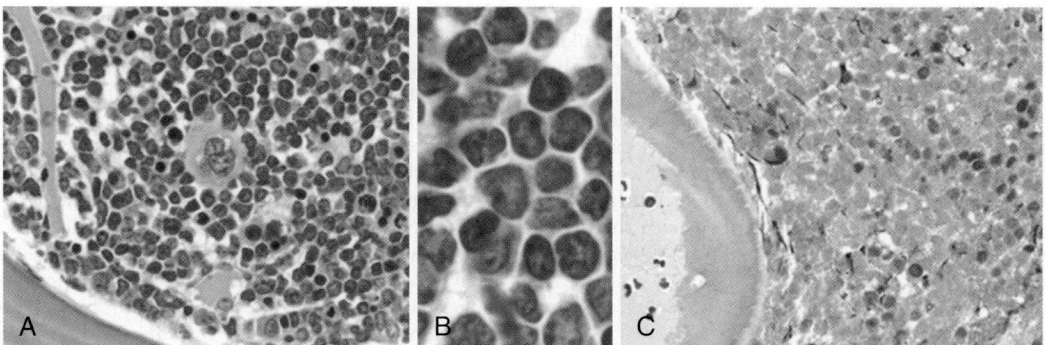

Fig. 66.2 MORPHOLOGIC FEATURES OF ACUTE LYMPHOBLASTIC LEUKEMIA IN THE BONE MARROW BIOPSY. (A) The findings in the bone marrow (BM) biopsy in acute lymphoblastic leukemia are varied, but frequently the biopsy is 100% cellular and packed with blasts. Sometimes there is some residual hematopoiesis with sparing of megakaryocytes as shown. (B) A high power of the lymphoblasts is shown, illustrating the fine, dispersed, and "blastic" chromatin pattern of the cells. Sometimes the BM can be hypocellular (not shown); however, the majority of the cells in such cases are blasts. (C) Sometimes there is necrosis. The necrotic cells are referred to as "ghost" cells. They may retain some of their antigen expression as identified by immunostains; however, if the entire biopsy shows necrosis, a diagnosis should be made from the findings in the blood or a repeat BM may be necessary. Other tumors can present with BM necrosis.

challenging or almost impossible. A repeat BM biopsy should be attempted and will usually provide diagnostic material. Some increase in reticulin fibrosis is present in 60% to 70% of ALL patients. When fibrosis is extensive, an aspirate cannot be obtained, limiting material available for ancillary studies such as flow cytometry and cytogenetics.

For these patients, the immunophenotyping can be performed by immunoperoxidase immunohistochemistry on the bone core biopsy. A second core can be obtained and submitted without fixation to the cytogenetic laboratory; evaluation can be performed from cells obtained from the disaggregation of the core.

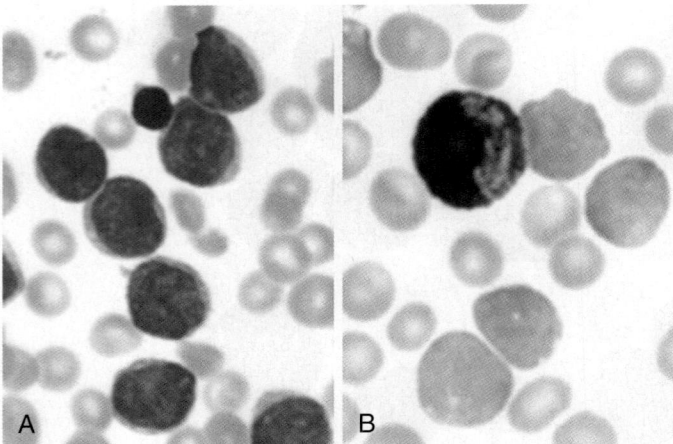

Fig. 66.3 CYTOCHEMISTRY IN ACUTE LYMPHOBLASTIC LEUKE-MIA. (A) The blasts in acute lymphoblastic leukemia are always myeloperoxidase reaction negative. (B) Compare the blasts with a single positively reactive granulocyte with a black–blue reaction product. Evaluating for nonspecific esterase reactivity (α-naphthyl acetate esterase, or α-naphthyl butyrate esterase) might also be performed when the blasts are difficult to distinguish from monoblasts.

Organs other than the BM can be frequently involved. Extramedullary or lymphomatous presentation is more common with T-acute lymphoblastic leukemia (T-ALL) than B-acute lymphoblastic leukemia (B-ALL). The cytomorphology of the malignant cells in extramedullary disease is similar to that described in the bone core biopsy. Lymph node involvement is usually diffuse but can be partial with sparing of the follicles.

CYTOCHEMISTRY

The use of cytochemistry to assign lineage has been largely replaced by flow cytometry evaluation of the leukemic blast immunophenotype. However, when available, the myeloperoxidase reaction (Fig. 66.3A and B) permits a rapid distinction from acute myeloid leukemia (AML). The reaction detects the myeloperoxidase enzyme in the primary granules of myeloblasts and is specific for the myeloid lineage. An acute leukemia in which 3% or more of the cells are myeloperoxidase positive is considered myeloid. There is excellent concordance between the myeloperoxidase reaction detected by cytochemistry and the myeloperoxidase molecule detected by flow cytometry. A block-like positivity has been described with the periodic acid-Schiff reaction that detects glycogen in almost 50% of ALL cases.

IMMUNOPHENOTYPE

Based on large cooperative group studies in Europe and the United States, the incidence of B-ALL ranges from 75% to 80% and T-ALL from 15% to 25%. B lymphoblasts cannot be distinguished from T lymphoblasts by morphology. Extensive immunophenotypic characterization is therefore required for the appropriate classification of ALL and indeed distinction from certain subtypes of AML. When adequate material is available, immunophenotyping should be performed using multicolor flow cytometry so that multiple antigens can be detected simultaneously on the lymphoblasts (Fig. 66.4). When interpreting the immunophenotypic data, it is important to remember that no single antigen is specific for any given lineage and multiple antigens need to be evaluated to establish the correct diagnosis. The panel of antibodies used for flow cytometry of a new leukemia and the pattern of expression seen in B-ALL and T-ALL are shown in Table 66.2. In addition, the combination of markers expressed on the

TABLE 66.2	Antigens Used for Immunophenotyping of Acute Lymphoblastic Leukemia[a]	
	Commonly Positive	**Variable Expression**
B-ALL	CD19[b]	CD20
	cCD22[b]	CD34
	cCD79a[b]	CD45
	Pax5[c]	CD13[d]
	CD10	CD33[d]
	sCD22	sIgM[e]
	CD24	CD58[d]
	TdT	CD38[d]
T-ALL	TdT	CD1a
	cCD3[f]	CD2
	CD7	sCD3
		CD4[g]
		CD5
		CD8[g]
		CD10
		CD34
		CD99
		CD19
		CD33[h]
		CD79a
		CD117[h]
		CD56
		CD13[h]

[a]Antigens are listed approximately in order of frequency.
[b]Almost always positive.
[c]Most specific for B lineage but can be positive in t(8;21) acute myeloid leukemia.
[d]Altered expression provides leukemia associated phenotype crucial for detection of minimal residual disease.
[e]Rarely present.
[f]Only marker considered lineage specific.
[g]Frequently coexpressed.
[h]Along with CD5 [lo], CD1a-, CD8-, the expression of these antigens is helpful in identifying early T-cell precursor acute lymphoblastic leukemia. For prognostic significance, please refer to discussion in text.
B-ALL, B-acute lymphoblastic leukemia; c, cytoplasmic; s, surface; T-ALL, T-acute lymphoblastic leukemia.

B or T lymphoblasts can be reflective of the stage of development at which the transformation happened (Table 66.3). Of note, expression of myeloid antigens is seen frequently in B-ALL and T-ALL, as is the expression of T-cell antigens in B-ALL and B-cell antigens in T-ALL. Expression of individual myeloid antigens should not be a deterrent to making the diagnosis of ALL. Of particular significance is the subgroup of T-ALL that lack CD1a, CD8, and CD5 but show expression of one or more myeloid or stem cell markers and have been recently designated as *early T-cell precursor ALL*. While these leukemias can have a gene expression profile and spectrum of genetic mutations that overlaps significantly with biphenotypic leukemia, most recent studies suggest improved outcomes using T-ALL therapy. It is therefore best to recognize this type of ALL as a type of T-ALL rather than mixed lineage leukemia. The criteria for diagnosis of acute leukemias of ambiguous lineage, which would include mixed phenotype acute leukemia, have been extensively revised in the current WHO classification.

CYTOGENETICS AND MOLECULAR GENETICS

Chromosomal abnormalities can be detected in almost 80% of B-ALLs and 70% of T-ALLs. Cytogenetic classification remains the single most important prognostic factor in both pediatric and adult ALL. Numerical abnormalities as well as structural abnormalities that disrupt the function of transcription factors involved in hematopoietic development and differentiation are common. These genetic abnormalities define the biology of the disease and have an impact

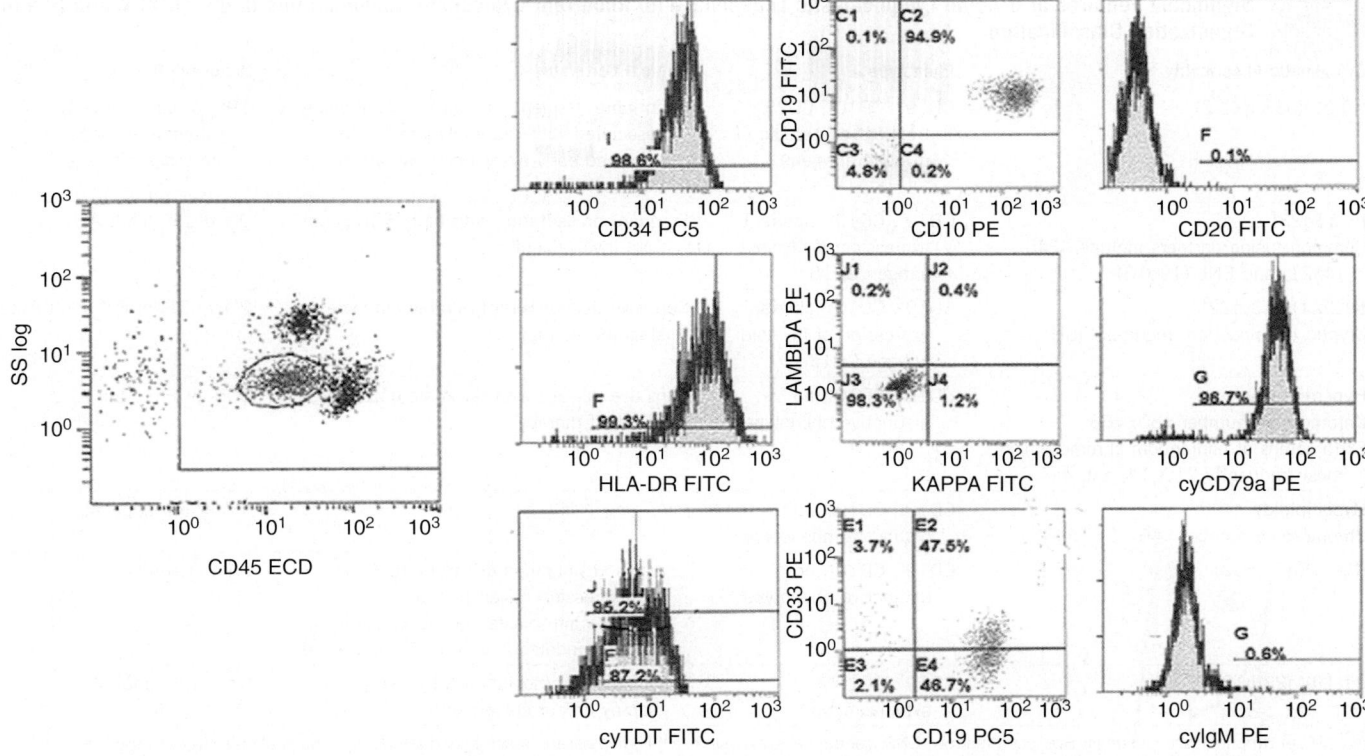

Fig. 66.4 AN EXAMPLE OF FLOW CYTOMETRIC EVALUATION IN A CASE OF B-ACUTE LYM-PHOBLASTIC LEUKEMIA. Selected histograms from a panel of markers used in the evaluation of acute lymphoblastic leukemia by flow cytometry are illustrated. The blasts are first identified by weak CD45 expression and low side scatter (*left histogram, circled population*). This is a useful gating strategy because it allows for an easy identification of the blast population and its separation from lymphocytes (with bright CD45) and nucleated red blood cells (with absent CD45 expression). Because no single antigen is specific for a lineage, multiple antigens are evaluated using multicolor flow cytometry. The phenotype illustrated is that of a common precursor B-acute lymphoblastic leukemia. In this case, the blasts are CD34$^+$, HLA-DR$^+$, TdT$^+$, CD19$^+$, CD10$^+$, CD20$^-$, cyCD79a$^+$, κ$^-$, λ$^-$, and cyIgμ$^-$. There is weak and partial expression of the myeloid marker CD33.

TABLE 66.3 Immunophenotypes of B and T-Lymphocyte Progenitors

B Lineage	CD10	CD19	CD22	CD79a	TdT	CyIgμ	
Early precursor (pro-B)	–	+	+	+	+	–	
Intermediate (common)	+	+	+	+	+	–	
Pre-B	+/–	+	+	+	+	+	
T Lineage	**CD1a**	**CD2**	**CD3**	**CD4**	**CD7**	**CD8**	**CD34**
ETP[a]	–	+/–	C	+/–	+/–	–	+
Pro-T	–	–	C	–	+	–	+/–
Pre-T	–	+	C	–	+	–	+–
Cortical T	+	+	C	+	+	+	–
Medullary T	–	+	C, S	[b]	+	[b]	–

[a]ETP ALL CD5-/lo, CD1a-, CD8- with stem cell myeloid markers, notably CD34, CD117, CD33, and CD13.
[b]Medullary T lymphocytes are positive for either CD4 or CD8, but not both.
C, Cytoplasmic; CyIgμ, cytoplasmic μ heavy chain; ETP, early T-cell precursor; S, surface; TdT, terminal deoxynucleotidyl transferase.

on treatment outcome. In addition, specific cytogenetic or molecular abnormalities are associated with unique phenotypic characteristics and are amenable to targeted therapy. Although Ph$^+$ ALL is the first subset of ALL to use a molecularly targeted TKI therapy as frontline treatment, it is likely that more genetically-defined entities will be targeted for specific therapy. This was recognized in the 2008 WHO classification with a specific discussion on lymphoblastic leukemia/ lymphoma with recurrent cytogenetic abnormalities (Table 66.4).

The ongoing revision of the WHO classification will build upon the framework established in 2008 to incorporate subsequent discoveries on molecular genetics of ALL in order to potentially identify groups of ALL likely to benefit from specific targeted therapy (see discussion on Philadelphia chromosome-like ALL (Ph-like ALL) later).

Hyperdiploidy, defined by the presence of more than 50 chromosomes, is seen in almost 25% of pediatric patients and 4% to 5% of adult ALL patients. In addition to routine karyotyping or fluorescence

TABLE 66.4   Significant Features of B-Acute Lymphoblastic Leukemia With Recurrent Cytogenetic Abnormalities in the 2008 World Health Organization Classification

Cytogenetic Abnormality	Phenotype	Clinical Correlates	Incidence #
t(9;22)(q33;q11.2)	CD19+, CD10+, CD25+; frequent expression of myeloid antigens	Seen more frequently in adults; traditionally associated with extremely poor outcome; improved early event-free survival with targeted therapy	19% of all adult ALL patients; incidence increases with age
t(v;11q23) Common fusion partners include AF4 (4q21) and ENL (19p13)	CD19+, CD10−; aberrant expression of myeloid antigen CD15	Frequent presentation with high WBC count, CNS involvement	9% of Ph− adult ALL
t(12;21)(p13;q22) Cryptic translocation; requires FISH	CD19+, CD10+; aberrant expression of myeloid antigen CD13	Sensitive disease with favorable outcome on standard therapy	2% to 3% of Ph− adult ALL
Hyperdiploidy Chromosome number >50, <66 Extra copies of nonrandom chromosomes, most frequently 21,X,14, and 4	CD19+, CD10+; no distinctive phenotype	Sensitive disease with favorable outcome on standard therapy	10% of Ph− adult ALL
Hypodiploidy Chromosome number <46	CD19+, CD10+; no distinctive phenotype	Poor prognosis	4% of Ph− adult ALL
t(5;14)(q31;q32)	CD19+, CD10+; no distinctive phenotype	Reactive eosinophilia driven by IL-3 overexpression driven by the translocation; blasts may be <20% in the BM and undetectable in peripheral blood	Rare in adults
t(1;19)(q23;p13.3)	CD19+, CD10+; cytoplasmic μ+	No significant association with response to therapy on current protocols	3% of Ph− adult ALL

ALL, Acute lymphoblastic leukemia; BM, bone marrow; CNS, central nervous system; FISH, fluorescent in situ hybridization; IL-3, interleukin-3; Ph, philadelphia chromosome; WBC, white blood cell.
Data from Moorman AV, Harrison CJ, Buck GA, et al, Adult Leukaemia Working Party, Medical Research Council/National Cancer Research Institute: Karyotype is an independent prognostic factor in adult acute lymphoblastic leukemia (ALL): analysis of cytogenetic data from patients treated on the Medical Research Council (MRC) UKALLXII/Eastern Cooperative Oncology Group (ECOG) 2993 trial. *Blood* 109:3189, 2007; and Pui CH, Relling MV, Downing JR: Acute lymphoblastic leukemia. *N Engl J Med* 350:1535, 2004.

in situ hybridization (FISH) analysis, hyperdiploid DNA content can be determined by flow cytometry using DNA-binding fluorescent dyes and corresponds to a DNA content between 1.16 and 1.6. However, some studies have demonstrated that hyperdiploidy resulting from duplication of specific chromosomes (4, 10, and 17) is a better indicator of a favorable prognosis than the actual ploidy or the DNA content. Careful analysis of the specific pattern of chromosomal gains and losses or flow cytometry peaks for DNA content is required to distinguish true hyperdiploid cases from near-haploid cases that have undergone endoreplication (vide infra). In contrast to hyperdiploidy, a hypodiploid karyotype is associated with an adverse prognosis. Hypodiploid ALL with near-diploid chromosome numbers (44–45) is associated with somewhat distinct biology (loss of sex chromosome, dicentric chromosomes, presence of recurrent cytogenetic abnormalities such as ETV6-RUNX1) and is associated with a better outcome. In contrast, presence of hypodiploidy with chromosome numbers less than 44 is invariably associated with poor outcome. The most common chromosome complements within the hypodiploid group are near haploid (24–31 chromosomes) and low hypodiploid (32–39 chromosomes), and are both associated with a poor outcome. Of note, low-hypodiploid ALL is frequently associated with germline *TP53* mutations and at least in a subset of cases appears to be a manifestation of Li–Fraumeni syndrome. Both near-haploid and low-hypodiploid ALL have activation of phosphatidylinositol 3-kinase (PI3K)/mammalian target of rapamycin (mTOR) and MEK-ERK signaling that can potentially be targeted by PI3K inhibitors.

A structural abnormality seen commonly in the pediatric age group but extremely rarely in the adult age group is a cryptic translocation, the t(12;21)(p13;q22) (*ETV6-RUNX1*). When present, it is associated with a favorable prognosis. Leukemias that harbor rearrangements of the mixed-lineage leukemia (*MLL*) gene at chromosome 11q23, most notably t(4;11)(q21;q23), present with high WBC counts and frequent CNS involvement, and are associated with poor clinical outcomes. Ph+ ALL associated with t(9;22)(q34;q11.2) is seen

in 25% of adults diagnosed with ALL. The translocation results in *BCR-ABL1* fusion and the resulting leukemia has a poor outcome without the inclusion of TKIs into frontline treatment. Intrachromosomal amplification of chromosome 21 (iAMP21) is defined as a gain of at least three copies of regions of chromosome 21 that include *RUNX1*. The abnormality seen in 2% of B-ALL patients is associated with an older age at diagnosis and poor outcome with standard-risk therapy. iAMP21 is usually the sole cytogenetic abnormality but can be seen in patients with Ph-like ALL (see later). In addition, use of technology to assess copy number variation has identified submicroscopic genomic alterations that have significant impact on the biology of B-ALL. These involve transcription factors such as *IKZF1* (Ikaros), *EBF*, and *PAX5*. The role of these transcription factors in B-cell development and the biology of B-ALL are discussed in greater detail in Chapter 64.

One of the most critical and clinically relevant discoveries with respect to ALL has been the description of high-risk ALL with a gene expression profile similar to that of Ph+ ALL but without the *BCR-ABL1* fusion gene. This subtype of leukemia is referred to as *Ph-like ALL* and the kinase-activating alterations are a result of a diverse group of genetic lesions that result in dysregulated cytokine receptor and tyrosine kinase signaling. The lesions can be grouped into a surprisingly small number of broad categories. The most frequent category involves *CRLF2* rearrangements that account for almost 50% of Ph-like ALLs. The rearrangements involve either translocation of *IGH2* at locus on chromosome 14q32 to *CRLF2* on Xp22.3/Yp11.3 (pseudoautosomal region 1), or a 320-kb interstitial deletion centromeric of *CRLF2* resulting in *P2RY8-CRLF2* fusion. *CRLF2* overexpression is frequently associated with activating mutations of *JAK1/ JAK2*, *IL7R*, or deletion of the JAK-STAT negative regulator *SH2B3*, resulting in activation of JAK-STAT signaling. JAK-STAT signaling activation also occurs in a second category of Ph-like ALL with *JAK2/EPOR* rearrangements. The third broad category of Ph-like ALL involves *ABL1*, *ABL2*, *CSF1R*, and *PDGRB*, described

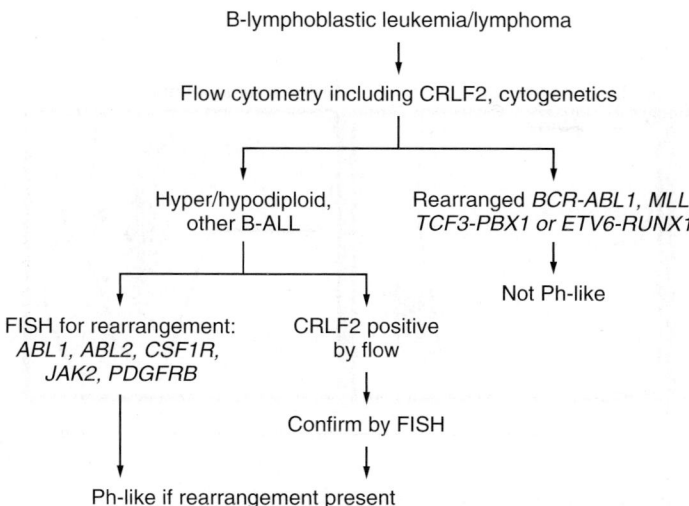

B-lymphoblastic leukemia/lymphoma

↓

Flow cytometry including CRLF2, cytogenetics

Hyper/hypodiploid, other B-ALL

Rearranged *BCR-ABL1, MLL, TCF3-PBX1* or *ETV6-RUNX1*

Not Ph-like

FISH for rearrangement: *ABL1, ABL2, CSF1R, JAK2, PDGFRB*

CRLF2 positive by flow

↓

Confirm by FISH

Ph-like if rearrangement present

Fig. 66.5 ALGORITHM TO EVALUATE FOR PHILADELPHIA CHROMOSOME-LIKE ACUTE LYMPHOBLASTIC LEUKEMIA. Initial evaluation includes standard karyotype analysis to exclude cases with *BCR-ABL1, MLL, TCF3-PBX1, ETV6-RUNX1* rearrangements. Flow cytometry for *CRLF2* can identify as many as 50% of Philadelphia chromosome-like (Ph-like) acute lymphoblastic leukemia. In the remaining cases FISH analysis can be used to identify recurrent rearrangements that contribute to a Ph-like gene expression profile. However, some cases will require additional analysis by next-generation sequencing. *B-ALL*, B-acute lymphoblastic leukemia; *FISH*, fluorescence in situ hybridization; (*Modified from Roberts KG, Li Y, Payne-Turner D, et al: Targetable kinase-activating lesions in Ph-like acute lymphoblastic leukemia. N Engl J Med 371:1005, 2014.*)

together as *ABL1* class rearrangements. In addition, other kinases such as *NTRK3, PTK2B,* and *TYK2* have also been shown to be involved in rearrangements in sporadic cases. As preclinical studies as well as case reports continue to document dramatic responses to targeted therapy for this group of patients, it is imperative that these lesions be identified prospectively. Because a wide variety of lesions result in a Ph-like phenotype, the laboratory diagnosis of Ph-like ALL remains a challenge. One approach to work-up of Ph-like ALL is highlighted in Fig. 66.5.

Similar to B-ALL, translocations involving transcription factors are common in T-ALL. The most commonly involved genes include *HOX11* and *HOX11L2*. Other genes that have been described to be involved in T-ALL are *MYC, TAL1, LMO2,* and *LYL1*. Similar to t(12;21), translocations involving the *TAL1* gene are cryptic and require detection by molecular techniques. Activating mutations of the *NOTCH1* gene are detected in almost 50% of ALL patients. Although activating mutations of *NOTCH1* appear to be associated with disease pathogenesis, they do not appear to be associated with an adverse prognosis in the majority of studies; in fact, some pediatric studies suggest that NOTCH1-mutated T-ALL may have a relatively favorable response to current treatment regimens. Deletions of the *CDKN2A* gene on chromosome 9p are also particularly frequent as are mutations in the *FBXW7* gene, but neither has clear prognostic significance as single abnormalities. The significance of these mutations remains an area of active research.

DIFFERENTIAL DIAGNOSIS

ALL blasts can be easily distinguished from the reactive lymphocytes seen in viral infections because of the precursor phenotype of these cells. Low to weak expression of CD45 and expression of one or more precursor antigens such as TdT or CD34 is useful. In addition, precursor T-ALL cells express only cytoplasmic CD3 and no surface CD3, and B-ALLs frequently lack expression of CD20 while being CD19 positive. As mentioned previously, ALL cells can have some

cytoplasmic vacuolation and need to be distinguished from leukemic presentation of Burkitt lymphoma (BL). Unlike ALL, BL cells are mature B cells with bright surface Ig expression, very strong CD20 expression, and no expression of CD34. Diagnosis of BL is confirmed by the presence of an *MYC* translocation using FISH or cytogenetics. Other entities that require distinction from ALL depend on the age of presentation. In the pediatric age group, ALL blasts need to be distinguished from hematogones. Hematogones are normal B-cell precursors present within the BM. These are more abundant in childhood and decrease with increasing age. Hematogones may also be increased during hematopoietic regeneration, particularly after chemotherapy or BM engraftment after stem cell transplant. Hematogones possess a distinct pattern of antigen expression that recapitulates progressive B-cell maturation. This is reflected in progressive loss of antigens such as CD34, TdT, and CD10 and acquisition of CD20 and surface Ig expression (Fig. 66.6). Other diseases that need to be morphologically distinguished from ALL include small blue cell tumors, including Ewing sarcoma, neuroblastoma, and medulloblastoma. Ancillary studies, including immunophenotyping and cytogenetics, are helpful in making the distinction. In older adults, entities that can morphologically mimic ALL include blastoid mantle cell lymphoma, chronic lymphocytic leukemia, and prolymphocytic leukemia. These latter are all mature B-cell malignancies that can be distinguished from ALL based on the mature B-cell phenotype, including consistent expression of CD20 and surface Igs.

PROGNOSIS

Prognostication based on clinical and biologic risk factors has been useful in making informed decisions about postremission treatment options. Established risk factors for a poor prognosis with current chemotherapeutic approaches include age older than 60 years, elevated WBC count at diagnosis (>30,000/μL for B-cell ALL;>100,000/μL for T-cell ALL), pro–B-cell or early T-cell immunophenotype, and cytogenetics (t[4;11][q21;q23] and other *MLL* rearrangements, hypodiploidy, or a complex karyotype). The presence of the Philadelphia chromosome, t(9;22)(q34;q11.2) resulting in the *BCR-ABL* fusion gene, was previously associated with very poor treatment outcomes. Recent addition of ABL kinase inhibitors (molecularly targeted therapy), discussed in detail later, has improved the prognosis for these patients. Time to achievement of complete remission (CR) longer than 4 weeks has also been associated with a poor clinical outcome (Table 66.5).

Although different study groups have used slightly different variations of these risk factors, the presence of any one of the following is generally accepted as high risk (HR): high WBC count at diagnosis (>30,000/μL in B-cell ALL or >100,000/μL in T-cell ALL); cytogenetic abnormalities [hypodiploidy, t(4;11), t(9;22)]; age older than 60 years; pro–B-cell phenotype; and time to remission longer than 4 weeks. All other patients are considered standard risk (SR).

Nevertheless, despite being labeled as SR, up to 40% to 50% of these adults eventually relapse. Thus, there is a need for refinement of prognostic markers for ALL patients. Recently, an early T-cell phenotype, the expression of CD20+ and several recently described genetic mutations (*IKAROS, CRLF2,* and *JAK2*; reviewed earlier in this chapter) have been identified as being associated with adverse outcomes from retrospective analyses.

MINIMAL RESIDUAL DISEASE

The identification and measurement of MRD (below the level of morphologic disease detection) using leukemia clone-specific quantitative polymerase chain reaction (PCR) and flow cytometry is an independent prognostic factor that is now being used to guide postremission therapies in many pediatric and some adult ALL treatment studies. In a study that directly compared MRD detection by PCR and flow cytometry in 1375 samples from 227 patients, the results were consistent in 97% of cases. In general, these techniques have

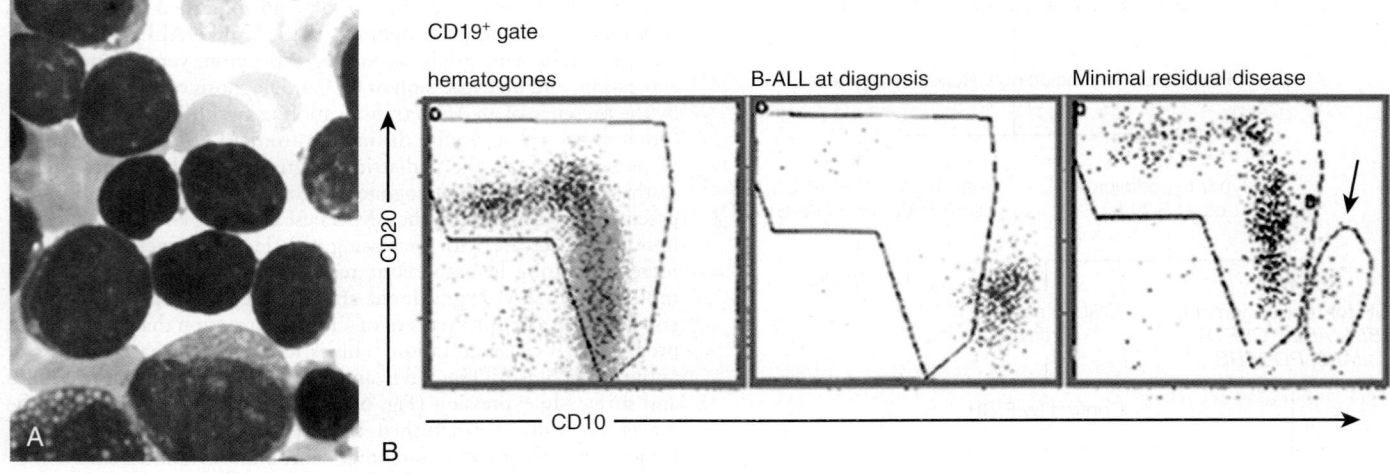

Fig. 66.6 HEMATOGONES AND FLOW CYTOMETRIC EVALUATION OF MINIMAL RESIDUAL DISEASE. Hematogones are nonmalignant immature precursor B cells that are present in the bone marrow (BM). They are more commonly seen in pediatric patients but can be seen in adults during BM regeneration or associated with other conditions. (A) They can be difficult to distinguish morphologically from malignant lymphoblasts because the cytologic features overlap significantly. (B) Unlike malignant lymphoblasts, hematogones exhibit a spectrum of maturation that can be seen, for example, by analyzing CD10 and CD20 expression on CD19+ cells *(left histogram)*. Hematogones are CD10+, but as CD20 is expressed, CD10 is diminished. Lymphoblasts, on the other hand, frequently exhibit maturation arrest and over- or underexpression of markers. They can also exhibit aberrant markers. In the *middle histogram*, the B lymphoblasts from the initial diagnosis specimen can be seen *(red)*, and the CD10 and CD20 expression is outside the normal hematogone range, with overexpression of CD10 and absence of CD20. This pattern can be used to identify minimal residual disease *(right histogram)* and distinguish regenerative hematogones *(black)* from residual or recurrent blasts *(red)* after therapy. Multiple markers and parameters are usually used to study posttherapy specimens in this way. *B-ALL,* B-acute lymphoblastic leukemia.

TABLE 66.5	Markers for Poor Prognosis in Adult Acute Lymphoblastic Leukemia
Established Risk Factors	
Age	>60 years
Presenting WBC count	>30,000/μL (B-cell ALL); >100,000/μL (T-cell ALL)
Immunophenotype	Pro-B cell; early T cell[a]
Cytogenetics	t(4;11)(q21;q23) and other *MLL* rearrangements t(9;22)(q34;q11.2) – Philadelphia chromosome Hypodiploidy (<44 chromosomes) Complex (>5 abnormalities)
Therapy response	Time to complete remission >4 weeks
MRD	≥0.01% at 3–6 months after initiation of therapy[b]
Emerging Risk Factors	
Immunophenotype	CD20
Molecular	BAALC FUS ERG IKZF1[c] Ph-like ALL

[a]Initial report characterizing ETP ALL showed a poor outcome. However, subsequent studies have shown variable association with response to therapy.
[b]Different studies have used different time points for MRD assessment.
[c]Focal deletions in IKZF1 are present in up to 70% of Ph-like ALL. However, IKZF1 deletions are associated with adverse outcome irrespective of association with Ph-like phenotype.
ALL, Acute lymphoblastic leukemia; ETP, early T-cell precursor; MRD, minimal residual disease; Ph, philadelphia chromosome; WBC, white blood cell.

not yet been widely standardized; however, the majority of studies demonstrate that MRD detection during early postremission therapy is a reliable and independent predictor of relapse. Recently, pediatric studies have confirmed that achieving lower levels of MRD also have prognostic significance, with rates of relapse being higher in those with MRD greater than 0.01% by PCR (calculated using a ratio of the clone-specific IgH or T-cell receptor gene rearrangement/control gene such as glyceraldehyde 3-phosphate dehydrogenase) compared to those with MRD of less than 0.01%. The optimal time point for outcome prognostication based on MRD measurements varies from study to study; undoubtedly, some of this variability is the result of differences in the PCR technique used, the sensitivity of detection of MRD of the individual assay, the treatment intensity, and the population being studied. While MRD assessment after induction has been the primary time point for prognostication and allocation of risk-adapted postremission therapy in pediatric ALL (and to a lesser degree in adults), more recent data suggest that additional MRD assessments during postremission therapy at weeks 16–22 can further refine prognostic information and help to delineate further therapy. In a study of 142 adult ALL patients, those with MRD greater than 0.01% after consolidation were eligible for transplant and those with MRD less than 0.01% received maintenance therapy. The 5-year overall survival (OS) rate was significantly higher for patients with MRD less than 0.01% or negative status postconsolidation (75% versus 33%). A subsequent GMALL study incorporated autologous hematopoietic stem cell transplant (aHSCT) for all patients with molecular disease after consolidation. For patients that remained MRD positive after consolidation, the subgroup who underwent aHSCT achieved significantly higher rates of CR at 5 years (66% versus 12%), and this trended towards higher rates of OS (54% versus 33%) compared with those that did not undergo aHSCT. Based on these findings, the majority of studies indicate that MRD detection anywhere from 4–20 weeks from initiation of treatment is highly predictive of relapse. Thus current studies are using novel approaches to try to eradicate MRD during early remission or stratifying

MRD-positive patients to early intensification with aSCT to try to improve survival for these patients at very HR for relapse. Recent data from the ALL-SCT-BFM 2003 study showed that MRD can also be reliably assessed after aHSCT as a predictor for relapse. Further data from these studies will help elucidate the optimal timing of MRD assessments and the appropriate management response.

TREATMENT OF ACUTE LYMPHOBLASTIC LEUKEMIA

Combination chemotherapy is the cornerstone of ALL management. In the 1960s, investigators at the National Institutes of Health designed multidrug chemotherapy regimens given over many different courses for pediatric ALL patients. A similar approach was then introduced for adults with ALL. The Berlin–Frankfurt–Muenster (BFM) group in the 1980s conducted pioneering studies and showed that an intensive multidrug induction and consolidation chemotherapy followed by delayed intensification led to improvement in survival in the majority of children. These regimens combine drugs with varying mechanisms of action at different doses, often in complex schedules, which have largely evolved empirically. Only a few of these drugs have been tested individually in randomized clinical trials in adults with ALL; therefore, the relative contribution of each of the drugs in a multidrug regimen to the overall outcome is difficult to assess. Because there is an increased propensity for CNS involvement in ALL patients, all treatment regimens must also include CNS prophylaxis with intrathecal chemotherapy with or without cranial radiation.

The therapy for ALL is typically divided into three phases: (1) the remission induction phase, (2) remission consolidation or intensification, and (3) the maintenance (or continuation) phase. The remission induction and consolidation phases typically involve blocks of monthly treatment for 6–8 months followed by long-term maintenance, which is given for up to 3 years; thus the treatment of ALL is long and challenging, and requires tremendous attention to detail, compliance, and support. Because of these challenges and the relative rarity and biologic heterogeneity of the disease, it is recommended that patients are referred to larger academic centers for evaluation and treatment to ensure the best possible survival rates. In the ensuing sections, the various components of treatment are reviewed. Special attention to the treatment of certain disease subsets are addressed because treatment of ALL is becoming increasingly based on its heterogeneity and the ability to adapt therapy to each of these subsets.

Effective chemotherapy regimens must be supplemented with adequate supportive care measures to obtain the best patient outcomes. Given the highly immunosuppressive nature of ALL treatment regimens, prophylaxis for *Pneumocystis carinii* with trimethoprim–sulfamethoxazole should be initiated early during treatment and continue throughout the consolidation and maintenance phases of chemotherapy. It is also reasonable to consider antifungal and antiviral prophylaxis during periods of neutropenia. Consideration may be given to antibacterial prophylaxis during periods of neutropenia. Fluoroquinolones such as levofloxacin are the preferred agent, although the optimal antibiotic choice should depend on local bacterial resistance patterns. Neutropenic fever in this group of patients must be treated as a medical emergency with immediate institution of intravenous (IV) antibiotics after obtaining the necessary cultures.

In an attempt to decrease the duration of neutropenia and improve remission rates, several groups have studied the role of granulocyte colony-stimulating factor (G-CSF) or granulocyte-macrophage colony-stimulating factor (GM-CSF) during induction therapy. In the CALGB 9111 trial, 198 adults with untreated ALL were randomized to receive G-CSF (beginning 4 days after the start of induction until neutrophil recovery) versus placebo. The median time to neutrophil recovery (≥1000/μL for 2 days) significantly shortened to 16 days in the G-CSF arm compared with 22 days in the placebo arm. The duration of hospitalization was also significantly shorter in the G-CSF arm. There was a trend toward increased CR rate in the G-CSF arm. However, the infectious complications, disease-free survival (DFS), and OS were similar in the two arms. Thomas and colleagues randomized 236 ALL patients treated on the LALA-94 trial to receive G-CSF, GM-CSF, or no CSF. Use of G-CSF was associated with a significant decrease in time to neutrophil recovery, duration of hospitalization, and infections that were grade 3 or higher. Thus use of G-CSF can allow for faster hematopoietic recovery, especially in older adult patients, and may decrease infectious complications; however, the prophylactic use of G-CSF has not been uniformly adopted, and many studies simply follow standard guidelines for use of growth factors in the setting of neutropenic fever.

All patients should be monitored carefully for tumor lysis syndromes, especially those with risk factors such as elevated WBC counts, renal dysfunction, and elevated LDH at presentation. Patients must be provided adequate hydration and prophylaxis or treatment for hyperuricemia with allopurinol for the first week of induction. Rasburicase, a urate oxidase, can be considered for the treatment of hyperuricemia in cases with high proliferation rates.

REMISSION INDUCTION

The aim of induction therapy is to achieve maximal reduction of the leukemic burden to result in morphologic remission (<5% blasts with trilineage hematopoiesis) and normalization of the blood counts, with as little toxicity as possible. This is typically achieved using combination chemotherapy consisting of four or five systemically administered drugs and intrathecal chemotherapy over a period of approximately 3–4 weeks. Most current ALL induction regimens in adults are modeled after pediatric regimens, and include a prolonged course of oral corticosteroid (prednisone or dexamethasone), weekly vincristine, and either weekly or pulsed anthracycline (doxorubicin, daunorubicin, or mitoxantrone). Many groups (CALGB, French Group for Research in Adult Acute Lymphoblastic Leukemia [GRAALL] 2003, and BFM) have also used twice-weekly L-asparaginase as part of induction therapy and some have added cyclophosphamide (MD Anderson, GRAALL 2003, and GMALL 07/2003, CALGB 8811, and CALGB 19802). With the current treatment regimens, very high CR rates in adults with ALL have been achieved in the range of 84% to 94% (Table 66.6). There have been few randomized comparisons between these different induction regimens; therefore the choice of the regimen should depend on the treating physician's experience with a particular regimen. Most ALL regimens are designed to optimally deliver a variety of chemotherapeutic agents; thus an entire treatment program should be selected at the time of diagnosis based on the patient's performance status and biologic risk factors. Whenever possible, these patients should be referred to centers that offer expertise in the treatment of ALL and where enrollment into clinical trials is available. Once a specific regimen has been selected, the goal (and challenge) is for both the medical team and the patient to adhere to the recommended treatments, which are arduous and lengthy in duration.

Traditionally, prednisone was the corticosteroid of choice during induction therapy for ALL trials. Studies in pediatric patients have shown lower relapse rates but higher toxicity (more sepsis, higher incidence of osteonecrosis) with dexamethasone. Dexamethasone penetrates the blood–brain barrier effectively and therefore may offer more direct CNS protection than prednisone. Comparative studies of prednisone versus dexamethasone have not been performed in adults, and some groups have incorporated prednisone (CALGB 10403, GRAALL 2003, and BFM); others have incorporated dexamethasone (CALGB 10102, MD Anderson, and GMALL 07/2003) during the induction cycle. Anthracyclines form an important part of induction therapy. In an early trial from the CALGB (7612), patients were randomized to receive vincristine, prednisone, and L-asparaginase with or without daunorubicin. Significant improvements in CR rates and remission duration were noted with the addition of daunorubicin; anthracyclines have since become standard components of induction chemotherapy in adult and pediatric ALL. Different anthracyclines (doxorubicin, daunorubicin, and mitoxantrone) are thought to be clinically equivalent and, to date, dose

TABLE 66.6   Clinical Trials With Various Chemotherapy Regimens for Adult Acute Lymphoblastic Leukemia

Trial	Patients (n)	Age in Years, Median (Range)	CR Rate (%)	Disease-Free Survival	Overall Survival	Comments
CALGB 8811[1]	197	32 (16–80)	85	46% at 3 years	36 months (median)	Five-drug induction regimen based on pediatric trials with earlier and more intensive L-asparaginase
CALGB 9111[2]	198	35 (16–83)	85	40% at 3 years	23 months (median)	Patients randomized to G-CSF vs. placebo; G-CSF significantly decreased time to neutrophil recovery and CR rate with no effect on DFS, OS, or toxicities
MDACC hyper-CVAD[3]	288	40 (15–92)	92	38% at 5 years	32 months (median)	Long-term follow-up results of hyper-CVAD regimen; regimen does not include asparaginase
GMALL 05/93[4]	1163	35 (15–65)	83		35% at 5 years	
GMALL 07/2003[5]	713	34 (15–55)	89		54% at 5 years	Risk-adapted SCT for HR and very HR groups
LALA 94[6]	922	33 (18–79)	84	30% at 5 years	23 months (median)	CR rate similar between IDA and DNR arms; significantly higher TRM with IDA; improved DFS for the IDA arm for patients receiving only chemotherapy; for SR patients, intensive consolidation did not affect outcomes
JALSG ALL-93[7]	263	31 (15–59)	78	30% at 6 years	33% at 6 years	Doxorubicin dose intensity did not improve outcomes; during maintenance phase, early sequential intensification compared with intermittent intensification did not affect DFS
JALSG ALL-97[8]	404	38 (15–64)	74	33% at 5 years	32% at 5 years	Induction and maintenance based on CALGB 8811; dose-intensive doxorubicin during consolidation did not improve outcomes
GIMEMA 0288[9]	778	28 (12–60)	82	33% at 9 years	29% at 9 years	Addition of cyclophosphamide to induction did not influence CR rate or survival; responders to prednisone pretreatment had favorable outcomes
MRC UKALLXII/ ECOG E2993[10]	1646 (Ph⁻)	(15–64)	90		43% at 5 years	Largest ALL trial to date; in a donor vs. no-donor analysis, those with a donor had improved OS and lower relapse rate; ASCT cannot replace consolidation or maintenance chemotherapy in any risk group
PETHEMA ALL-93[11]	222 high-risk ALL	27 (15–50)	82	35% at 5 years	34% at 5 years	Did not show beneficial effect of aSCT compared with ASCT or chemotherapy
GRAALL-2003[12]	225 Ph- ALL	31 (15–60)	94	59% at 3.5 years	60% at 3.5 years	Pediatric-inspired treatment regimen; in a historical comparison, significant increases in CR, EFS, and OS rates compared with LALA-94 trial; OS was improved for patients younger than 45 years only

ALL, Acute lymphoblastic leukemia; aSCT, allogeneic stem cell transplantation; ASCT, autologous stem cell transplantation; CALGB, Cancer And Leukemia Group B; CR, complete remission; CVAD, cyclophosphamide, vincristine, adriamycin, and dexamethasone; DFS, disease-free survival; DNR, daunorubicin; G-CSF, granulocyte colony-stimulating factor; HR, high risk; IDA, idarubicin; OS, overall survival; Ph, philadelphia chromosome; SCT, stem cell transplantation; SR, standard risk; TRM, transplant-related mortality.

intensification of anthracycline during induction has been tested in a variety of prospective clinical trials but has not been shown to definitely improve already high CR rates or to result in significant benefits in DFS. Addition of pulsed cyclophosphamide to induction chemotherapy has been studied with conflicting results. In the CALGB 8811 trial, addition of cyclophosphamide to the induction regimen was shown to lead to improved responses compared with historical control participants. However, in a prospective, randomized Italian GIMEMA 0288 study, the addition of cyclophosphamide did not influence CR rate or survival.

L-asparaginase (asparaginase) is also an important component of ALL therapy and has been incorporated into most ALL trials beginning with induction. ALL cells are unable to produce asparagine and are dependent on plasma levels of this amino acid for protein synthesis. Depletion of asparagine results in inhibition of protein synthesis and subsequent apoptotic leukemic cell death. Traditionally, native enzyme derived from *Escherichia coli* has been used. However, this preparation can be immunogenic, leading to hypersensitivity reactions and development of cross-reacting antibodies; this preparation, while still used elsewhere, is no longer available for administration in the United States. Polyethylene glycosylated (PEG)–asparaginase, formed by covalently attaching PEG to the native *E. coli* enzyme, has been developed and offers lower immunogenicity and a longer half-life. Douer and colleagues treated 25 newly diagnosed adult ALL patients (median age: 27 years; range: 17–55 years) with the adult ALL BFM protocol in which 14 injections of *E. coli* asparaginase were replaced by a single dose of pegaspargase (2000 IU/m^2 IV) on day 16 of induction therapy. After the single dose, asparagine deamination was complete in all patients after 2 hours and in 100%, 81%, and 44% on days 14, 21, and 28, respectively. No allergic reactions or pancreatitis was observed, and a CR was achieved in 24 of the 25 patients. The CALGB 9511 trial used pegaspargase (2000 IU/m^2 subcutaneously, two doses during induction and two during first intensification) as part of the five-drug induction regimen. Of the 85 evaluable patients, those with effective asparagine depletion (defined by enzyme levels >0.03 U/mL plasma for 14 consecutive days after pegaspargase administration) had improved DFS and OS compared with those without effective asparagine deletion. Thus, use of pegaspargase is generally safe and effective in adults, and has replaced native L-asparaginase as the agent for asparagine depletion. In 2011 the Food and Drug Administration (FDA) approved Erwinaze (asparaginase *Erwinia chrysanthemi*) to treat ALL patients who develop a hypersensitivity reaction to *E. coli*-derived asparaginase and pegaspargase. 25,000 u/m^2 of erwinia asparaginase given every 48 hours for six doses (for every one dose of pegasparaginase) has demonstrated safety and results in effective asparagine depletion in pediatric ALL. Patients receiving *Erwinia* asparaginase are still at risk for known toxicities of asparaginase, including bleeding, clotting, transaminitis, and pancreatitis. To avoid systemic toxicities, a novel preparation of L-asparaginase in which L-asparaginase is encapsulated within red blood cells (GRASPA [erythrocytes encapsulating L-asparaginase]) has been developed and is in early clinical development in Europe.

One of the regimens that is widely used in the United States and that also results in high CR rates of approximately 90% is the hyper-CVAD (cyclophosphamide, vincristine, adriamycin, and dexamethasone) regimen developed at the MD Anderson Cancer Center. The hyper-CVAD regimen differs from the pulsed weekly therapy developed by the pediatric groups and consists of four cycles of intensive infusional cyclophosphamide, vincristine, doxorubicin, and dexamethasone alternating with four cycles of high-dose methotrexate and high-dose cytarabine for a total of eight intensive treatment cycles.

Because CD20 is expressed on 20% to 40% of pre-B lymphoblasts and has been noted to be associated with adverse prognosis, the investigators at MD Anderson subsequently added rituximab to a modified hyper-CVAD regimen for patients with CD20 expression greater than or equal to 20%. In younger patients (≤60 years of age), rituximab improved 3-year OS to 75% compared with 47% in the historical control participants; however, no difference was seen for older adults. The GMALL has substantiated these results and rituximab is now routinely used with these regimens.

Some groups have also instituted a 5–7-day steroid prophase before starting the induction therapy. This results in gentle cytoreduction and reduces the risk of tumor lysis. The achievement of rapid cytoreduction during this steroid prophase has also been shown to be of prognostic value in several studies.

In summary, although all of the currently employed induction regimens in adults with ALL now routinely result in very high CR rates of 80% to 90%, none of them has yet translated into the 80% to 85% DFS rates that are routinely achieved in pediatric ALL. In adult ALL, DFS generally has been reported to be at 40% to 45% at 3 years and 30% to 35% at 5 years (see Table 66.6). Thus the main problem with the current treatment programs in adult ALL is disease relapse from the emergence of resistant disease and not in the failure to achieve CR.

POSTREMISSION THERAPY

As mentioned earlier, 80% to 90% of adults with previously untreated ALL achieve CR with induction chemotherapy. However, all patients relapse if no further chemotherapy is given. This underscores the need for effective postremission management strategies for these patients in first CR (CR1). As described earlier, adult patients with ALL have traditionally been stratified into SR or HR.

The type of recommended postremission strategy is to be based on the risk (risk-adapted approach), which implies more aggressive therapeutic approaches for HR groups compared with the SR group. There have been three tested approaches for postremission therapies: (1) postremission chemotherapy modules followed by long-term maintenance chemotherapy; (2) alloSCT; and least frequently, (3) autologous stem cell transplantation (ASCT). Studies using these postremission strategies are reviewed later.

The optimal postremission strategy for SR adult patients is not clear. Conventionally, consolidation and maintenance chemotherapy has been the recommendation for this group of patients, given lower potential for toxicities and up to 40% to 60% survival at 5 years with this approach. Postremission chemotherapy typically consists of a variety of non–cross-resistant chemotherapeutic agents administered in treatment "modules" for a total of 6–8 months after achievement of remission. The postremission modules are typically 4–6 weeks in length and are modeled after successful pediatric regimens and often consist of consolidation module(s), interim maintenance modules that often focus on CNS prophylaxis (described in more detail below), and a late intensification module(s), which is often quite similar to the induction chemotherapy course. The specific drugs and the sequence or combinations in which they used are different for each protocol but typically include cyclophosphamide, L-asparaginase (or pegasparaginase), methotrexate, cytarabine, 6-mercaptopurine, vincristine, and doxorubicin. Many of these protocols have evolved empirically with few randomized trials evaluating the impact of any of the modifications that have been developed (see Table 66.6).

A different approach to postremission therapy has been taken by the MD Anderson Cancer Center, which have reported long-term results of the hyper-CVAD regimen (also listed in Table 66.6). As described earlier in the induction section, patients received alternating cycles of hyperfractionated cyclophosphamide, vincristine, adriamycin, and dexamethasone hyper-CVAD (courses 1, 3, 5, and 7) alternating with high-dose methotrexate and cytarabine (courses 2, 4, 6, and 8) followed by maintenance therapy for 2 years with 6-mercaptopurine, methotrexate, vincristine, and prednisone (POMP). They identified the following factors to be independent poor prognostic factors for survival: older age, Ph$^+$ disease, leukocytosis, thrombocytopenia, poor performance status, and hepatomegaly. The 5-year OS for the good-risk (risk score: 0–1), intermediate risk (risk score: 2–3), and poor-risk groups (risk score: ≥4) were 62%, 34%, and 5%, respectively.

In summary, despite attempts to intensify postremission therapy with high doses of cytarabine and anthracycline, the OS rate of patients in all of the studies published in the past decade is

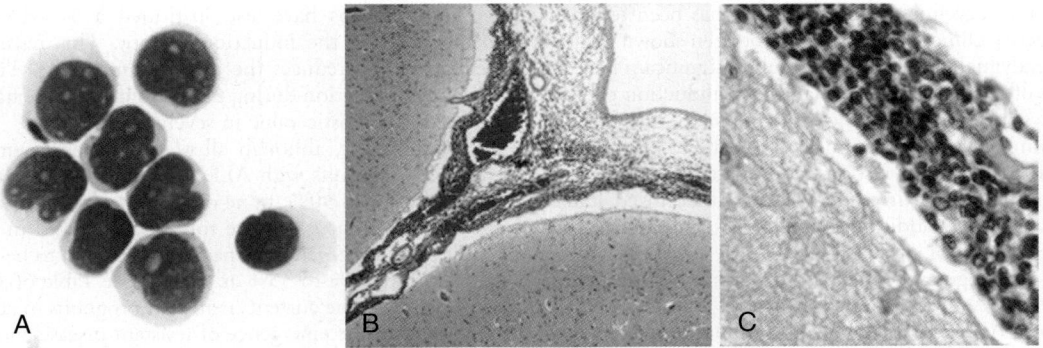

Fig. 66.7 CEREBROSPINAL FLUID AND CENTRAL NERVOUS SYSTEM DISEASE. Blasts in the cerebrospinal fluid can be identified on a cytospin preparation. (A) They have similar cytologic features as the blasts in the blood or bone marrow aspirate. Histologic section of the brain is illustrated from a patient with acute lymphoblastic leukemia and leukemic meningitis. (B) The sections show blasts within the leptomeninges (higher power, C).

approximately 30% to 50%, depending on risk factors and treatment approach. Notably, adults older than the age of 60 years have uniformly fared poorly with an OS below 10%. Table 66.6 summarizes the major treatment questions, therapeutic approach, and results of several of the recent large prospective cooperative group trials in the United States and Europe.

CENTRAL NERVOUS SYSTEM DISEASE: PROPHYLAXIS AND TREATMENT

Involvement of the CNS (Fig. 66.7) is uncommon at the time of diagnosis, with most series reporting it at less than 10%. However, because many patients with CNS involvement may not be referred for clinical trial enrollment, this may be an underestimate of the true rate. In the MRC UKALL XII/ECOG E2993 trial, of the 1508 eligible patients, 77 (5%) had CNS involvement at diagnosis. Similarly, the French group reported a 7% (104 out of 1493 patients) incidence of CNS disease at diagnosis. Risk factors for CNS disease at diagnosis have varied in different studies. In the French trial (LALA-87 and LALA-94), risk factors included mediastinal mass associated with precursor T-cell immunophenotype, lymphadenopathy, higher hemoglobin level, and absence of the Philadelphia chromosome. In the MRC trial, the risk factors included a higher WBC count, precursor T-cell immunophenotype, and mediastinal mass. The presence of CNS disease at diagnosis has been shown not to affect the CR rate. The French group also reported no significant difference in the OS in patients with and without CNS disease at diagnosis. However, in the MRC trial, the OS at 5 years was lower in the CNS disease group (29% versus 38%; $p = .03$), and they also reported that patients with CNS disease at diagnosis were twice as likely to relapse in the CNS. In the French study, younger age (<30 years), male gender, absence of the Ph chromosome, achievement of CR with one course, and use of transplant as postremission therapy had favorable impact on OS for patients presenting with CNS disease at diagnosis.

Induction therapy of ALL usually includes lumbar punctures with introduction of intrathecal chemotherapy during the first weeks of therapy. For those presenting with CNS disease at diagnosis or in whom CNS disease develops later in the course of the treatment, immediate intensified CNS treatment is imperative. These patients should receive intrathecal chemotherapy (intrathecal methotrexate alone or together with cytarabine and steroid [triple intrathecal therapy]) twice weekly until clearing of cerebrospinal fluid along with initiation of systemic chemotherapy. Cranial irradiation (1800 cGy given in 10 daily fractions of 180 cGy per fraction) is considered necessary for the successful treatment of CNS disease with cranial nerve involvement.

CNS prophylaxis is an essential component of therapy for all patients given the high incidence (30% to 40%) of CNS relapse if the CNS prophylaxis is omitted. Now with the universal adoption of CNS prophylaxis in the treatment regimens, the rates of CNS relapse have decreased substantially. CNS prophylaxis is typically administered by multiple rounds of intrathecal chemotherapy that are staggered over the entire treatment duration. In addition, the use of high-dose methotrexate and cytarabine also provides for CNS prophylaxis because both agents penetrate the blood–brain barrier. The intensive use of high-dose systemic methotrexate and frequent intrathecal therapy has often replaced the more traditional combination of CNS irradiation and intrathecal therapy that were the hallmarks of the earlier ALL regimens. This non–radiation-containing approach has resulted in effective CNS protection, with rates of CNS relapse now routinely reported as occurring in fewer than 5% to 10% of cases. Adolescents and young adults (AYAs) treated on pediatric regimens with more intensive CNS prophylaxis have reported CNS relapse rates as low as 1%. The omission of cranial irradiation may prevent neurocognitive damage in adults. Although this has not been demonstrated in adult studies, definitive evidence from pediatric studies indicates that avoidance of cranial irradiation may prevent declines in cognitive function.

MAINTENANCE THERAPY

The goal of maintenance treatment is to prevent disease relapse by elimination of leukemia clones by long-term exposure to cytotoxic drugs. One of the commonly used regimens uses daily 6-mercaptopurine and weekly oral methotrexate with monthly vincristine and prednisone (POMP regimen). Some groups replaced prednisone with dexamethasone. The duration of maintenance treatment is generally 2–3 years (2 years for women and 3 years for men). Similar to the other components of adult ALL regimens, the adoption of long-term maintenance therapy is based upon the benefit of maintenance therapy that has been demonstrated in pediatric trials.

Although the benefit of maintenance therapy in adult trials has not been demonstrated in randomized trials, it has been shown that omission of maintenance treatment leads to worse clinical outcomes. In a CALGB study, 164 newly diagnosed ALL patients were randomized to receive daunorubicin or mitoxantrone during induction followed by four cycles of consolidation. No maintenance therapy was planned. There were significantly more relapses noted in this study, with median remission duration of only 10–12 months. The study was stopped earlier than planned because remission duration was shorter than in historical control participants who had received maintenance therapy. Similar results were obtained by the Dutch–Belgian Haemato-Oncology Cooperative Group (HOVON), which treated 130 ALL patients with induction followed by three cycles of consolidation. No maintenance therapy was given. The estimated 5-year OS and DFS were only 22% and 28%, respectively. Pediatric regimens routinely incorporate CNS prophylaxis during the maintenance phase. Pediatric studies have also reported favorable impact on DFS of achieving adequate myelosuppression with the chemotherapy drugs during the maintenance phase. Thus, it appears that careful adjustment of the doses of the oral agents used during maintenance therapy to achieve optimal yet safe myelosuppression improves treatment outcomes.

ALLOGENEIC STEM CELL TRANSPLANT IN FIRST COMPLETE REMISSION

Despite attempts to improve DFS in adult ALL, OS with the standard chemotherapy regimens described earlier has been "fixed" at about 35% to 45% for the past decade. Thus, several groups have evaluated the role of treatment intensification with transplant (both aSCT and ASCT) as postremission therapy and compared the outcomes with the traditional chemotherapy approaches described previously. Conventionally, an aSCT has been reserved as the standard recommendation for only HR patients in CR1. In one of the earliest randomized trials to investigate the role of allogeneic transplant, the French LALA-87 study, patients in CR1 were assigned to a donor group (if they had an HLA-matched related donor); the remaining patients (no-donor group) were randomized to ASCT versus chemotherapy. In this study, patients with HR ALL (defined as the presence of Philadelphia chromosome, or null leukemia [defined by a CD10, CD20-immunophenotype], undifferentiated leukemia, or common leukemia with at least one adverse prognosis factor such as age older than 35 years, WBC count greater than 30,000/μL, or time to CR longer than 4 weeks) benefitted from aSCT. For the HR group, 5-year OS was 44% in the donor arm ($n = 41$), which was significantly better than the 20% in the no-donor arm ($n = 55$; $p = .03$). The outcome of the SR group was not improved with aSCT (5-year OS of 51% in the donor arm versus 45% in the no-donor arm). Similar results were seen in a follow-up of LALA-94 trials with benefit of aSCT in the HR group. In contrast, the Program Español de Tratamiento en (PETHEMA) ALL-93 trial failed to show benefit of aSCT in HR ALL patients.

In the MRC UKALLXII/ECOG E2993 trial, all patients (age <50 years or <55 years after 2003) in CR1, irrespective of risk status, were assigned to aSCT if they had an HLA-compatible sibling donor. All other patients were randomized to consolidation or maintenance therapy, or to an ASCT. In this largest adult ALL trial to date, 1646 Ph-negative patients were enrolled; 1484 (90%) achieved CR1. After excluding patients who were older than 55 years of age and those without available HLA-typed siblings, 1031 CR1 patients (55% SR; 45% HR) were HLA typed. In a "genetic randomization" approach using donor ($n = 443$) versus no-donor ($n = 588$) analysis, OS benefit was seen for the donor arm when all patients were considered (5-year OS, 53% versus 45%; $p = .01$). In a subgroup analysis, the survival benefit of transplant was restricted to patients who were younger than 35 years of age. For patients older than 35 years of age or with adverse cytogenetics, OS was not better than with standard chemotherapy because of transplant-related toxicities, which resulted in early deaths.

In a report by the Dutch–Belgian HOVON group, patients younger than 50–55 years in CR1 were offered an aSCT. In a donor ($n = 96$) versus no-donor ($n = 161$) analysis for all patients, 5-year OS was 61% for the donor arm compared with 47% in the no-donor arm ($p = .08$). In subset analysis, the survival benefit of transplant was restricted to SR patients, which were those without any of the following HR features: presence of a high WBC count at diagnosis (>30,000/μL in B-ALL or >100,000/μL in T-ALL), cytogenetic abnormalities (t[4;11], t[1;19], t[9;22]), pro–B-cell immunophenotype, and CR achievement longer than 4 weeks from start of induction.

A meta-analysis of seven studies (with 1274 patients) that prospectively assessed OS using genetic randomization based on donor availability reported significantly better OS in the donor group versus the no-donor groups (hazard ratio: 1.29; $p = .037$), which was more pronounced in patients with HR features.

Alternative Stem Cell Sources; Alternative Preparative Regimens for Allogeneic Stem Cell Transplantation

Matched sibling donors (MSDs) remain the preferred modality for the stem cell source (Table 66.7). For patients lacking an MSD, a matched unrelated donor (MUD) or an alternative donor source (e.g., umbilical cord blood [UCB]) should be pursued. In a Center for International Blood and Marrow Transplant Research (CIBMTR) registry study, outcomes of 169 patients with ALL in CR1 who underwent unrelated donor (URD) transplants between 1995 and 2004 were analyzed. A total of 41% were HLA well matched, 41% partially HLA matched, and 18% HLA mismatched. The majority (93%) of the patients had at least one HR feature. One-year transplant-related mortality (TRM) was high at 36%, and TRM at 5 years was 42%. The relapse rate at 5 years was 20%, with 5-year DFS and OS of 38% and 39%, respectively. Factors associated with worse survival included WBC greater than 100×10^9/L, time to CR1 longer than 8 weeks, cytomegalovirus seropositivity, HLA mismatching, and T-cell depletion. The Minnesota group recently reported outcomes of myeloablative aSCT for ALL patients transplanted at their center and compared retrospectively the outcomes with respect to different donor sources. In an analysis restricted to 91 adult patients who received aSCT in CR1 or CR2 from 1990 to 2005, there was no difference between the allogeneic donor sources (matched related donor versus matched URD versus UCB donor) for OS, DFS, or TRM. Similarly, in the ALL-SCT-BFM 2003 study of children and adolescents, no difference was observed between matched related donor sources and at least 9 out of 10 MUD sources.

Because the majority of older adults are not candidates for a myeloablative aSCT, reduced-intensity conditioning (RIC) approaches have been explored in this patient population (Table 66.8). The Seattle group recently reported outcomes of aSCT using nonmyeloablative conditioning in 51 patients with ALL (median age: 56 years), half of whom were Ph positive. For the Ph-negative group, the 3-year OS for those transplanted in CR1 was 52%. The incidence of chronic graft-versus-host disease, however, was high at 44%. A recent registry study examined the efficacy of RIC in 93 ALL patients and compared it with 1428 ALL patients receiving myeloablative conditioning for aSCT using either a sibling or unrelated donor in CR1/CR2. Interestingly, the TRM at 3 years was similar between the RIC and myeloablative regimens (32% versus 33%, respectively). The relapse rate at 3 years was slightly higher in the RIC arm, although this was not statistically significant (35% versus 26%; $p = .08$). The OS at 3 years was similar between the two groups (38% for RIC arm versus 43% for myeloablative arm, $p = .39$). This was a retrospective registry study; however, it provides evidence that RIC regimens can lead to similar survival in adults with ALL as aSCT with a more intensive, myeloablative conditioning regimen. This is particularly compelling because the median age was significantly older for those receiving RIC (median age in RIC arm: 45 years versus 28 years for myeloablative arm). The group from Minnesota has also reported encouraging results with UCB donor transplantation using a RIC regimen. Eighteen adults (median age: 49 years; range: 24–68 years) with high-risk ALL (majority Ph+ ALL) received a cord blood transplant using a RIC conditioning regimen and reported 3-year OS, TRM, and relapse rates of 49%, 28%, and 33%, respectively. Notably, patients in CR1 had a TRM of only 8% with no events after 6 months. These results with UCB donor transplantation are promising and compare favorably to conventional aSCT with relatively low TRM in this high-risk population. Thus RIC-based aSCT regimens with alternative donor sources should be considered for older adults in prospective clinical trials.

In summary, aSCT is a curative option for patients with ALL and can be considered the standard recommendation for patients with a good performance status but with adverse disease risk factors in CR1. There have been significant improvements in transplantation techniques (better supportive care, refinement of preparative regimens, and uses of alternative donors as a source of stem cells) that are

| TABLE 66.7 | Clinical Trials Evaluating Role of Myeloablative Allogeneic Stem Cell Transplant in Acute Lymphoblastic Leukemia |

Trial	Patients (n)	Age in Years, Median (Range)	Conditioning Regimen/ Donor	TRM	DFS/OS	Comments
GOELAL02[13]	41 (HR)	34 (15–52)	Etoposide/ cyclophosphamide/ TBI (12 Gy in six fractions) MSD	15%	DFS: 75% at 6 years; OS: 75% at 6 years	Showed improved survival with aSCT compared with ASCT
LALA 94[6]	100 (HR ALL excluding Ph+ ALL)	33 (15–55) for the entire study cohort of 922 patients	Cyclophosphamide/ TBI (10 Gy as a single dose or 12 Gy in six fractions) MRD	18% at 3 years	3-year DFS: 47%	For HR ALL, aSCT was superior to an ASCT
PETHEMA-93[11]	222 HR patient underwent MSD (if available); if not, randomized to ASCT vs. chemotherapy	27 (15–50)	Cyclophosphamide/ TBI (12 Gy in six fractions) MSD		5-year OS: 35%	No benefit of an MSD transplant for HR patients (compared with ASCT or chemotherapy only approach)
MRC UKALLXII/ ECOG E2993[10]	Patients assigned to aSCT if an MSD available (donor group); those without donors randomized to ASCT vs. chemotherapy	15–64	Etoposide/TBI (13.2 Gy in six fractions) MSD	NRM HR (36% donor; 14% no-donor); SR (20% donor; 7% no donor)	5-year OS: HR (41% donor, 35% no donor) SR (62% donor vs. 52% donor)	Beneficial effect of all-SCT limited to SR group only; relapse rate decreased with aSCT in both HR and SR groups
HOVON[14]	ALL in CR1 according to sibling donor vs. no-donor comparison HR: 46 donor; 73 no donor SR: 50 donor; 88 no donor	Donor 31 (16–55)	Cyclophosphamide/ TBI (12 Gy in six fractions) MRD	HR: NRM at 5 years (15% donor vs. 4% no-donor) SR: NRM at 5 years (16% donor vs. 2% no-donor, $p = .01$)	HR: OS at 5 years (53% donor vs. 41% no donor) SR: OS at 5 years (69% donor vs. 49% no donor, $p = .05$)	Similar to the MRC UKALLXII/ECOG E2993 trial, benefit of aSCT seems limited to SR patients

ALL, Acute lymphoblastic leukemia; aSCT, allogeneic stem cell transplantation; ASCT, autologous stem cell transplantation; CR1, first complete remission; DFS, disease-free survival; HR, high risk; MRD, minimal residual disease; MSD, matched sibling donor; NRM, non-relapse mortality; OS, overall survival; Ph, philadelphia chromosome; SCT, stem cell transplantation; SR, standard risk; TBI, total-body irradiation; TRM, transplant-related mortality.

resulting in greater availability and improved transplant outcomes. At the same time, the TRM and mortality are significant, and aSCT has largely been offered only to patients younger than 60 years of age because of the poor tolerance of older adults to standard myeloablative transplant preparative regimens. Prospective incorporation of MRD evaluation may refine the ability to risk-stratify patients who are at HR of relapse and might benefit from aSCT in CR1. However, the benefit of a SCT for MRD-positive patients remains to be proven and has only been studied prospectively in a single study to date. Conversely, patients who were MRD negative in CR1 may best be treated by chemotherapy alone. Overall, the role of aSCT in CR1 merits further study, and it is important to refer these patients to clinical trials exploring such approaches.

Autologous Stem Cell Transplantation

ASCT in CR1 has also been studied prospectively in several clinical trials. Dhedin and colleagues reviewed the data from the French LALA 85, 87, and 94 trials and compared the outcomes of patients in CR1 who were randomized to chemotherapy versus ASCT. There was no improvement in DFS or OS with the use of ASCT compared with postremission chemotherapy, but there was a lower incidence of

relapse at 10 years (66% versus 78%; $p = .05$). In the MRC UKALLXII/ECOG E2993 trial, 456 patients were randomized to chemotherapy versus ASCT in CR1. Patients randomized to chemotherapy had significantly better 5-year event-free survival (EFS) (41% versus 32%; $p = .02$) and OS (46% versus 37%; $p = .03$). Thus, outside of a clinical trial, an ASCT cannot be recommended for ALL patients.

THERAPY FOR SPECIFIC DISEASE SUBSETS

Philadelphia Chromosome-Positive Acute Lymphoblastic Leukemia

The Philadelphia chromosome [t(9;22)(q34;q11)] is the most common cytogenetic abnormality in adult ALL, and its incidence increases with age. Among patients older than 60 years, 40% to 50% have the Philadelphia chromosome. Before the introduction of molecularly targeted therapy, Ph+ ALL was associated with lower remission rates and a very poor prognosis, with a median survival time of only approximately 9 months.

With the introduction of therapy using TKIs targeted to the aberrant BCR-ABL protein, the outcome of Ph+ ALL has improved

TABLE 66.8	Clinical Trials Evaluating Role of Reduced-Intensity Conditioning Allogeneic Stem Cell Transplant in Acute Lymphoblastic Leukemia					
Trial	Number of Patients	Age in Years, Median (Range)	Conditioning Regimen/Donor	Mortality	DFS/OS	Comments
Arnold[15]	22 (11 Ph⁺)	38 (21–58)	Fludarabine/busulfan +/– ATG MSD or MUD	TRM: 45%	Median survival: 354 days	High TRM of the group; all patients with aGVHD had CR indicating toward GVL effect
Martino[16]	27 (11 Ph⁺)	50 (18–63)	Fludarabine/melphalan (most cases) MSD or MUD	2-year TRM: 23%	2-year OS: 31%	100-day acute grade II–IV GVHD: 48%; cGVHD 72% (extensive in 39%)
Hamaki[17]	33 (14 Ph⁺)	55 (17–68)	Different RIC regimens MSD or MUD	TRM: 27%	1-year OS: 39.6%	Grade II–IV aGVHD: 45%; cGVHD: 64%
Mohty[18]	97 (37 Ph⁺)	38 (17–65)	Different RIC regimens MSD or MUD	NRM: 28% (for those transplanted in CR1: 18%)	2-year OS: 31% (for those transplanted in CR1: 52%)	Three factors associated with improved OS:CR1 at time of transplant, chronic GVHD, and woman donor
Stein[19]	24 (10 Ph⁺)	47.5 (23–68)	Fludarabine/melphalan MSD or MUD	NRM at 2 years: 21.5%	OS at 2-years: 61.5%	75% aGVHD (62% grade II–IV aGVHD) 86% cGVHD (62% extensive)
Bachanova[20]	22 (14 Ph⁺)	49 (24–68)	Fludarabine/cyclophosphamide/ TBI 200 cGy MRD (n = 4) or umbilical cord blood donor graft (n = 18)	TRM at 3 years: 27%	OS at 3 years: 50% (for CR1: 81%)	3-year OS for those in CR1 81% vs. 15% for those in CR2 or more (p < .01). For CR1: 8% TRM
Ram[21]	51 (25 Ph⁺)	56 (8–69)	Fludarabine/TBI 200 cGy MSD or MUD	NRM at 3 years: 28%	OS at 3-years: 34%	Grade II–IV aGVHD: 53% Chronic extensive GVHD: 42%

aGVHD, Acute graft-versus-host disease; cGVHD, chronic graft-versus-host disease; ATG, anti-thymocyte globulin; CR1, first complete remission; CR2, second complete remission; DFS, disease-free survival; GVHD, graft-versus-host disease; GVL, graft-versus-leukemia; MSD, matched sibling donor; MUD, matched unrelated donor; NRM, non-relapse mortality; OS, overall survival; Ph⁺, philadelphia chromosome positive; RIC, reduced-intensity conditioning; TBI, total-body irradiation; TRM, transplant-related mortality.

substantially and has been the major treatment advance for adults with ALL in the past two decades. Imatinib, the first targeted TKI developed for use in Ph⁺ leukemias, has been combined with multi-agent chemotherapy by various groups and this has substantially improved both CR rates and DFS (Table 66.9).

The MD Anderson Cancer Center was the first to report on the combination of imatinib with chemotherapy (hyper-CVAD). They used imatinib 400 mg/day on days 1 to 14 of each of the intensive chemotherapy courses, followed by imatinib at a dose of 600 mg daily during the maintenance phase, with monthly vincristine and prednisone, and then imatinib indefinitely. Thomas and colleagues recently reported long-term results of the Hyper-CVAD–Imatinib trial. The 3-year CR duration and OS rates were significantly superior in the hyper-CVAD–imatinib arm compared with historical control participants treated with hyper-CVAD alone (68% versus 24% and 54% versus 15%, respectively; p < .001). The Japanese have also reported impressive improvements compared to their control participants. In the JALSG ALL202 trial, imatinib, 600 mg/day, was added to standard induction followed by alternating cycles of high-dose methotrexate and high-dose cytarabine and single agent imatinib 600 mg/day. Later maintenance therapy with imatinib 600 mg/day with monthly vincristine and prednisone was given. In a recent update, they reported results on 103 patients with Ph⁺ ALL with a 97% CR rate and 3-year OS of 57%, both of which were significantly better than in historical control participants.

Older adults with Ph⁺ ALL have also demonstrated improved survival with the addition of imatinib to reduced-intensity chemotherapy regimens. Ottmann and colleagues reported for the German study group in which older adults (>55 years of age) Ph⁺ ALL patients were randomized to receive induction cycle with imatinib alone (n = 28) versus combination chemotherapy (n = 27). The CR rate was 96% in the imatinib arm, which was significantly better than the CR rate of 50% in the chemotherapy alone arm. This is the first prospective randomized controlled trial comparing imatinib with chemotherapy and clearly showed the superiority of the imatinib arm. There was no difference in the two arms with respect to DFS and OS, likely due to the fact that all patients received imatinib-based consolidation or maintenance therapy. The Italian GIMEMA group treated 30 Ph⁺ ALL patients (median age: 69 years; range: 61–83 years) with 7-day steroid pretreatment followed by induction treatment with only imatinib (800 mg/day) plus steroids. Impressively, all 29 evaluable patients achieved CR with 1-year DFS and OS of 48% and 74%, respectively.

There is general consensus that early TKI therapy is crucial, and most current treatment protocols include chemotherapy with continuous TKI therapy. In general, the TKI has been started with induction chemotherapy and continues throughout postremission and maintenance therapy.

Despite these significant advances in the treatment of Ph⁺ ALL, relapses are still major challenges. Resistance to imatinib develops and

TABLE 66.9   Clinical Trials With Tyrosine Kinase Inhibitor Plus Chemotherapy for Adult Philadelphia Chromosome-Positive Acute Lymphoblastic Leukemia

Trial	Patients (n)	Age in Years, Median (Range)	CR Rate	Disease-Free Survival	Overall Survival	Comments
MDACC Hyper-CVAD Imatinib[22,23]	54	51 (17–84)	93%	68% at 3 years	In de novo patients 40 years of age or younger: 3-year OS was 90% with aSCT (n = 10) vs. 33% without aSCT (n = 6), p = .05	First report of the combination of chemotherapy with a TKI Imatinib 400 mg/day on days 1–14 of induction; 600 mg continuously during courses 2–8; 600 mg during 2 years of maintenance therapy with monthly vincristine–prednisone; then imatinib indefinitely; allo-SCT in CR1 as feasible
JALSG ALL202[24–26]	103	45 (15–64)	97%	For those younger than age 55 years, 54 of 74 patients in CR1 who had aSCT, only 13% relapsed; among the 20/74 patients in CR1 who did not undergo SCT, 90% relapsed	57% at 3 years For patients younger than age 55 years, OS at 3 years was 75.0% for the transplanted group vs. 36.4% for the nontransplanted group	Standard induction plus imatinib 600 mg/day followed by alternating cycles of high-dose methotrexate and high-dose cytarabine and imatinib 600 mg/day; imatinib 600 mg/day with monthly vincristine–prednisone for maintenance
GRAAPH-2003[27,28]	45	45 (16–59)	96%	43% at 4 years	52% at 4 years The 4-year OS in the aSCT, ASCT, and no SCT groups were 55%, 80%, and 25%, respectively	Imatinib was started with consolidation in good early responders (corticosensitive and chemosensitive ALL) or during the induction course in poor early responders
GMALL[29]	47 (alternating imatinib and chemotherapy)	46 (21–65)	NA because only CR patients were eligible	52% at 2 years	36% at 2 years	Coadministration of imatinib with induction cycle 2 led to CR rate of 95% and molecular CR rate of 52% of patients compared with 19% (significantly worse) in patients in the alternating treatment cohort
	45 (concurrent imatinib and chemotherapy starting after induction I)	41 (19–63)	95%	61% at 2 years	43% at 2 years	
GMALL[30]	28 (imatinib arm)	66 (54–79)	96%	30% at 1.5 years	57% at 1.5 years	Patients older than age 55 years with de novo ALL and not eligible for aSCT; randomized to single-agent imatinib induction versus. multi-agent chemotherapy induction; subsequent consolidation or maintenance with imatinib plus chemotherapy for all patients
	27 (chemotherapy arm)	68 (58–78)	50% (significantly inferior to imatinib arm)	35% at 1.5 years	41% at 1.5 years	

TABLE 66.9	Clinical Trials With Tyrosine Kinase Inhibitor Plus Chemotherapy for Adult Philadelphia Chromosome-Positive Acute Lymphoblastic Leukemia—cont'd					
Trial	Patients (n)	Age in Years, Median (Range)	CR Rate	Disease-Free Survival	Overall Survival	Comments
GIMEMA[31]	29	69 (61–83)	100%	48% at 1 year	74% at 1 year	7-day steroid pretreatment followed by induction treatment with imatinib (800 mg/day) plus steroids
NILG protocol 09/00[32]	59	45 (20–66)	92%	39% at 5 years	38% at 5 years	Imatinib (600 mg/day) was added to each chemotherapy course for 7 consecutive days, starting from day 15 of chemotherapy course 1 and from 3 days before chemotherapy during courses 2 to 8.
UKALLXII/ ECOG2993[33]	175	Not reported	92%	54% at 3 years	42% at 3 years	Outcomes (CR, DFS, and OS) were significantly better compared with the historical preimatinib cohort; for the imatinib group, 3-year OS for patients who received aSCT was 59% vs. 28% for those who did not receive aSCT
PACE[34]	32	62	41%	7% at 12 months	40% at 12 months	Ponatinib is active in Ph+ ALL with T135I mutation
EWALL-PH-02[35]	36	66	97%	89% at median follow up of 7 months		
CALGB 10001[36]	58	45	8 patients converted from MMR to CMR after transplant	Median DFS 5.9 months after auto-HSCT	Median OS 4.8 years. 47% OS with allo-HSCT versus 42% OS with auto-HSCT	TRM associated with auto-SCT occurred in one (5%) of 19 patients, while TRM associated with allo-SCT occurred in 3 (20%) of 15 patients

ALL, Acute lymphoblastic leukemia; aSCT, allogeneic stem cell transplantation; ASCT, autologous stem cell transplantation; CMR, complete molecular response; CR, complete remission; CR1, first complete remission; DFS, disease-free survival; HSCT, hematopoietic stem cell transplantation; MMR, major molecular response; NA, not applicable; OS, overall survival; Ph+, philadelphia chromosome positive; SCT, stem cell transplantation; TKI, tyrosine kinase inhibitor; TRM, treatment–related mortality.

most frequently results from the emergence of a resistant clone with ABL kinase domain mutations. These kinase domain mutations cause conformational changes in the ABL protein that prevent effective binding. Other potential mechanisms of resistance that have been described include reduced intracellular availability of imatinib and activation of alternative signaling pathways such as the Src-kinase pathways. Second-generation TKIs, dasatinib and nilotinib, are more potent kinase inhibitors and are also effective against many imatinib-resistant mutations (although not the T315I mutation). In addition, dasatinib has been shown to penetrate the CNS and thus may be particularly effective in Ph+ ALL.

Dasatinib has been tested in several prospective trials for previously untreated Ph+ ALL. MD Anderson Cancer Center investigators evaluated hyper-CVAD plus dasatinib in newly diagnosed Ph+ ALL patients. Dasatinib 100 mg/day was given for the first 14 days of each of eight cycles of hyper-CVAD. The study was amended to allow dasatinib 100 mg/day for 14 days during cycle 1, and then 70 mg/day continuously during subsequent cycles. Maintenance chemotherapy consisted of daily dasatinib 100 mg/day with monthly vincristine and prednisone for 2 years followed by dasatinib

indefinitely. The median age of the 35 patients studied was 53 years (range: 21–79 years); 94% achieved CR. Of the patients who achieved CR, 61% of patients achieved complete molecular remission, meaning that there was no detectable MRD using quantitative PCR for BCR-ABL. In a recent update to the hyper-CVAD and dasatinib study, the MD Anderson Cancer Center group reported that 24% patients underwent aSCT (16% in CR1; 8% CR2), and 3-year DFS and OS for the entire cohort were 49% and 62%, respectively.

Foa and colleagues reported the results of the GIMEMA LAL1205 study in which dasatinib monotherapy (70 mg twice daily) with steroids was investigated for frontline treatment of 53 adult Ph+ ALL patients (median age: 54 years). All patients achieved a complete hematologic response, and there were no induction deaths. BCR-ABL transcript levels decreased rapidly during induction therapy, and the percentage of patients achieving BCR-ABL levels below 0.001% increased from 23% at day 22 to 52% at day 85. aSCT in CR1 was performed in 18 (34%) patients. At 20 months, the OS was 69% and DFS was 51%. BCR-ABL levels of less than 0.001% at day 85 correlated with DFS. These results with dasatinib without any cytotoxic chemotherapy are encouraging but demonstrated that single-agent dasatinib is not sufficient to cure this disease. In a subsequent trial, the GIMEMA LAL1509, if patients did not achieve complete molecular response after a prolonged 84-day induction with dasatinib and steroids, they received more intensive combination chemotherapy and/or allogeneic transplantation. At day 85, 58 out of 60 (97%) patients achieved a complete hematologic remission; however, only 11 (18.6%) patients achieved a complete molecular remission (CMR) with TKI plus steroid induction, suggesting that dasatinib and steroids are insufficient to achieve a molecular remission in most patients and that additional postremission intensification is needed. Using this stratified treatment approach, the DFS was 62% with 18 months of follow-up and OS was 69%. Nilotinib is also a second-generation TKI that that has been evaluated as frontline therapy. In a prospective, single arm phase II trial, induction treatment consisted of vincristine, daunorubicin, oral prednisolone, and nilotinib (400 mg orally twice daily). Patients in CR received either five courses of consolidation followed by 2-year maintenance therapy or an aSCT, depending on donor availability. Nilotinib was administered from day 8 of induction continuously until the end of maintenance or aSCT. Patients achieved a complete hematologic remission in 45 out of 50 (90%) cases. More than 70% of patients received aSCT. Estimated DFS and OS at 2 years were 71% and 66%, respectively, similar to rates observed with other TKIs. A subsequent study, EWALL-PH02, in patients greater than 55 years old evaluated nilotinib as induction therapy with vincristine and dexamethasone followed by consolidation cycles with further chemotherapy added. Patients achieved a CR with induction in 35 out of 36 (97%) cases. In addition, 30% of patients were in a molecular remission after induction. Although these results are similar to other studies with dasatinib, most of the current trials in Ph+ ALL have incorporated dasatinib in the frontline therapy because of its potential advantage over nilotinib with respect to CNS penetration.

Ponatinib is a third-generation ABL kinase inhibitor with the ability to inactivate the T315I mutant ABL kinase, which has been the most commonly occurring mutation at time of relapse in Ph+ ALL, and is approved for relapsed disease based on data from the PACE trial. In the chronic myeloid leukemia blast phase/Ph+ ALL cohort, 37% (11 out of 30) of patients who were resistant or intolerant to second-generation TKIs and 27% (6 out of 22) of patients with T315I mutations achieved a major hematologic remission. Recently the MD Anderson Cancer Center has reported preliminary results from a phase II study of ponatinib with hyperCVAD in newly diagnosed Ph+ ALL. Thirty five (95%) patients achieved major molecular remission and 26 (70%) complete molecular remission. The median time to MMR and CMR were 3 and 10 weeks, respectively. Several patients received alternative TKI therapy due to vascular toxicities. Further definition of the incidence of serious vascular events with ponatinib in the frontline treatment setting of Ph+ ALL is required; thus at this time the use of ponatinib as initial therapy in Ph+ ALL remains investigational.

Role of Transplantation for Philadelphia Chromosome Positive Acute Lymphoblastic Leukemia in the Era of Tyrosine Kinase Inhibitor-Based Therapy

aSCT in CR1 was the only curative treatment option for Ph+ ALL in the pre-TKI era. Although the addition of TKI therapy has significantly improved the outcome of Ph+ ALL, many recent studies have also highlighted the continued role of aSCT for Ph+ ALL. In an update of the hyper-CVAD-imatinib protocol, the MD Anderson Cancer Center group reported that in a subgroup of patients younger than 40 years of age, the 3-year OS was 90% with an aSCT compared with 33% without aSCT (p = .05). In the Japanese study, aSCT was performed in the CR1 in 54 of the 74 CR1 patients younger than 55 years of age. Relapse occurred in 13% (7 out of 54) of the transplanted patients compared with 90% (18 out of 20) in those who were not transplanted. Similarly, OS at 3 years was 75% for the transplanted group versus 36% for the nontransplanted group.

Similar results have been reported in preliminary form by the MRC UKALLXII/ECOG E2993 trial group. In this study, 175 Ph+ ALL patients received imatinib plus chemotherapy (2003 onward). The authors reported that 44% of the patients were able to receive an aSCT per protocol, a number much higher than the 28% who were able to receive aSCT in the preimatinib era of this study (1993–2003). For the imatinib cohort, the 3-year OS for patients who received protocol aSCT was 59% versus 28% for those who did not receive aSCT. In a recent update of the GMALL study, 219 of 335 (66%) Ph+ ALL patients treated with an imatinib-based chemotherapy regimen underwent aSCT in CR1. For the transplanted patients, the median OS was 57% after 3 years and 52% after 7 years compared with the dismal outcome of the nontransplanted group (3-year OS of only 14%). Similarly, the GRAAPH2005 study from the GRAAL group showed that patients who received imatinib-based therapy and aSCT had a 4-year OS of 76%, whereas the OS was 33% for those that received imatinib maintenance alone. These studies provide a strong rationale for the continued recommendation for an aSCT in CR1 for Ph+ ALL patients.

While ASCTs (as described previously) have not demonstrated efficacy overall in ALL, a study from the CALGB (10001) suggests that this may be an effective approach for Ph+ ALL. A combination of imatinib and chemotherapy induction and postremission CNS intensification was followed by allogeneic or autologous transplant (if no sibling donor available) in newly diagnosed Ph+ ALL. Nineteen patients subsequently received autologous transplantation in CR1. The OS with a median follow-up of 6 years was not reached and the median DFS was 3.5 years compared with 4.1 years (not statistically different) in the 15 patients who received allogeneic SCT in CR1. The authors concluded that autologous transplantation represents a safe and effective alternative to allogeneic transplant in Ph+ ALL without a donor.

The role and duration of TKI therapy after transplant is currently an area of active investigation. Wassmann and colleagues (GMALL) treated 27 Ph+ ALL patients with imatinib upon detection of MRD after SCT. Approximately 50% of patients achieved a molecular remission after a median of 1.5 months and these patients had a significantly longer time to progression (28.6 months versus 3.6 months; p < .001) and OS (2-year OS, 80% versus 23%; p < .001) compared with those who had persistent BCR-ABL1 transcript levels. The German group also reported results of a randomized study that compared prophylactic (n = 26) versus preemptive (after detection of BCR-ABL1 transcripts, n = 29) imatinib after aSCT for Ph+ ALL. Imatinib was discontinued early in more than half the patients in both groups, mostly because of gastrointestinal toxicity. Prophylactic administration of imatinib significantly reduced the incidence of molecular relapse after the aSCT. However, the OS was similar in the two arms (5-year OS: 75% to 80%), suggesting that imatinib can be effective either prophylactically after aSCT or based on molecular relapse. At the present time, it appears that continuing TKI therapy after transplant is an appropriate strategy. Studies evaluating MRD may provide guidance with the question of duration of posttransplant TKI therapy. The CALGB 10701 study, which includes 1 year of maintenance dasatinib after transplant, has recently completed accrual and will provide further data to address this issue.

In summary, during the last decade the addition of TKIs to combination chemotherapy has resulted in significant improvement in DFS and OS for both younger and older adults with Ph+ ALL. High complete molecular remission rates can now be achieved and have been demonstrated to be associated with improved outcomes. While allogeneic SCT remains the current treatment of choice for eligible patients, the next generation of studies in Ph+ ALL may help to define the role of transplantation when complete molecular remissions are achieved with combination TKI and chemotherapy alone.

BURKITT LYMPHOMA/LEUKEMIA

BL is a mature B-cell lymphoma with an extremely short doubling time that often presents in extranodal sites or as acute leukemia.

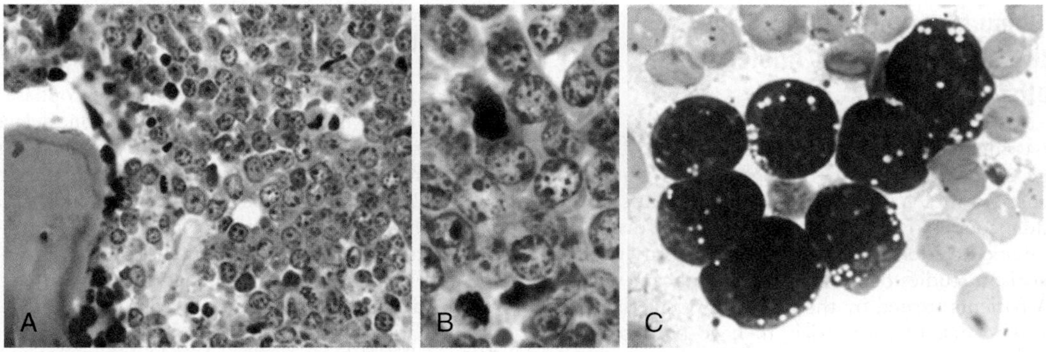

Fig. 66.8 BURKITT LEUKEMIA/LYMPHOMA (A–C). Bone marrow biopsy and aspirate features of Burkitt leukemia/lymphoma are illustrated. The bone marrow (or lymph node) will show sheets of highly proliferating intermediate-sized neoplastic cells with a syncytial appearance. The cells are monotonous but have a stippled intermediate chromatin pattern with multiple small nucleoli. (C) On the aspirate, the Burkitt cells have an intermediate size, a denser chromatin than lymphoblasts, and deeply blue cytoplasm with prominent vacuoles.

Thus a brief description of the therapy is warranted in this chapter. Morphologically (Fig. 66.8), the malignant cells are intermediate in size, have round nuclei with small nucleoli, are intensely basophilic, and frequently have vacuolated cytoplasms. In a BM biopsy and in tissue sections, the tumor is classically described as having a "starry sky" appearance because of the presence of multiple tingible body macrophages with phagocytized cellular debris. Immunophenotypically, the tumor cells express moderate to strong levels of surface immunoglobulin M with light chain restriction, indicating origin of the tumor from a mature B cell. The tumor cells also universally express the B-cell antigens CD19 and CD20, and germinal center associated markers such as CD10 and BCL6. Unlike B-ALL, BL cells do not express CD34 or TdT. The genetic basis of the disease is the underlying MYC translocation at band 8q24 to either the Ig heavy chain region on chromosome 14 or less commonly at the lambda (22q11) or kappa (2p12) loci.

Prompt diagnosis and recognition of this entity is essential because this is now a highly curable leukemia (in the range of 65% to 80% in recent trials); however, failure to institute appropriate therapy at diagnosis for Burkitt lymphoma/leukemia results in emergence of early resistance and dismal outcomes. Traditional CHOP (cyclophosphamide, hydroxydaunomycin, vincristine [Oncovin], and prednisone) chemotherapy is inadequate and should not be used. Treatment should be initiated quickly and consists of aggressive combination chemotherapy with CNS prophylaxis. These patients are at HR for the development of tumor lysis syndrome; therefore aggressive hydration and administration of allopurinol and/or rasburicase is important. All current regimens rely on short intensive courses of chemotherapy that incorporate fractionated doses of alkylating agents, high doses of methotrexate and cytarabine, and intensive intrathecal prophylaxis. In the United States, commonly used regimens include CODOX-M/IVAC, CALGB 9251, and hyper-CVAD. With these regimens, approximately 80% achieve CR, and 2-year survival is around 60% to 70%. In the CALGB 9251 trial, 52% of the patients were alive and in continuous CR at a median follow-up of 5.1 years. Because Burkitt lymphoma/leukemia has a predisposition for CNS involvement, aggressive CNS-directed therapy is essential and typically consists of intrathecal administration of methotrexate, cytarabine, and hydrocortisone. Recurrence after the first 2 years rarely occurs; therefore maintenance therapy has not been shown to be beneficial and is not recommended.

Because of the strong expression of CD20 in mature B-cell ALL, several groups have incorporated rituximab into the frontline chemotherapy regimen with impressive further improvements in survival. The hyper-CVAD–rituximab regimen was reported in 31 patients with newly diagnosed Burkitt lymphoma/leukemia with a CR rate of 86% and a 3-year survival rate of 89%. Similarly, the addition of rituximab to the treatment in both the GMALL and CALGB

TABLE 66.10	Outcomes of Adolescent and Young Adult Patients Treated With Pediatric Intensive Regimens: Several Examples of Recent Trials		
	ALL-96 (PETHEMA)[37]	DFCI adult ALL 01-175.[38]	C10403 (US Intergroup)[39]
Patient Population			
Patients (n)	81	92	318
Median age (range)	20 years (15–30)	28 years (18–50)	24 years (17–39)
Gender	Male: 62%	Male: 61%	Male: 61%
Immunophenotype	Precursor B and T-ALL	Precursor B and T-ALL	Precursor B and T-ALL
Outcomes			
EFS	61% (6 year)	58% (4 year)	66% (2 year)
OS	69% (6 year)	67% (4 year)	78% (2 year)

ALL, Acute lymphoblastic leukemia; EFS, event-free survival; OS, overall survival.

regimens has proven feasible with OS of 91% (3 years) and 79% (2 years), respectively. Based on these exciting improvements in survival, the addition of anti-CD20 targeting to frontline therapies for BL is now considered the standard of care.

ADOLESCENTS AND YOUNG ADULTS WITH ACUTE LYMPHOBLASTIC LEUKEMIA: THE INTERSECTION BETWEEN PEDIATRIC AND ADULT CARE

Evaluation of the outcomes of young adult patients, here defined as patients between the ages of 15 and 39 years, presents specific challenges. Because of community referral patterns, these patients may be treated by either pediatric or adult oncologists. As such, the treating physician may view a patient in this age group either as an older child or as a younger adult. The oncologist will choose a regimen most appropriate for the population usually seen by that particular physician. A number of comparisons of the clinical outcome of adolescents enrolled on adult and pediatric clinical trials (Table 66.10) have resulted in interesting observations about what that appropriate treatment regimen should be and have guided the design of a number of prospective clinical trials designed specifically for AYAs with ALL.

Retrospective Comparison of Pediatric and Adult Cooperative Group Trials in Adolescents and Young Adults

The retrospective comparisons summarized in Table 66.10 were performed by large cooperative groups throughout the world and examined the outcome of the AYA patients aged 15–21 years treated on pediatric or adult cooperative group trials for newly diagnosed ALL that were conducted contemporaneously. The majority of these retrospective comparison studies demonstrated a significant survival advantage for AYA patients treated by the pediatric versus the adult cooperative group. The first of these trials to have been reported highlights many of the interesting questions posed by these comparisons and is reviewed briefly here. The CALGB and the Children's Cancer Group (CCG) examined the outcome of 321 AYA patients between 16 and 20 years of age treated on consecutive trials from 1988 to 2001. The two patient groups were well matched for biologic features, including immunophenotype and cytogenetics. Although the age range was the same in both groups examined, the median age of the patients in the CALGB studies was 19 years compared with 16 years for the CCG patients. CR rates were identical—90% for both CALGB and CCG AYAs. However, CCG AYAs had a 63% EFS at 7 years and 67% OS at 7 years in contrast to the CALGB AYAs, in which the 7-year EFS was only 34%. A difference in pattern of relapse was also noted. The incidence of CNS relapses was significantly higher in CALGB AYAs (11%) compared with the CCG AYAs (1.4%; $p < .001$).

Since the initial report of these findings in 2000, multiple national European cooperative groups have reported similar results with improvement in the outcome of AYAs treated on pediatric compared with adult protocols, and these are summarized in Table 66.10. Although the treatment approaches differ among countries, several treatment themes have emerged as being potentially important. Pediatric studies throughout the world use considerably more treatment with nonmyelosuppressive drugs, including glucocorticoids (both dexamethasone and prednisone), vincristine, and L-asparaginase. CNS prophylaxis is typically administered earlier, with a greater frequency, and for a more prolonged period during pediatric group trials. Finally, long-term maintenance therapy was also continued for a longer period in pediatric cooperative group trials. Based on additional retrospective data from Finland and the MD Anderson Cancer Center, it appears that treating patients in a uniform fashion by an experienced group of physicians and nurses is also a very important component in the successful treatment of young adults with ALL.

To begin to address the many unanswered questions that have been raised by the retrospective comparison trials and to determine whether AYA patients treated by adult hematologists and oncologists can achieve similarly improved outcomes to the pediatricians for this age group, prospective cooperative group trials are being conducted in North America and in Europe. Early results from several of these trials have recently been reported. The PETHEMA Protocol ALL-96 addressed the toxicity and results of a pediatric-based protocol in 35 adolescent (age: 15–18 years) and 46 young adults (age: 19–30 years) with SR ALL. In this trial, patients received a standard five-drug, 5-week induction course followed by two cycles of early consolidation, maintenance with monthly reinforcement cycles for 1 year after remission, and standard maintenance chemotherapy for up to 2 years after CR. The AYAs were well matched for pretreatment characteristics. The CR rate was 98%, and with a median follow-up of 4.2 years, the 6-year EFS and OS were 61% and 69%, respectively. The only significant predictor of poor EFS for the entire group was a slow response to initial induction therapy (>10% blasts remaining in BM aspirate done on day 14 of induction therapy). Thus the investigators concluded that a pediatric regimen was tolerable and efficacious in AYAs with ALL up to the age of 30 years.

Two pilot studies from French adult cooperative groups have also demonstrated the feasibility of using modified pediatric-inspired regimens in adults with ALL, but the age range of these studies

extends well into the middle years of adult life. In the French Acute Lymphoblastic Leukemia Pediatric group (FRALLE) study, 28 Ph⁻ adult ALL patients 16–57 years old were treated on the FRALLE 2000 protocol consisting of a prednisone prophase, four-drug induction including L-asparaginase, consolidation, delayed intensification, and maintenance chemotherapy. Four-year DFS was 90% versus 47% seen in matched historical control participants. In the GRAALL 2003 study, 225 Ph⁻ ALL patients 15–60 years old (median: 31 years) were treated between 2003 and 2005 with five-drug induction, dose-intense consolidation, delayed intensification, and 2-year maintenance therapy. Notably, aSCT for patients younger than 55 years was recommended in this trial and makes interpretation of this trial more problematic. The CR rate was 93.5%. Among the 139 CR patients, 71 actually underwent transplantation in CR1 and were censored at the time of transplant. At 42 months, EFS was 55% versus 41% when comparing patients from an earlier French trial, the LALA-94, and the OS was 61%, significantly better than the 41% OS observed in the LALA-94 trial ($p < .001$). The benefit of the GRAALL approach was not statistically significant in patients older than 45 years of age because of a significant increase in treatment-related mortality of 23% compared with 5% treatment-related mortality for patients younger than 45 years old. The investigators concluded that the use of a pediatric-inspired regimen in adults up to 45 years of age was tolerable and markedly improved outcome for "younger" adults with ALL. This regimen included older adults up to the age of 60 years and used only a modified pediatric regimen that did not use the dose intensity of corticosteroids, asparaginase, and vincristine that are routinely used in current pediatric regimens. Another difference from the pediatric regimens is that all patients in these trials still received prophylactic cranial irradiation. Also, the majority of CR1 patients actually underwent aSCT, which is not the approach used by pediatric groups. Thus any interpretation of the contribution of the "chemotherapy" intensification component of these trials to DFS is very difficult to assess.

The Dana-Farber Cancer Institute (DFCI) consortium has also extended its successful pediatric regimen to older patients 18–50 years old. The trial design here was a true pediatric approach with intensification of *Escherichia coli* L-asparaginase, glucocorticoids, and vincristine for patients up to 50 years old; aSCT was not routinely recommended. A total of 92 patients, with a median age of 28 years (range: 18–50 years) were evaluable. Seventy nine patients (85%) achieved a CR after 1 month of intensive induction therapy. With a median follow-up time of 4.5 years, the 4-year DFS rate for all patients was 69% and the OS rate 67%. For the 74 patients with Ph⁻ ALL, DFS was 71%, and OS was 70%.

The largest prospective trial to evaluate the feasibility of using a pediatric regimen in AYA patients treated by adult medical hematologists and oncologists is ongoing in North America (CALGB-10403). The United States adult and pediatric cooperative groups are currently enrolling a total of 300 young adults aged between16 and 39 years on a prospective phase II trial (CALGB-10403) that uses one treatment arm of a successful Children's Oncology Group (COG) protocol for adolescents (and HR children with ALL). Early results from this trial also suggest both the feasibility of use of an intensive pediatric regimen in young adults and significant improvement in EFS of 66% and OS of 79% compared with historical controls. Longer follow-up is required to substantiate these promising early results.

These prospective trials are demonstrating that it is possible to achieve significant improvements in outcome for AYAs with ALL, although many challenges remain to ensure access to care, to minimize treatment toxicity, and to develop and follow specific survivorship monitoring plans. As stated previously, the successful outcome of a patient with ALL is, largely, based on the ability of both the medical team and the patient to adhere to the rigorous and lengthy regimens that currently remain the gold standard of care. The next generation of studies, linked to important biologic, psychosocial, and pharmacologic correlates, will result in further insights into optimizing the comprehensive approach to treatment and follow-up for this significant group of patients with ALL, and may be the next step to achieving the high cure rate and successful transition back to "normal" life now routinely achieved in children with ALL. In particular, due to significant pharmacogenomic variability and age-related changes in drug metabolism, further evaluation and potential dose modifications of some of the agents including glucocorticoids, vincristine, and asparaginase, crucial to the successful outcomes of children, will need to be addressed in future studies of AYA and older adults with ALL in order to optimize these regimens for these populations Enrollment in clinical trials, which has led to the survival rates now approaching more than 90% in pediatric ALL, will be the key to making progress in survival rates for both younger and older adults with ALL.

Comparison of Pediatric-Inspired Regimens With Allogeneic Transplant for Adolescents and Young Adults

Given these very encouraging improvements in outcome for AYAs with ALL using intensified pediatric regimens, the role of aSCT in CR1 has been reexamined in a recently presented retrospective comparison study. The International Bone Marrow Transplant Registry (IBMTR) examined outcomes of patients 18–50 years old who were treated during 2002–2011 on the DFCI intensive pediatric regimen described above ($n = 108$) compared with registry patients who received aSCT in CR1 using HLA matched related or unrelated donors ($n = 422$). These investigators reported significantly better outcomes for patients receiving the intensive pediatric approach compared to transplant (HR: 3.12; $p < .0001$). Overall, treatment using a pediatric-inspired regimen for young adults with ALL appears to result in significantly improved survival compared to aSCT in CR1. Similarly, data from the GRAALL pediatric-inspired protocols GRAALL 2003 and 2005 showed that there was no difference in relapse, nonrelapse mortality, or relapse-free survival (RFS) overall in patients that went onto aSCT compared to those that did not undergo transplant. However, aSCT did result in a longer RFS in patients that were MRD positive after induction chemotherapy, suggesting there is a select HR group of patients that still benefit from transplant.

OLDER ADULTS WITH ACUTE LYMPHOBLASTIC LEUKEMIA

Older adults (generally defined as >60 years old) constitute a challenging subset of ALL patients with worse prognosis reported in many studies compared with their younger counterparts. Most studies demonstrate that adults older than 60 years old have survival rates below 15%. Various factors contribute to the poor outcome of these patients, both patient related (e.g., the presence of comorbidities, less likely to be eligible for aSCT, poor tolerance of intensive chemotherapies) and disease related (more likely to have unfavorable disease characteristics such as the presence of Philadelphia chromosome). It is important to note that many large clinical trials have excluded patients older than 60 years of age; therefore clinical outcome data for this group are sparse. Annino and colleagues reviewed the results of 679 older adult patients (variably defined as older than 50 to older than 65 years of age, depending on the study) from 19 studies and reported a CR rate of 59% (range: 31% to 85%) with an early mortality rate of 23% (range: 7.5% to 50%) and 2-year OS of 15% to 19%, all of which are inferior to younger ALL patients. With hyper-CVAD regimens, the CR rate and 3-year survival for patients 60 years of age or older ($n = 58$) were 88% and 29%, respectively. In a pooled analysis of six consecutive CALGB clinical trials, the CR rate and 3-year survival for patients 60 years of age or older ($n = 197$) were 61% and 15%, respectively.

Sancho and colleagues reported results of the Spanish PETHEMA-ALL 96 trial looking specifically at the outcomes of Ph⁻ ALL patients who were 55 years of age or older. They initially treated 10 patients with an induction regimen consisting of vincristine, daunorubicin, prednisone, asparaginase, and cyclophosphamide. However, 7 of the 10 patients died during induction. Asparaginase

and cyclophosphamide were then omitted from the induction cycle, and 23 additional patients were treated with a CR rate of 70%; the induction death rate was reduced to 22%. The 2-year DFS and OS for the entire series were 46% and 39%, respectively.

Because most patients in this age group may not be eligible for conventional myeloablative aSCT, consideration should be given for RIC-based aSCT. Initial results with the use of RIC conditioning have been favorable, and long-term data are awaited (see earlier section on allogeneic stem cell transplant).

Many novel agents are being evaluated for this group of patients given the poor prognosis with the currently available therapies. To date, with the exception of TKI-based therapy for Ph⁺ ALL in older adults, none have resulted in improved outcomes. The GRAALL-SA1 randomized phase II trial compared the efficacy and toxicity of pegylated liposomal doxorubicin (Peg-Dox) versus continuous-infusion doxorubicin (CI-Dox) in patients 55 years of age and older with Ph⁻ ALL. Use of Peg-Dox led to significant lower toxicities; however, there was a trend toward a lower CR rate, more refractory disease, and higher relapse rate in the Peg-Dox arm compared with CI-Dox arm. Other newer agents approved for relapsed disease, including liposomal vincristine and the bispecific antibody blinatumomab, are being tested in frontline therapy for older adults with ALL; these trials are currently ongoing. Single-agent activity of these agents in the relapsed setting is described later in more detail in the novel therapies section. Consideration should be given to enrollment of older adults into these new frontline therapies given the lack of progress with dose intensification of traditional agents. Management of older adult patients with Ph⁺ ALL is discussed in the Ph⁺ ALL section; the incorporation of TKIs into frontline therapy has already made significant improvements in DFS for these high-risk patients.

RELAPSED ACUTE LYMPHOBLASTIC LEUKEMIA

As described earlier, with standard therapies for ALL, long-term DFS is only around 30% to 40%. Thus the majority of patients with ALL relapse despite the administration of postremission treatment. Postrelapse therapies will lead to a second CR (CR2) in 30% to 40% of patients with a 5-year OS of only around 10%. An aSCT is the only chance for long-term cure in these patients and must be considered for all patients.

In the largest report of relapsed adult ALL patients to date, Fielding and colleagues analyzed the outcomes of relapsed adult ALL patients who were treated in the MRC UKALLXII/ECOG E2993 trial. Of the 1508 evaluable patients, 1372 (91%) achieved CR1, of whom 609 (44% of the CR1 patients) relapsed at a median of 11 months. The 5-year OS was only 7% for the relapsed patients, which was significantly worse compared with 38% for the newly diagnosed ALL patients in this study. The median OS for the relapsed patients was 5.5 months. The sites of the relapses were BM alone (86%), CNS alone (4%), BM plus CNS (5%), and other extramedullary sites (4%). The majority of the relapses (81%) occurred within 2 years of diagnosis. In this series, none of the 55 patients who had CNS involvement at relapse were alive at 5 years. Receiving aSCT after relapse led to significant improved outcomes compared with chemotherapy alone (5-year OS, 23% for matched sibling SCT versus 4% for the chemotherapy-alone arm).

Tavernier and colleagues reported outcomes of 421 ALL patients who experienced first relapse after treatment on the French LALA-94 trial. A CR2 was achieved in 44% patients with a median DFS of 5.2 months and median OS of 6.3 months. Factors associated with favorable outcome after relapse included transplant performed in CR2, CR1 of longer than 1 year, and platelet count greater than 100,000/μL at relapse. The outcomes after relapse were not influenced by risk stratification at diagnosis or the treatment received during first CR. An aSCT was performed in 24% ($n = 99$) of the relapsing patients (in CR2 [$n = 61$] or with active disease at the time of SCT [$n = 38$], directly as a salvage therapy after relapse [$n = 14$], or after failure of salvage regimen [$n = 24$]). Median OS from an aSCT was 6.7 months with 5-year OS of 25% with a significantly higher OS at 3 years after aSCT in CR2 compared with those with active disease at the time of SCT.

Oriol and colleagues reported the outcomes of 263 ALL patients in first relapse treated in four consecutive PETHEMA trials. CR2 was achieved in 45% of patients, a rate similar to that in the French LALA trials. The median OS after relapse was 4.5 months, with a 5-year OS of 10%. Factors associated with a favorable outcome after relapse included age younger than 30 years and CR1 duration of longer than 2 years. The best subgroup of patients was younger than 30 years of age with CR1 longer than 2 years in which the 5-year DFS and OS were 53% and 38%, respectively.

Vincristine is an important component of ALL treatment. In preclinical models, encapsulation of vincristine into sphingomyelin liposomes or "sphingosomes" has been shown to lead to increased efficacy without increased neurotoxicity compared with conventional vincristine. Sphingosomal vincristine administered every 2 weeks in relapsed or refractory ALL reported an overall response rate of 14%. A weekly schedule resulted in a higher CR rate of 19% overall, and 29% in first salvage treatment. Based on an improved toxicity profile and comparable efficacy in relapsed/refractory (RR) ALL, particularly as a single agent, in 2012 the FDA approved vincristine sulfate liposome injection (VSLI) for the treatment of adult patients with Ph-negative ALL in second or greater relapse or whose disease has progressed following two or more antileukemia therapies. An ongoing international phase III trial is examining the benefit of liposomal vincristine as frontline therapy of older adults with ALL.

Blinatumomab is a novel bispecific T-cell–engaging antibody targeted against CD3 on T cells and CD19 on leukemia B cells. When blinatumomab concurrently binds CD3 and CD19, the T cells are activated and directed to CD19-expressing target B cells, resulting in a cytotoxic T-cell response. Among 189 patients with relapsed/refractory ALL treated with blinatumomab, 43% achieved CR or CR with incomplete recovery of counts (CRi), and 82% became MRD negative. Patients that achieved MRD negativity had higher RFS and OS, 6.9 and 11.5 months, respectively, compared to patients in CR with MRD, 2.3 and 6.7 months respectively. The FDA granted accelerated approval for the use of blinatumomab in relapsed/refractory ALL in 2014. A small trial of blinatumomab for relapsed Ph+ ALL has also been completed; however, at the present time, this agent is only approved for Ph- B-cell ALL.

Nelarabine is a prodrug that is demethylated by adenosine deaminase to the deoxyguanosine analog (ara-G). T lymphoblasts are sensitive to the cytotoxic effects of nelarabine, and this drug has been studied in T-cell ALL in the relapsed or refractory setting. DeAngelo and colleagues treated 26 patients with T-cell ALL and 13 patients with T-cell lymphoblastic lymphoma with nelarabine. The median age was 34 years (range: 16–66 years). The CR rate was 31% with a 1-year OS of 28%. Neurotoxicity was seen in many patients. Nelarabine is currently approved in the United States for both pediatric and adult patients with T-cell ALL and T-cell lymphoblastic lymphoma who have failed at least two chemotherapeutic regimens. The COG has recently completed a study evaluating the addition of nelarabine to the frontline setting for T-ALL, but longer follow-up will be needed to evaluate its impact on progression-free survival.

Despite the approval of these new agents, patients with relapsed ALL continue to be a challenging subgroup of patients, and additional novel therapies (see later discussion) may improve outcomes by improving CR2 rates and increasing the percentage of patients who could be candidates for aSCT. Importantly, these agents are now entering trials in the frontline setting with the hope that they will decrease relapse rates, obviate the need for rescue therapy, and improve OS in ALL.

NOVEL THERAPIES

Chemotherapy

Many new agents are being investigated for patients with ALL, both in the relapsed and frontline setting. Clofarabine is a purine nucleoside analog that is currently approved by the FDA for the treatment of pediatric patients with relapsed or refractory ALL who have failed two prior regimens. The response rate CR, CR with incomplete recovery of platelets (CRp), and partial response (PR) in pediatric ALL is approximately 30%. Response rates in the adult population appear to be considerably lower and may be associated with significant toxicity. Kantarjian and colleagues reported 17% response rate (CR, CRp, PR) with single-agent clofarabine in adults with relapsed or refractory ALL. Based on the modest single-agent activity, studies evaluating the role of the combination of clofarabine with cytarabine or cyclophosphamide are being conducted. The Southwest Oncology Group Study S0530 was a phase II trial of a combination of clofarabine and cytarabine for relapsed or refractory ALL patients ($n = 37$) and demonstrated a response rate of 17% (CR/CRp), which was not better than that reported as a single agent. The COG is now testing the addition of clofarabine to frontline therapy in an attempt to improve the outcomes for high-risk children and adolescents.

(Table 66.11) CD22 is a commonly expressed antigen on the precursor B-cell lymphoblast cell surface that is internalized upon ligand binding, which makes it an attractive target for monoclonal antibodies and antibody drug conjugates. Epratuzumab, a humanized monoclonal antibody against CD22, also has activity in a subset of patients with ALL. In a COG pilot study, epratuzumab in combination with standard reinduction chemotherapy was evaluated in 15 pediatric patients with relapsed ALL. There was rapid clearing of surface CD22 antigen, and 9 out of 15 patients achieved a CR. In adult patients epratuzumab has been combined with cytarabine and clofarabine in relapsed/refractory precursor B-ALL. Thirteen out of 29 patients responded and five patients had MRD assessments, of which one achieved a significant molecular remission. The rate of response with epratuzumab, clofarabine, and cytarabine appeared to be greater than historical control of clofarabine and cytarabine (SWOG S0530); however, long-term DFS and OS data are not yet available. Given its modest initial response rates, the field has moved onto the evaluation of anti-CD22 conjugates, described briefly here.

Inotuzumab ozogamicin, a CD22 monoclonal antibody attached to immunotoxin calicheamicin, has shown activity in non-Hodgkin lymphoma and is currently being evaluated in ALL patients. Inotuzumab has demonstrated response rates of up to 80% in relapsed/refractory ALL and 78% of responding patients became MRD negative. Veno-occlusive disease and transaminitis are toxicities suggesting off-target drug effects that will need to be evaluated further. Longer clinical follow-up data are expected from ongoing trials regarding DFS and OS. In particular, a randomized phase III trial comparing inotuzumab to salvage chemotherapy in patients with relapsed/refractory ALL to determine efficacy and OS will serve as a registration trial for this antibody conjugate. Frontline introduction of this agent is also being tested. Inotuzumab, in combination with low-dose chemotherapy (cyclophosphamide, vincristine, cytarabine, methotrexate, dexamethasone, rituximab) is being evaluated in newly diagnosed and relapsed older adult (>60 years of age) ALL patients. Preliminary feasibility and efficacy data from an ongoing trial at the MD Anderson Cancer Center were recently reported. In 26 treatment-naive patients, 25 achieved a CR or CRp (overall response rate: 96%) and MRD negativity with 86% progression-free survival and 81% OS at 1 year.

Moxetumomab pasudotox is another antibody–drug conjugate that consists of an anti-CD22 monoclonal antibody fused to a truncated form of *Pseudomonas* exotoxin A. In a phase I dose–escalation study, 21 pediatric patients with relapsed or refractory ALL were enrolled. The drug was well tolerated. In this heavily pretreated patient population (median number of prior therapies: four), preliminary efficacy results are encouraging with hematologic improvement in 41% and CR in 24% of the patients. Moxetumomab is currently under investigation in children and young adults with relapsed/refractory CD22+ ALL, as well as adults with relapsed/refractory ALL.

Coltuximab ravtansine (CoR) or SAR3419 is an anti-CD19 monoclonal antibody linked to the tubulin inhibitor maytansinoid

DM4, which demonstrated efficacy in vitro and in vivo in ALL, as well as safety in a lymphoma phase I study. The results of a phase II trial of CoR in relapsed/refractory adult B-ALL are awaited.

Combotox is constructed from two antibody–drug conjugates, consisting of a monoclonal anti-CD19 antibody and an anti-CD22 antibody conjugated to the toxin deglycosylated ricin A chain in equal parts. In relapsed/refractory pediatric pre-B-ALL only 18% of patients achieved a CR; however, 35% had a greater than 95% decrease in their peripheral blood blast counts. In adults Combotox reduced the leukemic disease burden in all patients, but no CRs were observed. In an ALL xenograft model Combotox acted synergistically with cytarabine, leading to a phase I trial of Combotox and cytarabine in adults with relapsed/refractory ALL.

In addition to the relapsed/refractory disease setting, antibody-based therapies are also being investigated for MRD. Blinatumomab was initially evaluated in MRD positive B-ALL after induction or molecularly relapsed disease. Eighty percent of patients achieved a molecular remission, including 57% of patients who had never previously been MRD negative. Based on these promising results, a United States Intergroup Trial, ECOG 1910, is comparing blinatumomab plus chemotherapy to chemotherapy alone in adults with newly diagnosed B-ALL. Another study in older adult patients, SWOG 1318, will investigate blinatumomab and POMP (prednisone, vincristine, methotrexate, 6-mercaptopurine) chemotherapy in newly diagnosed Ph$^-$ ALL and dasatinib, prednisone and blinatumomab for newly diagnosed Ph$^+$ ALL.

Although less prevalent than CD19 or CD22 antigen expression, 70% of all (both precursor B-cell and precursor T-cell) ALL patients express CD52. Alemtuzumab, a humanized anti-CD52 monoclonal antibody, has been evaluated in ALL as an agent for eradication of MRD during postremission therapy. Alemtuzumab decreased MRD and improved DFS compared to chemotherapy alone in adult ALL. However, alemtuzumab failed to demonstrate significant activity in relapsed/refractory pediatric ALL. Additional studies have been conducted with alemtuzumab and other agents in order to further assess their role in frontline therapy of ALL (CALGB 10102) and have demonstrated feasibility; outcome data have not yet been formally reported.

Immunotherapy

Chimeric Antigen Receptor T Cells

Potentially one of the most exciting breakthroughs in ALL therapy is the development and early results from trials evaluating chimeric antigen receptor (CAR)-T cells (Table 66.11).

CAR-T cells are genetically engineered autologous T cells that express antigen receptors that result in recognition and killing of targeted malignant cells. In ALL, the CAR-T cells contain antibody-binding domains of single-chain variable fragments linked to T-cell-stimulating moieties, most commonly CD3ζ with either CD28 or CD137 (41BB) costimulatory domains. The chimeric receptor CTL019 binds CD19 on malignant B cells and leads to tyrosine kinase-mediated activation of the T cell through the CD3ζ-chain portion and costimulatory activity of CD137 or CD28. Investigators at the University of Pennsylvania treated 25 pediatric and five adult patients with relapsed/refractory ALL with anti-CD19-CD137/CD3ζ CAR-T cells. CRs were achieved in 90% of patients. Two patients also achieved CNS remission without evidence of disease recurrence at 6 months. The probability of CAR-T cell persistence at 6 months was 68%. B-cell aplasia continued as long as CTL019 cells persisted; however, increased rates of infection were not reported. After a limited 6-month follow-up the EFS was 67% and OS 78%, suggesting promise compared to standard salvage chemotherapy. Investigators at the Memorial Sloan Kettering Cancer Center (MSKCC) treated 24 relapsed/refractory adult B-ALL patients with CD19-specific CD28/CD3ζ CAR-T cells. Prior to CAR-T cell treatment, of 22 evaluable patients, 10 were MRD positive and 12 had morphologic evidence of disease. Overall, 91% responded to CAR-T

cells, and 90% of these patients were MRD negative. Six patients remain in remission after 1 year. Three out of five patients that relapsed received repeat CAR-T cell infusion and two of these patients regained CR. Cell levels expanded and peaked at 1–2 weeks and were low or undetectable by 2–3 months.

In both studies all responding patients experienced cytokine-release syndrome (CRS). CRS timing correlated with peak T-cell expansion and severity correlated with disease burden prior to treatment and appears to be mediated by release of interleukin-6 (IL-6) and other inflammatory cytokines. MSKCC defined severe CRS (sCRS) requiring treatment for fevers for greater than or equal to 3 consecutive days and at least one clinical sign of toxicity such as hypotension requiring a vasopressor, or hypoxia, or neurologic symptoms (confusion, obtundation, and seizures). Neurologic toxicities were also common, ranging from delirium during CRS to encephalopathy independent of CRS; however, the pathophysiology of this is unclear. Recently, CAR-T investigators have successfully employed tocilizumab, an anti-IL-6 antibody to treat and reverse the symptoms associated with CRS. Several patients received T cells of donor origin after prior allogeneic stem cell transplant; interestingly, no graft-versus-host disease occurred following CAR-T cell infusions in either study.

Philadelphia Chromosome Positive Acute Lymphoblastic Leukemia

Bosutinib 500 mg daily has been found to be safe in relapsed/refractory Ph$^+$ ALL, with diarrhea being the most common toxicity. However, further investigation is required to assess efficacy. Other agents, such as the dual BCR-ABL/LYN TKI INNO-406 and the aurora kinase inhibitor MK-0457, have also been evaluated in Ph$^+$ ALL, but demonstrated limited efficacy. ABL001 is an allosteric BCR-ABL inhibitor that mimics the myristoylated N-terminus of the kinase domain by occupying its vacant binding site, thus restoring the negative regulation of the kinase activity. ABL001 is currently being investigated in a phase I study as a single agent and was also developed to be dosed with nilotinib.

Philadelphia Chromosome-Like Acute Lymphoblastic Leukemia

There has been an increasing understanding of the molecular biology of ALL, which may translate into newer therapeutic options. Mullighan and colleagues reported loss of the *IKZF1* gene on 7p12, which encodes the early lymphoid transcription factor Ikaros in 84% of BCR-ABL–positive ALL and in 28% of BCR-ABL–negative B-cell ALL. An *IKZF1* deletion was reported in 63% of 83 adult Ph$^+$ ALL patients treated in various GIMEMA trials. The presence of the deletion of the *IKZF1* gene has been associated with poor prognosis, with worse DFS and increased relapse risk. Patients with *IKZF1* alteration have a gene expression profile similar to that of Ph$^+$ ALL (Ph-like ALL described earlier), and one-third of such patients have rearrangements of the lymphoid cytokine receptor gene *CRLF2*, either alone or with mutations of the Janus kinase (JAK) genes *JAK1* and *JAK2*. This has been further identified in pediatric and young adult ALL patients. Among 1725 B-ALL cases analyzed, the prevalence of Ph-like ALL increased from 10% in children to 27% in young adults. Kinase activating mutations in *ABL1*, *ABL2*, *CRLF2*, *CSF1R*, *EPOR*, *JAK2*, and *PDGFRB* were found in 91% of Ph-like ALL cases observed. *CRLF2* mutations were present in up to 60% of young adults and 55% of patients with *CRLF2* mutations had concurrent JAK mutations, most commonly in *JAK2*. Twelve patients with *ABL*, *JAK2*, or *PDGFR* mutations were ultimately treated with dasatinib, imatinib, or ruxolitinib, and achieved rapid and sustained responses. This provides rationale to test ABL and JAK inhibitors as a targeted strategy for this group of patients.

Targeting Intracellular Signaling Pathways

The *NOTCH1* gene encodes a transmembrane receptor protein that drives stem cell commitment to T-cell differentiation. *NOTCH1*

TABLE
66.11   **Novel Immunotherapies in Relapsed/Refractory Acute Lymphoblastic Leukemia**

Trial	Cell Surface Antigen Target and Agent	Class	Disease Status	n	CR (%)	MRD Negativity[a] (%)	Survival Outcomes
	CD19						
	Blinatumomab	Bispecific T-cell–engaging antibody					
Topp M[40]			MRD+ or relapsed	21		16 (80)	RFS: 61% at 33 months
Topp M[41]			RR	189	81 (43)	60 (82)	Median RFS: 5.9 months Median OS: 6.1 months
	CAR-T cells	CAR-T cells					
Maude S[42]			Pediatric/adult RR	25/5	27 (90)	22 (81)	EFS: 67% OS: 78% at 6 months
Park J[43]			RR	24	20 (91)	18 (90)	RFS 30% at 12 months Median OS: 9 months
	CD22						
Wayne A[44]	Moxetumomab pasudotox	Antibody–drug conjugate	Pediatric RR	12	3 (25)		
	Inotuzumab ozogamicin	Antibody–drug conjugate					
Kantarjian H[45]			Pediatric/adult RR	49	28 (57)		Median DOR: 6.3 months Median OS; 7.9 months
O'Brien S[46]			RR	34	18 (53)		Median OS: 6.3 months
Advani A[47]			RR	35	23 (66)	18 (78)	Median OS: 7.4 months
	CD19 and CD22						
	Combotox	Combined antibody–drug conjugate					
Herrera L[48]			Pediatric RR ALL	17	3 (18)		
Schindler J[49]			Adult RR ALL	17	0 (0)		Xenograft models demonstrate survival benefit

[a]MRD in ALL refers to the presence of leukemic cells below the threshold of detection by conventional morphologic methods. Patients who achieved a CR by morphologic assessment alone can potentially harbor a large number of leukemic cells in the bone marrow.
Current multicolor flow cytometry or PCR methods can detect leukemic cells at a sensitivity threshold of $<1 \times 10^{-4}$ (<0.01%) bone marrow mononuclear cells.
ALL, Acute lymphoblastic leukemia; CAR-T cell, chimeric antigen receptor-T cell; CR, complete remission; DOR, duration of response; EFS, event-free survival; MRD, minimal residual disease; OS, overall survival; RFS, relapse-free survival; RR, relapsed/refractory ALL; SCT, stem cell transplantation.

activation occurs in more than 50% of patients with precursor T-cell ALL and has been used as a therapeutic target. γ-Secretase is required for *NOTCH1* proteolytic activation. The γ-secretase inhibitor, MK-052, caused high rates of gastrointestinal toxicity and failed to induce responses in relapsed/refractory T-ALL. In addition to Notch, γ-secretase affects other substrates, suggesting that the drug likely has off-target effects. Another γ-secretase inhibitor, PF-03084014, is currently under investigation in a phase I trial. The anti-NOTCH1 receptor monoclonal antibody demcizumab may avoid the toxicities of γ-secretase inhibitors and warrants investigation. In vitro data demonstrated that NOTCH1 is a key driver in the mTOR pathway and c-MYC serves an intermediary between NOTCH1 and mTOR, suggesting that mTOR inhibition alone or with NOTCH1 inhibition may also be highly relevant for T-ALL.

The PI3K/AKT/mTOR pathway is also thought to be active in Ph+ and Ph− B-ALL. As a single agent, the rapalogue sirolimus only resulted in stable disease in relapsed/refractory pediatric ALL. Temsirolimus, everolimus, and sirolimus are each under investigation in combination with chemotherapy in relapsed/refractory ALL. BEZ-235 is a dual inhibitor of PI3K and mTORC1/mTORC2, which in vitro in T- and B-ALL, including Ph+ cells, caused cell cycle arrest and apoptosis, and acted synergistically with chemotherapy. In a phase I trial of BEZ-235 in relapsed/refractory acute leukemias, one out of 10 ALL patients achieved a CR and two additional patients had improvement in blood counts. Similar to rapalogues, this agent may be more effective in combination with chemotherapy.

Epigenetic Modulation

MLL gene rearrangements at position 11q23 occur in approximately 10% of ALL, AML, or MLL, and are associated with an aggressive disease course. MLL gene mutations result in oncogenic fusion proteins that associate with disruption of telomeric silencing 1-like (DOT1L), leading to hypermethylation and activation of MLL target genes that drive leukemogenesis. The DOT1L inhibitor, EPZ5676, is currently being evaluated in a phase I trial in relapsed/refractory acute leukemias. In a preliminary report, four out of 28 patients responded to treatment.

Bone Marrow Microenvironment

AMD11070 is an orally available, small molecule inhibitor of CXC-chemokine receptor 4 and has been studied in ALL cell lines and mouse models as an agent to eradicate leukemic cells that are otherwise protected by stromal elements. Mice with murine Ph+ ALL survived significantly longer when treated with a combination of nilotinib and AMD11070. Similarly, a combination of vincristine and AMD11070 showed encouraging responses.

SURVIVORSHIP

Although fewer specific data are available on long-term complications of survivors of young adults with ALL, the long-term complications of successful treatment of children with ALL have been well described and include neurocognitive and neurologic dysfunction, endocrine and metabolic abnormalities (including obesity), bone toxicity (osteonecrosis), cardiac toxicity, and secondary malignancies. To guide the frequency and focus of medical visits and the ordering of appropriate surveillance tests, comprehensive guidelines have been published in many countries, including North America, where guidelines created by the COG, titled "Long-Term Follow-up Guidelines for Survivors of Childhood, Adolescent and Young Adult Cancers" are available at http://www.survivorshipguidelines.org and should be adopted by the adult oncology community.

FUTURE DIRECTIONS

ALL is a heterogeneous group of diseases with varied clinical outcomes, depending on molecular, cytogenetic, and clinical characterization. There have been significant advances in our understanding of the molecular pathogenesis of this disease, which should translate into effective targeted therapies and better patient outcomes. Given the rarity of this disease, it is strongly recommended that patients be referred to centers of expertise, and it is crucial that patients be enrolled in clinical trials designed to evaluate subset-specific therapies to improve survival.

SUGGESTED READINGS

EPIDEMIOLOGY, CLASSIFICATION AND PROGNOSIS

Borowitz MJ, Chan JKC: B-lymphoblastic leukaemia/lymphoma with recurrent genetic abnormalities. In Swerdlow SH, Camp E, Harris NL, et al, editors: *WHO classification of tumors of haematopoietic and lymphoid tissues*, Lyon, France, 2008, IARC, p 171.

Fielding AK, Richards SM, Chopra R, et al: Outcome of 609 adults after relapse of acute lymphoblastic leukemia (ALL); an MRC UKALL12/ECOG 2993 study. *Blood* 109:944, 2007.

Gale KB, Ford AM, Repp R, et al: Backtracking leukemia to birth: identification of clonotypic gene fusion sequences in neonatal blood spots. *Proc Natl Acad Sci USA* 94:13950, 1997.

Moorman AV, Chilton L, Wilkinson J, et al: A population-based cytogenetic study of adults with acute lymphoblastic leukemia. *Blood* 115:206, 2010.

Mullighan CG, Su X, Zhang J, et al: Deletion of IKZF1 and prognosis in acute lymphoblastic leukemia. *N Engl J Med* 360:470, 2009.

Roberts KG, Li Y, Payne-Turner D, et al: Targetable kinase-activating lesions in Ph-like acute lymphoblastic leukemia. *N Engl J Med* 371:1005, 2014.

Wetzler M, Dodge RK, Mrozek K, et al: Prospective karyotype analysis in adult acute lymphoblastic leukemia: the cancer and leukemia Group B experience. *Blood* 93:3983, 1999.

CLINICAL SIGNIFICANCE OF MRD

Bassan R, Spinelli O, Oldani E, et al: Improved risk classification for risk-specific therapy based on the molecular study of minimal residual disease (MRD) in adult acute lymphoblastic leukemia (ALL). *Blood* 113:4153, 2009.

Campana D: Minimal residual disease in acute lymphoblastic leukemia. *Hematology Am Soc Hematol Educ Program* 2010:7, 2010.

Gökbuget N, Kneba M, Raff T, et al: Adult patients with acute lymphoblastic leukemia and molecular failure display a poor prognosis and are candidates for stem cell transplantation and targeted therapies. *Blood* 120:1868, 2012.

HEMATOPOIETIC STEM CELL TRANSPLANTATION

Bachanova V, Verneris MR, DeFor T, et al: Prolonged survival in adults with acute lymphoblastic leukemia after reduced-intensity conditioning with cord blood or sibling donor transplantation. *Blood* 113:2902, 2009.

Cornelissen JJ, van der Holt B, Verhoef GE, et al: Myeloablative allogeneic versus autologous stem cell transplantation in adult patients with acute lymphoblastic leukemia in first remission: a prospective sibling donor versus no-donor comparison. *Blood* 113:1375, 2009.

Dhedin N, Dombret H, Thomas X, et al: Autologous stem cell transplantation in adults with acute lymphoblastic leukemia in first complete remission: analysis of the LALA-85, -87 and -94 trials. *Leukemia* 20:336, 2006.

Goldstone AH, Richards SM, Lazarus HM, et al: In adults with standard-risk acute lymphoblastic leukemia, the greatest benefit is achieved from a matched sibling allogeneic transplantation in first complete remission, and an autologous transplantation is less effective than conventional consolidation/maintenance chemotherapy in all patients: final results of the International ALL Trial (MRC UKALL XII/ECOG E2993). *Blood* 111:1827, 2008.

Marks DI, Wang T, Perez WS, et al: The outcome of full-intensity and reduced-intensity conditioning matched sibling or unrelated donor transplantation in adults with Philadelphia chromosome-negative acute lymphoblastic leukemia in first and second complete remission. *Blood* 116:366, 2010.

Tomblyn MB, Arora M, Baker KS, et al: Myeloablative hematopoietic cell transplantation for acute lymphoblastic leukemia: analysis of graft sources and long-term outcome. *J Clin Oncol* 27:3634, 2009.

STANDARD TREATMENT REGIMENS

Kantarjian HM, O'Brien S, Smith TL, et al: Results of treatment with hyper-CVAD, a dose-intensive regimen, in adult acute lymphocytic leukemia. *J Clin Oncol* 18:547, 2000.

Larson RA, Dodge RK, Burns CP, et al: A five-drug remission induction regimen with intensive consolidation for adults with acute lymphoblastic leukemia: cancer and leukemia group B study 8811. *Blood* 85:2025, 1995.

Lazarus HM, Richards SM, Chopra R, et al: Central nervous system involvement in adult acute lymphoblastic leukemia at diagnosis: results from the international ALL trial MRC UKALL XII/ECOG E2993. *Blood* 108:465, 2006.

Vignetti M, Fazi P, Cimino G, et al: Imatinib plus steroids induces complete remissions and prolonged survival in elderly Philadelphia chromosome-positive patients with acute lymphoblastic leukemia without additional chemotherapy: results of the Gruppo Italiano Malattie Ematologiche dell'Adulto (GIMEMA) LAL0201-B protocol. *Blood* 109:3676, 2007.

Rowe JM, Buck G, Burnett AK, et al: Induction therapy for adults with acute lymphoblastic leukemia: results of more than 1500 patients from the international ALL trial: MRC UKALL XII/ECOG E2993. *Blood* 106:3760, 2005.

Salzer WL, Asselin B, Supko JG, et al: Erwinia asparaginase achieves therapeutic activity after pegasparagase allergy: a report from the Children's Oncology Group. *Blood* 122:507, 2013.

Thomas X, Boiron JM, Huguet F, et al: Outcome of treatment in adults with acute lymphoblastic leukemia: analysis of the LALA-94 trial. *J Clin Oncol* 22:4075, 2004.

ADOLESCENT AND YOUNG ADULTS

DeAngelo DJ, Dahlberg S, Silverman LB, et al: A Multicenter Phase II Study Using a Dose Intensified Pediatric Regimen in Adults with Untreated Acute Lymphoblastic Leukemia [abstract]. *Blood* 110:Abstract 587, 2007.

Huguet F, Leguay T, Raffoux E, et al: Pediatric-inspired therapy in adults with Philadelphia chromosome-negative acute lymphoblastic leukemia: the GRAALL-2003 study. *J Clin Oncol* 27:911, 2009.

Ribera JM, Oriol A, Sanz MA, et al: Comparison of the results of the treatment of adolescents and young adults with standard-risk acute lymphoblastic leukemia with the Programa Espanol de Tratamiento en Hematologia pediatric-based protocol ALL-96. *J Clin Oncol* 26:1843, 2008.

Stock W, La M, Sanford B, et al: What determines the outcomes for adolescents and young adults with acute lymphoblastic leukemia treated on cooperative group protocols? A comparison of Children's Cancer Group and Cancer and Leukemia Group B studies. *Blood* 112:1646, 2008.

PH⁺ ALL

Cortes JE, Kim DW, Pinilla-Ibarz J, et al: A phase 2 trial of ponatinib in Philadelphia chromosome positive leukemias. *N Engl J Med* 369:1783, 2013.

Foa R, Vitale A, Vignetti M, et al: Dasatinib as first-line treatment for adult patients with Philadelphia chromosome-positive acute lymphoblastic leukemia. *Blood* 118:6521, 2011.

Ravandi F, O'Brien S, Thomas D, et al: First report of phase 2 study of dasatinib with hyper-CVAD for the frontline treatment of patients with Philadelphia chromosome-positive (Ph+) acute lymphoblastic leukemia. *Blood* 116:2070, 2010.

Thomas DA, Faderl S, Cortes J, et al: Treatment of Philadelphia chromosome-positive acute lymphocytic leukemia with hyper-CVAD and imatinib mesylate. *Blood* 103:4396, 2004.

Vignetti M, Fazi P, Cimino G, et al: Imatinib plus steroids induces complete remissions and prolonged survival in elderly Philadelphia chromosome-positive patients with acute lymphoblastic leukemia without additional chemotherapy: results of the Gruppo Italiano Malattie Ematologiche dell'Adulto (GIMEMA) LAL0201-B protocol. *Blood* 109:3676, 2007.

Wetzler M, Watson D, Stock W, et al: Autologous transplantation for Philadelphia chromosome positive acute lymphoblastic leukemia achieves outcomes similar to allogeneic stem cell transplantation: Results of CALGB Study 10001 (Alliance). *Haematologica* 99:111, 2014.

Yanada M, Takeuchi J, Sugiura I, et al: High complete remission rate and promising outcome by combination of imatinib and chemotherapy for newly diagnosed BCR-ABL-positive acute lymphoblastic leukemia: a phase II study by the Japan Adult Leukemia Study Group. *J Clin Oncol* 24:460, 2006.

BURKITT LYMPHOMA/LEUKEMIA

Dunleavy K, Pittaluga S, Shovlin M, et al: Low-intensity therapy in adults with Burkitt's lymphoma. *N Engl J Med* 369:1915, 2013.

Kenkre VP, Stock W: Burkitt lymphoma/leukemia: improving prognosis. *Clin Lymphoma Myeloma* 9:S231, 2009.

Rizzieri D, Johnson J, Byrd J, et al: improved efficacy using rituximab and brief duration, high intensity chemotherapy with filgrastim support for Burkitt or aggressive lymphomas: cancer and Leukemia Group B study 10002. *Br J Haematol* 165:102, 2014.

Thomas DA, Cortes J, O'Brien S, et al: Hyper-CVAD program in Burkitt's-type adult acute lymphoblastic leukemia. *J Clin Oncol* 17:2461, 1999.

RELAPSED DISEASE AND NOVEL THERAPIES

Collins-Underwood J, Mullighan C: Genomic profiling of high risk acute lymphoblastic leukemia. *Leukemia* 24:1676–1685, 2010.

DeAngelo DJ, Yu D, Johnson JL, et al: Nelarabine induces complete remissions in adults with relapsed or refractory T-lineage acute lymphoblastic leukemia or lymphoblastic lymphoma: Cancer and Leukemia Group B study 19801. *Blood* 109:5136, 2007.

Kantarjian H, Thomas D, Jorgensen J, et al: Inotuzumab ozogamicin, an anti-CD22-calecheamicin conjugate, for refractory and relapsed acute lymphocytic leukaemia: a phase 2 study. *Lancet Oncol* 13:403, 2012.

Maude S, Frey N, Shaw P, et al: Chimeric antigen receptor T cells for sustained remissions in leukemia. *N Engl J Med* 371:1507, 2014.

O'Brien S, Schiller G, Lister J, et al: High-dose vincristine sulfate liposome injection for advanced, relapsed, and refractory adult Philadelphia chromosome–negative acute lymphoblastic leukemia. *J Clin Oncol* 31:676, 2013.

Park J, Riviere I, Wang X, et al: CD19-targeted 19-28z CAR modified autologous T cells induce high rates of complete remission and durable responses in adult patients with relapsed, refractory B-cell ALL. *Blood* 124(21):Abstract 382, 2014.

Roberts KG, Mullighan CG: Genomics in acute lymphoblastic leukaemia: insights and treatment implications. *Nat Rev Clin Oncol* 12:344, 2015.

Topp MS, Gökbuget N, Stein AS, et al: Safety and activity of blinatumomab for adult patients with relapsed or refractory B-precursor acute lymphoblastic leukaemia: a multicentre, single-arm, phase 2 study. *Lancet Oncol* 16:57, 2014.

Weng AP, Ferrando AA, Lee W, et al: Activating mutations of NOTCH1 in human T cell acute lymphoblastic leukemia. *Science* 306:269, 2004.

REFERENCES

For the complete list of references, log on to www.expertconsult.com.

Chronic myeloid leukemia (CML) is a hematopoietic malignancy originating from transformation of a primitive hematopoietic cell. Without treatment, CML progresses from an initial chronic phase (CP), characterized by marrow hyperplasia and increased numbers of circulating differentiated myeloid cells, to more advanced phases of disease (accelerated phase [AP] and blast crisis [BC]) marked by a block in differentiation, accumulation of blasts, and depletion of normal hematopoietic cells, especially white blood cells (WBCs) and platelets. CML was the first malignant disease found to be consistently associated with a specific cytogenetic abnormality, the Philadelphia chromosome (Ph), resulting in the formation of the *BCR-ABL* fusion oncogene. Study of the *BCR-ABL* gene has not only led to sensitive methods to detect residual disease and predict outcome, but has also yielded highly effective "targeted" therapies aimed at inhibiting abnormal tyrosine kinase activity resulting from the *BCR-ABL* fusion oncogene. In addition, CML was one of the first diseases demonstrated to be curable by hematopoietic cell transplantation (HCT). Thus, CML has become the model for "tailored" therapy, in which various treatments can be escalated on the basis of molecular response.

ETIOLOGY/EPIDEMIOLOGY/GENETICS

CML was recognized as a distinct entity, associated with massive splenomegaly and leukocytosis without other explanations, in the mid-1800s. The modern history of CML was initiated by Nowell and Hungerford in 1960. They used newly developed techniques to detect a small chromosome in metaphase preparations of marrow cells from CML patients. This abnormal chromosome was the first consistent chromosomal abnormality in human malignancies and was termed the *Philadelphia chromosome* after the city of its discovery. Rowley showed that the Philadelphia chromosome resulted from a translocation between chromosomes 9 and 22 [t(9;22)(q34;q11)] (Fig. 67.1). The genes involved in this translocation were cloned in the 1980s, and the t(9;22) translocation was shown to result from the fusion of the breakpoint cluster region (*BCR*) gene on chromosome 22 to the Abelson leukemia virus (*ABL*) gene on chromosome 9, with formation of the *BCR-ABL* fusion oncogene. This oncogene codes for a constitutively active cytoplasmic tyrosine kinase, which is the principal cause of the CP of CML. Until the 1970s, CML was regarded as an incurable and inevitably lethal disorder. It was then recognized that selected patients can be cured by allogeneic HCT. However, transplantation therapy for CML is limited by donor availability and the risk for life-threatening toxicity. More recently, imatinib mesylate and other tyrosine kinase inhibitors (TKIs), which specifically block the enzymatic action of the abnormal tyrosine kinase coded by the fusion oncogene, have resulted in a high rate of remission and improved survival in CML patients.

CML is the most common of the myeloproliferative diseases and represents 15% to 20% of all new leukemia cases. The annual incidence of CML is 1 to 1.5 cases per 100,000 population per year. The median age at diagnosis is 67 years and the incidence sharply rises with age. The disease occurs slightly more often in men than in women. CML may occur in children, but only approximately 10% of cases occur in individuals between 5 and 20 years of age, representing only 3% of all childhood leukemias. Concordance of disease is not observed between identical twins. Persons exposed to high-dose irradiation, including survivors of atomic bombing, have a

significantly increased risk for leukemia. High-dose irradiation of myeloid cell lines in vitro induces the expression of *BCR-ABL* transcripts indistinguishable from those that characterize CML. The *BCR-ABL* gene can be detected at low levels in a proportion of healthy individuals using a very sensitive polymerase chain reaction (PCR) assay. These findings suggest that the fusion gene develops relatively frequently in hematopoietic cells, but only infrequently leads to leukemia development. The mechanism by which the Ph chromosome is first formed and the time required for progression to overt disease are unknown.

PATHOPHYSIOLOGY

CML is generally believed to develop from transformation of a primitive hematopoietic stem cell (HSC) by the *BCR-ABL* fusion gene. The progeny of transformed HSCs have a proliferative advantage over normal hematopoietic cells, thus allowing the Ph-positive clone to gradually displace residual normal hematopoiesis. The translocation is found in cells of myeloid, erythroid, megakaryocytic, and B-lymphoid origin, consistent with a HSC origin of the disease. Hematopoietic expansion in patients with CP disease primarily involves an increase in myeloid cell mass, related to an expansion of mature cells, as well as increased numbers of precursor and progenitor cells. In CP, the leukemic cells are minimally invasive and are primarily located in hematopoietic tissues including the blood, bone marrow, spleen, and liver. The proliferative advantage of the malignant clone may be related to enhanced responsiveness to hematopoietic growth factors and/or reduced response to inhibitory factors. CML progenitors also demonstrate altered adhesion to marrow stromal cells and extracellular matrix. Altered microenvironmental interactions may contribute to another feature of CML, which is abnormal progenitor trafficking with increased numbers of circulating progenitors and extramedullary hematopoiesis. Several observations indicate that although the Ph-positive clone displaces normal hematopoiesis, it does not destroy residual normal stem cells. For example, Ph-negative progenitors can be seen after cultures of CML cells in vitro are selected on the basis of cell surface phenotype, and can be identified in the blood after high-dose chemotherapy. As described later in the Therapy section, treatment with agents such as interferon (IFN) or TKIs can result in restoration of Ph-negative hematopoiesis in CML patients.

The *BCR-ABL* gene originates from a chromosomal translocation that results in the fusion of the *ABL* gene on chromosome 9 and the *BCR* gene on chromosome 22. The translocation is related to a break in *ABL* upstream of exon a2 and in the major breakpoint cluster region of the *BCR* gene. This leads to juxtaposition of a 5′ portion of *BCR* and a 3′ portion of *ABL* on a shortened chromosome 22 (the derivative 22q-, or Ph). The resulting messenger RNA (mRNA) usually contains one of two *BCR-ABL* junctions, designated e13a2 (formerly b2a2) and e14a2 (or b3a2). Both *BCR-ABL* mRNA molecules are translated into a 210-kD fusion protein, referred to as *p210BCR-ABL*. Rarely, other variant breakpoints and fusions can give rise to full-length, functionally oncogenic BCR-ABL proteins, notably p190BCR-ABL (associated with an e1a2 mRNA junction) and p230BCR-ABL (associated with an e19a2 mRNA junction). Of patients with CML who have a normal-appearing karyotype, one-third have a cytogenetically occult *BCR-ABL* gene, usually located on

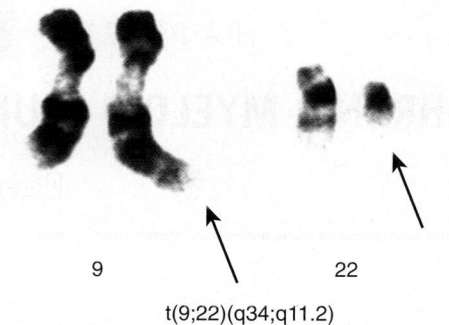

9   22

t(9;22)(q34;q11.2)

Fig. 67.1 PARTIAL KARYOTYPE SHOWING THE t(9;22)(q34;q11). The Philadelphia chromosome is the derivative chromosome 22 *(right arrow)*.

a normal-appearing chromosome 22 but occasionally on chromosome 9. In the remaining patients with Ph-negative, *BCR-ABL*-negative disease, the molecular basis of leukemia is not known.

Some studies have suggested that pathogenesis of CML may be a multistep process, with development of clonal hematopoiesis preceding the t(9;22) translocation. However, there is substantial evidence to suggest that the generation of a classic *BCR-ABL* fusion gene in a HSC is sufficient to initiate CML. Expression of *BCR-ABL* has been shown to transform mouse fibroblast cell lines, growth factor-dependent hematopoietic cell lines, and primary murine bone marrow cells. Expression of *BCR-ABL* in human CD34$^+$ cells also causes increased proliferation, reduced apoptosis, and altered adhesion and migration, mimicking alterations seen in progenitor cells from CML patients. Transplantation of murine bone marrow cells made to ectopically express the *BCR-ABL* gene by retroviral transduction induces a myeloproliferative disorder (MPD) that closely resembles human CML with increased numbers of peripheral blood cells (with a predominance of granulocytes), splenomegaly, and extramedullary hematopoiesis, although the disease is much more fulminant than human CML. Initial development of transgenic and knock-in mouse models of CML was problematic. It appears to be crucial to express this oncogene in the proper cell type. Expression of *BCR-ABL* in B-cell lymphocytic and megakaryocytic precursors resulted in the development of B-acute lymphocytic leukemia and megakaryocytic myeloproliferative syndrome. Specific expression of the oncogene in HSCs through a stem cell leukemia enhancer to regulate expression induces development of a CML-like disease.

The *ABL* gene encodes a nonreceptor tyrosine kinase that is expressed in most tissues. Mice with homozygous disruption of the *ABL* gene demonstrate increased perinatal mortality, lymphopenia, and osteoporosis, and are smaller, with abnormal head and eye development. The *BCR* gene also encodes a signaling protein that contains multiple modular domains. Although *BCR*-deficient mice develop normally, their neutrophils produce excess levels of oxygen metabolites following activation. The normally regulated tyrosine kinase activity of the ABL protein is constitutively activated by the juxtaposition of N-terminal *BCR* sequences. BCR acts by promoting protein dimerization, leading to phosphorylation of tyrosine residues in the kinase-activation loops and leading to constitutive activation of kinase activity. The fusion of *BCR* sequences to *ABL* also adds new regulatory domains/motifs to ABL, such as the growth factor receptor-bound protein 2 (GRB2) SH2-binding site. The uncontrolled kinase activity of *BCR-ABL* and enhanced interaction with a variety of effector proteins lead to deregulation of cell signaling mechanisms that regulate proliferation. The ABL protein is located in both the nucleus and the cytoplasm, and shuttles between these two compartments, whereas the BCR-ABL protein is exclusively cytoplasmic and localizes to the cytoskeleton, where it appears to contribute to adhesion and migration abnormalities.

The structure of the BCR-ABL protein and the biochemical pathways affected have been extensively studied. However, most such interactions have been studied only in cell lines and conditions of forced overexpression. Their existence in primary leukemia cells and relevance to CML pathogenesis is not certain. The murine

transduction–transplantation CML model has been helpful in studying the role of BCR-ABL domains and signaling interaction in primary hematopoietic cells in vivo. The ABL tyrosine kinase is crucial for oncogenic transformation. Mice that express a form of *BCR-ABL* with a point mutation in the ATP-binding site of ABL that inhibits its kinase activity do not develop leukemia, suggesting that the ABL kinase activity is essential for BCR-ABL leukemogenesis in vivo. The success of kinase inhibitor therapy for CML provides further proof of the importance of kinase activity in maintenance of human disease. Other important domains in BCR-ABL also regulate the kinase activity of ABL or connect to other downstream signaling pathways. The N-terminal coiled-coil oligomerization domain of BCR is an important activator of ABL kinase activity, and also promotes the association of BCR-ABL with F-actin fibers. Phosphorylation of BCR at tyrosine 177 generates a GRB2-binding site, which is important for RAS activation. Mutation of the tyrosine-177 residue of *BCR-ABL* to phenylalanine (Y177F) largely abolishes its ability to bind GRB2, without affecting the kinase activity of ABL. The Y177F mutant has a greatly reduced ability to induce MPD in mice. A tyrosine phosphorylation site in the activation loop of the ABL kinase domain and the SH2 domain of ABL also contribute to RAS activation. Mutations in the SH2 domain of ABL and a Y1294F point mutation reduce the ability of BCR-ABL to induce a CML-like MPD in mice. The C-terminal region of ABL is required for the proper function of normal ABL. However, deletion of the ABL actin-binding domain was reported to not affect the ability of BCR-ABL to induce CML-like MPD in mice, suggesting that this domain may be dispensable for BCR-ABL–mediated leukemogenesis. Certain BCR-ABL domains may have complementary or overlapping functions. Many signaling proteins become phosphorylated in BCR-ABL–expressing cells and/or interact with BCR-ABL through various functional domains. These interactions in turn activate signaling through mechanisms including RAS, phosphatidylinositol 3-kinase, AKT, JNK, and SRC family kinases, protein phosphatase, signal transducers and activators of transcription, nuclear factor-κB, and MYC. BCR-ABL also induces expression of cytokines such as interleukin-3, granulocyte colony-stimulating factor (G-CSF), and granulocyte-macrophage colony-stimulating factor.

Progression to AP and BC is associated with an increase in immature blast cells that may be located within hematopoietic tissues or may infiltrate a number of extramedullary sites, including lymph nodes, skin, soft tissue, and the CNS. A number of molecular mechanisms, rather than a single gene defect, are likely to underlie the arrest of maturation, enhanced proliferation and survival, and increased tissue invasiveness that characterize BC CML. Increased level of *BCR-ABL* expression is a common feature and appears to be a key factor in the development of features of BC, through effects on cell signaling and on transcription and translation of important regulatory genes. Additional cytogenetic and molecular changes are also frequently seen during progression. It appears that genetic instability in CML may be induced by several factors, including increased oxidative stress, reduced DNA repair, or reduced DNA damage checkpoint signaling response. Genetic changes observed in leukemic cells from blast-phase CML patients include nonrandom cytogenetic changes such as ++8, ++Ph, ++19, and I(17)q; point mutations in *TP53*, *RB*, and *CDKN2A* (p16^{INK4A}); and overexpression of *EVI1* and *MYC*. Additional chromosome translocations are also observed, such as t(3;21)(q26;q22), which generates *AML1-EVI1*. Other CML-associated fusion genes include *AML1-ETO*, resulting from the t(8;21)(q22;q22) translocation; *NUP98-HOXA9*, resulting from the t(7;11)(p15;p15) translocation; and *CBFβ-SMMHC*, which results from inv(16)(p13;q22). These observations suggest that the block in myeloid differentiation in BC may involve cooperation between *BCR-ABL* and defects in hematopoietic transcriptional regulators. Gene expression analyses suggest that the progression of CML from CP to advanced phase is associated with gene expression changes occurring early in AP before the accumulation of increased numbers of leukemia blast cells. Especially noteworthy and potentially significant in the progression program are deregulation of the WNT/β-catenin pathway, decreased expression of *JUNB* and *FOS*, and

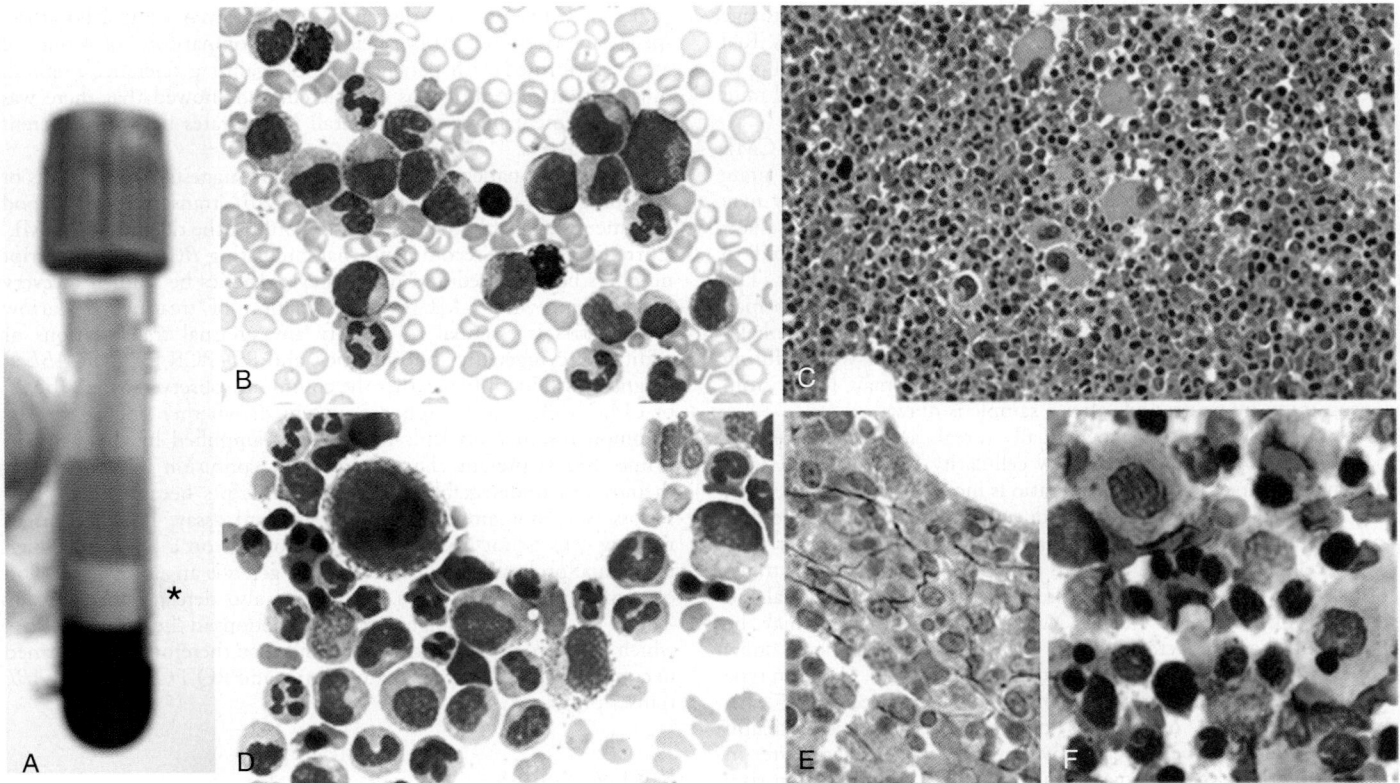

Fig. 67.2 CHRONIC MYELOID LEUKEMIA, PERIPHERAL BLOOD TUBE, AND IMAGES OF BLOOD SMEAR AND BONE MARROW BIOPSY AND ASPIRATE IN CHRONIC PHASE. (A) The spun tube of peripheral blood (ethylenediaminetetraacetic acid collected) is from a patient with chronic-phase chronic myeloid leukemia who presented with a white blood cell count of about 600 K/µL. Note the markedly expanded "buffy coat" layer *(asterisk)* due to the severe leukocytosis. (B) Peripheral smear showing marked leukocytosis due to a granulocytic proliferation of all stages with particularly increased myelocytes and absolute basophilia. (C) Bone core biopsy illustrating markedly hypercellular marrow due to granulocytic proliferation and increased small hypolobated megakaryocytes. (D) Bone marrow aspirate showing the same granulocytic proliferation and small, "dwarf" megakaryocytes. Mild fibrosis as seen on reticulin stain (E), and pseudo-Gaucher cells (F).

alternative kinase deregulation. Other studies suggest that the granulocyte/macrophage progenitor (GMP) pool is expanded in patients with blast-phase CML, and that these cells have increased levels of *BCR-ABL* expression and increased WNT signaling activity that may lead to increased self-renewal capacity, transforming GMP cells into leukemic stem cells.[1,2]

CLINICAL FEATURES

History

Most CML patients (>90%) present in CP. CML is often diagnosed incidentally during routine examination or examination for another illness. Symptoms usually include fatigue, weight loss, bone pain, sweating, and abdominal discomfort and early satiety related to splenomegaly. Symptoms are generally gradual in onset over weeks to months. Uncommon presenting symptoms include those related to leukostasis, acute abdominal pain related to splenic infarction, priapism, and hypermetabolism, hyperuricemia, and gouty arthritis.

Physical Examination

Physical examination may detect pallor and splenomegaly. In the past, the incidence of splenomegaly was often greater than 90% at diagnosis, but this has been decreasing in frequency since the disease is being diagnosed earlier.

Laboratory Manifestations

Laboratory findings at presentation generally include leukocytosis, thrombocytosis, and anemia (Fig. 67.2). The total leukocyte count is always elevated at the time of diagnosis and is usually over 25×10^9/L. The WBC count rises progressively if patients are left untreated. Striking cyclic variations in WBC counts have been described in rare patients. Differential counts reveal granulocytes at all stages of differentiation in peripheral blood cells. Circulating granulocytes are usually normal in appearance. The blast percentage is between 0.5% and 10%. Neutrophil alkaline phosphatase activity is low or absent in more than 90% of patients. However, activity can increase in response to infection, inflammation, and reduction of counts by treatment. Functional abnormalities of neutrophils are mild and are not associated with predisposition to infection. Although the proportion of eosinophils is usually not increased, the absolute eosinophil count is usually increased. The absolute basophil count is almost always increased in CML. The proportion of basophils is usually less than 15% in CP patients, although rarely this may be higher. In contrast to mastocytosis, hyperhistaminemia is uncommon. The absolute lymphocyte count is increased as a result of an increase in T but not B cells.

The platelet count is elevated in 50% of patients at the time of diagnosis. The platelet count may increase during the course of CP. Platelet dysfunction may occur, but disorders of thrombosis and hemorrhage are rare. Thrombocytopenia is rare at diagnosis and usually is a sign of progression toward AP. A deficiency in the second wave of aggregation to epinephrine is the most common abnormality and is associated with deficiency of adenine nucleotides in the storage pool. The hematocrit is decreased in most patients at diagnosis. Red cells tend to show only mild alterations with increased variability of size and shape. Small numbers of nucleated red blood cells and mild reticulocytosis may be seen.

Chemical abnormalities seen in patients with untreated CML include hyperuricemia and hyperuricosuria. The formation of urate stones is common, and patients with underlying susceptibility may develop acute gouty arthritis or urate nephropathy. Patients have increased serum levels of vitamin B_{12}-binding capacity related to release of transcobalamin I and II from mature neutrophils. The serum B_{12} level in CML is an average of 10-fold higher than normal. Serum lactate dehydrogenase is elevated in CML. Pseudohyperkalemia may be seen related to release of potassium from WBCs during clotting. Spurious hypoglycemia or hypoxemia may result from consumption by neutrophils after a sample is drawn.

Examination of the marrow usually reveals a very hypercellular marrow, with 75% to 90% marrow cellularity (see Fig. 67.2C and D). The granulocytic-to-erythroid ratio is increased to 10:1 to 30:1, with increased granulopoiesis and reduced erythropoiesis. Eosinophils and basophils may be increased. Blasts usually represent fewer than 5% of cells. The presence of more than 10% blasts indicates transformation to AP. Megakaryocytes are typically smaller than usual and may have hypolobated nuclei. Megakaryocyte numbers may be normal or slightly decreased, but 40% to 50% of patients show moderate-to-extensive proliferation of megakaryocytes. Collagen type III detected by silver staining is typically increased (see Fig. 67.2E). Approximately half of patients demonstrate increased reticulin fibrosis, which may be associated with increased megakaryocytes in marrow. Increased fibrosis may be associated with larger spleen size, anemia, and increased blasts in blood and marrow. Pseudo-Gaucher cells and sea-blue histiocytes, secondary to increased marrow cell turnover, may be seen in 30% of specimens (see H5eC69, Fig. 67.2F). The spleen shows enlargement related to infiltration of the cords of the red pulp with granulocytes at different stages of maturation. The liver may show infiltration with granulocytic cells in the portal areas and hepatic sinusoids.

Cytogenetic examination shows t(9;22)(q34;q11) and Ph chromosome in more than 90% of patients. Additional chromosomal abnormalities besides the Philadelphia chromosome are seen at diagnosis in 20% of patients including –Y and +8, and have not been shown to affect disease course. Variant Ph chromosomes are seen in 5% of patients, with complex rearrangement involving exchange of material with an additional chromosome besides chromosomes 9 and 22. In a small proportion of patients cryptic or complex translocations can be detected by fluorescence in situ hybridization (FISH) or PCR assays. The methodology used for identifying BCR-ABL transcripts has evolved over the years. Initially it was possible only to identify the presence or absence of BCR-ABL transcripts by either single-step amplification or a two-step "nested" amplification with internal primers to increase the sensitivity. Real-time quantitative PCR (RQ-PCR) provides an accurate measure of the total leukemia cell mass, and the degree to which BCR-ABL transcripts are reduced by therapy correlates with progression-free survival (PFS). A consensus meeting at the National Institutes of Health in October 2005 made suggestions for (A) harmonizing the different methodologies for measuring BCR-ABL transcripts in patients with CML undergoing treatment and using a conversion factor whereby individual laboratories can express BCR-ABL transcript levels on an internationally agreed scale; (B) using serial quantitative-PCR results rather than bone marrow cytogenetics or FISH for the BCR-ABL gene to monitor individual patients responding to treatment; and (C) detecting and reporting Ph-positive subpopulations bearing BCR-ABL kinase domain mutations. An international scale for comparison of BCR-ABL mRNA levels has been subsequently developed and implemented to facilitate common interpretation of data derived from individual laboratories and comparison of clinical studies, as well as to guide clinical decision. BCR-ABL values generated by different laboratories were aligned to the international scale such that major molecular response (MMR) was defined as BCR-ABL

values of 0.1% or less. Alignment was achieved using laboratory-specific conversion factors calculated by comparisons of results of assays performed with patient samples against a reference method. A validation procedure was completed, and showed that there was good agreement between the overall MMR rates between different validated assays.[3]

In any new patient whose blood count suggests the diagnosis of a chronic MPD, the detection of BCR-ABL transcripts in a blood specimen is probably the best way to confirm the diagnosis of CML. Current guidelines recommend that circulating BCR-ABL transcript numbers be measured and marrow cytogenetics be studied in every new patient with CML before initiation of treatment. Marrow cytogenetics is essential to identify any unusual translocations or additional cytogenetic abnormalities, and RQ-PCR for BCR-ABL at diagnosis will identify whether the commonly observed e13a2 (b2a2) or e14a2 (b3a2) transcripts are present or whether one of the less common fusion transcripts that are not amplified by the standard primer sets is present. This can prevent confusion if a patient on therapy has undetectable BCR-ABL transcripts because their transcripts were not amplified in the standard assay. If collection of marrow cells is not feasible, FISH performed on a blood specimen using dual probes for the BCR and ABL genes is an alternate method of confirming the diagnosis. FISH may also detect cytogenetically "silent" BCR-ABL rearrangements and deletions in the derivative 9q+, which have prognostic significance, and may therefore be performed in conjunction with marrow cytogenetics and RQ-PCR for BCR-ABL transcripts.

Natural History

The natural history of CML, determined more than 75 years ago, suggests a median survival from diagnosis of approximately 3 years. Without therapy, CML evolves from a CP to an AP, and eventually to BC. In approximately 25% of patients, there is no intervening AP between CP and BC (Table 67.1). Median survival times have been significantly prolonged with therapy (discussed later in the Therapy section). Following the introduction of imatinib treatment, a dramatic decrease in CML deaths was seen in age-adjusted death data from the US Surveillance Epidemiology and End Results (http://seer.cancer.gov/statistics/).[4] Long-term follow-up of CML patients who achieved complete cytogenetic response (CCR) 2 years after starting imatinib treatment showed that CML-related deaths are uncommon and survival is not statistically significantly different from that of the general population.[5]

Accelerated Phase

In general, AP is characterized by symptoms of fever, night sweats, weight loss, and bone pain, difficulty in controlling counts using conventional therapy, increased numbers of blasts and early myeloid cells in marrow and peripheral blood, and evidence of karyotypic evolution (Fig. 67.3). The World Health Organization classification defines AP of CML as one or more of the following changes: (A) 10% to 19% myeloblasts in peripheral blood or bone marrow; (B) peripheral blood basophils higher than 20%; (C) persistent thrombocytopenia, less than 100×10^9/L; (D) persistent thrombocytosis, more than 1000×10^9/L unrelated to therapy; (E) increasing WBC count and increasing spleen size unresponsive to therapy; and/or (F) evidence of clonal evolution. The most common cytogenetic changes associated with disease evolution are an additional Ph chromosome, trisomy 8, isochrome I(17q), and trisomy 19.

Blast Crisis

The blast phase of CML resembles acute leukemia. BC is defined as having more than 20% blasts in the bone marrow or peripheral blood, the presence of large aggregates and clusters of blasts in the bone marrow biopsy, or the development of extramedullary blastic infiltrates. In approximately two-thirds of patients, the blasts have a myeloid or undifferentiated-like phenotype, whereas in the remaining third the blasts appear more lymphoid-like. Immunophenotypic analysis is recommended to characterize the nature of the blasts (Fig. 67.4). Extramedullary BC most commonly affects the skin, lymph nodes, spleen, bone, or CNS, but it may occur elsewhere and may be of myeloid or lymphoid lineage.

TABLE 67.1	WHO Criteria for Accelerated and Blast Phases of Chronic Myeloid Leukemia
Accelerated phase	Diagnosis can be made if one or more of the following is present: Blasts 10% to 19% of peripheral blood white cells or bone marrow cells Peripheral blood basophils at least 20% Persistent thrombocytopenia (<100 × 10⁹/L) unrelated to therapy, or persistent thrombocytosis (>1000 × 10⁹/L) unresponsive to therapy Increasing spleen size and increasing WBC count unresponsive to therapy Cytogenetic evidence of clonal evolution (i.e., the appearance of an additional genetic abnormality that was not present in the initial specimen at the time of diagnosis of CP CML) Megakaryocytic proliferation in sizable sheets and clusters, associated with marked reticulin or collagen fibrosis, and/or severe granulocytic dysplasia, should be considered as suggestive of AP CML. (These findings have not yet been analyzed in large clinical studies; thus, it is not clear whether they are independent criteria for AP. They often occur simultaneously with one or more of the other features listed.)
Blast crisis	Diagnosis can be made if one or more of following is present: Blasts 20% or more of peripheral WBCs or bone marrow cells Extramedullary blast proliferation Large foci or clusters of blasts in bone marrow biopsy

AP, Accelerated phase; CML, chronic myeloid leukemia; CP, chronic phase; WBC, white blood cell.

PROGNOSIS

A number of prognostic scoring systems have been developed with the goal of predicting the length of CP in individual patients. The best-known and most widely used index was developed by Sokal and colleagues. An algorithm was identified using spleen size, percentage of circulating blasts, platelet count, and age as prognostic factors for CP patients. However, the Sokal scale was based on therapies available at that time (busulfan [BU], splenectomy), and newer systems for patients treated with IFN subsequently resulted in newer prognostic scoring systems. These scales, however, may have limited predictive value in the age of TKIs.

Approximately 20% of patients with CML have deletions of chromosomal material of varying size on the derivative 9q+. These deletions presumably occur at the same time as the formation of the Ph chromosome, and are thus not considered to be additional clonal changes as would be suggestive of AP disease. Patients with der 9q+ have a worse prognosis if they receive IFN therapy; it is unclear whether or not such deletions have a poor prognosis in patients receiving imatinib therapy.

Population-based studies investigating CML mortality in the imatinib era are now becoming available. They show that the pattern of mortality in CML patients related to high Sokal scores has become similar to those of intermediate scores induced by the use of imatinib in CP-CML patients.[4]

THERAPY

Definitions of Response to Treatment

Hematologic, cytogenetic, and molecular responses to treatment in CML have been defined (Table 67.2). A complete hematologic response (CHR) is defined as the achievement of normal WBC and platelet counts and normal differential, along with the disappearance of all symptoms and signs of CML. A partial hematologic response is defined as a decrease in the WBC count to less than 50% of the pretreatment level or the normalization of the WBC count accompanied by persistent splenomegaly or immature cells in the peripheral blood. A CCR is defined as the absence of Ph⁺ metaphases in marrow cells, along with partial cytogenetic response as 1% to 34% Ph⁺ metaphases. Major cytogenetic remission (MCR) combines the percentages of complete and partial response. There is now increasing reliance on BCR-ABL mRNA levels for assessment of response. According to the international scale for comparison of BCR-ABL mRNA levels, a MMR is defined as a value of 0.1% or less.[3] Lack of detection of BCR-ABL mRNA is referred to as a complete molecular response (CMR). Since the ability to detect BCR-ABL mRNA depends on the sensitivity of the PCR assay, there is now consensus

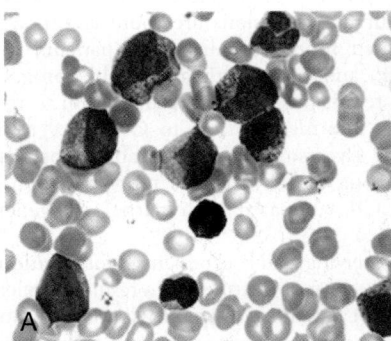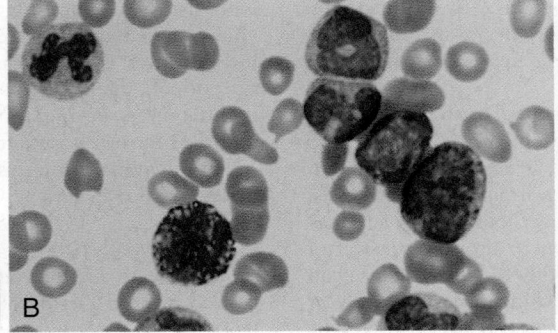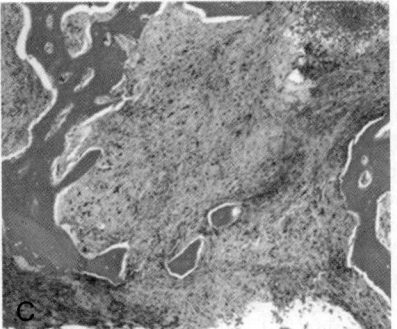

Fig. 67.3 CHRONIC MYELOID LEUKEMIA, ACCELERATED PHASE. (A) Peripheral smear showing increased immaturity in a case in which blasts were more than 10% of circulating leukocytes. (B) Peripheral smear illustrating increased basophils in a case in which basophils were more than 20% of circulating leukocytes. (C) Bone core biopsy showing increased fibrosis and small dysplastic megakaryocyte. These findings are suggestive of accelerated phase.

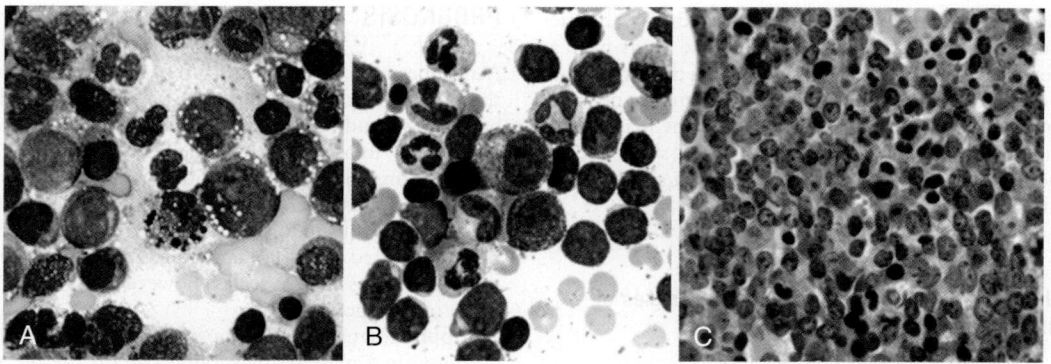

Fig. 67.4 CHRONIC MYELOID LEUKEMIA, BLAST PHASE. (A) Bone marrow aspirate showing myeloid blast phase associated with t(9;22) and inv(16). Note abnormal eosinophil *(center)*. (B) Bone marrow aspirate showing lymphoid blast phase in the background of residual chronic myeloid leukemia. (C) Bone core biopsy illustrating focal blast phase.

TABLE 67.2	Response Definition and Monitoring		
Hematologic Response	**Cytogenetic Response**	**Molecular Response**	
Complete: platelet count <450 × 10⁹/L; WBC count <10 × 10⁹/L; differential without immature granulocytes and with less than 5% basophils; nonpalpable spleen	Complete: Ph⁺ 0 Major: Ph⁺ 1–35% Minor: Ph⁺ 36–65% Minimal: Ph⁺ 66–95% None: Ph⁺ <95%	Complete: *BCR-ABL* transcripts nonquantifiable and nondetectableᵃ Major: ≤0.10%	

BCR-ABL to control gene ratio according to the proposed international scale for measuring molecular response, with a standardized "baseline", as established in the IRIS trial, taken to represent 100% on the international scale, and a 3-log reduction from the standardized baseline (major molecular response) fixed at 0.10%.
ᵃQualified by the limit of sensitivity of the polymerase chain reaction assay employed. ABL, Abelson leukemia virus; BCR, breakpoint cluster region; Ph⁺, Philadelphia chromosome positive; WBC, white blood cell.

that CMR be defined based on assay sensitivity (e.g., CMR⁴·⁰, where *BCR-ABL* mRNA levels are 0.01% or 4.0-log reduced).

Chemotherapy

BU chemotherapy for CML was introduced in the 1950s. BU was administered in doses of 4–6 mg/day and then held when the WBC count fell to 30 × 10⁹/L. The drug effect could persist for weeks, and the counts could fall further after therapy was discontinued. BU therapy was associated with serious adverse effects, including prolonged aplasia, pulmonary fibrosis, and a syndrome simulating adrenal insufficiency.

Treatment with hydroxyurea (HU) was started as an alternative to BU. HU therapy is usually initiated at doses of 1–6 g/day in an attempt to lower counts. HU administered at doses of 1–2 g/day is then used to maintain blood counts in the normal range. HU is less toxic than BU. Its major adverse effect is reversible marrow suppression. In randomized trials, HU was shown to prolong survival of patients with CP CML when compared with BU therapy. Median survival of HU-treated patients was 5 years compared with 3.75-year median survival of BU-treated patients. Because neither drug results in significant selective suppression of the Ph⁺ clone, the aim of therapy with these agents is to control disease and symptoms. HU is now commonly used to achieve control of counts simultaneous with, or prior to, initiation of treatment with imatinib or other disease-specific therapies.

Several other chemotherapeutic agents can be used to reduce the white cell counts in CML. Low-dose cytosine arabinoside can be used either as an intermittent bolus or as a daily infusion to control disease in cases where neither HU nor BU is proving useful. Cytosine arabinoside has also been used in combination with other agents, including IFN and imatinib in an attempt to enhance response.

Hyperuricemia and hyperuricosuria are frequently encountered problems in newly diagnosed and relapsed CML patients. Allopurinol given at a dose of 300 mg daily and adequate hydration should be started before initiating treatment. Allopurinol should be discontinued after the WBC count has been controlled.

Interferon

Pioneering observational studies initiated in the 1980s by investigators at the MD Anderson Cancer Center provided evidence for efficacy of IFN in CML and indicated a 70% to 80% probability of complete hematologic remission in selected CML patients. Initial research involved the use of human leukocyte IFN, but subsequent clinical studies used recombinant human IFN-α (rIFN-α). Recombinant IFN-γ (rIFN-γ) has been shown to be relatively ineffective for CML. The potential mechanisms by which IFN works in CML are not understood but may include inhibition of increased proliferation, correction of the adhesion defect of the malignant progenitor in CML, or stimulating an immune response to CML. Rates for complete and partial cytogenetic remissions range from 0% to 38%. Evidence exists for a dose–response relationship, with IFN doses of 4–5 million units/m²/day more likely to achieve remission (and toxicity) than lower doses. The pegylated form of IFN, designed to have a longer half-life in the blood, may be associated with increased efficacy. Durable remissions are more common in young patients, those treated soon after diagnosis, patients with less advanced stage disease, and those with a favorable prognostic outlook. Hematologic remissions usually occur within 1 to 3 months after starting IFN. The median time to CCR is 9 to 18 months but may occur after 4 years of therapy. Durable cytogenetic responses, some lasting as long as 10 years, are more common in patients who achieve a CCR compared with partial cytogenetic remission.

Virtually all patients receiving IFN experience constitutional adverse effects, and discontinuation of treatment as a result of toxicity is necessary for 4% to 18% of patients compared with 1% of those receiving HU. Acute adverse effects are generally mild to moderate and include influenza-like symptoms such as fever, chills, and malaise. A constellation of other more severe acute reactions and chronic complications can occur. Overall, the mechanisms underlying the toxic effects are not well understood, but adverse effects are usually dose and duration dependent.

Randomized studies show an improvement in survival rates in patients receiving IFN compared with patients receiving BU or HU. An Italian multicenter study randomly assigned 218 patients to receive IFN and 104 patients to receive HU or BU (the control group). Cytogenetic remissions were significantly more common in the IFN group. After a median follow-up of 68 months, the observed 6-year survival rate was 50% for IFN-treated patients and 29% for controls, with median survivals of 72 and 52 months, respectively. The time for progression from CP to accelerated or blast phase was lengthened from 45 months to more than 72 months. In a German multicenter study, 622 patients were randomized to receive IFN, BU, or HU. The 5-year survival rate in the IFN group (59%) exceeded that of the BU group (32%) but was not significantly higher than that of the HU group (44%). Much of the discrepancy between the Italian and German findings can be explained by differences in case mix and treatment regimens. Two other randomized trials also showed benefit for IFN treatment compared with chemotherapy. The UK Medical Research Council randomly assigned 293 patients to receive IFN and 294 patients to receive HU or BU. The 5-year survival rate was 52% for the IFN group and 34% for the control group. A Japanese randomized control trial compared IFN (80 patients) with BU (79 patients). Hematologic and cytogenetic remission rates did not differ significantly. After a median follow-up of 50 months, the predicted 5-year survival rate was 54% for patients receiving IFN and 32% for those receiving BU.

The added value of combining IFN with cytosine arabinoside was shown in a French multicenter trial, wherein 360 patients were randomly assigned to receive IFN combined with cytosine arabinoside (20 mg/m^2/day for 10 days) and 361 patients to receive only IFN. After 3 years, the survival rate was 86% with IFN and cytosine arabinoside and 79% with IFN alone. The rate of hematologic response was higher in the IFN–cytosine arabinoside group than in the IFN group. Major cytogenetic responses were observed 12 months after randomization in 41% of patients treated with IFN-cytosine arabinoside and in 24% of patients treated with IFN only.

Thus, accumulated evidence from randomized trials suggests that IFN improves survival in CP patients with favorable features compared with BU and HU. Metaanalysis suggests that the pooled 5-year survival rate is 57% (50–59%) for IFN and 42% (29–44%) for chemotherapy, which results from a delay in the onset of BC. The controlled trials suggest that IFN increases life expectancy by a median of approximately 20 months compared with BU and HU. There is no direct evidence that IFN has a greater impact on survival than does HU for patients who are in the later stages of CP (e.g., more than 1 year after diagnosis) or for those who are more ill (e.g., more than 10% to 30% blasts in peripheral blood). Adding cytosine arabinoside to IFN appears to add further survival benefit but also increases toxicity. Although IFN clearly is beneficial in patients with CML patients, benefit is limited by low levels of cytogenetic response and considerable toxicity. As discussed later, the use of IFN in the modern treatment of CML patients has been replaced by use of imatinib and other TKIs.

Tyrosine Kinase Inhibitor Treatment

Because the tyrosine kinase activity of BCR-ABL plays a critical role in cellular transformation, it is an attractive target for inhibition. The introduction of TKIs into clinical practice has dramatically changed CML treatment. TKI therapy, now the mainstay of treatment, is remarkably effective for CP CML, inducing remissions in most patients and leading to excellent survival. TKI resistance can occur, especially in AP and BC CML, usually as a result of tyrosine kinase domain point mutations. Resistance to imatinib can often be treated by "second-generation" TKIs dasatinib or nilotinib, and there is evidence that these drugs may be even more effective than imatinib for front-line treatment of CML. Molecular endpoints that correlate with long-term outcomes have been developed and have been incorporated into guidelines to monitor response to TKIs treatment.

Imatinib Mesylate

Imatinib mesylate is a small, 2-phenylaminopyrimidine molecule that inhibits the kinase activity of all proteins that contain ABL, ABL-related gene (ARG) protein, or platelet-derived growth factor receptor, as well as the KIT receptor, at micromole concentrations.[6] Imatinib is a competitive inhibitor that acts at the ATP-binding site in the kinase domain to inhibit the normal binding of ATP and blocks the ability of BCR-ABL to phosphorylate tyrosine residues on its substrates (Fig. 67.5).

Initial phase I and phase II trials established that imatinib was well tolerated and induced hematologic as well as cytogenetic response in the majority of patients with CP CML in whom other treatments had failed.[7] In a phase II study, 532 CP patients who were refractory to or intolerant of IFN-α were treated with imatinib at a dose of 400 mg daily. A CHR was achieved in 95% of patients, MCR in 60% of patients, and CCR in 41% of patients. With a median follow-up of 18 months, the estimated PFS was 89%. Only 2% of patients discontinued therapy because of adverse events.

Subsequently the International Randomized Interferon and STI571 (IRIS) study compared imatinib at 400 mg daily with IFN-α plus cytosine arabinoside in 1106 newly diagnosed patients in first CP. This study was closed with the conclusion that imatinib is the initial nontransplant treatment of choice for patients with newly diagnosed CP CML. This conclusion was based primarily on a higher rate of disease progression in the patient group receiving IFN plus cytosine arabinoside. In the initial report from this study, after a median follow-up of 19 months, the estimated rate of an MCR at 18 months was 87.1% (95% confidence interval [CI]: 84.1–90.0) in the imatinib group and 34.7% (95% CI: 29.3–40.0) in the IFN plus cytosine arabinoside group (p < .001).[8] The estimated rates of CCR were 76.2% (95% CI: 72.5–79.9) and 14.5% (95% CI: 10.5 18.5), respectively (p < .001). At 18 months, the estimated rate of freedom from progression to AP or BC CML was 96.7% in the imatinib group and 91.5% in the IFN group (p < .001). Imatinib was better tolerated than combination therapy. In a subsequent 60-month follow-up report for this study, the estimated cumulative incidence rate of CHR, MCR, and CCR for patients on first-line imatinib was 98%, 92%, and 87% at 60 months (Fig. 67.6). Only 7% of patients progressed to advanced phase, and the estimated overall survival (OS) was 89%. Crossover between arms was permitted for treatment failure, and 382 (69%) of 553 patients originally allocated to the IFN/cytarabine arm crossed over to the imatinib arm at a median of 60 months from start of treatment. The main reason for crossover from IFN to imatinib was intolerance of treatment, but reasons also included disease progression and failure to achieve hematologic or cytogenetic response. During the 6th year of study treatment, there were no further reports of disease progression and the toxicity profile remained unchanged. Of all patients randomized to receive imatinib and still on study treatment, 63% showed CCR at last assessment. The estimated event-free survival (EFS) at 6 years was 83%, and the estimated OS was 88%.[9]

A dose of 400 mg of imatinib daily is currently the standard dose for initiating therapy in newly diagnosed CP patients. Nonrandomized studies suggested that patients receiving initial therapy with 800 mg imatinib daily will achieve CCR more rapidly than patients receiving standard 400-mg daily doses. The Tyrosine Kinase Inhibitor Optimization and Selectivity study compared imatinib 800 mg/day (n = 319) to 400 mg/day (n = 157). Higher dose imatinib provided faster response CCR rates at 6 months (57% vs. 45%, respectively), but there was no significant difference between the arms at 12 months (70% vs. 66%, respectively) or 24 months (76% in both groups). Similarly, no difference in EFS, PFS, or OS was seen. However, a subset of patients who can tolerate higher doses of imatinib, without interruptions for side effects, can have a better response.[10]

Cumulative response estimates do not take into account patients who have left the study for a variety of reasons. It is also clear that the results of imatinib therapy in the community setting are less favorable. Thus, only 55% of patients treated with first-line imatinib

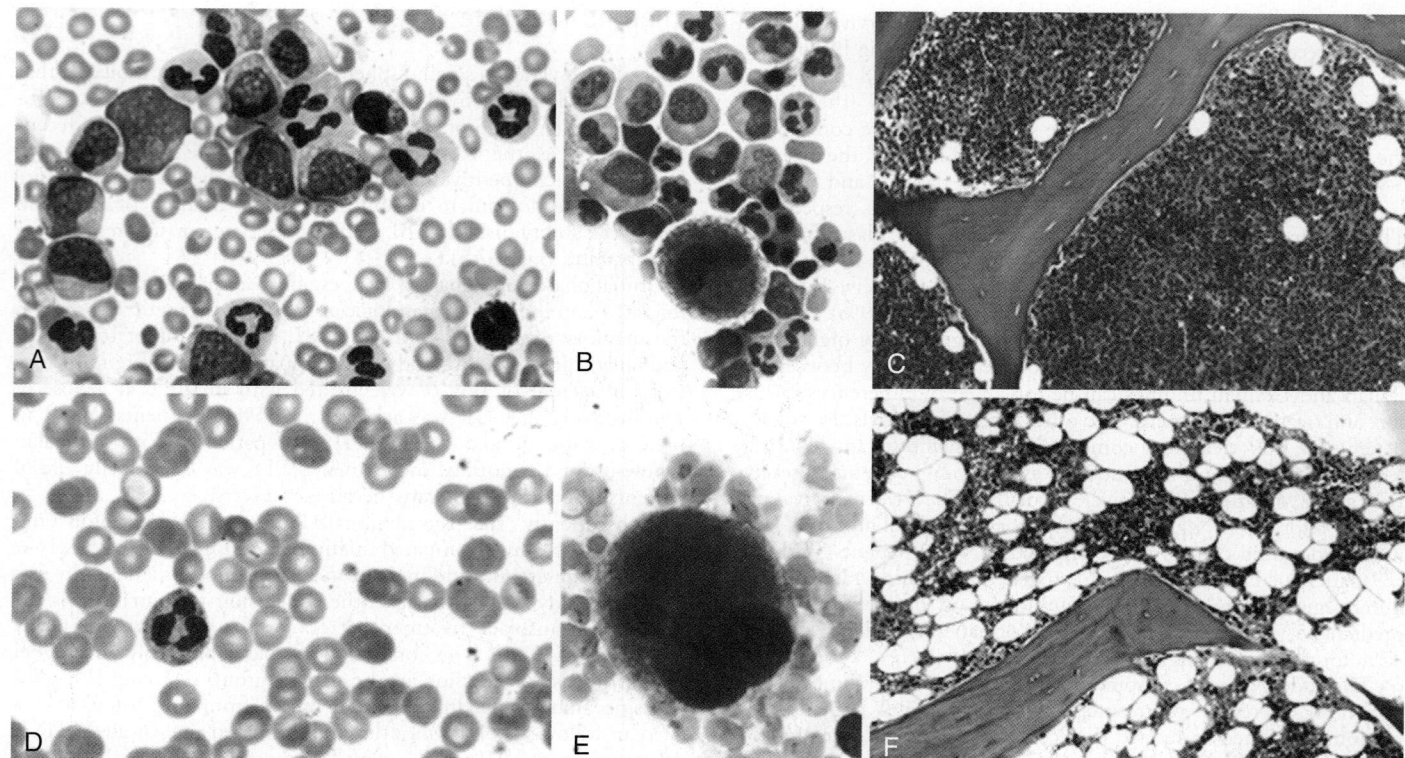

Fig. 67.5 CHRONIC MYELOID LEUKEMIA, BEFORE AND 3 MONTHS AFTER IMATINIB THERAPY. Chronic-phase chronic myeloid leukemia, as seen in the peripheral blood (A), aspirate (B), and biopsy (C), and after 3 months of imatinib therapy (D–F). Note normalization of white cell count (D), megakaryocyte size (E), and marrow cellularity (F).

in the IRIS study were still receiving imatinib at follow-up of 8 years, while the remainder had discontinued therapy as a result of inadequate therapeutic effect or toxicity. A report from the Hammersmith Hospital, which defined imatinib failure more broadly than the IRIS study as discontinuation of drug for any reason, including toxicity as well as a lack of major cytogenetic response, calculated 5 years EFS at only 63%.[11]

Comparison of health-related quality of life (QOL) of imatinib-treated patients and the general population indicated marked impairments of QOL in younger patients, especially between 18 and 39 years of age, related to physical and emotional problems. Women had worse QOL than men. The most frequently reported symptom was fatigue. Patients older than 60 years had a QOL similar to that of the general population.[12]

Prognostic Indicators

Pretreatment risk factors can predict the likelihood of achieving and maintaining response to imatinib. At 60 months, the estimated risk for disease progression was significantly higher for patients with a higher pretreatment Sokal score (estimated rates for high-risk, intermediate-risk, and low-risk groups of 17%, 8%, and 3%, respectively; $p < .002$).

The achievement of certain milestones of response can also predict prognosis. For example, patients who do not experience a CHR response by 3 months of treatment, any cytogenetic response by 6 months, or a major cytogenetic response by 12 months do poorly in comparison with patients achieving these milestones. Reduction of BCR-ABL levels observed with cytogenetic and quantitative PCR monitoring is also predictive of prognosis (Fig. 67.7). A landmark analysis indicated that at 60 months, 97% of the patients (95% CI: 94–99) who had achieved CCR at 12 months after the initiation of imatinib treatment ($n = 350$) had not progressed to AP or BC

(see Fig. 67.7). For patients who did not have a MCR within 12 months ($n = 73$), the estimate was 81% (95% CI: 70–92; $p < .001$). Of interest, the Sokal score was not predictive of risk for disease progression in patients who had a CCR (95%, 95%, and 99% in the high-risk, intermediate-risk, and low-risk groups, respectively; $p = .20$). The prognostic significance of molecular responses at 6, 12, and 18 months in predicting EFS and time to progression to AP/BC at 7 years was evaluated in the IRIS cohort. Patients with BCR-ABL mRNA levels >10% at 6 months and >1% at 12 months using the international scale had inferior EFS and higher rates of progression compared with all other molecular response groups. Conversely, patients who achieved MMR (BCR-ABL [IS] <0.1%) by 18 months enjoyed durable responses, with no progression, 95% EFS, and only 3% probability of loss of complete cytogenetic remission (CCyR) at 7 years.[13] In an analysis from the Hammersmith group, patients with BCR-ABL mRNA levels >9.84% at 3 months had significantly lower 8-year probabilities of OS (56.9% vs. 93.3%; $p < .001$), PFS, cumulative incidence of CCyR, and CMR than those with higher levels. Similarly, BCR-ABL mRNA levels >1.67% at 6 months and >0.53% at 12 months also identified patients at increased risk for progression.[14] These results indicate a strong association between the degree of reduction of BCR-ABL transcript numbers and long-term clinical outcome, and have led to the adoption of time-dependent molecular response measurements in determining optimal response to therapy. The European Leukemia Net criteria consider an optimal response for survival, as well as deeper responses allowing treatment-free remission, to include BCR-ABL transcript levels <10% at 3 months, <1% at 6 months, <0.1% at 1 year, and <0.01% subsequently. Molecular monitoring should include mutational analysis in case of failure. Recent retrospective analyses have shown that the dynamics of the early molecular response may be a more important prognostic indicator than the molecular response at 3 months, but requires monthly monitoring following initiation of treatment.

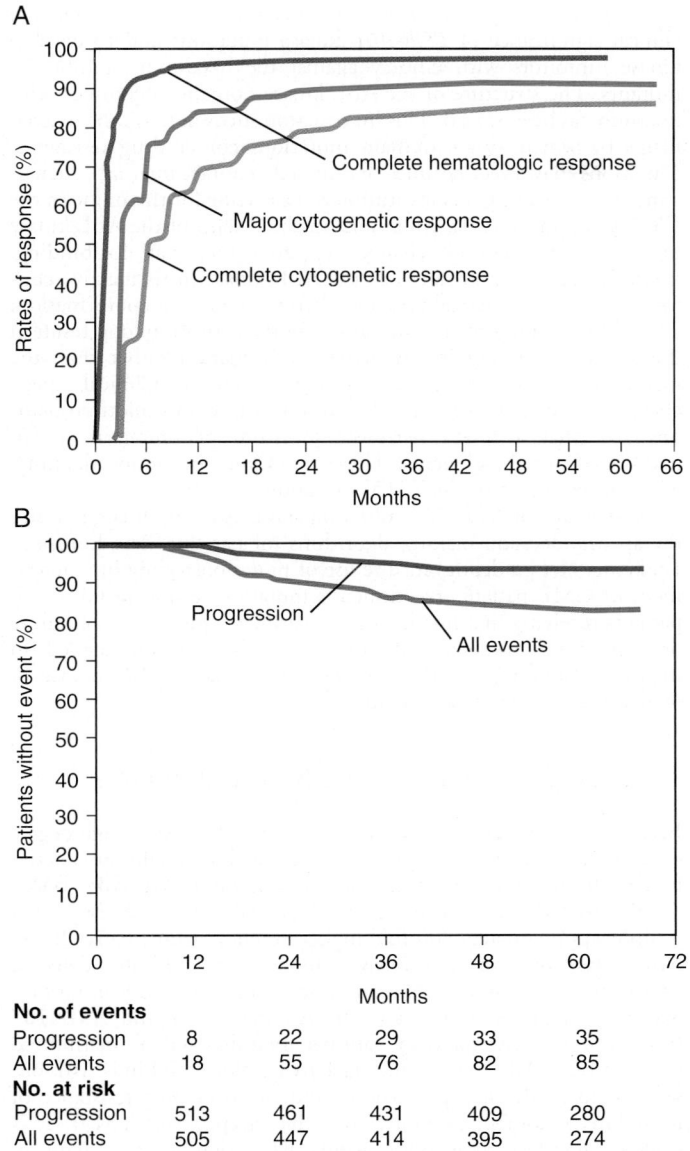

No. of events

Progression	8	22	29	33	35
All events	18	55	76	82	85

No. at risk

Progression	513	461	431	409	280
All events	505	447	414	395	274

Fig. 67.6 RESPONSE OF NEWLY DIAGNOSED CHRONIC MYELOID LEUKEMIA PATIENTS TO IMATINIB MESYLATE BASED ON 5 YEARS' FOLLOW-UP ON THE INTERNATIONAL RANDOMIZED INTERFERON AND STI571 (IRIS) STUDY. (A) Kaplan–Meier estimates of the cumulative best response to initial imatinib therapy. (B) Kaplan–Meier estimates of the rates of event-free survival and progression to the accelerated phase or blast crisis of chronic myeloid leukemia for patients receiving imatinib. *(Data from Druker BJ, Guilhot F, O'Brien SG, et al: Five-year follow-up of patients receiving imatinib for chronic myeloid leukemia. N Engl J Med 355:2408, 2006.)*

Lack of adherence to medication is a major underlying reason for failure of treatment. It has been reported, on multivariate analysis, that in CML patients treated with imatinib for some years, the adherence rate and failure to achieve a MMR were the only independent predictors for loss of CCR and discontinuation of imatinib, and poor adherence may be the predominant reason for inability to obtain adequate molecular responses.[15,16]

Results of Treatment in Accelerated Phase and Blast Crisis

A phase II study in AP patients enrolled 235 patients. Some hematologic response was seen in 82% of patients, with 34% of patients

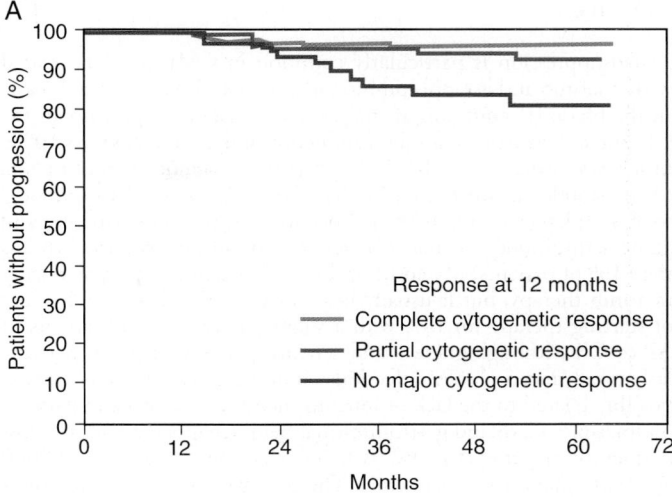

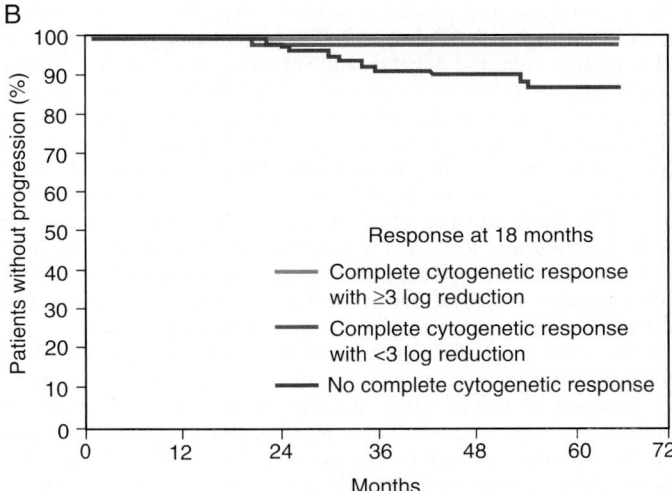

Fig. 67.7 EVENT-FREE SURVIVAL OF NEWLY DIAGNOSED CHRONIC MYELOID LEUKEMIA PATIENTS TREATED WITH IMATINIB MESYLATE AFTER 7 YEARS' FOLLOW-UP ON THE INTERNATIONAL RANDOMIZED INTERFERON AND STI571 (IRIS) STUDY BASED ON MOLECULAR RESPONSE AT 6- (A), 12- (B), AND 18-MONTH (C) LANDMARKS. *(Data from Hughes TP, Hochhaus A, Branford S, et al: Long-term prognostic significance of early molecular response to imatinib in newly diagnosed chronic myeloid leukemia: An analysis from the International Randomized Study of Interferon and STI571 (IRIS). Blood 116:3758, 2010.)*

achieving a CHR. A major cytogenetic response occurred in 24% of patients, with 17% complete responses (CRs). Estimated 12-month PFS and OS rates were 59% and 74%, respectively.

A phase II study of 260 patients in myeloid BC who were treated with imatinib showed an overall response rate of 52%, with sustained hematologic responses lasting at least 4 weeks in 31% of patients. Eight percent of patients achieved a complete remission with peripheral blood recovery. Another 4% of patients cleared their marrows to less than 5% blasts but did not meet the criteria for CR because of persistent cytopenias. Eighteen percent of patients either "returned" to CP or had partial responses. Major cytogenetic responses were seen in 16% of patients, with 7% having CCRs. The median survival was 7 months. These results compare favorably with historical controls treated with chemotherapy for myeloid BC in which the median survival is approximately 3 months. In patients with Ph-positive ALL, 29 out of 48 (60%) responded to a single agent, imatinib. However, the duration of response was relatively short, with a median estimated time to disease progression of only 2 months.

Toxicity

Myelosuppression is particularly common in CML patients treated with imatinib and is more common in patients with advanced disease. In the phase III randomized trial of newly diagnosed patients in the CP, grade 3 neutropenia (absolute neutrophil count [ANC] <1000/mm^3) was experienced by 11% of patients, grade 4 neutropenia (ANC <500/mm^3) occurred in 2% of patients, grade 3 thrombocytopenia (platelets <50,000/mm^3) occurred in 6.9% of patients, and grade 4 thrombocytopenia (platelets <10,000/mm^3) occurred in less than 1% of patients. Myelosuppression can occur at any time during imatinib therapy, but it usually begins within the first 2 to 4 weeks of starting therapy for BC, with a slightly later onset in patients in AP or CP. Although grade 3 and 4 neutropenia is frequent, particularly in advanced phases, infectious complications are relatively rare, possibly related to the lack of mucous membrane damage in patients on imatinib. CNS and gastrointestinal hemorrhages may occur, most frequently in patients in BC with platelet counts less than 20,000 and with uncontrolled leukemia. The primary goal in treating otherwise healthy patients in CP is to avoid the risk for potentially dangerous neutropenia and platelet transfusion dependence. For patients with BC or high-risk AP disease (>15% blasts), a suggested approach is to balance risks and benefits, and support patients with a platelet count under 10,000/mm^3 or under 50,000/mm^3 with clinically evident bleeding with platelet transfusions. In the event of clinically significant bleeding, imatinib should be held immediately until the bleeding is controlled. In patients whose ANC is less than 500/mm^3, imatinib should be continued if the marrow is hypercellular or if there are >30% blasts. In cases where the marrow is hypocellular and the ANC is <500/mm^3 for 2 to 4 weeks, imatinib may be held, the dose may be reduced, or myeloid growth factors can be used. Concurrent administration of growth factors and imatinib is well tolerated, and patients have not experienced a greater rate of relapse.[17]

The most common nonhematologic adverse events related to imatinib were nausea, muscle cramps, fluid retention, diarrhea, musculoskeletal pain, fatigue, and skin rashes. Only a minority of patients experienced grade 3 or 4 toxicity, and there was a low rate of discontinuance of therapy because of toxicity of 5%, 3%, and 2% in the phase II studies for BC, AP, and CP, respectively. The higher rate of severe toxicity in patients with advanced-phase disease may relate to the higher doses administered or to the poorer underlying health of patients. Most adverse effects can be managed successfully with supportive measures. Some toxicities (e.g., mild skin rashes, mild elevations of transaminases, bone pain, and arthralgias) may improve spontaneously despite continued therapy at the same dosage.

Imatinib Resistance

Both de novo and acquired resistance have been observed in imatinib-treated CML patients. The most commonly described mechanisms associated with resistance are point mutations in the *BCR-ABL* gene that prevent imatinib from inhibiting kinase activity and *BCR-ABL* gene amplification. *BCR-ABL*-independent mechanisms may also play a role in imatinib resistance in some patients. Activation of the SRC family kinase, LYN, has been demonstrated in cells from patients with acquired imatinib resistance. The Sawyers group, in an original study of nine patients who relapsed on imatinib treatment, detected *BCR-ABL* gene amplification in three patients and kinase domain mutations in six. Relapse was associated with reactivation of BCR-ABL kinase activity. Subsequent studies have shown that there are >90 different amino acid substitutions detected in imatinib-resistant patients (see Fig. 67.1), occurring with varying frequency.[18] The different mutations conferred varying degrees of imatinib resistance. In patients with stable CP disease, detection of mutations correlated with subsequent disease progression. Mutations have been found in some patients before the start of treatment, supporting a model in which preexisting *BCR-ABL* mutations that confer imatinib resistance acquire a selective clonal growth advantage during imatinib treatment.

Intensive efforts have been made to characterize the biologic and clinical significance of *BCR-ABL* kinase mutations and to develop kinase inhibitors with efficacy against the maximum number of mutants. The structure of the ABL kinase domain in complex with imatinib has been solved. This information sheds light on the mechanisms by which kinase domain mutations confer drug resistance. Mutations may affect residues that directly contact imatinib, such as a mutation resulting in substitution of isoleucine for threonine in the T315 position (T315I). Mutations in the P-loop of the ABL kinase prevent conformational changes required for imatinib binding. Imatinib captures and stabilizes the ABL kinase in its inactive conformation, but is sterically excluded from the active conformation. The M351T mutation and mutations in the activation loop result in the kinase remaining in the active conformation rather than the inactive conformation required for imatinib binding. Clinical experience with the second-generation TKIs dasatinib and nilotinib demonstrates that a much narrower spectrum of mutations retain insensitivity to these agents. These mutations are nonoverlapping, with the exception of the T315I mutation.

Knowledge of *BCR-ABL* mutation status is being integrated into therapeutic decision-making algorithms for patients. The European Leukemia Net guidelines for the use of mutation testing in management of CML patients recommends mutation testing in CP CML patients receiving first-line imatinib treatment only in case of failure or suboptimal response. Mutation analysis is recommended in imatinib-resistant patients receiving an alternative TKI in case of hematologic or cytogenetic failure.[18]

Second-Generation Tyrosine Kinase Inhibitors

Because the active conformations of ABL and SRC bear a high degree of structural similarity, compounds with SRC kinase inhibitory activity have been evaluated against native and mutant BCR-ABL. BMS-354825 (dasatinib, Sprycel) is a dual SRC-ABL kinase inhibitor that exhibits approximately 300-fold higher potency against native BCR-ABL. Dasatinib can effectively inhibit most clinically detected BCR-ABL kinase domain mutants at low nanomolar concentrations, with the notable exception of T315I. Another compound, AMN107 (nilotinib) was generated by rational modification of imatinib to enhance BCR-ABL kinase binding activity. Nilotinib binds ABL but with significantly increased avidity and can overcome resistance of most kinase domain mutants, with the exception of T315I. It is evident, however, that both agents have significant activity in imatinib-resistant CML. Of note, responses occurred in patients with and without BCR-ABL kinase domain mutations at trial entry, with the exception of patients with the T315I mutation. Responses in CP and, to a lesser extent, in AP have been stable. In contrast, many patients with myeloid and all patients with lymphoid BC or Ph-positive ALL have relapsed. These data are similar to the results of the initial studies with imatinib and indicate that once the disease has progressed beyond the CP, TKI-based monotherapy is not sufficient to induce lasting responses. Both dasatinib and nilotinib are approved for the treatment of patients with CML that is resistant to imatinib and those who are intolerant to the drug. Both agents are quite effective in resistant disease, yielding CCR in approximately 50% of CP cases (for cases who discontinue imatinib because of drug intolerance, the CCR rates are >70%).

Because of this strong clinical activity, both drugs have been tried as first-line therapy in newly diagnosed CP CML. Two single-center trials of dasatinib and nilotinib have been performed at the MD Anderson Cancer Center. At 18 to 24 months, both agents showed a similarly small but consistent benefit in CCR over historical controls treated on imatinib trials. An Italian phase II study of nilotinib in newly diagnosed CP cases showed a similarly high rate of CCR of >90% after 12 months of therapy. Dasatinib and nilotinib were compared with imatinib for front-line treatment of CP CML. The Dasatinib Versus Imatinib Study in Treatment-Naïve CML (DASISION) study tested 100 mg dasatinib daily versus 400 mg imatinib daily.[19] The Evaluating Nilotinib Efficacy and Safety in Clinical Trials

Newly Diagnosed Patients (ENESTnd) study compared two nilotinib doses (400 mg twice daily and 300 mg twice daily) with imatinib 400 mg daily.[20] Both studies found the experimental arms (dasatinib and nilotinib) to be superior to imatinib in achieving the primary endpoints (dasatinib: CCR by 12 months; nilotinib: MMR at 12 months). Patients treated with nilotinib had a significantly reduced risk for progression. Based on these results, both nilotinib and dasatinib were approved for front-line therapy of newly diagnosed CP CML patients in the United States (US) in 2010.

Bosutinib, another dual Src/Abl kinase inhibitor, has also shown potent activity against CML and was approved for the treatment of CP, AP, and BC CML by the US Food and Drug Administration (FDA) in 2012. Bosutinib overcomes the majority of imatinib-resistant BCR-ABL mutations except the T315I and V299L mutations. Bosutinib shows activity against certain mutations conferring resistance to dasatinib (e.g., F317L) and nilotinib (e.g., F359V). The recommended dose is 500 mg orally, taken once daily with food. The toxicity profile of Bosutinib differs from other approved TKIs in CML, possibly due to the minimal activity against platelet-derived growth factor receptor and KIT. The most common nonhematological adverse events are gastrointestinal, including diarrhea, nausea, vomiting and abdominal pain, predominantly occurring within the first 4 weeks of treatment and generally resolving spontaneously, and ALT elevations. Bosutinib provides an important additional treatment of CML patients previously treated with one or more TKIs, for whom imatinib, nilotinib, and dasatinib are not appropriate options.

The choice of TKI in newly diagnosed patients remains open to debate. Dasatinib and nilotinib are associated with faster and deeper reduction in leukemia burden. On the other hand, no differences in OS have been observed yet, although follow-up is required and long-term data from randomized clinical studies are needed to confirm the initial findings. Imatinib is less expensive, and there is longer experience with its use. A direct comparison between nilotinib and dasatinib has not been performed. Since their overall efficacy appears to be similar, the selection may be based primarily on side effect profile and convenience. Dasatinib treatment is associated with higher rates of myelosuppression and hemorrhage, and with pericardial and pleural effusion. In contrast, nilotinib can induce an increase in pancreatic enzymes, although radiographic/clinical pancreatitis is rarely noted. Hyperglycemia and hyperbilirubinemia are observed in some nilotinib-treated patients. More recent data suggest a risk for severe peripheral arterial occlusive disease and other cardiovascular events, including cerebral ischemia and myocardial infarction, in patients receiving nilotinib. Skin rash is also a prominent side effect of nilotinib therapy, but this is usually moderate and/or resolves spontaneously. Severe, uncontrolled diabetes and past pancreatitis may be considered as risk factors for nilotinib use, whereas patients with a history of hypertension, asthma, pneumonia, gastrointestinal bleeding, chronic obstructive pulmonary disease, congestive heart failure, vascular disease, autoimmune disorders, or concomitant aspirin use may be at increased risk for pleural and pericardial effusions, bleeding, and infection with dasatinib. For the choice of the second- or third-line TKI, mutational analyses, the occurrence of adverse events related to treatment, and coexisting patient pathologies are important considerations.

Drugs Targeting the T315I Mutation

The fact that the T315I mutant is not responsive to either dasatinib or nilotinib and that this mutant has been detected in some patients with acquired resistance to dasatinib and nilotinib underscores the need for drugs with T315I inhibitory activity.[21] Ponatinib is a multitargeted kinase inhibitor active against all BCR-ABL mutants, including T315I. In a phase I study, more than 50% of patients in CP, mostly patients in whom two or more TKIs had failed, attained CCR.[21] The CCR rate was 92% in patients with the T315I mutation. Responses were less frequent and stable in patients with advanced disease. This was confirmed in a phase II study where 51% of patients resistant to or intolerant of second-generation TKIs and 70% of

patients with the T315I BCR-ABL mutation experienced a major cytogenetic response. However, 1 year after its accelerated approval by the US FDA, a high number of vascular occlusive events, both arterial and venous thromboembolic events, began to be reported, leading to the US FDA placing a partial clinical hold on the drug. The hold was lifted following dose-reduction recommendations, but use is currently restricted to patients with the T315I mutation or for whom no alternative TKI is available.

Omacetaxine mepesuccinate is a semisynthetic formulation of homoharringtonine, an alkaloid extracted from various Cephalotaxus species.[22] It has a distinct mechanism of action related to inhibition of protein synthesis—interfering with initial protein elongation—leading to decreased levels of proteins important for leukemia cell survival, including BCR-ABL MYC and MCL1. Omacetaxine is approved for the treatment of adult patients with CP or AP CML with resistance or intolerance to two or more TKIs. Of 111 CP or AP CML patients who received two or more prior TKIs, major cytogenetic response was achieved in 18% of patients with CP, with median response duration of 12.5 months and major hematologic response in 14% of patients with AP, with a median response duration of 4.7 months. Omacetaxine is supplied as a single-use vial for parenteral administration. Common adverse reactions included thrombocytopenia, anemia, neutropenia, diarrhea, nausea, fatigue, asthenia, injection site reaction, pyrexia, and infection.

Residual Disease in Patients Treated With Tyrosine Kinase Inhibitors

Currently, reverse-transcriptase PCR (RT-PCR) is the most sensitive method for detecting low numbers of BCR-ABL transcripts in a patient after apparently successful HCT. Most patients who have been treated with imatinib and have responded well continue to demonstrate evidence of residual disease using sensitive PCR assays. Recent updates of clinical trials of imatinib in CP CML patients indicate that an increasing proportion of patients appear to enter molecular remission over time, including some patients achieving a PCR-undetectable status. However, even patients with negative PCR (so-called CMR) may still have significant numbers of residual malignant cells. Several groups have identified BCR-ABL–expressing leukemia stem cells in patients with sustained undetectable molecular residual remission. Patients with undetectable minimal residual disease (MRD) after imatinib therapy continued to have BCR-ABL rearrangement detectable at the genomic level, indicating persistence of residual leukemic cells not detected by RT-PCR. It is important to note that residual leukemic cells with leukemia-initiating capacity have been shown to persist in CML patients in sustained molecular remission on imatinib.[23] Together, these data suggest that imatinib alone may not be capable of eradicating the leukemic cell clone, and at present, patients are recommended to continue medication indefinitely, outside of investigational studies as described later.

Discontinuation of Tyrosine Kinase Inhibitor Treatment

Discontinuation of imatinib has emerged as an investigational approach for patients with CP CML with undetectable MRD. A pilot study of imatinib discontinuation in patients in CMR for 2 years indicated that half of the patients experienced molecular relapse within 6 months of treatment discontinuation, but that the remaining patients did not develop molecular relapses with an extended follow-up of 4 years. These results were confirmed in the multicenter STIM study, in which 40 out of 69 patients (61%) lost CMR within the first 6 months, and the probability of persistent CMR at 12 months was 41%.[24] Comparable results were reported in the Australian TWISTER study, which used very similar entry criteria. At 24 months, the actuarial estimate of stable treatment-free remission was 47.1%. Most relapses occurred within 6 months of stopping imatinib, and no relapses beyond 27 months were seen. The multicenter

According to STIM (A-STIM) study evaluated whether the loss of MMR, defined as <0.1% BCR-ABL (IS), was a safe and clinically relevant measure for defining molecular relapse after imatinib discontinuation. Eighty patients with CP-CML in prolonged CMR were studied. Cumulative MMR loss was 36% at 24 months, whereas probability of losing CMR was higher. Fluctuation of *BCR-ABL* transcript levels below the MMR threshold was observed in 31% of patients. Treatment-free remission was estimated as 61% at 36 months. These results suggest that loss of MMR is a practical and safe criterion for restarting therapy after treatment discontinuation in CML patients with prolonged CMR.

Management of Pregnancy in CML Patients

Imatinib therapy has been associated with a constellation of rare congenital malformations and spontaneous abortions. All couples should be counselled on the risks associated with pregnancy whilst receiving TKI therapy. At the time of diagnosis, fertility preservation should be discussed with both male and female patients of childbearing potential. Patients should be counselled regarding fertility options such as semen cryopreservation, oocyte retrieval and storage, and embryo cryopreservation because of potential deleterious effects of TKIs on gonadal function and fertility. Pregnancy in CML presents specific management challenges, and requires a multidisciplinary approach with close collaboration with the obstetricians. Management of patients who become pregnant whilst receiving TKI therapy requires balancing risks to the fetus of continuing therapy versus risks to the patient from treatment interruption and loss of disease control. Patients presenting with CP CML during pregnancy could safely continue their pregnancy to term and be successfully managed with leukapheresis during the first and subsequent trimesters, and introduction of IFN in the second trimester onwards if needed. Patients presenting in advanced phase disease should consider elective termination of pregnancy in order to commence induction chemotherapy and/or a TKI.[25]

Allogeneic Hematopoietic Cell Transplantation

Allogeneic HCT is a well-established treatment for CML, associated with the possibility of long-term disease-free survival, but has largely been replaced as an initial curative strategy as a result of the success of TKI treatment of CML.

The Seattle team reported initial results of HLA-matched sibling donor hematopoietic cell transplants performed as therapy for 10 CML patients in 1982, and subsequently published a larger study on 167 patients transplanted from matched siblings through 1983. Long-term follow-up demonstrates that approximately 40% of patients transplanted in CP nearly 20 years ago are surviving. HCT became the first curative treatment in CML. Data from 4267 recipients of matched sibling transplants reported to the Center for International Blood and Marrow Transplant Research (CIBMTR) between 1994 and 1999 show a probability of survival of 69% ± 2% for 2876 patients transplanted within the first year from diagnosis, and 57% ± 3% for 1391 patients transplanted more than 1 year from diagnosis. Contemporary results from selected single institutions continue to demonstrate excellent outcomes with HCT, in part because of advances in preparative regimens, supportive care, and HLA typing for unrelated donors (Fig. 67.8). For example, the Seattle group, using a preparative regimen of targeted BU plus cyclophosphamide (CY) in 131 consecutive CP CML patients, reported survival at 3 years posttransplant of 86%, with 87% of surviving patients molecularly negative for *BCR-ABL*.

The outcome of allogeneic HCT in CML is influenced by many factors, including the phase of disease, type of donor used (related or unrelated), the source of the stem cell product (marrow or peripheral blood), and the age of the patient. Outcomes are superior for HCT in CP compared with advanced phases of disease. In a Seattle analysis of 58 patients with AP CML who received transplants from

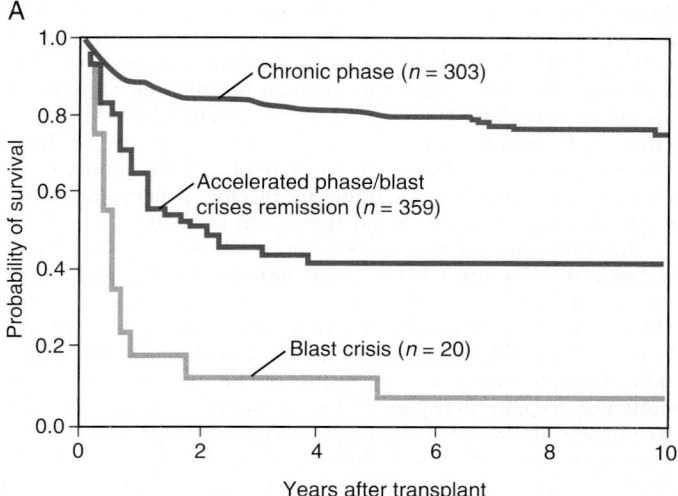

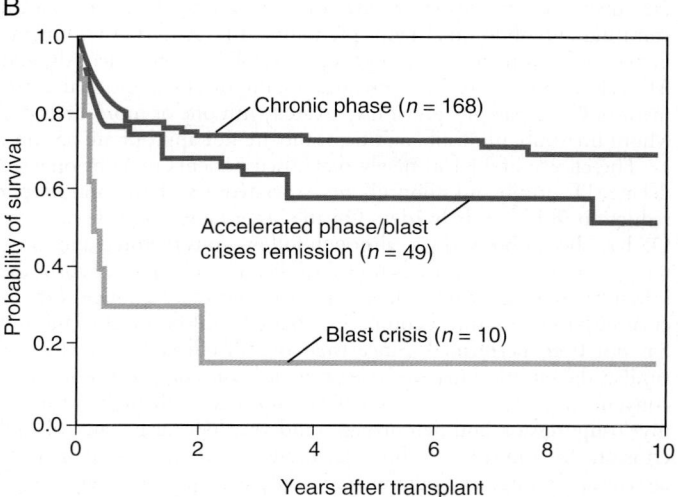

Fig. 67.8 Probability of survival following (A) related donor transplantation and (B) unrelated donor transplantation for chronic myeloid leukemia, chronic phase, accelerated phase, and blast crisis performed after 1992, at the Fred Hutchinson Cancer Research Center, Seattle.

HLA-identical siblings, the 4-year probabilities of survival and EFS were 49% and 43%, respectively, and the probability of relapse was 12%. The outcome of transplantation for patients in BC is poor, with a high rate of disease recurrence and transplant-related deaths with EFSs of 43%, 18%, and 11% at 100 days, 1 year, and 3 years, respectively. Before the development of imatinib, only a small proportion of patients with blast-phase CML (generally, patients with lymphoid BC) could achieve a hematologic remission with chemotherapy. Response rates of patients with CML in blast phase to imatinib are considerably higher than those seen with conventional chemotherapy. These responses tend to be short, particularly in the setting of lymphoid BC. The German CML Study Group reported 3-year respective OS rates in selected high-risk CP, imatinib-failure CP, and AP/BP patients after allogeneic HCT of 88%, 94%, and 59%, supporting its use as a second-line treatment following TKI failure.

Preparative regimens have improved incrementally. The majority of patients treated in the early 1980s received a preparative regimen of 120 mg/kg CY, followed by total-body irradiation (TBI). Tutschka and colleagues later described the use of 16 mg/kg BU administered over 4 days combined with 60 mg/kg CY on each of 2 successive days, in myeloid malignancies. In 1988 a randomized trial of BU/CY versus CY/12 Gy TBI in myeloid malignancies showed no differences between the CY/TBI and BU/CY treatment groups in survival at 3 years (80%), relapse (13%), or EFS (68% for CY/TBI and 71% for BU/CY). Updated results showed OS of 78% at 10 years with BU/CY versus 64% with CY/TBI. The absorption and metabolism of BU varies considerably from patient to patient, and BU assays were incorporated into transplant trials. Patients with a steady-state BU concentration less than the median value (<917 ng/mL) of the cohort had a significantly higher risk for disease recurrence and worse OS than those with levels greater than 917 ng/mL. A subsequent report of 131 consecutive CML CP patients who received transplants from HLA-identical relatives showed a 3-year survival of 86%, a relapse rate of only 8%, and a nonrelapse mortality rate of 14%. Surprisingly, there were no significant differences in outcome related to patient age up to 65 years of age.

Only approximately one-third of patients have HLA-matched family members to serve as donors. Although early results with matched unrelated donor transplantation in CML showed results somewhat poorer than those seen with matched siblings, advances in donor selection, graft-versus-host disease (GVHD) prophylaxis, and supportive care have resulted in continued improvements in outcome. Thus, in many institutions results following unrelated transplants are almost equivalent to those seen with matched siblings (with a caveat that unrelated donor transplants have a lower age patient exclusion), and registry data of multiple centers report 65% survival at 5 years among younger patients transplanted within a year of diagnosis.

Marrow was used as the stem cell source in all initial transplant studies. Two large randomized trials involving a variety of hematologic malignancies have shown that use of filgrastim (G-CSF)-mobilized peripheral blood hematopoietic cells leads to more rapid myeloid and platelet recovery when compared with marrow, with no significant difference in acute or chronic GVHD and an OS advantage. Although there was a trend toward improved survival in CML patients with the use of peripheral blood, it should be noted that these studies were not prospectively designed to address the role of peripheral blood versus marrow for individual disease states. Furthermore, the results of a randomized study of CP CML showed no statistically significant differences in outcome between the marrow and peripheral blood groups, although relapse rates were lower in the peripheral blood group and chronic GVHD occurrence was higher compared with patients transplanted with marrow.

Several studies have shown that an increased interval from diagnosis to transplant is associated with a worse transplant outcome for patients treated in CP. No single cause of failure is markedly increased with delay; rather there is a modest effect of delay on relapse rate and nonrelapse mortality. A CIBMTR report suggested that exposure to low-dose BU led to a worse outcome with subsequent transplantation. Reports have suggested that exposure to IFN might worsen the outcome of unrelated donor transplant, but data on the effect of IFN on matched sibling transplantation were less clear. In a recent German report, the 5-year survival rate from transplant was 46% for the 50 patients who received IFN within the last 90 days before transplant and 71% for the 36 patients who did not. These observations suggest that IFN should be avoided, if possible, in the months immediately preceding allogeneic HCT.

The form of GVHD prophylaxis used in treatment regimens also influences the outcome of transplantation for CML, especially in CP. Although successful in reducing the incidence of GVHD, T-cell depletion in CML was associated with high rates of graft failure and relapse, leading to poorer disease-free and OS. These findings illustrated the critical role of the graft-versus-leukemia (GVL) effect in eradicating CML following allogeneic transplantation. Because of these observations, T-cell depletion was largely abandoned as a method to control GVHD in CML transplants. However, there has been renewed interest in the possibility of preventing GVHD without loss of a GVL effect by combining T-cell depletion with an intensified conditioning regimen and delayed reinfusion of viable donor lymphocytes.

Several studies have investigated the effect of prior imatinib and transplant outcomes. Early reports warned of an increase in regimen-related toxicity and mortality, especially from hepatic causes. Larger studies have failed to show a deleterious effect of pretransplant imatinib (Fig. 67.9). A study of only CML patients showed no difference in regimen-related mortality, survival, or relapse between 140 patients who received imatinib versus 200 historical controls. Curiously, in a few studies, the incidence of chronic GVHD has been significantly lower in patients receiving imatinib before transplant. However, an analysis from the CIBMTR of CML patients undergoing allogeneic transplantation showed that the cumulative incidence rates of acute and chronic GVHD and treatment-related mortality were not affected by pre-HCT IM exposure. On multivariate analysis conventional prognostic indicators remained the strongest determinants of transplant outcomes.[26] The biology underlying this effect is unknown. Allogeneic transplantation appears to be an effective treatment for T315I-mutated leukemias, providing acceptable survival rates with long-term control of the malignancy without detectable residual disease in some cases.[27]

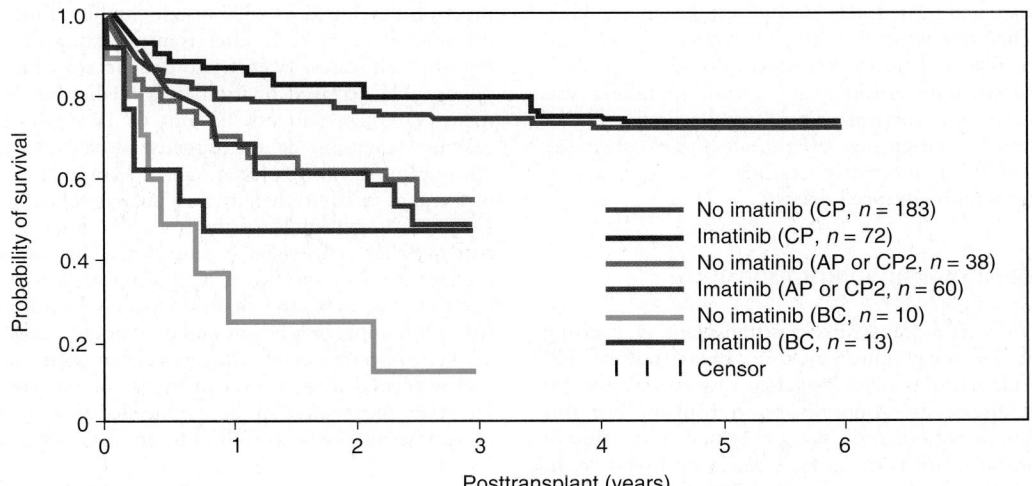

Fig. 67.9 EFFECT OF PRIOR TREATMENT WITH IMATINIB ON OVERALL SURVIVAL AFTER TRANSPLANTATION. *AP*, Accelerated phase; *BC*, blast crisis; *CP*, chronic phase; *CP2*, a return to chronic phase after treatment for accelerated phase or blast crisis disease. (*Data from Oehler VG, Gooley T, Snyder DS, et al: The effects of imatinib mesylate treatment before allogeneic transplantation for chronic myeloid leukemia.* Blood *109:1782, 2007.*)

Graft Versus Leukemia Effect in Chronic Myeloid Leukemia

Although evidence for a GVL effect can be found in many settings, nowhere is it as strong as in the setting of allogeneic HCT therapy for CML. Evidence in support of such an effect includes the following: the higher rates of relapse following syngeneic and T-cell–depleted transplants compared with unmodified allogeneic transplants; the close association between the development of acute and chronic GVHD and freedom from relapse following non-T-cell–depleted transplants; and the high response rate to donor lymphocyte infusions (DLIs) to treat posttransplant relapse (range: 50–100%), which is higher than in any other malignancy. The markedly increased relapse rates seen with T-cell depletion indicate a role for T cells in GVL. T-cell targets might include minor histocompatibility antigens shared by most cells in the body, thus accounting for the association of GVL with GVHD. Alternatively, there may be polymorphic minor histocompatibility antigens, with expression limited to hematopoietic tissue. A third possible category of targets for the GVL effect in CML is the overexpression of protein targets in CML cells. Understanding the cells and their targets responsible for the potent GVL effect seen in CML will be critical to the development of more effective, less toxic transplant-based therapies in the future.

Reduced-Intensity Conditioning

Reduced-intensity conditioning (RIC) or nonablative transplant approaches have been introduced with the aim of avoiding the toxicities of high-dose preparative regimens while retaining GVL effects. These approaches are of particular relevance for patients with CML because their median age at diagnosis is 67 years. Using a preparative regimen consisting only of 200-cGy TBI, and GVHD prophylaxis using cyclosporine and mycophenolate mofetil, McSweeney and colleagues reported CMRs in five out of nine patients transplanted for CML in CP ($n = 6$) or AP ($n = 3$). The other four patients rejected their grafts. By adding 30 mg/m^2 fludarabine pretransplant, graft rejection has been eliminated as a problem following matched sibling transplantation. Or and colleagues recently reported similar encouraging results using a preparative regimen of fludarabine, low-dose BU, and antithymocyte globulin. The MD Anderson Cancer Center group reported outcomes of 64 CML patients with advanced-phase disease (80% beyond first CP), not eligible for myeloablative preparative regimens because of older age or comorbid conditions, who received transplants with fludarabine-based reduced intensity conditioning regimens (matched related, $n = 30$; one antigen-mismatched related, $n = 4$; matched unrelated, $n = 30$).[28] At 5 years, the OS and PFS were 33% and 20%, and treatment-related mortality was 48%. In multivariate analysis, only disease stage at time of HSCT was significantly predictive for survival. These results indicate that reduced-intensity transplantation may offer a safe and effective way to treat CML in the CP, but alternative treatment strategies need to be explored in patients with advanced disease.

Residual Disease Posttransplantation

The detection of BCR-ABL transcripts posttransplant is a strong predictor of relapse following transplantation. In a study of 346 patients after transplantation, 40% of patients were positive for BCR-ABL residual disease at 3 months posttransplant, but this finding was not predictive of outcome, suggesting that eradication of the CML clone posttransplant takes an extended period of time. In contrast, at 6 or 12 months posttransplant, 27% of patients were BCR-ABL positive and at this time the assay was a powerful predictor of outcome, as only 3% of PCR-negative patients eventually relapsed compared with 42% of PCR-positive patients. The predictive power of PCR detection of BCR-ABL among longer term survivors is somewhat weaker. At 18 months posttransplant, 1% of 289

BCR-ABL-negative patients subsequently relapsed compared with 14% of 90 BCR-ABL-positive patients. The advent of reliable quantitative PCR testing further refined risk prediction of BCR-ABL detection. Olavarria and colleagues studied 138 transplant patients at 3 to 5 months posttransplant and were able to define patients as having a low risk for relapse (16%), an intermediate risk (43%), or a high risk (86%) based on BCR-ABL quantification. Further studies have confirmed the importance of quantitative BCR-ABL monitoring of minimal residual disease after transplantation for CML, which offers an obvious opportunity for early intervention for patients with residual or recurring disease.

Treatment of Posttransplant Relapse

The pace of disease progression after posttransplant relapse is variable; some patients remain low-level PCR positive for BCR-ABL for years without relapsing, and some relapse with low levels of Ph$^+$ metaphases and remain stable for many years. An appreciation of the likely tempo of progression is thus important when considering treatment intervention options.

An increasing number of potential interventions are available for relapsing disease. IFN can produce both clinical and cytogenetic remissions in patients who have relapsed after transplantation. Results with IFN appear better if treatment is initiated at the time of cytogenetic relapse instead of waiting until hematologic relapse. A large number of studies now demonstrate cytogenetic CR rates of 50% to 100% in patients treated with DLI for clinically relapsed CP CML. Response rates tend to be higher for patients treated earlier at the time of cytogenetic relapse and lower for patients in AP. The two major complications of DLI are transient marrow failure and the development of GVHD. Marrow failure only occurs in patients treated in hematologic relapse. Treatment earlier in the course of relapse can avoid this complication. The overall incidence of GVHD following DLI is approximately 50% in most series. It has since been reported that large numbers of T cells are tolerated with less GVHD if administered in a fractionated fashion rather than as a single bulk dose. A recent report from the European Group for Blood and Marrow Transplantation provides further support for starting at lower doses of lymphocytes and escalating dosage as required.

Imatinib mesylate has been shown to be active as posttransplant therapy. In a report of 128 patients who were treated with imatinib for posttransplant relapse, an overall response rate of 79% was seen, with CHR seen in 100% of patients in CP, 83% in AP, and 43% in BC. CCR was seen in 29% of patients. Recurrence of GVHD was seen in 18%, and granulocytopenia requiring dose adjustments of imatinib developed in 43% of patients. Imatinib appears to be well tolerated if given early after transplantation to prevent relapse in high-risk Ph$^+$ cases. Twenty two patients with Ph$^+$ ALL or advanced-phase CML received imatinib at a median of 28 days postengraftment. Of these patients, 17 out of 19 adults and all 3 children tolerated imatinib at the targeted dose (400 mg/day for adults, 260 mg/m^2/day for children), and 19 completed the planned course of 1 year of imatinib therapy. At a median follow-up of approximately 1½ years, 12 out of 15 of the Ph$^+$ ALL and 5 out of 7 of the CML patients were in molecular remission. The use of TKI early posttransplant appears to be safe and effective in reducing relapse in CP CML, but less effective in advanced CML. Administration of TKIs with DLIs appears to be safe and does not increase the risk of GVHD. Two retrospective analyses suggested that posttransplant TKI therapy was associated with a lower incidence of extensive chronic GVHD. However, prospective studies are needed to determine the benefit of posttransplant TKIs, as well as to optimize TKI dose and duration.

Indications for Allogeneic Transplant in the TKI Era

In the period before the advent of TKIs, allogeneic transplant was the front-line treatment of choice for CML, especially for younger patients. With the firm establishment of imatinib and other TKIs as front-line therapy for CML with excellent outcomes on long-term follow-up, the number of patients undergoing allogeneic transplantation has declined dramatically. Currently, allogeneic transplantation is a preferred treatment for patients in whom a second-generation TKI has failed, patients with TKI-resistant mutations such as T315I, and patients in AP or blast phase CML. The MD Anderson Cancer Center group reported outcomes of imatinib-resistant CML patients (CP, $n = 34$; AP, $n = 9$; and BC, $n = 4$) who underwent allogeneic transplantation. Nineteen patients (40%) had *BCR-ABL* mutations, 15 of whom had advanced disease. Thirty two patients (68%) had a MMR after transplantation, with a 2-year EFS of 36% and 58% for the mutant and nonmutant groups, and a 2-year OS of 44% and 76%, respectively. These results confirm the effectiveness of transplantation as salvage treatment for TKI-resistant patients.[29] Since patients with mutations are more likely to develop advanced disease and have worse outcomes after transplantation, this procedure should be considered early for patients with poor response to a second-generation TKI. Major or CCR to TKI therapy was associated with better posttransplant outcome, supporting the use of TKIs to reduce disease burden before allogenic HCT for AP and BC CML.

Autologous Transplantation

The rationale for autologous transplantation in CML was provided by experimental and clinical evidence for persistence of polyclonal Ph⁻ progenitors capable of reconstituting hematopoiesis in CML patients. This is most dramatically demonstrated by the high rate of cytogenetic and molecular response in CML patients treated with TKIs. Furthermore, it was shown that transplantation of autologous cells may allow restoration of Ph hematopoiesis. Initial studies carried out using unmanipulated autologous marrow or blood cells indicated that autologous transplantation could reestablish CP in patients with advanced disease and induce cytogenetic responses in a small proportion of CML CP patients. Subsequent studies indicated that depletion of Ph⁺ progenitors by ex vivo graft manipulation was associated with cytogenetic remission posttransplant. Another approach to depleting malignant cells from the graft was to treat patients before harvesting marrow or peripheral blood for transplantation, also called *in vivo purging*. However, remissions following autologous transplantation were usually of short duration. In addition, the procedure was often associated with significant toxicity and delayed recovery. Although the compiled results of 200 autologous transplants at eight different centers in Europe and North America indicated a possibility of improved survival, it is not possible to make any definite conclusions in the absence of controlled clinical trials. A meta-analysis of six trials in which patients were randomly allocated to receive autologous HCT or an IFN-based regimen did not show an advantage for HCT.

Autologous HCT fell out of favor in view of the excellent results of TKI treatment in CML patients. Collection of peripheral blood stem cells from patients responsive to TKIs may form the framework of any future attempts to perform autologous transplantation in CML, and is well tolerated and results in more consistent achievement of Ph⁻ collections. However, additional strategies are needed to further deplete leukemia cells and to improve therapy for residual disease posttransplant. At this point, autologous HCT for CML should be limited to investigational trials for patients who lack allogeneic donors and for those in whom TKIs have failed.

TREATMENT OF CML PATIENTS WITH ADVANCED DISEASE

The incidence of BC has been significantly reduced following the advent of TKI treatment compared with the pre-TKI era. The German CML study IV, a five-arm study of imatinib-based treatments, reported an 8-year cumulative BC incidence of 5.6 % compared with 12% to 62% in studies preceding the TKI era. The highest incidence of BC occurs in the first year after diagnosis. Treatment of CML patients with advanced disease depends on previous therapy,

---

Management of the Newly Diagnosed Chronic Myeloid Leukemia Patient

What should be the initial management for CML patients? After years of clinical research, we know (A) imatinib is remarkably effective for patients treated in CP, because more than 85% of patients obtain a CCR and approximately 70% of cases remain in CCR at 5 years of follow-up; (B) second-generation TKIs, dasatinib and nilotinib, used as first-line treatment for CP CML, may be even more effective, resulting in faster and more profound reduction in BCR-ABL levels; (C) allogeneic transplantation is generally associated with 10-year survival rates of 70% or better for younger patients in early CP; and (D) outcome for patients receiving TKI treatment can be effectively monitored by sensitive RT-PCR assays.

Imatinib has become the initial treatment of choice for patients with CML. For patients diagnosed during CP, imatinib is a reasonable first choice of therapy. However, in view of the association between cytogenetic and molecular responses on imatinib and survival, it is reasonable to suggest that the faster and deeper reduction in disease burden using the second-generation agents may reduce the risk for progression when compared with imatinib. The tolerability of the newer agents appears to be comparable with imatinib, although long-term effects of treatment are a potential concern. It is notable that differences in overall survival have not been observed as yet. In addition, low-risk CP patients demonstrate excellent survival with imatinib, and imatinib is considerably less expensive than the newer agents and a generic form will soon be available, reducing costs further. Careful monitoring of imatinib response could potentially identify the subset of patients who will benefit from second-generation TKI treatment. An alternative strategy to universal first-line use of second-generation TKIs was tested in the Australian Therapeutic Intensification in De Novo Leukemia II study, which used imatinib to treat CML first-line, with selective nilotinib switching based on failure to achieve targeted reduction in BCR-ABL levels at designated time points. This approach was associated with excellent molecular response and survival, supporting the feasibility of this approach. At present, the choice of first-line TKI is dependent on individual preference based on risk group, toxicity profile, dosing schedule, and economic factors.

For patients with CP disease, tyrosine kinase treatment can be initiated with simultaneous workup of family donors and unrelated donors. Criteria for failure or suboptimal response have been developed. Certainly, the failure of imatinib treatment to achieve a CHR at 3 months of treatment, lack of any cytogenetic response by 6 months, or lack of a major cytogenetic response by 12 months is an indication to switch therapy. By a conservative approach, patients should achieve a CCR by 18 months of therapy. Similarly, BCR-ABL mRNA levels greater than 10% at 6 months and greater than 1% at 12 months (using the international scale) are indicators to switch treatment. Patients who relapse after a CCR, especially those with ABL point mutations, should consider alternative therapy, including transplant. For patients diagnosed in accelerated phase or in blast crisis, initial treatment with dasatinib results in better responses than those seen with imatinib, but in general these responses tend to be short-lived; thus advanced-phase patients should consider transplantation as soon as possible.

---

the type of BC (myeloid or lymphoid), and whether or not HCT is possible. Allogeneic HCT remains the only curative option for patients with available matched donors who are able to tolerate the procedure. The best results are achieved if the patient returns to CP, especially with significant cytogenetic or molecular improvement prior to transplant. All TKIs except nilotinib are approved for the treatment of BC. Hematologic and cytogenetic responses with single-agent TKIs are achieved in about 50% and 12%, respectively, the 1-year overall response ranges from 25% to 49%, and median survival from 6 to 11.8 months. The combination of dasatinib and the hyperCVAD regimen has shown efficacy in relapsed Ph⁺ ALL or lymphoid BC of CML (CML-LB). The overall response rate was 91%, with 71% of patients achieving CR, and 21% CR with incomplete platelet recovery. Grades 3 and 4 toxicities included hemorrhage, pleural and pericardial effusions, and infections. The 3-year OS of patients with CML-LB was 70%, with 68% remaining in CR at 3 years. Therefore long-term leukemia-free survival is possible in CML-LB patients even without allogeneic HCT.

REFERENCES

1. Perrotti D, Jamieson C, Goldman J, et al: Chronic myeloid leukemia: Mechanisms of blastic transformation. *J Clin Invest* 120:2254, 2010.
2. Goldman JM, Melo JV: Chronic myeloid leukemia—Advances in biology and new approaches to treatment. *N Engl J Med* 349:1451, 2003.
3. Branford S, Fletcher L, Cross NC, et al: Desirable performance characteristics for BCR-ABL measurement on an international reporting scale to allow consistent interpretation of individual patient response and comparison of response rates between clinical trials. *Blood* 112:3330, 2008.
4. Corm S, Roche L, Micol JB, et al: Changes in the dynamics of the excess mortality rate in chronic phase-chronic myeloid leukemia over 1990–2007: A population study. *Blood* 118:4331, 2011.
5. Gambacorti-Passerini C, Antolini L, Mahon FX, et al: Multicenter independent assessment of outcomes in chronic myeloid leukemia patients treated with imatinib. *J Natl Cancer Inst* 103:553, 2011.
6. Druker B, Tamura S, Buchdunger E, et al: Effects of a selective inhibitor of the Abl tyrosine kinase on the growth of Bcr-Abl positive cells. *Nat Med* 2:561, 1996.
7. Druker BJ, Talpaz M, Resta DJ, et al: Efficacy and safety of a specific inhibitor of the BCR-ABL tyrosine kinase in chronic myeloid leukemia. *N Engl J Med* 344:1031, 2001.
8. O'Brien SG, Guilhot F, Larson RA, et al: Imatinib compared with interferon and low-dose cytarabine for newly diagnosed chronic-phase chronic myeloid leukemia. *N Engl J Med* 348:994, 2003.
9. Hochhaus A, O'Brien SG, Guilhot F, et al: Six-year follow-up of patients receiving imatinib for the first-line treatment of chronic myeloid leukemia. *Leukemia* 23:1054, 2009.
10. Cortes JE, Baccarani M, Guilhot F, et al: Phase III, randomized, open-label study of daily imatinib mesylate 400 mg versus 800 mg in patients with newly diagnosed, previously untreated chronic myeloid leukemia in chronic phase using molecular end points: Tyrosine kinase inhibitor optimization and selectivity study. *J Clin Oncol* 28:424, 2010.
11. de Lavallade H, Apperley JF, Khorashad JS, et al: Imatinib for newly diagnosed patients with chronic myeloid leukemia: Incidence of sustained responses in an intention-to-treat analysis. *J Clin Oncol* 26:3358, 2008.
12. Efficace F, Baccarani M, Breccia M, et al: Health-related quality of life in chronic myeloid leukemia patients receiving long-term therapy with imatinib compared with the general population. *Blood* 118:4554, 2011.
13. Hughes TP, Hochhaus A, Branford S, et al: Long-term prognostic significance of early molecular response to imatinib in newly diagnosed chronic myeloid leukemia: An analysis from the International Randomized Study of Interferon and STI571 (IRIS). *Blood* 116:3758, 2010.
14. Marin D, Ibrahim AR, Lucas C, et al: Assessment of BCR-ABL1 Transcript levels at 3 months is the only requirement for predicting outcome for patients with chronic myeloid leukemia treated with tyrosine kinase inhibitors. *J Clin Oncol* 30:232, 2012.
15. Baccarani M, Deininger MW, Rosti G, et al: (2013) European LeukemiaNet recommendations for the management of chronic myeloid leukemia. *Blood* 122(6):872–884, 2013.
16. Marin D, Bazeos A, Mahon FX, et al: Adherence is the critical factor for achieving molecular responses in patients with chronic myeloid leukemia who achieve complete cytogenetic responses on imatinib. *J Clin Oncol* 28:2381, 2011.
17. Deininger MW, O'Brien SG, Ford JM, et al: Practical management of patients with chronic myeloid leukemia receiving imatinib. *J Clin Oncol* 21:1637, 2003.
18. Soverini S, Hochhaus A, Nicolini FE, et al: BCR-ABL kinase domain mutation analysis in chronic myeloid leukemia patients treated with tyrosine kinase inhibitors: Recommendations from an expert panel on behalf of European LeukemiaNet. *Blood* 118:1208, 2011.
19. Kantarjian H, Shah NP, Hochhaus A, et al: Dasatinib versus imatinib in newly diagnosed chronic-phase chronic myeloid leukemia. *N Engl J Med* 362:2260, 2010.
20. Saglio G, Kim DW, Issaragrisil S, et al: Nilotinib versus imatinib for newly diagnosed chronic myeloid leukemia. *N Engl J Med* 362:2251, 2010.
21. Berman E: Where exactly does ponatinib fit in chronic myelogenous leukemia? *J Natl Compr Canc Netw* 12:1615–1620, 2014.
22. Alvandi F, Kwitkowski VE, Ko CW, et al: U.S. Food and Drug Administration approval summary: omacetaxine mepesuccinate as treatment for chronic myeloid leukemia. *Oncologist* 19:94–99, 2014.
23. Chu S, McDonald T, Lin A, et al: Persistence of leukemia stem cells in chronic myelogenous leukemia patients in prolonged remission with imatinib treatment. *Blood* 118:5565, 2011.
24. Mahon FX, Rea D, Guilhot J, et al: Discontinuation of imatinib in patients with chronic myeloid leukaemia who have maintained complete molecular remission for at least 2 years: The prospective, multicentre Stop Imatinib (STIM) trial. *Lancet Oncol* 11:1029, 2010.
25. Palani R, Milojkovic D, Apperley JF: Managing pregnancy in chronic myeloid leukaemia. *Ann Hematol* 94(Suppl 2):S167–S176, 2015.
26. Khoury HJ, Kukreja M, Goldman JM, et al: Prognostic factors for outcomes in allogeneic transplantation for CML in the imatinib era: A CIBMTR analysis. *Bone Marrow Transplant* 2011.
27. Basak G, Torosian T, Snarski E, et al: Hematopoietic stem cell transplantation for T315I-mutated chronic myelogenous leukemia. *Ann Transplant* 15:68, 2010.
28. Kebriaei P, Detry MA, Giralt S, et al: Long-term follow-up of allogeneic hematopoietic stem-cell transplantation with reduced-intensity conditioning for patients with chronic myeloid leukemia. *Blood* 110:3456, 2007.
29. Jabbour E, Cortes J, Santos FP, et al: Results of allogeneic hematopoietic stem cell transplantation for chronic myelogenous leukemia patients who failed tyrosine kinase inhibitors after developing BCR-ABL1 kinase domain mutations. *Blood* 117:3641, 2011.

CHAPTER 68

THE POLYCYTHEMIAS

Marina Kremyanskaya, Vesna Najfeld, John Mascarenhas, and Ronald Hoffman

Under normal conditions, the red blood cell (RBC) mass in humans is tightly controlled and remains relatively constant in a given individual. The numbers of senescent RBCs lost daily are replaced by newly formed ones by a carefully controlled network of growth factors and progenitor cells. Erythropoiesis can be augmented by a variety of stimuli that increase the delivery of oxygen to tissues. This delicate balance can be disturbed by various pathologic conditions and can result in either reduced numbers of RBCs (anemia) or excessive numbers of RBCs (polycythemia). Hematocrit values over 49% in males and 48% in females are abnormal and require further evaluation to determine if the patient has an absolute increase in their RBC mass and if investigation of its cause should be pursued. The RBC mass is increased if it is greater than 125% above that expected for sex and body mass. The measurement of the RBC mass is a diagnostic study that is now available at a dwindling number of tertiary care centers, making other diagnostic studies pivotal in evaluating patients with elevated hematocrit levels. Polycythemic states can be caused by a variety of disorders that can be attributed to several pathophysiologic mechanisms. Determination of the etiology of an individual's polycythemia is a critical step in defining the patient's appropriate prognosis and treatment plan. Primary polycythemias are the result of innate abnormalities involving hematopoietic progenitors and stem cells that lead to constitutive overproduction of RBCs, which are accompanied by low erythropoietin (EPO) levels. By contrast, secondary polycythemias are the consequence of a number of conditions that lead to increased EPO production, which acts on normal progenitors to overproduce RBCs. In a small number of patients, the cause of erythrocytosis cannot be determined; these patients are classified as having idiopathic erythrocytosis.

ERYTHROPOIESIS

RBC production can be influenced by numerous factors, including nutrients, growth factors, numbers and function of bone marrow (BM) progenitor and precursor cells, and cellular receptors and transcription factors. EPO is considered to be the physiologic regulator of the terminal phases of erythropoiesis. Alterations in its production are followed by adjustments in the rate of formation of RBCs. In humans, EPO production is controlled by the relative supply of oxygen to the kidneys, the major site of EPO production. In states of severe hypoxia, EPO production can be increased up to 1000-fold. In a healthy person after phlebotomy, EPO excretion increases, and an inverse logarithmic relationship between hematocrit and EPO excretion rates exists. Patients with secondary erythrocytosis caused by chronic hypoxia have either normal or increased basal EPO values, but they also have increased values after reduction of the hematocrit to normal levels by phlebotomy. By contrast, EPO excretion is invariably subnormal in patients with polycythemia vera (PV), which demonstrates that this disorder is not a result of excessive EPO production.

ERYTHROPOIETIN, OXYGEN SENSING, AND HYPOXIA-INDUCIBLE FACTOR

Under normal conditions, EPO production is mediated by a reduced oxygen content, termed *hypoxemia*, which leads to decreased oxygen delivery to tissues. Regulation of oxygen homeostasis is critical to survival. In humans, oxygen sensing occurs at many levels, leading to both acute and chronic adaptation. The acute reduction of the availability of oxygen leads to the initiation of a cascade of adaptive events that sets in place compensatory events to correct the lack of oxygen supply. Low oxygen levels, or hypoxia (60 mmHg), in humans cause oxygen-sensing chemosensory cells to undergo rapid membrane depolarization within seconds, leading to the production of action potentials, influx of calcium ions, and release of the neurotransmitters that result in stimulation of the brain stem that controls the respiratory and cardiovascular systems. These chemosensory cells are found within the glomus cells of the carotid body located at the bifurcation of the internal and external carotid arteries. The released neurotransmitters activate the nerve endings of the carotid body sensory nerve to convey to the CNS signals that command ventilation to fight hypoxia, resulting in an increase of the lung ventilation rate and restoration of normal oxygen tension to vital organs. In addition, there are changes in blood pressure and heart rate to maximize oxygen delivery. The carotid body is the organ with the greatest blood flow within the body. Activation of the carotid body results in the sensation of breathlessness experienced by individuals at high altitudes. During chronic hypoxia when the carotid body is permanently active, there is marked enlargement of the carotid body because of an increase in capillaries and a marked reduction in the mean distance from the capillaries to the edge of the chemoreceptor cells.

In response to chronic hypoxia, multiple compensatory mechanisms come into play over several days within the kidneys, the major site of EPO production. Hypoxic stimulation results in production of hypoxia-inducible factor-1 (HIF-1), the major factor responsible for transcriptional activation of the *EPO* gene.[1] The HIF transcriptional system is a master regulator of the hypoxic response controlling a large number of genes in multiple cell types. HIF-1 is a heterodimeric protein consisting of HIF-1α and HIF-1β, which is required for normal development of the heart, blood vessels, and blood cells. The levels of HIF-1α increase exponentially as the oxygen concentration declines. As the key mediator of cellular oxygen maintenance, HIF-1 facilitates body oxygen delivery and responses to oxygen deprivation by regulating the expression of gene products that are involved in cellular energy metabolism and glucose transport, angiogenesis, erythropoiesis and iron metabolism, pH regulation, apoptosis, cell proliferation, and cell–cell and cell–matrix interactions. Classic HIF target genes include phosphoglycerate kinase, glucose transporter-1, vascular endothelial growth factor (VEGF), and EPO. The HIF proteins are members of the Per–ARNT–Sim family of heterodimeric basic helix–loop–helix transcription factors (Fig. 68.1).

In contrast to the constitutively expressed, HIF-1β subunits, HIF-1α is an oxygen-labile protein that becomes stabilized in response to hypoxia. HIF-1α mRNA and protein levels are induced by hypoxia, and HIF-1α protein levels decay rapidly with return to normoxia. The posttranslational regulation of HIF-1α protein accounts for the majority of the regulation of this gene. Normoxia-induced, ubiquitin-mediated degradation of the HIF-1α protein is the major regulator of HIF-1α levels, thereby reducing the stimulus for additional EPO production. The targeting and subsequent polyubiquitination of HIF-1α require the von Hippel-Lindau (VHL) protein, oxygen, and three different iron-requiring proline hydroxylase (PHD) enzymes (see Fig. 68.1). The PHD proteins exist in three

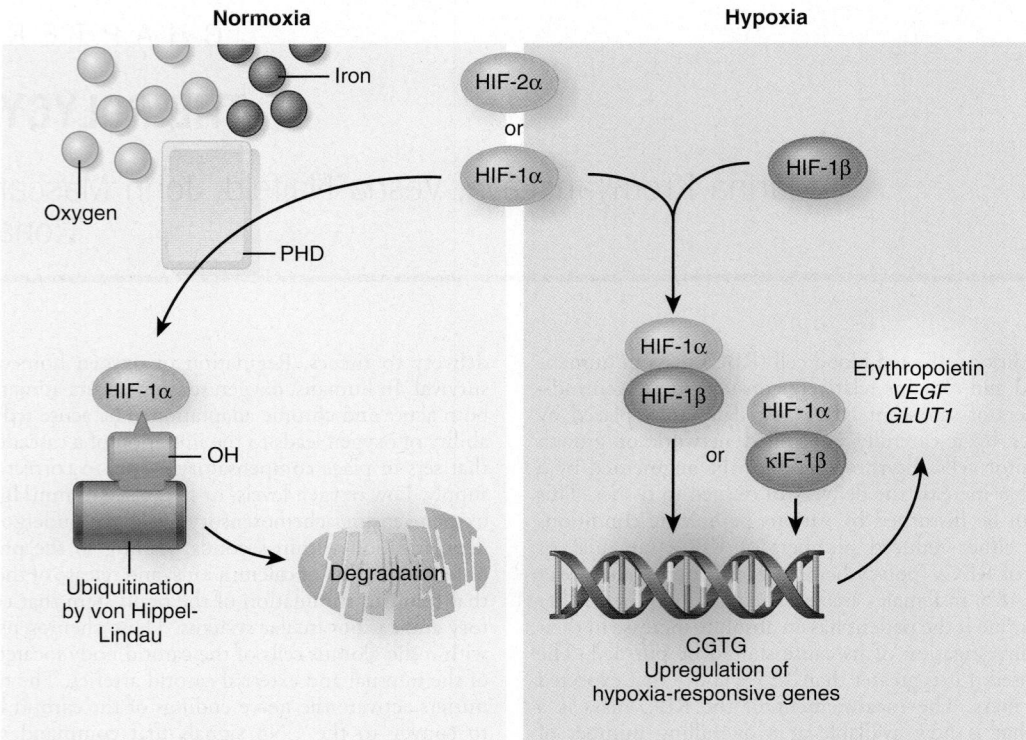

Fig. 68.1 SCHEMATIC REPRESENTATION OF THE RELATIONSHIP BETWEEN HYPOXIA SENSING AND ERYTHROPOIETIN PRODUCTION. *GLUT*, Glucose transporter 1; *HIF*, hypoxia-inducible factor; *PHD*, proline hydroxylase; *VEGF*, vascular endothelial growth factor.

isoforms, PHD1, PHD2, and PHD3. HIF-1α is hydroxylated by all three isoforms but primarily by PHD2. The prolyl hydroxylation of HIF-1α is necessary for the binding of HIF-1α to VHL, which is the substrate-recognition subunit of an E3 ubiquitin-protein ligase. Different parts of the HIF-1α chains have different functions. The N-terminus part of HIF-1α is involved in DNA binding and dimerization, and the C-terminus portion has regulatory functions. One domain at the C-terminus influences transcriptional activity without affecting HIF-1α protein levels, and the other region, termed the oxygen-dependent degradation domain (ODD), affects protein abundance. The ODD is divided into an N-terminus and a C-terminus subdomain. The VHL protein physically interacts with the ODD of HIF-1α, targeting it for ubiquitination and destruction by the proteasome. Iron-chelating drugs can also block the interaction of HIF-1α with the VHL protein, suggesting a role for iron in the degradation of HIF-1α.

Under normoxic conditions, hydroxylation of HIF-1α is essential for HIF proteolytic degradation by promoting interaction with the VHL tumor-suppressor protein through hydrogen bonding to the hydroxy proline-binding pocket in the VHL-β domain. As oxygen levels decrease, hydroxylation of HIF decreases, and HIF-1α then no longer binds VHL. As a result, it becomes stabilized, dimerizes with HIF-1β, and activates transcription of target genes. The activity of PHDs depends on the availability of molecular oxygen, which qualifies these enzymes as oxygen sensors. In addition, these dioxygenases require 2-oxyglutarate as a cosubstrate and vitamin C to keep their central nonheme iron in the ferrous state. Although PHD-2 appears to be the hydroxylase that is essential for HIF-1α degradation under normoxic conditions, PHD-3 is important for hydroxylation of HIF-1α during reoxygenation. Different effects of individual PHDs on HIF-1α and HIF-2α hydroxylation indicate that the stability of individual HIF-1α subunits and their target gene expression might be affected by tissue- and cell-type differences in PHD expression and activity levels. The activity of PHDs can be modulated by mitochondrial reactive oxygen species, implicating mitochondria in oxygen sensing. Another protein termed HIF-2α has been identified that

under hypoxic conditions dimerizes with HIF-1β and activates the transcription of a set of target genes that overlap with the target genes regulated by HIF-1α/HIF-1β heterodimers. HIF-1α is expressed by all nucleated cells, but HIF-2α is expressed by specific cell types, including vascular endothelial cells, renal interstitial cells, hepatocytes, cardiomyocytes, and astrocytes. HIF-2α appears to play a critical role in regulating EPO production in adult mammals, and HIF-1α is also important during yolk sac erythropoiesis. HIF-1 also controls the absorption and delivery of iron to the BM through its repression of hepcidin and activation of genes encoding transferrin and the transferrin receptor.

VHL syndrome is a hereditary cancer syndrome that is associated with exaggerated responses to hypoxia caused by posttranslational abnormalities in HIF. VHL syndrome is characterized by a propensity for developing clear-cell renal carcinomas, retinal hemangioblastomas, cerebellar and spinal hemangiomas, pancreatic and renal cysts, islet cell tumors of the pancreas, and pheochromocytomas.[2] The tumors result from somatic mutations that cause a loss of heterozygosity (LOH) of the *VHL* gene. VHL disease affects approximately 1 in 35,000 individuals and is transmitted in an autosomal dominant manner. Individuals with VHL disease carry one wild-type (WT) *VHL* allele and one inactivated *VHL* allele. This inactivation can occur by somatic mutation or hypermethylation. Tumor or cyst development is linked to somatic inactivation or loss of the remaining WT *VHL* allele. Approximately 20–37% of VHL patients have large or partial germ-line deletions, 23–27% have nonsense or frame-shift mutations, and 30–35% have missense mutations. More than 150 different *VHL* mutations linked to VHL disease have been reported. The tumors linked to *VHL* inactivation are often highly vascular and can produce angiogenic factors such as VEGF. In addition, renal cell carcinoma, cerebellar hemangioblastomas, and pheochromocytomas have been associated with paraneoplastic erythrocytosis caused by overproduction of EPO. Overproduction of HIF-inducible mRNAs is the hallmark of VHL protein defective cells. Genotype–phenotype correlates in VHL disease suggest that VHL has functions independent of HIF regulation that might play a role in tumor formation.

VHL protein has other binding partners, including atypical protein kinase C and a family of deubiquitinating enzymes called *VHL-interacting deubiquitinating enzymes 1 and 2*. In addition, VHL has been involved in numerous cellular processes, including regulation of extracellular matrix, cytoskeleton stability, cell cycle control, and differentiation. VHL disease is not associated with erythrocytosis.

THE ERYTHROPOIETIN RECEPTOR

Interaction of EPO with the EPO receptor (EPOR) present on the erythroid progenitor and precursor cells leads to its homodimerization, resulting in (1) stimulation of cell division, (2) differentiation by induction of erythroid-specific gene expression, and (3) prevention of erythroid progenitor and precursor cell apoptosis. EPOR is a member of the type I cytokine receptor superfamily. Signal transduction through the receptor is initiated by ligand binding, which induces dimerization of EPOR monomers. The predominant signaling cascade activated by EPOR and other cytokine receptors is the Janus-activated kinase (JAK)/signal transducer and activator of transcription (STAT) pathway. JAK tyrosine kinases are constitutively associated with the membrane proximal regions of cytokine receptor cytoplasmic domains and are activated by receptor dimerization. The EPOR associates predominantly with JAK2. JAK2 binds to EPOR in the endoplasmic reticulum and acts as a chaperone protein transporting the EPOR to the plasma membrane. Immediately after EPO binding, JAK2 phosphorylates itself and the EPOR on multiple tyrosine residues in its cytoplasmic domain, thus creating a platform for the recruitment and activation of multiple key signaling regulators. One of such proteins is STAT5. JAK2–STAT5 signaling plays an essential role in EPO/EPOR-mediated regulation of erythropoiesis. Consistent with their essential roles in erythropoiesis, EPO-, EPOR- and JAK2-deficient mice die embryonically from severe anemia.

The C-terminal cytoplasmic portion of the EPOR also possesses a negative regulatory domain. Hematopoietic cell phosphatase (HCP; also known as *SHP-1* or *PTP N6*) interacts with this portion of the EPOR and downregulates signal transduction by promoting dephosphorylation (Fig. 68.2). Inactivation of the HCP-binding site leads to prolonged phosphorylation of JAK2–STAT5. Another negative regulator of erythropoiesis, suppressor of cytokine signaling-3 (SOCS-3), binds to the cytoplasmic portion of the EPOR and suppresses EPO-dependent JAK2–STAT5 signaling. Thus, deletion of the distal C-terminal cytoplasmic portion of the EPOR abolishes negative regulatory elements and results in increased proliferation of erythroid progenitor cells. Mutations in the *EPOR* gene have been observed in some patients with primary familial and congenital polycythemia (PFCP) and are occasionally found in erythroleukemia (see Fig. 68.2). Such secondary growth factors as insulin-like growth factor-1 (IGF-1) and the components of the renin–angiotensin system (RAS) may also influence the production of RBCs.

THE RENIN–ANGIOTENSIN SYSTEM AND HEMATOPOIESIS

The RAS regulates fluid and electrolyte homeostasis and blood pressure, and has been hypothesized to also play a role in the regulation of erythropoiesis. The primary function of angiotensin during development is the regulation of tissue growth and differentiation. Angiotensin II (AngII) is a ligand for two distinct receptors, type 1 and type 2 (AT1 and AT2). AT1 appears to play a major role in the regulation of cell proliferation.[3]

The RAS was first postulated to influence erythropoiesis in the 1980s after the use of angiotensin-converting enzyme (ACE) inhibitors to treat hypertension was shown to result in anemia. In animals, increased blood levels of renin (a major regulator of AngII synthesis) were found to result in elevated serum EPO levels and erythrocytosis. In humans, the infusion of AngII in healthy volunteers increased serum EPO levels by 35% or higher via activation of the AngII type I receptor, and ACE inhibitors significantly decrease plasma EPO levels by as much as 20–30%. The pathway underlying AngII-driven EPO secretion is unknown. However, some investigators have suggested that AngII modulates renal EPO production through changes in renal perfusion and sodium reabsorption. This hypothesis is based on the presumption that reduced oxygen pressure in the kidneys triggers HIF-1α to induce release of EPO. AngII also directly stimulates proliferation of hematopoietic progenitors in vitro, and inhibition of this effect with ACE inhibitors induces apoptosis of erythroid progenitors in renal transplantation patients. ACE-1 knockout mice develop a normocytic anemia that can be fully reversed by infusion of AngII. ACE-related anemia is most pronounced in patients with renal insufficiency or end-stage renal disease and in patients who have

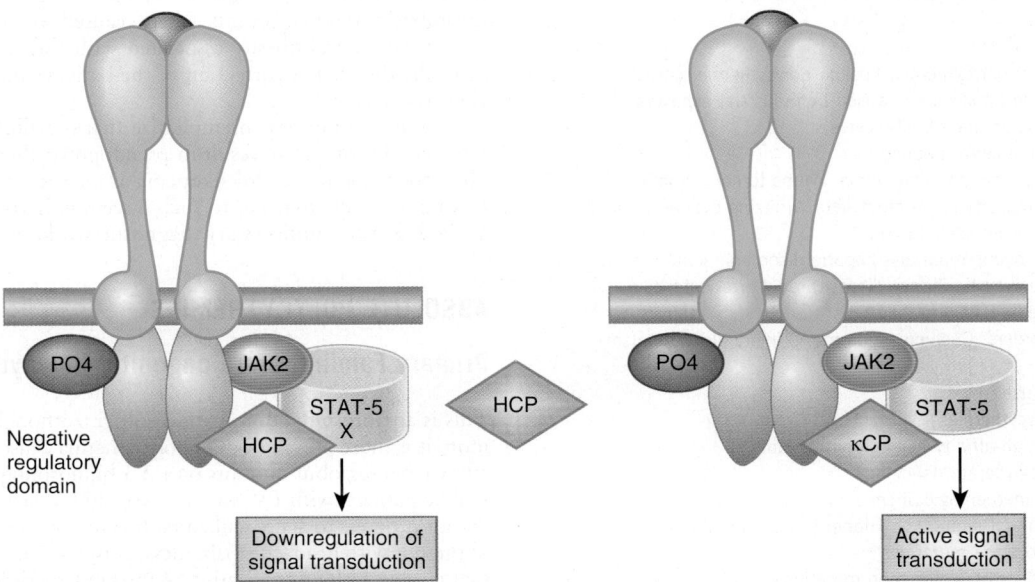

Fig. 68.2 SCHEMATIC REPRESENTATION OF THE ERYTHROPOIETIN RECEPTOR AND THE DEFECT IN THE RECEPTOR UNDERLYING PRIMARY FAMILIAL AND CONGENITAL POLYCYTHEMIA. *HCP*, Hematopoietic cell phosphatase; *JAK*, Janus kinase; *STAT*, signal transducer and activator of transcription.

received a renal allograft. The pathogenesis of this anemia is not clear, but reduced levels of circulating EPO are not solely responsible, suggesting that there might be other contributing factors. The AT1 receptor is present on erythroid progenitors, and its ligand, AngII, augments EPO stimulation of erythropoiesis. The involvement of JAK2 kinase in AngII signaling suggests that this signal transduction pathway mediated by EPO and AngII might overlap. Postrenal transplant erythrocytosis likely can be accounted for by activation of the RAS.

DEFINITION AND CLASSIFICATION OF POLYCYTHEMIA

The term *polycythemia* is a literal translation from Greek, meaning "too many cells in the blood," and refers to an increase in the RBC mass; it is frequently used interchangeably with the term *erythrocytosis*. Polycythemia may be due to a myriad of causes (Table 68.1). The polycythemias can be classified as relative and absolute. Relative polycythemia is a disorder in which the patient characteristically has a modest elevation of the hematocrit level without an elevated RBC mass but rather because of contraction of the plasma volume. The absolute polycythemias are accompanied by an actual increase in the circulating RBC mass. Polycythemias can also be classified according to the responsiveness of their erythroid progenitor cells to growth factors or the circulating levels of such growth factors. Primary polycythemias are characterized by increased sensitivity of the erythroid progenitors to regulatory growth factors as a result of acquired

TABLE 68.1	**Differential Diagnosis of the Polycythemias**

Relative or Spurious Polycythemia
1. Decreased plasma volume—reduced fluid intake, marked loss of body fluids (diaphoresis, vomiting, diarrhea, "third spacing")
2. Gaisböck syndrome
3. Overfilling of blood in collection vacuum tubes

Absolute Polycythemia
1. Secondary polycythemia
A. Acquired
Hypoxia
   • Pulmonary disease
   • Cyanotic congenital heart disease
   • Hypoventilation syndromes: sleep apnea, Pickwickian syndrome
   • High altitude
   • Smokers' polycythemia, hookah polycythemia, carbon monoxide intoxication caused by industrial exposure
Postrenal transplantation erythrocytosis
Aberrant erythropoietin production
   • Tumors: renal cell carcinoma, Wilms tumor, hepatic carcinoma, uterine leiomyomata, virilizing ovarian tumors, vascular cerebellar tumors
   • Miscellaneous renal and hepatic disorders: solitary renal cysts, polycystic kidney disease, renal artery stenosis hydronephrosis, viral hepatitis
Endocrine disorders: Cushing syndrome, primary aldosteronism
Androgen use
Erythropoietin use
B. Congenital polycythemias
   • Abnormal high-affinity hemoglobin variants
   • Bisphosphoglycerate deficiency
   • Congenital methemoglobinemia
   • Chuvash polycythemia (von Hippel-Lindau mutations)
   • Prolyl hydroxylase mutations
   • Hypoxia-inducible factor gene mutations
2. Primary polycythemias
   • Primary congenital and familial polycythemia
   • Polycythemia vera

somatic or inherited germ-line mutations expressed by hematopoietic progenitor cells (HPCs). In contrast, secondary polycythemias are characterized by an increase in regulatory growth factors, primarily EPO, and normal responsiveness of their erythroid progenitors to these growth factors. These conditions can usually be distinguished by in vitro assays of erythroid progenitor cells, quantitation of serum EPO levels, and detection of somatic *JAK2* mutations. In a small number of patients, the cause of erythrocytosis cannot be determined; these patients are classified as having idiopathic erythrocytosis.

RELATIVE POLYCYTHEMIA

Individuals with a modestly increased venous hematocrit level that is not accompanied by an increased RBC mass are frequently thought to be polycythemic by imprecise yet widely accepted medical practice. Frequently, these individuals are thought to be polycythemic owing to the lack of appreciation by a clinician of what constitutes the upper limit of normal values for a hematocrit (49% in males and 48% in females). Such individuals frequently prove not to have an absolute polycythemia as defined by an actual increase in the measured RBC mass. *Relative* or *spurious polycythemia* is a term used to describe an elevation of the hematocrit level either caused by an acute transient state of hemoconcentration associated with intravascular fluid depletion or a chronic sustained relative polycythemia caused by contraction of the plasma volume (see Table 68.1).

Transient polycythemias may be a result of acute depletion of the plasma volume from a variety of disorders, including protracted vomiting or diarrhea, plasma loss from external burns, sudden cold exposure or protracted exercise, insensible fluid loss from fever, sepsis, diabetic ketoacidosis, or acute ethanol intoxication. These elevations of hematocrit can be easily corrected by appropriate replacement of intravascular fluids.

Gaisböck syndrome, first described in 1905, is a condition observed mainly in obese, hypertensive, middle-aged, male smokers. Alcohol, diuretics, obesity, hypoxia, psychologic stress, and excess catecholamine secretion have been identified as possible causes of relative polycythemia. Such individuals can have a chronic modest-to-moderate elevation of the hematocrit level associated with a normal RBC mass and low plasma volume, which has been attributed to reduced venous compliance, or they can have a high normal RBC mass with either a normal or slightly decreased plasma volume. The primary significance of the identification of a patient with relative polycythemia is the recognition of the increased risk of developing thrombotic vascular events likely caused by excessive smoking, hypertension, and obesity associated with this disease. Treatment is generally directed at correction of the patient's underlying cardiovascular risk factors.

It is also important to emphasize that overfilling of blood collection vacuum tubes can result in pseudopolycythemia, pseudothrombocytopenia, and pseudoleukopenia as a result of inadequate sample mixing. Careful attention to such a seemingly trivial detail can help avoid expensive, unnecessary diagnostic workups.

ABSOLUTE POLYCYTHEMIAS

Primary Familial and Congenital Polycythemia

This is an autosomal dominant disorder. Although PFCP is uncommon, it is more prevalent than polycythemia caused by high-oxygen–affinity hemoglobin mutants or a 2,3-biphosphoglycerate deficiency. Unlike patients with PV, patients with PFCP lack splenomegaly and do not progress to acute leukemia. It is not unusual for these patients to present with headaches, dizziness, epistaxis, and exertional dyspnea that resolve with normalization of the hematocrit level.[4] An increased incidence of cardiovascular events and premature morbidity and mortality has been reported in some affected members, but many appear to have a benign clinical course. Although clinical symptoms are relieved by phlebotomy, the increased risk of cardiovascular morbidity is not corrected by maintaining a normal hematocrit. Characteristic laboratory findings are (1) an increased hematocrit and RBC mass without an increased leukocyte or platelet count, (2) an absence of an activating mutation of *JAK2*, (3) a normal hemoglobin–oxygen dissociation curve, (4) low serum EPO levels, and (5) in vitro hypersensitivity of erythroid progenitors to EPO. Even though PFCP is present at birth, many affected patients are incidentally diagnosed later in life after the performance of routine blood counts or when evaluated in the context of multiple family members having polycythemia. It is of interest that one individual so affected was an accomplished cross-country skier who had won medals at the Olympic Games. Numerous mutations of the EPOR associated with PFCP have been described, leading to a loss in the negative regulatory domain of the EPOR.

The physiologic basis for EPO-mediated activation of erythropoiesis is as follows: EPO activates its receptor by conformational changes of its dimers, leading to initiation of an erythroid-specific cascade of events. The first signal is initiated by the binding of a tyrosine kinase to the EPOR and its phosphorylation and activation of a transcription factor, STAT5, which regulates erythroid-specific genes. This "on" signal is negated by dephosphorylation of the EPOR by HCP, that is, the "off" signal. Truncation of the EPOR leads to a loss in the negative regulatory domain of the EPOR, a binding site for HCP, leading to a gain-of-function mutation of the EPOR (see Fig. 68.2). In addition, the negative regulation of erythropoiesis by SOCS-3, cytokine-inducible SH2 domain containing protein (CIS), and Src homology region 2 domain-containing phosphatase-1 (SHP-1) is presumed to contribute to the underlying cause of PFCP.

Alternative explanations for the increased sensitivity of erythroid progenitors to EPO of patients with PFCP have been proposed. EPOR downregulation provides another mechanism by which EPO desensitization can occur. EPOR downregulation is a complex process that involves EPOR-induced internalization or ubiquitination and degradation by proteasomes. EPO-induced receptor internalization is an efficient means of rapidly reducing EPO responsiveness. This process is mediated by binding of the EPOR to the p85 subunit of phosphatidylinositol 3-kinase (PI3K) but does not involve its kinase activity as the PI3K inhibitor wortmannin does not impair EPOR internalization. All of the truncated mutants associated with PFCP are associated with failure to internalize the EPOR, contributing to prolonged signaling through the EPOR. The EPOR degradation process removes all of the phosphorylated tyrosine residues in the intracellular domain of the receptor, thereby preventing further signal transduction. The remaining part of the EPO–EPOR complex is then internalized and degraded by lysosomes. The E3 ligase B-transducin repeat containing protein-1 (B-Trcp-1) is responsible for EPOR ubiquitination and degradation. Mutations in *B-Trcp-1* abolish EPOR ubiquitination and degradation, making cells expressing the EPORs hypersensitive to EPO. Each of the *PFCP* mutations involving the EPOR results in loss of the binding site for B-Trcp-1. These findings suggest that the EPO hypersensitivity in PFCP might not only be attributable to a failure to recruit negative regulators such as phosphatases to inactivate JAK2, but that these mutant receptors are defective in EPO-induced receptor downregulation.

The effect of a truncated EPOR is not always predictable. Some patients who inherit an EPOR mutation are not polycythemic. This observation suggests that undefined environmental or genetic factors may mask the development of polycythemia. Also, the heterogeneity of the polycythemic phenotype observed in a PFCP animal model appears to be strain dependent. This indicates that gene modifiers or epigenetic factors may mask the development of the full PFCP phenotype. Recently, four different rearrangements of the EPOR have been observed in Philadelphia chromosome-like (Ph-like) acute lymphoblastic leukemia (ALL) B cells. Normal B cells do not express the EPOR, but the EPOR has been described in ETV6-RUNX1–positive ALL blast cells. All of these rearrangements are different from those observed in PFCP but result in truncation of the cytoplasmic tail of the EPOR at residues similar to those mutated in PFCP, with preservation of the proximal tyrosine essential for receptor activation and loss of distal regulatory residues. This leads to dysregulated EPOR expression, hypersensitivity to EPO stimulation, and heightened JAK–STAT activation. Expression of truncated EPOR in murine B-cell progenitors leads to the development of ALL in vivo (see Chapters 64 and 66). Several observations suggest that the EPOR mutations in human leukemic cells in Ph-like ALL are driver mutations that are acquired during early stages of leukemogenesis and are logical targets for therapeutic targeting with JAK2 inhibitors.

Mutations of genes encoding proteins other than the EPOR account for most cases of PFCP. Mutations of the EPOR have been found in only 10–20% of subjects with PFCP. Additional disease-causing genes and their mutations have yet to be identified. In patients with erythrocytosis who are *JAK2V617F* negative and do not have a *JAK2* exon 12 mutation, and who have life-long erythrocytosis associated with a low serum EPO level, sequencing of the EPOR should be pursued.

SECONDARY POLYCYTHEMIAS

Secondary polycythemias can be either congenital or acquired (see Table 68.1). Conditions leading to hypoxia, such as high altitude, cyanotic heart disease, or chronic lung disease, may result in physiologic polycythemia mediated by increased levels of EPO. There are marked variations in EPO levels and subsequent erythroid response in the face of chronic hypoxia, suggesting that some of these factors may be genetically determined. The same degree of renal tissue hypoxia may induce substantially different levels of EPO production in response to high altitude. It is likely that these individual variations are a function of genetic differences in hypoxia sensing and the hypoxia response pathways. For purposes of simplicity and clinical diagnostic usefulness, the secondary polycythemic disorders are divided into those that are acquired and those that are congenital. It should be kept in mind that this division, although useful for differential diagnosis, is artificial. Patients with inherited germ-line mutations, for instance, can develop an EPO-secreting pheochromocytoma or renal cell cancer, and a patient with PV can smoke and have chronic obstructive pulmonary disease (COPD). In other instances, polycythemia caused by a germ-line mutation can be masked by an acquired environmental factor or another gene-modifying mutation.

Acquired Secondary Polycythemias

Polycythemias of Cyanotic Heart Disease and Pulmonary Disease

Patients with cyanotic heart disease and pulmonary disease frequently have arterial hypoxemia, leading to increased production of EPO and polycythemia. Excessive EPO production occurs when the PaO_2 is sustained below 67 mmHg as a result of severely impaired pulmonary mechanics. Because patients with severe pulmonary disease and secondary erythrocytosis frequently have elevated plasma volumes, the degree of elevation of the hematocrit level may be modest. Hematocrit levels as high as 65% or rarely 75% have, however, been reported. Moderate elevations of hematocrit have been estimated to occur in 20% of patients with COPD. Polycythemia in this setting can contribute to pulmonary hypertension, pulmonary endothelial cell dysfunction, reduced cerebral blood flow, hyperuricemia, gout, and an increased risk of venous thromboembolic disease.

Why some patients with pulmonary disease and congenital heart disease develop polycythemia but others do not is not clear. Increased oxygen-carrying capacity may improve oxygen delivery; however, it is not obvious at what hematocrit level the resultant elevation in blood viscosity impairs blood flow to the tissues, leading to a reduction in oxygen uptake. In addition, oxygen uptake to the tissues is markedly influenced by whole blood volume. Thus, whereas the optimal hematocrit level for oxygen delivery is about 45% in normovolemic subjects, it rises to over 60% in hypervolemic states, likely as a result of engorgement of the vascular bed and a decrease in peripheral resistance. Furthermore, chronic exposure to hypoxia leads to respiratory alkalosis that in turn promotes the synthesis of 2,3-bisphosphoglycerate (2,3-BPG), facilitating increased oxygen delivery to tissues.

The practical relevance of an elevated hematocrit level in this clinical situation is whether and at what level it is harmful or beneficial. An extremely elevated hematocrit level may be detrimental to optimal oxygen delivery. Extreme but not moderate polycythemia caused by chronic hypoxia may affect systemic vascular function by altering blood viscosity, vessel wall shear stress, reduced endothelial cell–derived nitric oxide release, and increasing the secretion of endothelin. Although it is widely accepted that polycythemic pediatric patients with cyanotic heart disease are at an increased risk for developing cerebrovascular accidents, the literature provides conflicting data as relates to the prevalence of such events among adults. A 10–13.6% prevalence of stroke and transient ischemic attacks (TIAs) has been reported in a cohort of adult patients with cyanotic heart disease, but others have claimed that such events are rare.

Iron deficiency occurs in more than 30% because of the total depletion of iron stores to support erythropoiesis. Microcytic RBCs are, however, rarely found, and despite the iron deficiency, these patients frequently have normal mean corpuscular volumes and high mean corpuscular hemoglobin concentrations, which might maximize the amount of hemoglobin within an individual RBC, thereby maximizing oxygen delivery. In the past, compensatory erythrocytosis was thought to lead to an increased plasma viscosity, leading to a compromised microcirculation, resulting in such symptoms as headache, sluggish mentation, dizziness, blurry vision, muscle weakness, or paresthesias. In reality, such symptoms are rare in patients with chronic compensated secondary erythrocytosis, and the secondary erythrocytosis is viewed as a physiologically desirable response to chronic hypoxia. The symptoms delineated above are likely attributable to decreased tissue oxygen delivery rather than hyperviscosity.

The treatment of hyperviscosity secondary to erythrocytosis in cyanotic heart disease with prophylactic phlebotomy is rarely used. In fact, phlebotomy has been reported to have harmful rather than beneficial effects in adults with cyanotic congenital heart disease. Because almost one-third of these patients are iron deficient even though their RBC indices do not reflect this, routine assessment of the patient's iron status is suggested with gradual supplementation with sufficient iron to attain appropriate compensatory levels of erythropoiesis but avoiding excessive sudden increases in the degree of erythrocytosis. The present evidence indicates that prophylactic phlebotomy promotes the development of iron deficiency, decreases exercise tolerance, and increases the number of cerebrovascular events. Currently, experts in this field recommend that phlebotomy should be restricted to individuals with symptoms with extreme erythrocytosis (hematocrit >65%) and preoperatively to improve hemostasis. Clinical data to justify these recommendations are lacking. Phlebotomy should be followed by the infusion of an equal volume of fluids to maintain intravascular volume and blood flow, as well as to provide a dilutional effect to reduce the hematocrit level. Hydroxyurea therapy has been used occasionally to reduce erythropoiesis in this situation to reduce the need for phlebotomy, but little evidence exists for this approach. The superiority of hydroxyurea therapy versus phlebotomy therapy has not been documented. Hydroxyurea might act not only by suppressing RBC production but also by promoting macrocytic RBC formation, thereby increasing RBC deformability and decreasing RBC adhesiveness.

Chronic oxygen therapy in patients with severe COPD has resulted in relief of hypoxia and a modest reduction in hematocrit levels. Pharmacologic interventions, including theophylline, inhaled nitric oxide, sildenafil, or antagonism of the renin–angiotensin pathway with losartin, may also reduce the degree of pulmonary hypertension or secondary erythrocytosis.

Obstructive Sleep Apnea–Induced Polycythemia

Obstructive sleep apnea syndrome is characterized by repetitive episodes of partial or complete obstruction of airflow during sleep. Common symptoms include loud snoring and breathing pauses observed by a bed partner, feelings of nonrefreshing sleep, and excess daytime sleeping. Although the evidence is largely anecdotal, secondary polycythemia is a widely recognized complication of long-standing sleep apnea, being found in 5–10% of those with nocturnal apnea and hypopnea. Similarly, 25% of those with unexplained polycythemia are subsequently found to have sleep apnea. The mechanism by which sleep apnea causes polycythemia is unclear. Differences in EPO levels between normoxic and hypoxemic patients referred for suspected sleep apnea have not been documented. Obstructive sleep apnea is also associated with an increased risk of developing cardiovascular diseases, including systemic hypertension, pulmonary hypertension, cardiac arrhythmias, atherosclerosis, ischemic heart disease, and stroke. Intermittent hypoxia is thought to be a major cause of cardiovascular complications. These patients undergo repeated episodes of hypoxia and normoxia. The hypoxia leads to ischemia, and the reoxygenation causes a sudden increase of oxygen. This reoxygenation phase results in the production of reactive oxygen species and the promotion of oxidative stress, leading to an inflammatory response and the development of vascular complications.

Conversely, PV may induce central sleep apnea by decreasing cerebral blood flow to diencephalic respiratory centers, and patients so affected can have complete resolution of their sleep disorder with normalization of their blood counts.

Pickwickian Syndrome and Polycythemia

Pickwickian syndrome or obesity–hypoventilation syndrome, seen in morbidly obese individuals, is characterized by chronic hypoxemia and hypercapnia caused by alveolar hypoventilation, with a resultant increase in EPO production, polycythemia, and cor pulmonale. The three principal causes are the high cost of the work of respiration in morbidly obese individuals, dysfunction of the respiratory centers, and repeated episodes of nocturnal obstructive apnea. Effective treatments include surgically induced weight loss, nasal continuous positive airway pressure ventilation, and the respiratory stimulant medroxyprogesterone acetate.

Polycythemia Caused by High Altitude

Polycythemia caused by the hypoxic conditions encountered by high-altitude dwellers would appear at first glance to represent a universal adaptive process to altitude. High altitude results in hyperventilation, alkalosis, and shifting of the O_2 dissociation curve to the left, leading to the impaired release of O_2 from hemoglobin and ultimately tissue hypoxia. This tissue hypoxia results in markedly increased EPO production, leading to increased plasma iron turnover, reticulocytosis, and a rising hematocrit level. Residents of the Andes Mountains who live 4200 m above sea level frequently have 30% higher hematocrit levels than individuals living at sea level.

People native to high altitudes (highlanders) live in a hypobaric hypoxic environment characterized by a low ambient partial pressure of oxygen. In response to this environment, they develop alveolar hypoxia, hypoxemia, and polycythemia. Healthy highlanders develop pulmonary hypertension, right ventricular hypertrophy, and an increased amount of smooth muscle cells in the distal pulmonary arterial branches, which leads to increased pulmonary vascular resistance and pulmonary artery pressure compared with individuals living at sea level. The importance of these structural changes in the pulmonary vasculature in highlanders is confirmed by the slow decline of pulmonary artery pressure, which is normalized after living for 2 years at sea level. Despite these adaptive changes, healthy highlanders are able to perform physical activities similar to or often even more strenuous than those living at sea level. In fact, there are differences in ventilation rates between athletes performing at sea level and those at high altitudes. Ventilation rates of athletes increase normally during exercise at sea level, but relative hypoventilation occurs in highlanders. This relative hypoventilation is characteristic of Andean natives and has been ascribed to desensitization of the carotid bodies to the hypoxic stimulus. The erythrocytosis observed in individuals who reside at high altitudes for relatively short periods of time (days) can also be attributed in part to excessive water loss and contraction of the plasma volume. Total acclimatization of an individual who moves from sea level to a high altitude may actually require years. Individuals who reside at sea level and are acutely exposed to high altitudes are at increased risks of developing deep venous thrombosis, pulmonary infarction, retinal hemorrhage, and ischemic digits because of increased blood viscosity. High-altitude climbers frequently combat these problems by intravenous administration of isotonic saline, with considerable success.

The chronic responses of various ethnic and racial groups to high altitudes are quite variable. Andean natives, known as the Quechua and Ayamara Indians, experience a gradual increase in their hemoglobin levels with age. In addition, hemoglobin values are almost 10% higher in those living at 5500 m above sea level than in those living at 4355 m above sea level. Curiously, their Tibetan and Ethiopian counterparts living at similar altitudes do not respond to the resultant chronic hypoxia by increasing their hematocrits. It has been suggested that high levels of nitrous oxide in the exhaled breath of Tibetans may improve oxygen delivery by inducing vasodilatation and increasing blood flow to tissues, thus making the compensatory increased RBC volume unnecessary. Interestingly, Tibetans and Ethiopians have lived much longer as mountain dwellers than the Quechua or Ayamara Indians, suggesting that extreme elevation of the RBC mass is a maladaptation that Tibetans and Ethiopians have avoided by adopting more physiologic compensatory mechanisms. Many residents of the Tibetan plateau reside at elevations exceeding 4000 m and experience oxygen concentrations that are about 40% lower than experienced at sea level. Human adaptation to a high-altitude environment has been believed to be the result of advantageous genetic mutations and selective pressure.[5] These genetic adaptations are shared by common ancestors within East Asian but not Central and South Asian populations and confer characteristics including adaptation to hypoxia, the absence of CMS, and high offspring survival rates. Polymorphisms in the EPAS1 gene that encodes HIF-2α, and the EGLN1 gene, which encodes PHD2, have been positively selected and have been shown to be associated with the key adaptive features in Tibetans. The putative advantageous haplotypes of EGLN1 and EPAS1 have revealed negative correlations with hemoglobin levels in Tibetans compared with lowlander Han Chinese. Tibetans do not exhibit increased hemoglobin levels at high altitude. A high-frequency missense mutation in the EGLN1 gene, which encodes PHD2, contributes to this adaptive response. A variant in EGLN1, c.[12C>G; 380G>C], has been shown to contribute functionally to the Tibetan high-altitude phenotype. PHD2 triggers the degradation of hypoxia-inducible factors (HIFs). The PHD2 p.[Asp4Glu; Cys127Ser] variant exhibits a lower Km value for oxygen, suggesting that it promotes increased HIF degradation under hypoxic conditions. Whereas hypoxia stimulates the proliferation of WT erythroid progenitors, the proliferation of progenitors with the c.[12C>G; 380G>C] mutation in EGLN1 is significantly impaired under hypoxic culture conditions. The c.[12C>G; 380G>C] mutation abrogates hypoxia-induced and HIF-mediated augmentation of erythropoiesis, which provides a molecular mechanism for the observed protection of Tibetans from polycythemia at high altitude.

This individual variability of elevation of serum EPO levels in high-altitude dwellers and the resultant increase in RBC mass appears widespread. For example, acclimatization to moderately high altitudes when combined with low-altitude training (so-called *living high, training low*) improves sea-level performance in endurance athletes, in part because of the erythropoietic effects of altitude exposure. This substantial individual variability in response to all forms of altitude training correlates with improved athletic performance and with elevation of EPO levels. A large component of this individual variability appears to be related to differences in the peak and rate of decay of the increase in EPO in response to altitude exposure. These observations suggest that genetically determined variables account for individual responses to hypoxia.

Chronic mountain sickness (CMS) is a pathological loss of adaptation to altitude. CMS is a clinical syndrome that occurs in native or lifelong residents living above 2500 m. Anecdotal reports of families or people being particularly susceptible to CMS are frequently cited as evidence that certain individuals have an innate susceptibility to develop CMS. It is characterized by excessive erythrocytosis (females, Hb >19 g/dL; males, Hb >21 g/dL); severe hypoxemia; and in some cases, moderate or severe pulmonary hypertension that may lead to the development of cor pulmonale and congestive heart failure. The clinical picture of CMS gradually disappears after descending to lower altitudes and reappears after returning to high altitudes. The prevalence of CMS is higher in men than women and increases with altitude, aging, associated lung disease, history of smoking, and air pollution. CMS is a public health problem in mountainous regions of the world living above 2500 m. In China alone, 80 million people live above that altitude, but in South America, 35 million people live above 2500 m. The CMS phenotype has been associated with a single-nucleotide polymorphism (SNP) in the Sentrin-specific Protease 1 (SENP1) gene.[6] The SENP1 gene encodes for a protease that regulates the function of hypoxia-relevant transcription factors such as HIF and GATA, and thus might have an erythropoietic regulatory role in CMS through modulation of the expression of EPO or EPOR. Fibroblasts obtained from CMS patients express less SNEP1 protein than their healthy counterparts under hypoxic conditions. SENP1 has been shown to regulate EPO production by regulating the stability of HIF1α during hypoxia, and indeed SENP1$^{-/-}$ mice die of anemia during early life. SENP1 also mediates a positive-feedback loop under hypoxic conditions that is responsible for VEGF production and angiogenesis. The major mechanism underlying the development of CMS is relative alveolar hypoventilation. Healthy highlanders characteristically hyperventilate. A gradual decline in the rate of alveolar ventilation in these individuals leads to progressive loss of adaptation to chronic hypoxia and the development of CMS. The main components of this syndrome include (1) alveolar hypoventilation leading to relative hypercapnia and increasing hypoxemia; (2) excessive polycythemia leading to increased blood viscosity and expansion of the total lung blood volume; (3) pulmonary hypertension and right ventricular hypertrophy that may evolve to hypoxic cor pulmonale and heart failure; and (4) neuropsychiatric symptoms, including sleep disorders, headache, dizziness, and mental fatigue. Physical examination reveals cyanosis of the nail beds, ears, and lips in contrast to the ruddy color that is characteristic of a healthy highlander. In some cases, the face is almost black, and the mucosa and conjunctiva are dark red. The fingers are frequently clubbed, and auscultation of the heart reveals an increased pulmonary second sound. The patients are frequently hypertensive and have evidence of heart failure. Chest radiographic and electrocardiographic findings are characteristic of right atrial and right ventricular hypertrophy. Criteria for the diagnosis of CMS have been published and are useful in identifying CMS patients as well as monitoring their response to treatment.

The definitive treatment for CMS is descent to lower altitudes or sea level. The degree of polycythemia decreases after a few weeks or months, and eventually the hematocrit level returns to sea-level values. Pulmonary hypertension and right ventricular hypertrophy gradually resolve and disappear after 1–2 years of living at sea level. Phlebotomy or isovolemic hemodilution can reduce the excessive erythrocytosis and hyperviscosity, improve oxygenation and leads to relief from symptoms. Due to its transient effects, phlebotomy is not a long-term treatment for CMS. A variety of drugs has also been evaluated for the treatment of patients with CMS. Ten weeks of the respiratory stimulant medroxyprogesterone acetate at doses of 60 mg/day led to a reduction of the hematocrit level from 60% to 52% and an increase in arterial oxygen saturation from 84% to 90% in 17 highlanders with CMS. Medroxyprogesterone use, however, was associated with a loss of libido in men and therefore is infrequently used in this population. Therapy with almitrine, a respiratory stimulant, or enalapril, an ACE inhibitor (10 mg/day for 30 days), has resulted in even more modest reductions of hematocrit levels. Therapy with acetazolamide is the most useful treatment for CMS.

Acetazolamide therapy has been evaluated in two double-blind, placebo-controlled, randomized clinical trials of patients with CMS. Acetazolamide is an inhibitor of carbonic anhydrase and stimulates ventilation by promoting the development of metabolic acidosis. Furthermore, acetazolamide reduces renal EPO production. Patients with CMS were randomized to receive placebo or acetazolamide therapy at a dose of 250 or 500 mg/day for 21 days. Drug therapy at both doses of acetazolamide resulted in reduction of hematocrit levels by 7% ($p < .001$) and serum EPO levels by 50–67% ($p < .1$), with an increase in nocturnal oxygen saturation levels of 5% ($p < .01$). Presently, 250 mg of acetazolamide daily appears to be an inexpensive, nontoxic, and effective therapy for CMS.

Smokers' Polycythemia or Carbon Monoxide-Induced Polycythemia

Smoking is the most common cause of secondary polycythemia. Those affected have a carboxyhemoglobin-induced increase in RBC mass or decrease in plasma volume, either of which is reversible with smoking cessation. Excessive carbon monoxide exposure can also be attributed to exposure to industrial emissions and automobile exhaust. Carbon monoxide binds to hemoglobin with a more than 200-times greater affinity than oxygen, resulting in not only occupation of one of the heme groups of hemoglobin but also an increase in the O_2 affinity by the remaining heme group. Individuals smoking even one pack of cigarettes a day frequently have elevated hematocrit levels. These patients characteristically have normal blood gases and elevation of carboxyhemoglobin levels, resulting in a reduction in $P_{50}O_2$. The elevation of the hematocrit level is reversed with interruption of the smoking behavior. Increased hematocrit levels have been observed in 3–5% of heavy smokers. Although these patients are not immune to thrombotic complications, the number of thromboembolic events is lower than in patients with PV. Polycythemia has also been reported to be associated with hookah use. A hookah is an oriental pipe containing tobacco often mixed with molasses and fruit flavors connected by a long flexible tube that draws the smoke to the bowl of water. Hookah use exposes the user to generous amounts of carbon monoxide, resulting in erythrocytosis.

Postrenal Transplantation Erythrocytosis

Postrenal transplantation erythrocytosis (PTE) is defined as a persistently elevated hematocrit level greater than 51% after renal transplantation without an elevation of the WBC count or platelet count. PTE is a potentially dangerous condition found in approximately 10–15% of renal allograft recipients. PTE usually develops within 8–24 months after a successful renal transplantation and resolves spontaneously within 2 years in about 25% of patients despite persistently good renal allograft function. PTE is more common in males and may recur in the same patient after a second successful renal transplantation. Factors that increase the likelihood of its development are a lack of EPO therapy before transplantation, a history of smoking, diabetes mellitus, transplant-related renal artery stenosis, retention of the native kidney, low serum ferritin levels, and normal or high pretransplantation EPO levels. PTE is also more frequent in patients who do not experience rejection. There is some evidence that the use of cyclosporine as an immunosuppressive agent is associated with increased risk of PTE. At higher hematocrit levels (usually >60%), thrombotic events may complicate the clinical course of patients with PTE.

Approximately 60% of patients with PTE experience malaise, headache, plethora, lethargy, and dizziness. In addition, from 10% to 20% develop thromboembolic complications involving either arteries or veins. Retention of the native kidney is essential for the development of PTE in most cases. Although the transplanted kidney produces EPO under normal regulatory mechanisms, the native kidney overproduces EPO despite the development of erythrocytosis.

Frequently, the PTE resolves with removal of the native kidney. Plasma EPO levels can be normal or high in patients with PTE

The molecular basis of PTE remains unclear; AngII is believed, however, to play an important role in its pathogenesis by sustaining the secretion of EPO. Growing evidence indicates that increased AT1R expression makes erythroid progenitor cells hypersensitive to AngII. Furthermore, AngII can modulate release of erythropoietic stimulatory factors, including EPO and IGF-1. Androgens are thought to play a role in the development of the syndrome. Androgens can directly affect erythroid progenitor cells or stimulate EPO production or actually the RAS. Treatment of patients with PTE includes intermittent phlebotomy or administration of drugs. The ACE inhibitor enalapril suppresses the renin–angiotensin pathway and virtually eliminates the need for therapeutic phlebotomy in these patients. Maximal reduction of hemoglobin levels is evident 6 months after starting therapy with either ACE inhibitor or angiotensin receptor blockers. Some patients are exquisitely sensitive to these medications and may become severely anemic. The AT1R antagonist losartan has been shown to be as effective in treating PTE as are ACE inhibitors. Therapy is usually begun at hematocrit levels above 55% with the hope of maintaining hematocrit levels below 50% to reduce the risk of thrombosis. Furthermore, the ACE inhibitor fosinopril in an open-label crossover trial with theophylline was shown to produce a dramatic reduction in hematocrits in patients with PTE (51.3–43.7%; $p < .005$). Low doses of ramipril, another ACE inhibitor, normalized the hematocrit level in 26 out of 27 patients with PTE after a mean of 127 days of therapy.

Polycythemia Accompanying Kidney and Liver Diseases and Neoplastic Disorders

Polycythemia has been reported in association with kidney diseases such as renal cell carcinoma, renal artery stenosis, hydronephrosis, Wilms tumor, and polycystic kidney disease, paragangliomas, and pituitary adenomas. Renal tumors account for approximately one-third of cases of tumor-associated polycythemias. The tumor tissue has been demonstrated to produce excessive amounts of EPO, and the erythrocytosis resolves with surgical resections of the tumor. The mechanisms underlying the activation of the *EPO* gene have been related to somatic mutations of the *VHL* gene in clear-cell renal carcinomas. Clear-cell carcinoma is associated with erythrocytosis and high serum EPO levels caused by increased expression of EPO mRNA, HIF-1α, and HIF-2α. These abnormalities were related to a point mutation in the *VHL* gene that impaired the bindings of HIF-1α to VHL, leading to its accumulation and increased production of EPO. Polycythemia is also a well-described paraneoplastic manifestation of hepatocellular carcinoma in 2.5–10% of patients and is again caused by the production of EPO by the tumor. Polycythemia in hepatoma patients is strongly related to tumor burden and elevated α-fetoprotein levels. Polycythemia has also been associated with cerebellar hemangioblastomas and very large uterine fibromas. In tumor-associated erythrocytosis, EPO production has been shown to be autonomous of hypoxic stimuli. Paragangliomas are tumors arising from extraadrenal paraganglial neural crest cells. Most paragangliomas arise retroperitoneally or within the peritoneal cavity and are associated with high EPO levels and erythrocytosis. After tumor resection, reduction of the EPO levels and erythrocytosis occurs. Germ-line mutations involving two Krebs cycle enzymes, fumarate hydratase and succinate dehydrogenase, have been implicated in the hereditary paraganglioma–pheochromocytoma syndrome. In tumors deficient in these enzymes fumarate and succinate accumulate, which inhibits PHD, leading to accumulation of HIF-1α and eventually resulting in erythrocytosis. In another patient with a paraganglioma who did not have the inherited syndrome but had extreme erythrocytosis, a germ-line mutation in *PHD2* was demonstrated. In this patient's tumor, tumor analysis showed LOH with the mutant allele predominating, which was associated with a loss of function. The degradation of both HIF-1α and HIF-2α was decreased. These data indicate that PHD2 can act as a tumor suppressor gene. The tumor suppressor activity of PHD2 has also been reported in sporadic endometrial, breast, and pancreatic cancers, with inactivating mutations ultimately leading to the increased production of growth factors that contribute to tumor growth. Two plasma cell dyscrasias, POEMS (**P**olyneuropathy, **O**rganomegaly, **E**ndocrinopathy, **M**onoclonal protein, **S**kin changes) syndrome and TEMPI (**T**elangiectasias, **E**rythrocytosis with elevated erythropoietin levels, **M**onoclonal gammopathy of unknown significance [MGUS], **P**erinephric fluid collections, and **I**ntrapulmonary shunting syndrome) have been recently been reported to be associated with erythrocytosis. Treatment is directed at the underlying disease. In TEMPI syndrome, the most effective treatment has been bortezomib, which suggests that TEMPI syndrome is a consequence of the abnormal plasma cell clone.

Polycythemia in Endocrine Disorders

Polycythemia is also associated with Cushing syndrome, acromegaly, and primary aldosteronism. Secondary polycythemia can also be seen in 24% of older hypogonadal men receiving long-term androgen-replacement therapy and a significant number of competitive athletes taking anabolic steroids. For instance, in a small study of professional bodybuilders, 67% of those examined had hematocrit levels above 50%. The effectiveness of drug screening in athletic competitions is demonstrated by the very low rate of positive test results for androgens (<2% of 170,000 tests) on random testing at the Olympic Games and other international events. Despite previous assertions regarding increased EPO excretion after androgen therapy, none of the athletes examined had elevated levels of EPO. Recombinant human EPO has also been abused by athletes competing in endurance sports and can be detected by analyzing the individual's hematocrit level, reticulocyte count, percentage of macrocytic RBCs, serum EPO level, serum transferrin receptor level, and electrophoretic mobility of the EPO molecule (recombinant EPO is less negatively charged than endogenous EPO).

Congenital Secondary Polycythemias

High-Oxygen-Affinity Hemoglobins and Bisphosphoglycerate Deficiency

More than 100 mutations of hemoglobin lead to increased oxygen affinity and thus decreased oxygen delivery and compensatory polycythemia (see Chapter 43). These mutations involve either the α- or β-chain globin chains.[7] Such polycythemias are usually well tolerated in young patients but may lead to thrombotic complications in older patients. High-oxygen–affinity hemoglobin variants are transmitted as autosomal dominants. Phlebotomy therapy of such patients has been reported to not be of any beneficial value and has been shown to decrease exercise tolerance. The best test to detect high-oxygen–affinity hemoglobin relies on the determination of hemoglobin dissociation kinetics and P_{50} (partial pressure of O_2 at which hemoglobin is 50% oxygenated). If cooximetry is not available, the P_{50} can be mathematically estimated from a venous blood gas measurement by using a computer algorithm, which is available online.

Whereas a $P_{50}O_2$ below 17 mmHg is indicative of a mutant hemoglobin with high oxygen affinity, a level above 35 mmHg is strongly suggestive of a mutant hemoglobin with a low oxygen affinity. Hemoglobin electrophoresis is not a reliable screen to rule out such a hemoglobin mutation because only about half of these mutants are electrophoretically distinguishable. Hemoglobin electrophoresis will reveal the presence of an abnormal hemoglobin only if the mutation leads to a change in electrical charge. If such a charge differential is not present, high-performance liquid chromatography or mass spectrometry followed by polymerase chain reaction (PCR)-directed sequencing will be required to establish the diagnosis.

A rare cause of congenital polycythemia is 2,3-bisphosphoglycerate (2,3-BPG; previously known as *2,3-DPG*) deficiency (see Chapter 44). 2,3-BPG is synthesized in RBCs and binds to hemoglobin, thereby reducing its affinity for oxygen. An absence of 2,3-BPG

therefore leads to increased affinity of hemoglobin for oxygen, resulting in a lifelong hypoxic stimulus and erythrocytosis.

Congenital methemoglobinemias, whether caused by cytochrome b5 reductase mutations or globin mutations, may be associated with mild polycythemia (see Chapter 43). When hemoglobin is oxidized to methemoglobin, all of the four subunits of the tetramer may be affected, eliminating the oxygen transport capacity of hemoglobin.

Hypoxia-Inducible Factor Pathway Mutations Leading to Erythrocytosis

Alterations of a number of proteins in the HIF pathway have been shown to lead to increased EPO production and erythrocytosis (see Fig. 68.1). Chuvash polycythemia (CP) is an autosomal recessive disorder associated with germ-line mutations of *VHL* and erythrocytosis. CP was first described in the mid-1970s and is endemic in the Chuvash population of the Russian republic. The serum EPO concentration in affected individuals is elevated compared with healthy first-degree family members, although some patients may have normal serum EPO levels. They also have elevated levels of VEGF and plasminogen activator inhibitor-1. The erythroid progenitors of patients with CP are also hypersensitive to EPO; thus, CP has characteristics of both primary and secondary polycythemias. A homozygous missense mutation in the *VHL* gene, VHL598C→T mutation, has been identified in CP patients. The disorder is characterized by high hemoglobin levels (usually >20 g/L), increased plasma EPO levels, varicose veins, vertebral hemangiomas, low blood pressure, and an elevated concentration of VEGF. The defective *VHL* gene product is not capable of promoting the ubiquitin-mediated degradation of HIF-1α and HIF-2α, thereby leading to increased levels of both of these proteins and increased elaboration of EPO. The CP-VHL mutants have been shown to affect EPO signaling in erythroid progenitor cells of patients with CP. JAK2 phosphorylation of STAT5 triggers not only erythroid progenitor development but also a negative feedback mechanism by transactivating the expression of SOCS family members, which bind and inhibit activated JAKs by promoting their ubiquination and protosomal degradation. The CP mutation causes conformational changes, leading to a tight CP–VHL–SOCS-1 association, thereby slowing phosphorylated JAK2 degradation. These events lead to hyperactivation of the JAK2–STAT pathway in erythroid progenitor cells, causing their hypersensitivity to EPO, which likely contributes to the excessive erythrocytosis characteristic of CP. Inheritance occurs as an autosomal recessive, and the frequency of the allele has been estimated to be at 0.057 in the Chuvash population. Several other similar types of mutations in VHL have been described that have been observed in a variety of other ethnic groups. A number of heterozygotes with erythrocytosis have been reported, which can likely be accounted for by an as yet undiscovered additional defect. CP is associated with a high mortality rate from thrombotic and hemorrhagic vascular complications. Most patients complain of chronic headache, fatigue, and/or lower extremity pain, and are noted to have lower blood pressures. Cerebrovascular events are especially common causes of death. The median age of death from cerebrovascular events is 42 years. Estimated survival to age 65 years is 29% for individuals with CP and 64% for age-matched community members. There is a perfect genotype–phenotypic correlation, with all patients with CP being homozygotes for the mutation. Interestingly, heterozygous carriers do not develop erythrocytosis but do have lower blood pressures and do not seem to be at increased risk for tumors, which contrasts with patients with VHL syndrome. Patients with CP also have larger livers, spleens, and kidneys than control patients, which has been attributed to enhanced cellular proliferation caused by HIF-2α suppression of p21Cip1.

Germ-line mutations of *VHL* alleles have been reported in several patients with apparent congenital polycythemia that had no evidence of developing a tumor; some of these subjects had germ-line mutations of both *VHL* alleles. Other subjects with congenital polycythemia of various ethnicities, including Pakistanis, Punjabis, African–Americans, and whites, harboring homozygosity for the CP

VHL mutation or double heterozygosity for CP and other *VHL* mutations, have been found. The VHL598C→T mutation has been shown to originate in a single haplotype in the Chuvash patients, as well as in whites, Asian Indians, and one African–American individual. Homozygosity of this mutation appears to be the most common genetic defect leading to congenital polycythemia. The mutation originated from a single founder 12,000–51,000 years ago. This suggests that such wide dissemination from the original founder may be associated with some survival advantage for heterozygotes carrying this mutation. Such an advantage might be related to a subtle improvement of iron metabolism, erythropoiesis, embryonic development, energy metabolism, or some other yet unknown effect.

VHL mutations are likely the most common cause of congenital polycythemias, greatly exceeding the number of patients with hemoglobin chain mutations. In point of fact, in one study of more than 200 unrelated subjects with apparently congenital polycythemia, none had a 2,3-BPG deficiency, two had a globin mutation (Hgb Vanderbilt, and Hemoglobin San Diego), and 12 had *EPOR* mutations to account for their polycythemia. By contrast, when 50 patients were examined for the *VHL* mutation, 22 had *VHL* mutations, most of them being the CP *VHL* mutation, occurring either homozygously or in combination with another *VHL* mutation. The failure of patients with CP to develop VHL syndrome tumors is consistent with the concept that dysregulation of H1F-1α and VEGF are not sufficient to cause tumors. A cluster of patients with clinical features identical to patients with CP has been documented on the island of Ischia in the Bay of Naples, Italy. All of these patients also had the VHL598C→T mutation. Twelve of the 14 patients were homozygotes, and two were heterozygotes. The homozygotes had symptoms identical to patients in Chuvashia with this mutation. Unlike heterozygotes in Chuvashia, the heterozygotes from Ischia developed erythrocytosis associated with high EPO levels, which raises the possibility that genetic alterations of additional components of the oxygen-sensing pathway other than VHL may contribute to the development of erythrocytosis in the Italian patients. The disorder in Ischia has a gene frequency even higher than that in Chuvashia, with 14% of the population estimated to be heterozygotes, which has led to the suggestion that heterozygotes have a survival advantage, perhaps caused by heterozygosity conferring protection from developing anemia.

The Chuvash mutation has also been shown to have a profound effect on the cardiopulmonary system. Patients with CP have significant abnormalities of cardiopulmonary physiology, including elevated basal ventilation rates and increased pulmonary vascular tone, with extremely high ventilatory rates and heightened pulmonary vasoconstriction and heart rates in response to acute hypoxia. These observations indicate that the VHL–HIF pathway might also play a central role in calibrating the pulmonary system to hypoxic challenges. Such undesirable exaggerated hypoxic responses and the resulting elevated pulmonary vascular hypertension may contribute to the morbidity and mortality associated with CP. Increased expression of endothelin-1 has been documented in patients with CP. Endothelin-1 has been associated with the development of hypoxia-related pulmonary hypertension. Endothelin-1 receptor inhibitors might therefore be useful in reversing the associated pulmonary hypertension in these patients. Treatment strategies for patients with CP have included phlebotomy, aspirin, and occasionally chemotherapy. Most patients are treated empirically with phlebotomy therapy, but at present it remains unknown if this approach reduces the incidence of thrombotic incidences or improves the quality of life.

Additional genetic abnormalities of oxygen sensing have been reported that lead to familial polycythemia. A heterozygous C-to-G change at base 950 of the coding sequence of *PHD2* (*P317R* mutation) was first detected in all three affected family members with this syndrome. Hydroxylation of HIF-1 by PHD2 facilitates its interaction with VHL, thereby favoring its ubiquitination and degradation by the proteosome.[8] The failure of *PHD2 P317R* to bind HIF-1 and HIF-2α and promote HIF hydroxylase activity ultimately leads to increased HIF-1 and EPO levels, resulting in the development of erythrocytosis. The *PHD2 P317R* mutation is inherited as an autosomal dominant trait in contrast to the CP defect, which is an

autosomal recessive disorder. Polycythemic patients with *PHD2 P317R* do not have any evidence of tumors characteristic of the VHL syndrome. Additional mutations in *PHD2* have been reported that lead to erythrocytosis. All of these mutations are germ-line and heterozygous, encoding predicted mutant full-length PHD2 proteins. A series of HIF-2α gain-of-function mutations have also been reported to lead to familial erythrocytosis. These mutations lead to weakened bonds between PHD2 and HIF-1α, resulting in less hydroxylation of HIF-1α and subsequent recognition of HIF-1α by VHL. Many of these patients present in their twenties, although patients have also been diagnosed in their fifties with erythrocytosis associated with high EPO levels. All patients have heterozygous mutations, suggesting that one allele is sufficient to cause erythrocytosis. It is not unusual for patients to have a clinical history of thrombotic disorders, but there does not appear to be an increased incidence of cancer.

Neonatal Polycythemia

Because of the high oxygen affinity of fetal hemoglobin, many neonates have markedly elevated hematocrit levels. Babies with hematocrit levels over 65% have more neurologic and functional impairments, and are more likely to be born to diabetic mothers. Although phlebotomy has been recommended, there is little evidence that it has been beneficial for these babies.

Drug-Induced Erythrocytosis

The administration of EPO, corticosteroids, or androgens to an excessive degree has each been associated with reversible erythrocytosis. Androgens have been shown to simulate EPO production and to directly affect erythroid progenitor cells. Approximately 5% of patients receiving long-term testosterone therapy for testosterone-deficiency syndrome develop erythrocytosis. Androgens activate HIF-1 and HIF-1-regulated gene expression, leading to increased expression of VEGF and presumably EPO. Rarely, erythrocytosis can be the presenting manifestation of Cushing syndrome. Blood doping refers to the use of EPO to increase the RBC mass and enhance oxygen delivery with the hope of increasing endurance performance in athletes. A monitoring of an athlete's hematologic profile longitudinally provides some insight into the likelihood of blood doping playing a role in the development of erythrocytosis

The development of paradoxical polycythemia in three patients with VHL syndrome and CNS or retinal hemangioblastomas treated with a VEGF receptor inhibitor has been reported. The cause of these phenomena remains unknown. In addition, reversible paradoxical erythrocytosis has been reported with the use of VEGF tyrosine kinase inhibitors, including sunitinib, sorafenib, axitinib, pazopanin, and the anti-VEGF monoclonal antibody bevacizumab, primarily in patients with renal cell carcinomas. These patients become symptomatic due to fatigue, pruritis, myalgias, headaches, and malignant hypertension. The cause of the erythrocytosis associated with these drugs has been attributed to either elevation of EPO levels or sensitization of erythroid cells to EPO. The erythrocytosis in this situation can be controlled with phlebotomy therapy with relief of symptoms.

POLYCYTHEMIA VERA

PV is a clonal, chronic, progressive myeloproliferative neoplasm (MPN) often of insidious onset characterized by an absolute increase in RBC mass and often by leukocytosis, thrombocytosis, and splenomegaly. PV leads to excessive proliferation of erythroid, myeloid, and megakaryocytic elements within the BM. Vaquez first described this clinical entity in 1892, noting the characteristic physical findings. At the turn of this century, Cabot and Osler independently associated the name PV with this clinical disorder.

PV differs from many other hematologic malignancies in that prolonged survival is enjoyed by most patients if the excessive production of RBCs and platelets can be controlled. This prolonged survival, however, can be punctuated by the development of other syndromes,

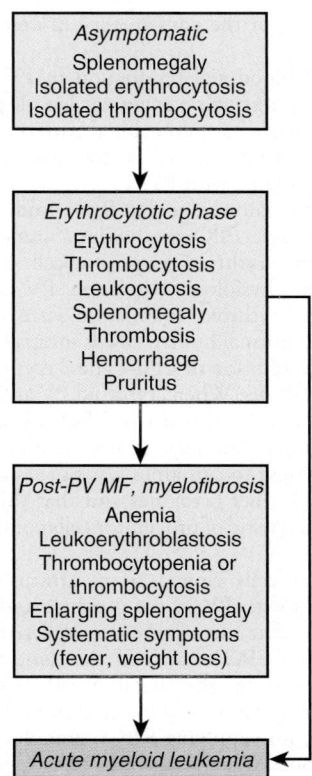

Fig. 68.3 EVOLUTION OF POLYCYTHEMIA VERA. *MF,* Myelofibrosis; *PV,* polycythemia vera.

such as myelofibrosis (MF), termed *post-PV MF,* and acute leukemia (Fig. 68.3). Frequently, patients present asymptomatically to a physician only to find that they have splenomegaly, isolated erythrocytosis, or thrombocytosis. Left untreated, these patients will become symptomatic owing to the excessive production of RBCs, platelets, or both, leading to arterial or venous thromboses, aquagenic pruritus, and symptoms caused by increasing splenomegaly. After a number of years, the erythrocytotic phase of the disease frequently becomes inactive, and the patient may no longer have the sequelae of excessive RBC production. Subsequently, these patients can develop post-PV MF, which is frequently indistinguishable from another MPN, primary MF (PMF). Finally, a significant proportion of these patients will go on to develop acute myeloid leukemia (AML). Only a limited number of patients undergo this orderly transition; many patients transition from the polycythemic phase directly into an acute leukemia or a myelodysplastic disorder.[9]

The transition from one phase of this MPN to another is not necessarily unidirectional. About 10–15% of patients with *JAK2V617F*-positive essential thrombocythemia eventually develop erythrocytosis and are reclassified as having PV. A number of cases of presumed PMF either spontaneously or after chemotherapy have been described where the patient develops erythrocytosis and a syndrome that is virtually indistinguishable from de novo PV. The constantly changing clinical picture of this malignant hematologic disorder requires careful observation and treatment to deal with the numerous problems that can be encountered.

Epidemiology

PV is the most common primary polycythemia. Incidence rates (IRs) have been reported to be around 2.8 per 100,000 persons per year. It is important to emphasize that no or very few population-based estimates of the prevalence of this disorder are presently available. Actual determination of its prevalence has been a difficult process because of the need in the past to pursue an extensive diagnostic

evaluation to differentiate this disorder from other causes of spurious or absolute erythrocytosis. The diagnosis of PV has been simplified by the identification of PV-associated mutations (*JAK2V617F* and *JAK2* exon 12 mutations), permitting for the first time molecular epidemiologic studies. The prevalence of the *JAK2V617F* mutation in a normal population in Denmark was recently determined to be 0.2%, with 63% of these individuals not having a previously detected hematological malignancy. The presence of the mutation was associated with increasing age, male sex, and a lower cumulative survival. Recently available 2001–2012 data from the Surveillance, Epidemiology and End Results (SEER) Program from the US National Cancer Institute provided new insight into the IR of the MPNs. This study utilized the WHO Diagnostic Criteria and for the last 5 years of the study *JAK2V617F* testing was included. The age adjusted IR of PV and essential thrombocythemia (ET) were 10.9 and 9.4 per 1 million per year, respectively. The IR for PMF was 3.1. In order to grasp the magnitude of the IR of these various MPNs, the IR of CML was 3.3, demonstrating that the IR of these Ph⁻ MPNs were sevenfold higher than CML. Both PV and PMF were more frequent in males while the IR for ET was greater in females. Several groups have reported that 50% of patients with a splanchnic vein thrombosis without an overt MPN are *JAK2V617F* positive and that more than 50% of these individuals subsequently develop an MPN. However, the incidence of the mutation with unprovoked thromboembolism in the more usual sites (deep venous thrombosis involving the leg veins or pulmonary embolism) ranges between 0.2 and 1.0%. Such data have led to the conclusion that systematic screening for *JAK2V617* in such a patient population is not warranted.

The prevalence of PV has been reported by several investigators to be higher among American Jews and lower among African–Americans and Hispanics. The reported lower incidence in African–Americans might reflect a referral bias characteristic of centers with research interest in MPN because the authors, when practicing in several large urban areas, have observed a considerable number of African–Americans with MPNs, including PV. The incidence of the disorder is greater among Ashkenazi Jews, who originate from eastern and central Europe, than among Arabs and Sephardic Jews. Interestingly, extremely low occurrence rates have been reported from Japan. These findings suggest that important genetic factors might be involved in the biogenesis of this disorder. The importance of genetic factors in the origin of this disease is further emphasized by reports of multiple cases of *JAK2V617F* or *JAK2* exon 12 mutation-positive and -negative MPN, including PV, within multiple generations of a number of families. These forms of familial PV must be distinguished from PFCP, CP, and polycythemia associated with mutations in the HIF pathway. The reports of families in which multiple members have PV first raised the possibility that a genetic predisposition to acquire such mutations exists in these families that is inherited in an autosomal dominant pattern with decreased penetrance. Clinical analyses of affected family members confirmed that they have clonal hematopoiesis and that their clinical manifestations are identical to patients with sporadic PV. In a large population study from Sweden, the ratives of MPN patients were shown to have a significantly increased risk of developing a Ph⁻ MPN and possibly chronic myeloid leukemia.[10] It was estimated that first-degree relatives of MPN patients have a five- to sevenfold greater risk of developing an MPN, again supporting the hypothesis that common strong susceptibility genes predispose one to develop PV, essential thrombocytosis (ET), PMF, and possibly CML.

One notable exception to the low prevalence of PV in Japan has been the higher incidence observed among populations exposed to atomic bomb explosions. The possibility that radiation exposure is an etiologic factor in the generation of PV was also raised by the observation in the United States of four cases of PV 10–20 years after the Smokey nuclear weapons test in which 3000 military observers were exposed. An epidemiologic investigation that focused on occupational exposure among petroleum refinery and chemical plant workers has revealed an increased incidence of PV relative to the general population. In this study, the increased incidence of PV was linked to similar increases in the frequency of multiple myeloma and non-Hodgkin lymphoma, suggesting involvement of a putative environmental toxin that may have broad hematopoietic toxicity. The possibility of environmental factors contributing to the development of PV was recently raised by the identification of a cluster of patients with *JAK2V617F*-positive PV in an area of Eastern Pennsylvania that contained numerous sources of hazardous materials including, waste coal power plants and United States Environmental Protection Agency Superfund sites. What possible environmental factors might contribute to this fourfold increase in the number of PV cases is currently the subject of intense investigation.

In several large studies, 5% of patients with PV were younger than 40 years of age, 1% were younger than 25 years at diagnosis, and 0.1% were younger than 20 years. Small numbers of patients with PV have been reported who presented during childhood. Interestingly, females comprise the majority of PV patients diagnosed before the age of 40 years, suggesting a unique risk factor for developing the disease at early age.[11] These young female patients tend to present with unique complications such as abdominal venous thrombosis and their risk of transformation to MF or AML is similar to older patients.

The *JAK2V617F* mutation has a prevalence of 0.1–0.2% in the general population. These individuals usually have an allele burden of less than 10%. Some these patients have an undiagnosed MPN or represent an early molecular stage of a MPN, which will evolve over time. Those normal individuals with an allele burden of <2% likely have a latent form of an MPN.

Pathobiology

Considerable speculation has centered on the pathobiology of the erythrocytosis that characterizes PV. The expanded RBC mass in PV patients is due to a two- to threefold increase in the production of RBCs by a hyperplastic BM and is not attributable to prolongation of the RBC lifespan. Granulocyte and platelet production are also increased in this disorder. This overly exuberant production of all cellular elements of the blood suggests that the basic defect resides at the level of the pluripotent hematopoietic stem cell (HSC).

Serum EPO levels have been shown to be subnormal in patients with PV, elevated in many but not all cases of secondary erythrocytosis, and normal in patients with relative polycythemia, indicating that PV cannot be an abnormality of EPO production.

In 1951, Dameshek postulated that chronic myeloid leukemia, PV, essential thrombocythemia, and PMF were related disorders, which he called *myeloproliferative disorders*, but are now termed *MPNs* because of the evidence that these disorders are hematologic malignancies.

Since the mid-1970s, data have accumulated that conclusively demonstrate PV to be the result of a neoplastic proliferation of hematopoietic cells. The cellular origin of the disorder was first established by the analysis of glucose-6-phosphate dehydrogenase (G6PD) isoenzymes in African–American women who were heterozygous for this X-linked gene. This approach was based on the random irreversible inactivation of one X chromosome in each female somatic cell during embryogenesis. Inactivation of the same X chromosome occurs in the progeny of these cells. A normal African–American female heterozygous for G6PD will therefore have approximately equal populations of BM cells with a different G6PD isoenzyme. The G6PD isoenzymes can be readily distinguished by electrophoretic methods.

This approach was exploited in a seminal study by Adamson and coworkers in an effort to determine the cellular origin of PV. They presumed that cells comprising a tumor that arises from a single cell in a G6PD heterozygote would express a single isoenzyme type, but a neoplasm originating from multiple cells would express both isoenzyme types. These investigators found that circulating RBCs, granulocytes, and platelets obtained from African–American female patients who were G6PD heterozygotes express the same isoenzyme, but skin and cultured BM fibroblasts obtained from these same patients demonstrate both isoenzymes. They concluded that PV represented a clonal proliferation of neoplastic HSCs and was not

multicellular in origin or the consequence of excessive proliferation of normal HSCs.

The clonality of blood cell production in PV has subsequently been confirmed using restriction fragment length polymorphisms of the active X chromosome. A monoclonal pattern of X chromosome inactivation has been defined in RBCs, granulocytes, monocytes, and platelets in female patients with PV.

On the basis of the knowledge that RBC production in PV is not associated with excessive EPO production, numerous investigators hypothesized that the erythroid progenitor cell in this disorder was no longer subject to physiologic regulators. PV BM can form substantial numbers of erythroid colonies in vitro in the absence of exogenous EPO, but normal human BM is incapable of forming such colonies without the addition of EPO. These erythroid colonies were termed *endogenous colonies*. When erythroid PV and normal BM were subsequently assayed in the presence of EPO, PV BM was characterized by a higher cloning efficiency. Additional observations suggested that the altered response to cytokines was not restricted to EPO but included a variety of other cytokines and that this cytokine hypersensitivity was characteristic of progenitor cells committed to a variety of other lineages.

In addition, BM cells cloned from African–American female G6PD heterozygotes with PV in the presence and absence of exogenous EPO revealed that the erythroid colonies that formed in the absence of exogenous EPO contained the same G6PD isoenzyme type as that expressed by peripheral blood elements. Thus, the so-called *endogenous erythroid colonies* arose from the abnormal clone that was responsible for supplying RBCs, granulocytes, and platelets to the peripheral blood. When exogenous EPO was added, increasing numbers of colonies were formed containing cellular elements expressing the other G6PD isoenzymes; presumably, these colonies originated from cells not involved in the malignant process. Similarly, small numbers of granulocyte–macrophage colonies not originating from the PV clone were also observed in these assays. These data collectively indicate the existence of malignant and nonmalignant populations of HPCs in PV BM. The relative frequency of the neoplastic clone in relation to normal progenitor cells was further examined by Adamson and coworkers, who, by monitoring the proportion of neoplastic erythroid clones and their numeric relationship to normal clones over a period of several years, showed disease progression to be associated with a significant decline in the frequency of normal progenitor cells and increasing proportion of the neoplastic clone. Erythroid progenitor cells from PV patients are, in fact, abnormally sensitive to the actions of this EPO. This increased responsiveness allows these cells to form colonies in the presence of small amounts of EPO. Most PV patients possess two distinct populations of erythroid progenitor cells: a normally EPO-responsive population and a population of cells similar in proliferative and maturational behavior in vitro but requiring little or no EPO. These investigators suggested that the proliferation of the normal progenitor cells in vivo was at a disadvantage. A number of investigators have demonstrated that the increased responsiveness of these BM progenitor populations extends to their responses to other cytokines, including SCF, IL-3, GM-CSF, and IGF-1.

Identification of *JAK2V617F* Mutation in PV

For more than two decades a number of research groups searched for the genetic defect underlying PV. Most groups predicted that this defect involved the signaling pathways downstream of the EPOR. These pathways include the tyrosine kinase JAK2 and the transcriptional signal transducers and activators of transcription, STAT3 and STAT5. The initial discovery of a mutation was predicated on a somewhat simplistic yet revealing set of experiments performed by Vainchenker and colleagues in France.[12] They observed that the inhibition of JAK2 by a small molecule (AG490) or by small interfering RNA (siRNA) reduced EPO-independent colony formation by PV BM mononuclear cells. This observation prompted them to directly sequence JAK2 in the hematopoietic cells of PV patients and

A

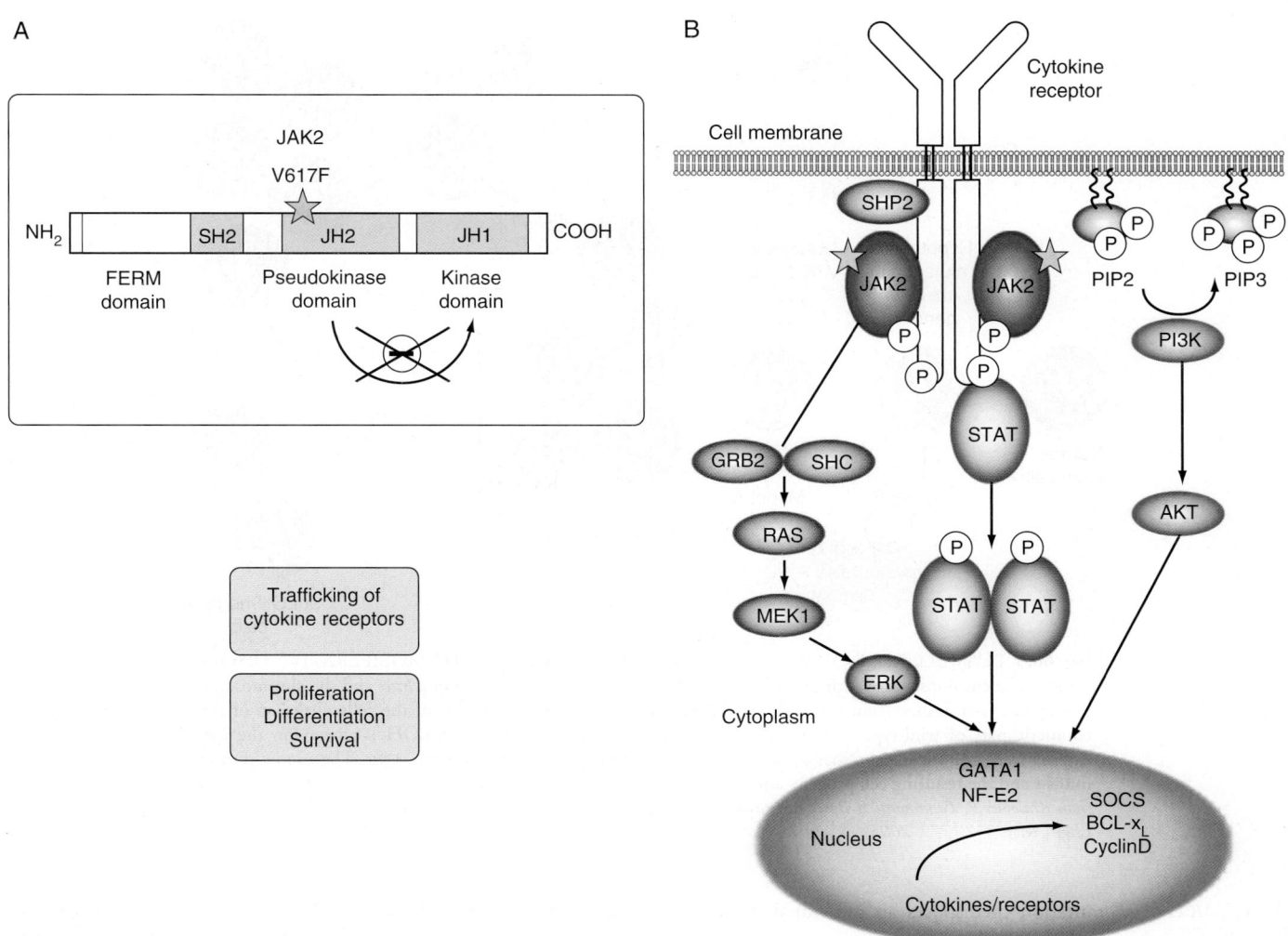

B

Fig. 68.4 *JAK2V617F* SIGNALING IN MYELOPROLIFERATIVE DISORDERS. (A) Structure of *JAK2V617F*: the mutation is located in pseudokinase JAK JH2 and disrupts the autoinhibition of this regulatory domain. Consequently, the tyrosine kinase corresponding to the JH1 domain is constitutively activated. (B) In the presence of a homodimeric cytokine receptor (e.g., erythropoietin receptor), the two *JAK2V617F* proteins bound to the intracellular domain of the receptor transphosphorylate its tyrosine residues. In turn, STAT5, PI3K, and RAS signaling pathways are activated, leading to the downstream modulation of transcription and protein levels for cell cycle, proliferation, and apoptosis-related factors. *Bcl-X_L*, B-cell lymphoma-extra large; *ERK*, extracellular signal-related kinase; *GATA*, GATA-binding factor; *GRB*, growth factor receptor-bound protein; *JAK*, Janus kinase; *JH2*, JAK homology domain 2; *MEK1*, dual specificity mitogen-activated protein kinase kinase 1; *NF*, nuclear factor; *P*, Phosphate; *PI3K*, phosphatidylinositol 3-kinase; *PIP2* and *PIP3*, phosphatidylinositol bi- and triphosphate; *RAS*, renin–angiotensin system; *SH2*, src homology 2; *SOCS*, suppressor of cytokine signaling; STAT, signal transducer and activator of transcription. *(From Delhommeau F, Pisani DF, James C, et al: Oncogenic mechanisms in myeloproliferative disorders. Cell Mol Life Sci 6363:2939, 2006.)*

to discover a single recurrent point mutation. A guanine-to-thymine mutation was observed that resulted in a substitution of valine to phenylalanine at codon 617 within the pseudokinase domain (JH2) of *JAK2* (*JAK2V617F*; Fig. 68.4). These findings were quickly confirmed by several different groups. Kralovics et al[13] had previously identified a region of LOH on chromosome 9p in PV and identified a 6.2-Mbp region common to all PV patients screened. Because this region contained *JAK2*, with its known role in erythropoiesis, it was screened for mutations and the same *JAK2V617F* mutation identified. Three other groups targeted *JAK2* as part of a global sequencing screen of tyrosine kinases and phosphatases in MPNs. *JAK2V617F* is an acquired somatic mutation present exclusively in hematopoietic cells. All patients with PV have a population of erythroid progenitor cells that are homozygous for the mutation. Using quantitative PCR, patients can be divided into those with a low allele burden of *JAK2V617F* in granulocytes (<50%) and patients with a

higher burden of *JAK2V617F* (>50%). A subset of patients with PV are homozygous for *JAK2V617F*, which is the result of mitotic recombination and duplication of the mutant allele (Fig. 68.5). The occurrence of mitotic recombination has been observed during the clinical course of individual patients, leading to *JAK2V617F* heterozygous patients becoming homozygous over time. The concept of the conversion of *JAK2V617F* low burden to high burden is further supported by the observation that the median duration of disease at the time of evaluation was 48 months in high-burden PV patients compared with 23 months in low-burden PV. These observations are consistent with a multistep pathogenesis of PV. The first step consists of the acquisition of *JAK2V617F*, which results in a low allele burden of *JAK2V617F*, followed by a second step, homologous recombination, that leads to *JAK2V617F* homozygous progenitor cells and eventually granulocytes with a high burden of *JAK2V617F*. It remains unknown at present if a lesion occurring before acquisition

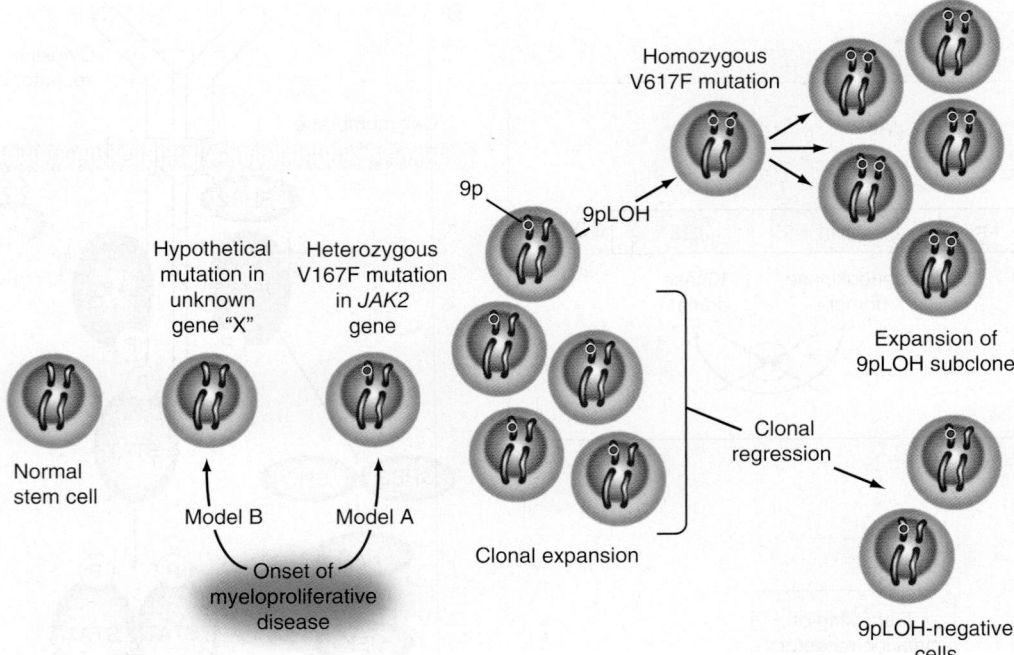

Fig. 68.5 POSSIBLE ROLE OF *JAK2V617F* IN THE BIOLOGY OF MYELOPROLIFERATIVE DISORDERS. The chromosome 9 with the wild-type *JAK2* sequence (G) is depicted in *white*, and the chromosome 9 with the G–T transversion (T) is shown in *red*. *Circles* symbolize the nuclei of the cells. Deletion of the telomeric part of wild-type chromosome 9p as a potential mechanism for 9pLOH is shown on the *left*. Alternatively, mitotic recombination could also result in 9pLOH, shown on the *right*. The events during mitosis and the resulting cell progeny after mitotic recombination of chromosome 9p are also shown. (*Adapted from Kralovics R, Passamonti F, Buser AS, et al: A gain-of-function mutation of JAK2 in myeloproliferative disorders. N Engl J Med 352:1779, 2005.*)

of the *JAK2V617F* mutation predisposes an individual to acquire *JAK2V617F*.

The mutational frequency of *JAKV617F* in PV is greater than 95% of cases. Approximately 50–60% of patients with ET and PMF are also *JAK2V617F* positive. ET is distinguished from PV by being associated with a low allele burden. In the overwhelming majority of cases, PV is characterized by a population of *JAK2V617F* homozygous colonies with some heterozygous and WT colonies. By contrast, in ET, there are few homozygous colonies, with the majority being heterozygous or WT. The majority of ET and PMF patients who are negative for *JAK2V617F* have clonal hematopoiesis, which indicates that these *JAK2V617F* diseases likely are the consequences of other genetic events including mutations in the thrombopoietin receptor, MPL, or calreticulin, which are discussed in Chapters 69 and 70. The *JAK2V617F* allele has also been observed in a limited number of patients with chronic myelomonocytic leukemia, myelodysplastic syndromes (MDS), refractory anemia with ringed sideroblasts and thrombocytosis, and AML, although most *JAK2V617F* mutations in AML occur in patients with a preceding diagnosis of PV, ET, or PMF. *JAK2V617F* is an acquired somatic mutation, does not appear in nonhematopoietic cells, and has not been detected in patients with secondary erythrocytosis. Moreover, *JAK2V617F* has not been observed in lymphoid malignancies, although other mutations in *JAK2* have been identified in 10% of patients with pediatric high-risk ALL.

Other *JAK2* Mutations in Polycythemia Vera

Other mutations of *JAK2* associated with erythrocytosis, however, can also constitutively activate JAK2 kinase activity. Several gain-of-function mutations affecting *JAK2* exon 12 within an area immediately adjacent to the pseudokinase domain of *JAK2V617F*-negative patients have been identified in 2.5–3.4% of PV patients and

approximately 30% of *JAK2V617F*-negative PV cases. To date, >40 different such mutations have been identified. Two-thirds of patients with a *JAK2* exon 12 mutation presented with an isolated erythrocytosis and distinctive BM morphology, and had reduced serum EPO levels, but the remainder of patients have erythrocytosis plus leukocytosis, thrombocytosis, or both. These exon 12 mutations perturb the autoinhibitory domain of *JAK2*. *JAK2* exon 12 mutations have not been reported in patients with ET or PMF, but have been occasionally observed in patients with refractory anemia and ringed sideroblasts associated with thrombocytosis. Erythroid colonies cloned from their blood samples in the absence of exogenous EPO were most frequently heterozygous for the mutation, with homozygous colonies only rarely occurring, but colonies homozygous for the mutation occur in most PV patients with *JAK2V617F*, suggesting that a *JAK2* exon 12 mutation results in a stronger activation of the JAK2-mediated intracellular signaling pathways. Patients with exon 12 mutations can develop thrombotic episodes and can evolve into PV-related MF or acute leukemia. In several series, approximately 2.7% of patients with a clinical syndrome that resembles PV have been observed who have a WT JAK2. The existence of such patients may be the result of several factors, including limited sensitivity of the assay used for genotyping; prior treatment with interferon (IFN), which might eliminate the *JAK2* mutations; or lack of efforts to exclude inherited genetic disorders associated with erythrocytosis that have been described in this chapter. Alternatively, additional acquired genetic lesions that have yet to be described may be responsible for the disease phenotype.

JAK2V617F Is Likely Not the Disease-Initiating Event in Polycythemia Vera

Despite data generated using a variety of mouse models suggesting that *JAK2V617F* might be sufficient for the development of PV, increasing evidence shows that PV is not solely initiated by *JAK2V617F*. The fact that *JAK2V617F* has been identified in patients with three phenotypically related but clinically distinct MPNs suggests that additional genetic or epigenetic events likely contribute to the phenotypic divergence of these disorders. These differing disease phenotypes have been hypothesized to be caused by striking differences in the degree to which the mutation activates the JAK-STAT pathway. Mutant *JAK2* activates multiple cytokine receptor-associated pathways, including STAT1 and STAT5, which can have competing consequences. STAT1 appears to be activated in association with *JAK2V617F* ET but not PV. Inhibition of STAT1 in ET progenitor cells enhances erythropoiesis, indicating that in ET, the phospo-STAT1 response to *JAK2V617F* constrains erythropoiesis and promotes megakaryocytic differentiation, but in PV, the reduced pSTAT1 response removes the break on erythropoiesis, allowing enhanced erythropoiesis to occur.

The role of *JAK2V617F* in the underlying pathogenesis of PV has been extensively explored using either restricted fragment length polymorphism analysis or the presence of marker cytogenetic abnormalities in patients with MPNs. The percentage of granulocytes and platelets that are *JAK2V617F* positive is often lower than the percentage of granulocytes belonging to the malignant clone. In addition, these marker cytogenetic abnormalities may occur before or after the acquisition of *JAK2V617F*. Furthermore *JAK2V617F*-negative erythroid colonies have been cloned in vitro in the absence of the addition of EPO, a hallmark of PV, indicating the presence of an undefined molecular lesion that precedes the *JAK2V617* mutation.

Several investigators have reported families in which multiple members have MPNs, including PV, ET, PMF, and CML, and have analyzed the *JAK2V617F* and *CALR* status of family members. The families with multiple members with MPNs have been analyzed for mutational status. In affected patients the *JAK2V617F* mutation was the most commonly acquired followed by *CALR* exon 9 mutations, with no *MPL W515L/K* mutations being detected. Interestingly, in some families, both *JAK2V617F*-positive and -negative members with MPN were observed. A small number of relatives who were *JAK2V617F* negative and did not have a diagnosis of PV, ET, or PMF had hematopoietic cells that formed endogenous erythroid colonies in vitro. Disease evolution can be highly variable within families presenting with the same type of MPN. These results suggest that an as yet unidentified genetic event, either germ-line or somatic, might contribute to the pathogenesis of PV, ET, and PMF, regardless of *JAK2* mutational status, and that there may be "initiating events" that precede the acquisition of *JAK2V617F* in these disorders. Acquired mutations of the ten–eleven translocation 2 gene (*TET2*), which are discussed in greater detail in Chapter 70, were studied in these families to determine if it was a gene that played a role in PV before acquisition of *JAK2V617F*. These acquired *TET2* mutations occurred in approximately 12% of patients with sporadic MPNs. The frequency and types of *TET2* mutations in patients with familial MPNs were similar to that observed in sporadic MPNs. As a whole, 20% of the family members with *JAK2V617F* MPNs have *TET2* mutations, and 17% of *JAK2V617F*-negative members had a MPN with a *TET2* mutation. In addition, the *TET2* mutation may occur either before or after the acquisition of *JAK2V617F*. When *JAK2V617F* coexisted with *TET2*, the *TET2* allele burden varied from 20% to 60%. Different *TET2* mutations were observed in affected members of the same family and were shown to be acquired, indicating that *TET2* mutations were not a major predisposing factor to either sporadic or familial MPNS. Familial clustering of MPNs supports the evidence that the pathologic phenotype is driven by yet to be defined susceptibility genes.

Evidence has accumulated from epidemiological and familial studies that indicate that common low-penetrance factors present in the general population contribute to the risk of developing an MPN and possibly to the phenotype of the particular MPN. The germ-line constitutive *JAK2* haplotype, called GGCC or 46/1, has been shown to be a susceptibility factor for the development of *JAK2V617F*-positive PV.[14] The *JAK2* 46/1 haplotype is also weakly associated with exon 12 *JAK2* PV, *MPL W515* MPNs, as well as MPNs that lack

MPL mutations. How this *JAK2* SNP promotes the development of *JAK2V617F* MPNs remains the subject of great speculation, but two hypotheses have been proposed: (1) hypermutability of the chromosome region facilitates the acquisition of somatic mutation; or (2) the JAK2 SNP confers a selective proliferative advantage, the so-called *fertile ground hypothesis*. Recently, germ-line polymorphisms in the *TERT* gene have also been reported to predispose to *JAK2V617F*-positive and -negative sporadic and familial MPNs. The predisposition was far stronger in familial than sporadic MPNs, suggesting that low-penetrance variants might be responsible for the familial clustering of MPNs. Two additional SNPs involving TERT and HBS1L/MYB were shown to have a stronger association with MPN populations with *CALR* or *MPL* mutations that lacked *JAK2V617F*.[15] Reduced expression of MYB has been linked to ET-like disease in several animal models. In *JAK2V617F/JAK2V617F*-positive individuals, the reduced MYB associated with the MYB SNP favored the development of an ET phenotype. In addition, polymorphisms of the glucocorticoid receptor have been associated with PV and PMF but not ET.

In the MPNs, acquisition of mutations in either *TET2* or *JAK2* may occur first, but those patients that acquire *JAK2V617F* first are more likely to develop PV. The concept that the MPN phenotype is the consequence of the order of mutational acquisition was first proposed by Ortmann and coworkers.[16] *JAK2* and *TET2* mutations each occurred first in 50% of patients. *JAK2V617F* homozygosity was not required for acquisition of a *TET2* mutation to occur. *JAK2* first patients were more likely to present with PV, were younger, more sensitive to ruxolitinib treatment, and were more likely to suffer from a thrombotic event than those individuals who acquired a *TET2* mutation initially. These data indicate that the order of acquisition of mutations might influence the clinical phenotype of the resultant MPN. *TET2* mutations have been shown to result in expansion of the malignant clone in elderly persons with normal blood counts, and in murine studies, a double-mutant *TET2–JAK2* clone was out competed by its *TET2* single-mutant ancestor. In mice, expression of *JAK2 V617F* but not TET2 resulted in increased erythropoiesis. A *TET2*-inactivating mutation but not *JAK2V617F* leads to hematopoietic stem cell expansion. The report by Ortmann and coworkers suggests that in patients who acquire TET2 first, TET2 single-mutant hematopoietic stem and progenitor cells expand but do not give rise to excess differentiated megakaryocytic and erythroid cells until a *JAK2* mutation is acquired. By contrast, in patients who acquire JAK2 first, *JAK2* single-mutant hematopoietic stem and progenitor cells generate increased numbers of megakaryocytic and erythroid cells, and stem cell numbers only expand after acquisition of a *TET2* mutation. This model is consistent with the earlier clinical presentation of patients who first acquire a *JAK2* mutation since they more rapidly generate excess megakaryocytic and erythroid cells. The initial *TET2* mutation may modify the epigenetic program of HSCs and progenitor cells, and thus alter the consequences of the second mutation. A prior mutation of *TET2* alters the transcriptional consequences of *JAK2 V617F* in a cell-intrinsic manner and prevents *JAK2 V617F* from upregulating stem and progenitor cell proliferation.

The *JAK2V617F* Mutation Is Present in Hematopoietic Stem Cells in Polycythemia Vera

Previous studies had demonstrated that the majority of patients with PV had clonal involvement of multiple lineages, including myeloid, erythroid, and lymphoid cells. These results suggested that PV originates in hematopoietic progenitors with the ability to differentiate into multiple lineages. In addition, LOH at 9p24, known to correspond to homozygous *JAK2V617F* mutations, can be identified in both myeloid and lymphoid cells in some patients with PV, further suggesting that the underlying mutations occur in progenitor cells with the ability to differentiate into multiple hematopoietic lineages.

The *JAK2V617F* mutation has been detected in hematopoietic colony-forming cells and more mature progeny, such as neutrophils and platelets. Populations of cells enriched for HSCs, common myeloid progenitors (CMPs), granulocyte–macrophage progenitors (GMPs), and megakaryocytic–erythroid progenitors (MEPs) from patients with PV have been analyzed for the presence of the JAK2V617F mutation. JAK2V617F was detected in HSCs, CMPs, GMPs, and MEPs from patients with PV, supporting that PV is a disorder that arises in HSCs and involves the myeloid, erythroid, and megakaryocytic lineages. These data indicate that JAK2V617F in PV originates in lymphomyeloid progenitor cells.[17] Analyses of hematopoietic cells from PV patients has suggested that JAK2V617F amplifies the terminal stages of hematopoiesis but not the more primitive hematopoietic stem/progenitor cells. In mouse models, however, JAK2V617F has been shown to lead to the amplification of both stem and progenitor cells, providing them with a competitive advantage compared with their normal counterpart through increased cell cycling and a reduced rate of apoptosis resulting in the emergence of the MPN phenotype. JAK2V617F may give only a subtle advantage, which will require several years for mutated stem and progenitor cells to predominate in humans over their normal counterparts. In man, other mutations such as ASXL1, DNMT3a, and TET2 may further alter the biology of the JAK2V617F-mutated clone in a manner that affects phenotype as well as disease evolution.

Structural and Functional Aspects of JAK2V617F-Mediated Transformation

The JAK2V617F mutation occurs within the JH2 domain of JAK2, which has significant homology to the kinase domain of JAK2 (JH1) but lacks catalytic activity (see Fig. 68.4). The JH2 domain exerts an inhibitory effect on JAK2 kinase activity, and the V617F mutation is predicted to disrupt this inhibition. In vitro kinase assays with JAK2V617F and WT JAK2 have revealed that JAK2V617F has greatly increased kinase activity, as assessed by autophosphorylation and by substrate phosphorylation. Ectopic expression of JAK2V617F in either epithelial or hemopoietic cell lines results in autophosphorylation of mutant JAK2, but not the WT JAK2, and activation of downstream signaling events. BAF3 or FDCP cell lines expressing the EPOR and engineered to stably express JAK2V617F are largely independent of the addition of exogenous growth factors and are hypersensitive to EPO. Coexpression of JAK2V617F and a homodimeric type 1 cytokine receptor (EPOR, TPOR, or G-CSFR) facilitates the transformation of cells to growth factor independence, suggesting that the mutant JAK2 requires a receptor scaffold to be active. This contrasts with the effects of the TEL-JAK2 fusion gene, which can readily transform cells on its own, presumably because of the strong homodimerization effects of the TEL moiety. Ectopic expression of JAK2V617F can also sensitize cells to the effects of IGF1, a characteristic feature of PV progenitors.

Expression of JAK2V617F in hematopoietic cells activates intracellular signaling pathways downstream of the EPOR, including STAT5, STAT3, the MAP kinase pathway, and the PI3K–Akt pathway. STAT5 is normally phosphorylated by the cytokine receptor–JAK2 complex, and phosphorylated STAT5 then translocates to the nucleus and activates the transcription of target genes. The target genes of STAT5 include Bcl-X$_L$, an important antiapoptotic protein known to be expressed in increased levels in PV proerythroblasts. The possibility that STAT5-mediated activation of Bcl-X$_L$ is important in the pathogenesis of PV was suggested by observations that expression of either constitutively active STAT-5 or Bcl-X$_L$ resulted in spontaneous erythroid colony formation. Furthermore, the degree of apoptosis can also be altered by p53 levels. JAK2V617F appears to functionally inactivate p53 by upregulating MDM2, an E3 ubiquitin ligase, thereby decreasing the degree of apoptosis. In addition, cells expressing JAK2V617F display constitutive activation of the MAP kinase pathway (as assessed by phosphorylation of ERK), and of the PI3K pathway (as assessed by phosphorylation of AKT). Furthermore, JAK2 has been shown to play a role in cellular MPL trafficking. Decreased expression of MPL on the cell surface of platelets and Mks is an established feature of PV and MF. Lower expression of MPL

on the cell surface of platelets and Mks in MPNs has been reported to be due to both a reduction in the recycling and maturation of the receptor as well as an increase in MPL proteasomal degradation mediated by JAK2V617F protein. Furthermore, JAK2V617F and activated STAT5 have been shown to increase the expression of 6 phosphofructokinase/fructose-2,6 bisphosphatase 3 (PFKFB3), which controls glycolytic flux through 6-6-phosphofructo-1-kinase. PFKB3 is required for JAK2V617F-dependent lactate production, oxidative metabolic activity, and glucose activity, thereby promoting cell proliferation. It is important to note that many other oncogenic tyrosine kinases activate the same signal transduction pathways, and the role and requirement for each of these signaling pathways in the transformation of hematopoietic cells by JAK2V617F remain unknown. Although once thought to reside strictly in the cytoplasm of cells, a growing body of evidence indicates that both JAK1 and JAK2 are present in the nucleus of certain cells under conditions associated with high rates of cell proliferation. Nuclear JAKs have been reported to affect gene expression by activating other transcription factors besides STATs and influencing epigenetic events by phosphorylating H3 and activating global gene expression. JAK2V617F may alter chromatin structure by selectively phosphorylating the arginine methyltransferase PRMT5, impairing PRMT5 methyltransferase activity by negatively affecting its association with methylsome protein 50. Reduced PRMT5 activity increases HPC proliferation and promotes erythroid differentiation.

Many PV patients have a low burden of JAK2V617F, as assessed by DNA sequencing, suggesting that there is either a subpopulation of cells that are homozygous for JAK2V617F mixed with WT cells or a clonal population of cells with one WT copy of JAK2 and one mutant copy of JAK2. In PV, data from clonality or quantitative JAK2V617F assessment and from colony assays suggest that most PV patients have a subpopulation of cells homozygous for JAK2V617F, but in ET, clonal progenitor cells are heterozygous for JAK2V617F. It is therefore important to determine whether the WT allele can interfere with the ability of JAK2V617F to constitutively signal in the heterozygous state and whether there is an effect of gene dosage on the activation of signal transduction pathways. Transient coexpression of WT JAK2 does not interfere with the ability of JAK2V617F to autophosphorylate even when WT JAK2 is expressed at higher levels than the mutant kinase. This suggests that JAK2V617F kinase activity is unaffected by coexpression of WT JAK2. In contrast, when JAK2V617F and WT JAK2 were coexpressed in Ba/F3 cells, cytokine-independent growth was attenuated, suggesting in this cellular context that WT JAK2 is able to interfere with JAK2V617F-mediated transformation. SOCS proteins bind to the JH1 catalytic loop and target JAK2 for degradation.[18] SOCS-1 and SOCS-3 bind to the catalytic groove belonging to JAK2 and inhibit its catalytic activity. SOCS-3 binds to EPOR and JAK2 to inhibit EPOR signaling. SOCS proteins inhibit JAK2 by functioning as E3 ubiquitin ligases. Although SOCS-1, SOCS-2, and SOCS-3 inhibit phosphorylation of WT JAK2, they are incapable of blocking phosphorylation of JAK2V617F. On the basis of their findings, SOCS-3 appears to be unable to inactivate JAK2V617, and SOCS-3 itself is not degraded but accumulates and actually promotes the further phosphorylation of JAK2V617F. Such dysregulation likely enhances JAK2V617F-induced cell proliferation and prolongs signaling. These data have been suggested as an explanation for why JAK2V617F hematopoiesis predominates in PV heterozygotes. Low levels of JAK2V617F signaling in JAK2V617F heterozygotes likely induce SOCS-3, which would downregulate JAK2 WT signaling and enhance signaling by JAK2V617F, permitting the malignant clone to predominate.

Additional Mutations Associated With Polycythemia Vera

After the application of whole-genome assays (comparative genomic hybridization and SNPs) as well as whole-genome sequencing, an increasing number of mutations have been observed in patients with Philadelphia chromosome-negative MPNs. These mutations are not unique to any of the MPNs and are associated with AML and MDS.[19] Four of these genes—EZH2, ASXL, DNMT3a, and TET2—participate in the epigenetic control of transcription and are discussed in greater detail in Chapter 70. EZH2 mutations occur in 3% of PV patients, 7–16% of PV patients have TET2 mutations, and 5–7% have mutations of DNMT3a; ASXL mutations are rare in PV (<7%). Each of these mutations may precede JAK2V617F, but the converse may also occur. Each of these mutations are far less frequent in PV and ET than PMF, supporting that these events may combine to generate a more accelerated phase of the classic MPN that phenotypically presents as MF. In addition to epigenetic regulators, mutations in genes that encode proteins that participate in the process of splicing immature mRNA have also been described in MPNs, specifically SF3B1, SRSF2, and U2AF1. SF3B1 mutations are mostly found in PMF where they cluster within exons 12–16. Alterations in SRSF2 are mostly found in PMF and MPN evolved to AML. U2AF1 mutations are detected in up to 15% of PMF cases, but are not present in ET or PV patients. IDH1/2, IKZF deletions, NRAS/KRAS, p53 mutations, and RUNX1 mutations rarely occur in PV but are all associated with transformation of an underlying MPN such as PV to acute leukemia.[18]

The Hypercoagulable State That Characterizes Polycythemia Vera

Thrombosis is a major cause of morbidity and mortality in PV patients. These thrombotic events are most frequently microcirculatory and arterial, but venous thromboses are also of important clinical significance. The increased risk for thrombosis can be attributed to abnormalities in the vessel wall, blood cell components, and the dynamics of blood flow. A number of risk factors for thrombosis have been investigated, but most of them are not firmly established.

In the European Collaboration on Low-Dose Aspirin in Polycythemia Vera (ECLAP) study, the incidence of cardiovascular complications was higher in patients older than 65 years (5.0% of patients per year; hazard ratio [HR]: 2.0; 95% confidence interval [CI]: 1.22–3.29; $p < .006$) or with a history of thrombosis (4.93% of patients per year; HR: 1.96; 95% CI: 1.29–2.97; $p = .0017$). Patients both with a history of thrombosis and older than 65 years had the highest risk of developing additional cardiovascular events (10.9% of patients per year; HR: 4.35; 95% CI: 2.95–6.41; $p < .0001$).[20] These data confirm previous findings that increasing age and history of thrombosis are the two most important prognostic factors for the development of vascular complications.

This information does not negate the increased incidence of thrombotic incidents also observed in younger patients with this disorder. In a series of 58 PV patients younger than 40 years of age, a disturbingly high incidence of life-threatening thrombotic events was observed. In fact, seven of the 10 patients in this series who died during the period of observation died from thrombotic events—four from Budd-Chiari syndrome (BCS), one from a pulmonary embolism, and two from cerebral thrombosis. Therefore, although a significant factor, preexisting atherosclerotic disease is not the sole etiologic factor in the genesis of thrombosis in PV. Analysis of the ECLAP study identified smoking in addition to older age as an important risk factor for major thrombosis. A retrospective study of 450 patients with PV demonstrated that hypertension and tobacco use were associated with arterial thrombosis ($p < .02$) and diabetes mellitus was associated with venous thrombosis ($p = .002$).

The principal hemorrheologic abnormality in PV is an elevated whole blood viscosity. The blood viscosity in PV is higher than that of normal control participants at all shear rates. In a retrospective analysis of PV patients with histories of vascular thrombosis, a strong correlation in univariate analysis between hematocrit level and the development of thrombotic episodes, including many cerebrovascular occlusions, was demonstrated. Cerebral blood flow is reduced in patients with PV in whom the hematocrit level is 53–62%. These abnormalities were observed even in patients with hematocrits at the lower levels of normal, that is, 46–52%. Reductions in cerebral blood flow are correctable with phlebotomy. Reduction of the hematocrit by relatively small amounts frequently led to substantial improvements in whole blood viscosity and cerebral blood flow. Some PV patients apparently still maintain a higher than normal whole blood viscosity despite the normalization of the hematocrit, suggesting that an increase in hematocrit may not be the only factor responsible for increased blood viscosity. There appear to be important gender differences as related to the location of thromboses in PV patients. Women appear to have a higher incidence of thromboses within the abdominal cavity involving the portal, mesenteric, or hepatic vessels but a comparable rate of other vascular complications. Several groups have reported that patients with splanchnic vein thromboses frequently have endothelial cells that are affected by JAK2V617F, suggesting that in such individuals, their MPN might originate not at the level of the HSC but rather at the level of a hemangioblast, from which myeloid and endothelial cells originate. Such JAK2V61F-positive endothelial cells have been shown to exhibit a high efficiency of adhering to normal mononuclear cells, thereby likely leading to an increased risk of thrombosis.

A number of possible explanations have been suggested for the observed relationship between hematocrit level and the development of thrombotic events in PV patients. Platelet adhesion and thrombus formation on the vascular subendothelium are determined in part by the rate at which platelets are transported to the vascular surface. In a polycythemic condition in which increased numbers of RBCs are present, a greater number of intercellular collisions between RBCs and platelets occurs. These collisions could lead to increased platelet movement in a direction perpendicular to blood flow. This facilitation of platelet transport to the vessel wall may be an important factor in the development of thrombosis. An alternative explanation for the association between hematocrit level and the risk of thrombosis is based on the knowledge that blood viscosity is particularly sensitive to hematocrit levels. Increased hematocrits lead to increased blood viscosity, in turn leading to increased peripheral vascular resistance and an actual reduction in blood flow to a variety of organs, predisposing them to the development of thrombosis. The issue of hematocrits and thrombosis in PV has been prospectively investigated in an analysis of 1638 patients enrolled in the ECLAP study. In this prospective study, despite recommendations of maintaining hematocrit levels lower than 45%, only 50% of patients achieved this target during the follow-up, and 10% had hematocrit levels above 50%. These different hematocrit values were not associated with different thrombotic outcomes as assessed using univariate and multivariable analysis. However, in a recent prospective randomized clinical trial of 365 patients with PV, it was shown that patients with hematocrit maintained at less than 45% had a lower incidence of cardiovascular events compared with patients whose hematocrits were maintained at 45–50% (4.4% vs. 10.9%; $p = .02$). The group with lower hematocrit also had lower death rates from cardiovascular events or major thrombosis.[21] This study confirmed the need for strict hematocrit control in PV patients.

Additional factors have been implicated in the development of thrombosis in PV patients. Almost all patients with PV are iron deficient. Decreased RBC deformability has been said to accompany iron deficiency, leading to increased blood viscosity and a decreased ability of RBCs to pass through small-bore polycarbonate filters. This increased membrane stiffness, however, might be counterbalanced by the effect of a reduced RBC size on the adherence of blood platelets to arteriolar subendothelium. RBC size is a major determinant of platelet adherence, with larger RBCs leading to increased platelet adherence and smaller RBCs to decreased platelet adherence. Whether the increased membrane stiffness associated with iron deficiency is counterbalanced by the decreased platelet adherence associated with smaller RBCs is yet to be determined.

Inflammation may be another predictor of thrombosis in patients with PV. In a retrospective study patients with increased inflammation as evidenced by an increased C-reactive protein (CRP) had significantly greater risk for thrombosis based on a multivariant analysis that adjusted for age, sex, ET, or PV diagnosis, cardiovascular risk factors, and JAK2V617F mutation status.

Thrombocytosis and qualitative platelet abnormalities occur frequently and are likely to be important contributory factors to the development of thrombosis. Some investigators have implicated uncontrolled thrombocytosis as a cause of thrombosis in these patients, but this relationship has not been confirmed by others. Increased plasma and urinary thromboxane production has been linked to increased platelet activation in these patients. A low-dose aspirin regimen selective for inhibition of platelet cyclooxygenase has been found to suppress increased thromboxane production in vivo and to clinically benefit patients with PV. Furthermore, elevated levels of serum VEGF and plasma TPO have been observed in patients with PV. These growth factors have been shown to lead to platelet activation.

Despite conflicting data, no clear clinical relationship between platelet number or function and the incidence of hemorrhage or thrombosis in PV patients has been delineated. An argument in favor of a role of elevated platelet numbers in the genesis of thrombosis in PV and ET is the observation in patients with ET that a reduction of excessive platelet numbers with the use of hydroxyurea is associated with a reduction in the risk of developing thrombotic events. However, this should not be taken as evidence that the reduction in developing additional vascular events was caused by platelet count normalization alone; very likely, it may be related to the suppression by hydroxyurea of each of three myeloid lineages. In line with this interpretation are the results of a randomized study performed by the Medical Research Council in the United Kingdom (PT-01) in which patients with ET were randomized to receive either hydroxyurea or anagrelide therapy. This study showed that hydroxyurea therapy rather than anagrelide, a selective platelet number-reducing drug, was associated with a reduction in the number of arterial thrombotic events, especially in *JAK2V617F* patients. In this study the rate of thrombosis in PV patients during follow-up did not vary according to different platelet numbers. Select patients with PV have, however, been afforded prompt resolution of vascular complications such as erythromelalgia or TIAs after institution of platelet antiaggregating agents or cytoreduction. It is important to emphasize that erythromelalgia does not resolve in PV patients with phlebotomy alone or with anticoagulation, but requires the use of platelet antiaggregating agents or reduction of platelet numbers. What distinguishes the clinical courses of these patients from those of others is unknown. These reports, coupled with the knowledge of abnormal thromboxane metabolism of platelets in PV, provide substance to the belief that platelets contribute to the generation of the thrombotic and hemorrhagic tendencies observed in PV. Although a number of clinical assessments of platelet function have been used to identify patients who are potentially at a high risk of developing a life-threatening hemorrhagic or thrombotic event, the results of these studies to date have been very disappointing. It appears that the etiology of thrombosis and hemorrhage in PV is multifactorial, and that the available tools are inadequate to identify patients at highest risk.

An elevation of WBC number occurs in 50–60% of PV patients, which may also have a detrimental effect on the rheology of the microcirculation in PV. An analysis of the ECLAP database showed that a baseline WBC count above $15,000 \times 10^6$ L^{-1} was associated with the development of major arterial events, mainly myocardial infarction. A retrospective study of 459 patients with PV showed a significant association between baseline leukocyte count $>15 \times 10^9$/L and venous thrombotic events during a median follow up of 64 months. Similar results were shown in two additional studies in patients with ET. Activated leukocytes may release proteases and oxygen radicals that alter endothelial cells and platelets so as to favor the development of a prothrombotic state. A series of markers of leukocyte activation, including expression of membrane CD11b and leukocyte alkaline phosphatase antigen, cellular elastase content, plasma elastase levels, and myeloperoxidase levels, are elevated in patients with PV. Limited and conflicting data are available as to whether or not there is a correlation between the presence of platelet–leukocyte interactions and thrombotic events. Increased expression of leukocyte adhesion molecules increases the adhesion of leukocytes to platelets and the endothelium. These cell-to-cell interactions

stimulate the activation of endothelial cells and platelets, and induce the release from activated leukocytes reactive oxygen species as well as proteases that are capable of impairing a number of hemostatic processes. Platelet–leukocyte aggregates are increased in number in PV and are associated with an increased propensity to thrombose. In addition, the prothrombotic state in PV has been attributed to an acquired resistance to the naturally occurring anticoagulant, protein C, which is associated with reduced levels of protein S. The loss of protein S in PV patients is especially profound in those with a high *JAK2V617F* allele burden, but its cause remains unknown, although some have speculated that it is the consequence of the degradation of protein S by the increased levels of neutrophil elastase.

JAK2V617F allele burden has also been implicated as a potential risk factor for thrombosis. In a prospective study of 173 patients with PV that were followed for a median of 24 months, patients with a *JAK2V617F* allele burden of >75% had a sevenfold increased risk of thrombosis compared with patients with an allele burden of <25%. However, another prospective study comparing patients with an allele burden of <50% versus <50% did not confirm the association between *JAK2V617F* allele burden and thrombotic risk. In a retrospective study of 186 patients with MPN, individuals harboring the *JAK2V617F* mutation were at highest risk for VTE. *JAK2* allele burdens higher than 20% identified patients with a sevenfold increased risk of VTE but not arterial thrombosis. More studies are needed to clearly establish higher *JAK2V617F* allele burden as a risk factor for thrombosis.

Clearly, the thrombotic tendencies in PV are multifactorial and in the future it is likely that the thrombotic risk will be assessed on an individual basis, taking into account many of the factors mentioned previously.

Polycythemia Vera and the Risk of Hemorrhage

Patients with PV are also at an increased risk of developing life-threatening hemorrhagic complications. Abnormalities in platelet function and number have been implicated as the cause of this hemorrhagic tendency. Qualitative platelet abnormalities frequently found in these patients include platelet hypofunction, as demonstrated by defective in vitro platelet aggregation, acquired storage pool disease, and platelet membrane defects, and increased platelet reactivity, as demonstrated by enhanced platelet aggregation, increased plasma β-thromboglobulin levels, and shortened platelet survival. With platelet counts greater than 1000×10^9 L^{-1}, the development of acquired von Willebrand syndrome has been reported and is associated with life-threatening hemorrhagic episodes.

Post-Polycythemia Vera Myelofibrosis and Acute Myeloid Leukemia

A major cause of morbidity and mortality in PV results from the transition from the polycythemic phase of the disease to post-PV MF and to acute leukemia. Post-PV MF is characterized by cytopenias, MF, and extramedullary hematopoiesis. In a variety of MPNs, the fibroblastic component of the BM has been shown not to be directly involved in the malignant process but to be a reactive event to the neoplastic clone. Several investigators have suggested that the release of growth factors, particularly VEGF, fibroblast growth factor, transforming growth factor-β, lipocalin, and tumor necrosis factor-α from myeloid cells are responsible for the marrow fibroblastic proliferation, increased marrow microvessel density, osteosclerosis, as well as the systemic symptoms observed in patients with PV-related MF. Whether the use of any particular therapeutic agents for treatment of PV accelerates the development of PV related MF remains hotly debated, although it is well established that the use of alkylating agents such as piprobroman or chlorambucil increases the risk of developing acute leukemia. It remains a source of debate if treatment with hydroxyurea increases the risk of developing MF or AML. The bulk of evidence does not support a clear leukemogenic role for this drug that is the standard of care for high-risk PV patients. Nevertheless, as a cautionary principle, it is wise to consider carefully the use of this agent in very young patients, in those carrying cytogenetic abnormalities, and in patients previously exposed to alkylating agents. In a report in which patients were treated exclusively with hydroxyurea with an average follow-up of 16.3 years, the cumulative incidence of AML/MDS was 7.3%, 10.7%, and 16.6% at 10, 15, and 20 years, respectively, and was significantly lower than in patients treated with the alkylating agent piprobroman.[22] However, patients treated with hydroxyurea had a greater chance of developing MF (at 20 years, 31.6% vs. 21.3%). Whether hydroxyurea really is leukemogenic is difficult to say from this study. The possibility exists that these rates of evolution reported with hydroxyurea use merely reflect the natural history of the disease.

Genetic studies of paired samples before and after leukemic transformation have suggested there are at least two distinct routes for leukemic transformation that are operational. Some patients who present with a *JAK2V617F/MPL* mutation-positive MPN progress to *JAK2V617F/MPL* mutation-positive AML that is associated with the acquisition of additional genetic alterations. A second, more complex, route to AML from MPN has been described in which *JAK2V617F/MPL* mutation-positive MPN is followed by *JAK2V617F/MPL* mutation-negative AML. Clonality studies using X-chromosome inactivation in informative females demonstrated that *JAK2V617F/MPL* mutation-positive MPN and *JAK2V617F/MPL* mutation-negative AML are clonally related, consistent with transformation of an antecedent, pre-*JAK2V617F/MPL* mutation mutant clone that can progress to AML. Patients with *JAK2V617F*-positive MPN who developed *JAK2V617F*-negative leukemias had a shorter time between the diagnosis of the original MPN and the leukemic transformation (3 + 2 vs. 10 + 7 years, respectively) than patients with *JAK2V617F*-positive leukemias. SNP array analysis has shown that genomic alterations occur at an increased frequency during the period of blastic transformation and that no single gene or molecular pathway is sufficient to cause transformation. A surprising correlation has been observed between the phenotype of the preceding MPN and the *JAK2* mutational status of the leukemic blasts after transformation. In contrast to *JAK2* WT AML in this setting, evolution to *JAK2V617F*-positive leukemia is invariably preceded by a myelofibrotic transformation of ET/PV or *JAK2V617F*-positive PMF. Because of these observations, myelofibrotic transformation of ET or PV is thought by many to represent an accelerated phase of the initial MPN preceded by genetic changes that result in evolution to MF and eventually leukemia. *JAK2* WT leukemia, by contrast, usually arises in patients with chronic-phase PV or ET that do not undergo evolution to MF. Some have suggested that these leukemias are therapy related. The reversion from *JAK2V617F* to WT *JAK2* in these leukemias has been shown not to be caused by homologous recombination. Two models have been proposed to account for the clonal relationship between *JAK2* WT AML and its preceding MPN: (1) both the chronic MPN and the AML arise from a shared pre-*JAK2V617F* founder clone; and (2) the chronic MPN and the AML arise from two independent stem cells. It remains possible that each model is viable and operates in different individual patients. Mutations in *CALR*, *JAK2*, *TP53*, *IDH2*, and *ASXL1* are frequent events in AML, which evolves from a prior MPN, while mutations in *NPM1*, cohesin complex members, *FLT3*, and *CEBPA*, which are common events in de novo AML, are rarely, if ever, observed in post-MPN AML. These data provide genetic evidence that post-MPN AML is a distinct disease from classical AML with a unique mutational profile and molecular pathogenesis and that lack of response to AML chemotherapy regimens reflects the divergent biology of post-MPN AML. Important differences in the mutational spectrum of *JAK2V617F* and *JAK2*-WT in post-MPN AML have been observed. *TP53* mutations are frequent, cooccurring events in patients with *JAK2V617F* mutations but not in patients with *CALR* mutations. In patients with cooccurring *JAK2V617F* and *TP53* mutations, the *JAK2/Tp53* mutant clone dominates, consistent with potent cooperativity in vivo and with a dominant role in inducing transformation from the chronic *JAK2V617F*-positive MPN to AML. By contrast, mutations

in members of the RAS pathway, *SRSF2*, and in *ASXL1* were more common in *JAK2* WT post-MPN AML, and these mutations often were present as subclonal disease alleles at the time of transformation, suggesting they are not rate limiting in the transformation from MPN to AML.

CLINICAL MANIFESTATIONS

The principal clinical manifestations of PV can largely be attributed to the excessive production of cells belonging to each of the myeloid lineages affected by the malignant process, including RBCs, platelets, and WBCs. With the implementation of laboratory tests during annual physical examinations, increasing numbers of people are being diagnosed with PV before the symptoms related to this neoplastic process become apparent. Symptomatic patients with PV may present to a physician with a myriad of nonspecific complaints, including headaches, weakness, pruritus, dizziness, excessive sweating, visual disturbances, paresthesias, joint symptoms, abdominal distress, a thrombotic or hemorrhagic episode, and weight loss. Thrombosis is a frequent presenting event. Two-thirds of such thrombotic events occur either at presentation or before diagnosis and the remainder most often during the first 10 years of follow-up. At diagnosis, one-third of patients have already lost 10% of their body weight, presumably secondary to the hypermetabolism associated with this disorder, and complaints of fatigue are common. Arthropathies are frequently observed and are largely caused by the clinical manifestations of gout. The hyperproliferative BM state characteristic of PV and the increased nucleoprotein degradation are contributory factors in the development of hyperuricemia.

The principal findings on physical examination of a patient with PV include ruddy cyanosis, conjunctival plethora, hepatomegaly, splenomegaly, and hypertension.

Untreated patients are at particularly high risk for thrombotic and hemorrhagic events. In several large series of patients with PV, thrombosis was the cause of death in 30–40% of patients. Arterial thrombotic events account for two-thirds of such events, with venous thrombotic events representing the remainder. Ischemic stroke, myocardial infarction, and TIAs are the most common arterial thrombotic events. Patients may also present with deep venous thrombosis in the lower extremities, pulmonary embolism, or peripheral vascular occlusions. The cumulative rate of thrombosis ranges from 2.5% to 5% per patient per year. The prevalence of thrombosis at diagnosis ranges from 34% to 39%. It is not unusual for patients with PV to develop thromboses at unusual anatomic sites; in particular, thromboses are relatively frequent in the splanchnic veins, including the splenic, hepatic, portal, and mesenteric vessels or cerebral sinus veins, thrombosis of the vena cava, and intraventricular thrombosis. A particularly serious thrombotic event associated with PV is BCS, which results from hepatic venous or inferior vena caval thrombosis and obstruction. These events lead to hepatic venous outflow obstruction, increased hepatic sinusoidal pressure, and portal hypertension. Portal venous perfusion of the liver is frequently reduced, leading to portal venous thrombosis and hypoxic damage of liver parenchymal cells. This cascade of events results in centrilobular hepatic necrosis, centrilobular fibrosis, and nodular regenerative fibrosis, which culminates in the development of cirrhosis of the liver. The cause of BCS can be identified in 75% of cases, including hereditary and acquired prothrombotic disorders, trauma, and infection. PV account for 10–40% of all cases of BCS. Paroxysmal nocturnal hemoglobinuria is also a frequent cause of BCS. Because BM cells from 87% of patients with idiopathic BCS form erythroid colonies in the absence of EPO, such patients were in the past believed to have a forme fruste of an MPN. The identification of these latent MPNs, without elevated blood counts, has been facilitated by screening for *JAK2V617F*. These patients tend to be younger and female, and to have normal blood counts caused by hemodilution and hypersplenism, which mask an elevated RBC mass. Many of these patients (37%) also have another predisposing factor for thrombosis such as exposure to oral contraceptives, antiphospholipid antibodies, factor V Leiden, or protein C deficiency. The *JAK2V617F* mutation has been reported in 32.7% patients of 831 patients with an idiopathic splanchnic vein thrombosis. The mutation was present in 49% of patients at diagnosis of the idiopathic form of splanchnic vein thrombosis, of which 60% were diagnosed as having a coexisting MPN; more than 52% of the remaining patients went on to develop an MPN after a median of 49 months. *JAK2V617F* was detected in 45% of patients with BCS, and at least in one series, neither exon 12 *JAK2* mutations nor *MPL* mutations were observed. Furthermore, additional patients (6.9%) who have idiopathic splanchnic vein thrombosis have a BM histopathologic picture diagnostic of an MPN but are *JAK2V617F* negative. The diagnostic value of low serum EPO level in BCS has been questioned because elevated levels have been attributed in *JAK2V617F*-positive patients with necrotic liver tissue.

There are fulminant, acute, subacute, and chronic forms of BCS. These clinical manifestations depend on the extent and rapidity of hepatic vein occlusion and the development of venous collaterals to decompress the venous sinusoids. One should always consider a diagnosis of BCS in any patient with an MPN with ascites, upper abdominal pain, and liver function abnormalities. This syndrome is characterized by hepatosplenomegaly, ascites, edema of the peripheral extremities, and distention of superficial abdominal veins caused by resultant portal hypertension. Routine biochemical determinations of hepatocellular function and injury are frequently of little diagnostic value in patients with suspected BCS. Doppler ultrasonography is the best tool for screening patients for BCS. This test has a sensitivity and specificity of 85%. Characteristic findings include an absence of flow in the hepatic veins or nonvisualization of the hepatic vein. Contrast-enhanced computed tomography scanning and magnetic resonance imaging (MRI) are useful in better defining the hepatic venous anatomy. Hepatic venous and inferior vena caval catheterization is a key diagnostic procedure indicating the sites of venous obstruction. The diagnosis can be definitively made by a spider web pattern on hepatic venography. Transjugular liver biopsy specimens usually reveal intense congestion and cellular atrophy.

It has been emphasized that patients with PV can present with portal or hepatic vein thrombosis with normal hemoglobin or hematocrit values. Such patients may have leukocytosis, thrombocytosis, or splenomegaly. Screening for the *JAK2* mutation should be systematically carried out in such situations and may substitute for BM examinations in individuals who are *JAK2V617F* positive. In patients with an idiopathic form of splanchnic vein thrombosis but who are *JAK2V617F* negative, a BM aspirate and biopsy are recommended to exclude the possibility of a *JAK2V617F*-negative MPN. Gastrointestinal bleeding or an increase in plasma volume that is a consequence of splenomegaly often accounts for the normal blood counts in such patients with BCS. The factors operational in the PV patient that lead to the development of hepatic vein thrombosis are believed to be multiple. Whereas splenomegaly causes increased portal blood flow, extramedullary hematopoiesis within the hepatic sinusoids frequently obstructs hepatic blood flow, and *JAK2V617F*-positive endothelial cells might affect adhesion to monocytes, leading to aggregation of blood elements. These processes are surely important contributory factors in addition to the other previously discussed risk factors that lead to the development of thrombosis in this patient population.

Neurologic abnormalities occur in almost 60–80% of untreated or poorly controlled PV patients and include TIAs, cerebral infarction, cerebral hemorrhage, fluctuating dementia, confusional states, and choreic syndromes. PV associated chorea has been reported as a presenting complaint, primarily in older females, which typically involves the orolingual or appendicular musculature and often resolves with phlebotomy or cytoreductive therapy. In addition, complaints of dizziness, paresthesias, visual disturbances, tinnitus, and headaches have been attributed to the increased blood viscosity and reduced cerebral blood flow caused by erythrocytosis. The transient neurologic symptoms can also be the consequence of small infarcts in the region of the basal ganglia, which can be detected by computed tomography. These small infarcts are known as *lacunae* and result from the occlusion of small penetrating arteries, which are

particularly susceptible to thrombosis. Cerebrovascular thrombosis occurs more often in PV patients than in the general population. Symptoms caused by intermittent carotid or vertebral basilar artery insufficiency (or both) occur so frequently in PV that it is suggested that every patient with focal cerebrovascular insufficiency should at least have a complete blood count test to exclude the diagnosis of an underlying MPN.

Thrombosis of the dural sinus or cerebral veins (CVT) is an uncommon form of stroke, usually affecting young individuals. CVT represents about 0.5–1% of all strokes. While 3.8% of CVT patients are diagnosed with MPNs, 0.4% of MPN patients have a CVT during their clinical course. Headache, generally indicative of an increase in intracranial pressure, is the most common symptom in CVT. Clinical manifestations of CVT may also depend on the location of the thrombosis. The superior sagittal sinus is most commonly involved, which may lead to headache, increased intracranial pressure, and papilledema. A motor deficit, sometimes with seizures, can also occur. Scalp edema and dilated scalp veins may be seen on examination. For lateral sinus thromboses, symptoms related to an underlying condition (middle-ear infection) may be noted, including constitutional symptoms, fever, and ear discharge. Pain in the ear or mastoid region and headache are typical. Hemianopia, contralateral weakness, and aphasia may sometimes be seen owing to cortical involvement. Approximately 16% of patients with CVT have thrombosis of the deep cerebral venous system (internal cerebral vein, vein of Galen, and straight sinus), which can lead to thalamic or basal ganglial infarction. Cavernous sinus thrombosis is usually associated with a primary infectious etiology involving a focus in the face, throat, mouth, ear, or sinuses. Aseptic cavernous sinus thrombosis is an extremely rare phenomenon that has been reported in patients with PV. These patients present with monocular blindness and the characteristic features of ipsilateral cavernous sinus thrombosis, and only retrospectively is the diagnosis of PV made. Therefore, patients found to have this symptom complex who have no known infectious predisposing causes should be carefully evaluated to rule out this diagnosis. The most sensitive diagnostic technique is MRI in combination with magnetic resonance venography.

Thrombosis of large-caliber arteries is a relatively rare event in PV patients, but there have been case reports of thromboses within the chambers of the heart, leading to refractory congestive heart failure and acute aortic occlusion. Such catastrophic thrombotic events in the heart or large vessels would suggest that cardiac catheterization be performed with some caution.

PV frequently manifests with symptoms caused by peripheral vascular disease. In these cases, patients may first be seen by surgeons or dermatologists. Intense redness or cyanosis of the digits with or without burning, classic erythromelalgia, digital ischemia with palpable pulses, or thrombophlebitis without another known cause may be the presenting symptoms.

Erythromelalgia is characterized by burning pain in the digits, an objective sensation of increased temperature, and relief by cooling. PV is the most common cause of erythromelalgia and is one of the few disorders in which digital ischemia with or without ulceration may exist in the presence of palpable pulses. Other disorders that can lead to this abnormality include embolism, trauma, cutaneous infarction, neuritis, infection, and various types of arteritis. Painful and ulcerating toes and fingers have frequently been observed to be presenting symptoms in patients with PV. The likelihood that arterial insufficiency is the cause of such ulceration is quite small in patients who have a palpable dorsalis pedis and posterior tibialis pulses; in this situation, the possibility of an underlying hematologic disorder such as PV should be entertained. Foot pain at rest is a distressing but not widely recognized symptom of PV. In patients with this complaint, peripheral pulses are of normal character, and cutaneous circulation appears to be adequate. The pain is most severe at night, is dull in nature, and occurs primarily in the feet or legs. These symptoms have been shown to be the results of platelet activation and aggregation in vivo, which preferentially occur in arterioles. If untreated, erythromelalgia can progress to ischemic acrocyanosis or gangrene. Phlebotomy alone in PV does not improve erythromelalgia. These symptoms can be abolished by reducing the platelet counts to normal levels and can be rapidly reversed after the institution of antiplatelet aggregation therapy but not coumadin. Therefore, the cause of erythromelalgia appears to be closely linked to abnormal arachidonic acid metabolism that occurs within platelets in this disorder.

Retrospective reviews have revealed a higher than expected number of patients with PV and pulmonary hypertension. Proposed etiologies include direct obstruction of pulmonary arteries by circulating megakaryocytes, extramedullary hematopoiesis in the pulmonary parenchyma, smooth muscle hyperplasia induced by release of PDGF from activated platelets, chronic disseminated intravascular coagulation, and unrecognized recurrent pulmonary emboli. The diagnosis of pulmonary hypertension is made, on average, 9.5 years after the diagnosis of the underlying MPN and is associated with a poor prognosis, with death usually occurring as a result of congestive heart failure or pneumonia. Although anecdotal reports have claimed improvements in patients' pulmonary artery pressure with control of the underlying disease, others have not found any change in serial measurements of 11 patients' pulmonary arterial pressures despite good disease control. Recently, ruxolitinib therapy has been reported to result in improved outcomes, pulmonary and echocardiographic findings, as well as correction of cytokine dysregulation in MPN patients with pulmonary hypertension.

As many as 30–40% of patients with PV experience some sort of hemorrhagic event, which can be relatively trivial, such as epistaxis or gingival hemorrhage, or can be life-threatening, such as gastrointestinal hemorrhage or hematomas involving vital organs. The gastrointestinal tract is a frequent site of hemorrhagic complications because patients with PV are predisposed to portal vein thrombosis and resultant variceal bleeding and peptic ulcer disease. Gastroduodenal erosions and ulcers, and *Helicobacter pylori* infection are all significantly more common in PV patients than in control patients with dyspepsia. This may be partly attributable to altered mucosal blood flow as a result of increased plasma viscosity or increased histamine release caused by peripheral blood basophilia. Cerebral hemorrhage is a common cause of morbidity and mortality. Bleeding events frequently occur with the use of aspirin or other nonsteroidal antiinflammatory agents; an association between the hemorrhage and the use of high doses of these platelet-paralyzing drugs has been made in almost one-third of such instances. Low-dose aspirin therapy has, however, been reported not to lead to an increased incidence of life-threatening hemorrhagic events. Spontaneous bleeding in patients with PV is relatively rare, although spontaneous retropharyngeal hematomas leading to acute upper airway obstruction or hematomas in the groin or retroperitoneum have been reported.

Patients with PV who undergo surgical procedures are at a very high risk of developing postoperative complications. In one series of 62 major operations on 54 patients with PV, postoperative complications occurred in 49% of patients; 52% of complications were from hemorrhage, 18% from thrombosis, and 14% from hemorrhage and thrombosis. The postoperative mortality rate in this patient population was 18%. In another series of 15 patients, five had serious complications secondary to thrombosis and hemorrhage. A study by an Italian group retrospectively evaluated 311 surgical interventions in 105 patients with PV and 150 with ET: 24 arterial or venous thromboses (7.7%), 23 major hemorrhages (7.3%), and five surgery-related deaths (1.6%) were observed within 3 months of the procedure. PV patients with uncontrolled erythrocytosis before surgery have been shown to have the highest complication rate. Patients with inadequately controlled disease had a 79% incidence of complications, but in those with adequate hematologic control before surgery, the rate of perioperative and postoperative complications was reduced to 28%. In addition, the duration of disease control was an important factor in decreasing surgical risk; a prolonged period of effective disease control before surgery reduced the complication rate to 5%. Complication rates after surgery can therefore be dramatically reduced by appropriate therapeutic interventions with normalization of blood counts. The chief deterrent to such an approach has been the failure by physicians to recognize the risk associated with PV in the surgical setting.

Another situation that puts patients with PV and ET at high risk for thrombosis is pregnancy. Maternal and fetal complications have been reported. Specifically, the rate of fetal loss is higher than that of the general population.

Generalized pruritus occurs in approximately 40% of cases of PV. Water contact, such as during showers or bathing, induces attacks of intolerable pruritus. There appears to be no clear relationship between the degree of the pruritus and severity of the disease, and 20% of patients continue to experience itching despite reduction of their hematocrits to normal levels. Aquagenic pruritus is significantly more common among *JAK2V617F* homozygous patients than heterozygotes. The degree of pruritus is so severe in some patients that they are unable to tolerate bathing at all and find it necessary to substitute gentle skin swabbing or to simply not bathe. The etiology of the pruritus in PV remains uncertain. Several groups have attempted to implicate elevated blood and urine histamine levels in its pathobiology. A strong correlation between skin mast cell numbers and the severity of itching has been demonstrated, and mast cells in PV have been shown to be *JAK2V617F* positive. However, the failure of the pruritus to respond to antihistamine therapy in many patients suggests that abnormally high histamine levels probably do not constitute the sole factor in its development.

Iron deficiency has also been implicated as a factor contributing to pruritus in PV patients who are almost invariably iron deficient. Iron-substitution therapy has resulted in symptomatic improvement, but this approach is less than optimal because it frequently results in uncontrollable erythrocytosis. Ruxolitinib therapy has been reported to be effective in alleviating the patient's aquagenic pruritis in 80% of patients.

The development of post-PV MF was increased with prolonged duration of disease and is directly related to the duration of long-term follow-up, but the influence of the modality used to treat the initial PV phase of the disease on the rate of transformation to this more accelerated form of the disease remains uncertain. Post-PV MF should be considered the natural evolution of PV. Criteria for the diagnosis of post-PV MF have been established (Table 68.2) and can be used as a guide for documenting this transition in disease phenotype, which in reality represents a point in the continuum of PV. For patients with disease duration greater than 10 years, the hazard ratio was 15.24 (95% CI: 4.22–55.06; $p < .0001$). The median interval between the diagnosis of PV and the development of post-PV MF is 13 years. Post-PV MF is characterized by (1) increasing splenomegaly;

TABLE 68.2 | **International Working Group for Myelofibrosis Research and Recommended Treatment Criteria for Post-Polycythemia Vera Myelofibrosis**

Required Criteria

1. Documentation of a previous diagnosis of polycythemia vera as defined by the WHO criteria
2. Bone marrow fibrosis grade 2–3 (on 0–3 scale) or grade 3–4 (on 0–4 scale)

Additional Criteria (Two Are Required)

1. Anemia or sustained loss of requirement of either phlebotomy (in the absence of cytoreductive therapy) or cytoreductive treatment for erythrocytosis
2. A leukoerythroblastic peripheral blood picture
3. Increasing splenomegaly defined as either an increase in palpable splenomegaly of ≥5 cm (distance of the tip of the spleen from the left costal margin) or the appearance of a newly palpable splenomegaly
4. Development of ≥one of three constitutional symptoms: >10% weight loss in 6 months, night sweats, unexplained fever (>37.5°C)

WHO, World Health Organization.
Adapted from Proposed criteria for the diagnosis of post-polycythemia vera and post-essential thrombocythemia myelofibrosis: A consensus statement from the international working group for myelofibrosis research and treatment. *Leukemia* 22:437, 2008.

(2) teardrop RBC morphology; (3) extensive BM fibrosis; (4) a leukoerythroblastic blood picture, systemic symptoms including fatigue, weight loss, night sweats, bone pain, and fevers; and (5) anemia and or thrombocytopenia. The patients may be entirely asymptomatic but often complain of fatigue, dizziness, weight loss, and anorexia. Splenomegaly can lead to abdominal pain caused by repeated splenic infarcts and to early satiety caused by mechanical obstruction of the upper gastrointestinal tract. Patients with post-PV MF are virtually all *JAK2V617F* positive and characteristically have high *JAK2V617F* allele burdens.

The anemia that characterizes post-PV MF is primarily a result of splenic pooling, ineffective erythropoiesis, hemolysis, and extramedullary production of RBCs with a shortened RBC survival. Patients positive for *JAK2V617F* are less likely to require blood transfusions but have a poorer survival. Occasionally, the anemia is exacerbated by folate or iron deficiency. Before assuming that a patient has entered post-PV MF, it is prudent to assess BM iron stores. Replacement therapy with iron may lead to the resurgence of erythropoiesis and prevent the faulty categorization of disease progression.

Bleeding abnormalities caused by thrombocytopenia or qualitative platelet abnormalities are especially common during this phase of the disease. Frequent instances of epistaxis or ecchymoses occur, and gastrointestinal hemorrhage caused by esophageal varices arising from portal hypertension is a recurrent problem. The majority of hemorrhagic events are minor in nature. Frequently, patients have generalized wasting characterized by progressive asthenia and weight loss. Severe hyperuricemia, leading to secondary gout or uric acid nephropathy, may also complicate the clinical course.

The median survival for patients with post-PV MF is 5.7 years. Patients with post-PV MF are at a high risk for the development of acute leukemia. Of patients who develop post-PV MF, approximately 18% will undergo leukemic transformation after 3 years and likely a greater number with longer follow-up.

The leukemic transformation of PV has been extensively described. The possibility, that a relationship exists between the therapeutic modality used during the erythrocytotic phase and the frequency of development of acute leukemia, has been a point of heated discussion. Some of the controversy surrounding this question was formerly caused by a lack of understanding of the basic origins of PV. Clinical hematologists in the 1950s and 1960s frequently thought of PV as a benign hematologic abnormality and believed that therapeutic interventions either with alkylating agents or radiotherapy were solely responsible for the development of acute leukemia. That concept has proved erroneous, and PV, similar to the other MPNs, has been shown to be a clonal malignant hematologic disorder. The evolution to acute leukemia can therefore be thought of as a natural consequence of this malignant disorder, which can be accentuated by the therapeutic interventions already discussed. In fact, 25% of patients who develop acute leukemia have never been exposed to any form of cytotoxic therapy.

Further insight into the relationship between acute leukemia and PV has been best provided by the results of the PV Study Group (PVSG), which described a randomized trial comparing the use of phlebotomy, chlorambucil, and ^{32}P for the treatment of this disorder. The incidence of acute leukemia was approximately 1.5% in patients treated with phlebotomy alone, 17.5% in patients treated with chlorambucil, and 10.9% in patients treated with ^{32}P after over 15 years of follow-up. The incidence of acute leukemia in the patients treated with phlebotomy alone is therefore much higher than that expected in a normal age-matched control group, again indicating that leukemia is a natural evolutionary event in the clinical course of an individual with PV. The incidence of acute leukemia can be increased, however, by the institution of therapy with either alkylating agents or [32]P. The time course for the development of acute leukemia appears to be dependent on the treatment used to control the polycythemia. The development of acute leukemia in patients treated with phlebotomy in the PVSG trial was limited to the first 5 years of treatment, suggesting that the development of acute leukemia is not solely attributable to the prolongation of survival. In contrast, analysis of the hazard function was virtually flat for

patients treated with chlorambucil from years 2 to 7 after randomization; however, the risk for acute leukemia became alarmingly high after 10 years of study, suggesting that the risk of acute leukemia increases with time even after the drug has been stopped. One half of the cases of acute leukemia in the chlorambucil arm occurred during the first 5 years, with the remainder equally split between the second and third 5-year periods. In contrast, 60% of the cases of acute leukemia in the group treated with radioactive phosphorus occurred 6–10 years after randomization. Of particular concern is the high incidence of leukemia recently reported in patients who were initially treated with radioactive phosphorous or busulphan and then switched to maintenance therapy with hydroxyurea, previously believed to be a nonleukemogenic agent. These findings suggest that a combination of an alkylating agent, busulphan, piprobroman, or melphalan, and another chemotherapeutic agent (hydroxyurea) may particularly increase the risk of leukemia. Approximately 30–50% of patients with PV who develop acute leukemia have previously entered the post-PV MF phase. In contrast, approximately 50% of patients progress directly from the erythrocytotic phase to acute leukemia. The phenotype of the leukemic phase that characterize the leukemic cells is overwhelmingly myeloid, although rare cases of lymphoblastic and biphenotypic leukemias have been reported. Patients with *JAK2V617F*-positive MPN are also at a higher risk of developing both additional hematologic malignancies and solid tumors. The SNPs for TERT, which is a susceptibility factor for familial and sporadic MPNS, have also been shown to be associated with a variety of solid tumors. The presence of this SNP predisposes to the development of MPNS and the cooccurrence of solid tumors, especially in patients receiving cytoreductive therapy. Some investigators have suggested that prolonged cytoreductive therapy be avoided in patients with the TERT polymorphism. In addition, low-grade lymphoproliferative disorders such as chronic lymphocytic leukemia and MGUS have been shown to coexist in patients with a variety of MPNs, including PV, and not to have an adverse effect on prognosis.

In some instances, a preleukemic phase characterized by refractory anemia with excess blasts has been described. In fact, half of such cases of acute leukemia in one series were preceded by a myelodysplastic disorder.

LABORATORY MANIFESTATIONS

Laboratory evaluation of patients with erythrocytosis involves the careful use of a broad range of diagnostic studies. These studies must be used in a rational manner or the evaluation can become extremely costly. Because PV is a panmyelosis, the overwhelming number of patients has elevated hematocrits, WBC counts, and platelet counts. The diagnosis of PV has been greatly simplified by the discovery of the *JAK2V617F* mutation, which is present in more than 90% of PV patients. Hematocrit values greater than 49% in males and greater than 48% in females are abnormal and require further evaluation. Documentation of the absolute increase in RBC mass is rarely required and is a test that is available at smaller and smaller numbers of institutions. A hematocrit value greater than 60% in men or greater than 55% in women is almost always associated with an absolute erythrocytosis. Occasionally, an elevated RBC mass can actually be present in the face of a normal hematocrit value. In cases of splenomegaly caused by portal hypertension, an expanded plasma volume may mask an elevated RBC mass. In addition, iron deficiency can also lead to a normalization of the hematocrit in PV, making the diagnosis difficult. PV is associated with a 20–30% frequency of peptic ulcers and gastritis, which can be associated with blood loss. In this situation, thrombocytosis may be exacerbated as a consequence of the iron deficiency. Iron supplementation is not necessary to make a diagnosis of an MPN because of the availability of molecular diagnostic studies. Administration of iron to such patients must be performed carefully to avoid a rapid increase in RBC mass, which can be associated with a high risk of thrombosis.

Leukocytosis is present in approximately two-thirds of cases and seems to be proportional to the burden of *JAK2V617F*. Thrombocytosis is observed in 50% of cases. Abnormalities of RBC, WBC, and platelet morphology are frequently observed. The morphologic RBC changes observed during the erythrocytotic phases are characteristic of iron deficiency and include microcytosis, hypochromia, and frequently polychromatophilia. Some anisocytosis and poikilocytosis can be seen as well. Fetal hemoglobin levels and the number of RBCs containing fetal hemoglobin, known as *F cells*, may be increased. The WBCs are characterized by normal morphology, although the numbers of basophils, eosinophils, and immature myeloid forms can be increased. Platelet morphology is also quite striking in PV. Frequently, megathrombocytes (platelets the sizes of RBCs) are seen on the peripheral blood smear. Patients frequently have platelet counts of less than 1×10^6 mm^{-3}, but it is not unusual to observe a patient with a platelet count higher than this value. PV-related MF is characterized by a leukoerythroblastic blood picture, with the appearance in the peripheral blood of dacryocytes or teardrop RBCs, myelocytes, metamyelocytes, and (rarely) blasts and promyelocytes in addition to nucleated RBCs in the peripheral blood.

Platelet aggregation studies do not correlate frequently with the risk of bleeding episodes. The most common abnormalities are decreased primary and secondary aggregation to either or both epinephrine and adenosine diphosphate, and decreased response to collagen with generally a normal response to arachidonic acid. An abnormal platelet storage pool disease is a characteristic feature and is caused by abnormal platelet activation. Prothrombin times (PT) and partial thromboplastin times (aPTT), as well as fibrinogen levels, are usually normal. Profound abnormalities of the PT and aPTT, however, are frequently reported. This is largely a laboratory artifact caused by the extreme erythrocytosis, which results in a relatively smaller volume of plasma being present in the whole blood sample. Coagulation assays are performed on blood anticoagulated with sodium citrate, and the citrate concentration in the anticoagulant is calibrated to chelate the plasma calcium and inhibit coagulation reactions. All coagulation assays include the addition of calcium chloride to neutralize the excess citrate and provide free calcium to mediate coagulation reactions. In patients with extreme erythrocytosis, the ratio of citrate in the collection tube to the volume of plasma is too high; therefore, excess citrate is present, and the standard amount of calcium chloride added during the performance of the PT and aPTT is insufficient to neutralize the excessive citrate, and the coagulation assays are frequently and factually prolonged. To avoid this problem, the clinician should calculate the relative amount of plasma compared with the normal amount and remove the corresponding volume of sodium citrate from the blood collection tube. Normal values can then be confidently anticipated in patients with erythrocytosis. A shortened fibrinogen half-life has been detected in some patients with PV and a significantly increased fractional catabolic rate of the plasma fibrinogen pool per day. In addition, elevated platelet β-thromboglobulin and plasma β-thromboglobulin levels are observed. The constellation of findings is indicative of increased platelet turnover. Prothrombin fragments F1 and 2, thrombin–antithrombin complex, and D-dimer levels are frequently elevated in PV patients. These are enzyme–inhibitor complexes or byproducts of active thrombosis that serve as a biochemical signature of the hypercoagulable state that characterizes PV.

Acquired von Willebrand syndrome occurs frequently in patients with PV and ET with over 1×10^6/L platelet numbers. This syndrome is characterized by a normal or prolonged bleeding time, normal factor VIII level, and normal von Willebrand factor (vWF) antigen level, but abnormal vWF ristocetin cofactor actively associated with a decrease or absence of large vWF multimers. This acquired defect resembles type II vWF disease. Because the molecular size of vWF is a major determinant of its adhesive function and the larger multimers are most active in achieving hemostasis, the deficiency of large vWF multimers is associated with a bleeding tendency. The decrease in the frequency of large vWF multimers occurs in patients with platelet counts over 1000×10^9 L^{-1}. This abnormality has been reported not only with patients with severe thrombocytosis caused by MPN, but also in patients with reactive thrombocytosis. An inverse correlation between the proportion of large vWF multimers and platelet numbers has been observed. In addition, normalization of the platelet count is accompanied by restoration of a normal vWF multimer pattern. These findings suggest that thrombocytosis of any etiology may favor the adsorption of larger forms of vWF multimers onto platelet membranes, resulting in their removal from the circulation and subsequent degradation by platelet-associated proteases. Although patients with MPN frequently have bleeding tendencies, this is not the case in secondary thrombocytosis, possibly because of the limited periods of extreme thrombocytosis observed in such patients. Patients with PV with clinical courses punctuated by hemorrhagic events, extreme thrombocytosis, and acquired von Willebrand syndrome should not receive aspirin therapy if they are having a thrombotic episode but should be phlebotomized, and platelet-reduction therapy should be initiated. Patients with PV and acquired von Willebrand syndrome have recurrent bleeding from mucous membranes and the digestive tract, and easy bruisability. These symptoms frequently resolve with normalization of the platelet count.

Deficiencies of one or more natural anticoagulants as well as the antiphospholipid antibody syndrome have been observed in patients with PV and thrombosis. These studies indicate that either familial or acquired antithrombin III deficiency, protein C or S deficiency, factor V Leiden mutation, or the prothrombin G gene mutation may contribute to the hypercoagulable state observed in PV. Of note, although hyperhomocysteinemia caused by deficiency of cobalamin or folate can be found in 32–56% of PV patients, there is no agreement as to its role in the genesis of thrombotic episodes. Such inherited disorders associated with the erythrocytosis of PV provide a scenario that frequently favors thrombosis in affected individuals. In attempting to determine if a patient with PV and an active thrombosis has such an inherited predisposition, it is important to be aware that proteins C and S as well as antithrombin III levels can be low in patients with an ongoing acute thrombosis or liver cirrhosis. Normal prothrombin and factor VII levels in such patients eliminate liver cirrhosis as a cause of the reduction of these circulating anticoagulants. Individuals with inherited prethrombotic conditions frequently have levels of specific proteins below 10–20% of normal during periods of active thrombosis.

The leukocyte alkaline phosphatase activity level is elevated in 70% of patients. Moreover, recent data indicate an increase of neutrophil elastase levels in granulocytes and in plasma that correlates with *JAK2* mutational status. Whereas serum vitamin B$_{12}$ concentrations have been found to be elevated in 40% of patients, serum vitamin B$_{12}$-binding proteins are elevated in 70% of patients. Hyperuricemia occurs in an overwhelming number of patients, and elevated histamine levels are also frequently observed. BM aspirates and biopsies obtained at the time of diagnosis of patients with PV are hypercellular and display characteristic erythroid, granulocytic, and megakaryocytic hyperplasia. The cellular elements (Fig. 68.6) are frequently morphologically normal. Iron stores are almost uniformly absent in pretreatment biopsy specimens. Significant increases in BM reticulin may be present in biopsies obtained early in the course but also may develop during the erythrocytotic phase and may be present for long periods before the onset of the post-PV MF. It is important to emphasize that individuals may have considerable BM fibrosis, which occurs as a consequence of the underlying MPN. The presence of minimal BM fibrosis should not be considered a harbinger of the development of post-PV MF. In patients with post-PV MF, a moderate-to-marked increase in reticulin fiber is observed, either simultaneously with or within 1 year of this clinical transformation.

Several investigators have attempted to use BM biopsy morphology as a differential diagnostic tool to differentiate between PV and secondary forms of erythrocytosis. The marked hypercellularity, erythroid and megakaryocytic hyperplasia with pleiomorphic enlarged megakaryocytes that are the hallmarks of MPNs are useful parameters for identifying such individuals (see Fig. 68.6). It is imperative to use the BM biopsy rather than the aspirate specimens for this purpose. It has been suggested that those PV patients with minor BM fibrosis

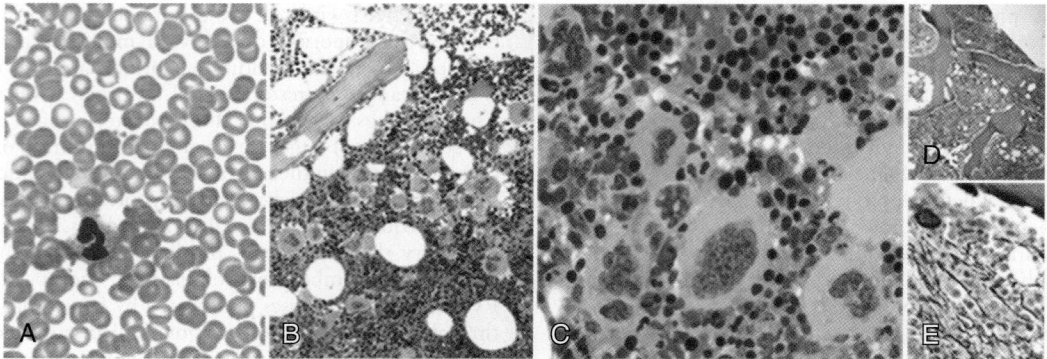

Fig. 68.6 PHOTOMICROGRAPH OF BONE MARROW BIOPSY OBTAINED FROM A PATIENT WITH POLYCYTHEMIA VERA IN MYELOFIBROTIC PHASE DEMONSTRATING HYPERCELLULARITY AND INCREASED NUMBER OF MEGAKARYOCYTES (×160).

are at an increased risk to develop a thrombotic episode or to evolve into post-PV MF but not acute leukemia during the course of their disease.

The pathologic appearance of the spleen in PV depends on the stage of the disease at which the organ is examined. Spleens from patients in the erythrocytotic phase of the disease are characterized by striking congestion with mature erythrocytes. Small numbers of hematopoietic precursor cells are frequently present. By contrast, spleens examined during the PV-related MF phase are characterized by prominent numbers of foci of extramedullary hematopoiesis, with representation of all BM precursor elements.

Allele-specific PCR methods can be used to detect the *JAK2V617F* or a *JAK2* exon 12 mutation in approximately 95% of patients with PV. The very high frequency of *JAK2V617F* in PV has dramatically improved our ability to diagnose this disease. Patients with isolated erythrocytosis associated with normal neutrophil and platelet counts but low serum EPO levels and the formation of erythroid colonies by peripheral blood mononuclear cells in the absence of EPO in vitro are the characteristic phenotype of patients with the exon 12 mutation. BM biopsies from these patients were slightly hypercellular with isolated erythroid hyperplasia. Megakaryocytes were morphologically normal and not clustered. The exon 12 mutations were frequently present at low levels in granulocyte DNA but were readily identifiable in endogenous erythroid colonies generated in vitro. Because granulocyte involvement with *JAK2* exon 12 mutations is low, it is important to sequence DNA from BM cells or from endogenous erythroid colonies generated in vitro to make this diagnosis. At diagnosis, serum EPO levels in PV are either reduced or at the lower limits of normal. Even after normalization of the hematocrit, the serum EPO level in PV remains low in two thirds of patients.

Arterial blood gas measurements are frequently performed to rule out hypoxia as a cause of erythrocytosis. In PV with extreme thrombocytosis, such routine measurements can prove to be misleading. Spurious hypoxemia can frequently be attributed to either significant leukocytosis or thrombocytosis caused by in vitro consumption of oxygen, the so-called *platelet and leukocyte larceny*. In this situation, pulse oximetry can be a useful tool for establishing the patient's true oxygenation status.

CYTOGENETIC ABNORMALITIES

The occurrence of nonrandom cytogenetic abnormalities in PV is anticipated because this is a feature of most hematologic malignancies. Such abnormalities have been observed without a single characteristic abnormality defined; the most frequent abnormalities are the gain of chromosome 9 as well as 9p, deletion of the long arm of chromosome 20, gain of the long arms of chromosome 1, trisomy 8, and deletion of chromosome 13 (Fig. 68.7). Balanced translocations are rarely observed in PV. At diagnosis, approximately 28% of patients have a recurrent clonal chromosome marker.

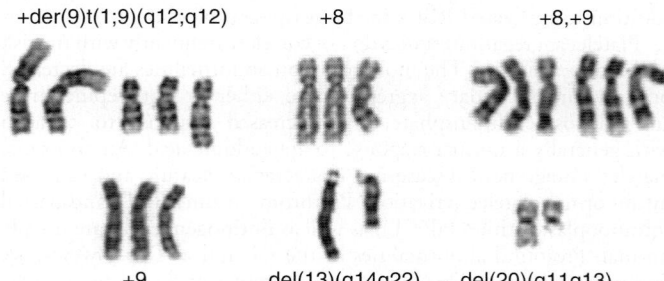

Fig. 68.7 Most frequent chromosomal abnormalities associated with polycythemia vera at diagnosis include *(top row)* a gain of derivative(9)t(1;9), resulting in three copies of the long arms of chromosome 1 and three copies of the long arms of chromosome 9, including Janus kinase 2; gain of chromosome 8 and simultaneous gain of both chromosomes 8 and 9 *(bottom row)*; gain of chromosome 9 alone; interstitial deletion of chromosome 13; and interstitial deletion of chromosome 20.

Interphase fluorescence in situ hybridization (FISH) testing with 12 probes for loci most frequently associated with PV and other Ph⁻ MPNs occasionally identifies cryptic +9p, del(20q) or del(13q) abnormalities and thus may increase the frequency of detecting a chromosomal rearrangement at diagnosis to 29–30%.[23] However, interphase FISH (I-FISH) does not appear to significantly increase the detection rate in untreated patients. Among 452 patients with PV cytogenetically studied at the authors' institution between 1984 and April 2011, 28% had cytogenetic abnormalities at diagnosis. I-FISH studies alone (without cytogenetic examination) using an MPN panel of 12 probes revealed that 29% of patients had genomic changes (Fig. 68.8). The frequency of detection of cytogenetic abnormalities in PV increases over time, with 35–55% of patients having clonal cytogenetic abnormalities after extended follow-up and more than 80% of those patients in whom acute leukemia eventually develops. Progression from a normal to an abnormal karyotype is an important adverse prognostic parameter.

Trisomy of the long arms of chromosome 1 is a recurrent abnormality present in about 4–6% of patients with PV with an abnormal karyotype. This abnormality has also been described in PMF and other myeloid malignancies. Specifically, 70% of patients with post-PV MF develop trisomy 1q as a result of unbalanced translocations. Trisomy 1q rarely occurs alone and is most frequently found translocated to another chromosome, creating an unbalanced +1q translocation. The recipient chromosome most frequently involved is chromosome 6 followed by chromosome 9. Jumping translocations are rare cytogenetic phenomenon whereby a part of one chromosome is translocated to several recipient chromosomes, creating multiple related clones within a single patient. Jumping 1q in MPN occurs in 4.2% of cytogenetically abnormal MPN; 86% of such patients

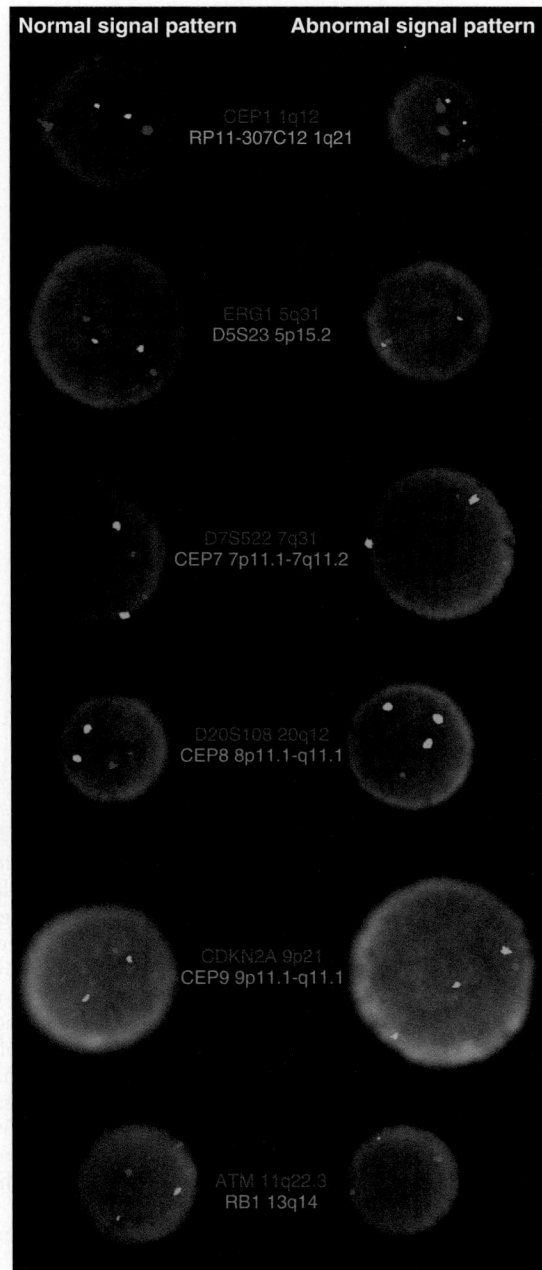

Fig. 68.8 Myeloproliferative neoplasm fluorescence in situ hybridization (FISH) panel includes 12 loci on eight different chromosomes for detection of the most frequent chromosomal rearrangements when cytogenetics are either not available or in conjunction with conventional cytogenetics for detection of cryptic abnormalities. Discrepancy in frequency of abnormality detected by interphase FISH and conventional cytogenetics are present and often suggest a proliferative advantage of the abnormal clone.

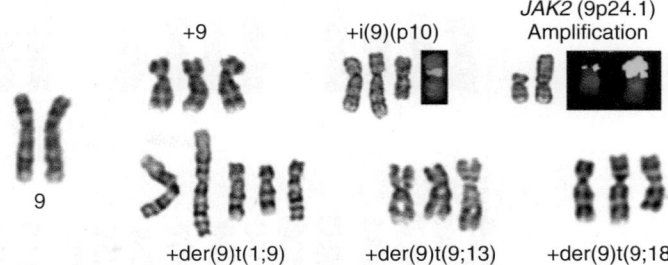

Fig. 68.9 NUMEROUS CHROMOSOMAL ABNORMALITIES RESULTING IN TRISOMY, TETRASOMY, OR AMPLIFICATION OF THE SHORT ARMS OF CHROMOSOME 9. *JAK2,* Janus kinase 2.

cells but not in lymphoid cells. The genetic consequences of trisomy 8 are unclear, although recent studies have suggested a role for microRNAs that are localized on chromosome 8. MicroRNAs are small noncoding RNAs ($\approx$19–25 nucleotides in length) that act as regulators of gene expression by inducing translational inhibition and cleavage of target mRNAs.

Trisomy 9 and gain of the short arms of chromosome 9 is most frequently and almost exclusively observed in PV. There are three types of 9p abnormalities in PV: (1) about 30% of patients have uniparental disomy of the 9p region; (2) numerical gain, such as different chromosomal rearrangements that contribute to trisomy, tetrasomy, or amplification of 9p; and (3) unbalanced translocations, of which the most frequent, +der(9)t(1;9), results in a trisomy of both 9p and 1q, and appears to be a relatively specific abnormality in PV patients (Fig. 68.9). This rearrangement provides an extra copy of mutated *JAK2.* Trisomy 9p and three copies of mutated *JAK2* are rare recurrent abnormalities resulting from unbalanced chromosome 9 translocations such as der(18)t(9;18)(p13;p11)/der(9;18)(p10;q10). I-FISH has been used to detect cryptic chromosome 9 rearrangements. FISH has uncovered chromosome 9 rearrangements in 53% of patients with abnormal FISH patterns, indicating that a gain of 9p is the most frequent genomic alteration in PV. The association between the trisomy of 9p and PV was one of the keys to the identification of the *JAK2V617F* mutation. Cytogenetic studies of 9p and LOH indicate that the LOH is attributable to mitotic recombination. The prognostic significance of +9/+9p is still unknown.

Interstitial deletions of the long arms of chromosome 13 are not specific for PV and are more frequently observed in PMF than in PV. About 1–13% of cytogenetically abnormal patients with PV have del(13q). Among patients with del(13q), about 91% have breakpoints in 13q12-14 to q21-22 regions. Fine FISH mapping has defined the commonly deleted region to 13q13.3-q14.3 encompassing Rb1 and two microsatellite loci, D13S319 and D13S25. Cryptic del(13q) occurs and is easily identified with the FISH method. Deletions are heterogeneous and may involve one, two, or all three loci, including Rb1.

Del(20)(q11q13), an interstitial deletion of the long arm of chromosome 20, is the second most common cytogenetic abnormality in PV (Fig. 68.10). Del(20)(q11q13) is not diagnostic of PV because it also occurs in PMF and ET, as well as in MDS and AML. Heterogeneity of the breakpoints is suggested by the observation that two minimally deleted regions (MDRs) characterize different disorders. A 2.7-Mb region spanning D20S10-8 (proximal) and D20S481 (distal) is identified in Ph⁻ MPN, and a 2.6-Mb region spanning R52161 (proximal) and Wi-12515 (distal) is found in other malignancies. Two commonly deleted regions (CDR), CDR1 spanning 2.4 Mb between bands 20q11.23 and 20q12, and CDR2 encompassing 1.8 Mb within 20q13.12, have been identified. The commonly retained region (CRR)1 spans 1.9 Mb within 20q11.21 and CRR2 encompasses 2.5 Mb within 20q13.33. High-resolution genotyping has not revealed any somatic copy-neutral LOH within these regions. Investigations to date of candidate genes within the deleted segments have failed to identify any mutations within deleted segments. In contrast, haploinsufficiency of the *L3MBTL1* gene, the

progress to AML after an average of 8 months, suggesting that 1q jumping translocations are associated with both disease progression and poor prognosis.

Gain of chromosome 8 is a recurrent abnormality not only in Ph⁻ MPN, but it is also one of the three most frequent abnormalities in MDS and is present in 10% of patients with malignant hematopoietic disorders of both myeloid and lymphoid lineages. The prognostic significance in PV is unknown. Some patients with PV with trisomy 8 do not acquire other abnormalities after 20 years. The simultaneous presence of both +8 and +9 is PV specific, and is observed in 3–4% of PV cases; it is rarely seen in other hematologic malignancies. In PV, trisomy 8 has been demonstrated in myeloid

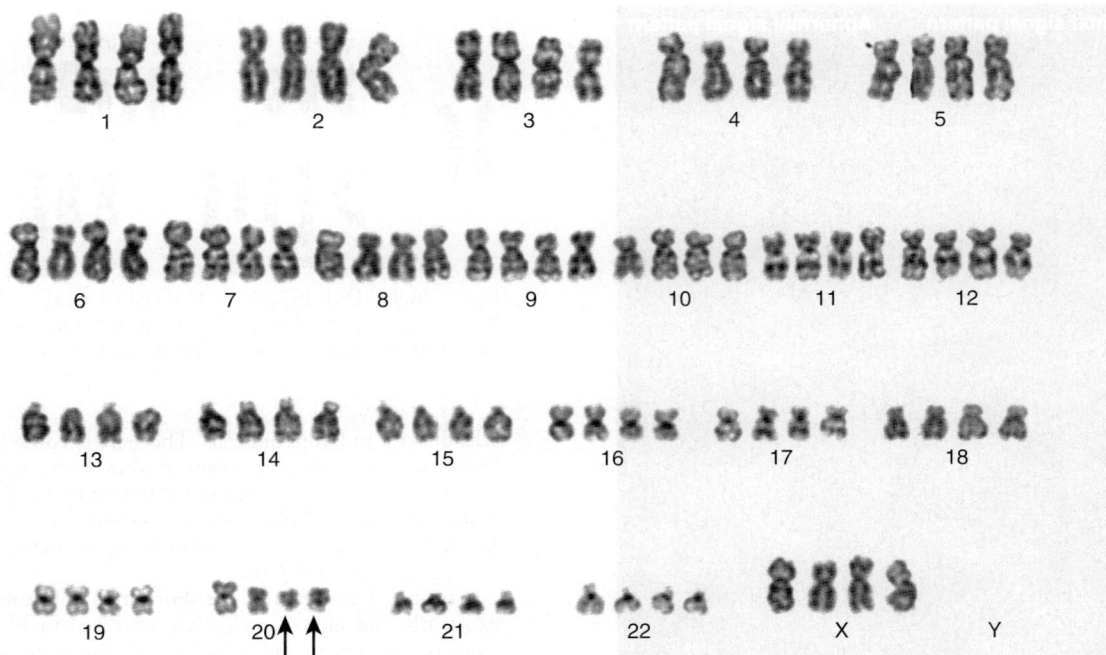

Fig. 68.10 A karyotype from a dividing megakaryocyte showing (*arrows*) two copies of deleted 20q in a cell with 92 chromosomes.

human homolog of the *Drosophila* L(3)MBT polycomb group tumor suppressor gene located on the 20q12 within a region commonly deleted in several myeloid malignancies, may play a role in erythropoiesis in PV. Downregulation of *L3MBTL1* expression in primary hematopoietic stem progenitor cells (HSPCs) causes enhanced commitment to and acceleration of erythroid differentiation. Moreover, overexpression of *L3MBTL1* in primary hematopoietic CD34+ cells as well as in 20q cell lines limits erythroid differentiation. Therefore, haploinsufficiency of *L3MBTL1* may contribute to erythroid differentiation in PV. It has also been demonstrated that *L3MBTL1* is important for the normal progression of cells through mitosis because both overexpression and loss of activity can affect cell division. There is evidence that 20q deletions may impair the release of granulocytes into the peripheral blood. Some patients with PV and 20q deletion in BM cells have cytogenetically normal peripheral blood granulocytes, which has been attributed to del(20q) cells being preferentially retained or destroyed in the BM. The significance of this abnormality remains unknown because it may be dormant for many years before cells with del(20q) gain proliferative advantage. It is important to emphasize, however, that patients with del(20q) have been observed without further karyotypic instability for more than 10 years.

Other rare recurrent chromosomal abnormalities may occur at the onset of the disease or are associated with disease progression. Both interstitial deletions of the long arms of chromosomes 5 and 7 have been reported at diagnosis and are associated with disease progression. Loss of P53 as a result of del(17p) or other chromosomal rearrangements is a rare finding in PV and appears to be related to disease progression. Del(17p) is not PV specific because it is found in many other myeloid malignancies.

Chromosome abnormalities including +8, +9, and del(20) (q11q13) are related to the biogenesis of the disease rather than occurring as a consequence of the chemotherapy. However, in some patients an abnormal clone (abnormalities of chromosome 5, 7, or 17) appears to develop as a consequence of exposure to chemotherapeutic agents. Some investigators have suggested that patients with cytogenetic abnormalities at diagnosis have a statistically significant poorer survival rate than those in whom a normal karyotype is observed. This influence of cytogenetic abnormalities on prognosis has, however, not been verified.

DIFFERENTIAL DIAGNOSIS

In most patients, establishing the cause leading to erythrocytosis is not difficult. Initially, it is critical to be certain that one is dealing with a patient with absolute erythrocytosis. A hematocrit level greater than 60% on several occasions in men or greater than 55% in women, however, is certainly associated with an elevated RBC mass. Testing for *JAK2V617F* and *JAK2* exon 12 mutations can be extremely useful in diagnosing PV and is now a standard practice to make a diagnosis in any patient who is suspected of having PV. The presence of splenomegaly is an important finding on clinical examination, and adjunctive laboratory findings include normal arterial oxygen saturation, elevated leukocyte alkaline phosphatase activity, and *JAK2V617F* assays. Splenic sizing by ultrasonography can be useful in documenting splenic enlargement when the spleen is not palpable by physical examination.

It is initially important to differentiate PV from the large number of other causes of secondary erythrocytosis. Characteristically, the patient with PV will present with erythrocytosis, leukocytosis, thrombocytosis, and splenomegaly, and is positive for *JAK2V617F*. The BM biopsy shows hypercellularity with trilineage hyperplasia. In individuals who lack a mutated *JAK2*, it is important to determine the SaO_2 using an arterial blood gas, the carboxyhemoglobin level, and the $P_{50}O_2$ in patients with other family members with erythrocytosis to exclude obvious causes of secondary erythrocytosis. Because smokers' polycythemia is the most frequent cause of erythrocytosis, it is wise to measure carboxyhemoglobin levels early on in the investigation. In addition, a PaO_2 greater than 67 mmHg or an O_2 saturation greater than 95%, as quantitated on an arterial blood gas, is helpful in ruling out hypoxic conditions that lead to erythrocytosis. In patients with intermittent hypoxia, such as sleep apnea syndrome or alveolar hypoventilation caused by obesity, such blood gas determinations can be normal. A low $P_{50}O_2$ is indicative of a hemoglobin mutant with high O_2 affinity, leading to tissue hypoxia and erythrocytosis. Patients with PV characteristically exhibit serum EPO levels below the 95% CIs for the range observed in normal control participants. It is not unusual to have a normal EPO level in some patients with hypoxic causes of secondary erythrocytosis, unless the hypoxia exists over an extended period of time. A normal EPO level cannot be used to exclude a hypoxic cause of erythrocytosis. EPO

TABLE 68.3	World Health Organization Criteria for Polycythemia Vera[24]

2016 WHO Diagnostic Criteria for PV

Major criteria:

1. Hemoglobin >16.5 g/dL in men, 16 g/dL in women, or hematocrit >49% (men), >48% women or increased RCM)[a]
2. BM biopsy showing hypercellularity for age with trilineage growth (panmyelosis) including prominent erythroid, granulocytic, and megakaryocytic proliferation with pleomorphic, mature megakaryocytes
3. Presence of *JAK2V617F* or *JAK2* exon 12 mutation

Minor criteria:

1. Serum EPO level less than the reference range for normal

Diagnosis requires meeting either all three major criteria or the first two major criteria and the minor criterion

[a]More than 25% above mean normal predicted value.
BM, Bone marrow; EPO, erythropoietin; PV, polycythemia vera; RCM, red cell mass; WHO, World Health Organization.
Data from Arber DA, Orazi A, Hasserjian R, et al: The 2016 revision to the World Health Organization classification of myeloid neoplasms and acute leukemia. *Blood* 127:2391, 2016.

measurements do, however, remain an important diagnostic tool. Elevation of EPO levels in the face of erythrocytosis is indicative of a hypoxic cause of secondary erythrocytosis, but extremely low levels of EPO (<4 mIU/mL) are virtually diagnostic of PV.

Incorporating a mutational screen into the algorithm for investigating a case of suspected polycythemia will help to streamline the diagnosis of PV, although the presence of a *JAK2* mutation alone does not distinguish PV from PMF or ET. Clinical criteria for the diagnosis of PV have been defined by the World Health Organization (WHO), which serves as a uniform platform with which to diagnose PV. It is important, however, for the clinician to realize that some patients undoubtedly have an MPN disorder resembling PV but do not fulfill all the diagnostic criteria of the PVSG or the WHO. The criteria for the diagnosis of PV, including the use of the *JAK2V617* assay and histopathologic parameters, have been provided by the WHO (Table 68.3).[24] These criteria are the consensus of many experts working in this field.

There will always be unusual cases with clinical characteristics that cannot be pigeonholed into a particular diagnostic category. If these patients have serious symptoms, the individual physician must make treatment decisions on the basis of the risk–benefit ratio for that patient.

A particularly difficult dilemma occurs when evaluating patients with isolated pure erythrocytosis. These patients have elevated RBC masses, normal WBC counts, normal platelet counts, no evidence of splenomegaly, and no evidence of any recognizable cause of secondary erythrocytosis. Clearly, some of these patients have *JAK2V617F*-positive PV or mutations of exon 12 *JAK2*, leading to isolated erythrocytosis. The PFCPs are caused by truncation of the EPOR, characterized by increased sensitivity of erythroid progenitor cells to EPO, and can be easily distinguished from PV. These patients frequently present in childhood, and this disorder is characterized by isolated erythrocytosis that is associated with an increased risk of thrombotic events. There is a strong family history of polycythemia. The BM progenitor cells are hypersensitive to EPO, yet no colonies form in the absence of EPO. The patient with profound erythrocytosis who is negative for *JAK2V617F* as well as exon 12 *JAK2* mutations and does not have erythrocytosis caused by smoking, cyanotic heart disease, an EPO-secreting tumor,, sleep apnea, or resides at a high altitude remains a diagnostic dilemma. All patients should have a good family and drug history, an arterial oxygen saturation study and a carboxyhemoglobin measurement, and measurement or calculation of p50, and quantitation of 2,3BPG and serum EPO levels. If these studies are unrewarding, these patients should then be investigated for mutations in the hypoxia-responsive element of the human *EPO* gene, HIF-2α and HIF-1α, VHL, PHD1,2,3, STAT5, LNK,

and TET2. Some of these tests can be performed by commercial laboratories, but often one will have to contact an academic reference laboratory to complete such an extensive investigative effort (www.mayomedicallaboratories.com/articles/features/erythrocytosis/testing).

PV must also be differentiated from the other MPNs, such as CML, ET, and PMF. Such classification has major prognostic implications and influences important therapeutic decisions, including the use of tyrosine kinase inhibitors. With the distinctive cytogenetic abnormalities and molecular genetic abnormalities that are unique to CML (Philadelphia chromosome, *BCR-ABL* gene fusion), these two disorders should not be difficult to differentiate. Occasional patients with an MPN have been shown to have both *JAK2V617F* as well as *BCR-ABL*; whether this unusual occurrence that takes place in two different clones and thereby represents two independent MPNs or a single clone and is caused by the predisposition of such patients to acquire mutations in their hematopoietic cells is a subject of speculation.

Patients with PMF can present with abnormalities that are virtually indistinguishable from those of patients with PV-related MF. Almost 50% of PMF are *JAK2V617F* positive, but more than 90% of patients with post-PV MF are *JAK2V617F* positive. The survival of patients with the latter disorder is much shorter than that of patients with the former condition. Unusual patients with PMF may actually develop PV after iron supplementation or the institution of chemotherapy. ET with a borderline elevated hematocrit and PV with marked thrombocytosis can easily be confused. When the RBC mass is used as a definitive diagnostic test, a distinction between ET and the erythrocytotic phase of PV is usually readily apparent. This measurement is not widely available and can also be normal or actually low in patients with PV who are iron deficient because of bleeding or excessive phlebotomy. Campbell and coworkers have used sensitive PCR-based methods to assess the *JAK2* mutational states in 806 patients with ET. The mutation was present in more than 50% of patients with ET. *JAK2V617F*-positive ET patients were characterized by multiple features that resembled those of patients with PV, including higher hemoglobin levels, higher WBC counts, more prominent BM erythroid and granulocytic hyperplasia, a higher incidence of venous but not arterial thrombosis, low serum EPO levels, and lower serum ferritin levels. Surprisingly, *JAK2V617F*-negative patients who likely had calreticulin mutations had higher platelet counts. Furthermore, *JAK2V617F*-positive ET patients had a higher probability of developing PV with long follow-up. Acquisition of homozygosity for the *JAK2V617* caused by homologous recombination is likely the critical event in the development of PV in *JAK2V617F* ET patients. Homozygosity for *JAK2V617F* occurs in at least 30% of patients with PV but is extremely rare in ET.

PROGNOSIS

The prognosis of a patient with PV depends on the nature and severity of the complications that occur during the clinical course of that particular patient's disorder. In addition, an individual patient's prognosis depends on the duration of the erythrocytotic phase or the time to transition to post-PV MF or acute leukemia. Survival is also influenced by whether appropriate treatment is instituted during the erythrocytotic phase of the illness. Patients who have uncontrolled erythrocytosis are at an extremely high risk for the development of thromboses. The median survival time from the onset of symptoms has been reported in a study that is over four decades old to be as short as 1.5 years in untreated patients, but this number seems excessive because of the relatively large number of patients who are diagnosed during routine examinations and are asymptomatic for prolonged periods of time. Determination of the optimal management of patients with PV has been a difficult task because the disease, when treated, is associated with a survival period of approximately 17 years. Studies of new potential therapeutic interventions therefore require prospective studies with prolonged follow-up times before

TABLE 68.4	Risk Stratification in Polycythemia Vera Based on Thrombotic Risk		
Risk Category	**Age >60 Years or History of Thrombosis**	**Cardiovascular Risk Factors[a]**	
Low	No	No	
Intermediate	No	Yes	
High	Yes		

[a]Hypertension, hypercholesterolemia, diabetes, and smoking (see text). Extreme thrombocytosis (platelet count >1500 × 10^9 L^{-1}) is a risk factor for bleeding. Its role as a risk factor for thrombosis is uncertain. An increasing leukocyte count has been identified as a novel risk factor for thrombosis, but confirmation is required.
Data from Finazzi G, Barbui T: How I treat patients with polycythemia vera. *Blood* 109:5104, 2007.

meaningful results can be generated determining their ability to improve upon overall survival.

Increasing age and history of vascular events have consistently proven to be independent predictors of developing additional thromboses in patients with PV. In the ECLAP trial, the incidence of cardiovascular complications was higher in patients older than 69 years of age, patients with a history of thrombosis, and patients with WBC counts higher than 15,000 × 10^9 L^{-1}. Conventional cardiovascular risk factors, including hypertension, hyperlipidemia, diabetes, and smoking, are assumed to be associated with the same relative risk of developing thrombosis in PV patients as that observed in the general population. Although practicing hematologists are frequently concerned about elevated platelet counts in PV patients, several reports have failed to show any association between platelet count and thrombotic events, suggesting that therapies in PV targeting reduction of platelet numbers are ill conceived.

These data have led to stratification of therapy in patients with PV based on clearly identifiable risk factors (Table 68.4) of developing additional thrombotic events. The development of acute leukemia was a relatively rare event in PV, occurring in 22 out of 1638 patients in the ECLAP observational study after a median of 8.4 years from the time of diagnosis. Older age as well as treatment with alkylating agents was associated with a four- to eightfold increased risk of developing AML or MDS compared with patients treated with phlebotomy alone, hydroxyurea, or IFN. The effect of *JAK2V617F* allele frequency on the prognosis of PV patients has been examined. More than 95% of patients with PV are *JAK2V617F* positive, and their mutational load can be determined by allele-specific PCR. Approximately 30% of PV patients have a high *JAK2V617F* burden (>50%), and the remainder have a lower burden (<50%), with the small numbers being WT. Some investigators, but not all, have reported that high burdens of *JAK2V617F* in PV patients are associated with larger splenic volumes, more frequent aquagenic pruritus, a higher incidence of thrombotic events, and a higher rate of evolution into MF and acute leukemia.

High leukocyte counts (>15,000 × 10^9/L) at the time of diagnosis have been identified as another independent predictor of developing a major thrombosis in PV patients. In addition, others have suggested that this parameter is predictive of evolution to MF and AML and an overall inferior survival time.

In a study of more than 1500 patients with PV, risk factors for survival included advanced age, leukocytosis, venous thrombosis, and abnormal karyotype. Median survival was 23 years in the absence of advanced age and leukocytosis, and 9 years with the presence of both of these risk factors. In another study of 327 patients with PV from France and Sweden, multivariable analysis identified age >70 years, leukocyte count >13 × 10^9/L, and thrombosis at diagnosis as risk factors for survival. Patients with two or more of these risk factors had a 10-year relative survival of 26%, as opposed to patients with zero or one risk factors, who had a 10-year survival of 84% and 59%, respectively.

The choice of therapeutic agents used to treat the erythrocytotic phase of disease clearly influences patient outcomes. The use of alkylating agents is associated with an established risk for leukemic transformation or evolution to MDS. Clearly, this risk is also associated with increased duration of the disease. The effect of hydroxyurea on leukemic transformation rates is limited, if any. In addition, the influence of long-term IFN therapy on disease outcomes is not at present clearly defined.

THERAPY

The cumulative duration of survival for PV patients treated with modern strategies is between 15 and 17 years. Despite the implementation of standard therapeutic strategies, the mortality rate of PV patients is increased by 1.84 compared with age- and sex-matched populations. The primary goals of treatment are to reduce the risk for thrombosis, ameliorate the PV symptom burden, and prevent evolution to MF and/or AML. Unfortunately, current therapies are not effective for this latter purpose, and controlling blood counts may have less of an effect than anticipated. The European Leukemia Net (ELN) expert panel defined a complete response as a hematocrit less than 45% without phlebotomy, platelet count less than 400 × 10^9/L, leukocyte count less than 10 × 10^9/L, normal spleen size, and no disease-related symptoms.[25] However, in a study of 261 patients with PV who were given hydroxyurea (HU) and followed up for a median of 4.4 years, no association was observed between achieving an ELN or a hematocrit response and better survival or fewer vascular complications. No particular platelet or leukocyte count could be shown to be protective against thrombosis. The ELN response criteria were updated in 2013, but they have not been validated to predict survival or progression to MF or AML. Therapy is also stratified based on the presumed risk of an individual patient to develop additional thrombotic episodes, with low-risk patients being treated with phlebotomy therapy alone plus a therapy directed toward paralysis of platelet function and high-risk patients receiving not only phlebotomy plus antiplatelet therapy but also some form of myelosuppressive therapy (hydroxyurea, IFN, busulfan, melphalan, ruxolitinib). At present, the therapeutic goals are to reduce the risk of thrombosis by normalizing the hematocrit levels to 45% (some experts advocate reducing the hematocrit to 42% in females) based on a randomized prospective study that demonstrated a decreased risk of cardiovascular morbidity and mortality with a goal hematocrit of less than 45% compared to 45–50%.[21] Previous studies have indicated a lack of a relationship between thrombocytosis at diagnosis or during the period of follow-up with thrombotic complications. Whether therapy should be directed at normalization of platelets remains uncertain at present and should not be pursued unless within the context of a clinical trial. Extreme thrombocytosis (>1 × 10^9/L), if associated with spontaneous hemorrhage, is an indication for normalization of platelet numbers. Phlebotomy therapy alone is the standard of care for low-risk PV patients (see box on General Principles of Therapy).

A series of studies, although completed more than 30 years ago, by the Polycythemia Vera Study Group answered several very important questions regarding the efficacy and associated complications of particular therapeutic modalities. These investigations have aided in the identification of optimal therapy for individual patients, which must be selected on the basis of age and comorbid disease status to minimize treatment-related complications.

The first PVSG randomized trial (01 trial) evaluated three treatment strategies: (1) phlebotomy alone to maintain the hematocrit level at less than 45%; (2) intravenous ^{32}P at 2.3 mCi/m^2 repeated every 12 weeks, if needed (maximum, 5 mCi per dose) supplemented by phlebotomy to maintain the hematocrit level at less than 45%; and (3) myelosuppression with chlorambucil 10 mg/day orally for 6 weeks and then daily on alternate months with necessary dose reductions and supplemental phlebotomy. More than 400 patients were randomly assigned to this protocol. The median survival duration from entry into the study until death was 9.1 years for patients treated with chlorambucil, 10.9 years for those treated with ^{32}P, and 12.6 years for the phlebotomy group. Long-term survival was inferior for patients treated with chlorambucil compared with those treated with

General Principles of Therapy

1. The etiology of erythrocytosis must be correctly categorized to be certain the patient has polycythemia vera (PV). This will avoid inappropriate exposure of patients with nonmalignant disorders to the adverse effects of myelosuppresive agents. To this end, a major contribution is played by incorporating molecular marker testing (*JAK2V617F* and exon 12 *JAK2* mutational determinations) in the diagnostic workup, and in this way, early phases of PV can be recognized as well. In individuals with erythrocytosis without a *JAK2* mutation, search for causes of secondary causes of erythrocytocytosis as well as inherited disorders that lead to erythrocytosis, which includes mutations in *EPOR*, *VHL*, *PHD2*, *HIF-1* and *HIF-2*.
2. Therapy should be individualized.
3. Initially, the hematocrit should be reduced to 45% as soon as possible. The speed of phlebotomy will depend on patients' general medical conditions (250–500 mL every other day). Elderly patients with compromised cardiovascular or pulmonary systems should be more carefully phlebotomized (twice a week), or smaller volumes of blood should be removed.
4. Hematocrit levels should be maintained at 45%.
5. The use of chemotherapeutic agents should be avoided in low-risk PV patients, and treatment with hydroxyurea or interferon (IFN) or ruxolitinib should be reserved for high-risk patients. Be on the lookout for toxicities from each of these agents.
6. Hyperuricemia is treated with allopurinol (100–300 mg/day).
7. Pruritus may be improved with PV-directed therapy (phlebotomyhydroxyurea or IFN). Empiric therapy with antihistamines can be useful in selected patients. Selective serotonin uptake inhibitors (paroxetine 20 mg/day or fluoxetine 10 mg/day) or phototherapy can also be of use. Dramatic relief, however, can be achieved in almost all cases with the institution of ruxolitinib. Due to cost, ruxolitinib therapy should be reserved for individuals with pruritis not relieved by less costly strategies.
8. Elective surgery or dental procedures should be delayed until hematocrit levels have been normalized for more than 2 months. Aspirin should be withdrawn at least 1 week before surgery. If emergency surgery is contemplated, phlebotomy and cytapheresis should be pursued.
9. Women and men who are contemplating having children should be treated by phlebotomy plus low-dose aspirin therapy (81 mg/day) or with IFN-α to avoid teratogenic effects of chemotherapy. Such avoidance will also prevent deleterious effects on fertility. During pregnancy, therapy is frequently not necessary; if it is, phlebotomy plus low-dose aspirin should be exclusively used. If phlebotomy control is inadequate, treatment with IFN-α should be pursued.

[32]P or phlebotomy. An early finding was the appearance during the first 5 years of a significant excess of deaths from acute leukemia in the chlorambucil arm, which reached 17% after 15 years of follow-up. As a result, the chlorambucil arm was discontinued, and patients were assigned randomly to one of the other two arms. Even though no statistical difference in overall survival between ^{32}P and phlebotomy alone was apparent through the first 10 years, the morbidity and mortality associated with each type of therapy were attributable to distinctly different causes. Thrombosis as a cause of death was much more frequent in the phlebotomy-only group during the first 5–7 years of follow-up. Analyses of factors associated with thrombosis revealed that the performance of phlebotomy, the rate of phlebotomy, advancing age, and history of previous thrombosis were statistically significant factors predictive of this outcome. Historical studies have raised concerns about therapy with phlebotomy alone. The need for more than four therapeutic phlebotomies a year in the phlebotomy-alone arm was associated with an increased thrombotic risk. This led to the belief that frequent phlebotomy requirements were detrimental and necessitated cytoreductive therapy. However, overall survival and risk of evolution to MF and AML were lower in the phlebotomy alone arm. Certain concerns about phlebotomy may be unfounded. Iron deficiency is a consequence of repeated therapeutic phlebotomy; but in fact, it should be viewed as a therapeutic goal to further limit erythropoiesis. Although iron deficiency can be associated with a number of clinical signs and symptoms, including glossitis, dysphagia, cheilosis, koilonychia, fatigue, global weakness, cognitive deficits, neuromuscular disturbances, and pica syndrome, these rarely prompt treatment discontinuation. In contrast, the use of ^{32}P led to a lower rate of thrombosis during the first 5 years, but the incidences of leukemias, lymphomas, and nonhematologic malignancies increased during the next 5 years to nearly 10%. After a 15-year period of observation, the incidences of leukemia and lymphoma in the chlorambucil group had risen to 17%. A statistically significant increase in skin and gastrointestinal cancers occurred in the [32]P- and chlorambucil-treated cohorts compared with the group treated with phlebotomy alone (see box on Algorithm for Management of Patients With Polycythemia Vera). Based on these studies, therapy with chlorambucil and ^{32}P are no longer recommended.

Impetus for the use of nonchemotherapeutic agents for the treatment of PV was provided by an extensive natural history study of 1213 patients reported by the Gruppo Italiano Studio Policitemia. They showed that the age- and gender-standardized mortality rate of patients with PV was 1.7-times greater than the mortality rate of control participants in the general Italian population. In addition, four times as many patients who had previously received ^{32}P, alkylating agents, or hydroxyurea died of cancer compared with patients treated with phlebotomy alone. When this group combined the total number of deaths and the number of nonfatal myocardial infarctions and strokes, they found an unsatisfactory risk-to-benefit profile in patients treated with chemotherapeutic agents and suggested that antithrombotic strategies, such as low-dose aspirin, be carefully evaluated for use in the care of patients with PV.

PV platelets are known to have a generalized abnormality of arachidonate metabolism that is characterized by enhanced synthesis of thromboxane A_2, which likely reflects stimuli to platelet activation. The exact mechanism responsible for enhanced platelet synthesis of thromboxane A_2 in PV remains unknown and requires further investigation. A low-dose aspirin regimen (50 mg/day for 7–14 days) has been shown to suppress more than 80% of the excretion of the metabolites of thromboxane A_2. A pilot study was performed in which the toxicity of low-dose aspirin therapy in PV patients was evaluated. A very low-dose aspirin regimen (40 mg/day) was chosen to prevent thrombosis yet minimize the risk of bleeding. After follow-up of the low-dose aspirin treatment group and control group, low-dose therapy was shown not to be associated with an increased incidence of bleeding complications. Aspirin therapy was well tolerated and was associated with complete inhibition of platelet cyclooxygenase activity. A large, randomized, placebo-controlled clinical trial testing the risk-to-benefit ratio of low-dose aspirin therapy in preventing thrombotic episodes in PV has been completed. Treatment with low-dose aspirin (100 mg/day) compared with placebo reduced the risk of the combined end points of nonfatal myocardial infarction, nonfatal stroke, pulmonary embolism, major venous thrombosis, or death from cardiovascular courses. Overall mortality and cardiovascular mortality, however, was not reduced significantly by aspirin therapy. Importantly, the incidence of major bleeding episodes was not significantly increased in the aspirin group. It is important to emphasize that patients require aggressive phlebotomy therapy to the appropriate target hematocrit levels as well as the appropriate use of myelosuppressive agents as primary therapy, with the addition of aspirin serving as an adjunct to this strategy. The conclusions of this study have been questioned by several investigators. In addition, a retrospective analysis performed by independent investigators of the 630 patients treated by the ECLAP group has concluded that low-dose aspirin therapy in PV patients was associated with a statistically nonsignificant reduction in the risk of fatal thrombotic episodes without an increased risk of bleeding.[26] This meta-analysis is surely not a ringing endorsement of the widespread use of aspirin therapy, which is a strategy that has been indiscriminately used worldwide to treat such patients. Because it is unlikely that the value of aspirin therapy will be examined in a properly powered randomized trial, it is suggested that since aspirin therapy is a relatively innocuous therapy it should be used in high-risk patients judiciously.

Algorithm for Management of Patients With Polycythemia Vera

Low-Risk Young Patients (Age <60 Years) and No History of Thrombosis, Platelet Count <1.5 × 10⁶ mm⁻³

Phlebotomy + low-dose aspirin (81 mg/day) to maintain hematocrit lower than 45%. Aspirin should not be used in patients with histories of a hemorrhagic episode or with extreme thrombocytosis (>1.5 × 10^6 mm⁻³) or acquired von Willebrand syndrome.

↓

Thrombosis or hemorrhage
Systemic symptoms
Severe pruritus refractory to histamine antagonists
Painful splenomegaly

↓

Hydroxyurea 15–20 mg/kg (unless age <40 years, pregnant, intolerant to hydroxyurea; consider pegylated interferon [IFN])

↓

Pegylated IFN 45–180 µg/week or IFN-α - (3 × 10⁶ units three times a week; alter dose depending on response and toxicity) or ruxolitinib 10 mg twice daily and titrate dose depending on the response. →

In a patient with a prior thrombosis or a history of bleeding due to acquired von Willebrand's syndrome, normalization of platelet numbers is necessary. If platelet control is inadequate or the patient cannot tolerate interferon, one option is the use of anagrelide. In this case, supplemental phlebotomy is required to maintain hematocrit lower than 45%, and the use of hydroxyurea should be considered, especially if the patient continues to have thrombotic episodes.

↓

If the patient has increasing splenomegaly, systemic symptoms, or repeated thromboses despite adequate dose of hydroxyurea (2–3 g/day) or if unable to tolerate hydroxyurea, start ruxolitinib 10 mg twice daily and titrate up or down based on hematologic parameters
For patients unable to tolerate ruxolitinib or resistant to it, start low doses of busulphan or melphalan, which should be administered until the blood counts are normalized. Therapy should be then discontinued since patients frequently enjoy drug-free prolonged remissions lasting months. Therapy should only be reinstituted at the time the blood counts begin to be elevated again. Such therapy with alkylating agents should be rarely used in young patients. It should be mentioned that the sequential use of hydroxyurea and alkylating agents may be associated with an increased risk of leukemia. Supplemental phlebotomy may be required.

Painful splenomegaly

↓

Patients should be treated with ruxolitinib
If unable to tolerate or insufficient response
Splenectomy + continued systemic therapy

↓

High-risk patients (age >60 years), previous thrombosis, platelet count >1.5 × 10⁶ mm⁻³
Phlebotomy to hematocrit of 45%
Aspirin (81 mg/day) to be given only in patients with platelet counts <1.5 × 10⁶ mm⁻²
Myelosuppressive therapy with hydroxyurea 30 mg/kg orally for 1 week
Then 15–20 mg/kg

↓

If patient continues to have thrombotic episodes and has extreme thrombocytosis or cannot tolerate hydroxyurea
Consider pegylated IFN 45–180 µg/week, anagrelide, or ruxolitinib 10 mg twice daily, or add intermittent busulphan or melphalan (in older patients).
If on busulphan or melphalan, stop when blood counts are normalized or platelet count is lower than 300,000 mm⁻³.
Occasional supplemental phlebotomy if hematocrit is >45%; when patient relapses (patient is symptomatic) initiate busulphan therapy again at same dose.

Patient Age >70 Years

Phlebotomy + low-dose aspirin + hydroxyurea

↓

No response or poor compliance
Ruxolitinib, melphalan, or busulfan.

However, it should be avoided in patients with extremely high platelet counts who are at risk for hemorrhage.

After the disappointing results experienced with the alkylating agent chlorambucil, the PVSG began a nonrandomized phase II investigation of hydroxyurea, an S-phase–specific ribonucleotide reductase inhibitor. The hope was that this agent would be nonleukemogenic. Of 53 patients with PV treated with hydroxyurea who had never received other forms of myelosuppression, after follow-up for a median period of 8.6 years and a maximum follow-up of 795 weeks, 5.4% developed acute leukemia compared with 1.5% of patients treated with phlebotomy alone on the original PVSG randomized study.

In a comparable trial from Israel, 71 patients were treated with hydroxyurea for a mean duration of 7.3 years. Remarkably, the incidence of thrombosis was only 6%, indicating the potential of hydroxyurea to lower the incidence of thrombosis in patients with PV, confirming an observation previously made by another group. The incidence of leukemia in the Israeli trial was 5.6%. In another retrospective series, the incidence of acute leukemia and myelodysplasia in patients with PV treated with hydroxyurea alone was 6.9%. In patients treated first with busulphan and then hydroxyurea, the rate of acute leukemia and myelodysplasia was 13.8%. Twenty two patients developed AML and MDS in the ECLAP study that enrolled 1638 patients. AML and MDS were diagnosed after a median of 8.4 years from the diagnosis of PV; the variable associated with progression was older age, but overall disease duration (>10 years) failed to reach statistical significance. Exposure to P^{32}, busulphan, and pipobroman but not hydroxyurea alone had an independent role in producing an excess risk for progression to AML and MDS compared with treatment with phlebotomy or IFN. The potential leukemia-promoting potential of hydroxyurea has been readdressed in two additional studies. Kiladjian and coworkers[26] reported the results of a randomized trial of hydroxyurea versus piprobroman that was initiated in 1980; the overall survival was 20.3 years in the hydroxyurea-treated group compared with 15.4 years for the patients treated with piprobroman. The incidence of AML and MDS in the piprobroman group was dramatically higher, which is not unexpected because pipobroman is an alkylating agent. This trial was designed with a cross-over option, but 93 patients only received piprobroman. The incidence of AML and MDS in the patient group that only received hydroxyurea was 7.3%, 10.7%, and 16.6% at 10, 15, and 20 years, respectively. Since there was not a control arm treated with phlebotomy alone, one cannot determine if this rate of evolution to AML/MDS represents the natural history of PV or a possible limited leukemogenic effect of hydroxyurea. Interestingly, no difference in the incidence of vascular events was seen between the two arms. This same question was again addressed in a nested case–control study performed in Sweden.[27] The most important observation was that 25% of patients with various MPNs (68% had PV) who evolved to AML and MDS had not been exposed to any chemotherapeutic agent, indicating that the risk of leukemic evolution was higher than had been previously appreciated. The use of radioactive phosphorous and alkylating agents, but not hydroxyurea, was associated with a higher rate of AML and MDS. These reports indicate that nontreatment-related factors play a major role in the development of AML and MDS, and the contribution of hydroxyurea based on the best available evidence is at best minimal. These data and the ease of administration make hydroxyurea a very useful chemotherapeutic agent in older, high-risk patients with disease that cannot be controlled with phlebotomy alone. Excessive myelosuppression, macrocytosis, hypersegmentation of polymorphonuclear leukocytes, cutaneous actinic keratosis, squamous cell carcinoma of the skin, hyperpigmentation of the skin and nail beds, stomatitis, painful leg ulcers, creatinine elevations, and jaundice have been attributed to the use of hydroxyurea. Aphthous and leg ulcers occur in 9% of patients, usually after approximately 10 months of therapy (see Fig. 68.11).[28] Rarely, cycling of platelet and leukocyte counts but not RBCs occurs while patients are being treated with hydroxyurea. In this situation, the authors have maintained patients on a fixed dose of hydroxyurea rather than chasing cycling platelet counts. In addition, the use of

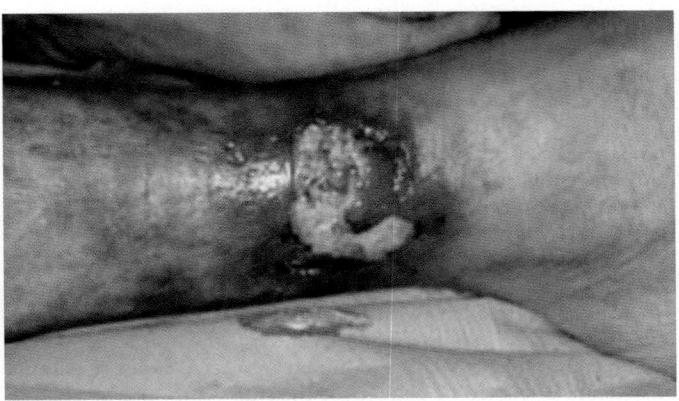

Fig. 68.11 EXAMPLE OF A HYDROXYUREA-INDUCED LEG ULCER. *(From Soutou B, Aractingi S: Myeloproliferative disorder therapy: Assessment and management of adverse events: A dermatologist's perspective. Hematol Oncol 27:11, 2009.)*

hydroxyurea requires patient compliance and careful monitoring of blood counts to avoid the sequelae of excessive myelosuppression.

Some clinical investigators have suggested that a program of phlebotomy alone with low-dose aspirin is the most appropriate for younger patients who have not experienced a cerebrovascular or cardiovascular event.

Anagrelide, a selective inhibitor of platelet production, has been used to treat uncontrolled thrombocytosis not responsive to hydroxyurea in PV patients with thrombotic or hemorrhagic complications. This agent appears to be nonleukemogenic and acts by impairing megakaryocyte maturation. Its use leads to a selective reduction in platelet numbers, and it has been effective in patients refractory to hydroxyurea and IFN. This drug does not effectively control the erythrocytosis and leukocytosis or systemic symptoms associated with PV, and therefore is best used as a supplement to phlebotomy therapy. The time to complete response generally ranges between 17 and 25 days. The dose of anagrelide required to control thrombocytosis remains constant over time in most patients. When anagrelide is discontinued, platelet counts returned to pretreatment levels within 5–7 days. The simultaneous administration of anagrelide and low-dose aspirin has been reported to lead to a significant increase in bleeding manifestations. Clinicians presume that the effects of anagrelide observed in ET patients will be relevant to patients with PV. This assumption has not been tested in a randomized clinical trial. Anagrelide therapy should be reserved for patients with recent thromboses (e.g., stroke, migraines, erythromelalgia) and with thrombocytosis that cannot be controlled with IFN, hydroxyurea, or ruxolitinib therapy alone. It can also be used in combination with hydroxyurea to minimize adverse events that accompany the use of each drug alone. Anagrelide should not be used in pregnant patients because it can easily cross the placenta, leading to adverse effects on the platelet count of the fetus.

Approximately 15–20% of patients treated with anagrelide discontinue the medication because of nonmyelosuppressive side effects. The spectrum of adverse effects involved neurologic (headaches and dizziness), cardiac (vasodilatation, fluid retention, congestive heart failure, palpitations, and tachycardia), and gastrointestinal (nausea) toxicities. These toxicities reflect the novel mechanism of action of anagrelide as a cyclic nucleotide phosphodiesterase inhibitor. Anagrelide should be used with caution in patients with known or suspected cardiac disease because of its ability to promote fluid retention. Because many patients with PV are elderly, careful attention to fluid status should be maintained to avoid slipping into congestive heart failure after the initiation of anagrelide.

IFN-α therapy has been explored for several decades for the treatment of PV patients, but its positive effects have been more greatly appreciated during the past 7–12 years.[29] Its effects on myeloid malignancies are likely the consequence of its broad range of biologic activities, including direct effects on malignant cells, enhancement of antitumor immune responses, induction of proapoptotic genes, inhibition of angiogenesis, and promotion of the cycling of dormant malignant stem cells. Because of the recent development of "targeted" therapies, the use of IFN has been dramatically reduced over the past decade. The increasing awareness of the numerous mutations beyond those involving *JAK2* suggest, however, that such an approach using target-specific agents is not universally effective. This awareness provided the rationale for the use of an agent such as IFN-α that might be especially useful for the treatment of a disease in which multiple genetic, epigenetic, and environmental factors contribute to its origin and progression. IFN-α promotes apoptosis of a variety of tumor cell types. The induction of apoptosis by IFN-α involves the activation of a number of IFN-stimulated genes that mediate this response. Gene expression studies have identified more than 15 IFN-stimulated genes with proapoptotic functions. Although these IFN-stimulated genes alone are probably not sufficient to induce apoptosis, their cumulative effects likely result in apoptosis. Type 1 IFNs suppress the ability of normal human HPCs to proliferate in vitro in the presence of cytokine combinations. IFN-α acts directly against HPCs; this inhibitory activity has been documented using CD34+ cell populations. PV CD34+ cells are more sensitive to the inhibitory effects of IFN-α than normal HPCs.

The ability of type 1 IFNs to inhibit HPC proliferation and maturation has been documented to occur independently of the STAT pathway. Type 1 IFNs activate the p38 MAP kinase, a proline-directed serine/threonine kinase that is required for IFN-stimulated gene transcription through IFN-sensitive response elements (IRSE). The pharmacologic blockade of p38 in IFN-treated PV HPCs reverses the inhibitory effects of IFN-α. Activation of p38 MAP kinase results in mitochondrial translocation of the proapoptotic protein Bax, leading to the induction of apoptosis.

IFN has also been shown to be able to affect HSC behavior. High levels of IFN-α induce murine HSCs to exit from a normally quiescent state and to transiently proliferate. Several studies using either primary PV CD34+ cells or murine models of *JAK2V617*-positive PV have provided evidence that IFN-α is able to selectively deplete malignant PV stem cells. In the United States, the pioneering study by Silver in 1988 documented the clinical effectiveness of IFN-α in controlling erythrocytosis as well as pruritus and other constitutional symptoms in PV patients, and Austrian and French groups reported during the same period evidence that IFN-α was also effective in reducing thrombocytosis in ET patients. A number of clinical trials have been performed subsequently using several different commercial preparations of IFN. In almost all PV and ET trials, IFN-α therapy rapidly normalized platelet numbers and corrected the degree of leukocytosis and erythrocytosis, allowing reduction in the requirement for phlebotomies within a few months. In both diseases, an objective hematologic response was observed in about 80% of patients, including complete freedom from phlebotomies in PV in 60% of patients. In addition, IFN-α was also able to reduce PV-associated pruritus in a significant number of patients and appears to be an effective drug for this purpose. However, toxicity associated with IFN-α therapy was not trivial, leading to the discontinuation of treatment in almost 25% of patients. A pegylated form of IFN has been used with increasing frequency to treat patients with a variety of MPNs with great success. This form of IFN can be administered once weekly, and its use is associated with a more favorable toxicity profile. Several phase II studies using peg-IFNα-2a in PV and ET showed similarly impressive hematologic response rates compared with standard IFN-α, but with less associated toxicity (<10% of patients discontinued therapy during the first year of therapy). In addition, these studies showed for the first time evidence of significant molecular responses, as documented by a clear reduction in the *JAK2V617F* allele burden after IFN-α treatment. Overall, the two clinical trials with peg-IFNα-2a showed a meaningful and progressive reduction in the *JAK2V617F* allele burden in about 70% of PV and 40% of ET patients. Importantly, the *JAK2V617F* mutation became undetectable (with 1% sensitivity PCR assays) in 24% of PV patients in the French PVN-1 study after about 3 years' median follow-up, and in 14% and 6% of PV and ET patients, respectively, in the United States study after about 2 years' median follow-up. Combining both studies, 12 out of 64 (19%) PV patients achieved a molecular complete response (MCR). Of note, many of these MCRs occurred after the 12th month of treatment, but hematologic responses occurred within a few weeks. Prolonged exposure (>12 months) to peg-IFNα-2a seems to be an important factor in achieving MCR. The reduction in the *JAK2V617F* allele burden was not influenced by the cumulative dose of peg-IFNα-2a in the PVN-1 study, but toxicity was clearly dose dependent in the United States study. Taken together, these results indicate that peg-IFNα-2a therapy is best initiated at very low doses that are gradually increased until hematologic response is achieved; this strategy avoids cessation of therapy and allows sufficient exposure to the drug to allow for the achievement of a molecular response. These results are in agreement with studies from Denmark, showing major molecular responses in PV after long-term treatment with IFNα-2b that could persist after IFN-α was discontinued. Finally, several who achieved MCR in the PVN-1 study have maintained this response after peg-IFNα-2a was discontinued (≤30 months after discontinuation), with none experiencing hematologic relapse. Such long-term clinical and molecular responses after the discontinuation of treatment have previously been reported after IFN-α therapy in MPN patients, an effect that has not been reported with other currently available therapies. It is important to emphasize that the elimination of *JAK2V617F* in this setting is not necessarily indicative of cure of the MPN, and that clinical implications of these molecular responses remain uncertain and require validation. It has been shown that molecular relapse can rapidly occur after IFN-α discontinuation in some cases. In one patient with a biclonal *JAK2V617F/TET2*-mutated PV, peg-IFNα-2a treatment did not affect the *TET2*-mutated cells, but the *JAK2V617F* clone was eradicated. Nevertheless, prolonged periods of time (≤40 months, personal unpublished data) during which the patient remained in complete hematologic remission without any cytoreductive therapy after peg-IFNα-2a withdrawal was observed in several patients of the PVN-1 study even though low levels of the *JAK2V617F* allele (≈5%) were still detected. Such results suggests that despite the disease not being eradicated, long-term exposure to peg-IFNα-2a was sufficient to modify the clinical expression of the MPN for a sustained period of time.

In addition to clinical, hematologic, and MCRs achieved in a significant proportion of PV and ET patients, IFN-α therapy has also been shown recently to reverse BM histopathologic abnormalities in selected cases of both PV and PMF. Thus, IFN-α seems to be a drug able to deplete PV stem cells, and induce complete resolution of all clinical, biologic, and morphologic abnormalities in selected MPN patients, raising the hope that a curative outcome might be possible in a limited subset of such patients. These observations lead one to question the validity of the current therapeutic strategies for PV and ET patients in which myelosuppressive therapy is exclusively used in subpopulations of patients at high risk for developing additional thrombotic events

IFN is not a leukemogenic drug but it is also not an innocuous agent, necessitating careful follow-up of patients receiving such treatment. Initially, many patients experience flu-like symptoms, which are controllable with acetaminophen or aspirin. Such symptoms usually resolve spontaneously after several months of therapy. More serious side effects, including excessive suppression of blood counts, irritability, high fevers, severe asthenia, reversible lower extremity bilateral neuritis, retinopathy, hypothyroidism, depression, sarcoidosis, and left-sided heart failure have been reported and may require cessation of IFN-α therapy. Exacerbation of depression and other psychiatric manifestations are serious potential side effects of IFN, and it should probably not be used in patients with history of clinically significant psychiatric conditions. Patients and family members should be counseled to watch for subtle evidence of depression, mood swings, and personality changes and to immediately report their concerns to the treating physician. The use of IFN should also be avoided in patients with any history of autoimmune diseases and new development of autoimmune disorders should be high on the

differential diagnosis of patients being treated with any formulation of IFN. The role of pegylated IFN therapy versus hydroxyurea therapy or pegylated IFN versus ruxolitinib will be defined only after the performance of a randomized phase III trial in newly diagnosed high-risk ET and PV patients. Two randomized multicenter trials comparing IFN and hydroxyurea are currently ongoing and will hopefully establish differences in terms of efficacy and tolerability of the two medications.

The use of small-molecule inhibitors of JAK1/2 ruxolitinib was first approved in the United States in 2011 for the treatment of advanced forms of MF, and most recently in 2015 was approved for the treatment of patients with PV that are intolerant or resistant to HU. In a phase III study (RESPONSE trial), hydroxyurea resistant or intolerant patients were randomized to receive either ruxolitinib or standard care.[30] To be eligible for the study entry patients had to have splenomegaly with a spleen volume of at least 450 cm³ and ongoing phlebotomy requirements, and be resistant to or intolerant of hydroxyurea according to the standardized criteria. Standard care was selected by the investigator and included hydroxyurea. Patients receiving standard therapy were able to cross over to ruxolitinib if they failed to achieve the primary end point by 32 weeks. The primary end point was achievement of hematocrit control and reduction in spleen size (at least 35% by MRI). This was achieved in 21% of patients in the ruxolitinib arm versus 1% of patients in the standard therapy arm. Hematocrit control was achieved in 60% of patients receiving ruxolitinib and 20% of patients receiving standard therapy, and 38% of patients in the ruxolitinib arm met the reduction in spleen end point versus 1% of patients in the standard therapy arm. By week 80, almost 60% of patients treated with ruxolitinib had normalization of their platelet counts. Patients on ruxolitinib enjoyed improvement in such PV-related symptoms as pruritus, headaches, fatigue, and night sweats. The mean change in *JAK2V617F* allele burden from baseline to week 32 was 12.2% in the ruxolitinib group and 1.2% in the standard therapy group. Based on an analysis after 80 weeks of follow-up, there was a suggestion that those patients receiving ruxolitinib had a reduced incidence of serious thrombotic events but that ruxolitinib therapy did not affect progression to MF and AML; these conclusions are not well substantiated since the study was not powered to examine these events. It also did not provide information on correction of the BM histopathological findings and chromosomal abnormalities in patients treated with ruxolitinib. In general, ruxolitinib was well tolerated with 85% of patients remaining on ruxolitinib at 81 weeks. The most common nonhematological adverse event was diarrhea, while the hematological toxicity included anemia, lymphopenia, and thrombocytopenia. In addition the rates of nonmelanoma skin cancer were higher in the ruxolitinib arm compared with those patients receiving standard therapy. An increase in infectious complications was observed on ruxolitinib treatment, specifically herpes zoster infection. This has also been observed in MF patients treated with ruxolitinib. Cases of tuberculosis activation, toxoplasmosis, and other atypical infections have been reported in ruxolitinib-treated patients. The increased number of infections has been attributed to the inhibition of both T- and NK-cell function by ruxolitinib.

Pruritus in PV patients occurs on exposure to sudden body cooling, especially after a warm bath, and is experienced by as many as 40–60% of patients treated with phlebotomy. Aquagenic pruritus in MPN patients and in patients without an associated malignancy has been associated with lactose intolerance. In some instances, multiple family members are affected, suggesting that genetic factors might predispose individuals to this symptom. In some studies, basophils and mast cells have been shown to be involved with *JAK2V617F* in patients with aquagenic pruritus and PV, likely leading to the elaboration of mediators that lead to itching. The frequency of pruritus appears to be somewhat lower in patients treated with myelosuppressive agents. This observation is related to the probable relationship between pruritus and degranulation of tissue mast cells and circulating basophils. Aged transgenic mice expressing *JAK2V617F* suffer from pruritis and the massive accumulation of mast cells in the skin. Cultured mast cells from these mice exhibited enhanced proliferative signals, relative resistance to cell death upon growth factor deprivation, and a growth advantage over control cells under suboptimal growth conditions. A JAK inhibitor was shown to reduce mast cell numbers and alleviate pruritus in *JAK2V617F* transgenic mice. Some uncontrolled studies have attributed pruritus to hyperhistaminemia or severe iron deficiency, with relief associated with the use of histamine antagonists or ferrous sulfate. Iron replacement is frequently not possible because it can lead to dangerous elevations of the RBC mass. In a number of instances, however, iron replacement has been possible with disease control with IFN-α. The association between pruritus and tissue infiltration by mast cells would appear to explain the response of occasional patients to photochemotherapy with psoralens and ultraviolet irradiation. In addition, 80% of patients with pruritus have been reported to respond to the selective serotonin uptake inhibitors paroxetine or fluoxetine. Other effective options include anticonvulsant drugs such as pregabalin. Ruxolitinib and other JAK inhibitors both in PV and PMF have a remarkable effect on reducing the severity of intractable pruritus that not infrequently affects PV patients. These drugs appear to be much more effective in treating this particular symptom of PV compared with both hydroxyurea and IFN, but in occasional patients this effect, unfortunately, is not sustained.

BCS is a catastrophic illness that can lead to significant morbidity and mortality in patients with PV. Patients with MPN are at a high risk of developing this syndrome. Independently, the use of oral contraceptive pills and congenital and acquired thrombophilic factors are involved in its development. A number of cases of hepatic vein thrombosis have been reported in nonpolycythemic women taking oral contraceptives. Although no data are available, one must be concerned about the use of oral contraceptives in women with PV.

The optimal approach to the problem of BCS is obviously preventive and involves maintenance of normal blood values in the patient with PV. When BCS develops, the prognosis without treatment is dismal. The goals of therapy are to prevent further propagation of thrombus, relieve the intense hepatic congestion, and manage the severe ascites that often plague these patients. If untreated, these patients often have a slowly progressive course, with deterioration and death occurring within 3.5 years. Spontaneous resolution of the hepatic vein occlusion rarely occurs. There are no prospective randomized trials of anticoagulation in BCS, but retrospective studies suggest a survival benefit. Anticoagulation should be continued indefinitely unless there is a contraindication. Typically, low-molecular–weight heparin (LMWH) is used as the initial treatment with subsequent switch to warfarin. New oral anticoagulants that act by direct thrombin or factor Xa inhibition are being increasingly used for various prophylactic and therapeutic indications, but their use for these patients should be avoided until more reversal agents become available and the experience of using them becomes more widespread. The use of thrombolytic therapy directly in the thrombosed vein is infrequent due to the lack of data and potentially high risk of bleeding Angioplasty with or without the use of stents attempts to restore hepatic blood flow and is often used if anticoagulation is not successful, and should be considered if liver function is deteriorating despite therapeutic anticoagulation. The overall success rate is about 95%, with a low periprocedural complications rate. The clinical deterioration of patients with BCS results from damage to the hepatocytes from necrosis associated with marked elevation in sinusoidal pressure coupled with ischemia from reduced hepatic arteriole perfusion. The only rational therapeutic intervention, therefore, involves some sort of portal vein decompression to achieve an effective reduction of sinusoidal pressure. Portosystemic shunting such as transjugular intrahepatic portosystemic shunt (TIPS) has been used extensively to treat refractory portal hypertension. Recent data show good long-term outcomes when using TIPS, and it is now considered standard management if anticoagulation or angioplasty are not successful, or if patients have high-risk disease. It has been shown that about a third of patients with BCS require TIPS placement. One-year survival in a recent large UK single-center study was 97% and 5-year survival 72%. Procedure-related complications are frequent but mortality rates are low.

Liver transplantation is a potential option for treatment of PV BCS patients with continued hepatic decompensation. The indications for liver transplantation are cirrhosis, fulminant hepatic failure, and failure of a portosystemic shunt. The overall actuarial survival at 1 year was 76% and was 68% at 10 years. Because PV is a slowly progressive disease, transplantation should not be withheld from these patients. Pretransplant predictors of mortality based on a multivariable analysis were impaired renal function and a history of a shunt. The hematologic consequences of polycythemia must be aggressively treated in the posttransplantation setting; hepatic vein occlusion may reoccur in the transplanted liver.

Therapy of CVT and sinuses includes anticoagulation with heparin to arrest the thrombotic process and to prevent pulmonary embolism. LMWH should be started as soon as the diagnosis is confirmed even in the presence of hemorrhagic infarcts. After the acute phase, life-long oral anticoagulant therapy is recommended. There is currently no available evidence from randomized clinical trials regarding the efficacy or safety of thrombolytic therapy.

The performance of any surgical procedures on patients with PV is, as previously discussed, accompanied by excessively high morbidity and mortality. Elective surgery should not be contemplated unless the patient's hematologic values have been normalized for several months. The longer the hematologic control has been in effect, the lower the incidence of postoperative complications. If emergency surgery is required, the patient should be phlebotomized rapidly until a normal hematocrit is reached, and platelets should be available in case excessive perioperative or postoperative bleeding occurs. After emergency or elective surgery, the patient should be mobilized as soon as possible, and strong consideration should be given to anticoagulation with LMWH unless the patient has some contraindication. Dental extractions can also result in excessive hemorrhage and should not be performed unless the patient is under strict hematologic control.

Perhaps the most difficult and frustrating period encountered during the clinical course of a patient with PV is the development of post-PV MF. The origins, manifestations, and management options are discussed in detail in Chapter 70.

Limited information is available concerning the treatment of patients who develop acute leukemia after PV. The overwhelming majority of such cases involve myeloid leukemias. The leukemia is frequently preceded by post-PV MF but not always. Patients with post-PV MF and acute leukemia frequently have greater than 20% blasts in the peripheral blood but far fewer blast cells in the BM, which has led to a hypothesis that the leukemia originates from an extramedullary site, particularly the spleen. These cases tend to have a more indolent course, but patients with a greater degree of BM infiltration have a more highly proliferative form of leukemia that is associated with an even more aggressive course. The optimal treatment of such patients is unknown. In elderly adults with significant comorbidities, the choice not to institute chemotherapy is a reasonable option. These patients are frequently elderly, and poor results with standard regimens have been reported. Patients rarely achieve a complete remission but rather return to a clinical condition that resembles their original MPN for limited periods of time. In a retrospective analysis on 23 patients with leukemic transformation of PV, the median patient age was 68 years, and leukemia developed a median of 12.8 years from the diagnosis of PV. Twelve of the 14 patients in whom cytogenetic analyses were performed had complex cytogenetic abnormalities associated with high-risk leukemias. Fifteen patients were treated with palliative measures and had a median survival of 2.5 months. Of the eight patients treated with standard induction therapy, one obtained a complete remission, and seven died without obtaining a response. The median survival time of these chemotherapy-treated patients was 5.6 months. The median survival time of the entire cohort of 23 patients was 2.9 months. This poor outcome is likely the result of clinical and biologic features of the acute leukemia, advanced patient age, unfavorable cytogenetics, and patient comorbidities associated with advanced age. Selected patients are likely to tolerate and have a favorable outcome with allogeneic stem cell transplantation and reduced-intensity conditioning. In fact, the only long-term survival with post-PV leukemia has been observed in patients receiving allogeneic stem cell transplantation. Whether the patients should receive some form of induction chemotherapy before receiving conditioning therapy for preparation of the transplant or proceed directly to transplant is a decision that varies from patient to patient and from center to center. Most patients with PV-related acute leukemia should be considered candidates for experimental therapeutic strategies. Recently, promising results with the use of DNA hypomethylating agents such as decitabine or azacitidine alone or in combination with ruxolitinib have been reported, with 50–60% of patients achieving clinically significant responses persisting for 6–24 months in the majority of cases. These chemotherapeutic regimens can frequently be administered as an outpatient but require treatment for at least six monthly cycles before clinical responses can be evaluated. Although many of these patients do not achieve true complete remissions, their prolonged survival and quality of life, at least based upon single-institutional studies, appears to be superior to that achieved with standard induction chemotherapy. The use of hypomethylating agents, JAK2 inhibitors, or both is now being explored as bridging therapies before patients receive allogeneic transplants.

PV occurs frequently during childbearing years. A discussion of contraception options is imperative because the use of oral contraceptive pills may be associated with an increased risk of deep venous thrombosis as well as splanchnic vein thrombosis. It seems prudent to entertain alternative forms of contraception with such individuals. Discontinuation of hydroxyurea in both men and women desiring to have a child is recommended. Hydroxyurea is capable of inducing azoospermia in men, frequently limiting their ability to father a child. Pregnancy is itself a prothrombotic condition. PV in a pregnant individual has been reported to lead to an increased incidence of fetal wastage, with 30% of pregnancies in PV patients terminating in spontaneous abortions. In addition, preeclampsia occurs more frequently in these women. A team approach requiring close communication between an obstetrician skilled in providing care for high-risk pregnancies and the responsible hematologist provides the optimal integration of care to the mother and the child. Pregnancy in PV patients is frequently associated with a gradual normalization of blood values, and it is not unusual for a woman who has required extensive therapy for control of her disease to no longer require phlebotomies during pregnancy. Delivery appears not to be complicated by excessive hemorrhage, but the postpartum period carries an increased risk of venous thrombosis. Although some degree of hematocrit level normalization can be explained by expansion of the plasma volume or by nutritional deficiencies that occur during pregnancy, it is unlikely that these factors can be solely responsible. It seems more reasonable to assume that the high estrogen levels characteristic of pregnancy suppress erythropoiesis. After completion of the pregnancies, the patients' hematologic values slowly drift back to their previously elevated values in parallel with the return to normal estrogen levels. Because pregnancy is usually associated with spontaneous control of the polycythemic state, no specific therapy is required except for careful observation. If needed, therapy should be limited to phlebotomy and low-dose aspirin therapy because of the mutagenic effects of chemotherapeutic agents. Aggressive treatment of hypertension is imperative, as well as attention to the risk of developing preeclampsia and toxemia, which should be treated in a standard fashion. In individuals with a history of repeated spontaneous abortions associated with placental infarction, consideration should be given to low-dose aspirin with LMWH therapy, making sure that these agents are discontinued at the time of delivery to avoid the risk of excessive hemorrhage. If this approach is not successful, IFN therapy is suggested because it is not known to be leukemogenic or teratogenic and does not cross the placenta. In the puerperium, thromboprophylaxis with 6 weeks of LMWH therapy is recommended. Aggressive intervention with hematocrit levels maintained below 45% and aspirin therapy with LMWH is associated with a positive outcome for the pregnancy. Breastfeeding is recommended if the mother is receiving therapy with heparin or Coumadin as long as the baby receives adequate supplementation with vitamin

K. Rapid mobilization of the mother after delivery is of great importance.

Because PV is ultimately a stem cell disorder, it should be possible to achieve a cure with stem cell transplantation. Thus far, the majority of patients undergoing allogeneic stem cell transplantation have been relatively young and have been transplanted after evolution to MF, MDS, or acute leukemia. Transplantation during the polycythemia phase of the disease is rarely appropriate.

FUTURE DIRECTIONS

The discovery of *JAK2V617F* mutations has led to a more comprehensive understanding of the pathophysiology of the MPNs, including PV. There is no question that the diagnostic tests for *JAK2V617F* and exon 12 mutations of *JAK2*, as well as mutations in *VHL*, *HIF-1*, *HIF-2*, the *EPOR*, and *PHD* have revolutionized the diagnostic approach to patients with erythrocytosis. PV is a stem cell disease that will ultimately require curative therapies at a minimum to deplete or eliminate malignant stem cells if curative small-molecule therapies are to become a reality. Before the *JAK2V617F* allele burden is used as a biomarker for outcomes of novel therapeutic approaches to treat patients with PV, studies are needed to determine the extent of reduction of allele burden that would be predictive of altering the natural history of PV and eliminating complications from thrombotic episodes or evolution to MF or acute leukemia. The use of drugs affecting only JAK2 are unlikely to be curative because multiple genetic and epigenetic events likely contribute to the origins and progression of PV. Randomized clinical trials of combinations of drugs, rather than single drugs, and comparing these outcomes with the standard of care are more likely to lead to significant advances in improving the natural history of PV patients.

REFERENCES

1. Haase VH: Regulation of erythropoiesis by hypoxia-inducible factors. *Blood Rev* 27:41–53, 2013.
2. McMullin MF: HIF pathway mutations and erythrocytosis. *Expert Rev Hematol* 3:93–101, 2010.
3. Vlahakos DV, Marathias KP, Madias NE: The role of the renin-angiotensin system in the regulation of erythropoiesis. *Am J Kidney Dis* 56:558–565, 2010.
4. Huang LJ, Shen YM, Bulut GB: Advances in understanding the pathogenesis of primary familial and congenital polycythaemia. *Br J Haematol* 148:844–852, 2010.
5. Lorenzo FR, Huff C, Myllymaki M, et al: A genetic mechanism for Tibetan high-altitude adaptation. *Nat Genet* 46:951–956, 2014.
6. Villafuerte FC: New genetic and physiological factors for excessive erythrocytosis and Chronic Mountain Sickness. *J Appl Physiol (1985)* 119:1481–1486, 2015.
7. Bento C, Percy MJ, Gardie B, et al: Genetic basis of congenital erythrocytosis: mutation update and online databases. *Hum Mutat* 35:15–26, 2014.
8. Albiero E, Ruggeri M, Fortuna S, et al: Isolated erythrocytosis: study of 67 patients and identification of three novel germ-line mutations in the prolyl hydroxylase domain protein 2 (PHD2) gene. *Haematologica* 97:123–127, 2012.
9. Stein BL, Oh ST, Berenzon D, et al: Polycythemia Vera: An Appraisal of the Biology and Management 10 Years After the Discovery of JAK2 V617F. *J Clin Oncol* 33:3953–3960, 2015.
10. Landgren O, Goldin LR, Kristinsson SY, et al: Increased risks of polycythemia vera, essential thrombocythemia, and myelofibrosis among 24,577 first-degree relatives of 11,039 patients with myeloproliferative neoplasms in Sweden. *Blood* 112:2199–2204, 2008.
11. Stein BL, Saraf S, Sobol U, et al: Age-related differences in disease characteristics and clinical outcomes in polycythemia vera. *Leuk Lymphoma* 54:1989–1995, 2013.

12. James C, Ugo V, Le Couedic JP, et al: A unique clonal JAK2 mutation leading to constitutive signalling causes polycythaemia vera. *Nature* 434:1144–1148, 2005.

13. Kralovics R, Passamonti F, Buser AS, et al: A gain-of-function mutation of JAK2 in myeloproliferative disorders. *N Engl J Med* 352:1779–1790, 2005.

14. Jones AV, Chase A, Silver RT, et al: JAK2 haplotype is a major risk factor for the development of myeloproliferative neoplasms. *Nat Genet* 41:446–449, 2009.

15. Tapper W, Jones AV, Kralovics R, et al: Genetic variation at MECOM, TERT, JAK2 and HBS1L-MYB predisposes to myeloproliferative neoplasms. *Nat Commun* 6:6691, 2015.

16. Ortmann CA, Kent DG, Nangalia J, et al: Effect of mutation order on myeloproliferative neoplasms. *N Engl J Med* 372:601–612, 2015.

17. Jamieson CH, Gotlib J, Durocher JA, et al: The JAK2 V617F mutation occurs in hematopoietic stem cells in polycythemia vera and predisposes toward erythroid differentiation. *Proc Natl Acad Sci USA* 103:6224–6229, 2006.

18. Rampal R, Ahn J, Abdel-Wahab O, et al: Genomic and functional analysis of leukemic transformation of myeloproliferative neoplasms. *Proc Natl Acad Sci USA* 111:E5401–E5410, 2014.

19. Wang L, Swierczek SI, Drummond J, et al: Whole-exome sequencing of polycythemia vera revealed novel driver genes and somatic mutation shared by T cells and granulocytes. *Leukemia* 28:935–938, 2014.

20. Landolfi R, Marchioli R, Kutti J, et al: Efficacy and safety of low-dose aspirin in polycythemia vera. *N Engl J Med* 350:114–124, 2004.

21. Marchioli R, Finazzi G, Specchia G, et al: Cardiovascular events and intensity of treatment in polycythemia vera. *N Engl J Med* 368:22–33, 2013.

22. Kiladjian JJ, Chevret S, Dosquet C, et al: Treatment of polycythemia vera with hydroxyurea and pipobroman: final results of a randomized trial initiated in 1980. *J Clin Oncol* 29:3907–3913, 2011.

23. Najfeld V, Montella L, Scalise A, et al: Exploring polycythaemia vera with fluorescence in situ hybridization: additional cryptic 9p is the most frequent abnormality detected. *Br J Haematol* 119:558–566, 2002.

24. Arber DA, Orazi A, Hasserjian R, et al: The 2016 revision to the World Health Organization classification of myeloid neoplasms and acute leukemia. *Blood* 127:2391–2405, 2016.

25. Barosi G, Mesa R, Finazzi G, et al: Revised response criteria for polycythemia vera and essential thrombocythemia: an ELN and IWG-MRT consensus project. *Blood* 121:4778–4781, 2013.

26. Sergueeva AI, Miasnikova GY, Polyakova LA, et al: Complications in children and adolescents with Chuvash polycythemia. *Blood* 125:414–415, 2015.

27. Bjorkholm M, Derolf AR, Hultcrantz M, et al: Treatment-related risk factors for transformation to acute myeloid leukemia and myelodysplastic syndromes in myeloproliferative neoplasms. *J Clin Oncol* 29:2410–2415, 2011.

28. Soutou B, Aractingi S: Myeloproliferative disorder therapy: assessment and management of adverse events–a dermatologist's perspective. *Hematol Oncol* 27(Suppl 1):11–13, 2009.

29. Stein BL, Tiu RV: Biological rationale and clinical use of interferon in the classical BCR-ABL-negative myeloproliferative neoplasms. *J Interferon Cytokine Res* 33:145–153, 2013.

30. Vannucchi AM, Kiladjian JJ, Griesshammer M, et al: Ruxolitinib versus standard therapy for the treatment of polycythemia vera. *N Engl J Med* 372:426–435, 2015.

CHAPTER 69

ESSENTIAL THROMBOCYTHEMIA

John Mascarenhas, Camelia Iancu-Rubin, Marina Kremyanskaya, Vesna Najfeld, and Ronald Hoffman

Essential thrombocythemia (ET) is a chronic myeloproliferative neoplasm (MPN) characterized by platelet counts in excess of 450 × 10^9/L, profound bone marrow (BM) megakaryocyte hyperplasia, leukocytosis, splenomegaly, a clinical course punctuated by hemorrhagic and/ or thrombotic episodes, and possible evolution to myelofibrosis (MF) and acute leukemia. ET is a clinically heterogeneous disorder, with more than half of patients meeting the criteria for diagnosis being asymptomatic at presentation. ET was first described in 1934 by Epstein and Goedel, who described a patient with an elevated platelet count who had repeated hemorrhagic episodes.

EPIDEMIOLOGY

The true incidence of ET is unknown because extensive epidemiologic studies are not available. The incidence of ET has been estimated to be approximately 1.5–2.4 patients per 100,000 populations annually. A Swedish study a indicated that first-degree relatives of patients with an MPN, including ET, had a five- to sevenfold increased risk of developing an MPN, supporting the concept that there is a strong genetic predilection. ET occurs in individuals with a median age of 67–73 years. To gain additional insight into the patterns of occurrence of MPNs by age, sex, race/ethnicity, and susceptible populations, and provide a population-based assessment of patient survival, Srour and coworkers[12] used data from the Surveillance, Epidemiology and End Results (SEER) Program from the National Cancer Institute in the United States to better assess the incidence of MPNs in the United States from 2001 to 2012. Importantly, during part of this period of time the use of mutational analyses in making the diagnosis of MPNs became widespread. There were 31,904 MPN cases diagnosed among residents of 18 SEER registries evaluated. The age-adjusted incidence rates (IRs) were as follows: polycythemia vera (PV) 10.9 per 1 million patient years), ET (9.6), chronic myeloid leukemia (CML; 3.3), and primary myelofibrosis (PMF; 3.1). ET was the only MPN with a significantly lower IR among males than females; the average age at diagnosis was 68 years. The female predominance was most pronounced in individuals less than 60 years of age. Surprisingly, the IR of ET was 18% higher among blacks than non-Hispanic whites; ET was associated with a female predominance among non-Hispanic whites, white Hispanics, blacks and Asian–Pacific islanders, suggesting shared gender-specific risk factor(s) across these racial/ethnic groups.

The incidence patterns observed by Srour and coworkers[12] support inherent differences in susceptibility to developing an MPN. This study is of importance, since it represents the first step in appreciating the potential of molecular diagnostics on improving our understanding of the epidemiology of the MPNs. Future studies will need to include not only JAK2V617F analyses, but also documentation of mutations in calreticulin (*CALR*) and the thrombopoietin receptor (*MPL*). These data suggest that ET is a relatively common hematological malignancy that has an especially significant impact on women.

Recently, several groups have identified shared susceptibility genes that predispose individuals to develop one of the MPNs. The Janus kinase 2 (*JAK2*) mutations (*V617F* and exon 14 mutations) are not acquired randomly, but arise preferentially on a specific *JAK2*

haplotype (46/1). The *JAK2* 46/1 haplotype has been shown not only to predispose to *JAK2V617F*-positive ET, but also to ET harboring *MPL* and *CALR* mutations, again indicating that genetic factors play a role in the susceptibility to develop ET. Tapper and coworkers[13] also identified an additional two single-nucleotide polymorphisms (SNPs), rs12339666 within *JAK2* and rs2201862, 153 kb downstream of the DS1 and EVI1 complex locus protein EVI1 (*MECOM*), which were associated with *JAK2V617F*-negative MPNs. Two additional SNPs, rs2736100 in telomerase reverse transcriptase (*TERT*) and rs9376092 between *HBS1L* and *MYB*, were associated with *JAK2V617F*-positive MPNs. The SNP between *HBS1L* and *MYB*, rs9376092, however, had a stronger effect on MPNs associated with *CALR* and/or *MPL* mutations, whereas in *JAK2V617F*-positive cases rs9376092 was associated with ET rather than PV. These investigators demonstrated that the candidate risk allele at rs9376092, which had a strong association with ET, was associated with reduced *MYB*. Prior functional analyses had shown that mice expressing low levels of MYB develop a transplantable ET-like disease. These findings indicate that multiple germ-line variants predispose to the development of each of the MPNs and link constitutional differences in *MYB* expression, in particular to ET.

ET has rarely been reported in the pediatric age group. The incidence of ET in childhood has been reported to be approximately 1 per 10^7 population, which is 60-times less than that in adults. Approximately 30% of children with this disorder experience thrombotic or hemorrhagic complications at diagnosis or later in their course, and 50% have splenomegaly. Mutations in one of the established MPN driver genes *JAK2*, *CALR*, or *MPL* were present in a lower percentage of pediatric cases (34%) compared with adult MPN patients (90%). The subgroup of patients without a detectable driver mutation tended to have higher platelet counts compared with patients with mutations.

Several families with multiple members having ET have been described. The prevalence of the *JAK2V617F* mutation in familial cases of MPN has been analyzed in 72 families, including 174 patients (68 with ET). The *JAK2* mutation was found in half of patients with ET, and a similar proportion as observed in sporadic, nonfamilial cases. Among 46 families with at least two cases of PV, ET, or PMF, the *JAK2* mutation was absent in six families, heterogeneously distributed in 18, and present in all patients with MPN in 22. Thus, the *JAK2* mutation does not seem to be required for the development of ET or other MPNs, and this familial clustering cannot be accounted for by the prevalence of the *JAK2* 46/1 haplotype. In familial MPNs, *CALR* mutations can also be somatically acquired and are associated with an ET or PMF phenotype.

PATHOBIOLOGY

ET is a clonal hematological malignancy originating at the level of the hematopoietic stem cell. The thrombocytosis that characterizes ET is caused by increased platelet production by megakaryocytes. Effective platelet production is increased as much as 10-fold and is associated with an increase in megakaryocyte clustering, volume, nuclear lobe number, and nuclear ploidy.

ET is typically a clonal hematopoietic disorder originating at the level of the pluripotent hematopoietic stem cell. A significant proportion of nonclonally derived leukocytes exist in addition to the clonally derived population of leukocytes in patients with ET. In one study of 42 patients with ET, 31 patients exhibited clonality of at least one hematopoietic lineage, but the remaining 11 patients had polyclonal origin of all lineages studied. The biogenesis of polyclonal ET remains ill defined. It is possible that small numbers of normal hematopoietic stem cells account for this admixture of nonclonal populations. It has been reported by several groups that ET patients with polyclonal hematopoiesis have fewer thrombotic complications. Interestingly, in some patients, monoclonality of hematopoiesis is restricted to platelets despite the polyclonal origin of the other lineages. Other studies, however, have indicated a common origin of granulocytes, platelets, and B lymphocytes in this disorder. Such studies raise the possibility that the malignant transformation leading to ET occurs at a number of cellular stages along the hematopoietic cellular hierarchy.

Increased numbers of megakaryocyte progenitor cells are present in the BM and the peripheral blood of patients with ET. These data support the concept that the principal abnormality is an expansion of the progenitor cell pool. In addition, progenitor cells were noted to either be hypersensitive or independent of the addition of exogenous cytokines, including interleukin (IL)-3, IL-6, and thrombopoietin. A second subpopulation of colony-forming unit–megakaryocyte (CFU-MK) assayed from patients with ET remained dependent on the addition of exogenous cytokines.

This hypersensitivity of ET progenitor cells to a variety of cytokines is due to the clonal acquisition of driver mutations (*JAK2*, *MPL*, or *CALR*) that activate the JAK-STAT signaling pathway, allowing hematopoiesis to occur in the absence of exogenous cytokines. The *JAK2V617F* mutation occurs in 50–60% of ET patients while recurrent *CALR* mutations occur in 25% of patients and 3–5% have *MPL* mutations. The patients with ET who lack such driver mutations are said to be "triple negative".

JAK2 is a cytoplasmic tyrosine kinase that plays a key role in mediating intracellular signaling from a variety of growth factors, including IL-3, erythropoietin, granulocyte-macrophage colony-stimulating factor (GM-CSF), granulocyte colony-stimulating factor (G-CSF), and thrombopoietin. Coexpression of *JAK2V617F* with a homodimeric type 1 cytokine receptor (including erythropoietin, thrombopoietin, or G-CSF) is necessary for hormone activation of JAK-STAT (signal transducer and activator of transcription) signaling pathways and for hematopoietic cell proliferation to become growth factor independent. The *JAK2V617F* mutation is present in ET patients with both clonal and polyclonal hematopoiesis. Patients with clonal hematopoiesis have a higher *JAK2V617F* allele burden (26%) than patients with polyclonal hematopoiesis (16%). The relative size of the *JAK2V617F* clone is often small and remains stable over time in patients with both clonal and polyclonal hematopoiesis. Although an allele burden higher than 50% indicating the presence of granulocytes homozygous for *JAK2V617F* has been found in 70% of PV patients, it has been observed less frequently in ET patients. All PV patients have assayable erythroid colonies that are homozygous for *JAK2V617F*, even in PV patients with a low burden of *JAK2V617F*. By contrast, hematopoietic colonies cloned from ET patients are only occasionally *JAK2V617F* homozygous, unlike the case of PV. The transition from *JAK2* heterozygous to homozygous progenitors is a consequence of homologous recombination. These studies suggest that such an event is characteristic of PV but rarely occurs in ET. If such an event occurred in ET, it would likely lead to a transition from an ET phenotype to a PV phenotype.

STATs are activated downstream to *JAK2V617F*. STAT3 is a pivotal regulator of megakaryocytopoiesis, which might provide an explanation for its exclusive upregulation in ET. To further examine the differences between hematopoiesis in *JAK2V617F* ET and PV, the gene expression changes in *JAK2V617F*-heterozygous erythroid colonies have been examined. Erythroblasts from ET patients were characterized by enhanced expression of genes associated with interferon (IFN) signaling and phosho-STAT1 compared with PV erythroblasts.[5] STAT1 is essential for IFN-γ signaling. Increased STAT1 in normal CD34+ cells has been shown to favor megakaryocytic but

reduce erythroid differentiation, creating a differentiation pattern that resembles ET. Furthermore, inhibition of STAT1 signaling in ET hematopoietic progenitor cells led to enhanced erythropoiesis and reduced megakaryocytopoiesis. These studies suggest that in ET, *JAK2V617F* induces simultaneous activation of STAT5 and STAT1 pathways, but in PV, the relative reduced levels of phospho-STAT1 reduces a brake, favoring more profound erythropoiesis.

Thrombopoietin is the primary physiologic regulator of thrombopoiesis. This growth factor acts by binding to its cell surface receptor, MPL. MPL is expressed by CD34+ hematopoietic stem and progenitor cells, MKs, and platelets. Normal or slightly elevated thrombopoietin levels have been observed in patients with ET. Furthermore, expression of the thrombopoietin receptor and its mRNA has been shown to be dramatically reduced in the platelets of patients with ET. Thrombopoietin serum levels are controlled by platelet mass through MPL-mediated thrombopoietin uptake and degradation. The reduced platelet MPL expression occurs not only in ET but also in PV and PMF, and has been shown to be a downstream event of *JAK2V617F*, which promotes the proteasomal degradation of MPL. The reduced MPL likely results in the decreased capacity of platelets to absorb thrombopoietin, contributing to the increased megakaryocyte mass and thrombocytosis. The mutations in thrombopoietin receptor, *MPLW515L* and *MPL515K*, are present in approximately 3–5% of patients with ET. About 60% of patients with *MPL* mutations have the *W515L* mutation and 40% the *W515K* mutation. The mutant allele burden is greater than 50% in 50% of *W515K* patients compared with 17% of *W515L* patients. The most prevalent *MPL* mutations in ET occur on tryptophan 515, an amino acid that maintains MPL in an inactive form in the absence of cytokines. Rarely in ET patients another *MPL* mutation, *S505N*, located in the exon 10 domain that encodes the transmembrane domain of MPL and induces dimerization of the transmembrane helix in an active confirmation, serves as a driver mutation. The *MPL* mutations occurring in ET trigger conformational changes in the receptor, bringing in close proximity two molecules of bound JAK2 for transphosphorylation and activation of the JAK-STAT signaling cascade. The loss of tryptophan but not the acquisition of a particular residue induces the constitutive activation of MPL. More than 50% of patients with *MPL* mutant alleles are also *JAK2V617F* positive. In ET, both *JAK2V617F* and *MPL* mutations arise preferentially on a specific constitutional *JAK2* 46/1 haplotype. Two hypotheses have been proposed to account for this predilection: 46/1 is inherently genetically more unstable (hypermutability hypothesis) or 46/1 confers a growth advantage that favors the predominance of *JAK2V617F* hematopoiesis (fertile ground hypothesis). The association of *MPL* mutations with the *JAK2* 46/1 haplotype strongly favors the hypermutability hypothesis rather than the fertile ground hypothesis. The presence of *MPLW515K* mutations in ET patients are associated with lower hemoglobin levels and higher platelet counts, as well as preferential expansion of the numbers of megakaryocytes at the expense of erythroid precursors, as observed in BM biopsy specimens.

Mutations in the *CALR* gene occur in 25% of ET patients and rarely occur together with mutations of *JAK2* or *MPL*. *CALR* mutations have been observed exclusively in ET and MF patients but not PV. The wild-type *CALR* gene encodes for an evolutionarily conserved, multifunctional protein involved in multiple cellular processes ranging from calcium homeostasis and protein folding in the endoplasmic reticulum, to apoptotic cell death clearance and cellular adhesion. The *CALR* mutations identified in MPN mainly consist of deletions (i.e., type I) or insertions (i.e., type II) occurring within the exon 9, which create a novel epitope in the C-terminal domain of the protein. Despite the heterogeneity of these mutations, the new C-terminus sequence is identical and results in the loss of the KDEL domain, which is critical for CALR retention in the endoplasmic reticulum and its ability to regulate calcium homeostasis. The original studies describing *CALR* mutations in MPN indicated that such a uniform defect may confer a proliferative advantage to the malignant cells via activation of the JAK-STAT pathway. Mutations of *CALR* are found almost exclusively in patients with MF and ET, the two MPN entities in which MK hyperplasia is a hallmark of the disease.

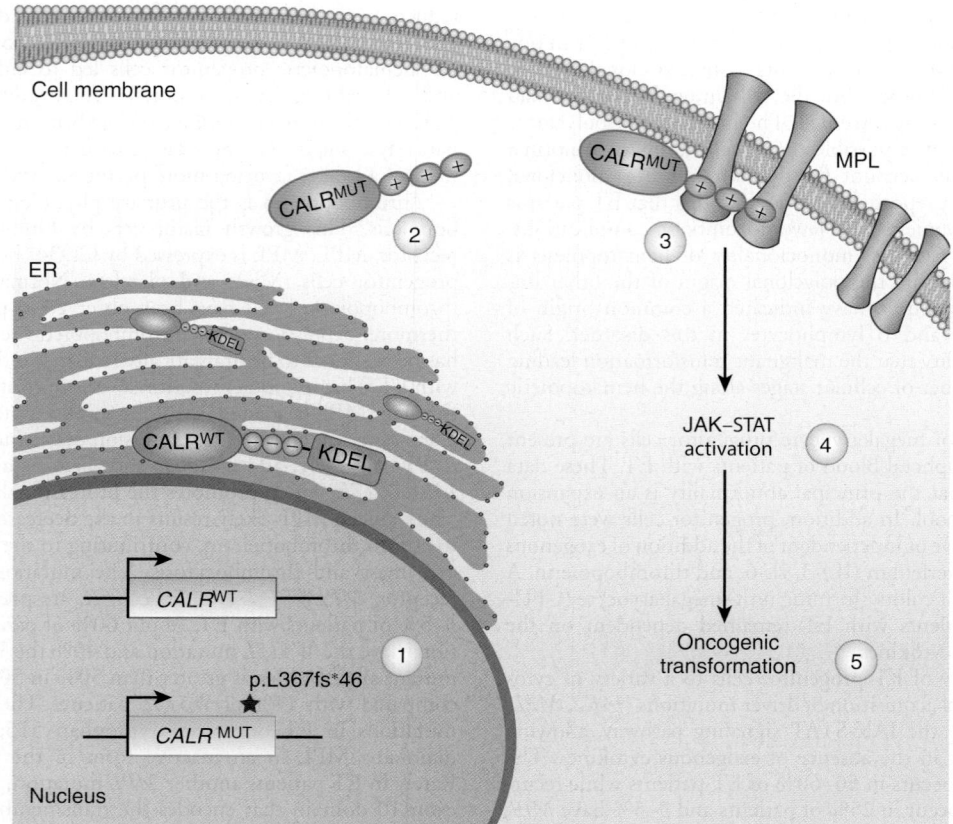

Fig. 69.1 SCHEMATIC REPRESENTATION OF THE POTENTIAL MECHANISM OF ACTION OF MUTATED CALRETICULIN. Deletions (type I mutations) or insertions (type II mutations) occurring in the exon 9 of *CALR* gene (1) result in a novel epitope in the C-terminus of the protein which lacks the ER-retention signal (KDEL) and is positively charged compared with the negatively charged wild-type protein (2). The mutated *CALR* is capable of binding MPL (3), which, in turn, activates the JAK-STAT signaling pathway (4), thus providing proliferative advantage of the malignant clone (5). *CALR*, Calreticulin; *ER*, endoplasmic reticulum; *JAK-STAT*, Janus-activated kinase–signal transducer and activator of transcription; *MPL*, thrombopoietin receptor. *(From Stanley RF, Steidl U: Cancer Disc 6:344, 2016.)*

Intriguingly, the expression of both wild-type and mutated *CALR* is restricted to MK lineage, implying a role for *CALR* in normal MK biology. By corroborating these observations, a series of subsequent reports have shed light into the mechanisms responsible for the mutated *CALR* ability to induce MK hyperplasia and thrombocytosis in MPN. Thus, four independent laboratories have demonstrated that the oncogenic activity of mutated *CALR* is mediated by MPL, which is critical for both HSC and MK lineage development. Thus, mutant CALR expressed by hematopoietic cells in vitro or in vivo in mouse models binds and activates MPL, but not other type I hematopoietic cytokine receptors. This, in turn, leads to JAK-STAT pathway activation, resulting in the development of thrombocytosis and an ET-like phenotype. Interestingly, in vivo overexpression of either of the mutation variants (type I, deletion; or type II, insertion) induces thrombocytosis and constitutively activates MPL and JAK-STAT signaling. Yet, while type II mutations favor MK proliferation, type I mutations confer clonal dominance of HSC, resulting in splenomegaly, BM hypocellularity, and fibrosis, a phenotype reminiscent of "post-ET" MF. These findings mirror the clinical observations in which type I mutations are prevalent in MF patients while type II mutations are frequent in ET patients. Moreover, CD34+ hematopoietic progenitors from ET patients harboring the type II *CALR* mutation are capable of forming spontaneous CFU-MK, validating the initial suggestions that mutated *CALR* confers cytokine-independent cell growth.

Elegant molecular and biochemical studies dissecting the interaction between mutant *CALR* and *MPL* and its downstream consequences revealed that the N-glycosylation sites of the MPL extracellular domain are required for its activation by mutated *CALR* and is independent of thrombopoietin binding site. Furthermore, mutated *CALR* translocates to the cell surface and acts in an autocrine manner in binding and activating MPL. Although the exact mechanisms by which the mutated *CALR* binds MPL remain under investigation, preliminary evidence suggests that the oncogenic properties of the mutated *CALR* can be attributed to the positive electrostatic charge of the novel peptide, which may be responsible not only for the physical interaction with MPL, but also for other cellular functions involving the normally negatively charged portion of the protein (Fig. 69.1).

The clinical phenotype of patients with *JAK2*-mutated and *CALR*-mutated ET differ. The presence of mutated *CALR*, which occurs in 25% of patients with ET and is mutually exclusive of mutations in *JAK2* and *MPL*, is associated with a younger age, male predominance, higher platelet count, lower hemoglobin level, and a lower risk of thrombotic complications. Investigators have recently demonstrated that the lower thrombotic rate in *CALR*+ ET may in part be due to reduced leukocyte activation compared with *JAK2V617F*-positive counterparts.

Occasional cases of ET are associated with loss-of-function *Lnk* (SH2B3) mutations. In mouse models, the inhibitory adaptor protein Lnk has been shown to be associated with downmodulation of erythropoietin and thrombopoietin signaling. Lnk can bind to wild-type *JAK2*, *JAK2V617F*, wild-type MPL, and *MPLW515L*. Lnk levels are upregulated and correlate with an increase in the *JAK2V617F* allele burden in MPN patients. In *JAK2V617F*-positive ET, Lnk mRNA expression is upregulated and serves to modulate

JAK2V617F-mediated cell regulation. Thrombopoietin-mediated signaling regulates Lnk expression at both the mRNA and protein levels. Furthermore, acquired *Lnk* mutations have been observed in less than 1% of ET. The inactivating *Lnk* mutations in ET patients result in JAK-STAT activation, leading to high levels of STAT3 and STAT5 activation.

Recently, Cabagnois and coworkers used whole-exome sequencing and next-generation sequencing targeting *JAK2* and *MPL* with the intent of detecting additional mutations in triple-negative ET patients. They found several signaling mutations including *JAK2V617F* at very low allele frequency, as well as additional mutations such as: *LNK* mutation, *MPL-S505N*, *MPL-W515R*, and *MPL-S204P*. *MPL-S204P* and *MPL-Y591N* were shown to be weak gain-of-function mutants increasing MPL signaling and conferring either thrombopoietin hypersensitivity or independence to expressing cells, but with a low efficiency. These data demonstrate that some clonal, noncanonical *MPL* gain-of-function mutations are associated with triple-negative cases of ET. In the triple-negative patients in whom these mutations were not detected, a number had clonal while the others had polyclonal hematopoiesis, suggesting that certain patients with triple-negative ET cannot be classified as having an MPN and should be evaluated for inherited forms of thrombocytosis that will be discussed later.

With the development of whole-exome sequencing, mutations in epigenetic regulators (such as *TET2*, *DNMT3A*, *ASXL1*, *EZH2*, and isocitrate dehydrogenase [*IDH*]*1/IDH2*) and in spliceosome components (such as *SRSF2*, *U2AF1*, and *SF3B1*) have been shown to be present in MPN patients with *JAK2/MPL/CALR* mutations. Other mutations were also directly associated with leukemic progression, such as *p53*, *RUNX1*, *CBL*, and deletion in *IKAROS*. Several of these mutations can occur in the same patient, and most frequently *SRSF2* can occur with *TET2*, *ASXL1* or *IDH* mutations. In contrast to *MPN* driver mutations, which are rare in other myeloid malignancies, these additional mutations are not specific to MPNs and are found with a higher frequency in patients with MDS and in MDS/MPN overlap syndromes, such as chronic myelomonocytic leukemia as well as AML. Biologic studies and mouse models have shown that these additional mutations may cooperate with the *MPN* driver mutations to favor clonal dominance (*TET2* or *DNMT3A*), to modify disease phenotype, or to promote either progression to MF or leukemic transformation (*ASXL1*, *IDH1/2*, *EZH2*, and *TP53*).

The ten–eleven translocation (*TET2*) gene encodes for a hydroxylase that is able to hydroxylate methylated cytosine. These mutations result in loss of function, leading to increased DNA methylation and a reduction in hydroxymethyl cytosine. *TET2* mutations occur in 11% of ET patients. Mutations in *TET2* can occur either before or after mutations of *JA2V617F* or *MPL*. Mutations in the gene for IDH occur in 0.9% of ET patients and can functionally lead to similar effects as *TET2* mutations on DNA methylation. Furthermore, disrupting mutations of *ASXL*, which occur in 36% of PMF patients, are infrequent in ET, as are mutations of *CBL* or *EZH2*.

Furthermore, the transcription factor NF-E2 has been shown to be overexpressed in the cells of patients with MPNs independent of the presence or absence of *JAK2V617F*. NF-E2 acts as an epigenetic transcriptional regulator and chromatin modifier. Genetically engineered mice that overexpress NF-E2 have been created and are characterized by extreme thrombocytosis and leukocytosis, normal hemoglobin levels, and BM hypercellularity, a clinical picture similar to that observed in ET patients.

The cause of the increased risk of developing hemorrhagic and thrombotic events associated with ET remains the subject of investigation. Thrombotic complications occur most frequently in patients older than age 60 years; patients with a history of a thrombotic event; and individuals with cardiovascular risk factors, including tobacco use, hypertension, or diabetes mellitus, but hemorrhagic events occur almost exclusively in individuals with extremely high platelet counts (>1000 × 10^9/L).[4] In addition, leukocytosis (>11,0000/L) and *JAK2V617F* positivity have been associated with the development of arterial thrombosis. Platelet counts in excess of 1000 × 10^9/L are associated with a lower risk of developing arterial thromboses.

The incidence of thrombotic events in ET patients ranges from 1.5% to 6.6% per patient-year. The thrombotic events in ET are largely arterial, but venous thromboses also occur not infrequently. *JAK2V617F*-positive ET patients compared with patients with a *CALR* mutation or those who are triple negative have a higher risk of developing thrombotic events, but a dose-dependent correlation between allele burden and the development of clinical symptoms has not been demonstrated. The age-related differences in the frequency of these events have been attributed to the coexistence of vascular disease in older patients. Many investigators have struggled to identify ET patients who are at the greatest risk of developing thrombotic episodes. Recently, a new thrombotic scoring system has been developed by investigators on both sides of the Atlantic.[1] In the latest iteration of this risk stratification schema four categories were delineated: very low risk (no thrombosis history, age ≤60 years, and *JAK2* unmutated); low risk (no thrombosis history, age ≤60 years, and *JAK2* mutated); intermediate risk (no thrombosis history, age >60 years, and *JAK2* unmutated) and high risk (thrombosis history, age >60 years, and *JAK2* mutation). How to personalize therapy based upon such a schema remains problematic and to date untested.[2]

Some progress has been made in defining the relationship between platelet numbers and the risks for thrombotic and hemorrhagic events in ET. In a randomized trial of patients at a high risk of developing a thrombotic event (>60 years of age, a history of a thrombotic episode, or both), the reduction of platelet numbers was highly effective in preventing additional thrombotic events (Fig. 69.2).[5] Furthermore, the incidence of thrombotic events has been shown to be closely correlated with the duration of thrombocytosis in a case–control study. Unfortunately, there has been difficulty in defining what particular target platelet count should serve as an endpoint for myelosuppressive therapies to maximally reduce the degree of thrombotic risk. Many investigators have provided data that indicate that interactions between platelets and activated leukocytes participate in the thrombotic risk of ET patients, suggesting to some that normalization of leukocyte numbers should also be a therapeutic endpoint.

Several groups have now confirmed that the degree and duration of bleeding in ET patients is correlated with platelet numbers. The clinical spectrum of bleeding in ET patients closely resembles that observed in von Willebrand disease. Several groups have now shown that high platelet counts (>1000 × 10^9/L) are associated with an acquired form of von Willebrand syndrome, and that reduction of platelet numbers is associated with correction of the von Willebrand syndrome-like abnormalities and cessation of bleeding episodes. The mean platelet count in patients with ET and acquired von Willebrand disease is 2050 ± 1107 × 10^9/L. An increase in the number of

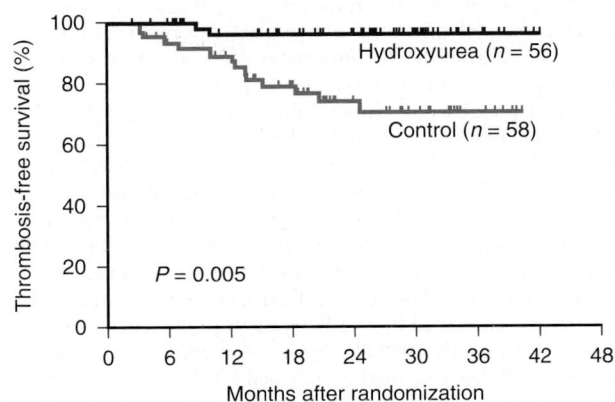

Fig. 69.2 PROBABILITY OF THROMBOSIS-FREE SURVIVAL IN 114 PATIENTS WITH ESSENTIAL THROMBOCYTHEMIA TREATED WITH HYDROXYUREA OR LEFT UNTREATED. *(From Cortelazzo S, Finazzi G, Ruggeri M, et al: Hydroxyurea for patients with essential thrombocythemia and a high risk of thrombosis. N Engl J Med 332:1132, 1995.)*

circulating platelets appears to favor the adsorption of larger von Willebrand multimers onto platelet membranes, resulting in their removal from the circulation and their subsequent degradation.

Platelets in patients with ET have been known for a considerable time to be qualitatively abnormal. Although both increased and decreased platelet reactivity has been described, these findings have not been definitively associated with thrombohemorrhagic complications with two noteworthy exceptions—erythromelalgia, in which the prompt relief of symptoms by cyclooxygenase inhibitors provides direct evidence that prostaglandins play a role in the development of vascular occlusion, and acquired von Willebrand syndrome, which is a major cause of bleeding in patients with ET.

Abnormal platelet aggregation has been reported in 35–100% of patients with ET. The majority of such studies have used conventional platelet aggregation studies performed on platelet-rich plasma. The simultaneous measurement of platelet aggregation and adenosine triphosphate–dense granule release by whole-blood platelet lumiaggregometry has been used to study platelet function in ET patients with the hope of identifying patients at a risk of developing thrombosis. A prospective analysis of large cohorts of patients has not been performed to confirm the utility of such assays. Platelets derived from patients with ET and PV have been shown to contain a large proportion of immature platelets that have been recently released from the BM. Such immature platelets have increased hemostatic activity, as demonstrated by a heightened response to thrombin and greater expression of P-selectin. Hydroxyurea has been shown to be capable of reducing the number of immature platelets in ET, which might partly be responsible for the reduced thrombotic risk associated with its use.

Abnormal aggregation studies have not been successful in predicting the incidence of episodes of hemorrhage or thrombosis. In ET, platelet aggregation is classically defective in response to epinephrine, adenosine diphosphate (ADP), and collagen but is usually normal with arachidonic acid and ristocetin. Characteristically, in ET, the first wave of aggregation is diminished, and the second wave of aggregation is absent in response to epinephrine. Interestingly, preincubation of ET platelets with thrombopoietin partly corrects the impaired aggregation in response to epinephrine, ADP, and collagen. An acquired form of platelet storage pool disease occurs frequently in ET. Platelet α-granule content and the release of the content of granules are abnormal, resulting in elevated plasma levels of platelet factor-4 and β-thromboglobulin.

Numerous individual functional platelet abnormalities have been demonstrated. A defect in the metabolism of arachidonic acid by lipoxygenase has been documented, as have decreased numbers of platelet receptors for prostaglandin D_2 and adrenergic receptors for epinephrine. Platelets from patients with thrombotic episodes have been found to be capable of increased generation of thromboxanes and to have an increased affinity for fibrinogen. Elevations in β-thromboglobulin and serum thromboxane levels in ET patients are validated indices of enhanced in vivo platelet activation and possibly thrombin generation. Such abnormalities are not present in patients with secondary thrombocytosis and may provide some explanation for the high incidence of thrombosis associated with ET. The antithrombotic activity of aspirin has been attributed to its ability to permanently and selectively inactivate platelet cyclooxygenase-1 (COX-1), thereby blocking thromboxane biosynthesis. This action has served as the rationale for the widespread use of aspirin in ET patients for thrombosis prophylaxis in the absence of valid controlled clinical trials. COX-2 has been shown to be overexpressed by the megakaryocytes and platelets of ET patients; COX-2 can also contribute to the enhanced biosynthesis of thromboxanes in ET. Low-dose aspirin can only partially correct this enhanced thromboxane synthesis, likely because of the increased COX-2 activity associated with the increased rate of platelet generation associated with ET, providing the rationale for the use of more aggressive aspirin scheduling or the addition of thromboxane receptor A_2 antagonists to reduce the incidence of thrombotic events. Although laboratory data indicate a rationale for twice-daily dosing of aspirin, prospective clinical data for this approach are lacking.

The platelet activation observed in ET has also been linked to Src, which is a nonreceptor tyrosine kinase particularly abundant in platelets. In thrombin-stimulated platelets, Src kinase is required for platelet aggregation. This preactivation of Src that is characteristic of ET and the related platelet hyperactivity is likely to account for the hypercoagulable state that is emblematic of ET. Recent in vitro studies also implicate *JAK2V617F*-driven heparinase overexpression in ET as a novel thrombotic mechanism. Heparinase has previously been shown to complex and enhance the activity of tissue factor, resulting in activation of the coagulation cascade.

Microvascular thrombosis causing digital or central nervous system ischemia leads to a variety of clinical syndromes closely associated with ET. The survival of platelets in ET patients with erythromelalgia and thrombosis has been shown to be reduced. Thrombosis in this setting is associated with an increased platelet turnover. Treatment of erythromelalgia with aspirin increased mean platelet survival from 4.0 ± 0.3 days to 6.9 ± 0.4 days and was associated with a significant elevation of platelet numbers. These findings suggest that erythromelalgia results from platelet-mediated thrombosis of the arterial microvasculature of the extremities. Complete correction of this ischemic circulatory defect is associated with the use of platelet cyclooxygenase inhibitors, such as aspirin and indomethacin. Agents that do not inhibit platelet cyclooxygenase, such as coumadin, sodium salicylate, dipyridamole, sulfinpyrazone, and ticlopidine, are not active in the treatment of this disorder.

One intriguing explanation for the increased risk of thrombosis in patients with ET has been the observation that the total amount of thrombin generated on the platelet surfaces of patients with ET is markedly greater than that generated on the platelet surfaces of normal control participants or patients with reactive thrombocytosis. The molecular basis of this abnormality has not been defined. Increased numbers of platelet microparticles, as well as increased platelet–neutrophil and platelet–monocyte complexes, have been observed in patients with ET. Platelet microparticles support thrombin generation and leukocyte activation. Increased numbers of platelet microparticles have been associated with the development of vascular thrombosis.

Recently, in vivo leukocyte activation has been shown to occur in ET and to be associated with signs of activation of both the coagulation cascade and endothelial cells. Such platelet and leukocyte activation may play a role in the generation of the prethrombotic state that characterizes ET. Interestingly, the presence of the *JAK2* mutation is associated with a greater degree of platelet and leukocyte activation. Activated neutrophils are able to bind platelets, which triggers the expression of tissue factor, as well as endothelial cell activation and damage. From a clinical point of view, several studies have demonstrated that an increased leukocyte count ($>11,000 \times 10^9$) in patients with ET is an independent risk factor for developing arterial thrombosis, especially myocardial infarction, and is associated with an inferior survival rate. Therefore, an important role for leukocytes in the pathogenesis of thrombosis in ET is becoming more evident. Direct involvement of endothelial cells of MPN patients by *JAK2V617F* has been reported by several groups, which might lead to endothelial dysfunction in subsets of MPN patients, further enhancing the thrombotic predisposition to the development of splanchnic vein thromboses.

CLINICAL MANIFESTATIONS

The presenting symptoms of patients with ET are quite variable. Many patients (12–67%) reach medical attention fortuitously as a result of the extreme degree of thrombocytosis detected when obtaining a routine blood cell count. Most patients present with symptoms related to small- or large-vessel thrombosis, or minor bleeding. The thrombotic events at diagnosis and during follow-up occurred at rates of 10–29% and 8–31%, respectively. In general, arterial events predominate over venous events. Presentation with a major bleeding episode is unusual. Neurologic complications are common. Table 69.1 lists representative neurologic complaints, of which headache

TABLE 69.1	Frequency of Neurologic Complaints Associated With Essential Thrombocythemia	
Manifestations		**Patients** *(n)*
Headache		13
Paresthesias		10
Posterior cerebral circulatory ischemia		9
Anterior cerebral circulatory ischemia		6
Visual disturbances		6
Epileptic seizures		2
Total number of patients		33

Data from Jabaily J, Iland HJ, Laszlo J, et al: Neurologic manifestations of essential thrombocythemia. *Ann Intern Med* 99:513, 1983.

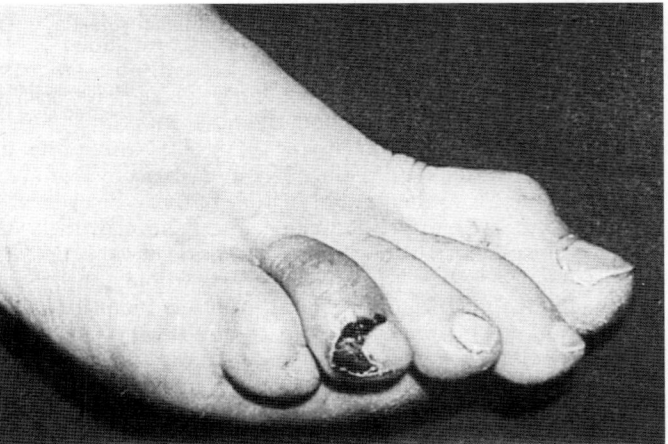

Fig. 69.3 GANGRENE OF THE TOE IN A PATIENT WITH ESSENTIAL THROMBOCYTHEMIA.

was the most common, with paresthesias of the extremities a close second. There was an extremely high incidence of transient ischemic attacks involving both the anterior and posterior cerebral circulation. These attacks have a sudden onset, last for a few moments, and are frequently associated with a pulsatile headache. The various symptoms occur sequentially rather than simultaneously and can be preceded or followed by erythromelalgia. Transient neurologic symptoms include unsteadiness, dysarthria, dysphoria, motor hemiparesis, scintillating scotomas, amaurosis fugax, vertigo, dizziness, migraine-like symptoms, syncope, and seizures. The syndrome is caused by platelet-mediated ischemia and thrombosis in end-arterial microvasculature. It is not unusual for these symptoms to eventually progress to definitive cerebral infarcts.

Microvascular circulatory insufficiency involving the toes and fingers is frequent. Such events can lead to digital pain, enhanced by warmth; distal-extremity gangrene; and classic erythromelalgia. The term *erythromelalgia* refers to a syndrome of redness and burning pain in the extremities. Erythromelalgia, which is characterized by a burning pain and a dusky congestion of swollen extremities, is usually preceded by paresthesias. Cold provides relief to these symptoms, and heat intensifies the symptoms. Patients prefer to wear shoes or slippers without socks and elevate their feet. These symptoms may progress in intensity and lead to peeling of the skin in affected appendages or affected toes or fingers, which then may become cold and ischemic with a dark purplish tinge. Erythromelalgia symptoms are asymmetric in the majority of cases. Symptoms related to coronary artery disease or transient ischemic attacks may precede or accompany the onset of erythromelalgia. Occasionally, hemorrhagic episodes may occur in patients experiencing erythromelalgia. Platelet counts in patients with erythromelalgia are frequently below $1000 \times 10^9/L$. The relief of such pain for several days after a single dose of aspirin is diagnostic of erythromelalgia. The specific microvascular syndrome of erythromelalgia is readily explained by platelet-mediated arteriolar inflammation and occlusive thrombosis leading to acrocyanosis and even gangrene. Skin biopsies from affected sites reveal arteriolar lesions without involvement of venules, capillaries, or nerves. The arteriolar endothelial cells are swollen and the vessel walls thickened by cellular swelling and deposition of intracellular material. Compared with atherosclerotic circulatory obstruction, arterial pulses in patients with erythromelalgia remain normal. Other patients develop platelet-mediated acral inflammation and arterial thrombosis, which can progress to ischemic acrocyanosis or necrosis of fingers, toes, and, rarely, the tip of the nose (Fig. 69.3).

Although thrombosis of the microvasculature is generally more frequent, thrombosis of large veins and arteries in patients with ET still occurs commonly. Patient symptoms frequently occur related to large-vessel thrombosis, mostly in the arteries of the legs, the coronary arteries, and the renal arteries. Involvement of the carotid, mesenteric, and subclavian arteries is frequent, and patients characteristically have venous thromboses involving the splenic vein, hepatic veins, or veins of the legs and pelvis. Unexplained thrombosis of the hepatic veins leads to Budd-Chiari syndrome, and thrombosis of the renal vein can

result in the development of nephrotic syndrome. Splanchnic vein thromboses occur predominantly in young women with ET. Patients with this complication are at a high risk of having a poor survival because of hepatic failure or transformation to MF or acute leukemia. It is worth noting that a fraction of patients with idiopathic splanchnic vein thrombosis may present with normal or near-normal blood counts but have an occult MPN based on genetic or histopathologic abnormalities. In a review of more than 800 patients with splanchnic vein thrombosis without a diagnosis of an MPN, a mean of 32.7% of patients were *JAK2V617F* positive. More than 50% of these patients were subsequently diagnosed with an MPN. In addition, 2.6% of patients with a cerebral sinus and vein thrombosis were also shown to be *JAK2V617F* positive. These studies suggest that all cases of splanchnic vein thrombosis and likely cerebral sinus and vein thrombosis should be tested for *JAK2V617F* to identify patients with an occult MPN. Occasional patients with idiopathic splanchnic vein thromboses with *CALR* mutations have been reported. In those patients who are *JAK2V617F* negative it is prudent to also search for *CALR* mutations. Priapism is a rare complication of ET, presumably caused by platelet sludging in the corpus cavernosum. In addition, myocardial ischemia and infarction associated with normal coronary angiograms has been reported in patients with ET, as has a high incidence of anginal symptoms. Acute renal failure has been observed after thrombosis of renal arteries and veins in patients with ET. Pulmonary hypertension secondary to alveolar capillary plugging by platelets and megakaryocytes has also been reported in patients with ET.

Hemorrhagic events occur in 3–11% of patients with ET; the primary site of bleeding is the gastrointestinal tract. Other sites of bleeding may be the skin, eyes, urinary tract, gums, tooth sockets (after extraction), joints, or brain. A high incidence of bleeding episodes during the immediate postoperative period is likely caused by postsurgical thrombocytosis and the development of acquired von Willebrand syndrome or the use of antithrombotic prophylaxis therapy. Bleeding is closely correlated with a significant increase in platelet counts in excess of $1500 \times 10^9/L$ and is associated with pseudohyperkalemia. It is important to emphasize that individual patients can experience both thrombotic and hemorrhagic episodes.

Appreciation of the risk of developing thrombohemorrhagic events in asymptomatic patients with ET who are younger than 40 years of age is imprecise at best. Such patients are thought to be at a low risk of developing thrombotic episodes unless they have experienced a prior thrombotic episode or have associated cardiovascular risk factors. The most common thrombotic complications include migraine headaches in 20% and erythromelalgia in 5% of the patients. Life-threatening hemorrhagic episodes are rare. The degree of leukocytosis has been suggested by some investigators to be useful in discriminating between young patients with a low or high risk to develop a thrombotic episode.

TABLE
69.2
Risk Stratification in Essential Thrombocythemia Based on Thrombotic Risk[a]

Risk Category	Age >60 Years or History of Thrombosis	Cardiovascular Risk Factors
Low	No	No
Intermediate	No	Yes
High	Yes	Yes

[a]Cardiovascular risk factors: hypertension, hypercholesterolemia, diabetes, smoking, and congestive heart failure. Extreme thrombocytosis (platelet count >1500 × 10^9/L) is a risk factor for bleeding. Its role as a risk factor for thrombosis in essential thrombocythemia is uncertain.
Data from Finazzi G, Barbui T: Risk-adapted therapy in essential thrombocythemia and polycythemia vera. *Blood Rev* 19:243, 2005.

A meta-analysis has revealed that the *JAK2V617* mutation is associated with a twofold higher risk of developing either a venous or arterial thrombosis but does not influence the risk of suffering from a hemorrhagic event. Regardless, it is conceivable that the significantly more advanced age and elevated hematocrit and leukocyte levels in mutation-positive patients might contribute to the apparent association between *JAK2V617F* and thrombosis reported in some studies.

Patients with ET who are older than 60 years of age who have had a prior thrombotic event have a greater risk of developing additional thrombotic events (Table 69.2). By contrast, the incidence of thrombotic and hemorrhagic complications in asymptomatic patients with ET who are younger than 60 years of age who have platelet counts of less than 1500 × 10^9/L has been shown to be comparable to a normal control population. Gender, hypertension, diabetes mellitus, hypercholesterolemia, and smoking have been shown to be independent risk factors for developing arterial thrombotic complications in ET (see Table 69.2). Screening of patients for other acquired and inherited thrombophilic states may identify patients at an even higher risk for both arterial and venous thrombotic events.

Pregnancy is not contraindicated in patients with ET. The outcome of pregnancy in patients with ET has been the subject of intense investigation. The rate of having a successful pregnancy is 61% compared with an 85–90% rate in normal women. The rate of spontaneous abortions ranges from 39–44% compared with the miscarriage rate of 10–15% in normal pregnancies. Placental infarction is often responsible for intrauterine fetal growth retardation (5%). Abruptio placenta has been reported in 3.6% of cases, a rate that is higher than that observed in the general population (1%). Major thrombotic episodes occur in 3% of these pregnancies while major bleeding episodes occur in 2% of cases. These rates are higher than that observed in the overall population of pregnant women. Baseline platelet count is not predictive of pregnancy outcome. ET patients with the *JAK2V617F* mutation have been reported to be at a higher risk of developing complications with pregnancy. In the postpartum period, the platelet counts return to their earlier levels, and rebound thrombocytosis may occur in some patients. This is thought to increase the probability of vascular complications during this period to a level similar to that observed in other conditions of thrombophilia.

In the large majority of cases, the fetal losses in pregnant ET women occur during the first trimester. A previous history of spontaneous abortion may be the greatest risk factor for the development of subsequent spontaneous abortions.

Physical examination findings are relatively unremarkable in patients with ET. Most patients are not severely ill at diagnosis, with a median Karnofsky score of 90% being reported in one series. Splenomegaly is detectable in 40–50% of patients, and approximately 20% have hepatomegaly. During the course of the disorder, a further increase in the degree of hepatosplenomegaly may be observed in patients who are developing post-ET MF. Recently, skin manifestations of the MPN have been reported to be relatively common, ranging from paraneoplastic lesions, including vascular, neutrophilic

plaques, and unexplained dermatoses. Rarely, vascular changes result in microcirculatory flow abnormalities, leading to a vasculitis resulting in classic purpura that may progress to skin necrosis. This should be distinguished from leg ulcers that occur in patients being treated with hydroxyurea. Occasionally, patients also develop pyoderma gangrenosum or Sweet syndrome.

LABORATORY MANIFESTATIONS

The hallmark of ET is a sustained and unexplained elevation of the platelet count (≥450 × 10^9/L). Accompanying leukocytosis is a common finding. A leukoerythroblastic blood picture, as well as teardrop-shaped RBCs are not features of ET but are suggestive of an early form of MF. Mild eosinophilia (>400/mm^3) and basophilia (>100/mm^3) have been reported in more than one-third of patients.

The most common morphologic abnormalities are variations in RBC size and shape and the presence of megathrombocytes (Fig. 69.3). The BM is usually normocellular or slightly hypercellular without a significant increase in granulopoiesis or erythropoiesis. Increased numbers of enlarged megakaryocytes with hyperlobulated or deeply folded nuclei that cluster in small groups along sinuses are the hallmarks of ET (see Fig. 69.4). Reticulin fibrosis is not significantly evident. A great deal of controversy currently surrounds distinguishing "true ET" from an early prefibrotic form of MF (prePMF) in which the BM is characteristically hypercellular with pronounced proliferation of granulocytes and reduced erythroid precursors. The megakaryocytes are increased in number but are loosely clustered or located along the endosteal bone surface. The megakaryocytes contain hyperchromatic, hypolobulated bulbous, or irregularly folded nuclei with an abnormal nuclear-to-cytoplasmic ratio. The histopathologic criteria for this form of prePMF have been combined with clinical criteria (minor criteria) by the World Health Organization (WHO). The 2016 criteria for the diagnosis of ET and preMF are particularly useful (Table 69.3). These new criteria are heavily dependent on mutational analyses. The *JAK2V617F* mutation occurs in 50–60% of ET patients, while recurrent mutations in *CALR* mutations occur in 25% of patients and 3–5% have *MPL* mutations. Approximately 25% of patients harbor mutated *CALR* as either a type I (52-bp del) or type II (5-bp insertion).

The patients with ET who lack such driver mutations are said to be "triple negative" (Table 69.3). Based on the 2016 WHO Diagnostic Criteria, the presence of modest BM reticulin fibrosis does not exclude the diagnosis of ET. Although select hematopathologists can reproducibly distinguish ET from prePMF, it remains uncertain whether this distinction is broadly applicable. In 70–80% of ET patients, iron stores were present in the BM, albeit at reduced levels. Almost all patients have normal serum ferritin levels. The absence of iron stores in 30% of patients may merely be an epiphenomenon of a chronic MPN and not truly reflective of an iron deficiency state. Platelet aggregation study results are frequently abnormal, most often demonstrate an impaired aggregation response to epinephrine, ADP, and collagen but not to arachidonic acid and ristocetin. Spontaneous platelet aggregation has been reported to occur frequently in such patients, but this has not been a universal finding.

Approximately 25% of patients with ET have been reported to have elevated uric acid levels at diagnosis. The average value of the serum potassium at diagnosis is usually within the normal range, although 23% of patients have been reported to have pseudohyperkalemia, caused by the degranulation of platelets when in vitro clotting releases potassium. Both excessive numbers of RBCs and leukocytes can also be associated with these phenomena. The pseudohyperkalemia can be documented by measuring plasma instead of serum potassium levels and the lack of electrocardiographic findings associated with true hyperkalemia. Pseudohypoxemia has also been observed in ET patients with extreme degrees of thrombocytosis. Acquired von Willebrand syndrome is associated almost uniformly with a platelet count greater than 1500 × 10^9/L, a prolonged bleeding time, normal factor VIII coagulant activity, and a normal von Willebrand antigen level

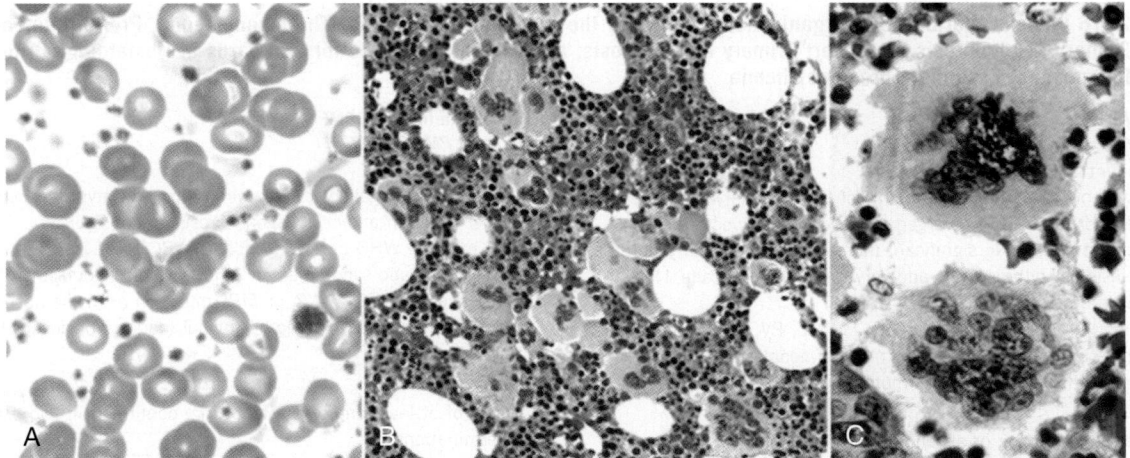

Fig. 69.4 ESSENTIAL THROMBOCYTHEMIA: PERIPHERAL BLOOD SMEAR AND BONE MARROW BIOPSY. The peripheral blood smear in essential thrombocythemia (ET) shows a marked thrombocytosis with anisocytosis (varying sizes) of the platelets (A). The bone marrow (B) is hypercellular and exhibits a marked proliferation of large and giant megakaryocytes in loose clusters with other hematopoietic elements in the background. The large megakaryocytes (C) tend to be extensively lobulated.

but decreased von Willebrand factor–ristocetin cofactor activity and collagen binding activity, as well as a decrease or absence of large von Willebrand factor multimers simulating a type II von Willebrand disorder. The serum vitamin B_{12} level can be increased in 25% of cases.

In ET, BM karyotypes are characteristically normal. The absence of the Philadelphia chromosome and the *BCR-ABL* rearrangement excludes the diagnosis of CML, which is important to consider when evaluating a new case of thrombocytosis. Rare patients share two molecular markers of MPNs (*JAK2V617F* and *BCR/ABL*). Aneuploidy is seen in the minority of cases at diagnosis. In fact, ET is associated with a definite chromosomal abnormality in only 7.8% of cases, but with disease progression there is an increased risk of aneuploidy. Specific chromosome abnormalities associated with ET have not been described, but abnormalities observed in PV and PMF, as well as in myelodysplastic syndrome (MDS), such as trisomy 1q, deletions of 5q, 13q, and 20q, trisomy 8, as well as monosomal karyotypes, have been reported. Many nonspecific chromosomal rearrangements have also been observed such as a complex karyotype, presence of a marker chromosome, and unusual translocations. Molecular cytogenetic studies in ET have not been performed extensively. In one reported study, addition of fluorescence in situ hybridization increased detection of chromosomally abnormal clones by 15%. However, in 21 patients studied with oligoarray comparative genomic hybridization, one additional patient with deletion 13q was identified compared with conventional cytogenetics. Leukemic transformation of ET is characterized by the development of an abnormal karyotype in 60–100% of patients. Consistent chromosomal abnormalities associated with ET progression in *JAK2V617F*-positive patients are der(1)t(1;9) and der(1;7)(q10;p10). Of the eight reported ET patients with der(1;7), five received previous chemotherapy (chlorambucil, hydroxyurea, pipobroman, melphalan, cytosine arabinoside, anthracycline), and six transformed to acute leukemia. Although der(1)t(1;9) is a consistent nonrandom rearrangement associated with de novo PV and with PV progression, four ET patients had der(1)t(1;9) with different breakpoints (p13;p13) and (q10;p10). In ET, similar to PV, PMF, and other myeloid disorders, formation of trisomy 1q alone or subsequent formation of jumping +1q translocations should be considered as a clonal marker associated with disease progression or transformation to AML. As has been previously mentioned, approximately 50% of ET patients are *JAK2V617F* positive, with only 4% having a high allele burden. Approximately 3–5% of patients have activating *MPL* mutations. Approximately 25% of patients harbor mutated *CALR* as either a type I (52-bp deletion) or type II (5-bp insertion).

DIFFERENTIAL DIAGNOSIS

There are numerous causes of primary, secondary, and spurious forms of thrombocytosis. A listing of the conditions that can lead to thrombocytosis is provided in Table 69.4. Primary thrombocytosis includes both acquired and hereditary forms. In acquired forms of primary thrombocytosis, the genetic abnormalities are present exclusively in hematopoietic cells, but in the hereditary forms, these underlying defects can be detected in both somatic and germ-line cells, and are inherited. The discovery of *JAK2*, *MPL*, and *CALR* mutations has provided definitive diagnostic tools with which to diagnose the MPNs, including ET. These mutations, however, can be found only in approximately 75% of ET patients. Hence, it is reasonable to consider *JAK2V617F* analysis and search for a mutation in *CALR* or *MPL* when evaluating patients with otherwise unexplained thrombocytosis. A positive test result indicates an underlying MPN. However, further investigations, including a BM biopsy (see Table 69.3) as well as cytogenetic analyses, are still required to differentiate ET from the other chronic MPNs, as well as from MDS presenting with thrombocytosis, such as the 5q syndrome and refractory anemia with ring sideroblasts and thrombocytosis (RARS-T; see Table 69.3) and prePMF.

For those patients who present with thrombocytosis who are triple negative for driver mutations, the first step in determining the cause of thrombocytosis is to exclude reactive forms of thrombocytosis. The causes of secondary or reactive forms of thrombocytosis are numerous, but the most common causes are infection, inflammation, hemolysis, severe exercise, malignancy, hyposplenism, and other causes of an acute-phase response (see Table 69.4). In a hospital population, patients with extreme thrombocytosis ($>1000 \times 10^9/L$) are not particularly rare in adult or pediatric patient populations. Examination of the blood smear is important to avoid confusion with so-called *pseudothrombocytosis*. This occurs in a number of conditions in which platelet-sized particles of red or white blood cell fragments (CLL, TTP, hemoglobin H disease), schistocytes, microspherocytosis, and cryoglobulinemia are erroneously enumerated as platelets by automatic particle counters. Confirmation of increased numbers of platelets by examination of the peripheral smear will avoid misdiagnosis and unnecessary clinical evaluation.

Whereas reactive thrombocytosis accounts for more than 88–97% of cases, thrombocytosis caused by an MPN accounts for only a minority of cases. Reactive thrombocytosis is more common in all age groups, except those in the eighth decade and older. Thrombotic and hemorrhagic events infrequently occur in patients with reactive thrombocytosis. These findings are in contrast to the enhanced risk

TABLE 69.3	2016 Revised World Health Organization Criteria for the Diagnosis of Essential Thrombocythemia, Pre-fibrotic Form of Primary Myelofibrosis, and Overt Primary Myelofibrosis, and British Committee for Standards in Hematology Criteria for Diagnosis of Essential Thrombocythemia

WHO ET Criteria
Major Criteria

1. Platelet count ≥450 × 10⁹/L
2. BM biopsy showing proliferation mainly of the megakaryocyte lineage with increased numbers of enlarged, mature megakaryocytes with hyperlobulated nuclei. No significant increase or left shift in neutrophil granulopoiesis or erythropoiesis and very rarely minor (grade 1) increase in reticulin fibers
3. Not meeting WHO criteria for *BCR-ABL1⁺* CML, PV, PMF, myelodysplastic syndromes, or other myeloid neoplasms
4. Presence of *JAK2, CALR,* or *MPL* mutation

Minor Criteria

Presence of a clonal marker or absence of evidence for reactive thrombocytosis

Diagnosis of ET requires meeting all four major criteria or the first three major criteria and the minor criterion

WHO Criteria for Pre-Fibrotic Form of Primary Myelofibrosis
WHO prePMF Criteria
Major Criteria

1. Megakaryocytic proliferation and atypia, without reticulin fibrosis >grade 1ᵃ, accompanied by increased age-adjusted BM cellularity, granulocytic proliferation, and often decreased erythropoiesis
2. Not meeting the WHO criteria for *BCR-ABL1⁺* CML, PV, ET, myelodysplastic syndromes, or other myeloid neoplasms
3. Presence of *JAK2, CALR,* or *MPL* mutation, or in the absence of these mutations, presence of another clonal marker,ᵇ or absence of minor reactive BM reticulin fibrosisᶜ

Minor Criteria

Presence of at least one of the following, confirmed in two consecutive determinations:

a. Anemia not attributed to a comorbid condition
b. Leukocytosis ≥11 × 10⁹/L
c. Palpable splenomegaly
d. LDH increased to above upper normal limit of institutional reference range

Diagnosis of prePMF requires meeting all three major criteria, and at least one minor criterion

- ᵃSee Table 69.8.
- ᵇIn the absence of any of the three major clonal mutations, the search for the most frequent accompanying mutations (e.g., *ASXL1, EZH2, TET2, IDH1/IDH2, SRSF2, SF3B1*) are of help in determining the clonal nature of the disease.
- ᶜMinor (grade 1) reticulin fibrosis secondary to infection, autoimmune disorder or other chronic inflammatory conditions, hairy cell leukemia or other lymphoid neoplasm, metastatic malignancy, or toxic (chronic) myelopathies.

WHO Criteria for Overt PMF
WHO Overt PMF Criteria
Major Criteria

1. Presence of megakaryocytic proliferation and atypia, accompanied by either reticulin and/or collagen fibrosis grades 2 or 3ᵃ
2. Not meeting WHO criteria for ET, PV, *BCR-ABL1⁺* CML, myelodysplastic syndromes, or other myeloid neoplasms
3. Presence of *JAK2, CALR,* or *MPL* mutation or in the absence of these mutations, presence of another clonal marker,ᵇ or absence of reactive myelofibrosisᶜ

Minor Criteria

Presence of at least one of the following, confirmed in two consecutive determinations:

a. Anemia not attributed to a comorbid condition
b. Leukocytosis ≥11 × 10⁹/L
c. Palpable splenomegaly
d. LDH increased to above upper normal limit of institutional reference range
e. Leukoerythroblastosis

Diagnosis of overt PMF requires meeting all three major criteria, and at least one minor criterion

- ᵃSee Table 69.8.
- ᵇIn the absence of any of the three major clonal mutations, the search for the most frequent accompanying mutations (e.g., *ASXL1, EZH2, TET2, IDH1/IDH2, SRSF2, SF3B1*) are of help in determining the clonal nature of the disease.
- BM fibrosis secondary to infection, autoimmune disorder, or other chronic inflammatory conditions, hairy cell leukemia or other lymphoid neoplasm, metastatic malignancy, or toxic (chronic) myelopathies.

British Committee for Standards in Hematology Criteria for Diagnosis of Essential Thrombocythemia

Requires A1–A3 or A1 + A3–A5

A1: Sustained platelet count >450 × 10⁹/L
A2: Presence of an acquired pathogenic mutation (e.g., in *JAK2* or *MPL*)
A3: No other myeloid malignancy, especially PV, PMF, CML, or MDS
A4: No reactive cause for thrombocytosis and normal iron stores
A5: BM aspirate and trephine biopsy showing increased megakaryocyte numbers displaying a spectrum of morphology with predominant large megakaryocytes with hyperlobated nuclei and abundant cytoplasm

BM, Bone marrow; CML, chronic myeloid leukemia; JAK2, Janus kinase 2; MDS, myelodysplastic syndrome; MPL, thrombopoietin receptor; PMF, primary myelofibrosis; PV, polycythemia vera.
From Harrison et al: *Br. J Haemotol* 149:352, 2010.

of these two complications in patients with ET. This relatively high frequency of extreme thrombocytosis in an acute-care hospital emphasizes the need for caution in making a diagnosis of ET (Table 69.5). A number of groups have shown that reactive thrombocytosis may be a consequence of the elaboration of known cytokines in response to the underlying inflammatory or neoplastic disorder, and are accompanied by an elevated erythrocyte sedimentation rate or a high C-reactive protein (CRP). Elevated levels of IL-1, IL-6, GM-CSF, G-CSF, and thrombopoietin have been detected in such patient populations and frequently in individuals with thrombocytosis caused by an underlying MPN. Elevation of thrombopoietin levels has not only been found in patients with reactive thrombocytosis but also in patients with ET. IL-6–induced thrombocytosis is mediated

in part by secondary thrombopoietin production by the liver in inflammatory disorders and malignant diseases. CRP is an acute-phase reactant, the hepatic synthesis of which is mediated by IL-6. CRP levels are high in patients with high levels of IL-6. In one series, whereas 81% of patients with reactive thrombocytosis had elevated IL-6 or CRP levels, patients with uncomplicated thrombocytosis secondary to an MPN had undetectable IL-6 levels. Low levels of both IL-6 and CRP are strongly indicative of the thrombocytosis being the consequence of an underlying MPN.

Both familial forms of thrombocytosis and thrombocytosis that accompanies hematologic malignancies are examples of primary thrombocytoses. The MPNs are characterized by clonal hematopoiesis, but in the familial forms of thrombocytosis, hematopoiesis

TABLE 69.4 Conditions Associated With Thrombocytosis

Primary Thrombocytosis

Malignancies
  Essential thrombocythemia
  Polycythemia vera
  Primary myelofibrosis
  Chronic myeloid leukemia
  Refractory anemia with ringed sideroblasts and thrombocytosis
  Chronic myelomonocytic leukemia
  MDS/MPN overlap
Familial thrombocythemia (inherited mutations in thrombopoietin or thrombopoietin receptor)

Secondary (Reactive) Thrombocytosis

Blood loss or iron deficiency
  Infection
  Inflammation
  Disseminated malignancy
  Hemolysis
  Drug therapy
  Hyposplenism
  Cytokine administration

Spurious Thrombocytosis

Schistocytes
Cytoplasmic fragmentation of neoplastic cells
Cryoglobulinemia
Bacteria

MDS, Myelodysplastic syndrome; MPN, myeloproliferative neoplasm.

TABLE 69.5 Clinical and Laboratory Features Helpful in Distinguishing Essential Thrombocythemia From Reactive Thrombocytosis[a]

Feature	ET	RT
Chronic platelet increase	+	−
Known causes of RT	−	+
Thrombosis or hemorrhage	+	−
Splenomegaly	+	−
BM reticulin fibrosis	+	−
BM megakaryocyte clusters	+	−
Abnormal cytogenetics	+	−
Increased acute phase reactants	−	+
Spontaneous colony formation[b]	+	−
JAK2V617F mutation	+	−

[a]Acute phase reactants include C-reactive protein and fibrinogen.
[b]Erythroid colonies.
BM, Bone marrow; ET, essential thrombocythemia; RT, reactive thrombocytosis.
Modified from Tefferi A, Hoagland HC: Issues in the diagnosis and management of primary thrombocythemia. *Mayo Clin Proc* 69:651, 1994.

is polyclonal. An abnormality of thrombopoietin production or of the thrombopoietin receptor has been documented to be the basis of these inherited disorders leading to thrombocytosis. Because the median age of diagnosis of patients with these familial forms of thrombocytosis is 17 years, these disorders should be carefully considered in all *JAK2V617F-*, *MPLW515L-*, and *MPL515K*-negative children with multiple family members with thrombocytosis.

Several different mutations have been reported in families in which excessive thrombocytosis has been attributed to increased thrombopoietin production.[8] A Dutch family with 11 family members and a Japanese family with eight family members were reported with a hereditary form of thrombocytosis that was inherited as an autosomal dominant. The thrombopoietin receptor in the Dutch family was normal, yet there was a G-to-C transversion in the splice donor site of intron 3 of the thrombopoietin gene. All of the affected members of the Dutch family were shown to have elevated thrombopoietin levels. In this family, a point mutation in the thrombopoietin gene was believed to lead to systemic overproduction of thrombopoietin, leading to a familial form of thrombocytosis. This was the first example of a human disease caused by increased efficiency of mRNA production. Actually, the translation of full-length thrombopoietin is almost completely inhibited by the presence in the 5′ untranslated region of seven AUG codons, which create seven upstream open reading frames (uORFs). These uORFs are potent inhibitors of translation, and mutations in this area cause thrombocytosis by eliminating the normal physiological inhibition of thrombopoietin mRNA translation. Additional families with thrombocytosis caused by a similar genetic mechanism have been identified.

Hereditary mutations of *MPL* can either result in loss of function and thrombocytopenia, or in gain of function and thrombocythemia, and are important models to analyze the mechanism of c-Mpl activity. Familial thrombocytosis has been attributed to germ-line mutations of *MPL* (*MPL-S505N*, *MPL-K39N*, and *MPL-P106L*). *MPL-S505N* was first described in a Japanese pedigree of familial thrombocytosis that is inherited in an autosomal dominant fashion. This disorder has been attributed to a dominant-positive activating mutation of the cellular receptor of MPL. Eight additional Italian families with thrombocytosis and MPL-S505N have been identified. In these individuals hematopoiesis is polyclonal. Etheridge and coworkers recently described a novel, autosomal dominant germ-line mutation that causes familial ET resulting from a single-nucleotide substitution, generating the mutant kinase *JAK2R564Q*. Their data indicate that this mutation leads to isolated thrombocytosis. Mild thrombocytosis was observed as well as polyclonal hematopoiesis. Furthermore, increased activation of JAK2 was confirmed in the platelets of *JAK2R564Q*-positive family members compared with those without the mutation

A polymorphism of the thrombopoietin receptor (MPL Baltimore, MPL-K39N) that is accompanied by thrombocytosis has also been described. This germ-line polymorphism is caused by a single-nucleotide substitution that results in a lysine-to-asparagine (K39N) substitution in the ligand-binding domain of MPL. The polymorphism occurs exclusively in African–Americans and appears to have an autosomal dominant pattern of inheritance with incomplete penetrance because some heterozygotes have normal platelet counts while others have thrombocytosis. Approximately 7% of African–Americans are heterozygous for MPLK39N. The mutation in the homozygous state is associated with extreme thrombocytosis with a reduced expression of platelet MPL, which has been proposed to affect the receptor's ability to bind thrombopoietin, resulting in its reduced clearance and increased stimulation of megakaryocytopoiesis. *MPL-P106L* is another germ-line mutation associated with thrombocytosis that has been found in 3.3% of Arabs. It leads to severe thrombocytosis in homozygotes and occasionally to mild thrombocytosis in heterozygotes. In the families described with this germ-line mutation, extreme thrombocytosis was associated with homozygosity and the mode of inheritance is regarded as being autosomal recessive with possible mild manifestations occurring in heterozygotes.

Subjects with familial forms of thrombocytosis are characteristically diagnosed at earlier ages than patients with ET, and appear to have similar risks for thrombotic and hemorrhagic complications. These disorders were initially considered to be associated with a benign clinical course, but follow-up of such families for longer periods of time has corrected this misperception. Overall, 23 members of a Dutch and a Polish family with a form of thrombocytosis attributed to excessive thrombopoietin production were shown to have similar thrombotic and hemorrhagic complications as individuals with ET. Also, these family members experienced vasomotor symptoms, including erythromelalgia and Raynaud phenomena, which responded to aspirin therapy but not hydroxyurea therapy. Furthermore, many of these patients developed splenomegaly as well as BM histopathologic findings that resemble an MPN, including BM hypercellularity, clustering of megakaryocytes, and a mild increase in BM fibrosis. Surprisingly, more prolonged follow-up of members of the Dutch family due to overproduction of thrombopoietin have revealed progression to symptomatic MF in one individual and progression to acute leukemia in a second family member. The patient with acute leukemia had not received any chemotherapeutic agents, and evaluation of the strength of the relationship between this high thrombopoietin condition and the development of acute leukemia requires further investigation of these families. Similarly, patients with an activating mutation of MPL, MPL-S505N, also have a high incidence of major thrombotic events, including stroke, myocardial infarction, and Budd-Chiari syndrome. In adult patients, overt BM reticulin and collagen fibrosis associated with mild reductions in hemoglobin levels have been observed, but differences in platelet counts, incidence in thrombotic episodes, or splenomegaly have not been observed when one compares these individuals with ET patients. In women with MPL-S505N, hematopoiesis was polyclonal, and the mutation was observed not only in hematopoietic tissues but also other somatic tissues. Family members who are affected by this mutation appear to have a significantly shorter survival time than nonaffected family members who did not have thrombocytosis, with affected individuals dying most frequently of thrombotic events or complications of MF. By contrast, individuals with either MPL-K39N or MPL-P106L, which both involve the extracellular domain of MPL, affecting its ability to bind thrombopoietin, were not observed to have an increased risk for thrombosis, splenomegaly, or BM fibrosis.

Table 69.3 outlines the 2016 WHO criteria for the diagnosis of ET that incorporates JAK2V7617F, CALR and MPL mutational analyses. RBC mass and plasma volume studies, if available, are sometimes helpful in differentiating between JAK2V617F-positive ET with borderline elevated hematocrits from patients with PV, but such patients likely represent a continuum of evolution of a JAK2V617F-positive hematologic malignancy. BM karyotypic analysis or studies of the BCR-ABL fusion gene are imperative in every patient to exclude the diagnosis of CML or to detect another clonal hematologic malignancy. This step is necessary because the natural history of these disorders is very different, and early therapeutic intervention with specific medical therapy for CML, such as a BCR-ABL tyrosine kinase inhibitor is essential.

Occasionally, ET may be distinguished from RARS-T. These patients present with thrombocytosis that is associated with a moderate-to-severe anemia and frequently splenomegaly. Their BMs are characterized by the morphologic features of ET and the presence of more than 15% ringed sideroblasts. This entity likely represents a heterogeneous, poorly defined disorder that includes a spectrum of conditions sharing features of an MPN and a myelodysplastic disorder. This entity is associated with JAK2V617F in 58% of reported patients, MPLW515 mutation in 7% of reported patients, and CALR mutation in <5% of patients. Occasional patients with thrombocytosis and increased ringed sideroblasts but without anemia have also been described. Patients with RARS-T have a similar prognosis as ET patients. RARS-T has been recently shown to be associated with somatic mutations of SF3B1, a gene encoding a core component of the RNA splicing machinery. RARS-T therefore likely results from a combination of SF3B1 and JAK2 or MPL mutations. About 25% of patients with RARS-T have wild-type SF3B1, suggesting that other molecular defects can be associated with RARS-T.

Because patients with preMF frequently present with thrombocytosis, this form of PMF can frequently be difficult to distinguish from ET. This early form of PMF was previously referred to as a prefibrotic form of PMF. In prePMF, nucleated RBCs, teardrop-shaped RBCs, immature myeloid cells, and megathrombocytes are observed in the peripheral blood. In the BM biopsy, the megakaryocytes are markedly abnormal, a morphologic finding that is helpful in distinguishing this entity from ET. In prePMF, the megakaryocytes often appear in clusters adjacent to the sinusoids; deviations in the nuclear cytoplasmic ratio in the megakaryocytes are observed with abnormal patterns of chromatin clumping, and plump clouds similar to a balloon-shaped lobulation of the nuclei are observed associated with minimal fibrosis or even absent reticulin fibrosis during this stage of PMF.

The presence of clonal hematopoiesis, at least in one lineage, quickly establishes the diagnosis of ET. Unfortunately, techniques to study clonality are currently not widely available and are restricted to the evaluation of female patients. Such studies may be particularly useful in young female patients with thrombocytosis. Probes for a variety of genes on the X chromosome can be informative for clonal analysis of blood cell production in more than 72% of female Americans. In such patients, analysis of restriction fragment length polymorphisms can be used to establish a pattern of clonal hematopoiesis, which is indicative of a hematologic malignancy and established the diagnosis of ET in a young female patient with thrombocytosis who was lacking a driver mutation. Polyclonal hematopoiesis is found in all cases of reactive and familial thrombocytosis. Polyclonal hematopoiesis, however, does not exclude the diagnosis of ET because in several series almost one-third of patients who met the clinical criteria for ET had polyclonal hematopoiesis in all studied lineages. The biogenesis of this polyclonal form of ET is poorly understood. Initial studies, however, have suggested that women with polyclonal hematopoiesis may have fewer thrombotic complications than those with clonal hematopoiesis.

At times, it is impossible to define the cause of an individual patient's thrombocytosis. In an asymptomatic patient, follow-up to determine whether the degree of thrombocytosis increases is warranted. If additional clues to the cause of the thrombocytosis are subsequently revealed, a diagnosis will become apparent. Some reassurance is provided by reports of larger cohorts of patients, each with platelet counts of greater than 1000×10^9/L, which have been followed for years. Virtually none of the patients with reactive thrombocytosis developed a cerebrovascular accident, thrombophlebitis, or a peripheral arterial thrombosis.

PROGNOSIS

The probability that a patient with ET will survive 10 years ranges from 64% to 80%. In a large study from Spain with extensive follow-up, there was no substantial difference between the probability of survival of patients with ET and that of a control population. However, a study of 322 consecutive patients seen at the Mayo Clinic and followed for a median follow-up of 13.6 years showed a different pattern. Survival of patients with ET was similar to that of the control population during the first decade of disease, but the survival became significantly worse thereafter. Multivariable analysis identified an age at diagnosis of 60 years or older, leukocytosis (>15,000/µl), previous venous thrombosis, tobacco use, and diabetes mellitus as independent predictors of poor survival. The risk of developing leukemia or MF was low in the first 10 years (1.4% and 3.8%, respectively) but increased substantially in the second (8.1% and 19.9%, respectively) and third (24.0% and 28.9%, respectively) decades of the disease. The presence of the JAK2V617F mutation did not influence either survival or the rate of leukemic transformation in this analysis. The rate of leukemic transformation was higher in patients with platelet counts above 1000×10^9/L and abnormal hemoglobin levels. The development of MF was heralded by the appearance of immature myeloid precursors and dacryocytes in the blood smear, and increased serum lactate dehydrogenase levels followed by a reduction in platelet numbers and progressive splenomegaly. The presence of CALR, which occurs in 15–25% of patients with ET and is mutually exclusive with mutations in JAK2 and MPL, is associated with younger age, male sex and higher platelet counts, lower hemoglobin levels, and a lower risk of thrombotic complications.

The International Prognostic Score for Essential Thrombocythemia (IPSET) was developed from the retrospective review of clinical outcome of 891 patients with ET diagnosed by WHO criteria in which age ≥60 years, leukocyte count $\geq 11 \times 10^9$/L, and history of thrombosis were determined to have prognostic significance for survival, with weighted values of 2, 1, and 1 points, respectively.[1] The IPSET categories of low (no points), intermediate (1–2 points), or high (3–4 points) had corresponding median survivals of not yet reached, 24.5 years, and 13.8 years, respectively. Analysis of this

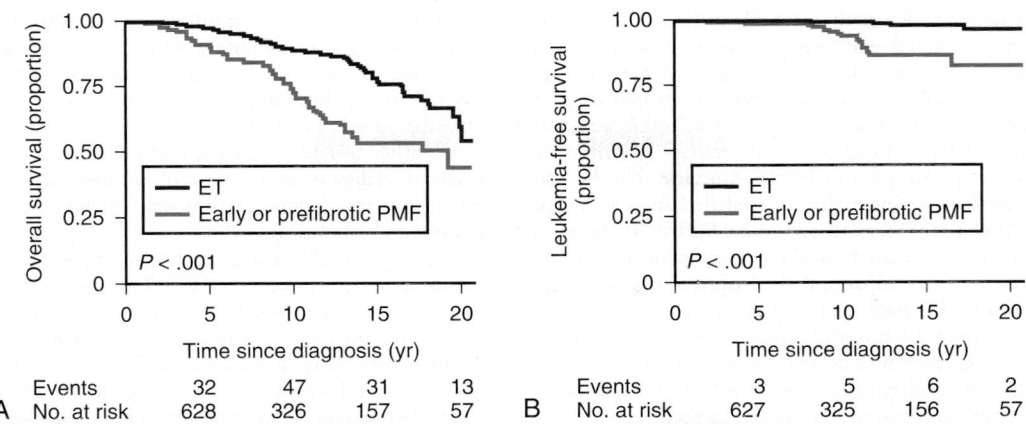

Fig. 69.5 Overall (A) and leukemia-free (B) survival of patients with true ET versus early or PMF. ET, Essential thrombocythemia; PMF, prefibrotic primary myelofibrosis. *(Data from Barbui T, Thiele J, Passamonti F, et al: Survival and disease progression in essential thrombocythemia are significantly influenced by accurate morphologic diagnosis: An international study.* J Clin Oncol *29:3179, 2011.)*

cohort for thrombotic risk determined age >60 years (1 point), history of thrombosis (2 points), presence of cardiovascular risk factors (1 point; diabetes, hypertension, smoking) and the presence of mutated *JAK2* (2 points) as independent risk factors. Low-risk (0–1 points), intermediate-risk (2 points), and high-risk (3+) categories were associated with 1.03%, 2.35% and 3.56%/year risk of thrombosis, respectively.[9]

A major determinant of the prognosis of a patient with a presumptive diagnosis of ET depends on the discrimination of whether such patients actually have true ET or an early form of MF based on histopathologic and clinical criteria adopted by the WHO (see Table 69.3).[14] In a group of 891 patients with a prior diagnosis of ET with BM biopsies evaluated retrospectively histopathologically, 16% were reclassified as having prePMF. Thrombosis rates and *JAK2V617F* positivity were similar in the two groups. However, patients with prePMF had higher leukocyte counts, lower hemoglobin levels, higher platelet counts, higher lactic dehydrogenase levels, greater numbers of circulating CD34[+] cells, and a greater incidence of palpable splenomegaly than patients with true ET. Survival was reported to be significantly inferior for those patients with pre PMF compared with patients with histopathologically validated ET (Fig. 69.5). In one series with a median follow-up of approximately 7 years, the median survival of patients with ET ranged from 16 to 21 years, and the survival of the patients with the preMF ranged from 10.8 to 14.4 years, with the majority of deaths being attributed to progression to overt PMF and acute leukemia. Although the patients with ET enjoyed a more favorable outcome, the 15-year cumulative incidences of overt MF and acute leukemia were still 9.3% and 2.1%, respectively, emphasizing the seriousness of this diagnosis, especially in younger patients.

Death of ET patients predominantly results from thrombotic complications, but transformation to AML is an important cause of mortality. The phenotype of the blast cell can be myeloid, myelomonocytic, megakaryocytic, of mixed lineage, or even lymphoblastic. According to the data mentioned earlier, the risk of patients with ET transforming into acute leukemia is greater than that of normal individuals. This is a phenomenon shared with the other MPN. The risk of developing acute leukemia after treatment with hydroxyurea alone has been reported to increase only slightly (3–4%), but the sequential use of hydroxyurea with other cytotoxic agents, such as busulfan or pipobroman, significantly increases the risk of developing a secondary leukemia.

The development of acute leukemia is often associated with a deletion of the short arm of chromosome 17, which is most frequently deleted in hydroxyurea-treated patients, but a trisomy of the long arm of chromosome 1 and monosomy 7q has been observed in patients treated with pipobroman. These cytogenetic abnormalities are believed to be induced by the use of these chemotherapeutic agents.

TABLE 69.6 Risk Factors for Thrombosis in 100 Patients With Essential Thrombocythemia

Risk Factor	Incidence of Thrombosis (% Patient-Year)	Relative Risk (95% CI)	*p*
Age (years)			
<40	1.7	1.0[a]	
40–60	6.3	3.9 (0.7–21.5)	NS
>60	15.1	10.3 (2.1–51.5)	< .001
Previous Thrombosis			
No	3.4	1.0[a]	< .0005
Yes	31.4	13.0 (4.1–1.5)	

[a]Reference category.
CI, Confidence interval; NS, not significant.
Data from Finazzi G, Barbui T: Risk-adapted therapy in essential thrombocythemia and polycythemia vera. *Blood Rev* 19:243, 2005.

The median survival after the development of myelodysplasia or leukemic transformation is 4 months. Acute leukemia, which develops after ET, is frequently refractory to standard induction chemotherapy but has been recently reported to be responsive to hypomethylating agents, including 5-azacytidine and decitabine. Because allogeneic stem cell transplantation can be curative, rapid referral to a transplant center is recommended if the patient has an appropriate performance status and an allogeneic stem cell donor is available.

THERAPY

The goal in treating patients with ET is to prevent additional thrombotic and hemorrhagic events without increasing the risk of transformation to post-ET MF, MDS, or AML. Both age (>60 years of age) and history of a prior thrombosis are widely accepted predictors of a patient developing additional thrombotic events during follow-up (Table 69.6). Other predictors of cardiovascular morbidity include a history of smoking, hypertension, obesity, diabetes mellitus, and congestive heart failure, and a white blood cell count greater than 11×10^9/L. Ironically, patients with platelet counts greater than 1000×10^9/L have a lower risk of developing an arterial thrombosis and a higher risk of bleeding. These parameters have been widely used by clinicians to stratify ET patients according to their risk for developing additional thrombotic events. Such stratification strategies have been used to make treatment decisions to reduce the platelet count. It is important to emphasize that such risk factors have been identified based on retrospective analyses of registries of ET patients that have largely not been created using modern molecular and histopathologic diagnostic tools. Using such patient-stratification strategies, patients have been placed into high-, intermediate-, or low-risk groups based on their predicted risk of developing an additional life-threatening thrombotic event. This strategy is uniformly implemented throughout Europe and North America. The benefit of this strategy is based on a single clinical trial that indicated that the reduction of platelet numbers to less than 600×10^9/L with hydroxyurea therapy was associated with a reduction of developing additional thrombotic events compared with a control group (see Fig. 69.2). This study involved a total of 114 patients, and the median follow-up period was only 27 months. Greater degrees of platelet suppression have not been shown to be associated with further reduction in the possibility of developing a thrombotic episode, which in hydroxyurea-treated high-risk patients has been reported to be 1.66% patients per year. Although the implementation of such a strategy is widely accepted, it is important to be aware that this approach is not based on robust data that one associates with modern-day evidence-based medicine. In fact, in several studies, an elevated leukocyte count of above 11×10^9/L has been more closely associated with the risk of developing additional thromboses than the degree of elevation of the platelet count. These conflicting reports in the literature among experts in this field make it increasingly more difficult to be dogmatic about who to treat with platelet-lowering agents and what the target platelet count should be. The risk stratification of patients should not be ignored, and patients with a life-threatening thrombosis or disabling symptoms because of microcirculatory problems should receive drugs that lower the platelet count. If a patient of any age has excessive thrombocytosis and a thrombotic or hemorrhagic event, that patient must be treated. However, for asymptomatic ET patients in so-called *high-risk categories*, the decision to embark upon a strategy including platelet-lowering agents is in reality a murky one that is more based on personal treatment decisions rather than volumes of data.

The treatment of asymptomatic low-risk patients with ET is controversial and remains largely problematic, yet greater insight into the management of such patients has recently been gained. Management of ET patients with life-threatening hemorrhagic or thrombotic episodes is more straightforward. Life-threatening thrombotic events require platelet pheresis in combination with the institution of myelosuppressive therapy. In this situation, immediate physical removal of large numbers of platelets is preferred because chemotherapeutic agents generally require 18–20 days before platelet counts can be reduced to normal levels. It is recommended to reduce the platelet count to 500,000/mm³ by each platelet pheresis and suggested that achievement of such a goal requires the passage of two blood volumes over a 3–4-hour period.

Such a therapeutic approach has been used to treat acutely ill patients with problems such as cerebrovascular accidents, myocardial infarction, transient ischemic attacks, or life-threatening gastrointestinal hemorrhage. Long-term platelet pheresis is an ineffective means of controlling thrombocytosis, presumably because of the rapid rate of production of platelets. Therefore, most clinicians begin by administering a chemotherapeutic agent that has a rapid onset of action, such as hydroxyurea at doses of 2–4 g/day, simultaneously with the institution of platelet pheresis. The dose of hydroxyurea requires close monitoring with appropriate reduction of dose to avoid excessive myelosuppression.

In patients found to have ET and who are clearly symptomatic and fall into the high-risk group, little controversy exists as to the need for lowering platelet numbers. The large number of thrombotic complications that occur in patients with ET who smoke points to the urgent need for smoking cessation. Most investigators try to normalize the platelet count or reach a platelet count at which the symptoms of the high-risk patient resolve. Although major bleeding episodes requiring hospitalizations are rare, patients with extreme thrombocytosis ($>1500 \times 10^9$/L), acquired von Willebrand syndrome, and history of hemorrhagic episode are clearly at risk for developing additional bleeding complications. These patients require reduction of the increased platelet numbers to the normal range with use of a variety of agents, including hydroxyurea, anagrelide, or IFN-α. According to some authors, such patients should avoid exposure to aspirin even if they have hemorrhagic complications and thrombotic episodes simultaneously.

Another situation that requires treatment is discomfort caused by erythromelalgia or progression of erythromelalgia to frank gangrene. Such patients respond within days to low-dose aspirin therapy or platelet-reduction therapy.

During the 1980s and 1990s, hydroxyurea became the drug of choice for the treatment of ET. The impetus for this practice was based on the knowledge that agents such as ^{32}P and alkylating agents such as melphalan and busulfan were leukemogenic. The popularity of the ribonucleoside reductase inhibitor, hydroxyurea, for the management of ET was due to the belief in the early 1970s that it was nonleukemogenic. Hydroxyurea can be administered at a dose of 15 mg/kg initially, with adjustment of the dose to maintain a platelet count (at the least) below 600×10^9/L without inducing significant neutropenia. After the agent is started, frequent monitoring of blood counts is mandatory to avoid the development of neutropenia until the maintenance dose is determined. The use of this drug in a high-risk group of patients with reduction of platelet numbers to less than 600×10^9/L has resulted in reduction of thrombotic events compared with a control population. The reduction of platelet numbers to this level did not entirely eliminate the occurrence of additional thrombotic episodes.

Hydroxyurea use is associated with some toxicity, including dose-related neutropenia, fever, nausea, stomatitis, hair loss, nail discoloration, and lower extremity and oral ulcerations, as well as increased risk of developing squamous cell carcinoma of the skin. Many of these problems resolve with withdrawal of the drug or dose reduction, but leg ulcers can be persistent, sometimes requiring skin grafting. These ulcers typically heal within 1–9 months of cessation of therapy. Such leg ulcers have been reported to occur in 9% of patients treated with hydroxyurea and are an indication for immediate discontinuation of therapy and elimination of any rechallenge with the drug. Hydroxyurea is also not universally successful in controlling the thrombocytosis; resistance to hydroxyurea has been reported in 11–17% of cases. The criteria for defining resistance or intolerance to hydroxyurea have been established by an International Working Group. They include a platelet count greater than 600×10^9/L after at least 2 g/day of hydroxyurea (2.5 g/day in patients with a body weight >80 kg); platelet count greater than 400×10^9/L and WBC less than 2500/mm³ or hemoglobin less than 10 g/dL at any dose of hydroxyurea; presence of leg ulcers or other unacceptable mucocutaneous manifestations at any dose of hydroxyurea; and hydroxyurea-related fever. In such situations, hydroxyurea can be substituted for (or combined with) other platelet-lowering agents. These criteria for hydroxyurea resistance are imperfect because they do not include the development of a thrombotic event while on therapy, which is the central goal of therapy. Whether such patients who develop a new thrombosis would benefit from use of another therapeutic agent has not been explored.

The risk of evolving to acute leukemia is extremely low in untreated ET patients. More recent prospective studies both in ET and PV have confirmed that hydroxyurea therapy is associated with a low incidence of leukemic transformation when used alone (<5%) and with long-term follow-up ($\leq$14 years). However, the leukemic risk increased significantly when the drug is used before or after treatment with alkylating agents, particularly busulfan. One can conclude from these studies that hydroxyurea therapy alone is less leukemogenic than alkylating agents or ^{32}P alone, but a small increased risk for the development of leukemia secondary to its use cannot be completely excluded. Of concern is the observation that a high proportion of AML and MDS occurring in ET patients treated with hydroxyurea alone have morphologic, cytogenetic, and molecular characteristics of the 17p deletion syndrome. These patients are reported to have a typical form of dysgranulopoiesis characterized by hypolobulated polymorphonuclear leukocytes with small vacuoles in neutrophils and *p53* mutations.

An alternative to hydroxyurea is therapy with anagrelide. Data on the use of anagrelide in ET suggest that it is nonleukemogenic. When considering the risk-to-benefit ratio, one can conclude that hydroxyurea therapy is a first-line therapy for ET patients at a high risk of developing an additional thrombosis, including those older than 60 years of age or with a history of a thrombotic episode or with significant other cardiovascular risk factors. Such nonleukemogenic drugs as IFN-α, anagrelide, or pegylated IFN appear to be good choices in symptomatic patients younger than 40 years of age.

Anagrelide is a member of the imidazo(2,1-b)quinazolin-2-1 series of compounds. When studied in humans, it was noted that anagrelide in small doses produced thrombocytopenia. The drug acts primarily by reducing megakaryocyte size and ploidy, and decreasing megakaryocyte proliferation. Anagrelide therefore appears to lower platelet counts, primarily by interfering with the development of megakaryocytes. Anagrelide suppresses megakaryocytopoiesis by selectively reducing the expression levels of GATA-1, FLI-1, NFE-2, and FOG-1 in cells belonging to the megakaryocytic lineage. The effects of anagrelide do not involve thrombopoietin-mediated signal transduction events. GATA-1 and FOG-1 play critical roles in megakaryocytic differentiation. Anagrelide in low doses is effective in lowering the platelet count in 93% of patients. Most importantly, it is effective despite resistance to prior therapies. Resistance to anagrelide therapy has not been documented, but occasionally patients have been observed to require extraordinarily high doses to control the excessive thrombocytosis. The recommended initial dose is 0.5 mg orally two to four times a day. The dose should be increased by 0.5 mg/week to control thrombocythemia. The dose of anagrelide should not exceed 10 mg/day or a 2-mg/dose. Excessive use will result in predictable thrombocytopenia and increase the likelihood of side effects. The median maintenance dose in patients with ET is 2 mg/day administered in divided doses. Data on more than 3000 patients with a variety of MPNs complicated by extreme thrombocytosis are available. In addition, follow-up of more than 500 patients for more than 5 years had been reported. Anagrelide has been shown to be an effective drug in the treatment of ET, resulting in a median time to response of 2.5–4 weeks. An effect on platelet numbers is usually noted in 6–10 days. Anagrelide leads to a reduction in hematocrit in 25–36% of patients, but it has no effect on white blood cell numbers, systemic symptoms, or the degree of splenomegaly. Anagrelide use in 1700 patients reduced the incidence of thrombohemorrhagic episodes related to thrombocytosis associated with MPNs from 0.66 symptoms per patient before therapy to 0.07 symptoms per patient after 28–30 months of therapy.

The most common side effects of anagrelide resulted from its vasodilatory and positive inotropic actions. These effects resulted in complaints of headache, dizziness, fluid retention, palpitations, and high-output cardiac failure. The vasodilatory effect leads to reduced renal blood flow, resulting in fluid retention. In addition, gastrointestinal complications, such as nausea, abdominal pain, and diarrhea, are prominent. These side effects usually develop within 2 weeks of initiation of therapy and frequently diminish in severity or resolve within 2 weeks of continued therapy. Because of its ability to promote fluid retention and the development of tachyarrhythmias, anagrelide therapy should be used with caution in patients with cardiac disease and should be administered carefully to elderly patients. If congestive heart failure or arrhythmias other than tachycardia develop, anagrelide therapy should be discontinued. Prolonged anagrelide therapy may be associated with a potentially irreversible drug-induced cardiomyopathy that is reminiscent of tachycardia-induced cardiomyopathy. Dose reduction can be used to lessen the degree of tachycardia or fluid retention. Before the institution of anagrelide, it is recommended that a basic cardiac evaluation be performed, including an assessment of cardiac risk factors, a careful cardiac history, and an electrocardiogram, which can be used as a baseline if the patient develops rhythm disturbances. Although most adverse effects are mild or moderate, in one series, therapy was discontinued in 16% of patients because of intolerable side effects, especially headache, nausea, fluid retention, and, rarely, frank congestive heart failure. Anagrelide has no mutagenic activity, but its use is not currently

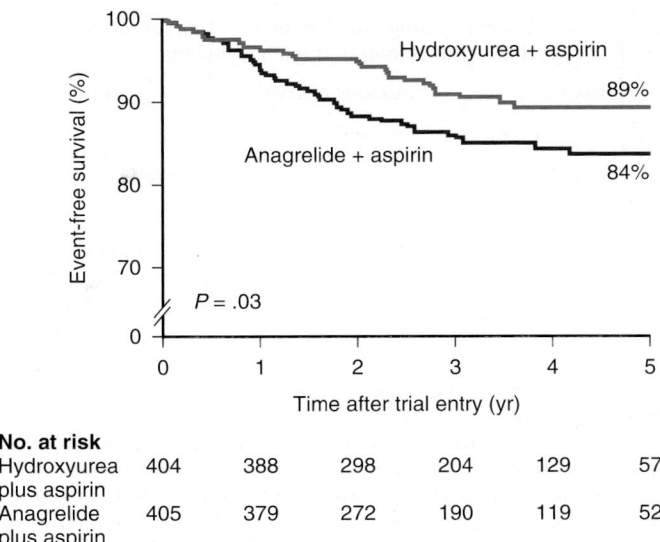

Fig. 69.6 EVENT-FREE SURVIVAL IN A HYDROXYUREA-TREATED GROUP COMPARED WITH AN ANAGRELIDE-TREATED GROUP. Primary end points were arterial or venous thrombosis, serious hemorrhage, or death from any of these causes. *(From Harrison CN, Campbell PJ, Buck G, et al: Hydroxyurea compared with anagrelide in high-risk essential thrombocythemia. N Engl J Med 353:33, 2005.)*

advised during pregnancy. Because of its small molecular weight, it is believed to be capable of crossing the placenta and thus may lead to fetal thrombocytopenia. Anagrelide appears to be a suitable drug for the treatment of young, symptomatic patients with ET and for those who are resistant or refractory to front-line treatment with hydroxyurea.

Hydroxyurea and anagrelide have been compared in a large randomized trial of 809 "high-risk" patients with ET in combination with low-dose aspirin (75–100 mg/day).[7] The dose of each cytoreductive agent was titrated to achieve a platelet count $<400 \times 10^9$/L and long-term control was attained in each treatment arm. Overall, patients randomized to anagrelide (and aspirin) were more likely to reach the composite primary endpoint of major thrombosis (arterial or venous), major hemorrhage, or death from vascular causes ($p = .03$; Fig. 69.6). When individual endpoints were assessed, arterial thrombosis, major hemorrhage, and the development of MF were all significantly more frequent in patients treated with anagrelide (7% vs. 2%; $p = .004$, .008, and .01, respectively). Anagrelide and aspirin seemed to offer at least partial protection from thrombosis because the prevalence of thrombotic events (8% at 2 years) was significantly less than that observed in the control arm of a previous study (28%). Intriguingly, the number of venous thromboses was less frequent in patients treated with anagrelide ($p = .006$). In addition, patients with *JAK2V617F*-positive ET were more sensitive to therapy with hydroxyurea but not anagrelide. Recent analyses of anagrelide-treated ET patients indicate responsiveness irrespective of driver mutation status. In long-term follow-up of 67 patients with ET treated with anagrelide, therapy-related anemia was more frequent in *CALR*-mutated patients without differences in thrombotic rates among the four molecular subtypes. Also, the incidence of discontinuation of anagrelide therapy because of drug-related adverse events was significantly greater than that observed with patients receiving hydroxyurea. Based on this large randomized study, hydroxyurea is presently considered first-line therapy for patients with high-risk ET (Table 69.7). Although equivalent control of the platelet count was achieved with both agents, hydroxyurea proved superior, perhaps because of its ability to reduce not only platelet numbers but also leukocyte numbers, which have been associated with thrombosis in ET patients. In addition, the combination of anagrelide and low-dose aspirin was associated with a higher incidence of bleeding episodes, suggesting

TABLE 69.7	Choice of Drugs for Treatment of Patients With High-Risk Essential Thrombocythemia	
Age (years)	Treatment of Choice	Second Line
<50	Interferon	Anagrelide Hydroxyurea
50–75	Hydroxyurea	Interferon Anagrelide
>75	Hydroxyurea	Anagrelide Busulfan

that aspirin therapy might be best avoided in patients being treated with anagrelide.

The ANAHYDRET study was a prospective, randomized, non-inferiority study comparing hydroxyurea to anagrelide treatment in 259 patients with treatment-naïve, high-risk ET (WHO diagnosis confirmed).[6] Anagrelide was determined to be noninferior to hydroxyurea based on equivalent rates of thrombotic (arterial and venous) and hemorrhagic (major and minor) complications. A criticism of this study was the low rate of aspirin use in this study of approximately 28% in both arms and the lack of date indicating relative rates of transformation to MF.

IFN-α has been used to treat the MPN associated thrombocytosis since the 1990s. IFN-α acts by directly inhibiting megakaryocyte colony formation and secondarily by inhibiting the expression of thrombopoietic-stimulating cytokines, such as GM-CSF, G-CSF, IL-3, and IL-11 and by stimulating the production of negative regulators of megakaryocytopoiesis, such as IL-1ra (receptor agonist) and macrophage inflammatory protein 1 (MIP-1a). IFN-α inhibits thrombopoiesis by suppressing thrombopoietin-induced phosphorylation of the JAK2 substrates, MPL and STAT5. Furthermore, IFN-α also induces the production of suppressor of cytokine signalling-1, which inhibits thrombopoietin-mediated cell proliferation. In a total of 212 patients treated with IFN-α in a total of 11 different clinical trials, a response rate of approximately 90% was reported. Therapy was administered to outpatients, most frequently at an initial dose of 3 million units daily, and usually produced a rapid decrease in platelets within 2 months. The mean time to complete response with a daily dose of 3 million units daily was about 3 months. IFN-α was effective in patients who had received other chemotherapeutic agents and in patients resistant to conventional cytotoxic drugs. In the majority of patients, the IFN dose required to maintain a normal platelet count during maintenance therapy was lower than the induction dose. In one study, 61% of patients required 3 million units three times a week, 15% once a week, and 24% daily. In addition, sustained remissions that persisted for 3–36 months were achieved with IFN-α therapy in 9–16% of patients. IFN-α is reported to be nonmutagenic and does not cross the placenta, making it a useful drug for the treatment of the symptomatic pregnant patient with ET. Reduction in platelet numbers with IFN results in a marked improvement in clinical symptoms. Toxicity, especially in older patients, the need for parenteral administration, and cost limit the usefulness of IFN-α. Side effects include flu-like symptoms during induction therapy, such as fever, bone and muscle pain, fatigue, lethargy, and depression. Symptoms are frequently controlled with acetaminophen. Long-term administration of IFN-α can result in mild weight loss; alopecia; retinal abnormalities; rarely, a reversible form of sarcoidosis and a reversible form of left-sided heart failure; and the development of autoimmune conditions, including thyroiditis leading to hypothyroidism and autoimmune hemolytic anemia. Patients may develop neutralizing antibodies to recombinant IFN, leading to a concomitant rise in platelet numbers. Approximately 25% of IFN therapy-treated ET patients discontinued therapy due to poor compliance or limiting side effects.

A semisynthetic protein polymer conjugate of IFN-α2b, pegylated IFN (peg-IFNα-2b), was anticipated to be superior to unmodified IFN as related to its adverse event profile and efficacy when used to treat ET patients. This formulation of IFN provides prolonged activity that permits once-weekly dosing. Normalization of blood counts occurred after a median time of 2–3 months; 12% of patients discontinued therapy because of inability to tolerate the drug, and 17% did not achieve normalization of their platelet counts. The majority of side effects were WHO grade 1 or 2, although some encountered grade 3 toxicity, primarily fatigue and flu-like symptoms. More importantly, no thromboembolic or hemorrhagic complications occurred during the period of treatment, although 12 thrombotic events occurred in 42 patients (24%) in the 24 months before the institution of therapy. This form of IFN, however, appears to lead to a similar frequency and severity of side effects during long-term use as experienced with conventional IFN. Interestingly, the use of another pegylated form of IFN (peg-IFNα-2a) in patients with PV was able to decrease the percentage of mutated JAK2 allele in 24 out of 27 treated patients from a mean of 49% to a mean of 27%.[10] The use of this form of IFN appeared to be associated with fewer side effects than standard forms of IFN or peg-IFNα-2b. This form of pegylated IFN has been used to treat approximately 40 patients with ET, with more than 75% of patients achieving a complete hematologic remission. Almost 40% of patients with JAK2V617F-positive ET had a reduction in their JAK2V617F allele burden, with occasional patients no longer having detectable JAK2V617F, leading to their being classified as having achieved a complete molecular remission. Although hematologic remissions were frequently achieved after 3 months of therapy, the effects on JAK2V617F were observed after 6 months of treatment. Most patients were successfully treated with 45–90 μg/weekly, and 22% of patients ceased therapy because of toxicity. Surprisingly, the hematologic and molecular responses persist for a number of months after discontinuation of therapy, suggesting that intermittent therapy may be an acceptable means of chronically administering this drug. More recently, molecular responses in a cohort of 31 CALR+ ET patients treated with peg-IFNα-2b were reported with a baseline allelic frequency of 41% reduced to 26% and two complete responses. Patients with additional subclonal mutations (TET2, ASXL1, IDH2, and TP53) were less likely to achieve molecular responses. This is consistent with the finding that patients harboring concurrent mutated JAK2 and TET2 can still have evidence of persistent TET2, despite complete response of JAK2V617F after peg-IFNα-2b therapy.

No data indicating whether IFN therapy delays or prevents the evolution to MF are available. To gain a more comprehensive assessment of the clinical usefulness of IFN-α, a prospective clinical trial comparing IFN-α with hydroxyurea in patients with ET is underway at numerous sites in North America and Europe. Until the results of this trial are available, IFN-α or anagrelide should be considered as reasonable alternatives to hydroxyurea in a patient younger than 40 years of age who has had a previous thrombotic episode (see Table 69.7), but which drug is the standard of care in so-called high-risk patients will require data emanating from the randomized trial. A number of small-molecule inhibitors of JAK2 have been evaluated for the treatment of ET patients. These agents reproducibly lower platelet counts, but the definition of the appropriate role of such agents in the treatment of ET patients will require their careful evaluation in well-controlled clinical trials.

The use of platelet antiaggregating agents remains an important area of investigation. Patients with ET have an increased predisposition to hemorrhage, which is likely potentiated by the use of drugs that affect platelet function. Transient ischemic attacks and erythromelalgia associated with ET respond rapidly to aspirin alone. In erythromelalgia, symptoms disappear for 2–4 days after administration of a single dose of aspirin. Although these agents surely have a role in the treatment of these specific complications, their use should be pursued with extreme caution because of the increased risk of hemorrhage. Low-dose aspirin therapy has been uniformly recommended for virtually all patients with ET independent of their risk of developing a thrombotic event. These recommendations are somewhat surprising because they are based on two clinical trials of the effects of low-dose aspirin therapy in PV patients, and such a trial with aspirin has never been performed with a population of ET

TABLE 69.8 Outcome in Patients With Low-Risk Essential Thrombocythemia Followed With Careful Observation or Treated With Antiplatelet Therapy

	Observation (848 Person-Years)		Antiplatelet Therapy (802 Person-Years)		
	Events (n)	Incidence Rate (95% CI)	Events (n)	Incidence Rate (95% CI)	p
Thrombosis (arterial and venous)	15	17.7 (107–29.3)	17	21.2 (13.2–34.1)	.6
Arterial thrombosis	8	9.4 (4.7–18.9)	13	16.2 (9.4–27.9)	.2
Venous thrombosis	7	8.2 (3.9–17.3)	4	4.9 (1.9–13.3)	.4
Bleeding	5	6.0 (2.5–14.5)	10	12.6 (6.8–23.4)	.09

From Alvarez-Larrán A, Cervantes F, Pereira A, et al: Observation versus antiplatelet therapy as primary prophylaxis for thrombosis in low-risk essential thrombocythemia. *Blood* 116:1205, 2010.

patients. An independent analysis of the data from these two trials by the Cochrane Collaboration indicated that the use of low-dose aspirin therapy was associated with a statistically nonsignificant reduction in the risk of fatal thrombotic events and was not associated with an increased risk of bleeding episodes. Furthermore, after a retrospective study of 198 patients with low-risk ET, Alvarez-Larrán et al concluded that antiplatelet therapy did not reduce the incidence of thrombotic events and might increase the bleeding risk if platelet counts are greater than 1000×10^9/L or aspirin is used in patients with a bleeding history (Table 69.8). Most recently, a retrospective study of 433 patients (*CALR* = 271, *JAK2V617F* = 162) with low-risk ET receiving aspirin demonstrated no significant reduction in thrombotic complications, but rather an increase in hemorrhagic complications in the *CALR*-mutated cohort (12.9 vs. 1.8 ×1000 patient-years, $p = .03$. Interestingly, the presence of *JAK2V617F* and cardiovascular risk factors were associated with higher risk of thrombosis, which was reduced with administration of aspirin, and time to cytoreductive therapy was shorter in the *CALR*-mutated cohort compared with the *JAK2V617F* cohort of ET patients.

Aspirin should be used with caution in patients with peptic ulcer disease. Such patients who require aspirin benefit from the concurrent use of a proton pump inhibitor such as omeprazole rather than switching them to clopidogrel. This more critical evaluation of the evidence supporting the indiscriminate use of aspirin therapy in ET patients requires serious reconsideration of this practice. In patients who absolutely require aspirin therapy, one should avoid the simultaneous administration of aspirin with a nonsteroidal antiinflammatory drug (NSAID) such as ibuprofen or naproxen, because such NSAIDs are known to compete with aspirin for a common binding site on COX-1 that prevents aspirin from gaining access to and acetylating its target serine. Low-dose aspirin therapy must be restricted to patients with platelet counts of less than 1500×10^9/L and not be used in patients receiving anagrelide therapy unless they have experienced an arterial thrombotic event. The diagnosis of acquired von Willebrand syndrome should be excluded before aspirin use and considered a contraindication to the use of aspirin. Whether all patients with low-risk ET should be uniformly treated with aspirin remains speculative because prospective randomized clinical trials including appropriate numbers of patients so as to assure the resolution of this dilemma have not been completed to date.

A continuing clinical controversy revolves around the question of whether any treatment is indicated in patients with ET in whom the platelet count elevation is initially detected fortuitously and who remain largely asymptomatic. In a retrospective study of 99 consecutive low-risk ET patients (age <60 years) who presented with extreme thrombocytosis (platelet count >1000×10^9/L) but without a previous history of thrombohemorrhagic complications, the incidence of major thrombosis and hemorrhagic events was shown to be similar during follow-up to those who were treated with prophylactic cytoreductive therapy and those who did not receive such therapy. If the clinician feels compelled to use some therapeutic intervention in young, asymptomatic patients, low-dose aspirin (81 mg/day) appears to be effective in the treatment of microvascular complications, and its use is associated with limited toxicity. Still, it seems reasonable to withhold therapy in younger, asymptomatic patients until the

development of a clinically significant thrombotic or hemorrhagic event. Patients older than 60 years of age with other significant risk factors for cardiovascular complications are probably best served by immediate institution of therapy.

The management of pregnant patients with ET remains problematic. The major goal of any therapeutic intervention in pregnant patients with ET should be the prevention of the vasoocclusive events that lead to placental infarction; intrauterine fetal growth retardation; and, in some cases, fetal death. Patients with *JAK2V617F*-positive ET are at a higher risk of developing such complications. In one large series, there was no significant relationship between the fetal outcome and the degree of maternal thrombocytosis or the presence of disease complications. In this series, there were no instances of excessive bleeding or other related complications during delivery. This group did not recommend the use of therapeutic platelet pheresis and, in fact, claimed that specific therapy (aspirin, heparin, or platelet pheresis) did not alter the clinical course. Low-dose aspirin (81 mg/day), because of its profound effect on events involving the microcirculation such as erythromelalgia and transient ischemic events, has been used with increasing frequency in pregnant patients during the first and second trimesters. Low-dose aspirin therapy is safe in pregnant women. It is recommended that aspirin be discontinued at least 1 week before delivery to avoid bleeding complications such as an epidural hematoma during delivery or during the postpartum period. Because of the high risk of bleeding in patients with platelet counts greater than 1000×10^9/L with acquired von Willebrand syndrome, aspirin therapy is contraindicated. There is limited experience reported in the literature with aspirin therapy alone, and although the results are promising, the sample size is too small to confirm a beneficial effect. The observed true birth rate, however, was 75% in those receiving aspirin compared with 43% in the group in the literature who received no therapy. Aspirin therapy has, however, recently been found to be ineffective in preventing complications in *JAK2V617F*-positive pregnant ET patients. Chemotherapeutic drugs should be avoided during the period of conception and especially during the first trimester. Both hydroxyurea and busulfan are known teratogens in animal models. In addition, busulfan and hydroxyurea reduce fertility in men. Because the greatest risk of thrombosis is postpartum, thrombosis prophylaxis should be initiated in the form of low-molecular–weight heparin and low-dose aspirin after delivery, unless the patient is hemorrhaging for approximately 8 weeks. These measures should be continued for 6 weeks. Mothers receiving IFN, anagrelide, or hydroxyurea should refrain from breastfeeding.

IFN-α therapy is not known to be leukemogenic or teratogenic, and because it does not cross the placenta, its use may be considered during pregnancy. The manufacturers of IFN-α still advise that IFN-α not be used during pregnancy because adverse effects on the fetus cannot be ruled out. The effect of IFN-α on male fertility remains uncertain. Anagrelide therapy should be avoided in pregnant patients because of its potential to lead to fetal thrombocytopenia.

Hormone-replacement therapy including oral contraceptives and estrogen-replacement hormone therapy remains controversial in patients with ET. Each of these agents in the normal population is associated with an increased incidence of arterial and venous thrombosis. Intuitively, it would seem wise to avoid such agents in patients with ET who are already at an increased risk of developing thrombosis. Gangat et al retrospectively reviewed the consequences of such hormonal interventions in 305 women. Oral contraceptive therapy was associated with a high incidence of venous thrombosis occurring within the abdominal cavity, but estrogen-replacement hormone therapy in menopausal women did not appear to be associated with an increased incidence of thrombosis. This observation is surprising and might be a consequence of the limited numbers of patients included within this study.

If a patient with ET develops a thrombotic episode, anticoagulation with low-molecular–weight heparin and then transition to an oral anticoagulant is recommended. The thrombotic episode places a patient into a high-risk group in which myelosuppressive therapy is clearly indicated. Whether patients should have life-long anticoagulation or should receive only 6–12 months of anticoagulation after they are in a complete hematologic remission has not been investigated in a systematic fashion. Because the data necessary to make this decision are not available, this decision can only be made at the discretion of the treating physician. Antiplatelet therapy has been shown to reduce the risks of deep venous thrombosis and pulmonary embolism in a variety of high-risk groups. In patients who have a new thrombosis while they are in complete hematologic remission and are optimally anticoagulated, some consideration should be given to adding low-dose aspirin if the risk of hemorrhage is not excessive.

Lastly, consensus response criteria have been updated recently to allow for more uniform reporting of therapeutic response within clinical trials (Table 69.9). Standardized response categories were created by a working group formed by the ELN and IWG-MRT in 2013 in an attempt to incorporate symptom response with clinical, hematologic, and histologic response criteria in order to ultimately enhance the evaluation of novel therapies tested in clinical trials.[3] It is important to note that these response criteria have not been validated in a prospective fashion and their utility in the management of an individual patient with ET in the clinic is uncertain.

FUTURE DIRECTIONS

ET is a hematologic malignancy with its own distinct clinical manifestations and associated complications. Better means of identifying patients at risk for developing fatal thrombotic or hemorrhagic complications are necessary to provide the basis with which to develop the optimal care of such patients. The ability to reduce the incidence of thrombohemorrhagic episodes with cytoreductive therapy in high-risk patients is well established.

Multiinstitutional studies comparing the efficacy of such promising agents as IFN-α or pegylated IFN for the treatment of high-risk patients compared with hydroxyurea are currently being pursued and initial results are anticipated in 2017. The use of low-dose aspirin therapy to reduce the number of episodes of erythromelalgia and transient ischemic attacks is widely practiced, but whether aspirin therapy should be indiscriminately used remains a subject of dispute that will only be resolved with the completion of appropriately powered clinical trials. Another pressing question that requires resolution is the degree of reduction of platelet or leukocyte numbers required for optimal management of ET patients.

The report of 18 patients with high-risk, treatment-refractory ET treated with imetelstat, a 13-mer oligonucleotide competitive inhibitor of telomerase, was recently published indicating a novel MPN therapeutic approach. The rationale for this prospective clinical trial was based on laboratory findings of selective inhibition of malignant megakaryopoiesis compared with megakaryocytes isolated from normal controls after in vitro exposure to imetelstat. In this open label, phase II study, the complete hematologic remission was 89% and reductions in driver mutation allele burden (JAK2, MPL, CALR) were observed (median reduction of JAK2V617F of 59% at 12 months and reductions in CALR and MPL allele burden of 15–60%. Grade 3 neutropenia was seen in 22% of treated patients, and low-grade reversible transaminitis was seen in the majority of patients. The role of this infusional agent administered every 3 weeks in the

treatment of ET is yet to be determined and currently MF is the focus of ongoing clinical investigation.

Finally, the discovery of the JAK2V617F, MPL, and CALR mutations have already had a major impact on disease classification during routine clinical practice. Diagnostic strategies have now incorporated screening for these driver mutations. This new understanding of the molecular pathogenesis of MPN has led to the development of novel targeted therapies. The use of specific JAK2 inhibitors for ET patients should be carefully studied in well-controlled clinical trials in which significant endpoints such as incidence of thrombosis, hemorrhage, and transformation to MF and acute leukemia are incorporated. This is critical because the degree of reduction of platelet numbers has not served as a suitable biomarker for the development of these complications (see box on Personal Approach to Therapy of Essential Thrombocythemia).

TABLE 69.9   Response Criteria for Essential Thrombocythemia

	Criteria
Complete Remission	
A	Durable[a] resolution of disease-related signs including palpable hepatosplenomegaly, large symptoms improvement,[b] AND
B	Durable[a] peripheral blood count remission, defined as: platelet count ≤400 ×10⁹/L, WBC count <10 × 10⁹/L, absence of leukoerythroblastosis, AND
C	Without signs of progressive disease, and absence of any hemorrhagic or thrombotic events, AND
D	Bone marrow histological remission defined as disappearance of megakaryocyte hyperplasia and absence of >grade 1 reticulin fibrosis.
Partial Remission	
A	Durable[a] resolution of disease-related signs including palpable hepatosplenomegaly, and large symptoms improvement, AND
B	Durable[a] peripheral blood count remission, defined as: platelet count ≤400 × 10⁹/L, WBC count <10 × 10⁹/L, absence of leukoerythroblastosis, AND
C	Without signs of progressive disease, and absence of any hemorrhagic or thrombotic events, AND
D	Without bone marrow histological remission, defined as the persistence of megakaryocyte hyperplasia
No response	Any response that does not satisfy partial remission
Progressive disease	Transformation into PV, post-ET myelofibrosis, myelodysplastic syndrome or acute leukemia[c]

Molecular response is not required for assignment as complete response or partial response. Molecular response evaluation requires analysis in peripheral blood granulocytes. Complete response is defined as eradication of a preexisting abnormality. Partial response applies only to patients with at least 20% mutant allele burden at baseline. Partial response is defined as ≥50% decrease in allele burden.
[a]Lasting at least 12 weeks.
[b]Large symptom improvement (≥10-point decrease) in MPN-SAF TSS.[10]
[c]For the diagnosis of PV see World Health Organization criteria (WHO)[13]; for the diagnosis of post-ET myelofibrosis, see the IWG-MRT criteria[12]; for the diagnosis of myelodysplastic syndrome and acute leukemia, see WHO criteria.[13]
ET, Essential thrombocythemia; PV, polycythemia vera; WBC, white blood cell.
From Barosi G, Mesa R, Finazzi G, et al: Response criteria for polycythemia vera and essential thrombocythemia: an ELN and IWG-MRT consensus project. Blood 121:4778, 2013.

Personal Approach to Therapy of Essential Thrombocythemia

The optimal therapy for all patients with essential thrombocythemia (ET) remains uncertain. Therapy is geared toward interventions to reduce the potential for developing thrombotic episodes. Patients with the greatest risk of developing a thrombus have a number of characteristics, including age 60 years or older, history of a thrombotic event, leukocytosis (platelet count ≥11,000 × 10^9/L), and cardiovascular risk factors (hypertension, hypercholesterolemia, diabetes mellitus, obesity). Patients with ET or a prefibrotic form of MF can frequently present with elevated platelet counts and are treated in a similar fashion by us. No known therapy is commercially available that is capable of reversing the bone marrow (BM) fibrosis in such patients or delaying or eliminating evolution to myelofibrosis (MF). Certain concepts, however, apply to all patients. All patients with ET should stop smoking to minimize the risk factors associated with atherosclerotic disease. Indiscriminant use of high doses of nonsteroidal antiinflammatory drugs should be avoided because this practice can lead to an increased risk of hemorrhage. Use of such agents is particularly frequent in elderly patients in whom ET is common. In patients with a life-threatening thrombotic or hemorrhagic episode, plateletpheresis should be initiated in addition to starting them on hydroxyurea therapy.

In high-risk patients, cytoreductive therapy has been shown to lessen the chance of developing additional thrombotic events with the reduction of extreme thrombocytosis to platelet counts below 600,000 × 10^9/L. High-risk patients include patients older than 60 years of age and patients with a history of a previous thrombotic episode, including erythromelalgia, transient ischemic attacks, or large-vessel thrombosis. Even though this treatment philosophy has been considered common practice, the recommendation to treat patients older than the age of 60 years who have not experienced a thrombotic episode with cytoreductive therapy is not based on robust data from multiple randomized trials. Asymptomatic high-risk patients without cardiovascular risk factors may not necessarily benefit from this treatment, and the decision on how to treat them should be based on individual assessment.

At present, no therapy is indicated in asymptomatic patients younger than 60 years of age. If a patient has a platelet count greater than or equal to 1500 × 10^9/L and acquired von Willebrand syndrome with bleeding symptoms, platelet-reduction therapy is indicated to avoid the high risk of hemorrhage. In totally asymptomatic patients with platelet counts greater than 1500 × 10^9/L, we frequently observe the patients and do not feel compelled to treat them. Patients with acquired von Willebrand syndrome should clearly avoid the use of aspirin.

In patients requiring platelet reduction therapy, the choice among the use of anagrelide, interferon (IFN)-α, pegylated IFN, or hydroxyurea therapy is based on patient age, ease of administration, and drug-related toxicity. Randomized trials comparing these treatments in high-risk patients are ongoing. Until the results are available, we use the following strategy. In patients older than 50 years, hydroxyurea therapy is the treatment of choice, but in younger patients, we prefer to initiate therapy with IFN-α. IFN therapy should be avoided in patients with a history of depression, autoimmune disorders, or retinitis. If the patient cannot tolerate IFN-α or it is not available, we feel comfortable treating symptomatic patients younger than 50 years of age with anagrelide or hydroxyurea. Although we remain concerned about the leukemogenic potential of hydroxyurea, the risk appears to be low if not associated with the prior use of an alkylating agent. The development of malleolar ulcers is a frequent complication of hydroxyurea treatment and is a signal for the elimination of hydroxyurea as a therapeutic agent for that particular patient.

Patients who initially receive hydroxyurea and no longer respond to this agent or experience toxicity and require another agent should not receive an alkylating agent. This sequence of administration is associated with an extremely high risk of leukemic transformation. Patients who have had a trial of hydroxyurea and require further treatment should receive either anagrelide, IFN-α, or pegylated IFN. Doses of each of these agents required for disease control will, of course, be dependent on the target platelet level that one hopes to achieve. Strict control to a platelet count of lower than 600 × 10^9/L does not appear to be necessary. In these patients, the addition of low-dose aspirin (81 mg/day) should be considered; it is less clear to us if patients who achieve better platelet control with cytoreductive therapy should also be so treated. However, in studies from Europe addressing this question in polycythemia vera, the approach of combining aspirin with cytoreduction therapy appears to minimize thrombotic complications. The use of anagrelide and aspirin in combination should be avoided because of the high risk of a hemorrhage. In patients with thrombotic episodes, especially episodes involving the microcirculation or large vessels, we administer low-dose aspirin (81 mg/day). This dose of aspirin does increase the number of bleeding episodes to a modest degree but is effective in the treatment of thrombotic events. This low-dose aspirin therapy is given in addition to an agent, which reduces platelet numbers.

Hydroxyurea can be started at a dose of 1 g/day and then adjusted to achieve the target platelet count (≤600 × 10^9/L) without developing leukopenia. Anagrelide is initiated at 0.5 mg twice daily and increased by 0.5 mg/day every 5–7 days if platelet counts do not begin to drop. The usual dose to achieve platelet number control is 2.0–2.5 mg/day. Alternatively, combination therapy with anagrelide and hydroxyurea may be considered. Some patients do not tolerate either hydroxyurea or anagrelide. In this patient group, IFN-α therapy is initiated at 3 million units three times per week subcutaneously, or consideration to therapy with a pegylated form of interferon (peg-IFNα-2a) should be given. Busulfan at 4 mg/day for 2-week courses every time the platelet count rises above the normal range is another therapeutic option. Busulfan therapy is typically reserved for patients older than 70 years.

Complications even in young, otherwise healthy patients with platelet counts greater than 2000 × 10^9/L are unusual. However, these marked elevations of platelet numbers can be anxiety-provoking situations for the patient and the clinician.

In certain situations, in young, low-risk patients, treatment should be instituted. Surgery can increase the risk of thrombosis, and the use of antiinflammatory agents can increase the risk of bleeding postoperatively. Under these circumstances, the platelet count should be lowered to the normal range. In pregnant patients with ET, low-dose aspirin therapy is the first treatment option. If the patient develops symptoms as a result of thrombosis, platelet reduction therapy is necessary, and IFN-α therapy is the treatment of choice.

In a patient with ET and a serious acute hemorrhagic event, the site of bleeding should be determined immediately, and any antiplatelet-aggregating agents should be stopped. Although the platelet count may be high, these platelets should be considered to be qualitatively abnormal, leading to defective hemostasis. The patient may have acquired von Willebrand syndrome. In patients with acquired von Willebrand syndrome, desmopressin (DDAVP) or factor VIII concentrates containing von Willebrand factor can be used immediately at the same time chemotherapy is being administered. If acquired von Willebrand syndrome is not present, the transfusion of normal platelets is suggested. In patients with persistent hemorrhage, immediate reduction of the platelet count can be achieved by platelet pheresis. If this approach fails, some consideration to the use of activated factor VIIa should be given. Hydroxyurea at 2–4 g/day for 3–5 days should be administered immediately and then reduced to 1 g/day. All patients receiving hydroxyurea should be monitored for the onset of granulocytopenia or thrombocytopenia. Reduction of platelet counts is usually observed within 3–5 days of hydroxyurea treatment.

In contrast, patients with acute arterial thrombosis require immediate institution of platelet antiaggregating agents. Aspirin at a dose of 81 mg/day is suggested. Patients with erythromelalgia or transient ischemic attacks will have a rapid cessation of symptoms after the use of low-dose aspirin. In a patient with a life-threatening arterial thrombosis, the platelet count should be lowered with either a combination of apheresis and hydroxyurea or with hydroxyurea alone, depending on the severity of the event. If the arterial thrombosis involves the microcirculation and is not life threatening (transient ischemic attacks or erythromelalgia), immediate low-dose aspirin therapy is indicated, and platelet-reduction therapy (hydroxyurea, anagrelide, or IFN-α) can be initiated using a standard dose and schedule.

REFERENCES

1. Barbui T, Finazzi G, Carobbio A, et al: Development and validation of an International Prognostic Score of thrombosis in World Health Organization-essential thrombocythemia (IPSET-thrombosis). *Blood* 120(26):5128–5133, 2012.

2. Barbui T, Vannucchi AM, Buxhofer-Ausch V: Practice-relevant revision of IPSET-thrombosis based on 1019 patients with WHO-defined essential thrombocythemia. *Blood Cancer J.* 5:e369, 2015.

3. Barosi G, Mesa R, Finazzi G, et al: Revised response criteria for polycythemia vera and essential thrombocythemia: an ELN and IWG-MRT consensus project. *Blood* 121(23):4778–4781, 2013.

4. Carobbio A, Thiele J, Passamonti F, et al: Risk factors for arterial and venous thrombosis in WHO-defined essential thrombocythemia: an international study of 891 patients. *Blood* 117:5857, 2011.

5. Cortelazzo S, Finazzi G, Ruggeri M, et al: Hydroxyurea for patients with essential thrombocythemia and a high risk of thrombosis. *N Engl J Med* 332:1132, 1995.

6. Gisslinger H, Gotic M, Holowiecki J, et al: Anagrelide compared with hydroxyurea in WHO-classified essential thrombocythemia: the ANAHYDRET Study, a randomized controlled trial. *Blood* 121(10):1720–1728, 2013.

7. Harrison CN, Campbell PJ, Buck G, et al: United Kingdom Medical Research Council Primary Thrombocythemia 1 Study. Hydroxyurea compared with anagrelide in high-risk essential thrombocythemia. *N Engl J Med* 353:33, 2005.

8. Karow A, Nienhold R, Lundberg P, et al: Mutational profile of childhood myeloproliferative neoplasms. *Leukemia* 29(12):2407–2409, 2015.

9. Passamonti F, Thiele J, Girodon F, et al: A prognostic model to predict survival in 867 World Health Organization-defined essential thrombocythemia at diagnosis: a study by the International Working Group on Myelofibrosis Research and Treatment. *Blood* 120(6):1197–1201, 2012.

10. Quintás-Cardama A, Kantarjian H, Manshouri T, et al: Pegylated interferon alfa-2a yields high rates of hematologic and molecular response in patients with advanced essential thrombocythemia and polycythemia vera. *J Clin Oncol* 27:5418, 2009.

11. Rumi E, Pietra D, Ferretti V, et al: JAK2 or CALR mutation status defines subtypes of essential thrombocythemia with substantially different clinical course and outcomes. *Blood* 123(10):1544–1551, 2014.

12. Srour SA, Devesa SS, Morton LM, et al: Incidence and patient survival of myeloproliferative neoplasms and myelodysplastic/myeloproliferative neoplasms in the United States, 2001-12. *Br J Haematol* 2016. doi: 10.1111/bjh.14061.

13. Tapper W, Jones AV, Kralovics R, et al: Genetic variation at MECOM, TERT, JAK2 and HBS1L-MYB predisposes to myeloproliferative neoplasms. *Nat Commun* 6:6691, 2015. doi: 10.1038/ncomms7691.

14. Thiele J, Kvasnicka HM, Müllauer L, et al: Essential thrombocythemia versus early primary myelofibrosis: a multicenter study to validate the WHO classification. *Blood* 117:5710–5718, 2011.

John Mascarenhas, Vesna Najfeld, Marina Kremyanskaya, Alla Keyzner, Mohamed E. Salama, and Ronald Hoffman

Primary myelofibrosis (PMF) is a chronic, malignant hematologic disorder characterized by splenomegaly, cytopenias, systemic symptoms, leukoerythroblastosis, teardrop poikilocytosis (i.e., dacryocytes), ineffective hematopoiesis associated with megakaryocytic hyperplasia and dysplastic megakaryocytopoiesis, and the acquisition of a variety of driver mutations (*JAK2V617F*, calreticulin exon 9 [*CALR*], and the thrombopoietin receptor, *MPL515L/K*) along with varying degrees of bone marrow (BM) fibrosis, increased BM microvessel density, and extramedullary hematopoiesis (EMH). The dysplastic megakaryocytes and clonal populations of myeloid cells elaborate cytokines that are responsible for the development of BM fibrosis. Fibrosis of the BM is not unique to PMF and may accompany many other disorders (Table 70.1). The terms *postpolycythemia vera (PV) myelofibrosis (post-PV MF)* and *postessential thrombocythemia (ET) myelofibrosis (post-ET MF)* have been developed to classify MF that is preceded by a history of PV or ET. In PMF, the BM fibrosis occurs in response to the progeny of a clonal proliferation of hematopoietic stem cells (HSCs). In 1951, Dameshek included PMF among a group of related disorders that he termed *myeloproliferative disorders* (MPDs). This hypothesis was largely based on clinical observations of patients with PV, chronic myeloid leukemia (CML), and ET who developed BM fibrosis and a clinical picture resembling PMF. Dameshek also noticed that each of these MPDs frequently evolve over time, changing their clinical phenotype, and frequently terminate in a leukemic phase. In 2008, the World Health Organization (WHO) modified the terminology of MPDs to myeloproliferative neoplasms (MPNs) to correctly reflect their malignant nature.[1]

EPIDEMIOLOGY

Few epidemiologic studies are available to estimate the incidence of PMF. Previously published reports indicate an annual incidence rate in European, Australian, and North American localities ranging from 0.5 to 1.3 cases per 100,000 persons. The annual incidence rate of PMF in Olmstead County (MN, USA) was reported to be 1.33 cases per 100,000 persons, and in southeast England (UK), the annual incidence has been reported to be 0.37 per 100,000 persons. In Japan, PMF is considered a rare disorder. The incidence of MF among survivors who were 10,000 m or less from the hypocenter of the atomic bomb explosion at Hiroshima, however, was 18 times the incidence reported from the remainder of Japan. These patients became symptomatic an average of 6 years after the bomb blast. Such data indicate a strong link between excessive radiation exposure and development of PMF, which is further substantiated by the high incidence of MF in patients who have received the contrast material Thorotrast (which contains ^{232}Th, a radioactive element with a half-life of 1.41×10^{10} years). Thorotrast is taken up and retained indefinitely by cells of the reticuloendothelial system, which results in continuous irradiation of the liver, spleen, lymph nodes, and BM. Chronic exposure to several industrial solvents, including benzene and toluene, has also been associated with the development of PMF. Unlike PV, where clusters of patients have been identified in Eastern Pennsylvania, raising the concern for possible environmental effects of waste-coal and Superfund sites, there are no definitive epidemiologic studies supporting environmental exposures in PMF. PMF has been reported as a complication of chronic benzene poisoning since

the chemical was first used in the leather and shoe industries during the 1930s and 1940s. The average age at diagnosis of PMF is approximately 65 years, and most patients are diagnosed between 50 and 69 years of age. In several series, men have been affected more frequently than women, but others have failed to confirm this male predominance. Rarely, PMF has been reported in the pediatric age group. Evidence of genetic transmission exists: a higher incidence has been reported in Ashkenazi Jews than in Arabs, who both live in Northern Israel, and families where multiple members who suffer from a number of the MPNs including PMF have been identified.

PMF is a clonal hematologic malignancy originating in primitive hematopoietic cells capable of producing lymphoid and myeloid cells, while the BM fibrosis represents a secondary reaction of BM stromal cells. The ability of primitive human hematopoietic cells to engraft sublethally irradiated immunodeficient mice is the standard surrogate *in vivo* assay for human HSCs. PMF CD34$^+$ cells are capable of engrafting non-obese non-diabetic/severe combined immune deficient (NOD/SCID) mice and generating myeloid and B cells that are clonal, *JAK2V617F* positive, and carry a patient-specific marker chromosomal abnormality.[2] The differentiation program of PMF CD34$^+$ cells after transplant into NOD/SCID mice was also remarkably different from that of normal CD34$^+$ cells, producing greater numbers of CD34$^+$, CD33$^+$, and CD41$^+$ cells but fewer CD19$^+$ cells. This predisposition to produce greater numbers of megakaryocytes has been further explored by incubating PMF, PV, and CD34$^+$ cells in vitro in the presence of stem cell factor and thrombopoietin. PMF CD34$^+$ cells displayed a far greater proliferative capacity and produced greater numbers of megakaryocytes that were characterized by a resistance to undergo apoptosis in vitro caused by overexpression of the antiapoptotic factor B-cell lymphoma-extra large (Bcl-XL). The megakaryocyte hyperplasia in PMF, therefore, could be accounted for by two factors—an increased ability of CD34$^+$ cells to generate megakaryocytes and the accumulation of megakaryocytes caused by Bcl-xL overexpression. Although Bcl-xL overexpression has been linked to *JAK2V617F*, PMF megakaryocyte Bcl-xL overexpression also occurred to a similar degree in megakaryocytes generated from CD34$^+$ cells isolated from individuals with both *JAK2V617F*-positive and -negative disease. The role of megakaryocytes in the development of fibrosis in PMF is further supported by megakaryocytic hyperplasia with dysplastic or necrotic megakaryocytes that characterizes this disorder; by the increased circulating megakaryocytes and megakaryocyte progenitors that are present in PMF; by the association of BM fibrosis and acute megakaryocytic leukemia; and by the presence of MF in gray platelet syndrome, an inherited disorder of platelet α-granules. Ineffective megakaryocytopoiesis in PMF has been hypothesized to lead to the liberation of excessive amounts of such growth factors, leading to BM fibroblast proliferation and collagen synthesis. PMF platelet-derived growth factor (PDGF) and transforming growth factor-β (TGF-β) levels have been found to be 2.0–3.0-fold and 1.5–3.0-fold higher, respectively, in PMF than in normal control participants, but fibroblast growth factor (FGF) levels in PMF were similar to those of control platelets. The roles of PDGF and TGF-β in the biogenesis of PMF probably are not restricted to promoting fibroblastic proliferation, but are also related to the effect of these two growth factors on synthesis, secretion, and degradation of extracellular matrix components. TGF-β enhances fibronectin and collagens types I, III, and IV, as well as chondroitin or dermatan

TABLE 70.1	Conditions Associated With Myelofibrosis

Nonmalignant Conditions

Infections: tuberculosis, histoplasmosis
Renal osteodystrophy
Vitamin D deficiency
Hypoparathyroidism
Hyperparathyroidism
Gray platelet syndrome
Systemic lupus erythematosus
Scleroderma
Radiation exposure
Osteopetrosis
Paget disease
Benzene exposure
Thorotrast exposure
Gaucher disease
Primary autoimmune myelofibrosis

Malignant Disorders

Primary myelofibrosis
Other chronic myeloproliferative disorders: polycythemia vera, chronic
    myeloid leukemia, essential thrombocythemia
Acute myelofibrosis
Acute myeloid leukemia
Acute lymphocytic leukemia
Hairy cell leukemia
Hodgkin lymphoma
Myelodysplasia with myelofibrosis
Multiple myeloma
Systemic mastocytosis
Non-Hodgkin lymphoma
Carcinomas: breast, lung, prostate, stomach

sulphate and proteoglycan gene expression. TGF-β decreases the synthesis of various collagenase-like enzymes that degrade extracellular matrices while at the same time stimulating the synthesis of protease inhibitors such as plasminogen activator inhibitor 1. The net effect of these complex interactions is the accumulation of extracellular matrix, which probably contributes to further progression of fibrosis. Additional growth factors including lipocalin 2 (LCN2), which is elaborated by myelocytes and promyelocytes, have been implicated in the development of progressive fibrosis in PMF. Basic FGF (bFGF) is a potent angiogenic factor and is a mitogen for human BM stromal cells. Elevated platelet, megakaryocyte, and serum bFGF levels have been reported in PMF patients with progressive fibrosis. bFGF may be released or leaked from dysplastic and necrotic PMF megakaryocytes or platelets. These findings suggest that bFGF may also contribute to the progressive fibrosis and pronounced angiogenesis frequently observed in PMF. The mechanism by which the pathologic release of growth factors from megakaryocytes occurs in PMF remains unknown. Investigators have suggested that impaired megakaryocyte emperipolesis might lead to this liberation of fibrogenic cytokines. *Emperipolesis* is defined as the random entry of hematopoietic cells into the cytoplasm of megakaryocytes. Impaired emperipolesis of neutrophils and eosinophils in PMF and resultant liberation of myeloperoxidase-positive granules by the engulfed neutrophils has been reported. The degree of emperipolesis in PMF BM biopsies has been shown to be correlated with the degree of BM fibrosis. Abnormal P-selectin distribution in megakaryocytes has been suggested to account for the selective sequestration of granulocytes by PMF megakaryocytes.[3]

The development of extensive fibrosis of the BM in PMF is frequently preceded by an asymptomatic phase of the disease of variable duration characterized by a hypercellular marrow with megakaryocytic hyperplasia and atypia and minimal fibrosis (prefibrotic phase of MF). Reversal of MF has been observed after allogeneic stem cell transplantation (aSCT) and infrequently seen occasionally after

long-term administration of interferon (IFN). Such findings indicate that the BM fibrosis in PMF is not irreversible and is clearly a secondary consequence of the neoplastic cellular proliferation.

Many of the peripheral blood abnormalities associated with PMF may be attributed to the EMH that is characteristic of this disorder. CD34+ cells in PMF are constitutively mobilized and exit from the BM; because of abnormal trafficking patterns, they are filtered out by the spleen, accumulate progressively, and continue to proliferate. Ultimately, there is an unequal distribution of CD34+ cells, with a twofold greater number being present in the spleen than the BM. The EMH within the spleen is characterized by disturbances of splenic architecture, including an increased presence of megakaryocytes and their progenitor cells. Intravascular hematopoiesis within the sinusoids of the BM is a conspicuous finding in PMF. The characteristic changes of the BM vascular architecture consist of increased quantities of collagen type IV deposits associated with increased BM microvessel density, resulting in increased blood flow. The excessively dilated BM sinusoids in PMF contain prominent intraluminal foci of hematopoiesis. This increase in BM microvessel density in PMF has been confirmed using immunohistochemical methods and has been shown to correlate with increased spleen size and to be an independent risk factor for overall survival (OS). Vessels from patients with PMF are frequently markedly abnormal and appear as localized vascular nests consisting of numerous short vessels that are highly branched and tortuous. The increased BM microvessel density in PMF is probably mediated by megakaryocyte α-granule constituents. A number of angiogenic growth factors, including bFGF and vascular endothelial growth factor (VEGF), have been implicated as causative factors of the increased BM microvessel density observed in the BMs of PMF patients. Elevated serum VEGF levels have been reported in PMF, and increased expression of bFGF has been reported in PMF megakaryocytes and platelets. Osteosclerosis is a prominent clinical feature of many patients, with PMF frequently manifesting itself as bone pain. The osteosclerosis is a consequence of cytokines produced by the malignant BM cells or stroma conditioned and activated by an interaction with PMF cells. PMF-associated osteosclerosis can be reversed after aSCT with the establishment of normal hematopoiesis. Studies of both PMF patients and animal models of PMF indicate that both TGF-β and stromal cell-derived osteoprotegerin, a member of the TNF receptor family, play pivotal roles in the development of osteosclerosis. Osteoprotegerin is a decoy receptor for the receptor activator of the nuclear factor kappa-B ligand (RANKL). RANKL is a transmembrane protein expressed on the cell surface of osteoblasts that can be cleaved into a soluble form by proteases. Both soluble and membrane-bound RANKL attach to RANK, a cell receptor expressed by osteoclast precursors to stimulate osteoclastogenesis. RANKL and osteoprotegerin are positive and negative regulators of osteoclast differentiation, respectively. Osteoprotegerin can reduce the production of osteoclasts by inhibiting the differentiation of osteoclast progenitor cells into mature osteoclasts, leading to the development of osteosclerosis. In patients with PMF, it remains unknown if the degree of osteosclerosis is corrected with increased levels of osteoprotegerin.

Elevated thrombopoietin levels have been observed in patients with PMF. This unanticipated elevation of plasma thrombopoietin levels is not caused by enhanced production of thrombopoietin messenger RNA (mRNA) by BM fibroblasts or BM cells, but is likely caused by the reduced expression of the thrombopoietin receptor by the platelets and megakaryocytes of PMF patients, leading to decreased clearance of thrombopoietin. In ET and PMF, platelets and megakaryocytes are characterized by lower MPL protein levels and most of the receptors are immature. Endo-H–sensitive activated *JAK2* has been shown to strongly promote cell surface localization and enhance protein levels of MPL. This effect has been shown to be caused by stabilization of the mature endoglycosidase H-resistant form of the receptor. The reduced expression of MPL has also been linked to *JAK2V617F*, leading to receptor ubiquitinylation and degradation by proteasomal and lysosomal pathways. Platelet MPL levels can be restored by treatment with proteasome inhibitors or *JAK2* inhibitors. By contrast, the persistence of MPL expression by progenitor or stem cells has been linked to the development of myeloproliferation. These observations support a model where a decrease in MPL mass in platelets and megakaryocytes results in increased thrombopoietin levels, which acts on the primitive stems cells contributing to the development of myeloproliferation

Vannucchi and colleagues studied mutant mice with reduced expression of the transcription factor GATA1 to further define the role of megakaryocytes and the development of BM fibrosis. Mutations in the GATA1 functional pathway in human PMF have not been described. However, at the protein level, a large number of the megakaryocytes in the BM of PMF patients are GATA1 negative, suggesting that whatever the genetic defect leading to PMF is, it involves the pathway that affects the posttranscriptional or posttranslational regulation of GATA1 in megakaryocytes

Megakaryocytes are not the only cells capable of releasing cytokines that promote BM fibrosis. Levels of macrophage colony-stimulating factor, a cytokine that regulates macrophage development and proliferation, are elevated in the serum of PMF patients. Monocytes and macrophages from patients with PMF can produce greater quantities of TGF-β and interleukin-1 (IL-1) than those from normal control participants. IL-1 and TGF-β are fibroblast mitogens that induce extracellular matrix protein production. Monocyte adhesion to extracellular matrix proteins has been shown to lead to the overproduction of IL-1 and TGF-β by PMF monocytes. Monocyte adhesion through the adhesion molecule, CD44, appears to be involved in the induction of fibrogenic cytokines by mediating the interaction between monocytes and accumulated extracellular matrix protein deposits. The proinflammatory transcriptional factor nuclear factor kappa-B (NFκB) plays a pivotal role in the elaboration of IL-1 and TGF-β in the activation of NFκB monocytes and that of PMF patients. These investigators suggest that NFκB stimulates TGF-β production by influencing intracellular IL-1 levels, and may serve as another potential therapeutic target for the treatment of PMF. Abnormal cytokine expression in PMF is thought to represent an inflammatory response to the disease phenotype that contributes not only to the development of BM fibrosis, osteosclerosis, and increased BM microvessel density, but also PMF-associated constitutional symptoms including weight loss, anorexia, pruritus, bone pain, and night sweats. Elevated levels of IL-8 and IL-2R have been closely correlated with the presence of constitutional symptoms, the requirement for red blood cell (RBC) transfusions, and leukocytosis, as well as inferior OS and leukemia-free survival. These observations raise the possibility that mutational events leading to the malignant transformation of hematopoietic cells in PMF may also lead to activation of transcriptional programs that promote hematopoietic cell survival and disease progression. The elevation of a variety of cytokines may therefore not only be responsible for the numerous epiphenomena that occur as a consequence of the presence of these malignant cells, but also act on the malignant clone affecting the proliferation and differentiation in differing microenvironments characteristic of the BM and various extramedullary sites, including the spleen. Ultimately, this may increase the risk of disease progression or leukemic transformation.

When PMF mononuclear cells are cloned in semisolid media, erythroid and megakaryocyte colony formation occurs in the absence of added exogenous cytokines, a finding common to other MPNs. These findings suggest that possible genetic mutations activating several intracellular signaling pathways responsible for normal hematopoiesis might account for this autonomous in vitro hematopoiesis. In addition to a population of autonomous proliferating megakaryocyte progenitor cells, a second and more common population remains dependent on the addition of exogenous growth factors. The search for the genetic mutations that accounted for the autonomous hematopoiesis that characterizes each of the MPNs culminated in the discovery of a gain-of-function mutation of an autoinhibitory domain of the JAK family of protein tyrosine kinases, which is involved in cytokine receptor signalling.[4] The *JAK2V617F* mutation leads to ongoing phosphorylation activity, which can then bind to a cytokine receptor and promote signal transducer and activator of transcription (STAT) recruitment. This mutation is the likely cause of

the hypersensitivity to cytokines that characterizes hematopoietic progenitors from each of the MPN. In a mouse BM transplant model, BM cells transduced with *JAK2V617F* results in a clinical phenotype that closely resembles PV, including erythrocytosis, EMH, and BM fibrosis. Although >90% of patients with PV are *JAK2V617F* positive, approximately 50% of PMF patients harbor this mutation. The *JAK2V617F* mutation is homozygous in 13% of patients with PMF but in 30% of patients with PV. Homozygosity has been attributed to homologous recombination. Homozygosity of *JAK2V617F* in PMF patients is associated with a more frequent occurrence of unfavorable cytogenetic abnormalities. There are conflicting data as to whether the clinical course of patients with *JAK2V617F*-positive and *JAK2V617F*-negative PMF differ. Additional somatic mutations have been identified in patients with PMF that likely play a role in the biogenesis of PMF. A mutation in the transmembrane domain of the thrombopoietin receptor (*cMPL*) has been documented in 9% of patients with *JAK2V617F*-negative PMF (*MPL W515L* or *MPL W515K*).[5] *MPL 515L*, *MPL 515K*, and MPL wild-type (WT) alleles can coexist in the same patient. Furthermore, 30% of PMF patients with mutations in *cMPL* also have the *JAK2V617F* mutation. By studying archival material, the burden of *MPL 515L*, *MPK 515K*, and *JAK2V617F* in PMF patients has been shown to remain constant throughout the clinical course of patients with PMF. In a murine BM transplant assay, expression of *MPL W515L* but not WT *MPL* resulted in a rapidly progressive, fully penetrable, lethal MPN (18 days) characterized by marked thrombocytosis, leukocytosis, splenomegaly, hepatomegaly, BM megakaryocytic hyperplasia, and BM fibrosis but not erythrocytosis. These data have suggested that the MPL mutation favors the development of thrombocytosis but the *JAK2V617F* mutation favors the development of erythrocytosis. PMF patients with *MPL 515L/K* PMF compared with *MPL* WT PMF are older, present with more severe anemia, and are more likely to require transfusional support. The genetic origins of PMF likely represent the culmination of multiple genetic and possibly epigenetic events.

Further insight into the phenotypic heterogeneity of *JAK2V617F*-positive and -negative MPNs has recently been provided. Immunohistochemical analyses of BM have shown that PV is characterized by increased expression of phosphorylated STAT3 and STAT5 protein, but PMF is characterized by reduced expression of STAT3 and STAT5. This expression pattern was independent of *JAK2V617F* status. Such observations suggest that additional or alternative molecular events occur in PMF and PV that might play a role in the development of their distinctive clinical phenotypes.

In 2013, mutations in *CALR* were reported by two separate laboratory groups. *CALR* is located on chromosome 19p13.2 and encodes for a calcium-binding protein with multiple functions including protein folding/chaperoning, cell proliferation and motility, phagocytosis, apoptosis, and calcium homeostasis. CALR can be localized to the endoplasmic reticulum, nucleus, extracellular matrix and membrane. *CALR* exon 9 frameshift mutations result in a mutant calreticulin protein with a novel calcium-binding/endoplasmic reticulum retention motif C-terminus. These insertion/deletion mutations (>50 reported) occurring in exon 9 of *CALR* and are found at a frequency of approximately 25% in ET and PMF patients, and appear to be mutually exclusive with *JAK2* and *MPL* mutations (frequency of approximately 75% of *JAK2/MPL* WT). Type 1 (52-bp deletion) and type 2 (5-bp insertion) mutations constitute 80% of the reported mutations in *JAK2*-negative MPN patients. Retrospective studies implicate the presence of *CALR* mutations in PMF patients with higher platelet counts, lower hemoglobin and leukocyte counts, less risk of thrombosis, and better overall prognosis than patients with *JAK2V617F*. Initial studies also appear to implicate a worse prognosis for type 2 *CALR* mutants compared with type 1. Additionally, studies have now shown that *CALR* mutant MF patients also have upregulated JAK-STAT signaling, and are also responsive to the effects of JAK2 inhibitor treatment.

The exact pathobiologic link between *CALR* mutation and the dysregulated JAK-STAT pathway is the subject of intense investigation. Chachoua and colleagues have recently shown that neither expression of the mutant C-terminus alone nor expression of *CALR* lacking the C-terminus leads to cytokine-independent growth, suggesting that the novel C-terminus is necessary (but not sufficient) for transformation. They found that the oncogenic activity of mutant *CALR* is not encoded within a specific sequence or domain of the mutant C-terminus, but that the positive electrostatic charge of the mutant C-terminus was critical for its transforming capacity. Mutagenizing all 18 lysine/arginine residues (positively charged) within the C-terminus to a neutral glycine residue abrogated *CALR-del52* transformation activity. In contrast, mutagenizing the 18 nonlysine/arginine residues within the C-terminus to glycine did not affect transforming activity, a remarkable finding considering that, in this mutant, 50% of the amino acids have been modified, Using coimmunoprecipitation assays, Elf et al found that mutant *CALR*, but not WT *CALR*, physically interacted with MPL, and that neither the mutant C-terminus alone nor mutant *CALR* lacking the C-terminus can bind to MPL. This suggests that the tertiary structure of mutant *CALR* is required for binding to MPL.

Approximately 10% of PMF patients lack any of the three driver mutations. However, recently Milosevic-Feenstra and coworkers identified noncanonical *MPL* mutations by whole-exon sequencing in eight out of 70 (11.4%) and *JAK2* mutations in five out of 57 (8.8%) patients with triple-negative ET and PMF. All mutations were heterozygous. The mutations in *MPL* and *JAK2* were mutually exclusive. Evidence for clonal disease was lacking in 50% of these triple-negative cases and the presence of germ-line mutations indicated that some of these individuals likely had a hereditary rather than an acquired MPN-like disorder. Based upon these findings, sequencing of all coding exons of *MPL* and *JAK2* during the diagnostic work-up of ET and PMF patients who are triple negative is recommended.

A growing list of additional mutations have been identified in PMF patients over the past several years, providing further insight into the complex molecular pathology of this disease.[6] Many of these mutations impact the epigenome and can coexist in PMF CD34[+] cells. None of the genetic or epigenetic lesions identified thus far are specific to PMF, clearly aid in prognostication, or appear to be disease-initiating events. Table 70.2 lists the molecular lesions that have been characterized in patients with PMF.

Translocation ten-eleven oncogene family member 2 (TET2), located on chromosome 4q24, has been identified in many myeloid malignancies at a frequency of approximately 15%. Acquired somatic

mutations throughout the 11 exons of this gene result in compromised catalytic activity of an α-ketoglutarate-dependent enzyme responsible for oxidation of 5-methylcytosine (5mC) to 5-hydroxymethylcytosine (5hmC) in DNA. Low levels of 5hmC result in a hypermethylation phenotype at CpG sites in various DNA promoter regions. *TET2* mRNA has been found to be highly expressed in Lin[−], Sca-1[+], c-Kit[hi] murine multipotent progenitor cells isolated from the BM and thymus. This expression pattern was maintained in myeloid progenitor cells but low in mature granulocytes. Moreover, in patient samples, when compared with normal samples, low 5hmC levels correlated with a significant decrease in DNA hypermethylation, supporting a role of *TET2* loss of function leading to DNA hypermethylation. It is currently believed that *TET2* mutations result in loss of function and lead to the accumulation of 5mC in DNA, promoting DNA hypermethylation that may inhibit cells from differentiating beyond a HSC-like state. In vitro studies reveal that TET2 deficiency restrains hematopoietic cells from normal differentiation patterns and skews differentiation in favor of the monocyte/macrophage lineage with transgenic animals, with knockout of *TET2* having a phenotype resembling chronic myelomonocytic leukemia. Somatic, recurrent *TET2* mutations have been reported in normal elderly individuals with acquired clonal hematopoiesis. Alterations in *TET2* that include base substitutions, out-of-frame insertions or deletions, and splice site mutations have been shown to occur in 15–20% of PMF patients. Such mutations are more common in older patients. In families with multiple family members having an MPN, all *TET2* mutations were almost universally acquired, and their incidence was similar to that of patients with sporadic PMF. Clonal analysis studies in MPN patient samples failed to define a consistent temporal sequence of acquisition of *TET2* mutations with respect to *JAK2* mutations and can occur late in the progression of MPNs. These two genetic events appear to occur independently. *TET2* mutational status in PMF patients does not appear to provide a new prognostic marker. *TET2* mutations can be found in PMF patients with and without the *JAK2V617F* mutation, and do not influence rate of thrombosis, leukemic transformation, or OS.

Isocitrate dehydrogenase 1 and 2 (*IDH1/2*), located on chromosome 2q33.3 and 15q26.1, respectively, encode NADP[+]-dependent enzymes that catalyze the oxidative decarboxylation of isocitrate to α-ketoglutarate. Mutant IDH forms preferentially transform α-ketoglutarate to 2-hydroxyglutarate and appear to promote tumorigenesis by inducing hypoxia-inducible factor 1α (HIF-1α).

TABLE 70.2 Acquired Genetic Lesions Identified in Patients With Primary Myelofibrosis

Gene	Location	Mutation	Frequency
Janus kinase 2 (*JAK2*)	9p24 exon 14 9p24 exon 12	*JAK2V617F*	65% Infrequent
Calreticulin (*CALR*)	19p13.2 exon 9	Type 1 (52 bp del) and Type 2 (5 bp in)	25%
Ten-eleven translocation 2 (*TET2*)	4q24		17%
Serine/arginine-rich splicing factor 2 (*SRSF2*)	17q25.1		17%
U2 small nuclear RNA auxillary factor 1 (*U2AF1*)	21q22.3		16%
DNA methyltransferase 3 alpha (*DNMT3a*)	2p23		15%
Enhancer of zeste homolog 2 (*EZH2*)	7q36.1		13%
Myeloproliferative leukemia virus (*MPL*)	1p34 exon 10	*MPL W515L/K*	5%-10%
Casitas B-lineage lymphoma (*CBL*)	11q23.3	Exons 8 and 9	6%
Splicing factor 3B unit 1 (*SF3B1*)	2q33.1		6%
Isocitrate dehydrogenase (*IDH1* and *2*)	2q33.3/15q26.1		4%
Lymphocyte specific adapter protein (*LNK*)	12q24		Infrequent
Ikaros family zinc finger 1 (*IKZF1*)	7p12		Infrequent
Additional sex Combs-like 1 (*ASXL1*)	20q11.1		Infrequent

IDH1/2 mutations are found at a frequency of approximately 4% in PMF and can coexist with mutations in *JAK2*, *MPL*, and *TET2*. The specific IDH mutant variants seen in MPNs (*IDH1 R132C*, *IDH1 R132S*, *IDH2 R140Q*) all affect arginine residues. *IDH1/2* mutations are not predictive of survival in PMF but do have prognostic significance in multivariate analysis in blast-phase disease. It is not yet clear if different IDH mutation variants carry different biologic or prognostic consequences in PMF. A significant association between *IDH1/2* mutation and absence of the 46/1 *JAK2* haplotype has been observed, and supports a theory that PMF patients that are nullizygous for the 46/1 haplotype are more susceptible to acquiring additional molecular lesions that contribute to a poor prognosis.

The additional sex combs-like 1 (*ASXL1*) gene is located on chromosome 20q11.1 and is responsible for encoding an enhancer of the trithorax group (trxG) and polycomb repressive complex (PcG). The PcG proteins (repress) and trxG proteins (activate) regulate gene expression of homeotic genes, such as *Hox* genes via histone methylation. *ASXL1* mutations result in loss of PRC2-mediated H3 lysine (H3K27me3) trimethylation. *ASXL* mutations have been identified in various myeloid malignancies and are in highest frequency in myelodysplastic syndrome (MDS) and CMML patients. In a study of 64 MPN cases, *ASXL1* mutations were found in five MPN patients (three with PMF), all of whom were negative for the *JAK2* mutation. *ASXL1* mutations can be found in the MPN HSC, suggesting acquisition early in the pathogenesis of MPNs. *ASXL1* mutations are associated with an adverse outcome and leukemic transformation in PMF patients.

The Casitas B-lineage lymphoma (*CBL*) proto-oncogene is located on chromosome 11q23.3 and is believed to play a role in the maintenance of the hematopoietic pluripotent stem cell pool. CBL has the capacity to downregulate and upregulate tyrosine kinase activity by either serving as an adaptor protein or recruiting downstream targets of the pathway or by activation of E3 ubiquitin protein ligase activity and the subsequent recycling of the receptor through internalization of the receptor/ligand complex or lysosomal-directed destruction. *CBL* mutations were first appreciated in MPNs in the setting of mutational screening of acquired uniparental disomy of chromosome 11q, with a total of 27 CBL variants identified in MPNs. Within a cohort of 579 MPN patients screened, three patients with PMF were identified with CBL mutations at an overall frequency of 6%. The majority of the CBL mutations identified were located in the RING or linker domains, resulting in impaired ubiquitin ligase activity. Additionally, the oncogenic activity of selected CBL mutant variants was tested in vitro by monitoring its ability to confer growth factor independence to the IL-3-dependent cell line 32D and by its ability to enhance the proliferation of transformed cells overexpressing WT *FLT3*.

Ikaros is a Kruppel-like zinc finger transcription factor that has pleiotropic functions important in the development of normal hematopoiesis and is encoded by the Ikaros family zinc finger 1 (*IKZF1*) gene located at 7p.12. Mutations involving *IKZF1* have been identified as a molecular event leading to transformation of chronic-phase MPNs to blast-phase disease, and appears to occur after the acquisition of *JAK2V617F*. The mutational frequency in chronic-phase MPN is very low at 0.2%, in contrast to 21% of blast-phase MPN patients, and is highly associated with del7p. The potential effects of an *IKZF1* mutation was studied in mouse primary progenitor cells by creating *IKZF1* deficiency with small hairpin RNA technology, which was associated with cytokine hypersensitivity and increased p-STAT5 expression.

The enhancer of zeste homolog 2 (*EZH2*) gene located on chromosome 7q36.1 encodes the catalytic subunit of the histone methyltransferase polycomb repressor complex 2 (PRC2), and mutations in this gene have also been described in MPN patients. PRC2 is a multiprotein enzyme complex (EZH2, SUz12, EED, and YY1) responsible for the trimethylation of lysine 27 on histone H3 (H3K27me3). Additionally, PRC2 can recruit other polycomb complexes, DNA methyltransferases (DNMTs), and histone deacetylases to the gene site, resulting in chromatin compaction and additional repressive activity. Upregulation of *EZH2* gene expression has

been documented in MPNs, most frequently in PMF patients, suggesting a potential role of tumor suppressor gene silencing as a mechanism in disease progression. In a study of 614 patients with myeloid malignancies, 42 cases were found to have a total of 49 *EZH2* mutations. Thirty PMF patients were analyzed in this cohort, and 13% were found to have an *EZH2* mutation. Microarray and single-nucleotide polymorphism (SNP) analysis did not show an association with copy number alterations or uniparental disomy. Because of small patient numbers and short follow-up, it has not been possible to gauge the true prognostic significance of mutated *EZH2* in PMF. Retrospective studies using archived MPN BM samples to assess for *EZH2* mutations have also not been shown to have prognostic significance in PMF.

The use of next-generation sequencing of 104 genes from a cohort of 197 MPN patients by Skoda et al has provided insight into the impact of clonal evolution on clinical phenotype. Somatic mutations were observed in 90% of patient samples in which approximately 40% harbored mutations other than *JAK2V617F* and *CALR*. *JAK2V616F* was the most common mutation (69%), followed by *CALR* (15%), *TET2* (12%), *ASXL1* (5%) and *DNMT3A* (5%). The presence of two or more acquired somatic mutations portended a poor outcome and increased risk of leukemic transformation. By contrast, none of the patients with a sole mutation in *JAK2*, *MPL*, or *CALR* evolved to AML. However, the rate of acquisition of new mutations was very low when assayed from serial samples (two mutations detected during a total follow-up of 133 patient-years). The majority of mutations were present at low allelic levels from the time of diagnosis, and in the case of *p53*, rapid evolution to blast phase occurred with loss of the WT allele. Mutations in *p53* were frequently present in a heterozygous state for a prolonged period of time, but the loss of the WT allele either by chromosomal deletion or uniparental disomy was associated with leukemic transformation. These data argue against the concepts of hypermutability and genomic instability in MF. These data also support a complex clonal architecture in MPNs, where some individuals may develop biclonal disease and others develop a linear acquisition pattern. In general, mutations in *TET2* and *DNMT3A* appeared earlier in the disease course, whereas mutations in *ASXL1*, *EZH2*, and *IDH1* were often acquired after *JAK2V617F*. The authors provide a model for clonal evolution of MPNs and influence on disease course and risk of transformation to leukemia (Fig. 70.1).

The number of hematopoietic progenitor cells constitutively mobilized into the blood of PMF patients is dramatically increased. The number of $CD34^+$ cells present in the peripheral blood in PMF is 360 times greater than in normal control participants and 18–30 times higher than in patients with PV or ET. These findings are so striking that some investigators have suggested that the quantitation of $CD34^+$ cells in the peripheral blood might serve as a means of discriminating PMF from other MPNs. A level of 15×10^6 $CD34^+$ cells/L in peripheral blood allows differentiation of PMF from PV and ET. The numbers of circulating $CD34^+$ cells tend to increase as the disease progresses, and there is a close correlation between patients presenting with more than 300×10^6 $CD34^+$ cells/L of peripheral blood and imminent evolution to leukemia. These findings suggest that PMF $CD34^+$ cell trafficking abnormality is caused by the inability of these cells to be retained within the BM or their premature release into the peripheral blood.

PMF is characterized not only by the constitutive mobilization of $CD34^+$ hematopoietic cells, but also endothelial progenitor cells into the peripheral blood. Endothelial progenitor cell mobilization predominates during the prefibrotic phase of PMF, while hematopoietic stem/progenitor cell mobilization occurs characteristically in more clinically advanced phases of the disease. This dysregulation of stem cell trafficking likely ultimately leads to the seeding of extramedullary sites with primitive hematopoietic and endothelial cells, which results in the production of EMH within the liver and spleen, as well as a variety of other organs. Several proteolytic pathways have been documented to play a role in cytokine-mediated stem cell mobilization. Proteases released by activated neutrophils cleave vascular adhesion molecule-1 (VCAM-1) expressed by stromal cells, leading

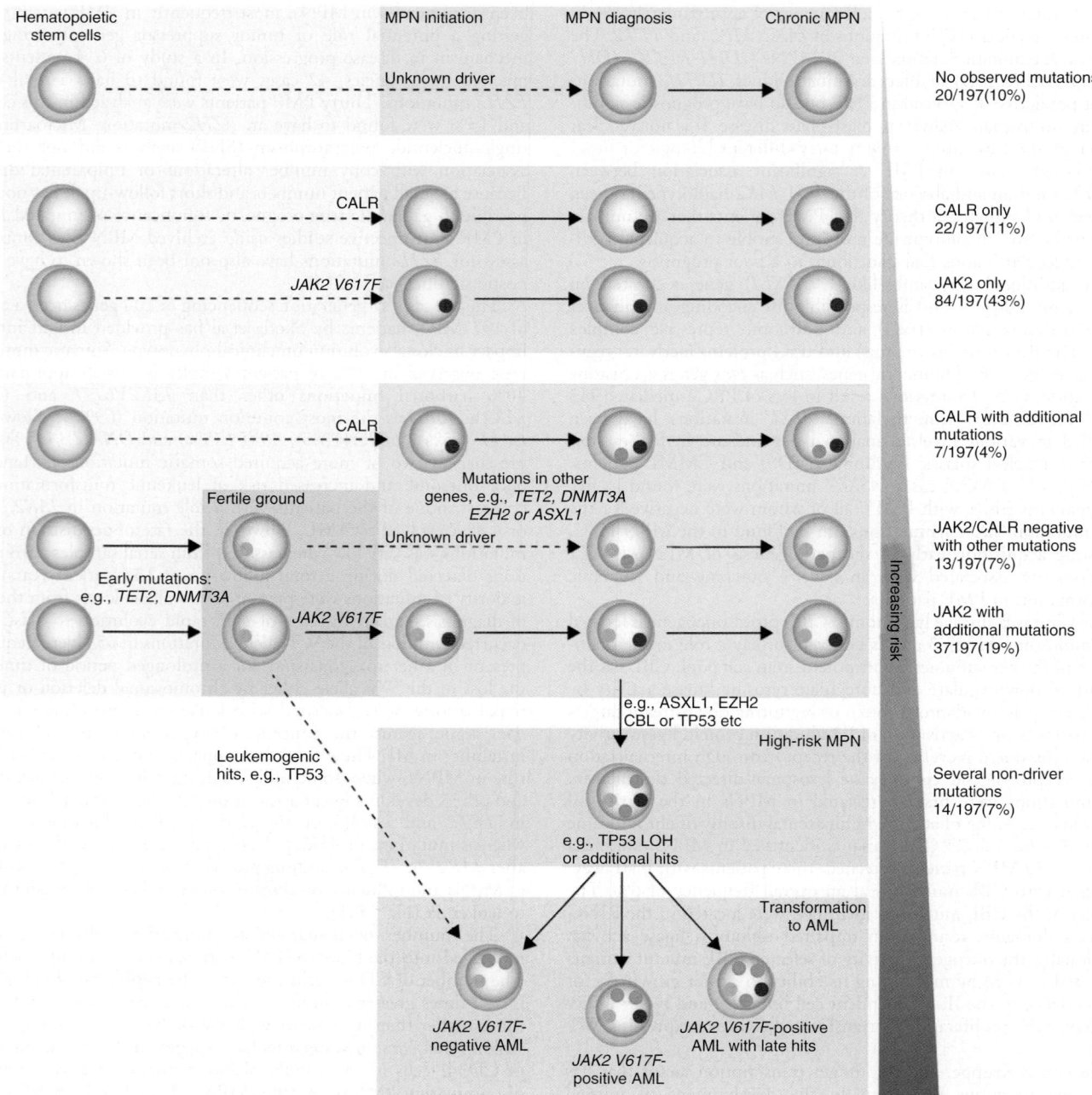

Fig. 70.1 MODEL OF MYELOPROLIFERATIVE DISEASE EVOLUTION AND RISK STRATIFICA-TION IN CORRELATION TO MUTATIONAL EVENTS. In 10% of myeloproliferative (MPN) patients a driver mutation (*JAK2, MPL, CALR*) is not detected. In approximately 50–60% of MPN patients, either *JAK2V617F* or *CALR* are found, and this group collectively has a favorable prognosis with a low risk of evolution to acute myeloid leukemia (AML). In patients with mutated *CALR*, additional molecular events appear to occur after this initiating event, whereas in the majority of patients with mutated *JAK2*, similar somatic mutations appear to occur prior to the acquisition of *JAK2V617F*. The presence of additional somatic mutations correlates with increased risk of disease evolution and acquisition of *TP53* mutation is associated with development of *JAK2*-mutated or wild-type *AML*. In model 1 (A), the two phases of disease are phylogenetically related, having arisen from a shared (pre-*JAK2*) founder clone, but in model 2 (B), the two phases of disease are clonally unrelated, reflecting transformation of independent stem cells. *AML*, Acute myeloid leukemia; *HSC*, hematopoietic stem cell. *(From Lundberg et al: Clonal evolution and clinical correlates of somatic mutations in myeloproliferative neoplasms.* Blood *123:2220, 2014.)*

to the disruption of a key adhesive interaction between VCAM-1 and very late antigen-4 (VLA-4) expressed by HSCs and progenitor cells. The interaction between stromal cell–, endothelial cell–, and osteoblast-derived stromal cell–derived factor-1 (SDF-1 or CXCL12) and the CXC chemokine receptor-4 (CXCR-4) expressed by HSCs

and progenitor cells is also believed to determine patterns of stem cell trafficking. Proteases, including neutrophil elastase, soluble matrix metalloproteinase-9 (MMP-9), and cell-bound MMP-9, have been shown to play a role in the constitutive mobilization of CD34+ cells that occurs in PMF patients. The concentrations of soluble VCAM-1, a degradation product of VCAM-1, is elevated in the plasma of PMF patients, and these levels correlate with the absolute numbers of CD34$^+$ cells in the peripheral blood. In addition, these elevated levels of proteases have been shown to be responsible for degradation of the chemokine CXCL12, which plays a role in retention of CD34$^+$ cells within the BM because the degradations products lack the ability to attract CD34$^+$ cells, thereby favoring their mobilization. By contrast, the amount of intact CXCL12 present within the spleen is increased, likely favoring the homing and localization of HPC/HSC to extramedullary sites such as the spleen. Furthermore, CXCR-4 expression by PMF CD34$^+$ cells is epigenetically downregulated, which may account for altered CXCL12–CXCR-4 interactions, participating in CD34$^+$ cell mobilization. This downregulation of CXCR4 expression can be reversed in vitro by treatment with chromatin-modifying agents. Furthermore, the expression levels of CXCR4 were significantly lower in patients with a high burden of *JAK2V617F* (allele frequency: 75%) compared with patients with low-burden *JAK2V617F*, suggesting the dependence of gene expression on the frequency of the mutated allele. Similar degrees of CD34$^+$ cell mobilization are observed in post-ET and post-PV MF, as occurs in PMF. In PV patients, Passamonti and coworkers have demonstrated a relationship between *JAK2V617F* allele burden and the degree of constitutive mobilization of CD34$^+$ cells, suggesting that such mobilization may be a consequence of the transition from *JAK2V617F* heterozygosity to homozygosity that is accompanied by granulocyte activation. Drugs that target the proteases responsible for constitutive CD34$^+$ cell mobilization may present a possible strategy to prevent the establishment of extramedullary sites of hematopoiesis in patients with PMF.

The kinetics of engraftment of normal stem cells after aSCT in PMF patients and the slow regression of fibrosis after transplant lead one to question if the distorted BM architecture associated with fibrosis in PMF actually disrupts the functions of the BM microenvironment. In PMF patients, normal stem cells engraft after transplant and hematopoietic cell recovery occurs before the BM fibrosis has resolved. These observations raise some questions concerning the prospects for success with strategies for the treatment of patients with PMF that are directed solely toward reversing the BM fibrosis rather than eliminating the malignant clone and its progeny. Furthermore, in mouse models of MF, inhibition of TGF-β1 was capable of preventing the development of BM fibrosis but did not rescue animals from a fatal MPN.

CLINICAL MANIFESTATIONS

Table 70.3 lists the symptoms and physical findings of patients with PMF at presentation.

Approximately 25% of patients are entirely asymptomatic and come to medical attention because of an enlarged spleen detected during routine physical examination or because of an abnormal blood cell count or peripheral blood smear. The most common symptom in PMF is fatigue, which in the majority of patients affects the quality of daily life and social activities. Fatigue may be the result of anemia, which leads to the associated complaints of weakness, dyspnea on exertion, and palpitations. But when patients were questioned with the aid of specific questionnaires, fatigue was found to be a significant burden even in patients who were not anemic. The presence of anemia, splenomegaly, and other features associated with advanced disease favors the development of higher levels of fatigue. Other nonspecific constitutional symptoms, including fever, night sweats, pruritus, bone pain, and weight loss, are present at diagnosis in 20–50% of patients with PMF and are more frequent in older patients.

With enlargement of the spleen, various syndromes characterized by abdominal discomfort emerge. Pressure of the spleen on the stomach may lead to delayed gastric emptying and early satiety. Patients may merely complain of a dull, heavy sensation in the left upper quadrant. Pain of extreme severity, simulating an acute abdominal emergency, is produced by splenic infarction. Pressure of the spleen on the colon or small bowel may be responsible of severe, disabling diarrhea.

TABLE 70.3	Summary of Symptoms and Physical Findings of Patients With Primary Myelofibrosis Detected at Diagnosis	
Symptom or Finding		**Incidence (%)**
Asymptomatic		16–30
Fatigue		47–71
Fever		5–15
Weight loss		7–39
Night sweats		6–21
Symptoms due to enlarged spleen		11–48
Bleeding		5–20
Gout or renal stones		6–13
Pallor		60
Petechiae or ecchymoses		15–20
Splenomegaly		89–99
Hepatomegaly		39–70
Peripheral edema		13
Evidence of portal hypertension		2–6
Lymphadenopathy		1–10
Jaundice		0–4

Thrombotic episodes are rarely a presenting feature of the disease but may occur during its course, with a probability of 9.6% at 5 years, a rate higher than in the control general population. Thromboses may be venous (cerebral venous sinus thrombosis, splanchnic vein thrombosis, deep venous thrombosis, pulmonary thromboembolism) or arterial (stroke, transient ischemic attacks, retinal artery occlusion, myocardial infarction, angina pectoris, and peripheral arterial disease). The cellular phase of PMF with thrombocytosis and presence of cardiovascular risk factors such as hypertension, smoking, hypercholesterolemia, and diabetes are independent predictors of thrombosis.[7] The prefibrotic phase of MF as defined by WHO criteria is associated with a higher thrombotic risk than that observed in ET patients. After splenectomy, the rate of thrombosis increases and is associated with the development of thrombocytosis after the procedure. A systematic review of *JAK2V617F*-positive PMF patients failed to clearly define a statistically significant increased risk of thrombosis in this population.

Bleeding problems may complicate the clinical course of PMF patients and range from petechiae and ecchymoses, to life-threatening issues such as uncontrollable esophageal variceal bleeding. Bleeding can be a direct result of thrombocytopenia or impaired platelet function. Bleeding may be only initially encountered during a surgical procedure such as splenectomy; in this case, the bleeding diathesis may result from inapparent disseminated intravascular coagulopathy and has the potential for catastrophic consequences.

Occurrence of isolated sites of ectopic sites of EMH occur particularly in the pulmonary, gastrointestinal, central nervous, and genitourinary systems. EMH can rarely occur in the skin, manifesting as nontender, occasionally pruritic red, pink, or violaceous plaques, papules, or hemangioma-like nodules. These dermal infiltrates, when biopsied, are composed of combinations of myeloid, erythroid, and megakaryocytic cells. Patients with nonsplenic EMH, depending on the location, can present with cough, headache, or paralysis resulting from "brain tumors or spinal cord tumors," small-bowel obstruction, or intractable ascites from ectopic implants of hematopoietic tissue in the gut or peritoneum. Ascites occurring in a patient with PMF may result from peritoneal or mesenteric implants of EMH or from portal hypertension. If the ascites result from peritoneal implants, the fluid is always exudative and sterile, and frequently contains myeloid, erythroid, and megakaryocytic elements. Such cytologic studies should routinely be performed on ascitic or pleural fluid obtained from patients with PMF. Table 70.3 lists the prominent physical findings in patients with PMF.[8] Splenomegaly serves as the hallmark of the disease. Its extent may vary, but massive splenomegaly, with the organ occupying the entire left side of the abdomen and extending into the pelvis, may occur in 35% of patients. Hepatomegaly occurs in almost 70% of cases, and lymphadenopathy is observed in 10–20%, but the degree of nodal enlargement is frequently only moderate. Other important physical findings include pallor, signs of cachexia peripheral edema, jaundice, and bony tenderness. Acute monoarticular inflammation caused by secondary gout is seen in 6% of patients.

Portal hypertension may occur and is a result of massive increases in hepatic blood flow and intrahepatic obstruction. Clinical features of portal hypertension, such as ascites or esophageal varices, occur in 9–18% of patients with PMF. Occasionally, cirrhosis or evidence of thrombosis of the portal or hepatic veins has been reported. In patients with portal hypertension, thrombotic lesions in small- or medium-sized portal veins and in extrahepatic portal veins were observed. Nodular regenerative liver hyperplasia occurred in 14.6% of cases and correlated closely with the presence of portal vein lesions.

Rarely, the development of PMF can be preceded by the appearance of multiple cutaneous edematous plaques and nodules characteristic of Sweet syndrome, a cutaneous process occurring in response to a number of hematologic malignancies. Pyoderma gangrenosum has been reported to be associated with PMF, and atypical pyoderma gangrenosum is reported to be a complication at splenectomy incision.

PMF may be associated with the development of pulmonary hypertension. These patients present with progressive dyspnea, signs of biventricular heart failure, and rapidly increasing hepatosplenomegaly. An elevation in pulmonary artery pressure can be documented by transthoracic Doppler echocardiography and right-heart catheterization. Many of these patients succumb to cardiopulmonary complications within 18 months of the documentation of pulmonary artery hypertension. The development of pulmonary artery hypertension can be attributed to thromboembolic disease, EMH diffusely involving the lung, or pulmonary fibrosis due to the elaboration of fibrogenic cytokines from dysfunctional circulating megakaryocytes and platelets. BM fibrosis also occurs in patients with primary pulmonary hypertension and can be associated with anemia and thrombocytopenia. These patients can be distinguished from patients with PMF by their lack of high levels of circulating CD34[+] cells, teardrop RBCs, hematopoietic cell clonality, and absence of molecular markers such as *JAK2V617F*, *CALR*, or *MPL* mutations.

The nephrotic syndrome can occasionally be associated with PMF. Renal EMH is a constant finding in these cases, but renal biopsy may also reveal a picture of mesangioproliferative glomerulopathy or membranous glomerulonephritis. Immunocomplex deposition with subepithelial electron-dense deposits caused by immunodysfunction of PMF has been proposed as the pathogenetic explanation for this association.

PMF may be associated with preexisting or simultaneously appearing autoimmune diseases, such as systemic lupus erythematosus (SLE), scleroderma, primary biliary cirrhosis, ulcerative colitis, polyarteritis nodosa, or juvenile rheumatoid arthritis. These nonmalignant autoimmune forms of MF are most commonly associated with SLE. These patients characteristically are young females who have cytopenias and BM fibrosis, but have a limited degree of splenomegaly and only mild numbers of teardrop RBC and immature myeloid cells in the peripheral blood. Circulating immune complexes and autoantibodies in SLE are thought to act on the megakaryocyte Fc-receptors and release growth factors, which are known to induce collagen production.

Patients with autoimmune MF frequently have a positive direct antiglobulin test result and antinuclear antibodies (ANAs) but are negative for MPN-associated genetic markers. They also lack marker cytogenetic abnormalities

LABORATORY MANIFESTATIONS

Careful examination of the peripheral blood smear and BM (Fig. 70.2) permits ready diagnosis of PMF. Leukoerythroblastosis with teardrop RBCs strongly suggests this diagnosis. The leukoerythroblastic condition is characterized by the presence of nucleated RBCs and immature myeloid elements in 96% of cases. Megathrombocytes and megakaryocytic fragments are frequent findings. The number of teardrop erythrocytes (i.e., dacryocytes) decreases after splenectomy or institution of chemotherapy, which has led some to suggest that splenic fibrosis causes the development of these RBC changes. In approximately 60% of patients, hemoglobin levels drop to less than 10 g/dL. The degree of anemia is not infrequently difficult to estimate by hemoglobin or hematocrit determinations because individuals with large spleens often have expanded plasma volumes and apparent anemia, which is largely dilutional in nature. Most patients have normochromic normocytic RBC indices. The anemia may be caused by decreased production due to erythroid hypoplasia or ineffective erythropoiesis and shortened RBC survival. The cause of the hemolytic anemia is usually multifactorial, with contributions from hypersplenism, a defect in RBCs resembling paroxysmal nocturnal hemoglobinuria, and antierythrocyte autoantibodies.

Hypochromic microcytic anemia resulting from iron deficiency secondary to blood loss may develop in 5% of PMF patients. Blood loss may be caused by leaking esophageal varices, duodenal ulceration, or intravascular hemolysis. Occasionally, a patient with PMF may develop an occult malignancy or a site of EMH within the gastrointestinal tract, which may serve as a bleeding source. Unexplained microcytosis (mean corpuscular volume <80 fL) has been reported as a laboratory feature in PMF and in general has not been shown to have prognostic relevance. Macrocytic anemia may complicate PMF. Folic acid absorption is normal in these patients, and folic acid deficiency probably results from increased use.

Leukopenia can occur in 13–25% of patients, and leukocytosis is seen in one third. Occasional blast cells and granulocytes with the pseudo–Pelger-Huët anomaly are frequent findings. The leukocyte alkaline phosphatase score is high in more than half of patients but low in about one third. Platelet counts of less than 100,000/mm[3] are observed in 31% of patients, and platelet counts of more than 800,000/mm[3] have been observed in 12%. In the prefibrotic phase of the disease, almost 90% of patients had platelet counts greater than 500,000/mm[3]. Defective platelet function is common, and platelets frequently do not respond to collagen or epinephrine. A variety of qualitative platelet anomalies have been documented as abnormal using automated platelet function analyzers such as the platelet function analyzer PF100 or light transmission platelet aggregometry. In 15% of patients, abnormalities suggestive of ongoing DIC are found, including decreased platelet numbers, decreased levels of factor V and VIII, and increased fibrin-split products. Usually, when DIC occurs in PMF, it produces no symptoms and unfortunately may only become clinically apparent after surgical intervention. Associated liver dysfunction may also be a contributory factor to prolongation of the prothrombin time. In addition, patients with a prefibrotic form of MF with extreme thrombocytosis can develop acquired form of Von Willebrand disease, which is not infrequently associated with bleeding.

Additional laboratory abnormalities are quite common. In one series, lactic acid levels were elevated in 95% of patients, bilirubin levels in 40%, uric acid in 60%, and alkaline phosphate and serum glutamic oxaloacetic transaminase levels in 50%. Patients with PMF have decreased levels of total cholesterol. The ratio of high-density lipoprotein cholesterol to low-density lipoprotein cholesterol is diminished.

A variety of immunologic abnormalities have been reported in PMF, including the presence of ANAs, elevated rheumatoid factor titers, direct Coombs test positivity, lupus-type circulating anticoagulants, hypocomplementemia, BM lymphoid nodules, and increased circulating immune complexes. In one series of 50 patients with PMF, increased quantities of circulating immune complexes were detected in 39% and found to be associated with increased disease activity, as

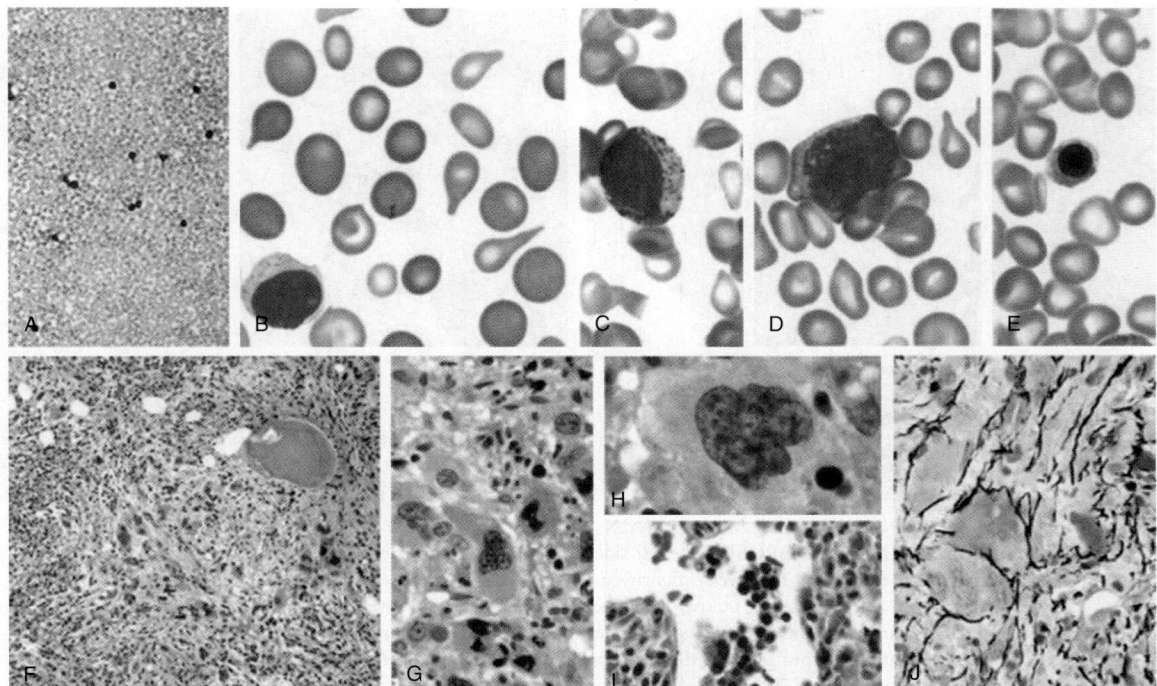

Fig. 70.2 PRIMARY MYELOFIBROSIS. Peripheral blood and bone marrow (BM) biopsy. The leukocyte count can vary in primary myelofibrosis from leukopenia to marked leukocytosis. In the case illustrated, the count was normal (A). However, the smear showed numerous dacryocytes, or teardrop forms (B), and a leukoerythroblastic picture (C–E), which is the presence leukoblasts or immature granulocytic precursors (C), including myeloblasts (D), and circulating nucleated red blood cells or erythroblasts (E). The BM biopsy is frequently hypercellular (F) and comprised of an atypical megakaryocytic and granulocytic proliferation (G) in which some of the megakaryocytes have atypical and pyknotic nuclei. Other megakaryocytes (H) are considered to have nuclei that are "cloud-like". The BM biopsy frequently shows sinusoidal hematopoiesis (I) and significant fibrosis, as illustrated by a reticulin stain (J).

manifested by increased transfusion requirements, bone pain, and fever. Some investigators have suggested that abnormalities of the complement system may be important in the disease progression of PMF, and others have hypothesized that low levels of C3 may predispose these patients to develop serious bacterial infections. A remarkably high incidence of monoclonal gammopathies has been reported in PMF, with such benign gammopathies occurring in 8–10% of patients in some series. A number of cases of the simultaneous occurrence of a plasma cell or B-cell dyscrasia and PMF have been reported.

Successful BM aspiration is unusual, accomplished in 5–10% of cases, with the tap completely dry in 50% of cases. A BM biopsy is necessary in all cases for the diagnosis and monitoring of the disease. The amount of residual hematopoietic cellular tissue and the degree of BM fibrosis are the key elements that should be assessed. Most BM biopsies in PMF are hypercellular and are remarkable for increased numbers of megakaryocytes. BM fibrosis and osteosclerosis were seen in 67% and 54% of cases, respectively. The characteristic morphologic features include patchiness of hematopoietic cellularity and reticulin fibrosis, some microscopic fields being cellular and others depleted of hematopoietic cells. The amount of reticulin may vary from field to field. Megakaryocytes are increased in number and are often arranged around and within the sinuses and not always clustered in groups. They are large with irregular, roundish, cloudlike nuclei, and distended BM sinusoids frequently containing intravascular hematopoiesis. BM biopsies reveal a substantial increase in vascularity. BM microvessels are more tortuous and branched than observed in normal control participants. The increased microvessel density is correlated with increased VEGF expression by megakaryocytes (Fig. 70.3A and B). A rare histologic variant of PMF is the so-called *MF with fatty BM*, in which the BM is characterized by myeloid hypoplasia associated with fairly complete fatty substitution,

mimicking the BM of aplastic anemia. These patients frequently have areas of clusters of densely aggregated hematopoietic elements exhibiting the histopathologic characteristics of PMF and large numbers of hematopoietic progenitors circulating in their peripheral blood. This variant of PMF is likely caused by the abnormal trafficking of hematopoietic cells from the BM to extramedullary sites, consistent with the osteosclerosis observed in patients with PMF, increased thickness of some bone units with new lamellae, and focal areas of woven bone. There is a net decrease in osteoclast number and conversion of trabecular pillars into plates.

Progressive fibrosis is frequently observed in patients who did not have maximal MF at the time of the initial biopsy. Thiele and colleagues[7] have described an early prefibrotic subtype of PMF with no or minimal BM reticulin fibrosis and another phase with conspicuous fibrosis and osteosclerotic changes of the BM. Based on a careful histomorphometric evaluation of the BM, a progressive fibroosteosclerotic process during the evolution of the disease that is paralleled by an increase in numbers of small megakaryocytes with irregular perimeters and megakaryocytes with naked nuclei has been observed. The clinical and morphologic findings of patients with the prefibrotic stage of PMF have been further characterized. Although a steady progression to BM fibrosis has been demonstrated in patients with the prefibrotic phase, fibrosis may remain static or diminish in the more advanced stages of PMF.

Different scoring systems for pathologically grading BM cellularity and fibrosis have been used with the aim of staging and documenting progression of the disease. The European consensus classification, the importance of age-dependent decrease in cellularity, was recognized (Table 70.4). Grading of MF was simplified by using four easily reproducible categories, including differentiation between reticulin and collagen. A consensus was reached that the density of fibers must be assessed in relation to the hematopoietic tissue. This feature is

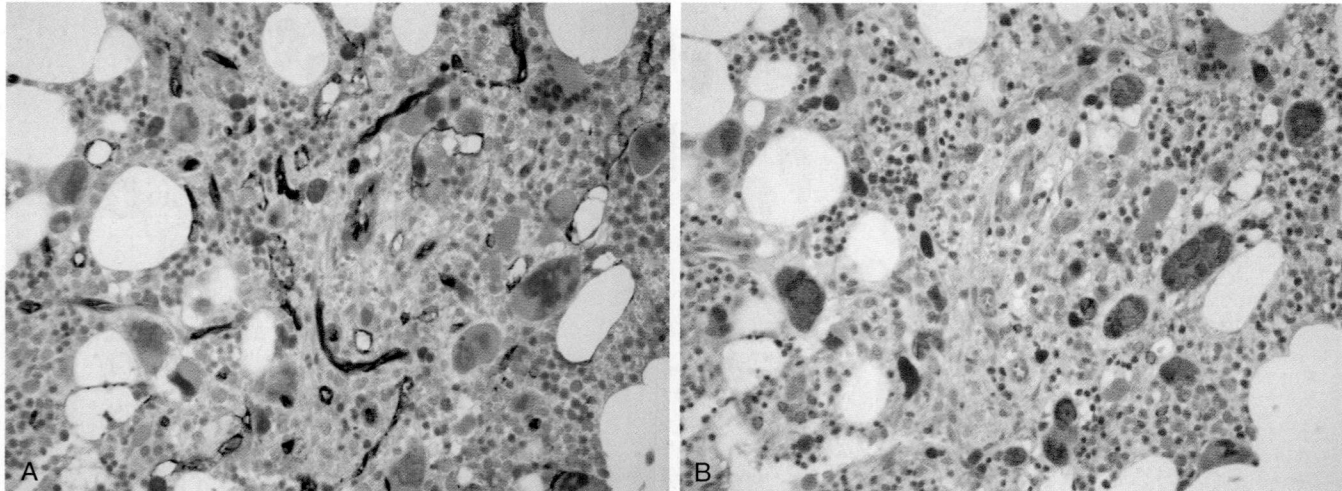

Fig. 70.3 IMMUNOHISTOCHEMICAL STAIN OF BONE MARROW BIOPSY FROM A PATIENT WITH PRIMARY MYELOFIBROSIS. The left side shows immunohistochemical stain for CD34 antibody, which highlights the increased microvessel density, as noted with the increased number of vascular structures with the lumen. Please note also the increased number of scattered CD34$^+$ myeloid blasts that are highlighted with granular staining (A). The right side shows immunohistochemical stain for vascular endothelial growth factor (VEGF)C antibody from a matched area of the bone marrow biopsy from the same patient. Note the increased expression of VEGF, as indicated by the brown staining in the cytoplasm of the dysplastic mega-karyocytes (B).

TABLE 70.4	Grading of Myelofibrosis According to the European Consensus Criteria	
Grading	**Description**[a]	
MF-0	Scattered linear reticulin with no intersections (cross-overs) corresponding to normal bone marrow	
MF-1	Loose network of reticulin with many intersections, especially in perivascular areas	
MF-2	Diffuse and dense increase in reticulin with extensive intersections, occasionally with focal bundles of collagen, focal osteosclerosis, or both	
MF-3	Diffuse and dense increase in reticulin with extensive intersections and coarse bundles of collagen, often associated with osteosclerosis	

[a]The quality of the reticulin stain should be assessed by detection of normal staining in vessel walls as internal control. The degree of myelofibrosis should be assessed by disregarding lymphoid nodules and vessels and disregarding fibers framing adipocytes. Areas of prominent scleredema or scarring should be included in the overall grading of myelofibrosis. Fiber density should be assessed in hematopoietic areas.
MF, Myelofibrosis.
Data from Thiele J, Kvasnicka HM, Facchetti F, et al: European consensus on grading bone marrow fibrosis and assessment of cellularity. *Haematologica* 90:1128, 2005.

especially important to avoid a false impression of reduced fiber content in fatty or edematous BM samples after treatment. The progression of BM fibrosis in PMF is accompanied by the expression of subsets of collagenases that is independent of *JAK2V617F* status.

Morphologic examination of the spleen frequently reveals follicular atrophy in the white pulp (Fig. 70.4A) with foci of EMH in the sinusoids of the red pulp (Fig. 70.4B) where megakaryocytes, myeloid elements, and nucleated erythroid elements are seen. The extramedullary hematopoietic cells belonging to each of the myeloid lineages can be distributed in the spleen diffusely or be limited to macronodules. The predominance of immature granulocytic forms is associated with an especially poor prognosis. Pathologic examination of the liver reveals hematopoietic cellular elements within the sinusoids (see E-Slide VM03954). Sinusoidal dilatation is a common finding, as well as prominent intrahepatocyte and Kupffer cell hemosiderin deposition. A marked increase in the hepatic reticulin network has also been observed.

Approximately 30–50% of patients with PMF have karyotypic abnormalities at diagnosis. It is important to perform appropriate cytogenetic analyses to exclude rare cases of chronic myelogenous leukemia with associated BM fibrosis. Because of BM fibrosis, it is often difficult to obtain optimal numbers of metaphase cells for cytogenetic analysis. In the past, a substantial percentage of patients with PMF had a "dry tap" or were uninformative, thereby making cytogenetic analysis challenging. Although cytogenetic analysis of PMF remains time consuming and laborious, cytogenetic studies are now informative in about 99% of patients from unstimulated peripheral blood specimens. This success is due to the presence of large numbers of immature mitotic hematopoietic cells (including CD34$^+$ cells) present in the peripheral blood combined with the use of an MPN interphase FISH panel that allows for essentially all PMF patients to be examined for the most frequent cytogenomic changes (Fig. 70.5). There is a high concordance rate (92%) between conventional cytogenetics and interphase FISH for the 12 most frequent chromosomal abnormalities detected in PMF.

Among the Philadelphia chromosome-negative MPNs, PMF has the highest rate of chromosomal abnormalities at diagnosis. Deletions of the long arms of chromosomes 13 and 20, trisomy 8, and abnormalities of chromosomes 1, 7, and 9 constitute more than 80% of all chromosomal abnormalities detected in PMF (see Fig. 70.5). None of these lesions are specific for PMF because they are also detected in PV, ET, MDS, and other myeloid malignancies. Deletion of the long arm of chromosome 13 is substantially more frequent in PMF than in PV. Fine FISH mapping has defined the commonly deleted region to 13q13.3-q14.3 encompassing *RB1*, *D13S319*, and *D13S25* loci. As mentioned in Chapter 68, del(20q) and +9/+9p are more frequent in PV than in PMF. Multiple copies of 9p result in trisomy/tetrasomy or amplification of *JAK2*, and each of these abnormalities has been reported in PMF. A 2.7-Mb region on chromosome 20 spanning *D20S108* (proximal) and *D20S481* (distal) is deleted in all Philadelphia chromosome-negative MPNs. A different region is deleted in other myeloid malignancies, but a common 1.6-kb region may constitute the major site responsible for loss of heterozygosity.

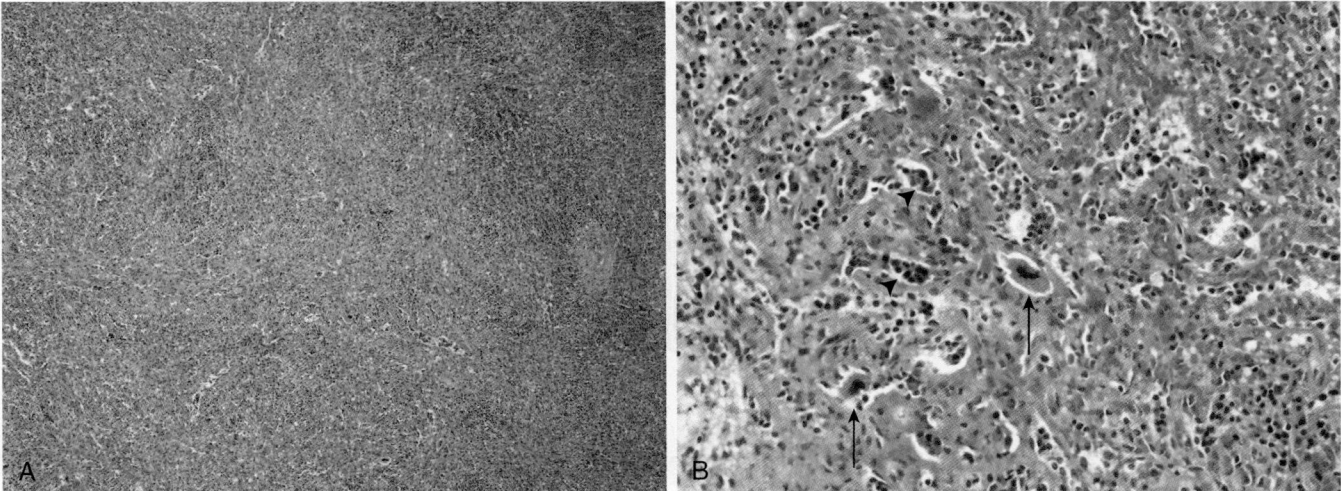

Fig. 70.4 SPLEEN MORPHOLOGY IN PRIMARY MYELOFIBROSIS. The left side shows low-power magnification of spleen tissue from a patient with PMF with expanded red pulp and reduced-to-absent white pulp (A). The right sides shows higher power magnification with extramedullary hematopoiesis with intra-sinusoidal dysplastic megakaryocytes *(blocked arrows)*, and erythroid progenitor clusters *(arrowheads)* along with scattered myeloid cells (B).

With disease progression from PV/ET to MF, the frequency of cytogenetic abnormalities increases to 70% to 90%. The types of chromosomal abnormalities observed in these cases are similar to those seen at diagnosis of PV/ET or PMF, but through subclonal evolution they may become very complex. The number of genomic alterations is more than two or three times greater in the blast phase as in the chronic phase. Specific regions on 12p (*ETV6*), 17p (*P53*), and on 21q (*RUNX1*) are frequently altered and associated with disease progression.

The use of comparative genomic hybridization techniques suggest that genomic aberrations are much more common than has been previously indicated by conventional cytogenetic analysis and occur in the majority of cases. Gains of 9p were the most frequent finding, occurring in 50% of patients, suggesting that genes on 9p may play a crucial role in the pathogenesis of PMF.

The performance of mutational studies is a critical step in making a definitive diagnosis of PMF. In PMF, the proportion of patients with the *JAK2V617F* mutation in granulocytes has been reported to range from 35% to 95%. The detection rate for *JAK2V617F* is much higher for patients with post-PV MF (91%) than PMF (45%) or post-ET MF (39%). In PV, a high burden of *JAK2V617F* allele has been associated with an increased rate of evolution to MF. Such wide differences in the mutational frequencies can be attributed to the different sensitivity of the techniques used to detect the mutation and to differences in the case mix of the reported series (i.e., proportion of primary and secondary PMF cases). *JAK2V617F* in PMF is associated with an older patient age at diagnosis and a history of thrombosis or pruritus. A common *JAK2* germ-line haplotype (46/1) that is identified by the rs12343867 SNP was found to influence susceptibility to develop PMF regardless of *JAK2* mutational status.

Gain-of-function mutations of the thrombopoietin receptor, *MPL W515L* and *MPL W515K*, are present in approximately 5% of patients with PMF, 1% of patients with ET, but no patients with PV. *MPL* mutations may occur concurrently with *JAK2V617F*, suggesting that these alleles may have functional complementation in MPN. In all cases, the *MPL W515K/L* allele burden occurs in excess of the *JAK2V617F* allele. In contrast to de novo acute myeloid leukemia (AML), mutations in the receptor tyrosine kinases *KIT*, *FMS*, and *FLT3* have not been documented in PMF, and the spectrum of mutations seen at time of leukemic transformation from PMF also differ in that mutations in *JAK2*, *SRSF2*, *TET2*, *IDH1/2*, and *ASXL1* are more common.

The number of circulating cells expressing the CD34 antigen, a phenotypic marker of hematopoietic stem and progenitor cells as well as endothelial cells, in patients with PMF has been reported to be more than 300-times higher than in normal volunteers and 18–30-times higher than in patients with PV or ET. The clinical utility of the cytofluorimetric measurement of CD34$^+$ cells as a diagnostic marker of PMF is hampered by the observation that a small number of subjects with PMF exhibit a normal number of CD34$^+$ cells in the peripheral blood. Cases with very mild disease or absent or slight reticulin BM fibrosis account for the majority of such patients. High values of CD34$^+$ cells (>200 × 10^6/L) have been proposed as an indicator of an accelerated phase of the disease.

The characteristic radiographic features of PMF include a diffuse increase in bone density and increased prominence of the bony trabeculae. This increased bone density may be patchy and can produce a mottled appearance. Such abnormalities have been reported in 25–66% of patients with PMF.

Noninvasive imaging of BM is a promising means of evaluating the BM cellularity and distribution in PMF. Magnetic resonance imaging (MRI) can portray the conversion or reconversion of fatty to cellular BM. Fibrotic BM is easily distinguished from cellular BM by its strikingly low signal intensity with all pulse signals. The BM patterns in the proximal femurs of PMF patients have been reported to be correlated with the clinical severity of the disease. BM MRI has been used to differentiate PMF from ET, where the BM adipose tissue is preserved, but in PMF, the adiposity of the BM is reduced.

DIFFERENTIAL DIAGNOSIS

A patient with hepatosplenomegaly, peripheral cytopenias, teardrop poikilocytosis, leukoerythroblastosis, and BM fibrosis probably has PMF, but other disorders may also lead to this clinical picture (see Table 70.1 and Fig. 70.6). The WHO diagnostic criteria were revised, incorporating testing for *JAK2V617F* and activating *MPL* mutations, as well as greater emphasis on histomorphologic criteria, which allow one to distinguish early phases of PMF from ET (Table 70.5). The WHO criteria are based on the recognition of a prefibrotic form of PMF without reticulin fibrosis and that the primary diagnostic features of PMF are increased megakaryocyte numbers, megakaryocyte morphology, and abnormalities of granulocyte mutation. Secondary MF frequently occurs in patients with lymphoma or metastatic carcinoma of the stomach, prostate, lung, or breast. The clinician should

Chromosomal Findings Associated With a Favorable Prognosis

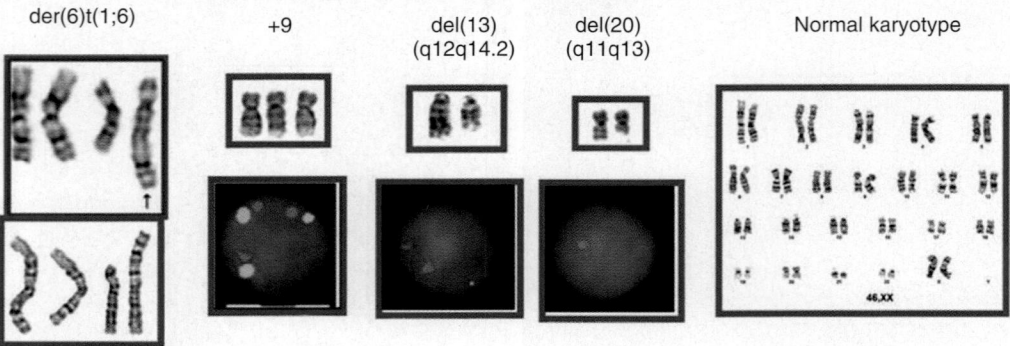

Chromosomal Findings Associated With an Unfavorable Prognosis

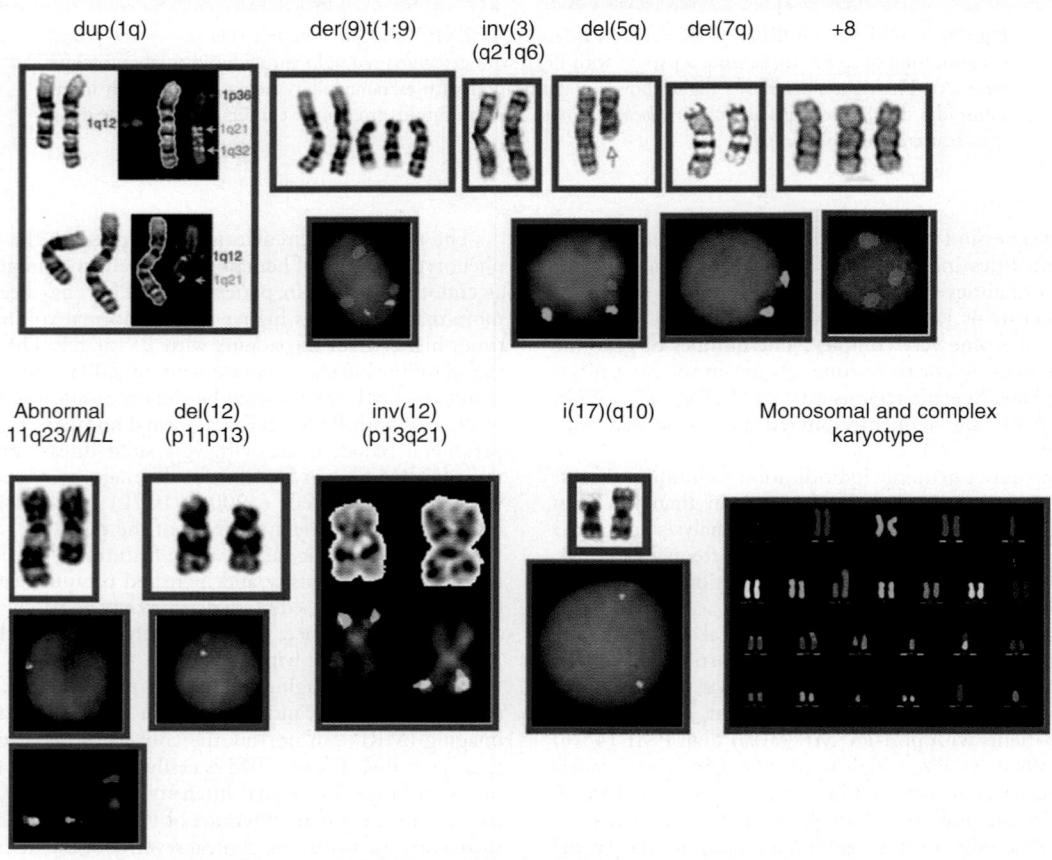

Fig. 70.5 CYTOGENETIC FINDINGS IN PRIMARY MYELOFIBROSIS. The *top row* shows chromosomal abnormalities and corresponding interphase fluorescence in situ hybridization (FISH) findings associated with a favorable prognosis. They include unbalanced translocations between chromosomes 1 and 6 (both the short and long arms of chromosome 6) resulting in a gain of 1q, sole abnormality of chromosomes 9, 13, and 20, as well as the normal karyotype. Abnormalities include a gain of chromosome 9 and interstitial deletions of the long arm of chromosome 13 and 20. Note, that gain of 1q and jumping 1q is associated with disease progression to acute myeloid leukemia. The *bottom row* shows chromosomal abnormalities and corresponding interphase nuclei after FISH studies associated with an unfavorable prognosis. They include duplication and trisomy 1q. The most frequent abnormality associated with polycythemia vera-related primary myelofibrosis (PMF) is der (9)t(1;9), resulting in a gain of 1q *(red)* and 9p. Inversion of chromosome 3, -5/del(5q) *(red)*, and -7/del(7q) *(red)* are rare in PMF, as are rearrangement of 11q23 and deletion of the short arms of chromosome 12. Sole trisomy 8 is a frequent abnormality associated with PMF, and rearrangements of 12q are almost exclusively identified in PMF. The chromosomal abnormalities associated with the most dismal prognosis are heterozygous 17p loss *(red)* and monosomal or complex karyotype.

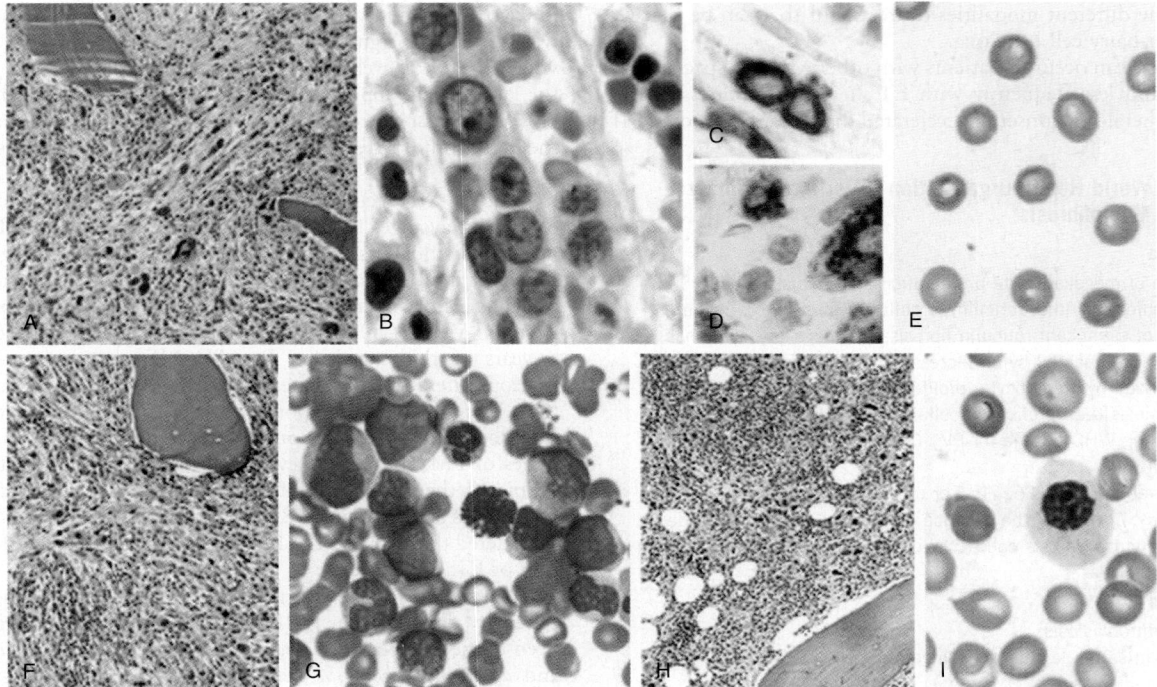

Fig. 70.6 DIFFERENTIAL DIAGNOSTIC CONSIDERATIONS IN PRIMARY MYELOFIBROSIS. (A–E) Acute panmyelosis with myelofibrosis (APMF). (F and G) Chronic myelogenous leukemia (CML) in an advance phase with fibrosis. (H and I) Myelodysplastic syndrome (MDS) with fibrosis. The bone marrow (BM) biopsy of APMF, CML in advanced phase with fibrosis, and MDS with fibrosis can all look similar to PMF at low power (A, F, and H). In APMF, the distinction from PMF is made in part by seeing increased immature cells on the biopsy (B) interspersed with other hematopoietic precursors. These are usually CD34+ (C), but in contrast to acute megakaryoblastic leukemia are usually CD61− (D). In addition, the peripheral blood usually shows pancytopenia with neither teardrop red blood cells nor leukoerythroblastosis (E). Although the biopsy of CML presenting in an advanced phase can resemble PMF (F), the peripheral blood usually shows classic granulocytosis with left shift and basophilia (G). In the case illustrated, the 30-year-old female patient had fibrotic BM (F) but presented with a white blood cell count of 148,000/L showing a full spectrum of granulocytes, increased blasts (22%), and basophilia. P210 *BCR/ABL1* was demonstrated. The bone marrow biopsy in MDS with fibrosis has small megakaryocytes (H), but dysplasia is otherwise difficult to evaluate in the absence of an aspirate, and one must rely on the peripheral blood to identify dysplasia, as in the severely dysplastic neutrophil (F).

be extremely careful in making the diagnosis of PMF in a patient who has a history of a primary neoplasm. Demonstration of carcinoma cells in the BM establishes that metastatic carcinoma is the cause of the BM fibrosis (Fig. 70.7A and B). The finding of blastic or lytic bone lesions in patients with MF suggests the presence of an underlying carcinoma. Disseminated tuberculosis and histoplasmosis have been associated with the development of secondary MF. Caseating or noncaseating granulomas observed on BM biopsy suggest the presence of these infectious disorders. Identification of the causative organisms by culture techniques should be pursued.

A number of other primary hematologic disorders can also be accompanied by BM fibrosis (see Table 70.1). A variety of overlap syndromes that share features of both PMF and MDS have been reported and are seen frequently in clinical practice. These so-called *overlap syndromes* have pathologic and clinical features of both MPN and MDS, and are characterized by BM hypercellularity, dysplasia of various myeloid lineages, and proliferative features, as well as ineffective hematopoiesis, modest hepatosplenomegaly, and some degree of BM fibrosis. These patients are occasionally *JAK2V617F* positive and frequently have *TET2* mutations. Such patients frequently present with cytopenias and are at a high risk of developing acute leukemia. These cases indicate the limitations of adhering to strict disease classifications and underscore that a continuum exists between MPNs and MDS. The peripheral blood and BM findings that allow differentiation of these disorders can be enhanced by *JAK2V617F, MPL W515L/K* and *CALR* mutational analyses. Patients with the variant

MDS with MF frequently present with cytopenias and have dysplastic cellular abnormalities indistinguishable from those of other patients with myelodysplasia. Their BMs, however, are characterized by the presence of BM fibrosis and a striking megakaryocytic hyperplasia, with a predominance of small hypolobulated forms, in some cases surrounding fibrosis. Reticulocytopenia is characteristic of these patients, as are teardrop RBCs and a clinical picture of leukoerythroblastosis. Unlike patients with PMF, patients with myelodysplasia and BM fibrosis do not have hepatic or splenic enlargement extending more than 3 cm below the costal margin. The OS time of patients with this variant of MDS has been reported to be 30 months, with death resulting from the effects of cytopenias or transformation to acute leukemia. Additional studies have indicated that the presence of MF in patients with myelodysplasia was associated with a particularly short survival time (9.6 months) compared with patients with myelodysplasia without fibrosis (17.4 months).

Hairy cell leukemia can also be confused with PMF. In one study, five out of 61 patients who had originally been diagnosed as having PMF were shown retrospectively to have had hairy cell leukemia. Hairy cell leukemia can present as pancytopenia with splenomegaly and is associated with a dry BM tap. In one series, BM reticulin content was increased in 26 out of 29 patients with hairy cell leukemia. The presence of hairy mononuclear cells possessing tartrate-resistant acid phosphatase or the appropriate phenotype in the peripheral blood or BM should facilitate differentiation of PMF from hairy cell leukemia (see Chapter 78). This exercise is important because of the different modalities of treatment that can be successfully used for hairy cell leukemia.

BM fibrosis can occur in patients with other MPNs, especially PV and CML, and less frequently with ET. In CML, progressive BM fibrosis may herald the onset of accelerated disease or blast crisis. MF

TABLE 70.5	World Health Organization Criteria for Primary Myelofibrosis[a]

Major Criteria

1. Presence of megakaryocyte proliferation and atypia,[b] usually accompanied by either reticulin or collagen fibrosis, or, in the absence of significant reticulin fibrosis, the megakaryocyte changes must be accompanied by an increased bone marrow cellularity characterized by granulocytic proliferation and often decreased erythropoiesis (i.e., prefibrotic cellular-phase disease)
2. Not meeting WHO criteria for PV,[c] CML,[d] MDS,[e] or other myeloid neoplasm
3. Demonstration of *JAK2617V>F* or other clonal marker (e.g., *MPL515W>L/K*), or in the absence of a clonal marker, no evidence of bone marrow fibrosis caused by underlying inflammatory or other neoplastic diseases[f]

Minor Criteria

1. Leukoerythroblastosis[g]
2. Increase in serum lactate dehydrogenase level[g]
3. Anemia[g]
4. Palpable splenomegaly[g]

[a]Diagnosis requires meeting all three major criteria and two minor criteria.
[b]Small-to-large megakaryocytes with an aberrant nuclear-to-cytoplasmic ratio and hyperchromatic, bulbous, or irregularly folded nuclei and dense clustering.
[c]Requires the failure of iron-replacement therapy to increase hemoglobin level to the polycythemia vera range in the presence of decreased serum ferritin. Exclusion of polycythemia vera is based on hemoglobin and hematocrit levels. Red blood cell mass measurement is not required.
[d]Requires the absence of *BCR-ABL*.
[e]Requires the absence of dyserythropoiesis and dysgranulopoiesis.
[f]Secondary to infection, autoimmune disorder or other chronic inflammatory condition, hairy cell leukemia or other lymphoid neoplasm, metastatic malignancy, or toxic (chronic) myelopathies. It should be noted that patients with conditions associated with reactive myelofibrosis are not immune to primary myelofibrosis, and the diagnosis should be considered in such cases if other criteria are met.
[g]Degree of abnormality could be borderline or marked.
CML, Chronic myeloid leukemia; MDS, myelodysplastic syndrome; PV, polycythemia vera; WHO, World Health Organization.
Data from Tefferi A, Thiele J, Orazi A, et al: Proposals and rationale for revision of the World Health Organization diagnostic criteria for polycythemia vera, essential thrombocythemia, and primary myelofibrosis: Recommendations from an ad hoc international expert panel. *Blood* 110:1092, 2007.

in CML occurs in two distinct patterns, one in which patients present with CML and significant associated BM fibrosis, and a second in which the MF develops late in the course of the CML. The MF in the latter group appears at a mean of 36 months after the diagnosis of CML, is associated with a mean survival time of 4.9 months from the detection of MF, and therefore represents an ominous prognostic sign.

Post-PV MF occurs in 5–15% of patients with PV. This transition occurs, on average, 10 years after the initial diagnosis of PV is made, but in individual cases it may appear after shorter or longer intervals. PMF is clinically indistinguishable from post-PV MF except for the previous history of erythrocytosis in the latter group. Of patients with post-PV MF, 25–50% develop leukemia, and 70% are dead within 3 years of this transition. Post-PV MF represents a transitional myeloproliferative syndrome with relatively grave prognostic implications. MF has also been reported after ET. These investigators claimed that these patients did not represent individuals with prefibrotic stages of PMF but rather evolution of patients with true ET. They estimated the probability of developing such a complication to be 3% 5 years after diagnosis, 8% at 10 years, and 15% at 15 years, and considered this evolution to BM fibrosis a major long-term complication of ET.

Acute panmyelosis with myelofibrosis (APMF) represents a clinical entity distinct from PMF (see Fig. 70.6). This disorder has also been termed *acute MF, acute myelosclerosis, acute megakaryocytic MF,* and *acute myelodysplasia with MF.* APMF is exceedingly rare and corresponds to less than 1% of the cases of AML. Patients characteristically present with pancytopenia, fever, absence of clinically significant splenomegaly, minimal or absent teardrop poikilocytosis, and fibrotic BM. The BM is characterized by the appearance of immature myeloid cells and blast cells, which frequently express megakaryocytic phenotypic properties. Survival ranges from 1 to 9 months after diagnosis. Its distinction from PMF is important because aggressive chemotherapy and possibly SCT are the treatments of choice. Up to 12% of patients who present with MF have been reported to have an underlying autoimmune disorder such as SLE, although in the authors' clinical practice, this is an extraordinary rare event. Primary autoimmune MF (primary AIMF) likely represents a distinct clinicopathologic syndrome unrelated to other well-defined autoimmune disorders. Eight diagnostic criteria for AIMF, including grade 3 or 4 reticulin fibrosis in the BM, lack of clustered or atypical megakaryocytes, lack of dysplasia or eosinophilia or basophilia, lymphoid infiltration of the BM, lack of osteosclerosis, absent or mild splenomegaly, presence of autoantibodies, and absence of disorders associated with MF, have been outlined. Autoimmune MF occurs predominantly in females with a broad clinical spectrum. Patients

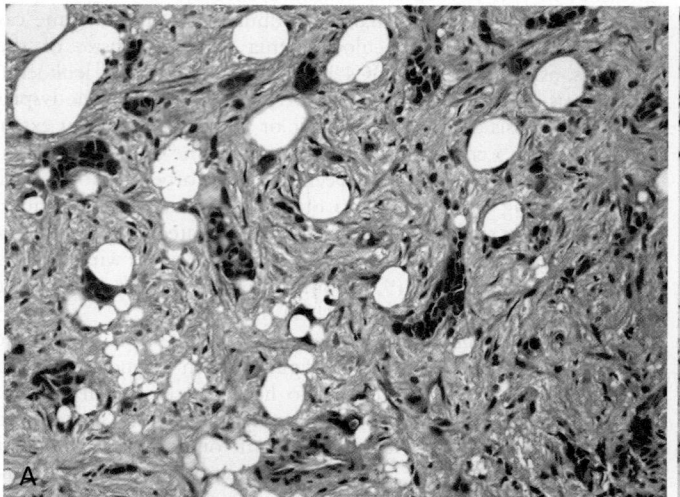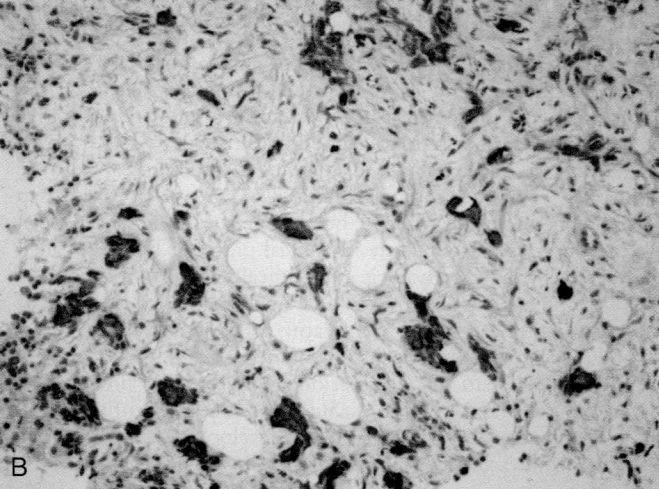

Fig. 70.7 Metastatic carcinoma to the bone marrow often is associated with bone marrow fibrosis as noted in this hematoxylin and eosin-stained section with clusters of carcinoma cells (A) that are highlighted by cytokeratin immunostain (B).

may present with MF in the setting of established SLE or in patients with minimal manifestations of an autoimmune disorder, as in primary AIMF. The presence of teardrop erythrocytes or leukoerythroblastosis in a patient with lupus suggests autoimmune MF. Such patients universally have a positive ANA test result or an elevated anti-DNA titer. Because the physical manifestations of an autoimmune disease may not be evident, all patients with MF should have an ANA test to exclude an autoimmune etiology. Primary AIMF patients lack MPN mutations such as *JAK2V617F, MPL W515L/K,* and *CALR,* or marker cytogenetic abnormalities consistent with polyclonal rather than clonal hematopoiesis

PROGNOSIS

The median OS period from the time of diagnosis of PMF varies from series to series but is approximately 6–7 years (Fig. 70.8). The primary causes of death include infection, leukemic transformation, heart failure, bleeding, hepatic failure caused by EMH of the liver, portal hypertension, renal failure, pulmonary embolism, and complications occurring following aSCT. The incidence of acute leukemia as a terminal event ranges from 5% to 22%, (Fig. 70.9). Approximately half of the patients who develop acute leukemia have not received previous treatment with alkylating agents or radiotherapy, indicating that the evolution into acute leukemia is part of the natural history of PMF. The actuarial cumulative risk of death from leukemic

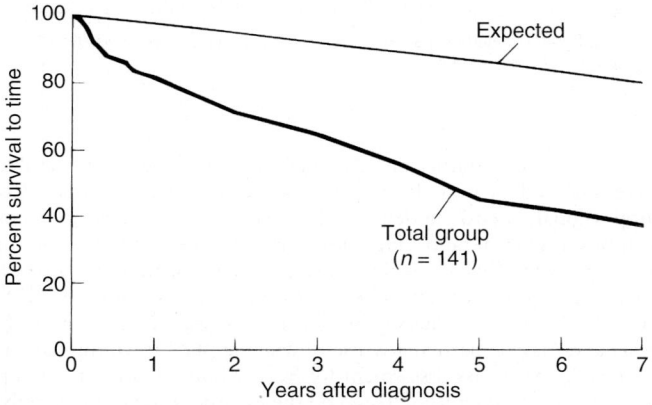

Fig. 70.8 OVERALL SURVIVAL FROM THE TIME OF DIAGNOSIS OF 141 PATIENTS WITH PRIMARY MYELOFIBROSIS. *(Data from Silverstein MN:* Agnogenic myeloid metaplasia, *Acton, MA, 1975, Publishing Sciences Group, p 197.)*

transformation at 1 and 5 years after diagnosis has been reported to be 2% and 16%, respectively. Immunologic and morphologic characterization of the blast cell phenotypes comprising these leukemias reveals that a typical myeloid phenotype is most commonly detected; other cell lineages, such as megakaryocytic, erythroid, lymphoid, and even stem cell phenotype, may also be involved, leading to the existence of mixed myeloid and hybrid transformations. Megakaryoblastic transformations have been detected in one-third of cases in one series, an incidence higher than that found in de novo AML. In 50% of cases of *JAK2V617F* MPNs, the blast cells that represent the progeny of the leukemia initiating clone are *JAK2V617F* negative, suggesting that the leukemia originates from a clone distinct from the *JAK2V617F*-positive clone. This coexistent *JAK2V617F*-negative clone appears to have a higher propensity to undergo leukemic transformation. *JAK2V617F* therefore does not appear to be a prerequisite for leukemic transformation of MPNs, suggesting that additional genetic and epigenetic events are required for full transformation to occur. SNP array analysis has shown that genomic alterations occur at an increased frequency during the period of blastic transformation and that no single gene or molecular pathway is sufficient to cause transformation. Acquisition of somatic mutations in *TET2, IDH, TP53,* and *ASXL1* have all been implicated as genetic events leading to leukemic transformation in MF patients.

A surprising correlation has been observed between the phenotype of the preceding MPN and the *JAK2* mutational status of the leukemic blasts after transformation. In contrast to *JAK2* WT AML in this setting, evolution to leukemias with *JAK2V617F*-positive blast cells is invariably preceded by the evolution of ET or PV to MF. Because of these observations, myelofibrotic transformation of ET or PV likely represents an accelerated phase of the initial MPN preceded by genetic changes that result in evolution to MF and eventually leukemia. *JAK2* WT leukemia, by contrast, usually arises in patients with chronic-phase PV or ET who have not evolved to MF. Some have suggested that these leukemias are therapy related and are the consequence of the administration of myelosuppressive agents administered during the chronic phase. The reversion from *JAK2V617F* to WT *JAK2* in these leukemias is not due to homologous recombination. Two models have previously been proposed to account for the clonal relationship between *JAK2* WT AML and its preceding MPN: (1) Both the chronic MPN and the AML arise from a shared pre-*JAK2V617F* founder clone, and (2) the chronic MPN and AML arise from two independent stem cells. A more recent model proposed by Lundberg and colleagues also reflects similar models incorporating new understanding of phylogenetic ordering of mutated *JAK2* and *CALR* with respect to additional acquired somatic mutations (see Fig. 70.1).[8] It remains possible that each model is viable and operates in different individual patients. Survival after blast transformation is limited, a phenomenon that is probably a result of patient age and

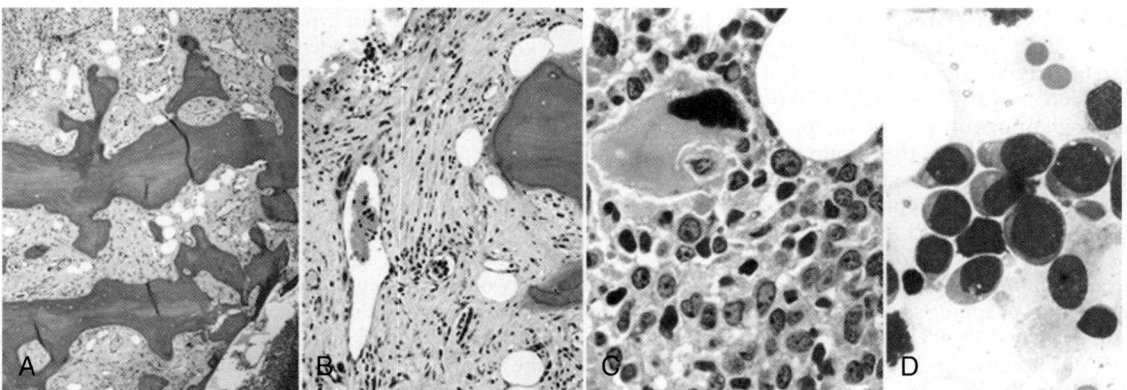

Fig. 70.9 DISEASE PROGRESSION IN PRIMARY MYELOFIBROSIS. Marked osteosclerosis (A and B) and acute leukemia (C and D). In some patients, primary myelofibrosis progresses to severe osteosclerosis, in which there is markedly thickened and irregular bone formation (A) and a bone marrow space that is fibrotic and nearly depleted of hematopoietic elements (B). A terminal transformation to acute leukemia (C and D) occurs in 5–22% of cases.

TABLE 70.6	Prognostic Scoring Systems for Primary Myelofibrosis			
Risk Factor	Lille	IPSS	DIPSS	DIPSS Plus
Anemia (hemoglobin)	X (<10 g/dL)	X (<10 g/dL)	X (<10 g/dL)	X (<10 g/dL)
Leukocytosis (white blood cell count)	X (<4 or >30 × 10⁹/L)	X (>25 × 10⁹/L)	X (>25 × 10⁹/L)	X (>25 × 10⁹/L)
Peripheral blood blasts		X (≥1%)	X (≥1%)	X (≥1%)
Constitutional symptoms		X	X	X
Age (years)		X (>65)	X (adjusted for age)	X
Karyotype				X (unfavorableᵃ)
Platelet				X (<100 × 10⁹/L)
Transfusion status				X

ᵃUnfavorable karyotype includes complex or sole or two abnormalities that include +8, –7/7q–, i7/7q–, i(17q), –5/5q–, 12p–, inv(3), or 11q23 rearrangements.
DIPSS, Dynamic international prognostic scoring system; IPSS, international prognostic scoring system.

the aggressive biology of these leukemias. Leukemic transformation of PMF has been reported to be fatal in 98% of patients after a median of 2.6 months. Successful leukemia remission induction therapy in these patients is an extremely rare event. Patients should optimally be sent for aSCT before leukemic transformation. Leukemia-free survival in PMF has been shown to be significantly worse in the presence of a triple-negative mutational status, compared with patients with *CALR*-, *JAK2*-, or *MPL*-mutated status. Conversely, CALR-mutated patients were at lower risk of leukemic transformation compared with triple-negative and *JAK2*-mutated cases, but not when compared with *MPL*-mutated cases.

The clinical and biologic parameters that are characteristic of patients at diagnosis have been used to identify subgroups of patients with different prognoses. Some investigators have suggested that there are two subpopulations of patients with PMF; short-lived and long-lived subpopulations of patients. These efforts are of importance in identifying which patients have a limited survival and should proceed with aSCT in a timely fashion or in selecting groups of MF patients with a similar prognosis for participation in clinical trials. Each of these efforts have uniformly shown that patients with anemia at presentation have a shorter survival. Dupriez and associates developed an extremely simple scoring system, the Lille scoring system, based on two adverse prognostic factors—hemoglobin level less than 10 g/dL and WBC count less than 4000/mm³ or more than 30,000/mm³, and were able to stratify patients into three groups. The low-risk (zero factors), intermediate-risk (one factor), and high-risk (two factors) groups were associated with median survival times of 93, 26, and 13 months, respectively. Other scoring systems that use simple clinical hematologic parameters have been subsequently proposed.

The International Working Group for Myelofibrosis Research and Treatment (IWG-MRT) have developed an international prognostic scoring systems (IPSS) based on the clinical characteristics of 1054 patients diagnosed with PMF.[9] Tables 70.6 and 70.7 compare four validated prognostic scoring systems for patients with PMF. The overall median survival for this group was 69 months, and multivariate analysis identified an age greater than 65 years, the presence of constitutional symptoms, hemoglobin below 10 g/dL, leukocyte count above 25 × 10⁹/L, and 1% or greater peripheral blood blasts as significant risk factors. The sum of the risk factors allows for allocation into discrete risk groups. Four risk groups can be discerned with nonoverlapping survival curves based on this model with median survivals of 135, 95, 48, and 27 months for low (0), intermediate-1 (1), intermediate-2 (2), and high-risk (3–5) groups, respectively. Although the presence of *JAK2V617F* was associated with age greater than 65 years, it did not influence survival in this study. The presence of cytogenetic abnormalities influenced the survival of the intermediate-risk groups only. Subsequently, a cohort of 525 PMF patients was followed over time to assess the prognostic influence of the five IPSS clinical variables acquired during the

TABLE 70.7	Median Survival of Each Risk Group in Four Prognostic Scoring Systems for Primary Myelofibrosis			
Risk Group	Lille	IPSS	DIPSS	DIPSS Plus
Low	93 months	135 months	Not reached	185 months
Intermediate-1	26 months	95 months	170 months	78 months
Intermediate-2		48 months	48 months	35 months
High	13 months	27 months	18 months	16 months

DIPSS, Dynamic international prognostic scoring system; IPSS, international prognostic scoring system.

course of disease rather than at presentation. The IPSS variables were analyzed as time-dependent covariates in a multivariate Cox proportional hazard model. Anemia was found to have the most significant hazard ratio (HR) for survival. The advantage of this dynamic IPSS (DIPSS) is its ability to assess real-time prognosis as a patient acquires different clinical features. An age-adjusted DIPSS (aaDIPSS) was also proposed for patients younger than the age of 65 years and may be particularly useful when applied to young patients in the context of risk assessment for SCT. More recently, an attempt to further refine the DIPSS based on the incorporation of unfavorable karyotype, platelet count below 100 × 10⁹/L and transfusional status within the scoring system was reported. A poorer, leukemia-free survival was predicted by the presence of thrombocytopenia or an unfavorable karyotype with a 10-year risk of 31% (HR: 3.3; 95% confidence interval: 1.9–5.6).

Substantial progress has been made during the past few years to allow for the use of cytogenetics as a prognostic indicator. Initially, a group at the MD Anderson Cancer Center performed a retrospective analysis of 256 patients (36% had an abnormal karyotype) and determined that baseline cytogenetic status was useful in predicting survival. Deletions of chromosomes 13 and 20 or trisomy 9 alone or in the presence of other abnormalities were associated with a median survival time similar to those with a normal karyotype (63 and 46 months, respectively). By contrast, abnormalities of chromosomes 5 or 7, or three or more abnormalities were associated with a median survival time of 15 months. In a larger study from the Mayo Clinic, a two-tier cytogenetic risk stratification after a median follow-up of 4 years was developed. Because cytogenetic analysis is not yet incorporated in the IPSS, the following cytogenetic current schema should be carefully considered. Patients with favorable karyotype include chromosome del(13q), del(20q), trisomy 9, alone other single abnormalities, two abnormalities excluding unfavorable types of abnormalities, and a normal karyotype. The 5-year survival rate was 51% with a median survival of 5.2 years observed for patients in the group with favorable karyotypes. Although derivative 1;6 resulting in 1q gain has been considered a favorable prognostic finding, gain of chromosome 1q, which occurs in 22% of PMF patients, has been reported to be associated with disease progression, and jumping 1q translocations have been observed to be associated with imminent transformation to AML. In PMF, the region on chromosome 1 that is most frequently duplicated or occurring in trisomy is between 1q21-32 and 1q32-44 band regions (see Fig. 70.5). The 5-year survival for patients with an unfavorable karyotype, including trisomy 8, abnormalities of chromosomes 5 or 7, inversion of chromosome 3, isochromosome 17q, deletion 12p or 11q23 rearrangement, as well as two abnormalities including an unfavorable abnormality and a complex karyotype, was 8% with a median survival of 2 years. Moreover, multivariable analysis demonstrated that karyotype and platelet count ($<100 \times 10^9/L$) but not the IPSS status predicted leukemia-free survival. The 5-year leukemic transformation rates for patients with an unfavorable versus favorable karyotype were 46% and 7%, respectively ($p < .0001$). The widespread implementation of this cytogenetically-based scoring system requires more extensive validation. A new cytogenetic risk category, monosomal karyotype (MK), also defines an unfavorable risk category. An MK is defined as having two or more autosomal monosomies or a single autosomal monosomy associated with at least one structural abnormality. This is a rare cytogenetic change associated with median survival of 6 months and a 2-year leukemic transformation rate of 29.4%. At diagnosis of PMF, detection of MK is associated with extremely poor overall and leukemia-free survival.

The mutational profile of a MF patient has also been shown to have prognostic significance. Four risk groups based on mutational status of the driver mutations involving *JAK2*, *MPL*, and *CALR* have been shown to predict different overall and leukemia-free survival. MF patients with *CALR*-positive, *JAK2V617F*-positive, *MPL*-positive, or "triple-negative" disease have a mean OS of 17.7 years, 9.2 years, 9.1 years, and 3.2 years, respectively. In fact, the incorporation of these molecular markers into modern risk-adapted treatment stratification has been proposed by some investigators. Additionally, MF patients harboring both *CALR* and *ASXL1* mutations have been shown to have a good prognosis compared with patients harboring an *ASXL1* mutation alone.

Most studies have indicated that the OS of patients with *JAK2V617F*-positive and -negative PMF are similar; however, patients with *JAK2V617F*-positive disease and a low allele burden (<25%) have been shown to have a shorter survival time. In addition, mutations in *MPL* or *TET2* do not appear to influence overall or leukemia-free survival. A number of investigators have attempted to correlate the presence of a variety of additional mutations with disease outcomes. See Table 70.2 for a list of documented recurrent acquired mutations associated with MF. *EZH2* mutations have been identified in 6% of patients with PMF, 3% of PV patients, 3% of patients with post-PV MF, and 9.4% of patients with post-ET MF. More than 40% of the patients with *EZH2* mutations were *JAK2V617F*-positive, 6% have a *TET2* mutation, and, 22% harbored an *ASXL* mutation. Concurrent *EZH2* mutations and *MPL* mutations have not been observed. *EZH2* mutations are usually present at the diagnosis of chronic MPN and are maintained universally in the leukemic blasts at the time of transformation to AML. *EZH2*-mutated patients are characterized by more profound leukocytosis and larger spleens, and have a higher percentage of blasts. The survival of patients with *EZH2* mutations was clearly inferior because they are clustered in patients with high-risk IPSS scores. In addition, IDH mutations, albeit rare in PMF patients, have been associated with inferior survival in *JAK2V617F*-positive patients, raising the possibility of the cooperation between *IDH* mutations and *JAK2V617F* in leukemic transformation.

Therapy

The treatment of the PMF patient was thought until recently to be largely a futile exercise, but with reports of curative nonmyeloablative (MA) aSCT for a subpopulation of PMF patients, and the approval of a small-molecule JAK2 inhibitor that is effective in reducing the degree of splenomegaly and alleviating systemic symptoms, therapy for PMF patients has become much more effective. The therapeutic strategies employed for an individual patient are currently based on an assessment of the patient's clinical characteristics, performance status, and prognosis estimated using one of the prognostic scoring systems described above. A conservative approach to management is generally recommended for low-risk patients, with observation of asymptomatic patients and therapeutic intervention reserved for patients with intermediate/high-risk disease or individuals with especially burdensome symptoms.[10]

In general, therapy is indicated for PMF patients with the following conditions: symptoms attributable to anemia, pressure symptoms related to splenomegaly, bleeding problems, life-threatening thrombocytopenia, significant hyperuricemia, bone pain, systemic symptoms (fevers, night sweats, and weight loss), and portal hypertension and life-threatening gastrointestinal bleeding. Hyperuricemia should be aggressively treated in all patients with PMF. Hydration and chronic administration of allopurinol (300 mg/day) are suggested.

Patients with the prefibrotic form of MF or low-risk MF, particularly if they are young, are particularly challenging for most physicians. These patients are largely asymptomatic but are at a risk of their disease eventually evolving to a symptomatic form of MF or acute leukemia. Many patients are eager to entertain options that might prevent the evolution of such disease but at present there is no data to indicate that any approach can successively achieve this goal. Also aSCT is not an option for such patients due to the morbidity and mortality associated with its implementation. During the last decade several investigators have promoted IFN-α therapy as an agent that might be capable of delaying disease progression by decreasing the rate of fibrosis if administered chronically during the early course of this disease. Others have not reported such effects in patients with more advanced phases of the disease. In one series, only four of 11 patients were able to complete 1 year of therapy; the other seven patients discontinued the drug because of unacceptable toxicity or the development of severe cytopenias. A clinically significant improvement (degree of BM fibrosis, osteosclerosis, or angiogenesis) was not observed in any of these patients. A small phase II pilot study in PMF patients demonstrated responses in patients with a prefibrotic form of PMF treated with low doses of IFN-α-2b over an extended period (median duration: 3 years). Four patients with *JAK2V617F*-positive PMF were followed over time, and although each had clinical responses, only one had a significant reduction in mutant allele burden. The drug was generally well tolerated at doses between 1 and 2 million units weekly, and responses in the BM included reduction in the degree of reticulin fibrosis and abnormal cellular morphology. Eleven patients with PMF were treated with a pegylated form of IFN-α-2b (PEG-IFN-α-2b) at starting dose between 2 and 3 μg/kg/week; only a single patient responded. Although the pegylated form of this drug allows for weekly injections, the toxicity profile was found to be similar to the standard formulation and for many patients limited the duration of therapy. The most common grade 3/4 toxicity was fatigue and thrombocytopenia. Because of the recent encouraging results reported with PEG-IFN-α-2a (Pegasys) in PV patients, this form of IFN-α has also been evaluated in MF patients. The French Groupe d'Etudes des Myelofibrosis (GEM) and France Intergroupe des Syndromes Myeloproliferatifs conducted a study of 18 patients with PMF and post-ET/PV MF treated with Pegasys. Of the four PMF patients included in this study, one had a complete response, two had a minor response, and one had no response. Responses were associated with improvement in the degree of anemia, leukocytosis, and thrombocytosis, but not splenomegaly, and appeared to be irrespective of JAK2 status. Comprehensive reviews of the literature suggest that modest benefits may be derived from IFN-α therapy for PMF after patients have entered the more advanced phases of the disease. Further large randomized studies are warranted in patients with the prefibrotic phase of PMF to determine the effects of this modality of treatment on disease-free survival, OS, quality of life, and progression to more advanced phases of PMF or evolution to acute leukemia. Before such trials are completed, IFN therapy at any phase of PMF should be considered an experimental form of therapy and not embarked upon unless the patient is participating in a clinical trial.[11]

Treatment of the Anemic Patient

Anemia is a common problem in patients with PMF. It is usually multifactorial in origin; contributing factors are folate deficiency, iron deficiency, ineffective erythropoiesis, erythroid hypoplasia, increased clearance, and hemolysis. Patients with documented nutritional deficiencies should receive folate, iron supplementation, or both. Transfusion therapy with packed RBCs is clearly indicated in patients who are symptomatic from their anemia. Chronic transfusion therapy is frequently required, and the clinician should try to attain a hemoglobin level at which symptoms resolve. Long-term transfusion therapy potentially may lead to the development of iron-overload syndrome. It remains unclear if iron chelation provides a meaningful clinical benefit to patients with MF and the justification of the use of this therapy has mostly been extrapolated from the MDS literature and case reports. Low-dose dexamethasone has been reported to be useful in the treatment of patients with transfusion-dependent PMF.

Corticosteroids (e.g., prednisone 1 mg/kg/day taken orally) have also been successfully used for treatment of the hemolytic anemia associated with PMF. Other therapeutic options for PMF-associated hemolytic anemia can include therapy with intravenous immunoglobulins and recombinant human erythropoietin-α (rHuEPO). Recently, retrospective analysis of single-agent prednisone therapy for 30 intermediate-2 or high-risk PMF patients with anemia/thrombocytopenia was published. The initial dose was 0.5–1 mg/kg daily, with tapering to the minimum effective dose in responders. Twelve patients (40%) achieved an anemia response by IWG-MRT criteria. The median response duration was 12.3 months. Patients with constitutional symptoms or >2% circulating blasts had a lower response rate. Median survival from the initiation of prednisone therapy was significantly longer in anemia responders (5.0 years vs. 1.5 years, $p = .002$). Additional information that supports the use of corticosteroids for the treatment of MF-related anemia is derived from a prospective clinical trial that was constructed to evaluate the efficacy of the immunomodulatory agent, pomalidomide. This study surprisingly revealed that prednisone alone can induce significant responses in unselected MF patients with severe anemia. In this randomized study, the active control arm that included 21 patients consisted of prednisone (30 mg/day during the first 28-day cycle, 15 mg/day the second cycle, 15 mg every other day the third cycle) plus placebo (up to 12 cycles). Overall, four out of 16 (25%) patients assigned to the control arm who completed three cycles of treatment achieved anemia response according to the IWG-MRT criteria. Three of the four responses were short-lived, lasting between 2.3 and 5.5 months. These data are similar to our own experience indicating that prednisone therapy can improve the anemia and thrombocytopenia associated with PMF even after the failure of standard therapies.

It is important to be aware that the hemolytic anemia in patients with PMF may also rarely be a consequence of a coexisting secondary form of paroxysmal nocturnal hemoglobinuria that can be responsive to eculizumab therapy (see Chapter 32). Furthermore, patients with PMF who receive multiple transfusions are candidates for developing delayed hemolytic transfusion reactions that occasionally may be severe and persistent. The direct antiglobulin test result is usually positive in this setting. It is generally believed that additional transfusions in these patients with delayed hemolytic transfusion reactions should be avoided if possible.

Anemia caused by erythroid cell hypoplasia as well as ineffective erythropoiesis in PMF may respond to anabolic steroids. A good response, as defined by a decrease or total avoidance of transfusion therapy, occurs in about 20–40% of patients. A course of 3–6 months of androgen therapy is indicated to identify responsive patients, but the development of hepatic dysfunction or virilizing side effects may limit long-term androgen administration. Patients with associated chromosomal abnormalities have been reported to be less likely to respond to androgen therapy. Danazol, a synthetic attenuated androgen, has also been useful in reducing the requirement for RBC transfusion support and correction of thrombocytopenia in 20–40% of treated patients in several series. Variables associated with response were lack of transfusion requirement and higher hemoglobin levels. The experience with the use of rHuEPO in PMF has been reviewed by Cervantes and colleagues in a total of 51 patients, documenting that 28 (55%) of these patients responded to rHuEPO treatment, including 16 complete and 12 partial responses. Endogenous serum EPO levels inappropriately low for the degree of anemia is predictive of a favorable response to rHuEPO. Serum EPO levels below 125 U/L were found to be associated with a favorable response to rHuEPO therapy. Responses can be associated with a limited enlargement of the spleen.

The use of darbepoetin, a novel hyperglycosylated erythropoiesis-stimulating protein, has been reported in 20 PMF patients. With an initial weekly dose of 150 µg, increased to 300 µg, when no response was observed after 4–8 weeks, eight patients (40%) responded to treatment, including six complete and two partial responses, and five maintained their response after a median follow-up of 12 months (range: 4–22 months). The median time to response was 2 months. Univariate analysis indicated that older age was the only factor associated with a favorable response to treatment ($p < .006$). None of the patients with elevated serum EPO levels responded. Treatment was usually well tolerated, and patients can be successfully switched from rHuEPO to darbepoetin.

Multiple trials have explored the use of thalidomide in the treatment of anemia in PMF based on the drug's antiangiogenic, immunomodulatory, and antiinflammatory actions. A pooled analysis of five small phase II studies indicated that 29% of patients with moderate to severe anemia experience an increase in hemoglobin or reduction or elimination of blood transfusion requirements with thalidomide therapy at a standard dose of 200–800 mg/day. Nevertheless, most of the patients treated with these doses had adverse effects that resulted in an attrition rate of greater than 50% after 3 months. Moreover, increases of WBC numbers or platelet counts were frequently reported to be associated with such serious adverse events as pericardial effusions secondary to myeloid metaplasia. Using a dose-escalation design and starting with a low dose of thalidomide (50 mg/day), 31% of patients with transfusion-dependent anemia were reported to experience a response after treatment. A combination of low-dose thalidomide (50 mg/day) with prednisone has been reported to be a better-tolerated regimen and equally or more effective than standard-dose treatment. This regimen also had a significant effect on the degree of thrombocytopenia and resulted in a reduction in the degree of splenomegaly in almost 10% of the patients. These responses were frequently maintained after therapy was halted. Higher doses of thalidomide were not more effective than lower doses. A prospective phase IIB, randomized, double-blind, multicenter trial compared therapy with 200–400 mg of thalidomide with placebo and documented that in the thalidomide group, only 10 out of 26 patients completed 6 months of treatment and that no difference was observed between the thalidomide and placebo groups as regards to improvement of hemoglobin levels or reduction of the number of RBC transfusion required. In addition, experience with thalidomide therapy in a two-stage phase II dose-escalation trial in 44 patients with advanced PMF has been reported. Starting at 200 mg/day and increasing to 800 mg as tolerated, the median tolerated dose was 400 mg for a median duration of 3 months, and 20% of the patients experienced improvement in their degree of anemia (21% became transfusion independent). A more potent thalidomide analog, lenalidomide, was evaluated in 68 symptomatic patients with PMF at two institutions. Oral lenalidomide was administered at a dose of 10 mg/day if the platelet count was greater than 100,000/mm³ or at a dose of 5 mg/day if the platelet count was less than 100,000/mm³ for 3–4 months. The overall response rates were 22% for patients with anemia, 33% for patients with splenomegaly, and 50% for thrombocytopenia. Several patients normalized their hemoglobin levels or became RBC transfusion independent. The most common associated toxicities were grade 3 and 4 neutropenia and thrombocytopenia, which occurred in approximately 30% of patients but resolved with discontinuation of therapy. In several patients with del(5)(q31)-associated PMF or post-PV MF, lenalidomide therapy was associated with reduction of the numbers of cells with a marker chromosome as assayed by FISH and reduction of the *JAK2V617F* burden. Lenalidomide therapy in combination with prednisone therapy in PMF has been evaluated in a phase II trial within the Eastern Cooperative Oncology Group and appears to be modestly active and myelosuppressive. Forty two MF patients with anemia were treated with lenalidomide at 10 mg/day in combination with a 3-month prednisone taper. Grade 3 and higher myelotoxicity was noted in 88% of patients, and a response rate of 23% by IWG-MRT was obtained (19% clinical improvement in anemia or 10% clinical improvement in spleen size). Whether either of these immunomodulatory drugs (IMiDs) is superior to the other is the subject of speculation, which would require a large randomized clinical trial. The mechanism by which these agents achieve these clinical responses also remains of larger speculation.

Because IMiDs as a class have shown activity in MF and their use is often undermined by neurotoxicity or myelosuppression, recent interest in the structurally related but more potent pomalidomide in the treatment of MF-associated anemia has led to the completion of several early-phase studies and a randomized phase III study. The first study to evaluate the response of pomalidomide in MF was a phase II randomized, double-blind, placebo-controlled adaptive design study with four treatment arms. This study reported an overall response in anemia of 24% (10 patients), and 15 of these patients achieved transfusion independence that was durable at 7.5 months. Pomalidomide at 0.5 mg/day with or without a prednisone taper was found to have better anemia responses with less toxicity compared with pomalidomide at 2 mg/day with or without prednisone. Grade 3/4 myelosuppression and neurotoxicity were not frequent adverse events. A single-center phase II study of low-dose pomalidomide was conducted at Mayo Clinic. A cohort of 58 patients were treated with pomalidomide at 0.5 mg/day. Of the 42 transfusion-dependent *JAK2V617F*-positive MF patients, 10 had significant responses in anemia, with nine patients achieving transfusion independence. Although there were no spleen responses, a 58% response in thrombocytopenia for those with baseline platelets below 100×10^9 cells/L was noted. The anemia response was predicted by peripheral blood basophilia within the first month of therapy and the absence of massive splenomegaly, and was restricted to MF patients who were *JAK2V617F* positive. Pomalidomide was also evaluated in a dose-escalation phase I/II setting with the purpose of determining if higher doses of pomalidomide were more effective in reversing the anemia associated with MF. Doses of 3 mg/day given for 21 out of 28 consecutive days were found to be the maximum tolerated dose, and myelosuppression the dose-limiting toxicity without any added response in anemia. The placebo-controlled, randomized, phase III RESUME trial compared pomalidomide at 0.5 mg/day with prednisone with an opportunity to cross over, and were enrolled both *JAK2* mutated and WT MF patients with documented anemia. The primary endpoint of anemia response was not met in this large global trial; however, 21% of patients achieved clinical improvement in platelet count. Whether this trial would have had positive results if eligibility had been restricted to MF patients with *JAK2V617F* and limited splenomegaly, remains conjecture. The responses to prednisone therapy in anemic MF patients have been previously discussed and raise the possibility that this was not the appropriate control group in this randomized pomalidomide study.

Treatment of Spleen-Related and Systemic Symptoms

Pressure symptoms caused by splenic enlargement have been treated historically with cytotoxic chemotherapy. Busulfan, melphalan, and hydroxyurea have each been used for this purpose. A significant reduction in spleen size with relief of pressure symptoms occurs in occasional patients receiving chemotherapy.[4] Responses are unfortunately short lived, lasting a median of only 4.5 months. Only 16%

of patients with long-term maintenance therapy enjoy sustained relief of symptoms. Hematologic toxicity often necessitates cessation of therapy. Inhibition of the activated JAK-STAT pathway is an attractive therapeutic target in PMF and has led to the development of oral small-molecule inhibitors. Ruxolitinib, a selective JAK1 and JAK2 tyrosine kinase inhibitor, was approved in 2011 for the treatment of patients with MF; this is the first drug approved by the United States Food and Drug Administration (US FDA) where the indication for use is intermediate- or high-risk MF. The phase I/II study determined the optimal starting dose of 15 mg twice daily, and that thrombocytopenia and worsening anemia were dose-limiting toxicities. A dose-dependent suppression of phospho-STAT3 was seen in both WT and mutated *JAK2* patients treated with ruxolitinib, demonstrating that drug activity does not discriminate between mutated and WT *JAK2* in its inhibitory activity. Fifty two percent of treated patients achieved a greater than 50% reduction in splenomegaly for greater than 12 months, which was irrespective of their *JAK2* mutational status. The debilitating symptoms associated with MF were dramatically improved, and this was correlated with reduction in inflammatory cytokines believed to be mediated through inhibition of JAK1 signaling. This compound was then evaluated in two randomized phase III trials, COMFORT 1 (United States, Canada, and Australia), in which ruxolitinib therapy was compared with a placebo control, and COMFORT 2 trial (Europe), in which ruxolitinib therapy was compared with the best available therapy.[12,13] The results of each of these trials are remarkably similar, and each trial was adequately powered. Patients with intermediate-2 or high-risk MF as assessed using the IPSS were eligible regardless of *JAK2* mutational status. All patients had platelet counts over 100×10^9/L and had a spleen palpated at least 5 cm below the left costal margin. In COMFORT 1, the primary endpoint of 35% or greater reduction in spleen volume was met at 24 weeks in 41.9% of the ruxolitinib-treated cohort and only 0.7% in the placebo group. This response was maintained 48 weeks or more in 67% of treated patients. Fig. 70.10 shows the percent change in spleen volume from baseline at week 24 for individual patients on both arms of this trial and depicts the contrast of spleen reduction in ruxolitinib-treated patients compared with the majority of patients in the placebo arm who had an increase in spleen volume. There were 13 deaths in the ruxolitinib arm and 24 deaths in the placebo arm, revealing a modest survival benefit for MF patients treated with ruxolitinib. Although grade 3/4 anemia and

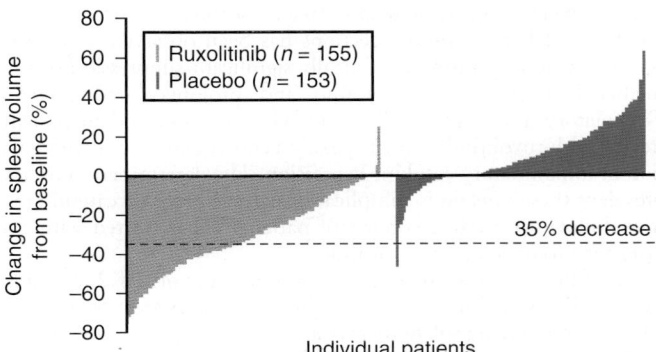

Fig. 70.10 REDUCTION IN SPLENIC VOLUME WITH RUXOLITINIB THERAPY IN THE COMFORT I TRIAL. The waterfall plot shows the percent change from baseline in spleen volume at week 24 (in 139 patients in the ruxolitinib group and 106 in the placebo group) or at the last evaluation before week 24 (in 16 patients in the ruxolitinib group and 47 in the placebo group). Data for one patient with a missing baseline value are not included on the graph. Most patients in the ruxolitinib group (150 out of 155) had a reduction in spleen volume, but most patients in the placebo group had either an increase in spleen volume (102 out of 153 patients) or no change (15 out of 153 patients). *(From Verstovsek S, Mesa RA, Gotlib J, et al: A double-blind, placebo-controlled trial of ruxolitinib for myelofibrosis. N Engl J Med 366:799, 2012.)*

thrombocytopenia were frequent in the ruxolitinib arm (45.2% and 12.9%, respectively), discontinuation for these events was extremely rare. The primary endpoint in the COMFORT-2 trial was met at 48 weeks, with 28% of patients in the ruxolitinib arm and 0% in the BAT arm achieving at least a 35% reduction in spleen volume. The mean length of palpable spleen decreased by 56% at 48 weeks compared with an increase of 4% in the BAT arm. Sophisticated disease-specific quality-of-life tools were used to evaluate the effects of ruxolitinib therapy on the systemic symptoms that have been presumed to be a consequence of the increased elaboration of inflammatory cytokines modulated by JAK1 signaling. The effects of ruxolitinib were, however, limited in that reversal of histomorphologic abnormalities, including BM fibrosis or osteosclerosis, significant reduction in the *JAK2V617F* allele burden, and loss of marker cytogenetic abnormalities indicating that the underlying malignant potential of PMF is not affected by this therapy. In addition, abrupt discontinuation of ruxolitinib therapy was associated with rapid return to baseline levels of splenomegaly and severity of the systemic symptoms that at times can be disabling. More gradual tapering of this agent or the use of a short steroid taper is recommended to avoid this complication. Ruxolitinib is an important agent for the palliation of symptomatic splenomegaly and the debilitating symptoms seen in patients with PMF. The survival data from the COMFORT 1 trial, although modest, are intriguing and suggest that even if an appreciable impact on abnormal BM histopathology or molecular or cytogenetic responses is not seen with ruxolitinib, pharmacologic suppression of the JAK pathway decreases the risk of death, perhaps simply by improving the overall performance status, and reversing cancer cachexia of an individual. The use of ruxolitinib has been demonstrated to be safe is patients with a minimum platelet count of 50×10^9/L. The need to treat patients who are asymptomatic with limited splenomegaly is not apparent since treatment does not appear to affect the underlying malignant disorder. With a median follow-up of 3 years, the mature results of the COMFORT-1 trial demonstrate a durable response in spleen reduction and symptom improvement in those subjects that remain on treatment. The absence of new/unexpected toxicities or late-onset emergent hematologic adverse events was also appreciated. However, it should be noted that a 50% discontinuation rate was reported in the arm originally randomized to ruxolitnib, and the potential for leukemic transformation with sites of extramedullary leukemia have also been reported. Patients treated with ruxolitinib have been noted to have an increased incidence of infectious complications, including toxoplasmosis, cryptoccocal pneumonia, reactivation of latent herpes simplex virus and hepatitis B, and disseminated tuberculosis. An almost threefold increase in the incidence of herpes zoster infections has been observed, suggesting that the drug may promote clinically significant suppression of cell-mediated immunity. A profound and prolonged reduction in T-regulatory and natural killer cells has been observed in patients treated with ruxolitinib, which is likely a consequence of downregulation of inflammatory cytokine expression. The determination of how prevalent these infectious complications are will require careful long-term follow-up of large cohorts of patients being treated with this drug for prolonged periods of time.

A number of other small-molecule inhibitors of JAK2 are under various phases of clinical development, and all appear to be generally effective in reducing splenomegaly and improving symptom burden. It is important to note that none of the currently tested JAK2 inhibitors have been shown to clearly achieve complete BM pathologic responses or induce cytogenetic/molecular remissions. Additionally, data to support the superiority of one agent over another do not exist. Momelotinib (JAK1/JAK2 inhibitor) and pacritinib (JAK2/FLT3 inhibitor) are currently being evaluated in phase III registration trials, and have the potential to be used as either first-line agents in ruxolitinib-naïve patients with significant baseline cytopenias, or as second-line agents for patients experiencing ruxolitinib-associated cytopenias or loss of clinical response. These agents have different target specificities and toxicity profiles, and require further evaluation in mature clinical trials to ultimately determine their utility in comparison to ruxolitinib.

Phase I/II data of momelotinib (CYT387, Gilead) in patients with MF is notable for the potential durable anemia response reported (70% transfusion independence). Headache and elevated lipase levels were determined to be the dose limiting toxicities of momelotinib treatment. Pacritinib (SB1518, CTI Biopharma) has been evaluated in a phase I/II trial in which treatment-emergent myelosuppression was limited and appears to be effective in safely reducing splenomegaly in patients with low baseline platelet levels. The results of the phase III PERSIST-1 trial were recently presented and confirmed the beneficial effects of this JAK2/FLT3 inhibitor in 327 ruxolitinib-naïve, intermediate/high-risk MF patients with any baseline platelet count. Compared with the best available therapy arms (excluding ruxolitinib), pacritinib was superior in achieving the primary endpoint of spleen reduction (19.1% vs. 4.7%) without a significant increase in hematologic toxicity. Gastrointestinal toxicity was more frequently observed with pacritinib therapy (diarrhea 50%) but mostly grade 1/2 and not a frequent reason for drug discontinuation. Additionally, RBC transfusion independence was achieved in 25% of transfusion-dependent patients at baseline. Fedratinib (SAR302503, Sanofi Aventis) was a selective JAK2 inhibitor with positive results reported in two phase III trials conducted in MF patients, but was unfortunately found to be associated with the emergence of Wernicke encephalopathy in several patients. This drug is no longer in clinical development and joins several other JAK2 inhibitors that are no longer being tested due to concerns regarding treatment-related toxicity such as XL019, AZD1480, and BMS-911543.

Splenic irradiation has frequently been used in the past for treatment of the painful large-spleen syndrome, but is now considered a last-resort option with the approval of JAK1/2 inhibitor therapy. Irradiation in fractions of 0.15–1 Gy administered daily or by an intermittent fractionation schedule (i.e., two or three times a week) to a total dose per treatment course of 2.5–6.5 Gy may be effective. Responses are transient, lasting an average of 3.5 months, and hematopoietic toxicity is frequently significant. Splenic irradiation is especially useful for treatment of splenic pain of sudden onset and for treatment of ascites caused by implants of hematopoietic tissue. Radiation therapy should be considered as a temporary measure to be used in patients who are too ill to tolerate splenectomy or chemotherapy. Splenic irradiation is limited by myelosuppression with significant prolonged cytopenias, which is not predictable and is not correlated with the doses of radiation administered.

Radiotherapy offers a viable treatment option and sometimes may be the therapy of choice for the treatment of patients with symptomatic hepatomegaly, peritoneal and pleural implants or pulmonary infiltration leading to ascites or pleural effusions, and EMH in vital organs leading to organ dysfunction. Because of the inherent sensitivity of myeloid tissue to radiation and profound BM suppression that may occur after irradiation, therapy is usually initiated at low doses (20–25 cGy/day), with modification of the dose as the clinical situation dictates. An alternative approach using intraperitoneal administration of cytosine arabinoside has been used to treat ascites in PMF. Low-dose, single-fraction, whole-lung radiotherapy has also been useful in treating pulmonary artery hypertension associated with PMF.

Splenectomy remains a viable option even in the face of the recent availability of JAK2 inhibitors in patients with hemolysis, thrombocytopenia, painful splenomegaly, recurrent splenic infarction, and portal hypertension refractory to other therapeutic modalities or in individuals with leukopenia or thrombocytopenia that prevents one from resorting to therapy with chemotherapeutic agents or a JAK2 inhibitor. Splenectomy in patients with PMF is associated with a postoperative morbidity rate of 15–30% and a mortality rate of almost 10%. The appropriate implementation of splenectomy can result in the improved quality of life of PMF patients who frequently do not have other therapeutic options available. Because splenectomy is associated with significant morbidity and mortality, the physician should only resort to this strategy if thrombocytopenia, anemia, or symptomatic splenomegaly is unresponsive to less invasive approaches such as JAK2 inhibitor treatment. Progressive hepatomegaly and marked thrombocytosis occurred, respectively, in 16% and 22% of patients after splenectomy and can be controlled with ruxolitinib therapy.

Allogeneic Stem Cell Transplantation

aSCT is a potentially curative option in patients with PMF who have an appropriate donor available. Successful transplantation is associated with gradual resolution of BM fibrosis, reduction in splenomegaly, and normalization of hematopoiesis (see box on Algorithm for Selection of Appropriate Patients for Stem Cell Transplantation Stratified According to Risk Status).

Most of our understanding of the role of aSCT in primary and post-PV/ET MF with conventional MA conditioning regimens comes from two retrospective series of transplants with more than 50 patients performed between 1979 and 2002. The median age of transplanted patients was 42 and 43 years; treatment-related mortality (TRM) was 27% and 33%, with 5-year survival of 47% and 58%, respectively. The 5-year probability of treatment failure caused by nonengraftment, relapse or persistent disease after transplantation was 36%, and the failure of sustained engraftment was 10.7%, which occurred solely in patients receiving BM transplants from mismatched or unrelated donors. The probability of grade III–IV acute graft-versus-host disease (GVHD) was 33% and 21%, and extensive chronic GVHD was 35% and 50%, respectively. Older age and factors associated with more advanced disease (Hg <10, increased number of RBC transfusions, presence of osteomyelosclerosis, increased number of clonal abnormalities) adversely affected the outcome. The Seattle group has updated their 15-year experience with 95 PMF and post-PV/ET MF patients who received MA busulfan and/or TBI-containing regimens. The 7-year actual survival rate was 61%, although 10% of patients died of recurrent or a persistent disease. Non-TBI–containing regimen of targeted busulfan/cytoxan resulted in an improved probability of survival of 68%. These retrospective reports of MA allo-HSCT in PMF provided evidence that engraftment can be achieved and that a complete and durable remission of the disease can occur in approximately 50% of patients. However, owing to the poor transplant outcomes in older patients, enrollment to this procedure represents a major therapeutic dilemma in PMF patients who are primarily diagnosed at ages in excess of 60 years.

The advent of non-MA, reduced-intensity conditioning (RIC) regimens for aSCT has resulted in decreased TRM and has expanded the use of this treatment modality to older patients. Rondelli and coworkers provided one of the initial retrospective reports on the outcome of 21 intermediate- to high-risk PMF patients (without leukemic transformation) with a median age of 54 years (range: 27–68 years) who underwent RIC preparation and utilized a peripheral blood stem cell (PBSC) source in 18 cases and related donors in 18 cases. This trial was conducted at multiple institutions belonging to the MPD-Research Consortium (MPD-RC). Predominantly fludarabine-based RIC regimens allowed engraftment in all but one patient with TRM of 10% and 2-year OS rates of 87%. Durable remission was achieved in 17 out of 18 patients alive 12–122 months (median: 31 months) after transplant. Three patients relapsed, with two of them able to achieve remission following second transplantation and donor lymphocyte infusion. Thirty three percent of patients developed acute GVHD grades II–IV (9% grade III–IV), and 72% developed chronic GVHD, with 44% being extensive.

Recent CIBMTR retrospective data derived from an analysis of 223 patients who underwent RIC fludarabine-based allogeneic transplantation between 1997 and 2010 showed the probability of 5-year survival to be 47%. Donor type was the only significant factor to impact survival, with 5-year OS in the related donor arm of 56% versus matched unrelated donor of 48% and mismatched unrelated donor of 34%. A trend toward decreased mortality was observed in patients with low/intermediate-1 DIPSS score versus intermediate-2/high-risk DIPSS.

The use of RIC PBSC transplantation in patients with advanced MF has been evaluated prospectively in two phase II trials by the European Group for Blood and Marrow Transplantation (EBMT)

and MPD-RC. An EBMT trial included 103 MF patients transplanted from related (n = 33) or unrelated donors (n = 70), with 21% of donors having at least one allele or antigen mismatch using a fludarabine/busulfan/ATG regimen. Although all but two patients achieved initial engraftment, secondary graft failure or poor graft function occurred in 11% of patients. The estimated 5-year event-free survival (EFS) and OS was 51% and 67%, respectively. One-year nonrelapse mortality was 16%—similar among related and unrelated donor transplants but significantly higher in mismatched transplants (38% vs. 12%). One third of patients developed grade II–IV acute GVHD (11% grade III–IV), with half of patients affected by chronic GVHD (24% extensive). Relapse rate/treatment failure at 3 and 5 years was 22% and 29%, respectively. As can be seen in Fig. 70.11, age over 55 years, human leukocyte antigen (HLA) mismatching, and advanced disease are associated with decreased PFS and OS. However, even in this high-risk group, the OS was approximately 40%. Remarkably, patients younger than 55 years of age had a 5-year OS rate of 82%. Elimination of JAK2V617F after transplant was associated with a reduced incidence of relapse.

The prospective, multicenter phase II MPD-RC 101 trial included two parallel cohorts of patients: related donors (n = 32, 94% HLA matched) and unrelated donors (n = 34, 74% HLA matched). Fludarabine/melphalan was used as a conditioning regimen with rabbit anti-thymocyte globulin (rATG) added in the unrelated donor group. Patient characteristics were similar in the two groups, with 63 out of 66 patients having intermediate- to high-risk disease based on Lille score. After a median of 25 months follow-up, OS was 75% (median not reached) in the related donor cohort and 32% (median: 6 months) in the unrelated donor. Nonrelapse mortality at 59% was significantly higher in the unrelated group compared with 22% in the related group. Graft failure occurred in 36% (24% primary) of unrelated transplants and 6% (3% primary) of related. The unrelated cohort had double the rate of severe acute GVHD grade III–IV (21% vs. 12%) but comparable rates of chronic GVHD (38% vs. 36%), including extensive form (20% vs. 25%). Patients who were able to achieve sustained stem cell engraftment experienced an overall response rate of 93% in the related group and 69% in the unrelated group, with only four patients experiencing progression of disease. Neither disease diagnosis (primary or secondary MF), HLA mismatch, presence of JAK2V617F mutation, nor age >57 years showed a statistically significant effect on survival. The only factor that correlated with improved survival was related donor type, as seen in Fig. 70.12. The low/intermediate-1–risk patients in the unrelated group had better survival than the intermediate-2/high-risk patients, whereas there was no difference in survival between these two DIPSS groups in the related group.

The German group has analyzed the effect of multiple risk factors related to patient, disease, and transplant characteristics on survival after RIC SCT and developed a predictive model based on three risk factors: age ≥57, JAK2 WT status, and presence of constitutional symptoms. Five-year OS in the absence of any risk factors was 90%. The presence of one or two risk factors reduced 5-year OS to 74% and 51%, respectively. Patients who had all three risk factors did extremely poorly after RIC SCT, with a 1-year OS of 25%. Despite inferior outcomes in older patients, SCT is feasible, as demonstrated by a retrospective study of aSCT of 30 PMF patients between the ages of 60 and 78 (median: 65) years transplanted at four major United States academic centers with 3-year OS and PFS rates of 45% and 40%, respectively.

One of the limitations of widely applying aSCT to more patients with PMF is the lack of access to appropriate donors. Takagi and coworkers from Japan reported surprisingly positive results with umbilical cord blood (UCB) grafts for RIC allogeneic transplantation in adults (median age: 57.5 years) with various hematologic disorders associated with extensive BM fibrosis (PMF, post-MPN AML, and MDS-related AML). The estimated probability of survival at 4 years for this group was 28.6%, which is modest but considerably superior to that which would be anticipated with presently available chemotherapy regimens for such high-risk disease. Retrospective analysis of 35 high-risk MF patients (20% blast-phase myelofibrosis, median

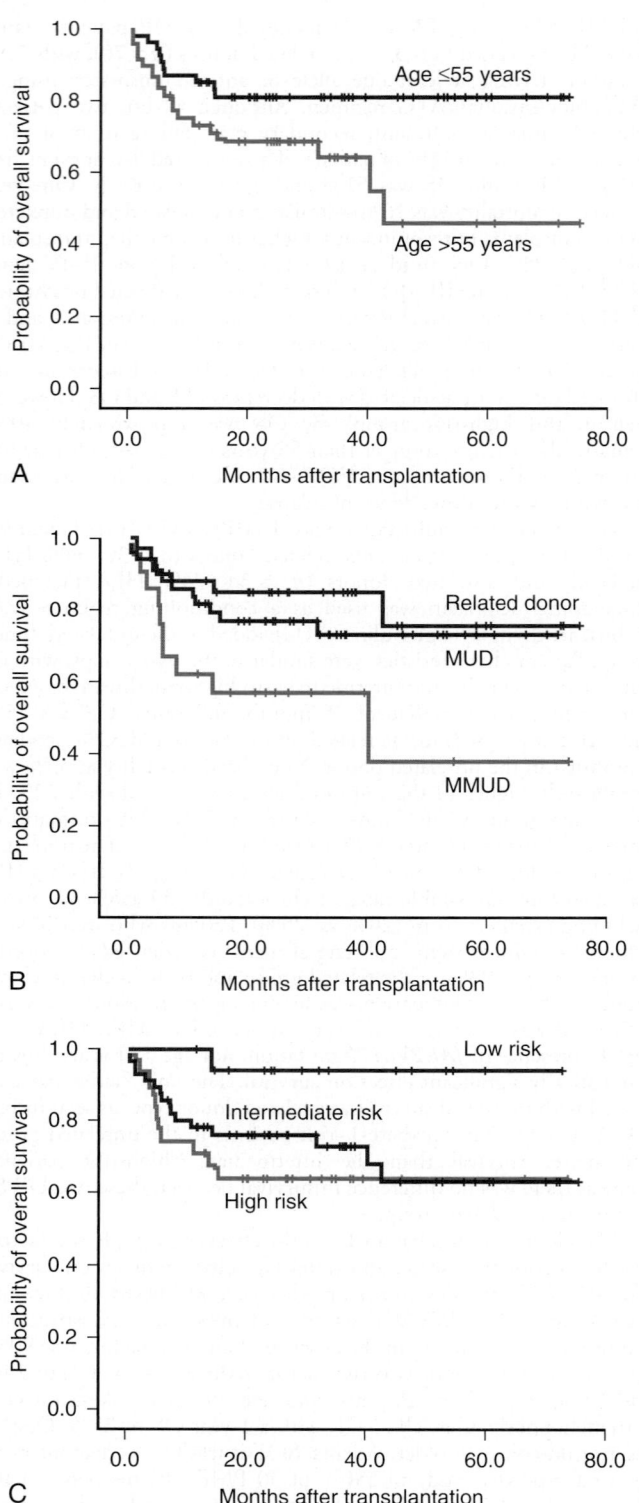

Fig. 70.11 Survival of patients with myelofibrosis after reduced-intensity allogeneic stem cell transplantation according to age (A), donor (B), and Lille risk profile (C). *MMUD*, mismatched unrelated donor; *MUD*, matched unrelated donor.

age: 54 years) who underwent UCB transplantation reported to Eurocord showed a 2-year OS and EFS of 44% and 30%, respectively. Conditioning using TBI, cyclophosphamide and fludarabine was associated with the best results in terms of blood count recovery and EFS. These studies provide the rationale for the further evaluation of RIC allogeneic transplant for eligible PMF patients lacking an HLA-matched sibling or unrelated donor with the use of alternative sources of grafts such as UCB or possibly haploidentical donors.

Occasionally, patients with PMF after allogeneic transplant can experience relapse of their underlying disease, failure of engraftment, or graft failure. Relapse can frequently be treated with donor lymphocyte infusions. Second RIC allogeneic transplants should be considered for individuals who do not respond to donor lymphocyte infusions or experience difficulty with engraftment or late graft failure. In *JAK2V617F*-positive patients, monitoring allele burden following SCT can help predict patients at risk for relapse and prompt early intervention. The feasibility of utilizing aSCT as the front-line therapy for all intermediate- and high-risk patients is limited by the presence of competing comorbidities or a poor performance status due to the systemic effects of the underlying PMF. Although the JAK2 inhibitors are largely palliative, they do reduce the degree of splenomegaly and often improve the performance status of such patients, frequently resulting in weight gain, and improve their candidacy for transplant. The reported outcomes with JAK2 inhibitor therapy as a component of the conditioning regimen for allogeneic transplantation have resulted in conflicting results, and will require rigorous testing to determine its effect on immediate and long-term survival and transplant-related complications. This approach is currently being evaluated within the MPD-RC as a phase II trial of preconditioning ruxolitinib treatment (MPD-RC 114).

The fact that allogeneic RIC transplant is curative in appropriate patients is undeniable, and the improvements in the design of conditioning regimens and supportive therapy make this a viable first-line approach for individuals with HLA-matched donors and advanced disease. Whether such an approach should also be implemented in patients with earlier phases of the disease is a point of contention that requires further careful investigation. This decision is especially important in young patients with early forms of PMF because their disease is likely to eventually progress, and the best results with allogeneic transplant have been reported in lower risk patients, especially if they do not have a related donor. The flaw in the argument to proceed with immediate transplant in young patients with early PMF is the exposure to significant mortality and morbidity in a patient population that frequently can anticipate a decade or more of a good-quality life with no or minimal therapeutic interventions. New molecular markers such as *JAK2V617F*, *EZH2*, *ASXL1*, and *CALR* mutations will help further refine risk stratification and likely better guide treatment decision.

Many unresolved issues remain to be clarified concerning the optimal strategy for aSCT in PMF. The need for splenectomy before aSCT remains a major issue. Splenectomy before aHSCT in PMF results in faster hematopoietic recovery but at the cost of potentially prolonged and complicated postoperative recovery. Although some analyses suggest improved survival with pretransplant splenectomy, it has also been associated with a potential increased risk of relapse. Moreover, even extensive splenomegaly (>30-cm longitudinal size by computed tomography scan) does not appear to prolong hematologic reconstitution after transplant.

The establishment of valid complete remission criteria of PMF after aSCT remains a major issue because the conventional criteria for response after aSCT are often influenced by GVHD, infections, or poor graft function, and cannot be used. Conversely, normal blood counts and disappearance of disease-related symptoms do not exclude residual disease. In *JAK2V617F*-positive patients, the mutational allele burden following transplantation may serve as a surrogate parameter for complete remission assessment and as a guide for instituting adoptive immunotherapy.

Investigational Therapeutic Options

The identification of various epigenetic defects in PMF has provided novel therapeutic targets, and preclinical studies are actively being translated into early-phase clinical trials. This class of agents leads to accumulation of acetylated histones, which in turn leads to increased tumor-suppressor gene expression. The DNA methyltransferase inhibitor 5-azacitidine has been evaluated in a phase II study in 34 MF patients. The overall response rate was 24% after a median of 5

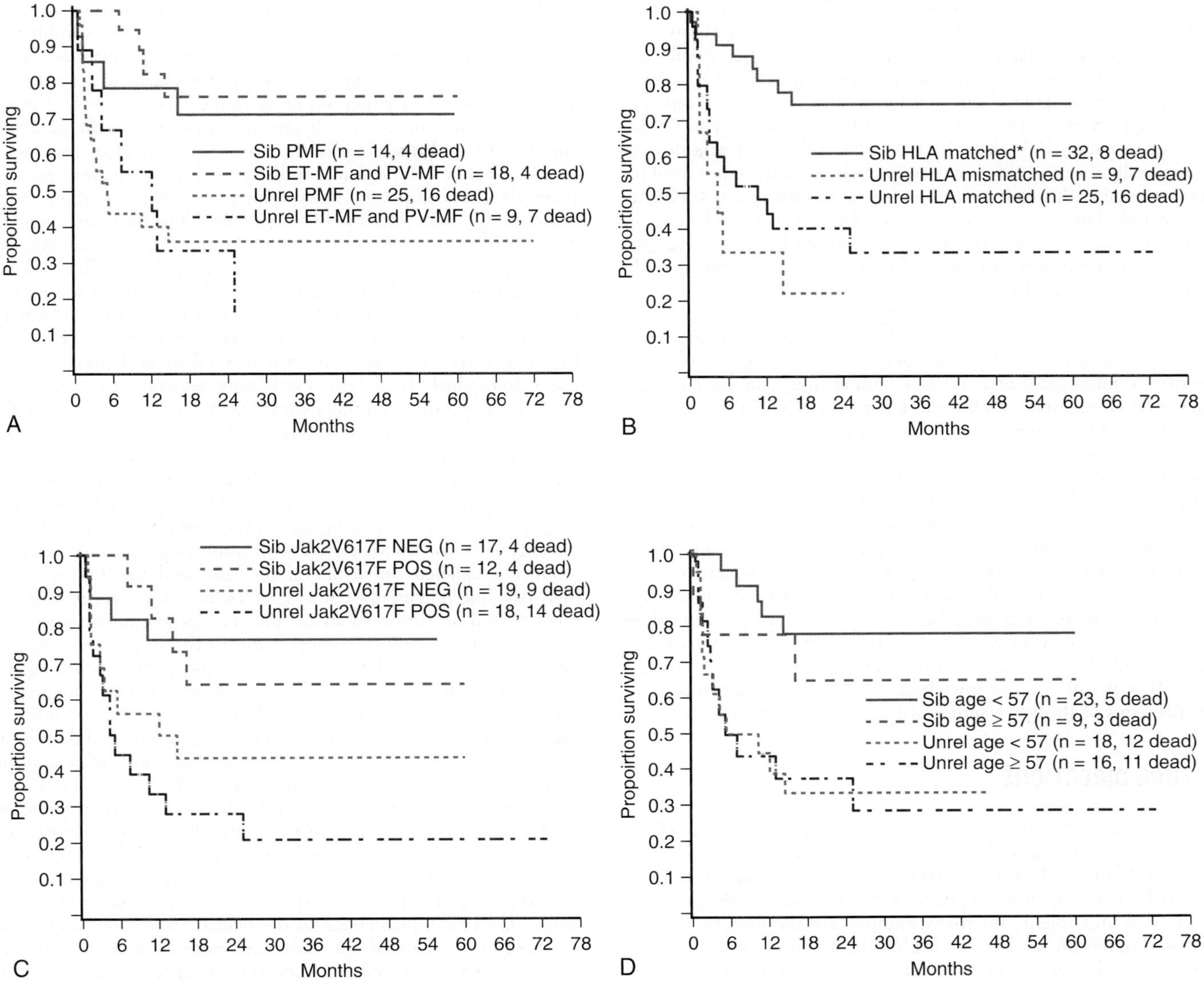

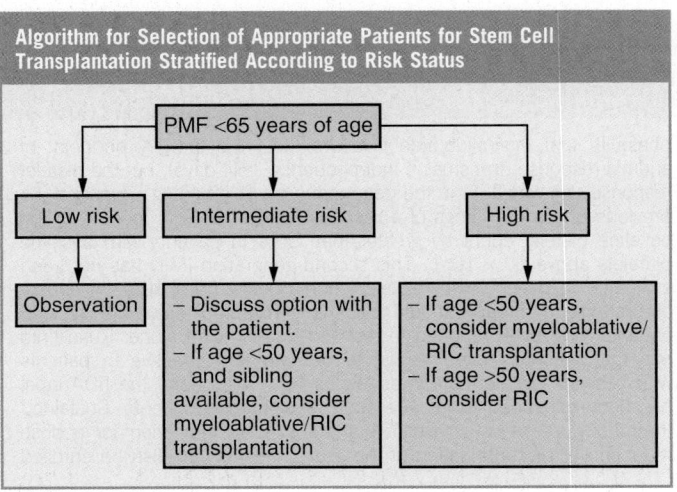

Fig. 70.12 Survival for patients with myelofibrosis after receiving reduced-intensity allogeneic hematopoietic stem cell transplantation was worse in the unrelated donor cohort compared with the related donor cohort irrespective of diagnosis subtype, degree of HLA matching, *JAK2* mutational status, and age. Final results from the multicenter phase II MPD-RC 101 trial. *ET-MF*, essential thrombocythemia myelofibrosis; *HLA*, human leukocyte antigen; *NEG*, negative; *PMF*, primary myelofibrosis; *POS*, positive; *PV-MF*, polycythemia vera myelofibrosis. (*Data from Rondelli et al: MPD-RC 101 prospective study of reduced-intensity allogeneic hematopoietic stem cell transplantation in patients with myelofibrosis. Blood 124:1183, 2014.*)

Algorithm for Selection of Appropriate Patients for Stem Cell Transplantation Stratified According to Risk Status

PMF <65 years of age

- Low risk
  - Observation
- Intermediate risk
  - Discuss option with the patient.
  - If age <50 years, and sibling available, consider myeloablative/RIC transplantation
- High risk
  - If age <50 years, consider myeloablative/RIC transplantation
  - If age >50 years, consider RIC

months of treatment, and grade 3/4 myelosuppression was seen in 29% of patients, requiring dose reduction in 47% of the cases. Interestingly, there was no difference in global hypomethylation between responders and nonresponders. This finding could argue that the mechanism of action of this drug in responding MF patients may not be directly through induction of DNA promoter site demethylation. Studies designed to evaluate the methylation status of specific genes thought to be silenced by this epigenetic modification (e.g., $p15^{INK4b}$ and $p16^{INK4a}$) need to be done in the future. A modified 5-day course of 5-azacitidine was also tested in a group of 10 MF patients, and was found to have even less of a response rate than the full 7-day course. Case series highlight the potential role of decitabine in the treatment of MF in blast phase, and initial reports of subcutaneous low-dose decitabine in advanced MF also appears to hold promise and is currently being evaluated in larger studies. LBH589 (panobinostat) is a potent pan-deacetylase inhibitor that has also been evaluated in PMF patients in two separate trials with thrombocytopenia as the dose-limiting toxicity and the demonstration of a signal of clinical activity that is associated with enhanced histone acetyla-tion. A report of the results of long-term administration of low-dose panobinostat in MF patients demonstrated the potential to alleviate constitutional symptoms, reduce splenomegaly, improve anemia, eliminate peripheral blood leukoerythroblastosis, reduce BM reticulin and collagen fibrosis, and restore normal BM morphology in a small number of patients. A phase II study of panobinostat at a dose of 25 mg orally thrice weekly is currently ongoing, and studies combin-ing this agent with ruxolitinib are ongoing, and the results are highly anticipated. The therapeutic potential for the use of chromatin-modifying agents for the treatment of PMF patients is an exciting approach and requires further careful evaluation in ongoing, well-designed clinical studies.

A novel and exciting therapeutic approach to the treatment of MF was recently reported by the Mayo Clinic group, in which a pilot study at this single institution was conducted evaluating an infusional telomerase inhibitor. Imetelstat is a 13-mer lipid conjugated oligo-nucleotide competitive inhibitor of telomerase RNA (hTR) resulting in telomere shortening and cell cycle arrest and apoptosis. Thirty three patients were treated either with weekly infusion and then every 3 weeks infusion or every 3 weeks from the start. The majority of patients discontinued due to suboptimal response or progressive disease, and three patients died on study. However, after a median of five cycles of treatment, seven responses were documented (four complete response and three partial response; three complete molecu-lar responses) and appeared to be durable for a median of >9 months). Additionally, anemia responses ($n = 4$) and 50% reduction in spleen size ($n = 9$) were reported. The occurrence of transaminitis was a cause initially for temporary study hold and now a large multicenter phase II trial will evaluate imetelstat in MF patients and molecular determinants of therapy response will be prospectively assessed.

FUTURE DIRECTIONS

More rational therapies for PMF are evolving from increased understanding of the cellular and molecular biologic abnormali-ties underlying PMF. Studies defining the relative contributions of acquired genetic mutations, epigenetic events, as well as the influence of the BM and splenic microenvironment on the origins of PMF, disease progression, and events leading to leukemic transformation are ongoing. Because PMF originates at the level of the HSC, the identification of novel drugs that eliminate such malignant stem cells is likely the most direct route to potentially curative pharmacologic strategies. Also, further delineation of the therapeutic potential of IFN as well as histone deacetylase inhibitor therapies must be pursued to define their potential use in the management of PMF patients. The evaluation of the use of combinations of active agents, including the JAK2 inhibitors, TGF-β inhibitors, IMiDS, histone deacetylase inhibitors, telomerase inhibitors, and pegylated forms of

IFN are anticipated to lead to significant clinical improvements in the outcomes of PMF patients. The evaluation of these combination therapies will certainly require the use of novel strategies for the design of clinical trials that will evaluate the effects of several active agents administered either simultaneously or sequentially. Overall, the implementation of any therapeutic approach by the practicing community of hematologists should only occur after evidence is provided by the completion of well-planned and adequately powered phase III trials comparing the experimental approach to the standard of care. aSCT with RIC and PBSC grafts remains the only potentially curative therapy available for patients under 70 years of age with an acceptable performance status and a suitable available donor. Although there is a reluctance to expose PMF patients to the risks of aSCT, if their underlying disorder is associated with a sufficiently poor prognosis, this risk appears to be warranted. Because early forms of PMF are associated with survival of well over a decade, many individuals have been even more reluctant to expose such patients to experimental therapeutic agents or aSCT. Unfortunately, progression to more advanced forms of MF is anticipated in younger patients. Exploration of therapeutic agents that can delay or even prevent disease progression or identification of the appropriate role of SCT in this low-risk group will require additional study. Such trials will be time consuming due to the prolonged survival of such patients with low-risk disease. The decision to proceed to transplant requires a detailed discussion of the risks and benefits of such a high-risk but potentially curative procedure. The recent establish-ment of multiinstitutional cooperative groups to evaluate such novel therapies and treatment strategies for PMF patients has met the need of insuring rapid evaluation of candidate therapeutic agents. No single institution has sufficient numbers of patients to perform this ever-growing number of required investigative efforts. Only with the completion of such rigorous evaluations of individual therapeutic strategies will one be able to determine the value of a continu-ously growing number of potentially active agents used alone or in combination. Each new therapy will likely be evaluated using not only a number of clinical endpoints, but also surrogate biomarkers and consideration of the immediate and long-term toxicities associ-ated with their use documented. Independently developed objective criteria by which responses to experimental therapeutic agents can be judged must be implemented for the evaluation of promising agents. Furthermore, quality-of-life tools have become more widely used in the evaluation of such experimental therapeutic agents. Because it is likely that a large number of such agents will be evaluated in patients with PMF in the future, it is recommended that a uniform standard be adopted so that the relative efficacy of any new thera-peutic approach can be more easily judged. The integration of these new classes of agents can also be incorporated into the conditioning regimens that are used before aSCT; this approach will also likely contribute to significant improvements in outcomes in PMF patients undergoing aSCT.

How Should PMF Patients With Thrombocytopenia Be Treated?

Platelet Count 50–100 × 10⁹/L:

It is important to be certain that vitamin B_{12} or folate deficiencies and/or sustained suppression from prior chemotherapeutic agents have not contributing to the development of a low platelet count. Chemothera-peutic agents such as hydroxyurea can be used in patients with marked splenomegaly, which can result in an improvement in the platelet count as the spleen volume is reduced. Patients can also be treated with thalidomide or lenalidomide in combination with prednisone. These first-generation immunomodulatory drugs (IMiDs) can sometimes improve cytopenias and reduce splenomegaly in primary myelofibrosis (PMF) patients, and in some cases, this response can persist even after drug discontinuation. Lenalidomide can induce cytopenias to a greater extent than thalidomide, which needs to be taken into consideration before this agent is used in the thrombocytopenic patient. In a randomized

phase III trial, pomalidomide failed to meet the primary endpoint of anemia response (transfusion independence: ≥84 days), but the platelet response rate was 22% in the treatment arm. This finding supported the previous phase II findings of a response rate of 58% in increasing the baseline platelet count by greater than 50% in patients with baseline platelets above 50×10^9/L. This second-generation IMiD has not been evaluated in patients with platelet counts below 50×10^9/L. A course of prednisone therapy should also be considered, since 30–40% of patients have been reported to respond to this agent alone. Ruxolitinib has more recently been shown to be safe and effective in patients with baseline platelet counts as low as 50×10^9/L, and the FDA label has been expanded to include such myelofibrosis patients. Sustained thrombocytopenia with ruxolitinib therapy is an indication for a dose reduction or discontinuation of the drug. Patients can also be enrolled

How Should PMF Patients With Thrombocytopenia Be Treated?—cont'd

in other JAK2 inhibitor clinical trials in which reduced platelet counts are acceptable (such as the PERSIST-2 phase III pacritinib trial) or in clinical trials with other agents in development. If thrombocytopenia worsens with the current treatment plan, then proceed with the strategy outlined below.

Platelet Count 20–50 × 10⁹/L:

Thalidomide or lenalidomide in combination with prednisone can be used to correct anemia in these PMF patients but rarely improve the platelet counts in a clinically meaningful way. Most clinical trials involving a variety of therapeutic agents including JAK2 inhibitors will require baseline platelets above 50×10^9/L. In patients who are experiencing life-threatening bleeding, in addition to aggressive immediate platelet transfusions, splenectomy is a reasonable therapeutic option.

Platelet Count <20 × 10⁹/L

The treatment choices are truly limited for these patients. Intervention is also dependent on the clinical picture, with emphasis on addressing bleeding. Supportive therapy with frequent platelet transfusions is a possibility, but it is likely not sustainable in the long term. It is our practice to transfuse if the platelet count is below 10×10^9/L unless there is no evidence of mucosal bleeding or life-threatening hemorrhage. Occasionally, patients may have an improvement in the degree of thrombocytopenia with steroids. About 20–30% of patients with severe thrombocytopenia will have significant improvement in platelet counts after a splenectomy. Aggressive platelet transfusional support is necessary before, during, and after splenectomy in many cases. However, splenectomy in patients with PMF is associated with a postoperative morbidity rate of 15–30% and a mortality rate close to 10%. These numbers, however, are highly dependent on the institutional experience and the operating surgeon. Splenectomy can also result in extramedullary hematopoiesis in the liver, causing hepatomegaly, which may require the administration of judicious amount of chemotherapeutic agents (hydroxyurea, busulfan, cladribine) or a JAK2 inhibitor. Severe thrombocytopenia is an adverse prognostic feature. Such patients who are eligible for stem cell transplantation (SCT) and have available donors should be considered for transplantation. Thrombopoietin mimetics have been associated with increased bone marrow fibrosis when used for the treatment of immune thrombocytopenia purpura and have not been evaluated in the setting of PMF-associated thrombocytopenia. Additionally, patients with extreme thrombocytopenia and signs of leukemic transformation can be considered for therapy with decitabine or azacytidine with aggressive platelet transfusional support, and then ideally should proceed to allogeneic SCT if a donor is available and the patient's performance status is appropriate.

Which Patients Should Be Considered for Allogeneic Hematopoietic Stem Cell Transplantation?

Allogeneic stem cell transplantation (aSCT) is the only potential curative treatment option for primary myelofibrosis (PMF). Patients with poor risk features and decreased probability for survival should be considered for SCT because of the not insignificant risk of transplant-related morbidity and mortality. All patients younger than 70 years of age and their siblings should be human leukocyte antigen typed at the time of diagnosis to determine if there is a potential match. Patients between the ages of 65 and 70 years with available related donors should be evaluated based on their performance status and presence of comorbid conditions. Patients younger than 70 years of age with good performance status and available donors (either related or fully matched unrelated) should be encouraged to undergo evaluation for SCT soon after the diagnosis and preferably within a clinical trial. Patients with high- or intermediate-risk disease with available donors should consider transplantation before developing debilitating symptoms or significant worsening in their performance status. Patients with low-risk disease can be closely monitored without intervention but should proceed to transplantation with evidence of disease progression. For patients with available donors but poor performance status because of symptoms of myelofibrosis, a course of treatment with ruxolitinib can be considered with a goal of improvement in performance status associated with reduction of splenomegaly and constitutional symptoms. These patients may become more viable transplant candidates with this pretransplant treatment approach. Splenectomy before transplant is not essential to ensure adequate engraftment. Currently, SCT using reduced-intensity conditioning regimens, haploidentical donors, and cord blood grafts are being actively evaluated.

Which PMF Patients Are Appropriate for JAK2 Inhibitor Therapy?

Not all primary myelofibrosis (PMF) patients require treatment with JAK2 inhibitor therapy. Patients with symptomatic splenomegaly or debilitating myelofibrosis (MF)-related symptoms are potential candidates for treatment with ruxolitinib. Inhibition of JAK1/2 is associated with myelosuppression and could further compromise existing cytopenias. In patients with isolated splenomegaly and adequate blood counts, a course of hydroxyurea should be considered. If the patient fails hydroxyurea or has debilitating symptoms, then ruxolitinib would be the appropriate agent. Ruxolitinib is currently approved for patients with intermediate- and high-risk MF, and has yet to be explored in cases of symptomatic patients with low-risk disease. Additionally, the use of this drug is not advised in MF patients with platelet counts below 50×10^9/L. Whether Ruxolitinib should be used in patients with poor performance status before allogeneic stem cell transplantation (SCT) as a means to improve their performance status and promote weight gain in an attempt to optimize them for SCT, is under prospective evaluation within the MPD-Research Consortium. Although the COMFORT 1 trial reported a modest improvement in survival at a median of 51 weeks of treatment with ruxolitinib, the exact mechanism that underlies this survival benefit remains, and this agent should not be given with the primary goal of disease process modification and promoting increased survival. Patients started on ruxolitinib need to have frequent monitoring of blood counts, and if discontinued, the dose should be either tapered or a pulse of concurrent steroid therapy considered to avoid the rapid reappearance of systemic symptoms and splenomegaly, which can occur at times.

How Does Characterizing the Mutational Profile of a PMF Patient Influence Care?

Assessing the status of the primary myelofibrosis driver mutations *JAK2*, *MPL*, and *CALR* can help refine prognostication and influence therapeutic decision-making. Retrospective studies suggest that molecular risk stratification can further refine the individual risk for leukemic transformation and shortened overall survival. Patients with triple-negative status (lacking mutations of *JAK2*, *MPL*, and *CALR*) or with an *ASXL1* mutation are at highest risk for a poor outcome and should be evaluated for early stem cell transplantation (SCT) or experimental therapy, even if they are assessed to have low-risk disease by conventional risk-stratification tools. Such patients should be sent for transplant at the earliest time of evidence of disease evolution. Proposed molecular stratification tools have recently been proposed but not yet validated in prospective trials. It is also important to remember that *JAK2* wild type status, and *MPL*- and *CALR*-mutated patients respond equally well to ruxolitinib therapy. The characterization of nearly 20 recurrent gene mutations in PMF patients has been reported by various groups and implicates a complex and heterogeneous molecular pathophysiology that will likely not allow for a single therapeutic target drug approach. Whether the presence of certain gene mutations will ultimately predict for therapeutic response with differing agents has yet to be shown. The presence of these mutations can also be used to detect minimal residual disease after SCT

REFERENCES

1. Swerdlow SH, Campo E, Harris NL, et al: *WHO classification of tumours of haematopoietic and lymphoid tissues*, ed 4, 2008.
2. Tefferi A: Novel mutations and their functional and clinical relevance in myeloproliferative neoplasms: JAK2, MPL, TET2, ASXL1, CBL, IDH and IKZF1. *Leukemia* 24:1128, 2010.
3. Schmitt A, Jouault H, Guichard J, et al: Pathologic interaction between megakaryocytes and polymorphonuclear leukocytes in myelofibrosis. *Blood* 96:1342, 2000.
4. James C, Ugo V, Le Couédic JP, et al: A unique clonal JAK2 mutation leading to constitutive signalling causes polycythaemia vera. *Nature* 434:1144, 2005.
5. Pardanani AD, Levine RL, Lasho T, et al: MPL515 mutations in myeloproliferative and other myeloid disorders: a study of 1182 patients. *Blood* 108:3472, 2006.
6. Nangalia J, Massie CE, Baxter EJ, et al: Somatic CALR mutations in myeloproliferative neoplasms with nonmutated JAK2. *N Engl J Med* 369(25):2391, 2013.
7. Thiele J, Kvasnicka HM, Werden C, et al: Idiopathic primary osteomyelofibrosis: a clinico-pathological study on 208 patients with special emphasis on evolution of disease features, differentiation from essential thrombocythemia and variables of prognostic impact. *Leuk Lymphoma* 22:303, 1996.
8. Lundberg P, Karow A, Nienhold R, et al: Clonal evolution and clinical correlates of somatic mutations in myeloproliferative neoplasms. *Blood* 123(14):2220, 2014.
9. Cervantes F, Dupriez B, Pereira A, et al: New prognostic scoring system for primary myelofibrosis based on a study of the International Working Group for Myelofibrosis Research and Treatment. *Blood* 113:2895, 2009.
10. Tefferi A: How I treat myelofibrosis. *Blood* 117:3494, 2011.
11. Kiladjian JJ, Mesa RA, Hoffman R: The renaissance of interferon therapy for the treatment of myeloid malignancies. *Blood* 117:4706, 2011.
12. Verstovsek S, Mesa RA, Gotlib J, et al: A double-blind, placebo-controlled trial of ruxolitinib for myelofibrosis. *N Engl J Med* 366:799, 2012.
13. Harrison C, Kiladjian JJ, Al-Ali HK, et al: JAK inhibition with ruxolitinib versus best available therapy for myelofibrosis. *N Engl J Med* 366:787, 2012.

CHAPTER 71

EOSINOPHILIA, EOSINOPHIL-ASSOCIATED DISEASES, EOSINOPHILIC LEUKEMIAS, AND THE HYPEREOSINOPHILIC SYNDROMES

Peter Valent, Andreas Reiter, and Jason Gotlib

Eosinophils are highly specialized granulocytic effector cells that produce and store numerous biologically active mediators, including cytotoxic proteins, lipid mediators, chemotactic peptides, and cytokines (Table 71.1). Under various pathologic conditions, blood eosinophils transmigrate through the endothelial layer and invade various target organs, where they secrete their products into the surrounding tissues, thereby triggering inflammation, toxic damage, and tissue remodeling.[1] Since their initial characterization by Paul Ehrlich in 1879, eosinophilic granulocytes have been implicated in a growing number of systemic diseases and conditions characterized by blood and/or tissue eosinophilia (Table 71.2). During the past few years, researchers have also gained a better understanding of the unique features and functions of activated eosinophils, and of the specific roles some of their granule proteins and inducible lipid mediators may play in the pathogenesis of allergic, parasitic, neoplastic, and other diseases.[1] In addition, recognition of the eosinophil as a major proinflammatory and tissue-remodeling effector cell has fueled a surge of interest in this granulocyte in recent years.

Studies of the biochemistry, biologic activities, and tissue localization of distinct enzymatic and nonenzymatic cationic proteins derived from eosinophils have provided convincing evidence for their role in the pathogenesis of inflammation and tissue damage in eosinophil-associated diseases. The five cationic granule proteins that may play a role in eosinophil-related pathologies include two major basic proteins (MBP-1, MBP-2), eosinophil peroxidase (EPX), and two ribonucleases, namely eosinophil cationic protein (ECP) and eosinophil-derived neurotoxin (EDN; see Table 71.1). Eosinophils also have the capacity to express toxic oxidative intermediates and other mediators of inflammation, as well as mediators of thrombosis and fibrosis. In addition, eosinophils are a rich source of DNA traps that may facilitate fibrin deposition as well as the killing of microbial invaders.[2] A clinically important aspect is that the various mediators produced and released by (activated) eosinophils often act together to trigger thrombosis and tissue damage, especially when eosinophil expansion and activation is chronic and "treatment-resistant".

The process of determining the cause of eosinophilia is often frustrating for both the physician and the patient, and in many instances, the resulting diagnosis is "eosinophilia of unknown etiology". Depending on laboratory standards and local guidelines, eosinophilia is defined as more than 450–500 eosinophils/μL blood, confirmed by visual microscopy. Diurnal variations in eosinophil counts are well documented, with minimum numbers appearing early in the morning and greatest numbers appearing late at night, mirroring circadian rhythms in adrenal corticosteroids. Although these variations are usually limited to a certain extent, basal eosinophil counts should be routinely measured during daytime. Transient mild eosinophilia is commonly seen in allergic reactions, during and shortly after a bacterial infection, and in many other reactive states. Sometimes, transient eosinophilia may be substantial or even excessive. Such transient (<4 weeks) form of reactive eosinophilia per se, if present, is considered harmless in most instances, but should prompt the physician to search for certain underlying diseases, such as an occult allergy or an unrecognized infection.

Eosinophil disorders and related syndromes are a heterogeneous group of diseases characterized by marked expansion and persistent accumulation of eosinophils in the peripheral blood (PB) and other organ systems. In general, eosinophil disorders can be divided into (A) neoplastic states where eosinophils are found to be monoclonal, and (B) reactive states where eosinophil expansion is considered to be "poly-clonal" and triggered by eosinotropic cytokines, such as interleukin-5 (IL-5).[3] In both instances, hypereosinophilia (HE), defined by a persistent eosinophil count of $\geq 1.5 \times 10^4$/L blood, is typically present. Depending on the underlying disease and other factors, the HE state may or may not be accompanied by specific (HE-mediated) organ damage, also referred to as *hypereosinophilic syndrome* (HES). In many instances, HES-related organ damage manifests as overt thromboembolism (thrombosis) or fibrosis. In other patients, organ damage is associated with less specific findings, and may involve the skin, gastrointestinal (GI) tract, or the CNS. Based on the underlying condition, both HE and HES can be divided into familial, primary (neoplastic), and secondary (reactive) forms (Table 71.3).[3] Apart from these classical forms of HES, more specific syndromes associated with HE and HE-related organopathy have been described. Some of these syndromes are associated with a genetic (germ-line) defect, whereas others are accompanied by distinct immunological abnormalities (Table 71.4A). Finally, HE may develop in the context of organ-restricted inflammatory conditions such as eosinophilic pneumonia or eosinophilic colitis (Table 71.4B).

A thorough examination of all clinical and laboratory parameters, including radiologic and imaging studies, bone marrow (BM) investigations, cytogenetics, and molecular studies, are required in order to establish the correct diagnosis (underlying disease and organ damage) in patients with initially unexplained HE.[3] The current chapter provides an overview on the epidemiology, pathogenesis, course, prognosis, and clinical features of various eosinophil disorders. We also discuss recent developments in the field and the impact of molecular markers and targets. In addition, this chapter provides diagnostic algorithms and recommendations for the management and treatment of patients with eosinophil disorders.

EPIDEMIOLOGY

Little is known about the prevalence and incidence of primary eosinophil disorders (eosinophil neoplasms) and HE-related syndromes, including HES. Based on the available literature, most eosinophil neoplasms and all types of HES are rare, and the same holds true for other HE-related conditions, such as the Gleich syndrome or Churg-Strauss syndrome (CSS). In an attempt to estimate the incidence of HES, data collected by the Surveillance, Epidemiology and End Results (SEER) database, sponsored by the National Cancer Institute, have been reviewed. A crude incidence of 0.035 cases per 100,000 person-years was found, and the male-to-female ratio was reported to be 1.47 to 1. The average age at diagnosis was 52.5 years, and the peak incidence was recorded in individuals aged 65–74 years. Childhood cases of HES have been reported but are very rare. Unfortunately, all these data have serious limitations and

TABLE 71.1   Eosinophil-Derived Molecules and Their Potential Role in Health and Disease

Eosinophil Product/Molecule	Relevant Function(s)	Eosinophil Product/Molecule	Relevant Function(s)
Eosinophil-Related Enzymes		**Growth Factors/Cytokines**	
Nonspecific esterase	Cytotoxic effects (microbes and tissue cells)	Interleukin-1-α (IL-1α)	Endothelial activation, inflammation
Catalase	Cytotoxic effects (microbes and tissue cells)	Interleukin-2 (IL-2)	Activation of T lymphocytes
Acid phosphatase	Cytotoxic effects (microbes and tissue cells)	Interleukin-3 (IL-3)	Amplification of eosinophil accumulation/activation and basophil activation
Lysophospholipase	Tissue inflammation	Interleukin-4 (IL-4)	B-cell maturation and mast cell differentiation
Phospholipase D	Migration, adhesion, vesicle transport, secretion	Interleukin-5 (IL-5)	Amplification of eosinophil accumulation/activation
Hexosaminidase	Tissue inflammation and tissue remodeling	Interleukin-6 (IL-6)	Lymphocyte maturation
Arylsulphatase B	Lysosomal hydrolase	Interleukin-13 (IL-13)	Bronchial hyperreactivity, mucus production, B-cell maturation
5-Lipoxygenase	Leukotriene production, angiogenesis	GM-CSF	Leukocyte/eosinophil accumulation/activation
Leukotriene C4 synthase	Leukotriene production	TGF-α	Fibrosis, growth inhibition
Cyclooxygenase	Prostaglandin production	TGF-β	Fibrosis, growth inhibition
Histaminase	Histamine degradation	TNF-α	Endothelial activation, inflammation, cachexia
Eosinophil Basic Proteins		Oncostatin-M (OSM)	Fibrosis, angiogenesis, paracrine mobilization of eosinophils via upregulated SDF-1 production in fibroblasts
Eosinophil peroxidase (EPX)	Cytotoxic effects (parasites, microbes, tissue cells)	**Lipid Membrane-Derived Substances**	
Major basic protein-1 (MBP-1)	Cytotoxic effects (parasites, microbes, tissue cells)	PAF	Bronchoconstriction, edema formation
Major basic protein-2 (MBP-2)	Cytotoxic effects (parasites, microbes, tissue cells)	TXB2	Platelet aggregation
Eosinophil cationic protein (ECP)	Cytotoxic effects, mucus secretion, fibrosis	LTC4	Mucus secretion
Eosinophil-derived neurotoxin (EDN)	Cytotoxic effects (antiviral, RNase activity)	15-HETE	Diverse effects on blood and tissue cells
Chemokines		PGE1 and PGE2	Diverse effects on platelets, endothelial cells, fibroblasts and other tissue cells
Interleukin-8 (IL-8)	Leukocyte recruitment and activation	**Antifibrinolytic Mediators**	
MIP-1-alpha (CCL3)	Leukocyte recruitment and activation	PAI-2	Antifibrinolytic and prothrombotic
RANTES (CCL5)	Leukocyte recruitment and activation	Extracellular DNA traps	Fibrin deposition, antibacterial effect
Eotaxin (CCL11)	Further eosinophil recruitment		

CCL, chemokine (C-C motif) ligand; GM-CSF, granulocyte/macrophage colony-stimulating factor; LTC4, leukotriene C4; MIP-1-alpha, macrophage inflammatory protein-1-alpha; PAF, platelet-activating factor; PAI-2, plasminogen activator inhibitor-2; RANTES, regulated on activation, normal T-cell expressed and secreted; TGF, transforming growth factor; TNF, tumor necrosis factor; TXB2, thromboxane B2.

TABLE 71.2   Conditions Associated With Eosinophilia

Reactive Conditions

Helminth infections (filariasis, toxocariasis, schistosomiasis, trichinosis, onchocerciasis, fascioliasis, strongyloidiasis, ascariasis, hookworm, echinococcus/hydatid disease)

Fungal infections (aspergillosis, coccidioidomycosis, cryptococcosis)

Scabies and other infestations

Bacterial infections (convalescent phase of pneumococcal pneumonia, chlamydial pneumonia, scarlet fever, other bacterial infections)

Viral infections (HIV infection, chronic active hepatitis)

Allergic reactions (asthma, rhinitis, bronchitis, urticaria,

Atopic diseases (atopic asthma, atopic dermatitis)

Drug reactions (allergic, toxic)

Administration of IL-2, IL-3, or GM-CSF

Autoimmune diseases/connective tissue diseases/vasculitis (Sjögren syndrome, rheumatoid arthritis, lupus erythematodes, hypersensitivity vasculitis, bullous pemphigoid, others)

Acute and chronic graft-versus-host disease

Angioblastic lymphoid hyperplasia (Kimura disease)

Lymphocytic/lymphoid variant HES (HES$_L$)

Endocrinologic Conditions

Addison disease

Neoplastic Conditions Involving the Hematopoietic System

Myeloid neoplasms

Mast cell neoplasms

Lymphoid neoplasms

Paraneoplastic Conditions

Solid tumors/malignancy

Lymphoproliferative neoplasms (B- or T-cell lymphoma, Hodgkin disease)

Langerhans cell histiocytosis

Idiopathic Forms

Idiopathic eosinophilia[a]

HE of uncertain (undetermined) significance (HE$_{US}$)

Idiopathic hypereosinophilic syndrome (HES$_I$)

Hereditary HE of unknown etiology

[a]Idiopathic mild eosinophilia (500–1500 eosinophils/μL blood = less than HE) of unknown etiology.

HE, Hypereosinophilia; HES, hypereosinophilic syndrome; HES$_I$, idiopathic HES; HES$_L$, lymphoid variant HES; HE$_{US}$, hypereosinophilia of undetermined (unknown) clinical significance; GM-CSF, granulocyte-macrophage colony-stimulating factor; HIV, human immunodeficiency virus; IL-2, interleukin-2; IL-3, interleukin-3.

TABLE
71.3

TABLE 71.3 Classification of Hypereosinophilia and Hypereosinophilic Syndromes

HE Variant	Abbreviation	Associated HES Variant
Familial/hereditary HE	HE$_{FA}$	Familial HES = HES$_F$
HE of undetermined/ Unknown Significance	HE$_{US}$[a]	Idiopathic HES = HES$_I$[a]
Neoplastic/primary HE	HE$_N$	Neoplastic HES = HES$_N$
Reactive/secondary HE	HE$_R$	Reactive HES = HES$_R$ Lymphocytic variant = HES$_L$[b]

[a]In patients with HE$_{US}$, the presence of HES is excluded by definition; as soon as HES is diagnosed in a patient with HE$_{US}$, the diagnosis changes to HES$_I$, unless an underlying etiology (condition/disease) is also found.
[b]HES$_L$ is regarded a special variant of HES$_R$.
HE, Hypereosinophilia; HES, hypereosinophilic syndrome; HES$_F$, familial HES; HES$_I$, idiopathic HES; HES$_L$, lymphocytic variant HES; HES$_N$, primary (neoplastic) HES; HES$_R$, reactive HES; HE$_{US}$, hypereosinophilia of undetermined (unknown) clinical significance.

TABLE 71.4A Rare HES-Like Syndromes Accompanied by Hypereosinophilia

Syndrome	Characteristic Features and Laboratory Abnormalities
Gleich syndrome	Cyclic recurrent angioedema, fever, weight gain, elevated polyclonal IgM, increased IL-5 production, evidence of clonal T cells (CD3⁻ T cells)[a]
Churg-Strauss syndrome (CSS) = eosinophilic granulomatosis with polyangiitis (EGPA)	Stage I: Asthma and rhinosinusitis (isolated) Stage II: Eosinophilic phase (HES-like) Stage III: Vasculitic phase defined by necrotizing (small-vessel) vasculitis and HE with pulmonary infiltrates and/or neuropathy (ANCA+ and ANCA− subvariants).
Eosinophilia myalgia syndrome (EMS)	Severe myalgia ± fever (flu-like), edema, fatigue, weight loss, neurologic symptoms, skin abnormalities Epidemic cases have been reported to result from exposure to L-tryptophan (toxic oil syndrome).
Eosinophilic fasciitis (EF) = Shulman syndrome	Scleroderma-like condition with painful swelling of the skin and chronic induration (limbs and trunk) as well as laboratory signs of systemic inflammation
Omenn syndrome (OS)	Severe combined immunodeficiency (SCID) with well-populated lymphatic organs (OS paradox) Autosomal recessive genetic (pediatric) disease (recurrent mutations in RAG1 or RAG2) Clinical findings: erythroderma, hepatosplenomegaly, lymphadenopathy, increased IgE, diarrhea, weight loss (GVHD-like condition with autoreactive T cells)
Hyper-IgE syndrome (HIES)	Hereditary immunodeficiency syndrome with elevated IgE, recurrent severe infections, often with skin eczema and facial anomalies Known recurrent gene mutations: Autosomal dominant variant: STAT3 mutations Autosomal recessive variant: DOCK8 mutations PGM3 mutations

[a]EGPA/CSS with clonal T cells is often regarded as special variant of lymphoid variant HES (HES$_L$).
ANCA, Anti-neutrophil cytoplasmic antibodies; DOCK8, dedicator of cytokinesis 8; GVHD, graft-versus-host disease; HE, hypereosinophilia; HES, hypereosinophilic syndrome; IgE, immunoglobulin E; PGM3, phosphoglucomutase 3; RAG, recombination-activating gene; STAT3, signal transducer and activator of transcription-3.

TABLE 71.4B Organ-restricted (Inflammatory) Conditions Accompanied by Eosinophilia

Eosinophilic gastrointestinal disorders (EGIDs)
    Eosinophilic esophagitis
    Eosinophilic gastritis
    Eosinophilic gastroenteritis
    Eosinophilic colitis
Eosinophilic pancreatitis
Eosinophilic hepatitis
Eosinophilic ascites
Pulmonary eosinophilic syndromes
    Eosinophilic asthma
    Eosinophilic bronchitis
    Eosinophilic pneumonia
    Eosinophil pleuritis
Eosinophilic nephritis
Eosinophilic cystitis
Eosinophilic endometritis and myometritis
Eosinophilic mastitis
Eosinophilic ocular disorders
Eosinophilic myocarditis
Eosinophilic synovitis
Skin diseases/conditions associated with eosinophilia[a]
    Allergic contact dermatitis
    Atopic dermatitis
    Drug reactions
    Bullous pemphigoid and pemphigoid variants
    Eosinophilic cellulitis (Wells syndrome)
    Radiotherapy-related eruptions associated with eosinophilia
    Eosinophilic pustular folliculitis
    Infestations (parasitic) and infections (bacterial, viral, fungal) involving the skin
    Mycosis fungoides
    Pachydermatous eosinophilic dermatitis
Kimura disease (skin and lymph nodes)
Eosinophilic panniculitis

[a]Many other skin abnormalities can be accompanied by eosinophilia, especially when a systemic inflammatory disease process is present and triggers eosinophilia.

emphasize the need for more comprehensive epidemiologic studies using currently available diagnostic criteria and robust registries. A complicating issue is that HES may coexist with an underlying primary eosinophil disorder, a lymphoma, but also an allergy or another reactive condition.[3] In eosinophilic leukemia presenting with the *FIP1L1-PDGFRA* fusion gene (*F/P*), a clear male predominance is found. As a consequence, any HES registry including patients with *F/P*+ eosinophilic leukemia and/or other *F/P*+ myeloproliferative neoplasms (MPNs) with eosinophilia (MPN-eo) will report on an overall male predominance of HES, even if other HES types are evenly distributed in males and females. Indeed, no clear gender predominance has been reported in other groups of HE or HES. Familial forms of HE and HES have been described, but are very rare. In these cases, a hyper-immunoglobulin (Ig)E syndrome or Omenn syndrome (OS) have to be excluded. No cases of familial *F/P*+ leukemia have been reported to date.

MORPHOLOGY AND PHENOTYPE OF EOSINOPHILS

Eosinophils contain three granule populations, namely (1) electron-dense, round, primary progranules present mainly at the promyelocyte and myelocyte stages, (2) specific (secondary) eosinophilic granules with an electron-dense crystalloid core, specifically found in mature eosinophils, and (3) small-sized granules, which may contain catalase, acid phosphatase, and arylsulfatase.[1] The large, specific granule is the major source of cytotoxic and proinflammatory cationic proteins. Eosinophils also contain lipid bodies that may serve as a source of eosinophil eicosanoide-forming enzymes, including 5-lipoxygenase, leukotriene C4 synthase, and cyclooxygenase (see Table 71.1).

The immunophenotype of human eosinophils is well established and may assist in eosinophil detection and enumeration by flow cytometry. In common with all leukocytes, eosinophils express leukosialin (CD43), the homing cell adhesion molecule HCAM (CD44), and the pan-leukocyte tyrosine phosphatase C (CD45).[5] In addition, eosinophils express several myeloid differentiation antigens, including LFA-1 (CD11a/CD18) and Siglec-3 (CD33). These cell surface antigens are also expressed on other myeloid cells, including monocytes and basophils. However, a few cell surface structures are largely restricted to eosinophils and thus serve as cell-specific markers through which eosinophils can be detected and isolated. One of these markers is Siglec-8, an inhibitory receptor that, when crosslinked, mediates eosinophil apoptosis.[6] Apart from eosinophils, basophils also display Siglec-8 (Fig. 71.1). Eosinophils also express several cytokine receptors, such as the IL-5 receptor, granulocyte-macrophage colony-stimulating factor (GM-CSF) receptor, and IL-3 receptor. Moreover, eosinophils exhibit diverse chemokine receptors, including eotaxin receptors and CXC-chemokine receptor 4 (CXCR4), a receptor for stromal cell-derived factor (SDF)-1 (Table 71.5). Finally, eosinophils express diverse complement receptors (CRs), such as CR3 (CD11b/CD18) and C5aR (CD88), adhesion receptors, and immunoglobulin (Fc) receptors. Several of these cell surface markers have been considered as potential targets of therapy. However, no aberrantly expressed or disease-specific markers for neoplastic eosinophils or reactive eosinophils have been identified yet. Several studies have shown that eosinophils in HES patients may express increased amounts of CD11b, CD16, CD25, or/and HLA-DR. However, overexpression of these antigens is not disease-specific.

Apart from cell surface antigens, eosinophils also express more or less specific marker antigens in their cytoplasm by which these cells can be detected in various tissues by immunohistochemistry (IHC). Useful eosinophil IHC stains include ECP, EPX, and MBP (Fig. 71.2A). Depending on the condition and underlying neoplasm, these antibodies may also react with (immature) basophils. Otherwise, however, the staining reaction appears to be largely specific for eosinophil granulocytes. Another important aspect is that some of the eosinophil proteins, like MBP, can be detected in tissue sections as deposit material after complete degranulation of eosinophils and even after their subsequent destruction (disappearance), which is often seen in the context of chronic HE-related tissue damage (HES).[7] Therefore, the definition of tissue HE includes not only the detection of a local eosinophil (cellular) infiltrate, but also the presence of eosinophil protein deposits, even in the absence of eosinophil infiltrates.

Eosinophils from the PB and tissues of patients with HE may differ from their normal counterparts by morphologic, biochemical, and functional characteristics. The most important morphologic distinction is that between immature and mature eosinophils. In most instances, this distinction is a straightforward approach, as immature forms exhibit distinct nuclear and cytoplasmic morphologic features (Fig. 71.2B and C). However, sometimes the distinction may be challenging, especially in reactive states with massive inflammation and in certain myeloid neoplasms. In immature myeloid neoplasms, eosinophil precursor cells may exhibit dark basophilic granules that must not be confused with the specific granules of blood basophils. These immature eosinophils may also be misinterpreted as mixed-lineage cells.

Immature eosinophils also differ from mature eosinophils in several other aspects, including density, nuclear shape, protein composition, and cell surface antigens. A difficult task is to differentiate normal eosinophils from activated (sometimes immature) eosinophils in reactive states. In previous years, researchers focused on cell density. In particular, a distinction was made between the "normodense" (normal-density) and the "hypodense" (light-density) eosinophil. The blood of normal individuals contains less than 10% eosinophils with densities less than 1.082 g/mL, whereas patients with eosinophilia can have markedly increased numbers of hypodense cells. Hypodense eosinophils appear to be cytokine-activated cells that are characterized

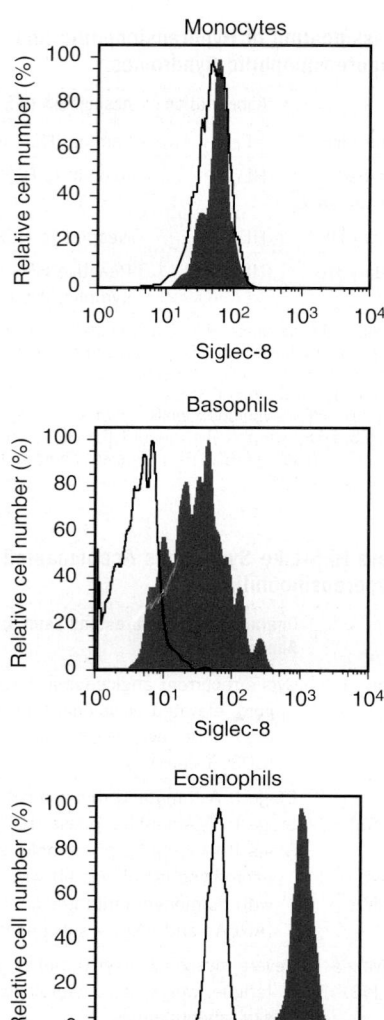

Fig. 71.1 EXPRESSION OF SIGLEC-8 ON PERIPHERAL BLOOD EOSINOPHILS. Peripheral blood cells were obtained from a patient suffering from a myeloproliferative neoplasm with eosinophilia (MNP-eo). Cells were stained with an antibody against Siglec-8, as well as antibodies against CD203c (for basophil detection) and CD14 (for monocyte detection), and analyzed by multicolor flow cytometry. As visible, Siglec-8 is expressed on eosinophils (detected by their characteristic side-scatter properties and autofluorescence) as well as on blood basophils, whereas monocytes (like most other leukocytes) lack Siglec-8.

by increased vacuolization, decreased granule size, decreased content of granule cationic proteins, and increased numbers of cytoplasmic lipid bodies. The numbers of surface receptors for a variety of eosinophil agonists, including complement components, immunoglobulins, and PAF, are expressed at higher levels by hypodense eosinophils. Functionally, hypodense eosinophils show increased metabolic activity and oxygen consumption, an increased capacity for the synthesis and secretion of LTC4 and certain cytokines, enhanced chemotaxis, and augmented cytotoxicity. So far, no clear relationship between the percentage of hypodense eosinophils and the etiology of eosinophilic disorders has been established. The percentage of these cells increases in most reactive forms of HE and HES, but also in patients with primary HES. Ultrastructurally, HES eosinophils may show a selective loss of secondary granule components (crystalloid MBP-containing core or granular matrix, or both), a decreased number and size of granules, and increased numbers of cytoplasmic lipid bodies and tubulovesicular structures that may be involved in eosinophil secretion during the process of piecemeal degranulation.

TABLE 71.5	Receptors and Ligands Regulating Growth and Function of Eosinophils	
Receptor (R) on Eosinophils	**Ligand**	**Effects on Eosinophils**
IL-2RA/CD25[a]	IL-2	Activation?[a] Migration?[a]
IL-3R/CD123 + CD131	IL-3	Differentiation, survival, adhesion, migration, activation, priming
IL-4R/CD124	IL-4	Priming for effects of chemotaxins
IL-5R/CD125 + CD131	IL-5	Differentiation, survival, adhesion, migration, activation, priming
GM-CSFR/CD116 + CD131	GM-CSF	Differentiation, survival, adhesion, migration, activation, priming
IL-10R	IL-10	Inhibitory (activation, survival)
IL-12R	IL-12	Inhibitory (activation)
IL-13R	IL-13	Unknown
CD4	IL-16 (LCF)	Activation, priming
IL-25R	IL-25	Survival, activation
IL-27R	IL-27	Survival, activation
IL-33R/ST2	IL-33	Activation, survival
VEGFR-1/FLT-1	VEGF	Chemotaxis, activation
Tie-2/TEK	Angiopoietin-1	Chemotaxis, activation?
PDGFRA/B	PDGF	Activation and growth?
FGFR	FGF	Activation?
TGFββ1R	TGFβ1	Inhibitory (differentiation)
TGFβ2R	TGFβ2	Inhibitory (differentiation)
IFN-α-R	IFN-α	Inhibitory (growth)
IFN-γ-R	IFN-γ	Inhibitory (growth, migration)
CCR3 (CD193)	RANTES (CCL5)	Chemotaxis, activation
	MCP-3 (CCL7)	Chemotaxis, activation
	MCP-4 (CCL13)	Chemotaxis, activation
	Eotaxin-1 (CCL11)	Chemotaxis, activation
	Eotaxin-2 (CCL24)	Chemotaxis, activation
	Eotaxin-3 (CCL26)	Chemotaxis, activation
CXCR4 (CD184)	SDF-1 (CXCL12)	Chemotaxis
PAF-R	PAF	Chemotaxis, activation
C5aR (CD88)	C5a	Chemotaxis, activation
TLR1, 4, 7, 9, 10	Toll-like R-ligands	Survival, activation
Corticosteroid R	Corticosteroids	Inhibitory (activation)

[a]Eosinophils derived from patients with hypereosinophilic syndromes (activated eosinophils) may express CD25. However, the role of CD25 in eosinophil function remains unknown.
CCL, Chemokine ligand; CCR, chemokine receptor; FGF, fibroblast growth factor; GM-CSF, granulocyte-macrophage colony-stimulating factor; IFN, interferon; IL, interleukin; LCF, lymphocyte chemoattractant factor; MCP, monocyte chemotactic protein; PAF, platelet-activating factor; PDGF, platelet-derived growth factor; TGF, transforming growth factor; VEGF, vascular endothelial growth factor.

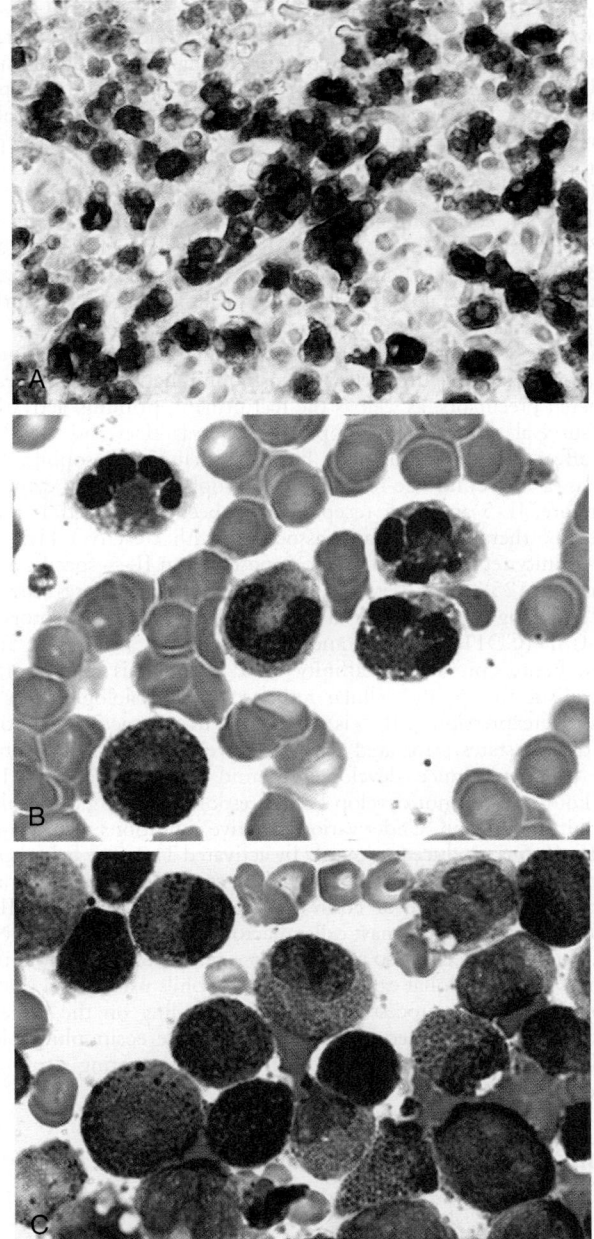

Fig. 71.2 IMMUNOHISTOCHEMICAL AND MORPHOLOGIC PROPERTIES OF NEOPLASTIC EOSINOPHILS. (A) Expression of major basic protein (MBP) in neoplastic eosinophils in a patient suffering from a myeloid neoplasm with eosinophilia. Paraffin-embedded bone marrow sections were stained with an antibody against MBP by indirect immunohistochemistry. (B) Wright-Giemsa-stained bone marrow smear in a patient with chronic eosinophilic leukemia. Note the presence of atypical eosinophils, some of which contain multi-lobed nuclei. (C) Wright-Giemsa-stained bone marrow smear in a patient with an acute eosinophilic leukemia. As visible, the smear contains a mixture of immature and mature eosinophils. Some of the immature eosinophils exhibit a blast-like morphology. Other immature forms contain "basophilic" dark-blue granules, but these cells still belong to the eosinophil lineage.

ORIGIN, DIFFERENTIATION, RECRUITMENT, AND ACTIVATION OF EOSINOPHILS

Eosinophilopoiesis

Eosinophils originate from pluripotent and granulocyte-committed, CD34+, hematopoietic progenitor cells that are detectable in the BM,

in the PB, and various extramedullary organs. Eosinophil development from their multipotent and lineage-restricted progenitors is controlled by a network of transcription factors, including GATA-1, GATA-2, C/EBP-A, and C/EBP-E. Lineage-specific signaling as well as transcription factor expression is controlled by a network of cytokines and cytokine receptors. In fact, eosinophils develop from their progenitors in response to T-cell–derived growth factors, including IL-3, GM-CSF, and IL-5. The most potent and specific eosinophilopoietic growth factor is IL-5. Eosinophils are derived from multipotent or bipotent colony-forming progenitor cell units (CFUs). Bipotent CFUs giving rise to eosinophils and basophils (CFU-eo/ba) are frequently detected in the BM and PB in healthy individuals, as well as in various disease states.[8] By contrast, progenitor cells selectively giving rise to eosinophils and mast cells (CFU-eo/mast) are very rare. At an early stage of progenitor cell development, eosinophil-committed progenitors exhibit CD34 and CD38, and coexpress receptors for IL-3, GM-CSF, and IL-5. Later, CD34 is diminished, whereas the interleukin receptors continue to be expressed, and several additional, functionally important cell surface antigens are acquired by maturing eosinophils.

IL-3, GM-CSF, and IL-5 promote eosinophil differentiation in hematopoietic progenitor cells and eosinophil maturation of lineage-restricted precursors, as well as the recruitment, priming, activation, and survival of mature eosinophils.[9] Whereas IL-3 and GM-CSF also affect other hematopoietic lineages, including basophils, IL-5 acts as a more lineage-restricted (eosinophil-targeting) cytokine. Therefore, IL-5 and IL-5 receptors have been recognized as major targets of therapy in diseases associated with (reactive) HE. The high-affinity receptor for IL-5 is composed of an IL-5–specific alpha chain (CD125) and a beta chain (CD131) that mediates intracellular signaling and is shared also by the high-affinity receptors for GM-CSF (CD116/CD131) and IL-3 (CD123/CD131; see Table 71.5). Expression of high-affinity IL-5 receptors is an important prerequisite for specific cellular responses to "physiologic doses" of IL-5. Overexpression of IL-5 is observed in many reactive conditions and disease states associated with (reactive) HE. Correspondingly, IL-5 transgenic mice develop profound eosinophilia, and IL-5 knockout mice do not develop HE in response to allergic stimuli or a helminth infection. Under various reactive conditions accompanied by HE, IL-5 is produced primarily by activated Th2-type helper cells. However, although activated T cells are considered a primary and most important source of eosinophilopoietic cytokines, like IL-5, other cell types, such as mast cells, macrophages, natural killer (NK) cells, and stromal cells, also produce these cytokines. In myeloid neoplasms with HE, clonal expansion of eosinophils usually is a growth factor-independent process. Moreover, depending on the underlying disease, neoplastic eosinophils may produce eosinophilopoietic cytokines in an autocrine manner, thereby augmenting tissue and blood HE.

Mobilization and Migration of Eosinophils to Sites of Inflammation

In healthy individuals as well as in reactive states, eosinophils circulate only briefly in the PB, and then transit to extravascular sites. Depending on environmental factors and demand, eosinophils localize preferentially in tissues and organs exposed to external environments, principally the submucosal membranes and loose connective tissues of the skin, GI tract, genital tract, and lungs. During an acute or chronic inflammatory process, larger numbers of eosinophils may be recruited actively into local tissue sites.[9] The mobilization of eosinophils from the vasculature into (vascularized) tissues is a multistep process that involves their rolling on vascular endothelial cells and their subsequent adhesion to endothelium via L-selectin, followed by binding to intercellular adhesion molecule-1 (ICAM-1 = CD54) through a CD18/CD11a/b-dependent mechanism.[4] Expression of selectins on endothelial cells is triggered by histamine and other mediators, whereas expression of ICAM-1 on endothelial cells is induced by various proinflammatory cytokines, such as tumor necrosis factor-α (TNF-α). As both histamine and TNF-α are produced and are rapidly provided by (activated) mast cells, these cells are considered to play a crucial role in eosinophil recruitment in various allergic and other inflammatory reactions. However, the recruitment of eosinophils is a complex process involving many different mechanisms and molecules, such as E-selectin, endothelial-leukocyte adhesion molecule 1 (ELAM-1 = CD62E) or vascular cell

adhesion molecule-1 (VCAM-1 = CD106).[4] Selective recruitment of eosinophils is mediated by adhesion to VCAM-1 via the β1 integrin very late activation antigen-4 (VLA-4 = CD49d/CD29), which is expressed by eosinophils but not by blood neutrophils.

Eosinophil migration is regulated by several different chemotactic factors, including various chemokines (SDF-1, eotaxins, IL-8, regulated on activation, normal T-cell expressed and secreted [RANTES], and others), the complement fragment C5a, platelet-activating factor (PAF), and several eosinotropic cytokines, such as IL-5 or GM-CSF, which also prime eosinophils for enhanced migratory responses to PAF and IL-8. In addition, IL-2, leukotriene B4, and the lymphocyte chemoattractant factor (LCF = IL-16) can induce eosinophil migration. At least for neoplastic eosinophils, a most potent chemoattractant appears to be SDF-1, a stromal cell-derived chemokine that binds to CXCR4 (CD184) on normal and neoplastic eosinophils.[10] Other potent chemoattractants for (neoplastic) eosinophils are the eotaxins (eotaxin-1, -2, -3) that bind to and signal through the chemokine receptor CCR3 (CD193; see Table 71.5).[9] Depending on the underlying disease, the cell type(s) involved, and the presence of comorbidities (triggering, e.g., local or systemic inflammation) all these chemotactic factors may act together to trigger eosinophil recruitment and accumulation in the affected (often inflamed) tissue sites. Likewise, in several reactive conditions, IL-5 and eotaxin reportedly cooperate locally to promote eosinophil migration and tissue HE.

The primary source of eosinophil chemotactic factors often remains unknown. In many disease states accompanied by HE, eosinophil chemotactic factors may be produced by microenvironmental cells, including fibroblasts, endothelial cells, macrophages, and mast cells. Several of these chemotaxins, like SDF-1, are produced by stromal cells in a paracrine fashion. For example, in neoplastic eosinophils, the *F/P* mutant triggers expression and release of oncostatin M (OSM), which in turn induces fibroblast and endothelial cell proliferation but also the expression and release of SDF-1 from these cells, thereby augmenting the accumulation of additional eosinophils.[11] In this regard, it is noteworthy that the SDF-1 receptor CXCR4 is not only expressed on mature eosinophils, but also on pluripotent stem cells and eosinophil-committed precursor cells. Depending on the type of underlying neoplasm, eosinophil chemotactic cytokines may also be produced in an autocrine manner.

Role of Mast Cells in Eosinophil Recruitment and Accumulation

In various inflammatory and allergic reactions, several different interactions between eosinophils and mast cells have been postulated. For example, mast cells provide the immediate stimuli upon activation to initiate allergic inflammation, resulting in eosinophil recruitment during the later phases following an allergen encounter. In addition, mast cells and eosinophils are often increased in numbers in allergic reactions, but also in nonallergic inflammatory conditions and even in neoplastic states. Both cell types express a similar profile of chemotactic receptors, such as CCR3, and both respond to eotaxins and RANTES (CCL5), leading to their recruitment into local tissue sites. Mast cells and eosinophils also interact with each other via cell–cell contact and through several different soluble mediators. Likewise, mast cell-derived heparin binds and stabilizes various chemokines, including the eotaxins. In addition, mast cells are a source of various cytokines involved in the regulation of eosinophil adhesion, migration, and function. As previously mentioned, mast cells express and release histamine and TNF-α, and thereby facilitate eosinophil recruitment. Mast cell proteases appear to have a dual action on eosinophil functions. Mast cell-derived chymase suppresses eosinophil apoptosis and induces the release of IL-6 and various chemokines (CXCL1, CXCL8, CCL2) from eosinophils. Beta-tryptase, on the other hand, can cleave eotaxin and RANTES, and thereby may limit eosinophil chemotaxis. Apart from these interactions, eosinophils and mast cells may sometimes also derive from the same stem or progenitor cell compartment, and therefore may express the same driver mutant, which has been documented for cases of *F/P+* chronic eosinophilic leukemia (CEL) with accompanying mast cell expansion, as well as for patients with *KIT D816V+* systemic mastocytosis (SM) with concomitant HE. Therefore, mast cells and eosinophils may often appear as a dual target cell population, both in reactive and neoplastic states, which is a critical point when considering the development of specific therapies. For example, simultaneous downregulation of eosinophil and mast cell activation might be achieved by certain inhibitory surface molecules, such as CD300a or Siglec-8.[12] Several other target receptors, such as Siglec-3 (CD33) are expressed on eosinophils, mast cells, and basophils. In *F/P+* cases, imatinib can induce apoptosis in both eosinophils and mast cells, as both cell types express the mutant platelet-derived growth factor receptor (PDGFR) target in this neoplasm.

MONITORING OF EOSINOPHIL NUMBERS AND ACTIVITY IN HEALTH AND DISEASE

In the PB, eosinophils can easily be measured by microscopy or flow cytometry based on their characteristic side scatter properties and their autofluorescence. In case of atypical (immature) cells or questionable results, immunophenotyping can be performed to confirm the presence of eosinophils. In tissue sections, the quantification of eosinophils is a more difficult task that makes routine clinical evaluations somewhat impractical. Alternative approaches such as analysis of tissue secretions from affected organs (e.g., bronchoalveolar lavage [BAL]) have been used with success in evaluating local eosinophil numbers and function in asthma. In addition to routine histochemical identification and enumeration of eosinophils and the immunochemical localization of secreted eosinophil granule cationic proteins in tissue biopsies, two other methods have been employed to demonstrate and monitor eosinophil activation and involvement, (1) the identification of activated eosinophils by staining with anti-ECP antibody EG2 recognizing a secreted (deglycosylated) form of the protein, and (2) measurement of eosinophil granule proteins, such as MBP or ECP by radioimmunoassay (RIA) or enzyme-linked immunosorbent assay in various body fluids, including serum, plasma, urine, sputum, nasal lavage, and BAL. Indeed, these antigens may serve as reliable biomarkers of eosinophil involvement and activation in allergic, parasitic, and inflammatory diseases. In addition, treatment responses can be demonstrated and measured with these assays.

ETIOLOGY AND PATHOBIOLOGY OF HE

In patients with documented HE, four etiologies have to be considered: (1) myeloid (and rarely myeloid/lymphoid) neoplasms where eosinophils are usually derived from neoplastic stem and progenitor cells, (2) lymphoid neoplasms or nonhematopoietic (solid) tumors where HE is a paraneoplastic phenomenon, (3) reactive conditions, such as an allergy, infection or an autoimmune disease where HE is a reactive process, and (4) rare syndromes accompanied by HE, including rare inherited disorders (see Table 71.4A).[3] In patients with clonal (primary) HE, eosinophils and their progenitors often display rearrangements in *PDGFRA*, *PDGFRB*, or *FGFR1* genes.[13] Therefore, the World Health Organization (WHO) has employed these mutations as primary criteria to describe (classify) hematopoietic neoplasms accompanied by HE (Table 71.6).[14] The resulting "fusion proteins" act as prooncogenic drivers and are considered to contribute to cytokine-independent differentiation of eosinophil progenitor cells. The most frequently detected molecular abnormality is the *F/P* fusion gene, a mutant gene created by an 800-kb interstitial deletion on chromosome 4q12. The fusion gene is detectable by polymerase chain reaction (PCR) as well as by fluorescence in situ hybridization (FISH; deleted *CHIC2* gene) but not by conventional karyotyping. However, conventional cytogenetics may reveal translocations, deletions, or inversions on chromosome 5q31-33, indicating rearrangements of *PDGFRB*, or abnormalities on chromosome band

TABLE 71.6	Molecular Classification of Eosinophil-Related Neoplasms Proposed by the WHO and Related Molecular and Cytogenetic Defects[a]

1. Myeloid and lymphoid neoplasms with eosinophilia and abnormalities of *PDGFRA*, *PDGFRB* or *FGFR1*
   Myeloid and lymphoid neoplasms with *PDGFRA* rearrangement
   Most common variant: *FIP1L1-PDGFRA+* CEL
   Myeloid neoplasms with *PDGFRB* rearrangement
   Most common variant: *ETV6-PDGFRB+* leukemia (aCML, CMML or others)
   Myeloid and lymphoid neoplasms with *FGFR1* rearrangement
   Most common variant: *ZMYM2-FGFR1+* disease

2. Chronic eosinophilic leukemia, not otherwise specified
   BCR-ABL1 and abnormalities in *PDGFRA*, *PDGFRB*, or *FGFR1* are excluded
   Other MPN-related molecular lesions, such as *JAK2* mutations, or certain cytogenetic defects, such as +8 or i(17q), support the diagnosis of CEL

3. WHO-defined myeloid neoplasms with HE, not included in "1" or "2"
   a. Ph+ (*BCR-ABL1+*) chronic myeloid leukemia (CML-eo)
   b. *JAK2 V617F+* myeloproliferative neoplasms (MPN-eo)
   c. *KIT D816V+* systemic mastocytosis (SM-eo)
   d. *CBFβ*-fusion gene-related acute myeloid leukemia (AML-eo/M4-eo)
   e. Myelodysplastic syndromes with HE (MDS-eo)
   f. Other WHO-defined myeloid neoplasms with HE

[a]The table refers to the WHO classification of eosinophil neoplasm.[14]
aCML, Atypical chronic myeloid leukemia; CEL, chronic eosinophilic leukemia; CMML, chronic myelomonocytic leukemia; FGFR, fibroblast growth factor receptor; HE, hypereosinophilia; MDS, myelodysplastic syndrome; MPN, myeloproliferative neoplasm; PDGFR, platelet-derived growth factor receptor; Ph+, Philadelphia chromosome positive; SM, systemic mastocytosis; WHO, World Health Organisation.

8p11-12, indicating a rearrangement of the *FGFR1* gene. From a clinical point of view, it is of great importance to screen for these rearrangements in all patients using the correct techniques, as many of them, including *F/P*, are responsive to imatinib or other tyrosine kinase inhibitors (TKIs). However, clonal HE may also be triggered by other mutations, including *BCR-ABL1*, rearranged *JAK2* or *FLT3*, or *KIT* D816V.[14] In a substantial subset of patients with MPN-eo, no mutation is found.

In paraneoplastic and reactive states, HE is usually triggered by eosinophilopoietic cytokines, including IL-5, IL-3, or GM-CSF. These cytokines, especially IL-5, may be detected in the serum of these patients and are considered to be produced by activated T cells or other activated immune cells. In a few patients with HE and HES, activated (clonal) T cells are detectable by phenotyping and PCR, but no underlying lymphoma or other underlying condition is found. In these cases, the lymphoid variant of HES (HES$_L$) is diagnosed.[15] In some of these patients, an overt T-cell lymphoma or Sézary syndrome may develop in the follow-up. A number of different reactive conditions and disorders, including helminth infections, fungal infections, autoimmune disorders, allergies, or drug reactions, can lead to reactive HE and reactive HES (HES$_R$). These conditions are listed in Table 71.2.

Pathogenesis of Eosinophil-Associated End-Organ Damage in Patients With HES

Regardless of the underlying etiology (neoplastic or reactive), sustained HE may lead to typical end-organ damage defined as HES. Even in patients with idiopathic HE, such organ damage may occur and is then called *idiopathic HES* (HES$_I$).[3] However, not all patients presenting with HE develop organ damage even if followed over a longer time period. For example, patients with an underlying allergic disease, an inherited disorder accompanied by HE, or those with organ-specific HE syndromes, such as eosinophilic pneumonia, usually fail to develop the cardiac damage seen in patients with typical HES. When neither an underlying disease nor HE-related organ damage is found, the diagnosis HE of undetermined significance (HE$_{US}$) is established.[3] In general, the risk of HES is lower in reactive forms of HE, especially when the underlying disease can be treated successfully. Correspondingly, IL-5 transgenic mice with massive HE do not develop significant end-organ damage, suggesting that other factors (in addition to IL-5) are likely necessary for the occurrence of a HE-related organ damage. In patients with an underlying MPN or other underlying myeloid neoplasm, the risk of HE-related organ damage (HES) is relatively high. The highest risk is found in patients with mutations in *PDGFR* genes. Likewise, most untreated patients with *F/P*+ MPN-eo or CEL may develop HES with cardiac involvement over time. Additional risk factors may also contribute in these patients: these factors include, among others, an additional prothrombophilic state, late detection of the disease, and late initiation of specific (anti-CEL) therapy. There may also be a certain genetic predisposition for early occurrence of tissue HE in patients with *F/P*+ CEL (*F/P*+ MPN-eo). In particular, the severity (extent) of tissue HE seems to correlate with a polymorphic variant (SNP in the 5′-UTR) in the *IL-5RA* gene.[16] However, it remains unclear whether this SNP predisposes to HES development or progression, and thus is relevant clinically. Today, the general recommendation is to initiate therapy with imatinib early in all *F/P*+ patients, regardless of genetic, molecular or other factors, in order to prevent any HES occurrence as well as disease progression (to acute leukemia).

A number of different organ systems are affected in patients with HES. The most common manifestations are summarized in Table 71.7. Although multiple organ systems are involved and the manifestation patterns are quite complex with varying courses and outcomes, some common pathogenetic factors have been described. One common feature is the mobilization of the tissue microenvironment by eosinophil-derived mediators and cytokines, which leads to tissue remodeling, fibrosis, and increased angiogenesis. Another common factor is tissue inflammation, which is typically triggered by eosinophil-derived cytokines and chemokines. Finally, HE-related organopathies may often result from direct cytotoxic damage that is induced by the various toxic mediators produced and released by (reactive and neoplastic) eosinophils. With regard to thrombosis, several different eosinophil-derived mediators have been implicated, including TNF-α, plasminogen activator inhibitors (PAIs), and eosinophil-derived DNA traps (see Table 71.1).[17] In addition, ECPs have the capacity to alter thrombomodulin activity. A number of different compounds produced by eosinophils, including cationic proteins and various cytokines, may induce fibrosis. Among these cytokines, OSM may play a particular role as a HES-related profibrogenic cytokine.[11] HE-related neoangiogenesis may be triggered by IL-8, OSM, and vascular endothelial growth factor (VEGF). All these cytokines are produced and secreted by normal/reactive and also by neoplastic eosinophils. However, neoplastic eosinophils produce some of these cytokines in excess over their normal counterparts. For example, *F/P*+ eosinophils express and release huge amounts of OSM, IL-8, and VEGF. The *F/P* mutant induces the production and secretion of these mediators in neoplastic cells in a STAT5-dependent manner. Concerning the mobilization of the microenvironment in various organs in patients with HES, a most critical *F/P* target gene may be *OSM*. Notably, OSM initiates not only fibrosis and angiogenesis by triggering fibroblast proliferation and tube formation in endothelial cells, but also by inducing the production of multiple cytokines and chemokines in stromal cells. Among these mediators are IL-8, SDF-1, and other chemotactic factors that can recruit additional CXCR4+ precursor cells and eosinophils to local tissue sites.[11]

An unresolved question is why HE-related fibrosis and thrombosis affect certain tissues and organs, including the heart, whereas the same organs are spared by other thrombophilia-inducing MPN types,

TABLE 71.7 End-Organ Damage Typically Observed in Patients With Hypereosinophilic Syndrome

Cardiac
Intramural thrombi
Valve regurgitation
Constrictive pericarditis
Endomyocardial fibrosis
Myocarditis
Cardiomyopathy

Neurologic
Fatigue
Thromboembolism and stroke
Peripheral neuropathy
Central nervous system dysfunction and dementia
Paresthesias and/or sensory deficits
Epilepsy

Dermatologic
Angioedema
Urticaria
Papular and/or nodular lesions
Mucosal ulcers
Vesicobullous lesions
Microthrombi

Pulmonary
Pulmonary infiltrates
Pulmonary thromboembolism
Pneumonitis
Fibrosis
Pleural effusion

Ocular
Microthrombi
Vasculitis
Retinal arteritis

Connective Tissue
Arthralgias
Effusions
Polyarthritis
Raynaud phenomenon
Digital necrosis

Gastrointestinal
Ascites
Diarrhea
Gastritis
Colitis
Cholangitis

such as the *JAK2*-mutated variants. One explanation may be that eosinophils invade heart and lung tissues via "physiologic" routes, which may not be the case in other MPNs where HE usually does not occur. An additional explanation may be that eosinophil-derived mediators are toxic to certain (tissue-specific) cell types such as cardiomyocytes. Indeed, as noted earlier, eosinophils express a number of different cationic proteins capable of inducing endothelial and endocardial damage and neurotoxicity. In addition, the eosinophil has the capacity to generate reactive oxidative species that can augment tissue damage.

DEFINITION AND CLASSIFICATION OF HE AND HES

The term HES was initially proposed for a syndrome characterized by idiopathic HE and HE-related organ damage, as well as by exclusion of various conditions and diseases that are typically accompanied by HE. More recently, the definition of HES has been refined as any type of HE (not just idiopathic) associated with typical HE-related end-organ damage.[3] According to the proposal of an international working group on eosinophil disorders (ICOG-EO), the term HES should be reserved for clinical syndromes fulfilling HES criteria, but not for underlying (hematologic) malignancies or immunological disorders presenting with HE.[3] In other words, the diagnosis HES must prompt the physician to search for (detect) an underlying (HES-triggering) disease. Accordingly, the final diagnosis is either idiopathic HES or HES based on a recognized underlying disorder, and both need to be documented in the final diagnosis. In previous WHO classifications, the term HES was sometimes used as a synonym of CEL, and sometimes to discriminate CEL from other less well-defined myeloid neoplasms with HE. However, in the 2008 edition of the WHO monograph, the term HES was no longer recommended as a synonym of WHO-defined neoplasms, a distinction that is in agreement with the proposal of the ICON group and the proposal of the ICOG-EO group.[3]

Definition of HE

HE is currently defined as a persistent, microscopically confirmed increase in PB eosinophils above $1.5 \times 10^4/L$. In previous definitions, persistent eosinophilia over 6 months was required to establish the diagnosis HE. However, based on improved diagnostics and treatment, and the necessity to introduce such treatment rapidly to avoid organ damage, the proposed definition of HE has recently been revised to a 4-week observation interval by the ICOG-EO group.[3] The term "tissue HE" has also been proposed by several experts, and it may be useful to apply it in certain conditions, especially in the context of (to demonstrate) HE-related organ damage (HES). However, isolated tissue HE (without blood HE) is rare, and the documentation of tissue HE often requires special immunostains directed against eosinophil granule proteins.[7] Therefore, the presence of tissue HE is often overlooked or is not documented, and PB HE clearly remains the key diagnostic marker in daily practice. In some of these patients, criteria for blood HE are not met, but molecular and clinical signs are strongly indicative of a particular eosinophil disorder with or without accompanying HES. These patients should be followed closely, as they may progress to an overt eosinophil disease (neoplasm) over time. The same holds true for WHO-based neoplasms presenting with *PDGFR* or *FGFR1* fusion genes without overt HE.[14]

Diagnostic Algorithm

When arriving at the provisional diagnostic "checkpoint" HE, two critical questions have to be addressed in order to approach to a final diagnosis: (1) is there any underlying disease or condition triggering HE? *and* (2) are there clinical signs and symptoms or laboratory abnormalities that point to the presence of HE-induced organ damage, so that the additional diagnosis of HES can be established? For example, the hematologic work-up in a patient with HE revealed CEL, and staging investigations showed endocardial thrombus formation: the final diagnosis in this patient is CEL with concomitant primary HES (HES$_N$). A diagnostic algorithm is shown in Fig. 71.3. In patients with typical HES and typical clinical manifestation, histopathologic evaluation is generally not warranted to confirm the presence of tissue HE. However, in patients with rare or atypical manifestations, such as renal failure, isolated myocarditis or bloody diarrhea, a tissue biopsy is required to document the presence of tissue HE and to confirm HE-induced organ damage, so that the diagnosis HES can be

established. The demonstration of extensive extracellular deposition of eosinophil-derived proteins supports the conclusion the organ damage is "HE-related".[7]

Classification of HE and HES

The classification of HE and HES is essentially based on the related disease and underlying etiology. Accordingly, HE and HES are both divided into a familial variant (HE$_F$, HES$_F$), a primary/neoplastic form (HE$_N$, HES$_N$), and reactive entities (HE$_R$, HES$_R$; see Table 71.3).[3] In a smaller fraction of patients, the etiology of HE and HES remains uncertain or two different causative factors are detected. When the etiology of HE remains uncertain after a thorough investigation and appropriate testing and no organ damage is detected, the final diagnosis is HE of uncertain (undetermined) significance (HE$_{US}$); and if HES is diagnosed, but no underlying disease is detected, the final diagnosis is idiopathic HES (HES$_I$).[3]

In general, four major groups of underlying disorders (conditions) have to be considered in HE (HES) patients: (1) myeloid (and rarely myeloid/lymphoid) neoplasms including eosinophilic leukemias (HE$_N$; HES$_N$), (2) lymphoid or nonhematopoietic neoplasms (paraneoplastic HE, a special variant of HE$_R$), (3) common allergic, reactive, or immunologic conditions (HE$_R$ and HES$_R$), and (4) clinically defined, rare syndromes and conditions accompanied by HE, including rare inherited disorders and organ-restricted inflammatory diseases with tissue HE.[3,17] Overall, the classification of HE/HES remains an important step in the diagnostic algorithm (Fig. 71.3). Using generally accepted criteria and parameters, this approach should lead to a final diagnosis concerning the presence or absence of HES and the presence or absence of an underlying disease.

CLINICAL MANIFESTATIONS OF HES IN VARIOUS ORGAN SYSTEMS AND DIFFERENTIAL DIAGNOSIS

Depending on the type of disease and other factors, a number of different organ systems may be involved in patients with HES. The most commonly involved organs are the skin, lungs, GI tract, heart, and the CNS (see Table 71.7). In some patients, the relationship between HE and the typical clinical signs and symptoms are pathognomonic, whereas in other cases a tissue biopsy may be required to confirm HE-related organopathy.

Cardiac Manifestations in Patients With HES

Prior to the advent of improved diagnostics and management, and novel therapeutic approaches, cardiac disease was the leading cause of morbidity and mortality in patients with HES. Endomyocardial thrombosis and fibrosis are often documented in HES$_N$, particularly in association with the *F/P* fusion gene, but are also seen in other variants of HES, including tropical forms induced by (persistent) parasitic infections and other reactive forms of HES. A thorough cardiac evaluation including an ECG and echocardiogram is mandatory in all patients with HE, and cardiac magnetic resonance imaging (MRI) may be helpful in distinguishing a HE-related cardiac disease from other etiologies. In uncertain cases, troponin levels and B-type natriuretic peptide levels may be helpful parameters. An endomyocardial biopsy may be required in some of these patients in order to establish the definitive diagnosis, but biopsies are usually not performed in daily practice.

The cardiac damage seen in HES usually progresses from early necrotic changes through thrombosis and fibrosis. The presence of eosinophils in the myocardium is always abnormal and highly suggestive of eosinophil-mediated organopathy. Identical forms of cardiac pathology can develop in patients with HES forms of diverse etiologies, including tropical eosinophilias caused by parasitic infections, drug reactions, eosinophilic leukemias, MPN-eo, solid tumors,

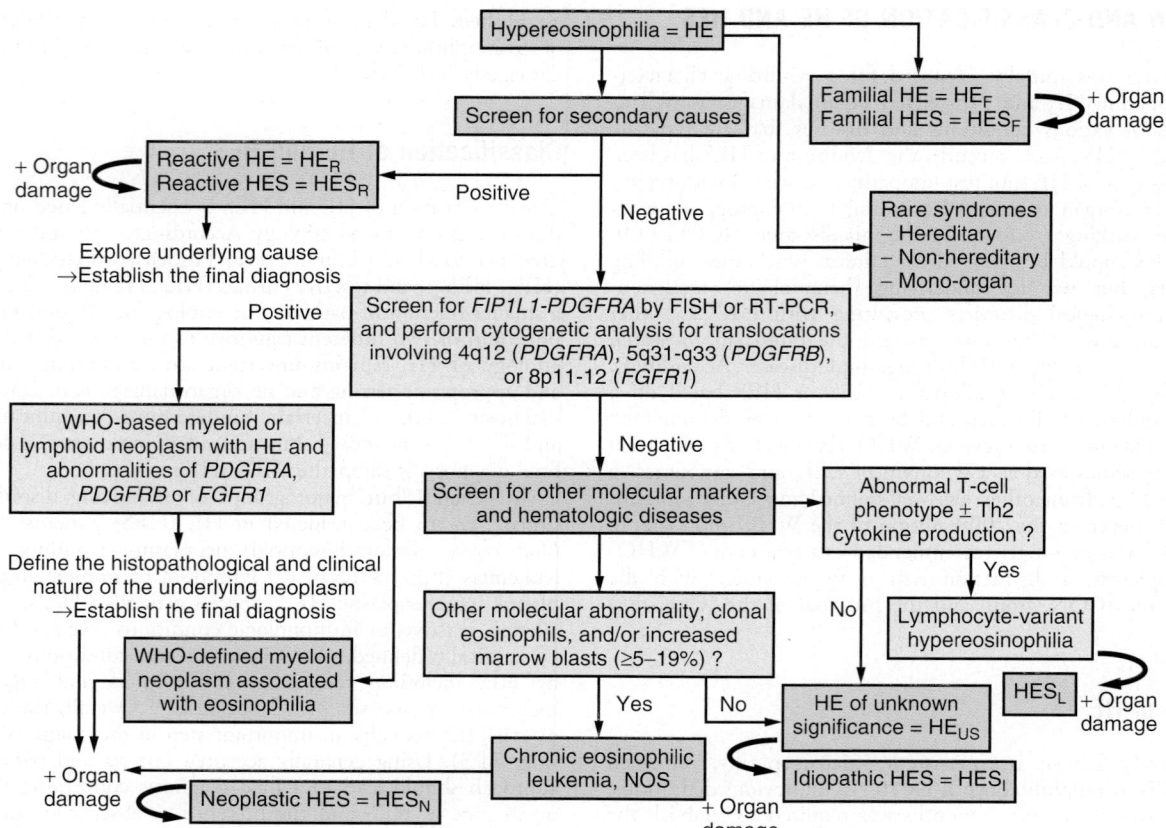

Fig. 71.3 DIAGNOSTIC ALGORITHM FOR PATIENTS WITH EOSINOPHIL DISORDERS. The first important step in the algorithm is to confirm the presence of HE, defined by a persistent (>4 weeks) increase in eosinophils above 1500/μL blood. The next important question is whether HE is reactive (HE_R) or neoplastic (clonal = HE_N) in nature. In patients with HE_N, WHO criteria should be applied in order to define the underlying molecular lesion. In addition, morphologic and histopathologic criteria are used to arrive at a final diagnosis regarding the underlying disease. In patients with HE_R, an underlying disease must also be defined. In both groups of patients, the next important question is whether (or not) HE-related organ damage is present. If such organopathy is found, it is appropriate to diagnose the (additional) presence of HES. According to the underlying etiology (disease), HES is classified again into HES_R and HES_N. In some patients with HES, a clonal T-cell population, but no lymphoproliferative disease, is detected. In these patients, the HES_L variant is diagnosed. If no clonal T cells and no underlying reactive or neoplastic condition is detected in a patient with HES, the (provisional) diagnosis of an HES_I is established. If no underlying disease and no HES is detected, the patient has HE_{US} by definition. Familial cases of HE or HES are very rare, and the same holds true for hereditary syndromes and mono-organ syndromes accompanied by HE. HE, Hypereosinophilia; HES, hypereosinophilic syndrome; HES_F, familial HES; HES_I, idiopathic HES; HES_L, lymphoid variant of HES; HES_N, primary (neoplastic) HES; HES_R, reactive HES; HE_{US}, HE of undermined (unknown) significance; *WHO*, World Health Organisation.

CSS and lymphomas. However, some of these patients may never go on to develop cardiac involvement, suggesting that disease manifestation likely involves as yet undefined factors required for HE-related tissue damage. The histopathology of cardiac involvement in HES is well characterized and can evolve through three sequentially defined stages in which eosinophils and eosinophil-derived mediators may be involved. These include (1) an initial acute necrotic stage of short duration (a few weeks) involving active endomyocarditis, (2) a later thrombotic stage (several months) with mural thrombus formation over endocardial lesions, and (3) a late fibrotic stage (after approximately 2 years of illness) with development of endomyocardial fibrosis. The early necrotic stage of cardiac disease is usually not recognized clinically. Echocardiography and angiography may fail to detect abnormalities at this early stage because ventricular thickening has not yet occurred and endomyocardial biopsies, generally from the right ventricle, are required to make the correct diagnosis of cardiac involvement. In the second stage, thrombi form over the damaged endocardium in either of the ventricles or the atrium,

generally with sparing of the aortic and pulmonary valves. Progressive scarring at sites of mural thrombus formation ultimately leads to the late fibrotic stage, with endomyocardial fibrosis resulting in a restrictive cardiomyopathy and mitral or/and tricuspid valve regurgitation (see Table 71.7). The more common clinical manifestations in the later progressive stages of endomyocardial fibrosis include dyspnea, chest pain, signs of left or right ventricular congestive heart failure, or both, murmurs from mitral valve regurgitation, cardiomegaly, and T-wave inversions. Most patients who progress to this stage of HES-related cardiopathy have echocardiographic abnormalities, with thickening of the left ventricular wall being a common finding. However, electrocardiographic and MRI changes in these patients are not specific to HES. Differential diagnoses include infectious etiologies (endomyocarditis), CSS, autoimmune disorders such as rheumatoid arthritis, Marfan syndrome, thyroid disorders, and ischemic heart disease. Although various imaging techniques are helpful in evaluating HES-related cardiopathy, endomyocardial biopsy from the right and left ventricle remains a gold standard in diagnostic evaluation in patients with HE-related cardiopathy.

Pulmonary Manifestations

Approximately 50% of HES patients have pulmonary involvement, with the most common symptom being a chronic and persistent (nonproductive) cough. In order to confirm pulmonary manifestation in HES, a number of studies may be helpful, including pulmonary function tests, chest radiography and/or CT scan, and bronchoscopy with BAL studies and a tissue biopsy if necessary. The physiologic basis of pulmonary involvement in HES remains unknown. As in the heart, several different eosinophil-derived (cytotoxic and stroma-targeting) mediators and cytokines may act together to induce tissue damage and tissue remodeling, as well as fibrosis and thrombosis. Some of the pulmonary features may also reflect changes secondary to congestive heart failure. Although bronchospasm has been noted in some patients, full-blown asthma is rare in HES patients. Transudative pleural effusions are mostly seen in patients with frank congestive heart failure. In contrast to chronic eosinophilic pneumonia, the pulmonary infiltrates seen in HES patients are either diffuse or focal, without any preference for particular regions of the lung. Pulmonary infiltrates in HES often clear with prednisone treatment, but not all patients are responders. Pulmonary fibrosis is rare, but can develop in patients with endomyocardial fibrosis. The differential diagnosis of HES$_R$ with pulmonary involvement includes drug allergy, CSS, chronic eosinophilic pneumonia, severe allergic bronchial asthma with eosinophilia, allergic bronchopulmonary aspergillosis, and other eosinophilic lung infections.

Cutaneous Manifestations

The skin is frequently involved in HES, with cutaneous lesions present in over 50% of all cases. In these patients, the cutaneous lesions fall into three categories: (1) angioedematous and urticarial lesions; (2) erythematous, pruritic papules and nodules; and (3) mucosal ulcerations (see Table 71.7).[18] Patients with angioedema and urticaria are more likely to have a benign disease that is responsive to corticosteroids, without the development of cardiac or neurologic symptoms. A subgroup of patients with cyclical angioedema and eosinophilia are considered to have a syndrome (episodic angioedema with eosinophilia = Gleich syndrome) that is distinct from classical HES. These patients have a disorder with recurrent attacks of angioedema and urticaria accompanied by fever and weight gain. In HES patients with papular or nodular lesions, dermal biopsies usually show mixed cellular infiltrates, including eosinophils, without signs of vasculitis. Perivascular eosinophilic infiltrates are also found in these lesions. In a group of HES patients with skin involvement, the erythematous pruritic eruptions and indurated papules and nodules may respond to psoralen and ultraviolet light A. In other patients with HES-associated pruritus, the nodular lesions may respond to dapsone and corticosteroids. Oral sodium cromoglycate (cromolyn sodium), administered before meals, has also been reported to be efficacious, although neither dapsone nor cromolyn is able to reduce eosinophil counts in the blood. Severe and sometimes incapacitating mucocutaneous ulcerations may be a prodrome to HES and indicate a subset of HES patients with a poor prognosis. These lesions can appear at multiple sites, including the mouth, nose, pharynx, penis, esophagus, stomach, and anus. The lesions can flare up independently of other clinical manifestations of HES. Biopsies of the ulcerative lesions usually show mixed cellular infiltrates, without a predominance of eosinophils or any evidence of vasculitis or microthrombi. These ulcers are usually resistant to treatment with corticosteroids, colchicine, and hydroxyurea (HU), but they usually respond to interferon-α (IFN-α), with complete and durable remissions in most patients. There are a number of differential diagnoses that have to be considered in HES patients with suspected skin involvement, including drug reactions, local infections, and atopic eczema.

Neurologic Manifestations

Neurologic involvement is quite common in HES, affecting approximately 50% of all patients. In these cases, three different types of manifestations have been described. The first form of neurologic involvement is caused by thromboemboli, which may originate from intracardiac thrombi in the left ventricle but may also develop locally in cerebral vessels. Some of these thromboembolic episodes may occur before an overt cardiac manifestation has been documented. Patients with thrombotic complications may experience embolic strokes or transient ischemic attacks that may be multiple and recurrent, and these episodes may occur even though the patient is adequately anticoagulated. The second type of neurologic manifestation is primary diffuse CNS involvement. These patients may variably exhibit changes in behavior, confusion, ataxia, and loss of memory. The third neurologic abnormality noted in HES is the development of peripheral neuropathy, which can occur in approximately 50% of HES patients exhibiting neurologic involvement. This includes symmetric or asymmetric sensory polyneuropathies, including sensory deficits, painful paresthesias, or mixed sensory and motor defects (see Table 71.7). These neuropathies may improve with corticosteroid administration or other treatments, and may be stable or continue to progress despite therapy, or may improve or even resolve with time. The histopathology of the involved nerves usually shows varying degrees of axonal loss, without evidence of vasculitis or direct or peripheral eosinophil infiltration. Whether eosinophil-derived EDN and/or ECP, known to cause neurotoxicity in experimental animals, are involved in the development of neuropathies in HES remains unknown. Based on immunohistochemical studies, these proteins are not detectable at the sites of ongoing neuropathology in HES patients. All in all, the etiology of HES-related neuropathy remains poorly defined. Differential diagnoses of HES-related neuropathies are manifold and include, among others, neurodegenerative disorders, multiple sclerosis, and CNS infections.

Gastrointestinal Manifestations

Compared to lung or skin, GI tract involvement is less common in patients with HES. Although any form of HES can present with GI tract manifestation, GI tract symptoms are mostly recorded in patients with HES$_R$ or the idiopathic form of HES. In these patients, a wide variety of symptoms and findings have been described, including abdominal pain, vomiting, diarrhea, or ulcerative disease, but also ascites or an overt colitis (see Table 71.7). These patients may also report bloody diarrhea and weight loss. Histologically, GI tract involvement with HES is characterized by an infiltration of the mucosa and submucosa with eosinophils. Immunohistochemical examination may reveal a huge infiltration with eosinophils as well as extensive deposition of extracellular eosinophil proteins in the gastric mucosa. In most patients with reactive HES, the GI tract disease component responds to treatment with oral corticosteroids. Differential diagnoses of GI tract involvement with HES include localized (organ-restricted) inflammatory disorders, such as eosinophilic esophagitis, eosinophilic gastroenteritis, eosinophilic colitis, autoimmune diseases, chronic inflammatory bowel disease, GI infections, GI tract lymphomas, and GI tract involvement in patients with SM. Especially in patients with SM, the underlying disease is often overlooked, since neoplastic mast cells are outnumbered by the infiltrating eosinophils. In these cases, the use of mast cell-related immunohistochemical markers, such as tryptase, KIT (CD117), or CD25, may be helpful to diagnose an underlying SM.

Hematologic Manifestations and BM Involvement

In HES patients suffering from an underlying myeloid neoplasm (HE$_N$, HES$_N$), the BM is almost always involved. In these patients, the BM is often hypercellular and shows a substantial increase in eosinophil numbers. In addition, alterations in the BM microenvironment, including neoangiogenesis and BM fibrosis, is usually detected in these patients. Depending on the underlying neoplasm, other hematopoietic lineages may also be affected and may show typical morphological or phenotypic aberrations. Depending on the underlying neoplasm, eosinophils may be mature or (rather) immature cells (Fig. 71.2B and C). The BM is also affected in patients with reactive or idiopathic HES. However, in these patients eosinophils are usually mature cells and no major alterations in the BM microenvironment or abnormalities in other hematopoietic lineages are found.

Apart from eosinophilic leukemias, a number of different underlying BM neoplasms may be identified, such as a MPN, myelodysplastic syndrome (MDS), MDS/MPN overlap syndrome, acute myeloid leukemia (AML), or, rarely, a lymphoid malignancy.[17] In these patients, various blood count abnormalities may be present, such as neutrophilia, monocytosis, basophilia, thrombocytosis, a left-shifted white blood count, or an increase in blasts. In some cases, anemia or/ and thrombocytopenia with or without increased blast cells or dysplasia is found, consistent with the diagnosis of an overt MDS, a MDS/MPN overlap syndrome, or AML. In rare cases, a stem cell neoplasm with involvement of both the myeloid and lymphoid lineage is detected. In these patients, an *FGFR1*-rearranged neoplasm (previously referred to as *8p11 myeloproliferative syndrome* or *stem cell leukemia/lymphoma syndrome*) may be diagnosed.[13] The prognosis is poor in these patients. In some patients with CEL, a massive leukocytosis is found. In these cases, eosinophilia of more than 90% may be seen, and total leukocyte counts may exceed 50,000 or even 100,000/mm[3]. Extremely high leukocyte (eosinophil) counts are more commonly seen in patients with HES$_N$ in the context of CEL and are considered to be associated with a more unfavorable prognosis. Blood smears from patients with HES$_R$ and HES$_I$ generally show more or less normal, mature eosinophil morphologies, including typical bilobed nuclei and granule-rich cytoplasm. However, hypodense eosinophils and eosinophilic precursor cells may be recorded, although less commonly, and eosinophils may also exhibit morphologic abnormalities, including nuclear hypersegmentation, decreased size and/or numbers of secondary granules, and cytoplasmic vacuolization. Mast cells may be increased in number in HES patients, especially in *F/P*+ cases, where these cells usually belong to the neoplastic clone. The presence of myeloblasts and/or dysplastic findings in the PB may suggest AML or MDS. Splenomegaly is present in a substantial subset of patients with HES, mostly in those with an underlying myeloid neoplasm, but sometimes also in cases with a reactive form of HES or idiopathic HES. In patients with markedly enlarged spleens, hypersplenism may develop and may contribute to thrombocytopenia and anemia. In these patients, splenic pain induced by capsular distention or infarction are well-known complications.

Underlying Hematologic Disorders and Differential Diagnoses

Although various hematologic neoplasms may be accompanied by eosinophilia, only a few of these are associated with persistent HE (HE$_N$) and HE-related organ damage (= HES$_N$). For example, mild-to-moderate eosinophilia may be detected in Philadelphia chromosome-positive (Ph[+]; BCR-ABL1[+]) chronic myelogenous leukemia (CML) and various Ph[−] MPNs, but marked HE is unusual and HES is rarely found in these patients. However, in a few patients with CML or MPNs, excessive HE may develop. In these patients, HE is usually responsive to BCR-ABL1 kinase inhibitors in CML, and to conventional cytostatic drugs, such as HU or IFN-α, in MPN. In a few myeloid neoplasms substantial or even excessive HE is a typical finding. These malignancies include the rare variant of acute eosinophilic leukemia (AEL), the more common variant of CEL that is often associated with a *F/P* fusion gene, and other forms or CEL or MPN-eo with rearrangements involving *PDGFRA*, *PDGFRB*, or *FGFR1*.[13] Other patients with CEL may fulfill the criteria of the WHO category CEL, NOS (see Table 71.6).[14] Rarely, HE$_N$ is found in patients with MDS. In most cases with dysplastic BM and HE,

however, additional signs of myeloproliferation are found, consistent with a diagnosis of a MDS/MPN overlap syndrome or frank MPN. Another myeloid neoplasm that is often accompanied by HE is SM.[19] In fact, HE$_N$ is frequently seen in patients with advanced SM, including aggressive SM and mast cell leukemia (see Table 71.6). Most of these patients develop HE without HE-related organ damage (HES). In rare cases, lymphoid neoplasms may also present with HE. In these patients, a T-cell lymphoma is most commonly detected as underlying disease during initial staging investigations or during follow-up. In most patients with T-cell lymphomas accompanied by HE, eosinophils are nonclonal cells. By contrast, in patients with fusions involving *FGFR1*, where stem cells are considered to give rise to malignant cells, both eosinophils and lymphocytes are clonally involved. The prognosis in these patients is grave.

Several different concepts by which to classify eosinophil neoplasms have been proposed in the recent past.[20] The WHO has classified eosinophil-related disorders according to the presence of certain molecular lesions, including abnormalities in the *PDGFR* or *FGFR* genes (see Table 71.6).[14] The advantage of this approach is that it refers to molecular targets of therapy. As a result, therapeutic decisions may be directly based on a WHO-based diagnosis. However, independent of the clinical presentation and markers, the WHO classification has to be complemented by a final histopathologic diagnosis, which in turn is based on thorough morphologic, histopathologic, and immunohistochemical studies of the BM.[3,17] Based on a proposal of the ICOG-EO group,[3] the following underlying neoplasms have to be delineated (see Table 71.8A):

Acute Eosinophilic Leukemia

This type of leukemia is defined by HE, more than 19% (≥20%) myeloblasts and greater than 29% (≥30%) eosinophils in BM smears (see Table 71.8A).[3] Other classical types of MPN and CML must be excluded. AEL is an extremely rare disease. Eosinophils in these patients may be quite immature, hypogranulated cells, or represent a

TABLE 71.8A	Histopathologic Classification and Criteria of Eosinophilic Leukemias and Other Myeloid Neoplasms Presenting With Hypereosinophilia		
Neoplasm(s)		**Abbreviation**	**Definition/Criteria**
i.	Acute eosinophilic leukemia	AEL	HE and eosinophils ≥30% and myeloblasts ≥20%
ii.	Chronic eosinophilic leukemia	CEL[a]	HE and eosinophils ≥30% and myeloblasts <20% and no underlying stem cell-, myeloid or lymphoid neoplasm found
iii.	Other myeloid neoplasm (MN) or stem cell neoplasm with HE: MPN-eo, MDS-eo, SM-eo,	MN-eo	MN or stem cell neoplasm by WHO or FAB criteria and HE, but eosinophils <30%

The histopathological classification of eosinophil disorders assists the WHO-based delineation of neoplasms presenting with eosinophilia (HE). In a first step, the diagnosis is based on the WHO definition as molecular and cytogenetic abnormalities are examined. In a second step, the final histomorphologically defined diagnosis needs to be established using the criteria depicted in this table.[3] Values for eosinophils and blast cells refer to the bone marrow smear. In rare cases (acute leukemia), eosinophils may be quite immature and may escape conventional morphological identification. In these cases, immunophenotyping or electron microscopy may be required.

[a]In order to diagnose CEL, the following cytogenetic and molecular defects have to be excluded as primary reason of HE: BCR-ABL1, inv(16), t(16;16), JAK2 V617F.

FAB, French–American–British Cooperative Study Group; HE, Hypereosinophilia; MDS, myelodysplastic syndromes; MPN, myeloproliferative neoplasm; WHO, World Health Organization.

mixture of mature and immature eosinophils. In some of these patients, a prodrome of MDS or MPN without HE occurs. In addition, *F/P+* patients with CEL or *F/P+* MPN-eo may progress to AEL during their terminal phase. However, no (other) recurrent cytogenetic or molecular marker has been identified in AEL patients. The clinical course in AEL is unfavorable. Chemotherapy and stem cell transplantation are usually recommended. Major differential diagnoses are AML M4-eo with inv16, CEL with signs of progression, and SM-AHN-eo (e.g., SM-AML-eo).

Chronic Eosinophilic Leukemia

In patients with CEL, eosinophils comprise ≥30% of all nucleated BM cells and/or blood leukocytes. As per definition, patients with CEL have overt HE_N and less than 20% myeloblasts in their BM and/or blood smears (see Table 71.8A).[3] Usually, blast counts are below 5%. In most patients, neoplastic cells exhibit rearrangements (mutations) in genes coding for *PDGFRA*, *PDGFRB*, or *FGFR1*. Therefore, most patients also fit into the WHO category of "myeloid or lymphoid neoplasms associated with eosinophilia and abnormalities of *PDGFRA*, *PDGFRB*, or *FGFR1*". Other BM neoplasms need to be excluded by BM examination. Major differential diagnoses include AEL, MPN-eo, MPN/MDS-eo, SM-eo, SM-AHN-eo, and reactive forms of HE/HES. Progression from CEL to AEL is an extremely rare event. However, in untreated patients with *PDGFR* mutations and those with *FGFR1* mutations, progression of CEL to AEL or even AML may occur. The prognosis in CEL depends largely on the molecular lesions detected. In patients with CEL exhibiting *PDGFR* mutations, the prognosis is excellent, as in most cases the disease responds to imatinib. By contrast, in patients with *FGFR1* mutations, the diagnosis is dismal, even when treated with chemotherapy and early allogeneic hematopoietic stem cell transplantation (HSCT) should be considered.

MPN-eo, MPN/MDS-eo, MDS-eo, and SM-eo

The exact nomenclature of myeloid or mast cell neoplasms with marked eosinophilia (HE) is still under debate.[20] The ICOG-EO group has recently proposed the use of the appendix "-eo" for patients in whom HE_N is detected but criteria of AEL or CEL are not met.[3] In fact, in these patients an underlying MPN, MPN/MDS, MDS, or SM is diagnosed, and HE is present. However, eosinophils comprise less than 30% of all nucleated BM and PB leukocytes. In patients with MPN-eo, MPN/MDS-eo, or MDS-eo, HE may be detected at diagnosis or may develop during the follow-up period. In a small group of patients, mutant forms of *PDGFRs* or the *FGFR* are found. In other patients, karyotype abnormalities are detected, but *PDGFR* or *FGFR* mutants are not found. The molecular mechanisms underlying HE development in these patients usually remains unknown. Differential diagnoses include Ph+ CML, CEL, AEL, and SM-AHN-eo. The overall prognosis depends on the underlying neoplasm, especially on blast cell counts, karyotypes and the expression of *PDGFR* or *FGFR1* mutants. Therefore, it is important to apply all markers and diagnostic tests in order to define the exact final diagnosis. In MDS and MPN/MDS, the presence of eosinophilia is an independent prognostic factor and indicative of poor survival, especially when HE is accompanied by blood basophilia.[21] Treatment of patients depends largely on the type of underlying malignancy, but also on the presence of distinct molecular lesions and targets. In advanced stages of the disease, a complex karyotype and complex mutational patterns are often found. These patients are candidates for intensive treatment, including HSCT.

Lymphoid Neoplasms, Lymphomas

A number of different lymphomas may produce eosinophilia, mostly through the generation of eosinophilopoietic cytokines in neoplastic

TABLE 71.8B	Hematopoietic Neoplasms Accompanied by Eosinophilia

Neoplasms in Which Eosinophils Are Likely To Be Clonal Cells

Acute eosinophilic leukemia (AEL)

Chronic eosinophilic leukemia (CEL)

Acute myeloid leukemia with inv(16) (FAB AML M4eo)

Chronic myeloid leukemia (CML – *BCR-ABL1+*)

Myeloid neoplasms with *PDGFR* abnormalities (WHO types)

Hematopoietic neoplasms with *FGFR1* abnormalities (WHO types)

Smoldering systemic mastocytosis

Aggressive systemic mastocytosis (ASM)

Mast cell leukemia (MCL)

SM-AHN (SM-CEL)

Neoplasms in Which Eosinophils May or May Not Be Part of The Malignant Clone

Other myeloproliferative neoplasms (MPN) with eosinophilia[a]

Myelodysplastic syndromes (MDS) with eosinophilia

Other MDS/MPN overlap syndromes with eosinophilia[a]

Indolent systemic mastocytosis

Neoplasms in Which Eosinophils Usually Are Not Part of the Malignant Clone

Hodgkin disease

B- or T-cell non-Hodgkin lymphoma

Acute lymphoblastic leukemia (ALL)

Chronic lymphocytic leukemia (CLL)

Langerhans cell histiocytosis

[a]Other MPN or MPN/MDS: neoplasms where no abnormalities in the *PDGFR* or *FGFR1* genes are detectable.

AHN, Associated hematologic neoplasm; FAB, French–American–British Cooperative Study Group; SM, systemic mastocytosis; WHO, World Health Organisation.

cells. An exception is the 8p11 myeloproliferative syndrome (*FGFR1*-rearranged neoplasm), where eosinophils are derived from the malignant clone even if the primary tumor was classified as a lymphoma.[13] Most lymphoma patients with paracrine HE also suffer from a (peripheral) T-cell non-Hodgkin lymphoma (NHL). In these patients, clonal T cells are considered the primary source of eosinophilopoietic cytokines, such as IL-5. A prephase of HES_L or HE_{US} may be present in these patients. The prognosis of patients with peripheral T-cell NHLs is poor, even when treated with chemotherapy, such as cyclophosphamide, hydroxydaunomycin, vincristine (Oncovin), and prednisone. Therefore, allogeneic HSCT is usually recommended for these patients, provided that the patient has an acceptable performance status and a suitable donor is available, and the same holds true for lymphoma patients presenting with an *FGFR1* rearrangement. Relapsing disease after HSCT has an extremely poor outcome. These patients are treated with investigational agents and palliative cytoreduction. A summary of BM neoplasms presenting with HE is provided in Table 71.8B.

Reactive, Immunologic and Paraneoplastic Conditions associated With HE

A number of different nonhematologic malignancies may be accompanied by HE. These include, among others, solid tumors of the GI tract, adenocarcinomas of the lung, carcinomas in other internal organs, skin cancer, urogenital malignancies, and stromal cell-derived tumors. In several of these patients, the cancer cells or the cancer-related microenvironment (e.g., fibroblasts) may produce eosinophilopoietic cytokines. In many cases, PB HE but also tissue eosinophilia (tissue HE) may be recorded. In some of these cancer patients, the tumor cells are tightly surrounded and sometimes even outnumbered by the infiltrating eosinophils. So far, it remains unknown whether tissue HE and eosinophil-derived mediators contributes to tumor formation (through neoangiogenesis or tissue remodeling) or even hinder tumor formation in these patients. As mentioned earlier, lymphomas may also be accompanied by reactive/paracrine HE.

A number of different immunologic and other reactive conditions can cause reactive HE (HE$_R$). These include infectious diseases (e.g., helminth infections, HIV, and certain fungal infections), allergic disorders (e.g., asthma, food allergy, atopic dermatitis, and drug reactions), chronic inflammatory reactions, and autoimmune processes (see Table 71.2).[17] Treatment of the underlying disease is usually followed by resolution of HE$_R$, thereby confirming the etiology of HE. In most reactive conditions, HE is triggered by cytokines derived from activated immune cells, such as T cells or mast cells. In some of these patients, an underlying disease is not detectable, but clonal T lymphocytes and/or lymphocytes with an aberrant surface immunophenotype are present. In such cases, HE-related organ damage may also be seen, which leads to the diagnosis of the lymphoid variant of HES (HES$_L$).[15]

Specific Syndromes and Conditions Associated With HE

Several specific conditions and syndromes defined by HE and organ damage may fulfill the criteria of a HES, but based on traditional views and their unique etiologies, these syndromes are still regarded as distinct entities that should be discriminated from the classical HES variants. In the future, however, most or all of these syndromes may be regarded as a special form of HES. These syndromes include, among others, episodic angioedema and eosinophilia (Gleich syndrome), CSS, eosinophilia myalgia syndrome (EMS), OS, and hyper-IgE syndrome (see Table 71.4A).

Gleich syndrome is characterized by recurrent angioedema associated with eosinophilia (HE), elevated serum cytokine (IL-5) levels, and increased (polyclonal) IgM production.[22] The episodes of angioedema and eosinophilia typically occur at monthly intervals and often resolve spontaneously without therapy. Patients with Gleich syndrome may suffer from fever and increasing body weight. The clinical course is usually benign without involvement of internal organs, thereby contrasting the typical HES variants. In a subset of patients, the symptoms and HE persist. These patients usually respond to low-dose corticosteroids. So far, little is known about the pathogenesis of Gleich syndrome. Several lines of evidence suggest that multiple cell types are involved, including neutrophils, mast cells, eosinophils, and T lymphocytes. Whereas most of these cells are considered to be cytokine-mobilized cells, T cells are often found to be clonal in these patients. In fact, in many patients with Gleich syndrome, T-cell phenotyping reveals an abnormal phenotype of CD4$^+$ lymphocytes, with decreased or absent CD3 expression (see Table 71.4A).[22] In addition, in several of these patients a clonal T-cell receptor rearrangement has been found. Therefore, Gleich syndrome has also been considered as a special (cycling) subvariant of HES$_L$.

CSS, also known as *eosinophilic granulomatosis with polyangiitis* (EGPA), is defined by a disseminated necrotizing vasculitis that is accompanied by asthma and (tissue) eosinophilia (HE).[23] CSS is a small-vessel vasculitis characterized by the formation of extravascular granulomas and the production of antineutrophil cytoplasmic antibodies (ANCA). Both, tissue HE and the ANCAs produced in these cases are considered to play an active role in the pathogenesis of CSS. However, the exact etiology of CSS remains unknown. More recent data suggest that CSS/EGPA may be a Th2-mediated disease. Clinically, CSS develops in three distinct phases: the initial (early) phase is characterized by asthma and rhinosinusitis, the eosinophilic phase is defined by HE$_R$ and HE-related organ involvement, and the late ("vasculitic") phase is defined by clinical manifestations originating from the small-vessel vasculitis (see Table 71.4A). CSS is a systemic disease that may affect a number of different organ systems, including the lungs, skin, kidneys, nerves, and heart. Criteria for CSS have been proposed by various expert groups. According to the American College of Rheumatology, the following criteria define CSS: asthma, eosinophilia (>10%), neuropathy (mononeuropathy or

polyneuropathy), pulmonary infiltrates, paranasal sinus abnormalities, and extravascular eosinophil infiltrates on tissue biopsies. When four out of these six criteria apply, the diagnosis CSS can be established. Based on the considerable clinical overlap with classical HES variants, CSS is also regarded as a special HES variant, defined by an ANCA+ vasculitis. The prognosis of patients with CSS depends on a number of clinical variables, including lung involvement, duration of disease, and response to therapy. Treatment of patients with CSS is based on the individual situation in each case and the presence or absence of prognostic factors. A combination of high-dose corticosteroids and cyclophosphamide remains a standard for treatment. More recently, antibody-based drugs, such as rituximab or mepolizumab, have been proposed as therapeutic alternatives and should be considered in cases resistant to cyclophosphamide.

EMS is a flu-like condition defined by recurrent episodes of myalgia and persistent eosinophilia. In many patients, neurological symptoms and skin abnormalities are found. In addition, patients may suffer from fever, weight loss, edema, and severe fatigue. The etiology of EMS remains uncertain. A clue to pathogenesis was the detection or a relationship between EMS and exposure to contaminated L-tryptophan or rapeseed oil (toxic oil syndrome). EMS is an incurable disease, but fatal cases are rare. As in Gleich syndrome and CSS, the clinical overlap with HES is obvious, and many experts believe that EMS could be regarded as a special subvariant of HES.

Eosinophilic fasciitis (EF) is a scleroderma-like syndrome with HE, polyclonal hypergammaglobulinemia, and signs of systemic inflammation. The etiology of EF remains unknown, but most authors regard EF as an immunologic hyperreactivity disorder manifesting in the skin. Painful swelling of the skin with progressive induration and thickening of the skin and soft tissues of the limbs and trunk are typical clinical findings. Corticosteroids are usually prescribed and have been shown to be efficacious in EF patients. In a subset of patients, spontaneous improvement is found. Again, based on clinical findings and HE, it is difficult to differentiate between EF and skin involvement in HES$_R$.

OS is a rare, autosomal recessive form of severe combined immunodeficiency (SCID) associated with leukocytosis, HE, elevated IgE levels, and a high mortality rate. Recognition in early childhood is required in order to initiate life-saving therapy. OS is caused by hypomorphic missense-mutations in the recombination-activating genes *RAG1* and *RAG2* (see Table 71.4A). Unlike patients with typical SCID, patients with OS have well-populated lymphatic organs and usually suffer from diarrhea, hepatosplenomegaly, lymphadenopathy, and weight loss. In addition, severe erythroderma, increased IgE levels, and eosinophilia are found in most cases. HE and inflammation observed in these patients may result from the activity of clonally expanded T cells, which are predominantly of the Th2 type. Overall, the disease presents very similar to a graft-versus-host reaction, which is due to patients producing T cells with limited recombination ability (mutant *RAG* genes) and a specific affinity for self-antigens, making them autoreactive T lymphocytes. Other SCID-related mutations may also lead to an OS-like disease, including certain mutations in the *IL-7 receptor* (*IL-7R*) gene. The treatment of choice in OS is allogeneic HSCT. For patients who cannot be transplanted or need a bridging therapy prior to allogeneic HSCT, cyclosporine A (CSA) may be considered.

Hyper-IgE syndromes (HIES) are a group of rare hereditary immunodeficiency syndromes characterized by elevated IgE levels, severe recurrent infections, and HE. In many cases, skin eczema and facial anomalies are found. So far, little is known about the pathogenesis of the HIES. The disease can manifest as an autosomal dominant or autosomal recessive variant. Several different genes may be affected. In the autosomal dominant variant, *STAT3* mutations are most commonly described. Since STAT3 acts as a key transcription factor downstream of multiple cytokine receptors regulating diverse immunologic responses, impaired STAT3 function is likely to cause immunodeficiency. In the autosomal recessive HIES variants, mutations in *DOCK8* and, less commonly, in the phosphoglucomutase 3 (*PGM3*) gene, have been reported (see Table 71.4A). The natural course of HIES patients is variable, but overall the long-term prognosis is poor. Therefore, early allogeneic HSCT should be considered whenever possible.

Organ-Restricted HE Syndromes

There are other clinical conditions and syndromes accompanied by HE-related organ damage that cannot be classified (diagnosed) as typical HES. A special group of such disorders are organ-restricted inflammatory conditions, such as eosinophilic colitis, eosinophilic pneumonia, or eosinophilic esophagitis (see Table 71.4B). In these patients, cytokine production and disease manifestations are typically restricted to one single-organ system, in contrast to the classical forms of HES and most of the above-described specific syndromes. The etiology of these organ-restricted HE syndromes remains largely unknown. In many instances, infectious or toxic agents or specific allergens are felt to play a pathogenetic role. In addition, genetic or epigenetic factors may contribute to disease manifestations. Depending on disease severity, suspected etiology, and presence of comorbidities, a treatment-plan is established. In many cases, corticosteroids are prescribed. In those with suspected allergy, additional drugs, such as antihistamines or leukotriene antagonists, have been recommended. The prognosis is variable and depends largely on the underlying etiology and response to treatment. Most patients respond to corticosteroids. In some patients, an underlying (initially unrecognized) systemic disease, infectious disease, or local tumor is diagnosed during follow-up. In these patients, the prognosis and treatment depends on the type and stage of the underlying disease.

TREATMENT ALGORITHM, TREATMENT OPTIONS AND PROGNOSIS

When establishing the management plan for a patient with HE, several important questions have to be addressed. First, the final diagnosis concerning the presence or absence of HES, and the presence and nature of the underlying disease, if present, has to be firmly established. Second, it is important to decide whether the patient needs symptomatic or/and interventional therapy. In some of these HE patients, a wait-and-watch strategy may be acceptable, whereas in other cases (when HES is diagnosed) specific therapy needs to be introduced quickly. Finally, the optimal treatment plan and most useful drugs need to be defined. The type of therapy varies depending on the underlying condition and the type of HES.[24]

Primary Management and Algorithm

In many cases, treatment of HES is a straightforward approach. For example, reactive HES is often managed (and resolved) quite easily by treating the underlying disease, such as a helminth infection or an autoimmune disease. In cases with idiopathic HE or HES and those with advanced or aggressive disease, however, treatment should always be performed in collaboration with a specialized center and in an interdisciplinary approach involving hematologists, immunologists, pathologists, and/or laboratory specialists, as needed.

In patients with HE_{US} and HE_{F}, it seems appropriate to follow the patient without treatment provided there are no signs or symptoms of eosinophil-related organ damage despite careful medical monitoring. However, both HE_{US} and HE_{F} must be regarded as provisional diagnoses, and in both conditions organ damage may develop over time. In addition, a hematologic or other underlying disease may be detected during follow-up of these cases. In the reactive form of HES, it is important to define and to treat the underlying condition. Additional symptomatic therapy, often in the form of corticosteroids, may be required to control eosinophil activation in these patients, especially when eosinophil counts are high or/and cells undergo rapid lysis, which may occur during treatment with cytotoxic drugs.[24]

In the past, most patients with HES received corticosteroids as front-line therapy. However, this strategy has changed with more extensive knowledge about the pathogenesis of HE and HES etiologies, and the advent of novel drugs such as PDGFR-targeting TKIs. Notably, today, front-line therapy is largely dependent on the underlying disease and the molecular targets detectable in neoplastic cells.[24] In patients in whom eosinophils display mutated forms of PDGFRs, imatinib is considered standard front-line therapy. By contrast, in patients with idiopathic HES (HES_{I}) and those with HES_{L}, corticosteroids remain standard front-line therapy. However, there are also patients in whom an initial staging and grading and/or molecular studies suggest that neither steroids nor imatinib will work. These cases include, among others, patients with an advanced myeloid neoplasm without a *PDGFR* mutation (e.g., AML-eo, MDS-eo, or SM-eo) and patients with rearranged *FGFR* genes. In many of these cases, the primary treatment plan includes intensive chemotherapy and allogeneic HSCT.

All in all, a number of different therapeutic approaches for the treatment of HES and of the underlying (eosinophil) disorder(s) detected in these patients are available. In the following sections, these treatment approaches are briefly reviewed and discussed.

Corticosteroids

In patients with idiopathic HES (HES_{I}) and HES_{L}, corticosteroids are considered standard front-line therapy. By contrast, in patients with HES_{R} and HES_{N}, corticosteroids should only be considered as an adjunct to more specific treatment, in order to stop eosinophil activation and eosinophil recruitment as early as possible. In patients with a (suspected) infection, diabetes mellitus, an ulcerative GI tract disease, or arterial hypertension, corticosteroids should be administered with caution and with recognition of potential side effects and the related risk. In patients with HES_{I} and HES_{L}, corticosteroid therapy, usually in form of prednisone at 1 mg/kg/ day (initial dose) is usually effective in reducing eosinophil counts to normal levels, with overall response rates of >75% in HES_{I}. In contrast, most patients with HES_{N} do not respond to corticosteroid therapy.

The mechanisms of action by which corticosteroids suppress HE in HES_{I} and HES_{L} patients are only partly understood. Steroids act through specific corticosteroid receptors that are present in the cytoplasm of eosinophils and eosinophil precursor cells, but also in the cytoplasm of T lymphocytes and mast cells. It has also been described that steroids effectively block the production of various eosinotropic cytokines by T lymphocytes. In addition, corticosteroids effectively counteract T-cell expansion. Based on these effects, corticosteroids may act directly and indirectly to block HE in HES patients, namely by (1) inducing growth inhibition and apoptosis of eosinophils and their precursor cells, by (2) directly blocking eosinophil recruitment and migration, and by (3) inhibiting the production and release of eosinophilopoietic cytokines by T lymphocytes and other immune cells.

As mentioned earlier, long-term treatment with steroids is associated with a risk of (severe) side effects. Therefore, steroids should be tapered down (and discontinued) whenever possible, especially in cases with HES_{R} and HES_{N}. However, in many patients with HES_{I}, maintenance therapy with corticosteroids is required to control disease activity. In these patients, the steroid dose applied should be reduced to a minimum. In fact, even though corticosteroids are "natural" substances and very effective in reducing eosinophil counts in HES_{I}, chronic use of steroids is associated with the risk of serious adverse events and long-term toxicity. Once reduction of the eosinophil count to below 1500/mm³ and symptom control have been achieved, the corticosteroid dose should be tapered. Increases in eosinophil numbers on a prednisone dose greater than 10 mg daily and/or reappearance of symptoms or signs of organ damage are indications for the addition of other agents to the steroid regimen. A number of different drugs may be useful as steroid-sparing agents in patients with HES. These drugs include, among others, conventional cytostatic agents such as HU or cyclophosphamide, IFN-α, and the IL-5-targeting antibody mepolizumab.[25]

Conventional Cytoreduction and Chemotherapy

Several studies have shown that HU (0.5–2 g/day), is efficacious in steroid-nonresponsive patients with HES, including those with HES_I and HES_N. In patients with HES_I, HU is administered as an alternative drug or in conjunction with corticosteroids as a steroid-sparing medication. A typical starting dose is 500–1000 mg daily. In combination with corticosteroids, the overall response rate exceeds 50%. Eosinophil counts begin to decrease 7–14 days after starting HU treatment. Depending on the dose, HU may induce cytopenias. Otherwise, HU is usually well tolerated unless very high doses are administered, and is therefore also used as a palliative drug in HES_N patients resistant to targeted drugs and chemotherapy. However, not all patients with HES may respond to HU. Historically, a number of cytotoxic agents have been used to treat HES refractory to steroids and HU, including vincristine, etoposide (VP-16), and chlorambucil. However, each of these agents can produce cytopenias and other side effects, and their use should be limited to select patients with HES in whom neoplastic cells develop resistance against other agents including HU. In patients with advanced, resistant CEL or AEL, but also in patients with AML-eo, other advanced myeloid neoplasms with *FGFR1* rearrangement (8p11 myeloproliferative syndrome), intensive polychemotherapy and allogeneic HSCT are usually recommended. These chemotherapy regimens are usually the same as applied in patients with refractory leukemias without HE/HES. Chemotherapy before allogeneic HSCT is often a preferable initial approach for two reasons: first, debulking may result in remission, and patients in remission have in general a better overall outcome after allogeneic HSCT. In addition, chemotherapy can provide some indication as to whether a patient can tolerate intensive therapy. On the other hand, multiple cycles of chemotherapy increase the risk of infections, which may be problematic in the context of a planned allogeneic HSCT.

Interferon-α

IFN-α has been used for the treatment of HES for more than 25 years, both as monotherapy and in combination with other agents. A number of studies have shown that this type of therapy can successfully counteract HE and HES in patients in whom treatment with prednisone and HU has failed. Response rates to IFN-α vary depending on the underlying disease and dose, but may be approximately 50% when used as monotherapy and 75% in combination with other agents. Usually, therapy is initiated at a dose of 1 million units three times a week, and is titrated up to 4 million units three times weekly. In the responding patients, eosinophil counts decrease, and improvement in splenomegaly and hepatomegaly has been reported. Moreover, the risk of cardiac and thromboembolic complications can be reduced by treatment with IFN-α. Finally, mucosal ulcerative lesions and other skin manifestations may substantially improve. The unprocessed and the pegylated form of IFN-α may be equally effective. However, despite efficacy, the administration of IFN-α is problematic because of side effects. These side effects are often dose dependent and include fever, a flu-like syndrome, fatigue, impotence, depression, suicidal ideation, and psychosis. In addition, IFN-α therapy may lead to exacerbations of autoimmune disorders, such as autoimmune thyroiditis, psoriasis, ulcerative colitis, and others, but also to exacerbation of depression or other psychiatric diseases. Other serious adverse events observed with IFN-α include excessive suppression of blood counts, retinopathy, sarcoidosis, and left-sided heart failure. All these (potential) side effects have to be taken into account, especially when prescribing IFN-α on a long-term basis at relatively high doses. On the other hand, IFN-α is non-mutagenic and is considered a drug that can be prescribed even during pregnancy. The mechanism of action of IFN-α is not well understood. Receptors for this cytokine are expressed on multipotent hematopoietic progenitor cells, eosinophil-committed precursors, and mature blood eosinophils. Therefore, in contrast to corticosteroids, IFN-α works in HES patients with diverse etiologies, including HES_L, but also in HES_N and even in HES_I. IFN-α inhibits eosinophil activation and the release of various toxic mediators from eosinophils. However, IFN-α may also exert an antiinflammatory effect on other cell types that may contribute to tissue damage in HES.

Cyclosporine A (CSA)

CSA, an immunosuppressant that interferes with multiple functions and growth of immunocompetent T lymphocytes, has been reported to be effective in a subset of patients with HES. The goal of CSA treatment in HES is to inhibit production of eosinophilopoietic cytokines, including IL-5, by T cells in these patients. CSA has been used as a single agent or in conjunction with low-dose corticosteroids. In those with steroid-sensitive disease, CSA may act as a steroid-sparing agent. However, good responses may only be seen in distinct variants of HES, namely those HES variants where T-cell activation is a causative etiology. Another important point is that efficacy has so far only been described for CSA in short-term–treated HES patients (10 months), whereas long-term efficacy has not been determined so far. In each case, the side effects and immunosuppressive effects of CSA have to be taken into account. In patients with HES_N, CSA should not be administered.

Targeted Treatment Approaches Using Tyrosine Kinase Inhibitors

Several different oncogenic kinases have been detected in primary eosinophilic disorders (mostly CEL and MPN-eo) and serve as targets of therapy.[13] The most relevant and most frequent target kinase detectable in patients with CEL is *F/P*. This fusion gene product is a target of imatinib and also sensitive to other TKIs, such as nilotinib, dasatinib, PKC412 (midostaurin), or ponatinib. A number of other oncoproteins may also serve as targets of imatinib and are detectable in primary eosinophil disorders. Most of these fusion genes involve *PDGFRA* or *PDGFRB*, whereas *FGFR1* mutants are imatinib resistant. The hematologic benefit of imatinib in *F/P*-positive neoplasms and *PDGFRB*-rearranged neoplasms has been confirmed in several clinical trials.[26,27] Therefore, imatinib is regarded as standard first-line therapy in these patients. Given the poor prognosis in patients with overt organ damage (HES_N), patients with an *F/P*+ neoplasm or another mutation involving *PDGFRA* or *PDGFRB* genes should be treated with imatinib, even in the absence of end-organ damage, in order to prevent any HES occurrence. Although the optimal dosing strategy for imatinib has not been fully defined, a number of studies have shown that a daily dose of 100 mg appears to be sufficient to induce complete hematologic and molecular remission in most patients.[26] Moreover, 100 mg imatinib/day appears to be a safe approach in all patients, including those who suffer from cardiac involvement. Therefore, 100 mg/day is regarded a standard dose of initial therapy with imatinib in *F/P*+ CEL. However, in a few patients with *PDGFRA*- or *PDGFRB*-rearranged neoplasms, higher doses of imatinib (400 mg daily) are required to induce a durable remission. In those who enter a hematologic and molecular remission, imatinib is usually maintained, as discontinuation is often followed by a relapse.[28] However, it remains unknown whether all patients need to continue on their initial dose on a life-long basis. In fact, it has been described that many of these patients do not relapse when lowering the dose of imatinib or even when imatinib is discontinued. In other patients, however, resistance against imatinib may occur. In relapsing patients, *F/P* point mutations associated with decreased (or loss of) drug-binding capacity may be detected. For these patients, novel TKIs, such as sorafenib, nilotinib, midostaurin, or ponatinib may be considered. The most commonly detected mutant, T674I, is sensitive in vitro to a number of different TKIs, including PKC412, sorafenib, and ponatinib. Other secondary mutations in *F/P*+ disease, such as D842V, are very rare. However, once these secondary mutations occur during treatment with multiple TKIs, they usually exhibit pan-resistance. In fact, durable responses to TKIs with either the T674I or D842V mutation are not generally observed, and especially the *F/P* D842V mutant is resistant to almost all available TKIs. More recently, it has been described that ponatinib can kill neoplastic eosinophils exhibiting all types of *F/P* mutations *in vitro* at clinically achievable drug concentrations. Whether this also holds true *in vivo* in patients with TKI-resistant CEL or acute leukemias exhibiting this *F/P* mutant, presently remains unknown. Another approach in patients with TKI-resistant eosinophil neoplasms is to apply cytoreductive agents (IFN-α, HU) or experimental drugs. In patients who transform to an acute leukemia, polychemotherapy and allogeneic HSCT is usually recommended.

A number of different markers have been proposed for the monitoring of treatment responses in patients with *F/P+* CEL. A close hematologic follow-up is recommended for the first weeks of therapy, where a rapid decline in eosinophils (and leukocytes) is usually observed, and is regarded a good prognostic sign. After a few months, the BM should be examined in order to document and confirm the hematologic response. A complete remission is obtained in most patients, even if the initial BM revealed marked involvement at diagnosis, including fibrosis and/or increased blast cells. In patients with a complete hematologic remission, molecular monitoring and a repeat PCR and FISH analysis is recommended in order to define the molecular response. Quantitative measurement of the *F/P* mRNA burden by reverse-transcriptase-PCR is available in many centers and can be employed to define the depth of the remission. In those with an initially elevated serum tryptase, serial determinations of tryptase are also useful to document the response to imatinib or other TKIs. Finally, in those with end-organ damage, including cardiac disease, reinvestigation of all involved organ systems is recommended to demonstrate potential reversion of end-organ damage. In high-risk patients (e.g., cardiac history), echocardiography and troponin as well as B-type natriuretic peptide levels before initiating therapy may be recommended to gauge the potential risk.

Although imatinib and other TKI therapies in CEL patients is generally well tolerated, all these agents can produce severe side effects. Even imatinib may produce severe side effects, especially when applied to HES patients with cardiopathy at 400 mg daily. In fact, in a few cases severe left ventricular dysfunction has been reported soon after initiation of imatinib therapy. Therefore, close monitoring of these patients is recommended during this time period and prophylactic steroids (during the first week of treatment) should be considered. The second- and third-generation TKIs used to treat CML and CEL may also produce severe side effects, and many of them may affect the cardiovascular system or metabolic parameters, which is relevant clinically in the context of HES. The most relevant side effects of dasatinib are pleural and pericardial effusion, and the most relevant adverse events observed with nilotinib and ponatinib are arterial occlusive events that may occur as a result of a rapidly progressive form of atherosclerosis. In the case of nilotinib, increasing fasting glucose levels and cholesterol levels have been documented during therapy.

Targeted Antibodies

A number of targeted antibodies and antibody–toxin conjugates have been considered for patients with HE-related disorders and HES.[29] These antibodies are either directed against (neoplastic) eosinophils and their precursor cells or against eosinotropic cytokines, such as IL-5. Antieosinophil antibodies are considered useful in neoplastic states and should ideally be directed against both eosinophils and their precursor cells, or even neoplastic stem cells. One such antibody is alemtuzumab. This humanized antibody is directed against CD52 (= Campath-1), a surface receptor expressed on neoplastic stem cells in various leukemias as well as on eosinophils and their precursor cells. Alemtuzumab therapy in patients with drug-resistant eosinophil disorders has been reported in a limited number of studies. In about 80–90% of the patients the drug induced remission. However, in over 80% of these patients relapses occurred after cessation of therapy. In addition, alemtuzumab produced substantial side effects, including severe hematological toxicity with subsequent opportunistic infections. Several other antibodies directed against cell

surface receptors expressed by eosinophils are currently in preclinical development. The epidermal growth factor-like modul-containing, mucin-like hormone receptor 1 (EMR1) is expressed specifically on human blood eosinophils and may serve as a potential target of therapy. A novel, humanized afucosylated anti-EMR1 IgG1 antibody has recently been shown to augment NK cell-mediated killing of eosinophil granulocytes. Benralizumab is an antibody directed against the IL-5 receptor on eosinophils and their precursor cells. So far, benralizumab has been tested in normal subjects and patients with asthma, and is currently being tested in patients with HES. BM studies have shown that this antibody induces a remarkable depletion of eosinophils and their precursor cells. It is noteworthy that the IL-5 receptor is also expressed on basophils, albeit at lower levels. Another interesting target receptor is Siglec-8. This antigen is expressed on eosinophils and mast cells, but not on neoplastic stem cells. Remarkably, Siglec-8 crosslinking induces eosinophil apoptosis and inhibits IgE-mediated mast cell activation, thereby providing a common mechanism to limit inflammation caused by the coexistence and functional interactions of these cells.[6] Whether this concept is clinically effective, remains at present unknown. Since Siglec-8 is not expressed on immature eosinophilic progenitor cells or neoplastic stem cells, the drug may not be useful in eosinophil malignancies. By contrast, Siglec-3 (CD33), another established drug target, is displayed by normal and neoplastic eosinophils and even by neoplastic stem cells. Gemtuzumab ozogamicin is a humanized CD33 antibody conjugated with calicheamicin. Although the drug is highly effective in targeting myeloid cells and their progenitors in AML, the drug has been withdrawn from the market because of toxicity issues. However, when used at limited doses and at reasonable time intervals, the toxicity of such antibodies may be acceptable.

Another approach is to target eosinotropic cytokines using specific antibodies, which is a strategy that is recommended for patients with reactive HE and HES (HES$_R$) as well as HES$_L$, where overproduction of such cytokines is known to play a pathogenetic role. These agents include antibodies directed against IL-5, against eotaxin, or other cytokine agonists. Mepolizumab is a fully humanized IgG1 antibody that binds IL-5 and prevents its binding to the IL-5 receptor alpha chain.[29] In 2008 a randomized, double-blind, placebo-controlled trial showed that mepolizumab is effective as a corticosteroid-sparing agent in patients with severe (drug-resistant) HES$_R$.[25] Adverse events were tolerable and similar in the treated and in the placebo groups. Mepolizumab has been recently FDA approved for the treatment of eosinophilic asthma and tested in HES patients in clinical trials. Reslizumab is a humanized IgG4 anti IL-5 antibody that is currently being tested in clinical trials for eosinophilic esophagitis and in pediatric patients for eosinophilic asthma, but it has not been studied in the context of HES.[29] Initial results suggest that the drug is effective in reducing eosinophil counts and clinical symptoms. Bertilimumab is a human anti-eotaxin-1 antibody that is currently being tested in a phase II clinical trial for ulcerative colitis, but has not been tested yet in HES patients. Together, more controlled clinical trials in HES patients are needed in order to learn which antibodies directed against eosinophilic receptors and eosinotropic cytokines are most effective in patients with primary or reactive eosinophil disorders and HES.

Leukapheresis

Leukapheresis has no defined role in the management of HES. However, leukapheresis may be useful in emergency situations for patients with excessively high eosinophil counts. Since cell counts rebound rapidly to pretreatment levels, such a maneuver should always be combined with cytoreductive therapy in order to keep eosinophil counts under control.

Anticoagulation and Antiplatelet Agents

Thromboembolic complications may be life-threatening in HES patients. Therefore, prophylactic anticoagulation may be considered in patients with HES, especially in those in whom the risk for thromboembolic complications is high, such as in patients with a *F/P+* disease, cardiac involvement, or neurologic symptoms. In patients with overt HES and associated thromboembolic events, anticoagulation is a standard approach. Commonly used agents are warfarin, antiplatelet agents, and heparin. The efficacy of these drugs has not been formally established in HES, and some of the patients may continue to have thrombotic events, despite adequate anticoagulation. Therefore, it is always important to also treat the underlying disease if possible, in order to stop the thromboembolic state.

Splenectomy

Splenectomy is usually not required in patients with MPN-eo, AEL, or CEL. However, in rare cases, splenomegaly has been performed to correct hypersplenism-related cytopenias, or to avoid splenic infarction and pain induced by capsular distention.

Allogeneic Hematopoietic Stem Cell Transplantation

Although the experience with allogeneic HSCT in patients with advanced BM neoplasms accompanied by HE (with or without HES) is quite limited, allogeneic HSCT should be considered in certain groups of patients, especially those who are (1) young and fit, (2) have a suitable transplant donor, and (3) have a progressive and treatment-resistant form of an underlying myeloid or lymphoid neoplasm. More or less definitive indications in this regard include *FGFR1*-rearranged neoplasms, drug-resistant cases of AEL or CEL, chemotherapy-resistant peripheral T-cell lymphomas accompanied by HE/HES, and treatment-resistant (progressive) cases of MPN-eo, AML-eo, or MDS-eo. If possible, debulking therapy should be introduced prior to conditioning and HSCT, especially when the burden of neoplastic cells is high or excessive. Such debulking may be performed with polychemotherapy or with experimental drugs. Several but not all transplanted patients may enter a complete remission. Transplant-related mortality rates may not be higher compared with age-matched patients with other advanced hematopoietic neoplasms. As in other BM neoplasms, age, comorbidities, and the disease status are major risk factors concerning survival and transplant-related mortality. In this regard, it should be noted that the presence of HES-related organ damage, such as overt cardiomyopathy or thromboembolism, but also neuropathies or GI disease, may count as relevant comorbidities, and if severe in nature, may represent a contraindication to allogeneic HSCT. In those who are successfully transplanted, the clinical course may be complicated by graft-versus-host disease requiring treatment with corticosteroids, cyclosporin-A, or/and other immunosuppressive drugs. Little is known about long-term outcomes after allogeneic HSCT. In smaller case series and single cases reports, long-term survivors have been described. However, relapses have also been reported in most groups of patients.

Cardiac Surgery

In a subset of patients with HES, surgical intervention of cardiac lesions is required. Interestingly, such intervention does not appear to carry a major risk for disease recurrence at the operative sites. Indications for surgery include a significant compromise of valvular function and the presence of a clinically significant thrombotic mass. Cardiac surgery has the capacity to provide a substantial clinical and quality-of-life benefit in these patients. In fact, successful mitral valve and/or tricuspid valve repair or replacements have been reported in HES patients in several studies. For mitral valve replacements, mechanical valves have proven problematic because of recurrent thrombosis despite adequate anticoagulation, suggesting the use of porcine valves whenever possible. HES patients who have received valve replacements have generally experienced long-term

improvement in cardiac function, provided the underlying disease and the related HE can be kept under control.

SUMMARY AND FUTURE PERSPECTIVES

The diagnosis, classification, and management of patients with persistent HE remains a challenge in clinical practice, especially when no underlying disease is identified and/or HE-related organ damage (HES) develops. Because of disease heterogeneity and the power and specificity of novel markers and targets, each case needs to be investigated and managed using the full battery of diagnostic markers and assays, and according to contemporary diagnostic and therapeutic algorithms.[3,14] Depending on the overall situation, initial investigations include BM studies (histology, cytology, and cytogenetics with FISH), molecular analyses, immunologic parameters, and a complete staging of all potentially involved end-organ systems. In benign disease variants, the course can sometimes be monitored without specific treatment. However, in patients with (1) advanced hematopoietic neoplasms, (2) overt HE-related end-organ damage (HES), (3) an active underlying (systemic) immunologic, infectious, or allergic disease, (4) evidence of a specific clinical syndrome with systemic organ involvement, or (5) organ-restricted marked inflammation associated with eosinophilia, such as eosinophilic colitis or eosinophilic pneumonia, specific treatment needs to be initiated. In reactive conditions, symptomatic treatment and corticosteroids are usually administered. In addition, it is of utmost importance to treat and eradicate (or control) the underlying disease, such as a NHL, helminth infection or IgE-dependent allergy, in these patients. Such treatment is often followed by complete resolution of reactive HE and of the related HES. In treatment-resistant patients in whom reactive eosinophilia is likely to be triggered by eosinophilotropic cytokines such as IL-5, anti-cytokine therapy, such as mepolizumab, may be considered. This drug has shown promising results in patients with steroid-resistant reactive HES and other HE-related conditions, such as eosinophilic esophagitis. In advanced hematopoietic neoplasms, treatment with targeted drugs or less specific cytoreductive agents is recommended. In *F/P+* patients and those with related *PDGFR* fusion genes, imatinib is an undisputable standard of therapy. For patients with imatinib-resistant *F/P+* CEL or MPN-eo, MPN-eo without a *PDGFR* mutant, or HE-related malignancies expressing *FGFR1* or *JAK2* fusion genes, novel TKIs are available. In patients in whom secondary mutations in *F/P* are detectable, novel PDGFR-targeting TKIs such as ponatinib may work. In cases with *FGFR1*-rearranged neoplasms, novel FGFR blockers may overcome resistance, and in patients with *JAK2*-mutated MPN-eo, ruxolitinib may elicit clinically meaningful responses. In rapidly progressive and/or drug-resistant cases, high-dose chemotherapy and allogeneic HSCT need to be considered. In patients who are TKI resistant and not eligible for allogeneic HSCT, HU, other cytostatic agents, or IFN-α serve as palliative drugs. Current research aims at exploring the evolution of HES and at defining mechanisms regulating the development of HE-mediated end-organ damage, which should lead to more selective and improved therapies in the future. Clinically relevant targets for these efforts are likely to include (1) neoplastic stem cells producing eosinophil neoplasms such as CEL or MPN-eo, (2) molecular targets created specifically by neoplastic cells, such as mutant forms of *PDGFRs* or *FGFRs*, (3) eosinophilotropic cytokines and their receptors, (4) underlying T-cell clones triggering eosinophil expansion and/or activation through production of eosinopoietic cytokines, (5) adhesion receptors and other molecules mediating eosinophil homing and redistribution, such as VLA-4, and (6) signaling molecules responsible for cytokine-dependent or -independent eosinophil proliferation, migration, adhesion, or/and activation. Another aim for the future is to better understand cellular interactions and related molecular mechanisms underlying HE-induced organ damage (HES) in various organ systems. There is hope that an improved knowledge of mechanisms regulating end-organ damage will lead to the development of new treatment concepts and better therapies for patients with HES.

REFERENCES

1. Kita H: Eosinophils: multifaceted biological properties and roles in health and disease. *Immunol Rev* 242:161, 2011.
2. Yousefi S, Simon D, Simon HU: Eosinophil extracellular DNA traps: molecular mechanisms and potential roles in disease. *Curr Opin Immunol* 24:736, 2012.
3. Valent P, Klion AD, Horny HP, et al: Contemporary consensus proposal on criteria and classification of eosinophilic disorders and related syndromes. *J Allergy Clin Immunol* 130:607, 2012.
4. Bochner BS, Schleimer RP: Mast cells, basophils, and eosinophils: distinct but overlapping pathways for recruitment. *Immunol Rev* 179:5, 2001.
5. Valent P: The phenotype of human eosinophils, basophils, and mast cells. *J Allergy Clin Immunol* 94:1177, 1994.
6. Bochner BS: Siglec-8 on human eosinophils and mast cells, and Siglec-F on murine eosinophils, are functionally related inhibitory receptors. *Clin Exp Allergy* 39:317, 2009.
7. Tai PC, Ackerman SJ, Spry CJ, et al: Deposits of eosinophil granule proteins in cardiac tissues of patients with eosinophilic endomyocardial disease. *Lancet* 1:643, 1987.
8. Gauvreau GM, Ellis AK, Denburg JA: Haemopoietic processes in allergic disease: eosinophil/basophil development. *Clin Exp Allergy* 39:1297, 2009.
9. Lampinen M, Carlson M, Håkansson LD, et al: Cytokine-regulated accumulation of eosinophils in inflammatory disease. *Allergy* 59:793, 2004.
10. Sadovnik I, Lierman E, Peter B, et al: Identification of Ponatinib as a potent inhibitor of growth, migration, and activation of neoplastic eosinophils carrying FIP1L1-PDGFRA. *Exp Hematol* 42:282, 2014.
11. Hoermann G, Cerny-Reiterer S, Sadovnik I, et al: Oncostatin M is a FIP1L1/PDGFRA-dependent mediator of cytokine production in chronic eosinophilic leukemia. *Allergy* 68:713, 2013.
12. Kiwamoto T, Kawasaki N, Paulson JC, et al: Siglec-8 as a drugable target to treat eosinophil and mast cell-associated conditions. *Pharmacol Ther* 135:327, 2012.
13. Cross NC, Reiter A: Fibroblast growth factor receptor and platelet-derived growth factor receptor abnormalities in eosinophilic myeloproliferative disorders. *Acta Haematol* 119:199, 2008.
14. Gotlib J: World Health Organization-defined eosinophilic disorders: 2015 update on diagnosis, risk stratification, and management. *Am J Hematol* 90:1077, 2015.
15. Roufosse F, Garaud S, de Leval L: Lymphoproliferative disorders associated with hypereosinophilia. *Semin Hematol* 49:138, 2012.
16. Burgstaller S1, Kreil S, Waghorn K, et al: The severity of FIP1L1-PDGFRA-positive chronic eosinophilic leukaemia is associated with polymorphic variation at the IL5RA locus. *Leukemia* 21:2428, 2007.
17. Valent P, Gleich GJ, Reiter A, et al: Pathogenesis and classification of eosinophil disorders: a review of recent developments in the field. *Expert Rev Hematol* 5:157, 2012.
18. Plötz SG, Hüttig B, Aigner B, et al: Clinical overview of cutaneous features in hypereosinophilic syndrome. *Curr Allergy Asthma Rep* 12:85, 2012.
19. Gotlib J, Akin C: Mast cells and eosinophils in mastocytosis, chronic eosinophilic leukemia, and non-clonal disorders. *Semin Hematol* 49:128, 2012.
20. Valent P, Horny HP, Bochner BS, et al: Controversies and open questions in the definitions and classification of the hypereosinophilic syndromes and eosinophilic leukemias. *Semin Hematol* 49:171, 2012.
21. Wimazal F, Germing U, Kundi M, et al: Evaluation of the prognostic significance of eosinophilia and basophilia in a larger cohort of patients with myelodysplastic syndromes. *Cancer* 116:2372, 2010.
22. Gleich GJ, Schroeter AL, Marcoux JP, et al: Episodic angioedema associated with eosinophilia. *N Engl J Med* 310:1621, 1984.
23. Vaglio A, Moosig F, Zwerina J: Churg-Strauss syndrome: update on pathophysiology and treatment. *Curr Opin Rheumatol* 24:24, 2012.
24. Schwartz LB, Sheikh J, Singh A: Current strategies in the management of hypereosinophilic syndrome, including mepolizumab. *Curr Med Res Opin* 26:1933, 2010.
25. Rothenberg ME, Klion AD, Roufosse FE, et al: Treatment of patients with the hypereosinophilic syndrome with mepolizumab. *N Engl J Med* 358:1215, 2008.
26. Jovanovic JV, Score J, Waghorn K, et al: Low-dose imatinib mesylate leads to rapid induction of major molecular responses and achievement of complete molecular remission in FIP1L1-PDGFRA-positive chronic eosinophilic leukemia. *Blood* 109:4635, 2007.
27. Apperley JF, Gardembas M, Melo J, et al: Response to imatinib mesylate in patients with chronic myeloproliferative diseases with rearrangements of the platelet-derived growth factor receptor beta. *N Engl J Med* 347:481, 2002.
28. Klion AD, Robyn J, Maric I, et al: Relapse following discontinuation of imatinib mesylate therapy for FIP1L1/PDGFRA-positive chronic eosinophilic leukemia: implications for optimal dosing. *Blood* 110:3552, 2007.
29. Radonjic-Hoesli S, Valent P, Klion AD, et al: Novel targeted therapies for eosinophil-associated diseases and allergy. *Annu Rev Pharmacol Toxicol* 55:633, 2015.

CHAPTER 72

MAST CELLS AND MASTOCYTOSIS

Jason Gotlib, Hans-Peter Horny, and Peter Valent

INTRODUCTION

The year 2015 marked a century since the death of Paul Ehrlich, who used his 1878 doctoral thesis to characterize a new cell type—the mast cell (MC)—based on its reactivity to aniline dyes and the metachromatic appearance of its cytoplasmic granules.[1] He referred to MCs as *Mastzellen* and he speculated that their intracellular granules contained phagocytosed materials or nutrients. Ehrlich also described a close relationship in tissues between MCs and blood vessels, nerves, gland excretory ducts, as well as their proximity within the environment of tumors and chronic inflammation. In 1894, the pathobiologic association of MCs with lesions of urticaria pigmentosa was reported, and from the 1930s forward, basic incremental discoveries about normal MC functions were made. Their capacity to undergo degranulation in response to various stimuli, their source of histamine and heparin, and their important role in anaphylaxis was examined.[2]

Perturbations of MC growth and function may lead to mastocytosis, a condition defined by pathologic expansion and accumulation of MCs in diverse tissues such as the skin, bone marrow (BM), spleen, liver, lymph nodes, and gastrointestinal tract. In 1949 the first case report of systemic mastocytosis (SM) was published. Later, between 1950 and 1980, several different subtypes of SM were described, including a leukemic variant termed *mast cell leukemia* (MCL). The first classification of mastocytosis was created by the Kiel group of pathologists, and in 1991 the first consensus classification was published. Criteria for SM and other variants of the disease were established between 1990 and 2000. In 2000 these criteria were discussed by a consensus group and were employed to establish a robust consensus classification of mastocytosis,[3] that was adopted by the World Health Organization (WHO) in 2001 and also in 2008.[4] In consecutive years, the consensus group published treatment response criteria and established a widely accepted update of the classification of mastocytosis in 2007.[5] In this updated classification, the smoldering state is defined as a separate category of SM which was confirmed by the WHO in 2016. In 2002 the European Competence Network on Mastocytosis (ECNM) was founded. Since then, the ECNM has facilitated basic science and translational research dealing with mastocytosis and related MC disorders. This chapter provides an overview of normal MC physiology and highlights contemporary issues related to the classification, diagnosis, and treatment of SM.

ORIGIN AND DEVELOPMENT OF MAST CELLS

The marrow origin of MCs was first demonstrated by engrafting BM cells into irradiated mice. Human MCs can be generated from a CD34+ hematopoietic progenitor cell in response to stimulation with stem cell factor (SCF). In vitro MC differentiation models showed that circulating MC progenitors express CD13, CD34, and KIT, but lack CD14 and CD17.[6] MC progenitors are released from the BM into the circulation in a primitive state and undergo terminal maturation and differentiation after their migration to tissues. Although shared histomorphologic and biologic features of MCs and basophils include cytoplasmic basophilic granules, expression of high-affinity immunoglobulin (Ig)E receptors (FcεRI), and release of histamine upon stimulation, basophils exhibit several distinctive characteristics. Basophils circulate as mature cells, which are incapable

of proliferation, and subsequently undergo apoptosis after their recruitment and activation in the tissues. Differential expression of the transcription factor CCAAT-enhancer-binding protein (CEBP)α may be a primary determinant of whether development is skewed toward basophil progenitors (CEBPα present) or MC progenitors (CEBPα absent). Although eosinophils and basophils have been found to share a common bipotential progenitor in humans, definitive data for a similar progenitor giving rise to both basophils and MCs are lacking. Rather, based on colony assays, MCs are directly derived from multilineage and lineage-restricted progenitors, but not from such a bi-potent precursor cell.[6] In line with this observation, evidence against a bilineage basophil/MC progenitor also came from tracking lineage involvement of *KIT* D816V in patients with SM, where *KIT* D816V was only found in basophils in a small subset of patients, namely those with multilineage involvement of the mutation. In addition, when highly enriched by cell sorting, neither mature blood basophils nor mature blood monocytes give rise to MCs in vitro.[6]

KIT and Stem Cell Factor (KIT Ligand)

KIT

Kit is the cellular homolog of the *v-Kit* oncogene of the Hardy-Zuckerman 4 feline sarcoma virus. The human *KIT* gene on chromosome 4q11–12 was found to be allelic to the white spotting locus (*W*) in mice, in which over 30 mutations have been identified. The common theme of mutant alleles at the *W* locus is decreased kit kinase activity either through missense mutations that generate kinase-defective kit (e.g., W^{42} [*kit* D790N]; W^{37} [*kit* E582K]; W^v [*kit* T660M]; and W^{41} [*kit* V831M]) or decreased expression of kit on the cell surface (e.g., the *W* allele, caused by a 78-amino acid deletion that involves the transmembrane region of the kit protein).

Double mutants at the murine *W* locus not only result in markedly decreased MC numbers, but also in pleiotropic phenotypes, including white coat color/spotting, sterility, and anemia, that respectively relate to the failure of melanocytes, germ cells, and hematopoietic progenitors to migrate and/or proliferate effectively during development. Heterozygosity or homozygosity for the different alleles at the *W* locus results in variable phenotypic effects on hematopoiesis, pigmentation, and fertility. Mutations at the *W* locus can also result in abnormalities of the interstitial pacemaker cells of Cajal, leading to functional gut abnormalities, such as megacolon. Intriguingly, some of these clinical correlates can also be seen in patients undergoing long-term treatment with a strong KIT inhibitor, like imatinib: these individuals can develop MC deficiency, depigmented skin areas, cytopenias, and fertility problems.

KIT is a member of the type III receptor tyrosine kinases (TKs) that also include platelet-derived growth factor receptor (PDGFR)-α and -β, FMS-like tyrosine kinase-3 (FLT3), vascular endothelial growth factor receptor 2 (VEGFR2), and the receptor for macrophage colony-stimulating factor (FMS).[7] These TKs share common structural motifs including an extracellular domain containing five Ig-like motifs that bind their specific ligands, a short transmembrane (TM) domain that anchors KIT to the cell membrane, a cytoplasmic TK domain that is split by an insert sequence into ATP-binding and phosphotransferase regions, and a juxtamembrane (JM) domain that lies between the TM and TK domains. KIT is expressed on hematopoietic stem/progenitor cells and is also essential for gametogenesis and melanogenesis. KIT expression is lost when hematopoietic cells undergo differentiation. However, the exception is MCs, which retain persistent and high-level expression of KIT (CD117). This can be exploited for the purposes of MC identification by immunohistochemistry and/or flow immunophenotyping (in conjunction with other surface and cytoplasmic markers).

The two major splice variants of KIT differ by the presence or absence of four amino acids (GNNK) at the extracellular JM region. In NIH3T3 cells, the GNNK$^-$ isoform induced loss of contact inhibition, anchorage-independent growth, and tumorigenicity in mice, whereas the GNNK$^+$ isoform did not exhibit most of these characteristics. Also, despite similar binding of SCF to KIT, the GNNK$^-$ isoform displayed more rapid and extensive tyrosine autophosphorylation and faster internalization. Preferential expression of the GNNK isoform has been noted in small cohorts of patients with SM and germ cell tumors, but larger series are needed to determine the relevance of these KIT isoforms to disease pathogenesis.

Stem Cell Factor

SCF (KIT ligand) was identified by three groups in 1990 as the principal growth and differentiation factor for human MCs. In fact, SCF was found to induce MC differentiation from CD34$^+$ cells or blood/BM mononuclear cells. SCF is produced by fibroblasts and endothelial cells, and promotes the proliferation, differentiation, survival, and migration of hematopoietic progenitors, melanocytes, MCs, and germ cells.

Loss-of-function mutations at the *Sl* (steel) locus on chromosome 10 in mice were found to phenocopy mutations at the *W* locus. Ultimately, the gene product of the *Sl* locus was found to be the ligand for kit, SCF. In the case of mutations affecting the *W* (kit) locus, transplantation of BM cells from congenic +/+ mice into *W/W^v* mice corrected MC deficiency and anemia, consistent with an intrinsic progenitor/stem cell defect. In contrast, skin and BM engraftment experiments demonstrated that mutations at the *Sl* locus were cell extrinsic (e.g., microenvironmental) in nature. When skin from either *W/W^v* or *Sl/Sl^d* mice was transplanted onto the backs of congenic +/+ mice, MCs were capable of engrafting the skin from *W/W^v* mice but not the skin from *Sl/Sl^d* mice. In addition, hematologic abnormalities in *Sl/Sl^d* mice failed to correct with transplantation of BM cells from congenic +/+ animals. These experiments formally established that SCF is a physiologically relevant ligand of kit and that development is critically dependent on this ligand-receptor interaction. Therefore SCF has also been termed *mast cell growth factor*.

Alternative splicing results in two isoforms of membrane-bound SCF with different susceptibility to proteolytic cleavage: a longer isoform that retains exon 6 and contains a cleavage site that results in soluble SCF, and a shorter isoform lacking the cleavage site, which remains membrane-bound and serves as a stem cell homing receptor in the BM niche. Both the membrane-bound and soluble form of SCF (which exists in a homodimeric confirmation) are capable of binding to and inducing homodimerization of KIT, which, in turn, leads to autophosphorylation of tyrosine residues located in intracellular portions of the molecule. A cascade of signaling events ensues via downstream effector molecules, including Src kinases, c-Jun N-terminal kinase (Jnk), mitogen-activated protein (MAP) kinases, and the Janus-activated kinase (JAK)-signal transducer and activator of transcription and phosphatidylinositol 3-kinase (PI3K)/AKT pathways. In addition to promoting MC differentiation and survival, SCF can regulate MC adhesion to extracellular matrix proteins as well as mediator release via IgE-dependent and IgE-independent mechanisms. Likewise, when applied at relatively high concentrations for 90 min, SCF is capable of directly inducing mediator secretion from human MCs. Whereas in mice several different cytokines are involved in the regulation of growth and activation of MCs, SCF seems to be a rather specific cytokine for human MCs. Other studies

have shown that certain cytokines or hormonal factors exert inhibitory effects on MCs (e.g., interferon [IFN]-γ), and some cytokine pairs counterbalance each other's effects (e.g., T-helper 2 [Th2] cytokine interleukin [IL]-4 vs. regulatory T cell cytokine TGF-β1) on MC homeostasis. Expression of the death receptor tumor necrosis factor–related apoptosis-inducing ligand and inhibitor receptors CD300a and Siglec-8 may also contribute to downregulation of MC activation, survival, and IgE-mediated responses.

MAST CELL ACTIVATION AND FUNCTION

MCs commonly reside at the interface between the host and environment, usually in the skin, or in the mucosa lining the lungs or gastrointestinal tract. Migration and homing of MCs to various sites is regulated by the interaction between surface expression of numerous types of chemokine receptors (e.g., CXC chemokine receptor 2) and integrins (e.g., $\alpha4\beta7$, $\alpha4\beta1$) on MCs to tissue-specific endothelial binding sites such as mucosal vascular address in cell adhesion molecule-1 (MAdCAM-1) and vascular cell adhesion molecule-1 (VCAM-1). In addition to playing a primary role in mediating allergic responses and inflammation, MCs act as one arm of the adaptive immune system by playing a role in host defense against pathogens such as bacteria, fungi, and viruses.

MCs serve as a rich source of a variety of biologically active molecules (Table 72.1). These include preformed mediators such as vasoactive amines (histamine), anionic proteoglycans (heparin, chrondroitin sulfate), and proteases (tryptase, chymase, and carboxypeptidase).[2] Activated MCs also contribute to de novo synthesis of lipid-derived mediators that constitute the slow-reacting substance of anaphylaxis (SRS-A). These mediators include lipoxygenase-derived metabolites of arachidonic acid—the cysteinyl leukotrienes LTC4,

TABLE 72.1	Human Mast Cell Cell–Derived Mediators	
Class	**Mediators**	**Physiologic Effects**
Preformed mediators	Histamine, serotonin, heparin, neutral proteases (tryptase and chymase, carboxypeptidase, cathepsin G), major basic protein, acid hydrolases, peroxidase, phospholipases	Vasodilation, vasoconstriction, angiogenesis, mitogenesis, pain, protein processing/degradation, lipid/proteoglycan hydrolysis, arachidonic acid generation, tissue damage and repair, inflammation
Lipid mediators	LTB4, LTC4, PGE2, PGD2, PAF	Leukocyte chemotaxis, vasoconstriction, bronchoconstriction, platelet activation, vasodilation
Cytokines	TNF-α, TGF-β, IFN-α, IFN-β, IL-1α, IL-1β, IL-5, IL-6, IL-13 IL-16, IL-18	Inflammation, leukocyte migration/proliferation
Chemokines	IL-8 (CXCL8), I-309 (CCL-1), MCP-1 (CCL2), MIP-1αS (CCL3), MIP1β (CCL4), MCP-3 (CCL7), RANTES (CCL5), eotaxin (CCL11), MCAF (MCP-1)	Chemoattraction and tissue infiltration of leukocytes
Growth factors	SCF, M-CSF, GM-CSF, bFGF, VEGF, NGF, PDGF	Growth of various cell types, vasodilation, neovascularization, angiogenesis

The mediators in the table are examples only. In addition, many mediators are identified in mouse mast cells, human mast cell lines or primary cultures of human mast cells and may not be produced in vivo.
From Metcalfe DD: Mast cells and mastocytosis. *Blood* 112:946, 2008.[2]

LTD4, and LTE4, and cyclooxygenase-derived prostaglandin (PG) D2. These substances are involved in mediating vasodilation and vasopermeability, smooth muscle constriction, mucus secretion, and other proinflammatory sequelae. IgE- and non–IgE–dependent mechanisms (e.g., IgG, complement [C3a, C5a], neuropeptides, narcotics, physical stimuli, and activation of Toll-like receptors by bacterial products) can induce MCs to release a variety of cytokines (e.g., TNF-α, macrophage inflammatory protein [MIP]-1α and -1β, monocyte chemoattractant protein [MCP]-1, IFN-α, β, and γ, and various interleukins) and growth factors (see Table 72.1) that are implicated in the aforementioned physiologic roles of inflammation, allergic responses, and host defense. MCs mediate early-phase (e.g., anaphylaxis, acute asthma) and late-phase allergic responses, as well as non–type I hypersensitivity reactions through their proinflammatory mediators. Furthermore, MCs mediate upregulation of Th2 responses and allergen-specific IgE biosynthesis, which contribute to host defense against parasitic infections. MCs have also been implicated in the pathogenesis of various nonallergic conditions such as infectious or autoimmune diseases (e.g., multiple sclerosis, psoriasis, rheumatoid arthritis, inflammatory bowel disease), and also in repair after tissue injury, such as wound healing, thrombolysis, or tissue remodeling.

Coupling of MCs and eosinophils often occurs in the same tissue niches in allergic/inflammatory and neoplastic disorders such as eosinophilic esophagitis, chronic gastritis, gastrointestinal neoplasms, parasitic infections, and inflammatory bowel disease.[8] MCs can initiate the allergic inflammatory cascade, resulting in recruitment of eosinophils during the later phases of an allergen encounter. Both MCs and eosinophils express CCR3 and respond to eotaxins and RANTES (CCL5), leading to recruitment of both cell types into inflamed tissue. Moreover, MC-derived heparin can bind and stabilize eotaxins. In addition, MCs and eosinophils can interact with each other through soluble mediators or via direct cell-to-cell contact. At least in the murine system, MCs can also be induced to produce IL-3 and IL-5, which can potentiate eosinophil recruitment in tissues. The two principle MC-derived proteases exert dual actions on eosinophils. For example, MC-derived chymase suppresses eosinophil apoptosis and induces release of IL-6, CXCL8, CCL2, and CXCL1 from eosinophils. In contrast, β-tryptase can cleave eotaxin and RANTES, and can limit eosinophil chemotaxis. Eosinophils in turn produce SCF, which can attract more tissue MCs and protect them from apoptosis.

IgE-mediated hypersensitivity reactions (e.g., allergic rhinitis or asthma, anaphylaxis) are mediated by binding of allergen-specific IgE to the high-affinity FcεRI receptor, which is constitutively expressed at a high level on MCs. Engagement of FcεRI leads to its inclusion in lipid rafts, and phosphorylation of its β- and γ-chain immunoreceptor tyrosine-based activation motifs (ITAMs) by Lyn kinase and subsequent activation of Syk kinase through its binding to the ITAMs.[9] These proximal signaling events also activate Fyn kinase, which is important for phosphorylation of the adaptor protein Gab2 and activation of the PI3K pathway. Lyn kinase also regulates phosphorylation of the protein scaffolds LAT and NTAL, which coordinate multiple signaling pathways including Ras/MAP kinase, TEC family kinases, and PLCγ activation. PLCγ, in turn, is a critical mediator of MC cytokine production and degranulation. Experimental data indicate that the functions of KIT and FcεRI in MCs are interdependent. It has been observed that SCF enhances FcεRI-mediated MC degranulation, and that phosphorylation of the membrane adaptor molecule NTAL is a crucial link between the signaling cascades following KIT activation and FcεRI aggregation. In addition, BTK is a mediator of FcεRI-mediated MC degranulation and plays a critical role in the amplification of FcεRI activation by KIT.

TOOLS TO STUDY HUMAN MAST CELLS

The challenges of studying MCs relate to heterogeneity in their morphology and function between different species, and also within

different tissues of the same organism. Although several techniques, including flow cytometry-based cell sorting, exist for ex vivo isolation of BM MCs, yields are typically low, reflecting the low numbers of MCs in the BM and the difficulties in isolating them from other tissues, such as the lung. Ex vivo generation of human cord blood–derived or peripheral blood–derived MCs from their CD34+ or CD133+ progenitor cells using SCF and IL-6, can generate large numbers of functionally mature MCs that can be interrogated for various types of biologic investigations. Many studies of MCs and/ or mastocytosis have relied on MC lines such as the SCF-dependent cell lines LAD1/LAD2, derived from patients with MC sarcoma with KIT D816V (this cell line actually has normal KIT despite its origin, and is SCF dependent); the LUVA cell line (derived from CD34+ cells, growth factor–independent, normal KIT, and tendency to lose FcεRI expression with long-term culture); and the SCF-independent human mast cell line HMC-1 derived from a patient with MCL. Two HMC-1 subclones are available—HMC-1.1, which contains the KIT V560G mutation, and HMC-1.2, which expresses both KIT V560G and D816V. Both clones have been useful for in vitro evaluation of the differential sensitivity of different small-molecule inhibitors of KIT. None of these human MC lines, however, express both a functional IgE receptor and KIT D816V. However, more recently, a human cord blood–derived cell line that is SCF dependent and FcεRI+ (ROSA^KIT WT), and that converts to SCF independence and tumorigenic growth with transfection by KIT D816V (ROSA^KIT D816V), has been established, and should be a useful tool for studying the biology and pharmacologic aspects of mastocytosis.[10]

Mouse Models to Study Human Mastocytosis

A number of murine models of mastocytosis are available, including several transgenic models and xenotransplantation models. First, all the cell lines described earlier have been applied successfully in xenotransplantation models. In most instances, NSG mice were employed. In addition, several transgenic models have been established. In one model, transgenic mice harboring a fusion transgene consisting of the 571-bp primate chymase gene (Δ571-bchm) promoter fragment and the human Kit proto-oncogene cDNA with the codon 816 Asp→Val substitution were generated. These mice were found to slowly develop a MC disease-like condition with focal accumulations of MCs in the spleen and other organs, resembling indolent SM (ISM). In another model, a transgenic mouse exhibiting murine KIT D814V was established. These mice developed gastrointestinal MC accumulations. Both models may not reflect all aspects of the human disease, but may be helpful in basic science.

FIP1L1-PDGFRA- and NPM-ALK-Based Murine Models

Expression of the FIP1L1-PDGFRA fusion alone in murine BM cells was not sufficient to cause eosinophilia, but only a general myeloproliferative disease. However, overexpression of IL-5 together with FIP1L1-PDGFRA produced typical features closely resembling HES, including tissue infiltration by eosinophils. However, a phenotype of mastocytosis in addition to eosinophilia developed in another murine model by introducing FIP1L1-PDGFRA into hematopoietic stem cells and progenitors with T-cell overexpression of IL-5. Transplantation of NPM-ALK (nucleophosmin-anaplastic lymphoma kinase)–transduced progenitors into normal mice or IL-9–transgenic mice without NPM-ALK each result in MC hyperplasia; however, both "single-hit" models are insufficient to generate a histopathologic picture of SM. SM is only observed when NPM-ALK is transduced into mouse BM progenitors of lethally irradiated IL-9 transgenic mice. Similar to the model of FIP1L1-PDGFRA and IL-5, this model of the NPM-ALK fusion and IL-9 highlights the biologic interdependence of a fusion oncogene and cytokine-related pathways in promoting the full expression of neoplastic MC growth.

Germline Susceptibility to Mast Cell Disorders and Familial Mastocytosis

In general, mastocytosis behaves as an acquired, somatic disease. However, a few familial cases have been reported. In most of these families, a *KIT* mutation (various codons affected) can be detected in the germline. However, in a few families, the *KIT* mutation was only expressed in hematopoietic cells, but not in the germline of the affected individuals, suggesting that predisposing germline factors may contribute to disease development. However, so far, little is known about what gene polymorphisms serve as susceptibility alleles. In one study, polymorphisms within certain cytokine genes have been identified as exerting a potential predisposition to development of SM. In particular, a polymorphism in the promoter of the *IL-13* gene, −1112C/T, was significantly more frequent in SM patients versus both cutaneous mastocytosis (CM) patients and healthy controls. In addition −1112C/T was associated with increased serum tryptase levels and adult-onset disease. MCs express IL-13 receptors and IL-13–containing medium provides enhanced support for the growth of MCs. However, it remains unclear how −1112C/T relates to these specific biologic findings. In contradistinction to the IL-13 −1112C/T germline allele, the *IL-4α* chain receptor Q576 polymorphism was associated with more limited forms of mastocytosis. IL-4 modulates the growth and differentiation of MCs, and induces IgE receptor expression in MCs. Polymorphisms in the IL4 receptor have been implicated in allergic and inflammatory conditions. In a study of patients with cutaneous and systemic forms of mastocytosis, this polymorphic allele was significantly more associated with cutaneous disease, childhood-onset disease, and lower levels of serum tryptase and soluble CD117. The Q576 polymorphism in the *IL4α* chain receptor therefore appears to protect against MC hyperplasia and more aggressive forms of the disease. The Asp358Ala polymorphism in the *IL-6* receptor was associated with a 2.5-fold lower risk for mastocytosis compared with those with the AC or CC genotypes. However, no association was found between the *IL-6* 174G/C polymorphism and increased susceptibility to SM.

EPIDEMIOLOGY AND CLASSIFICATION OF MASTOCYTOSIS

In 2008, SM was included in the WHO category of myeloproliferative neoplasms (MPNs).[4] However, based on the complex clinical picture, biology and pathology, SM has been again defined by the WHO as a separate unique myeloid neoplasm in 2016. SM is an orphan disease and sparse data exist regarding its incidence or other epidemiologic features. A slight male predominance has been observed, and in one study, the median age at time of SM diagnosis was 55 years. A retrospective study from Denmark that canvassed the years from 1997 to 2010 estimated the incidence of SM at 0.89 per 100,000 persons per year, with an estimated prevalence of 9.59 per 100,000 individuals. A Dutch analysis estimated the prevalence of ISM to be 13 cases per 100,000 inhabitants.

The first diagnostic checkpoint is to distinguish SM from CM, which is characterized by predominant skin involvement. Criteria to diagnose SM are not fulfilled in these patients. However, in rare cases with CM, a discrete involvement of the BM by clonal cells may be detected, and serum tryptase levels may be slightly elevated. SM primarily occurs in adults, whereas CM is more common in children and its natural history is typically defined by spontaneous resolution of skin lesions usually at the time of puberty. CM variants include urticaria pigmentosa/maculopapular CM, diffuse CM, and solitary mastocytoma of the skin. In the overwhelmingly majority of adults with cutaneous involvement, systemic disease (SM) is diagnosed. However, absence of skin lesions does not exclude the presence of SM. Skin involvement occurs in over 80% of all patients with adult SM. However, sometimes, no BM examination is performed for some time, especially when the patient has not been referred to a hematologist. In such cases, cutaneous lesions are referred to as *mastocytosis in the skin* (MIS).

Diagnostic criteria for SM were initially formulated by a working group of MC disease experts at a consensus conference in Vienna in 2000,[3] and adopted by the WHO in both 2001 and 2008.[4] In the 2008 WHO Classification of hematolymphoid neoplasms, mastocytosis was classified as one of the disease subtypes under the major category of "Myeloproliferative Neoplasms (MPNs)". However, in the revised 2016 WHO classification, mastocytosis is now classified as its own major category distinct from MPNs. Minimal diagnostic criteria for SM requires at least one major plus one minor criterion, or at least three minor criteria (Table 72.2). The major criterion is the presence of multifocal dense aggregates of MCs (>15 MCs in aggregates) in sections of BM or other extracutaneous organ(s); minor criteria include: (1) >25% of the MCs in the infiltrate or in the BM smear are of spindle shape or of otherwise atypical morphology; (2) activating mutation at codon 816 in the *KIT* gene in an extracutaneous organ; (3) expression of CD2 and/or CD25 in/on MCs; and 4) serum tryptase level >20 ng/mL, unless there is an associated myeloid disorder that makes this parameter not valid.

SM is further divided into several subtypes that reflect the presence or absence of certain clinical or laboratory findings (Tables 72.3 and 72.4). The most common form of SM in adults is ISM, characterized by a slightly to markedly increased burden of neoplastic MCs in the BM and/or other extracutaneous organ(s). By definition, ISM patients do not exhibit MC-related organ damage or an associated hematologic disorder, and life expectancy in this variant is similar to that of an age-matched healthy population (Fig. 72.1).[11] However, ISM patients often experience mediator symptoms related to MC degranulation (e.g., flushing, pruritis, diarrhea, abdominal cramping, neuropsychiatric complaints). Although triggers may not always be identifiable, known provokers of MC activation and/or anaphylaxis include non-IgE and IgE-mediated causes: physical or emotional stress, exercise, hot or cold temperature stimuli, medications such as aspirin, NSAIDs, opioid analgesics, or antibiotics, alcohol, radiocontrast dye, and IgE-mediated allergies. One critical comorbidity is Hymenoptera venom allergy. In particular, these patients are at high risk of developing severe or even fatal anaphylaxis upon exposure to the venom. Cutaneous involvement usually develops in conjunction with the ISM subtype, both in younger individuals as well as in older patients. Bony disease (e.g., localized bone pain, diffuse osteopenia, osteoporosis with or without pathologic fractures, osteosclerosis) is also well described in ISM, but can cause morbid complications across the spectrum of SM variants.

In the 2008 WHO classification, smoldering SM (SSM) was designated as a subvariant of ISM. However, based on the current

TABLE 72.2	World Health Organization Diagnostic Criteria for Systemic Mastocytosis[a]
Major criterion	Multifocal dense infiltrates of mast cells (>15 mast cells in aggregates) detected in sections of bone marrow and/or other extracutaneous organ(s)
Minor criteria	a. In biopsy sections of bone marrow or other extracutaneous organs, >25% of the mast cells in the infiltrate are spindle shaped or have atypical morphology or, of all mast cells in bone marrow aspirate smears, >25% are immature or atypical b. Detection of an activating point mutation at codon 816 in *KIT* in bone marrow, blood, or another extracutaneous organ c. Mast cells in bone marrow, blood, or other extracutaneous organs express CD2 and/or CD25 in addition to normal mast cell markers d. Serum total tryptase persistently exceeds 20 ng/mL (unless there is an associated clonal myeloid disorder, in which case this parameter is not valid)

[a]Requires at least 1 major + 1 minor criteria or 3 minor criteria.

TABLE 72.3	2016 World Health Organization Variants of Mastocytosis

1. Cutaneous mastocytosis (CM)
   a. Maculopapular CM
   b. Diffuse CM
   c. Mastocytoma of skin
2. Indolent systemic mastocytosis (ISM)
   a. Isolated bone marrow mastocytosis
3. Smoldering systemic mastocytosis (SSM)
4. Systemic mastocytosis with an associated hematologic neoplasm (SM-AHN)*
   a. SM-MDS
   b. SM-MPN (e.g. PV, ET, MF, CML)
   c. SM-MDS/MPN (e.g. CMML, MDS/MPN-unclassified)
   d. SM-CEL
   e. SM-AML
   f. SM-lymphoid neoplasm (e.g. NHL, CLL, multiple myeloma)
5. Aggressive systemic mastocytosis (ASM)
6. Mast cell leukemia (MCL)
   a. Aleukemic MCL
7. Mast cell sarcoma (MCS)

*SM-AHN is a new term that may be used in lieu of, or interchangeably with the previously used term, SM-AHNMD (systemic mastocytosis with an associated non-mast cell lineage disease).
AML, Acute myeloid leukemia; CEL, chronic eosinophilic leukemia; CLL, chronic lymphocytic leukemia; CML, chronic myeloid leukemia; CMML, chronic myelomonocytic leukemia; ET, essential thrombocythemia; MDS, myelodysplastic syndrome; MF, myelofibrosis; MPN, myeloproliferative neoplasm; NHL, non–Hodgkin lymphoma; PV, polycythemia vera.

TABLE 72.4	2016 World Health Organization Diagnostic Criteria for Variants of (Systemic) Mastocytosis

1. **Indolent systemic mastocytosis (ISM):** Meets criteria for SM. No "B" or "C" findings. No evidence of associated clonal hematologic malignancy/disorder. In this variant, the mast cell burden is usually low; skin lesions are almost invariably present.
   - *Bone marrow mastocytosis:* As above, with bone marrow involvement, but no skin lesions.
2. **Smoldering systemic mastocytosis (SSM):** Meets criteria for SM. Two or more "B" findings and no "C" findings.
3. **Systemic mastocytosis with an associated hematologic neoplasm (SM-AHN)*:** Meets criteria for SM and criteria for an associated hematologic neoplasm (MDS, MPN, MDS/MPN, CEL, AML, lymphoma, or other hematologic neoplasm that meets the criteria for a distinct entity in the WHO classification).
3. **Aggressive systemic mastocytosis (ASM):** Meets criteria for SM. One or more "C" findings. No associated clonal hematologic neoplasm. No evidence of mast cell leukemia.
4. **Mast cell leukemia (MCL):** Meets criteria for SM. Bone marrow biopsy shows diffuse infiltration, usually interstitial pattern, by atypical, immature mast cells. Bone marrow aspirate smears show 20% or more mast cells. Cases in which <10% of circulating WBCs are mast cells are referred to as 'aleukemic mast cell leukemia'.
5. **Mast cell sarcoma (MCS):** Unifocal mast cell tumor. No evidence of SM. No skin lesions. Destructive growth pattern. High-grade cytology.

*SM-AHN is a new term that may be used in lieu of, or interchangeably with the previously used term, SM-AHNMD (systemic mastocytosis with an associated non-mast cell lineage disease).
AML, Acute myeloid leukemia; CEL, chronic eosinophiic leukemia; MDS, myelodysplastic syndrome; MPN, myeloproliferative neoplasm; WBC, white blood cell; WHO, World Health Organization.

classification proposed by the consensus group, SSM is now included in the revised 2016 WHO classification as a separate variant of SM, which is meaningful because these patients exhibit a higher chance of progression to more advanced disease. SSM is defined by two or more "B" findings (Table 72.5), e.g., (1) hepatomegaly without impairment of liver function, and/or palpable splenomegaly without hypersplenism, and/or lymphadenopathy on palpation or imaging; (2) BM MC burden >30% and serum tryptase level >200 ng/mL; and (3) signs of dysplasia or myeloproliferation, in non-MC lineage(s), but insufficient criteria for definitive diagnosis of an additional hematopoietic neoplasm, with normal or only slightly abnormal blood counts. Compared with ISM, SSM patients often exhibit clonal multilineage involvement of the *KIT* D816V mutation, which is also a prognostically relevant variable.

SM with an associated hematologic neoplasm (SM-AHN) comprises 30% of SM variants, although this figure may vary because of referral patterns. In the revised 2016 WHO classification, the term "SM-AHN" can be used interchangeably with or in lieu of the prior term "SM-AHNMD" (SM with an associated hematologic non-mast cell lineage disease). The vast majority of AHNs are myeloid neoplasms: myelodysplastic syndrome (MDS), MPNs, MDS/MPN overlap disorders such as chronic myelomonocytic leukemia (CMML) or MDS/MPN-unclassified, chronic eosinophilic leukemia (CEL), and acute myeloid leukemia (AML).[12] Rarely, lymphoid neoplasms such as chronic lymphocytic leukemia, myeloma, or lymphomas have been found in association with SM. Identifying a concomitant myeloid neoplasm may depend on several factors, including the expertise of the evaluating pathologist, and whether one disease is masked by the presence of another. For example, in cases of SM-AML, MC aggregates may only be unmasked after induction chemotherapy with achievement of BM hypoplasia, because neoplastic MCs may persist after such therapy. Distinguishing nonhematologic or hematologic organ damage because of the SM component versus the associated myeloid disease can be very difficult, if not impossible, in some patients. Even when a biopsy of the involved extramedullary organ is analyzed to elucidate the burden of neoplastic MCs versus associated myeloid neoplasm, it is sometimes impossible to define the relative impact of the SM versus AHN component on organ

TABLE 72.5	"B" Findings: Indication of High Mast Cell Burden

1. Infiltration grade (mast cells) greater than 30% in bone marrow in histology and serum total tryptase levels greater than 200 ng/mL
2. Hypercellular marrow with loss of fat cells, discrete signs of dysmyelopoiesis without substantial cytopenias, and without WHO criteria for an MDS or MPN
3. Organomegaly: palpable hepatomegaly, splenomegaly, or lymphadenopathy (on CT or ultrasound) greater than 2 cm without impaired organ function

MDS, Myelodysplastic syndrome; MPN, myeloproliferative neoplasm; WHO, World Health Organization.

dysfunction, especially when both disease components are of an aggressive type.

Although the prognosis of SM-AHN frequently relates to the AHN component, the burden of SM as well as the type and stage of the associated myeloid neoplasm need to be considered on an individual basis. Treatment plans are tailored to the histopathologic and molecular findings and the clinical sequelae that are felt to be attributable to each disease component. A commonly cited therapeutic approach has been to treat the SM component as if the myeloid neoplasm were not present, and to treat the myeloid neoplasm as if SM were not present. Because the *KIT* D816V mutation may be present in the cells belonging to both disease compartments, small molecule inhibitors of dysregulated KIT may provide benefit for both the SM and AHN in selected cases.

Aggressive systemic mastocytosis (ASM) comprises 5%–10% of SM variants and is defined by one or more "C findings" (Table 72.6) reflecting organ dysfunction because of neoplastic MC infiltrates. Examples of C findings include marked cytopenias because of extensive BM involvement (defined by an absolute neutrophil count

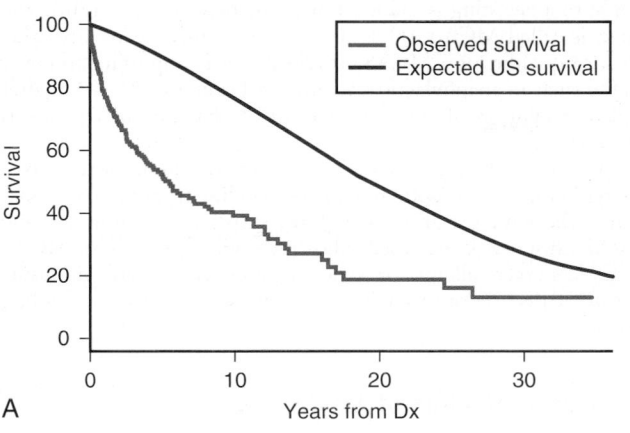

Expected US survival compared to all systemic mastocytosis patients

A

Years from Dx

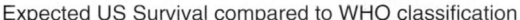

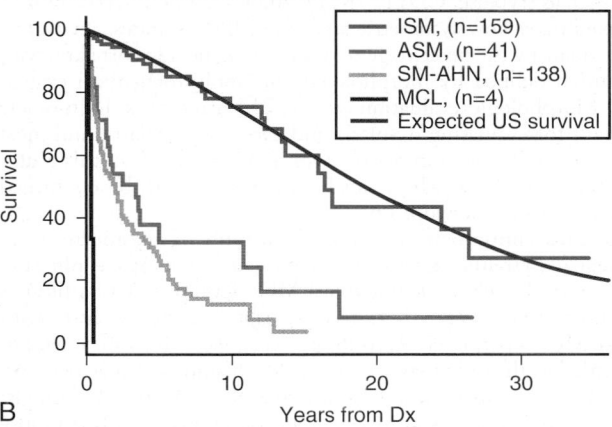

Expected US Survival compared to WHO classification

B

Years from Dx

Fig. 72.1 SURVIVAL OF SYSTEMIC MASTOCYTOSIS PATIENTS. (A) The observed Kaplan-Meier survival for systemic mastocytosis patients *(red)* compared with the expected survival of the age- and sex-matched US population *(blue)*. (B) The observed Kaplan-Meier survival for patients with systemic mastocytosis, classified by disease subtypes ISM *(red)*, ASM *(green)*, SM-AHN *(yellow)*, and MCL *(purple)* compared with the expected survival of the age- and sex-matched US population *(blue)*. *ASM,* Aggressive systemic mastocytosis; *ISM,* indolent systemic mastocytosis; *MCL,* mast cell leukemia; *SM-AHN,* systemic mastocytosis with an associated hematologic neoplasm; *US,* United States; *WHO,* World Health Organization.

TABLE 72.6	"C" Findings: Indication of Organ Damage Attributable to Neoplastic Mast Cell Infiltration

1. Cytopenia(s): Absolute neutrophil count <1000/µL or hemoglobin <10 g/dL or platelets <100,000/µL
2. Hepatomegaly with ascites and/or impaired liver function
3. Palpable splenomegaly with hypersplenism
4. Malabsorption with hypoalbuminemia and weight loss
5. Skeletal lesions: large-sized osteolyses or severe osteoporosis causing pathologic fractures
6. Life-threatening organopathy in other organ systems that is definitively caused by an infiltration of the tissue by neoplastic mast cells

nuclei, metachromatic blasts, and mitotic figures. In MCL, circulating MCs (≥10% of nucleated cells) may be found; however, the aleukemic MCL variant (<10% MCs in the peripheral blood) is more common. MCL may arise de novo or progress from less advanced forms of SM, such as ASM with elevated MC counts on the BM aspirate.[13] MCL typically has a dismal prognosis with a life expectancy of 6 months or less in most patients (see Fig. 72.1).[11,13,14] However, a chronic form of MCL has also been described, wherein patients meet histopathologic criteria for the disease, but without C findings (see later).[13] In these cases, MCs tend to show a more mature morphology. However, even those with the initially more indolent form of (chronic) MCL are expected to show progression over time with development of organ damage (transformation to acute MCL) and limited survival.

MC sarcoma (MCS) is a rare MC tumor that can invade local tissues and has a high potential to develop advanced systemic disease with a fulminant course. In particular, most if not all patients with MCS progress to MCL within a relatively short time period. Extracutaneous mastocytoma is another rare SM variant that typically follows a benign course.

Well-differentiated SM (WDSM) is a more recently described, rare variant of SM that is not yet formally recognized by the WHO (see later for histopathologic characteristics). The major reason for this is that the well-differentiated (WD) morphology of MCs can be found in all WHO subvariants of SM, including ISM, ASM, and MCL. Therefore the WD phenotype should be used as a descriptive term to complement the WHO diagnosis rather than as a tool to formulate a new entity.

Mast Cell Activation Syndromes

During the past few years, diagnostic criteria have been formulated for mast cell activation syndromes (MCAS), which are clinical conditions defined by MC activation but are not regarded as subtypes of SM (Table 72.7).[15] Patients with MCAS exhibit symptoms (e.g., anaphylaxis) and/or biochemical evidence of massive MC degranulation, with an event-related increase in serum tryptase. Other mediators produced by MCs may also increase during anaphylaxis. These mediators include plasma histamine, 24-h urine *N*-methylhistamine, PGD2 or metabolite 11-beta PGF2. Several different variants of MCAS have been described (Table 72.8). In patients with reactive MCAS, an underlying allergy is most commonly detected, whereas no signs of MC clonality are found. By contrast, in patients with primary (clonal) MCAS, MC monoclonality can be demonstrated. In these patients, MCs in the BM may be increased, often with atypical morphology, and evidence for their clonality can be established by identification of *KIT* D816V or cell surface expression of CD25. In patients with primary MCAS, there are two subsets of patients. One group of patients fulfills the criteria of an underlying MC disease, usually in form of SM (criteria to diagnose SM are fulfilled). In the second group of patients, the burden of MCs is very low, and despite the documented presence of clonal MCs, neither SM nor CM can be diagnosed. In these patients, one or two minor

[ANC] <1 × 10^9/L, hemoglobin <10 g/dL, and/or platelet count <100 × 10^9/L) and/or hypersplenism; hepatomegaly with liver dysfunction, and/or portal hypertension or ascites; hypoalbuminemia, which may relate to liver dysfunction and/or gut infiltration by neoplastic MCs; weight loss; and severe bone disease manifested by significant osteopenia and/or pathologic fractures. In a majority of patients with ASM, the percentage of MCs in the BM smear is below 5%, which is a favorable prognostic sign. Notably, in the less frequent ASM patients in whom MCs comprise ≥5% of all nucleated BM cells on a Giemsa-stained BM smear, the prognosis is poor, as many of these patients progress and transform to MCL or an ASM-AHN. Therefore these patients have recently been described as ASM in transformation (ASM-t; see later also under diagnostic evaluation of mastocytosis).[13] As soon as the percentage of MCs in these patients increase to ≥20% in the BM smear, the diagnosis changes to MCL.

MCL is a very rare form of SM (~1% of SM variants) and is defined by MCs comprising ≥20% of nucleated cells on BM aspirate smears. On the core biopsy, MCs form a diffuse, compact infiltrate with usually low levels of fibrosis. High-grade cytologic features of MCs can be observed in MCL, including multilobed or clefted

TABLE
72.7
Criteria for the Diagnosis of Mast Cell Activation

A. Typical symptoms (see below)
B. Increase in serum total tryptase by at least 20% above baseline plus 2 ng/mL during or within 4 h after a symptomatic period
C. Response of clinical symptoms to histamine receptor blockers or MC-targeting agents, e.g., cromolyn

Typical Symptoms

Flushing
Pruritis
Urticaria
Angioedema
Nasal congestion
Nasal pruritis
Wheezing
Throat swelling
Headache
Hypotension
Diarrhea

MC, Mast cell.
Modified from Valent P, Akin C, Arock M, et al: Definitions, criteria and global classification of mast cell disorders with special reference to mast cell activation syndromes: a consensus protocol. *Int Arch Allergy Immunol* 157:215, 2015.

TABLE
72.8
Classification of Mast Cell Activation Syndromes

Category and Variants	Proposed Criteria
Primary MCAS = (mono) clonal MCAS Mastocytosis Primary MCAS without evidence of mastocytosis	MCA criteria fulfilled and MC (mono) clonality proven (CD25⁺ MC and/or *KIT* D816V)ᵃ
Secondary MCAS Allergy Other underlying disorderᵇ	MCA criteria fulfilled and criteria for the diagnosis of allergy or other diseases that can produce MCA fulfilled as well
Idiopathic MCASᶜ	MCA criteria fulfilled, but no disease that could lead to MCA diagnosed

ᵃCD25⁺ MCs plus *KIT* D816V detectable, or *KIT* D816V detectable, but MCs cannot be demonstrated to express CD25.
ᵇDisorders associated with MCA include autoimmune diseases, certain bacterial infections, and some adverse drug reactions.
ᶜIdiopathic MCAS is a final diagnosis but needs an extensive workup in order to exclude all potential underlying conditions. Idiopathic and secondary MCA episodes may occur at different time points in the same patient.
MC, Mast cell; MCA, mast cell activation; MCAS, mast cell activation syndrome.
From Valent P, Akin C, Arock M, et al. Definitions, criteria and global classification of mast cell disorders with special reference to mast cell activation syndromes: a consensus protocol. *Int Arch Allergy Immunol* 157:215, 2012.

SM criteria are typically present. However, at the time of diagnosis, a diagnosis of an underlying MC disease cannot be established.[16] In both instances, the diagnosis is primary (clonal) MCAS. Because of the very low numbers of MCs, techniques to enrich for MCs and/or use of sensitive techniques to detect *KIT* D816V (e.g., allele-specific PCR) may be necessary to detect neoplastic MCs in these patients. Currently, there is no evidence that these two entities are "prodromal" SM conditions with a defined rate of progression to systemic MC disease. If neither an underlying allergy nor another underlying reactive process nor a clonal population of MCs can be detected in an MCAS patient, the final diagnosis is idiopathic MCAS.[15] Criteria for MCAS include an event-related increase in serum tryptase, typical clinical symptoms, and response of these symptoms to drugs targeting MC activation, MC-derived mediators, or their specific receptors.[15] All three MCAS criteria must be fulfilled to characterize the condition as MCAS. The minimal increase in tryptase is defined by the following formula: 20% of baseline plus absolute 2 ng/mL. Example: if in

an SM patient with 100 ng/mL baseline tryptase, an anaphylactic response to a bee sting is followed by an increase to 150 ng/mL, the reaction is called MCA (100 + 20 + 3 = 123; this means any value above 123 qualifies as a MCAS criterion).[15] It is important to know that after such an anaphylactic reaction, it takes at least 24–48 h (after complete resolution of symptoms) until the baseline of tryptase is again reached.

In patients with IgE-mediated hymenoptera venom anaphylaxis, particularly individuals with an elevated baseline tryptase level (separate from the acute rise after a sting), the suspicion for an underlying clonal MC disorder is increased. The differential diagnosis for MCAS includes less severe allergic or toxic reactions, endocrinologic disorders, cardiac diseases or severe infectious diseases (septicemia) leading to shock.

Diagnostic Evaluation of Mastocytosis

Tissue biopsy in conjunction with clinical and pathology expertise are critical in establishing the diagnosis of SM. BM MC burden is best quantified by morphologic analysis and immunohistochemical stains such as tryptase, CD117 (KIT), and CD25 on the core biopsy. Multiparameter flow cytometric analysis of BM aspirates can also be used to quantify the percentage of MCs, and generally correlates with SM burden defined by morphologic/immunohistochemical evaluation.[16] Morphologic evaluation of the BM aspirate is additionally important for evaluating dysplasia and excess myeloblasts, and most relevant to MCL, the number of atypical MCs. Based on this evaluation, the presence of MCL can be excluded or can be confirmed during the diagnostic work-up.

The most important morphologic feature of mastocytosis, in particular its systemic variants, is the presence of compact infiltrates consisting of densely packed atypical MCs. Compact MC infiltrates are almost never detected in reactive states, even in those with marked MC hyperplasia. Accordingly, compact MC infiltrates can be regarded as the only major criterion for diagnosis of mastocytosis, which also underlines the important role of the hematopathologist in making these diagnoses. Investigation of an adequate BM biopsy trephine specimen is crucial to assess or exclude a diagnosis of SM. In most patients a few compact infiltrates can be identified even by using conventional stains like Giemsa-Wright or toluidine blue, which both facilitate detection of the pathognomonic metachromatic granules. The MCs are round or spindle shaped, and often exhibit at least some hypogranulation. The nuclei are round or elongated depending on the shape of the cell. Prominent nucleoli are not seen. Almost always such compact infiltrates also contain mature eosinophils, histiocytes, and sometimes large follicle-like aggregates of lymphocytes that are polyclonal in nature. Reticulin fiber density is always increased with the exception of a few very small but diagnostic infiltrates. Larger compact and mixed infiltrates often show patchy collagen fibrosis. The degree of reticulin fibrosis in most cases of MCL is low, which can be used as a criterion that allows one to distinguish MCL from aggressive SM, which usually exhibits marked reticulin or even collagen fibrosis (Fig. 72.2). Immunohistochemistry should be performed in all cases in order to enumerate the numbers of loosely scattered MCs and to detect small but diagnostic compact infiltrates. The degree of MC infiltration should always be documented by the hematopathologist: it is recommended to refer to the section area and to the overall cellularity in this respect. This enables monitoring of the disease during and after therapy. MCs almost always coexpress tryptase and CD117; in most SM cases, MCs also aberrantly express CD25, whereas aberrant expression of other antigens such as CD2 is more rarely encountered and therefore of minor diagnostic importance (Fig. 72.3). Interestingly, it could be shown that MCs may lose immunohistochemically detectable tryptase expression during or after therapy with TK inhibitors such as midostaurin, and MCs in cases of intestinal involvement by SM may lack tryptase expression at diagnosis (e.g., incomplete immunophenotype). However, it can be stated definitively that a cell lacking expression of CD117 (KIT) cannot be a MC. Although

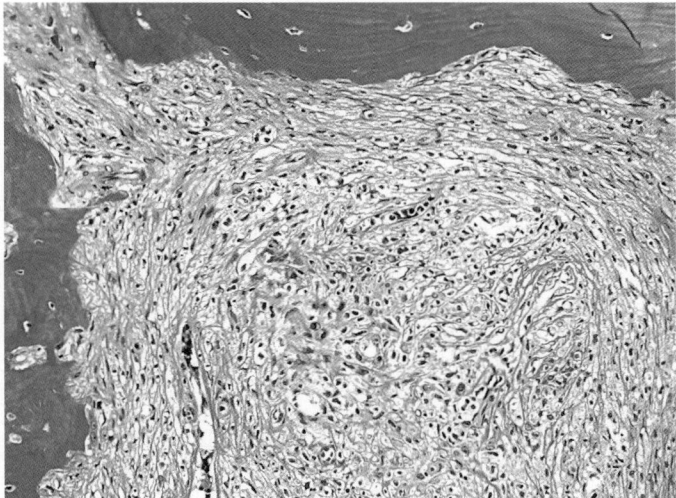

Fig. 72.2 AGGRESSIVE SYSTEMIC MASTOCYTOSIS. Core biopsy, hematoxylin and eosin stain. Extremely hypercellular bone marrow with subtotal depletion of fat cells and normal blood cell precursors. Packed infiltration by atypical hypogranulated spindle-shaped mast cells that are embedded in a dense fibrotic stroma is the typical finding in aggressive systemic mastocytosis (ASM). However, only the presence of C-finding(s) qualifies such cases to be subtyped as ASM. Similar pictures can be seen in smoldering systemic mastocytosis with B-findings. Note that the morphologic features of nonspecific fibrosis or granulation tissue may be very similar and appropriate immunostaining is necessary to confirm the diagnosis of SM.

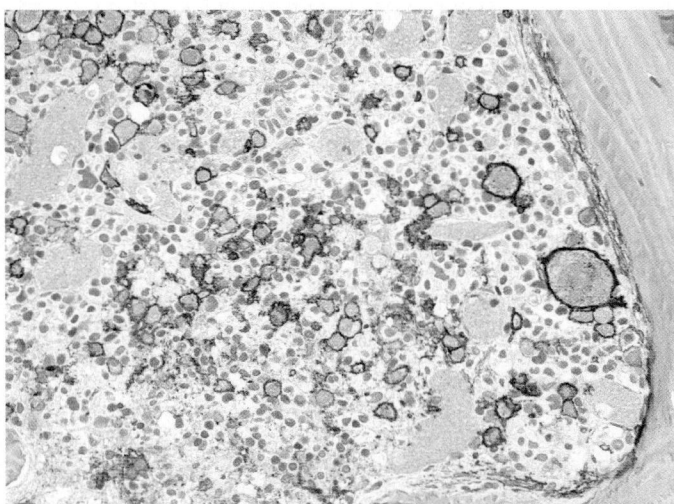

Fig. 72.3 ACUTE MAST CELL LEUKEMIA WITH CD30 EXPRESSION. Core biopsy with positive staining of mast cells for surface CD30. Bone marrow section shows extreme hypercellularity with diffuse-packed infiltration by atypical round mast cells coexpressing tryptase and CD117 (not depicted). A significant number of the mast cells stain positive by an antibody against CD30, among them a few multinucleated giant cells that resemble Reed-Sternberg cells. A diagnosis of Hodgkin lymphoma should not be established in such cases.

ISM and isolated mastocytosis of the BM usually show a minor degree of BM involvement with multifocal compact infiltrates (<10% of the section area), smoldering and aggressive SM but also MCL usually exhibit a more diffuse or packed infiltration occupying more than 30% and up to 100% of the section area. Regarding morphologic and immunophenotypical features of MCs in SM, a broad spectrum of differential diagnoses should be considered.

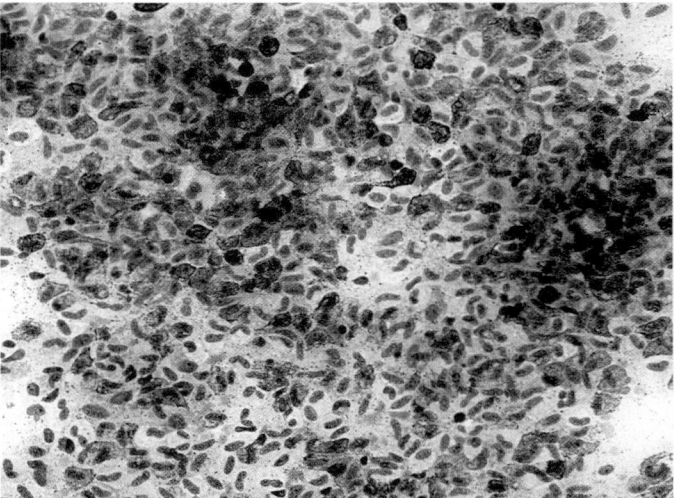

Fig. 72.4 CHRONIC MAST CELL LEUKEMIA (BY CLINICAL BEHAVIOR). Bone marrow aspirate (Pappenheim stain) shows a very unusual picture with an extreme increase of spindle-shaped and often slightly hypogranulated mast cells. Note their elongated nuclei. Nucleoli are inconspicuous. Mast cell number is almost 100% and a diagnosis of mast cell leukemia can easily be established. The prolonged survival of this patient and the unique cytomorphologic aspect qualifies this case to be subtyped as chronic mast cell leukemia.

The following list only contains the main entities and is therefore incomplete:

1. monocytic leukemias (clear cell feature + CD14)
2. histiocytoses (clear cell feature + CD68)
3. clear-cell carcinomas (clear cell feature)
4. basophilic leukemias (metachromatic granules + tryptase)
5. myelomastocytic leukemia (metachromatic granules + tryptase + CD117)
6. Hodgkin lymphoma (CD30)
7. hairy cell leukemia (clear cell feature + CD25)

Evaluation of blood and BM smears is crucial for both identification and subtyping of MCL and separation of MCL from a recently described subtype of ASM, namely ASM-t (see earlier). In almost all patients with ISM and SSM, but also in most cases with ASM, the MC numbers in BM smears are lower than 5%, in ISM and SSM usually even below 1%. Crushed particles with higher numbers of MCs must not be considered in this respect. In a few patients with ASM the number of MCs is unusually high, exceeding 5% but not 19% of all nucleated cells. It is this subgroup of patients that bears a worse prognosis but do not fulfill criteria for MCL and have therefore been termed ASM-t.

Cytomorphologic findings in SM include atypically shaped MCs with spindled appearance (type I) on the one hand and round immature MCs with bilobated or monocytoid nuclei on the other (type II). Atypical type I MCs are usually encountered in ISM, SSM, and often also in ASM, but also in isolated mastocytosis of the BM (BMM), whereas atypical type II MCs dominate the picture in most cases of MCL, and are often found also in patients with ASM and ASM-t. Exceedingly rare cases of MCL with predominance of spindle-shaped cells of type I are associated with a relatively good prognosis and the disease accordingly has been termed *chronic MCL* (see earlier) (Fig. 72.4). There is one peculiar phenotypic variant of SM termed *well-differentiated SM* (; see earlier) that consists exclusively of round hypergranular-appearing MCs that form the typical cohesive clusters in BM smears. Such MC clusters are not seen in all of the subvariants of SM. The feature of well-differentiated SM has been encountered in almost all defined subvariants of SM including

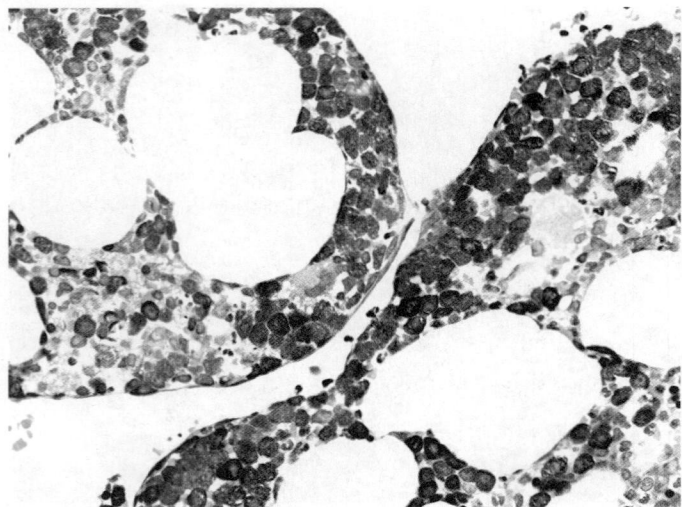

Fig. 72.5 WELL-DIFFERENTIATED SYSTEMIC MASTOCYTOSIS. Core biopsy, Giemsa stain. Bone marrow shows aggregates of exclusively round mast cells with an abundance of metachromatic granules. This is the typical phenotypical appearance of a well-differentiated systemic mastocytosis. The disease was otherwise subtyped as indolent systemic mastocytosis with skin involvement but missing *KIT* D816V mutation and also lack of CD25 expression by the mast cells (not depicted).

MCL. Well-differentiated SM usually lacks aberrant expression of CD25 and does also not show the typical activating point mutations at codon 816 of *KIT* (Fig. 72.5).

CD30 (Ki-1) is a cytoplasmic and membrane-bound antigen expressed by neoplastic cells in Hodgkin lymphoma and anaplastic large-cell lymphoma. Recently, however, CD30 has also been shown to be expressed by neoplastic MCs in SM.[17] Although the antigen was originally reported as an immunohistochemical marker that is primarily expressed in the cytoplasm of MCs in more advanced forms of SM, other studies have detected CD30 by immunohistochemistry in less advanced forms of MC disease, including CM, as well as ISM and SSM. CD30 is not only expressed in the cytoplasm of neoplastic MCs but also on the cell surface, which has clinical implications as a CD30 antibody-toxin conjugate is available and is currently being tested in patients with advanced SM.

Serum Tryptase Level

Tryptase is considered to be a most reliable and robust initial parameter with which to screen patients with suspected SM.[18,19] Tryptase is a serine protease primarily produced by MCs, and to a lesser extent by mature basophils and myeloid progenitors. Commercially available ELISA-based assays measure total serum tryptase levels which consist of both mature tryptase (β-tryptase) and protryptases (e.g., α-tryptase). The basal serum tryptase level reflects the MC burden in healthy individuals as well as in patients with SM, whereas the event-related (further) increase in tryptase is a marker of MC activation. β-tryptase is stored in MCs and released together with all other granular substances upon degranulation/anaphylaxis (tryptase levels peak 1–2 h after degranulation event and return to baseline after 24–48 h). The α-tryptase form is constitutively produced by MCs and thus more reflects the total burden of MCs. For many centers, the upper normal reference range for the serum tryptase level is 10 or 11.4 ng/mL. However, healthy individuals may exhibit levels in the range of 5–15 ng/mL or higher, which may be confounded by the association between advancing age and increasing serum tryptase levels. Although a serum tryptase level >20 ng/mL serves as a minor diagnostic criterion for SM, a minority of patients with histopathologically proven SM can exhibit values lower than this threshold. In adult patients with MIS or hymenoptera allergy, a serum tryptase level >20 ng/mL is suggestive of the presence of SM. Conversely, patients with CM usually exhibit a serum tryptase level <20 ng/mL, or it may be within normal range. Other medical conditions besides SM and anaphylaxis that can produce an elevated tryptase level include renal failure, chronic helminth infections (MC hyperplasia), SCF treatment, and myeloid neoplasms, including MDS, MPN, AML, and CEL—notably patients with the *FIP1L1-PDGFRA* fusion gene.

Although there is a close correlation between high tryptase levels and advanced SM, serum tryptase levels do not necessarily reflect the aggressiveness of the disease. Likewise, SSM is partially defined by a very high serum tryptase level exceeding 200 ng/mL, and in many of these cases, progression dose not occur for many years. Contrasting the smoldering state, most patients with typical ISM have lower serum tryptase levels, although enzyme levels can vary widely among patients according to the MC burden. Patients with ASM and MCL may exhibit serum tryptase levels in the several-hundred range to over 1000 ng/mL. In many of these patients, serum basal tryptase levels increase rapidly over time (in contrast to ISM and SSM). Although discordances can exist between the serum tryptase level and the degree of MC infiltration of the marrow and other organs, it is the most useful and widely available biomarker that can be used to assess changes in the MC burden in response to cytoreductive therapy.

Clinical Manifestations

Organomegaly

Splenomegaly and hepatomegaly, without associated organ damage, have traditionally been referred to as "B" findings and are one of the defining features of SSM. Similarly, SM-related substantial (palpable, >2 cm) lymphadenopathy has been included in the category of "B" findings. Organomegaly by itself does not indicate inexorable progression to advanced SM or organ damage. However, even in the absence of organ damage, symptomatic splenomegaly may warrant therapeutic intervention similar to patients with myelofibrosis or other hematologic neoplasms.

Nonhematologic Organ Damage

The challenge of defining response parameters related to hepatic function is several-fold. First, for patients with SM with associated myeloid neoplasm, it is unclear whether liver dysfunction is related to the SM or the accompanying myeloid disease. Concomitant diseases such as MPN or MDS/MPN such as CMML, CEL, or AML may (also) involve the liver and result in a hepatitis-like syndrome or obstructive liver disease. It is unknown what level of liver involvement by MC consistently results in liver dysfunction. Liver biopsy is sometimes performed and may help to assess the grade and extent of liver involvement by SM. Although liver biopsy may be informative, the potential information gleaned from the procedure must be weighed against potential complications such as bleeding, especially in the setting of severe thrombocytopenia and/or coagulopathy.

Hypoalbuminemia is an adverse prognostic factor for overall survival (OS) in SM[3,11]; it can reflect worsening synthetic function of the liver, and/or worsening nutritional status or even malabsorption because of gastrointestinal infiltration by neoplastic MCs. The development of ascites in SM usually reflects aggressive liver disease and may be accompanied not only by hepatomegaly but also by abnormal liver function test, often with an elevated alkaline phosphatase and/or portal hypertension. More uncommonly, ascites may develop without evidence for liver disease, or in conjunction with massive abdominal lymphadenopathy. Similar to ascites, pleural effusions may develop in advanced SM, although it is an uncommon event. Every attempt should be made to establish that the ascites or pleural effusion is related to SM and/or the associated myeloid neoplasm, including evaluation of MC content. Other causes of effusion should be excluded including infection, heart failure, and drugs such as dasatinib that have been used to treat advanced SM.

Hematologic Organ Involvement

The etiology of cytopenias in advanced SM includes compromise of normal marrow reserve by infiltration with neoplastic MCs (often seen in ASM and MCL), ineffective hematopoiesis in the context of SM with an associated myeloid neoplasm, hypersplenism, and other causes such as recent myelosuppressive therapy or gastrointestinal bleeding. The coexistence of another myeloid neoplasm (AHN) often makes it difficult to ascertain the specific cause of the low blood counts. This distinction is not relevant to ISM, where the relatively lower MC burden is not expected to contribute to the development of cytopenias.

Molecular Features of SM

Following the discovery of the somatic *KIT* D816V mutation in MC neoplasms in the mid-1990s,[20] it has become evident that this molecular abnormality is found in approximately 80% to 90% of SM patients. *KIT* D816V serves as a minor diagnostic criterion for the disease, and is considered a major driver of SM pathogenesis. Rare codon 816 variants such as D816F/H/I/Y have also been described and are considered functionally equivalent to D816V. Mutations affecting codon 816 are located in exon 17 and affect the second TK domain (TK2) that contains the phosphotransferase site and activation loop of KIT. Other mutations that have been identified in exon 17, for example in cases of ASM and MC sarcoma, include D820G and N822K. *KIT* mutations in exons 8–9 of the extracellular region (del419, S451C, ITD 502–503) and the TM region (exon 10; e.g., F522C), and JM domain (exon 11; e.g., V560G/I) comprise some of the additional rare mutations in *KIT* that have been observed (Fig. 72.6).[21] With a few exceptions (e.g., V559I), mutations affecting these domains are more likely to exhibit sensitivity to imatinib, whereas codon 816 variants are imatinib resistant. Contrary to other SM subtypes, MCL less frequently exhibits the *KIT* D816V mutation; in a review of MCL, D816V was found in 13 of 28 (46%) evaluable patients. MCL patients may exhibit other variants within *KIT*, or sequencing of the entire *KIT* gene may reveal no mutations. Increasingly sensitive assays, such as allele-specific quantitative PCR for *KIT* D816V, are now available and can detect *KIT* D816V in the peripheral blood of almost all adult patients with SM. Where available, it has been recommended that such sensitive assays be used as a valuable screening test for patients with suspected SM.[19] However, a low MC burden or the presence of other rare *KIT* or non-*KIT* mutations could lead to negative results; therefore a full workup with BM biopsy is warranted in typical cases where clinical symptoms and findings are highly suggestive of the presence of SM.

In a large cohort of pediatric mastocytosis patients, 36% exhibited *KIT* D816V mutations, and three (6%) patients had other codon 816 mutations (D816Y [*n* = 2] and D816I [*n* = 1]). Another 42% demonstrated *KIT* mutations outside exon 17, with half of these being located in exons 8 and 9 (D417-418, D419Y, C443Y, S476I, ITD502-503, K509I) and exon 11 (D572A). When these data were combined with a cohort from Dubreil and colleagues, 76% of the pediatric patients were found to have alterations in *KIT*, all of which resulted in constitutive activation of the TK. Multiple families with hereditary mastocytosis, typically manifesting as cutaneous disease, were found to have germline *KIT* mutations, including K509I, A533D, N822I, M835K, S849I, or deletion of amino acids 419 or 559–560).

SM-AHN cases commonly harbor molecular abnormalities related to the myeloid disease component in addition to *KIT* D816V. For example, *JAK2* V617F has been found in SM with myelofibrosis; *BCR-ABL1* in rare cases of concurrent SM-CML; and in SM-AML,

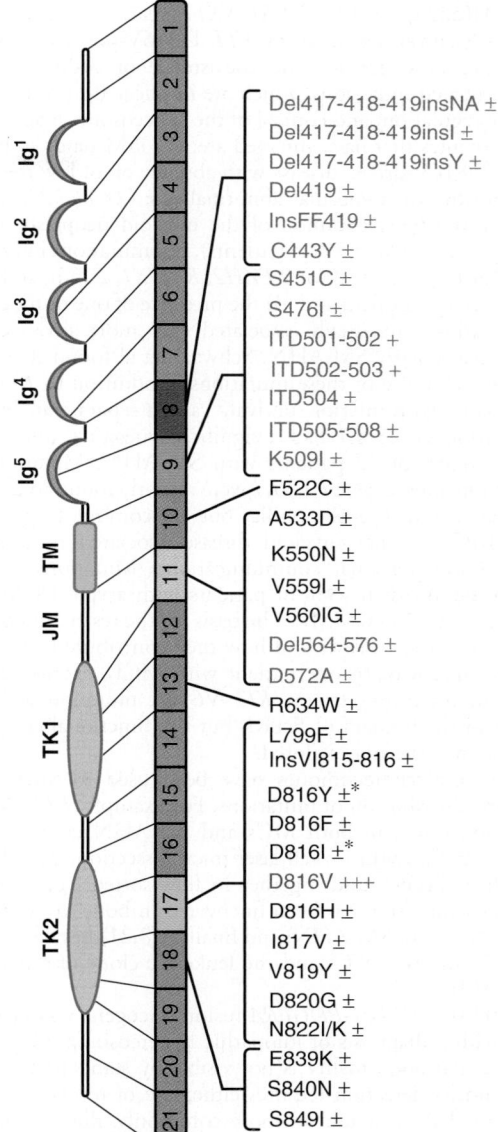

Fig. 72.6 STRUCTURE OF THE *KIT* GENE AND MUTATIONS IN MASTOCYTOSIS. Representation of the structure of *KIT*, illustrating the localization of the more frequently observed mutations in the *KIT* sequence in pediatric and adult patients with mastocytosis. The receptor is presented under its monomeric form, whereas its WT counterpart dimerizes upon ligation with SCF before being activated in normal cells. In children, the *KIT* D816V PTD mutant (in red) is found in nearly 30% of the patients, whereas the ECD mutants (in blue) are found in nearly 40% of the affected children, the most frequent being the deletion 419. In adults, depending of the category of mastocytosis, the *KIT* D816V mutant *(in red)* is found in at least 80% of all patients. The complete list of *KIT* mutants retrieved in the literature for mastocytosis is depicted here. In children, the structure of *KIT* is found WT in ~25% of the patients analyzed, whereas in adults, *KIT* is found WT in <20% of all patients analyzed so far. Some of the mutations are found only in a very few number of patients. The symbols indicate the following: ±, mutation found in <10% of the pediatric or adult patients; +, mutations found in 1%–5% of pediatric patients; ++, mutation found in 5%–20% of pediatric patients; +++, mutation found in ~30% of pediatric patients and in >80% of all adult patients. *Mutation also found in children at low frequency. *Del,* Deletion; *ECD,* extracellular domain; *Ig,* immunoglobulin; *Ins,* insertion; *ITD,* internal tandem duplication; *JM,* juxtamembrane domain; *KI,* kinase insert; *PTD,* phosphotransferase domain; *TK,* tyrosine kinase; *TM,* transmembrane domain. *(From Arock M, Sotlar K, Akin C, et al: KIT mutation analysis in mast cell neoplasms: recommendations of the European Competence Network on Mastocytosis. Leukemia 29:1223, 2015.)*[21]

the t(8;21)(q22;q22) *RUNX1/RUNX1T* rearrangement is a well-known association. In cases of *KIT* D816V-positive SM, several reports have now detailed the coexistence of additional myeloid neoplasm-related mutations, which are implicated in differentiation, epigenetic regulation, and control of the spliceosome machinery. The common themes that have emerged are: (1) ISM tends to be more a pure *KIT* D816V-driven disease with absence of, or low frequency of additional (known) molecular abnormalities; (2) *TET2*, *SRSF2*, and *ASXL1* are the most common of the myeloid neoplasm-associated mutated genes (~20%–35% of patients), but mutations in *DNMT3A*, *CBL*, *K/NRAS*, *UA2F1*, *ZRSF2 EZH2*, *RUNX1*, *ETV6*, and *SETBP1* have also been identified; and (3) the presence of one or more of these genes mutations are usually associated with more advanced disease subtypes, particularly SM-AHN. Schwaab et al found that the presence of one or more of these mutations in addition to *KIT* D816V was associated with inferior survival,[22] and a separate analysis found that mutation of *ASXL1* had a significant negative impact on OS among a cohort of 62 patients with SM-AHN. Mutations in the ethanolamine kinase gene *ETNK1* were recently found to be enriched in SM patients with eosinophilia, but are commonly present with *KIT* D816V or other myeloid disease-associated mutations (Dr. Andreas Reiter, personal communication). Mutations in *ETNK1* were also identified in ~9% of patients with atypical CML and in <5% of patients with CMML. The basis for the restriction of *ETNK1* mutations to these diseases and how they contribute to their pathogenesis is unknown. In one patient with MCL, exome sequencing revealed an imatinib-resistant *KIT* V654A mutation as well as a mutation in the β-chain of FcεRI, but the functional consequences of this variant were not explored.

Special research techniques have been used to interrogate the cell-specific distribution of mutations. For example, *KIT* D816V has been demonstrated in both MCs and the AHN component (e.g., monocytes in CMML) by cell laser microdissection; *TET2* and *KIT* D816V have been found together in flow-sorted MCs; the *SRSF2* P95 hotspot mutation has been uncovered in both MCs and monocytes from a case of SM-AHN; and finally, t(8;21) has been identified by FISH in the BM MCs and the leukemic clone of a patient with SM and AML.

In 2003 the *FIP1L1-PDGFRA* fusion oncogene was identified in patients with a diagnosis of idiopathic hypereosinophilic syndrome. This molecular abnormality is not visible by standard chromosome analysis and its detection requires either use of reverse-transcriptase polymerase chain reaction or, more commonly, fluorescence in situ hybridization (FISH). Because this genetic lesion results from an interstitial 800-kb deletion on chromosome 4q12, which removes a segment of DNA involving the *CHIC2* gene, the diagnostic test is referred to as "FISH for the *CHIC2* deletion." Patients with *FIP1L1-PDGFRA*-associated eosinophilia present with features of a myeloproliferative disorder: splenomegaly, hypercellular BMs, and clinicopathologic characteristics that overlap with SM, including increased numbers of abnormal-appearing BM MCs, marrow fibrosis, and elevated serum tryptase levels. However, although *FIP1L1-PDGFRA*–positive myeloid neoplasms may exhibit increased numbers of BM MCs, they usually form interstitial or loose clusters, and this disease entity is not considered a subtype of SM by the WHO. However, in a smaller subset of patients, criteria for SM may be fulfilled even if a *KIT* mutation is not detected. Notably, in almost all cases with *FIP1L1-PDGFRA*–positive myeloid neoplasms, including those who have SM-CEL, MCs do not exhibit *KIT* D816V, even if they express CD25. Although the *FIP1L1-PDGFRA* genetic abnormality was once considered mutually exclusive of *KIT* D816V, rare cases with both mutations have now been reported, including their coexistence in tryptase-positive microdissected MCs.

Investigators identified a set of clinical and laboratory features that could reliably distinguish patients with *KIT* D816V-positive SM with eosinophilia from individuals with the *FIP1L1-PDGFRA*–positive myeloid neoplasms with eosinophilia (Table 72.9).[23] These criteria may be particularly useful when molecular testing is not readily available. In the D816V *KIT*-positive group, gastrointestinal symptoms, urticaria pigmentosa, thrombocytosis, median serum tryptase

TABLE 72.9	Clinicopathologic Features of Eosinophilia-Associated *FIP1L1-PDGFRA*–Rearranged Myeloid Neoplasms Versus *KIT* D816V-Positive Systemic Mastocytosis	
Features	**FIP1L1-PDGFRA– Rearranged**	**KIT D816V–Positive**
Gender	Overwhelmingly male	Less gender skewing
Bone marrow mast cell aggregates	Loose clusters/ interstitial	Dense aggregates
AEC/tryptase ratio	>100	≤100
Treatment	Imatinib sensitive	Imatinib-resistant; second-generation TKIs (e.g., midostaurin)
Symptom profile	Cardiac/pulmonary	Gastrointestinal/urticaria pigmentosa/anaphylaxis
Vitamin B$_{12}$ level	Elevated	Often normal

AEC, Absolute eosinophil count; TKI, tyrosine kinase inhibitor.
Modified from Maric I, Robyn J, Metcalfe DD, et al: KIT D816V-associated systemic mastocytosis with eosinophilia and FIP1L1/PDGFRA-associated chronic eosinophilic leukemia are distinct entities. *J Allergy Clin Immunol* 120(3):680-687, 2007.

value, and the presence of dense MC aggregates in the BM were statistically significantly increased or more frequently represented compared with patients with the *FIP1L1-PDGFRA* gene fusion. Conversely, male sex, cardiac and pulmonary symptoms, median peak absolute eosinophil count, the eosinophil to tryptase ratio, and elevated serum B$_{12}$ levels were higher or more common in the group with *FIP1L1-PDGFRA*. A scoring system incorporating these clinical and laboratory parameters could reliably predict whether patients with peripheral eosinophilia and increased marrow MC burden carried the *FIP1L1-PDGFRA* gene fusion or the *KIT* D816V mutation, which is important for guiding targeted therapy options.[23] Treatment of *FIP1L1-PDGFRA*–positive myeloid neoplasms associated with eosinophilia is discussed in Chapter 71.

Additional Diagnostic Studies

In all patients with symptomatic SM, a thorough work-up for allergies, including total and specific IgE levels, should be performed. Biochemical studies to evaluate for MC activation/mediator release include 24-h urine evaluation of *N*-methylhistamine, prostaglandin D2, or 11-B-prostaglandin F2. Bleeding diatheses have been reported in patients with MCAS or SM, and increased heparin levels can be found in patients with SM or MC activation. Dual energy x-ray absorptiometry (DEXA) scans should be undertaken to screen for osteoporosis, and plain x-ray films (e.g., metastatic skeletal survey) are used to evaluate osteolytic lesions and/or pathologic fractures. MC-related gastrointestinal symptoms such as diarrhea and signs of malabsorption (e.g., hypoalbuminemia and weight loss) can be evaluated with endoscopy/colonoscopy with biopsy using appropriate immunohistochemical stains (e.g., CD117, tryptase, CD25, and CD3 as a control T-cell marker) to highlight abnormal MCs. Ultrasonography, CT and/or MRI of the abdomen/pelvis (with or without volumetric imaging) are utilized to determine the presence and extent of B and C findings such as hepato/splenomegaly, portal hypertension, ascites, and lymphadenopathy.

Diagnostic Decision Making

In patients presenting with MC activation symptoms or anaphylaxis without signs of cutaneous involvement, and a normal or elevated serum tryptase level, the diagnostic workup is centered on establishing whether WHO diagnostic criteria for SM are met (Fig. 72.7). If these criteria are not satisfied, a workup is performed to rule out or diagnose MCAS, and to document (other) primary and secondary causes of MC expansion or MC activation.

In adult patients with cutaneous MC lesions, the large majority of such patients will ultimately be found to have SM according to WHO diagnostic criteria. A BM biopsy is generally recommended in these patients to establish a diagnosis of SM (see Fig. 72.7). In patients with modest elevations of the serum tryptase level, mild or no symptomology, nor evidence of blood count abnormalities or other signs of organ damage, diagnostic testing may not elicit short-term changes in management even if SM is found. However, given the differences in OS between adult CM and SM, and the fact that only those with SM may develop severe bone disease (osteoporosis) requiring therapy staging investigations should be extended in SM, BM analysis can be very helpful as an initial "forensic" assessment of these potential disease trajectories. Children with skin lesions rarely have systemic disease. Therefore a BM biopsy is generally not recommended in children unless the serum tryptase level is unusually high

or progressively increasing, or organomegaly and/or blood count abnormalities emerge.

Survival and Prognostic Factors

In a Mayo series of 342 patients with SM (46% ISM, 12% ASM, 40% SM-AHN, 1% MCL), life expectancy in ISM was similar to age- and sex-matched normal controls.[11] In contrast, median OS (and leukemia-free survival) was inferior in patients with more advanced forms of SM. For example, the median OS was 41 months and 24 months, respectively for ASM ($n = 41$ patients) and SM-AHN ($n = 138$ patients), and only 2 months for MCL ($n = 4$) patients. In a multivariate analysis, independent adverse prognostic factors included advanced age, weight loss, anemia, thrombocytopenia, hypoalbuminemia, and excess BM blasts.[11] In addition to an increased percentage of MCs on marrow aspirate smears, Spanish investigators found that

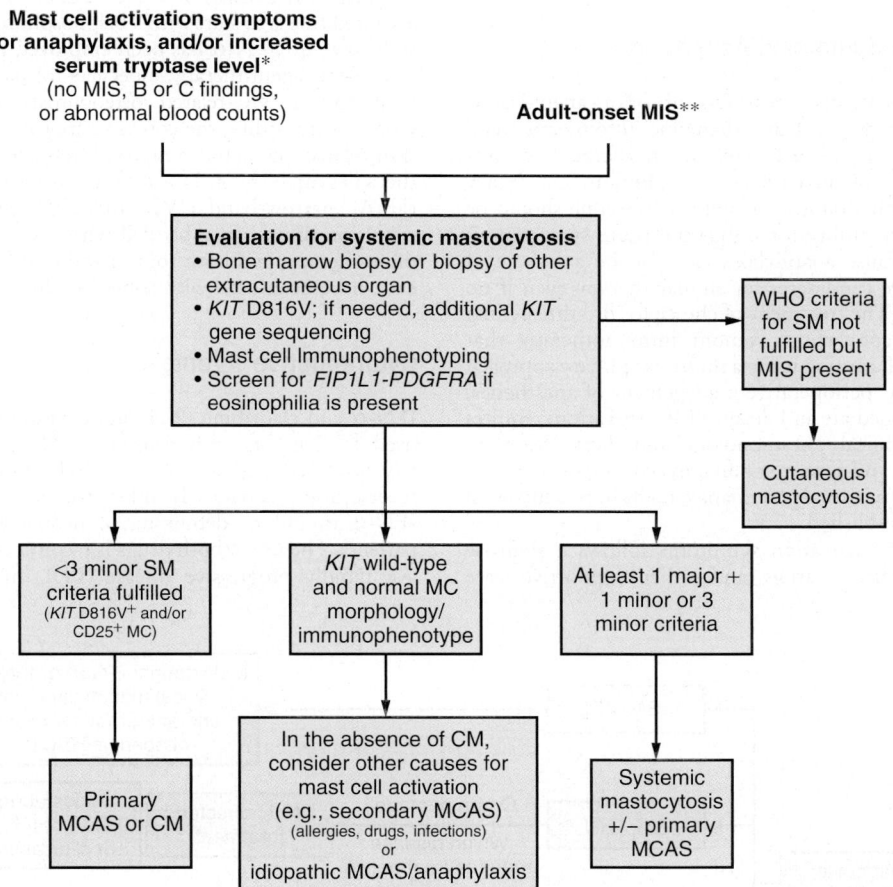

Fig. 72.7 DIAGNOSTIC DECISION PATHWAYS FOR PATIENTS WITH MAST CELL ACTIVATION SYMPTOMS OR ADULT-ONSET MASTOCYTOSIS IN THE SKIN. For patients with mast cell activation symptoms or anaphylaxis (and/or increased serum tryptase level), or adult-onset MIS, screening to assess whether the diagnostic criteria for SM are met should be the first diagnostic checkpoint. For patients not meeting criteria for SM, evaluation for MCAS (primary vs. secondary vs. idiopathic) and idiopathic anaphylaxis is the next phase of evaluation. Patients with MIS for whom no signs of SM can be found may be categorized as cutaneous mastocytosis. *The serum tryptase level may be below the 20 ng/mL threshold, or only transiently elevated. **Although an evaluation for systemic mastocytosis is generally recommended in adults with MIS with no blood count abnormalities or organ dysfunction, and a normal or mildly increased serum tryptase level, the value of performing a bone marrow biopsy should be discussed with the patient. *MC,* Mast cell; *MCAS,* mast cell activation syndrome; *MIS,* mastocytosis in the skin; *SM,* systemic mastocytosis; *PDGFRA,* platelet-derived growth factor receptor A; *WHO,* World Health Organization. *(Adapted from:Pardanani A: How I treat patients with indolent and smoldering mastocytosis (rare conditions but difficult to manage). Blood 2013;121:3085, 2013; Valent P, Akin C, Arock M, et al: Definitions, criteria and global classification of mast cell disorders with special reference to mast cell activation syndromes: a consensus protocol. Int Arch Allergy Immunol 157:215, 2012.)*

multilineage involvement of the *KIT* D816V mutation in more than just MCs (e.g., other myeloid lineages, and sometimes lymphoid cells) is a poor prognostic factor and leads to an increased risk of progression to advanced SM.[24] Many of these patients may suffer from overt SSM. In patients with SM, eosinophilia was also associated with inferior outcomes in one study, and was prognostically neutral in another series. SM patients with eosinophilia tend to suffer from SSM, ASM, or MCL, but even in ISM, eosinophilia may be detected.

TREATMENT

Therapy of mastocytosis centers on addressing symptoms related to MC activation (in all categories), and using cytoreductive agents to reverse organ damage caused by neoplastic MC infiltrates in advanced SM. Fig. 72.8 provides a treatment algorithm for indolent versus advanced stages of SM and the broad therapeutic strategies that are available based on the presence of mediator symptoms, organ damage, and a concomitant AHN.

Mast Cell Activation Symptoms/Anaphylaxis

All adult mastocytosis patients, regardless of prior anaphylactic events, should carry two doses of an adrenaline autoinjector (and should be instructed in its safe use, e.g., by an allergist) to treat potential future episodes of anaphylaxis. In addition, emergency medicines such as diphenhydramine or oral prednisolone should be considered, although their utility for mitigating acute symptoms is less well-established. Because anaphylaxis can also be a feature of MCAS, these patients are candidates for similar therapy even if no overt SM was diagnosed. The treatment of choice for life-threatening Hymenoptera allergy/anaphylaxis is venom immunotherapy that should be undertaken with caution using a multidisciplinary approach led by allergists. Similarly, perioperative management of anesthetics, which can precipitate immediate and delayed MC activation, requires consultation with the surgical, anesthesiology, and allergy teams to minimize the occurrence and severity of anaphylaxis. General guidelines regarding anesthesia and analgesic management in patients with mastocytosis have been published.

The treatment of MC activation symptoms follows a stepwise approach using antimediator drugs and other supportive care measures.[25] These medications include H1-histamine blockers for flushing and pruritis, and H2-histamine blockers for SM-related gastrointestinal (GI) symptomatology such as diarrhea, abdominal discomfort/cramping, and peptic ulcer disease. Leukotriene antagonists such as Montelukast are commonly added to H1-histamine blockers for persistent flushing and pruritis. In rare cases, aspirin can be a alternative therapy for refractory flushing, but needs to be used with caution because of its ability to precipitate MC activation, bleeding tendency, and GI tract ulcerative disease. In general, however, aspirin is not recommended for use in SM. Although the MC stabilizer sodium cromoglycate (Gastrocrom) is geared to persistent GI symptoms such as diarrhea, proton pump inhibitors may be specifically useful for patients with refractory GERD/peptic ulcer disease. Alternative treatments that have been used for refractory mediator symptoms include the off-label antihistamine/MC stabilizer ketotifen, and the anti-IgE antibody omalizumab, which has also been used for anaphylaxis, as well as asthma. Although bisphosphonates (alendronate 70 mg q week; risedronate 35 mg q week; pamidronic acid 90 mg intravenously (IV) q 4 weeks; and zoledronic acid 4 mg IV q 4 weeks) are recommended for bony disease, reports of their use in SM primarily consists of single cases or small cases series. A generally accepted rule is to start with a bisphosphonate when the T-score drops to below −2.[5] IFN-α has been employed with bisphosphonates and/or as single agent therapy, especially for patients with refractory bony pain and/or MC-related osteoporosis and pathologic fractures. Concerns regarding the cosmetic appearance of cutaneous lesions or skin-related mediator symptoms refractory to the aforementioned therapies can be helped for a limited period of time with phototherapy (UVA₁, narrow-band UVB, and UVA plus psoralen). In addition, occlusion dressings embedded with topical steroids with or without phototherapy, and both topical and oral forms of sodium cromoglycate, have been used with some benefit.

Cytoreductive Agents

IFN-α and cladribine (2-chlorodeoxyadenosine) have typically been used for patients with progressive SSM and for cytoreduction in advanced SM patients (ASM, MCL, and SM-AHN) to reduce or reverse organ damage. In most instances, cladribine is favored over IFN-α to induce debulking of neoplastic MCs in advanced SM patients. The use of both drugs is recommended to treat patients with less rapidly progressive disease (PD). In addition, cladribine and

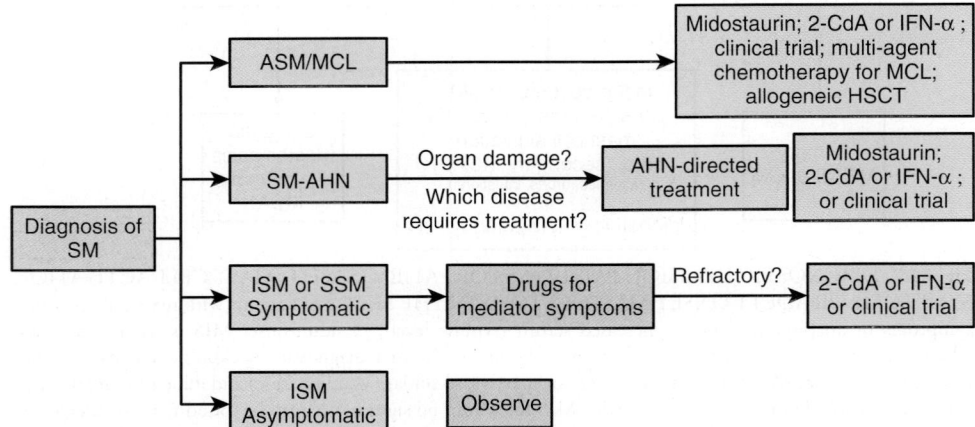

Fig. 72.8 TREATMENT OPTIONS BASED ON SUBTYPE OF SYSTEMIC MASTOCYTOSIS. Treatment options are listed based on subvariant of SM (indolent vs. advanced forms of disease), whether organ damage is considered related to SM or the associated myeloid neoplasm in patients with SM-AHN, and whether cytoreductive therapy may need to be considered in patients with ISM and refractory mediator symptoms. *2-CdA*, 2-Chlorodeoxyadenosine; *ASM*, aggressive systemic mastocytosis; *HSCT*, hematopoietic stem cell transplantation; *ISM*, indolent systemic mastocytosis; *IFN-α*, interferon-α; *MCL*, mast cell leukemia; *SM*, systemic mastocytosis; *SM-AHN*, systemic mastocytosis with an associated hematologic neoplasm; *SSM*, smoldering systemic mastocytosis.

IFN-α are sometimes used to control mediator symptoms, especially when these symptoms are refractory to conventional antimediator-type drugs. In addition, low-dose IFN-α has been suggested for ISM patients with drug-resistant osteoporosis. Otherwise, however, these agents are not recommended for use in ISM or SSM. In patients with rapidly progressive ASM or MCL, more intensive therapy is usually recommended, whereas cladribine alone or IFN-α alone are insufficient to control rapid disease expansion or transformation in SM.

Interferon-α

IFN-α has been used as monotherapy or in combination with corticosteroids, mostly in patients with ASM with slow progression or mono-organ involvement. For example, the drug works effectively in patients with ASM with liver involvement and ascites. Prednisone or prednisolone 0.5–1 mg/kg is initiated with IFN-α (or as a lead-in dose for several days prior) in order to improve its efficacy and tolerability, and tapered over 2–3 months if feasible. In some patients with severe and persistent mediator symptoms or organ damage that is particularly responsive to corticosteroids, a longer term maintenance dose (e.g., ≤10 mg daily) may be required. IFN-α dosing has been variable between studies and an optimal dose has not been identified. Starting doses have ranged from 1 million units (MU)/day to 3 MU three times weekly, with median total weekly maintenance doses in the range of 15–30 MU. Because of the (low) risk of anaphylactic reactions, consideration should be given to hospitalization of patients during the first days of treatment, if possible.

In the Mayo experience with IFN-α (with or without prednisone),[25] 21 of 40 evaluable patients responded (53%); response rates by subgroup were: six of 10 ISM, six of 10 ASM, and nine of 20 SM-AHN. The 21 responses consisted of one complete remission (CR), six major responses (MRs), and 14 partial responses (PRs). The median duration of response (DOR) was 12 months (range, 1–67) with no statistical difference between responders and nonresponders regarding use of prednisone or the median weekly dose of IFN-α. However, the absence of mediator-related symptoms was associated with a significantly lower response rate.

In the French experience with 20 SM patients (four ISM and 16 ASM), IFN-α-2b was initiated at 1 MU daily and progressively increased as tolerated up to 5 MU/m² daily. Among the 13 patients treated for at least 6 months (mean daily dose: 3.2 MU daily), all had partial or complete resolution of systemic or cutaneous disease manifestations and/or MC mediator levels, but no significant reduction in BM MC burden. The lack of a substantive effect on tumor load and rapid relapse in four responding patients after drug withdrawal suggests that IFN-α exerts a cytostatic effect on MCs.

Responses to IFN-α primarily include amelioration of MC mediator symptoms and associated laboratory markers of MC activation such as levels of histamine or its metabolites. Single cases and small case series, in addition to the aggregate data from the aforementioned larger trials, indicate variable potential to ameliorate skin lesions, osteoporosis, and C findings such as cytopenias, hepato/splenomegaly with liver dysfunction and/or ascites, and weight loss. Toxicities associated with IFN-α such as flu-like symptoms, myelosuppression, transaminitis, hypothyroidism, depression, and bone pain are not uncommon, and result in a moderate proportion of patients requiring dose-reduction or drug discontinuation.

Cladribine

Cladribine has been used off-label across a spectrum of SM subtypes. In 2013 cladribine received orphan designation (not marketing authorization) for the treatment of SM in Europe. Following an initial report indicating that cladribine could elicit improvement of mediator symptoms, urticaria pigmentosa lesions, and reduction of MC burden and the serum tryptase level, Kluin-Nelemans and colleagues published a series of 10 patients, including 3 with ISM, 1 SSM, 3 SM-AHN, and 3 ASM. Cladribine was administered for 5 days every 4–8 weeks at a dose of 0.10–0.13 mg/kg over 2 h IV. Among 9 evaluable patients (1 discontinued because of toxicoderma), the drug elicited improvement in symptoms, and a decrease (often rapid) in urticaria pigmentosa lesions, MC burden, serum tryptase levels, and urine metabolites of MC activation.

In the Mayo Clinic experience,[25] cladribine was administered for 5 days at a dose of 5 mg/m²/day (or 0.13–0.17 mg/kg/day) for 5 days IV. A median of 3 cycles (range, 1–9) was administered. The overall response rate was 12 of 22 (55%), consisting of 1 CR, 7 MR, and 4 PR. Responses were observed in 5 of 9 ISM, 1 of 2 ASM, and 6 of 11 SM-AHN patients. Improvement in mediator symptoms, organomegaly, C-findings (e.g., ascites, anemia), and markers of MC burden and/or activation (e.g., serum tryptase level and MC-derived urine metabolites) were observed. The median response duration was 11 months, and inferior outcomes were predicted by leukocytosis, monocytosis, and circulating immature myeloid cells, the latter remaining significant in a multivariate analysis.

The long-term French experience with cladribine in both indolent ($n = 36$) and advanced ($n = 32$) SM patients was recently published.[26] Cladribine was administered as an infusion or subcutaneously at a dose of 0.14 mg/kg, for 1–5 days, every 4–12 weeks. A median of 3.7 courses was administered (range, 1–9). The overall response rate was 72%, split between 92% and 50% for indolent and advanced disease, respectively. Among patients with advanced SM, the respective CR, MR, and PR rates were 0%, 37.5%, and 12.5%. Significant decreases in serum tryptase levels was only observed in ISM patients, and changes in BM MC burden were only evaluated in nine patients, precluding a substantive conclusion regarding this endpoint. Median durations of response were 3.71 (range, 0.1–8) and 2.47 (range, 0.5–8.6) years for indolent and advanced SM, respectively. Lymphopenia (82%), neutropenia (47%), and opportunistic infections (13%) were the most common grade 3/4 adverse events. Although cladribine has activity in selected patients with SM, its use in subjects with indolent disease (even those with refractory mediator symptoms) needs to be approached very cautiously because of the potential for substantial high-grade toxicities in these individuals who otherwise exhibit similar survival to age-matched controls.

Tyrosine Kinase Inhibitors

Dasatinib

Multikinase inhibitors with activity against KIT have been evaluated in patients with advanced SM. Dasatinib is a dual SRC/ABL kinase inhibitor that is used as front-line treatment of chronic myelogenous leukemia, or as second- or third-line therapy for patients with intolerance to, or resistance to imatinib (or nilotinib). Dasatinib exerts relatively weak inhibition of KIT D816V and has a short half-life. A case series and a phase II trial of dasatinib (140 mg total daily dose) revealed limited activity in SM. In the phase II trial of 33 patients (ISM, $n = 18$; ASM, $n = 9$; SM-AHN), 11 (33%) responded. Two complete responses were recorded in patients who were negative for the *KIT* D816V mutation, including a patient with *JAK2* V617F-positive SM-PMF and a patient with SM-CEL. The other 9 responses provided symptomatic benefit only, without clinically significant reductions in either BM MC burden or serum tryptase levels. In the context of the CML experience, (which may also pertain to the treatment of SM), side effects of dasatinib have included pleural and pericardial effusions, cytopenias, an increased risk of bleeding, as well as immunosuppression.

Imatinib

Imatinib is currently the only US Food and Drug Administration–approved drug for SM and is indicated for adult patients with ASM without the *KIT* D816V mutation or with unknown *KIT* mutational status. The general utility of imatinib in SM is therefore limited given the high prevalence of the *KIT* D816V mutation, and the increasing sensitivity and widespread use of assays that can detect this molecular abnormality. Although imatinib lacks activity against KIT D816V in vitro and in vivo, it has led to clinical benefit in patients with alternative *KIT* mutations or wild-type *KIT*. For example, imatinib has elicited excellent responses in cases of the well-differentiated SM variant with either the F522C TM *KIT* mutation[27] or wild-type *KIT*; in a patient with familial SM carrying the germline *KIT* K509I mutation; with deletion of codon 419 in exon 8 of *KIT* in pediatric CM; and in a case of MCL with mutation in exon 9 (p.A502_Y503dup). It is also noteworthy that long-term treatment with imatinib (400 mg/day) is associated with an almost complete MC deficiency, which may be of clinical relevance in reactive (nonclonal) MCAS and other MC-dependent diseases.

Masitinib

Masitinib (AB1010), is an inhibitor of Lyn, Fyn, PDGFR-α/β, and wild-type KIT. After an initial study II trial in patients with ISM or CM with symptoms unresponsive to prior therapy, masitinib was studied in a phase III, randomized, double-bind trial of 135 patients with ISM or SSM (108 subjects formally satisfied the WHO criteria for SM). Subjects were randomized to oral masitinib (6 mg/kg daily in two daily doses) or placebo. The primary end-point of the study was based on a 75% or more improvement in one or more symptom categories: pruritis, flushing, depression, or fatigue. Of the patients taking masitinib, 18.7% achieved this endpoint compared to 7.4% of patients taking placebo. At week 24, there was an 18% decrease in the serum tryptase level in the masitinib arm versus an increase of 2.2% in the placebo arm (*P* <.0001). Also, urticaria pigmentosa lesions on masitinib therapy decreased by an average body surface area of 12.3% versus an increase of 15.9% for the placebo group. Masitinib-associated clinical benefits were generally sustained during a two-year extension period. Although treatment was generally well tolerated, there was an excess incidence of diarrhea, rash, and asthenia in 9%, 6%, and 4% of patients, respectively, in the masitinib group. In addition, 24% of patients in the masitinib arm discontinued therapy because of an adverse event, compared with 10% in the placebo arm. For these patients with lower-risk disease who have a normal life expectancy, these side effects need to be weighed against the potential benefits of the drug in alleviating SM-related symptoms.

Midostaurin

Midostaurin (*N*-benzoylstaurosporine; PKC412) is an inhibitor of multiple TKs including wild-type and D816V-mutated KIT, FLT3, PDGFR-α/β, FGFR1, and VEGFR2. In Ba/F3 cells transformed by *KIT* D816V, the IC_{50} of midostaurin was 30–40 nM compared with greater than 1 μM with imatinib. A PR with midostaurin in a patient with MCL and an associated MDS/MPN, and encouraging responses in a phase II trial of 26 patients with advanced SM led to a global, multicenter, open-label trial of midostaurin (100 mg twice daily on 28-day continuous cycles) in patients with ASM, MCL, and SM-AHN.[28]

The trial employed a steering committee and central pathology review to adjudicate eligibility, response, and histopathology. Among 89 evaluable patients, the ORR was 60%, of which 75% were MRs. Responses in organ damage (e.g., normalization of cytopenias/red blood cell or platelet transfusion dependence) and liver function abnormalities, hypoalbuminemia) were observed regardless of *KIT* D816V status, prior therapy, or the presence of an AHN. The median best reduction in serum tryptase level was −58%. In addition, the median change in BM MC burden was −59%, and 57% of patients had a ≥50% reduction in BM MCs. After a median follow-up of 26 months, the median DOR and median OS were 24.1 and 28.7 months, respectively. Median OS in responders was 44.4 months compared with 15.4 months in nonresponders. Of the 16 patients with MCL, 8 responded, including 7 MR (44%); among MCL

patients, the median DOR was not reached, with three MRs ongoing at 49, 33, and 19 months at the time of data cut-off. The median OS was 9.4 months among all patients with MCL, but was not reached among responding MCL patients. In addition, the hazard for death was reduced by 95% in MCL responders versus nonresponders. Symptoms and quality of life, measured by the Memorial Symptom Assessment Scale (MSAS) and Short-Form 12 (SF-12) survey, respectively, were significantly improved with midostaurin treatment. Improved symptoms and quality of life may relate to the ability of midostaurin to block IgE-dependent mediator release from MCs in vitro. The drug was generally well tolerated with a manageable toxicity profile consisting mostly of gastrointestinal side effects, including nausea and vomiting, primarily grade 1–2 in nature. These data support further exploration of midostaurin in combination with other agents with activity in advanced SM (e.g., cladribine), and evaluation of the drug in ISM patients with refractory MC activation symptoms.

Other Agents

Phase I/II trials of denileukin diftitox, everolimus (RAD001), daclizumab, thalidomide, and lenalidomide have shown limited or no activity in small numbers of SM patients. Hydroxyurea has been used to control leukocytosis and splenomegaly in patients with a concurrent AHN such as MPN, CEL/HES, or MDS/MPN. Multiagent, intensive chemotherapy is usually reserved for patients with MCL, especially for patients with kinetically active disease, but the results thus far have been disappointing. Anthracycline plus cytarabine-based induction chemotherapy is the standard of care for patients with AML who are suitable for high-intensity therapy, including those in whom SM is also present. In such cases, treatment of the AML almost always takes priority, and the finding of the *KIT* D816V mutation may provide an opportunity to consider the addition of KIT inhibitors such as dasatinib or midostaurin to the induction, consolidation, and/or maintenance phases of treatment. However, the safety and efficacy of this approach has yet to be validated in the context of clinical trials. Other agents have shown activity against *KIT* D816V-mutated MCs in vitro, including the multikinase/KIT inhibitor EXEL-0862, heat shock protein 90 inhibitor STA-9090, proteasome inhibitor MG132, BCL-2 inhibitor obatoclax, hypomethylating agents azacitidine and decitabine, and the alkaloid omacetaxine mepesuccinate (homoharringtonine). However, clinical trial data regarding their activity in patients have not yet been published. Finally, several antibodies and antibody-drug conjugates have been considered for use in advanced SM. For example, the anti-CD30 antibody-drug conjugate brentuximab vedotin induces growth inhibition and apoptosis of CD30+ MCs. A clinical trial testing brentuximab has recently been initiated in the United States. Other agents that may be useful for the eradication of neoplastic MCs and possibly also neoplastic stem cells, include CD33, CD44, CD52, and CD123 monoclonal antibodies.

Allogeneic Hematopoietic Stem Cell Transplantation

Until recently, the role of hematopoietic stem cell transplantation (HSCT) in advanced SM remained poorly characterized, and only on a limited number of case reports and series had appeared. In a large, multicenter retrospective analysis published in 2014, Ustun and colleagues evaluated the outcomes of 57 SM patients (SM-AHN, *n* = 38 [AML = 20]; ASM, *n* = 7; and MCL, *n* = 12) who underwent allogeneic HSCT.[29] Donor types consisted of HLA-matched identical (*n* = 34) and unrelated (*n* = 17) donors, umbilical cord blood (*n* = 2), and haploidentical (*n* = 1), and three unknown. Responses were observed in 70% of patients, including a 16% CR rate. The remaining 30% of responses were split between stable disease (21%) and primary refractory disease (9%). All 38 patients with SM-AHN achieved CR regarding the AHN component, but 10 subsequently relapsed with AHN, and half of these patients died.

The median OS for all patients at 3 years was 57%, consisting of 74% for patients with SM-AHN, and 43% and 17% for ASM and MCL patients, respectively. The strongest risk factor for a poor OS was a diagnosis of MCL. In addition, inferior survival was observed in patients undergoing reduced-intensity versus fully myeloablative conditioning. However, patient age, donor age, donor type (sibling or unrelated donor), graft source (BM or peripheral HSCT, *KIT* mutation status, karyotype), and total-body irradiation used in myeloablative conditioning had no impact on overall or progression-free survival. Treatment-related mortality at 6 months and 1 year was 11% and 20%, respectively, and was highest in MCL patients. Although a prospective trial is needed to better define the role of HSCT in advanced SM, these data suggest that transplantation can provide extended survival in selected patients, particularly for patients with SM-AHN.

Response Criteria for Advanced SM

Response criteria for advanced SM were first published in 2003 and reiterated in a consensus conference report in 2007.[5] In this system, evaluation of clinical evidence of organ damage, or "C" findings, was the foundation for distinguishing levels of response. Changes in BM MC burden, serum tryptase level, and hepatosplenomegaly were additionally employed to subcategorize levels of MR. These original criteria or their modified version have been used to adjudicate responses in clinical trials of new agents.

According to prior consensus response criteria, a MR is defined as normalization of one or more "C" findings. In turn, MR is divided into three subcategories: (1) complete remission (resolution of abnormal MC infiltrates in organs, decrease of serum tryptase below 20 ng/mL, and disappearance of SM-associated organomegaly); (2) incomplete remission (decrease of MC infiltrates and/or serum tryptase level, and/or visible regression of organomegaly by >50%), and (3) pure clinical response (without decrease of MC infiltrates, serum tryptase level, or organomegaly). A PR is defined as incomplete regression of one or more "C" findings (good PR; >50% regression of one or more "C" findings; and minor response, ≤50% regression). Progression of one or more "C" findings even in the presence of an improvement of other "C" findings defines PD.

Several shortcomings emerged regarding these SM response criteria. First, achievement of an "MR" is permitted in patients with baseline laboratory values just outside of the normal reference range. Second, responses in C-findings such as ascites, weight loss, and bone lesions are often difficult to quantify. Third, criteria for baseline red blood cell and platelet transfusion dependence were not codified. Lastly, the minimal DOR was not clearly defined, although a minimum response duration of 8 weeks has been incorporated ad hoc into many trials.

In order to overcome these challenges, and to generate response criteria that can be adopted across clinical trials, the International Working Group for Myeloproliferative Neoplasms Research and Treatment (IWG-MRT) and the ECNM established revised response criteria for advanced SM that better characterize nonhematologic and hematologic organ damage findings, and lend more specificity and quantitation to evaluation of clinical and histopathologic improvement.[30] First, a minimum of grade 2 (according to NCI Common Terminology Criteria version 4.03) hematologic or nonhematologic organ damage was required to be considered eligible for organ damage adjudication. Resolution of one or more nonhematologic or hematologic organ damage findings without concomitant worsening of other eligible organ damage was defined as "clinical improvement" (CI). Response categories of CR and PR were defined based on the percent reduction of (1) the burden of neoplastic MCs in the BM (and/or extracutaneous organ) and (2) the serum tryptase level. In addition to changes in MC burden and serum tryptase level, achievement of a PR or CR requires that patients also meet criteria for resolution of at least one or all CI findings, respectively. For additional clinical relevance, the duration of CI and histopathologic response need to be maintained for at least 12 weeks. The criteria for stable disease, PD, and loss of response were also detailed in the report.

FUTURE DIRECTIONS

Several clinical and translational initiatives are being pursued in MC disease and should reach fruition in the near future. Given the relatively low incidence of SM, efforts are currently being led by the ECNM to combine patient data from multiple collaborators into a central registry (e.g., such data should be useful in generating prognostic variables to help risk stratify patient outcomes). Efforts are also underway to validate SM-specific patient-reported outcome tools to qualitatively and quantitatively measure patients' symptom burden and quality of life. Regulatory health agencies are increasingly focused on these patient measures for drug approval, and validated patient-reported outcomes are critical for stringent adjudication of treatment-related changes in the context of placebo-controlled, double-blind study designs.

Clinical trials are under development to investigate targets and pathways relevant to MC pathobiology. Novel approaches include use of the anti-CD30 antibody-drug immunoconjugate brentuximab vedotin, JAK inhibitors (e.g., ruxolitinib), PI3K inhibitors, and BTK inhibitors such as ibrutinib. In addition, new selective inhibitors of *KIT* D816V entered phase I trials in 2016. Other agents that merit investigation include inhibitors of BCL-2, agonist antibodies against inhibitory receptors such as siglec-8 in order to induce MC apoptosis, and antibodies against other newly described aberrant markers on neoplastic MCs, such as CD123 (IL-3 receptor-α). Biologic correlates of therapeutic response such as changes in *KIT* mutant allele burden, circulating tumor DNA, and cytokine profiles are now being incorporated into trials. Transcriptome and proteomic profiling of purified MCs and AHN cell populations are compelling translational objectives for future protocols.

REFERENCES

1. Ehrlich P: *Beitrage zur theorie und praxis der histologischen färbung [thesis]*, Leipzig, Germany, 1878, University of Leipzig.
2. Metcalfe DD: Mast cells and mastocytosis. *Blood* 112(4):946–956, 2008.
3. Valent P, Horny HP, Escribano L, et al: Diagnostic criteria and classification of mastocytosis: a consensus proposal. *Leuk Res* 25(7):603–625, 2001.
4. Horny HP, Akin C, Metcalfe DD, et al: Mastocytosis. In Swerdlow SH, Campo E, Harris NL, et al, editors: *WHO Classification of Tumors of Hematopoietic and Lymphoid Tissues*, Lyon, 2008, International Agency for Research and Cancer (IARC), pp 54–63.
5. Valent P, Akin C, Escribano L, et al: Standards and standardization in mastocytosis: consensus statements on diagnostics, treatment recommendations and response criteria. *Eur J Clin Invest* 37(6):435–453, 2007.
6. Agis H, Willheim M, Sperr WR, et al: Monocytes do not make mast cells when cultured in the presence of SCF. Characterization of the circulating mast cell progenitor as a c-kit+, CD34+, Ly-, CD14-, CD17-, colony-forming cell. *J Immunol* 151(8):4221–4227, 1993.
7. Reilly JT: Class III receptor tyrosine kinases: role in leukaemogenesis. *Br J Haematol* 116(4):744–757, 2002.
8. Gotlib J, Akin C: Mast cells and eosinophils in mastocytosis, chronic eosinophilic leukemia, and non-clonal disorders. *Semin Hematol* 49(2):128–137, 2012.
9. Gilfillan AM, Rivera J: The tyrosine kinase network regulating mast cell activation. *Immunol Rev* 228(1):149–169, 2009.
10. Saleh R, Wedeh G, Herrmann H, et al: A new human mast cell line expressing a functional IgE receptor converts to tumorigenic growth by KIT D816V transfection. *Blood* 124(1):111–120, 2014.
11. Lim KH, Tefferi A, Lasho TL, et al: Systemic mastocytosis in 342 consecutive adults: survival studies and prognostic factors. *Blood* 113(23):5727–5736, 2009.
12. Pardanani A, Lim KH, Lasho TL, et al: Prognostically relevant breakdown of 123 patients with systemic mastocytosis associated with other myeloid malignancies. *Blood* 114(18):3769–3772, 2009.

13. Valent P, Sotlar K, Sperr WR, et al: Refined diagnostic criteria and classification of mast cell leukemia (MCL) and myelomastocytic leukemia (MML): a consensus proposal. *Ann Oncol* 25(9):1691–1700, 2014.

14. Georgin-Lavialle S, Lhermitte L, Dubreuil P, et al: Mast cell leukemia. *Blood* 121(8):1285–1295, 2013.

15. Valent P, Akin C, Arock M, et al: Definitions, criteria and global classification of mast cell disorders with special reference to mast cell activation syndromes: a consensus protocol. *Int Arch Allergy Immunol* 157(3):215–225, 2012.

16. Escribano L, Diaz-Augustin B, López A, et al: Immunophenotypic analysis of mast cells in mastocytosis: when and how to do it. Proposals of the Spanish Network on Mastocytosis (REMA). *Cytometry B Clin Cytom* 58(1):1–8, 2004.

17. Sotlar K, Cerny-Reiterer S, Petat-Dutter K, et al: Aberrant expression of CD30 in neoplastic mast cells in high-grade mastocytosis. *Mod Pathol* 24(4):585–595, 2011.

18. Schwartz LB, Sakai K, Bradford TR, et al: The alpha form of human tryptase is the predominant type present in blood at baseline in normal subjects and is elevated in those with systemic mastocytosis. *J Clin Invest* 96(6):2702–2710, 1995.

19. Valent P, Escribano L, Broesby-Olsen S, et al: Proposed diagnostic algorithm for patients with suspected mastocytosis: a proposal of the European Competence Network on Mastocytosis. *Allergy* 69(10):1267–1274, 2014.

20. Nagata H, Worobec AS, Oh CK, et al: Identification of a point mutation in the catalytic domain of the protooncogene c-kit in the peripheral blood mononuclear cells of patients who have mastocytosis with an associated hematologic disorder. *Proc Natl Acad Sci USA* 92(23):10560–10564, 1995.

21. Arock M, Sotlar K, Akin C, et al: KIT mutation analysis in mast cell neoplasms: recommendations of the European Competence Network on Mastocytosis. *Leukemia* 29:1223, 2015.

22. Schwaab J, Schnittger S, Sotlar K, et al: Comprehensive mutational profiling in advanced systemic mastocytosis. *Blood* 122(14):2460–2466, 2013.

23. Maric I, Robyn J, Metcalfe DD, et al: KIT D816V-associated systemic mastocytosis with eosinophilia and FIP1L1/PDGFRA-associated chronic eosinophilic leukemia are distinct entities. *J Allergy Clin Immunol* 120(3):680–687, 2007.

24. Garcia-Montero AC, Jara-Acevedo M, Teodosio C, et al: KIT mutation in mast cells and other bone marrow haematopoietic cell lineages in systemic mast cell disorders: a prospective study of the Spanish Network on Mastocytosis (REMA) in a series of 113 patients. *Blood* 108(7):2366–2372, 2006.

25. Pardanani A: Systemic mastocytosis in adults: 2015 update on diagnosis, risk stratification, and management. *Am J Hematol* 90(3):250–262, 2015.

26. Barete S, Lortholary O, Damaj G, et al: Long-term efficacy and safety of cladribine (2-CdA) in adult patients with mastocytosis. *Blood* 126(8):1009–1016, 2015.

27. Akin C, Fumo G, Yavuz AS, et al: A novel form of mastocytosis associated with a transmembrane c-kit mutation and response to imatinib. *Blood* 103(8):3222–3225, 2004.

28. Gotlib J, Kluin-Nelemans HC, George TI, et al: Efficacy and safety of midostaurin in advanced systemic mastocytosis. *N Engl J Med* 374(26):2530–2541, 2016.

29. Ustun C, Reiter A, Scott BL, et al: Hematopoietic stem-cell transplantation for advanced systemic mastocytosis. *J Clin Oncol* 32(29):3264–3274, 2014.

30. Gotlib J, Pardanani A, Akin C, et al: International Working Group-Myeloproliferative Neoplasms Research and Treatment (IWG-MRT) & European Competence Network on Mastocytosis (ECNM) consensus response criteria in advanced systemic mastocytosis. *Blood* 121(13):2393–2401, 2013.

THE PATHOLOGIC BASIS FOR THE CLASSIFICATION OF NON-HODGKIN AND HODGKIN LYMPHOMAS

Elaine S. Jaffe, Stefania Pittaluga, and John Anastasi

INTRODUCTION AND HISTORICAL BACKGROUND

The classification of malignant lymphomas has undergone significant changes over the past 50 years. The current approach is based on the integration of morphologic, phenotypic, genetic, and clinical features that allows the identification of distinct disease entities (See box on Principles of the Classification of Lymphomas). This practical approach to lymphoma categorization was initially proposed by the International Lymphoma Study Group in 1994 and formed the basis of the Revised European-American Classification of lymphoid neoplasm (REAL). It was then adopted by the World Health Organization (WHO) classification of neoplasm of the hematopoietic and lymphoid tissues, published in 2001, updated in 2008 and revised again in 2016 (Table 73.1).[1,2] The WHO classification represents a significant achievement in terms of cooperation, communication and consensus among pathologists, hematologists, and oncologists. Furthermore, it recognizes that any classification system to be viable and applicable should evolve and incorporate new data resulting from emerging technologies in the field of hematopathology such as results from genome-wide large-scale sequencing studies. These studies have led to the identifications of new prognostic and diagnostic categories, and provide insight into therapeutic targets based on a better understanding of molecular mechanisms of transformation. This chapter will focus on the classification of neoplasms derived from mature B cells, T cells, and natural killer (NK) cells with emphasis on malignant lymphoma. We provide a framework for the subsequent chapters on Hodgkin and non-Hodgkin lymphomas in reviewing the major entities according to the WHO classification.

MATURE B-CELL NEOPLASMS

Chronic Lymphocytic Leukemia/Small Lymphocytic Lymphoma

Chronic lymphocytic leukemia/small lymphocytic lymphoma (CLL/SLL) usually presents in adults with generalized lymphadenopathy, frequent bone marrow and peripheral blood involvement, and often hepatosplenomegaly. Presentation as leukemia, that is, CLL, is more common than as lymphoma, SLL. Even in patients with a lymphomatous presentation, careful examination of the blood may reveal a circulating monoclonal B-cell component. Nevertheless, there are some patients who will present with generalized adenopathy, and whereas progression to CLL is frequent, it does not necessarily occur in all cases.

The increased sensitivity of immunophenotypic/molecular methodologies has resulted in the detection of clonal lymphoid proliferations with a CLL phenotype in the general population, even in the absence of clinical lymphocytosis, a condition now designated monoclonal B-cell lymphocytosis (MBL) (Box on Early Events in Lymphoid Neoplasia). The International Workshop on CLL proposed new diagnostic criteria that were then included in the WHO classification of 2008. Recent studies have distinguished between high count and low count MBL, with a count of monoclonal B cells greater than 5.0 $\times 10^3$/L being more clinically significant.[4] Similar to peripheral blood, small clonal populations with a CLL phenotype can be detected in

lymph nodes as an incidental finding, and appear to represent a tissue counterpart of MBL.[5] Histologically, the lymph node involved by CLL/SLL shows diffuse architectural effacement (Fig. 73.1), although occasional residual naked germinal centers can be observed. The predominant cell type is a small lymphocyte with clumped chromatin, but a spectrum of nuclear morphology is usually seen. Pseudofollicular growth centers or proliferation centers are present in the majority of cases and contain a spectrum of cells ranging from small lymphocytes to prolymphocytes and paraimmunoblasts. The prolymphocytes and paraimmunoblasts have more dispersed chromatin and more prominent nucleoli usually centrally placed. The presence of proliferation centers is also a helpful criterion in the differential diagnosis with mantle cell lymphoma (MCL), which may show otherwise some overlapping features with CLL. If needed, immunophenotypic studies can be helpful in this differential diagnosis.

CLL/SLL is characterized by CD5[+], CD23[+], LEF1[+] B cells expressing dim CD20, and usually dim surface immunoglobulin (sIg). Cyclin D1 is negative, in contrast to MCL. CLL has been shown to have a greater degree of heterogeneity biologically and different subgroups have been identified based on immunoglobulin heavy chain mutational status, cytogenetics, ZAP-70 expression, and CD38 expression. The latter two have been used as partial surrogate markers for the mutational status. ZAP-70 expression correlates with an unmutated status and poorer prognosis. In fact, ZAP-70 expression has been suggested to be more clinically relevant than mutation status, when the two markers are discordant. The use of CD38 as surrogate marker for mutational status is less useful, but its high expression is also associated with a poor prognosis. Recently, recurrent somatic mutations have been identified in a subset of CLL patients using whole-genome and exome sequencing techniques, and some of them have been associated with clinical outcome and may be useful in the future for risk stratification.[6] Deletions at 17p, or mutations in TP53 correlate with more aggressive course.[7]

Histologic transformation over time may occur in CLL, a phenomenon known as Richter syndrome. Short of progression to diffuse large B-cell lymphoma (DLBCL), lymph nodes may show an increased number of prolymphocytes and paraimmunoblasts, sometimes referred to as "accelerated phase". Two forms of Richter transformation with features of classic Hodgkin lymphoma (CHL) have been described. In Type I, Reed–Sternberg (RS) cells and mononuclear variants are seen in a background of small round B lymphocytes, consistent with CLL. The process lacks the rich inflammatory background characteristic of CHL, such as eosinophils, plasma cells, and histiocytes. In other instances, referred to as Type II, the histologic pattern is that of typical CHL, which may be diagnosed at a site not involved by CLL. There is a relatively high incidence of positivity for Epstein-Barr virus (EBV) in both Type I and Type II cases. Treatment with immunosuppressive agents such as fludarabine appears to increase risk.

Lymphoplasmacytic Lymphoma

The definition of lymphoplasmacytic lymphoma (LPL) and its relationship to other B-cell lymphomas associated with plasmacytoid differentiation and monoclonal gammopathy has been clarified in recent years. LPL is frequently, but not invariably, associated with

TABLE 73.1	World Health Organization Classification of Lymphomas[a]

Mature B-Cell Neoplasms
Chronic Lymphocytic Leukemia/Small Lymphocytic Lymphoma
B-cell prolymphocytic leukemia
Splenic B-cell marginal zone lymphoma
Hairy cell leukemia
Splenic B-cell lymphoma/leukemia, unclassifiable
    Splenic diffuse red pulp small B-cell lymphoma
    Hairy cell leukemia-variant
Lymphoplasmacytic lymphoma
    Waldenström macroglobulinemia
Heavy Chain Diseases
    Alpha heavy chain disease
    Gamma heavy chain disease
    Mu heavy chain disease
Plasma Cell Myeloma
Solitary plasmacytoma of bone
Extraosseous plasmacytoma
Extranodal Marginal Zone Lymphoma of Mucosa-Associated Lymphoid Tissue (MALT Lymphoma)
Nodal Marginal zone lymphoma
    Pediatric nodal marginal zone lymphoma
Follicular Lymphoma
    Pediatric-type follicular lymphoma
Primary cutaneous follicle center lymphoma
Mantle Cell Lymphoma
Diffuse Large B-Cell Lymphoma (DLBCL), NOS
    T-cell/histiocyte–rich large B-cell lymphoma
    Primary DLBCL of the CNS
    Primary cutaneous DLBCL, leg type
    EBV-positive DLBCL
    DLBCL associated with chronic inflammation
Lymphomatoid granulomatosis
Primary mediastinal (thymic) large B-cell lymphoma
Intravascular large B-cell lymphoma
ALK-positive large B-cell lymphoma
Plasmablastic lymphoma
HHV8-positive diffuse large B-cell lymphoma & primary effusion lymphoma
Burkitt lymphoma
	High grade B-cell lymphomas, with *MYC* and *BCL2* and/or *BCL6* rearrangements
	B-cell lymphoma unclassifiable, with features intermediate between diffuse large B-cell lymphoma and classic Hodgkin lymphoma
	Mature T-Cell and NK-Cell Neoplasms
	T-cell prolymphocytic leukemia
	T-cell large granular lymphocytic leukemia
	Chronic lymphoproliferative disorder of NK-cells
	Aggressive NK leukemia
	Systemic EBV-positive T-cell lymphoma of childhood
	Hydroa vacciniforme-like lymphoma
	Adult T-cell leukemia/lymphoma
	Extranodal NK/T-cell lymphoma, nasal type
	Enteropathy-associated T-cell lymphoma
	Monomorphic epitheliotropic intestinal T-cell lymphoma
	Hepatosplenic T-cell lymphoma
	Subcutaneous panniculitis-like T-cell lymphoma
	Mycosis Fungoides
	Sézary syndrome
	Primary cutaneous CD30-positive T-cell lymphoproliferative disorders
	    Lymphoid papulosis
	    Primary cutaneous anaplastic large cell lymphoma
	Primary cutaneous gamma-delta T-cell lymphoma
	Primary cutaneous CD8-positive aggressive epidermotropic cytotoxic T-cell lymphoma
	Primary cutaneous CD4-positive small/medium T-cell lymphoproliferative disease
	Peripheral T-Cell Lymphoma, NOS
	Angioimmunoblastic T-Cell Lymphoma
	Anaplastic Large Cell Lymphoma, ALK-Positive
	Anaplastic large cell lymphoma, ALK-negative
	Hodgkin Lymphoma
	Nodular Lymphocyte Predominant Hodgkin Lymphoma
	Classic Hodgkin Lymphoma
	Nodular Sclerosis Hodgkin Lymphoma
	Lymphocyte-rich classic Hodgkin lymphoma
	Mixed cellularity classic Hodgkin lymphoma
	Lymphocyte-depleted classic Hodgkin lymphoma

[a]Most common entities are underlined. Provisional entities are in italics. Some rare entities or variants are omitted. (See reference 2 for complete list.)
ALK, Anaplastic lymphoma kinase; CNS, central nervous system; EBV, Epstein-Barr virus; HHV-8, human herpesvirus-8; NK, natural killer; NOS, not otherwise specified.

Principles of the Classification of Lymphomas Based on the Revised European-American Classification of Lymphoid Neoplasm/World Health Organization Classifications

- Each disease is defined as a distinct entity based on a constellation of morphologic, clinical, and biologic features.
- The cell of origin is the starting point of disease definition.
- Some lymphoid neoplasms can be identified by routine morphologic approaches. However, for most diseases, knowledge of the immunophenotype and molecular genetics/cytogenetics plays an important role in differential diagnosis.
- A disease-based approach to classification facilitates discovery of molecular pathogenesis
- The sites of presentation and involvement are important clues to underlying biologic distinctions. Extranodal lymphomas differ in many respects from their nodal counterparts.
- Many lymphoma entities display a range in cytologic grade and clinical aggressiveness, making it difficult to stratify lymphomas according to clinical behavior. A number of prognostic factors influence clinical outcome, including stage, international prognostic index, cytologic grade, gene expression profile, secondary genetic events, and the host environment.

Early Events in Lymphoid Neoplasia

- In recent years, there has been a greater appreciation of early events in lymphoid neoplasia.
- These early lesions can in some ways be considered equivalent to benign neoplasms in the epithelial system, and require special management approaches.
- These are clonal proliferations of B cells or T cells that carry genetic aberrations associated with specific forms of lymphoid neoplasia: CLL, multiple myeloma, follicular lymphoma, and mantle cell lymphoma.
- Examples include: MGUS, MBL, follicular lymphoma in situ, and mantle cell lymphoma in situ; lymphomatoid papulosis, patch stage of mycosis fungoides, primary cutaneous CD4+ small medium T-cell lymphoproliferative disease.
- Early lesions appear to lack the secondary and tertiary "hits" seen in lymphoid neoplasms that are clinically significant, and most patients have a very low risk of clinical progression.
- Challenges for the future are:
  - to define the precise genetic features that distinguish early lesions from lymphoma
  - to assess the risk of clinical progression
  - to determine how these patients should be managed clinically

CLL, Chronic lymphocytic leukemia; MBL, monoclonal B-cell lymphocytosis; MGUS, monoclonal gammopathy of undetermined significance.

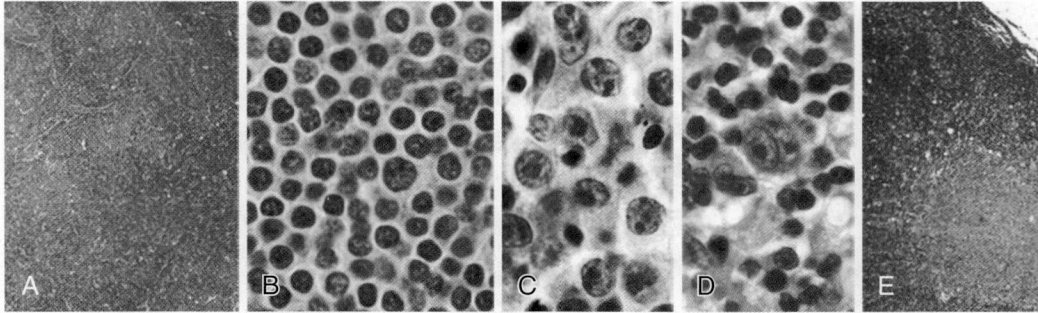

Fig. 73.1 SMALL LYMPHOCYTIC LYMPHOMA. Low-power view (A) illustrates a diffuse effacement of the lymph node. A monotonous population of small lymphocytes is seen at higher power (B). These have fairly round nuclear contours, condensed nuclear chromatin, and inconspicuous or absent nucleoli. Only rare larger cells are present. Small lymphocytic lymphoma can transform to large cell lymphoma (C) and occasionally to Hodgkin lymphoma (D). Patients can also develop worsening lymphadenopathy from viral infections such as herpes simplex virus, in which the node typically shows focal necrosis (E).

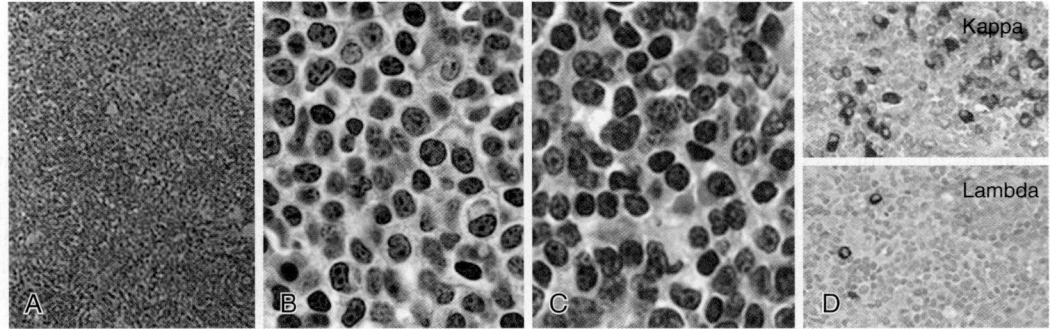

Fig. 73.2 LYMPHOPLASMACYTIC LYMPHOMA (LPL). Lymphoplasmacytic lymphoma and Waldenström macroglobulinemia have nearly identical morphology. There is a diffuse infiltrate (A) of small lymphocytes that have plasmacytoid features or interspersed plasma cells ((B), bone marrow; (C), lymph node). Intranuclear inclusions can sometimes be seen. Evaluation for κ and λ by immunohistochemical stains can demonstrate clonality in the plasma cells and plasmacytoid lymphocytes (D).

Waldenström macroglobulinemia (WM). The 2008 WHO classification adopted the approach advocated at the second international workshop on WM, which defined WM as the presence of an, immunoglobulin M (IgM) monoclonal gammopathy of any concentration associated with bone marrow involvement by LPL.[8] Hence LPL and WM are not synonymous, with WM defying a subset of LPL.

More recently recurrent mutations in MYD88 (L265P) have been identified in greater than 90% of WM patients and are highly associated with LPL, but infrequently seen in other B-cell lymphomas with plasmacytoid features, such as marginal zone lymphomas.[9] In addition, nonsense and frameshift mutations involving CXC-chemokine receptor 4, similar to those occurring in warts hypogammaglobulinemia infections myelokathexis (WHIM) patients, were reported and are associated with heavy disease burden.

LPL is a disease of adult life that usually presents with bone marrow involvement, and sometimes with nodal and splenic involvement (splenomegaly), vague constitutional symptoms, and anemia. (see Chapter 87) The tumor consists of a diffuse proliferation of small lymphocytes, plasmacytoid lymphocytes, and plasma cells, with or without Dutcher bodies (Fig. 73.2). The growth pattern is often interfollicular, with sparing of the sinuses. The cells have surface and cytoplasmic immunoglobulin (Ig), usually of IgM type, usually lack IgD, and express B-cell–associated antigens (CD19, 20, 22, 79a). They are usually negative for CD5 and CD10. CD25 or CD11c may be weakly expressed in some cases. The lack of CD5 and the presence of strong cytoplasmic Ig are useful in distinction from CLL. The postulated normal counterpart is thought to be a postfollicular medullary cord B-cell–based in part on the presence of somatic mutations in the Ig heavy and light-chain variable region genes.

Mantle Cell Lymphoma

MCL is a distinct entity that has been more precisely defined in recent years through the integration of immunophenotypic, molecular genetic, and clinicopathologic studies.[3] The molecular hallmark of MCL is the t(11;14)(q13;q32) involving Cyclin D1 (*CCND1*) and the *IGH* gene. Cyclin D1 overexpression is believed to be essential in the pathogenesis of MCL. However, rare variants negative for Cyclin D1 with similar immunomorphology and gene expression signature have been identified, and most often have translocations involving *CCND2*. Sox11 is overexpressed in most Cyclin D1 positive and negative cases.[10] The postulated normal counterpart is the CD5+ "naive" B cell, sIgM+ and sIgD+, which can be found in the peripheral blood and in the mantle of reactive germinal centers. Mutational analysis of the rearranged immunoglobulin variable region genes shows few or no somatic mutations; however, similarly to CLL a subset of MCL have mutated *IG* genes.

Recently, because of the widespread use of immunohistochemistry, early involvement of lymph node by cells carrying t(11;14) translocation with subsequent overexpression of Cyclin D1 has been documented in several cases, referred to as "in situ MCL". Most often these represent an incidental finding, but some cases will eventually progress to overt MCL.[5] In some cases, in situ MCL is detected in a lymph node involved by another lymphoma type, such as follicular lymphoma. The risk of progression of in situ MCL is difficult to ascertain, as the number of reported cases is few. The preferred term in the revised WHO classification is "in situ mantle cell neoplasia". In a recent multicentric retrospective study, it was noted that the expression of Sox11 was more frequently associated with progression

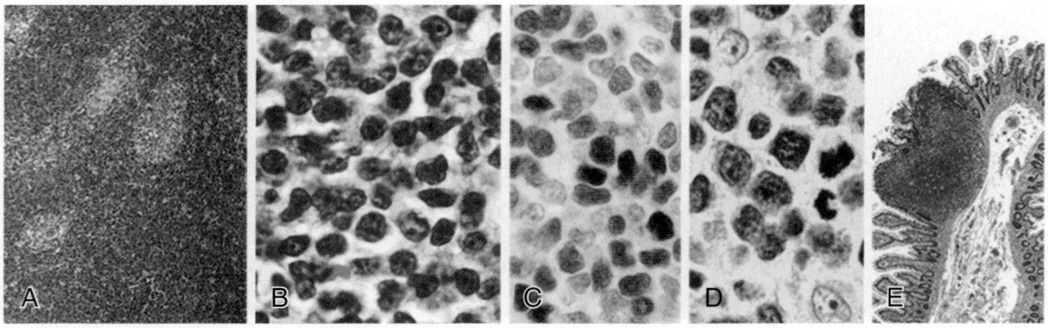

Fig. 73.3 MANTLE CELL LYMPHOMA. At low power, mantle cell lymphoma (MCL) can show a diffuse, vaguely nodular, or mantle zone pattern. In the latter, the neoplastic mantle zones are expanded and can become confluent leaving "naked" germinal centers (A). At higher power, the lymphoma cells are small or slightly enlarged (B). They have irregular nuclear contours, especially compared with small lymphocytic lymphoma, and they have dense chromatin. Typically, cases are positive for cyclin D1 expression (C), which is related to the t(11;14) involving IgH and *CCND1*. Some cases can develop a "blastoid" transformation (D), although some cases can present as a "blastoid" variant. Such cases are characterized by cells with an intermediate size, a high mitotic rate, and finely dispersed "blastic" chromatin. Sometimes when the "blastoid" cases develop a leukemic phase, they can be difficult to distinguish morphologically from acute lymphoblastic leukemia. In such cases, flow immunophenotyping is needed to resolve the differential diagnosis. MCL can also present with gastrointestinal involvement (E) as in lymphomatoid papulosis.

to MCL, since the majority of in situ cases lacked Sox11 expression. Also, similar to follicular lymphoma in situ, a distinction should be made between partial involvement by mantle cell lymphoma with a mantle zone pattern and in situ MCL. The latter refers to a reactive lymph node with Cyclin D1 positive cells limited to an otherwise normal appearing follicle mantle; these cases tend not to progress and should not be labeled as lymphomas.

Another newly identified variant is an indolent form of MCL characterized by a leukemic phase without nodal disease, but often with long standing splenomegaly. These patients have an indolent clinical course and do not appear to require aggressive chemotherapy. These cases carry t(11;14) with few additional chromosomal abnormalities and lack expression of Sox11 in contrast to conventional MCL.

MCL occurs in adults (median age 62), with a high male-to-female ratio. Most patients present with advanced stage at diagnosis. Common sites of involvement include lymph nodes, spleen, bone marrow, and lymphoid tissue of Waldeyer ring. Gastrointestinal (GI) tract involvement is frequent and is associated with the picture of lymphomatous polyposis.

The hallmark of MCL is a very monotonous cellular composition. In the typical case, the cells are slightly larger than a normal lymphocyte with finely clumped chromatin, scant cytoplasm, and inconspicuous nucleoli (Fig. 73.3). The nuclear contour is usually irregular or cleaved. Some cytologic variants, blastoid (blastic) and pleomorphic, tend to be associated with a more aggressive course, and adverse biologic features, such as tetraploidy or p53 mutation/deletion. The proliferation rate was previously identified as prognostically important based on scoring of Ki67-positive cells. More recently gene expression profiling (GEP), using genes involved in cell cycle progression and DNA synthesis, has identified a proliferation signature that delineates cohorts with varied prognosis. These correlate to some extent with cytologic subtype. For example, the blastoid variant has a high proliferation rate, utilizing both KI-67 and GEP.

Follicular Lymphoma

Follicular lymphoma (FL) is the most common subtype of non-Hodgkin lymphoma within the United States and accounts for approximately 45% of all newly diagnosed cases. It has a peak incidence in the fifth and sixth decades, and is rare under the age of 20. Men and women are equally affected. FL is less common in black and Asian populations. Most patients have stage 3 or 4 disease at

diagnosis, with generalized lymphadenopathy. Staging evaluation will usually detect bone marrow involvement. Approximately 10% of patients will have circulating malignant cells. However, careful immunophenotypic or molecular analyses may disclose peripheral blood involvement in a higher proportion of patients. A more accurate prognostic index than the international prognostic index (IPI), the follicular lymphoma international prognostic index, has been proposed for FL, and has been widely adopted.

The natural history of the disease is associated with histologic progression in both pattern and cell type (Fig. 73.4). A heterogeneous cytologic composition is one of the hallmarks of FL. Usually, all of the follicle center cells are represented, but in varying proportions. It should be stressed that the variation in cytologic grade is a continuum, and therefore precise morphologic criteria for subclassification are difficult to establish.

According to the WHO classification, all low-grade FL are combined into a single category, Grade 1–2, all containing overall a predominance of centrocytes with fewer than 15 centroblasts/high power field (hpf). FL grade 3 (with >15 centroblasts/hpf) is further subdivided in 3A and 3B based on the presence or absence of centrocytes in the background.

The vast majority of FL (approximately 85%) are associated with a t(14;18) involving rearrangement of the *BCL2* gene. This translocation appears to result in constitutive expression of BCL2 protein, which is capable of inhibiting apoptosis in lymphoid cells. The cells of FL accumulate and are at risk to acquire secondary mutations, which may be associated with histologic progression. It has been postulated that the *BCL2/JH* translocation occurs during immunoglobulin gene rearrangement in the bone marrow at the pre-B cell stage of development. This fact might contribute to the difficulty in eradicating the neoplastic clone with chemotherapy.

Biologically, the pathogenesis of most cases of FL grade 3B differs from that of FL grades 1–2/3A, in lacking the BCL2/IGH, but also differs from diffuse large B-cell lymphoma, in having a low incidence of BCL6 aberrations.[11] These data provide a biologic explanation for the greater curability of grade 3B FL with aggressive therapy, although some studies have not found support for this hypothesis. Differences in diagnostic criteria might account for this apparent discrepancy, and the correlation between grade 3A versus 3B, and molecular alterations is imprecise. Other phenotypic variants appear to have prognostic significance, such as FL negative for CD10 but positive for MUM1/IRF4. These cases are usually of higher grade and interestingly also lack the *BCL2* translocation. Evolution towards a molecularly defined classification of FL is a possibility for the future.

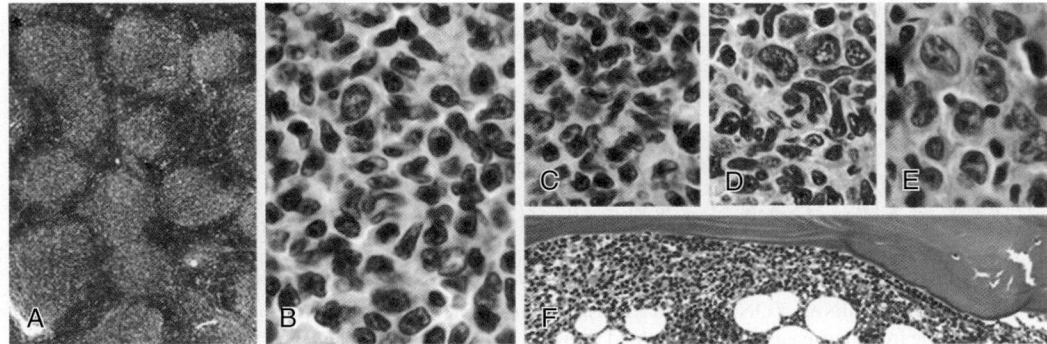

Fig. 73.4 FOLLICULAR LYMPHOMA (FL). Follicular lymphoma (FL) shows effacement of the normal lymph node architecture because of an accumulation of neoplastic lymphoid follicles that lack the features of reactive follicles (A). They are crowded, show back-to-back localization, lack distinct mantle zones, and show no polarity. The lymphoma cells are highly irregular (B) with elongated, twisted, or clefted nuclear contours and dense chromatin. FL is typically graded into grade 1 or 2 (1/2; C, D), or 3 (E), depending on the number of large cells seen at higher power (see text). FL typically involves the bone marrow with lymphoma cells spreading along the bone (F). This localization is termed "paratrabecular."

The phenomenon of localization of FL cells to isolated germinal centers within a lymph node has been termed FL in situ.[5] The revised WHO classification proposes in situ follicular neoplasia as a preferred term. The likelihood of evolution to clinically significant FL is low for these patients, if there is no other evidence of disease at the time of diagnosis. Indeed, this translocation can be found in the peripheral blood and lymphoid organs of healthy individuals, and suggests that the *BCL2/JH* translocation is necessary but not sufficient for the development of FL. "FL in situ" or in situ follicular neoplasia should be distinguished from partial involvement by FL. In the true "in situ" lesion clusters of B cells strongly positive for CD10 and BCL2 are localized to germinal centers in an otherwise reactive lymph node. It often represents an incidental finding, in a lymph node biopsied for other reasons.

The 2008 WHO classification recognizes other lymphomas of follicle center derivation that may resemble nodal FL, but exhibit significant differences either clinically or biologically.[12] These include diffuse follicular FL, pediatric forms of FL, primary intestinal FL and cutaneous lymphomas of follicle center cell derivation. Intestinal FL, most often presenting in the duodenum, is associated with the BCL2/IGH translocation, but usually presents as isolated mucosal polyps with a low risk of dissemination.[5] FL in the pediatric age group is histologically diverse. Most nodal cases are cytologically high grade, composed of blastoid cells, but are usually localized, and may be cured in a number of instances with surgical excision. This so-called pediatric type of FL may also be seen in adults more rarely, and shows a strong male predominance. Another form of FL seen in children and young adults is associated with translocations involving IRF4, and shows overexpression of MUM1 by immunohistochemistry. These cases frequently present in Waldeyer ring.[13]

There are rare variants of FL with a mainly diffuse growth pattern. These often present as bulky localized inguinal masses, and lack the BCL2 translocation but often have deletions at 1p36.[12] Primary cutaneous follicle center lymphoma, which also frequently lacks the *BCL2* translocation and BCL2 expression, is now considered by the WHO classification as a separate entity.[2] They usually present in the head or upper trunk, and can be managed conservatively with local approaches. However, when BCL2 expression is detected, the possibility that this may represent a secondary site of involvement should be considered.

Extranodal Marginal-Zone Lymphoma of Mucosa-Associated Lymphoid Tissue Type

Most lymphomas of marginal-zone derivation present in extranodal sites and have the histopathologic and clinical features identified by

Isaacson and Wright as part of the spectrum of mucosa-associated lymphoid tissue (MALT) lymphomas. MALT lymphomas are characterized by a heterogeneous cellular composition that includes marginal-zone or centrocyte-like cells, monocytoid B cells, small lymphocytes, and plasma cells (Fig. 73.5A). In most cases, large transformed cells are infrequent. Reactive germinal centers are nearly always present. When follicular colonization occurs, the process may simulate follicular lymphoma. Clonality is confirmed by molecular and or immunohistochemical studies.

MALT lymphomas have been described in nearly every anatomic site but are most frequent in the stomach, lung, thyroid, salivary gland, and lacrimal gland. Other less common sites of involvement include the orbit, breast, conjunctiva, bladder and kidney, and thymus gland. Widespread nodal involvement is infrequent, as is marrow involvement. The clinical course is usually quite indolent, and many patients are asymptomatic. MALT lymphomas tend to relapse in other MALT-associated sites.

MALT lymphomas of the salivary gland and thyroid are usually associated with a history of autoimmune diseases. Helicobacter gastritis is frequent in most patients with gastric MALT lymphomas. Other infectious agents have been described in MALT lymphomas involving skin (*Borrelia burgdorferi*), ocular adnexae (*Chlamydia psittaci*), and small intestine (*Campylobacter jejuni*); however, in this latter group a causal relationship has not yet been demonstrated. Chronic antigen stimulation is critical to both the development of a MALT lymphoma and the maintenance of the neoplastic state. Indeed, in some cases antibiotic therapy and the eradication of *Helicobacter pylori* has led to the spontaneous remission of gastric MALT lymphoma in cases lacking genetic aberrations.

By immunophenotype MALT lymphomas are positive for B-cell–associated antigens CD19, CD20, and CD22, but are negative for CD5 and CD10. The absence of cyclin D1 is useful in ruling out MCL, especially in intestinal disease. Rare cases of MALT lymphoma have been reported to be CD5-positive, and in some but not all instances this has been associated with more aggressive disease. The clinical significance of increased transformed cells is still uncertain, and no formal grading system exists for MALT lymphoma. The putative cell of origin of MALT lymphoma is a postgerminal center B-cell.

MALT lymphomas also have several recurring cytogenetic abnormalities, including t(11;18)(q21;q21), t(1;14)(p22;q32), t(14;18)(q32;q21), t(3;14)(q27;q32), and t(3;14)(p14.1;q32), which are observed with variable frequency, often depending upon the anatomic site. Although several genes are involved in these translocations, at least three of them, (t(11;18), t(1;14), and t(14;18), share a common pathway, which leads to the activation of NF-κB and its downstream targets. By genome–wide DNA profiling integrated with GEP,

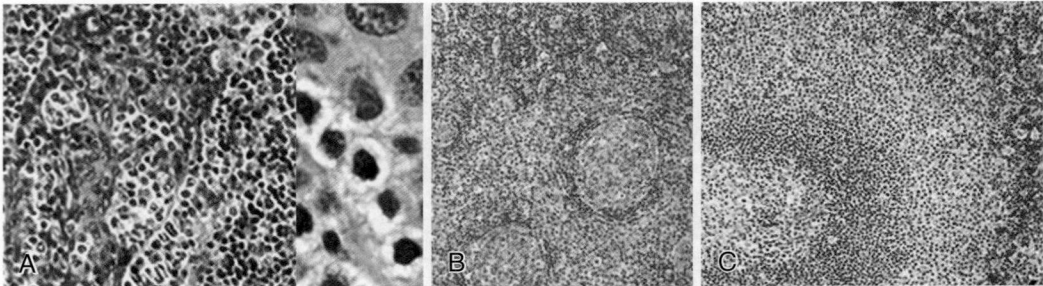

Fig. 73.5 MARGINAL ZONE LYMPHOMA. Marginal zone lymphomas commonly occur at extranodal sites arising from mucosa-associated lymphoid tissue (MALT). MALT lymphomas typically infiltrate or invade into epithelial structures, resulting in "lymphoepithelial lesions" (A). They are composed of small to intermediate-sized cells with abundant clear cytoplasms (A, *detail*). The normal lymph node does not have a marginal zone, but primary nodal marginal zone lymphomas (NMZL) can occur. They infiltrate the node in what would be a marginal zone pattern with an expansion of cells peripheral to mantle zone (B). The spleen does have a normal marginal zone, and this can give rise to a splenic marginal zone lymphoma (SMZL). Early on, these show expansion of the marginal zone areas (C) but later can become more diffuse, infiltrating the red pulp. In the case illustrated, the spleen weighed 1700 g.

differences were detected among the three different main types of marginal zone lymphomas lending support to the current WHO classification, which separates these three entities.[14]

Nodal Marginal-Zone B-Cell Lymphoma

Nodal marginal zone lymphoma (NMZL) is a primary nodal disease, which resembles other marginal zone lymphomas, extranodal or splenic types. These patients often present with bone marrow involvement, and tend to have a more aggressive clinical course than those with extranodal MALT. The neoplastic proliferation is polymorphous and composed of monocytoid B cells, plasmacytoid cells, with interspersed large blast-like cells. There is an expansion of the marginal-zone area, often with preservation of the nodal architecture (see Fig. 73.5B). The mantle zone may be intact, attenuated, or effaced. The immunophenotype is similar to other MZL, that is, CD20-positive, CD10-negative, CD5-negative, with variable expression of IgD (weak to negative). Because there are no precise immunophenotypic or genotypic markers of NMZL, the diagnosis is sometimes one of exclusion. The differential diagnosis with LPL may be problematic; however, the MYD88 (L265P) somatic mutation is detected infrequently in MZL lymphomas and its presence should raise the possibility of LPL. More stringent criteria are needed to separate these two entities. A variant of nodal MZL occurs in children; these cases show a striking male predominance, present with localized disease, and can be managed with local therapies.[1]

Splenic Marginal-Zone Lymphoma

Splenic marginal-zone lymphoma (SMZL) presents in adults and is slightly more frequent in females than males. The clinical presentation is splenomegaly, usually without peripheral lymphadenopathy. The majority of patients have marrow involvement, but there is usually only a modest lymphocytosis, with elevations in the lymphocyte count usually less than that seen in CLL. Some evidence of plasmacytoid differentiation may be seen and patients may have a small M component. The abundant pale cytoplasm evident in tissue sections may also be seen in blood smears. The course is indolent, and splenectomy may be followed by a prolonged remission.

Histologically, the spleen shows expansion of the white pulp, but usually some infiltration of the red pulp is also present (see Fig. 73.5C). A characteristic biphasic pattern in the neoplastic white pulp has been described, with the neoplastic cells surrounding regressed follicles. The immunophenotype of these cells resembles that of other marginal-zone B-cell lymphomas; however, IgD expression is more

frequently observed. Progression to diffuse large B-cell lymphoma can be seen.

Although the molecular pathogenesis of SMZL has not been fully delineated, a frequent cytogenetic alteration involving deletions of the region 7q(22-32) has been reported.[15] Mutations in *NOTCH2* are the most common event but other genes in the NOTCH pathway may be targeted.[16] Many of the affected genes appear to play a role in marginal zone B-cell development. The differential diagnosis of SMZL includes other unspecified B-cell lymphomas of the spleen, including splenic lymphoma with villous lymphocytes (SLVL), and hairy cell variant. The latter have been grouped together under splenic B-cell lymphoma/leukemia unclassifiable, and the interrelationship among these disorders is not fully resolved.

Diffuse Large B-Cell Lymphoma, Not Otherwise Specified

DLBCL is one of the more common subtypes of non-Hodgkin lymphoma, representing up to 40% of cases. It has an aggressive natural history but responds well to chemotherapy. The complete remission rate with modern regimens is 75% to 80%, with long-term disease-free survival approaching 50% or more in most series. This lymphoma may present in lymph nodes or in extranodal sites. Frequent extranodal sites of involvement include bone, skin, thyroid, GI tract, and lung.

DLBCL represents one of the most heterogeneous categories in the WHO, and attempts to identify prognostic groups based on morphology and phenotype have shown limited usefulness and reproducibility (Boxon Varied Basis for the Recognition of Diverse Entities). To address these issues, DLBCLs were among the first cases to be analyzed by complementary DNA (cDNA) array technology, and more recently also by genome-wide analysis.[17] By GEP three groups were identified based on the differential expression of a large set of genes, namely germinal center-like group (GCB), activated B-cell–like group (ABC), and primary mediastinal (thymic) large B-cell lymphoma (PMBL). PMBL is now recognized as a separate entity, and adaptations in GEP now allow profiling of formalin fixed paraffin-embedded (FFPE) biopsies.[18] The ABC subtype frequently exhibits mutations in the BCR-signaling and NF-κB pathways providing new insight in the pathogenesis of DLBCL and new potential therapeutic targets.[19] Recurrent mutations in the GCB type of DLBCL appear to target histone-modifying genes.[17] Somatic mutations in *EZH2* also have been identified in FL, another tumor of germinal center derivation.

DLBCLs are composed of large, transformed lymphoid cells with nuclei at least twice the size of a small lymphocyte (Fig. 73.6). The

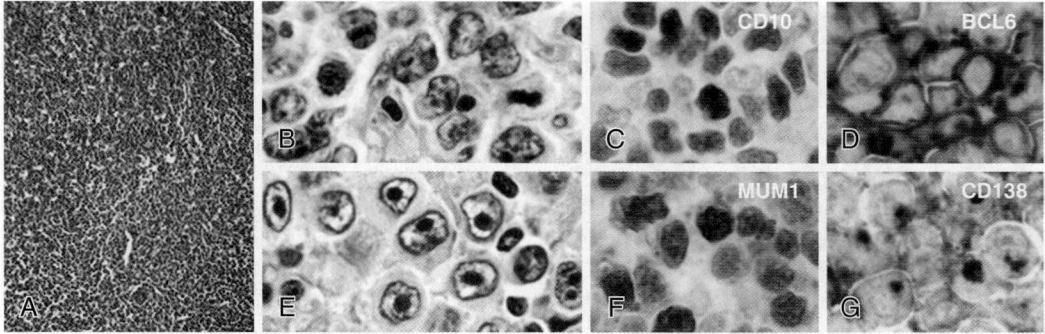

Fig. 73.6 DIFFUSE LARGE B-CELL LYMPHOMA. The low-power illustration demonstrates the diffuse nature of the process (A). At high power (B), there are sheets of large cells. Those with a vesicular nuclear chromatin and variable numbers of nucleoli along the nuclear membrane are referred to as centroblasts. These typically have a germinal center gene expression profile and a germinal center immunophenotype with expression of CD10 and BCL6 (C and D). Those cases composed of large cells with a single prominent nucleolus (E) are called immunoblastic and commonly have an activated B-cell (ABC) gene expression profile and an ABC phenotype with expression of MUM-1, CD138 (F and G), and IFR-4. The correlation of morphology and immunophenotype is not always exact.

Varied Basis for the Recognition of Diverse Entities Among Aggressive B-Cell Neoplasms

- Cell of origin, in part as determined by gene expression profiling
  Activated B cell versus germinal center B cell
  Thymic B cell of PMBL
- Clinical factors
  Anatomic site, e.g., CNS, mediastinum, intravascular
  Advanced age, background of chronic inflammation
- Etiologic factors
  EBV, HHV-8
- Molecular pathogenesis
  BCL6, C-MYC, ALK, BCL2, MYD88 (translocations, amplification, mutation)

CNS, Central nervous system; EBV, Epstein-Barr virus; HHV-8, human herpesvirus-8; PMBL, primary mediastinal large B cell lymphoma;

---

nuclei generally have vesicular chromatin, prominent nucleoli, and basophilic cytoplasm, resembling the centroblasts of the normal germinal center. The immunoblastic variant is characterized by cells with prominent central nucleoli, and abundant deeply staining cytoplasm. Although there is no absolute correlation between morphology and GEP, the majority of centroblastic DLBCL falls into the GCB group, and the majority of immunoblastic into the ABC group.

Algorithms based on immunophenotype have been proposed as surrogates for cDNA microarray using CD10/BCL6 positivity for GCB and MUM1/IRF-4 for ABC with the addition of BCL2 in combination with IPI and may improve the stratification of DLBCL. Because of emerging differences in the treatment of GCB versus ABC (or non-GCB) DLBCL, it is recommended to include the subtype by integrating GEP and/or immunohistochemistry (IHC) results in the report with clarification of the method used and the type of algorithm. As noted, newer GEP methods may be applicable to FFPE material.[18]

Diffuse Large B-Cell Lymphomas, Other Variants and Subtypes.

The spectrum of aggressive B-cell lymphomas has broadened in recent years, incorporating new entities based on unique clinical features such as age or anatomic site, viral pathogenesis (EBV, human herpesvirus [HHV]-8), or distinctive pathologic features.[20] *T cell/histiocyte–rich large B-cell lymphoma (THRLBCL)* has distinctive morphologic and clinical features. It is associated with aggressive clinical behavior, and often presents with advanced stage and bone marrow involvement. The relevance of the microenvironment and recruitment mechanism of the inflammatory cells, which are the main histologic component, has been the focus of recent studies.[21]

The WHO classification recognizes that some lymphomas arising in certain anatomic sites may have distinctive features both clinically and biologically. Among these are *primary DLBCL of the central nervous system (CNS)* and *DLBCL of the testis*. DLBCLs in these sanctuary sites differ at the genomic level from usual nodal DLBCL.[22,23] Both primary CNS DLBCL and intraocular large B-cell lymphomas commonly have mutations in MYD88.

Primary cutaneous DLBCL, leg type, has a GEP resembling the ABC type of DLBCL, presents most often in older adult females, and generally has an aggressive clinical course. As with nodal DLBCL, BCL2 expression is an adverse prognostic factor.

EBV-positive DLBCL was a provisional entity in the 2008 WHO classification, and was first recognized in the older adult.[24] More recent studies have shown a wider age distribution. Decreased immune surveillance in the older adult, or a tolerogenic immune microenvironment may facilitate tumor development.[25] The morphologic spectrum is broad, but most cases have a prominent inflammatory background. The prognosis in the older adult is poor but younger patients have a good outcome. EBV-positive DLBCL should be distinguished from EBV-positive mucocutaneous ulcer, which affects mainly cutaneous sites, and often has a self-limited clinical course. These lesions arise in a setting of decreased immune surveillance, most often in the elderly, and frequently with iatrogenic immune suppression.

Lymphomatoid granulomatosis is an EBV-positive B-cell lymphoproliferative disorder (LPD) associated with an inflammatory background rich in T cells. The lung is nearly always involved, with skin, kidney, liver and brain being frequently affected as well. *DLBCL associated with chronic inflammation* was first described in association with chronic pyothorax, but now has been associated with EBV-driven large B-cell proliferations in diverse clinical settings, usually associated with a confined anatomic space and a background of chronic inflammation. These cases appear to have a good prognosis if successfully resected.

There are several LPDs associated with HHV-8/Kaposi sarcoma–associated herpesvirus (KSHV). These include *primary effusion lymphoma (PEL)* and *multicentric Castleman disease (MCD)*. The cells of PEL are usually coinfected with EBV, and the disease is most often diagnosed in the setting of human immunodeficiency virus (HIV) infection and immunosuppression. While pleural or peritoneal effusions are most common, extracavitary PEL can present as a tumor mass, usually in extranodal sites. PEL has a phenotype resembling that of terminally differentiated B-cells, i.e., plasmablastic (Fig. 73.7).

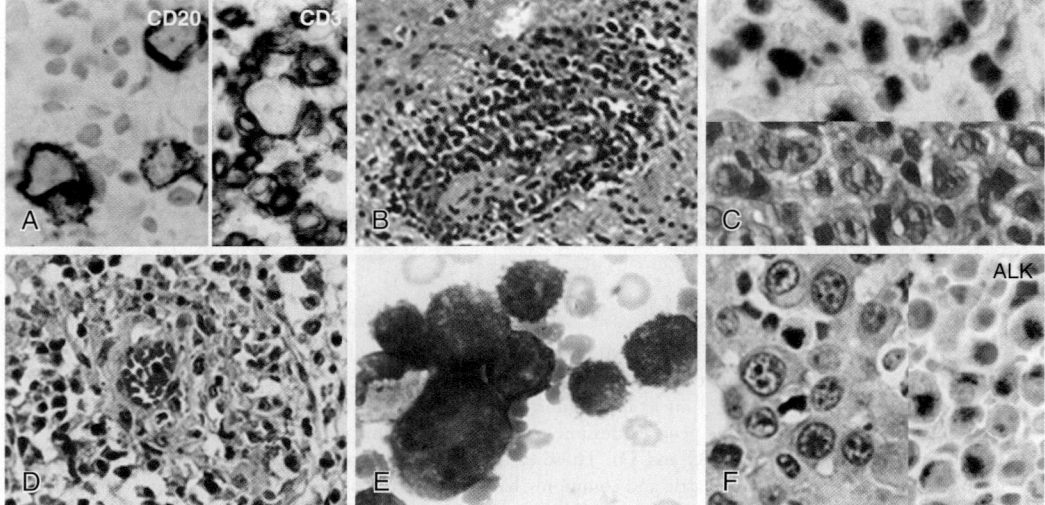

Fig. 73.7 DIFFUSE LARGE B-CELL LYMPHOMA, VARIANTS AND SUBTYPES. T-cell/histiocyte–rich large B-cell lymphoma is illustrated in (A), where a CD20 immunostain *(right)* identifies scattered large B cells, which are associated with a prominent background of small reactive T cells (CD3; *left*). Sometimes there are numerous histiocytes in the background or an admixture of reactive T cells and histiocytes. Primary diffuse large B-cell lymphoma (DLBCL) of the central nervous system usually shows a perivascular distribution (B). Epstein-Barr virus (EBV)–positive DLBCL can have variable morphologic features. The illustrated case is monomorphic and composed of large cells, which are positive for EBV-encoded RNA (EBER) (C, *bottom* and *top*). Lymphomatoid granulomatosis (D) also has a perivascular distribution and is composed of a mix of malignant large EBV-positive B cells and reactive T cells. Primary effusion lymphoma is usually diagnosed from cytologic preparations (E) and by flow cytometric and molecular techniques. Although the tumor cells do not generally form masses, extracavitary primary effusion lymphoma can present as a tumor mass, usually in extranodal sites. ALK-positive large B-cell lymphomas are rare, and show ALK positivity as a consequence of a translocation of *ALK* (F). *ALK,* Anaplastic lymphoma kinase; *RNA,* ribonucleic acid.

Two other lymphomas with a plasmablastic phenotype include *plasmablastic lymphoma (PBL),* and *anaplastic lymphoma kinase (ALK)-positive large B-cell lymphoma.* PBL is usually positive for EBV, most often extranodal, and associated with immunosuppression from either HIV infection or advanced age. Recent studies have identified a high incidence of MYC translocation in PBL.[26] ALK-positive large B-cell lymphomas show overexpression of ALK, usually as a consequence of translocation. They mainly affect older individuals, but can occur at any age. Interestingly, IgA is most often expressed.

Intravascular Large B-Cell Lymphoma

Intravascular large B-cell lymphoma is a rare form of DLBCL characterized by the presence of lymphoma cells only in the lumens of small vessels, particularly capillaries. These cells are nearly always of B-cell phenotype, often with aberrant expression of CD5 (Fig. 73.8). The tumor cells are large, with vesicular nuclei and prominent nucleoli, resembling centroblasts or immunoblasts. Lymph node involvement is rare, and the tumor presents in extranodal sites, most readily diagnosed in the skin. Neurologic symptoms associated with plugging of small vessels in the CNS are common. The disease is often not diagnosed until autopsy, because of the lack of definitive radiologic or clinical evidence of disease, and diverse symptomatology.

Primary Mediastinal (Thymic) Large B-Cell Lymphoma

Primary mediastinal large B-cell lymphoma (PMBL) has emerged in recent years as a distinct clinicopathologic entity, typically arising in young women, with a peak incidence in the fourth decade. Patients present with a mediastinal mass, with frequent superior vena cava syndrome. Regional lymph nodes may be involved but spread to distant nodal sites is uncommon. Frequent extranodal sites of involvement, particularly at relapse, include the liver, kidneys, adrenal glands, ovaries, GI tract, and central nervous system.

Histologically, PMBL is characterized by fine compartmentalizing sclerosis, and large lymphoid cells with abundant pale cytoplasm (see Fig. 73.8B). An origin from medullary thymic B cells is proposed. The cells express CD20 and CD79a, but do not express surface Ig. Recently, expression of the *MAL* gene has been detected in PMBL and not in other DLBCLs.[27] PMBL usually lack rearrangement for *BCL2, BCL6*; however, *REL* amplification is a common feature. A common cytogenetic abnormality seen in approximately 50% of cases includes gains in 9p, which may be associated with amplification of *JAK2* and *PDL1/PDL2* as well as translocations involving MHC class II transactivator (*CIITA*). Recently, gene expression profiling studies have found that PMBL bears a distinct molecular signature that differs from that of other DLBCLs and shares features of CHL; however, the same signature is not restricted to mediastinal sites since it can also be detected in other DLBCL-not otherwise specified (NOS) at nonmediastinal sites.

B-Cell Lymphoma, Unclassifiable, With Features Intermediate Between Diffuse Large B-Cell Lymphoma and Classic Hodgkin Lymphoma

This lymphoma is sometimes referred to as mediastinal gray zone lymphoma, since the mediastinum is the most common site of presentation. A close relationship between PMBL and CHL was supported by gene expression profiling. TRAF1 expression and c-REL amplification were also seen in both types of neoplasms and could be detected with suitable immunohistochemical studies.

Gray zone lymphomas are more common in males than females, present with bulky mediastinal masses, and appear to have a more aggressive clinical course than PMBL or CHL. A recent study using

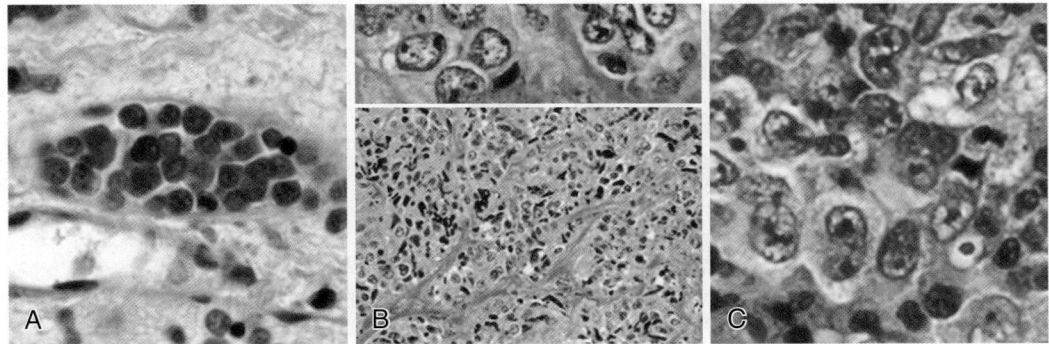

Fig. 73.8 DIFFUSE LARGE B-CELL LYMPHOMA VARIANTS (INTRAVASCULAR, MEDIASTINAL, GRAY ZONE). In intravascular lymphoma, also known as angiotropic lymphoma, the large B cells are confined to the lumens of small vessels (A). Paradoxically, they do not spread to the blood. Primary mediastinal (thymic) large B-cell lymphoma typically shows large B cells in a finely sclerotic background (B, *top* and *bottom*). So-called "gray zone lymphoma" has features intermediate between large B-cell lymphoma and Hodgkin lymphoma. In the case illustrated (C), the male patient presented with a mediastinal mass. The cells were CD30+ and only variably positive for CD45 as in Hodgkin lymphoma, but they were strongly and uniformly positive for CD20 and PAX5. They also strongly expressed the B-cell transcription factors OCT2 and BOB1.

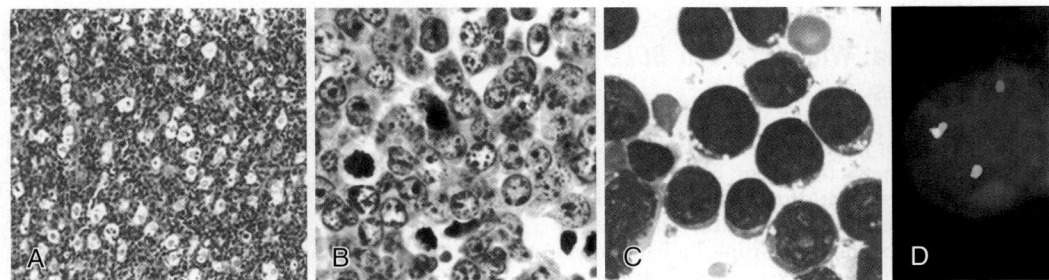

Fig. 73.9 BURKITT LYMPHOMA. At low power, Burkitt lymphoma gives a classic "starry sky" appearance because of numerous histiocytes or tingible body macrophages with clear cytoplasm *(stars)*, in a background of darkly stained tumor cells (A). At high power, the cells exhibit a very high mitotic rate and are intermediate in size with finely clumped nuclear chromatin (B). On a Wright-stained touch preparation or in the blood or bone marrow aspirate, the cells also have a characteristic appearance with deep blue cytoplasm typically with vacuoles (C). Fluorescence in situ hybridization with a probe that spans *MYC* will show a break-apart signal (D) indicating that *MYC* has translocated to a partner chromosome.

methylation profiling identified gray zone lymphomas as having a signature distinct from both CHL and PMBL. However, by fluorescence in situ hybridization, gray zone lymphomas, PBMCL and CHL share a number of common cytogenetic aberrations including gains at 2p16.1 (*REL/BCL11A* locus), 9p24.1 (*JAK2/PDL2)* and rearrangements of 16p13.13 (*CIITA*). It is not clear how these patients should be approached therapeutically, but they appear to benefit from combined modality therapy (systemic chemotherapy and radiation).

Burkitt Lymphoma

Burkitt lymphoma (BL) is most common in children and accounts for up to one-third of all pediatric lymphomas in the United States. It is the most rapidly growing of all lymphomas, with 100% of the cells in cell cycle at any time. It usually presents in extranodal sites. In nonendemic regions, such as the United States, frequent sites of presentation are the ileocecal region, ovaries, kidneys, or breasts. Jaw presentations, as well as involvement of other facial bones, are common in African or endemic cases and are seen occasionally in nonendemic regions. Bone marrow involvement is a poor prognostic sign.

BL is one of the more common tumors associated with HIV. It can present at any time during the clinical course. In some patients

with HIV infection, BL may be the initial acquired immunodeficiency syndrome-defining illness.

The pathogenesis of BL is related to the translocations involving the *MYC* oncogene, which are seen in virtually 100% of cases and often constitute the sole karyotypic abnormality. Most cases involve the IG heavy-chain gene on chromosome 14, and less frequently the light-chain genes on chromosomes 2 and 22. In endemic BL, genomic instability is thought to be promoted by Plasmodium infection.[28] EBV is closely linked to BL in endemic regions but is less frequently seen (15%–20%) in sporadic cases. In other regions, characterized by low socioeconomic status and EBV infection at an early age, BL is often EBV-positive, in the range of 50% to 70%. These data support the concept that the EBV is a cofactor for the development of BL. Cytologically, BL is monomorphic (Fig. 73.9). The cells are medium in size with round nuclei, moderately clumped chromatin, and multiple (2–5) basophilic nucleoli. The cytoplasm is deeply basophilic and moderately abundant. These cells contain cytoplasmic lipid vacuoles, which are probably a manifestation of the high rate of proliferation and high rate of spontaneous cell death. The starry sky pattern characteristic of BL is a manifestation of the numerous benign macrophages that have ingested karyorrhectic or apoptotic tumor cells.

BL has a mature B cell phenotype. The cells express CD19, CD20, CD22, CD79a, and monoclonal surface Ig, nearly always IgM.

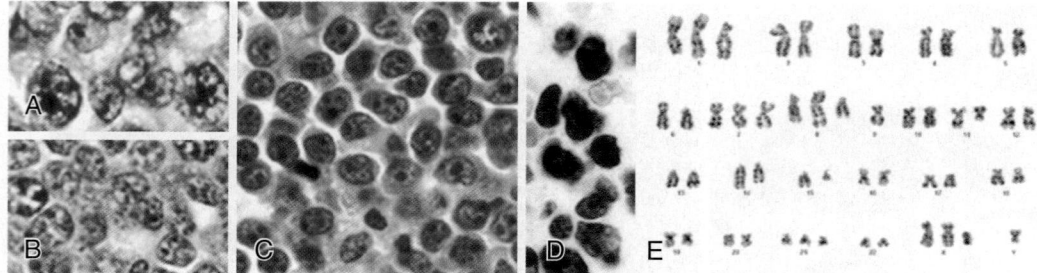

Fig. 73.10 B-CELL LYMPHOMA, UNCLASSIFIABLE WITH FEATURES INTERMEDIATE BETWEEN DIFFUSE LARGE B-CELL LYMPHOMA AND BURKITT LYMPHOMA. Examples of diffuse large B-cell lymphoma (DLBCL) (A) and Burkitt lymphoma (BL) (B) are for comparison. In (C), the lymphoma cells are intermediate in size and not as large as the DLBCL but without the typical characteristics of BL cells. The cells had a high Ki67 rate (D) and a B-cell phenotype with CD10 and BCL2 expression (not shown). The karyotype had a t(14;18) as in follicular lymphoma, *MYC* translocation as in BL, but was complex with multiple aberrations. (E). The karyotype was as follows: 51,XY,+X,+1,dup(1)(q32q44),der(1)del(1)(p21p36.3) dup(1)(q32q44),t(6;8)(p21.1;q24.1),+7,+del(?8) (p11.2p23),der(8)i(8)(q10)t(8;11)(q24.1;q13),9,der(11) t(8;11)(q24.1;q13), t(14;15)(q32;q15), t(14;18)(q32;q21.3),+21,+mar[13]/46,XY[1]. *(The karyotype was kindly provided by Dr. Yanming Zhan of Northwestern University.)*

CD10 is positive in nearly all cases, and CD5, CD23, and BCL2 are consistently negative.

High Grade B-Cell Lymphoma, With *MYC* and *BCL2* and/or *BCL6* Rearrangements

Historically, it has been difficult for pathologists to distinguish some DLBCL with a very high growth fraction from BL with atypical cytology. In addition, there are cases that carry a C-*MYC* translocation, but carry additional cytogenetic abnormalities, most often involving *BCL2* or *BCL6*. These double hit and triple hit lymphomas have a very aggressive clinical course, and will be separately delineated in the revised WHO classification[29] (Fig. 73.10). The clinical impact of *MYC* overexpression in DLBCL has not been fully resolved; in some series, it has been associated with a more aggressive clinical course. For the time being, an otherwise typical DLBCL with a C-*MYC* translocation should still be classified as DLBCL. Cases of BL with atypical cytologic features, are retained under the heading of BL, and have a better prognosis when treated appropriately.

T AND NATURAL KILLER-CELL LYMPHOMAS

Overview of the Classification of T-Cell Neoplasms

Although the definition of precursor T-cell or lymphoblastic neoplasms is straightforward, the classification of peripheral T-cell lymphomas has been controversial. These are uncommon, representing less than 15% of all non-Hodgkin lymphomas. Most previously published classification schemes for the malignant lymphomas in the United States or Europe have been based on B-cell malignancies, as these are far more common than their T-cell counterparts. T-cell and NK-cell lymphomas show significant variation in incidence in different geographic regions and racial populations.

The classification of T-cell and NK-cell neoplasms proposed by the WHO emphasizes a multiparameter approach, integrating morphologic, immunophenotypic, genetic, and clinical features. Clinical features play particular importance in the subclassification of these tumors, in part caused by the lack of specificity of other parameters (See Box on Natural Killer and T-cell Subsets).

In contrast to B-cell lymphomas, specific immunophenotypic profiles are not associated with most T-cell lymphoma subtypes. Although certain antigens are commonly associated with specific disease entities, these associations are not entirely disease-specific. Presently, specific genetic features have not been identified for many of the T-cell and NK-cell neoplasms, although there are few exceptions.

Natural Killer and T-Cell Subsets and the Classification of Peripheral T-Cell and Natural Killer-Cell Neoplasms	
Innate Immune System	**Adaptive Immune System**
Does not require antigen sensitization	Characterized by specificity and memory
NK-cells, NK/T-cells, γδ T-cells	Effector and memory T-cells
Cell-mediated cytotoxicity	Act principally through cytokines and chemokines
Mainly cutaneous and other extranodal sites	Mainly nodal lymphomas
Children and adults	More often in adults
NK, Natural killer.	

Angioimmunoblastic T-Cell Lymphoma

Angioimmunoblastic T-cell lymphoma (AITL) was initially proposed as an abnormal immune reaction or form of atypical lymphoid hyperplasia with a high risk of progression to malignant lymphoma. Because the majority of cases show clonal rearrangements of T-cell receptor genes, it is now regarded as a variant of T-cell lymphoma. The median survival is generally less than 5 years.

AITL presents in adults; most patients have generalized lymphadenopathy, hepatosplenomegaly, skin rash, and prominent constitutional symptoms. There is usually polyclonal hypergammaglobulinemia and other hematologic abnormalities such as Coombs-positive hemolytic anemia. Rituximab has been used in some recent clinical trials, in an attempt to control some of the effects of B-cell hyperactivity in this disease. Patients may also show evidence of immunodeficiency with recurrent opportunistic infections that may ultimately lead to their demise.

The nodal architecture is generally effaced, but peripheral sinuses are often open and even dilated. At low power, there is usually a striking proliferation of high endothelial venules (HEV) with prominent arborization (Fig. 73.11). Follicles are typically regressed, but there is a proliferation of dendritic cells around HEV. The atypical T-cells have clear cytoplasm, and are associated with small lymphocytes, immunoblasts, plasma cells, and histiocytes. The abnormal cells are usually positive for CD3, CD4, CD10, and CD279 (PD-1), a phenotype characteristic of follicular T-helper cells. This relationship is also confirmed by recent gene expression profiling data. CXC-chemokine ligand 13, a chemokine involved in B-cell trafficking into the germinal centers, is also expressed is in AITL.

EBV-positive large B-cell blasts, sometimes with Reed–Sternberg (RS) like features, are nearly always present in the background, and

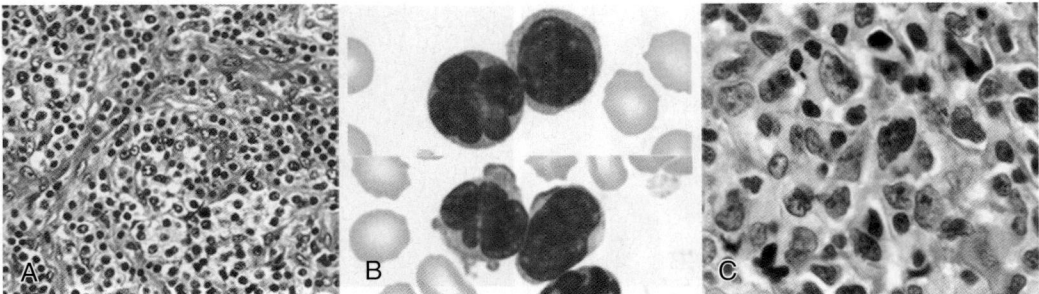

Fig. 73.11 PERIPHERAL T-CELL LYMPHOMAS. In angioimmunoblastic T-cell lymphoma, the lymph node shows effacement with an arborizing vascular proliferation of postcapillary venules and clustered large cells with clear cytoplasm in the background of plasma cells, immunoblasts, and small lymphocytes (A). The peripheral blood in adult T-cell leukemia/lymphoma has classic "flower-cells" (B). Peripheral T-cell lymphoma, not otherwise specified is heterogeneous, but typically there is a mixture of small and large neoplastic T cells (C).

progression to EBV-positive DLBCL has been reported in rare cases. Atypical B-cell proliferations that are negative for EBV also occur, presumably related to the T-helper follicular function of the neoplastic cells in promoting the activation and migration of bystander B cells. However, the exact role of EBV in AITL remains uncertain. Recently recurrent mutations have been reported in AITL; these include mutations in *IDH2*, *TET2*, and *RHOA*.

The biologic spectrum of AITL is greater than previously thought and other entities related to follicular T-helper cells are considered within the same group. Indeed, peripheral T-cell lymphoma (PTCL)-NOS, follicular variant shares some of the underlying genetic changes and has overlapping gene expression profile characteristics. These changes will be reflected in the updated version of the WHO classification.[30]

Adult T-Cell Leukemia/Lymphoma

Adult T-cell leukemia/lymphoma (ATL) is a distinct clinicopathologic entity associated with the retrovirus human T-lymphotropic virus-1 (HTLV-1), which is found clonally integrated in the T cells. HTLV-1 infection is endemic in Southwestern Japan and in the Caribbean basin. The disease has a long latency, and affected individuals are usually exposed to the virus very early in life. The virus may be transmitted in breast milk, and through exposure to blood and blood products. The cumulative incidence of ATL is estimated to be 2.5% among HTLV-1 carriers.

The median age of affected individuals is 45 years. Patients may present with leukemia or with generalized lymphadenopathy. Other clinical findings include lymphadenopathy, hepatosplenomegaly, lytic bone lesions, and hypercalcemia. Cutaneous involvement is seen in the majority of patients. The acute form of the disease is associated with a poor prognosis and a median survival of less than 2 years. Complete remissions may be obtained but the relapse rate is nearly 100%.

Chronic and smoldering forms of the disease are seen less commonly, and are associated with minimal lymphadenopathy. The predominant clinical manifestation is skin rash, with only small numbers of atypical cells in the peripheral blood.

The cytologic spectrum of ATL is extremely diverse (see Fig. 73.11B). The cells are often markedly polylobated, and have been referred to as flower cells. Peripheral blood involvement is very common, but often in the absence of bone marrow disease. Immunophenotypically, the neoplastic cells are positive for mature T cell antigens, such as CD2, CD3, and CD5; they are typically CD4/CD25-positive, a phenotype that resembles regulatory T (Treg) cells. Some cases express FoxP3, but usually in a minority of tumor cells. The function of the tumor cells as Treg cells may correlate with the associated immunodeficiency.

Peripheral T-Cell Lymphomas, Not Otherwise Specified

PTCL, NOS is a diagnosis of exclusion and is admittedly a heterogeneous category with most cases being nodal in origin. Therefore, not unexpectedly the cytologic spectrum is very broad.[30] (see Fig. 73.11C). An inflammatory background is frequent, consisting of eosinophils, plasma cells, and histiocytes. If the epithelioid histiocytes are numerous and clustered, the neoplasm fulfils the criteria for the *lymphoepithelioid cell variant* of PTCL. The *T-zone variant* is composed of small to medium-sized cells that preferentially involve the paracortical regions of the lymph node.

Clinically, PTCL, NOS most often presents in adults with generalized lymphadenopathy, hepatosplenomegaly, and frequent bone marrow involvement. Constitutional symptoms, including fever and night sweats, are common, as is pruritus. The clinical course is aggressive, although complete remissions may be obtained with combination chemotherapy. However, the relapse rate is higher than in aggressive B-cell lymphomas, including DLBCL.

PTCL, NOS, as defined in the WHO classification, remains heterogeneous. It is likely that individual clinicopathologic entities will be delineated in the future from this broad group of malignancies. Thus far immunophenotypic criteria have not been helpful in delineating subtypes. Most cases have a mature T-cell phenotype, and express one of the major subset antigens: CD4 greater than CD8. These are not clonal markers, and antigen expression can change over time. Loss of one of the pan T-cell antigens (CD3, CD5, CD2, or CD7) is seen in 75% of cases, with CD7 most frequently being absent. GEP studies have shown some cases with a profile resembling AITL. Cases with a high proliferation signature appear to have a more aggressive clinical course, but GEP has not led to the delineation of distinctive subtypes as independent entities.

Anaplastic Large Cell Lymphoma, ALK-Positive

Anaplastic large cell lymphoma (ALCL) is characterized by pleomorphic or monomorphic cells, which have a propensity to invade lymphoid sinuses (Fig. 73.12). Because of the sinusoidal location of the tumor cells, and their lobulated nuclear appearance, this disease when first observed was suspected to be of histiocytic origin. A consistent feature is the strong expression of CD30 antigen, a diagnostic hallmark. However, CD30 expression is not specific for ALCL and can be seen in a variety of conditions, including of course, CHL. Systemic ALCL is associated with a characteristic chromosomal translocation, t(2;5)(p23;q35) involving *NPM/ALK* genes, respectively. A number of variant translocations have been identified that involve partners other than *NPM*. All lead to overexpression of *ALK*, although the cellular distribution of ALK varies according to the gene partner.

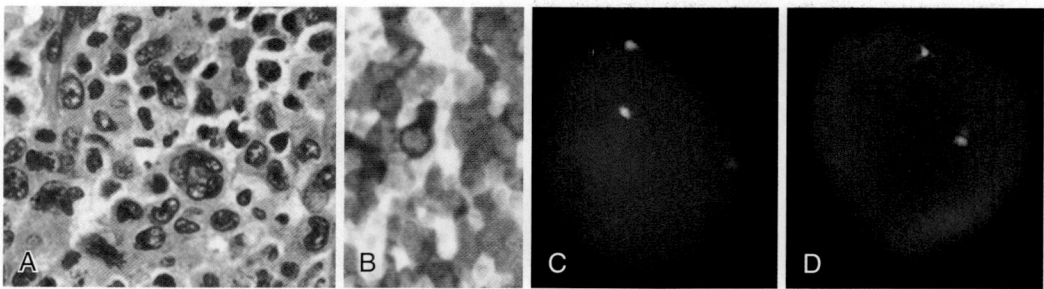

Fig. 73.12 ANAPLASTIC LARGE CELL LYMPHOMA. Anaplastic large cell lymphoma can show a wide spectrum in cell size, and there is a small cell variant in addition to the more typical common form. The cells (A) include "wreath cells" *(center)* and "hallmark cells" *(bottom right)*. (B), The presence of ALK staining with nuclear and cytoplasmic localization *(right)* is associated with the t(2;5). A translocation of ALK can be identified with a break-apart probe that spans *ALK* but is split when *ALK* is translocated to one of a number of partners. A cell with a translocated *ALK* is pictured in (C) and a normal cell in (D). *ALK,* Anaplastic lymphoma kinase.

The cells of classic ALCL have large, often lobulated nuclei with small basophilic nucleoli, so called hallmark cells. The cytoplasm is usually abundant, amphophilic, and there are distinct cytoplasmic borders. A prominent Golgi region is generally visible. Small cell and lymphohistiocytic variants constitute part of the entity, and appear to be associated with a more aggressive clinical course.

The cells exhibit an aberrant phenotype with loss of many of the T-cell associated antigens. Both CD3 and CD5 are negative in greater than 50% of cases. CD2 and CD4 are positive in the majority of cases. CD8 is usually negative. ALCL cells, despite the CD4-positive/CD8-negative phenotype, exhibit positivity for the cytotoxic associated antigens TIA-1, granzyme B, and perforin. In addition, clusterin is generally present in ALCL and represents another useful diagnostic marker. By molecular studies, in most of the cases, a T-cell receptor rearrangement is found, confirming a T-cell origin.

ALCL is most common in children and young adults, with a marked male predominance noted. Although most patients present with nodal disease, a high incidence of extranodal involvement has been reported (involving skin, bone, and soft tissue). Approximately 75% of cases present with advanced-stage and systemic symptoms. Although these lymphomas have an aggressive natural clinical history, they respond well to chemotherapy. Overall survival and disease-free survival are significantly better among ALK-positive versus ALK-negative cases. Both ALK+ and ALK ALCL have a better prognosis than other PTCLs, with a plateau in the survival curve seen in both groups.[31]

Anaplastic Large Cell Lymphoma, ALK-Negative

It has been controversial whether ALCL negative for ALK is a separate entity or part of the spectrum of PTCL, NOS. Part of the controversy relates to the lack of absolute criteria to recognize these cases. They should be morphologically (i.e., sinusoidal and cohesive growth pattern, presence of hallmark cells) and phenotypically similar to ALK+ ALCL, with strong CD30 expression. A cytotoxic phenotype is common but is not essential. They occur in an older age group than the ALK+, and as noted earlier, appear to have a better prognosis than other PTCL, NOS. Recent molecular/cytogenetic studies have identified candidate genes *TP63* and *DUSP22*; the latter is associated with a more favorable outcome. Both ALK+ and ALK ALCL appear to share activation of the JAK/STAT pathway.

Primary Cutaneous Anaplastic Large Cell Lymphoma

The primary cutaneous form of ALCL is closely related to lymphomatoid papulosis, and differs clinically, immunophenotypically, and at the molecular level from the systemic form. Lymphomatoid

papulosis (LYP) and cutaneous ALCL are part of the spectrum of CD30-positive cutaneous T-cell lymphoproliferative diseases. Small lesions are likely to regress. Patients with large tumor masses may develop disseminated disease with lymph node involvement. However, primary cutaneous ALCL is a more indolent disease than other T-cell lymphomas of the skin. Because the skin nodules may show spontaneous regression, usually a period of observation is warranted before the institution of any chemotherapy. Cutaneous ALCL is CD30-positive but ALK-negative, lacking translocations involving the *ALK* gene. However, recent studies have identified rearrangements of *DUSP22* in a subset of cutaneous ALCL.

Mycosis Fungoides/Sézary Syndrome

Mycosis fungoides/Sézary syndrome (MF/SS) are now regarded as separate diseases, but are closely related and often considered together from a clinical and biologic standpoint.[32] Both are primary cutaneous T-cell malignancies derived from mature CD4 positive skin-homing T cells. Skin involvement may be manifested as multiple cutaneous plaques or nodules (Fig. 73.13). SS is characterized by erythroderma and a leukemic phase. Lymphadenopathy is usually not present at presentation and, when identified, is associated with a poor prognosis. In early stages, enlarged lymph nodes may only show changes (Category I). If malignant cells are present in significant numbers and are associated with architectural effacement (Category II or III), the prognosis is significantly worse.

Cytologically, the small cells of MF demonstrate cerebriform nuclei with clumped chromatin, inconspicuous nucleoli, and sparse cytoplasm. Epidermotropism is usually a prominent feature. SS presents with exfoliative erythroderma and circulating cerebriform lymphocytes known as Sezary cells. The typical phenotype is CD2+, CD3+, CD5+, CD4+, and CD8. However, CD8-positive variants of MF have been described, and are more common in children. The absence of CD7 is a constant feature but may also be seen in reactive conditions, and therefore is of limited diagnostic value. Aberrant expression of other T-cell antigens may be seen but mainly occurs in the advanced (tumor) stages. Inactivation of p16 (*CDKN2A*) and *PTEN* has been identified in some cases and may be associated with disease progression.

Subcutaneous Panniculitis-Like T-Cell Lymphoma

Subcutaneous panniculitis-like T-cell lymphoma (SPTCL) usually presents with subcutaneous nodules, primarily affecting the extremities and trunk. The nodules range in size from 0.5 cm to several centimeters in diameter. In its early stages the infiltrate may appear deceptively benign, and lesions are often misdiagnosed as panniculitis. However, histologic progression usually occurs and subsequent

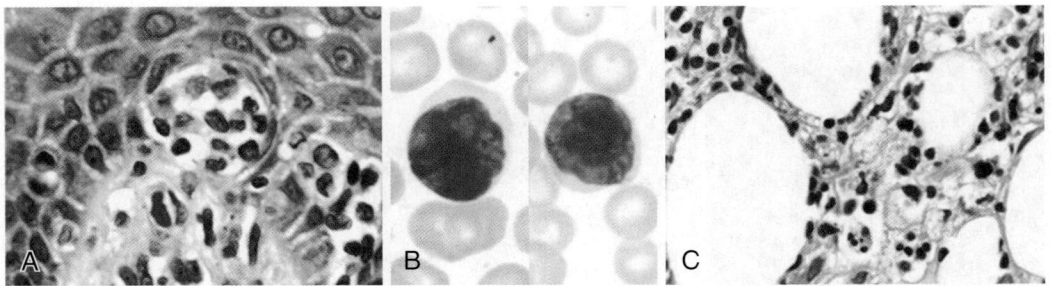

Fig. 73.13 CUTANEOUS T-CELL LYMPHOMAS: MYCOSIS FUNGOIDES/SÉZARY SYNDROME AND SUBCUTANEOUS PANNICULITIS-LIKE T-CELL LYMPHOMA. In mycosis fungoides, there is a dermal infiltrate with some malignant T cells infiltrating into the epithelium (Pautrier microabscesses) (A). Sézary cells with convoluted nuclear folding are seen in (B). The peripheral nuclear outline is fairly rounded, but the internal nuclear detail shows complex nuclear folding giving rise to a convoluted and cerebriform look. A case of subcutaneous panniculitis-like T-cell lymphoma is illustrated and shows an abnormal lymphoid infiltrate in the subcutaneous fat (C). Fat necrosis is usually evident.

biopsies show more pronounced cytologic atypia, permitting the diagnosis of malignant lymphoma.

Atypical lymphoid cells rim individual fat cells. Admixed reactive histiocytes are frequently present, particularly in areas of fat infiltration and destruction. Vascular invasion may be seen in some cases, and necrosis and karyorrhexis are common (see Fig. 73.13C).

The neoplastic cells are CD8-positive T alpha-beta cells, with tumors composed of gamma-delta T-cells now included under primary cutaneous gamma-delta T-cell lymphomas. The cells display an activated cytotoxic immunophenotype (positive for TIA-1, granzyme-B, and perforin). These proteins may be responsible for the cellular destruction seen in these tumors

A hemophagocytic syndrome is less often seen in SPTCL than in panniculitis-like tumors of gamma-delta T-cell derivation, but whenever seen, is associated with an adverse prognosis.[33] Patients present with fever, pancytopenia, and hepatosplenomegaly. The cause of the hemophagocytic syndrome appears related to cytokine production by the malignant cells.

Primary Cutaneous Gamma-Delta T-Cell Lymphoma

Primary cutaneous gamma-delta T-cell lymphoma is considered a distinct entity, which can involve the subcutis, the dermis, or with epidermal infiltration. These are clinically aggressive tumors. The cells have a cytotoxic phenotype, and like normal gamma delta T-cells, lack CD5, are positive for TCR-gamma and express cytotoxic molecules. They may be CD8-positive, or more often, double negative for CD4 and CD8. It is important to rule out MF and LYP before rendering a diagnosis of primary cutaneous gamma-delta T cell lymphoma, since there are newly recognized forms of LYP that share morphologic and phenotypic features. While skin is the most common presenting site, lymphomas of gamma delta T-cell origin can present in other mainly extranodal sites. The cells are invariably EBV-negative, and show clonal rearrangement of T-cell receptor genes.

Primary Cutaneous CD8-Positive Aggressive Epidermotropic Cytotoxic T-Cell Lymphoma and Primary Cutaneous CD4-Positive Small/Medium T-Cell Lymphoproliferative Disorder

Primary cutaneous CD8-positive aggressive epidermotropic cytotoxic T-cell lymphoma is an aggressive cutaneous neoplasm that shares many clinical features with primary cutaneous gamma delta T-cell lymphomas, but is derived from cytotoxic alpha-beta T cells. As the term implies, the neoplastic cells show prominent epidermotropism.

Primary cutaneous CD4-positive small/medium T-cell lymphoproliferative disorder (LPD) most often presents with localized skin lesions. It is associated with an excellent prognosis, and requires only limited localized therapy, unless multiple skin lesions are present. The term LPD rather than lymphoma is used, reflecting the indolent nature of the proliferation. The lesions are rich in B cells, and the proliferating T cells have a T_{FH} phenotype, with clonality usually evident by molecular testing.

Enteropathy-Associated T-Cell Lymphoma

Two variants of Enteropathy-associated T-cell lymphoma (EATL) were recognized in the WHO 2008, EATL Type I and Type II. The classic Type I form of EATL, is associated with either overt or clinically silent gluten-sensitive enteropathy, and is largely seen in patients of European extraction, whereas the Type II form has a more worldwide distribution. In recognition of its distinction from EATL Type I, the proposed term in the revised WHO classification is "monomorphic epitheliotropic intestinal T-cell lymphoma." Patients usually present with abdominal symptoms, including pain, small bowel perforation, and associated peritonitis. The clinical course is aggressive, and most patients have multifocal intestinal disease.[30,34]

In EATL, Type I, the cytologic composition is somewhat varied; the neoplastic cells show prominent invasion of the mucosa and are cytotoxic T cells most often of alpha-beta origin. The cells also express the homing receptor CD103 (HML-1) (Fig. 73.14). Cells with anaplastic features positive for CD30 may be present. In EATL, Type I, the adjacent small bowel usually shows villous atrophy associated with celiac disease. In EATL Type II, (now monomorphic epitheliotropic intestinal T-cell lymphoma), the infiltrate is monomorphic and composed of medium-sized cells with clear cytoplasm showing prominent epitheliotropism. They are CD56-positive, CD8-positive, and most often of gamma-delta T-cell derivation. An association with celiac disease is seen only rarely, and this form of intestinal lymphoma is relatively common in Asia. Both EATL Types I and II share some genetic aberrations, including chromosomal gains on 9q33–34 as well as activating mutations involving the JAK/STAT pathway.

Other PTCL can present with intestinal disease, and should be distinguished from EATL. These include the EBV-positive extranodal T/NK cell lymphomas, PTCL, NOS, and a rare indolent form of T-cell lymphoproliferative disorder of the GI tract.[35]

Hepatosplenic T-Cell Lymphoma

Hepatosplenic T-cell lymphoma (HSTCL) presents with marked hepatosplenomegaly in the absence of lymphadenopathy. The great

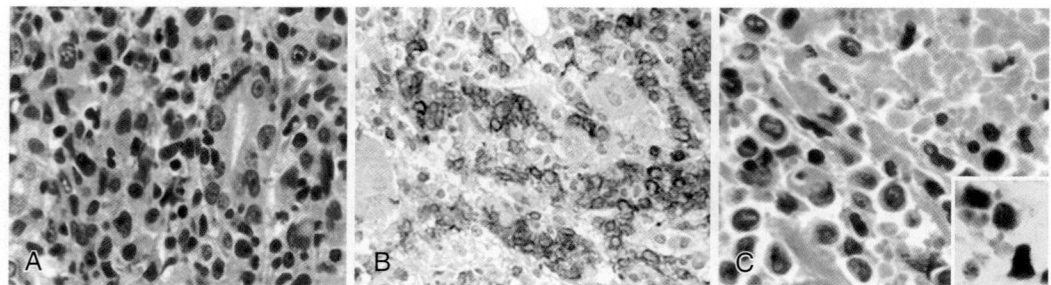

Fig. 73.14 OTHER T-CELL AND NATURAL KILLER-CELL LYMPHOMAS. In enteropathy-associated T-cell lymphoma (A), there is an abnormal T-lymphoid proliferation with infiltration into the gastrointestinal glandular elements *(center right)*. Hepatosplenic gamma delta T-cell lymphoma in the bone marrow is illustrated with a CD2 stain showing the characteristic sinusoidal distribution (B). Extranodal natural killer cell/T-cell lymphoma typically has marked necrosis (C). The malignant cells are Epstein-Barr virus (EBV)–positive by in situ hybridization for EBV encoded RNA *(insert)*. *RNA,* ribonucleic acid.

majority of cases are of gamma-delta T-cell origin. Most patients are male, with a peak incidence in young adults. Although patients may respond initially to chemotherapy, relapse has been seen in the vast majority of cases, and the median survival is less than 3 years. Rare long-term survival has been seen following allogeneic hematopoietic cell transplantation.

The cells of HSTCL are usually moderate in size, with a rim of pale cytoplasm. The nuclear chromatin is loosely condensed, with small inconspicuous nucleoli. The pattern of infiltration mimics the homing pattern of gamma-delta T cells with marked sinusoidal infiltration in liver and spleen. Abnormal cells are usually present in the sinusoids of the bone marrow but may be difficult to identify without immunohistochemical stains. The neoplastic cells also have a phenotype that resembles that of normal resting gamma-delta T cells. They are often negative for both CD4 and CD8, although CD8 may be expressed in some cases. CD56 is typically positive. The neoplastic cells express markers associated with cytotoxic T cells, such as TIA-1. However, perforin and granzyme B are usually negative, suggesting that these cells are not activated. Isochromosome 7q is a consistent cytogenetic abnormality, and is often seen in association with trisomy 8. In addition, activating mutations involving STAT5B and less frequently STAT3 have been described.[36]

Extranodal Natural Killer/T-Cell Lymphoma, Nasal-Type

Extranodal NK/T-cell lymphoma, nasal type, is a distinct clinicopathologic entity highly associated with EBV. It is much more common in Asians than in Europeans.[34] Clusters of the disease also have been reported in Central and South America in individuals of Native American heritage, suggesting that ethnic background i.e., genetic risk factors, may play a role in the pathogenesis of these lymphomas. It affects adults (median age 50) and the most common clinical presentation is a destructive nasal or midline facial lesion. Palatal destruction, orbital swelling, and edema may be prominent. NK/T-cell lymphomas have been reported in other extranodal sites, including skin, soft tissue, testis, upper respiratory tract, and GI tract. The clinical course is usually aggressive, with a slightly improved median survival in patients with localized disease, in which local radiation therapy may be useful.[37] A hemophagocytic syndrome is a common clinical complication, and adversely affects survival.

Extranodal NK/T-cell lymphoma, nasal type, is characterized by a broad cytologic spectrum (see Fig. 73.14C). Although the cells express some T cell-associated antigens, most commonly CD2, other T-cell markers, such as surface CD3, are usually absent. The cells express cytoplasmic CD3, but lack T-cell receptor gene rearrangement. In support of an NK-cell origin the cells are usually CD56-positive, but do not express CD57 or CD16. EBV is positive in 100% of cases by in situ hybridization.

Aggressive NK-cell leukemia is a closely related entity. It presents at a younger age than extranodal NK/T-cell lymphoma, is associated with systemic disease, and a fulminant clinical course. It has a similar phenotype, EBV association, and epidemiology.

There are other EBV+ T-cell and NK-cell proliferations that are seen mainly in children. These include *systemic EBV+ T-cell lymphoma, hydroa vacciniforme-like lymphoma, and mosquito bite allergy,* the latter usually being derived from NK-cells. All are seen most often in Asian children but are also reported in Central and South America, in individuals of Native American origin. The latter two conditions affect mainly the skin and have a more indolent clinical course, whereas the systemic disease has a very aggressive clinical course with survival measured in weeks. Systemic EBV+ T-cell lymphoma may arise in a background of chronic active EBV-infection.

Hodgkin Lymphomas

Hodgkin and non-Hodgkin lymphoma have long been regarded as distinct disease entities based on their differences in pathology, phenotype, clinical features, and response to therapy. It is now accepted that the malignant cell of HL is an altered B cell. Therefore, it is not surprising that both biologic and clinical overlaps should occur between these two lymphoma groups, as also shown by GEP in PMBL and cell lines derived from CHL. Although we have become aware of this closer relationship from the histogenetic point of view (hence the name Hodgkin lymphoma), these disorders are still treated with different modalities.

The diagnosis of CHL depends on the identification of Hodgkin and Reed-Sternberg (HRS) cells in an appropriate inflammatory background composed of small T lymphocytes, plasma cells, histiocytes, and granulocytes (often eosinophils). All cases of CHL share certain immunophenotypic and genotypic features. Neoplastic cells are CD30+, CD15+/−, CD45−, and EMA−. Expression of B-cell–associated antigens is seen in up to 75% of cases. However, when present, CD20 staining is weaker than that seen in normal B cells with variable in intensity among individual tumor cells. CD79a is usually negative. IG and T-cell receptor genes are usually germline, caused by the paucity of tumor cells in the inflammatory background, but using microdissection and polymerase chain reaction (PCR) amplification clonal rearrangement of the Ig genes can generally be shown. In addition, the presence of somatic mutations indicates transit through the germinal center.

Sufficient evidence has emerged in recent years to warrant the recognition of nodular lymphocyte-predominant HL (NLPHL) as a distinct entity. Although it resembles other types of HL in having a minority of putative neoplastic cells on a background of benign inflammatory cells, it differs morphologically, immunophenotypically, and clinically from classic HL. The preferred term of Hodgkin lymphoma over Hodgkin disease reflects current knowledge concerning the nature of the neoplastic cell as a lymphocyte.

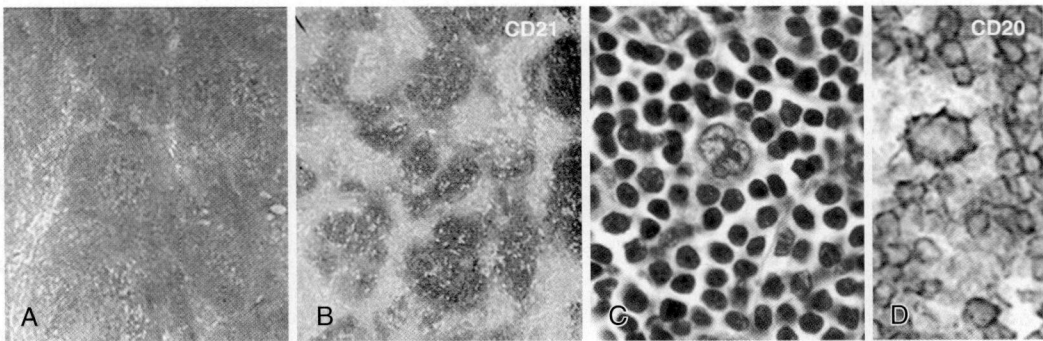

Fig. 73.15 NODULAR LYMPHOCYTE PREDOMINANT HODGKIN LYMPHOMA. Low-power illustration shows vague expansile nodules that efface the lymph node architecture (A). The nodules can be accentuated with a stain for follicular dendritic cells, CD21 (B). The neoplastic cells are the so-called "LP" cells (previously called "L&H" cells or "popcorn" cells) (C). Unlike the neoplastic cells of classic Hodgkin lymphoma, these LP cells stain brightly for CD20 (D) and are typically CD45+, CD30−, and CD15−.

Nodular Lymphocyte-Predominant Hodgkin Lymphoma

NLPHL usually has a nodular growth pattern, with or without diffuse areas; it is rarely purely diffuse (Fig. 73.15). Nodularity may be more easily recognized using immunohistologic stains with anti–B-cell or antifollicular dendritic cell (FDC) antibodies. Progressively transformed germinal centers are often seen in partially involved lymph nodes or other lymph node sites. The atypical cells have vesicular, polylobated nuclei, and small nucleoli. These had been called lymphocytic and/or histiocytic (L&H) cells, or "popcorn" cells, but the term LP cell is now preferred. Although these cells may be very numerous, usually no diagnostic HRS cells are found. The background is predominantly lymphocytes with or without epithelioid histiocyte clusters. Plasma cells are infrequent, and eosinophils and neutrophils are rarely seen. Occasionally sclerosis may cause lesions to resemble nodular sclerosis.

The atypical cells are CD45+-expressing B-cell–associated antigens (CD19, 20, 22, 79a), CDw75+, EMA+/− CD15−, CD30−/+ and usually SIg− by routine techniques, although one study reported light-chain restriction. Neoplastic cells positive for IgD are more often found in young males. J chain has been demonstrated in many cases. Small lymphocytes in the nodules are predominantly B cells with a mantle-zone phenotype. However, numerous T cells are present, with T cells positive for CD57 and PD-1 (CD279) surrounding the LP cells. The proportion of T cells tends to increase over time in sequential biopsies. A prominent meshwork of FDC is present within the nodules. LP cells, when isolated by microdissection, have clonally rearranged Ig genes with evidence of somatic hypermutation.

NLPHL occurs at all ages, in adults more commonly than in children, and in males more than in females. It usually involves peripheral lymph nodes, with sparing of the mediastinum. It is usually localized at diagnosis, but may be rarely disseminated. Survival is long, with or without treatment, for localized cases. However, when disseminated the prognosis is often poor. Patients with advanced stage disease may benefit from treatment regimens used for aggressive B-cell lymphomas. Late relapses have been reported to be more common than in other types of HL; it may be associated with, or progress to, large B-cell lymphoma. Progression to a process resembling T-cell/histiocyte rich large B-cell lymphoma may also been seen, and recent data suggest that these diseases may be different ends of a spectrum, with a close biologic relationship.[38]

Classic Hodgkin Lymphoma, Nodular Sclerosis

This variant is most common in adolescents and young adults, but can occur at any age; female cases equal or exceed those in males. The mediastinum is commonly involved; stage and bulk of disease have prognostic importance. Nodular sclerosis classical Hodgkin lymphoma (NSCHL) is often curable; however, in long-term survivors the risk of secondary malignancies is increased, especially in those receiving both radiation and chemotherapy. NSCHL of the mediastinum is thought to be closely related to PMBL, and both types of tumors can be seen in the same patient, either as composite malignancy, or sequentially.[39]

The tumor has at least a partially nodular pattern, with fibrous bands separating the nodules in most cases (Fig. 73.16). Diffuse areas may be present, as is necrosis. The characteristic cell is the lacunar-type RS cell, which may be very numerous. Diagnostic RS cells are usually also present. The background contains lymphocytes, histiocytes, plasma cells, eosinophils, and neutrophils. It can be graded according to the proportion of the tumor cells and the presence of necrosis: Grades I and II. However, grading is considered optional. The immunophenotype and genotype are characteristic of CHL. However, EBV is infrequently positive, less than 15% of cases.

Classic Hodgkin Lymphoma, Mixed Cellularity

Patients are usually adults; males outnumber females and the stage is often advanced. The course is moderately aggressive but is often curable. Classic Hodgkin lymphoma, mixed cellularity (CHLMC) has a bimodal age distribution, with a peak in young children, and again in older adults. It is often EBV-positive, seen in up to 75% of cases. Both CHLMC and the lymphocyte depleted form can be associated with underlying HIV-infection. The infiltrate is diffuse, without band-forming sclerosis, although fine interstitial fibrosis may be present (see Fig. 73.16C). HRS cells are of the classic type.

Classic Hodgkin Lymphoma, Lymphocyte Depletion

This is the least common variant of CHL and is most common in older people, in HIV-positive individuals, and in nonindustrialized countries. It frequently presents with abdominal lymphadenopathy, spleen, liver, and bone marrow involvement, without peripheral adenopathy. The stage is usually advanced at diagnosis. It shares many features with CHLMC, and appears to represent a continuum with this variant, associated with more frequent neoplastic cells and fewer normal T cells. The infiltrate is diffuse and often appears hypocellular, owing to the presence of diffuse fibrosis and necrosis. Relative to the number of normal lymphocytes there are large numbers of HRS cells and occasional bizarre 'sarcomatous' variants, with a paucity of other inflammatory cells. The immunophenotype is characteristic of CHL. Since the histologic differential diagnosis often includes B or T-large-cell lymphoma or ALCL, immunohistochemistry should be performed in most cases. EBV is positive in the majority of cases.

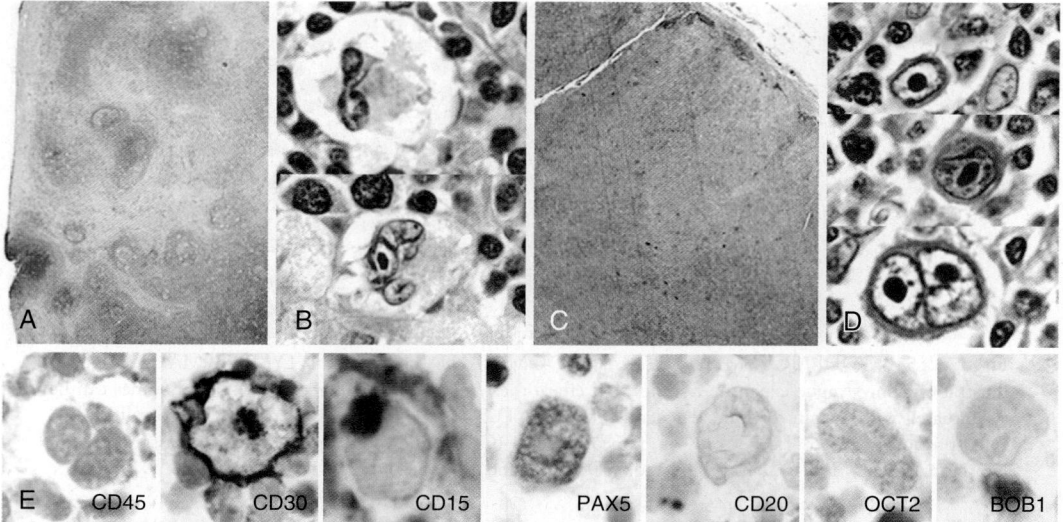

Fig. 73.16 CLASSIC HODGKIN LYMPHOMA, NODULAR SCLEROSIS, AND MIXED CELLULARITY SUBTYPES. In nodular sclerosis Hodgkin Lymphoma, broad bands of sclerosis typically divide the lymph node into cellular nodules (A). The nodules contain a mixed cellular infiltrate and scattered neoplastic cells with lobular nuclei and retracted cytoplasm (B). In mixed cellularity Hodgkin lymphoma, the lymph node is usually diffusely effaced with only fine fibrosis (C). Classic mononuclear, binuclear, and multinuclear Hodgkin and Reed-Sternberg cells are present (D). Both the lacunar and Hodgkin and Reed-Sternberg cells are typically CD45, CD30⁺, CD15⁺, weakly PAX5⁺, and CD20.The B-cell transcription factors OCT2 and BOB1 are variable but often negative (E).

Classic Hodgkin Lymphoma, Lymphocyte-Rich

This type of CHL may be nodular or diffuse and contains relatively infrequent HRS cells, which are of the classic type, rather than the LP variants seen in NLPHL. There are infrequent eosinophils or plasma cells. In the nodular form the HRS cells are seen at the periphery of B cell–rich nodules, mainly in the marginal zone. The neoplastic cells have the immunophenotype of classic HRS cells, but morphologically may be difficult to distinguish from LP cells in some cases. Thus, in the past many cases were misdiagnosed as NLPHL. The genetic features are similar to those of the other variants of CHL. Patients usually present with localized disease, and tend to be older than patients with NLPHL.

REFERENCES

1. Jaffe ES, Harris NL, Stein H, et al: Classification of lymphoid neoplasms: the microscope as a tool for disease discovery. *Blood* 112(12):4384–4399, 2008.
2. Swerdlow SH, Campo E, Pileri SA, et al: The 2016 revision of the World Health Organization classification of lymphoid neoplasms. *Blood* 127(20):2375–2390, 2016.
3. Jares P, Colomer D, Campo E: Molecular pathogenesis of mantle cell lymphoma. *J Clin Invest* 122(10):3416–3423, 2012.
4. Strati P, Shanafelt TD: Monoclonal B-cell lymphocytosis and early-stage chronic lymphocytic leukemia: diagnosis, natural history, and risk stratification. *Blood* 126(4):454–462, 2015.
5. Ganapathi KA, Pittaluga S, Odejide OO, et al: Early lymphoid lesions: conceptual, diagnostic and clinical challenges. *Haematologica* 99(9):1421–1432, 2014.
6. Puente XS, Pinyol M, Quesada V, et al: Whole-genome sequencing identifies recurrent mutations in chronic lymphocytic leukaemia. *Nature* 475(7354):101–105, 2011.
7. Hallek M: Chronic lymphocytic leukemia: 2015 update on diagnosis, risk stratification, and treatment. *Am J Hematol* 90(5):446–460, 2015.
8. Owen RG, Treon SP, Al-Katib A, et al: Clinicopathological definition of Waldenstrom's macroglobulinemia: consensus panel recommendations from the Second International Workshop on Waldenstrom's Macroglobulinemia. *Semin Oncol* 30(2):110–115, 2003.
9. Treon SP, Hunter ZR, Castillo JJ, et al: Waldenstrom macroglobulinemia. *Hematol Oncol Clin North Am* 28(5):945–970, 2014.
10. Soldini D, Valera A, Sole C, et al: Assessment of SOX11 expression in routine lymphoma tissue sections: characterization of new monoclonal antibodies for diagnosis of mantle cell lymphoma. *Am J Surg Pathol* 38(1):86–93, 2014.
11. Horn H, Schmelter C, Leich E, et al: Follicular lymphoma grade 3B is a distinct neoplasm according to cytogenetic and immunohistochemical profiles. *Haematologica* 96(9):1327–1334, 2011.
12. Jaffe ES: Follicular lymphomas: a tapestry of common and contrasting threads. *Haematologica* 98(8):1163–1165, 2013.
13. Salaverria I, Philipp C, Oschlies I, et al: Translocations activating IRF4 identify a subtype of germinal center-derived B-cell lymphoma affecting predominantly children and young adults. *Blood* 118(1):139–147, 2011.
14. Rinaldi A, Mian M, Chigrinova E, et al: Genome-wide DNA profiling of marginal zone lymphomas identifies subtype-specific lesions with an impact on the clinical outcome. *Blood* 117(5):1595–1604, 2011.
15. Watkins AJ, Huang Y, Ye H, et al: Splenic marginal zone lymphoma: characterization of 7q deletion and its value in diagnosis. *J Pathol* 220(4):461–474, 2010.
16. Rossi D, Trifonov V, Fangazio M, et al: The coding genome of splenic marginal zone lymphoma: activation of NOTCH2 and other pathways regulating marginal zone development. *J Exp Med* 209(9):1537–1551, 2012.
17. Morin RD, Mendez-Lago M, Mungall AJ, et al: Frequent mutation of histone-modifying genes in non-Hodgkin lymphoma. *Nature* 476(7360):298–303, 2011.
18. Scott DW, Wright GW, Williams PM, et al: Determining cell-of-origin subtypes of diffuse large B-cell lymphoma using gene expression in formalin-fixed paraffin-embedded tissue. *Blood* 123(8):1214–1217, 2014.
19. Wilson WH, Young RM, Schmitz R, et al: Targeting B cell receptor signaling with ibrutinib in diffuse large B cell lymphoma. *Nat Med* 21(8):922–926, 2015.
20. Xie Y, Pittaluga S, Jaffe ES: The histological classification of diffuse large B-cell lymphomas. *Semin Hematol* 52(2):57–66, 2015.

21. Van Loo P, Tousseyn T, Vanhentenrijk V, et al: T-cell/histiocyte-rich large B-cell lymphoma shows transcriptional features suggestive of a tolerogenic host immune response. *Haematologica* 95(3):440–448, 2010.

22. Vater I, Montesinos-Rongen M, Schlesner M, et al: The mutational pattern of primary lymphoma of the central nervous system determined by whole-exome sequencing. *Leukemia* 29(3):677–685, 2015.

23. Twa DD, Mottok A, Chan FC, et al: Recurrent genomic rearrangements in primary testicular lymphoma. *J Pathol* 236(2):136–141, 2015.

24. Dojcinov SD, Venkataraman G, Pittaluga S, et al: Age-related EBV-associated lymphoproliferative disorders in the Western population: a spectrum of reactive lymphoid hyperplasia and lymphoma. *Blood* 117(18):4726–4735, 2011.

25. Nicolae A, Pittaluga S, Abdullah S, et al: EBV-positive large B-cell lymphomas in young patients: a nodal lymphoma with evidence for a tolerogenic immune environment. *Blood* 126(7):863–872, 2015.

26. Valera A, Balague O, Colomo L, et al: IG/MYC rearrangements are the main cytogenetic alteration in plasmablastic lymphomas. *Am J Surg Pathol* 34(11):1686–1694, 2010.

27. Steidl C, Gascoyne RD: The molecular pathogenesis of primary mediastinal large B-cell lymphoma. *Blood* 118(10):2659–2669, 2011.

28. Robbiani DF, Deroubaix S, Feldhahn N, et al: Plasmodium infection promotes genomic instability and AID-dependent B cell lymphoma. *Cell* 162(4):727–737, 2015.

29. Swerdlow SH: Diagnosis of 'double hit' diffuse large B-cell lymphoma and B-cell lymphoma, unclassifiable, with features intermediate between DLBCL and Burkitt lymphoma: when and how, FISH versus IHC. *Hematology Am Soc Hematol Educ Program* 2014(1):90–99, 2014.

30. Attygalle AD, Cabecadas J, Gaulard P, et al: Peripheral T-cell and NK-cell lymphomas and their mimics; taking a step forward—report on the lymphoma workshop of the XVIth meeting of the European Association for Haematopathology and the Society for Hematopathology. *Histopathology* 64(2):171–199, 2014.

31. Vose J, Armitage J, Weisenburger D: International peripheral T-cell and natural killer/T-cell lymphoma study: pathology findings and clinical outcomes. *J Clin Oncol* 26(25):4124–4130, 2008.

32. Hwang ST, Janik JE, Jaffe ES, et al: Mycosis fungoides and Sezary syndrome. *Lancet* 371(9616):945–957, 2008.

33. Willemze R, Jansen PM, Cerroni L, et al: Subcutaneous panniculitis-like T-cell lymphoma: definition, classification, and prognostic factors: an EORTC Cutaneous Lymphoma Group Study of 83 cases. *Blood* 111(2):838–845, 2008.

34. Swerdlow SH, Jaffe ES, Brousset P, et al: Cytotoxic T-cell and NK-cell Lymphomas: Current Questions and Controversies. *Am J Surg Pathol* 38(10):e60–e71, 2014.

35. Perry AM, Warnke RA, Hu Q, et al: Indolent T-cell lymphoproliferative disease of the gastrointestinal tract. *Blood* 122(22):3599–3606, 2013.

36. Nicolae A, Xi L, Pittaluga S, et al: Frequent STAT5B mutations in gammadelta hepatosplenic T-cell lymphomas. *Leukemia* 28(11):2244–2248, 2014.

37. Au WY, Weisenburger DD, Intragumtornchai T, et al: Clinical differences between nasal and extranasal natural killer/T-cell lymphoma: a study of 136 cases from the International Peripheral T-Cell Lymphoma Project. *Blood* 113(17):3931–3937, 2009.

38. Hartmann S, Doring C, Jakobus C, et al: Nodular lymphocyte predominant Hodgkin lymphoma and T cell/histiocyte rich large B cell lymphoma - endpoints of a spectrum of one disease? *PLoS ONE* 8(11):e78812, 2013.

39. Harris NL: Shades of gray between large B-cell lymphomas and Hodgkin lymphomas: differential diagnosis and biological implications. *Mod Pathol* 26(Suppl 1):S57–S70, 2013.

CHAPTER 74

ORIGIN OF HODGKIN LYMPHOMA

Ralf Küppers

INTRODUCTION

More than 150 years ago, Thomas Hodgkin described several cases of a lymphoproliferative disease, later named Hodgkin disease. For a long time this malignancy, now called *Hodgkin lymphoma* (HL), has been one of the most enigmatic forms of lymphomas. This is due to several key features of the disease: First, the pathognomonic and suspected tumor cells of HL, the mononuclear Hodgkin and the bi- or multinucleated large Reed-Sternberg cells, are very rare in the tumor tissue, often accounting for only about 1% of the cells. Thus the molecular analysis of these cells was hampered until methods became available to isolate these cells by microdissection from tissue sections. Second, the Hodgkin and Reed-Sternberg (HRS) cells have a very unusual immunophenotype that does not resemble any normal cell in the hematopoietic system. Therefore immunophenotyping, which was very informative in revealing the cellular derivation of most other lymphoid malignancies, did not help to uncover the cellular origin of HRS cells. Third, only a few cell lines could be established from patients with HL, these lines were rather heterogeneous, and for hardly any of these lines was the derivation from the HRS cells in the patient unequivocally shown. Hence it was initially difficult to draw firm conclusions from the study of such lines. Although HL still harbors many secrets, exciting novel insights into the cellular origin of the HRS cells and the pathogenetic processes in their generation have been obtained in recent years, which will be discussed in this chapter.

CLASSIFICATION OF HODGKIN LYMPHOMA

HL is subdivided into classical HL, which accounts for about 95% of cases, and nodular lymphocyte predominant HL (NLPHL). The tumor cells are called *HRS cells* in classical HL and *lymphocyte predominant (LP)* cells in NLPHL (until recently the tumor cells in NLPHL were called *lymphocytic and histiocytic [L&H] cells*). Classical HL and NLPHL differ in the histologic picture, the morphology and immunophenotype of the tumor cells, and multiple clinical features. Classical HL is further subdivided into four subforms: nodular sclerosis, mixed cellularity, lymphocyte-rich classical, and lymphocyte depletion HL. Again, differences in the histologic picture and HRS cell morphology are the basis for this subtyping (see Chapter 73 for a detailed description).

B-cell Development and Differentiation

Because we now know that HRS and LP cells are derived from B cells (see later), a brief outline of B-cell development and differentiation is given first. B cells are generated in the bone marrow from hematopoietic stem cells in a multistep developmental process. The key determinant for B-cell development is the generation of a functional B-cell receptor (BCR) that is composed of two identical immunoglobulin (Ig) heavy chains and two identical light chains, the latter of which can be of the κ or λ type. B-cell development is initiated when common lymphoid progenitors undergo gene rearrangements at the Ig gene heavy chain locus. The variable part of the antibody heavy chain is composed of three gene segments: variable (V), diversity (D), and joining (J). First, a randomly selected D_H gene segment

is rearranged to one J_H gene segment. In the next step, a V_H gene segment is rearranged to a D_H-J_H joint. A heavy chain can be expressed and the developmental stage of a pre-B cell is reached if the rearrangement is in-frame and productive. In the next step, V_κ to J_κ rearrangements occur to generate a κ light chain. If this is not successful, V gene rearrangement processes take place at the λ light chain locus. B cells expressing a functional (and nonautoreactive) BCR are released into the periphery and express their BCR as IgM and IgD receptors—that is, two different classes of the heavy chain constant region. The first D_H-J_H rearrangements are not completely specific for B-lineage cells, but $V_H D_H J_H$ rearrangements and light chain gene rearrangements are highly specific for B cells. Thus their detection in a cell unequivocally defines that cell as a B cell. Moreover, because of the availability of multiple V, D, and J gene segments and additional diversity generated at the joining sites of the rearranging gene segments, a V(D)J rearrangement (in particular for the heavy chain locus) is unique for each B cell and thus can be used as a clonal marker for B cells deriving from the same mature B cell.

If B cells are activated through binding of antigen to their BCR and through cognate help from T-helper cells, the cells undergo a T-dependent immune response in specific histologic structures, the germinal centers (GC), in lymph nodes or other secondary lymphoid organs. In these follicles, activated B cells undergo massive clonal expansion and further diversify their BCR through two processes: somatic hypermutation and class switching. The process of somatic hypermutation introduces point mutations and some deletions and duplications at a very high rate into the Ig heavy and light chain V region genes. This randomly modifies amino acids in the V regions, and in a selection process involving follicular dendritic cells and follicular T-helper cells, B cells expressing mutated BCR with increased affinity to the stimulating antigen are positively selected, whereas B cells acquiring unfavorable mutations undergo apoptosis within the GC microenvironment (Fig. 74.1). Unfavorable mutations include clearly destructive mutations, such as nonsense mutations and deletions or duplications causing reading frame-shifts that prevent expression of a BCR as such. Other disadvantageous replacement mutations still allow BCR expression, but reduce the affinity to the antigen. After multiple rounds of proliferation, mutation, and selection, positively selected B cells expressing a high-affinity BCR differentiate into long-lived memory B cells or plasma cells and exit the GC. Many GC B cells also undergo class switching before they are selected into the memory or plasma cell pool. In class switching, the originally expressed Cμ and Cδ heavy chain constant region genes (encoding IgM and IgD, respectively) are replaced by downstream located Cγ, Cα, or Cε genes, encoding IgG, IgA, and IgE heavy chains, respectively, so that antibodies with altered effector functions are generated. At all stages of their development, B lineage cells are selected for expression of the appropriate BCR, and cells failing this selection are eliminated.

Cellular Origin of Lymphocyte Predominant Cells in Nodular Lymphocyte Predominant Hodgkin Lymphoma

LP cells in NLPHL express multiple typical B cell markers, such as the surface molecules CD20 and CD79 and the transcription factors PAX5, OCT-2, and BOB1 (Table 74.1).[1] LP cells mostly lack expression of markers of other hematopoietic cell lineages, thus their

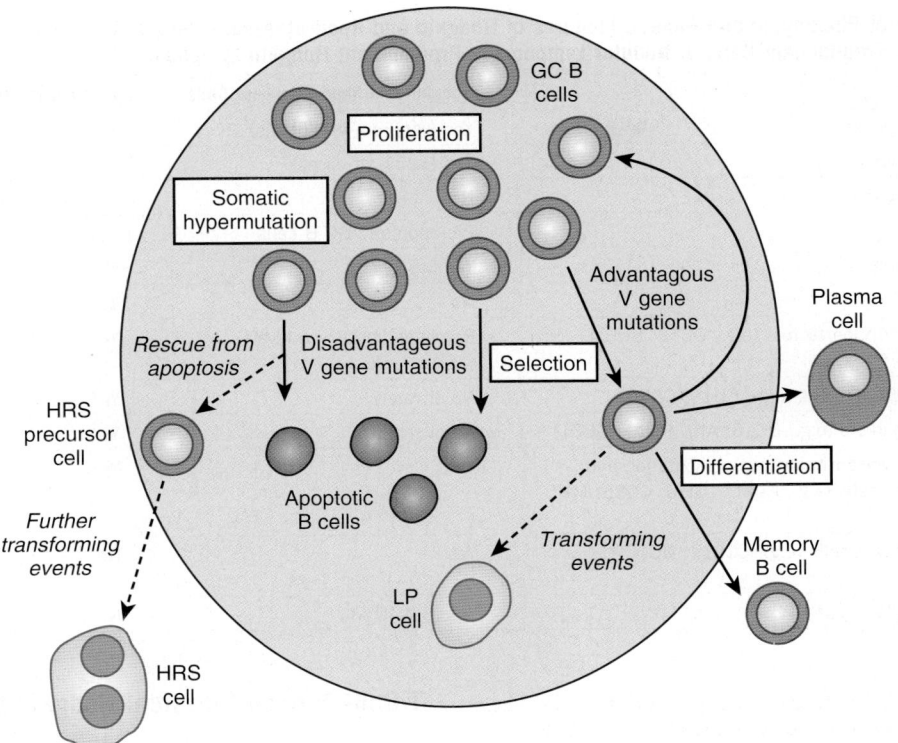

Fig. 74.1 THE GERMINAL CENTER REACTION AND A SCENARIO FOR HODGKIN AND REED-STERNBERG AND LYMPHOCYTE PREDOMINANT CELL DERIVATION. Antigen-activated B cells that receive costimulatory signals from T-helper cells establish germinal center (GC) reactions in T-dependent humoral immune responses. In the GC, the activated B cells undergo massive clonal expansion in the dark zone. The proliferating GC B cells are called *centroblasts*. In the centroblasts, the process of somatic hypermutation is activated, which introduces somatic mutations at a very high rate into rearranged Ig V genes. Centroblasts migrate into the light zone and become resting centrocytes. Centrocytes are then selected based on their BCR. Most Ig V gene mutations will be disadvantageous (e.g., when they cause premature stop codons or lead to amino acid changes that reduce the affinity of the BCR to the immunizing antigen) and will cause apoptotic death of the respective B cells. GC B cells acquiring affinity-increasing mutations will be positively selected by interaction with T-helper cells and follicular dendritic cells (not shown). Positively selected centrocytes may either return to the dark zone for further rounds of proliferation, mutation, and selection, or they differentiate into memory B cells or plasma cells and exit the GC. LP cells of NLPHL express functional Ig V genes and proliferate in a follicular microenvironment resembling GC. Thus these cells are likely derived from selected GC B cells. HRS cells in classical HL often carry destructive Ig V gene mutations, indicating that they derive from GC B cells that normally would have undergone apoptosis (i.e., preapoptotic GC B cells). Initial transforming events in HRS cell pathogenesis might have occurred already at a pre–GC B cell differentiation stage, or they might happen in the GC. In EBV-positive cases, EBV is a good candidate for a factor that allows GC B cells with destructive Ig V gene mutations to escape from apoptosis.

immunophenotype suggests a B-cell origin. Moreover, LP cells are located in follicular structures in close association with follicular dendritic cells and GC-type T-helper cells, suggesting a close relationship with GC B cells. Indeed, LP cells express the transcription factor BCL6, the main regulator of the GC B cell differentiation program. They also express activation-induced cytidine deaminase (AID), an enzyme that regulates somatic hypermutation and class switching in GC B cells. Thus all of these phenotypic features point to a GC B cell origin of LP cells (Table 74.1), and this was further corroborated at the genetic level when clonally rearranged and productive Ig V region genes were amplified from isolated LP cells. These rearrangements were always somatically mutated. In some cases, intraclonal diversity of V region genes was observed, indicating ongoing somatic hypermutation during clonal expansion. Therefore the Ig V gene analysis further strongly supported a GC B cell origin of LP cells (Fig. 74.1). The detection of the same V gene rearrangements in all LP cells of a given NLPHL case was also important because this firmly established for the first time the monoclonality of the LP cells, a hallmark for tumor cells. A gene expression profiling study of primary LP cells indicated that LP cells have partly downregulated a fraction

of typical B cell genes and that their gene expression pattern indicates a relationship to late GC B cells on the way to becoming post-GC memory B cells.[2]

Cellular Origin of Hodgkin and Reed-Sternberg Cells in Classical Hodgkin Lymphoma

As mentioned earlier, HRS cells show a peculiar immunophenotype that does not resemble any normal hematopoietic cell type. HRS cells express markers of different cell lineages in a fraction or even most cases, including B cell genes (e.g., PAX5, IRF4), T cell genes (e.g., NOTCH-1, GATA3), natural killer cell genes (ID2), myeloid genes (e.g., CD15, CSF1R), and dendritic cell markers (e.g., CCL17, fascin, restin) (Table 74.1).[1,3,4] Therefore immunohistochemical studies could not resolve the cellular origin of HRS cells. In addition, the first cell lines established from patients with HL and presumed to be derived from HRS cells were either of B-cell origin, T-cell, or nonlymphoid origin (discussed in further detail later). The origin of HRS cells was finally clarified when HRS cells microdissected from

TABLE 74.1 Comparison of Phenotypic and Genetic Features of Hodgkin and Reed-Sternberg Cells of Classical Hodgkin Lymphoma and Lymphocyte Predominant Cells of Nodular Lymphocyte Predominant Hodgkin Lymphoma

Feature	Hodgkin and Reed-Sternberg Cells	Lymphocyte Predominant Cells
Somatically mutated Ig V genes	Yes (very rare exceptions)	Yes
Crippling Ig V gene mutations	Yes (>25% of cases)	No
Ongoing somatic hypermutation	No	Yes (moderately)
Presumed cellular origin	Pre-apoptotic GC B cells	Positively selected, mutating GC B cells
Rare cases with a T-cell origin	Yes (<5%)	No
B-cell receptor expression	No	Yes
Expression of B-cell transcription factors (e.g., OCT2, BOB.1, PU.1, PAX5, E2A)	Rarely and/or at low levels	Yes
Expression of B-cell surface antigens (e.g., CD19, CD20)	No or rarely	Yes
Expression of GC B cell markers (e.g., BCL6, AID, HGAL, GCET)	No or rarely	Yes
Expression of molecules involved in antigen presentation and interaction with T-helper cells (e.g., CD40, CD80, CD86, MHC class II)	Yes	Yes
Expression of markers of nonB cells (e.g., CCL17, NOTCH1, GATA3, ID2, CSFR1)	Yes	No
EBV infection of tumor cells	Yes (30–40%)	No

tissue sections were analyzed for rearranged Ig V region genes. These studies revealed that HRS cells in nearly all cases carry clonal Ig heavy and light chain gene rearrangements.[1,5] Because such rearrangements are highly specific for B cells, this established their B-cell nature. Moreover, with rare exceptions, the rearranged V region genes were highly mutated, pointing to a derivation from GC or post-GC B cells.[1,5] Intraclonal V gene diversity was not observed, showing that the process of somatic hypermutation is no longer active in these cells. There is also indication that many HRS cell clones underwent class-switch recombination, a further antigen-driven and B cell–specific process. Thus, these genetic features of the rearranged Ig genes unequivocally demonstrate that the HRS cells are derived from mature B cells that had been activated by antigen. Although some initial studies reported polyclonality of HRS cells, these results could not be verified, and additional analyses firmly established the monoclonality of the HRS cells in a given case.

Surprisingly, in about a quarter of the cases of classical HL, the Ig V gene rearrangements carried clearly destructive mutations that rendered originally functional V region genes nonfunctional.[1,5] Such "crippling" mutations included deletions and insertions causing loss of the correct reading frame, as well as nonsense mutations. As discussed earlier, destructive mutations regularly happen in mutating GC B cells, but this normally results very efficiently in the removal of the cells by apoptosis. Thus, it is highly likely that the GC B cells that acquired the destructive mutations already carried some transforming events that allowed them to escape apoptosis (Fig. 74.1). Of note, most disadvantageous mutations that cause apoptosis of normal GC B cells are likely replacement mutations that reduce affinity to the antigen or interfere with the proper folding and/or pairing of the Ig heavy and light chains. These mutations cannot be easily recognized by looking at the V gene sequences. Thus, the clearly crippling mutations likely represent only the "tip of the iceberg," and we have speculated that HRS cells, as a rule, derive from the pool of pre-apoptotic GC B cells (Fig. 74.1).[1,5] Rare cases of classical HL with unmutated V region genes have also been described. In such cases, the HRS cells may stem from pre-GC B cells. However, because GC B cells acquire their apoptosis proneness upon entering the GC even before starting to undergo hypermutation, it is also conceivable that such cases may originate from GC founder cells.

Decisive steps in HL pathogenesis, therefore, become effective or take place in GC B cells. Thus, although some final transforming events may well occur when HRS precursor cells have already left the GC microenvironment, for the reasons discussed earlier, classical HL is considered as a GC B cell–derived malignancy.

T Cell–Derived Classical Hodgkin Lymphoma

The observation that in a fraction of cases the HRS cells express several T cell markers (e.g., CD3, granzyme B, perforin, T cell intracellular antigen 1) prompted studies aimed to clarify whether in such cases the HRS cells might derive from T cells. Analysis of HRS cells from several cases with T cell marker expression showed that most of these cases nevertheless are B cell–derived. However, several cases were identified that lacked Ig V gene rearrangements and that showed clonal T-cell receptor gene rearrangements.[6,7] Thus, these cases have a T cell origin. Because the cellular origin of a lymphoma clone is a key factor for current lymphoma classification, it is a matter of debate whether lymphomas with HRS cells of T cell origin should be called *HL* or whether they should be considered a rare, separate type of T-cell lymphoma. Given that these cases are very rare (likely accounting for less than 5% of classical HL) because it is currently not possible to identify them by immunohistochemistry, and because it is unclear whether such cases differ in their clinical behavior from B cell–derived classical HL, there is currently no easy way to resolve this issue. Notably, in gene expression studies of HL cell lines, HDLM-2 (a T cell–derived HL cell line) clustered more closely to B cell–derived HL cell lines than to other T-cell lymphoma lines, suggesting that B cell– and T cell–derived HRS cells have a similar gene expression pattern.

Hodgkin Lymphoma Cell Lines

Tumor cell lines are valuable tools for detailed genetic, biochemical, and functional studies of a malignancy. Thus, there have been many attempts to establish such lines from patients with HL. However, this has proved to be a very difficult task, and less than 10 HL cell lines exist. A main reason for the difficulty in growing HRS or LP cells in culture is most likely their dependence on survival signals from the cellular microenvironment in the disease-affected lymph nodes. Of note, all of the existing HL lines are derived from patients at end-stage and were not established from lymph nodes, but rather from peripheral blood, bone marrow, or pleural effusions. This suggests that only when the HRS cells have become independent from the lymph node microenvironment in the patient do they also have a chance to survive in suspension culture. The existing and available HL lines are L428, L540, L591, L1236, KM-H2, HDLM-2, UHO-1, SUP-HD1, and DEV (Table 74.2). Most lines are of B-cell origin, but HDLM2 and L540 are T cell–derived. L591 is the only HL line that is Epstein-Barr

	TABLE 74.2	Characteristics of Hodgkin Lymphoma Cell Lines[a]			
Cell Line	Hodgkin Lymphoma Subtype	Cellular Origin	Known Genetic Lesions in Oncogenes or Tumor Suppressor Genes	Remarks	
L428	Classical	B cell	B2M, NFKBIA, NFKBIE, PTPN1, SOCS1, TP53		
L540	Classical	T cell	PTPN1		
L591	Classical	B cell		Only EBV-positive line	
L1236	Classical	B cell	CD95, PTPN1, SOCS1, TNFAIP3, TP53	Only line with proven origin from HRS cells in patient	
KM-H2	Classical	B cell	CIITA (translocation), CYLD, NFKBIA, TNFAIP3		
HDLM-2	Classical	T cell	SOCS1, TNFAIP3, TNFSF7, TNFSF9, TP53, UTX		
UHO-1	Classical	B cell	PTPN1, TNFAIP3, TRAF3		
SUP-HD1	Classical	B cell	PTPN1, PTPN2, TNFAIP3		
DEV	NLPHL	B cell	B2M, BCL6 (translocation), SOCS1		

[a]A few additional lines have been published (HO, ZO, HD-70, HKB-1), but these have not been used in published studies in recent years, so it is unclear to the author whether they still exist, and very little is known about their phenotypic, functional, and genetic features.

virus (EBV)–positive. Among primary cases of classical HL, approximately 30% to 40% show EBV infection of the HRS cells (see further details later). Notably, L591 cells do not have the typical EBV gene expression pattern of primary EBV-infected HRS cells, which should be kept in mind when using this line for gene expression or functional studies. The DEV line was originally reported as being derived from a case of classical HL, but subsequent more detailed phenotypic and gene expression studies indicated that this is indeed the only existing cell line from a patient with NLPHL. Although the phenotype and genotype of these lines fits well with their presumed origin from HRS cells (or LP cells in the case of DEV), L1236 is the only cell line that the derivation from the HRS cell clone of the patient from which it was established was unequivocally proven. In 1998 a line from a pediatric patient with HL was established (HKB-1), but no further studies with this line were reported. Originally, the CO line was also published as an HL cell line. However, later studies showed that this line represents a cell culture contamination. Also the HD-Myz line was for a long time considered to be a classical HL cell line. However, it was later discovered that the phenotype of the line differs in key aspects from the phenotype of the primary HRS cells of the respective patient. Even more important, HD-Myz lacks Ig- and T-cell receptor gene rearrangements and is presumably of myeloid origin. Considering that all informative HL cases studied in detail for a lymphoid origin have turned out to be B cell–derived, or in rare cases T cell–derived, the nonlymphoid origin of HD-Myz argues against its derivation from HRS cells; thus this line should no longer be used as a model for HL.

Although the HL cell lines are a valuable (and practically the only) tool for functional studies with HRS cells, it needs to be taken into consideration that the cells are adapted to growth in suspension culture in the absence of their normal microenvironment. Indeed, a comparison of the gene expression pattern of primary HRS cells and classical HL cell lines revealed more than one thousand differentially expressed genes, including many genes regulating the extracellular matrix, proliferation, and chemokine production and signaling.[8]

Relationship Between Hodgkin Cells and Reed-Sternberg Cells

The population of HRS cells is always composed of a mixture of mononuclear Hodgkin cells and bi- or multinucleated Reed-Sternberg cells. It is thus an intriguing question how these two types of cells are related to each other. It was proposed that fusion of two independent cells might be involved in the generation of Reed-Sternberg cells from Hodgkin cells. It was also discussed whether the whole HRS cell clone could derive from a cell fusion (e.g., a fusion of a B cell with a non-B cell). Such a scenario was attractive because it might

have provided an explanation for the mixed immunophenotype and the usually aneuploid karyotype of the HRS cells. However, generation of the HRS cell clone through fusion of two separate cells was excluded by molecular studies.[9] Indeed, there is now firm evidence from studies of HL cell lines that Reed-Sternberg cells develop from mononuclear Hodgkin cells through a process of incomplete cytokinesis.[10] When Hodgkin cells attempt to undergo cell division, the final separation of the daughter cells often fails, and these cells undergo refusion, giving rise to a binucleated Reed-Sternberg cell.[10] Reed-Sternberg cells have little further proliferative potential, so that the mononuclear Hodgkin cells are the principal proliferative compartment of the HRS cell clone.

Potential Hodgkin and Reed-Sternberg Precursor or Stem Cells

Another interesting question is whether the rare CD30[+] HRS cells represent the whole tumor cell clone in the HL tissue or whether further tumor clone members are present among the smaller, CD30[–] cells in the microenvironment. In a single-cell Ig V gene analysis of EBV-positive HRS cells and EBV-infected CD30-negative cells, it was found that the HRS cells and the small CD30[–] EBV-infected B cells carried distinct V gene rearrangements in nearly all instances.[11] Because EBV infection of HRS cells is a clonal event, so that in EBV[+] HL cases all members of the tumor clone should carry the virus, this finding was taken as an argument that the HRS cell clone does not have additional members among CD30-negative lymphocytes.

In several types of tumors, cancer stem cells were identified. These cells are defined as rare cells that have a particular proliferative potential and that sustain the tumor clone, whereas the bulk of the tumor clone lacks the potential to regrow to a full tumor. One study described the existence of HRS precursor cells in HL that fulfill at least some key features of cancer stem cells. In that work, it was reported that CD20[+]BCR[+]CD30[–] cells belonging to the HRS cell clone exist in the peripheral blood of patients with HL and that these cells express the stem cell marker aldehyde dehydrogenase.[12] However, this finding was criticized because the markers for a clonal relationship between the HRS and non-HRS cells were unreliable and even argued, in part, against a relationship of the cells.[13] Moreover, a previous highly sensitive study that searched for HRS clone members in the peripheral blood failed to identify such cells.[14] Thus there is currently no convincing evidence for the existence of CD20[+]BCR[+] HRS stem cells. In any case, it needs to be considered that HRS cells carry clonal and somatically mutated Ig V gene rearrangements; thus if HRS stem cells exist, they must be mature GC-derived B cells that carry the same Ig gene rearrangements and mutation pattern as the HRS cells.

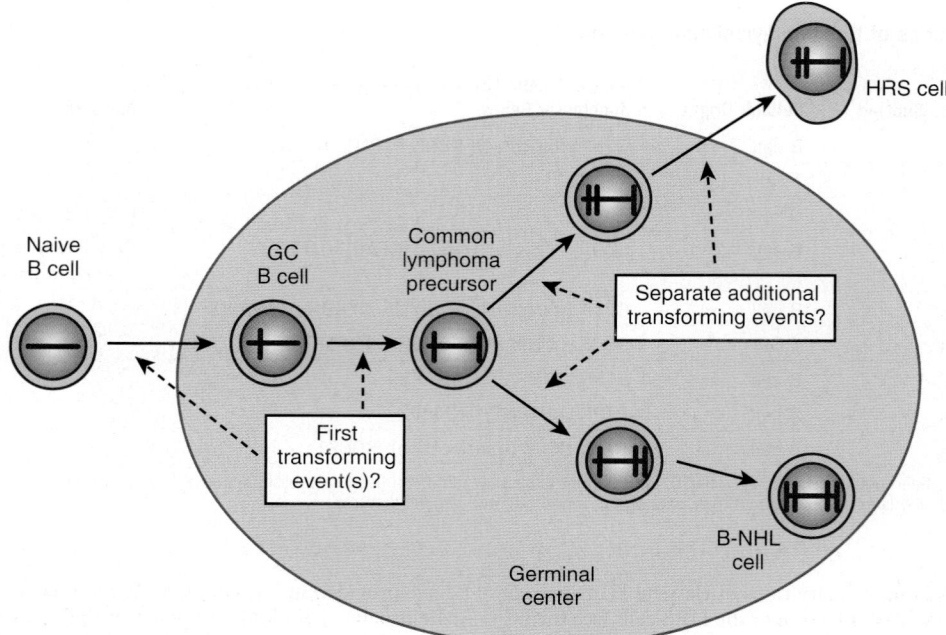

Fig. 74.2 SCENARIO FOR THE GENERATION OF COMPOSITE LYMPHOMAS. Composite lymphomas are very rare combinations of two distinct lymphomas, often a classical HL and an NHL. Detailed molecular analysis of rearranged Ig V genes in several combined HL and B-cell derived NHL revealed that, in most instances, the two lymphomas are clonally related. Notably, the pattern of both shared and distinct V gene mutations in the majority of these cases revealed that the two lymphomas share a common precursor, but developed separately from this precursor. The direct clonal relationship of HRS cells with typical GC B cell–derived NHL is a further strong argument for a GC derivation of HRS cells. The horizontal line within the cells indicates an Ig V region gene; the vertical lines indicate somatic Ig V gene mutations. *(Modified from Bräuninger A, Hansmann ML, Strickler JG, et al: Identification of common germinal center B-cell precursors in two patients with both Hodgkin's disease and non-Hodgkin's lymphoma.* New Engl J Med *340:1239, 1999.)*

The issue of potential subpopulations among the HRS cell clone with specific features in terms of proliferative potential and chemotherapy resistance was also addressed by searching for *side population cells,* which are defined as cells that extrude the Hoechst dye 33342, usually because they express drug transporters of the ABC family, such as the multidrug resistance 1 gene. In several types of tumors, side population cells were shown to share features with cancer stem cells (e.g., increased proliferative potential and chemotherapy resistance). Side population cells were indeed detected at low frequency (about 0.5% of cells) in some HL cell lines, and these cells showed increased resistance to chemotherapeutic drugs.[15,16] The side population cells had the phenotype of small Hodgkin cells and they were positive for CD30 and negative for CD19 and CD20. Hence these cells are different from the cells identified earlier as potential HRS stem cells. Notably, side population cells were able to reestablish the full HRS cell clone upon subcloning. However, not all HL cell lines showed side population cells,[15,16] arguing against a general role of these cells in the maintenance of the HRS cell clone. Moreover, although side population cells were also identified in cell suspensions of HL lymph nodes, it remains to be clarified whether these cells belong to the HRS cell clone. Thus, there are exciting developments regarding the potential existence of subpopulations among the HRS cell clones with specific biologic features, but additional studies are needed to characterize these cells and reveal their relevance for the HRS clone in vivo.

Lessons From Composite Lymphomas

Composite lymphomas are very rare lymphomas in which two distinct lymphomas, often an HL and a non-Hodgkin lymphoma (NHL), occur in the same patient. In a strict definition of composite lymphoma, this happens concurrently, but there are also cases where an HL may occur either before or after an NHL in the same patient. There are a few cases where the two lymphomas are not related to each other and hence represent the chance occurrence of two unrelated malignancies developing in parallel in a patient. However, in most composite and sequential HL and NHL that have been molecularly studied for their clonal relationship, it was found that the lymphomas share a common origin, even in instances where sequential lymphomas occurred several years apart from each other.[17] The detailed study of the rearranged Ig V genes of such cases revealed that although, in many cases, the clonally related V region genes of the lymphomas share a number of somatic mutations, there are often additional mutations that were present only in the HRS cells and others only in the NHL B cells.[17] This showed that the two lymphomas have a common precursor, most likely a mutating GC B cell, and that the two lymphomas most likely developed from two distinct members of the GC B cell clone (Fig. 74.2). Thus these composite lymphomas usually do not represent the transformation of one lymphoma into the other but, rather, the parallel development of the two malignant clones from a common, premalignant precursor cell. It is likely that some transforming events were already present in the common precursor, but distinct daughter cells of this GC B cell later acquired different mutations, leading to the generation of the two distinct B-cell malignancies (Fig. 74.2). Therefore composite lymphomas are intriguing models to study the multistep transformation process in lymphomagenesis. In initial studies of several composite lymphomas for shared and distinct transforming events, examples for such genetic lesions were indeed identified.

A further important aspect of the molecular studies of composite lymphomas is that they provide further evidence for the derivation of HRS cells in classical HL from GC B cells, because the clonal relationship with shared and distinct somatic Ig V gene mutations of an HRS cell clone and a typical GC B cell–derived lymphoma (e.g., follicular lymphoma or diffuse large B-cell lymphoma) strongly supports a common GC B-cell origin of both malignancies.

The Role of Epstein-Barr Virus in Classical Hodgkin Lymphoma

In about 40% of cases of classical HL in the Western world, and in about 90% of childhood HL cases in Central and Southern America, HRS cells are infected by EBV. Molecular analyses of EBV$^+$ cases showed that EBV infection of HRS cells is a clonal event (i.e., EBV infected or was already present in the founder cell of the HRS cell clone). EBV-positive HRS cells typically show a latency II gene expression pattern characterized by expression of the EBV nuclear antigen 1 (EBNA1) and the two latent membrane proteins 1 and 2a (LMP1 and LMP2a, respectively). EBNA1 is essential for the replication of the EBV episome in proliferating cells. LMP1 is an oncogene, and one of its main functions is to cause constitutive NFκB activation by mimicking an activated CD40 receptor. LMP2a has a cytoplasmic motif that resembles the signaling motif of the BCR. LMP2a can, on the one hand, diminish BCR signaling by recruiting BCR signaling components away from the BCR, but on the other hand, it mimics a tonic BCR signal. Strikingly, all HRS cell clones with clearly destructive Ig V gene mutations that prevent the expression of a BCR were found to be EBV-positive.[18] Hence it appears that in GC B cell precursors of HRS cells that acquired BCR-destructive mutations, EBV is essential to rescue these cells from apoptosis upon loss of BCR expression. This scenario is supported by studies showing that EBV can rescue BCR-deficient GC B cells from apoptosis, and that LMP2a has an important role in this process.[19] Whether the BCR-mimicking function is still important in the established HRS cell clone is unclear. The downregulation of most components of BCR signaling in HRS cells indicates that LMP2a does not have this role in the established HRS cell clone.

Genetic Lesions in Hodgkin and Reed-Sternberg and Lymphocyte Predominant Cells

The molecular analysis of HRS and LP cells for genetic lesions is hampered by the rarity of these cells. Nevertheless, we are now aware of a number of transforming events, especially for HRS cells. The recognition of constitutive activity of the NFκB transcription factor, which is normally only transiently activated in lymphocytes, prompted studies of whether gene mutations cause this deregulated activity. Inactivating mutations in the gene NFKBIA, which encodes the main inhibitor of NFκB (i.e., IκBα) were detected in 10% to 20% of cases of classical HL (Fig. 74.3).[1] Also, mutations in the NFKBIE gene were found. Genomic gains of the REL gene, encoding one of the NFκB factors, are present in about 40% of classical HL. Inactivating mutations in TNFAIP3, a further negative regulator of NFκB, were detected in 40% of HRS cell clones.[20,21] Interestingly, most cases with TNFAIP3 mutations were EBV-negative,[21] suggesting that EBV infection and TNFAIP3 mutations are alternative mechanisms in HL pathogenesis, thereby further supporting a pathogenetic role of EBV in HL development. Reestablishing wild-type TNFAIP3 in HL cell lines reduced NFκB activity and survival, establishing that TNFAIP3 functions as a tumor suppressor gene in this lymphoma.[21] For CYLD, another tumor suppressor gene and negative regulator of NFκB, inactivating mutations were found in one HL cell line, but not in several primary cases of HL studied, indicating that mutations in this gene also occur in HRS cells, albeit at a low frequency. Rare mutations were recently also found in TRAF3, a negative regulator of the noncanonical NFκB pathway. Finally, the NIK kinase gene (MAP3K4), encoding a major activating factor for the noncanonical NFκB pathway, shows gains in 20% of classical HL.

Although LP cells of NLPHL also show constitutive NFκB activity,[2] no destructive mutations were found in TNFAIP3 and NFKBIA in these cells, and LP cells are not infected by EBV. In some NLPHL REL gains were found. Thus, the mechanisms causing NFκB activation in HRS and LP cells are largely different.

A second signaling pathway that shows constitutive activity in HRS cells and mutations in various pathway members is the JAK/STAT pathway, the main pathway for cytokine signaling. Upon activation of cytokine receptors, JAK kinases bind to the receptors and become activated. The activated JAKs then phosphorylate and thereby activate STAT factors, which upon phosphorylation and dimerization translocate into the nucleus and function as transcription factors. Frequent genomic gains of JAK2 and also rare translocations involving this gene have been detected in HRS cells. However, activating point mutations in the JAK2 gene, although they are frequent in other types of hematologic diseases, are absent in HRS cells. SOCS1, a main inhibitor of this signaling pathway, is inactivated by somatic mutations in the HRS cells in about 40% of cases of classical HL.[22] Recently, destructive mutations in the PTPN1 gene were detected in HRS cells in 20% of cases.[23] PTPN1 is a phosphatase that, among other functions, negatively regulates STAT activity.

Notably, the genomic region on 9p24, which harbors the JAK2 gene and shows gains in HRS cells, also encompasses the gene JMJD2C that encodes a histone demethylase, and the programmed death 1 (PD-1) ligand genes PD-L1 and PD-L2.[24,25] PD-1 ligands inhibit PD-1–expressing T cells and may contribute to the immunosuppressive microenvironment in HL.[24] A functional role of JMJD2C in HRS cells is indicated from the finding that downregulation of its expression in HL cell lines is toxic for these cells.[25] Thus, a single genetic lesion, the genomic gain on 9p24, affects four genes with pathogenetic roles in HRS cells.

Because disturbed apoptosis seems to be a key aspect of classical HL pathogenesis, numerous regulators of apoptosis were also studied in HL cell lines and/or primary HRS cells. Mutations in the TP53 gene were found in three HL cell lines and a few primary cases.[26] Mutations in the CD95 gene were found in less than 10% of cases, and no mutations were found in the CD95 signaling components CASP8, CASP10, and FADD.[26] Moreover, no mutations were detected in the proapoptotic gene BAD; mutations in ATM are also very rare.[26]

Chromosomal translocations, usually involving one of the Ig loci and an oncogene, are a hallmark of most B cell lymphomas. Also in classical HL, chromosomal breaks involving the Ig loci were detected by fluorescence in situ hybridization in about 20% of cases. However, the translocation partners are in most cases unknown. In a few instances, BCL2, BCL3, BCL6, or MYC were identified as partners of the translocations. This also includes composite lymphomas where the clonally related classical HL and the B cell NHL were found to carry the identical translocation—for example, a BCL2-IgH translocation in a composite classical HL/follicular lymphoma.[17] Notably, Ig locus–associated translocations usually function by causing deregulated expression of the translocated oncogene that has been brought under the control of the Ig regulatory elements, which are active in normal B cells and B cell NHL. Because the Ig loci are largely silenced in HRS cells, it is still unclear whether the partner genes of Ig locus–associated translocations in HRS cells are still active and pathogenetically relevant. Perhaps the translocations were important during early stages of HRS cell pathogenesis, when the lymphoma precursor cells still had a B-cell gene expression program, but became less important during later stages of the multistep transformation process. Alternatively, it should also be considered that translocations might function by mechanisms other than Ig enhancer–driven oncogene overexpression (e.g., promoter replacement or tumor suppressor gene inactivation).

HRS cells show a heterogeneous pattern of major histocompatibility complex (MHC) class I and II expression. Recurrent translocations involving the MHC class II transactivator gene CIITA were found in about 15% of classical HL.[27] These translocations involved heterogeneous partner genes and seemed to function by impairing CIITA function and hence dampening MHC class II expression. The MHC class I component β-2-microglobulin (B2M) is mutated in more than half of classical HL according to a recent study.[28] Downmodulation of MHC class I is often a strategy of cancer cells to evade attack by cytotoxic T cells.

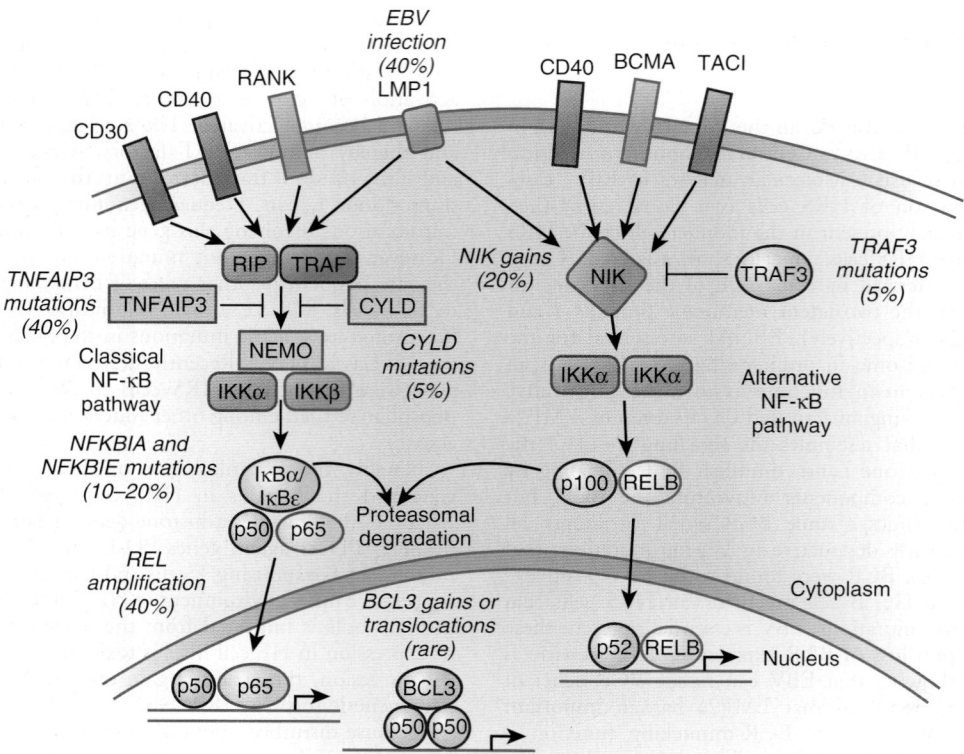

Fig. 74.3 MECHANISM OF NFκB ACTIVATION IN HODGKIN AND REED-STERNBERG CELLS. A classical and an alternative NFκB signaling pathway are distinguished. In the classical NFκB pathway stimulation of numerous receptors (e.g., RANK, CD30, and CD40) leads via TNF receptor–associated factors (TRAFs) and other associated factors, such as the receptor-interacting protein (RIP), to activation of the IKK complex. The IKK complex is composed of IKKα, IKKβ, and NEMO. The activated IKK complex phosphorylates the NFκB inhibitors IκBα and IκBε that are encoded by the NFKBIA and NFKBIE genes, respectively. The phosphorylation marks the IκB factors for ubiquitinylation and subsequent proteasomal degradation. Thus the NFκB transcription factors (e.g., p50/p65 or p50/REL heterodimers) are no longer retained in the cytoplasm and translocate into the nucleus where they activate multiple genes. The signal transduction from TRAFs/RIP to the IKK complex can be inhibited by A20/TNFAIP3, which removes activating ubiquitins from RIP and TRAFs and additionally links ubiquitins to these molecules to mark them for proteasomal degradation. In the alternative NFκB pathway, activation of receptors such as BCMA, CD40, and TACI causes stimulation of the kinase NIK (encoded by the MAP3K4 gene), which then activates an IKKα complex. Activated IKKα processes p100 precursors to p52 molecules that translocate as active p52/RELB NFκB heterodimers into the nucleus. HRS cells show constitutive activity of the classical and alternative NFκB signaling pathways. This activity is mediated by diverse mechanisms, including receptor signaling through CD40, RANK, BCMA, and TACI; genomic REL and MAP3K4 amplifications; destructive mutations in the TNFAIP3, NFKBIA, and NFKBIE genes; and signaling through the EBV-encoded latent membrane protein 1. HRS cells may also harbor nuclear BCL3/(p50)₂ complexes, and in a few cases the strong BCL3 expression appears to be mediated by genomic gains or chromosomal translocations of this gene. In rare instances, inactivating mutations in the inhibitory factors TRAF3 and CYLD have been found. *(Modified and updated from Küppers R: The biology of Hodgkin's lymphoma.* Nat Rev Cancer 9:15, 2009.)

For LP cells of NLPHL, few genetic lesions are known. SOCS1 mutations occur frequently in LP cells, and translocations involving the BCL6 gene are often found in these cells.[29,30] BCL6 encodes a transcription factor that orchestrates the GC B-cell differentiation program and that has an oncogenic function when constitutively expressed in B cells. A study published in 2016 identified highly recurrent mutations in the serine/threonine kinase SGK1, the phosphatase DUSP2, and the AP-1 transcription factor JUNB in LP cells.[29]

FUTURE DIRECTIONS

It is now firmly established that HRS and LP cells stem from mature B cells. A few cases with features of classical HL and a T-cell origin of the HRS cells exist. HRS cells in classical HL appear to derive

from crippled GC B cells, whereas LP cells likely originate from antigen-selected GC B cells. HRS cells show deregulated activation of multiple signaling pathways, and numerous genetic lesions have been identified that contribute to the deregulated activation of the NFκB and JAK/STAT pathways. HRS cells show a nearly complete loss of the B-cell gene expression program.[3] As normal GC B cells are stringently selected to express a functional, high affinity BCR, the lost B-cell phenotype may be related to the origin of HRS cells from preapoptotic GC B cells: by losing the B cell–typical gene expression program, the HRS cell precursors may escape from the pressure to undergo apoptosis as "failed B cells." It has been speculated that transient hypoxic conditions in the GC may contribute to the initial "dedifferentiation" of the HRS precursor cells, because exposing human B cells to hypoxia induces several phenotypic changes in these cells toward an HRS cell phenotype. It should, however, be noted that further distinct subpopulations of GC B cells are currently being recognized (e.g., CD30+ GC B cells), and it will be important to take these novel findings into consideration for a refinement of the cellular origin of HRS and LP cells.

The recent molecular biologic findings about HRS cells also offer some explanations for the typical and rather unique immunophenotypic heterogeneity of the HRS cells between cases and also among HRS cells of a given clone. The heterogeneity is likely due in part to different combinations of transforming events between HL cases. Moreover, the coexpression of multiple master regulators of different hematopoietic cell lineages (e.g., PAX5, ID2, NOTCH1) within one HRS cell clone may cause major fluctuations in gene expression between clone members by fluctuation of the competing transcription factors. Finally, because HRS cells are intimately interacting with multiple types of cells in their microenvironment, both by cellular interactions and through cytokines and chemokines, variations in the direct surrounding of HRS cells may cause differences in gene expression in these cells.

Further work is needed to fully understand the transforming events that lead to the generation of malignant HRS and LP cell clones, but with the availability of new methods, such as massive parallel sequencing of tumor genomes, it can be expected that major progresses will be made in the near future.

Finally, the recent detection of cell-free DNA presumably derived from HRS cells in the blood plasma of patients with HL[30] offers exciting novel possibilities to monitor the disease, and this tumor-specific DNA may become a useful biomarker.

REFERENCES

1. Küppers R, Engert A, Hansmann M-L: Hodgkin lymphoma. *J Clin Invest* 122(10):3439–3447, 2012.
2. Brune V, Tiacci E, Pfeil I, et al: Origin and pathogenesis of nodular lymphocyte-predominant Hodgkin lymphoma as revealed by global gene expression analysis. *J Exp Med* 205(10):2251–2268, 2008.
3. Schwering I, Bräuninger A, Klein U, et al: Loss of the B-lineage-specific gene expression program in Hodgkin and Reed-Sternberg cells of Hodgkin lymphoma. *Blood* 101(4):1505–1512, 2003.
4. Lamprecht B, Walter K, Kreher S, et al: Derepression of an endogenous long terminal repeat activates the CSF1R proto-oncogene in human lymphoma. *Nat Med* 16(5):571–579, 2010.
5. Kanzler H, Küppers R, Hansmann ML, et al: Hodgkin and Reed-Sternberg cells in Hodgkin's disease represent the outgrowth of a dominant tumor clone derived from (crippled) germinal center B cells. *J Exp Med* 184(4):1495–1505, 1996.
6. Müschen M, Rajewsky K, Bräuninger A, et al: Rare occurrence of classical Hodgkin's disease as a T cell lymphoma. *J Exp Med* 191(2):387–394, 2000.
7. Seitz V, Hummel M, Marafioti T, et al: Detection of clonal T-cell receptor gamma-chain gene rearrangements in Reed-Sternberg cells of classic Hodgkin disease. *Blood* 95(10):3020–3024, 2000.
8. Tiacci E, Döring C, Brune V, et al: Analyzing primary Hodgkin and Reed-Sternberg cells to capture the molecular and cellular pathogenesis of classical Hodgkin lymphoma. *Blood* 120(23):4609–4620, 2012.
9. Küppers R, Bräuninger A, Müschen M, et al: Evidence that Hodgkin and Reed-Sternberg cells in Hodgkin disease do not represent cell fusions. *Blood* 97(3):818–821, 2001.
10. Rengstl B, Newrzela S, Heinrich T, et al: Incomplete cytokinesis and re-fusion of small mononucleated Hodgkin cells lead to giant multinucleated Reed-Sternberg cells. *Proc Natl Acad Sci USA* 110(51):20729–20734, 2013.
11. Spieker T, Kurth J, Küppers R, et al: Molecular single-cell analysis of the clonal relationship of small Epstein-Barr virus-infected cells and Epstein-Barr virus-harboring Hodgkin and Reed/Sternberg cells in Hodgkin disease. *Blood* 96(9):3133–3138, 2000.
12. Jones RJ, Gocke CD, Kasamon YL, et al: Circulating clonotypic B cells in classic Hodgkin lymphoma. *Blood* 113(23):5920–5926, 2009.
13. Küppers R: Clonogenic B cells in classic Hodgkin lymphoma. *Blood* 114(18):3970–3971, 2009.
14. Vockerodt M, Soares M, Kanzler H, et al: Detection of clonal Hodgkin and Reed-Sternberg cells with identical somatically mutated and rearranged VH genes in different biopsies in relapsed Hodgkin's disease. *Blood* 92(8):2899–2907, 1998.
15. Nakashima M, Ishii Y, Watanabe M, et al: The side population, as a precursor of Hodgkin and Reed-Sternberg cells and a target for nuclear factor-kappaB inhibitors in Hodgkin's lymphoma. *Cancer Sci* 101(11):2490–2496, 2010.
16. Shafer JA, Cruz CR, Leen AM, et al: Antigen-specific cytotoxic T lymphocytes can target chemoresistant side-population tumor cells in Hodgkin lymphoma. *Leuk Lymphoma* 51(5):870–880, 2010.
17. Küppers R, Dührsen U, Hansmann ML: Pathogenesis, diagnosis, and treatment of composite lymphomas. *Lancet Oncol* 15(10):e435–e446, 2014.
18. Bräuninger A, Schmitz R, Bechtel D, et al: Küppers R. Molecular biology of Hodgkin and Reed/Sternberg cells in Hodgkin's lymphoma. *Int J Cancer* 118(8):1853–1861, 2006.
19. Mancao C, Hammerschmidt W: Epstein-Barr virus latent membrane protein 2A is a B-cell receptor mimic and essential for B-cell survival. *Blood* 110(10):3715–3721, 2007.
20. Kato M, Sanada M, Kato I, et al: Frequent inactivation of A20 in B-cell lymphomas. *Nature* 459(7247):712–716, 2009.
21. Schmitz R, Hansmann ML, Bohle V, et al: TNFAIP3 (A20) is a tumor suppressor gene in Hodgkin lymphoma and primary mediastinal B cell lymphoma. *J Exp Med* 206(5):981–989, 2009.
22. Weniger MA, Melzner I, Menz CK, et al: Mutations of the tumor suppressor gene SOCS-1 in classical Hodgkin lymphoma are frequent and associated with nuclear phospho-STAT5 accumulation. *Oncogene* 25(18):2679–2684, 2006.
23. Gunawardana J, Chan FC, Telenius A, et al: Recurrent somatic mutations of PTPN1 in primary mediastinal B cell lymphoma and Hodgkin lymphoma. *Nat Genet* 46(4):329–335, 2014.
24. Green MR, Monti S, Rodig SJ, et al: Integrative analysis reveals selective 9p24.1 amplification, increased PD-1 ligand expression, and further induction via JAK2 in nodular sclerosing Hodgkin lymphoma and primary mediastinal large B-cell lymphoma. *Blood* 116(17):3268–3277, 2010.
25. Rui L, Emre NC, Kruhlak MJ, et al: Cooperative epigenetic modulation by cancer amplicon genes. *Cancer Cell* 18(6):590–605, 2010.
26. Schmitz R, Stanelle J, Hansmann M-L, et al: Pathogenesis of classical and lymphocyte-predominant Hodgkin lymphoma. *Annu Rev Pathol* 4:151–174, 2009.
27. Steidl C, Shah SP, Woolcock BW, et al: MHC class II transactivator CIITA is a recurrent gene fusion partner in lymphoid cancers. *Nature* 471(7338):377–381, 2011.
28. Reichel J, Chadburn A, Rubinstein PG, et al: Flow-sorting and exome sequencing reveals the oncogenome of primary Hodgkin and Reed-Sternberg cells. *Blood* 125(7):1061–1072, 2015.
29. Hartmann S, Schuhmacher B, Rausch T, et al: Highly recurrent mutations of *SGK1*, *DUSP2* and *JUNB* in nodular lymphocyte predominant Hodgkin lymphoma. *Leukemia* 30(4):844–853, 2016.
30. Vandenberghe P, Wlodarska I, Tousseyn T, et al: Non-invasive detection of genomic imbalances in Hodgkin/Reed-Sternberg cells in early and advanced stage Hodgkin's lymphoma by sequencing of circulating cell-free DNA: a technical proof-of-principle study. *Lancet Haematology* 2:e55–e65, 2015.

HODGKIN LYMPHOMA: CLINICAL MANIFESTATIONS, STAGING, AND THERAPY

Katy Smith, April Chiu, Rahul Parikh, Joachim Yahalom, and Anas Younes

Hodgkin lymphoma (HL) is an uncommon lymphoproliferative malignancy arising from B cells. It can affect all age groups but is most common in young adults. HL is the first adult malignancy to demonstrate the curative potential of combination chemotherapy. Today more than 80% of patients with newly diagnosed HL can now expect to be cured of their disease.

The challenge now, particularly since many affected patients are young, is not only to improve cure rates further, but also to minimize the risk of long-term complications of treatment, which can impact quality of life and survival. Accordingly HL provides a very important clinical model for ongoing cancer research involving both the development of novel targeted agents and the study of late effects of cancer therapy.

Traditionally the choice of frontline therapy for HL has been determined by clinical stage and prognostic factors. A combined modality approach with chemotherapy and radiotherapy remains the standard of care for those with early-stage disease, whereas chemotherapy alone is routinely used for those presenting with more advanced clinical features. The availability of highly effective chemotherapy combinations and sensitive imaging tests has allowed the development of less toxic therapeutic strategies for those with limited disease. This includes the implementation of involved-field radiotherapy (IFRT), and more recently involved-site radiotherapy (ISRT), and a reduction in the number of chemotherapy cycles. This more focused treatment delivery has allowed efficacy to be preserved while exposure to unnecessary toxicity is reduced.

The management of HL continues to evolve. Positron emission tomography (PET) imaging has emerged as a useful tool for assessing response and to guide further therapy that may allow radiation therapy (RT)–free regimens. This, coupled with ongoing research to identify better biologic prognostic factors, is likely to allow for a more accurate risk-adapted approach to management, with the future treatment of patients with HL being tailored to the needs of the individual. In addition, improved understanding of the molecular mechanisms underlying HL has hastened the development of more effective, and often less toxic, targeted therapies for use either as monotherapy or in combination with traditional chemotherapy to augment efficacy and decrease overall toxicity.

EPIDEMIOLOGY AND ETIOLOGY

Incidence and Age of Onset

HL is a rare B-cell malignancy accounting for less than 1% of all cancers with approximately 9200 new cases diagnosed in the United States and approximately 5500 new cases diagnosed in Europe each year. The incidence of HL varies with economic status and geographic location. In developed countries it is associated with a bimodal age of onset distribution, with an early, larger, peak occurring in young adults aged between 20 and 40 years and a second, smaller, peak occurring in those over 55 years. In contrast, in developing countries, the disease predominantly occurs in childhood, with the incidence decreasing with age. Overall, men are affected slightly more frequently than women (1.3 : 1).

Etiology

The exact cause of HL remains unknown and clearly defined risk factors for the development of the disease are lacking. However, certain associations with its development have been identified. Although a clear genetic cause has not been established, familial susceptibility has been suggested by both an apparent increased risk among siblings of patients with HL, as well as concordance for HL observed in monozygotic twins. Increased maternal education, early birth order, low number of siblings and single-family dwellings in childhood have all also been positively associated with the occurrence of HL in younger patients.

Epstein-Barr virus (EBV)–positive Reed-Sternberg (RS) cells are found in approximately 40% of patients with HL using modern molecular techniques, mostly in cases of mixed cellularity classic HL (MCCHL) and lymphocyte-depleted classic HL (LDCHL), with reduced frequency observed in nodular sclerosis classic HL (NSCHL) and lymphocyte-rich classic Hodgkin Lymphoma (LRCHL). The incidence of HL among those with a past history of EBV infection appears to be higher than those without previous exposure. EBV may play a role in promoting RS survival and has been associated with the increased production of molecules that are involved in mechanisms of immune escape, in turn influencing the microenvironment that supports HL development.

The incidence of HL is higher in patients with human immunodeficiency virus (HIV) infection, suggesting a potential contributory role for immune suppression and reinforcing the likelihood of there being an important immune component underlying HL pathogenesis (see Special Considerations: Hodgkin Lymphoma in Patients with HIV Infection section, later).

PATHOBIOLOGY OF HODGKIN LYMPHOMA

The World Health Organization (WHO) classifies HL into two distinct disease types: classic HL (cHL), representing 95% of all cases, and nodular lymphocyte-predominant HL (NLPHL), accounting for only 5%. Both cHL and NLPHL are neoplasms composed of a minor component of atypical large neoplastic cells, usually accounting for <10% of all cells that are present in a reactive nonneoplastic background. However, based on their distinct clinical and molecular genetic features, it is now evident that cHL and NLPHL are two biologically distinct entities. Within cHL, four histologic subtypes are recognized based on the morphology of the neoplastic cells, composition of the nonneoplastic infiltrate, and overall nodal architecture: nodular sclerosing (NSCHL), mixed cellularity (MCCHL), lymphocyte-depleted (LDCHL) and lymphocyte-rich (LRCHL). Of these, NSCHL predominates, accounting for 70% of cases of cHL in Europe and the United States (Table 75.1). The rate of NSCHL, however, varies with geographic location and socioeconomic status and is much lower in developing countries, where MCCHL predominates. Furthermore, NSCHL occurs less frequently in patients infected with HIV, among whom the more common presenting subtype, again, is MCCHL (see Special Considerations: Hodgkin Lymphoma in Patients with HIV Infection section, later).

Nodular Lymphocyte-Predominant Hodgkin Lymphoma

Typical cases of NLPHL show partial or complete nodal architectural effacement by a macronodular proliferation (Fig. 75.1A), where the nodules are composed of scattered neoplastic cells termed *lymphocyte-predominant (LP) cells*, formerly known as L&H cells. LP cells are large with single folded or multilobulated nucleus with distinct but smaller nucleoli than RS cells. Because of their highly complex nuclear lobation, they have also been widely referred to as "popcorn cells" (see Fig. 75.1B). The background nonneoplastic infiltrate is composed of predominantly small B cells and a variable number of histiocytes. Mixed inflammatory cells such as eosinophils and neutrophils are rare to absent.

LP cells typically express B-cell markers including CD20 (see Fig. 75.1C), PAX-5, and CD79a. In addition, LP cells consistently express CD45, and the B-cell transcriptional factors OCT-2 and BOB.1, that are usually not expressed by RS cells. In contrast to RS cells, LP cells typically lack CD15 and CD30 expression. In keeping with their germinal center B-cell origin, LP cells are consistently positive for BCL6, although CD10 is usually not expressed. They express EMA (epithelial membrane antigen) in approximately 50% of the cases,

and variably express IRF4/MUM1. EBV-encoded RNA (EBER) and latent membrane protein-1 (LMP1) are consistently negative.

The nodules in NLPHL are typically supported by an expanded meshwork of follicular dendritic cells that can be highlighted by CD21 and CD35, and populated by small B cells that are positive for immunoglobulin (Ig) M and IgD. There are a variable number of T cells, a significant proportion of which is positive for CD4, CD57, and programmed cell death protein 1 (PD-1) which frequently form rosettes around the LP cells (see Fig. 75.1D).

Genetic studies performed on microdissected LP cells show clonally rearranged Ig genes with high load of somatic mutations in the variable region, indicating the presence of ongoing mutations and consistent with germinal center B-cell derivation of NLPHL. In contrast to cHL, the Ig rearrangement is functional with detectable Ig mRNA transcripts.

Classic Hodgkin Lymphoma

cHL is characterized by the presence of RS cells and their morphologic variants in a reactive background composed of mixed inflammatory cells (except in lymphocyte-rich variant). *Classic (diagnostic) RS cells* are large binucleated or multinucleated cells with pale chromatin, distinct nuclear membrane, single prominent eosinophilic, inclusion-like nucleolus in each nuclear lobe, and abundant amphophilic cytoplasm (Fig. 75.2A). Mononuclear variants with otherwise similar cytonuclear features are termed *Hodgkin cells* (see Fig. 75.2B). *Mummified cells* are degenerated RS and Hodgkin cells with pyknotic nuclei and condensed cytoplasm (see Fig. 75.2C). These variants are usually seen in various proportions in all four subtypes of cHL. In addition, *lacunar cells* are characteristic of nodular sclerosis cHL but usually not other subtypes, which have abundant pale cytoplasm that frequently retracts in formalin fixed tissue, creating an empty space (lacunae) around the cells (see Fig. 75.2D).

NSCHL is characterized by sclerotic nodal capsule and presence of collagenous bands traversing through the nodal parenchyma,

TABLE 75.1	Frequency of Histologic Subtypes of Hodgkin Lymphoma According to the 2008 WHO Classification	
Classic Hodgkin Lymphoma (cHL)		95%
• Nodular sclerosis classic Hodgkin lymphoma (NSCHL)		70%
• Mixed cellularity classic Hodgkin lymphoma (MCCHL)		20–25%
• Lymphocyte-rich classic Hodgkin lymphoma (LRCHL)		5%
• Lymphocyte-depleted classic Hodgkin lymphoma (LDCHL)		<1%
Nodular Lymphocyte Predominant Hodgkin Lymphoma (NLPHL)		5%

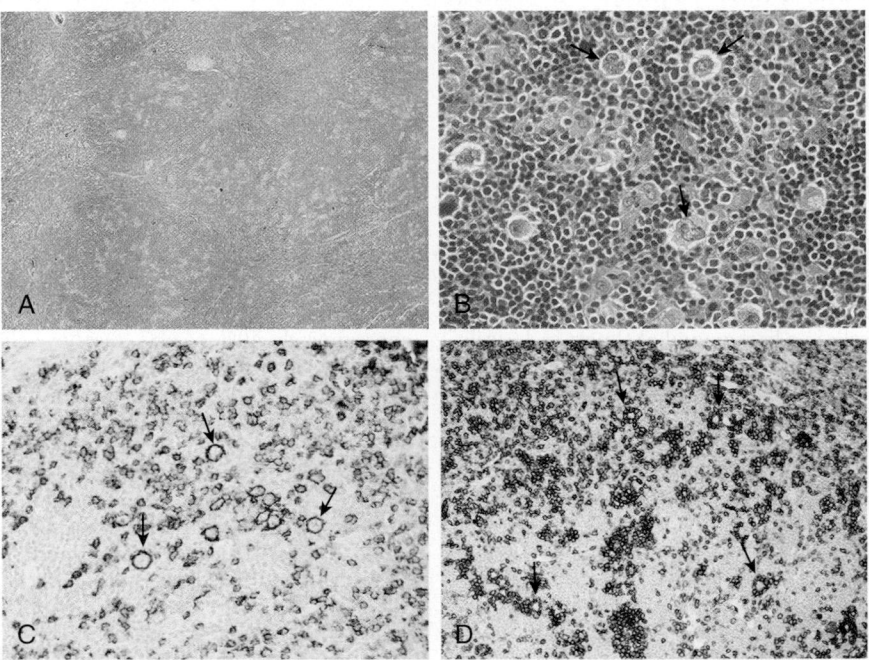

Fig. 75.1 A CASE OF NODULAR LYMPHOCYTE–PREDOMINANT HODGKIN LYMPHOMA. The lymph node architecture is effaced by multiple expansile nodules with mottled appearance (A). Within the nodules there are scattered atypical large cells (lymphocyte-predominant [LP] cells) with single folded or multilobated nucleus with distinct but relatively small nucleoli (B). The LP cells are positive for CD20 *(arrows)* with similar strong expression intensity as background small reactive B cells (C). The background infiltrate is composed of numerous programmed cell death protein 1 (PD-1)–positive T cells that frequently form rosettes *(arrows)* around the LP cells (D).

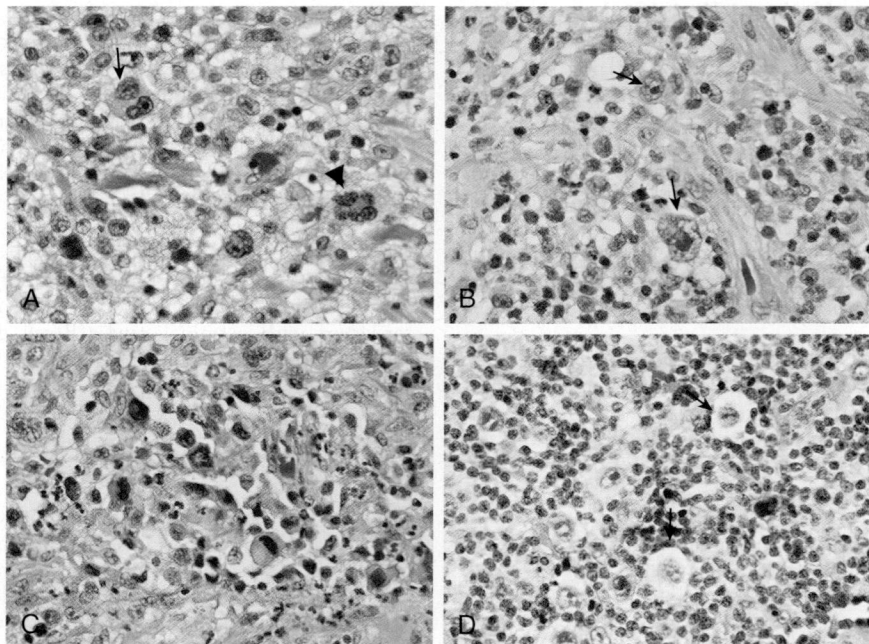

Fig. 75.2 MORPHOLOGIC VARIATIONS OF REED-STERNBERG (RS) CELLS IN CLASSIC HODGKIN LYMPHOMA (cHL). The diagnostic RS cells (A) are large binucleated *(arrow)* or multinucleated cells *(arrowhead)* with distinct nuclear membrane, prominent nucleolus in each nuclear lobe, and abundant amphophilic cytoplasm. Hodgkin cells are mononuclear variants of RS cells with similar cytonuclear features (B); numerous eosinophils and granulocytes are noted in the background. Mummified cells are degenerated RS and Hodgkin cells with pyknotic nuclei and condensed cytoplasm (C). Lacunar cells, characteristic of nodular sclerosis cHL, have abundant pale cytoplasm which frequently retracts in formalin fixed tissue (D).

imparting a prominent nodular pattern (Fig. 75.3A). Within the nodules there are a variable number of RS cells and variants, especially lacunar cells, with a background of mixed inflammatory cells composed of a variable proportion of small lymphocytes, histiocytes, plasma cells, eosinophils, and neutrophils. The RS cells and variants may be singly dispersed or form confluent aggregates/sheets.

In *MCCHL* the lymph node architecture is usually diffusely obliterated, although an interfollicular pattern may be seen in early involvement. In contrast to NSCHL, the nodal capsule is not thickened and there are no collagenous bands of fibrosis (see Fig. 75.3B). RS cells and variants are usually easily identified and dispersed throughout the nodal tissue in a mixed inflammatory background. In comparison to NSCHL, MCCHL is more often associated with higher stage disease and EBV positivity, and is more likely seen in the HIV-infected patient population.

LRCHL is a relatively recently defined subtype of cHL characterized by the presence of RS cells in a background of almost exclusively small lymphocytes, with a paucity or absence of eosinophils and neutrophils. The vast majority of the cases exhibit nodular growth pattern, although a rare diffuse variant has also been described. In the vast majority of the cases the affected lymph node is obliterated by multiple expansile nodules with expanded mantle zones and regressed, eccentrically located residual germinal centers (see Fig. 75.3C).

LDCHL is exceedingly rare (<1% of cHL) with a highly variable histologic appearance, but in all cases characterized by a relative predominance of RS cells in comparison to the background lymphocytes. Some cases are characterized by scattered RS cells in a diffusely fibrotic background containing histiocytes, fibroblasts, and few lymphocytes. In others, sheets of bizarre, pleomorphic, or anaplastic-appearing RS cells are present, imparting a sarcomatous appearance (see Fig. 75.3D).

The immunophenotypic profile of RS cells in all cHL subtypes is similar. RS cells are strongly positive for CD30 with membranous and Golgi pattern in nearly all cases (Fig. 75.4A), and CD15 with variable staining intensity in approximately 80% of the cases (see Fig.

75.4B). Consistent with their B-cell derivation, RS cells express PAX-5 in almost all cases (95%) but with weaker intensity when compared with the surrounding nonneoplastic small B cells (see Fig. 75.4C). However, in keeping with their defective B-cell program, RS cells lack Ig production as evidenced by absence of J chain, and are negative for most other B cell–associated antigens: CD20 (expressed in only 20%–30% of cases; often only in a subset of RS cells with weak/variable intensity), CD19, and CD79a; as well as B-cell transcriptional factors OCT-2 and BOB.1 (each expressed in 10% of cases; coexpression is rare). RS cells are almost always positive for IRF4/MUM1 and negative for CD45 and EMA, features that may help distinguish cHL from NLPHL. Expression of other hematopoietic lineage–associated markers, such as T cells (CD4, granzyme B), dendritic cells (fascin, CCL17), and myeloid cells (colony stimulating factor 1 receptor and α_1-antitrypsin) is also often present. EBV LMP1 and/or EBER expression (see Fig. 75.4D) by RS cells is seen in approximately 40% of cHL cases overall in Western countries, but mostly in MCCHL and LDCHL and less frequently in NSCHL and LRCHL. However, an association with EBV is seen in up to 90% of cHL cases in developing countries and nearly all cases in the HIV patient population.

The nonneoplastic background lymphocytes, with the exception of LRCHL, are composed of predominantly T cells with marked predominance of CD4-positive cells that coexpress CD25 and FOXP3, consistent with immunosuppressive regulatory T-cells (TReg). In addition there is a significant population of TH2 cells. TReg and TH2 cells are attracted by cytokines (CCL5, CCL17, and CCL22) secreted by RS cells. In HIV-infected patients there is often a predominance of CD8-positive T cells. In contrast to NLPHL, CD57-positive T cells are not increased in number in cHL.

Polymerase chain reaction studies performed on RS cells procured by microdissection demonstrated that in the vast majority of cHL cases (>98%), the RS cells harbor clonal IgH gene rearrangement. The rearranged IgH shows a high load of somatic hypermutation in the variable region without evidence of ongoing mutation, consistent with germinal center or postgerminal center B-cell derivation. Rare

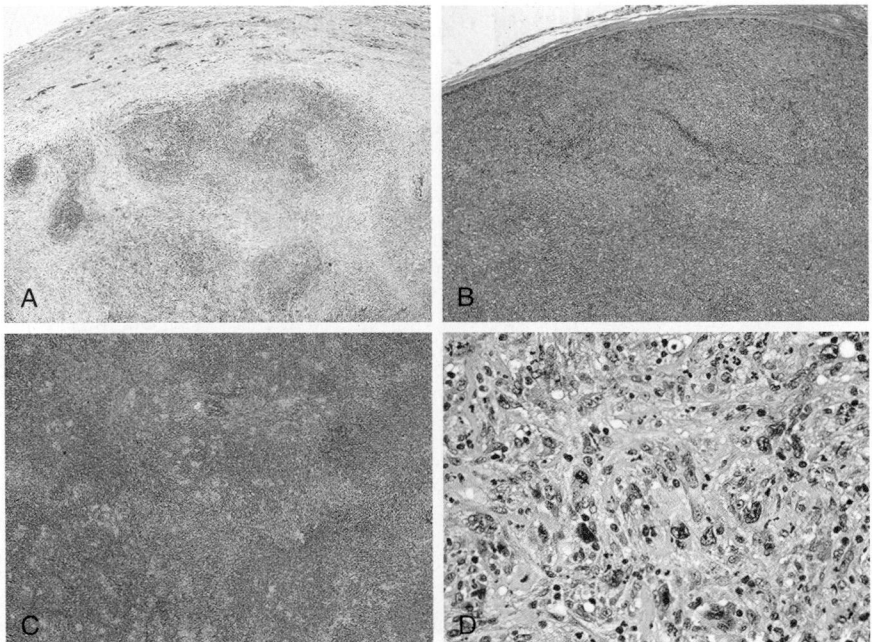

Fig. 75.3 HISTOLOGIC PATTERNS OF CLASSIC HODGKIN LYMPHOMA (cHL) SUBTYPES. Nodular sclerosis cHL characteristically shows multinodular pattern on low magnification, where the nodules are surrounded by broad collagenous bands. The nodal capsule is markedly sclerotic (A). In mixed cellularity cHL, the lymph node architecture is diffusely obliterated by the neoplastic infiltrate. The nodal capsule is not sclerotic and there are no collagenous bands of fibrosis (B). A case of lymphocyte-rich cHL where the affected lymph node is obliterated by multiple expansile nodules, with strikingly similar morphologic appearance to nodular lymphocyte predominant Hodgkin lymphoma (C). A case of lymphocyte-depleted cHL with presence of numerous pleomorphic/anaplastic appearing Reed-Sternberg (RS) cells (D).

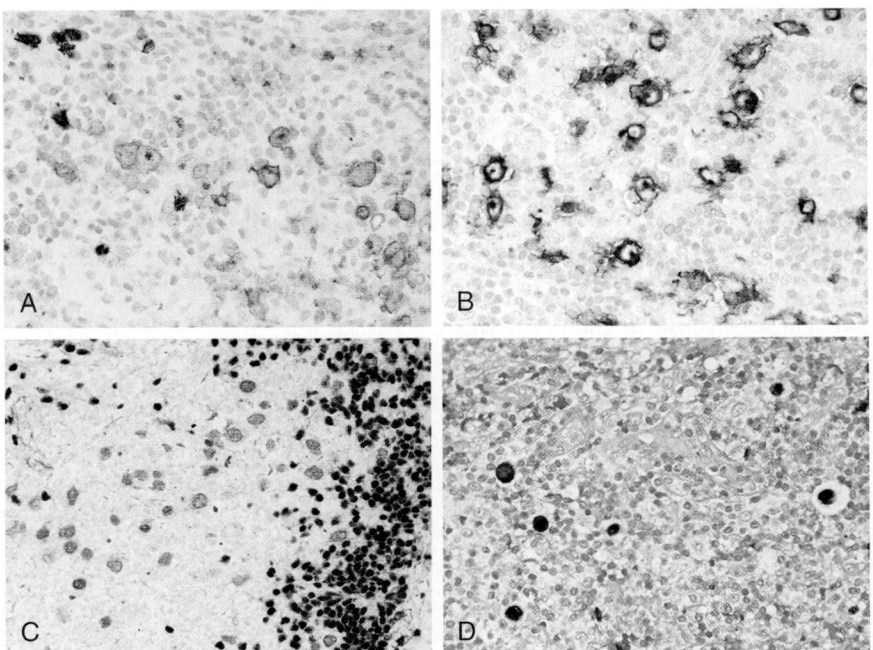

Fig. 75.4 IMMUNOPHENOTYPIC PROFILE OF REED-STERNBERG (RS) CELLS IN CLASSIC HODGKIN LYMPHOMA. The RS cells and variants are positive for CD15 (A) and CD30 (B), with characteristic membranous staining and Golgi accentuation. These cells are positive for PAX-5, but with weaker intensity in comparison to background small reactive B cells (C). The RS cells are positive for Epstein-Barr virus (EBV) as demonstrated by in situ hybridization for EBV-encoded RNA/EBV-encoded RNA (EBER) (D).

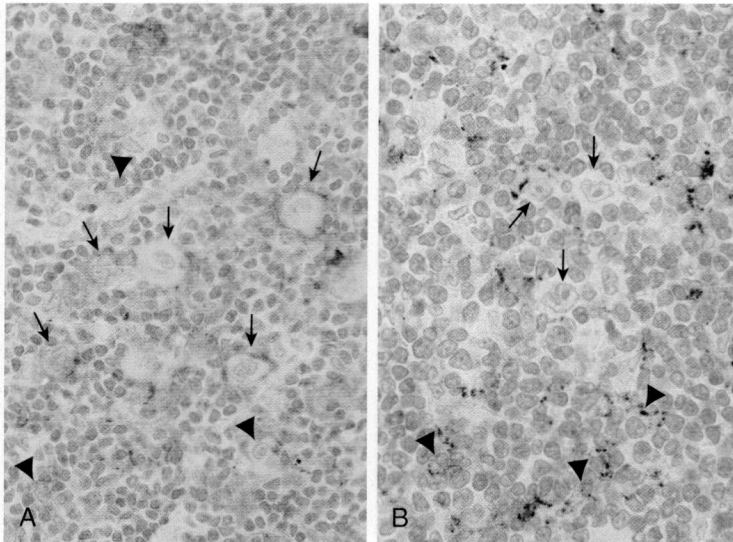

Fig. 75.5 IMMUNOHISTOCHEMICAL ANALYSIS OF PDL-1 EXPRESSION IN CLASSIC HODGKIN LYMPHOMA (cHL) AND NODULAR LYMPHOCYTE-PREDOMINANT HODGKIN LYMPHOMA (NLPHL). (A) A case of nodular sclerosis cHL showing distinct membranous expression for PDL-1 by Reed-Sternberg (RS) cells *(arrows)*. PDL-1 also highlights cell processes of tumor-infiltrating histiocytes *(arrowheads)* with granular staining pattern. (B) A case of nodular lymphocyte predominant Hodgkin lymphoma showing lymphocyte predominant (LP) cells *(arrows)* are negative for PDL-1, whereas the background tumor-infiltrating histiocytes *(arrowheads)* are highlighted by PDL-1 with granular pattern of staining by their cell processes.

cases harboring T-cell receptor gene rearrangements have also been documented. Genetic structural alterations that modulate the tumor microenvironment have also been observed. For example, 9p24.1 amplification leads to enhanced PDL-1 expression by RS cells, which inhibit T-cell effector functions by binding to PD-1 on T cells, enhancing survival of the RS cells (Fig. 75.5).[1]

DIAGNOSIS AND STAGING

Diagnosis

The definitive diagnosis of HL must be made pathologically via excision biopsy of an affected lymph node or other suspected organ. Core needle biopsy is deemed inferior to excision biopsy because of the unique architecture of the lymph node in HL that comprises a relatively dilute population of malignant cells. The presence of RS cells in cHL, and LP cells in NLPHL in tissue biopsy, provides the basis for discriminating between these two major diagnostic subtypes, with immunophenotypic profiling representing a crucial adjunct for all new cases of HL (see Pathobiology of HL section, earlier).

Staging

Stage of disease is the major determinant of prognosis for patients with newly diagnosed HL, and accurate assessment is paramount when deciding upon optimal therapy. The current staging system used for patients with HL is the Cotswold-modified Ann Arbor classification system (Table 75.2).

More recently, in 2014, the Lugano classification proposed further modifications to the evaluation, staging, and response assessment of patients with HL: as well as further defining the criteria for and significance of extranodal disease involvement, the group heralded integrated PET/computed tomography (CT) as the "gold standard" for the staging of ^{18}F-2-deoxyglucose (FDG)–avid lymphomas and reinforced its recommendation as an effective response assessment tool both early on during treatment and at the end of treatment to establish remission status.[2] CT (neck, chest, abdomen, pelvis) alone

TABLE 75.2 **Cotswold-Modified Ann Arbor Staging System for Hodgkin Lymphoma**

Stage	Criteria
I	Disease affecting a single lymph node region or lymphoid structure (e.g., spleen, thymus, Waldeyer ring).
II	Disease affecting two or more discrete lymph node regions confined to the same side of the diaphragm.
II	Disease affecting two or more discrete lymph node regions or lymphoid structures on both sides of the diaphragm.
IV	Disease that has spread to one or more extranodal site (that does not meet the criteria for E) or extralymphatic structure including involvement of the bone marrow, liver, or lungs.

Designation	Criteria
A	Absence of B symptoms[a]
B	Presence of B symptoms[a]
S	Involvement of the spleen
E	Single extranodal site or involvement of an extranodal site that is contiguous to an involved nodal region.
X	Bulky disease as defined as >1/3 mediastinum at its widest part or a nodal mass >10 cm at its greatest diameter.

[a]B symptoms: constitutional symptoms including night sweats, fevers, or weight loss (>10% over 6 months).

should only be performed if integrated PET/CT is unavailable. In selected cases with mediastinal involvement, chest x-ray (CXR) may still be indicated at staging, to determine whether or not criteria for bulky disease are met.

Bone marrow involvement occurs in <5% of patients with HL at diagnosis. Until recently, following pathologic diagnosis with excisional node biopsy, a bone marrow biopsy was also required as part of routine staging for all patients with newly diagnosed HL. However, because of the high sensitivity of PET/CT for bone marrow involvement, bone marrow biopsy is no longer mandated for the routine staging of patients with newly diagnosed HL, unless PET/CT imaging is unavailable.[2]

In addition to excisional node biopsy and staging with PET/CT, assessment of the peripheral blood represents an important part of the diagnostic workup for patients with newly diagnosed HL with particular respect to risk stratification and treatment choice. Complete blood count, erythrocyte sedimentation rate (ESR), and serum biochemistry including C-reactive protein, alkaline phosphatase, lactate dehydrogenase, liver function tests, renal function tests, and albumin are required as part of standard care, and screening for HIV and hepatitis is strongly advised. In addition, given the potentially damaging effects of chemotherapy and RT, certain pretreatment investigations including cardiac and pulmonary function tests, thyroid function tests, reproductive counseling, and serum pregnancy testing, may also be warranted in selected patients.

As advances continue to be made with regards to imaging modality, molecular profiling, and improved disease characterization, further modifications to the current staging approach for patients with HL are expected. However, at present, the principles of the Cotswold-modified Ann Arbor staging system still apply and provide the backbone for management decisions and clinical trial design worldwide.

CLINICAL FEATURES

The importance of an accurate clinical history in facilitating the management of patients with HL should not be underestimated. Certain symptoms may provide clues as to the likely stage of disease or lead to further investigations that might identify additional sites of disease. This may result in important treatment modifications. An accurate past medical history, particularly with regards to lung, heart, and kidney function, is also crucial in highlighting those organs that might benefit from further investigation before commencing therapy, to ensure that treatment choices are both effective and safe for the individual.

Systemic symptoms that are known to influence prognosis in patients with HL include night sweats, fever, and weight loss. These constitutional symptoms have come to be known as "B symptoms" and their importance in HL is reflected by their inclusion as key components of the Cotswold-modified Ann Arbor staging system (see Staging section, earlier). B symptoms are a presenting feature in approximately 30% of patients with HL and may predate lymphadenopathy in some cases. Fever in HL may take any form, from continuous low-grade pyrexia to intermittent spikes exceeding 38°C (101°F), whereas night sweats are typically drenching. A particular type of fever that is considered characteristic of HL historically, is the Pel-Ebstein fever, which typically follows a swinging pattern, occurring on a daily basis for many weeks, with intermittent afebrile periods occurring between episodes. In reality, however, this phenomenon features rarely in the modern clinical setting. B symptoms may occur in isolation or simultaneously, and incidence tends to increase with more advanced disease.

Other well-described clinical features associated with HL include fatigue, chronic pruritus, which may be an early sign of disease in up to 15% of patients, and the presence of a pain localized to the site of involved lymphadenopathy that is precipitated by the consumption of alcohol.

PROGNOSTIC FACTORS, RISK STRATIFICATION, AND TREATMENT GROUPS

Prognostic factors have helped to predict the likely outcome for individual patients with HL at diagnosis. Clinical stage, presence of systemic symptoms, and tumor burden continue to be important prognostic factors in HL, and, in addition to disease histology and anatomic stage, are widely used for risk stratification and subsequent selection of appropriate initial therapy.

HL patients have traditionally been divided into two distinct prognostic groups according to clinical stage at diagnosis: early-stage disease, accounting for 45% of newly diagnosed patients, and advanced-stage disease, accounting for 55% of newly diagnosed patients.

Early Stage Disease

The category of early-stage HL includes patients with stages I or II. Early-stage disease may also include patients with B symptoms, bulky disease, or extension to adjacent sites. Limited stage disease is usually confined to nodes above the diaphragm nodes and less frequently presents in only subdiaphragmatic sites.

Data from large clinical studies in which HL patients with variable disease characteristics were treated uniformly and closely followed have allowed additional prognostic factors to be identified. These additional prognostic factors have led to the more accurate stratification of early-stage disease into early "favorable" and early "unfavorable" disease subgroups, with regards to outcome. Early stage I or II HL is considered "favorable" if it is limited to an area above the diaphragm and is not associated with other risk factors. Early stage I or II HL is considered "unfavorable" in the presence of other risk factors related to age, tumor burden, ESR, and number of involved nodal areas (Table 75.3).

The criteria for early-unfavorable stage HL vary slightly according to international cooperative group. Since 1982 the European Organization for Research and Treatment of Cancer (EORTC) has defined early-unfavorable HL as clinical stage I–IIA disease with one or more of the following: age greater than 50 years; ESR >50 mm/h in the absence of symptoms; ESR >30 mm/h in the presence of B symptoms; large mediastinal mass. The German Hodgkin Study Group (GHSG), however, refined these criteria in 1988 to include clinical stage I–IIA patients with any of the following risk factors: mediastinal mass greater than one-third of the maximum thoracic diameter; greater than three affected nodal areas; elevated ESR and localized extranodal disease infiltration. Early-unfavorable disease is often also referred to as Intermediate stage disease and these terms may be used interchangeably (see Table 75.3). Thus, early-stage HL is a heterogeneous group and treatment algorithms have been developed for different subgroups based on these prognostic factors and response criteria (see Treatment of Early-Stage Hodgkin Lymphoma section, later).

Advanced-Stage Disease

The criteria for advanced-stage HL again vary slightly according to international cooperative group. Whereas the EORTC defines advanced stage as those patients with clinical stage III–IV disease only, the GHSG also includes those patients with clinical stage IIB disease and a large mediastinal mass and/or extranodal disease involvement in their definition (see Table 75.3).

Following the identification of more specific and more widely applicable prognostic factors, the International Prognostic Score (IPS) was developed as an internationally accepted means of distinguishing those patients with newly diagnosed advanced HL who might be cured by standard treatment, and therefore avoid overtreatment, from those in whom standard treatment might fail. In 1998 based on a multivariate analysis of survival data from 5141 patients with newly diagnosed advanced HL treated between 1983 and 1992, seven adverse prognostic factors were identified as being statistically meaningful when predicting 5-year freedom from progression (FFP) and overall survival (OS): age ≥45 years, male sex, albumin <40 g/L, hemoglobin <10.5 g/dL, Ann Arbor stage IV, leucocytosis ≥15 × 10^9/L, and lymphocyte count <0.6 × 10^9/L. Five-year FFP was 84% for those patients with no adverse prognostic factors, and each additional factor reduced FFP by 7%, with four to seven factors

TABLE 75.3   Prognostic Factors in Early and Advanced-Stage Hodgkin Lymphoma

Prognostic Group	EORTC	GHSG	NCCN
Early-favorable	CS I-II without risk factors (supra-diaphragmatic)	CS I-II without risk factors	CS IA-IIA without risk factors
Early-unfavorable (Intermediate)	CS I-II with ≥1 risk factor (supra-diaphragmatic)	CS I-IIA with ≥1 risk factor C/D but not A/B	CS I-II with ≥1 risk factor
Advanced	CS III-IV	CS IIB with risk factors A/B CS III/IV	CS III-IV
Prognostic factors	(A) Bulky mediastinal mass[a] (B) Age ≥50 years (C) Elevated ESR (>50 mm/h without B symptoms; >30 mm/h with B symptoms[b]) (D) ≥4 nodal areas (out of 5 supra-diaphragmatic EORTC areas)	(A) Bulky mediastinal mass[a] (B) Extranodal disease (>1 lesion) (C) Elevated ESR (>50 mm/h without B symptoms; >30 mm/h with B symptoms[b]) (D) ≥3 nodal areas (out of 11 GHSG areas)	(A) Bulky mediastinal mass[a] (B) Bulk >10 cm (C) Elevated ESR (>50 mm/h without B symptoms) (D) B symptoms (E) ≥4 nodal areas (out of 17 Ann Arbor regions)

[a]Bulky mediastinal mass: ratio ≥0.035 of the maximum horizontal chest diameter (EORTC); ratio ≥1/3 of the maximum horizontal chest diameter (GHSG); ratio >1/3 of the maximum horizontal chest diameter (NCCN).
[b]B symptoms: night-sweats, fever, weight loss (unexplained, >10% over 6 months).
CS, Clinical stage; EORTC, European Organization for Research and Treatment of Cancer; ESR, estimated sedimentation rate; GHSG, German Hodgkin Study Group; NCCN, National Comprehensive Cancer Network.

TABLE 75.4   International Prognostic Score (IPS) for Advanced Hodgkin Lymphoma

No of Prognostic Factors	% of patients	5-year FFP (%)	5-year OS (%)
0–1 (low-risk)	29	79	90
2–3 (intermediate-risk)	52	64	80
4–7 (high-risk)	19	47	59

FFP, Freedom from progression; OS, overall survival.

TABLE 75.5   Standard Treatment Approach According to Prognostic Group

Early-favorable HL	Combined modality therapy • 2–4 cycles of chemotherapy followed by involved-field radiotherapy
Early-unfavorable HL (intermediate-stage)	Combined modality therapy • 4–6 cycles of chemotherapy followed by involved-field radiotherapy
Advanced HL	Extensive chemotherapy • 6–8 cycles of chemotherapy ± consolidation with localized radiotherapy

representing an FFP of 40%.[3] Three risk groups were established as a result, allowing therapy to be chosen according to these specific clinical characteristics, with the consensus being that higher risk patients should receive more intensive therapy (Table 75.4).

Treatment According to Prognostic Group

The stratification of patients with newly diagnosed HL into early-favorable, early-unfavorable, or advanced prognostic groups, has allowed initial treatment of these individuals to be risk-adapted. The treatment approach for those with early-favorable disease typically involves combined modality therapy, with two to four cycles of chemotherapy followed by IFRT. For early-unfavorable disease the treatment approach is similar, but with four to six cycles of chemotherapy usually being administered before RT. For advanced disease a more aggressive approach is adopted with six to eight cycles of combination chemotherapy alone, followed by consolidative localized RT in selected cases (Table 75.5).

The importance of clinical prognostic factors in predicting outcome and directing treatment for individuals with newly diagnosed HL is well established, and has undoubtedly contributed to the huge advances observed in HL over the past two decades. However, despite high cure rates, up to 30% of patients will still relapse. Furthermore, a significant proportion of those who are cured of their disease will go on to develop serious complications of treatment later on in life. Therefore the identification of additional, and more specific, biologic markers is needed to better discriminate these individuals according to their unique risk profiles, with the subsequent delivery of therapy that is personalized. Response-adapted tailoring of treatment with PET (discussed later) and gene expression profiling of primary tumor tissue are two approaches currently being investigated for this role.

TREATMENT OF EARLY-STAGE HODGKIN LYMPHOMA

Early-Stage Nodular Lymphocyte-Predominant Hodgkin Lymphoma

Traditionally, patients with NLPHL present with localized, early-stage peripheral lymphadenopathy, and are less likely to present with B symptoms, bulky disease, or mediastinal involvement. The behavior of this disease entity contrasts favorably to cHL, and its clinical behavior is more comparable to that of an indolent non-HL. A retrospective matched-pair analysis from the GHSG of 394 patients with NLPHL (compared with 7904 patients with cHL) confirmed these findings and validated the improved prognosis (tumor control and OS) of this disease entity. In addition, the European Task Force on Lymphoma (ETFL) conducted an analysis comprising 219 patients with histologically confirmed NLPHL. Both analyses revealed that B symptoms, bulky/extranodal disease, increased ESR and lactate dehydrogenase, and involvement of three or more nodal areas were less frequently found in NLPHL than in cHL.

For localized asymptomatic nonbulky NLPHL, ISRT alone is the preferred treatment. For the rare patient with localized NLPHL who presents with B symptoms or bulky disease, ISRT remains a consolidation treatment after initial rituximab and/or chemotherapy.

Early-Stage Classic Hodgkin Lymphoma

Recent strategies for the management of early-stage cHL have continued to focus on optimizing treatment by minimizing the extent of both chemotherapy and RT while maintaining the excellent cure rate and still reducing short- and long-term risk of complications. These approaches are based on the distinction between the amounts of treatment required in early-favorable patients compared with that required for optimal outcome in early-unfavorable patients. The risk factors that are used by different study groups to define early-stage HL subgroups are listed in Table 75.4. All criteria include the presence of a large mediastinal mass and B symptoms and use the principal that favorable disease should not have any of the risk factors listed (see Prognostic Factors, Risk Stratification, and Treatment Groups: Early-Stage Disease section, earlier).

The most comprehensive and powerful studies attempting reduction of treatment for early stage HL were published by the GHSG. In the HD10 randomized trial of 1370 patients with favorable disease, as few as two cycles of ABVD (adriamycin, bleomycin, vinblastine, and dacarbazine) followed by 20 Gy IFRT resulted in OS of 96.6% and freedom from treatment failure (FFTF) of 91.2% at 5 years. The minimal combined modality approach has become the standard of care for patients with early-stage favorable HL. HD10 was one of the first large studies to show that reduction of treatment intensity of both chemotherapy and RT did not reduce efficacy, but toxicity was decreased and side-effects of treatment were fewer. The next step of the GHSG to reduce treatment was by testing the possible elimination of either bleomycin or dacarbazine or both from ABVD ×2 followed by IFRT (HD13 trial), but was not successful and data suggested that if using only two cycles of ABVD, both bleomycin and dacarbazine should remain part of the regimen.

In unfavorable early-stage patients the GHSG HD11 trial randomized 1397 patients between four cycles of ABVD and four cycles of baseline BEACOPP (bleomycin, etoposide, doxorubicin, cyclophosphamide, vincristine, procarbazine, and prednisolone), and each chemotherapy arm was followed by either 30 Gy or 20 Gy IFRT. Four cycles of ABVD followed by IFRT of 30 Gy resulted in a 5-year FFTF of 85.3% and OS of 94.3% and was less toxic than baseline BEACOPP. Most groups recommend this approach of ABVD ×4 followed by IFRT of 30 Gy as the standard of care. It should be noted, however, that patients with a combination of bulky disease and B symptoms were not included in GHSG unfavorable early-stage programs and were referred to advanced-stage disease studies.

Another approach studied by the GHSG for patients ≤60 years who are eligible for a more intensive treatment involved using two cycles of escalated BEACOPP followed by two cycles of ABVD and 30 Gy IFRT (HD14 trial). After a median follow-up of 43 months, FFTF with this protocol was superior in comparison with four cycles of ABVD followed by 30 Gy IFRT, but an advantage in OS could not be shown.

Ultimately the standard practice for patients with unfavorable-risk early-stage HL is four cycles of chemotherapy followed by IFRT (30 Gy). Some current clinical trials are exploring new combinations of new chemotherapy combinations that include brentuximab vedotin (BV) and reduced radiation doses to explore even more effective therapies.

Response-Adapted Treatment Approach

In the era of FDG-PET imaging for assessment of metabolic response to induction chemotherapy, the need for consolidation RT has been challenged in two important recent trials.

The EORTC H10 trial, which used modern-involved node RT (INRT) techniques, randomized (both favorable and unfavorable risk) patients to chemotherapy alone versus combined modality treatment (CMT) for those with a negative FDG-PET after two cycles of ABVD. The outcomes appeared to be excellent (in terms of OS) in both arms of patients who received chemotherapy alone or CMT.[4] This study enrolled 1137 patients and after 34 events, an interim analysis found an unacceptably high rate of treatment failures in the chemotherapy alone group, subsequently mandating its closure.[4] The most favorable subgroup of patients in this study, who had a negative early PET scan after two cycles of ABVD only, experienced an inferior

1-year progression-free survival (PFS) of 94.5% (versus 100% in CMT arm). As per the statistical analysis plan for this noninferiority study, the primary endpoint will take place approximately 6.5 years after recruitment, with additional long-term analyses of OS, to be carried out after a median follow-up of 10 and 20 years.

Also, emerging data from the UK National Cancer Research Institute (NCRI) RAPID trial shows that early-stage HL patients with a favorable PET-based response after three cycles of chemotherapy may have an excellent prognosis without consolidation RT.[5] This study randomized 420 PET-negative patients (after three cycles of ABVD) to receive IFRT versus no further treatment. After a median follow-up of 45 months, this noninferiority trial revealed no difference in OS, but slightly, although not statistically significant, higher 3-year PFS (intention to treat analysis) in patients receiving IFRT (93.8% versus 90.7%), where a margin of ≤7% PFS difference was deemed acceptable.[5] Because 26 of 211 patients randomized to receive consolidation RT died from unrelated causes, but were scored as events within the RT arm, this raised the observation arm under the margin of noninferiority. When an "as-treated" analysis was performed, the 3-year PFS was 97% for CMT versus 90.7% for chemotherapy alone (hazard ratio [HR] = 2.39, p = .03).[5]

More recently, in 2015, the Cochrane Hematological Malignancies Group conducted a systematic review of randomized controlled trials that addressed the issue of whether PET-adapted therapy in individuals with HL results in better PFS (OS was not available in these very recent studies). In 1480 patients analyzed, PFS was shorter in participants with PET-adapted therapy (without RT) than in those receiving standard treatment with RT (HR 2.38; 95% confidence interval [CI] 1.62 to 3.50; p < .0001). This difference was also apparent in comparisons of participants receiving no additional RT (PET-adapted therapy) versus RT (standard therapy) (HR 1.86; 95% CI 1.07 to 3.23; p = .03) and in those receiving chemotherapy but no RT (PET-adapted therapy) versus standard RT (HR 3.00; 95% CI 1.75 to 5.14; p < .0001). Based on the data, the authors could assume that of 1000 individuals receiving PET-adapted treatment over 4 years, 222 individuals would experience disease progression or death compared with 100 of 1000 individuals receiving standard treatment.

TREATMENT OF ADVANCED-STAGE HODGKIN LYMPHOMA

The improved outlook for patients with advanced-stage HL (stages IIB–IV) over recent decades is largely attributed to the global drive to develop front-line chemotherapy regimens in which improved efficacy is coupled with reduced treatment-associated toxicity. The identification of adverse prognostic factors at diagnosis has been instrumental to this cause, in allowing more appropriate stratification of patients at baseline into groups in which therapy is risk-adapted. In addition, the use of the IPS over the years to further subdivide patients with advanced HL into more specific prognostic groups, each with significantly different FFP rates, has paved the way for a more preferable treatment approach that aims to achieve cure without exposing the individual to the unnecessary risks associated with overtreatment (see Prognostic Factors, Risk Stratification, and Treatment Groups section, earlier). In the 1960s the development of the drug combination MOPP (nitrogen mustard, vincristine [oncovin], procarbazine and prednisolone) was a pioneering step in the effective treatment of patients with advanced HL. With a complete remission (CR) rate of up to 80% and cure in more than 50% of patients, this regimen was heralded as revolutionary at the time not only within the field of lymphoma, in which patients with advanced HL had previously been considered incurable, but also for oncology as a whole; it was the first chemotherapy combination to be associated with cancer cure.[6]

Today, the most widely used regimens are ABVD (adriamycin, bleomycin, vinblastine, and dacarbazine) and BEACOPP (bleomycin, etoposide, doxorubicin, cyclophosphamide, vincristine, procarbazine, and prednisolone) (Table 75.6).

TABLE 75.6	Standard Chemotherapy Regimens for the Treatment of Advanced Hodgkin Lymphoma		
Regimen	Drugs	Route	Schedule
ABVD	Adriamycin 25 mg/m²	IV	Day 1 and 15
	Bleomycin 10 mg/m²	IV	Day 1 and 15
	Vinblastine 6 mg/m²	IV	Day 1 and 15
	Dacarbazine 375 mg/m²	IV	Day 1 and 15
			Every 28 days
BEACOPP (escalated)	Bleomycin 10 mg/m²	IV	Day 8
	Etoposide 200 mg/m²	IV	Day 1–3
	Adriamycin 35 mg/m²	IV	Day 1
	Cyclophosphamide 1250 mg/m²	IV	Day 1
	Vincristine 1.4 mg/m²	IV	Day 8
	Procabazine 100 mg/m²	PO	Days 1–7
	Prednisolone 40 mg/m²	PO	Days 1–14
	G-CSF	SC	From day 8
			Every 21 days

G-CSF, Granulocyte colony-stimulating factor.

ABVD

Despite the initial success of MOPP chemotherapy, failure to achieve initial remission continued to be a problem in up to 20% of patients with advanced HL and of those patients who *were* successfully treated with MOPP, a third still relapsed. Furthermore, as a result of prolonged exposure to alkylating agents, significant toxicities including secondary leukemias, myelodysplasia, and sterility had emerged with this regimen.

In 1975, in an initial attempt to treat patients with relapsed HL, the ABVD drug combination was developed by Bonadonna and colleagues.[6a] An early randomized control study directly comparing MOPP with ABVD for patients with advanced HL showed comparable CR rates between the two groups (76% versus 75%) and crossover carried out for progressive disease or for relapse after initial remission successfully demonstrated an absence of cross-resistance between the two regimens. As a result, ABVD was highlighted as an appropriate second-line option for those in whom initial MOPP therapy had failed.

In 1986, because of this success, the same group went on to investigate the potential role for ABVD in the first-line setting by comparing standard MOPP therapy with an alternating regimen of MOPP and ABVD in patients with stage IV HL who were chemotherapy-naive. The alternating MOPP/ABVD regimen was found to be superior to MOPP alone with regards to CR rate (88.9% vs. 74.4%), FFP (64.6% vs. 35.9% at 8 years, $p < .005$), relapse-free survival (72.6% vs. 45.1%), OS (83.9% vs. 63.9%, $p < .06$), and survival of complete responders (94.8% vs. 77.1%). Furthermore, in this landmark study there was no observed increase in associated major toxicity in the MOPP/ABVD arm.

A number of randomized trials were subsequently carried out to further investigate the role of ABVD for the upfront treatment of patients with advanced HL either by itself, or in combination with MOPP. In 1992 results from a pivotal multicenter trial conducted by the Cancer and Leukemia Group (CALGB), comparing six to eight cycles of MOPP alone, six to eight cycles of ABVD alone, and 12 alternating cycles of MOPP and ABVD, showed superior complete response rates (MOPP 67%, ABVD 82%, MOPP/ABVD 83%, $p = .006$) and 5-year failure-free survival rates (MOPP 50%, ABVD 61%, MOPP/ABVD 65%, $p = .02$) in both the ABVD and ABVD/MOPP arms compared with MOPP alone. Although subsequent analysis showed no significant difference between either of the ABVD-containing regimens and MOPP with regards to OS, the ABVD-alone arm was consistently shown to be significantly less myelotoxic than either of the regimens containing MOPP.[7]

Additional studies comparing hybrid regimens of MOPP and ABVD (given concurrently) with alternating cycles of MOPP and ABVD also demonstrated equivalent survival with either approach.[8,9]

Furthermore, in one study comparing a modified hybrid of MOPP/ABV with ABVD alone, not only were similar OS rates seen (OS ABVD 82% versus MOPP/ABV 81%), but pulmonary toxicity, hematologic toxicity, treatment-related death, and secondary malignancies were also shown to be significantly less in the ABVD-alone arm.[10] The conclusion was that ABVD was not only at least as effective as the standard of care at that time, but also easier to administer and safer. These data subsequently led to the international approval of six to eight cycles of ABVD as the new standard of care for the frontline treatment of patients with newly diagnosed advanced HL (see Table 75.6).

Although one of the main attractions of ABVD is its ability to maintain excellent OS without unnecessarily exposing the patient to the toxicity associated with alkylating agents, bleomycin-induced pulmonary toxicity remains an important problem for some individuals. For this reason, alternative drug combinations utilizing agents that have previously shown promise in the setting of relapsed HL have also been developed for the frontline treatment of patients with advanced HL and of these, etoposide-based regimens have emerged as acceptable substitutes.

BEACOPP

The relationship between chemotherapy dose and tumor response is well established. In 1992 the GHSG conducted a pilot study investigating whether treatment response and outcome could be improved by dose intensification in patients with newly diagnosed advanced HL. Dose intensification was achieved by reducing the duration over which the same treatment was administered and adding etoposide. As a result, the BEACOPP regimen (bleomycin, etoposide, doxorubicin, cyclophosphamide, vincristine, procarbazine, and prednisolone) was developed with encouraging results in preliminary studies.[11] The subsequent randomized HD9 trial, in 2009, comparing COPP/ABVD with standard-dose BEACOPP and escalated BEACOPP in patients aged 15–65 years with stage IIB, III, and IV HL, showed significantly improved FFTF and OS rates with BEACOPP compared with COPP/ABVD, with the best results observed with escalated BEACOPP (OS 91% escalated BEACOPP vs. 88% standard BEACOPP vs. 83% COPP/ABVD, $p < .002$). The rate of early progression was also significantly lower in the escalated BEACOPP arm (2% escalated BEACOPP vs. 8% standard BEACOPP vs. 10% COPP/ABVD, $p < .001$). Because of the superior outcomes observed with both BEACOPP regimens, the COPP/ABVD arm in this study was closed at interim analysis. The improved outcome seen with escalated BEACOPP in the HD9 study was substantiated by long-term follow-up analysis at 10 years.[12]

Despite the success demonstrated by escalated BEACOPP in the HD9 trial, longer-term complications including the development of myelodysplastic syndrome and secondary acute myeloid leukemia (AML) occurred more frequently when compared with standard BEACOPP and COPP/ABVD. In addition, acute hematologic toxicity, including anemia and thrombocytopenia, was also greater in the escalated BEACOPP arm, with blood product support being required more frequently. The increased toxicity observed with escalated BEACOPP provided the rationale for the GHSG to investigate the efficacy and toxicity of a time-intensified, rather than dose-intensified, variant of BEACOPP for patients with advanced HL. In their pilot study, standard dose BEACOPP (i.e., nonescalated) was administered over a reduced cycle duration of 14 days, as opposed to 21 days, along with granulocyte colony-stimulating factor (G-CSF) support. Results showed that although acute leukopenia, thrombocytopenia, and anemia were moderate with BEACOPP-14, the severity appeared to be less than that observed previously with escalated BEACOPP, while efficacy was maintained. This led to a multicenter, noninferiority randomized study (HD15 trial) in which 2182 patients with newly diagnosed advanced HL, aged between 18 and 60 years, were assigned to receive either eight cycles of escalated BEACOPP, six cycles of escalated BEACOPP, or eight cycles of BEACOPP-14, followed by PET-directed RT. The aim of the study was to establish the optimal number of cycles required to sustain efficacy while reducing toxicity to an acceptable level. FFTF at 5 years was sequentially superior with six cycles of escalated BEACOPP (89.9%) and eight cycles of BEACOPP-14 (85.4%) when compared with eight cycles of escalated BEACOPP (84.4%), as was OS (95.3% for 6× escBEACOPP vs. 94.5% for 8× BEACOPP-14 and 91.9% for 8× escBEACOPP). Furthermore, eight cycles of escalated BEACOPP was associated with a higher mortality rate when compared with either six cycles of escalated BEACOPP or eight cycles of BEACOPP-14 (7.5% vs. 4.6% and 5.2%, respectively), as well as an increased frequency of secondary malignancies (1.8% vs. 0.7% and 1.1%, respectively). It was concluded that overall, in patients younger than 60 years, six cycles of escalated BEACOPP followed by PET-directed RT was more effective and less toxic. This regimen was subsequently adopted as standard of care for patients with newly diagnosed advanced HL in Europe.

ABVD Versus Escalated BEACOPP

ABVD and escalated BEACOPP are internationally accepted as appropriate first-line treatments for patients with newly diagnosed advanced HL, but which of these approaches is optimal remains under debate. Although ABVD is more widely used in the Unites States, escalated BEACOPP tends to be the more favored approach in Europe.

A number of studies have directly compared these two strategies, not only in an attempt to establish superiority of one over the other in terms of OS, but also to identify specific subgroups of patients with advanced HL who might benefit more from a more intensive, or indeed less intensive, treatment approach.

A randomized study carried out by the EORTC in 2012 investigated whether patients with high-risk advanced disease (IPS ≥3) were likely to achieve greater benefit with a more intensive upfront regimen comprising four cycles of escalated BEACOPP followed by four cycles of standard BEACOPP or eight cycles of ABVD. Initial results of this study showed no significant difference in event-free survival (EFS) or OS between the two treatment groups at a median follow-up of 3.9 years.[13] Relapse rates were higher with ABVD, but the frequency of early discontinuations was greater with escalated BEACOPP. More recently, in 2014, Mournier and colleagues[13a] published results from the LYSA H34 trial, a parallel study investigating the same two regimens but in patients with advanced HL deemed to be at lower-risk (IPS 0–2). At a median follow-up of 5.5 years, PFS was significantly better in the BEACOPP arm (93% vs. 75%, p = .007), but OS was comparable (99% vs. 92%, p = .06). Again, fewer relapses were observed with BEACOPP.

Although greater response rates and improved PFS have been well demonstrated with escalated BEACOPP across a number of studies, making it an attractive option for many, its toxicity profile is not insignificant and should be carefully considered. Whether the treatment-related risks associated with this regimen can be justified in all patients remains controversial, particularly when effective salvage strategies with stem cell transplantation exist for patients who subsequently relapse. It is this argument that has led others to favor the use of the less aggressive ABVD approach first for patients with advanced HL.

In 2011 Viviani and colleagues reported results from a trial directly comparing frontline ABVD with escalated BEACOPP in patients with unfavorable or advanced HL (stage IIB, III, or IV, or IPI score ≥3). Following this, patients with residual or progressive disease went on to receive high-dose chemotherapy (HDCT) and autologous stem cell transplant (ASCT). Escalated BEACOPP (eBEACOPP) was found to be superior to ABVD with respect to duration of first remission (PFS at 7 years 85% vs. 73%, respectively, p = .004). Interestingly however, after completion of treatment overall, it emerged that salvage HDCT was sufficient to achieve comparable 7-year EFS and OS rates between the two groups, regardless of which initial chemotherapy regimen was administered (EFS 78% eBEACOPP vs. 71% ABVD, p = .15; OS eBEACOPP 89% vs.

84% ABVD, p = .39).[14] Thus, although treatment with BEACOPP resulted in better initial tumor control, the long-term outcome of the two regimens appeared to be the same, suggesting that neither was superior overall. It is important to note, however, that in this study initial ABVD was associated with significantly less treatment-related toxicity, including infertility and secondary malignancy, compared with escalated BEACOPP. Overall then, if the aim of treatment in this patient population is to achieve cure with minimal toxic risk, then a less aggressive frontline approach of ABVD seems reasonable, reserving more intense treatment with HDCT and ASCT for those with refractory or relapsed disease. For those with more adverse prognostic risk, however, more intense treatment with escalated BEACOPP may be warranted upfront. One potential strategy, which is currently being explored in clinical studies, includes reducing the total number of cycles of escalated BEACOPP and using interim-PET assessment to guide ongoing risk-adapted treatment. The overall goal is to maintain optimal disease control while limiting toxicity by restricting exposure to only those with high-risk disease in whom it may be better justified from a risk-benefit perspective. The role of interim-PET in this setting is discussed in more detail later (see New Directions in the Treatment of Advanced HL).

At present, ABVD and escalated BEACOPP are both considered acceptable strategies for the initial treatment of patients with advanced HL and are each currently recommended as standard of care.

Consolidation Approaches in Advanced Hodgkin Lymphoma

Consolidative Radiotherapy

Consolidation is frequently adopted following initial chemotherapy to augment response and to prevent progression of disease at residual sites. The role of consolidative RT for patients with advanced HL who achieve complete response or partial response (PR) following initial chemotherapy has been widely investigated in clinical trials, but a clear survival benefit has not been demonstrated. Some have pointed to small sample sizes in randomized studies as a reason for this. In an attempt to draw valid conclusions from the available data, Loeffler et al conducted a large metaanalysis of all studies comparing chemotherapy alone versus combined modality treatment (n = 1740). Combined modality treatment did not reduce rate of relapse in patients with stage IV disease and was, overall, associated with significantly inferior long-term survival compared with chemotherapy alone.

In 2003 an important prospective randomized study investigating the use of IFRT after chemotherapy for patients with previously untreated advanced HL was published by the EORTC. In this study of 739 patients, those achieving CR after initial treatment with MOPP-ABV (n = 421) were randomized to receive either IFRT to all originally involved nodal and extranodal sites or no further treatment. At a median follow-up of 79 months, IFRT was not shown to improve 5-year EFS or OS in those already achieving a CR after initial chemotherapy compared with observation alone (EFS 79% vs. 84%, respectively, p = .35; OS 85% vs. 91%, respectively, p = .07). However, benefit with consolidative IFRT was observed in those only achieving a PR after initial chemotherapy and interestingly, the overall outcome of these patients matched that of the group who achieved a CR (5-year EFS 79% and OS 87%). This observation suggests a potential role for consolidative RT in this subgroup of patients. Further evaluation is needed, however, and at present the exact subgroups of patients who are likely to consistently benefit from this modality have still not been fully established.

The use of more intensive first-line chemotherapy has led to more durable responses, and as such, the need for consolidation RT has come into question for patients with advanced HL. The increasing use of PET to assess early response and potentially direct ongoing treatment may further question its role. However, importantly, PET-directed management may also clarify those patients with localized bulky disease who may benefit from irradiation. In the GHSG HD15 trial, following six to eight cycles of standard BEACOPP chemotherapy, patients with residual PET-positive disease received IFRT. PFS at 1 year was 96% for the PET-negative patients who did not receive IFRT and 85% for the PET-positive group who did receive IFRT ($p = .011$), suggesting a possible role for consolidative RT in this subgroup.

Before any sound conclusions can be made, however, long-term follow-up data from these prospective randomized trials are needed to better evaluate the risks and benefits of adjuvant RT after initial chemotherapy in this patient population, particularly when considering the late toxicities that are associated with its use, including secondary malignancy within the treated field and cardiovascular disease (see Long-Term Complications of Treatment in Hodgkin Lymphoma section, later).

Consolidative Autologous Transplant

The function of ASCT to enhance outcome in patients with advanced HL immediately following standard chemotherapy has been investigated in a number of clinical studies. However, no survival benefit with this approach has been demonstrated. Instead, current practice is to reserve high-dose chemotherapy and ASCT for those patients who have either progressed through, or relapsed after, first-line therapy (see Relapsed and Refractory Hodgkin Lymphoma section, later).

New Directions in the Treatment of Advanced Hodgkin Lymphoma

Interim PET

The identification of reliable and consistent risk factors is crucial for the future development of more specific, and therefore more successful, treatment approaches for patients with advanced HL, in which therapy is tailored to the needs of the individual. Interim PET analysis early on during first-line chemotherapy is being widely investigated as a potential means of enhancing this risk-directed approach by allowing initial therapy to be modified according to response.

The significance of residual FDG-avid disease during treatment for patients with advanced HL has been well described: In an early prospective study of patients with newly diagnosed advanced HL, a positive PET following two cycles of standard ABVD was associated with a 2-year PFS of 12.8% compared with 95% for those achieving a PET-negative response ($p < .0001$). Furthermore, in multivariate analyses interim PET was found to be more predictive of outcome than IPS score ($p < .0001$).[15] These early observations have been reproduced in parallel studies using escalated BEACOPP.

Clinical studies have since explored the role of interim PET as a tool for directing early, response-based, treatment modifications and have attempted to investigate the effect of this on patient outcome. In a retrospective analysis by Gallamini et al in 2011,[15a] the outcome of patients remaining PET-positive following two cycles of standard ABVD, who went on to receive treatment intensification with BEACOPP, was better than that of ABVD-treated historic controls. In a contrasting study by Avigdor et al in 2010,[15b] patients achieving a PET-negative remission following two cycles of escalated BEACOPP underwent deescalation of treatment to ABVD and in this group, despite attenuation of treatment, the 4-year PFS was maintained at 87%, implying that in this PET-negative population similar efficacy can be achieved with a less toxic approach.

At present two large randomized control trials are underway to further determine the role of PET-directed therapy in the future management of patients with advanced HL. The RATHL trial (Response Adapted Therapy using FDG-PET Imaging in Advanced Hodgkin Lymphoma), conducted by the UK NCRI, is evaluating intensification of therapy with BEACOPP in patients who remain

TABLE 75.7	Deauville 5-Point Scale for the Interpretation of Interim and End of Treatment FDG-PET Imaging in Patients with Hodgkin Lymphoma	
FDG-PET Uptake		**Deauville Score**
No uptake above background		1
Uptake equal to or below mediastinum		2
Uptake higher than mediastinum but equal to or lower than liver		3
Uptake moderately higher than liver		4
Uptake significantly higher than liver and/or presence of new lesions		5
New areas of uptake/New FDG-PET avid lesions		X

FDG, ^{18}F-2-deoxyglucose; PET, positron emission tomography.

PET-positive after two cycles of initial ABVD, while the GHSG's HD18 trial is evaluating the effect of reducing therapy from eight cycles of escalated BEACOPP to four cycles of escalated BEACOPP in patients who are interim PET-negative. Results of both of these trials are eagerly awaited.

Collectively, these data have indicated that early interim PET is a powerful predictor of treatment failure for patients with advanced HL and may effectively discriminate individuals with different risk profiles and therefore different treatment needs. The recent Lugano Classification recommends PET/CT as standard practice for response assessment in all patients with FDG-avid HL both at the end of treatment and early on during treatment using the highly reproducible Deauville 5-point scale[2] (Table 75.7). At interim analysis, a score of 1 or 2 represents complete metabolic response, whereas a score of 4 or 5 represents partial metabolic response. A score of 3 may or may not reflect a favorable prognosis depending on the timing of assessment, clinical background, and treatment used. At the end of treatment, residual disease denoted by a score of 4 or 5 represents treatment failure.

The strategy of subsequently utilizing PET response to deescalate ongoing treatment in the best responders to avoid late toxicity, or to intensify treatment in patients with suboptimal response, holds great potential for the future management of patients with advanced HL; however, at present this approach still remains investigational. Long-term prospective data from randomized clinical trials are crucial to evaluate the impact of PET-directed alteration of therapy on OS, before it is considered standard of care for this patient population.

Novel Therapies in Advanced Hodgkin Lymphoma

Although effective, the intensification of chemotherapy based on improved risk-stratification techniques may not be appropriate for all patients with HL. The development of novel targeted therapies has recently led to important advances in cancer care by allowing the provision of effective specific biologic agents which are not associated with the same toxic complications as traditional chemotherapy. This approach may be particularly beneficial for those with less favorable performance scores in whom traditional doses of intensive chemotherapy are deemed intolerable. One approach, which is currently being evaluated to further improve outcomes in patients with advanced HL, is the incorporation of novel targeted agents into less intense frontline chemotherapy regimens.

The recent success of BV in the treatment of relapsed/refractory HL (see Relapsed and Refractory Hodgkin Lymphoma section, later) has prompted efforts to explore its role when combined with standard chemotherapy in the upfront treatment of newly diagnosed advanced HL. In a phase I safety study including patients with newly diagnosed, treatment-naive advanced HL, escalating doses of Brentuximab Vedotin were added to either an ABVD or modified-AVD backbone (without bleomycin) for up to six cycles. The maximum tolerated dose (MTD) of brentuximab when combined with ABVD or AVD was 1.2 mg/kg. In this study CR was achieved in 95% of those receiving brentuximab plus ABVD and 96% of those receiving brentuximab plus AVD. Although a manageable toxicity profile was observed with brentuximab and AVD, an unacceptable level of pulmonary toxicity was associated with brentuximab and ABVD, exceeding that of ABVD alone, and, as a result, this combination was contraindicated. In contrast, no toxic pulmonary effects were observed with the brentuximab and AVD regimen.[16] A randomized phase III trial comparing BV and AVD with standard ABVD alone is currently ongoing (ECHELON-1). Similar studies investigating the combination of BV with BEACOPP-like regimens are also underway. Furthermore, the incorporation of other novel agents including rituximab and lenalidomide into frontline chemotherapy for patients with advanced HL is also being explored.

In summary, the current standard of care for the upfront treatment of patients with advanced HL includes initial chemotherapy, generally with ABVD or escalated BEACOPP. A clear role for consolidative RT has not been established. The future standard of care for patients with advanced HL is likely to be shaped by both PET-directed therapy, in which treatment is modified according to risk, and the incorporation of novel targeted agents into frontline chemotherapy regimens, with the overall aim of achieving cure while limiting exposure to unnecessary treatment-related toxicity. As a result, it is anticipated that the overall outcome for patients with advanced HL will continue to improve.

RELAPSED AND REFRACTORY HODGKIN LYMPHOMA

Although the vast majority of patients with newly diagnosed HL achieve a remission after first-line therapy, around 10% will have refractory disease (defined as progression or nonresponse during initial treatment or within 90 days of completing treatment). In addition, of those achieving initial cure, approximately 30% will relapse. Further remissions can be achieved for these patients with salvage therapy, for which the optimal choice depends on a combination of factors including the patient's stage of disease at relapse, their prior therapies, and their risk factor profile.

Prognostic Factors in Relapsed or Refractory Hodgkin Lymphoma

A number of risk factors for refractory disease or relapse following initial therapy have been identified for patients with HL. In two large retrospective analyses conducted by the GHSG, poor performance score at the time of progression, age greater than 50 years, and failure to achieve a temporary remission on first-line treatment were highlighted as significant predictors of adverse outcome for patients with primary refractory HL: in addition, time to first relapse, clinical stage III or IV disease at relapse, and anemia (hemoglobin <12 g/L males or <10.5 females) were considered significant predictors of adverse outcome for patients with relapsed HL.[17,18] Of these prognostic factors, performance status at relapse, advanced stage at relapse, and time to relapse appear to be consistently associated with poor risk across studies, but prospective confirmation of these is still needed.

Treatment of Relapsed or Refractory Hodgkin Lymphoma

For a select group of patients with favorable criteria who experience localized relapse at previously nonirradiated sites, treatment with salvage RT alone may be effective. More commonly, however, the role for radiation in the management of relapsed HL is limited to the treatment of either localized residual disease following salvage chemotherapy or localized late recurrence (>12 months) as part of planned consolidation. For a subset of other patients who relapse after primary chemotherapy, salvage chemotherapy alone with various, more intensive, second-line regimens can achieve further responses, although these responses are often suboptimal and the long-term

disease-free survival in these patients is often bleak, particularly for those with unfavorable prognostic factors.

The treatment of choice for the majority of patients with relapsed HL, or with refractory disease that has not responded to initial chemotherapy, is cytoreduction with salvage chemotherapy followed by high-dose salvage chemotherapy (HDCT) and ASCT. With modern-day transplant techniques and improved peritransplant management, the rate of early transplant-related mortality with ASCT has fallen from as high as 20% previously to <5% and, as such, ASCT is considered a safer and more accessible treatment option for a wider group of patients. As described later, favorable remissions and improved outcomes have been observed with HDCT followed by ASCT, compared with conventional salvage strategies and, as a result, this approach remains the standard of care for the initial treatment of patients with relapsed or refractory HL.

Salvage Chemotherapy and HDCT Before ASCT

The goal of cytoreduction with salvage chemotherapy and preparative HDCT conditioning before ASCT is to achieve high response rates and a minimal disease state, while maintaining an acceptable toxicity profile, without compromising subsequent stem cell mobilization. A number of second-line salvage chemotherapy combinations are currently in use, but because of a lack of randomized data comparing these regimens, there is no consensus as to which is optimal. Common regimens include DHAP (dexamethasone, cisplatin, cytarabine), ICE (ifosfamide, carboplatin, etoposide), GVD (gemcitabine, vinorelbine, liposomal doxorubicin), ESHAP (etoposide, methylprednisolone, cytarabine, cisplatin), mini-BEAM (carmustine, etoposide, cytarabine, melphalan) and dexa-BEAM (dexamethasone, carmustine, etoposide, cytarabine, melphalan), with patients typically receiving two to three cycles of therapy before proceeding to ASCT. Of these regimens, the greatest experience has been reported with DHAP, mini-BEAM, and dexa-BEAM in the context of randomized control trials assessing ASCT, with similarly high response rates being observed with each combination.[19–21] Although there is no evidence to suggest superiority of one salvage regimen over another with regards to efficacy, greater toxicity and impaired peripheral blood stem cell mobilization have been reported with melphalan-containing combinations.

HDCT and ASCT

The advantage of HDCT followed by ASCT over standard chemotherapy alone has been demonstrated in a number of studies. In 1997 Yuen and colleagues compared the outcome of patients receiving high-dose etoposide, cyclophosphamide, and total body irradiation (TBI) or carmustine followed by ASCT, with a matched conventional salvage group who received chemotherapy alone. At 4 years of follow-up a clear improvement was seen in those who underwent transplant with regards to OS, EFS, and FFP over chemotherapy alone (OS 54% vs. 47%, $p = .25$; EFS 53% vs. 27%, $p < .01$, FFP 62% vs. 32%, $p < .01$).

Two key randomized control trials (RCTs) have supported the superior role of HDCT followed by ASCT over conventional salvage therapy and have been integral to establishing this approach as the standard of care for patients with relapsed or refractory HL: In a comparison of high-dose BEAM chemotherapy plus autologous transplant versus standard-dose mini-BEAM chemotherapy alone, the British National Lymphoma Investigation (BNLI) group demonstrated significant differences in EFS and PFS in favor of BEAM followed by autologous transplant (53% vs. 10%).[19] In a larger trial conducted by the GHSG/EBMT, 161 patients with relapsed or refractory HL were randomized to receive either four cycles of dexa-BEAM or two cycles of dexa-BEAM followed by two further cycles of high-dose BEAM and ASCT. In chemosensitive patients, FFTF at 3 years was significantly better for those proceeding to HDCT and ASCT (55%) compared with standard chemotherapy alone (34%,

$p = .019$), although there was no significant difference in OS between the two groups.[20]

Intensification of HDCT

Although HDCT followed by ASCT has become standard practice for the management of patients with relapsed or refractory HL, the intensity of treatment that is required has not been fully determined. Following cytoreduction with salvage chemotherapy, high-dose chemotherapy can be intensified by delivering an additional course of treatment over a shorter period of time, before proceeding to a standard myeloablative regimen and ASCT, so-called sequential HDCT. Whether or not this approach improves outcome, particularly for those patients who achieve less than a complete response (CR) post–salvage therapy, is unclear. In a randomized control trial performed by the GHSG, EORTC, and EBMT intergroup, the impact of sequential HDCT was evaluated. Patients with relapsed HL who had responded to two cycles of DHAP were randomly assigned either standard HDCT with BEAM followed by ASCT or sequential high-dose cyclophosphamide, methotrexate, and etoposide before BEAM and ASCT. There was no significant difference between the two arms with regards to FFTF or OS, but sequential HDCT was associated with greater toxicity.[21] Sequential HDCT has therefore not replaced standard HDCT before ASCT in the treatment of patients with relapsed or refractory HL, although further work evaluating its role is ongoing.

Another intensification approach being investigated for patients with refractory HL or with unfavorable risk is tandem autologous transplantation, in which two courses of HDCT are each followed by a transplant of the patient's own peripheral blood stem cells. In the large multicenter H96 trial led by the GELA, patients were risk-stratified as follows: high-risk patients with primary refractory disease or at least two risk factors (time to relapse <12 months, stage III–IV disease at relapse or relapse in previously irradiated sites) underwent tandem ASCT whereas intermediate-risk patients with one risk factor underwent single ASCT only. Five-year OS was 85% in the intermediate-risk group and 57% in the high-risk tandem transplant group, an improvement on 30% previously reported in this poor-risk population. Randomized control trials are needed to establish the true value of tandem autologous transplant for patients with relapsed or refractory HL.

Despite the intensity of salvage chemotherapy before ASCT, up to 40% of patients will not attain a response.[19–21] Whether subsequent ASCT is of benefit to these chemoresistant individuals remains unclear because of a lack of randomized data in the literature. Second attempts to achieve responses that are good enough to support subsequent ASCT have been made using other non–cross-resistant agents, but this appears to be effective in only a proportion of patients and the overall outcome of these individuals tends to be unfavorable compared with those who respond to salvage chemotherapy initially.

Role of PET Post–Salvage Therapy and Before ASCT

Emerging data on the role of PET imaging as a means of assessing response post–salvage chemotherapy have reinforced the importance of achieving a second complete response before transplantation and may be of particular benefit for these refractory patients in guiding more appropriate ongoing treatment.

The prognostic value of PET before HSCT and ASCT has been investigated in clinical studies. In a large prospective analysis from Memorial Sloan Kettering Cancer Center (MSKCC) identifying prognostic factors for patients with relapsed or refractory HL undergoing transplant, 153 patients with chemosensitive disease to ICE salvage therapy received HDCT and ASCT. Response was assessed by CT and functional imaging (gallium or FDG-PET) both before and after salvage therapy. Normalization of functional imaging (FI) after salvage therapy was identified as being strongly predictive of outcome: 5-year EFS was 75% in FI-negative patients versus 31% in FI-positive patients ($p < .0001$).[22]

In a phase II trial from the same institution, the importance of achieving PET-negativity before ASCT was reinforced further and the potential of this to guide ongoing treatment was suggested: Patients achieving a negative PET following initial salvage therapy with ICE proceeded to ASCT, whereas those remaining PET-positive (38%) went on to receive a second course of salvage therapy with non–cross-resistant gemcitabine, vinorelbine, and liposomal doxorubicin (GVD). Those responding to GVD (26/33) then also proceeded to HDCT and ASCT. At a median follow-up of 51 months, patients with negative PET scans before ASCT (either after one or two lines of salvage therapy) had an improved EFS of >80% compared with 28.6% in those who were PET-positive ($p < .001$). Furthermore, of those patients undergoing a second salvage attempt with GVD, 52% achieved a negative PET scan and the outcome of these patients was comparable to those who were PET-negative post–initial ICE.[23]

In summary, these data demonstrate the benefit of achieving PET negativity before ASCT. As such, despite still being investigational, there is mounting evidence to support a formal role for PET post–salvage chemotherapy as a predictive biomarker for directing further treatment in this relapsed/refractory population of patients: For those with a negative PET following salvage therapy, in whom a complete response is confirmed, HDCT followed by ASCT remains standard of care. However, for those with suboptimal response or evidence of disease progression by PET criteria following initial salvage therapy, it may be more appropriate to attempt further salvage approaches first, with ASCT being reserved for those in whom a successful second response is achieved. Validation of this approach, however, is required before it can be considered standard and, at present, the use of interim PET-guided treatment should be restricted to clinical trials.

Treatment Options for Patients Who Relapse Following ASCT

Although durable remissions have been reported following ASCT, approximately 40% of these individuals will experience further recurrence of their disease. Patients who experience relapse after ASCT often have a poor prognosis with mean survival estimated at just over 2 years. For these individuals, the treatment options are limited, with focus typically on achieving palliative control of disease and keeping treatment-related toxicity to a minimum, rather than on cure.

Further responses can be observed with single-agent chemotherapy including gemcitabine, vinorelbine, or bendamustine, but remissions are often not durable. IFRT may be of benefit for patients with localized relapse at previously uninvolved sites, particularly for those in whom further HDCT and ASCT is not deemed appropriate. The aim of RT in this setting is to extend disease control to delay the need for palliative chemotherapy. A more common role for RT in the peritransplant setting, however, is as adjuvant therapy, either directly before or after ASCT, to consolidate the responses achieved with HDCT and ASCT.

In a highly selected group of patients who relapse after first ASCT, a second autologous transplant may also be considered. This approach tends to be restricted to those relapsing more than 1 year after first ASCT, although data defining a clear role for second autograft are lacking. Another approach is to consider a reduced-intensity allogeneic stem cell transplant.

Allogeneic Transplant

Allogeneic stem cell transplantation (aSCT) may be offered as a means of salvage therapy for a specific group of patients with relapsed or progressive disease following ASCT. The benefits of aSCT over autologous include the advantage of using a disease-free graft and the ability to exploit a "graft versus lymphoma" effect as a direct result of acquisitioning a new immune system from a healthy donor.

The challenge of aSCT is to generate sufficient immunosuppression to permit donor engraftment, while reducing treatment-related toxicity to a minimum. Early attempts with myeloablative conditioning regimens in this patient population were associated with unacceptable rates of treatment-related mortality. As such, reduced-intensity, nonmyeloablative conditioning before aSCT, has been adopted as a more appropriate alternative.

In 2012 results of the largest prospective phase II study to date (HDR-ALLO study) were published by the EBMT and the Grupo Espanol de Linfomas/Trasplante de Medula Osea (GEL/TAMO). In this study the role of reduced-intensity aSCT was investigated in 92 patients with relapsed or refractory HL. Fourteen patients died as a result of refractory, and subsequently progressive, disease, with 78 proceeding to reduced-intensity aSCT. The PFS of these patients was 48% at 1 year and 24% at 4 years, with an OS of 71% at 1 year and 43% at 4 years. A nonrelapse mortality (NRM) rate of 8% at 100 days and 15% at 1 year was observed. Interestingly, chronic graft-versus-host disease (GVHD) was associated with lower rates of relapse and improved PFS.

For those who relapse after aSCT, donor-lymphocyte infusion (DLI) has been attempted as a salvage strategy to enhance the graft-versus-lymphoma effect with the aim of preventing relapse. In the HDR-ALLO study described earlier, DLI was administered to half of the patients who relapsed following aSCT. This was associated with an overall response rate (ORR) of 40% and a median time to progression of 7 months. Evidence for the use of DLI in this setting, however, remains limited.

These data suggest that aSCT has the potential to achieve relatively long-term remissions in selected, heavily pretreated, patients with HL who relapse following ASCT and that with a reduced-intensity approach NRM is substantially reduced. In this sense its use may be extended to greater number of patients than previously assumed. The prognosis of these individuals, however, remains extremely poor. A key concern with this approach is the relatively high risk of relapse, which continues to be the main cause of failure and represents the major on-going therapeutic hurdle.

Robust evidence to support a clear role for these potential strategies in the treatment of those with multiply relapsed HL is lacking and the absence of randomized studies has prevented a standard of care from being identified. Patients with relapsed or refractory disease following ASCT have unaddressed clinical needs and, as such, enrollment into well-designed clinical trials evaluating novel agents should be encouraged for all these individuals where possible. One such agent that has shown striking success over recent years and which, at present, remains the only drug approved by the US Food and Drug Administration (FDA) for this indication is BV.

Brentuximab Vedotin

The cell surface antigen CD30 is highly expressed on Hodgkin and Reed-Sternberg (HRS) cells. The efficacy of agents targeting CD30 has been extensively investigated for patients with relapsed and refractory HL. Brentuximab vedotin (SGN-35) is an antibody-drug conjugate (ADC) comprising an anti-CD30 monoclonal antibody conjugated to antitubulin monomethyl auristatin E (MMAE). The impressive activity demonstrated by BV in the preclinical setting has been matched by its marked efficacy in phase I and II clinical trials.

An initial phase I dose-escalation study in patients with relapsed or refractory CD30-positive hematologic cancers showed that BV is associated with a favorable safety profile and established 1.8 mg/kg every 3 weeks as the MTD. Significant efficacy was also observed in this study: tumor regression was demonstrated in 86% of patients, with a median durable response of 9.7 months.[24]

In a pivotal phase II trial of 102 patients with CD30-positive relapsed or refractory HL who had failed ASCT the safety and efficacy of BV was evaluated further.[25] ORR was 75%, with 34% of patients achieving a complete response. The median duration of response was 20.5 months. Peripheral neuropathy, nausea, fatigue, neutropenia, and diarrhea were the most common treatment-related toxicities. As a result of this study, in 2011 BV was the first drug to be approved

by the US FDA for the treatment of patients with relapsed or refractory HL following ASCT.

More recently, a potential role for BV as maintenance therapy following ASCT has also been suggested: Initial data from the international randomized AETHERA trial, presented in abstract form at the 2014 American Society of Hematology (ASH) Annual Meeting, show significantly improved PFS following the administration of BV every 3 weeks for up to 12 months after ASCT versus placebo in patients with high-risk relapsed or refractory HL.

On the back of its success in the relapsed/refractory setting, BV is now being evaluated in the frontline setting in combination with standard chemotherapy and results so far are promising, particularly in the advanced disease setting[16] (see New Directions in the Treatment of Advanced Hodgkin Lymphoma: Novel Therapies section, earlier).

NOVEL AGENTS

The approval of BV as standard of care for patients with relapsed HL following autologous transplantation has improved the survival in this challenging patient population. The success of BV has paved the way for the development of a number of other novel therapeutics for the treatment of relapsed or refractory HL, including immune checkpoint inhibitors, epigenetic therapeutics, and other small molecules, with promising clinical activity being demonstrated so far (Fig. 75.6).

PD-1/PDL-1 Checkpoint Inhibitors

PD-1 (programmed cell death protein 1) is a cell surface receptor that is expressed on T regulatory and activated T cells (CD4 and CD8), activated B cells and NK cells. PD-1 binds PDL-1 and PDL-2, two ligands that are expressed by antigen-presenting cells and several cancer cells, including RS cells in HL (see Fig. 75.5). The PD-1/PDL-1/2 interaction inhibits kinases that are normally involved in T-cell activation. In this way the PD-1 pathway serves as a checkpoint to restrict T-cell–mediated immune responses, enabling tumor cells to evade immune detection. Inhibitors of PD-1, which block PD-1/PDL-1/2 engagement, may enhance T-cell immunity and prevent immune evasion by tumor cells, leading to effective cancer cell death.

Remarkable single-agent activity in patients with relapsed HL has been demonstrated with nivolumab, a specific monoclonal antibody directed against PD-1. Preliminary data from an ongoing trial evaluating the safety and efficacy of this agent in heavily pretreated patients with HL were recently published. Of 23 enrolled patients, 78% had failed prior ASCT and 78% had failed prior treatment with BV. Overall response rate following nivolumab therapy was 87% (95% CI, 66–97), with 17% achieving a CR and 70% achieving a PR. PFS survival at 24 weeks was 86% (95% CI, 62–95). Drug-related adverse events were reported in 78% of patients and none of these were greater than grade 3 toxicity (22%).[26]

PD-1 blockade with another monoclonal antibody, pembrolizumab, is also under clinical development for patients with relapsed HL after BV failure and preliminary results from a phase Ib study, which were recently presented at the 2014 ASH Annual Meeting, are encouraging.

The striking therapeutic activity and tolerability of PD-1 inhibitors suggests real potential for their inclusion in the future standard of care treatment of patients with relapsed or refractory HL, either as single-agent therapy or in combination with other agents. Long-term data, however, are awaited.

Histone Deacetylase Inhibitors

Histone deacetylase (HDAC) inhibitors are a class of agents that bring about tumor response in two distinct ways: by directly inhibiting tumor cell proliferation as a result of inducing cell cycle arrest

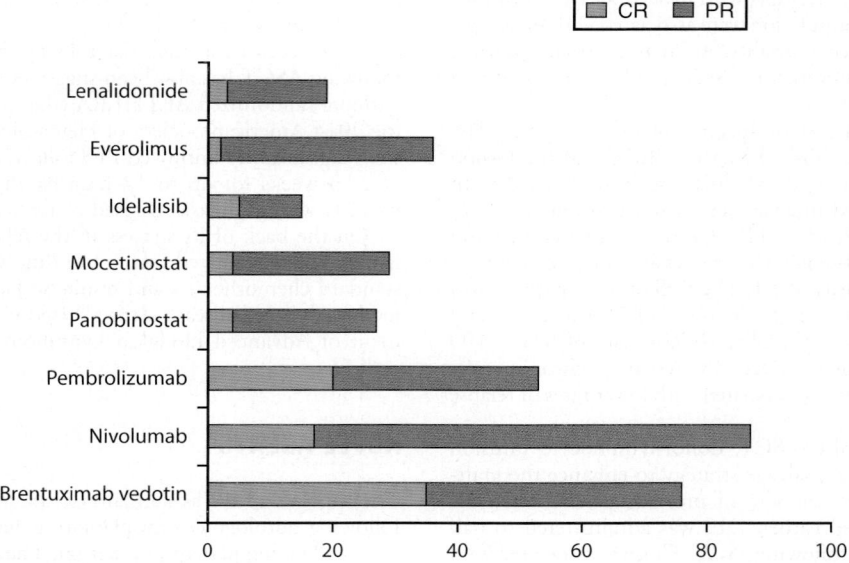

Fig. 75.6 RESPONSE RATES OF CURRENT NOVEL AGENTS UNDER INVESTIGATION FOR THE TREATMENT OF PATIENTS WITH RELAPSED OR REFRACTORY HODGKIN LYMPHOMA. *CR,* Complete response; *PR,* partial response.

and apoptosis via epigenetic effects on gene expression, and by interfering with T-cell chemotaxis in the tumor microenvironment and, in turn, indirectly generating a favorable antitumor immune response. As such, HDAC inhibitors have attracted much interest as potential agents for the treatment of patients with relapsed/refractory HL and, based on promising preclinical data, several, including panobinostat, mocetinostat, vorinostat, and entinostat are currently under clinical investigation.

In the largest phase II prospective international study of 129 heavily pretreated patients with HL who failed prior ASCT, the activity and safety of panobinostat (LBH 589) was explored. ORR was 27% (*n* = 35), of which 23% (*n* = 30) were partial responses and 4% (*n* = 5) were complete responses. Tumor reduction was observed in 74% of patients, and the median duration of response (DOR) was 6.9 months. Median PFS was 6.1 months, with an estimated 1-year OS of 78%. Common grade 1 and 2 toxicities included diarrhea, nausea, vomiting, and fatigue, and common grade 3 and 4 toxicities included thrombocytopenia, anemia, and neutropenia, which were all manageable.[27] In a similar population of 51 patients with relapsed or refractory HL, mocetinostat (MGCD0103), an oral isotype-selective HDAC inhibitor has also demonstrated single-agent activity (ORR 27%) with acceptable toxicity.[28]

PI3K/mTOR Pathway Inhibitors

The PI3K/AKT/mTOR intracellular signaling pathway plays an integral role in cell cycle regulation of metabolism, survival, and immunity and its aberrant activation, leading to increased proliferation and reduced apoptosis, has been implicated in a number of malignancies, including HL. Components of this pathway have therefore become attractive targets for anticancer therapeutic intervention.

Idelalisib (GS-1101 or CAL1011), an oral selective PI3K-delta inhibitor, has been shown, via the inhibition of AKT phosphorylation, to attenuate pathway signaling and induce apoptosis in cellular models of relapsed HL. Furthermore, in the clinical setting, promising efficacy and manageable toxicity have been demonstrated by targeting the downstream mTOR kinase: in a phase II study everolimus, an oral mTOR inhibitor, was associated with an ORR of 42% in 57 patients with heavily pretreated HL, with a median PFS of 9 months.[29]

More recently, the synergistic effect of combining an mTOR inhibitor with an HDAC inhibitor has been explored in the clinical

setting, following compelling preclinical data. In 2013 Oki et al[29a] published results from a phase I study evaluating the safety and efficacy of panobinostat plus everolimus in patients with relapsed or refractory HL and non-HL. Of the 14 patients with HL the ORR was 43% with a CR of 15%; however, in this study, thrombocytopenia was highlighted as a significant dose-limiting toxicity, suggesting that although this combination is effective, future studies are needed to explore how the tolerability of this approach may be improved.

Immunomodulators

A phase II multicenter study evaluating the efficacy of lenalidomide has provided preliminary evidence supporting the activity of this known, small molecule, immunomodulatory agent in patients with relapsed and refractory HL. In this study of 36 evaluable patients with a median of four prior therapies, the ORR was 19% and treatment was well tolerated.[30] The combination of lenalidomide with conventional chemotherapy or with other novel agents might also be considered a viable treatment approach in the future.

In summary, drug development continues to be an attractive and exciting area of clinical research in HL and future directions are likely to focus on how best to incorporate these agents into current treatment approaches. The effect of combining already established novel agents, such as BV, with first- and second-line chemotherapy is already being evaluated and the investigation of other biologics, either as mono or dual therapy, is also expected to continue. As a result, new treatment strategies are anticipated with the overall aim being to improve the survival of patients with HL even further, in the most tolerable way possible.

SPECIAL CONSIDERATIONS

Hodgkin Lymphoma in the Elderly

The number of patients living with cancer over the age of 60 years is increasing. The outcome of elderly patients with HL may differ significantly because of the heterogeneity of this population with regards to life expectancy, premorbid performance status, and comorbidity. Establishing optimal treatment is therefore challenging, particularly because older patients do not tend to be well represented in large clinical trials caused by tight exclusion criteria that often render them ineligible for enrollment. Data therefore are not necessarily representative of the general elderly population.

In 2005 Engert and colleagues[30a] from the GHSG published the results of a comprehensive retrospective analysis of 4251 patients with HL showing that acute treatment-related toxicity was higher in older patients compared with those under the age of 60 years. In addition, elderly patients with HL had a worse outcome with respect to FFTF (60% vs. 80%) and OS (65% vs. 90%), which was attributed to both increased mortality during treatment as well as the fact that significantly fewer elderly patients were able to tolerate the intended full dose of therapy (75% vs. 91%).

It is recommended that elderly patients without significant comorbidity and with a good performance status should be treated according to the current standard of care for younger individuals, on a risk-adapted basis, according to stage, with curative intent. Treatment-related toxicity and mortality may, however, occur more frequently. In 2005 a prospective randomized trial (H9-elderly), again conducted by the GHSG, compared standard-dose BEACOPP with COPP-ABVD in patients with newly diagnosed advanced HL. Disease-specific FFTF at 5 years was superior with standard-dose BEACOPP (74% vs. 55%, $p = .13$), but survival was not significantly different between the two treatment groups because of a higher rate of treatment-related mortality in the more intensive BEACOPP regimen compared with COPP-ABVD (21% vs. 8%). BEACOPP is therefore not recommended for elderly patients. More recently, in 2013, the North American intergroup reported results from the E2496 randomized trial investigating the efficacy and tolerability of ABVD and another combination, Stanford V (adriamycin, vinblastine, vincristine, bleomycin, nitrogen mustard, etoposide, prednisolone), in advanced-stage HL patients aged ≥60 years. Toxicities were comparable between the two age groups except for bleomycin lung toxicity which occurred more frequently in the elderly population receiving ABVD. Overall treatment-related mortality was 9% among older HL patients versus 0.3% in those less than 60 years old ($p < .001$). Outcome was significantly poorer in the elderly population with respect to 5-year failure-free survival and 5-year OS (5-year FFS 48% vs. 74%, $p < .002$; OS 58% vs. 90%, $p < .0001$), although there was no significant difference in time-to-progression (TTP) (5-year TTP 68% vs. 78%).

For elderly patients with poorer performance status, either caused by frailty or the presence of significant comorbidity, standard chemotherapy is not usually considered appropriate. Alternative, reduced intensity regimens such as VEPEMB (vinblastine, cyclophosphamide, procarbazine, prednisone, etoposide, mitoxantrone, and bleomycin) and, more recently, PVAG (prednisone, vinblastine, doxorubicin, gemcitabine) may be considered, although clear recommendations have not been established because of a lack of randomized data in this patient population. For relapsed disease, oral-based palliative chemotherapy with lomustine (CCNU) has been shown to prolong disease control in some cases. The potential role of less-toxic novel targeted therapies, such as BV, is also under current evaluation for the treatment of elderly patients with HL.

Hodgkin Lymphoma During Pregnancy

Given that the early incidence peak of HL coincides with childbearing age its management during pregnancy should assume special consideration. Lymphoma is the fourth commonest malignancy presenting in pregnancy and, of these, HL occurs most frequently. The diagnosis of HL during pregnancy matches that of the background population; lymph node biopsy can be performed safely either under local or general anesthetic. Clearly, however, traditional staging methods for patients with newly diagnosed HL who are pregnant need to be adapted. To avoid the risks associated with radiation exposure to the fetus, radiologic evaluation via chest x-ray with abdominal shielding, abdominal ultrasound, or magnetic resonance imaging, is recommended rather than CT or PET. Routine blood work and bone marrow biopsy are also indicated, as per standard practice. This modified approach to staging during pregnancy is

considered sufficient to allow appropriate ongoing management decisions, at least until more comprehensive imaging can be completed following delivery.

Consensus regarding the optimal treatment for pregnant patients with HL varies. The risk of spontaneous abortion and congenital malformations secondary to cytotoxic treatments and/or RT is known to be highest in the first trimester. Although risk decreases as pregnancy continues, the exact extent of risk during this period has not been clearly established and long-term complications are unknown. This is largely caused by the lack of data that exists as a result of small patient numbers. Thus whether chemotherapy should be started or not during pregnancy requires cautious evaluation of the risks to the unborn fetus versus the risks to maternal survival as a result of postponing treatment. Low-risk, asymptomatic patients may be monitored closely, with treatment being delayed until either the end of the first trimester or until delivery if diagnosis occurs later on during the pregnancy. For patients with bulky or symptomatic disease that requires treatment, however, single agent anthracyclines or vinca-alkaloids are deemed acceptable first choices, escalating to combined chemotherapy, usually with ABVD, following delivery or during the second or third trimester if there is evidence of progressive disease. In this latter subgroup of patients, however, the option of therapeutic abortion should be discussed with the patient and family to ensure all decisions made are informed. Traditionally, RT has not been advised during pregnancy; however, advancing techniques in this area have led to reduced fetal risk and, as such, it may be considered for selected individuals.

Hodgkin Lymphoma in Patients With HIV Infection

The incidence of HL is approximately 10-fold higher among HIV-positive individuals compared with those who are HIV-negative, and HL remains the most common non-AIDS defining malignancy. The vast majority of cases are associated with concurrent EBV infection, implicating a causative role for EBV in the pathogenesis HL in HIV-positive patients.

HL occurring in HIV-infected patients typically presents with more advanced disease, often with extranodal involvement and the presence of B symptoms. In contrast to HL presenting in HIV-negative patients, the mixed cellularity histologic subtype tends to predominate in this group.

In the past, before the arrival of highly active antiretroviral therapy (HAART), the treatment of HIV-associated HL was challenging, particularly in view of the immunosuppressed state. Less intense combination chemotherapy regimens were attempted, but response was often suboptimal and overall prognosis was poor.

Since the widespread use of HAART, however, the treatment of patients with HIV-associated HL has evolved and the outcome of these patients has significantly improved. Interestingly, despite improved outcome, the incidence of HL in HIV-positive patients has increased in the post-HAART era when compared with the start of the HIV epidemic. It has been postulated that improved CD4 counts, as a direct result of antiretroviral therapy, have allowed the restoration of a more competent immune microenvironment in which newly-populating CD4+ T cells are able to support underlying mechanisms of tumor development. To reinforce this, a pathologic shift has also been observed following the advent of HAART therapy, with the nodular-sclerosing subtype of HL now appearing more frequently among HIV-positive patients, mirroring the histologic distribution of cHL usually seen among the HIV-negative background population.

This concept has important implications when considering effective treatment for these patients. The enhanced immune environment following HAART has allowed more intensive regimens to be tested, and to good effect. As such, the current recommendation is to treat newly diagnosed cases of HL in HIV-infected patients with curative intent, using the same treatment approaches that have been adopted as standard of care for those without HIV infection. With modern HIV management, the OS of patients with HIV-associated HL is similar to that of the background, HIV-negative, population.

LONG-TERM COMPLICATIONS OF TREATMENT IN HODGKIN LYMPHOMA

The high cure rate associated with HL translates to a significant proportion of patients who are at increased risk for a range of long-term sequelae of treatment. Data on the cumulative incidence of cause-specific mortality in HL survivors show that although the rate of lymphoma-related deaths plateaus after the first 10–15 years following therapy, the rate of death because of late complications continues to rise.

The management of late toxicities associated with chemotherapy and/or RT is often more challenging than acute, with effects in some cases being irreversible and life threatening. Long-term treatment-related complications in patients previously treated for HL include hypothyroidism, peripheral neuropathy, gonadal dysfunction, secondary malignancy, and cardiovascular disease. Of these, secondary malignancy and cardiovascular complications occur most frequently, with risk continuing even beyond 25 years from diagnosis, and represent the two most common entities determining quality of life, long-term morbidity, and mortality in this patient population.

Secondary Malignancy

It is well described that intensive RT with extended field size and certain chemotherapy agents, such as cyclophosphamide, nitrogen mustard, procarbazine, and etoposide may increase the risk of developing secondary malignancies. Solid tumors appear to account for the majority of cases of secondary malignancy, with breast cancer, lung cancer, and gastrointestinal cancer occurring most frequently. This risk has been shown to be significantly greater among patients treated for HL during childhood or during teenage years. Among the female population, secondary breast cancer predominates, with extended radiation field size and the administration of RT to those under the age of 30 years representing the two most significant risk factors. Time to development of breast cancer is usually about 10–15 years. Therefore for all female patients receiving radiation to the mediastinum or axillae, annual breast screening with mammography is recommended 8–10 years after treatment or from the age of 40 years, whichever occurs first.

The risk of secondary hematologic malignancy, including leukemia and myelodysplasia, has been particularly associated with prior exposure to alkylating chemotherapy, especially when delivered in combination with large-field RT. Although this risk has fallen with the use of more modern chemotherapy, the exact choice of regimen still appears to be significant, with the incidence of AML or myelodysplasia being significantly greater among those treated with more intensive chemotherapy, such as BEACOPP, than with ABVD.[12,14] Time to development of treatment-related leukemia after HL is about 3–5 years, and the prognosis of these patients is poor, with an estimated OS of 7.2 months.

Cardiovascular Disease

The risk of cardiovascular disease may be three- to fivefold increased in survivors of HL compared with the general population. Cardiac complications tend to present approximately 10–15 years after exposure, although actual disease onset may in fact be well before this, given the lack of early symptoms in many cases. The association between anthracycline-based chemotherapy and cardiac toxicity is well established and is particularly relevant to the setting of HL given the chemotherapy combinations currently used in standard practice. Anthracycline-induced cardiac toxicity typically manifests as arrhythmias or congestive cardiac failure as a result of ventricular dysfunction secondary to direct myocardial damage. The severity of cardiac toxicity is directly correlated to the cumulative dose that is delivered and, as such, both individual dosage and the number of cycles are significant considerations when planning treatment. Radiation exposure has also been implicated in the development of late cardiac diseases including coronary artery disease, valvular dysfunction, myocardial dysfunction, pericarditis, and conduction defects, and radiation-related cardiac toxicity remains a major factor compromising overall outcome in HL survivors. Optimal screening methods for cardiovascular disease are not clearly established and therefore close monitoring of these patients is warranted, including strict control of cardiac risk factors (including hypertension, diabetes, hypercholesterolemia, and smoking).

Gonadal Dysfunction

A number of agents used in the treatment of HL can result in gonadal dysfunction, which is of particular relevance given the young age of this patient population. Pelvic RT and intensive alkylating-based frontline chemotherapy regimens such as MOPP and escalated BEACOPP have been shown to induce male and female sterility whereas the risk is reduced with baseline BEACOPP and reduced further still with less aggressive combinations such as ABVD where it is usually only transient. Unsurprisingly, however, the risk rises significantly among patients with relapsed or refractory disease following high-dose salvage chemotherapy. It is therefore recommended that all patients with newly diagnosed HL, who are of reproductive age, should be offered fertility preservation before commencing therapy.

The significance of long-term sequelae following treatment for HL has become more apparent over recent years given the growing number of young survivors. However, it is important to remember that a significant proportion of the data surrounding late effects relate to patients who were treated with chemotherapy and RT approaches that no longer feature in current practice. Increased awareness of long-term complications can account for many of the important treatment modifications which have been made over the past two decades, and provides the current rationale for ongoing development with regards to novel agents as well as RT technique. Current and future follow-up approaches for these individuals requires vigilance, focusing on strategies that enable both early detection and primary prevention wherever possible for the impact of these sequelae to be reduced. Guidelines for the optimal monitoring of adult HL survivors 5 years out of treatment have been issued by the National Comprehensive Cancer Network (NCCN).

CONCLUSION

The treatment of HL over the last 50 years has been one of the great success stories in oncology. Developments in combination chemotherapy and its use in association with RT have resulted in cure rates of greater than 80%, for a disease that was once usually fatal. For some patients, however, cure is still unachievable, and for others, survival is limited by late complications of cancer therapy. At present, the key objective in the ongoing management of HL is to increase efficacy without increasing the risk of unnecessary toxicity. Future approaches to management, not only in the relapsed and refractory setting, but also at earlier stages of disease are going to involve the use of targeted therapies. The best example so far is brentuximab vedotin, the first FDA-approved drug for HL since 1977, and its success is likely to revolutionize treatment. As more specific targets emerge based on advances in molecular tumor biology, further antibody and small molecule targeting, including for example PD-1 inhibitors, are likely to be developed. In addition, PET-directed approaches and the identification of more specific predictive biomarkers should help define which patients need more, or less, intensive treatments. The future management of HL is therefore likely to shift toward an approach that is no longer according to prognostic group, but rather according to the specific needs of the individual. This marks a pivotal moment in the treatment of a disease for which the development of new drugs had, until recently, remained static for more than 30 years.

REFERENCES

1. Green MR, Monti S, Rodig SJ, et al: Integrative analysis reveals selective 9p24.1 amplification, increased PD-1 ligand expression, and further induction via JAK2 in nodular sclerosing Hodgkin lymphoma and primary mediastinal large B-cell lymphoma. *Blood* 116(17):3268–3277, 2010.

2. Cheson BD, Fisher RI, Barrington SF, et al: Recommendations for initial evaluation, staging, and response assessment of Hodgkin and non-Hodgkin lymphoma: the Lugano classification. *J Clin Oncol* 32(27):3059–3068, 2014.

3. Hasenclever D, Diehl V: A prognostic score for advanced Hodgkin's disease. International Prognostic Factors Project on Advanced Hodgkin's Disease. *N Engl J Med* 339(21):1506–1514, 1998.

4. Raemaekers JMM, André MPE, Federico M, et al: Omitting radiotherapy in early positron emission tomography-negative stage I/II Hodgkin lymphoma is associated with an increased risk of early relapse: Clinical results of the preplanned interim analysis of the randomized EORTC/LYSA/FIL H10 trial. *J Clin Oncol* 32(12):1188–1194, 2014.

5. Radford J, Barrington S, Counsell N, et al: Involved field radiotherapy versus no further treatment in patients with clinical stages IA and IIA Hodgkin lymphoma and a 'negative' PET scan after 3 cycles ABVD: Results of the UK NCRI RAPID Trial. *Blood* 120:547, 2012.

6. Longo DL, Young RC, Wesley M, et al: Twenty years of MOPP therapy for Hodgkin's disease. *J Clin Oncol* 4(9):1295–1306, 1986.

6a. Bonadonna G, Zucali R, Monfardini S, et al: Combination chemotherapy of Hodgkin's disease with adriamycin, blemycin, vinblastine, and imidazole carboxamide versus MOPP. *Cancer* 1975:252–259, 1975.

7. Canellos GP, Anderson JR, Propert KJ, et al: Chemotherapy of advanced Hodgkin's disease with MOPP, ABVD, or MOPP alternating with ABVD. *N Engl J Med* 327(21):1478–1484, 1992.

8. Viviani S, Bonadonna G, Santoro A, et al: Alternating versus hybrid MOPP and ABVD combinations in advanced Hodgkin's disease: ten-year results. *J Clin Oncol* 14(5):1421–1430, 1996.

9. Connors JM, Klimo P, Adams G, et al: Treatment of advanced Hodgkin's disease with chemotherapy–comparison of MOPP/ABV hybrid regimen with alternating courses of MOPP and ABVD: a report from the National Cancer Institute of Canada clinical trials group. *J Clin Oncol* 15(4):1638–1645, 1997.

10. Duggan DB, Petroni GR, Johnson JL, et al: Randomized comparison of ABVD and MOPP/ABV hybrid for the treatment of advanced Hodgkin's disease: report of an intergroup trial. *J Clin Oncol* 21(4):607–614, 2003.

11. Diehl V, Sieber M, Rüffer U, et al: BEACOPP: an intensified chemotherapy regimen in advanced Hodgkin's disease. The German Hodgkin's Lymphoma Study Group. *Ann Oncol* 8(2):143–148, 1997.

12. Engert A, Diehl V, Franklin J, et al: Escalated-dose BEACOPP in the treatment of patients with advanced-stage Hodgkin's lymphoma: 10 years of follow-up of the GHSG HD9 study. *J Clin Oncol* 27(27):4548–4554, 2009.

13. Carde PP, Karrasch M, Fortpied C, et al: ABVD (8 cycles) versus BEACOPP (4 escalated cycles => 4 baseline) in stage III-IV high-risk Hodgkin lymphoma (HL): First results of EORTC 20012 Intergroup randomized phase III clinical trial. *J Clin Oncol* 30(Suppl 15s), 2012. Abstract 8002.

13a. Mournier N, Brice P, Bologna S, et al: Lymphoma Study Association (LYSA): ABVD (8 cycles) versus BEACOPP (4 escalated cycles ≥ 4 baseline): final results in stage III-IV low-risk Hodgkin lymphoma (IPS 0-2) of the LYSA H34 randomized trial. *Ann Oncol* 25(8):1622–1628, 2014.

14. Viviani S, Zinzani PL, Rambaldi A, et al: ABVD versus BEACOPP for Hodgkin's lymphoma when high-dose salvage is planned. *N Engl J Med* 365(3):203–212, 2011.

15. Gallamini A, Hutchings M, Rigacci L, et al: Early interim 2-[^{18}F]fluoro-2-deoxy-D-glucose positron emission tomography is prognostically superior to international prognostic score in advanced-stage Hodgkin's lymphoma: a report from a joint Italian-Danish study. *J Clin Oncol* 25(24):3746–3752, 2007.

15a. Gallamini A, Patti C, Viviani S, et al: Gruppo Italiano Terapie Innovative nei Linfomi (GITIL): Early chemotherapy intensification with BEACOPP in advanced-stage Hodgkin lymphoma patients with a interim-PET positive after two ABVD courses. *Br J Haematol* 152(5):551–560, 2011.

15b. Avigdor A, Bulvik S, Levi I, et al: Two cycles of escalated BEACOPP followed by four cycles of ABVD utilizing early-interim PET/CT scan is an effective regimen for advanced high-risk Hodgkin's lymphoma. *Ann Oncol* 21(1):126–132, 2010.

16. Batlevi CL, Younes A: Novel therapy for Hodgkin lymphoma. *Hematology Am Soc Hematol Educ Program* 2013:394–399, 2013.

17. Josting A, Rueffer U, Franklin J, et al: Prognostic factors and treatment outcome in primary progressive Hodgkin lymphoma: a report from the German Hodgkin Lymphoma Study Group. *Blood* 96(4):1280–1286, 2000.

18. Josting A, Franklin J, May M, et al: New prognostic score based on treatment outcome of patients with relapsed Hodgkin's lymphoma registered in the database of the German Hodgkin's lymphoma study group. *J Clin Oncol* 20(1):221–230, 2002.

19. Linch DC, Winfield D, Goldstone AH, et al: Dose intensification with autologous bone-marrow transplantation in relapsed and resistant Hodgkin's disease: results of a BNLI randomised trial. *Lancet* 341(8852):1051–1054, 1993.

20. Schmitz N, Pfistner B, Sextro M, et al: Aggressive conventional chemotherapy compared with high-dose chemotherapy with autologous haemopoietic stem-cell transplantation for relapsed chemosensitive Hodgkin's disease: a randomised trial. *Lancet* 359(9323):2065–2071, 2002.

21. Josting A, Müller H, Borchmann P, et al: Dose intensity of chemotherapy in patients with relapsed Hodgkin's lymphoma. *J Clin Oncol* 28(34):5074–5080, 2010.

22. Moskowitz AJ, Yahalom J, Kewalramani T, et al: Pretransplantation functional imaging predicts outcome following autologous stem cell transplantation for relapsed and refractory Hodgkin lymphoma. *Blood* 116(23):4934–4937, 2010.

23. Moskowitz CH, Matasar MJ, Zelenetz AD, et al: Normalization of pre-ASCT, FDG-PET imaging with second-line, non-cross-resistant, chemotherapy programs improves event-free survival in patients with Hodgkin lymphoma. *Blood* 119(7):1665–1670, 2012.

24. Younes A, Bartlett NL, Leonard JP, et al: Brentuximab vedotin (SGN-35) for relapsed CD30-positive lymphomas. *N Engl J Med* 363(19):1812–1821, 2010.

25. Younes A, Gopal AK, Smith SE, et al: Results of a pivotal phase II study of brentuximab vedotin for patients with relapsed or refractory Hodgkin's lymphoma. *J Clin Oncol* 30(18):2183–2189, 2012.

26. Ansell SM, Lesokhin AM, Borrello I, et al: PD-1 blockade with nivolumab in relapsed or refractory Hodgkin's lymphoma. *N Engl J Med* 372(4):311–319, 2015.

27. Younes A, Sureda A, Ben-Yehuda D, et al: Panobinostat in patients with relapsed/refractory Hodgkin's lymphoma after autologous stem-cell transplantation: results of a phase II study. *J Clin Oncol* 30(18):2197–2203, 2012.

28. Younes A, Oki Y, Bociek RG, et al: Mocetinostat for relapsed classical Hodgkin's lymphoma: an open-label, single-arm, phase 2 trial. *Lancet Oncol* 12(13):1222–1228, 2011.

29. Johnston PB, Pinter–Brown L, Rogerio J, et al: Everolimus for Relapsed/Refractory Classical Hodgkin Lymphoma: Multicenter, Open-Label, Single-Arm, Phase 2 Study. *ASH Annual Meeting Abstracts* 120(21):2740, 2012.

29a. Oki Y, Buglio D, Fanale M, et al: Phase I study of panobinostat plus everolimus in patients with relapsed or refractory lymphoma. *Clin Cancer Res* 29(24):6882–6890, 2013.

30. Fehniger TA, Larson S, Trinkaus K, et al: A phase 2 multicenter study of lenalidomide in relapsed or refractory classical Hodgkin lymphoma. *Blood* 118(19):5119–5125, 2011.

30a. Engert A, Ballova V, Haverkamp H, et al: Hodgkin's lymphoma in elderly patients: a comprehensive retrospective analysis from the German Hodgkin's Study Group. *J Clin Oncol* 23(22):5052–5060, 2005.

CHAPTER 76

ORIGIN OF NON-HODGKIN LYMPHOMA

Matthew S. McKinney and Sandeep S. Dave

Over the past two decades, discoveries in basic immunology and the pathogenesis of malignancies have significantly advanced our understanding of the origin of lymphoid neoplasms. These diseases have been reexamined and grouped based on recurrent chromosomal rearrangements, histologic patterns, and gene expression profiles. The multiple revisions to the World Health Organization's classification schemes for lymphomas reflect this progress. As with other cancers, lymphoma development is dependent upon acquisition of mutations, DNA copy number changes, recurrent cytogenetic rearrangements, and epigenetic dysregulation of gene expression involving oncogenic and tumor suppressor pathways. Many of these derangements occur as a result of disordered genetic recombination and somatic hypermutation (SHM) events intended to support adaptive immunity. Also, analysis of molecular features of lymphomas compared with normal lymphocyte compartments provides clues to the events driving their pathogenesis.

An evolving understanding of the steps involved in lymphoid development has provided further insights into the development of this diverse group of malignancies because most non-Hodgkin lymphomas (NHLs) reflect stages of lymphoid development. The application of gene expression profiling (GEP) and massively parallel high-throughput sequencing, as well as a better appreciation of the contribution of microRNAs (miRNAs) and epigenetic alterations to lymphoma pathogenesis, have shed new light on the mechanisms underlying lymphomagenesis. Correlation of these findings with the clinical outcomes has further refined prediction of outcome, and has suggested targets for novel therapies.

This chapter reviews the most common NHL subtypes, focusing on common B cell lymphoma subtypes, with regard to classification using prevailing views regarding genetic or genomic classification of these disorders. Additionally, insights regarding pathogenesis, prognosis, and possible therapeutic targets gleaned from genomic approaches are discussed.

OVERVIEW OF B-CELL LYMPHOMAS

Greater than 85% of NHL cases have a B-cell phenotype. With rare exception, B-cell lymphomas represent immortalized, "frozen" stages of B-cell development and the underlying molecular features of B-cell tumors reflect biologic features found in analogous normal B-cell compartments. Understanding factors governing regulation of B-cell compartments that mirror B-cell NHL subtypes is thus crucial to comprehending the driving forces behind lymphoma development (Fig. 76.1).

The goal of early B-cell development is to produce mature B cells expressing surface immunoglobulin M (IgM) that can efficiently recognize cognate antigen. After this is accomplished, B cells develop along pathways involving germinal center (GC), mantle, and marginal zones in lymphoid organs where they encounter antigens in association with activated antigen-presenting cells (APCs). Differentiation of mature B cells into plasma cells after SHM is the final step in B-cell development and is critical to the development of effective humoral immunity. Antibody diversity is accomplished through the process of somatic V(D)J recombination at the pro–B cell stage via recombinase activating genes (RAG1 and RAG2) followed by trafficking to GCs where they proliferate rapidly with dividing times of 6 to 8 hours. High-affinity B-cell clones produced in part via

activation-induced cytidine deaminase (AID) expression and SHM are favored because of protection from apoptosis. Through this mechanism, protective antibodies are produced at the risk of exposing antigen-stimulated B cells to genetic lesions caused by the molecular machinery utilized to create V(D)J recombination and SHM. Many NHLs exhibit translocations of driver oncogenes to highly active Ig loci, implying that recombination events intended to produce high-affinity antibodies are misdirected and instead produce immortalized B cells representing stages of B-cell development. Furthermore, mutations in oncogenes or tumor suppressors frequently occur in a pattern consistent with SHM at these loci. When considered together with the recurrent chromosomal rearrangements noted in NHL, this confirms the notion that these neoplasms stem from mature B cells that have entered (or are poised to enter) GCs.

Subsets of NHL recapitulate this pattern of normal B-cell differentiation at the histologic, molecular, and genomic levels and serve as a template for the classification of these diseases. This template can be applied to the entire spectrum of B-cell neoplasms, suggesting that NHLs form as a result of genetic alterations developed along this process. B-cell differentiation must be carefully choreographed at the molecular and genomic level because the expression of the RAG genes and AID cause DNA strand breaks and put the nascent lymphocyte at risk of oncogene overexpression and tumor suppressor deletion. Moreover, a coordinated regulation of gene expression is required to allow such genomic revision without triggering reflexive, protective apoptotic pathways and to allow appropriate B-cell differentiation. GC B cells highly express BCL6, and its functions are critically important to regulation of cell survival and differentiation. Targets of BCL6 also include cell cycle regulators (p21, p27) and TP53, which may overall work to facilitate cell cycle progression in the face of ongoing AID-mediated DNA strand breaks. BCL6 also represses PRDM1/Blimp1 and serves to prevent plasmacytic differentiation. Plasma cell differentiation is mediated by upregulation of IRF4 and nuclear factor kappa-B (NFκB), which establish characteristic regulatory programs.

Genetic lesions altering these pathways are found recurrently in NHL. BCL6 rearrangements occur in diffuse large B-cell lymphoma (DLBCL) and other lymphomas, and constitutively active NFκB signaling is associated specifically with aggressive phenotypes of DLBCL. Translocations and or mutations of BCL2, which is expressed at very low levels in GCs, occur in almost all follicular lymphomas (FLs) and illustrate the dangers of aberrant recombination events in the GCs because BCL2 translocation appears to be a primary event in the formation of these tumors. Recent analyses of whole genome/exome/transcriptome sequencing data have confirmed the frequent presence of these genetic lesions and have illuminated other pathways driving lymphomagenesis. In GC-derived B cell lymphomas, mutations in EZH2, a member of the polycomb group (PcG), occur frequently. In these tumors, EZH2 mutations result in aberrant histone methylation with resultant dysregulated control of gene expression and result in GC hyperplasia in mouse models. This process appears to enhance lymphomagenesis due to an acquired inability of GC B cells to differentiate and appropriately complete maturation and thus become transformed in a state of reflecting GC B cells (Fig. 76.2). A similar role for GC regulation has been defined for genes in the sphingosine-1-phosphate receptor2 (S1PR-2) signaling pathway. Genes encoding mediators of this pathway such as S1PR, P2RY8 and GNA13 are frequently mutated in GC B-derived lymphomas and

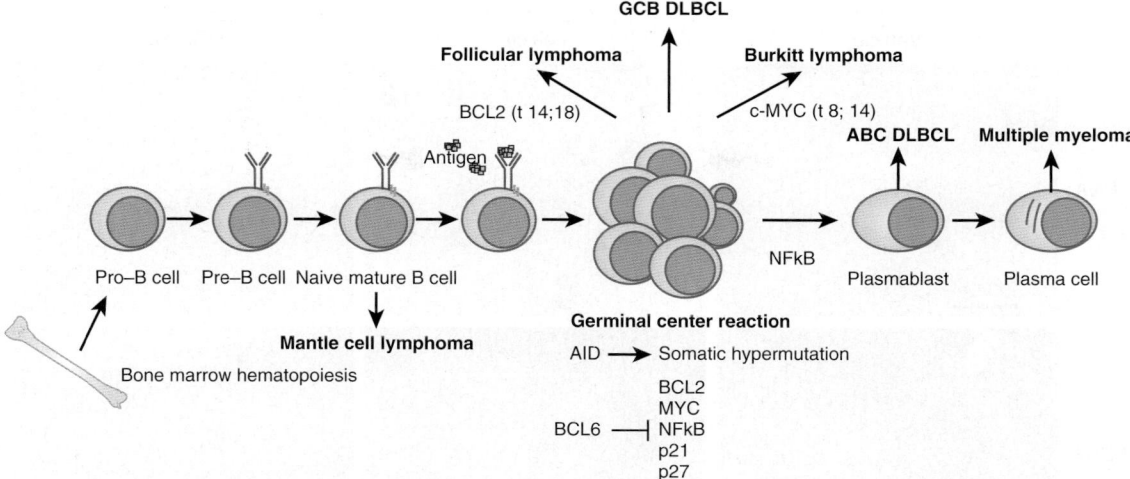

Fig. 76.1 CLASSIFICATION OF COMMON NON-HODGKIN LYMPHOMAS (NHLs) IN RELATION TO B-CELL DEVELOPMENT IN GERMINAL CENTERS (GCs). Hematopoiesis results in B cell precursors that ultimately produce immunoglobulin M (IgM) that recognize cognate antigen via activation of recombinase activating genes (*RAG1* and *RAG2*) and a GC reaction occurs. A regulatory program relying on BCL6 regulation of cell proliferation and apoptosis occurs at this point, and rearrangements presumed to occur along this course result in post-GC lymphomas, including follicular lymphoma, Burkitt lymphoma, and diffuse large B-cell lymphoma (DLBCL). The underlying molecular biology of NHL subsets (and other lymphoid neoplasms) reflects the GC step and other stages of B-cell development. For example, gene profiling of DLBCL reveals that whereas activated B cell–like (ABC) DLBCL reflects the plasmablast stage along normal B-cell development, multiple myeloma expression profiles more consistent with differentiated plasma cell origin.

result in dissemination of GC cells within lymph nodes. Thus, derangements in several different genes can result in abnormal GC homeostasis and drive lymphoma formation; thus is a novel paradigm whereby dysregulation of B cell differentiation leads to transformation and lymphoma.

Regulation of antigen stimulation of the B-cell receptor (BCR) is also important in both B-cell maturation and the development of NHL. The BCR consists of a multimeric signaling complex, including CD79A and CD79B, which acts through the immunoreceptor tyrosine activation motif on CD79B and leads to a cascade of molecular events involving SYK and BTK signaling. The end-result of this cascade is an increase in cellular proliferation through activation of NFκB target genes and other cellular machinery. Almost all NHLs express surface Ig, suggesting that functional BCR signaling is important at some point in the process of lymphoma formation. Analysis of Ig SHM patterns in lymphoma samples further suggests that antigen-induced selective pressure is important in the pathogenesis of NHL. The antigen(s) involved in this process are unknown, and it is also unclear whether ongoing antigen stimulation is important in subsets of NHL.

Epidemiologic studies have bolstered the argument that chronic immune activation and inflammation are connected with NHL development; these data also suggest that immune surveillance also plays a role in the origin of NHL. DLBCL and Burkitt lymphoma (BL) occur more frequently in immunocompromised hosts and are often Epstein-Barr virus (EBV)–positive. HIV/AIDS is a significant risk factor for post-GC neoplasms, and this risk is attenuated with the use of highly active antiretroviral therapy. For example, the risk of central nervous system lymphomas is increased more than 1000-fold in patients with AIDS. NHL also occurs more frequently in acquired or inherited immunodeficiencies such as common variable immunodeficiency and severe combined immunodeficiency and with solid organ and hemopoietic transplantation. Other clinical situations in which chronic infection or inflammation occurs have also been linked to NHL. Gastric MALT (*Helicobacter pylori*), hepatosplenic T-cell lymphoma (associated with infliximab use), and thyroid NHL (Hashimoto thyroiditis) are specific instances in which the development of lymphoid malignancy can be traced to chronic inflammation, either of microbial or autoimmune etiology. Finally, a

critical association with EBV has been noted for posttransplant lymphoproliferative disorder, a disease that occurs in the setting of organ transplantation and immunosuppression targeting cellular immunity.

Beyond these factors, the contributions of other modifiable risk factors and heredity appear to play only a small role in NHL development. Several environmental factors (pesticides, Agent Orange, radiation exposure) have been implicated in NHL, but the associations between these agents and lymphomagenesis are difficult to prove and the effect size of these factors appears to be relatively small. Pesticide exposure does appear to have a dose-effect relationship with regard to NHL pathogenesis and has been linked to recurrent t(14;18) cytogenetic rearrangements that are noted in DLBCL and FL, but the percentage of cases linked to pesticide exposure in these entities is very low. Likewise, several genetic linkage studies have found associations between several genes and the development of various lymphoma subtypes, but the role of variations in these pathways in lymphomagenesis has not been validated. Thus, there does appear to be inherited or modifiable risk factors that likely conspire with other acquired genetic/molecular lesions in the origin of lymphoma.

And so, factors related to abnormal immune surveillance, chronic inflammation, external exposures and host factors conspire to produce genetic/molecular lesions involved in lymphoma formation and progression. The remainder of this review will focus on current knowledge of biologic features of individual NHL subtypes.

DIFFUSE LARGE B-CELL LYMPHOMA

Diffuse large B-cell lymphoma is the most common subtype of NHL (~25% of all NHL) and is responsible for more patient deaths than any other form of lymphoma. This entity often presents at an advanced stage, and around 50% of all patients fail to respond long-term to standard chemotherapy programs; the vast majority of those patients will eventually succumb to their disease. Even prior to the availability of gene expression profiling technology, it was clear clinically (based on tumor morphology, immunohistochemical staining, and patient outcomes) that DLBCL is a heterogeneous disease.

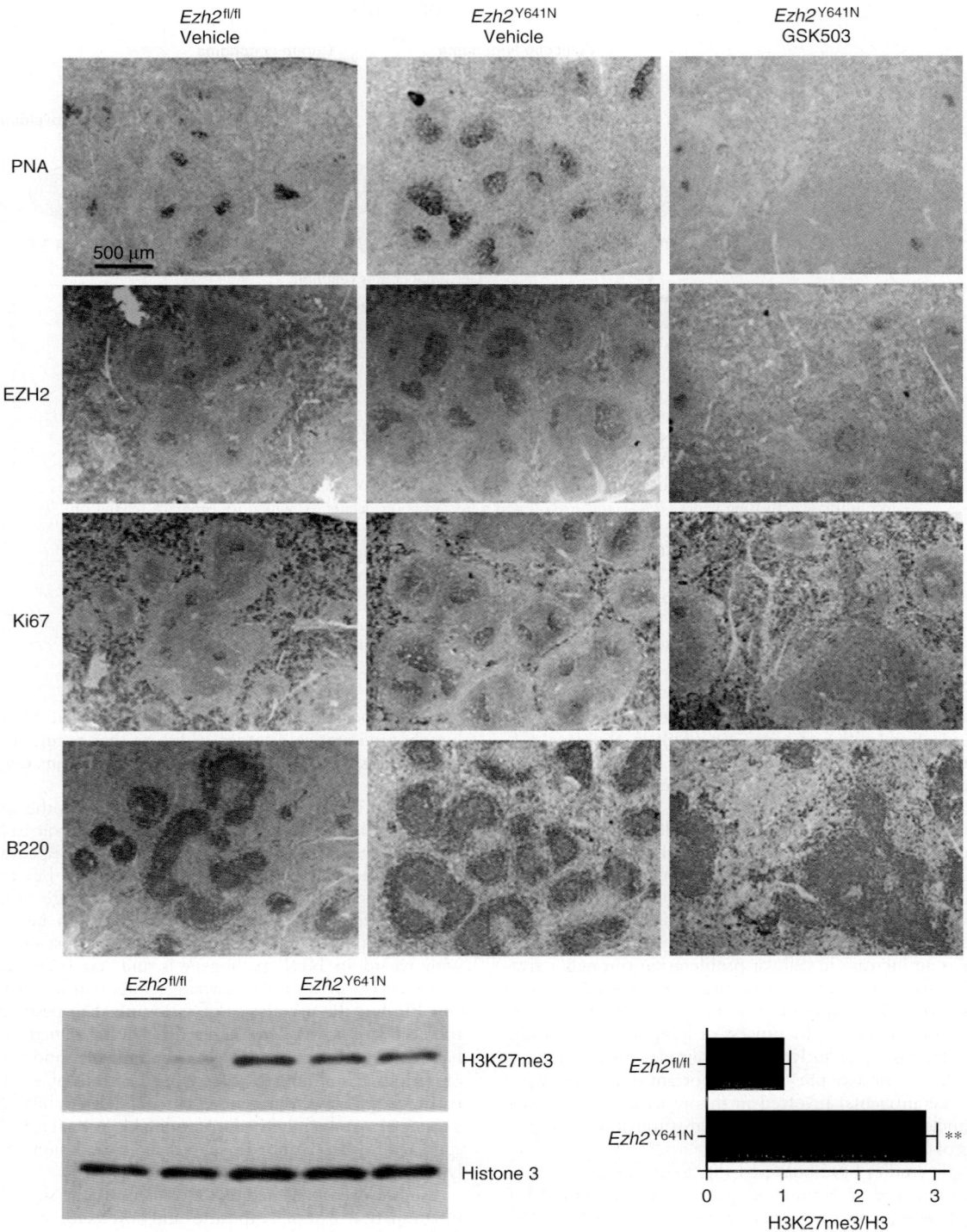

Fig. 76.2 EXPANSION OF GERMINAL CENTERS WITH EZH2 MUTATION CONFERRING INCREASE HISTONE 3 LYSINE 36 TRIMETHYLATION (H3K36ME3). *Upper* color panels depict histologic staining as indicated by row (PNA, EZH2, Ki67, B220) of murine mouse model bearing wild type versus mutant (Y641N) EZH2 with or without exposure to EZH2 inhibitor GSK503. Panels at *bottom* depict H3K36me3 levels according to EZH2 mutational status. *(See Beguelin, W: EZH2 is required for germinal center formation and somatic EZH2 mutations promote lymphoid transformation. Cancer Cell 23: 677, 2013.)*

Advances in molecular biology and genomic technologies have clarified the basis for some of this observed heterogeneity, and it has become clear that DLBCL comprises a diverse group of lymphomas that have distinct cellular origins, recurrent gene mutations, and chromosomal rearrangements that dictate their behavior. It is also clear that the stromal environment appears to play a key role in the development and progression of DLBCL, as with other cancers.

GENE EXPRESSION PROFILES DEFINE DIFFUSE LARGE B-CELL LYMPHOMA SUBTYPES

GEP has identified GC B cell–like (GCB) and activated B cell–like (ABC) DLBCL subsets that express gene signatures that mimic GCs and activated B cells (Fig. 76.3; Table 76.1). Roughly 30%

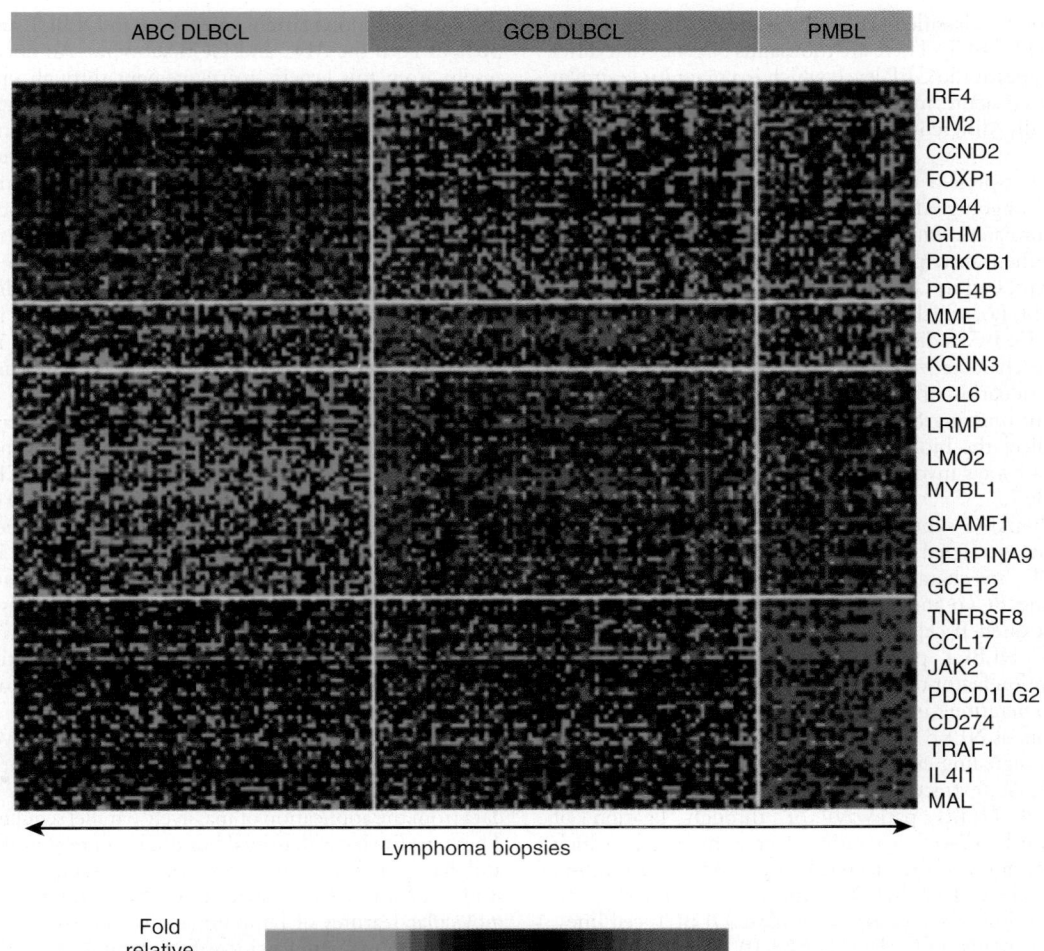

| ABC DLBCL | GCB DLBCL | PMBL |

IRF4
PIM2
CCND2
FOXP1
CD44
IGHM
PRKCB1
PDE4B
MME
CR2
KCNN3
BCL6
LRMP
LMO2
MYBL1
SLAMF1
SERPINA9
GCET2
TNFRSF8
CCL17
JAK2
PDCD1LG2
CD274
TRAF1
IL4I1
MAL

Lymphoma biopsies

Fold relative expression   0.25x   0.5x   1x   2x   4x

Fig. 76.3 GENES CHARACTERISTICALLY EXPRESSED BY SUBGROUPS OF DIFFUSE LARGE B-CELL LYMPHOMA (DLBCL). Activated B-cell–like (ABC) DLBCL, germinal center B cell–like (GCB) DLBCL, and primary mediastinal B-cell lymphoma (PMBL). Each column represents gene expression data from a single DLBCL biopsy sample, and each row represents expression of a single gene. Relative gene expression is indicated according to the color scale shown. *(From Alizadeh, AA: Distinct types of diffuse large B-cell lymphoma identified by gene expression profiling.* Nature *403:503, 2000.)*

TABLE 76.1 Frequency of Recurrent Genetic Aberrations in Diffuse Large B-Cell Lymphoma Subtypes

Genetic Feature	ABC DLBCL	GCB DLBCL	PMBL	Notes
BCL2 translocation t(14;18)	0%	40%–50%	20%	Alternatively translocated to light chain loci 5–10% of time
BCL2 amplification	34%	10%	16%	
BCL6 translocation t(3;V) (q27;V)	25%	10%	20%	Variable translocation partners (14q32, 2p11, 22q11, 4p11, 6p21, 11q23)
3q amplification	25%	0%	<5%	
9q24 amplification	5%	0%	45%	
PRDM1/PRDM1 deletion/ mutation	25%	0%	Unknown	
REL amplification	0	15%	25%	
Recurrent mutation	*CARD11, MYD88, CD79B*	*EZH2, GNA13, BCL2*	*PTPN1, SOCS1, STAT6*	
MYC rearrangement t(8;14) (q24;q32)	5%–10% of all DLBCLs	25%–30% occur with t(14;18)(q32;q21)		

ABC, Activated B cell–like; DLCBL, diffuse large B-cell lymphoma; GCB, germinal center B cell–like;mPMBL, primary mediastinal B-cell lymphoma
Compiled from Iqbal J: Distinctive patterns of BCL6 molecular alterations and their functional consequences in different subgroups of diffuse large B-cell lymphoma. *Leukemia* 21:2332, 2007; Iqbal J, Neppalli VT, Wright G, et al: BCL2 expression is a prognostic marker for the activated B cell–like type of diffuse large B-cell lymphoma. *J Clin Oncol* 24:961, 2006; Iqbal J, Weisenburger DD, Greiner TC, et al: Molecular signatures to improve diagnosis in peripheral T-cell lymphoma and prognostication in angioimmunoblastic T-cell lymphoma. *Blood* 115:1026, 2010; Pasqualucci L. Inactivation of the *PRDM1*/BLIMP1 gene in diffuse large B cell lymphoma. *J Exp Med* 203:311, 2006; and Tam W: Mutational analysis of *PRDM1* indicates a tumor-suppressor role in diffuse large B-cell lymphomas. *Blood* 107:4090, 2006.

of DLBCLs cannot be classified using this system and have been deemed unclassified DLBCL. There are thousands of genes that differ between these subtypes at the GEP level, which is a magnitude similar to that seen between acute myeloid and lymphoblastic leukemias that have profoundly different mechanisms of origin and natural histories.

GC B DLBCLs express a characteristic spectrum of genes and exhibit evidence of ongoing AID-mediated SHM as well as a histologic phenotype consistent with GC origin. BCL6 and LMO2 are both important to the transcriptional program of GCs and are commensurately overexpressed in GCB DLBCLs. Conversely, PRDM1 is downregulated by BCL6, which results in decreased PRDM1 activity in GCs, and GCB DLBCLs display a similar pattern. Histologically, GCB DLBCLs are characterized by CD10 expression and lack of IRF4 expression. Evaluation of Ig loci within GCB DLBCLs has also revealed evidence of ongoing SHM, which is further evidence that GCB DLBCLs reflect the biology of normal GC B cells and that dysregulation of pathways involved in GC formation might lead to this subset of DLBCL.

Alternatively, the ABC subtype of DLBCL expresses a post-GC phenotype but appears trapped just before differentiation into plasma cells. ABC DLBCLs are characterized by downregulation of many GC genes, including BCL6 and LMO2, and by expression of genes associated with activated B cells and plasma cells. One of the hallmarks of the ABC DLBCL phenotype is upregulation of NFκB. NFκB is a transcription factor that targets a number of gene programs governing cell proliferation, immortality, and angiogenesis within NHLs. The effectors of NFκB signaling exist in inactive form in the cytosol and require signaling either through MAPK/ERK (mitogen-activated protein kinase/extracellular signal-regulated kinase) signaling (the canonical NFκB pathway) or through ligation of CD40–LTbR–BAFF-R (B-cell activating factor receptor), which results in phosphorylation of the inactive complex and translocation of either the p50–RelA or p52–Rel B complexes to the nucleus and subsequent transcription of target genes. In ABC DLBCL cell lines, a signaling complex involving CARD11, BCL10, and MALT1 (the CBM complex) constitutively activates NFκB signaling and selective knock-down of any of the components of this complex using RNAi or small molecule inhibitors is lethal to ABC cell lines. Interestingly, a few GCB cell lines also demonstrate activation of NFκB and mutations in the NFκB pathway, which might confer sensitivity to inhibition of this pathway in those tumors. The mechanisms by which DLBCLs acquire and maintain constitutive NFκB activity are still being elucidated and may provide insights into the origin and into possible treatments for this entity.

Primary mediastinal B-cell lymphoma (PMBL) represents a distinct subset of patients that have sometimes been classified as DLBCL. PMBL was originally identified based on the clinical characteristics of the disease. Patients with PMBL are generally young (third or fourth decades of life), predominantly women, and present with a large mediastinal mass; outcomes with chemoimmunotherapy for PMBL are generally superior to those with other subtypes of DLBCL. GEP studies revealed that PMBL can be clearly delineated from ABC and GCB, subtypes. Indeed, by gene expression, PMBL appears similar to Hodgkin lymphoma with many shared features in both diseases, including the expression of CD30 (Fig. 76.4). Both diseases also express genes associated with JAK (Janus-activated kinase)–STAT (signal transducer and activator of transcription) signaling as well as targets of the NFκB pathway.

Molecular Pathogenesis of Diffuse Large B-Cell Lymphoma

Investigation of the molecular landscape of DLBCL has revealed a set of recurrent cytogenetic and molecular abnormalities associated with pathogenesis. Chromosomal translocations involving BCL6, BCL2, and MYC (v-myc myelocytomatosis viral oncogene homolog) occur frequently in DLBCL, and these translocations appear to be specific to cell-of-origin phenotype. 3q27 rearrangement with Ig gene partners is

the most common rearrangement seen in DLBCL and occurs in about 30% of both the ABC and GCB subtypes. An oncogenic phenotype results from this genetic rearrangement through upregulation of the BCL6 gene. Additional mutations in the transcriptional regulatory program of BCL6 may also occur with alternative translocation. Notably, BCL6 translocations appear to not be sufficient for lymphoma formation as evidenced by mice bearing t(3;14) translocations that develop NHL at a low rate. BCL2 translocations occur in a minority of GCB DLBCLs but are not seen in the ABC phenotype; this mirrors the situation in FL, in which BCL2 overexpression is associated with disordered GC transit. MYC rearrangements additionally occur in DLBCL (~10% to 15% of cases), sometimes with rearrangements of BCL2, BCL6, or both. These tumors, sometimes termed double-hit lymphomas, display an aggressive phenotype seemingly intermediate between BL and DLBCL.

Oncogenic mutations and areas of chromosomal amplification or deletion also appear important in the pathogenesis of DLBCL. Upregulation of c-REL occurs in about 20% of GCB tumors through amplification of the 2p locus. Amplification of MYC and BCL2 may also occur through this mechanism. TP53 mutations and SHM of other loci, including PIM1, BCL6, and MYC, also appear to contribute to lymphoma formation and progression. Mutations in CARD11 causing constitutive NFκB activation have been described in a subset of both ABC and GCB DLBCLs and appear to drive oncogenesis in these tumors. Overall, the patterns of gene mutation and recurrent cytogenetic abnormalities add further complexity to the classification of DLBCLs.

The genetic mutational landscapes of genes involved in DLBCL pathogenesis have also been reported. Most recently, several groups have reported analyses of whole-genome, exome, or transcriptome data from the application of massively parallel sequencing in DLBCLs. These studies have identified hundreds of novel mutations in DLBCL and have further defined patterns of mutational overlap through studies of mutual exclusivity (Fig. 76.5). Interestingly, some of the molecular features of lymphoma subtypes such as activation of the NFκB signaling pathway identified through gene expression profiling been shown to correlate with specific mutations in DLBCL cancer genes. Inactivating mutations of PRDM1 and mutation in genes regulating NFκB signaling (TNFAIP3, MYD88, CARD11) have been noted in ABC DLBCL subtypes. CD79B and BCL2 have also been found to harbor mutations in DLBCL and other NHLs. A series that performed RNA sequencing on 127 NHL samples (including 83 DLBCL tumors) found 651 coding single nucleotide variants (cSNVs), many of which were not previously documented in malignancies. Truncating deletions in tumor suppressor genes (TP53, TNFRSF14, CREBBP) were among the most significantly mutated genes and other heavily mutated genes not previously known to be involved in DLBCL pathogenesis (including MLL2, BTG1, EZH2 and GNA13). MLL2 contained cSNVs in 26% of tumors and most often occurred as a heterozygous defect, and sometimes multiple mutations occurred in trans fashion. MLL2 functions as a H3K4-specific methyltransferase responsible for regulation of transcription of developmental genes. Ostensibly, MLL2 might serve to deregulate genes involved in differentiation or development and act in conjunction with other oncogenes to facilitate NHL. Other groups have confirmed mutations in MLL2 and other genes (CREBBP/EP300) that coordinate chromatin acetylation, leading to the hypothesis that mutations in histone-modifying genes lead to DLBCL and other NHLs. Further work is needed to dissect the mechanism(s) by which the various molecular lesions in individual tumors cause lymphoma formation and this will perhaps also improve our understanding of normal lymphocyte biology while providing new tools for lymphoma diagnosis and treatment.

The Tumor Microenvironment and Diffuse Large B-Cell Lymphoma

The complexities of antigen presentation and recognition and regulation of B-cell proliferation that occur in GCs suggest that the

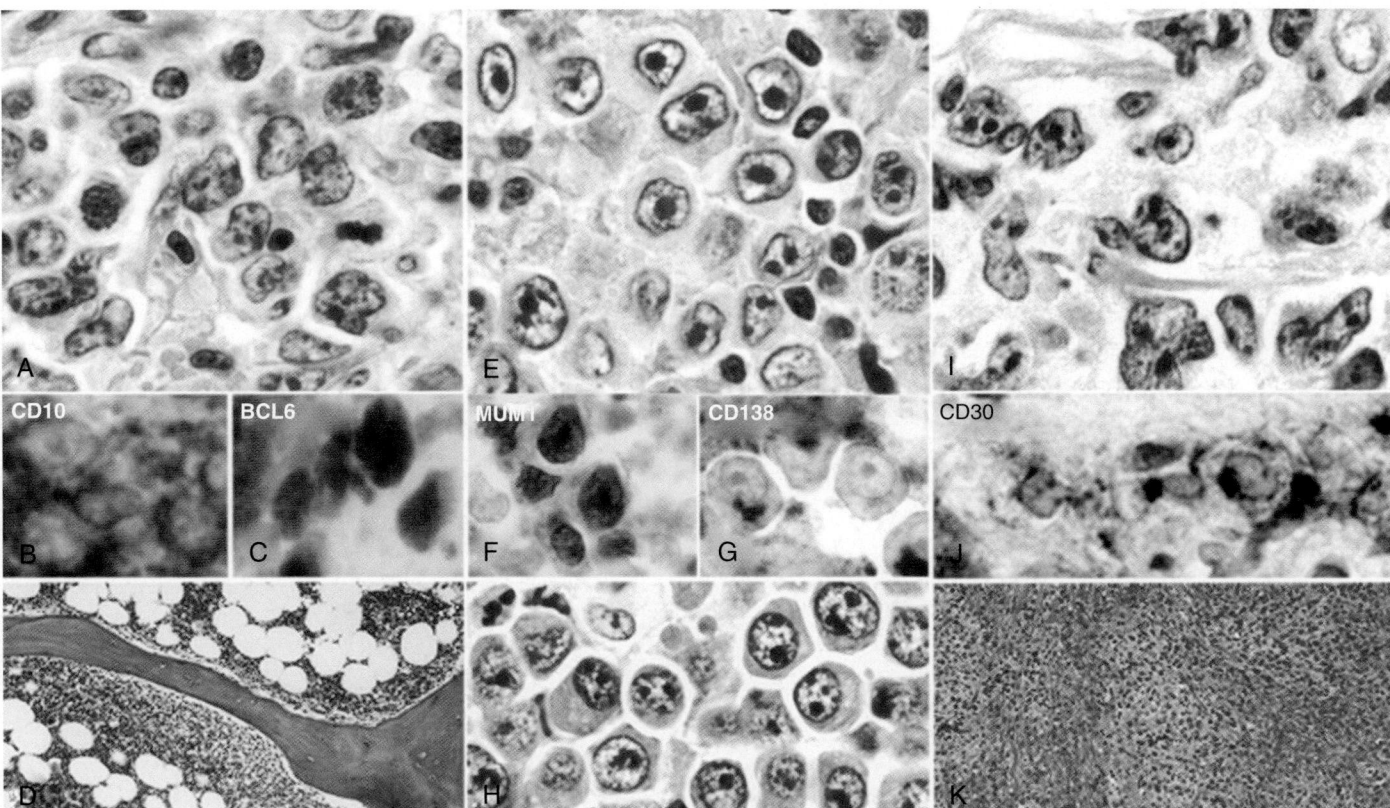

Fig. 76.4 THREE TYPES OF DIFFUSE LARGE B-CELL LYMPHOMA DELINEATED BY HISTO-LOGIC PATTERNS. Germinal center B cell–like (GCB), activated B-cell–type, and primary mediastinal B-cell lymphoma (PMBCL) type. GCB, or germinal center (GC)–derived large B-cell lymphomas usually have a centroblastic morphology (A), are CD20$^+$, and express the GC markers CD10 (B) and BCL6 (C). In this case, the patient's staging bone marrow (D) showed paratrabecular involvement by small cleaved cells (centrocytes), indicating that the large B-cell lymphoma likely arose from a lower grade follicular lymphoma. Activated B cell–like large B-cell lymphoma can sometime have an immunoblastic morphology (E) and can typically express MUM1 (F) and CD138 (G). These post-GC cell types of lymphomas can also have a plasmablastic morphology (H), as sometimes seen in HIV-related cases. PMBCLs are frequently composed of multilobated centroblasts (I). They are typically CD45$^+$, CD20$^+$, and usually CD30$^+$ (J) but CD15-negative. Surface immunoglobulin may be negative on such cases. PMBL is commonly associated with fibrosis, which is present in broad bands (K) or surrounding individual cells (as in I).

microenvironment may play a role in the origin and progression of DLBCL. Tumor-infiltrating T cells have been correlated with longer survival in patients with DLBCL, and failure of immune editing is likely responsible for the increase in NHL in HIV-positive and immunosuppressed persons. Gene expression profiling has been used to define stromal elements related to DLBCL progression. In one series, hierarchical clustering was used to define three groups among DLBCL samples by GEP. Clusters identifying gene signature termed *oxidative phosphorylation, BCR proliferation,* and *host response* were identified; notably, the host response group exhibited gene expression profiles associated with T and natural killer cells, dendritic cells, and macrophages. This work illustrates that patterns of stromal involvement in DLBCL could play a key role in pathogenesis. In another series involving biopsy specimens from 414 patients treated with chemotherapy and immunochemotherapy, two gene signatures characterizing patterns of tumor stroma best predicted survival. Improved survival was noted with a pattern that included genes associated with the extracellular matrix and histiocytic infiltration. The converse was true for gene profiles correlating to angiogenesis because these were associated with far worse overall survival.

Although it is not known what roles distinct lymph node subsets play in the pathogenesis of lymphoma, it is clear from these studies that the tumor microenvironment plays a role in the origin of NHL.

Conclusions

Diffuse large B-cell lymphoma represents a heterogeneous group of B-cell neoplasms with a distinct underlying biology, prognosis, and response to therapy. Recent genomic approaches to studying DLBCL have identified a number of interesting potential targets for better prognostic stratification and treatment of patients afflicted with this disease. More work is needed to this end and to better understand the origin of DLBCL and the role of stromal factors in disease progression.

BURKITT LYMPHOMA

Burkitt lymphoma (BL) is a highly aggressive lymphoma entity characterized by a high mitotic rate, extranodal spread, and early death, but it is frequently curable with high-intensity multi-agent chemotherapy. It was first described more than 50 years ago as a disease in young Africans in association with EBV infection. Since then, sporadic and immunodeficiency-related forms of the disease have been described. Subsequent work has shown that translocation of the *MYC* gene on chromosome 8q24 to the Ig locus occurs in virtually all cases of BL (see Figs. 76.6 and 76.7 for an overview of BL). Given the high prevalence of *MYC* rearrangements and the high

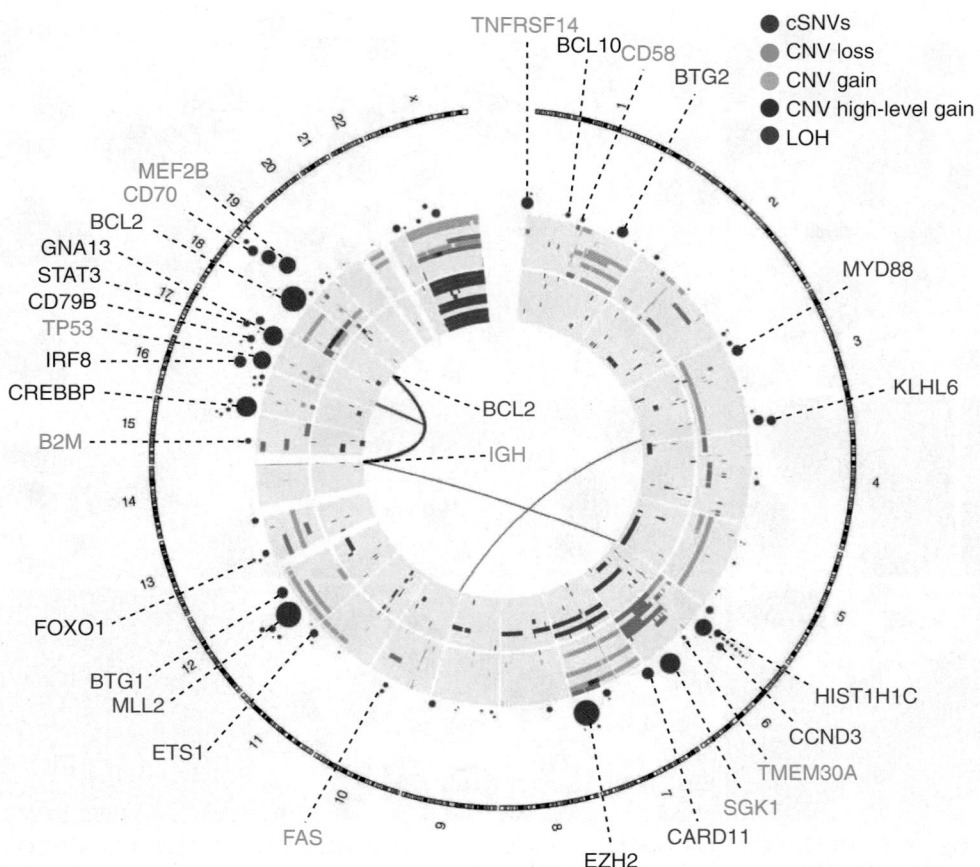

Fig. 76.5 GENOMIC EVENTS IN DIFFUSE LARGE B CELL LYMPHOMA AND FOLLICULAR LYMPHOMA. CIRCOS plot of coding single nucleotide variant (cSNVs), copy number variation (CNV) and loss of heterozygosity (LOH) in DLBCL and FL cases plotted by gene (chromosomal) annotation. *(From Morin:* Nature *476:298, 2011.)*

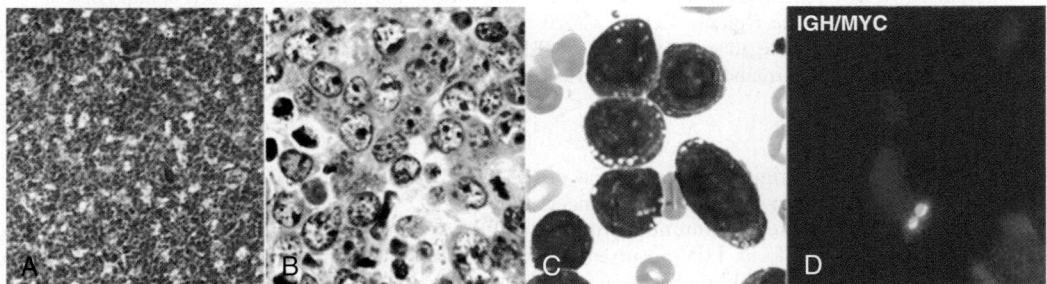

Fig. 76.6 BURKITT LYMPHOMA (BL). (A) A case of BL illustrated at low power showing the "starry sky" appearance. This appearance is attributable to the dense proliferating cells producing the "dark sky," and the scattered lighter-staining tingible body macrophages ("stars") phagocytizing dying cells. (B) Higher magnification image illustrating the syncytia of intermediate-sized cells with coarse chromatin and multiple nucleoli. Note the tingible body macrophage with abundant light cytoplasm and ingested debris *(center bottom)*. (C) Burkitt cells as seen on a Wright-stained bone marrow aspirate in a patient with BL. Notice deep blue cytoplasm with numerous vacuoles. (D) Fluorescence in situ hybridization with probes to MYC and immunoglobulin h (IgH) illustrate the IgH–MYC fusion. *(Courtesy Dr. Yanming Zhang, University of Chicago.)*

cure rates observed with chemotherapy, many have studied BL as a model for other B-cell lymphomas.

BL tumors typically display the immunophenotypic characteristics of GC B cells, and genetic and genomic studies have reinforced this notion of GC origin. Additionally, in virtually all cases, rearrangements are found between the MYC locus and one of the Ig genes, most commonly with the IgH locus at 14q32.33 in more than 80% of cases. Alternative rearrangements involving MYC and the κ or λ

light chain regions are also noted in a minority of cases. Two different patterns of rearrangement and SHM have been noted among the three types of BL. In endemic BL, chromosome 14 breakpoints can be mapped to J$_H$ regions, indicating *RAG1-* or *RAG2*-mediated rearrangement occurring at the pro-B cell stage. In contrast, sporadic and immunodeficiency-related BL often demonstrate SHM and rearrangement at chromosome 14 breakpoints related in Ig switch regions; this is consistent with GC or memory B-cell origin.

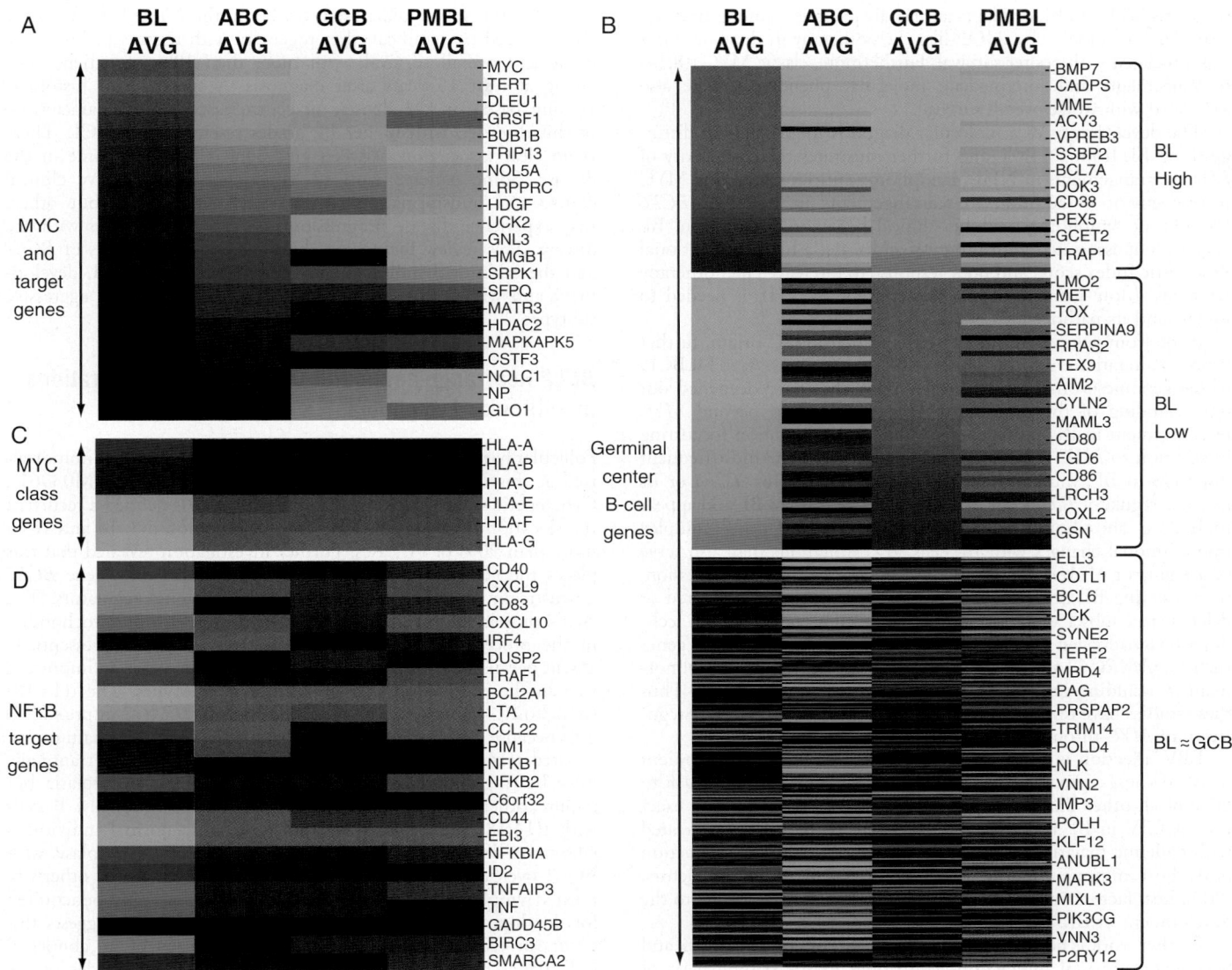

Fig. 76.7 Relative expression of genes that distinguish Burkitt lymphoma (BL) from subgroups of diffuse large B-cell lymphoma (DLBCL)—activated B cell–like (ABC) DLBCL, germinal center B (GCB) DLBCL, and primary mediastinal B-cell lymphoma (PMBL)—is categorized into gene expression signatures: c-myc and its target genes (A); genes that are expressed in normal germinal center (GC) B cells (B) and are expressed more highly (BL-high), less highly (BL-low), or equivalently (BL–GCB) in BL than in GCB DLBCL; major histocompatibility class I genes (C); and genes targeted by the nuclear factor kappa-B (NFκB) signaling pathway (D). GC B-cell signature genes are those that were overexpressed in normal GC B cells, compared with blood B cells. The "BL-high" genes were expressed at levels twice as high in BL as in GCB DLBCL ($p < .001$). The "BL-low" genes were expressed at levels twice as high in GCB DLBCL as in BL ($p < .001$). The expression levels of the "BL–GCB" genes did not differ significantly between the two lymphoma subtypes. *(From Dave SS, Fu K, Wright GW, et al: Lymphoma/Leukemia Molecular Profiling Project: Molecular diagnosis of Burkitt's lymphoma. N Engl J Med 354:2431, 2006.)*

Translocations placing MYC downstream of Ig genes result in massive gene upregulation and oncogenesis by dysregulation of multiple pathways. In normal B cells, MYC regulates B-cell proliferation and differentiation and is tightly regulated by multiple mechanisms, including posttranslational modifications and transcriptional autoregulation and by other factors, including a careful balance of interactions with regulatory proteins. Under normal circumstances, MYC also induces a number of proapoptotic cellular mechanisms, which are then perturbed when MYC is overexpressed by the robust Ig gene promoters existing in GC B cells. Constitutive induction of MYC expression in GCs via the upstream Ig gene promoter then confers a neoplastic phenotype. Highlighting the complexities of MYC in this setting, even brief reversal of MYC overexpression may induce a reversion of tumors to a benign phenotype; this implies that

c-*MYC*–Ig rearrangements might serve as the "switch" that drives BL formation in the context of GCs.

Recently, GEP has further examined the role of MYC in BL and revealed insights into the similarities and differences between BL and other GCB-origin NHLs. This work has further defined the differences between BL and DLBCLs carrying MYC rearrangements because these entities can be difficult to distinguish on histopathologic grounds alone. Although BL is characterized by gene expression profiles consistent with GC origin, a group of genes found in GCB DLBCL, including *LMO2, BCL2, CD80,* and *CD86,* are expressed only weakly in BL. BLs also express low amounts of NFκB and major histocompatibility class I molecules compared with DLBCL. These data also serve to allow the diagnostic distinction of BLs on molecular grounds. In two large studies, a fraction of DLBCLs were classified as BL in instances when there was DLBCL–BL overlap, causing disagreement among pathologists. The outcome with CHOP-like chemotherapy in these instances was associated with poorer survival. Furthermore, classic MYC t(8;14) rearrangements and intermediate molecular phenotypes were also associated with worse overall survival.

The development of a molecular diagnosis for BL aids in distinguishing BL from DLBCL and further illustrates the complexity of *MYC* rearrangements in NHL. Lymphoma entities containing MYC rearrangement in addition to rearrangements in *BCL2* or *BCL6* (double hit lymphomas) exhibit clinical behavior distant from BL and is often associated with progressive disease, a high International Prognostic Index score, and poor response to intensive chemotherapy regimens. More work regarding this subtype of NHL is needed to understand its pathogenesis.

Aside from gene expression patterns related to GC origin, further genomic alterations may contribute to BL pathogenesis. As in DLBCL, whole genome/exome/transcriptome approaches have deepened our understanding of the importance of genetic lesions beyond *MYC* rearrangement in BL pathogenesis. While *MYC* mutation (occurring in addition to *MYC* rearrangement) appears to be the most frequent mutation in BL, mutations in the transcription factor *TCF3* or its negative regulator *ID3* occur in the majority of cases of BL and appear to lead to phosphoinositol-3-kinase activation and other complex transcriptional changes with BL cells. *ID3* mutations may also serve as a regulator of *MYC* and directly influence cell cycle progression, thus fostering BL development. *TP53* is frequently also mutated or deleted in a subset of BL tumors. High throughput genomic techniques have revealed many other novel BL cancer mutations in genes such as *SMARCA2* and *CCND3* and recurrent copy number abnormalities including gains of 1q and 18q and deletion of 19p13. Thus these studies have revealed molecular complexity beyond the dysregulation of *MYC* through cytogenetic rearrangement.

EBV infection is also thought to play a role in the development of BL because virtually 100% of cases of endemic BL and 30% to 50% of all other BLs are associated with EBV positivity. The exact role of EBV in BL is unclear. Endemic BL is frequently associated with endemic malaria, which further suggests a complex interaction of the host immune response with microorganisms and other factors. Other host factors or genomic changes may further contribute to the development of BL.

Further work is needed to define what other genomic changes and host–environmental interactions contribute to the pathogenesis of BL. Ongoing studies seeking to define the entire spectrum of molecular, immunologic, genomic, and epigenetic changes associated with BL pathogenesis may further elucidate this process.

FOLLICULAR LYMPHOMA

Follicular lymphoma is a low-grade B-cell neoplasm that is also characterized by recurrent chromosomal rearrangements involving the IgH locus. It is the most common indolent NHL with more than 16,000 adults diagnosed yearly in the United States. It is characterized by significant heterogeneity with regards to histologic grade and overall survival, with more than 10% of patients surviving at least 15 years after diagnosis. A spectrum of histologic grading based on the density of centroblasts is also characteristic of this disorder, with higher FL grades resembling DLBCL. There is no clear association between grade and clinical outcome in the disease. Some patients with FL experience an aggressive clinical course and transformation to aggressive lymphomas, but others may experience disease progression only after many years with the disease. This review focuses on the classic rearrangements of *BCL2* and the additional molecular changes associated with FL development and with histologic transformation of FL to more aggressive subtypes.

BCL2 Rearrangements and Other Genomic Alterations in Follicular Lymphoma

Follicular lymphoma arises from GC B cells that have been immortalized at this stage of B-cell differentiation (see E-Slide VM03961). Cytogenetic studies performed in the early 1970s defined a recurrent translocation involving the long arms of chromosomes 14 and 18 in more than 90% of FL cases. Further investigation revealed that this places the gene encoding the important antiapoptotic gene *BCL2* downstream of the Ig heavy chain transcriptional regulators. The BCL2 protein inhibits the release of cytochrome c from mitochondria in the process of apoptosis. In normal GCs, *BCL2* is essentially absent because selection of B-cell clones via apoptosis is an important step in the production of high-affinity Ig idiotypes. The t(14;18) (q32.3;q21.3) appears to be mediated by *RAG1/RAG2* in pre-GC B cells because *BCL2* is most often found juxtaposed to J chain exons. Isolated t(14;18) is not sufficient to induce FL because transgenic mice bearing this translocation develop lymphoid hyperplasia but require other genetic lesions to develop FL. Additionally, B cells with t(14;18) can be isolated from apparently normal individuals who never develop lymphoma, and in situ follicular hyperplasia with BCL2 overexpression has been noted on examination of otherwise normal lymph nodes. This suggests that other lesions must be acquired for development of FL; a preponderance of evidence suggests this occurs in GCs. Histologically, FL is characterized by an abnormal follicular architecture containing neoplastic cells. The follicles loosely resemble GCs but usually lack an appreciable mantle zone. The follicles generally occur in close proximity to follicular T-helper cells expressing CD3, CD4, CD57, PD1, and CXCL13. FL usually exhibits a CD10+BCL6+IRF8+ GC-like phenotype in association with ongoing SHM, confirming GC or post-GC origin (Fig. 76.8). One obvious hypothesis is that BCL2 overexpression dysregulates apoptosis such that GC transition and SHM result in further genomic and epigenomic changes that result in FL. This framework might need to be reexamined in the small proportion of FL cases that do not express BCL2.

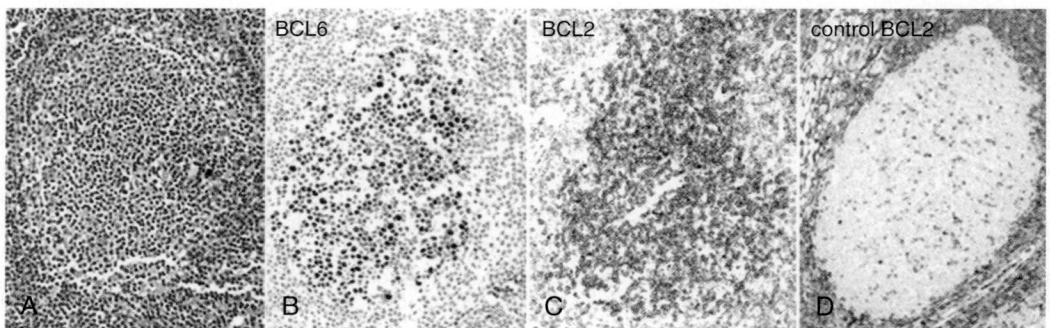

Fig. 76.8 FOLLICULAR LYMPHOMA (FL). Details from a case of FL, grade 1 of 3 associated with t(14;18) (q32;q21). Malignant follicle (A) with immunohistochemical stains for the germinal center marker, BCL6 (B), and BCL2 (C). Note the overexpression of BCL2 compared with a reactive follicle (D).

Although BCL2 is thought to have a critical role in development of FL, nearly 30% of grade 3A and a majority of grade 3B FLs are t(14;18) negative. Alternative rearrangements involving the κ or λ light chains and *BCL2* may occur, but many t(14;18) FLs do not express BCL2. These entities express a post-GC CD10-IRF4-phenotype with 3q27/*BCL6* rearrangements and are associated with lower chemotherapy response rates as well as worse overall survival compared with t(14;18)-positive FLs. It is not clear how this subset of FL evolves from normal B cells, but this immunophenotype suggests a late- or post-GC origin. GEP and analysis of miRNA profiles of FL confirm this association. Leich et al analyzed gene expression profiles of 184 grade I-3A FLs, of which 17 were t(14;18) negative (six of these rearrangement-negative FLs still overexpressed BCL2). Analysis of this data showed enrichment of signatures associated with activated B cells, including NFκB signaling, and those associated with cell cycle, proliferation, and the tumor microenvironment. A study involving a similar cohort showed that a pattern of 17 miRNAs was differentially expressed between translocation positive and negative phenotypes. A group of five miRNAs was found to be downregulated in the t(14;18) group, and this correlated with overexpression of genes related to proliferation, apoptosis, and differentiation. Thus evidence for a post-GCB origin of t(14;18) translocation–negative FLs exists at the gene expression level. Further work is needed to fully understand how BCL2-negative FL develops.

Similar work with BCL2-positive FL has revealed the additional steps required for FL development after t(14;18). Conventional cytogenetic studies in FL reveal recurrent duplications of 1p36 and 6q and gains of chromosomes 2, 8, 17, 21, and X. Additionally, SHM appears to affect glycosylation status of surface Ig, implicating BCR signaling in FL pathogenesis. As in DLBCL, FL is characterized by frequent mutations in genes involved in epigenetic regulation of gene expression including *ARID1A, MLL3, CREBBP* as well as other genes involved in cellular proliferation and avoidance of apoptosis such as *TP53, MCL1* and *TNFRSF14*.

Further genomic changes and host factors have also been delineated for DLBCL arising from FL. Histologic transformation is associated with further mutations or deletions in *TP53* and *p16* and appears to occur by distinct mechanisms involving either clonal evolution or transformation of a putative progenitor FL stem cell. Acquired rearrangement of the MYC oncogene can also occur and has been associated with an aggressive plasmablastic phenotype. Stromal factors with FL tumors also likely play a key role in FL propagation and have been studied as having prognostic consequence in FL as well.

Tumor Microenvironment and Survival in Follicular Lymphoma

Just as the lymphoid microenvironment is integral to the formation and function of GCs and immune factors predict survival in DLBCL, FL development appears to depend on stromal factors and the host immune response. In the largest study examining this relationship Dave et al performed gene expression analysis using whole-genome microarrays on 191 FL specimens with the goal of determining genomic predictors of survival. Genes identified were stratified into two groups based on correlation of expression with patient outcome (gene sets associated with good prognosis or poor prognosis). Hierarchical clustering then identified five survival gene sets within each of these groups; analysis revealed that a combination of two gene sets (immune response-1 and immune response-2) formed the best model for prediction of survival. Interestingly, immune response-1 consists of genes (*CD7, CD8B1, ITK, LEF1, STAT4*) associated with specific T-cell populations and macrophages. Conversely, immune response-2 consisted of genes found in dendritic cells and macrophages and was devoid of genes expressed by T-cell subsets (Fig. 76.9). Comparison with T-cell genes suggested a complex relationship with immune response-1 rather than a simple preponderance of T cells in the tumor biopsy.

Several hypotheses can be generated regarding the implication of these findings in FL biology. Given the relationship of genes involved in the immune response to survival, a direct impact of T-cell effector subsets in FL tumors could be one conclusion. Conversely, poor-risk tumors may be those that have become independent of FL follicles and therefore are more aggressive; this may be reflected in the variability of the immune response gene signatures seen across FLs. The

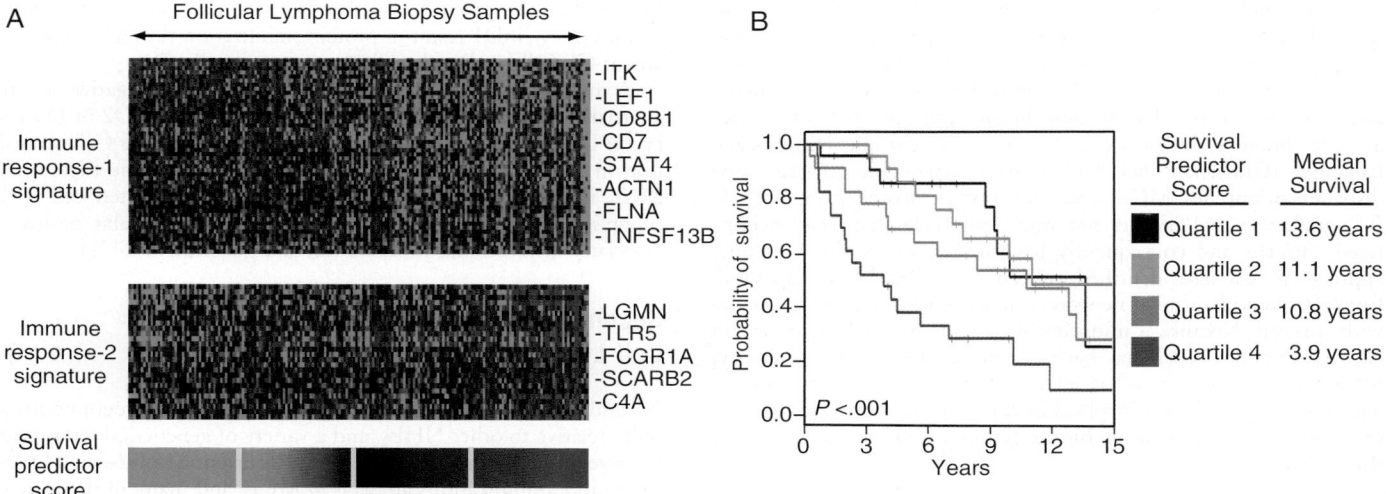

Fig. 76.9 SURVIVAL IN FOLLICULAR LYMPHOMA (FL) CAN BE PREDICTED USING FEATURES OF THE TUMOR MICROENVIRONMENT. (A) Two sets of coordinately expressed genes, termed the *immune response-1* and *immune response-2 signatures*, are associated with survival in FL. The expression pattern of each gene in these two signatures is shown for FL biopsy samples. Expression of the immune response-1 signature is associated with favorable survival after diagnosis, and expression of the immune response-2 signature is associated with adverse survival. These signatures are combined into a multivariate model of survival that generates a survival predictor score for each patient. Patients are ranked according to this survival predictor and divided into four equal quartiles as shown. (B) Kaplan-Meier plot of overall survival of patients in the four quartiles of the survival predictor. (*A, see Dave SS, Wright G, Tan B, et al: Prediction of survival in follicular lymphoma based on molecular features of tumor-infiltrating immune cells. N Engl J Med 351:2159, 2004.*)

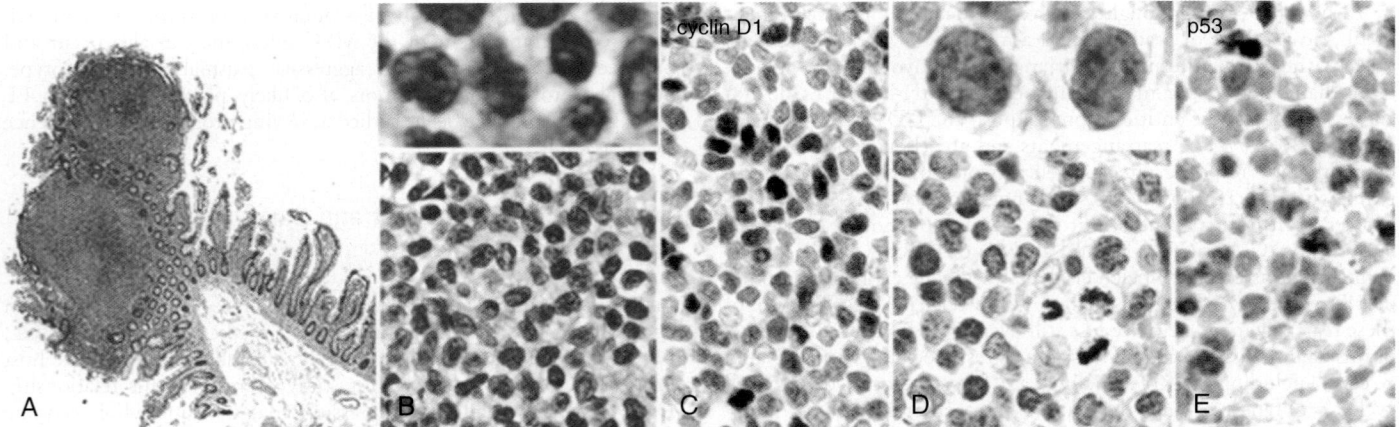

Fig. 76.10 MANTLE CELL LYMPHOMA (MCL). (A) A case of MCL presenting as lymphomatoid polyposis. (B) The lymphoma cells are small to intermediate in size and have irregular nuclear contours and condensed nuclear chromatin. The cells were CD19+, monoclonal B cells with λ light chain restriction, coexpression of CD5, FMC-7, and lack of CD23. C, The cells showed cyclin D1 expression by immunohistochemical staining. The t(11;14)(q13;q32) was detected by conventional cytogenetic analysis. (D) In comparison, the blastoid variant of MCL has larger cells with a high mitotic rate and fine chromatin. (E) These cases frequently overexpress p53 and are associated with a complex karyotype, including t(11;14).

impact of immune factors has been seen in other studies as well because survival may depend on FoxP3+ regulatory T-cell subsets, infiltration of macrophages, and the peripheral total monocyte count. Further work is needed to more clearly identify how the FL microenvironment impacts FL development and progression and to clarify whether manipulation of the immune compartment may be used therapeutically.

MANTLE CELL LYMPHOMA

Mantle cell lymphoma (MCL) is characterized by the chromosomal translocation t(11;14)q13;q32, which places cyclin D1 under the transcriptional control of the IgH promoter. MCL is predominantly a disease of elderly men and is characterized by a rather short median survival of 5 to 7 years. Histologic evaluation divides MCL into classic and blastoid variants, with the blastoid subtype having worse survival. Subgroups can also be defined on the basis of somatic mutations in the IgH loci because Ig-mutated tumors tend to have a more indolent disease as is the case with chronic lymphocytic leukemia (CLL), another CD5+ neoplasm. This suggests two disparate origins for MCL with one subtype arising from pre-GC B lymphocytes and another stemming from cells that have encountered antigens and consequently have undergone SHM. Genomic approaches have also identified molecular profiles delineating MCL from histologically similar neoplasms and identified factors associated with survival. Notably, a minority of patients with MCL are cyclin D1-negative, and GEP has been useful in identifying this entity; further work in this area has identified numerous genomic lesions and molecular pathways involved in MCL. Herein the pathogenesis of MCL is reviewed focusing on the genomic and molecular basis of this disease.

Cyclin D1 and Mantle Cell Lymphoma

The genetic hallmark of MCL, the t(11;14) (q13; q32) translocation, juxtaposes the *CCND1* gene to the IgH locus, leading to overexpression of the cell cycle regulator cyclin D1. The three D-type cyclins (D1, D2, and D3) play an important role in cellular proliferation by propelling cells from G_1 to S phase of the cell cycle. Each forms heterodimers with the cyclin-dependent kinases CDK4 and CDK6, thus forming active kinase complexes. These complexes inactivate retinoblastoma protein (Rb) and bind to p27kip1, which functions

to facilitate cell entry into the S phase of the cell cycle and consequent proliferation.

Cyclin D1 is not expressed in normal lymphocytes, and t(11;14) thus represents a pathogenic event in the origin of MCL. The gene encoding cyclin D1 *(CCND1)* consists of five exons that are alternatively spliced into two isoforms, cyclin D1a and D1b. Cyclin D1b does not appear to play a role in MCL. The proliferative capacity of MCL tumors appears closely tied to the degree of cyclin D1a overexpression. MCLs carry mutations in the 3′ untranslated region of *CCND1* that serve to stabilize cyclinD1a transcripts by removing miRNA (miR15/16) binding sites and deleting mRNA destabilizing elements. These sequences usually result in cyclin D1a being an unstable entity, with a half-life of less than 1 hour, but in MCL these deletions or mutations result in cyclin D1a accumulation and increased cellular proliferation. Additional mutations in the translated regions of cyclinD1 result in protein stabilization through the blockade of GSK3β-mediated nuclear export of cyclin D1.

A minority of patients with MCL are cyclin D1-negative and are alternatively characterized by overexpression of cyclin D2 or D3 and cyclin D2. These derangements serve to deregulate the G_1–S transition in a manner similar to t(11;14) and highlight the theme that MCL is a disease created by cyclin complex–mediated cell cycle progression aided by upregulation of several molecular pathways associated with cellular proliferation and genomic instability.

Secondary Genomic Alterations in Mantle Cell Lymphoma

Beyond t(11;14), MCL is characterized by extensive genomic instability relative to other NHLs, and a variety of genetic lesions appears to drive proliferation of these tumors. Recurrent chromosomal losses, gains, and amplifications are seen in MCL, and many of these affect a large proportion of cases. Secondary genetic instability may occur as a result of aberrant DNA replication in the setting of deregulated S phase transition mediated by cyclinD1–CD4-complexes. Acquired lesions in genes mediating cellular response to DNA damage and microtubule dynamics may contribute to the accumulation of these alterations as well.

Many (30%–50%) of MCL cases are characterized by mutations or deletions in the DNA damage response pathway mediated by ATM and TP53 or modifiers of this pathway such as MDM2 and p14/ARF. *ATM* is often mutated with loss of the other chromosomal allele. TP53 may also be downregulated in these tumors via similar mechanisms, and overexpression of TP53-negative regulators MDM2 and MDM4 also occurs via copy number amplification (examples of MCL histology with cyclin D1 and p53 staining are shown in Fig. 76.10). These overall serve to deregulate important cellular machinery involved in DNA damage repair, apoptosis, and cell cycle arrest, leading to increased cell cycle progression and proliferation in MCL. Further deletions at 9p21 occur frequently in MCL and serve to enhance cell cycle progression and block apoptosis. The 9p21 locus encodes p16(INK4a) and p14(ARF), which function as tumor suppressors. p16(INK4a) inhibits CDK 4/6 complex binding to cyclin D1, which results in decreased cell cycle progression. Deletion of p16(INK4a) in the setting of t(11;14) enhances proliferation in MCL and has been associated with worse overall survival. The function of p14(ARF) in MCL pathogenesis is less clear, but p14(ARF) blocks MDM2-mediated TP53 ubiquitination; p14(ARF) has other effects on cellular proliferation that usually work in a homeostatic pattern. Interestingly, cyclin D1 levels and INK4a/ARF deletions both correlate to a MCL proliferation signature created using GEP. Using a similar strategy, cyclin D1 expression levels and the presence of INK4a/ARF deletion have been used to create a predictor of overall survival using a cohort of patients with MCL. Survival among groups stratified by this approach varies widely (from 6–7 years to <10 months), which confirms the importance of involvement of genes involved with the cell cycle and proliferation in MCL. This parallels the experience noted with histologic markers of tumor proliferation because Ki-67 (a marker of actively dividing cells) and the presence of blastoid features have previously been shown to correlate with worse outcomes.

When considered together, the recurrent deletions and mutations noted in MCL illustrate the importance of unchecked cell cycle progression in this disorder. DNA instability is another hallmark of MCL that appears to result from the blockade of cell cycle checkpoints in the setting of ongoing DNA damage. These factors are intertwined in a complicated fashion in MCL and further work to upregulate several diverse molecular pathways involved in cellular proliferation and survival.

Molecular Pathways and Profiles in Mantle Cell Lymphoma

A variety of molecular pathways have recently been described as being active in MCL. These include signaling pathways facilitating cellular proliferation, avoidance of apoptosis, evasion of immune editing, and cellular microenvironment interactions. As in other NHLs, GEP has been used to define a molecular diagnosis of MCL and identify genes and molecular pathways involved in its pathogenesis.

Genomic approaches identify a subset of MCL that is cyclin D1-negative and has features similar to other CD5+ B-cell neoplasms such as CLL. Although such cases are indistinguishable by histologic analysis, GEP demonstrates that these tumors express gene signatures that are otherwise nearly identical to cyclin D1+ MCL but lack the classic t(11;14) rearrangement. Overexpression of other D cyclins (cyclin D2 or D3) via rearrangement, amplification, or other mechanisms is found in many of these cases; this is consistent with the underlying theme that MCL is a disease of disordered cell cycle progression. Using a similar approach, *SOX11* has been identified as a sensitive and specific marker of MCL regardless of cyclinD1 expression status. *SOX11* encodes an HMG-box transcription factor that regulates embryogenesis and is important in neural development. Because greater than 90% of MCL specimens overexpress *SOX11* and this finding is rare in histologically similar NHLs, *SOX11* is a potentially useful marker for improving the diagnosis of MCL. *SOX11* has also been incorporated into prognostic models of MCL using histologic, clinical, and GEP data. Reports regarding the clinical significance of *SOX11* have been conflicting. Thus further work is needed to understand the molecular mechanisms underlying *SOX11* expression in MCL and the implications in this disease.

Mantle cell lymphoma has also been characterized by expression of several molecular pathways that enhance cellular proliferation and

metabolism and are tightly intertwined with abnormalities in cell cycle regulation (Fig. 76.11). *Wnt 3* is a consistently overexpressed gene in MCL, and abnormal Wnt signaling may be one way that MCLs bypass negative feedback loops controlling differentiation. Proliferation in MCLs may also depend on Wnt-B-catenin signaling, but the impact of this pathway on patient survival or as a therapeutic target in MCL is unknown. Similar to ABC DLBCLs, the NFκB pathway is also active in MCL, and crosstalk between proliferation signaling between this pathway PI3K/AKT/mTOR and cell cycle signaling also appears to be important. Importantly, phosphatase and tensin homologue (PTEN), a molecule that has important roles in providing negative feedback to the mTOR pathway is also commonly deleted or acquires loss of function mutations in MCL. Taken together, these facts reinforce that abnormalities in several diverse signaling pathways are required beyond t(11;14) for MCL to form. Further work is needed to define how to use these findings to build better prognostic models in this disease, and studies investigating the therapeutic utility of targeting these pathways are beginning.

OTHER NON-HODGKIN LYMPHOMAS

Gene expression profiling and high-throughput sequencing have been applied to other lymphomas in manners similar to the subtypes already described. Important discoveries regarding other NHLs such as marginal zone lymphomas, lymphoplasmacytic lymphoma, and peripheral T-cell lymphomas (PTCLs) have refined our understanding of how these diseases develop. Recurrent mutations in genes and involvement of molecular pathways governing control of apoptosis, cellular proliferation, and metabolism are recurrent themes in these NHL subtypes as well as those described earlier. In addition to being found in DLBCLs, *MYD88* L265P mutations have been reported in virtually all cases of lymphoplasmacytic lymphoma (Waldenström macroglobulinemia) and may serve (along with *CXCR4* mutations) as a marker to differentiate this disease from other indolent lymphomas. *NOTCH2* mutations have been noted in a subset of marginal zone lymphomas and have been found in DLBCLs and other NHLs. Gene clusters have also been developed for T-cell lymphomas and identify PTCL subtypes such as angioimmunoblastic T-cell lymphoma (AITL) and hepatosplenic T cell lymphoma as distinct molecular entities as compared with other PTCLs; this work also has shown upregulation of genes involved in NFκB signaling in AITL. A subset of PTCL is characterized by t(2;5) (p23;q35), which joins the anaplastic lymphoma kinase-1 gene *(ALK)* next to *NPM-1* at 5q35. This creates an aberrant tyrosine kinase that appears to have a number of downstream transforming effects. ALK positivity is generally associated with response to cytotoxic chemotherapy in PTCL; however, better molecular predictors of response are needed. Whereas NFκB gene signature expression also correlates to improved survival in PTCL, tumors that exhibit increased markers of proliferation are associated with poor outcomes, as in other NHLs. High throughput genomic sequencing approaches have also revealed distinct patterns of somatic tumor mutations in PTCL subsets compared with B cell lymphomas. A recurrent mutation in *RHOA* (RHOA G17V), a small GTPase involved in regulation of actin polymerization and stress fiber formation occurs in both PTCL subtypes and AITL and appears to correlate with gene signatures of NFκB and MAP kinase activation, although the exact oncogenic role of RHOA in these tumors is unknown. Additionally, activating mutations in mediators of T cell receptor (TCR) signaling including FYN kinase have been reported and point toward an oncogenic role for constitutively active TCR signaling in these lymphomas. Further studies are needed to define the roles of these mutations in T cell lymphogenesis.

FUTURE DIRECTIONS

Non-Hodgkin lymphoma represents a complex group of related neoplasms that have quite disparate molecular characteristics. Given

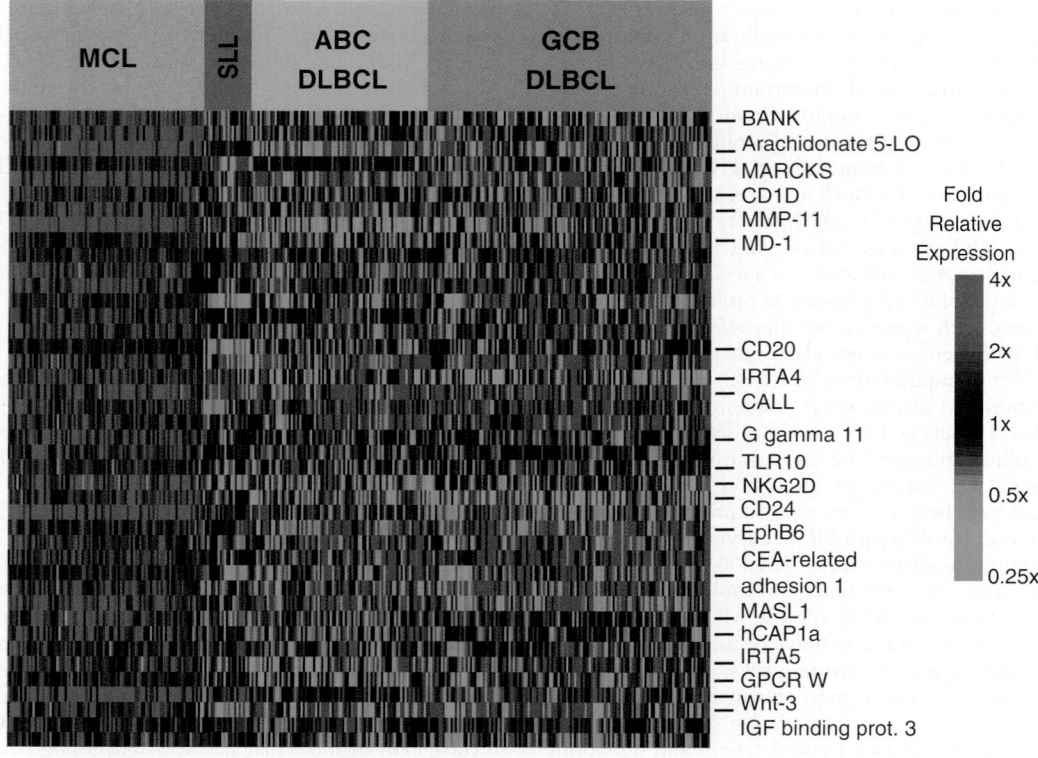

Lymphoma Biopsies

Fig. 76.11 HIERARCHICAL CLUSTERING OF EXPRESSION MEASUREMENTS FROM 42 MANTLE CELL LYMPHOMA (MCL) SIGNATURE GENES THAT ARE MORE HIGHLY EXPRESSED IN MCL SAMPLES COMPARED WITH SMALL LYMPHOCYTIC LYMPHOMA (SLL), ACTIVATED B CELL–LIKE (ABC) DIFFUSE LARGE B-CELL LYMPHOMA (DLBCL), AND GERMINAL CENTER B (GCB) DLBCL SAMPLES. Each column represents a single lymphoma specimen, and each row represents expression of a single gene. *Red squares* indicate increased expression, and *green squares* indicate decreased expression relative to the median expression level according to the color scale shown. *(From Fu K, Weisenburger DD, Greiner TC, et al: Lymphoma/Leukemia Molecular Profiling Project: Cyclin D1-negative mantle cell lymphoma: A clinicopathologic study based on gene expression profiling.* Blood *106:4315, 2005 and Rosenwald A, Wright G, Wiestner A, et al: The proliferation gene expression signature is a quantitative integrator of oncogenic events that predicts survival in mantle cell lymphoma.* Cancer Cell *3:185, 2003.)*

the lack of modifiable risk factors and varied prognosis with standard treatment (chemoimmunotherapy), a better understanding of the processes driving NHL is needed. Advances in technology have recently allowed whole-genomic surveys to identify the role of altered genetics, transcription, and epigenetic regulation as contributors to the observed lymphoma phenotypes. This work will serve as the starting point for the unraveling of new diagnostic and prognostic markers, as well as therapeutic targets in a group of diseases in which such options are urgently needed.

SUGGESTED READINGS

Alizadeh AA: Distinct types of diffuse large B-cell lymphoma identified by gene expression profiling. *Nature* 403:503, 2000.

Bakhshi A, Jensen JP, Goldman P, et al: Cloning the chromosomal breakpoint of t(14;18) human lymphomas: Clustering around JH on chromosome 14 and near a transcriptional unit on 18. *Cell* 41:899, 1985.

Bea S, Zettl A, Wright G, et al: Lymphoma/Leukemia Molecular Profiling Project: Diffuse large B-cell lymphoma subgroups have distinct genetic profiles that influence tumor biology and improve gene-expression-based survival prediction. *Blood* 106:3183, 2005.

Dave SS, Fu K, Wright GW, et al: Lymphoma/Leukemia Molecular Profiling Project: Molecular diagnosis of Burkitt's lymphoma. *N Engl J Med* 354:2431, 2006.

Dave SS, Wright G, Tan B, et al: Prediction of survival in follicular lymphoma based on molecular features of tumor-infiltrating immune cells. *N Engl J Med* 351:2159, 2004.

de Boer CJ, van Krieken JH, Kluin-Nelemans HC, et al: Cyclin D1 messenger RNA overexpression as a marker for mantle cell lymphoma. *Oncogene* 10:1833, 1995.

Dolken G, Illerhaus G, Hirt C, et al: BCL2/JH rearrangements in circulating B cells of healthy blood donors and patients with nonmalignant diseases. *J Clin Oncol* 14:1333, 1996.

Fisher SG, Fisher RI: The epidemiology of non-Hodgkin's lymphoma. *Oncogene* 23:6524, 2004.

Fu K, Weisenburger DD, Greiner TC, et al: Lymphoma/Leukemia Molecular Profiling Project: Cyclin D1-negative mantle cell lymphoma: A clinicopathologic study based on gene expression profiling. *Blood* 106:4315, 2005.

Gracias DT, Katsikis PD: MicroRNAs: Key components of immune regulation. *Adv Exp Med Biol* 780:15, 2011.

Iqbal J: Distinctive patterns of BCL6 molecular alterations and their functional consequences in different subgroups of diffuse large B-cell lymphoma. *Leukemia* 21:2332, 2007.

Iqbal J, Neppalli VT, Wright G, et al: BCL2 expression is a prognostic marker for the activated B-cell-like type of diffuse large B-cell lymphoma. *J Clin Oncol* 24:961, 2006.

Iqbal J, Wright G, Wang C, et al: Gene expression signatures delineate biological and prognostic subgroups in peripheral T-cell lymphoma. *Blood* 123(19):2915–2923, 2014.

Jardin F, Gaulard P, Buchonnet G, et al: Follicular lymphoma without t(14;18) and with BCL6 rearrangement: A lymphoma subtype with distinct pathological, molecular and clinical characteristics. *Leukemia* 16:2309, 2002.

Jost PJ, Ruland J: Aberrant NF-kappaB signaling in lymphoma: Mechanisms, consequences, and therapeutic implications. *Blood* 109:2700, 2007.

Kucuk C, Jiang B, Hu X, et al: Activating mutations of STAT5B and STAT3 in lymphomas derived from gammadelta-T or NK cells. *Nat Commun* 6:6025, 2015.

Leich E, Zamo A, Horn H, et al: MicroRNA profiles of t(14;18)-negative follicular lymphoma support a late germinal center B-cell phenotype. *Blood* 118:5550, 2011.

Lenz G, Nagel I, Siebert R, et al: Aberrant immunoglobulin class switch recombination and switch translocations in activated B cell-like diffuse large B cell lymphoma. *J Exp Med* 204:633, 2007.

Lenz G, Wright G, Dave SS, et al: Lymphoma/Leukemia Molecular Profiling Project: Stromal gene signatures in large-B-cell lymphomas. *N Engl J Med* 359:2313, 2008.

Magrath I: Epidemiology: Clues to the pathogenesis of Burkitt lymphoma. *Br J Haematol* 156:744, 2012.

McHeyzer-Williams M, Okitsu S, Wang N, et al: Molecular programming of B cell memory. *Nat Rev Immunol* 12:24, 2011.

Morin RD, Mendez-Lago M, Mungall AJ, et al: Frequent mutation of histone-modifying genes in non-Hodgkin lymphoma. *Nature* 476:298, 2011.

Pasqualucci L: Inactivation of the PRDM1/BLIMP1 gene in diffuse large B cell lymphoma. *J Exp Med* 203:311, 2006.

Rosebeck S, Rehman AO, Lucas PC, et al: From MALT lymphoma to the CBM signalosome: Three decades of discovery. *Cell Cycle* 10:2485, 2011.

Rosenwald A: The use of molecular profiling to predict survival after chemotherapy for diffuse large-B-cell lymphoma. *N Engl J Med* 346:1937, 2002.

Rosenwald A, Wright G, Leroy K, et al: Molecular diagnosis of primary mediastinal B cell lymphoma identifies a clinically favorable subgroup of diffuse large B cell lymphoma related to Hodgkin lymphoma. *J Exp Med* 198:851, 2003.

Rosenwald A, Wright G, Wiestner A, et al: The proliferation gene expression signature is a quantitative integrator of oncogenic events that predicts survival in mantle cell lymphoma. *Cancer Cell* 3:185, 2003.

Roschewski M, Staudt LM, Wilson WH: Diffuse large B-cell lymphoma-treatment approaches in the molecular era. *Nat Rev Clin Oncol* 11(1):12–23, 2014.

Schaffner C, Idler I, Stilgenbauer S, et al: Mantle cell lymphoma is characterized by inactivation of the ATM gene. *Proc Natl Acad Sci USA* 97:2773, 2000.

Tam W: Mutational analysis of PRDM1 indicates a tumor-suppressor role in diffuse large-B-cell lymphomas. *Blood* 107:4090, 2006.

Volpe G, Vitolo U, Carbone A, et al: Molecular heterogeneity of B-lineage diffuse large cell lymphoma. *Genes Chromosomes Cancer* 16:21, 1996.

Wang LD, Clark MR: B-cell antigen-receptor signalling in lymphocyte development. *Immunology* 110:411, 2003.

Weinstock DM, Dalla-Favera R, Gascoyne RD, et al: A roadmap for discovery and translation in lymphoma. *Blood* 125(13):2175–2177, 2015.

CHAPTER 77

CHRONIC LYMPHOCYTIC LEUKEMIA

Farrukh T. Awan and John C. Byrd

Over the past several decades, major advances have been realized in terms of improved understanding of the pathophysiology and therapeutic options for chronic lymphocytic leukemia (CLL). The plethora of information about CLL has increased dramatically and made management of what was a relatively straightforward disease quite complex but more rewarding. The authors herein provide a reference source focused on critical issues in routine clinical management of CLL.

EPIDEMIOLOGY

CLL is one of the most common types of leukemia in the Western Hemisphere. Surveillance, Epidemiology, and End Results (program and database) (SEER) estimates for 2015 indicate that approximately 14,620 patients (9940 men and 4678 women) were diagnosed in the United States and that 4650 patients died from CLL. The median age at diagnosis for CLL was 71 years from 2008–2012, according to the SEER database. The incidence of CLL increases proportionately by decade, as shown in Fig. 77.1. This figure illustrates that CLL is a very uncommon diagnosis before 45 years of age and infrequent (30% of total patients diagnosed) in patients before 65 years of age. The age-adjusted incidence rate was 4.5 per 100,000 men and women per year; 0.6% of men and women born from 2010–2012 are expected to be diagnosed with CLL during their lifetime. The estimated survival after diagnosis at 5 years is 81.7%, which explains the estimated prevalence of 126,299 patients currently living with CLL in the United States. Similar to other types of leukemia, the risk of dying from disease-specific causes increases proportionately with increasing age. Another analysis of the SEER database comparing outcome of elderly patients with CLL with age- and sex-matched healthy control participants demonstrated that CLL has the greatest impact on survival in the most elderly group of patients. However, even for patients diagnosed with CLL before the age of 50 years, Montserrat and colleagues demonstrated that the median expected life span is only 12.3 years compared with 31.2 years in age-matched control participants. Thus, CLL is a significant health problem affecting all ages of patients with this disease.

CLL is more common in men than women. Women diagnosed with CLL have 5- and 10-year overall survival (OS) rates that exceed those of men. CLL is most common in whites and decreases in frequency in a descending order among Blacks, Hispanics, American Indians and Native Alaskans, and Asians and Pacific Islanders, respectively. While adverse outcome based upon race has been reported, this has not been uniformly confirmed in other studies. The rarity of CLL among Asians and Pacific Islanders persists even in immigrants from these areas who have migrated to the Western Hemisphere. This implicates a possible genetic predisposition to the development of CLL. The relationship of environmental factors such as exposure to benzene and other chemicals to the development of CLL is not clearly defined. However, CLL is recognized as a service-connected illness among Vietnam War veterans who were exposed to Agent Orange. Occupational or environmental exposure to radiation does not appear to predispose patients to a higher risk of developing CLL. For example, although the frequency of acute myeloid leukemia (AML), chronic myeloid leukemia (CML), and acute lymphoblastic leukemia (ALL) were increased among survivors of the atomic bomb at Hiroshima, an increase in CLL was not appreciated. The recently reported large International Lymphoma Epidemiology Consortium non-Hodgkin lymphoma Subtypes Project (InterLymph Study), identified multiple factors that were associated with the presence of CLL; including 1) family history of a first degree relative with hematologic malignancy including lymphomas, leukemias, and myeloma; 2) a history of working or living on a farm; 3) hairdressers, and 4) a history of hepatitis C infection. Protective factors included a history of allergies, blood transfusions, sun exposure, and smoking.

FAMILIAL CHRONIC LYMPHOCYTIC LEUKEMIA

Up to 10% of CLL patients have a first- or second-degree relative with CLL, making CLL one of the most common types of malignancy with familial predisposition. Newer studies identifying an even higher frequency of monoclonal B-cell lymphocytosis (MBL) in these families provides further evidence of inheritance in a subset of patients. Unlike other types of familial cancer, it is very uncommon for CLL patients to have large pedigrees with many affected distant relatives throughout an extensive family tree. Rather, the more common finding is for most patients to have one or two first- or second-degree relatives with this diagnosis. Large case-control studies concluded that the risk ratio (RR) for first-degree relatives of CLL probands to also have CLL was higher than that for most other cancers. Although the average RR for all cancers in a U.S. study was approximately 2.1, CLL showed an RR of 5.0, the fourth highest of all cancers. Relatives of patients with CLL also appear to have a higher frequency of other lymphoproliferative disorders and autoimmune diseases. Unlike a variety of other cancers that have known predisposing genes, identification of divergent genes in CLL has been generally unsuccessful. Multiple association studies have identified numerous putative genes, polymorphisms and genetic factors including death-associated protein kinase (DAPK) and LEU7 (CD57), IRF4, BAK, CD38, CD5, TNF-α and others, but weak evidence for linkage and conclusive studies demonstrating a strong mechanistic contribution to pathogenesis are lacking. The role of anticipation in identifying other family members has been reported by several groups; patients with such a family history are generally diagnosed a median of 10 years earlier than other patients. However, other clinical features of CLL at diagnosis do not appear to be different. Thus, patients with familial CLL do not appear to be genetically or clinically different from individuals with sporadic CLL.

PATHOBIOLOGY

The complexity of the biology of CLL has become increasingly apparent, as insight into these processes has expanded. Despite these advances, many questions remain unsolved, including (1) the cell of origin from which CLL is derived, (2) the existence of a CLL stem cell as occurs in other leukemias, (3) the biologic etiology of the divergent natural histories of immunoglobulin heavy chain variable regions (IGHV)-mutated versus unmutated CLL, and (4) the existence and identification of infectious or other naturally occurring antigens that may drive the appearance of B-cell clone. Nonetheless, significant advances in our understanding of the roles of cytogenetics, immunology, and other relevant biologic markers in predicting the natural history, disease progression and response to therapy in CLL

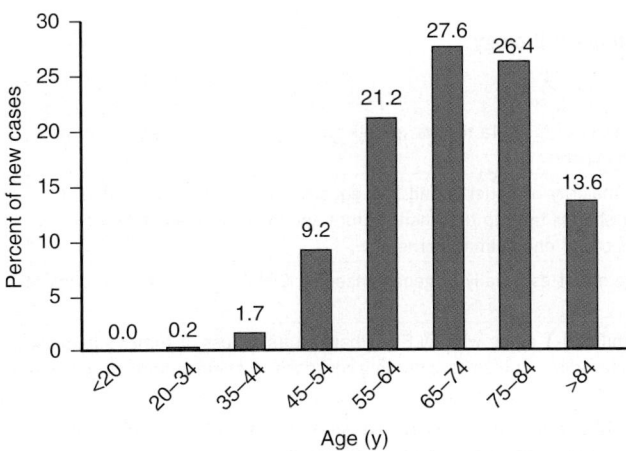

Fig. 77.1 GRAPH SHOWING THAT CHRONIC LYMPHOCYTIC LEUKEMIA IS A VERY UNCOMMON DIAGNOSIS BEFORE AGE 45 YEARS AND INFREQUENT (<30% OF TOTAL PATIENTS DIAGNOSED) BEFORE AGE 65 YEARS.

make an understanding of the basic biology of CLL increasingly relevant and important to clinicians caring for CLL patients.

For many years, CLL was believed to represent a single disease that had a varied natural history. Basic research focused on understanding (1) the normal cell of origin from which CLL is derived; (2) the function of the B-cell receptor (BCR) in CLL; (3) the maturational point in B-cell development at which CLL occurs; (4) the relevance and contribution of a self- or acquired-antigen to driving the disease; and (5) the role of the microenvironment in disease development and progression. All of these observations are important scientific areas of active, ongoing study, and readers are referred to several recent definitive reviews for further information on the basic biology of CLL. The biology and genetics covered within this chapter focus predominantly on areas relevant to clinicians who care for patients with CLL.

B-CELL RECEPTOR PATHWAY AND ITS ROLE IN PATHOGENESIS

Modulation of the BCR plays an integral part in the development and maturation of B cells. Its constitutive activation through antigen dependent or independent signaling provides an important survival signal for the propagation of CLL B cells. Signal transduction occurs through a variety of kinases including LYN, PI3K, SYK and Bruton tyrosine kinase (BTK) with resultant phosphorylation of phospholipase C (PLC)-$\gamma 2$ and induction of downstream second messengers that further modulate cell survival regulators. These kinases can now be effectively pharmacologically targeted, which results in abrogation of the survival signal leading to B-cell apoptosis. Combinations of these inhibitors with existing and novel therapeutic agents have the potential to change the natural history of the disease.

X-linked agammaglobulinemia is a disease characterized by a severe immunodeficient state that results from deficient BTK. Characterization of this defect and its resultant impact on causing severe impairments in B-cell development and humoral immunity has been critical to our understanding of CLL disease biology. Activating mutations of BTK have not been identified in CLL or other cancers but CLL B cells tend to have higher levels of BTK that can be induced through the BCR signaling pathway. Ibrutinib is the first in class BTK inhibitor that efficiently targets BTK and results in significant abrogation of downstream survival signaling transduced through this pathway and results in the inhibition of cell survival and proliferation. Similarly, both SYK and PI3K can be induced by activation of BCR pathway. The PI3-kinase isoform delta inhibitor idelalisib and syk inhibitors have been shown to antagonize these survival signals and result in clinically meaningful disease responses.

IGHV Mutational Status

Two seminal manuscripts in 1999 demonstrated that the IGHV gene had undergone somatic mutation, indicating that the patient's CLL arose after this point in B-cell maturation, in 60% of CLL patients at diagnosis. Detailed epigenetic studies examining the methylation changes occurring in normal B cells during development have subsequently suggested that immunoglobulin mutational analysis may indicate simply where in normal B-cell development transformation occurred. In an attempt to identify surrogate genes associated with IGHV-unmutated disease, ZAP-70 overexpression was identified. The majority of IGHV-unmutated CLL cells have ZAP-70 expression and demonstrate evidence of syk activation and other essential BCR downstream activation signals after ligation of surface immunoglobulin M (sIgM) that is related to overexpression of this protein. In contrast, virtually all IGHV-mutated patients lack significant ZAP-70 expression and do not signal after ligation by sIgM, but can often weakly signal through other alternative BCRs. Thus, although gene expression profiling demonstrates all CLL cells to be most closely related to memory B cells, IGHV-unmutated and IGHV-mutated CLL cells differ significantly with respect to their ability to transduce intracellular signals after sIgM ligation. A common repertoire of mutational changes among CLL patients has also been documented that differs significantly from that found in the normal adult B-cell repertoire. These studies have prompted the hypothesis that CLL may represent an antigen-driven disease. Targeting BCR signaling based on this has already resulted in the development of several therapeutic agents directed against signaling pathways downstream of the BCR.

Defective Apoptosis

Since its initial description and early characterization, CLL has been considered a disease of slow accumulation of tumor cells caused by disrupted or defective apoptosis. Multiple studies have demonstrated that CLL cells overexpress several antiapoptotic proteins, including BCL2, MCL1, Bak, and X-linked inactivator of apoptosis protein, and have diminished expression of compensatory proapoptotic proteins such as Bax. Overexpression of BCL2 and MCL1 and an increase of the ratio of these proteins to Bax have correlated not only with disrupted apoptosis but also shortened OS and poor response to therapy. Studies have demonstrated that CLL cells are characterized by constitutive activation of several antiapoptotic transcription factors, including nuclear factor kappa-B (NFκB), nuclear factor of activated T cells, and signal transducer and activator of transcription 3. Each of these transcription factors can influence one or more of the antiapoptotic proteins that promote survival in vivo. The source of activation of these different transcription factors is not completely defined but may be partly attributable to autocrine and paracrine networks involving B-cell activation factor (BAFF), a proliferation inducing ligand vascular endothelial growth factor, interleukin-4 (IL-4), and CD40. CLL cells are also maintained through contact with stromal cells (bone marrow [BM] and dendritic) and similar nurse cells through a complex interface of adhesion molecules and stromal survival factors such as stromal cell–derived factor. The importance of the in vivo environment to CLL survival is supported by the increase in apoptosis when CLL cells are cultured in vitro.

Genetic Abnormalities

Detailed study of the genetics of CLL has been hindered by the inability to effectively induce proliferation of tumor cells for standard

TABLE 77.1   Summary of Important Prognostic Markers and Their Role in Disease Biology

Prognostic Markers	Frequency (%)	Putative Role in Disease Biology
Del17p/loss of Tp53	~7–10	Loss of p53 protein and decreased levels of miR34a results in cell cycle dysfunction. Predicts for poor response to treatment and worse survival
Del11q	~18–20	Results in ATM gene deletion in the majority of patients and subsequently a lack of repair of double-stranded DNA breaks. Predicts for shorter time to treatment failure and survival. Impact may be overcome with the use of alkylator based chemoimmunotherapy.
Trisomy 12	~16–20	Impact maybe through a gene dosage effect especially of genes encoding CDK4 and MDM2. Predicts for intermediate risk disease
Del13q	~55–60	Results in the loss of miR-15a and miR-16-1 along with DLEU7 that results in loss of tumor suppressor activity. Generally associated with favorable outcomes including response to chemoimmunotherapy and survival
NOTCH1 mutation	~10	Constitutive activation of NOTCH1 results in increased cell survival and resistance to apoptosis and predicts for inferior response to rituximab and shorter treatment-free interval
SF3B1 mutation	~9–18	Mutually exclusive with NOTCH1 mutations. May cause abnormal transcription and splicing events. Associated with rapid disease progression
BIRC3 mutation	~5	Associated with unmutated IGHV, a shorter treatment-free interval and del11q. mutually exclusive with Tp53 mutations
MYD88 mutation	~3–13	Important adapter of the IL-1 and toll-like receptor pathway. Gain of function mutations result in increased cytokine production and activation of the NFκB pathway. Associated with improved survival

ATM, Ataxia-telangiectasia–mutations; IGHV, immunoglobulin heavy chain variable region; IL, interleukin; MYD88, myeloid differentiation primary response 88; SF3B1, NA splicing factor 3B, subunit 1

metaphase cytogenetic analysis and the poor response of CLL cells to B-cell mitogens. Nonetheless, several cytogenetic studies identified a variety of deletions, including del(11q22.3), del(17p13.1), del(13q14), and del(6q21-q23), as well as trisomy 12, as common abnormalities in CLL. The frequency of these abnormalities has been further refined through the use of fluorescence in situ hybridization (FISH) of interphase cells, which does not require isolation of dividing cells. These studies have demonstrated that del(13q14) is by far the most common cytogenetic abnormality in CLL followed by trisomy 12, del(11q22.3), del(17p13.1), and del(6q22.3). Stimulation of CLL cells with CpG oligonucleotides plus IL-4 or CD40 confirmed the prevalence of these abnormalities and identified unbalanced translocations not generally observed with traditional metaphase cytogenetics. The prognostic implications of these unbalanced translocations appear to be significant. Similarly, the complexity of karyotype appears to be a poor prognostic factor in CLL. Interestingly, balanced translocations, which are more frequently observed in ALL and AML, are generally not observed in CLL.

The presence of recurrent deletions in CLL suggests the possibility of unique tumor suppressor genes in these different regions. This was confirmed by the discovery of miR15 and miR16, two noncoding microRNAs, in the deleted region of 13q14. Noncoding RNAs range in size from 21–25 nucleotides and represent a newly recognized class of gene products whose function is to silence genes through binding to the 3′-untranslated region of specific genes to inhibit translation. It was later shown that miR16 regulates expression of BCL2, which is overexpressed in CLL and other B-cell lymphoproliferative disorders. Multiple different studies have associated specific miR expression with rapid disease progression, fludarabine resistance, and poor prognosis. In addition, miR34a has been directly related to the adverse outcome associated with p53 dysfunction. Further study of miRs in CLL is under way to elucidate their role in the pathogenesis and progression of CLL.

Recurring Mutations in Chronic Lymphocytic Leukemia

Until the advent of whole-exon and whole-genomic sequencing, CLL was not typically associated with recurring mutations early in the

pathogenesis of the disease. Probably best characterized are p53 mutations, which occur in up to 10% of patients at diagnosis, often in conjunction with deletion of the alternative allele (at 17p13.1 loci) that is associated with rapid disease progression and poor survival. With treatment and subsequent relapse, the frequency of p53 mutations continues to increase proportionately and is most common in patients with Richter transformation. Thus, p53 mutations are considered by most to be a secondary abnormality in CLL associated with progression. Nonetheless, p53 mutations or deletions have significant impact on consideration of treatment of CLL, and the 2008 International Workshop on CLL (IWCLL) criteria recommended that patients with p53 mutations with deletions be treated in a different manner than other CLL patients. Although detailed studies of ataxia-telangiectasia–mutations (ATM) have been performed, the impact of this abnormality is less well defined, in particular as it relates to treatment response. Other recurring mutations in CLL, including SF3B1, NOTCH1, MYD88, XPO1, and ERK1 have been described with varying clinical significance. With continued sequencing studies, more abnormalities will likely be appreciated. A summary of important genetic abnormalities and their impact is provided in Table 77.1.

Immune and Microenvironmental Features

The importance of progressive immune suppression with progression of CLL has become appreciated in both human forms of CLL and murine models of this disease. The absolute number of T cells and natural killer (NK) cells in CLL patients at diagnosis has been shown to predict OS. In particular, expansion of suppressive T-regulatory cells has been documented as patients approach the time when they require therapy. Similarly, the importance of microenvironmental compartments of CLL such as lymph nodes and BM, where stromal cells provide proliferative signals as well as survival signals to protect CLL cells from apoptosis, has been recognized. Based on this work, biomarkers involving measurable chemokines which are responsible for T-cell recruitment to the microenvironment have been identified. Given the link of these stimuli to BCR signaling, inhibitory molecules directed at kinases involved in this interaction can now target these pathways.

CLINICAL MANIFESTATIONS

At diagnosis, most CLL patients do not have clinical manifestations associated with their disease. For early stage CLL patients, the diagnosis is often identified as part of routine blood tests for evaluation of an unrelated problem such as an infection, kidney stones, or during a preoperative assessment in which an elevated leukocyte count is noted with increased mature lymphocytes observed. For a much smaller subset of patients with CLL, presentation of disease occurs as a consequence of fatigue, weight loss, early satiety (from spleen enlargement), petechiae (from low platelets), or new palpable lymph nodes. Patients with symptomatic CLL at diagnosis represent only 15% of those seen, corresponding to the more indolent nature of this disease at diagnosis. With additional follow-up, the majority of CLL patients will eventually manifest symptoms of the disease that ultimately lead to the need for treatment. The most common symptoms associated with progression include increasing fatigue (as a consequence of anemia and cytokines elaborated by the involved tissues), increasing lymph node and spleen size, worsening hematologic parameters (anemia and thrombocytopenia), and rarely infiltration of other organs (kidney, lung, pleural space, skin) that necessitates initiation of treatment to palliate symptoms. Symptoms generally associated with CLL progression are night sweats, fevers, and weight loss. These are generally suggestive of Richter transformation.

Separate from direct CLL progression, the disease is also immunosuppressive, and with more advanced disease, an increase in infections is generally observed. This represents a major morbidity of CLL and is a leading contribution to mortality associated with this disease. Other manifestations of immune suppression, including higher rate of secondary malignancies and autoimmune complications.

DIAGNOSIS AND LABORATORY MANIFESTATIONS

The diagnosis of CLL, as defined by the IWCLL 2008 criteria, requires an absolute malignant B-cell lymphocyte count of greater than 5000/μL that coexpress CD5 and CD23 on immunophenotyping. Morphologically, the lymphocytes appear mature with fewer than 55% prolymphocytes (Fig. 77.2A–E). The BM aspirate smear if done, should show greater than 30% of all nucleated cells to be lymphoid, or the BM core biopsy shows lymphoid infiltrates consistent with CLL (Fig. 77.2F–G). The overall cellularity is normocellular or hypercellular. Immunophenotyping reveals a predominant B-cell monoclonal population coexpressing the B-cell markers CD19, CD20, and CD23 and the T-cell antigen CD5 in the absence of other pan-T cell markers (see later section). In some cases, a hypocellular marrow can be present as an artifact of marrow aspiration.

Patients may present with tumor cells immunophenotypically consistent with CLL but have predominantly lymph node disease without a peripheral B-cell lymphocyte count of 5000/μL despite BM involvement. Although these patients are considered to have small lymphocytic lymphoma (SLL) and not true CLL by the National Cancer Institute criteria, the most recent World Health Organization classification considers such SLL patients to have CLL, given the similar immunophenotypic features, genetic findings, natural history, and complications of these two diseases. The clinical management of SLL patients should be similar to CLL with respect to diagnostic testing and treatment.

The recent increase in diagnostic blood testing for other B-cell lymphoid cancers has led to recognition of a clinical precursor to CLL called MBL. Patients with MBL have circulating peripheral B cells immunophenotypically consistent with CLL but do not have enlarged lymph nodes, a malignant lymphocyte count greater than 5000/μL, or cytopenias. The frequency of MBL increases with age; 0.3% of patients younger than the age of 40 years have MBL compared with 2.1% of 40- to 60-year-old patients and 5.2% of 60- to 90-year-old patients. The frequency of MBL in family members of patients with a first-degree relative with CLL is significantly higher in both young and older patients. With the new IWCLL 2008 definition of CLL requiring 5000/μL malignant B lymphocytes, more cases of MBL

Initial Evaluation of Young Patients With Chronic Lymphocytic Leukemia

Only 10% of patients diagnosed with CLL are younger than 50 years of age, and these patients often present a diagnostic and therapeutic dilemma to hematologists initially evaluating them. The great majority of patients diagnosed before the age of 50 years will have early-stage CLL with a slightly higher predisposition to a prior first-generation relative with this disease. In addition, these patients are generally of a higher economic status or have chronic fatigue or medical illnesses for which they have been undergoing routine blood testing, leading to diagnosis of CLL. When the diagnosis of CLL is made, these younger patients have a more challenging time understanding how the disease will impact them. For patients with no symptoms referable to CLL, we generally discuss complications of the disease during the first visit and have a detailed discussion regarding assessment of genetic risk factors predisposing to early disease progression, including select interphase chromosomal abnormalities (del[17p13.1] and del[11q22.3]) and IGHV mutational status (unmutated). During this time, it is important to counsel patients that identification of high-risk genomic features can actually increase anxiety because no treatment intervention is indicated in the absence of symptoms, regardless of genomic profile, outside of a clinical trial. In our experience, the great majority of patients desire this testing. Despite the potential benefit of allogeneic stem cell transplantation in younger patients with CLL, we generally mention this only as one treatment option used in this disease and do not pursue consultation or tissue typing of patients or siblings until patients are truly symptomatic from their disease. We provide considerable discussion about the promising but early data with kinase inhibitors currently approved and other promising novel molecules and therapies available in clinical trials. During the second visit 4 to 6 weeks later, we review the results of these prognostic factors and answer additional questions that have arisen. Ultimately, the majority of patients have low-risk disease, and knowing this allows patients to take partial control of their disease and move on with their lives. Serial assessment of the psychologic well-being of patients with CLL during this first year is incredibly important. At no place during the evaluation do we refer to CLL as being a good or favorable leukemia. In our experience, the most common reason for dissatisfaction toward the initial hematology evaluation is lack of explanation of the disease process or the minimization of CLL as a "good leukemia to have."

For young patients presenting with other chronic medical problems who are asymptomatic from their CLL, we follow the approach outlined earlier. More commonly, these patients have fatigue, mild anemia, or other symptoms that could be attributable to the CLL. In addition, this group is more commonly overweight or obese. In either setting, it is important to first think like an internist and pursue other causes for symptoms potentially attributable to CLL. In particular, encouragement of both weight loss and a fixed exercise plan should be encouraged for fatigue and often improve quality of life and in other medical comorbidities. In some cases here, methylphenidate can be effective for the management of CLL related fatigue. It is very important to note that younger patients with CLL can often go a decade or more without therapy and early treatment of this patient group in the absence of symptoms still offers no proven long-term advantage. For this reason, our group remains very conservative on starting therapy for young patients with CLL unless they have high-risk disease and are treated on a clinical trial.

have been recognized than in the past with many patients being downstaged from early CLL to MBL. Similar to the relationship of monoclonal gammopathy of undetermined significance and multiple myeloma, it appears that only a small proportion of patients with MBL develop overt CLL over time. Whereas genetic features such as IGHV mutational status and cytogenetic abnormalities may predict progression of CLL, it is unclear if these tests bear any relevance to predicting MBL progression to CLL. For this reason, we generally do not perform these tests in MBL patients. Interestingly, these patients have many of the long-term complications of CLL related to immune suppression including a higher frequency of infections and also secondary malignancies. We therefore approach the initial counseling of these patients similar to newly diagnosed CLL patients with respect to interventions (vaccines and education) to minimize these

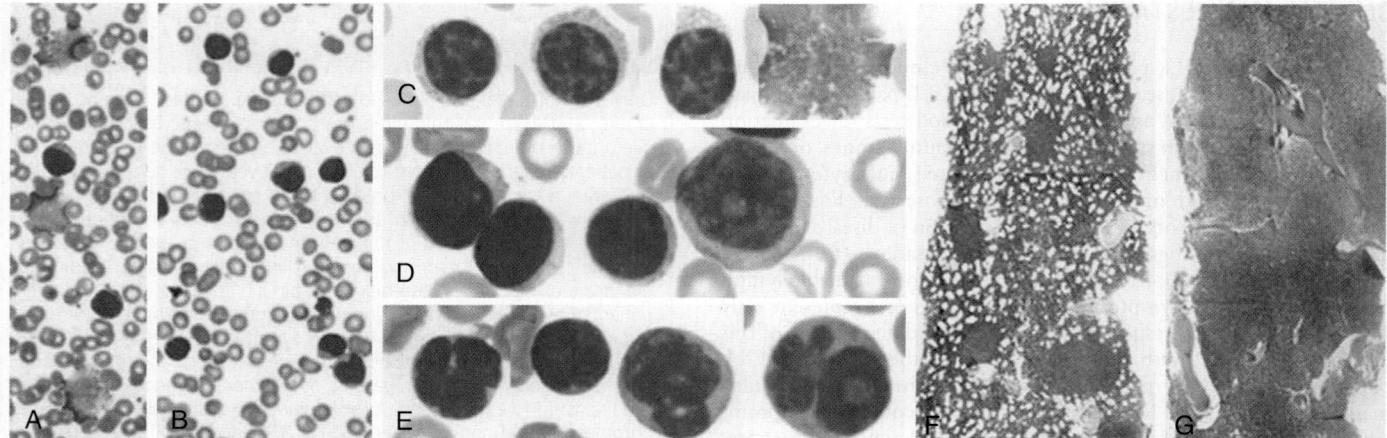

Fig. 77.2 CHRONIC LYMPHOCYTIC LEUKEMIA (CLL). The peripheral blood smear (A) typically shows lymphocytosis and increased smudge cells as a result of the fragility of the CLL cells (see also smudge cell in C, *right side*). These can be avoided by making a preparation of blood and bovine serum albumin (22%) at a ratio of 11 drops of blood and 1 drop of albumin before preparing the slide (B). Cytologic features of CLL cells differ. Classic cells have a small nucleus with a "soccer ball" chromatin pattern (C). Some cases have increased large cells, or prolymphocytes, with more open chromatin and prominent "punched-out" nucleoli (D; prolymphocyte, *right side*). Other cases, sometimes referred to as "atypical," have clefted cells and large cells (E). The bone marrow can show nodular infiltrates of CLL cells (F), an interstitial infiltrate, or a diffuse infiltrate (G).

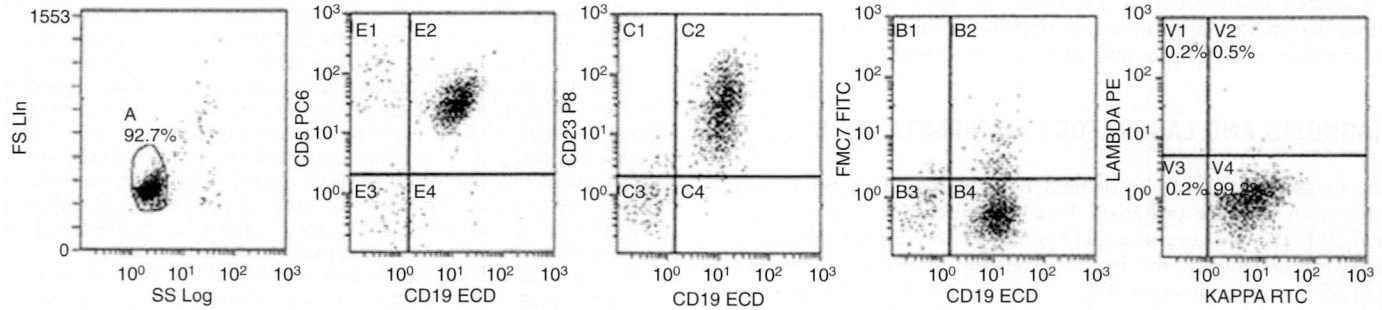

Fig. 77.3 FLOW IMMUNOPHENOTYPING IN CHRONIC LYMPHOCYTIC LEUKEMIA (CLL). Flow data in a typical case of CLL. The clonal B cells are CD19+ with κ light chain restriction (weak to moderately intense), with coexpression of CD5 and CD23, but lack of FMC-7. The cells were CD38-negative.

TABLE 77.2	Diseases That Can Mimic Chronic Lymphocytic Leukemia

- Follicular lymphoma
- Mantle cell lymphoma
- Marginal zone lymphoma
- Hairy cell leukemia
- Acute lymphoblastic leukemia
- T-cell prolymphocytic leukemia
- Large granular natural killer or T-cell leukemia

complications. We also continue to follow these patients with yearly blood counts and exams.

LABORATORY MANIFESTATIONS

For many years, the diagnosis of CLL was made based on morphologic examination of the peripheral blood smear, which demonstrated mature lymphocytes with an abundance of smudge cells. Despite rigorous morphology, many diseases can mimic CLL in both appearance and clinical presentation, as summarized in Table 77.2, resulting in incorrect diagnoses. With the advent of new, more effective tar-

geted therapies for CLL and other related diseases listed in Table 77.2, determining the correct diagnosis is of great importance. Flow cytometry, or immunophenotyping is now the standard approach to establish the diagnosis of CLL (Fig. 77.3, for example). The diagnosis of CLL relies on immunophenotypic confirmation, and flow cytometry should therefore be performed on all CLL patients at diagnosis. CLL cells have a relatively consistent immunophenotype, which differentiates CLL from mantle cell lymphoma, hairy cell leukemia, follicular lymphoma, marginal zone lymphoma, and other indolent B-cell malignancies. Specifically, CLL cells express a variety of B-cell markers, including dim sIg, CD19, dim CD20, CD200, and CD23, as well as the pan T-cell marker CD5. Kappa or λ restriction is always present, establishing the presence of a clonal B-cell population, although sIg expression may be so dim that light chain restriction may be difficult to determine. In contrast, the presence of CD10, FMC7, or CD79b (all typically absent on CLL cells) or bright expression of CD11c, CD20, or CD25 (all typically dim on CLL cells) suggests an alternative low-grade B-cell lymphoproliferative malignancy. Expression of CD5 without CD200 or CD23 suggests mantle cell lymphoma, and FISH for t(11;14) should be performed to exclude mantle cell lymphoma. Some genetic subsets of CLL are predisposed to variant antigen expression, particularly patients with trisomy 12. Repeating immunophenotyping after the initial diagnosis is not required unless there is a suspicion of transformation to a more aggressive histology or there is a need to assess

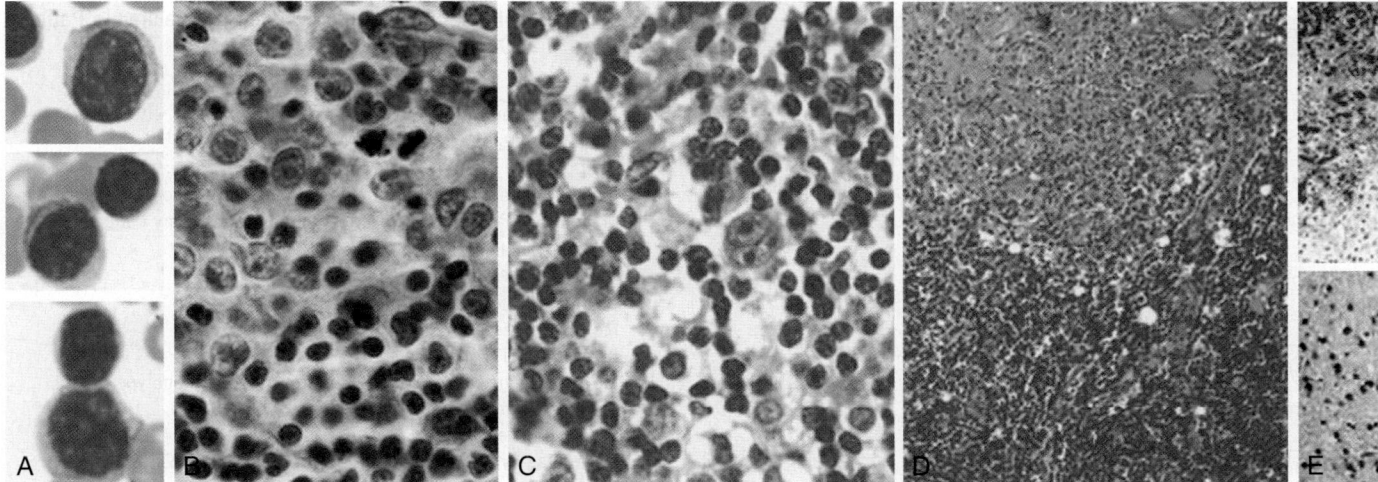

Fig. 77.4 TRANSFORMATION IN CHRONIC LYMPHOCYTIC LEUKEMIA (CLL). Some patients with CLL develop increasing numbers of prolymphocytes (A) and a "prolymphocytic transformation." A Richter transformation indicates evolution to a large-cell lymphoma (B; large cells, *upper left,* residual CLL, *lower right*). Occasionally, cases can transform to Hodgkin lymphoma (i.e., the Hodgkin variant of Richter syndrome) (C). With the use of fludarabine and other immunosuppressants, patient can also develop Epstein-Barr virus–related lymphadenopathies or lymphadenopathies with large areas of necrosis caused by herpes simplex virus (HSV). The case illustrated in (D) and (E) had both (E; *upper panel* shows an immunostain of HSV-1/2, and lower is *Epstein-Barr virus*—encoded small RNAs in situ hybridization).

BM response or antigen expression for an antibody directed therapeutic agent. Transformation of CLL (Fig. 77.4A–C) to either prolymphocytic leukemia (PLL) or large cell lymphoma (Richter transformation) is often associated with immunophenotypic drift, where CD5 is lost and FMC7 expression is acquired. In addition, expression of CD20 and surface immunoglobulins typically become brighter in PLL or Richter transformation. Although the morphologic appearance of prolymphocytes or large lymphoid cells in blood, BM, or lymph nodes is typically adequate to make the diagnosis of transformation, flow cytometry may be useful in cases when morphologic findings are less clear.

Patients with CLL often present with no symptoms, with the diagnosis being made as a consequence of asymptomatic enlarged lymph nodes or splenomegaly detected on physical examination or routine blood work done for another cause. Other patients present with symptoms of BM replacement (fatigue, dyspnea, or petechiae secondary to anemia and thrombocytopenia), symptomatic lymphadenopathy or hepatosplenomegaly, autoimmune complications (hemolytic anemia or idiopathic thrombocytopenic purpura), or B symptoms (fevers, night sweats, and weight loss). A small proportion of CLL patients will have pulmonary infiltrates at diagnosis that are representative of CLL involvement in some cases and active infection in others.

In addition to blood and BM lymphocytosis, a few abnormal laboratory findings are commonly observed in CLL. Neutropenia, anemia, and thrombocytopenia can develop as a consequence of BM infiltration or myelosuppressive therapy administered to eliminate the leukemia. A positive direct antibody, or Coombs, test result is observed in approximately 10% to 25% of CLL patients at some time during the course of the disease. Similarly, autoimmune thrombocytopenia or neutropenia may be present, although other causes such as BM replacement or chemotherapy effect are much more common and should be excluded. Pure red blood cell (RBC) aplasia can sometimes be observed with isolated anemia and absence of RBC precursor cells. Hypogammaglobulinemia is common in CLL and becomes more frequent and marked as the disease progresses. In contrast, hypercalcemia and markedly elevated lactate dehydrogenase (LDH) are not common in CLL and suggest Richter transformation. Clearly, a wide spectrum of presentations exists for patients with CLL.

When Do We Consider a Transplant Evaluation in Chronic Lymphocytic Leukemia?

With the introduction of nonmyeloablative stem cell transplantation, the morbidity and mortality associated with this therapy in CLL has decreased, and this option thereby was extended to young and older patients alike. In addition, extended follow up at several transplant series suggested that prolonged remissions could occur with this treatment approach, potentially providing the only curative therapeutic option for this disease. However, with the availability of newer and more effective therapeutic options such as the kinase inhibitors and soon to be approved BCL2 inhibitor, the indications for transplant have declined tremendously over the past few years. In general, we do not consider detailed discussion of transplant or referral for asymptomatic patients. When patients become symptomatic and require therapy for their CLL, we briefly discuss the role of stem cell transplantation (SCT) as a potentially curative option. Approximately 50% of patients with CLL are 75 years of age or younger, have acceptable end-organ function, and lack comorbidities when symptomatic disease develops. This CLL patient group may benefit from an allogeneic transplant consultation. However, this group can potentially attain a long-term disease control state with the administration of kinase inhibitors. Moreover, the use of kinase inhibitors does not result in a significant number of complete responses and SCT in patients with residual disease generally results in a higher incidence of relapses. Autologous transplant in CLL offers no opportunity for cure and is associated with treatment-related myelodysplastic syndrome (MDS)/AML. For patients without del(17p13.1) who attain a complete remission (CR) with initial chemotherapy, we do not consider a consolidative SCT. For patients treated with ibrutinib, SCT can be considered, although it is not our preference for young healthy patients with del17p and complex karyotype in complete or good partial response since these patients typically have the worst outcomes even in the era of kinase inhibitor therapy. However, we do not consider this approach until the patient is 1 to 2 years into treatment with kinase inhibitors. The impressive and sustained disease control afforded by kinase inhibitors and the possibility of more effective and potentially curative and less toxic therapeutic alternatives like chimeric antigen T cell (CAR-T cells) have significantly limited the role of SCT for the routine management of patients with CLL.

TABLE 77.3	Rai Staging System		
Rai Stage at Diagnosis		Percent of Patients Never Requiring Chronic Lymphocytic Leukemia Therapy	Expected Survival in Months From Initial Diagnosis
0 - Lymphocytosis >5 × 10⁹/L only		59	150
1 - Lymph node enlargement		21	101
2 - Spleen or liver enlargement		23	71
3 - Anemia with hemoglobin <11 g/dL		5	19
4 - Thrombocytopenia <100 × 10¹²/L		0	19

Adapted from Rai KR, Sawitsky A, Cronkite EP, et al. Clinical staging of chronic lymphocytic leukemia, *Blood* 46:219, 1975.

PROGNOSIS

Historically, patients with CLL have been staged using either the Rai (Table 77.3) or Binet system. Both of these discriminate CLL by the sites of disease and degree of cytopenias induced by BM replacement by the leukemia. Patients can be categorized into three groups on the basis of these features. According to the modified Rai criteria, patients in the low-risk group (stage 0) have lymphocytosis without any other abnormality; patients in the intermediate-risk group (stages I and II) have, in addition to their lymphocytosis, enlarged lymph nodes, spleen, or liver; and patients in the high-risk group (stages III and IV) have anemia (hemoglobin <11.0 g/dL) or thrombocytopenia (platelets <100 × 10⁹/L). The median survival times for the Rai low-, intermediate-, and high-risk groups are similar to those of Binet stages A, B, and C: 12+, 8, and 2 years (see Table 77.2). For early-stage patients with CLL (Rai low- and intermediate-stage and Binet stages A and B), a significant range of time to developing symptoms of CLL exists. The lack of survival advantage with early treatment, the observation that a subset of CLL patients will never require therapy, and the varied natural history of the disease have driven research efforts in CLL to identify specific biologic or clinical prognostic factors that predict time to progression.

Although lymphadenopathy is a common clinical feature of CLL and is incorporated into both major clinical staging systems, computed tomography (CT) scans are not commonly used to determine staging or to evaluate response to therapy outside of clinical trials. However, several studies have examined whether the incorporation of CT scans in initial staging or response evaluation may affect the ability to predict disease progression at diagnosis and assessment of clinical response to therapy. Although a few reports have suggested that such studies may help predict disease progression, studies done serially at the time of treatment and for response show that CT scans generally do not impact assessment of response, progression-free survival (PFS), or OS. In addition, CT scan identification of new nodal areas do not impact decisions for retreatment. Thus, routine CT scans should not be performed for staging and response evaluation in CLL. Similarly, positron emission tomography (PET) scans appear to be sensitive for Richter transformation, with a high negative predictive value, but specificity is poor. We generally use these studies to identify patients who warrant biopsy for Richter transformation and to localize where to biopsy.

With recent advances in the molecular biology of CLL, some prognostic factors such as BM infiltration pattern, which requires an invasive procedure at diagnosis, have not maintained their usefulness in predicting disease progression. Prognostic features outside of the traditional staging systems outlined earlier relative to daily practice are summarized later (Table 77.4).

TABLE 77.4	Evaluation of Chronic Lymphocytic Leukemia Patients at Diagnosis

History
- B symptom and fatigue assessment
- Infectious history assessment
- Occupational assessment for chemical exposure
- Familial history of CLL and lymphoproliferative disorders
- Preventive interventions for infections and secondary cancers

Physical Examination
Laboratory Assessment
- CBC with differential
- Morphology assessment of lymphocytes
- Chemistry, LFT enzymes, LDH
- Flow cytometry assessment to confirm immunophenotype of CLL
- Serum immunoglobulins
- Serum β₂M levels
- Interphase cytogenetics for del(17p13.1), del(11q22.3), del(13q14), del(6q21), and trisomy 12
- IGHV mutational analysis
- Stimulated metaphase karyotype (if available)

Selected Tests Under Certain Circumstances
- DAT, haptoglobin, reticulocyte count if anemia present
- CT scan if unexplained abdominal pain or enlargement present
- PET scan or biopsy (or both) if large nodal mass present
- BM aspirate and biopsy if cytopenias present
- Familial counseling if first-degree relative with CLL

Teaching
- Varicella zoster identification instruction
- Skin cancer identification
- Disease education (Leukemia and Lymphoma Society)

BM, Bone marrow; CBC, complete blood count; CLL, chronic lymphocytic leukemia; CT, computed tomography; DAT, direct antiglobulin test; IGHV, immunoglobulin heavy chain variable region; LDH, lactate dehydrogenase; LFT, liver function test; PET, positron emission tomography.

Thymidine Kinase Activity and β₂-Microglobulin

Thymidine kinase is an enzyme involved in the salvage pathway of DNA synthesis and its levels correlate with proliferative activity. Elevated thymidine kinase activity (TKA) has been observed to be predictive of early progression in a subgroup of untreated patients with smoldering CLL. β₂-Microglobulin (β₂M) is an extracellular protein component of the human leukocyte antigen (HLA) class I complex. β₂M has been shown to have significant prognostic relevance in lymphoma and multiple myeloma patients and correlates with disease burden in CLL patients. Hallek and colleagues examined 113 CLL and immunocytoma patients for β₂M levels and TKA and demonstrated that elevated TKA and β₂M both were independent predictors of shortened PFS. Keating et al confirmed the prognostic value of β₂M in CLL patients, reporting that an elevated level was associated with a significantly shorter survival time for both untreated and previously treated patients. In their studies, elevated β₂M levels were observed in patients with high tumor burden and extensive BM infiltration. In addition to disease progression, both β₂M and TKA have been associated with short duration of remission and inferior survival after treatment.

IGHV Mutational Status

Although the malignant CLL cell morphologically resembles a mature lymphocyte, genetic, immunologic, and phenotypic studies suggest that this cell is better designated as either a pregerminal or postgerminal B cell. Somatic mutations in the first and second complementarity-determining regions (CDR1 and CDR2) of the IGHV genes are thought to occur in the germinal centers. Examination of IGHV genes in patient cells suggests that there may be two subsets of CLL: leukemias whose cell of origin has successfully traversed the germinal center, resulting in the mutated IGHV phenotype, and leukemias that are derived from naive B cells with the unmutated (germline) IGHV sequence. Whereas approximately 60% of CLL patients have cells with mutated IGHV genes (<98% identity to germline), the remaining patients have cells exhibiting unmutated IGHV (≥98% sequence identity with germline), typical of pregerminal B cells. The prognostic significance of the absence of IGHV gene mutations is substantial, with studies uniformly noting an inferior survival and high tendency to require early treatment in this patient subset. A CLL Research Consortium study examined the impact of IGHV mutation in 307 untreated CLL patients enrolled in a prospective tissue collection study. A total of 53% of these patients exhibited unmutated IGHV genes, and this population had a significantly shorter median time to initial therapy (3.5 years) than those with mutated IGHV (9.2 years; $p < .001$).

Because of the difficulties in determining IGHV gene mutational status, researchers have sought surrogate markers for this parameter. Correlation between the absence of IGHV gene mutations and elevated expression of the cell surface molecule CD38 on CLL cells has been noted. In another report, ZAP-70 expression was shown to correlate with IGHV gene mutational status. ZAP-70 is a T-cell receptor–associated tyrosine kinase that is aberrantly expressed in CLL cells, and ZAP-70 expression is generally found in patients with unmutated IGHV but not in patients with mutated IGHV. These two associated biomarkers appear to be linked directly to the difference in the behavior between these two genetic subtypes of CLL and are discussed independently. Other surrogate markers for the mutational status of the IGHV gene have been reported, including methylation and subsequent silencing of TWIST2, a transcription factor that negatively regulates p53. TWIST2 methylation and silencing are preferentially observed in IGHV-mutated CLL cases. Elevated levels of lipoprotein lipase and related genes have been noted in patients with IGHV-unmutated disease. In addition, it has been reported that IGHV-mutated CLL cells have long telomeres with low telomerase activity, but IGHV-unmutated patients have short telomeres with high telomerase activity. The extreme shortening of telomeres and elevated telomerase activity are associated with both genetic instability and disrupted apoptosis in other diseases, suggesting that a similar process occurs in IGHV-unmutated CLL cells. Finally, distinct gene and microRNA (miRNA) expression profiles have also been correlated with IGHV gene mutational status.

CD38 Expression

Retrospective studies have shown that CD38 is an independent prognostic marker in CLL, demonstrating that high CD38 expression is associated with both a shorter time from diagnosis to treatment and inferior survival. CD38 functional studies using CD31 and plexin B1 transfected fibroblasts have provided a biologic explanation for this observation. CD38 interaction with its ligand, CD31, in the presence of IL-2 results in upregulation of the survival receptor CD100 exclusively on proliferating CLL cells. This occurs with concomitant downmodulation of CD72, a negative regulator of immune response. The interaction between CD38 and CD100 on CLL cells and CD31 and plexin B1, respectively, on transfected fibroblasts results in enhanced survival and growth of CLL cells. Furthermore, the presence of nurse-like cells in CLL patients expressing high levels of CD31 and plexin B1 corroborates the interplay of CD38 and CD31 and provides further evidence of activation of circulating CD38-positive CLL cells by the microenvironment. This finding provides an explanation for the aggressive nature of these CLL clones.

ZAP-70

ZAP-70 expression was identified as another surrogate marker for IGHV gene mutational status by a cDNA microarray analysis of untreated CLL patients. Functional studies in ZAP-70–positive cases have shown that BCR ligation leads to increased phosphorylation of cytosolic proteins (Syk, BLNK, PLCγ), calcium mobilization, degradation of IκB, and ultimately NFκB target gene activation. Despite clear data showing that ZAP-70 is a prognostic marker, the reproducibility of this assay across laboratories has been problematic. Inconsistent measurement of ZAP-70 may be the cause of this lack of reproducibility because ZAP-70 is a labile protein, and laboratories have used different methods and reagents. Given the challenges of measuring ZAP-70 protein accurately, others have attempted to identify alternative markers or more stable readouts of ZAP-70 expression. For example, methylation of select regions in the proximal 5′ region of the ZAP-70 gene has been shown to correlate closely with expression of ZAP-70 and to be correlated with treatment outcome. Overall, despite the apparent usefulness of ZAP-70 in research laboratories for discriminating CLL patients at high risk for progression, this test is of limited utility for routine clinical practice.

CD49d Expression

CD49d is a surface subunit of the integrin heterodimer that is involved in promoting survival of the CLL cells through microenvironment derived growth signals. CD49d can be used as a reliable predictive marker of aggressive disease course and inferior survival is associated with ≥30% cells expressing CD49d by flow cytometry.

Other Prognostic Markers

Various other markers have been used for predicting the disease course of CLL patients. Elevated serum LDH levels are associated with aggressive disease and with the development of Richter syndrome and prolymphocytic lymphoma. Similarly, patients with a lymphocyte doubling time of 12 months or less have been shown to have a worse overall and treatment-free survival. Other markers include soluble factors including CD23, CD44, VCAM-1, CD27, and MMP-9, IL-6 and IL-8, etc. However, none of these biomarkers are routinely used in clinical practice.

MicroRNAs (miR) are noncoding RNAs that are 19–25 nucleotides in length and modulate mRNA translation and synthesis of various proteins. Various microRNAs have been validated as useful CLL prognostic markers, especially miR-15a and miR-16-1 which were the first to be identified as being underexpressed in CLL B-cells. Deletion of chromosome 13q14 decreases their transcription and increases the expression of the antiapoptotic BCL2 protein. Similarly, miR-34c is affected by del11q23 and regulates the expression of ZAP-70 and other proteins involved in the Tp53 pathway. MiR mass array profiles have also been found to be predictive of disease progression, fludarabine resistance and clinical outcomes.

Chromosomal Aberrations

Conventional metaphase karyotype analysis can identify chromosomal aberrations in only 20% to 50% of CLL cases because of the low in vitro mitotic activity of CLL cells. Abnormalities noted in descending frequency of occurrence include trisomy 12; deletions at 13q14; structural aberrations of 14q32; and deletions of 11q, 17p, and 6q. In addition, a complex karyotype (three or more abnormalities) occurs in approximately 15% of patients and is predictive of rapid disease progression, Richter transformation, and inferior survival. The use of CD40L or the combination of IL-2 and CpG for B-cell stimulation has revealed translocations in 33 of 96 patients (34%). These translocations were both balanced and unbalanced, occurring at 13q14, 11(q21q25), 14q32, or regions also seen in lymphomas such as 1(p32p36), 1(q21q25), 2(p11p13), 6(p11p12), 6(p21p25), and 18q21. The presence of such translocations defines a prognostic subgroup of patients with a significantly shorter median time from diagnosis to requiring therapy (24 vs. 106 months) and

OS (94 vs. 346 months) as compared with those without translocations. The frequency of such translocations in untreated patients is less common, suggesting that such transactions accumulate with disease progression.

Given the limitation of standard or stimulated karyotype analysis, interphase FISH has become the state-of-the-art technique for accurately distinguishing genetic subtypes of CLL. The largest study of interphase FISH resulted in improved sensitivity to detect partial trisomies (12q12, 3q27, 8q24), deletions (13q14, 11q22-23, 6q21, 6q27, 17p13), and translocations (band 14q32) in more than 80% of all cases. In a large study of 325 patients by Dohner and colleagues, a hierarchical model consisting of five cytogenetic subgroups was constructed on the basis of regression analysis of CLL patients with chromosomal aberrations. Patients with a 17p deletion had the shortest median survival time (32 months) and the shortest treatment-free interval (TFI, months); patients with an 11q deletion followed closely with 79 months and 13 months, respectively. Whereas the favorable 13q14 deletion group had a long TFI of 92 months and a median survival of 133 months, the group without detectable chromosomal anomalies and those with trisomy 12 fell into the intermediate group with median survival of 111 and 114 months, respectively, and TFI of 33 and 49 months, respectively. According to this pivotal study, CLL patients are prioritized in a hierarchical order (deletion 17p13 > deletion 11q22-q23 > trisomy 12 > no aberration > deletion 13q14). The hierarchical model of cytogenetic abnormalities in predicting disease progression by FISH has been further confirmed by other studies. Of interest, patients with high-risk interphase cytogenetic abnormalities or other complex abnormalities are almost always found to have IGHV-unmutated CLL.

Mutational Analysis

Numerous recurrent mutations and or deletions have been described in CLL that are often associated with IGHV mutational status. While the majority of these mutations do not impact the clinical outcome of CLL patients, several including p53, ATM, NOTCH1, SF3B1, XPO1, and BIRC3 have been shown to predict time to initiation of treatment and also overall survival. Outside of p53 mutations, the frequency of these mutations are often low and therefore prevent definitive independent determination of their impact on outcome with respect to other features. The presence of several other mutations including ERK1, BRAF, and MYD88 have served as a rationale for therapeutic targeting with novel agents that are U.S Food and Drug Administration (FDA) approved or are being evaluated in clinical trials. However, none of these drugs have been shown to be effective in CLL. Despite routine mutational tests being available, it is not our practice to examine these broadly at diagnosis or at time of treatment. The exception to this is p53 mutations for which there may be value although their independence of del(17)(p13.1) as a negative biomarker has only rarely been demonstrated because of the common association of these two aberrations.

TREATMENT

Initiation of Treatment of Newly Diagnosed or Previously Untreated Patients

Many patients are incidentally diagnosed with CLL on routine complete blood count examination and are asymptomatic with a normal hemoglobin and platelet count at the time of initial diagnosis. Expectant observation without therapy is the standard practice for such asymptomatic patients, and patients receive treatment only when their disease progresses. This practice is based on several studies that failed to show an improvement in OS when early therapeutic intervention with chlorambucil was administered to asymptomatic patients. A metaanalysis of 2048 patients participating in six trials demonstrated no difference in death rate between patients who were randomized to early therapy (42.6%) and those with treatment

How Should Staging and Biomarkers Be Used for Treatment Decisions in Chronic Lymphocytic Leukemia Patients?

Our understanding of the biology of CLL has improved dramatically, and many relevant biomarkers are now available for predicting when CLL patients will clinically progress. However, no study to date has demonstrated that earlier treatment will alter the natural history of the patient in even the higher risk groups with high progression rates. Therefore, at the present time, the use of staging and predictive biomarkers should be used only to provide patients with information relative to the expected course of their disease. Outside of a clinical trial, these results should never be used to initiate therapy in patients with asymptomatic disease or as an indication for treatment. Before performing predictive tests, a detailed discussion with the patient of how these tests will be used should occur and the option of not performing them should be provided. In a subset of patients, significant anxiety can be produced by identifying high-risk features for which observation, without therapeutic intervention, remains the standard of care. Table 77.4 provides an example of the initial evaluation provided by our group when seeing a newly diagnosed patient. Because lymphocyte-doubling time is a prognostic feature in the progression of CLL, our approach is to follow patients every 3 months during the first year following diagnosis; if little change in clinical or laboratory parameters occurs at this point, we extend this time period to every 6 months in the absence of new complaints.

deferred (41.6%). Thus, patients with asymptomatic or early-stage disease derive no therapeutic benefit from early alkylating agent therapy. However, in these studies, chlorambucil was administered as initial therapy, and chlorambucil achieves complete response (CR) in few patients. Similarly, fludarabine when used early for patients who do not meet the conventional criteria for treatment resulted in higher response rate but failed to demonstrate a survival advantage. A recently completed trial from the German CLL study group of high risk CLL patients did not demonstrate an advantage of even more aggressive chemoimmunotherapy with fludarabine, cyclophosphamide, and rituximab in improving overall survival. It is now well-established that CLL undergoes genetic clonal evolution over time with greater frequency in IGHV-unmutated CLL, resulting in increasing resistance to therapy. Thus, the issue of early treatment needs to be reconsidered, particularly in patients with high-risk biological or molecular markers predicting a poor long-term prognosis, such as IGHV-unmutated disease and especially with the advent of kinase inhibitors that may be associated with limited toxicities.

To establish uniform clinical practice standards and ensure reproducible eligibility criteria for entrance into clinical studies, the IWCLL established guidelines for initiation of treatment. Indications to begin therapy included nonautoimmune cytopenias (Rai stage III and IV), bulky or symptomatic lymphadenopathy or hepatosplenomegaly, disease-related B symptoms or fatigue, extreme lymphocytosis (>300 × 10^9/L) or a rapid lymphocyte-doubling time, and autoimmune hemolytic anemia (AIHA) or thrombocytopenia not controlled with steroids. A rapidly rising lymphocyte doubling time was recently removed from the National Comprehensive Cancer Network (NCCN) criteria as an indication to treat as it commits many patients to earlier intervention, which may not be necessary in the absence of other symptoms. It is imperative to determine if a patient's symptoms are attributable to CLL or a comorbid medical condition because constitutional symptoms such as fatigue are nonspecific and can be attributed to many causes in elderly patients with comorbid illnesses. In addition to the official IWCLL 2008 criteria for therapy, an increasing frequency of infections and slowly progressive anemia are other indications that can aid the practicing physician in deciding when to initiate therapy in patients with CLL. A summary of the IWCLL 2008 guidelines for treatment is provided in Table 77.5 with some minimal modifications used by our group.

A useful paradigm for clinical practice is to institute treatment in CLL only for cytopenias or directly referable symptoms. When treatment is necessary, a variety of agents have been examined in clinical trials (outlined below). Previously identified biomarkers are used in

TABLE 77.5	Modified Indications for Treatment of Chronic Lymphocytic Leukemia

- Grade 2 or greater fatigue limiting life activities
- B symptoms persisting for ≥2 weeks
- Lymph nodes >10 cm or progressively enlarging lymph nodes causing symptoms
- Spleen or liver with progressive enlargement or causing symptoms
- Anemia (hemoglobin <11 g/dL) referable to CLL
- Thrombocytopenia (platelets <100 × 10^{12}/L) referable to CLL or ITP poorly responsive to traditional therapy
- Severe paraneoplastic (e.g., insect hypersensitivity, vasculitis, myositis) process related to CLL not responsive to traditional therapies

CLL, chronic lymphocytic leukemia; ITP, idiopathic thrombocytopenic purpura.

selecting the initial treatment for CLL. In addition, several studies have shown that CLL patients older than 70 years of age or who have multiple comorbid illnesses do not benefit from fludarabine-containing regimens, which should be factored into treatment algorithms. Below, we summarize the findings of clinical studies of different treatments for CLL; where such data exist, we integrate genomic biomarkers as well as clinical features, including age and comorbid illnesses. Different therapies are outlined below with attention to details related to their initial use in previously untreated CLL. Because many of these regimens were also developed in relapsed CLL patients, these data will be reviewed and later referred to in the section Treatment of Patients With Relapsed Chronic Lymphocytic Leukemia.

Cytotoxic Chemotherapy

Alkylating Agents

Chlorambucil and other alkylating agents have served as first-line therapy for CLL for many decades, and chlorambucil is still given as first-line therapy for some patients, particularly older patients and patients who cannot tolerate purine analog therapy. Chlorambucil is generally administered as a single pulse dose 40 mg/m^2 orally (PO) every 28 days with or without concomitant steroid therapy, although alternative dosing schedules are used, particularly in Europe. Chlorambucil is typically given without steroid therapy because the addition of steroids to alkylating agent therapy has not been shown to improve survival. Although a high-dose continuous dosing schedule of 15 mg/day PO has been evaluated in several large European studies and led to results superior to those of pulse therapy, high-dose therapy is associated with greater myelosuppression and frequently requires dose reduction, particularly in older or more fragile patients in whom chlorambucil is typically considered. Although high-dose therapy may be more effective if maximal cytoreduction is desired, the less intensive pulse dosing schedule should generally be used outside the setting of a clinical trial. Because most studies of alkylating agent therapy predated widespread use of cytogenetic and biologic risk factors, data on the effect of biomarkers on predicting response to chlorambucil are limited. However, the existing data indicate that patients with del(11q22.3) or del(17p13.1) have a lower response rate and a shorter duration of remission to chlorambucil compared with patients without these abnormalities. The primary advantages of chlorambucil are its well-established toxicity profile and its low cost; its primary disadvantages are its low CR rate, even in previously untreated patients, and the small possibility of developing myelodysplasia with extended therapy. Although not typically given as a single agent to younger patients, its use should be considered in older patients and other patients who may not tolerate more intensive chemotherapy based regimens. Given the benefit of the chimeric monoclonal anti-CD20 antibody rituximab as part of chemoimmunotherapy regimens with fludarabine, several studies have been performed combining chlorambucil with rituximab, ofatumumab and

the novel type II monoclonal anti-CD20 antibody obinutuzumab. (Both obinutuzumab and ofatumumab are discussed later in this chapter.)

Bendamustine

Although typically classified as a bifunctional alkylator, bendamustine has an uncertain mechanism of action. Although the drug predominantly promotes cytotoxicity by inducing DNA damage and the generation of reactive oxygen species, bendamustine displays a distinct pattern of activity unrelated to other DNA-alkylating agents but closest to melphalan. Unlike other alkylating agents, bendamustine activates a base excision DNA repair pathway rather than an alkyltransferase DNA repair mechanism. Studies of bendamustine in a variety of solid tumors, non-Hodgkin lymphoma (NHL), multiple myeloma, Hodgkin disease, and CLL have shown single agent activity. Bendamustine has been widely used in East Germany and several European countries for decades and was approved by the U.S. Food and Drug Administration (FDA) for treatment of CLL in 2008. This was based on a well-controlled, randomized phase III study comparing bendamustine 100 mg/m^2 intravenous (IV) on days 1 and 2 with chlorambucil 0.8 mg/kg PO on days 1 and 15 every 4 weeks for six cycles. A total of 319 patients were enrolled with an overall response rate (ORR) of 68% and 31% CR with bendamustine versus 31% ORR and 2% CR with chlorambucil treatment ($p < .0001$). The median PFS was significantly better ($p < .0001$) with bendamustine (21.6 vs. 8.3 months) than chlorambucil. Grade 3/4 hematologic toxicity and severe infections (grades 3–4) occurred more commonly with bendamustine. Overall, this study and others that have followed showed that bendamustine is well tolerated in young and old CLL patients. This agent has been effectively combined with rituximab and will be discussed later in this chapter.

Combination Chemotherapy With Alkylating Agents

A variety of trials combining alkylating agents and other cytotoxic agents have been performed. A phase III Eastern Cooperative Oncology Group (ECOG) study of chlorambucil and prednisone (CP) with or without vincristine (CVP) demonstrated no benefit in PFS for the CVP arm. The French CLL group showed that a modified cyclophosphamide, Adriamycin, vincristine, prednisone (CHOP) regimen was superior to CVP and achieved similar results as fludarabine monotherapy. A metaanalysis compared alkylating agent-based combination regimens with a single-agent regimen based on an alkylating agent and demonstrated no survival benefit. Given that alkylating agent–based combination regimens are associated with more toxicity and show no benefit over fludarabine-based therapy, there is a limited role for combination alkylator-based therapy in the routine management of patients with CLL. In the relapse setting, although salvage lymphoma regimens such as CHOP-R; rituximab, ifosfamide, carboplatin, and etoposide (R-ICE); and etoposide, methylprednisolone, cytarabine, cisplatin, and rituximab (ESHAP-R) are used to treat CLL, clinical studies of these regimens in CLL are lacking, and the utility of these regimens is undefined.

Purine Analogs

The introduction of purine analogs in the 1980s by Grever and later Keating revolutionized CLL therapy, and fludarabine has demonstrated significant clinical efficacy in both relapsed and previously untreated CLL. Pentostatin was the first nucleoside analog that demonstrated clinical activity in CLL and related B-cell lymphoproliferative disorders; however, subsequent phase II studies showed modest activity, limiting further trials of this agent. Given its more favorable myelosuppression profile compared with other nucleoside analogs, pentostatin has been combined with other agents and shown favorable clinical activity and toxicity in selected populations. Two other nucleoside analogs, fludarabine and cladribine, were subsequently found to be clinically active in CLL. Phase II–III studies of cladribine monotherapy achieved similar clinical responses as alkylating agent–based treatment but were associated with more cytopenias and immune suppression. The FDA approved fludarabine for the treatment of CLL, and thus most studies of purine analog–based therapy in CLL have focused on fludarabine. The remainder of this section focuses predominantly on clinical trials of fludarabine.

Fludarabine was initially approved by the FDA for alkylating agent–resistant CLL in 1991 based on two phase II studies demonstrating a high response rate to fludarabine in this patient subset, prompting several additional trials of fludarabine as monotherapy in relapsed and previously untreated CLL. After the observation of high response rates and a 33% CR rate in previously untreated CLL by Keating and colleagues, several large prospective randomized studies in previously untreated CLL patients compared alkylating agent–based regimens with fludarabine. These studies collectively established fludarabine as an accepted standard first-line therapy for CLL based on improved response rates and PFS. A multicenter European study randomized 196 evaluable patients to fludarabine or cyclophosphamide, doxorubicin, and prednisone (CAP). The ORR favored fludarabine (60% vs. 44%), and this benefit was observed in both relapsed ($n = 96$; 48% vs. 27%) and previously untreated ($n = 100$; 71% vs. 60%) patients, although the difference was not statistically significant in the untreated group. Fludarabine achieved a longer median duration of response than did CAP, with a tendency toward longer OS in previously untreated patients. A randomized, multicenter American study confirmed these findings in 509 previously untreated CLL patients. Patients were randomized to receive fludarabine 25 mg/m^2 IV daily for 5 days every 28 days, chlorambucil 40 mg/m^2 PO every 28 days, or fludarabine 20 mg/m^2 daily for 5 days and chlorambucil 20 mg/m^2 PO every 28 days, for up to 12 cycles. Patients who failed to respond or relapsed were allowed to cross over to the other arm. The combination arm was closed because of excessive toxicity. Fludarabine achieved a superior CR rate, ORR, median duration of remission, and median duration of PFS (20%, 63%, 25 months, 20 months, respectively) than did chlorambucil (4%, 37%, 14 months, 14 months, respectively). However, there was no statistically significant difference in OS even after 10 years of follow up (66 vs. 56 months), possibly because of the crossover design. A multicenter French study randomized 938 patients with previously untreated Binet stage B and C CLL to fludarabine, CHOP, or CAP. Although fludarabine achieved better response rates than CAP, OS (67–70 months) was identical for all three treatment groups. Thus, single-agent fludarabine achieves superior response rates and duration of PFS than alkylating agent–based regimens. The impact of prognostic factors on response rates and duration of PFS to fludarabine was recently examined; patients with high-risk cytogenetic abnormalities, including del(11q22.3) and del(17p13.1), have significantly shorter PFS in response to fludarabine-based therapy than patients with other cytogenetic abnormalities.

However, the benefit of fludarabine does not apply to patients older than the age of 65 years. A phase III trial by the German CLL Study Group randomized 193 previously untreated CLL patients older than 65 years to fludarabine 25 mg/m^2 IV for 5 days every 28 days for six cycles or chlorambucil 0.4–0.8 mg/kg PO every 15 days for 12 months. Fludarabine achieved higher OR (72% vs. 51%) and CR rates (7% vs. 0%) and longer time to treatment failure (19 vs. 18 months). However, PFS was similar in both arms (19 months vs. 18 months), and OS was 46 months for fludarabine compared with 64 months for chlorambucil arm ($p = .15$). Thus, the results achieved in younger patients do not necessarily apply to older patients with comorbid diseases or who otherwise cannot tolerate more aggressive therapies.

Combining Fludarabine With Alkylating Agent Therapy

Fludarabine was combined with cyclophosphamide (Flu/Cy) in three randomized phase III studies, based on two promising pilot studies

in previously untreated CLL patients, with the goal of improving response rates and hopefully long-term survival. The German CLL Study Group randomized 375 previously untreated patients (age younger than 65 years) to standard fludarabine or Flu/Cy (fludarabine 30 mg/m^2 IV and cyclophosphamide 250 mg/m^2 IV daily for 3 days) every 28 days for six cycles. The ORR (94% vs. 83%), CR rate (24% vs. 7%), median PFS (48 vs. 20 months), and duration of treatment-free survival (37 vs. 25 months) all favored Flu/Cy, although there were more patients with cytopenias in the combination arm. Furthermore, no difference in OS was observed. ECOG randomized 278 patients to single-agent fludarabine or fludarabine 25 mg/m^2 on days 1–5, cyclophosphamide 600 mg/m^2 on day 1, and granulocyte colony-stimulating factor (G-CSF) support every 28 days for six cycles. Flu/Cy therapy achieved a superior ORR (74% vs. 59%), rates of CR (23% vs. 5%), and duration of PFS (32 vs. 19 months), although no OS advantage was observed. The United Kingdom LRF CLL4 study randomized 777 patients to oral chlorambucil, fludarabine, or Flu/Cy. Patients randomized to Flu/Cy enjoyed superior ORR, CR rates, and 5-year PFS rates (94%, 39%, and 33%, respectively) as compared with patients who received chlorambucil (72%, 7%, and 9%, respectively) or fludarabine (80%, 15%, and 14%, respectively).

These three large, prospective, randomized, multicenter studies in the United States and Europe have clearly demonstrated that Flu/Cy therapy is associated with better response rates and duration of PFS than single-agent fludarabine. However, no OS advantage for upfront Flu/Cy has been observed to date. Although toxicity has generally been manageable, greater hematologic toxicity has been observed with Flu/Cy. In addition, patients older than 65 or 70 years, who make up the majority of CLL patients receiving therapy in clinical practice, have either been excluded or minimally represented in these trials. Further studies are needed to determine if Flu/Cy is as well tolerated and active in older patients as it is in younger patients. Finally, of these patients, long-term follow up is required to determine the duration of remission, OS, and the incidence of potential late complications such as therapy-related myeloid neoplasia (tr-MN) to fully assess the utility of the Flu/Cy regimen. Indeed, the U.S. Intergroup study of Flu/Cy versus Flu suggested an increased risk of tr-MN in the Flu/Cy arm. Examination of outcome by cytogenetic risk groups showed that patients with high-risk cytogenetic abnormalities, including del(17p13.1), had a significantly shorter remission than patients in the groups with good- or intermediate-risk cytogenetic findings. Therefore, the addition of alkylating agents to fludarabine does not appear to alter the poor prognosis associated with high-risk cytogenetic abnormalities except for patients with del(11q22.3).

Rituximab

Rituximab is a chimeric murine monoclonal antibody that targets the CD20 antigen on the surface of normal and malignant B-lymphocytes, and is the best studied and most widely used monoclonal antibody for the treatment of CLL and B-NHL. CD20, a calcium channel that interacts with the BCR complex, is an ideal target, because CD20 is expressed in 90% to 100% of cases of CLL and B-NHL and is only minimally internalized or shed. Rituximab induces antibody-dependent cellular cytotoxicity (ADCC) and complement-dependent cytotoxicity (CDC), activates caspase 3, and induces apoptosis in CLL and B-NHL cells. These multiple mechanisms of action likely contribute to rituximab's effectiveness in CLL.

In phase I clinical studies in indolent B-NHL rituximab, 375 mg/m^2 IV was administered weekly for four doses, although the dose and length of treatment were empirically determined. The pivotal phase II trial of rituximab was pursued in 166 patients with relapsed or refractory indolent B-NHL, including SLL. Although an ORR of 60% was achieved in indolent follicle center B-NHL, only four of 30 patients (13%) with SLL/CLL responded. Similarly, disappointing results were obtained in several other small studies. Responses in each of these studies were predominantly in the blood and nodal compartment with little improvement in BM disease. In contrast, two trials in which higher doses of rituximab weekly (≤ 2250 mg/m^2 per dose) or in which rituximab was administered thrice weekly (at 375 mg/m^2) to relapsed CLL patients showed improved response rates with response duration approaching that achieved in follicular B-NHL. These studies established a role for single-agent rituximab in patients with relapsed CLL and led to combination therapy with other agents.

In contrast to studies in relapsed CLL, weekly single-agent rituximab demonstrated greater clinical efficacy when given to patients with previously untreated SLL/CLL. Forty-four previously untreated patients with SLL/CLL received 4-weekly doses of rituximab 375 mg/m^2; the ORR after the first course of rituximab was 51% (CR 4%). Twenty-eight patients with stable or responsive disease received additional 4-week courses of rituximab every 6 months for up to four cycles. However, there was only a modest increase in ORR (58%) and CR rates (9%), and the median duration of PFS of 19 months was shorter than the 36- to 40-month median duration of PFS reported by the same investigators using the same regimen in previously untreated patients with follicle center B-NHL. Nonetheless, this response duration compared favorably with the response duration achieved with fludarabine in the upfront setting, suggesting that rituximab is active and may have a role in the upfront therapy of SLL/CLL.

Rituximab is selective for the B-cell antigen CD20 and therefore has a relatively favorable toxicity profile. Toxicity associated with infusion of this agent commonly occurs with the first infusion of rituximab and may be greater in patients with CLL compared with patients with NHL. These symptoms generally include fever, rigors, transient hypoxemia, dyspnea, and hypotension, which are partly caused by an inflammatory cytokine release syndrome. Although poorly understood, CLL patients with platelet counts less than 50×10^{12}/L may experience transient, severe thrombocytopenia associated with this infusional toxicity and may require platelet transfusions with the first one or two doses of rituximab. Patients with preexisting thrombocytopenia should therefore have a posttherapy platelet count after the first one or two doses of rituximab. Another uncommon but potentially severe toxicity is a tumor lysis syndrome, which is generally observed in patients with a high circulating peripheral lymphocyte count with CLL variants. Such patients should receive prophylactic allopurinol, hydration, and careful observation, and inpatient monitoring before administration of rituximab can be considered for the highest risk patients. Patients who develop tumor lysis syndrome after the first dose of rituximab can safely receive subsequent doses, especially after the number of circulating CLL cells is reduced. Other rare toxicities with rituximab therapy include delayed neutropenia, hepatitis B reactivation, skin toxicity, interstitial pneumonitis, serum sickness, and progressive multifocal encephalopathy. Patients with prior hepatitis B exposure, as indicated by positive serologies, should receive rituximab only if viral load testing indicates no active disease. Such patients should undergo regular viral load monitoring during and after completion of rituximab therapy, and prophylactic antiviral therapy may be considered to reduce the likelihood of viral reactivation. Patients who develop profound neutropenia, pulmonary, or skin toxicity with rituximab should not be challenged with repeated dosing. In general, rituximab is a very well-tolerated therapy, making it ideal for use in combination with other agents in patients with CLL.

Phase II Studies of Rituximab Chemoimmunotherapy

Given its activity and toxicity profile, rituximab has been combined with cytotoxic chemotherapy in the treatment of CLL, and clinical trials have examined several such chemoimmunotherapy regimens. Studies of chemoimmunotherapy in CLL have focused primarily on fludarabine-based combinations because of the established role of fludarabine therapy in this disease. The approval of bendamustine and potentially its unique mechanism of action has led to combination therapy with bendamustine and rituximab. Finally, given the recent recognition that elderly patients do not benefit from

fludarabine-containing regimens, several trials have also combined rituximab with chlorambucil with promising results. Alternative regimens, including FCR–mitoxantrone (FCR-M) and pentostatin, rituximab, and cyclophosphamide (PCR), have been published and used in CLL but are unlikely to be building blocks for improvement in CLL therapy in the future and are therefore not described later.

Fludarabine and Rituximab

The Cancer and Leukemia Group B (CALGB) 9712 study randomized 104 previously untreated CLL patients to sequential or concurrent fludarabine and rituximab (FR) therapy. Patients received standard fludarabine 25 mg/m^2 days 1–5 every 4 weeks for six cycles with or without concurrent rituximab 375 mg/m^2 on day 1 of each cycle with an additional dose on day 4 of cycle 1. Patients in both arms received rituximab 375 mg/m^2 weekly for four doses beginning 2 months after completion of fludarabine; thus patients in the concurrent arm received 11 total doses of rituximab compared with four in the sequential arm. Patients receiving concurrent FR therapy enjoyed a superior CR rate (47% vs. 28%) and ORR (90% vs. 77%) as compared with patients in the sequential arm. Retrospective comparison to a fludarabine only–containing treatment study performed previously by CALGB demonstrated improved PFS and OS for patients enrolled in the concurrent arm. Analysis of prognostic cytogenetic abnormalities demonstrated that patients with del(11q22.3) and del(17p13.1) have a shorter duration of response to FR. A recent update of this study with a median follow up of 117 months showed that the median OS was 85 months with 71% of patients alive at 5 years. The median PFS was 42 months with 27% progression-free at 5 years. Importantly, an estimated 13% of patients remained free of progression after almost 10 years of follow-up. IGHV-mutated disease status was favorably associated with extended PFS and OS, but not having high-risk cytogenetic abnormality was also associated with a favorable OS. Notably, there were no cases of tr-MN occurring before relapse contrasting with prior studies with fludarabine- and alkylator-containing regimens.

Fludarabine, Cyclophosphamide, and Rituximab

The most favorable phase II results with chemoimmunotherapy have been reported by the MD Anderson group with a combination FCR regimen in both previously treated and untreated CLL. A total of 177 evaluable patients with previously treated CLL received fludarabine 25 mg/m^2 and cyclophosphamide 250 mg/m^2 on days 2–4 of cycle 1 and on days 1–3 of cycles 2–6 in addition to rituximab 375 mg/m^2 on day 1 of cycle 1 and 500 mg/m^2 on day 1 of cycles 2–6. An ORR of 73% with a 25% CR rate and 16% nodular PR rate was reported, and 12 of 37 patients (32%) in CR achieved molecular remission. The same authors administered FCR to 300 previously untreated CLL patients; the ORR was 95%, with 72% of patients attaining a CR. Six-year PFS was 51%, and OS was 77%. Features associated with poor response included high β_2M levels, del(17p13.1), age older than 70 years, and white blood cell count elevation above 150×10^9/L. Late infectious or other complications were uncommon except for tr-MN, which occurred in 9% of patients. The outcome of patients with tr-MN was poor irrespective of treatment. In a multivariate analysis of patients receiving fludarabine-based therapy at MD Anderson, FCR therapy was significantly associated with improved survival, thereby validating the experience with FR, suggesting that rituximab therapy was improving OS. Moreover, patients with mutated IGHV with a low β2M level did not experience any relapse of their disease after 10 years suggesting that a subset of patients can achieve long-term remissions and potentially cure.

The benefit of adding rituximab to FC was confirmed by the German CLL study group, which randomized 817 physically fit, previously untreated CLL patients, ages 30–81 years, to fludarabine 25 mg/m^2 on days 1–3 and cyclophosphamide 250 mg/m^2 IV on days 1–3, with or without rituximab 375 mg/m^2 day 0 of cycle 1 and 500 mg/m^2 day 1 of cycles 2–6 every 28 days for six cycles. A total of 761 patients were evaluable for response. FCR induced higher OR (95 vs. 88%) and CR rates (44 vs. 22%) than FC. Median PFS was 32.8 months for FC and 51.8 months for FCR, and the largest benefit for FCR was observed in Binet stage A and B patients. The OS rate at 37.7 months favored FCR over FC (84% vs. 79%; $p = .01$). FCR resulted in more grade 3 and grade 4 neutropenia (34% vs. 21%) and leukopenia (24% vs. 12%), but there was no difference in the number of severe infections or treatment-related deaths between the two arms. As with other chemoimmunotherapy trials in CLL, neutropenia was more common with FCR than FC. Emerging from this study were numerous biologic correlative studies showing the most predictive test of long-term PFS and OS was attainment of a minimal residual disease (MRD)–negative state using high-sensitivity flow cytometry. In addition, patients with unmutated IGHV disease had a shorter PFS and OS with both FCR and FC, although rituximab appeared to benefit both treatment groups. All groups based upon cytogenetic analysis benefited from rituximab with the exception of the del(17p13.1) and normal karyotype patients, who had similar outcomes to FC or FCR treatment. An update of this study demonstrated that IGHV-mutated CLL have the similar long-term disease free plateau suggestive of potential cure than after earlier follow up than the MD Anderson series. Thus, even in the age of new targeted therapy, FCR must be strongly considered as a therapeutic option for the younger patient group with IGHV-mutated disease given the potential for cure with combined chemoimmunotherapy.

Bendamustine and Rituximab

Based on promising single agent activity of bendamustine in previously treated CLL and in vitro studies demonstrating synergy between bendamustine and rituximab, the German CLL Study Group examined the feasibility and safety of this combination in a phase II study in 78 relapsed CLL patients. Bendamustine was administered at a dose of 70 mg/m^2 days 1 and 2 and rituximab at 375 mg/m^2 on day 0 of cycle 1 and 500 mg/m^2 on day 1 of cycles 2–6. Using an intent-to-treat analysis, the ORR was 59% with a CR of 9%. The median PFS was 14.7 months. Response was poor (7%) in the del(17p) patients. Severe infections occurred in 13% of patients. Grade 3 or grade 4 neutropenia, thrombocytopenia, and anemia were documented in 23%, 28%, and 17% of patients, respectively.

A follow-up study (CLL2M) included a total of 117 symptomatic, previously untreated CLL patients who were treated with bendamustine (90 mg/m^2 on days 1 and 2) and rituximab (375 mg/m^2 in cycle 1 and 500 mg/m^2 in cycle 2–6). Treatment was administered every 28 days for up to six cycles. Demographics of the patients included a median age of 64 years with 48% having Binet C disease. The ORR was 91%, and the CR was 33%. After 18 months, 76% of patients were still in remission, and median PFS had not been reached at the time of the report. The treatment was well tolerated with cytopenias and infections being most problematic. Treatment-related mortality (TRM) was 2.6%. Patients with all cytogenetic groups based upon cytogenetic analyses except for del(17p13.1) responded favorably. Based on these encouraging phase II data, the German CLL Study Group conducted a phase III study comparing bendamustine/fludarabine (BR) with FCR (CLL10) in previously untreated, physically fit CLL patients. FCR therapy demonstrated an improved CR (39% vs. 30%) and PFS (median 55 months vs. 41%) as compared with BR but OS was similar after an early follow up. FCR was associated with significantly higher risk of neutropenia, thrombocytopenia, and infections. However, early data in the favorable IGHV-mutated patients has not suggested that a similar disease-free plateau exists with BR as with FCR. Thus, it is our practice in the current era of kinase inhibitor therapy to use FCR when considering chemoimmunotherapy with intent of pursuing extended DFS and potential for patients to be off therapy for an extended period of time.

Chlorambucil and Anti-CD20 Antibodies

Based on the success of chemoimmunotherapy and the potential absence of benefit of nucleoside analogs in elderly CLL patients, Hillmen and colleagues initiated a study in 100 elderly, previously untreated CLL patients combining rituximab (day 1; 375 mg/m^2 IV cycle 1, 500 mg/m^2 cycles 2–6) and chlorambucil (days 1–7; 10 mg/

m^2/day PO) every 28 days for six cycles. Patients were permitted to receive six additional cycles of chlorambucil if they had evidence of continuing clinical response after six cycles. The median age was 70 years. The OR rate on an intent-to-treat analysis was 82%, with nine patients achieving a CR, 58 patients achieved a partial response (PR), 15 patients achieved a nodular PR (nPR), and 11 patients had stable disease. The median PFS to date is 23.5 months. The response rate in this study was significantly higher than patients receiving chlorambucil alone in the CLL4 study, suggesting a benefit of adding rituximab. A second Italian phase II study using a similar combination of chlorambucil and rituximab together demonstrated a similar favorable response data. Based on these phase II studies, a randomized phase III study comparing chlorambucil (Chl) versus chlorambucil with either rituximab (Chl-R) or the human monoclonal antibody which binds to CD20, obinutuzumab (Chl-O) was conducted by the German CLL Study Group. In this CLL11 trial the Chl-O had higher ORR (78% vs. 65% vs 31%) and CR rates (20% vs. 7% vs. 0%) in Chl-O versus Chl-R versus Chl arms respectively. Similarly, PFS was also improved significantly with Chl-O (median 26 months vs. 16 months vs. 11 months). Importantly, Chl-O was able to induce a higher proportion of MRD-negative responses when compared with Chl-R. Chl-O was associated with higher incidence of infusion reactions and cytopenias but the incidence of infections was similar in all three groups. In a similar study, ofatumumab in combination with chlorambucil was compared with chlorambucil alone in previously untreated patients and demonstrated a significantly prolonged median PFS of 22 months versus 13 months. Based on these results both obinutuzumab and the fully human monoclonal antibody for CD20, ofatumumab were approved in combination with chlorambucil for the treatment of patients with untreated CLL who would not otherwise be candidates for conventional chemotherapy.

Alemtuzumab

Alemtuzumab is a humanized monoclonal antibody against CD52, a cell-surface glycopeptide expressed by virtually all human lymphocytes, monocytes, and macrophages, a small subset of granulocytes, but not erythrocytes, platelets, or hematopoietic stem cells. CD52 is

---

What Is the Role of Anti-CD20 Antibodies in Chronic Lymphocytic Leukemia?

Studies of rituximab have demonstrated modest single-agent clinical activity in both previously untreated CLL patients using the weekly dosing schedule and in the relapsed state using more intensive dosing regimens. Rituximab does not have activity against CLL with del(17p13.1). For this reason, rituximab monotherapy is generally used in either of these settings only if more definitive therapy cannot be administered because of other comorbid conditions. Rituximab's greatest contribution is to combination therapy both in symptomatic, previously untreated CLL patients and relapsed patients receiving the FR or FCR regimen, particularly in younger patients. Phase III studies have demonstrated the clear benefit of chemoimmunotherapy over traditional chemotherapy alone and have established chemoimmunotherapy as the standard of care for CLL. Several other studies have combined rituximab with other therapies such as bendamustine, chlorambucil, and pentostatin–cyclophosphamide that might be more tolerable to older patients. Inclusion of rituximab in alternative chemoimmunotherapy regimens for patients not appropriate for chemotherapy-containing regimens is reasonable. Multiple other CD20 targeting agents including especially obinutuzumab, however have been reported to have demonstrated superiority over rituximab. Although several studies of maintenance rituximab have been published after completion of chemoimmunotherapy, the benefit of this is uncertain. These studies were performed mostly in patients with low-risk disease who would ordinarily be expected to respond well to conventional therapy. Similar results have also been reported with ofatumumab suggesting a slight benefit in patients relapsing after chemoimmunotherapy. At this time, maintenance rituximab or other CD20 antibody in CLL cannot be justified and should not be used outside of the context of a clinical trial.

expressed on all CLL cells and indolent B-NHL cells. Alemtuzumab has been demonstrated to mediate apoptosis, CDC, and ADCC of CLL cells in vitro. CD52 is not shed, internalized, or modulated and is therefore an ideal antigen for targeted immunotherapy. However, the ubiquitous expression of CD52 on normal lymphocytes and monocytes is predictive of the increased neutropenia, lymphopenia, and infectious complications observed with alemtuzumab therapy. Alemtuzumab has modest efficacy in patients with relapsed disease including patients with del17p disease but not in patients with bulky lymphadenopathy (>5 cm). Responses are better and more durable when it was used in patients with previously untreated disease and comparable with other CD20 antibodies when used in combination with chlorambucil. Similarly, the combination of alemtuzumab with chemotherapy resulted in improved responses but with significantly higher toxicities. Alemtuzumab is not marketed in the U.S. anymore for CLL but is available from the manufacturer on request. Given its infrequent use, the discussion on alemtuzumab has been curtailed and readers are referred to previous editions of this chapter.

What is the Role of Ibrutinib in the Initial Management of Patients With Del(17p13.1)?

Conventional chemotherapy has limited benefit in the initial treatment of patients with del(17p13.1) deletion with the median PFS being in the range of 11–14 months. Limited and early data from the use of ibrutinib has been extremely promising and ibrutinib use has resulted in an ORR of up to 97% in this high-risk group of patients. Responses were rapid and deepened with time and resulted in a PFS at 24-months of 82%. This compares extremely well with historic data with alternative agents used for patients with del(17p.13) and along with activity observed in patients with relapsed disease, resulted in the approval of ibrutinib for patients with del(17p13.1).

TREATMENT OF PATIENTS WITH RELAPSED CHRONIC LYMPHOCYTIC LEUKEMIA

The approach to reinitiating therapy for CLL patients who have relapsed after initial therapy is similar to that applied to the assessment for initial therapy. Patients need not receive therapy at the first sign of relapse. Rather, patients should have an indication for treatment, as discussed earlier. Patients should have repeat interphase FISH analysis of the peripheral blood or a BM aspirate because patients may acquire additional cytogenetic abnormalities, most notably del(17p13.1), as their CLL becomes more advanced. The incidence of del(17p13.1) increases from 5% in patients at initial diagnosis to nearly half of heavily treated patients with advanced CLL, and acquisition of this abnormality has profound implications on treatment, as will be discussed later. IGHV mutational analysis does not need to be performed if such information has been obtained previously because a patient's IGHV mutational status does not change with time. A BM analysis should be performed if cytopenias are present to confirm that CLL is the cause and to exclude other potential causes of cytopenias such as transformed lymphoma, prolonged BM toxicity from prior therapy, or development of treatment-related myelodysplasia. Patients should be treated according to the indications outlined in Table 77.5. Multiple novel agents have now been approved and more are in the advanced stages of development. The treatment for relapsed disease will continue to evolve with time. In general, therapy is moving away from chemoimmunotherapy to better tolerated targeted oral agents especially for patients older than 70 years of age and those with multiple comorbid conditions.

Agents Targeting B-Cell Receptor Signaling Pathways

BCR signaling and microenvironmental signals are now known to be important in both proliferation and protection of CLL cells in BM

and nodal sites. These findings prompted the introduction of several novel, orally available kinase inhibitors. In particular, agents targeting the δ isoform of PI3-kinase and BTK have shown very promising clinical activity and, importantly, durability of remission over time in refractory CLL patients. Early results from these trials led to the approval of both ibrutinib and idelalisib for the treatment of patients with relapsed CLL. Moreover, ibrutinib was also approved for treatment of patients with del17p disease. The results of these studies are summarized later.

Ibrutinib

Ibrutinib is a potent, irreversible, covalent inhibitor of BTK. BTK is a tyrosine kinase in the Tec family of tyrosine kinases and is an essential element of the BCR signaling pathway. Genetic knockout or inactivation of BTK in mice produces predominantly a B-cell defect with absent B1 lymphocytes, diminished B cells, and disrupted BCR signaling. Mutations in BTK in humans result in a more profound humoral immune defect with absent B cells, immunoglobulins, and an increased incidence of infections. Preclinical work with ibrutinib demonstrated disruption of BCR signaling and in vivo activity in spontaneous canine lymphoma models with documented targeted inhibition of BTK. Preclinical trials demonstrated that ibrutinib promotes apoptosis of CLL cells, inhibits activation of PI3-kinase, ERK1, and NFκB by external microenvironment signals, and also prevents CLL proliferation.

Collectively, these preclinical studies prompted phase I/II studies with ibrutinib in NHL and CLL. The phase I study of ibrutinib was completed at two dose levels above where BTK inhibition occurred without obtaining a maximum tolerated dose. At the highest dose, toxicity was quite mild, including grade 1/2 nausea, diarrhea, infections, rash, and fatigue. Activity was seen at all doses, including in 9 of 16 CLL/SLL patients. A subsequent trial used the 420 mg daily oral dose of ibrutinib and demonstrated an ORR of 71% with an additional 20% of patients experiencing PR with lymphocytosis (PR+L). The PR+L state observed with ibrutinib does not appear to predict for inferior PFS. Importantly, the responses seen with ibrutinib are sustained and resulted in a PFS of 69% at 30 months. Responses to ibrutinib also tend to improve with time and after a median follow up of 2-years CR rates improved from 2% to 7%. Responses were also seen in patients with del17p who had an ORR of 55.9% with a median duration of response of 25 months. This compares favorably with historical comparison with either cyclin-dependent kinase inhibitors or other conventional therapies used in the past for patients with del17p. Patients with previously untreated CLL also appear to benefit from ibrutinib monotherapy with an ORR of 71% and 13% PR+L. PFS was 96% at 2 years. Ibrutinib was also well tolerated and the most common side effects were diarrhea, nausea, and fatigue. A subsequent randomized study comparing ibrutinib with ofatumumab in relapsed CLL confirmed the benefits of ibrutinib with an improved response rate, PFS and OS. However, these studies also demonstrated a higher incidence of both minor bleeding possibly caused by a collagen-mediated platelet aggregation defect and atrial fibrillation with ibrutinib. Ibrutinib should therefore be used with caution in patients receiving concurrent anticoagulation with warfarin and patients should be taken off treatment for 3–7 days before and after surgical procedures. Patients experience a progressive decline in the incidence of infectious complications with continued use of ibrutinib and do not require routine antimicrobial prophylaxis. There is also subjective improvements in stress, depressive symptoms, fatigue, and quality-of-life in patients.

Since treatment with ibrutinib does not result in CRs in the majority of patients, at this time it is recommended that treatment be continued indefinitely until disease progression or unacceptable toxicity, since ibrutinib discontinuation in heavily pretreated patients often results in rapid disease progression. Development of resistance has been rare but whole-exome sequencing has identified a cysteine-to-serine mutation in BTK at the binding site of ibrutinib and three distinct mutations in PLCγ2. Functional analysis revealed that the C481S mutation of BTK results in a protein that is only reversibly inhibited by ibrutinib. The R665W and L845F mutations in PLCγ2 are both potentially gain-of-function mutations that lead to autonomous B-cell–receptor activity. To improve the depth of response, ibrutinib is being combined with various other agents like rituximab and BR or FCR. This has resulted in higher response rates but improvements in PFS are yet to be demonstrated. The combination of ibrutinib and rituximab in patients with high-risk CLL was generally well-tolerated and resulted in an OR rate of 95% and a PFS of 78% at 18 months in all patients, and 72% in patients with del17p. A randomized phase III trial comparing BR + placebo with BR + ibrutinib in patients with relapsed CLL demonstrated a significant improvement in PFS in the ibrutinib arm. From preliminary reports, PFS at 18 months was 79% for the BR + ibrutinib arm and 24% in the BR + placebo arm. Therapy was generally well tolerated with a slightly higher percentage of patients in the ibrutinib arm discontinuing therapy. These promising results have resulted in the initiation of two pivotal trials for the initial treatment of patients with CLL. The ECOG (ECOG 1912) trial is for patients younger than 70 years of age and is comparing patients treated with either FCR or ibrutinib + rituximab. The Alliance (A041202) trial is for patients ≥65 years of age and is comparing BR versus ibrutinib + rituximab versus ibrutinib alone. Participation in these trials is strongly encouraged and they have the potential to change the treatment paradigms for this disease.

Idelalisib

Idelalisib (GS1101, CAL-101) is an orally bioavailable, isoform specific, PI3-kinase-δ inhibitor that, at therapeutic levels obtained in patients, does not inhibit other isoforms of PI3-kinase. Genetic mouse models knocking out PI3-kinase-δ demonstrate predominantly a B-cell defect, absent B1 lymphocytes, and disrupted BCR signaling. Preclinical studies demonstrated that idelalisib promotes the apoptosis of CLL cells via a PI3-kinase-δ pathway and inhibits signals from the microenvironment that protects CLL cells from apoptosis. Based in part on these data, a phase I study in healthy volunteers showed this agent to be well tolerated, and subsequently a large phase I study in NHL, CLL, multiple myeloma, and AML was undertaken. Idelalisib was active at all dose levels tested, with the dose-limiting toxicity being reversible transaminitis that generally occurs during the first 2 months of therapy in approximately 5% to 20% of patients, depending on histology. Although patients with NHL experienced a higher incidence of transaminitis, the cause of which is poorly understood, the incidence of transaminitis was less than 5% in CLL patients. In a phase I trial of 54 patients, with relapsed/refractory high-risk CLL patients, idelalisib resulted in an ORR of 72 percent (including PR+L). The median PFS was 15.8 months. Therapy was generally well-tolerated with the most commonly observed grade ≥3 adverse events being pneumonia in 20%, neutropenic fever in 11% and diarrhea in 6% of the patients. Subsequent studies have been undertaken with idelalisib combining it with rituximab, ofatumumab, obinutuzumab and bendamustine/rituximab, showing that combination therapy with idelalisib is feasible. The combination of idelalisib and rituximab was also compared with rituximab and placebo in a phase III trial and resulted in an ORR of 81% versus 13% and PFS at 1 year in excess of 90% versus 5.5 months in the rituximab and placebo arm respectively. Serious toxicities observed with idelalisib were similar to the ones observed with the single agent. Based on these results, idelalisib was approved in combination with rituximab for the treatment of patients with relapsed CLL who would not be considered suitable for conventional chemotherapy.

Ofatumumab in Relapsed Chronic Lymphocytic Leukemia

Ofatumumab is a fully human type I anti-CD20 monoclonal antibody that was initially approved for the treatment of CLL in late 2009. In vitro, it has improved CDC, ADCC, and direct killing (with cross-linking), compared with rituximab. Ofatumumab has a different binding epitope of CD20 than rituximab, binding to both the small and large extracellular loops of CD20, and a slower off rate as well. Ofatumumab is able to kill rituximab-resistant CLL cells caused by its greater induction of CDC and its ability to kill cells with low CD20 expression, which may be relevant given the limited CD20 expression by CLL cells. Based on these promising data, a phase I/II study of ofatumumab, given at doses of 500–2000 weekly for four doses in 33 relapsed or refractory CLL patients, demonstrated that it is generally well tolerated even at higher doses. Ofatumumab was active, with an ORR of 50% in the cohort treated at 2000 mg. Infusion-related adverse events were similar to those reported with rituximab and decreased after the first infusion. Infections were fairly common, occurring in 51% of patients, including one fatal infection. These results prompted a pivotal, single-arm study of ofatumumab administered as eight weekly infusions of ofatumumab followed by 4 monthly infusions. Patients received 300 mg as the first dose to minimize infusion-related reactions, and the dose was increased to 2000 mg for all subsequent infusions. Patients included in this study were required to be fludarabine-refractory and also alemtuzumab-refractory (FA-refractory group; n = 95) or to have bulky lymphadenopathy larger than 5 cm (BF-refractory group; n = 111). The ORR, as assessed by an independent review committee, was 51% for the FA-refractory group and 44% for the BR-refractory group, with two CRs observed in the BF-refractory group. All other responses were partial. The median duration of response was 5.7 months in the FA-refractory group and 6.0 months in the BF-refractory group with most patients progressing during treatment. The median PFS was 5.5 months in both the FA-refractory and BF-refractory groups. Median OS was 14.2 months and 17.4 months, respectively. For rituximab-treated (n = 117), rituximab-refractory (n = 98), and rituximab-naive (n = 89) patients, the OR rates were 43%, 44%, and 53%, respectively; median PFS was 5.3, 5.5, and 5.6 months, respectively; and median OS was 15.5, 15.5, and 20.2 months, respectively. Thus, prior exposure to rituximab did not affect the response to ofatumumab.

The presence of del(17p13.1) was associated with a lower response rate and shorter median PFS in both patient groups (37% vs. 56% and 3.3 months vs. 5.5 months in FA-refractory group; 22% vs. 49% and 3.8 vs. 5.6 months in BF-refractory group). Thus, in contrast to rituximab, ofatumumab is active as a single agent in del(17p13.1) CLL but has less activity as compared with alemtuzumab. Toxicity included infusion-related reactions, infections, and cytopenias. This trial led to accelerated approval of ofatumumab for the treatment of patients with fludarabine- and alemtuzumab-refractory CLL, however, a phase III study of ofatumumab versus physician's choice of therapy in bulky, fludarabine-refractory CLL has preliminarily not documented a significant improvement in PFS. Determination of the clinical superiority of ofatumumab over rituximab will require randomized trials comparing equivalent doses and as a result the use of ofatumumab has been limited in CLL. In addition, the approval of BCR signaling inhibitors has further diminished the use of this option in salvage therapy of CLL.

Other Emerging Therapeutic Modalities for Chronic Lymphocytic Leukemia

Several other promising therapeutics are in late phase II/III clinical trials for CLL. Those with documented activity in this disease that have potential to be approved for use in CLL are described here.

BCL2 Inhibitors

The BCL2 antiapoptotic protein is overexpressed in CLL and has been shown to disrupt apoptosis of CLL cells. Although the BCL2 antisense molecule genasense did not meet the bar for regulatory approval in CLL, attempts to target BCL2 with small molecule inhibitors have proceeded. Another potent inhibitor of BCL2, navitoclax (formerly ABT263), demonstrated single agent activity in relapsed CLL with a target specific (BCL-XL) dose-limiting toxicity of profound thrombocytopenia. A second-generation oral BCL2 inhibitor venetoclax (ABT-199) that lacks off-target effects on BCL-XL is currently being evaluated in clinical trials and has shown impressive activity with deep remissions in patients with relapsed and refractory CLL including those who have del17p. Therapy with venetoclax has been complicated by the development of episodes of fulminant tumor lysis syndrome especially in patients with high burden of disease and mitigation strategies have been developed to improve its safety and reduce the incidence of hyperacute tumor lysis. Early results have demonstrated impressive activity of this agent in patients with relapsed disease with an ORR of 88% with 31% CRs including in patients with del17p. Venetoclax use also resulted in deep MRD-responses that have persisted for sustained periods. It was generally well tolerated and the most common adverse events were cytopenias. Multiple studies are currently ongoing to further establish the role of venetoclax as monotherapy or in combination with other agents for patients with CLL.

Chimeric Antigen Receptor T-Cell Therapy

To date, efforts at directing T-cell immune suppression toward the tumor cells have been relatively limited. A major development has been preclinical and early phase I studies demonstrating that ex vivo transfected T cells with chimeric T-cell receptors bearing both CD3 and also a B-cell–specific antigen (most often CD19) have great potential to eradicate established B-cell tumors after administration into both xenograft models and, recently, patients with refractory CLL. Even though chimeric antigen receptor T cell (CAR-T) therapy has preliminarily shown deep and durable responses, toxicity remains a major concern and it continues to require significant development and optimization before this can be readily administered widely.

Lenalidomide

Lenalidomide (Revlimid), is an immunomodulatory drug that is a more potent analog of thalidomide. Lenalidomide is approved for marketing in multiple myeloma and transfusion-dependent myelodysplasia. Lenalidomide has clinical activity in a variety of other malignancies, including CLL. Two initial studies examining either an intermittent 25 mg PO daily for 21 days or 5 mg with dose escalation to 10 mg PO as tolerated given as continuous therapy were pursued initially in relapsed CLL. The higher dose, intermittent schedule was active with an ORR of 47% and 9% CR. Major side effects of therapy were cytopenias, rash, and tumor flare, which in some cases can be life threatening. The continuous, low-dose regimen had a 32% intent-to-treat ORR with a 7% CR rate. Toxicity was less with this schedule but still included cytopenias in most. On the basis of these promising phase II clinical studies, a large, multicenter trial randomizing patients to low-dose (10 mg) or high-dose (25 mg) lenalidomide was undertaken, which was halted early because of life-threatening adverse events in patients receiving the higher dose of therapy. Subsequent studies have shown that lower doses of lenalidomide administered as continuous treatment in patients with relapsed CLL are feasible. These data have prompted several single agent studies in symptomatic, previously untreated CLL in which the clinical activity has ranged from an ORR of 56% to 65% with up to 10% CR. Most provocative of these studies was the observation that lenalidomide reversed the hypogammaglobulinemia observed in CLL patients. PFS with this treatment is approximately 2 years. Associated toxicity, includes tumor flare, cytopenias, rash, and infection, but these events are manageable. Lenalidomide was subsequently combined with other agents, most notably anti-CD20 antibodies such as rituximab and ofatumumab, or used as consolidation therapy after purine analog or bendamustine-based induction therapy. Antibody combination therapy diminished the tumor flare but was associated with increased cytopenias. Similarly, lenalidomide as consolidation therapy after PCR-based treatment, appeared to potentially extend PFS over that previously seen with PCR alone. Unfortunately, a pivotal trial comparing chlorambucil with lenalidomide was halted because of higher mortality observed in elderly patients on the lenalidomide arm. No obvious cause of the increased mortality has been identified. This has significantly limited the prospects of further development of this agent in CLL. However, lenalidomide has profound immunologic effects in patients

with CLL and the immune modulatory effects could be used as a strategy for earlier control of the disease or as an adjuvant to vaccine-based approaches. Because of its relative modest activity in heavily pretreated patients, other alternatives for first-line therapy, and the potential for life-threatening tumor flare and other toxicities associated with lenalidomide, this agent should only be considered as part of a well-designed clinical trial despite its FDA approval for other indications (MDS and multiple myeloma).

Other Agents

Therapeutic antibodies or small modular immune pharmaceuticals targeting surface antigens, including CD19 (Xm5574), CD37 (otlertuzumab, IMGN529, and MAb 37.1), and BAFF-R (VAY736), are under development. In addition, therapeutic agents targeting signal transduction pathways (HSP-90 inhibitors, Syk inhibitors, AKT inhibitors, ILK inhibitors, NFκB inhibitors, and PP2A activating agents) are in early clinical development. Finally, agents targeting epigenetic events or innate immune activation (CpG oligonucleotides or IL-21) have promising data to support their ongoing early clinical investigation.

Stem Cell Transplantation

For many years, autologous and allogeneic SCT was extensively used for treatment of CLL late in the course of the disease. However, trials of SCT have indicated that patients with multiply relapsed and chemotherapy-resistant disease are at highest risk for both relapse and TRM. In addition, many patients with heavily treated CLL cannot be adequately cytoreduced or disease control cannot be maintained for a sufficient period of time to obtain insurance approval and find a suitable allogeneic donor, producing a selection bias that often excludes patients with the most refractory or aggressive disease from actually receiving a SCT. The recognition that patients with poor prognostic features such as del(11q22.3) and del(17p13.1) and patients who fail to achieve CR after receiving regimens such as FCR have a short remission duration, had prompted many transplant centers to consider earlier application of allogeneic SCT as therapy for CLL, including its use as consolidation treatment after induction therapy for the highest risk patients. The timing of SCT has been thrown into a bigger conundrum with long-term disease control seen in patients with relapsed disease including patients with high risk disease receiving ibrutinib. Recent data has identified a subgroup of patients with a complex karyotype that have a shorter PFS despite kinase inhibitor therapy. Referral of such high-risk CLL patients at the time of treatment to an experienced transplant center for evaluation, potential tissue typing of the patient and his or her siblings, and initiation of an unrelated donor search (if needed) should be considered. Although autologous SCT has been used historically as a treatment for CLL, nonmyeloablative allogeneic SCT is the preferred modality for most patients requiring a transplant unless a suitable allogeneic donor is not available. Autologous SCT is no longer used in CLL because of a lack of a survival advantage, only modest benefit in PFS, and a high risk of tr-MN with this modality. Therefore, autologous SCT is not reviewed in this chapter.

Myeloablative Allogeneic Stem Cell Transplantation

The use of an allogeneic donor provides an immunologic graft-versus-leukemia (GVL) effect for patients with CLL. Limited data suggest that total body irradiation (TBI)-containing conditioning regimens are superior to chemotherapy-only regimens in CLL transplant patients. A small study of 25 patients demonstrated a 100-day TRM of 57% in patients who received busulfan and cyclophosphamide (Bu/Cy; $n = 7$), compared with 17% for patients who received a TBI-containing regimen ($n = 18$). Five-year actuarial survival was 56% for 14 patients transplanted with TBI regimens during

1992–1999. A study of Cy/TBI in 28 CLL patients observed a 100-day TRM of 11%. Five-year PFS and OS were 78% and 78% for chemosensitive patients compared with 26% and 31% for refractory patients.

A retrospective European Society for Blood and Marrow Transplantation (EBMT) study of 135 patients showed 54% 3-year OS and 40% 100-day TRM. The International Bone Marrow Transplant Registry Database (IBMTR) reported similar findings, with 45% 3-year OS and 30% 100-day TRM in 242 patients. The high TRM may be explained in part by the late stage of the disease in many of these patients. Median time from diagnosis to SCT was 41 and 46 months in these two studies, and 37% of patients in the EBMT study were chemorefractory before transplant. In a Canadian study of allogeneic SCT in 30 CLL patients, the 5-year EFS and OS were both 39%, with 48% for patients with sibling donors. The role of unrelated donor allogeneic SCT was examined by a multicenter study of 38 patients, 92% of whom received TBI. Five-year PFS and OS were 30% and 33%, and TRM was 38%. Although there are no prospective randomized studies, a retrospective comparison showed a 3-year DFS of 57% for allogeneic SCT versus 24% for purged autologous SCT. Finally, allogeneic SCT appears to overcome the adverse prognosis associated with an unmutated IGHV; an analysis of 34 CLL patients who underwent SCT found that only two of 14 patients who received allogeneic SCT relapsed, compared with 13 of 20 patients who underwent autologous SCT. Thus, myeloablative allogeneic SCT may provide superior DFS to patients with CLL compared with autologous SCT. Although the 3-year DFS after allogeneic SCT is approximately 50%, longer follow up is needed to determine if the disease remissions are durable. However, this DFS advantage is offset by significantly higher TRM, thus limiting the use of allogeneic SCT in CLL. Limited data indicate that Bu/Cy may be particularly toxic in this population; by contrast, TBI regimens have acceptable TRM. To preserve the immunologic GVL effect while reducing TRM, the focus of clinical SCT practice in CLL has turned to nonmyeloablative or reduced-intensity allogeneic SCT.

Nonmyeloablative Allogeneic Stem Cell Therapy

Ideally, the goal is to harness the GVL effect of allogeneic SCT for patients with CLL while reducing TRM from acute graft-versus-host-disease (GVHD), acute infection, and organ toxicity associated with myeloablative conditioning. Fludarabine, busulfan, and ATG were administered to 30 German CLL patients; the stem cell source was a matched related ($n = 15$) or unrelated ($n = 15$) donor. Grade 2–4 acute GVHD was observed in 56% of patients and 75% developed chronic GVHD. Responses were seen in 93% of patients, with 40% achieving CR. Of note, it took up to 2 years for patients to achieve CR, suggesting a GVL effect. All patients achieved a molecular CR by PCR, but only six patients were in continued molecular CR after a median follow up of 2 years. Two-year TRM, PFS, and OS were 15%, 67%, and 72%, respectively. The EBMT retrospectively examined 77 CLL patients who received a variety of nonmyeloablative conditioning regimens, followed by allogeneic SCT. The 1-year TRM was 18%, and the 2-year probability of relapse was 31%. Two-year DFS and OS were 56% and 72%, respectively. Nineteen patients received donor lymphocyte infusions (DLIs) for relapse or incomplete donor chimerism, but only seven responded to DLI (37%). Unfortunately, this study was complicated by the heterogeneity of conditioning regimens and the use of ATG or Campath-1H for T-cell depletion of the grafts in 40% of patients. A retrospective analysis of 73 CLL patients who underwent nonmyeloablative SCT and 82 patients who underwent myeloablative allogeneic SCT showed that the TRM was significantly reduced in the former group, with a hazard ratio of 0.4; however, there was no difference in EFS or OS between the two groups.

Sixty-four patients received 200 cGy of TBI, with ($n = 53$) or without ($n = 11$) fludarabine followed by an allogeneic SCT from a related ($n = 44$) or unrelated ($n = 20$) donor. The 2-year DFS and OS were 52% and 60%, respectively, and the 2-year TRM was 22%. The incidence of relapse at 2 years was 26%, and the mortality

because of relapse was 18%. Finally, a British study of 41 CLL patients who received fludarabine, melphalan, and alemtuzumab followed by an allogeneic SCT from a related ($n = 24$) or unrelated ($n = 17$) donor observed a 2-year OS and TRM of 51% and 26%. Eleven patients (27%) relapsed and received escalated DLIs, but only three patients had a sustained response to DLI. Five patients (12%) died of relapsed disease.

Given the approval and outstanding results observed with agents that target BCR signaling, the actual timing of transplantation in CLL has been questioned. Our own practice is to not consider reduced intensity allogeneic transplant for CLL in patients unless they have relapsed after ibrutinib. An exception to this is the younger patient with a complex karyotype receiving ibrutinib where transplant might be considered as part of consolidation therapy given the high risk of eventual relapse. Further follow up on outcome of the kinase inhibitors will be required before definitive recommendations can be made to where transplant should be considered in CLL

Management of Chronic Lymphocytic Leukemia in Specialized Centers

Given the recent advent of prognostic markers and treatment options in CLL, a recent study that examined the impact of physician expertise on patient outcomes in CLL has shown that disease-specific expertise made significant differences in outcomes across all aspects of patient care from prognostic evaluation to choice of therapy. These findings suggest that the expertise of the physician caring for the patient with CLL/SLL is an independent prognostic variable that may not be related to the number of patients he or she manages. We therefore recommend that all patients with newly diagnosed CLL/SLL should be managed in consultation with a CLL expert at a tertiary care center with access to the most recent molecular diagnostic tools.

SPECIAL CLINICAL SCENARIOS IN CHRONIC LYMPHOCYTIC LEUKEMIA

Young Patients (Younger Than 50 Years of Age) With Chronic Lymphocytic Leukemia

As mentioned previously, CLL is a disease of elderly adults, with only 10% of patients being younger than the age of 50 years at diagnosis. Although CLL patients live for a prolonged period of time, young patients without comorbid illnesses have a great potential to have their lives significantly shortened by the disease, irrespective of their cytogenetic abnormalities. In addition, stress associated with job performance, insurance coverage maintenance, and disease-related symptoms are most significant in this age group. Special attention to psychosocial issues related to CLL should occur early during the course of the disease to allow patients to maintain or resume their normal lifestyles as soon as possible. In the absence of impending need for therapy, our approach is generally not to empirically pursue HLA typing or examine transplant options before the development of symptomatic disease. When therapy is initiated for this group of patients, aggressive intervention to promote prolonged remission duration is always compared with prolonged disease control state with the use of kinase inhibitors. SCT and/or CAR-T–cell therapy is generally considered for patients in this age group who have high-risk cytogenetic abnormalities in first remission and for all patients who relapse after initial therapy unless high-risk cytogenetic abnormalities are not present and a CR is attained.

Patients With Fludarabine-Refractory Chronic Lymphocytic Leukemia

Fludarabine-refractory CLL is generally considered to exist if a patient has not responded to a fludarabine-based therapy or relapses within

6 months of completing such a regimen. Several retrospective studies have documented a short survival time (9–12 months) and a particularly high frequency of both bacterial and opportunistic infections in this patient population. With the introduction of chemoimmunotherapy as initial therapy, another poor prognostic group includes patients relapsing within 2 years of FCR- or FR-based therapy. These patients have a significantly shorter PFS with subsequent therapies. Other therapeutic agents such as bendamustine, ofatumumab, and alemtuzumab have been evaluated in this setting and have modest activity and produce relatively short remissions. Newer kinase inhibitors have resulted in impressive responses and PFS and are the recommended therapeutic option for the vast majority of patients with relapsed disease. Currently there is no consensus about the management of patients relapsing after kinase inhibitor therapy and these patients should be considered for participation on clinical trials. The complexities of complications, poor therapeutic options, and acute features of this advanced form of CLL can put great strain on the patient, family members, and general hematologist alike. Referral of such patients to tertiary CLL centers for access to clinical trials and treatment of these specialized needs should be considered for patients with fludarabine-refractory, short remission after chemoimmunotherapy and relapsed disease after kinase inhibitors.

Patients Relapsing After Kinase Inhibitors

The use of kinase inhibitors has significantly transformed the management of CLL, and patients are now experiencing prolonged progression-free intervals. Less than 5% of patients with previously untreated disease who have been treated with ibrutinib in the frontline setting have experienced disease progression at 3-years of follow-up. However, a larger proportion of patients have disease progression when they were treated with either ibrutinib or idelalisib in the relapsed setting. The majority of these patients have high-risk disease and have failed prior chemoimmunotherapy based treatments. Moreover, patients also experience transient disease flares if they have to temporarily hold therapy for routine surgical or unrelated medical procedures. There is limited data to guide management of these patients and multiple trials are currently underway to address these issues. Early experience with these patients indicate that switching kinase inhibitors for progressive disease is a feasible option in a subset of these patients. Similarly, there is no direct comparative data comparing the efficacy of these agents and a formal recommendation cannot be made regarding the choice for initial kinase inhibitor therapy. Therapy should be tailored to patient needs and comorbid conditions and special consideration should be made for patients who require long-term anticoagulation in which idelalisib might be a better option, and for patients with lung, liver, or gastrointestinal issues in whom ibrutinib might be more suitable.

Richter Syndrome

Richter syndrome (RS), the development of high-grade lymphoma in patients with CLL, was described by Maurice Richter in 1928. Over the years, the classification of RS has expanded to include lymphoid malignancies such as Hodgkin disease, lymphoblastic lymphoma, PLL, and hairy cell leukemia (see Fig. 77.4A–C). Incidence estimates range from 2.8% to 10.7%. Recent studies have suggested that the development of RS may be related to the evolution of an abnormal clone unrelated to the underlying CLL clone. Clearly identifiable risk factors for the development of RS are lacking, and its development has been shown to be independent of disease stage, duration of disease, type of therapy, or response to therapy. However, the presence of diffuse lymphomatous involvement, advanced Rai stage, IGHV-unmutated disease, ZAP-70 expression, high LDH, del(17p13.1), high serum β_2M levels, and recently NOTCH1 mutations may predict the development of RS. RS is characterized by sudden onset of B symptoms (fever, night sweats, weight loss) and rapidly progressive lymphadenopathy at any anatomic site. Rarely, the lymphomatous clone may arise from the bone or an extranodal site. Laboratory abnormalities including anemia, neutropenia, and thrombocytopenia which may be caused by large-cell transformation in the BM. A rapid increase in the serum LDH is seen in the majority of patients. The diagnosis is generally made after examining the histology of a rapidly enlarging lymph node, which typically reveals large-cell lymphoma. PET scans can be helpful in these patients to localize the most hypermetabolic node for biopsy. Historically, RS has been treated with regimens similar to those used for the treatment of large-cell lymphomas involving multiple agents such as methotrexate, doxorubicin, cyclophosphamide, vincristine, prednisone, bleomycin, dexamethasone, cytarabine, and cisplatin (e.g., methotrexate with leucovorin rescue, doxorubicin, cyclophosphamide, vincristine, prednisone, and bleomycin [MACOP-B], CHOP-B, dexamethasone, high-dose cytarabine [ara-C], and cisplatin [Platinol] and vincristine, doxorubicin, dexamethasone [VAD]) in combination with rituximab. Other regimens incorporating oxaliplatin have been reported, although their benefit in RS is uncertain over traditional lymphoma regimens. Our institution prefers dose-adjusted infusional therapy (R-EPOCH) for the initial treatment of these patients. The duration of response and the OS rates are dismal, with most patients likely to die within 6 months of their diagnosis despite aggressive therapy. Long-term remissions and survival have been reported in a few patients after allogeneic SCT, but this approach is associated with a high TRM. When Richter transformation occurs, treatment on a clinical trial and consolidation with allogeneic SCT is the preferred treatment.

Similar to RS, prolymphocytic transformation (PT) occurs in fewer than 10% of patients with CLL. PT is characterized by the appearance of large, immature prolymphocytes in the peripheral blood, which make up >55% of the peripheral circulating malignant lymphoid cells. These patients may be older with advanced disease and have more pronounced lymphadenopathy and splenomegaly. PT is associated with a poor outcome, with limited survival beyond 1 year. These patients often have del(17p13.1) but do appear to respond to many of the newer therapies coming forward for treatment of CLL. Allogeneic SCT may also be used as a potentially curative therapeutic option.

Hodgkin lymphoma can also manifest as a form of RS and may have a better outcome provided patients are treated appropriately. Identification of this diagnosis can sometimes be challenging because of its localization to the bone marrow, lower standardized uptake value (SUV) readings on PET scan, and also more insidious onset as compared with the diffuse large B-cell lymphoma (DLBCL) presentation of RS. Hodgkin lymphoma disease in the setting of CLL can be treated as de novo disease with some individuals attaining long-term remissions. Unlike DLBCL transformation of CLL to RS where reduced intensity allogeneic SCT is recommended, we generally do not pursue this in individuals with Hodgkin lymphoma transformation.

Secondary Malignancies in Chronic Lymphocytic Leukemia

Chronic lymphocytic leukemia is associated with an increased risk of secondary malignancies. These include not only hematologic malignancies such as MDS and AML associated with the use of chemotherapeutic agents but also solid tumors such as Kaposi sarcoma, malignant melanoma, and laryngeal and lung cancers. The increased incidence of secondary malignancies may be attributable to multiple reasons, including the immune dysfunction associated with CLL, the frequent infectious complications, the carcinogenic side effects of the various chemotherapeutic agents, and the increased and close medical surveillance that patients with CLL receive from trained oncologists.

Hypersensitivity in Chronic Lymphocytic Leukemia to Mosquitoes and Insect Bites and Treatment

Patients with chronic lymphocytic leukemia commonly exhibit an exaggerated cutaneous response to insect bites. This was first reported in 1965 by Robert Weed, who documented a hypersensitivity reaction to insect bites in 8 of 97 patients with CLL over a 13-year period. The reaction is characterized histologically by the presence of a dermal infiltrate composed of a mixed population of T and B cells, eosinophils, and eosinophilic granule protein. The extent of eosinophilic degranulation may also correlate with the severity of symptoms. Clinically, these patients present with recurrent, painful, bullous eruptions that may be traced to an insect bite in some instances. In limited cases, we have also observed that CLL patients have hypersensitivity to bed bugs, and this should be considered in the differential diagnosis. Identification and avoidance of known triggers may be useful in some cases, but most patients are unable to identify the inciting exposure. Treatment with a short course of steroids is usually effective, but these patients frequently relapse and may require multiple courses of therapy. Dapsone and chlorambucil may also be useful in severe, recurrent cases.

Other cutaneous conditions are also common in CLL patients, with up to 45% reporting some form of skin involvement. These include petechial, purpural, or ecchymotic lesions related to thrombocytopenia; infectious eruptions such as herpes simplex and zoster; and direct leukemic involvement in fewer than 10% of all patients with advanced disease.

INFECTIONS IN PATIENTS WITH CHRONIC LYMPHOCYTIC LEUKEMIA

Infectious complications remain the leading cause of morbidity and mortality in patients with CLL. The incidence of infectious complications has been estimated to be as high as 80% with a mortality rate of approximately 60%. Various factors contribute to the increased incidence of infectious complications in CLL, the most important being progressive disease affecting host immunity through an impaired antibody response and hypogammaglobulinemia; weakened host cellular immune responses, including impaired macrophage function; a decrease in T-regulatory cells; and, finally, the acquired defects after immunosuppressive chemotherapy.

Recent studies have examined predictors of acquiring severe infections in patients with CLL. In their retrospective analysis of infection-related mortality in 280 patients, advanced age, clinical stage B or C disease, unmutated IGHV, and positive CD38 status have been identified as independent predictors of both shorter time to first infection and infection-related mortality. Other risk factors that may also have an impact on development of infections include type of initial therapy and development of renal insufficiency.

Historically, sinopulmonary infections from encapsulated bacteria such as *Streptococcus pneumoniae* and *Haemophilus influenzae* have been the most common cause of infectious complications in patients with CLL. With the recent use of more potent cytotoxic chemotherapy and the resultant profound myelosuppression, an increased frequency of severe pulmonary infections, bacteremia, and gram-negative infections has been reported. Infections caused by atypical organisms such as *Listeria monocytogenes, Nocardia* spp., *Mycobacterium* spp., and *Neisseria meningitidis* are relatively infrequent in patients who receive conventional chemotherapy. Treatment for presumed infection should be initiated empirically in CLL patients who develop fever because fever in CLL patients usually indicates an active infection. Therapy should be tailored to the particular organ involved and the sensitivity of the organism. Prophylactic antibiotics can be initiated for debilitated patients with high-risk disease and significant immune dysfunction.

Viral infections are also commonly encountered in CLL patients (see Fig. 77.3D–E). Herpesvirus infections are especially common in patients treated with nucleoside analogs and alemtuzumab. Chronic, indolent oropharyngeal and circumoral herpes simplex virus (HSV) outbreaks are more frequent than aggressive, disseminated visceral disease. Reactivation of Epstein-Barr virus (EBV) has been implicated in some cases of Richter transformation. Other viruses may cause severe systemic disease in patients with CLL. Varicella zoster virus can cause herpes zoster, herpetic neuralgia, and rarely meningoencephalitis, parvovirus B19 can cause severe polyarthritis and pure

RBC aplasia, and JC polyoma virus has been implicated in the development of progressive multifocal leukoencephalopathy. Management of these infections depends on early recognition of disseminated viral disease, timely initiation of antiviral therapy in cases of HSV and EBV, and a low threshold for the introduction of prophylactic acyclovir and supportive therapy. All patients should be provided instructions to identify the signs and symptoms of herpes virus infection at the time of diagnosis of CLL.

Fungal infections are not typically observed in CLL in the absence of treatment with corticosteroids or other immunosuppressive therapy for autoimmune complications arising from CLL. Cryptococcal meningitis, pneumonia, and fungemia are well-recognized events in patients with CLL and are associated with significant morbidity and mortality. More cases of *P. carinii* pneumonia, systemic candidiasis, and aspergillosis have been reported since the advent of combination nucleoside analog therapy with steroids. Treatment of the infection is dictated by the identification of the particular organism. Trimethoprim–sulfamethoxazole is routinely used as effective prophylaxis against *P. carinii* infections, especially during and immediately after the use of nucleoside analogs or alemtuzumab. Fungal prophylaxis with posaconazole may also be used during protracted therapy with high-dose steroids to avoid invasive aspergillosis.

Prophylactic Strategies for Infections

Routine use of prophylactic antibiotics is generally not used for CLL despite the higher frequency of infections observed in patients with this disease. Early recognition of signs and symptoms of infection and prompt initiation of empiric broad-spectrum antibiotics is probably a more feasible and cost-effective approach. When chemoimmunotherapy is used that includes a nucleoside analog or alemtuzumab therapy, prophylaxis for herpes simplex and varicella zoster should be used, particularly in older patients. Trimethoprim–sulfamethoxazole (or other alternative *P. carinii* pneumonia prophylaxis) should also be administered in this setting. Fortunately, kinase inhibitors result in continued decline in the incidence of infectious complications with ongoing therapy, primarily as a result of better disease control and routine prophylactic antibiotics are either not required or can be tapered off in the majority of patients.

Hypogammaglobulinemia is virtually always present in advanced CLL, and several studies have examined whether IV immunoglobulin (IVIG) replacement therapy can reduce the incidence and severity of infectious complications. Patients receiving IVIG in a double-blind, placebo-controlled trial experienced significantly fewer bacterial infections than the placebo group. The therapy was well tolerated with few adverse reactions, but there was no observed benefit in terms of preventing viral or fungal infections. However, other studies have shown an almost 50% reduction in the number of serious infections per year with IVIG infusions. Limited data support the use of IVIG at a higher dose of 600 mg/kg every 4 weeks to reduce the number and severity of respiratory infections. However, the prohibitive cost of IVIG therapy and the fact that it has not been shown to prolong survival argues against its empiric use in all patients. IVIG should be used judiciously and reserved for patients with advanced disease and recurrent infections. The usual dose used is 200–400 mg/kg every 4–6 weeks as needed, with the aim of keeping the trough serum IgG concentration greater than 500 mg/dL. Our group routinely uses this strategy for refractory patients or those who have more than two infections requiring hospitalization during 1 year.

Among the strategies for preventing infections in this patient population is immunization. CLL patients, however, typically respond poorly to pneumococcal and influenza vaccines. Advanced age, advanced disease stage, hypogammaglobulinemia, and low levels of soluble CD23 influence the rate of responses to immunizations. Soluble CD23, a degradation product of membrane-bound CD23, is involved in several aspects of B-cell activation and proliferation and has a synergistic effect on histamine release. Histamine has a direct inhibitory effect on immunoglobulin production by B cells in vitro via histamine type-2 (H2) receptors and acts as an immune regulatory factor that can be modulated by H2 receptor antagonists. Thus, responses to vaccines may be further enhanced by adjuvant treatment with H2 blockers. Studies have shown that response to protein-conjugated vaccines may be enhanced by ranitidine in CLL patients to as much as 90% compared with 43% in the control group. Unfortunately, this response is not seen with polysaccharide vaccines. Other studies have indicated that protein-conjugated vaccines may be more immunogenic, as shown by a more significant immune response to *Haemophilus influenzae* type b conjugate vaccine than to plain polysaccharide antigen. In light of the paucity of data on an appropriate immunization schedule, we suggest a modified immunization plan based on the recommendations of the Advisory Committee on Immunization Practices. This includes use of Prevnar-13 for pneumococcal prophylaxis and avoiding live vaccines, including the varicella zoster virus.

Growth factors such as G-CSF or granulocyte macrophage colony-stimulating factor can be used prophylactically in high-risk, severely neutropenic patients to shorten the duration and severity of neutropenia.

AUTOIMMUNE COMPLICATIONS OF CHRONIC LYMPHOCYTIC LEUKEMIA

Patients with CLL have a greater predisposition to develop autoimmune hematologic complications, including AIHA, idiopathic thrombocytopenia purpura (ITP), and pure RBC aplasia. AIHA occurs in up to 37% of CLL patients at some time during the course of their disease. A small proportion (10–15%) of patients may present with AIHA at diagnosis. AIHA can have a varied presentation, with patients developing signs of anemia, including weakness, lethargy, dyspnea on exertion, and dizziness over a period of months. Examination may reveal pallor, jaundice, hepatosplenomegaly, and lymphadenopathy. Hemolysis can cause mild to moderate indirect hyperbilirubinemia, elevated LDH levels, and hemoglobinuria. The direct antiglobulin Coombs test result is positive in up to 74% of patients with CLL, but not all patients develop hemolysis. Most of the antibodies produced are warm reactive, but patients can occasionally present with cold agglutination syndrome. The antibodies are mostly polyclonal and usually a product of normal B cells rather than the leukemic clone.

In contrast to the high frequency of AIHA in CLL, ITP or ITP and AIHA, or Evans syndrome, occurs less frequently in CLL. These events can occur throughout the entire course of CLL and are much more difficult to diagnose because of the absence of multiple implicating laboratory features as seen with AIHA. Given the small number of patients with AIHA, there are no data from controlled trials to guide the management of AIHA. Glucocorticoids have been used since the 1940s and are considered the first line of therapy. Most patients will respond to prednisone at a dose of 1 mg/kg for 10–14 days followed by a slow taper over 2–3 months, depending on the extent of hemolysis. ORRs of up to 90%, with 65% CRs, have been reported with the use of steroids. Unfortunately, approximately 60% of patients relapse when steroid therapy is stopped. Rituximab 375 mg/m^2 weekly for 4 weeks is often effective for steroid-resistant AIHA or ITP and if steroid withdrawal is not possible. Because of the long-term morbidity of prolonged steroid administration in CLL and data demonstrating benefit to concurrent steroids and rituximab for rapid withdrawal of corticosteroids in ITP, our group gives these two agents concurrently at diagnosis of ITP or AIHA unless contraindicated (e.g., hepatitis B). IVIG, the next line of treatment, induces responses in 40% of patients for both AIHA and ITP. Thrombopoietin agonists are effective for refractory ITP in CLL and could also be considered at this time. Cyclosporine A (CSA) at 5 mg/kg per day given in divided doses twice daily has been used for refractory AIHA and ITP of CLL. The dose should be adjusted to maintain a serum level of around 100–150 µg/dL. Other treatment modalities include splenectomy or splenic irradiation, alkylating agents, or therapy (FCR or FR directed at the disease if active). Treatment of the underlying CLL is generally required for long-term control of autoimmune cytopenias. However, our practice is to first control the autoimmune process with steroids or other therapies before considering treatment of the underlying CLL. Supportive therapy with periodic RBC transfusions is also important in the management of AIHA. Ibrutinib has also been shown to reduce the incidence of autoimmune complications in patients who initiate therapy for progressive disease and provides an exciting option for these patients. Unfortunately, ibrutinib has not been shown to be effective when treating active AIHA.

Pure RBC aplasia (PRCA) is a relatively rare T-cell–dependent complication associated with CLL, with an incidence as high as 6% having been reported. PRCA was first described by Dameshek and colleagues in 1967. It is characterized by a hypoproliferative anemia that can be detected even in early-stage CLL patients and is thought to be caused by the cytotoxic effects of suppressor T cells on erythroid progenitor cells. Increased numbers of cells coexpressing CD3, CD8, and CD57 have been shown to gradually accumulate in the BM of patients with PRCA. Abeloff and Waterbury described the first remission of PRCA with cyclophosphamide therapy in 1974, and Chikkappa and colleagues described the first case of response to CSA. Subsequent larger studies have shown a response rate as high as 63% with 300 mg/day of oral CSA. Mild reversible nephrotoxicity may warrant dose adjustment in some patients. Most patients exhibit a response by having reticulocytosis within the first 10–14 days of the initiation of therapy, but maximal response may occur on average after 10 weeks. Steroid therapy at a dose of 1 mg/kg per day of prednisone remains the first line of treatment. If a response is not obtained in 4 weeks, CSA should be added to the regimen. Other agents that have shown promising activity in treating PRCA include rituximab, IVIG, alemtuzumab, and antithymocyte globulin. Packed RBC transfusions are usually indicated in patients who are clinically symptomatic from severe anemia.

A number of other complications, most of which are autoimmune in nature, have been reported in patients with CLL. These complications include paraneoplastic pemphigus, angioedema caused by acquired C1-inhibitor deficiency, and nephrotic syndrome. As a result of autoimmune involvement of various organs, patients with CLL may have abnormal serum chemistry profiles and liver function tests.

FUTURE DIRECTIONS

Advances in the understanding of molecular events associated with CLL over the past 2 decades has resulted into new diagnostic tests that allow better assessment of initial prognosis and also treatment assignments. In addition, multiple new therapies have been identified, and progress is being made to extend remission duration, clarify mechanisms of resistance, develop stopping rules for therapies and improve the quality of life of CLL patients. In addition, medications and interventions to overcome complications that arise from CLL have also been introduced. Overall, the future for patients with CLL remains brighter based on such efforts and likely will continue to improve with additional laboratory and clinical research. In particular, the use of kinase inhibitors have transformed treatment approaches and the outcome of patients with CLL which will likely alter the natural history of the disease.

FINANCIAL SUPPORT

This work was supported by the National Cancer Institute P01 CA95426, R01 CA095241, the American Cancer Society, the Leukemia and Lymphoma Society, the Lymphoma Research Foundation and the D. Warren Brown Foundation.

SUGGESTED READINGS

Awan FT, Byrd JC: New strategies in chronic lymphocytic leukemia: shifting treatment paradigms. *Clin Cancer Res* 20:5869, 2014.

Awan FT, Hillmen P, Hellmann A, et al: A randomized, open-label, multi-centre, phase 2/3 study to evaluate the safety and efficacy of lumiliximab in combination with fludarabine, cyclophosphamide and rituximab versus fludarabine, cyclophosphamide and rituximab alone in subjects with relapsed chronic lymphocytic leukaemia. *Br J Haematol* 167:466–477, 2014.

Badoux XC, Keating MJ, Wang X, et al: Fludarabine, cyclophosphamide, and rituximab chemoimmunotherapy is highly effective treatment for relapsed patients with CLL. *Blood* 117:3016, 2011.

Badoux XC, Keating MJ, Wen S, et al: Lenalidomide as initial therapy of elderly patients with chronic lymphocytic leukemia. *Blood* 118:3489, 2011.

Burger JA, Tedeschi A, Barr PM, et al: Ibrutinib as initial therapy for patients with chronic lymphocytic leukemia. *N Engl J Med* 373(25):2425–2437, 2015.

Byrd JC, Brown JR, O'Brien S, et al: Ibrutinib versus ofatumumab in previously treated chronic lymphoid leukemia. *N Engl J Med* 371:213–223, 2014.

Byrd JC, Furman RR, Coutre SE, et al: Three-year follow-up of treatment-naïve and previously treated patients with CLL and SLL receiving single-agent ibrutinib. *Blood* 125:2497–2506, 2015.

Byrd JC, Furman RR, Coutre SE, et al: Targeting BTK with ibrutinib in relapsed chronic lymphocytic leukemia. *N Engl J Med* 369:32–42, 2013.

Chen CI, Bergsagel PL, Paul H, et al: Single-agent lenalidomide in the treatment of previously untreated chronic lymphocytic leukemia. *J Clin Oncol* 29:1175, 2011.

Crowther-Swanepoel D, Corre T, Lloyd A, et al: Inherited genetic susceptibility to monoclonal B-cell lymphocytosis. *Blood* 116:5957, 2010.

Döhner H, Stilgenbauer S, Benner A, et al: Genomic aberrations and survival in chronic lymphocytic leukemia. *N Engl J Med* 343(26):1910–1916, 2000.

Dreger P, Döhner H, Ritgen M, et al: German CLL Study Group: Allogeneic stem cell transplantation provides durable disease control in poor-risk chronic lymphocytic leukemia: long-term clinical and MRD results of the German CLL Study Group CLL3X trial. *Blood* 116:2438, 2010.

Eichhorst BF, Busch R, Stilgenbauer S, et al: German CLL Study Group (GCLLSG): First-line therapy with fludarabine compared with chlorambucil does not result in a major benefit for elderly patients with advanced chronic lymphocytic leukemia. *Blood* 114:3382, 2009.

Eichhorst BF, Fischer K, Fink AM, et al: German CLL Study Group (GCLLSG): Limited clinical relevance of imaging techniques in the follow-up of patients with advanced chronic lymphocytic leukemia: results of a meta-analysis. *Blood* 117:1817, 2011.

Fabbri M, Bottoni A, Shimizu M, et al: Association of a microRNA/TP53 feedback circuitry with pathogenesis and outcome of B-cell chronic lymphocytic leukemia. *JAMA* 305:59, 2011.

Fabbri G: Dalla-favera R. The molecular pathogenesis of chronic lymphocytic leukaemia. *Nat Rev Cancer* 16(3):145–162, 2016.

Fischer K, Cramer P, Busch R, et al: Bendamustine combined with rituximab in patients with relapsed and/or refractory chronic lymphocytic leukemia: A multicenter phase II trial of the German Chronic Lymphocytic Leukemia Study Group. *J Clin Oncol* 29:3559, 2011.

Goede V, Fischer K, Busch R, et al: Obinutuzumab plus chlorambucil in patients with CLL and coexisting conditions. *N Engl J Med* 370(12):1101–1110, 2014.

Hallek M, Cheson BD, Catovsky D, et al: International Workshop on Chronic Lymphocytic Leukemia: Guidelines for the diagnosis and treatment of chronic lymphocytic leukemia: a report from the International Workshop on Chronic Lymphocytic Leukemia updating the National Cancer Institute-Working Group 1996 guidelines. *Blood* 111:5446, 2008.

Hallek M, Fischer K, Fingerle-Rowson G, et al: International Group of Investigators; German Chronic Lymphocytic Leukaemia Study Group: Addition of rituximab to fludarabine and cyclophosphamide in patients with chronic lymphocytic leukaemia: a randomised, open-label, phase 3 trial. *Lancet* 376:1164, 2010.

Herishanu Y, Pérez-Galán P, Liu D, et al: The lymph node microenvironment promotes B-cell receptor signaling, NF-kappaB activation, and tumor proliferation in chronic lymphocytic leukemia. *Blood* 117:563, 2011.

Keating MJ, O'Brien S, Albitar M, et al: Early results of a chemoimmunotherapy regimen of fludarabine, cyclophosphamide, and rituximab as initial therapy for chronic lymphocytic leukemia. *J Clin Oncol* 23(18):4079–4088, 2005.

Kikushige Y, Ishikawa F, Miyamoto T, et al: Self-renewing hematopoietic stem cell is the primary target in pathogenesis of human chronic lymphocytic leukemia. *Cancer Cell* 20:246, 2011.

Knauf WU, Lissichkov T, Aldaoud A, et al: Phase III randomized study of bendamustine compared with chlorambucil in previously untreated patients with chronic lymphocytic leukemia. *J Clin Oncol* 27:4378, 2009.

O'Brien S, Furman RR, Coutre SE, et al: Ibrutinib as initial therapy for elderly patients with chronic lymphocytic leukaemia or small lymphocytic lymphoma: an open-label, multicentre, phase 1b/2 trial. *Lancet Oncol* 15:48–58, 2014.

Parikh SA, Strati P, Tsang M, et al: Should IGHV status and FISH testing be performed in all CLL patients at diagnosis? A systematic review and meta-analysis. *Blood* 127(14):1752–1760, 2016.

Puente XS, Pinyol M, Quesada V, et al: Whole-genome sequencing identifies recurrent mutations in chronic lymphocytic leukaemia. *Nature* 475:101, 2011.

Robak T, Dmoszynska A, Solal-Céligny P, et al: Rituximab plus fludarabine and cyclophosphamide prolongs progression-free survival compared with fludarabine and cyclophosphamide alone in previously treated chronic lymphocytic leukemia. *J Clin Oncol* 28:1756, 2010.

Rogers KA, Ruppert AS, Bingman A, et al: Incidence and description of autoimmune cytopenias during treatment with ibrutinib for chronic lymphocytic leukemia. *Leukemia* 30:346–350, 2016.

Shanafelt TD, Drake MT, Maurer MJ, et al: Vitamin D insufficiency and prognosis in chronic lymphocytic leukemia. *Blood* 117:1492, 2011.

Sorror ML, Storer BE, Sandmaier BM, et al: Five-year follow-up of patients with advanced chronic lymphocytic leukemia treated with allogeneic hematopoietic cell transplantation after nonmyeloablative conditioning. *J Clin Oncol* 26:4912, 2008.

Stilgenbauer S, Zenz T, Winkler D, et al: German Chronic Lymphocytic Leukemia Study; Subcutaneous alemtuzumab in fludarabine-refractory chronic lymphocytic leukemia: clinical results and prognostic marker analyses from the CLL2H study of the German Chronic Lymphocytic Leukemia Study Group. *J Clin Oncol* 27:3994, 2009.

Tam CS, Keating MJ: Chemoimmunotherapy of chronic lymphocytic leukemia. *Nat Rev Clin Oncol* 7:521, 2010.

Tam CS, O'Brien S, Wierda W, et al: Long-term results of the fludarabine, cyclophosphamide, and rituximab regimen as initial therapy of chronic lymphocytic leukemia. *Blood* 112:975, 2008.

Wierda WG, Kipps TJ, Mayer J, et al: Hx-CD20-406 Study Investigators: Ofatumumab as single-agent CD20 immunotherapy in fludarabine-refractory chronic lymphocytic leukemia. *J Clin Oncol* 28:1749, 2010.

Wierda WG, O'Brien S, Wang X, et al: Multivariable model for time to first treatment in patients with chronic lymphocytic leukemia. *J Clin Oncol* 29:4088, 2011.

Woyach JA, Ruppert AS, Heerema NA, et al: Chemoimmunotherapy with fludarabine and rituximab produces extended overall survival and progression-free survival in chronic lymphocytic leukemia: long-term follow-up of CALGB study 9712. *J Clin Oncol* 29:1349, 2011.

Woyach JA, Furman RR, Liu TM, et al: Resistance mechanisms for the Bruton's tyrosine kinase inhibitor ibrutinib. *N Engl J Med* 370:2286–2294, 2014.

Zenz T, Eichhorst B, Busch R, et al: TP53 mutation and survival in chronic lymphocytic leukemia. *J Clin Oncol* 28:4473, 2010.

Zenz T, Mertens D, Küppers R, et al: From pathogenesis to treatment of chronic lymphocytic leukemia. *Nat Rev Cancer* 10:37, 2010.

INTRODUCTION

Hairy cell leukemia (HCL) is one of the diseases exemplifying the importance of the application of appropriate diagnostic techniques and treatment strategies to obtain the best treatment outcomes for the individual patient.[1] The disease was first described by Bouroncle and colleagues in 1958. The term *hairy cell leukemia* was first used to describe the disorder by Schreck and Donnelly in 1966 and is derived from the observation of hair-like projections from mononuclear cells giving rise to a frayed cell surface appearance.

The evolution of therapeutic strategies in patients with HCL over the past 25 years has led to a significant change in the natural history of the disease. Using the currently available drugs, the majority of patients with this disease achieve complete response (CR), and the published survival curves from several large series are similar to those for appropriate age-matched individuals without the disease. At the same time, recent research efforts have led to a better understanding of the molecular mechanisms responsible for the disease pathogenesis. Several studies, using modern techniques, have demonstrated the persistence of minimal residual disease (MRD) after therapy with nucleoside analogs in the majority of patients without consensus on the significance of such MRD. The role of monoclonal antibodies, naked or conjugated with toxins, in the management of HCL, as well as their ability to eradicate MRD, is under investigation. The possibility of such strategies of chemoimmunotherapy leading to further improvements in the outcome of patients with HCL needs to be further investigated.

EPIDEMIOLOGY

HCL is an uncommon lymphoid malignancy, accounting for only 2% of lymphoid leukemias, with approximately 600 to 800 new patients diagnosed each year in the United States.[1] The disease is more common in whites and occurs more frequently in men than women by a ratio of 4 : 1.[1] The median age at diagnosis is reported by most studies to be 50 to 59 years. However, it is possible that the disease is underreported in the older population. The Swedish Cancer Registry has maintained records on the incidence of the disease for several decades and has shown a stable incidence since the 1980s. It reports the median age at diagnosis of 62 years, suggesting less rigid diagnostic efforts in older patients.

HCL has been diagnosed in patients aged in their 20s and 30s but is exceptionally rare in children. Using data from the 17 population-based cancer registry areas in the United States, the National Cancer Institute's Surveillance Epidemiology and End Results program reported that the incidence of the disease was stable in the decades between 1978 and 2004 with a rapid rise in age-specific incidence ratios until approximately age 40 years and then at a slower pace beyond that age.

ETIOLOGY AND CELL OF ORIGIN

Several reports have suggested an association between development of HCL and exposure to benzene, organophosphorus insecticides, and other solvents. However, such association has not been confirmed by other reports. Exposure to radiation, wood dust, or agricultural chemicals, and a previous history of infectious mononucleosis have also been suggested as predisposing factors, but a direct, causal association has not been established with any of these or other factors.

Morphologically and phenotypically, the cells in HCL have no resemblance to any of the normal stages of B-cell development and maturation; past studies have debated the cell of origin. Initially, because of morphologic and functional similarities between hairy cells and cells of the monocyte/macrophage system, HCL tumor cells were thought to be derived from a cell transformed from the reticuloendothelium. Korsmeyer demonstrated the rearrangement of the B-cell receptor (BCR) immunoglobulin genes in HCL, demonstrating for the first time the B-cell origin of the disease. Recently, several studies have increased our understanding of the cell of origin in HCL allowing for a better description of pathogenic mechanisms responsible for its development.[2]

In lymphoid cells, the analysis of the immunoglobulin variable region genes provides a tool for the delineation of the clonal history of cells at which lymphoid neoplasms originate, identifying whether antigen encountered by a normal mature B cell has resulted in somatic mutation (Fig. 78.1). This process occurs within the germinal centers (GCs) of lymph tissues and may be associated with isotype switching. The enzyme activation–induced cytidine deaminase (AICD) is critical for both processes. Tumor cells from various B-cell malignancies are arrested at a number of stages along normal B-cell differentiation, conserving the immunogenetic characteristics of the stage-specific cell. The analysis of immunoglobulin variable gene regions can provide information about whether the cell of origin has undergone somatic mutation and isotype switching. Several reports have clearly demonstrated that in more than 85% of patients with HCL, the tumor cells express switched immunoglobulin isotypes, and their rearranged variable region genes have undergone somatic mutations.[3] Furthermore, HCL cells express AICD, the enzyme that is critical for both processes.[3] This suggests that the cell of origin in the majority of HCL cases has transited through the GCs of peripheral lymphoid tissue having undergone the GC reaction.[2] Of interest, in about 40% of cases of HCL, the leukemia cells express multiple immunoglobulin heavy chain isotypes, with dominance of immunoglobulin G3 (IgG3) but only a single light chain, suggesting that clonally related multiple isotypes coexist in single hairy cells. Therefore, this subset of the disease may be arrested at a point after isotype switching and before exit from the GC. However, other lines of evidence suggest a post-GC origin.[2]

Arons and colleagues have provided evidence that in the majority of patients with classic HCL (83% of 102 cases), the cell of origin is post-GC with a mutated immunoglobulin heavy chain variable region.[4] This is contrasted with historic data for patients with chronic lymphocytic leukemia, in which case, about half of the time the cell of origin is unmutated. They also reported higher usage of certain immunoglobulin gene families and a difference in mutational frequency among these genes.[4] Furthermore, by demonstrating that the mutations fulfilled predefined characteristics of a canonic and nonrandom event, Arons and colleagues provided further evidence suggestive of an antigen-driven process.

The post-GC origin of HCL is supported by gene expression profiling studies comparing HCL cells with cells from other lymphoid neoplasms, as well as with naive and memory B cells.[5] HCL patients displayed a homogeneous pattern of gene expression that was clearly distinct from other B-cell lymphomas and was related to post-GC

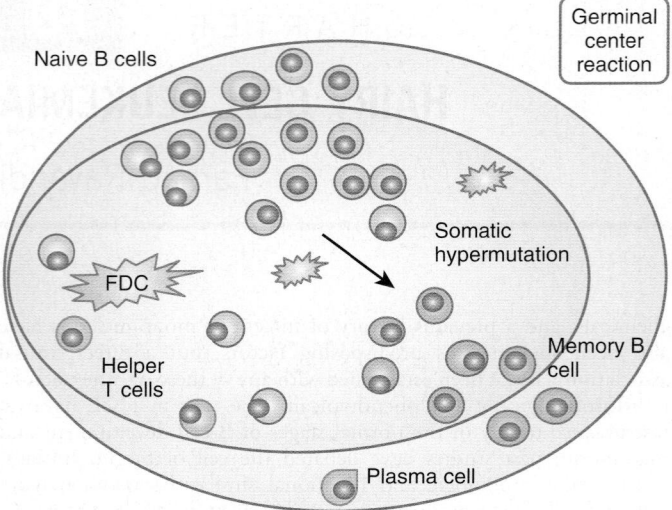

Fig. 78.1 GERMINAL CENTER REACTION. The process of somatic hypermutation and isotypic switch in the germinal center.

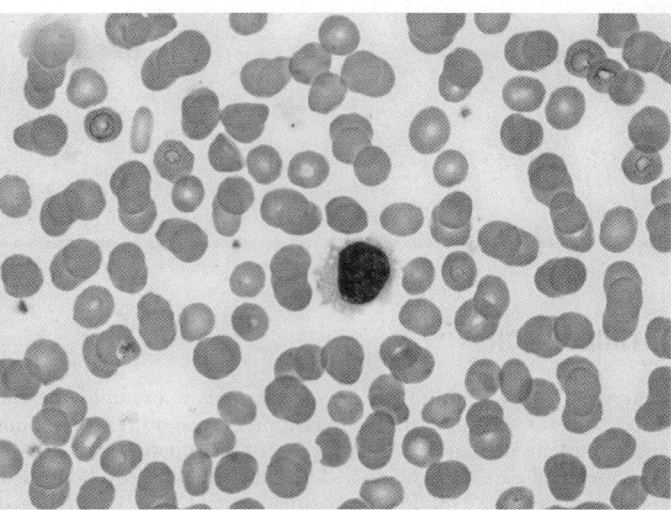

Fig. 78.2 PHOTOMICROGRAPH OF A HAIRY CELL IN THE PERIPHERAL BLOOD. *(Provided by Jeffrey Jorgensen, Department of Hematopathology, UTMDACC.)*

memory B cells.[5] Other investigators have reported this remarkably stable genome in HCL. Furthermore, when compared with memory B cells, HCL cells had a remarkable conservation of proliferation, apoptosis, and DNA metabolism programs but differed significantly in the expression of genes controlling cell adhesion and response to chemokines.[5] Against the hypothesis of a memory B-cell origin is the lack of expression by hairy cells of the memory B-cell marker, CD27. However, CD27-negative memory B cells have been described in humans, and hairy cells may lose this marker as a result of the neoplastic transformation.

As lymph node involvement in HCL is uncommon, the post-GC cell of origin is likely to originate from the spleen or the bone marrow, sites involved by the disease almost invariably. A number of reports have suggested that HCL may originate from the B cells of the splenic marginal zone (SMZ). Normal SMZ B cells are mainly memory B cells. Vanhentenrijk and colleagues, using comparative expressed sequence hybridization studies, demonstrated that hairy cells had an expression profile consistent with a splenic expression signature that most likely reflected the expression profile of spleen-specific components, such as the sinusoidal lining cells from the red pulp and the marginal zone B cells from the white pulp.

Recently, Tiacci and colleagues reported the presence of *BRAF* V600E mutations in each of 47 patients with HCL and no mutations in the cells from patients with 195 peripheral B-cell lymphomas or leukemias.[6] Using whole-genome sequencing they identified, in an index patient, five missense somatic clonal mutations, including a heterozygous mutation in *BRAF* that resulted in a BRAF V600E variant protein.[6] Since *BRAF* V600F is known to be oncogenic in other tumors, Tiacci and colleagues focused on this mutation and analyzed the subsequent 46 cases as well as the patients with other lymphomas. They also demonstrated expression of phosphorylated MEK and extracellular signal-related kinase (ERK), showing constitutive activation of the RAF-MEK-ERK mitogen-activated protein kinase pathway in HCL.[6] This discovery has potential significance in the understanding of the pathogenic mechanisms of HCL; its applications in diagnosis and treatment of this disease are likely to increase with further research.

CLINICAL PRESENTATION AND DIAGNOSIS

Typically, the majority of patients present with pancytopenia and splenomegaly with the associated fatigue, left upper quadrant abdominal pain, fever and infections, and/or bleeding problems (Table 78.1). Common presenting features include significant anemia, seen in up to 85% of patients, thrombocytopenia in about 60% to

TABLE 78.1	Initial Workup of a Patient With Suspected Hairy Cell Leukemia

History and physical examination
Complete blood count with differential counts
Review of peripheral blood smear
Serum chemistries
Bone marrow aspirate and biopsy with immunostains
Immunophenotyping by flow cytometry of peripheral blood and bone marrow
? Serum soluble markers such as CD25 and CD22
? Immune status analysis with CD4/CD8 lymphocyte subsets
Appropriate imaging, if febrile, to rule out infections

80%, and leukopenia in 60% of patients; these cytopenias can be severe and life-threatening and are likely multifactorial, with hypersplenism and marrow infiltration being the more important contributors. Monocytopenia is a characteristic finding. Circulating hairy cells are typically scant in most patients and frequently absent. Hairy cells are small- and medium-sized lymphoid cells with an oval or indented (bean-shaped) nucleus with homogeneous chromatin that is less clumped than normal B cells (Fig. 78.2).[1] Nucleoli are typically absent or inconspicuous and the cytoplasm abundant and pale blue in color with circumferential "hairy" projections. Electron micrographs of hairy cells clearly demonstrate their distinctive and complex surface features with multiple surface folds and clusters of short microvilli, creating an appearance unique to hairy cells (Fig. 78.3).

Bone marrow involvement can be interstitial or patchy with the infiltrate characterized by widely spaced nuclei because of the abundant cytoplasm, giving rise to the commonly described "fried egg" appearance (Fig. 78.4).[1] Occasionally, an increase in the bone marrow reticulin fibrosis, as well as significant loss of the hematopoietic elements, leads to a "dry tap." Bone marrow fibrosis is caused by the production and assembly of a fibronectin matrix by hairy cells and the deposition of fine reticulin fibers (mainly composed of type III collagen fibrils) by fibroblasts.[2] Hairy cells express isoenzyme 5 of acid phosphatase, which imparts resistance to treatment with tartaric acid, with virtually all cases being positive for tartrate-resistant acid phosphatase (TRAP) (Fig. 78.5). Combined expression of DBA44 and TRAP by immunohistochemical analysis is highly specific and useful for arriving at the diagnosis. More recently, immunostaining for annexin A1 (ANAX1) has been reported to be very specific for HCL.[7] ANAX1 can be used to distinguish HCL from its variant form and from other lymphoid neoplasms such as SMZ lymphoma

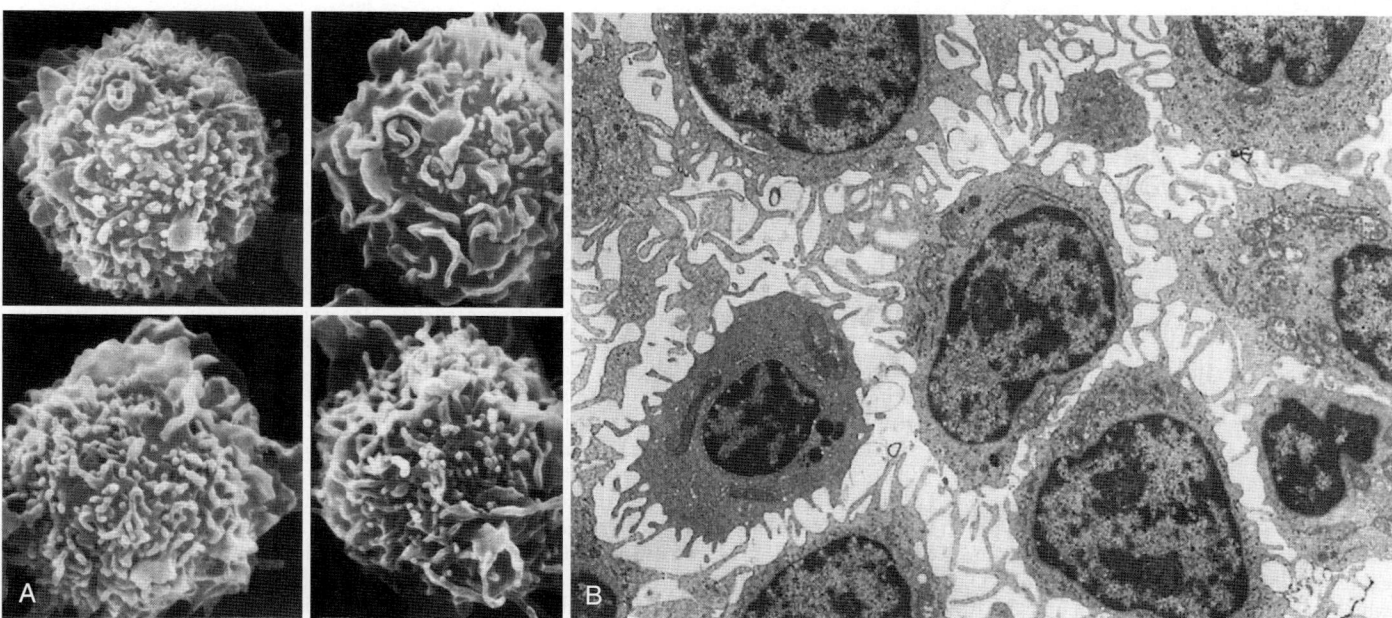

Fig. 78.3 ELECTRON MICROGRAPH OF HAIRY CELLS. (A) Ruffles and folds on the surface. (B) Hair-like projections from the cytoplasm. *(Used with permission from Aaron Polliack, Emeritus Professor of Hematology, Hadassah University Hospital, Hebrew University Medical School, Jerusalem, Israel.)*

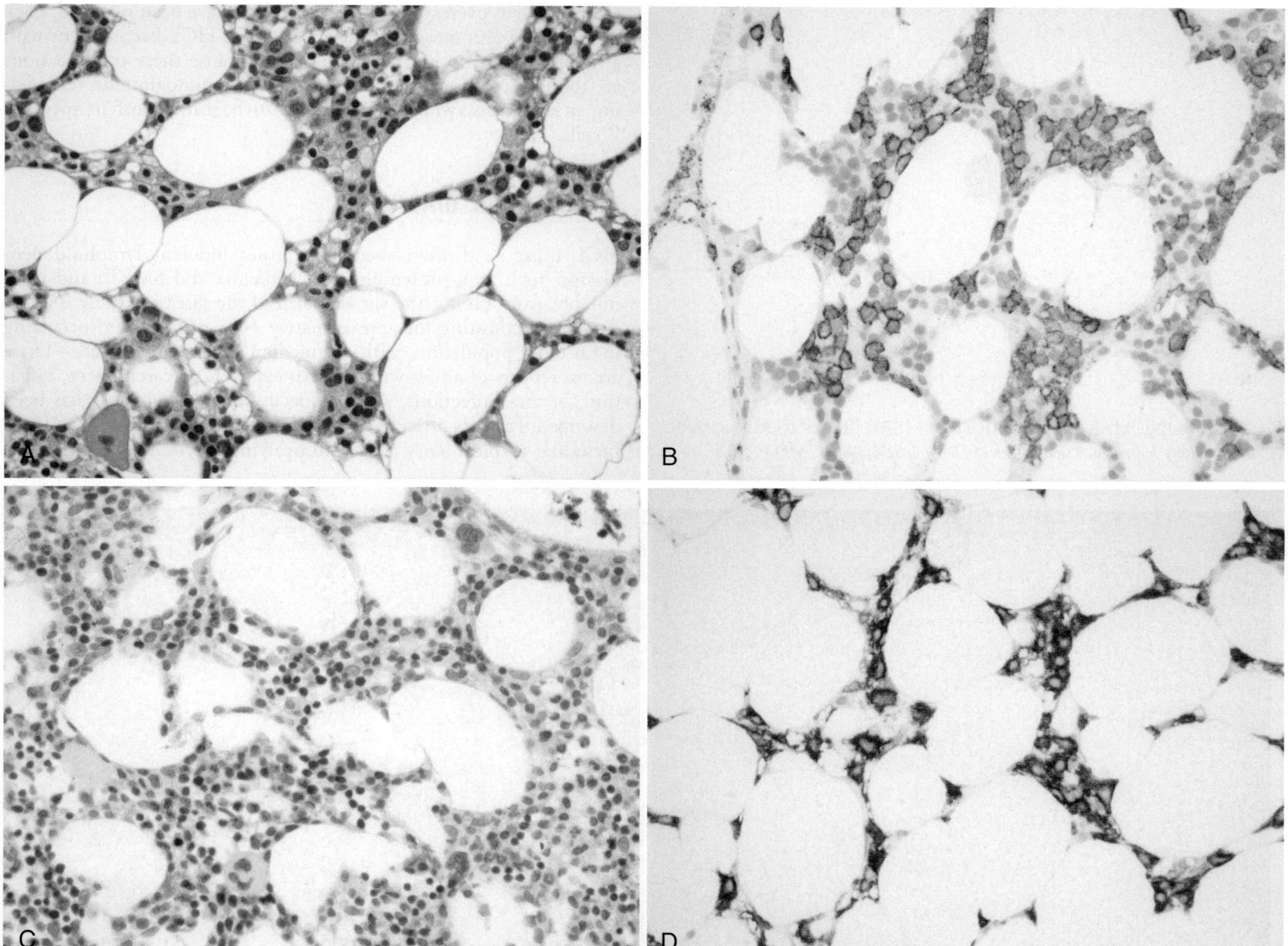

Fig. 78.4 BONE MARROW FINDINGS IN HAIRY CELL LEUKEMIA. (A) Bone marrow biopsy (Hematoxylin & eosin stain ×400). (B) Bone marrow biopsy (CD20 stain ×400). (C) Bone marrow biopsy (Annexin A1 stain ×400). (D) Bone marrow biopsy (CD11c stain ×400). *(Provided by Jeffrey Jorgensen, Department of Hematopathology, UTMDACC.)*

(SMZL).[1,7] Cyclin D1 (encoded by *CCND1* gene) is frequently expressed, but this is not secondary to translocation involving *CCND1*, unlike mantle cell lymphoma. In a proportion of patients, the bone marrow is hypocellular with the loss of hematopoietic elements, which can result in an erroneous diagnosis of aplastic anemia. Immunostaining for antigens such as CD20 may be helpful to detect the abnormal B-cell infiltrate, hence prompting more specific stains for HCL.[1]

HCL cells have a characteristic immunophenotype with flow cytometry being an important element of diagnostic evaluation in this disease (see Table 78.1). Hairy cells strongly express CD45 and gate within the monocytic region when analyzed by CD45 versus side scatter, which is typically devoid of monocytes. They exhibit a mature B-cell phenotype and commonly express one or more heavy chains and monotypic light chains (κ and λ light chains in equal numbers of patients). They express B-cell associated antigens CD19, CD20, CD22, FMC7, and CD79b but typically lack CD5, CD10 (positive in about 10%), and CD23 (positive in about 20%) expression. No single marker is specific for distinguishing HCL from other B-cell neoplasms; however, the antigens CD11c, CD103, CD123, as well as the interleukin (IL)-2 receptor α-subunit (CD25), are typically expressed in HCL. Bright expression of CD22 and CD20 is also seen, which can be important therapeutically. Among the patients evaluated in one study, CD52 was also universally expressed.

Splenic enlargement is present in the majority of patients and can be massive in about 20% of cases. Splenic involvement is characterized by diffuse infiltration of the red pulp cords and sinuses, with atrophy and replacement of white pulp. Blood-filled sinuses lined by hairy cells (often referred to as *pseudosinuses* or *red blood lakes*) are often a prominent but not pathognomonic finding (Fig. 78.6).[1] Significant lymphadenopathy is uncommon and present only in the advanced stages of the disease. When involved, the lymph node enlargement is largely confined to the abdominal and retroperitoneal nodes. The infiltrates are distributed in the interfollicular and paracortical areas of the nodes and may extend through the capsule to the surrounding adipose tissue. Hepatomegaly is much less frequent, occurring in up to a third of patients. However, the liver is almost always involved with a mononuclear cell infiltrate in the sinusoids, portal areas, or both. Unusual sites of disease involvement have been reported, including mediastinal and paravertebral masses, skeletal lytic lesions, pleural effusions and ascites, as well as involvement of skin, eye, the central nervous system, and the gastrointestinal tract. Other notable clinical features include a predisposition to infections and an uncommon association with autoimmune disorders such as polyarteritis nodosa, vasculitis, and rheumatoid arthritis.

Several cytogenetic abnormalities have been reported in HCL but no single abnormality is present consistently. Few cytogenetic studies have been reported because of the rarity of the disease, difficulty in obtaining marrow samples, and low responsiveness of hairy cells to common mitogens. In the reported series, chromosomes 1, 2, 5, 6, 11, 14, 19, and 20 are most frequently involved, with chromosome 5 and 14 abnormalities predominating. Deletions and mutations of p53, as well as overexpression of cyclin D1, have been reported. Lack of reciprocal chromosomal translocations in HCL is consistent with a memory B-cell origin of the disease, because these translocations are thought to arise from mistakes in the immunoglobulin remodeling mechanisms, which are believed to be turned off in memory B cells.[2]

DIFFERENTIAL DIAGNOSIS

HCL must be distinguished from other indolent lymphoid neoplasms, such as B-prolymphocytic leukemia and SMZL, and most notably, from HCLv, the variant form of the disease. HCLv is a rare disorder accounting for approximately 10% of cases and occurring in an older population, with the median age being 71 years.[8] There are no reports of an association with exposure to carcinogens, radiation, or viral infections, and no specific underlying cause has been described. Patients often have an elevated WBC count ($>10 \times 10^9$/L) including atypical hairy cells with prolymphocytic features and lack

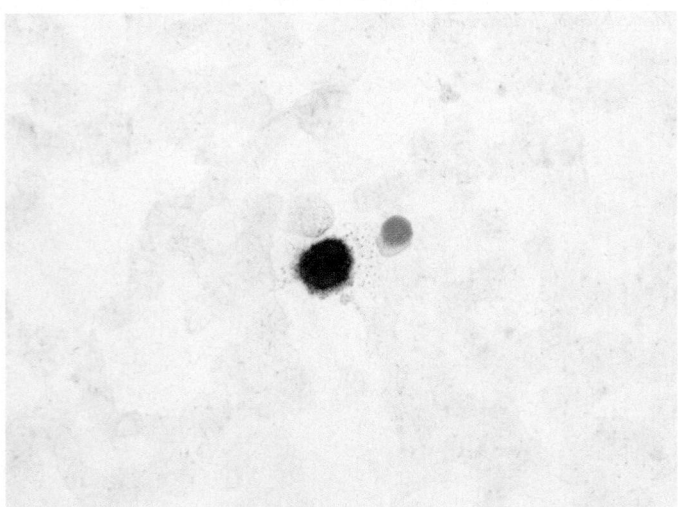

Fig. 78.5 BONE MARROW ASPIRATE SMEAR (TRAP STAIN ×1000). *(Courtesy Jeffrey Jorgensen, Department of Hematopathology, UTMDACC.)*

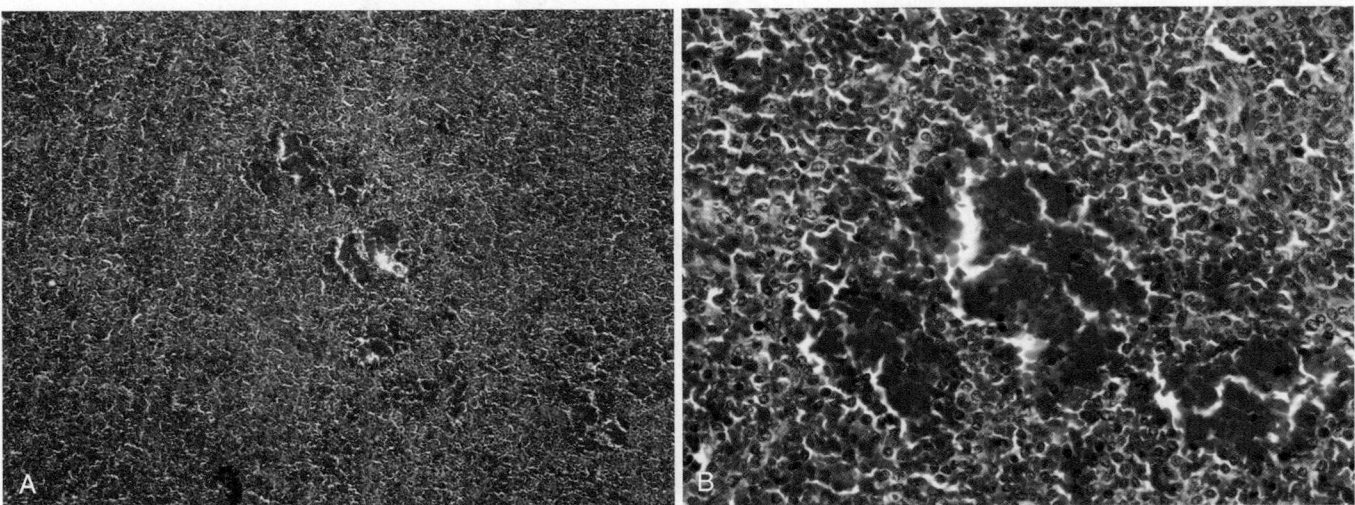

Fig. 78.6 PATHOLOGIC FINDINGS IN THE SPLEEN. (A) Hematoxylin and eosin (H&E) stain (×100). (B) H&E stain (×400). *(Provided by Roberto Miranda, Department of Hematopathology, UTMDACC.)*

TABLE 78.2	Immunophenotype of Hairy Cell Leukemia and Other Indolent Lymphoid Neoplasms								
Disease	sIg	CD5	CD10	CD11c	CD20	CD22	CD23	CD25	CD103
HCL	+/−	−/+	−	++	+	+	−/+	+	++
CLL	+/−	++	−	−/+	+/−	−/+	++	−/+	−
B-PLL	++	+	−	−/+	+/−	+	+/−	−	−
HCLv	+/−	−	−	++	+	+	−	−	−/+
MCL	+	++	−	−	+	+	−/+	−	−
SMZL	+	−/+	−/+	+	+	+/−	−/+	−	−
FL	+	−	+	−	++	+	−/+	−	−

B-PLL, B-prolymphocytic leukemia; CLL, chronic lymphocytic leukemia; FL, follicular lymphoma; HCLv, variant form of hairy cell leukemia; MCL, mantle cell lymphoma; sIg, surface immunoglobulin; SMZL, splenic marginal zone lymphoma.

monocytopenia. Splenomegaly and cytopenias are present in the majority of patients, and the pattern of bone marrow and splenic involvement is similar to HCL and different from prolymphocytic leukemia and SMZL. The immunophenotypic expression of various lymphoid markers is also different in these disorders, with HCLv lacking CD25 expression, further assisting diagnosis (Table 78.2). Another aid in distinguishing HCL from HCLv is CD123 expression, which is positive in the former and negative in the latter. A number of chromosomal abnormalities, including translocations, have been reported in a few cases. Although HCLv has some similarities to HCL, the two conditions differ in a number of features, most notably being HCLv's lack of responsiveness to classic HCL therapies. As such, it is important to distinguish the two and consider them as separate diseases. HCL and HCLv have different immunoglobulin heavy (IGH) chain gene repertoires and somatic hypermutation patterns.[4] A recent report also suggested that high expression levels of AICD can distinguish HCL from HCLv, as well as from SMZL. However, the same group was unable to find distinct cytogenetic events to distinguish HCL from its variant, using high-resolution genomic profiling. Most recently, *BRAF* V600F mutations have been shown to occur exclusively in HCL samples and not in those from patients with HCLv and SMZL.

SMZL (previously referred to as *splenic lymphoma with villous lymphocytes [SLVL]*) exhibits some of the clinical and morphologic features of HCL but typically has a more prominent peripheral blood involvement, lacks TRAP expression, and has a different immunophenotype, including absence of expression of CD25 and CD103. HCL should be distinguished from other indolent lymphoid neoplasms such as chronic lymphocytic leukemia, prolymphocytic leukemia, and follicular lymphomas, but this distinction is typically easily made using the characteristic morphologic and immunotypic findings characteristic of these disorders (see Table 78.2). Other disorders that should be included in the differential diagnosis include aplastic anemia, primary myelofibrosis, and systemic mast cell disorders.

TREATMENT

Indications for Therapy

HCL has an indolent course, with some patients surviving many years without receiving therapy and others not requiring further therapy despite persistence of residual morphologic evidence of the disease after the initial treatment.[9] Therefore a watch-and-wait strategy may be appropriate in the initial management of patients with limited or no manifestations of the disease. Disease progression that necessitates therapy is commonly evident by the development of progressive cytopenias and their associated complications, such as infections, bleeding, and progressive fatigue. No specific criteria for therapy have been established, but generally treatment is indicated when the patient has significant cytopenias, symptomatic organomegaly or adenopathy, infections, or constitutional symptoms such as fever, night sweats, or fatigue. Typical blood counts warranting therapy

include an absolute neutrophil count $<1.0 \times 10^9/L$, a platelet count $<100 \times 10^9/L$, and/or a hemoglobin <12.0 g/dL.

Historic Aspects of Therapy

Progress in the treatment of patients with HCL over the last 25 years has been significant, with survival curves now approaching those of age-matched cohorts without the disease. Before the introduction of interferon (IFN)-α, splenectomy was used effectively to treat patients with HCL. Although splenectomy does not result in morphologic remissions in the bone marrow, the peripheral blood counts are normalized in up to 70% of patients. Progression of disease can be expected in about 45% within 5 years. Furthermore, there is an associated morbidity and mortality with the procedure. As such, splenectomy is no longer performed in this disease except in rare, selected patients.

The first report of effective treatment of HCL with IFN-α described several patients with progressive disease who received daily doses of 3 million units. Three patients achieved CR with the other four having partial responses (PR). The activity of IFN-α in HCL was further confirmed by several large trials reporting CR rates of 4% to 30% and PR rates of 43% to 86%. Even in patients achieving a CR, careful morphologic examination of the bone marrow revealed residual hairy cells. With further follow up of patients treated with IFN-α, it is clear that a significant proportion will relapse and require further therapy. However, the same authors reported that a number of patients remaining alive after a 10-year follow up had not required further therapy with interferon. The median failure-free survival reported by these and other investigators ranges from 6 to 25 months. A number of predictors of outcome have been evaluated, with expression of CD5 reported as a predictor of poor response.

The precise mechanism of action of IFN-α in HCL is unknown and may be related to the reduced production of a number of cytokines such as granulocyte colony-stimulating factor, granulocyte-macrophage colony-stimulating factor, IL-3, and IL-6. Others have demonstrated that IFN-α can mediate apoptosis of hairy cells through the effects of tumor necrosis factor-α.

Treatment with IFN-α is associated with significant toxicity including flu-like symptoms, anorexia, fatigue, nausea and vomiting, diarrhea, skin rash, peripheral neuropathy, and central nervous system dysfunction (such as depression and memory loss). This and the introduction of nucleoside analogs that are generally more effective in achieving responses has led to the use of interferon being limited to rare cases and special circumstances.

Purine Nucleoside Analogs

Although there are no specific guidelines for the treatment of HCL, monotherapy with cladribine or pentostatin is the current established standard. Furthermore, despite the lack of a comparative study, a substantial number of data suggest that both drugs are equally effective in terms of response rate and durability.[10] The use of nucleoside

TABLE 78.3	Selected Published Reports of Cladribine Therapy for Hairy Cell Leukemia			
Reference	Evaluable Patients (n)	CR (%)	PR (%)	OR (%)
Intravenous Daily Administration (Continuous or Pulsed)				
Saven[15]	349	91	7	98
Goodman[16]	207	95	5	100
Tallman	50	80	18	98
Chadha[17]	85	79	21	100
Hoffman	49	76	24	100
Seymore[18]	46	78	11	89
Dearden	45	84	16	100
Juliusson	16	75	0	75
Zinzani[a]	21	81	19	100
Jehn	44	98	2	100
Robak[b,13]	132	76	19	95
Intravenous Weekly Administration				
Lauria	30	73	27	100
Zinzani[a]	16	81	19	100
Robak[b,13]	57	72	19	91
Subcutaneous Administration				
Juliusson[14]	73	81	13	94
Forconi[19]	58	72	19	91

[a]Reports from the same publication.
[b]Numbers reported for the two arms of a randomized study.
CR, Complete response; OR, overall response; PR, partial response.

TABLE 78.4	Alternative Dose and Schedules of Cladribine Therapy Reported in the Literature		
Study	Dosing	Route of Administration	Responses
Saven[15]	0.1 mg/kg/day × 7 days	Continuous IV infusion	CR: 91%; PR: 7%
Juliusson[14]	3.4 mg/m²/day × 7 days	Subcutaneous injection	CR: 75% after 1 cycle, 85% after 2 cycles
Robak[13]	0.12 mg/kg/day × 5 days	2-hour IV bolus	CR: 76%; PR: 19%
Robak[13]	0.12 mg/kg/week × 6 weeks	2 hour IV bolus	CR: 72%; PR: 19%
Chacko	0.15 mg/kg/week × 6 weeks	3 hour IV infusion	CR: 100%
Lauria[12]	0.15 mg/kg/week × 6 weeks	2 hour IV bolus	CR: 76%; PR: 24%
Von Rohr	0.14 mg/kg/day × 5 days	Subcutaneous injection	CR: 76%; PR: 21%

CR, Complete response; IV, intravenous; PR, partial response.

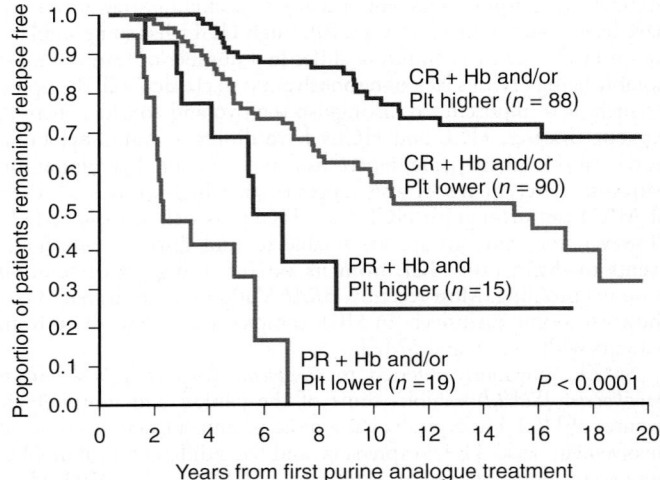

Fig. 78.7 LONG-TERM FOLLOW UP OF PATIENTS TREATED WITH NUCLEOSIDE ANALOG MONOTHERAPY. Excellent outcome for the majority, and significantly better relapse-free survival for patients achieving complete (CR) versus partial response (PR) with initial therapy. *(Else M, Dearden CE, Matutes E, et al: Long-term follow-up of 233 patients with hairy cell leukaemia, treated initially with pentostatin or cladribine, at a median of 16 years from diagnosis. Br J Haematol 145:733, 2009.)*

analogs in treating lymphoid neoplasms can be traced back to the observation that children with the deficiency of the enzyme adenine deaminase (ADA) developed severe combined immunodeficiency. The accumulation of the triphosphorylated form of deoxyadenosine (dependent on the action of the enzyme deoxycitidine kinase [DCK]) is thought to be responsible for the lack of lymphocyte development. Similarly, after treatment with purine nucleoside analogs, the accumulation of deoxyadenosine triphosphate results in DNA strand breaks, inhibition of DNA repair, and apoptosis preferentially in lymphoid cells, rich in DCK and low in 5′ nucleotidase (the enzyme responsible for degrading deoxyadenosine monophosphate).

Cladribine is a purine nucleoside analog resistant to deamination by ADA. It accumulates in lymphocytes rich in DCK and inhibits ribonucleotide reductase, impairing DNA synthesis and repair. Cladribine has been very effective for the initial therapy of HCL, with overall response rates ranging from 75% to 100% after a single course of the drug (Table 78.3). Piro and colleagues first reported 12 patients with HCL who received cladribine 0.1 mg/kg per day by intravenous continuous infusion for 7 days.[11] Eleven patients achieved CR, and one had PR.[11] Since then, other dose, routes of administration, and schedules of the drug have been used effectively (see Table 78.3 and Table 78.4). Weekly administration was evaluated in severely neutropenic patients in a pilot study in an effort to produce a less toxic strategy.[12] The authors reported a 73% CR rate, with an overall response rate of 100%. However, only 16% developed severe neutropenia and 8% infections.[12] In a more recent report, 132 patients with untreated HCL were randomized to receive cladribine either on 5 consecutive days or a novel schedule of six weekly doses.[13] The response rates, overall response rates, progression-free, overall survival, and incidence of grade 3 and 4 infections were the same in the two arms.[13] The subcutaneous route was also evaluated after the initial demonstration that similar plasma levels to those seen with the intravenous route can be achieved subcutaneously. Juliusson and colleagues treated 73 patients with cladribine administered as a subcutaneous daily injection for 7 days and reported a CR rate of 75% after one course and 81% after two courses.[14]

Despite the very high response rate to cladribine, responses are not universal and a significant proportion of patients relapse. Saven and colleagues reported the long-term outcome of 358 patients with HCL who were followed for a median of 52 months.[15] Of these patients, 26% relapsed after a median of 29 months.[15] The same group reported on 209 patients treated with cladribine with a follow-up period of at least 7 years.[16] Although the overall response rate was 100%, 76 (37%) patients relapsed after their first course of cladribine with a median time to relapse of 42 months.[16] Notably, the time to treatment failure curve did not show a plateau, indicating that the treatment is probably not "curative."[16] Outcome of patients achieving CR with their initial therapy is better than those achieving PR (Fig. 78.7). More recent publications have confirmed the high response rate of patients with HCL treated with cladribine and have provided long-term follow-up data.[17] Jehn and colleagues described a 12-year follow up of 44 patients (including 11 with prior therapy before receiving cladribine) who received cladribine at the originally reported dose and schedule. The CR rate was 98%, and with a median follow up of 8.5 years (range 0.1–12.2), 17 patients had relapsed. Eight of nine patients retreated with cladribine responded again. The overall survival at 12 years was 79%. Zinzani and colleagues reported the long-term outcome of 37 patients treated with one of two regimens of cladribine. Twenty-one patients received cladribine by a 2-hour infusion for 5 days, whereas 16 patients were treated with a once-weekly schedule for 5 weeks. A CR rate of 81% with an overall response rate of 100% was reported, with no difference between the two schedules. After a median follow up of 122 months (range 54–156), the overall relapse rate was about 30% for both groups. The projected 13-year overall and relapse-free survival rates were 96% and 52%, respectively. Investigators at Northwestern University treated 86 consecutive patients with cladribine and reported a CR rate of 79%, as well as a PR rate of 21%.[17] The progression-free survival after 12 years was 54%. After a median follow up of 9.7 years (range 0.3–13.8), 31 patients (36%) relapsed.[17] Of these, 23 were treated with a second course of cladribine; 12 (52%) achieved CR, and 7 (30%) achieved PR. The overall survival after 12 years was 87%.[17] The authors suggested that the lower CR rate in this study was caused by their more stringent criteria for response, which included a requirement for resolution of splenomegaly and lymphadenopathy by computed tomography scan as criteria for CR.[17]

Similar excellent responses have been achieved using pentostatin (Table 78.5). Overall CR rates of 44% to 89% have been reported with pentostatin administered intravenously at a dose of 2–4 mg/m^2 every 2 weeks. Spiers and colleagues were the first to report that a nucleoside analog (pentostatin) was capable of producing CRs in patients with HCL. The activity of pentostatin in HCL was confirmed in a number of larger studies by several investigators. Grever and colleagues conducted a large, randomized clinical trial comparing pentostatin with IFN-α in patients with previously untreated HCL.[20] Patients were randomized to receive either IFN-α 3 million units subcutaneously three times per week or pentostatin 4 mg/m^2 intravenously every 2 weeks.[20] Patients who did not respond to initial treatment were crossed over. Confirmed complete and overall response rates were reported for 76% and 79% of patients treated with pentostatin, respectively, as compared with 11% and 38% of those treated with IFN-α.[20] Response rates were significantly higher ($p < .0001$), and relapse-free survival was significantly longer with pentostatin than with interferon ($p < .0001$).[20] Furthermore, patients who were initially assigned to receive interferon were frequently crossed over to pentostatin therapy, achieving a CR rate of 66%. In a follow-up report, Flinn and colleagues described the long-term outcome of 241 patients who were treated with pentostatin either as initial therapy or after failure of IFN-α.[21] The 5- and 10-year event-free survival rates were 85% and 67% respectively (Fig. 78.8). Other investigators have reported long-term follow-up data on patients treated with pentostatin. Maloisel and colleagues reported outcome of 230 evaluable patients with HCL treated with pentostatin, including 84 with pentostatin as the initial agent. They reported a CR rate of

79%, with an overall response rate of 96%. With a median follow up of 63.5 months, 34 (15%) of 220 responding patients had relapsed. The estimated 5- and 10-year disease-free survival was 88% and 69%, respectively, and the estimated 5-year overall survival was 89%.

There are no prospective trials comparing the efficacy and durability of response between cladribine and pentostatin. Dearden and colleagues examined the outcome of the patients with the two agents at their institution and reported that 82% of 165 patients treated with pentostatin achieved a CR compared with 84% of 45 patients treated with cladribine. Relapse rates were 24% with pentostatin and 29% with cladribine after median follow up of 71 and 45 months, respectively. These relapse rates suggest a longer remission duration with pentostatin. However, with further follow up, there appears to be no difference between the two agents with regard to disease-free survival (Fig. 78.9A). Further follow-up data of these cohorts of patients have been reported.[10] With a median follow up of 16 years, there was no significant difference in the outcome of the patients treated with the two drugs. After relapse or nonresponse, patients could be successfully retreated with pentostatin or cladribine but

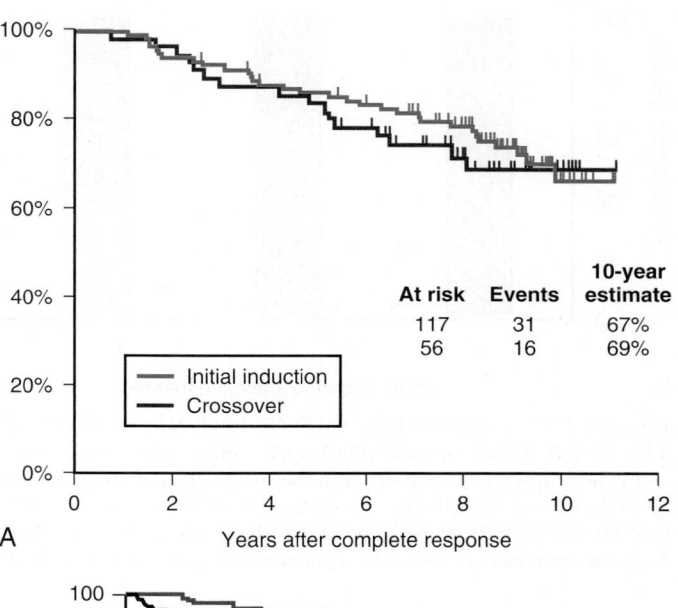

A

Years after complete response

	At risk	Events	10-year estimate
Initial induction	117	31	67%
Crossover	56	16	69%

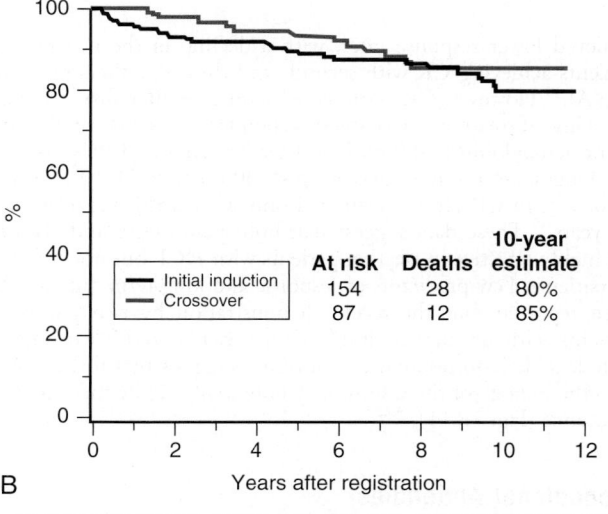

B

Years after registration

	At risk	Deaths	10-year estimate
Initial induction	154	28	80%
Crossover	87	12	85%

Fig. 78.8 LONG-TERM FOLLOW UP OF PATIENTS TREATED WITH PENTOSTATIN FOR THEIR INITIAL THERAPY OR FOLLOWING FAILURE OF INTERFERON-α AS A PART OF THE RANDOMIZED INTERGROUP STUDY. (A) Relapse-free survival by phase of treatment. (B) Overall survival by phase of treatment. *(Flinn IW, Kopecky KJ, Foucar MK, et al: Long-term follow-up of remission duration, mortality, and second malignancies in hairy cell leukemia patients treated with pentostatin. Blood 96:2981, 2000.)*

TABLE 78.5	Selected Published Reports of Pentostatin Therapy for Hairy Cell Leukemia			
Reference	Evaluable Patients (*n*)	CR (%)	PR (%)	OR (%)
Kraut	23	87	4	91
Johnston	28	89	11	100
Dearden	165	82	15	97
Catovsky	148	74	22	96
Grever[20]	154	76	3	79
Rafel	78	72	16	88
Ribeiro	49	44	52	96
Maloisel	230	79	17	96

CR, Complete response; PR, partial response; OR, overall response.

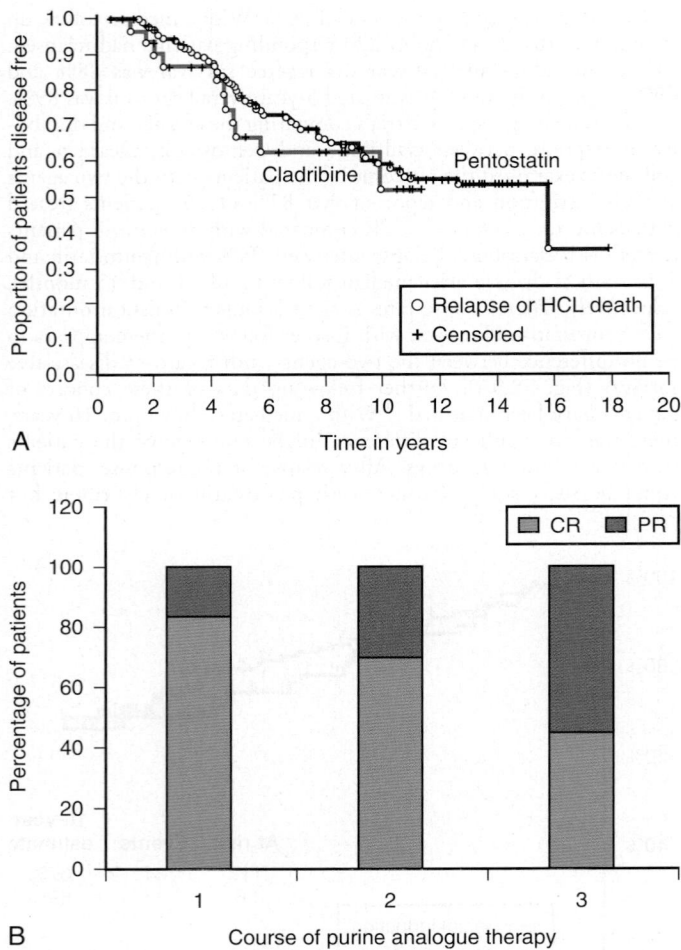

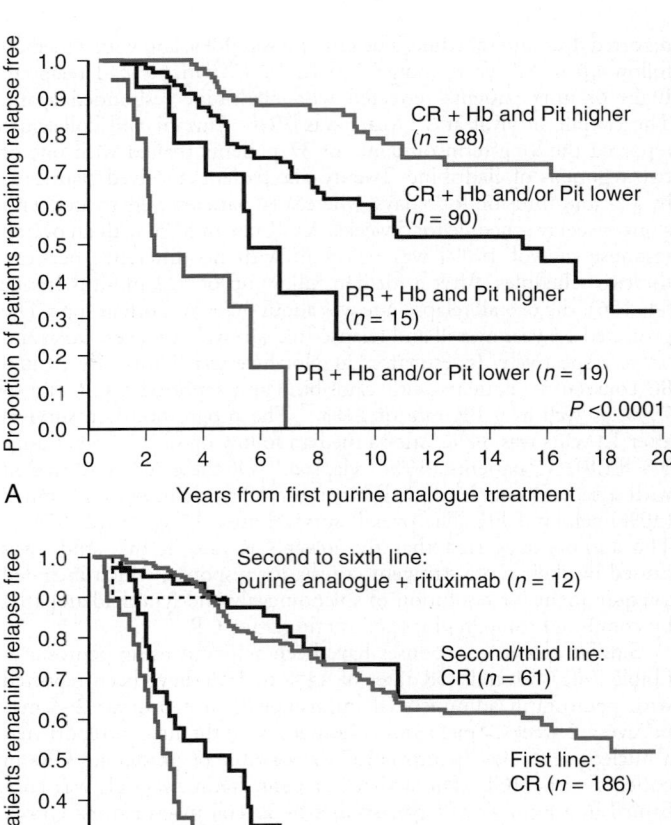

Fig. 78.9 LONG-TERM FOLLOW UP OF PATIENTS TREATED AT THE ROYAL MARSDEN HOSPITAL. (A) Patients who received either cladribine or pentostatin as their initial therapy. (B) Proportion of patients achieving CR and PR with first-, second-, and third-line therapy. *CR, HCL,* hairy cell leukemia; *PR,* partial response. *(Else MA, Ruchlemer R, Osuji N, et al: Long remissions in hairy cell leukemia with purine analogs. Cancer 104:2442, 2005.)*

Fig. 78.10 (A) Relapse-free survival after initial therapy with nucleoside analogs by initial response and blood counts. (B) Relapse-free survival analyzed by line of therapy and response to treatment. Complete responses (CR) were equally durable, whether achieved at first-, second-, or third-line single-agent treatment. *PR,* Partial response. *(Else MA, Ruchlemer R, Osuji N, et al: Long remissions in hairy cell leukemia with purine analogs. Cancer 104:2442, 2005; and Else M, Dearden CE, Matutes E, et al: Long-term follow-up of 233 patients with hairy cell leukaemia, treated initially with pentostatin or cladribine, at a median of 16 years from diagnosis. Br J Haematol 145:733, 2009.)*

achieved lower response rates, with a decline in the proportion of patients achieving CR with second- and third-line therapy (see Fig. 78.9A).[10] However, CRs were equally durable after first, second, or third line of treatment. Complete responders and those with pretreatment hemoglobin >10.0 g/dL and platelet count >100 × 10⁹/L had the longest relapse-free survival ($p < .0001$) (Fig. 78.10).[10] Patients who were in CR after 5 years had only a 25% risk for relapsing by 15 years.[10] These data suggest that both pentostatin and cladribine are highly effective in treating patients with HCL but not curative in all patients. Few predictors of response and long-term outcome have been reported, but the recent demonstration by two groups that patients with unmutated IGH chain variable *(IGHV)* region gene were less likely to respond to cladribine suggests that further insight into the biology of the disease may potentially clarify mechanisms of resistance (Fig. 78.11).[19,22]

Monoclonal Antibodies

Several therapeutic options are now available for patients with relapsed HCL. The efficacy of the monoclonal antibody rituximab in treating these patients has been suggested by a number of studies (Table 78.6). Rituximab is a monoclonal antibody directed against the pan–B-cell antigen (CD20), which is heavily expressed on the surface of hairy cells. Nieva and colleagues reported their experience with 4 weekly doses of rituximab in 24 patients with HCL who

had failed prior treatment with cladribine. The overall response rate was 26%, with 13% CR and 13% PR. No unusual toxicity was reported. Lauria and colleagues treated 10 patients with relapsed/progressed HCL with 4 weekly doses of rituximab and reported one CR and four PR (overall response rate of 50%). Hagberg and colleagues treated 11 patients with HCL (including three previously untreated patients) with the same regimen of rituximab for 4 weeks. The response rate was 64%, with six CRs and one PR (including one CR in an untreated patient). The Swiss Group for Clinical Cancer Research reported their study of 4 weekly doses of rituximab in 26 patients with relapsed/progressed HCL, showing an 80% response rate, with 32% achieving CR. Thomas and colleagues used an extended regimen of rituximab 375 mg/m² weekly for eight doses to treat 15 patients with relapsed/refractory HCL and reported a response rate of 80%, including eight (52%) CR, two (13%) CR with residual marrow disease, and two (13%) PR.[23]

Rituximab has been evaluated in a sequential strategy to improve responses in patients with HCL after treatment with cladribine.[24] Rituximab has also been used concomitantly to treat patients with refractory disease with reported excellent responses suggesting a

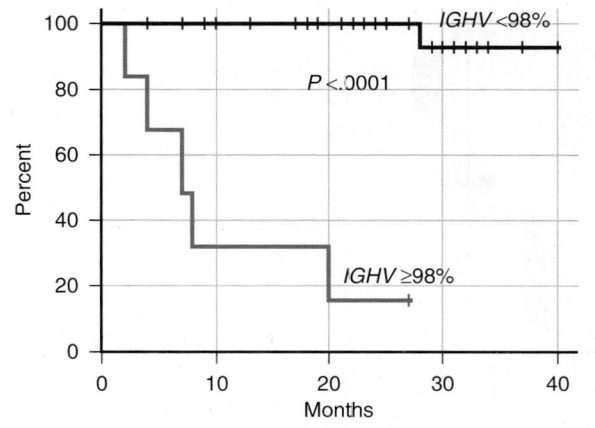

IGHV homology	Events/N	Median EFS	P
<98% ≥98%	1/52 5/6	Not reached 7.5 months	<.0001

A

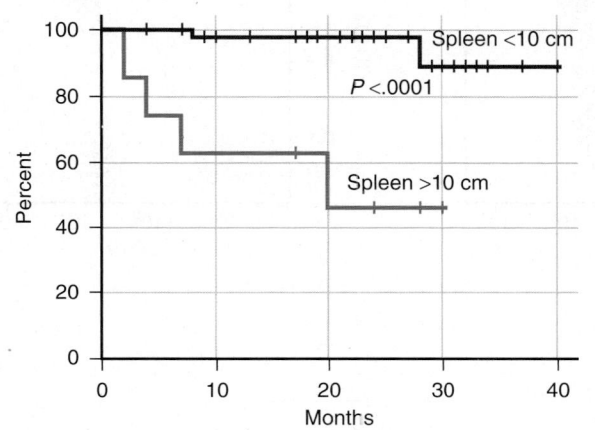

Spleen b.c.m.	Events/N	Median EFS	P
<10 cm ≥10 cm	2/50 4/8	Not reached 20 months	<.0001

B

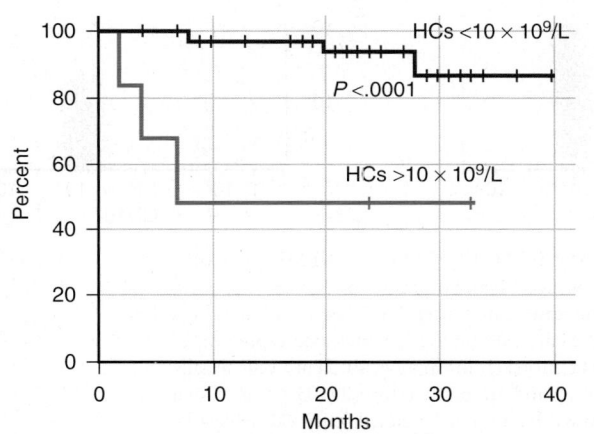

HCs	Events/N	Median EFS	P
<10 × 10⁹/L ≥10 × 10⁹/L	3/52 3/6	Not reached 8 months	<.0001

C

Fig. 78.11 PREDICTING RESPONSE AND OUTCOME OF THERAPY WITH CLADRIBINE BY ASSESSING *IGHV* MUTATIONAL STATUS (AS WELL AS BY SPLENOMEGALY AND LEUKOCYTOSIS). *EFS,* Event-free survival; *HCs,* hairy cells; *IGHV,* immunoglobulin heavy chain variable.

TABLE 78.6	Selected Published Reports of Rituximab Therapy for Hairy Cell Leukemia				
Reference	Patients (*n*)	No Prior Therapy (*n*)	CR (%) (Untreated)	PR (%)	OR (%)
Lauria	10	0	10	40	50
Hagberg	11	3	55 (33)	10	65
Nieva	24	0	13	13	26
Thomas[23]	15	0	66	13	80
Zenhausern	25	0	32	48	80

CR, Complete response; OR, overall response; PR, partial response.

possible synergy. The investigators from the Royal Marsden NHS Trust treated 18 patients with either pentostatin (*n* = 12) or cladribine (*n* = 6) in combination with rituximab after a median of two (range, 1–6) prior treatments and reported a CR rate of 89%. Toxicity with the combination was minimal, and with a median follow up of 36 months, all 16 patients who had achieved CR remained in CR.

Other monoclonal antibody–based therapies have developed and are under investigation. BL22 is a recombinant immunotoxin containing the variable domains of the anti-CD22 monoclonal antibody RFB4 fused to a truncated pseudomonas endotoxin A.[25] In a dose-escalation study, 16 patients who were resistant to cladribine were treated with BL22 by intravenous infusion every other day for a total of three doses.[25] Response included 11 CR and 2 PR. The three nonresponders either had preexisting neutralizing antibodies or received low doses of the immunotoxin.[25] Toxicity included a cytokine-release syndrome and development of a reversible hemolytic-uremic syndrome in two patients.[25] In a larger phase I follow-up study of 46 patients with previously treated CD22+ lymphoid malignancies, including 31 with HCL, 61% achieved a CR and 19% experienced a PR, further demonstrating the activity of this agent in HCL. Neutralizing antibodies occurred in 11 (24%) of 46 patients (all HCL), and a reversible hemolytic uremic syndrome requiring plasmapheresis was observed in 1 patient with NHL during cycle 1 and in 4 patients with HCL during cycle 2 or 3. The median duration for CR was 36 months (range, 5–66 months). The maximum tolerated dose (MTD) was established at 40 µg/kg every other day × three doses. More recently, the results of a phase 2 study of the same drug in 36 patients with relapsed or refractory HCL was published.[26] Patients received BL22 at the MTD on cycle 1. Those achieving hematologic remission were observed while the others were retreated at 30 µg/kg every other day for three doses every 4 weeks beginning at least 8 weeks after cycle 1. The response after one cycle (CR, 25%; PR, 25%) improved when 56% were retreated (CR, 47%; PR, 25%).[26] A modified version of this agent, moxetumomab pasudotox (or HA22), has a superior affinity for CD22 and is under clinical development.

CD52 is also expressed on the surface of hairy cells, and an anecdotal report of a response to alemtuzumab has recently been published.

Minimal Residual Disease and Its Significance

Despite excellent responses, there is a definite relapse rate associated with therapy of HCL with both cladribine and pentostatin, and the relapse-free survival does not appear to plateau.[10] Wheaton and colleagues were the first to note that detection of MRD by immunohistochemistry (using anti-CD45RO, anti-CD20, and DBA.44) in paraffin-embedded bone marrow sections of 39 patients with HCL in CR after receiving cladribine was predictive of relapse.[27] More sensitive methods of MRD detection such as immunophenotyping using multiparameter flow cytometry, as well as analysis of antigen receptor genes by polymerase chain reaction (PCR) using consensus or clone-specific primers, have been evaluated recently and can be used to monitor the disease course (Fig. 78.12).[24,28,29] Other

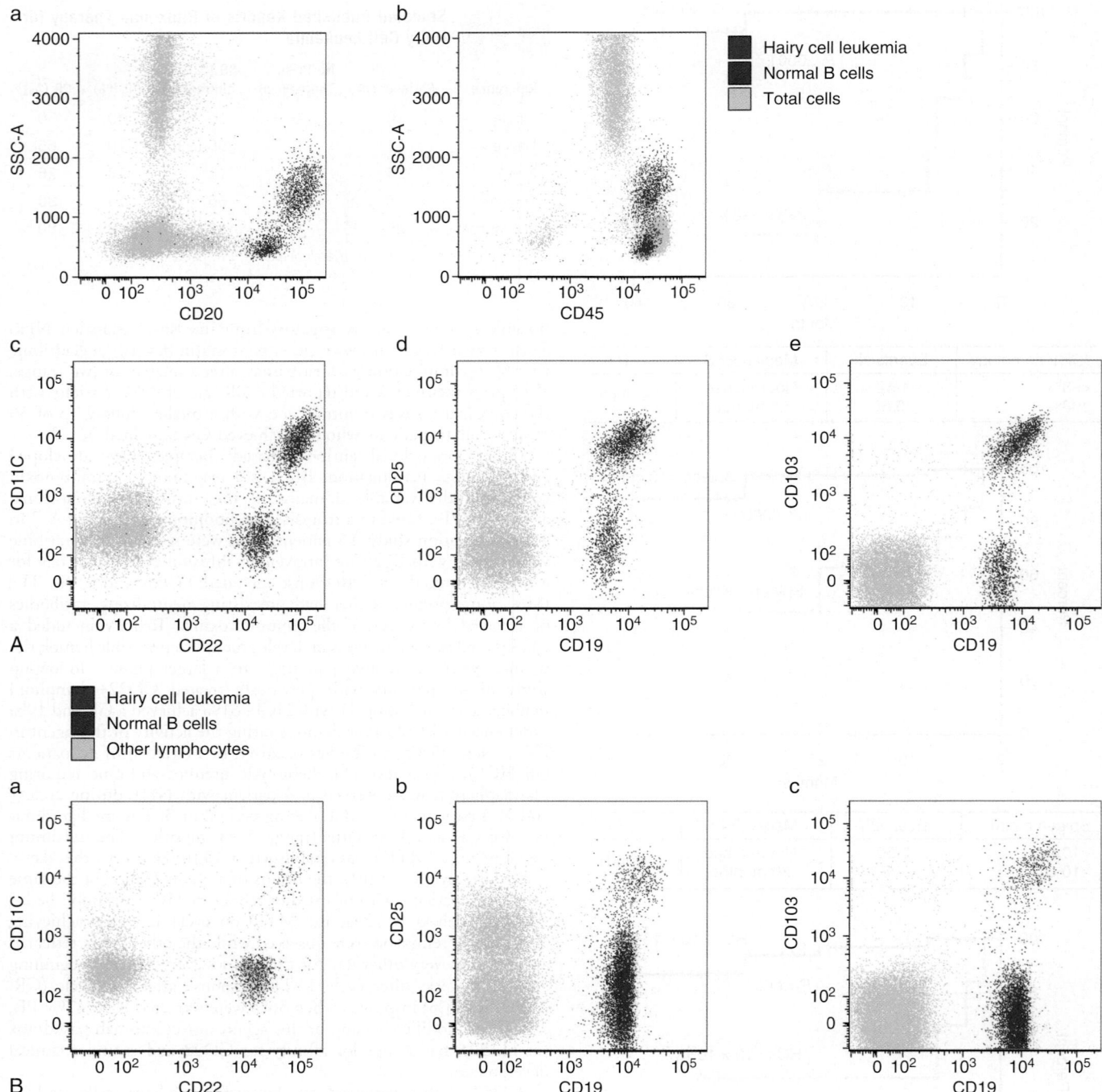

Fig. 78.12 MONITORING MINIMAL RESIDUAL DISEASE IN HAIRY CELL LEUKEMIA. (A) Total nucleated cells in a hemodilute bone marrow aspirate (*a* and *b*); total lymphocytes (*c* to *e*). Hairy cells (*red,* about 6% of total cellularity and 12% of lymphocytes) show increased side scatter (SSC) because of their high cytoplasmic complexity, compared with normal B cells *(blue)*. Hairy cells often show increased expression of CD20 *(a)*. On CD45 versus SSC gating plots *(b),* they may be mistaken for monocytes. Hairy cells usually show bright expression of CD11c and CD22 *(c)* and CD25 *(d)* and are positive for CD103 *(e)*. (B) Total lymphocytes from a posttherapy bone marrow aspirate, positive for minimal residual hairy cell leukemia, accounting for about 0.6% of total cellularity. Hairy cells (*red)* can be easily distinguished from normal B cells *(blue),* particularly on the basis of their bright expression of CD11c *(a)* and CD25 *(b)* and positivity for CD103 *(c)*. In *a,* 30,000 total cells were collected; in *b* and *c,* 100,000. *(Courtesy Jeffrey Jorgensen, Department of Hematopathology, UTMDACC.)*

markers of the disease, such as serum-soluble CD25, CD22, and CD307, have been evaluated and shown to be reliable for disease monitoring.[30]

Rituximab has been evaluated for eradication of MRD assessed by flow cytometry and consensus primer PCR; whether such elimination of MRD can translate to a longer relapse-free survival is unclear.[9,24] Sigal and colleagues reported that patients with HCL may harbor MRD and even morphologically evident disease many years after initial therapy without experiencing overt relapse, raising the question of whether eradication of MRD should be the goal of therapy in HCL.[9] However, several studies have suggested that patients who achieve a morphologic CR have a better outcome than those with lesser responses. Whether this can be extrapolated to complete eradication of detectable disease remains to be established.

Treatment of Disease Relapse

Despite the success of the nucleoside analogs in achieving generally durable responses in the majority of patients, they are not considered to be curative, with about 40% of patients relapsing by 10 years after treatment.[10] Second and third courses of nucleoside analogs have been used, either with the same or the alternate agent used to treat relapsing disease. However, CRs are less frequent with subsequent courses. Because a single course of cladribine or pentostatin can suppress CD4+ lymphocytes for a substantial period of time, concerns about the use of multiple courses of these agents have been raised.[18]

Rituximab has the advantage of sparing T-lymphocytes and has shown significant activity in patients with relapsed disease (see Table 78.6). However, the overall response rate is relatively low, particularly in studies using only 4 weekly doses of rituximab. Recent studies of combination therapy with rituximab and nucleoside analogs have reported high response rates, improved activity in variant HCL, and second CR durations longer than the first CR achieved with nucleoside analogs alone.[31,32] Immunotoxins such as BL22 and HA22 have been studied in cases of relapsed disease, produce high responses, and have limited toxicity; however, they are not, as yet, widely available. Bendamustine, a novel molecule with structural features of both an alkylating agent and a purine nucleoside analog, has been used by one group for the treatment of relapsed and refractory disease. Anecdotal reports have circulated about the use of other agents such as alemtuzumab. BCRs signaling kinase inhibitors such as ibrutinib have shown significant promise in the treatment of a number of lymphoid neoplasms and are being investigated in patients with relapsed disease and HCLv.[33] The identification of BRAF V600F as a universal aberration in patients with HCL and the availability of BRAF inhibitors for the treatment of solid tumors such as melanoma led to the investigation of this agent in patients with relapsed HCL with promising early reports.[34] The BRAF mutation, BRAFV600E constitutively activates the mitogen activated kinase pathway in virtually all patients with HCL. Two phase II trials of the BRAF inhibitor, vemurafenib, have been reported.[35] The treated patients had relapsed or were refractory to treatment with purine analogs. The drug was administered orally at a dose of 960 mgms orally twice a day for 16 to 18 weeks. The overall response rate was 96% to 100% with a CR rate of 35% to 42% All patients had evidence of MRD at the end of treatment. The progression-free survival rate was 73% and the overall survival was 91%. Myelosuppression was minimal and the most common adverse effects were rash, arthralgias or arthritis. These studies suggest that BRAF inhibitors are promising agents for HCL patients that are unresponsive or refractory to purine analogs. The role of these agents in treating patients with HCL will need further studies and longer follow up.

Incidence of Second Malignancies

Early studies suggested an association between HCL and development of second malignancies, but this link is controversial and has been refuted by other reports. The reported second cancers include melanoma, prostate cancer, gastrointestinal cancers, and non-Hodgkin lymphomas. Whether these second malignancies are related to the primary disease itself or to its treatment has also been debated. A number of long-term studies of patients treated with pentostatin or cladribine have not shown a statistically significant increased risk for second malignancies. It remains unclear whether the immunosuppressive effects of nucleoside analogs play a role in such susceptibility to developing a second malignancy or whether disease-related factors or perhaps increased monitoring of these patients are important.

FUTURE DIRECTIONS

Over the past decade, success in the treatment of HCL has led to diminished interest in developing new therapeutic strategies for treating this uncommon leukemia, with research confined to a few specialized centers interested in the biology and pathogenesis of this disease. Recent reports unraveling the biologic and molecular aspects of the disease have kindled a significant resurgence of interest.[2] Further studies into other aspects of the disease, such as the role of microenvironment, BCR signaling, and the complex interaction of various signaling pathways will likely provide better therapeutic tools and strategies.[2]

REFERENCES

1. Foucar K, Falini B, Catovsky D, et al: Hairy cell leukemia. In Swerdlow SH, Campo E, Harris NL, editors: *WHO classification of tumors of haematopoietic and lymphoid tissues*, ed 4, Lyon, 2008, International Agency for Research on Cancer (IARC).
2. Tiacci E, Liso A, Piris M, et al: Evolving concepts in the pathogenesis of hairy-cell leukaemia. *Nat Rev Cancer* 6:437, 2006.
3. Forconi F, Sahota SS, Raspadori D, et al: Hairy cell leukemia: at the crossroad of somatic mutation and isotype switch. *Blood* 104:3312, 2004.
4. Arons E, Roth L, Sapolsky J, et al: Evidence of canonical somatic hypermutation in hairy cell leukemia. *Blood* 117:4844, 2011.
5. Basso K, Liso A, Tiacci E, et al: Gene expression profiling of hairy cell leukemia reveals a phenotype related to memory B cells with altered expression of chemokine and adhesion receptors. *J Exp Med* 199:59, 2004.
6. Tiacci E, Trifonov V, Schiavoni G, et al: BRAF mutations in hairy-cell leukemia. *N Engl J Med* 364:2305, 2011.
7. Falini B, Tiacci E, Liso A, et al: Simple diagnostic assay for hairy cell leukaemia by immunocytochemical detection of annexin A1 (ANXA1). *Lancet* 363:1869, 2004.
8. Matutes E, Wotherspoon A, Brito-Babapulle V, et al: The natural history and clinico-pathological features of the variant form of hairy cell leukemia. *Leukemia* 15:184, 2001.
9. Sigal DS, Sharpe R, Burian C, et al: Very long-term eradication of minimal residual disease in patients with hairy cell leukemia after a single course of cladribine. *Blood* 115:1893, 2010.
10. Else M, Dearden CE, Matutes E, et al: Long-term follow-up of 233 patients with hairy cell leukaemia, treated initially with pentostatin or cladribine, at a median of 16 years from diagnosis. *Br J Haematol* 145:733, 2009.
11. Piro LD, Carrera CJ, Carson DA, et al: Lasting remissions in hairy-cell leukemia induced by a single infusion of 2-chlorodeoxyadenosine. *N Engl J Med* 322:1117, 1990.
12. Lauria F, Bocchia M, Marotta G, et al: Weekly administration of 2-chlorodeoxyadenosine in patients with hairy-cell leukemia: a new treatment schedule effective and safer in preventing infectious complications. *Blood* 89:1838, 1997.
13. Robak T, Jamroziak K, Gora-Tybor J, et al: Cladribine in a weekly versus daily schedule for untreated active hairy cell leukemia: final report from the Polish Adult Leukemia Group (PALG) of a prospective, randomized, multicenter trial. *Blood* 109:3672, 2007.

14. Juliusson G, Heldal D, Hippe E, et al: Subcutaneous injections of 2-chlorodeoxyadenosine for symptomatic hairy cell leukemia. *J Clin Oncol* 13:989, 1995.

15. Saven A, Burian C, Koziol JA, et al: Long-term follow-up of patients with hairy cell leukemia after cladribine treatment. *Blood* 92:1918, 1998.

16. Goodman GR, Burian C, Koziol JA, et al: Extended follow-up of patients with hairy cell leukemia after treatment with cladribine. *J Clin Oncol* 21:891, 2003.

17. Chadha P, Rademaker AW, Mendiratta P, et al: Treatment of hairy cell leukemia with 2-chlorodeoxyadenosine (2-CdA): long-term follow-up of the Northwestern University experience. *Blood* 106:241, 2005.

18. Seymour JF, Kurzrock R, Freireich EJ, et al: 2-chlorodeoxyadenosine induces durable remissions and prolonged suppression of CD4+ lymphocyte counts in patients with hairy cell leukemia. *Blood* 83:2906, 1994.

19. Forconi F, Sozzi E, Cencini E, et al: Hairy cell leukemias with unmutated IGHV genes define the minor subset refractory to single-agent cladribine and with more aggressive behavior. *Blood* 114:4696, 2009.

20. Grever M, Kopecky K, Foucar MK, et al: Randomized comparison of pentostatin versus interferon alfa-2a in previously untreated patients with hairy cell leukemia: an intergroup study. *J Clin Oncol* 13:974, 1995.

21. Flinn IW, Kopecky KJ, Foucar MK, et al: Long-term follow-up of remission duration, mortality, and second malignancies in hairy cell leukemia patients treated with pentostatin. *Blood* 96:2981, 2000.

22. Arons E, Suntum T, Stetler-Stevenson M, et al: VH4-34+ hairy cell leukemia, a new variant with poor prognosis despite standard therapy. *Blood* 114:4687, 2009.

23. Thomas DA, O'Brien S, Bueso-Ramos C, et al: Rituximab in relapsed or refractory hairy cell leukemia. *Blood* 102:3906, 2003.

24. Ravandi F, Jorgensen JL, O'Brien SM, et al: Eradication of minimal residual disease in hairy cell leukemia. *Blood* 107:4658, 2006.

25. Kreitman RJ, Wilson WH, Bergeron K, et al: Efficacy of the anti-CD22 recombinant immunotoxin BL22 in chemotherapy-resistant hairy-cell leukemia. *N Engl J Med* 345:241, 2001.

26. Kreitman RJ, Stetler-Stevenson M, Margulies I, et al: Phase II trial of recombinant immunotoxin RFB4(dsFv)-PE38 (BL22) in patients with hairy cell leukemia. *J Clin Oncol* 27:2983, 2009.

27. Wheaton S, Tallman MS, Hakimian D, et al: Minimal residual disease may predict bone marrow relapse in patients with hairy cell leukemia treated with 2-chlorodeoxyadenosine. *Blood* 87:1556, 1996.

28. Sausville JE, Salloum RG, Sorbara L, et al: Minimal residual disease detection in hairy cell leukemia: Comparison of flow cytometric immunophenotyping with clonal analysis using consensus primer polymerase chain reaction for the heavy chain gene. *Am J Clin Pathol* 119:213, 2003.

29. Arons E, Margulies I, Sorbara L, et al: Minimal residual disease in hairy cell leukemia patients assessed by clone-specific polymerase chain reaction. *Clin Cancer Res* 12:2804, 2006.

30. Ravandi F, O'Brien S, Jorgensen J, et al: Phase II study of cladribine followed by rituximab in patients with hairy cell leukemia. *Blood* 118:3818, 2011.

31. Else M, Dearden CE, Matutes E, et al: Rituximab with pentostatin or cladribine: an effective combination treatment for hairy cell leukemia after disease recurrence. *Leuk Lymphoma* 52:75, 2011.

32. Kreitman R, Wilson W, Calvo KR, et al: Cladribine with immediate rituximab for the treatment of patients with variant hairy cell leukemia. *Clin Cancer Res* 19:6873, 2013.

33. Sivina M, Kreitman R, Arons E, et al: The bruton tyrosine kinase inhibitor (PCI-32765) blocks hairy cell leukemia survival, proliferation and B cell receptor signaling: a new therapeutic approach. *Br J Haematol* 166:177, 2014.

34. Pettirossi V, Santi A, Imperi E, et al: BRAF inhibitors reverse the unique molecular signature and phenotype of hairy cell leukemia and exert potent antileukemic activity. *Blood* 125:1207, 2015.

35. Tiacci E1, Park JH, et al: Targeting Mutant BRAF in Relapsed or Refractory Hairy-Cell Leukemia. *N Engl J Med* 373(18):1733–1747, 2015.

MARGINAL ZONE LYMPHOMAS (EXTRANODAL/MALT, SPLENIC, AND NODAL)

Carlos A. Ramos

The term *marginal zone* refers to a histologic compartment located at the periphery of lymphoid follicles immediately outside their mantle zone.[1] The marginal zone is especially evident in the spleen, although identical areas have been observed in other lymphoid structures, including mesenteric lymph nodes and mucosa-associated lymphoid tissue (MALT) (Fig. 79.1).[2] Ordinarily, it is composed predominantly of B cells that are slightly larger than mantle zone lymphocytes and strongly positive for surface immunoglobulin (Ig) M, but weakly positive for IgD (in contrast to mantle zone cells, which are strongly positive for IgD).[3] Marginal zone B lymphocytes are thought to be involved in fast protective responses against pathogenic encapsulated bacteria that do not trigger classical T-cell–dependent humoral immunity.[4] They are also assumed to be the physiologic counterpart of a group of non-Hodgkin lymphomas (NHL) that are currently referred to as *marginal zone lymphomas (MZLs).*

Although MZLs share a common denomination, arising from histologic similarities, new genetic findings and longer follow-up studies have established that the currently recognized subtypes of MZLs, initially described in the Revised European-American Lymphoma (REAL) classification, are different diseases.[5] In the most recent WHO classification of tumors of the hematopoietic and lymphoid tissues,[6] these disorders comprise three distinct entities: extranodal MZL of MALT type (ENMZL), splenic MZL (SMZL) and nodal MZL (NMZL). Immunoproliferative small intestinal disease (IPSID), formerly known as alpha heavy chain (or Seligmann) disease, has been recently recognized as a variant of ENMZL.[7] In aggregate, MZLs represent approximately 10% of all NHL.[8] Clinically, they behave indolently and have a prolonged course. Therefore, management strategies share similarity with other low-grade lymphomas,[9] although specific biologic characteristics and particular pathophysiologic mechanisms determine unique therapeutic approaches in some of the subtypes. This chapter will summarize the clinical characteristics and current management strategies for the different types of MZL.

INITIAL EVALUATION OF MARGINAL ZONE LYMPHOMA

As for other lymphomas, biopsy of an adequate amount of tissue with review by a hematopathologist with expertise in the field is essential to establish the diagnosis. Excisional or incisional biopsies of a lymph node or suspicious mass, obtained by endoscopic or conventional means, are preferred. In patients without easily accessible nodes or masses, computed tomography (CT) or ultrasound-guided core needle biopsy is usually well tolerated and may be adequate for diagnosis. Fine-needle aspiration is not appropriate for diagnosis; sufficient material must be obtained for proper histologic examination and required immunophenotypic and genetic studies.

Physical examination with special attention to peripheral lymph nodes and the abdomen should be performed. Initial laboratory evaluation should include a complete blood count (cytopenias may be evidence of marrow infiltration or of autoimmunity) with evaluation of a peripheral blood smear (to exclude leukemic involvement) and basic biochemical studies, including lactate dehydrogenase (LDH) level, which is an important prognostic factor and a potential indicator of transformation from indolent to aggressive lymphoma.

Antiglobulin tests and reticulocyte count may be useful to rule out autoimmune hemolytic anemia. Serum protein electrophoresis and immunofixation may demonstrate a monoclonal immunoglobulin. β_2-microglobulin levels may have prognostic value[10] as in other indolent lymphomas. Viral hepatitis (B and C) and HIV studies to exclude coexisting infections that affect therapeutic approaches should be obtained.

Depending on the primary site of disease, specific procedures may be indicated. Gastrointestinal MZLs may require repeat staging endoscopies, during which an adequate number of biopsies should be obtained. For gastric ENMZL, the European Gastro-Intestinal Lymphoma Study (EGILS) group recommends a mapping procedure with a minimum of 10 biopsies taken from visible lesions and additional ones from macroscopically normal mucosa; the same procedure should be repeated to assess treatment response.[11–17] Because endoscopic biopsies are not transmural, endoscopic ultrasound (EUS) is a useful way to assess the depth of involvement, which has prognostic implications.[12–17] For head primaries, such as ocular adnexal ENMZL, appropriate directed examination and imaging studies (CT or magnetic resonance) are indicated.

STAGING OF MARGINAL ZONE LYMPHOMA

Imaging studies of the chest, abdomen, and pelvis, usually CT scans, should be obtained to adequately stage the disease. Positron emission tomography (PET) scan has been increasingly used for staging and evaluation of response to therapy in NHL, but it may be less useful in MZL because up to 60% of these lymphomas may be PET-negative, especially in early-stage gastric ENZML.[18] Some MZL series, however, document a PET-positivity rate of up to 80%,[19–23] with better detection rates seen for head and neck and bronchial versus gastric or ocular MZL.[24] Also for staging and, occasionally, for diagnostic purposes, bone marrow biopsy and aspirate are usually advocated, even in cases in which the likelihood of systemic disease is low, because any positive result has important implications for therapy.

Staging of MZL is similar to that of other lymphomas; the Ann Arbor system, or an adapted version,[25] is used most frequently (Table 79.1). Nonetheless, specific staging systems have been adopted for particular sites. Gastrointestinal MZL is often staged according to a modified Ann Arbor scheme, commonly known as the Lugano staging system,[26] which incorporates indices corresponding to depth of mucosal invasion and proximity of affected lymph nodes to the primary lesion (see Table 79.1). Of note, the Lugano system has no stage III, and its stage IIE may refer to lesions that extend by contiguity to adjacent organs and not necessarily to secondary involvement of lymph nodes. Recently, arguing that the dissemination patterns of extranodal lymphomas are essentially different from those of primary nodal lymphomas, the EGILS group has proposed a new staging system (the Paris staging system)[27] that is based on the TNM scheme used for solid tumors (see Table 79.1). The International Society for Cutaneous Lymphomas (ISCL) and the cutaneous lymphoma task force of the European Organization of Research and Treatment of Cancer (EORTC) have also recently suggested a new, TNM-based staging system for cutaneous lymphomas other than mycosis

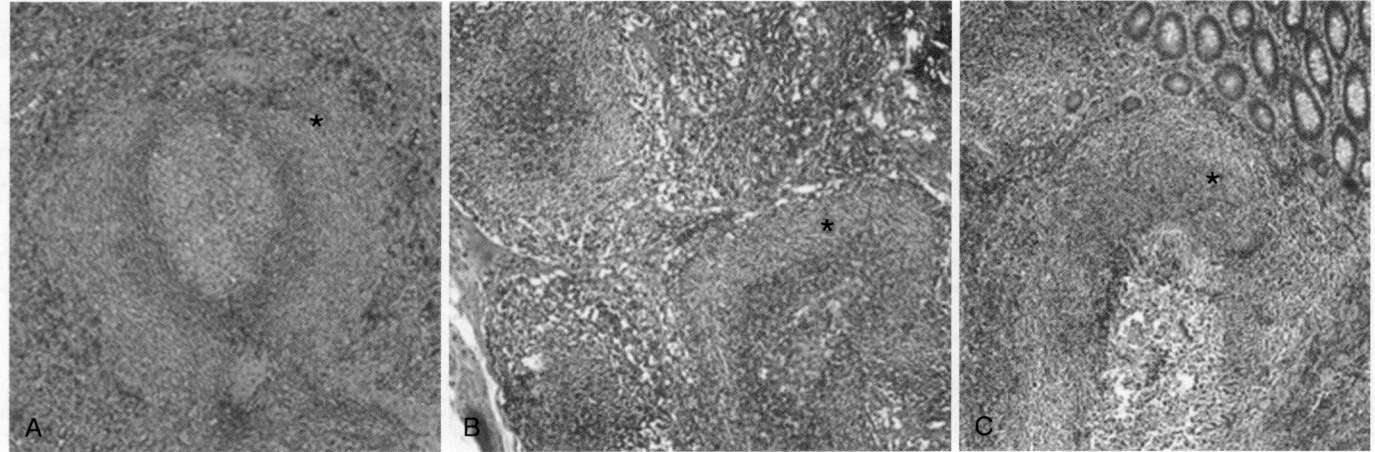

Fig. 79.1 NORMAL MARGINAL ZONE CELLS. (A) Marginal zone cells are seen most readily in sections from the normal spleen. The splenic white pulp typically has three distinctive layers: the germinal center, the mantle zone, and external to this, the marginal zone (see *asterisk*). (B) Marginal zone cells are not usually seen in lymph nodes, but for some reason are sometimes present in mesenteric lymph nodes (see *asterisk*). They have a similar appearance to those in the spleen. (C) In the gastrointestinal tract, the lymphoid tissue in Peyer's patches is believed to have a marginal zone equivalent (see *asterisk*). The cells are again external to the mantle zone and are believed to traffic between the epithelium and the lymphoid follicle.

TABLE 79.1	Staging Systems for Gastrointestinal Lymphomas			
Adapted Ann Arbor System[25]	Lugano System[26]	Paris System[27]	Areas Involved[a]	
IE1	I₁	T1 N0 M0	Mucosa to submucosa	
IE2	I₂	T2 N0 M0	To muscularis propria or subserosa	
		T3 N0 M0	To serosa	
	IIE	T4 N0 M0	To adjacent organs	
IIE1	II₁	T1–4 N1 M0	Regional lymph nodes[b]	
IIE2	II₂	T1–4 N2 M0	Nonregional abdominal lymph nodes	
IIIE	IV	T1–4 N3 M0	Extraabdominal lymph nodes	
IV		T1–4 N0–3 M1	Distant organs	
		B1	Bone marrow	

[a]In case of more than one visible lesion synchronously originating in the gastrointestinal tract, select the characteristics of the more advanced lesion.
[b]Anatomic designation of lymph nodes as *regional* according to site: (a) stomach: perigastric nodes and those located along the ramifications of the celiac artery (i.e., left gastric artery, common hepatic artery, splenic artery); (b) duodenum: pancreaticoduodenal, pyloric, hepatic, and superior mesenteric nodes; (c) jejunum/ileum: mesenteric nodes and, for the terminal ileum only, the ileocolic as well as the posterior cecal nodes; (d) colorectum: pericolic and perirectal nodes and those located along the ileocolic, right, middle, and left colic, inferior mesenteric, superior rectal, and internal iliac arteries.

fungoides and Sézary syndrome,[28] which may be used for the cutaneous forms of ENMZL.

EXTRANODAL MARGINAL ZONE LYMPHOMA OF MALT TYPE

Epidemiology and Manifestations

ENMZL is the most frequent of the MZL subtypes, accounting for approximately 8% of all NHL.[8] A recent analysis of Surveillance, Epidemiology, and End Results (SEER) data quotes a yearly incidence rate of 1.59 per 100,000 adults in the United States.[29] The median age of presentation is around 60, with a wide range spanning from the third to the ninth decades, and there is a slight female predominance (55%).[30] In contrast to most other indolent lymphomas, ENMZL frequently presents at a localized stage (≈40% stage I and ≈30% stage II), and the risk for systemic dissemination is low (albeit variable depending on primary location), which has important implications for the choice of therapy.

The most commonly affected primary site is the mucosa of the gastrointestinal tract, in particular the stomach (approximately 44% of all ENMZL cases) followed by the small intestine (≈7%). Ocular structures are also frequently involved (≈12%), namely, the orbit (≈40% of all ocular adnexal ENMZL), the conjunctiva (35%–40%), the lacrimal glands (10%–15%), and the eyelids (≈10%).[31] Other commonly affected sites include the bronchial mucosa (≈11% of all ENMZL cases), the skin (≈9%), the salivary glands (≈6%), and the thyroid gland (≈6%). More rarely reported sites are Waldeyer pharyngeal lymphoid ring, breast, liver, pancreas, urogenital tract, and central nervous system.[32–35] Findings at presentation depend on the specific organ affected. Gastric ENMZL may lead to dyspepsia, epigastric pain, nausea, anorexia, and manifestations of gastrointestinal bleeding.[36] Conjunctival ENMZL often forms a painless nodule or plaque that has a "salmon-pink patch" appearance and can be associated with erythema, chemosis, and foreign-body sensation.[37] Primary cutaneous ENMZL frequently presents as multiple red to violaceous papules, plaques, or nodules, most often on the trunk or extremities, in particular the arms, which very uncommonly ulcerate.[38] Salivary and lacrimal gland ENMZL are often preceded by sicca syndrome, with xerostomia or xerophthalmia. B symptoms are uncommon (≈15% of cases).[32]

IPSID usually affects young adults, with no gender predominance, and is seen most commonly in the Middle East and Northern Africa, usually in low socioeconomic status populations.[39] The disease affects the proximal small bowel diffusely and generally presents with a malabsorption syndrome, with steatorrhea, hypocalcemia, weight loss, abdominal pain, and fever. Cases involving the stomach, the colon, and very rarely, the respiratory tract have been described.[7]

Pathobiology and Differential Diagnosis

Etiology

ENMZL is strongly associated with chronic antigenic stimulation, including that deriving from chronic bacterial infections[15,17,40–59] or autoimmune disorders[60–64] (Table 79.2), although the strength of this correlation for some primary sites of disease is discordant among studies, suggesting a possible geographic variation. The common assumption about this association is that continual immune stimulation by bacterial or self-antigens leads to expansion of lymphoid elements in the connective tissue adjacent to the epithelium involved, initially leading to a process of reactive lymphoid hyperplasia. Persistent lymphocytic activation and proliferation predisposes to the accumulation of genetic errors that ultimately may result in antigen-independent growth and, consequently, lymphoma emergence.[65,66] The histologic distinction between the reactive inflammatory process associated with chronic infection (or autoimmunity) and lymphoma proper may be difficult, in which case demonstration of immunoglobulin gene monoclonality by molecular studies may aid in establishing the diagnosis of lymphoma.[67]

Histology

ENMZL is composed predominantly of morphologically heterogeneous small B cells.[67] These resemble a spectrum spanning from small lymphocytes with scant cytoplasm to slightly larger cells with nuclei

TABLE 79.2	Chronic Antigenic Stimulation and Extranodal Marginal Zone Lymphoma	
Bacterial Infections		
Organism	**Site**	**Prevalence (%)**
Helicobacter pylori[15,17,41,42,43]	Stomach	72–100
Campylobacter jejuni[44]	Intestine (IPSID)	≈70
Chlamydophila psittaci[45,46,47,48,49,50,51,52,53,54,55]	Conjunctiva	0–89
Borrelia burgdorferi[56,57,58,59]	Skin	0–42
Autoimmune Disorders		
Disease	**Site**	**Relative Risk**
Hashimoto thyroiditis[a][61,62]	Thyroid	67–80
Sjögren syndrome[60,63,64]	Salivary and lacrimal glands	6.6–30.6

[a]Estimated by assuming cases of thyroid histiocytic lymphoma were ENMZL because these were published before the REAL classification.

similar to those of centrocytes and having relatively abundant pale cytoplasm (leading possibly to a monocytoid appearance). These cells are located in the outer zone of reactive lymphoid follicles, extend into the interfollicular region, and may sometimes colonize the germinal centers. Larger, immunoblast- or centroblast-like cells may be present in small numbers, but an abundance of these should raise suspicion for diffuse large B-cell lymphoma (DLBCL), which requires different management. According to the newest WHO classification, the term *high-grade MALT lymphoma*, denoting the presence of sheets of transformed cells, should not be used and instead these tumors should be diagnosed as DLBCL.

Often there are lymphoid infiltrates invading and destroying glandular structures, with eosinophilic degeneration of epithelial cells (so-called lymphoepithelioid lesions), which are strongly suggestive, albeit not pathognomonic, of progression to lymphoma in cases where the differential diagnosis with reactive lymphoid hyperplasia is in doubt (Fig. 79.2). Plasmacytic differentiation is frequent, especially in association with cutaneous, thyroid, and intestinal (IPSID) ENMZL and may pose differential diagnosis problems with lymphoplasmacytic lymphoma. These plasmacytoid cells often contain periodic acid–Schiff (PAS)–positive inclusions, known as Dutcher or Russell bodies, depending on whether they are located over the nucleus or in the cytoplasm, respectively.[68]

In gastric ENMZL, histology also plays an important role in establishing the diagnosis of *Helicobacter pylori* infection. All biopsy samples should have sections appropriately stained for its detection (see Fig. 79.2D). Because proton pump inhibitors (PPIs) may decrease the sensitivity of detection, patients should stop taking these medications for at least 2 weeks before biopsies are obtained.[69,70]

Immunophenotype

ENMZL cells display common pan–B-cell markers, such as CD19 and CD20. They are also usually positive for the complement receptors CD21 and CD35, antigens that are shared with follicular dendritic cells, and also for CD79a. Plasmacytoid cells can be CD138-positive. Helpful in the differential diagnosis with other indolent lymphomas, ENMZL are usually CD5-negative (in contrast to chronic lymphocytic leukemia/small lymphocytic lymphoma [CLL/SLL] and mantle cell lymphoma [MCL]), CD23-negative (in contrast to CLL/SLL), CD10-negative (in contrast to follicular lymphoma [FL]), and cyclin D1-negative (in contrast to MCL). They

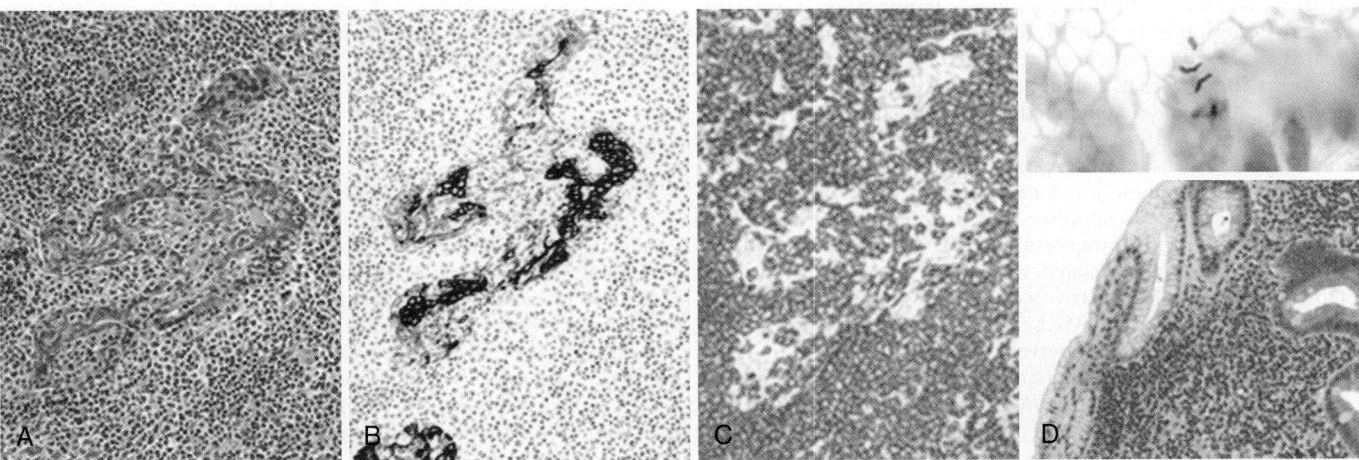

Fig. 79.2 EXTRANODAL MARGINAL ZONE LYMPHOMAS OF MUCOSA-ASSOCIATED LYMPHOID TISSUE (MALT LYMPHOMAS). A–C, An example of a MALT lymphoma in the parotid gland is illustrated with various stains. The glandular tissue is overrun by lymphoid cells, which disrupt and destroy the gland. The resulting structure is referred to as a *lymphoepithelial lesion* (A). These can be more clearly identified with a keratin stain (B) and with a B-cell stain such as CD20 (C), which illustrate the glandular remnant and the B-cell proliferation. (D) MALT lymphoma of the stomach is commonly associated with *H. pylori* infection, which can be identified by special stains *(top)*.

TABLE 79.3	Frequency of Common Genetic Aberrations in Extranodal Marginal Zone Lymphoma According to Primary Site of Disease					
	Genetic Abnormality[33,34,71] Genes Involved[77]					
	t(11;18)(q21;q21) BIRC3/MALT1	t(14;18)(q32;q21) IGH@/MALT1	t(1;14)(p22;q32) IGH@/BCL10	t(3;14)(p14.1;q32) IGH@/FOXP1	+3[a] NFKBIZ, BCL6, FOXP1, ...	+18[a] BCL2, NFATC1, ...
Primary Site						
Lung	36–53	6–10	2–7	0	13–20	7
Intestine (non-IPSID)	13–56	0	0–13	0	75	13–25
Stomach	6–26	1–5	0	0	11–18	6–29
Ocular adnexa	3–10	0–25	0	0–20	30–38	14–26
Salivary glands	0–5	0–16	0–2	0	8–55	8–19
Skin	0–4	0–14	0	0–10	20	4
Thyroid	0–17	0	0	0–50	11–17	0–22

All values expressed as percentages of cases.
[a]Mostly partial trisomies. Data summarized based on references noted.

are also negative for BCL6, which may be helpful to exclude transformation to DLBCL. Except for IPSID, in which tumor cells express a truncated alpha heavy chain without any light chain, most ENMZL are typically positive for IgM or, less commonly, IgA or IgG, with light chain restriction. IgD expression is usually negative or very weak. These immunoglobulins may be secreted, especially when there is significant plasmacytic differentiation, and can give rise to a monoclonal band in the serum protein electrophoresis. The truncated heavy chains of IPSID usually do not appear as a monoclonal band because they comigrate with other serum proteins but can be detected with anti–alpha heavy chain antibodies on immunofixation.

Genetics

Specific chromosomal aberrations have been associated with ENMZL, the frequency of which depends strongly on the primary site of disease (Table 79.3).[33,34,71] These abnormalities can be detected by conventional cytogenetics in metaphase plates or through fluorescent in situ hybridization (FISH) of interphase nuclei using specific probes. The most commonly observed abnormality is the t(11;18)(q21;q21), which fuses the BIRC3 (baculoviral inhibitor of apoptosis repeat containing 3, also known as API2, or apoptosis inhibitor-2 protein) and MALT1 (MALT lymphoma translocation-1 protein) genes in chromosomes 11 and 18, respectively, leading to expression of a BIRC3-MALT1 chimeric protein.[72] The native MALT1 is part of a protein complex that includes the BCL10 protein (B-cell lymphoma protein 10) and that indirectly leads to nuclear factor kappa-B (NFκB) activation, a process under strict control by several upstream factors. Expression of the fusion protein leads to constitutive activation of NFκB via canonic[73] and noncanonic[74] pathways, which in turn leads to resistance to apoptosis and uncontrolled proliferation. The t(11;18) has a special prognostic significance in gastric ENMZL, because its presence is associated with worse response to antibiotherapy,[75] which is at least partly because of its higher prevalence in H. pylori–negative gastric ENMZL.[76]

Another, less frequently observed, abnormality is the t(14;18)(q32;q21). This translocation is different from that observed in follicular lymphoma, which involves the BCL2 gene, and instead brings the MALT1 gene under the influence of the immunoglobulin heavy chain gene promoter (IGH@), leading to overexpression of MALT1 and, through mechanisms akin to those of t(11;18), constitutive activation of NFκB. The t(1;14)(p22;q32) is seen even more rarely and causes overexpression of the BCL10 gene, which is placed under control of the IGH@ promoter, and, in turn, activation of the same pathways affected by MALT1. A fourth translocation, t(3;14)(p14.1;q32), described mostly in ocular, cutaneous, and thyroid ENMZL, involves the FOXP1 (forkhead box protein P1) transcription factor and the

heavy chain promoter.[78] Although FOXP1 is overexpressed in these tumors, its exact significance in their biology is unknown.

Apart from the translocations described, all believed to be mutually exclusive, ENMZL has also been associated with gains of genetic material, in particular partial trisomies of chromosomes 3 (including regions affecting FOXP1, NFKBIZ [NFκB inhibitor zeta], and BCL6) and 18 (affecting NFATC1 [nuclear factor of activated T cells, cytoplasmic, calcineurin-dependent 1], and BCL2). Gains at 6p25 and losses at 6q (affecting TNFAIP3 [tumor necrosis factor, α-induced protein 3])[79,80] and 1p have also been reported.[77]

Consistent with a postgerminal center B-cell origin, ENMZL have rearranged immunoglobulin genes that display somatic hypermutation of their variable regions.[81] In the case of IPSID, there are deletions of the alpha heavy chain gene in the VH and CH1 regions, which result in the production of an abnormal heavy chain that cannot bind light chains to form a complete immunoglobulin molecule.[82]

Therapy for Early-Stage (I/II) Disease

Given its rarity, there are no randomized controlled trials defining the optimal treatment for ENMZL. Most recommendations arise from consensus panels based on data from retrospective or uncontrolled prospective trials. The most extensive body of data has been gathered on gastric ENMZL.

Gastric Extranodal Marginal Zone Lymphoma

This form of ENMZL has a strong association with active H. pylori infection. If histologic analysis of the gastric biopsies obtained during staging endoscopy fails to demonstrate H. pylori, noninvasive methods, such as breath tests, stool antigen test, or serology, should be used to exclude the infection. Although not necessarily a marker of active infection, the presence of antibodies against H. pylori in an individual not previously treated for this bacterium implicates it in the pathogenesis of the lymphoma.

The focus of therapy for H. pylori–positive disease is on eradication of the infection with one of the currently recommended regimens for this purpose. These commonly combine a PPI and clarithromycin with a second antibiotic, usually amoxicillin or metronidazole (triple therapy), but this is an issue in flux as resistance to clarithromycin is increasing in several regions.[83] Alternatively, quadruple therapy with a PPI, bismuth, tetracycline, and metronidazole can be used. Most authors recommend 10–14 days of treatment because of data suggesting better results than with 7-day courses. According to some authorities, eradication of H. pylori should be confirmed with an appropriate test, such as the urea breath test, at least 4 weeks after finishing antibiotherapy and 2 weeks after discontinuing PPI.[83] Pooled data from several prospective and retrospective studies suggest more than 90% eradication rates after initial antibiotherapy.[84] Persistent infection should be treated with a different course of antibiotics, preferably guided by sensitivity tests, because the same data suggest an eradication rate close to 100% after second- or third-line treatments. Repeat endoscopy with biopsies should be obtained 3 months after completion of antibacterial therapy to assess tumor response and also to allow histologic confirmation of *H. pylori* eradication. If *H. pylori* is still detected, a different antibiotic combination should be tried and the patient reassessed as mentioned previously.[9,11]

Responses to therapy are classified according to biopsy findings on endoscopy. Complete histologic response (complete remission [CR]) should be confirmed by a second endoscopy 3 months later and is managed by observation and regular follow up thereafter as clinically indicated. The presence of small residual lymphoid aggregates early after *H. pylori* eradication, corresponding to a category of *probable minimal residual disease* in the French Study Group of Adult Lymphomas (GELA) grading system for posttreatment evaluation, should also be managed as CR.[85] In some cases, these lymphoid aggregates have been shown to harbor cells with the same monoclonal rearrangements of the original tumor.[86] Nevertheless, these patients do not seem to have an increased risk for relapse and most will have evidence of complete response in a subsequent evaluation.[87]

Patients with overt residual (partial remission [PR]) or stable disease, as long as asymptomatic, can also be managed conservatively, with observation or antibiotherapy as appropriate, for several months. Of interest, responses may occur as late as more than 18 months after completion of antibiotic therapy.[43,87] Progressive or symptomatic disease should be managed with local therapy, with radiotherapy being preferred. Despite its established efficacy in disease control, gastrectomy, because of its immediate morbidity and long-term metabolic complications, is currently reserved for management of rare complications such as perforation or bleeding that cannot be controlled endoscopically.[9,11]

A recent meta-analysis of 1436 patients with early stage (IE-IIE1) *H. pylori*–positive disease on prospective or retrospective studies estimates an overall CR rate of 78% after eradication of *H. pylori*,[88] but with individual study remission rates anywhere from 47% to 100%.[15,17,41–43,86,89–113] On univariate analysis of available data from the same studies, adverse risk factors for achieving remission included the presence of t(11;18), stage greater than IE1, proximal (body or fundus) location of lesions, and Western (versus Asian) residence. No good evidence is available to support adjuvant chemotherapy after anti–*H. pylori* treatment as a means to prevent recurrence in localized gastric MALT lymphomas, although this has only been formally addressed with an additional single agent (chlorambucil).[114]

The management of early-stage *H. pylori*–negative disease is controversial, with some groups suggesting involved field radiation therapy or, if radiation therapy is contraindicated, systemic therapy with rituximab as initial treatment,[9] whereas others propose a trial of anti-*Helicobacter* therapy.[11] The rationale for the latter derives from anecdotal reports of CR in *H. pylori*–negative gastric ENMZL patients who were treated exclusively with antibacterials,[115] with a metaanalysis suggesting a response rate of up to 19%.[116] These patients are assumed to have been infected with *H. pylori* that was missed by diagnostic tests or with a different species of *Helicobacter*, several of which have been recently recognized.[117,118]

Responses to radiation therapy are excellent, with some series reporting CR rates of up to 100% with total doses as low as 30 Gy.[119,120] Recurrence rate is very low in these patients, but follow up is limited for most series reported.

The optimal follow-up schedule is unknown, although most recommend periodic endoscopies every 3–6 months for the first 5 years and yearly thereafter.[9,11] Long-term follow-up data in patients with complete remission after *H. pylori* eradication document a 7.2% relapse rate overall (2.2% per year).[88] Some of these relapses were associated with *H. pylori* recurrence, and responses to retreatment

for *H. pylori* were seen. Whether most complete remissions equate to cures is a question that will require longer follow-up studies. An additional argument in favor of periodic endoscopies is that *H. pylori* may be associated with an increased risk for gastric adenocarcinoma.[121]

Molecular studies should not be done routinely in follow-up biopsy samples, outside of a research protocol. Several studies have shown that molecular disease, defined by the presence of residual t(11;18) or monoclonal immunoglobulin as evidenced by PCR methods, may still be detected even with complete pathologic remissions.[100,122,123] However, this finding is not associated with an increased relapse rate and thus is not currently helpful for clinical management.

Ocular Extranodal Marginal Zone Lymphoma

Localized forms of ocular adnexal ENMZL are most frequently managed with radiation therapy, with treatment specifics dependent on the exact location of the tumor in the orbit. Reported responses are very good, with CR rates of 83%–100%.[124–133] Local recurrence rates vary between 0% and 17%, and distant recurrences can occur up to 25% over 10 years, although disease-specific survival approaches 100% in most series. The exact site of presentation correlates with the risk for systemic recurrence, the lowest being for conjunctival and the highest for eyelid primaries.[31] Long-term complications, such as cataract formation and xerophthalmia, occur in approximately half the patients.[134]

Based on the success of antibiotherapy for *H. pylori*–associated ENMZL and reports of the presence of *Chlamydophila psittaci* (by PCR, immunofluorescence, or electron microscopy) in ocular tissues of patients affected by ocular adnexal ENMZL, a course of an anti-chlamydial antibiotic has been evaluated as initial management for these patients.[45–55] A few of these studies have reported PR or CR in a significant fraction of these patients, with a recent prospective study documenting an overall response rate (CR+PR) of 65% and suggesting improved response rate and progression-free survival in patients in whom *C. psittaci* eradication was documented.[50] However, the recommendation to treat with a tetracycline at initial diagnosis is still controversial because the reported rates of association with *C. psittaci* are highly variable—some studies suggest prevalences as high as 80%, whereas others are not able to detect the organism in any of the patients. A meta-analysis has suggested that the benefit of antibiotherapy may be restricted to specific geographic areas and, even then, is likely to be limited.[135]

Cutaneous Extranodal Marginal Zone Lymphoma

Results for both surgical excision and radiation therapy for limited disease are comparable, with CR rates approaching 100%. Both approaches have a relapse rate (usually limited to the skin) of around 45%. Encouraging results have also been obtained with intralesional injection of rituximab or α-interferon.[38]

Studies from Europe have suggested an association between *Borrelia burgdorferi* infection and ENMZL of the skin, although this has not been reproduced in Asian and American studies.[56–59] In view of this, similar to ocular lymphoma, it has been suggested that a course of a tetracycline may be a reasonable first approach, especially in locations where the association has been documented or when infection by *B. burgdorferi* is detected.

IPSID

Antibiotherapy (varying from single-agent tetracycline to triple-antibiotic therapy with ampicillin, metronidazole, and tetracycline, or an *H. pylori* regimen)[136–139] has long been recognized as being able to induce CR in early-stage disease. Recently, IPSID has been associated with chronic infection with *Campylobacter jejuni*.[44] Therefore treatment of early disease is directed at bacterial eradication. Historic rates of remission vary between 30% and 70%, depending on the study. Maximal responses may take more than 5 months of therapy, and relapses occur in a fraction of patients.

Other Extranodal Marginal Zone Lymphoma

Early-stage ENMZL in other primary sites is managed in a similar way to ocular adnexal or cutaneous forms. When feasible, surgery can be potentially curative and often may be done with primary diagnostic intent. If full resection is achieved, these patients may be observed. Otherwise, for sites not amenable to surgery or if there is residual disease after surgical excision (i.e., positive margins), radiation therapy is the usual preferred approach. If radiation is contraindicated and the patient is asymptomatic, observation is an option. Otherwise, systemic therapy as for advanced stage, preferably one with minimal toxicity, is appropriate.[9,140]

Therapy for Advanced-Stage (III/IV) Disease

The data regarding management of advanced-stage disease are also limited, because most large treatment series with long-term follow-up aggregate all indolent lymphomas and include only a small fraction of patients with MZL among other more frequent histologies. Thus most treatment approaches have been modeled after those for FL (see Chapter 80), and indeed the most common recommendation is that advanced ENMZL be managed as advanced FL.[9] In any case, there is some suggestion that responses may be better, possibly because of a usually lower burden of disease. Eligible patients should be included whenever possible in clinical trials.

As in other indolent lymphomas, extensive disease is likely incurable with current approaches, which together with a generally slow pace of progression means that systemic treatment is not always indicated. Because no benefit in survival has been demonstrated with early systemic treatment of asymptomatic disease, unless a treatable etiology has been identified, initial management of asymptomatic patients with expectant observation is acceptable. While on this watch-and-wait approach, patients should be reassessed approximately every 3 months with history, physical examination, complete blood counts, basic chemistry, and LDH. Any new symptoms or findings suggestive of transformation should be investigated with a repeat biopsy to rule it out. Routine repeat imaging studies are controversial but often used.

Indications for initiating systemic treatment include symptomatic disease caused by mass effect or effusion, risk for local compressive disease, bulky lymphadenopathy, symptomatic splenomegaly, B symptoms, cytopenias arising from bone marrow involvement, or rapid disease progression. Although unlikely to contribute to regression of established advanced disease, treatment of an underlying infection associated with the lymphoma (such as *H. pylori* for primary gastric ENMZL and *C. jejuni* for IPSID) is advisable to remove any inciting factor. Otherwise, as already mentioned, the same treatment approaches used for FL (see Chapter 80) are usually followed for ENMZL. Nonetheless, a few studies specifically addressing MZL are worth reviewing here.

Rituximab

Given its low toxicity, single-agent immunotherapy with rituximab has generated a lot of interest in the management of advanced disease. Two series of approximately 30 patients each, pooling early- and advanced-stage ENMZL, have reported overall response rates of around 75%,[141,142] with up to 48% CR in patients without previous therapy. In one of the series, median time to treatment failure was 22 versus 12 months in chemotherapy-naive versus non-naive patients, respectively.[141] Rituximab has activity in t(11;18)–positive disease.[142]

Alkylating Agents

Single-agent alkylators have also been used in this setting. A study of 24 patients with gastric ENMZL (stages IE or IV) treated with daily oral chlorambucil or cyclophosphamide for 12–24 months showed a CR rate of 75%, with the remaining patients achieving PR.[143] Remissions were durable in approximately half of the patients after a median follow-up time of 45 months. Another study of 21 patients (stages I to IV) treated with continuous alkylating drugs documented a CR rate of 42% and 89% in t(11;18)–positive and t(11;18)–negative disease, respectively.[144] After a median follow up of 7.5 years, CR was sustained in all patients with translocation-negative disease, but in only one patient otherwise.

The combination of rituximab and chlorambucil has produced an impressive 100% CR rate in 13 patients with t(11;18)–positive gastric ENMZL (stages I to IV).[145] No relapses were observed after a median follow-up of 24 months in this report but long-term data were not available.

This combination has been studied in a randomized controlled trial versus each single agent in 393 patients not responding or not suitable for local therapy.[146,147] CR rate, and 5-year event-free and progression-free survival were better with the combination, but 5-year overall survival was 90% in the whole population, without significant differences between the three arms.

Purine Analogues

The purine analogue cladribine has also been used as single-agent therapy in a series of 25 patients (stages I to IV), and CR was obtained in 84% of them. After a median follow-up time of 80 months, seven patients experienced disease relapse.[148] Of note, one of the patients treated developed a myelodysplastic syndrome immediately after the third infusion of the drug.[149] Another purine analogue, fludarabine, has been used in combination with rituximab to treat a series of 22 patients (stages I to IV).[150] At the end of treatment (three cycles, with some patients requiring six), 90% of patients achieved CR. The progression-free survival rate at 2 years in patients with gastric and extragastric ENMZL was 100% and 89%, respectively. Both purine analogues seem to have activity in t(11;18)–positive gastric ENMZL.

Other Single Agents

Other single chemotherapeutic agents whose use has been reported in ENMZL include oxaliplatin, bendamustine, bortezomib, and vorinostat. In a study of 16 patients (stages I to IV) treated with oxaliplatin, a CR rate of 56% with a median time to response of 4 months was observed.[151] Responses to bendamustine (with or without rituximab) have been documented in patients with relapsed/refractory indolent lymphomas, a small fraction of which were ENMZL[152,153]; a retrospective series of 14 ENMZL patients reported 10 CR and three PR with the combination of bendamustine and rituximab.[154] Other studies of patients with relapsed, multiply treated indolent lymphomas report encouraging responses to bortezomib (two cases with PR out of two patients)[155] and vorinostat (one CR and one PR out of nine patients).[156] Long-term follow up is not available; therefore, the role of these agents as first-line therapy has not been established.

Combination Chemotherapy

Combination chemotherapy regimens reported in ENMZL patients include CVP (cyclophosphamide, vincristine, and prednisone) followed by radiation therapy,[157] FM (fludarabine and mitoxantrone),[158] CHOP (cyclophosphamide, hydroxydaunomycin, vincristine [Oncovin], and prednisone) followed by CVP,[159] MCP (mitoxantrone, chlorambucil, and prednisone),[160] R-CHOP (rituximab, cyclophosphamide, hydroxydaunomycin, vincristine [Oncovin], and prednisone) and R-CNOP (rituximab, cyclophosphamide, mitoxantrone [Novantrone], vincristine [Oncovin], and prednisone).[161] These regimens have mostly been used in patients who were believed to have more aggressive disease. CR rates vary from 61% to 100%, with relapse rates reaching up to 36% on long-term follow-up. Advanced/transformed IPSID has usually been treated with combination chemotherapy, such as CHOP.[7,162]

Radioimmunotherapy

Radioisotope-conjugated forms of anti-CD20 antibodies (ibritumomab and tositumomab) have also been used both as first-line[163] therapy (eight CRs and one PR in nine patients with ocular adnexal ENMZL) and for relapsed disease[164,165] (three CRs and three PRs in six patients with ocular adnexal ENMZL; four CRs and one PR in six patients with a variety of primary sites). The combination of conventional radiation therapy and rituximab has been studied for early-stage follicular lymphoma.[166] There are no published studies of its use on ENMZL.

Therapy for Relapsed Disease

Limited relapses can be retreated, if feasible, with local therapy. Otherwise, treatment considerations are similar to those described for advanced disease. Symptomatic, relapsed extensive disease will usually require an alternative regimen to those previously used.

The role of hematopoietic stem cell transplantation is controversial because most series do not directly address ENMZL and thus most recommendations are again extrapolated from studies of FL.[167–171] Given that most young patients with relapsed systemic ENMZL are likely to succumb to complications of their disease, considering them for allogeneic stem cell transplantation is reasonable, although this should preferably take place on a clinical trial. Encouraging results have also recently been reported with high-dose therapy and autologous stem cell transplantation specifically for MZL.[172]

Prognosis

Overall, prognosis of limited stage ENMZL is excellent, as mentioned in each of the treatment subsections. Even for advanced disease, the expected lymphoma-specific survival at 5 years is close to 90%, with some series showing survivals similar to those of early disease. A recent retrospective analysis of SEER data lists the best 5-year overall survivals for cutaneous (88%), ocular (83%) and thyroid (85%) forms, and worst for genitourinary (76%), intestinal (69%), and central nervous system (71%) forms.[29] As in other indolent lymphomas, transformation to aggressive forms (DLBCL) can occur, but this is thought to be a rare event (less than 10% of cases) associated with acquisition of additional genetic abnormalities.[35] Regardless, even patients in CR after first-line therapy can develop DLBCL. For instance, 0.05% of individuals with gastric ENMZL who underwent successful antibiotic treatment had evidence of DLBCL between 6 months and 2 years after achieving remission.[88] On the other hand, untreated IPSID tends to evolve to large-cell transformation.[7,162]

As for other lymphomas, the International Prognostic Index (IPI)[173] (see Chapter 82) predicts outcomes, with reported 5-year overall survivals of >90%, 70%–80%, and 40%–50% for patients with low, low-intermediate/high-intermediate, and high-risk scores, respectively.[30] Nonetheless, the utility of the IPI in ENMZL has been disputed.[174] One of the main criticisms to its use in patients with indolent lymphomas is that prognostic subgroups do not have a good discriminating power, because most patients are assigned to the favorable outcome groups and only very few patients are allocated to the adverse prognostic groups.[175] To circumvent this issue, modifications of the original IPI have been proposed in some cases,[176] but none has been universally adopted.

Suggested Treatment Approach to Extranodal Marginal Zone Lymphoma

Stage I/II

Gastric H. pylori–Positive
- Antibiotic therapy
- Repeat endoscopy in 3–6 months
- If still *H. Pylori*–positive and no progression, alternative antibiotic therapy
- Repeat endoscopy in 3 months

Nongastric, Gastric H. pylori–Negative or Not Responding to Antibiotic Therapy
- Antibiotic trial for stage I gastric, ocular, or cutaneous?
- Involved field radiation therapy (30 Gy)

Stage III/IV or Relapsed After Antibiotic and Radiation Therapy
- Expectant observation until indication to treat
- Rituximab ± single-agent alkylator/purine analogue or combination chemotherapy (CVP/FND)

The recent explosion of genomic analysis of these neoplasms has also led to a plethora of findings that have been shown to have prognostic significance in ENMZL. For instance, the expression of FOXP1 in tumors predicts poor prognosis and transformation to diffuse large B-cell lymphoma.[177] Although these findings are not yet incorporated into clinical practice, as they become more widely available, they may be useful for risk stratification and therapeutic decisions (see box on Suggested Treatment Approach to Extranodal Marginal Zone Lymphoma).

SPLENIC MARGINAL ZONE LYMPHOMA

Epidemiology and Manifestations

SMZL (Fig. 79.3; E-Slide VM03955) is a rare disease, corresponding to <1% of all NHL,[8] with a yearly incidence rate of 0.25 per 100,000 adults in the United States according to SEER data.[29] The median age at diagnosis is around 65, but as with ENMZL, the age range is wide and there may be a slight female predominance. The vast majority of patients present with advanced-stage disease involving the spleen (with splenomegaly in more than 80% of patients), abdominal (mainly splenic hilar) lymph nodes, and in 83%–94% of patients, the bone marrow.[178–181] Peripheral lymphadenopathy is, however, uncommon. Liver involvement is seen in up to one-fourth of patients, and rarely other nonhematopoietic sites can also be involved. B symptoms occur in approximately 25%–60% of patients, depending on the series.[179,180]

Circulating villous lymphocytes (with short polar villi) can be seen in approximately two-thirds of patients (see Fig. 79.3B) and frank lymphocytosis in up to one-half. This has led to a prior designation of *splenic lymphoma with villous lymphocytes* being given to a specific presentation of this disorder and explains why the disease was called *SMZL with or without villous lymphocytes* in a previous version of the WHO classification. Anemia is seen in about one-half to two-thirds and thrombocytopenia in one-fifth of cases, which can be the result of bone marrow involvement or an autoimmune process (seen in approximately 15% of patients). Between 25% and 40% of patients have a low-level circulating monoclonal immunoglobulin (mostly IgM),[180] and in a few patients, especially in those with active hepatitis C virus (HCV) infection, mixed cryoglobulins can be demonstrated, which can be associated with vasculitis.[182,183]

Pathobiology and Differential Diagnosis

Etiology

Approximately 10%–20% of SMZL patients from European series have evidence of HCV infection,[178,181] and a significant fraction of

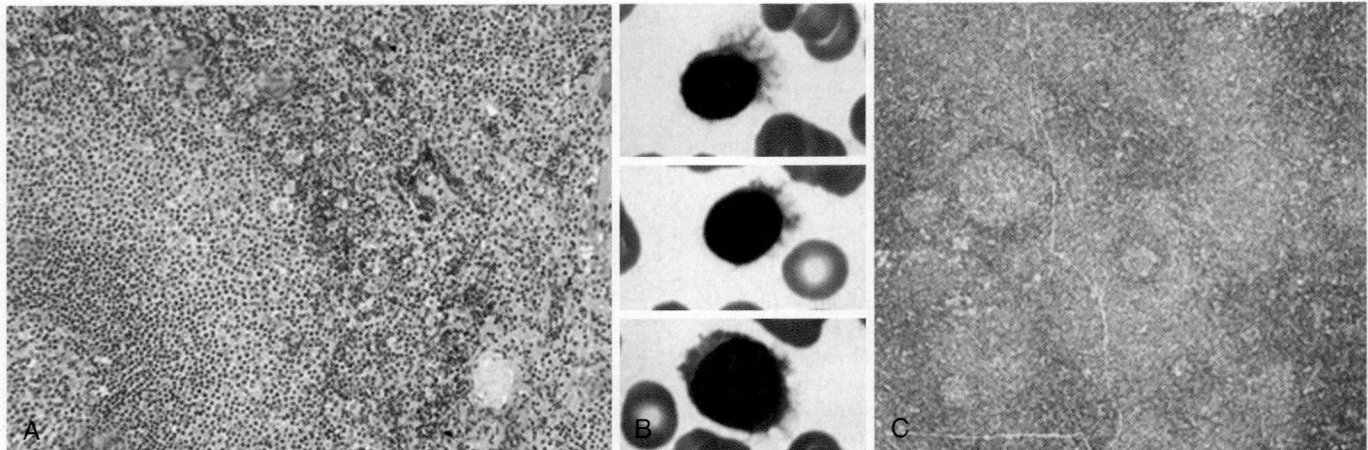

Fig. 79.3 SPLENIC MARGINAL ZONE LYMPHOMA, VILLOUS LYMPHOCYTES, AND PRIMARY NODAL MARGINAL ZONE LYMPHOMA. (A) Splenic marginal zone lymphoma is characterized by an expansion of the marginal zone cells (*left*) and their spilling into the red pulp (*right*). (B) These cells can also become leukemic and can be recognized on the peripheral blood smear. Note the polar distribution of the cytoplasmic projections. (C) Primary nodal marginal zone lymphoma is rare, and involvement of a node by extranodal disease must always be ruled out. NMZL is histologically characterized by an expansion of marginal zone cells (formerly referred to as monocytoid B cells) in between reactive germinal centers.

these patients can achieve CR after successful treatment of the infection.[183,184] This raises the possibility that, like ENMZL, this disease is associated with chronic antigenic stimulation. However, no other infections have been described in clear connection to SMZL, despite a suggested association with *Plasmodium*,[185] and thus the etiology of most cases is unknown.

Histology

The classic histology of SMZL includes a population of small lymphocytes that surrounds or replaces the germinal centers of the lymphoid follicles of the white pulp, effacing their mantle zone, and progressively merging peripherally with larger, marginal zone–like cells.[186] These cells expand to the interfollicular zones and invariably invade the red pulp (see Fig. 79.3A). A few scattered lymphoblasts are usually present, and as in ENMZL, plasmacytic differentiation can occur. Bone marrow involvement usually gives rise to nodular interstitial lymphoid infiltrates that resemble the histology of the spleen, although the cell types are usually admixed, without distinct zones. Peripheral blood involvement is typically associated with lymphocytes that have short polar villi (see Fig. 79.3B), as mentioned earlier, although the villi may be absent.

Immunophenotype

The phenotype of SMZL is similar to that of ENMZL (see earlier), but in contrast to the latter, SMZL is usually IgD-positive. The same differential diagnosis considerations apply; additionally, because this disease behaves as a chronic B-cell leukemia, it is of interest that SMZL is negative for annexin A1 and CD25 and usually negative for CD103 (in contrast to hairy cell leukemia).[186] Rare cases may be CD5-positive.[187]

Genetics

A substantial amount of genetic data on SMZL has been accumulated during the last decade. A recent review of 330 patients with SMZL documented del(7q) (affecting different loci in regions q21 to q36) as the most frequent cytogenetic abnormality (≈40% of patients).[181] Gains of genetic material from chromosomes 3 (≈25%), 8 (≈10%), and 12 (≈8%) were also seen frequently. Translocations involving

14q32, different from those seen in ENMZL, occurred in 12% of patients. The translocation t(11;18) was not seen in SMZL. More than 50% of cases had three or more cytogenetic aberrations. Deletions of 8p and 17p (TP53) have been seen in approximately 15% of cases analyzed with DNA microarrays.[77] The biologic significance of these chromosomal abnormalities is unclear at this point, although there are ongoing efforts at clarifying it.[188]

Approximately 50%–60% of SMZL have evidence of somatic hypermutation of the immunoglobulin genes,[181,188–190] and there is some evidence that, similar to CLL, these cases may have better overall prognosis.[189] Both mutated and unmutated tumors display bias in variable region usage, with predominance of VH1-2 family genes. Intraclonal variation has also been described, which suggests the presence of ongoing mutational events in these lymphomas.[191]

In contrast to hairy cell leukemia, the V600E BRAF variant has not been detected in SMZL.[192] In addition, the L265P MYD88 mutation commonly observed in Waldenström macroglobulinemia/lymphoplasmacytic lymphoma is rare in SMZL.[193] These findings may help distinguish these disorders when the diagnosis is in doubt.

Therapy

Because SMZL behaves indolently, in asymptomatic patients without significant or progressive cytopenias, expectant observation is a reasonable approach. The 5-year overall survival rate of 32 patients with asymptomatic SMZL who never received treatment was 86% in one published series.[194] In another series, 10 out of 14 untreated patients were alive between 1 and 6 years after diagnosis.[195]

Indications for lymphoma treatment are similar to those for advanced-stage ENMZL, including symptomatic splenomegaly. As for other forms of MZL, there are no data from randomized trials guiding selection of therapy, and most recommendations come from consensus opinions of experts in the field.[9]

Anti-HCV Therapy

In patients with evidence of active HCV infection, anti-HCV therapy is recommended. A study of the effects of interferon-α (IFN-α) in SMZL showed eight complete and one partial hematologic responses in nine HCV-positive patients after clearance of HCV (with two of them requiring addition of ribavirin), versus no responses in six HCV-negative individuals.[184] One patient in CR treated initially only with IFN-α had a relapse of the lymphoma with detectable levels of HCV RNA; treatment with IFN-α and ribavirin resulted in second complete virologic and hematologic responses. Given that newer anti-HCV drugs are less toxic and more effective than IFN-α, these may become first choice for these patients. Of note, evidence of monoclonal immunoglobulin gene rearrangement may persist after successful treatment of HCV and SMZL.[183]

Rituximab

Rituximab has been used as single agent or in combination with chemotherapeutic drugs in symptomatic HCV-negative patients or in those whose disease did not respond to anti-HCV treatment. The response rate to single-agent rituximab in a retrospective subseries of 25 patients with splenic and nonsplenic MZL was 88%, which compared favorably with that of 11 patients who received chemotherapy alone (55%).[196] In two other retrospective studies, rituximab was found to be an effective therapy in 90%–95% patients with SMZL, with reduction in splenomegaly and improvement in blood counts.[197,198] Because of its low toxicity, single agent rituximab is often proposed as initial therapy for symptomatic SMZL.

Splenectomy

Before rituximab was widely available and studied in SMZL, splenectomy was frequently used as first-line therapy. A benefit of this procedure, which may be done for diagnostic purposes in patients with localized disease, is the usual improvement of cytopenias occurring as a result of hypersplenism. Precise response rates to splenectomy are difficult to ascertain. All of 25 patients in a series treated with splenectomy alone had responses, including two CRs.[10] Most responses were durable: only eight of these 25 patients experienced disease progression on long-term follow up, with a median time to progression of 32 months (with a range of 4–137 months).[199] Moreover, all of 16 patients treated with first-line splenectomy in an earlier series had good responses, most likely partial (complete responses could not be assessed because of a lack of bone marrow assessment after treatment); two patients progressed subsequently.[195] Finally, another series of 28 patients documented a 5-year overall survival of 71% after splenectomy; no CRs were reported.[194] Although an effective procedure with very low operative mortality, splenectomy is associated with a long-term increased risk of infection and sepsis, and possibly a hypercoagulable state with potential cardiovascular complications.[200] On the other hand, retrospective analysis of SEER data showed no advantage of splenectomy over other treatment approaches for SMZL.[201] Given these considerations, the role of therapeutic splenectomy in SMZL has been questioned.[202,203]

Chemotherapy

Single alkylating agents (chlorambucil or cyclophosphamide) have also been used for treatment of SMZL. Most series are very small, but all report a significant fraction of responses, albeit mostly partial. Fludarabine has produced encouraging results also,[204,205] but the efficacy of cladribine is controversial.[206,207] The use of combination chemotherapy (including CVP and CHOP) has also been reported, but differences between CHOP (or CHOP-like) therapy and other less-intensive regimens could not be demonstrated.[180] In a subseries of 19 patients treated with chemotherapy alone, the 5-year overall survival rate was 64%.[194]

Radiation Therapy

In patients ineligible for any of the aforementioned therapies, radiation therapy to the spleen can be used for symptomatic control. Even

Suggested Treatment Approach to Splenic Marginal Zone Lymphoma
HCV-Positive
• Anti-HCV therapy
HCV-Negative (or Not Responding to Anti-HCV Therapy) or Relapsed
• Expectant observation until indication to treat
• Rituximab
• Splenectomy?
• Rituximab + single-agent alkylator/purine analogue or combination chemotherapy (CVP/FND)
• If contraindication to splenectomy and systemic therapy, low-dose splenic irradiation

low-dose radiation (around 4 Gy) can result in resolution of splenomegaly and correction of cytopenias,[208] at least temporarily.

Although it is tempting to compare the results of observation, splenectomy and systemic therapy, this is not prudent. All published series have considerable selection bias, because patients who are believed to have more aggressive disease have been usually offered more-intensive therapies.

Prognosis

Reported 5-year overall survival rates vary from 65%–78%,[180,194] with a median survival of 10.4 years.[10] The Italian Lymphoma Intergroup (ILI) has proposed a prognostic model using hemoglobin less than 12 g/dL, LDH higher than normal, and albumin less than 3.5 g/dL as risk factors.[178] Low-risk (no factors), intermediate-risk (one factor), and high-risk (two or more factors) patients have 5-year overall survivals of 83%, 72%, and 56%, respectively. Shorter survival has been associated with CD38 expression, unmutated variable region immunoglobulin genes, and expression of a specific set of NFκB pathway genes (by gene expression array).[188] The presence of both del(8p) and del(17p) involving TP53 is associated with worse prognosis, although isolated deletion 17p is not.[77] Transformation to aggressive lymphoma may occur in around 10% of cases[10] (see box on Suggested Treatment Approach to SMZL).

NODAL MARGINAL ZONE LYMPHOMA

Epidemiology and Manifestations

NMZL represents approximately 2% of all NHL, corresponding to a yearly incidence rate of 0.83 per 100,000 adults in the United States according to SEER data. The reported incidence of NMZL has increased significantly over the previous decade,[29] but it is unclear whether this is the result of a true increase in the number of cases or of an increased recognition of this entity. The diagnosis requires the absence of extranodal or splenic disease, the presence of which makes ENMZL and SMZL more likely. The median age at presentation is around 60, and in most series there is a slight female predominance. Most patients present with asymptomatic lymphadenopathy, most often in peripheral lymph nodes (especially cervical and inguinal), which is frequently associated with mediastinal or abdominal involvement. The most recent series report the presence of B symptoms in less than 20% of patients.[32,179,209–213] Except in three of the published series,[210–212] the majority of patients present with stage III or IV disease (approximately 70%–80% of cases), with bone marrow involvement detected in up to two-thirds of cases. Anemia and thrombocytopenia have been described in up to 30% and 10% of cases, respectively. A monoclonal IgM is seen in approximately 10% of patients. A pediatric form, with excellent prognosis, has been recognized, reported in 2003.[214]

Pathobiology and Differential Diagnosis

Etiology

As with SMZL, some series have reported an association with HCV in up to one-fourth of NMZL cases, but with a strong geographic variation (mostly Italian and Spanish series).[209,210,212,213] No other clear association has been described.

Histology and Immunophenotype

The histology and immunophenotype of NMZL resembles that of ENMZL or SMZL (see Fig. 79.3C).[215] The frequent presence of monocytoid B cells explains why this disease has been previously called *monocytoid B-cell lymphoma*[216] and *NMZL with or without monocytoid B cells*. A primary ENMZL should always be ruled out with appropriate studies (such as endoscopy) because 30%–40% of cases presenting as NMZL may in fact represent nodal dissemination of an ENMZL of MALT type.[217,218]

Genetics

Complex genetic abnormalities are usually observed in NMZL, with the most frequent being partial trisomies of chromosomes 3 and 18, affecting the same regions as in ENMZL. None of the characteristic translocations of ENMZL are seen in NMZL, however.[77] Furthermore, del(7q) is also not observed. More than 75% of cases have mutated immunoglobulin genes.[210,219] Of interest, different VH immunoglobulin gene segments are predominantly involved in HCV-positive and HCV-negative patients, raising the possibility that distinct antigens drive different underlying chronic immune stimulation processes.[220]

Therapy

Few data are available to guide treatment of NMZL, and most recommendations are extrapolated from the management of FL.[9] As in other indolent lymphomas, expectant observation is appropriate for asymptomatic patients. Radiation therapy may be curative for early disease. Symptomatic advanced disease can be managed with the same general approach described for advanced ENMZL, although there is usually a tendency to use combination chemoimmunotherapy identical to that for FL as first-line treatment because of the generally worse outcomes with NMZL as compared with ENMZL.

Prognosis

Most series report worse prognosis for NMZL when compared with the other forms of MZL.[32] Overall survival rates at 5 years vary from 55% to 70% in most series, except for those containing a greater proportion of early-stage disease, which report 5-year survivals of up to 80%. Five-year progression-free survival is around 30%. Relapse in extranodal sites is rare. As in other lymphomas, the IPI correlates with outcomes, as does the Follicular Lymphoma International Prognostic Index (FLIPI)[221] (see Chapter 80). In a series of 47 patients, those with low-, intermediate-, and poor-risk FLIPI scores had a 5-year overall survival of approximately 90%, 70% and 35%, respectively.[209]

SUGGESTED READINGS

Al-Saleem T, Al-Mondhiry H: Immunoproliferative small intestinal disease (IPSID): a model for mature B-cell neoplasms. *Blood* 105:2274, 2005.

Armitage JO, Weisenburger DD: New approach to classifying non-Hodgkin's lymphomas: clinical features of the major histologic subtypes. Non-Hodgkin's Lymphoma Classification Project. *J Clin Oncol* 16:2780, 1998.

Berger F, Felman P, Thieblemont C, et al: Non-MALT marginal zone B-cell lymphomas: a description of clinical presentation and outcome in 124 patients. *Blood* 95:1950, 2000.

Chacon JI, Mollejo M, Munoz E, et al: Splenic marginal zone lymphoma: clinical characteristics and prognostic factors in a series of 60 patients. *Blood* 100:1648, 2002.

Craig VJ, Arnold I, Gerke C, et al: Gastric MALT lymphoma B cells express polyreactive, somatically mutated immunoglobulins. *Blood* 115:581, 2010.

Escalon MP, Champlin RE, Saliba RM, et al: Nonmyeloablative allogeneic hematopoietic transplantation: a promising salvage therapy for patients with non-Hodgkin's lymphoma whose disease has failed a prior autologous transplantation. *J Clin Oncol* 22:2419, 2004.

Fischbach W, Goebeler ME, Ruskone-Fourmestraux A, et al: Most patients with minimal histological residuals of gastric MALT lymphoma after successful eradication of *Helicobacter pylori* can be managed safely by a watch and wait strategy: experience from a large international series. *Gut* 56:1685, 2007.

Hancock BW, Qian W, Linch D, et al: Chlorambucil versus observation after anti-*Helicobacter* therapy in gastric MALT lymphomas: results of the international randomised LY03 trial. *Br J Haematol* 144:367, 2009.

Hermine O, Lefrere F, Bronowicki JP, et al: Regression of splenic lymphoma with villous lymphocytes after treatment of hepatitis C virus infection. *N Engl J Med* 347:89, 2002.

Ho L, Davis RE, Conne B, et al: MALT1 and the API2-MALT1 fusion act between CD40 and IKK and confer NF-κ B-dependent proliferative advantage and resistance against FAS-induced cell death in B cells. *Blood* 105:2891, 2005.

Husain A, Roberts D, Pro B, et al: Meta-analyses of the association between *Chlamydia psittaci* and ocular adnexal lymphoma and the response of ocular adnexal lymphoma to antibiotics. *Cancer* 110:809, 2007.

Lecuit M, Abachin E, Martin A, et al: Immunoproliferative small intestinal disease associated with *Campylobacter jejuni*. *N Engl J Med* 350:239, 2004.

Liu H, Ruskon-Fourmestraux A, Lavergne-Slove A, et al: Resistance of t(11;18) positive gastric mucosa-associated lymphoid tissue lymphoma to *Helicobacter pylori* eradication therapy. *Lancet* 357:39, 2001.

Malfertheiner P, Megraud F, O'Morain C, et al: Current concepts in the management of *Helicobacter pylori* infection: the Maastricht III Consensus Report. *Gut* 56:772, 2007.

Nathwani BN, Anderson JR, Armitage JO, et al: Marginal zone B-cell lymphoma: a clinical comparison of nodal and mucosa-associated lymphoid tissue types. Non-Hodgkin's Lymphoma Classification Project. *J Clin Oncol* 17:2486, 1999.

Olszewski AJ, Castillo JJ: Survival of patients with marginal zone lymphoma: analysis of the Surveillance, Epidemiology, and End Results database. *Cancer* 119:629, 2013.

Rinaldi A, Mian M, Chigrinova E, et al: Genome-wide DNA profiling of marginal zone lymphomas identifies subtype-specific lesions with an impact on the clinical outcome. *Blood* 117:1595, 2011.

Rosebeck S, Madden L, Jin X, et al: Cleavage of NIK by the API2-MALT1 fusion oncoprotein leads to noncanonical NF-κB activation. *Science* 331:468, 2011.

Ruskone-Fourmestraux A, Fischbach W, Aleman BM, et al: EGILS consensus report. Gastric extranodal marginal zone B-cell lymphoma of MALT. *Gut* 60:747, 2011.

Salido M, Baro C, Oscier D, et al: Cytogenetic aberrations and their prognostic value in a series of 330 splenic marginal zone B-cell lymphomas: a multicenter study of the Splenic B-Cell Lymphoma Group. *Blood* 116:1479, 2010.

Schechter NR, Portlock CS, Yahalom J: Treatment of mucosa-associated lymphoid tissue lymphoma of the stomach with radiation alone. *J Clin Oncol* 16:1916, 1998.

Seligmann M, Danon F, Hurez D, et al: Alpha-chain disease: a new immunoglobulin abnormality. *Science* 162:1396, 1968.

Senff NJ, Noordijk EM, Kim YH, et al: European Organization for Research and Treatment of Cancer and International Society for Cutaneous

Lymphoma consensus recommendations for the management of cutaneous B-cell lymphomas. *Blood* 112:1600, 2008.

Smedby KE, Vajdic CM, Falster M, et al: Autoimmune disorders and risk of non-Hodgkin lymphoma subtypes: a pooled analysis within the InterLymph Consortium. *Blood* 111:4029, 2008.

Stefanovic A, Lossos IS: Extranodal marginal zone lymphoma of the ocular adnexa. *Blood* 114:501, 2009.

Swerdlow SH, Campo E, Harris NL, et al, editors: *WHO classification of tumours of haematopoietic and lymphoid tissues*, Lyon, 2008, International Agency for Research on Cancer.

Weill JC, Weller S, Reynaud CA: Human marginal zone B cells. *Annu Rev Immunol* 27:267, 2009.

Zelenetz AD, Abramson JS, Advani RH, et al: NCCN Clinical Practice Guidelines in Oncology: non-Hodgkin's lymphomas. *J Natl Compr Canc Netw* 8:288, 2010.

Zucca E, Bertoni F, Roggero E, et al: Molecular analysis of the progression from *Helicobacter pylori*-associated chronic gastritis to mucosa-associated lymphoid-tissue lymphoma of the stomach. *N Engl J Med* 338:804, 1998.

Zullo A, Hassan C, Cristofari F, et al: Effects of *Helicobacter pylori* eradication on early stage gastric mucosa-associated lymphoid tissue lymphoma. *Clin Gastroenterol Hepatol* 8:105, 2010.

REFERENCES

For the complete list of references, log on to www.expertconsult.com.

CHAPTER 80

CLINICAL MANIFESTATIONS, STAGING, AND TREATMENT OF FOLLICULAR LYMPHOMA

John G. Gribben

Non-Hodgkin lymphoma (NHL) refers to all malignancies of the lymphoid system with the exception of Hodgkin lymphoma. Development of the lymphoid system is a highly regulated process, characterized by differential expression of a number of cell-surface and intracytoplasmic proteins and antigen receptor gene rearrangements, somatic hypermutation, and class switching. Dysregulation of this orderly process can result in humoral deficiency, autoimmunity, or malignancy. The indolent B-cell lymphomas are mature peripheral B-cell neoplasms that exclude those diseases associated with an aggressive clinical course. Despite differences in cell of origin, molecular biology, clinical presentation, and clinical course, the indolent lymphomas share common features, including frequent localization to the principal lymphoid organs, a propensity for bone marrow (BM) infiltration and leukemic presentation, and generally an indolent clinical course. The classification of NHLs has been a challenge for pathologists as well as practicing physicians. A number of classifications have been proposed over the years, leading to considerable confusion and difficulty in comparison of outcomes of clinical trials performed using different pathologic classifications. The World Health Organization (WHO) lymphoma classification lists nearly 100 different types of lymphoid neoplasm.[1] This classification uses all available information such as morphology, cytochemistry, immunophenotype, and molecular genetics as well as clinical features. The WHO classification does not include the terminology *indolent lymphoma*. This is a clinical and not a pathologic term and defines those lymphomas that tend to grow and spread slowly and produce few symptoms (http://www.nih.gov). Indolent lymphomas represent 35% to 40% of NHLs, and follicular lymphoma (FL) is the most common of the indolent lymphomas.

EPIDEMIOLOGY

It is estimated that in 2016 more than 72,500 cases of NHL will be diagnosed in the United States and more than 20,000 patients will die of their disease, making NHL the seventh most common cancer and the fifth most common cause of death from cancer (http://seer.cancer.gov/statfacts/html/nhl.html). NHL is extremely heterogeneous in its molecular pathophysiology, histology, and clinical course, and there are major differences in the incidence of subtypes in different geographic locations and among different racial and ethnic populations. This difference in geographic distribution is particularly striking for FL and in the Western world, FL is the second most common lymphoma, comprising approximately 20% of all NHLs. The incidence of FL in the United States is approximately 3.18 cases per 100,000 persons per year and in Europe is approximately 2.18 cases per 100,000 persons per year.[2] The incidence of FL and other indolent lymphomas is shown in Table 80.1. The incidence appears stable over time. There is no strong sex preponderance, but the incidence in whites is approximately twice that of black and Asian populations and the disease appears less common in Central and South America. The incidence increases with age and the median age of diagnosis is 65 years. Although most cases are sporadic, there is an increased incidence in family members of affected individuals, with a relative risk of 2.3 for siblings of patients.[3] Differentiation of complex environmental factors from true inherited factors remains

difficult. The complexity of the epidemiology of NHL mirrors the complexity of the disease and the complexity of the immune system. Since lymphomas do not constitute a single disease, it should come as no surprise that there is no single etiologic factor. The influence on immune dysregulation of viruses, chemicals, radiation, diet, and aging remains unclear. Immune suppression leads to increased incidence of aggressive lymphomas, but not usually indolent lymphomas. FL typically presents in middle age and in the older adult, and the median age at diagnosis is 60 years. There is a slight female preponderance.[2]

PATHOGENESIS

FL (Fig. 80.1) is derived from germinal center B cells and maintains the gene expression profile of this stage of differentiation.[4] FL cells express CD19, CD20, CD22, and surface immunoglobulin and 60% express CD10. A hallmark of the disease is the chromosomal translocation t(14.18) contributing to overexpression of the antiapoptotic protein BCL2. Morphologically the disease is composed of a mixture of centrocytes and centroblasts. The WHO third edition pathologic classification recommended grading in grades 1–3 according to the number of centroblasts (0–5, 6–15, and >15 per high-power field, respectively). Grade 3 was further subdivided into 3A (centrocytes still present) and 3B (sheets of centroblasts). An increased percentage of centroblasts is predictive of poor outcome. A problem with this classification is that it is poorly reproducible among pathologists. It is also clear that there are no major biologic or clinical differences between grades 1 and 2, whereas grade 3B FL is biologically distinct from grades 1–3A, with features suggesting a close relationship to diffuse large B-cell lymphoma (DLBCL).[5] These considerations led to the recommendation to group together FL grade 1–3A as FL and create a new category called FL3B. However, the gene signature in FL3B is closer to FL than to DLBCL.[6] The final classification combined FL grades 1 and 2 into one category (FL1–2 of 3) and made the distinction between FL3A and FL3B optional rather than mandatory.[7] The fourth edition of the WHO classification recognizes some distinctive clinical and genetic subtypes of FL, including primary duodenal FL and the pediatric type of FL that lacks the t(14:18) and usually presents with localized disease. Several variants of FL that lack the t(14;18) have some distinctive features, e.g., predominantly diffuse FL with deletions of 1p36 that presents with localized bulky disease in the inguinal region. The gene expression profiles of FL cases with and without t(14;18) show some differences, with t(14;18)–negative FL resembling activated late-stage germinal center B cells.[8]

Although 85% of patients with FL have the t(14;18), the pathogenesis of FL remains poorly understood. Recent studies have demonstrated frequent secondary genetic alterations including genomic gains, losses, and mutations, particularly inactivating mutations of the *MLL2* gene, which occurred in 89% of FL cases examined,[9] as well as in the *EPHA7, TNFRSF14* and *EZH2* genes. The major mutations seen in FL are shown in Table 80.2. A notable feature of these findings is that many of the mutated genes are involved in transcriptional regulation. It is likely that posttranscriptional modification of histones is of key importance in germinal center B cells and that the deregulated histone modification caused by these mutations

Incidence Rates Per 100,000 of the Indolent Lymphomas (Ref)

	All	Male	Female
Non-hodgkin lymphoma	32.2	40.2	25.9
Follicular lymphoma	3.6	3.9	3.3
Small B lymphocytic lymphoma/Chronic lymphocytic leukemia/	6.6	7.9	4.6
Lymphoplasmacytic lymphoma	0.6	0.8	0.5
Mantle cell lymphoma	0.8	1.3	0.4
Marginal zone lymphoma	2.0	2.1	1.9

From SEER data base https://seer.cancer.gov/csr/1975_2013/browse_csr.php?sectionSEL=19&pageSEL=sect_19_table.26.html (accessed January 29, 2017)

Mutations in Follicular Lymphoma

Gene Name	Abbreviation	Location	Frequency at Diagnosis
Myeloid/lymphoid or mixed-lineage leukemia 2	MLL2	12q	89%
CREB binding protein	CREBBP	16p	33%
Tumor necrosis factor receptor superfamily member 14	TNFRSF14	1p	25%
E1A binding protein p300	EP300	22q	15%
Myocyte enhancer factor 2B	MEF2B	19p	13%
Enhancer of zeste homolog 2	EZH2	7q	11%

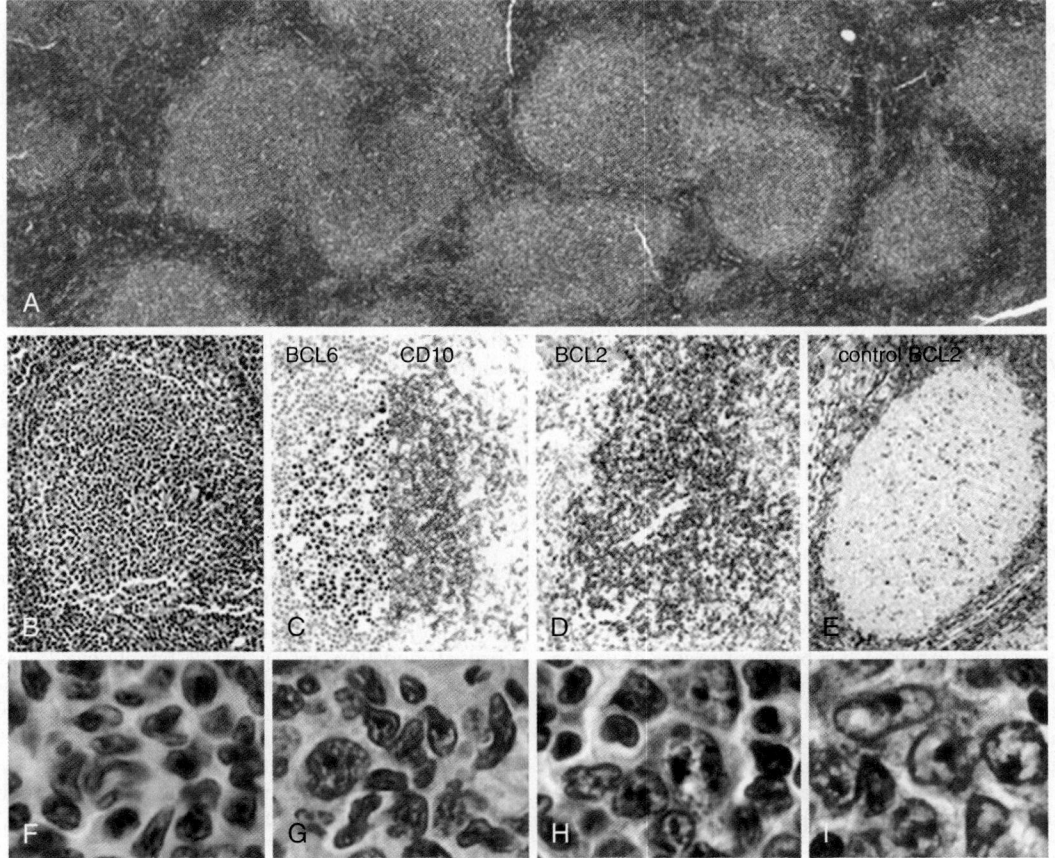

Fig. 80.1 FOLLICULAR LYMPHOMA: MORPHOLOGIC AND IMMUNOPHENOTYPIC FINDINGS. (A) Low-power photomicrograph illustrates a lymph node involved by follicular lymphoma. The lymphoma cells grow in nodules or follicles that resemble the normal lymphoid follicles of a reactive lymph node. However, in the lymphomatous growth, the follicles are crowded, show back-to-back localization, and lack many of the features of their reactive counterparts. At higher power (B), the neoplastic follicles lack mantle zones, and the normal polarization of small and large germinal center cells (centrocytes and centroblasts, respectively), which occurs because of the cellular response to antigenic stimulation as it sweeps thorough the follicle. (C) The neoplastic follicles stain for the germinal center markers, BCL6 and CD10; however, they overexpress BCL2 (D) caused by the associated translocation t(14;18) involving the *IgH* gene and *BCL2*. BCL2 is not much expressed in normal germinal center B cells (E, control for comparison). Follicular lymphoma is graded by the number of large neoplastic cells (centroblasts) present among the smaller neoplastic cells (centrocytes) (F–I). The grading system is not entirely accurate, but provides some framework for subclassifying cases morphologically. Only 0–5 centroblasts per average field is grade 1 (F); between 6 and 15 is grade 2 (G); and greater than 15 is grade 3A (H). Grades 1 and 2 are now considered together. When most of the cells in the neoplastic follicles are centroblasts without centrocytes the case is considered grade 3B (I) (see text).

is likely to result in reduced acetylation and enhanced methylation, which will act as a driver event in the development of FL. Attention has also been paid recently to the complex interaction between the malignant B cell, the host,[10] and the tumor microenvironment.[4,11,12]

CLINICAL PRESENTATION

The majority of patients present with lymphadenopathy in one or more sites. Patients with FL often present with a long history of having noted painless increased lymph nodes (LN) over a number of years before presentation. Lymphadenopathy may wax and wane and spontaneous remissions can occur, albeit rarely.[13] Disease transformation to a more aggressive histologic type is a common terminal event.[14]

Extranodal disease is relatively common and can affect any organ. The most common sites of extranodal disease include the BM, skin, gastrointestinal tract, and bone. Symptoms may be nonspecific or related to the site of disease involvement. Many patients are asymptomatic, but some, particularly those with bulky disease may present with B symptoms defined as fever, drenching sweats, or weight loss of more than 10% of body weight. Patients may present with evidence of bowel obstruction from intraabdominal lymphadenopathy, and retroperitoneal disease may manifest as obstructive uropathy. Inguinal disease may cause compression of the venous system with deep venous thrombosis. Central nervous system involvement can occur, but is uncommon in FL.

DIAGNOSIS OF FOLLICULAR LYMPHOMA

Suggested guidelines for the diagnosis of lymphomas have been outlined by the National Comprehensive Cancer Network (guidelines available at http://www.nccn.org/) and by the European Society for Medical Oncology.[15] In all cases possible, diagnosis should be confirmed by excisional biopsy of an accessible LN with review by an expert hematopathologist with expertise in lymphoma diagnosis. In patients without easily accessible peripheral nodes, computed tomography (CT) or ultrasound-guided biopsy are typically well tolerated. Fine-needle aspiration is not appropriate for diagnosis in these conditions and sufficient material must be obtained for immunophenotyping and genetic studies as required for diagnosis and assay for prognostic markers. Where possible consent should be obtained for the procurement and storage of use of excess tissue from LN biopsies at the time of presentation and at each subsequent relapse of disease for research purposes to investigate the molecular biology of these diseases as new technologies and findings become available.

Initial essential investigations are shown in Table 80.3. Physical examination should include careful examination of all peripheral LN groups including the cervical, surpaclavicular, axillary, and inguinal chains and examination of the Waldeyer ring. Abdominal examination should focus on evaluation of any intraabdominal masses, with particular attention paid to detection of enlargement of the liver or spleen. The skin should be carefully examined. Patients may present with pleural or pericardial effusions, although this is less common than in the aggressive lymphomas. Laboratory investigations should include a complete blood count to evaluate for cytopenias, which may be evidence of BM infiltration or of autoimmunity. A white blood count with differential and examination of the peripheral blood smear may elucidate leukemic involvement with disease. Baseline electrolytes including calcium and phosphate, creatinine, and liver function tests are important to determine organ dysfunction that may be related to direct infiltration by lymphoma. Elevation of lactate dehydrogenase (LDH) is an important prognostic factor and may be a useful indicator of transformation from indolent to aggressive lymphoma. Hepatitis B testing is essential as patients will likely require subsequent treatment with anti-CD20 monoclonal antibody therapy.

Staging workup also includes a CT scan of the chest, abdomen, and pelvis. Particular attention should be paid to sites of bulk disease and to the number of involved sites. BM biopsy provides essential

TABLE 80.3	Initial Evaluation of Follicular Lymphoma

Physical examination with attention to peripheral nodes, abdomen
Complete blood count, evaluation of peripheral blood
Liver function tests; LDH; β_2-microglobulin
CT scans of chest, abdomen, pelvis, (PET scan if indicated)
LN biopsy with review by an expert lymphoma histopathologist
Bone marrow biopsy/aspirate
Other studies as indicated

CT, Computed tomography; LDH, lactate dehydrogenase; LN, lymph node; PET, positron emission tomography.

TABLE 80.4	Ann Arbor Staging	
Stage	**Criteria**	
I	Involvement of 1 lymph node (I) or 1 extralymphatic organ or site (IE)	
II	Involvement of ≥2 lymph nodes on same side of diaphragm (II) or localized extralymphatic organ or site and ≥1 involved lymph node on same side of diaphragm (IIE)	
III	Involvement of lymph nodes on both sides of diaphragm (III) or same side with localized involvement of extralymphatic site (IIIE), spleen (IIIS), or both (IIIS+E)	
IV	Diffuse or disseminated involvement of 1 extralymphatic organ or tissues with or without lymph node enlargement	

information and should be performed routinely as it is required for staging of disease. Although the yield of bilateral BM biopsy is moderately higher (15%) than that of unilateral biopsy, this is not now usually performed. Liver biopsy may be indicated based upon abnormal imaging or laboratory testing.

STAGING

The staging of NHL uses the Ann Arbor Classification (Table 80.4). CT scans have replaced lymphangiography. The impact of whole-body positron emission tomography (PET), which is included in the revised guidelines for aggressive lymphomas,[16] has been much less studied in the indolent lymphomas. There is considerable heterogeneity in uptake of fluorine-18 fluorodeoxyglucose based upon histology, but PET demonstrates 94% sensitivity and 100% specificity for staging in FL.[17] Although there is insufficient data yet to recommend PET scans routinely in patients with FL, these can be useful to direct biopsy in cases where transformation is suspected.

NATURAL HISTORY

Until recently there was little evidence that the natural history of FL had changed over the last 30 years from the median survival of 10 years from diagnosis.[18] The survival of patients with FL presenting at St. Bartholomew's Hospital is shown in Fig. 80.2. There is clear evidence that the introduction of monoclonal antibodies in combination with chemotherapy has finally led to an improvement in survival, with the result that the median survival is now increased to 12–14 years.[19,20] The clinical course is extremely variable, with some patients having an extremely aggressive course and death within 1 year, while others may live for more than 20 years and never require therapy. There is therefore a need for prognostic markers that can help identify those patients who will have a good or poor prognosis. The follicular lymphoma international prognostic index (FLIPI) is a five-factor prognostic index based upon the clinical characteristics age, stage, number of nodal sites, hemoglobin, and LDH level (Table 80.5), and

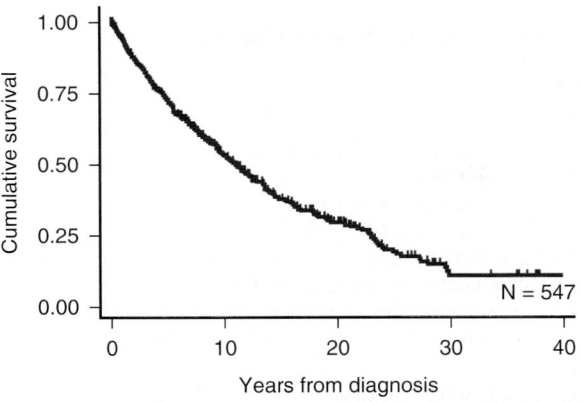

Fig. 80.2 OVERALL PROBABILITY OF SURVIVAL OF PATIENTS WITH FOLLICULAR LYMPHOMA TREATED AT ST. BARTHOLOMEW'S HOSPITAL.

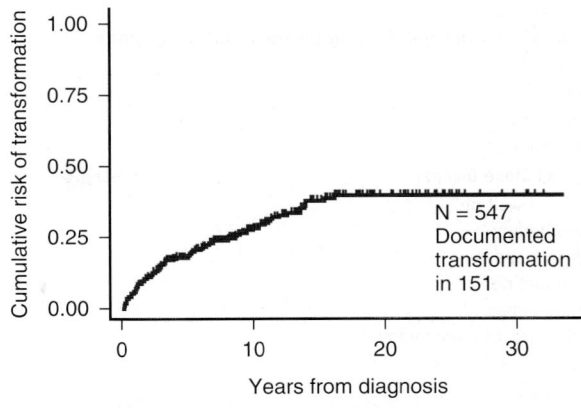

Fig. 80.3 PROBABILITY OF RISK OF TRANSFORMATION OF PATIENTS WITH FOLLICULAR LYMPHOMA.

TABLE 80.5	Factors Having Prognostic Significance in the Follicular Lymphoma International Prognostic Index (FLIPI),[21] and FLIPI2[22]		
FLIPI			
Parameter	Adverse Factor	HR	
Age	≥60 y	2.38	
Ann Arbor stage	III–IV	2.00	
Hemoglobin level	<120 g/L	1.55	
Serum LDH level	>ULN	1.50	
Number of nodal sites	>4	1.39	
FLIPI2			
Parameter	Adverse Factor	HR (in Final Model)	
β2-microglobulin	>ULN	1.5	
BM involvement	BM involvement with disease	1.59	
Hemoglobin level	<120 g/L	1.51	
Largest diameter of LN	>6 cm	1.66	
Age	>60y	1.38	

BM, Bone marrow; HR, hazard ratio; LDH, lactate dehydrogenase; LN, lymph node; ULN, upper limit of normal.

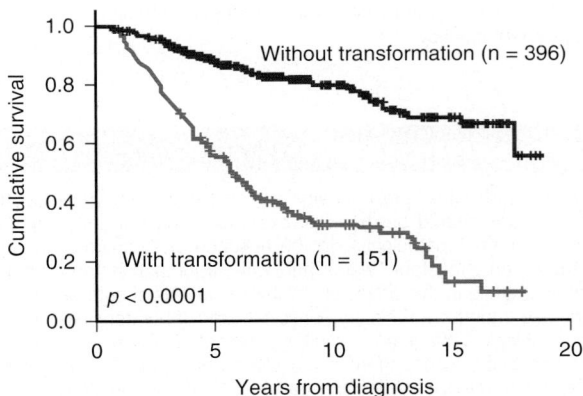

Fig. 80.4 OVERALL PROBABILITY OF SURVIVAL OF PATIENTS WITH FOLLICULAR LYMPHOMA WHO HAVE AND HAVE NOT UNDERGONE HISTOLOGIC TRANSFORMATION.

defines three prognostic risk groups of an almost equal numbers of patients.[21] This tool is useful in assessing the likely need for early treatment of patients and potential outcome, as well as in comparing the outcomes of different clinical trials. A revised FLIPI2 (incorporating β2-microglobulin, diameter of largest LN, BM involvement, and hemoglobin level) may better discriminate the outcome for patients requiring treatment, with 5-year overall survival of 96% for low-risk patients, 80% for intermediate-risk, and 50% for high-risk patients.[22]

An important factor for the prognosis of FL is whether patients undergo histologic transformation.[14] The actuarial risk of FL undergoing histologic transformation in the database of the patients treated at St. Bartholomew's Hospital is shown in Fig. 80.3 and the survival of patients with and without transformation is shown in Fig. 80.4. Despite a considerable body of information on the pathologic and molecular events associated with histologic transformation the pathogenesis of transformation remains elusive and the molecular events that have been identified have not been translated into changes in clinical practice. A major focus of research is the attempt to identify patients at high risk of transformation early in their clinical course, but this is not yet possible. The outcome of patients who undergo transformation after already having received multiple lines of therapy remains poor, but for those patients who undergo transformation and who receive their first therapy for the transformed disease, the use of chemoimmunotherapy has led to a significant improvement in the prognosis of patients.

TREATMENT OF FOLLICULAR LYMPHOMA

For most cases of FL the goal of therapy has been to maintain the best quality of life and treat only when patients develop symptoms. Any alteration to this approach requires demonstration of improved survival with early institution of therapy, or identification of criteria that define patients sufficiently "high-risk" to merit early therapy. There are many available therapies and no consensus on an optimal first-line or relapse treatment. Despite the lack of any data demonstrating benefit for early therapy, patients are being treated earlier in their disease course. There is no clear cut treatment pathway for patients with FL and although we have a good evidence base to decide on a particular treatment, there are little or no data regarding the optimal sequencing of treatment approaches in this disease. In the absence of such data, treatment choices remain empiric and should always involve discussion regarding patient choice and the goal of therapy. This is becoming even more complicated because many novel agents are either approved or in clinical studies, particularly, novel monoclonal antibodies and agents that alter the B-cell receptor signaling pathways or antiapoptotic pathways. The impact of these new agents on practice will be dependent upon the results of the ongoing clinical trials.

Multiple treatment approaches exist for advanced stage low-grade lymphomas and these patients are best treated in the setting of clinical trials. Options range from a "watch and wait" expectant management approach, to single agent chemotherapy or monoclonal antibody therapy with rituximab, to combination chemoimmunotherapy, with use of autologous or allogeneic stem cell transplantation (SCT) (Table 80.6). Patients remaining on an expectant course should be followed every 3–6 months for 5 years and then annually if stable,

TABLE 80.6   Treatment Strategies for Indolent Lymphomas

Localized Disease
Radiotherapy
"Watchful waiting"

Advanced Stage Disease
"Watchful waiting"
Chemotherapy
Alkylating agents
Bendamustine
Purine analogs
Combination chemotherapy
Monoclonal antibodies
Unconjugated
Conjugated—radioimmunoconjugates and immunotoxins
Chemotherapy + monoclonal antibodies (chemoimmunotherapy)
High-dose chemotherapy plus autologous/allogeneic stem cell
   transplantation
Reduced intensity conditioning allogeneic transplantation.
Palliative radiotherapy

TABLE 80.7   Criteria for Delaying Treatment

GELF[26]
All of the following

- Maximum diameter of disease <7 cm
- Fewer than 3 nodal sites
- Absence of systemic symptoms
- Spleen <16 cm on CT
- No significant effusions
- No risk of local compressive symptoms
- No circulating lymphoma cells or marrow compromise
  (Hb ≤10 g/dL, WBC <1.5 or platelets <100,000/dL)

BNLI[27]
Absence of all of the following

- B symptoms or pruritus
- Rapid generalized disease progression
- Marrow compromise (Hb ≤10 g/dL, WBC <3.0 or platelets
  <100,000/dL)
- Life-threatening organ involvement
- Renal infiltration
- Bone lesions

BNLI, British National Lymphoma Investigation; CT, Computed tomography; GELF, Groupe pour l'Etude de Lymphome Folliculaire; Hb, hemoglobin; WBC, white blood cells.

Management of Follicular Lymphoma

Patients most often present with asymptomatic lymphadenopathy. The diagnosis should be made by excisional biopsy and reviewed by an expert hematopathologist. In the absence of symptoms requiring treatment, an expectant "watch and wait" approach is the treatment of choice. While in this phase of treatment patients should be followed every 3–6 months for history, physical, and laboratory examination with radiologic restaging as clinically indicated. Once a decision to treat has been made, there is no clear treatment algorithm and a number of treatment options are available. The treatment goal, whether palliative or potentially with curative intent, is dependent upon the age and performance status of patients. Enrollment in a clinical trial should be the treatment of choice. For younger patients in whom high-dose therapy may be indicated later in their disease course, it is best to avoid profoundly myelotoxic regimens. Rituximab maintenance therapy in first remission given 2-monthly for two years has been demonstrated to improve progression-free, but not overall survival. The role of maintenance therapy in first remission using interferon-α remains controversial. The choice of therapy after first relapse is also dependent upon the goal of therapy, but is also dependent upon the previous therapy given, response, and duration of response. Autologous or allogeneic stem cell transplantation has a role to play in selected younger patients with this disease.

with history, physical exam, and blood counts including LDH. Special attention should be paid to any change in symptoms that might be suggestive of transformation as these are an indication for a repeat biopsy to examine for histologic evidence to confirm transformation. Repeat scanning is not routinely performed unless this is indicated by symptoms or signs.

Since there is no clearly defined treatment algorithm for most patients with FL, eligible patients should be included whenever possible in clinical trials. This ensures delivery of optimal care and helps inform design of subsequent trials, hopefully leading to cure. Information on available clinical trials can be found at http://www.clinicaltrials.gov.

WHEN TO INSTITUTE THERAPY

Stage I–II Disease

Involved site radiation therapy is the preferred treatment for the approximately 10% of patients who present with limited stage, nonbulky disease. Treatment with photons, electrons, or protons may all be appropriate depending on clinical circumstances. This treatment option is offered with curative potential[23] but has to be weighed against the potential toxicity in terms of the radiation therapy to other tissues. In patients with large tumor burden or with other adverse risk factors, systemic therapy is indicated. There is no proven role of radiation consolidation therapy.

Bulky Stage II and Stage II/IV Disease

Expectant management is the treatment of choice for asymptomatic patients with low-bulk disease until clear indications for initiation of treatment are seen, except for those patients enrolled in a clinical trial assessing the impact of early therapy. This approach is based upon the demonstration of no survival advantage for institution of immediate treatment compared with deferred treatment until time of progression.[24] Three randomized trials, performed in the pre–rituximab era, confirmed no survival benefit for early therapy.[25–27] In the National Cancer Institute study in 104 newly diagnosed patients with FL, deferred treatment was compared with immediate treatment with ProMACE-MOPP followed by total nodal irradiation. An updated analysis of this data is long overdue, but there was no difference in overall survival (OS) between the two arms at the time of the last analysis.[25] The Groupe pour l'Etude de Lymphome Folliculaire (GELF) used defined criteria for patients for whom immediate therapy was not felt to be indicated (Table 80.7) and randomized 193 patients to deferred treatment or to receive prednimustine 200 mg/m² per day for 5 days per month for 18 months or IFN-α 5 million units (MU)/day for 3 months followed by 5 MU three times per week for 15 months.[26] The median OS time was not reached and was the same in all three arms of the study. The British National Lymphoma Investigation (BNLI)[27] compared treatment in 309 patients with asymptomatic advanced-stage, indolent lymphoma in whom 158 patients were randomized to receive immediate therapy with oral chlorambucil 10 mg per day continuously and 151 patients were randomized to deferred treatment until disease progression (see Table 80.7). In both arms, local radiotherapy to symptomatic nodes was allowed. There was no difference in OS or cause-specific survival between the two groups with median follow up of 16 years. A subsequent multicenter study examined whether rituximab could delay the need for chemotherapy or radiotherapy

TABLE 80.8   Chemotherapy Regimens in Indolent Lymphomas

BR (Every 28 Days) Bendamustine 120 mg/m^2 days 1 and 2 Rituximab 375 mg/m^2 IV day 1	**ProMACE-MOPP** Cycles repeated every 28 days
CVP-R (Every 21 Days) Cyclophosphamide 750 mg/m^2 IV on day 1 Vincristine1.4 mg/m^2, up to a maximal dose of 2 mg IV, on day 1 Prednisone 40 mg/m^2 daily PO days 1–5 Rituximab 375 mg/m^2 IV day 1[32]	***Day 1*** Cyclophosphamide 650 mg/m^2 IV Doxorubicin 25 mg/m^2 IV Etoposide 120 mg/m^2 IV Prednisone 60 mg/m^2 orally daily days 1–14
R-CHOP (Every 21 Days) Cyclophosphamide 750 mg/m^2 IV on day 1 Doxorubicin 50 mg/m^2 IV on day 1 Vincristine1.4 mg/m^2, up to a maximal dose of 2 mg IV, on day 1 Prednisone 100 mg daily orally on days 1–5 Rituximab 375 mg/m^2 IV on day 1 of each therapy cycle[33] or by alternate schedule[34]	***Day 8*** Mechlorethamine 6 mg/m^2 IV Vincristine 1.4 mg/m^2 (maximum 2 mg) IV on day 8 Procarbazine 100 mg/m^2 orally daily days 8–14 ***Day 15*** Methotrexate 500 mg/m^2 IV on day 15 with leucovorin 50 mg/m^2 orally every 6 hours for four doses beginning 24 hours after methotrexate
CNOP (Every 21 Days) Cyclophosphamide 750 mg/m^2 IV on day 1 Mitoxantrone 10 mg/m^2 IV on day 1 Vincristine1.4 mg/m^2, up to a maximal dose of 2 mg IV, on day 1 Prednisone 50 mg/m^2 daily orally on days 1–5	**R-Hyper-CVAD (Every 21 Days)[36]** ***Cycles 1, 3, 5 and 7*** Rituxuimab 375 mg/m^2 IV on day 1 Cyclophosphamide (with mesna) 300 mg/m^2 IV over 3 hours every 12 hours on days 2–4 (total 6 doses) Vincristine 1.4 mg/m^2 (maximum 2 mg) IV on days 5 and 12 Doxorubicin 16.6 mg/m^2 IV by continuous infusion on days 5–7 Dexamethasone 40 mg/day PO/IV on days 2–5 and days 12–15.
R-CHVP-IFN (Every 28 Days for 6 Months, Then Every 2 Months for 6 Months).[35] Cyclophosphamide 600 mg/m^2 Doxorubicin 25 mg/m^2 Etoposide 100 mg/m^2 on day 1 (replaces original teniposide 60 mg/m^2 on day 1) Prednisolone 40 mg/m^2 on days 1–5 Interferon-α 5–3 times a week Patients being treated with R-CHVP also received 375 mg/m^2 of rituximab IV on day 1 of each therapy cycle for 6 cycles	***Cycles 2,4, 6 and 8*** Rituxuimab 375 mg/m^2 IV on day 1 Methotrexate 200 mg/m^2 IV over 2 hours, followed by 800 mg/m^2 IV continuous infusion over 22 hours on day 2 Leucovorin 50 mg PO starting 12 hours after completion of methotrexate infusion, followed by 15 mg PO every 6 hours for 8 dosed until the methotrexate level is less than 0.1 µM/L. Cytarabine 3000 mg/m^2 IV over 2 hours every 12 hours on days 3 and 4 (4 doses total)
FMD (Every 28 Days) Fludarabine 25 mg/m^2 IV on day 1–3 Mitoxantrone 10 mg/m^2 IV on day 1 Dexamethasone 20 mg /day PO days 1–5 Patients being treated with R-FMD also received 375 mg/m^2 of rituximab IV on day 1 of each therapy cycle	**Rituximab Monotherapy** Rituximab 375 mg/m^2 weekly for 4 weeks

compared with watchful waiting.[28] A total of 463 patients were randomly assigned to watchful waiting, rituximab 375 mg/m^2 weekly for 4 weeks (rituximab induction), or rituximab induction followed by a maintenance schedule of 12 further infusions given at 2-monthly intervals for 2 years (maintenance rituximab). The rituximab induction arm was closed early and the study continued to accrue to the other two arms. There was a significant difference in the time to start of next treatment, with 46% of watchful waiting patients still not needing treatment at 3 years compared with 88% in the maintenance rituximab group (p <.0001) and 78% in the rituximab induction group.

A major clinical trial question is whether identification of clinical or molecular risk factors can guide which patients are candidates for early therapy. A survival predictor score has also been developed from gene expression profiling studies.[4] The results from this study suggest that the molecular determinants of biologic heterogeneity are already present in the diagnostic LN biopsies rather than by the later acquisition of secondary genetic changes. A major component of the gene expression prognostic signature is related to immune cells in the tumor microenvironment.[11,12,29] Whereas it is to be hoped that in the future guidelines for treatment will be based upon clinical staging systems, genetic profiles, and immune response signatures, it has not yet been established which factors help us to decide who should have immediate therapy. This may well have practical implications since it has been demonstrated that patients who progress within 2 years of diagnosis have poorer outcome[30] and might well benefit from earlier institution of treatment.

Although there are little available data to suggest that we should change our practice of "watch and wait" for the asymptomatic low-bulk patients, data suggest that this practice is becoming much less common in the United States.[31] The National Lymphocare study is a prospective observational study designed to assess presentation, prognosis, treatment, and clinical outcomes in newly diagnosed FL. The treating physician determines management according to clinical judgment with no prescribed treatment regimen and data regarding histology, stage, therapy, response, relapse, and death are recorded. Among 2708 patients enrolled at 265 centers, only 17.7% of patients were initially observed and of these, 22% received active therapy within 1 year and 31% within 2 years, the majority with chemoimmunotherapy. This observation is in stark contrast to the data from the BNLI study which demonstrated that, when censored for non-lymphoma death, 19% of patients and 40% of those older than 70 years who were randomized to expectant management still did not require therapy at 10 years.[27]

TREATMENT APPROACHES

Treatment is indicated in patients with symptomatic disease, bulky lymphadenopathy and/or splenomegaly, risk of local compressive disease, marrow compromise, or steady progression of disease. Once indicated, numerous treatment approaches are available (Table 80.8). The concept that the approach can be to "do nothing" or discuss an approach with considerable morbidity and mortality even including

TABLE 80.9 Studies of Rituximab Maintenance Therapy in Indolent Lymphomas

Trial	Disease Setting	Diseases Included	Previous Therapy
ECOG[37]	1st line	Follicular Small lymphocytic	CVP
SAKK[38]	1st line Relapsed/refractory	Follicular Mantle cell	Rituximab
EORTC[39]	Relapsed/refractory	Follicular	CHOP vs R-CHOP
GLSG[40]	Relapsed/refractory	Follicular Mantle cell	FCM vs. R-FCM
LYM-5[41]	Relapsed/refractory	Follicular Small lymphocytic	Rituximab

CHOP, Cyclophosphamide, adriamycin, vincristine, prednisone; CVP, cyclophosphamide, vincristine, prednisone; FCM, fludarabine, cyclophosphamide, mitoxantrone; R-CHOP, rituximab plus CHOP; R-FCM, rituximab plus FCM.

approaches such as SCT is a confusing one for the newly diagnosed patient (as well as for the physician) and considerable consultation time is required to review available treatment approaches. Staging of response in FL is by the revised response criteria.[16] Depending on the treatment approach used, restaging after two to three cycles of therapy can be useful to ensure responsiveness, and the patient is then fully restaged after completion of therapy. Whereas curative approaches are being sought in aggressive lymphomas, the failure to achieve complete remission (CR) or complete eradication of disease does not have the same implication in FL as in aggressive lymphomas and depending upon the goal of therapy a partial remission (PR) may be a sufficient response to alleviate symptoms. The more commonly used regimens in indolent lymphomas are shown in Table 80.9.[32–41]

In the absence of a clear standard of care with curative potential, optimal first-line treatment remains enrolment in randomized clinical trials wherever possible. In the National Lymphocare study,[42] academic sites are more likely than community sites to treat patients on clinical trials (12% versus 4%), but it is lamentable that only 6% of patients were enrolled in clinical trials. For patients who are not eligible for or who refuse entry into clinical trials, there is data demonstrating higher response rates and longer duration of responses, and perhaps improved survival with chemoimmunotherapy. Many investigators favor alkylator over fludarabine-based regimens for FL, based upon concerns regarding the ability to obtain stem cells for later use for autologous SCT (ASCT) in fludarabine-treated patients.[43] It is suggested that more aggressive first-line therapy should be offered to patients who progress within 1 year of presentation, since these patients have a worse outcome.[26] Older adult patients or those with poor performance status may remain candidates for single-agent chlorambucil, although this is given most often in combination with rituximab. Single-agent rituximab therapy is appropriate for patients who choose to avoid chemotherapy and is a reasonable treatment choice based upon the results of clinical trials of standard or prolonged induction with or without maintenance therapy with rituximab. Although data suggest a survival advantage with the use of interferon (IFN)-α in combination with chemotherapy, this is associated with a significant side effect profile and this agent is now rarely used. Optimal results are seen when radioimmunoconjugates are used earlier in the disease course. On the basis of results showing no benefit for ASCT, there is no indication for the use of high dose therapy and SCT in first remission in FL unless as part of a clinical trial.

Chemoimmunotherapy is now the treatment of choice for FL. No randomized trials demonstrate a benefit for the addition of anthracyclines, but cyclophosphamide, adriamycin, vincristine, prednisone, and rituximab (R-CHOP) is heavily favored over cyclophosphamide, vincristine, prednisone, and rituximab (CVP-R) or fludarabine-based regimens. Following demonstration of improved outcome using bendamustine plus rituximab (BR) compared with R-CHOP[44] or to fludarabine plus rituximab,[45] the use of BR has greatly increased. BR also has improved tolerability and can be given without the

complication of hair loss. Choice to initiate therapy was associated with FLIPI, stage, and grade but FLIPI was not associated with decision to use a specific treatment approach. In the Lymphocare study, significant regional and center differences are observed and strongly suggest that physician preference is the predominant factor that drives initial therapy. For example, initial "watch and wait" was used in 31% of patients in the Northeast, but in 13% of patients in the Southeast, whereas fludarabine-based chemoimmunotherapy was used in 18% of patients in the Southwest and in only 3% of patients in the Northeast.

Alkylating Agents

The alkylating agents, chlorambucil and cyclophosphamide, with or without prednisone and CVP or CHOP, and other alkylator-based combination chemotherapy regimens have been the standard of therapy for decades. Single-agent alkylators at different doses and schedules produce overall response (OR) rates of 50% to 75% in FL.[46,47] Comparable response rates, but higher CR rates with longer progression-free survival (PFS) are seen with CVP compared with chlorambucil, but have no survival advantage.[48,49] The addition of anthracyclines has not improved the response rate or duration of the response,[50,51] but its use may be associated with a lower risk of histologic transformation.[25,52] This finding has yet to be confirmed, particularly in the era of chemoimmunotherapy.

Purine Analogues

The purine analogues have been studied extensively in various types of indolent lymphoma. Fludarabine monotherapy produces response rates of 65% to 84%, with 37% to 47% CR in previously untreated patients with FL.[53] In a randomized trial of 381 previously untreated indolent lymphoma patients CR rates were higher with fludarabine than CVP.[54] Fludarabine combinations result in increased response rates, with 89% CR rate in an Eastern Cooperative Oncology Group (ECOG) trial combining fludarabine and cyclophosphamide,[55] while fludarabine and mitoxantrone (FM), produced a 91% overall response rate (ORR), 43% CR and 2-year disease-free survival (DFS) of 63%.[56] A higher CR rate was seen with FM (68%) compared with CHOP (42%) in a randomized trial.[57] The use of alkylator-based regimens or purine analog–based regimens appears to vary geographically, suggesting personal preference for the use of regimens in which the clinician has experience, rather than alterations of practice based on the results of the published studies.

Bendamustine

Bendamustine is a potent alkylating agent that has been demonstrated to have substantial efficacy in NHL patients, including those with FL. Bendamustine is highly effective in rituximab-refractory FL and in patients whose disease is refractory to other alkylating agents. It has also demonstrated considerable efficacy in previously untreated FL, both alone and in combination with rituximab or other chemotherapeutic agents.[58,59] Increased understanding of the mechanisms of action of bendamustine and the efficacy of bendamustine in combination with rituximab in newly diagnosed or relapsed/refractory FL[44,45,58] has led to investigation of other combinations. Ongoing studies are examining bendamustine with other agents.

Biologic Therapy

IFN-α is approved by the Food and Drug Administration (FDA) for the treatment of advanced stage FL in combination with anthracycline-based chemotherapy, based upon improved survival in clinical trials,[21,60,61] and meta-analysis of phase III trial data.[62] IFN-α was more widely used in Europe than the United States, where it is felt

TABLE 80.10	Randomized Trials of Chemotherapy Versus Chemoimmunotherapy					
Study	Treatment, Number of Patients	Median FU, Months	OR %	CR %	Median TTF, Months	OS %
M39021[32]	CVP, 159	53	57	10	15	77
	R-CVP, 162		81	41	34	83
					$p < .0001$	$p = .0290$
GLSG[33]	CHOP, 205	18	90	17	29	90
	R-CHOP, 223		96	20	NR	95
					$p < .001$	$p = .016$
M39023[79]	MCP, 96	47	75	25	26	74
	R-MCP, 105		92	50	NR	87
					$p < .0001$	$p = .0096$
FL2000[80]	CHVP-IFN, 183	42	73	63	46	84
	R-CHVP-IFN 175		84	X	67	91
					$p < .0001$	$p = .029$

CHOP, Cyclophosphamide, adriamycin, vincristine, prednisone; CVP, cyclophosphamide, vincristine, prednisone; CHVP-IFN, cyclophosphamide, doxorubicin, teniposide, prednisone, IFN-α; CR, complete remission; FU, follow-up; MCP, MCP received a combination of mitoxantrone 8 mg/m^2 intravenously on days 1 and 2, chlorambucil 3 $\times$ 3 mg/m^2 orally on days 1 to 5, and prednisolone 25 mg/m^2 orally on days 1 to 5; NR, no response; OR, overall response; R-CHOP, rituximab plus CHOP; R-CHVP-IFN, rituximab plus CHVP-IFN; R-CVP, rituximab plus CVP; R-MCP, rituximab plus MCP; TTF, time to treatment failure.

that its toxicity profile outweighs potential benefit. In the Southwest Oncology Group (SWOG) study,[63] 571 patients with stage III and IV indolent lymphoma were treated with ProMACE-MOPP and 279 responding patients were randomized to 24 months of observation versus treatment with IFN-α. No statistically significant difference in PFS or OS was observed between observation and IFN-α groups at 4 years.

Monoclonal Antibody Therapy

Monoclonal antibodies remain the most exciting agents to emerge in the treatment of indolent lymphomas. The most widely used monoclonal antibody is rituximab, a chimeric unconjugated antibody against the CD20-antigen licensed by the FDA[64] and the European Agency for the Evaluation of Medicinal Products[65] for treatment of patients with relapsed or refractory, CD20-positive low-grade or FL; for the first-line treatment of CD20-positive FL in combination with CVP chemotherapy; and for the treatment of CD20-positive low-grade NHL in patients with stable disease or who achieve a PR or CR following first-line treatment with CVP chemotherapy. The use of this agent has a profound effect in finally leading to improvement in patient survival in FL.[19,20,66]

Following phase I studies,[67] rituximab at a dose of 375 mg/m^2 weekly for 4 weeks was selected for the pivotal phase II trial[68] and although this remains the standard dose, the optimal dose and schedule of rituximab is still unknown. In relapsed patients with FL OR to rituximab monotherapy was 60% with a median PFS for responders of 13 months. Factors associated with lower response rates include chemoresistant disease,[68] bulky disease,[69] and treatment late in the disease course.[70] OR was 73% in previously untreated patients with low-bulk disease,[71] and some of these patients needed no further treatment and had no evidence of polymerase chain reaction (PCR) detectable minimal residual disease (MRD) after 7 years.[72] Extended use with 8 weeks instead of 4 is associated with improvement in OR and duration of response.[73] Comparable or even longer durations of response have been observed with retreatment.[74]

A number of trials in front-line and in relapsed/refractory patients have investigated the potential benefits of extended or maintenance rituximab treatment[37–41,75,76] and all demonstrated prolonged time to progression in patients receiving maintenance rituximab (see Table 80.9). The results from the E1496 randomized trial from ECOG and Cancer and Leukemia Group B comparing CVP alone to CVP followed by rituximab in patients with advanced-stage FL demonstrated that addition of rituximab maintenance significantly improved OS,[37] and led to FDA approval for rituximab therapy

in patients responding to CVP chemotherapy. The results of the primary rituximab and maintenance (PRIMA) study demonstrated an advantage in PFS for maintenance rituximab therapy offered after initial chemoimmunotherapy.[76] The study remains too premature to determine whether this will have an impact on OS and questions remain as to whether this should be standard of care.[77]

Chemoimmunotherapy

In a phase II study, 40 patients with indolent lymphoma were treated with six infusions of rituximab (375 mg/m^2 per dose) in combination with six doses of CHOP chemotherapy (R-CHOP),[34] and OR was 95%, with 55% CR. In a phase II study of 40 patients with indolent lymphomas, rituximab in combination with fludarabine produced OR of 90%, with 80% CR, with similar response rates in treatment-naive and previously treated patients.[78]

A number of randomized trials show a benefit for the use of rituximab with chemotherapy compared with chemotherapy alone (Table 80.10).[32,33,39,79,80] Each study showed an improvement in time to treatment failure and more recent follow-up data suggests improved OS in patients treated with chemoimmunotherapy compared with chemotherapy alone. A meta-analysis of these trials demonstrates that OS, OR and disease control are significantly better in those on chemoimmunotherapy compared with chemotherapy for FL and mantle cell lymphoma (MCL).[81] Data from the German low grade study group (GLSG) suggest that it is the addition of rituximab that has led to the recent improvement in survival of patients with FL.[20] An independently assessed analysis of the clinical benefits provided by rituximab in relation to cost concluded that it is highly-cost effective.[82]

The largest FL trial reported is the PRIMA study.[76] This study enrolled 1217 patients to receive initial chemoimmunotherapy from three possible regimens, but of note 75% received R-CHOP. All patients had fulfilled the criteria for treatment and 80% had FLIPI intermediate or high-risk features. Responding patients were randomized to receive no further therapy or to receive 12 doses (every 8 weeks) for two years.

Patients who received rituximab maintenance therapy had significantly better rates of 3-year PFS than did those who received observation (75% versus 58%) and the benefit to maintenance was observed in all FLIPI groups. Time to next treatment was also longer in the maintenance group than in the observation group. There were increased toxicities in the maintenance group, with most being infections, but these were largely self-limiting.

The type II anti-CD20 monoclonal antibody obinutuzumab is approved for use in combination with bendamustine for patients who are refractory to or relapse early after use with rituximab containing regimens and showed improved outcome in the Gallium study comparing obinutuzumab plus chemotherapy head-to-head with rituximab plus chemotherapy (NCT01332968).

Conjugated Radio-Labeled Monoclonal Antibody Therapy

Complexing a radioisotope to a monoclonal antibody (radioimmunoconjugate) might be expected to improve efficacy over antibody therapy alone. Tositumomab complexes [131]Iodine to the anti-B1 antibody and has been studied extensively in the treatment of heavily pretreated,[83] untreated,[84] and for retreatment of indolent lymphomas.[85] Best responses are seen in previously untreated patients with FL treated with a single treatment course with tositumomab in whom there was a 95% OR, 75% CR, and 80% of assessable patients achieved eradication of PCR detectable MRD patients.[84] Median PFS was 6.1 years, with 40 patients remaining in remission for 4.3–7.7 years and no cases of myelodysplastic syndrome were observed. A SWOG study investigated chemoimmunotherapy with six cycles of CHOP chemotherapy followed 4–8 weeks later by tositumomab in 90 patients with previously untreated, advanced-stage FL.[86] The OR was 91%, including 69% CR and at median follow-up time of 5.1 years, the estimated 5-year OS was 87%, and PFS 67%, 23% better than CHOP alone on previous SWOG protocols. Ibritumomab Tiuxetan is a ^{90}Y-labeled anti-CD20 antibody and produced OR of 74% and 15% CR in 57 FL patients refractory to rituximab.[88] Toxicity is primarily hematologic, with nadir counts occurring at 7–9 weeks and lasting approximately 1–4 weeks. The risk of hematologic toxicity increased with dose delivered and with degree of baseline BM lymphoma involvement.[89] An acceptable safety profile was observed in relapsed patients with less than 25% lymphoma marrow involvement, adequate marrow reserve, platelets greater than 100,000 cells/μL, and neutrophils greater than 1500 cells/μL.

High Dose Therapy as Consolidation of First Remission

The role of high dose therapy and ASCT in patients with FL during first remission was explored in phase II trials,[90,91] and in three phase III randomized trials.[35,87,92] The GLSG trial[92] recruited 307 previously untreated patients up to 60 years of age and patients who responded after induction chemotherapy with two cycles of CHOP or mitoxantrone-chlorambucil-prednisone (MCP) and were randomized to ASCT or IFN-α maintenance. Among 240 evaluable patients, the 5-year PFS was 64.7% for ASCT, and 33.3% in the IFN-α arm ($p < .0001$). Acute toxicity was higher in the ASCT group, but early mortality was below 2.5% in both study arms. Longer follow-up is necessary to determine the effect of ASCT on OS. In the Groupe Ouest-Est des Leucémies Aigües et des Maladies du Sang study, 172 patients newly diagnosed with advanced FL were randomized either to cyclophosphamide, doxorubicin, teniposide, prednisone (CHVP), and IFN-α or to high-dose therapy followed by purged ASCT.[87] Patients treated with high-dose therapy had a higher response rate than patients who received chemotherapy and IFN-α (81% versus 69%, $p = .045$) and a longer median PFS (not reached versus 45 months), but this did not translate into a better OS because of an excess of secondary malignancies after transplantation. A subgroup of patients with a significantly higher event-free survival rate ASCT could be identified using the FLIPI. The GELF94 study enrolled 401 previously untreated patients with advanced-stage FL who were randomized to receive CHVP plus IFN-α compared with four courses of CHOP followed by HDT with total body irradiation (TBI) and ASCT and overall response (OR) rates were similar in both groups (79% and 78% respectively) and 87% of eligible patients underwent ASCT. Intent-to-treat analysis after a median follow up of 7.5 years showed no difference between the two arms for OS ($p = .53$) or PFS ($p = .11$). Long-term follow up demonstrated no statistically significant benefit in favor of first-line

ASCT in patients with FL, which the investigators conclude, should be reserved for relapsed patients. A meta-analysis concluded that high-dose therapy and ASCT does not improve overall survival in FL.[93] In view of these results, ASCT should be used in first remission only in the setting of clinical trials.

TREATMENT OF RELAPSED INDOLENT LYMPHOMA

The treatment options after relapse remain the same as for first-line therapy (see Table 80.6), and relapsed patients should ideally be treated in clinical trials. Agents approved for rituximab refractory disease include idelalisib and obinutuzumab. Relapsed asymptomatic disease is not necessarily an indication for treatment and patients can again be managed expectantly. A number of factors must be taken into account in planning therapy and it is not possible to define treatment at relapse without considering the goal of therapy (palliative versus potentially curative) performance status, previous therapy, response, and duration of response. Single-agent rituximab is approved for relapsed lymphoma and is widely used in this setting. A multicenter randomized trial in relapsed patients has demonstrated a survival advantage for chemoimmunotherapy with CHOP-R or CHOP followed by rituximab compared with CHOP alone, and a further benefit for rituximab maintenance therapy.[39] For younger patients who are suitable candidates for either ASCT or reduced intensity conditioning (RIC) allogeneic transplantation, referral to a transplant center should be considered early to discuss the potential role and timing of transplantation. Best results are seen when transplantation is considered sufficiently early in the course of disease that patients have not already become chemorefractory. High-dose therapy and ASCT remains an effective treatment approach for younger patients with chemoresponsive relapsed disease, SCT approaches must be considered in the context of the improving results that are being seen with novel salvage therapies.

The Role of Transplant in Relapsed Indolent Lymphomas

Unlike aggressive lymphomas, the use of high-dose chemotherapy with ASCT in the treatment of FL has not yet been fully established. The rationale for considering transplantation is that the disease is incurable using standard approaches, young patients with FL will die of their disease, and promising results have been observed in a number of phase II studies.[94–96] Detection of MRD has been a useful surrogate marker for tracking long-term PFS in patients examining the autologous stem cells or serial samples after transplantation.[96–100] A major concern relates to the risk of development of secondary myelodysplasia/acute myeloid leukemia.[101] The European Bone Marrow Transplant Registry (EBMTR) sponsored CUP (conventional chemotherapy, unpurged, purged autograft) study is the only prospective randomized trial to assess the role of ASCT in patients with relapsed FL.[102] The results of the study suggest a PFS and OS advantage of ASCT over conventional chemotherapy, with 4-year OS of 46% for the chemotherapy arm, versus 71% for the unpurged and 77% for the purged ASCT arms. The study was closed early because of slow accrual with 140 of the planned 250 patients accrued and only 89 randomized.

Novel Agents

There are a large number of novel approaches that are being studied in patients with FL. Recently approved agents for FL include idelalisib[103] and obinutuzumab, the first type II glycoengineered and humanized monoclonal anti-CD20 antibody.[104] Other agents under investigation include novel monoclonal antibodies, immunomodulatory agents, and novel kinase inhibitors. Combinations of monoclonal antibodies are being explored, such as combining anti-CD20 with anti-CD22 antibodies.[105] Kinases involved in the B-cell receptor signaling pathway are logical targets for therapy in FL. In addition, idelalisib is approved for the treatment of rituximab-refractory follicular lymphoma and clinical trial data has been presented for kinase inhibitors that target Bruton tyrosine kinase (BTK),[106,107] and spleen tyrosine kinase (SYK).[108] Novel agents are being examined in combination with monoclonal antibodies and chemotherapy. Since a hallmark of FL is overexpression of BCL2, this protein is also a logical target for small molecule inhibitors that can inhibit the antiapoptotic activity of BCL2. Clinical responses have been observed in the phase I study examining the efficacy of navitoclax in lymphoid malignancies.[109] The next generation agent venetoclax is now approved in chronic lymphocytic leukemia and clinical trials are ongoing in FL, both alone and in combinations.

Allogeneic Bone Marrow Transplant

There is a trend towards increasing use of allogeneic SCT (aSCT) in the management of indolent lymphomas. In a report of the International Bone Marrow Transplant Registry (IBMTR), results after SCT are described for 904 patients with FL.[110] Among these patients, 176 patients underwent aSCT, 131 patients underwent ASCT using purged stem cells and 597 using purged autologous stem cells. The treatment related mortality (TRM) in these three groups was 30%, 14% and 8% respectively. Disease recurrence occurred in 21%, 43% and 58% and 5-year overall survival was 51%, 62% and 55% respectively. The use of TBI containing regimens was associated with increased TRM but decreased risk of relapse. The use of aSCT was associated with increased TRM, but significantly lower risk of disease recurrence in keeping with a graft versus lymphoma effect in this disease. Trends suggest that outcomes are improving and this is highly likely to continue with the increased use of reduced intensity conditioning regimens that have become used increasingly since the time this registry data was collated. Long-term PFS has been observed after aSCT even in patients with refractory FL.[111] In 29 patients with FL, 11 of whom had refractory disease, the nonrelapse mortality was 24% and there was a 23% incidence of relapse. The 5-year OS was 58% with 53% event-free survival. A group of patients with very poor outcome are those patients who have relapsed after previous ASCT. The outcome following myeloablative aSCT of 114 such patients has been reported from the IBMTR.[112] The treatment related mortality was 22% and the probability of disease progression was 52% at 3 years. The use of TBI conditioning regimens and achievement of CR at the time of aSCT were associated with improved outcome. The use of reduced intensity conditioning regimens appears to be associated with improved outcome. In 20 such patients, there was only one treatment related mortality from fungal infection and the 3-year PFS was an excellent 95%.[113] The outcome following reduced intensity conditioning transplant regimen incorporating alemtuzumab immunosuppressive therapy has been reported for 81 patients with lymphoma and included 41 with low-grade, 37 with high/intermediate-grade and 10 patients with MCL, 31 of whom had relapsed following previous ASCT.[114] Patients received a conditioning regimen consisting of alemtuzumab, fludarabine, and melphalan, and received short course cyclosporin as graft-versus-host disease (GVHD) prophylaxis. The use of this conditioning regimen was associated with a low incidence of GVHD and the treatment related mortality was decreased in patients with low-grade compared with higher grade histology. The 3-year PFS was 65% for patients with low-grade lymphoma, 50% for patients with MCL and 34% for high-grade lymphoma ($p = .002$). Donor lymphocyte infusion (DLI) was given to 36 patients, 21 for relapsed or persistent disease and 15 for persistence of mixed chimerism. The use of DLI to treat relapse after aSCT is solely dependent upon the existence of a graft versus lymphoma effect. In seven patients with FL and small lymphocytic lymphoma who had relapsed after prior aSCT, six patients responded and four maintained CR for 43–89 months. The effectiveness of DLI to treat relapse after aSCT provides very strong evidence for a graft versus lymphoma effect that can be exploited in indolent lymphomas.[114,115] The role of RIC aSCT has been evaluated by Cancer and Leukemia Group B in a phase II study to evaluate the safety and efficacy in patients with recurrent low-grade B-cell malignancies, including 16 patients with FL.[116] The 3-year TRM was 9% and the 3-year OS was 81%. The incidence of grade II–IV acute GVHD was 29%, and extensive chronic GVHD was 18%.

SUGGESTED READINGS

Dave SS, Wright G, Tab B, et al: Prediction of survival in follicular lymphoma based on molecular features of tumor-infiltrating immune cells. *N Engl J Med* 351:2159–2169, *2004.*

Friedberg JW, Byrtek M, Link BK, et al: Effectiveness of first-line management strategies for stage I follicular lymphoma: analysis of the National LymphoCare Study. *J Clin Oncol* 30:3368–3375, 2012.

Gopal AK, Kahl BS, de Vos S, et al: PI3Kdelta inhibition by idelalisib in patients with relapsed indolent lymphoma. *N Engl J Med* 370:*1008–1018,* 2014.

Kridel R, Sehn LH, Gascoyne RD: Pathogenesis of follicular lymphoma. *J Clin Invest* 122:3424–3431, 2012.

Okosun J, Bodor C, Wang J, et al: Integrated genomic analysis identifies recurrent mutations and evolution patterns driving the initiation and progression of follicular lymphoma. *Nat Genet* 46:176–181, 2014.

Salles G, Seymour JF, Offner F, et al: Rituximab maintenance for 2 years in patients with high tumour burden follicular lymphoma responding to rituximab plus chemotherapy (PRIMA): a phase 3, randomised controlled trial. *Lancet* 377:42–51, 2011.

REFERENCES

For the complete list of references, log on to www.expertconsult.com.

CHAPTER 81

MANTLE CELL LYMPHOMA

Vijaya Raj Bhatt, Roberto Ferro Valdes, and Julie M. Vose

INTRODUCTION

Mantle cell lymphoma (MCL) is a distinct subtype of mature B-cell non-Hodgkin lymphoma (NHL) that accounts for 5–10% of all NHL. Although a subset of patients with MCL may have an indolent course, MCL is generally an aggressive NHL. In the 1970s, the Kiel classification used the terminology *centrocytic lymphoma* to describe MCL, whereas Berard and Dorfman categorized it as *lymphocytic lymphoma of intermediate differentiation*. In the 1980s, the term *mantle zone lymphoma* was used to denote a distinct subtype of MCL characterized by the proliferation of atypical small lymphoid cells with wide mantles around benign germinal centers (GCs). In the Revised European-American Lymphoma classification in 1994 and later in 2001 and 2008, the WHO classification of tumors of hematopoietic and lymphoid tissues recognized MCL as a distinct disease under mature B-cell lymphomas. With the recognition as a distinct entity, in recent years, significant progress has been made toward understanding the underlying pathogenesis of MCL and translating that knowledge to design more effective therapies.[1]

EPIDEMIOLOGY

MCL is two- to sevenfold more common in men than women and almost twofold more common in whites than African Americans. The average age at diagnosis varies between 60 and 70 years. The annual incidence is approximately 4 to 8 cases per million population in the United States and Europe.

PATHOBIOLOGY

MCL, characterized by an alteration in the regulation of the cell-cycle, demonstrates cyclin D1 overexpression and increased replication. The tumor cells also demonstrate decreased response to DNA damage and resistance to apoptosis. The tumor cells originate from pre-B cells in the bone marrow that can follow at least two different molecular pathways of development.

The classical MCL originates from a naive B cell that has not entered the follicular GC, but has SOX11 expression, lambda light chain restriction, and limited or no immunoglobulin heavy chain variable (IgVH) somatic mutations. SOX11 expression is associated with the activation of histone marks and absence of DNA methylation. The second subset of MCL, an indolent form typically limited to peripheral blood and spleen, originates from post-GC B cells. This MCL subset has frequent IgVH mutations, typically lacks SOX11 expression, and has kappa light chain restriction. A few studies have demonstrated a correlation between SOX11 expression and aggressive tumors with high serum levels of lactate dehydrogenase (LDH) and high Ki-67 index. Conversely, SOX11-negative MCL may occasionally acquire complex karyotype and TP53 alterations and transform into aggressive tumor (Fig. 81.1).

Genetic Alteration of Proliferative Pathways

The three most common recurrent mutations in MCL involve CCND1 (also known as Cyclin D1, BCL1, or PRAD1), TP53, and ataxia telangiectasia mutated (ATM) genes. The vast majority of MCL have the reciprocal translocation, t(11;14) (q13;q23), which juxtaposes CCND1 gene to the immunoglobin heavy-chain locus. The consequent overexpression of CCND1 gene located at 11q13 encodes cyclin D1 protein. Cyclin D1 protein, which is not expressed in normal lymphocytes, is expressed in virtually all MCL, and at a lower level in Burkitt lymphoma and acute lymphoblastic lymphoma (ALL). A few cells with t(11;14) have been found in the blood of 1–2% of healthy individuals. Therefore, cyclin D1 overexpression is not sufficient for the transformation of normal B cells to MCL, rather it is thought to represent an early genetic event. Interestingly, the close physical proximity of the chromosomal regions of the IgVH and CCND1 loci in the nucleus of immature lymphoid B cells may facilitate the occurrence of recurrent translocations. Furthermore, colocalization and interaction of IgVH-CCND1 chromosomal segment and a transcription factor called *nucleolin* near the perinucleolar area leads to the transcription of cyclin D1 protein. Cyclin D1 protein then regulates the G1 phase by binding to cyclin-dependent kinase (CDK) 4 and CDK6. The cyclin D1-CDK complex phosphorylates retinoblastoma 1 (RB1) resulting in a release of E2F transcription factor, and transition of a cell from G1 to S phase. Additionally, the CDKN2A gene on chromosome 9p, which regulates INK4a protein, is deleted in 20–30% of highly proliferating MCL. The INK4a protein inhibits CDK4 and CDK6, and thus maintains the RB1 protein in its active, antiproliferative state. INK4a is frequently deleted in MCL and cooperates with CCND1 gene. Therefore, the CDKN2A-INK4a-CDK4-RB1 pathway is dysregulated in patients with MCL, particularly those with blastoid histology.[2]

Recent studies have described cyclin D1-negative MCL cases that demonstrate pathologic features and gene expression profile similar to cyclin D1-positive MCL. Cyclin D1-negative MCL is associated with the dysregulation in the expression of the following genes, often due to epigenetic changes: overexpression of cyclin D2 or D3; decreased CDK inhibitor 1B (CDKI1B or p27); upregulation of cyclin E; or inactivation of RB gene. CDKI1B protein regulates the cell progression from G1 to S phase by inhibiting the cyclin E/CDK2 complex (the latter also inactivates the RB protein). Although the diagnosis of cyclin D1-negative MCL is uncommon and requires caution, these cases highlight the relevance of the oncogenic dysregulation of the cell cycle, especially of the G1 phase in the pathogenesis of MCL.

Antiapoptotic and Prosurvival Pathways

Some patients with aggressive MCL, particularly the blastoid variant, have an increased number of chromosomal abnormalities, such as complex karyotype and tetraploidy. The accumulation of chromosomal abnormalities suggests alterations in the DNA damage response pathways. TP53 mutation and deletion or point mutation of the ATM gene (located at 11q22-q23) are recurrent mutations in MCL. TP53 mutations, associated with alterations of 17p chromosomal segment, are present in 10% to 28% of MCL cases. These point mutations are frequently missense mutations that compromise normal p53 expression. The TP53 tumor suppressor gene normally regulates the cell cycle, DNA repair, apoptosis, senescence, and autophagy through transcription-dependent and independent pathways. Disruption in TP53-dependent apoptosis has also been linked to deletion, mutation, or silencing of BIM and NOXA genes. The

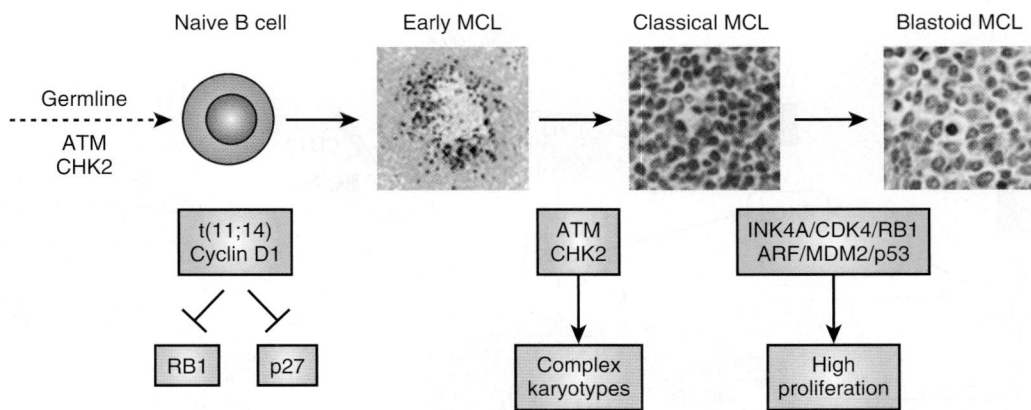

Fig. 81.1 PROPOSED MODEL OF MOLECULAR PATHOGENESIS IN THE DEVELOPMENT AND PROGRESSION OF MANTLE CELL LYMPHOMA. Germline mutation of ataxia telangiectasia mutated (ATM) or cell cycle checkpoint kinase 2 (CHK2) genes may facilitate the early development of mantle cell lymphoma (MCL). The translocation t(11;14)(q13;q23), which occurs in an immature B cell results in the constitutive overexpression of CCND1 gene, initiation of the B-cell transformation process, and clonal B-cell expansion in the mantle zone of lymphoid follicles. Acquired alterations of DNA damage response pathways may facilitate genomic instability, acquisition of additional genetic changes, and the development of classical MCL. The accumulation of further chromosomal abnormalities involving proliferative pathways, complex karyotypes, tetraploidization, and 17p/TP53 alterations lead to more proliferative and aggressive variants of MCL. *(From Jares P, Colomer D, Campo E: Genetic and molecular pathogenesis of mantle cell lymphoma: perspectives for new targeted therapeutics.* Nat Rev Cancer *7:750, 2007.)*

latter two genes transcribe proapoptotic proteins important in Bax/Bak-mediated cytochrome C release, which is essential to apoptosis. TP53 expression is also inhibited by the binding of PAX5 transcription factor to the TP53 promoter. PAX5 is upregulated by SOX11 in a significant number of patients with MCL. PAX5 represses PRDM1/BLIMP1 and negatively regulates differentiation of early lymphoid progenitors to plasma cells. Therefore, the SOX11-PAX5-PRDM1/BLIMP1 axis suppresses B-cell differentiation to plasma cells and plays an important role in the pathogenesis of MCL. MDM2 is another protein overexpressed in about 16% of MCL and mediates polyubiquitination and degradation of p53. This function of MDM2 protein is prevented by ARF protein, also known as p14 (encoded by CDKN2A gene); however, the homozygous deletion of the CDKN2A gene in MCL allows MDM2-mediated degradation of TP53 and dysregulation of apoptotic pathways.

Inactivation of the ATM gene, detected in about 40% of MCL, facilitates genomic instability by impairing responses to DNA damage. Intriguingly, the inactivation of ATM, perhaps an early phenomenon in MCL, is not commonly seen in other lymphomas except in T-cell prolymphocytic leukemia. ATM encodes the PI3K protein, which phosphorylates p53, promoting its stabilization and transcriptional activation, therefore leading to cell cycle arrest, DNA repair, or apoptosis. Consequently, inactivation of ATM causes genomic instability by inactivation of p53. Despite having similar pathogenic significance, ATM mutations do not impact overall survival, whereas TP53 mutations do predict for worse survival. In addition, ATM may play a role in activation of the nuclear factor kappaB (NFκB) by phosphorylation of the NFκB inhibitor, IkappaB. The NFκB signaling regulates transcription factors that activate numerous genes involved in cell survival, apoptosis, and cell migration. Its persistent activity is associated with tumor formation, tumor growth, metastasis, and drug resistance in B-cell lymphomas and other cancers. Notably, the PI3K-AKT pathway is upstream of the mammalian target of rapamycin (mTOR), which in turn is upstream of cyclin D1, CDKI1B, and other regulatory proteins. Conversely, CHK2 and CHK1 are kinases downstream of ATM and prevent cell cycle progression in response to ATM. Downregulation or mutations of CHK2 and CHK1 are also commonly seen in MCL.

Wnt canonical and Sonic Hedgehog (SHH) pathways are also altered in MCL. The Wnt canonical pathway via β-catenin, important for normal cell growth and development, is constitutively activated in a subset of MCL and may promote tumor growth. Similarly,

SHH-GLI signaling molecules such as PTCH and SMO receptors as well as GLI1 and GLI2 transcription factors are expressed in MCL and may contribute to the proliferation of MCL.

Lastly, dysregulation of the B-cell receptor (BCR), a key player of normal B-cell differentiation and development, is involved in the pathogenesis of MCL. Activation of BCR-associated kinases, including spleen tyrosine kinase (SYK), Bruton tyrosine kinase (BTK), and protein kinase C-beta (PKC-β) is observed in MCL. BTK, a member of the Tec family of nonreceptor protein tyrosine kinases, has a well-defined role in the constitutively activated BCR signaling pathway in MCL. Amplification and overexpression of SYK have been found in a subset of MCL. SYK, LYN, and BTK are frequently phosphorylated in MCL, suggesting activation of the BCR pathway. Therefore, the BCR pathway appears to contribute to the growth and survival of MCL cells. The signaling pathways that contribute to the pathogenesis are summarized in Fig. 81.2.

CLINICAL MANIFESTATIONS

The early symptoms usually include fever, night sweats, unexplained weight loss, lymphadenopathy, and splenomegaly. Typically, the majority of patients present at an advanced stage (III or IV) with lymphadenopathy, hepatomegaly, splenomegaly, and bone marrow involvement. Splenomegaly is noted in 40% of patients, and approximately 50% of patients present with circulating lymphoma cells. MCL also tends to involve extranodal sites, especially in the gastrointestinal (GI) tract. Involvement of the GI tract, frequently in the form of lymphomatous polyposis, can be detected in up to 90% of patients; however, many patients do not have any pertinent GI symptoms. During disease progression, MCL can infiltrate other organs including the respiratory tract, breast, or orbit. Involvement of the central nervous system (CNS) is rare but may be relatively more common with blastoid MCL and relapsed disease.

LABORATORY MANIFESTATIONS

Cytopenias are typically present secondary to bone marrow involvement, whereas autoimmune cytopenias are rare. Elevation of LDH and uric acid correlates with tumor burden. Liver function tests may be abnormal if there is hepatic involvement. Other findings include

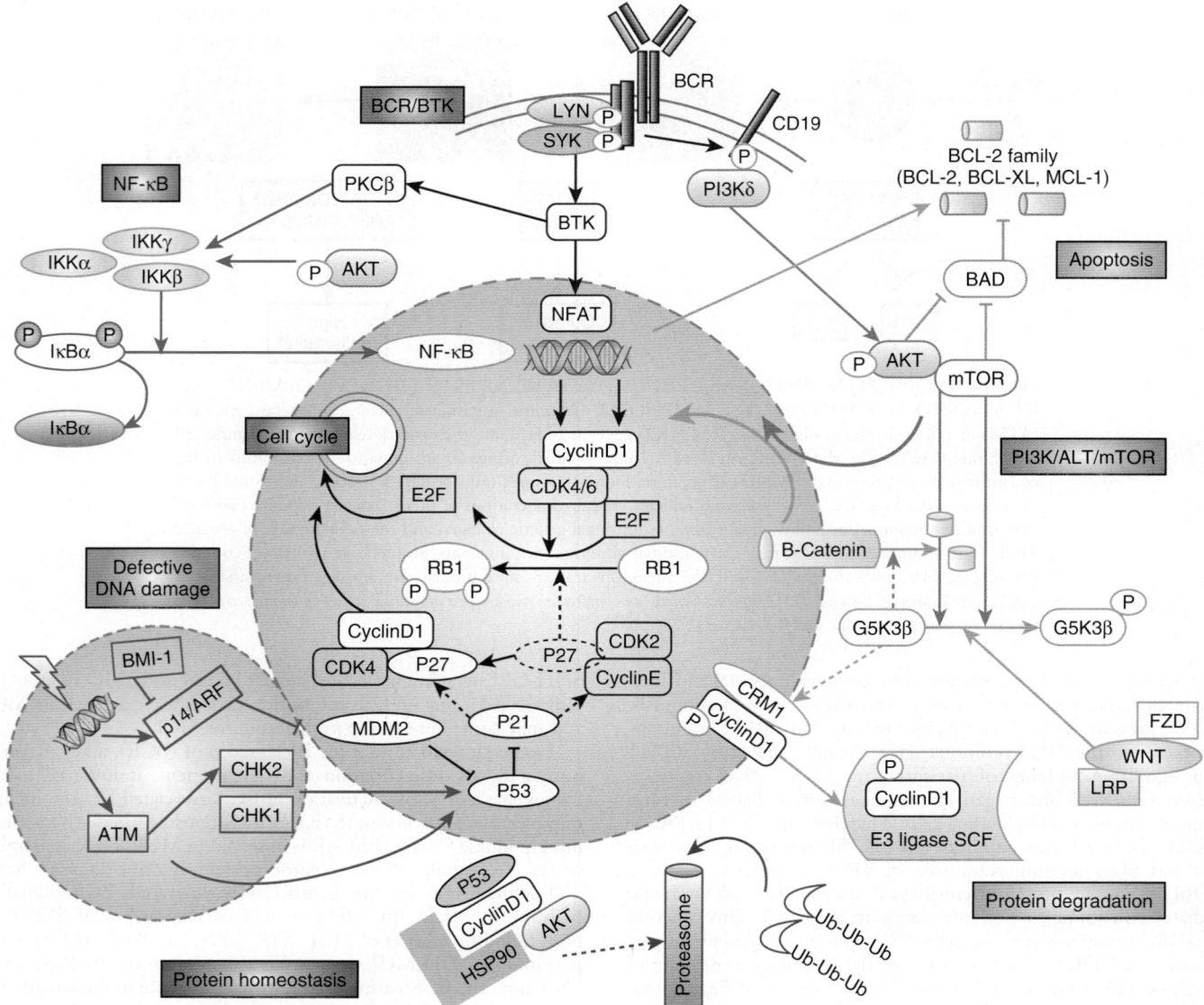

Fig. 81.2 THE SIGNALING PATHWAYS CONTRIBUTING TO MANTLE CELL LYMPHOMA PATHOGENESIS. CCND1 translocation and mutation of TP53 and ataxia telangiectasia mutated (ATM) genes are common genetic alterations involved in the pathogenesis of mantle cell lymphoma (MCL). Cyclin D1 protein regulates the G1 phase by binding to cyclin-dependent kinase (CDK) 4 and CDK6. The cyclin D1-CDK complex phosphorylates retinoblastoma 1 (RB1) resulting in release of E2F transcription factor and transition of a cell from G1 to S phase. Other major abnormalities include inactivation of the ATM, and cell cycle checkpoint kinase (CHK) 1 and 2 genes; MDM2-mediated degradation of TP53; activation of B cell receptor-associated kinases and constitutive activation of nuclear factor kappaB (NFκB), PI3K/AKT/mammalian target of rapamycin (mTOR), Wnt canonical, and Sonic Hedgehog (SHH) pathways.

elevated beta 2-microglobulin, and rarely hypogammaglobulinemia or monoclonal gammopathy.

Histologically, the 2008 WHO classification[3] describes classical MCL as a monomorphic proliferation of small- to medium-sized lymphoid cells with an irregular nuclear border, dispersed chromatin, and inconspicuous nucleoli. The architectural patterns may include a vaguely nodular, diffuse, mantle zone, or rarely follicular growth pattern. Infrequent cases, referred to as in situ MCL, may exclusively involve the inner mantle zones or narrow mantles. Histologic transformation to large B-cell lymphoma does not occur; however, MCL can have several morphologic variants including aggressive blastoid and pleomorphic variants (Fig. 81.3; E-Slide VM03960).

1. Blastoid variant: lymphoma cells have a high mitotic rate (20–30 per 10 high-power fields) and dispersed chromatin; frequently resembles lymphoblasts.

2. Pleomorphic variant: cells have different forms including frequent large cells, pale cytoplasm, oval to irregular nuclear border, and often prominent nucleoli.

3. Small cell variant: cells are small and round with clumped chromatin; frequently resembles small lymphocytic lymphoma (SLL).

4. Marginal zone-like variant: this variant has clusters of marginal zone-like or monocytoid B cells with abundant pale cytoplasm.

DIAGNOSIS

The diagnosis of MCL is based on the morphologic, immunophenotypic, and genetic features evaluated on biopsied tissue. The inclusion of immunophenotyping increased the diagnostic consensus between expert hematopathologists in the International Non-Hodgkin

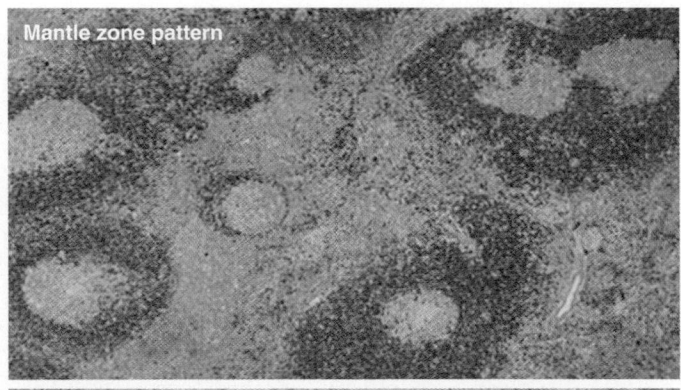

Mantle zone pattern

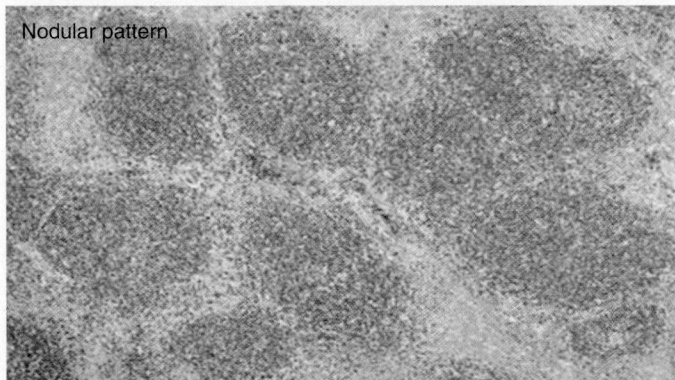

Nodular pattern

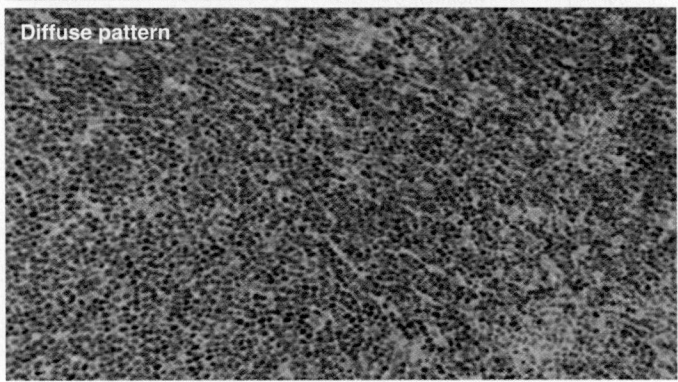

Diffuse pattern

Fig. 81.3 HISTOPATHOLOGY OF MANTLE CELL LYMPHOMA.

Lymphoma Classification project from 77% (based on histology) to 87%. The characteristic immunophenotypic features of MCL include expression of the B cell–associated antigens CD19, CD20, CD22, and CD79a and aberrant expression of the T cell–associated antigens CD5 and CD43, and a lack of expression of CD3, CD10, and CD23. The identification of t(11;14)(q13;q32) and CCND1 oncogene can further aid to the diagnostic accuracy.[3] The presence of CCND1 oncogene is revealed most accurately in stains of formalin-fixed, paraffin-embedded lymph nodes or soft tissue. Nonetheless, the cyclin D1 overexpression can also be seen in a subset of patients with ALL, Burkitt lymphoma, hairy cell leukemia and multiple myeloma. The t(11;14) is seen in more than half of patients on karyotyping and in virtually all the patients screened with fluorescence in situ hybridization. In patients with cyclin D1-negative MCL, overexpression of cyclin D2, cyclin D3, or SOX11 can help in establishing the diagnosis. However, cyclin D2 is also overexpressed in patients with chronic lymphocytic leukemia and lymphoplasmacytic lymphoma, and cyclin D3 can be overexpressed in the vast majority of B-cell malignancies. Overexpression of SOX11, present in more than 90% of the patients with MCL, can also be seen in ALL, T-cell prolymphocytic leukemia, and Burkitt lymphoma. However, these other entities are usually easier to differentiate by clinicopathologic and other criteria; therefore, SOX11 is a very useful tool in cyclin D1-negative cases.

Differential Diagnosis

MCL should be differentiated from other B-cell NHL, particularly SLL/chronic lymphocytic leukemia, lymphoplasmacytic lymphoma, marginal-zone lymphoma, and follicular lymphoma. Additionally, with minimal differentiation, the blastoid variant MCL may resemble B-cell ALL and acute myeloid leukemia. Immunophenotypic markers are helpful in differentiating MCL (CD5+, CD10−, CD19+, CD23−, FMC+) from SLL/chronic lymphocytic leukemia (CD5+, CD10−, CD19+, CD23+, FMC−), and follicular lymphoma (CD5−, CD10+, CD19+). In CD5 negative or cyclin D1-negative MCL, careful exclusion of other lymphomas via detection of overexpression of cyclin D2, cyclin D3 or SOX11 and gene expression profiling may help in the diagnosis.

Staging

Staging procedures include a complete blood count, comprehensive metabolic panel, lactate dehydrogenase, evaluation of a bone marrow biopsy, and computed tomography (CT) of chest, abdomen, and pelvis. Although endoscopies of upper and lower GI tracts are frequently positive, such evaluation did not change management in a retrospective study. MCL has low to intermediate avidity for fluorodeoxyglucose (FDG); however, the blastoid variant is more FDG avid. Nonetheless, an integrated FDG positron emission tomography (PET) and CT scan is frequently utilized for staging of patients with MCL. Lumbar puncture is not routinely performed but should be done in patients with neurologic symptoms. Multigated acquisition scan or echocardiography is often performed prior to the use of anthracycline; however, their role in asymptomatic patients without cardiac disease is unclear. Hepatitis B serologies are performed prior to the use of rituximab because of a risk of reactivation.

THERAPY

MCL combines the worst features of both follicular lymphoma (noncurability) and diffuse large B-cell lymphoma (aggressive course). A paucity of randomized controlled trials consequent to disease rarity has resulted in a lack of standard therapy. Therapy options range from wait-and-watch strategy in select asymptomatic patients to intensified chemotherapy followed by upfront high-dose chemotherapy (HDT) and autologous hematopoietic stem cell transplant (ASCT) in young fit patients.[1] When a decision has been made to start treatment, several chemoimmunotherapy regimens are available: alkylator-based (cyclophosphamide, vincristine, and prednisone, CVP), anthracycline-based (cyclophosphamide, doxorubicin, vincristine and prednisone, CHOP), fludarabine-based (fludarabine, cyclophosphamide, mitoxantrone, FCM), bendamustine-based (bendamustine and rituximab, BR) as well as cytarabine-, and methotrexate-based (cyclophosphamide, vincristine, doxorubicin and dexamethasone alternating with cytarabine and methotrexate, Hyper-CVAD/MA) regimens, almost always combined with rituximab in the current era (Tables 81.1 and 81.2). More recently, attempts to incorporate bortezomib in upfront therapy have shown promising results. With conventional chemotherapy such as rituximab and CHOP (R-CHOP), the median remission duration is 1.5–3 years; consequently, many experts prefer upfront intensive therapy in younger patients. However, no single strategy is conclusively superior to the other in terms of an overall survival (OS). Blastoid-variant MCL has particularly poor prognosis with few long-term survivors, but histology is often not utilized in selecting therapies. Nonetheless, young patients with blastoid-variant MCL may benefit from intensified therapy and upfront ASCT. Ultimately, therapy selection has to be based on age and performance

TABLE 81.1   Outcomes of Nonintensive Rituximab-Based Therapy Utilized in Mantle Cell Lymphoma

Author, Year	Number of Patients	Therapy	CR (%)	EFS/PFS	OS (%)
Howard, 2002[4]	40	R-CHOP	48%	16.6 months median	-
Forstpointer, 2004[5]	48	R-FCM vs. FCM	29% vs. 0%	4 vs. 8 months median (p = .38)	Not reached at a median follow-up of ~18 months vs. 11 months (p = .004)
Lenz, 2005[6]	122	R-CHOP vs. CHOP	34% vs. 7%, p < .001	Median time to treatment failure (21 vs. 14 months, p = .013) but similar PFS (p = .31)	76% at 2 years (p = .93)
Herold, 2008[7]	44	R-MCP[a]	32%	26% at 50 months	56% at 50 months
Ruan, 2011[8]	36	R-CHOP + Bortezomib	72%	44% at 2 years	86% at 2 years
Spurgeon, 2011[9]	31	R-cladribine	61%	37 months median	85 months median
Grant, 2011[10]	26	DA-R-EPOCH and idiotype vaccine	92%	24 months median	104 months median
Kluin-Nelemans, 2012[11]	485	R-CHOP vs. FCR[b]	34% vs. 40%, p = .1[c]	–	47% vs. 62% at 4 years, p = .005
Smith, 2012[12]	56	R-CHOP followed by ^{90}Y ibritumomab	55%	34 months median TTF	73% at 5 years
Dunleavy, 2012[13]	43	Bortezomib + DA-R-EPOCH	–	50% at 4 years	80% at 4 years
Rummel, 2013[14]	94 MCL/549 NHL	BR vs. R-CHOP	40% vs. 30%, p = .02 (for entire cohort)	Median of 35 vs. 22 months, p = .004	Similar
Visco, 2013[15]	20	Rituximab, bendamustine and cytarabine	95%	95% at 2 years	–
Flinn, 2014[16]	74 MCL/447 NHL	BR vs. R-CHOP/R-CVP	50% vs. 27%	–	–

[a]R-MCP was not superior to MCP but the study population was small (*n* = 90).
[b]Second randomization to maintenance rituximab or interferon alpha demonstrated reduction of the risk of progression or death by 45% with rituximab. Rituximab maintenance improved OS among patients who had responded to R-CHOP.
[c]Overall response rate was 86% vs. 78% for R-CHOP vs. FCR (*p* = 0.06).
BR, Bendamustine and rituximab; CHOP, cyclophosphamide, doxorubicin, vincristine and prednisone; CR, complete remission; DA-R-EPOCH, dose-adjusted etoposide, cyclophosphamide and doxorubicin along with prednisone, vincristine and rituximab; EFS, event-free survival; FCM, fludarabine, cyclophosphamide, mitoxantrone; FCR, fludarabine, cyclophosphamide and rituximab; PFS, progression-free survival; OS, overall survival; R, rituximab; R-CHOP, rituximab and CHOP; R-CVP, rituximab, cyclophosphamide, vincristine, and prednisone; RDHAP, rituximab, cisplatin, cytarabine, and dexamethasone; R-FCM, rituximab and FCM; R-Hyper-CVAD/R-MA, rituximab, cyclophosphamide, vincristine, doxorubicin, and dexamethasone alternating with rituximab, cytarabine, and methotrexate; R-MCP, rituximab, mitoxantrone, chlormabucil and prednisolone.

status of the patient, the presence of comorbidities, the individual's goals of care as well as the preferences of the patient and physician (Fig. 81.4).

Wait-and-Watch Strategy

The approach of watchful waiting, as utilized in other indolent lymphomas, has been advocated by some investigators in select patients with MCL. This recommendation is supported by a study from Weill Cornell Medical College among 97 patients with MCL, which compared the outcomes between early treatment and observation groups. Among the observation group, the median time to treatment was 12 months (4 to 128 months). Patients in the observation group had better performance status and were more likely to have lower-risk standard International Prognostic Index scores than the early treatment group. The study demonstrated that a delay in initiation of therapy did not influence OS in a multivariate analysis.[34] Good outcomes with initial wait-and-watch approach were demonstrated in other studies from the United Kingdom and Sweden. Although these retrospective studies may have limitations, the wait-and-watch strategy is reasonable in asymptomatic older patients, who emphasize on delaying the use of noncurative therapy to preserve the quality of life.

Stage I and II A (Nonbulky) Disease

MCL generally presents with stage III/IV disease with diffuse lymphadenopathy and involvement of blood, bone marrow, and spleen; stage I and II disease at presentation is uncommon. A retrospective study from Vancouver among stage I/II MCL patients (*n* = 26) demonstrated an improvement of progression-free survival (PFS) and possibly OS with the addition of radiotherapy to chemotherapy; however, this study had several limitations including small sample size, retrospective single-center study, and use of suboptimal chemotherapy. Another study from Sweden demonstrated a 3-year OS of 93% with curative intent radiotherapy among 43 patients with stage I–II MCL.[35] A large study based on Surveillance, Epidemiology, and End Results (SEER) database also demonstrated improvement in OS with the use of upfront radiotherapy.[36] For these reasons, the 2015 National Comprehensive Cancer Network (NCCN) guidelines for MCL support the use of radiotherapy (30–36 Gy) alone or combination with chemoimmunotherapy with or without radiotherapy for stage I/II MCL.

Role of Rituximab

Although the incorporation of rituximab to chemotherapy has improved the outcomes of MCL, the effects are not as profound as

TABLE 81.2	Outcomes of Intensive Therapy Utilized in Mantle Cell Lymphoma				
Author, Year	Number of Patients	Therapy	CR with induction therapy (%)	EFS/PFS	OS (%)
Khouri, 1998[17]	45	Hyper-CVAD/MA, then SCT	38	72% vs. 17% at 3 years for previously untreated vs. treated	92% vs. 25% at 3 years for previously untreated vs. treated
Romaguera, 2000[18]	25	Hyper-CVAD/MA	68	Median of 15 months	–
Gianni, 2003[19]	28	CHOP like, then R-HDT/ASCT	100 after ASCT	79% at 4.5 years	89% at 4.5 years
de Guibert, 2006[20]	24	R-DHAP, then HDT/ASCT	92	65% at 3 years	69% at 3 years
Epner, 2007[21]	49	R-Hyper-CVAD/R-MA	58	63% at 2 years	76% at 2 years
Ritchie, 2007[22]	13	R-Hyper-CVAD/R-MA	92	92% at 3 years	92% at 3 years
Dreger, 2007[23]	34	CHOP, then R-HDT/ASCT	94 after ASCT	83% at 4 years	87% at 4 years
Damon, 2009[24]	78	R-Methotrexate- augmented CHOP+ HDT/ASCT	69 after ASCT	56% at 5 years	64% at 5 years
van 't Veer, 2009[25]	87	R-CHOP/high-dose cytarabine, then HDT/ASCT	43%	36% FFS at 4 years	66% at 4 years
Gressin, 2010[26]	113	(R)VAD+C with vs. without ASCT	46	62% vs. 6% at 3 years	81% vs. 47% at 3 years
Romaguera, 2010[27]	97	R-Hyper-CVAD/R-MA	87	TTF 43% at 8 years	56% at 8 years
Chang, 2011[28]	30	VcR-CVAD, then maintenance rituximab	77	63% at 3 years	86% at 3 years
Merli, 2012[29]	63	R-Hyper-CVAD/R-MA	72	61% at 5 years	73% at 5 years
Geisler, 2012[30]	160	R+Maxi-CHOP/cytarabine, then HDT/ASCT	54	43% at 10 years	58% at 10 years
Ahmadi, 2012[31]	44	R-Hyper-CVAD/MA, then rituximab maintenance or HDT/ASCT	91	Median of 3.5 years[a]	Median of >4.1 years
Hermine, 2012[32]	455	R-CHOP vs. CHOP/R-DHAP, then HDT/ASCT [b]	40% vs. 54%, p = .0003	TTF 46 months vs. 88 months, p = .038[c]	Not reached vs. 82 months, p = .045[c]
Delarue, 2013[33]	60	CHOP-(R)/R-DHAP, then HDT/ASCT	57	64% at 5 years	75% at 5 years

[a]Median PFS of 2.3 years for R-Hyper-CVAD only vs. 3.9 years for R-Hyper-CVAD and rituximab maintenance, and 4.5 years for R-Hyper-CVAD and HDT/ASCT
[b]CHOP/R-DHAP included three cycles of each chemoregimen, followed by high-dose cytarabine containing myeloablative regimen; in R-CHOP group, high-dose therapy did not include cytarabine.
[c]Median follow-up was 51 months
ASCT, Autologous stem cell transplantation; BEAM/ BEAC, carmustine, etoposide, cytarabine, and melphalan/cyclophosphamide; CHOP, cyclophosphamide, doxorubicin, vincristine, and prednisone; CR, complete remission; EFS, event-free survival; FFS, failure-free survival; HDT, high-dose chemotherapy; Hyper-CVAD/MA, cyclophosphamide, vincristine, doxorubicin, and dexamethasone, alternating with methotrexate and cytarabine; Maxi-CHOP, dose-intensified CHOP; OS, overall survival; PFS, progression-free survival; R, rituximab; RDHAP, rituximab, cisplatin, cytarabine, and dexamethasone; VAD+C,vincristine, doxorubicin, dexamethasone, chlorambucil; SCT, stem cell transplantation; TTF, time to treatment failure; VcR-CVAD, bortezomib, rituximab, cyclophosphamide, doxorubicin, vincristine, dexamethasone.

seen in other CD20$^+$ B-cell lymphomas. In one of the earliest studies (n = 40), R-CHOP resulted in an overall response rate of 96%, complete response rate of 48%, and median PFS of 16.6 months. Patients who achieved a molecular remission (n = 9, 36%), did not have improved PFS (16.5 vs. 18.8 months, p = .51) compared with patients without molecular remission. However, the study may have been underpowered due to a small sample size.[4] Another larger study (n = 122) demonstrated a higher overall response rate (94% vs. 75%, p = .005), complete remission rate (34% vs. 7%, p < .001), and median time to treatment failure (21 vs. 14 months, p = .013), but similar PFS (p = .31) with R-CHOP, compared with CHOP.[6] In the third study (n = 48), R-FCM resulted in a similar overall response rate (58% vs. 46%, p = .28) and median PFS (8 vs. 4 months, p = .38), but improved median OS (not reached vs. 11 months, p = .004) compared with FCM.[5] In a large Nordic Lymphoma Group observational study, rituximab use was an independent predictor of improved OS.[35] The moderate benefit with incorporation of rituximab has led to its widespread use in MCL with most of the recent trials utilizing rituximab-based chemoimmunotherapy.

Low Intensity Therapy

Older patients (~65 years or more) or patients who have major comorbidities, poor performance status, or a preference for a nonaggressive approach, are treated with a low intensity chemotherapy

regimen. Several therapy options are available as listed in Table 81.1; however, BR as well as R-CHOP are the two most commonly utilized regimens in newly diagnosed MCL. R-CHOP results in an overall response rate of approximately 90% with a complete remission in about one-third of patients. In various studies, median PFS has ranged from 16 to 22 months, whereas median OS were 76% at 2 years and 47% at 4 years. Recent studies have demonstrated a more favorable outcome with BR, as compared with R-CHOP in patients with indolent NHL including MCL. In a large randomized phase III noninferiority trial, BR resulted in a higher complete response rate (40% vs. 30%, p = .02) and median PFS (35 vs. 22 months, p = .004) compared with R-CHOP among patients with MCL. Additionally, BR was associated with lower risk for hematologic and other toxicities (except erythematous or allergic skin rash).[14] In another study, BR was found to be noninferior to R-CHOP/R-CVP; among patients with MCL, complete response rate was 50% vs. 27% for BR vs. R-CHOP/R-CVP, respectively. BR was associated with a higher risk of vomiting (higher use of aprepitant in R-CHOP group), drug hypersensitivity (use of prednisone in R-CHOP/R-CVP), and a lower risk of neuropathy and alopecia. Grade III/IV lymphopenia was more common with BR, whereas the use of R-CHOP was associated with a higher risk of grade III/IV neutropenia and greater utilization of granulocyte colony stimulating factor.[16] Given better tolerance and at least equivalent outcomes, many experts prefer BR over R-CHOP particularly in older patients. A recent phase 3 trial has demonstrated improved median PFS (30 vs. 16 months) and 4-year OS (64% vs.

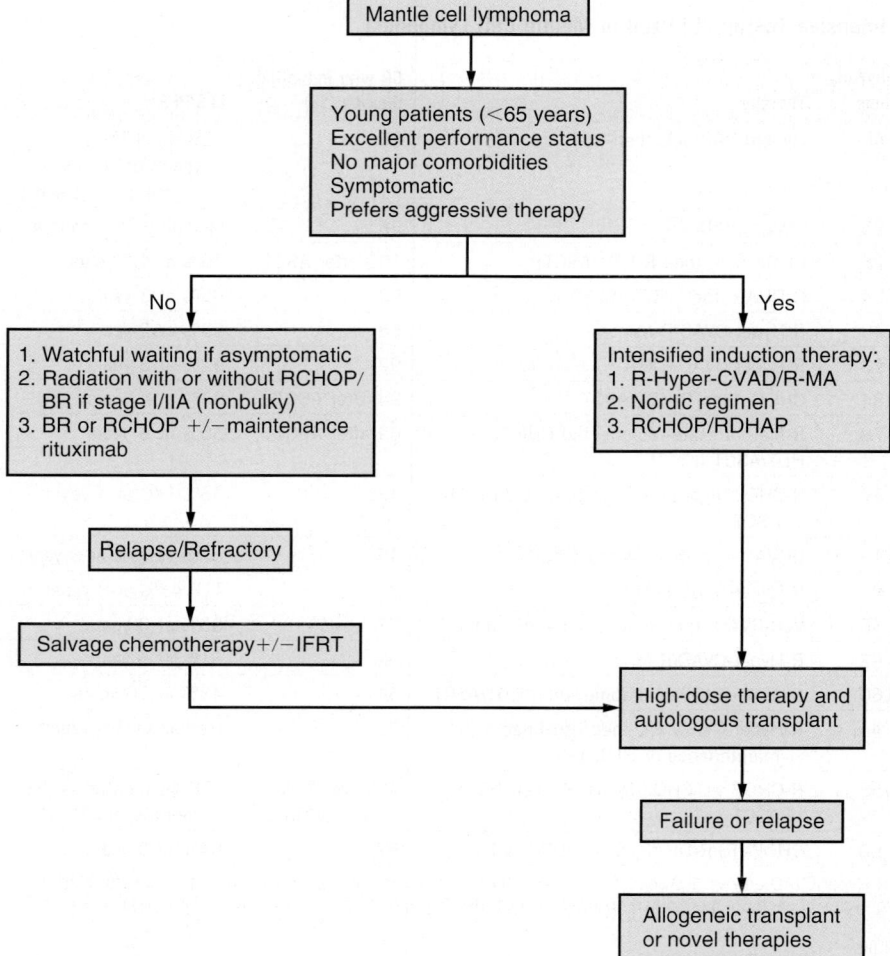

Fig. 81.4 Algorithm for management of mantle cell lymphoma outside of a trial. *BR,* Bendamustine and rituximab; *CHOP,* cyclophosphamide, doxorubicin, vincristine and prednisone; *IFRT,* involved field radiotherapy; *R-CHOP,* rituximab and CHOP; *RDHAP,* rituximab, cisplatin, cytarabine, and dexamethasone; *R-Hyper-CVAD/R-MA,* rituximab, cyclophosphamide, vincristine, doxorubicin, and dexamethasone alternating with rituximab, cytarabine, and methotrexate.

54%) with bortezomib replacing vincristine in R-CHOP, as compared with R-CHOP.[37] The addition of bortezomib to R-CHOP and the use of ^{90}Y ibritumomab after R-CHOP have also shown promising results. Similarly, dose-adjusted infusional R-EPOCH (rituximab, etoposide, prednisone, vincristine, cyclophosphamide, and doxorubicin) with idiotype vaccine or bortezomib have resulted in excellent survival rates.

Upfront Intensified Therapy and Autologous Stem Cell Transplantation

Several studies have demonstrated improved outcomes with upfront intensified therapy and HDT/ASCT in young symptomatic patients with MCL. In the European MCL network randomized trial conducted in the pre-rituximab era, the use of myeloablative radiochemotherapy and ASCT versus α-interferon maintenance following CHOP-like regimen improved median PFS (39 vs. 17 months, $p = .01$) without OS benefit (83% vs. 77% at 3 years, $p = 0.18$) in 122 patients with MCL ≤65 years old in the first complete remission.[38] In the rituximab era, several nonrandomized prospective and retrospective studies have demonstrated better survival outcomes with intensified therapy and HDT/ASCT compared with historical controls. The second Nordic MCL trial among untreated patients with MCL <66 years ($n = 160$) utilized a phase II protocol

with dose-intensified induction immunochemotherapy with maxi-CHOP-R (dose-intensified R-CHOP), alternating with rituximab and high-dose cytarabine, followed by HDT and rituximab-in vivo purged ASCT among the responders. This resulted in a 6-year OS and event-free survival (EFS) of 70% and 56%, respectively, with a higher proportion of molecular response rate (92% vs. 38%, $p < .001$) compared with a historical control in the first Nordic MCL trial.[39] Cancer and Leukemia Group B (CALGB) 59909 study demonstrated a five-year PFS and OS of 56% and 64%, respectively, among patients with MCL up to the age of 69 years ($n = 78$) who were treated with cytarabine- and methotrexate-based immunochemotherapy followed by HDT/ASCT.[24] Several other studies have demonstrated excellent outcomes with rituximab-based chemotherapy such as R-Hyper-CVAD or R-CHOP/RDHAP (rituximab, cisplatin, cytarabine and dexamethasone) and HDT/ASCT (Table 81.2).

Although these studies demonstrate improved PFS with HDT/ASCT consolidation, the optimal induction therapy is unclear. To determine the value of induction therapy an NCCN NHL database study compared the outcomes of patients with MCL <65 years treated with several chemotherapy regimens. This study demonstrated a worse 3-year PFS with R-CHOP alone (18%) compared with R-Hyper-CVAD (58%, $p < .001$), R-CHOP and HDT/ASCT (56%, $p < .001$), and R-Hyper-CVAD and HDT/ASCT (55%, $p = .004$). PFS did not differ between the latter three groups. The 3-year OS was similar between R-CHOP alone (69%), R-Hyper-CVAD (85%,

TABLE 81.3   Outcomes of Therapy Utilized in Relapsed/Refractory Mantle Cell Lymphoma

Author, Year	Number of patients	Therapy	ORR (%)	EFS/PFS	OS (%)
Rummel, 2005[47]	16	Rituximab, bendamustine	75	18 months	NA
Robinson, 2008[48]	66	Rituximab, bendamustine	92	23 months	NA
Inwards, 2008[49]	24	Cladribine	46	~5 months	~22 months
Goy, 2009[50]	141	Bortezomib	32	~6 months	~23 months
O'Connor, 2009[51]	40	Bortezomib	47[a]	~5 months [a]	NA
Wang, 2009[52]	32	Yttrium-90-Ibritumomab Tiuxetan	31	6 months	21 months
Baiocchi, 2011[53]	14	Rituximab, bortezomib	29	~2 months	NA
Lamm, 2011[54]	16	Rituximab, bortezomib, dexamethasone	81	12 months	38 months
Ansell, 2011[55]	69	Rituximab, temsirolimus	59	TTP ~9 months	29 months
Witzig, 2011	57	Lenalidomide	42	~6 months	NA
Wang, 2012[56]	44	Rituximab, lenalidomide	57	11 months	24 months
Zaja, 2012[57]	33	Lenalidomide and dexamethasone	52	12 months	20 months
Renner, 2012[58]	35	Everolimus	20	~5 months	
Visco, 2013[15]	20	Rituximab, bendamustine, and cytarabine	80	70% at 2 years	-
Wang, 2013[43]	111	Ibrutinib	68	~14 months	58% at 18 months
Kahl, 2014[59]	40	Idelalisib	40	~4 months; 22% at 1 year	NA

[a]No difference in outcomes between relapsed and refractory patients.
EFS, Event-free survival; NA, not available; ORR, overall response rate; OS, overall survival; PFS, progression-free survival; TTP, time to progression

$p < .07$), and R-CHOP and HDT/ASCT (87%, $p < .20$). Multivariable analysis revealed that R-CHOP alone had worse OS compared with R-Hyper-CVAD, but not to R-CHOP and HDT/ASCT.[40] Similarly, the type of induction therapy or the timing of therapy did not predict OS in 118 patients with MCL treated with HDT/ASCT in another study. The use of R-Hyper-CVAD, compared with R-CHOP-like therapy, improved PFS for the entire MCL cohort ($p = .01$) but not among transplant recipients ($p = .26$).[41] These studies indicate that intensive induction therapy such as R-Hyper-CVAD may be preferred to R-CHOP among patients who are not planned to undergo HDT/ASCT consolidation; however, the choice of initial therapy may not make a significant difference in OS of patients who are scheduled to undergo HDT/ASCT.

The use of rituximab during or after HDT/ASCT and incorporation of bortezomib to induction or conditioning regimen have demonstrated promising results. In a study, the use of pre-emptive rituximab therapy (375 mg/m^2 weekly for 4 weeks) for molecular relapse after upfront HDT/ASCT resulted in re-induction of molecular remission in 92%, and median molecular and clinical relapse-free survivals of 1.5 and 3.7 years, respectively.[42] Rituximab maintenance after R-Hyper-CVAD or upfront HDT/ASCT may also improve PFS. The use of rituximab frequently increases the risk of neutropenia and hypogammaglobulinemia; however, this may not necessarily translate to a substantially increased risk of major infections.

Central Nervous System Prophylaxis

The incidence of CNS involvement at diagnosis and the role of primary CNS prophylaxis in MCL are controversial. In relapsed MCL, CNS involvement is noted in up to 5–20% of patients, particularly with blastoid variant, and portends a poor prognosis. CNS-penetrating agents such as high-dose methotrexate and cytarabine, with or without intrathecal chemotherapy, may provide sufficient CNS prophylaxis in patients undergoing intensive therapies. In other patients with high-risk features such as blastoid morphology or presence of neurologic symptoms, some centers perform lumbar puncture and utilize intrathecal methotrexate or high-dose systemic methotrexate.

Relapsed or Refractory MCL

The vast majority of patients with MCL will relapse and require subsequent therapies. The choice of therapy in relapsed or refractory MCL depends on the upfront chemotherapy regimen, outcomes with initial therapy, performance status, comorbidities, and desired goals. Several options are available including ibrutinib as well as bortezomib, bendamustine, lenalidomide, or temsirolimus, frequently combined with rituximab (Table 81.3). Ibrutinib received an accelerated approval in November 2013 based on a phase II study of relapsed or refractory MCL ($n = 111$), which demonstrated an overall response rate of 68% with an OS of 58% at 18 months.[43] Given its oral route of administration and tolerability, ibrutinib is increasingly utilized as the preferred option in relapsed or refractory MCL. However, other regimens appear to be equally efficacious and may be used as an alternative or as third-line options. Patients who have not undergone upfront HDT/ASCT may benefit from HDT/ASCT after salvage therapy. In one study, the use of HDT/ASCT demonstrated a median EFS and OS of 36% and 65%, respectively.[44] In this setting, the use of R-Hyper-CVAD salvage therapy prior to HDT/ASCT may result in lower relapse rates but similar PFS and OS.[45] Another study demonstrated a promising result with ^{131}I-tositumomab prior to HDT/ASCT with a complete response rate of 91% and 3-year PFS and OS of 61% and 93%, respectively, highlighting the radiosensitive nature of MCL.[46]

Allogeneic Stem Cell Transplantation

Although allogeneic stem cell transplantation (alloSCT) is potentially curative, lack of large-scale randomized trials and high transplant-related mortality (TRM) has limited enthusiasm toward the use of alloSCT in MCL. Nonetheless, alloSCT should be considered in young and fit patients with MCL with multiple relapsed disease or ASCT failure. The outcomes of alloSCT have been compared with those of ASCT in a few studies. In retrospective studies, alloSCT, compared with ASCT, is associated with higher TRM, lower relapse, and similar OS. In a study of 97 patients with MCL, the alloSCT group, compared with the ASCT group, was younger, more heavily pretreated, and less likely to be in first complete remission. AlloSCT versus ASCT resulted in a greater mortality at 100 days (19% vs. 0%, $p < .01$), numerically lower but statistically similar relapse rate (21% vs. 56%, $p = .11$) and similar OS (49% vs. 47%, $p = .51$) at 5 years.[45] Similarly, in a Center for International Blood and Marrow Transplant Research (CIBMTR) study of chemosensitive patients with MCL ($n = 519$), reduced intensity conditioning (RIC) alloSCT, compared with ASCT, resulted in lower relapse/progression, which was offset by a higher nonrelapse mortality (NRM); hence, the 5-year OS was similar between the two groups. ASCT in first complete remission was associated with the highest OS and PFS confirming the results of prior studies of upfront HDT/ASCT.[60] The comparable OS with alloSCT, compared with ASCT, in these studies also demonstrates the efficacy of disease control with alloSCT in patients with multiple relapses. In clinical practice, therefore, alloSCT may be utilized in heavily pretreated patients.

RIC has been explored with a hope to reduce TRM and expand alloSCT to older patients or patients with other comorbidities. In a study, 70 patients with relapsed and refractory MCL including prior ASCT failures (34%) underwent RIC alloSCT, mainly with alemtuzumab-containing regimens. NRM, cumulative risk of relapse, PFS, and OS were 21%, 65%, 14%, and 37%, respectively, at 5 years. Among patients who relapsed, donor lymphocyte infusion (DLI) or a second RIC alloSCT resulted in a complete remission rate of 73%.[61] In another study of 33 relapsed and patients with refractory MCL, nonmyeloablative conditioning with fludarabine and 2 Gy total body irradiation was associated with an overall response rate of 85%, 2-year NRM, disease-free survival, and OS of 24%, 60%, and 65% respectively.[62] Hence, RIC and nonmyeloablative alloSCT along with DLI for relapse may be reasonable options in patients who are not candidates for myeloablative alloSCT.

PROGNOSIS

As discussed previously, complete remission is seen in up to two-third of patients with MCL, particularly with upfront intensive therapy; however, almost all patients will relapse and develop resistance to chemotherapy over time. Although the prognosis for newly diagnosed patients has improved over the last decades, the OS compares unfavorably with the more frequent NHLs such as follicular lymphoma and diffuse large B-cell lymphoma. A small subset of patients may follow a more indolent clinical course in the beginning, and these patients may have a clinical history that resembles a chronic lymphocytic leukemia.

Prior studies have identified several adverse prognostic factors, which include eastern cooperative oncology group (ECOG) performance status (PS) ≥ 2, age >65 years, elevated LDH, elevated serum beta$_2$-microglobulin, hemoglobin level <12 g/dL, advanced stage, involvement of peripheral blood or extranodal sites ≥ 2, high cell proliferation rate (Ki-67, mitotic index or proliferation signature), blastoid variant histology, deletion or mutation of TP53, and secondary chromosomal aberrations (the presence of gain 3q, 12q and 13q and losses of 6q, 9p, 11q, and 17p).[63] More recent studies have demonstrated that the MCL international prognostic index (MIPI), based on age, ECOG PS, LDH, and white blood cell count, is one of the most important prognostic factors in MCL. In a large study, MIPI categorized MCL patients into low risk (0–3 scores; OS not reached at a median follow-up of 32 months), intermediate risk (4–5 scores; median OS of 51 months), and high risk (6–11 scores; median OS of 29 months) categories with a significant difference in OS (Fig. 81.5). MIPI separated the survival curves better than IPI utilized for diffuse large B-cell lymphoma or follicular lymphoma (FLIPI). Cell proliferation (Ki-67), but not number of mitoses per square millimeter, was an independent prognostic score.[64] Ki-67 and MIPI have been shown to independently predict PFS and OS in other studies also. Prognosis may also be influenced by disease status at ASCT or alloSCT, achievement of molecular remission after therapy, moderate or strong expression of PIM1 (a serine/threonine kinase and proto-oncogene), and number of prior therapies before HDT/ASCT or alloSCT. In the modern era, molecular diagnostics such as gene

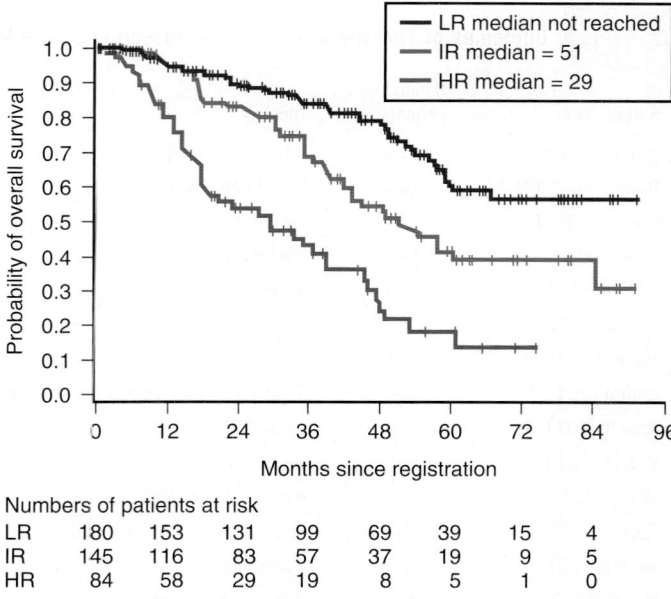

Fig. 81.5 PROGNOSTIC GROUPS STRATIFIED ACCORDING TO THE MANTLE CELL INTERNATIONAL PROGNOSTIC INDEX. *HR,* High risk; *IR,* intermediate risk; *LR,* low risk.

expression profiling, genome-wide miRNA profiling as well as a limited-gene model (based on five genes RAN, MYC, TNFRSF10B, POLE2, and SLC29A2) may also provide meaningful prognostic information; however, the lack of commercial testing and standardization, as well as high cost limit their use in clinical practice.

FUTURE DIRECTIONS

Since the recognition of MCL as a separate entity there has been significant advancement in the understanding of tumor biology, diagnostic, prognostic, and treatment approaches. This has resulted in a significant improvement in OS of patients with MCL at a population level, with approximately half of the patients in the United States surviving beyond 5 years in recent years.[65] A few studies have demonstrated poor prognosis of blastoid-variant MCL. Intensified therapy including upfront ASCT may overcome this poor prognosis, which needs further exploration in prospective studies. The roles of radiotherapy and CNS prophylaxis are currently not well established and should be investigated. Integration of clinical parameters and gene expression profiling has a potential to improve prognostication. Such prognostication may identify an indolent subgroup that can be observed, as well as an aggressive subgroup that may be better served with upfront intensive therapy. A development of prognosis-directed therapy is an ideal goal. Molecular markers such as t(11;14), clonal immunoglobulin heavy chain gene rearrangements, and SOX11 gene expression may be used to identify minimal residual disease. Although the correlation is not consistent, molecular remission has been correlated with long-term remission and PFS. Molecular relapse may precede clinical relapse and has been utilized to guide preemptive therapy, as discussed above. If confirmed in other prospective trials, minimal residual disease-based therapies may be utilized to improve PFS in the future. Elderly patients and patients with comorbidities generally have poor outcomes and should be enrolled in clinical trials of novel well-tolerated agents. Novel agents such as ibrutinib, idelalisib, lenalidomide, and bortezomib have shown promising results; their integration in upfront therapies has a potential to further improve outcomes with initial therapy. Improved prognostic tools, incorporation of minimal residual disease based preemptive therapy, translation of molecular tumor biology to bedside in the form of novel therapies, and integration of such therapies to upfront traditional chemoimmunotherapy regimens offer a potential to change the therapeutic landscape of MCL.

Pathogenesis

- Mantle cell lymphoma (MCL) is characterized by alterations in proliferative, antiapoptotic and prosurvival pathways.
- The vast majority of MCL have the reciprocal translocation, t(11;14) (q13,q23), which juxtaposes the CCND1 gene to the immunoglobin heavy-chain locus. TP53 and ATM genes are other commonly mutated genes.
- Aggressive cases, particularly the blastoid variant, have an increased number of chromosomal abnormalities and complex karyotype.
- Dysregulation of the B cell receptor has also been implicated in the pathogenesis of MCL.

Diagnosis

- The majority of patients present at an advanced stage (III or IV) with lymphadenopathy, hepatomegaly, splenomegaly, and involvement of bone marrow and extranodal sites, especially the gastrointestinal tract.
- Morphologic findings include monomorphic proliferation of small to medium-sized lymphoid cells with irregular nuclear border, dispersed chromatin, and inconspicuous nucleoli.
- Histologic transformation to large B-cell lymphoma does not occur; however, MCL can have several morphological variants such as blastoid and pleomorphic variants.
- The characteristic immunophenotypic features (CD5$^+$, CD10$^-$, CD19$^+$, CD23$^-$, FMC$^+$) and the identification of t(11;14)(q13;q32) or cyclin D1 overexpression improve diagnostic accuracy.

- Staging procedure includes a bone marrow biopsy and CT or PET-CT of chest, abdomen, and pelvis; however, lumbar puncture is not routinely performed. Although endoscopies of upper and lower gastrointestinal tracts are frequently positive, such evaluation may not change management.

Therapy and Prognosis

- MCL combines the worst features of both indolent lymphoma (noncurability) and aggressive lymphoma (aggressive course).
- Therapeutic strategy is not standardized and may include wait-and-watch strategy in select asymptomatic patients, rituximab-based immunochemotherapy (BR or R-CHOP) in older patients, and intensified chemotherapy such as R-Hyper-CVAD followed by upfront high-dose chemotherapy and autologous hematopoietic stem cell transplant in young fit patients.
- Recent studies have demonstrated improved response rate and less toxicity with BR, as compared with R-CHOP.
- Ibrutinib has emerged as an excellent option for the management of relapsed or refractory MCL. Other salvage therapy includes bortezomib, bendamustine, lenalidomide, or temsirolimus frequently combined with rituximab.
- Ki-67 level and MIPI (based on age, ECOG PS, LDH and white blood cell count) are two of the most important prognostic factors in MCL.
- Recent advances in the therapy of MCL have improved the OS at a population level, with approximately half of the patients in the United States surviving beyond 5 years in recent years.

SUGGESTED READINGS

Abrahamsson A, Albertsson-Lindblad A, Brown PN, et al: Real world data on primary treatment for mantle cell lymphoma: a Nordic Lymphoma Group observational study. *Blood* 124(8):1288–1295, 2014.

Andersen NS, Pedersen LB, Laurell A, et al: Pre-emptive treatment with rituximab of molecular relapse after autologous stem cell transplantation in mantle cell lymphoma. *J Clin Oncol* 27(26):4365–4370, 2009.

Budde LE, Guthrie KA, Till BG, et al: Mantle cell lymphoma international prognostic index but not pretransplantation induction regimen predicts survival for patients with mantle-cell lymphoma receiving high-dose therapy and autologous stem-cell transplantation. *J Clin Oncol* 29(22):3023–3029, 2011.

Caballero D, Campo E, Lopez-Guillermo A, et al: Clinical practice guidelines for diagnosis, treatment, and follow-up of patients with mantle cell lymphoma. Recommendations from the GEL/TAMO Spanish Cooperative Group. *Ann Hematol* 92(9):1151–1179, 2013.

Chandran R, Gardiner SK, Simon M, et al: Survival trends in mantle cell lymphoma in the United States over 16 years 1992-2007. *Leuk Lymphoma* 53(8):1488–1493, 2012.

Cook G, Smith GM, Kirkland K, et al: Outcome following Reduced-Intensity Allogeneic Stem Cell Transplantation (RIC AlloSCT) for relapsed and refractory mantle cell lymphoma (MCL): a study of the British Society for Blood and Marrow Transplantation. *Biol Blood Marrow Transplant* 16(10):1419–1427, 2010.

Damon LE, Johnson JL, Niedzwiecki D, et al: Immunochemotherapy and autologous stem-cell transplantation for untreated patients with mantle-cell lymphoma: CALGB 59909. *J Clin Oncol* 27(36):6101–6108, 2009.

Dreyling M, Lenz G, Hoster E, et al: Early consolidation by myeloablative radiochemotherapy followed by autologous stem cell transplantation in first remission significantly prolongs progression-free survival in mantle-cell lymphoma: results of a prospective randomized trial of the European MCL Network. *Blood* 105(7):2677–2684, 2005.

Fenske TS, Zhang MJ, Carreras J, et al: Autologous or reduced-intensity conditioning allogeneic hematopoietic cell transplantation for chemotherapy-sensitive mantle-cell lymphoma: analysis of transplantation timing and modality. *J Clin Oncol* 32(4):273–281, 2014.

Flinn IW, van der Jagt R, Kahl BS, et al: Randomized trial of bendamustine-rituximab or R-CHOP/R-CVP in first-line treatment of indolent NHL or MCL: the BRIGHT study. *Blood* 123(19):2944–2952, 2014.

Forstpointner R, Dreyling M, Repp R, et al: The addition of rituximab to a combination of fludarabine, cyclophosphamide, mitoxantrone (FCM) significantly increases the response rate and prolongs survival as compared with FCM alone in patients with relapsed and refractory follicular and mantle cell lymphomas: results of a prospective randomized study of the German Low-Grade Lymphoma Study Group. *Blood* 104(10):3064–3071, 2004.

Ganti AK, Bierman PJ, Lynch JC, et al: Hematopoietic stem cell transplantation in mantle cell lymphoma. *Ann Oncol* 16(4):618–624, 2005.

Geisler CH, Kolstad A, Laurell A, et al: Long-term progression-free survival of mantle cell lymphoma after intensive front-line immunochemotherapy with in vivo-purged stem cell rescue: a nonrandomized phase 2 multicenter study by the Nordic Lymphoma Group. *Blood* 112(7):2687–2693, 2008.

Gopal AK, Rajendran JG, Petersdorf SH, et al: High-dose chemo-radioimmunotherapy with autologous stem cell support for relapsed mantle cell lymphoma. *Blood* 99(9):3158–3162, 2002.

Guru Murthy GS, Venkitachalam R, Mehta P: Effect of radiotherapy on the survival of patients with stage I and stage II mantle cell lymphoma: analysis of the Surveillance, Epidemiology and End Results database. *Clin Lymphoma Myeloma Leuk* 14(Suppl):S90–S95, 2014.

Hoster E, Dreyling M, Klapper W, et al: A new prognostic index (MIPI) for patients with advanced-stage mantle cell lymphoma. *Blood* 111(2):558–565, 2008.

Howard OM, Gribben JG, Neuberg DS, et al: Rituximab and CHOP induction therapy for newly diagnosed mantle-cell lymphoma: molecular complete responses are not predictive of progression-free survival. *J Clin Oncol* 20(5):1288–1294, 2002.

Jares P, Colomer D, Campo E: Genetic and molecular pathogenesis of mantle cell lymphoma: perspectives for new targeted therapeutics. *Nat Rev Cancer* 7(10):750–762, 2007.

LaCasce AS, Vandergrift JL, Rodriguez MA, et al: Comparative outcome of initial therapy for younger patients with mantle cell lymphoma: an analysis from the NCCN NHL Database. *Blood* 119(9):2093–2099, 2012.

Lenz G, Dreyling M, Hoster E, et al: Immunochemotherapy with rituximab and cyclophosphamide, doxorubicin, vincristine, and prednisone significantly improves response and time to treatment failure, but not long-term outcome in patients with previously untreated mantle cell lymphoma: results of a prospective randomized trial of the German Low Grade Lymphoma Study Group (GLSG). *J Clin Oncol* 23(9):1984–1992, 2005.

Maris MB, Sandmaier BM, Storer BE, et al: Allogeneic hematopoietic cell transplantation after fludarabine and 2 Gy total body irradiation for relapsed and refractory mantle cell lymphoma. *Blood* 104(12):3535–3542, 2004.

Martin P, Chadburn A, Christos P, et al: Outcome of deferred initial therapy in mantle-cell lymphoma. *J Clin Oncol* 27(8):1209–1213, 2009.

Robak T, Huang H, Jin J, et al: Bortezomib-based therapy for newly diagnosed mantle-cell lymphoma. *N Engl J Med* 372(10):944–953, 2015.

Rummel MJ, Niederle N, Maschmeyer G, et al: Bendamustine plus rituximab versus CHOP plus rituximab as first-line treatment for patients with indolent and mantle-cell lymphomas: an open-label, multicentre, randomised, phase 3 non-inferiority trial. *Lancet* 381(9873):1203–1210, 2013.

Swerdlow SH, Campo E, Harris NL, et al: *WHO Classification of Tumours of Haematopoietic and Lymphoid Tissues. Primary mediastinal (thymic) large B-cell lymphoma*, Lyon, France, 2008, IARC Press, pp 250–251.

Vose JM: Mantle cell lymphoma: 2013 Update on diagnosis, risk-stratification, and clinical management. *Am J Hematol* 88(12):1082–1088, 2013.

Vose JM, Bierman PJ, Weisenburger DD, et al: Autologous hematopoietic stem cell transplantation for mantle cell lymphoma. *Biol Blood Marrow Transplant* 6(6):640–645, 2000.

Wang ML, Rule S, Martin P, et al: Targeting BTK with ibrutinib in relapsed or refractory mantle-cell lymphoma. *N Engl J Med* 369(6):507–516, 2013.

REFERENCES

For the complete list of references, log on to www.expertconsult.com.

DIAGNOSIS AND TREATMENT OF DIFFUSE LARGE B-CELL LYMPHOMA AND BURKITT LYMPHOMA

Kieron Dunleavy and Wyndham H. Wilson

Diffuse large B-cell lymphoma (DLBCL) and Burkitt lymphoma (BL) are the most common types of aggressive B-cell lymphoma. Although they share many clinical and biologic features, the approach to their management is different; therefore, an accurate histologic diagnosis is of utmost importance. There have been several recent therapeutic advances in the management of these diseases, and both DLBCL and BL have high cure rates with current treatment approaches. Therefore, it is imperative to promptly evaluate patients with these diseases and expeditiously institute appropriate therapy.

DIFFUSE LARGE B-CELL LYMPHOMA

Epidemiology

DLBCL is the most prevalent histologic subtype of non-Hodgkin lymphoma (NHL) (of which there are approximately 72,000 new cases in the United States each year) and comprises 30% to 40% of these diseases. Although the median age at diagnosis is in the seventh decade of life, DLBCL affects children and adults of all ages, and it is slightly more common in males than females. Though the etiology of DLBCL is unknown in most cases, it can arise from transformation of an indolent lymphoma. A history of immunodeficiency is a significant risk factor, and individuals who are human immunodeficiency virus (HIV) positive have in the range of 100 times higher incidence of developing DLBCL over those who do not have HIV.

Pathobiology

The pathobiology of DLBCL is very heterogeneous, and within DLBCL, there are several morphologic variants that include centroblastic, immunoblastic, T-cell rich or histiocyte-rich, (see E-Slide VM03959) and anaplastic subtypes. Recent progress using techniques such as molecular profiling and other high-resolution genetic technologies are further advancing this taxonomy. There are also several clinical-pathologic variants of DLBCL. Primary mediastinal B-cell lymphoma (PMBL), for example, commonly presents in young women and usually remains localized to the mediastinum (Fig. 82.1). Primary central nervous system lymphoma (PCNSL) is another rare subtype of DLBCL that rarely disseminates to extraneural sites and is much more commonly observed in HIV-positive individuals. It is important to recognize that DLBCL can also arise as a result of histologic transformation from an indolent lymphoma. Although this differentiation may not affect treatment choice initially, it will affect prognosis and natural history, and therefore needs to be recognized at diagnosis.[1]

The neoplastic cells of DLBCL express pan B-cell markers, including CD20, and surface or cytoplasmic immunoglobulin is often demonstrated. CD10, BCL6, and IRF4/MUM1 are variably expressed, and the proliferation index as measured by Ki67 staining is typically high. Approximately 30% of cases show abnormalities involving the BCL6 gene, and translocation of the BCL2 gene, a hallmark of follicular lymphoma, is present in 20% to 30% of cases. Approximately 10% of cases of DLBCL harbor a t(8:14) MYC translocation, and recently, several groups have demonstrated that

this confers a much worse prognosis compared with MYC-negative cases when CHOP-type (cyclophosphamide, doxorubicin [Novantrone], vincristine [Oncovin], and prednisone) regimens are used.

Recently, gene expression profiling has defined a new molecular taxonomy for DLBCL. Morphologically indistinguishable tumors can show marked heterogeneity in gene expression, and these patterns of expression may be classified into signatures that correspond to the cellular origin of the lymphoma according to its stage of B-cell differentiation; on the basis of these signatures, DLBCL can be divided into at least three different subtypes: germinal center B-cell (GCB)-like, activated B-cell (ABC)-like, and primary mediastinal B-cell lymphoma (PMBL).[2] Importantly, these subtypes of DLBCL have disparate outcomes following standard therapy with the ABC subtype having an inferior survival in many retrospective studies.[3]

Clinical Features

The clinical presentation of DLBCL is variable and depends on a number of factors, including histology, patient age, and immune status. The disease typically presents with lymphadenopathy that can range from relatively asymptomatic to causing pain (Fig. 82.2), causing organ compromise such as ureteral obstruction or spinal cord compression. The involvement of bone marrow (BM) is much less frequent than with indolent lymphomas and is present in approximately 20% of cases.

Patients may have constitutional manifestations from the production of inflammatory molecules and a variety of other cytokines and chemokines produced by the lymphoma cells or host tissues. Such manifestations include weight loss, malaise, fevers, night sweats, and loss of appetite. Of these, unexplained weight loss of more than 10% of body weight and temperature higher than 38°C as well as drenching night sweats are referred to as "B" symptoms.

Investigation

History and Physical Examination

Patients should be questioned about systemic symptoms, and their performance status should be assessed (Table 82.1). It is important to determine if there is a history of potential causative factors such as prior malignancy, chemotherapy or radiation treatment, or autoimmune or immunodeficiency diseases. A history of infection with or exposure to various pathogens, including HIV and hepatitis B and C, should be excluded. A detailed physical examination should be performed with particular attention to lymph node (LN) regions. Skin involvement by DLBCL is rare (Fig. 82.3).

An accurate histologic diagnosis is imperative to determine the patient's prognosis and treatment; therefore, the single most important diagnostic test is a technically adequate and properly evaluated excisional tissue biopsy. With few exceptions, fine-needle aspiration is inadequate for diagnosis. Aggressive lymphoma should be diagnosed by an experienced hematopathologist familiar with the nuances and pitfalls of lymphoma diagnosis.

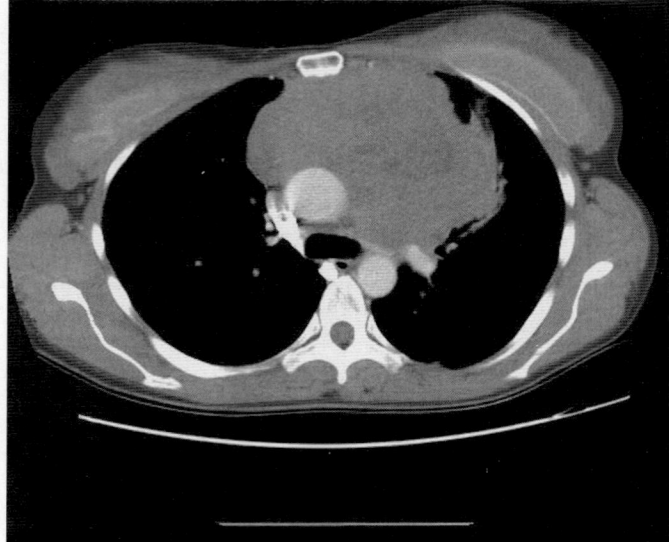

Fig. 82.1 COMPUTED TOMOGRAPHY SCAN OF THE CHEST SHOWING A LARGE 17-CM ANTERIOR MEDIASTINAL MASS. A biopsy was consistent with primary mediastinal B-cell lymphoma.

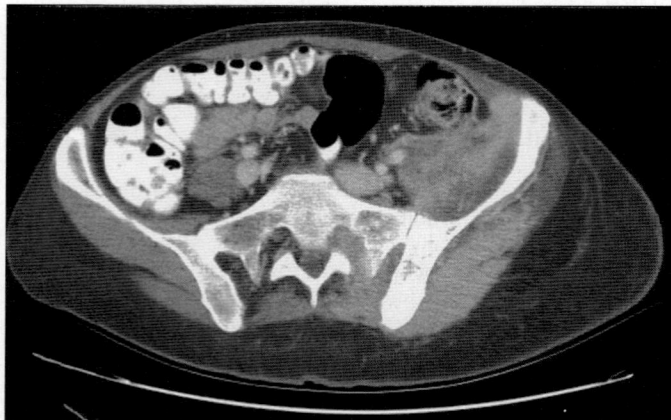

Fig. 82.2 COMPUTED TOMOGRAPHY SCAN OF THE ABDOMEN SHOWING A LARGE LEFT-SIDED PSOAS MASS. A biopsy was consistent with diffuse large B-cell lymphoma.

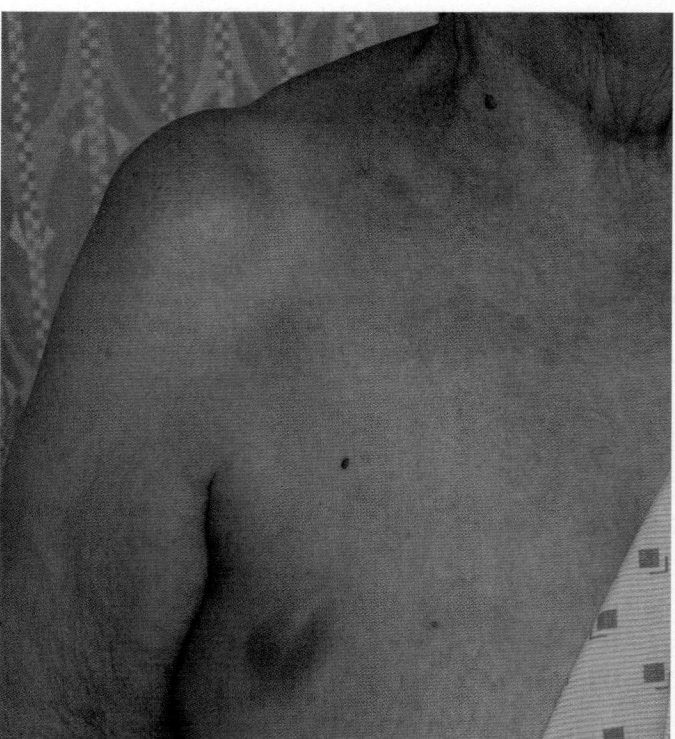

Fig. 82.3 INFILTRATION OF THE RIGHT LOWER ANTERIOR CHEST WALL WITH DIFFUSE LARGE B-CELL LYMPHOMA.

Hepatitis B Prophylaxis and Therapy During Lymphoma Treatment

There is a risk of hepatitis B reactivation both from chemotherapy and rituximab, and this is a potentially fatal complication. We check hepatitis serology (hepatitis B surface antigen [HBsAg], hepatitis B surface antibody [anti-HBs], and hepatitis B core antibody [anti-HBc]) in all patients at diagnosis. Patients with active hepatitis B receive antiviral medication and liver function tests (LFTs) and hepatitis B viral loads are monitored closely. Patients with a history of hepatitis B infection should either receive antiviral prophylaxis or have the hepatitis B viral load monitored very closely (ideally on each cycle) with a low threshold to commence antiviral medications.

TABLE 82.1	Eastern Co-operative Group Performance Scale
Performance Status	**Definition**
0	Asymptomatic
1	Symptomatic but fully ambulatory
2	Symptomatic and in bed <50% of the day
3	Symptomatic and in bed >50% of the day
4	Bedridden

Laboratory Investigations

Laboratory tests should include a complete blood count; serum chemistry, including lactate dehydrogenase (LDH); and HIV and hepatitis serology tests (Table 82.2). The latter should be included due to the importance of identifying patients with active hepatitis and a history of hepatitis B because they will likely require treatment with antivirals, monitoring, or both (see box on Hepatitis B Prophylaxis and Therapy During Lymphoma Treatment). Epstein-Barr virus (EBV) viral loads may also be useful in specific lymphomas such as posttransplant lymphoproliferative disorders (PTLDs) and EBV-positive DLBCL of elderly adults. An elevated LDH level has adverse prognostic implications for patients with DLBCL.

Imaging and Staging

It is important to determine sites of disease involvement; therefore, imaging studies should include computed tomography (CT) scanning of the chest, abdomen, and pelvis as well as fludeoxyglucose positron emission tomography (FDG-PET) scanning in most cases. The use of other imaging modalities depends on the clinical presentation and sites of disease. For example, if central nervous system (CNS) involvement is highly suspected, evaluation of the head by CT or magnetic resonance imaging (MRI) may be indicated. Involvement of the bone is best evaluated by MRI and PET scans.

Because involvement of the BM may impact management, it should be assessed in all patients with DLBCL by a BM aspirate and biopsy. Patients at increased risk of CNS involvement should undergo lumbar puncture with evaluation of the cerebrospinal fluid (CSF) by cytology and flow cytometry.[4] Specifically, clinical presentations with several extranodal sites and elevated LDH level as well as particular

TABLE 82.2   Staging Evaluation for Diffuse Large B-Cell Lymphoma

All Patients	As Clinically Indicated
History and physical examination	Other viral studies
CBC and chemistry (including LDH)	CT or MRI of the head
HIV and hepatitis B and C serology	Body PET scan
Chest radiograph	Additional imaging
CT scan of the chest, abdomen, and pelvis	CSF evaluation by cytology or flow cytometry
BM aspirate and biopsy	Other tests indicated by results of staging

BM, Bone marrow; CBC, complete blood count; CSF, cerebrospinal fluid; CT, computed tomography; LDH, lactate dehydrogenase; MRI, magnetic resonance imaging; PET, positron emission tomography.

Intrathecal Prophylaxis in Diffuse Large B-Cell Lymphoma

In DLBCL, the role of intrathecal prophylaxis to prevent CNS recurrence is controversial and poorly studied, and there are several different approaches. Our approach is as follows. All patients at risk for CNS disease undergo a lumbar puncture at diagnosis, and CSF is checked by cytology and flow cytometry; if the results are positive, patients receive active treatment of the CNS. We administer intrathecal prophylaxis to all patients who fulfill either of the following criteria:
1. Two or more extranodal sites of disease involvement and an elevated LDH level.
2. Certain extranodal sites of involvement that have been associated with an increased risk of CNS spread such as BM and testis.
We use intrathecal methotrexate at a dose of 12 mg. We commence prophylaxis on cycle 3 day 1 and administer it on days 1 and 5 of cycles 3 through 6.

TABLE 82.3   Ann Arbor Staging System for Lymphomas

Stage[a]	Cotswold Modification of Arbor Classification
I	Involvement of a single LN region or lymphoid structure
II	Involvement of two or more LN regions on the same side of the diaphragm (the mediastinum is considered a single site, but the hilar LNs are considered bilaterally); the number of atomic sites should be indicated by a subscript (e.g., II_3)
III	Involvement of LN regions on both sides of the diaphragm: III_1 (with or without involvement of splenic hilar, celiac, or portal nodes) and III_2 (with involvement of paraaortic, iliac, and mesenteric nodes
IV	Involvement of one or more extranodal sites in addition to a site for which the designation E has been used

[a]All cases are subclassified to indicate the absence (A) or presence (B) of the systemic symptoms of significant fever (>38.0°C [100.4°F]), night sweats, and unexplained weight loss exceeding 10% of normal body weight within the previous 6 months. The clinical stage (CS) denotes the stage as determined by all diagnostic examinations and a single diagnostic biopsy only. In the Ann Arbor classification, the term *pathologic stage* (PS) is used if a second biopsy of any kind has been obtained, whether the result was negative or positive. In the Cotswold modification, the PS is determined by laparotomy; X designates bulky disease (widening of the mediastinum by more than one-third or the presence of a nodal mass >10 cm), and E designates involvement of a single extranodal site that is contiguous or proximal to the known nodal site.
LN, Lymph node.

TABLE 82.4   Revised International Prognostic Index (R-IPI)[a]

No. of IPI Factors	IPI Score	Outcome	Overall Survival (%)
0	0	Very good	94
1–2	1–2	Good	79
3, 4, or 5	3–5	Poor	55

[a]One point is given for the presence of each of the following characteristics: age older than 60 years, elevated serum LDH level, ECOG performance status ≥2, Ann Arbor stage III or IV, and more than two extranodal sites.
ECOG, Eastern Cooperative Oncology Group; IPI, International Prognostic Index; LDH, lactate dehydrogenase
From Sehn LH, Berry B, Chhanabhai M, et al: The revised International Prognostic Index is a better predictor of outcome than the standard IPI for patients with diffuse large B-cell lymphoma treated with R-CHOP. *Blood* 109:1857, 2007.

---

sites such as the testis and BM are associated with an increased risk of CNS disease, and intrathecal prophylaxis should be considered (see box on Intrathecal Prophylaxis in Diffuse Large B-Cell Lymphoma).

DLBCL is staged according to the Ann Arbor staging system (Table 82.3), which was originally developed for Hodgkin lymphoma (HL). However, because of the heterogeneity and hematogenous pattern of dissemination in NHL, in contrast to contiguous LN spread with HL, the staging system has more limited value. At the same time, important modifications to the Ann Arbor staging system made at the Cotswold Conference have made it more applicable to NHL.[5]

Prognosis

To identify prognostic factors in NHL, an international project to correlate clinical variables and outcome in 2031 patients with untreated aggressive lymphoma was undertaken. The following parameters were associated with inferior outcome: age older than 60 years, Ann Arbor stage III or IV disease, serum LDH level above normal range, Eastern Co-operative Oncology Group (ECOG) performance status of two or higher, and involvement of two or more extranodal sites. A clinical prognostic model, termed the International Prognostic Index (IPI), was developed using these five factors. In this model, one point was allocated for each feature and nicely stratified patients into four groups with 5-year survivals of 73%, 51%, 43%, and 26% for zero or one, two, three, and four or five risk factors, respectively, with CHOP-based treatment. Based on this model, the IPI has become the standard in DLBCL for assessing clinical prognosis and treatment stratification within and comparison between clinical trials. Recently, a revised prognostic model for R-CHOP, termed *Revised-IPI*, was published (Table 82.4).[6]

Although not yet routinely performed in aggressive NHL, gene expression profiling is emerging as an important prognostic tool. In DLBCL, overall survival is different in each group and in many studies superior in patients with the GCB compared with the ABC subtype. Using gene expression profiling, a molecular prognostic model of survival, independent of the IPI, has been developed for R-CHOP–treated DLBCL. In routine clinical practice, it has not been feasible to perform gene expression profiling and immunohistochemistry algorithms to predict cell of origin have been used up until now. While these have been somewhat helpful, they have demonstrated varying degrees of concordance with microarray results, limiting their usefulness. Therefore novel assays to more accurately predict cell of origin are needed and in that regard, the recent 20-gene predictor assay developed by the Lymphoma and Leukemia Molecular Profiling Project (LLMPP) is promising and potentially widely applicable (Fig. 82.4).

This increased understanding of the heterogeneous biology of DLBCL has led to the investigation of strategies and novel agents that have selective activity within molecular subtypes and sets the stage for an era of precision medicine in DLBCL therapeutics, where therapy can be ascribed based on molecular phenotype.[5] This offers the chance of improving the curability of DLBCL, particularly in the activated B-cell subtype where standard approaches are inadequate for the majority of patients.

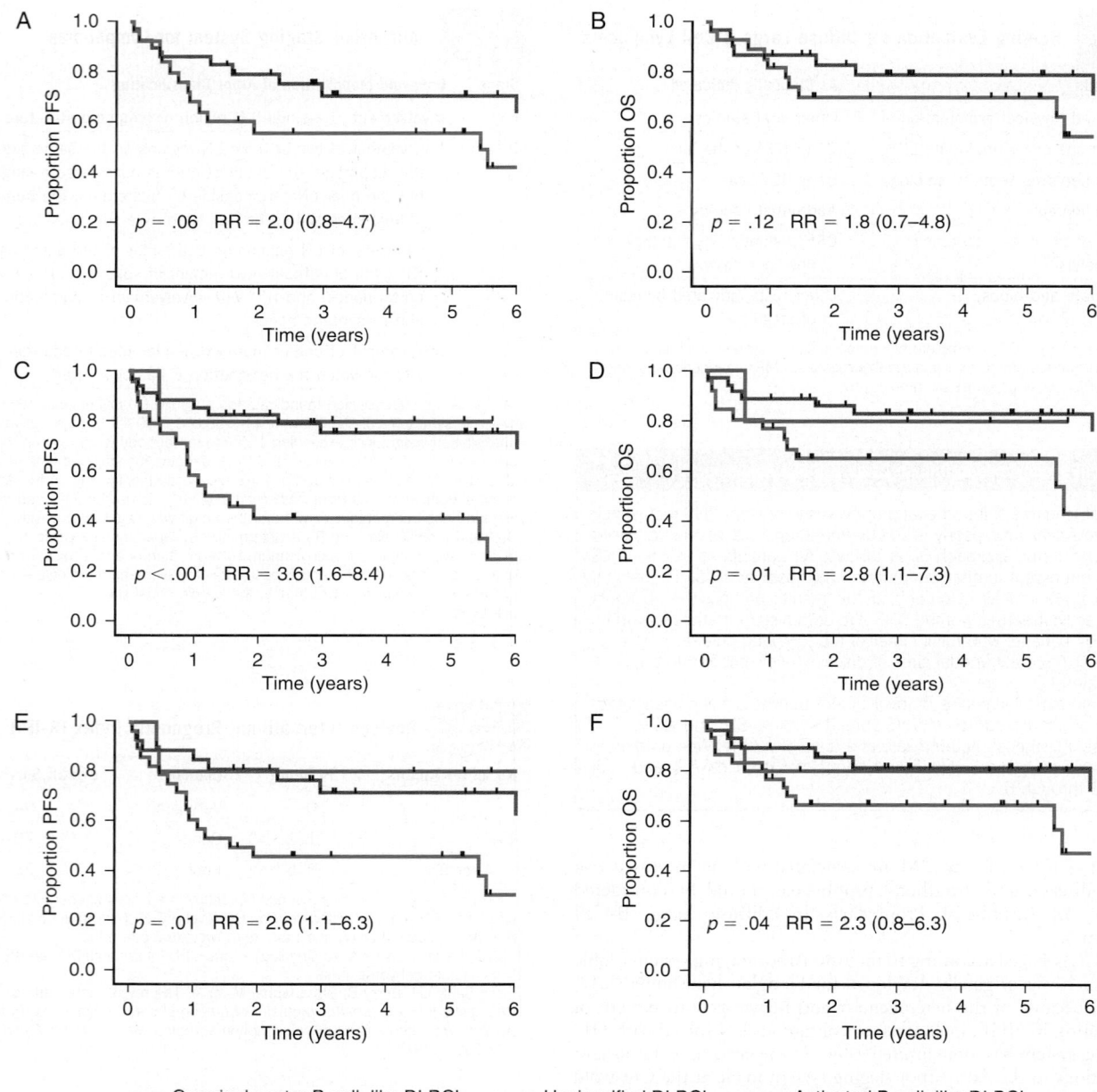

Germinal center B-cell–like DLBCL — Unclassified DLBCL — Activated B-cell–like DLBCL

Fig. 82.4 PATIENTS WITH DIFFUSE LARGE B-CELL LYMPHOMA (DLBCL) OUTCOMES FOLLOWING R-CHOP ACCORDING TO CELL ORIGIN (COO; IN THE INDEPENDENT VALIDATION COHORT). (A) Progression-free survival (PFS) for COO assignment using the "Hans" algorithm. (B) Overall survival (OS) for COO assignment using the "Hans" algorithm. (C) PFS in the COO groups as determined by the Lymph2Cx assay. (D) OS in the COO groups as determined by the Lymph2Cx assay. (E) PFS in the COO groups determined by the gold-standard method applying the previously described model to gene expression on frozen tissue (FT). (F) OS in the COO groups determined by the gold-standard method. The p-values are from log-rank tests comparing the activated B-cell (ABC) and germinal center B-cell (GCB) groups. The log-rank tests are one sided in the direction of greater hazard for ABC. RR, relative risk (with the 95% confidence interval in brackets) associated with the ABC group compared with the GCB group. *(Republished with permission of the American Society of Hematology from Scott DW, Wright GW, Williams PM, Lih CJ, Walsh W, Jaffe ES, et al: Determining cell-of-origin subtypes of diffuse large B-cell lymphoma using gene expression in formalin-fixed paraffin-embedded tissue. Blood 123:1214, 2014. Permission conveyed through Copyright Clearance Center.)*

Treatment

The mainstay of treatment for DLBCL is systemic chemotherapy; radiation treatment alone is inadequate and associated with high recurrence rates. For early stage disease, whether or not radiation treatment adds benefit to chemotherapy has been controversial. Based on a randomized study that showed a survival advantage of limited course CHOP plus involved field radiation compared with full course CHOP in early stage (I/II) aggressive lymphoma, combined modality therapy became the standard. However, longer patient follow-up showed a convergence of the overall survival curves because of late systemic relapses in the combined modality arm, thus reopening the debate on radiation. In this regard, a prospective Groupe d'Etude des Lymphomes de l'Adulte (GELA) study randomized elderly patients with favorable early stage aggressive lymphoma to receive CHOP alone (four cycles) or CHOP plus radiation, and found that combined modality therapy was not superior to chemotherapy alone. Given these results and the improved outcome of R-CHOP, it is difficult to justify the routine use of radiation in early stage disease.

A possible exception to the omission of radiation is in the treatment of primary mediastinal DLBCL (PMBL), depending on the chemotherapy regimen. In a study of 50 untreated patients with PMBL who received MACOP-B (methotrexate, ARA-C [Cytarabine], cyclophosphamide, vincristine, prednisone, and bleomycin) followed by radiation, 66% had persistently positive gallium scans after chemotherapy, suggesting active disease. After consolidation radiotherapy, however, only 19% of patients had a positive gallium scan, and 80% were event-free at 39 months of median follow-up. This important study suggested that radiotherapy was necessary after chemotherapy in PMBL. Furthermore, historical evidence indicated that dose-intense regimens such as MACOP-B or VACOP-B (etoposide, doxorubicin, cyclophosphamide, vincristine, prednisone, and bleomycin) were superior to CHOP for PMBL, raising yet another question about the optimal chemotherapy for this disease. Although the addition of rituximab to CHOP has improved the outcome for patients with DLBCL, there remains a high proportion of patients who do not achieve remission with R-CHOP, and require mediastinal radiation. Recent results with the pharmacodynamically dose-adjusted regimen of doxorubicin, vincristine, and etoposide infused over 96 hours with bolus intravenous cyclophosphamide, rituximab, and oral prednisone (DA-EPOCH-R) challenge the need for radiation in PMBL as in a prospective study of 53 patients, 93% were event-free with DA-EPOCH-R alone[7] (see box on Treatment of Primary Mediastinal B-Cell Lymphoma). These results suggest that regimens such as DA-EPOCH-R obviate the need for radiation in a high proportion of patients with PMBL, thus eliminating the risk of long-term toxicities such as secondary malignancies and heart disease. An ongoing study by the International Extranodal Lymphoma Study Group (IELSG) is testing if mediastinal radiation can be omitted in patients who have a negative FDG-PET scan at the end of therapy.[8]

Today, most newly diagnosed patients with DLBCL receive rituximab in combination with a chemotherapy backbone consisting of cyclophosphamide, doxorubicin, vincristine, and prednisone (CHOP) (Fig. 82.5). This backbone has been used since the early 1970s when doxorubicin was added to cyclophosphamide, vincristine, and prednisone (CVP) and CHOP became the first curative regimen in DLBCL, highlighting the critical role of anthracyclines. Later on, in an attempt to improve upon the results with CHOP, subsequent studies focused on the empiric addition of drugs to the regimen. However, this did not improve survival, as evidenced in a pivotal randomized study comparing CHOP to second and third generation regimens, where there was no evidence of superiority with the latter approaches, but there was much higher toxicity. Later on, other groups such as The Deutsche Studiengruppe für Hochmaligne Non-Hodgkin' Lymphome (DSHNHL) also made attempts to improve the outcomes that had been observed following CHOP. They carried out four-arm studies of CHOP where they tested different schedules of the regimen (every 14 versus every 21 days) with or without etoposide (CHOEP) in both older (>60 years) and younger (≤60 years) patients. While CHOEP-21 benefited patients

Treatment of Primary Mediastinal B-Cell Lymphoma

Patients with a diagnosis of PMBL undergo routine CT staging of chest, abdomen, and pelvis. We administer six cycles of DA-EPOCH-R. After four cycles of therapy, we repeat CT staging, and after six cycles, we perform CTs and an FDG-PET scan. If patients have responded and the posttherapy PET scan result is negative, we repeat CT scans every few months. If the FDG-PET result is positive, we attempt to perform a biopsy, and if there is residual disease, patients undergo mediastinal radiation treatment. If the FDG-PET result is suspicious (low SUV values), we repeat it in 4 to 6 weeks. If at this time, the result becomes negative, patients go into routine follow-up, and if it remains abnormal, we perform a biopsy and administer radiation if the biopsy confirms residual disease.

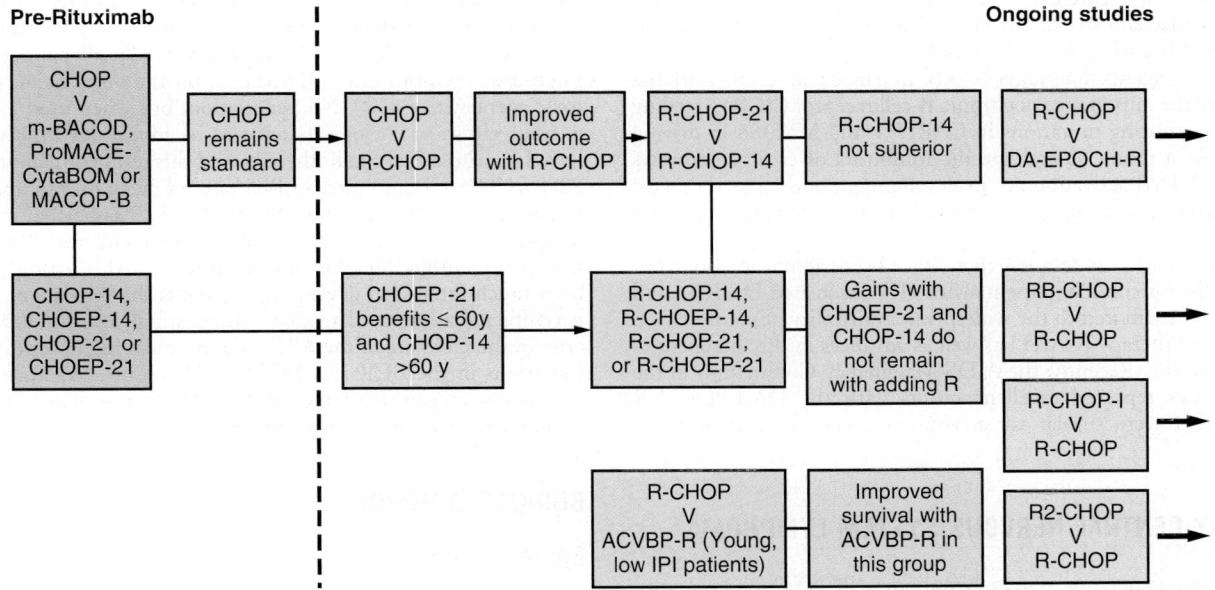

Fig. 82.5 EVOLUTION OF DIFFUSE LARGE B-CELL LYMPHOMA (DLBCL) THERAPEUTICS. Schema of progress in DLBCL clinical trials over the past 30 years. This schema shows selected randomized studies in DLBCL from the pre- to post-rituximab eras and within molecular subtypes of DLBCL. *ACVBP,* Dose-intensified doxorubicin, cyclophosphamide, vindesine, bleomycin, and prednisone; *CHOP,* cyclophosphamide, doxorubicin, vincristine, and prednisone; *CHOEP,* CHOP with etoposide; *m-BACOD,* methotrexate, bleomycin, doxorubicin, cyclophosphamide, vincristine, dexamethasone; *R-CHOP-I,* R-CHOP ibrutinib; *R2-CHOP,* R-CHOP with lenalidomide (Revlimid); *RB-CHOP,* R-CHOP with bortezomib, in non–germinal center B-cell DLBCL.[5]

≤60 years and CHOP-14 benefited patients >60 years, these survival gains did not remain significant with the addition of rituximab, (following on from a GELA study that showed a survival advantage in older patients treated with R-CHOP versus CHOP). The RICOVER-60 study was a randomized comparison in elderly patients of six versus eight cycles of CHOP-14, with or without rituximab. Although the DSHNHL found no significant differences in survival between the two groups, they reached the conclusion that R-CHOP-14 should be adapted as the new standard based on historical comparisons in this population. Subsequently, however, two randomized studies, one in all age groups (≥18 years) and the other in older patients (>60 years), showed no benefit of R-CHOP-14 over R-CHOP-21.[9,10] Therefore, R-CHOP-21 remains the standard.

Others have investigated the use of increased dose intensity approaches as an alternative to R-CHOP. Rituximab with doxorubicin, cyclophosphamide, vindesine, bleomycin, and prednisone (R-ACVBP) was compared to R-CHOP-21 in a randomized study performed by the GELA group in patients under 60 years with an age-adjusted international prognostic index score of 1.[11] While the R-ACVBP arm showed an improved progression free-survival (PFS) (87% versus 73%), the significant hematologic toxicity of the regimen confines its use to younger patients and it is not feasible for most patients with DLBCL who are over the age of 65 years. This restricts the potential of approaches like R-ACVBP to replace R-CHOP as the universal platform for this disease. Other intensive approaches such as using autologous stem cell transplantation in the upfront setting have been tried but they have never shown a clear benefit over R-CHOP alone and are associated with much higher toxicity.[12] Another increased dose-intensity regimen is dose-adjusted etoposide, prednisone, vincristine, cyclophosphamide, and doxorubicin with rituximab (DA-EPOCH-R).[13] Following on from the promising activity of DA-EPOCH-R in DLBCL in NCI and multicenter Cancer and Leukemia Group B (CALGB) single-arm studies, a randomized study comparing it to R-CHOP recently completed accrual and results are awaited.[14] This study aims to investigate if there are differential outcomes in DLBCL sub-types in R-CHOP or DA-EPOCH-R treated patients.

The appreciation that distinct subtypes of DLBCL have "targetable" pathways has led to novel drug development in DLBCL. In particular, in DLBCL of the ABC subtype, the understanding of various mechanisms of NFκB activation in ABC DLBCL has evolved significantly paving the way for the development of several new classes of agents that target NFκB. In particular, recent work has underlined the importance of chronic B-cell receptor (BCR) signaling as well as activating mutations in CARD11 and MYD88 in driving NFκB.[15] As a result, several specific inhibitors of critical pathways that drive NFκB activation are in development and large scale randomized trials evaluating ibrutnib and lenalidomide particularly, are ongoing.

Over the past few decades, there have been significant improvements in the outcome of patients with HIV-associated DLBCL, and these can be attributed to the widespread availability of combination antiretroviral therapy (CART) as well as advances in the therapeutics of these diseases. Recently, the AIDS Malignancy Consortium in the United States reported excellent results with the DA-EPOCH-R regimen that were similar to survival outcomes in HIV-negative DLBCL.

PRIMARY CENTRAL NERVOUS SYSTEM LYMPHOMA

Primary central nervous system lymphoma (PCNSL) is a rare and highly aggressive lymphoma confined to the CNS and is of diffuse large B-cell histology in over 90% of cases. Its unique radiographic findings present challenges in evaluation. The incidence of PCNSL is particularly high in the setting of HIV infection, in which it often presents with multifocal disease and is virtually always associated with EBV. In contrast, PCNSL in HIV-negative patients often presents with solitary intracranial masses and is almost never associated with EBV (Fig. 82.6).

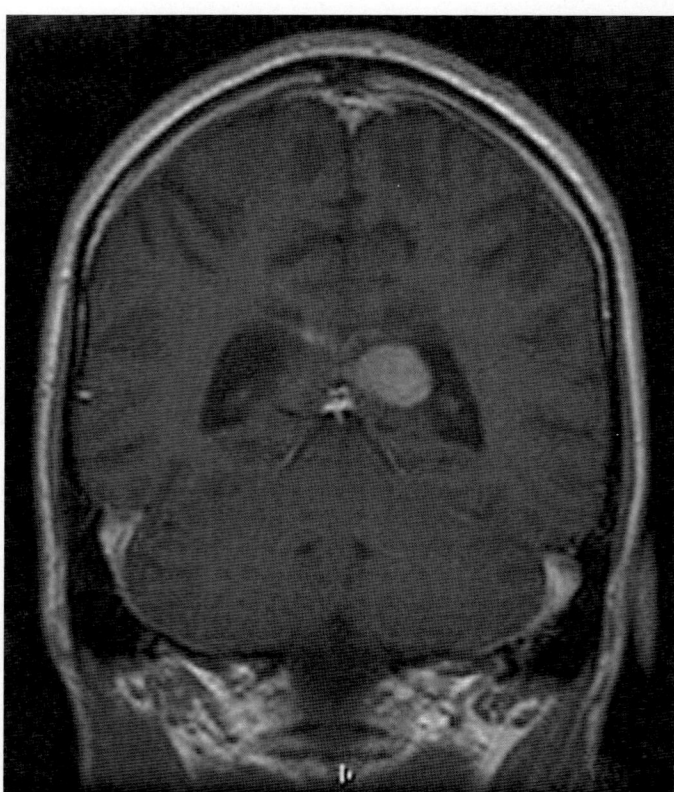

Fig. 82.6 THIS GADOLINIUM-ENHANCED MAGNETIC RESONANCE IMAGING SCAN OF THE BRAIN SHOWS AN ENHANCING INFILTRATIVE MASS IN THE MAJOR FORCEPS OF THE CORPUS CALLOSUM. A biopsy was consistent with primary central nervous system lymphoma.

Treatment of PCNSL differs from systemic DLBCL because many chemotherapy agents do not adequately penetrate the blood-brain barrier. Radiotherapy has been a mainstay of treatment because it is effective and sidestepped the limitations of chemotherapy, but responses are usually short lived, and virtually all patients relapse. High-dose methotrexate (HD-MTX), on the other hand, is a cytotoxic agent with good CNS penetration, but when used alone, PFS is relatively short. A logical step was to administer HD-MTX followed by whole-brain radiotherapy, and this resulted in an impressive 82% to 88% CR and median PFS rates of 32 to 40 months. Unfortunately, such combined modality treatment is associated with severe long-term neurotoxicity and recently, a high incidence of late relapses has been identified for this disease entity. For this reason, there has been much interest in developing regimens that obviate or defer the need for radiation until relapse.[16] Interestingly, most DLBCLs that arise in the CNS are of the ABC subtype and a high proportion have mutations in the BCR and MYD88. Therefore, there is interest in pursuing strategies that target BCR signaling as well as using immunomodulatory agents in these diseases.

BURKITT LYMPHOMA

Epidemiology

BL mostly occurs in the first two decades of life, is more common in males, and accounts for some 2% of all lymphomas. There are three recognized clinical variants, and they vary in whom they affect and how they present, and they also have morphologic and biologic differences. Endemic BL occurs in equatorial Africa and Papua New Guinea, peaks in incidence in 4- to 7-year–old children, and is predominantly a male disease. Sporadic BL presents worldwide and is the most common variant in the Western world. It typically affects

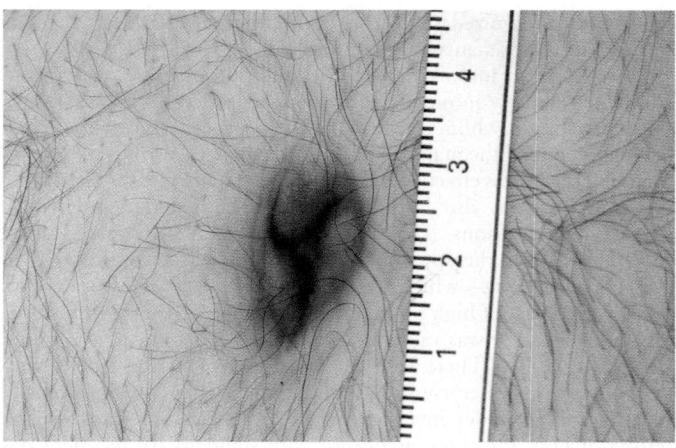

Fig. 82.7 BURKITT LYMPHOMA (BL) INVOLVING THE UMBILI-CUS. This is an 18-year old man who presented with a history of abdominal pain. Computed tomography scan demonstrated a large intraabdominal mass extending up to the umbilicus, and a biopsy revealed it to be BL.

children and young adults and is more commonly observed in boys. Immunodeficiency-associated BL occurs in association with HIV infection and is approximately 1000 times more common in HIV-infected individuals.

Pathobiology

BL is highly aggressive and characterized by an extremely high proliferation fraction and a high fraction of apoptosis, and this accounts for its "starry sky" appearance (see E-Slide VM03958). Although a leukemic phase of BL can occur in patients with advanced disease, it is very rare for BL to present purely as acute leukemia. Biologically, BL is derived from a GCB cell as indicated by its CD20$^+$, CD10$^+$, and TdT-negative immunohistochemical profile and gene expression profiling. The neoplastic cells are usually negative or weakly positive for BCL2. Although EBV is virtually always detected in endemic BL, it is only present in 25% to 40% of sporadic and immunodeficiency-associated cases.

Although virtually all cases of BL have MYC translocations, usually at 8q24 to the IG heavy chain region, MYC translocations are not specific for BL and can be found in other aggressive B-cell lymphomas (Fig. 82.7). BL has a unique gene expression signature that is molecularly distinct from that of DLBCL. Studies have demonstrated that some cases of DLBCL by histology have gene expression profiles consistent with BL. Given that BL does not respond well to CHOP-based treatments, this distinction by molecular profiling is important, and gene expression profiling may be useful in rare cases that would otherwise be diagnosed as DLBCL. Additionally, there are cases with a profile intermediate between that of DLBCL and BL; these cases typically harbor MYC and have a poor outcome with CHOP-based regimens.

Clinical Features

The clinical presentation of BL is variable and depends on the epidemiologic subtype as well as other factors. In endemic BL, it is common for patients to present with jaw and other facial disease, and other extranodal sites of involvement include the ileocecum, gonads, kidneys, and breasts. The ileocecal area is the most common site of disease involvement in sporadic BL (Fig. 82.8), and jaw involvement is very rare. In immunodeficiency-associated BL, involvement of the ileocecum, LNs, and BM is commonly observed. Patients often present with advanced stage and bulky disease caused by the short doubling time of the tumor, and it is common for patients to develop tumor lysis syndrome (TLS) after the institution of therapy.

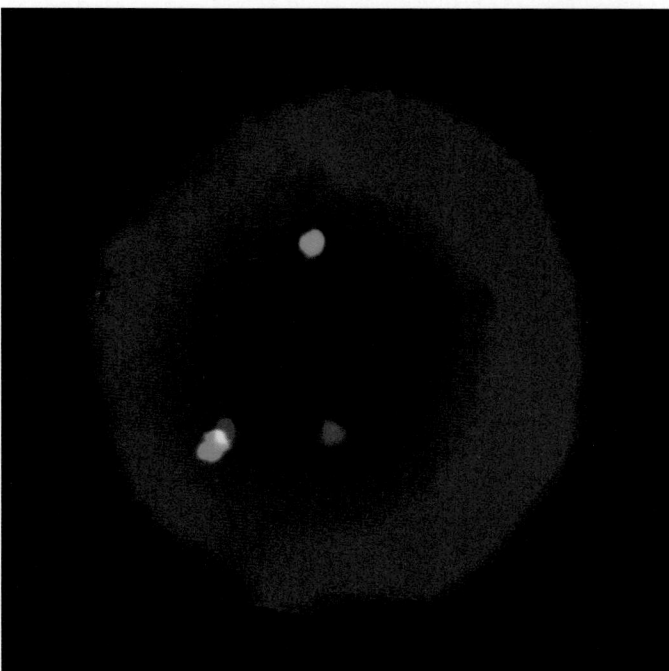

Fig. 82.8 FLUORESCENT IN SITU HYBRIDIZATION SHOWING AN MYC TRANSLOCATION IN A PATIENT WITH DIFFUSE LARGE B-CELL LYMPHOMA. This is a break apart probe (LSI-MYC) with one normal (fused) signal and one abnormal (separated green and red) signal indicating a translocation involving MYC.

Investigation

History and Physical Examination and Laboratory Investigations

Similar to patients with DLBCL, a detailed history and physical examination is required, and the diagnosis of BL should be made by an experienced hematopathologist. Given its association with HIV infection, it is imperative to perform an HIV test at diagnosis and to check hepatitis serologies.

Imaging and Staging

As with DLBCL, imaging studies should include chest radiography and CT scanning of the chest, abdomen, and pelvis. The need for additional imaging studies depends on the clinical presentation. A BM aspirate and biopsy should be performed in all patients, and depending on clinical presentation, patients should undergo a lumbar puncture with evaluation of the CSF by cytology and flow cytometry. Although BL in adults is staged according to the Ann Arbor staging system, the Murphy staging system is often used in children.

Prognosis

Age, large tumor volume, and CNS involvement have been associated with a poor prognosis in the past. Although early studies demonstrated that HIV-positive patients with BL had a worse outcome, this has not been the case with newer treatment approaches.

Treatment

BL is a systemic disease and requires chemotherapy for all disease stages. Importantly, locoregional radiation does not improve survival and should be avoided. Although older studies demonstrated that surgical resection of abdominal disease improved outcome, indicating the importance of tumor volume, more effective and risk-adapted treatments have made surgical resection unnecessary except for specific complications such as obstruction, perforation, fistula, or bleeding.

Early treatment strategies for BL were modeled on acute lymphoblastic leukemia (ALL) regimens that used dose-intense and prolonged treatment with induction, consolidation, and maintenance phases. These approaches stand in contrast to the significantly less dose-intense regimens used in adults with "intermediate-grade" lymphoma, such as CHOP and CHOP-based regimens, that only produced a 50% to 60% event-free survival (EFS). Although dose intensity and dose density are important treatment components for BL, later studies indicated that shorter treatment durations were equally effective. Furthermore, the recognition that tumor volume is an important prognostic feature led to the use of risk adaptive approaches and a further reduction in treatment for patients with early stage disease. Several biologic characteristics of BL have helped guide treatment strategies, including its high proliferative fraction. It has been recognized for years that BL is sensitive to multiple chemotherapy classes, and in endemic BL, cures were occasionally achieved with single-agent cyclophosphamide. Despite initial sensitivity, however, patients frequently relapsed, particularly those with higher volume disease. This apparent dichotomy can potentially be explained by the high tumor proliferation rate, resulting in "kinetic" failure. One strategy to overcome "kinetic" failure is to increase the dose density through frequent chemotherapy administration, a strategy used in most current BL regimens. Another strategy is to increase the fractional cell kill or efficacy of chemotherapy, thereby reducing the number of tumor cells that can survive and proliferate between cycles. Hence, BL regimens commonly use multiple chemotherapy agents in high doses and alternating cycles. They typically include anthracyclines, epipodophyllotoxins, vinca alkaloids, and alkylators, as well as methotrexate and cytarabine, which are cell cycle active agents and take advantage of the high tumor proliferation. These agents, however, are administered in a variety of combinations and schedule, indicating the empiric nature of the actual combinations.

The risks of TLS and propensity for CNS dissemination in BL also have important treatment implications. All patients should receive TLS prophylaxis during the first cycle and undergo close monitoring of their electrolytes. The high risk of CNS involvement has prompted the use in the past of relatively high-dose intravenous methotrexate and cytarabine, both of which have CNS penetration, and intrathecal administration of these drugs. An important advance has been to reduce intrathecal treatment and eliminate whole-brain radiation for prophylaxis, which has significantly reduced CNS toxicity. A study published by the FAB/LMB demonstrated that patients with early stage BL had a high cure rate and very low rate of CNS relapse without the use of intrathecal chemotherapy.[17]

There are multiple highly effective regimens for BL; however, because of the rarity of the disease (there are only 1200 new cases in the United States each year) there are no good comparative studies of different therapies in BL. A variety of dose-intense short-duration regimens have achieved durable CRs in a high proportion of patients. Included in these are the French LMB and German Berlin-Frankfurt-Munster (BFM) protocols and the National Cancer Institute CODOX-M/IVAC (cyclophosphamide, vincristine, doxorubicin, and HD-MTX alternating with ifosfamide, etoposide, and high-dose cytarabine; intrathecal methotrexate and cytarabine are also administered) regimen. These regimens are similar in their drug composition, short cycle length, and CNS prophylaxis. Although most BL occurs in children, Magrath and colleagues demonstrated that adults have a similar disease outcome when treated with the same regimen and reported cure rates approximately 90%. Other groups have confirmed the efficacy of this regimen albeit with lower survival rates. In the United Kingdom, Mead and colleagues reported an overall EFS of 65% at 2 years. The hyper-CVAD regimen has also been tested in BL with good results (recently with the addition of rituximab). Rituximab is typically used in this disease, and early

reports of randomized studies in both children and adults demonstrate that it adds a survival advantage.

Toxicity is an important clinical limitation of these regimens in adults, particularly in older patients and in patients who are immunosuppressed, in whom severe morbidity and even mortality occur. Therefore, one of the major therapeutic challenges in BL is to develop therapies that are as effective in achieving high cure rates as "standard" regimens but that also improve the therapeutic index and reduce toxicity complications. This approach has been investigated using EPOCH-R-based therapy in BL. Based on the efficacy of the regimen in a DLBCL study—which suggested that DA-EPOCH overcomes the adverse effect of high proliferation, likely because of its infusional schedule—a study was undertaken in BL and demonstrated a high PFS of over 90%.[18] There were very low rates of TLS and other toxicities compared with conventional BL regimens and this low-intensity therapy is now under investigation in a multi-center study. In the setting of HIV infection, a concern with standard BL regimens has been toxicity and less toxic appear to be more appropriate.[18,19]

SALVAGE THERAPY

The salvage treatment of relapsed DLBCL should be approached in an individual manner because the choice of treatment is influenced by the time to recurrence, prior therapy, medical condition, and the potential for cure. Although most relapsed aggressive lymphomas require combination chemotherapy for adequate disease control, it is important to recognize that patients with local disease may be salvaged with radiation therapy. Examples include primary mediastinal DLBCL, which can remain local even at relapse, and PTLDs, which may have an isolated resistant EBV clone after chemotherapy.

A variety of active salvage chemotherapy regimens are available for relapsed or refractory DLBCL. Platinum-containing regimens, such as ESHAP (etoposide, methylprednisolone, cytosine arabinoside, and platinum) and ICE (ifosfamid, carboplatin, and etoposide), are currently among the most widely used salvage treatment. It is a commonly held notion that salvage treatment should include different agents from past treatment to avoid drug resistance. Recent evidence indicates, however, that sensitivity to apoptosis is a central cause of drug resistance and that drug-specific mechanisms are less important. Hence, salvage regimens developed around the most active upfront agents should show high activity. The addition of rituximab appears to enhance the activity of salvage regimens as demonstrated by results with R-ICE (rituximab, ifosfamid, carboplatin, and etoposide) and ICE, which showed CRs of 53% and 27%, respectively.

Patients with chemotherapy-sensitive disease have the best outcome with ASCT, and this is recommended at initial relapse; in the pre-rituximab era, this approach yielded overall survival (OS) and EFS rates in the range of 40% to 50% and 30% to 40%, respectively. However, the improvement in upfront curability of DLBCL because of immunochemotherapy has diminished the efficacy of ASCT at relapse, which was recently demonstrated in the CORAL study, in which the 3-year EFS of patients who had initially received rituximab was merely 21% after ASCT. Of course, patients with chemotherapy-resistant disease do poorly with ASCT and should be considered for experimental treatments such as allogeneic SCT. Recently, in B-cell lymphoproliferative disorders, chimeric antigen receptor T-cell therapy has been investigated in many different relapsed/refractory settings and has shown some promising activity in DLBCL.[20]

The outcome for patients with BL who relapse after or progress during initial therapy is extremely poor, and there are no standard approaches that have been associated with good outcomes; therefore, experimental approaches should be considered.

Late Complications of Treatment and Follow-up

It is important to recognize that successful treatment may be associated with late complications that may not appear for decades. Among the major late-term complications are secondary malignancies, ischemic heart disease, anthracycline-related cardiotoxicity, and radiation- or bleomycin-induced pulmonary toxicity. The risk of developing myelodysplastic disorders and acute myeloid leukemia is related to alkylator and topoisomerase inhibitor use and is enhanced by radiation. Radiation therapy increases the risk of malignancy in the treatment region, particularly breast cancer in women and lung cancer in smokers. Indeed, it is imperative to consider late-term toxicity when selecting treatment.

A general guideline for follow-up after initial therapy involves visits every 3 or 4 months for 2 years, and every 6 months or annually thereafter. During these visits, examination of the LN areas, abdomen, thyroid, and skin is important. CT scans are recommended in early follow-up but it is important to note that they are associated with a relatively high radiation exposure and projected risks and should not be used unnecessarily or for a prolonged amount of time. PET scans are not recommended for routine follow-up because the high rate of false-positive scans is unlikely to offset the value of early detection. Routine laboratory studies with blood counts, liver function tests, and LD should be performed. Thyroid-stimulating hormone levels should be monitored annually in patients who received neck radiotherapy. Mammography for women should begin 10 years from the diagnosis of lymphoma or at age 40 years, whichever comes first.

FUTURE DIRECTIONS

Over recent years, we have made significant advances in elucidating the molecular biology of DLBCL and BL, and this has led to an era of enhanced and exciting drug discovery. In DLBCL in particular, many critical pathways and novel mutations have been identified, and many small molecule inhibitors are being investigated and in development as a result of these advances. For example, in the ABC subtype of DLBCL, recent work has identified that chronic active B-cell receptor signaling is an important mechanism of ABC tumor cell survival; to test this clinically, studies in patients with ABC DLBCL are in progress targeting specific components of this pathway. In BL, cure rates are very high with conventional approaches, and the challenge for the future is to further develop strategies that maintain the efficacy of "standard" treatment but with much less toxicity. Recently, the discovery of novel mutations in BL has set the stage for the investigation of small molecule inhibitors in this disease also.[21] To advance the therapeutics of these diseases, it is critical to wisely choose which drugs should be developed and incorporated into upfront clinical trials and to pair drug development with understanding of tumor biology.

REFERENCES

1. Sehn LH, Gascoyne RD: Diffuse large B-cell lymphoma: optimizing outcome in the context of clinical and biologic heterogeneity. *Blood* 125:22, 2015.
2. Scott DW, Wright GW, Williams PM, et al: Determining cell-of-origin subtypes of diffuse large B-cell lymphoma using gene expression in formalin-fixed paraffin-embedded tissue. *Blood* 123(8):1214–1217, 2014.
3. Lenz G, Wright G, Dave SS, et al: Stromal gene signatures in large-B-cell lymphomas. *N Engl J Med* 359(22):2313–2323, 2008.
4. Wilson WH, Bromberg JE, Stetler-Stevenson M, et al: Detection and outcome of occult leptomeningeal disease in diffuse large B-cell lymphoma and Burkitt lymphoma. *Haematologica* 99(7):1228–1235, 2014.
5. Dunleavy K, Roschewski M, Wilson WH: Precision treatment of distinct molecular subtypes of diffuse large B-cell lymphoma: ascribing treatment based on the molecular phenotype. *Clin Cancer Res* 20(20):5182–5193, 2014.
6. Zhou Z, Sehn LH, Rademaker AW, et al: An enhanced International Prognostic Index (NCCN-IPI) for patients with diffuse large B-cell lymphoma treated in the rituximab era. *Blood* 123(6):837–842, 2014.
7. Dunleavy K, Pittaluga S, Maeda LS, et al: Dose-adjusted EPOCH-rituximab therapy in primary mediastinal B-cell lymphoma. *New Engl J Med* 368(15):1408–1416, 2013.
8. Martelli M, Ceriani L, Zucca E, et al: [18F]fluorodeoxyglucose positron emission tomography predicts survival after chemoimmunotherapy for primary mediastinal large B-cell lymphoma: results of the International Extranodal Lymphoma Study Group IELSG-26 Study. *J Clin Oncol* 32(17):1769–1775, 2014.
9. Cunningham D, Hawkes EA, Jack A, et al: Rituximab plus cyclophosphamide, doxorubicin, vincristine, and prednisolone in patients with newly diagnosed diffuse large B-cell non-Hodgkin lymphoma: a phase 3 comparison of dose intensification with 14-day versus 21-day cycles. *Lancet* 381(9880):1817–1826, 2013.
10. Delarue R, Tilly H, Mounier N, et al: Dose-dense rituximab-CHOP compared with standard rituximab-CHOP in elderly patients with diffuse large B-cell lymphoma (the LNH03-6B study): a randomised phase 3 trial. *Lancet Oncol* 14(6):525–533, 2013.
11. Récher C, Coiffier B, Haioun C, et al: Intensified chemotherapy with ACVBP plus rituximab versus standard CHOP plus rituximab for the treatment of diffuse large B-cell lymphoma (LNH03-2B): an open-label randomised phase 3 trial. *Lancet* 378(9806):1858–1867, 2011.
12. Holte H, Leppa S, Bjorkholm M, et al: Dose-densified chemoimmunotherapy followed by systemic central nervous system prophylaxis for younger high-risk diffuse large B-cell/follicular grade 3 lymphoma patients: results of a phase II Nordic Lymphoma Group study. *Ann Oncol* 2012.
13. Wilson WH, Grossbard ML, Pittaluga S, et al: Dose-adjusted EPOCH chemotherapy for untreated large B-cell lymphomas: a pharmacodynamic approach with high efficacy. *Blood* 99(8):2685–2693, 2002.
14. Wilson WH, Dunleavy K, Pittaluga S, et al: Phase II study of dose-adjusted EPOCH and rituximab in untreated diffuse large B-cell lymphoma with analysis of germinal center and post-germinal center biomarkers. *J Clin Oncol* 26(16):2717–2724, 2008.
15. Davis RE, Ngo VN, Lenz G, et al: Chronic active B-cell-receptor signaling in diffuse large B-cell lymphoma. *Nature* 463(7277):88–92, 2010.
16. Rubenstein JL, Hsi ED, Johnson JL, et al: Intensive chemotherapy and immunotherapy in patients with newly diagnosed primary CNS lymphoma: CALGB 50202 (Alliance 50202). *J Clin Oncol* 31(25):3061–3068, 2013.
17. Gerrard M, Cairo MS, Weston C, et al: Excellent survival following two courses of COPAD chemotherapy in children and adolescents with resected localized B-cell non-Hodgkin's lymphoma: results of the FAB/LMB 96 international study. *Br J Haematol* 141(6):840–847, 2008.
18. Dunleavy K, Pittaluga S, Shovlin M, et al: Low-intensity therapy in adults with Burkitt's lymphoma. *N Engl J Med* 369(20):1915–1925, 2013.
19. Noy A, Lee JY, Cesarman E, et al: AMC 048: modified CODOX-M/IVAC-rituximab is safe and effective for HIV-associated Burkitt lymphoma. *Blood* 126(2):160–166, 2015.
20. Kochenderfer JN, Dudley ME, Kassim SH, et al: Chemotherapy-refractory diffuse large B-cell lymphoma and indolent B-cell malignancies can be effectively treated with autologous T cells expressing an anti-CD19 chimeric antigen receptor. *J Clin Oncol* 33(6):540–549, 2015.
21. Basso K, Dalla-Favera R: Germinal centres and B cell lymphomagenesis. *Nat Rev Immunol* 15(3):172–184, 2015.

CHAPTER 83

VIRUS-ASSOCIATED LYMPHOMA

Jennifer A. Kanakry and Richard F. Ambinder

There are five well-characterized human viruses that are generally accepted as important in lymphomagenesis (Table 83.1). These viruses may infect tumor cells (or their progenitors) or may act at a distance. The genomes of Epstein-Barr virus (EBV), Kaposi sarcoma–associated herpesvirus (KSHV, also known as *human herpesvirus 8* [HHV-8]), and human T-lymphotropic virus-1 (HTLV-1) are present in tumor cells. The viral genes expressed in tumor cells modulate cellular metabolism, proliferation, and cell death. By contrast, the human immunodeficiency virus (HIV) genome is generally not detected in tumor cells. Whether hepatitis C virus (HCV) genomes are present in lymphoma cells remains a subject of controversy.

Although viral infection plays a role in the pathogenesis of some lymphomas, lymphomagenesis is unusual. Only a small subset of infected people develops lymphoma. Furthermore, although primary viral infection may be followed by lymphomagenesis within days or weeks in exceptional circumstances, most lymphomas arise years or decades after primary infection, speaking to the role of cofactors in the development of malignancy. Indeed the term *adult* in adult T-cell leukemia/lymphoma (ATL) reflects the time lag between HTLV-1 infection in infancy and the evolution to malignancy. Geography and associated environmental exposures, host genetic factors, and immune status all modify risk.

Aspects of the biology and epidemiology of each of these viruses and their relationship with lymphomagenesis are reviewed in this chapter. In addition, clinically important and distinctive features of diagnosis and treatment of the associated lymphomas are presented.

EPSTEIN-BARR VIRUS

Viral Biology

EBV is a gammaherpesvirus transmitted mainly through saliva.[1,2] After primary infection, some of the infected cells are driven to proliferate and thereby spread infection throughout the B-cell compartment. Ultimately, in the normal host, there is an immune response that controls infection and eradicates virus-infected proliferating cells. Thereafter the viral genome is harbored mainly in resting memory B lymphocytes that persist for life. These B cells that harbor virus elude immune surveillance in part because of their very restricted viral gene expression, such that few viral antigens are presented. Occasionally there is activation of viral lytic gene expression (occurring at least in some instances in concert with plasma cell differentiation), leading to production of infectious virions that may infect other B cells. T cell–mediated immune function keeps such proliferation in check.[3]

In vitro, EBV immortalizes B cells such that they grow indefinitely as lymphoblastoid cell lines (LCLs) (Fig. 83.1). LCLs are tumorigenic in immunodeficient mice. In LCLs, viral genomes are present as circular, double-stranded deoxyribonucleic acid (DNA) episomes within the nucleus. The viral proteins required for immortalization include Epstein-Barr virus nuclear antigen-1 (EBNA1), a sequence-specific DNA-binding protein important in the maintenance of the viral episome; EBNA2, a transcription factor that has many effects similar to those of activated Notch receptors; and latent membrane protein-1 (LMP1), a constitutively activated member of the tumor necrosis factor receptor superfamily, which most closely resembles CD40.[4] LMP1 activates the nuclear factor-κB (NFκB) pathway,

which modulates cell proliferation and apoptosis.[5] Several other EBV proteins are also required for immortalization. Although EBV immortalization of B cells in vitro may offer some insights into tumorigenesis, some caution is required in using LCL as a tumor model. Most EBV tumors, including tumors of B-lineage cells, do not express many of the viral genes required for lymphocyte immortalization. The only tumors that express the full complement of viral proteins required for immortalization are those that arise in the most profoundly immunocompromised patients (organ or hematopoietic transplant recipients, patients with congenital immunodeficiency, or patients with far-advanced acquired immunodeficiency syndrome [AIDS]). Thus in posttransplant lymphoproliferative disorder (PTLD), tumor cells may resemble LCL in expressing many viral latency genes in association with normal karyotype (and few mutations of the cellular genome). It has been suggested that there is an inverse relationship between cellular mutations and viral gene expression in tumors.[6]

EBV gene expression may directly drive proliferation or inhibit apoptotic pathways, as illustrated by lymphocyte immortalization. However, viral gene expression may also perturb normal lymphocyte biology. Thus LMP1 expression upregulates activation induced (cytidine) deaminase expression, which facilitates somatic hypermutation and immunoglobulin class switching.[7] LMP1 expression may also be important in the conversion of naïve B cells to postgerminal center memory B cells. LMP2A allows B cells that lack normal immunoglobulin expression to escape regulatory checkpoints and survive.[8]

Epidemiology of Viral Infection

EBV infection is ubiquitous. The vast majority of adults are infected worldwide. Primary infection is most often asymptomatic, especially when it occurs in childhood.[9] Primary infection may be associated with the syndrome of infectious mononucleosis. Symptomatic primary infection occurs more frequently in older children and in adults than in younger children. Other possible determinants of symptomatic primary infection include genetic factors and possibly the size of the viral inoculum.

Strain differences in EBV are well recognized.[10] However, the importance of these strain differences with regard to lymphomagenesis remains poorly understood. There is general agreement that the type 1 strain EBV is most common worldwide and in tumors. The type 2 strain virus has been identified in some African Burkitt lymphoma (BL) and in some AIDS-associated lymphoma. The type 1 strain virus is more efficient at lymphocyte immortalization in vitro and lymphomagenesis in mouse models. The two strains of virus differ mainly in the *EBNA2* gene, but differences are recognized in some other viral proteins as well.[11] Variations in the regulatory regions or coding regions of a variety of other genes, including *EBNA1, LMP1,* and *ZTA,* have been recognized and suggested to play a role in lymphomagenesis. A simple classification of latent viral gene expression recognizes three patterns, as shown in Table 83.2.

Epstein-Barr Virus Detection in Clinical Specimens

The sensitivity of polymerase chain reaction (PCR) makes detection of viral DNA straightforward, but the ubiquity of EBV infection, as

TABLE 83.1	Viruses and Lymphomagenesis	
Virus	Viral Genome in Tumor Cell	Lymphoma Type
EBV	Episomal	B, T, NK
KSHV	Episomal	B
HTLV-1	Integrated	T
HIV-1	Absent	B
HCV	Uncertain	B

EBV, Epstein-Barr virus; HCV, hepatitis C virus; HIV-1, human immunodeficiency virus type 1; HTLV-1, human T-lymphotropic virus-1; KSHV, Kaposi sarcoma–associated herpesvirus; NK, natural killer.

TABLE 83.2	Patterns of Epstein-Barr Virus Gene Expression in Latency			
Latency	EBNA1	EBNA2, EBNA3A, EBNA3B, EBNA3C	LMP1	LMP2A
I	+			
II	+		+	+
III	+	+	+	+

EBNA1, Epstein-Barr virus nuclear antigen 1; EBV, Epstein-Barr virus; LMP1, latent membrane protein 1.

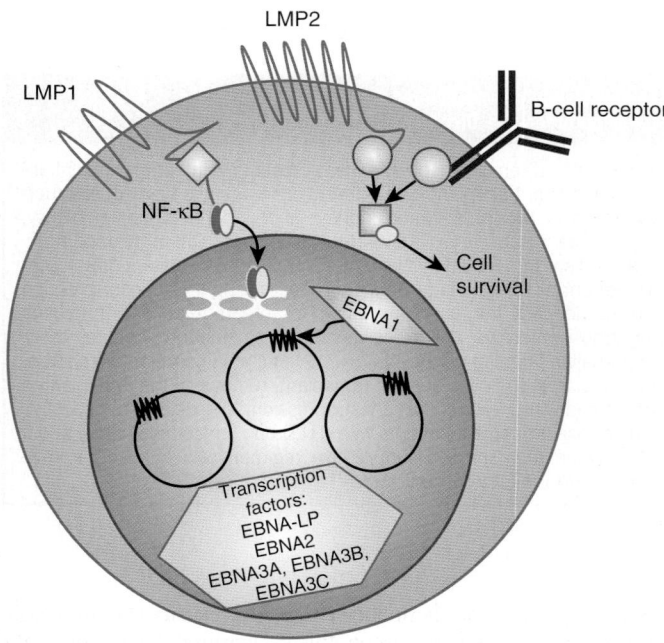

Fig. 83.1 EPSTEIN-BARR VIRUS (EBV)–IMMORTALIZED B CELL. Normal B cells are readily immortalized in vitro with EBV. These cells express EBV nuclear and membrane proteins. The nuclear proteins include a protein expressed in all EBV-associated tumors, Epstein-Barr virus nuclear antigen 1 (EBNA1). This protein is required for episomal maintenance. Other viral nuclear proteins expressed are transcription factors. These include EBNA-LP, EBNA2, EBNA3A, EBNA3B, and EBNA3C. Two membrane proteins are expressed: latent membrane protein 1 (LMP1), which activates nuclear factor-κB (NFκB) pathways, and LMP2A, which mimics B-cell receptor (immunoglobulin) signaling.

well as the persistence of B cells that harbor EBV in all seropositive individuals, means that EBV DNA is readily detected in many specimens that include normal lymphocytes. Thus the diagnosis of an EBV association in general requires viral detection specifically in tumor cells. Techniques for viral DNA detection by fluorescence in

situ hybridization or related techniques, although greatly improved in recent years, remain the purview of research laboratories and are generally not readily applicable to clinical specimens. This reflects the relatively low copy number of the viral genome in tumor cells, typically 1–200 copies per cell. In contrast, in situ hybridization for the EBV-encoded ribonucleic acids (RNAs) has emerged as a clinical laboratory standard.[12] These RNAs are polymerase 3 transcripts that are expressed at very high copy number (perhaps millions of copies per cell) in latently infected cells. The functions of these RNAs are disputed, but their use for the detection of virus in a variety of tissue specimens is generally accepted.

Viral antigens are detected by immunohistochemistry. In clinical laboratories, immunohistochemistry for LMP1 is commonly employed and is sensitive for the detection of EBV in Hodgkin lymphoma (HL). In a variety of other EBV-associated B- and T-cell malignancies, expression of LMP1 is more variable. Thus failure to detect LMP1 expression does not exclude the presence of EBV, except perhaps in HL. In principle, detection of EBNA1 should be universally applicable, although the low level of antigen expression and the cross-reactivity of available monoclonal antibodies have prevented immunohistochemistry for this antigen from emerging as a standard tool.

Association With Particular Types of Lymphoma

Some lymphoma types are nearly 100% EBV associated, including endemic BL, extranodal natural killer (NK)/T-cell lymphoma of the nasal type, early PTLD, lymphomatoid granulomatosis, diffuse large B-cell lymphoma (DLBCL) associated with chronic inflammation, EBV-positive DLBCL of older adults, and AIDS primary central nervous system (CNS) lymphoma (PCNSL).[13–16] Other lymphoma types are variably EBV associated. These include classic HL, PTLDs occurring many months or years after transplantation, and systemic AIDS-related lymphoma.

Some lymphoma types appear never or almost never to be EBV associated, including most indolent B-cell lymphomas, although there is growing evidence that exceptions do exist, particularly in the setting of immunocompromise. Nodular lymphocyte predominant HL was historically thought to always be EBV negative, but a recent pathologic review of over 300 cases suggests that 3%–5% are EBV positive.[17] Low-grade lymphomas such as EBV-positive mucosa-associated lymphoid tissue (MALT) lymphomas have been reported in patients with congenital immunodeficiencies.[18] Whereas low-grade lymphomas that arise posttransplant are not considered to be PTLD in the current classification, it is interesting to note that cases of EBV-positive, indolent B-cell lymphomas, particularly MALT lymphomas with a predilection to involve the subcutaneous or soft tissues, have been reported in transplant patients.[19,20] Thus the spectrum of EBV-associated lymphomas continues to expand, and the presence of EBV might be an indication to consider an underlying immune defect in the patient.

Other lymphomas are typically not EBV associated but have the interesting feature of being associated with EBV upon transformation or upon development of de novo secondary lymphomas. Chronic lymphocytic leukemia (CLL) is a low-grade lymphoma that is not EBV positive; however, CLL can rarely transform to HL, and these transformed, clonally related lymphomas are often EBV positive.[21] In angioimmunoblastic T-cell lymphoma (AITL) and other peripheral T-cell lymphomas, EBV-positive polyclonal proliferations of atypical B cells that have the appearance of Hodgkin and Reed-Sternberg cells can be present in the background of the tumor.[22] A rare but consistently described phenomenon in AITL is the subsequent development of EBV-positive DLBCL.[23] The role of EBV in the setting of transformation or secondary lymphomagenesis remains to be defined.

Table 83.3 lists the lymphomas that have been associated with EBV, associated cofactors, viral antigen expression, and an estimate of the percentage of tumors within each lymphoma subtype that harbor viral genomes. The table serves to illustrate the range of EBV

TABLE 83.3	Epstein-Barr Virus-Associated Lymphoma				
Type	Cofactors	Viral Gene Expression	Approximate Percentage EBV Associated	Comment	
PTLD	Immunosuppression, allograft	Latency II or III	50%–95%	Early days/months after transplantat are more commonly associated with EBV	
Sporadic BL		Latency I	20% in the United States	Higher in Latin America	
Endemic BL	Malaria	Latency I	>95%		
AIDS BL	HIV	Latency I	30%		
HL		Latency II	30% in the United States	Higher percentage in mixed cellularity, in males, in Hispanics	
AIDS PCNSL	HIV	Latency II or III	>95%		
Extranodal NK/T-cell lymphoma, nasal type	More common in Asia	Latency II	>95%		
AIDS PEL	HIV and KSHV	Latency I	>75%	Rare cases of PEL in HIV-negative patients are typically EBV negative	
Lymphomatoid granulomatosis	Immunocompromise	Latency II	>90%		
Methotrexate-associated lymphoma	Methotrexate treatment	Latency III	>95%	May regress with withdrawal of methotrexate	

AIDS, Acquired immunodeficiency syndrome; BL, Burkitt lymphoma; EBV, Epstein-Barr virus; HIV, human immunodeficiency virus; HL, Hodgkin lymphoma; KSHV, Kaposi sarcoma–associated herpesvirus; NK, natural killer; PCNSL, primary central nervous system lymphoma; PEL, primary effusion lymphoma; PTLD, posttransplantation lymphoproliferative disorder.

lymphomas as well as host features that increase risk, but it is not meant to be comprehensive.

Posttransplantation Lymphoproliferative Disorder

PTLD is a group of lymphoproliferative disorders ranging from polyclonal lymphoid hyperplasia to lymphomas that arise in patients after solid organ or hematopoietic stem cell transplant (HSCT).[24] PTLD, especially in the first few months after transplant, is highly associated with EBV (Fig. 83.2A, B). EBV gene expression in PTLD corresponds to latencies II and III.[25] Broad expression of viral proteins is seen only in immunosuppressed hosts, reflecting that many of these proteins are immunogenic and commonly targeted by cytotoxic T cells.

B cells that harbor EBV are able to proliferate in the setting of posttransplant immunosuppression, at least in part because of decreased T-cell surveillance.[26] HSCT patients who receive grafts that have been T-cell depleted develop EBV-associated PTLD at very high rates. Treatment of rejection in solid organ transplant recipients with agents such as the monoclonal antibody OKT3, which targets CD3+ cells, is associated with markedly increased risk for PTLD.[27] Treatment strategies such as the use of rituximab and infusion of EBV-specific cytotoxic T cells have been quite effective in treating or preventing PTLD (see box on Epstein-Barr Virus–Associated Positive Posttransplant Lymphoproliferative Disorder).

Hodgkin Lymphoma

Approximately 30% of classical HL tumors in the United States and Europe are EBV associated (Fig. 83.2C, D).[29,30] Epidemiologic studies in Denmark and Sweden suggest that individuals with a history of symptomatic infectious mononucleosis are at increased risk for EBV-associated HL, but not for EBV-negative HL or other lymphomas.[31] The period of risk peaks at about 2 years but continues to be elevated for at least 10 years after symptomatic mononucleosis.

Higher EBV associations are seen in Latin America, Africa, and parts of Asia. Factors associated with EBV tumor positivity include

> **Epstein-Barr Virus–Associated Positive Posttransplant Lymphoproliferative Disorder**
>
> A 55-year-old renal transplant patient presents with acute renal failure 5 months after transplant. She is found on imaging to have an obstructing mass in the transplanted kidney. She undergoes kidney biopsy, and Epstein-Barr virus (EBV)–positive posttransplant lymphoproliferative disorder (PTLD) involving the transplanted organ is diagnosed. Treatment options include rituximab; decreasing immunosuppression (acknowledging the associated risk for organ rejection); changing immunosuppressive agents—switching a calcineurin inhibitor for a mammalian target of rapamycin (mTOR) inhibitor; combination chemotherapy; or, in the case of renal transplant, removal of the transplanted organ and withdrawal of immunosuppression. In a recent retrospective study, renal transplant patients with PTLD had a response rate of about 30% when their immunosuppressive regimen was changed from a calcineurin inhibitor to rapamycin.[28]

mixed cellularity and lymphocyte-depleted classic HL histologic subtypes, male sex, low socioeconomic background, history of symptomatic infectious mononucleosis, and Hispanic ethnicity.[29,32,33] Organ and hematopoietic stem cell transplant recipients, patients with primary immunodeficiencies, and HIV-positive patients are more likely to develop HL than the general population, and approximately 90% of the tumors in these settings are EBV associated.[34]

The EBV gene expression pattern in HL is latency II, even when HL occurs in immunocompromised populations.[35] LMP1 and LMP2A may mimic signaling of B-cell receptors and thus protect B cells lacking functional immunoglobulin expression from apoptotic signaling. Approximately 20% of HL lack productive immunoglobulin gene rearrangements. These tumors appear to be exclusively EBV associated.

The EBV association of HL may have prognostic significance because it has been associated with poorer survival in older patients in several reports.[30] Patients with EBV-positive HL quite reliably have EBV DNA detected in cell-free blood (plasma or serum) in the setting of active disease.[36–38] Thus plasma EBV DNA is a potential tumor

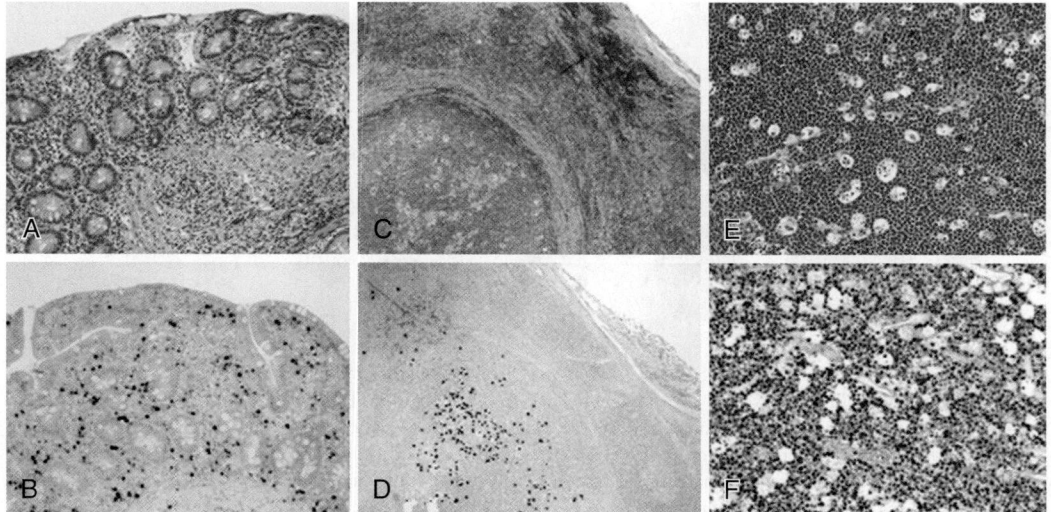

Fig. 83.2 EXAMPLES OF EPSTEIN-BARR VIRUS (EBV)–RELATED LYMPHOMAS. Posttransplant lymphoproliferative disorder (PTLD), polymorphic type, EBV positive occurring in the gastrointestinal tract of a 15-month-old girl following an orthotopic liver transplant (A and B). There was a mildly atypical lymphocytic infiltrate in the duodenal mucosa composed of small lymphocytes, plasma cells, and occasional large cells (A). The infiltrate was EBV positive, as demonstrated by in situ hybridization for Epstein-Barr–encoded RNA (EBER) (B). Hodgkin lymphoma, nodular sclerosing type, EBV positive (C and D). The hematoxylin and eosin–stained section shows a portion of a lymph node from a cervical lymph node biopsy of an 8-year-old girl. There are bands of sclerosis forming a cellular nodule, and within the nodule there are a mixed inflammatory infiltrate and scattered large cells with contracted cytoplasm consistent with lacunar cells (C). The immunophenotype of these cells was that of classic Hodgkin lymphoma, and the cells were EBER positive (D). EBV is seen more frequently in mixed-cellularity Hodgkin lymphoma but can be seen in 10%–40% of cases of nodular sclerosing type. It is even more frequent in cases associated with human immunodeficiency virus (HIV; see text) and in resource-poor regions. Burkitt lymphoma, sporadic type, EBV positive (E and F). A section of the cervical lymph node biopsy of a 9-year-old girl with a rapidly enlarging neck mass is shown. The section illustrates the classic morphologic features of Burkitt lymphoma with a "starry sky" appearance, sheets of intermediate-sized cells with multiple small nucleoli and high mitotic rate. The cells were virtually all EBER positive (F). EBV can be seen in about 20%–30% of cases of sporadic Burkitt lymphoma and is essentially always positive in endemic cases.

marker in EBV-positive HL, and elevated EBV DNA in plasma prior to therapy has been associated with inferior failure-free survival in one study, even on multivariate analysis.[36] In addition, elevated EBV DNA in plasma after completion of first-line therapy for HL was also associated with inferior failure-free survival in this study.[36]

Currently treatment regimens for EBV-positive HL do not differ from those used for EBV-negative HL. However, novel treatment strategies involving adoptive therapy with autologous EBV-specific T cells targeting type II latency LMP antigens appear to be associated with durable complete responses and low toxicity in some patients with EBV-positive HL, even in the setting of relapsed/refractory disease.[39]

Burkitt Lymphoma

Endemic BL is nearly 100% associated with EBV, whereas sporadic and HIV-associated BL are much more variably EBV associated (see Table 83.3 and Fig. 83.2E, F).[40] Viral expression is latency I (i.e., EBNA1 is the only viral protein consistently expressed). The defining feature of BL is a translocation between c-Myc on chromosome 8 and one of the immunoglobulin genes on chromosome 2, 14, or 22. It has been generally presumed that falciparum malaria is a cofactor in endemic BL, and the distribution of BL in Africa corresponds to the distribution of holoendemic malaria. However, little is understood of the pathogenesis or interaction between these infectious cofactors. The characteristic presentation of BL is different in the endemic versus sporadic settings, but there is no evidence to link these presentations specifically with the virus. The virus-tumor association

does not currently guide diagnosis, therapy, or estimation of prognosis.

Diffuse, Large B-Cell Lymphoma Associated With Chronic Inflammation

EBV-associated lymphomas sometimes arise in the setting of long-standing chronic inflammation.[15] This was first described in Japanese patients with a remote history of pulmonary tuberculosis treated with thoracoplasty with resulting chronic pyothorax. These patients developed EBV-associated DLBCL of the pleural lining and associated lung tissue decades after thoracoplasty. Similar cases of aggressive, EBV-associated B-cell lymphomas have been reported to arise in patients at the sites of chronic inflammation associated with various implants, surgical mesh, or in the lung after chronic empyema.

KAPOSI SARCOMA–ASSOCIATED HERPESVIRUS

Virus and Tumor Epidemiology

KSHV (HHV-8) is a gammaherpesvirus that, unlike EBV, has a low prevalence worldwide.[41] The virus is endemic in certain areas, such as in sub-Saharan Africa and the Middle East, and has an intermediate prevalence in Mediterranean countries. Transmission is believed to be predominately through saliva. Similar to EBV, KSHV latently infects B cells, and viral genes that promote cell survival are implicated in lymphomagenesis.

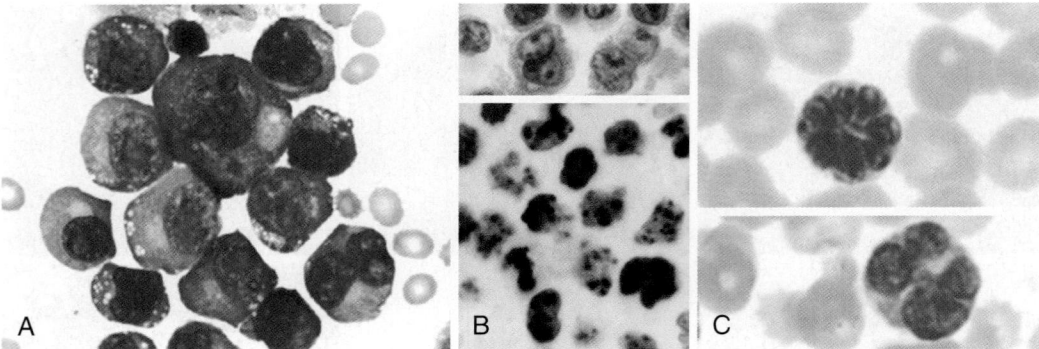

Fig. 83.3 EXAMPLES OF KAPOSI SARCOMA–ASSOCIATED HERPESVIRUS (KSHV)–AND HUMAN T-LYMPHOTROPIC VIRUS-1 (HTLV-1)–ASSOCIATED LYMPHOPROLIFERATIVE DISEASE. Primary effusion lymphoma (A and B). (A) The pleural tap had a high cell count, and the cytospin preparation revealed a markedly pleomorphic cell population with large and giant cells with deep-blue cytoplasm. (B) A cell block was prepared *(top)* so that in situ hybridization studies could be performed. These studies showed the cells to be KSHV positive by immunohistochemistry for latency associated nuclear antigen-1 (LANA-1) *(bottom)* and EBV positive by EBER in situ hybridization (not shown). (C) Adult T-cell leukemia/lymphoma in a patient who was HTLV-1 positive. The peripheral smear showed the classic "flower" cells. *EBER,* Epstein-Barr–encoded RNA. *(A and B, courtesy Dr. Elizabeth Hyjek, University of Chicago.)*

KSHV was discovered in Kaposi sarcoma but is also present in rare lymphoproliferative diseases, including primary effusion lymphoma (PEL) (Fig. 83.3A, B) and multicentric Castleman disease (MCD).[16,42] Other KSHV-positive lymphomas have been characterized, all of which tend to occur in severely immunocompromised individuals and carry a poor prognosis.[43] One exception is germinotropic lymphoproliferative disorder, a KSHV-positive, EBV-positive tumor that carries a good prognosis in the HIV-negative setting.[44,45] PEL occurs almost exclusively in HIV-positive patients, particularly in men who have sex with men, and typically when CD4 counts are less than 100/mm^3. However, PEL has been reported very rarely in solid organ transplant patients and elderly men with some degree of immunocompromise.[46] KSHV is always present in PEL. In HIV patients with PEL, tumor cells are usually dually infected with EBV as well. By contrast, HIV-negative PEL is usually EBV-negative. KSHV-associated MCD, although much more common in HIV-infected populations, also occurs in the general population.

MCD is a KSHV-associated, immunoglobulin M (IgM) λ–producing, nonclonal lymphoproliferative disorder typically involving the mantle zone of lymph nodes and the spleen. The KSHV-positive cells in MCD are always EBV negative. These cells express a broad range of KSHV lytic antigens, and high KSHV copy numbers are reported in plasma. Evolution into or coassociation with an aggressive lymphoma, often of plasmablastic phenotype, is not uncommon. Within the HIV population, nearly all cases of MCD are KSHV-associated; this viral association is not as strong among HIV-negative MCD patients. High expression of viral interleukin-6 (IL-6) is thought to contribute to the systemic inflammation seen in this disorder.[47] The KSHV-associated lymphomas that arise in association with MCD are not nodal equivalents of PEL; rather, these plasmablastic lymphomas (see E-Slide VM03957) are uniformly EBV negative and express IgM λ.[16]

Diagnostic and Therapeutic Considerations

The requisite finding in PEL is a lymphomatous effusion, which can be pleural, pericardial, or peritoneal, without associated lymphadenopathy or masses, arising in the setting of immunocompromise. Often, patients with HIV/AIDS will present with PEL in addition to other KSHV-associated diseases, such as Kaposi sarcoma and MCD, so thorough evaluation and staging should be undertaken at diagnosis. On cytologic examination, the PEL tumor cells are large with prominent nucleoli. The effusion cells are clonal B cells with

CD45 positivity but typically lack other specific B-cell lineage markers, although CD30 and CD38 positivity can be seen. BCL6 mutations are frequently detected. Tumor cells always harbor KSHV, as demonstrated by staining for KSHV-associated latency-associated nuclear antigen-1. In MCD, there is characteristically λ light chain restriction.[48] This does not reflect clonality as assessed by study of immunoglobulin DNA rearrangements. Rather, it reflects a tendency for the virus to selectively infect cells expressing λ or to selectively drive such cells to proliferate.

Treatment of PEL is most commonly combination chemotherapy, although novel approaches such as intracavitary cidofovir have been reported to be successful in rare cases.[49] Outcomes remain quite poor. Treatment of MCD with targeted therapies has been more successful, including the use of rituximab and IL-6 inhibition.[50,51] Siltuximab, a monoclonal antibody against human IL-6, is now approved in the United States for HIV-negative patients with KSHV-negative MCD, but it has not been studied clinically in those with virus-associated MCD.[52] Antivirals such as ganciclovir and valganciclovir have shown clinical activity in MCD, because viral lytic replication is a feature of this disease.[53] Rituximab plus liposomal doxorubicin has been shown to be associated with high rates of clinical response in HIV-associated MCD, with minimal increased risk of worsening concurrent Kaposi sarcoma lesions during therapy.[54]

HUMAN T-LYMPHOTROPIC VIRUS-1

Viral Biology

HTLV-1 is a retrovirus with a single-stranded RNA genome. Following infection there is reverse transcription and integration of proviral DNA into the host genome. HTLV-1 infects a variety of cell types but persists in the subset of CD4$^+$ T lymphocytes that are regulatory T cells.[55] Viral infection within the host is spread from cell to cell through direct cell-to-cell contact. As with EBV, the proliferation of HTLV-1–infected lymphocytes plays a central role in ensuring viral persistence.

The HTLV-1 protein Tax is also a mediator of immune dysregulation, T-lymphocyte immortalization, and transformation (Fig. 83.4).[56,57] Tax affects NFκB and the serine/threonine kinase AKT pathways with diverse proliferative and antiapoptotic effects. As with some of the immunodominant EBV antigens expressed in proliferating lymphocytes, Tax expression is targeted by cytotoxic T cells. Another viral protein, Hbz, suppresses Tax expression, allowing

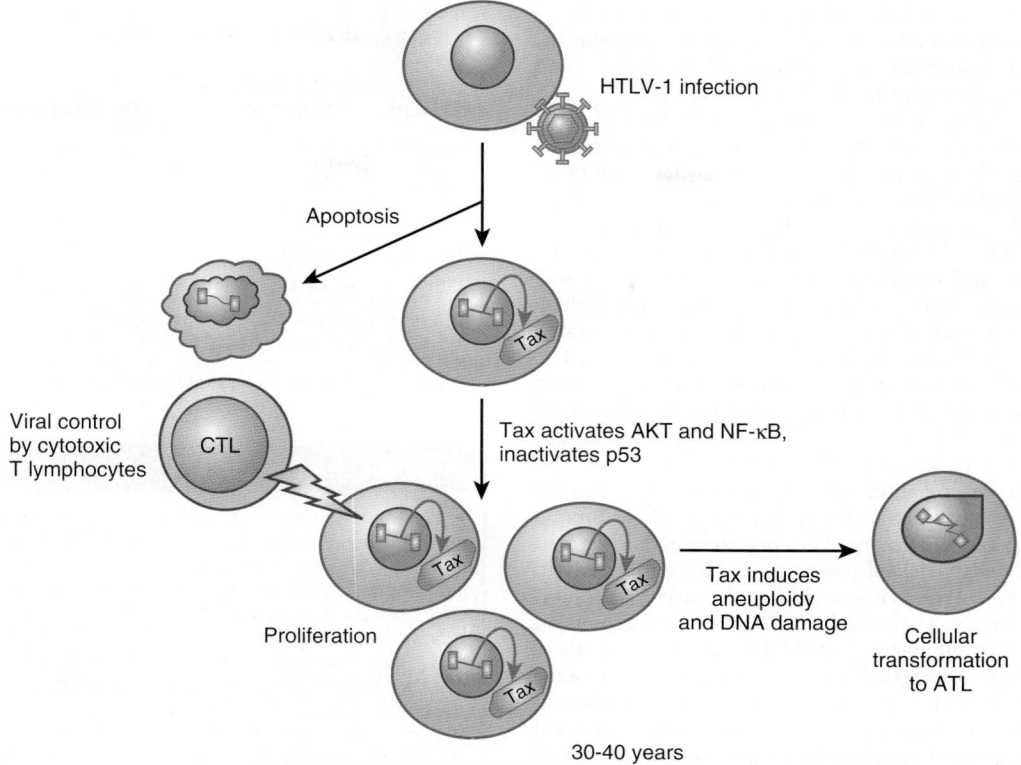

Fig. 83.4 HUMAN T-LYMPHOTROPIC VIRUS-1 (HTLV-1) AND THE EVOLUTION OF ADULT T-CELL LEUKEMIA/LYMPHOMA. Following HTLV-1 infection, many cells undergo apoptosis, but some infected CD4+ T cells are driven to proliferate by the effects of Tax on the nuclear factor-κB (NFκB) pathway and on the AKT pathway. Tax is also suggested to result in inactivation of p53, aneuploidy, and deoxyribonucleic acid (DNA) damage. Over many decades, malignancy evolves.

transformed T cells to elude immune surveillance.[57] Tax interferes with various DNA repair pathways and induces reactive oxygen species, facilitating the development of aneuploidy.[56,58] Tax leads to functional inactivation of p53 and may interfere with the spindle assembly checkpoint that normally operates in mitosis to preserve euploidy.

Epidemiology of Viral Infection and Adult T-Cell Leukemia/Lymphoma

HTLV-1 is endemic in particular regions of Japan, Africa, South America, and some Caribbean islands.[58,59] As assessed by seroprevalence, rates up to 37% are found on the southwestern Japanese islands of Shikoku, Kyushu, and Okinawa, whereas most other areas of Japan have an intermediate prevalence of 1%–5%. In the United States, the incidence in blood donors is 0.025%. It has been estimated that about 20 million individuals are infected worldwide. The major mode of transmission in endemic areas is from mother to child in breast milk, although infection is also transmitted through sexual intercourse, transfusion of cellular blood products, and the sharing of needles and syringes. Evidence has been presented that HTLV-1 infection persists in association with certain human leukocyte antigen (HLA) types and may be more readily transmitted from mother to child when these HLA types are shared.

ATL is more common in men than in women and typically presents in the fourth or fifth decade of life. Perhaps as a function of the long latency period, cases of ATL following blood transfusion or needle sharing are vanishingly rare. The lifetime risk for ATL has been estimated to be in excess of 6% in men who are HTLV-1 carriers in an endemic region of Japan, although in other settings the risk may be much lower.[60] As with EBV, the subset of the infected population that develops lymphoma is quite small.

Adult T-Cell Leukemia/Lymphoma Diagnostic Considerations

There is a spectrum of ATL.[61] In the acute leukemic subtype of ATL, comprising around 60% of cases, leukocytosis, diffuse lymphoadenopathy, and hypercalcemia are common. The classic findings on a peripheral blood smear are lymphocytes with flower-shaped nuclei (Fig. 83.3C). Twenty percent of patients with ATL present with a lymphomatous subtype dominated by lymphadenopathy and hepatosplenomegaly. Cutaneous infiltration, lytic bone lesions, malignant effusions, and involvement of the CNS and other extranodal sites are not uncommon.[57] There are also chronic and smoldering subtypes that behave much more indolently and may in some cases not require treatment upon diagnosis. Across all subtypes, presentations reflecting immune dysfunction such as strongyloidiasis with dissemination, *Pneumocystis jiroveci* pneumonia (PJP), mycobacterium, or cryptococcal infection are common. The immune dysfunction seen in patients with ATL may be due to the fact that the leukemic cells have a regulatory T-cell phenotype that fosters an immunosuppressive environment.

Histologically ATL shows lymph node effacement by large, atypical T cells usually expressing CD4+, CD25+, and CD52+, with variable CD30 and CD15 expression. Aneuploidy is consistent, although characteristic cytogenetic abnormalities have not been identified. Serologic analysis confirms the presence of HTLV-1 infection.[61]

Therapies Specific to HTLV-1 ATL

The leukemic and lymphomatous forms of ATL are aggressive and are associated with poor responses to chemotherapy, high relapse rates, and low overall survival. In a phase III randomized trial in Japan, researchers compared two multiagent chemotherapy regimens (vincristine, cyclophosphamide, doxorubicin [Adriamycin], and prednisone [VCAP], doxorubicin [Adriamycin], ranimustine, and prednisone [AMP], and vindesine, etoposide, carboplatin, and prednisone [VECP] [together, VCAP-AMP-VECP] to cyclophosphamide, hydroxydaunomycin (doxorubicin), Oncovin (vincristine), and prednisone [together, CHOP-14]) in patients with poor prognosis ATL.[62] VCAP-AMP-VECP was associated with higher complete response rates, with a trend toward improved overall survival, although the toxicity of this regimen is significant, and the treatment as planned was not tolerated by the majority of patients. In a randomized, phase II study, patients with newly diagnosed aggressive ATL were treated with VCAP-AMP-VECP with or without the humanized anti–CC chemokine receptor 4 antibody mogamulizimab.[63] Although patients treated with the chemotherapy–antibody combination had higher complete response rates that were deemed to be clinically significant, infections, severe skin rashes, and other adverse events were also more common in the combination arm. Several antivirals used in the treatment of HIV infection have activity against HTLV-1. Among them are zidovudine and lamivudine. The combination of interferon (IFN) and zidovudine has yielded promising results, particularly in the leukemic subtype.[61] Proteasome and histone deacetylase inhibitors have attracted interest. Given high CD25 and CD52 expression in ATL, the efficacy of monoclonal antibodies aimed against these two receptors has been investigated. Thus far, alemtuzumab, an anti-CD52 monoclonal antibody, may have some activity in ATL based on small phase II studies and case reports.[64,65] Arsenic trioxide combined with IFN-α has been shown to induce remissions in relapsed, refractory patients with ATL, although durable responses were limited. In a trial of 20 patients with ATL, all-*trans* retinoic acid was used, with 40% achieving remission. Allogeneic hematopoietic transplant has been increasingly recognized as an effective therapy for ATL.[66,67]

HIV-ASSOCIATED LYMPHOMAS

Viral Biology and Pathogenesis

HIV-1 is a retrovirus that infects CD4+ T cells and monocytes.[68] It appears to establish a lifelong reservoir in CD4+ T cells.[69] Viral infection may lead to cell death or establishment of latency in resting cells. HIV infection is spread either through new rounds of virion production with cellular infection or cell–cell fusion. There is no evidence to suggest that infected cells are driven to proliferate. This is in contrast to HTLV-1 and EBV, where proliferation of infected cells appears to play a key role in establishing the long-term viral reservoir and perhaps in mediating lymphomagenesis. The lymphomas that are increased in HIV-infected patients (Table 83.4) are of B-cell lineage, and many are associated with EBV, KSHV, or both (see Table 83.4).

There is no substantial evidence that HIV infection of B cells is important in the pathogenesis of these lymphomas. Rather, it appears that the HIV infection compromises cellular immunity, decreasing immune surveillance of EBV- and KSHV-infected B cells. In addition, HIV infection stimulates proliferation of B lymphocytes and perhaps genetic aberrations in the proliferating cells.[70] Many possible mechanisms have been invoked, including (1) direct stimulation of B cells by HIV antigens or antigens associated with opportunistic infection; (2) stimulation of B cells by cellular proteins (CD40 ligand) incorporated into the HIV virion, leading to expression of activation-induced deaminase, an enzyme that mediates double-stranded DNA breaks; and (3) dysregulation of B cells as a consequence of T-cell dysfunction.[16,70,71]

There is also some evidence that host biology may contribute to lymphomagenesis. In particular, there are a variety of genetic polymorphisms that influence susceptibility to HIV-1 infection, such as CCR5-Δ32.[72,73] Individuals who are homozygous for this polymorphism are much less likely than others to be infected by HIV. Some evidence has emerged to suggest that, in heterozygotes who are

TABLE 83.4	HIV-Associated Lymphoma		
Lymphoma	CD4 Association (cells/mm³)	EBV Association (%)	Other Cofactors
PCNSL	<50	>95%	
DLBCL	Variable	40%	
BL	>100	30%	
HL	>100	90%	
PEL	<100	>75%	KSHV

BL, Burkitt lymphoma; DLBCL, diffuse large B-cell lymphoma; EBV, Epstein-Barr virus; HIV, human immunodeficiency virus; HL, Hodgkin lymphoma; KSHV, Kaposi sarcoma–associated herpesvirus; PCNSL, primary central nervous system lymphoma; PEL, primary effusion lymphoma.

HIV Hodgkin Lymphoma

A 42-year-old human immunodeficiency virus (HIV)–positive patient, on highly active antiretroviral therapy (HAART) with a CD4 count of 324 cells/mm³ and undetectable viral load, presents with fever, weight loss, and a palpable axillary lymph node. Hodgkin lymphoma (HL) is diagnosed on excisional biopsy, and Epstein-Barr virus (EBV) positivity is demonstrated by EBV-encoded RNA (EBER) in the Reed-Sternberg tumor cells. Although he lacks additional lymphadenopathy, a bone marrow biopsy is performed, and it shows involvement by HL. He has stage IVB disease. *Pneumocystis jiroveci* pneumonia prophylaxis is started despite an adequate CD4 count in anticipation of chemotherapy. His HAART regimen is reviewed for potential antiviral-chemotherapy drug interactions. He receives six cycles of full-dose, first-line chemotherapy and achieves a complete remission.

---

infected, HIV progression is slowed, and there is less likelihood of lymphomagenesis.

Epidemiology

Lymphoma is increased in all HIV risk groups, in contrast to Kaposi sarcoma, which is rarely seen in injection drug users (or in hemophiliacs in an earlier era).[74] There is a well-established relationship between CD4+ cells per cubic millimeter overall and the risk for lymphoma, but the relationship is complex and differs among lymphomas (see Table 83.4).

The incidence of non-Hodgkin lymphoma (NHL) in the HIV population, particularly PCNSL (Fig. 83.5A–C), has decreased with the widespread use of highly active antiretroviral therapy (HAART), although patients with HIV on HAART still carry an increased risk for lymphoma compared with the HIV-negative population.[75,76] In the HAART era, patients with HIV on average have higher CD4+ counts (often >100 cells/mm³) when diagnosed with lymphoma as compared with the pre-HAART era. Among patients with HIV with very low CD4+ counts,[75] NHLs are still seen at rates similar to the pre-HAART era. Patients with HIV are now living much longer because of effective antiretroviral regimens and decreased rates of opportunistic infection. As a result, malignancy has emerged as the major cause of mortality in HIV populations with access to antiretroviral therapy.[77,78]

With the widespread use of HAART, the incidence of HL in HIV-seropositive patients has not declined; patients with CD4+ counts between 150 and 199 cells/mm³ actually have higher risk for HIV-associated HL than patients with CD4+ counts of less than 50 cells/mm³.[79]

Diagnostic Considerations Specific to Lymphoma in Patients With HIV

Lymphomas in patients with HIV infection are more likely to present with B symptoms such as fever and night sweats, as well as advanced

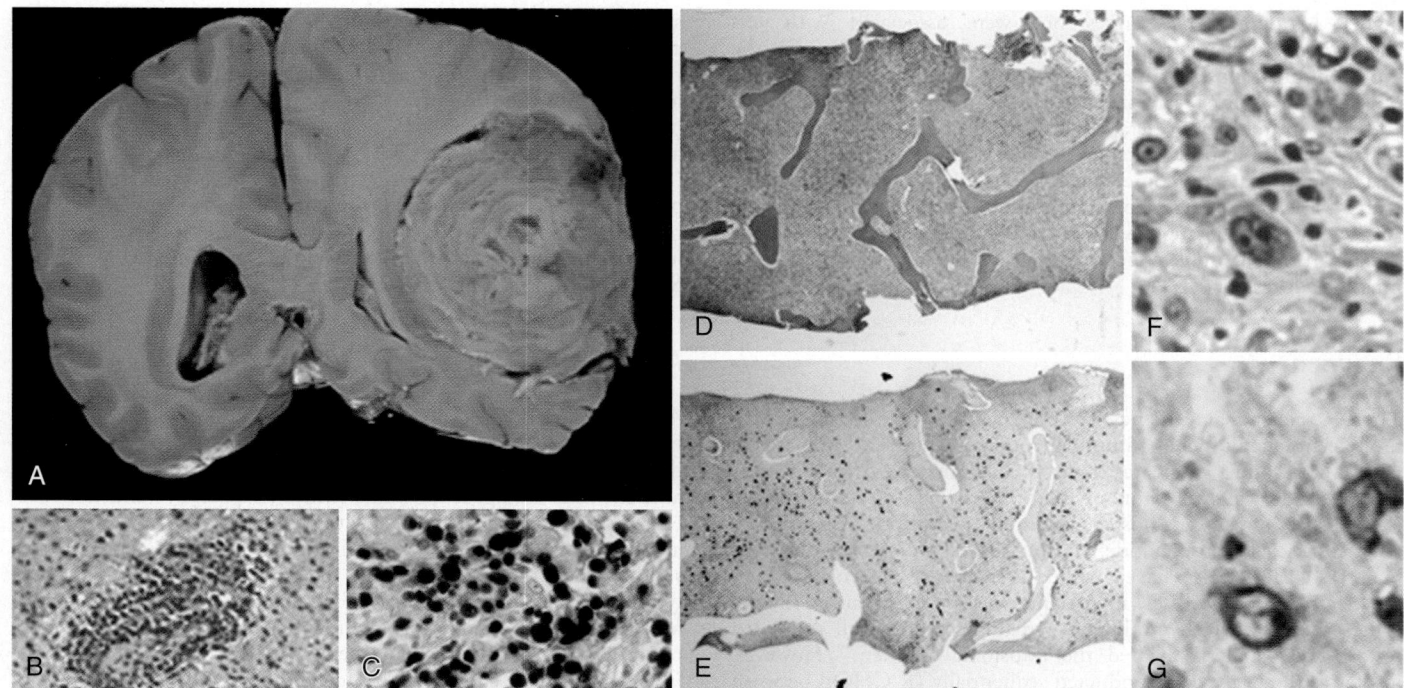

Fig. 83.5 EXAMPLES OF HUMAN IMMUNODEFICIENCY VIRUS (HIV)–RELATED LYMPHOMAS. Primary central nervous system (CNS) lymphoma in HIV-positive patients (A–C). Gross appearance (coronal section) of the brain from an autopsy of a 24-year-old HIV-positive female patient with temporoparietal mass due to a primary CNS lymphoma (A). The patient died as a result of uncal and cingulate herniation. (B) Biopsy section from another patient showing a perivascular infiltrate of large lymphoma cells. This is the typical pattern of involvement by CNS lymphoma. The cells were shown to be CD20+ B cells and were EBER positive (C). A diagnosis can be made without biopsy when magnetic resonance imaging studies show characteristic features and EBV is demonstrated in the cerebrospinal fluid by polymerase chain reaction (see box on AIDS Primary Central Nervous System Lymphoma). Hodgkin lymphoma extensively involving the bone marrow in an HIV-positive patient with stage IVB disease (D–G). The bone marrow biopsy was entirely replaced with Hodgkin lymphoma associated with dense sclerosis (D). An EBER study shows scattered positive cells throughout the marrow (E), corresponding to the Hodgkin and Reed-Sternberg cells (F), which were CD30+ as illustrated (G). Hodgkin lymphoma infrequently involves the bone marrow in HIV-negative cases, but some HIV-positive patients can first present with extensive bone marrow disease (see box on HIV Hodgkin Lymphoma). *(A, courtesy Dr. Peter Pytel, University of Chicago.)*

stage, including bone marrow, extranodal, and CNS involvement. Thus the approach to diagnosis is somewhat different from the approach in the HIV-negative patient.

Unexplained fever and sweats in an HIV-seropositive patient, even in the absence of lymphadenopathy, are sufficient to warrant consideration of HL. Patterns of disease involvement also differ in HIV-infected patients. Contiguous spread so characteristic of classic HL in other settings is less common in HIV HL, and bone marrow–only presentations of HL are not uncommon (Fig. 83.5D–G).

Patients with HIV-associated NHL have higher rates of extranodal involvement, including bone marrow and CNS disease, as well as higher-stage disease and more aggressive tumors on average.[80] Therefore, it is recommended that all HIV-seropositive patients with aggressive NHL undergo a diagnostic lumbar puncture. The routine use of CNS intrathecal chemotherapy prophylaxis in all HIV-seropositive patients with NHL is controversial but reasonable and typically is done in particularly high-risk patients, such as those with BL, marrow or testicular involvement, or extranodal disease.

Imaging is often more difficult to interpret in patients with HIV than in other settings. Lymphadenopathy associated with HIV infection or opportunistic infection is common, and the presumption that enlarged lymph nodes reflect the presence of lymphoma in patients with known lymphoma or a history of lymphoma is not as safe as in other settings. Positron emission tomography–computed tomography (PET-CT), although useful, must also be interpreted with caution insofar as HIV infection itself, opportunistic infection,

and immune reconstitution following the initiation of antiretroviral therapy are all associated with signal on metabolic imaging with fluorodeoxyglucose.

CD4+ counts can help to guide evaluation insofar as CD4+ counts of greater than 300 cells/mm^3 are typically associated with BL or HL,[81] whereas these diagnoses would be unlikely in patients with very low CD4+ counts of less than 50 cells/mm^3 (see box on AIDS PCNSL).[82]

AIDS PRIMARY CENTRAL NERVOUS SYSTEM LYMPHOMA

In AIDS PCNSL, EBV PCR of the cerebrospinal fluid is positive approximately 90% of the time and rarely positive in patients with AIDS but without PCNSL. When EBV is detected in the cerebrospinal fluid of a patient with AIDS, coupled with characteristic magnetic resonance imaging findings, this is sufficient to diagnose AIDS PCNSL without a confirmatory brain biopsy.

Treatment

Aggressive chemotherapy for HIV-associated lymphoma was initially associated with morbidity and mortality related to immunocompromise. A phase III randomized study identified a reduced-dose regimen as preferable to standard dose.[83] Lower doses were not associated with higher lymphoma cure rates but were associated with less chemotherapy-related morbidity and mortality. However, with the evolution of supportive care, including PJP prophylaxis and neutrophil growth factors, tolerance of chemotherapy improved. With effective antiretroviral therapy, long-term outcomes improved as well.[84,85] With full-dose therapies, some evidence emerged to suggest that stage-for-stage outcomes might be as good or better in patients with HIV-associated lymphoma compared with those without HIV.[86] At the outset of therapy, a series of questions related to the chemotherapy regimen, dose, concomitant HAART, and supportive care must be addressed.

Regimen

There is general agreement that the inclusion of rituximab with multiagent chemotherapy improves outcome, at least in patients with $CD4^+$ counts of greater than 50 cells/mm[3]. Rituximab, cyclophosphamide, hydroxydaunomycin, vincristine, and prednisone (R-CHOP) and dose-adjusted, infusional etoposide, prednisone, vincristine, cyclophosphamide, and hydroxydaunomycin with rituximab (DA-EPOCH-R) have emerged as standard regimens.[87,88] As in the treatment of DLBCL, in patients without HIV infection, the value of infusional chemotherapy remains controversial. A pooled retrospective analysis favored the infusional regimen.[89] However, insofar as the trials were conducted sequentially (R-CHOP between 1998 and 2002, and R-EPOCH between 2002 and 2006), it is difficult to exclude other factors, such as the availability of better antiretroviral agents, improvements in supportive care, or changes in the population studied.

BL typically requires more intensive treatment regimens than those used for DLBCL.[90] Thus there has been concern about using these regimens in the HIV-seropositive population. A small retrospective study of cyclophosphamide, vincristine (Oncovin), doxorubicin, and methotrexate (CODOX-M)/ifosfamide, etoposide, and cytarabine (IVAC) for BL that included 14 patients with HIV showed HIV-seropositive patients to have similar progression-free survival, overall survival, and complete response rates as compared with the HIV-negative patients with BL. In a multicenter retrospective study, HIV-positive patients with BL treated with rituximab plus CODOX-M/IVAC had better progression-free and overall survival with no increase in toxicity as compared with HIV-positive patients who received CODOX-M/IVAC without rituximab.[91] In a prospective Spanish study, HIV-seropositive and HIV-seronegative patients with BL were treated with six cycles of intensive chemotherapy and rituximab and were found to have comparable outcomes, regardless of HIV status.[92] In this study all HIV-seropositive patients were required to be on HAART to enroll, and the majority had $CD4^+$ counts of greater than 200 cells/mm[3]. Granulocyte colony-stimulating factor support was used throughout chemotherapy cycles, as well as PJP and other antimicrobial prophylaxis. Differences in induction-related mortality, duration of neutropenia, progression-free survival, or overall survival were not detected, although HIV-seropositive patients did have significantly more severe mucositis and infectious complications.

Dose

Most would agree that dose reduction is appropriate in patients with low $CD4^+$ count (<100 cells/mm[3]), history of ongoing opportunistic infection, performance status below 75%, or compromised organ function. Some regimens begin with a 50% dose reduction in cyclophosphamide for a $CD4^+$ count of less than 100 cells/mm[3] with a built-in dose escalation for the next cycle if well tolerated.[84,88]

Chemotherapy regimens of varying intensity depending on $CD4^+$ count, performance status, and International Prognostic Index score have been studied, including a comparison of low-dose CHOP with standard-dose CHOP, with no differences found in overall

survival based on the intensity of the chemotherapy regimen.[86] In patients with very low $CD4^+$ counts, low-dose chemotherapy is a reasonable treatment option, while maintaining the possibility of long-term disease-free survival in some. In a recent uncontrolled prospective study where HIV-positive patients with BL were given a shortened course of EPOCH with a double dose of rituximab (SC-EPOCH-RR), freedom from progression and overall survival outcomes were favorable and comparable to those seen in HIV-negative patients treated with the standard DA-EPOCH-R, with less toxicity and lower cumulative doses of chemotherapy in the SC-EPOCH-RR group.[93]

Antiretroviral Therapy

A few key special issues in considering concurrent antiretroviral and lymphoma therapy include concerns about shared toxicities, drug–drug interactions, and risk for inability to comply with consistent antiretroviral dosing. Zidovudine is myelosuppressive and can exacerbate pancytopenia associated with lymphoma therapy. If patients are already on a zidovudine-containing regimen, it is generally possible to substitute an alternative regimen before the initiation of lymphoma therapy. Many antiretroviral agents alter the metabolism of drugs used in lymphoma treatment. This has been a particular concern when infusional chemotherapy regimens are used, and some investigators have chosen to stop chemotherapy before initiation of such regimens.[84] However, in trials involving infusional chemotherapy that allowed patients already on a stable antiretroviral regimen to remain on that regimen during lymphoma treatment, major problems were not noted.[88] Nausea and vomiting associated with chemotherapy regimens may interfere with regular antiviral dosing. Intermittent antiretroviral therapy raises concerns about the development of a resistant strain of HIV. Because of the concern that initiation of antiretroviral therapy with cytotoxic chemotherapy might result in such resistance, many recommend delaying initiation of antiretroviral therapy until an appropriate regimen to control nausea and vomiting is established. Stopping antiretroviral therapy also carries with it some risks. When antiretroviral therapy includes drugs with different half-lives, stopping treatment may result in the longest-lived agent being present in the absence of other antiretroviral agents. This is particularly an issue for long-lived nonnucleoside reverse transcriptase inhibitors. Even a single dose of such agents in the absence of other antiretroviral agents may lead to resistance to that class of agents. Thus when an interruption of antiretroviral therapy is planned, specific strategies have been advocated, including a "staggered stop" or a change to a regimen with components that have similar half-lives.[94]

For patients already on antiretroviral treatment at the time of lymphoma diagnosis, the particulars of the regimen should be considered during the pretreatment evaluation. Atazanavir and indinavir are associated with hyperbilirubinemia as a result of UGT1A1 inhibition.[94] This is an unconjugated hyperbilirubinemia similar to that occurring with Gilbert syndrome. Elevated total bilirubin in such patients is not indicative of hepatic involvement or other serious hepatic dysfunction and should not guide decisions about chemotherapy dose adjustments. Ritonavir inhibits the clearance of midazolam, phenytoin, and voriconazole and other agents metabolized by the cytochrome P-450 CYP3A4 pathway.

Supportive Care

Although PJP prophylaxis is recommended only when the $CD4^+$ count is less than 200 cells/mm[3] for patients with HIV not receiving cytotoxic chemotherapy, prophylaxis is universally recommended for patients with HIV receiving cytotoxic chemotherapy. The following are also commonly used: fungal prophylaxis with fluconazole; herpes simplex and varicella prophylaxis with acyclovir, valacyclovir, or famciclovir; quinolone prophylaxis when neutrophil counts fall below 1000 cells/mm[3]; and granulocyte growth factors.

Bone Marrow Transplant in Patients With HIV

Autologous bone marrow transplant has been successful in HIV-seropositive patients with NHL, with these patients having adequate stem cell mobilization, nonrelapse mortality rates comparable to those for HIV-negative patients, count recovery within 2 weeks of stem cell rescue, and maintained control of HIV viral loads and CD4+ counts after high-dose chemotherapy.[95,96] There have also been successful reduced-intensity allogeneic bone marrow transplants in HIV-seropositive patients, making the possibilities for treating HIV patients with NHL even more vast, even in those patients with chemotherapy-resistant disease (see box on Autologous Bone Marrow Transplant in an HIV-Seropositive Hodgkin Lymphoma Patient).[97,98] Outcomes of patients with HIV undergoing allogeneic bone marrow transplant have improved in the post-HAART era.[99,100] The first national trial of allogeneic bone marrow transplant for patients with HIV and hematologic malignancy is ongoing. The role of transplant in curing HIV is an area of active investigation, including cell engineering strategies to render cells resistant to HIV.

HEPATITIS C VIRUS

Viral Biology and B-Lymphocyte Proliferation

HCV is an enveloped, positive-stranded RNA virus.[101,102] Infection involves interactions between E2, a viral structural protein with two hypervariable regions, and a cellular protein CD81 present on hepatocytes and B lymphocytes. A polyprotein is translated from viral RNA and is cleaved by cellular and viral proteases, including NS3, to yield proteins required for viral replication. The RNA-dependent RNA polymerase that replicates the viral genome lacks proofreading capacity, thus generating genetic heterogeneity among viral progeny. Viral replication occurs predominantly in hepatocytes, but viral RNA and NS3 have also been detected in B cells, although HCV replication in B cells remains controversial.[103]

Chronic infection can be associated with mixed cryoglobulinemia, a systemic immune disease that results from clonal expansion of B cells producing an IgM autoantibody against IgG, leading to deposition of immune complexes on endothelial surfaces and resulting in inflammation.[104] In this setting of B-cell proliferation, some patients develop B-cell NHL, which is classically of low-grade histology. Several hypotheses have been advanced with regard to how HCV might drive B-cell proliferation. There is controversy as to whether infection of B cells plays any role in this process. A lymphoma cell line that produces infectious HCV has been reported. Even in the absence of infection of B cells, interaction of the HCV E2 protein with CD81 on B cells may drive B-cell proliferation or lower the threshold for other B-cell stimuli to drive proliferation. Immunoglobulin signaling may be activated by immunoglobulin–virus complexes, and Toll-like receptor 7 signaling may be activated by viral RNA. Finally, it is noted that E2 binding triggers expression of activation-induced deaminase, an enzyme that is important in generating somatic hypermutation and that has also been implicated

in mediating mutations thought to play a role in DLBCL lymphomagenesis.[102]

Epidemiology of Viral Infection and Associated Lymphoma

The association between HCV and lymphoma was first recognized in patients with HCV-associated type II mixed cryoglobulinemia, an autoimmune extrahepatic manifestation of HCV infection, although it is now recognized that patients with HCV but without type II mixed cryoglobulinemia also show a predisposition to B-NHL.[105] In systematic reviews, approximately 13%–18% of B-cell lymphomas are associated with HCV infection.[106,107] Most commonly, these lymphomas are histologically indolent subtypes, with splenic marginal zone lymphoma (MZL), nongastric MALT, and lymphoplasmacytic lymphoma more often seen in association with HCV than aggressive histologies such as DLBCL.[108–111] In cases of HCV-associated DLBCL, histologic transformation should be considered because studies have demonstrated that DLBCL in this setting more frequently has evolved out of low-grade lymphoma as compared with HCV-negative patients with DLBCL.[112] For example, in Taiwan, the rate of chronic HCV infection in patients with NHL was 11%, 10-fold higher than in the general Taiwanese population.[113] Among HCV-infected patients with lymphoma, nodal and splenic MZL, but not MALT lymphomas, were increased. The HCV–lymphoma association is more apparent in some countries than in others, with the association being established most clearly in Italy and Japan. Several studies in regions or countries where HCV infection is less prevalent have failed to identify any association with lymphoma.[114–116] In the United States, data from the National Cancer Institute Surveillance, Epidemiology, and End Results registry and the Department of Veterans Affairs have demonstrated a small but significant increase in B-NHL risk with HCV infection.[109,117]

Further evidence in support of an etiologic relationship comes from studies in which successful treatment of HCV was followed by lymphoma regression.[118] The most dramatic illustration comes from patients with splenic lymphoma with villous lymphocytes treated with ribavirin and IFN. Furthermore, clearance of HCV infection has been shown to reduce the incidence of B-NHL, with cumulative incidence of lymphoma among patients with a sustained virologic response of 0% at 15 years, as compared with 2.6% at 15 years among both nonresponders and untreated patients.[119] However, the mechanisms by which chronic HCV infection contributes to lymphomagenesis remain largely undefined, although hypotheses include an indirect role related to B-cell activation and proliferation in the setting of chronic antigenic stimulation.[120]

Certain HCV genotypes may confer increased risk for NHL, with genotypes 2a/III and 2b/IV seen more frequently in the HCV-seropositive patients who develop NHL. However, there is no clear association between genotype and NHL risk, and varying responses to antiviral therapy by genotype further complicate these analyses.

Diagnostic and Prognostic Considerations

In contrast to EBV-, KSHV-, or HTLV-1–associated tumors, there is no established role for studies demonstrating HCV nucleic acid or protein in tumor cells. Thus serologic study and measurement of HCV copy number are the only tools available for inferring an association. We recommend checking HCV serologic characteristics in all patients with B-cell lymphomas most commonly associated with chronic HCV infection.[118] In addition, screening patients with chronic HCV for a monoclonal gammopathy and cryoglobulinemia may be of benefit to identify patients at highest risk for malignant transformation. Elevated serum γ-globulin levels have been found to be a predictor of NHL among patients with type II mixed cryoglobulinemia.[121] In patients who are HCV seropositive, HCV RNA is evaluated in plasma. There seems to be a predilection of HCV-associated lymphomas to involve extranodal sites, particularly the liver and salivary glands, as well as the spleen.[122] Unusual presentations of low-grade HCV-associated lymphomas have been described, including subcutaneous "lipoma-like" MALT lymphoma predominantly in elderly, HCV-positive women.[123] An HCV prognostic score, comprised of poor performance status, hypoalbuminemia, and high HCV-RNA viral load, effectively risk stratified patients into three groups with significantly different progression-free and overall survival outcomes.[124]

Therapy

In patients with indolent lymphomas and untreated HCV infection, antiviral treatment with pegylated IFN-α and ribavirin may obviate the need for cytotoxic chemotherapy and should be considered as an initial therapeutic strategy. Tumor regression with antiviral therapy was first reported in 2002 and is now further supported by subsequent reports.[118] In a recent cohort study from Italy, antiviral treatment resulting in virologic response was shown to be effective as first-line treatment for indolent HCV-associated lymphomas, with not only high overall response rates but also a survival advantage on multivariate analysis.[125] Since 2011, new antiviral agents have become available, notably protease inhibitors specific for the HCV protease. Likelihood of response to older therapy is a function of viral genotype, host genetics (*IL28R* polymorphisms play a critical role in response to protease inhibitors), and other factors. The field is rapidly evolving, and colleagues with specific expertise in appropriate antiviral approaches should be consulted.[101] In general, treatment of the underlying HCV is favored in chronically infected patients who develop indolent lymphoma, given the potential for tumor regression with antiviral therapy, as well as the theoretical reduction in relapse that might accompany virologic responses.

Rituximab has posed an interesting dilemma for the treatment of patients with HCV and lymphoma. It has been reported that HCV plasma RNA increases following rituximab treatment, and there is certainly the possibility that elimination of B cells for 3–18 months following treatment may compromise humoral responses to the evolution of HCV quasispecies. However, in studies to date, overall survival is not inferior.[126] Similarly, combination chemotherapy is safe in patients with HCV infection.[127] Rituximab does not seem to increase the risk of hepatotoxicity with anthracycline-based chemotherapy regimens.[124] Rituximab is specifically recommended for the treatment of HCV-associated cryoglobulinemia (although, as in the treatment of Waldenström macroglobulinemia, it must be appreciated that the initial response to rituximab may be an increase in the IgM paraprotein level, necessitating plasmapheresis). Unlike in cases of indolent lymphoma, where antiviral therapy alone may be sufficient, rituximab-containing multiagent chemotherapy regimens are recommended for HCV-associated DLBCL, and attempts to concomitantly treat with antivirals are generally not advised, given the added risks of cytopenias and hepatotoxicity.

Aspects of Therapy

With regard to the use of rituximab to treat B-cell lymphomas in patients with HCV, overall survival is not inferior, although there do appear to be increased rates of hepatotoxicity and rises in HCV viral load during therapy. Similarly, combination chemotherapy is safe in patients with HCV infection, although HCV RNA levels can rise during treatment. Interestingly, patients with HCV and splenic MZL have had regression of their tumors with treatment for HCV infection with IFN-α and ribavirin, an effect not seen in HCV-negative patients with splenic MZL treated with the same regimen.

FUTURE DIRECTIONS

In this chapter, a variety of virus-associated lymphomas and lymphoproliferative diseases have been reviewed. For most of these lymphomas, standard antiviral drugs do not have a role in treatment. There are several exceptions, however, and these are worth highlighting. Antiviral therapy for HCV-associated splenic lymphoma with villous lymphocytes is accepted as a standard approach and likely has a role in the treatment of other HCV-associated indolent lymphomas. Similarly, ganciclovir or valganciclovir appears to have a role in the management of MCD associated with KSHV in patients with HIV. Of course, in addition, there is an established role for antiretroviral therapy in the treatment of patients with HIV patients and malignancy. There are virus-targeted therapies that are broadly accepted as standard, including adoptive immunotherapy with EBV-specific T cells for PTLD. The use of targeted T cells also has promise in other settings, including EBV-associated HL. Other virus-targeted therapies are being developed. Some involve vaccination; others involve induction of viral genes in tumor cells, rendering them more susceptible to pharmacologic treatment. Finally, it may ultimately be possible to prevent some kinds of lymphoma by preventing viral infection or altering the host response to viral infection.

SUGGESTED READINGS

Balsalobre P, Diez-Martin JL, Re A, et al: Autologous stem-cell transplantation in patients with HIV-related lymphoma. *J Clin Oncol* 27:2192, 2009.

Barta SK, Lee JY, Kaplan LD, et al: Pooled analysis of AIDS malignancy consortium trials evaluating rituximab plus CHOP or infusional EPOCH chemotherapy in HIV-associated non-Hodgkin lymphoma. *Cancer* 118:3977, 2012.

Bazarbachi A, Suarez F, Fields P, et al: How I treat adult T-cell leukemia/lymphoma. *Blood* 118:1736, 2011.

Bower M, Newsom-Davis T, Naresh K, et al: Clinical features and outcome in HIV-associated multicentric Castleman's disease. *J Clin Oncol* 29:2481, 2011.

Carbone A, Cesarman E, Spina M, et al: HIV-associated lymphomas and gamma-herpesviruses. *Blood* 113:1213, 2009.

Choi I, Tanosaki R, Uike N, et al: Long-term outcomes after hematopoietic SCT for adult T-cell leukemia/lymphoma: results of prospective trials. *Bone Marrow Transplant* 46:116, 2011.

Chuang SS, Liao YL, Chang ST, et al: Hepatitis C virus infection is significantly associated with malignant lymphoma in Taiwan, particularly with nodal and splenic marginal zone lymphomas. *J Clin Pathol* 63:595, 2010.

Engels EA, Pfeiffer RM, Landgren O, et al: Immunologic and virologic predictors of AIDS-related non-Hodgkin lymphoma in the highly active antiretroviral therapy era. *J Acquir Immune Defic Syndr* 54:78, 2010.

Epeldegui M, Hung YP, McQuay A, et al: Infection of human B cells with Epstein-Barr virus results in the expression of somatic hypermutation-inducing molecules and in the accrual of oncogene mutations. *Mol Immunol* 44:934, 2007.

Evens AM, Roy R, Sterrenberg D, et al: Post-transplantation lymphoproliferative disorders: diagnosis, prognosis, and current approaches to therapy. *Curr Oncol Rep* 12:383, 2010.

Giordano TP, Henderson L, Landgren O, et al: Risk of non-Hodgkin lymphoma and lymphoproliferative precursor diseases in US veterans with hepatitis C virus. *JAMA* 297:2010, 2007.

Guech-Ongey M, Simard EP, Anderson WF, et al: AIDS-related Burkitt lymphoma in the United States: what do age and CD4 lymphocyte patterns tell us about etiology and/or biology? *Blood* 116:5600, 2010.

Heslop HE, Slobod KS, Pule MA, et al: Long-term outcome of EBV-specific T-cell infusions to prevent or treat EBV-related lymphoproliferative disease in transplant recipients. *Blood* 115:925, 2010.

Hishizawa M, Kanda J, Utsunomiya A, et al: Transplantation of allogeneic hematopoietic stem cells for adult T-cell leukemia: a nationwide retrospective study. *Blood* 116:1369, 2010.

Ito M, Kusunoki H, Mochida K, et al: HCV infection and B-cell lymphomagenesis. *Adv Hematol* 2011:835314, 2011.

Jaffe ES, Campo E, Swerdlow SH, et al: The 2008 WHO classification of lymphoid neoplasms and beyond: evolving concepts and practical applications. *Blood* 117:5019, 2011.

Keegan TH, Glaser SL, Clarke CA, et al: Epstein-Barr virus as a marker of survival after Hodgkin's lymphoma: a population-based study. *J Clin Oncol* 23:7604, 2005.

Kelly GL, Rickinson AB: Burkitt lymphoma: revisiting the pathogenesis of a virus-associated malignancy. *Hematology Am Soc Hematol Educ Program* 2007:277, 2007.

Kitahata MM, Achenbach CJ, Saag MS: Age at cancer diagnosis among persons with AIDS. *Ann Intern Med* 154:642, 2011.

Levine AM: HIV-associated lymphoma. *Blood* 115:2986, 2010.

Libra M, Polesel J, Russo AE, et al: Extrahepatic disorders of HCV infection: a distinct entity of B-cell neoplasia? *Int J Oncol* 36:1331, 2010.

Matsuoka M, Jeang KT: Human T-cell leukaemia virus type 1 (HTLV-1) infectivity and cellular transformation. *Nat Rev Cancer* 7:270, 2007.

Matsuoka M, Jeang KT: Human T-cell leukemia virus type 1 (HTLV-1) and leukemic transformation: viral infectivity, Tax, HBZ and therapy. *Oncogene* 30:1379, 2011.

Moore PS, Chang Y: KSHV: forgotten but not gone. *Blood* 117:6973, 2011.

Ratner L, Harrington W, Feng X, et al: Human T cell leukemia virus reactivation with progression of adult T-cell leukemia-lymphoma. *PLoS ONE* 4:e4420, 2009.

Rudek MA, Flexner C, Ambinder RF: Use of antineoplastic agents in patients with cancer who have HIV/AIDS. *Lancet Oncol* 12:905, 2011.

Savoldo B, Goss JA, Hammer MM, et al: Treatment of solid organ transplant recipients with autologous Epstein Barr virus-specific cytotoxic T lymphocytes (CTLs). *Blood* 108:2942, 2006.

Sparano JA, Lee JY, Kaplan LD, et al: Rituximab plus concurrent infusional EPOCH chemotherapy is highly effective in HIV-associated B-cell non-Hodgkin lymphoma. *Blood* 115:3008, 2010.

Uldrick TS, Polizzotto MN, Aleman K, et al: High-dose zidovudine plus valganciclovir for Kaposi sarcoma herpesvirus-associated multicentric Castleman disease: a pilot study of virus-activated cytotoxic therapy. *Blood* 117:6977, 2011.

Vereide DT, Sugden B: Lymphomas differ in their dependence on Epstein-Barr virus. *Blood* 117:1977, 2011.

REFERENCES

For the complete list of references, log on to www.expertconsult.com.

CHAPTER 84

MALIGNANT LYMPHOMAS IN CHILDHOOD

Kara M. Kelly, Birgit Burkhardt, and Catherine M. Bollard

Malignant lymphomas are the third most common malignancy among children and adolescents.[1–3] Among children <15 years of age, non-Hodgkin lymphoma (NHL) is more frequent; however, in patients up to 18 years of age, Hodgkin lymphoma (HL) is predominant. NHLs in children are usually extranodal, diffuse, high-grade tumors, whereas low- and intermediate-grade nodal lymphomas predominate in adults. These differences are speculated to reflect maturational changes in the function and composition of the immune system.[2] The different histologies explain in part the differing clinical features, disease course, and treatment strategies used in adults and children.

The differences in treatment approach and disease subtypes are less striking in adults and children with HL. However, there are significant challenges in the management of children with HL. These primarily comprise the sequelae of therapy, such as radiation-induced bone growth abnormalities, endocrine dysfunction, and chemotherapy-related sterility. Of greater concern are the radiation- and chemotherapy-related second malignancies and late cardiac deaths. Current trials are examining ways to reduce the toxicity of therapy without compromising the excellent outcome generally achieved.

NON-HODGKIN LYMPHOMA

Epidemiology

The incidence of NHL increases steadily throughout life, in contrast to Hodgkin disease, which has a bimodal age distribution peaking in early and late adulthood.[2] Although NHLs may occur at any age in childhood, they are infrequent among children younger than 3 years of age; the median age at presentation is approximately 10 years. NHL is two to three times more frequent in boys than in girls and is almost twice as common in whites as in African Americans. The reasons for these differences have yet to be determined.[4]

Specific populations at risk for the development of NHL include those with either congenital or acquired immunodeficiency conditions.[5] Inherited immunodeficiency syndromes include Wiskott-Aldrich syndrome, X-linked lymphoproliferative syndrome (XLP), and ataxia telangiectasia (AT). The recognition of these syndromes in children with newly diagnosed NHL is important for appropriate therapeutic design. For example, involved field irradiation and radiomimetics should be avoided in children with AT. Additionally, children with AT are at increased risk for the development of cyclophosphamide-induced hemorrhagic cystitis; therefore, they should receive vigorous hydration and uroprotectants (e.g., mesna) when administering any dose of cyclophosphamide. XLP should be considered in any male with a high-grade B-cell lymphoma who either develops a late recurrence (second occurrence) of a high-grade B-cell lymphoma or has a brother with either a high-grade B-cell lymphoma or fatal infectious mononucleosis. Children with acquired immunodeficiency conditions predisposing them to the development of NHL include those who have received posttransplant immunosuppressive therapy and those with acquired immunodeficiency syndrome (AIDS).

There are differences in both the incidence and proportion of histologic subtypes in different parts of the world. For example, the NHLs are very rare in Japan but occur quite frequently in equatorial Africa. Burkitt lymphoma, which accounts for about one-half of all childhood cancers in equatorial Africa, is the predominant NHL

histologic subtype in both equatorial Africa and northeastern Brazil.[6] There are also geographic differences in both the clinical and biologic features of certain NHL subtypes.[7,8]

Classification

After Thomas Hodgkin described the disease bearing his name in 1832, various schemes emerged to classify the tumors now collectively referred to as the NHLs. Several classification schemes were developed on the basis of histopathologic features and the putative cell of origin. In an attempt to reduce the confusion of multiple classification schemes, the National Cancer Institute (NCI) sponsored a workshop to design a single classification scheme for clinical use. This scheme, published in 1982 and referred to as the NCI Working Formulation, was widely accepted for almost two decades. In the Working Formulation, the NHLs of childhood are predominantly diffuse high-grade tumors and can be divided among three major subgroups: lymphoblastic, small noncleaved cell, and large-cell lymphomas.

In the past decade, additional classification schemes were designed to improve upon the NCI Working Formulation. Because of the problems associated with attempts to classify lymphoid neoplasms into categories based on presumed normal cell counterparts, the International Lymphoma Study Group proposed a classification system for lymphoid neoplasms[9] predicated on a practical approach to categorizing these diseases using available immunologic and molecular genetic techniques in addition to the standard morphologic criteria. This Revised European-American Classification of Lymphoid Neoplasms (REAL Classification) has been endorsed by many of the world's leading lymphoma pathologists and has served as the basis for the World Health Organization (WHO) classification of hematopoietic and lymphoid tumors.[10] Both the REAL and WHO classification systems include related lymphoid leukemias and recognize that NHL and acute lymphoblastic leukemia (ALL) represent different stages of evolution within specific morphologically and immunologically defined disease categories, an observation recognized by clinicians caring for children with lymphoid neoplasms and reflected in current clinical practice, which prescribes similar therapies for lymphomas and leukemias of related phenotype.

In the REAL and WHO classification systems, NHLs are classified on the basis of phenotype (B lineage vs. T lineage vs. natural killer [NK] cell lineage) and differentiation (precursor vs. mature). Hence, NHLs that occur commonly in children appear in three major categories: lymphoblastic lymphoma (LBL; precursor B-cell lymphoma and precursor T-cell lymphoma), mature B-cell NHL (Burkitt and Burkitt-like lymphoma and diffuse, large B-cell lymphoma [DLBCL]), and anaplastic large-cell lymphoma (ALCL; mature T-cell or null-cell types). The current version of the WHO classification introduced pediatric follicular lymphoma, marginal zone lymphoma, and gray zone lymphoma. The clinical and biologic characteristics of NHL in children are summarized in Table 84.1 and illustrated in Fig. 84.1A–C.

Lymphoblastic Lymphoma

Whether LBL and ALL are two clinical presentations of the same disease or two different diseases is the subject of ongoing discussion.

Patients with a mass and less than 25% bone marrow (BM) lymphoblasts are designated as having LBL, whereas patients with at least 25% BM involvement have ALL. In contrast to ALL, more than 75% of patients with LBL demonstrate a precursor T-cell immunophenotype (T-LBL), with the remainder showing a precursor B-cell immunophenotype (pB-LBL).[11–13]

TABLE 84.1	Characteristics of Non-Hodgkin Lymphoma in Children		
Subtype	Proportion of Cases in BFM Studies (%)[11]	Phenotype	Primary Site
Lymphoblastic	26	T cell; B cell	Mediastinum or head and neck; lymph nodes, skin, soft tissue, bone
Burkitt	49	B cell	Abdomen or head and neck
DLBCL	13	B cell	Lymph nodes, mediastinum, abdomen, head and neck
ALCL	13	T cell indeterminate	Mediastinum, abdomen, head and neck, bone, soft tissue, or skin

ALCL, Anaplastic large-cell lymphoma; BFM, Berlin-Frankfurt-Münster; DLBCL, diffuse large B-cell lymphoma; Ig, immunoglobulin.

Epidemiology

LBL constitutes 22% to 28% of childhood NHL. There is a 2 : 1 male predominance for LBL, but the incidence of LBL remains constant across the pediatric age group for both boys and girls.[14]

Pathobiology

LBL arises from precursor T or B lymphoblasts at varying stages of differentiation. The morphology is similar to that of ALL, with lymphoblasts of small or medium size and with scant cytoplasm, round or convoluted nuclei, fine chromatin, and indistinct or small nucleoli. Immunophenotyping shows terminal deoxynucleotidyl transferase (TdT) positivity. T-LBL are usually positive for CD7 and surface or cytoplasmic CD3, with variable expression of CD2, CD5, CD1a, CD4, and CD8. Staining for TdT, CD3, myeloperoxidase, and a B-cell marker–like pax5 or CD79a are recommended parts of a resource-saving diagnostic staining panel.[15] CD10 expression is more frequent in T-LBL (40%) than in T-ALL (less than 10%), possibly related to maturational stage, with T-ALL more frequently demonstrating an immature phenotype.[13,16,17] B-lineage markers are positive in pB-LBL. Unlike ALL, there are no known cytogenetic prognostic factors for LBL. Recurrent cytogenetic anomalies are seen in about half of childhood T-ALL but have not been well-defined in T-LBL. Literature is scarce regarding typical chromosomal aberrations for T-LBL. The commonest chromosomal translocations for both T-LBL and T-ALL involve the T-cell receptor (*TCR*) gene loci at chromosome 14q11 or 7q34, resulting in the juxtaposition of an oncogenic partner gene with the regulatory region of one of the *TCR* gene loci and subsequent deregulation of a reciprocal partner gene, such as *TAL1*, *MYC*, *HOXA* gene cluster, and *MYB*. Certain molecular genetic alterations were analyzed in relevant patient series of pediatric T-LBL, including NOTCH1, FBXW7 mutations, alterations of chromosome 9p containing *CDKN2A/CDKN2B* loci, and chromosome 6q.[18,19] Prospective systematic validation is required to evaluate whether one of these markers or a combination of molecular

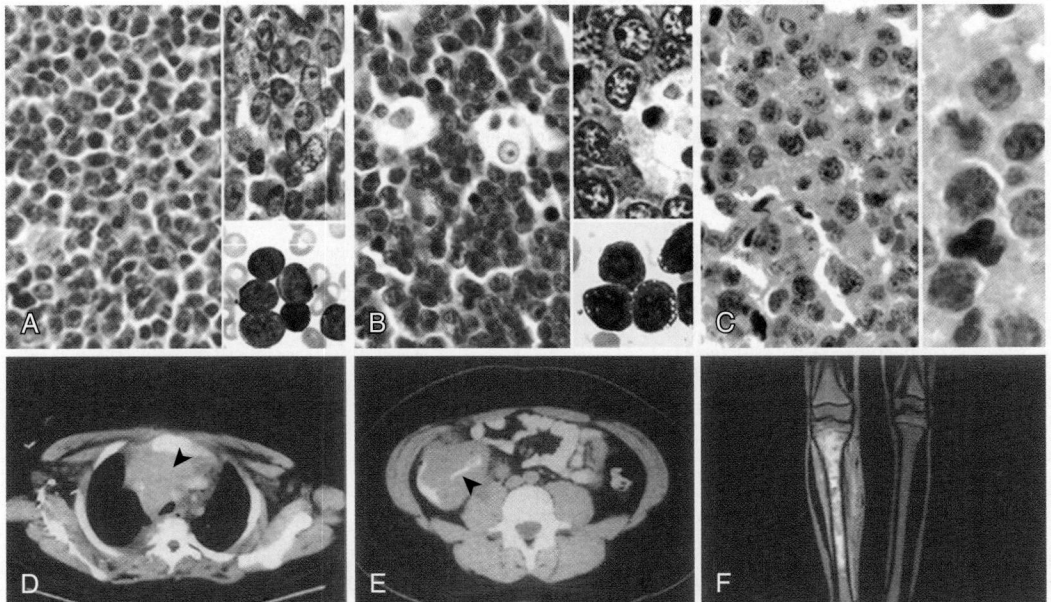

Fig. 84.1 HISTOLOGIC AND CLINICAL FEATURES OF THE NON-HODGKIN LYMPHOMAS OF CHILDHOOD. The *upper panels* demonstrate the appearance in hematoxylin and eosin–stained sections of (A) lymphoblastic lymphoma, (B) Burkitt lymphoma, and (C) anaplastic large cell lymphoma. The *insets* in (A) and (B) demonstrate the appearance of Wright's-stained specimens of the L3 blasts of Burkitt lymphoma and the L1 blasts of lymphoblastic lymphoma, respectively. The *lower panels* show common clinical presentations of the two histologic subtypes of lymphoma: (D) airway compression by lymphoblastic lymphoma of the anterior mediastinum on computed tomography of the chest and (E) encasement of the bowel lumen by Burkitt lymphoma visualized by abdominal computed tomography, and (F) tibial bone disease in primary lymphoma of the bone. (*Reproduced, in part, with permission from Sandlund JT, Downing JR, Crist WM: Non-Hodgkin's lymphoma in childhood,* N Engl J *Med 334:1238, 1996.*)

markers are of stable prognostic relevance and can be used to optimize current treatment stratification systems.

Clinical Manifestations

The clinical features at presentation vary with primary site and extent of disease spread. Almost all patients with T-LBL present with an anterior mediastinal mass that may cause respiratory symptoms, airway compromise, dysphagia, or superior vena cava syndrome (see Fig. 84.1D). Pleural effusions are common (75%), and lymphadenopathy above the diaphragm is frequent. Bone, skin, BM, central nervous system (CNS), abdominal organs, other lymph nodes, and occasionally testes may also be involved. Children with B-LBL are less likely to present with a mediastinal mass, but there is a higher frequency of cutaneous, soft tissue, or bone involvement with pB-LBL.[20–23] CNS involvement at diagnosis is seen in 4% to 5% of patients with LBL.[22,24]

Differential Diagnosis

LBL is distinguished from ALL by having less than 25% BM involvement and from myeloid malignancies being positive for TdT and T- or B-cell markers and negative for myeloperoxidase. T-LBL and pB-LBL are differentiated by flow cytometry. In cases of insufficient biopsy material or incomplete diagnostic staining, LBL cases are sometimes misdiagnosed (for example, as Ewing sarcoma or other small-, round-, blue-cell tumors).

Prognosis (Staging)

After obtaining malignant effusion or tissue diagnosis, staging is performed with imaging (ultrasound and magnetic resonance imaging or computed tomography [CT] of neck, chest, abdomen, and pelvis), bilateral BM evaluation, and lumbar puncture. Bone scans are done only if clinically indicated. Childhood NHL, including LBL, is most commonly staged using the Murphy classification (Table 84.2) and the analogue Revised International Pediatric Non-Hodgkin Lymphoma Staging System.[25,25a]

With current therapies based on ALL protocols, LBL has a long-term survival greater than 90% in low-stage disease and greater than 80% in advanced-stage disease[26] (Table 84.3). The Children's Oncology Group (COG) demonstrated that minimal disseminated disease at diagnosis has prognostic value, as indicated by flow cytometric evidence of tumor cells in BM. In 99 children with T-LBL treated in the A5971 study, 2-year event-free survival (EFS) was 68.1% ± 11.1% for patients with ≥1% T-LBL cells in BM by flow cytometry,

TABLE 84.2   Staging of Non-Hodgkin Lymphoma

Stage I

A single tumor (extranodal) or involvement of a single anatomic area (nodal), with the exclusion of the mediastinum and abdomen

Stage II

A single tumor (extranodal) with regional node involvement

Two or more nodal areas on the same side of the diaphragm

Two single (extranodal) tumors, with or without regional node involvement on the same side of the diaphragm

A primary gastrointestinal tract tumor (usually in the ileocecal area), with or without involvement of associated mesenteric nodes, that is completely resectable

Stage III

Two single tumors (extranodal) on opposite sides of the diaphragm

Two or more nodal areas above and below the diaphragm

Any primary intrathoracic tumor (mediastinal, pleural, or thymic)

Extensive primary intraabdominal disease

Any paraspinal or epidural tumor, whether or not other sites are involved

Stage IV

Any of the above findings with initial involvement of the central nervous system, bone marrow, or both

Based on the classification proposed by Murphy SB, Fairclough DL, Hutchison RE, Berard CW: Non-Hodgkin's lymphomas of childhood: an analysis of the histology, staging, and response to treatment of 338 cases at a single institution. *J Clin Oncol* 7:186, 1989.

TABLE 84.3   Outcomes for Lymphoblastic Lymphoma

Trial	Age	Stage	Treatment	Number of Patients	pEFS
LMT81[31]	9 yr (0.9–16)	I–IV	Mod. LSA2-L2	84	75 ± 3%
CCG502[32]	9 yr (0.5–19)	I–IV	Mod. LSA2-L2 vs. ADCOMP	143 138	74% 64%
POG8704[33]	10 yr (5–15)	III/IV	L-Asp-negative vs.	83	64 ± 6%
			L-Asp-positive	84	78 ± 5%
NHL-BFM90[26]	9 yr (1–16)	I–IV	ALL-BFM	105	90%
NHL-BFM95[34]	8 yr (0.2–19)	III/IV	BFM	169	78 ± 3%
EORTC 58881[35]	8 yr (0–16)	I–IV	BFM-based	119	78 ± 3%
COG pilot[36]	n.d.	III/IV	Mod. LSA2-L2	85	78 ± 5%
LNH92[37]	8 yr (0–<16)	I–IV	Mod. LSA2-L2	55	69 ± 6%
St. Jude 13[38]	n.d.	III/V	T-ALL	41	83 ± 6%
pB EORTC[22]	7 yr	I–IV	Mod. LMT, BFM	53	82%
POG 9404[39]	50% <10 yr	III/IV	Mod. DFCI ALL with HDMTX; without HDMTX	66; 71	82 ± 5% 88 ± 4%
COG A 5971[40]	7 yr (1–25)	I/II	CCG BFM	56	90%
COG A5971[41]	10 yr	III/IV	NHL-BFM95 MTX without HDMTX intensification without intensification	257 total	85 ± 4% 83 ± 4% 83 ± 4% 83 ± 4%

ALL, Acute lymphoblastic leukemia; Asp, asparaginase; BFM, Berlin-Frankfurt-Münster; CCG, Children's Cancer Group; DFCI, Dana-Faber Cancer Institute; EFS, event-free survival; EORTC, European Organisation for Research and Treatment of Cancer; HDMTX, high-dose methotrexate; mod, modified; MTX, methotrexate; n.d., no data; NHL, Non-Hodgkin lymphoma; pB-LBL, precursor B-cell lymphoblastic lymphoma; POG, Pediatric Oncology Group; T-ALL, T-cell acute lymphoblastic leukemia; T-LBL, T-cell lymphoblastic lymphoma.

as compared with 90.7% ± 4.4% for patients with lower degree of marrow involvement.[27] Minimal disseminated disease at diagnosis was associated with an increased likelihood of BM or distant recurrence but not local recurrence. In NHL-BFM trials, adolescent girls with T-LBL had poorer outcomes than adolescent boys despite similar presenting characteristics. In 45 adolescents with T-LBL, the 5-year EFS was 57% for girls and 92% for boys (*p* = .004). This sex difference was not observed in children less than 15 years old in NHL-BFM trials.[28] One adult study of T-cell ALL has demonstrated poorer outcomes in females than in males,[29] but a prognostic impact of sex has not been found in other pediatric or adult studies of LBL. Whereas adolescent age itself has not been established as a poor prognostic factor as it has for ALL, adult outcomes of LBL are inferior to pediatric outcomes.[30]

Therapy

Two potentially life-threatening situations requiring urgent intervention must be considered in children with LBL: (1) mediastinal tumor with airway obstruction or superior vena cava syndrome and (2) tumor lysis syndrome. Owing to the cardiac and respiratory risks of anesthesia or sedation in children with a large mediastinal mass, the least invasive procedure should be chosen to establish a tissue diagnosis. In children with relevant pleural effusion, pleural puncture and morphologic combined with immunologic diagnostics by flow cytometry allow adequate diagnosis. In children with peripheral lymphadenopathy, lymph node biopsy under local anesthesia may be possible. In children who cannot tolerate a procedure, pretreatment with steroids may be necessary to stabilize the patient. Because pretreatment may diminish the ability to accurately diagnose a patient, a tissue diagnosis should be obtained as soon as it is possible to do so safely. Tumor lysis syndrome is characterized by metabolic consequences of the breakdown of lymphoma cells causing renal failure if severe. Hyperuricemia, hyperkalemia, and hyperphosphatemia must be aggressively managed by hyperhydration, rasburicase, and/or allopurinol, as well as close monitoring. Children with NHL can also present with epidural masses and associated neurologic deficits caused by spinal cord compression. If the diagnosis is known, chemotherapy should be started as soon as possible. If the diagnosis is not known, or if there is a sluggish response to chemotherapy, low-dose radiation therapy may be considered in consultation with a radiation oncologist.

ALL treatment strategies achieved favorable outcome in LBL and are accepted as standard treatment as, for example, the Berlin-Frankfurt-Münster (BFM) combination chemotherapy with induction, consolidation, and maintenance phases lasting a total of 24 months with 90% 5-year EFS.[26] Even patients with stages III and IV LBL had good outcomes on ALL-type therapy.[39,42] This ALL-like therapy has now become standard for LBL (Table 84.3). CNS prophylaxis is needed for LBL, but chemotherapy prophylaxis has not proven inferior to prophylactic cranial irradiation in CNS-negative patients, even those with advanced-stage disease.[22,34,38] Additionally, the Pediatric Oncology Group did not demonstrate a survival advantage of high-dose methotrexate for T-LBL, although its utility in T-ALL is still being evaluated.[39]

Burkitt Lymphoma

Burkitt lymphoma (BL) was first described in Uganda by Dennis Burkitt in the 1950s.[43] First thought to be endemic to equatorial Africa, it was subsequently observed in Europe and North America. The WHO classification recognizes three variants: (1) sporadic BL, occurring throughout the world and more common in children, adolescents, and young adults; (2) endemic BL, occurring primarily in sub-Saharan Africa and New Guinea, with some unique clinical features but morphologically identical to sporadic BL; and (3) immunodeficiency-associated BL, observed primarily in patients with HIV and less commonly in the setting of other immunodeficiencies. The WHO and REAL classifications also recognize the controversial entity of Burkitt-like lymphoma, with features intermediate between

BL and DLBCL (gray zone lymphoma). Burkitt-like lymphoma is rare in children, and the clinical value of this classification is unclear. When there is marrow involvement, it is designated Burkitt leukemia (French-American-British [FAB] classification L3 leukemia) but is treated similarly to BL.[10,44]

Epidemiology

Sporadic BL constitutes approximately 50%% of childhood NHL and is much commoner in boys than in girls (4 : 1 ratio), with a peak incidence between 5 and 14 years of age.[11,14] Endemic BL associated with Epstein-Barr virus (EBV) in more than 85% of cases accounts for approximately half of all childhood cancers in equatorial Africa. In contrast, sporadic BL is most common in the United States and Europe and is associated with EBV in only 10% to 15% of cases.[45,46]

Pathobiology

BL is composed of monomorphic, small, noncleaved cells with round nuclei, clumped chromatin, and basophilic cytoplasm. A high uniform proliferation index is seen, with the Ki-67 positivity approaching 100%. The classic "starry sky" appearance of BL seen under low-power microscopy is caused by tingible body macrophages scattered among malignant cells. BL cells show mature B-cell features and usually express surface immunoglobulins. B-cell markers such as CD19, CD20, and CD22 are usually present, and the majority express CD10 (common acute lymphoblastic leukemia antigen). BL is negative for TdT and BCL2. CD21, the EBV receptor, is more commonly seen in endemic BL than in sporadic BL.

Characteristic chromosomal translocations suggest that BL develops from genetic aberrations during somatic hypermutation or attempted immunoglobulin class switching in a B-cell precursor. These translocations, usually t(8;14) or infrequently t(8;22) or t(2;8), juxtapose the *c-myc* gene (involved in cellular proliferation) with immunoglobulin locus regulatory elements, resulting in *c-myc* overexpression. In sporadic cases, the predominant chromosome 8 breakpoints usually occur within the *c-myc* gene, whereas they are upstream of the gene in endemic cases. For the rare event of *c-myc*–negative BL, characteristic aberrations of chromosome 11q characterized by interstitial gains, including 11q23.2–11q23.3 and telomeric losses of 11q24.1-qter, were reported.[47] Other cytogenetic abnormalities, such as gain of 7q and deletion of 13q, are uncommon.[48,49] Recently published large-scale next-generation sequencing studies unveiled sets of recurrently mutated genes in tumor cells of pediatric and adult patients with B-NHL and introduced functionally related inhibitor of DNA 3 (*ID3*), transcription factor 3 (*TCF3*), and cyclin D3 (*CCND3*) as potential drivers of BL lymphomagenesis.[50-52]

Clinical Manifestations

BL is an extremely fast-growing malignancy. The most common primary sites of sporadic BL are the abdomen and the lymph nodes of the head and neck.[53,54] Abdominal disease presentation, often associated with nausea, vomiting, and abdominal pain, carries a risk of intestinal perforation, obstruction, and gastrointestinal bleeding. Abdominal lymphoma often arises from the distal ileum, causing intestinal obstruction secondary to intussusception or compression by an expanding mass encasing the bowel (Fig. 84.1E). BL can involve testes, bone, skin, BM, and CNS. CNS involvement at diagnosis, occurring in about 9% of patients, is associated with a worse outcome.[24] Endemic BL frequently involves the abdomen, jaw, paraspinal region, orbit, and CNS.

Differential Diagnosis

In DLBCL, another mature B-cell lymphoma, the cells are usually larger, and additional cytogenetic abnormalities such as BCL-6 gene rearrangements or t(14;18) may be seen, although these abnormalities are more common in adult DLBCL. Ki-67 staining in less than 95% of the cells or positivity for BCL2 are helpful in excluding a diagnosis of BL. Burkitt-like lymphoma is a controversial diagnosis with some morphologic features more similar to DLBCL, including larger cells, but commonly with *c-myc* translocations and a clinical behavior

TABLE 84.4	French Society of Pediatric Oncology Risk Group Classification of Mature B-Cell Lymphomas	
Group	**Extent of Disease**	
Group A	Completely resected stage I	
	Completely resected abdominal stage II	
Group B	Nonresected stages I and II	
	Any stage III	
	CNS-negative stage IV with BM involvement 5% to 25%	
Group C	CNS-positive stage IV	
	Stage IV with BM involvement ≥25% (mature B-cell ALL)	

ALL, Acute lymphoblastic leukemia; BM, bone marrow; CNS, central nervous system.

TABLE 84.5	Berlin-Frankfurt-Münster Risk Group Classification of Mature B-Cell Lymphomas	
Risk Group	**Resection Status**	**Stage and Initial Serum LDH Level**
R1	Complete	
R2	Incomplete	Stages I + II
		Stage III and LDH <500 U/L
R3	Incomplete	Stage III and LDH ≥500 U/L but <1000 U/L
		Stage IV/B-AL and LDH <1000 U/L and CNS-negative
R4	Incomplete	Stage III and LDH ≥1000 U/L
		Stage IV/B-AL and LDH ≥1000 U/L and CNS-negative
R4 CNS+	Incomplete	Stage IV/B-AL and CNS-positive

B-AL, Burkitt leukemia with ≥25% blasts in the bone marrow; BFM, Berlin-Frankfurt-Münster; BM, bone marrow; CNS, central nervous system; LDH, lactate dehydrogenase.

similar to that of classic BL.[55,56] TdT negativity is helpful in distinguishing BL from B-LBL.

Prognosis (Staging)

The risk group classification developed by the French Society of Pediatric Oncology (SFOP) is widely used in current protocols incorporating risk-adapted therapy (Table 84.4). This system accounts for the adverse prognosis associated with CNS or BM involvement and whether localized disease has been resected. Patients with localized or CNS-negative advanced-stage BL have greater than 90% long-term survival with current therapies.[57] Combined CNS and BM involvement and suboptimal response to initial cytoreduction are also associated with worse prognosis, and poor responders are often stratified to more intensive chemotherapy in current regimens.[58] High lactate dehydrogenase (LDH) at diagnosis also carries a worse prognosis and is frequently incorporated in risk classification schemes, such as that of the BFM group (Table 84.5).[59] Age greater than 15 years has a worse outcome for mature B-cell malignancies, but this may be due primarily to DLBCL rather than to BL.

Therapy

Tumor lysis syndrome must be anticipated as a major risk in newly diagnosed BL. To help prevent this complication, children at risk should be vigorously hydrated (3–4 L/m²/day with D5 1/4 NaCl and 40 mEq/L NaHCO₃; there should be no added potassium) and started on allopurinol, a xanthine oxidase inhibitor. The urine pH should be maintained at about 7.0; at a more alkaline pH, phosphorus is less soluble, and at a more acidic pH, uric acid is less soluble. In some cases, mannitol followed by furosemide is required to maintain urine output. Uricolytic agents (e.g., uricozyme), which has been used for many years in Europe, directly cleaves the uric acid molecule and results in a precipitous drop in serum uric acid levels within a

few hours. The use of uricolytic agents (e.g., urate oxidase, uricase, rasburicase) has proven to be superior to allopurinol to reduce the level of serum uric acid rapidly and improve renal function. Rasburicase has significantly reduced the need for hemodialysis consequent upon tumor lysis syndrome. Recent protocols incorporate a prophase of reduced intensity to decrease the risk of severe tumor lysis syndrome.[60] In the setting of abdominal BL, intestinal perforation, obstruction, or gastrointestinal bleeding may not occur until after the initiation of chemotherapy as the lymphoma begins to regress.

Localized, resected mature B-cell NHL (including both BL and DLBCL) could be cured without significant toxicity by two courses of chemotherapy.[59,61–63] Advanced-stage BL requires aggressive combination chemotherapy with CNS prophylaxis (Table 84.6). Cyclophosphamide, methotrexate, and cytarabine at high doses have been used most recently, with or without anthracyclines and epipodophyllotoxins. Therapy should be started as quickly as possible upon presentation because this tumor grows very rapidly, and subsequent cycles should be administered in an intensive fashion as soon as recovery from the last cycle occurs. CNS prophylaxis is needed because without it approximately 30% to 50% of patients will relapse in the CNS,[64] whereas 6% to 11% develop CNS relapse if adequate prophylaxis is given.[24] CNS prophylaxis includes high-dose methotrexate and cytarabine to penetrate the CNS, together with intensive intrathecal chemotherapy. Risk-adapted therapy used in the FAB/LMB-96 study and the NHL-BFM95 study conferred an excellent EFS in advanced-stage patients.[58–60] Treatment intensity was escalated on the basis of tumor burden and response to therapy. These are the best published outcomes to date, but these regimens have significant hematologic toxicity. Researchers in both the FAB/LMB-96 study and the NHL-BFM 95 study successfully reduced therapy for low- and intermediate-risk patients without a compromise in survival. However, both studies failed to safely reduce the intensity of therapy for patients with advanced stages of disease.

Rituximab is a mouse/human chimeric monoclonal antibody against CD20, highly expressed in BL and DLBCL. In adults, the addition of rituximab to cyclophosphamide, doxorubicin, vincristine, and prednisone (CHOP) chemotherapy is beneficial for DLBCL and has been given safely in combination with intensive BL therapy. In children, single-agent rituximab showed activity for BL in a phase II window study for newly diagnosed patients,[65] and the COG showed the safety of adding rituximab to the LMB backbone for the treatment of BL.[66,67] Current clinical trials address the question whether rituximab added to standard chemotherapy can improve the EFS of patients with advanced disease.

Local radiation therapy has no role in BL, because it is chemosensitive and often diffuse. CNS radiation has been used in the past for CNS involvement at diagnosis but did not show an impact on outcome in this group. Surgery is no longer routinely used for BL. However, patients with localized disease who undergo resection at diagnosis are eligible for reduced chemotherapy as noted above.

Diffuse Large B-Cell Lymphoma

DLBCL includes a heterogeneous group of neoplasms of transformed B cells, accounting for 10% to 13% of pediatric NHL.[11] DLBCL has some distinctive biologic and clinical features, described in more detail below.[68] DLBCL involving the mediastinum needs to be distinguished from primary mediastinal large B-cell lymphoma (PMBCL), which represents a distinct subtype of B-NHL in the WHO classification. In addition, the current version of the WHO classification introduced pediatric follicular lymphoma, marginal zone lymphoma, and gray zone lymphoma.

Epidemiology

The incidence of DLBCL increases with age, being commoner in the second decade of life.[14,69] It is rare in children younger than 4 years of age. Although commoner in boys than girls in a 2:1 ratio, the sex difference is less than in BL. PMBCL is more common in adolescents, with no sex difference.[68,70]

TABLE 84.6 Outcomes for Burkitt Lymphoma and Diffuse Large B-Cell Lymphoma

Trial	Arm	Patients	Number of Courses	EFS (%)
Limited Disease				
LMB89[57]	A	10%	2	98%
FAB-LMB96[62]	A	144	2	98%
NHL-BFM95[59]	R1	10%	2	94%
AIEOP LNH92[63]	R1	9%	3	100%
JACLS NHL-98[61]	A	19%	2	100%
Intermediate Disease				
LMB89[57]	B	69%	6	92%
FAB-LMB96[60]	B arm 1	164	5	n.a.
	B arm 1	163	4	n.a.
	B arm 3	167	5	n.a.
	B arm 3	163	4	n.a.
NHL-BFM95[59]	R2	46%	5	94%
	R3	16%	6	85%
AIEOP LNH92[63]	R2	38%	5	87%
	R2/R3 with insufficient response	30% of R2 and 55% of R3	7	n.a.
JACLS NHL-98[61]	B	25%	5	100%
	C	30%	7	75%
Advanced Disease				
LMB89[57]	C	22%	9	84%
FAB-LMB96[58]	C CNS-negative stand.	52	9	94%
	C CNS-negative red.	51	6	86%
	C CNS-positive stand.	44	9	84%
	C CNS-positive red.	43	6	72%
NHL-BFM95[59]	R4	28%	7	81%
AIEOP LNH92[63]	R3	53%	7	75%
	R2/R3 with insufficient response	30% of R2 and 55% of R3	7	n.a.
JACLS NHL-98[61]	D	26% (18/69)	7	66%

AIEOP, Associazione Italiana di Ematologia e Oncologia Pediatrica; CCG, Children's Cancer Group; EFS, event-free survival; JACLS, Japan Association of Childhood Leukemia Study; LMB, Lymphome Malins de Burkitt; n.a., not available; NHL-BFM, Non-Hodgkin lymphoma Berlin-Frankfurt-Münster; red., reduced; stand., standard.

Pathobiology

Most pediatric DLBCL cases have a germinal center mature B-cell phenotype.[69] Nuclei are usually more than twice the size of normal lymphocytes. They express pan–B-cell antigens, including CD19, CD20, CD22, and CD79a, with or without surface immunoglobulin. Most express CD10 and BCL6, and approximately 40% express BCL2. However, breaks or translocations in *BCL2* and *BCL6* are rare in pediatric DLBCL. Unlike adult DLBCL, pediatric cases rarely demonstrate the t(14;18) translocation.[68,69] Gene profiling has led to subclassification of adult cases into germinal center B-cell–like, activated B-cell–like, and type 3 (not belonging to the first two groups) phenotypes. The great majority of children have the germinal center B-cell–like phenotype.[69,71] Interestingly, this phenotype has a better prognosis in adults, and childhood DLBCL outcomes are better than adult outcomes. Morphologic variants of DLBCL include centroblastic, immunoblastic, anaplastic, and T-cell/histiocyte-rich variants.[72] Although DLBCL is clearly heterogeneous, the clinical value of these distinctions is unclear in children.

PMBCL is thought to originate from medullary thymic B cells. B-lineage antigens and CD30 are often positive, but surface immunoglobulin and human leukocyte antigen (HLA) classes I and II molecules are absent or incompletely expressed.[68] *MYC*, *BCL2*, and *BCL6* genes are not rearranged. PMBCL is associated with gains in chromosome 9p (involving *JAK2*) and 2p (involving c-*rel*). They commonly demonstrate inactivation of *SOCS1*.[73,74] Variable degrees of sclerosis occur in PMBCL,[75] as well as occasional lymphocytes, eosinophils, and Reed-Sternberg–like cells, sometimes leading to confusion with HL.

Clinical Manifestations

DLBCL is often more localized than BL and is less likely to involve the BM or CNS.[24] Nodal disease is commoner in DLBCL than in BL, but extranodal disease is frequent. Common sites of involvement include the head and neck, abdomen, mediastinum, and bone. PMBCL is locally invasive and frequently associated with superior vena cava syndrome or airway compression. Pleural or pericardial effusions are present in approximately 40% of PMBCL cases,[75] and kidney metastases are frequent.[68]

Differential Diagnosis

The differential diagnosis of DLBCL encompasses BL, B-LBL, and nodular lymphocyte predominant HL. BL is distinguished from DLBCL by morphology, although atypical BL shows more pleomorphism than typical BL. BCL2 negativity, high cell proliferation, and translocations involving c-*myc* may suggest BL but are not definitive. DLBCL, with its mature phenotype, differs from B-LBL by a lack of TdT expression. DLBCL and nodular lymphocyte predominant HL share some similar features and derive from a common B-cell clone. DLBCL may represent the clonal progression of nodular lymphocyte predominant HL. PMBCL can also be confused with HL, and an adequate biopsy is essential for diagnosis. PMBCL and other DLBCL are distinguished clinically because PBMCL typically reside within the thymic area, whereas mediastinal DLBCL usually involve mediastinal lymph nodes.

Prognosis (Staging)

The Murphy classification is used to stage DLBCL.[76] There is no difference in outcomes between BL and DLBCL based on histology, and the treatment is identical in children.[68] Outcomes for pediatric DLBCL are superior to those for adults, with 5-year overall survival (OS) of 90% for current therapies. Adolescent girls fared worse than adolescent boys with DLBCL on NHL-BFM protocols.[28] BCL2 expression is not an unfavorable prognostic factor in children with DLBCL, in contrast to adults with DLBCL.[69] Prognosis is poorer for children and adolescents with PMBCL (5-year EFS of 65% to 75%).[48,75] In the setting of PMBCL, LDH of 500 U/L or more has a worse prognosis.[75] For adult patients with PMBCL, favorable outcome was reported using a dose-adjusted EPOCH-rituximab regimen with continuous infusions of etoposide, doxorubicin, vincristine, and bolus administrations of cyclophosphamide and prednisone.[77] In a small pediatric series, similar excellent results were observed, but they require systematic prospective validation.[78]

Therapy

In children, all mature B-cell lymphomas are usually treated similarly with good results. Despite biologic and clinical differences, BL therapy is effective in DLBCL (Table 84.6).[68] Risk-adapted therapy with LMB (SFOP) or B-NHL (BFM) backbones consists of short, dose-intense courses of chemotherapy including steroids, vincristine, high-dose methotrexate, cyclophosphamide, doxorubicin, cytarabine, etoposide, and intrathecal chemotherapy.[42,57,60,79] As described for BL, risk-adapted therapy based on FAB/LMB-96 and NHL-BFM 95 are also the current standard of care for childhood DLBCL.[57,59,60] Rituximab can improve adult outcomes for DLBCL when added to CHOP or CHOP-like therapy, but the benefit has not been proven in children.[80–82] Adult data suggest that rituximab may allow diminished use of agents with serious acute or late toxicities, warranting further study.[80] Having evolved from BL regimens, DLBCL treatment has traditionally included intrathecal chemotherapy for CNS prophylaxis. Because the risk of CNS involvement is lower for DLBCL than for BL, it is unclear if CNS-directed therapy should be as intensive.[24,68] Local radiation has no role in frontline DLBCL therapy.[68] As mentioned above, the optimal treatment strategy for PMBCL has not been established yet, but might be influenced by the preliminary favorable results with DA-R-EPOCH.

Anaplastic Large Cell Lymphoma

Epidemiology

Most childhood NHLs previously classified as large-cell lymphomas fall into the category of ALCL in the REAL and WHO classifications. This entity was first described in 1985 as a clinicopathologic variant of large-cell lymphoma with a predilection for young patients.[83]

Pathobiology

ALCL are characterized by the proliferation of large, pleomorphic cells with one or more prominent nucleoli (Fig. 84.2). The cells preferentially involve lymph node sinuses and extranodal sites (notably skin, bone, and soft tissue), where they grow in a cohesive pattern. The cells express epithelial membrane antigen and CD30 (Ki-1) antigen, a 120-kDa membrane-bound molecule that is a member of the tumor necrosis factor receptor superfamily, previously found in association with Hodgkin disease. A soluble (88-kDa) form of the CD30 molecule is found at high levels in the serum of nearly all patients with ALCL.[84] Marked elevation of soluble CD30 levels in patients with ALCL correlates with higher risk of relapse, and soluble CD30 levels correlate with clinical disease status, returning to normal with attainment of complete remission and increasing with disease recurrence.

The ALCL are associated with chromosomal rearrangements involving the long arm of chromosome 5 at position q35.[85] In most cases, this translocation includes material from chromosome 2p23 [t(2;5)(p23;q35)], resulting in the fusion of the nucleophosmin (*NPM*) nucleolar phosphoprotein gene on chromosome 5q35 to anaplastic lymphoma kinase (*ALK*), a tyrosine kinase gene

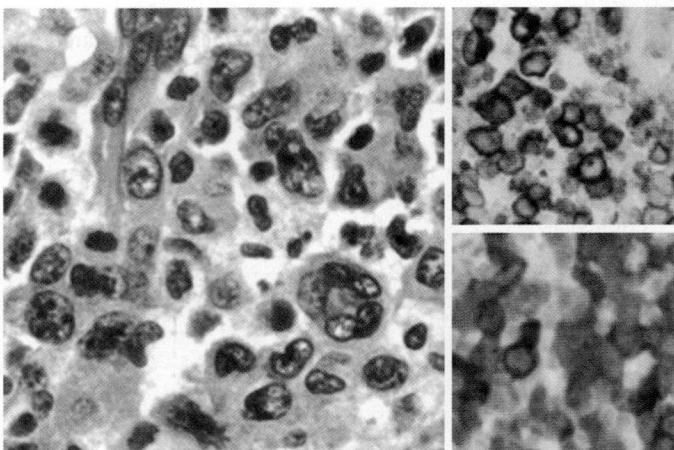

Fig. 84.2 HISTOLOGIC AND IMMUNOPHENOTYPIC FEATURES OF ANAPLASTIC LARGE-CELL LYMPHOMA. The section shows anaplastic cells including a "wreath cell" and a staining pattern with bright CD30 (Ki-1) positivity *(top right)* and anaplastic lymphoma kinase (ALK) positivity *(bottom right)*. The nuclear and cytoplasmic staining by ALK would predict that the case has the t(2;5) translocation.

on chromosome 2p23. The hybrid protein produced from the translocation links the amino terminus of NPM with the catalytic domain of ALK.[86] Deregulated expression of the truncated ALK may contribute to malignant transformation. The chimeric NPM-ALK protein is clearly oncogenic, perhaps through triggering of antiapoptotic signals via phosphatidylinositol 3-kinase/Akt, although secondary molecular events may be required for lymphomagenesis.

Immunologic and molecular biologic studies reveal that most cases of Ki-1+ ALCL are derived from activated T cells, although non-T, non-B cell (null cell) cases, and more rarely B cell cases, occur.[87] On the basis of extended testing for T-cell antigens and examination of the configuration of T-cell receptor genes, many "null" cell cases are, in fact, T-lineage neoplasms, although a minority may be derived from NK cells.[88] The diagnosis of ALCL can be difficult, and many cases are initially misdiagnosed as Hodgkin disease. Molecular techniques (reverse-transcriptase polymerase chain reaction [RT-PCR] to detect the fusion gene produced of the t(2;5) in many cases of ALCL confirms the diagnosis. Variant translocations where *ALK* is involved with other partner genes on other chromosomes limit the application of RT-PCR for diagnosis. However, the t(2;5) results in the expression of the NPM-ALK fusion protein, whereas the variant translocations result in upregulation of *ALK*. The ALK1 monoclonal antibody recognizing the formalin-resistant epitope of both the NPM-ALK chimeric protein and normal ALK thus serves as a useful diagnostic reagent for identifying cases of ALCL. It should be noted that the distribution of ALK staining varies, depending on the translocation. Further, ALK expression is a feature of inflammatory myofibroblastic tumors; however, confusion with ALCL can be minimized by testing for other hematopoietic markers, and the distinction is not usually difficult for experienced pathologists.

Clinical Manifestations

ALCL is rare, accounting for approximately 8% to 13% of childhood NHLs and roughly 30% to 40% of the pediatric large-cell lymphomas. Approximately one-third of the cases present with localized disease, whereas the majority have advanced disease at presentation, although BM and CNS involvement is uncommon.[89] A rare leukemic presentation of ALCL possibly associated with the small-cell variant of ALCL has been described. Systemic symptoms (fevers, weight loss) are frequently present in advanced-stage disease. Cutaneous (spontaneously regressing) lesions sometimes accompany disease at other sites, but skin involvement is not universal.[83] A variety of presenting sites—both nodal and extranodal—can occur, including the

TABLE 84.7	Outcomes for Anaplastic Large-Cell Lymphoma			
Protocol	Number of Subjects	Stage	Regimen	EFS
POG 8314 and 8719[90]	72	I–II (resected)	CHOP with or without maintenance	88% (5 yr)[a]
CCG 5941[91]	86	Nonlocalized	Multiagent with maintenance	68% (5 yr)
NHL-BFM 90[92]	9	I–II (resected)	Multiagent, risk-adapted (short-pulse B-NHL type therapy)	100% (5 yr)
	65	II (nonresected)–III		73% (5 yr)
	14	IV and multifocal bone involvement		79% (5 yr)
ALCL-99[93]	225	I–IV	Multiagent, risk-adapted, 3–6 cycles chemotherapy	81% (3 yr) (100% EFS in complete resection patients
COG ANHL0131[94]	125	III or IV	APO versus APV	74% (3 yr) in APO group 79% (3 yr) in APV group

[a]ALCL and diffuse large B-cell lymphoma combined.
ALCL, Anaplastic large cell lymphoma; APO, doxorubicin, prednisone, vincristine, methotrexate, 6-mercaptopurine; APV, doxorubicin, prednisone, vinblastine, methotrexate, 6-mercaptopurine; BFM, Berlin-Frankfurt-Münster; CCG, Children's Cancer Group; CHOP, cyclophosphamide, doxorubicin, vincristine, prednisone; EFS, event-free survival; NHL, Non-Hodgkin lymphoma; POG, Pediatric Oncology Group.

mediastinum, gastrointestinal tract, and bone. Further, tumors may invade adjacent structures and be associated with ascites and other intraabdominal sites of disease, including kidney, liver, and lymph nodes. The outcome of children with ALCL in most series has been good (with survival ranging from 70% to 85%), albeit inferior to that of children with BL and DLBCL (Table 84.7).

Diagnosis and Differential Diagnosis

Immunophenotyping and immunohistochemistry are critical for the definitive diagnosis of ALCL. The typical ALCL immunophenotype is CD30+CD15−CD45+, in contrast to HL, which is typically CD30+CD15+. Over 60% of cases of ALCL express one or more T-cell antigens (CD3+, CD43, or CD45RO), and ALK protein is detected in most cases (over 60%).

Prognosis (Staging)

The disease stage of ALCL is determined according to the staging system described by Murphy (Table 84.2).[25] As for other types of childhood NHL, stages I and II are considered limited-stage disease, whereas stage III represents advanced-stage disease. Stage IV is reserved for children with BM or CNS involvement. For elderly patients with cutaneous CD30+ ALCL, the 5-year disease-free survival (DFS) appears to be determined by the extent of limb involvement; however, this has not been shown in children, possibly owing to the fact that primary cutaneous ALCL is rare in the pediatric population.[95]

For systemic ALCL, studies have suggested that the stage of disease may be more important than the expression of the ALK protein. The European Intergroup for Childhood Non-Hodgkin Lymphoma defined three factors (mediastinal involvement, visceral involvement, and skin lesions) associated with poorer prognosis in childhood ALCL.[93] This group conducted a multivariate analysis (merging preexisting databases from BFM, SFOP, and United Kingdom Children's Cancer Study Group studies) and identified poor prognosis (one or more risk factors) and standard risk groups with 5-year PFS of 61% and 89%, respectively. However, it is important to note that this study was not done as a prospective collaborative study. In contrast, the Children's Cancer Group Study 5941 researchers reported that only BM involvement significantly changed the 5-year survival rate.[91]

The presence of ALK autoantibodies appears to be associated with decreased clinical risk factors and lower clinical stage, resulting in a lower cumulative incidence of relapses.[96] There is no correlation between outcome and the ALK translocation type. However, recently, the SFOP group showed that, for patients with ALK+ ALCL, the presence of a small-cell or lymphohistiocytic component is associated with a worse prognosis.[97]

Therapy

The optimal treatment approach for patients with ALCL has yet to be determined, as evidenced by a wide range of successful treatment strategies. In the United States, children with advanced stage CD30+ ALCL are generally treated with non-ALCL large-cell lymphoma regimens, with long-term EFS rates ranging from 60% to 75%[90–93] (Table 84.7). In a randomized trial performed by the POG, addition of intermediate-dose methotrexate and high-dose cytarabine did not improve upon the 70% 4-year EFS achieved with doxorubicin, prednisone, vincristine, methotrexate, and 6-mercaptopurine (APO) alone.[98] The BFM reported 3-year EFS of about 80% using a BL-based strategy.[92] Regimens designed specifically for children with CD30+ ALCL have been developed by the SFOP and German study groups.[99] The SFOP also reported the successful salvage of patients with ALCL with the weekly administration of single-agent vinblastine.[100]

The impact of incorporating vinblastine into two different front-line treatments for ALCL (the BFM B-cell approach [multinational European trial] and APO [COG trial in the United States]) was then studied in randomized fashion. In the European study, patients receiving the vinblastine plus chemotherapy regimen had a better EFS in the first year after therapy (91%) than those not receiving vinblastine (74%); however, at 2 years of follow-up, EFS was 73% for both groups.[101] Similarly, the researchers in the COG ANHL0131 study evaluated whether a maintenance regimen including vinblastine compared with APO alone would result in superior EFS. Postinduction patients were randomized to receive APO with vincristine every 3 weeks or a regimen that substituted vincristine with weekly vinblastine (APV). In this study of 125 patients, no difference was observed between the patients randomized to the APO versus APV arms in either EFS (3-year EFS 74% vs. 79%; $p = .68$) or overall survival (OS 84% vs. 86%; $p = .87$).[94]

In addition, the European study also showed that infusing methotrexate 1 g/m² over 24 hours was comparable to 3 g/m² over 3-hour infusions without intrathecal methotrexate.[102] However, 3 g/m² of methotrexate had less toxicity. Other studies have come to no firm conclusions. For example, (1) the POG-9317 trial demonstrated no benefit of adding methotrexate and high-dose cytarabine to 52 weeks of their APO (doxorubicin, prednisone, and vincristine) regimen,[98] and (2) the CCG-5941 study, which evaluated a more intensive induction and consolidation with maintenance for a 1-year total duration of therapy again had similar outcomes, but with significant hematologic toxicity.[92]

Targeted therapy options are important areas of investigation for future studies because crizotinib, an ALK inhibitor, has had outstanding results in pediatric phase I studies in children with ALCL, showing a nearly 100% response rate and minimal toxicity.[103]

In addition, with the remarkable activity of brentuximab vedotin (tubulin inhibitor-conjugated monoclonal anti-CD30) in ALCL,[104] this has led the COG researchers to pursue testing the efficacy and toxicity of adding these two targeted biologic agents with standard ALCL-99 chemotherapy in pediatric patients newly diagnosed with ALCL (ANHL12P1).

Relapsed Non-Hodgkin Lymphoma Management

There is no standard treatment for relapsed NHL. Treatment usually consists of intensive chemotherapy to induce a complete or partial response, followed by autologous or allogeneic stem cell transplant. Recent studies suggest that allogeneic transplant may be more effective than autologous transplant for relapsed NHL, particularly for LBL.[105] Outcomes are significantly better for patients with complete remission prior to transplant. Radiation may be useful prior to transplant in selected patients with an incomplete response to chemotherapy.

Outcomes vary by histologic subtype. Relapsed BL and DLBCL are often chemoresistant, and survival is only 10% to 20%. The COG used rituximab, ifosfamide, carboplatin, and etoposide for salvage therapy in this population, achieving a 60% response rate (complete and partial).[106] Patients who achieve a complete remission should proceed to stem cell transplant. Relapsed LBL is also frequently chemoresistant, and reported survival is 10% to 40%.[107-109] Salvage regimens used for ALL may be employed for LBL, and nelarabine has demonstrated a 40% response rate in this setting for T-ALL and T-LBL in a phase II COG study.[110] Survival for relapsed ALCL is better than for other NHLs, reaching 40% to 60%.[28,107,111] Vinblastine monotherapy as salvage therapy resulted in a complete remission rate of 83% in one study.[112] Brentuximab vedotin, an antibody against CD30, has been used successfully in adults with relapsed ALCL but has not been well-studied in children yet.[113] Crizotinib, an ALK inhibitor, has also shown promise in adults in early clinical trials for patients with relapsed ALCL and has shown remarkable results in phase I studies in children.[103] Autologous transplant has been used successfully for some patients, but allogeneic transplant may have better outcomes and is preferred for patients with BM or CNS involvement, early relapse, and CD30+ ALCL.[28,105,114]

Posttransplant Lymphoproliferative Disease

Posttransplant lymphoproliferative disease (PTLD) is discussed in other chapters in this book. Therefore, this section serves merely to summarize the issues specific for the pediatric population. The major pediatric populations where PTLD is seen most frequently are patients with congenital immune deficiencies or patients after BM or solid organ transplant (SOT). Further, stem cell transplant recipients with underlying immunodeficiencies such as Wiskott-Aldrich syndrome represent an independent risk group for EBV-associated lymphoproliferative disease (LPD).[115] Patients with primary, congenital immunodeficiencies such as X-linked agammaglobulinemia and AT have an incidence of EBV-associated LPD ranging from 0.7% to 15%.[116] The incidence of PTLD after SOT is higher in children than in the adult population. The disease is heterogeneous, but in children it is most frequently of B-cell origin and EBV-associated. In the United States, approximately 150 new cases are diagnosed in children each year.

Numerous therapeutic approaches to PTLD have been explored in children, but generally there has been a paucity of multicenter collaborative studies for this disease. Withdrawal or reduction of immunosuppression is often considered as firstline therapy for PTLD, but the choice depends on whether the patient has a recovering immune system sufficient to eradicate EBV-infected B cells and on stage and disease histology. For the pediatric hematopoietic stem cell transplant (HSCT) patient, strategies have included reduction in immune suppression, rituximab,[117] donor lymphocyte infusions,[118] and EBV-specific T-cell direct therapy.[119] The advantage of T cell–based therapies over antibody therapy is that EBV-specific T-cell immune reconstitution is restored, thus reducing the risk for disease recurrence. Responses to donor-derived EBV-specific T-cell therapies developed at multiple centers for pediatric patients range from 70% to 85%.[119,120] Immune-based therapies are generally preferred in this population because the use of chemotherapy in patients with LPD post-HSCT is associated with high mortality rates secondary to increased infectious complications.[121] However, hydroxyurea- and immune-based therapies may be an option for patients with CNS disease.[122] After SOT, modalities such as radiotherapy or surgical resection for localized LPD can result in complete remission. One study evaluated the efficacy of low-dose cyclophosphamide and prednisone for pediatric patients with PTLD after SOT. Efforts at reducing the immune suppression had failed in all patients, and all had received six cycles. The 2-year EFS and OS were 67% and 73%, respectively.[123] Subsequently, in a phase II study (COG-ANHL0221), the COG evaluated the addition of the CD20 monoclonal antibody to the previously reported regimen of low-dose cyclophosphamide and prednisone regimen (http://clinicaltrials.gov/show/NCT00066469). All patients had refractory PTLD after SOT or CD20+EBV+ PTLD in pediatric patients following SOT. The study showed that the addition of the CD20 monoclonal antibody to the previously reported regimen of low-dose cyclophosphamide and prednisone had EFS and OS of 71% and 83%, respectively.[124] Therefore, to build on the success of this first cooperative group trial for PTLD, the COG now propose to administer "off-the-shelf" third-party allogeneic latent membrane protein cytotoxic T lymphocytes (EBV/LMP-CTLs)[125] to determine its safety and efficacy in combination with rituximab in patients with PTLD post-SOT. This would represent the first multicenter study of its kind combining antibody therapy with off-the-shelf antigen-specific T-cell therapy for this disease. Finally, for patients refractory to these low-dose regimens or patients with definitive features of malignancy, standard lymphoma chemotherapeutic regimens are used, depending on histological subtype (e.g., BL- vs. DLBCL- vs. HL-directed therapy).

HODGKIN LYMPHOMA

Epidemiology

HL comprises 10% of all lymphomas and approximately 10% of pediatric cancers[2] and has a bimodal incidence, with one peak at 15–34 years of age and a second peak in the sixth decade of life. In children, the highest peak is among 15–19-year-olds (29 per million per year) and is least frequent in children under 5 years of age. There is an age-dependent sex predominance, with a male predominance in children under 5 years old (male:female ratio of 5.3 : 1) and a slight female predominance in children aged 15–19 years (male:female ratio of 0.8 : 1). HL (especially the nodular sclerosing subtype) is classically associated with higher socioeconomic status, increased incidence in single-family homes, smaller family sizes, and a higher level of maternal education. In contrast, mixed cellularity HL is inversely related to socioeconomic status. It is commonly postulated that delayed exposure to some environmental antigen may trigger development of HL, and that higher rates of certain childhood infections (e.g., varicella, measles, mumps, rubella) are negatively associated with HL development.[126] HL has been shown to have a genetic predisposition, although this is incompletely understood. Siblings of patients with HL have a two- to ninefold increased risk of developing HL. There is also an increased risk among parent-child pairs, though not between spouses, supporting a genetic rather than a uniquely environmental predisposition. Environmental factors are nevertheless involved in HL. Approximately 40% of all HL cases in economically developed countries harbor EBV in the Hodgkin and Reed-Sternberg (HRS) cells. EBV positivity of the malignant HRS populations is more common in children under 10 years of age and is highly associated with childhood HL with mixed cellularity subtype (approximately 80% of cases), characteristically seen in developing countries.

The EBV protein LMP1 may be the key in the oncogenic process because it can elicit B-lymphocyte transformation in vitro.[127]

There is also a relationship between the development of HL and cell-mediated immune deficiency, with an increased incidence in patients with HIV,[128] patients on chronic immunosuppressive therapy following SOT, and common variable immune deficiency. It remains unclear whether the underlying immune deficiency commonly seen in HL is primary, secondary, or both.[127]

Pathobiology

HL is generally considered to be slow-growing with a tendency to spread to contiguous lymph nodes. Only in advanced stages is there evidence of blood vessel invasion and spread to more distant organs.[129] Over the past 30 years, significant advances have been made in the treatment of pediatric HL, such that over 85% of children are cured with chemotherapy and/or radiation even with stage III/IV disease.

HL is notable for the characteristic B cell–derived HRS cells found in a background of an inflammatory microenvironment usually comprising regulatory T cells, Th2 T cells, macrophages, and eosinophils. The REAL and WHO classification systems identify two main subtypes: classical HL and lymphocyte-predominant HL. Classical HL accounts for the majority of cases in adolescents and young adults and is characterized by HRS cells that are usually CD15+ and CD30+. HRS cells do not express B-cell markers such as CD19 and CD79A, although CD20 is expressed in approximately 5% to 10% of cases. Mixed cellularity HL accounts for approximately one-third of cases diagnosed in children younger than 10 years old. The histopathology shows frequent HRS cells on a background of normal reactive immune cells, including T lymphocytes, plasma cells, eosinophils, macrophages, and histiocytes. Lymphocyte-predominant HL and lymphocyte-rich classical HL may both have nodular appearances, but the former is more commonly CD15− and usually has strong CD20 and CD45 positivity, thus distinguishing it from classical HL.[130]

Clinical Manifestations

The majority of pediatric patients with HL present with painless, firm, "rubbery" lymphadenopathy, most commonly in the cervical/supraclavicular regions. Over 70% of adolescents and young adults present with mediastinal disease, which can be asymptomatic. This presentation is less frequent in younger children, possibly related to a lower incidence of nodular sclerosis HL and a greater frequency of mixed cellularity or lymphocyte-predominant HL in this group. Approximately one-fourth of patients present with systemic "B" symptoms, including fevers, weight loss, and drenching night sweats. The majority of pediatric patients presenting with HL have stages I–III disease (involvement of lymph nodes and/or the spleen only) with a minority (approximately 15%) presenting with stage IV disease (noncontiguous extranodal involvement such as BM, lung, liver, and/or bone).

Staging

Pediatric HL is staged using the Ann Arbor staging system (with subsets A and B used for the absence or presence of B symptoms, respectively).[131] Briefly, stage I involves a single lymph node region. Stage II involves two or more lymph node regions on the same side of the diaphragm. Stage III involves lymph node regions above and below the diaphragm. For stages I–III, if there is extension to an adjacent extralymphatic region/organ, then this is designated E (for example, stage IIE). For stage III, if there is splenic involvement, this is designated stage IIIS. Finally, for Stage IV disease, there is noncontiguous involvement of one or more extralymphatic organs or tissues with or without involvement of associated lymph nodes.

Treatment

Despite the excellent outcomes for children with HL, there is still no ideal therapeutic approach. Generally, combination chemotherapy with low-dose involved-field radiation is used with varying intensities and durations, usually depending on disease stage and prognostic factors such as disease bulk and B symptoms. However, studies of late effects in these patients[132] have fueled cooperative groups in particular to explore regimens with decreased radiation and/or chemotherapy doses, especially for children with low-risk disease. Risk stratification for treatment assignment varies considerably between the pediatric HL research groups, thus limiting comparisons between trial results. The general consensus, however, is that chemotherapy should be given to all patients with HL, with or without radiation. The exception to this approach is patients with stage I, completely resected, nodular lymphocyte-predominant HL, who can achieve cure with surgery alone.[133]

Chemotherapeutic agents used for the initial treatment of pediatric HL are similar to those used in adults and include alkylating agents, corticosteroids, vinca alkaloids, antimetabolites, doxorubicin, bleomycin, dacarbazine, and etoposide. However, doxorubicin (or Adriamycin) is associated with cardiac toxicity; bleomycin can lead to pulmonary fibrosis; and alkylators may impair fertility. Therefore, many cooperative group studies have developed hybrid regimens using lower cumulative doses of alkylators, doxorubicin, and bleomycin, especially for low-risk (stages I–IIA, no bulk, no B symptoms) and intermediate-risk (all stages I and II patients not classified as early stage; stage IIIA; and variably stage IVA) disease. Results of clinical trials conducted by the major international pediatric HL study groups are summarized in Table 84.8. Trials differ by the use of chemotherapy regimens of varying dose intensity, as well as the criteria for omission of radiotherapy. The German Society of Pediatric Oncology, and now in conjunction with other European pediatric oncology centers (Euronet Consortium), has investigated OEPA (vincristine, etoposide, prednisone, doxorubicin) for low risk groups and OEPA with COPDac (cyclophosphamide, vincristine, prednisone, dacarbazine) for intermediate- and high-risk groups.[134] In North America, the COG has primarily evaluated ABVE-PC (doxorubicin, bleomycin, vincristine, etoposide, prednisone, cyclophosphamide) and its derivatives across the risk groups.[135–138]

Radiotherapy use varies considerably. In the only recent large randomized trial to evaluate omission of radiotherapy, the COG reported that radiotherapy may be safely omitted in intermediate-risk patients who have a rapid reduction in tumor dimensions by CT after two cycles of chemotherapy.[142,143] The European consortium has omitted radiotherapy for low-risk patients achieving a complete response after two cycles of OEPA.[134] The utility of response by positron emission tomography (PET) has been evaluated in trials recently completed or in progress by all the major groups. In general, pediatric radiotherapy approaches use lower doses (15–25 Gy) and fields (involved field or node).

Therapies targeting CD30, a transmembrane glycoprotein that is present on Reed-Sternberg cells but is not expressed in most normal tissue, have been an area of significant interest as a means of improving efficacy and replacing agents with long-term toxicities. Brentuximab vedotin is an antibody drug conjugate composed of a monoclonal anti-CD30 antibody linked to the antimitotic agent monomethyl auristatin E. In a phase II study evaluating brentuximab vedotin in relapsed HL, the overall response rate was 75%, with complete remission achieved in 34%.[144] Incorporation of brentuximab vedotin in frontline chemotherapy regimens is currently under investigation in a phase II trial of pediatric high-risk HL by the Stanford, St. Jude, Dana-Farber Cancer Institute consortium and a randomized phase III trial by the COG.

Management of Relapsed Hodgkin's Lymphoma

For patients who relapse, response depends on whether they had favorable disease at diagnosis and whether the relapse is confined to

TABLE 84.8	Treatment Outcomes for Pediatric Low-Risk Hodgkin Lymphoma				
Study	**Number of Subjects**	**Risk Group**	**Treatment**	**Radiation (Gy)**	**EFS or DFS; OS (yr)**
Children's Oncology Group					
CCG5942[139]	215	IA, IB, IIA without adverse features (bulk, hilar adenopathy, >3 nodal regions)	COPP/ABV ×4	CR after cycle 4: randomized to 21, IF vs none; PR: 21, IF	IF: 97.1% None: 89.1% (p = .001); IF: 100%, None: 95.9% (p = .5) (10 yr)
POG9426[138]	294	IA, IIA, IIIA (no bulk)	DBVE ×2–4 (based on response after cycle 2)	25.5, IF	86.2%; 97.4% (8 yr)
AHOD0431[137]	287	IA, IIA (no bulk)	AVPC ×3	CR after cycle 3: none PR: 21, IF	79.8%; 99.6% (4 yr)
German Society of Pediatric Oncology					
GPOH[134]	195	IA, IB, IIA	OEPA (males) OPPA (females) ×2	CR after cycle 2: no RT; PR after cycle 2: 20–30, IF	92%; 99.5% (5 yr)
French Society of Pediatric Oncology (SFOP)					
MDH-90[140]	202	IA, IB, IIA, IIB	VBVP × (OPPA ×1–2 if PR after cycle 4)	20–40, IF	91.1%, 97.5% (5 yr)
Stanford, Dana-Farber, and St. Jude Consortium					
Stanford, Dana-Farber, and St. Jude Consortium[144a]	110	IA, IB, IIA, IIB no bulk, no E	VAMP ×4	15–22.5, IF	89.4%; 96.1% (10 yr)
Stanford, Dana-Farber, and St. Jude Consortium[141]	88	IA, IIA, <3 nodal sites, no bulk, no E	VAMP ×4	CR after 2 cycles: no RT; PR after cycle 2: 25.5 IF	CR: 89.4%, PR: 92.5% (2 yr)

ABV, Doxorubicin, bleomycin, and vinblastine; *AVPC*, doxorubicin, vincristine, prednisone, and cyclophosphamide; *CCG*, Children's Cancer Group; *COPP*, cyclophosphamide, vincristine, procarbazine, and prednisone; *CR*, complete response; *DBVE*, doxorubicin, bleomycin, vincristine, and etoposide; *DFS*, disease-free survival; *EFS*, event-free survival; *IF*, involved field; *OEPA*, vincristine, etoposide, prednisone, and doxorubicin; *OPPA*, vincristine, procarbazine, prednisone, and doxorubicin; *OS*, overall survival; *POG*, Pediatric Oncology Group; *PR*, partial response; *VAMP*, vincristine, doxorubicin, methotrexate, and prednisone; *VBVD*, vinblastine, bleomycin, etoposide, and prednisone.

an area of initial involvement after chemotherapy and no radiation. Time to relapse and response to reinduction therapy are strong predictors of outcome.[145] These patients can generally be salvaged with chemotherapy and involved-field radiation therapy, and results are very acceptable even without HSCT. For all other patients, treatment of refractory, progressive, or relapsed disease includes induction chemotherapy with multiple chemotherapeutic agents not generally used in the initial therapy (e.g., gemcitabine, vinorelbine, carboplatin/cisplatin, ifosfamide, and more recently brentuximab vedotin, alone or currently being investigated in combination with gemcitabine or bendamustine), followed by high-dose chemotherapy and autologous stem cell rescue. Conditioning regimens are generally alkylator-based,[146] and the frequently reported regimens are CBV (cyclophosphamide, carmustine, and etoposide), BEAM (carmustine, etoposide, cytosine arabinoside, and melphalan), and BEAC (carmustine, etoposide, cytarabine, and cyclophosphamide).[147–149] None of these conditioning regimens produce a superior outcome in pediatric patients, and CVB and BEAM remain the most widely used. The role of local radiation therapy either before or after HSCT is still unclear, although total body irradiation is now generally not used.[150,151] Although an overall DFS of approximately 50% is consistently reported with this approach, the reported range is 20% to 60% because outcomes are related to prognostic factors such as disease burden and chemosensitivity.[147,148,152,153]

The role of allogeneic HSCT has also been investigated for patients with relapsed/refractory HL, although never in a prospective, randomized manner.[154] The use of submyeloablative regimens (generally fludarabine-based) may reduce transplant-related mortality rates while still achieving a graft-versus-lymphoma effect in patients with lymphoma receiving allografts, and it warrants further investigation in the pediatric population.[155,156]

Among the more promising approaches to activating therapeutic antitumor immunity in HL is the blockade of the immune checkpoint, programmed cell death protein 1 (PD-1) pathway. Classical HL is characterized by HRS cells surrounded by an extensive but ineffective inflammatory cell infiltrate. Increased PD-1 expression by T lymphocytes in the microenvironment and increased PD-1 ligand expression by HRS cells allow evasion of T cell–mediated destruction of HRS cells. Blocking the interaction between PD-1 and its ligands through the administration of PD-1–blocking antibodies can result in T-cell activation and a more florid tissue inflammatory response.[157] Nivolumab is associated with a high objective response rate of 87% among heavily pretreated patients with HL.[158] Another anti–PD-1 drug, pembrolizumab, was associated with a 66% response rate in a similar cohort of patients. Researchers are now investigating these agents in conjunction with other targeted therapies, including brentuximab vedotin. Finally, investigational therapies such as targeted T-cell therapies are being explored for pediatric HL patients associated with EBV either as adjuvant therapy after transplant or for relapsed disease.[159,160]

In summary, most children with HL are initially treated with risk-adapted chemotherapy alone or in combination with low-dose involved-field or involved-node radiotherapy involving carefully designed radiation fields to achieve local disease control while minimizing bystander organ toxicity. Especially for low-risk patients, some studies suggest that the overall survival for patients receiving chemotherapy alone may be similar to that for patients receiving chemotherapy plus radiotherapy, despite possible differences in EFS. This is owing to the fact that it is usually possible to salvage relapse after initial therapy.[161] If salvage therapy for such patients can be targeted and relatively nontoxic (e.g., by using novel agents such as brentuximab),[162] then using a less intense initial regimen may be appropriate. Currently, however, salvage therapy for the majority of patients is typically more toxic and can lead to an unacceptable incidence of late events such as cardiac toxicities and secondary malignancies.[163] Therefore, strategies using a less intense frontline regimen should be investigated only within the context of a clinical trial. Researchers in future clinical studies therefore will attempt to address this important issue by evaluating the prognostic significance of achieving PET-negative disease after one or two cycles of chemotherapy and the use of frontline brentuximab to replace more toxic modalities such as bleomycin and radiation therapy.

RARE SUBTYPES OF LYMPHOMA

Other subtypes that are observed rarely in children deserve mention, but the rarity of these neoplasms in children make generalizations and therapeutic recommendations difficult. Follicular lymphomas (characterized by the arrangement of malignant cells in aggregates separated by normal cells), which account for approximately 30% of adult NHLs, are extremely rare in children. Children with follicular lymphomas tend to present with cervical lymph node involvement (although primary tumors of the testis have been reported[164]) with early-stage disease and have an excellent prognosis.[165,166] Unlike most cases of follicular lymphoma in adults, where aberrant expression of BCL2 [usually as a result of the t(14;18) translocation] is thought to play an important role in lymphomagenesis, the majority of cases of follicular lymphomas in children demonstrate neither the t(14;18) translocation nor BCL2 expression. BCL2 expression appears to occur more frequently in older children and is associated with advanced-stage disease at presentation and a more aggressive clinical course.[165]

Marginal zone B-cell lymphomas arising in mucosa-associated lymphoid tissue can arise in extranodal sites. They tend to present with localized disease and infrequently disseminate. NK cell lymphoma and NK-like T-cell lymphomas usually involve the upper aerodigestive tract (midline lethal granuloma, angiocentric T-cell lymphoma), but they can present in the skin as well.[167–169] They are rare in children, follow a very aggressive clinical course, and are often fatal, but they may respond to high-dose chemotherapy with stem cell transplant.[169] Peripheral T-cell lymphomas include a variety of neoplasms that have not yet been further specified. These lymphomas are rare in children but in advanced stage at presentation, often in association with systemic symptoms; hemophagocytic syndrome is common; and an aggressive course is the rule.

FUTURE DIRECTIONS

Although there have been dramatic improvements in the treatment of children with NHL and HL over the past 25 years, approximately 25% of children with these tumors still relapse or fail to respond to initial therapy. Additionally, late effects such as anthracycline-related cardiomyopathy, secondary malignancies such as epipodophyllotoxin-related acute myeloid leukemia, and endocrine abnormalities such as cyclophosphamide-related azoospermia remain a concern.[163,170] Thus, a major task is to develop treatment strategies that provide a cure for the remaining 25% while reducing treatment-related morbidity. Several approaches appear promising.

The identification of both clinical and biologic features at the time of diagnosis that predict treatment failure will enable investigators to refine existing risk-adapted therapeutic approaches. Strategies to be considered for children at high risk for treatment failure include the intensification of existing regimens and the incorporation of new active or novel agents. More intensive therapy may require either autologous or allogeneic hematopoietic stem cell support. The administration of colony-stimulating factors may be necessary in

some cases, although its role in therapy remains controversial. Novel approaches include the incorporation of immunotherapeutic agents into multiagent chemotherapy regimens. For example, there is increasing experience with the anti-CD20 antibody rituximab in pediatric patients with B-cell lymphomas.[65] A radiolabeled form of this product (Yttrium-90; Zevalin) has also yielded promising preliminary results in children.[171] CD30+ lymphomas such as ALCL, mediastinal B-large cell lymphoma, and HL are also candidates for CD30 antibody therapy. Novel immunotherapeutic approaches include the use of surface protein–specific cytotoxic T lymphocytes; this approach is effective in the prevention and treatment of EBV-related PTLD, NHL, and HL.[119,125] Agents targeting specific molecular lesions (e.g., the ALK inhibitor for ALCL) are promising and are already in phase I studies in children, and the implementation of anti-idiotype and antisense strategies are also being studied.

The continued investigation of molecular abnormalities and pathogenic mechanisms of malignant transformation associated with childhood lymphomas is essential. Microchip gene arrays have already identified clinically relevant subtypes of large B-cell lymphomas in adults.[172] Gene array analyses of BL, ALCL, and T-lymphoblastic disease have also been reported.[173] Similar studies are ongoing for childhood lymphomas, and preliminary results for T-lymphoblastic leukemia/lymphoma have been published.[174] Flow-sorting tissue for HRS and intratumor T cells and optimizing low-input exome sequencing are beginning to overcome the limitations of genomic evaluation in HL.[175] Comprehensive molecular characterization of childhood lymphomas may help to further refine disease classification, provide a means of detecting minimal residual disease (MRD) during clinical remission, and enhance assessment of early response.[176] Monitoring is facilitated by the finding that the level of MRD in the peripheral blood is comparable to that in the BM in children presenting with advanced-stage lymphomas. Additionally, a more complete understanding of the molecular pathogenesis of pediatric HL and NHLs will provide clues to new and better treatments directed toward tumor-specific molecular lesions.

SUGGESTED READINGS

Ansell SM, Lesokhin AM, Borrello I, et al: PD-1 blockade with nivolumab in relapsed or refractory Hodgkin's lymphoma. *N Engl J Med* 372:311, 2015.

Attarbaschi A, Beishuizen A, Mann G, et al: Children and adolescents with follicular lymphoma have an excellent prognosis with either limited chemotherapy or with a "watch and wait" strategy after complete resection. *Ann Hematol* 92:1537, 2013.

Bollard CM, Rooney CM, Heslop HE: T-cell therapy in the treatment of post-transplant lymphoproliferative disease. *Nat Rev Clin Oncol* 9:510, 2012.

Bollard CM, Gottschalk S, Torrano V, et al: Sustained complete responses in patients with lymphoma receiving autologous cytotoxic T lymphocytes targeting Epstein-Barr virus latent membrane proteins. *J Clin Oncol* 32:798, 2014.

Bonn BR, Rohde M, Zimmermann M, et al: Incidence and prognostic relevance of genetic variations in T-cell lymphoblastic lymphoma in childhood and adolescence. *Blood* 121:3153, 2013.

Burkhardt B, Oschlies I, Klapper W, et al: Non-Hodgkin's lymphoma in adolescents: experiences in 378 adolescent NHL patients treated according to pediatric NHL-BFM protocols. *Leukemia* 25:153, 2011.

Burkhardt B, Reiter A, Landmann E, et al: Poor outcome for children and adolescents with progressive disease or relapse of lymphoblastic lymphoma: a report from the Berlin-Frankfurt-Muenster Group. *J Clin Oncol* 27:3363, 2009.

Burkhardt B, Woessmann W, Zimmermann M, et al: Impact of cranial radiotherapy on central nervous system prophylaxis in children and adolescents with central nervous system-negative stage III or IV lymphoblastic lymphoma. *J Clin Oncol* 24:491, 2006.

Campo E, Swerdlow SH, Harris NL, et al: The 2008 WHO classification of lymphoid neoplasms and beyond: evolving concepts and practical applications. *Blood* 117:5019, 2011.

Castellino SM, Geiger AM, Mertens AC, et al: Morbidity and mortality in long-term survivors of Hodgkin lymphoma: a report from the Childhood Cancer Survivor Study. *Blood* 117:1806, 2011.

Ducassou S, Ferlay C, Bergeron C, et al: Clinical presentation, evolution, and prognosis of precursor B-cell lymphoblastic lymphoma in trials LMT96, EORTC 58881, and EORTC 58951. *Br J Haematol* 152:441, 2011.

Dunleavy K, Pittaluga S, Maeda LS, et al: Dose-adjusted EPOCH-rituximab therapy in primary mediastinal B-cell lymphoma. *N Engl J Med* 368:1408, 2013.

Friedman DL, Chen L, Wolden S, et al: Dose-intensive response-based chemotherapy and radiation therapy for children and adolescents with newly diagnosed intermediate-risk Hodgkin lymphoma: a report from the Children's Oncology Group Study AHOD0031. *J Clin Oncol* 32:3651, 2014.

Gambacorti-Passerini C, Messa C, Pogliani EM: Crizotinib in anaplastic large-cell lymphoma. *N Engl J Med* 364:775, 2011.

Goldman S, Smith L, Anderson JR, et al: Rituximab and FAB/LMB 96 chemotherapy in children with stage III/IV B-cell non-Hodgkin lymphoma: a Children's Oncology Group report. *Leukemia* 27:1174, 2013.

Gross TG, Orjuela MA, Perkins SL, et al: Low-dose chemotherapy and rituximab for posttransplant lymphoproliferative disease (PTLD): a Children's Oncology Group report. *Am J Transplant* 12:3069, 2012.

Lamant L, McCarthy K, d'Amore E, et al: Prognostic impact of morphologic and phenotypic features of childhood ALK-positive anaplastic large-cell lymphoma: results of the ALCL99 study. *J Clin Oncol* 29:4669, 2011.

Le Deley MC, Rosolen A, Williams DM, et al: Vinblastine in children and adolescents with high-risk anaplastic large-cell lymphoma: results of the randomized ALCL99-vinblastine trial. *J Clin Oncol* 28:3987, 2010.

Mauz-Körholz C, Hasenclever D, Dorffel W, et al: Procarbazine-free OEPA-COPDAC chemotherapy in boys and standard OPPA-COPP in girls have comparable effectiveness in pediatric Hodgkin's lymphoma: the GPOH-HD-2002 study. *J Clin Oncol* 28:3680, 2010.

Meinhardt A, Burkhardt B, Zimmermann M, et al: Phase II window study on rituximab in newly diagnosed pediatric mature B-cell non-Hodgkin's lymphoma and Burkitt leukemia. *J Clin Oncol* 28:3115, 2010.

Minard-Colin V, Brugières L, Reiter A, et al: Non-Hodgkin lymphoma in children and adolescents: progress through effective collaboration, current knowledge, and challenges ahead. *J Clin Oncol* 33:2963, 2015.

Oschlies I, Klapper W, Zimmermann M, et al: Diffuse large B-cell lymphoma in pediatric patients belongs predominantly to the germinal-center type B-cell lymphomas: a clinicopathologic analysis of cases included in the German BFM (Berlin-Frankfurt-Münster) Multicenter Trial. *Blood* 107:4047, 2006.

Patte C, Auperin A, Gerrard M, et al: Results of the randomized international FAB/LMB96 trial for intermediate risk B-cell non-Hodgkin lymphoma in children and adolescents: it is possible to reduce treatment for the early responding patients. *Blood* 109:2773, 2007.

Poirel HA, Cairo MS, Heerema NA, et al: Specific cytogenetic abnormalities are associated with a significantly inferior outcome in children and adolescents with mature B-cell non-Hodgkin's lymphoma: results of the FAB/LMB 96 international study. *Leukemia* 23:323, 2009.

Pro B, Advani R, Brice P, et al: Brentuximab vedotin (SGN-35) in patients with relapsed or refractory systemic anaplastic large-cell lymphoma: results of a phase II study. *J Clin Oncol* 30:2190, 2012.

Salzburg J, Burkhardt B, Zimmermann M, et al: Prevalence, clinical pattern, and outcome of CNS involvement in childhood and adolescent non-Hodgkin's lymphoma differ by non-Hodgkin's lymphoma subtype: a Berlin-Frankfurt-Münster Group Report. *J Clin Oncol* 25:3915, 2007.

Sandlund JT, Downing JR, Crist WM: Non-Hodgkin's lymphoma in childhood. *N Engl J Med* 334:1238, 1996.

Schmitz R, Young RM, Ceribelli M, et al: Burkitt lymphoma pathogenesis and therapeutic targets from structural and functional genomics. *Nature* 490:116, 2012.

Schwartz CL, Constine LS, Villaluna D, et al: A risk-adapted, response-based approach using ABVE-PC for children and adolescents with intermediate- and high-risk Hodgkin lymphoma: the results of P9425. *Blood* 114:2051, 2009.

Woessmann W, Seidemann K, Mann G, et al: The impact of the methotrexate administration schedule and dose in the treatment of children and adolescents with B-cell neoplasms: a report of the BFM Group Study NHL-BFM95. *Blood* 105:948, 2005.

Wolden SL, Chen L, Kelly KM, et al: Long-term results of CCG 5942: a randomized comparison of chemotherapy with and without radiotherapy for children with Hodgkin's lymphoma—a report from the Children's Oncology Group. *J Clin Oncol* 30:3174, 2012.

Younes A, Bartlett NL, Leonard JP, et al: Brentuximab vedotin (SGN-35) for relapsed CD30-positive lymphomas. *N Engl J Med* 363:1812, 2010.

REFERENCES

For the complete list of references, log on to www.expertconsult.com.

Owen A. O'Connor, Govind Bhagat, Karthik A. Ganapathi, Jason Kaplan, Paolo Corradini, Joan Guitart, Steven T. Rosen, and Timothy M. Kuzel

The T-cell lymphomas are a heterogeneous group of diseases. They are generally divided into those that predominantly arise within the skin, and are thus referred to as the *cutaneous T-cell lymphomas* (CTCLs), and those that do not primarily arise in the skin, namely, the mature or peripheral T-cell lymphomas (PTCLs). Like the B-cell malignancies, each of these subcategories of T-cell lymphoma can be divided into indolent and aggressive diseases, each associated with its own characteristic biology and treatment principles. Although CTCL is considered a mature T-cell lymphoma, these diseases are for the most part indolent in nature. They are characterized by a variety of clinical entities, each with its own unique biology and presentation. The mature or peripheral T-cell lymphomas typically arise in lymph nodes, extranodal sites, or with a leukemic disease, and are for the most part very aggressive diseases. The separation of the T-cell lymphomas into cutaneous or noncutaneous is largely intended to highlight some of the general differences in behavior, although clearly there is overlap. Some forms of CTCL can involve nodal and extranodal sites, and some forms of PTCL can involve the skin. Given the marked differences in biology, clinical behavior, and treatment of these two categories of T-cell lymphoma, in this chapter we have organized them into different sections.

THE PERIPHERAL T-CELL LYMPHOMAS (NONCUTANEOUS)

The mature or peripheral T-cell lymphomas are a heterogeneous group of diseases. Most PTCL entities are highly aggressive diseases that respond poorly to conventional chemotherapy. Among the most common subtypes are PTCL, not otherwise specified (NOS), angioimmunoblastic T-cell lymphoma (AITL), and the anaplastic large-cell lymphomas (ALCLs). Although these diseases are considered to carry an unfavorable prognosis compared with their B-cell counterparts, select molecular entities, such as anaplastic lymphoma kinase (ALK)-positive ALCLs, are associated with a highly favorable prognosis, comparable to or better than diffuse large B-cell lymphoma (DLBCL).

It is estimated that there were approximately 66,360 cases of non-Hodgkin lymphoma (NHL) in the United States in 2011, of which the T-cell lymphomas account for approximately 5%–10% of all cases. The median age at diagnosis is 59 years, which is lower than the median age of 66 for patients with NHL in general. Like other forms of lymphoma, T-cell lymphomas are diseases of older adults, with approximately 40% of cases occurring between the ages of 55 and 74 years, and only about 5% of cases occurring after the age of 85 years. Between 2004 and 2008, Surveillance Epidemiology and End Results (SEER) reported the age-adjusted incidence rate of T-cell lymphoma as approximately 1.8 per 100,000 men and women. The incidence rates among all races in males and females are approximately 2.3 and 1.4 per 100,000 individuals, respectively, in contrast to 24 and 16.5 cases per 100,000 males and females, respectively, for NHL. The disease is almost twice as frequent in males as females. In general, PTCLs are far more common in Asia. For example, the International Peripheral T-Cell and Natural Killer/T-Cell Lymphoma Study noted that T-cell lymphomas accounted for only 5%–10% of all NHL cases in Western countries and about 10%–20% in Asian countries. Rudiger et al have reported that the frequency of PTCL in Vancouver (Canada), for example, was roughly 1.6%, compared with the 18.3% frequency in Hong Kong.

Although rare in the West, subtypes of PTCL are not uncommon in the Eastern hemisphere and in Central and South America. Geographic and ethnic variability have been cited as reasons for the differences in the prevalence of some types of PTCL. Exposure to certain infectious or environmental agents is thought to account for some of the geographic variation, especially with regard to human T-lymphotropic virus-1 (HTLV-1) infection and occurrence of adult T-cell leukemia/lymphoma (ATLL), as well as Epstein-Barr virus (EBV) infection and the development of natural killer (NK)/T-cell lymphoma (NKTCL) in Asia, the Caribbean, and Central and South America. Globally the three most common subtypes of PTCL are PTCL-NOS (25.9%), AITL (18.5%), and ALCL (12%). PTCL-NOS is recognized as being slightly more common in North America, with a lower incidence in Europe and Asia, whereas AITL appears to be more common in Europe compared with Asia or North America. Enteropathy-associated T-cell lymphoma (EATL) is associated with celiac disease, which itself is associated with human leukocyte antigens DQ2 or DQ8, both being more common in European populations. Similarly, EBV-associated lymphomas are primarily seen in Japan, Korea, and northern China, as well as immigrant populations from South America in North America. These data suggest that there may be a variety of both genetic and environmental factors that may predispose to T-cell lymphomas, many of which are only now being identified in larger epidemiologic studies.

Classification

The classification of PTCLs has evolved substantially over the past several decades. Older classification schemes failed to incorporate all the necessary immunophenotypic, cytogenetic, morphologic, and clinical data to subclassify these diseases, as now presented in the context of the World Health Organization (WHO) classification system. The WHO classification published in 2008 recognizes more than 22 different subtypes of T-cell lymphoma distributed among four different subcategories. As shown in Table 85.1 and Fig. 85.1, these subcategories are divided into nodal, extranodal, cutaneous, and leukemic, each based on the predominant clinical behavior of that disease entity.

The nodal group consists of PTCL-NOS, which is the most common subtype of PTCL, accounting for roughly one-quarter of all PTCL cases. Other subtypes include ALCL and AITL. In ALCL there is a significant impact of specific cytogenetic features on prognosis. The ALK-positive forms of ALCL (Fig. 85.2), which are characterized by the nucleophosmin (NPM)-ALK translocation [t(2;5)] have a highly favorable prognosis, whereas those variants that are ALK negative carry a relatively poor prognosis. Other than the presence of the ALK translocation as determined by fluorescence in situ hybridization (FISH), there is no way to differentiate these diseases on strictly morphologic or immunophenotypic grounds. As such, the appropriate therapeutic recommendations for these two diseases obligatorily involve an understanding of this specific cytogenetic feature. Each of these ALCL variants accounts for about 5%–6% of all cases of PTCL. Similarly, it is often a significant diagnostic challenge to discriminate ALK-negative ALCL from PTCL-NOS.

TABLE 85.1	WHO Classification of the Mature T-Cell Lymphomas
Leukemic	T-cell prolymphocytic leukemia
	T-cell large granular lymphocytic leukemia
	Aggressive NK-cell leukemia
	Indolent large granular NK-cell lymphoproliferative disorder (provisional)
	Adult T-cell leukemia (HTLV-1, ATL)
Extranodal	Extranodal NK/T-cell lymphoma, nasal type
	Enteropathy-associated T-cell lymphoma
	Monomorphic epitheliotropic intestinal T-cell lymphoma
	Hepatosplenic T-cell lymphoma
	Subcutaneous panniculitis-like T-cell lymphoma (αβT-cell lineage only)
	Primary cutaneous γδ T-cell lymphoma
Nodal	ALCL, systemic or cutaneous
	ALCL:ALK positive [t(2;5)]
	ALCL:ALK negative
	AITL
	PTCL-NOS
Cutaneous	Mycosis fungoides/Sézary syndrome
	Primary cutaneous CD30+ T-cell LPD LyP and primary cutaneous ALCL
	Primary cutaneous CD4+ small/medium T-cell lymphoma (provisional)
	Primary cutaneous CD8+ aggressive epidermotropic cytotoxic T-cell lymphoma (provisional)
Other	Systemic EBV-positive T-cell LPD of childhood
	Hydroa vacciniforme–like lymphoma

AITL, Angioimmunoblastic T-cell lymphoma; ALCL, anaplastic large-cell lymphoma; ALK, anaplastic lymphoma kinase; ATL, adult T-cell leukemia/lymphoma; EBV, Epstein-Barr virus; HTLV-1, human T-lymphotropic virus-1; LPD, lymphoproliferative disease; LyP, lymphomatoid papulosis; NK, natural killer; NOS, not otherwise specified; PTCL, peripheral T-cell lymphoma; WHO, World Health Organization.

AITL is the second most common subtype of PTCL, accounting for about 18%–19% of all cases of PTCL. It, uniquely, can also be associated with an EBV-infected clonal B-cell population.

The extranodal subtypes of PTCL are associated with their own unique clinical behavior. This subcategory can include very rare and aggressive diseases such as hepatosplenic T-cell lymphoma (HSTL). Normal T cells express either of the two dimeric forms of the T-cell receptor (TCR) protein on their surface, αβ and γδ. Approximately 95% of all PTCLs possess TCR proteins with the αβ heterodimer, whereas the γδ T-cell lymphomas, like the majority of HSTLs and certain types of intestinal T-cell lymphomas and CTCLs, possess a TCR composed of the γδ chains. HSTLs are thought to be derived from a primitive γδ T-cell that has a penchant for infiltrating the liver and spleen. EATL accounts for 5%–10% of all PTCL cases. EATL is highly associated with celiac disease, which itself is far more prevalent in Europe. As a result, EATL accounts for only about 6% of all PTCL cases in North America, about 10% in Europe, and less than 2% in Asia, where celiac disease is very uncommon. Subcutaneous panniculitis-like T-cell lymphoma is another subtype of extranodal PTCL. It accounts for less than 1% of all cases of PTCL and is associated with a very aggressive course and resistance to chemotherapy. The immunophenotype of this lymphoma is CD3 and CD8 positive and CD4 negative. This rare form of lymphoma is often misdiagnosed, frequently being confused with the panniculitic-like lesions seen in lupus. It usually presents with subcutaneous nodules that may be indurated or necrotic, rendering the diagnosis challenging.

The leukemic subtypes of T-cell lymphoma largely consist of ATLL, which is commonly associated with the HTLV-1 retrovirus. The immunophenotype is typically CD3 and CD5 positive, CD7 negative, with positivity for CD4 and CD25 in the majority of cases. ATLL is associated with clonal integration of HTLV-1 in neoplastic T cells in 100% of cases. Typically the interval between viral infection and onset of lymphoma is long, on the order of 10–40 years, with usually less than 5% of infected individuals actually developing ATLL. The disease is typically very aggressive, often involving the bone marrow and lymph nodes, although smoldering and chronic forms of ATLL do exist and are often managed differently.

Pathobiology

The PTCLs comprise many rare subsets of NHLs that arise from post-thymic T cells or NK cells, which can occur at nodal or extranodal sites. Over recent years there has been some progress in disease characterization and classification. Unlike B-NHLs, the pathogenesis of PTCL is poorly understood, and the cell of origin of many PTCL entities is unknown at present. Progress in understanding the etiology of PTCL and the associated pathogenetic molecular alterations is hampered by the rarity and heterogeneous nature of this disease.

Peripheral T-Cell Lymphoma, Not Otherwise Specified

PTCL-NOS is the most common subtype of PTCL, accounting for 20%–30% of all PTCLs occurring worldwide. It is a clinically heterogeneous entity that comprises cases lacking morphologic (Fig. 85.3) and phenotypic features of other PTCL subtypes, and is associated with poor survival. Early gene expression profiling studies were able to differentiate PTCL from T-lymphoblastic leukemia and distinguish certain entities based on different signaling pathways. More recent studies suggest a relationship with either activated helper CD4+ or cytotoxic CD8+ T cells, with lymphomas manifesting expression profiles similar to the latter being associated with inferior survival. PTCL-NOS lack specific cytogenetic abnormalities, although complex cytogenetic aberrations have been associated with a poor prognosis. Recurrent gains of chromosome 7q that target cyclin-dependent kinase 6 and 8q involving the MYC locus have been reported. A recurrent translocation t(5:9)(q33:32) resulting in the fusion of the IL-2–inducible T-cell kinase (ITK) gene with the spleen tyrosine kinase (SYK) gene has been identified in a subset of PTCL-NOS. Interestingly, transgenic mice expressing the ITK-SYK fusion transcript develop a T-cell lymphoma mimicking the human disease. Additionally, overexpression of total and phosphorylated Syk tyrosine kinase, even in the absence of SYK translocations, raises the possibility of Syk being a therapeutic target in this disease.

Translocations involving the interferon regulatory factor-4 (IRF4) gene have been identified in a small subset of PTCL-NOS. However, like Syk, IRF4 overexpression in PTCL-NOS can be seen in the absence of IRF4 rearrangement as a consequence of a CD30/nuclear factor kappa-B (NFκB) positive feedback mechanism, at least in certain cases, suggesting a role for CD30 and/or NFκB inhibitors in disease subsets.

Next-generation sequencing analyses have identified recurrent rearrangements of the TP53 family member, TP63, with TBL1XR1 or ATXN1 genes in PTCL-NOS, resulting in the expression of an oncogenic mutant p63 protein, which is associated with adverse clinical outcomes. Recent gene expression profiling of a large cohort of PTCLs identified two subgroups of PTCL-NOS based on expression of GATA3 (required for T-helper type 2 cell [Th2] development and function) and TBX21 (required for T-helper type 1 cell [Th1] development and function). The GATA3 subgroup, enriched in MYC, phosphatidylinositol 3-kinase (PI3K), and β-catenin gene signatures, was associated with an inferior outcome. The TBX21 subgroup, enriched in interferon-gamma (IFN-γ)-induced and NF-κB gene signatures, overall, had a more favorable clinical outcome, except for cases exhibiting a cytotoxic T-cell signature. Targeted mutation analysis has uncovered coexisting TET2 and DNMT3A mutations in a significant proportion of PTCL-NOS, suggesting roles for the modification of the T-cell epigenome in disease pathogenesis and the use of demethylating agents as potential therapy. Recent whole-exome sequencing of PTCL

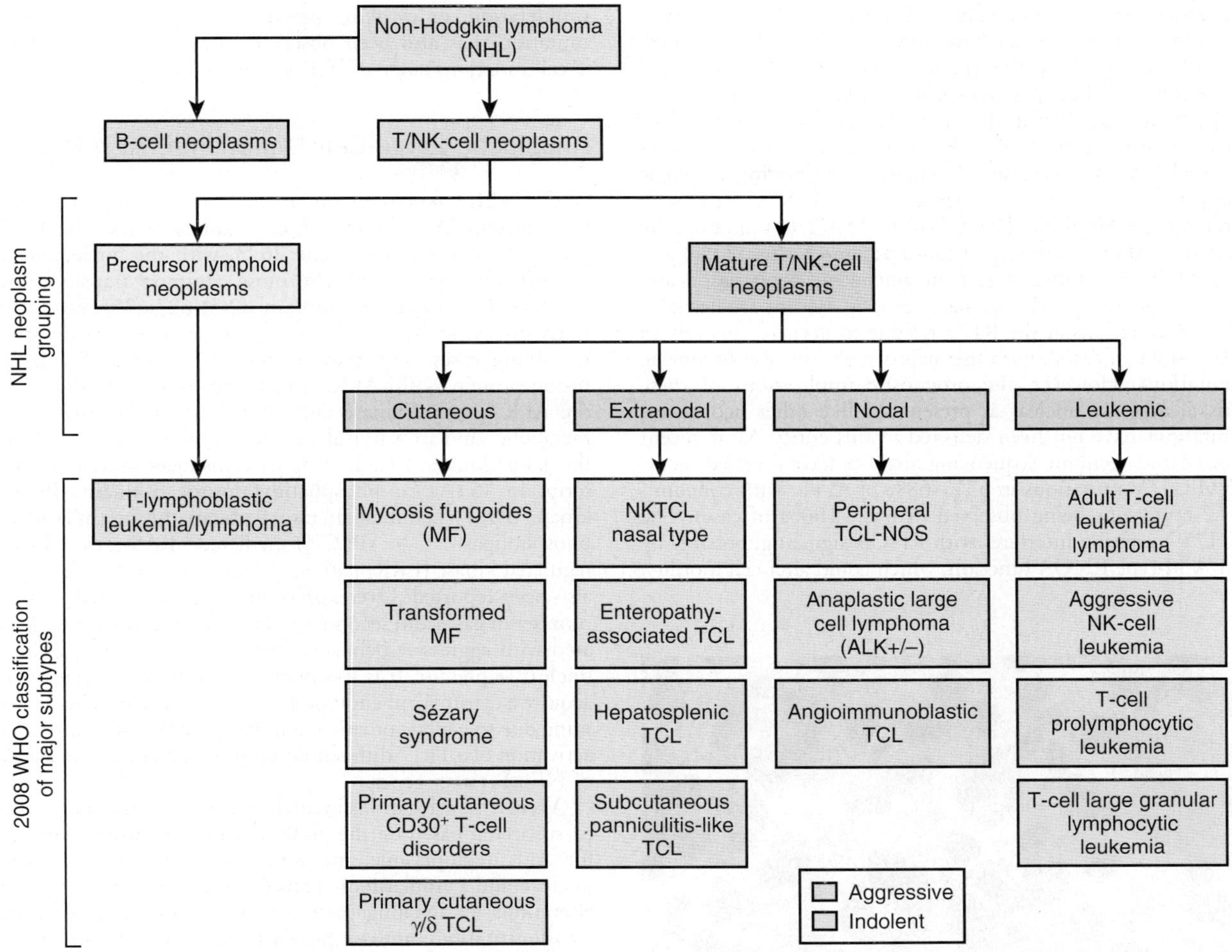

Non-Hodgkin lymphoma (NHL)

→ B-cell neoplasms

→ T/NK-cell neoplasms

NHL neoplasm grouping

Precursor lymphoid neoplasms

Mature T/NK-cell neoplasms

→ Cutaneous
→ Extranodal
→ Nodal
→ Leukemic

2008 WHO classification of major subtypes

T-lymphoblastic leukemia/lymphoma

Cutaneous:
- Mycosis fungoides (MF)
- Transformed MF
- Sézary syndrome
- Primary cutaneous CD30+ T-cell disorders
- Primary cutaneous γ/δ TCL

Extranodal:
- NKTCL nasal type
- Enteropathy-associated TCL
- Hepatosplenic TCL
- Subcutaneous panniculitis-like TCL

Nodal:
- Peripheral TCL-NOS
- Anaplastic large cell lymphoma (ALK+/−)
- Angioimmunoblastic TCL

Leukemic:
- Adult T-cell leukemia/lymphoma
- Aggressive NK-cell leukemia
- T-cell prolymphocytic leukemia
- T-cell large granular lymphocytic leukemia

☐ Aggressive
☐ Indolent

Fig. 85.1 WHO CLASSIFICATION OF THE MATURE T-CELL NEOPLASMS. *NK*, Natural killer; *NOS*, not otherwise specified; *TCL*, T-cell lymphoma.

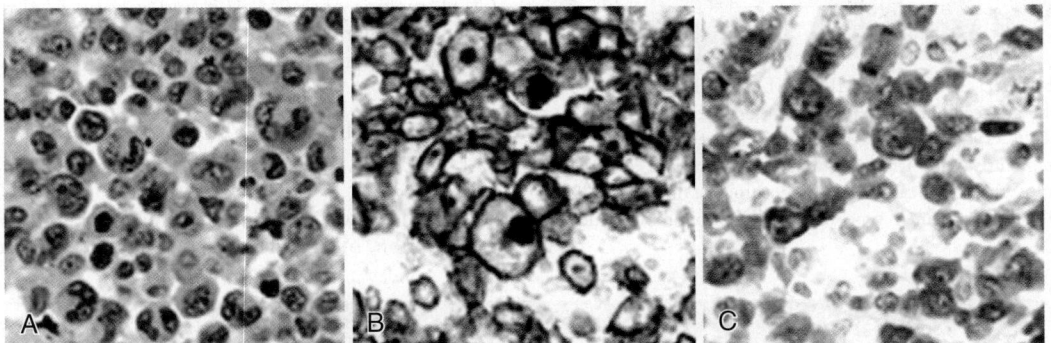

Fig. 85.2 ANAPLASTIC LARGE-CELL LYMPHOMA. Anaplastic large-cell lymphoma has variable morphologic features but is typically composed of large, highly irregular "anaplastic" cells, which include giant cells sometimes with a wreath-like or horseshoe-shape nuclei, and "hallmark" cells, which are cells with a folded up nucleus with an embryo shape (A). The cells are typically brightly CD30+ (B). ALK1 staining with cytoplasmic and nuclear localization (C) is associated with the t(2;5)(p23;q35) translocation, whereas other patterns are associated with the variant translocations (C). Whether *ALK1*-negative cases should be considered as a separate group or classified together with peripheral T-cell lymphoma not otherwise specified is somewhat debatable (see text).

has revealed recurrent mutations in *RHOA* and *FYN* in a small subset of PTCL-NOS, but their prognostic import is currently unknown.

Angioimmunoblastic T-Cell Lymphoma

AITL is the second-most common PTCL subtype worldwide that has a characteristic clinical presentation, often manifesting features of immune dysregulation, which is derived from T-follicular helper (T_{FH}) cells, based on phenotypic features and overexpression of genes characteristic of normal T_{FH} cells (Fig. 85.4). Early gene expression profiling studies could not reliably distinguish between AITL and subsets of PTCL-NOS. However, recent studies have shown a unique genetic signature for AITL, including four prognostically relevant subsets; those displaying a B-cell, monocytic, cytotoxic, or p53-induced target gene signature, with cases exhibiting the B-cell signature associated with a more favorable outcome. Recurrent gains of chromosomes 3q, 5q, and 21 have been noted in AITL, although the genes affected by these abnormalities remain unknown. Mutations of genes involved in epigenetic processes have been observed in AITL more frequently than in the other PTCLs. Inactivating *TET2* mutations are observed in 33%–76% of AITL and 38% of PTCL-NOS, especially in cases expressing T$_{FH}$ markers, suggesting a biologic relationship between AITL and a subset of PTCL-NOS exhibiting the T$_{FH}$ phenotype. Similar to PTCL-NOS, *DNMT3A* mutations are also detected in AITL, with a significant fraction of cases (73%) also harboring *TET2* mutations, suggesting oncogenic cooperation and epigenetic deregulation in disease pathogenesis. Recent studies have shown *IDH2* mutations at the R172 residue to occur exclusively in AITL (20%–45% of cases), with the majority of cases also harboring *TET2* mutations. However, the prognostic implications of these alterations, if any, are unclear at present. Unlike other neoplasms, *IDH1* mutations have not been detected in this entity. More recent whole-exome and -genome sequencing analyses have revealed recurrent *RHOA* G17V mutations in 53%–68% of AITL, with concomitant *TET2* mutations being observed in 65%–100% of cases. The *RHOA* G17V mutation interferes with RHOA signaling, possibly by inhibiting wild-type RHOA function, which could alter cell motility,

proliferation, or cytokine signaling. A low frequency of recurrent mutations has also been observed in genes that impact important T-cell functions such as TCR signaling (*CD28*, *FYN*).

Anaplastic Large-Cell Lymphoma, ALK-Positive

ALCL, ALK+ represents one of the few subtypes of PTCL defined by recurrent chromosomal translocations. These involve the *ALK* gene located on chromosome 2p23, with the nucleophosmin gene (*NPM*), on 5q35, being the most common translocation partner (55%–85% of cases), resulting in t(2;5)(p23;q35); variant translocations involving *ALK* and other partner genes are detected in the remaining cases. The translocation t(2;5)(p23;q35) results in the fusion protein NPM-ALK, which leads to constitutive activation of the ALK tyrosine kinase and alterations in downstream signaling, metabolic, and prosurvival pathways, among others. These include the Janus kinase 3 (JAK3)/signal transducer and activator of transcription (STAT)3, phosphatidylinositol 3-kinase (PI3K)/protein kinase (AKT)/mammalian target of rapamycin (mTOR), and the phospholipase C-γ (PLC-γ)-mediated RAS-extracellular signal-regulated kinase (ERK) pathways. Activation of Notch1 signaling has also been reported. Overexpression of *MYC* is noted in a significant number of cases and secondary *MYC* translocations have been associated with aggressive behavior. The cell of origin of ALCL, ALK+ is unclear at present. It is speculated that different T-cell subsets could acquire a cytotoxic phenotype as a consequence of cellular reprogramming due to genetic or epigenetic aberrations, and some tumors show activation of a Th17 differentiation program and increased expression of NF-κB target genes.

Variant translocations involving ALK and other partner genes can be suspected based on the pattern of immunohistochemical staining for ALK (cytoplasmic, membranous, or nucleolar instead of the nuclear and cytoplasmic). Pathologic consequences and molecular alterations in signaling pathways as a consequence of variant *ALK* translocations are not completely understood yet, but partial overlap with gene expression profiles of *NPM-ALK* has been described.

While differences in gene expression profiles between certain morphologic subtypes of ALCL, ALK+ have been reported, array CGH analysis of *NPM-ALK* and variant *ALK* translocations have revealed similar recurrent secondary genetic abnormalities including gains at 17p and losses at 4q and 11q.

Anaplastic Large-Cell Lymphoma, ALK-Negative (ALCL, ALK–)

ALCL, ALK– was considered a provisional entity in the WHO 2008 classification, but recent studies suggest it to be a unique subtype of

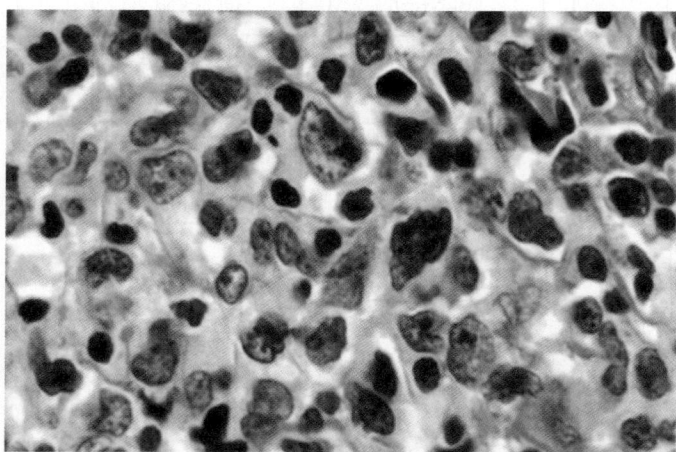

Fig. 85.3 PERIPHERAL T-CELL LYMPHOMA NOT OTHERWISE SPECIFIED. Peripheral T-cell lymphoma not otherwise specified is morphologically heterogeneous. Typically, cases have a spectrum of small-to-large lymphoma cells, frequently with irregular nuclear borders and sometimes with clear cytoplasm. Other cases can have a predominance of small or large cells. Features of the other defined types of T-cell lymphoma should be lacking.

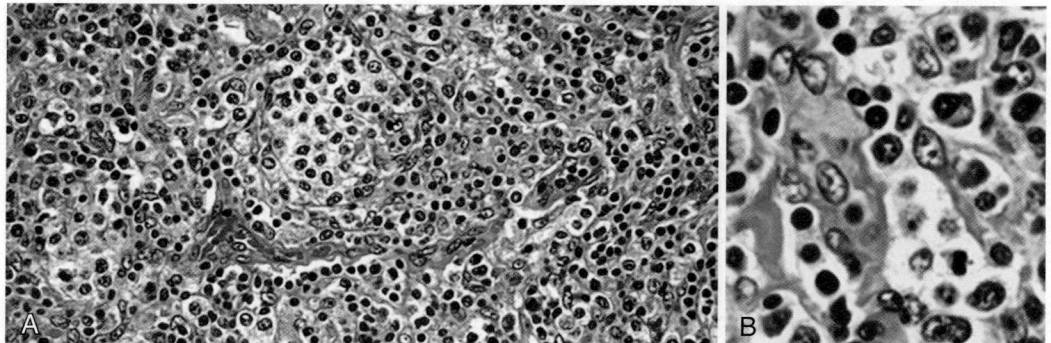

Fig. 85.4 ANGIOIMMUNOBLASTIC T-CELL LYMPHOMA. A prominent feature of angioimmunoblastic T-cell lymphoma is the prominent vasculature in the background. The vessels usually show branching and prominent endothelial cells (A). The cellular composition is a mix of plasma cells, immunoblasts, and small lymphocytes; the lymphoma cells can be of intermediate or large size, and they tend to cluster and exhibit clear cytoplasm (A, B). Some cases can develop a superimposed Epstein-Barr virus-driven large B-cell lymphoma.

PTCL. While it shares morphologic and immunophenotypic features with ALCL, ALK+, including CD30 expression, it characteristically lacks *ALK* translocations, occurs in older individuals, and has a poorer prognosis. Additionally, a subset of PTCL-NOS can express CD30 and distinguishing ALCL, ALK– from these lesions can be challenging. Refined, supervised gene expression analysis could reliably differentiate ALCL, ALK– from PTCL-NOS and metaanalysis of the transcriptional profiles of a large series of PTCLs revealed a three-gene model, comprising *TNFRSF8*, *BATF3*, and *TMOD1*, that could accurately separate ALCL, ALK– from PTCL-NOS. Recently, an enrichment of MYC, IRF4 targets, mTOR and PI3K pathway gene signatures were described in ALCL, ALK–, while hypoxia-inducible factor 1-α targets, interleukin (IL)-10-induced genes and H/K-ras–induced genes appear enriched in ALCL, ALK+.

Array comparative genomic hybridization (CGH) analysis of ALCL, ALK+ and ALCL, ALK– has highlighted differences in secondary genetic aberrations between the two subtypes, and differential expression of microRNAs. Genome-wide single-nucleotide polymorphism profiling has shown recurrent losses of 17p13.3–p12 (*TP53*) and 6q21 (*PRDM1*) at a significantly higher frequency in ALCL, ALK– compared with ALCL, ALK+. In addition to loss, *PRDM1* mutations were also detected in a subset of ALCL, ALK– cases, and loss of either *PRDM1* and/or *TP53* conferred a worse prognosis.

Next-generation sequencing analysis has identified a recurrent balanced translocation t(6;7)(p25.3;q32.3) in 10% of ALCL, ALK–, leading to juxtaposition of the *DUSP22* phosphatase gene (6p25.3) with the fragile site *FRA7H* (7q32.3) locus, resulting in the downregulation of *DUSP22* and upregulation of *MIR29* microRNAs on 7q32.3. Mutually exclusive and recurrent rearrangements of *DUSP22* and *TP63* have been identified in 30% and 8% of ALCL, ALK–, respectively, and differences in morphology and phenotype have been reported for the different subsets. Cases with *DUSP22* rearrangements have a significantly better prognosis compared with those with *TP63* rearrangements. Recent whole-exome sequencing analysis of ALCL, ALK– identified recurrent and concurrent mutations in *JAK1* and *STAT3*. Interestingly, a subset of cases lacking mutations in either JAK1 or STAT3 harbored chimeric fusion proteins involving NF-κB2 and tyrosine kinases ROS1 and TYK2, which result in constitutive STAT3 activation. Hence, activation of the STAT3 pathway may represent a common and critical event in the pathogenesis of ALCL, ALK– and possibly a therapeutic target.

Enteropathy-Associated T-Cell Lymphoma

EATL is a rare subtype of PTCL, accounting for 5%–10% of PTCLs, that is derived from small intestinal intraepithelial lymphocytes. Although two types of EATL were recognized in the 2008 WHO classification, EATL types I and II, recent studies have suggested distinct differences between these entities and proposed to designate EATL type II as "monomorphic epitheliotropic intestinal T-cell lymphoma" (MEITL). EATL type I, now simply referred to as EATL, occurs in individuals with celiac disease and is associated with the HLA DQ2 or DQ8 haplotypes. Homozygosity for HLA-DQ2 has been shown to increase the risk of developing EATL. Refractory celiac disease (RCD), especially RCD type II, is considered a precursor of at least a subset of EATL. Cytogenetic analysis of RCD II has shown recurrent gains of chromosome 1q22–q44, a feature shared with EATL, indicating early acquisition of chromosome 1q abnormalities in the pathogenesis of EATL.

Genomic analyses of EATL have revealed additional recurrent chromosome abnormalities. Gains or amplifications of chromosome 9q34 are the most frequent (40%–58%), but recurrent gains at 5q and 7q and losses of 8p, 9p, and 13q have also been reported. The pattern of aberrations suggests at least two subtypes of EATL. Segmental amplifications of the chromosome 9q31.3-qter region, encompassing known protooncogenes (e.g. *NOTCH1*, *ABL1*, *VAV*), or, alternatively, deletions at 16q12.1 have been reported in greater than 80% of EATLs, while a small subset exhibit allelic imbalances at 3q27.

MEITL has a wider geographic distribution than EATL and it appears to be more common in Asians and Hispanics. Serologic evidence of celiac disease is lacking in the vast majority of cases and the morphology is distinct from EATL. Recent studies from Asia have reported 23%–78% of MEITLs to manifest the TCRγδ phenotype, and a lack of TCR expression has been described in up to a third of cases. On comparing genomic profiles of EATL and MEITL, mutually exclusive segmental amplifications of 9q31.3-qter and deletions of 16q12.1 have been detected in both disease types, with gains of 1q and 5q occurring more frequently in EATL and gains of the *MYC* locus (8q24) more often observed in MEITL. These data suggest the possibility of common as well as distinct genetic alterations associated with the pathogenesis of the two subtypes of intestinal T-cell lymphomas.

Hepatosplenic T-Cell Lymphoma

HSTL is a rare subtype of PTCL that has been associated with underlying immune dysfunction (Fig. 85.5). It is most commonly of γδ T-cell lineage; however, lymphomas bearing the αβ TCR have been described, as have occasional cases lacking surface TCR. Isochromosome 7q [i(7)(q10)] is reported to be a frequent recurrent chromosomal aberration, but specific abnormalities of particular genes have not been defined. Of interest, i(7)(q10) has been detected in hepatosplenic T-cell lymphoma irrespective of the phenotype (γδ

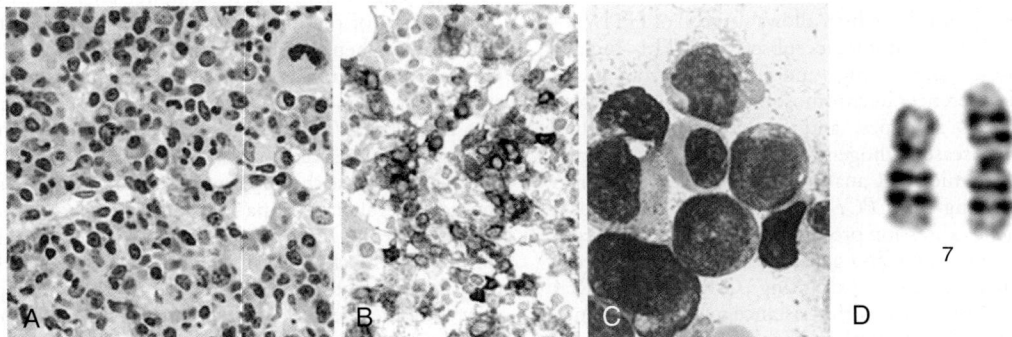

Fig. 85.5 HEPATOSPLENIC T-CELL LYMPHOMA. Hepatosplenic γδ T-cell lymphoma is commonly diagnosed from a bone marrow biopsy specimen in a patient being evaluated for hepatosplenomegaly. The bone marrow typically shows a subtle lymphoid infiltrate (A), which becomes more evident with a T-cell stain such as CD3 (B). This highlights the classic sinusoidal distribution of the lymphoma. Lymphoma cells may be seen in the circulation or in the marrow aspirate and can resemble monocytes or blasts (C). The lymphoma is typically associated with isochromosome 7q, as illustrated in the partial karyotype (D).

or αβ). Moreover, an increase in the number of 7q signals, often accompanied by trisomy 8, has been associated with disease progression. The gene expression profile of HSTL appears distinct from other types of PTCL and is characterized by overexpression of NK cell-associated molecules such as killer cell immunoglobulin (Ig)-like receptor (KIR) genes and killer lectin-like receptors. Mutually exclusive *STAT5B* and *STAT3* mutations have been reported in a subset of HSTL cases.

Extranodal Natural Killer/T-Cell Lymphoma

Extranodal NK/T-cell lymphoma (ENKTCL) is an aggressive PTCL associated with clonal episomal EBV infection of NK or T cells. It is less common in the western hemisphere but it has a significantly higher incidence in Asia, excluding Japan. It occurs most commonly in the nasopharynx (nasal type) and less frequently at other anatomic sites (extranasal). Cooperating genetic and environmental factors are likely to play roles in disease pathogenesis. Gene expression profiling of ENKTCL has revealed overexpression of cytotoxic proteins (granzyme H) and PDGFRA. Early studies showed recurrent deletions of chromosome 6q21–25 in ENKTCL and array CGH analysis detected recurrent gains of 2q, and losses of 6q16.1–q27 and 11q22.3–q23.3, with loss of potential tumor suppressor genes *PRDM1*, *ATG5*, and *AIM1* located on 6q12–25. Oligonucleotide array CGH and functional studies have identified *FOXO3* in addition to *PRDM1* (*BLIMP1*) as candidate tumor suppressor genes located at 6q21. Analysis of a small cohort of ENKTCL cases described recurrent loss of 8p11.23 in 46% cases, which was associated with an adverse prognosis. Genetic analysis of this locus showed recurrent mutations in *ADAM3A*, a metalloproteinase family member. Recent studies have shown *JAK3* and *STAT3* mutations resulting in the constitutive activation of these transcription factors as well as loss of *PTPRK* on 6q22, which can also lead to STAT3 activation. These findings suggest a role for JAK-STAT signaling in the pathogenesis of ENKTCL. Similar to other types of PTCLs, mutations in epigenetic modifier genes are also frequent in this disease.

Human T-Lymphotropic Virus-1–Associated Adult T-Cell Leukemia/Lymphoma

HTLV-1 is a retrovirus endemic in Japan, central Africa, Iran and the Caribbean basin. HTLV-1 infection is transmitted via infected T cells present in body fluids, especially breast milk and semen, and blood of carriers of the HTLV-1 provirus. HTLV-1 infection leads to the clonal expansion and immortalization of CD4$^+$ T cells. Disease pathogenesis involves viral and host factors. A variety of viral proteins cooperate in cellular transformation, including Tax and HBZ, which modulate multiple signal transduction pathways (CREB/ATF, NF-κB, JAK-STAT, mTOR-AKT). This leads to deregulated cytokine production and impairment of host immunity, which allows survival of HTLV-1–infected lymphocytes. Clinicopathologic subsets of ATLL include leukemic, lymphomatous, smoldering, and chronic. Array CGH studies have identified differences in chromosome alterations between acute and lymphomatous subtypes, and have suggested distinct oncogenic pathways in disease pathogenesis. Single-nucleotide polymorphism array and genomic PCR analysis have revealed rearrangements at 10p11.2 involving the *EPC1* gene locus and *ASXL2* as a partner fusion gene. Gene expression profiling has uncovered dysregulation of *MYC*, *REL-1*, and *NOTCH-1* genes, all known to be upregulated by the Tax protein. Cases exhibiting C-REL and IRF4 overexpression have been associated with resistance to antiviral agents. Somatic gain-of-function *CCR4* mutations have been reported in 26% of ATLL, leading to enhanced activation of the PI3K/AKT pathway. Hyperactivity of PI3K secondary to inhibition of protein phosphatases is known to play an important role in ATLL pathogenesis and has been linked to the formation of the characteristic multilobated "flower-like" nuclei in tumor cells. Recent comprehensive genomic analysis of a large series of ATLL samples identified mutations or alterations in T-cell

receptor signaling and NF-κB pathway genes, as well as defects in immunosurveillance mechanisms.

Clinical Manifestations

PTCLs, with the exclusion of CTCL, recapitulate the general presentation of aggressive NHL, which can vary depending on histologic features, patient age, and immune status. PTCL generally presents with lymphadenopathy, and patients can range from being asymptomatic to presenting in extremis with diverse symptoms and significant end-organ compromise. PTCL can present as discrete nodal, extranodal, leukemic, or cutaneous disease, or with any combination of these involved sites. An extranodal presentation is common in PTCL and often contributes to a delay in the diagnosis. When compared with aggressive B-cell lymphomas, patients with PTCL tend to present with more advanced disease, a poorer performance status, and frequently B symptoms. Patients may have constitutional manifestations because of the production of inflammatory cytokines and chemokines produced by the lymphoma cells and host tissues. Paraneoplastic syndromes, including eosinophilia, hemophagocytic syndrome, and autoimmune phenomena, have been well described in different PTCL subtypes. For example, AITL is often characterized by systemic symptoms, skin rash, organomegaly, hypergammaglobulinemia, and hemolytic anemia. It affects older adults, and patients frequently present with peripheral lymphadenopathy, hepatosplenomegaly, skin rash, and constitutional symptoms. In contrast, hepatosplenic T-cell lymphoma, which often occurs in young adults, is characterized by marked hepatosplenomegaly and bone marrow involvement.

Laboratory Manifestations

Laboratory tests should include a complete blood count, serum chemistry determination (including lactate dehydrogenase [LDH]), titers, and viral studies, including HTLV-1 status and EBV in appropriate cases. The level of β$_2$-microglobulin is usually normal compared with that found with the B-cell lymphomas. Peripheral blood flow cytometry and bone marrow biopsy can be helpful in understanding the extent of disease.

Differential Diagnosis

Accuracy in the diagnosis of PTCLs more often than not requires the consensus of hematopathologists with a specific expertise in this field. Diagnosis is based on examination of peripheral blood or tissue biopsy specimens for histologic features supplemented by detailed immunohistochemistry, flow cytometry, cytogenetics, and molecular genetics. Expert hematopathologic review is essential for the correct classification of the different subtypes, given the often poor concordance among hematopathologists in matching the diagnosis. Detailed clinical information is essential for the hematopathologist to make the correct diagnosis. For example, in patients from Japan, information regarding HTLV-1 status is essential to aiding the pathologist in distinguishing between lymph node involvement due to PTCL-NOS and ATL. Because this disease also occurs in the West, HTLV-1 status should be evaluated in patients at high risk for the disease or from endemic areas. Other diagnoses such as AITL and EATL are often clarified by the clinical information. For cases in which it is difficult to distinguish between different entities, gene expression profiling may become helpful in the future for confirming the correct diagnosis.

Prognostic Factors

The majority of PTCLs are associated with a very poor prognosis compared with their B-cell counterparts (Fig. 85.6). Treatment

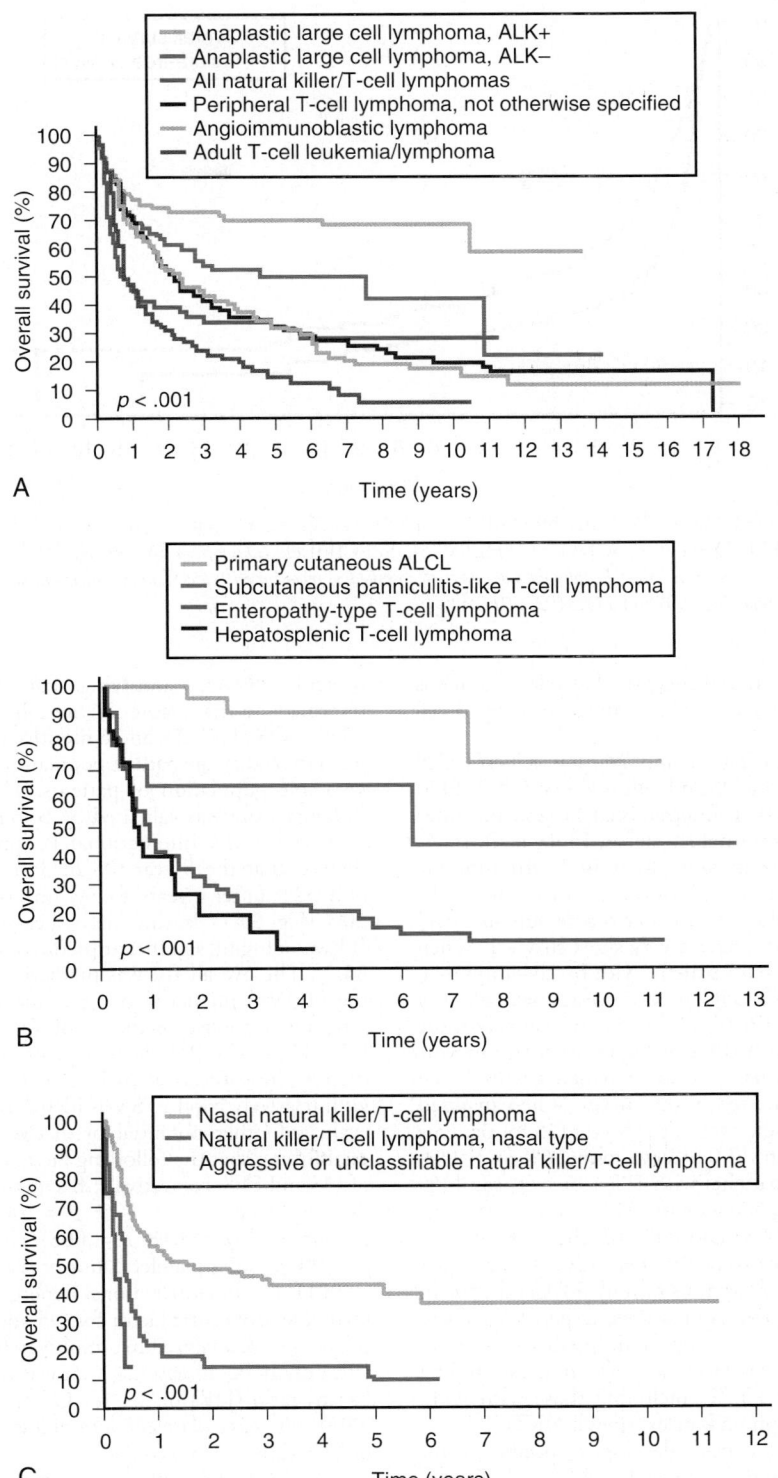

Fig. 85.6 (A) Overall survival of patients with the common subtypes of peripheral T-cell lymphoma (PTCL). (B) Overall survival of patients with less common subtypes of PTCL. (C) Overall survival of patients with natural killer/T-cell lymphoma. *(Data from Vose J, Armitage J, Weisenburger D: International peripheral T-cell and natural killer/T-cell lymphoma study: Pathology findings and clinical outcomes.* J Clin Oncol *26:4124, 2008.)*

outcomes for PTCL patients are substantially inferior to those for their B-cell lymphoma counterparts. Lymphomas derived from the T-cell lineage have been shown to be an independent negative prognostic factor. The adverse prognosis of patients with relapsed or refractory PTCL has been highlighted in a recent experience from the British Columbia Cancer Agency (BCCA). In this series, the BCCA identified 153 patients who relapsed or progressed after primary therapy. They identified 153 patients with a variety of PTCL

subtypes including PTCL-NOS, AITL, ALK+ and ALK– T-cell lymphomas. The median time from diagnosis to relapse or progression of disease after primary therapy was 6.7 months. The median overall survival (OS) and second progression-free survival were only 5.5 and 3.1 months, respectively, which was only marginally improved if those patients went on to receive subsequent chemotherapy. This experience underscores the poor performance of conventional treatment regimens in the treatment of the disease, highlights the

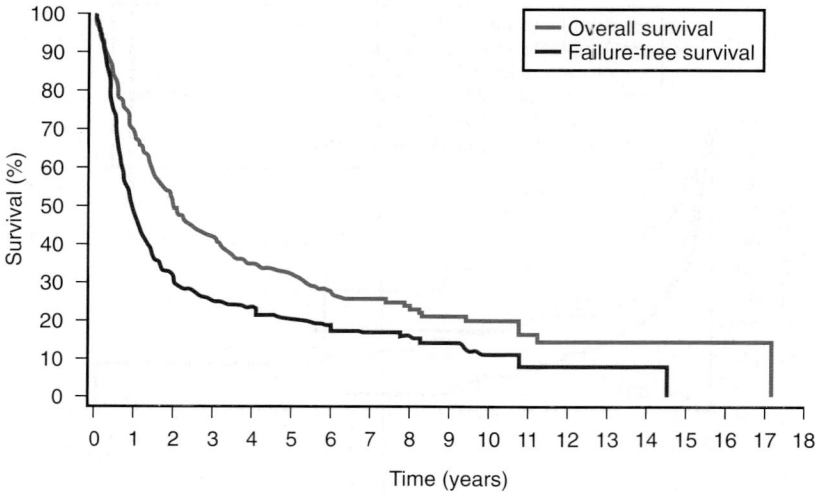

Fig. 85.7 OVERALL SURVIVAL AND FAILURE-FREE SURVIVAL OF 340 PATIENTS WITH PERIPH-ERAL T-CELL LYMPHOMA NOT OTHERWISE SPECIFIED. *(Data from Weisenburger DD, Savage KJ, Harris NL, et al: Peripheral T-cell lymphoma, not otherwise specified: A report of 340 cases from the International Peripheral T-cell Lymphoma Project.* Blood *117:3402, 2011.)*

importance of first-line treatment, and suggests that relapse alone is a profoundly adverse prognostic feature, in contrast to many B-cell lymphomas.

The International Peripheral T-Cell and Natural Killer/T-Cell Lymphoma study reported that the OS and failure-free survival (FFS) at 10–15 years was only 10%. The International Prognostic Index (IPI), which is based on age, performance status, LDH level, stage, and extranodal involvement, appears to be useful in determining the prognosis for certain PTCL subtypes. However, even patients in the best risk categories (IPI 0 or 1) do not have a favorable outcome, and patients in the high-risk categories have a very short survival. When compared with the IPI curves seen for patients with B-cell lymphoma, the curves seen for patients with T-cell lymphoma essentially identify two risk categories, those with IPI 0 or 1 having a relatively more favorable outcome, and those with IPI 2 or higher with an unfavorable outcome. In contrast to what is seen in patients with B-cell lymphoma, there is limited separation of the curves. When analyzed as a function of the histopathologic subset, the 5-year OS for patients with PTCL-NOS and AITL with IPI 0 or 1 was only 56% and 50%, respectively, whereas for those patients with IPI 4 or 5 it was 11% and 25%, respectively. Among patients with ALCL, the 5-year survival for IPI 0 or 1 is roughly 90% and 74% for the ALK-positive and ALK-negative patients, respectively. Patients with IPI 2 or higher have a poor outcome, with 5-year survivals of only 33% and 13% in the ALK-positive and ALK-negative populations, respectively. These observations confirm that IPI is an important predictor even in ALK-positive ALCL. The IPI has been less useful in stratifying patients with other subtypes of PTCL, including those with ATL, EATL, hepatosplenic T-cell lymphoma, or extranasal NKTCL.

Other prognostic models have been developed specifically for patients with PTCL. The Prognostic Index for PTCL (PIT) was developed based on risk factors that include age, LDH level, performance status, and bone marrow involvement. When applied to a PTCL-NOS population, the PIT stratified patients into more distinct prognostic groups compared with the IPI. Of 322 patients studied, 20% had no adverse features, 34% had one, and 20% had three or more. The 5-year OS for the most favorable subgroup with no adverse prognostic features was 62% compared with 18% for patients with three or four prognostic factors. Despite improved stratification, the so-called *favorable-risk population* of patients with PTCL still had a strikingly poor outcome.

Efforts to improve on the more traditional clinically based scoring systems have been proposed. The Bologna scoring system was developed integrating both patient-specific and tumor-specific characteristics (age >60 years, performance status, LDH level, and Ki-67

protein ≥80%), stratifying patients into low-risk (score 1), intermediate-risk (score 2), and high-risk disease (score 3), with median OS of 37, 23, and 6 months, respectively. Although the scores seem to stratify the patient population, it is clear that there is no really favorable population of patients. The prognostic capability of the Bologna score was validated by Briones et al.

Recently the International Peripheral Lymphoma Study (IPLS) showed that the 5-year OS of 340 patients with PTCL-NOS was only 32% (after 3 years' follow-up), whereas the 5-year FFS was only 20% (Fig. 85.7). In this analysis, each of the prognostic factors in the IPI was a highly significant predictor of OS and FFS ($p < .001$) (Fig. 85.8). The overall IPI was predictive of both OS and FFS, whereas the PIT was predictive of only survival. Bone marrow involvement was not a robust predictor of OS ($p = .03$) or FFS ($p = .06$) (Fig. 85.9). The PIT did not prove to be superior to the IPI in predicting the survival of patients with PTCL-NOS. Only one group with relatively good FFS was identified using both models. The IPLS evaluated other potential predictive factors by univariate analysis, establishing that the following factors were adverse prognostic factors of OS and FFS, respectively: B symptoms ($p = .004$; $p = .014$), bulky disease ≥10 cm ($p = .005$; $p = .004$), elevated serum C-reactive protein level ($p = .018$; $p = .008$), circulating tumor cells ($p < .001$; $p < .001$), and a platelet count of less than 150×10^9/L ($p < .001$; $p < .001$). For unclear reasons, hypergammaglobulinemia fell out as a favorable prognostic factor for OS and FFS ($p = .04$; $p = .03$). When the data were analyzed in a multivariate analysis, after controlling for IPI, only bulky disease ≥10 cm was still predictive of survival with a hazard ratio (HR) of 2.1 for OS ($p = .019$) and 2.5 for FFS ($p = .003$), whereas a platelet count of less than 150×10^9/L was predictive of FFS (HR = 1.6, $p = .016$).

The IPLS also explored the impact of several pathologic features that were associated with inferior OS and FFS, including the following: Ki-67 index more than 25%, the presence of transformed tumor cells more than 70%, significant numbers of EBV-positive B cells (Epstein-Barr–encoded ribonucleic acid [EBER] 3–4⁺), and CD56 and CD30 expression by more than 20% on tumor cells. EBV positivity was predictive of an adverse survival only in patients younger than 60 years and was independent of a history of immunosuppressive therapy or autoimmune disorders. Factors that appeared to be favorably associated with improved OS and FFS included lymphoepithelioid (Lennert) variant and background CD8⁺ T cells constituting more than 10% of the population. Several clinicopathologic factors were identified to be of prognostic significance by univariate analysis, but only bulky disease (>10 cm) and thrombocytopenia (<150 × 10⁹ cells/L) were predictive of OS.

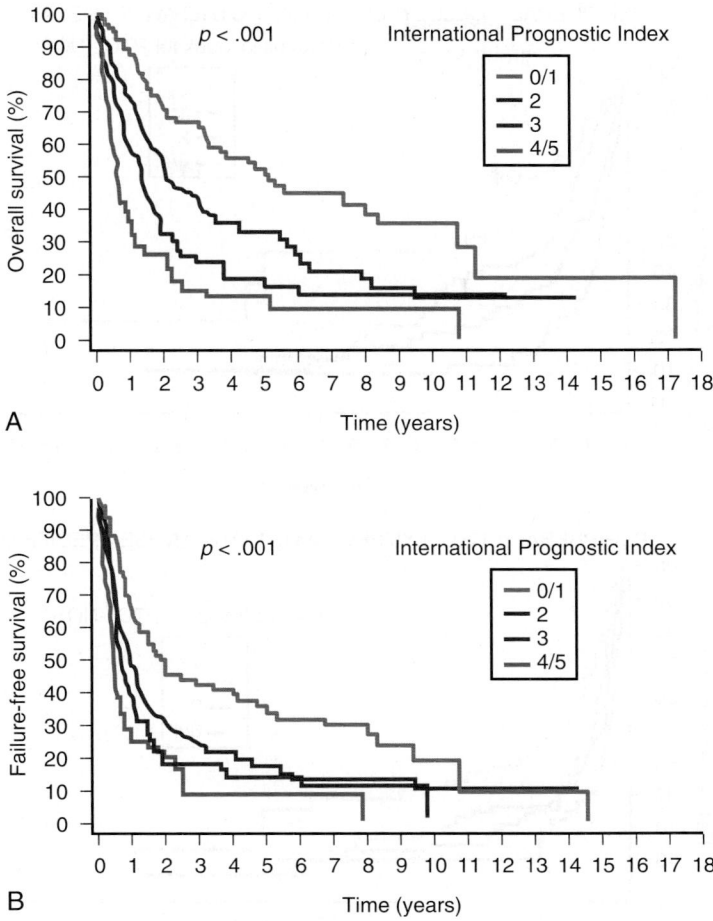

Fig. 85.8 OVERALL SURVIVAL (A) AND FAILURE-FREE SURVIVAL (B) OF 315 PATIENTS WITH PERIPHERAL T-CELL LYMPHOMA NOT OTHERWISE SPECIFIED ACCORDING TO THE INTERNATIONAL PROGNOSTIC INDEX. *(Data from Weisenburger DD, Savage KJ, Harris NL, et al: Peripheral T-cell lymphoma, not otherwise specified: A report of 340 cases from the International Peripheral T-cell Lymphoma Project.* Blood *117:3402, 2011.)*

Probably the most important prognostic factor for any subtype of PTCL is the presence or absence of ALK in ALCL. The OS of ALK-positive ALCL is substantially better than that seen for ALK-negative ALCL (71% ± 6% vs. 15% ± 11%, respectively). However, within the good prognostic category of ALK-positive ALCL, survival was 94% ± 5% for the low/low-intermediate risk group (age-adjusted IPI 0–1) and 41% ± 12% for the high/high-intermediate risk group (age-adjusted IPI ≥2). Multivariate analysis identified ALK expression and the IPI as independent variables that were able to predict survival among T/null primary, systemic ALCL.

More recently, recognizing the biologic and clinical heterogeneity of PTCL, investigators have begun to develop subtype-specific prognostic models. Although potentially interesting, these models still need to be validated in large studies.

Therapy

Standard of Care

CHOP-Like Therapy in Mature T-Cell Lymphomas

Treatment approaches employed for patients with PTCL have largely mirrored the strategies employed for the treatment of DLBCL. Consequently, CHOP (cyclophosphamide, hydroxydaunomycin, vincristine [Oncovin], and prednisone) has emerged as the "standard of care" despite disappointing outcomes. The milestone Southwest Oncology Group (SWOG) trial that compared CHOP with the second- and third-generation dose-intensive regimens in aggressive

lymphoma established that CHOP exhibited the same efficacy and less toxicity than the other regimens. This landmark trial was based on the use of a histopathologic classification system when immunophenotyping was not yet routinely applied to all cases. Unfortunately, there are no large randomized prospective studies that compare the benefit of anthracycline-based therapies to other combination regimens in PTCL.

Conventional front-line chemotherapy such as CHOP has led to disappointing results in patients with T-cell lymphomas. Analysis of the data as a function of the primary PTCL subtypes revealed that only ALCL with the t(2;5) translocation (NPM-ALK fusion protein) had an equivalent or superior prognosis compared with patients with DLBCL. The LNH87 study conducted by the Groupe d'Etudes des Lymphomes de l'Adulte showed that the use of anthracycline-containing chemotherapy regimens in T- and B-cell lymphomas were able to induce the complete remission (CR) in 54% versus 63% of the patients, with an OS of 41% and 53%, and an event-free survival (EFS) of 33% and 42%, respectively. The same group published the results of the LNH84 study, in which they employed a dose-intense consolidation. Again, although there was no difference in the response rate (RR), patients with T-cell lymphomas relapsed more frequently and earlier compared with patients with B-cell lymphoma. More recently the CHOEP regimen (cyclophosphamide, hydroxydaunomycin, vincristine [Oncovin], etoposide, and prednisone) was retrospectively studied by the German High-Grade Non-Hodgkin Lymphoma Study Group in 343 patients with T-cell lymphoma, including PTCL-NOS, ALCL, and AITL, who had been included in seven German high-grade phase II or III aggressive NHL treatment

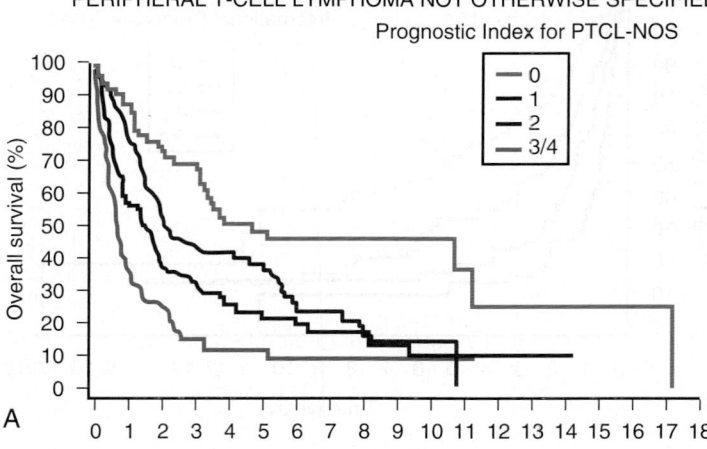

PERIPHERAL T-CELL LYMPHOMA NOT OTHERWISE SPECIFIED

Prognostic Index for PTCL-NOS

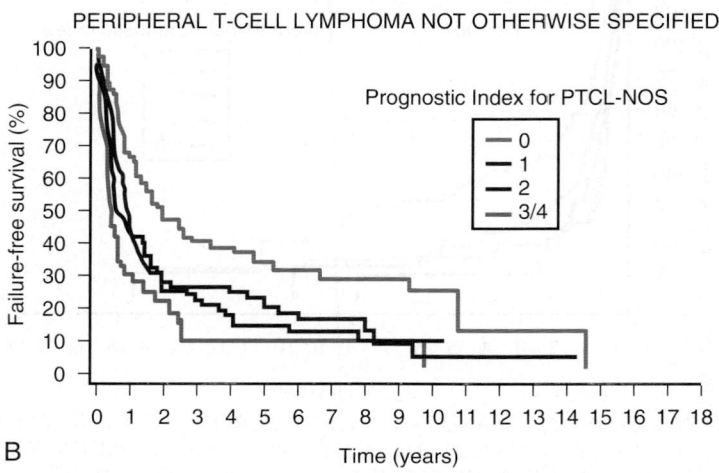

PERIPHERAL T-CELL LYMPHOMA NOT OTHERWISE SPECIFIED

Prognostic Index for PTCL-NOS

Fig. 85.9 OVERALL SURVIVAL (A) AND FAILURE-FREE SURVIVAL (B) OF 315 PATIENTS WITH PERIPHERAL T-CELL LYMPHOMA NOT OTHERWISE SPECIFIED ACCORDING TO THE PROGNOSTIC INDEX. *PTCL-NOS*, Peripheral T-cell lymphoma not otherwise specified. *(Data from Weisenburger DD, Savage KJ, Harris NL, et al: Peripheral T-cell lymphoma, not otherwise specified: A report of 340 cases from the International Peripheral T-cell Lymphoma Project.* Blood *117:3402, 2011.)*

studies. The main purpose was to determine whether the addition of etoposide or shortening of the interval of chemotherapy from 3 weeks to 2 weeks affected survival. In older adult patients, neither shortening the interval nor the addition of etoposide improved the EFS and OS.

A recent literature review and meta-analysis reported a CR rate of 52% achieved with CHOP/CHOP-like regimens (excluding ALK-positive ALCL), with an estimated 5-year OS of only 35% in PTCL. This is in contrast to the 65% or better long-term survival frequently reported in DLBCL. Select studies reporting on the activity of various combination regimens in PTCL are presented in Table 85.2.

Anaplastic Large-Cell Lymphoma

ALCL is a unique subtype of an aggressive mature T-cell lymphoma that carries a highly favorable prognosis, especially for patients with who carry the *ALK* translocation [the NPM-ALK; t(2:5)] with IPI 1 or 2 disease. Virtually all cases of ALCL express CD30, and about half of the patients with this disease harbor the t(2;5)(p21;q35) translocation. This chromosomal aberration leads to fusion of the *NPM* gene with the ALK tyrosine kinase, leading to its constitutive activation. The presence of the *ALK* translocation confers a highly favorable prognosis, and determination of ALK's status by FISH is imperative in all cases of ALCL, especially those in which the differential diagnosis also includes PTCL-NOS. The National Comprehensive Cancer Network guidelines recommend standard CHOP-based chemotherapy for these patients, sometimes combined with radiation for bulky disease, which typically produces remission rates

close to 80%. Patients who experience relapse of their disease generally exhibit the same poor prognosis as patients with other subtypes of PTCL. Patients with ALK-negative ALCL carry the same poor prognosis as other subtypes of mature T-cell lymphoma, and may be suitable candidates for clinical trials in both the upfront and relapsed settings.

Nasal NKTCL: Combined-Modality Versus Single-Modality Approaches

Radiotherapy is considered the most active treatment for early-stage nasal NKTCL. For patients with limited stage IE or stage IE disease without any adverse factors, radiotherapy alone should be pursued with curative intent. Radiation produces complete RR of up to 70%; however, approximately 50% of patients who receive radiation alone will relapse, with about 25% of patients experiencing a systemic relapse. Hence, the addition of chemotherapy is intended to reduce the risk or recurrence, and is essential for advanced stages of nasal and extranasal NKTCL. For patients with extensive stage I and II disease, radiotherapy followed by consolidation with chemotherapy is commonly used. Because of the intrinsic drug resistance frequently seen in this disease, chemotherapy is not recommended as primary treatment in early-stage nasal NKTCL. Extranodal NKTCL is generally refractory to CHOP-based chemotherapy and is often associated with the expression of multidrug resistance (MDR) genes.

Despite the benefit of radiotherapy in this disease, a uniformly accepted standard of care has yet to be identified. Recently a phase

TABLE 85.2 Summary of Retrospective Up-Front Studies in Peripheral T-Cell Lymphoma

Regimen	PTCL Subtypes	n	CR (%)	OS
Anthracycline based	NK/T nasal	24	66.7	Not reported
Anthracycline based	PTCL-NOS	24	69.6	2 years: 63%
	NK/T nasal	51	56.0	2 years: 43%
Anthracycline based	PTCL-combined	174	49.0	4 years: 38%
	PTCL-NOS	95	47.0	4 years: 32%
	ALCL	30	69.0	
	AITL	22	37.0	
	NK/T nasal	14	46.0	
	EATL	12	27.0	
CHOP-like	AITL	33	60.6	5 years: 36%
CHOP type ± RT	NK/T nasal	7	28.6	
CMT	NK/T nasal	61	65.6	5 years: 41%
CHOP ± RT	PTCL-combined	78	52.6	5 years: 36%
	ALCL	13	69.2	
	PTCL-NOS	31	51.6	
	AITL	5	40.0	
	NK/T nasal	25	52.0	
Anthracycline based	PTCL-combined	66	62.0	5 years: 55%
	ALCL	19	79.0	
	PTCL-NOS	28	60.7	
	AITL	7	28.6	
Adriamycin based	Non-ALCL PTCL	96		5 years: 26%
Anthracycline based + RT	NK/T nasal	47	65.9	
CHOP based	NK/T nasal local	18	50.0	5 years: 15%
CHOP based + RT	NK/T nasal local	27	74.1	5 years: 59%
CHOP based	NK/T nasal systemic	10	60.0	5 years: 30%
CHOP based + RT	NK/T nasal systemic	10	30.0	5 years: 20%
CHOP type	PTCL-Nos	117	64.1	5 years: 35%
	ALCL	33	55.0	5 years: 43%
	AITL	10	70.0	5 years: 36%
	NK/T nasal	17	73.0	5 years: 24%
	EATL	9	33.0	5 years: 22%
CT + RT	NK/T nasal	16		5 years: 42%
CT	NK/T nasal	15		5 years: 20%
CHOP	Non-ALCL PTCL	24	58.0	3 years: 43%
CHOP intensive	Non-ALCL PTCL	52	59.0	3 years: 49%
CHOP/COPBLAM-V + RT	NK/T nasal	16	37.5	5 years: 59%
RT	NK/T nasal	33	52.0	5 years: 76%
CHOP type	PTCL-combined	125	53.0	5 years: 43%
	ALCL	21	71.0	5 years: 61%
	PTCL-NOS	70	55.0	5 years: 45%
	AITL	34	36.0	5 years: 28%
CHOP based + RT	NK/T nasal	71	84.5	5 years: 76%
CHOP alone	NK/T nasal	3	33.3	
Anthracycline-based	PTCL-NOS	340		5 years: 32%
	ALK-negative	72		5 years: 49%
	ALCL	243		5 years: 32%
	AITL	136		5 years: 42%
	NK/T nasal	62		3 years: 20%
	EATL			

AITL, Angioimmunoblastic T-cell lymphoma; ALCL, anaplastic large-cell lymphoma; CHOP, cyclophosphamide, hydroxydaunomycin, vincristine (Oncovin), and prednisone; CMT, combined modality therapy; COPBLAM-V, cyclophosphamide, vincristine (Oncovin), prednisone, bleomycin, doxorubicin (Adriamycin), and procarbazine; CR, complete remission; CT, chemotherapy; EATL, enteropathy-associated T-cell lymphoma; NK, natural killer; NOS, not otherwise specified; OS, overall survival, PTCL, peripheral T-cell lymphoma; RT, radiotherapy.

I/II study using concurrent chemotherapy and radiotherapy was reported. Patients were treated concurrently with radiotherapy and chemotherapy, which included carboplatin, etoposide, ifosfamide, and dexamethasone. Among the 26 patients reported, the objective response rate (ORR) was 81% with 77% CR. The most common grade 3 nonhematologic toxicity was mucositis (30% of patients), which was attributed to the radiotherapy. With a median follow-up of 32 months, the study reported a 2-year OS of 78%, which compares very favorably with the historical control group, which received radiotherapy alone (45%). Increasingly, many physicians are considering combined-modality therapy as the best upfront treatment for this disease, despite the potentially significant associated toxicity.

Newer approaches for patients with advanced NKTCLs have explored integrating L-asparaginase into a dexamethasone (steroid), methotrexate, ifosfamide, and etoposide-based backbone (SMILE). Yong et al treated 18 patients that were refractory to CHOP with L-asparaginase, vincristine, dexamethasone, and involved field radiotherapy. The ORR was 83.3%, with 10 (55.6%) of the patients achieving CR, and five (27.8%) achieving partial response (PR). The 5-year OS rate was 55.6%. Results of the preliminary clinical study indicated that the L-asparaginase–based salvage regimens significantly improved the RR and 5-year survival rate. A prospective phase II trial has been reported with the SMILE regimen in patients with newly diagnosed stage IV or relapsed refractory NKTCLs. Among the 39 patients treated, 29 (74%) completed the planned treatment. The responses included 15 patients in CR and 14 in PR, with early deaths due to infection in four patients. Infection was the most commonly observed toxicity, seen in 41% of the patients. Based on these studies, we conclude that L-asparaginase may have a role either in the upfront setting or for patients with relapsed or refractory disease.

Efforts to find approaches with a more favorable safety profile have led to the development of regimens built on drugs that are not affected by P-glycoprotein. The GELOX regimen (gemcitabine, oxaliplatin, and L-asparaginase) with involved field radiotherapy sandwiched between chemotherapy was studied in patients with stage IE/IIE extranodal NKTCL (EN-NKTCL) by the Chinese. The prospective study reported a ORR of 96.3% with a 74% rate of CR. Grade 3 or 4 toxicities were minimal, and no treatment-related deaths occurred. The rates of 2-year OS and PFS were both 86%, with patients achieving a CR doing substantially better than patients not in CR. These data, while now being studied in larger patient populations, is promising, and may afford a new and improved approach to patients with EN-NKTCL.

Adult T-Cell Leukemia/Lymphoma: Role of Antiviral Agents

The results of traditional chemotherapy in patients with ATL, like in other forms of PTCL, have been uniformly poor, leading to a consensus recommendation to enroll patients when possible in a clinical trial in either the upfront or relapsed or refractory setting. This recommendation is relevant for patients with most subtypes of PTCL. Although there is again no standard of care for these patients, the general sentiment is that CHOP-based chemotherapy regimens are inadequate. Owing to the comparatively higher incidence of ATL in Japan, many studies regarding the management of ATL come from Asia. The Japanese evaluated a complex combination regimen of VCAP (vincristine, cyclophosphamide, doxorubicin [Adriamycin], and prednisone), AMP (doxorubicin [Adriamycin], ranimustine [MCNU], and prednisone), and VECP (vindesine, etoposide, carboplatin, and prednisone) against CHOP-14 in ATL. A total of 118 patients were enrolled in the trial and treated with either six courses of VCAP-AMP-VECP every 4 weeks or eight courses of biweekly CHOP. The CR rate was higher in the VCAP-AMP-VECP arm than in the CHOP-14 arm (40% vs. 25%, respectively), and the progression-free survival (PFS) at 1 year was 28% in the VCAP-AMP-VECP arm compared with 16% in the CHOP arm. The OS at 3 years was 24% in the VCAP-AMP-VECP arm and 13% in the CHOP arm. Overall, the toxicity in the VCAP-AMP-VECP arm was

higher than in the CHOP-14 arm, with substantially more grade 3 or 4 cytopenias in the VCAP-AMP-VECP arm, which included three toxic deaths. Because most patients with ATL do not have curable disease when treated with these chemotherapy regimens, it is reasonable to consider allogeneic stem cell transplantation (aSCT) in patients who show responses to chemotherapy. Although this experience is very limited, there is some suggestion that there may be benefit in some patients.

Infection with HTLV-1 can cause ATL. Nineteen patients with acute or lymphomatous forms of ATL were treated with oral zidovudine (200 mg five times daily) and IFN-α (Intron A; 5–10 million units subcutaneously each day). Seven of these patients either relapsed or were refractory to combination chemotherapy. Major responses were achieved in 58% of the patients (11 of 19), including CR in 26% (5 of 19). Four patients in whom prior cytotoxic therapy had failed experienced major responses, two of which were CRs. Six patients have survived for more than 12 months, with the longest remission since the discontinuation of treatment lasting more than 59 months. A recent metaanalysis evaluated 116 patients with acute ATL, 18 patients with chronic ATL, 11 patients with smoldering ATL, and 100 patients with ATL lymphoma. The 5-year OS rates were 46% for 75 patients who received first-line antiviral therapy ($p = .004$), 20% for the 77 patients who received first-line chemotherapy, and 12% for the 55 patients who received first-line chemotherapy followed by antiviral therapy. The metaanalysis suggested that patients with acute, chronic, and smoldering ATL significantly benefited from first-line antiviral therapy, whereas patients with ATL lymphoma experienced a better outcome with chemotherapy. In acute ATL, 82% of patients were alive at 5 years with antiviral therapy, and 100% of patients with chronic and smoldering ATL were alive at 5 years. Multivariate analysis showed that first-line antiviral therapy significantly improved OS (HR = 0.47; 95% CI, 0.27–0.83; $p = .021$). Prospective studies are warranted to better define the role of antiviral therapy in treatment of ATL.

Given the activity of the anti-cc chemokine receptor 4 antibody (CCR4) mogamulizumab in ATL, a randomized phase II study explored integration of the biological into the mLSG15 regimen (the VCAMP/AMP/VECP regimen discussed earlier). Fifty-three patients with acute, lymphomatous, and chronic ATL were randomized to the mLSG15 ($n = 24$) or mLSG15 plus mogamulizumab ($n = 29$) regimens. The respective ORR and CR rates were 86% and 52% in the mogamulizumab-containing arm, and 75% and 33% in the sLSG15 alone arm. While the PFS was improved in the mogamulizumab arm (8.5 vs. 6.3 months), there was no difference in OS. In addition, there was substantially more toxicity in the antibody-containing arm, raising issues regarding how best to optimally integrate novel drugs such as mogamulizumab into standard cytotoxic regimens like mLSG15.

Angioimmunoblastic T-Cell Lymphoma: The Role of Cyclosporin and Rituximab

AITL is one of the most common forms of PTCL, with peculiar clinical and pathologic features. Although the normal counterpart has been recently identified as the T_{FH} cell, the nonneoplastic cells typically represent the quantitatively major component of AITL. Clinically the manifestations of the disease reflect a dysregulated immune and/or inflammatory response rather than being the direct complication of aberrant tumor growth, supporting the concept of a paraneoplastic immunologic dysfunction. Despite the use of different intensive anthracycline-based chemotherapies, AITL is an aggressive disease compared with other PTCLs, for which the optimal therapeutic strategy is still not defined. Given the considerable immune dysregulation present in AITL, the possible role of cyclosporine A (CsA) has been investigated in a small number of patients. Twelve patients were treated with the immunomodulatory CsA, 10 of whom had failed prior therapy with either chemotherapy and/or steroids (one to two prior regimens). Two patients were untreated because of age or comorbid conditions. Three patients achieved CR and five a PR for an overall RR of 67%, suggesting a possible role for CsA in this setting. In AITL, symptoms linked to B-lymphocyte activation

Treatment of Peripheral T-Cell Lymphoma

Given that the mature T-cell lymphomas are relatively rare diseases, there is a lack of large randomized clinical trials comparing the "standard" CHOP (cyclophosphamide, hydroxydaunomycin, vincristine [Oncovin], and prednisone) and CHOP-like regimens to other more intensified chemotherapy strategies, or even other novel drug platforms. Our approach involves tailoring the treatment to the specific histologic subtype and age of the patient. From the outset, we send HLA typing for possible allogeneic stem cell transplant, assuming the patient is eligible, and request immunohistochemical staining of the primary tissue for CD30. Where possible, we preferentially try to put all patients on a clinical trial. For the majority of peripheral T-cell lymphomas, our standard initial approach is to use an etoposide-based regimen (CHOEP [cyclophosphamide, hydroxydaunomycin, vincristine (Oncovin), etoposide, and prednisone] or EPOCH [etoposide, prednisone, vincristine (Oncovin), cyclophosphamide, and hydroxydaunomycin]), especially for young patients or older adult patients with an excellent performance status. As alluded to earlier, there are some data to suggest a reduced failure-free interval and higher complete response rate. For patients with a poor performance status or older adult patients, standard CHOP administered on an every-21-day basis for six to eight cycles would be our preferred recommendation. In select cases, where an older adult patient is not a candidate for combination chemotherapy and requires palliative care, we have successfully used single-agent gemcitabine to obtain disease control and improve performance status. Those patients who attain a complete remission are usually referred for an autologous stem cell transplant. Those patients who do not attain a complete remission with standard front-line chemotherapy are typically referred for treatment with one of the drugs recently approved by the Food and Drug Administration for patients with relapsed or refractory disease, including pralatrexate, romidepsin, belinostat, or brentuximab vedotin (if CD30+), or clinical studies exploring the merits of these agents in combination. For patients who relapse or are refractory to front-line and beyond therapy, we typically consider allogeneic stem cell transplant, assuming they are transplant eligible and have an appropriate human leukocyte antigen match.

are common, and variable numbers of CD20+ large B-blasts, often infected by EBV virus, are found in the neoplastic tissues. It has recently been suggested that the disruption of putative B- and T-cell interactions and/or depletion of the EBV reservoir by anti-CD20 monoclonal antibody (rituximab) might improve clinical outcome observed with conventional chemotherapy. Twenty five newly diagnosed patients were treated in a phase II study with eight cycles of rituximab plus chemotherapy (R-CHOP21). The complete RR was 44%, the 2-year PFS rate was 42%, and OS was 62%. This trial showed no clear benefit of adding rituximab to conventional chemotherapy (see box on Treatment of Peripheral T-Cell Lymphoma).

Role of Stem Cell Transplantation in Treatment

Because of the poor outcomes often seen with conventional chemotherapy in patients with PTCL, many investigators have explored high-dose chemotherapy followed by autologous or aSCT as front-line therapy and in patients who have relapsed. Despite the growing number of reports, one must keep in mind a number of limitations associated with these reports: (1) most of the studies are retrospective; (2) randomized trials comparing chemotherapy and SCT have not been published to date; (3) many prospective studies of autologous SCT include both front-line treatment and relapsed patients with diverse subtypes of PTCL, making the results difficult to interpret.

High-Dose Chemotherapy and Autologous Stem Cell Transplantation

High-dose chemotherapy followed by autologous SCT is currently accepted as the treatment of choice for patients with relapsed

aggressive B-cell lymphomas, resulting in 40%–50% long-term disease-free survival. The role of autologous SCT in PTCL is less clear, and whether or not autografting during first or subsequent remissions may be of clinical benefit remains uncertain.

Autologous SCT is usually performed as front-line consolidation therapy for young patients with PTCL. In this setting there are several prospective and retrospective studies evaluating this approach (see Table 85.1).

In a retrospective analysis, the Japan registry demonstrated that long-term outcome of PTCL was better in patients transplanted during first CR or partial remission (PR) than those not in remission (5-year OS, 72.9% vs. 45.8%; progression-free survival [PFS], 73.1% vs. 42.2%). The British Society of Bone Marrow Transplantation (BSBMT) and Stanford University reported similar data. The 2-year OS and PFS were 62% and 59%, respectively, for patients receiving autologous SCT as consolidation during first CR[3]. The Spanish group published a retrospective analysis of 74 patients undergoing autologous SCT after the achievement of CR with front-line anthracycline-based induction chemotherapy. After a median follow-up of 67 months, 5-year OS and PFS were 68% and 63%, respectively, and the main cause of death was disease progression. After a multivariate analysis, only the PIT score was significantly associated with OS and PFS. Although data about ALK expression were lacking, patients affected by ALCL had a significantly better outcome compared with other PTCL subtypes. The same authors published the results of a prospective study in 26 high-risk nodal PTCL patients, excluding those with ALK-positive ALCL. The patients who were positron emission tomography positive after three cycles of dose-escalated CHOP (MegaCHOP) received salvage chemotherapy followed by autologous SCT. After a median follow-up of 35 months, the 3-year OS and PFS of the entire cohort of patients were 73% and 56%, respectively, whereas those patients who were rescued by high-dose chemotherapy achieved a 2-year disease-free survival of 63%.

An Italian multicenter prospective study employed high-dose sequential chemotherapy followed by autologous SCT as front-line therapy in 62 patients with high-risk PTCL (stage III–IV and/or age-adjusted IPI >1) including 19 ALK-positive ALCL patients. On an intent-to-treat analysis, only 46 of 62 patients (74%) completed the whole program. Progressive disease during the induction phase was the main obstacle for proceeding to autologous SCT and the main reason for treatment failure. The high progression rate led to disappointing 12-year OS and EFS curves (34% and 30%, respectively). However, in the cohort of patients who did undergo autologous SCT, the RR was high: 89% of these patients achieved a CR. As in the Spanish study, patients with ALCL had the most favorable OS and EFS (62% and 54%, respectively, compared with 21% and 18%, respectively, of non-ALCL). On the other hand, when patients with PTCL-NOS were in CR at the time of transplant, the EFS was 62% versus 10% for those not in CR. The CR status remained a significant predictor of long-term outcome in multivariate analysis.

The German group published the results of a prospective multicenter study employing myeloablative doses of cyclophosphamide and total-body irradiation as the conditioning regimen for 83 ALK-negative ALCL patients who were at least in PR after six cycles of CHOP. Similar to the Italian data, 34% of patients did not complete the study because of progressive disease. The estimated 3-year OS was 71% for patients who received an autologous SCT compared with 11% for those who did not. A large registry study from the Swedish group confirmed a survival advantage for those patients who received an autologous SCT as front-line consolidation therapy. In this study, ALK-positive ALCL patients were excluded. Also after multivariate analysis, front-line ASCT was associated with a favorable PFS and OS compared with the cohort treated without autologous SCT. Of note, the addition of etoposide to CHOP chemotherapy was associated with a higher PFS in patients younger than 60 years, but this was not true for OS.

Although most of the published data include different histologic subtypes of PTCL, efforts have been made to define the role of autologous SCT in specific subtypes of PTCL. Some studies have focused on the results obtained with PTCL-NOS and ALCL patients, emphasizing that the histologic subtype can influence the outcome after autologous SCT. The Toronto group compared relapsed and refractory PTCL patients with those achieved with DLBCL patients, who were transplanted for the same indication over the same period of time. The 3-year OS and EFS were 48% and 37%, respectively, for PTCL patients, compared with 53% and 42%, respectively, for DLBCL patients. Nevertheless, a significantly different outcome has been reported when the subtypes of PTCL were analyzed individually. Patients with PTCL NOS had an inferior EFS (3-year EFS, 23%) when compared with patients with DLBCL. By contrast, patients with ALCL exhibited similar outcomes to patients with DLBCL. These results are consistent with data from a retrospective study performed at the Memorial Sloan-Kettering Cancer Center that reported a 5-year PFS of 24% for relapsed or refractory ALK-negative ALCL. The more favorable prognosis of ALCL after autologous SCT was confirmed by Northern Europe Investigators.

AITL patients have a median survival of 18 months after conventional chemotherapy, with less than 50% of the patients achieving a CR. A retrospective analysis of the European Group for Blood and Marrow Transplantation (EBMT) of autologous SCT in 146 AITL patients demonstrated an OS and PFS of 59% and 42%, respectively, at 4 years. PFS was longer in patients who received an autologous SCT in CR, 56% at 4 years, compared with 23% in the case of patients with chemotherapy-refractory disease.

EATL is another very poor prognosis PTCL subgroup, commonly associated with celiac disease. Because of its rarity, very few data on EATL treatment are available. In a prospective observational study using ASCT as front-line treatment, 5-year OS was 60% versus 22% for patients treated with standard chemotherapy. A retrospective study from EBMT confirmed these results on a cohort of 44 patients affected by EATL and treated with autologous SCT with a 4-year PFS and OS of 54% and 59%, respectively. Being in first CR or PR at the time of autologous SCT was associated with a trend for better survival compared with patients with a less favorable disease status (4-year OS 66% vs. 36%, $p = .062$).

Besides the differences in outcomes based on histologic subtypes and induction therapies, a common feature of PTCLs is that only two thirds of young patients are able to undergo the final autografting phase with a satisfactory disease response.

To increase the number of patients undergoing autologous SCT in CR or at least PR, some trials were designed with a more intense pretransplant phase. The Nordic Lymphoma Group included a dose-dense induction phase for 160 PTCL patients. After six cycles of CHOEP every 2 weeks, 85% of patients achieved CR and 70% proceeded with autologous SCT at last follow-up. Five-year OS and PFS were 50% and 43%, respectively. A Spanish group used alternating CHOP and ESHAP (etoposide, methylprednisolone, cytarabine, cisplatin) during the induction phase of 41 ALK-negative patients: 58% of the patients were in CR or PR after the induction phase, but only 41% underwent autologous SCT. More recently, the Italian Lymphoma Foundation performed an intensive front-line induction chemotherapy before transplant in young PTCL patients (excluding ALK-positive ALCL cases). Two cycles of CHOP plus alemtuzumab were followed by two cycles of HyperCHidam (methotrexate followed by hyperfractionated cyclophosphamide and cytarabin). Patients achieving a CR or PR received consolidation therapy with an autologous SCT or aSCT (in case of a compatible donor). With an intent-to-treat analysis, the 4-year PFS and OS were 44% and 49%, respectively. In fact, a clinical response was obtained in 62% of the study cohort, highlighting the need for more effective induction therapy for PTCLs.

Finally, the prognosis of PTCL patients seems poor when autologous SCT is used in patients with relapsed disease, where long-term remissions have been observed in less than one third of patients. Those who benefit the most are patients with ALK-positive ALCL in CR at time of transplant or those with a low IPI. A registry analysis from the Center for International Blood and Marrow Transplant Research (CIBMTR) confirmed these results. One hundred and fifteen patients received autologous SCT as front-line consolidation

therapy ($n = 40$) or as a component of a subsequent course of therapy ($n = 75$), with survival outcomes in favor of the front-line group: 3-year PFS of 58% versus 50% and 3-year OS of 70% versus 53%. Patients affected by ALCL were an exception. In this group, autologous SCT after first CR was still associated with good survival outcomes (3-year PFS 50% and OS 74%). Of note, ALK status was not available for these analyses.

In conclusion, the role of autologous SCT for the therapy of patients with PTCL may be summarized as follows: (1) young patients affected by PTCL appear to have an advantage when receiving an autologous SCT while in first CR; (2) ALK-positive ALCL patients have a more favorable outcome after autologous SCT, but they also do well with conventional chemotherapy, allowing this strategy to be possibly delayed to the salvage setting; (3) clinical protocols should be designed with more innovative pretransplant therapies in order to achieve optimal disease control prior to transplantation and thereby increasing the number of patients who are eligible to receive an autologous SCT.

Allogeneic Stem Cell Transplantation

aSCT has been most frequently used in PTCL patients with progressive or refractory disease after several courses of chemotherapy or in the case of relapse after an autologous SCT. This strategy is associated with the infusion of a lymphoma-free graft and the generation of a potentially active graft-versus-lymphoma (GvL) effect. Survival after myeloablative aSCT has been hampered by the high nonrelapse mortality (NRM) caused by graft-versus-host disease, infections, and acute organ toxicities.

Retrospective comparative analyses of autologous SCT versus aSCT in PTCL suffer the limitation of significant selection bias. In fact, patients receiving aSCT usually had more advanced disease, more prior lines of therapy, and/or bone marrow involvement. However, these studies have demonstrated that aSCT is associated with a lower relapse risk compared with autologous SCT, but also with a higher NRM, which offsets the survival benefit. The results of aSCT as a therapeutic strategy are listed in Table 85.2. A small retrospective comparative study conducted by the Spanish Lymphoma/Autologous Bone Marrow Transplant Study Group (GELTAMO) compared the outcome of patients receiving autologous SCT ($n = 29$) versus aSCT ($n = 7$) for PTCL. The 3-year OS was 39% and 29% for autologous SCT and aSCT, respectively. However, the majority of patients in the group receiving allogeneic grafts in CR died because of transplant-related complications. In 2006 a Japanese group published the first large analysis on the outcome of PTCL after myeloablative aSCT from matched related and unrelated donors. Kim and colleagues recently compared outcomes of patients affected by PTCL treated with autologous SCT ($n = 135$) versus myeloablative or reduced-intensity conditioning (RIC) aSCT ($n = 96$). No differences in survival was noted between the two groups (5-year OS 46% vs. 48%, $p = .34$), even though the aSCT group had more unfavorable features than the autologous SCT group in terms of prior courses of therapy and disease status at the time of transplant. Of note, despite a higher NRM, aSCT was able to induce a prolonged OS in 40% of patients who had chemorefractory disease, showing the efficacy of this salvage strategy for that group of PTCL patients that cannot achieve a response with standard chemotherapy. Similarly, Smith and colleagues compared 241 PTCL patients who received an autologous SCT ($n = 115$) or aSCT ($n = 126$). Also in this study, the two groups were different in terms of prior courses of therapy, chemosensitive disease, and histologic subtypes. In fact, the aSCT group had more unfavorable features including a lower number of ALCL patients. Two interesting results emerged from this study: the first was to confirm that performing a transplant (either autologous or allogeneic) later during the course of disease (after two or more prior courses of therapy) was associated with a threefold increased risk of relapse, fivefold increased risk of overall mortality, and a sevenfold risk of NRM; the second one was that autologous SCT at relapse was beneficial for those patients affected by ALCL (ALK status was not available) with superior overall survival compared with aSCT.

During the last 15 years, RIC regimens have been increasingly used in patients with relapsed lymphomas in order to reduce NRM, thus making this strategy feasible in older adults or heavily pretreated patients. In 2004 one of the first reports of RIC aSCT in PTCL patients reported that 56% of patients were alive and in CR after 1.4 years. The first prospective study evaluated the outcome of 17 relapsed PTCL patients after a fludarabine-based RIC regimen: 14 of 17 enrolled patients were alive (12 in CR) after a median follow-up of 28 months, with an estimated 3-year NRM, OS, and PFS of 6%, 81%, and 64%, respectively.

In this study, there were some data suggesting the existence of a GvL effect, based on the following observations: (1) the achievement of durable responses with aSCT in patients who had already failed a prior autologous SCT; and (2) the demonstration of clinical responses to donor lymphocyte infusions. These preliminary results were supported by a larger Italian multicenter retrospective study with a longer follow-up. In this study, the 5-year outcomes showed a NRM, OS, and PFS of 12%, 50%, and 40%, respectively, and a plateau in the survival curves after 36 months, suggesting a probable cure for these patients. Following multivariate analysis, being older than 45 years and having refractory disease were independent prognostic factors, highlighting that timing of an aSCT can significantly influence the final outcome. Similarly, in a French retrospective study of 77 PTCL patients receiving aSCT with both RIC or myeloablative conditioning regimens, those patients with chemosensitive disease or with less than two prior courses of chemotherapy at the time of transplant experienced better survival outcomes.

In both the Italian and French studies, survival was not significantly different among the histologic subtypes of T-cell lymphoma (of note, the ALK mutational majority of the ALCL patients was unknown), although patients with AITL did slightly better. In support of this finding, an EBMT retrospective analysis of 45 PTCL patients undergoing aSCT between 1998 and 2005 had a relapse risk of 20% at 3 years, with a PFS of 53% and an OS of 64%.

Several studies have reported survival outcomes of aSCT for PTCL patients when employed as front-line consolidation therapy. The only prospective study of this strategy showed encouraging 4-year PFS and OS of 69% using a RIC regimen and an HLA-compatible donor. Other retrospective studies have confirmed these data with a 2-year PFS and OS between 35%–65% and 40%–75%, respectively.

In conclusion, aSCT can be offered in relapsed and refractory PTCL based on the following observations: (1) in all studies survival curves seem to reach a plateau after 24–36 months, suggesting the potential curability of the disease; (2) delaying aSCT too long from the time of diagnosis may significantly compromise the outcome, thus aSCT should be performed during a chemosensitive relapse; (3) RIC regimens have increased the feasibility of performing aSCT by reducing NRM, and aSCT may be used in older and heavily pretreated patients. Hopefully in the future we will see if the combination of new agents with aSCT can improve the outcomes of a significant proportion of patients with refractory disease.

Emerging New Drugs for PTCL

There is little question that one of the most promising new areas in PTCL research is new drug development. Over the past several years, four new drugs, all with relatively unique mechanisms of action, have been approved for the treatment of patients with relapsed or refractory disease. These drugs, which all now have substantial data demonstrating their marked single-agent activity in these diseases, have created a unique opportunity to build non-CHOP–based platforms for treatment. In addition to the four drugs already approved, many new drugs are in various stages of clinical development, with very promising signals (Table 85.3). We will discuss some of these new agents and how they are beginning to change the treatment paradigms for PTCL.

Pralatrexate

Pralatrexate was the first drug approved for the treatment of patients with relapsed or refractory PTCL in 2009. Pralatrexate is a novel antifolate with very high affinity for the reduced folate carrier, designed to enhance its intracellular transport. The reduced folate carrier is an oncofetal protein expressed at relatively high levels on the surface of malignant cells. The carrier is responsible for transporting into the cell natural folate required for DNA biosynthesis. Pralatrexate, designed to have a high affinity for the folate receptors, is rapidly internalized into the cell, where it undergoes efficient polyglutamylation by the folylpolyglutamate synthase, which enhances the affinity of the drug for dihydrofolate reductase and increases its intracellular retention.

TABLE 85.3 Recent FDA-Approved and Emerging New Drugs in Peripheral T-Cell Lymphoma

Drug	Disease/No. of Patients	Overall Response Rate	Complete Response Rate	PFS/DOR
Pralatrexate (accelerated approval 2009)	Relapsed/refractory PTCL N = 111	29%	11%	Median DOR = 10.1 months
Romidepsin (accelerated approval 2011)	Relapsed/refractory PTCL N = 130	25%	15%	Median DOR = 17 months
Brentuximab vedotin (accelerated approval 2011)	CD30+ anaplastic large-cell lymphoma N = 58	86%	57%	Median DOR = 12.6 months
KW-0761	HTLV-1 ATL N = 27	13 of 26 (50%)	8 of 13 (61%)	PFS = 5.2 months
Bortezomib	Relapsed/refractory CTCL and PTCL N = 12	8 of 12 (67%) (2 patients with PTCL)	2 of 12 (17%) (1 of 2 patients with PTCL)	Not reported
Lenalidomide	Relapsed/refractory PTCL N = 10 (Zinzani) N = 24 (Dueck)	30% 30%	3 of 10 0 of 7	Not reported Median PFS 96 days
Alisertib	Relapsed/refractory PTCL N = 8	4 of 8 (50%)	2 of 4	Not reported

ATL, Adult T-cell leukemia/lymphoma; CTCL, cutaneous T-cell lymphoma; DOR, duration of response; FDA, Food and Drug Administration; HTLV-1, human T-lymphotropic virus-1; PFS, progression-free survival; PTCL, peripheral T-cell lymphoma.

A phase "II–I–II" study of pralatrexate in patients with relapsed or refractory NHL established the maximum tolerated dose as 30 mg/m² weekly for 6 of 7 consecutive weeks of treatment. The dose-limiting toxicity was determined to be mucositis, which was largely controlled with the addition of folic acid and vitamin B₁₂. These data revealed an ORR of 31% among the entire population of patients with both B- and T-cell lymphoma ($n = 48$ evaluable), of which eight patients obtained a CR. Among the 20 evaluable patients with B-cell lymphoma, the ORR was 5%, of which there were no CRs. Among the 26 evaluable patients with T-cell lymphoma, the ORR was 54%, of which there were eight CRs. All the CRs, many of which were very durable and included patients who had responded to prior methotrexate, were seen exclusively in patients with PTCL.

These data gave rise to a pivotal study of pralatrexate in patients with most subtypes of relapsed or refractory PTCL. The Pralatrexate in Patients With Relapsed or Refractory Peripheral T-Cell Lymphoma (PROPEL) study was an international, open-label, single-arm trial in which pralatrexate was administered at a dose of 30 mg/m² weekly for 6 of 7 consecutive weeks. At the time, it was the largest study ever conducted in this patient population. Of 115 patients enrolled, 111 were treated with pralatrexate. Overall, the patient population was very heavily pretreated, with the median number of prior therapies being 3, with a range of 1 to 12. Twenty percent of patients in PROPEL had received more than five lines of prior chemotherapy. Of all the new drug studies that have emerged recently, the PROPEL study accrued the greatest diversity of patients with PTCL including patients with blastic NK/T-cell lymphoma, ATLL, and transformed mycosis fungoides (MF), which are variably excluded from other studies. In addition, the PROPEL population was, to date, the most heavily treated population of the studies reported. The RR among the 109 evaluable patients was 29%, which included 12 CRs (11%), with an updated median duration of response of over 121 months. The most common grade 3 or 4 toxicities included thrombocytopenia and mucositis. These data led to pralatrexate becoming the first drug ever approved by the United States Food and Drug Administration (FDA) for PTCL, receiving accelerated approval in late 2009.

Detailed population pharmacokinetic and pharmacodynamics studies have demonstrated that two variables had the greatest impact on the risk of mucositis from pralatrexate, including: (1) area under the curve of exposure; and (2) pretreatment methylmalonic acid and homocysteine levels. These observations have given rise over the past few years to several modifications of drug administration. The first has involved the incorporation of leucovorin into the standard administration of pralatrexate. Given the profoundly greater affinity of pralatrexate for the reduced folate carrier, risks of mitigating efficacy with coadministration seem to be far less. Albeit early, these evolving experiences suggest that leucovorin after and prior to pralatrexate can markedly reduce the risk of mucositis, and in some cases allows for higher doses of the drug to be tolerated, at least in preclinical models. Similarly, the contribution of idiosyncratic AUC drug exposure has been addressed with a titrated dose-escalation approach (10 mg/m² week 1; 20 mg/m² week 2; and 30 mg/m² week 3, on a 4-week dosing basis), allowing for a tailoring of the dose to the idiosyncratic disposition of the drug in a given patient. These approaches, while preliminary in nature, are being studied in larger populations of patients.

Probably the greatest advances in recent years with not just pralatrexate, but all these agents emerging in PTCL, has been the emergence of both preclinical and clinical data confirming marked synergy with pralatrexate and other drugs, including gemcitabine, bortezomib, histone deacetylase (HDAC) inhibitors (HDACIs) such as romidepsin, and belinostat. Much of this preclinical experience has now been translated into early proof-of-principal clinical studies.

Histone Deacetylase Inhibitors

The HDACIs appear to exhibit a consistent pattern of activity in T-cell neoplasms, with little to no activity in B-cell lymphoid malignancies. Acetylation of histone proteins facilitates an open chromatin structure, leading to access by transcription factors and thus transcriptional activation. Conversely, HDACs facilitate deacetylation of chromatin, which leads to a closed chromatin structure and transcriptional silencing. Although the modulation of chromatin structure has been long postulated as one of the key mechanisms for HDACI activity, it is now widely recognized that these drugs are more appropriately recognized as more general protein deacetylase inhibitors. In this capacity, it is also recognized that HDACIs may functionally affect tumor cell growth and survival by modulating the posttranslational state of different proteins, which leads to activation or inactivation of various tumor suppressor genes or oncogenes. While it is not precisely known how or why this class of drugs work consistently in PTCL, overexpression of HDAC1, HDAC2, and HDAC6, as well as acetylated histone 4 (H4) have been seen in select subtypes of the disease.

To date, three HDAC inhibitors have been approved for the treatment of cancer, including: (1) vorinostat for the treatment of relapsed or refractory CTCL; (2) romidepsin approved for relapsed or refractory CTCL and PTCL; and (3) belinostat approved for the treatment of relapsed or refractory PTCL. The first HDACI approved for the treatment of cancer was vorinostat, or SAHA. Vorinostat is a hydroxamic acid derivative known to be a potent class 1–2 inhibitor of HDAC. Early developmental clinical studies performed with both intravenous and oral vorinostat demonstrated that the drug could inhibit HDACs, leading to accumulation of acetylated H3/H4. These studies also demonstrated that the drug was well tolerated for extended periods of time, with dose-limiting toxicities of fatigue, diarrhea, and anorexia for the oral formulations, and myelosuppression for the intravenous formulations. Expanded phase II experiences with vorinostat confirmed single-agent activity in HL-transformed lymphomas and CTCL. These data gave rise to pivotal studies in CTCL, leading to FDA approval in 2006.

Romidepsin is a potent macrolide HDAC inhibitor isolated from *Chromobacterium violaceum*. An early phase I–II trial demonstrated that romidepsin exhibited marked single-agent activity in patients with relapsed or refractory CTCL and PTCL. In fact, among 47 patients with relapsed or refractory PTCL, excluding patients with transformed MF and HTLV-1 ATL, which were included in the PROPEL study, an ORR of 38% was noted, including eight patients who attained a CR. The most common toxicities were very similar to those reported for vorinostat and included nausea, fatigue, and transient thrombocytopenia. The median duration of response was roughly 8.9 months, and responses were seen in most of the PTCL subtypes studied. These data gave rise to an international, open-label, pivotal phase II study of romidepsin in patients with relapsed or refractory PTCL who had received at least one line of prior therapy. Of the 131 patients enrolled, 130 had histologically confirmed PTCL. The median number of prior therapies was 1, with a range of 1 to 8. The ORR was 25%, which included 19 (15%) CRs, and the median duration of response was 17 months. These data led to a conditional approval of romidepsin in patients with relapsed or refractory PTCL by the FDA in June of 2011.

In 2014 belinostat became the third HDAC inhibitor approved for the treatment of cancer, specifically patients with relapsed or refractory PTCL. Belinostat is a hydroxamic-based pan class I and II HDAC inhibitor. It is currently approved for patients with relapsed or refractory PTCL who have received at least one line of prior therapy. The original phase II (CLN-6) trial included patients with various subtypes of T-cell lymphomas (TCLs; $n = 24$), and produced an ORR of 25% in relapsed/refractory PTCL. This activity was the basis for initiating the BELIEF study, where 129 patients with relapsed and refractory disease received belinostat. The median number of prior therapies was 2. The ORR was 26% (11% CR; 15% PR), with a PFS and OS of 1.6 and 7.9 months, respectively, and a median duration of response of 13.6 months. Forty-six percent of patients with AITL experienced a response.

Recent data have now suggested that pralatrexate potently synergizes with other HDAC inhibitors in models of T-cell lymphoma. These data are now being used as a rationale to support a multicenter phase I study that will define the maximum tolerated dose of this regimen, and then the tolerability and activity in a subpopulation of patients with PTCL.

Brentuximab Vedotin

Monoclonal antibodies have emerged as potentially important new therapeutic tools in the treatment of many subtypes of NHL. Monoclonal antibodies are now being developed against a host of other cell surface proteins, including the chemokine receptor CCR4, and other surface proteins such as CD4 and more recently CD30. CD30 (also known as *TNFRSF8*) is a 120-kD transmembrane protein of the tumor necrosis factor family and a known tumor marker found on many kinds of lymphoma. The receptor is found on the surface of only activated T cells, and some B cells. CD30 is found on virtually all cases of ALCL, and the majority of cases of Hodgkin lymphoma (HL), where it is seen on the surface of the Reed-Sternberg cell. It is also expressed by several nonlymphoid malignancies, including embryonal carcinoma and some cases of non–small–cell lung cancer. Clinical trials with the chimeric anti-CD30 monoclonal antibody were uniformly disappointing in patients with ALCL and HL. For example, among 38 patients with HL and 41 patients with ALCL treated with SGN-30, no responses were seen in patients with HL, whereas two patients with ALCL achieved a CR. Similar results have been reported with other anti-CD30 monoclonal antibodies.

Conjugation of small molecules to highly targeted monoclonal antibodies to create an antibody–drug conjugate offers a promising way to deliver highly toxic drugs to select populations of cells. The conjugation of a highly potent antimicrotubule agent, monomethyl auristatin E to the anti-CD30 monoclonal antibody creates a novel antibody–drug conjugate called *SGN-35*, or *brentuximab vedotin*. Clinical trials of this drug in patients with HL and ALCL have demonstrated remarkable activity in these CD30-expressing diseases. A pivotal trial of brentuximab vedotin in patients with relapsed or refractory ALCL produced an ORR of 86%, with a CR rate of 57%. These remissions were found to be very durable, with a median response duration of 12.6 months and a median duration of response among patients in CR of 13.2 months. The majority of patients enrolled in the study exhibited poor prognostic features: 72% of patients had ALK-negative ALCL, 63% of patients were refractory to front-line therapy, and 22% of patients had never responded to any prior therapy. These results recently led the FDA to grant accelerated approval to brentuximab vedotin in patients with ALCL. A subsequent experience in non-ALCL PTCL ($n = 35$ patients), essentially restricted to PTCL-NOS and AITL, revealed an ORR of 41% (24% with a CR), with a median PFS and duration of response of 2.6 months and 7.6 months, respectively. Ongoing studies are now exploring the benefits of this drug in combination with standard upfront chemotherapy regimens such as CHOP.

KW-0761

Another novel cell surface protein for which there is now a targeted drug is the CCR4 chemokine receptor, which is encoded by the *CCR4* gene. CCR4 has also recently been designated *CD194*. The CCR4 protein belongs to the G-protein–coupled receptor family and is a receptor for many different cytokines that influence the behavior of leukocytes. CCR4 is known to be expressed on Th2 cells and regulatory T cells. Several studies have demonstrated that CCR4 is expressed at relatively high levels on select T-cell neoplasms, including HTLV-1 ATLL. KW-0761 is a defucosylated humanized IgG1 anti-CCR4 monoclonal antibody that enhances antibody-dependent cellular cytotoxicity and has been evaluated in multicenter phase I and II studies in patients with relapsed, aggressive CCR4+ ATL.

Patients received intravenous infusions of KW-0761 once a week for 8 weeks at a dose of 1.0 mg/kg. The phase II study of KW-0761 was conducted in 28 patients with relapsed or refractory ATL. The overall RR was 50%, including eight complete responses, and the median PFS and OS were 5.2 and 13.7 months, respectively. The most common adverse events were infusion reactions (89%) and skin rashes (63%), which were manageable and reversible in all cases. Albeit relatively early, this study demonstrated clinically meaningful antitumor activity in patients with relapsed aggressive ATL, with an acceptable toxicity profile. Another study in 2014 evaluated 37 patients with relapsed CCR4+ PTCL. The authors noted objective responses for 35% of the patients including 14% with a CR. The ORR was 34% in patients with PTCL (three of 16 for PTCL-NOS, six of 12 for AITL, and one of one for ALCL, ALK negative). The median PFS and OS for patients with PTCL were 2 months (8.2 months for PTCL responders) and 14.2 months, respectively. Interestingly, the total ORR did not significantly correlate with CCR4 expression level. Further investigation of KW-0761 for treatment of ATL and other T-cell neoplasms are now warranted.

Miscellaneous Agents

The drugs mentioned earlier all represent agents that have been studied in a reasonable number of patients with T-cell lymphoma, and have been approved by regulatory agencies for select diseases. In addition to these there are other agents with very early and potentially promising signals of activity in PTCL.

Proteasome Inhibitors

The proteasome inhibitors, including bortezomib and carfilzomib, have marked activity in multiple myeloma and mantle cell lymphoma. Although the experience in PTCL is modest, 10 patients with CTCL and two with PTCL were treated with bortezomib at a dose of 1.3 mg/m² on a day 1, 4, 8, and 11 schedule. Although the ORR was reported to be 67%, dramatic responses were seen in patients with advanced CTCL, and one of the two patients with PTCL experienced a CR. Emerging data have now demonstrated that the proteasome inhibitors potently synergize with the HDACIs and pralatrexate, which is now leading to combination studies in patients with PTCL.

Immunomodulatory Drugs

Another novel class of drugs with a signal of activity in the T-cell lymphomas includes the immunomodulatory drug lenalidomide. This class of drugs is thought to increase the immunologic synapse by increasing NK cell activity against the lymphoma cells. In one report, lenalidomide was administered orally for 21 days on a 28-day cycle at a dose of 25 mg daily in 24 patients with relapsed or refractory PTCL with an ORR of 30% being reported (seven responses among 23 evaluable patients), with no CR. Responses were seen in patients with ALCL, AITL, and PTCL-NOS. The median PFS was 96 days. Similar results were reported among 10 patients with relapsed and refractory PTCL-NOS, where three CRs were reported.

Alisertib (Aurora A Kinase Inhibitor)

Preliminary reports from a phase II study of a novel aurora A kinase inhibitor, MLN8237/alisertib, in patients with aggressive NHL have recently demonstrated activity in patients with PTCL. An initial phase II trial of alisertib in patients with B- and T-cell lymphoma demonstrated an ORR of 27%, and in eight patients with PTCL, a RR of 50%. Recently, SWOG-1108 evaluated alisertib in 37 patients with PTCL in the relapsed and refractory setting. In this study, Barr et al reported two CRs and seven PRs, with an ORR of 24% and 33%, respectively, for the most common subtypes (PTCL-NOS, AITL, and ALCL). The LUMIERE trial, which is a phase III study of alisertib versus investigator's choice (pralatrexate, romidepsin, gemcitabine) in relapsed/refractory PTCL has recently closed and we eagerly await these results.

Bendamustine

The BENTLY trial evaluated bendamustine in 60 patients with relapsed or refractory PTCL. The ORR was 50%, including a CR rate of 28% and a PR rate of 22%. The drug showed consistent efficacy independent of major disease characteristics. The median

PFS and duration of response were 3.6 and 3.5 months, respectively.

Sorafenib

Sorafenib is a multikinase inhibitor that modulates multiple intracellular pathways, including PDGFR/VEGFR and MAP kinase signaling. One report evaluated sorafenib in 12 patients with T-cell lymphomas (three with PTCL and nine with CTCL). While the population was not that heavily treated (median number or prior treatments = 2), three achieved a CR and one underwent aSCT. The median EFS for the entire cohort was 3.5 months. At a median follow-up of 11.2 months, 10 patients were alive (83%) and disease stabilization or reduction was noted in 75% of patients.

Duvelisib

Duvelisib (IPI-145) is an oral inhibitor of PI3K-δ and -γ. Mutation in PI3K has been found to be a recurring finding across all of cancer biology, as this pathway plays a critical role regulating many cellular processes including cell survival, proliferation, and differentiation. PI3K-δ and PI3K-γ isoforms are preferentially expressed in leukocytes with distinct roles in T-cell function. A phase I trial of duvelisib was performed which included 16 patients with PTCL. The median number of prior therapies was four. Of the 31 patients evaluable, an ORR of 42% was observed and in PTCL, the ORR was 47%, with two CRs and five PRs.

Plitidepsin

Plitidepsin is a cyclic depsipeptide originally isolated from the tunicate *Aplidium albicans* and is commercially produced by chemical synthesis. It displays a broad spectrum of anticancer activities, including induction of apoptosis and G1/G2 cell cycle arrest. Plitidepsin has demonstrated reproducible activity against a variety of malignant cell lines, including leukemias and lymphomas. A phase II trial evaluated plitidepsin in 67 patients, which included 34 patients with relapsed/refractory noncutaneous PTCL. Of the 29 evaluable patients with noncutaneous PTCL, six patients demonstrated an objective response to plitidepsin (two CRs and four PRs; ORR = 20.7%) with a median PFS and duration of response of 1.6 and 2.2 months, respectively.

FUTURE DIRECTIONS

Over the past several years there has been a remarkable increase in our understanding of the diversity within the PTCLs. The appreciation that the mature T-cell lymphomas represent a vast spectrum of both indolent and aggressive subtypes, commonly associated with diverse clinical pictures with substantial global variation, has shaped how we now classify and think about these diseases. Even prognosticating the outcomes of patients with these diseases has become remarkably complicated, because each subtype of PTCL is now widely recognized as possessing its own unique clinical behavior and thus its own unique response to different therapeutic approaches. Eventually these prognostic models will be used to better risk-stratify patients at diagnosis, allowing physicians to institute an optimal treatment plan earlier, which may include ASCT for select patients and aSCT for those with relapsed or refractory disease.

Unquestionably, however, the increase in the number of new drugs available for the treatment of this group of diseases has begun to reshape our options when considering the management of patients with relapsed or refractory disease. As these new drugs are used with increasing frequency, each having significant single-agent activity in these traditionally chemotherapy-resistant diseases, the emergence of novel non-CHOP–based drug combinations will likely emerge. Perhaps most exciting is the recent demonstration that combinations of these agents are associated with marked synergy in the preclinical setting, including combinations of drugs such as pralatrexate and romidepsin, hypomethylating agents and HDAC inhibitors, and aurora A kinase inhibitors, and romidepsin, many of which are being translated to the clinical setting with early promise of tolerability and

marked activity. It is likely that a systematic analysis of agents with lineage-specific activity in PTCL will form the basis of novel, PTCL-specific treatment platforms that will create future non-CHOP–based opportunities for front-line care.

CUTANEOUS T-CELL LYMPHOMAS

This portion of the chapter focuses on the disorders that would be encompassed by the diagnosis *cutaneous T-cell lymphoma* (Table 85.4). The most common subtypes of CTCLs are the epidermotropic variants MF and the related leukemic variant, Sézary syndrome (SS).

Epidemiology

CTCLs account for 71% of the 3844 cutaneous lymphomas diagnosed in the United States between 2001 and 2010. MF and SS are the most common CTCL subtypes worldwide, constituting 54% of

TABLE 85.4	Comparison of EORTC and WHO Classifications of Primary Cutaneous Lymphoma
EORTC Classification	**WHO Classification**
Cutaneous T-Cell Lymphoma	
Indolent clinical behavior	Mycosis fungoides
Mycosis fungoides variants	Mycosis fungoides variants
Follicular mycosis fungoides	Follicular mycosis fungoides
Pagetoid reticulosis	Pagetoid reticulosis
CTCL, large cell, CD30+	Primary cutaneous CD30+ ALCL (CD30+ lymphoproliferative disease, including lymphomatoid papulosis)
Lymphomatoid papulosis	
Aggressive clinical behavior	
Sézary syndrome	Sézary syndrome
CTCL, large cell, CD30-	Peripheral T-cell lymphoma, unspecified (most); extranodal NK/T-cell lymphoma, nasal type
Provisional Entities	
CTCL, pleomorphic, small/medium sized	
Subcutaneous panniculitis-like T-cell lymphoma	Subcutaneous panniculitis-like T-cell lymphoma
Cutaneous B-Cell Lymphoma	
Indolent clinical behavior	Extranodal marginal zone B-cell lymphoma
Primary cutaneous immunocytoma (marginal zone B-cell lymphoma)	
Follicle center cell lymphoma (any grade)	
Intermediate clinical behavior	
Primary cutaneous large B-cell lymphoma of the leg	
Provisional Entities	
Primary cutaneous plasmacytoma	Plasmacytoma
Intravascular large B-cell lymphoma	Diffuse large B-cell lymphoma (intravascular)

ALCL, Anaplastic large-cell lymphoma; CTCL, cutaneous T-cell lymphoma; EORTC, European Organization for Research and Treatment of Cancer; NK, natural killer; WHO, World Health Organization.

the CTCLs and an annual incidence of approximately four cases per million people. MF and SS are the most common primary lymphomas involving the skin. Data collected from the SEER program showed a rapidly increasing incidence from 0.2 cases per 100,000 people in 1973 to 0.4 cases per 100,000 people in 1984. This increasing trend has stabilized in the last decade, with an incidence of 10.2 new annual cases per million during the period 2005–2009 (PMID: 24005876).

Whether this represented a true increase in incidence or was attributable to a better awareness and therefore more frequent recognition of this disease has not been resolved. Since that time the incidence rate of CTCL has stabilized at 0.36 cases per 100,000 persons, and the mortality rate has declined. The incidence of MF/SS increases with advancing age, as does the incidence of NHLs in general. The average age at presentation is approximately 50 years. Although cases in very young patients have been reported, most patients are at least 30 years of age. MF/SS is seen in all racial groups. There is a 1.6:1 ratio of African-Americans to whites and a 2.2:1 ratio of men to women with this disorder. MF is less common in the Asian population. Identification of clusters of CTCL in certain geographic regions has been reported using two distinct cancer registries (PMID: 25728286; PMID: 25046454).

Clusters of cases of MF/SS within families have been reported. An association with histocompatibility antigens AW31, AW32, B8, BW35, and DR5 has been described. However, a solid genetic predisposition or inherited genetic defect has not been demonstrated.

Pathobiology

The T lymphocyte is central to the body's ability to mount an immune response and is the precursor of neoplastic cells in MF/SS. Sézary cells respond to phytohemagglutinin and perform T-cell immunoregulatory functions similar to normal lymphocytes. The clonal nature of CTCL has been demonstrated by Southern blotting or polymerase chain reaction methods for analysis of the TCR.

The development of monoclonal antibodies directed against different T-cell antigens has allowed for more precise identification of surface markers on the malignant T cells. Most cases of MF and SS are comprised of the helper memory or effector T cells with a $CD4^+CD45RO^+$ phenotype. In most instances, the cells express the pan–T-cell antigens CD2 (the sheep erythrocyte receptor), CD3, and CD5. CD7 is a T-cell marker expressed in early differentiation, but usually absent in T-cell homing to the skin. Although benign conditions may show some downregulation of CD7, marked deletion of CD7 is commonly used by the pathologist as an ancillary confirmatory test for CTCL. Flow cytometry provides a sensitive method for detecting early peripheral blood involvement in patients by detection of $CD4^+CD26^-$ T-cell populations. A small subset of MF is characterized by the expression of CD8, a marker that is essentially never expressed in SS. Low expression of the α-chain component of the IL-2 receptor (CD25) is detected with heterogeneous expression by the malignant cells in less than half of the patients. The implication of this finding is of uncertain significance, because both activated T cells and immunoregulatory T cells can express CD25. Key signaling pathway alterations that affect MF and SS include Notch overexpression, Fas underexpression, and the association of PKC inhibition with apoptosis. Also of particular relevance is the observation of increased expression of programmed death-1 (PD-1) on SS cells, compared with $CD4^+$ cells from healthy volunteers and from MF patients, likely contributing to the impaired immunity (antitumor and antiinfectious) noted in SS patients. Overexpression of KIR3DL2 (CD158k) has also been observed in SS and advanced MF, and may assist in distinguishing CTCL cells from normal ones, but more important, it may have targeted therapeutic implications. Increased mRNA expression of *PLS3*, *DNM3*, and *TWIST1* have also been reported in most cases (PMID: 18033314).

Cytogenetic analyses have demonstrated numeric and structural chromosomal abnormalities in MF/SS, although usually in advanced-stage disease. Hyperdiploidy and complex karyotypes are common.

Nonrandom deletions of chromosomes 1p, 6, 8, 9p10q, and 17p have been reported, with gains in chromosome 17q and 4p occurring in more than 25% of cases. Regions of the genome that include genes encoding the TCR do not appear to be involved, suggesting that the genetic basis for malignant transformation in MF/SS appears to be different from that involved in other T-cell malignant disorders.

Modest data exist on the aberrant expression of oncogenes and suppressor genes in MF/SS. Loss of heterozygosity is identified in 30%–60% of patients, commonly at 9p, 10q, 1p, and 17p. Loss of heterozygosity in early stages of disease is associated with a threefold increase in mortality. Various mutations involving the Fas pathway are commonly seen from the early stages of lymphomagenesis, reflecting an initial accumulation of abnormal lymphocytes secondary to abnormal proapoptotic pathways. Mutant forms of the *p53* tumor suppressor gene are rarely observed, usually in tumor stage and large-cell transformation of MF. LYT-10, a member of the NFκB family of transcription factors associated with translocations in lymphoid malignancies, is rearranged in a small proportion of cases. However, *BCL2*, a gene whose rearrangement is characteristic of follicular B-cell lymphomas and which slows programmed cell death, is overexpressed in MF. Constitutive phosphorylation of STAT3 (a member of the transcription factor family that contributes to the diversity of cytokine responses) has been reported and suggests that these malignant T cells are activated. Altered expression or release of select cytokines or their receptors, including IL-1, IL-2R, IL-4, IL-5, IL-6, IL-7, IL-8, IL-12, and TGF-β receptor II, has been noted. IL-7 and IL-15 have been identified as growth factors for MF/SS and shown to regulate expression of the *BCL2* and *MYB* oncogenes and stimulate DNA binding of STAT proteins. NFκB has also been demonstrated to be constitutively activated in CTCL and leads to transcription of antiapoptotic genes (e.g., Bcl-2, cIAP1, and cIAP2), proinflammatory genes, and antiinflammatory genes, resulting in increased survival and the immunosuppressive nature of CTCLs. Constitutive activation of c-Jun N-terminal kinases (JNKs) and JAK may lead to elevated levels of VEGF, resulting in increased angiogenesis. Massive parallel targeted sequencing of a set of 524 genes from CTCL samples revealed frequent mutations of the NFκB, JAK/STAT, and PLC pathways. Three samples harbored mutations of *PLCG1*, the gene that encodes for phospholipase C, gamma 1. Further analysis of another cohort of samples from 42 CTCL patients revealed the presence of *PLCG1* S345F mutation in 19% of the cases and was associated with increased signaling of calcineurin/nuclear factor of activated T cells (NFAT). In vitro inhibition of PLC and calcineurin led to decreased cell proliferation and increased apoptosis in mutant cells. There is also evidence of the role of the mTOR-containing complex 1 (mTORC1) pathway in CTCL pathogenesis, along with evidence to support the beneficial role of its inhibition simultaneously with inhibition of MNK kinase. Various cancer-testis antigens, normally observed only in testicular germ cells, appear to be ectopically expressed in CTCL, as does B-lymphoid tyrosine kinase (Blk), a member of the Src kinase family, which is normally only expressed in B cells and thymocytes. Supporting the tumorigenic role of Blk, there was antitumor activity of dasatinib, a Src kinase inhibitor, within a Blk+ CTCL cell line and a xenograft mouse model. There is recent evidence suggesting that SS and MF may follow different molecular pathways with dysregulation of genes encoding c-Myc and c-Myc regulatory proteins commonly associated with SS but not with MF.

The cause of MF/SS remains unknown. It is considered to be a sporadic disease without compelling evidence of transmissibility. Several viruses have been implicated in the pathogenesis of MF/SS, including HTLV-1 and HTLV-2, herpes simplex virus, human herpesvirus 6, and EBV. However, a viral cause of MF/SS has not been proven, and no epidemiologic evidence supports these hypotheses (PMID: 23806159).

Investigators have suggested that prolonged antigenic stimulation via exposure to contact allergens or superantigen stimulation associated with infections may lead to enhanced immune responses, with subsequent mutations in apoptotic pathway leading directly or indirectly to the development of MF/SS. Sézary cells respond in vitro to superantigenic exotoxins, and colonization by *Staphylococcus aureus* may influence disease activity. Several reports suggested that exposure to metals or their salts, pesticides or herbicides, and organic solvents (halogenated or aromatic hydrocarbons) could be related to the development of MF/SS. However, two well-designed case-control studies have failed to support these observations.

Various theories have been advanced to explain the epidermotropism of malignant T cells in MF/SS. Organ-specific affinity to skin and other organs has been recognized in subsets of normal T cells. Homing of CTCL cells to the skin is probably mediated by more than one adhesion receptor mechanism. CTCL cells express cutaneous lymphocyte antigen, a skin-homing receptor that interacts with E-selectin expressed by dermal venules. Furthermore, the cutaneous lymphocyte antigens T lymphocytes also typically express the CCR4 chemokine receptor, which binds to chemokines produced by the skin, such as the CC-chemokine ligands 17 and 22. Peripheral blood mononuclear cells bind to cultured keratinocytes exposed to IFN-γ. The major histocompatibility complex class II proteins along with intercellular adhesion molecule 1 present on keratinocytes, and attract and bind lymphocytes. Additional chemokine receptors, such as CXC chemokine receptors 3 and 4, as well as unique integrins, have been shown to have corresponding ligands or integrin receptors on dermal Langerhans cells, suggesting a relationship between the malignant T cells and host immune cells. The chemokine receptor CCR4 is expressed by a spectrum of CTCL cells, and an anti-CCR4 monoclonal antibody has significant activity against these diseases.

An additional feature of MF/SS cells is the production of a cytokine profile consistent with Th2 cells. Th2 cells produce IL-4, IL-5, and IL-6, and they are inhibited by IFN-γ. The expression of immunomodulatory molecule IL-17 is also increased in MF and SS. Th2 cells are critical for stimulating antibody- and eosinophil-mediated responses. Hypergammaglobulinemia and eosinophilia are occasionally seen in advanced cases of MF/SS and are consistent with a Th2 profile. Stimulation of Th2 cells inhibits the Th1 subpopulation of lymphocytes involved in cell-mediated immunity. Progression of MF/SS is associated with immune suppression as a result of depletion of this T-cell subset. The Th2 cytokine profile may explain the decrease in tumor-infiltrating lymphocytes during tumor progression. In addition to the effect of cytokines secreted by the neoplastic cells, malignant CD4+ cells express antigens (e.g., Fas ligand) that may directly mediate elimination of the CD8+-infiltrating lymphocytes by induction of apoptosis. CD4+ T cells from MF skin lesions have an effector memory phenotype, whereas T cells from SS skin lesions display central memory characteristics with the expression of the lymph node chemoattractant CCR7, which is not expressed in MF.

Clinical Presentation

Alibert reported the first case of MF in 1806. His patient developed a skin eruption that progressed into mushroom-like tumors, prompting the term *mycosis fungoides*. Later in the 19th century, Bazin defined the three classic cutaneous phases (patch, plaque, and tumor stage) of the disease. The recognition of the clinical triad of intensely pruritic erythroderma, lymphadenopathy, and abnormal hyperconvoluted cells in the peripheral blood led to the description of SS.

MF is the prototype of CTCL observed in over 50% of CTCL cases. The initial course of patients with MF is usually indolent. Most patients give a history of antecedent skin lesions, usually nonspecific erythematous patches that can mimic eczema or psoriasis. In many cases, there is an orderly progression from limited patches to more generalized patches, plaques, tumors, and nodal or visceral involvement. However, some patients may present with extensive skin involvement and tumor lesions, whereas other patients have limited patch disease that remains unaltered for the patient's entire life. The characteristic patch lesion is typically well demarcated with fading edges, lightly erythematous, and scaly, with a predilection for sun-protected areas, such as the lower abdomen or buttocks (Fig. 85.10). The texture can vary from poikilodermatous atrophic cases to serpiginous annular lesions or markedly keratotic patches. Plaque lesions are more indurated, have fairly well-demarcated margins, and

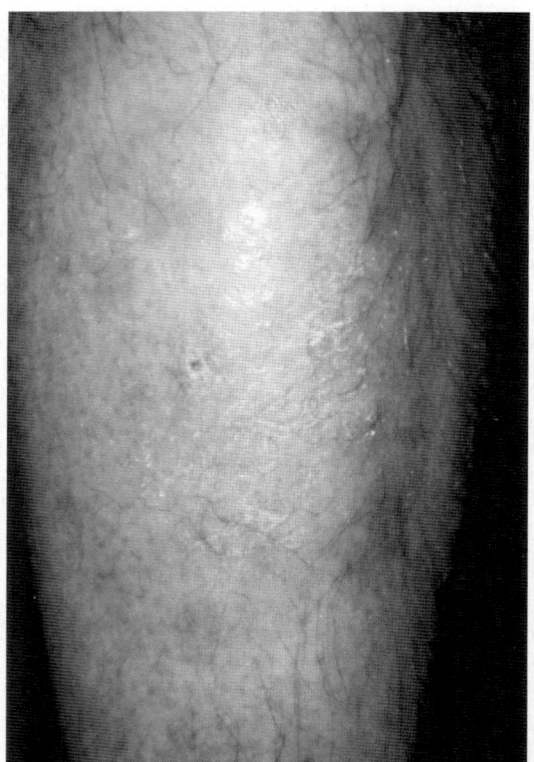

Fig. 85.10 ERYTHEMATOUS AND SCALY PATCH LESION OF MYCOSIS FUNGOIDES.

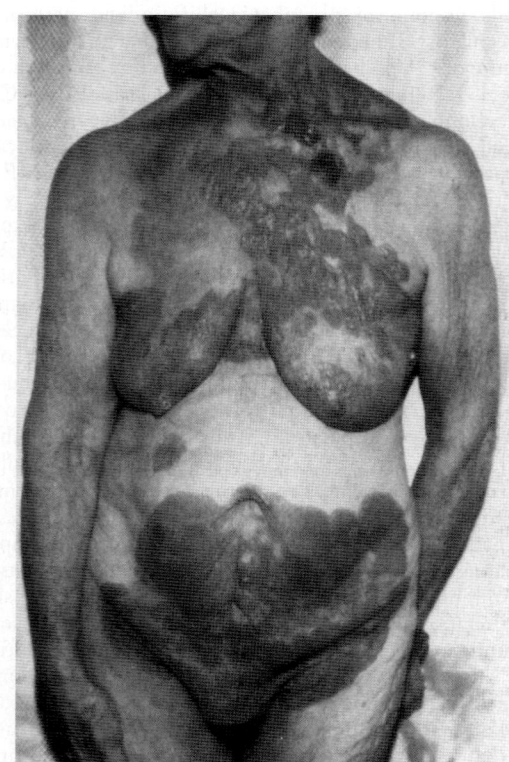

Fig. 85.11 PLAQUE LESION OF CUTANEOUS T-CELL LYMPHOMA.

some scaling (Fig. 85.11). Plaques can arise from patch lesions or previously uninvolved areas of skin. The distinction between a patch and a plaque is often subjective, with a low rate of interpersonal agreement among experts. Tumor lesions tend to appear in advanced cases, frequently associated with previous patches or plaques, and are commonly associated with histologic evidence and large-cell transformation. They can be located on any part of the body. Ulceration of these lesions is common, and secondary infection is a major cause of morbidity (Fig. 85.12). Tumors may be the initial presentation in a small percentage of patients (d'emblée presentation, Vidal and Brocq, 1889).

SS patients present with generalized desquamative erythroderma, pruritus, and circulating malignant cells. Peripheral blood usually shows a significant number or percentage of hyperconvoluted atypical lymphocytes (Fig. 85.13). Approximately 5%–10% of all newly reported cases of CTCL are SS. In its most advanced form, patients with SS suffer from alopecia, ectropion, leonine facies, hyperkeratosis, nail dystrophy, fissuring of the palms and soles, and severe pruritus and cutaneous pain. Many other entities can clinically mimic this disease, including drug eruptions, atopic dermatitis, contact dermatitis, and erythrodermic psoriasis. A number of variant presentations of CTCL are described in the following sections.

Cutaneous Lymphoid Dyscrasias (Clonal Dermatitis)

Cutaneous lymphoid dyscrasias or clonal dermatitis, which include a variety of lymphocyte-rich dermatoses, are often characterized by clonal T-lymphocyte proliferations that occasionally progress to bona fide mycosis fungoides. Clinically they exhibit a myriad of cutaneous presentations from poikiloderma (atrophic patches) to hyperpigmented areas resembling pigmented purpuric dermatosis or an acneiform presentation of follicular mucinosis.

The term *large-plaque parapsoriasis* has also been traditionally used for these types of poorly defined lesions that may evolve into MF. It most commonly consists of a few scattered, erythematous-to-brown plaques that are usually larger than 6 cm. There is a predilection for the buttocks and intertriginous areas. Histologic examination shows a superficial lymphocytic infiltrate with minimal nuclear atypia. Epidermotropism is scant or absent, and dermal fibrosis correlates with the chronicity of the process. Plaques can persist for decades before a frank evolution to MF occurs. Approximately 10%–30% of patients ultimately develop an overt malignant transformation. Large-plaque parapsoriasis is more likely to evolve into MF than small-plaque lesions.

Idiopathic Follicular Mucinosis

Follicular mucinosis is also considered a variant of cutaneous lymphoid dyscrasias that manifests with grouped erythematous follicular papules or boggy or indurated nodular plaques, notably devoid of hair (Fig. 85.14). There is a predilection for the head and neck area, especially the forehead, which has the highest density of pilosebaceous units. Histopathologic evaluation reveals cells in sebaceous glands often associated with destruction of hair follicle structures due to infiltration by a T-lymphocytic process. This idiopathic condition can evolve or be associated with folliculotropic MF. Even idiopathic cases

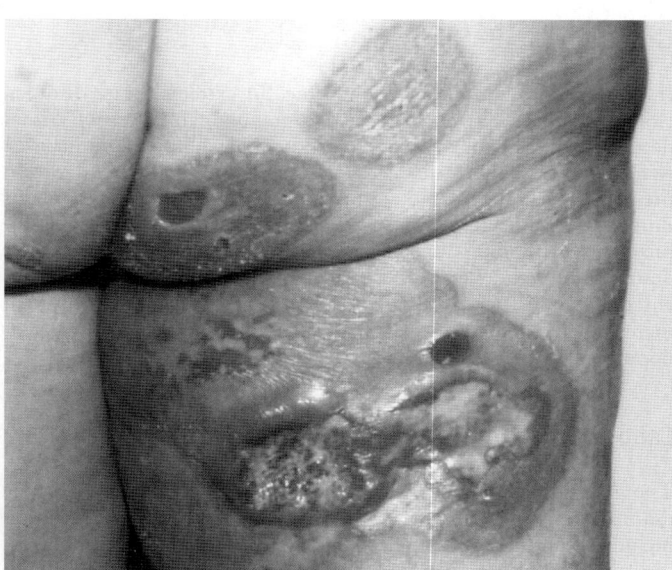

Fig. 85.12 ULCERATED TUMORS ARISING FROM MYCOSIS FUNGOIDES PLAQUES.

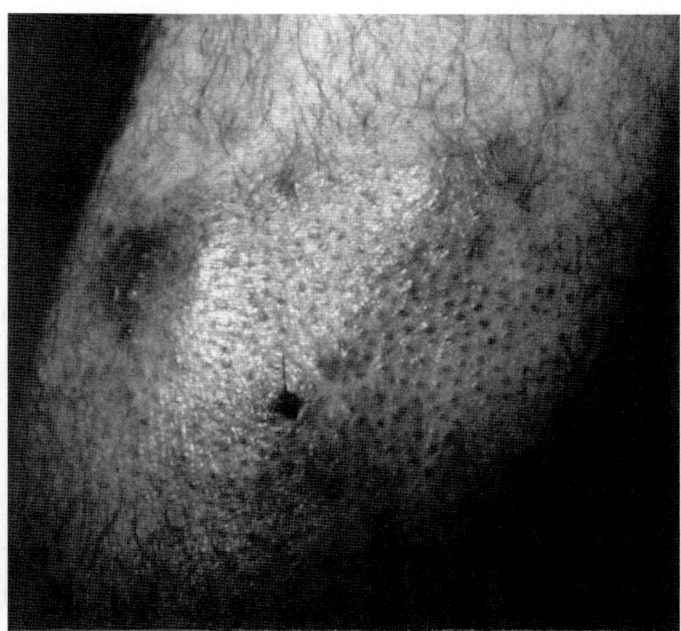

Fig. 85.14 FOLLICULAR MUCINOSIS SHOWING A PATCH OF ALOPECIA WITH FOLLICULAR PROMINENCE.

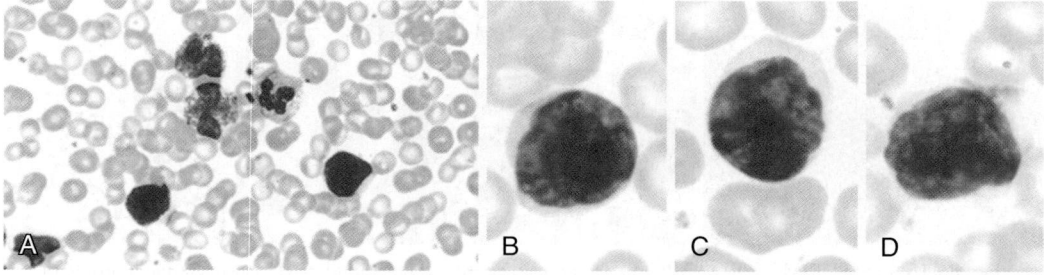

Fig. 85.13 SÉZARY CELLS. Peripheral smear (A) with Sézary cells associated with eosinophilia. Note the cerebriform nuclei with fine chromatin (B–D). The hyperconvoluted nature of the nuclei is evident as complex nuclear folds seen through the chromatin.

can be associated with clonal T-lymphocytic infiltration. In general, patients older than 40 years with a more generalized cutaneous involvement and a chronic course are more likely to develop associated MF. No cases of MF have been reported in children with alopecia mucinosa, although a few reports of HL have been reported in children with follicular mucinosis. Patients with folliculotropic MF and follicular mucinosis are reported to have a worse prognosis, stage for stage, which may be caused by inability of topical treatment to penetrate to the deeper layers of the process.

Lymphomatoid Papulosis

Lymphomatoid papulosis (LyP) is characterized by recurrent crops of self-healing, red-brown, centrally necrotic, asymptomatic papules and nodules (Fig. 85.15). This entity represents 10%–15% of all CTCL cases. Patients may have a few lesions or more than 100 at a time. Histologic evaluation reveals an atypical CD4$^+$ lymphocytic infiltrate with a variable mixed inflammatory infiltrate (Fig. 85.16). These may be primarily small cerebriform cells similar to those seen in MF (type B), but most often there are larger CD30$^+$ cells with prominent nucleoli resembling Reed-Sternberg cells (type A). A third variety of LyP (type C) with sheets of anaplastic large cells resembling CD30$^+$ large-cell lymphoma (CD30$^+$ LCL) has also been reported. Lately other subtypes have been reported. Type D, commonly seen in the pediatric population, is characterized by pagetoid or highly epidermotropic small atypical lymphocytes with CD8 expression. Such cases may be difficult to distinguish from pityriasis lichenoides acuta (PMID: 22688398).

Type E LyP is characterized by hemorrhagic and necrotic lesions often showing evidence of vasculitis on histological evaluation (PMID: 23026936).

The prognosis of these new subtypes is not different to the other subgroups. *TCR* gene rearrangement studies demonstrate a clonal

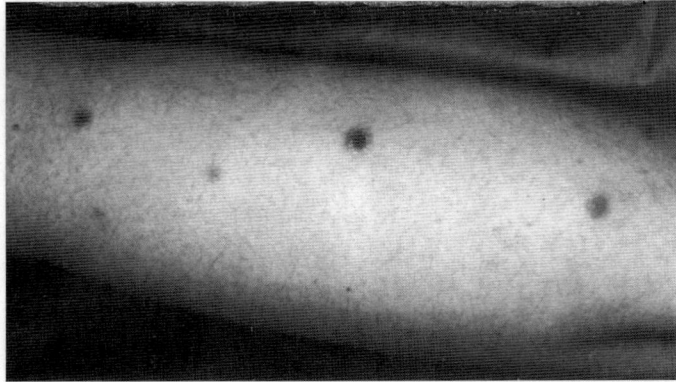

Fig. 85.15 LESIONS OF LYMPHOMATOID PAPULOSIS APPEAR IN CROPS AND CONSIST OF ULCERATED PAPULES AND SCARS.

origin. Although the typical course is usually indolent, spanning decades, approximately 15% of patients develop MF, HL, or NHL during their lifetime. A direct link between LyP, CTCL, and HL was demonstrated in a patient with the three lymphoproliferative disorders arising from a common T-cell clone, as shown by *TCR* gene studies.

Pagetoid Reticulosis

Pagetoid reticulosis (i.e., Woringer-Kolopp disease) is a rare condition affecting young adults. It typically manifests with a solitary, hyperkeratotic, often verrucous plaque on the lower limb. Biopsy results show atypical cerebriform lymphocytes with a perinuclear halo almost exclusively localized within the intraepidermal compartment. Extracutaneous dissemination is exceedingly rare. Most cases have a CD8$^+$ phenotype, although CD4$^+$ cases or double-negative (CD4$^+$/CD8) cases have been reported. Frequently the tumor cells express CD30, but *TCR* gene rearrangement study results are often negative. Whether pagetoid reticulosis should be considered a localized form of MF or a reactive pseudomalignant process is debatable. Although most cases have an indolent protracted course, generalized and sometimes aggressive variants have been reported. Cases presenting with a solitary lesion are extremely indolent and could be considered a reactive or pseudolymphomatous process. At the opposite end of the spectrum there are patients with extensive ulcerative plaques formerly known as *generalized pagetoid reticulosis* or *Ketron-Goodman disease* that are now diagnosed as the CD8$^+$ aggressive intraepidermal T-cell lymphoma.

Granulomatous Slack Skin

In granulomatous slack skin syndrome, an extremely rare disorder, clonal CD4$^+$ T cells elicit a reactive granulomatous response that destroys the elastic fibers, rendering skin slack, fibrotic, and inelastic (Fig. 85.17). Changes characteristic of MF are often found within the epidermis and papillary dermis, and the reticular dermis contains numerous histiocytes with multinucleated giant cells and elastophagocytosis. Some patients with granulomatous MF do not have destruction of the elastic fibers with slack skin changes. The differential diagnosis includes sarcoidosis and tuberculoid leprosy. An increased incidence of HL has been reported in this patient population.

Laboratory Manifestations

The gold standard in the diagnosis of MF/SS is light microscopic examination of a skin biopsy specimen. Characteristic findings include a band-like infiltrate involving the papillary dermis containing small, medium-sized, and occasionally large mononuclear cells with hyperchromatic, hyperconvoluted (cerebriform) nuclei, and

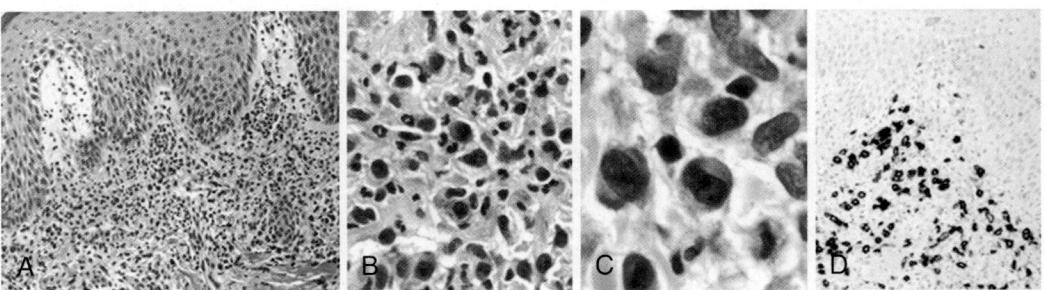

Fig. 85.16 LYMPHOMATOID PAPULOSIS. Low power (A) shows a moderately dense dermal infiltrate of lymphoid cells admixed with inflammatory cells, including neutrophils and eosinophils (B). The lymphoid cells are varied but include atypical large forms (C), which are brightly positive for CD30 (D). *(Courtesy Drs. Vesna Petrovic-Rosic and Mark Racz, University of Chicago.)*

variable numbers of admixed inflammatory cells often expanding into adnexal structures (hair follicles and sweat glands). Epidermal exocytosis of single or small clusters of neoplastic cells is a characteristic finding (Fig. 85.18A, C, and D). The presence of Pautrier microabscesses, defined as four or more atypical lymphocytes arranged in an aggregate in the epidermis, is classic but is seen in only a minority of cases. Reticular fibroplasia of the papillary dermis is also a common finding. Tumor-stage lesions demonstrate a more diffuse, superficial, and deep dermal infiltrate with fewer reactive cells and an absence of epidermotropism (Fig. 85.18B, E, and F). The malignant T-cell clone often evolves into large-cell morphology during tumor progression, although rare cases show large-cell morphology from the early patch lesions. The presence of large cells in a skin lesion should be distinguished from "large-cell transformation," which displays rapid skin, node, and visceral progression, is refractory to treatment, and is associated with poor survival. The histologic features in SS may be similar to those of MF. However, the cellular infiltrates in SS are more often monotonous, and epidermotropism may be absent.

Lymph node involvement initially involves the paracortical regions. Progression is associated with small-to-large clusters of atypical cells with preserved nodal architecture, followed by partial or total effacement of the node by neoplastic cells. Visceral involvement is a late clinical feature. Variable peripheral blood involvement can be demonstrated in all stages of skin disease, although it is most prevalent in patients with tumor or erythrodermic presentations. Patients with SS present with large numbers of circulating neoplastic cells, typically more than 1000 cells/mL (B2), but a lower count may be noted initially (B1). Bone marrow biopsy results are typically negative. However, some involvement may be detected by flow cytometry in many cases of SS or advanced MF but rarely influences management outside an investigational setting. A staging bone marrow aspirate and biopsy is not recommended, unless unexplained cytopenias are seen.

The malignant cells are typically CD3$^+$, CD4$^+$, CD45RO$^+$, CD8$^+$, and CD30$^+$ by immunohistochemical analysis. CD7 is not expressed by cells from the early disease stages. More aggressive variants and advanced forms of CTCL may have cells with multiple pan–T-cell antigen deletions, especially CD2, CD5, and even CD4. *TCR* genes are clonally rearranged and can be documented in most cases by Southern blotting or polymerase chain reaction assays when a sufficient malignant infiltrate exists.

Analysis of peripheral blood may reveal an elevated LDH level, mostly in patients with high-blood–burden SS and bulky advanced MF. Eosinophilia and hypergammaglobulinemia are occasionally observed in advanced SS. In addition, several reports of SS and other CTCL variants have been reported to be associated with B-cell lymphoproliferative conditions, or small peripheral B-cell clones or monoclonal gammopathy (PMID: 19481294). Elevated serum β_2-microglobulin and IL-2 receptor levels have also been observed in advanced cases.

Imaging studies for classic MF/SS are generally of modest utility. Computed tomographic scans of the chest, abdomen, or pelvis should be reserved for patients with SS, nodal involvement, or CTCL variants. In an investigational setting, electron microscopy, cytogenetics, and molecular analyses have shown that a higher percentage of patients have occult involvement of internal organs.

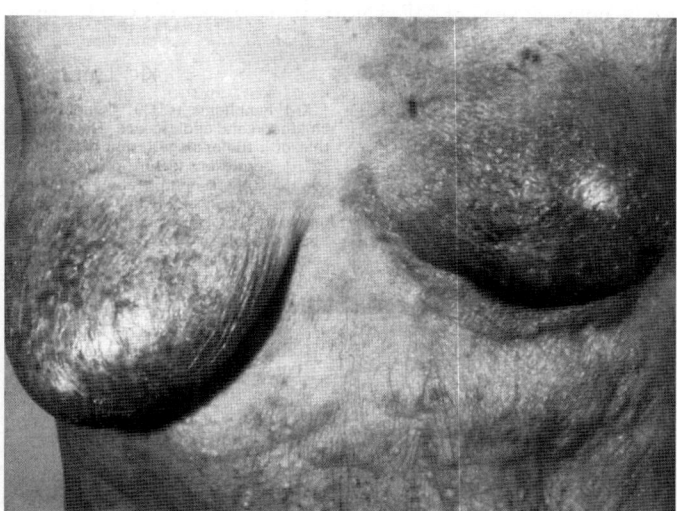

Fig. 85.17 LESIONS OF GRANULOMATOUS SLACK SKIN WITH DESTRUCTION OF THE DERMAL ELASTICITY.

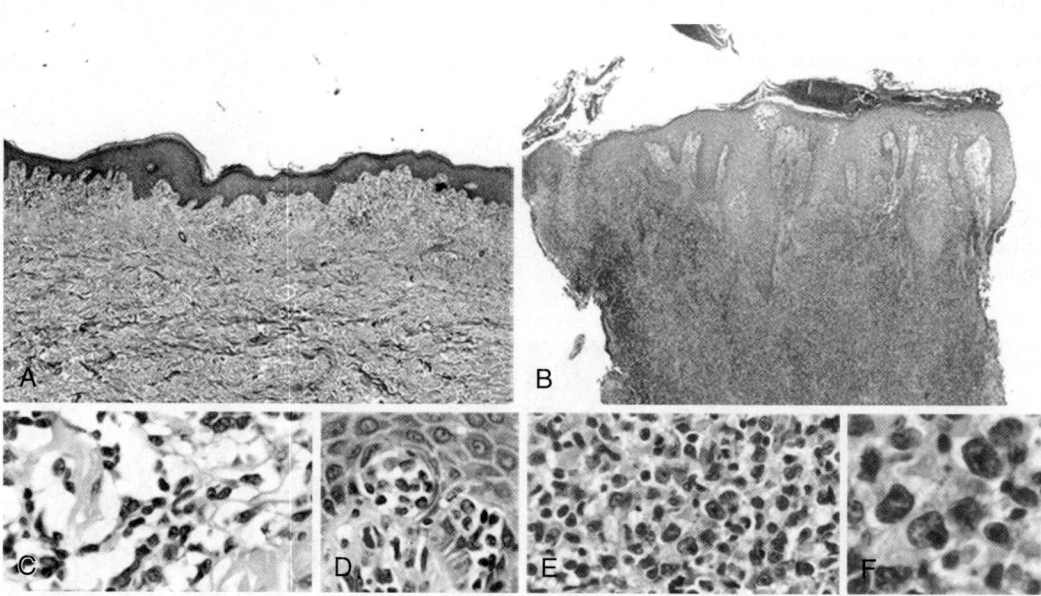

Fig. 85.18 MYCOSIS FUNGOIDES, PLAQUE STAGE, AND TRANSFORMED TUMOR STAGE. Plaque stage (A, C, D) demonstrates a band-like infiltrate (A, C) with some epidermotropism in the form of Pautrier microabscesses (D). In the tumor stage (B, E, F) there is a deep and dense infiltrate without significant epidermotropism. The cells are mostly large and atypical (E, F) and CD30$^+$ (not shown). *(Courtesy Drs. Vesna Petrovic-Rosic and Mark Racz, University of Chicago.)*

Differential Diagnosis

Primary CTCL represents a heterogeneous group of disorders with considerable variability in histologic characteristics, phenotype, and prognosis. The Kiel Classification, the Working Formulation, and the Revised European-American Lymphoma (REAL) classification system were developed for NHLs and were not designed to provide an adequate characterization of the spectrum of CTCLs. To address the deficiencies of the previously proposed systems, a more clinically useful classification was developed by the European Organization for Research and Treatment of Cancer (EORTC). WHO has proposed a classification with nearly 90% concordance with the EORTC classification (see Table 85.4). A number of other disorders in which malignant T cells infiltrate the skin should be distinguished from MF/SS. These disorders are discussed in the following sections.

CD30 Lymphoproliferative Disorders

CD30 lymphoproliferative disorders include LyP, primary cutaneous ALCL, and a spectrum of borderline cases. By definition, ALCL presents with single or multiple tumors measuring more than 2 cm and with a tendency for ulceration and steady growth. Borderline lesions are smaller but also tend to have a prolonged course, often with spontaneous resolution.

Lymphomatoid Papulosis

LyP is characterized by recurrent crops of self-healing, red-brown, centrally necrotic, asymptomatic papules and nodules. This entity represents 10%–15% of all CTCL cases. Patients may have a few lesions or more than 100 at a time. Histologic evaluation reveals an atypical CD4$^+$ lymphocytic infiltrate with a variable mixed inflammatory infiltrate. These may be primarily small cerebriform cells similar to those seen in MF (type B), but most often there are larger CD30$^+$ cells with prominent nucleoli resembling Reed-Sternberg cells (type A). A third variety of LyP (type C), also considered borderline ALCL, presents with sheets of large cells resembling CD30$^+$ large cells. *TCR* gene rearrangement studies demonstrate a clonal origin. Although the typical course is usually indolent, spanning decades, approximately 15% of patients develop MF, cutaneous ALCL, and very rarely HL or NHL during their lifetime. A direct link between LyP, CTCL, and HL was demonstrated in a patient with the three lymphoproliferative disorders arising from a common T-cell clone, as shown by *TCR* gene studies.

CD30$^+$ Cutaneous T-Cell Lymphoma

Primary cutaneous CD30$^+$ LCL typically occurs in adults presenting with solitary or localized (ulcerating) nodules or tumors (Fig. 85.19). Regional lymph node involvement is seen in 25% of patients at presentation. These primary cutaneous CD30$^+$ LCLs are probably closely related to LyP, regressing atypical histiocytosis, and primary cutaneous HL. The tumor has a favorable prognosis, and often complete or partial spontaneous regression occurs. This is in contrast to primary noncutaneous CD30$^+$ LCLs, which can be seen in children or adults and which carries a poor prognosis. These primary cutaneous lesions, in contrast to nodal or pediatric cases, have been shown to rarely have the chromosomal translocation t(2;5) associated with overexpression of ALK (ALK negative). Histopathology consists of diffuse nonepidermotropic infiltrates with cohesive sheets of large CD30$^+$ tumor cells (Fig. 85.20). In most instances, the tumor cells have anaplastic morphologic characteristics, showing round, oval, or irregularly shaped nuclei; prominent (eosinophilic) nucleoli; and abundant cytoplasm. Less commonly, the neoplastic cells have a pleomorphic or immunoblastic appearance. Reactive lymphocytes are often present, but infiltrating eosinophils are often less conspicuous. The immunophenotype of this disorder is characteristically CD4$^+$, with more than 75% of neoplastic cells expressing CD30. In contrast to the poor outcome of MF that has transformed to a CD30$^+$ large-cell variant, primary cutaneous CD30$^+$ LCLs are associated with an excellent prognosis. Radiotherapy is the preferred treatment for solitary or localized disease, with combination chemotherapy reserved for patients with generalized skin lesions or extracutaneous dissemination. Surgical excision may be adequate in many cases. In advanced cases, 5-year survival exceeds 30%.

CD30$^-$ Cutaneous T-Cell Lymphoma

These rare presentations often classified as CTCL, NOS, or d'emblée presentation, tend to have an aggressive clinical course. Patients present with localized or generalized plaques, nodules, or tumors.

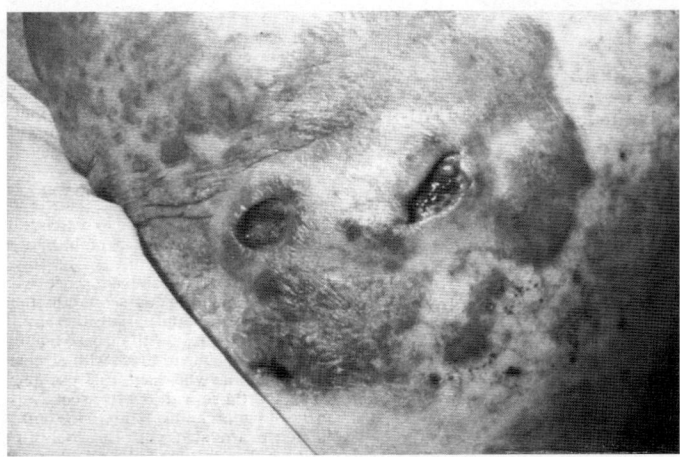

Fig. 85.19 LESIONS OF CD30$^+$ LARGE-CELL LYMPHOMA WITH ULCERATION.

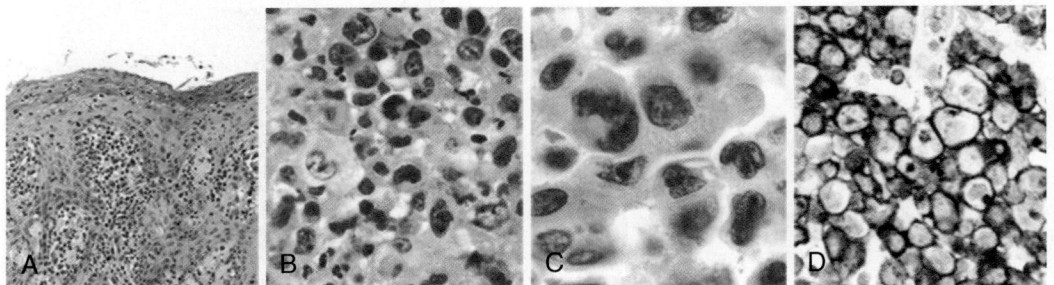

Fig. 85.20 CUTANEOUS ANAPLASTIC LARGE-CELL LYMPHOMA. Sheets of tumor cells are present in the dermis (A) and are associated with marked pseudoepitheliomatous hyperplasia. The cells are quite varied and bizarre (B), and frequently show abnormal "embryoid" shapes (C) constituting the "hallmark" cells. There is bright staining with CD30 (D). ALK staining (not shown) is typically negative.

Histopathologic evaluation demonstrates that infiltrates are nonepidermotropic, with variable numbers of medium-sized to large pleomorphic T cells with or without cerebriform nuclei and immunoblasts. The tumor cells are CD4$^+$, with CD30$^-$ expression restricted to a few scattered tumor cells. The infiltrate is often accompanied by a mixed infiltrate with reactive B cells and granulomatous or histiocytic component. Multiagent chemotherapy is used in most instances, with radiation therapy reserved for patients with localized disease. The 5-year survival rate is less than 20%.

Pleomorphic Small- or Medium-Sized Cutaneous T-Cell Lymphoma

Pleomorphic small- or medium-sized CTCL is a rare entity. Patients typically present with a single red-purplish nodule or tumor involving the head and neck regions. Rarely are multiple nodules noted. The neoplastic cells are accompanied by many reactive B cells and histiocytes, which has led to the hypothesis that they may arise from a follicular T-helper cell population expressing BCL6, PD-1, and CD10. Typically, CD30 is negative, and CD4 expression is strong. TCR should be positive. In our opinion, cases presenting with a single lesion should not be diagnosed as having lymphoma; despite its clonal nature, the prognosis is invariably benign. These lesions were called *pseudolymphomas* in the past without significant consequences. However, patients presenting with multiple lesions are part of the d'emblée presentation and should be approached more aggressively, including full staging and systemic therapy. Patients with more generalized disease have been treated with regimens used for indolent NHLs. Five-year survival rates are 100% in unilesional cases and exceed 60% in patients with more extensive disease.

Subcutaneous Panniculitis-Like T-Cell Lymphoma

Subcutaneous panniculitis-like T-cell lymphoma is a rare entity. Patients, typically younger and female, present with asymptomatic deep subcutaneous nonulcerated nodules and plaques involving the legs. Systemic symptoms are common, including fevers, fatigue, and anorexia. Overlapping or preceding signs of systemic lupus erythematosus or other autoimmune conditions are commonly observed. Histopathologic examination reveals a subcutaneous infiltrate with pleomorphic medium-sized T cells mixed with a reactive lymphoid infiltrate and some histiocytes. Tumor cell necrosis, karyorrhexis, and erythrophagocytosis are common findings. Differential diagnosis includes the frequently fatal but nonneoplastic cytophagic histiocytic panniculitis. Neoplastic infiltration of deep blood vessels can be noted in some cases. Immunophenotyping reveals postthymic T-cell markers with a CD8$^+$ phenotype and expression of cytotoxic markers such as TIA-1 and granzyme B. By definition the tumor cells are negative for EBV markers and lack expression of the γδ heterodimer. However, T-cell clonality including the γ- or β-gene is commonly identified. The prognosis is fairly good, with a 5-year survival rate over 80% with the exception of patients with a concurrent hemophagocytic syndrome (fevers, cytopenias). Cases in which the panniculitic findings coexist with systemic lupus erythematosus may behave in a clinically indolent fashion.

Primary Cutaneous γδ-T-Cell Lymphoma

Cutaneous γδ T-cell lymphoma is a rare condition that tends to present with extensive panniculitis-like plaques on the extremities with a tendency to ulcerate during the course of the disease. A subset of patients present with single lesions resembling an infectious process or with extensive chronic erythematous and scaly patches resembling MF. Several of our patients had comorbidities associated with immune suppression, including autoimmune conditions or other lymphoproliferative conditions or malignancies. Chronic antigen stimulation has been hypothesized to play a role in the pathogenesis

of cutaneous γδ T-cell lymphoma. Patients often present with a high level of LDH and constitutional symptoms and succumb to the disease, often associated with hemophagocytic syndrome. For the most part, all therapies have shown modest effectiveness. Sustained remissions have not resulted from radiation, immune therapy, or multiagent chemotherapy. However, a case with CR for 23 months following aSCT has been reported. Cytotoxic features such as necrosis, hemorrhage, and vasculitis are commonly encountered. The immunophenotype is characterized by CD4/CD8 double negativity (with some CD8$^+$ cases), lack of CD5 expression, and expression of cytotoxic granules.

Primary Cutaneous Aggressive Epidermotropic CD8$^+$ T-Cell Lymphoma

This extremely rare condition, formerly known as *generalized pagetoid reticulosis* or *Ketron-Goodman syndrome*, constitutes less than 1% of all cutaneous lymphomas. The term *Berti lymphoma* is often used to refer to this condition. Men are affected more commonly, and patients present with extensive erosive patches with frequent mucosal involvement. Occasionally the lesions are exophytic and hemorrhagic, resembling pyogenic granuloma. The course is invariable and rapidly fatal with exceptional cases reported surviving following ASCT. Histologically the infiltrate is markedly epidermotropic and adnexotropic, infiltrating into hair follicles and sweat glands, eventually becoming hemorrhagic and ulcerated. The cells are also of intermediate size, always expressing CD8 as well as other T-cell markers such as CD7 and CD45RO.

Extranasal Natural Killer/T-Cell Lymphoma

EBV-induced extranasal NKTCLs rarely appear in the skin as the initial site of presentation. This condition is mostly reported in Asia and Latin America with rare cases seen in the United States. Although occasional cases remain localized in the skin, most of these lymphomas eventually involve other sites such as the testes or the gastrointestinal tract. A careful ear, nose, and throat evaluation to rule out nasopharyngeal involvement is important. The lesions are mostly large ulcerated tumor lesions with hemorrhagic and necrotic appearance. Histologically the tumor is composed of a deep infiltrate with intermediate-sized lymphocytes with cytotoxic changes, hemorrhage, and necrotic debris. A histologic landmark is the presence of angiocentric and angiodestructive features. The immunophenotype is characterized by the expression of CD3ε in the cytoplasmic membrane, as well as CD56. Cytotoxic cytoplasmic granules are always identified, and EBV in the tumor cells can be demonstrated by the expression of EBER or LMP1. A lymphoproliferative disorder resembling hydroa vacciniforme has been reported almost exclusively in Latin America, especially in the Andes region, where the combination of high altitude with intense ultraviolet rays triggers this process, which is mostly seen in vulnerable indigenous patients. These patients present with facial edema, hepatosplenomegaly, and necrotizing hemorrhagic lesions triggered by sun exposure or an arthropod bite reactions. These conditions are associated with a very aggressive clinical course and patients often succumb to hemophagocytic syndrome. Multiagent chemotherapy has not been effective, and perhaps the only hope for these individuals is an ASCT.

Lymphomatoid Granulomatosis

Lymphomatoid granulomatosis is a rare multiorgan disease of the lungs, nasopharynx, joints, and peripheral and central nervous systems. Cutaneous involvement occurs in 25%–50% of patients. Although nodules are most common, some patients have nonspecific macules, papules, or ulceration. Histologic evaluation reveals an angiocentric, polymorphous infiltrate of atypical lymphocytes and histiocytes surrounding and invading blood vessels within the dermis.

Molecular and immunologic studies suggest a mature clonal helper T-cell process. However, reports have suggested a massive reactive T-cell infiltrate driven by a small number of clonal B cells.

EBV DNA sequences are frequently present, and their role in the pathogenesis of this disorder remains poorly defined. Although the clinical course is variable, the prognosis for patients with diffuse pulmonary involvement or evolution to high-grade lymphoma is poor, with a median survival of less than 2 years. Treatment depends on histologic findings and extent and location of disease, and may include corticosteroids, radiotherapy, and chemotherapy. IFN has shown significant activity against this disease. Related conditions include the recently reported EBV-induced mucocutaneous ulcer seen in immunosuppressed patients and B-cell lymphomas of older adults.

Adult T-Cell Leukemia

ATL is in most instances a rapidly progressive T-cell neoplasm expressing a helper phenotype that is described earlier in this chapter. It is endemic in southern Japan and the Caribbean islands, and is associated with the retrovirus HTLV-1. However, most HTLV-l–infected patients remain asymptomatic, and only 2%–4% develop ATL. The clinical presentation is polymorphous and can resemble MF or SS. Cutaneous lesions are variable, ranging from a rash simulating a viral exanthem, to annular lesions resembling erythema multiforme, to large tumors and plaques similar to MF (Fig. 85.21). Advanced stages of the disease, which affects a younger population than seen with MF, are characterized by visceral involvement, immunodeficiency, elevated LDH level, and hypercalcemia. Malignant lymphocytes often have convoluted or multilobed nuclei and can be detected in the peripheral blood in 75% of patients. The neoplastic T cells express high levels of the IL-2 receptor (CD25). For purposes of treatment and prognosis, it is wise to view ATL as a spectrum with two subgroups—acute and all others—with treatment, although inadequate, reserved for those with acute ATL. Therapeutic options include multiagent chemotherapy and antibody or recombinant toxins directed against the IL-2 receptor. Patients with acute ATL have poor survival rates, with a median duration of 4–6 months. Patients with disease that is not "acute" are considered to have "smoldering" disease and have lesions that may wax and wane in size and shape despite treatment.

Prognosis

The goals of treatment in MF are the relief of symptoms with improved quality of life, generally through prevention or delay in development of advanced skin disease and improvement in cosmetics. Despite some uncontrolled clinical trial results that have been reported to suggest "cures" in this disease, the general perception remains that this disease is not curable with standard therapies available today. The disease behaves similarly to other low-grade lymphomas, with periods of remission gradually becoming shorter with subsequent therapeutic interventions. Unlike B-cell low-grade lymphomas, however, advanced-stage MF is associated with a relatively short median life expectancy. Patients with significant nodal involvement (LN3 or LN4) or extensive skin involvement (T4) have median life expectancies of 30–55 months (Table 85.5). A driving force in the development of treatments for this disease is the goal of altering the natural history for this group of poor-prognosis patients. No clinical trial has determined that aggressive early therapy is better than sequential palliative approaches or investigational approaches, and new treatments continue to be developed and tested for these patients.

In 1979 the staging committee at an international workshop on MF proposed a staging system based on the international tumor-node-metastasis (TNM) system (see Table 85.5). This classification was based on the evaluation of 347 patients and a multivariate analysis of potential prognostic factors. This group identified several independent prognostic factors: extent of skin disease at diagnosis (T), type of lymph node (N) involvement, presence or absence of peripheral blood (PB) involvement, and presence or absence of visceral (M) involvement. In 2007 this staging system was revised by the International Society for Cutaneous Lymphomas (ISCL) and the EORTC to incorporate advances related to tumor cell biology and diagnostic techniques, including status of blood involvement, and to improve inter-investigator communication and development of standardized clinical trials (see Table 85.5). Investigators at the National Cancer Institute retrospectively analyzed 152 patients who underwent uniform pathologic staging. They were able to identify three distinct prognostic groups. Good-risk patients had plaque-only skin disease without lymph node, blood, or visceral involvement, and a median survival of more than 12 years. Less than 10% of patients with stage 1A (limited patch) and less than 30% with stage 1B (extensive patch or plaque) progress to more advanced disease. Intermediate-risk patients had skin tumors, erythroderma, or plaque disease with lymph node or blood involvement (but no visceral disease) and a median survival of 5 years. Poor-risk patients had visceral disease or complete effacement of lymph nodes by lymphoma, and a median survival of 2.5 years.

In addition to the classic TNM staging, implementation of techniques such as flow cytometry, cytogenetic analysis, and determination of nuclear contour indices may also improve diagnostic and prognostic specificity. Flow cytometry and cytogenetic analysis are complementary techniques. Flow cytometry allows the detection of cell populations with a normal (diploid) number of chromosomes versus abnormal (aneuploid) numbers, and cytogenetic analysis precisely identifies the individual chromosomal structure and number. Bunn et al demonstrated that in MF/SS the presence of aneuploidy during the clinical course was associated with more aggressive disease. Hyperdiploid cell clones were demonstrated in patients with large-cell histology, aggressive disease, and shortened survival time. Specific chromosomal deletions also influenced prognosis.

The nuclear contour index has been used by several groups in an effort to separate "benign" cutaneous lymphocytic disorders, such as LyP and pityriasis lichenoides, from MF/SS. Electron microscopy

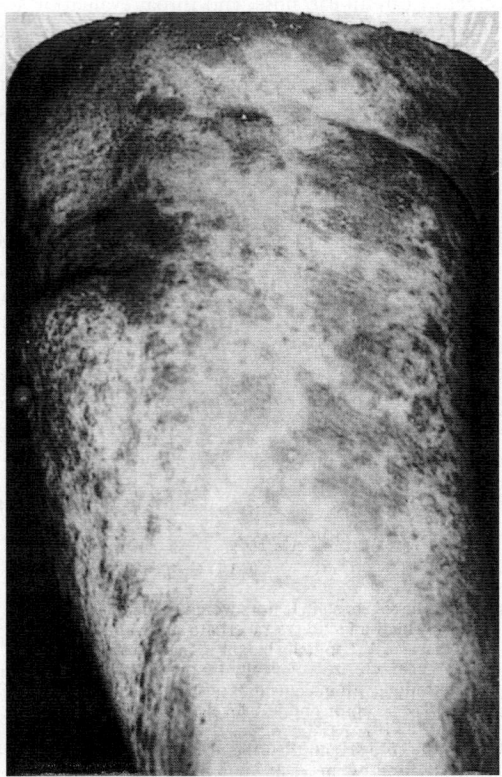

Fig. 85.21 SKIN LESIONS IN ADULT T-CELL LYMPHOMA/LEUKEMIA.

TABLE 85.5	ISCL/EORTC Revision to the Classification of MF and SS (Adaptation)

TNMB Stages

Skin

T_1	Limited patches, papules, and/or plaques covering <10% of the skin surface. May stratify into T_{1a} (patch only) vs T_{1b} (plaque ± patch).
T_2	Patches, papules or plaques covering ≥10% of skin surface. May stratify into T_{2a} (patch only) vs T_{2b} (plaque ± patch).
T_3	One or more tumors (≥1-cm diameter)
T_4	Confluence of erythema covering ≥80% body surface area

Node

N_0	No clinically abnormal peripheral lymph nodes; biopsy not required
N_1	Abnormal peripheral lymph nodes; histopathology Dutch grade 1 or NCI LN_{0-2}
N_2	Abnormal peripheral lymph nodes; histopathology Dutch grade 2 or NCI LN_3
N_3	Abnormal peripheral lymph nodes; histopathology Dutch grades 3–4 or NCI LN_4
N_x	Abnormal peripheral lymph nodes; no histologic confirmation

Visceral

M_0	No visceral organ involvement
M_1	Visceral involvement (must have pathology confirmation and involved organ should be specified)

Blood

B_0	Absence of significant blood involvement: ≤5% of peripheral blood lymphocytes are atypical (Sézary) cells
B_1	Low blood tumor burden: >5% of peripheral blood lymphocytes are atypical (Sézary) but does not meet the criteria for B_2
B2	High blood tumor burden: ≥1000/μL Sézary cells with positive clones

Clinical Staging

IA	T1, N0, M0, B0,1
IB	T2, N0, M0, B0,1
IIA	T1,2, N1,2, M0, B0,1
IIB	T3, N0–2, M0, B0,1
IIIA	T4, N0–2, M0, B0
IIIB	T4, N0–2, M0, B1
IVA_1	T1–4, N0–2, M0, B2
IVA_2	T1–4, N3, M0, B0–2
IVB	T1–4, N0–3, M1, B0–2

CTCL, Cutaneous T-cell lymphoma; EORTC, European Organization of Research and Treatment of Cancer; ISCL, International Society for Cutaneous Lymphomas; NCI LN, National Cancer Institute lymph node grading system; TNMB, tumor-node-metastasis-blood.

TABLE 85.6	Therapeutic Options for Mycosis Fungoides

Topical Therapy

Ultraviolet A with psoralen
Ultraviolet B
External beam radiation therapy
Total-skin electron beam radiation
Topical chemotherapy
Topical retinoids

Systemic Therapy

Photophoresis
Interferon-α
Oral retinoids
Targeted therapies
Single-agent chemotherapy
Combination chemotherapy
Stem cell transplantation
Investigational agents

from typical small, convoluted lymphocytes to larger lymphocytes, such as those associated with large-cell lymphoma, has been documented. Whether this conversion is secondary to prior therapeutic modalities used remains uncertain.

The gold standard for the diagnosis of MF is still routine histopathologic evaluation with adequate clinical correlation. Early lesions of MF are frequently accompanied by heavy infiltrates of benign reactive T cells, hampering the detection of abnormal T-cell clones by any laboratory method. Hence most adjuvant laboratory methods are not helpful at the precise time when they are most needed.

Therapy

Therapy can be conveniently divided into two approaches: topical (skin directed), such as psoralen plus ultraviolet A (PUVA), topical chemotherapy application (nitrogen mustard or carmustine), external beam radiotherapy, and total-skin electron beam radiotherapy, and systemic (skin and viscera directed), such as IFNs, oral or parenteral chemotherapy, photopheresis, oral retinoids, and investigational new compounds (Table 85.6). No studies have demonstrated that one topical therapy is more effective than another, and patient and investigator preference remains the most important discriminating factor governing choice. However, as the biology of the neoplastic cell has become better understood, it is clear that some therapies may actually have topical and systemic effects through alterations in the body's cytokine milieu and ability to mount a host response against the neoplastic cell. Furthermore, knowledge regarding signaling pathways in the neoplastic cells in MF/SS offers hope that future development of targeted treatment approaches will soon be available. Investigational approaches combining therapies also remains an active research strategy (see box on How We Manage Mycosis Fungoides/Sézary Syndrome).

Phototherapy

8-Methoxypsoralen (8-MOP) is a member of a family of photoactivated compounds (furocoumarin derivatives), which may inhibit DNA and RNA synthesis through formation of monofunctional or bifunctional thymine adducts, gene mutations, or sister chromatid exchanges. The cross-strand formed between DNA strands results in a halt in cell division, as well as oxidative damage to cytoplasmic organelles and cell membranes. These drugs are active only if the tissue containing the psoralen compound is exposed to ultraviolet A (UVA). The mechanism of cell cytotoxicity for many cancer therapies involves the induction of apoptosis. Yoo et al demonstrated that peripheral blood mononuclear cells from SS patients and controls

allows the calculation of a value based on the degree of nuclear folding; this nuclear contour index is significantly greater in patients with MF than in other benign conditions.

The density of epidermal Langerhans cells in biopsy samples, as determined by immunoperoxidase stains, has been identified as a prognostic feature. Epidermal Langerhans cells are necessary for antigen recognition and processing in the normal immune response. Patients with Langerhans cell densities greater than 90 cells/mm² had a significantly reduced risk for death from MF/SS compared with those with lower densities. There was no prognostic significance identified for the presence or absence of CD30⁺ cells. It has been noted that the presence of cytotoxic CD8⁺ T lymphocytes in the skin infiltrate is associated with a more favorable prognosis.

Occasionally patients may develop a more clinically aggressive lymphoma concurrent with a change in the histologic appearance of the neoplastic cells and the pace of their disease. This progression

How We Manage Mycosis Fungoides/Sézary Syndrome

There is no current accepted standard first-line approach or subsequent lines of therapy for patients with mycosis fungoides and Sézary syndrome. Published guidelines include active drugs/treatment approaches, but unfortunately few randomized trials have been completed to allow for comparative effectiveness. Our philosophy regarding management is to try to avoid the side effects of therapy being worse than the symptoms from the disease. Thus for patients with limited cutaneous only disease (stage I–IIa) we favor topical therapy alone with either limited topical steroid/drug applications for T1 stage disease (and for more extensive T2 stage disease our preference is ultraviolet light-based approaches, but other centers utilize topical chemotherapy or total skin electron beam radiation therapy). For patients with T2 thicker plaque disease we would consider a topical plus systemic therapy such as interferon (IFN) or targretin depending upon ages and comorbidities of patients. For patients with tumor stage or generalized erythroderma/Sézary syndrome, and visceral involvement (stages IIb–IVb) we would favor initially a systemic agent such as IFN or targretin with some topical agents, and total body ultraviolet light or extracorporeal photopheresis (Sézary), and limited radiation to tumors (stage IIb). If these approaches do not control disease we favor attempting any of the systemic chemotherapy drugs or ideally an appropriate clinical trial. For younger/healthier patients with heavily pretreated refractory disease we consider earlier use of allogeneic stem cell therapy.

exposed in vitro to PUVA undergo apoptosis. Unfortunately, normal and neoplastic lymphocytes were equally sensitive to the apoptosis induced by PUVA (as opposed to with psoralen alone). However, macrophages appeared to be resistant to apoptosis induction and phagocytized apoptotic lymphocytes (but not nonapoptotic lymphocytes). Apoptosis induction may be the ultimate end point yielding benefit, but an immunologic effect due to monocyte phagocytosis and antigen presentation resulting from effector cells may also be present.

Photochemotherapy units with UVA lamps emit a continuous spectrum of long UVA in the range of 320–400 nm with peak emission between 350 and 380 nm. Initial exposure times of patients to high-output UVA are based on the degree of pigmentation before therapy, history of ability to tan, and the output of the photochemotherapy units. Exposure times are increased with each treatment depending on the patient's response and evidence of erythema. The initial UVA dose is between 0.5 and 2.0 J/cm^2 and can be increased by approximately 0.5 J/cm^2 per treatment as tolerated. The psoralen compound is ingested 2 hours before the UVA exposure. Topical psoralen protocols are also available. UV-blocking glasses should be worn for 24 hours after administration of 8-MOP. Therapy is typically given three-times weekly until complete clearing occurs. The frequency of treatments can then be reduced, but some maintenance therapy (once every 2–4 weeks) may prolong the duration of remission. As data have emerged regarding the long-term risks of secondary skin malignancies after PUVA, the advisability of this maintenance therapy has been questioned.

Initial trials using PUVA benefited psoriasis patients. Clinical trials with PUVA for patients with MF soon followed. These studies all demonstrated high rates of remission in the early stage (patch or plaque stage of disease). The Scandinavian study group reported a 58% CR rate for these patients within 4–12 months of initiation of therapy. Maintenance therapy was associated with a remission duration of up to 53 months. In these early studies, the same group also reported a surprisingly high rate of objective remissions in tumor-stage patients of 83%. In a large series, 82 patients were followed for a median of 43 months. An ORR was observed in 95% of patients, with a 65% complete clearance rate. Ninety percent of these patients had early-stage disease (stage IA–IIA). A single patient with tumor-stage disease attained a short remission with PUVA alone. Two of six patients with generalized erythroderma cleared completely (no evidence of circulating neoplastic lymphocytes). Given the difficulty in treating advanced-stage patients with PUVA alone, we usually restrict

PUVA therapy to patients with stage IA–IIA disease (see Table 85.5), monitoring patients with tumor disease closely for progression.

Side effects associated with PUVA are quite tolerable. Nausea or vomiting due to psoralen ingestion is observed occasionally, and erythema, pruritus, and chronic dry skin are effects of the UVA damage. Long-term PUVA exposure has been associated with a number of delayed effects. These include dry skin, lichenification, keratosis, and rarely amyloid deposition in the skin. Most important is the late development of iatrogenic (basal and squamous) carcinomas, secondary malignant melanomas of the skin, and rarely cataract formation. Because the cumulative dose of PUVA is correlated with the risk for developing a second skin cancer, routine use of maintenance therapy may be less desirable, especially for patients with an excellent prognosis (stage IA). Despite these problems, the long remissions induced, the ease of administration, and the lack of interactions with other therapeutic modalities make PUVA an attractive early intervention.

Narrow-band UVB (wavelength of 311 nm) is emerging as a valid alternative to PUVA for patients with limited patch or plaque disease. Although probably not as effective as PUVA, initial studies reported RRs near 70%. The advantages of narrow-band UVB are that oral psoralen is not required and there may be less of a photocarcinogenic effect. The role for maintenance therapy has not been established.

UVA-1 is a modality of phototherapy that uses high-energy UVA1 (340–400 nm) output, which penetrates deep into the dermis. Resolution of tumor lesions has even been reported using this therapeutic approach. However, the reduction in circulating CD4$^+$ cells raises the possibility that chronic use of this modality could be immunosuppressive.

Radiation Therapy

The CTCLs have been shown to be radiosensitive. External-beam radiation adequately controls local areas of otherwise resistant MF or provides palliation in cases of bulky tumor lesions. Unfortunately, the cumulative dosage that can be given to patients over time is limited due to organ toxicity. Side effects consisting of leukopenia, thrombocytopenia, and radiation-induced dermatitis may prevent long-term therapy with other agents. Newer techniques involving total nodal irradiation, fractionated total-body irradiation, and limited fraction lesional irradiation all may have a role to play in the development of multimodality approaches to this disease. There has been little comparative research into methodology for external beam radiation that provides guidance to clinicians.

We recently reviewed our outcomes with a single fraction of external beam radiation, which was hypothesized to optimize convenience and minimize expense to patients. Two hundred and seventy individual lesions in 58 patients were primarily treated with more than 700 cGy (97%). With a mean follow-up of 41 months, 94.4% of lesions completely responded, and 3.7% partially responded. Predictors of poor response included lower extremity lesion, tumors, and lesions exhibiting large-cell transformation. Lesions treated with electron beams had a higher CR rate than those treated with photon beams. Cost estimates have suggested multifractionated radiation was 200% more expensive than the single fraction.

The limitations of external beam radiation led to increasing use of electron beam radiotherapy for cases of MF confined to the skin. Linear accelerator-generated electron beams are scattered by a penetrable plate placed at the collimator site. The energy of the electrons is reduced to 4–7 MeV and allows adequate field distribution. Because of this low energy level, the beam only penetrates the surface several millimeters to 1 cm into the dermis. Patients may be treated using six-field or rotational treatments. The total skin surface can be treated without significant internal organ toxicity. Most patients are able to tolerate total doses of approximately 3000–3600 cGy over an 8–10-week period.

An excellent review compared results of external beam therapy at Stanford University with those achieved in Hamilton, Ontario (Canada). The results cited in this paper reflect the extensive expertise of both centers in the delivery of this therapy and may not be applicable to centers where this approach is less frequently used. For patients with stage IA–IIA disease (see Table 85.5), almost 65%–95% of patients achieved a CR. Treatment delivered without adjuvant therapies is associated with a relatively high rate of relapse in patients of all stages except stage IA. Ten-year relapse-free survival rates at the two centers ranged from 33% to 52% for this good-prognosis group. However, for stage IB and more advanced disease, 10-year unmaintained remission rates were only 16% or less. Higher risk patients may be "induced" with external beam radiation and then placed on topical chemotherapy or systemic treatments such as extracorporeal photopheresis for "maintenance." Still the benefits of therapy may extend beyond crude estimates of relapse rates or survival. Patients with tumor lesions, generalized erythroderma, peripheral blood or nodal involvement, and even visceral spread can be successfully palliated with electron beam radiation therapy as well. Side effects, however, can be occasionally extreme, including scaling, dryness of skin, erythema, edematous extremities, telangiectasia formation, skin ulceration, and hair or sweat gland loss (usually transient but occasionally permanent). Careful radiation dosimetric techniques are required to ensure adequate skin treatment without excessive organ toxicity. We do not use electron beam radiotherapy early in the course of the disease because other topical therapies have been developed that yield similar RRs with less potential toxicity. The long duration of remissions observed in patients with stage IA disease does not equate with cure, because their life expectancy is essentially the same as age-matched controls, and these patients may simply have indolent biology. One group has reported their experience with multiple courses of therapy. Fifteen patients with relapsed MF a mean of 41 months after the initial course of electron beam therapy were retreated. All patients had received intervening therapies for disease control. Eleven of the 15 had a CR with their first cycle of radiation. The second course achieved six CRs and nine PRs. The median duration of the initial CR was 11 months. The median duration of CR to the second course of therapy was only 3 months, suggesting radiation resistance had developed between the first and second cycles in many patients. In general, toxicity was thought to be tolerable.

Topical Drug Therapy

The initial therapies for MF focused on treatment of the skin disease. Patients have long been known to benefit from the application of topical steroids. Zackheim et al reported a 63% complete RR with twice-daily applications in stage T1 patients but only a 25% complete RR in stage T2 patients. Novel approaches by dermatologists to apply chemotherapy topically to avoid systemic therapy complications have also been devised. Mechlorethamine hydrochloride was the first topical agent evaluated to demonstrate efficacy in MF. The solution used for topical application contains 10–20 mg of mechlorethamine dissolved in 50–100 mL of tap water (no vesicant activity at this low concentration). Although several methods may be used for administration, self-administration at home to the entire skin surface is preferred. The concentration may need to be varied depending on patient tolerance and sensitivity. The time to initial response is usually short, approximately 1–2 weeks, but long-term application is usually required to obtain the maximum response.

Several large studies have been completed demonstrating the benefit of mechlorethamine, especially in early-stage disease. One by Vonderheid et al reported their experience with topical mechlorethamine and found that it compared favorably with results achieved with electron beam treatment. CRs were seen in 80%, 68%, and 61% of patients with limited plaque, extensive plaque, and tumor lesions, respectively. The corresponding median duration of remissions was in excess of 15, 5, and 12 months, respectively. It is difficult to draw definite conclusions from these data, because many patients included in the analysis also received intravenous mechlorethamine or methotrexate, and some may have received radiation therapy. Several patients have relapsed as long as 8 years after the completion of therapy, suggesting that follow-up times must be long to compare

various topical therapies for early-stage disease. Hoppe et al confirmed these findings using an ointment-based (Aquaphor or polyethylene glycol) topical mechlorethamine, which may be associated with a lower incidence of cutaneous sensitivity. A mechlorethamine, 0.02%, gel preparation has been developed and, compared with the other preparations, has a longer stability and a consistent potency. It is also quick drying, greaseless, and developed under good manufacturing practices (not compounded in pharmacy). This gel preparation received FDA approval in 2013 for the treatment of previously treated stage IA/IB MF after a 12-month phase II multicenter randomized trial involving 260 subjects demonstrated noninferiority to mechlorethamine, 0.02%, ointment. Responses, as measured by the Composite Assessment of Index Lesion Severity (CAILS) score occurred in 58.5% of the patients on the gel arm and 47.7% of the patients receiving the ointment. Time to 50% RR was significantly earlier with the gel (26 weeks vs. 42 weeks; $p < .01$). Patients who tolerated therapy without achieving a CR were enrolled in a 7-month extension study assessing the efficacy and tolerability of a mechlorethamine, 0.04%, gel. Twenty six (26.5%) of the 98 patients who received treatment achieved confirmed CAILS responses including six CRs, and an additional 14 patients (14.3%) had their first response at their final visit, yielding an unconfirmed RR of 40.8%.

For early-stage disease, topical mechlorethamine offers an efficient, convenient (outpatient treatment), and relatively inexpensive treatment option. Side effects consist of delayed hypersensitivity in approximately 35% of patients, although ointment-based solutions appeared to offer a reduced risk for allergic contact dermatitis. Once hypersensitivity develops, patients can be desensitized by injecting minute daily doses of mechlorethamine over a period of several weeks. This should be done only in a medical setting with appropriate anaphylaxis precautions observed. Other investigators had difficulty replicating the results using this risky procedure, and topical desensitization has become much more common. Constantine et al propose that therapy should be transiently discontinued until clearance of the allergic dermatitis is achieved (using topical steroids if necessary). Then 0.01–0.1 mg per 100 mL of the drug should be applied daily for 1 week. If this dilution is tolerated, the dosage is doubled weekly until the dose achieved is often identical to the initial concentration that induced the hypersensitivity.

Some clinicians, however, believe that a mild hypersensitivity reaction may have beneficial antitumor effects. Ratner et al previously demonstrated that plaque lesions of MF cleared when exposed to topical doses of 2,4-dinitrochlorobenzene, a known universal inducer of delayed hypersensitivity responses. Anergic individuals failed to improve. Other known sensitizing agents yielded similar but less dramatic responses. Some hypersensitivity may be beneficial; the generalized erythroderma and pruritus are usually poorly tolerated when severe, however, and some alteration in therapy is required.

An increased risk for secondary skin cancers in patients receiving long-term mechlorethamine has been observed. Some physicians have expressed concern regarding the safety of family members or healthcare workers secondarily exposed to the topical solutions. Home treatment with topical mechlorethamine has been shown to result in aerosolized drug levels, which may result in mucous membrane or ocular irritation. However, we are unaware of any documented adverse outcomes and believe this to be a theoretical concern rather than a practical one.

Several other topical agents have been tested and shown to be of benefit in the treatment of MF, including cytarabine, dianhydrogalactitol, dacarbazine, guanazole, teniposide, hydroxyurea, thiotepa, and methotrexate. However, topical carmustine is the only one of these agents that has demonstrated clinical use. A stock solution is created with 300 mg carmustine in 150 mL of 95% ethanol (sufficient for 30 days of treatment). The patient then adds 5 mL of the 0.2% stock solution to 60 mL of room-temperature tap water. This solution can then be applied to the general body surface, with the exception of the head, genitals, palms, soles, and intertriginous zones, unless involved by disease. Applications are planned to occur daily for 2–6 months, if necessary. Brief exposures to double-dose solution can be used for resistant disease. Results in 188 patients with patch or plaque disease demonstrate efficacy similar to that of topical mechlorethamine. For limited patch disease, there was a failure-free rate of 90% at 3 years. For more extensive patch-stage disease, the freedom from treatment failure rate at 3 years was 62%. Some patients have been managed for as long as 10 years with topical carmustine. Side effects of contact dermatitis are less frequent with this agent, but systemic side effects, mainly leukopenia, are more common. This drug may be helpful for the treatment of patients who do not tolerate topical mechlorethamine, because there is no cross-sensitivity. A topical agent undergoing clinical investigation in a phase Ib multi-center, double-blind, placebo-controlled, randomized trial in early-stage CTCL patients is the hydroxamic acid HDAC inhibitor SHP-141. A 2014 update reported that six of the 18 patients enrolled had achieved a clinical objective response (>50% improvement by CAILS) and incremental weekly CAILS improvement throughout the dosing period. Time to response was noted to be as early as day 7. Skin biopsy histology revealed increased dermal acetylation, and pharmacokinetics results confirmed lack of SHP-141 peripheral blood exposure.

Hamminga et al performed one of the few prospective trials comparing total-skin electron beam radiation to topical mechlorethamine. A total of 42 patients with MF localized to the skin (no documented nodal or visceral involvement) were treated. Patients were not randomized to their treatment; rather, the physician based the decision on patient health, availability of the linear accelerator, and the distance the patient lived from the clinic. In patients with minimal skin disease, no difference in outcome was observed. In more advanced skin disease, a trend toward superior initial response was seen with electron beam therapy, but there was a high relapse rate in those patients, necessitating subsequent therapy.

Systemic Chemotherapy

Currently systemic chemotherapy is reserved for those patients with relapsed or refractory disease after topical interventions or for those patients with advanced nodal or visceral disease at presentation. Many of the patients treated with chemotherapy have also previously been treated with cytokine-based or other nontraditional chemotherapeutic agents before systemic chemotherapy is considered. With that in mind, a number of trials have been published reporting results using agents developed many years ago for other indications but still in use for the treatment of MF/SS today. Recently, novel agents are being increasingly studied for efficacy in MF/SS based upon a rationale developed with molecular or proteomic data. An example of such agents is the HDACI. Vorinostat (SAHA) has been approved by the FDA for the treatment of the cutaneous manifestations of CTCL in patients in whom bexarotene therapy (see Retinoids) has failed, and a related HDAC inhibitor, romidepsin (depsipeptide or FR901228), has been approved for the treatment of both CTCL and PTCL.

Approved Chemotherapy Agents for CTCL
Vorinostat 400 mg daily orally was tested in an open-label trial of 74 patients who had progressed on at least two prior systemic therapies. The ORR (skin only) was 29.5%, with 1 CR and 18 PRs. Common adverse events included diarrhea (49%) and fatigue (46%). Grade 3 events were less common but included fatigue (5%), deep venous thromboses/pulmonary emboli (5%), and thrombocytopenia (4%).

Reports from the National Cancer Institute with romidepsin have provided confirmatory results of the use of this class of agent for the treatment of patients with T-cell lymphomas, including some with MF/SS. In several phase I and II trials, 10 of 20 patients with MF/SS appeared to have had a PR. Two additional clinical trials demonstrated activity in CTCL. In a large, multicenter, open-label phase II trial of romidepsin, 96 patients with relapsed stage IB–IVA MF/SS (71% had stage IIB or higher) received standard dosing of 14 mg/m², on days 1, 8, and 15 every 28 days. Importantly in these trials, total disease burden, not just skin involvement, was assessed to determine the RRs. The overall RR was 34%, with 7% of patients

achieving a CR. The median response duration was 15 months. Common adverse events included nausea/vomiting in over 56% of patients, asthenia in 44%, and diarrhea in 14%, but again grade 3 toxicities were much less frequent, but also included fatigue in 6%. The HDACI have been linked to cardiac abnormalities and especially arrhythmias. However, in this large trial, events such as cardiac failure, atrioventricular block, and ventricular tachycardia were rare, occurring typically in less than 1% of patients. Avoiding other drugs that may also cause cardiac arrhythmias seems prudent in patients treated with HDACI. The second confirmatory trial was led by investigators at the National Cancer Institute. Seventy one patients (87% with stage IIB or higher) with heavily pretreated MF/SS (median four prior treatments) were treated with romidepsin at the same dose as described earlier. Again the overall RR was 34% with 6% CR. Although GI disturbances and fatigue were common in this trial in over 40% of patients, myelosuppression was seen more frequently, with 5%–10% of patients experiencing grade 3 neutropenia and thrombocytopenia. Cardiac arrhythmias were again uncommon, but T-wave/ST changes were seen in the majority of patients, and grade 1 QTc prolongation was seen in 10% of patients.

In general then, toxicity to romidepsin and vorinostat has included alterations in the cardiac conduction that could potentially predispose to arrhythmias, and treatment of patients has required ongoing telemetry monitoring in some trials, but no evidence for acute or chronic impairment in cardiac function has been noted. Vorinostat therapy led to drug-related grade 1 electrocardiographic changes in five patients and grade 2 in one patient. Therefore it appears safe to use these agents in the outpatient setting with a periodic assessment of cardiac rhythm and QTc interval with an electrocardiogram base.

Unfortunately, romidepsin has been shown to be a substrate for the MDR protein (a P-glycoprotein) and upregulates the expression of MDR1. Preliminary molecular analyses confirmed the upregulation of MDR1. These data suggest that when resistance to this agent develops, other chemotherapeutic drugs handled by MDR1 may be rendered ineffective. Several patients demonstrated increased surface expression of the CD25 component of the high-affinity IL-2 receptor after treatment. This protein is a target for denileukin diftitox (DD), discussed elsewhere in this chapter as a therapy for MF, suggesting that strategies for combination therapy approaches could be devised to enhance responses to both agents.

Approved Chemotherapy Agents for Cancer But not for CTCL
Older agents studied previously include alkylating agents such as chlorambucil or cisplatin, the microtubule inhibitors etoposide, vincristine, and vinblastine, or the antitumor antibiotics, such as bleomycin and doxorubicin. In general, the RRs are modest, and duration of response is typically less than 6 months.

McDonald and Bertino reported particularly good results with the antimetabolite methotrexate administered intravenously followed by oral citrovorum factor. Patients received 1–5 mg/kg of intravenous methotrexate every 5 days. If a patient tolerated the lowest dose, each subsequent dose was escalated. After five intravenous doses, patients were switched to oral methotrexate (25–50 mg) with oral citrovorum as weekly maintenance. All 11 patients achieved "good" or better clearing (>60%) for a median duration of 24 months. Mucositis and skin ulcerations were the most significant toxicity witnessed. Myelosuppression was mild in general. The related compound, trimetrexate has also been reported to be effective in treating CTCL.

As discussed previously, a newer folate analogue, pralatrexate, has also been shown to have substantial activity against PTCL. In early-phase trials several patients with CTCL were felt to benefit, and therefore a trial was designed specifically for MF/SS patients to identify an effective and tolerable dose. Starting with a dose de-escalation design at 30 mg/m²/week intravenously for 3 of 4 weeks, ultimately 15 mg/m²/week was identified as the recommended dosage for further exploration. Twenty nine patients received this dose for a median of four cycles, and the ORR was 45% (1 CR unconfirmed [CRu]/12 PR). No median response duration had been identified at the time of publication but ranged from 1 day to 372 days. Mucositis (17% grade 3), skin toxicity (7% grade 3), and fatigue (3% grade 3) were common with the use of this agent at the recommended dose. To date no comparison trials of pralatrexate to methotrexate have been performed to assess the relative cost and benefit differences.

Subsequently, the benefits of adding 5-fluorouracil to the methotrexate-based regimen, exploiting the synergy between these agents, were evaluated. The methotrexate was administered as a 24-hour continuous infusion at 60 mg/m². Immediately after this infusion, 5-flourouracil (20 mg/kg every 24 hours) was continuously infused for 36–48 hours. Oral citrovorum factor (10 mg/m²) was administered intravenously 6 hours after cessation of the methotrexate infusion and then orally for five additional doses. The methotrexate dose was escalated to a maximum of 120 mg/m², as allowed by toxicity and response. Ten patients were treated for an average duration of 33 months (range, 3–78 months). The number of cycles administered ranged from 5 to 45. All patients achieved a PR. Initial cycles were given every 5–8 days. Once a good response was achieved, cycles were administered every 3 months as maintenance. Other groups anecdotally reported success with low doses of oral methotrexate. In general these regimens appear to be fairly well tolerated.

The purine antimetabolites have been shown to be active in the treatment of MF/SS. These compounds do not have a single mechanism of action, but all ultimately interfere with intracellular regulation of deoxyribonucleotide pools and this imbalance partially explains the cytotoxicity. This family of drugs includes 2′-deoxycoformycin (DCF), fludarabine phosphate, and 2-chlorodeoxyadenosine (2-CdA).

DCF is a transition state inhibitor of adenosine deaminase. Inhibition of this enzyme, necessary for the conversion of adenosine to inosine, results in accumulation of 2-deoxy–ATP and subsequent inhibition of the enzyme ribonucleotide diphosphate reductase necessary for DNA synthesis in dividing cells. DCF is also effective against cells in the resting state, where ribonucleotide diphosphate reductase levels are barely detectable. It has been shown that deoxy-ATP accumulation in resting lymphocytes results in increased DNA strand breaks over time; this results in the activation of Ca^{2+}/Mg^{2+}-dependent endonuclease that produces double-stranded DNA breaks at internucleosomal regions and also activation of a poly-adenosine diphosphate (ADP)–ribose polymerase that consumes nicotinamide adenine dinucleotide and adenosine triphosphate (ATP). These perturbations lead to apoptotic cell death.

Fludarabine phosphate represents the fluorinated derivative of adenine arabinoside (ara-A). This compound was known to retain cytotoxic action against leukemias and was resistant to degradation by adenosine deaminase. Solubility was poor, however, unless the 5′-monophosphate derivative was used; hence, fludarabine monophosphate is the 5′-monophosphate form of F-ara-A. Similar to the mechanism of action of cytarabine or ara-A, fludarabine phosphate requires phosphorylation by deoxycytidine kinase to the active triphosphate metabolite F-ara-ATP. Again, this triphosphate derivative inhibits ribonucleotide reductase, resulting in nucleotide pool imbalances, which prevent DNA repair and ultimately cause apoptosis.

2-CdA represents another chemical modification of deoxyadenosine, which renders the drug resistant to adenosine deaminase. After activation by deoxycytidine kinase, the triphosphate derivative similarly inhibits ribonucleotide reductase and accumulates intracellularly, perturbing the deoxyribonucleotide pool balance, resulting in DNA damage and cell death.

Enzymes such as cytoplasmic 5′-nucleotidase catalyze the degradation of the active triphosphate derivatives discussed earlier. Cells with relatively greater levels of the activation enzymes versus degradation enzymes were identified as likely clinical targets. Lymphoid disorders make good targets for these agents because they contain high levels of deoxycytidine kinase and low levels of 5′-nucleotidase and depend on polymerase-α for DNA repair. Because it was known that T-lymphoblastoid cell lines were most sensitive to these drugs, it was thought that T-lymphocyte disorders would be sensitive in vivo to these agents.

TABLE 85.7	Response Rates Observed in Clinical Trials With Purine Antimetabolite Agents	
Drug	Overall Response Rate (%)	Reference
DCF	66	119
DCF	100	120
DCF	54	121
DCF	66	122
Fludarabine	18	123
2-CdA	28	124
2-CdA	38	125
2-CdA	18	126
2-CdA	100	127

2-CdA, 2-chlorodeoxyadenosine; DCF, 2′-deoxycoformycin.

A number of studies treating patients with MF/SS have been performed with these drugs. Table 85.7 shows the results in these studies. Four studies used DCF as a single agent at doses ranging from 3.75 to 10 mg/m² daily for three doses every 21–28 days. Twenty five patients with MF/SS were included in these studies; overall, three CRs (12%) and 12 PRs (48%) were documented. The fourth study represents the largest phase II experience reported for the treatment of MF/SS and other CTCLs. Twenty-seven eligible patients were treated for 3 consecutive days at 3.75 mg/m²/day. Essentially, 80% of the doses were delivered at 3.75 or 5.0 mg/m²/day. Twenty one of 24 response-evaluable patients had SS (14 patients), tumor-stage MF (six patients), or large-cell transformation of MF (one patient). Patients had failed a median of three prior treatments before enrollment. The overall RR for patients with MF/SS was 66% (five CRs and nine PRs). Most responses were short lived because the median duration of response in patients with tumor-stage disease was 2 months (range, 1–2 months) and the median duration of response in erythrodermic disease was 3.5 months (no range given, but two patients had responses of at least 17 months).

The use of fludarabine for the treatment of MF/SS has also been assessed in a single, large phase II trial by Von Hoff et al. They treated 33 patients who were good-risk disease (i.e., no prior systemic therapy) or poor-risk disease (i.e., prior systemic therapy) with fludarabine alone at doses of 25 and 18 mg/m² for the two groups, respectively. One complete response and five PRs were obtained for an overall RR of 18%.

2-CdA has been evaluated as a single agent for the treatment of MF/SS in 21 patients who had failed at least one prior therapy. There were three CRs and three PRs (overall RR of 29%). The median duration of response in this heavily pretreated group, however, was only 4 months. Three other groups have also reported results in small numbers of MF patients. A total of 21 patients were reported when the studies are pooled. Seven patients achieved responses, giving an overall ORR of 33%, remarkably similar to results from the prior large, single-institution study.

The similarity in mechanism of action of these compounds would suggest that toxicity associated with the various compounds would be similar. This has definitely not been the case, however. There are distinct differences in the spectrum of acute and chronic toxicities with these agents. DCF and fludarabine are associated with higher rates of nausea or vomiting and alopecia than commonly associated with 2-CdA. The most significant toxicities with DCF and fludarabine, however, are neurotoxicity and immunosuppression. Approximately 15% of patients developed sepsis, and 10% developed an opportunistic infection, such as disseminated toxoplasmosis, cytomegalovirus infection, Pneumocystis carinii pneumonia, atypical mycobacterial infection, and fungemia in studies. Another 15% developed severe neurotoxicity in the form of confusion, motor weakness, paresthesias, and CNS demyelination. Treatment with 2-CdA is extremely well tolerated initially but may result in somewhat greater myelosuppression than the other agents. This myelosuppression may even be more significant when the agent is used to treat T-lymphocyte disorders compared with B-cell diseases. In the study by Betticher et al, significant reductions in neutrophils and lymphocyte counts occurred in 46% and 41% of patients, respectively. In a study of 2-CdA, we reduced the days of therapy delivered by continuous infusion to 5 days from the usual 7 because of a perception that the toxicity, primarily prolonged thrombocytopenia, was unacceptable. These results suggest that patients treated with these agents should be carefully evaluated for infectious complications, especially opportunistic infections, and that prophylactic antibiotic therapy should be considered during and after therapy if significant immunosuppression is documented. In addition, one should carefully consider the value of continuing to administer cycles of therapy if there is no evidence of further improvement in clinical response, because of the risk for suddenly developing prolonged cytopenias that may limit future therapeutic approaches. In general it is not apparent that one purine antimetabolite is dramatically superior from these studies, although DCF has a slightly higher overall RR. It has been observed repeatedly in these studies that occasional patients with SS may have striking and durable responses to treatment, but ideally other agents emerging may allow for higher RRs with less toxicity in this population.

A relatively new class of antineoplastic agents, the proteasome inhibitors, also have activity in CTCL. In vitro activity of bortezomib has been demonstrated against CTCL cell lines, thought to be due to a decrease in NFκB expression observed, and this reduction resulted in marked increase in spontaneous apoptosis. These data formed the rationale for performing a clinical trial. Zinzani et al reported a small phase II trial of 10 evaluable patients with stage IV or greater MF. In this limited sample, there was one CR and six PR observed, with a range of response durations of 7–14 months at the time of the report. Toxicity was as expected, with nearly 20% of patients experiencing grade 3 neutropenia and thrombocytopenia. Additional studies are ongoing with this agent in combination with other agents for histologically aggressive T-cell lymphomas.

Combination chemotherapy has often been employed for MF/SS patients with advanced disease at presentation or with progression. Usually alkylating agents are used, in combination with doxorubicin or vinca alkaloids. Response rates of 80%–100% have been achieved, with longer durations of remission than observed with single-agent therapy. There have been no trials comparing different aggressive combination regimens. High RRs with perhaps less toxicity have been observed in treating other NHLs using infusional combination regimens such as EPOCH (etoposide, prednisone, vincristine [Oncovin], cyclophosphamide, and hydroxydaunomycin). A trial in CTCL suggested comparable activity to a bolus schedule, with greater risk for febrile neutropenia and bacteremia associated with indwelling catheters required for the infusion.

It is our philosophy that this disease behaves similarly to other low-grade lymphomas (e.g., B-cell type), with periods of remission becoming shorter with subsequent therapeutic interventions. However, as noted, advanced-stage MF is associated with a relatively short median life expectancy. Patients with significant nodal involvement or extensive skin disease (T4 in particular) have median life expectancies of 30–55 months. A driving force in the development of treatments for this disease is the goal of altering the natural history for this group of poor-prognosis patients, or for delaying the development of poor-prognosis disease. There is no clinical trial of any modality that has demonstrated a survival benefit compared with a control group. Kaye et al demonstrated more than a decade ago that combination chemotherapy (and total-skin electron beam radiation therapy) did not provide a more favorable survival or even clinically significant delays in time to recurrence for patients, compared with standard palliative, less aggressive therapies. New drugs or approaches are still being developed with the goal of altering the disease state in poor-prognosis patients.

Because of the pressing need to identify new strategies to provide more durable remissions or even curative therapy for advanced CTCL, new drugs continue to be tested. On the basis of the clinical evidence of possible activity in early-phase testing, several drugs have been evaluated. In a phase II trial of 44 patients with relapsed MF or PTCL (unspecified), a dose of gemcitabine was administered at 1200 mg/m² over 30 minutes for 3 weeks every 28 days. There were five (11%) CRs and 26 (59%) PRs (overall RR, 70.5%). The median duration of response ranged from 15 months for CRs to 10 months for those patients with PR. There appeared to be no difference in response type between patients with MF and PTCL. In a second trial at the MD Anderson Cancer Center with gemcitabine administered similarly but at a dose of 1000 mg/m², investigators documented a 68% overall RR (17 of 25), with two patients developing a CR. Toxicity included myelosuppression in the majority of patients and development of a hemolytic uremic syndrome in two older adult patients. Most recently, gemcitabine was studied as a first-line systemic treatment in 27 patients with stage T3 or T4 MF/SS. The overall RR was 70% (19 of 27), with six CRs. The median time to progression was 10 months. Toxicity was generally mild.

The camptothecins are a family of compounds that inhibit topoisomerase I, an enzyme required for unwinding strands of DNA for transcription and replication. In early-phase testing it was recognized that the administration of 9-aminocamptothecin (9-AC) by continuous infusion was required to maintain a drug concentration above a threshold level, which coupled with duration of exposure was important to ensure adequate inhibition of the target enzyme. In these studies at appropriate concentrations, activity was identified in NHLs, and it was therefore evaluated in MF/SS. We undertook a trial of intravenous 9-AC in patients with MF/SS. The trial was prematurely closed after 12 patients received 30 cycles. There were two PRs (17%) in a heavily pretreated population of patients; however, six of the 12 patients (50%) developed indwelling catheter infections, and three patients died 4–8 weeks after the last dose of 9-AC. The toxicity was deemed too excessive to justify this dose, route, and schedule of administration. This study nicely demonstrates the hazards of chemotherapy in this patient population, including the underlying risk for infection and the relative contraindication to indwelling catheters (hence a bias toward agents administered as short infusions through peripheral catheters, or oral agents, and the importance of prophylactic antibiotics if excessive invasive procedures are anticipated).

Another drug empirically tested for the treatment of MF/SS is pegylated doxorubicin based on the historic activity of doxorubicin against NHLs. The process of encapsulating the doxorubicin in pegylated liposomes creates stable, long circulating carriers of the drug that result in greater tumor cell uptake versus normal cell uptake. This may reduce normal cardiotoxicity and myelosuppression. The drug is approved for use against Kaposi sarcoma but has been evaluated in a small group of patients with MF in Europe. Six patients in this pilot study received pegylated liposomal doxorubicin at 20 mg/m² every 4 weeks. Four patients achieved a CR and one other patient achieved a PR. The overall RR was 83%. The median duration of response was not reported. Grade 3 adverse events were few and included one patient with lymphopenia and two with anemia. No other severe adverse effects were noted. A larger retrospective multicenter report of this agent administered intravenously at 20–40 mg/m² every 2–3 weeks in 34 patients has also been conducted. Overall, 15 patients achieved a CR and 15 achieved a PR (RR of 88%), with EFS of 12 months. Toxicity was similarly manageable.

The ability to biopsy skin lesions for studies of tumor cells in MF/SS has resulted in this disease being a favorable setting for the evaluation of candidate therapeutic agents and exploration of rational therapeutic development. These studies have allowed investigators to test new drugs at appropriate dosages with a correct schedule of administration, and to generate, prove, or refute hypotheses regarding mechanism of action or resistance. A number of studies of such agents have been completed and may lead to further drug testing in search of enhanced therapeutic activity in MF or perhaps achieve cure of MF.

An example of such an achievement has been the work with temozolomide for the treatment of MF/SS. This agent is an oral imidazotetrazine that has activity in solid tumors, such as brain tumors and melanoma. It has been determined that mechanisms of resistance to this agent include expression of high levels of the scavenger protein O^6-alkylguanine-DNA alkyltransferase (AGT) in tumor cells. This protein is implicated in the recognition and repair of alkylator-induced DNA damage introduced by chloroethylnitrosourea (e.g., bis-chloroethylnitrosourea [BCNU]) or methylating agents (temozolomide). The presence of the AGT protein imparts resistance by removing toxic lesions formed at the O^6 position of guanine. Chloroethylnitrosourea cross-links are prevented from forming by the removal of the chloroethyl lesion from the O^6 position before rearrangement or by reaction with the intermediate, $1,O^6$-ethanoguanine, to form a cross-link between DNA and the repair protein. The AGT protein is inactivated in the process. Studies evaluating AGT levels in patients with brain tumors receiving BCNU therapy support the role of AGT in resistance to chloroethylating and methylating agents. Retrospective and prospective human studies have demonstrated a correlation between AGT concentration and clinical outcome after treatment with BCNU.

Because of the unique sensitivity of MF to topical BCNU, we were interested in exploring levels of AGT in a variety of patients with various stages of MF/SS. Patients with patch or plaque lesions expressed low levels of the AGT protein compared with a number of controls with reactive dermatitis, and the level of AGT increased correlating with the stage of MF/SS (i.e., patients with malignant lymphocytes harvested from peripheral blood or involved lymph nodes had higher levels of AGT than those with patch or plaque lesions). Given these data, we initiated a prospective trial of temozolomide in relapsed patients with MF/SS, correlating response to levels of AGT and other known resistance proteins (such as the family DNA mismatch repair proteins).

Twenty-six patients with relapsed heavily pretreated stage IB–IVB disease were evaluated. The overall RR was 27%, with two complete responders. Median disease-free survival was 4 months. We hypothesized that the optimal phenotype that would predict for good response to therapy would be low levels of AGT combined with normal levels of several DNA mismatch repair proteins. Interestingly, hypermethylation of these DNA repair proteins has been reported to result in silencing of the genes and to correlate with lack of the proteins as assessed by immunohistochemical techniques in patients with MF. This hypermethylation may be more prevalent in more advanced tumor lesions and suggests that a propensity for mutations may precede clinical progression. It also suggests that patients might benefit from treatment with a demethylating agent in combination with temozolomide. Unfortunately, in the trial above, pretreatment levels of O^6-methylguanine-DNA methyltransferase (MGMT) and the mismatch repair genes mutL homolog 1 (*MLH1*)/mutS homolog 2 (*MSH2*) were not predictive of response to temozolomide.

Role of Stem Cell Transplantation

The natural evolution of the use of chemotherapy for this disease has been to use dose-intensified approaches with hematopoietic reconstitution with autologous or allogeneic bone marrow or stem cells. There are few reports in the literature of such treatment programs in well-designed prospective clinical trials.

Given the propensity of Sézary cells to be detectable despite a lack of clinical evidence even in early-stage disease if sophisticated molecular techniques are used, it is likely that reinfusion of neoplastic cells may occur with autologous bone marrow transplantation. The lack of dramatic benefit in low-grade B-cell lymphomas for autologous bone marrow transplantation similarly suggests that this approach will not benefit patients. We had a very limited experience with autologous bone marrow and SCT at our center and abandoned it, because of rapid progression of disease, in favor of aSCT.

aSCT has been presumed to be curative in small percentages of patients with low-grade B-cell lymphomas, and this approach has

now been investigated in the small subset of young MF/SS patients with HLA-identical siblings or HLA-matched unrelated donors who have poor-prognosis disease and have demonstrated relapse or resistance to IFNs, chemotherapy, and topical therapies. In an early study, a single patient treated with cyclophosphamide and total body irradiation was reported to achieve CR after aSCT, but relapse occurred by day 70, necessitating additional therapy. The patient remained in CR and was alive at least 6 years after the transplantation. In light of this, we and others have begun to explore this approach in patients with MF/SS who are young and have matched donors available. We have used as grafts marrow-derived stem cells enriched with peripheral blood–derived stem cells or peripheral blood stem cells only. We believe that in appropriate patients this approach should continue to be explored; older patients may benefit from strategies involving the use of RIC regimens that involve less myeloablative preparative regimens and rely on the effects of the donor marrow to create a GvL effect for disease control. Molina et al reported promising data using ASCT for patients with refractory MF/SS. Each of the seven patients treated had failed a median of seven therapies. Although one patient received a myeloablative conditioning regimen, five received a RIC regimen consisting of fludarabine and melphalan. Each of the patients achieved a clinical remission and resolution of molecular and cytogenetic evidence of the disease. After a median follow-up of 56 months, six of the eight patients were alive and free of evidence of lymphoma. The other two patients died of transplant-related complications. This small study provided the impetus to further develop ASCT strategies for the treatment of advanced CTCL refractory to standard therapies at many centers.

A metaanalysis from reports before 2008 of 20 allogeneic and 19 ASCTs was reported by Wu et al and includes some of the patients described here. The majority of patients in both groups received myeloablative chemotherapy and total-skin electron beam as preparative regimens, with the remainder in the aSCT group receiving RIC regimens. In the ASCT group EFS was only 20% at 1 year and 0% at 5 years, statistically significantly less the 65% and 60%, respectively, in the aSCT group. Overall survival was also significantly better in the ASCT group, confirming our impressions regarding the limitations of ASCT for this disease.

Since this metaanalysis was published, two larger single-institution or multiinstitution reports have been published. A European group reported the outcomes on 60 patients with MF/SS (36 of 24) who received either a matched related donor (mRD) or matched unrelated donor (mUD; 45 of 15) ASCT. Survival at 3 years was 54%. A multivariate analysis suggested that recipients of mRD ASCT had better progression-free and overall survival than patients receiving mUD ASCT transplants, and reduced-intensity transplants had less NRM without increased relapse of disease.

A single-institution trial in the United States reported the outcome of 19 patients treated with total-skin electron beam and nonmyeloablative ASCT in advanced MF/SS. The complete RR was 58%. Relapse was sometimes treated with reduced immunosuppression or donor lymphocyte infusions. With a median follow-up of 19 months, the median overall survival had not been reached.

Other Established Treatments for CTCL

Extracorporeal Photopheresis

An adaptation of the use of psoralen with UVA called *extracorporeal photopheresis* has been described by Edelson et al. Patients ingest 0.6 mg/kg of oral 8-MOP before a treatment. The treatment consists of routine leukapheresis with isolation of the mononuclear cell fraction. The cells are then exposed to UVA ex vivo within a special chamber inside the pheresis device. In the initial report, Edelson et al documented an 88.5% loss of lymphocyte viability compared with control patients treated with the drug alone. Overall, 64% of patients responded to therapy, with the best results in those with generalized erythroderma and, presumably, higher circulating Sézary cell levels. The mechanism is not thought to be directly cytotoxic, but rather to induce a host immune response to the reinfused altered Sézary cells, possibly through activation of circulating dendritic cells. This theory would explain the findings of some investigators that patients without leukemic involvement do poorly with such therapy. This treatment modality has resulted in the best results in SS patients with erythroderma of short duration and with adequate CD8+ blood counts.

Several other groups have reported their experiences with photopheresis. When the data are analyzed on an intent-to-treat basis, overall RRs of 36%–52% were observed. Only 12%–18% achieved CR. These investigators attempted to wean patients from therapy as clearing of lesions was documented. Ultimately, most responders developed recurrent disease. Many trials are underway combining extracorporeal photopheresis with other active modalities.

Toxicity is mild and includes occasional nausea, erythematous flares, and temperature elevations. Patients may develop hypotension during leukapheresis, which usually responds to saline infusions.

Interferons

IFN-α is an active agent for the treatment of MF. Dosages and routes of administration have differed among studies. Initially, high-dose IFN was used, with maximum doses of 36–50 million International Units (IU). Bunn et al and Olsen et al independently demonstrated complete RRs of 10%–27% in heavily pretreated patients. The duration of response was only 5.5 months. Later trials of untreated patients with doses of 3–18 million IU given subcutaneously daily have demonstrated RRs of 80%–92%. From all these studies, it appears that a reasonable and tolerable single-agent dose is 12 million IU/m² administered subcutaneously daily. We recommend starting at 3 million IU and gradually increasing as treatment is tolerated by the patient.

In a single trial, the results of treatment of 16 refractory CTCL patients with IFN-γ were reported. Five patients experienced PRs (RR, 31%) with a median duration of 10 months (range, 3–32+ months).

Side effects of all IFNs are dose dependent. Most common adverse effects are constitutional symptoms, consisting of fever, chills, myalgias, malaise, and anorexia. Rarely, cytopenias, elevations of liver function test results, renal dysfunction, cardiac dysfunction, or changes in mental status can be seen. Patients need to be monitored closely while on IFN.

A retrospective analysis of a CTCL database, including 198 MF/SS patients undergoing systemic therapies, revealed a median time to next treatment for single- or multiagent chemotherapy of 3.9 months (95% CI, 3.2–5.1), compared with 8.7 months for IFN-α (95% CI, 6.0–18.0, $p < .00001$). This study suggests that the use of conventional chemotherapy regimens should be delayed until other options are exhausted.

Retinoids

Vitamin A and its natural and synthetic analogues are known as *retinoids*. These compounds have diverse biologic effects, influencing differentiation and proliferation of a number of structures during development. In addition, some compounds have been shown to influence immune function. Clinically, a number of approved formulations have demonstrated efficacy in MF and SS.

Many of the trials of retinoids for MF/SS were performed decades ago with limited patient numbers. Treatment with isotretinoin (13-*cis*-retinoic acid), a nonaromatic retinoid, has been associated with clinical benefit in a number of trials. Overall objective responses have been described in 33 of 56 patients treated in three clinical trials. A monoaromatic retinoid compound, etretinate, did not achieve similar results when tested as monotherapy for MF in several trials but did show efficacy in a trial for the treatment of parapsoriasis en plaques. A polyaromatic retinoid demonstrated efficacy in a small trial. Objective responses were observed in three of six patients (one CR and two PRs).

Vitamin A Derivatives Not Approved for CTCL

There has been a resurgence of interest in retinoids for the treatment of hematologic malignancies with the approval of all-*trans* retinoic acid (ATRA) for acute promyelocytic leukemia. ATRA has been studied in 33 patients with relapsed MF who had not had prior exposure to oral retinoids. Patients received 45 mg/m² daily in two divided doses for up to 2 years. In 29 evaluable patients, five responses were observed (one CR, four PRs) for an ORR of 17% with a median duration of response of 4.5 months. Another seven patients (24%) had stable disease. The most common toxicities included headache (37%) and mucous membrane dryness (80%). Only one patient experienced severe elevation of lipid levels. ATRA works through binding to specific retinoic acid receptors (RARs; RAR family α, β, and γ), which then bind to retinoic acid response elements located upstream of gene promoters, providing transcriptional control of proteins.

Approved Vitamin A Derivatives for CTCL

A second family of receptors, the retinoid X family of receptors (RXR), has been identified. Bexarotene is a synthetic retinoid that selectively binds this family of receptors. Unfortunately, as is the case with the retinoids that bind the RAR family of receptors, the expression of which genes that are altered to achieve the clinical benefits observed remains unknown. This compound has been tested in separate trials of early- and advanced-stage patients. At the 300 mg/m² dosage daily (dose recommended by the FDA), 54% of the 94 advanced-stage patients in an open-label phase II study responded to therapy (2% CRs). The median duration of response was 299 days. The early disease trial showed similar RRs. The toxicity spectrum is somewhat different from the RAR-specific retinoids, including more frequent severe elevations of lipid levels (although rarely associated with pancreatitis), hypothyroidism, and less frequent headaches and dry mucous membranes. The compound can also be used topically. A phase I/II trial of the topical bexarotene demonstrated a 63% RR (21% clinical CRs) in primarily early-stage patients with lesional application. Toxicity was mostly local irritation with erythema.

The favorable toxicity profile has led to a number of combination modality trials using retinoids. Some of these small trials have combined retinoids with IFN-α and have reported RRs of 40%–50%. Combinations of retinoids with PUVA have been suggested to result in clinical benefit in less time with less exposure to ultraviolet radiation. These experiences have been generally limited and often uncontrolled, making definitive conclusions impossible. Larger randomized trials are needed to determine if routine use of such combinations should be undertaken outside of an investigational trial.

Monoclonal Antibodies

Targeted therapy has become a reality for the treatment of many types of cancer, including MF/SS. Although the most common approach has been with the use of antibodies that target antigens expressed by the tumor cells (e.g., rituximab), another class of compounds known as *recombinant fusion proteins* has been developed, the prototype being DD, for the treatment of CTCL.

Approved Monoclonal Antibodies for Cutaneous T-Cell Lymphoma

DD is a single-chain protein in which the receptor-binding domain of native diphtheria toxin is replaced by the sequences encoding the *IL-2* gene (CD25). Once this molecule binds to the high-affinity IL-2 receptor, the fusion toxin is internalized by receptor-mediated endocytosis and is proteolytically cleaved within endosomes to liberate the free ADP-ribosyl transferase activity of diphtheria toxin into the cytosol, where it then inhibits protein synthesis.

In early phase I studies with DD, the RR of CTCL patients who demonstrated at least 20% expression of the IL-2 receptor was 30%. A phase III study comparing various dose levels of DD demonstrated a similar RR, but there was significant toxicity that led to a high dropout rate (constitutional symptoms, infusional reactions such as hypotension, chest pain or dyspnea, and a vascular leak syndrome). Based on this trial the drug was approved for the treatment of relapsed/refractory CD25-expressing CTCL.

Recently, two dose levels of DD were compared with placebo in patients with stage IA–III disease. This clinical trial is one of the larger studies conducted in MF/SS to date and provides interesting information because it is one of the few to include a placebo control arm. Overall, 144 patients were enrolled, all with 20% or higher expression of CD25 on a skin biopsy specimen and randomized in a 1:1:1 fashion to either 18 μg/kg DD, 9 μg/kg DD, or the placebo, with the primary endpoint being overall RR. The RRs were 49.1%, 37.85%, and 15.9%, respectively, and both DD dose arms were statistically superior to the placebo. PFS (median >2 years) in the DD arms was also superior compared with placebo (median 4 months). Moderately severe and severe adverse events were both greater in the DD arms than placebo, but there was no dose effect with regard to safety.

Because of the toxicity spectrum of DD, we limit the use of this agent to patients who have failed several systemic agents (often bexarotene and IFN) previously and have more threatening disease such as the presence of skin tumors or nodal involvement. It is important to note that the pivotal trials did not allow concomitant use of corticosteroids to prevent nausea and infusional reactions. Subsequently, a retrospective case review of patients pretreated with corticosteroids suggested a more favorable toxicity profile and a RR of nearly 60%. The nature of the trial limited the conclusions to be drawn but suggested that aggressive pretreatment with steroids made this drug easier to administer to patients with advanced relapsed MF. However, this drug is currently not available. A newer version of the drug has been developed with improved manufacturing characteristics, but is only now entering clinical trials to determine if these changes have altered clinical activity.

Approved Targeted Agents for Cancer But Not for Cutaneous T-Cell Lymphoma

Targeted therapies against unique tumor antigens continue to be tested, such as the recombinant DNA-derived humanized monoclonal antibody alemtuzumab. This antibody is directed against CD52, which is present on the surface of normal and malignant B and T cells, and presumably works through antibody-dependent cellular cytotoxicity and activation of complement-dependent cytolysis, but may also induce apoptosis without complement activation. A number of trials of this agent in various stages of MF/SS have been reported. The initial phase II study using alemtuzumab in 50 patients with low-grade NHL, including eight patients with MF, demonstrated a 50% RR in MF (four of eight patients, two CR). In a phase II multicenter study of 22 patients with advanced MF ($n = 15$) and SS ($n = 7$) refractory to PUVA, radiotherapy, or systemic chemotherapy, intravenous treatment with 30 mg alemtuzumab three times a week for 12 weeks resulted in an ORR of 55%, with 32% of patients in CR and 23% in PR. Higher RRs were demonstrated in patients with erythroderma and those with fewer previous treatment regimens. Both patients with tumor-stage disease had progressive disease on alemtuzumab. Kennedy et al studied the efficacy of alemtuzumab in CTCL patients (stage IIB–IV) and demonstrated a PR in three (38%), with infectious complications in seven of eight patients. Two of the responders had SS, and these findings support our perspective that alemtuzumab may be most helpful in patients with erythrodermic MF and SS. We then conducted a trial in 19 heavily pretreated patients with erythrodermic MF or frank SS. In this trial the patients received a variety of subcutaneous, intravenous, or both routes of administration. The overall RR was 84% (47% CR and 37% PR). Median PFS was 6 months, but median overall survival was 41 months despite the advanced-stage disease and extensive prior therapy. We did not experience the dramatic infectious or cardiac events some investigators have reported, likely because of the routine inclusion of prophylactic antiviral, antifungal, and antipneumocystis agents. A multicenter retrospective analysis of 39 patients with advanced MF ($n = 6$) or SS ($n = 23$) indicated that the SS patients experienced a higher RR and longer median time to progression, an observation

that could be explained by findings from another study suggesting that alemtuzumab depletes all T cells in the blood but only the central memory T cells of the skin.

Another target of therapy for MF/SS is CD30. As noted earlier, this antigen is expressed in a variety of malignancies, including advanced HL, ALCL, and often the lesions of tumor-stage or transformed MF (tMF). As previously discussed, brentuximab vedotin (SGN-35) is an antibody to CD30 conjugated via a highly stable protease-cleavable linker to a derivative of auristatin E (monomethyl auristatin E), which inhibits microtubules and induces apoptosis in target cells. It has been approved for the treatment of relapsed HL and systemic ALCL that express CD30. There are now efforts underway to determine its efficacy in primary cutaneous ALCL and MF. Several preliminary studies have been reported. Investigators at Stanford led a trial of this molecule in MF/SS with all levels of expression of CD30. At the time of the preliminary report, 15 patients with MF/SS (13 stage IIB–IV MF/SS, nine with large-cell transformation) were included. Seven of the patients had less than 10% CD30 expression, seven had 10%–50% expression, and one had more than 50% expression by immunohistochemical analysis. An objective response was observed in 60% of the patients and in all cohorts by expression level of CD30. Toxicity was generally mild, including fatigue, peripheral neuropathy, rash, and infusion reactions. Two patients with pretreatment expression of CD30 developed antigen loss during treatment. In a phase II trial, in which SGN-35 was administered at 1.8 mg/kg every 3 weeks for up to eight cycles to 19 heavily pretreated MF/SS patients with variable CD30 expression, an ORR of 68% and median EFS of 27 weeks were reported. In another phase II trial involving 48 relapsed/refractory CD30+ CTCL patients (including patients with PC-ALCL, LyP, and MF) who received SGN-35, a 71% ORR was reported (100% ORR among the PC-ALCL and LyP patients). Neither of these studies demonstrated a correlation between response to SGN-35 and degree of CD30 expression, and response was noted even among cases with minimal expression of CD30. AEs observed in both studies included peripheral neuropathy, rash, diarrhea, and fatigue. Currently, patients with relapsed CD30+ MF or PC-ALCL are being enrolled in a multicenter, open-label phase III trial, which compares BV to physician's choice of either bexarotene or methotrexate (ClinicalTrials.gov identifier: NCT01578499).

Investigational Approaches

Because of the chronic relapsing nature of MF, new therapies with different mechanisms of action are needed to circumvent tumor resistance. A variety of such approaches are under investigation. These include the use of existing or newly developed retinoid compounds or combinations of retinoids with other agents. Other combination modalities under study include retinoids, IFNs, and chemotherapy or radiation therapy, and total-skin electron beam radiotherapy followed by photopheresis or chemotherapy. Given the lack of benefits of combination chemotherapy and radiotherapy previously, the role of such approaches should remain investigational. Another less toxic combination approach has been the simultaneous administration of IFN and phototherapy. An overall RR of 92% has been observed with this combination in all stages of patients, many of whom had been previously treated with other therapies.

Another approach to the therapy of this disease has involved new drugs to exploit the biologic characteristics of these neoplastic cells. For example, Notch signaling has been shown to be dysregulated in a variety of T-lymphocyte neoplasms. It has also been shown that Notch1 is expressed in tumor cells in many advanced-stage patients with MF/SS. There are specific inhibitors of Notch signaling that induce apoptosis in MF/SS cell lines, and this is an elegant example of how these molecular breakthroughs could be exploited to develop new approaches to the treatment of this disease. Other examples of recent or ongoing efforts to target aberrant molecular pathways in CTCL include clinical trials involving the use of PI3K inhibition and selective inhibition of nuclear export (ClinicalTrials.gov identifier:

NCT02314247). Direct targeting of surface receptors of the neoplastic cells with monoclonal antibodies continues to represent a common investigative approach, with a number of new molecules described later.

Anti-CCR4 Monoclonal Antibody

As already discussed, KW-0761 (mogamulizumab) is a humanized defucosylated anti-CCR4 monoclonal antibody that has been approved in Japan for the treatment of ATL. CCR4, often expressed by CTCL cells, contributes to the skin-homing ability of the CTLC cells. Defucosylation of the Fc region of the agent allows for a greater binding affinity to the Fcγ receptor of effector cells, resulting in antibody-dependent cell-mediated cytotoxicity (ADCC). Among 21 MF and 17 SS patients in a phase I/II multicenter study, KW-0761 0.1 mg/kg, 0.3 mg/kg or 1 mg/kg administered weekly resulted in an overall RR of 37% in the total intention-to-treat population. Interestingly, when measured by immunohistochemistry on skin biopsy samples and flow cytometric analysis of peripheral blood, CCR4 expression did not correlate with response to therapy. Ishii et al observed that the degree of KW-0761-mediated ADCC against ATL cells was determined primarily by the number of effector NK cells present rather than by the amount of CCR4 present on the ATL surface. These observations may support the study of NK cell quantification as a biomarker of efficacy of KW-0761 and may support the study of the combination of KW-0761 with an NK cell-enhancing immunomodulatory drug such as lenalidomide. KW-0761 was also evaluated in a multicenter phase II study of 37 relapsed PTCL or CTCL (*n* = 8) patients who received the drug weekly at 1.0 mg/kg for 8 weeks. Overall, there was a 35% RR and a median PFS of 3 months, and among the eight CTCL patients, three had a PR, four had stable disease (SD), and one progressed. AEs consisted of cytopenias, pyrexia, and skin disorders. A phase III multicenter trial is currently enrolling relapsed/refractory CTCL patients for randomization to KW-0761 or vorinostat (ClinicalTrials.gov identifier: NCT01728805).

Anti-CD3ε Immunotoxin

Resimmune (A-dmDT390-bisFv[UCHT1]) is a recombinant anti-CD3ε immunotoxin that is composed of the catalytic and translocation domains of diphtheria toxin fused to two antihuman CD3ε Fv fragments. In a phase I study the agent was administered to 25 CTCL patients, most of whom had been previously treated, at doses ranging from 2.5 to 11.25 μg/kg intravenously twice daily for 4 consecutive days. Nine patients (36%) experienced a response, four of which were complete (16%). The durations of the CRs were 72+, 72+, 60+, and 38+ months. Some patients in this study slowly converted from PR to CR even after receiving treatment. Patients with a lower tumor burden were more likely to respond. AEs were mild to moderate and included fevers, chills, hypotension, hypoalbuminemia, edema, hypophosphatemia, viral reactivation, and transaminitis. The phase II portion of this study is actively enrolling patients.

Anti-KIR3DL2 Therapy

As already mentioned, KIR3DL2 (CD158k) represents a unique cell surface target among the malignant CD4+ T cells from SS patients and tMF patients. KIR3DL2, which belongs to the inhibitory KIR family and is normally detectable on a minor subset of NK cells and on a rare subset of CD3+CD8+ circulating T cells, has ligand specificity for HLA-A3 and HLA-A11 through a peptide-specific interaction and for HLA-B27 homodimer through peptide-independent recognition. CpG oligodeoxynucleotides have been shown to act as a ligand to KIR3DL2 on NK cells as well as on Sézary cells, resulting in downmodulation of KIR3DL2 from the cell surface and induction of cytokine release. Among malignant CD4+ cells of SS and tMF,

KIR3DL2 acts as an inhibitory coreceptor by its ability to downmodulate CD3-dependent early signaling events and may be responsible for maintaining a high circulating malignant cell burden by preventing activation-induced cell death.

In support of the clinical investigation of the humanized anti-KIR3DL2 antibody, IPH4102, as a treatment for SS and tMF, Marie-Cardine et al demonstrated a correlation between KIR3DL2 expression and TCR-Vβ clonality on circulating CD4+ T cells from 32 SS patients (Spearman r = 0.6609, *p* < .0001). Among blood samples from 35 healthy volunteers, CD4+KIR3DL2+ T cells comprised 1.4%. Among six SS patient samples, costaining with IPH4102 bound to R-Phycoerythrin and anti-TCR-VB antibody showed consistent and homogeneous staining of the Sézary cells. A small population of TCR-negative cells stained positive for IPH4102, reflecting the normal NK cell population. ADCC and antibody-dependent PMN-mediated cytotoxicity, using allogeneic NK cells, were demonstrated using an SS cell line treated with IPH4102. Complement-dependent cytotoxicity, however, was not observed. In vivo antitumor efficacy was demonstrated in patient-derived xenograft murine models with solid and disseminated disease, with tumor reduction and improvement in survival demonstrated. Furthermore, IPH4102 showed in vitro ADCC among patient samples when using autologous NK cells. Lastly, despite that NK cells express KIR3DL2, the NK cells were spared from the cytotoxic effects of IPH4102 in this study, whereas alemtuzumab led to the elimination of NK cells. Altogether, this series of experiments demonstrate that Sézary cells are sensitive to ADCC mediated by IPH4102 through KIR3DL2 targeting at their surface; circulating NK cells of SS patients are functional and able to mediate potent IPH4102-directed ADCC; and IPH4102 antitumor activity is selectively targeted against KIR3DL2-expressing tumor cells and spares NK effectors. IPH4102 has received orphan drug designation by the European Commission for the treatment of CTCL, and a phase I trial is expected to start in the near future.

Anti-PD-1/PD-L1 Therapy

Given the established role of multiple forms of immunotherapy, such as IFN, extracorporeal photophoresis, and aSCT, in the treatment of CTCL, and the mounting supportive preclinical data, the investigation of the use of anti–PD-1/PDL1 therapy for CTCL is warranted. Conceptually, checkpoint blockade therapy differs from more traditional forms of immunotherapy, such as IFN-α and high-dose IL-2, by blocking the inhibitory controls (i.e., PD-1) of T cells rather than inducing brief periods of immunostimulation. This approach may overcome immunosuppression and thereby lead to more durable control of disease and improved survival. High expression of PD-1 has been noted among CD4+ T cells from SS patients, compared with the cells of early-stage MF patients and healthy donors in multiple studies. In vitro antibody blockade of PD-1 and PD-L1 from peripheral blood mononuclear cells of CTCL patients resulted in increased production of IFN-γ, a cytokine associated with Th1 antitumor immunity. The cytolytic activity of PD-L1–specific T cells against PD-L1–positive human CTCL cells and the lack of activity against PD-L1–negative human CTCL cells have also been demonstrated, but the use of PD-L1 as a predictive biomarker of response has not been validated. In immunophenotyping studies of freshly isolated malignant CD4+ T cells and tumor-infiltrating CD8+ T cells from CTCL patients, both cell lines displayed enhanced expression of PD-1 and other immune checkpoint proteins, consistent with immune exhaustion and suggestive that checkpoint blockade therapy may be beneficial in these patients. Recently presented data regarding the relationship between the mutational burden of some malignancies and response to anti–PD-1 antibody therapy support the investigation of mutational burden, directly assessed by sequencing or indirectly assessed by mismatch repair status, as a predictive marker to anti–PD-1/PD-L1 therapy in CTCL. In a phase I study of anti–PD-1 antibody nivolumab to treat hematologic malignancies, PRs were observed in two of 13 MF patients, while some others experienced stable disease. Currently, a phase II study is enrolling relapsed/refractory MF/SS patients to receive the anti–PD-1 antibody pembolizumab (ClinicalTrials.gov identifier NCT02243579).

FUTURE DIRECTIONS

Knowledge of the unique cytokine milieu associated with these neoplastic T cells has led to trials testing cytokines that may inhibit the growth of these cells, such as IL-12 or IL-2. Vaccine approaches may be practical.

Significant amounts of basic and practical research have been performed in an attempt to control this disease, and future treatment approaches will likely depend on further understanding of the molecular and genetic bases of these disorders. We hope that one of the strategies under development or study will lead to treatments that can control the disease and symptomatic effects, or even cure this neoplasm in the majority of afflicted patients.

SUGGESTED READINGS

Boddicker RL, et al: The oncogenic transcription factor IRF4 is regulated by a novel CD30/NF-kappaB positive feedback loop in peripheral T-cell lymphoma. *Blood* 2015.

Bunn PA, Jr, Schechter GP, Jaffe E, et al: Clinical course of retrovirus-associated adult T-cell lymphoma in the United States. *N Engl J Med* 309:257, 1983.

Cairns RA, Iqbal J, Lemonnier F, et al: IDH2 mutations are frequent in angioimmunoblastic T-cell lymphoma. *Blood* 119:1901, 2012.

Coiffier B, Pro B, Prince HM, et al: Results from a pivotal, open-label, phase II study of romidepsin in relapsed or refractory peripheral T-cell lymphoma after prior systemic therapy. *J Clin Oncol* 30:631, 2012.

Corradini P, Tarella C, Zallio F, et al: Long-term follow-up of patients with peripheral T-cell lymphomas treated up-front with high-dose chemotherapy followed by autologous stem cell transplantation. *Leukemia* 20:1533, 2006.

Couronne L, Bastard C, Bernard OA: TET2 and DNMT3A mutations in human T-cell lymphoma. *N Engl J Med* 366:95, 2012.

Cuadros M, Dave SS, Jaffe ES, et al: Identification of a proliferation signature related to survival in nodal peripheral T-cell lymphomas. *J Clin Oncol* 25:3321, 2007.

Feldman AL, Sun DX, Law ME, et al: Overexpression of Syk tyrosine kinase in peripheral T-cell lymphomas. *Leukemia* 22:1139, 2008.

Gallamini A, Stelitano C, Calvi R, et al: Peripheral T-cell lymphoma unspecified (PTCL-U): a new prognostic model from a retrospective multicentric clinical study. *Blood* 103:2474, 2004.

Ghez D, Danu A, Ribrag V: Investigational drugs for T-cell lymphoma. *Expert Opin Investig Drugs* 25(2):171–181, 2016.

Hayat MJ, Howlader N, Reichman ME, et al: Cancer statistics, trends, and multiple primary cancer analyses from the Surveillance, Epidemiology, and End Results (SEER) Program. *Oncologist* 12:20, 2007.

Horwitz SM, Kim YH, Foss F, et al: Identification of an active, well-tolerated dose of pralatrexate in patients with relapsed or refractory cutaneous T-cell lymphoma. *Blood* 119:4115, 2012.

Iqbal J, et al: Gene expression signatures delineate biological and prognostic subgroups in peripheral T-cell lymphoma. *Blood* 123(19):2915–2923, 2014.

Iqbal J, Weisenburger DD, Greiner TC, et al: Molecular signatures to improve diagnosis in peripheral T-cell lymphoma and prognostication in angioimmunoblastic T-cell lymphoma. *Blood* 115:1026, 2010.

Iqbal J, Wright G, Wang C, et al: Gene expression signatures delineate biological and prognostic subgroups in peripheral T-cell lymphoma. *Blood* 123(19):2915–2923, 2014.

Ishida T, et al: Dose intensified chemotherapy alone or in combination with mogamulizumab in newly diagnosed aggressive adult T-cell leukemia-lymphoma: Randomized Phase II study. *Br J Hematology* 169(5):672–682, 2015.

Kataoka K, et al: Integrated molecular analysis of adult T cell leukemia/lymphoma. *Nat Genet* 47(11):1304–1315, 2015.

Kaye FJ, Bunn PA, Jr, Steinberg SM, et al: A randomized trial comparing combination electron-beam radiation and chemotherapy with topical therapy in the initial treatment of mycosis fungoides. *N Engl J Med* 321:1784, 1989.

Mercadal S, Briones J, Xicoy B, et al: Intensive chemotherapy (high-dose CHOP/ESHAP regimen) followed by autologous stem-cell transplantation in previously untreated patients with peripheral T-cell lymphoma. *Ann Oncol* 19:958, 2008.

O'Connor OA, Heaney ML, Schwartz L, et al: Clinical experience with intravenous and oral formulations of the novel histone deacetylase inhibitor suberoylanilide hydroxamic acid in patients with advanced hematologic malignancies. *J Clin Oncol* 24:166, 2006.

O'Connor OA, Horwitz S, Hamlin P, et al: Phase II-I-II study of two different doses and schedules of pralatrexate, a high-affinity substrate for the reduced folate carrier, in patients with relapsed or refractory lymphoma reveals marked activity in T-cell malignancies. *J Clin Oncol* 27:4357, 2009.

O'Connor OA, Pro B, Pinter-Brown L, et al: Pralatrexate in patients with relapsed or refractory peripheral T-cell lymphoma: results from the pivotal PROPEL study. *J Clin Oncol* 29:1182, 2011.

Odejide O, et al: A targeted mutational landscape of angioimmunoblastic T-cell lymphoma. *Blood* 123(9):1293–1296, 2014.

Olsen E, Kim YH, Kuzel T, et al: Vorinostat (suberoylanilide hydroxamic acid, SAHA) is clinically active in advanced cutaneous T-cell lymphoma (CTCL): Results of a phase IIb trial. ASCO annual meeting proceedings part I. *J Clin Oncol* 24:7500, 2006.

Parrilla Castellar ER, et al: ALK-negative anaplastic large cell lymphoma is a genetically heterogeneous disease with widely disparate clinical outcomes. *Blood* 124(9):1473–1480, 2014.

Pechloff K, Holch J, Ferch U, et al: The fusion kinase ITK-SYK mimics a T cell receptor signal and drives oncogenesis in conditional mouse models of peripheral T cell lymphoma. *J Exp Med* 207:1031, 2010.

Piekarz RL, Frye R, Turner M, et al: Phase II multi-institutional trial of the histone deacetylase inhibitor romidepsin as monotherapy for patients with cutaneous T-cell lymphoma. *J Clin Oncol* 27:5410, 2009.

Prince HM, Duvic M, Martin A, et al: Phase III placebo-controlled trial of denileukin diftitox for patients with cutaneous T-cell lymphoma. *J Clin Oncol* 28:1870, 2010.

Quivoron C, Couronné L, Della Valle V, et al: TET2 inactivation results in pleiotropic hematopoietic abnormalities in mouse and is a recurrent event during human lymphomagenesis. *Cancer Cell* 20:25, 2011.

Reimer P, Rüdiger T, Geissinger E, et al: Autologous stem-cell transplantation as first-line therapy in peripheral T-cell lymphomas: results of a prospective multicenter study. *J Clin Oncol* 27:106, 2009.

Scarisbrick JJ: New drugs in cutaneous T-cell lymphomas. *Curr Opin Oncol* 28(5):384–389, 2016.

Schmitz N, Trümper L, Ziepert M, et al: Treatment and prognosis of mature T-cell and NK-cell lymphoma: an analysis of patients with T-cell lymphoma treated in studies of the German High-Grade Non-Hodgkin Lymphoma Study Group. *Blood* 116:3418, 2010.

Sharma M, Pro B: Bone Marrow Transplantation for Peripheral T-Cell Non-Hodgkins' Lymphoma in First Remission. *Curr Treat Options Oncol* 16(7):34, 2015.

Siegel RS, Pandolfino T, Guitart J, et al: Primary cutaneous T-cell lymphoma: review and current concepts. *J Clin Oncol* 18:2908, 2000.

Vose J, Armitage J, Weisenburger D: International peripheral T-cell and natural killer/T-cell lymphoma study: pathology findings and clinical outcomes. *J Clin Oncol* 26:4124, 2008.

Wang T, et al: GATA-3 expression identifies a high-risk subset of PTCL, NOS with distinct molecular and clinical features. *Blood* 123(19):3007–3015, 2014.

Weisenburger DD, et al: Peripheral T-cell lymphoma, not otherwise specified: a report of 340 cases from the International Peripheral T-cell Lymphoma Project. *Blood* 117(12):3402–3408, 2011.

Whittaker S, Hoppe R, Prince HM: How I treat mycosis fungoides and Sézary syndrome. *Blood* 127(25):3142–3153, 2016.

Willemze R, Beljaards RC: Spectrum of primary cutaneous CD30 (Ki-1)-positive lymphoproliferative disorders. A proposal for classification and guidelines for management and treatment. *J Am Acad Dermatol* 28:973, 1993.

Willemze R, Kerl H, Sterry W, et al: EORTC classification for primary cutaneous lymphomas: a proposal from the Cutaneous Lymphoma Study Group of the European Organization for Research and Treatment of Cancer. *Blood* 90:354, 1997.

Wu P, Kim YH, Lavori PW, et al: A meta-analysis of patients receiving allogeneic or autologous hematopoietic stem cell transplant in mycosis fungoides and Sézary syndrome. *Biol Blood Marrow Transplant* 15:982, 2009.

Yamaguchi M, Kwong YL, Kim WS, et al: Phase II study of SMILE chemotherapy for newly diagnosed stage IV, relapsed, or refractory extranodal natural killer (NK)/T-cell lymphoma, nasal type: the NK-Cell Tumor Study Group study. *J Clin Oncol* 29:4410, 2011.

Yoo HY, et al: A recurrent inactivating mutation in RHOA GTPase in angioimmunoblastic T cell lymphoma. *Nat Genet* 46(4):371–375, 2014.

Zinzani PL, Baliva G, Magagnoli M, et al: Gemcitabine treatment in pretreated cutaneous T-cell lymphoma: experience in 44 patients. *J Clin Oncol* 18:2603, 2000.

Zinzani PL, Bonthapally V, Huebner D, et al: Panoptic clinical review of the current and future treatment of relapsed/refractory T-cell lymphomas: Peripheral T-cell lymphomas. *Crit Rev Oncol Hematol* 99:214–227, 2016.

PLASMA CELL NEOPLASMS

Nikhil C. Munshi and Sundar Jagannath

Multiple myeloma (MM) is a malignancy involving terminally differentiated plasma cells. It includes a spectrum of plasma cell disorders ranging from monoclonal gammopathy of unknown significance (MGUS), a relatively benign condition to smoldering multiple myeloma (SMM), as well as the symptomatic malignant disorder MM, and its more aggressive form, plasma cell leukemia with circulating myeloma cells in the blood (Table 86.1). Various other plasma cell disorders belong to the same group of conditions, including Castleman disease, heavy chain disease, and Waldenström macroglobulinemia. MM is characterized by the presence of clonal plasma cells and production in the majority of cases of a monoclonal immunoglobulin (Ig) and/or its fragment with subsequent involvement or effects on organ function. Because there are five classes of immunoglobulins, the dysfunctional plasma cells can produce any one of the five immunoglobulin subtypes, including IgG, IgA, IgM, IgD, and IgE. Infrequently, heavy-chain components of the immunoglobulin are not produced by the myeloma cells, and the disease manifests as production and secretion of κ or λ light chains only. Very rarely, myeloma fails to produce a significant amount of protein and manifests as a nonsecretory MM. With the availability of a high-sensitivity, free light-chain assay, the frequency of true nonsecretory MM has significantly decreased.

EPIDEMIOLOGY

MM accounts for 1.8% of all malignancies and is the second most common hematologic malignancy. The prevalence of MM was around 95,688 in 2013, and it was estimated that 30,330 men and women (11,400 men and 9120 women) would be diagnosed with and 12,650 men and women would die as a result of myeloma in 2016. It is a disease involving a relatively older population with a median age at diagnosis of 69 years and median age at death of 74 years (Fig. 86.1A). Less than 5% of patients at diagnosis are younger than age 40 years. Myeloma is more frequent in men than in women and in African American than in white persons in the United States (Fig. 86.1B). The incidence of MM in African American males is approximately 15.7 per 100,000 per year as compared with 11.5 per 100,000 per year in African American females. The corresponding incidence rates are 7.7 and 4.5 per 100,000 in white males and females, respectively. A recent survey of MGUS in the US population showed a significantly higher prevalence of MGUS in African Americans (3.7%) as compared with white (2.3%) ($p = .001$) or Hispanic (1.8%) populations. Although the Asian population has a lower incidence of myeloma than their white counterparts, ethnic groups such as Hawaiians, female Hispanics, female American Indians from New Mexico, and Alaskan natives experience higher incidence rates than those of the US white population from the same geographic regions. Although there has been an increase in the incidence of MM, it is primarily attributed to better detection and surveillance of the disease as well as the overall aging of the population worldwide. Moreover, there has been an improvement in the overall survival (OS) of patients with MM from 3 to 7 years and longer.

HISTORICAL ASPECTS

The first published clinical description of a patient with myeloma was by Dr. Henry Bence Jones in 1850. He described a patient, Thomas Alexander McBean, who presented with symptoms of fatigue, diffuse bone pain, and urinary frequency. Urinalysis showed a urinary protein with a peculiar heat property (now called *Bence Jones proteins*). The disease was given the name *multiple myeloma* by Rustizky in 1873 following his observation of multiple bone lesions in a similar patient. A larger review of this disease by Kahler in 1889 led to its being called *Kahler disease,* especially in Europe. Subsequently, investigative advances defined the disease further with descriptions of plasma cell and x-ray abnormalities in 1900 by Wright, of bone marrow aspiration in 1929, of electrophoresis in 1937, and of immunoelectrophoresis identifying the heavy and light chains in 1953, confirming the monoclonality of immunoglobulins in this disease. In recent years, recurrent chromosomal translocations have defined subgroups of patients with myeloma, and gene expression profiling and proteomic studies are providing a greater molecular understanding of the disease. Similarly, the influence of bone marrow microenvironment on myeloma cell growth and survival has been explored and led to the identification of novel therapeutic targets. The first randomized study in myeloma compared urethane with placebo and indicated that the survival of patients receiving urethane was inferior to that observed with a placebo. Progress in myeloma therapy started with first successful use of a chemotherapeutic agent in myeloma with racemic mixture of D- and L-phenylalanine mustards (sarcolysine) in 1958 by Blokhin and colleagues; use of melphalan in 1962 by Bergsagel and colleagues; use of high doses of glucocorticoids in 1967; and subsequently use of melphalan in combination with prednisone (MP), which is used even today. With the use of high-dose therapy (HDT) with melphalan by McElwain and Powles in 1983, complete remissions (CRs) were achieved in a proportion of patients, and the identification of novel agents such as thalidomide and its immunomodulatory analogue lenalidomide and pomalidomide, as well as the proteasome inhibitor bortezomib and carfilzomib during the last 15 years targeting both myeloma cells and the bone marrow microenvironment, has further improved responses and OS.

PATHOBIOLOGY

MM, as with a number of other malignancies, remains a disease that is initiated and sustained by genomic changes that promote uncontrolled proliferative advantages to the tumor cells. Myeloma represents the classic multistep transformation process with an initial premalignant stage, MGUS, demonstrating a number of recurrent cytogenetic abnormalities as well as gene expression changes (Table 86.2). It is well documented that all MM develops from MGUS, suggesting that the initial event required for transformation to MGUS provides the first step in a multistep process.[1]

Cytogenetics

MM is characterized by a significant molecular and genomic heterogeneity affecting tumor clones. Karyotypes in MM are usually complex, with both number and structural chromosomal abnormalities observed[2] (see Chapter 56). Although chromosomal abnormalities using conventional cytogenetics in newly diagnosed patients are detected in only 30% to 50% of patients, owing to the low proliferative activity of MM cells, in advanced stages when cells usually have a higher proliferative index, a greater number of abnormalities are

TABLE 86.1   Diagnostic Criteria for Multiple Myeloma, Myeloma Variants, and Monoclonal Gammopathy of Unknown Significance

Monoclonal Gammopathy of Undetermined Significance (MGUS) or Monoclonal Gammopathy, Unattributed/Unassociated (MG[u])

M protein in serum <30 g/L
Bone marrow clonal plasma cells <10%
No evidence of other B-cell proliferative disorders
No myeloma-related organ or tissue impairment (no end-organ damage, including bone lesions)

Asymptomatic Myeloma (Smoldering Myeloma)

M protein in serum >30 g/L and/or
Bone marrow clonal plasma cell ≥10% to 60%
No related organ or tissue impairment (no end-organ damage, including bone lesions) or symptoms

Symptomatic Multiple Myeloma (MM)

M protein in serum and/or urine[a]
Bone marrow (clonal) plasma cells[a] or plasmacytoma
Related organ or tissue impairment (end-organ damage, including bone lesions)

Solitary Plasmacytoma of Bone

No M protein in serum and/or urine[b]
Single area of bone destruction caused by clonal plasma cells
Bone marrow not consistent with MM
Normal skeletal survey (and MRI of spine and pelvis if done)
No related organ or tissue impairment (no end-organ damage other than solitary bone lesion)[b]

Nonsecretory Myeloma

No M protein in serum and/or urine with immunofixation
Bone marrow clonal plasmacytosis ≥10% or plasmacytoma
Related organ or tissue impairment (end-organ damage, including bone lesions)

Extramedullary Plasmacytoma

No M protein in serum and/or urine[c]
Extramedullary tumor of clonal plasma cells
Normal bone marrow
Normal skeletal survey
No related organ or tissue impairment (end-organ damage including bone lesions)

Multiple Solitary Plasmacytomas (Recurrent or Not)

No M protein in serum and/or urine[d]
More than one localized area of bone destruction or extramedullary tumor of clonal plasma cells that may be recurrent
Normal bone marrow
Normal skeletal survey and MRI of spine and pelvis if done
No related organ or tissue impairment (no end-organ damage other than the localized bone lesions)

Myeloma-Related Organ or Tissue Impairment (End-Organ Damage)

Calcium levels increased: serum calcium >0–25 mmol/L above the upper limit of normal or >2–75 mmol/L
Renal insufficiency: creatinine >173 mmol/L
Anemia: Hemoglobin 2 g/dL below the lower limit of normal or hemoglobin <10 g/dL
Bone lesions: Lytic lesions or osteoporosis with compression fractures (MRI or CT may clarify)
Other: Symptomatic hyperviscosity, amyloidosis, recurrent bacterial infections (more than two episodes in 12 mo)

[a]If flow cytometry is performed, most plasma cells (>90%) will show a neoplastic phenotype.
[b]A small M component may sometimes be present.
[c]A small M component may sometimes be present.
[d]A small M component may sometimes be present.
CT, Computed tomography; MRI, magnetic resonance imaging.

TABLE 86.2   Recurrent Cytogenetic Changes in Myeloma

Common Cytogenetic Alterations		
Chromosomal Abnormality	Patients (%)	Genes Involved
Hyperdiploidy	50–60	Unclear
Hypodiploid	20	Unclear
Pseudodiploid	15	Unclear
del(17p)	8	p53
t(4;14)	15	FGFR3, MMSET
t(11;14)	20	Cyclin D1
t(14;16)	3	c-MAF
t(14;20)	1	MAFB
t(6p25 or 6p21;14)	1	IRF4 or CCND3
t(8;14)	5	c-Myc
t(9;14)	<1%	PAX5
del(13 or 13q)	50%	Unclear
Recently Identified Alterations		
1q+	35%	
1p–	30%	
5q+	50%	
12p–	10%	

identified. Importantly, using fluorescence in situ hybridization (FISH) as well as flow cytometry–based DNA aneuploidy analysis, genomic alterations are observed in over 90% of the patients with MM. These results suggest that the normal cytogenetics observed in the majority of the patients is derived from normal cellular components of the bone marrow and not from the cells belonging to the myeloma clone. Although detection of karyotypic changes in MGUS and SMM is extremely low, again owing to very low frequency of proliferating cells in these indolent conditions, with the use of FISH, up to 50% of the patients with MGUS and SMM have genomic alterations.

The most prominent cytogenetic abnormality identified is hyperdiploidy and recurrent translocations involving 14q32 region, which contains the *IgH* gene, the λ light chain region on chromosome 22, or the κ light-chain genes on chromosome 2, suggesting that these abnormalities may be an early important event in the development of plasma cell disorders. IgH translocation has been confirmed using FISH analysis in approximately 47% of patients with MGUS and over 70% of patients with MM, the λ light chain region in 17% of patients with MM, and the κ light-chain genes in a very small number of patients. The frequency of various common translocations in MM is provided in Table 86.2.

Hyperdiploidy

Almost half of patients with MM have a hyperdiploid karyotype (>46 chromosomes), whereas less than one-fourth of the patients have a hypodiploid karyotype (<46 chromosomes). Hyperdiploid MM is a relatively homogeneous group, with a median quartile of 54 chromosomes involving nonrandom gains. Interestingly, trisomies mostly involve odd-numbered chromosomes: 3, 5, 7, 9, 11, 15, 19, and 21. The structural abnormalities observed in MM are not exclusive for nonhyperdiploid MM, because they are also observed in hyperdiploid patients along with the hyperdiploid changes. Of note, most (if not all) of the human myeloma cell lines are derived from patients with the nonhyperdiploid genomic changes, which may reflect the difference in proliferative potential between these two categories. Hyperdiploidy has been reported to be associated with a better prognosis based upon retrospective analyses. This has been confirmed more

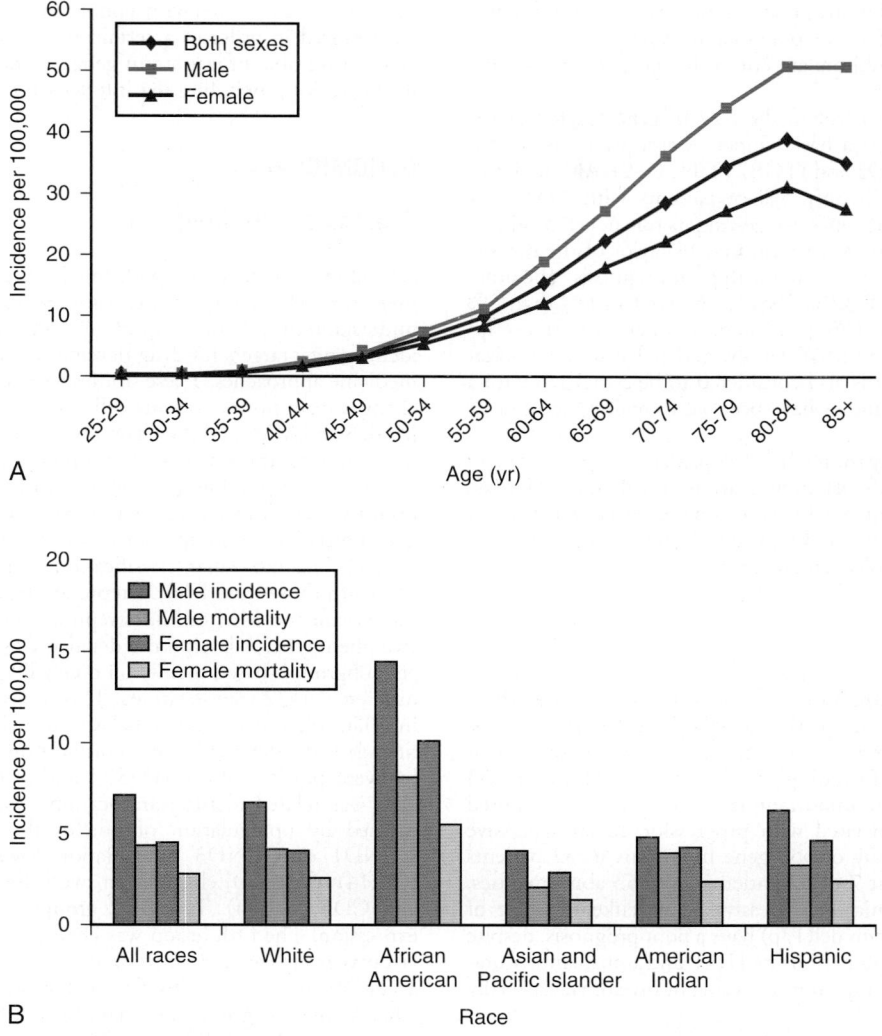

Fig. 86.1 (A) Multiple myeloma (MM) average annual age- and gender-specific incidence per 100,000 in the United States in 2009. (B) MM average annual race-specific incidence per 100,000 in the United States in 2009. Increase in incidence is noted with advancing age; the incidence is greater in males than in females; and a higher incidence is observed in African American than in white populations.

recently using an interphase FISH approach to define ploidy. However, a study by the International Myeloma Foundation (IFM) showed that hyperdiploidy was not an independent prognostic factor; rather, it was associated with a lower incidence of other independent poor risk features, such as del(13), t(4;14), and del(17p).[3]

Translocations Involving 14q32

Chromosomal region 14q32 has been identified as a recurrent site of translocations in myeloma. Unlike mantle cell lymphoma, where the IgH breakpoint is near the site targeted by VDJ recombination, the breakpoint on 14q32 in MM is located within the IgH or the switch region. In all, over 25 different chromosomal regions have been involved in translocations involving 14q32 region; the major translocation partners are 4p16, 6p21, 11q13, 16q23, and 20q11. The t(11;14)(q13;q32) translocation is present in approximately 20% of patients with myeloma and involves the cyclin D1 gene[4] (Table 86.2). Although this translocation leads to upregulation of cyclin D1, its role in oncogenesis is unknown. Despite known molecular functions of cyclin D1 in the cell-cycle and cellular proliferation, the t(11;14) myelomas have a low proliferative index, appearing morphologically as small mature plasma cells or lymphoplasmacytic cells expressing CD20. Initial studies suggested a better survival outcome in patients

with this translocation; however, larger studies have failed to confirm this observation.

The t(4;14)(p16;q32) is a cryptic translocation not easily detectable by conventional karyotyping. It leads to a unique dysregulation of two genes located at the 4p16 region; the gene for fibroblast growth factor receptor 3 (FGFR3) located on the telomeric side of the breakpoint and MM SET domain gene (MMSET) located on the centromeric side (Table 86.2). The translocation leads to the molecular activation of FGFR3 gene transcription. FGFR3 is one of the four high-affinity tyrosine kinase receptors for FGF and mediates signaling, resulting in signal transducer and activator of transcription 3 (STAT3) phosphorylation and activation of the mitogen-activated protein kinase (MAPK) pathway (Table 86.2). It is not expressed in normal plasma cells and is shown to have oncogenic potential in both in vitro and in vivo studies. Interestingly, about one-third of the patients with t(4;14) do not overexpress FGFR3. The translocation also generates a novel chimeric IGH-MMSET gene by disrupting the MMSET gene within its first intron. MMSET plays a crucial role in chromatin remodeling as well as in transformation in MM.

Several studies have confirmed that a poor prognosis is associated with the t(4;14); however, some of the newer therapies, such as bortezomib, are able to overcome the poor outcomes associated with t(4;14). It is interesting to note that genetic studies using FISH have identified the presence of del(13) in at least 85% of the patients with t(4;14). The reasons for this strong association are so far unknown. Both FGFR3 and MMSET are potential therapeutic targets, and several tyrosine kinase inhibitors are currently being tested in order to inhibit FGFR3 function.

The t(14;16)(q32;q23) involves the *c-MAF* gene located at the 16q23 breakpoint. c-Maf is a basic zipper transcription factor that positively regulates cyclin D2 and ITGB7 (Table 86.2). Although this translocation is reported in only 5% of patients with MM, it is observed in 25% of MM cell lines, suggesting its role in cell proliferation as well as its association with aggressive behavior of the disease. t(14;16) is considered to be associated with poor prognosis. The other translocation partner of 14q32 is 20q11, observed in less than 5% patients. It dysregulates *MAFB* expression, another basic transcription factor belonging to the MAF family, and it has as yet unclear molecular consequences. It is also considered to be associated with a poor outcome; however, studies have been very small because of its infrequent occurrence.

Although c-Myc is increasingly being considered to play a role in myeloma pathobiology, t(8;14) translocations involving c-Myc are rare, unlike Burkitt lymphoma, where it is considered a classic feature. Almost 20% of patients with 14q32 translocation have other partners with unclear clinical or molecular significance.

Deletion 17p

Loss of the short arm of chromosome 17 [del(17p)] has been described in about 10% of patients with early-stage MM. The deletion involves the major part of the short arm of chromosome 17 with consequent loss of a number of genes, including *p53* (Table 86.2). However, p53 abnormalities represent an important late event, mostly acquired during evolution and associated with progression to an aggressive form of the disease. A study of *p53* gene mutations in 52 patients with myeloma showed that 7 of 52 patients had p53 abnormalities, all with an advanced, clinically aggressive acute/leukemic stage of MM. Patients presenting with del(17p) have a poor prognosis, despite the use of novel agent combinations or HDT and transplant. Mutations of the *TP53* gene are uncommon events in myeloma, especially at diagnosis.[3]

Deletion 13q14

Deletion of chromosome 13 or part of its long arm is detected in approximately 15% to 20% of the patients by conventional cytogenetics and by interphase FISH in 50% of the patients. Interestingly, del(13q) is also detected in 50% of patients with MGUS by FISH, predominantly in a small subpopulation of cells, indicating that it is a secondary genetic event occurring after initial clonal expansion. Although the retinoblastoma gene is present in the deleted region, the exact molecular consequence of del(13q) has not yet been ascertained. A number of studies, especially with conventional agents as well as HDT, have identified del (13q) to be a poor prognostic feature in myeloma; however, recent studies have identified that there is an association between del (13q) and t(4;14), and in absence of t(4;14), del(13q) by itself is not associated with a poor prognosis, especially with the use of novel agents.[3] However, del(13q) detected by conventional cytogenetics is still considered a poor prognostic feature. Interestingly, del(13q) is also common in chronic lymphocytic leukemia but does not confer an adverse prognosis.

Abnormalities of the 1q Region

Recent studies have reported the biologic role and prognostic implications of a gain of 1q. In fact, this is one of the most frequently reported cytogenetic abnormalities in MM, being described in about one-third of the patients. This abnormality has also been reported in a number of other hematologic and solid tumors. A gain of the 1q21 chromosomal region or overexpression of the *CKS1B* gene located in this region is associated with a poor outcome; however, further studies are required in order to ascertain the clear prognostic impact of 1q gains. A number of important genes in addition to *CKSB* are located in this region, including the interleukin 6 (IL-6) receptor.[3]

GENOMICS

Expression Profiling

Several investigators have performed expression profiling of CD138+ myeloma cells using high-density microarrays in order to better understand the pathobiology of myeloma, develop prognostic models, identify new targets for drug development, and develop personalized medicine approaches. These studies have identified sequential genetic changes from normal plasma cells to plasma cells from patients with MGUS and MM, and they have provided clues to the molecular basis for malignant transformation and potential therapeutic targets.

Expression profiling in combination with cytogenetic changes has been used to classify myeloma in order both to identify phenotypic and molecular subgroups as well as to develop a prognostic scoring system. The molecular classification compared profiles from MM cells with those from MGUS representing an initial indolent form of the disease and MM cell lines representing cells with a more aggressive phenotype. A later, more detailed classification identified different subgroups, based mainly on cyclin D gene expression and on the different 14q32 translocations. This molecular classification, refined in 2006, identified seven subclasses of myeloma. In this model, the first class was defined by the translocation t(4;14) and was identified by overexpression of the MMSET and/or FGFR3 genes. The second class was related to the translocation t(14;16) or t(14;20) and was defined by upregulation of one of the MAF genes. Cases with CCND1 or CCND3 upregulation [owing to the translocations t(11;14) or t(6;14)] clustered in two different classes, CD1 (class 3) and CD2 (class 4). The CD2 group was characterized by CD20 expression. The fifth group was characterized by hyperdiploidy. The last two groups were characterized by a low incidence of bone disease, according to low Dickkopf-related protein 1 (DKK1) expression, whereas the last group was characterized by increased expression of genes involved in proliferation. This molecular classification has been further modified by the Dutch-Belgian Hemato-Oncology Group (HOVON) group. This analysis did not confirm the "low bone disease" group, but three other subgroups were identified: one group characterized by overexpression of cancer testis antigen genes, another group defined by overexpression of positive regulators of the nuclear factor-κB (NFκB) pathway, and a third subgroup enriched for "myeloid" genes (unclear significance).[5] Various prognostic signatures have also been developed using these expression profile data to identify high-risk disease. RNA sequencing is now replacing microarray-based expression profiling, providing additional genomic correlates including transcriptome modifiers and splicing.

Copy Number Alteration

DNA-based high-throughput techniques such as array comparative genomic hybridization (CGH) and high-density single-nucleotide polymorphism (SNP) arrays have identified recurrent copy number alterations (CNAs). These studies have identified significant molecular heterogeneity (Fig. 86.2).[6] CNAs have been observed in 98% of 192 newly diagnosed patients with MM. Two distinct groups were observed. One group of patients showed a hyperdiploid phenotype with gains of chromosomes 3, 5, 7, 9, 11, 15, 18, 19, and 21 and/or loss of chromosomes 13, 22, and X (in female cases). The second group is characterized by gain or loss of subchromosomal region. These include deletion of 1p, 6q, 8p, 12p, 14q, 16p, 16q, and 20p as well as amplification of 1q and 6p. The genomic heterogeneity observed within the hyperdiploid group is driven by the presence of either gain of copies of chromosome 1q and/or chromosome 11, chromosome 13 loss, or chromosome 5 gain. Subclasses of

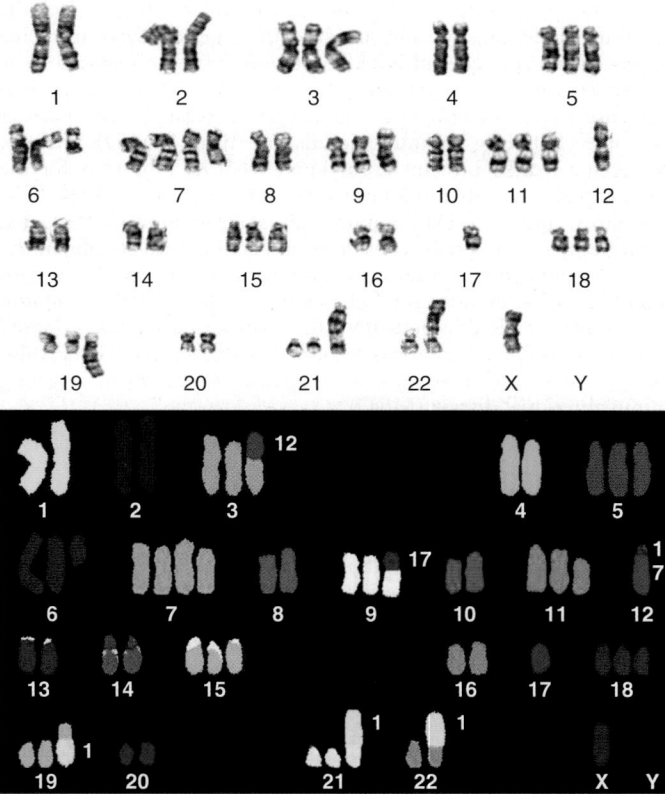

Fig. 86.2 UNSUPERVISED HIERARCHIC CLUSTERING OF SINGLE-NUCLEOTIDE POLYMORPHISM (SNP) ARRAY–BASED DATA IN 192 PATIENT SAMPLES. Each column represents a patient, and SNPs are arranged from 1p(tel) to Xq(tel) from *top* to *bottom* so that copy number changes are depicted from *top* to *bottom* for each chromosome. *Red* suggests gain of copy number, and *blue* suggests loss of copy number (*upper*). (A) Recurrence of copy number abnormalities (CNAs) across 192 patients with multiple myeloma (MM) in chromosomal order. *Red* or *blue bars* denote gain or loss of chromosome material *(lower)*. The figure identifies recurrent areas of gains and losses in MM with identification of genomic subgroups and potential therapeutic targets. *(Adapted from Avet-Loiseau H, Li C, Magrangeas F, et al: Prognostic significance of copy-number alterations in multiple myeloma.* J Clin Oncol *27:4585, 2009.)*

hyperdiploid patients with MM and their correlation with gene expression profiles provide a basis for identifying therapeutically targetable genes. The molecular basis of this genomic heterogeneity may stem from uncontrolled recombination activity that may drive continued acquisition of genomic changes.

To identify genetic events underlying the genesis and progression of MM, a high-resolution analysis of recurrent CNAs using array CGH and expression profiles was prepared from a collection of MM cell lines and outcome-annotated clinical specimens.[7] Attesting to the molecular heterogeneity of MM, distinct genomic subtypes along with 87 discrete minimal common regions within recurrent and highly focal CNAs were identified. The genes residing in these regions provide a genomic framework to understand the biology of MM as well as to identify potential therapeutic targets.

Transcriptome Modifiers

Alternate splicing is an important posttranslational modification that allows production of multiple protein isoforms, and over 90% of human genes undergo alternative splicing. The spliced isoform frequency varies between tissues, and these protein isoforms may have related, distinct, or even opposing functions. Changes in alternative splicing have been reported in myeloma cells compared with normal

plasma cells, and these changes have been correlated with an effect on overall clinical outcome.

MicroRNAs (miRNAs or miRs) are a class of small noncoding RNAs that cleave specific targeted transcripts inhibiting translational of specific genes. Differences in the expression patterns of miRNAs have been observed between MM and MGUS. For example, miR-32, and miR-17-92, are overexpressed only in MM, whereas miR-21, miR-106b-25, and miR-181a/b show similar expression patterns in both MM and MGUS but are highly expressed compared with normal plasma cells, providing a possible clue to events underlying progression from MGUS to MM. miRs 15a/16 are present on chromosome 13, and their downregulation is described in a subset of MM. Although this does not strictly correlate with chromosome 13 deletion, which is observed in almost half of the patients with MM, a potential effect of these miRs on MM cell proliferation has been described. A similar attempt at correlating observed cytogenetic changes and their effects on miR expression has identified overexpression of miR-let-7e, miR-125-5p, and miR-99b in patients with t(4;14) translocation and miR-1 and miR-133a in patients with t(14;16) MM. A causal relationship between changes in these miR expression patterns and their effects on target genes and eventual phenotypic changes in MM still needs to be established.[8] As in gene expression profiling, miRNA expression profiling also identifies subgroups with different clinical outcomes, highlighting a significant role of miRNAs in determining MM biology and its possible role as a therapeutic target. An integrated analysis of mRNA and miR profiling has been used to identify regulatory networks that combine miRNA-mRNA pairs that may drive the behavior of tumor cells. One such network combines p53-MDM2 expression with the downregulation of miR-192, miR-194, and miR-215 in a subset of patients with MM. Such analyses might explain some of the observed genomic changes in myelomagenesis and its progression. Further studies have reported a role for miR-21, miR-29, and miR-34a in supporting myeloma cell and survival, suggesting their potential as novel therapeutic targets. Efforts to combine various genomic changes to develop an integrated oncogenomic model are being pursued. A recent study has described feedforward loops integrating miRNA, transcription factor, and gene. One such dysregulated circuit in MM includes c-Myc/miR-23b/Sp1, which has potential for therapeutic targeting.

Epigenomic Alterations

The importance of epigenetic regulation in MM was established by the finding that a lysine methyltransferase (MMSET) was rearranged and activated in poor prognosis t(4;14)-associated MM. Additional studies in MM have begun to further describe epigenomic events, including DNA methylation, histone modifications, and other aberrations of chromatin, that affect MM proliferation and survival. This area of research has gained added importance with approval of the first histone deacetylase (HDAC) inhibitor for the treatment of MM.

A genome-wide methylation profile has identified hypomethylation as a characteristic that distinguishes nonmalignant from malignant plasma cells.[9] Different methylation patterns have been observed in MGUS and MM cells, explaining their distinct gene expression patterns and the behavior of myeloma cells. Similarly, the differential or downregulated expression of genes involved in cell–cell signaling and cell adhesion by plasma cell leukemia cells has been attributed to remethylation of the family of genes. The downregulated expression of adhesion genes might explain the independence of plasma cell leukemia cells from interactions with bone marrow stromal cells (BMSCs), leading to their release into the circulation. Epigenetic changes modulating myeloma cell growth and survival genes have also been reported. For example, methylation of p16, a negative cell-cycle regulator, is reported as an early event in MGUS. p16 methylation, however, has not been shown to be predictive of OS in a larger cohort study. A recent study combining DNA methylation and gene expression profiling identified hypermethylated *GPX3, RBP1, SPARC,* and *TGFBI* genes to be associated with significantly shorter OS, independent of other high-risk features.

Chromatin regulators have become an important target in understanding myeloma biology and as potential therapeutic targets. Bromodomain-containing protein 4 (BRD4) is a widely expressed transcriptional coactivator and has been identified as a regulatory factor for c-Myc expression in myeloma. JQ1, an inhibitor of BRD4, induces antiproliferative effects associated with cell-cycle arrest and cellular senescence. Although the prognostic impact of epigenomic changes has still not been studied in detail, it has already provided various therapeutic targets, including HDAC inhibitors or enhancer of zeste homolog 2 (EZH2) inhibitor.

Sequencing

The availability of next-generation sequencing (NGS) has revealed a complex and evolving genomic structure in myeloma. Three large independent studies (*n* = 733 patients) have described the mutational landscape in myeloma (Table 86.3). These studies failed to identify a universal driver mutation, but they revealed recurrent lower-frequency mutations in KRAS, NRAS, FAM46C, DIS3, BRAF, and TP53. Mutations in NRAS, KRAS, and BRAF all affect the MAPK pathway, with overall perturbation of this pathway occurring in around half of the patients. Specific mutations (ataxia telangiectasia mutated [ATM], ataxia telangiectasia and Rad3-related protein [ATR], TP53, CCND1), their mutational load, and copy number abnormalities have been used as markers of prognosis in myeloma.

NGS studies have confirmed that at the time of diagnosis, patients have a number of coexistent clones. Some mutations are in all the cells (clonal), whereas others are in a subset of cells (subclonal). Importantly, the clonal and subclonal content changes and evolves over time. Using sequential samples from the same patient, four distinct patterns of clonal evolution have been observed (linear, branching, no change, and differential clonal response) (Fig. 86.3). This information can now be exploited in the clinic. Because the genomic characteristics continue to evolve in a patient, repeated reassessment over time may be required.

Besides prognostication, the mutational profile is beginning to be used to guide therapy and to develop a personalized medicine approach. The presence of NRAS mutations has been reported to be associated with a poor response to bortezomib, whereas interferon regulatory factor 4 (*IRF4*) mutations are associated with a better outcome following immunomodulatory drug (IMiD) therapy. Mitogen-activated protein kinase kinase (MEK) inhibitors for the MAPK pathway, BRAF inhibitor for B-RAF mutations, ATR/ATM inhibitors, and CCND1 inhibitors are some examples of adapted strategies that can now be considered in patients with specific mutations. Vemurafenib was effective in a patient with myeloma with V600E BRAF mutation. Similarly, a larger study of a MEK inhibitor, trametinib, in RAS-mutated/MAPK pathway–activated relapsed refractory myeloma has shown encouraging efficacy. NGS data is also being used to accurately evaluate responses to treatment targeting minimal residual disease (MRD).

MICROENVIRONMENT AND SIGNALING

Myeloma cells interact with BMSCs, leading to both local cytokine production and both cytokine-mediated and adhesion-mediated signaling changes. The adhesion of the MM cell to the BMSC is mediated by the interaction of the adhesion molecules expressed by myeloma cells (Table 86.3) with BMSCs and extracellular matrix proteins. Adhesion and associated signaling changes affect the migration and localization of the myeloma cells in the bone marrow. Moreover, proliferative/antiapoptotic signaling cascades activated within MM cells as a result of these interactions include phosphatidylinositol 3-kinase (PI3K)/Akt, Ras/Raf/MAPK, MEK/extracellular signal-related kinase (ERK), Janus kinase 2 (JAK2)/STAT3, and NFκB. These pathways lead to MM cell growth, survival, and development of drug resistance (Fig. 86.4).[10] For example, syndecan-1, a cell surface transmembrane heparan sulfate proteoglycan present on MM cells, interacts with type I collagen and regulates the growth of MM cells; it also mediates increased osteoclast (OC) activity. Elevated

		Prevalence in Bolli et al (*n* = 67 Patients)	Prevalence in Lohr et al (*n* = 203 Patients)
Gene	**Function/Pathway**		
NRAS	MAP kinase pathway	25% (17/67)	20% (40/203)
KRAS	MAP kinase pathway	25% (17/67)	23% (52/203)
TP53	Tumor suppressor protein	15% (10/67)	8% (18/203)
DIS3[a]	Exosome endoribonuclease Recurrently mutated in NHDMM	1,5 % (1/67)	11% (23/203)
FAM46C	Unknown Recurrently mutated in HDMM	12% (8/67)	11% (24/203)
BRAF	MAP kinase pathway	15% (10/67) V600E in 3/10	6% (12/203)
SF3B1	RNA splicing machinery	3% (2/67)	1.5% (3/203)
CYLD	NFκB inhibitors	3% (2/67)	2.5 % (5/203)
TRAF3	NFκB inhibitors	3% (2/67)	5.5% (11/203)
ROBO1	Transmembrane receptor, MET signaling	7% (5/67)	2% (4/203)
EGR1	Transcription factor	6% (4/67)	3.5% (7/203)
SP140	Antigene response in mature B cells	7% (5/67)	4.4% (9/203)
LTB	Lymphoid development	4.5% (3/67)	1% (2/203)
RASA2	MAP kinase pathway suppressor of RAS function	3% (2/67)	3% (6/203)
FAT3	Cadherin superfamily member	7% (5/67)	4.4% (9/203)
CCND1	Cell-cycle progression	3% (2/67)	3% (6/203)

TABLE 86.3   Recurrent Mutated Genes in Multiple Myeloma

[a]The differences observed in the two studies are due to a small representation of patients harboring immunoglobulin H translocation in the study of Bolli et al, with *DIS3* mutations being significantly associated with NHDMM.
MAP, Mitogen-activated protein; NFκB, nuclear factor-κB.

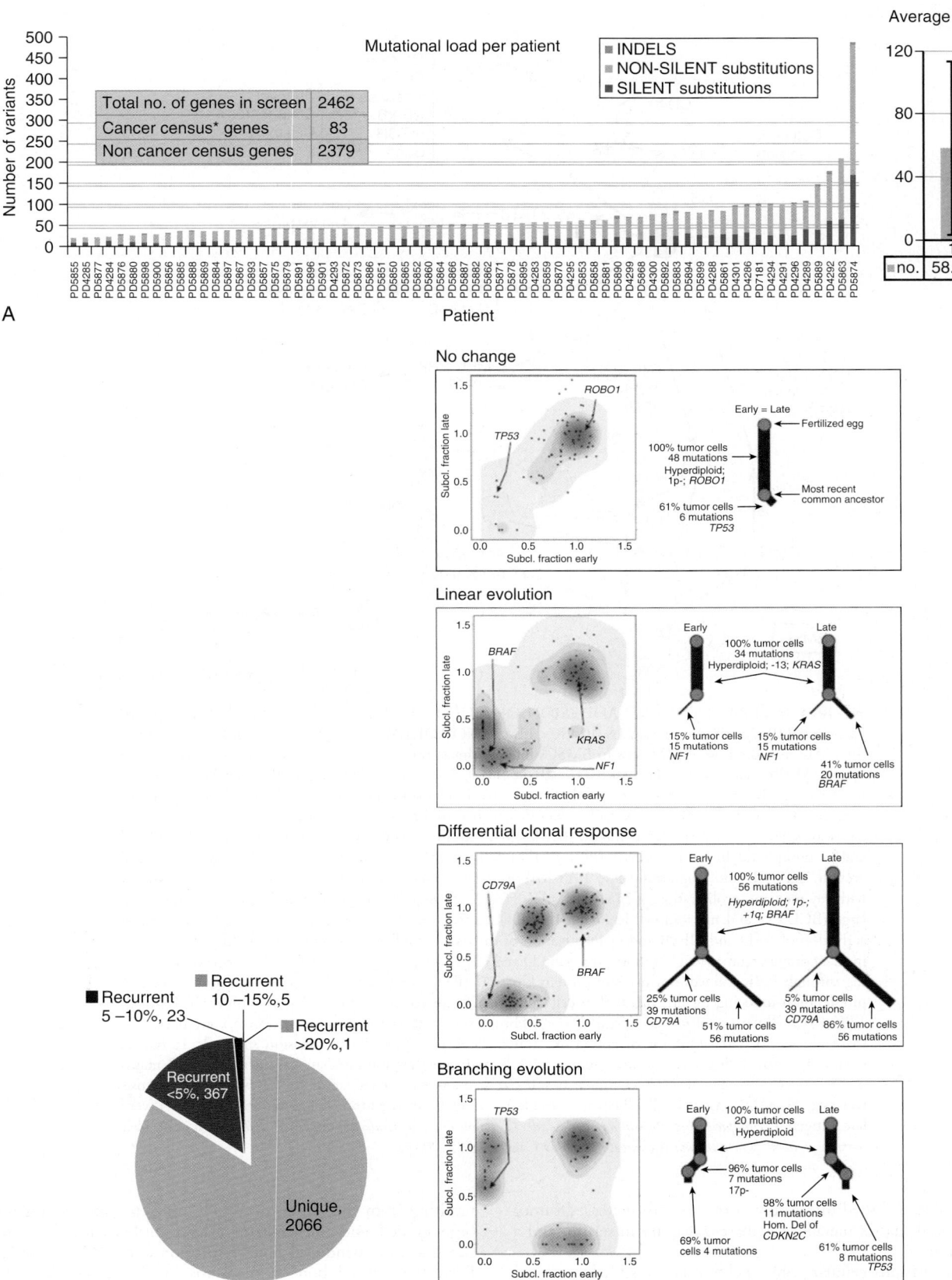

Fig. 86.3 (A) Total number of validated somatic variants for each patient in the cohort *(top left)*, average number of somatic variants per patients *(top right)*, and frequency of unique and recurrent mutations *(bottom left)*. Two-dimensional density plots show the clustering of the fraction of tumor cells carrying each mutation *(black dots)* at each time point (x = early sample, y = late sample; increasing intensity of *red* indicates the location of a high posterior probability of a cluster). *Right:* Phylograms representing the clonal composition of the tumor at each time point, where the length of each branch is proportional to the size of the clone (i.e., the number of variants) and the width to its clonality (i.e., the proportion of cells bearing each variant).

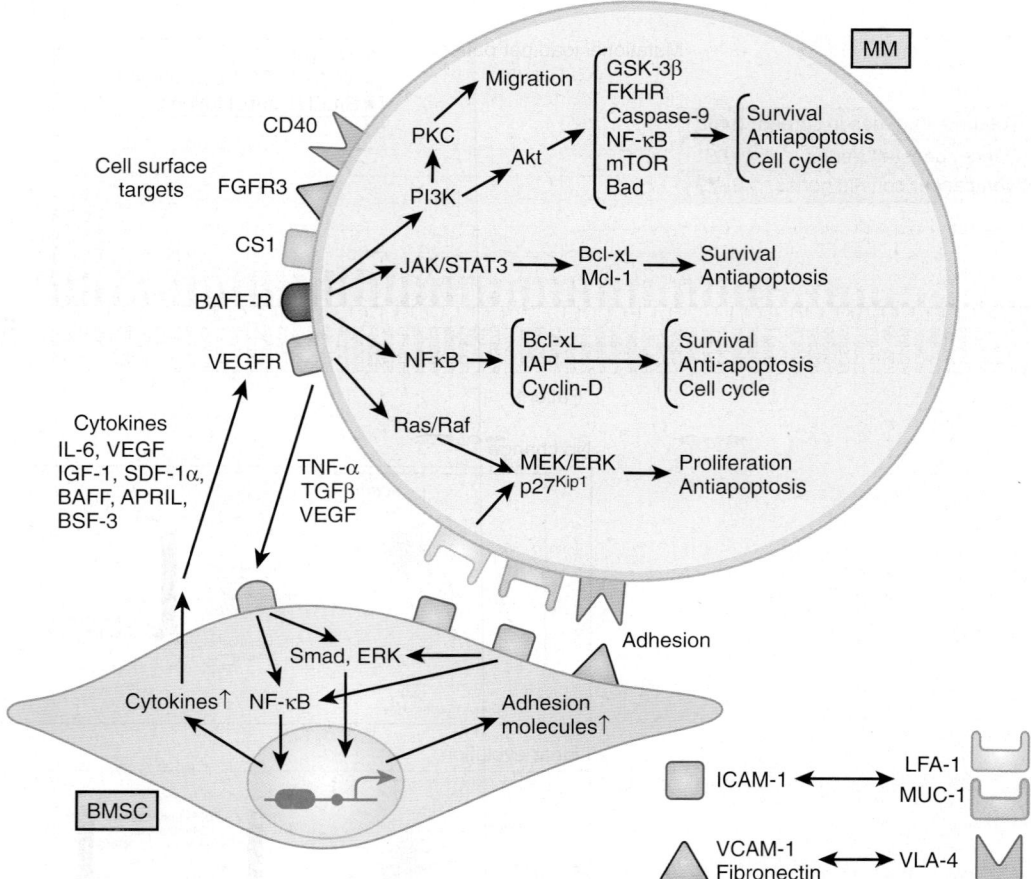

Fig. 86.4 INTERACTION AND ADHESION OF MULTIPLE MYELOMA (MM) CELLS TO BONE MARROW (BM) STROMAL CELLS (BMSCs) LEADS TO ADHESION- AND CYTOKINE-MEDIATED SIGNALING. Binding of MM cells to BMSCs induces the activation of p42/p44 mitogen-activated protein kinase (MAPK) and nuclear factor-κB (NFκB) in BMSCs. The activation of NFκB upregulates adhesion molecules on BMSCs. Cytokines secreted through this interaction, including interleukin 6 (IL-6), tumor necrosis factor-α (TNF-α), and vascular endothelial growth factor (VEGF), activate the main signaling pathways (p42/p44 MAPK, Janus kinase [JAK]/signal transducer and activator of transcription 3 [STAT3] and/or phosphatidylinositol 3-kinase [PI3K]/AKT) and their downstream targets, which triggers MM cell growth, survival, and migration. The RAS/RAF/mitogen-activated protein kinase kinase (MEK)/MAPK pathway mediates proliferation of MM cells. JAK/STAT3, along with upregulation of B cell lymphoma extra large (BCL-XL) and myeloid cell leukemia-1 (MCL1), mediates survival. PI3K/AKT, through downstream activation of BAD and NFκB and/or inactivation of caspase-9, mediates antiapoptosis. NFκB and forkhead in rhabdomyosarcoma (FKHR) modulate cyclin D and KIP1, thereby regulating cell-cycle progression. Signaling through PI3K induces downstream protein kinase C (PKC) activity and MM cell migration. *APRIL,* A proliferation-inducing ligand; *BAFF-R,* B cell–activating factor receptor; *BSF-3,* B-cell stimulating factor 3; *ERK,* Extracellular signal-related kinase; *FGFR3,* fibroblast growth factor receptor 3; *GSK-3β,* glycogen synthase kinase 3β; *IAP,* inhibitor of apoptosis protein; *ICAM-1,* intercellular adhesion molecule 1; *IGF-1,* insulin-like growth factor 1; *IL,* interleukin; *LFA-1,* lymphocyte function-associated antigen 1; *mTOR,* mammalian target of rapamycin; *MUC-1,* mucin 1; *SDF-1α,* stromal cell–derived factor 1α; *TNF-α,* tumor-necrosis factor-α; *VCAM-1,* vascular cell adhesion molecule 1; *VEGF,* vascular endothelial growth factor; *VLA-4,* very late antigen 4. *(Adapted from Hideshima T, Mitsiades C, Tonon G, et al: Understanding MM pathogenesis in the bone marrow to identify new therapeutic targets.* Nat Rev Cancer *7:585, 2007.)*

levels of syndecan-1 shed into serum correlate with increased tumor mass, decreased matrix metalloproteinase-9 activity in serum, and a poor prognosis.

There are various cellular components that constitute the bone marrow milieu, including OCs, osteoblasts (OBs), endothelial cells, and immune cells, each contributing distinctly to the overall effect of the microenvironment. For example, the cross-talk between tumor cells and components of the bone marrow comprised of OCs and OBs help propagate not only the development of osteolytic lesions but also survival and proliferation of MM cells. Several cytokines and signaling pathways have been identified as important mediators in the disruption of the OC–OB axis.[11] Impaired osteoblastogenesis

resulting from the release of WNT inhibitors such as DKK1 have been studied, and a neutralizing DKK1 antibody has been shown to suppress tumor-induced bone resorption and MM growth in vivo. Restoring normal bone homeostasis by disrupting this cross-talk represents a potential strategy to create a hostile niche for tumor growth. Similarly, endothelial cell proliferation and increased angiogenesis play a prominent role in MM. Compared with normal bone marrow, increased bone marrow microvessel density (MVD) has been observed in MGUS and MM. There is a stage-related increase in bone marrow MVD that is also correlated with prognosis. Both vascular endothelial growth factor (VEGF) and hepatocyte growth factor (HGF) have been reported to be angiogenic factors expressed by MM cells. These results also suggest angiogenesis as a potential therapeutic target and explain in part the efficacy of thalidomide and lenalidomide.

Activation of NFκB has been observed in MM cells, especially following their interaction with BMSCs. A number of abnormalities contributing to the dysregulation of NFκB and constitutive activation of the noncanonical NFκB pathway have been described.[10] The NFκB pathway can be activated either by deletion of NFκB inhibitors (such as TRAF3 or CYLD) or by activation of NFκB activators (such as NFκB–inducing kinase [NIK] or CD40). Inactivating mutations of TRAF3 and/or elevated expression of NIK by genomic alterations or protein stabilization have been described and may explain mechanisms whereby MM cells achieve autonomy from the bone marrow microenvironment.

CYTOKINES

Myeloma cell growth, survival, antiapoptosis, and drug resistance are in part mediated by a number of cytokines produced by MM cells as well as BMSCs. In fact, the production of cytokines is significantly modulated by MM–BMSC interactions and includes IL-6, insulin-like growth factor 1 (IGF-1), VEGF, tumor necrosis factor-α (TNF-α), transforming growth factor-β (TGF-β), IL-17, IL-21, C-X-C motif chemokine 12 ligand (CXCL-12), and others.[10]

Interleukin 6

IL-6 is one of the most important cytokines mediating both growth and survival of MM cells. IL-6 plays an important role in the terminal differentiation and also the proliferation of normal plasmablasts. The IL-6 receptor is composed of an α chain (gp80) and a signal-transducing β chain (gp130), which are expressed by MM cells. IL-6 binding to its receptor activates Ras/RAF/MEK/ERK, JAK/STAT, and PI3K/AKT signaling pathways, mediating growth, survival, and drug resistance. The major source of IL-6 production is the bone marrow stroma, with myeloma cells contributing to a lesser extent. IL-6 production is induced by MM–BMSC interactions as well as by other cytokines, including TNF-α and VEGF, present within the bone marrow milieu. IL-6 acts mainly in a paracrine fashion but also has, to some extent, autocrine activity. IL-6 has a number of other activities, including being responsible for a number of symptoms observed in patients, induces anemia and thrombocytosis, induces regulatory T cells (Tregs) as well as T helper 17 (Th17) cells with associated immunosuppression, and mediates enhanced bone resorption by OCs. Additionally, IL-6 promotes thrombosis without affecting fibrinolysis. It induces a prothrombotic state by increasing the expression of fibrinogen, factor VIII, and von Willebrand factor; increases the production of platelets; and activates endothelial cells. Importantly, it confers resistance to antitumor agents especially dexamethasone. Myeloma cells shed IL-6Rα and soluble IL-6R, which can transduce the response of myeloma cells to IL-6. High serum levels of IL-6 as well as IL-6R are predictive of a poor prognosis. Both IL-6 and IL-6R are thus therapeutic targets, and antibodies targeting them are in advanced stages of clinical development.

Insulin-Like Growth Factor 1

IGF-1, similar to IL-6, is a mitogenic factor secreted by myeloma cells and mediates growth and survival of myeloma cells through activation of the PI3K and MAPK signaling pathways. IGF-1 receptor is expressed by myeloma cells, and binding of IGF-1 to its receptor activates both signaling pathways. IGF-1 also mediates adhesion and migration of myeloma cells via β₁-integrin and upregulates FLIP, XIAP, and A1/Bfl1, thereby further enhancing tumor cell growth and survival. A number of IGF-binding proteins have been described that modulate IGF-1 activity. These molecular and signaling changes collectively lead to induction of drug resistance, especially to

dexamethasone and to a greater extent than that observed with IL-6. These results have provided evidence for IGF-1 as an important therapeutic target.

Vascular Endothelial Growth Factor

VEGF is produced predominantly by myeloma cells, and its expression is enhanced by MM–BMSC interaction as well as by IL-6 and CD40 activation. It has only modest proliferative effects on myeloma cells, but it is the major factor affecting myeloma cell migration as well as angiogenesis. VEGF mediates part of its activity via Flt-1 phosphorylation and downstream activation of MEK and protein kinase Cα (PKCα) signaling. Although these data suggest VEGF as a potential target, specific anti-VEGF therapeutics have not yet yielded significant clinical responses in myeloma.

Transforming Growth Factor-β

TGF-β does not have a direct effect on myeloma cells, but it has a number of activities that indirectly affect the clinical presentation of patients with myeloma. It is produced by MM cells and induces secretion of IL-6 by BMSCs. Importantly, it induces immunosuppression characteristic of myeloma and may also affect normal plasma cell development and function, thereby contributing to suppressed background immunoglobulin production in myeloma. It is also a major cytokine that affects Th cell development, especially Tregs and Th17 cells.

Interleukin 17 and Proinflammatory Cytokines

Elevated levels of Th17 cells, along with increased levels of serum IL-17 and associated proinflammatory cytokines IL-21, IL-22, and IL-23, are observed in patients with myeloma. IL-17 has multiple effects in myeloma, including induction of myeloma cell growth; suppression of immune function, especially in association with IL-22; and induction of bone disease by increasing OC number and function. IL-17 also induces IL-6 production by BMSCs, thereby augmenting its myeloma growth-inducing effects. IL-17 triggers phosphorylation of JAK1, STAT3, and ERK1/2. TNF-α upregulates expression of both IL-21 and of IL-21 receptor (IL-21R), and IL-21 induces proliferation and inhibits apoptosis of myeloma cells independent of IL-6 signaling.

Other Cytokines and Chemokines

Tumor Necrosis Factor-α

TNF-α is primarily a mediator of inflammation. It is produced by myeloma cells and has no significant direct effect on myeloma cells. However, it induces IL-6 production by BMSCs. Antibodies specifically targeting TNF-α have not shown clinical activity. CXCL-12 (SDF-1) is expressed by BMSCs, and its receptor CXCR4 is expressed by myeloma cells. It induces only a minimal proliferative effect; however, it plays a more important role in mediating migration. HGF, through its receptor c-Met expressed on the majority of myeloma cells, promotes cell invasion, migration, and proliferation. It also induces differentiation and proliferation of OCs and increases bone resorption in patients with myeloma.

IMMUNE ENVIRONMENT

Significant immune dysfunction is observed in patients with MM involving both T-cell and B-cell function as well as abnormalities in dendritic cell (DC), natural killer (NK) cell, and natural killer T (NKT) cell activity.[12–14] Researchers in a recent study described the importance of antigen-driven selection in the pathogenesis of MGUS. Those researchers investigated the increased association of MGUS in patients with Gaucher disease and showed that the clonal immunoglobulin in patients with Gaucher disease was reactive against lysoglucosylceramide, which is markedly elevated in these patients. Additionally, 33% of patients with sporadic MGUS also have clonal immunoglobulins specific for the lysolipids and lysophosphatidylcholine. These data were confirmed in mouse models of Gaucher disease–associated MGUS. Furthermore, these investigators also identified a novel type II NKT cell–mediated pathway for glucosphingolipid-mediated dysregulation of humoral immunity to account for the increased risk of B-cell malignancies observed in Gaucher disease.

T Cells

Significant phenotypic and functional aberrations in both CD4+ and CD8+ T cells have been observed in patients with both MGUS and MM. In MM, impaired action of virus-specific CD8+ cells, particularly against influenza and Epstein-Barr virus, has been reported. Hyperactive T cells associated with impaired T-cell receptor (TCR) signaling and increased sensitivity to costimulatory signals have been reported. In fact, further abnormalities of the TCR variable β-chain repertoire have been observed following chemotherapy in patients with MM. Reductions in CD4+ T-cell numbers and CD4+/CD8+ T-cell ratio are observed in the peripheral blood of patients with MM. Persistent proliferative activity of both CD4+ and CD8+ T cells has been observed in both patients with MGUS and patients with MM. This activity plays a possible role in controlling tumor cell growth and survival. Overall hyperactivity, clonal expansion, and homeostatic proliferation of T-cell activity has been observed. Moreover, CD4+ and CD8+ T cells from the bone marrow of patients with MGUS are able to mount a stronger immune response against autologous MGUS plasma cells than T cells from the bone marrow of patients with MM, suggesting the role of the immune system in controlling plasma cell growth in MGUS and loss of immune surveillance in MM. Although bone marrow T cells are dysfunctional in MM, these cells can be stimulated in vitro, leading to restored function. Tregs, the CD4+/CD25+ Th cells, specifically express forkhead box protein Foxp3 and actively suppress inappropriate immune responses, maintaining immune homeostasis. In MM, Tregs are lower in number and are dysfunctional, mediated by elevated IL-6, soluble IL-6R, and TGF-β levels. Another report suggests that, following short exposure to IL-2, purified Tregs from patients with MM are able to induce suppressive activity in vivo and in vitro. Lenalidomide, granulocyte colony-stimulating factor (G-CSF), and allogeneic stem cell transplant may directly or indirectly affect Tregs and may account for some of the observed variations in Treg number and function in patients with MM. Th17 cells specifically express the retinoic acid–related orphan receptor-γt and produce IL-17, which provides protection against certain bacterial, fungal, and viral infections. Development of Th17 cells is also determined by TGF-β and IL-6, which are upregulated in MM. In myeloma, an increased number of Th17 cells have been reported, which is associated with increased serum levels of IL-17 and other proinflammatory cytokines, such as IL-21, IL-22, and IL-23. These data support the hypothesis that myeloma cell growth suppresses immune function and induces osteoclastogenesis, supporting bone disease in MM. These effects make Th17 cells an important therapeutic target in MM. γδ T cells possess a distinct TCR and represent a small subset of T cells that is involved in generating an antimyeloma response. γδ T cells are considered a bridge between innate and adaptive immunity and are able to kill major histocompatibility complex class I chain–related protein A (MICA)-positive MM cells via the NKG2D (an NK cell–triggering receptor) pathway. Interestingly, MICA expression is significantly higher in plasma cells from patients with MGUS. Bisphosphonates have been shown to activate γδ T cells, which may in part explain their weak antimyeloma activity. As in other malignancies, expression of PD-1 is increased in T cells from patients with active myeloma. Moreover, myeloma cells express programmed death ligand 1 (PDL-1) at variable levels, along with PDL-1 by cells in bone marrow microenvironment, including plasmacytoid dendritic cells (pDCs) and myeloid-derived suppressor cells. These results partly explain the lack of antimyeloma immune response and provide a rationale for targeting this pathway using checkpoint inhibitors.

Significant B-cell and plasma cell dysfunction is observed in MM as represented by suppressed uninvolved immunoglobulins. For example, patients with IgA myeloma have suppression of serum IgG and IgM levels. This is not considered to be mediated by high levels of monoclonal paraprotein, because suppressed immunoglobulins have also been observed in patients with nonsecretory disease. An explanation for this observation remains elusive; however, suppressed uninvolved immunoglobulins predispose patients to infectious complication because they reduce the patient's ability to generate a specific humoral immune response to infections and/or vaccinations. For example, in a study of the serologic responses to vaccinations against influenza, Streptococcus pneumoniae, and Haemophilus influenzae in 52 patients with MM, researchers reported that only 19% developed protective antibody titer levels against influenza, 39% against S. pneumoniae (39%), and 41% against H. influenzae type b. These observations suggest the necessity to define suitable immunization protocols for patients with MM and the need to study the humoral and cellular responses following vaccination in terms of clinical efficacy, magnitude, and duration of response. Both B- and T-cell immune function are also affected by the therapeutic agents themselves with a further increase in the risk of infectious complications, such as the increased risk of herpes zoster virus infection following bortezomib treatment or bacterial infections following dexamethasone use. Recovery of uninvolved immunoglobulins to normal levels following effective therapy has been associated with both improved survival and protection from infectious complications.

Alteration in NK cell number has been observed in MM and is correlated with disease burden; for example, high numbers of NK cells have been observed in patients with a low tumor burden. NK cells are considered to have a potential therapeutic role, and the immunomodulatory drugs (thalidomide, lenalidomide, and pomalidomide) enhance NK cell–mediated cytotoxicity against MM cells. Invariant NKT cells, which constitute an innate lymphocyte lineage with potential for a potent antitumor immune response through the production of Th1 cytokines, are functionally defective in MM; however, these cells can be cultured in vitro with restored function, suggesting the possibility of their adoptive transfer as a potential therapeutic strategy in MM.

DCs are important antigen-presenting cells that generate effective immune responses, including antitumor responses. DC dysfunction partly mediated by cytokines such as VEGF, IL-10, and TGF-β has been reported in MM. However, it is possible to improve the defective DC function by in vitro generation. A number of studies have used DC-based vaccination strategies, including vaccinations with DCs pulsed with the idiotype protein. DCs pulsed with MM antigen-directed peptides or MM cell lysate, and fusion of MM cells with DCs has been reported to lead to an antimyeloma immune responses following vaccination. Increased numbers and function of pDCs have been reported in the bone marrow microenvironment, which mediates the immune deficiency characteristic of MM and promotes MM cell growth, survival, and drug resistance. pDCs are resistant to novel therapies; however, they are being targeted using specific agents, including anti-IL-3R antibody and Toll-like receptors with CpG oligodeoxynucleotides, to both restore pDC immune function and abrogate pDC-induced MM cell growth.

CLINICAL MANIFESTATIONS

Patients with MM present with a number of signs and symptoms that are related to either marrow infiltration by plasma cells or manifestations of end-organ damage leading to renal dysfunction, bone lesions, and/or immunoparesis (Table 86.4). However, in up to 20% of the patients, MM may present with asymptomatic disease diagnosed on

TABLE 86.4	Clinical Features of Multiple Myeloma	
Bone Destruction		**Marrow Infiltration**
Pain		Anemia
Fractures		Bleeding tendency
Cord compression		**Reduced Globulins**
Radicular pain		Recurrent infections
Hypercalcemia		Pneumonia
Polyuria, polydipsia		**Cryoglobulins**
Nausea, vomiting		Raynaud's phenomenon
Renal Failure		Acrocyanosis
Nausea, vomiting		**Hyperviscosity**
Malaise, weakness		Shortness of breath
Amyloidosis		Transient ischemic attacks
Peripheral neuropathy		Deep vein thrombosis
Dependent edema		Retinal hemorrhage
Organomegaly		Epistaxis

the basis of routine blood work. The symptoms may also be related either to deposition of paraproteins in various organs as either light chain or amyloid deposits or to cytokines such as IL-6 or VEGF produced by the myeloma cells and/or the BMSCs. Owing to improvement in routine blood work and availability of sensitive tests, the clinical presentation in myeloma has changed over the last 25 years. Overall, patients are more frequently being diagnosed with asymptomatic disease rather than on the basis of presenting symptoms. For example, patients present less often with bone pain, pathologic fractures, renal failure, or hyperviscosity. Various clinical features of myeloma are summarized in Table 86.4.

Bone Disease

Almost two-thirds of patients with MM present with bone pain as their main symptom. The mechanism of bone involvement is multifactorial, including direct bone destruction by the unbalanced hyperactivity of OCs and suppression of osteoblastic activity. This is further accentuated by the cytokine milieu generated in the bone marrow microenvironment by interaction between myeloma cells and BMSCs, which includes IL-6, IL-1β, TNF-α, and macrophage inflammatory protein 1α.[11] A member of the TNF family, receptor activator of nuclear factor-κB ligand (RANKL), also plays an important role in OC growth and differentiation via its receptor located on OCs. RANKL is secreted by stromal cells and OBs and induces differentiation and maturation of OC progenitors. Osteoprotegerin (OPG) acts as a decoy receptor for RANKL and plays a significant role in the development of bone disease in myeloma. In myeloma, the soluble syndecan produced by myeloma cells occupies and sequesters OPG, leading to excess RANKL activity, which induces OC differentiation and proliferation with the development of lytic bone lesions. Importantly, myeloma cells also secrete DKK-1, which has OB inhibitory activity, leading to suppression of new bone formation and further contributing to bone disease in myeloma.[15] Thus DKK-1 has become an important therapeutic target to improve bone anabolic effects. These factors together lead to osteoporosis and lytic bone lesions. Additionally, direct infiltration of bone by myeloma cells also causes bone destruction. Overall, one observes pain that is aggravated on movement and also collapse of vertebrae leading to a decrease in height as well as symptoms of nerve compression. Besides pain, involvement of extremity and/or spine leads to lack of mobility and associated problems, including predisposition to thrombotic events.

Hypercalcemia

Hypercalcemia is observed in approximately 25% to 30% of patients with myeloma and is usually a manifestation of higher disease burden.

Its occurrence is related to bone involvement as well as production of various cytokines that lead to increased bone resorption and calcium release. Hypercalcemia manifests as mental status changes, lethargy, nausea and vomiting, and constipation. In extreme cases, a patient can also develop seizure activity. A normal serum calcium level in the presence of high paraprotein and/or low albumen level may require calculation or measurement of ionized calcium levels to assess true and effective serum calcium levels. Hypercalcemia can also induce renal failure caused by dehydration, and it is to be considered a hematologic emergency meriting prompt intervention.

Renal Failure

Renal insufficiency is a frequent and serious complication of myeloma that has a multifactorial etiology.[16] The most common and reversible cause of renal failure is light chain tubular cast deposition and/or light chain deposition disease (commonly associated with κ light chains). Similarly, proteins can be deposited as amyloid, predominantly involving λ light chains (specifically λ light chain subtype 6) with development of kidney failure. Amyloidosis is quite often associated with nephrotic syndrome range proteinuria. The proteinuria observed in patients with amyloid is more nonspecific, which differs from conditions with light chain cast nephropathy with predominantly excess of light chain excretion in the urine. Another common cause is hypercalcemia leading to osmotic diuresis and prerenal dysfunction associated with volume depletion. Additional mechanisms of renal failure in myeloma include renal calcium deposition with interstitial nephritis, use of nonsteroidal antiinflammatory drugs for pain control, hyperuricemia, intravenous contrast dye use for imaging purposes, chemotherapy-induced nephrotoxicity, and use of bisphosphonates. The development of light chain deposition disease has been reported to be associated with Tamm-Horsfall protein, which promotes heterotypic aggregation of light chains with deposition in the kidneys. Patients with renal failure are quite asymptomatic. However, when symptoms are present, they are predominately malaise, weakness, nausea, or vomiting.

Anemia

Anemia is another presenting symptom of myeloma and is symptomatically associated with fatigue and shortness of breath. The anemia usually is normochromic and normocytic and has a number of etiologic factors, including inadequate erythropoietin production caused by renal dysfunction, erythropoietin unresponsiveness predominantly caused by various cytokines produced by MM cells, dilution resulting from a significantly increased immunoglobulin level, and bone marrow infiltrative processes.[17] Part of the development of anemia may also be related to high IL-6 levels. In patients who have had a number of treatments, quite often anemia is related to repeated rounds of chemotherapy. Erythropoietin administration therefore is an important supportive measure for the symptomatic treatment of anemia in myeloma. In one study, improvement in hemoglobin was observed in 60% of treated patients, and responses were observed in those with low erythropoietin levels compared with normal or high levels (72% vs. 20%).

Neurologic Symptoms

Patients with MM present with a number of neurologic symptoms related either to direct involvement of the nervous system or the impact of cytokines and/or paraproteins on the nervous system. The most common abnormality is compression of the spinal cord and/or nerve roots giving rise to pain as well as various degrees of neurologic dysfunction, including paraplegia with loss of bladder and bowel control. Cord compression is considered a neurologic emergency requiring prompt intervention, which might allow complete recovery of function. In this setting, urgent MRI followed by radiotherapeutic and/or surgical intervention is warranted. Peripheral neuropathy is another common manifestation observed in almost one-third of the newly diagnosed patients if analyzed using sophisticated and sensitive methods. Peripheral neuropathy also can develop as a result of use of a number of therapeutic agents, such as thalidomide, bortezomib, and vincristine. Moreover, POEMS syndrome (polyneuropathy, organomegaly, endocrinopathy, monoclonal gammopathy, and skin changes) includes a prominent sensory neuropathy associated with sclerotic myeloma. Paraneoplastic central nervous system (CNS) manifestations have been reported occasionally in myeloma and are considered to be related to clonal immunoglobulin targeting various CNS cells and/or structure. The polyneuropathy in myeloma is due to multiple factors, including amyloid deposits, infiltrative processes with other protein deposits, metabolic causes related to hypercalcemia and/or hyperviscosity, immune processes, or cytokines effects. IgM-related neuropathy is well described in which a myelin-associated globulin (MAG) has been described in 50% of the patients. Presence of MAG provides diagnostic clues as well as a parameter to follow therapy. Traditionally, meningeal involvement has been described very rarely in myeloma; however, with prolonged survival with novel agents, it is being seen more frequently. This type of complication is usually observed with high-risk disease. Finally, intracranial plasmacytomas involving brain parenchyma, either from the skull or from the skull base, has been reported in advanced cases.

Hyperviscosity

Hyperviscosity is less frequent in myeloma than in Waldenström macroglobulinemia, where higher-molecular-weight IgM molecules frequently cause an increase in viscosity. In general, hyperviscosity in IgG myeloma is extremely uncommon. For hyperviscosity to develop, generally an IgG more than 10 g/dL, IgA more than 7 g/dL, and IgM more than 5 g/dL are required to cause symptomatology. Occasionally, certain physicochemical characteristics of immunoglobulin may lead to self-aggregating properties and induce viscosity even at a lower level. This has been reported with IgG3, which is more frequently associated with hyperviscosity than various other IgG myelomas. The commonly observed symptoms are related to circulatory decline of vital organ function, leading to complaints of headache, visual symptoms, shortness of breath, bleeding complications such as nosebleeds, and eventually mental status changes. The confirmation of viscosity can be obtained by measuring viscosity, which may exceed 4.0 centipoise (cP); however, symptoms at lower levels of viscosity have been observed. Therapy is instituted more on the basis of symptomatology than on absolute measured levels of viscosity and requires prompt institution of plasmapheresis with quick resolution of symptoms.

Infections

Infection is one of the most important causes of morbidity and a common cause of mortality in myeloma. Owing to compromised T- and B-cell function, patients with myeloma are at a significant high risk of developing recurrent bacterial as well as viral and fungal infections. As described earlier, various factors lead to inability of patients with myeloma to mount a humoral immune response.[18] The patients are susceptible to polysaccharide-encapsulated organisms as well as enteric gram-negative bacilli. Further susceptibility to infections also stems from a number of therapeutic interventions, especially corticosteroids. For example, fungal infection, most commonly oral thrush, is observed following high-dose dexamethasone-based therapy, whereas herpes zoster viral infection is observed frequently following bortezomib-based therapy. In both cases, prophylactic antibiotics or antivirals are indicated. A number of cases of therapy-induced activation of *Mycobacterium tuberculosis* in developing countries have been reported. The risk of infection is highest during the first 2 months of initiation of therapy, when both myeloma-related immunosuppression and therapy-related immunosuppression increase the

predisposition to infectious complication. Prompt diagnosis of infectious complications and quick institution of therapy, or preferably initial prophylactic measures, prevents major complications.

Coagulation Disorders

Both bone marrow suppression with cytopenias and coagulation abnormalities are observed in myeloma. Myeloma might be associated with both bleeding problems and thrombotic events. The coagulation abnormalities are related to high levels of a paraprotein that interferes with the normal coagulation pathways as well as platelet dysfunction caused by either decreased numbers and/or function. The coagulation abnormalities include an acquired deficiency of factor VIII. A hypercoaluable state is observed in 15% of patients with IgG myeloma and one-third of patients with IgA myeloma, and it is related to hyperviscosity, acquired activated protein C resistance, lupus-like anticoagulants with thromboembolic complications, acquired deficiency of protein S, and a therapy-related hypercoaluable state associated specifically with immunomodulatory agents such as thalidomide and lenalidomide. In the absence of prophylactic measures, such immunomodulatory agents have been reported to cause deep vein thrombosis (DVT) in 10% to 20% of patients, in whom the thrombotic risk increases with associated use of dexamethasone, other chemotherapeutic agents, and/or previous history of DVT or immobility.

Thrombocytosis is more frequently associated with myeloma than thrombocytopenia, driven mainly by the high levels of IL-6, which drives growth and maturation of megakaryocytes. Rarely, extensive bone marrow infiltration by myeloma cells, and more commonly repeated cycles of chemotherapy, leads to thrombocytopenia during the advanced stages of the disease.

Amyloidosis

Monoclonal proteins, specifically light chains, can be deposited in various organs as an insoluble fibrillar protein, amyloid, affecting organ dysfunction (see Chapter 88). Around 20% of patients with light-chain (AL) amyloidosis also have a concurrent diagnosis of MM, and all patients with AL amyloid have clonal light-chain production. Although clinically overt amyloidosis is observed less frequently in MM, intense investigation to identify amyloid deposits using fat pad biopsies, concurrent staining of bone marrow with Sudan black, and obtaining rectal biopsies can identify some level of amyloid deposit in almost one-third of patients. Patients with amyloid deposits can present with a number of features primarily related to organ damage, including renal and cardiac dysfunction and symptoms suggesting carpal tunnel syndrome. Classic presentations of advance amyloid include cutaneous fragility around the eyelids, with raccoon eyes and macroglossia. Patients with advanced amyloid with myeloma have a poor overall outcome; however, therapeutic intervention currently remains the same in patients with myeloma with amyloidosis.

LABORATORY MANIFESTATIONS

Investigations to Detect Clonality

Protein Electrophoresis

Serum protein electrophoresis is performed to quantitate the monoclonal proteins present in myeloma (Table 86.5).[19] In 70% of the patients, the monoclonal protein is IgG; in 20%, it is IgA; and in 5% to 10% of patients, it is light chains only. Less than 1% patients have a monoclonal protein that is IgD, IgE, or IgM or truly a nonsecretory myeloma. The identification of the exact type of paraprotein in both serum and urine requires immunofixation (Fig. 86.5). This should be performed at the time of initial diagnosis, and it needs to

<table>
<tr><td>

| TABLE 86.5 | **Evaluation of Patients With Multiple Myeloma** |
</td></tr>
</table>

Evaluation for Diagnosis
Evaluation for Monoclonal Protein

  Serum protein electrophoresis, immunofixation
  Quantitative immunoglobulin by nephelometric method
  24-Hour urine collection for electrophoresis and Bence Jones
    protein assessment and immunofixation
  Serum free light chain and ratio

Evaluation for Clonal Plasma Cells

Bone marrow aspirate and biopsy for
  Histology
  Clonality by immunostaining or flow cytometry by κ/λ staining
  Fine-needle aspiration of plasmacytoma if indicated

Evaluation for End-Organ Damage

  Hemogram to detect anemia
  Chemistry panel for renal function and calcium
  Radiologic evaluation: skeletal survey
  PET-CT or MRI as indicated for bone lesions or extramedullary
    disease

Evaluation for Risk Stratification

  β_2-Microglobulin and serum albumin for ISS stage
  Cytogenetics and fluorescence in situ hybridization on bone marrow
    sample
  LDH
  C-reactive protein

Other Investigations for Selected Patients

  Abdominal fat pad or rectal biopsy for amyloid
  Solitary lytic lesion biopsy
  Serum viscosity if IgM component or high IgA levels or serum M
    component >7 g/dL
  Immunofixation for IgD or IgE in select cases

CT, Computed tomography; Ig, immunoglobulin; ISS, International Staging System; LDH, lactate dehydrogenase; MRI, magnetic resonance imaging; PET, positron emission tomography.

be repeated to confirm achievement of a complete response. Patients who produce intact immunoglobulins can also produce excess light chain, giving a picture that is associated with both heavy and light chains; for example, a patient can have an IgG κ and a κ light-chain myeloma. Associated with the presence of a monoclonal protein, the uninvolved immunoglobulins are suppressed. For example, patients with IgG myeloma will have suppressed IgA and IgM. In a setting where all three immunoglobulins are suppressed, one should suspect either light-chain disease and/or the possibility of IgD or IgE MM. Very rarely, a biclonal or triclonal pattern of immunoglobulins is observed, more often with the same light chain but rarely with a different heterotypic light chain. This may suggest truly separate clones, especially with separate light chains. Quantitation of Bence Jones proteins in urine is still important, both for diagnosis of myeloma and for follow-up. It is important to note that a free light-chain measurement in the urine is not informative. Those patients with only a monoclonal protein in the urine require frequent 24-hour Bence Jones protein measurements during follow-up. Therapeutically, patients with each of the various types of immunoglobulins are treated with a similar type of therapy; however, patients with IgA myeloma appear to have an inferior survival. The immunoglobulin isotype remains constant in a given patient over the natural history of the disease; however, occasionally, a patient producing one immunoglobulin at the time of diagnosis, at relapse, or with advanced disease may present with only the same light chain as initially observed with the original immunoglobulin (light chain escape) or occasionally may become nonsecretory. Both the changes are reflective of the change in plasma cells to a more aggressive or undifferentiated form. As a result of the observed light-chain escape, patients without initial Bence Jones proteins initially detected in the urine will require periodic 24-hour urine Bence Jones protein measurements during follow-up.

The unique sequences that are observed with the idiotype protein (CDR3) have been used as a marker that specifically identifies a tumor cell clone and have been applied to a polymerase chain reaction–based methodology to detect MRD with high sensitivity. Early studies using such molecular methods for detecting MRD have

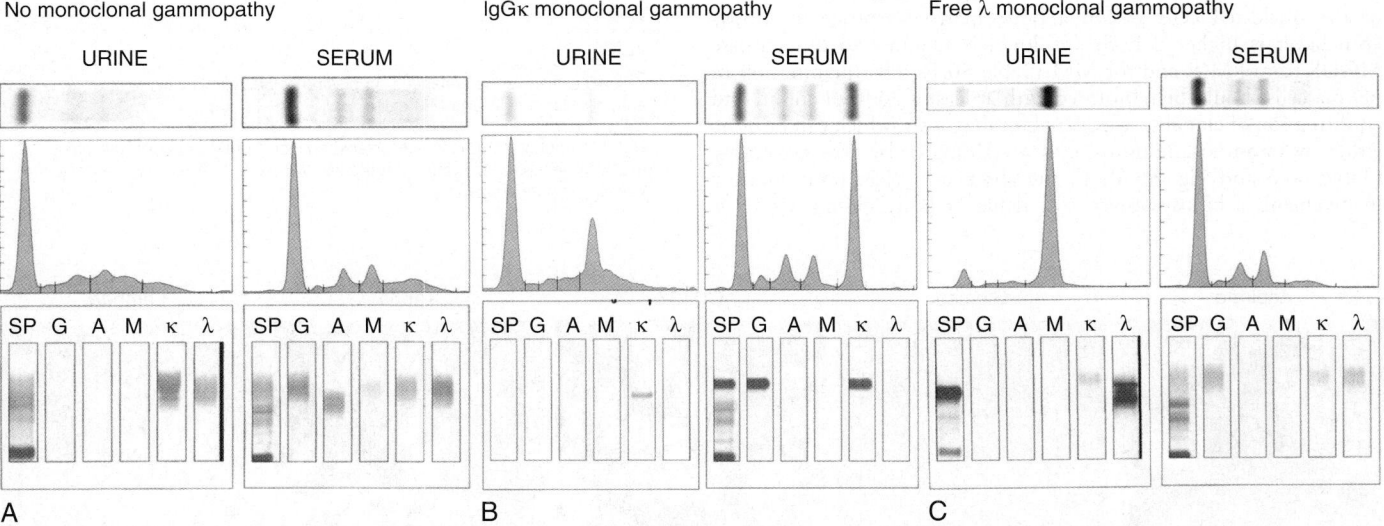

Fig. 86.5 REPRESENTATIVE PATTERNS OF SERUM ELECTROPHORESIS AND IMMUNOFIXATION. In each figure, the *upper panels* represent immunofixation patterns, the *middle panels* are the densitometric tracings of the gels, and the *lower panels* are agarose gels of urine sample *(left)* and serum *(right)*. (A) Normal pattern of serum and urine protein on electrophoresis. Because there are many different immunoglobulins in the serum, their differing mobilities in an electric field produce a broad peak. (B) In monoclonal gammopathies, the predominance of a product of a single cell produces a sharp peak. The immunofixation identifies the type of immunoglobulin, such as κ light chain in urine and IgGκ in serum. (C) In patients with light chain–only disease, a clonal band is observed only in urine, with no clear peak in serum, such as γ light chain in urine with no distinct immunofixation positivity in serum. *(Courtesy Dr. Neal I. Lindeman; used with permission.)*

identified those patients who achieve complete molecular remissions that are associated with improved overall outcome.

Serum Free Light Chains

This test measures serum light chains that are not associated with heavy chains. The presence of serum free light chains provides an additional marker and measurement of plasma cell proliferation, and its quantitation has been used to determine protein levels in a number of patients who were previously considered oligosecretory or nonsecretory. For example, 80% of patients with previously diagnosed nonsecretory myeloma have measurable serum free light chains. Routine use of serum free light chain measurements is indicated for diagnosis, response evaluation, and prognosis. As shown in patients with MGUS and SMM, serum free light chain ratio allows for identification of those patients with increased likelihood of progression to symptomatic myeloma. The measurement of serum free light chain does not replace the measurement of Bence Jones proteins in 24-hour urine collection.

A recently developed heavy/light chain assay allows identification and quantification of the different light chain types belonging to each immunoglobulin class (e.g., IgAκ and IgAλ) and allows calculation of ratios of monoclonal/polyclonal immunoglobulins (heavy/light chain ratio). In one study, heavy/light chain assays allowed quantification of monoclonal proteins not accurately measurable by SPEP or nephelometry, and the heavy/light chain ratio indicated the presence of disease in 8 of 31 patients who achieved CR and in sequential studies indicated evolving relapse in three patients before immunofixation became positive. The assay requires further validation before wider clinical use.

Bone Marrow Examination

Except for patients with solitary plasmacytoma, the presence of clonal plasma cells (>5%) is usually observed in all plasma cell disorders, and malignant plasma cells can be distinguished from normal plasma cells by monoclonal antibody staining and flow cytometry (Table 86.6).[20] Clonal plasma cell populations comprising 10% or greater of the nucleated cells within a bone marrow aspirate or biopsy (whichever is higher if both are done) is required to differentiate MGUS from SMM and for MM (Table 86.1). The quantitation of plasma cells should be performed with at least a 200-cell count, and confirmation of clonality is essential for diagnosis, which can be done either by immunostaining using κ/λ staining or by flow cytometry (Table 86.6 and Fig. 86.6). In the absence of clear bone marrow involvement, a biopsy-proven soft tissue or bony plasmacytoma is also adequate for diagnosis (Fig. 86.7). Cytogenetic and FISH studies should be performed on bone marrow samples at the time of diagnosis, and if initially confirmed as low-risk disease, then they should be repeated on bone marrow performed at the time of relapse. Although important for prognostication, cytogenetic or FISH study–identified abnormalities are not adequate for differentiating MM from MGUS or SMM. A seven-color flow cytometry panel is now also used with bone marrow samples to detect MRD.

Investigation to Detect End-Organ Damage

The diagnosis of a plasma cell disorder is based on the presence of a monoclonal protein and clonal plasma cells. However, the diagnosis

TABLE 86.6   Phenotypic Characterization of Plasma Cells

Adhesion Molecule	Normal Plasma Cells	MM Cells
CD138	+	+
CD19	+	−
CD28	−	−
CD38	+	+
CD40	+	+[a]
CD45	+	−[b]
CD27	−	+
CD11a	+	−
CD11b	−	−
CD44	+	+
CD54	+	+
CD56	−	+
CD58	−	+
LFA-1	−	−/+
RHAMM	−	+
VLA-4	+	+
VLA-5	+	+

[a]CCD40 expression is enhanced on plasma cell leukemia cells relative to normal plasma cells and MM cells.
[b]CD45 on immature myeloma cells.
LFA-1, Lymphocyte function-associated antigen 1; MM, multiple myeloma; RHAMM, receptor for hyaluronan-mediated motility; VLA-4, very late antigen 4; VLA-5, very late antigen 5.

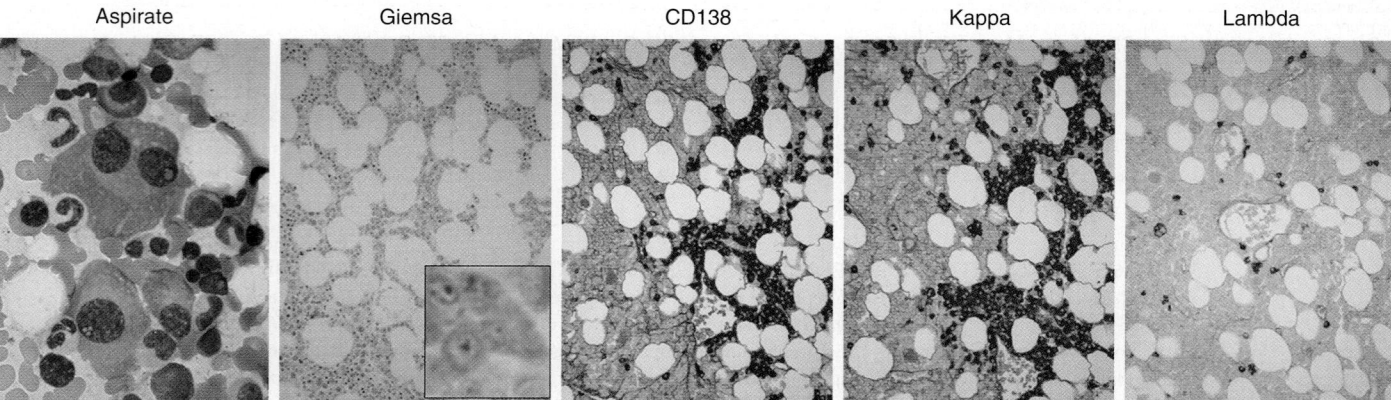

| Aspirate | Giemsa | CD138 | Kappa | Lambda |

Fig. 86.6 BONE MARROW EXAMINATION FROM A PATIENT WITH IMMUNOGLOBULIN Gκ MYELOMA SHOWING NEOPLASTIC PLASMA CELLS AT VARIOUS STAGES OF DIFFERENTIATION. The cells are CD138⁺, and κ light chain–positive but λ-negative. *(Courtesy Dr. Ruben Carrasco, M.D.; used with permission.)*

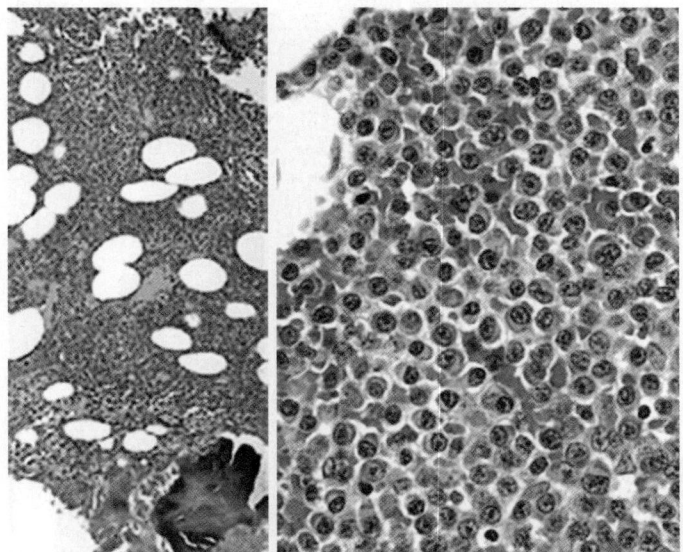

Fig. 86.7 MORPHOLOGIC SPECTRUM OF NEOPLASTIC PLASMA CELLS IN MULTIPLE MYELOMA. There is significant morphologic heterogeneity in the plasma cells, as seen on bone marrow aspirate (A–E) and biopsy (F and G). The plasma cells can sometimes be fairly normal appearing (A and F); they can be "lymphocyte-like" and difficult to distinguish from lymphoplasmacytic lymphoma (B and G); they frequently can exhibit cytologic atypia with prominent nucleoli and nuclear to cytoplasmic dyssynchrony (C and H); they can exhibit anaplastic features (D and I); and they can show "blastic" features (E and J). Myeloma can also evolve into leukemic phase (K) and can be associated with osteosclerosis (M), as sometimes seen in association with POEMS syndrome (polyneuropathy, organomegaly, endocrinopathy, monoclonal gammopathy, and skin changes).

of MGUS/SMM, which currently does not require therapeutic intervention, and active symptomatic MM, which needs treatment, is based on the detection of end-organ damage, which includes bone lesions, anemia, renal dysfunction, and hypercalcemia. The details of the diagnostic criteria are listed in Tables 86.7 and 86.8.[20]

Radiographic Evaluation

The standard evaluation of bone lesions in myeloma is by a skeletal survey that includes plain x-rays of the entire skeleton. The presence of characteristic lytic lesions is considered diagnostic for myeloma (Fig. 86.8). Rarely, in POEMS, bone lesions are osteosclerotic. The bone lesions do not always resolve following effective therapy. Because of the absence or suppression of osteoblastic activity, the bone scan is diagnostically not a useful investigative tool in myeloma. Almost all patients with myeloma have osteoporosis as a result of unbalanced osteoclastic activity. Bone mineral density (BMD) measurement by dual-energy x-ray absorptiometry helps identify osteoporosis and is consider a useful investigation. However, it is not uniformly used, because all patients with myeloma are known to have osteoporosis, and now all patients receive bisphosphonates, making the measurement of BMD irrelevant in therapeutic decision making. Details of various imaging modalities and their role in myeloma diagnostics are described in Table 86.9.

Magnetic resonance imaging (MRI), computed tomography (CT), and positron emission tomography (PET) are increasingly being used for patients with MM. An MRI scan allows assessment of the degree of bone marrow involvement and involvement of the spinal cord. One-third of the patients have generalized hyperintensity on MRI of the skeleton, another one-third have predominantly focal lesions within the background of a low level of bone marrow involvement, and the remaining one-third have a mixed picture with focal

---

TABLE 86.7 Bortezomib Regimens in Relapsed/Refractory Multiple Myeloma

Trial	Regimen	Number of Patients	ORR (%)	Median TTP (Mo)	Median OS
Richardson	Bortezomib (SUMMIT)	202	28	7	17 mo
Richardson	Bortezomib (APEX)	333	38	6.2	29.8 mo
	Dexamethasone	336	18	3.5	23.7 mo
Orlowski	Bortezomib	332	41	6.5	65% at 15 mo
	PLD + bortezomib	324	44	9.3	76% at 15 mo
Palumbo	VMPT	30	67	PFS 61% at 1 yr	84% at 1 yr

ORR, Overall response rate; OS, overall survival; PLD, pegylated liposomal doxorubicin; TTP, time to progression; VMPT, bortezomib-melphalan-prednisone-thalidomide.

TABLE 86.8 Bortezomib Regimens in Newly Diagnosed Multiple Myeloma

Trial	Regimen/Dose	Number of Patients	ORR (%)	Median TTP (Mo)	Median OS
Jagannath	VD	32	88	NA	87% at 1 yr
Harousseau	VD + SCT ×2	240	79	36	81 at 3 yr
	VAD + SCT ×2	242	63	30	77 at 3 yr
Neben	VAD + SCT ×2 + T	172	NA	35.7	84 at 3 yr
	PAD + SCT ×2 + V	182	NA	31.2	73 at 3 yr
Richardson	VRD	66	100	75% at 18 mo	97% at 18 mo
Cavo	VTD + SCT ×2 + VTD	236	93	68% at 3 yr	86% at 3 yr
	TD + SCT ×2 + TD	238	79	56% at 3 yr	84% at 3 yr
San Miguel	VMP	337	71	24	68.5% at 3 yr
	MP	331	35	16.6	54% at 3 yr

ORR, Overall response rate; OS, overall survival; MP, melphalan-prednisone; NA, not available; PAD, bortezomib-doxorubicin-dexamethasone; SCT, stem cell transplant; T, thalidomide; TD, thalidomide-dexamethasone; TTP, time to progression; V, bortezomib; VAD, vincristine-adriamycin-dexamethasone; VD, bortezomib-dexamethasone; VMP, bortezomib-melphalan-prednisone; VMPT, bortezomib-melphalan-prednisone-thalidomide; VRD, bortezomib-lenalidomide-dexamethasone; VTD, bortezomib-thalidomide-dexamethasone.

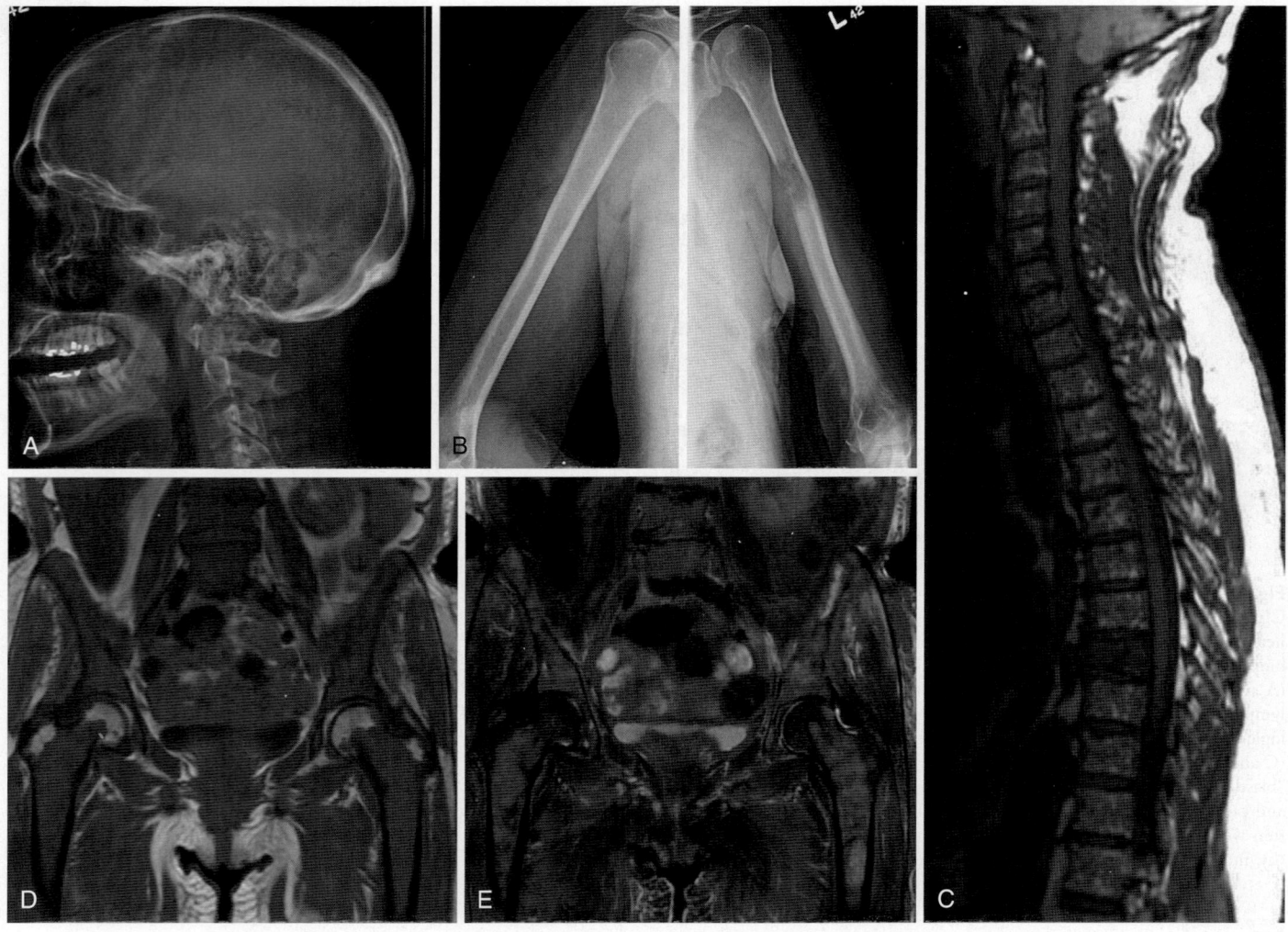

Fig. 86.8 TYPICAL SKELETAL CHANGES VISUALIZED ON ROENTGENOGRAMS. (A, B) Examples of "punched-out" lytic lesions in skull and humerus. (C, D) Magnetic resonance imaging pattern in multiple myeloma in spine and pelvis showing diffuse involvement with focal lesions.

TABLE 86.9	Imaging Modalities for Disease Assessment in Myeloma			
	Use	**Sensitivity/Specificity**	**False-Negatives**	**False-Positives**
Bone scan	• For diagnostic screening, except for multiple myeloma	Varies	• Pure osteolytic lesions	• Trauma • Inflammation • Benign tumor • Healing
X-ray	• Can clarify nonspecific findings on bone scan • Assesses risk of fracture • Possible follow-up of tumor response, but evidence of response takes considerable time to appear	Low sensitivity	• Low disease burden • Osteopenia	• Trauma • Inflammation • Benign tumor • Healing
CT	• For anatomic detail in axial skeleton • Possible follow-up of tumor response, but role is still undefined	High sensitivity	• Low disease burden	• Trauma • Inflammation • Benign tumor • Healing
MRI	• Detection of spinal cord compression • Can help distinguish benign from malignant vertebral compression fracture • Possible follow-up of tumor response, but role is still undefined	High sensitivity and specificity	• Lesion only in cortex	• Edema
PET scan	• May eventually become first-line screening test for bone metastases • Possible follow-up of tumor response, but role is still undefined	High specificity	• Lesion only in cortex	• After chemotherapy
Bone density	• Measure osteoporosis • Response to bisphosphonates	High specificity and sensitivity		• Age-related Osteoporosis

CT, Computed tomography; MRI, magnetic resonance imaging; PET, positron emission tomography.

lesions within the background of generalized involvement of the bone marrow. MRI is indicated in all patients with a suspected diagnosis of a solitary plasmacytoma and is indicated in SMM to identify any occult bone marrow involvement. Identification of multiple lesions not observed on a skeletal survey allows prediction of progression and early intervention.

In symptomatic myeloma, MRI is considered a routine evaluation to detect unsuspected focal lesions, to assess the extent of involvement of the bone marrow especially in the spine and pelvis, and to explore the possibility of cord compression. MRI is an important tool in patients with nonsecretory myeloma and becomes a critical method to evaluate response. Normalization of MRI findings after achieving

CR is a good prognostic feature and is being considered as one of the methods to better define a CR.

CT has been used to evaluate focal lesions in order to perform fine-needle biopsies for cytologic analysis. CT scans provide a better picture of the bone component and can also be used to judge the integrity of the bone. PET along with CT can be used to define extramedullary disease (EMD) as well as medullary lesions, and they complement MRI for follow-up of patients with nonsecretory myeloma (Fig. 86.9). Conversion of PET positivity to negativity has prognostic significance. In one prospective study of 192 patients, the presence at baseline of at least three focal lesions (FLs) detected by PET-CT, a standardized uptake value (SUV) >4.2, and EMD adversely

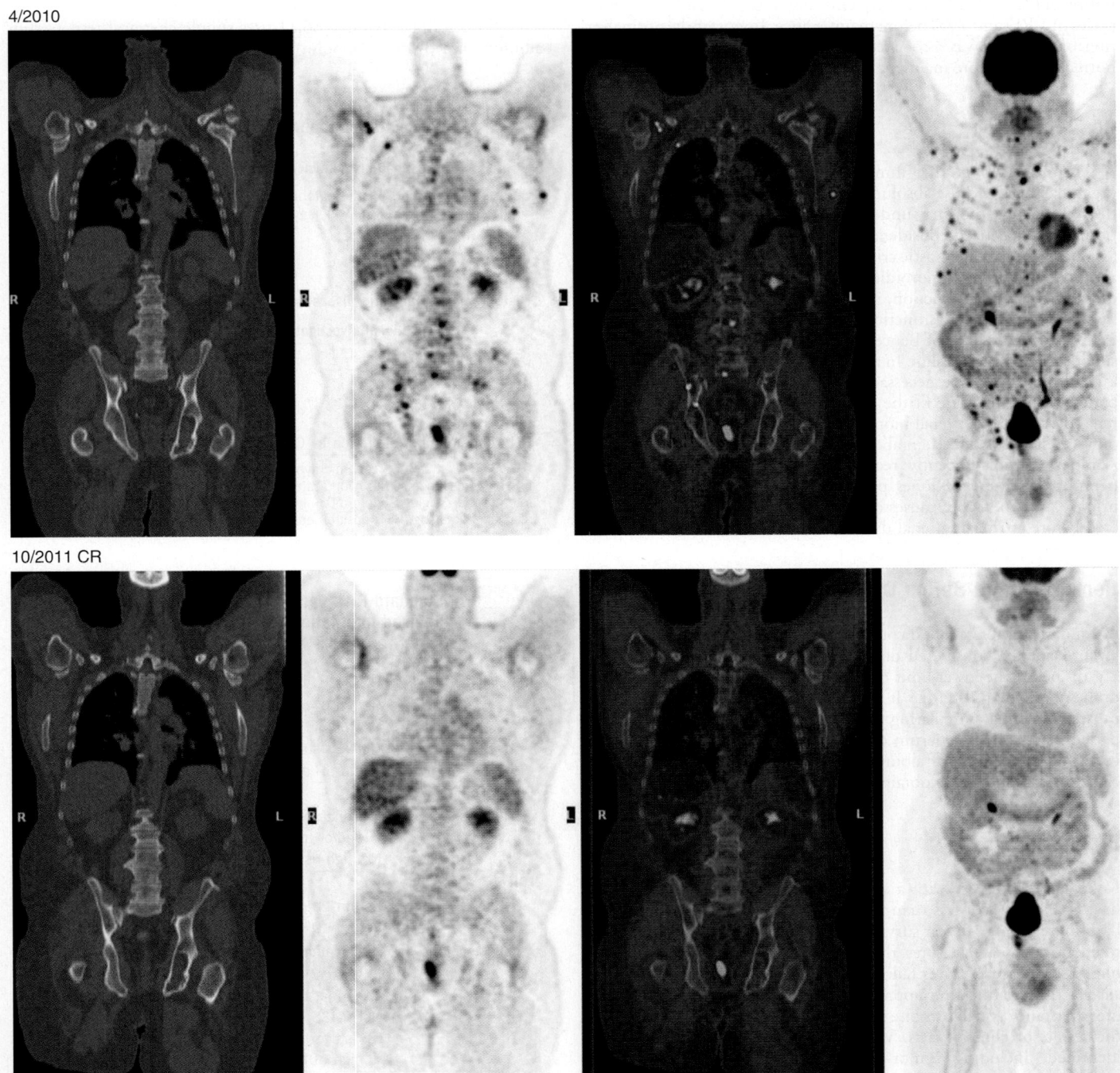

Fig. 86.9 POSITRON EMISSION TOMOGRAPHIC/COMPUTED TOMOGRAPHIC SCANS SHOWING MULTIPLE FLUORODEOXYGLUCOSE-AVID LESIONS IN SKELETON *(UPPER PANEL),* ALONG WITH THEIR RESOLUTION ON ACHIEVING COMPLETE REMISSION *(LOWER PANEL).*

affected the 4-year estimate of progression-free survival (PFS) ($\geq$3 FLs, 50%; SUV >4.2, 43%; presence of EMD, 28%). An SUV >4.2 and EMD was also correlated with a shorter OS (4-year OS rates 77% and 66%, respectively). In this study, posttherapy persistence of PET positivity for lesions predicted a poor outcome as compared with those with a negative PET-CT (PFS 66% and OS 89%).

A prospective evaluation of MRI and PET-CT at diagnosis and before maintenance therapy was performed in a subgroup of 134 patients with MM in the IFM/DFCI 2009 trial. At diagnosis, MRI was positive in 127 (94.7%) of 134 patients and PET-CT was positive in 122 (91%) of 134 patients, respectively ($p = .33$). Few patients achieved a normal MRI after three cycles of VRD before maintenance. Normalization of the MRI following three cycles of VRD and before maintenance had no prognostic value for both PFS and OS. Normalization of PET-CT was more frequently observed: 45% following three cycles of VRD and 79% before maintenance. Importantly, normalization of PET-CT was associated with an improvement in PFS, and normalization before maintenance was a predictor for improved OS.

Renal Function

A serum creatinine >173 mmol/L is considered to represent end-organ damage. Because absolute creatinine values do not incorporate the patient's age, they may underrepresent the extent of renal dysfunction. There has been consideration of using the creatinine clearance as a more optimal diagnostic criterion. Because patients with myeloma are older and other comorbidities such as diabetes and hypertension can also affect renal function, it is necessary to establish the relationship between renal dysfunction and the plasma cell disorder; for example, the presence of Bence Jones proteinuria may be required to support such a relationship. In the absence of Bence Jones proteinuria, a renal biopsy may be necessary. This may be even more critical in patients who otherwise fit the criteria for MGUS or SMM but have renal dysfunction. A renal biopsy is not required for all patients, but only when one is uncertain about the cause of the renal dysfunction. A biopsy is not currently required to document light chain cast nephropathy if Bence Jones protein is present as the predominant urinary protein. Other causes of renal dysfunction should be considered before attributing renal dysfunction to MM.

Hemogram and Serum Calcium

A standard complete blood count is performed to detect anemia. The level of anemia considered diagnostic of myeloma is a hemoglobin 2 g/dL below the lower limit of normal or the patient's baseline level or hemoglobin <10 g/dL. It is always necessary to exclude other causes of anemia. Circulating plasma cells are frequently observed in patients with MM. A serum calcium level should be measured and corrected to the level of albumin, or in occasional cases, an ionized calcium level should be obtained.

Prognosis

Myeloma is a disease with a varied outcome, with 20% of patients having a survival of less than 2 years, whereas over 40% of patients have more than a 10-year survival. Therefore it is critically important to identify disease features that allow one to identify low- versus high-risk disease to better tailor therapeutic interventions. Moreover, such a risk stratification approach permits the physician to predict life expectancy and allows one to develop metrics by which to evaluate the results of clinical trials. Various prognostic variables have been identified, including tumor-burden related factors such as β_2-microglobulin, more than three lytic bone lesions, hypercalcemia, and soluble IL-6 receptor; tumor biology–related factors such as cytogenetic/FISH-identified abnormalities, genomic changes, plasma cell labeling index, IgA myeloma, C-reactive protein, and lactate dehydrogenase (LDH); tumor microenvironment–related factors,

such as bone marrow MVD, serum soluble syndecan-1 levels, soluble CD16 levels, and bone marrow pDC numbers; patient-related factors, such as age, renal failure, albumin, and performance status; and treatment-related factors, such as achieving a CR or a very good partial response (VGPR) and the performance of tandem autologous transplants. Among these features, the International Staging System (ISS) uses serum albumin and β_2-microglobulin levels, cytogenetic/FISH changes, and newer genomic correlates of outcome that have been validated in a number of studies and are considered standard predictive markers. A short list of investigations to be performed for risk stratification of patients with MM is provided in Table 86.10.[21]

INTERNATIONAL STAGING SYSTEM

The ISS described in Table 86.11 uses simple chemical tests (serum albumin and β_2-microglobulin) to predict outcome.[22] ISS staging is

TABLE 86.10	Risk Stratification in Multiple Myeloma
Investigations Recommended for Risk Stratification	
Serum albumin and β_2-microglobulin to determine ISS stage	
Bone marrow examination for t(4;14), t(14;16), and del(17p) on identified PCs by FISH	
LDH	
Immunoglobulin type: IgA	
Histology: plasmablastic disease or plasma cell leukemia	
Additional Investigations for Risk Stratification	
Cytogenetics	
Gene expression profiling	
Labeling index	
MRI/PET scan	
DNA copy number alteration by CGH/SNP array	

CGH/SNP, Comparative genomic hybridization/single-nucleotide polymorphism; FISH, fluorescence in situ hybridization; IgA, immunoglobulin A; ISS, International Staging System; LDH, lactate dehydrogenase; MRI, magnetic resonance imaging; PET, positron emission tomography.

TABLE 86.11	Standard Risk Factors for Multiple Myeloma and the Revised International Staging System	
Prognostic Factor	**Criteria**	
ISS stage		
I	Serum β_2-microglobulin <3.5 mg/L, serum albumin $\geq$3.5 g/dL	
II	Not ISS stage I or III	
III	Serum β_2-microglobulin $\geq$5.5 mg/L	
CA by iFISH		
High risk	Presence of del(17p) and/or translocation t(4;14) and/or translocation t(14;16)	
Standard risk	No high-risk CA	
LDH		
Normal	Serum LDH below the upper limit of normal	
High	Serum LDH above the upper limit of normal	
A New Model for Risk Stratification for MM R-ISS stage		
I	ISS stage I and standard-risk CA by iFISH and normal LDH	
II	Not R-ISS stage I or III	
III	ISS stage III and either high-risk CA by iFISH or high LDH	

CA, Chromosomal abnormalities; iFISH, interphase fluorescence in situ hybridization; ISS, International Staging System; LDH, lactate dehydrogenase; MM, multiple myeloma; R-ISS, revised International Staging System.
From Greipp PR, San Miguel J, Durie BG, et al: International staging system for multiple myeloma. *J Clin Oncol* 23:3412, 2005.

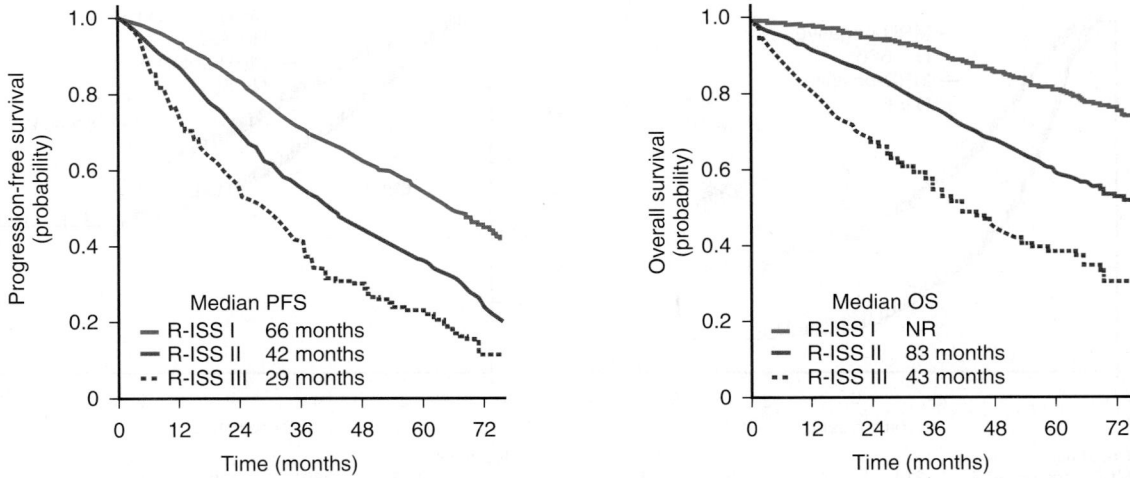

Fig. 86.10 REVISED INTERNATIONAL STAGING SYSTEM (R-ISS) INCORPORATING ISS, FLUO-RESCENCE IN SITU HYBRIDIZATION, AND LACTATE DEHYDROGENASE PREDICTS BOTH EVENT-FREE SURVIVAL *(LEFT PANEL)* AND OVERSALL SURVIVAL (OS; *RIGHT PANEL). NR,* Not reached; *PFS,* progression-free survival.

able to predict both event-free survival (EFS) and OS and is valid regardless of age, geographic region, study site, standard-dose therapy or HDT, method of albumin measurement, and use of novel agents. Although it is universally applicable, it does not include the genetic makeup of the myeloma cells and thus lacks an important biologic characteristic that drives the disease process.

Recent efforts have been made to combine multiple features to improve prognostication. Avet-Loiseau proposed a combination of β_2-microglobulin levels and cytogenetics to predict outcomes. A revised ISS that combines ISS staging with cytogenetic abnormalities (Table 86.11, Fig. 86.10) has been created. Walker et al combined recurrent molecular adverse features with the ISS and proposed an ISS mutation score to identify a high-risk patient.

Cytogenetics/FISH

Using conventional cytogenetics, detection of any abnormality is predictive of an adverse outcome. Of course, the recurrent chromosomal changes t(4;14) and t(14;16), as well as loss of 13q34 and 17p13, identified using traditional cytogenetic methods are associated with a poor prognosis. Hyperdiploidy and t(11;14) have been reported in some studies to predict a favorable outcome.

As described earlier, because of a low proliferative index, cytogenetic abnormalities are detected in only a small number of patients, and interphase FISH is used to detect specific genetic aberrations. Among these abnormalities, patients with t(4;14) (15% of the patients) have a poor prognosis. In some early studies, the use of bortezomib and lenalidomide has been shown to at least partly overcome the poor risk associated with this abnormality. The del(17p) observed in 8% to 10% of the patients remains a poor risk feature not overcome by novel therapies.[3] Although the *p53* gene resides in this region of the deletion, a clear biologic confirmation of its role is lacking. *p53* mutations have been detected in only a very small number of patients. In patients without t(4;14) or del17p, del(13) is not considered to predict a poor outcome. Moreover, the presence of del(13) is observed in patients with MGUS and SMM without clear correlation with clinical outcome. The findings raise questions about the role of del(13) in myeloma progression and its use in predicting prognosis. A combination of a high-risk feature such as a 17p13 deletion may coexist with trisomies of several chromosomes, a good risk feature. In a recent study by the IFM, researcheres reported that if patients have trisomy of 3 and 5 along with other poor-risk cytogenetics, their overall outcome may improve, whereas presence of trisomy 21 may further adversely affect the outcome. As shown in Table 86.2, newer additional chromosomal changes are being identified that are

predictive of clinical outcomes; gain of chromosome 1q and loss of 1p are considered to predict a poor outcome. Additional studies are needed to confirm their significance.

High-Throughput Genomic Studies

Additional analyses of genomic changes that drive the disease process have been performed using the high-throughput microarray profiling technique. CNAs have been studied using either SNP[6] or CGH[7] arrays, whereas expression of genes has been evaluated using expression profiling that covers the entire genome. These studies have been correlated to clinical outcomes.

The IFM-DFCI collaborative group has correlated CNA with survival outcomes in 192 newly diagnosed patients with MM who were uniformly treated. A univariate analysis identified amplifications of 1q and deletions of 1p, 12p, 14q, 16q, and 22q to be associated with a poor prognosis, whereas amplification of chromosomes 5, 9, 11, 15, and 19 was associated with a superior outcome. A multivariate analysis identified amp(1q23.3), amp(5q31.3), and del(12p13.31) as the most significant independent adverse markers ($p < .0001$). This model has been further validated in an independent cohort of 273 patients, confirming the utility of SNP profiling for prognostication.[6]

Using gene expression, profiling a 70-gene model has been proposed by the UAMS group.[23] This signature identifies three groups of patients: those with high-, intermediate-, and low-risk disease. Similarly, a 15-gene model classifying patients into two risk groups has been proposed by the IFM group.[24] Interestingly, there are no common genes between the two models. This likely is due to the different treatments received by the patient groups, differences in the platform used, and more likely the redundancy and overlapping functions of the genes regulating various pathways. A larger-scale study incorporating various genomic correlates will be required in the future to identify and validate signatures that can identify risk categories and response to therapies.

Minimal Residual Disease

Achieving a complete response has traditionally been considered an important prognostic indicator, and previous studies have indicated that achieving a VGPR is associated with a superior survival outcome. However, because the majority of patients achieving CR relapse, it is clear that substantial residual disease persists, requiring better methods to measure MRD. The large amount of recent data has demonstrated that an MRD-negative status can be achieved in a large proportion

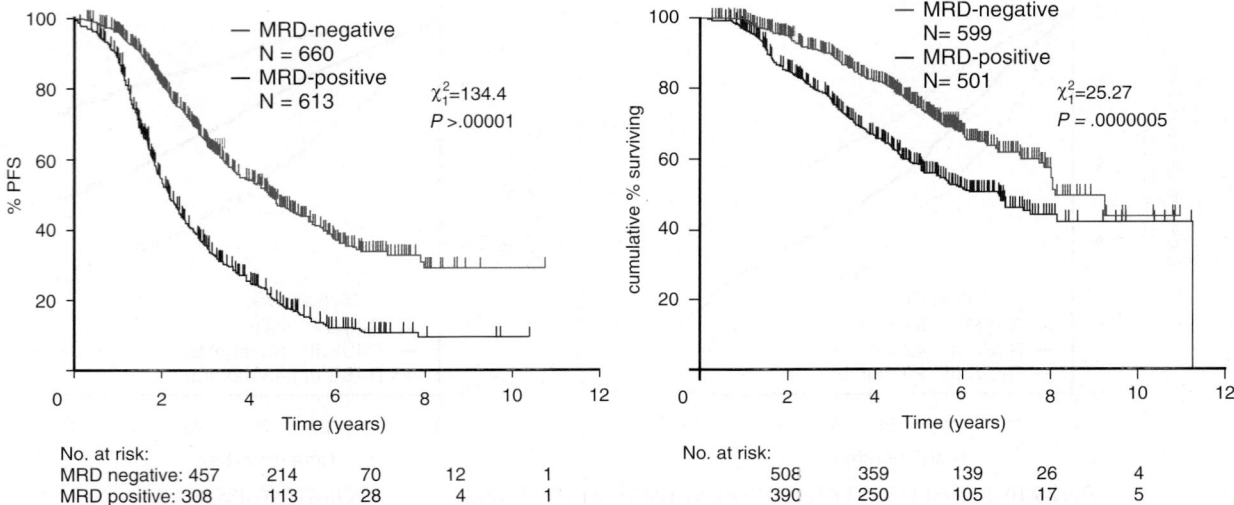

Fig. 86.11 KAPLAN-MEIER ESTIMATES OF PROGRESSION-FREE SURVIVAL (PFS; *LEFT*) AND OVERALL SURVIVAL (OS; *RIGHT*) IN PATIENTS ACVHIEVING MINIMAL RESIDUAL DISEASE (MRD)–NEGATIVE VERSUS MRD-POSITIVE STATUS. To evaluate the impact of achieving MRD-negative status on PFS and OS, 14 studies (*n* = 1273 subjects) provided data on the impact of MRD on PFS, and 12 studies (*n* = 1100) provided data on OS.

of patients. Two important methods used to measure MRD are multicolor flow cytometry and NGS. The latter has sensitivity of 1 cell in 10^6 bone marrow cells, which is required for best demonstration of a superior outcome in those patients achieving conventional CR. These studies and a meta-analysis clearly suggest significant improvement in both EFS and OS (Fig. 86.11) in those patients achieving MRD-negative status. The evolving consensus is that achieving MRD-negative status should become the ultimate goal of all therapeutic interventions.

DIFFERENTIAL DIAGNOSIS

The diagnosis of MM is based largely on laboratory investigations. No single symptom or group of symptoms is pathognomonic of MM. A significant number of patients remain asymptomatic, and the diagnosis is usually delayed. Most frequently, in a relatively asymptomatic patient, investigations are carried out because of increased total protein levels, proteinuria, renal dysfunction, and/or bone pain. An older patient with any of these features or unexplained back pain, anemia, or recurrent infection should be screened for myeloma. Unexplained and marked elevation of an erythrocyte sedimentation rate also warrants investigation. The diagnosis is pursued in two steps: first, the detection of a monoclonal protein and monoclonal plasma cells, and second, identification of end-organ damage. This is essential to differentiate early-stage plasma cell disorders such as MGUS or SMM from active symptomatic myeloma (Table 86.1). Once a diagnosis of MM is suspected, the investigations detailed in Table 86.5 are to be carried out. Detection of a monoclonal protein includes electrophoresis of serum proteins as well as 24-hour urine collection and serum-free light chain measurements. Both serum protein electrophoresis and quantitative immunoglobulins are required, and an immunofixation is important at the time of diagnosis to identify the type of paraprotein present. The bone marrow is examined for the presence of clonal plasma cells, mainly by histology but also importantly by immunostaining or flow cytometry using κ/λ staining (Table 86.6). Determination and quantitation of clonal plasma cells are required to differentiate SMM from MGUS (Table 86.1). Detailed investigations for evidence of organ damage should be undertaken to look for bony lesions, renal dysfunction, anemia, and hypercalcemia. In patients where hyperviscosity is suspected, besides measuring serum viscosity, a funduscopic examination is useful. Detailed diagnostic criteria are summarized in Table 86.1.[20]

TREATMENT

Treatment of underlying plasma cell neoplasm is warranted when an organ or tissue function is compromised. The damage or functional impairment of an organ can be caused by the underlying plasma cell clone or the monoclonal protein. The acronym *CRAB* (hypercalcemia, renal impairment, anemia, and bone disease) is helpful in this regard. Symptomatic hyperviscosity, amyloidosis, monoclonal immunoglobulin deposition disease, recurrent bacterial infections (more than two major infections), and progressive peripheral neuropathy are also indications for the initiation of treatment. The constellation of polyneuropathy, organomegaly, endocrinopathy, monoclonal gammopathy, and the skin changes in the setting of osteosclerotic myeloma (POEMS syndrome) may present a challenging diagnosis but is always an indication for treatment. In addition, the International Myeloma Working Group has defined the following events that warrant systemic therapy: (1) clonal bone marrow plasma cell percentage (aspirate or biopsy, whichever is higher) of 60% or above, (2) elevated serum free light chain 100 mg/L or greater associated with involved/uninvolved free light chain ratio ≤100, and/or (3) more than one focal lesion visualized by MRI. One or more osteolytic lesions >1 cm in size identified by CT or PET-CT, as well as lytic lesion(s) noted on skeletal surveys, is an acceptable indication to initiate therapy. Osteoporosis and compression fracture alone in the absence of lytic lesions with the latest imaging techniques is not a myeloma-defining event.

MGUS and SMM

MGUS is characterized by serum paraprotein <3 g/dL; bone marrow plasmacytosis <10%; and absence of amyloidosis, a solitary plasmacytoma, Waldenström macroglobulinemia, or a B-cell lymphoproliferative disorder (Table 86.1). Three distinct clinical subtypes of MGUS based on paraprotein have been described (non-IgM MGUS, IgM-MGUS, and light-chain MGUS). The diagnosis of MGUS is often incidental where a serum or urine protein electrophoresis and immunofixation are ordered as part of a battery of tests. The test may have been ordered for evaluation of elevated globulin in the serum, proteinuria, peripheral neuropathy, osteoporosis, immune disorders, or hypogammaglobulinemia.[25,26] The rate of progression of non-IgM MGUS to MM is 1% per year. These patients can be further risk stratified on the basis of a serum M spike level less than 1.5 g/dL,

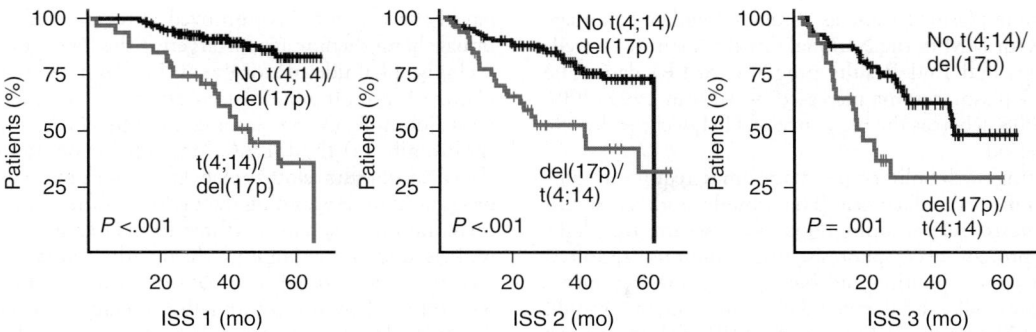

Fig. 86.12 KAPLAN-MEIER ESTIMATES OF LIKELIHOOD OF PROGRESSION TO MYELOMA FROM MONOCLONAL GAMMOPATHY OF UNKNOWN SIGNIFICANCE (MGUS) (A) OR SMOLDERING MULTIPLE MYELOMA (SMM) (B). Estimates are based on risk features identified in MGUS (M spike >1.5 g/dL, non–immunoglobulin G [non-IgG] paraprotein, and abnormal [Abn] free light-chain ratio [FLCR]) and in SMM (bone marrow [BM] with >10% plasma cells, M spike >3.0 g/dL, and Abn FLCR). *RR,* Relative risk.

IgG isotype, and normal serum free light chain ratio (Fig. 86.12). The presence of all these factors is associated with only a 2% chance of progression at 20 years after eliminating competing causes of death (low risk). If one of these factors is abnormal, patients will fall into the low intermediate-risk category, with 10% absolute risk of progression to myeloma at 20 years. Presence of two abnormal factors places the patients into the high intermediate-risk group; their absolute risk of progression to MM is 18% at 20 years. Finally, when all three risk factors are abnormal, the patient falls into a high-risk category with an absolute risk of progression of 27% at 20 years. IgM MGUS has a slightly higher rate of progression at 1.5% per year to Waldenström macroglobulinemia, chronic lymphocytic leukemia, AL amyloidosis and occasionally MM. MYD88 (L265P) is a recurrent mutation in Waldenström macroglobulinemia and is seen in 50% to 80% of cases of IgM MGUS. The presence of the MYD88 (L265P) is an independent predictor for progression to Waldenström macroglobulinemia or other lymphoproliferative disorder. The presence of both MYD88 mutation and serum M spike >1.5 g/dL at diagnosis identifies a subset of patients with a high risk for progression. Light chain MGUS is defined as Bence Jones proteinuria <0.5 g/24 hours and bone marrow <10% plasma cells; these patients have a 0.3% per year probability of progression to MM or light chain amyloidosis.

Non-IgM asymptomatic myeloma (smoldering myeloma) is characterized by bone marrow plasmacytosis 10% to 60% and/or serum paraprotein ≥3 g/dL but absence of myeloma-defining events or amyloidosis.[25] Asymptomatic myeloma is often diagnosed following a workup for an elevated total protein in the serum, proteinuria, or borderline anemia. It may also be discovered incidentally, like MGUS. It has been shown that every case of MM is preceded by detection of paraprotein by a minimum of 2 years or more. The rate of progression to MM is 10% per year for the first 5 years, 3% per year for the next 5 years, and 1% per year after 10 years. Because patients have no symptoms or related organ or tissue impairment, no treatment intervention is recommended. Several factors aid in categorizing patients into the different risk categories. Factors predictive of early progression include monoclonal spike ≥3 g/dL, bone marrow plasmacytosis ≥10%, and an abnormal free light chain ratio (>8 or <0.125). Presence of three or more of these factors identifies patients with a high risk for progression after a median of 2 years; presence of two of these variables identifies an intermediate-risk group with a median time to progression of 5 years; and presence of only one of these risk factors identifies a low-risk group with a median time to progression of 10 years. Other investigators have used other risk factors, such as aberrant plasma cell population ≥95% by flow cytometry, reduction in uninvolved globulins, evolving myeloma, and abnormal MRI findings, to stratify patients into different risk categories. Immunoparesis is also observed in MGUS and SMM. In one study, suppression of uninvolved immunoglobulin was observed in 25% of patients with MGUS (18% had decreased levels of only one

Ig, and 7% had low levels of two Igs) and 52% of patients with SMM (22% with one Ig, and 30% with both chains). In this analysis, immunoparesis was one of the independent predictors with a significant impact on PFS in MGUS and SMM. Light chain SMM is defined by the presence of Bence Jones proteinuria of ≥0.5 g/24 hours and bone marrow plasmacytosis ≥10%. These patients have a rate of progression to MM of 5% per year for 5 years, 3% per year for the next 5 years, and 2% per year after 10 years. IgM SMM has a cumulative probability of progressing to Waldenström macroglobulinemia, amyloidosis, or lymphoma of 6% at 1 year, 39% after 3 years, and 59% at 5 years (12% per year).

This information has been helpful in designing clinical trials to try to delay the progression to symptomatic MM for patients in a high-risk category. A single randomized trial by a Spanish group showed that early intervention with lenalidomide and dexamethasone in a high-risk group delays the time to progression and prevents the occurrence of renal failure or lytic bone disease. Moreover, by preventing complications, the study showed a survival advantage for early intervention. However, treatment intervention outside clinical trials is still not recommended for patients with asymptomatic myeloma. No benefit has been shown for early intervention as compared with treatment after the patient has progressed to symptomatic myeloma. Early intervention with thalidomide in asymptomatic myeloma has been reported to delay progression to symptomatic myeloma but was associated with peripheral neuropathy, and a survival benefit has not been shown in a randomized clinical trial.

Solitary Plasmacytoma: Medullary and Extramedullary

A diagnosis of solitary plasmacytoma requires fulfillment of each of the following criteria: histologic confirmation of clonal plasma cells at a single site; a negative bone marrow with absence of a clonal plasmacytosis; no distant bone involvement; and no anemia, hypercalcemia, or renal impairment (Table 86.1). The solitary plasmacytoma could present as a single bony lesion (medullary) or in soft tissue outside the bone (extramedullary). A solitary plasmacytoma of the bone is 40% more common than an extramedullary soft tissue plasmacytoma. Solitary plasmacytoma of the bone is most commonly encountered in the axial skeleton (skull, spine, pelvis, ribs, and sternum), accounting for 80% of cases; upper and lower extremities account for 15% of cases. Extramedullary soft tissue plasmacytomas are often associated with the mucosal area of the upper aerodigestive passages (80%).

Solitary plasmacytomas are rather uncommon and account for 6% of plasma cell neoplasms. The incidence is 0.3 per 100,000 person-years in United States. Similarly to MM, the incidence of solitary plasmacytomas increases with age; however, the median age of diagnosis was 62 years for extramedullary plasmacytomas and 65 years for solitary bone plasmacytoma as compared with median age of onset at 71 years for MM in the National Cancer Institute Surveillance, Epidemiology, and End Results program (SEER) data. The incidence of solitary plasmacytoma increased by 10% in 1999–2004 relative to 1992–2008, whereas the incidence of MM declined by 3% during the same period.

Patients presenting with solitary plasmacytomas require a complete workup to confirm the diagnosis. They should undergo serum protein electrophoresis, serum immunofixation, serum free light chain assay, urine protein electrophoresis, urine immunofixation, a diagnostic bone marrow aspiration and biopsy with flow cytometry to detect clonal plasma cells, and detailed skeletal imaging that should include either PET-CT or a skeletal survey and MRI of the spine and pelvis. One-third of the patients may present with a detectable monoclonal paraprotein in the serum or urine or both. Persistence of the monoclonal paraprotein after local treatment is predictive of a recurrence of MM. Patients with less than 10% plasma cells in the bone marrow biopsy may be managed with therapies directed against the solitary lesion initially. However, these patients will also progress to MM over the subsequent years of follow-up.

Solitary plasmacytomas are generally treated with local radiation therapy at a dose of 40–50 Gy. Depending upon the location, small extramedullary soft tissue plasmacytomas may be treated with excision biopsy alone. Solitary plasmacytomas of the bone may require surgical intervention for stabilization followed by local radiation therapy.

The disease-free survival at 10 years is 63% for patients with solitary plasmacytomas. The disease-specific survival seems to plateau at about 80% for extramedullary plasmacytomas, compared with 50% for solitary bone plasmacytomas. Less than one-third of solitary extramedullary plasmacytoma patients died as a result of myeloma, as compared with 58% of the patients with solitary bone plasmacytomas. Progression to myeloma generally occurs within 5 years from initial diagnosis. Patients presenting with medullary plasmacytomas, patients with persistence of a monoclonal paraprotein after treatment for the solitary plasmacytoma, patients with detectable low levels of clonal plasma cells in the bone marrow, patients between 40 and 60 years of age, and patients of African American descent are at higher risk for progression to MM. These patients should be followed closely for the next 5 years.

Symptomatic Myeloma

Patients presenting with symptoms caused by the myeloma tumor mass, such as anemia, lytic bone disease, hypercalcemia, or renal impairment (CRAB), require systemic therapy. Myeloma-defining events that warrant systemic therapy include a clonal bone marrow plasma cell percentage (aspirate or biopsy, whichever is higher) 60% or above, elevated serum free light chain 100 mg/L or greater associated with involved/uninvolved free light chain ratio ≤100, and/or more than one focal lesions on MRI studies. In addition, patients with a low tumor mass but with organ dysfunction caused by a paraprotein or immunodeficiency such as monoclonal immunoglobulin deposition disease or amyloidosis of an organ, progressive peripheral neuropathy, two are more serious infections (pneumonia, bacteremia) that require treatment. Related organ or tissue impairment also warrants initiation of systemic therapy.[20]

Front-line therapy for MM is often predicated on whether the patient is eligible, willing, and able to proceed with HDT and stem cell transplant. The treatment given before stem cell harvest and transplant is called induction therapy followed by consolidation with HDT and stem cell rescue. Patients not embarking on HDT are started on initial therapy for 9–18 months. Both groups of patients may subsequently receive maintenance therapy.

Induction Regimen/Initial Treatment

Tremendous progress has been made in the treatment of MM, with improvement in life expectancy. The availability of new drugs has paved the way for this improved outcome. This includes (1) traditional chemotherapy agents targeting the DNA, including melphalan, cyclophosphamide, doxorubicin, bendamustine, etoposide, and cisplatin; (2) immunomodulatory drugs thalidomide, lenalidomide, and pomalidomide; (3) proteasome inhibitors bortezomib, ixazomib, and carfilzomib; (4) the HDAC inhibitor panobinostat; and (5) monoclonal antibodies elotuzumab and daratumumab. There has been progress in understanding the biology of the disease. In every patient, there are multiple clones (three to five) at the time of diagnosis, as well as ongoing mutations during the course of the illness, and recurrences are caused by expansion of different clones (clonal tides) over time. Therefore combination therapy that includes drugs from different classes is likely to be more successful in eradicating the tumor. Achieving deep remission (CRs) predicts a better PFS. In addition, treatment should be tailored to tumor genetics, the age and frailty of the patient, comorbidities, and renal impairment.

TREATMENT OF NEWLY DIAGNOSED MYELOMA

Chemotherapy With Stem Cell–Sparing Agents

Patients considered for stem cell harvest are generally treated with combinations that are stem cell sparing. Before immunomodulatory agents and proteasome inhibitors became widely available, patients were treated with pulse dexamethasone alone or in combination with vincristine and adriamycin (VAD) and cyclophosphamide (CVAD or CVAMP; methylprednisolone substituted for dexamethasone). For more information, see box on Treatment of Newly Diagnosed Multiple Myeloma.

Dexamethasone

Glucocorticoids induce apoptosis in myeloma cells. Glucocorticoids induce IκB production, which then sequesters NFκB, resulting in downregulation of IL-6 and other inflammatory cytokines. Dexamethasone 40 mg is administered in a pulsed fashion for 4 days, starting on days 1, 9, and 17 for the first cycle. Some researchers have used this dose and schedule every 35 days, whereas others have given dexamethasone on days 1–4, every other cycle, on a 28-day schedule. Results achieved with pulsed dexamethasone alone compare well with those of VAD chemotherapy, and MP, with equivalent response rates and OS. Single-agent dexamethasone is no longer advocated as a treatment for newly diagnosed MM. However, under selected clinical situations, the use of pulsed dexamethasone is helpful in specific situations, including severe spinal cord compromise, hypercalcemia, and acute renal failure caused by light chain nephropathy. While patients are on intensive dexamethasone, close monitoring for hyperglycemia and antibiotic and prophylaxis against bacterial, *Pneumocystis carinii* pneumonia, and fungal infections are recommended. Weight gain, mood swings, insomnia, fluid retention, proximal myopathy, and steroid-induced psychosis are known side effects. Cataracts, osteoporosis, and avascular necrosis of the hips are some of the long-term consequences of steroid exposure.

Vincristine, Adriamycin, and Dexamethasone

Infusional therapy with vincristine and doxorubicin (Adriamycin) with pulsed dexamethasone is an effective stem cell–sparing induction regimen. Vincristine and doxorubicin are administered by continuous infusion at doses of 0.4 mg/day and 9 mg/m^2/day along with oral dexamethasone 40 mg/day for 4 days. Following six to nine cycles of VAD chemotherapy, the overall response rate (ORR) is 45% to 55%, and the CR rate is less than 5%. There are no differences in the median PFS (18 months) or OS (3 years) from those achieved with standard alkylating agent treatments (MP, VMCP/VBAP, VBMCP). However, if the induction therapy is followed by consolidation with high-dose melphalan and autologous stem cell transplant,

---

BOX 86.1 **Treatment of Newly Diagnosed Multiple Myeloma**

- Confirm patient has symptomatic myeloma. Patients with monoclonal gammopathy of unknown significance or smoldering multiple myeloma are not treated outside a clinical trial.
- Evaluate for risk stratification using International Staging System staging, fluorescence in situ hybridization/cytogenetic and biochemical testing to test renal function, and lactate dehydrogenase to develop long-term treatment plan as well as prognosis. Although initial treatment is not affected by risk category, a later consideration of more aggressive consolidation or use of allogeneic stem cell transplant in eligible patients can be considered in high-risk younger patients.
- Induction: Both transplant-eligible and transplant-ineligible patients can be treated with a triple-drug regimen (bortezomib and dexamethasone with lenalidomide [RVD], with thalidomide [VTD] or cyclophosphamide [VCD], OR other proteasome inhibitor (carfilzomib or ixazomib) in place of bortezomib, cyclophosphamide, thalidomide, dexamethasone [CTD]) for three to six cycles pretransplant or 9–12 months for transplant-ineligible patients. For transplant-ineligible patients, additional options include a two-drug regimen (dexamethsone with lenalidomide [RD], with bortezomib [VD] OR with thalidomide [TD]) OR melphalan-containing regimens, which include melphalan with prednisone (MP) in combination with any of the newer agents, MPT, MPV, or MPR.
- Selection of therapy should be influenced by patient characteristics.
  - Renal dysfunction: agents that can be considered for use are bortezomib, carfilzomib, cyclophosphamide, thalidomide, and dexamethasone (VCD or VTD)
  - Neuropathy: agents that can be considered for use are lenalidomide, carfilzomib cyclophosphamide, and dexamethasone.
  - Older-age patients: consider dose or schedule attenuation.
  - Convenience: use of oral versus intravenous agent regimen.
- Transplant-eligible patients can undergo a single autologous transplant with melphalan, with a second autologous transplant being optional, depending upon the overall response or on protocol participation.
- Maintenance: Following transplant or optimal induction therapy (to best response), patients can receive maintenance with thalidomide, lenalidomide, or bortezomib. For high-risk patients only, both bortezomib and lenalidomide or a thalidomide combination may be used. Selection can be influenced on the basis of the induction regimen.
- Improving complete response rates is a key goal of current trials, but patients can live a long time with residual paraprotein.

---

study and were noted to have equivalent antimyeloma activity. Cyclophosphamide is less stem cell toxic than melphalan. Cyclophosphamide in high doses (2 g/m² up to 6 g/m²) followed by filgrastim has been used for stem cell mobilization, whereas high doses of melphalan (200 mg/m²) are routinely used as the conditioning regimen in conjunction with an autologous stem cell transplant. There is a higher incidence of secondary leukemia associated with chronic melphalan therapy (up to 17% at 50 months), leading to abandonment of melphalan as maintenance therapy and limiting the exposure to 1 year or less.

Immunomodulatory Drugs

Currently, thalidomide, lenalidomide, and pomalidomide are the three IMiDs available for the treatment of MM. Recently, insights into the mechanism of action of IMiDs has been gained with the discovery of thalidomide-binding protein cereblon (CRBN). Human CRBN was originally identified as a candidate gene for an autosomal recessive form of mild mental retardation and is located on chromosome 3 at 3p26.2. CRBN is the substrate receptor of CUL4-RBX1-DDB1-CRBN also known as CRL4^{CRBN} E3 ubiquitin ligase. IMiDs bind CRBN and inhibit ubiquitination of endogenous CRL4^{CRBN} substrates, but unexpectedly IMiDs also repurpose the ligase to target new proteins for degradation. IMiDs induce degradation of the lymphoid transcription factors Ikaros (IKZF1) and Aiolos (IKZF3) and casein kinase 1α (CK1α). Degradation of Ikaros and Aiolos contributes to clinical efficacy in the treatment of MM, whereas degradation of CK1α is responsible for IMiD activity in 5q-associated myelodysplastic syndrome. Downregulation of Ikaros and Aiolos lead to specific and sequential downregulation of c-Myc followed by IRF4 and subsequent growth inhibition and apoptosis of myeloma cells. Drug resistance to IMiDs is associated with depletion of CRBN. Aiolos and Ikaros are transcriptional repressors of IL-2 in T cells. Thus IMiDs are able to increase the number of T cells and NK cells; there is polyfunctional T-cell activation with increased cytokine production by CD4 and CD8 T cells and reduction of the suppressive effects of Tregs on T-effector cells. There is increased expression of cytolysis genes granzyme B and perforin by CD8 T cells and NK cells.

Thalidomide

An international, randomized phase III trial has shown that thalidomide with dexamethasone (TD) is superior to dexamethasone alone for ORR (63% vs. 46%) and PFS (14.9 months vs. 6.5 months). There was no difference in efficacy between TD versus VAD as a pretransplant induction regimen. TD had a slightly inferior survival outcome compared with MP as first-line therapy in elderly patients. Thalidomide does not overcome poor prognostic genetic features. TD is no longer considered optimal treatment for newly diagnosed patients with MM. Thalidomide is generally prescribed at 200 mg daily. No maximally tolerated dose (MTD) has been defined; doses as high as 800 mg daily has been used. Major side effects of thalidomide include irreversible peripheral neuropathy that develops after exposure for a period of 6 months or longer. Other serious side effects include DVT and pulmonary embolism when combined with dexamethasone but does require thromboprophylaxis for patients without additional risk factors for developing DVT. Prophylaxis with a low-dose aspirin (81–100 mg) daily is adequate. Other clinically significant side effects include severe constipation, severe bradycardia, and skin rash. Results with thalidomide combinations in relapsed and newly diagnosed patients are summarized in Tables 86.12 and 86.13.

Thalidomide has been used in combination with other drugs in newly diagnosed patients with MM. Six large randomized clinical trials have been conducted combining melphalan and prednisone with or without thalidomide. Metaanalysis of these six large studies has shown MPT to be superior to MP alone: The ORR improved by 22% (59% vs. 37%); PFS improved by 5 months (20 months vs. 15

---

substantial improvement in the PFS and OS has been observed. Hair loss and the need for catheter placement to administer these vesicant agents are important limitations and require acceptance by the patient. It is also possible to administer the daily dose of vincristine and adriamycin as an intravenous push without loss of efficacy or increased toxicity.

Chemotherapy With Alkylating Agents

Alkylating agents melphalan and cyclophosphamide were introduced in the management of MM in the early 1960s. Since the time of introduction, they have continued to play a vital role in the treatment of myeloma. MP has been the gold standard of treatment. All new combinations are benchmarked against MP. MP has been given in different doses and schedules for a minimum of 9–18 months. Other agents such as cyclophosphamide, carmustine (BCNU), vincristine, and/or Adriamycin, have been successfully combined with MP (e.g., VBMCP, VBAP). Combination therapies improved the response rate but did not change the OS outcomes. MP has a response rate of 50% to 60%, a PFS of 18 months, and an OS of 30–36 months.

In the 1960s, single-agent oral cyclophosphamide and oral melphalan were compared head to head in a randomized, double-blind

TABLE 86.12   Thalidomide Regimens in Relapsed/Refractory Multiple Myeloma

Trial	Dose	Number of Patients	ORR (%)	Median PFS (Mo)	Median OS
Barlogie	100–800 mg	169	30	20% at 2 yr	48% at 2 yr
Yakoub-Agha	100 mg ± dex	205	14		68.8% at 1 yr
	400 mg ± dex	195	18		72.8% at 1 yr
Neben	100–400 mg	83	20.5	45% at 1 yr	86% at 1 yr
Palumbo	Thal-dex	120	51	11 mo	21 mo
Dimopoulos	Thal-dex	42	55	TTP 4.2 mo	12.6 mo
Kyriakou	CTD	52	79	34 at 2 yr	73% at 2 yr
Garcia-Sanz	CTD	71	57	57% at 2 yr	66% at 2 yr
Offidani	TAD	50	76	17 mo	≈62% at 2 yr

CTD, Cyclophosphamide-thalidomide-dexamethasone; Dex, Dexamethasone; ORR, Overall response rate; CS, overall survival; PFS, progression-free survival; TAD, thalidomide-adriamycin-dexamethasone; Thal, thalidomide.

TABLE 86.13   Thalidomide Regimens in Newly Diagnosed Multiple Myeloma

Trial	Randomization	Number of Patients	ORR (%)	Median PFS (Mo)	Median OS (Mo)
Rajkumar	TD	235	63	14.9	72% at 2 yr
	D	235	46	6.5	65% at 2 yr
Ludwig	TD	145	68	16.7	41.5
	MP	143	50	20.7	49.5
Lokhorst	TAD + SCT	268	71	34	51% at 5 yr
	VAD + SCT	268	57	25	50% at 5 yr
Palumbo	MPT	167	76	21.8	45
	MP	164	47.6	14.5	47.6
Facon	MPT	125	76	27.5	51.6
	MP	196	35	17.8	33.2
Hulin	MPT	113	62	24.1	44
	MP	116	31	18.5	29
Wijermans	MPT	165	66	33	40
	MP	168	45	21	31
Waage	MPT	182	57	15	29
	MP	175	40	14	32

D, Dexamethasone; MP, melphalan-prednisone; MPT, melphalan-prednisone-thalidomide; ORR, overall response rate; OS, overall survival; PFS, progression-free survival, SCT, stem cell transplant; TAD, thalidomide-doxorubicin-dexamethasone; TD, thalidomide-dexamethasone.

TABLE 86.14   Randomized Studies Comparing Melphalan-Prednisone–Related Regimens

Authors/Study	Regimen	Complete Response	Partial Response	PFS (Median Mo)	OS (Median Mo)
Morgan et al	CTD vs. CVAD	13% vs. 8%	82.5% vs. 71.2%		
San Miguel et al/VISTA[41]	MPV vs. MP	30% vs. 4% ($p < .001$)	71% vs. 35% ($p < .001$)	24[a] vs. 16.6 ($p < .001$)	Not reached vs. 43
Palumbo et al	MPRR vs. MP	18% vs. 5% ($p < .001$)	77% vs. 49% ($p < .001$)	Not reached vs. 13 ($p = .002$)	Not reached

[a]Time to progression.
CTD, Cyclophosphamide-thalidomide-dexamethasone; CVAD, Cyclophosphamide-vincristine-doxorubicin-dexamethasone; MP, melphalan-prednisone; MPRR, melphalan-prednisone-lenalidomide followed by lenalidomide maintenance; OS, overall survival; PFS, progression-free survival.

months); and OS by 6 months (39 months vs. 33 months) (Table 86.14). MPT is an acceptable front-line treatment for patients over the age of 65 years. Side effects were higher in the MPT arm; DVT occurred in 6% to 12% versus 1% to 4% of patients; peripheral neuropathy occurred in 6% to 23% of patients versus 0% to 5% of patients; and discontinuation of treatment occurred in 41% to 45% of patients versus 6% to 11% of patients compared with MP alone (Table 86.15).

Thalidomide, adriamycin, and dexamethasone (TAD) induction therapy followed by stem cell transplant and subsequent maintenance with thalidomide was noted to be superior to VAD induction followed by transplant and interferon maintenance in a large randomized trial by the HOVON Group.

Oral Regimens

Cyclophosphamide, thalidomide, and dexamethasone (CTD) was compared with infusional CVAD chemotherapy for patients eligible for HDT in a large, multicenter, randomized phase III trial conducted in the United Kingdom (MRC Myeloma IX Trial). The CTD regimen consisted of cyclophosphamide 500 mg weekly, thalidomide 100 mg daily, and dexamethasone 40 mg for 4 days every other week. The induction chemotherapy was given for a minimum of six cycles and up to nine cycles or until maximum response. The postinduction ORR was significantly higher with CTD versus CVAD (82.5% vs. 71.2%; $p < .0001$); likewise, CR rates were also higher with CTD (13% vs. 8.1%; $p = .0083$). This differential response was maintained following autologous stem cell transplant with regard to posttransplant CR (50% vs. 37.2%; $p = .00052$). With a median follow-up of 47 months, there was no difference in PFS or OS between the two groups. This establishes CTD as an acceptable induction therapy before transplant.

For elderly patients and patients otherwise ineligible for HDT, CTD was compared with MP. The dose of cyclophosphamide was 500 mg weekly, thalidomide 50 mg daily, and dexamethasone 20 mg for 4 days every other week. Both arms were oral regimens. CTD therapy was associated with a superior ORR (63.8% vs. 32.6%; $p < .0001$) and CR rate (13.1% vs. 2.4%) and VGPR (16.9% vs. 1.7%). After a median follow-up of 44 months, PFS and OS were similar between the groups. CTD was associated with higher rates of thromboembolic events, constipation, infection, and neuropathy. This study also illustrated that thalidomide was incapable of improving the outcome of patients with unfavorable genetic markers.

Lenalidomide

Lenalidomide and dexamethasone are an effective combination therapy for the treatment of previously untreated symptomatic myeloma patients. A large, open-label, phase III randomized trial comparing lenalidomide plus high-dose dexamethasone or lenalidomide plus weekly dexamethasone conducted by the Eastern Cooperative Oncology Group established lenalidomide and dexamethasone as a simple oral regimen that could be used as an induction therapy before transplant or as a first-line therapy without a stem cell transplant. Administration of lenalidomide 25 mg daily for 3 weeks on and 1 week off, along with dexamethasone 40 mg in a pulsed fashion (days 1–4, 9–12, and 17–20) for the first four cycles only (high-dose dexamethasone arm), gave a higher response rate of 79% compared with weekly dexamethasone 40 mg (low-dose dexamethasone arm; 60%); however, the high-dose dexamethasone arm was associated with a higher incidence of infections and venous thromboembolism and an inferior 1-year survival rate (87%) compared with the low-dose dexamethasone arm (1-year survival rate of 96%). However, with longer follow-up, there was no survival difference between the two arms.

In a large, open-label, international randomized clinical trial, 1623 patients who were transplant ineligible were randomly assigned to lenalidomide and dexamethasone (RD) administered as 28-day cycles until disease progression occurred (535 patients), to the same combination of RD for 72 weeks (18 cycles; 541 patients), or to MPT for 72 weeks (547 patients). The median PFS rates were 25.5 months with continuous RD, 20.7 months with 18 cycles of RD, and 21.2 months with MPT (hazard ratios for the risk of progression or death 0.724 for continuous RD vs. MPT and 0.704 for continuous RD vs. 18 cycles of RD; $p < .001$ for both comparisons). OS rates at 4 years were 59% with continuous RD, 56% with 18 cycles of RD, and 51% with MPT.

A retrospective case-control study done at a single institution by researchers who compared lenalidomide-dexamethasone with thalidomide-dexamethasone revealed that lenalidomide-dexamethasone was better tolerated, with a higher ORR (80% vs. 61%), higher VGPR (34% vs. 12%), improved PFS (27 months vs. 17 months), and improved OS. Addition of clarithromycin to lenalidomide and low-dose dexamethasone resulted in an ORR of 90%, a VGPR rate of 74%, and a CR for 39% of patients.

Thus the combination of lenalidomide and dexamethasone is an excellent induction regimen as first-line therapy for newly diagnosed patients with MM. Results with lenalidomide combinations in relapsed and newly diagnosed patients are summarized in Tables 86.16 and 86.17. Lenalidomide has also been combined with MP

TABLE 86.15	**MPT Versus MP: Efficacy in Newly Diagnosed Elderly Patients With Myeloma**

- Three trials (IFM99[a], IFM01[b], HOVON[c]) >RR, PFS, and OS
- Two trials (GIMEMA[d], Turkish[e]) >RR, PFS
- One trial (Nordic[f]) >RR

RR	64%	vs.	37%	(>27%)
CR	10%	vs.	2.5%	(>8 %)
PFS	20.3	vs.	14.9 mo	(6 mo) HR, 0.67
OS	39.3	vs.	32.7 mo	(>6 mo) HR, 0.82

- Thal maintenance in Italian, Nordic[f], HOVON[c]

[a]Facon T, Mary JY, Hulin C, et al: *Lancet* 370:1209, 2007.
[b]Hulin C, Facon T, Rodon P, et al: *J Clin Oncol* 27:3664, 2009.
[c]Wijermans P, Schaafsma M, Termorshuizen F, et al: *J Clin Oncol* 28:3160, 2010.
[d]Palumbo A, Bringhen S, Liberati AM, et al: *Blood* 112:3107, 2008.
[e]Beksac M, Haznedar R, Firatli-Tuglular T, et al: *Eur J Haematol* 86:16, 2011.
[f]Waage A, Gimsing P, Fayers P, et al: *Blood* 116:1405, 2010; Waage A, Palumbo AP, Fayers P, et al: *J Clin Oncol* 28:15S [abstract 8130], 2010; Kapoor P, Kumar S, Mandrekar SJ, et al: *Leukemia* 25:1195, 2011.
CR, Complete response; HR, hazard ratio; IFM, Intergroupe Francophone du Myélome; MP, melphalan-prednisone; MPT, melphalan-prednisolone-thalidomide; OS, overall survival; PFS, progression-free survival; RR, relapsed/refractory.

TABLE 86.16	**Lenalidomide Regimens in Relapsed/Refractory Multiple Myeloma**

Trial	Regimen/Dose	Number of Patients	ORR (%)	Median TTP (Mo)	Median OS
Weber	Len + Dex	177	61	11.1	30 mo
	Dex	176	20	4.7	20 mo
Dimpopoulos	Len + Dex	176	60	11.3	NR
	Dex	175	24	4.7	21 mo
Richardson	Len 30 mg once daily	67	18	7.7	28 mo
	Len 15 mg twice daily	35	14	3.9	27 mo
Richardson	VRD	36	61	7.7	37 mo
Knop	RAD	69	73	6.2	88% at 1 yr
Morgan	CRD	21	65	5.6	Approximately 80% at 1 yr

CRD, Lenalidomide-cyclophosphamide-dexamethasone; Dex, dexamethasone; Len, lenalidomide; NR, no response; ORR, Overall response rate; OS, overall survival; RAD, lenalidomide-adriamycin-dexamethasone; TTP, time to progression; VRD, bortezomib-lenalidomide-dexamethasone.

TABLE 86.17	Lenalidomide Regimens in Newly Diagnosed Multiple Myeloma				
Trial	Regimen	Number of Patients	ORR (%)	Median PFS (Mo)	Median OS
Rajkumar	RD/pulse Dex	21	91	59% at 2 yr	85% at 3 yr
	RD/pulse Dex + SCT	13		83% at 2 yr	92% at 3 yr
Niesvizky	BiRD	72	90	75% at 2 yr	86% at 1 yr
Rajkumar	RD	223	79	38% at 3 yr	87% at 2 yr
	Rd	222	68	43% at 3 yr	75% at 2 yr
Palumbo	MPR	54	81	92% at 1 yr	100% at 1 yr

BiRD, clarithromycin-lenalidomide-dexamethasone; Dex, dexamethasone; MPR, melphalan-prednisone-lenalidomide; ORR, Overall response rate; OS, overall survival; PFS, progression-free survival; RD,; Rd, lenalidomide-dexamethasone; SCT, stem cell transplant.

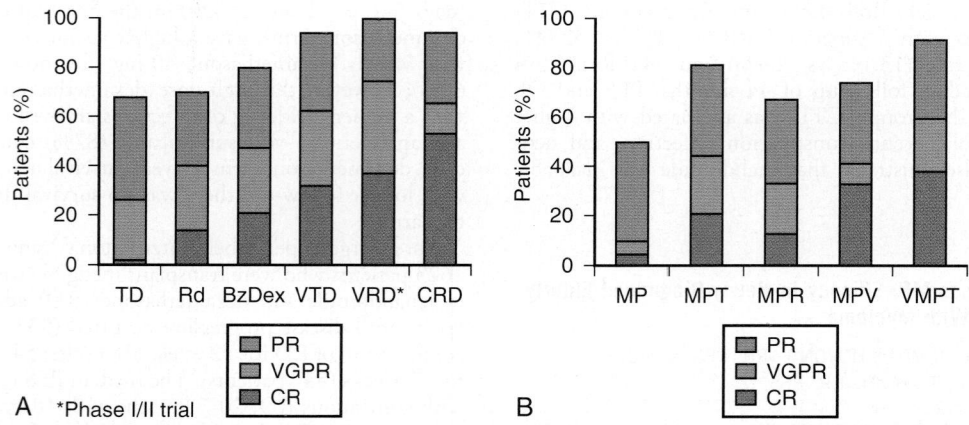

Fig. 86.13 PROGRESSIVE IMPROVEMENT IN RESPONSE TO COMBINATION THERAPIES INCORPORATING NEWER AGENTS. The partial response (PR), very good partial response (VGPR), and complete remission (CR) rates following induction therapy of newly diagnosed patients with multiple myeloma are plotted for a common novel agent combination selected from larger phases III and II studies. *Bz or V,* Bortezomib; *C,* carfilzomib; *D,* dexamethasone; *M,* melphalan; *P,* prednisone; *R,* lenalidomide; *T,* thalidomide.

with its continued use as maintenance, and as shown in Table 86.15, it provides a superior response and PFS to that of MP alone.

Bortezomib

Bortezomib, a boron-containing dipeptide, is the first proteasome inhibitor to be introduced for the treatment of MM. Bortezomib is a specific and reversible inhibitor of the 26S proteasome, binding to the chymotrypsin-like enzymatic site. The incomplete and transient inhibition of the proteasome results in apoptosis of myeloma cells by activation of both caspases 8 and 9 while sparing normal tissue. There is downregulation of NFκB in the myeloma cells, OCs, and the surrounding stromal cells. This results in decreased release of inflammatory cytokines such as IL-6 in the bone marrow milieu. Bortezomib not only arrests osteoclastic activity by reducing sRANKL and decreases CTX, and TRACP-5b but also induces OBs by decreasing serum DKK-1 as reflected by an increase in bone alkaline phosphatase and osteocalcin, regardless of treatment response.

Bortezomib as a single agent induces CR in 10% of patients and results in an ORR of 27% in newly diagnosed mm patients; bortezomib is not recommended as a monotherapy. Bortezomib and dexamethasone (B-D) is an excellent induction regimen with an ORR of 88% and CR+VGPR rate of 19% and one year survival of 87%. A randomized trial has shown B-D to be superior to VAD as an induction regimen with a higher CR rate (15% vs. 6%) and ORR (79% vs. 63%).[27] Following autologous stem cell transplant, there was a continued advantage for the B-D arm: CR/near-CR of 35% versus

18% and VGPR or better of 54% versus 37%. Median PFS was 36 months versus 30 months, and 3-year survival rates were 81% versus 77% with a median follow-up of 32 months. Results with bortezomib combination therapy including relapsed and newly diagnosed patients are summarized in Tables 86.7 and 86.8. Bortezomib has also been combined with melphalan and prednisone, and as shown in Table 86.15, after 5 years of follow-up, it provides ORR, CR, PFS, and OS superior to MP alone.

Combination of Three or Four Classes of Drugs

It is possible to combine drugs from different classes with nonoverlapping toxicities without compromising their dose to maximize their antitumor effect and eliminate potentially resistant clones to prolong remission duration. Generally, three-drug combinations have been shown to give the highest ORR and VGPR as compared with two-drug regimens (VCD, VRD, VTD).[28,29] Fig. 86.13 summarizes the results with two-, three-, and four-drug regimens and suggests improved responses and a higher incidence of CR using a three-drug regimen (RVD, VCD) with apparently no clear benefit of adding a fourth agent as yet. Similar results are also depicted in Fig. 86.13 with MP-based regimens. In the Southwest Oncology Group trial, 525 patients were randomly allocated to bortezomib, lenalidomide, and dexamethasone (VRD; 242 patients) or to lenalidomide and dexamethasone (RD; 229 patients). Patients randomized to VRD received eight 3-weekly cycles, and patients assigned to RD received six 28-day cycles. Patients from both arms were subsequently maintained on RD until progression. Patients randomized to the three-drug combination

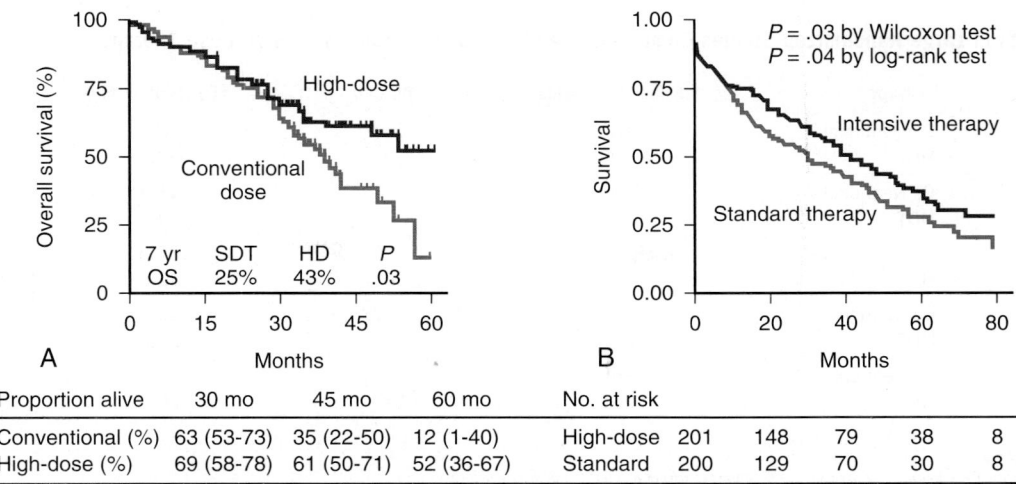

Fig. 86.14 COMPARATIVE TRIALS OF HIGH-DOSE THERAPY (HDT) WITH STANDARD-DOSE CHEMOTHERAPY (SDT). Intergroupe Francophone du Myélome (IFM-90; *left panel*) randomized trials with 200 patients randomized to SDT with VMCP-VBAP (vincristine, melphalan, cyclophosphamide, and prednisone and vincristine, carmustine, adriamycin, and prednisone) versus HDT with melphalan 140 mg/m^2 plus total body irradiation (800 cGy) and Medical Research Council (MRC-VII; *right panel*) trial with 401 patients randomized to SDT with doxorubicin, carmustine, cyclophosphamide, and melphalan or HDT with CVAD followed by melphalan 200 mg/m^2 and stem cell rescue. Significantly longer overall survival was noted with HDT in both studies. *HD,* High dose; *OS,* overall survival.

(VRD) had a better median PFS of 43 months than patients receiving two drugs (RD) with a median PFS of 30 months ($p = .0018$; HR, 0.712). Surprisingly, there was improvement in OS for the triplet regimen (VRD; median OS, 75 months) over the doublet regimen (RD; median OS, 64 months) with a hazard ratio of 0.7 and a p-value of .025.

High-Dose Therapy and Consolidation

Tim McElwain introduced high-dose intravenous melphalan for the treatment of MM in 1983. A dose–response effect for melphalan was quite evident in MM. In the 1980s and 1990s, HDT with stem cell support was increasingly used to treat younger patients (aged 65 years and under).

Source of Stem Cells

In the 1980s, bone marrow was harvested from the patient under general anesthesia. This approach has been completely supplanted by the use of peripheral blood stem/progenitor cells. Autologous bone marrow transplant was associated with delayed hematopoietic recovery by 1 week compared with mobilized blood stem cells, resulting in a higher transplant-related morbidity and mortality of 10% compared with 2% with peripheral blood progenitor cells. Stem cells can be mobilized with chemotherapy alone, chemotherapy and growth factor (G-CSF or granulocyte-macrophage colony-stimulating factor), or growth factors alone (G-CSF, G-CSF plus plerixafor). The degree of tumor cell contamination in the peripheral blood stem cell product has had no influence on transplant outcome. Ex vivo manipulations to eliminate tumor cells within the graft have not resulted in any improvement in the depth of response, PFS, or OS. It is preferable to use stem cell–sparing agents as induction therapy before stem cell harvest. Alkylating agent exposure and lenalidomide exposure should be limited to ensure adequate stem cell harvest and complete hematopoietic recovery posttransplant. It is preferable to collect stem cells after the achievement of best antitumor response to induction therapy to minimize tumor cell contamination.

AUTOLOGOUS STEM CELL TRANSPLANT

Single High-Dose Therapy With Stem Cell Transplant Rescue

Several prospective, randomized clinical trials were performed in the 1990s to define the role of HDT and stem cell transplant as a component of front-line therapy for patients with MM. In two studies (IFM 90[30] and MRC VII[31]), researchers reported the superiority of HDT and stem cell transplant with respect to response rate, PFS, and OS, which led to widespread use of HDT and stem cell transplant for patients up to the age of 65 years (Fig. 86.14).[32] However, there were other studies that did not show a survival advantage but did show improvements in the response rate and PFS. One such clinical trial was conducted by the French myeloma autograft group in patients between the ages of 55 and 65 years (MAG 90). That study showed a higher response rate (CR + MRD 36% vs. 20%) and a trend for improved PFS (EFS, 25.3 vs. 18.7 months; $p = .07$) in favor of the HDT arm, but no difference in OS. Researchers in a Spanish trial gave induction therapy with VBMCP/VBAD for four cycles at five week intervals, and subsequently responding patients were randomized between HDT and continuation of standard chemotherapy for eight additional cycles of VBMCP/VBAD. Although the HDT arm had a higher CR rate, there was no difference in PFS or OS. Another trial conducted in the United States also allowed for induction therapy, followed by randomization of all patients to a single autotransplant versus continued VBMCP therapy for 1 year. This study did not show a difference in OS between the two arms. In this study, the patients in the standard treatment arm were allowed to receive HDT and stem cell transplant following relapse. Results of five large randomized trials comparing SDT with HDT are summarized in Table 86.18.

In another randomized phase III trial with patients under the age of 56 years, investigatos evaluated the role of early versus late transplant (MAG 91). This study showed that there was no difference in OS. However, the investigators showed that early application of HDT resulted in prolonged PFS compared with the standard chemotherapy arm; the time without symptoms, additional treatment, and treatment toxicity were favorable when HDT was applied as part

TABLE 86.18   Results of Large Randomized Studies Comparing Standard-Dose Therapy With High-Dose Therapy

Authors	Therapy	Number of Patients	CR (%)	EFS (Median Mo)	OS (Median Mo)
Attal et al	Conventional	100	5[a]	18[a]	37[a]
	HDT	100	22	27	52
Fermand et al	Conventional	96	—	18.7[a]	50.4[b]
	HDT	94	—	24.3	55.3
Blade et al	Conventional	83	11[a]	34.3[a]	66.9[b]
	HDT	81	30	42.5	67.4
Child et al	Conventional	200	8.5[a]	19.6[a]	42.3[a]
	HDT	201	44	31.6	54.8
Barlogie et al	Conventional	255	15[b]	21[b]	53[b]
	HDT	261	17	25	58

[a]Significant difference.
[b]No significant difference.
CR, Complete remission; EFS, event-free survival; OS, overall survival; HDT, high-dose therapy.

TABLE 86.19   Single Versus Double Autologous Stem Cell Transplant for Newly Diagnosed MM

Study	ASCT	Number of Patients	CR (%)[a]	Median EFS (Mo)	Median OS (Mo)
Attal et al	Single	199	42[b]	25	48
			p = NS	p = .03	p = .01
(IFM94)	Double	200	50[b]	30	58
Fermand et al	Single	94	42[a]	No difference	No difference
			p = NS		
(MAG95)	Double	99	37[a]		
Sonneveld et al	Single	148	13	20	55
			p = .002	p = .02	p = NS
(HOVON24)	Double	155	28	22	50
Cavo et al	Single	115	35	Significant prolongation of EFS	59
(Bologna 96)	Double	113	p = NS	with double-SCT	p = NS
			48		73

[a]CR + minimum residual disease.
[b]CR + very good partial response.
ASCT, Autologous stem cell transplant; CR, complete remission; EFS, event-free survival; IFM, Intergroupe Francophone du Myélome; NS, not significant; OS, overall survival; SCT, stem cell transplant.

of the initial therapy. This allowed for flexibility in the timing of transplant to suit the patient's clinical situation and preference.

A metaanalysis of primary data obtained from the three French studies (IFM 90, MAG 90, and MAG 91) showed no difference in the OS between standard therapy and HDT arms. Likewise, authors of another metaanalysis using data culled from nine randomized clinical trials reported in the literature showed no survival benefit for HDT and stem cell transplant. These data are in direct contrast to the metaanalysis using the Swedish Cancer Registry and SEER data with improvement in 5-year relative survival ratios for younger patients primarily due to the introduction of HDT and stem cell transplant in the 1990s.

On the presumption that therapy with a single alkylating agent at MTD may not be adequate for disease eradication, Barlogie pioneered a tandem transplant approach as part of his total therapy approach for the treatment of MM in 1989 (Total Therapy 1) and reported promising results without increased treatment-related morbidity or mortality. Single HDT resulted in a CR rate well under 25% in most trials. These investigators tried to improve the results by providing a second consecutive high-dose melphalan and stem cell transplant (tandem transplant).

There have been four large randomized clinical trials comparing the role of tandem autotransplant against a single episode of HDT and stem cell transplant (Table 86.19). All four studies showed improvement in the depth of response (VGPR) following a tandem transplant, and three of the four studies showed improvement in PFS, but only one study showed an improvement in the OS. The French trial (IFM 94 [33]) showed the benefit of a second transplant only for patients not in VGPR or better after the first transplant. In the era of novel agents, a VGPR or better can be obtained before transplant, and therefore a second transplant is seldom used outside the setting of a clinical trial (Table 86.20).

In the era before introduction of novel agents, induction regimen had only a minimal role because CRs were uncommon (less than 5%) with high-dose dexamethasone or VAD chemotherapy. Thus HDT played a critical role in achieving favorable CR and VGPR rates and prolonged durability of unmaintained responses. The availability of novel agents has dramatically changed this paradigm. Novel agents have improved VGPR or better before stem cell transplant, allowing for posttransplant consolidation and maintenance. Whether novel agents can supplant HDT and stem cell transplant is an important question that has yet to be answered.

Induction Therapy With Novel Agents

Randomized clinical trials have shown that combined thalidomide and dexamethasone therapy is equivalent to VAD chemotherapy. The Dutch HOVON 50 trial researchers compared thalidomide during the induction phase and as maintenance following HDT and stem

TABLE 86.20	Single versus Tandem AutoTX							
			Age (yr)	Pat (n)	CR (%)	EFS (mo) 7-yr	OS (mo) 7-yr
Attal et al (NEJM 2003)	IFM94	Single	<61	199	42	25	48
		Tandem		200	50	30[a]	58[a]
						7-yr	7-yr
Cavo et al (J Clin Oncol 2007)	Bologna 96	Single	<61	163	33	23	65
		Tandem		158	47[a]	35[a]	71
Sonneveld et al (Haematologica 2007)	HOVON 24	Single	<66	148	13	21	55
		Tandem		156	32[a]	22[a]	50

[a]P Value significant.

cell transplant. TAD chemotherapy was superior to VAD chemotherapy on the basis of overall response and quality of response before and after HDT and stem cell transplant. In addition, maintenance with thalidomide improved the PFS and resulted in a trend toward improved OS. Lenalidomide and dexamethasone have been shown to be useful as an induction regimen before transplant. However, no formal randomized clinical trial has been performed comparing this combination with conventional chemotherapy. Exposure to lenalidomide should be limited to four to six cycles because it compromises stem cell mobilization.

French Study IFM 2005-1

B-D was superior to VAD chemotherapy as an induction regimen. There was improvement in CR and VGPR before and after transplant, and there was a trend for prolonged PFS but no difference in the OS.[27] The lack of impact on PFS and OS is perhaps a result of limited bortezomib exposure to a maximum of four cycles during the induction phase.

Combining bortezomib with immunomodulatory drugs further improves the outcome before and after stem cell transplant. In a large randomized clinical trial of 480 patients conducted by the GIMEMA Italian Myeloma Network, VTD was shown to be superior to PD for induction therapy and for consolidation after tandem transplant. VTD induction therapy significantly improved the rate of complete or near-complete response before the transplant. This higher response rate continued following tandem transplant and was further augmented by two cycles of VTD consolidation as opposed to TD posttransplant. This increase in the depth of response has translated to a superior PFS. However, there was increased neuropathy encountered by the patients in the VTD arm. The French investigators reduced the dose intensity of VTD and confirmed in another randomized trial that four cycles of VTD were superior to four cycles of B-D as an induction regimen before transplant.[34] There was less neuropathy, owing to the adjustment of bortezomib and thalidomide doses. The Spanish group compared TD, VTD, and multiagent chemotherapy as induction therapy and showed that VTD was superior following transplant. The patients were further randomized to maintenance therapy with VP versus VT, with no difference in outcome observed. Results of two large studies of HDT with over 7 and 12 years of follow-up are shown in Fig. 86.15, suggesting a possibility of a tail in the survival cure with over 10% to 20% of patients remaining disease-free or alive after 10 years, suggesting a possibility for long-term survival in myeloma.

Allogeneic Stem Cell Transplantation

Allogeneic stem cell transplant offers a potential for cure for patients with MM that is mediated by a graft-versus-myeloma effect, tumor-free graft, and potential for donor lymphocyte infusion to combat the residual or recurrent disease (Fig. 86.16). However, the role of allogeneic stem cell transplant in MM is limited. Patients are generally older (over 75% of the patients are over the age of 55 years), often presenting with comorbidities such as renal impairment, diastolic dysfunction of the heart, and restrictive lung disease. The underlying immunodeficiency associated with this disease is worsened by posttransplant immunosuppression, resulting in a high transplant-related mortality with standard myeloablative conditioning regimens. Relapse after allogeneic stem cell transplant contributes to the modest efficacy of this approach. Whereas it could be shown that there is a graft-versus-myeloma effect with sustained molecular remission, it has been difficult to induce graft-versus-myeloma effects while avoiding graft-versus-host disease (GVHD). There are no convincing survival data to support widespread use of allogeneic stem cell transplant outside a clinical trial.

There has been improvement in 6-month and 2-year survival rates since 1994 as compared with the prior era. This improvement reported by the European Bone Marrow Transplant Registry was attributed to better supportive care measures and patient selection. Reduced-intensity conditioning regimens, with reduction in immediate transplant-related mortality and stable engraftment, as well as use of peripheral blood progenitor cells from donors with their rapid engraftment kinetics, renewed interest in the use of allogeneic stem cell transplant for MM. Bensinger et al reported the long-term results of allogeneic transplant for MM at the Fred Hutchinson Cancer Research Center spanning 34 years. Among the 144 patients undergoing an ablative conditioning regimen, the 2-year nonrelapse transplant mortality was 55%; major causes of death included fungal and viral infections, acute respiratory distress syndrome, acute GVHD, and multiorgan failure. The 2-year non–transplant-related mortality was 18% among the recipients of nonablative conditioning regimens; the causes of death were mostly chronic GVHD and progressive disease. The 10-year OS was 15% for myeloablative regimens as compared with 35% for nonmyeloablative regimens. The incidence of acute GVHD was similar (65% ± 2%), but the incidence of extensive chronic GVHD was 27% for ablative regimens as compared with 67% for nonablative regimens (Table 86.21).

There have been several studies reported combining the tandem autologous transplant approach with "mini" allogeneic stem cell transplant. The Italian group reported superior outcomes for patients receiving an autograft-allograft protocol compared with patients receiving tandem autograft protocols.[35] After a median follow-up of 46 months, the median OS had not been reached for patients receiving auto-allotransplants as compared with 58 months for tandem autotransplants; the EFS rates were 43 and 33 months, respectively, for the two groups (Table 86.21). The French group subjected patients with high risk (β_2-microglobulin >3 mg/L and chromosome 13 deletion) to tandem auto-transplants or auto-allotransplant on the basis of availability of human leukocyte antigen–compatible sibling donors. On an intention-to-treat basis, there was no difference in EFS or OS with a trend for better OS in patients treated with tandem autologous stem cell transplants. In a recently completed BMT-CTN

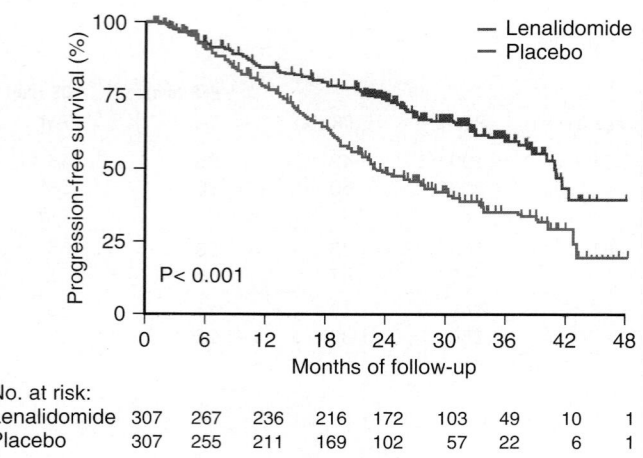

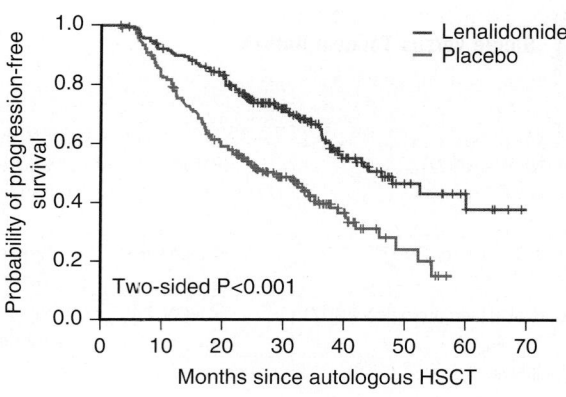

No. at risk:

Lenalidomide	307	267	236	216	172	103	49	10	1
Placebo	307	255	211	169	102	57	22	6	1

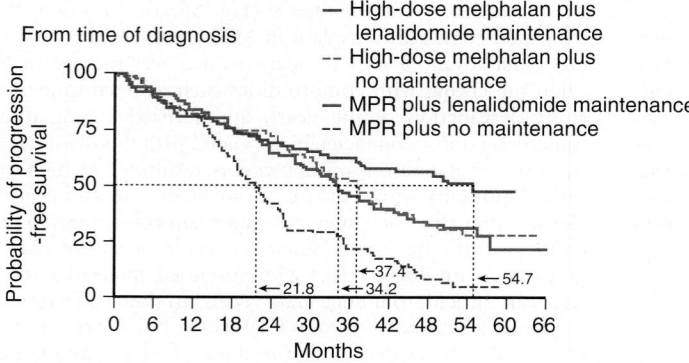

No. at risk:

High-dose melphalan plus lenalidomide maintenance	100	88	73	64	57	53	49	43	40	19	1
High-dose melphalan plus no maintenance	100	87	74	60	56	49	41	31	21	9	2
MPR plus lenalidomide maintenance	98	84	71	63	54	48	36	28	24	10	2
MPR plus no maintenance	104	87	77	55	36	26	18	14	7	2	0

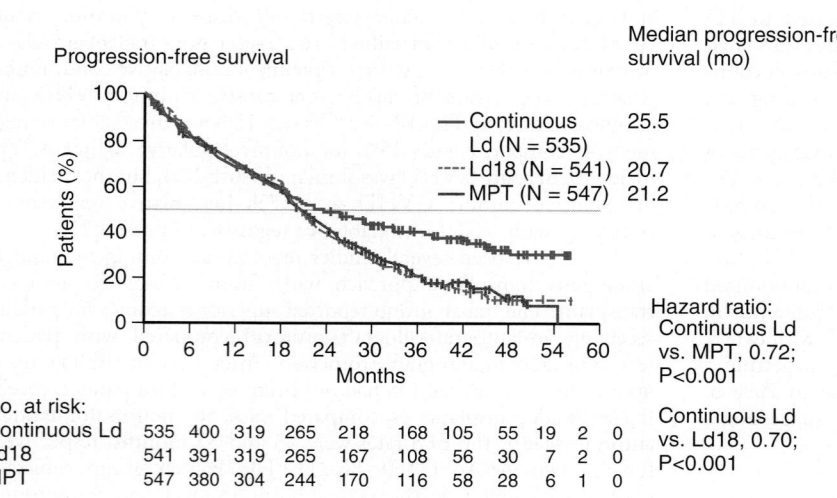

No. at risk:

Continuous Ld	535	400	319	265	218	168	105	55	19	2	0
Ld18	541	391	319	265	167	108	56	30	7	2	0
MPT	547	380	304	244	170	116	58	28	6	1	0

Median progression-free survival (mo)

Continuous Ld (N = 535) 25.5
Ld18 (N = 541) 20.7
MPT (N = 547) 21.2

Hazard ratio:
Continuous Ld vs. MPT, 0.72; P<0.001

Continuous Ld vs. Ld18, 0.70; P<0.001

Fig. 86.15 MAINTENANCE THERAPY PRO-LONGS PROGRESSION-FREE SURVIVAL (PFS). Lenalidomide maintenance improves PFS after hematopoietic stem cell transplant (HSCT). (A) Intergroupe Francophone du Myélome (IFM) trial. (B) Cancer and Leukemia Group B (CALGB) trial. (C) Lenalidomide maintenance improves PFS following standard chemotherapy (melphalan, prednisone, and lenalidomide [MPR]) or after high-dose therapy. (D) Improved PFS following continuous lenalidomide and dexamethasone (Ld) until progression versus Ld for 18 months or melphalan, prednisone, and thalidomide for 18 months. *MPT,* melpahalan, prednisone, and thalidomide; *Ld,* lenalidomide and weekly dexamethasone. *(Data from Attal M, Lauwers-Cances, Marit G, et al: lenalidomide maintenance after stem cell transplantation for multiple myeloma.* N Engl J Med *366:1782, 2012; McCarthy P, Owzar K, Hofmeister CC, et al: lenalidomide after stem cell transplantation for multiple myeloma.* N Engl J Med *366:1770, 2012; Palumbo A, Cavallo F, Gay F, et al: Autologous transplantation and maintenance therapy in multiple myeloma.* N Engl J Med *371:895, 2014; and Benboubker L, Dimopoulos MA, Dispenzieri A, et al: Lenalidomide and dexamethasone in transplant ineligible patients with myeloma.* N Engl J Med *371:906, 2014.)*

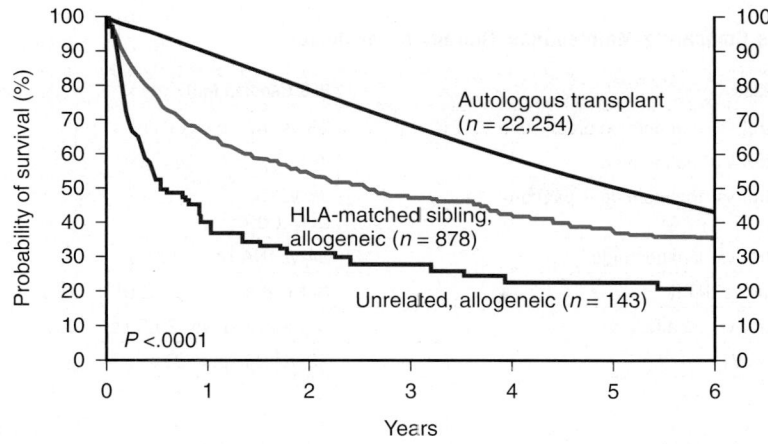

Fig. 86.16 CENTER FOR INTERNATIONAL BLOOD AND MARROW TRANSPLANT RESEARCH ANALYSIS OF MYELOMA TRANSPLANTS. Among 23,197 patients who received an autotransplant for multiple myeloma (MM) between 2000 and 2009, the 3-year probability of survival was 70% ± 1%. Allogeneic stem cell transplant for MM is reserved for patients with high-risk disease, and the majority of transplants were performed after an autologous hematopoietic cell transplant (HCT) with reduced-intensity or nonmyeloablative conditioning regimens. Among the 979 patients who received an allogeneic HCT between 2000 and 2009, the 3-year probabilities of survival were 51% ± 2% for the 827 recipients of human leukocyte antigen (HLA)–matched sibling donor grafts and 26% ± 2% for the 470 recipients of unrelated donor grafts. *(From Pasquini MD, Wang Z: CIBMTR summary slides, 2010. Adapted from http://www.cibmtr.org/.)*

TABLE 86.21 Studies of Myeloablative and Reduced-Intensity Allogeneic Stem Cell Transplant for Newly Diagnosed Myeloma

Authors	Number of Patients	TRM (%)	CR (%)	OS (Actuarial, Mo)	EFS (Actuarial, Mo)
Gahrton et al	162	41	44	28% at 84	45% at 60
Bensinger et al	80	44	36	20% at 54	24% at 54
Alyea et al	61[a]	5	28	40% at 36	20% at 38
Lee et al	45	36	64	3-Yr EFS 13%	Median 14 mo
Kroger et al	17	18	73	2-Yr PFS 55%	2-Yr OS 74%
Maloney et al	54	7	57	2-Yr DFS 56%	18-Mo OS 78%
Giralt et al	13	38	54	NA	NA
Bruno et al	58	7	55	Median 43 mo	Median >46 mo

[a]T cell depleted.
CR, Complete remission; DFS, disease-free survival; EFS, event-free survival; NA, not available; OS, overall survival; PFS, progression-free survival; TRM, treatment-related mortality.

trial in the United States, there was no difference in outcome between auto-/mini-allotransplant and tandem autologous transplant. In order to increase the effect of donor lymphocyte infusions against the tumor cells, vaccination strategies are currently being pursued.

Syngeneic Transplantation

Results of syngeneic transplant are superior to autologous transplant and allogeneic stem cell transplant. The results are better than autologous transplant because of lower relapse rates with twin transplant. This may be related to the lack of tumor cells in the graft and/or a graft-versus-myeloma effect without GVHD. The results of syngeneic transplant are also superior to allogeneic stem cell transplant on the basis of low transplant-related mortality and the absence of clinical GVHD. These conclusions were based on reports published by two large transplant registries (CIBMTR and EBMTR).

Maintenance

Maintenance therapy is the use of ongoing low-intensity chemotherapy to eliminate or suppress MRD over a prolonged period.

Maintenance therapy is administered when the disease is in remission, at either undetectable or low levels. The purpose of maintenance therapy is to prolong remission duration and thereby life expectancy. Maintenance therapy improves the quality of response, supporting the notion that an additional antitumor response during the maintenance phase will be beneficial. Immunomodulatory molecules are well suited for maintenance therapy because they can be administered orally at low doses for a prolonged period.[36]

The first two randomized trials published on thalidomide maintenance after autotransplant showed an improvement in PFS and OS. In the Total Therapy II trial, researchers randomized patients to thalidomide induction and a maintenance arm versus a no thalidomide arm; this study showed improvement in PFS and a delayed improvement in OS after 8 years of follow-up. In the HOVON 50 trial, patients were similarly randomized to thalidomide induction followed by thalidomide maintenance after transplant or VAD induction followed by interferon maintenance. This trial also showed improvement in PFS and OS for patients in the thalidomide arm. A meta-analysis of published results to date indicated a significant reduction of the risk for progression with thalidomide maintenance therapy. Outcome did not differ between trials that used thalidomide during the maintenance phase only and those that used thalidomide for both induction and maintenance treatment. The MRC IX trial

TABLE 86.22	Randomized Studies Comparing Maintenance Therapy in Myeloma		
Authors/Study	Regimen	PFS (Median Mo)	OS (Median Mo)
Spencer et al	Control vs. thalidomide/prednisone	23 vs. 42 ($p < .001$)	75 vs. 86 ($p = .004$)
Barlogie et al	Control vs. thalidomide	44%[a] vs. 57% ($p = .01$)	Not reached
Attal et al	Control vs. thalidomide + pamidronate	36 vs. 52 ($p = .009$)	77 vs. 87 ($p = .04$)
Attal et al	Control vs. lenalidomide	24 vs. NA ($p < .0001$)	80%[b] vs. 88%
Palumbo et al	MPRR vs. MPR	Not reached vs. 13.2 ($p = .002$)	Not reached
McCarthy et al	Control vs. lenalidomide	Not reached[c] vs. 25.5 ($p < .001$)	Not reached
Mateos et al	VP vs. VT	32 vs. 24 ($p = .01$)	Not reached

[a]5-year PFS rate.
[b]Survival after 3 years.
[c]Time to progression.
MPR, Melphalan-prednisone-lenalidomide; MPRR, melphalan-prednisone-lenalidomide followed by lenalidomide maintenance; NA, not available; OS, overall survival; PFS, progression-free survival; VP, bortezomib-prednisone; VT, bortezomib-thalidomide.

had an intensive therapy arm (stem cell transplant) and a nonintensive arm (no stem cell transplant); once the patients had completed the intensive or nonintensive treatment arm, they were randomized to receive thalidomide maintenance or no maintenance. There was improvement in PFS but no improvement in OS when the two groups were compared. Results of major randomized studies evaluating maintenance therapy are summarized in Table 86.22.

There have been three large randomized trials exploring the role of lenalidomide as maintenance therapy. Two of these studies were maintenance therapy after autologous stem cell transplant (CALGB and IFM), and the third study was in elderly patients receiving MP. All three studies showed improvement in PFS by 18 months; only the CALGB study showed improvement in OS. There appears to be a slightly increased risk of occurrence of a second malignancy when lenalidomide is administered along with melphalan immediately after HDT with melphalan. Lenalidomide therapy is also unable to alter the poor prognosis attributed to adverse cytogenetics or FISH results.

Bortezomib has also been used in the maintenance setting. Generally, bortezomib maintenance has been restricted to clinical trials in which bortezomib was also used during the induction phase of the treatment. Bortezomib maintenance seemingly improved the outcome in patients with high-risk cytogenetics or FISH results. Bortezomib is given less frequently in the maintenance setting; different studies have used different schedules of administration.

RELAPSED DISEASE

Relapse is defined as reappearance of signs and symptoms of the disease or signs of increasing disease and/or end-organ dysfunction that are related to the underlying myeloma.[37] Patients presenting with a symptomatic relapse require treatment intervention. Patients with rapidly rising paraprotein, doubling of the paraprotein within a short interval, also require treatment. Patients with asymptomatic biochemical relapse do not require treatment. Generally, serum M spike greater than 1 g/dL, Bence Jones proteinuria greater than 500 mg per day, or serum free light chain level greater than 200 mg/L would be a minimum requirement to consider intervention with systemic therapy. Occasionally, myeloma cells may become dedifferentiated or anaplastic and may produce only light chain components (Bence Jones escape phenomenon) or no paraprotein at all. These patients generally tend to have a more aggressive clinical course. The development of compression fractures and fractures at a site of previous lytic lesion per se does not constitute progression of myeloma. Development of hypercalcemia, progressive anemia, and new or worsening kidney function would merit prompt treatment intervention.

Currently, relapsed and refractory disease is defined as having failed three or more lines of prior therapy with previous exposure to all four classes of drugs (cytotoxic agents, immunomodulatory agents, proteasome inhibitors, and glucocorticoids) and progressing during the last line of therapy. These patients have a life expectancy less than 1 year.

There are several considerations in choosing the treatment for patients with relapsed myeloma.[37] These include disease-related factors such as slow, indolent, or single site of relapse or rapid and multiple sites of relapse. Patients with a single site of relapse may benefit from radiation treatment. Special considerations need to be given to patients presenting with extramedullary soft tissue plasmacytomas, CNS relapses, or plasma cell leukemia. Patients presenting with an elevated LDH, high β_2-microglobulin, del(17p), and multiple copies of 1q generally have a poor prognosis. Patients presenting with advanced age, poor performance status, renal impairment, and poor hematologic reserve or concurrent myelodysplastic syndrome from prior therapy present a great challenge. The choice of treatment is also predicated on prior drug exposure, whether the relapse is on or off therapy, and ongoing toxicity from prior therapy. For more information, see box on Treatment of Relapsed Multiple Myeloma.

Thalidomide

Thalidomide monotherapy was originally introduced for the treatment of advanced and refractory myeloma. In the initial phase II trial, thalidomide was administered at 200 mg daily with increments every 2 weeks up to 800 mg for 169 patients. A partial response or better was noted in 30% of patients with a 2-year EFS of 20% and OS of 48%. A phase III trial (OPTIMUM) compared dexamethasone with thalidomide monotherapy at 100 mg, 200 mg, and 400 mg daily doses. The median times to progression were 6, 7, 8, and 9.1 months, respectively. The response rates and the median survival were similar in all treatment groups. In a systematic review published by Glasmacher, partial responses or better in 30% of relapsed patients with 1-year survival of 60% were reported. Thalidomide has been combined successfully with other conventional chemotherapy agents as well as proteasome inhibitors for improved response rates and better disease control. Thalidomide is especially useful when a patient presents with renal impairment and cytopenias. It is also useful for palliation when combined with oral cyclophosphamide and prednisone in patients with a poor performance status.

Lenalidomide

In two large phase III randomized trials (MM 009, MM 010), lenalidomide and dexamethasone was found to be superior to dexamethasone in patients with relapsed myeloma after one to three lines of prior therapy. Updated results with a median follow-up of 48 months showed an ORR of 61%, median time to progression of 13.4

BOX 86.2	Treatment of Relapsed Multiple Myeloma

- Ensure patient has had relapse requiring intervention. A negative immunofixation test becoming positive is not an indication to initiate salvage therapy. A clear clinical relapse occurs with new or increased evidence of end-organ damage, and a substantial or aggressive biochemical relapse is defined by criteria for progressive disease.
- Selection of treatment depends on prior therapy received
  - Lenalidomide based
    - Initial treatment with bortezomib/thalidomide.
    - Underlying peripheral neuropathy
    - Lenalidomide used with caution in patients with renal dysfunction with appropriate dose adjustment
  - Bortezomib based
    - Initial treatment with immunomodulatory agents
    - Renal dysfunction
    - Poor hematopoietic reserve
    - Long response (>12 mo) to prior bortezomib
  - Thalidomide based
    - Prior bortezomib/lenalidomide
    - Renal impairment
    - Poor hematopoietic reserve
  - Chemotherapy with or without novel agent combination
    - Progressed on novel agents
    - Rapid, aggressive relapse with high lactate dehydrogenase and/or extramedullary plasmacytomas
  - Salvage transplant
    - In transplant-eligible patients, transplant needs to be considered if stem cell transplant was deferred at initial therapy or patient had a long remission (>3 yr) after first transplant or has poor hematopoietic reserve and stem cells are being stored. Transplant may also be considered as a way to reestablish hematopoiesis in select cases.
- Special considerations
  - Rapid, or multiple sites, or extramedullary sites: chemotherapy with or without novel agent combination
  - Central nervous system relapse - radiation therapy for localized disease, intrathecal chemotherapy for positive cerebrospinal fluid cytology, along with systemic therapy as indicated
  - Poor performance status and hematopoietic reserve - oral therapy with low-dose daily cyclophosphamide, thalidomide, and prednisone
  - Prior drug exposure and associated toxicity: consider presence of neuropathy, cytopenias, and renal dysfunction to decide on agents, their schedule, and dose
- Clinical trials
  - Consider enrolling patient on a clinical trial with a new drug

months, duration of response of 16 months, and OS of 38 months. Patients who had received more than one line of prior therapy had an ORR of 57%, and time to progression was 10.6 months. A median PFS of 9.5 months and OS of 31 months were reported. Patients with moderate or severe renal impairment developed more severe thrombocytopenia, required more frequent dose modifications, and had inferior survival outcomes. Prior exposure to thalidomide did not preclude responses to lenalidomide; however, patients who had relapsed or progressed on thalidomide had a lower response rate (under 50%) and a shorter time to progression (7 months). Lenalidomide can easily be combined with conventional chemotherapy as well as bortezomib. Combination therapy results in a higher response rate and better disease control.

Bortezomib

In a large phase II trial (SUMMIT) conducted with patients with relapsed and refractory MM, bortezomib monotherapy had an impressive ORR of 28%, including 10% CR or near-CR. The median time to progression was 7 months, the duration of response was 12.7 months, and the median survival time was 17 months.

Among patients with relapsed myeloma following one to three lines of prior therapy, bortezomib monotherapy had an ORR of 43%, a median time to progression of 6.2 months, a duration of response of 8 months, and a median survival of 30 months. Bortezomib monotherapy is less effective in patients who have received more than one line of prior therapy. Bortezomib is also synergistic when used in combination with other drugs, including alkylating agents, anthracyclines, immunomodulatory drugs, and dexamethasone. These combinations generally produce higher ORRs in the range of 50% to 80%, with an increasing duration of response and OS. Bortezomib plus pegylated liposomal doxorubicin was shown to be superior to monotherapy in a large randomized trial with an improved time to progression (9.3 vs. 6.5 months) and OS. Bortezomib also was recently administered as a subcutaneous injection. In a randomized trial comparing subcutaneous with intravenous administration, identical 42% response ratios were observed. The subcutaneous routes, however, had an improved safety profile, each with a reduced incidence of peripheral neuropathy (38% vs. 53% any grade, $p = .044$; 6% vs. 16% grade 3 or worse, $p = .026$).[38]

New Agents

Relapsed Myeloma

Several large phase II and phase III randomized clinical trials have been conducted in patients with relapsed myeloma. These studies have resulted in the approval of six new drugs for the treatment of relapsed myeloma since 2012, including three new drugs (panobinostat, ixazomib, and elotuzumab) for patients with one to three relapses and pomalidomide, carfilzomib, and daratumumab for those with more than three relapses or refractory myeloma (Tables 86.23, 86.24).

Carfilzomib is a selective and irreversible proteasome inhibitor of the chymotrypsin-like activity of the proteasome. It is administered intravenously. In a large, open-label, single-arm phase II study, 266 patients with relapsed myeloma progressing on the last therapy were treated with carfilzomib at 20 mg/m² during cycle 1 and thereafter at 27 mg/m² intravenously twice weekly for three of four weeks. Patients were refractory or intolerant to both bortezomib and lenalidomide. The ORR was 23.7% with a median duration of response of 7.8 months and a median OS of 15.6 months. Common adverse events included fatigue, anemia, and thrombocytopenia. A small proportion of patients (<5%) experienced grade 3 or 4 dyspnea, acute renal failure, and heart failure.

In the ENDEAVOR trial, dose-intense carfilzomib/dexamethasone (Kd) was more efficacious than bortezomib/dexamethasone (VD) with improvement in the ORR (77% vs. 63%) as well as doubling of CR rate (13% vs. 6%) and median PFS (18.7 months vs. 9.4 months). Because the median follow-up time was short (1 year), there was no survival advantage noted. Anemia, dyspnea, and cardiac failure were the most common grade 3/4 adverse events in the Kd group, whereas diarrhea and peripheral neuropathy were more common in the VD arm.

ASPIRE was a large, randomized phase III trial comparing carfilzomib, lenalidomide, and dexamethasone (KRd; 396 patients) with lenalidomide and dexamethasone (Rd; 396 patients) in patients with relapsed myeloma who had one to three prior treatments. PFS was significantly improved in the KRd arm compared with the Rd arm (26.3 months vs. 17.6 months; hazard ratio for progression or death, 0.69; $p = .0001$). The median OS was not reached in either group at the time of the interim analysis, but the 2-year OS survival rates were 73.3% in the KRd arm and 65.0% in the Rd arm (hazard ratio for death, 0.79; $p = .04$). The KRd arm had an ORR of 87.1% compared with 66.7% in the Rd arm ($p < .001$). There was an increased incidence of grade 3/4 adverse events such as hypokalemia, thrombocytopenia, hypertension, and cardiac failure in the KRd arm.

PANORAMA1 was a large, multicenter, international, randomized, placebo-controlled, double-blind phase III trial for patients with relapsed myeloma who had received between one and three regimens.

TABLE 86.23 Phase III Randomized Studies Evaluating Efficacy of Newer Agents

Key Outcomes	Aspire (KRd vs. Rd)	Endeavor (Kd vs. Vd)	Tourmaline-MM1 (IRd vs. Rd)		Eloquent-2 (ERd vs. Rd)	
Number of patients	396 vs. 396	464 vs. 465	360 vs. 362		321 vs. 325	
Median follow-up, mo	32.3	12.5	14.8	23	24.5	33
Median PFS, mo	26.3 vs. 17.6	18.7 vs. 9.4	20.6 vs. 14.7	20 vs. 15.9	19.4 vs. 14.9	—
HR, overall	0.69	0.53	0.74	0.82	0.70	0.73
HR, age ≥65 yr	0.85	Approximately 0.487	Approximately 0.843	—	0.65	—
HR, high-risk cytogenetics	0.70	0.65	0.54	—	0.65 [del(17p)] 0.53 [t(4;14)]	—
1-Yr relative improvement, PFS	Approximately 24%	Approximately 51%	Approximately 12%	—	19%	—
2-Yr relative improvement, PFS	Approximately 18%	—	—	Approximately 16%	52%	—
3-Yr relative improvement, PFS	Approximately 23%	—	—	—	—	44%
Median OS, mo	NE	NE	NE	—	43.7 vs. 39.6	—
HR	0.79	0.79	0.90	—	0.77	—
ORR (%)	87% vs. 67%	77% vs. 63%	78% vs. 72%	—	79% vs. 66%	—

ERd, Elotuzumab, lenalidomide and dexamethasone; HR, hazard ratio; Kd, carfilzomib and dexamethasone; KRd, carfilzomib, lenalidomide and dexamethasone; NE, not evaluable; ORR, overall response rate; OS, overall survival; PFS, progression-free survival; Rd, lenalidomide and dexamethasone.

TABLE 86.24 Phase II Studies Evaluating Novel Agents

Drug	Number of Patients	ORR	DOR (Mo)	PFS (Mo)
Single Agent				
Daratumumab	106	30%	7.6	3.7
Pomalidomide	108	18%	8.3	2.7
Carfilzomib	266	24%	7.8	3.7
Lenalidomide	222	26%	12.6	4.9
Bortezomib	202	27%	12.5	7
Doublets				
Len/Dex (RD)	704	61%	15.8	11.1
Pom/Dex	221	33%	10.7	4.2
Triplets				
Panobinostat + VD	768	60%	13.1	12
Elo + RD	646	80%	21	19.4
Ixazomib + RD	65	80%	20.5	20.6
CRD	792	85%	28.6	26.3

CRD, Lenalidomide-cyclophosphamide-dexamethasone; Dex, dexamethasone; DOR, duration of response; Elo, elotuzumab; Len, lenalidomide; ORR, overall response rate; PFS, progression-free survival; Pom, pomalidomide.

Patients were randomly assigned to receive panobinostat + BD (387 patients) or Placebo + BD (381 patients). The median PFS was 12 months for the panobinostat group and 8 months for the control group. The median follow-up was 6 months, and there was no difference in the OS at the time of publication of the results. There was an increased incidence of grade 3/4 adverse events such as thrombocytopenia, diarrhea, asthenia, or fatigue and peripheral neuropathy in the panobinostat arm.

TOURMALINE-MM1 was a phase III study comparing the oral proteasome inhibitors ixazomib, lenalidomide, and dexamethasone (IRd; 360 patients) with placebo, lenalidomide, and dexamethasone (Rd; 362 patients) in patients with relapsed/refractory myeloma who failed one to three regimens. After a median follow-up of 14.7 months, the IRd group had a PFS of 20.6 months compared with the placebo group, which had a PFS of 14.7 months (hazard ratio for disease progression or death in the ixazomib group, 0.74; $p = .01$).

The ORRs were 78% in the ixazomib group and 72% in the placebo group. The median OS has not been reached in either group after 23 months. Diarrhea, rash, and thrombocytopenia were the more common grade 3/4 adverse reactions associated with the IRd group compared with the placebo group.

Pomalidomide is a third-generation immunomodulatory molecule that is more potent than lenalidomide. In a multicenter, open-label, randomized phase II study, the efficacy and safety of pomalidomide with or without low-dose dexamethasone was studied in 221 patients who had relapsed myeloma after two or more lines of prior therapy and were progressing on the last therapy. The ORR was 33% for patients receiving pomalidomide and low-dose dexamethasone and 18% for patients receiving pomalidomide alone with median response durations of 8.3 and 10.7 months, median PFS rates of 4.2 and 2.7 months, and OS of 16.5 and 13.6 months, respectively. Refractoriness to lenalidomide or resistance to both lenalidomide and bortezomib did not affect the outcomes with pomalidomide and low-dose dexamethasone. Grade 3/4 neutropenia (41%), anemia (22%), and thrombocytopenia (19%), as well as pneumonia (22%), were the predominant adverse events encountered. An international, randomized, open-label phase III trial compared pomalidomide and low-dose dexamethasone with high-dose dexamethasone in patients with refractory myeloma after two lines of chemotherapy containing bortezomib and lenalidomide. A group of 302 patients was randomly assigned to receive pomalidomide and dexamethasone, and another group of 153 received high-dose dexamethasone alone. After a median follow-up of 10 months, the median PFS was 4 months for patients receiving pomalidomide and dexamethasone versus 1.9 months for high-dose dexamethasone alone. The most common grade 3/4 hematologic adverse events in the pomalidomide arm were neutropenia, anemia, and cytopenias. Nonhematologic adverse events (grade 3/4) included pneumonia and fatigue.

Elotuzumab is an immunostimulatory monoclonal antibody targeting signaling lymphocytic activation molecule F7 (SLAMF7). The drug showed activity in combination with lenalidomide and dexamethasone in a phase Ib-II study of patients with relapsed/refractory myeloma. Elotuzumab was further evaluated in an open-label, international, randomized, multicenter phase III trial known as the ELOQUENT-2 trial. The two arms of the trial consisted of elotuzumab, lenalidomide, and dexamethasone (ERd; 321 patients) and lenalidomide and dexamethasone (Rd; 325 patients). The rate of PFS at 1 year (after a median follow-up of 24.5 months) in the ERd group was 68%, as compared with 57% in the Rd group. Moreover, at 2 years, there was a 41% PFS advantage in the ERd group compared with 27% in the Rd group. The median PFS was 19.4 months in the ERd group versus 14.9 months in the Rd group (hazard ratio for progression or death in the elotuzumab group, 0.70; $p < .001$). ORRs varied between the two groups: 79% in the ERd group and 66% in the Rd group. Prespecified interim analysis for OS indicated a strong trend ($p = .0257$) in favor of the ERd arm compared with the Rd arm with early separation sustained over time (43.7 months vs. 39.6 months, respectively; hazard ratio, 0.77). Of the patients in the ERd group, 10% had infusion reactions. Other grade 3/4 adverse events in the ERd arm were lymphocytopenia and fatigue.

Daratumumab is a human anti-CD38 IgGκ monoclonal antibody that has recently been approved for patients who have had more than three relapses or refractory myeloma. Daratumumab binds CD38-expressing malignant plasma cells with high affinity and induces tumor cell death through diverse mechanisms of action, which include complement-dependent cytotoxicity; antibody–dependent, cell-mediated cytotoxicity; antibody-dependent cellular phagocytosis; and induction of apoptosis. Moreover, daratumumab suppresses Tregs and the actor enzyme activity-driven suppression of T cells via the adenosine signaling pathway. The ORR was 29% among 106 patients treated with daratumumab at 16 mg/kg; the median response duration was 7.4 months, PFS was 3.7 months, and OS was 17.5 months. Daratumumab was well tolerated; fatigue and anemia were the most common adverse events.

The POLLUX trial was a phase III study comparing daratumumab, lenalidomide, and dexamethasone (DRd; 286 patients) with lenalidomide and dexamethasone (Rd; 283 patients) in patients with relapsed/refractory myeloma. After a median follow-up of 13.5 months, the estimated median PFS was not reached in the DRd group compared with 18 months in the lenalidomide and dexamethasone group.

Other promising targets, agents, and stages of their clinical development are listed in Table 86.25. The optimal treatment of a relapsed patient requires ensuring that the patient's relapse requires intervention. The approach to therapy is dictated by whether the patient had a prior transplant or is a transplant candidate, and the selection of a possible drug depends on the prior therapy received. Additional selection criteria should consider patient characteristics such as age, risk factors, existing comorbidities such as renal failure, previous toxicities such as neuropathy, and patient convenience. Improving CR rates is a key goal of current trials in relapsed patients as well.

Bisphosphonates

Aminobisphosphonates, pamidronate, and zoledronate have been investigated in patients with myeloma and bone disease and have been shown to reduce skeletal complications and bone pain. Researchers in a number of older randomized studies looked at their efficacy in patients with existing bone lesions and evaluated the development of new skeletal-related events. In this regard, pamidronate 90 mg and zoledronic acid 4 mg are equipotent in reducing bone-related problems in MM; the infusion time for zoledronic acid is 15 minutes as compared with 1 to 2 hours for pamidronate. In a recent large study, MRC IX, investigators evaluated the efficacy of zoledronic acid in a randomized comparison with clodronate. This study included 1960 patients and confirmed the efficacy and superiority of zoledronic acid in preventing new skeletal-related events in patients both with and without existing bone lesions (Table 86.26), and it provided evidence that its continued use beyond 2 years was beneficial[39]; importantly, the study also suggested that zoledronic acid compared with clodronate, a first-generation bisphosphonate, improves OS, providing for the first time some evidence of its antimyeloma activity (Fig. 86.17).[40] A similar survival advantage has also been reported with pamidronate (21 vs. 14 months; $p = .041$) in patients receiving salvage chemotherapy and pamidronate versus chemotherapy alone. Pamidronate

administration alone has also been shown to produce responses or delays in disease progression in occasional patients. Bisphosphonates have multiple actions, including suppression of OC number and function, inhibition of IL-6 production by stromal cells, inhibition of farnesyl and geranyl-geranyl transferase activity, and immune effects via γ/δ T cells.

Two potential side effects of bisphosphonates have limited their very long-term use in the recent past; effects on renal function and development of osteonecrosis of the jaw (ONJ). ONJ is observed in patients with dental infections or procedures following its longer-term use. The frequency of these adverse events has been between 3% and 5%. In one study, 11 (3.8%) of 292 patients with MM developed ONJ. Patients receiving bisphosphonates require a thorough dental checkup before starting therapy and should have frequent dental follow-up with careful and conservative use of dental procedures. With these precautions, the frequency of ONJ has been reduced. Similarly, the measurement of renal function before each bisphosphonate dose and the adjustment of dose based on renal function also make use of bisphosphonates safer. A slower administration of bisphosphonates prevents or protects against the development of renal dysfunction. Most recently, the recommended duration of bisphosphonate has been 2 years, with reduction in frequency after that if patients enjoy a good remission. However, in the light of the recent MRC-IX study, this recommendation will require revision with the possible benefits of long-term use. Additional bone-directed targets and agents are in development that have the ability to further inhibit OC function (denosumab) and also to improve OB activity and with bone anabolic effects (DKK-1 - BHQ-880 and activin A -ACE-011). These agents are currently under clinical investigation in patients with MM.

FUTURE DIRECTIONS

Significant advances have occurred in the understanding of the pathobiology of MM, which have translated to development of novel therapeutics. Predictive in vitro and in vivo models have been developed to study growth and survival characteristics of MM cells in the context of the bone marrow microenvironment, but, more important, to preclinically evaluate efficacy of novel targeted agents. Similarly, there has been an explosion of genomic data covering various genomic correlates including expression profile, CNA, alternate splicing, miRNA, and now whole-genome and RNA sequencing with mutational analysis of expressed genes as well as noncoding regions. Understanding of mutational landscape, molecular drivers of the disease and patterns, and surrogates of genomic evolution are providing newer clues to the disease biology as well as novel therapeutic approaches. Evolving understanding of the epigenomic alterations that affect cell growth, survival, and development of drug resistance is providing clues for novel interventions. For example, there is already an HDAC inhibitor approved for therapy of relapsed myeloma. Moreover, MM cell proliferation is now considered to be dependent on the bromodomain and extraterminal (or "BET") domain family of bromodomain-containing proteins (BRD2, BRD3, and BRD4), which are novel therapeutic targets.

These model systems and improved understanding have led to new drug development, with 10 new agents approved for myeloma in the last 12 years and over 15 other novel agents in phase I or II studies. The genomic information is being integrated to develop more accurate risk stratification models and to develop personalized medicine to optimize response while avoiding toxicities. With these advances and use of combination of agents, there is a significant improvement in the achievement of CR, over 60% to 70% in some studies. This has led to validation of molecular MRD as an important new endpoint in myeloma with its incorporation into all clinical studies as well as exploration as an ultimate endpoint to achieve cure. Finally, because of these advances, the median survival of patients with MM has increased from 3 years to over 8–10 years, and in a number of individuals, it becomes a chronic disease with curative outcome predicted in a proportion of patients in the near future.

TABLE 86.25 Novel Targets in Myeloma, Agents, and Stages of Ongoing Clinical Trials

Target	Agent	Clinical Study Phase	Single Agent (S)/Combination (C)
Cell Surface Targets			
FGF, PDGF	(mAb) TKI258	I	S
CD38	mAb	I	S
CD40	SGN-40 (mAb)	I/II	S, C (lenalidomide)
	HCD122 (mAb)	I	S
CD56	huN901-DM1 (C-mAb)	I	S
CD138	BT062 (mAb-DM4)	I	S
RANKL	AMG162 (mAb)	I/II	S
MUC1	AR20.5 (mAb)	I/II	S
BAFFR	LY2127399 (mAb)	I/II	S
CD52	Alemtuzumab (mAb)	II	S
TRAIL	Apo2L/TRAIL (Apo2 ligand)	I	S
	Mapatumumab	I/II	S
IGF1/R	IGF1R CP-571 (mAb)	I	S
	EM164 (mAb)	I	S
IL6/R	CNTO328 (mAb)	II/III	S, C (bortezomib)
	Altizumab (mAb)	III	S
VEGF/R	Bevacizumab (mAb)	II	S
	SU5416	II	S
	Zactima (ZD6474)	II	S
DKK-1	BHQ-880	I/II	S
Activin A	ACC001	I/II	S
KIR	IPH101	I/II	S
CXCR3	AMD3100	II	C (bortezomib)
Intracytoplasmic and/or Nuclear Targets			
CDK	Alvocidib (NSC649890)	I	S
CDK and GSK3 AT7519M	I/II		S, C (bortezomib)
IKK	RTA402	I	S
Akt	Perofosine	III	C (bortezomib)
HDAC	Panabinostat	III	C (bortezomib)
	Vorinostat	II/III	C (bortezomib)
	Romidopsin	II/III	C (bortezomib)
Farnesyltransferase inhibitor	Tipifarnib (R115777)	II	S, C (bortezomib)
HSP90	KOS953	II	C (bortezomib)
	AUY922	II	C (bortezomib)
	IPI504	I/II	C (bortezomib)
Proteasome	Carfilzomib	II/III	S, C (lenalidomide)
	NPI-0052	I	S
	MLN9708	I	S
Mitochondria	GCS-100	I/II	C
mTOR	CCI-779 II	II	C (bortezomib)
	RAD001	II	C (lenalidomide, bortezomib)
	INK128	II	S
PKC	Enzastaurin	I/II	S, C (bortezomib)
Telomerase	GRN163L	I/II	S, C (bortezomib)

BAFFR, B cell–activating factor receptor; CDK, cyclin-dependent kinase; CXCR3, C-X-C motif chemokine receptor 3; DKK-1, Dickkopf-related protein 1; FGF, Fibroblast growth factor; GSK3, glycogen synthase kinase 3; HDAC, histone deacetylase; HSP90, heat shock protein 90; IGF1/R, insulin-like growth factor 1 receptor; IKK, inhibitor of nuclear factor-κB kinase; mAb, monoclonal antibody; IL6/R, interleukin-6 receptor; KIR, killer cell immunoglobulin-like receptor; mTOR, mammalian target of rapamycin; MUC1, mucin 1; PDGF, platelet-derived growth factor; PKC, protin kinase C; RANKL, receptor activator of nuclear factor-κB ligand; TRAIL, tumor necrosis factor–related apoptosis-inducing ligand; VEGF/R, vascular endothelial growth factor receptor.
Data collected from National Cancer Institute clinical trials website, Multiple Myeloma Research Foundation website, and International Myeloma Foundation website.

TABLE 86.26 Cumulative Annual Incidence of First and Subsequent Skeletal-Related Events for the Intention-to-Treat Populations Randomized to Zoledronic Acid Versus Clodronate

	Skeletal-Related Events		Incidence (95% CI)			
	Clodronic Acid (n = 979)	Zoledronic Acid (n = 981)	Clodronic Acid (n = 979)	Zoledronic Acid (n = 981)	Overall Difference (95% CI) Between Clodronic Acid and Zoledronic Acid[a]	p-Value for Preceding 12 Mo[b]
12 mo	451 (46%)	333 (34%)	0.43 (0.38–0.48)	0.33 (0.28–0.37)	0.11 (0.04–0.18)	0.0002
24 mo	93 (9%)	54 (6%)	0.60 (0.53–0.66)	0.42 (0.36–0.48)	0.18 (0.09–0.26)	0.0024
36 mo	28 (3%)	16 (2%)	0.69 (0.61–0.78)	0.47 (0.40–0.53)	0.23 (0.12–0.33)	0.0089

Data are number (%), unless otherwise indicated.
[a]$p < .0001$.
[b]Unadjusted p-value for the comparison of incidence of skeletal-related events in zoledronic acid group versus clodronic acid group per 12 months (e.g., 24-month p-value is for incidence between 12 months and 24 months).
CI, Confidence interval.

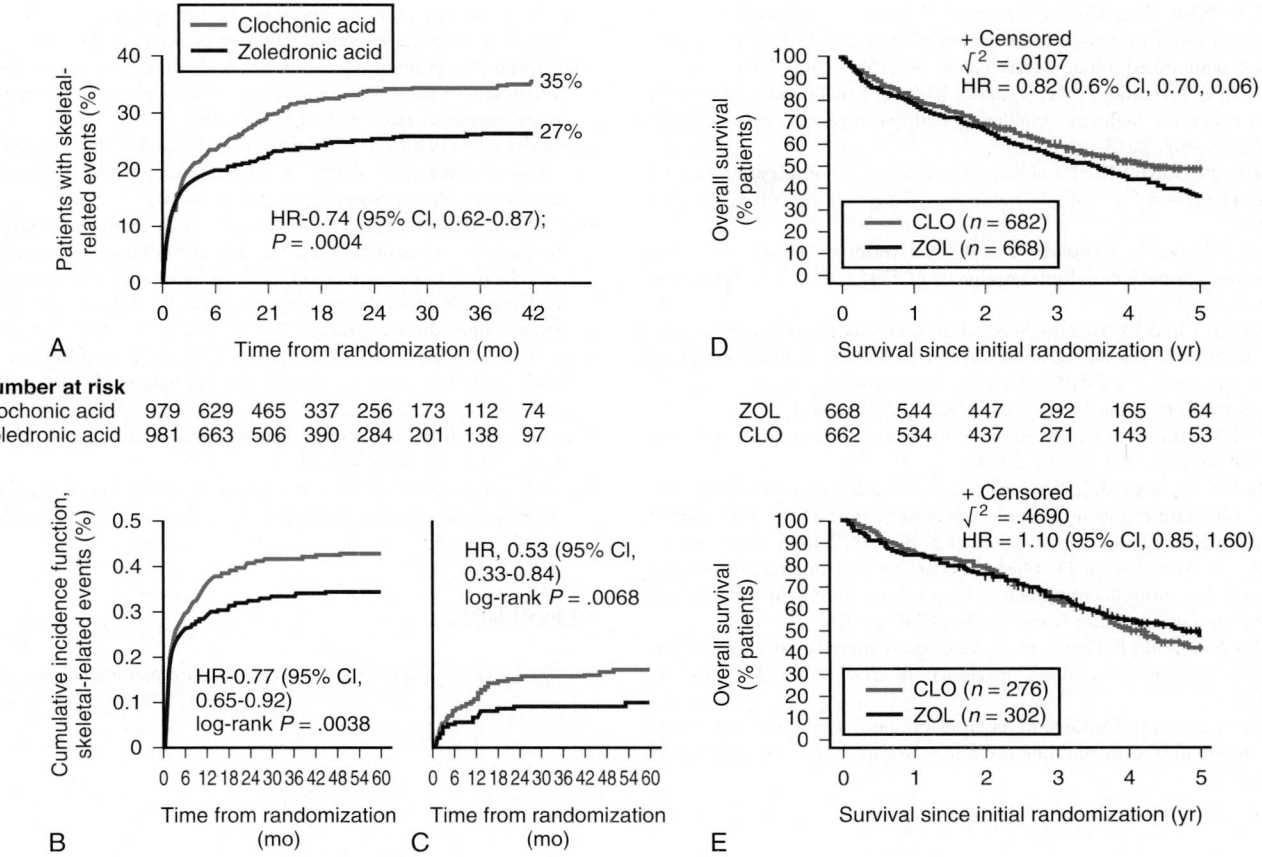

Fig. 86.17 Time to first skeletal-related event overall (A), in patients with bone lesions at baseline (B), and in patients without bone lesions at baseline (C). Cox proportional hazards *p*-value. Kaplan-Meier analyses of OS with zoledronic acid (ZOL) versus Clodronate (CLO) in patients with or without bone disease or other SRE at baseline. (D) Patients with bone disease or other SRE at baseline. (E) Patients without bone disease or other SRE at baseline. The benefit appears to be predominantly in those with prior SREs. *CI*, Confidence interval; *CLO*, clodronate; *HR*, hazard ratio; *OS*, overall survival; *SRE*, skeletal-related event; *ZOL*, zoledronic acid. *(Adapted from Morgan GJ, Child JA, Gregory WM, et al: Effects of zoledronic acid versus clodronic acid on skeletal morbidity in patients with newly diagnosed multiple myeloma (MRC Myeloma IX): Secondary outcomes from a randomised controlled trial.* Lancet Oncol *12:743, 2011; Morgan GJ, Davies FE, Gregory WM, et al: Effect of induction and maintenance plus long-term bisphosphonates on bone disease in patients with multiple myeloma: the Medical Research Council Myeloma IX trial.* Blood *119:5374, 2012.)*

SUGGESTED READINGS

Attal M, Lauwers-Cances V, Marit G, et al: Lenalidomide maintenance after stem-cell transplantation for multiple myeloma. *N Engl J Med* 366:1782–1791, 2012.

Avet-Loiseau H, Attal M, Campion L, et al: Long-term analysis of the IFM 99 trials for myeloma: cytogenetic abnormalities [t(4;14), del(17p), 1q gains] play a major role in defining long-term survival. *J Clin Oncol* 30:2012, 1949.

Avet-Loiseau H, Li C, Magrangeas F, et al: Prognostic significance of copy-number alterations in multiple myeloma. *J Clin Oncol* 27:4585, 2009.

Benboubker L, Dimopoulos MA, Dispenzieri A, et al: Lenalidomide and dexamethasone in transplant-ineligible patients with myeloma. *N Engl J Med* 371:906–917, 2014.

Bolli N, Avet-Loiseau H, Wedge DC, et al: Heterogeneity of genomic evolution and mutational profiles in multiple myeloma. *Nat Commun* 5:2997, 2014.

Broyl A, Hose D, Lokhorst H, et al: Gene expression profiling for molecular classification of multiple myeloma in newly diagnosed patients. *Blood* 116:2543–2553, 2010.

Bruno B, Rotta M, Patriarca F, et al: A comparison of allografting with autografting for newly diagnosed myeloma. *N Engl J Med* 356:1110, 2007.

Dimopoulos MA, Moreau P, Palumbo A, et al: Carfilzomib and dexamethasone versus bortezomib and dexamethasone for patients with relapsed or refractory multiple myeloma (ENDEAVOR): a randomised, phase 3, open-label, multicentre study. *Lancet Oncol* 17:27–38, 2016.

Dimopoulos M, Kyle R, Fermand JP, et al: Consensus recommendations for standard investigative workup: report of the International Myeloma Workshop Consensus Panel 3. *Blood* 117:4701–4705, 2011.

Hutchison CA, Batuman V, Behrens J, et al: The pathogenesis and diagnosis of acute kidney injury in multiple myeloma. *Nat Rev Nephrol* 8:43–51, 2012.

Koreth J, Cutler CS, Djulbegovic B, et al: High-dose therapy with single autologous transplantation versus chemotherapy for newly diagnosed multiple myeloma: a systematic review and meta-analysis of randomized controlled trials. *Biol Blood Marrow Transplant* 13:183, 2007.

Krönke J, Udeshi ND, Narla A, et al: Lenalidomide causes selective degradation of IKZF1 and IKZF3 in multiple myeloma cells. *Science* 343:301–305, 2014.

Landgren O, Kyle RA, Pfeiffer RM, et al: Monoclonal gammopathy of undetermined significance (MGUS) consistently precedes multiple myeloma: a prospective study. *Blood* 113:5412–5417, 2009.

Lokhorst HM, Plesner T, Laubach JP, et al: Targeting CD38 with daratumumab monotherapy in multiple myeloma. *N Engl J Med* 373:1207–1219, 2015.

Lonial S, Dimopoulos M, Palumbo A, et al: Elotuzumab therapy for relapsed or refractory multiple myeloma. *N Engl J Med* 373:621–631, 2015.

Lonial S, Weiss BM, Usmani SZ, et al: Daratumumab monotherapy in patients with treatment-refractory multiple myeloma (SIRIUS): an open-label, randomised, phase 2 trial. *Lancet* 387:1551–1560, 2016.

Mateos MV, Hernandez MT, Giraldo P, et al: Lenalidomide plus dexamethasone for high-risk smoldering multiple myeloma. *N Engl J Med* 369:438–447, 2013.

McCarthy PL, Owzar K, Hofmeister CC, et al: Lenalidomide after stem-cell transplantation for multiple myeloma. *N Engl J Med* 366:1770–1781, 2012.

Moreau P, Masszi T, Grzasko N, et al: Oral ixazomib, lenalidomide, and dexamethasone for multiple myeloma. *N Engl J Med* 374:1621–1634, 2016.

Morgan GJ, Child JA, Gregory WM, et al: Effects of zoledronic acid versus clodronic acid on skeletal morbidity in patients with newly diagnosed multiple myeloma (MRC Myeloma IX): secondary outcomes from a randomised controlled trial. *Lancet Oncol* 12:743, 2011.

Munshi NC, Anderson KC: Minimal residual disease in multiple myeloma. *J Clin Oncol* 31:2523–2526, 2013.

Munshi NC, Anderson KC, Bergsagel PL, et al: Consensus recommendations for risk stratification in multiple myeloma: report of the International Myeloma Workshop Consensus Panel 2. *Blood* 117:4696–4700, 2011.

Palumbo A, Avet-Loiseau H, Oliva S, et al: Revised international staging system for multiple myeloma: a report from International Myeloma Working Group. *J Clin Oncol* 33:2863–2869, 2015.

Palumbo A, Cavallo F, Gay F, et al: Autologous transplantation and maintenance therapy in multiple myeloma. *N Engl J Med* 371:895–905, 2014.

Palumbo A, Hajek R, Delforge M, et al: Continuous lenalidomide treatment for newly diagnosed multiple myeloma. *N Engl J Med* 366:1759–1769, 2012.

Raje N, Roodman GD: Advances in the biology and treatment of bone disease in multiple myeloma. *Clin Cancer Res* 17:1278, 2011.

Richardson PG, Hungria VT, Yoon SS, et al: Panobinostat plus bortezomib and dexamethasone in previously treated multiple myeloma: outcomes by prior treatment. *Blood* 127:713–721, 2016.

Richardson PG, Weller E, Lonial S, et al: Lenalidomide, bortezomib, and dexamethasone combination therapy in patients with newly diagnosed multiple myeloma. *Blood* 116:679–686, 2010.

Roussel M, Lauwers-Cances V, Robillard N, et al: Front-line transplantation program with lenalidomide, bortezomib, and dexamethasone combination as induction and consolidation followed by lenalidomide maintenance in patients with multiple myeloma: a phase II study by the Intergroupe Francophone du Myélome. *J Clin Oncol* 32:2712–2717, 2014.

Stewart AK, Rajkumar SV, Dimopoulos MA, et al: Carfilzomib, lenalidomide, and dexamethasone for relapsed multiple myeloma. *N Engl J Med* 372:142–152, 2015.

Szalat R, Munshi NC: Genomic heterogeneity in multiple myeloma. *Curr Opin Genet Dev* 30:56–65, 2015.

Szalat R, Munshi NC: Next-generation sequencing informing therapeutic decisions and personalized approaches. *Am Soc Clin Oncol Educ Book* 35:e442, 2016.

REFERENCES

For the complete list of references, log on to www.expertconsult.com.

WALDENSTRÖM MACROGLOBULINEMIA/ LYMPHOPLASMACYTIC LYMPHOMA

Steven P. Treon, Jorge J. Castillo, Zachary R. Hunter, and Giampaolo Merlini

Waldenström macroglobulinemia (WM) is a lymphoid neoplasm resulting from the accumulation, predominantly in the marrow, of a clonal population of lymphocytes, lymphoplasmacytic cells, and plasma cells, which secrete a monoclonal immunoglobulin (Ig) M.[1] WM corresponds to lymphoplasmacytic lymphoma (LPL) as defined in the Revised European-American Lymphoma (REAL) and World Health Organization classification systems.[2,3] Most cases of LPL are WM; less than 5% of cases are IgA-secreting, IgG-secreting, or nonsecreting LPL.

In 1944, Jan Waldenström, a Swedish physician-scientist, reported in *Acta Medica Scandinavica* three cases of a disease he presciently thought was related to myeloma but for the absence of bone involvement and the scarcity of plasma cells in the infiltrate of small lymphocytes. He noted the increase in plasma protein concentration, marked increased serum viscosity, exaggerated bleeding and retinal hemorrhages, and virtually every other feature of the disorder in his case descriptions. In collaboration with a colleague, he showed, using ultracentrifugation and electrophoresis, that the abundant abnormal protein had a molecular weight of approximately 1 million and was not an aggregate of smaller proteins. The disease, which he described with such thoroughness, was later named in his honor.

EPIDEMIOLOGY

The age-adjusted incidence rate of WM in the United States is 3.4 per 1 million among males and 1.7 per 1 million among females. It increases in incidence geometrically with age.[4,5] The incidence rate is higher among Americans of European descent. Americans of African descent represent approximately 5% of all patients.

Genetic factors play a role in the pathogenesis of WM. Approximately 20% of patients with WM are of Ashkenazi Jewish ethnic background.[6] Familial disease has been reported commonly, including multigenerational clustering of WM and other B-cell lymphoproliferative diseases.[7–10] Approximately 20% of 257 sequential patients with WM presenting to a tertiary referral center had a first-degree relative with either WM or another B-cell disorder.[9] Familial clustering of WM with other immunologic disorders, including hypogammaglobulinemia and hypergammaglobulinemia (particularly polyclonal IgM), autoantibody production (particularly to the thyroid), and manifestation of hyperactive B cells, has also been reported in relatives without WM.[9,10] Increased expression of the *BCL2* gene with enhanced survival has been observed in B cells from familial patients and their family members.[10]

The role of environmental factors is uncertain; however, but chronic antigenic stimulation from infections and certain drug or chemical exposures have been considered but have not reached a level of scientific certainty. Hepatitis C virus (HCV) infection was implicated in WM causality in some series, but no association was found in a study of 100 consecutive patients with WM in whom serologic and molecular diagnostic studies for HCV infection were performed.[11–13]

PATHOGENESIS

Nature of the WM Clone

Examination of the B-cell clone(s) found in the bone marrow (BM) of patients with WM reveals a range of differentiation, from small lymphocytes with large focal deposits of surface immunoglobulins, to lymphoplasmacytic cells, to mature plasma cells that contain intracytoplasmic IgM (Fig. 87.1).[14] Circulating clonal B cells are often detectable in patients with WM, though lymphocytosis is uncommon.[15,16] WM cells express the monoclonal IgM, and some clonal cells also express surface IgD.[17] The characteristic immunophenotypic profile of WM lymphoplasmacytic cells includes the expression of the pan–B-cell markers CD19, CD20 (including FMC7), CD22, and CD79.[17,18] Expression of CD5, CD10, and CD23 can be present in 10% to 20% of cases, and their presence does not exclude the diagnosis of WM.[19] In addition, multiparameter flow cytometric analysis has also identified CD25 and CD27 as being characteristic of the WM clone, and that a CD22^{dim}/CD25$^+$/CD27$^+$/IgM$^+$ population can be observed among clonal B lymphocytes in patients with IgM monoclonal gammopathy of undetermined significance (MGUS) who ultimately progress to WM.[20]

Somatic mutations in immunoglobulin genes are present with increased frequency of nonsynonymous versus silent mutations in complementarity-determining regions, along with somatic hypermutation, thereby supporting a postgerminal center derivation for the WM B-cell clone in most patients.[21,22] A strong preferential use of VH3/JH4 gene families without intraclonal variation, and without evidence for any isotype-switched transcripts, has also been shown.[23,24] Taken together, these data support an IgM$^+$ and/or IgM$^+$IgD$^+$ memory B-cell origin for most cases of WM.

In contrast to myeloma plasma cells, no recurrent translocations have been described in WM, which can help to distinguish IgM myeloma cases that often exhibit t11;14 translocations from WM.[25,26] Despite the absence of IgH translocations, recurrent chromosomal abnormalities are present in WM cells. These include deletions in chromosome 6q21–23 in 40% to 60% of patients with WM, with concordant gains in 6p in 41% of patients with 6q deletion.[27–30] In a series of 174 untreated patients with WM, 6q deletions, followed by trisomy 18, 13q deletions, 17p deletions, trisomy 4, and 11q deletions, were observed.[30] Deletion of 6q and trisomy 4 were associated with an adverse prognosis in this series. Because 6q deletions represent the most recurrent cytogenetic finding in WM cases, there has been great interest in identifying the region of minimal deletion and possible target genes within this region. Two putative gene candidates within this region include *TNFAIP3*, a negative regulator of nuclear factor-κB signaling (NFκB), and *PRDM1*, a master regulator of B-cell differentiation.[29,31] The removal of an NFκB-negative regulator is of particular interest because the phosphorylation and translocation of NFκB into the nucleus is a crucial event for WM cell survival.[32] The success of proteasome inhibitor therapy in WM has been postulated to occur because the degradation of negative regulators of NFκB, such as inhibitor of κ B (IκB), is blocked.[33,34]

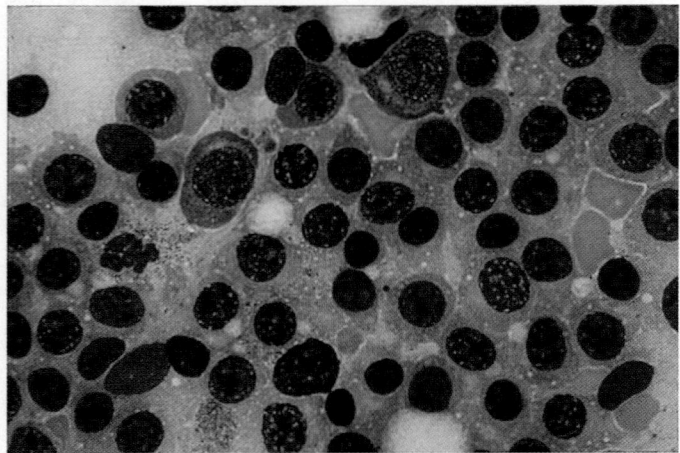

Fig. 87.1 MARROW FILM FROM A PATIENT WITH WALDEN-STRÖM MACROGLOBULINEMIA. Note infiltrate of mature lymphocytes, lymphoplasmacytic cells, and plasma cells. (*Used with permission from Marvin J. Stone, MD.*)

MUTATION IN MYD88

A highly recurrent somatic mutation *(MYD88^{L265P})* was first identified in patients with WM by whole genome sequencing (WGS) and confirmed by multiple studies through Sanger sequencing and/or allele-specific polymerase chain reaction (PCR) assays.[35–40] *MYD88^{L265P}* is expressed in 90% to 95% of WM cases when more sensitive allele-specific PCR is employed using both CD19-sorted and unsorted BM cells.[36–40] By comparison, MYD88^{L265P} was absent in myeloma samples, including IgM myeloma, and was expressed in a small subset (6% to 10%) of patients with marginal zone lymphoma, who surprisingly have WM-related features.[36–38,41] By PCR assays, 50% to 80% of patients with IgM MGUS also express *MYD88^{L265P}*, and expression of this mutation was associated with increased risk for malignant progression.[36–33,42] The presence of *MYD88^{L265P}* in patients with IgM MGUS suggests a role for this mutation as an early oncogenic driver, and other mutations and/or copy number alterations leading to abnormal gene expression are likely to promote disease progression.[29]

The impact of *MYD88^{L265P}* to growth and survival signaling in WM cells has been addressed in several studies (Fig. 87.2). Knockdown of *MYD88* decreased survival of *MYD88^{L265P}*-expressing WM cells, whereas survival was enhanced by knock-in of *MYD88^{L265P}* versus wild-type (WT) *MYD88*.[43] The discovery of a mutation in MYD88

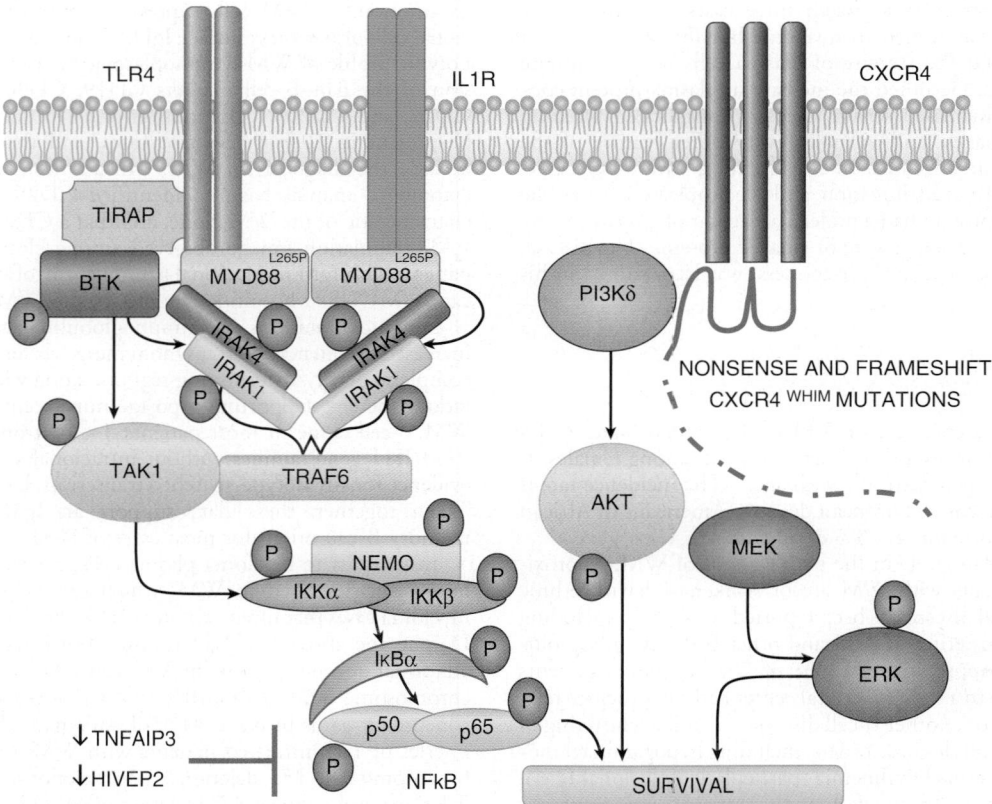

Fig. 87.2 *MYD88^{L265P}* AND *CXCR4^{WHIM}* MUTATIONS ARE HIGHLY PREVALENT IN PATIENTS WITH WALDENSTRÖM MACROGLOBULINEMIA AND TRIGGER TRANSCRIPTIONAL FACTORS THAT INCLUDE NFκB, AKT, AND ERK THAT SUPPORT THE GROWTH AND SURVIVAL OF LYMPHOPLASMACYTIC CELLS. BTK, Bruton's tyrosine kinase; CXCR4, C-X-C chemokine receptor type 4; ERK, Extracellular signal-regulated kinase; HIVEP2, human immunodeficiency virus type I enhancer binding protein 2; IKBα, nuclear factor of κ light polypeptide gene enhancer in B cells inhibitor α; IKK, inhibitor of nuclear factor-κB kinase; IL1R, interleukin-1 receptor; IRAK, interleukin receptor-associated kinase; MEK, mitogen-activated protein kinase kinase; NEMO, nuclear factor-κB essential modulator; NFκB, nuclear factor-κB; PI3Kδ, phosphoinositide 3-kinase δ; TAK1, transforming growth factor β-activated kinase 1; TIRAP, Toll-interleukin 1 receptor domain-containing adaptor protein; TLR4, Toll-like receptor 4; TNFAIP3, tumor necrosis factor α-induced protein 3; TRAF6, tumor necrosis factor α receptor-associated factor 6; WHIM, warts, hypogammaglobulinemia, infections, and myelokathexis syndrome.

is of significance, given its role as an adaptor molecule in Toll-like receptor (TLR) and interleukin-1 receptor (IL-1R) signaling.[44] All TLRs except for TLR3 use MYD88 to facilitate their signaling. Following TLR or IL-1R stimulation, MYD88 is recruited to the activated receptor complex as a homodimer, which then complexes with interleukin receptor-associated kinase 4 (IRAK4) and activates IRAK1 and IRAK2.[45–47] Tumor necrosis factor receptor-associated factor 6 is then activated by IRAK1, leading to NFκB activation via IκBα phosphorylation.[48] Use of inhibitors of the MYD88 pathway led to decreased IRAK1 and IκBα phosphorylation, as well as to survival of $MYD88^{L265P}$-expressing WM cells. These observations are of particular relevance to WM because NFκB signaling is important for WM growth and survival.[49] Bruton's tyrosine kinase (BTK) is also activated by $MYD88^{L265P}$.[43] Activated BTK coimmunoprecipitates with MYD88, which could be abrogated by use of a BTK inhibitor, and overexpression of $MYD88^{L265P}$ but not WT $MYD88$ triggers BTK activation. Knockdown of $MYD88$ by lentiviral transfection or use of a MYD88 homodimerization inhibitor also abrogated BTK activation in $MYD88^{L265P}$-mutated WM cells.

CXCR4 WHIM MUTATIONS

The second most common somatic mutation after $MYD88^{L265P}$ revealed by WGS was found in the C-terminus of the C-X-C chemokine receptor type 4 (CXCR4) receptor. These mutations are present in 30% to 35% of patients with WM, and they impact serine phosphorylation sites that regulate CXCR4 signaling by its only known ligand, SDF-1α (CXCL12).[29,50–52] The location of somatic mutations found in the C-terminus of $CXCR4$ in WM are similar to those observed in the germline of patients with WHIM (warts, hypogammaglobulinemia, infections, and myelokathexis) syndrome, a congenital immunodeficiency disorder characterized by chronic noncyclic neutropenia.[53] Patients with WHIM syndrome exhibit impaired CXCR4 receptor internalization following SDF-1α stimulation, which results in persistent CXCR4 activation and myelokathexis.[54]

In patients with WM, two classes of $CXCR4$ mutations occur in the C-terminus. These include nonsense $(CXCR4^{WHIM/NS})$ mutations that truncate the distal 15– to 20–amino acid region and frameshift $(CXCR4^{WHIM/FS})$ mutations that comprise a region of up to 40 amino acids in the C-terminal domain.[29,50] Nonsense and frameshift mutations are almost equally divided among patients with WM with CXCR4 somatic mutations, and over 30 different types of $CXCR4^{WHIM}$ mutations have been identified in patients with WM.[29,50] Preclinical studies with WM cells engineered to express nonsense and frameshift $CXCR4^{WHIM}$-mutated receptors have shown enhanced and sustained AKT and extracellular signal-regulated kinase signaling following SDF-1α relative to $CXCR4^{WT}$ (Fig. 87.2), as well as increased cell migration, adhesion, growth, and survival, and also drug resistance of WM cells.[51,55,56]

Other Somatic Events

Many copy number alterations have been revealed in patients with WM that impact growth and survival pathways. Frequent loss of $HIVEP2$ (80%) and $TNAIP3$ (50%) genes that are negative regulators of NFκB expression (Fig. 87.2), as well as LYN (70%) and $IBTK$ (40%) that modulate B-cell receptor signaling have been revealed by WGS.[29] WGS has also revealed common defects in chromatin remodeling, with somatic mutations in ARID1A present in 17% and loss of $ARID1B$ in 70% of patients with WM. Both $ARID1A$ and $ARID1B$ are members of the SWI/SNF family of proteins, and they are thought to exert their effects via p53 and cyclin-dependent kinase inhibitor 1A regulation. TP53 is mutated in 7% of sequenced WM genomes, whereas $PRDM2$ and $TOP1$ that participate in TP53-related signaling are deleted in 80% and 60% of patients with WM, respectively.[29] Taken together, somatic events that contribute to impaired DNA damage response are also common in WM.

IMPACT OF WM GENOMICS ON CLINICAL PRESENTATION

The importance of $MYD88$ and $CXCR4$ mutations in the clinical presentation of patients with WM was recently reported. Significantly higher BM involvement, serum IgM levels, and symptomatic disease requiring therapy, including hyperviscosity syndrome, were observed in those patients with $MYD88^{L265P}CXCR4^{WHIM/NS}$ mutations.[50] Patients with $MYD88^{L265P}CXCR4^{WHIM/FS}$ or $MYD88^{L265P}CXCR4^{WT}$ had intermediate BM and serum IgM levels; those with $MYD-88^{WT}CXCR4^{WT}$ showed the lowest BM disease burden. Fewer patients with $MYD88^{L265P}$ and $CXCR4^{WHIM/FS\ or\ NS}$ than with $MYD88^{L265P}CX-CR4^{WT}$ presented with adenopathy, further delineating differences in disease tropism based on $CXCR4$ status. Despite the more aggressive presentation associated with $CXCR4^{WHIM/NS}$ genotype, risk of death was not impacted by $CXCR4$ mutation status. Risk of death was found to be 10-fold higher in patients with the $MYD88^{WT}$ versus the $MYD88^{L265P}$ genotype.[50]

MARROW MICROENVIRONMENT

In patients with WM, increased numbers of mast cells are found in the BM, where they are usually admixed with tumor cell aggregates (Fig. 87.3).[14,18,57] The role of mast cells in WM has been investigated in one study in which coculture of primary autologous or mast cell lines with WM lymphoplasmacytic cells resulted in dose-dependent WM cell proliferation and/or tumor colony formation through CD40 ligand (CD40L) signaling.[57] WM cells release soluble CD27 (sCD27), which may be triggered by cleavage of membrane bound CD27 by matrix metalloproteinase 8.[58] sCD27 levels are elevated in the serum of patients with WM and follow disease burden in mice engrafted with WM cells, as well as in patients with WM.[59] sCD27 triggers the upregulation of CD40L as well as a proliferation-inducing ligand on mast cells derived from patients with WM, as well as mast cell lines through its receptor CD70. Modeling in mice treated with a CD70-blocking antibody shows inhibition of tumor cell growth,

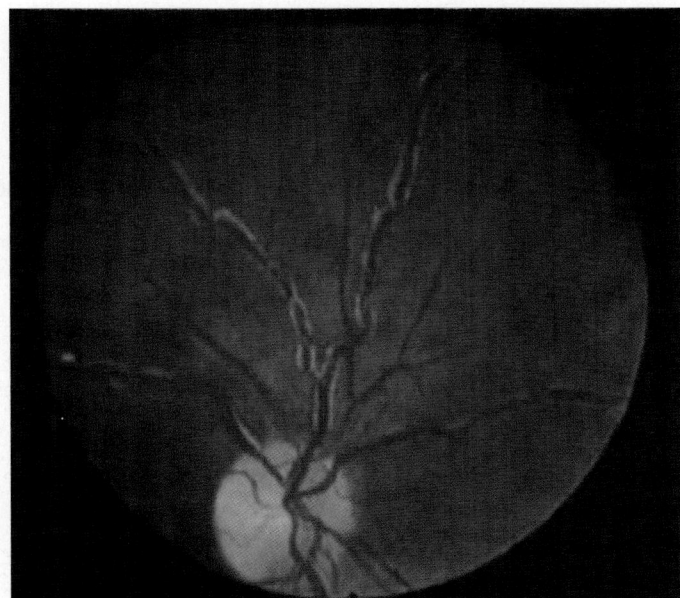

Fig. 87.3 FUNDUSCOPIC EXAMINATION OF A PATIENT WITH WALDENSTRÖM MACROGLOBULINEMIA WITH HYPERVISCOS-ITY-RELATED CHANGES, INCLUDING DILATED RETINAL VESSELS, HEMORRHAGES, AND "VENOUS SAUSAGING." The white material at the edge of the veins may be cryoglobulin. (*Used with permission from Marvin J. Stone, MD.*)

suggesting that WM cells require a microenvironmental support system for their growth and survival.[60] High levels of CXCR4 and very late antigen-4 (VLA-4) are expressed by WM cells.[59] In blocking experiment studies, CXCR4 was shown to support migration of WM cells, whereas VLA-4 contributed to adhesion of WM cells to BM stromal cells.[59]

CLINICAL FEATURES

Table 87.1 provides the clinical and laboratory features at the time of diagnosis of patients with WM in one large institutional study.[16]

TABLE 87.1	Clinical and Laboratory Findings for 356 Consecutive Newly Diagnosed Patients With Waldenström Macroglobulinemia		
	Median	Range	Normal Reference Range
Age (years)	58	32–91	NA
Sex (male/female)	215/141		NA
Marrow involvement (% of area on slide)	30	5–95	NA
Adenopathy (% of patients)	15		NA
Splenomegaly (% of patients)	10		NA
IgM (mg/dL)	2620	270–12,400	40–230
IgG (mg/dL)	674	80–2770	700–1600
IgA (mg/dL)	58	6–438	70–400
Serum viscosity (cp)	2.0	1.1–7.2	1.4–1.9
Hematocrit (%)	35	17–45	35–44
Platelet count (×10⁹/L)	275	42–675	155–410
White cell count (×10⁹/L)	6.4	1.7–22	3.8–9.2
β₂-M (mg/dL)	2.5	0.9–13.7	0–2.7
LDH (U/mL)	313	61–1701	313–618

β_2M, β_2-Microglobulin; cp, centipoise; Ig, immunoglobulin; LDH, lactate dehydrogenase; NA, not applicable.
Data from patients seen at the Dana-Farber Cancer Institute, Boston, MA.

Unlike most indolent lymphomas, splenomegaly and lymphadenopathy are uncommon (≤15%). Purpura is frequently associated with cryoglobulinemia and in rare circumstances with light-chain (AL) amyloidosis. Hemorrhagic and neuropathic manifestations are multifactorial (see "IgM-Related Neuropathy" section below). The morbidity associated with WM is caused by the co-occurrence of two main components: tissue infiltration by neoplastic cells and, importantly, the physicochemical and immunologic properties of the monoclonal IgM. As shown in Table 87.2, the monoclonal IgM can produce clinical manifestations through several different mechanisms related to its physicochemical properties, nonspecific interactions with other proteins, antibody activity, and tendency to deposit in tissues.[61–63]

MORBIDITY MEDIATED BY THE EFFECTS OF IGM

Hyperviscosity Syndrome

The increased plasma IgM levels lead to increased blood hyperviscosity and its complications.[64] The mechanisms behind the marked increase in the resistance to blood flow and the resulting impaired transit through the microcirculatory system are complex.[64–67] The main determinants are (1) a high concentration of monoclonal IgMs, which may form aggregates and may bind water through their carbohydrate component; and (2) the interaction of IgMs with blood cells. Monoclonal IgM increases red cell aggregation (rouleau formation) and red cell internal viscosity while reducing red cell deformability. The presence of cryoglobulins contributes to increasing blood viscosity, as well as to the tendency to induce erythrocyte aggregation. Serum viscosity is proportional to the IgM concentration up to 30 g/L, then increases sharply at higher levels. Increased plasma viscosity may also contribute to inappropriately low erythropoietin production, which is the major reason for anemia in these patients.[67] Renal synthesis of erythropoietin is inversely correlated with plasma viscosity. Clinical manifestations are related to circulatory disturbances that can best be appreciated by ophthalmoscopy, which shows distended and tortuous retinal veins, hemorrhages, and papilledema (Fig. 87.4).[68] Symptoms usually occur when the monoclonal IgM concentration exceeds 50 g/L or when serum viscosity is greater than 4.0 centipoises (cp), but there is individual variability, with some patients showing no evidence of hyperviscosity even at 10 cp.[64] The most common symptoms are oronasal mucosal bleeding, visual disturbances because of retinal bleeding, and dizziness that

TABLE 87.2	Physicochemical and Immunologic Properties of the Monoclonal Immunoglobulin M Protein in Waldenström Macroglobulinemia	
Properties of IgM Monoclonal Protein	Diagnostic Condition	Clinical Manifestations
Pentameric structure	Hyperviscosity	Headaches, blurred vision, epistaxis, retinal hemorrhages, leg cramps, impaired mentation, intracranial hemorrhage
Precipitation on cooling	Cryoglobulinemia (type I)	Raynaud phenomenon, acrocyanosis, ulcers, purpura, cold urticaria
Autoantibody activity to myelin-associated glycoprotein, ganglioside M₁, sulfatide moieties on peripheral nerve sheaths	Peripheral neuropathies	Sensorimotor neuropathies, painful neuropathies, ataxic gait, bilateral foot drop
Autoantibody activity to IgG	Cryoglobulinemia (type II)	Purpura, arthralgia, renal failure, sensorimotor neuropathies
Autoantibody activity to red blood cell antigens	Cold agglutinins	Hemolytic anemia, Raynaud phenomenon, acrocyanosis, livedo reticularis
Tissue deposition as amorphous aggregates	Organ dysfunction	Skin: bullous skin disease, papules, Schnitzler syndrome Gastrointestinal: diarrhea, malabsorption, bleeding Kidney: proteinuria, renal failure (light-chain component)
Tissue deposition as amyloid fibrils (light-chain component most commonly)	Organ dysfunction	Fatigue, weight loss, edema, hepatomegaly, macroglossia, organ dysfunction of involved organs (heart, kidney, liver, peripheral sensory and autonomic nerves)

IgM, Immunoglobulin M.

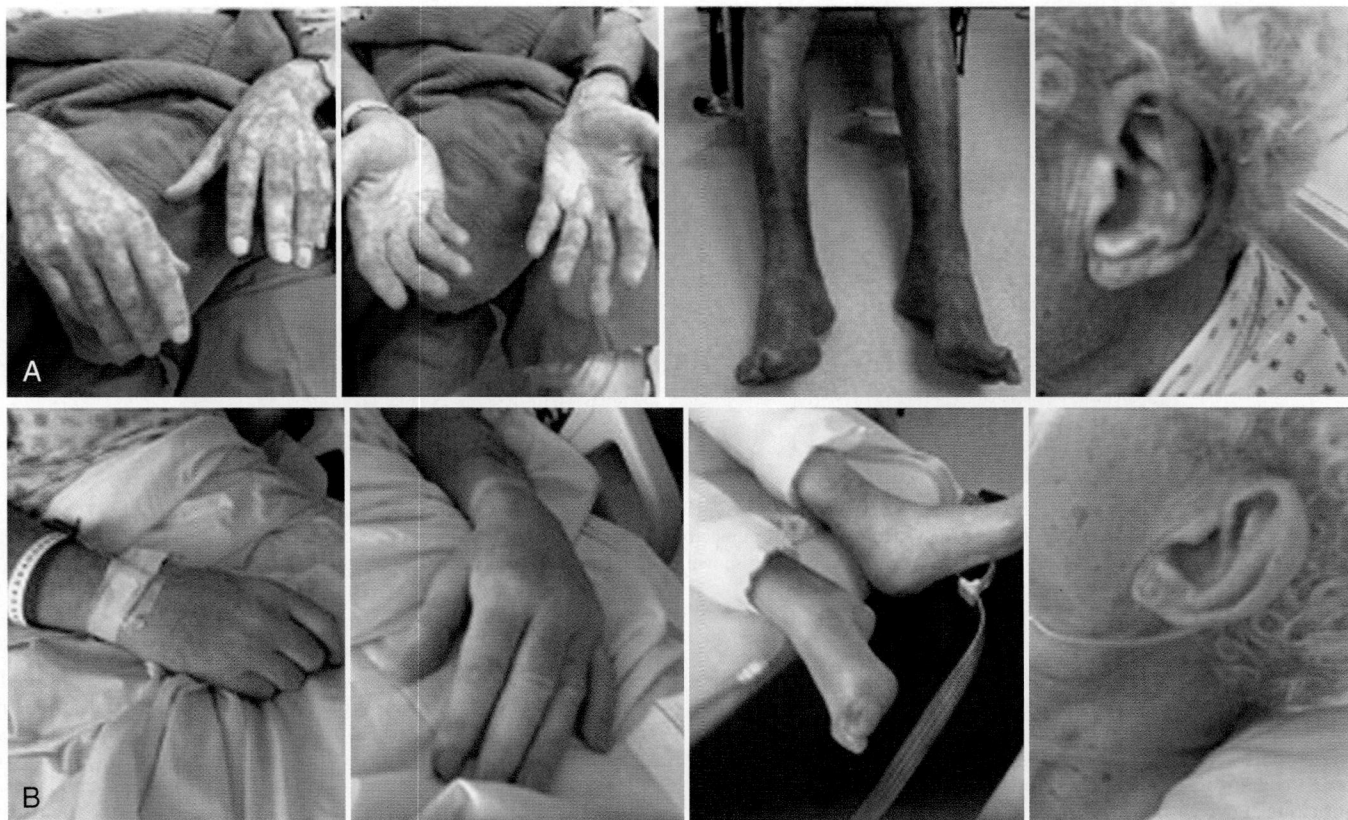

Fig. 87.4 CRYOGLOBULINEMIA MANIFESTING WITH SEVERE ACROCYANOSIS IN A PATIENT WITH WALDENSTRÖM MACROGLOBULINEMIA (A) BEFORE AND (B) FOLLOWING WARMING AND PLASMAPHERESIS.

rarely may lead to stupor or coma. Heart failure can be aggravated, particularly in the elderly, owing to increased blood viscosity, expanded plasma volume, and anemia. Inappropriate red cell transfusions can exacerbate hyperviscosity and may precipitate cardiac failure.

Cryoglobulinemia

The monoclonal IgM can behave as a type I cryoglobulin in up to 20% of patients, and it leads to no symptoms in most cases.[16,64,69,70] Cryoprecipitation is dependent mainly on the concentration of monoclonal IgM; for this reason, plasmapheresis or plasma exchange is commonly effective in this condition. Symptoms result from impaired blood flow in small vessels and include Raynaud phenomenon; acrocyanosis; necrosis of the regions most exposed to cold, such as the tips of the nose, ears, fingers, and toes (Fig. 87.5); malleolar ulcers; purpura; and cold urticaria. Renal manifestations are infrequent. Mixed cryoglobulins (type II) consisting of IgM-IgG complexes may be associated with HCV infection.[70]

Autoantibody Activity. Monoclonal IgM may exert its pathogenic effects through specific recognition of autologous antigens, the most notable being nerve constituents, immunoglobulin determinants, and red blood cell antigens.

IgM-Related Neuropathy. IgM-related peripheral neuropathy is common in patients with WM, with estimated prevalence rates of 5% to 40%.[71–73] Approximately 8% of idiopathic neuropathies are associated with a monoclonal gammopathy, with a preponderance of IgM (60%), followed by IgG (30%) and IgA (10%).[74,75] The nerve damage is mediated by diverse pathogenetic mechanisms: (1) IgM antibody activity toward nerve constituents causing demyelinating polyneuropathies; (2) endoneurial granulofibrillar deposits of IgM without antibody activity, associated with axonal polyneuropathy; (3) occasionally by tubular deposits in the endoneurium associated with IgM cryoglobulin; and, rarely, (4) amyloid deposits or neoplastic cell infiltration of nerve structures.[73,76]

Half of the patients with IgM neuropathy have a distinctive clinical syndrome that is associated with antibodies against a minor 100 kDa glycoprotein component of nerve known as the *myelin-associated glycoprotein* (MAG). Anti-MAG antibodies are generally monoclonal IgMκ and usually also exhibit reactivity with other glycoproteins or glycolipids that share antigenic determinants with MAG.[77–79] The anti–MAG-related neuropathy is typically distal and symmetrical, affecting both motor and sensory functions; it is slowly progressive with a long period of stability.[72,80] Most patients present with sensory complaints (paresthesias, aching discomfort, dysesthesias, or lancinating pains); imbalance and gait ataxia, owing to lack proprioception; and leg muscle atrophy in advanced stage. Patients with predominantly demyelinating sensory neuropathy in association with monoclonal IgM to gangliosides with disialosyl moieties, such as GD1b, GD3, GD2, GT1b, and GQ1b, have also been reported.[81,82] Anti-GD1b and anti-GQ1b antibodies were associated with sensory ataxic neuropathy. These antiganglioside monoclonal IgMs present core clinical features of chronic ataxic neuropathy sometimes associated with ophthalmoplegia and/or red blood cell cold agglutinating activity. The disialosyl epitope is also present on red blood cell glycophorins, thereby accounting for the red cell cold agglutinin activity of anti-Pr2 specificity.[83,84] Monoclonal IgM proteins that bind to gangliosides with a terminal trisaccharide moiety, including ganglioside M2 and GalNac-GD1A, are associated with chronic demyelinating neuropathy and severe sensory ataxia, unresponsive to glucocorticoids.[85] Antiganglioside IgM proteins may also cross-react with lipopolysaccharides of *Campylobacter jejuni*, an infection known to precipitate the Miller Fisher syndrome, a variant of Guillain-Barré

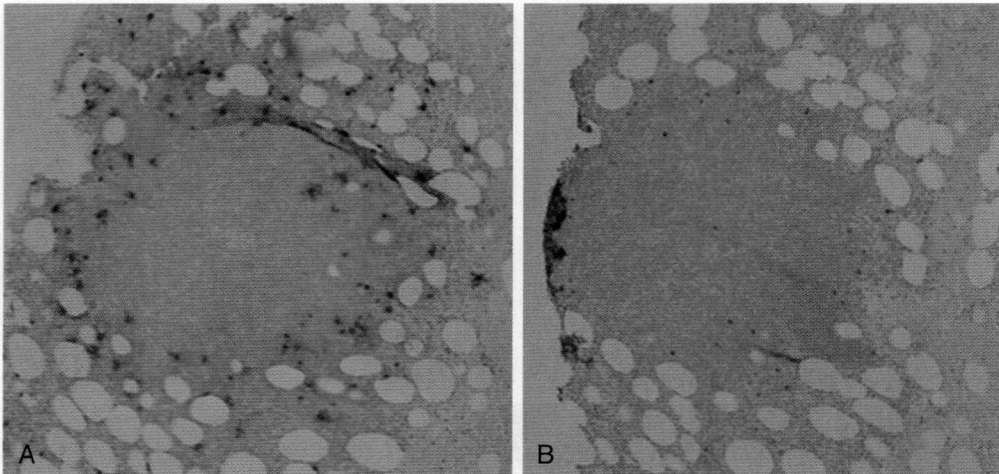

Fig. 87.5 MARROW CLOT SECTION. (A) Tryptase-staining mast cells surrounding a nodule of lympho-plasmacytic cells in a patient with Waldenström macroglobulinemia. (B) Mast cells in the same section exhibit strong CD40 ligand signaling, which has been shown to support (at least in part) the growth and survival of lymphoplasmacytic cells.

syndrome.[86] Thus molecular mimicry may play a role in this condition. Antisulfatide monoclonal IgM proteins, associated with sensory-sensorimotor neuropathy, have been detected in 5% of patients with IgM monoclonal gammopathy and neuropathy.[87] Motor neuron disease has been reported in patients with WM and monoclonal IgM with anti-GM$_1$ and sulfoglucuronyl paragloboside activity.[88] Polyneuropathy, organomegaly, endocrinopathy, M protein, and skin changes (the POEMS syndrome) are rare in patients with WM.[89]

Cold Agglutinin Hemolytic Anemia. Monoclonal IgMs may have cold agglutinin activity; they recognize specific red cell antigens at temperatures below 37°C, producing a chronic hemolytic anemia. This disorder occurs in less than 10% of patients with WM and is associated with cold agglutinin titers greater than 1:1000 in most cases.[90] The monoclonal component is usually an IgMκ and reacts most commonly with red cell I/i antigens, resulting in complement fixation and activation.[91,92] Mild to moderate chronic hemolytic anemia can be exacerbated after cold exposure. Hemoglobin levels usually remain above 70 g/L. The hemolysis is usually extravascular, mediated by removal of C3b opsonized red cells by the mononuclear phagocytes, primarily in the liver. Intravascular hemolysis from complement destruction of red blood cell membrane is infrequent. The agglutination of red cells in the skin circulation also causes Raynaud syndrome, acrocyanosis, and livedo reticularis. Macroglobulins with the properties of both cryoglobulins and cold agglutinins with anti-Pr specificity can occur. These properties may have as a common basis the binding of the sialic acid–containing carbohydrate present on red blood cell glycophorins and on Ig molecules. Several other macroglobulins with antibody activity toward autologous antigens (e.g., phospholipids, tissue and plasma proteins), and foreign ligands have also been described.

IgM Tissue Deposition. The monoclonal IgM can deposit in several tissues as amorphous aggregates. Linear deposition of monoclonal IgM along the skin basement membrane is associated with bullous skin disease.[93] Amorphous IgM deposits in the dermis result in IgM storage papules on the extensor surface of the extremities, referred to as *macroglobulinemia cutis*.[94] Deposition of monoclonal IgM in the lamina propria and/or submucosa of the intestine may be associated with diarrhea, malabsorption, and gastrointestinal bleeding.[95,96] Kidney involvement is less common and less severe in WM than in myeloma, probably because the amount of light chain that is excreted in the urine is generally less in WM than in myeloma and because of the absence of contributing factors, such as hypercalcemia.

Urinary cast nephropathy, however, has occurred in WM.[97] On the other hand, the IgM macromolecule is more susceptible to being trapped in the glomerular loops, where ultrafiltration presumably contributes to its precipitation, forming subendothelial deposits of aggregated IgM proteins that occlude the glomerular capillaries.[98] Mild and reversible proteinuria may result, and most patients are asymptomatic. The deposition of monoclonal light chain as fibrillar amyloid deposits (AL amyloidosis) is uncommon in patients with WM.[99] The clinical manifestations and prognosis are similar to those of other patients with AL amyloidosis, with involvement occurring in the heart (44%), kidneys (32%), liver (14%), lungs (10%), peripheral or autonomic nerves (38%), and soft tissues (18%). The incidence of cardiac and pulmonary involvement is higher in patients with monoclonal IgM than in those with other immunoglobulin isotypes. The association of WM with reactive amyloidosis has been documented rarely.[100,101] Simultaneous occurrence of fibrillary glomerulopathy, characterized by glomerular deposits of wide noncongophilic fibrils and amyloid deposits, has been described.[102]

Manifestations Related to Tissue Infiltration by Neoplastic Cells

Tissue infiltration by neoplastic cells is uncommon but can involve various organs and tissues, including the liver, spleen, lymph nodes, lungs, gastrointestinal tract, kidneys, skin, eyes, and central nervous system.

Lung. Pulmonary involvement in the form of masses, nodules, diffuse infiltrate, or pleural effusions is uncommon; the overall incidence of pulmonary and pleural findings is approximately 4%.[103–105] Cough is the most common presenting symptom, followed by dyspnea and chest pain. Chest radiographic findings include parenchymal infiltrates, confluent masses, and effusions.

Gastrointestinal Tract. Malabsorption, diarrhea, bleeding, or obstruction may indicate involvement of the gastrointestinal tract at the level of the stomach, duodenum, or small intestine.[106–109]

Renal System. In contrast to myeloma, infiltration of the kidney interstitium with lymphoplasmacytoid cell can occur in WM, and renal or perirenal masses are not uncommon.[110,111]

Skin. The skin can be the site of dense lymphoplasmacytic infiltrates, similar to those seen in the liver, spleen, and lymph nodes, forming cutaneous plaques and, rarely, nodules.[112] Chronic urticaria and IgM gammopathy are the two cardinal features of the Schnitzler syndrome, which is not usually associated initially with clinical features of WM, although evolution to WM is not uncommon.[113] Thus close follow-up of such patients is important.

Joints. Invasion of articular and periarticular structures by WM malignant cells is rarely reported.[114]

Eye. The neoplastic cells can infiltrate the periorbital structures, lacrimal gland, and retroorbital lymphoid tissues, resulting in ocular nerve palsies.[115,116]

Central Nervous System. Direct infiltration of the central nervous system by monoclonal lymphoplasmacytic cells as infiltrates or as tumors constitutes the rarely observed Bing-Neel syndrome, characterized clinically by confusion, memory loss, disorientation, and motor dysfunction (reviewed by Civit et al.[117]).

LABORATORY FINDINGS

Blood Abnormalities

Anemia is the most common finding in patients with symptomatic WM and is caused by a combination of factors: decrease in red cell survival, impaired erythropoiesis, moderate plasma volume expansion, hepcidin production leading to an iron reuse defect, and blood loss from the gastrointestinal tract.[16,118,119] Blood films are usually normocytic and normochromic, and rouleau formation is often pronounced. Mean red cell volume may be elevated spuriously owing to erythrocyte aggregation. In addition, the hemoglobin estimate can be inaccurate (i.e., falsely high) because of interaction between the monoclonal protein and the diluent used in some automated analyzers.[120] Leukocyte and platelet counts are usually within their reference ranges at presentation, although patients may occasionally present with severe thrombocytopenia. Monoclonal B lymphocytes expressing surface IgM and late-differentiation B-cell markers are uncommonly detected in blood by flow cytometry. A raised erythrocyte sedimentation rate is almost always present and may be the first clue to the presence of macroglobulinemia. The clotting abnormality detected most frequently is prolongation of thrombin time. AL amyloidosis should be suspected in all patients with nephrotic syndrome, cardiomyopathy, hepatomegaly, or peripheral neuropathy. Diagnosis requires the demonstration of green birefringence under polarized light of amyloid deposits stained with Congo red.

MARROW FINDINGS

Central to the diagnosis of WM is the demonstration, by trephine biopsy, of marrow infiltration by a lymphoplasmacytic cell population characterized by small lymphocytes with evidence of plasmacytoid and plasma cell maturation (Fig. 87.1).[1,14] The pattern of marrow infiltration may be diffuse, interstitial, or nodular, usually with an intertrabecular pattern of infiltration. A solely paratrabecular pattern of infiltration is unusual and should raise the possibility of follicular lymphoma.[1] The marrow cell immunophenotype should be confirmed by flow cytometry and/or immunohistochemistry. The cell immunoprofile sIgM+CD19+CD20+CD22+CD79+ is characteristic of WM.[14,120,121] Up to 20% of cases may express either CD5, CD10, or CD23.[19] In these cases, chronic lymphocytic leukemia and mantle cell lymphoma should be excluded. "Intranuclear" periodic acid-Schiff–positive inclusions (Dutcher-Fahey bodies)[122] consisting of IgM deposits in the perinuclear space, and sometimes in intranuclear vacuoles, may be seen occasionally in lymphoid cells. An increased number of mast cells, usually in association with the lymphoid aggregates, is commonly found, and their presence may help in differentiating WM from other B-cell lymphomas (see Fig. 87.3).[14] *MYD88^{L265P}* testing of BM samples has been incorporated

into many clinical laboratories and may help in clarifying the diagnosis of WM from other IgM-secreting entities.[35–39] The use of peripheral blood B cells may also permit determination of *MYD88^{L265P}* status by allele-specific PCR assays, particularly in untreated patients with WM.

IMMUNOLOGIC ABNORMALITIES

High-resolution electrophoresis combined with immunofixation of serum and urine is recommended for identification and characterization of the IgM monoclonal protein. The light chain of the monoclonal IgM is κ in 75% to 80% of patients. More than one M component may be present. The concentration of the serum monoclonal protein is very variable, but in most cases it lies within the range of 15–45 g/L. Densitometry should be adopted to determine IgM levels for serial evaluations because nephelometry is unreliable and shows large laboratory variation. The presence of cold agglutinins or cryoglobulins may affect determination of IgM levels, and therefore testing for cold agglutinins and cryoglobulins should be performed at diagnosis. If present, subsequent serum samples should be analyzed at 37°C for determination of serum monoclonal IgM level. Although Bence Jones proteinuria is frequently present, it exceeds 1 g/24 h in only 3% of cases. Whereas IgM levels are elevated in patients with WM, IgA and IgG levels are most often depressed and do not recover after successful treatment.[123]

SERUM VISCOSITY

Because of their large size (molecular weight almost 1 million), most IgM molecules are retained within the intravascular compartment and can exert an undue effect on serum viscosity.[64] Serum viscosity can be measured if the patient has signs or symptoms of hyperviscosity syndrome, though levels are often slow to be reported and erratic owing to a lack of standardization in most clinical laboratories.[16] As such, serum IgM levels may be more expedient and relied upon. Patients typically become symptomatic at serum viscosity levels of 4.0 cp and above, which relate to serum IgM levels above 6000 mg/dL.[124,125] Patients may be symptomatic at lower serum viscosity and IgM levels, and in these patients cryoglobulins may be present. Recurring nosebleeds, headaches, and visual disturbances are common symptoms in patients with symptomatic hyperviscosity.[16] Funduscopy is an important indicator of clinically relevant hyperviscosity. Among the first clinical signs of hyperviscosity are the appearance of peripheral and midperipheral dot- and blotlike hemorrhages in the retina, which are best appreciated with indirect ophthalmoscopy and scleral depression.[68] In more severe cases of hyperviscosity, dot, blot, and flame-shaped hemorrhages can appear in the macular area along with markedly dilated and tortuous veins with focal constrictions resulting in "venous sausaging," as well as papilledema (Fig. 87.4).

IMAGING

Magnetic resonance imaging (MRI) of the spine in conjunction with computed tomography (CT) of the abdomen and pelvis are useful in evaluating disease status.[126] Marrow involvement can be documented by MRI studies of the spine in more than 90% of patients; CT of the abdomen and pelvis demonstrates enlarged nodes in approximately 20% of patients with WM at diagnosis, but this proportion may be higher at relapse.[126]

LYMPH NODE BIOPSY

Lymph node biopsy may show preserved architecture or replacement by infiltration of neoplastic cells with lymphoplasmacytoid, lymphoplasmacytic, or polymorphous cytologic patterns.

TREATMENT

Initiating Treatment

As part of the Second International Workshop on Waldenström's Macroglobulinemia, a consensus panel was organized to recommend criteria for the initiation of therapy in patients with WM.[127] The panel recommended that initiation of therapy should not be based on the IgM level per se, because this may not correlate with the clinical manifestations of WM. The consensus panel did, however, agree that initiation of therapy is appropriate for patients with constitutional symptoms, such as recurrent fever, night sweats, fatigue as a consequence of anemia, or weight loss. Progressive symptomatic lymphadenopathy and/or splenomegaly provide additional reasons to begin therapy. Anemia with a hemoglobin value ≤10 g/dL or a platelet count ≤100 × 10⁹/L owing to marrow infiltration also justifies treatment. Certain complications, such as hyperviscosity syndrome, symptomatic sensorimotor peripheral neuropathy, systemic amyloidosis, renal insufficiency, or symptomatic cryoglobulinemia, may also be indications for therapy.[16,127]

Initial Therapy

The International Workshops on Waldenström's Macroglobulinemia have also formulated consensus recommendations for both initial therapy and therapy for refractory disease based on the best available evidence. The most recent recommendations emerged from the Seventh International Workshop on Waldenström's Macroglobulinemia.[128] Individual patient considerations, including the presence of cytopenias, need for more rapid disease control, age, and candidacy for autologous transplant therapy, should be taken into account in making the choice of the drugs to use. For patients who are candidates for autologous stem cell transplant (SCT), which typically is reserved for those patients younger than 70 years of age, the panel recommended that exposure to alkylating agents or nucleoside analogues should be limited. The use of nucleoside analogues should be approached cautiously in patients with WM because there appears to be an increased risk for the development of disease transformation as well as myelodysplasia and acute myelogenous leukemia.

Oral Alkylating Agents. Oral alkylating drugs, alone and in combination therapy with glucocorticoids, have been evaluated extensively in the treatment of WM. Chlorambucil has been administered on both a continuous (i.e., daily dose schedule) and an intermittent schedule. Patients receiving chlorambucil on a continuous schedule typically receive 0.1 mg/kg per day, whereas on the intermittent schedule patients typically receive 0.3 mg/kg for 7 days, every 6 weeks. In a prospective, randomized study, no significant difference in the overall response rate (ORR) between these schedules was observed,[129] although the median response duration was greater for patients receiving intermittent- versus continuous-dose chlorambucil (46 vs. 26 months). Despite the favorable median response duration in this study for use of the intermittent schedule, no difference in the median overall survival was observed. Moreover, an increased incidence for development of myelodysplasia and acute myelogenous leukemia with the intermittent (3 of 22 patients) versus the continuous (0 of 24 patients) chlorambucil schedule prompted the preference for use of continuous chlorambucil dosing. The use of glucocorticoids in combination with alkylating agent therapy has also been explored. Chlorambucil (8 mg/m²) plus prednisone (40 mg/m²) given orally for 10 days, every 6 weeks, resulted in a major response (i.e., reduction of IgM by more than 50%) in 72% of patients.[130] Alkylating agent regimens employing melphalan and cyclophosphamide in combination with glucocorticoids have also been examined.[131,132] This approach produced slightly higher ORRs and response durations, although the benefit of these more complex regimens over chlorambucil remains to be demonstrated. Pretreatment factors associated with shorter survival in the entire population of patients receiving single-agent chlorambucil were older than 60 years of age,

male sex, hemoglobin less than 10 g/dL, leukocytes less than 4 × 10⁹/L, and platelets less than 150 × 10⁹/L. Organomegaly, signs of hyperviscosity, renal failure, monoclonal IgM level, blood lymphocytosis, and percentage of marrow lymphoid cells were not significantly correlated with survival.[133] Additional factors to be taken into account in considering alkylating agent therapy for patients with WM include necessity for more rapid disease control, given the slow response, as well as consideration for preserving stem cells in patients who are candidates for autologous SCT. A large randomized study showed an inferior response rate and time to progression in patients with WM receiving chlorambucil versus fludarabine, as well as a higher incidence of secondary malignancies in the former. Neutropenia was more pronounced, however, in those patients on fludarabine.[134]

Nucleoside Analogue Therapy. Cladribine administered as a single agent by continuous intravenous infusion, by 2-hour daily infusion, or by subcutaneous bolus injections for 5–7 days has resulted in major responses in 40% to 90% of patients who received primary therapy, whereas in the previously treated patients, responses have ranged from 38% to 54%.[135–141] Median time to achievement of response in responding patients following cladribine ranged from 1.2 to 5 months. The ORR with daily infusion of fludarabine, administered mainly on 5-day schedules, in previously untreated and treated patients ranged from 38% to 100% and from 30% to 40%, respectively,[142–147] similar to the responses to cladribine. Median time to achievement of response for fludarabine (3–6 months) was also similar to cladribine. In general, response rates and durations of responses have been greater for patients receiving nucleoside analogues as initial therapy, although no difference in the ORR was reported in several studies in which both untreated and previously treated patients were enrolled.

Myelosuppression commonly occurs following prolonged exposure to either of the nucleoside analogues. A sustained decrease in both CD4⁺ and CD8⁺ T lymphocytes, measured 1 year following initiation of therapy, is notable.[135–137] Treatment-related mortality as a consequence of myelosuppression and/or opportunistic infections attributable to immunosuppression occurred in up to 5% of all treated patients in some series with nucleoside analogues.

Factors predicting a better response to nucleoside analogues include younger age at start of treatment (<70 years), higher pretreatment hemoglobin (>95 g/L), higher platelet count (>75 × 10⁹/L), disease relapsing off-therapy, and a long interval between firstline therapy and initiation of a nucleoside analogue in relapsing patients.[135,140,146] There are limited data on the use of an alternate nucleoside analogue in previously treated patients in whom disease relapsed or who had resistance when not on cladribine or fludarabine therapy.[148,149] Three (75%) of 4 patients responded to cladribine after progression following an unmaintained remission with fludarabine, whereas only 1 (10%) of 10 with disease resistant to fludarabine responded to cladribine.[148] A response to fludarabine has been reported in two (33%) of six patients and disease stabilization in the remaining patients, in spite of an inadequate response or progressive disease, following cladribine therapy.[149]

Harvesting autologous blood stem cells succeeded on the first attempt in 14 of 15 patients who did not receive nucleoside analogue therapy, as compared with 2 of 6 patients who received a nucleoside analogue.[150] A sevenfold increase in patients transforming to an aggressive lymphoma and a threefold increase in the development of myelodysplasia or acute myelogenous leukemia were observed among patients who received a nucleoside analogue versus other therapies for their WM.[151] A meta-analysis of several trials in which patients with WM were treated with nucleoside analogues included patients who had previously received an alkylating agent, and the results showed a crude incidence of approximately 8% of developing a disease transformation event and approximately 5% for developing myelodysplasia or acute myelogenous leukemia.[152] None of the risk factors—that is, sex, age, family history of WM, or B-cell malignancies, typical markers of tumor burden and prognosis, type of nucleoside analogue therapy (cladribine vs. fludarabine), time from diagnosis to nucleoside analogue use, nucleoside analogue treatment as primary or salvage therapy, or treatment with an oral alkylator (i.e., chlorambucil)—predicted the occurrence of transformation or development of myelodysplasia or acute myelogenous leukemia in patients treated with a nucleoside analogue.[152]

CD20-Directed Antibody Therapy. Rituximab is a chimeric monoclonal antibody that targets CD20, a widely expressed antigen on lymphoplasmacytic cells in WM.[153] Several retrospective and prospective studies have indicated that rituximab, when used at standard doses (i.e., 4 weekly infusions of 375 mg/m²/week) induced major responses in approximately 30% of previously treated and untreated patients.[154,155] Even patients who achieved minor responses benefited from rituximab by improved hemoglobin and platelet counts, as well as reduction of lymphadenopathy and/or splenomegaly.[154] The median time to treatment failure in these studies was found to range from 8 to 27+ months. Patients on an extended rituximab schedule consisting of 4 weekly courses at 375 mg/m² per week, repeated 3 months later by another 4-week course have demonstrated major response rates of approximately 45%, with time to progression estimates of 16+ to 29+ months.[156,157]

In many patients with WM, a transient increase or flare of the serum IgM may occur immediately following initiation of rituximab treatment.[156,158,159] Such an increase does not herald treatment failure, and most patients will return to their baseline serum IgM level by 12 weeks. Some patients continue to show a prolonged increase in IgM despite an apparent reduction in their marrow tumor cells. However, patients with baseline serum IgM levels >50 g/dL or serum viscosity >3.5 cp may be particularly at risk for a hyperviscosity-related event, and plasmapheresis should be considered in these patients in advance of rituximab therapy.[158] Because of the decreased likelihood of response in patients with higher IgM levels, as well as the possibility that serum IgM and blood viscosity levels may abruptly rise, rituximab monotherapy should not be used as sole therapy for the treatment of patients at risk for hyperviscosity symptoms.[128,156,157]

Time to response after rituximab is slow and exceeds 3 months on average. The time to best response in one study was 18 months.[157] Patients with baseline serum IgM levels <60 g/dL are more likely to respond, regardless of the underlying degree of marrow involvement by tumor cells.[156,157] An analysis of 52 patients who were treated with single-agent rituximab found the objective response rate was significantly lower in patients who had either low serum albumin (<35 g/L) or a serum monoclonal protein greater than 40 g/L.[160] The presence of both adverse prognostic factors was associated with a short time to progression (3.6 months). Patients who had normal serum albumin and relatively low serum monoclonal protein levels derived a substantial benefit from rituximab, with a time to progression exceeding 40 months.

A correlation between polymorphisms at position 158 in the FcγRIIIa receptor (CD16), an activating Fc receptor on important effector cells that mediate antibody-dependent, cell-mediated cytotoxicity, and rituximab response was observed in patients with WM.[161] Individuals may encode either the amino acid valine or phenylalanine at position 158 in the FcγRIIIa receptor. Patients with WM who carried the valine amino acid (either in a homozygous or heterozygous pattern) had a fourfold higher major response rate (i.e., 50% decline in serum IgM levels) to rituximab versus those patients who expressed phenylalanine in a homozygous pattern.

Proteasome Inhibitors. Both bortezomib and carfilzomib have been evaluated in prospective studies in patients with WM, though the latter only in combination therapy (discussed below). In a retrospective study, 10 patients with refractory or relapsed WM were treated with bortezomib administered intravenously at a dose of 1.3 mg/m² on days 1, 4, 8, and 11 in a 21-day cycle for a total of four cycles. Most patients had been exposed to all other active agents for WM, and eight patients had received three or more regimens. Six of these patients achieved a partial response that occurred after a median of 1 month. The median time to progression in the responding patients is expected to exceed 11 months. Peripheral neuropathy occurred in three patients, and one patient developed severe paralytic ileus.[162] In

a prospective study including 27 relapsed or refractory patients who received up to 8 cycles of bortezomib at 1.3 mg/m² on days 1, 4, 8, and 11, median serum IgM levels declined significantly, from 4.7 g/dL to 2.1 g/dL.[33] The ORR was 85%, with 10 and 13 patients achieving a minor (<25%) and major (<50%) decrease in IgM level, respectively. Responses occurred after a median of 1.4 months. The median time to progression for all responding patients in this study was 7.9 (range, 3–21.4+) months, and the most common grade III/IV toxicities were sensory neuropathies (22.2%), leukopenia (18.5%), neutropenia (14.8%), dizziness (11.1%), and thrombocytopenia (7.4%). Sensory neuropathies resolved or improved in nearly all patients following cessation of therapy. Twenty-seven patients with both untreated (44%) and previously treated (56%) disease received bortezomib, using the standard schedule until they either demonstrated progressive disease or two cycles beyond a complete response or stable disease.[163] The ORR was 78%, with major responses observed in 44% of patients. Sensory neuropathy occurred in 20 patients following two to four cycles of therapy. Among the 20 patients who developed a neuropathy, 14 showed resolution or improvement 2–13 months after therapy.

Combination Therapies. Because rituximab is not myelosuppressive, its use in combination with chemotherapy has been explored. A regimen of rituximab, cladribine, and cyclophosphamide in 17 previously untreated patients resulted in a partial response in 94% of patients with WM, including a complete response in 18%.[164] No patient had relapsed with a median follow-up of 21 months. The combination of rituximab and fludarabine was used in 43 patients, of whom 32 (75%) were previously untreated, which led to an ORR of 95.3%, with 83% of patients achieving a major response (i.e., 50% reduction in disease burden).[165] The median time to progression was 51.2 months in this series, and it was longer for those patients who were previously untreated and for those achieving a very good partial remission (i.e., 90% reduction in disease) or better. Hematologic toxicity was common: Grade 3 neutropenia and thrombocytopenia were observed in 27 and 4 patients, respectively. Two deaths occurred in this study as a result of pneumonia. Secondary malignancies, including transformation to aggressive lymphoma and development of myelodysplasia or acute myelogenous leukemia, were observed in six patients. The addition of rituximab to fludarabine and cyclophosphamide has also been explored in previously treated patients, and four of five patients had a response.[166] In another combination study, rituximab along with pentostatin and cyclophosphamide given to 13 patients with untreated and previously treated WM or LPL resulted in a major response in 77% of patients.[167] The combination of rituximab, dexamethasone, and cyclophosphamide was used as primary therapy to treat 72 patients with WM, among whom a major response was observed in 74% of patients, and the 2-year progression-free survival was 67%.[168] Therapy was well tolerated, although one patient died as a result of interstitial pneumonia.

Two studies have examined cyclophosphamide, doxorubicin, vincristine, and prednisone (CHOP) therapy in combination with rituximab (R-CHOP). In a randomized trial involving 69 patients, most of whom had WM, the addition of rituximab to CHOP resulted in a higher ORR (94% vs. 67%) and median time to progression (63 vs. 22 months) in comparison with patients treated with CHOP alone.[169] R-CHOP was also used in 13 patients with WM, 10 of whom had relapsed or refractory disease.[170] Among 13 evaluable patients, 10 patients achieved a major response (77%), including 3 complete and 7 partial remissions. Two other patients achieved a minor response. Patients in a retrospective study of symptomatic WM received either R-CHOP; rituximab, cyclophosphamide, vincristine, and prednisone (R-CVP); or cyclophosphamide, prednisone, and rituximab (R-CP). The patients were similar in most pretreatment variables, and the ORRs to therapy were comparable among all three treatment groups—R-CHOP (96%), R-CVP (88%), and R-CP (95%)—although there was a trend for more complete remissions among patients treated with R-CVP and R-CHOP.[171] Adverse events attributed to therapy showed a higher incidence for neutropenic fever and treatment-related neuropathy for R-CHOP and R-CVP versus

R-CP. The results of this study suggest that in patients with WM, the use of R-CP may provide treatment responses analogous to those of more intense cyclophosphamide-based regimens while minimizing treatment-related complications. The extended alkylator bendamustine has also been evaluated in combination with rituximab in both untreated and previously treated patients with WM. A randomized study by the German STiL Group examined bendamustine plus rituximab (Benda-R) versus R-CHOP in patients with untreated, indolent B-cell lymphomas including WM.[172] Patients with WM in this study showed similar overall responses (96% vs. 94%), though progression-free survival was significantly longer (69 vs. 29 months) in patients who received Benda-R versus R-CHOP. Treatment was also better tolerated in patients receiving Benda-R. In the relapsed or refractory setting, an ORR of 83% was observed with bendamustine in combination with a CD20 monoclonal antibody.[173] The median time to progression was 13 months in this study. Prolonged myelosuppression was more common in patients who had received prior nucleoside analogue therapy.

The use of two cycles of oral cyclophosphamide along with subcutaneous cladribine to 37 patients with previously untreated WM led to a partial response in 84% of patients, and the median duration of response was 36 months.[164] Fludarabine in combination with intravenous cyclophosphamide resulted in partial responses in 6 (55%) of 11 patients with WM with either primary refractory disease or who had relapsed on treatment.[174] The combination of fludarabine plus cyclophosphamide was also evaluated in 49 patients, 35 of whom were previously treated. Seventy-eight percent of the patients achieved a response, and the median time to treatment failure was 27 months.[175] Hematologic toxicity was frequent, and three patients died as a result of treatment-related toxicities. Two important findings in this study were the development of acute leukemia in two patients, histologic transformation to diffuse large B-cell lymphoma in one patient, and two cases of solid malignancies (prostate and melanoma), as well as failure to mobilize stem cells in four of six patients.

The combination of bortezomib, dexamethasone, and rituximab (BDR) as primary therapy in patients with WM resulted in an ORR of 96% and a major response rate of 83%.[176] The incidence of grade 3 neuropathy was approximately 30%, but this was reversible in most patients following discontinuation of therapy. An increased incidence of herpes zoster was also observed, prompting the prophylactic use of antiviral therapy. Alternative schedules for administration of bortezomib (i.e., once weekly at higher doses) in combination with rituximab in patients with WM have achieved ORRs of 80% to 90%.[177,178] The European Myeloma Network recently showed that transitioning bortezomib from twice-weekly intravenous dosing during the first cycle to weekly administration thereafter reduced grade 3 neuropathy to under 10% in patients treated with BDR.[179] There have been no studies addressing the safety and efficacy of subcutaneous bortezomib use in WM.

Carfilzomib, which is associated with a low risk of treatment-related peripheral neuropathy, has been evaluated in combination with rituximab and dexamethasone in patients with WM.[34] Carfilzomib was administered intravenously at 20 mg/m^2 (cycle 1), then 36 mg/m^2 (cycles 2–6), together with dexamethasone (20 mg) on days 1, 2, 8, and 9 as part of a 21-day cycle. As part of this regimen, rituximab 375 mg/m^2 was given on days 2 and 9 every 21 days. Maintenance therapy was given 8 weeks following induction therapy with intravenous carfilzomib (36 mg/m^2) and dexamethasone (20 mg) administered on days 1 and 2 and with rituximab 375 mg/m^2 on day 2 every 8 weeks for up to 8 cycles. The ORR with this regimen was 87.1% (1 complete response, 10 very good partial responses, 10 partial responses, and 6 minimal responses) and was not impacted by $MYD88^{L265P}$ or $CXCR4^{WHIM}$ mutation status. With a median follow-up of 15.4 months, 20 patients remained progression-free. Grade ≥2 toxicities included asymptomatic hyperlipasemia (41.9%), reversible neutropenia (12.9%), and cardiomyopathy in 1 patient (3.2%) with multiple risk factors. Grade 2 treatment-related neuropathy occurred in one patient (3.2%). Declines in serum IgA and IgG were common, and some patients required intravenous immunoglobulin therapy for recurring sinus and bronchial infections.

Novel Therapeutics. The use of ibrutinib was recently approved by the U.S. Food and Drug Administration for the treatment of symptomatic patients with WM. Ibrutinib targets BTK, a target of ibrutinib that is activated by $MYD88^{L265P}$.[43] In a multicenter study in which researchers examined the role of ibrutinib in previously treated (median 2 prior therapies, 40% refractory) patients with WM, the ORR was 87%.[180] Patients on this study received 420 mg per day of ibrutinib by mouth. Posttherapy median serum IgM levels declined from 3610 to 915 mg/dL; hemoglobin rose from 10.5 to 13.5 g/dL; and BM involvement declined from 60% to 30%. Decreased or resolved adenopathy was observed in 60% of patients with extramedullary disease, and five of nine patients with IgM-related peripheral neuropathy had symptomatic improvement. The 18-month estimates for progression-free and overall survival were 83% and 93%, respectively. Although major response rates were lower in patients with $MYD88^{wild-type}$ and $CXCR4^{WHIM}$ mutations, it is not recommended that genotyping be used to select which patients should be placed on ibrutinib until further data are available. Grade ≥2 treatment-related toxicities included neutropenia (25%) and thrombocytopenia (14%) that were more common in heavily pretreated patients, atrial fibrillation associated with a prior history of arrhythmia (5%), and bleeding associated with procedures and marine oil supplements (3%). Serum IgA and IgG levels were unchanged following treatment with ibrutinib, and treatment-related infections were infrequent.

Everolimus is an oral inhibitor of the mammalian target of rapamycin (mTOR) pathway that is active in WM. In a multicenter study, investigators examined everolimus in 60 previously treated patients and showed an ORR of 73%, with 50% of patients attaining a major response.[181] The median progression-free survival in this study was 21 months. Grade 3 or higher related toxicities were observed in 67% of patients, with cytopenias constituting the most common toxicity. Pulmonary toxicity occurred in 5% of patients, and dose reductions owing to toxicity occurred in 52% of patients. In a clinical trial in which researchers examined the activity of everolimus in 33 previously untreated patients with WM, serial BM biopsies were included in response assessment.[182] The ORR in this study was 72%, including partial or better responses in 60% of patients. However, discordance between serum IgM levels upon which consensus criteria for response are based and BM disease response was common, which complicated response assessment. In a few patients, discontinuation of everolimus led to rapid increases in serum IgM levels and symptomatic hyperviscosity. Grade ≥2 hematologic and nonhematologic toxicities in this study that were related to everolimus were predominately hematological, including anemia (40%), thrombocytopenia (12%), and neutropenia (18%). Nonhematologic toxicities included oral ulcerations (27%) that improved with oral dexamethasone swish and spit solution, as well as pneumonitis (15%), the latter leading to treatment discontinuation.

Maintenance Therapy. The outcome of rituximab-naïve patients who were either observed or received maintenance rituximab categorical responses was examined in a large retrospective study.[183] Categorical responses improved after induction therapy in 42% of patients who received maintenance rituximab versus 10% in patients in the observation group. Additionally, both progression-free (56.3 vs. 28.6 months) and overall (>120 vs. 116 months) survival were longer in patients who received maintenance rituximab. Improved progression-free survival was evident despite previous treatment status, induction with rituximab alone, or in combination therapy. Best serum IgM response was also lower, and hematocrit higher, in those patients who received maintenance rituximab. Among patients who received maintenance rituximab therapy, an increased number of infectious events, predominantly grade 1 or 2 sinusitis and bronchitis, was observed, along with lower serum IgA and IgG levels. A prospective study examining the role of maintenance rituximab has also been initiated by the German STiL Group.[184] In this study, patients received up to six cycles of bendamustine and rituximab, and responders were randomized to either observation or maintenance rituximab every 2 months for 2 years. Enrollment for this study is complete, and response outcome for maintenance rituximab therapy is awaited.

High-Dose Therapy and Stem Cell Transplant

The European Bone Marrow Transplant Registry (EBMT) reported the largest experience for both autologous as well as allogeneic SCT in WM.[185,186] Among 158 patients with WM receiving an autologous SCT, which included primarily relapsed or refractory patients, the 5-year progression-free and overall survival rates were 39.7% and 68.5%, respectively.[185] Nonrelapse mortality at 1 year was 3.8%. Chemorefractory disease and the number of prior lines of therapy at the time of the autologous SCT were the most important prognostic factors for progression-free and overall survival. In the allogeneic SCT experience from the EBMT, the long-term outcomes of 86 patients with WM were reported.[186] A total of 86 patients received an allograft following either myeloablative or reduced-intensity conditioning. The median age of patients in this series was 49 years, and 47 patients had undergone three or more previous lines of therapy. Eight patients failed prior autologous SCT. Fifty-nine patients (68.6%) had chemotherapy-sensitive disease at the time of allogeneic SCT. Nonrelapse mortality rates at 3 years were 33% for patients receiving a myeloablative transplant and 23% for those who received reduced-intensity conditioning. The ORR was 75.6%. The relapse rates at 3 years were 11% for myeloablative and 25% for reduced-intensity conditioning recipients. Five-year progression-free and overall survival for patients with WM who received a myeloablative allogeneic SCT were 56% and 62%, respectively, and for patients who received reduced intensity conditioning, the rates were 49% and 64%, respectively. The occurrence of chronic graft-versus-host disease was associated with improved progression-free survival and suggested the existence of a clinically relevant graft-versus-WM effect in this study.

Response Criteria in Waldenström Macroglobulinemia

Table 87.3 summarizes the response categories and criteria for progressive disease in WM based on the most recent consensus recommendations.[187] The term *overall response* is used to characterize all responses, including minor responses. *Major responses* include partial, very good partial, and complete responses. The attainment of very good partial or complete responses is associated with improved progression-free survival.[155,165,176,179,188] Response assessments in WM rely primarily on serum IgM or IgM paraprotein levels, though complete responses require disappearance of the IgM monoclonal protein, and resolution of evidence of BM and/or extramedullary disease.[187] An important concern with the use of IgM as a surrogate marker of disease is that it can fluctuate independent of tumor cell killing with some agents. By way of example, rituximab can induce a flare in serum IgM levels, whereas everolimus, bortezomib, and ibrutinib can suppress IgM levels independent of tumor cell killing in some patients, a phenomenon referred to as *IgM discordance*.[158,159,162,181,183,189] Moreover, with selective B cell–depleting agents such as rituximab and alemtuzumab, residual IgM-producing plasma cells are spared and persist, thus potentially skewing the relative response and assessment to treatment.[190] Soluble CD27 levels have been investigated as an alternative surrogate marker in WM, given their correlation with WM disease burden, and may remain a faithful marker of disease in patients experiencing a rituximab-related IgM flare, as well as after plasmapheresis.[60,191] The use of quantitative allele-specific PCR assays to assess serial MYD88[L265P] burden in patients with WM is also under investigation.[36,38]

Course and Prognosis

WM typically presents as an indolent disease. The presence of 6q deletions may have prognostic significance, although this is disputed.[20,21] Age is an important prognostic factor (>65 years),[192–194] but it is influenced by comorbidities. Anemia that reflects both marrow involvement and the serum level of the IgM monoclonal protein (because of the impact of IgM on intravascular fluid retention) has emerged as a strong adverse prognostic factor with hemoglobin levels of <9 to 12 g/dL associated with decreased survival in several series.[192–194] Other cytopenias also may be significant predictors of survival.[193] The precise level of cytopenias with prognostic significance has not been determined. Some series have identified a platelet count of <100 to 150 × 10^9/L and a granulocyte count of <1.5 × 10^9/L as independent prognostic factors.[193,194] The number of cytopenias in a given patient has been proposed as a prognostic factor.[193] Serum albumin levels also correlate with survival in patients

TABLE 87.3	Summary of Consensus Response Criteria for Waldenström Macroglobulinemia[187]	
Response Type	**Abbreviation**	**Criteria**
Complete response	CR	Absence of serum monoclonal IgM protein by immunofixation Normal serum IgM level Complete resolution of extramedullary disease (i.e., lymphadenopathy/splenomegaly if present at baseline) Morphologically normal bone marrow aspirate and trephine biopsy
Very good partial response	VGPR	Monoclonal IgM protein is detectable 90% reduction in serum IgM level from baseline or normalization of serum IgM level Complete resolution of extramedullary disease (i.e., lymphadenopathy/splenomegaly if present at baseline) No new signs or symptoms of active disease
Partial response	PR	Monoclonal IgM protein is detectable ≥50% but <90% reduction in serum IgM level from baseline Reduction in extramedullary disease (i.e., lymphadenopathy/splenomegaly if present at baseline) No new signs or symptoms of active disease
Minor response	MR	Monoclonal IgM protein is detectable ≥25% but <50% reduction in serum IgM level from baseline No new signs or symptoms of active disease
Stable disease	SD	Monoclonal IgM protein is detectable <25% reduction and <25% increase in serum IgM level from baseline No progression in extramedullary disease (i.e., lymphadenopathy/splenomegaly) No new signs or symptoms of active disease
Progressive disease	PD	>25% increase in serum IgM level from lowest nadir (requires confirmation) and/or progression in clinical features attributable to the disease

IgM, Immunoglobulin M.

TABLE 87.4   Prognostic Scoring Systems in Waldenström Macroglobulinemia

Study	Adverse Prognostic Factors	Number of Groups	Survival
Gobbi et al.[192]	Hgb <9 g/dL Age >70 years Weight loss Cryoglobulinemia	0–1 prognostic factors 2–4 prognostic factors	Median: 48 months Median: 80 months
Morel et al.[193]	Age ≥65 years Albumin <4 g/dL Number of cytopenias: Hgb <12 g/dL Platelets <150 × 10⁹/L WBC <4 × 10⁹/L	0–1 prognostic factors 2 prognostic factors 3–4 prognostic factors	5-year: 87% of patients 5-year: 62% 5-year: 25%
Dhodapkar et al.[194]	β_2M ≥3 g/dL Hgb <12 g/dL IgM <4 g/dL	β_2M <3 mg/dL + Hgb ≥12 g/dL β_2M <3 mg/dL + Hgb <12 g/dL β_2M ≥3 mg/dL + IgM ≥4 g/dL β_2M ≥3 mg/dL + IgM <4 g/dL	5-year: 87% of patients 5-year: 63% 5-year: 53% 5-year: 21%
Dimopoulos et al.[195]	Albumin ≤3.5 g/dL β_2M ≥3.5 mg/L	Albumin ≥3.5 g/dL + β_2M <3.5 mg/dL Albumin ≤3.5 g/dL + β_2M <3.5 or β_2M 3.5–5.5 mg/dL β_2M >5.5 mg/dL	Median: NR Median: 116 months Median: 54 months
Morel et al.[197]	Age >65 years Hgb <11.5 g/dL Platelets <100 × 10⁹/L β_2M >3 mg/L IgM >7 g/dL	0–1 prognostic factors (excluding age) 2 prognostic factors (or age >65 years) 3–5 prognostic factors	5 year: 87% of patients 5 year: 68% 5 year: 36%

β_2M, β_2-microbloulin; Hgb, hemoglobulin; IgM, immunoglobulin M; NR, not reported; WBC, white blood cell count.

with WM in some studies, using multivariate analyses.[193,195] Elevated serum β_2-microglobulin levels (>3–3.5 g/dL) have also been shown to have strong prognostic correlation in WM.[193–196] Several scoring systems have been proposed that are based on these analyses (Table 87.4), including the International Prognostic Scoring System for Waldenström macroglobulinemia (IPSSWM), which incorporates five adverse covariates: advanced age (>65 years), hemoglobin ≤11.5 g/dL, platelet count ≤100 × 10⁹/L, β_2-microglobulin >3 mg/L, and serum monoclonal protein concentration >7.0 g/dL.[197] Among 537 patients with WM evaluated in the development of IPSSWM, low-risk patients (27%) presented with no or one of the adverse characteristics and advanced age; intermediate-risk patients (38%) presented with two adverse characteristics or only advanced age; and high-risk patients (35%) presented with more than two adverse characteristics. Five-year survival rates for these three patient groups were 87%, 68%, and 36%, respectively. Importantly, the IPSS WM retained its prognostic significance in subgroups defined by age and treatment with alkylating agent and nucleoside analogues. Recent data from the Surveillance, Epidemiology, and End Results (SEER) database involving 7744 patients with WM showed that the relative survival of patients with WM has improved over time. Patients diagnosed during 2001–2010 had higher 5-year (78% vs. 67%) and 10-year (66% vs. 49%) relative survival rates versus patients diagnosed during 1980–2000. A Greek study that included 345 patients with WM failed to show any overall or cause-specific survival improvement in recent years, though the study might have been underpowered to detect any expected benefit.[196] A Swedish study of 1555 patients diagnosed with WM between 1980 and 2005 showed that the 5-year relative survival rate improved from 57% in 1980–1985 to 78% in 2001–2005.[198]

REFERENCES

For the complete list of references, log on to www.expertconsult.com.

SUGGESTED READINGS

Ansell SM, Hodge LS, Secreto FJ, et al: Activation of TAK1 by MYD88 L265P drives malignant B-cell growth in non-Hodgkin lymphoma. *Blood Cancer J* 4:e183, 2014.

Braggio E, Keats JJ, Leleu X, et al: Identification of copy number abnormalities and inactivating mutations in two negative regulators of nuclear factor-κB signaling pathways in Waldenström's macroglobulinemia. *Cancer Res* 69:3579, 2009.

Cao Y, Hunter ZR, Liu X, et al: The WHIM-like CXCR4^S338X somatic mutation activates AKT and ERK, and promotes resistance to ibrutinib and other agents used in the treatment of Waldenström's macroglobulinemia. *Leukemia* 29:169, 2015.

Castillo JJ, Olszewski A, Cronin AM, et al: Survival trends in Waldenström macroglobulinemia: an analysis of the Surveillance, Epidemiology and End Results database. *Blood* 123:3999, 2014.

Castillo JJ, Treon SP, Davids MS: Inhibition of the Bruton tyrosine kinase pathway in B-cell lymphoproliferative disorders. *Cancer J* 22:34, 2016.

Dimopoulos MA, Kastritis E, Owen RG, et al: Treatment recommendations for patients with Waldenström macroglobulinemia (WM) and related disorders: IWWM-7 consensus. *Blood* 124:1404, 2014.

Ho AW, Hatjiharissi E, Ciccarelli BT, et al: CD27-CD70 interactions in the pathogenesis of Waldenström macroglobulinemia. *Blood* 112:4683, 2008.

Hunter ZR, Xu L, Yang G, et al: The genomic landscape of Waldenstom's macroglobulinemia is characterized by highly recurring MYD88 and WHIM-like CXCR4 mutations, and small somatic deletions associated with B-cell lymphomagenesis. *Blood* 123:1637, 2014.

Jiménez C, Sebastián E, Del Carmen Chillón M, et al: MYD88 L265P is a marker highly characteristic of, but not restricted to, Waldenström's macroglobulinemia. *Leukemia* 27:1722, 2013.

Kastritis S, Kyrtsonis MC, Hatjiharissi E, et al: No significant improvement in the outcome of patients with Waldenström macroglobulinemia treated over the last 25 years. *Am J Hematol* 86:479, 2011.

Kristinsson SY, Eloranta S, Dickman PW, et al: Patterns of survival in lymphoplasmacytic lymphoma/Waldenström macroglobulinemia: a population based study of 1,555 patients diagnosed in Sweden from 1980 to 2005. *Am J Hematol* 88:60, 2013.

Kyle RA, Treon SP, Alexanian R, et al: Prognostic markers and criteria to initiate therapy in Waldenström's macroglobulinemia: consensus panel recommendations from the Second International Workshop on Waldenström's Macroglobulinemia. *Semin Oncol* 30:116, 2003.

Menke MN, Feke GT, McMeel JW, et al: Hyperviscosity-related retinopathy in Waldenström's macroglobulinemia. *Arch Ophthalmol* 124:1601, 2006.

Merlini G, Baldini L, Broglia C, et al: Prognostic factors in symptomatic Waldenström's macroglobulinemia. *Semin Oncol* 30:211, 2003.

Merlini G, Farhangi M, Osserman EF: Monoclonal immunoglobulins with antibody activity in myeloma, macroglobulinemia and related plasma cell dyscrasias. *Semin Oncol* 13:350, 1986.

Morel P, Duhamel A, Gobbi P, et al: International prognostic scoring system for Waldenström macroglobulinemia. *Blood* 113:4163, 2009.

Nobile-Orazio E, Marmiroli P, Baldini L, et al: Peripheral neuropathy in macroglobulinemia: incidence and antigen-specificity of M proteins. *Neurology* 37:1506, 1987.

Nguyen-Khac F, Lambert J, Chapiro E, et al: Chromosomal aberrations and their prognostic value in a series of 174 untreated patients with Waldenström's macroglobulinemia. *Haematologica* 98:649, 2013.

Owen RG, Treon SP, Al-Katib A, et al: Clinicopathological definition of Waldenström's macroglobulinemia: consensus panel recommendations from the Second International Workshop on Waldenström's Macroglobulinemia. *Semin Oncol* 30:110, 2003.

Poulain S, Roumier C, Decambron A, et al: MYD88 L265P mutation in Waldenström's macroglobulinemia. *Blood* 121:4504, 2013.

Roccaro A, Sacco A, Jiminez C, et al: C1013G/CXCR4 acts as a driver mutation of tumor progression and modulator of drug resistance in lymphoplasmacytic lymphoma. *Blood* 123:4120, 2014.

Stone MJ, Bogen SA: Evidence-based focused review of management of hyperviscosity syndrome. *Blood* 119:2205, 2012.

Swerdlow SH, Campo E, Harris NL, et al: *WHO classification of tumours of haematopoietic and lymphoid tissues*, ed 4, Lyon, France, 2008, IARC Press.

Treon SP, Hunter ZR, Aggarwal A, et al: Characterization of familial Waldenström's macroglobulinemia. *Ann Oncol* 17:488, 2006.

Treon SP, Xu L, Yang G, et al: MYD88 L265P somatic mutation in Waldenström's macroglobulinemia. *N Engl J Med* 367:826, 2012.

Treon SP, Cao Y, Xu L, et al: Somatic mutations in MYD88 and CXCR4 are determinants of clinical presentation and overall survival in Waldenström macroglobulinemia. *Blood* 123:2791, 2014.

Treon SP: How I treat Waldenström macroglobulinemia. *Blood* 126:721, 2015.

Treon SP, Tripsas CK, Meid K, et al: Ibrutinib in previously treated Waldenström's macroglobulinemia. *N Engl J Med* 372:1430, 2015.

Varettoni M, Arcaini L, Zibellini S, et al: Prevalence and clinical significance of the MYD88 L265P somatic mutation in Waldenström macroglobulinemia, and related lymphoid neoplasms. *Blood* 121:2522, 2013.

Xu L, Hunter Z, Yang G, et al: MYD88 L265P in Waldenström macroglobulinemia, immunoglobulin M monoclonal gammopathy, and other B-cell lymphoproliferative disorders using conventional and quantitative allele-specific polymerase chain reaction. *Blood* 121:2051, 2013.

Yang G, Zhou Y, Liu X, et al: A mutation in MYD88 (L265P) supports the survival of lymphoplasmacytic cells by activation of Bruton tyrosine kinase in Waldenström macroglobulinemia. *Blood* 122:1222, 2013.

IMMUNOGLOBULIN LIGHT CHAIN AMYLOIDOSIS (PRIMARY AMYLOIDOSIS)

Morie A. Gertz, Francis K. Buadi, Martha Q. Lacy, and Suzanne R. Hayman

Amyloidosis is defined as the clinical syndrome associated with deposition of amyloid. Amyloid in tissue is defined by its tinctorial properties of a homogeneous, eosinophilic, hyaline material when viewed by hematoxylin and eosin staining. Amyloid stains specifically with Congo red, demonstrating a deep pink amorphous composition. Although Congo red staining is the sine qua non for the diagnosis of amyloid, many pathology laboratories prefer the use of sulfated Alcian blue or crystal violet for screening. A second requirement is that the Congo red–positive histologic finding must demonstrate apple-green birefringence when observed under polarized light.

The term *amyloid* is a misnomer. The term was first used in 1838 by a German botanist because the tissue stained blue with iodine and was incorrectly thought to be starch-like, thus the terminology *amyloid*. In Vienna, Rokitansky believed that the material was not starch but rather of lipid composition and used the term *lardaceous degeneration* for amyloid. Both were incorrect because all forms of amyloid appear to be protein-derived.

By electron microscopy, amyloid has been shown to be fibrillar in origin with an approximate diameter of 9.5 nm and as being linear nonbranching and comprised of protofilaments (Fig. 88.1). The Congo red binding occurs because the protein misfolds from the physiologic configuration of the α-helix into a β-pleated sheet, which is directly responsible for its insolubility and resistance to proteolysis. Amyloid is highly resistant to solubilization unless it is subjected to the harshest denaturation conditions. This insolubility in physiologic solution likely contributes to amyloid's ability to disrupt normal organ function and leads to the clinical disease amyloidosis, the clinical syndrome associated with deposition of amyloid.

EPIDEMIOLOGY

The incidence of immunoglobulin light-chain amyloidosis is estimated to be approximately 8 per 1 million per year. It is the cause of death in 0.58 of 1000 recorded deaths and is responsible for 0.8% of end-stage renal disease. At Mayo Clinic, amyloid light-chain (AL) amyloidosis represents 9% of all patients seen with monoclonal gammopathies. AL amyloidosis represents 60% of all patients seen with amyloidosis. However, hereditary amyloidosis now accounts for 10% of patients, localized amyloidosis 8.5% of patients, senile systemic amyloidosis 18% of patients, and secondary amyloidosis 2.5% of patients. All these forms of amyloidosis have the same tinctorial properties in histologic section and must be distinguished using other techniques.

The cause of the plasma cell dyscrasia that underlies light-chain amyloidosis remains unknown. There does not appear to be a linkage to any specific occupation or toxic chemical exposure. No environmental agents have been linked to the development of amyloidosis. However, the Veterans Administration in the United States considers amyloidosis in a veteran who was exposed to Agent Orange during the Vietnam era to have a service-connected illness.

Amyloidosis may be systemic or localized. The localized forms generally do not require any systemic chemotherapy. The distinction is, therefore, important so that patients for whom chemotherapy will not benefit are not inappropriately subjected to this form of therapy. Localized amyloidosis can be suspected, usually based on the location

of the deposits, as discussed in the "Clinical Manifestations" section below.

Familial amyloidosis is, for most patients, caused by an inherited mutation of transthyretin (TTR). It is difficult to distinguish from light-chain amyloidosis because the clinical manifestations may be quite similar. Other inherited forms of amyloidosis have been associated with apolipoprotein A1 mutations, fibrinogen A α mutations, and mutations of gelsolin.

Secondary systemic amyloidosis is amyloidosis that is usually a consequence of a sustained inflammatory process. The frequency of symptomatic secondary systemic amyloidosis has been in sharp decline for the past decade. Previously, secondary systemic amyloidosis was a consequence of an uncontrolled inflammatory process, typically inflammatory polyarthropathies such as juvenile rheumatoid arthritis, psoriatic arthritis, or ankylosing spondylitis. Another cause was long-standing inflammatory bowel disease. Amyloidosis as a consequence of these inflammatory processes has fallen sharply with the introduction of biologic agents that function as inhibitors of interleukin-1, interleukin-6, and inhibitors of tumor necrosis factor α (TNF-α). The ability to control these sustained inflammatory processes has resulted in the sharp decline in the recognition of secondary systemic amyloidosis. Sporadic patients are seen with multiple cutaneous abscesses, usually as a result of subcutaneous injection of contaminated narcotics. Patients can also be seen with chronic infections related to paraplegia or quadriplegia. Rare patients with lifelong bronchiectasis related to cystic fibrosis can develop systemic amyloidosis. There are also forms of inherited secondary amyloidosis associated with familial inflammatory syndromes such as familial Mediterranean fever or mutations of the TNF receptor gene (so-called TNF receptor–associated periodic syndrome).

PATHOBIOLOGY OF THE DISEASE

In immunoglobulin light-chain amyloidosis, the immunoglobulin fragments have specific thermodynamic instability that causes them to misfold into the insoluble amyloid configuration. The injection of immunoglobulin light chains purified from the urine of patients with multiple myeloma will not produce amyloid when injected into mice. However, when the light chains are extracted from the urine of patients with light-chain amyloidosis and injected into mice, it will produce amyloid deposits and organ dysfunction, suggesting that the specifics of the immunoglobulin light chain are important in determining its propensity to misfold into amyloid. Monoclonal immunoglobulin light chains can be converted in vitro to amyloid by in vitro digestion with pepsin. Historically, before it was clearly understood that amyloidosis was derived from a plasma cell dyscrasia with the development of "toxic" immunoglobulin light chains, the term *primary amyloidosis* was used as a consequence of the lack of understanding of the pathophysiology. This term should be abandoned, and the term *immunoglobulin light-chain amyloidosis* or *AL amyloidosis* (amyloid light chain) should be used. Many forms of localized amyloidosis are also derived from immunoglobulin light chains, but there is no evidence of a systemic plasma cell dyscrasia, and systemic therapy is contraindicated. Virtually all patients with systemic AL amyloidosis have a demonstrable clonal plasma cell disorder. In

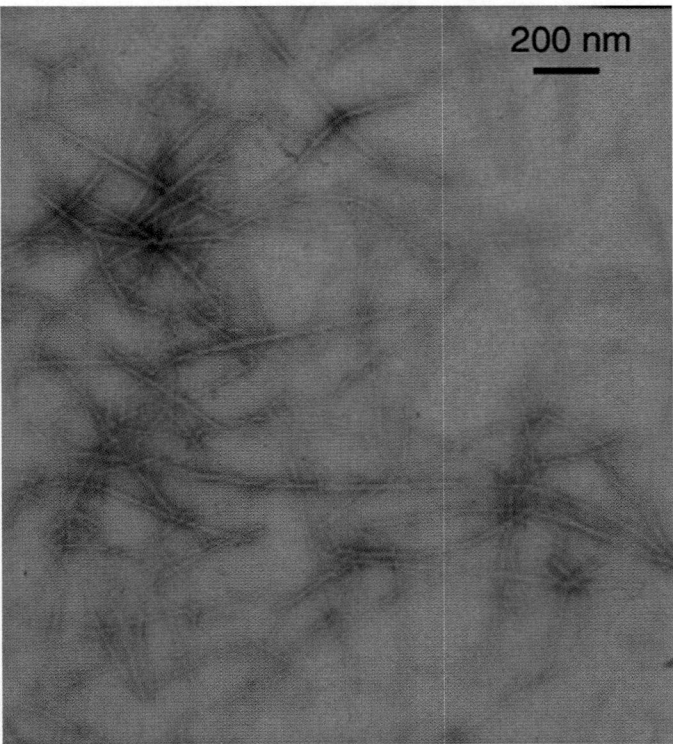

Fig. 88.1 ELECTRON MICROGRAPH DEMONSTRATING THE CLASSIC FIBRILS OF AMYLOID.

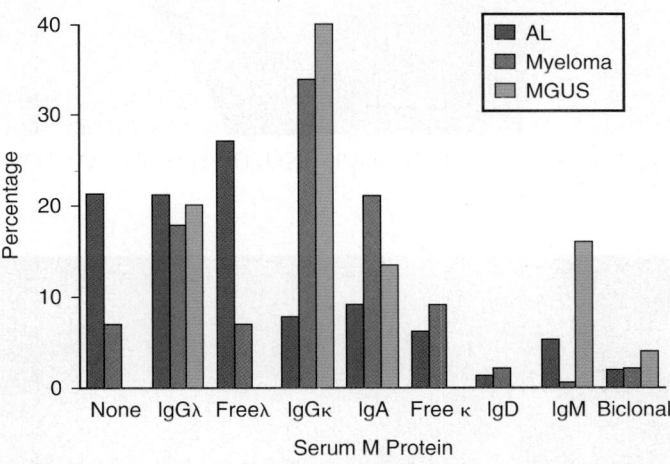

Fig. 88.2 DISTRIBUTION OF HEAVY- AND LIGHT-CHAIN PROTEINS IN MYELOMA, MONOCLONAL GAMMOPATHY OF UNDETERMINED SIGNIFICANCE, AND AMYLOID LIGHT-CHAIN AMYLOIDOSIS. *AL,* Amyloid light chain; *Ig,* Immunoglobulin; *MGUS,* monoclonal gammopathy of undetermined significance.

monoclonal gammopathy of undetermined significance (MGUS) and multiple myeloma, two-thirds of the immunoglobulin light chains are κ type. In AL amyloidosis, nearly three-fourths of the light chains are of λ origin (Fig. 88.2), suggesting that there is a greater propensity for λ light chains to misfold into amyloid configuration. The λ$_6$ subgroup of light chains is exclusively associated with amyloid deposition. There are also abnormalities in amyloid-associated germline gene use. A preferential use of variable lambda (VL) germline genes is noted for AL κ and AL λ patients. There is a significant correlation between the use of V λ$_6$ germline, 6a, and renal involvement as well as the λ$_3$ gene, 3r, with soft tissue AL. Identification of the clonal VL gene in AL has important implications regarding clinical outcome.

Chromosomal aberrations of the plasma cells in amyloidosis have also been recognized. Interphase fluorescence in situ hybridization (FISH) has detected a gain of 1q21, predicting a poor overall survival, and is an independent prognostic factor. Patients with t(11;14) have a longer median overall survival. Deletion 13q14 and hyperdiploidy are prognostically neutral.

The pathobiology of organ dysfunction associated with amyloidosis has long been assumed to be caused by the direct effect of amyloid protein deposition in tissues. However, there is increasing evidence that the light chains themselves have a toxic effect on tissues as a soluble mediator. A zebrafish model of human light-chain cardiotoxicity has demonstrated that injection of light chains results in impaired cardiac function, pericardial edema, and increased cell death. Mitogen-activated protein (MAP) kinase activation may mediate this cardiotoxicity, and p38 MAP kinase inhibition reduces cell death and improves cardiac function.

Amyloidosis and multiple myeloma both share the presence in the bone marrow of a clonal population of plasma cells. The number of plasma cells and the immunoglobulin light chains that they produce are both important for prognosis. Patients who have an increased number of plasma cells in the bone marrow with light-chain amyloidosis have a worse prognosis and a shorter overall survival, regardless of whether they manifest any of the clinical criteria associated with multiple myeloma, such as hypercalcemia, renal insufficiency, anemia, or destructive bone lesions. There appears to be no survival difference between patients who have an elevated plasma cell count in their bone marrow and whether they have overt symptoms of myeloma. The therapeutic import of this finding is still being investigated.

CLINICAL MANIFESTATIONS

Patient 1

Patient 1 is a 46-year-old man who, 10 months prior to diagnosis, began to develop cramping abdominal pain associated with an unexplained 45-lb weight loss. Four months later, he began to develop episodes of orthostatic syncope and was documented to have an orthostatic drop in blood pressure from systolic 110 mmHg in supine to 66 mmHg when standing. As a consequence of his abdominal cramping, the patient underwent endoscopy and colonoscopy. Biopsies were obtained from the duodenum, proximal jejunum, colon, and rectum, all of which demonstrated amyloid deposits. Subsequently, a bone marrow biopsy was performed that showed 4% clonal plasma cells. A subcutaneous fat aspirate was positive for amyloid. The plasma cells showed a CCND1/IgH fusion t(11;14). The patient's hemoglobin level was normal, as were his creatinine, alkaline phosphatase, and urinary protein. The patient had a λ free light chain level of 92.8 mg/L, κ free light chain of 10.9 mg/L, and a ratio of 0.12.

Comment on Patient 1

This patient presented with amyloid autonomic neuropathy, leading to gastrointestinal (GI) tract dysmotility and pain as well as orthostatic hypotension. There was clear-cut evidence of a low-grade plasma cell dyscrasia. Orthostatic hypotension causing lightheadedness is a very nonspecific complaint, and syncope owing to amyloid orthostatic hypotension is easily overlooked because of its infrequency.

Patient 2

A 61-year-old man with a known immunoglobulin G λ MGUS of 0.6 mg/dL was monitored on an annual basis with no change in the level of the monoclonal protein over a period of 3 years. He developed progressive fatigue and shortness of breath. He was evaluated by a cardiologist, and his echocardiogram showed thickening that was interpreted to be related to hypertension, with a normal ejection fraction. The patient was placed on lisinopril and did not improve. He returned and underwent catheterization with coronary angiography. His coronary arteries were normal, and he was diagnosed with deconditioning. His dyspnea continued, and he was referred to a pulmonologist, who recognized the long-standing monoclonal gammopathy and obtained light chain studies that showed a λ light chain of 41 mg/dL and κ of 10 mg/dL. The patient underwent a subcutaneous fat aspiration that demonstrated amyloid deposits, which, by mass spectroscopy, were found to be of λ origin. At this point, the patient had New York Heart Association class IV heart failure; he died within 3 months thereafter.

Comment on Patient 2

This case is an example of a classic failure to recognize that patients with monoclonal gammopathies should have amyloidosis included in the differential diagnosis. The fact that the monoclonal protein was stable would certainly argue against the development of multiple myeloma, but light-chain amyloidosis regularly occurs without any change in the M component over time. The failure to recognize the patient's progressive fatigue and shortness of breath as cardiac amyloid is not unusual. The echocardiographic findings of thickening were interpreted as being caused by hypertension, but, in fact, they were caused by infiltrative cardiomyopathy, and the cardiac catheterization and angiogram without an endomyocardial biopsy led to a missed diagnosis. Only an increased index of suspicion in patients with a known monoclonal protein allowed this diagnosis to be confirmed.

One of the major difficulties in the diagnosis of amyloidosis is that there is virtually no blood test or imaging study that is diagnostic of the disease. The most common symptoms associated with amyloidosis are fatigue, lower extremity edema (may be cardiac or renal), unexplained weight loss (often leading to search for occult malignancy), exertional dyspnea, orthostatic hypotension, and paresthesias. These symptoms are quite vague, and in a general medical practice, there are hundreds of disorders that are far more common and are responsible for light-chain amyloidosis. As noticed in Patient 2, the fatigue, which is often caused by early cardiac amyloid but is not associated with overt congestive heart failure, can be missed. Cardiac amyloidosis is a classic form of heart failure with preserved ejection fraction owing to the restrictive physiology associated with amyloidosis.

Edema in amyloidosis may be a manifestation of high right-sided filling pressures, leading to lower extremity edema, or it may be a consequence of renal involvement with the nephrotic syndrome (peripheral edema, hypoalbuminemia, hyperlipidemia, and proteinuria). Even when nephrotic range proteinuria is seen, amyloidosis, which is known to cause nephrotic syndrome in 10% of adults who are nondiabetic, is infrequently considered in the differential diagnosis, which would include minimal change glomerulopathy, as well as membranous and membranoproliferative glomerulopathy.

The physical findings that are known to be associated with light-chain amyloidosis include enlargement of the tongue (15%) (Fig. 88.3) and periorbital purpura (12%). These findings are highly specific when recognized. However, although they are highly specific, they lack sensitivity because nearly 80% of patients with amyloidosis lack both of these physical features. It is common for an enlarged tongue in amyloid to be misdiagnosed as suspect glossal cancer or a manifestation of acromegaly. Many patients with significant tongue enlargement needlessly undergo a painful and often hemorrhagic tongue biopsy, which could be avoided if the diagnosis was considered. Patients with enlargement of the tongue frequently have major indentations on the underside of their tongue from their teeth and from the continuous pressure that the tongue exerts against their lower jaw. The purpura is also quite specific, and the patient often will note the development of purpura simply by rubbing of the eyelids. However, these patients often undergo an evaluation for a coagulation disorder or are simply reassured that purpura is benign, and the physical findings do not trigger an investigation for light-chain amyloidosis (Fig. 88.4).

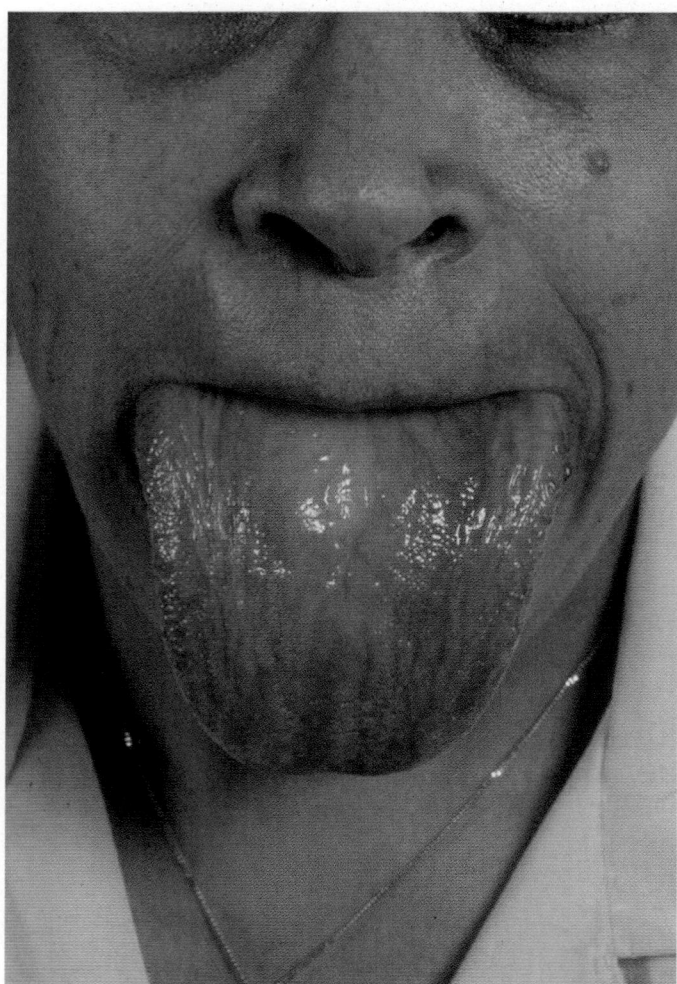

Fig. 88.3 ENLARGED TONGUE INFILTRATED BY AMYLOID DEPOSITS.

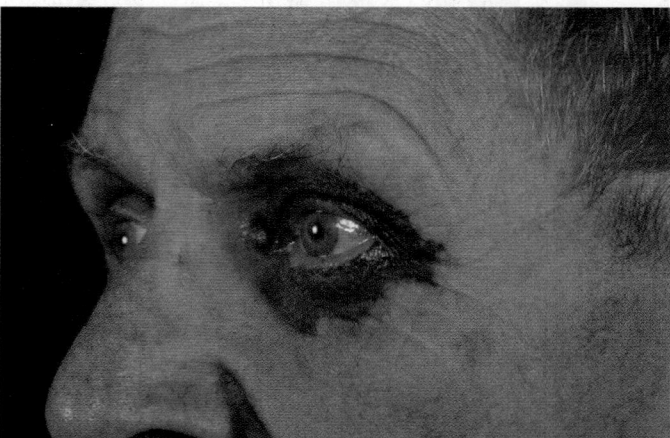

Fig. 88.4 CLASSIC AMYLOID PURPURA.

Hepatomegaly is seen in approximately 10% of patients with amyloidosis, but it is nonspecific, and imaging of the liver will show homogeneous enlargement without filling defects. Occasionally, patients will have widespread vascular amyloid that will result in claudication of the calf, buttock, upper extremities, and jaw. Occasionally, these patients will undergo temporal artery biopsy, which, when appropriately stained, will show amyloid. More often, these patients will be given an empiric diagnosis of polymyalgia rheumatica and be placed on corticosteroids without appropriate screening. The rarest physical finding in amyloidosis is periarticular infiltration of the synovium in the upper extremities, leading to the "shoulder pad" sign. This causes a continuous, chronic, low-grade pain caused by the periarticular infiltration. Diagnosis in this setting requires arthrocentesis and the demonstration of Congo red–positive deposits in the synovial fluid.

LABORATORY MANIFESTATIONS

If the symptoms of amyloidosis are so vague as not to be helpful and the physical findings are specific but not sensitive, when should a clinician suspect amyloidosis and aggressively pursue this rare disorder? Amyloidosis should be considered in any patient who presents with (1) nephrotic range proteinuria; (2) fatigue, which may have a cardiac basis, including heart failure with preserved ejection fraction or restrictive cardiomyopathy; (3) unexplained hepatomegaly; (4) a peripheral neuropathy resembling chronic inflammatory demyelinating polyneuropathy (CIDP); and (5) "atypical" multiple myeloma or MGUS with unexplained fatigue, weight loss, and edema. Consulting patients with any one of these five syndromes should lead to the placement of light-chain amyloid in the differential diagnosis, and screening should commence.

Because all patients with systemic immunoglobulin light-chain amyloidosis have a plasma cell dyscrasia, the initial step should be screening by performing immunofixation of the serum, immunofixation of the urine, and an immunoglobulin free light-chain assay. Results of one of these three tests will be abnormal in 99% of patients with light-chain amyloidosis. If results of these three tests are negative, the likelihood is that one of the following conditions exists: (1) The patient does not have amyloidosis; (2) the chance of immunoglobulin light-chain amyloidosis is only 1%; (3) the patient has systemic amyloidosis, but it is not of immunoglobulin light-chain origin (familial amyloid or senile systemic amyloid); or (4) the amyloidosis is localized.

Alternatively, if a patient with nephrotic range proteinuria has a monoclonal protein or an abnormal free light-chain ratio, the diagnosis, which often includes minimal change glomerulopathy and membranoproliferative glomerulopathy, suddenly shifts to either (1) myeloma cast nephropathy, (2) immunoglobulin light-chain amyloidosis of the kidney (Fig. 88.5), or (3) κ light-chain deposition disease of the kidney. In this situation, a kidney biopsy could be avoided by doing less invasive diagnostic testing.

In a patient with fatigue, weight loss, or dyspnea on exertion, the finding of an immunoglobulin abnormality raises the suspicion of amyloid. Evaluation can be redirected to include echocardiography with the specific inclusion of Doppler studies that accurately measure the restricted filling that occurs with amyloid infiltration (stiff heart syndrome). It may also include magnetic resonance imaging of the heart, which can show distinct endomyocardial enhancement following gadolinium injection, as well as myocardial nulling, which is specific for light-chain amyloidosis.

A patient with unexplained hepatomegaly who has a monoclonal protein can often avoid a liver biopsy, which rarely is associated with bleeding and occasionally with hepatic rupture. Fat aspiration is positive in over 75% of patients with hepatic amyloidosis.

In a patient with peripheral neuropathy who is found to have a monoclonal protein, consideration of amyloidosis in the differential diagnosis can prevent interventions such as plasma exchange or intravenous immunoglobulin infusions, which are ineffective in patients with light-chain amyloidosis but are often attempted in patients who have a monoclonal gammopathy and a peripheral neuropathy (presumed CIDP) if amyloidosis is not considered in the differential diagnosis.

All patients with MGUS need to be monitored for life for the development of myeloma and amyloidosis. Over 25 years, approximately 25% of patients will go on to develop a more serious plasma cell dyscrasia. In 21%, this represents multiple myeloma, but 4% of patients with MGUS will develop light-chain amyloidosis during the course of observation. If screening is limited to detection of changes consistent with multiple myeloma, such as anemia, bone pain, and hypercalcemia, amyloidosis will be overlooked because all three of these findings are unusual in light-chain amyloidosis. Patient 2, described above, was being followed by a hematologist for a monoclonal gammopathy, and when he developed fatigue in the absence of progressive anemia, amyloidosis was not considered.

Any patient with one of the five compatible clinical syndromes listed in Table 88.1 should be screened for monoclonal protein. If a monoclonal protein is not found, the likelihood of light-chain amyloidosis is very small. However, if a monoclonal gammopathy exists with an appropriate clinical syndrome, histologic demonstration of amyloid should be sought.

In patients who have renal, cardiac, hepatic, and peripheral nerve amyloid, biopsy of the affected organs has a very high sensitivity of demonstrating amyloid. However, these biopsies are not required if amyloid is considered in the differential diagnosis.

The first diagnostic studies that should be performed in patients with a compatible clinical syndrome and an immunoglobulin light-chain abnormality are a subcutaneous fat aspirate and a bone marrow biopsy. Subcutaneous fat aspirate in an experienced laboratory will demonstrate amyloid deposits in 75% of patients tested (Fig. 88.6). In a patient with light-chain amyloidosis, staining of the bone marrow biopsy for amyloid deposition in blood vessels is positive in 50%. A second advantage of the bone marrow biopsy is it provides the percentage of plasma cells in the bone marrow, which is prognostic and is an essential evaluation in patients with immunoglobulin light-chain abnormalities. When combining the subcutaneous fat aspirate and the bone marrow biopsy, nearly 85% of patients with light-chain amyloidosis will be identified. For the remaining 15%, direct biopsy of the involved organ would be indicated if the index of suspicion for light-chain amyloidosis remained high. Other centers have

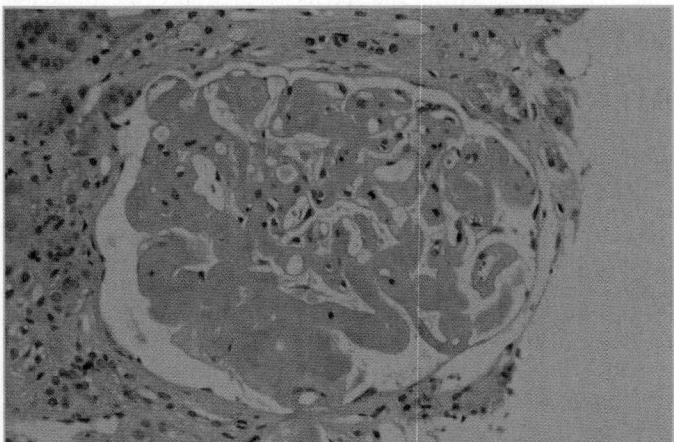

Fig. 88.5 RENAL BIOPSY SHOWING AMORPHOUS HYALINE MATERIAL CONSISTENT WITH AMYLOID. (Original magnification, ×1000.)

TABLE 88.1	Syndromes in Primary Amyloidosis
Syndrome	**Patients (%)**
Nephrotic or nephrotic and renal failure	30
Hepatomegaly	24
Congestive heart failure	22
Carpal tunnel	21
Neuropathy	17
Orthostatic hypotension	12

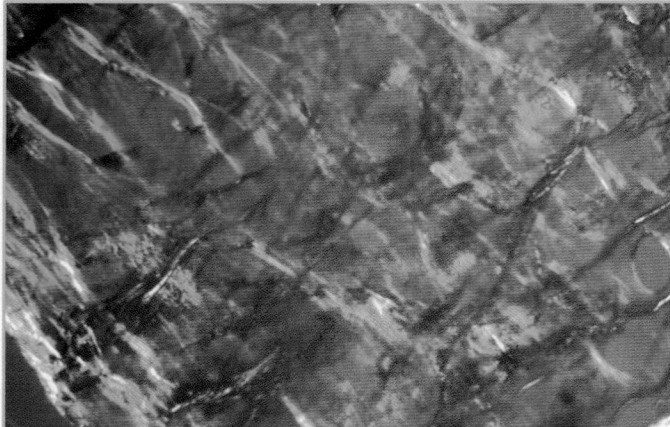

Fig. 88.6 FAT ASPIRATION. (Congo red stain; original magnification, ×1000.) Note preserved fat cell interstices.

TABLE 88.2	Nomenclature of Amyloidosis	
Protein	**Precursor**	**Clinical Characteristics**
AL or AH	Immunoglobulin light or heavy chain	Primary or localized; myeloma or macroglobulinemia associated
AA	SAA	Secondary or familial Mediterranean fever, familial periodic fever syndromes
ATTR	Transthyretin	Familial and senile
A fibrinogen	Fibrinogen	Familial renal amyloidosis (Ostertag type)
Aβ$_2$M	β$_2$-Microglobulin	Dialysis associated; carpal tunnel syndrome
Aβ	ABPP	Alzheimer disease
A Apo A-I/A-II	Apolipoprotein A-I Apolipoprotein A-II	Proteinuria Cardiac Neuropathy
A lysozyme	Lysozyme	GI tract Liver Renal
ALECT2	Renal	

AA, Amyloid A; *Aβ,* amyloid-β; *ABPP,* amyloid-β precursor protein; *Aβ$_2$M,* β$_2$-microglobulin-related amyloid; *AH,* amyloid heavy chain; *AL,* amyloid light chain; *ALECT2,* leukocyte chemotactic factor 2 amyloidosis; *Apo,* apolipoprotein; *ATTR,* transthyretin-related hereditary amyloidosis; *GI,* gastrointestinal; *SAA,* serum amyloid A.

reported success with biopsies of the minor submandibular salivary gland, skin biopsies, and endoscopic biopsies of the stomach. These procedures would be best undertaken in laboratories where there is extensive experience in the processing and staining of amyloid tissues.

Once amyloid has been demonstrated in histologic sections, it is imperative that the amyloid be typed to ensure it is of immunoglobulin light-chain origin because of the critical therapeutic implications. Although immunoglobulin light-chain amyloidosis is always associated with a monoclonal gammopathy, it is important to recognize that monoclonal gammopathies are common in the elderly population. On screening, 3% of adult patients over the age of 50 will have a monoclonal protein, and 5% of those over the age of 80 will have a monoclonal protein. Therefore, it is possible to have a positive biopsy for amyloid and a coincidental monoclonal protein when the amyloid itself is unrelated to immunoglobulin light-chain amyloidosis. Thus, when a pathologist reports amyloid-laden tissue, the task will not be complete until the specific type of amyloid is identified (Table 88.2). Historically immunohistochemistry was used to classify amyloid. This technique is being used less. First, the type of amyloid can be identified only if the appropriate antibodies are used. In patients with amyloid deposition, it would be very challenging to diagnose dialysis-related amyloid (β$_2$-microglobulin type), insulin-type amyloid (found at the sites of insulin injection in diabetics), keratin amyloid (seen in skin biopsies), or TTR amyloid (seen in senile systemic amyloid). Most laboratories are not equipped with such a broad panel of antibodies. Second, even when light-chain amyloidosis exists, the use of anti-κ and anti-λ antibodies frequently will not be able to identify the type of amyloid in tissue section. There are two widely held hypotheses for this lack of sensitivity of immunohistochemistry in AL amyloidosis.

The first hypothesis is a reflection of the immunoglobulin in amyloid deposits. The light chain in amyloid is usually not the intact immunoglobulin light chain but usually represents a fragment. The average AL is approximately 12 kDa, approximately half the molecular weight of an intact immunoglobulin light chain. In most of these proteins, the constant portion of the light chain has been deleted. Most commercial antisera used in immunohistochemistry recognize the constant portion of the immunoglobulin light chain and, therefore, have no recognizable binding sites on the AL, owing to the deletions its undergoes as it is deposited.

The second hypothesis is that the immunoglobulin light chain, by definition, has undergone misfolding as it assumes the amyloid configuration in tissues. This misfolding can lead to the loss of available epitopes on the protein surface that commercial antisera bind to. It is for these reasons that it is common for immunohistochemistry, even in light-chain amyloidosis, to be equivocal or difficult to distinguish from background staining. At Mayo Clinic, immunohistochemistry has been abandoned as a modality to diagnose the

type of amyloidosis. Currently laser capture microdissection with mass spectroscopic analysis of amyloid deposits has supplanted immunohistochemistry in our practice. Amyloid deposits can be excised by laser microdissection directly from a glass slide and then can undergo mass spectroscopic sequencing. The results are compared with a library of proteins stored in a database and then identified. Virtually all amyloid proteins contain serum amyloid P protein, apolipoprotein E, and vitronectin. These findings are confirmatory of amyloid but are ancillary proteins and are not the specific primary protein. In patients with amyloidosis, sequencing will identify the specific protein composition. In a survey of over 4000 tissues, light chains were detected by mass spectroscopic analysis in 61.68%, but 24.5% were transthyretin-related hereditary amyloidosis, 3.7% were amyloid A, 3.6% were leukocyte chemotactic factor 2 amyloidosis (ALECT2) (renal amyloidosis in Mexican and Indian patients), insulin 1% (localized in diabetic), and the remaining comprised <1%. Due to its high sensitivity and specificity, mass spectroscopy is now our technique of choice.

In a survey of 143 heart biopsies, of which 81 were TTR (familial or senile systemic amyloid), an M protein was found in 20 patients, and free light chain abnormality was found in 8 of the 81 patients, indicating that the finding of an immunoglobulin protein does not prove that amyloidosis is AL in origin. Because senile systemic amyloidosis is a disease that causes heart failure in the elderly, the finding of a high prevalence of immunoglobulin abnormalities as a coincidental observation is not unusual. Box 88.1 provides a list of the diagnostic tests needed to evaluate in patients for whom amyloidosis is established as a diagnosis.

Other required diagnostic studies in patients with amyloidosis include cardiac biomarkers, which are extensively discussed in the section below on prognosis and screening measurements of the coagulation system. A unique and highly specific finding, albeit limited to no more than 5% of patients with light chain amyloidosis, is the development of deficiency of coagulation factor X. This is usually recognized as prolongation of the prothrombin time. The underlying mechanism of factor X deficiency in amyloidosis is direct binding of factor X to the amyloid deposit itself, which can

- CBC
- Sodium, potassium, alkaline phosphatase, calcium, phosphorus, AST, bilirubin, creatinine, β_2-microglobulin, glucose, cholesterol, uric acid, thyroid profile
- Immunofixation; serum; immunofixation urine; nephelometric assay if immunoglobulin free light chains; immunoglobulins G, A, and M
- Troponin, NT-proBNP
- Factor X and prothrombin time
- Chest x-ray, EKG, echocardiogram with Doppler and strain imaging
- Cardiac MRI (optional selected situations)
- Bone marrow with FISH genetics, Congo red stain of marrow
- Fat aspiration
- Creatinine clearance

AST, Aspartate transaminase; *CBC*, complete blood count; *EKG*, electrocardiogram; *FISH*, fluorescence in situ hybridization; *NT-proBNP*, N-terminal pro-B-type natriuretic peptide; *MRI*, magnetic resonance imaging.

occasionally be associated with serious clinical bleeding and can complicate the systemic therapy of this disorder. If a prothrombin time is completely normal, it is not our habit to routinely screen for factor X deficiency, but any abnormality of the prothrombin time or international normalized ratio should lead to a screening for factor X deficiency, given its unique association with light chain amyloid. In our experience, factor X deficiency is most commonly seen in patients with hepatosplenic deposits of amyloid.

DIFFERENTIAL DIAGNOSIS

The path to the diagnosis of amyloid depends on the initial presentation. Many patients will present to a hematologist because of a monoclonal gammopathy and >10% plasma cells in the bone marrow, which will fulfill the diagnostic criteria for myeloma, even though the clinical manifestations and the drivers of outcome could all be related to amyloidosis. It therefore is incumbent upon practicing hematologists who see a patient with multiple myeloma or MGUS to inquire about progressive fatigue out of proportion to any anemia, intractable edema, unexplained elevation of the serum alkaline phosphatase, or the presence of a peripheral neuropathy. The index of suspicion should be heightened if the monoclonal gammopathy is of λ type relative to κ type because of the stronger association with light chain amyloidosis. Any of these findings should lead to staining of the bone marrow biopsy for Congo red and the performance of subcutaneous fat aspiration. If the fatigue is significant, echocardiography, specifically to look for amyloid, is indicated.

Conversely, any patient with a known cardiomyopathy should be screened with serum and urine immunofixation and immunoglobulin light-chain assay because a positive result will redirect the evaluation toward amyloidosis. Any patient with albuminuria and a light chain should not be assumed to have myeloma cast nephropathy. Rather, the pattern of the urinary protein, whether albumin-dominant or globulin-dominant, can help distinguish between the two syndromes. In a patient with a peripheral neuropathy and a monoclonal protein, it should not be assumed that this is MGUS neuropathy; rather, screening for amyloidosis, in the presence of associated autonomic neuropathy (rare in MGUS neuropathy, 20% of AL amyloidosis) or concomitant carpal tunnel syndrome (50% of amyloid neuropathy patients, uncommon in MGUS neuropathy) is required.

Excluding Localized Amyloidosis

Localized forms of amyloidosis are characterized by the presence of amyloid deposits in biopsy tissue without systemic organ dysfunction.

The typical sites associated with localized amyloidosis include skin, vocal cord, tracheobronchial tree, ureter, bladder, and urethra. Occasionally, GI biopsies, particularly polyps, or the edges of ulcers will show amyloid deposits and not be reflective of a systemic form of amyloidosis.

In some instances, mass spectroscopic analysis will demonstrate that the amyloid is not of immunoglobulin light-chain origin. However, there are a number of forms of localized amyloidosis that are of immunoglobulin light-chain origin but are not part of a systemic plasma cell dyscrasia. When a deposit is seen and is of light-chain origin but there is no evidence of a clonal plasma cell disorder in the bone marrow, and serum and urine immunofixation and light chain assays are normal, the index of suspicion should be that this is a localized form of amyloid for which systemic therapy is not indicated. Most forms of cutaneous amyloidosis do not require therapeutic intervention. Amyloidosis involving the vocal cords is most commonly treated by endoscopic resection of the deposits or yttrium-aluminium-garnet (YAG) laser vaporization of the deposits. Tracheobronchial amyloid deposits can be treated with laser vaporization of the deposits or, if the deposits extend beyond the reach of the bronchoscope, with external beam radiation, which has been reported to control the amyloid deposits successfully. Amyloids involving the ureter, bladder, and urethra are often diagnosed with a preoperative diagnosis of urothelial malignancy. Surgeons have often treated patients with ureteral resections for suspect transitional cell carcinoma only to find that amyloid is present. Bladder amyloid most commonly manifests with gross hematuria, and endoscopic resection will demonstrate amyloid deposits. Most patients can be controlled via cystoscopic resection and then surveillance. There are occasional patients who require subtotal cystectomy. There is experience with the use of instillation of dimethyl sulfoxide into the urinary bladder. Urethral amyloid can usually be treated with resection to prevent obstruction.

Systemic Forms of Amyloidosis Unrelated to Immunoglobulin Light Chain

The aging of the population is leading to increased recognition of senile systemic amyloidosis (formally known as *senile cardiac amyloidosis*). Autopsy studies in patients over the age of 90 shows that nearly one-third of patients have cardiac amyloid deposits, and approximately half of those deposits were responsible for clinically significant cardiac dysfunction. With the rising age of the population and increased application of echocardiography, it is expected that the recognition of senile systemic amyloid, also known as *native TTR amyloid* or *wild-type TTR amyloid,* will increase. Patients with this form of cardiac amyloidosis can develop congestive heart failure and commonly have conduction system abnormalities, including atrial fibrillation, first-degree heart block, and bundle branch block. The echocardiographic features are similar to those of light-chain amyloidosis, although extreme degrees of infiltration can be seen (septal thicknesses >20 mm), which are uncommon in light-chain amyloidosis. It should never be assumed that a patient with suspect cardiac amyloidosis has light-chain amyloidosis, particularly if the patient is over the age of 70. However, we have seen patients as young as 57 with senile systemic amyloidosis. Moreover, when patients are recognized by mass spectroscopy to have TTR cardiac amyloidosis, sequencing of the *TTR* gene is essential to exclude the possibility of a late-onset inherited form of amyloidosis. This is particularly the case because a specific mutation, ILE-122, is found in 4% of the African American population in the United States and is associated with the development of late-onset cardiac amyloidosis, and we have seen patients with inherited cardiac amyloidosis who have been inappropriately treated with systemic chemotherapy.

Familial amyloidosis represents a small but important subset of patients with systemic amyloidosis. The majority of cases are caused by mutations of TTR and can be recognized by identifying the TTR subunit by mass spectroscopy and by detection of the mutation by sequencing of the *TTR* gene using polymerase chain reaction

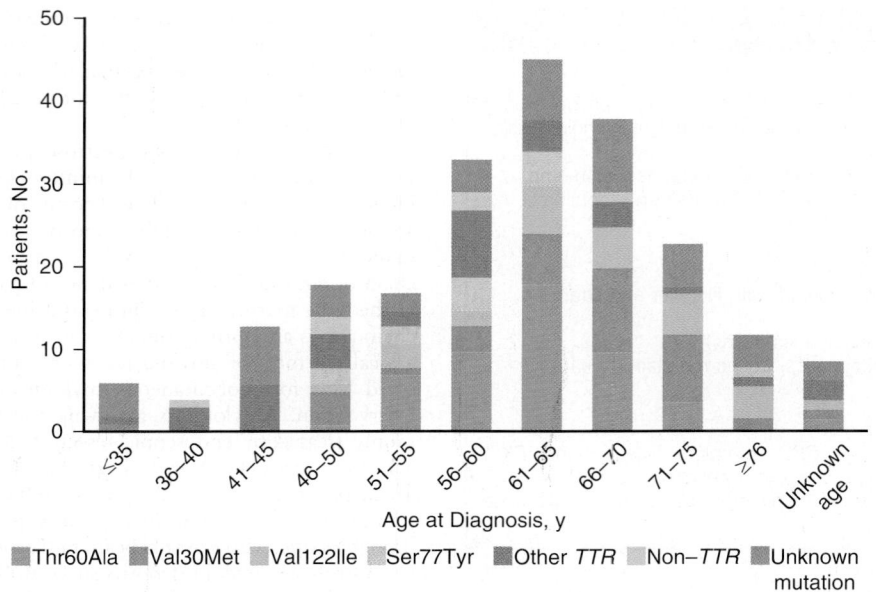

Fig. 88.7 TRANSTHYRETIN MUTATIONS SEEN AT MAYO CLINIC, BY AGE. *TTR,* Transthyretin.

amplification techniques (Fig. 88.7). Clinically, most patients present either with cardiac amyloid or with amyloid peripheral neuropathy and are not easily distinguished clinically from immunoglobulin light chain amyloid. Most of these patients will have no evidence of a systemic plasma cell dyscrasia. Only half of the patients in our practice actually have a positive family history for this autosomal dominantly inherited disorder. In many instances, this is simply because of a failure to recognize in a prior generation and misattribution of the etiology of cardiac death or neural disability.

There are forms of renal amyloidosis that are not immunoglobulin light chain in origin. The two most common are fibrinogen A α and ALECT2. Again, this requires mass spectroscopic identification of these subunit proteins to validate the diagnosis. The distinction for all forms of inherited amyloidosis are important because, in TTR amyloidosis, liver transplant has been demonstrated to be an effective technique; in other forms of non-TTR amyloidosis, organ transplant (renal transplant for apolipoprotein A1 amyloid renal failure) has been used for the management of renal and cardiac failure.

PROGNOSIS

The prognosis of immunoglobulin light-chain amyloidosis has been associated with abnormalities in lactate dehydrogenase, β_2-microglobulin, genetics, circulating plasma cells, the fraction of plasma cells in S-phase, and the serum amyloid P scanning technique. The simplest and most powerful assessments of prognosis revolve around the importance of cardiac amyloid in determining outcome.

The most common cause of death in patients with cardiac amyloidosis is cardiac failure or sudden death, presumed to be caused by arrhythmia. However, the most common cause of death in renal, hepatic, and peripheral nerve amyloid is also cardiac amyloid. The presence of cardiac amyloid predicts for the fraction of patients unable to complete 3 months of therapy and remains responsible for the 1-year mortality of amyloidosis of 40%, which has not changed in 25 years, is the major driver of outcome, and emphasizes why earlier diagnosis of cardiac amyloid is essential to improvement of outcomes for patients with this disease. In addition, the burden of plasma cells, as measured both in the bone marrow and by the levels of involved and uninvolved immunoglobulin light chains in the serum, is key in assessing prognosis. Box 88.2 gives the outcomes for the four stages of immunoglobulin light-chain amyloidosis, based on the measurement of cardiac troponin T, N-terminal pro-brain natriuretic peptide (NT-proBNP), and the difference between the involved

---

BOX 88.2   Amyloid Staging

Patients are assigned a score of 1 point for each of the following:
1. FLC-diff ≥18 mg/dL
2. cTnT ≥0.025 ng/mL
3. NT-proBNP ≥1800 pg/mL
   This creates stages I–IV with scores of 0–3 points, respectively
   Median Survival (months):
   I. 94.1
   II. 40.3
   III. 14
   IV. 5.8
       1. Difference between the involved and uninvolved serum light chain levels
       2. Cardiac troponin T
       3. N-terminal pro-brain natriuretic peptide

cTnT, Cardiac troponin T; *FLC-diff,* difference between involved and uninvolved free light chains; *NT-proBNP,* N-terminal pro-B-type natriuretic peptide.

---

and uninvolved serum free light-chain levels (Box 88.2). These three blood tests have been converted into a very convenient staging system with dramatic differences in prognosis and almost equal distribution of patients into the four stages. Fig. 88.8 shows posttransplant overall survival for the four stages in 444 patients. Other important prognostic features, which are not currently part of the staging system, include echocardiographic Doppler studies of diastolic performance and mitral deceleration time. Echocardiographic strain, which measures the rate at which myocardial shortening occurs, has also been shown to be a powerful measure of outcome. Others have described a systolic blood pressure of <90 mmHg as being adverse, but this has not been effectively incorporated into the current staging system for amyloidosis.

THERAPY

Before one can understand the various therapies, it is important to understand how to interpret response in patients with amyloidosis. In amyloidosis, because there is both a plasma cell dyscrasia and organ dysfunction related to amyloidosis, there are now response criteria for both hematologic and organ responses. Hematologic responses parallel response criteria that have been established for multiple myeloma

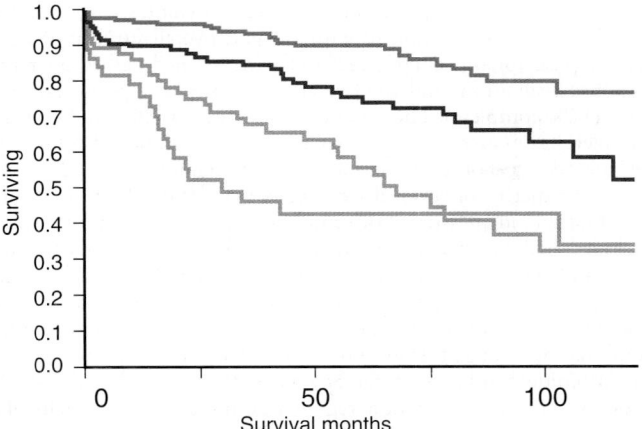

Fig. 88.8 SURVIVAL BY STAGE FOLLOWING STEM CELL TRANSPLANT. *Orange,* stage 1; *dark blue,* stage 2; *light blue,* stage 3; *pink,* stage 4.

and rely heavily on the measurement of the involved and uninvolved immunoglobulin free light chain.

The immunoglobulin free light-chain assay has been summarized earlier as being critical in the recognition of the disease; it has been described as being important in prognosis; and its serial measurement is the key to assessing hematologic response. In fact, when both an intact immunoglobulin is present and an abnormal involved free light chain is detected, the latter is more important prognostically than changes in the intact immunoglobulin and is given preference when interpreting responses in treated patients and for assessment of the role of salvage therapies. A complete hematologic response is defined as a negative serum and urine immunofixation, a normal free light-chain ratio, and a normal bone marrow examination. A very good partial response is now defined as a difference between involved and uninvolved free light chain of <40 mg/L. A partial response is a 50% reduction in the difference between involved and uninvolved serum free light-chain levels, and less than 50% decrease is considered stable disease. A cardiac response in amyloidosis is defined not by changes in the echocardiogram but by changes in the NT-proBNP. A decrease of NT-proBNP of 30% and at least 300 ng/L is considered a response. However, the NT-proBNP level must be >650 ng/L to be considered measurable. The definition of renal response is a 50% reduction in the amount of urinary protein loss over a 24-hour period. This reduction is associated with longer survival. A 75% reduction in proteinuria is associated with markedly prolonged survival.

The therapy for amyloidosis is both supportive care and systemic chemotherapy against the plasma cell dyscrasia. Supportive care for cardiac and renal amyloidosis includes diuretic therapy to help reduce the elevated filling pressures in both the right and left sides of the heart and reduce pulmonary edema, as well as to relieve symptomatic lower extremity edema. Diuretics are also required for the management of the lower extremity edema associated with nephrotic syndrome. Many cardiologists at Mayo Clinic believe that bumetanide is a superior diuretic to furosemide in patients with amyloidosis and prefer it. For refractory edema, the addition of metolazone can be useful, but it can result in serious hypokalemia when combined with furosemide or bumetanide. There is no evidence that the use of lisinopril, as has been applied in the nephrotic syndrome of diabetic nephropathy, plays any role in the management of renal amyloidosis. In addition, afterload reduction, shown to provide survival benefit in patients with ischemic cardiomyopathy, has not been shown to be beneficial in patients with amyloidosis and can significantly aggravate hypotension in patients with poor filling during diastole. Finally, a number of patients in our practice have shown significant deterioration with the addition of β-blockade, and these agents are avoided in our patients as well.

Management of amyloid orthostatic hypotension involves the use of both fludrocortisone and midodrine, which can help reduce

orthostatic syncope but are associated with both fluid retention and supine hypertension, making their use a challenge. The diarrhea associated with GI amyloid is also challenging. It is common for these patients to fail imodium therapy and loperamide. We frequently will use tincture of opium to manage this. In refractory instances where fecal incontinence is common, the placement of a diverting sigmoid colostomy has no impact on the diarrhea but can provide the patient important improved quality of life and social relief.

Chemotherapy Treatment for Light Chain Amyloidosis

The chemotherapy treatment of light-chain amyloidosis requires a determination of whether the patients are candidates for high-dose therapy with stem cell transplant or are best served with conventional chemotherapy regimens.

It is now 40 years since melphalan and prednisone treatment was shown to benefit patients with amyloidosis, and two randomized clinical trials comparing melphalan and prednisone with colchicine regimens demonstrated a response rate of 15% and a 50% increase in median survival in responders. Melphalan has a significant impact on survival in patients without heart failure. The best responses to melphalan-containing regimens are in patients with renal amyloid nephrotic syndrome and preserved renal function.

Dexamethasone in high doses of 40 mg on days 1–4, 9–12, and 17–20 was demonstrated in three individual studies to result in organ improvement in amyloid patients for whom melphalan-containing regimens had failed. Subsequently, the combination of melphalan and dexamethasone was introduced, showing a 50% 5-year survival rate, a hematologic complete response rate of 24%, and organ improvement in 43%. Oral melphalan and dexamethasone can be administered to virtually any patient with amyloidosis and should be considered the standard with which all other therapies are compared. There is a strong correlation between organ improvement and hematologic response. In patients who achieve a hematologic complete response, organ improvement has been seen in 87% of patients. Organ response rates are <15% in the patients who do not achieve a hematologic partial response.

The introduction of proteasome inhibitors and immunomodulatory agents has broadened the horizon for patients with amyloidosis. Initial experience with thalidomide demonstrated that the administration of immunomodulatory drugs to patients with amyloidosis cannot be implemented solely on the basis of experience with multiple myeloma. In an early study of 16 patients with AL amyloidosis treated with thalidomide, grade 3 or greater adverse events were noticed in 50% of patients, including exacerbation of neuropathy and heart failure. When thalidomide was combined with cyclophosphamide and dexamethasone, the hematologic response rates were high, but the toxicity was significant.

Lenalidomide has demonstrated activity in AL as a single agent and in combination with steroids and the alkylating agents cyclophosphamide and melphalan. Lenalidomide appears to be better tolerated than thalidomide but produces significant increases in the NT-proBNP and symptomatic exacerbations of cardiac symptoms. In a phase II trial of 35 patients, 8 of 13 evaluable subjects had a hematologic response, but the maximum tolerated dose of lenalidomide was only 15 mg. Lenalidomide has been used as salvage therapy in patients who have progressed after melphalan, dexamethasone, and bortezomib combinations. Melphalan, lenalidomide, and dexamethasone in a relapsed setting produced hematologic complete response rates in 42% of patients. A phase II trial at Mayo Clinic of cyclophosphamide, lenalidomide, and dexamethasone also produced response rates of 50%, with 7% showing a complete response. Myelosuppression with the combination of melphalan and lenalidomide is significant. Cardiac arrhythmias were seen in 33%.

As salvage therapy in relapsing disease, lenalidomide has been combined with cyclophosphamide and dexamethasone in 35 patients. The median number of treatment cycles was six, and the hematologic response rate was 60%; in those receiving at least four cycles, the response rate was 87%. A median overall survival of 37.8 months has been reported. In patients with amyloidosis, lenalidomide has been reported to worsen renal function even in patients whose amyloidosis spares the kidney. Recovery of renal function was reported in 44%. Lenalidomide salvage therapy after bortezomib achieves a hematologic response rate of 41%. Pomalidomide is a third-generation immunomodulatory drug with a toxicity profile that compares favorably with the other immunomodulatory drugs. In a single phase II trial, 29 patients previously treated received pomalidomide with a response rate of 38%. Three-fourths of the patients were alive at 1 year, and 56% were free of disease progression. The majority of these patients had previously received stem cell transplants, bortezomib, and thalidomide, indicating that this immunomodulatory drug is active and capable of producing durable remissions, albeit with significant toxicity.

Bortezomib

Bortezomib, which was the first proteasome inhibitor used for the treatment of amyloidosis, has the advantage of a rapid time to response and no modification required for renal dysfunction. In the first phase II trial, 14 of 18 patients with relapsed refractory AL amyloidosis had a hematologic response, with 16% achieving complete response. Schedules of weekly and twice-weekly bortezomib have been investigated with similar response rates and similar 1-year progression-free survival. The weekly form of bortezomib, however, does appear to have lower rates of treatment discontinuation and peripheral neuropathy. Bortezomib has been combined with dexamethasone with a hematologic response rate of 71%, complete in 25%. In previously untreated patients, bortezomib produces a complete response rate of 47%, although in one study the progression-free survival was only 5 months and the overall survival was 18.7 months, raising questions about how durable these responses are. Bortezomib has also been combined with stem cell transplant as induction therapy, as posttransplant consolidation therapy, and as part of the conditioning regimen. In a report of 19 patients for whom bortezomib was used after stem cell transplant to deepen the response, 67% of patients achieved a complete response, with organ responses in 60% using posttransplant consolidation with bortezomib. Data from 33 national centers were combined, with 94 patients having received bortezomib. A cardiac response was seen in 29% of patients. The NT-proBNP predicted survival. The median time to response was 7.5 weeks. Authors of a survey of European centers with 428 evaluable patients reported that bortezomib therapy achieved a lower difference between involved and uninvolved free light chains at the end of therapy compared with cyclophosphamide-thalidomide-dexamethasone, melphalan-dexamethasone, stem cell transplant, and cyclophosphamide-lenalidomide-dexamethasone.

Bortezomib had been combined with cyclophosphamide and dexamethasone. In a study of 17 patients, 10 of whom were therapy-naive, a response rate of 94% was achieved, 71% complete. A second cohort of 43 patients achieved a hematologic response rate of 81%, with 42% achieving a complete response and a 2-year progression-free survival of 67% for newly diagnosed patients.

Despite the promising published results with bortezomib, a prospective randomized trial conducted in Europe of bortezomib, melphalan, and dexamethasone (BMD) compared with melphalan and dexamethasone failed to show any difference in organ response rates or in progression-free or overall survival in the bortezomib-containing regimen; yet grade 3 toxicity was seen in 27% of patients receiving BMD compared with only 12% treated with melphalan and dexamethasone. Moreover, day 100 all-cause mortality was 7.5% in the BMD arm and only 2.5% in the melphalan dexamethasone lenalidomide. The hematologic response rate was higher in the BMD arm at 77% vs. 52% ($p = .045$). A compilation of 230 patients in Europe who received cyclophosphamide, bortezomib, and dexamethasone showed a high level of effectiveness in low-risk amyloidosis patients with an at least very good partial response rate of 56% and no deaths seen in stage I patients.

A European collaborative study of treatment outcomes in 346 patients with cardiac stage III AL amyloidosis was reported. In this cohort of patients with advanced cardiac amyloidosis, the median overall survival was 7 months with a 2-year overall survival of 29%. As is typical for this disease, 42% of patients died before their first response evaluation, and the overall hematologic response rate was 33% (12% complete). The overall survival rate was 88% at 2 years for complete responders, 53% for partial responders, and 22% for non-responders; 45% of responders achieved an organ response. The only factors predictive of survival were an NT-proBNP >8500 ng/L and a systolic blood pressure <100 mmHg. The regimens administered included melphalan and dexamethasone, alkylating agents thalidomide and dexamethasone, and bortezomib as well as lenalidomide combinations. Although this was not a prospective trial, the overall response rate for melphalan-dexamethasone-thalidomide-bortezomib combinations ranged from 60% to 64%. The response rate to lenalidomide combination therapy was 41% but included only 13 patients. The most common regimen administered was melphalan and dexamethasone, administered to 154 of the 286 patients evaluable for response.

Stem Cell Transplant

Unlike multiple myeloma, where visceral organ function tends to be normal with the exception of the kidney, and the bone marrow tends to be heavily involved, the converse is true in amyloidosis. In amyloidosis, the marrow shows minimal involvement, but organ dysfunction increases the morbidity as well as the mortality of high-dose chemotherapy and stem cell transplant. Ablative therapy can be more effective, and the response durability of patients who achieve a complete response is greater in amyloidosis than it is in multiple myeloma, the number one indication for autologous stem cell transplant in the United States. Stem cell transplant is not a suitable technique for patients with advanced cardiac disease, because these patients decompensate if they develop neutropenic infection during the phase of maximal immunosuppression. Careful patient selection becomes critical in ensuring a safe outcome for patients who undergo stem cell transplant. Over the past two decades, the treatment-related mortality associated with stem cell transplant has fallen from 10% to 2% because of improved supportive care and optimization of patient selection. As a general guideline, it has been our experience that patients whose NT-proBNP is >5000 pg/mL or whose troponin T is >0.06 ng/mL have too high a mortality associated with transplant and are better managed with standard-dosage chemotherapy, as outlined in the previous section. Systolic blood pressure >100 mmHg is also an important feature reflecting sufficient diastolic compliance to improve cardiac output during the stress of stem cell transplant. Patients who have stage III and stage IV cardiac amyloidosis are candidates for stem cell transplant if they fulfill the other criteria outlined.

At Mayo Clinic, approximately 20% of patients with newly diagnosed amyloidosis are eligible for high-dose melphalan. Melphalan 200 mg/m^2 and 140 mg/m^2 can both be used, but the response rates associated with lower-dose melphalan are decreased and may not be superior to the response rates reported with standard chemotherapies. The ability of stem cell transplant to produce a durable response is unmatched in the literature, with 43% of patients surviving 10 years or longer. Patients with more than two organs involved are oftentimes not considered adequate candidates for stem cell transplant, but some judgment is warranted because patients can have very mild involvement of three organs and be candidates, yet have advanced involvement of two organs and not be candidates (Fig. 88.9). The serum creatinine is predictive of the risk of requiring dialysis during the transplant, a major complication leading to serious morbidity. We are disinclined to perform transplant in renal amyloid patients whose serum creatinine is ≥1.8 mg/dL. Although age is not an absolute criterion, additional scrutiny is warranted above the age of 65. From January 1, 2013, through December 31, 2014, 85 amyloid patients underwent transplants; 35 were older than 65 years of age, and 11 were over age 70 years.

As with conventional chemotherapy, hematologic response is a predictor of survival, with complete responders having improved

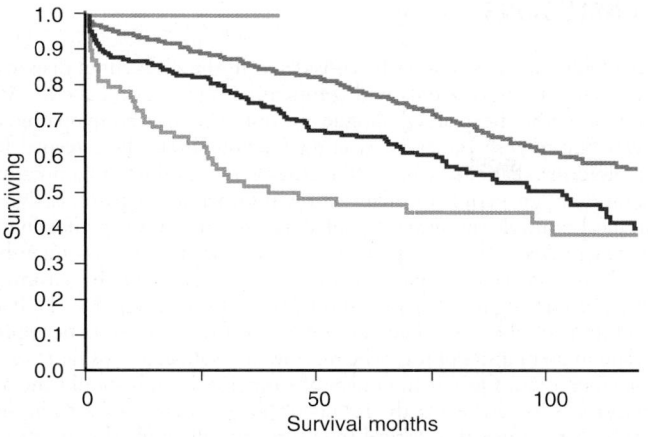

Fig. 88.9 SURVIVAL AFTER STEM CELL TRANSPLANT, BASED ON NUMBER OF ORGANS INVOLVED. *Pink,* Soft tissue only, no visceral involvement; *orange,* 1 organ; *dark blue,* 2 organs; *light blue,* >2 organs.

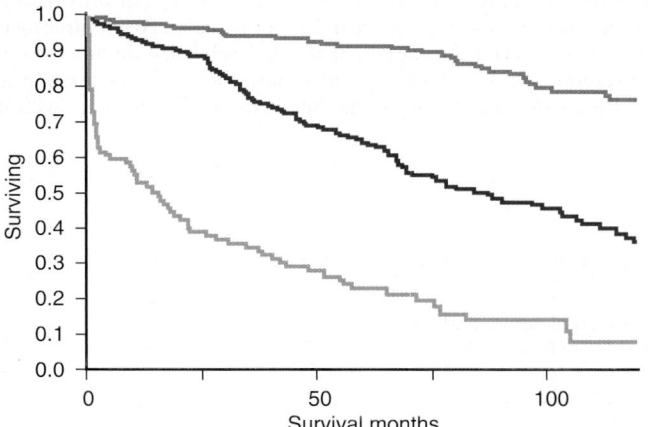

Fig. 88.10 SURVIVAL BY RESPONSE DEPTH. *Orange,* Complete response; *dark blue,* partial response; *light blue,* no response.

outcomes compared with very good partial responders and partial responders (Fig. 88.10). The depth of hematologic response required to achieve optimal outcomes is not well defined in amyloidosis, because highly amyloidogenic light chains can continue to deposit even if the levels are sharply reduced. Unlike myeloma (where the monoclonal protein is a surrogate for tumor mass), in amyloidosis, the monoclonal protein is itself the problem, and to completely disrupt deposition, one may hypothesize that nearly complete eradication of the protein from the serum is required. In amyloidosis, hematologic response is used as a surrogate for organ response, which is the only outcome that improves survival by the prevention of progressive organ failure.

Most published information on high-dose therapy and stem cell transplant in amyloidosis has used melphalan at doses ranging from 100 to 200 mg/m^2 as the standard. The Boston Medical Center reported 250 patients with AL amyloidosis who underwent high-dose melphalan and autologous stem cell rescue. Two-thirds were alive at a mean follow-up of 23 months, with a 3-month all-cause mortality of 14%. Febrile neutropenia, GI tract hemorrhage, and dialysis-dependent renal failure were unique toxicities associated with transplant. However, the Boston group has demonstrated an improved quality of life for patients who respond. We have published our experience with 434 patients with amyloidosis. The hematologic response rate among those patients was 75%. The complete response rate was 38%, and the organ response rate was 46%. The most important predictor of outcome was the depth of hematologic

response. Median survival was not reached for patients who achieved a complete response, whereas it was 107 months for those with partial remission and 32 months for nonresponders (Fig. 88.10). There is a significant impact of pretreatment NT-proBNP levels on outcome. We do not use chemomobilization to obtain stem cells. The low number of plasma cells in the bone marrow allows growth factor–only mobilization to achieve the requisite goal. Plerixafor is not routinely used to mobilize stem cells; it is used only in patients who do not achieve a peripheral blood CD34 count >10/μL. We also do not routinely use granulocyte colony-stimulating factor to support engraftment following transplant, owing to fluid retention that is seen, and we have observed no increase in bacteremia or hospital days after ceasing use of posttransplant growth factor support. Among amyloid patients, approximately 30% will complete the procedure without requiring hospitalization. Adjuvant therapy has been used in patients who are the recipients of stem cell transplants. Both thalidomide-dexamethasone and bortezomib-dexamethasone has been used to consolidate response after transplant, and it has been demonstrated that deepening of the response can be achieved.

It is difficult to obtain category A evidence in support of high-dose therapy and stem cell transplant for amyloidosis. The only prospective controlled trial enrolled 100 patients and did not demonstrate survival differences between the two groups, whether in a landmark analysis or on an intention-to-treat basis. This study has been called into question because of a 24% treatment-related mortality in the transplant group. A subsequent metaanalysis of high-dose therapy in patients with AL amyloidosis also could not identify a survival advantage with stem cell transplant. Boston University has reported a 10-year survival of 25% in their transplant population, compared with 4% prior to the advent of high-dose therapy. A case-matched control study done at Mayo Clinic matched 63 transplanted patients with 63 nontransplanted patients and showed a survival advantage for patients who received a stem cell transplant.

Organ Transplantation

Both cardiac and renal transplant have been performed in patients with AL amyloidosis. Criteria to be considered in selecting patients for solid organ transplant include amyloidosis confined only to the organ that is to be transplanted. Also the patient should either have achieved a complete hematologic response with therapy or be a candidate for therapy who has a high likelihood of producing a complete hematologic response and thereby obviate the possibility of recurrent amyloid in the transplanted organ.

Three patients were reported with AL amyloidosis who had cardiac involvement, and the time from symptomatic onset to the diagnosis of AL amyloidosis ranged from 12 to 24 months. The times from the onset of heart failure to orthotopic heart transplant in these three patients were 4, 5, and 7 months, respectively. The patients then underwent stem cell transplant at 13, 16, and 13 months, respectively; all three are alive at 23+, 35+, and 39 months, demonstrating that in highly selected patients, heart transplant in those with dominant cardiac involvement followed by subsequent stem cell transplant can result in survival benefit. Authors of a report of six patients who underwent heart transplant for cardiac amyloidosis at Stanford stated that all patients received chemotherapy in the interval between heart transplant and autologous stem cell transplant. Five patients were alive up to 25 months after heart transplant without evidence of recurrent cardiac amyloid deposition, but chemotherapy actually began as early as 32 days after cardiac transplant. The three patients are alive 19, 24, and 25 months posttransplant, respectively.

Renal transplant has also been reported. Nineteen patients with AL underwent renal transplant, comprising living donor transplants in eighteen and a cadaveric transplant in one, with a median follow-up of 41.4 months; 79% were alive, and five patients had cellular rejection. Recurrent amyloidosis was diagnosed by a kidney biopsy in only one patient, indicating that renal transplant can be successfully performed in patients with AL amyloidosis in complete hematologic response without a significant risk of recurrent amyloid when the primary hematologic disorder is controlled.

Nine cardiac transplants were reported from Boston, eight of whom subsequently received a stem cell transplant. Six of seven evaluable patients achieved a complete hematologic remission. One achieved a partial remission. At a median follow-up of 56 months, five of seven patients were alive without recurrent amyloid, comparable to patients who received heart transplants for nonamyloid heart disease. At Mayo Clinic, the median survival of patients who have received cardiac transplants for amyloid is approximately 50%, which is somewhat inferior to patients who receive hearts for cardiomyopathy without a systemic disorder. Eleven patients underwent heart transplant followed by autologous peripheral blood stem cell transplant. Two patients died as a result of transplant-related complications. Nine survived, but three died because of progressive amyloidosis. The 1- and 5-year survival rates were 82% and 65%, respectively. The median survival was 76 months from heart transplant and 57 months from stem cell transplant.

Organ transplant is a viable option for patients in whom complete suppression of light chain production can be achieved. Because of the shortage of organs, critical decisions regarding allocation must be made. Organ transplant has also been applied to familial amyloid polyneuropathy amyloidosis, usually combined with liver transplant. We have performed three cardiac transplants for familial amyloidosis, heart transplant for senile amyloid in 2 patients, heart-liver transplant for familial amyloid in 18 patients, and heart-liver-kidney transplant for familial amyloid in 4 patients.

CONCLUSIONS

Amyloidosis should always be considered in the differential diagnosis of a patient who presents with proteinuria and is nondiabetic. Any patient with unexplained fatigue or restrictive cardiomyopathy or heart failure with preserved ejection fraction should be screened for amyloidosis. Patients who fulfill criteria for chronic inflammatory demyelinating peripheral neuropathy, unexplained hepatomegaly, or atypical multiple myeloma should all be considered for the possibility of amyloidosis. When a patient with one of these five compatible syndromes is seen, screening with immunofixation of the serum or urine in a free light-chain assay should be performed (Fig. 88.11). If an immunoglobulin light-chain abnormality is found, it would be appropriate to do biopsies of the bone marrow and subcutaneous fat to stain for Congo red. Only if the index of suspicion is high should further biopsies be performed if the results of bone marrow and fat biopsies are both negative. It is critical to ensure that all amyloid deposits are typed. The gold standard is laser capture mass spectroscopy in an effort to ensure that all chemotherapy-treated amyloid is of immunoglobulin light chain origin. The prognosis of amyloidosis can be determined by measurements of the immunoglobulin free light chain, serum troponin, and NT-proBNP. We believe that stem cell transplant is the preferred technique for patients in whom it can be performed safely, but this should not be more than 20% of patients. For nontransplant candidates, melphalan-dexamethasone, melphalan-dexamethasone-bortezomib, and cyclophosphamide-bortezomib-dexamethasone are all legitimate options for induction therapy. For patients without

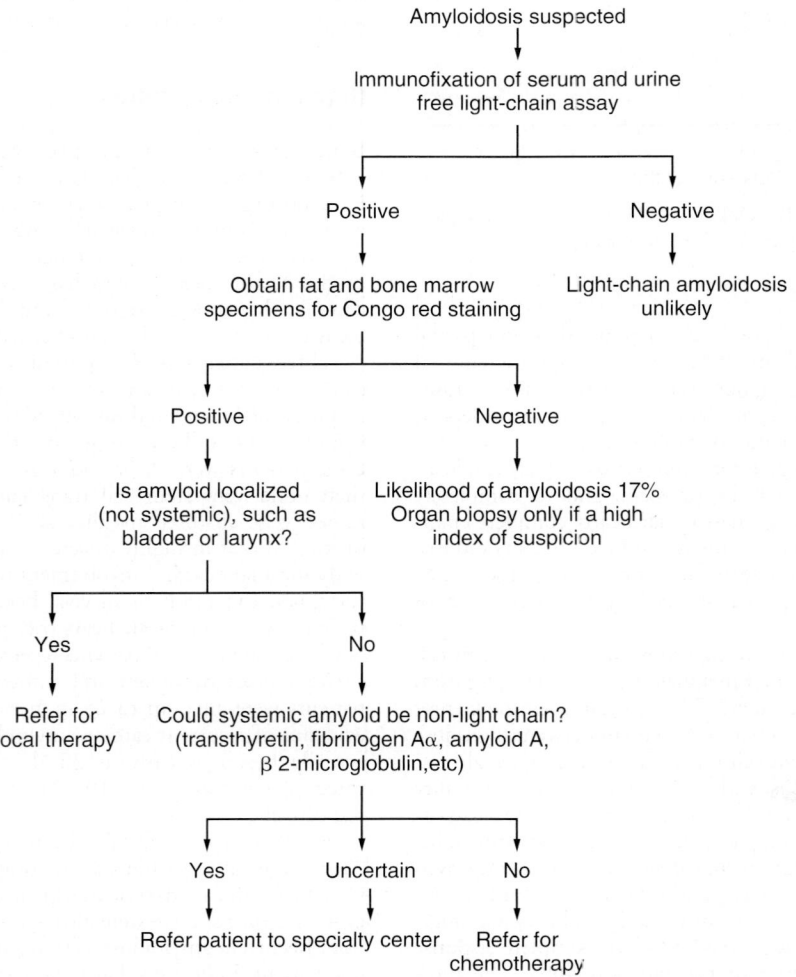

Fig. 88.11 DIAGNOSTIC ALGORITHM FOR USE WHEN AMYLOIDOSIS IS SUSPECTED.

TABLE 88.3	Active Nonchemotherapy Trials for Amyloidosis			
Drug	**Mechanism**	**Amyloidosis Type**	**Trial Registration Number**	**Comments**
Tafamidis	Misfolding interference	Mutant (Val122Ile) and wild-type TTR	NCT00935012	Double-blind, placebo-controlled trial
ALN-TTRSC	Suppress transthyretin expression	TTR wild type including cardiac involvement	NCT01994889, NCT01981837	None
ISIS-TTRRx	Suppress transthyretin expression	TTR neuropathy in ambulatory patients (use only one cane)	NCT01737398	Placebo-controlled
Doxycycline and tauroursodeoxycholic acid	Misfolding interference	TTR	NCT01171859	None
Doxycycline	Fibril disruption	AL and TTR	NCT01677286	None
NEOD001	Antibody-mediated fibril dissolution	AL	NCT01707264	None

AL, Light chain amyloid; *TTR,* transthyretin.

a response to their primary therapy, immunomodulatory drug–containing therapies such as melphalan-dexamethasone-lenalidomide, lenalidomide-dexamethasone, and cyclophosphamide-lenalidomide-dexamethasone are all appropriate combinations.

FUTURE DIRECTIONS AND SUMMARY

Some of the nonchemotherapy-based imitatives for amyloidosis treatment are listed in Table 88.3. Antibodies, small interfering RNA, and antisense oligonucleotides are all being explored. Combinations of anti–light-chain synthesis and therapies to prevent misfolding are likely the next generation of therapies.

SUGGESTED READINGS

Bhole MV, Sadler R, Ramasamy K: Serum-free light-chain assay: clinical utility and limitations. *Ann Clin Biochem* 51:528, 2014.

Chaulagain CP, Comenzo RL: New insights and modern treatment of AL amyloidosis. *Curr Hematol Malig Rep* 8:291, 2013.

Ericson S, Shah N, Liberman J, et al: Fatal bleeding due to acquired factor IX and X deficiency: a rare complication of primary amyloidosis; case report and review of the literature. *Clin Lymphoma Myeloma Leuk* 14:e81, 2014.

Fermand JP, Bridoux F, Kyle RA, et al: How I treat monoclonal gammopathy of renal significance (MGRS). *Blood* 122:3583, 2013.

Gertz MA: Immunoglobulin light chain amyloidosis: 2013 update on diagnosis, prognosis, and treatment. *Am J Hematol* 88:416, 2013.

Gertz MA, Dispenzieri A, Sher T: Pathophysiology and treatment of cardiac amyloidosis. *Nat Rev Cardiol* 12:91, 2015.

Gillmore JD, Hawkins PN: Pathophysiology and treatment of systemic amyloidosis. *Nat Rev Nephrol* 9:574, 2013.

Graziani MS, Merlini G: Serum free light chain analysis in the diagnosis and management of multiple myeloma and related conditions. *Expert Rev Mol Diagn* 14:55, 2014.

Jazbeh S, Said A, Haddad RY, et al: Renal amyloidosis. *Dis Mon* 60:489, 2014.

Mahmood S, Palladini G, Sanchorawala V, et al: Update on treatment of light chain amyloidosis. *Haematologica* 99:209, 2014.

Merlini G, Comenzo RL, Seldin DC, et al: Immunoglobulin light chain amyloidosis. *Expert Rev Hematol* 7:143, 2014.

Mollee P, Renaut P, Gottlieb D, et al: How to diagnose amyloidosis. *Intern Med J* 44:7, 2014.

Sachchithanantham S, Wechalekar AD: Imaging in systemic amyloidosis. *Br Med Bull* 107:41, 2013.

Sanchorawala V: High dose melphalan and autologous peripheral blood stem cell transplantation in AL amyloidosis. *Hematol Oncol Clin North Am* 28:1131, 2014.

Sayed RH, Hawkins PN, Lachmann HJ: Emerging treatments for amyloidosis. *Kidney Int* 87:516, 2015.

Shah G, Kaul E, Fallo S, et al: Bortezomib subcutaneous injection in combination regimens for myeloma or systemic light-chain amyloidosis: a retrospective chart review of response rates and toxicity in newly diagnosed patients. *Clin Ther* 35:1614, 2013.

Sher T, Gertz MA: Recent advances in the diagnosis and management of cardiac amyloidosis. *Future Cardiol* 10:131, 2014.

Ueda M, Ando Y: Recent advances in transthyretin amyloidosis therapy. *Transl Neurodegener* 3:19, 2014.

Weber N, Mollee P, Augustson B, et al: Management of systemic AL amyloidosis: recommendations of the Myeloma Foundation of Australia Medical and Scientific Advisory Group. *Intern Med J* 45:371, 2015.

Yusuf SW, Solhpour A, Banchs J, et al: Cardiac amyloidosis. *Expert Rev Cardiovasc Ther* 12:265, 2014.

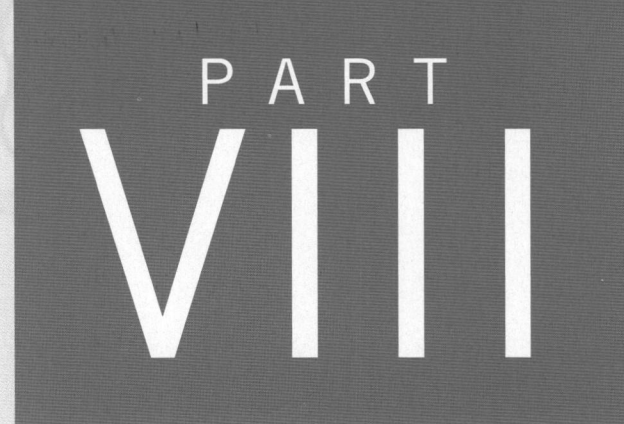

COMPREHENSIVE CARE OF PATIENTS WITH HEMATOLOGIC MALIGNANCIES

PART

VII

COMPREHENSIVE CARE OF PATIENTS
WITH HEMATOLOGIC MALIGNANCIES

Advances in the supportive care and treatment of hematologic malignancies have markedly improved the life expectancy of afflicted patients, but this progress is increasingly at the expense of developing a wider range of infectious complications often caused by drug-resistant organisms. The clinical approach to infections occurring among hematology patients involves understanding host immune system defects and anatomic barrier disruption that predispose patients to infection (Fig. 89.1). This chapter reviews specific hematologic conditions for their unique host defense defects and associated infections (Table 89.1) and the differential diagnoses of common infectious pathogens (Table 89.2). To demonstrate how periods of predictable anatomic defects combine with severe immune compromise, the prevention, diagnosis, and management strategies for infections occurring in the hematopoietic stem cell transplant (HSCT) recipient are presented as models.[1]

HEMATOLOGIC CONDITIONS PREDISPOSING TO INFECTION

Malignant Hematologic Disorders

Antineoplastic Therapy

During antineoplastic treatment, cytotoxic agents frequently are administered in combination with other immunosuppressive therapies, such as corticosteroids or radiation therapy. Several cytotoxic agents, notably methotrexate, cyclophosphamide, 6-mercaptopurine, and azathioprine, impair cell-mediated immunity. Many of the drugs themselves (e.g., cyclophosphamide) also impair humoral responses and produce quantitative phagocyte defects. Fludarabine, a major therapy for chronic lymphocytic leukemia (CLL), can produce prolonged and profound defects in cell-mediated immunity, thereby increasing susceptibility to *Pneumocystis*, yeast, and herpes group viruses (herpes simplex virus [HSV], varicella-zoster virus [VZV], and cytomegalovirus [CMV]).

The use of monoclonal antibody therapy for hematologic disorders results in dysfunction of particular aspects of the immune system.[2] Rituximab results in a sustained depletion of B lymphocytes for 6 to 9 months and has been specifically associated with reactivation of hepatitis B virus infection.[3] Alemtuzumab administration causes profound lymphopenia and an increased risk for a variety of viral and fungal infections.

Exogenous administration of glucocorticoids leads to increased susceptibility to infection. The degree of immunosuppression and the relative risk for infection depend on the dose and duration of use. The major effect of steroids on granulocyte function is a decrease in chemotactic activity. This accounts, in part, for the clinical observation that the signs and symptoms of severe infections may be masked or greatly reduced in patients receiving steroids. Steroids may enhance susceptibility to infection by means of negative effects on glucose homeostasis, wound healing, skin fragility, monocyte and lymphocyte function, production of cytokines, and humoral immune responses.

Radiation therapy has been associated with granulocyte dysfunction and delayed wound healing. Defects in cell-mediated immunity

may persist for more than 1 year after intensive radiation therapy or after HSCT.

Acute Leukemias

In patients with acute leukemias, a major cause of morbidity is infection due to drug-associated mucositis and therapy-induced neutropenia. Most infections occurring during neutropenia are bacterial, but patients with prolonged neutropenia are at additional risk for development of yeast and mold infections. Patients with acute leukemia who progress to advanced therapies, such as hematopoietic cell transplant, have added risk for infections associated with acquired deficiencies in cell-mediated and humoral immunity, such as *Pneumocystis jirovecii* and CMV infections.[1]

Chronic Leukemias

Patients with chronic myeloid leukemia do not have prominent host defense impairments, so infections are limited unless patients proceed to aggressive chemotherapy or HSCT. Host defense defects with tyrosine kinase inhibitors, such as imatinib or dasatinib, have not been well defined. Chemotherapy for blast crisis resembles therapy for acute leukemia. Patients with CLL are predisposed to infection because of immunodeficiency related to the leukemia itself (humoral and cellular immune dysfunction) and to therapy-related immunosuppression.[4] In early B-cell CLL, the infectious risk is mainly related to unbalanced immunoglobulin chain synthesis and resultant hypogammaglobulinemia. In patients with advanced CLL, particularly after the introduction of therapy with purine analogues and monoclonal agents (e.g., rituximab, alemtuzumab), neutropenia and defects in cell-mediated immunity are other factors predisposing to infection. The risk for infectious complications increases with the duration of CLL, reflecting the cumulative immunosuppression related to its treatment. The incidence of infection correlates with the serum levels of immunoglobulins (particularly IgG), which may be further impaired by use of anti-CD20 therapies.

Lymphomas

Hodgkin and non-Hodgkin lymphoma are commonly associated with impaired cell-mediated immunity. The degree of immune impairment may correlate with the extent of disease and often is compounded by administration of immunosuppressive therapy.[3] The intrinsic impairment of cell-mediated immunity in Hodgkin lymphoma can persist even after apparent cure. Splenectomy-related infections occur with sepsis caused by encapsulated bacterial organisms at a median of 22 months but sometimes many years after surgery.

Myelodysplastic Syndrome

Neutrophils and band forms from patients with myelodysplastic syndrome are functionally defective and probably are derived from a

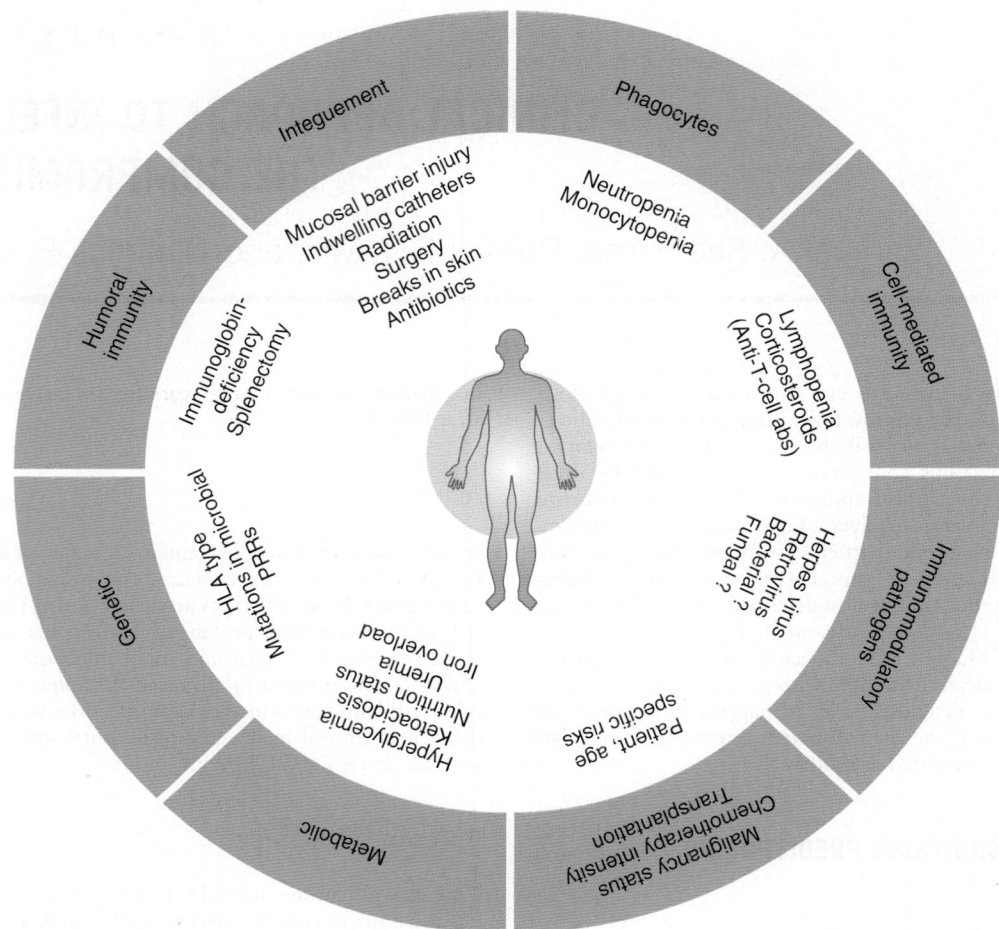

Fig. 89.1 CONSTELLATION OF FACTORS CONTRIBUTING TO INCREASED RISK FOR INFECTION IN IMMUNOCOMPROMISED HOSTS.

malignant clone of myeloid precursor cells. Neutrophils from patients with myelodysplastic syndrome have deficiencies in myeloperoxidase, elastase, and integrins. More than half of patients with myelodysplastic syndrome die within 3 years of diagnosis from infections, bleeding complications, or progression to acute leukemia.

Multiple Myeloma

Malignant plasma cells produce a variety of immunomodulatory molecules such as TGF-B that suppress B-cell function, so multiple myeloma is frequently associated with a variety of defects in humoral immunity.[5] Patients having myeloma with IgG paraprotein have an increased rate of catabolism of normal and clonal IgG. They also may have defects in complement and granulocyte function. Cell-mediated immunity is not impaired by the disease but is compromised by corticosteroids or cytotoxic therapy.

Uncommon Malignancies

Patients with hairy cell leukemia develop mycobacterial disease relatively often, especially infection with atypical mycobacteria. Reversal of host cellular immune defects with effective therapy can lead to rapid clinical response with eradication of mycobacterial infection.

Defects in cell-mediated immunity have been postulated to explain the incidence of infection caused by intracellular pathogens in patients with the relatively rare T-cell malignancies mycosis fungoides and T-cell CLL.

Nonmalignant Hematologic Disorders

Aplastic Anemia

This blood dyscrasia is associated with decreased peripheral blood cell counts due to marrow failure. Chronic neutropenia is the main cause of recurrent bacterial and fungal infections among patients. Periodontal infections are particularly common. Treatment of the underlying hematologic disease is required to stop recurrent infections and cure some chronic infections.

Paroxysmal Nocturnal Hemoglobinuria

Patients with paroxysmal nocturnal hemoglobinuria are at some increased risk for bacterial infection due to a deficiency of decay-accelerating factor on the membrane of neutrophils. Modest and progressive granulocytopenia, progression to aplasia or leukemia may compound these risks. Vaccination against meningococcus is required before treatment with the terminal complement inhibitor eculizumab.

Granulocytic Phagocyte Disorders

The clinical approach to infections in patients with granulocytic phagocyte disorders is specific to each of these disorders and is beyond the scope of this chapter. However, chronic granulomatous disease is discussed because patients with this congenital immunodeficiency

TABLE 89.1	Malignant and Select Nonmalignant Hematologic Diseases and Their Associated Infection-Predisposing Host Defects
Hematologic Condition	**Infection-Predisposing Host Defects**
Acute myeloid leukemia	Neutropenia; therapies such as dose-intensive chemotherapy and hematopoietic stem cell transplant may result in additional anatomic disruptions, cell-mediated defects, and humoral defects
Acute lymphocytic leukemia	Neutropenia; therapy effects similar to acute myeloid leukemia
Hairy cell leukemia	Neutropenia (also monocytopenia); abnormal humoral immunity; T-cell suppressing therapy
Chronic lymphocytic leukemia	Hypogammaglobulinemia; abnormal cell-mediated immunity
Chronic myeloid leukemia	No prominent host defects unless aggressive therapy, advanced stage, or postsplenectomy
Multiple myeloma	Hypogammaglobulinemia; other host defects may occur with aggressive therapy or advanced stage
Hodgkin/non-Hodgkin lymphomas	Abnormal cell-mediated immunity, therapy-related neutropenia, splenic dysfunction (if splenectomy or radiation)
Myelodysplastic syndromes	Functional or absolute neutropenia
Aplastic anemia	Neutropenia; abnormal cell-mediated immunity from immunosuppressive therapies (e.g., steroids, antithymocyte globulin, cyclosporine, hematopoietic stem cell transplantation)
Paroxysmal nocturnal hemoglobinuria	Deficient Fc receptor may contribute to abnormal cell-mediated immunity
Hemolytic states (thalassemia)	Gallstones may serve as a nidus for infection; splenic dysfunction or splenectomy
Sickle cell disease	Can be neutropenic with aplastic crisis; bone infarcts may serve as a nidus for infection; splenic dysfunction with poor complement activation and opsonization from autosplenectomy

TABLE 89.2	Host Defense Impairments and Their Associated Infectious Pathogens
Host Defense Defect	**Pathogen Categories**
Neutropenia	Enteric gram-negative organisms
	Gram-positive staphylococci and streptococci
	Anaerobes
	Yeast, particularly *Candida* species
	Molds, particularly *Aspergillus* species
Abnormal cell-mediated immunity	Atypical bacteria: *Legionella, Nocardia*
	Salmonella species
	Mycobacteria (*M. tuberculosis* and atypical mycobacteria)
	Disseminated infection from live bacilli Calmette-Guérin (BCG) vaccine
	Environmental fungi, including *Cryptococcus neoformans, Histoplasma capsulatum, Coccidioides immitis*
	Endogenous yeast, particularly *Candida* species
	Herpesviruses
	Infections from live-virus vaccines
	Pneumocystis jirovecii
	Toxoplasma gondii
	Cryptosporidium
	Strongyloides stercoralis
Immunoglobulin abnormalities	Gram-positive *Streptococcus pneumoniae, Staphylococcus aureus*
	Gram-negative *Haemophilus influenzae, Neisseria* species, enteric organisms
	Enteroviruses
	Disseminated infections from live-virus vaccines
	Giardia lamblia
Complement abnormalities C3, C5	Gram-positive *S. pneumoniae*, staphylococci
	Gram-negative *H. influenzae, Neisseria* species, enteric organisms
Complement abnormalities C5–C9	*Neisseria* species
Anatomic Disruption	**Pathogen Categories**
Oral cavity	α-Hemolytic streptococci, oral anaerobes
	Candida species
	Herpes simplex virus
Esophagus	*Candida* species,
	Herpes simplex virus, cytomegalovirus
Lower gastrointestinal tract	Enterococcus, gram-negative enteric organisms,
	Anaerobes (*Bacteroides fragilis, Clostridium perfringens*),
	Candida species, *Strongyloides stercoralis*
Skin (IV catheter)	Gram-positive staphylococci and streptococci, *Corynebacterium, Bacillus*
	Atypical mycobacteria
Urinary tract	Enterococcus,
	Gram-negative enteric organisms
	Candida species
Splenectomy	Encapsulated organisms: *S. pneumoniae, H. influenzae, Neisseria, Capnocytophaga canimorsus*
	Salmonella (especially sickle cell disease), *Babesia*

who survive into adulthood are at risk for severe infections. Chronic granulomatous disease is a heterogeneous group of disorders resulting from defective or malfunctioning oxidative metabolism capacity of phagocytes. Recurrent infections with bacteria and fungi are common and occasionally life threatening, despite optimal antimicrobial therapy. Infections with *Staphylococcus* species and *Aspergillus* species can be particularly aggressive.[6] Granulomata may form in response to infection, especially in the gastrointestinal (GI) and genitourinary tracts.

Erythrocyte Disorders

Glucose-6-phosphate dehydrogenase deficiency is a sex-linked disorder. Deficiency of this enzyme limits glucose metabolism through the hexose monophosphate shunt, resulting in an abnormal respiratory burst in neutrophils. Bacterial infections can occur if the deficiency is severe.

Hemoglobin Gene Variants

Patients with chronic hemolytic states may develop bilirubin gallstones, which can serve as a nidus for infection. Defects in cell-mediated immunity have been described in patients with thalassemia. Patients with sickle cell disease have an increased susceptibility to bacterial infections.[7] Defective alternative complement pathway function, especially in conjunction with asplenia, contributes to the propensity to bacterial infection. Splenic involution results in depressed synthesis of alternate pathway factor(s) of complement and decreased phagocytic clearance of bacteria. Phagocytosis of *Streptococcus pneumoniae* is abnormal, in part because of an inability to use the alternate pathway for C3 fixation as a means of opsonization. An increased risk for *Salmonella* infection appears to be unique to the sickle cell population. Suppurative arthritis can occur after repeated episodes of hemarthrosis among patients with sickle cell disease.

Coagulation Disorders

Hemophilias are sex-linked deficiencies of clotting factor VIII or IX. Septic arthritis should be considered in the differential diagnosis of any hemophiliac with repeated episodes of hemarthrosis whose articular signs and symptoms fail to improve quickly after administration of appropriate coagulation factor replacement. Hemophiliacs who have acquired infection with human immunodeficiency virus (HIV)-1 from plasma-derived factor replacement therapy may develop severe impairment of cell-mediated immunity after this retroviral infection progresses to acquired immunodeficiency syndrome (AIDS).

Blood Groups

The Duffy blood group antigen serves as a receptor for *Plasmodium vivax* to invade erythrocytes. Blood group O is associated with *Helicobacter pylori* infection and an associated increase in peptic ulceration because the Lewis (b) blood group antigen mediates *H. pylori* attachment to human gastric mucosa.

Host Defense Impairment and Associated Infection Issues

Neutropenia

Profound or absolute neutropenia can occur in patients with aplastic anemia or leukemia or from chemotherapy used for treatment of various malignant diseases. Infection rates increase when neutrophil counts fall below 1000/mm^3, but the patient is most at risk for spontaneous infection when the count is below 100/mm (Fig. 89.2). The patient who is neutropenic from cytotoxic therapy can serve as a basic model for predicting infections that could occur in other patients with qualitative or quantitative granulocyte defects.

Neutropenia predisposes to the development of bacterial and fungal infections but does not appear to increase the incidence or severity of viral and parasitic infections. Patients with profound and prolonged neutropenia who are at particular high risk for infection (e.g., cytopenic patients with acute myelogenous leukemia and severe mucositis following induction therapy) are likely to benefit from receiving prophylactic antimicrobials.[8,9] However, patients with moderate granulocytopenia (i.e., absolute granulocyte counts in the range from 500 to 2000/mm^3 that are not falling precipitously) should not receive prophylactic antimicrobial agents. Colony-stimulating factors (granulocyte colony-stimulating factor [G-CSF; pegylated filgrastim], granulocyte-macrophage colony-stimulating factor [GM-CSF, sargramostim]) are routinely used in the management of

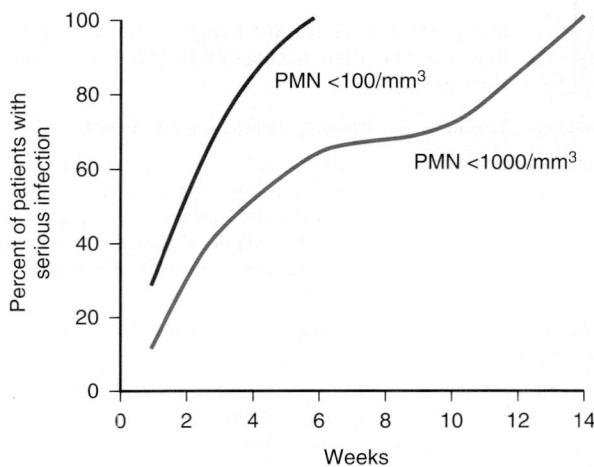

Fig. 89.2 RELATIONSHIP OF SEVERITY AND DURATION OF NEUTROPENIA TO THE RISK FOR DEVELOPING A SERIOUS INFECTION. *PMN,* Polymorphonuclear neutrophil. *(Courtesy GE Body.)*

hematologic disorders. A number of functional granulocyte parameters may be enhanced by G-CSF or GM-CSF, including enhanced per-cell phagocytosis, oxidative metabolism, microbicidal activity, and antibody-dependent cytotoxicity.[10] However, G-CSF or GM-CSF administration may decrease the motility of granulocytes, impair in vivo migration, and decrease bacteria-induced chemotaxis. The clinical significance of any of these effects remains to be established but is generally believed to be insignificant in light of the potency of these agents in shortening the depth and duration of therapy-induced neutropenia.

Defects in Cell-Mediated Immunity

Cellular immune dysfunction occurs in patients with lymphoid malignancies, in those with hematologic malignancies undergoing HSCT, and in patients with AIDS. The most frequently encountered pathogens are intracellular organisms because they can survive and even replicate inside macrophages in a nonimmune individual or in the absence of T-cell immunity. Specific pathogens associated with infection in patients with cell-mediated immunity include bacteria (including *Mycobacterium tuberculosis,* atypical mycobacteria, *Salmonella,* streptococci, *Legionella, Nocardia,* and *Listeria*); fungi (including the yeasts *Candida* and *Cryptococcus;* molds such as *Aspergillus;* endemic dimorphic fungi such as *Histoplasma* and *Coccidioides;* and *Pneumocystis*); viruses (including herpes group viruses [HSV, VZV, CMV] and respiratory viruses); and protozoa (*Toxoplasma gondii, Cryptosporidium,* and *Strongyloides stercoralis*).

Patients with defects in cell-mediated immunity or who are about to receive HSCT should undergo risk factor assessment for reactivation of tuberculosis. Patients with a known history of an untreated but positive Mantoux test or interferon-gamma release assay should receive prophylactic isoniazid to prevent reactivation and potential dissemination of tuberculosis. Patients without a prior Mantoux test but with risk factors for tuberculosis should undergo a screening test for latent tuberculosis before starting the conditioning regimen for HSCT.

Patients with defects in cell-mediated immunity are at risk for the development of disseminated infection due to live vaccines, even when the vaccine contains attenuated organisms. Accordingly, these patients should not receive vaccines containing bacillus Calmette-Guérin (BCG), vaccinia/smallpox, measles, mumps, rubella, yellow fever, or oral polio.[11] HSCT recipients are eligible for revaccination with some of the live virus vaccines 2 years after transplantation, provided the patient does not have graft-versus-host disease (GVHD) or is not receiving ongoing pharmacologic immunosuppression (see Chapter 110, Table 110.4).

Defects in the Humoral Immune System

Immunoglobulin and complement are components of the humoral immune system. Immunoglobulin and complement both have associated lytic and neutralizing activities. Patients with primary or secondary defects or deficiencies in humoral immunity are susceptible to recurrent pyogenic infections from polysaccharide-encapsulated bacteria, such as *Streptococcus pneumoniae*, *Haemophilus influenzae*, and *Neisseria* species. HSCT recipients who continue to receive immunosuppressants more than 100 days after transplantation should be given antimicrobial prophylaxis with coverage for encapsulated bacteria until immunosuppression is discontinued. Patients are also at risk for infections from enteroviruses and *Giardia lamblia*. Patients with low levels of circulating IgG may benefit from intravenous Ig (IVIg) infusions, although the benefit of using of IVIg infusions for routine prophylaxis must be weighed against the expense of this approach.

Abnormalities in Splenic Function

A number of hematologic disorders are complicated by either intrinsic splenic impairment or splenectomy. The spleen removes organisms from the blood that have been ineffectively opsonized by complement, serving an adjunctive role in fighting infection. It is involved in the regulation of the alternate complement pathway, and low levels of immunoglobulin and properdin have been reported in patients after splenectomy. Alternate pathway defects may be particularly important in patients with splenic dysfunction associated with sickle cell disease.

Asplenic or splenectomized patients are at increased risk for serious, frequently fulminant, bacterial infections, primarily for infections caused by *S. pneumoniae*, *H. influenzae*, *Neisseria*, *Babesia*, and *Capnocytophaga canimorsus*. The initial presentation of even overwhelming infection can be subtle, with fever often the only sign. Accordingly, all asplenic patients with underlying hematologic disease who present with fever should be managed initially as potentially septic. Overwhelming infection after splenectomy occurs in approximately 7% of postsplenectomy patients, with 50% of infection-related deaths occurring in the first 3 months. Prophylaxis against pneumococcal infection is used for asplenic patients who are small children or for those with increased immune impairment from malignant disease.

Pneumococcal, *H. influenzae* type b, and meningococcal vaccines should be administered to asplenic patients. Patients with an intact spleen may respond better to pneumococcal polysaccharide vaccine than do splenectomized patients, so immunization is recommended as early as possible before elective surgery. Additionally, immunization before splenectomy can result in protective pneumococcal antibody titers immediately after the operation. For patients with Hodgkin lymphoma, the antibody response to pneumococcal vaccine may not be affected by the timing of immunization relative to splenectomy. Immunizations reduce, but do not eliminate the risk for serious infection with encapsulated bacteria.

Anatomic Alterations in Host Defense

Immunocompromised patients frequently have disruptions in the skin and mucosa, which are important primary physical barriers against endogenous and exogenous sources of infections (Fig. 89.1). Disruption of skin and mucosa may result from invasion by malignant cells, from the effects of chemotherapy or radiation therapy, from use of invasive diagnostic or therapeutic procedures (e.g., intravenous catheters), and from the effects of local infections, such as oral HSV. Such alterations may provide a nidus for microbial colonization, a focus for localized infection, and a portal of entry for systemic invasion. Organisms associated with defects in skin or mucosal surfaces depend on the site of breakdown, local colonizing flora, and other factors. Gram-positive organisms are associated with isolated disruption of the skin from an indwelling intravenous catheter, usually with coagulase-negative staphylococci, but also with *Corynebacterium jeikeium*, *Bacillus* species, and occasionally atypical mycobacteria.

GI mucosal integrity is frequently disrupted by chemotherapeutic agents. Because the GI tract normally is colonized by a multitude of organisms, this state can lead to infection by streptococci, aerobic gram-negative enteric and anaerobic bacteria, and yeast. Mucosal damage can allow normal flora to invade and become pathogens. Lower GI ulcerations permit infections by *Bacteroides fragilis* or *Streptococcus bovis*. Oral lesions are associated with HSV reactivation, ulceration, and possible bloodstream infection with other common oral flora such as α-hemolytic streptococci.

The genitourinary tract mucosa may be disrupted by tumors, invasive procedures, or cytotoxic therapy, with subsequent colonization and the potential for local or invasive infection. The most common urinary tract pathogens are enteric gram-negative bacilli, enterococci, and *Candida albicans*. Viral reactivation is common, predominantly from adenovirus and polyomavirus (BK virus), but also from the herpesviruses (HSV and CMV).

The lung, genitourinary tract, biliary tract, and auditory canal are potential sites of mechanical obstruction, increasing the risk for localized infection. Obstruction may lead to stasis of local body fluids, with resultant overgrowth of potentially pathogenic colonizing organisms. Patients with chronic hemolytic states are prone to gallstones that can become a nidus for infection.

Anatomic alteration can predispose to infection simply by providing a nidus for growth of organisms. Many patients with sickle cell anemia and hemophilia have underlying anatomic abnormalities of the bones and joints as a result of vasoocclusive crises causing infarction of marrow, bony cortex, or synovium. In turn, these changes may predispose to infection such as osteomyelitis or arthritis. Decreased local blood flow and increased bacterial adherence may be other contributing factors. Foreign bodies, such as prosthetic devices, can lead to persistent infection after even transient bacteremia.

Infection in Patients With Acute Neutropenia or Lymphopenia Following Chemotherapy or Transplantation

This section outlines predictable infections that can present during acute profound neutropenia/lymphopenia.

Fever

Despite the specific prophylactic measures directed against common pathogens, many fevers occur in neutropenic patients after transplantation or chemotherapy. Fever can be divided into three categories: infectious fever with an obvious source, infectious fever without an obvious source, and noninfectious fever. Risk factor assessment should include knowledge of the temporal relationship to blood product infusions; recent exposure to contagious infection; degree of fever and whether the fever is accompanied by chills, rigors, or diaphoresis; and response to antipyretics. Symptom assessment should include evaluation to assess sinus drainage, sore throat, ear pain, cough, sputum production, shortness of breath, abdominal pain, diarrhea, rash, and dysuria.

The initial workup of fever in a patient with neutropenia, regardless of whether an infectious or noninfectious source is suspected, is identical and includes blood culture, culture of symptom-related sites (e.g., sputum, urine, with/without stool, with/without cerebrospinal fluid), review of medication list for potential contributors to drug fever, review of recent transfusions, chest radiograph, and computed tomography (CT) scan of any symptom-related body systems. When feasible, blood cultures should be drawn through an existing indwelling catheter as well as peripherally because this can facilitate the diagnosis of a catheter-related bloodstream infection compared with a bloodstream infection arising from a different source (e.g., the GI tract).[12]

Consensus guidelines on the management of patients with febrile neutropenia have been published.[13] Empiric antibiotics are recommended for all febrile patients with neutropenia, but the type of antibiotics and the site of administration (i.e., hospital vs. outpatient) depends on the severity of immunosuppression, expected duration of neutropenia, and factors related to the local epidemiology and resistance patterns (Fig. 89.3). Patients defined as low risk using the Multinational Association for Supportive Care in Cancer (MASCC) index can be treated as outpatients, whereas other patients are generally admitted for intravenous therapy.[14] Typical pathogens causing infection in this situation include Enterobacteriaceae, *Pseudomonas*, *Streptococcus*, and *Staphylococcus* spp. Thus antipseudomonal β-lactam antibiotics such as third-generation cephalosporins, piperacillin-tazobactam, and carbapenems are commonly employed as empiric

therapy.[15] Vancomycin is administered if staphylococcal disease is suspected or if the patient is clinically unstable while cultures are pending. Severely ill patients are often also treated with an aminoglycoside for the first 48 to 72 hours of illness, although data in support of this approach are lacking.

Therapeutic changes to the antimicrobial regimens are made in response to culture results, but the cultures are negative about 50% of the time (Fig. 89.3). If the patient becomes afebrile, therapy is usually continued for 7 days. Persistent fever after more than 72 hours of empiric therapy suggests an untreated infection. If the patient is recovering his or her neutrophil count, no additional changes in antibiotics are typically needed. However, the persistently neutropenic and febrile patient may have an occult fungal infection such as candidiasis or aspergillosis. Thus initiation of empiric antifungal therapy with antimold activity (e.g., amphotericin B, caspofungin, voriconazole) is usually begun in such a situation.

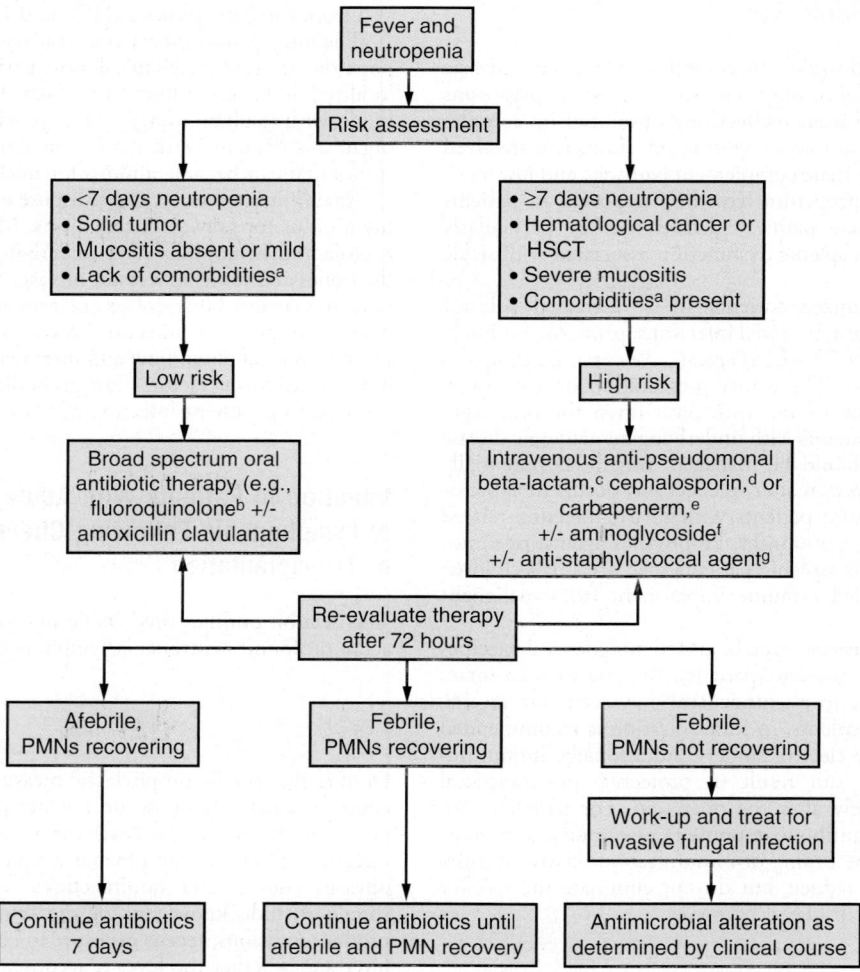

a   Hypotension, altered mental status, neurologic changes, respiratory failure, abdominal pain, hemorrhage, cardiac compromise or new arrythmia, catheter tunnel infection, extensive cellulitis, acute renal or liver failure
b   Institution sensitivity dependent, ciprofloxacin, levofloxacin, moxifloxacin
c   Drug selection and dosing institution-specific: piperacillin tazobactam, ticarcillin/clavulanate
d   Drug selection and dosing institution-specific: ceftazidime
e   imipenem, cefepime/cilastatin, meropenem, doripenem
f   Gentamin, tobramycin, or amikacin
g   Drug selection and institution institution-specific: vancomycin, linezolid, daptomycin, ceftaroline

Fig. 89.3 APPROACH TO PATIENT WITH FEVER AND NEUTROPENIA. *HSCT,* Hematopoietic stem cell transplant; *PMN,* polymorphonuclear neutrophil.

TABLE 89.3	Pulmonary Infiltrates and Their Association With Specific Infectious and Noninfectious Etiologies	
Radiologic Sign	**Differential Diagnosis**	
Interstitial infiltrates	Pulmonary edema	
	Diffuse alveolar damage	
	Idiopathic pneumonia syndrome	
	Respiratory viruses: respiratory syncytial virus, parainfluenza, influenza, adenovirus, enterovirus	
	Herpes viruses: cytomegalovirus, herpes simplex virus, varicella zoster virus, human herpes virus type 6	
	Pneumocystis pneumonia	
Focal airspace disease	Bacterial pneumonia	
	Fungal pneumonia	
Nodules	Fungal pneumonia (aspergillosis)	
	Nocardia	
	Legionella	
	Septic bacterial emboli	
	Mycobacterial infection (with cavitation)	
	Epstein-Barr virus lymphoproliferative disorder	
	Relapsed malignancy	
	Pulmonary embolism (pleural based)	
Halo sign or air crescent sign	Aspergillosis	

Two common anaerobic infections occur during neutropenia at sites where biopsy is difficult or contraindicated. Neutropenic enterocolitis, also known as typhlitis, manifests as fever, abdominal pain, and tenderness. CT scan of the abdomen shows signs of right-sided colonic and ileal inflammation.[16] Excessive soft-tissue swelling of the neck during mucositis can present as a Ludwig angina variant. Broadly active antianaerobic, aerobic, and possibly antifungal antimicrobial agents should be added for either of these clinical findings.

Pulmonary Infiltrates

Pulmonary infections are common in the immunocompromised host (see box on Approach to Pulmonary Infiltrates). Plain chest radiography is a good initial screen but lacks the sensitivity of CT, which generally provides more useful information in terms of characterizing the nature of an infiltrate and assists the pulmonologist in determining where to direct the bronchoscope for highest yield. A specific infectious and noninfectious differential diagnosis exists for certain radiologic signs (Table 89.3). For example, consolidative focal airspace disease is associated most typically with a bacterial pneumonia. A halo of interstitial changes around a pulmonary nodule or an air crescent above a pulmonary nodule is most likely due to aspergillosis (Fig. 89.4).[17] Although 90% of pulmonary nodules are due to fungal pneumonia (mainly aspergillosis), 10% have various etiologies, including septic bacterial emboli, *Nocardia, Legionella,* mycobacterial infection (with cavitation), Epstein-Barr virus (EBV)–related lymphoproliferative disease, relapsed malignancy, and pulmonary embolism (pleural based). Interstitial infiltrates can be caused by either respiratory viruses during the winter season (except for parainfluenza virus, which is nonseasonal), herpes viruses, *Pneumocystis,* edema, or idiopathic. A complete differential of causes of interstitial pneumonitis (a pulmonary syndrome often associated with HSCT) is given in Chapter 110.

Pulmonary and sinus infections from inhaled molds are more likely to occur as the duration of neutropenia lengthens, particularly beyond an initial 21-day window. For that reason, among HSCT recipients without graft failure, invasive tissue mold infections occur at a low rate (less than 3%) before engraftment because of the

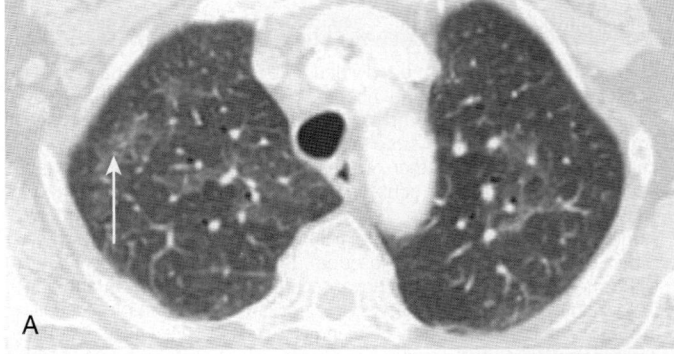
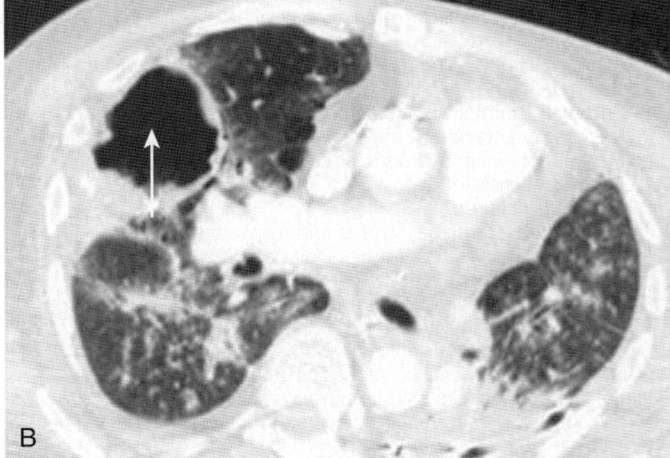
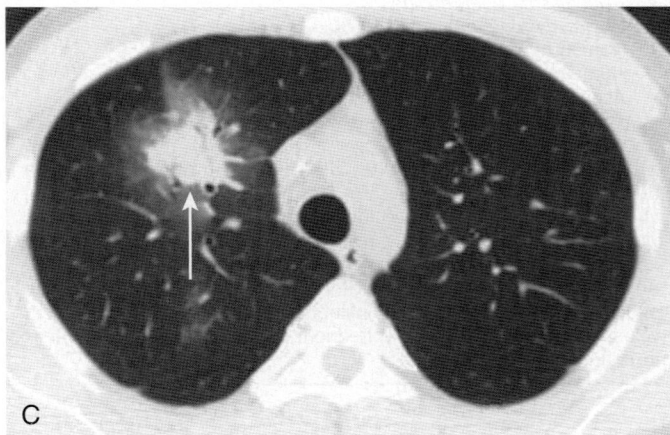

Fig. 89.4 COMPUTED TOMOGRAPHY SCAN EXAMPLES OF DIFFERENT PULMONARY INFILTRATES IN IMMUNOCOMPROMISED PATIENTS. (A) Diffuse ground-glass opacities in a patient with *Pneumocystis jirovecii* pneumonia. (B) Cavitary lung lesion in a patient with *Pseudomonas aeruginosa* pneumonia. (C) Lung nodule with halo sign due to *Aspergillus.* For each panel, the *arrow* points to involved pulmonary parenchyma.

environmental preventive measures taken for air filtration. However, if endogenous occult aspergillosis infections are present before HSCT, the infection can rapidly escalate when the immune system is profoundly suppressed by the preparative regimen. This phenomenon manifests as early invasive aspergillosis (before day 40). Therefore patients with hematologic malignancy at risk for occult mold infections in the lungs, sinuses, and at times, the oral cavity should have CT scans of the lungs and sinuses before the onset of any profoundly immunosuppressive regimens, such as HSCT and select nontransplantation regimens. High-risk patients may be given mold-active antifungal prophylaxis to either prevent or suppress invasive mold infections.

Approach to Pulmonary Infiltrates

Pulmonary infiltrates can be divided into three general categories: consolidative, interstitial, and nodular. A consolidative infiltrate may be bacterial, even polymicrobic, so sampling of the infiltrate through sputum or endotracheal tube suctioning for bacterial and fungal cultures is required. If either of these methods does not provide an adequate sample from a consolidative infiltrate, or if these methods do not lead to a diagnosis, "early" (within 72 hours) bronchoscopy is indicated. If interstitial or nodular infiltrates are not peripheral (i.e., within the range of the bronchoscope), they should also be evaluated with timely bronchoscopy. An advantage of bronchoscopy, in addition to the ability to obtain a deep specimen, is that the samples usually are sent for a broad range of diagnostic tests. These tests usually are ordered from preprinted order sheets, which reduce errors. Most preprinted order sheets for bronchoalveolar lavage fluid will test for the following:

- Cytology, with the attendant Fite and Gomori methenamine silver stains
- Bacterial (Gram) stain and aerobic culture
- Mycobacterial (acid-fast bacillus) stain and culture
- Fungal (potassium hydroxide or calcofluor) stain and culture
- *Nocardia* culture
- *Legionella* culture
- Viral cultures for herpes viruses and respiratory viruses
- Rapid test for cytomegalovirus (shell vial or polymerase chain reaction [PCR])
- Rapid test for respiratory viruses during respiratory virus season (pooled respiratory virus shell vial, respiratory syncytial virus antigen, influenza A/B antigen)

Optional tests that can be requested from bronchoalveolar lavage fluid, some at significant extra expense, include the following:

- Mycobacterial stain (requires separate 5 mL volume that cannot be used later for culture)
- *Mycoplasma pneumoniae* PCR
- *Chlamydia pneumoniae* PCR
- Human herpesvirus type 6 PCR
- Human metapneumovirus PCR
- *Aspergillus* galactomannan antigen
- Any of the above first-tier tests that your institution does not send on a routine basis (e.g., *Nocardia* or *Legionella*)

Invasive sampling may be the only definitive means for making a diagnosis of peripheral nodules. The two main options are percutaneous fine-needle aspiration or open lung biopsy (usually obtained through video-assisted thoracoscopic surgical procedure). In toto sampling of a lung nodule permits enough material for the whole range of the above diagnostic tests as well as histopathology. Of note, fewer lobectomies of unilateral pulmonary nodular infiltrates have been reported in recent years, probably a result of the frequent use of a broad range of less toxic antifungal medications.

Bacteria

Because bacterial infections cause significant morbidity and mortality in neutropenic patients, broad-spectrum antibacterial prophylaxis is often used during periods of profound neutropenia. The exact agents used vary, but typical agents include a quinolone (e.g., levofloxacin) or a β-lactam (e.g., cefpodoxime). Institutional protocols and resistance patterns drive selection of specific prophylactic agents. Oral prophylaxis regimens are generally discontinued and substituted with intravenous antibacterials with enhanced activity against *Pseudomonas aeruginosa* with the first onset of fever. The use of oral antibiotics among low-risk, neutropenic patients with fever is guided by the use of standardized scoring systems (e.g., MASCC index).[1]

Mucositis, with breakdown of oral and GI mucosal barriers, is common during this period. This condition can predispose to sepsis from bacterial and fungal organisms that typically colonize the GI tract. The most common serious infections occurring in neutropenic patients with mucositis are bacteremias due to viridans group streptococci and gram-negative bacilli. Such infections are particularly common during the first several weeks following HSCT, so broad-spectrum antimicrobial prophylaxis is generally given during this time period. The propensity of viridans streptococci to develop resistance to quinolones and gram-negative bacilli to be resistant to quinolones and β-lactams means that there is no perfect preventive regimen.

Central venous catheter placement through the skin can lead to blood infection from colonizing gram-positive skin organisms, despite sterile, operative placement of these catheters and antisepsis cleansing procedures.[18] Because the gram-positive bacteremias, including those caused by coagulase-negative *Staphylococcus* species, usually are not immediately life threatening, direct prophylactic coverage often is not immediately provided. During workup of a new fever, some treatment guidelines advocate the administration of vancomycin for several days until blood cultures demonstrate no gram-positive bacteremia. The use of antimicrobial-coated bloodstream catheters can be effective in reducing rates of catheter-related bloodstream infections.

Once a gram-positive bacterial infection is identified, vancomycin therapy is often used empirically until the susceptibility profile is available and targeted therapy can be provided. There are concerns about the efficacy of vancomycin in treating serious *S. aureus* infections because of relative or frank vancomycin resistance. Similarly, if the patient is known to be colonized with vancomycin-resistant enterococcus and the Gram stain indicates gram-positive organisms in chains, therapy for empiric vancomycin-resistant enterococcus is appropriate until the bacterial identification and susceptibility profile is available, usually with daptomycin or linezolid.

Once a gram-negative infection is identified, empiric therapy that includes *Pseudomonas* coverage is continued until the susceptibility profile is available. In the severely neutropenic host, serious gram-negative infections are often treated with combination therapy consisting of a β-lactam plus either an aminoglycoside or a quinolone depending on the antimicrobial sensitivity pattern and patient comorbidities.[15] However, data demonstrating the superiority of combination therapy over β-lactam monotherapy are lacking. The emergence of extended-spectrum β-lactamase producing gram-negative bacilli is a particular concern in patients with significant antimicrobial exposure as are the development of infections with pan-resistant organisms, such as multidrug-resistant *Acinetobacter baumannii* (see box on Treatment of Drug-Resistant Gram-Negative Bacilli). For many infections, the regimen then can be tailored to a single agent and continued for 2 weeks after the last positive culture in clinically responding patients. Therapy with a carbapenem resistant to β-lactamase hydrolysis is required if an organism is isolated that is known to have an inducible β-lactamase enzyme (e.g., *Enterobacter*).

For bloodstream infections, repeat blood cultures should be drawn after 2 to 3 days of effective therapy to ensure that sterilization of the bloodstream has been achieved. Persistently positive blood cultures suggest the development of a deep-seated or endovascular site of infection such as infective endocarditis or suppurative thrombophlebitis. When a bloodstream catheter is proven to be the source of the infection,[12,18] removal of the catheter may be required for most, but not all, infections. At the end of a 14-day treatment course beyond the last positive culture, the patient should be transitioned to an oral gram-negative prophylaxis regimen if still neutropenic.

Antimicrobial agents with anaerobic activity should be added for neutropenic enterocolitis, enlargement of neck soft tissues during mucositis (Ludwig angina variant), or culture-documented anaerobic infection. Infrequently, tuberculous and nontuberculous mycobacteria are responsible for infections in the bloodstream, catheters, and pulmonary tree. Infections of central catheters or catheter tunnels caused by rapidly growing atypical mycobacterial infections require a high index of suspicion, as well as specific culture media.[19] Organism identification and drug sensitivities may take several weeks. Tuberculous disease can be empirically treated based on risk factors. For patients without risk factors for tuberculosis, recovery of acid-fast bacilli will prompt therapy for suspected nontuberculous mycobacteria, usually with clarithromycin and either a quinolone or ethambutol until specific susceptibility information is available. Tailored therapy is often continued for a minimum of 3 to 6 months.

Treatment of Drug-Resistant Gram-Negative Bacilli

The widespread use of antibiotic prophylaxis among immunocompromised patients has been associated with the development of antimicrobial drug resistance, which is especially problematic among gram-negative bacilli. Drug-resistant organisms can colonize the GI tract for prolonged periods of time and emerge to cause serious infections during periods of neutropenia or other medical stress (e.g., following admission to the intensive care unit).

- *Pseudomonas aeruginosa* is the paradigm for drug resistance among gram-negative bacilli and often rapidly develops pan-resistance to antimicrobials. Serious pseudomonal infections are generally treated with two antimicrobial agents, although convincing data supporting this approach are lacking.
- Extended-spectrum β-lactamase (ESBL) production among Enterobacteriaceae such as *Escherichia coli* and *Klebsiella pneumoniae* renders these organisms resistant to non-carbapenem β-lactam antibiotics. Treatment is generally with a carbapenem (e.g., meropenem), although a quinolone can sometimes be used.
- The presence of a *Klebsiella pneumoniae* carbapenemase (KPC) can occur among species other than *K. pneumoniae* and creates resistance to all β-lactam antibiotics including carbapenems. Resistance to quinolones is also typical, so therapy is limited to the polymyxins (e.g., colistin), or to tigecycline and the aminoglycosides depending on the organism's antibiotic susceptibility pattern.
- Like *P. aeruginosa*, *A. baumannii* can develop resistance to all known antimicrobials via a variety of mechanisms. This generally occurs among critically ill patients following prolonged stays in the intensive care unit. Treatment options may include polymyxins and sulbactam, a β-lactamase inhibitor that possesses some activity against drug-resistant *Acinetobacter*.
- *Enterobacter, Serratia,* and *Citrobacter* species can elaborate an AmpC β-lactamase following initiation of β-lactam therapy, which can result in a relapsing infection following an initial response. Thus clinicians treating such infections with penicillins or cephalosporins should closely monitor patients for the emergence of resistance. If resistance does emerge, AmpC-producing organisms can be treated with a carbapenem.
- Patients with multidrug-resistant gram-negative infections should be cared for in such a manner as to minimize spread of these dangerous organisms to other patients. Compliance with infection control protocols is paramount.
- Knowledge of the local epidemiology and antibiogram are important for preemptive and empiric antibiotic choices, especially against gram-negative rods.
- A carefully designed and executed antibiotic stewardship program could curtail unnecessary antibiotic use, thereby decreasing antibiotic selection pressure with a resulting decrease in bacterial resistance rates.

Viruses

Neutropenia per se is not a major risk factor for developing viral infections but concomitant lymphopenia is common and does predispose to infections with a range of viruses.[20] Respiratory virus infections are seasonal, except for parainfluenza. A frequent pathogen with clinical significance is respiratory syncytial virus, although influenza, parainfluenza, adenovirus, enteroviruses, the herpesviruses (including HHV-6), human metapneumovirus, and rhinovirus also produce diffuse interstitial infiltrates and pneumonitis.[20] HHV-6 and human metapneumovirus are not recovered with the usual tests ordered at the time of bronchoscopy, so a high suspicion for infection is required to order specific PCR testing. Documented infection with RSV prompts contact and droplet isolation precautions. Treatment components may include aerosolized ribavirin, IVIg, and in some cases, monoclonal antibody therapy. However, proof of efficacy of these treatments remains elusive, and the disease can cause significant morbidity and mortality.[21] With respiratory syncytial virus infections, aerosolized ribavirin treatment appears safe, and trends of decreasing viral loads have been reported. Secondary graft failure or diffuse alveolar hemorrhage associated with parainfluenza virus infection has been sporadically reported following transplantation.

Patients with lymphopenia are susceptible to a range of herpes virus family infections. Herpes simplex reactivation infections typically manifest as oral or genital ulcers, although more widespread involvement can occur, and are treated with low doses of acyclovir adjusted for renal function (e.g., 5 mg/kg IV every 8 hours) or oral valacyclovir (1 g bid). Reactivation of VZV can be severe in immunosuppressed persons and is treated with higher doses of acyclovir (e.g., 10 mg/kg IV every 8 hours or oral valacyclovir, 1 g three times a day). Use of acyclovir to prevent reactivation of HSV will also prevent VZV reactivation. Because many patients have not been exposed to acyclovir chronically (except for patients previously treated with recurrent courses of acyclovir for frequent outbreaks of genital herpes), there is little reason to expect resistance to acyclovir. However, HSV infections that appear or persist through acyclovir prophylaxis should be considered acyclovir resistant until viral sensitivity testing can be performed, and consideration should be given to initiating treatment with foscarnet or cidofovir.[22] Reports of acyclovir-resistant varicella are extremely rare. Foscarnet infusions affect calcium homeostasis, so monitoring of ionized calcium and phosphorus levels is required during clinical use of the drug. The major side effect of cidofovir is renal toxicity, which can be reduced to some degree with probenecid and hydration. Clinically significant CMV infection can occur during neutropenia, but the antigenemia test cannot be used for diagnosis or monitoring of response to therapy in this situation, so DNA PCR methods are preferred in that setting.

Human herpesvirus type 6 (HHV-6) is ubiquitous, and reactivation commonly occurs in patients with significant immunosuppression. However, clinically significant disease due to HHV-6 occurs in only a small percentage of patients who have HHV-6 detected in their blood.[23] HHV-6 infection can manifest as fever or pancytopenia. Other recognized clinical syndromes include pneumonitis and encephalitis. Infection is diagnosed by quantitative PCR, although the exact levels of virus that indicate clinically significant disease are not known. Detection of virus in the first 3 weeks following transplantation may be associated with early skin maculopapular rash and acute GVHD, but it can also present without overt clinical symptoms. Prospective large-scale studies are needed to determine the role of HHV-6 infection. HHV-6 has 60% DNA homology with CMV, and treatment of documented infection usually is initiated with induction doses of foscarnet or ganciclovir. Responses to antiviral therapy are not universal, and benefits of foscarnet versus ganciclovir have not been determined.

Cidofovir, when combined with aggressive supportive measures, is considered an adjunct in treatment of BK and adenovirus-associated hemorrhagic cystitis. Similarly, cidofovir can be used to treat disseminated adenovirus infections typically three times a week at 1 mg/kg/day, along with probenecid and hyperhydration.

Fungi

Most yeast infections in immunosuppressed patients are caused by *Candida*.[24] Candidal organisms that colonize the mouth and gut proliferate when antibacterial agents suppress the coexisting bacterial flora population. Guidelines for the treatment of candidiasis have been issued.[25] Patients who are clinically stable generally can be treated with fluconazole unless there has been previous azole exposure or mold infection is also a concern. Unstable patients or those who have been receiving an azole are usually treated with an echinocandin. Prevention of candidemia among allogeneic HSCT recipients is generally achieved with fluconazole. However, fluconazole does not have activity against some nonalbicans *Candida* species (e.g., *C. glabrata, C. krusei*) and all molds (e.g., *Aspergillus, Fusarium,* the Mucorales species). Among patients colonized with yeast species other than *C. albicans* and among heavily pretreated patients who may have incubating mold infection, prophylaxis using a mold-active triazole (e.g., posaconazole) or an echinocandin is preferred.[26]

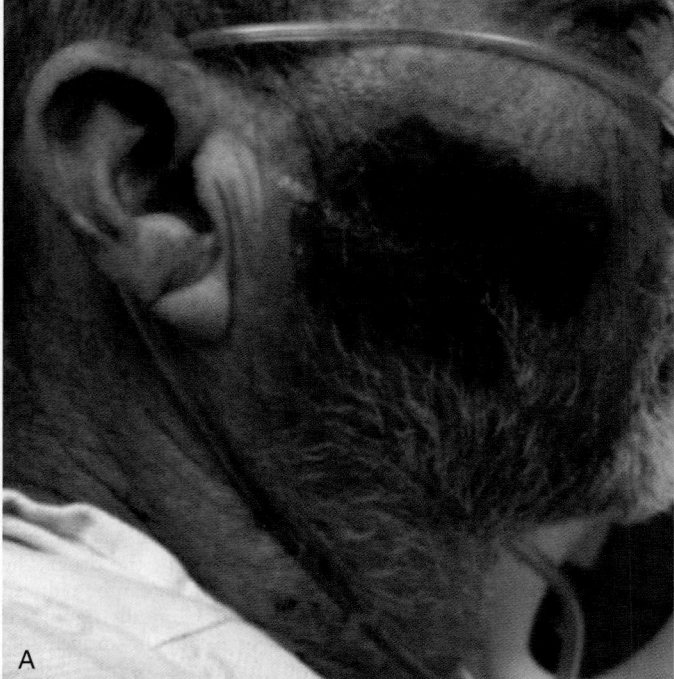

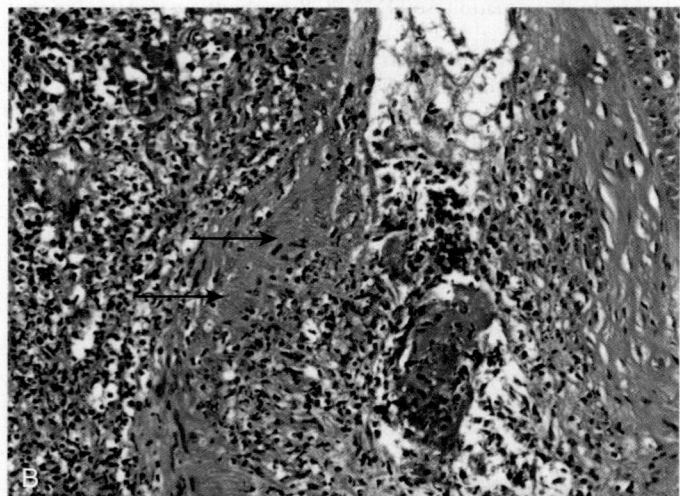

Fig. 89.5 EXAMPLES OF ASPERGILLOSIS. (A) Cutaneous aspergillosis in a patient with lymphoma treated with high-dose steroids. (B) Invasive aspergillosis with organism invading into blood vessel wall *(black arrows)*.

Although less common than *Candida* infections, mold infections in immunocompromised hosts are a significant source of mortality, with aspergillosis being the most common (Fig. 89.5). Because such infections are difficult to diagnose using standard microbiologic techniques, there has been significant interest in developing more effective screening tests. When used regularly, the serum *Aspergillus* galactomannan enzyme-linked immunosorbent assay (ELISA) may allow for earlier diagnosis of invasive aspergillosis in some patients.[27] The test is troubled by difficulties with both false-positive and false-negative results and thus needs to be interpreted as part of the overall clinical picture rather than as a stand-alone diagnostic tool. The development of a fungal infection in a patient receiving voriconazole should raise concern for mucormycosis, which is the second-most common mold infection in many transplant centers. Mucormycosis can rapidly disseminate through the lungs, sinuses, GI tract, and skin, which is uniformly fatal in patients with hematologic malignancies if not diagnosed early and aggressively treated.[28]

Although in vitro antifungal susceptibility testing for yeasts is not as well established as antibacterial testing, susceptibility from

The development of new antifungal drugs gives the clinician more options for prophylaxis and therapy than in previous years. There is an overall level of simplicity to the drug choices once their mechanisms of action are understood. The polyenes, including amphotericin products and the topical agent nystatin, attach onto ergosterol in the fungal cell membrane and are considered fungicidal, because cytoplasm leaks out, and individual cells die. The azoles, including fluconazole, itraconazole, voriconazole, and posaconazole, prevent the formation of new ergosterol. Azoles are considered fungistatic, because removal of the drug permits cell regrowth. Theoretically, use of an azole together with a polyene may have an overall static effect for an established infection as the ergosterol target for the fungicidal polyene is depleted. However, this combination may have advantages in terms of enhanced spectrum of activity. The echinocandins, including caspofungin, micafungin, and anidulafungin, prevent interaction of the catalytic and regulatory subunits of the β-glucan synthesis enzyme, so less β-glucan is formed for the cell wall. The scaffolding for the fungal cell wall is not maintained, and a dividing cell may burst open when trying to extend the new cell wall over daughter cells. The echinocandins are considered fungicidal for yeasts but fungistatic for molds, because drug activity is concentrated at only the tips of the extending hyphae with little effect on less metabolically active subapical compartments of the fungus. Combination therapy may have the most effect when a cell wall agent (an echinocandin) is used together with a cell membrane agent (a polyene or an azole). There is no role for three-drug therapy (an echinocandin, a polyene, and an azole). Aside from cases of cryptococcal meningitis, in which the importance of combination therapy is well established, the benefits of frontline use of combination antifungal for molds remain controversial, although active investigation continues in clinical trials. The value of combination regimens as salvage therapy for refractory mold infections remains uncertain.

bloodstream or invasive isolates can be helpful in the management of infections, especially if the patient will require transition to longer-term oral therapy. Long-term treatment with newer azoles may be valuable in responding patients. Echinocandins cannot be used to treat *Cryptococcus* or Mucorales as monotherapy, but there may be a role for echinocandin in combination treatment for Mucorales. Mucorales species are generally susceptible to amphotericin B and posaconazole and isavuconazole, although there are interspecies variations in susceptibility. In the case of mold infections, echinocandin agents may be fungistatic, rather than fungicidal, because interruption of fungal cell wall synthesis is limited to areas of hyphal branch points and growing hyphal tips. Because susceptibility testing for the echinocandin agents is of uncertain reliability, use of an echinocandin after the susceptibility profile has returned should be limited to non-neutropenic patients with uncomplicated candidemia. At present, the efficacy of combination drug therapy is unproven, but such therapy is often used in situations associated with high mortality. Clinical experience, but little clearly documented evidence, supports the value of extended combination antifungal therapy. Molds that often are resistant to amphotericin but may be susceptible to voriconazole or posaconazole include *Fusarium, Scedosporium* or *Pseudallescheria,* and *Trichosporon* (see box on Use of Antifungal Agents in Combination).

Malignancy-Associated Fever and Drug Fever

Although fever usually indicates the presence of infection, relapsing malignancy, autoimmune-granulomatous, collagen vascular diseases, or immunologic drug reactions can also be sources of fever in the immunocompromised host.[29] Malignancy or drug-associated fevers are the most common causes of persistent noninfectious fevers in cancer patients, but these are "diagnoses of exclusion" that require extensive clinical, radiographic, and microbiologic workup for occult infection until a noninfectious cause is considered most likely. All too often, patients receive escalating empiric broad-spectrum antibiotic therapy during this workup, which should be discouraged in clinically stable patients. Several clinical clues may favor a diagnosis of malignancy-associated fever, including (1) a prior history of fever at the time of initial malignancy diagnosis and (2) response of the fever to a trial of naproxen.[2] Patients with drug-associated fever often appear clinically well with relative bradycardia during periods of fever. Drug fevers typically develop 1 to 3 weeks after the start of a drug (β-lactams, sulfas, vancomycin, and phenytoin are among the most common inciting agents) and resolve, on average, within 48 hours of drug discontinuation unless the patient also has an accompanying rash. Drug-associated fever with rash and liver function test or complete blood count abnormalities (e.g., thrombocytopenia and eosinophilia) are often indicative of more severe reactions that should prompt immediate discontinuation or substitution of the likely offending medications.

INFECTION MANAGEMENT IN THE HEMATOPOIETIC STEM CELL TRANSPLANT RECIPIENT: A MODEL OF SEVERE IMMUNE DEFICIENCY

Infection is a major cause of morbidity and mortality in HSCT recipients. Such patients are susceptible to a wide range of infections, but the risk for a particular infection depends on a multitude of factors, including the type of transplantation, the length of time since transplantation, and the development of GVHD. A summary of common infections occurring in HSCT recipients is shown in Fig. 89.6.

Pretransplantation Prophylactic Techniques in Hematopoietic Stem Cell Transplant Recipients

Over the four decades during which HSCT has evolved, antimicrobial prophylaxis regimens have advanced to prevent common or high-risk infections.[3] This is balanced by problems associated with the preventive regimen, including toxicity, overgrowth of resistant organisms, and sometimes high cost. Algorithms for these preventive regimens evolve with changes in epidemiology, diagnostic methods, and new treatment agents for infections. Despite an overall preventive approach, infections still occur when a severe immune defect persists, when the infecting inoculum of organisms is large, when diagnostic methods are not sensitive enough for early detection, or when infecting agents overcome the effect of the antimicrobial agents. Measures taken to prevent infection in the preengraftment HSCT patient include pretransplantation serostatus blood workup, environmental measures to prevent infection (including frequent handwashing), and common sense.

Assessment of Pretransplantation Serostatus

Current pretransplant serologic testing of donor and recipient includes assaying for latent viruses (herpesvirus antibodies, hepatitis panels, and human T-cell lymphotropic virus antibodies [human T-lymphotropic virus I/II and HIV 1/2]) and syphilis. Antibody tests that are checked variably among individual transplantation centers include VZV, EBV, and *Toxoplasma*.

Herpes Simplex Virus

If the antibody test for HSV indicates prior infection or if the patient provides a clinical history of prior HSV infection (i.e., mucosal sores), latent infection exists and has the potential to reactivate during periods of T-cell suppression and neutropenia. This patient requires prophylactic medication (e.g., acyclovir or oral valacyclovir), which targets HSV for the neutropenic phase of transplantation. HSV lesions can appear as black scabs on the outside of the lips, white- to yellow-based ulcers when found on oral mucosa, or as an unusually severe exacerbation of mucositis or esophagitis. HSV prophylaxis administered until recovery from neutropenia may be helpful even in patients receiving nontransplantation chemotherapy such as acute leukemia induction therapy.

Cytomegalovirus

If the candidate is CMV seropositive before transplantation, the recipient should be followed with periodic (usually weekly) diagnostic

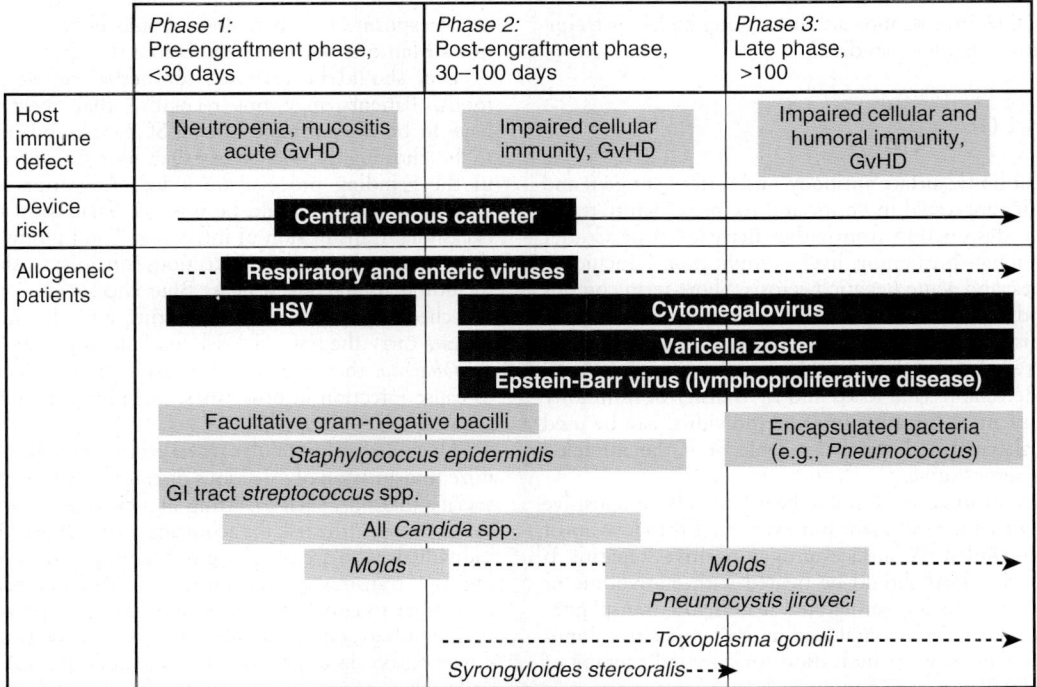

Fig. 89.6 TIMING OF INFECTIONS FOLLOWING HEMATOPOIETIC STEM CELL TRANSPLANT. *GI,* Gastrointestinal; *GVHD,* graft-versus-host disease; *HSV,* herpes simplex virus.

monitoring tests (e.g., pp65 antigenemia or PCR) for 10 to 20 weeks. No special measures are needed during neutropenia because a detectable circulating white count usually is necessary for reactivation of CMV. If the patient is CMV seronegative before transplantation but the donor is seropositive, the same monitoring algorithm used for the CMV-seropositive patient is needed.

If the donor and recipient are CMV seronegative before transplantation, infection through blood products is possible; therefore exclusive use of CMV-seronegative blood products or other means of preventing CMV seroconversion, such as leukocyte depletion by filtration, are recommended. CMV monitoring should be followed weekly, but the duration of this testing can be shortened by 50%, to 6 to 10 weeks, because late infection in seronegative recipients is uncommon.

Varicella, Human Herpes Virus Type 6, and Epstein-Barr Virus

A history of chickenpox is an adequate surrogate for performing the VZV antibody test. As an alternative to ordering varicella serology on every patient, the test could be ordered in patients with no history of varicella infection or vaccination.

Acyclovir used to prevent reactivation of HSV during neutropenia will also prevent occurrence of clinical VZV infection in most transplantation recipients. Later after transplantation, when acyclovir prophylaxis may have been discontinued, VZV reactivations usually are recognized by their characteristic dermatomal distribution, and treated using acyclovir or valacyclovir.

Serology for HHV-6 is not tested before transplantation because more than 95% of adults are seropositive for the virus. The transplantation recipient receiving minimal herpesvirus antiviral therapy during the transplantation procedure is at risk for reactivation of HHV-6. Whether the CMV-seronegative or HSV-seronegative recipient with a CMV-seronegative donor who ordinarily would receive no antiviral prophylaxis is at highest risk is not known. Additionally, the consequences of asymptomatic and untreated HHV-6 reactivation are not known.

The vast majority of adult patients undergoing transplantation and their donors are EBV seropositive. EBV reactivation is in the differential diagnosis of any new mass, such as enlarged nodes or lung nodules after transplantation (Chapter 52). Now that sensitive quantitative EBV viral load tests and effective treatments, such as rituximab, are available, investigators are monitoring high-risk recipients with quantitative viral load studies.[30]

Hepatitis B and C

Hepatitis B (core antibody, surface antibody, and surface antigen) and hepatitis C serologies are tested in donor and recipient before transplantation. Hepatic dysfunction from either hepatitis B or C after HSCT can lead to life-threatening liver complications, including venoocclusive disease and acute hepatic necrosis. Short-term complications are usually due to hepatitis B, whereas the long-term complication of cirrhosis is due to hepatitis C. The risk for hepatitis in the recipient can be reduced by antiviral therapy for recipients and donors who have detectable viral loads and by transfer of immunity from donor to recipient. A hepatitis-infected individual can be used as a donor if no alternative donor is available or if the intended recipient already is seropositive.

The risk for transmission is small when the hepatitis B–seropositive donor has an undetectable viral load; however, careful follow-up of recipients is recommended. A surface antigen-positive hepatitis B donor with a high viral load should be treated with lamivudine or another agent to reduce the circulating viral load before transplantation. High-circulating hepatitis C viral load in the seropositive donor for a seronegative recipient is an indication for antiviral therapy of the donor before HSCT.

If the potential recipient has serologic evidence of infection with hepatitis B or C before transplantation, viral load levels should be checked before and monitored after HSCT. High hepatitis B viral load (>10^5 copies/mL) is the most important risk factor for reactivation in patients positive for surface antigen undergoing HSCT. High-circulating hepatitis B viral load in the intended recipient is an indication for lamivudine. There is no evident correlation between hepatitis C genotype and type or severity of liver disease after transplantation.

Human Immunodeficiency Virus

A positive donor HIV test for a recipient candidate not known to be seropositive is a contraindication for donation. If the screening test for HIV is positive, a Western blot study should be completed to confirm the result because of the potential for false-positive testing.

Syphilis

If the indirect screening test for syphilis returns positive and is confirmed by a direct test, high-dose penicillin treatment should be given for 10 days after transplantation.

Toxoplasma

Historically, 15% of patients who undergo transplantation in the United States are seropositive for *Toxoplasma,* but this percentage may be higher for European centers. The risk for reactivation among seropositive patients is 2%, for an overall incidence of less than 1% of HSCT recipients. It is suspected that low-dose sulfa-based regimens, such as those used to prevent *Pneumocystis* pneumonia, may be effective in preventing *Toxoplasma.*

Review of Commonsense Measures to Prevent Infection

Commonsense measures that should be discussed before transplantation or aggressive nontransplantation chemotherapy include attention to diet, travel, crowds, and pets. Additionally, a history of family or social exposure to tuberculosis should be used to guide whether or not a Mantoux test is applied before therapy.

Diet should be reviewed for herbal supplements or restricted foods. Patients may not recognize that most supplements will have to be discontinued after HSCT. Ground meat products need to be thoroughly cooked so that bacteria, distributed onto meat in the grinding process, are killed. Any fruits or vegetables that cannot be peeled should be washed. Salad bars are associated with occasional transmission of infections. Food products or supplements that inherently contain infectious organisms should be avoided, including undercooked eggs. Blue cheeses have molds spiked into the cheese wheel as they are curing and should be avoided. Soft cheeses carry the potential risk for *Listeria* infection. Yogurt contains *Lactobacillus* that, rather than causing gut problems, has been found to cause infection in other sites, including the lungs after aspiration events.

There are no particular travel restrictions, but strategies to minimize transmission of infectious diseases have been summarized. Some social situations, such as sitting in a crowded movie theater or classroom, increase the risk for acquiring a viral illness. Turning away from individuals who are coughing or sneezing may be helpful in preventing the transmission of infections. Patients need instruction to remember to complete the cycle of infection prevention by washing their hands as soon as possible after being close to such an individual. Given outbreaks of noroviruses (Norwalk-like viruses) on cruise ships and other types of outbreaks (e.g., *Staphylococcus*) commonly associated with the close living quarters during this type of travel, cruise ships should be avoided.

Healthy dogs and cats are considered acceptable pets. However, the immunosuppressed patient should not be responsible for scooping cat litter because of potential *Toxoplasma* cyst exposure. Similarly, the patient should not play in sandboxes because these areas are concentrated sites that feral outdoor cats may use as litter boxes. Because reptiles of many sorts have been reported to be infected with *Salmonella,* patients should not touch these animals or the insides or outsides of their cages or tanks. The heated water of tropical fish tanks carry *Mycobacterium marinum. Cryptococcus* and *Chlamydophila* (formerly *Chlamydia) psittaci* can be transmitted from large pet birds.

Environmental Measures to Prevent Infection

Persons entering the patient's room to perform an examination or touch the patient (including visitors as well as health care workers) should wash their hands outside the room. Ideally, the institution will have handwashing sinks in the hallways outside patient rooms for this purpose. During respiratory virus season, the infection control department often adds extra signs to doorways and other places in the wards to remind visitors of the importance of handwashing. Staff and visitors without control of body secretions should not be permitted to have direct patient contact.

Some infectious situations require special isolation procedures. Contact isolation (gloves and gowns) is used for patients with adenovirus, methicillin-resistant *S. aureus,* or *Clostridium difficile* infection. Droplet precautions are added to contact precautions for respiratory virus or varicella infection. Carriers of vancomycin-resistant *Enterococcus* are placed in contact isolation until they meet defined criteria for discontinuation of isolation.

Laminar airflow is a cumbersome and expensive isolation technique that has been largely outmoded with advances in airflow and isolation technology as well as current antimicrobial therapy. Historically, it has been most commonly used for patients with aplastic anemia or those receiving T cell-depleted transplants.

High-efficiency particulate air (HEPA) filtration has replaced laminar airflow as the means for preventing infection through ventilation. With at least 12 air exchanges per hour, HEPA filters are capable of removing particles greater than 0.2 μm in diameter, such as mold spores. Patients often ask whether they should purchase portable HEPA filters for the home or apartment they will occupy after hospitalization. In the broadest sense, this is an extra measure that can be used on an individual basis. If portable HEPA filters are used, they should be obtained for each room that the patient will occupy during the day and night, and each unit should be sized for the individual room. A beneficial effect of HEPA filtration in the outpatient setting has not been demonstrated.

Infection in the Hematopoietic Stem Cell Transplant Recipient Preengraftment

The major risk factors for infection in the preengraftment period include drug-induced mucositis, profound neutropenia, and the presence of indwelling catheters. Thus the major infections observed in this period are due to bacteria that colonize the skin and GI tract (e.g., viridans group streptococci and gram-negative bacilli), *Candida,* and respiratory viruses, especially in the winter months (see Fig. 89.6). Reactivation of latent or partially treated fungal infections can also occur, with *Aspergillus* being well recognized. The propensity of patients to develop such infections has led to widespread use of prophylaxis with an antiviral, antibacterial, and antifungal agent during this time period.

Infection in the Hematopoietic Stem Cell Transplant Recipient After Engraftment

Once engraftment has occurred, the major risk factors for infection include immunosuppression used to treat GVHD and mechanical disruption of mucosal barriers, particular indwelling venous catheters. Viral infections that reactivate after engraftment often are related to defective T cell-mediated immunity and include CMV, adenovirus, and hepatitis viruses. Outpatient HSCT recipients inhale mold spores and *Pneumocystis* cysts from the environment, so common exogenously acquired infections include aspergillosis, mucormycosis, and *P. jirovecii* (previously *carinii*). Bacterial infections associated with defective cell-mediated immunity such as pneumococcosis, nocardiosis, and atypical mycobacterial disease can also occur in association with significant immunosuppression (Fig. 89.6).

Cytomegalovirus

CMV causes significant morbidity and mortality in transplant patients both directly and because of its immunosuppressive effects that predispose patients to concomitant or sequential infection with bacterial and fungal pathogens. Use of prophylactic ganciclovir at engraftment usually is avoided because it leads to myelosuppression and possibly a higher incidence of late CMV disease. Instead, the patient is treated with ganciclovir when weekly PCR or pp65 antigenemia monitoring test meets a positive threshold. Initial viral load levels do not predict disease. CMV infections are treated with an induction ganciclovir regimen followed by approximately 6 weeks of a maintenance regimen (half the induction dose). The duration of induction (1 to 3 weeks) varies by institution, but in general 1 week is used for low-grade infection, 2 weeks for high-grade infection, and 3 weeks for end-organ disease. A rising viral load, when checked weekly during the first month of preemptive therapy, signals the need for continued induction dosing or repeat induction dosing.

When the end-organ manifestation of CMV is pneumonitis (recovery of CMV from a deep lung specimen along with an interstitial infiltrate on chest radiograph), IVIg is added on an every-other-day basis for the duration of induction. When CMV manifests in an end organ other than the lungs, use of IVIg is not as clearly useful. Some centers add IVIg when the patient's total IgG level falls below 400 mg/dL. Dosing schedules vary from IVIg given once weekly for 3 weeks to every other day for the duration of induction, similar to therapy for pneumonitis. Ganciclovir resistance is uncommon, but when it occurs, foscarnet or cidofovir may be used.

Varicella-Zoster Virus

VZV reactivations from latency (zoster) usually are recognized by their characteristic dermatomal distribution. No temporal pattern is seen, viremia can occur concurrently, and multiple episodes are possible but uncommon. For patients who have been treated for a zoster episode after HSCT, some centers provide acyclovir prophylaxis until 1 year after HSCT. Less common VZV clinical manifestations that can result in severe infection and may require molecular testing or viral culture for diagnosis include hemorrhagic pneumonia, hepatitis, central nervous system disease, thrombocytopenia, and retinal necrosis.

HSCT recipients with a negative or unknown VZV disease history and a significant exposure to active varicella are susceptible to primary VZV infection. For these patients, varicella-zoster immune globulin should be provided within 96 hours of exposure. Patients with positive serology can become clinically reinfected after exposure and should be provided with acyclovir prophylaxis; however, such patients do not require varicella-zoster immune globulin.

Epstein-Barr Virus

EBV causes a spectrum of scenarios after stem cell transplantation, ranging from asymptomatic but detectable viremia, hemophagocytic syndrome, or posttransplant lymphoproliferative disorder (Chapter 52). The incidence of EBV-related complications is higher in mismatched donors, patients with T cell–depleted transplants, and patients receiving intensive immunosuppression (e.g., antithymocyte globulin). Posttransplant lymphoproliferative disorder after allogeneic stem cell transplantation most often is of donor origin. Quantitative EBV viral load diagnostic testing is relatively new and not standardized, so the algorithms for monitoring and initiation of treatment vary. Recognition of greater than 1000 viral copies/mL of blood requires investigation, repeated testing, and possibly treatment, especially in high-risk patients. Direct antiviral agents have limited impact on reducing detectable EBV viral loads. General treatment approaches involve reduction of immunosuppression and rituximab or donor lymphocyte infusion (see Chapter 52).

Invasive Mold Infections

Invasive fungal infections are among the most feared complications of HSCT both because of their high mortality rates and the difficulty in establishing a diagnosis.[4] Among HSCT recipients studied at autopsy, yeast and mold infections were common, seen in more than 25% of deaths. The probability of survival is higher in recent years, likely due to newer and more effective agents, as well as nonmyeloablative conditioning. Posaconazole has been shown to be effective in preventing invasive fungal infections during GVHD.[5] Mold spores may initiate a localized infection in the lungs or sinuses that, after intensive immunosuppression for GVHD, may disseminate to the skin, abdominal organs, or central nervous system. Treatment of central nervous system infections should include voriconazole, which attains cerebrospinal fluid levels approximately 50% those of plasma or central nervous system tissue levels approximately 200% those of plasma. Infection with Mucorales organisms tends to have later onset than infection with *Aspergillus* (after day 90).[4]

Pneumocystis

The most common presenting symptoms of *Pneumocystis* infection are dyspnea, cough, and fever. Diagnosis requires demonstration of the organism in silver-stained specimens (bronchoalveolar lavage or lung biopsy) although PCR testing of bronchoalveolar lavage fluid is becoming a more common diagnostic method. Disease occurs by both new infection and activation of latent infection. Most patients present between day 40 and day 80 after HSCT, but cases as early as day 12 and as late as 42 months after HSCT have been reported. Once lymphocyte function is more reconstituted, *Pneumocystis* infections are rare. Prophylaxis options include trimethoprim-sulfamethoxazole, aerosol or intravenous pentamidine, dapsone, and atovaquone. Among patients treated with dapsone after transplantation, increased red blood cell and platelet transfusion requirements are noted. Prophylaxis is generally discontinued 1 to 2 years after HSCT, or later if immunosuppression is ongoing.

Parasitic Infections

Toxoplasma gondii is a ubiquitous pathogen that causes significant morbidity and mortality. Although relatively uncommon, toxoplasmosis is recognized as a cause of cerebral, ocular, and lung disease in immunocompromised patients. Accurate diagnosis of this treatable infection is critical. PCR-based testing has become an adjunct method for diagnosis, occasionally replacing tissue biopsy, and can be used to monitor patients with positive anti-toxoplasma serology prior to transplant.

Infection Issues in the Late Posttransplantation Period

Encapsulated Organism Prophylaxis

Penicillin prophylaxis has decreased the incidence of infection-related morbidity and mortality from polysaccharide-encapsulated bacteria

(*S. pneumoniae*, *H. influenzae* type b, *Neisseria meningitidis*). Penicillin-resistant pneumococcal infection has been reported, prompting consideration of alternate prophylaxis, such as a change from penicillins to quinolones. Prophylaxis is generally discontinued 2 years after HSCT, or later if GVHD and immunosuppression are ongoing at the 2-year time point. Once the patient is ready for vaccinations, conjugate pneumococcal, meningococcal, and *H. influenzae* type b vaccines are given.

Vaccination

Recipients of HSCT frequently lose antibody responses to viral and bacterial pathogens previously targeted by childhood vaccination. Although practice varies among transplantation centers, killed-virus vaccines are often given at 1 year after HSCT and live-virus vaccines approximately 2 years after HSCT for patients without GVHD.[6] For adults, Tdap (formulation of reduced-antigen, combined diphtheria-tetanus-acellular pertussis vaccine) has replaced Td (diphtheria-tetanus booster vaccine) as a means for decreasing the adult reservoir of pertussis. For protection against hepatitis, the combined vaccine providing protection against both hepatitis A and B can be used. The efficacy of vaccination is influenced by the time elapsed since transplantation, the nature of the hematopoietic graft, the presence of GVHD, and the use of serial immunization. Guidelines have been published (Chapter 110, Table 110.4).

REFERENCES

1. Parody R, Martino R, Rovira M, et al: Severe infections after unrelated donor allogeneic hematopoietic stem cell transplantation in adults: Comparison of cord blood transplantation with peripheral blood and bone marrow transplantation. *Biol Blood Marrow Transplant* 12:748, 2006.
2. Koo S, Baden LR: Infectious complications associated with immunomodulating monoclonal antibodies used in the treatment of hematologic malignancy. *J Natl Compr Canc Netw* 6:213, 2008.
3. Gea-Banacloche JC: Rituximab-associated infections. *Semin Hematol* 47:198, 2010.
4. Morrison VA: Infectious complications of chronic lymphocytic leukaemia: Pathogenesis, spectrum of infection, preventive approaches. *Best Pract Res Clin Haematol* 23:153, 2010.
5. Pratt G, Goodyear O, Moss P: Immunodeficiency and immunotherapy in multiple myeloma. *Br J Haematol* 138:579, 2007.
6. Song E, Jaishankar GB, Saleh H, et al: Chronic granulomatous disease: A review of the infectious and inflammatory complications. *Clin Mol Allergy* 9:10, 2011.
7. Ramakrishnan M, Moisi JC, Klugman KP, et al: Increased risk of invasive bacterial infections in African people with sickle-cell disease: A systematic review and meta-analysis. *Lancet Infect Dis* 10:337, 2010.
8. Falagas ME, Vardakas KZ, Samonis G: Decreasing the incidence and impact of infections in neutropenic patients: Evidence from meta-analyses of randomized controlled trials. *Curr Med Res Opin* 24:235, 2008.
9. Engelhard D, Akova M, Boeckh MJ, et al: Bacterial infection prevention after hematopoietic cell transplantation. *Bone Marrow Transplant* 44:470, 2009.
10. Clark OA, Lyman GH, Castro AA, et al: Colony-stimulating factors for chemotherapy-induced febrile neutropenia: A meta-analysis of randomized controlled trials. *J Clin Oncol* 23:4214, 2005.
11. Ljungman P, Cordonnier C, Einsele H, et al: Vaccination of hematopoietic cell transplant recipients. *Bone Marrow Transplant* 44:526, 2009.
12. Mermel LA, Allon M, Bouza E, et al: Clinical practice guidelines for the diagnosis and management of intravascular catheter-related infection: 2009 update by the Infectious Diseases Society of America. *Clin Infect Dis* 49:45, 2009.
13. Freifeld AG, Bow EJ, Sepkowitz KA, et al: Clinical practice guideline for the use of antimicrobial agents in neutropenic patients with cancer:

2010 update by the Infectious Diseases Society of America. *Clin Infect Dis* 52:431, 2011.

14. Baskaran ND, Gan GG, Adeeba K: Applying the Multinational Association for Supportive Care in Cancer risk scoring in predicting outcome of febrile neutropenia patients in a cohort of patients. *Ann Hematol* 87:569, 2008.

15. Paul M, Yahav D, Bivas A, et al: Anti-pseudomonal beta-lactams for the initial, empirical, treatment of febrile neutropenia: Comparison of beta-lactams. *Cochrane Database Syst Rev* CD005197, 2010.

16. Blijlevens NM: Neutropenic enterocolitis: Challenges in diagnosis and treatment. *Clin Adv Hematol Oncol* 7:530, 2009.

17. Georgiadou SP, Sipsas NV, Marom EM, et al: The diagnostic value of halo and reversed halo signs for invasive mold infections in compromised hosts. *Clin Infect Dis* 52:1155, 2011.

18. O'Grady NP, Alexander M, Burns LA, et al: Guidelines for the prevention of intravascular catheter-related infections. *Clin Infect Dis* 52:e193, 2011.

19. Redelman-Sidi G, Sepkowitz KA: Rapidly growing mycobacteria infection in patients with cancer. *Clin Infect Dis* 51:434, 2010.

20. Kumar D: Emerging viruses in transplantation. *Curr Opin Infect Dis* 23:378, 2010.

21. Shah JN, Chemaly RF: Management of RSV infections in adult recipients of hematopoietic stem cell transplantation. *Blood* 117:2763, 2011.

22. Piret J, Boivin G: Resistance of herpes simplex viruses to nucleoside analogues: Mechanisms, prevalence, and management. *Antimicrob Agents Chemother* 55:472, 2011.

23. Agut H: Deciphering the clinical impact of acute human herpesvirus 6 (HHV-6) infections. *J Clin Virol* 52:171, 2011.

24. Kontoyiannis DP, Marr KA, Park BJ, et al: Prospective surveillance for invasive fungal infections in hematopoietic stem cell transplant recipients, 2001-2006: Overview of the Transplant-Associated Infection Surveillance Network (TRANSNET) database. *Clin Infect Dis* 50:1100, 2010.

25. Pappas PG, Kauffman CA, Andes D, et al: Clinical practice guidelines for the management of candidiasis: 2009 update by the Infectious Diseases Society of America. *Clin Infect Dis* 48:535, 2009.

26. Ullmann AJ, Lipton JH, Vesole DH, et al: Posaconazole or fluconazole for prophylaxis in severe graft-versus-host disease. *N Engl J Med* 356:347, 2007.

27. Wheat LJ, Walsh TJ: Diagnosis of invasive aspergillosis by galactomannan antigenemia detection using an enzyme immunoassay. *Eur J Clin Microbiol Infect Dis* 27:251, 2008.

28. Kontoyiannis DP, Lewis RE: How I treat mucormycosis. *Blood* 118:1224, 2011.

29. Zell JA, Chang JC: Neoplastic fever: A neglected paraneoplastic syndrome. *Support Care Cancer* 13:877, 2005.

30. Gulley ML, Tang W: Using Epstein-Barr viral load assays to diagnose, monitor, and prevent posttransplant lymphoproliferative disorder. *Clin Microbiol Rev* 23:366, 2010.

CHAPTER 90

PSYCHOSOCIAL ASPECTS OF HEMATOLOGIC DISORDERS

Matthew J. Gonzales, Dawn M. Gross, and Elizabeth Cooke

Major changes in the understanding and treatment of cancer have led to increased survival for people diagnosed with hematologic cancers. Regardless of the advances and concomitant survival increase, a diagnosis of a hematologic malignancy can have great impact on the psychosocial aspects of the lives of cancer survivors and their families. Diseases of the blood are perceived as serious and often fatal. Psychologic, existential, cognitive, social, and economic stressors are common experiences for cancer survivors. Despite the increasing attention by providers, policy makers, and the general public on long-term survivorship issues within the past 20 years, ongoing progress must continue to be made in identifying and testing interventions and services to meet the psychosocial aspects of quality cancer care for patients and their families.[1] Psychosocial interventions and services are those that enable patients, their families, and health care providers to optimize health care and health care outcomes by managing the psychologic, social, spiritual, and behavioral aspects of cancer and its consequences.

These psychosocial aspects may be intensified in patients with hematologic malignancies because of their association with an uncertain prognosis, a prolonged treatment course often involving numerous hospitalizations including periods of prolonged isolation, and the systemic nature of the diseases.[2] Involvement with a complex and fragmented health care system, the need for episodic and aggressive treatment, remissions and exacerbation of acute and distressing symptoms, functional limitations, family separation, financial burden, and role disruptions are a few of the issues that characterize the life of patients with hematologic malignancies, not to mention the threat to life imposed by these diagnoses. This chapter provides information on factors that affect psychosocial adjustment among patients with hematologic malignancies, the wide range of psychologic responses that are possible throughout the illness trajectory, and the efficacy of psychosocial interventions and services to minimize distress and promote adaptation. Some practical guidelines regarding patient management and identification of patients who may require formal psychiatric consultation are offered.

ACCOMPANYING TRENDS IN PSYCHOSOCIAL ISSUES

Within the past several decades there have been significant advances in oncology that have affected the psychosocial care of the cancer patient. The continued advances in quality-of-life research, survivorship, personalized medicine, patient-centered care, quality care initiatives; interest in the reduction of health care disparities, evidence-based medicine, and palliative medicine; and the increasing interest in psychosocial health for patients and caregivers are a few of the changes in cancer care.

Interest in health-related quality of life can be traced back to 1947 with the beginning of the first nonphysiologic outcome measure for cancer: the Karnofsky performance scale. Exponential growth in disease- and individual-specific tools for measurement of health-related quality of life continues to this day.[3,4] Since the beginning of the survivorship movement, there has been increasing growth in legislation, education, and advocacy for cancer survivors. The focus on personalized medicine coupled with an interest in decreasing health care disparities has incorporated the idea of tailoring interventions to the needs of individual patients.[5–7] The Institute of Medicine report the "Quality Chasm" has begun a dialogue of the patient-centered

view of medicine that is ongoing.[8–10] The emergence of palliative medicine, a new specialty that overlaps symptom management and end-of-life care with oncology specialists, has made an impact on improving symptoms in oncology patients.[11,12] The Institute of Medicine report *Cancer Care for the Whole Patient: Meeting Psychosocial Health Needs* lists 10 recommendations related to improving psychosocial health for patients and family members.[13]

CLINICAL COURSE OF HEMATOLOGIC MALIGNANCIES

The incidence, course, treatment, and survival for various hematologic malignancies vary widely, yet dramatic improvements in survival rates have been seen almost universally.

In contrast to treatment of many solid cancers, treatment of hematologic malignancies often involves intense regimens, highly technical therapies, lengthy hospitalizations, episodes of high infection risk, periods of unpredictability, and ongoing outpatient monitoring of the patient's condition. A number of patients respond to the curative attempts with long-term remission, remain well, and, after a period, are considered cured. However, some patients have an initial reduction in tumor burden in response to a curative attempt only to relapse at an unpredictable time later. Other patients begin treatment with a hope for a cure but their cancer does not dissipate often resulting in the individual's progressive decline. In some patients, the cancer is so advanced at the time of diagnoses that they experience a rapid progression of their disease. The remainder of this chapter proceeds through the common trajectories associated with hematologic malignancies including diagnosis, treatment, relapse, the end of life, and survivorship (Fig. 90.1).

Time of Diagnosis

Being diagnosed with a hematologic malignancy can be a devastating time of crisis. The time of diagnosis has been described by a cancer survivor as "a lightning bolt through a stop sign" or an existential plight.[14,15] It is a time of intense stress and likened to a personal disaster in the patient's and family's life.[15] Often these patients describe vague symptoms such as fatigue for weeks, even months, being treated in urgent care centers for presumed non–life-threatening illnesses, such as bronchitis or other uncomplicated infections. Families are often dismissed if they offer their concern, thus being unprepared and blind-sided by the ultimate diagnosis of an unexpected, catastrophic illness. More recent literature has continued to confirm the distress at diagnosis and advance the understanding to include potential psychiatric diagnosis such as depression and anxiety.[16]

The period from time of diagnosis through initiation of treatment is characterized by sometimes fast-paced medical evaluation and treatment, the development of new relationships with unfamiliar medical personnel, and the need to integrate a barrage of information that is at best frightening and confusing. Often patients with hematologic malignancies need immediate treatment intervention compared with those patients with solid tumors. But even with the advanced speed of information in this technologic age, patients have difficulty with information integration in a short period of time. Within the context of this anxiety-provoking situation, timely deci-

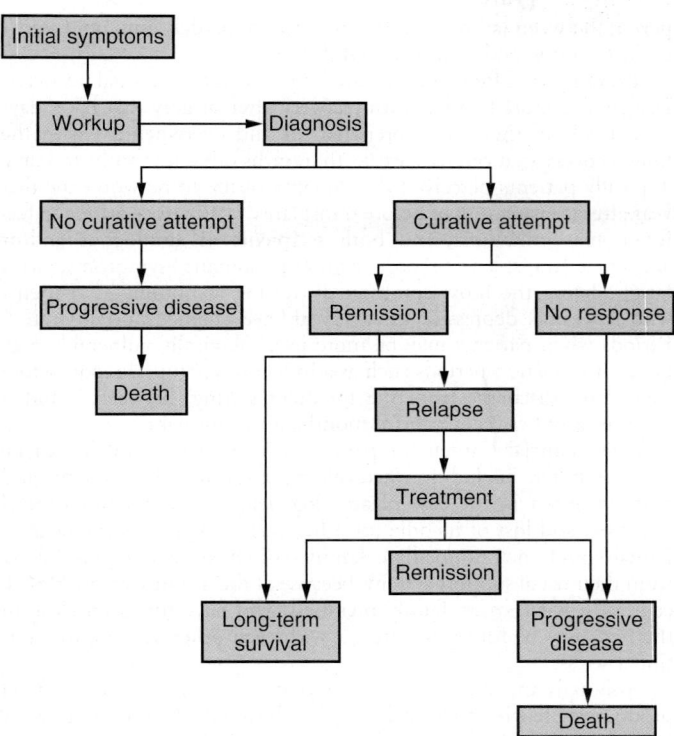

Fig. 90.1 CLINICAL COURSE OF A PATIENT WITH A HEMATO-LOGIC MALIGNANCY. *(Modified from Lesko LM: Hematopoietic dyscrasias. In Holland JC, editor:* Psychooncology, *New York, 1998, Oxford University Press, p 408.)*

BOX 90.1	Factors That May Predict Poor Coping in Patients With Cancer

Past psychiatric history
Compliance issues
Demographic factors such as younger age and female sex
Limited social support or difficult social relationships
Recent history of smoking cessation
Substance abuse history
Recent losses
Advanced disease
Uncontrolled symptoms
Pessimistic outlook on life
Multiple obligations
Avoidance coping (escape-avoidance, distancing, and denial)
Lower functional status
Higher regimen-related toxicity

sions must be made regarding treatment, and patients may feel tremendous responsibility, concern, and isolation during this period.

There are multiple personal and cultural factors that may profoundly influence the patient's response to the cancer diagnosis. Being aware of the patient's exposure to cancer in the past and the meaning of their cancer experience may provide an insight into response. Literature does indicate that preexisting issues such as symptoms, psychiatric history, gender, social and psychologic factors, disability and avoidance coping may influence the reaction to the time of diagnosis[17–20] Although extreme and sustained psychologic reactions as the first response to a cancer diagnosis are unusual, careful assessment of the nature of the patient's reaction remains important. Initial reactions often are predictive of later adaptation.[43] Early assessment by clinicians can help to identify people who are at risk for later adjustment problems and in greatest need of ongoing psychosocial support[21,22,27] (see Box 90.1). Because many clinicians are guarded about disclosing information until a firm diagnosis is established, patients may develop highly personal explanations that can be inaccurate and provoke intensely negative emotions. Ongoing involvement and consistent and repeated information from key health care providers help to minimize patients' uncertainty and the development of maladaptive coping strategies based on incomplete or inaccurate information.

Although the literature substantiates the devastating psychologic impact of a cancer diagnosis, it is also well documented that many patients cope effectively by embracing optimism. Also, contrary to the beliefs of many clinicians, denial has also been found to assist patients in coping effectively with a diagnosis of cancer, unless used to an excessive degree.[23] With the firm establishment of the cancer diagnosis, planning for treatment begins. If patients have been given a clear explanation of their condition while encouraged to maintain hope, the initial reaction of shock, fear, and desperation can give way to a sense of optimism. Health care providers have an important role in monitoring and possibly mediating psychosocial adjustment. Keeping patients informed and actively involved in their care and being aware of the unique meaning that people may associate with a

diagnosis of cancer are vital. Patients who have a pervasive and unyielding negative affect that persists long after the crisis of diagnosis may require ongoing psychosocial monitoring and referral for services and supportive interventions throughout their treatment and disease course.[24]

In addition, family assessment during this phase is vital. Levels of family distress, depression, and anxiety are mediated by the functioning of the family at the time of diagnosis.[24] Studies have shown that caregivers and families share similar rates of psychosocial angst.[24] Families who have open expression of feelings and actions have reported lower depression; however, those families who have dysfunctional problem-solving abilities have higher depression.[24] Also, anxiety within the family increases with unclear communication.[24] Both anxiety and depression are easy to assess in patients and family members, and timely referral for assistance during this period may lay a foundation of adequate coping throughout the patient's course of illness. During this time, many providers are conveying large amounts of information. It is not always easy for patients to differentiate the importance of each communication and prioritize their problem-solving behaviors. Consequently, providers must repeat information at each contact and inquire about the patients' and families' understanding of facts and treatment options. Often patients and families describe that they are in a state of numbness and that information is not really processed, understood, or comprehended.

Treatment

Psychosocial factors are critical parameters in considering which treatment is best for an individual patient. The development of a treatment plan should include information about all aspects of medical/surgical treatments as well as what is known about the psychosocial sequelae. Often patients react to a diagnosis of cancer with feelings of fear and helplessness. Patients look to the primary oncologist for a curative treatment that also can preserve their quality of life. Patients may feel vulnerable and believe that complete reliance on the oncologist is essential. Combating feelings of helplessness during this period can help patients alleviate painful anxiety and possible depression.[18] This is best done by a member of the health care team who has established a treatment alliance with the patient. The health care provider must make the patient feel like a partner in all aspects of care. This is especially true regarding decisions about treatment options. Giving information to patients and families often alleviates anxiety and uncertainty because patients feel more in control.

Active treatment of cancer usually initiates another acute phase of the cancer experience. It can occur while a patient is receiving treatment or as a complication of treatment. An important standard of clinical practice, based on extensive research, is to provide patients with information that will prepare them for what to expect during their treatment. Some providers wait until patients complain about potentially expected side effects. When this happens patients may become skeptical about the completeness or accuracy of any future information given by the person. This threat to undermine a trusting relationship has important implications for decision making, patient choice of care setting in the future, and recommendations made by patients to others who are seeking a source of cancer care.

Often during the treatment phase increasing burdens are placed on the immediate caregiver and family to support the patient's schedule for treatment, multiple admissions, and increasing dependency.[25] The patient may be unable to work, and financial stressors accumulate. Sensitivity and awareness by providers to social, economic, and relationship stresses are needed to assist with referral for social services and other psychologic assistance. Support groups with other patients, families and caregivers, can be helpful during this time. Evidence clearly indicates that sharing a common experience in a support group can have psychologic benefit.[26]

DECISION FOR HEMATOPOIETIC STEM CELL TRANSPLANTATION

Hematopoietic stem cell transplantation (HSCT) is increasingly becoming a standard treatment for many high-risk hematologic malignancies and nonmalignant diseases either as part of overall treatment or after relapse. The procedure for transplantation is complex and can cause intense psychologic distress and extreme social strain on the patient's caregiver, friends, and family members. Often the psychologic and social issues can be more challenging for the health care team than the medical issues. Because HSCT is an intense and distinctive experience for patients and families and has the potential to cause prolonged psychologic distress unlike other experiences with oncology patients, the issues unique to this population warrant a separate discussion.

HSCT patients may face unique physical and psychologic stresses consisting of recurrent infections, repeated hospitalizations, and social isolation for weeks to months during their initial recovery. Consequently a thorough pretransplant psychosocial evaluation is recommended to identify those patients at risk for development of psychosocial morbidity and to initiate timely interventions to optimize adaptation. Identified risk factors for psychosocial morbidity during and following transplant include previous psychiatric morbidity, pretransplant compliance issues, pretransplant physical and mental health problems, younger age, female sex, avoidant coping style, recent smoking cessation, lower functioning status on admission, problems with quality and presence of social support before transplant, perception of limited social support, and the presence of difficult relationships.[21,27]

The time of transplantation when the infusion of cells occurs can be a special moment for patients, with patients often referring to the date of transplant as a "birthday" or special anniversary date. Often family members are gathered at the bedside to celebrate the long-awaited event of the transplant. However, the weeks following transplant can be difficult psychologically. Factors that can affect psychologic distress and subsequent coping include persistent symptoms following transplant, increased regimen-related toxicity, slower physical recovery, low performance status, longer length of stay, graft-versus-host disease (GVHD), negative appraisal of the transplant experience, body image disturbance, fears of relapse and secondary malignancies,[27-29] The threat of death continues to be real, and patients experience social isolation, bodily discomfort, major body image changes, and a sense of loss of control. These issues lead to a myriad of emotions, including hope, anger, depression, anxiety, anticipation, guilt, and joy. Khan et al identified the following common psychiatric diagnoses with inpatient transplant patients: adjustment disorder (40%), depression (23%), generalized anxiety disorder (10%), acute psychotic disorder (10%), delirium (10%), and depressive psychosis (7%).[30] Kishi et al compared inpatient psychiatric consultations among transplant and nontransplant patients.[31] Transplant patients differed on several characteristics: more frequently white, less likely to have a previous psychiatric history, longer time

period between admission to consult, more delirium, and more socioeconomic and health-related distress.

Patients are often not prepared for the long, gradual recovery. Patients are more familiar with recovery after surgery that takes days to weeks, and they are unprepared for and overwhelmed with the long recovery that can take weeks to months or even months to years. Typically patients perceived their quality of life to be worse the first year after transplant than before transplant.[32] Patients continue to feel functional limitations, and both recipients of autologous and/or allogeneic transplants report common somatic symptoms, with fatigue being the most common distressing symptom.[33-35] Patients who experience depression the first year have a higher mortality rate.[36] Periods when patients may be more psychologically vulnerable may occur at transition periods such as admission workup, directly before transplant, discharge from the inpatient setting, between 3 and 5 months, and between 6 and 9 months posttransplant.

The financial burden for patients who undergo HSCT can be overwhelming, including medical expenses for the patient and marrow donor in the case of an allogeneic HSCT, potential travel expenses, and loss of income for other caregiving family members.[26] Patients and their immediate families often are geographically far from their usual support systems because of the distance to the HSCT center. In some cases, family members who have not been close in the past may be forced to interact with each other, leading to additional stress.

Although the literature is clear that most patients return to a productive life with high quality of life, during the first few years after transplantation, patients and family members may continue to experience physical and psychologic sequelae.[37] One study reported that 43% of long-term HSCT survivors with an average of 3.4 years after transplant had clinically significant global psychologic distress.[38] Despite this distress, only 50% of the patients received mental health services.[39]

Researchers have described the following factors as predictors of poorer quality of life in patients 1 to 5 years after transplant: diagnoses of anxiety and/or depression, younger age, long-term sequelae, chronic GVHD, unemployment, lower income, poor functional status, family/caregiver distress, and short follow-up by the treatment center.[32,33,39]

Patient and families are ready to put the experience behind them, only to discover that the experience of transplant has forever changed the patient's outlook, priorities, and family network. Fear of recurrence and feelings of uncertainty related to future relationships, work, and financial strain continue.[26] There is discordance between the patients' pre-HSCT expectations and the everyday symptoms that limit their physical abilities. Besides fatigue, which continues to be the dominant symptom, another distressing issue is cognitive dysfunction as patients return to the workplace or reenter school.[26] Educating patients about some expected common short-term side effects can reduce anxiety. Neurocognitive side effects of treatment can be long term in high-risk patients but are mostly temporary, including diminished concentration, short-term memory loss, decreased speed of information processing, and loss of effective problem-solving abilities. Sexuality issues are another area of great concern for patients in the posttransplant period. Barriers for discussion and lack of referrals for supportive services in this area may be related to the patient's embarrassment, the clinician's lack of knowledge, or the focus on other issues that may be interpreted as more critical. Common sexual issues after transplant include vaginal dryness and distressing menopausal symptoms in women and erectile dysfunction in men.[40]

Patients who experience physical symptoms after transplantation may be at risk for long-term psychologic distress.[25] Despite the fact that patients are followed by transplant physicians longer than patients with nonhematologic malignancies, this population often is referred back to primary care physicians 1 to 2 years after transplant. Primary care clinicians do not have the knowledge or experience to recognize physical complications related to the effects of chemotherapy, radiation, and GVHD, so ongoing communication between the providers and the transplant team and center is imperative.

Long-term effects may include persistent viral, bacterial, and fungal susceptibility, GVHD, dental caries, muscle atrophy, pneumonitis, gonadal dysfunction, sexual dysfunction, endocrine abnormalities, cataracts, ocular sicca syndrome, reduced bone mass, secondary malignancies, and cognitive dysfunction.[41] In addition to monitoring physical complications, the American Society for Blood and Marrow Transplantation (ASBMT) consensus statement recommends annual evaluation of patients' psychologic status. Health care providers must have a high level of vigilance to assess depression in both the patient and family caregiver years after transplant, with clinical assessments recommended annually after transplant. Studies of transplant survivors beyond 10 years indicate possible issues with returning to work, physical fitness, impairment in social functioning and family life, insurance denial, and continued symptoms such as pain, depression, muscle stiffness/cramps, memory/attention problems, sleep disorders, sexual issues, and incontinence.[42,43] In spite of the range of problems, only 9.8% of patients reported accessing psychologic support.[42]

The concept of posttraumatic growth (PTG) after transplantation has been evolving. By definition, the potential for PTG requires that patients experience a stressful event and then subsequently experience positive psychologic outcomes or benefits. As early as 1996, Fromm identified that positive sequelae are possible after transplantation, including the development of a new philosophy of life, greater appreciation of life, making changes in personal characteristics, and improving relationships with family and friends.[44] Potential predictors of PTG among posttransplant patients include good social support, little avoidance coping, younger age, less education, greater use of positive reinterpretation, problem solving, seeking alternative rewards, more stressful appraisal of the experience, and more negatively biased recall of pretransplant levels of psychologic distress.[22,45] Discussing the PTG potential with patients and making referrals for counseling to experienced clinicians who are aware of the potential for PTG are essential.

Although patients report long-term psychosocial effects after transplantation, they may be reluctant to accept help and fail to access psychologic resources and social support.[42] These patients must be encouraged to use resources and seek psychologic support, because this experience may impair the patients' and families' ability to cope with life after transplant. In an article about HSCT patients' experiences with a support group, Sherman et al identified the themes of meaning and changing of perspectives as patients expressed their struggles with redefining themselves, their priorities, and their values.[26] Some patients wanted to change their former values and behaviors. The support group experience may be therapeutic for patients who often do not have physical signs of transplant to the untrained eye but continue to experience increasing or unresolved psychologic and physical issues.[21,25] Sharing a common experience may encourage patients to believe that their symptoms and feelings are not unique and may decrease their feelings of isolation.

Immediate Period Following Diagnosis and Treatment

As the treatment and acute side effects improve and subside, patients often feel that the whirlwind has passed, only to be confronted with uneasy silence. Weeks and months of clinic and physician appointments, infusions, and admissions stop or trickle to a small stream of appointments. Families who have been functioning on a grinding schedule of crisis mode find the change almost paralyzing. Adding to this halt of activity, health care providers have a tendency to limit their contacts when the patients' physical status has stabilized. This is a critical time when psychosocial interventions and supportive services from other members of the health care team must be instituted for patients and family members to deal with the uncertainty and anxiety of waiting. Fears and anxieties change from fighting the disease to returning to life.[46] Because of less contact with the primary treatment hematologists, patients and families may perceive a withdrawal of support from the medical team. Long-term psychosocial health of the patient and family is affected by the meaning ascribed

to the cancer experience, fear of recurrence, support of the family, demographic factors, and financial stressors. This transition time is pivotal for patients' long-term quality of life. Surveillance with specific questions to access the need for referrals can have lasting outcomes.

Time of Relapse

The time of recurrence of cancer has been reported to be more distressing for patients and family members than the initial diagnosis. The recurrence of the disease can plunge the patient and family into despair and crisis as they realize that death may occur despite the ongoing fight to live. The psychosocial issues experienced by the person with cancer depend in part on the clinical course of the disease process. As the disease progresses, the person often reports an upsetting scenario that includes uncertainty, frequent pain, diminished functional ability, increased dependence, and disability.[47]

The development of a relapse after a disease-free interval can be especially devastating for patients and those close to them. The medical workup often is difficult and anxiety provoking, and psychosocial problems experienced at the time of diagnosis frequently resurface, often with greater intensity.[47] Shock and depression can accompany relapse and require patients and family members to reevaluate the future. In spite of the overwhelming nature of the psychosocial responses, however, most patients cope effectively with progressive disease. It is essential to recognize that intense emotions do not necessarily equate with maladaptive coping. Investigators studying quality of life in patients with cancer have demonstrated a clear relationship between a person's perception of their quality of life and the presence of discomfort.[48,49] As uncomfortable symptoms increase, perceived quality of life diminishes. An important goal in the psychosocial treatment of patients with advanced cancer is optimal symptom management.

An issue that repeatedly surfaces among patients, family members, and professional care providers is the use of aggressive treatment protocols in the presence of relapse and progressive disease. Currently there are newer agents that can induce remission even in the face of relapse. In addition, patients and families often request participation in experimental protocols, even when there is little likelihood of extending survival. Controversy continues about the efficacy of such therapies and the role health care providers can play in facilitating patients' choices about participating. Clear communication about treatment goals and expectations will assist in patient and family preparation.

Certain patients respond to investigational treatment with increased hope. It is vital to clarify the values, thoughts, and psychologic reactions of care providers, patients, and families to the delicate issues that evolve if individualized care with attention to the patient's psychosocial needs is to be provided.

Survivorship

The definition of a long-term survivor has evolved over time. Initially, individuals who had survived cancer-free for longer than 5 years were considered "survivors and cured." More recently the term *survivor* has been used to define individuals who have completed the acute phase of illness. Others use the term for all patients initially diagnosed with cancer. Some people would prefer changing the term to "thrivers," champions, or fighters.[50]

Successful treatment of hematologic malignancies has resulted in cure for many patients and progressively longer lives for others. However, longer survival is not without significant psychologic sequelae.[51-56] New treatments may result in unintended physical side effects such as infertility, treatment-related toxicity, persistent side effects, and organ system failure that can magnify and exacerbate the psychologic issues initially associated with diagnosis and treatment.[48,49,57] The overwhelming evidence from the literature involving survivors with hematologic malignancies is that, on average, most do very well after the initial adjustment in the first 1 to 3 years after treatment.[32,52] Most long-term HSCT survivors express satisfaction with their quality of life and describe themselves as productive, stable, and well adjusted without significant physical, functional, psychologic, and social problems related to their disease or HSCT treatment. However, there is a group of patients with a high rate of psychosocial morbidity who are vulnerable to ongoing and intermittent psychosocial distress. Empiric evidence showed that as many as 9% to 30% of long-term survivors with hematologic malignancies experience significant psychologic distress, including anxiety, depression, and posttraumatic distress symptoms.[53,55,58]

Psychologic aspects of survivorship may include concern over termination of treatment; fear of relapse; preoccupation with somatic symptoms; reentry into previous roles; lingering affinity with death; and financial, job, and insurance difficulties. These issues may manifest in a variety of ways, including denial of past illness, leading to medical compliance issues; ongoing problems with anxiety, panic, and depression; and inability to reenter or modify previous roles. Fear of recurrence by both patients and family members can severely affect quality of life.[48,59] In her classic article "The Enduring Seasons in Survival," Dow stated that the season of extended survival is dominated by fear of recurrence.[60] In fact, Baker et al showed in a group of cancer survivors that "being fearful my illness will return," "concern about relapsing," "fears about the future," and "difficulty making long-term plans" were a problem 68%, 60%, 58%, and 41% of the time, respectively.[33] Mellon and Northouse found that the strongest predictors of quality of life 1 to 5 years after treatment were concurrent family stressors, family social support, family member fear of recurrence, family meaning of the illness, and patient's employment status.[61]

There is increasing interest in patients' experiences with posttraumatic stress disorder (PTSD). Studies have consistently described a higher incidence of PTSD in patients with hematologic malignancies than in the average population.[62–64] Predictors of PTSD severity among patients with hematologic diagnosis include higher levels of distress and high avoidance coping coupled with low social support.[22] These researchers describe how providers can assess coping and presence of family support and potentially mitigate the effects of a distressing experience with the cancer diagnosis. Considerable evidence indicates that the wide range of surgical, chemotherapeutic, and radiation therapies leaves permanent damage to organs and physiologic functioning and disfigurement across the different hematologic diagnoses (Table 90.1). Health care providers should be mindful of psychologic sequelae among patients, even within the context of remission and a hopeful prognosis, and refer patients and family members to a mental health specialist for further evaluation, as needed.

Terminal Stage and End-of-Life Care

Technologic advances in health care have improved the potential for cure of many previously fatal hematologic malignancies. However, many patients still have disease that is unresponsive to treatment, continues to progress, and is considered incurable. When cure is acknowledged to be impossible and alternative efforts to combat the progress of disease are exhausted, patients are recognized as terminally ill or dying. In the past, experts had advocated for the pursuit of hospice care at this point in time foregoing further active treatment and shifting the emphasis of medical care to control of distressing symptoms and maintenance of quality of life at an optimal level.[59,65,66]

Over the past few years, the paradigm has shifted in the field of palliative care to initiating palliative care alongside curative treatment with the philosophy that it should be implemented across the illness trajectory. The ultimate goal is to improve the quality of life and facilitate relief of suffering over the course of one's illness.[67] In nonhematologic diseases such as severe heart failure or metastatic lung cancer, palliative care has been shown not only to improve quality of life but extend it.[11] The new World Health Organization definition states: "Palliative care is an approach to care which improves quality of life of patients and their families facing life-threatening illness,

TABLE 90.1	Long-Term Consequences of Therapies for Hematologic Cancers
Anxiety	
Depression	
Fear of recurrence	
Disfigurement	
Conditioned nausea and vomiting	
Unemployment	
Denial of life insurance	
Denial of health benefits	
Increase in life insurance rates	
Difficulty changing health care coverage	
Breakdown of marriage or relationship	
Decline in participation in leisure activities	
Diminution of support from others	
Disruption in sexual functioning	
Fertility	

through prevention, assessment and treatment of pain and other physical, psychologic, and spiritual problems."[68]

Palliative care began with the hospice movement. Since the concept of hospice was first introduced in England in the 1960s, hospice care has been recognized as the state-of-the-science end-of-life care, and hospice services are now available around the world. However, hospice care has not been integrated into the care of patients dying with hematologic malignancies.[69,70] Despite the strong emphasis on providing end-of-life care in accordance with patients' wishes and empiric studies showing that most terminal patients prefer spending their final days of life and dying at home, hematologic malignancy is the only diagnosis that has been repeatedly and consistently shown to predict hospital death.[71,72]

The reasons for such insufficiency have been attributed to many factors. Manitta et al in their article "Palliative Care and the Hemato-Oncologic Patient: Can We Live Together?" identified barriers between the expectations of two specialties: (1) the dying trajectory can be rapid with more unpredictability and more technology, (2) the various hematologic diagnoses are not uniform in response and treatment, (3) the goals of care can be unclear, (4) the focus on cure can preclude the focus on palliation, (5) lack of knowledge exists among hematologists about palliative care principles, and (6) the health care system does not encourage collaborative care.[73] Many of these issues are not unique to hematologic conditions, but are clearly challenges to be overcome. In our experience, one of the most significant barriers to initiation of hospice care for patients with hematologic malignancies is the ongoing need for blood product transfusions, which is often not provided by hospice agencies. Explorations around how much benefit these transfusions concretely provide are often helpful to bridging this gap. Additionally, partnering with insurance agencies to carve out blood products for ambulatory patients may be possible.

In addition to systematic barriers, personal barriers exist. Health care providers, first and foremost, must examine their own attitudes toward death and dying and avoid imposing their own values on patients and their families. Respecting patient and family wishes, appropriately managing and alleviating distressing symptoms, and providing care tailored to meeting patients' needs can help patients dying of hematologic malignancies reach the end of life with peace and dignity.

FACTORS THAT INFLUENCE PSYCHOSOCIAL ADJUSTMENT

Psychosocial responses to cancer vary widely and are influenced by several factors that clinicians should bear in mind when considering the responses of individual patients. A review of the literature points to key factors that may have an impact on psychosocial adjustment and include individual patient, environmental, and disease-related factors.

Individual Patient Factors

Demographics, comorbid conditions including previous psychiatric morbidity, and previous coping strategies have been consistently documented as important predictors for psychosocial adjustment. Female sex and younger age are important predictors for worse psychosocial adjustment and poorer quality of life for patients with hematologic malignancies.[21,74-76] As the population ages, there are more individuals diagnosed with cancer who already have comorbid diseases, which complicates treatment decisions and recovery.[77,78] Many individual patient factors are interrelated; for example, higher anxiety scores and worse quality of life outcomes have been observed in women more than in men. Poor quality of life after treatment has been associated with higher age of the recipient at the time of the transplant, poorer self-image, decreased cognitive functioning, and inability to return to work.[79,80] This makes it difficult to accurately predict psychosocial adjustment solely based on these factors.

One of the key predictors of psychosocial adjustment to cancer is the psychologic stability of the person before diagnosis. People with a history of poor psychosocial adjustment before development of cancer are at highest risk for psychologic decompensation and should be monitored closely throughout all phases of treatment.[27,81] This is particularly true of people with a history of a major psychiatric syndrome, psychiatric hospitalization, or both.[27]

Because a person's coping style is determined relatively early in life and tends to remain stable over time and across situations, it serves as a useful predictor of adjustment to cancer. Several investigators have identified specific personality characteristics, coping strategies, and life experiences that enhance or inhibit positive adjustment to cancer.[82,83] Empiric evidence demonstrates the beneficial impact of positive coping strategies and personality attributes on long-term survival.[84-86] Coping strategies found to be most effective include: having a "fighting spirit;" hopefulness and acceptance of the situation; a belief that life has purpose and coherence; and having a feeling of control over events. These strategies tend to result in active participation in treatment and engagement in daily life. By contrast, poor adjustment has been associated with avoidant coping strategies; anxious preoccupation and high distraction; prior negative sexual experiences; body image problems; and inhibition in discussing personal and sexual problems.[87] One study showed that patients who smoke are at higher risk for psychiatric morbidity, perhaps due to the potential development of depression and/or anxiety with withdrawal symptoms.[88] It is important to include smoking history in the patient's assessment of substance control use when preparing patients for treatment options.

Environmental Factors

Environmental factors include partner and family support as well as other forms of social support. The quality of spousal and family relationships has a significant impact on the psychologic health and even mortality of the patient.[89] Social support, network size, satisfaction with social support, and reliance on formal and informal social ties have consistently been found to influence a person's psychosocial adjustment to cancer.[71,72] The ability and availability of significant others in dealing with a diagnosis and discussion of treatment options can significantly affect the patient's view of himself or herself. Patients diagnosed with all types of life-threatening chronic disorders experience a heightened need for interpersonal support. Those who are able to maintain close connections with family and friends during the course of illness are more likely to cope effectively with the disease than are those who are not able to maintain such relationships.[69,86,90]

Often the transition out of the hospital posttransplant can be a fearful time for patients and families. Traditionally patients are not referred routinely to formal home nursing care at discharge. An initial home visit can be invaluable in assisting patients and families with the transition, in addition to identifying areas in which ongoing assistance is needed. Given changes in the current health care system, informal family caregivers are increasingly expected to serve as the major providers of care outside the hospital. Hence referral for home care can be of significant support.

Disease-Related Factors

Disease-related factors including the type of disease, side effects of treatment, and residual symptoms all greatly affect psychosocial adjustment. Different treatment modalities introduce varying degrees of side effects, symptoms, and impact on quality of life. Without exception, the greatest difficulties in psychosocial adjustment were observed among patients who underwent allogeneic HSCT, followed by autologous HSCT recipients, and then patients who received conventional or maintenance chemotherapy. The latter groups experienced the least impairment in quality of life and psychologic distress. Patients who underwent transplant also had more psychiatric morbidity if they experienced lower functional status and higher regimen-related toxicity.[27]

Time interval after treatment has been documented as an important predictor for psychosocial adjustment. Particularly, time since HSCT or completion of treatment was an important factor for facilitating psychosocial adjustment and improving quality of life. In general, during the first year after HSCT, patients perceived their physical and overall well-being as being at its worst, during which time they experienced more anxiety and total mood disturbance, and reported the highest degree of illness intrusiveness in every aspect of life.[32,57,91-95] With the passage of time, improvements in functional status, quality of life, levels of anxiety, depression, and satisfaction with life were frequently observed after transplant.

DIFFERENTIATING PSYCHIATRIC COMPLICATIONS FROM EXPECTED PSYCHOLOGIC RESPONSE

Living with a chronic illness often requires continuing care and management by a team of specialists. Use of supportive care services has been related to improved quality of life; therefore it is in the patient's best interest to access services needed for psychologic distress early in the continuum of care.[90] Care usually is provided through follow-up visits to ambulatory or outpatient clinics and consulting rooms, rather than through hospitalization. However, several barriers that may impair the outpatient cancer survivor from accessing health care services include economic and financial constraints.[96] Differentiating a psychiatric complication from expected psychologic responses is imperative.

Although any individual experiencing the crisis of a cancer diagnosis may become clinically depressed or experience a panic attack, most patients do not experience a diagnosable psychiatric condition. Currently the rates of adjustment disorder, depression, anxiety, and PTSD are 40%, 25%, 10%, and 5%, respectively. The ability of health care providers to distinguish expected reactions from more severe psychiatric complications is crucial.

Unfortunately, non–mental health providers often miss clinically relevant and severe psychiatric syndromes. Being knowledgeable about common symptoms of adjustment disorder, depression, anxiety, and PTSD are helpful. Table 90.2 provides a quick reference; also refer to the *Diagnostic and Statistical Manual of Mental Disorders*.

Another group of patients who are at high risk for developing adjustment problems includes those with coexisting severe mental illness including schizophrenia, bipolar disorder, schizoaffective disorder, and obsessive-compulsive disorder. Integrated care of psychiatry and oncology is the best option in treating these patients, first to stabilize the psychiatric illness and then to treat the cancer.[97,98] Good communication, empathy, listening skills, and providing emotional support are all skills that benefit these patients and specifically those

<table>
<tr><td colspan="4">**TABLE 90.2   Common Symptoms of Psychiatric Disorders**</td></tr>
</table>

Adjustment Disorder	Depression	Anxiety	Posttraumatic Stress Disorder
The development of emotional or behavioral symptoms in response to an identifiable stressor	Symptoms that are present for a 2-week period and a change from previous functioning	Excessive worry and anxiety for at least 6 months; the person finds it difficult not to worry	The person has been exposed to a traumatic event
1. Marked distress that is in excess of what would be expected for exposure to the stressor 2. Significant impairment in social or occupational functioning	1. Depressed mood most of the day 2. Marked diminished interest or pleasure 3. Significant weight loss or decrease or increase in appetite 4. Insomnia or hypersomnia 5. Psychomotor agitation or retardation 6. Fatigue 7. Feelings of worthlessness or guilt 8. Diminished ability to think or concentrate 9. Recurrent thoughts of death, suicidal ideation, or a plan for suicide	Anxiety and worry have to have three of the six following symptoms: 1. Restlessness 2. Fatigue 3. Difficulty concentrating 4. Irritability 5. Muscle tension 6. Sleep disturbance	1. Reexperiencing symptoms such as images, thoughts, and perceptions 2. Persistent avoidance of stimuli and numbing of general responsiveness 3. Persistent symptoms of increased arousal: sleep issues, anger or irritability, difficulty concentrating, hypervigilance, and exaggerated startle response

Data from American Psychiatric Association: *Diagnostic and statistical manual of mental disorders*, ed 4, Arlington, VA, 2000, American Psychiatric Association.

who have severe mental illness, who often have a history of disregard and neglect from providers.[99]

Most patients manifest transient psychologic symptoms that are responsive to support, reassurance, and information about what to expect regarding the cancer course and its treatment. Some require more aggressive psychotherapeutic interventions, such as pharmacotherapy and ongoing psychotherapy. The following guidelines can assist the clinician in identifying those patients who exhibit behavior suggesting the presence of a psychiatric syndrome.

General guidelines designed to assist in distinguishing patients who should be referred for evaluation by a trained psychiatric clinician include the following:

1. History of psychiatric hospitalization or significant psychiatric/personality disorder.
2. Persistent refusal, indecisiveness, or noncompliance with regard to needed treatment.
3. Persistent symptoms of anxiety and depression that are unresponsive to usual support from health care providers or family members; symptoms may present in the form of constant fear associated with treatment and procedures or excessive crying and feelings of hopelessness that worsen rather than improve with time.
4. Abrupt, unexplained change in mood or behavior.
5. Insomnia, anorexia, diminished energy out of proportion to expected treatment effects.
6. Persistent suicidal ideation.
7. Unusual or eccentric behavior or confusion (may be indicative of an organic mental disorder).
8. Excessive guilt and self-blame for illness.
9. Evidence of dysfunctional family coping or complex family issues.

After referral to a psychiatric specialist, one or a combination of therapeutic modalities may be used. Cancer and its treatment may precipitate an exacerbation of an underlying mental illness to which a patient was predisposed and that may require extensive treatment (e.g., hospitalization for a psychosis, ongoing pharmacotherapy, or psychotherapy). A discussion of these specialized forms of treatment is beyond the scope of this chapter. The reader is encouraged to consult an appropriate standard textbook.[100]

SCREENING FOR PSYCHOLOGIC DISTRESS

A number of tools have been developed to screen for psychologic distress, but adoption and consistent incorporation into clinical care has been slow.[101,102] Most recently, National Comprehensive Cancer Network (NCCN) guidelines have been updated to work towards implementing standard screening. Indeed these guidelines now clearly advocate for distress to be recognized, monitored, documented, and treated promptly at all stages of disease.[103] In a strong show of support for distress screening, the American College of Surgeons Commission on Cancer has required cancer centers to implement screening programs for psychosocial distress as a criterion for further accreditation.[104]

One tool that is easy to administer and that patients report as capturing their problems is the *distress thermometer*.[105] The term "*distress*" was selected as it was felt to be more acceptable and less stigmatizing than other related terms (e.g., psychiatric, psychosocial, emotional). The tool is similar to pain measurement scales that ask patients to rate their pain on a scale from 0 to 10, and consists of two parts. The first part is a picture of a thermometer, and patients are asked to mark their level of distress. A rating of 4 or above indicates that a patient has symptoms indicating a need for evaluation by a mental health professional and potentially has a need for referral for services. On the second part, the patient marks items that relate to his or her distress from a six-item problem list (Fig. 90.2).[105,106] Multiple studies have validated the use of this distress thermometer in various oncologic settings including stem cell transplant.[107,108] Lee et al found that the distress thermometer was a useful tool for screening transplant patients before admission.[108] Interestingly, pretransplant distress appeared to be highly predictive of distress following transplant and was a feasible marker to screen patients for distress.[108] Yet controversy remains about whether distress screening is of critical importance as is highlighted in a recent systematic review that found that the distress did not improve in screened patients as compared with those who received usual care.[109]

MANAGEMENT OF PSYCHOSOCIAL PROBLEMS

Interventions for these patients center on the uniqueness of the experience. In the initial phase of the experience, 50% of patients have psychologic distress, including both anxiety and depression.[106] A growing body of literature provides evidence that patients may experience PTSD.[110] Increased length of survival from time of diagnosis has highlighted the need for psychopharmacologic, psychotherapeutic, and cognitive and behaviorally oriented interventions to reduce distress, promote adjustment, and improve quality of life for patients with hematologic malignancies. Cognitive behavioral therapy is a promising intervention that has been used with transplant patients and shown to decrease PTSD symptoms and overall distress.[111] Because of the increasing complexity of patient care, a

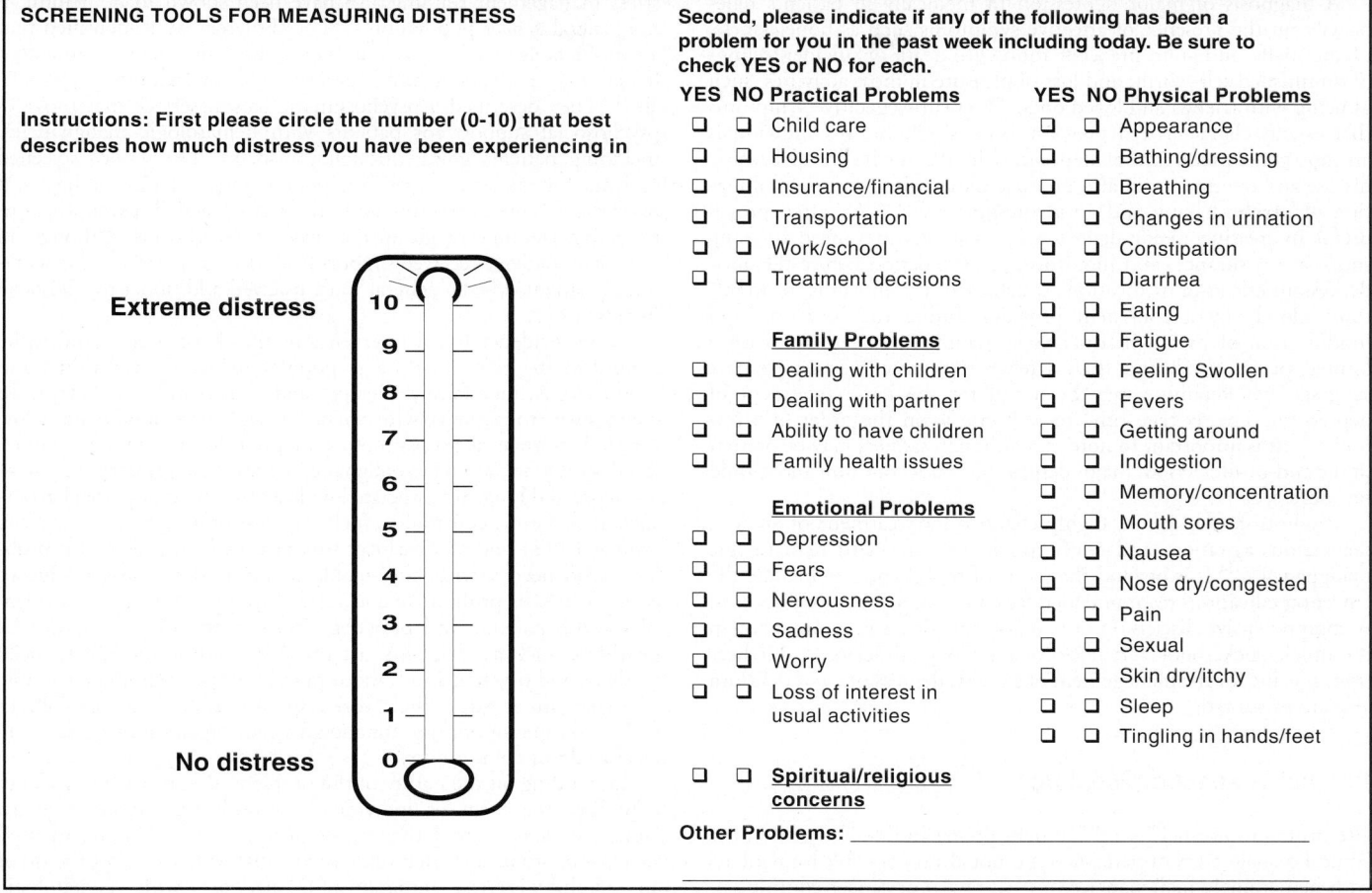

Fig. 90.2 NATIONAL COMPREHENSIVE CANCER NETWORK (NCCN) DISTRESS MANAGE-MENT GUIDELINE DIS-A-DISTRESS THERMOMETER. *(From National Comprehensive Cancer Network: The National Comprehensive Cancer Network 1.2005 Distress Management, the complete library of NCCN clinical practice guidelines in oncology (CD-ROM), Jenkintown, Pennsylvania, 2005, National Comprehensive Cancer Network.)*

multidisciplinary approach that includes regular avenues and options for communication about patient management and status updates is imperative. Numerous studies have documented the efficacy of a variety of modalities in managing psychosocial problems for such patients. Psychologic distress that can be managed effectively include anxiety and depression; sexual dysfunction; body image disturbances; noncompliance, pain, and neurologic complications such as delirium and dementia induced by brain metastasis or treatment; anticipatory and posttreatment nausea and vomiting; anorexia and feeding problems; and marital and family difficulties.

Pharmacologic Interventions

Pharmacotherapy, as an adjunct to one or more of the psychotherapies, can be an important aid in bringing psychologic symptoms under control. For patients with severe anxiety, factors other than a psychologic state must first be evaluated. Metabolic abnormalities, pain, hypoxia, and drug withdrawal states all can present as anxiety. Many common medications are associated with anxiety and depression. Medications such as steroids and antipsychotics, often used to control nausea, can cause anxiety characterized by agitation and motor restlessness. After medical or drug-induced causes for anxiety

are ruled out, an anxiolytic agent is the treatment of choice, except for patients who present with panic episodes, in whom selective serotonin reuptake inhibitors are most efficacious. Medications are most effective when used at adequate dosages and as standing orders. Use of these medications may assist the patient with participating in psychotherapy, which can provide more lasting control over psychologic symptoms. All pharmacologic treatments must be monitored for effectiveness and side effects.

Patients commonly demonstrate transient depressive symptoms at various points in the disease trajectory. In patients who exhibit prolonged or severe depressive symptoms, a major depressive illness must be considered. Depression can be related to a recurrence of past depressive disorder or the stress associated with treatment, or it can be a result of the illness process or treatment agents. Antidepressant medications are easily administered and are an effective treatment strategy. Disadvantages include the need for repeated visits to health care clinicians to monitor patient response and adjust the dosage, possible adverse side effects and medical reactions, potential use in suicide attempts, and the need for strict adherence to the medication schedule. Patients should be informed that most antidepressant medications must be taken for 4 to 6 weeks before a significant response is achieved. The clinician must be aware that patients at risk for suicide become more energized with medications and appear to look better long before their depressive feelings and suicidal thoughts are relieved. Careful monitoring of suicidal ideation should continue for weeks after the patient appears improved.

A diagnosis of major depression in medically ill patients relies heavily on the presence of affective symptoms such as hopelessness, crying spells, and guilt; preoccupation with death or suicide; feelings of diminished self-worth; and loss of pleasure in most activities, such as being with friends and loved ones. The neurovegetative symptoms that usually characterize depression in physically healthy individuals are not good predictors of depression in the medically ill because disease and treatment can also produce these symptoms. A combination of psychotherapy and antidepressant medication often proves useful in treating major depression.[112] Patients may need ongoing support, reassurance, and monitoring in the period before the antidepressant effects of medication are achieved. Patients must be monitored closely by a consistent provider during the initiation and modification of psychopharmacologic regimens. In patients with a limited prognosis shorter than a few weeks, recent emerging data suggests that ketamine may be useful for the rapid treatment of depression. The average time to response is on the order of a few hours.[113] It is important to note that although sadness may be present in the end-of-life period, major depression is not common and should be addressed.

Psychotropic drugs are highly effective for treatment of anxiety, depression, agitation, and confusion in patients with hematologic malignancies.[114] It is beyond the scope of this chapter to include the current medications recommended for common psychiatric disorders. A comprehensive discussion of psychotropic drugs is summarized in the quick pocketbook reference for oncology clinicians.[115] Medications specific for the management of anxiety, depression, and delirium also are presented.

Psychotherapeutic Modalities

"Returning to normal" is a prominent theme and desired goal in the clinical management of patients but is not always possible for patients with hematologic malignancies.[92,116] Survivors of cancer continue to face challenges with long-term physical and psychologic symptoms long after treatment has ended, and data indicate that they report more contact with mental health providers than do people without cancer.[96] The ASBMT released a joint statement recommending screening and preventive practices for long-term survivors of hematopoietic cell transplantation. The recommendation states that "a high level of vigilance for psychologic symptoms should be maintained. Clinical assessment is recommended throughout the recovery period, at six months, one year, and annually thereafter, with mental health professional counseling recommended for those with recognized deficits."[41] The number of intervention studies designed with the hematologic population is limited; however, growing interest in survivorship is changing the research climate in this area.

Support groups can provide a therapeutic experience for patients and family members. Initial evidence suggests that support groups may help reduce health care costs along with depression, mood disturbance, and psychiatric symptoms in patients.[117] Patients often feel alone in their distress and report that sharing a common experience normalizes their feelings, provides an avenue for emotional support, facilitates dialogue to problem solve, and offers opportunities to learn from other patients. Support groups facilitated by professionals such as social workers, nurses, or psychologists can provide a forum for health and psychologic education and provide patients with printed literature and online community-based resources. Sherman et al found that psychoeducational support groups facilitated by professionals were a helpful strategy for psychologic recovery in patients' post-HSCT.[26]

Other modalities have been shown to be effective with patients.[82,92] Studies have consistently shown that relaxation training with or without guided imagery or hypnosis may have some benefit with improving quality of life, symptom management, and

anxiety and depression management.[116,118,119] It is a skill taught to patients that takes minimal time. It does, however, require that patients be motivated to learn and practice new techniques as a way of coping. Cognitive therapy/reappraisal, problem solving, and stress management training also have been shown to be helpful in the general cancer population.[110,116,120] Fritzsche et al identified that a considerable need for psychotherapeutic treatment of inpatient hematology patients is best handled by mental health professionals.[119] They described a psychosomatic liaison service that provides psychosocial support for patients with hematologic malignancies, including patients going through transplant. The service screened patients for anxiety, depression, poor coping, quality of life, and psychosocial openness for support, and provided psychotherapy, relaxation training, or group therapy as interventions. Although all transplant patients received support from the team, 23% of the hematology patients on the general ward received additional psychosocial interventions.

Other evidence-based interventions that have been found to be helpful in the general oncology population include individual and group counseling, family therapy, and music and art therapy. In comparison to patients with solid cancers, there should be a low threshold for referral for psychosocial support for patients and families faced with a hematologic malignancy because the primary treatment is intense and long and associated with sensitivity to potential barriers such as economic constraints, including loss of insurance. It has been estimated that one of six cancer survivors with mental health problems who need services are unable to access those services due to cost.[96] If cost is prohibitive and referral to a psychologist is not feasible, both patients and providers must investigate other potential providers, such as chaplains, art therapists, music therapists, social workers, and psychiatric advanced practice nurses who might be able to see patients as part of their work responsibilities. Other possibilities include online support groups and advocacy organizations, including local wellness communities.

Depending on the nature of the problem, the treatment modality may take the form of individual psychotherapy, group therapy, family therapy, marital therapy, cognitive or behaviorally oriented therapy, or some combination.[13] Increasing evidence supports use of an aerobic exercise program for patients with hematologic malignancies.[121-123] Researchers have concluded that fatigue and loss of physical performance in patients undergoing HSCT may improve with exercise.[122] Others have found increased muscle strength with supervised weight bearing and lifting after allogeneic HSCT.[123] Table 90.3 outlines the major psychotherapeutic modalities and their advantages, goals, and indications.

FUTURE DIRECTIONS

The psychosocial issues faced by people diagnosed with and treated for hematologic malignancies are influenced by individual, environmental, and disease-related factors. Because involvement in decision making clearly is a positive aspect of current cancer therapies, great care should be taken to ensure that communication is timely, repeated, relevant, and consistent with the patient's needs, tolerance for information, and comprehension. A multidisciplinary approach is necessary to guarantee the communication of timely and essential information to patients and family members. Patients should be given the opportunity to speak with multiple members of the multidisciplinary treatment team and other patients who have experienced similar management and treatment protocols. Care should be taken to provide needed information from a variety of expert perspectives while respecting the unique characteristics, psychosocial profiles, needs, and desires of each individual. In treatment settings with limited resources, every effort should be made to enlist the help and support of providers and services that can assist patients with treatment decisions and their complex management. Referral to community resources and support services after discharge from the hospital often is helpful, even for patients who cope well with initial treatment.[124]

TABLE 90.3	Therapeutic Modalities Useful for Patients and Family Members		
Modality	Selected Indications	Goals and Advantages	Comments
Individual psychotherapy	Prolonged adverse reactions to diagnosis, treatment, and other aspects of chronic illness (e.g., anxiety, depression)	Supports patients and enhances ability to cope with distressing feelings Short-term therapy; focused and goal directed	Pharmacology and family involvement are useful adjuncts in some cases
Support groups	Patients desire contact with others who are experiencing chronic illness	Supports patient and enhances coping ability Patients benefit by observing coping strategies of others Usually does not involve a fee	Expands social network of patients with limited support systems
Family and marital therapy	Relationship problems secondary to illness (e.g., family tension, role changes, conflict, sexual problems)	Assists couples with clarifying problems and facilitates solving them together Addresses role changes in the family system	Problems, issues, and concerns about relationships including children can be addressed
Mind-body therapies, including progressive muscle relaxation, yoga, guided imagery, Reiki, meditation, hypnosis, and biofeedback	Patients desire assistance with control of pain, anxiety, anticipatory and posttreatment nausea and vomiting, fears associated with medical procedures	Increases sense of control and participation in treatment Individualized to meet patient's preferences and circumstances Time limited and goal directed Evaluated in terms of observable changes in symptoms and self-efficacy	Realistic goals should be stated explicitly (Some patients may view these therapies as a cancer cure)

Most patients undergoing cancer treatment, as well as their families, experience expected periods of psychologic turmoil that occur at transition points along the clinical course of cancer. In a small proportion of patients, more severe psychiatric complications may occur, warranting referral to a psychiatric specialist, including psychiatrists, social workers, psychologists, and psychiatric nurses. Screening for ongoing psychiatric problems must become standard care. A variety of psychotherapeutic modalities are useful for helping patients work through the expected psychologic responses to cancer as well as more severe responses.[15] Supportive psychotherapeutic measures should be used routinely because they minimize distress and enhance feelings of control and mastery over self and environment. For these reasons alone, their value in the care of patients with cancer is paramount.

Throughout the clinical course of cancer, the patient's relationship with health care providers and the presence of a supportive social network are important factors that can ensure successful management of the many physical and psychosocial demands imposed by a cancer diagnosis and treatment. As scientific inquiry continues to produce vast but sometimes conflicting information regarding etiology and treatment of cancers, concurrent research regarding the psychosocial aspects of hematologic malignancies is crucial. This line of inquiry will, at the very least, assist in promoting psychosocial well-being in patients and family members faced with an extreme and unexpected life crisis. At best, expanding the knowledge base relative to the psychosocial aspects of cancer may provide some "missing links" regarding psychosocial adaptation and quality of life and the impact of cancer on patients' survival. The Institute of Medicine report that recommends that all cancer care should ensure the provision of appropriate psychosocial health services, states that at a minimum, patients must be screened for emotional distress and evaluated for additional services.

SUGGESTED READINGS

Baker F, Denniston M, Smith T, et al: Adult cancer survivors: how are they faring? *Cancer* 104:2565, 2005.

Cooke L, Gemmill R, Kravits K, et al: Psychological issues of stem cell transplant. *Semin Oncol Nurs* 25:139, 2009.

Cooke L, Grant M, Eldredge D: Hematopoietic cell transplantation: the trajectory of quality of life. In Ezzone S, Schmit-Pokorny K, editors: *Blood and marrow stem cell transplantation*, ed 3, Sudbury, Mass, 2007, Jones & Bartlett Publishers, p 391.

Edwards B, Clarke V: The psychological impact of a cancer diagnosis on families: the influence of family functioning and patients' illness characteristics on depression and anxiety. *Psychooncology* 13:562, 2004.

Evan EE, Zeltzer LK: Psychosocial dimensions of cancer in adolescents and young adults. *Cancer* 107:1663, 2006.

Fleishman S, Greenberg D: Pharmacological interventions. In Holland J, Greenberg D, Hughes M, editors: *Quick reference for oncology clinicians: the psychiatric and psychological dimensions of cancer symptom management*, Charlottesville, Va, 2006, IPOS Press, p 26.

Fritzsche K, Struss Y, Stein B, et al: Psychosomatic liaison service in hematological oncology: need for psychotherapeutic interventions and their realization. *Hematol Oncol* 21:83, 2003.

Haylock PJ: The shifting paradigm of cancer care: The many needs of cancer survivors are starting to attract attention. *Am J Nurs* 106:16, 2006.

Hewitt M, Sheldon G, Stovall E: *From cancer patient to cancer survivor: lost in transition*, Washington, DC, 2006, National Academy Press.

Institute of Medicine (US) Committee on Psychosocial Services to Cancer Patients/Families in a Community Setting, Adler NE, Page AEK, editors: *Cancer care for the whole patient: meeting psychosocial health needs*, Washington DC, 2008, National Academies Press.

Jacobsen PB, Donovan KA, Trask PC, et al: Screening for psychologic distress in ambulatory cancer patients. *Cancer* 103:1494, 2005.

Jacobsen PB, Sadler IJ, Booth-Jones M, et al: Predictors of posttraumatic stress disorder symptomatology following bone marrow transplantation for cancer. *J Consult Clin Psychol* 70:235, 2002.

Jenks Kettmann JD, Altmaier EM: Social support and depression among bone marrow transplant patients. *J Health Psychol* 13:39, 2008.

Khan A, Irfan M, Shamsi T, et al: Psychiatric disorders in bone marrow transplant patients. *J Coll Physicians Surg Pak* 17:98, 2007.

Kishi Y, Meller WH, Swigart SE, et al: Are the patients with post-transplant psychiatric consultation different from other medical–surgical consultation inpatients? *Psychiatry Clin Neurosci* 59:19, 2005.

Lim JW, Zebrack B: Social networks and quality of life for long-term survivors of leukemia and lymphoma. *Support Care Cancer* 14:185, 2006.

Lorenz KA, Lynn J, Dy SM, et al: Evidence for improving palliative care at the end of life: a systematic review. *Ann Intern Med* 148:147, 2008.

Manitta VJ, Philip JAM, Cole-Sinclair MF: Palliative care and the hemato-oncological patient: can we live together? A review of the literature. *J Palliat Med* 13:1021, 2010.

McGrath P: End-of-life care for hematological malignancies: the 'technological imperative' and palliative care. *J Palliat Care* 18:39, 2002.

McQuellan R, Danhauer S: Psychosocial rehabilitation in cancer care. In Chang A, Ganz P, Hayes D, editors: *Oncology: an evidence-based approach*, New York, 2006, Springer Verlag, p 1942.

Mellon S, Northouse LL: Family survivorship and quality of life following a cancer diagnosis. *Res Nurs Health* 24:446, 2001.

Miovic M, Block S: Psychiatric disorders in advanced cancer. *Cancer* 110:2007, 1665.

Misono S, Weiss NS, Fann JR, et al: Incidence of suicide in persons with cancer. *J Clin Oncol* 26:4731, 2008.

Mosher CE, DuHamel KN, Rini CM, et al: Barriers to mental health service use among hematopoietic SCT survivors. *Bone Marrow Transplant* 45:570, 2010.

National Comprehensive Cancer Network: The National Comprehensive Cancer Network 1.2005 Distress Management, The Complete Library of NCCN Clinical Practice Guidelines in Oncology (CD-ROM), Jenkintown, PA, 2005, National Comprehensive Cancer Network.

Patrick DL, Engelberg RA, Curtis JR: Evaluating the quality of dying and death. *J Pain Symptom Manage* 22:717, 2001.

Sherman RS, Cooke E, Grant M: Dialogue among survivors of hematopoietic cell transplantation–Support-group themes. *J Psychosoc Oncol* 23:1, 2005.

Tang ST, McCorkle R: Determinants of place of death for terminal cancer patients. *Cancer Invest* 19:165, 2001.

Zabora J, BrintzenhofeSzoc K, Curbow B, et al: The prevalence of psychological distress by cancer site. *Psychooncology* 10:19, 2001.

REFERENCES

For the complete list of references, log on to www.expertconsult.com.

PAIN MANAGEMENT AND ANTIEMETIC THERAPY IN HEMATOLOGIC DISORDERS

Shane E. Peterson, Kathy J. Selvaggi, Bridget Fowler Scullion, and Craig D. Blinderman

Relieving pain in patients with hematologic disorders requires a multifaceted approach.[1,2] This chapter will provide the clinician with the tools to perform a systematic evaluation of the pain complaint and propose a rational, evidence-based, strategy. After the source and type of the pain has been identified and assessed, appropriate nonpharmacologic and pharmacologic therapies can be initiated. The approach to managing pain in hematologic disorders is largely based on the approach for managing cancer-related pain. We do not address the neurosurgical or anesthetic procedures for managing pain; those interested in these techniques are referred to several excellent reviews.[1–5] We will also review the pharmacologic strategies for managing nausea in patients with hematologic disorders undergoing treatment.

TAXONOMY OF PAIN

Although there is no one standardized classification system for cancer pain, several systems have been proposed. Cancer pain syndromes, and thus by analogy, pain syndromes in hematologic disorders, may be classified temporally, pathophysiologically, and etiologically, according to distinct clinical–anatomical entities, or any combination thereof. It is important to determine both the etiology and inferred pathophysiology in the assessment of the pain complaint because this may suggest the use of specific therapies. Pain can be categorized as *nociceptive* (somatic or visceral), *neuropathic*, or *idiopathic*.[6] Nociceptive pain is pain that is sustained predominantly by tissue injury or inflammation. Nociceptive somatic pain is described as sharp, aching, stabbing, throbbing, or pressure-like. Nociceptive visceral pain is poorly localized and is usually described as crampy pain (e.g., obstruction of hollow viscus) or as aching and stabbing (e.g., pain secondary to splenomegaly). Neuropathic pain is sustained by abnormal somatosensory processing in the peripheral or central nervous system (CNS). Sensations described as "burning," "shock-like," and "electrical" typically suggest neuropathic pain. On physical examination, patients may have allodynia (pain induced by nonpainful stimuli) and hyperalgesia (increased perception of painful stimuli). In the absence of evidence sufficient to label pain as either nociceptive or neuropathic, we may use the term *idiopathic*. However, in patients with hematologic disorders, this term should lead to additional workup and a search for an underlying etiology and pathophysiology.

EVALUATION OF THE PAIN COMPLAINT

Initial Evaluation

Effective pain management requires a comprehensive assessment of the patient's pain. The clinical presentation of a patient with chronic pain is very different from that of a patient in acute pain. The patient with chronic pain does not present with the common autonomic manifestations of acute pain (e.g., tachycardia, sweating, elevated blood pressure) or facial grimacing, but often is withdrawn, quiet, depressed, or irritable; moves very little spontaneously; and complains of discomfort when moved. When the pain is relieved, these patients often exhibit completely different behaviors, becoming mobile, engaged, and involved with other people. The first component in the assessment is to believe the patient's complaint.

Patient reports of pain are valid, reliable, and reproducible.[1] A variety of assessment tools that can be completed within 5–10 minutes are available.[1,7] The pain complaint should be characterized by a number of descriptors, including the pain location, intensity, quality, onset, and duration; location and patterns of radiation; and what relieves or exacerbates the pain and its functional consequences (including how the pain affects the patient's ability to sleep or eat and how it affects physical activity, relationships with others, emotions, and concentration). Most patients with chronic cancer pain also experience periodic flares of pain, or "breakthrough pain."[7,8] An important subtype of breakthrough pain is "incident pain," which is caused by voluntary activity. The initial evaluation should determine the extent to which the patient has breakthrough pain and if it is provoked by movement (nociceptive) or tends to be paroxysmal in nature (neuropathic). This subjective information, combined with the physical examination and diagnostic studies, may identify a specific pain syndrome and its implied pathophysiology.

In a patient with a hematologic disorder, the cause of pain may be the disease itself, the specific therapy for the disease, diagnostic procedures related to the disease, or unrelated disorders (Table 91.1). Splenomegaly, bone injury (e.g., infarction, infection, hemarthroses, and infiltration), leptomeningeal infiltration, and spinal cord compression frequently accompany hematologic diseases. Chemotherapy and radiation therapy can cause mucositis, typhlitis, hemorrhagic cystitis, and peripheral neuropathy; corticosteroid withdrawal may cause myalgias. Immunosuppression, caused by the diseases themselves or by the therapies used to treat them, may lead to painful infections such as perirectal abscesses, herpetic or candidal esophagitis, and herpes zoster. Patients with sickle cell disease have a number of causes for both acute and chronic pain (Table 91.2).

Distress, however, may arise from nonanatomic sources. The pain complaint may represent the patient's only means of expressing nonspecific feelings of distress to the physician. Chapman recognized three categories of this distress: anxiety, arising from fear of disfigurement or of uncontrollable pain, fear of loss of social position or of self-control, or fear of death; anger at the failure of the physicians to provide a cure; and depression from the loss of physical ability, a sense of helplessness, and the impact of financial problems. In addition to these psychological, social, and financial contributions, spiritual concerns may exacerbate any concomitant painful sensations.[9] Alleviating them may significantly reduce distress and decrease the need for pain medications or other interventions.

Sometimes there may be a disparity between the patient's expression of pain and the patient's family or friends' appreciation of the impact of the pain. The following observation may help to begin a conversation around this issue: "You seem to show a different perspective about the pain from those of your family and friends. Help me to understand *what the pain is like for you* and why you think your family and friends feel differently." Differences in cultural backgrounds may also affect the expression of pain, and thus may vary within a family, as well as in different families.[9]

TABLE 91.1	Common Pain Syndromes in Hematologic Malignancies	
Procedure-Related Pain		
Deep somatic pain	Bone marrow aspiration, biopsy, and harvest Headache following lumbar puncture	
Superficial somatic pain	Venepuncture (needle insertions) Central catheter placement/positioning	
Therapy-Related Pain		
Deep somatic pain	Bone marrow expansion and/or sensitization by granulocyte colony-stimulating factor, osteoporosis (e.g., from corticosteroids use), myalgias (e.g., from corticosteroid withdrawal), myopathy	
Superficial somatic pain	Oropharyngeal mucositis (e.g., from chemotherapy or radiotherapy)	
Visceral pain	Enteritis, typhlitis, hemorrhagic cystitis	
Neuropathic pain	Drug-related neuropathies (e.g., from chemotherapy agents)	
Headache	Drug related (e.g., due to tretinoin)	
Pain From Hematologic Malignancy		
Somatic pain	Bone infarct or necrosis, osteomyelitis, compression fracture, hemarthrosis	
Visceral pain	Tumor involvement, splenomegaly, lymphadenopathy, or lymphadenitis	
Neuropathic pain	Paraproteins with antimyelin properties, amyloid infiltration, peripheral nerve compression, spinal cord compression	
Mixed pain	Headache, meningeal infiltration or infection, brain metastasis, or primary tumor	

TABLE 91.2	Classification of Pain Syndromes in Sickle Cell Disease
Pain secondary to the disease itself	
Acute pain syndromes	
Acute chest syndrome	
Calculus cholecystitis (pigment stones)	
Hand–foot syndrome (in children)	
Hepatic crisis	
Priapism	
Pulmonary infarction	
Recurrent acute painful episode	
Splenic sequestration (in children)	
Chronic pain syndromes	
Arthropathies or arthritis	
Avascular necrosis	
Chronic osteomyelitis	
Intractable chronic pain	
Leg ulcers	
Neuropathic pain	
Pain secondary to therapy	
Loose prosthesis (in patients after arthroplasty for avascular necrosis)	
Opioid withdrawal	
Postoperative pain	
Pain caused by comorbid conditions	

Courtesy Ballas SK: Pain management of sickle cell disease. *Hematol Oncol Clin North Am* 19:785, 2005.

Continued Assessment

A standardized measurement tool, such as a verbal rating scale (VRS) or a visual analog scale (VAS), should be consistently used during follow-up visits.[1,7,10] These measurements are thought to be more accurate than mere qualitative descriptors, such as: "The pain is better." Using, for example, a scale of 0 (no pain) to 10 (the worst pain one can imagine), a decrease in pain intensity from 10 to 8 indicates that the patient could benefit from additional dose titration, but a decrease from 10 to 3 suggests that the current dose is effective. A pain goal should be assessed by asking the patient, "What level of pain would be acceptable to you?" The ongoing assessment should also pay attention to changes in the phenomenology of the pain, new occurrences of pain, or a change in the location of pain—all of which may suggest progression of disease in the patient with a hematologic disorder.

The successful outcome of pain therapy should be more than simply the lowering of pain intensity scores, but the impact on function, the minimization of side effects from treatment, and the prevention of opioid misuse. Passik and Weinreb developed a useful mnemonic device for the assessment of pain therapy in chronic nonmalignant pain known as the "4 As": analgesia, activities of daily living, adverse events, and aberrant drug-taking behaviors (e.g., repeated dose escalation or noncompliance, hoarding drugs, or acquiring drugs from other medical sources).[11] By focusing on these relevant domains in the continued assessment of the pain therapy, the clinician is able to determine if the therapy makes a true difference in the patient's life, stabilizes or improves psychosocial functioning, manages side effects, and provides a means of assessing for aberrant drug behaviors. Ultimately, the goal should be to lower the pain *to a level acceptable to the patient* and to improve the patient's level of functioning.

THERAPY DIRECTED AT THE UNDERLYING ETIOLOGY

A major component of pain therapy is to ameliorate the underlying cause of the pain, when possible. Surgery, chemotherapy, radiation therapy, immunosuppression, and antibiotics may all be used. Attention to patient comfort should be maintained regardless of the diagnostic or treatment interventions proposed.

NONPHARMACOLOGIC METHODS OF PAIN MANAGEMENT

Cognitive-Behavioral Interventions

Education and Reassurance

Patients with serious hematologic disorders are often required to undergo extensive diagnostic testing, which can include painful procedures. A rehearsal of the planned test or procedure, including a discussion (or view) of the appearance of the room and the length of time to be spent in the test apparatus, can minimize the patient's anxiety. Such explanations, offered preoperatively, lessen the need for postoperative medication and shorten the patient's hospital stay. If conscious sedation is not planned, a pleasant distraction may be helpful to divert attention from certain procedures (e.g., bone marrow aspiration or biopsy) that take place in the physician's office or in the patient's room. For example, a physician might present a patient with an electronic tablet–guided relaxation training session while the physician is preparing for a procedure. The patient is able to utilize the relaxation techniques recently acquired during the procedure in order to diminish pain.[12]

Hypnosis

Hypnosis can be a useful adjunct in the management of pain, including for patients undergoing painful procedures.[9] The hypnotic trance, a state of heightened and focused concentration, allows one to manipulate the perception of pain and diminish sleeplessness, anxiety, and anticipation of discomfort. Hypnotic training of patients with sickle cell anemia or hemophilia decreases the frequency and pain intensity of painful crises or bleeding episodes, respectively. In a controlled trial comparing hypnosis with cognitive-behavioral therapy in relieving mucositis after a bone marrow transplant, patients using hypnosis reported a significant reduction in pain control compared with patients who used cognitive-behavioral techniques.[12]

In the absence of a formal hypnotic induction, words used by a practitioner to describe procedures are very important. For example, suggesting that the numbness and coolness of a local anesthetic will persist may diminish the discomfort of a bone marrow biopsy. Using the phrase: "You will feel something; I'm not sure what you will feel because everyone feels this a little differently" in place of "This is going to hurt a lot!" gives the patient permission to alter the sensation and may also diminish the experience of pain.[13]

Meditation

Meditation has long been utilized as a method for controlling pain. Given the wide range of meditation practices and methods, it has historically been difficult to conduct evidence-based research into the effectiveness of medication. Some research has shown that using meditation to increase focus and clarity does improve pain symptoms and appears to correlate with decreased pharmacologic requirements.[14]

Cognitive-Behavioral Techniques and Counseling

The cognitive-behavioral approach addresses a number of psychosocial and behavioral factors that contribute to patients' experience of pain.[7,9,15] These techniques have demonstrated clinical utility for patients with a wide range of chronic pain syndromes. Psychological counseling as part of a multidisciplinary approach to pain treatment provides education, support, and skill development for patients with pain. It can improve patients' abilities to communicate their pain to health care personnel and may be effective in overcoming anxiety and depression. Spiritual counseling may help patients who have lost hope, can find no meaning in their lives, or believe they are being punished or have been forsaken by God.[9] They may interpret their pain in light of these feelings. Through counseling, they can regain a sense of worth and belonging. As they recast the pain in its true light, its intensity is often diminished.

Cutaneous Techniques

Acupuncture, massage, vibration, and applying cold or heat to the skin over injured areas are often very effective. Cold wraps, ice packs, or cold massage using a cup filled with water that has frozen into a solid piece of ice relieve the pain of muscles that are in spasm from nerve injury. Heat from heating pads, hot wraps, or paraffin treatments can soothe injured joints but should not be used over areas of vascular insufficiency.

EMLA, a cream containing two topical anesthetics (2.5% lidocaine and 2.5% prilocaine) is used, especially in children, to decrease the pain of superficial cutaneous procedures (e.g., venous cannulation or skin anesthesia before lumbar puncture, bone marrow aspiration, or biopsy).[9] In adults, it is used before access of implanted vascular access devices or CNS ports. To achieve anesthesia, the EMLA cream must be applied 1–1.5 hours before the planned procedure in a mound under a semipermeable dressing such as Opsite or Tegaderm. When EMLA is used as directed, methemoglobinemia has not been a problem even in infants as young as 3 months old. Skin blanching occurs, sometimes exceeding or equaling the frequency of that found with placebo moisturizing cream placed under the occlusive dressing. ELA-Max, a cream containing 4% lidocaine, is available over the counter and is an alternative to EMLA cream. Because it does not contain prilocaine, there is no risk of methemoglobinemia.

Lidocaine patches can be used over areas of hyperesthesia, as can occur in patients with postherpetic neuralgia (PHN) or nerve entrapment by vertebral body collapse.[9] The patch is applied to the affected area for no more than 12 consecutive hours a day and can be cut to size. Use should be avoided over areas of broken skin and in patients undergoing radiation therapy. Extended application of lidocaine patches has been safely applied for up to 24 hours/day for up to 4 days with minimal systemic absorption in healthy volunteers and in patients with PHN.

Neuromodulation

Transcutaneous electrical nerve stimulation (TENS) devices are indicated for patients with dermatomal pain, such as PHN or radiculopathy from spinal cord compression.[9,16] For optimal effect, a physiatrist or physical therapist familiar with the device should train the patient in its use. The efficacy of TENS therapy for patients with cancer pain remains controversial.

Radiation Therapy

Radiation therapy is commonly used in the management of painful bone lesions, spinal cord compression, bulky lymphadenopathy, and symptomatic splenomegaly in patients with hematologic malignancies.[9,17] Radiotherapy is the treatment of choice for local metastatic bone pain in most situations, although patients with underlying pathologic fractures may require surgical fixation before radiotherapy. Randomized trials have shown that single-fraction radiotherapy is as effective as multifraction radiotherapy in relieving pain caused by metastases. However, there are higher rates of retreatment, and single-fraction radiotherapy may not prevent pathological fractures or spinal cord compression.[17] In patients with poor performance status or a short life expectancy, a single dose (8 Gy) of radiation or a hypofractionated course (20 Gy/5 fractions) may be preferable and less burdensome.

Vertebroplasty and Kyphoplasty

Vertebroplasty and kyphoplasty are both minimally invasive techniques used to stabilize vertebral compression fractures and reduce pain. Vertebroplasty is a procedure in which bone cement, usually polymethylmethacrylate, is injected into the vertebral body. With kyphoplasty, a balloon is first inserted into the vertebral body followed by inflation and then deflation before cement is added. Balloon kyphoplasty has been shown to stabilize pathologic vertebral fractures caused by multiple myeloma and significantly reduce pain.[18]

Anesthetic Techniques

Trigger-point injections, nerve blocks, and neurolytic procedures are useful for acute and chronic localized pain. After excisional biopsy of an axillary lymph node, for example, a burning, constricting pain in the posterior arm and chest wall may develop; this pain is often promptly relieved by trigger-point injection.

Lymphoma or multiple myeloma may involve the spine and lead to vertebral collapse or pain from progressive disease that is refractory to antineoplastic therapy. Such pain is often particularly difficult to manage. Insertion of temporary or permanent indwelling epidural or intrathecal catheters to deliver opioids, local anesthetic agents, clonidine, or combinations of these and other agents can be very effective, especially in relieving lower thoracic or lumbar spine pain, as well as pelvic and lower extremity pain.[19] Reviews of the indications for and techniques of the anesthetic and neurolytic procedures are available.[4]

PHARMACOTHERAPY

Drugs useful for pain relief include nonopioid analgesics, opioids, and adjuvant analgesics. Most patients require a combination of medications for optimal pain relief (Fig. 91.1).[20]

WHO ANALGESIC LADDER

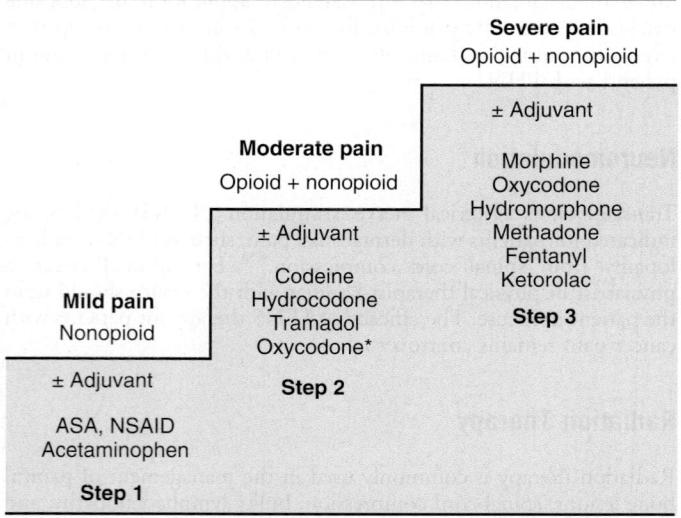

- Advance up the ladder if pain persists

Fig. 91.1 STRATEGY FOR PHARMACOLOGIC MANAGEMENT OF PAIN USING A MODIFIED (FOUR-STEP) WORLD HEALTH ORGANIZATIONANALGESIC LADDER. Multiagent therapy is usually required for optimal pain management. Patients with mild pain should be started on a nonopioid analgesic, and those with moderate pain should be started on a step 2 opioid. Many patients can benefit from the addition of a nonopioid to the opioid (e.g., for bone pain) or an adjuvant agent to the opioid (e.g., for neuropathic pain). If this combination does not produce adequate relief or the patient presents with severe pain, step 3 opioids should be begun initially. Toradol (Ketorolac) is a nonsteroidal antiinflammatory drug (NSAID) with the pain-relieving potency of a step 3 opioid. Many patients can benefit from the addition of nonopioid analgesics or adjuvants, if indicated. *Oxycodone in combination with products. It has been suggested that if opioids with nonopioid analgesics and adjuvants is unsuccessful in providing relief that an additional "4th step" of interventional/intraspinal delivery systems should be initiated.[20] *ASA*, Aspirin; *NSAID*, nonsteroidal antiinflammatory drug; *WHO*, World Health Organisation.

Management of Mild-to-Moderate Pain

Nonopioid analgesics should be given to patients with mild-to-moderate pain.[1,7] Aspirin and nonsteroidal antiinflammatory drugs (NSAIDs), including cyclooxygenase-2 (COX-2) inhibitors, are especially useful as antiinflammatory agents because they decrease local prostaglandin release through the inhibition of COX (although the mechanisms for their analgesic properties are not as clear).[21] Acetaminophen is an effective analgesic but only a weak antiinflammatory agent. Daily intake of acetaminophen should not exceed 4 g because of the potential hepatic toxicity (see box on Management of Severe Pain). It is important to prescribe an adequate dose of acetaminophen or NSAID at regular intervals, switching to another nonopioid analgesic only when maximal doses of the first have become ineffective.[21]

Ketorolac tromethamine (Toradol) is an NSAID of particular value in relieving moderate-to-severe acute pain.[22] A parenteral dose of 30 mg of ketorolac equals the pain-relieving potency of a parenteral dose of 15 mg of morphine, and acute toxicity is minimal if the total daily dose is under 100 mg. Oral ketorolac is considered less potent. Ketorolac has all of the side effects of the NSAIDs and is not recommended for use beyond 5 days because of an increased risk of renal toxicity. If that degree of pain relief is needed chronically, an opioid agent should be substituted.

Because NSAIDs can cause renal insufficiency in a significant number of patients, renal function should be assessed 1–2 weeks after initiation of any of these agents. NSAIDs should be used with caution in patients with a history of aspirin allergy or asthma because they can precipitate bronchospasm in as many as 20%. Significant edema can occur in patients with cirrhosis or congestive heart failure.[21] The relatively selective COX-2 inhibitors, such as meloxicam, celecoxib, and nabumetone, have been shown to cause similar gastrointestinal side effects as nonselective NSAIDs.[23] If NSAIDs are required in patients with a history of significant gastritis or ulcer disease, or who are older than 70 years, COX-2 inhibitors or a concomitant proton pump inhibitor should be considered. Cardiotoxicity is well described in the literature for COX-2 selective inhibitors.[24] Recently, the cardiac risk associated with traditional NSAIDs has been questioned. In a metaanalysis that included naproxen, ibuprofen, diclofenac, and several COX-2–specific inhibitors, ibuprofen and diclofenac demonstrated an increased risk of stroke. Diclofenac was also associated with an increased risk of cardiovascular death. Naproxen was not noted to increase risk in this study.[24] Nonopioid analgesics should be continued when opioid analgesics are added because they can potentiate the pain-relieving effect of the opioid (see Fig. 91.1).[25] However, when aspirin or acetaminophen is included in a fixed drug combination (e.g., Percodan, Percocet), toxicities may develop if the patient uses the medication more frequently than prescribed. The metabolism of salicylates is limited by the capacity of the hepatic microsomal system.[9] After it is saturated, salicylate levels are dependent on renal clearance. Small increases in maintenance doses can lead to serious salicylism. Patients with low albumin levels or acid urine are particularly susceptible to the development of salicylate toxicity.

Tramadol, which both weakly inhibits norepinephrine and serotonin reuptake, and weakly binds to μ-opioid receptors and has opioid-like side effects, can be used for mild-to-moderate pain. A dose of 100 mg is more effective than 60 mg of codeine. Tapentadol (Nucynta) also had both μ-receptor agonism and norepinephrine reuptake inhibition. Studied in moderate-to-severe acute postoperative pain, osteoarthritis, and low back pain, doses of 50–100 mg every 4–6 hours are comparable to oxycodone 10–15 mg every 4–6 hours with less nausea, vomiting, and constipation.

Management of Moderate-to-Severe Pain

Opioid therapy is the cornerstone of management of patients with moderate-to-severe pain.

In patients with acute moderate-to-severe pain (i.e., >4/10 on VRS), intravenous dosing should be started with the goal of rapid titration (see, for example, National Comprehensive Cancer Network [NCCN] guidelines for Adult Cancer Pain).[26] In opioid-naive patients, morphine 2–5 mg or its equivalent (see box on Relative Potencies of Commonly Used Opioids) should be dosed every 15 min (peak effect ~15 min). The patient should be reassessed for analgesic effect and side effects. If pain is not relieved, then the dose can be increased by 50%–100%; if the pain score decreases to an acceptable level, then the same dose can be continued and given as a standing dose "around the clock." Alternatively, a patient-controlled analgesia (PCA) can also be used in these situations and can provide the patient with significant control over their pain experience. Similarly, the PCA demand dose can be calculated over a 24-hour period to determine the "basal dose" of opioid the patient will need for stable analgesia. This can be provided as a basal rate on the PCA, or given the clinical situation, as a long-acting formulation equivalent to the amount of demand doses received. In opioid tolerant patients, a dose equivalent to 10%–20% of the patient's total 24-hour oral requirement should be administered as an intravenous bolus (see box on Relative Potencies of Commonly Used Opioids) and titrated, as above, every 15 minutes until pain is controlled and acceptable to the patient. For example, a patient receiving oxycodone sustained release 60 mg twice daily, should be prescribed morphine 5–10 mg intravenously every 15 minutes as needed (oxycodone 120 mg is approximately equivalent to 180 mg of oral morphine, or 60 mg of intravenous morphine; take 10%–20% of this dose). The long-acting opioid should be continued or converted to a continuous infusion, or given as a basal rate via a PCA.

Once the patient has an acceptable level of analgesia, this dose can be converted to a sustained release formulation, or to another equivalent long-acting opioid. If morphine is used, for example, the patient will need three times the parenteral dose that was effective. For example, a patient who requires 10 mg of morphine per hour (i.e., 240 mg/24 hours given intravenously) will need 720 mg/day of the oral sustained-release agent (240 mg every 8 hours). This can also be given orally as 360 mg every 12 hours. Short-acting immediate-release morphine should be available for rescue dosing at 10% of the total daily dose. For this patient, 60–90 mg every 3–4 hours is recommended. If the amount of opioid taken as a rescue dose is significant (>25% of the daily dose) for 1 or 2 days, the total dose of long-acting agent is adjusted upward accordingly.

In the outpatient setting, patients with chronic, moderate-to-severe pain can be treated with oral pain medications, e.g., morphine 5–15 mg (or an equianalgesic dose, e.g., oxycodone 5–10 mg), and titrated in a similar fashion. Note the peak effect of most oral opioids is approximately 60 minutes, so the patient should be reassessed 60 minutes following the dose for analgesic efficacy and side effects. The same strategy as above can be used for opioids-tolerant patients, i.e., 10–20% of the basal dose can be given for additional analgesia and titrated to effect.

Agents to prevent side effects should be started once opioids are initiated. All patients should be prescribed a stimulant laxative, e.g., senna (one or two tablets orally daily to twice daily, up to a maximum of eight pills per day), plus or minus a stool softener, e.g., colace 100 mg three times per day. If a more potent laxative effect is needed, lactulose (15–30 mL) or polyethylene glycol (17 g) is added. In opioid-naive patients, prochlorperazine (Compazine 10 mg taken orally two or three times daily) is prescribed as needed to treat nausea.

Opioid Analgesics

Patient Education

To ensure patient compliance with an opioid prescription, education of members of the health care team, the patient, and the family is often required to dispel the many misconceptions associated with opioid therapy.[9]

Fear of addiction is a common cause of inadequate prescribing of opioids and a barrier to their acceptance by patients.[9] Patient adherence can be improved by providing a full explanation of the differences between addiction and physical dependence, education regarding the appropriate use, storage, and disposal of opioid medications, and the risks factors for opioid misuse. Patients may also fear that if they take opioid medications for moderate pain, the medications will no longer be effective if more severe pain occurs. Because this fear, if unexpressed, can lead to undertreatment, the topic should be addressed even if the patient does not raise the question. A functional goal of therapy, such as returning to a favorite activity or reinstituting normal activities of everyday life, may enable the patient and the family to accept the opioid. Misconceptions about religious teachings may prevent health care personnel, patients, and their families from giving or accepting adequate pain medication. Catholics, for example, may not be aware of the church's position, as stated in the current catechism, that opioids may be used at the approach of death even if their use ultimately shortens the patient's life. The church does not consider this use of pain medication to be a means of suicide or euthanasia.[9]

Choice of Medication

Because a wide variety of medications are available, pharmacokinetic considerations and side-effect profiles should be considered when choosing opioid agents. Intermittent moderate-to-severe pain lasting hours to several days is amenable to oral analgesics with short half-lives (3–4 hours) with appropriate potency (e.g., immediate-release oxycodone, morphine, hydromorphone [Dilaudid], or oxymorphone

Relative Potencies of Commonly Used Opioids

Drug	Epidural	SC or IV (mg)	PO (mg)
Morphine	1	10	30
Codeine		130	200
Oxycodone		N/A	20
Hydromorphone	0.15	1.5	7.5
Methadone[a]		a	
Oxymorphone		1	10
Levorphanol		2	4
Fentanyl		0.1	N/A
Meperidine (Demerol)[b]		75	300

[a]Methadone is approximately half as potent orally as it is intravenously. It is usually not given SC because of local irritation. Standard equianalgesic tables do not reflect methadone's potency when used in repeated doses.
[b]Not recommended for patients with chronic pain.
IV, Intravenous; N/A, not applicable; PO, oral; SC, subcutaneous.

Conversions Between the Transdermal Fentanyl Patch and Morphine

Fentanyl (µg/hour)	Morphine (mg/24 hours)	
	Oral	IM or IV
25	50	17
50	100	33
75	150	50
100	200	67
125	250	83
150	300	100

IM, Intramuscular; IV, intravenous.
Data from Miaskowski C, Cleary J, Burney R, et al: Guideline for the management of cancer pain in adults and children, Aps clinical practice guidelines series, No.3. Glenview, IL, 2005, American Pain Society.

[Opana] when available). Severe pain of relatively constant intensity should be treated with oral sustained-release morphine or oxycodone taken every 8 or 12 hours,[1,7] hydromorphone (Exalgo) taken every 24 hours, oxymorphone (Opana ER) taken every 12 hours, hydrocodone (Zohydro ER, Hysingla ER) taken every 12 hours, methadone taken every 6–8 hours, or transdermal fentanyl renewed every 48–72 hours. Twelve- to 24-hour formulations of oral morphine (e.g., Kadian, Avinza) are also available; for patients unable to take pills, the capsule can be opened and the pellets sprinkled on food or suspended in water and given through a feeding tube[9] (see boxes on Relative Potencies of Commonly Used Opioids and Choice of Medication).

Practical Considerations When Using Opioids

Drugs with short half-lives should be used for "rescue doses" given for incident pain (i.e., pain with movement) and for between-dose pain exacerbations often referred to as "breakthrough pain." The dose of the rescue medication is usually calculated as 10%–20% of the total 24-hour dose, although there is no evidence for this heuristic.[27,28] For example, if a patient is receiving 300 mg of oral sustained-release morphine twice each day, the rescue dose is 10%–20% of 600 mg, which is 60–120 mg of short-acting morphine. Agents with short half-lives should also be used in elderly patients and in patients with impaired renal or hepatic function.[9] For patients with a history of drug abuse, agents with longer half-lives, such as methadone, are preferred.

There is considerable variability with respect to the side effect profile of the various opioids in each patient. Therefore it is often useful to switch to another agent if a patient is experiencing dose-limiting side effects with the initial opioid chosen. For example, if the patient on morphine experiences persistent or debilitating nausea, the rotation to another opioid at an equianalgesic dose should be considered (see box on Relative Potencies of Commonly Used Opioids). Because of incomplete crosstolerance, the initial dose for patients taking higher doses of opioids should be reduced by approximately 25%–50%. The short-acting rescue medication can provide relief if this initial dose does not prove adequate.

Methadone is increasingly used for patients with moderate-to-severe pain. It is by far the least expensive of the opioids; can be given by the oral, sublingual, rectal, intravenous, and epidural routes; and may have particular usefulness in patients with poor tolerance to other opioids. Methadone has anecdotally been used for neuropathic pain; however, recent clinical trials have not demonstrated this benefit.[29] Methadone is structurally unrelated to morphine and fentanyl, and can be used in the rare case of true allergy to these medications. It is also helpful when patients have neurotoxic side effects of other opioids. Methadone is a potent μ-opioid receptor agonist. The l-isomer has higher binding affinity for delta opioid receptors, which reduces tolerance, while the d-isomer has N-methyl-D-aspartate (NMDA) receptor antagonism and 5-hydroxytryptamine and norepinephrine reuptake blockade, which may be helpful in providing analgesia.[29] Patients with neuropathic pain and patients taking opioids chronically have increased levels of NMDA receptors in the dorsal horn of the spinal cord. NMDA antagonizes the activity of the opiate receptors. Blocking the NMDA receptors therefore enhances the analgesic effect of externally administered opioids. Ketamine, a pure NMDA antagonist, similarly enhances opioid efficacy but is associated with more cognitive side effects than methadone.

Methadone interacts with inducers and inhibitors of the cytochrome P450 system. It is extensively metabolized by CYP1A2, CYP3A4, and CYP2D6; the first two are induced by a number of drugs and other substances (e.g., cigarette smoke), and the last enzyme has a genetic polymorphism. Drug levels of desipramine and zidovudine increase when patients are receiving methadone. Drugs that lower the levels of methadone include phenytoin (by 50%), phenobarbital, carbamazepine, rifampicin, and risperidone, each of which has precipitated withdrawal symptoms.[30] Drugs that raise the serum methadone levels include ketoconazole, fluconazole, fluoxetine, and fluvoxamine. The selective serotonin reuptake inhibitors (SSRIs) (except venlafaxine) may raise methadone levels in CYP2D6 rapid metabolizers.

Methadone can cause prolongation of the QT interval. A mean methadone dose of 400 mg/day (standard deviation: 283 mg) was found in 17 patients with torsades de pointes. In an evaluation of reports of methadone-related adverse events to the US Food and Drug Administration (FDA), approximately 1% of the greater than 5000 reports were of QT prolongation or torsades de pointes. The median dose was 345 mg with a range of 29–1680 mg. Drugs that also prolong the QT interval, such as metoclopramide and olanzapine, should be used with caution in patients receiving significant doses of methadone. Gabapentin, the drug used most often as a neuropathic pain adjuvant, does not interact with methadone metabolism. There is insufficient evidence to recommend a screening interval or dose threshold for detecting methadone-induced QTc prolongation.[31]

Other difficulties with using methadone lie in its variable and long biologic half-life, and the controversy about its equianalgesic dosing range. Some studies have reported that the equianalgesic dose of morphine to methadone varies as the dose of morphine increases.[9] Dose ratios vary from 4:1 at morphine doses of 30–90 mg, to 6:1 at 90–300 mg, and to 8:1 at doses of more than 300 mg of morphine. Other studies report a ratio of 20:1 for doses of oral morphine equivalents greater than 1000 mg. Some physicians advise a 3-day conversion to methadone. On the first day, the dose of the old opioid is reduced by one-third, and one-third of the calculated dose of methadone is given; the second day, the dose of the remaining opioid is reduced by half, and the dose of methadone is only increased if the patient is experiencing moderate-to-severe pain; the third day, the old opioid is discontinued, and the standing dose of methadone is adjusted to reflect the rescue doses.[30] When converting patients directly from intravenous fentanyl to intravenous methadone, a conversion ratio of 25 μg/hour of fentanyl to 0.1 mg/hour of methadone has been found in a pilot study to be a safe and effective initial infusion rate.[32]

A relatively new opioid to the US market that is now available in both extended release and immediate release is oxymorphone. Oxymorphone extended release has been found to provide safe and effective pain relief for cancer pain.[33] Oxymorphone extended release is dosed twice daily and is about twice as potent as oxycodone.[34]

Levorphanol, which is chemically similar to dextromethorphan (an NMDA antagonist and cough suppressant), is a potent opioid that may be considered for patients with severe cancer pain. It was originally synthesized as an alternative to morphine more than 40 years ago. It has a greater potency than morphine, approximately five times as potent in its oral formulation. Analgesia is achieved through its agonistic activity at μ-, δ-, and κ-opioid receptors, as well as by its antagonism of NMDA receptors. Levorphanol can be given orally, intravenously, and subcutaneously.

Buprenorphine has long been used to treat patients with addiction as an alternative to methadone. It is available buccal/sublingually, intravenously, and now as a transdermal patch. Buprenorphine has been shown to be very effective in treating cancer pains (including neuropathic) and provides several important advantages over other opioids: It is associated with less cardiotoxicity (does not significantly prolong the QTc interval), respiratory depression, cognitive impairment, and constipation, and is one of the safer opioids to use in elderly patients or patients with renal dysfunction.[35]

Meperidine is eight to 10 times less potent than morphine and has a short duration of action, approximately 2–3 hours. Normeperidine, an active metabolite which induces dysphoria, is excitatory to the CNS and can cause agitation, tremors, myoclonus, and seizures, especially in high doses, with prolonged use or in renal failure.[9] Normeperidine has a half-life of 13–24 hours, which can lengthen with renal failure. The seizure incidence is further increased if the opioid antagonist naloxone (Narcan) must be given. Therefore meperidine is not recommended for use in patients with long-lasting moderate-to-severe pain.[1,7]

Routes of Delivery

Opioids can be delivered noninvasively (orally, rectally, transmucosally, or transdermally) or invasively (subcutaneously, intravenously, or by spinal infusion). For patients switched from one route to another such as oral or rectal to parenteral or spinal medication, or vice versa, the dose must be converted accordingly to avoid overdose or undertreatment (see box on Relative Potencies of Commonly Used Opioids).

Oral Route

Most patients can achieve excellent pain relief with short-acting and/or sustained-release oral opioid preparations. The typical onset of short-acting opioids via the oral route is 45 minutes to 1 hour, with a typical duration of action around 3–4 hours. When tablets and capsules are not feasible, many liquid forms are available in various concentrations. Some solutions do contain alcohol, which can be irritating to patients with oral lesions.

Rectal Route

Rectal opioids (i.e., morphine, oxymorphone, and hydromorphone) replace subcutaneous injections in patients who are suddenly unable to take oral medications. They have about the same potency and half-life as orally administered agents[9] and must therefore be administered frequently. Oxycodone has been shown to have a similar mean bioavailability but with a large interpatient variability but longer duration of activity (8 hours). Although not approved by the FDA, in single-dose bioavailability studies of sustained-release morphine preparations, despite delayed absorption from the rectal route, total morphine absorption over 24 hours was equivalent, whether the drug was given orally or rectally.[9]

Transdermal Route

The transdermal fentanyl patch delivers the lipophilic fentanyl into the fat-containing areas of the skin. The drug diffuses continuously from the patch's reservoir through a rate-controlling membrane and is absorbed from the skin depot into the bloodstream, where it is rapidly metabolized.[9] The onset of pain relief is delayed about 12 hours, and a relatively constant plasma concentration of fentanyl is not reached until about 14–20 hours after the initial patch is placed.[9] Liberal rescue medication must therefore be provided during the first 24 hours of use of the patch. Similarly if a patient develops signs of fentanyl overdose, naloxone (Narcan) must be given until the skin reservoir has become depleted. About 50% of the drug is still present 24 hours after patch removal. Converting patients from oral or parenteral medication to the patch is easily accomplished[9] (see box on Relative Potencies of Commonly Used Opioids). A new patch is applied every 72 hours, although up to 25% of patients require a new patch every 48 hours.

The transdermal system is an effective method of delivering pain relief for patients with a stable level of chronic moderate-to-severe pain, no oral route available, or no desire to take pills. Side effects include those caused by the contact adhesive along with those commonly associated with other opioids, but they may be better tolerated than those caused by morphine.

The transdermal system should not be used in patients with sepsis, those experiencing acute pain, those with markedly fluctuating opioid requirements, cachectic patients, or individuals with significant dermatologic insults (i.e., skin graft-versus-host disease [GVHD] or diffuse varicella). When the patient's temperature rises to 40°C, drug absorption from the skin can increase by as much as 35%. If hepatic function is impaired or sepsis or shock develops and blood flow to the liver decreases, plasma concentrations may rise sharply. Patients with cachexia lack the subcutaneous tissue necessary for formation of a drug reservoir. Lower doses may also be required in elderly patients and in those with respiratory insufficiency.

Transdermal buprenorphine (Butrans) patches have been shown to be safe and effective in patients with cancer pain.[36] They can be used alone or in combination with other opioids without reported problems, and unlike other opioids, which can cause a hyperalgesia effect from long-term use, buprenorphine has been described to exert an antihyperalgesic effect. A lack of immunosuppression and safety in renal insuffiency make buprenorphine ideal for the treatment of cancer patients. Due to the risk of QTc prolongation the transdermal patch carries an FDA warning against exceeding 20 µg per hour.

Transmucosal Route

Transmucosally administered fentanyl induces rapid analgesia with a short duration of effect (≈1 hour) and is an effective treatment in the management of breakthrough pain.[37] Oral transmucosal fentanyl citrate (Actiq), fentanyl buccal tablet (Fentora), fentanyl buccal soluble film (Onsolis), and fentanyl sublingual tablets (Abstral), as well as a fentanyl nasal spray (Lazanda) are the available transmucosal fentanyl products. They have been found to be both efficacious and safe in the treatment of cancer-related breakthrough pain.

Subcutaneous and Intravenous Routes

Subcutaneous or intravenous administration of opioids can provide pain relief in the shortest amount of time with minimal oversedation. The drugs can be delivered by portable infusion pump that is initiated or continued in the home.[9] Guidelines for their use are available. PCA systems for subcutaneous or intravenous drug delivery have the advantage of responding to the individual patient's threshold for pain while eliminating delays when nurses must administer supplemental medication. The pumps can administer a continuous fixed infusion of the opioid chosen and allow the patient to self-administer boluses of additional medication at frequencies chosen by the physician. By recording the additional amounts of self-administered medication,

the devices also facilitate the adjustment of the continuous dose required for pain relief.

Spinal Route

Epidural or intrathecal opioid infusions can be helpful for select patients. The infused opioids block pain transmission by binding to receptors in the dorsal horn of the spinal cord. Because the drug is being infused in close proximity to the spinal cord, only a small amount of opioid is needed, and the systemic side effects are reduced. Problems with this delivery system in patients who are not opioid naive include pruritus, respiratory depression, and sedation. If tolerance to the opioid develops and higher doses are required for relief, the incidence of side effects may approach that of systemically administered opioids.[38,39] Addition of local anesthetic or α-adrenergic agent (e.g., clonidine) or other agents[19] to the epidural opioid infusion allows for fairly rapid lowering of the opioid concentration and reestablishing opioid sensitivity but can cause hypotension.[40]

Management of Opioid-Related Side Effects

Sedation

The addition of 2.5–7.5 mg of dextroamphetamine or methylphenidate[9] (taken orally twice daily) has been shown to reduce opioid-induced sedation and at times allow for escalation of opioid doses without sedation. These medications also improve cognitive function and symptoms of depression. Methylphenidate may also enhance the analgesic effects of opioids.[9] They should be avoided in patients with anxiety, moderate-to-severe hypertension, agitation, thyrotoxicosis, tachyarrhythmias, severe angina pectoris, and closed-angle glaucoma. Modafinil (Provigil), a novel psychostimulant with a mechanism of action different than the amphetamine derivatives, which is approved for narcolepsy and fatigue related to multiple sclerosis, has also been found to be effective for opioid-related sedation.[9]

Constipation

Constipation is the most common opioid-induced side effect.[7] Laxatives should therefore be given routinely, not on an as-needed (PRN) basis,[1,7,9] to patients treated with any of the drugs listed in the box on Relative Potencies of Commonly Used Opioids. Detailed bowel preparation recommendations can be found, but no regimen has been studied in a controlled fashion. Commonly used stool softeners and stimulants include docusate sodium, senna, lactulose, and polyethylene glycol. A combination of a stool softener and laxative seems to be a rational choice for patients taking chronic opioids (e.g., docusate sodium with senna). Promotility agents most directly counter the mechanism of opioid-induced constipation. Bulk-forming laxatives such as psyllium and methylcellulose should be avoided because they increase stool volume without promoting peristaltic action. For refractory opioid-induced constipation, a trial of oral naloxone, methylnaltrexone, or alvimopan may be initiated.[9] These μ-opioid receptor antagonists (RAs) act locally to reverse the effects of opioids on the gut. There is minimal systemic absorption with oral naloxone and subsequently a low risk of precipitating opioid withdrawal or worsening pain at low-to-moderate doses (1.6–12 mg/day). Methylnaltrexone (administered subcutaneously)[9] and alvimopan (oral) do not cross the blood–brain barrier and therefore do not cause opioid withdrawal or worsening pain.

Nausea

Prochlorperazine (10 mg taken two or three times daily) or metoclopramide (10 mg taken three to four times daily) can prevent the nausea that occurs in most patients during the first days of opioid therapy. Relieving constipation or changing the opioid (e.g., from morphine to oxycodone) often eliminates the later development of nausea. Rarely, patients need oral or intravenous ondansetron (8 mg taken two or three times daily).

Respiratory Depression

Naloxone (Narcan), given intravenously, reverses opioid-induced respiratory depression, although repeated doses are often required.[9] Respiratory depression can occur in patients with mild-to-moderate pain during the initial use of opioids, although it is rare in patients with severe pain and in those chronically receiving opioids. Caution should be exercised before administering naloxone to patients who are chronically receiving opioids to avoid precipitation of severe pain and withdrawal. In such cases, it is inadvisable to administer the usual 0.4 mg/mL dose. Rather, 0.4 mg of naloxone should be diluted with 9 mL of saline and 1–2 mL (0.04–0.08 mg) of this dilute mixture given every 2–3 minutes until the patient is rousable and breathing at least 10 times/min. Do not give enough to fully waken the patient or withdrawal is likely to ensue.[1] In a comatose patient, endotracheal tube placement is recommended to prevent aspiration from the salivation and bronchial spasm that will be induced.[1] Naloxone should not be administered to an alert patient.

Adjuvant Analgesics

Adjuvant analgesics are a diverse class of medications, which typically have indications for conditions other than pain. They have analgesic properties and are often used when an opioid regimen alone is unable to provide sufficient analgesia or is associated with dose-limiting side effects.

Neuropathic Pain

Adjuvant agents for patients with neuropathic pain include anticonvulsants, antidepressants, α_2-adrenergic agonists, corticosteroids, topical agents, γ-aminobutyric acid (GABA) agonists, and NMDA RAs.[1,7,9,41] However, the analgesic antidepressants and anticonvulsants are typically preferred for treating neuropathic pain secondary to cancer.[42]

The anticonvulsants gabapentin (Neurontin) and pregabalin (Lyrica) have the fewest side effects and are very effective for patients with neuropathic pain from tumor, peripheral neuropathy from tumor or treatment, and PHN.[41] Despite their names, they have no effect on GABA receptors, but rather bind to the α-2-delta subunit of the N-type calcium channels in neurons within the dorsal horn, thus inhibiting calcium influx and diminishing neuronal hyperactivity. To minimize sedation, doses should be low at first (e.g., gabapentin 100 mg three times daily or 300 mg at bedtime; pregabalin 50 mg twice a day) and should be increased as tolerated every 3–5 days until analgesia is achieved. The effective dose of gabapentin varies between 900 and 3600 mg/day in divided doses and that of pregabalin is 150–300 mg twice a day. The pharmacokinetics of gabapentin are unique in that it has a ceiling effect related to a saturable transport mechanism in the gut, such that the effects of this drug may plateau during dose escalation.[42] The most common dose-limiting side effect is sedation. Gabapentin and pregabalin need to be renally dosed in patients with decreased creatinine clearance. Peripheral edema related to gabapentin or pregabalin may require diuretics. Pregabalin's gastrointestinal absorption is proportional to the dose throughout the effective dose range, making titration simpler. Other, generally less effective anticonvulsants used for neuropathic adjuvants include phenytoin, carbamazepine, lamotrigine, topiramate, and tiagabine.

The tricyclic antidepressants (TCAs; e.g., amitriptyline, nortriptyline) are effective agents for neuropathic pain.[9] The TCAs, when used as adjuvant analgesics, are effective faster and at lower doses than when they are used as antidepressants (e.g., amitriptyline is effective within 2–3 days at 50–100 mg/day). However, because of their anticholinergic side effects they should be started at doses of 10–25 mg

at bedtime and used with caution in elderly patients and in patients who have cardiac conduction abnormalities or bladder outlet obstruction. Combination therapy with gabapentin and nortriptyline has been shown to be more effective than either drug alone in patients with diabetic neuropathy and PHN.[43]

Selective serotonin and norepinephrine reuptake inhibitors (SSNRIs; e.g., venlafaxine and duloxetine) have been shown to be analgesic for a number of neuropathic pain syndromes. There is less evidence supporting the use of SSRIs for neuropathic pain.

Corticosteroids given epidurally, intravenously, or orally are useful as antineoplastics (e.g., in leukemia, lymphoma, and myeloma) and can also provide nonspecific relief for patients with spinal cord compression and plexus infiltrations. Doses of 16–100 mg of dexamethasone are needed to reduce vasogenic edema in spinal cord compression,[9] but lesser doses (6–20 mg/day) can be helpful in patients with plexus injuries. Patients must be monitored for the development of oral or esophageal candidiasis and steroid-induced delirium.

Bone Pain

Adjuvants for bone pain include NSAIDs, corticosteroids, bisphosphonates, receptor activator of nuclear factor κ-B ligand inhibitors (e.g., denosumab), and the radiopharmaceuticals strontium chloride (^{89}Sr) and samarium153-lexidronan.[9] Multiple studies have demonstrated the efficacy of bisphosphonates in reducing skeletal complications and pain from bone metastases.[9] Pamidronate and zoledronate are recommended for patients with multiple myeloma and other hematologic malignancies with painful bone lesions. Calcium and sometimes vitamin D supplementation (especially for denosumab) are often needed.[44] Also, the long-term use of bisphosphonates is associated with a small but meaningful risk of osteonecrosis of the jaw.[44] The limitations of radiopharmaceuticals include cost and cytopenias.[9] Given the limited evidence available, a recent Cochrane review did not support the use of calcitonin for control of pain from bone metastases.

Cannabinoids

Long used empirically for their analgesic and antiemetic properties in a wide range of illnesses, cannabis and cannabinoid therapies have been subjected to an increasingly large number of controlled clinical trials (of varying size and quality) over the last several decades.[45] Oral cannabis, used for breakthrough pain, was studied in a recent multicenter randomized controlled trial, involving 360 patients, who were started on a long-acting opioid. The study showed analgesic efficacy in the low and medium dose ranges, which were also well tolerated.[46] Inhaled cannabis, used for nausea and vomiting secondary to active cancer chemotherapy, was studied in three randomized controlled trials, involving 43 subjects in total, which demonstrated inhaled cannabis to be an efficacious antiemetic. Additional studies have provided evidence for its effect on spasticity, appetite stimulation, and insomnia.

SPECIFIC CLINICAL PROBLEMS

Oral Complications

Oral complications of chemotherapeutic and bone marrow transplant regimens can be frequent causes of pain. A thorough dental evaluation and prompt treatment of infections can minimize the discomfort arising from underlying periodontal disease and caries; secondary bacterial, viral, and fungal infections; and mucositis.[47] Preventive regimens include saline, sodium bicarbonate, chlorhexidine gluconate rinses, acyclovir, antifungals, and ice. Palifermin (recombinant human keratinocyte growth factor [KGF-1]) is used for the prevention and treatment of mucositis induced by conditioning regimens for hematopoietic stem cell transplants (SCT).[9] Amifostine is a thiol compound that is a selective cytoprotective agent approved for salivary gland protection in patients receiving radiation therapy.[48] The benefit of using colony-stimulating factors in the treatment of oral mucositis has been confirmed in at least four controlled trials.[49] They have not achieved widespread use, possibly because of their high cost.

Anesthetic cocktails composed of agents such as viscous lidocaine (Xylocaine), dyclonine hydrochloride, or a slurry of sucralfate, provide temporary relief from oral mucositis-related oral pain. A variety of mucosal-coating agents have been used to protect mucosal surfaces of the oral cavity including Orabase, Episil, oral antacids, and Gelclair. There is little evidence from randomized trials to support any benefit from these preparations. Gelclair, a bioadherent gel that adheres to the oral surface, creating a protective barrier for irritated tissue, showed a reduction in oral discomfort within 5–7 hours of initial treatment in an uncontrolled, open-label study of 30 hospice patients (only three of whom had chemotherapy-related mucositis).[50] The more severe cases, occurring in bone marrow transplant recipients, usually require infusional opioid therapy delivered by standard drip or PCA. Pilocarpine (5–10 mg three times daily 1 hour before meals) may improve xerostomia from neck irradiation. However, caution is warranted because of reported side effects of glaucoma and cardiac problems. Sugar-free hard candy is also useful for opioid-induced xerostomia and dysgeusia.

Postherpetic Neuralgia

PHN, defined as pain persisting beyond 4 months from the initial onset of the rash, can be a difficult problem for patients with hematologic disorders and has been the subject of several reviews. The anticonvulsant medications gabapentin, pregabalin, and valproic acid are especially useful in reducing the lancinating component of the various pain syndromes generated by this infection. A 2011 systemic review identified four placebo-controlled randomized trials, with two trials evaluating immediate-release gabapentin at doses between 1800 and 3600 mg daily showing benefit compared with placebo for the outcome of "much or very much improved" (38% vs. 20%).[51] Pregabalin in randomized studies with patients with PHN has shown improvement in sleep and decrease in pain at doses of 150–600 mg daily.[52] Because of the risks associated with physical dependence, tolerance, addiction, and overdose, many experts consider opioids as second- or third-line options for PHN.[53]

TCAs are effective for PHN.[54] One trial concluded that nortriptyline was better tolerated than amitriptyline.[55] Elderly patients, however, often do not tolerate the anticholinergic side effects, principally sedation and dry mouth, and therefore nortriptyline (Pamelor), a less anticholinergic TCA, may be useful in these patients. Topical lidocaine (5%) has been used for the relief of pain associated with postherpetic neuralgia; however, its role has not been established.[56] There are limited data on the efficacy of topical capsaicin (0.075%).[57] Available evidence of botulinum toxin injection for PNH has not been well studied, but available evidence suggests it is effective and well tolerated.[58] Patients with severe pain refractory to these therapies may benefit from a combination of intrathecal methylprednisolone and lidocaine.[59]

Sickle Cell Anemia

Patients with sickle cell anemia have chronic and episodic pain despite optimal medical therapy, and 60% of patients with sickle cell anemia will have an episode of severe pain each year. Chronic arthritic pain can be treated with physical therapy and full doses of antiarthritic medication, but some patients require low doses of chronic opioid therapy to maintain independent functioning. Several studies have confirmed the safety and efficacy of long-term opioids in the treatment of pain of nonmalignant origin. In some cases, joint replacement may be required.

When a patient with sickle cell anemia experiences pain, it is important to attempt to define the precise cause of the pain before attributing it to a vasoocclusive crisis. Acute vasoocclusive pain may occur along with the chronic pain caused by the long-term complications of compression fractures, avascular necrosis, arthropathies, fractures, avascular necroses, and leg ulcers.[60]

Treating patients with sickle cell pain is complex and requires understanding that much of the pain in adults with this illness is chronic with intermittent, recurring painful episodes. For mild pain, nonopioid therapy such as NSAIDs or acetaminophen with oxycodone or hydrocodone should be considered. However, because of possible compromise of renal blood flow in these patients and the risk of acute renal failure, NSAIDs should probably not be used beyond 5 days.[7] Uncontrolled severe pain accounts for more than 90% of hospital admissions in adults with sickle cell disease. Using short-acting analgesics on an "as-needed" basis exposes the patient to periods of insufficient analgesia, anticipation, and anxiety. Their repeated requests for medication to relieve their ongoing pain may be mistakenly interpreted as "drug-seeking behavior," and they may be unfairly stigmatized. Thus, intravenous analgesics should be started as a continuous infusion or with PCA. When adequate analgesia is obtained, a long-acting opioid or a sustained-release opioid may be initiated with intermittent use of rescue medication. In adult patients with frequent episodes of painful crisis, the use of long-acting opioid medications reduced visits to the emergency department and hospitalizations, and shortened the lengths of stay in hospital. Meperidine should be avoided in this population and has been associated with seizures in 1%–12% of these patients.

Patients With Opioid Addiction

In order to identify and treat patients with opioid addiction, the Food and Drug Administration Amendments Act (FDAAA) of 2007 established the requirement for postmarketing studies and mandated the implementation Risk Evaluation and Mitigation Strategies (REMS).[61] Statewide Prescription Drug Monitoring Programs (PDMP) were established to track patients with prescriptions for controlled substances from multiple practitioners (e.g., I-STOP in New York State). These systems allow the practitioner to easily reference which scripts a patient has filled from which practitioner. Many guidelines for treating non-malignant chronic pain with opioids exist. Patients with cancer are not immune to the risks of opioid misuse and some patients may have a history of substance abuse. It is important to screen all patients for a history of or ongoing substance misuse. Patients with risk factors should be managed more strictly with the use of medication management agreements, urine toxicology screening, pill counts and possibly more frequent visits with prescriptions for shorter durations.

Bone Marrow Transplantation

While some studies have reported pain after bone marrow transplantation, thought to be secondary to bone marrow expansion during the engraftment phase,[62] other studies have incidentally reported improvement in pain in patients with sickle cell disease after completion of successful bone marrow transplantation. While there are no studies that specifically look at pain outcomes, several studies report positive results. One study, which involved fifty children (26 with long-term follow-up) with stem cell transplants (SCT), reported that 22 of the children experienced no further episodes of pain after transplantation. It is notable that the age range was 4–14 years of age, which is likely to be too young to start developing the serious long-term effects of sickle cell disease.[63] Subsequent studies have demonstrated similar results in children who undergo SCT.[64] A recent study of adult patients with sickle cell disease who underwent SCT demonstrated that while these patients do continue to take opioids, they use them at lower doses. Pain in these

TABLE 91.3	Classification of Transplant-Related Pain Syndromes
Deep somatic pain	Bone marrow expansion and/or sensitization related to the engraftment, pneumonia, pleuritic, deep abscess
Superficial somatic pain	Oral ulcers and skin lesions associated with acute and chronic GVHD; superficial abscess, ocular lesions associated with chronic GVHD
Visceral pain	Gastrointestinal GVHD, neutropenic enterocolitis, visceral involvement by HZV and CMV
Neuropathic pain	HZV outbreak and PHN

CMV, Cytomegalovirus; GVHD, graft-versus-host disease; HZV, herpes zoster virus; PHN, postherpetic neuralgia.
Courtesy Niscola P et al: Pain syndromes in the setting of haematopoietic stem cell transplantation for haematological malignancies. *Bone Marrow Transplant* 41:757, 2008; doi:10.1038/bmt.2008.3.

patients is thought to be secondary to sickle cell disease injury prior to SCT.[65]

Graft-Versus-Host Disease

For patients who have undergone bone marrow transplantation, GVHD can be a significant problem. The usual triad of GVHD includes hepatitis, dermatitis, and gastroenteritis. Patients are usually unable to take oral, rectal, subcutaneous, or transdermal opioids because of the effects on the skin (GVHD), lining of the gastrointestinal tract (mucositis, infection, and GVHD), and thrombocytopenia. Polyarthritis and musculoskeletal manifestations can cause significant pain (Table 91.3). Therefore pain management with intravenous opioids is a necessity. The intestinal involvement that usually causes the most physical pain includes abdominal cramping and voluminous diarrhea. Treatment often begins with intravenous opioids given through a PCA pump. Addition of octreotide continuous infusion at 50–100 µg/hour intravenously or intermittent dosing at 500 µg subcutaneously every 8 hours may be effective in decreasing the volume of diarrhea and level of abdominal pain.[9]

Peripheral Neuropathy Caused by Chemotherapy Agents

Several chemotherapy agents used in the treatment of hematologic malignancies can cause painful sensory peripheral neuropathy. The vinca alkaloids, most notably vincristine, are neurotoxic, but they are not always associated with painful neuropathy. Thalidomide, lenalidomide, pomalidomide, bortezomib, carfilzomib, cisplatin, oxaliplatin, and paclitaxel are all commonly used agents that carry a significant risk of causing painful peripheral neuropathy. The most common mechanism of neuropathy is damage to the axons starting with the most distal branches and is a result of chemotherapy's ability to damage DNA replication, leading to apoptosis. The major manifestations are burning paresthesias of the hands and feet, and loss of reflexes. Paclitaxel also causes a motor neuropathy, which predominately affects proximal muscles.

Studies have evaluated numerous agents for prevention of painful peripheral neuropathy, although there have not been any magic bullets. Most of the research has focused on taxane and platinum-based chemotherapy agents. The American Society of Clinical Oncology (ASCO) has published a review of the available literature for prevention and treatment of chemotherapy-induced peripheral neuropathy (CIPN). Many vitamins and dietary supplements have been studied; however, most have not consistently shown benefit in larger randomized trials.[66] Specifically, the ASCO review indicates that acetyl-L-carnitine, vitamin E, all-*trans* retinoic acid, glutathione, and

calcium and magnesium infusions should not be utilized in the prevention of CIPN. Chemoprotectants have also not withstood scrutiny; amifostine, nimodipine, and others are not recommended. Although amitriptyline has not been shown to prevent CIPN, carbamazepine, oxcarbazepine, and venlafaxine have shown promise, although further evaluation is warranted.

Treatment of chemotherapy-induced painful peripheral neuropathy includes the usual agents used for patients with neuropathic pain from any etiology (i.e., anticonvulsants, TCAs, and occasionally tramadol or opioids). Duloxetine, a serotonin and norepinephrine reuptake inhibitor (SNRI), has been shown to improve CIPN at a dose of 60 mg daily.[67] In addition to treating these painful symptoms of neuropathy, the doses of the chemotherapy often require reduction or even discontinuation of therapy.

Problems in Elderly Patients

Pain management in elderly patients is a highly prevalent problem. It is complicated by difficulties in pain assessment and by the altered pharmacokinetics of opioids and of psychotropic adjuvant medications. Elderly patients may underreport pain because of misconceptions that pain is part of the aging process or fears of addiction.[68] Physicians may ascribe observed limitations in social contacts and physical activities to age-related changes when they are pain-induced limitations.

Elderly patients are particularly susceptible to the side effects of NSAIDs and opioids, and patients taking them should be monitored closely.[69] In elderly patients (70–89 years old), the volume of distribution for opioids is generally smaller, the drugs have longer plasma half-lives, and renal and hepatic clearances are decreased, all of which can prolong the duration of effect. The effective doses for these patients are half to one-fourth of those needed in younger patients. Drugs with short half-lives (e.g., morphine, oxycodone, hydromorphone) should be used, and initial doses should be low. Patients should be monitored carefully for the development of sedation or confusion, especially if they are receiving antihistaminic agents (e.g., famotidine, diphenhydramine), drugs with anticholinergic activity, or hypnotics.

Neuropathic pain syndromes are common in older adults, and the adjuvant analgesics gabapentin and pregabalin are often used. Common side effects include somnolence, dizziness, fatigue, and weight changes that can be problematic in the geriatric population.[70] Treatment should be initiated at 100 mg of gabapentin or 50 mg of pregabalin at bedtime, and close monitoring for side effects should occur before dose escalation. Acute urinary retention caused by opioids (especially in patients with prostatic hypertrophy) and the hypotension and tachycardia caused by tricyclic compounds can occur more frequently and be more clinically severe in this population. The starting dose of nortriptyline should be low (usually 10 mg at bedtime), and the dose should be slowly increased as tolerated. Treatment of opioid-related urinary retention may include generic Proscar (5 mg/day) in patients with benign prostatic hypertrophy and bethanechol (10–50 mg three times daily) to help increase bladder smooth muscle tone.

PATHOPHYSIOLOGY OF NAUSEA AND VOMITING

Nausea is the subjective sensation that precedes vomiting. It is caused by stimulation of one or more of four sites—the gastrointestinal tract, the vestibular system, the chemoreceptor trigger zone in the area postrema of the floor of the fourth ventricle, or higher centers in the CNS (Fig. 91.2). The gastrointestinal tract can activate the vomiting center by stimulation of mechanoreceptors or chemoreceptors on glossopharyngeal or vagal afferents (cranial nerves IX and X), or by release of serotonin from gut enterochromaffin cells, which in turn stimulates serotonin (5-HT3) receptors on vagal afferents. The vestibular system activates the vomiting center when stimulated by motion or disease (e.g., labyrinthitis) or when sensitized by

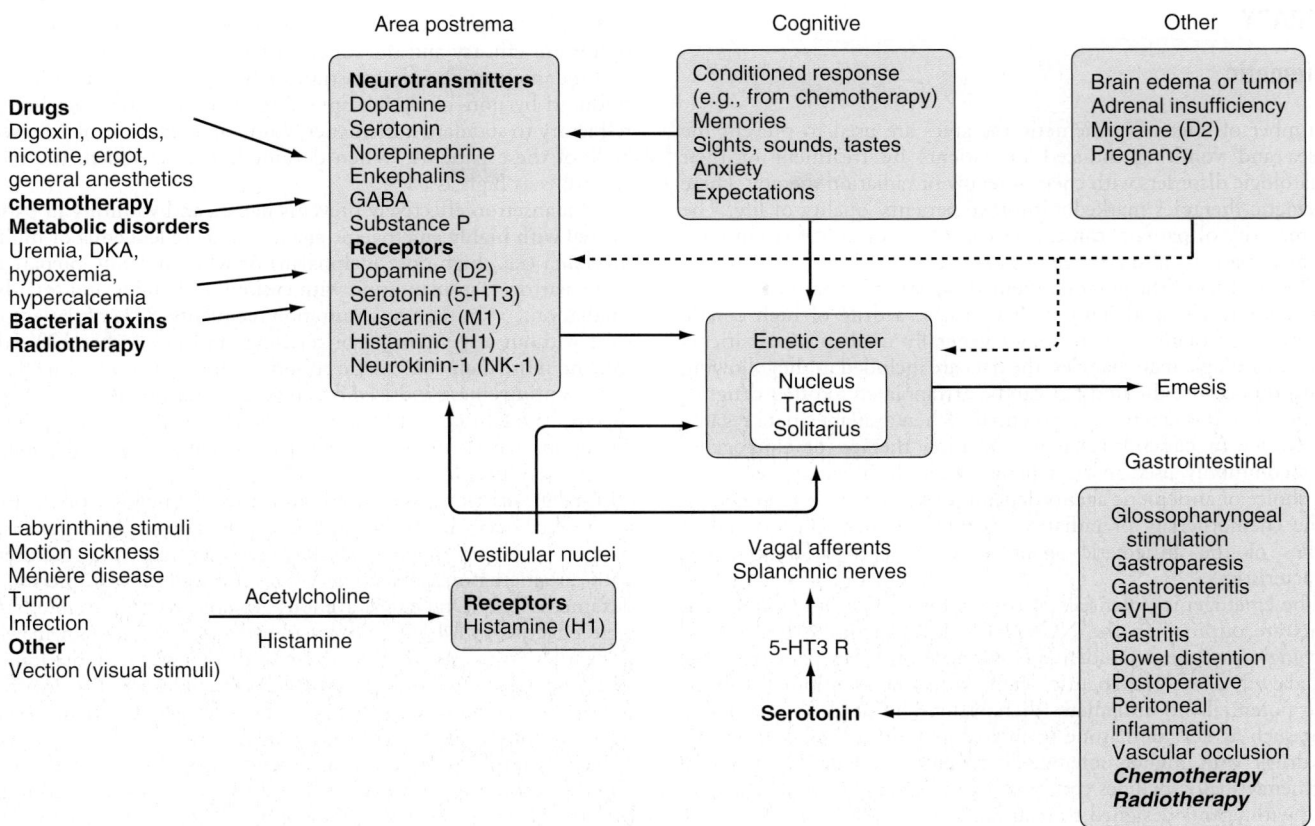

Fig. 91.2 PATHOPHYSIOLOGY OF NAUSEA AND VOMITING. *DKA,* Diabetic ketoacidosis; *GABA,* γ-aminobutyric acid; *GVHD,* graft-versus-host-disease; *5-HT3,* serotonin; *5-HT3 R,* serotonin receptor.

medication (e.g., opioids). Histamine (H1) and acetylcholine (M1) receptors are present on vestibular afferents. Endogenous or exogenous blood-borne toxins may activate chemoreceptors in the area postrema of the floor of the fourth ventricle via dopamine type 2 receptors. Finally, higher CNS centers may activate or inhibit the vomiting center. In addition, there may be direct activation of H1 receptors in the meninges secondary to increased intracranial pressure.

The means by which chemotherapy agents induce vomiting are still incompletely understood, but the most likely mechanism is believed to include stimulation of the chemoreceptor trigger zone.[9] Other causes of nausea and vomiting in hematologic patients include stimulation of the cerebral cortex, gastritis and gastroesophageal reflux disease, delayed gastric emptying, radiation enteritis, constipation, esophageal candidiasis, inner ear processes, hypoadrenalism, hypercalcemia, changes in taste and smell, and anticipatory nausea.[9]

Although the sites of emetic action of the chemotherapeutic agents have not been identified, blocking agents directed against type 3 serotonin receptors (5-HT3 receptors), dopamine (D2) receptors, and neurokinin (NK-1) receptors have been effective in inhibiting chemotherapy-induced nausea and vomiting (CINV).[9] Higher centers in the brain, such as the cortex, are also believed to be involved in producing anticipatory nausea and vomiting (ANV). Cognitive therapy, as well as antianxiety and amnesic agents, may provide effective antiemesis.

PATIENT ASSESSMENT

Risk factors for developing CINV include age younger than 60 years, female gender, history of motion sickness, and hyperemesis gravidarum.[9] Patients who have a history of alcohol intake of more than five alcoholic drinks per day (>100 g of alcohol) tend to have less nausea and vomiting. This has been studied carefully in patients

receiving high-dose cisplatin therapy but has been anecdotally observed in patients receiving other agents.

Anticipatory Nausea and Vomiting

ANV is believed to be a classic conditioned response.[9] Chemotherapy administration (the unconditioned stimulus) results in nausea and vomiting (the unconditioned response). Clinic sights, smells, and sounds are the conditioned stimuli. After frequent pairings of chemotherapy administration and the clinic's sights, smells, and sounds, the responses (nausea and vomiting) can be triggered in the absence of any chemotherapy by the clinic's sights, smells, or sounds, or simply by seeing clinic personnel even at a location distant from the site of treatment.

Patients who are at risk for developing ANV are those who have already experienced posttreatment nausea and vomiting. The risk of developing ANV increases with the increasing frequency, severity, and duration of the symptoms. Other possible predisposing factors include susceptibility to motion sickness, awareness of tastes or odors during infusions, younger age, lengthier infusions, greater autonomic sensitivity, and general anxiety or emotional distress.[9]

Acute and Delayed Chemotherapy-Induced Nausea and Vomiting

Acute CINV is defined as nausea, vomiting, or both occurring within 24 hours of administration of the agent. Although most drugs produce emesis 1–2 hours after they are given (in patients who have never before received chemotherapy), the onset of emesis from high-dose intravenous cyclophosphamide is delayed until 9–18 hours after treatment, and nausea and vomiting from high total doses of cisplatin can occur 24–72 hours later.

THERAPY

Antiemetic

A number of effective antiemetic therapies are used to prevent the nausea and vomiting induced in patients by treatment of their hematologic disorders with chemotherapy or radiation therapy. These antiemetic therapies markedly improve patients' quality of life. The vast majority of patients can expect complete control of vomiting,[71] and most patients also are free of nausea.

Most studies of the potent antiemetic agents have been conducted in patients receiving therapy with cisplatin, a drug of high emetic potential. Although cisplatin is not generally used to treat patients with hematologic malignancies, the data are included in the following discussion because the findings can be extrapolated to other drugs of equivalent or less emetogenic potential. When available, data regarding efficacy in patients receiving radiation therapy or emetogenic drugs commonly used to treat hematologic disorders are reviewed. The choice of antiemetic agents depends on the emetogenic potential of the chemotherapy or radiation therapy regimen, the side effect profiles of the antiemetic agents, and patient preferences and characteristics.

The emetogenic potentials of commonly used chemotherapeutic agents are outlined in the NCCN Clinical Practice Guidelines in Oncology Antiemesis Guideline (www.nccn.org). For patients being treated with chemotherapeutic agents with low or minimal emetogenic potential, no antiemetic therapy may be needed, or a single agent such as dexamethasone or metoclopramide may be sufficient. For drugs with higher emetogenic potential, standard antiemetic treatment usually includes combinations of several antiemetic agents along with agents designed to treat anxiety.

Combination Antiemetic

These combinations include a 5-HT3 RA such as ondansetron and a corticosteroid such as dexamethasone for moderately emetogenic regimens.[71] For highly emetogenic combination chemotherapy or regimens that include two moderately emetogenic agents, such as cyclophosphamide and adriamycin, an NK-1 inhibitor such as aprepitant should be added to the antiemetic combination.[71] Optional lorazepam may be added for anxiety-related symptoms. It is important to give antiemetic therapy before administering chemotherapy agents and to continue for about 24–72 hours after the drugs have been given to prevent emesis. Patient-specific factors and preferences regarding degree of alertness can help the health care provider choose an antiemetic regimen, as can the level of anxiety the provider observes in the patient. For instance, younger patients have a higher incidence of CINV and of metoclopramide-related acute dystonic reactions; trismus or torticollis was seen in only 2% of patients older than 30 years of age but in 27% of younger patients. Therefore even if they are receiving only moderately emetogenic therapy, they may require an antiemetic regimen for high-emetogenic drugs.[71] Younger patients find cannabinoids (e.g., Marinol) more effective than do older patients because they can better tolerate the side effects associated with the therapeutic doses of these agents. Elderly patients also have high risks of extrapyramidal side effects and are more susceptible to anticholinergic and sedating side effects. 5-HT3 RAs are therefore preferred to regimens containing metoclopramide and diphenhydramine.

The antiemetic evidence behind the utilization of different medications changes over time. We recommend utilizing the ASCO clinical practice guidelines for recommendations on combination antiemetic regimens: http://www.instituteforquality.org/practice-guidelines.

Serotonin Receptor Antagonists: Ondansetron, Granisetron, and Palonosetron

Ondansetron, granisetron, and palonosetron are the best studied of the 5-HT3 RAs. This class also includes the drugs dolasetron and tropisetron. Several studies of patients receiving regimens that included cyclophosphamide, methotrexate, or doxorubicin showed significant efficacy and the superiority of ondansetron over placebo.

Ondansetron also demonstrates efficacy in patients with emesis (induced by non–cisplatin-containing chemotherapy) that has been refractory to standard antiemetics, with complete control achieved in 50% of these patients. When dexamethasone is added, the rate of control is as high as 91%.

Ondansetron effectively prevents nausea and vomiting in patients treated with highly emetogenic agents for acute leukemia or multiple myeloma (i.e., high-dose melphalan) or who are being prepared for bone marrow transplantation with cyclophosphamide and total-body irradiation.[71,72] In the transplantation recipients, 83% of patient-days were without any vomiting or retching, and in another 10%, there were no more than two emetic episodes. Ondansetron is also effective in preventing emesis induced by single- or multiple-fraction radiation therapy.[9] Ondansetron is as effective as high-dose metoclopramide in preventing nausea induced by cisplatin, cyclophosphamide alone, or doxorubicin chemotherapy.

Oral granisetron has shown equivalence to ondansetron in studies of patients receiving cisplatin- or carboplatin-based regimens. In patients receiving moderately emetogenic therapy, oral granisetron with dexamethasone was as effective as intravenous ondansetron and dexamethasone. Oral or intravenous granisetron and dexamethasone were effective in a bone marrow transplantation program in which patients were treated with Cytoxan and total-body irradiation, and these agents, along with oral prochlorperazine, were also effective in patients undergoing peripheral blood SCT for which patients received Cytoxan, VP-16 or thiotepa, and cisplatin.

Palonosetron is a second-generation 5-HT3 RA with higher potency, stronger receptor-binding activity, and longer half-life than the other drugs in this class.[9] Palonosetron 0.25 mg intravenously has been studied in moderately and highly emetogenic chemotherapy. Several subgroup analyses of the registrational noninferiority trials have been reported in which palonosetron was superior. Palonosetron has been identified as the preferred 5-HT3 RA in prevention of nausea and vomiting from moderately emetogenic regimens. Ondansetron and the other 5-HT3 RAs have far fewer side effects than high-dose metoclopramide. Reports of extrapyramidal reactions are rare,[9] and sedation, dystonic reactions, akathisia (e.g., severe restlessness, "ants-in-the-pants" feeling), and tardive dyskinesias do not occur. Patients can develop constipation, mild headache, QT prolongation, and elevated levels of transaminases.

Corticosteroids

The mechanism of the antiemetic action of corticosteroids remains undefined. Corticosteroids are effective when used alone to prevent emesis induced by agents of moderate or low emetogenic potential.[71,72] They are also a useful component of antiemetic therapy regimens that include ondansetron, granisetron, aprepitant, or metoclopramide and add efficacy in randomized controlled trials.[71,72]

The recommended specific corticosteroid drug, dose, and duration of therapy has not been determined. Dexamethasone and methylprednisolone are the best-studied agents, but no trials have demonstrated the superiority of one corticosteroid over another. Using anecdotal evidence recommendations for dexamethasone 4-8 mg orally (PO) two to three times per day, methylprednisolone 16–32 mg PO two to three times per day, or prednisone 20–30 mg PO two to three times per day have all been suggested.

Metoclopramide

Metoclopramide is a substituted benzamide that promotes gastric motility and reduces the emetic activity of chemotherapy agents by blocking dopamine receptors (at low-to-moderate doses) and 5-HT3 receptors (at high doses) in the chemoreceptor trigger zone. Because of a more favorable side effect profile, 5-HT3 antagonists have replaced high-dose metoclopramide. At lower doses (5–10 mg orally or intravenously every 6 hours) metoclopramide is useful in treating mild-to-moderate and delayed nausea and vomiting. Delivery of the drug on a schedule that maintains adequate levels during expected emesis appears to be important.

The side effects, which may be caused by the interaction of metoclopramide with dopamine receptors, can be quite troublesome. They include akathisia, dystonic reactions (age related), sedation, and diarrhea. Benzodiazepines such as lorazepam and β-blockers such as propranolol can prevent or reverse the akathisia, and diphenhydramine or benztropine can prevent or reverse the dystonias. However, these agents induce additional side effects, including dry mouth and sedation. Short-term, high-dose metoclopramide or long-term use at usual doses has been associated with persistent and disabling movement disorders, especially tardive dyskinesias.

Neurokinin-1 Inhibitors

Substance P can cause emesis, and it appears to play a role in chemotherapy-related nausea and vomiting. Its effects are mediated through NK-1 receptors.[9] Agents that cross the blood–brain barrier and inhibit NK-1 activity (e.g., aprepitant, netupitant) are more effective than a 5-HT3 RA and dexamethasone alone in moderating acute chemotherapy-related nausea and vomiting, and they are particularly effective in decreasing delayed nausea and vomiting occurring after highly and moderately emetogenic chemotherapy (HEC and MEC).[9,71] Aprepitant is an inhibitor of CYP3A4 and therefore may cause elevation of chemotherapy agents primarily metabolized by this route; however, these elevations are not considered clinically significant, and there are no recommend dose adjustments. Aprepitant can cause significant decreases in the prolongation of the international normalized ratio induced by warfarin and increases the area under the curve of dexamethasone. The maximum dose of dexamethasone in combination with aprepitant is 12 mg. Fosaprepitant, the intravenous prodrug of aprepitant, has demonstrated equivalent efficacy to the 3-day oral regimen as a single dose at 150 mg on day 1. Oral netupitant has been studied in HEC and MEC regimens as part of a single-dose combination product with oral palonosetron. These studies have demonstrated similar safety and efficacy when compared with combination antiemetic therapy including aprepitant.[73]

Olanzapine

Olanzapine has been shown to improve control of both acute and delayed nausea and vomiting in HEC and MEC when used in combination with dexamethasone and a 5-HT3 RA. Olanzapine is also shown to be superior to standard antiemetics in the breakthrough CINV setting.[74]

Anticipatory Nausea and Vomiting

The treatment of ANV is best achieved through prevention with aggressive antiemetic therapy and treatment of anxiety with the appropriate agents (see Benzodiazepines). However, in patients for whom this approach has not been successful and in whom ANV develops, a variety of behavioral techniques have been helpful.[9] These include hypnosis, progressive muscle relaxation with guided imagery, systemic desensitization, and distraction. Results may be optimized if a therapist trained in these techniques works with the patient, but patients can use progressive muscle relaxation with guided imagery on their own.

Benzodiazepines

The benzodiazepine lorazepam has only mild antiemetic activity when used as a single agent. It is used frequently in the treatment and prevention of nausea and vomiting, particularly when anxiety is associated with the nausea and vomiting. It markedly decreases anxiety and the akathisia associated with metoclopramide therapy, and induces dose-related memory loss and marked sedation.

Cannabinoids

Currently two pharmaceutical tetrahydrocannabinol-containing agents are available via prescription. Nabilone and dronabinol are both FDA approved for the treatment of CINV. Synthetic cannabinoids are mostly reserved for patients with difficult-to-treat, refractory nausea and vomiting or as a rescue agent. Younger patients find cannabinoids more effective than do older patients, likely due to better tolerated side effects associated with the therapeutic doses of these agents. The cannabinoids cause ataxia, dry mouth, orthostatic hypotension and dizziness, euphoria (or dysphoria), and a feeling of being "high."[75]

Other Drugs

Other agents that are more active than placebo include the butyrophenones haloperidol and droperidol, and the phenothiazine prochlorperazine. These agents are less effective drugs than the agents previously mentioned, and all cause sedation. The butyrophenones produce dystonic reactions, akathisia, and occasionally hypotension. Scopolamine, a centrally acting anticholinergic, can be effective for patients with a vertiginous component to their nausea.

CONCLUSION

Pain remains one of the most distressing and debilitating symptoms in patients with hematological disorders. Whether secondary to the disease process, iatrogenic, diagnostic, or therapeutic interventions, or related complications, pain is frequently underappreciated and undertreated. A methodological approach to evaluate and manage pain is recommended. Knowledge of the wide range of pharmacologic and nonpharmacological interventions is essential for the clinician managing pain. Pain refractory to standard approaches should be referred to pain or palliative care specialists.

Nausea and vomiting are common side effects of chemotherapy and should be treated aggressively to assure patient comfort during the treatment of their hematologic illness. A number of targeted therapies exist and should be used based on the emetogenic potential of the agents used and the patient's clinical condition and comorbidities. Severe or refractory nausea should involve palliative care consultation.

REFERENCES

1. LeBlanc TW: Management of cancer pain. In DeVita VT, Lawrence TS, Rosenberg SA, et al, editors: *Devita, Hellman, and Rosenberg's cancer: principles and practice of oncology*, ed 10, Philadelphia, 2014, Lippincott Williams & Wilkins.
2. National Cancer Institute: *'Pain'*. N.p., 2015. Web. 12 Apr. 2015. <http://www.cancer.gov/cancertopics/pdq/supportivecare/pain/HealthProfessional>.
3. Strada EA, Portenoy RK: *Psychological, rehabilitative, and integrative therapies for cancer pain*. UpToDate online, Topic 14249 Version 19.0, (Accessed in 15.04.15.).
4. Kaplan R, Portenoy RK, *Cancer pain management: interventional therapies*. UpToDate online, Topic 14248, Version 23.0, (Accessed in 04.15.).
5. Blinderman CD: Management of cancer pain: optimal pharmacotherapy and the role of interventions. *Advances in Pain Management* 1(4):122–140, 2008.
6. Merskey H, Bogduk N: *Classification of chronic pain, second edition (revised), international association for the study of pain taxonomy*, Seattle, 2012, IASP Press. Updated May 22.
7. Miaskowski C, Cleary J, Burney R, et al: *Guideline for the management of cancer pain in adults and children, APS clinical practice guidelines series, No.3*, Glenview, IL, 2005, American Pain Society.
8. Zeppetella G, et al: Opioids for the management of breakthrough pain in cancer patients. *Cochrane Database Syst Rev* (10):CD004311, 2013.
9. Abrahm JL: *A physician's guide to pain and symptom management in cancer patients*, ed 2, Baltimore, 2005, Johns Hopkins University Press.
10. Jensen MP: The validity and reliability of pain measures in adults with cancer. *J Pain* 4:2–21, 2003.
11. Passik SD, et al: Managing chronic nonmalignant pain: overcoming obstacles to the use of opioids. *Adv Ther* 17(2):70–83, 2000.

12. Sheinfeld Gorin S, et al: Meta-analysis of psychosocial interventions to reduce pain in patients with cancer. *J Clin Oncol* 30(5):539–547, 2012.

13. Montgomery GH, et al: Hypnosis for cancer care: over 200 years young. *CA Cancer J Clin* 63(1):31–44, 2013.

14. Thomas JW, Cohen M: A methodological review of meditation research. *Front Psychiatry* 5:74, 2014.

15. Sheinfeld Gorin S, et al: Meta-analysis of psychosocial interventions to reduce pain in patients with cancer. *J Clin Oncol* 30(5):539–547, 2012.

16. Hurlow A, et al: Transcutaneous electric nerve stimulation (TENS) for cancer pain in adults. *Cochrane Database Syst Rev* (3):CD006276, 2012.

17. Sze WM, Shelley MD, Held I, et al: Palliation of metastatic bone pain: Single fraction versus multifraction radiotherapy—A systematic review of randomized trials. *Clin Oncol* 15:345, 2003.

18. Berenson J, Pfugmacher R, Jarzem P, et al: Balloon kyphoplasty versus non-surgical fracture management for treatment of painful vertebral body compression fractures in patients with cancer: A multicentre, randomized controlled trial. *Lancet Oncol* 12:225, 2011.

19. Stearns L, Boortz-Marx R, Du Pen S, et al: Intrathecal drug delivery for the management of cancer pain: A multidisciplinary consensus of best clinical practices. *J Support Oncol* 3:399, 2005.

20. Miguel R: Interventional treatment of cancer pain: the fourth step in the World Health Organization analgesic ladder? *Cancer Control* 7(2):149–156, 2000.

21. Rawlins MD, et al: Non-opioid analgesics. In Hanks G, Cherny NI, Christakis NA, editors: *Oxford textbook of palliative medicine*, ed 3, Oxford, UK, 2010, Oxford University Press, p 355.

22. Joishy SK, Walsh D: The opioid-sparing effects of intravenous ketorolac as an adjuvant analgesic in cancer pain: Application in bone metastases and the opioid bowel syndrome. *J Pain Symptom Manage* 16:334, 1998.

23. Vascular and upper gastrointestinal effects of non-steroidal anti-inflammatory drugs: meta-analyses of individual participant data from randomised trials. *Lancet* 382(9894):769–779, 2013.

24. Trelle S, Reichenbach S, Wandel S, et al: Cardiovascular safety of non-steroidal anti-inflammatory drugs: Network meta-analysis. *BMJ* 342:c7086, 2011.

25. McNicol E, et al: NSAIDS or paracetamol, alone or combined with opioids, for cancer pain. *Cochrane Database Syst Rev* (1):CD005180, 2005.

26. Swarm RA, Abernethy AP, et al: Adult cancer pain. *J Natl Compr Canc Netw* 11(8):992–1022, 2013.

27. Portenoy RK: Cancer pain management. *Clin Adv Hematol Oncol* 3:30, 2005.

28. Zeppetella G, et al: Opioids for the management of breakthrough pain in cancer patients. *Cochrane Database Syst Rev* (10):CD004311, 2013.

29. Nicholson AB: Methadone for cancer pain. *Cochrane Database Syst Rev* (4):CD003971, 2007.

30. Bruera E, Sweeney C: Methadone use in cancer patients with pain: A review. *J Pall Med* 5:127, 2002.

31. Pani PP, et al: QTc interval screening for cardiac risk in methadone treatment of opioid dependence. *Cochrane Database Syst Rev* (6):CD008939, 2013.

32. Santiago-Palma J, et al: Intravenous methadone in the management of chronic cancer pain: safe and effective starting doses when substituting methadone for fentanyl. *Cancer* 92(7):1919–1925, 2001.

33. Prommer E: Oxymorphone: a review. *Support Care Cancer* 14:109, 2006.

34. Gabrail NY, Dvergsten C, Ahdieh H: Establishing the dosage equivalency of oxymorphone extended release and oxycodone controlled release in patients with cancer pain: A randomized controlled study. *Curr Med Res Opin* 20:911, 2004.

35. Davis MP: Twelve reasons for considering buprenorphine as a frontline analgesic in the management of pain. *J Support Oncol* 10(6):209–219, 2012.

36. Schmidt-Hansen M, et al: Buprenorphine for treating cancer pain. *Cochrane Database Syst Rev* (3):CD009596, 2015.

37. Zeppetella G, Ribeiro MD: Opioids for the management of breakthrough pain in cancer patients. *Cochrane Database Syst Rev* (1):CD004311, 2006.

38. Smith TJ, et al: Use of an implantable drug delivery system for refractory chronic sickle cell pain. *Am J Hematol* 78(2):153–154, 2005.

39. Smith TJ, et al: Implantable drug delivery systems (IDDS) after failure of comprehensive medical management (CMM) can palliate symptoms in the most refractory cancer pain patients. *J Palliat Med* 8(4):736–742, 2005.

40. Swarm RA, Cousins MJ: Anaesthetic techniques for pain control. In Hanks G, Cherny NI, Christakis NA, et al, editors: *Oxford textbook of palliative medicine*, ed 3, Oxford, UK, 2010, Oxford University Press, p 390.

41. Portenoy RK: Adjuvant analgesics in pain management. In Hanks G, Cherny NI, Christakis NA, et al, editors: *Oxford textbook of palliative medicine*, ed 3, Oxford, UK, 2010, Oxford University Press, p 361.

42. McDonald A, Portenoy RK: How to use antidepressants and anticonvulsants as adjuvant analgesics in the treatment of neuropathic cancer pain. *J Support Oncol* 4:43, 2006.

43. Filron I, Bailey JM, Tu D, et al: Nortriptyline and gabapentin, alone and in combination for neuropathic pain: A double-blind, randomized controlled crossover trial. *Lancet* 374(9697):1252, 2009.

44. Kyle RA, Yee GC, Somerfield MR, et al: American Society of Clinical Oncology clinical practice guideline update on the role of bisphosphonates in multiple myeloma. *J Clin Oncol* 25:2464, 2007.

45. Hazekamp A, Grotenhermen F: Review on clinical studies with cannabis and cannabinoids 2005–2009. *Cannabinoids* 5:1–21, 2010.

46. Portenoy RK, et al: Nabiximols for opioid-treated cancer patients with poorly-controlled chronic pain: A randomized, placebo-controlled, graded-dose trial. *J Pain* 13:438–449, 2012.

47. Eliezer S, Fall-Dickson JM, Berger AM: Oral Complications. In DeVita VT, Lawrence TS, Rosenberg SA, editors: *Cancer:principles and practice of oncology*, ed 9, Philadelphia, 2011, Wolters Kluwer/Lipincott Williams and Wilkins, p 2337.

48. Sasse AD, Clark LG, Sasse EC, et al: Amifostine reduces side effects and improves complete response rate during radiotherapy: results of a meta-analyses. *Int J Radiat Oncol Biol Phys* 64:784, 2006.

49. Crawford J, Tomita DK, Mazanet R, et al: Reduction of oral mucositis by filgrastom (rmetHuG-CSF) in patients receiving chemotherapy. *Cytokines Cell Moll Ther* 5:187, 1999.

50. Innocenti M, Moscatelli G, Lopez S: Efficacy of gelclair in reducing pain in palliative care patients with oral lesions: preliminary findings from an open pilot study. *J Pain Symptom Manage* 24:456, 2002.

51. Moore RA, Wiffen PJ, Derry S, et al: Gabapentin for chronic neuropathic pain and fibromyalgia in adults. *Cochrane Database Syst Rev* (3):CD007938, 2011.

52. Sabatowski R, Galvez R, Cherry DA, et al: Pregabalin reduces pain and improves sleep and mood disturbances in patients with post-herpetic neuralgia: results of a randomized, placebo-controlled clinical trial. *Pain* 109:26, 2004.

53. Johnson RW, Rice AS: Clinical practice. Postherpetic neuralgia. *N Engl J Med* 371:1526, 2014.

54. Argoff CE: Review of current guidelines on the care of post herpetic neuralgia. *Post grad Med* 123:134, 2011.

55. Watson CP, Vernich L, Chipman M, et al: Nortriptyline versus amitriptyline in postherpetic neuralgia: a randomized trial. *Neurology* 51:1166, 1998.

56. Wolff RF, Bala MM, Westwood M, et al: 5% lidocaine-medicated plaster vs other relevant interventions and placebo for post herpetic neuralgia (PHN): a systemic review. *Acta Neurol Scand* 123:295, 2011.

57. Edelsberg JS, Lord C, Oster G: Systemic review and meta-analysis of efficacy, safety and tolerability data from randomized controlled trials of drugs used to treat postherpetic neuralgia. *Ann Pharmacother* 45:1483, 2011.

58. Apalla Z, Sotiriou E, Lallas A, et al: Botulinum toxin A in postherpetic neuralgia: A parallel, randomized, double-blind, single-dose, placebo-controlled trial. *Clin J Pain* 29:857, 2013.

59. Kotani N, Kushikata T, Hashimoto H, et al: Intrathecal methylprednisolone for intractable postherpetic neuralgia. *N Engl J Med* 343:1514, 2000.

60. Ballas SK: Pain management of sickle cell disease. *Hematol Oncol Clin North Am* 19:785, 2005.

61. Nelson L, et al: Curbing the opioid epidemic in the United States: the risk evaluation and mitigation strategy (REMS). *JAMA* 308(5):457–458, 2012.

62. Niscola P, et al: Pain syndromes in the setting of haematopoietic stem cell transplantation for haematological malignancies. *Bone Marrow Transplant* 41:757–764, 2008.

63. Walters MC, et al: Impact of bone marrow transplantation for symptomatic sickle cell disease: an interim report. *Blood* 95:1918–1924, 2000.

64. Walters MC, et al: Pulmonary, gonadal, and central nervous system status after bone marrow transplantation for sickle cell disease. *Biol Blood Marrow Transplant* 16(2):263–272, 2010.

65. Hsieh MM, et al: Nonmyeloablative HLA-matched sibling allogeneic hematopoietic stem cell transplantation for severe sickle cell phenotype. *JAMA* 312(1):48–56, 2014.

66. Hershman D, Lacchetti C, Dworkin RH, et al: Prevention and management of chemotherapy-induced peripheral neuropathy in survivors of adult cancers: American society of clinical oncology practice guideline. *J Clin Oncol* 32:1941–1967, 2014.

67. Lavoie Smith EM, Pang H, Cirrincione C, et al: Effect of duloxetine on pain, function, and quality of life among patients with chemotherapy-induced painful peripheral neuropathy: a randomized clinical trial. *JAMA* 309(13):1359–1367, 2013.

68. Culberson JW, Ziska M: Prescription drug misuse/abuse in the elderly. *Geriatrics* 63:22, 2008.

69. Gloth FM, 3rd.: Pharmacological management of persistent pain in older persons: focus on opioids and nonopioids. *J Pain* 12:S14, 2011.

70. Moore RA, Straube S, Wiffen PJ, et al: Pregabalin for acute and chronic pain in adults. *Cochrane Database Syst Rev* (3):CD007076, 2009.

71. Basch E, Prestrud AA, Hesketh PJ, et al: Antiemetics: American society of clinical oncology clinical practice guideline update. *J Clin Oncol* 29:4189–4198, 2011.

72. National Comprehensive Cancer Network: *Clinical practice guidelines in oncology: Antiemesis*, v.1.2015. Available at <www.ncc.org/professionals/physician_gls/pdf/antiemesis.pdf>. (Accessed April 15.04.15.).

73. Gralla RJ, Bosnjak SM, Hontsa A, et al: A phase III study evaluating the safety and efficacy of NEPA, a fixed-dose combination of netupitant and palonosetron, for prevention of chemotherapy-induced nausea and vomiting over repeated cycles of chemotherapy. *Ann Oncol* 25:1333–1339, 2014.

74. Hocking CM: Kichenadasse G. Olanzapine for chemotherapy-induced nausea and vomiting: a systematic review. *Support Care Cancer* 22(4):1143–1151, 2014.

75. Machado Rocha FC, et al: Therapeutic use of Cannabis sativa on chemotherapy-induced nausea and vomiting among cancer patients: systematic review and meta-analysis. *Eur J Cancer Care (Engl)* 17(5):431–443, 2008.

CHAPTER 92

PALLIATIVE CARE

Kristen G. Schaefer, Janet L. Abrahm, and Joanne Wolfe

Palliative care is an approach to care for children and adults provided by an interdisciplinary team with a focus on individual patient and family goals, values, preferences, and relief of suffering in the face of serious illness. In a seminal 2003 report,[1] and again in the recent "*Dying in America: Improving quality and honoring individual preferences near the end of life*",[2] the Institute of Medicine (IOM) defined the unique role of palliative care for children and adults with serious illness: "*Palliative care seeks to prevent or relieve the physical and emotional distress produced by a life-threatening medical condition or its treatment, to help patients with such conditions and their families live as normally as possible, and to provide them with timely and accurate information and support in decision making.*" The IOM report also outlined the need to improve patient access, education of health professionals, and research in palliative care (Table 92.1). In 2006, hospice and palliative medicine was accepted as a specialty by the American Board of Medical Specialties. In 2007, the Accreditation Council for Graduate Medical Education began accrediting fellowship programs, and the first qualifying examination in hospice and palliative medicine was given in 2008. Palliative care subspecialists provide clinical support in more complex situations and are also responsible for improving palliative care education, innovation and research, but all clinicians should integrate high-quality palliative care into their care of patients with serious illness.[3]

Palliative care practitioners have expertise in communication, in treatment of physical symptoms, and in relieving social, psychological, and spiritual and existential distress. Such care and assistance is not limited to people thought to be dying and should be available concurrently for patients receiving curative or life-prolonging treatments. Emerging evidence suggests that concurrent palliative care in serious illness can decrease costs and improve outcomes, and patient access to high-quality specialty-level palliative care is becoming the standard of care at most academic cancer centers[2,4] However, overall rates of referral to palliative care remain low, particularly for patients with hematologic malignancies.[5]

Recently published oncology consensus clinical guidelines[6] highlight the integral role of specialty-level palliative care throughout the cancer trajectory, and align with increasing public demand for better advance care planning and more timely referral to specialty-level palliative care and hospice.[2] This chapter will review core elements of palliative care for children and then for adults in each section, with specific attention to growing awareness and understanding of palliative care needs in patients with hematologic malignancies.

PEDIATRIC PALLIATIVE CARE: SPECIFIC ISSUES

I just wish that I had armfuls of time.

— *(4-year-old child)*[7]

Pediatric palliative care is an emerging frontier in the comprehensive care of children.[8] Specific issues related to palliative care for pediatric patients and their families include the following:[9]

- Smaller numbers of dying children than adults mean that there is less professional expertise and underrepresentation of children in palliative care protocols.

- The heterogeneity of illnesses, many rare, requires the involvement of many disciplines and specialists.
- Many children have genetic diseases, so there may be more than one affected child in a family.
- The time course of some illnesses can be extremely variable. Pediatric palliative care may extend over years, even decades.
- A broad developmental spectrum is represented, including changes in the individual child through time.
- The underlying principles and ethics of palliative care are universal across the life span. However, as in all specialties, children bring with them unique issues and dilemmas.
- A child or adolescent diagnosed with a life-threatening or life-limiting illness throws an assumed sequence out of order. A time of role reversal is expected, when children will care for dying parents. When parents instead find themselves watching their child face death, a sense of tragic absurdity prevails. Not only is time shortened, but its order is shattered. A child or adolescent with a life-threatening illness represents a premature separation to the family. Even before the child has become a differentiated individual through a natural developmental sequence, that child is wrenched away. There is little preparation for separation by death when a psychological separation has not yet been effected. The adolescent who is beginning to negotiate an independent existence is often the hardest to face when that "moving forward" is irreversibly halted, or at least disrupted. A child has not even had the time to begin to form life goals.
- The necessity for palliative care—the concept and the clinical approach—may emerge at different points in the illness trajectory, depending on the prognosis for the child, the decisions that must be made in choosing treatment options, and always, the management of pain and suffering in the provision of optimal quality of life. One of the foremost goals is to initiate palliative care for children earlier in the illness trajectory—in a proactive manner—so that effective care planning can be implemented. Care of the family, with a particular focus on the young siblings, is a priority.

COMMUNICATION

Good communication can dispel fears of abandonment. Breaking bad news and discussing prognosis with patients with advanced disease are occasions when clinicians can demonstrate their commitment to an ongoing partnership with patients and families. Conversations must demonstrate respect for cultural differences and the conviction that psychosocial and spiritual growth can occur even at the end of life. If done well, the groundwork will be laid for further discussions of patient hopes and fears, goals, values, and spiritual concerns that form the basis of decisions about resuscitation and artificial life support. These conversations should be documented in the medical record, and recorded as a physician order when possible, for example, a signed MOLST (Medical Order for Life-Sustaining Treatment) or POLST (Physician Order for Life-Sustaining Treatment) form.[2]

Communication with a child...

When I first heard my diagnosis, one question kept going around and around in my head: "How long do I have, Doc?"

— *(12-year-old child)*[7]

TABLE 92.1	Summary of the Institute of Medicine Report: *When Children Die: Improving Palliative and End-of-Life Care for Children and Their Families*

Improve Organization and Delivery of Care

Emphasis is placed on the development of care guidelines and protocols in all pediatric settings, the development of regional information programs and resources in rural areas, and policies and procedures for involving children in decision making

Reform Financing of Palliative Services and Hospice Care

Vast changes in public and private health coverage: add hospice, change eligibility rules, provide outlier payments, extend coverage for counseling family members and for bereavement follow-up

Better Prepare Health Professionals

Create educational experiences and curricula that will provide basic and advanced competence in palliative, end-of-life, and bereavement care

Strengthen Research Base for Effective Care

Emphases include appropriate quality-of-life measures, effective symptom management, impact of perinatal death on parents and siblings, impact of sudden death on family and professional caregivers, efficacy of bereavement interventions, models for provision of care, financing alternatives, effective strategies for educating professionals

From Institute of Medicine: *When children die: Improving palliative and end-of-life care for children and their families*, Washington, DC, 2003, National Academy Press.

Children with serious hematologic disorders have usually lived with the illness over a prolonged period of months or years. Their knowledge, understanding, and awareness of their precarious life situation is often profound, at physical, cognitive, and emotional levels.

The doctors think my bone marrow is fine for now—and for now is for now.

— *(8-year-old child)*[7]

The protective stance of the past stated that disclosure to the child of his or her prognosis (and even, in some instances, the diagnosis) would cause increased anxiety and fear. Since the 1980s, however, a shift toward open communication has been evident.[10] To shield the child from the truth may only heighten anxiety and cause the child to feel isolated, lonely, and unsure of whom to trust.

In communication with the life-threatened child at any juncture in the illness, the precedent for a climate that enables such honest interchange is created from the time of diagnosis. The individual child's competence and vulnerability serve as the context for decisions regarding disclosure at any point in the illness trajectory. Considerations about what or how much to tell include the child's age, cognitive and emotional maturity, family structure and functioning, cultural background, and history of loss.[7] These same factors apply at the end of life, with extreme sensitivity to how the parents have chosen to inform the child throughout the illness experience, how the child has understood and processed information up to this time, and what the child is now asking—implicitly and explicitly—about his or her situation.

For adult patients with advanced cancer, having had a discussion about end-of-life wishes with one's physician has been shown to correlate with less aggressive medical care near death, earlier hospice referrals, cost savings at the end of life, and improved bereavement adjustment for caregivers.[2] Furthermore, having had conversations about end-of-life wishes is not associated with higher rates of major depressive disorder or more worry. Proactive, direct communication with patients and their families about approaching and managing the end of life can be a satisfying and rewarding part of patient care. However, more training in palliative care clinical and communication skills is needed during hematology/oncology fellowship and in continuing medical education settings to ensure competency in these areas.

TABLE 92.2	Breaking Bad News

1. Make yourself, the patient, and the family comfortable
2. Find out what they know
3. Indicate that you are planning to tell them something that is unpleasant and may be disturbing
4. Find out whether they want to be told, or whether they want someone else to be told
5. Find out how much they want to know (i.e., the big picture versus all the details)
6. Tell them in words they can understand, allowing time for questions along the way
7. Respond to their feelings
8. Let them know that this is only the first of many discussions with you
9. Ask them to summarize what they heard you say; ask if they have further questions
10. Arrange your next meeting with them

From Abrahm JL: Update in palliative medicine and end-of-life care, *Annu Rev Med* 54:53, 2003; and Back A, Arnold R, Tulsky J: *Mastering communication with seriously ill patients: Balancing honesty with empathy and hope*, New York, 2009, Cambridge University Press.

Breaking Bad News

I just wanted to be told the truth and not too bluntly, but the truth nonetheless. So that I could make a decision myself, be able to accept it, decide what I was going to do about it.

— *Adult cancer patient seeking a second-opinion hematology-oncology consultation*[11]

Table 92.2 contains an outline of the suggested steps to take when breaking bad news.[12] For patients with advanced disease, the goal is to establish or strengthen trust, and reassure them that the physician is committed to caring for them even though their disease cannot be cured. To do this well, physicians need to believe that they have not failed the dying patient, even if medicine has.

Prognosis and Decision Making

Surveys of bereaved parents indicate that physician communication about prognosis is not optimal. At the same time, emerging data suggest that bereaved parents consider high-quality communication as the most important value when reflecting on physician quality of care.[2] Parents value clear information that is communicated sensitively and includes the child, when developmentally appropriate. When it comes to discussing prognosis, a majority of parents want as much information as possible.[13] Furthermore, although many parents find prognostic information about their child upsetting, they still want prognosis to be discussed. The data suggest, however, that parents are overly optimistic about the child's chances of cure in comparison to physicians, and this is especially true when the prognosis is uncertain. Being aware of these trends may help physicians to discuss prognosis with greater clarity.

One side of my head says: "Think optimistic." The other side says: "What if this treatment doesn't work?"

— *(11-year-old-child)*[7]

The child is often aware of the diminishing curative or life-prolonging options that he or she faces. It is at this time that the child may ask anxiously: "What if this medicine doesn't work? What will you give me next?" The child experiences a profound sense of loss of control. It is at this time that families are confronted with a series of decisions regarding the nature and intensity of medical interventions they wish to pursue. This process can be excruciating: they do not want their child to suffer more, yet they often cannot tolerate the thought of missing an opportunity for a cure or prolonged time. The physician and team's role shifts from leadership in recommending a curative treatment plan to the clarification of experimental and palliative options and consequences. In most instances, the parents make the decision; however, to varying degrees, when asked in a sensitive manner, children as young as 10 years of age are able and willing to talk about their experiences and end-of-life decisions.[8]

During the last decade there has been increased recognition of the child's participation in making treatment decisions. Crucial to this process is an assessment of the child's or adolescent's ability to appreciate the nature and consequences of a specific medical decision. This becomes particularly complex when the wishes of the child differ from those of the parents. Because actual assessment tools are only in the early stages of development, professionals must rely exclusively on their clinical judgment to assess children's understanding of the contingencies they are facing. This is often a juncture when input from members of the interdisciplinary team can be crucial: children often express their understanding, awareness, and thoughts about treatment options and living or dying to individuals other than their parents or primary physician.

The following example illustrates the remarkable capacity of a young child to address the transition towards end of life.

A 7-year-old girl told her parents that she was too tired to fight anymore, and that she wanted to give up. She added: "If I have to continue suffering, I would rather be in heaven." These statements were major determinants in the parents' choosing a palliative care plan without any further attempts at life-prolonging treatment. She went home on hospice care and died peacefully several weeks later.[7]

Adult patients and families also want to be prepared for the end of life, to be able to name someone to make decisions, know what to expect about their physical condition, have financial affairs in order, know that the physician is comfortable talking about death and dying, feel that the family is prepared for their death, have funeral arrangements in place, and have treatment preferences in writing.[12] For this to happen, patients must know how long they are likely to have left to live. For adults with refractory hematologic malignancy, prognostic uncertainty about when to stop therapy in pursuit of cure and when end-of-life begins can be a barrier to palliative care referral.[14]

The median survival of older adults with leukemia is not that different from advanced pancreatic cancer or stage IV lung cancer ... but we are stuck with this tail and so what do we do with that? We live on the tail, this 5% to 10% tail.
— *(Hematologic oncologist at an academic cancer center)*[15]

Although most patients report wanting prognostic information from their oncologist, patients with advanced refractory disease may not ask about their prognosis, and oncologists often do not initiate the discussion. In one recent observational study of patients after their first oncologic visit for a hematologic malignancy,[16] only half of patients were told unambiguous prognostic estimates for mortality or cure.

Discussions of prognosis can be very painful for clinicians, who may experience feelings of guilt, failure, or sadness. Clinicians interested in improving their skills may refer to practical educational handbooks and articles that outline how to discuss these issues both with patients who want to know their prognosis and with those who do not or are ambivalent.[17] Online resources for communication in serious illness training include the Center to Advance Palliative Care (capc.org) and VitalTalk (vitaltalk.org).

Impact on Hope

The rigors of treatment regimens and the physical and emotional demands of the complex care required for patients with advanced disease tend to isolate patients and their families and focus all their hopes on disease remission. They may have forgotten how to hope for anything else. Physicians and the teams they work with can help patients with advanced hematologic diseases develop new kinds of hope by encouraging them to reintegrate into activities that were meaningful before their disease began and they rearranged their lives around treatment schedules. Paradoxically, discussion about limited prognosis can lessen fears of abandonment and strengthen the trust patients have in the oncology team.[12] As disease progresses, despite ongoing treatment, patients who have begun to reengage in non–treatment-related activities and who have developed a broader relationship with their physicians are more likely to understand that the physician is not abandoning them when he or she says that the goals of treatment should be comfort.

CAREGIVERS

People who are not caregivers don't understand the continuous burden of the role ... the stress feels as if I'm constantly holding my breath.
— *(Family member about caring for a loved one with advanced disease)*[2]

Families and other nonprofessional caregivers, who provide the vast majority of care for patients with advanced cancer, are stressed by the patient's disability and degree of suffering, the lack of coordination of care, and underlying family, work, or financial pressures.[18] As many as 32% of these caregivers either have a major psychiatric condition (panic disorder, major depression, posttraumatic stress disorder, or generalized anxiety disorder) or access mental health services after the patient's diagnosis.[2] Caregivers are likely to need the support of many members of the team therefore to continue in their difficult role.

RELIEF OF SUFFERING

Suffering includes physical, psychological, social, and spiritual or existential dimensions.

Symptom Management in Children

Therapist: If you could choose one word to describe the time since your diagnosis, what would it be?
— *Child: PAIN.*[7]

Maintaining patient comfort is a critical issue throughout treatment, as well as during the end stages of life. Although effective pain control is a hallmark of palliative care, pain is only one of many distressing symptoms. The spectrum of physical symptoms includes (although it is not limited to) dyspnea, fatigue, seizures, loss of appetite, nausea and vomiting, constipation, and diarrhea. Early studies among bereaved parents or children who died of cancer indicate that optimal symptom management is still far from being achieved, even in major pediatric teaching centers,[19] and in one study more than 10% of parents had considered hastening their child's death; this was more likely if the child was in pain.[20] A recent study among children with advanced cancer confirmed high suffering from physical and psychosocial symptoms according to the children themselves.[21] Relief of a child's end-of-life distress may have long-lasting implications for bereaved parents, who are negatively affected by the child's experience of pain years beyond the death.

Psychologic symptoms such as depression and anxiety are also prevalent in children at the end of life.[19] Children also experience existential concerns. Creating opportunity for communication around these sources of distress involves using creative strategies that incorporate the developmental stage of the child. Strategies may involve verbal communication using open-ended questions such as "What are you hoping for?" and "What are you worried about?"

However, many children communicate best through nonverbal means such as artwork and music. Children may be more willing to "talk things over" with puppets or stuffed animals rather than real people. Importantly, euphemistic expressions about death can be confusing or even frightening (for instance, equating death with sleep may result in the child's being afraid of going to bed) and should be avoided.

Needless to say, parents of children with hematologic malignancies also experience distressing symptoms such as anxiety, depression, and spiritual and psychosocial concerns. Recognition of these by the pediatric clinician may serve families well while the child is alive and during bereavement.

Symptom Management in Adults

Patients with hematologic malignancies experience a high physical and psychologic symptom burden, similar to patients with metastatic solid tumors, especially during periods of treatment, when hospitalized, or with advanced disease.[22] Pain and antiemetic therapy for adults is reviewed elsewhere in this volume (see Chapter 91). Anxiety, depression, delirium, and control of symptoms occurring in the last days of life are reviewed subsequently.

Among social sources of distress are financial concerns and, with increasing debility, loss of independence and sense of contribution and efficacy. Worries about burdening the family or that the family will fail them when they really need them may lead patients to request physician-assisted suicide. Social workers are the key team members who can help alleviate or at least ameliorate these sources of distress, and can help the caregivers cope.

Physicians should also explore religious and spiritual concerns, and understand what rituals will be important at the end of life. Spiritual and existential distress occur when individuals are unable to find sources of meaning, hope, love, peace, comfort, strength, and connection in life, or when there is dissonance between their beliefs and what is happening to them. Patients who use "positive" religious coping (e.g., prayer, feeling a sense of connectedness to a religious community, having a positive relationship with God) have been found to have better mental health status, growth in the spiritual dimension with stress, and a better overall quality of life. Patients who use "negative" religious coping (e.g., ascribe their illness to a punishing God or one who has abandoned them) have a poorer quality of life.[23] Clinicians should therefore include either a formal or informal spiritual assessment for all patients diagnosed with serious illness.

PSYCHOLOGIC CONCERNS

Clinicians must assess and attend to patients' and families' psychosocial distress, including developmental issues, meaning and impact of illness, coping style, impact on sense of self, relationships, stressors, spiritual resources, economic circumstances, and physician–patient relationship; they must be able to distinguish normal human reactions of grief, sadness, despair, fear, anxiety, loss, and loneliness in patients facing the end of their lives, from clinical anxiety and depression.[24] Up to 50% (or more) of patients with advanced cancer meet criteria for a psychiatric disorder when the diagnosis of adjustment disorder is included.[25]

Anxiety and Depression

It is noteworthy that depression and anxiety are often not recognized as symptoms in children, and in many instances are inadequately addressed. Significant anxiety is found in approximately 25% of adult patients with cancer,[25] and anxiety symptoms can interfere with their ability to receive care. Patients with panic disorders, agitated depression, phobias, obsessive-compulsive disorder, delirium, posttraumatic stress disorder, or adjustment disorders can all present with anxiety. Anxiety in dying patients may arise from worries about the future (uncontrolled symptoms, family concerns, or concerns about death),

isolation from loved ones, sepsis, hypoxia, metabolic abnormalities, withdrawal from alcohol, opioids or benzodiazepines, drug reactions (e.g., akathisia from metoclopramide, phenothiazines, and butyrophenones; paradoxical agitation from benzodiazepines and olanzapine), and uncontrolled pain. Nonpharmacologic treatments, such as relaxation training, hypnosis, supportive psychotherapy, and counseling, are very effective. Pharmacologic treatments usually include benzodiazepines (e.g., the short-acting lorazepam, starting dose 0.5–2 mg every 8 hours as needed; or long-acting clonazepam, starting dose 0.25–0.5 mg orally (PO) two-times daily), selective serotonin reuptake inhibitors (SSRIs; see later), and, when there is evidence of delirium, neuroleptics (see later).

It is estimated that 5–26% of patients with advanced cancer meet criteria for a major depressive disorder, and patients with high symptom burden such as patients facing bone marrow transplantation are at higher risk.[25] It can be difficult to discern which patients with advanced disease are depressed or grieving. The usual somatic signs of depression or grief (e.g., anorexia, sleep disturbances, fatigue, or weight loss) are common in this population. Depressed patients, however, will be anhedonic and feel worthless, guilty, hopeless, or helpless. Grieving patients, in contrast, are very sad, but they are able to find happiness in some circumstances and can plan for the future.[25] Pain, a past or family history of substance abuse, depression, or bipolar illness are major risk factors for depression. Terminally ill patients responding "Yes" to the screening question "Are you depressed?" are very likely to be confirmed as depressed in a more comprehensive evaluation. Useful follow-up questions include "How do you see your future?" "What do you imagine is ahead for yourself with this illness?" "What aspects of your life do you feel most proud of? Most troubled by?"

As part of the treatment of depression, pain must be brought under control. Counseling can explore patient fears, provide emotional support, and help patients review their lives and find the meaning and areas of accomplishment in them. A variety of models of therapy are used, and none has been shown to be superior over the others. The psychostimulants dextroamphetamine and methylphenidate (2.5–5 mg, 8 AM and noon; maximum dose 60 mg daily) often act within a few days. The SSRIs are the first choice when immediate onset is not needed because they usually take several weeks to show effect. Useful agents include citalopram (Celexa) and paroxetine (Paxil; 10 mg PO daily initially; maximum 40 mg PO daily); escitalopram (Lexapro; 10 mg PO daily initially; maximum 20 mg PO daily); sertraline (Zoloft; 50 mg PO daily initially, maximum 200 mg PO daily); fluoxetine (5–10 mg PO daily initially; maximum 60 mg PO daily); and the serotonin–norepinephrine reuptake inhibitor venlafaxine (Effexor; 37.5 mg PO twice daily initially; maximum 225 mg PO daily). Venlafaxine inhibits norepinephrine, serotonin, and dopamine reuptake. Major side effects of the SSRIs include hyponatremia, sexual dysfunction or loss of libido, and gastrointestinal complaints (e.g., nausea, diarrhea, and foul-smelling flatus). Modafinil may also be an effective adjuvant agent to reduce SSRI-related sedation. The exact mechanism of action of mirtazapine (Remeron; 15 mg PO at bedtime initially; maximum 45 mg PO at bedtime) is unknown.

If the patient is expected to live longer than weeks to a few months, a stimulant and an SSRI should be started simultaneously, and the stimulant can be titrated off several weeks later. Tricyclic antidepressants are less useful in these patients because of their side-effect profile.

If the patient does not respond to first-line agents, a psychiatrist should be consulted. Referral to a psychiatrist is also necessary when the physician is unsure of the diagnosis; the patient is psychotic, confused, or delirious; the patient previously had a major psychiatric disorder; the patient is suicidal or requesting assisted suicide; or there are dysfunctional family dynamics.

Delirium

Delirium occurs in up to 80% of patients dying from advanced cancer and can cause distress and anxiety in caregivers.[12] Delirious patients can be agitated, hypoactive, or vacillate between the two. Symptoms of delirium include insomnia and daytime somnolence, nightmares, restlessness or agitation, irritability, distractibility, hypersensitivity to light and sound, anxiety, difficulty in concentrating or marshaling thoughts, fleeting illusions, hallucinations and delusions, emotional lability, attention deficits, and memory disturbances.

Validated delirium screening and severity tools are available, but a comprehensive psychiatric evaluation is recommended to exclude other disorders, such as anxiety, minor depression, anger, dementia, or psychosis. The cause of delirium is often never determined and is frequently multifactorial. Medications, especially opioids, nonsteroidal antiinflammatory drugs, and high-dose corticosteroids, commonly contribute. Opioid-induced central nervous system toxicities are more common in patients with renal dysfunction, on high doses of opioids for long periods of time, with impaired cognition before starting the opioids, with dehydration, or taking other psychoactive drugs. Other causes include metabolic abnormalities (hypercalcemia, hyperglycemia, or uremia), malnutrition, hypoxia, fever, infection, uncontrolled pain, hepatic failure, primary brain tumor, and brain metastases.

Treatment for delirium should begin while the underlying cause(s) are being treated. In addition to the medications listed in Table 92.3, it is helpful to make the patient's surroundings as familiar as possible, restore aids to hearing and sight if they are needed, reorient the patient frequently, and have family members, friends, or well-known caregivers present.

MANAGEMENT CONCERNS DURING THE LAST DAYS OF LIFE

Evidence suggests that children with advanced cancer who receive concurrent home-based palliative care have improved quality of life at the end of life and are more likely to die at home.[26] For some families, there is the possibility of planning ahead and choosing a setting for their child's death—home, hospice, or hospital. The child may express a preference about where he or she feels safe or prefers to be. Clear information about how the child is likely to die and professional support to validate the family's choice are crucial. Even more important is the explicitly stated "permission" from all members of the professional team that the family may change their choice freely at any time—that all options remain open and that no decision is irrevocable. In the past, siblings were rarely included in these discussions and were often inadequately prepared for the eventuality of a child dying at home. It is only recently that their voices are beginning to be heard.

The Dying Child

Therapist: Are you in any pain? Does anything hurt?
Child: My heart.
Therapist: Your heart?
Child: My heart is broken. I miss everybody.[7]

The distillation of anticipatory grief to its essence marks the imminence of death. At times imperceptibly, at other times dramatically, the child who has been living with the illness is transformed into a dying child.

The end point of the terminal phase is often marked by a turning inward on the part of the child, a pulling back from the external world. Cognitive and emotional horizons narrow, because all energy is needed simply for physical survival. A generalized irritability is not uncommon. The child may talk very little and may even retreat from physical contact. Although such withdrawal is not universal, a certain degree of quietness is almost always evident. The child is pulling into himself or herself, not away from others. This behavior is a normal and expectable precursor to death—a form of preparation for the ultimate separation that lies ahead.[7]

TABLE 92.3	Treatment of Delirium (Adult Patient)	
Drug	**Dose**	**Comment**
Typical and Atypical Antipsychotics		
Haloperidol	1–4 mg PO, or 0.5–2 mg SQ, IV qhs or bid to tid	Do not exceed 20 mg in 24 hours Can add the same dose q4h prn Maintain the patient on the effective dose (divided into a bid dose) for 3–4 days, then taper over 1 week, as tolerated Oral dose is 60–70% as potent as parenteral dose
Quetiapine	25–200 mg PO qhs	Particularly useful in elderly patients with evening delirium Start 25 mg hs for 3–4 days
Olanzapine	2.5–5 mg PO/SL	Start 2.5–5 mg PO/SL qhs to bid (2.5 mg for elderly patients); can use q 4–6 hours prn agitation Maintain the patient on the effective dose (divided into a bid dose), then taper over 2 weeks, as tolerated; also antiemetic
Aripiprazole	5 mg PO qd	Do not exceed 30 mg Does not prolong and may shorten QTc
Chlorpromazine	12.5–1000 mg PO/IV/PR	Sedating; may cause significant hypotension
Benzodiazepines[a]		
Lorazepam	0.5–1 mg q 1–2 hours	Add to antipsychotic for patients with an agitated delirium Tablets can be used PR for terminal delirium
Diazepam	5–10 pm PO bid	Useful PR for patients unable to take oral medication
Clonazepam	0.5–5 mg PO/SL bid to tid	Tablets have been used PR for terminal delirium; do not exceed 20 mg/24 hours
Midazolam	30–100 mg IV/SQ over 24 hours	IV drip or subcutaneous infusion for terminal delirium

[a]Caution: Any benzodiazepine may exacerbate delirium, especially in older adults (>70 years of age).

q, Every; hs, at bedtime; d, day; bid, twice a day; tid, three times a day; prn, as needed; IM, intramuscularly; IV, intravenously; PO, orally; SL, sublingual; PR, rectally; SL, sublingually; SQ, subcutaneously.

Modified from Abrahm JL: *A physician's guide to pain and symptom management in cancer patients*, ed 3, Baltimore, 2014, Johns Hopkins University Press; and Miovic M, Block S: Psychiatric disorders in advanced cancer. *Cancer* 110:1665, 2007.

TABLE 92.4	Treatment of Common Problems in the Final Days (Adult Patient)	
Problem	**Agent(s)**	**Routes, Doses**
Baseline pain	Concentrated oxycodone or morphine solution	PO/SL q4h around the clock; individualized
	Morphine or hydromorphone tablets	PR q4h; individualized
	Fentanyl[a]	Transdermal; individualized
	Methadone liquid	PO; individualized
	Acetaminophen, naproxen	PR tid to qid
	Dexamethasone (requires compounding)	PR daily to bid
Breakthrough pain	Concentrated oxycodone or morphine solution	PO or per gastric tube q4h around the clock; individualized
	Fentanyl[a]	Transmucosal (buccal, sublingual); individualized
"Death rattle"	Scopolamine	Transderm Scop patch 1–3q3 days; gel
	Hyoscyamine	0.125–0.25 SL tid to qid
	Glycopyrrolate	0.2–0.4 mg IV tid to qid or 1–2 mg po bid to tid
	Atropine	0.4 mg SL q4–6h
Dyspnea (anxiety)	Lorazepam	1 mg PO, SL, q2–4h
	Chlorpromazine	25 mg PO, PR q4–12h; or 12.5 mg IV q4–8h
Dyspnea (other)	Morphine/oxycodone	5–10 mg SL oral concentrate q2h
	Morphine	2–4 mg IV q1h
Nausea	Combinations of lorazepam, metoclopramide, dexamethasone, and/or haloperidol	PR q6h; compounded suppositories with desired agents (depending on presumed cause of nausea)
Anxiety	Lorazepam	1 mg PO, SL, q2–4h
	Diazepam suppository	5–10 mg PR daily

All liquid PO medications can be given per gastric tube.
[a]Fentanyl only for opioid tolerant patients.
h, Hour; IV, intravenously; PO, orally; PR, rectally; q, every; qid, four times a day; SL, sublingually; tid, three times a day.
Modified from Abrahm JL: *A physician's guide to pain and symptom management in cancer patients,* ed 3, Baltimore, 2014, Johns Hopkins University Press.

Adults

Common physical symptoms that occur in the last week to days before an adult's death from cancer include pain (70%), noisy or moist breathing (60%), urinary incontinence or retention, dyspnea, and nausea and vomiting.[12] Patients may also experience fatigue. Hunger and thirst are unusual. Treatments for problems at the end of life are reviewed in Table 92.4. Patient and family wishes and options about the setting for end-of-life care should be explored. Some evidence suggests that patients with cancer who die at home have better quality of life, and their caregivers have better bereavement outcomes than cancer patients who die in the hospital. However, given the potentially high symptom burden in the final moments of life, such as bleeding or dyspnea, more research is needed to understand barriers to hospice care and patient and family outcomes in hematologic malignancies.[27]

HOSPICE PROGRAMS

In the four weeks prior to his death, my father lived under the care of five different institutions in two states. Only the last place, the hospice, appeared willing or able to provide care and comfort to a man who was obviously at the end of his life.[2]
— (Bereaved family member)

In the United States, most hospice care takes place in the home, although patients can be admitted to nursing homes for brief periods (usually 5 days) to provide a respite for the family caregivers, or to the hospital (usually for up to 14 days) if symptoms cannot be controlled at home. Early referral to hospice programs improves outcomes, and in many cases hospice care is the only effective way to support these patients and families at home at the end of life. The Medicare Hospice Benefit does not require a do not resuscitate status, but it does require that the attending physician and the hospice medical director certify that the patient has a prognosis of 6 months or less to live if the disease follows its usual course. Medicare

reimburses hospice programs about $186 per day per patient (as of fiscal year 2013) to provide the routine care described in Table 92.5. Therefore, the cost of transfusions typically required for many patients with hematologic malignancies, even at the end of life, may make it difficult for hospice programs to enroll patients insured by Medicare alone. Other insurance programs may allow their patients to receive transfusions and hospice care. Notably, many children are not referred to hospice because their illness experience is inconsistent with hospice specifications—prognosis is uncertain; there is a blending of goals, which can result in more costly health care; and providers lack pediatric expertise. Importantly, the Patient Protection and Affordable Care Act now requires state Medicaid programs to allow children with a life-limiting illness to receive both hospice care and curative treatments concurrently; the full effect of this change remains to be seen.

BEREAVEMENT

Bereavement follow-up by the professional team is an intrinsic component of comprehensive pediatric palliative care. Bereaved families often express the sentiment of a double loss: loss of their child and loss of their oncology team whom they have known and trusted, often over months and years. Parental grief has been recognized as more intense and longer lasting than other types of grief. Contact from a team member after the child's death can assuage the family's sense of abandonment and the palliative care team can serve a crucial preventive role by identifying families at particular risk for prolonged grief disorders and identifying resources for them.

Each bereaved person's loss is unique, but many people manifest similar symptoms of grief, some of which become less persistent as they rebuild their lives. Recurrent intense symptoms typically occur at the anniversary of the death of the patient but can occur at unpredictable times, induced by reminders of the deceased. Survivors appreciate calls or letters from the patient's physician and nurses. For patients enrolled in hospice programs, a formal bereavement program is offered for the family throughout the first year after the patient's

TABLE 92.5	Specialty Level Palliative Care Versus Hospice Care	
Palliative Care	**Hospice Care**
Interdisciplinary Model of Care	***Interdisciplinary Program of Care***

• Clinical specialty, offers expert:
  • Symptom management and communication
  • Psychosocial and spiritual care
  • Inpatient, outpatient and home care consultations to the primary team
  • Coordination of care among treating teams
	• Medicare hospice benefit, delivers:
	  • Symptom management and communication
	  • Psychosocial and spiritual care
	  • Home, inpatient, or respite care in a nursing home under the direction of the patient's physician
	  • Continuity with referring care team

Eligibility	***Eligibility***
• Any patient with serious or life-threatening illness • Any stage the illness • Concurrent with curative or disease-directed therapies	• Estimated 6 months or less prognosis • Eligible for Medicare or secondary insurance • Focus is quality not life prolongation
Interdisciplinary Consult Team	***Interdisciplinary Care Team***
Palliative care physicians, advance practice nurses, physician assistants, nurses, social workers, chaplains, and bereavement counselors and others	Hospice medical director (physician), advance practice nurses, physician assistants, nurses, social workers, home health aides, chaplains, volunteers, administrative personnel, medical consultants, occupational therapists, physical therapists, speech therapists, and bereavement counselors.

death. After the formal program ends, the bereaved are welcome to continue to participate in any bereavement activities that have been meaningful to them.

At the time of death, survivors may seem numb, confused, or dazed and experience disbelief. By the second month after the death, yearning has replaced disbelief. During the next months, disbelief, depressed mood, and yearning decline gradually, and by 6 months after the death, most people will have accepted the reality of the death and are beginning to think about reengaging in relationships and work, discovering new meaning and purpose. Siblings are especially vulnerable in the year following a child's death.[28] By a year or two, most survivors have accommodated to their loss. They become aware of the changes that must be made if they are to resume old relationships and responsibilities, or to establish new ones and risk recurrent loss.

About 10–20% of survivors, however, suffer either from depression and/or from a symptom complex previously called *complicated grief*, now identified as *prolonged grief disorder*.[12] Patients with depression manifest symptoms of sadness, anhedonia, and psychomotor retardation, but they are not yearning for the deceased or unable to accept the death. Depressed survivors benefit from counseling and consideration of pharmacologic treatment. Patients with prolonged grief disorder, in contrast, have grief symptoms that last beyond 6 months and cause functional impairments. Such patients are at increased risk for medical and psychiatric illness and should be referred for psychiatric or spiritual counseling. Persons at higher risk for this disorder include those with a history of attachment disorders (childhood abuse, childhood separation anxiety), aversion to lifestyle changes, being unprepared for the death and unsupported after it, and a particularly interdependent relationship with the deceased.

SELF-CARE FOR CLINICIANS

Even while providing steady care for the patient and family, professional caregivers are often experiencing their own distress in a sort of parallel process. The professional often feels anguish and helplessness in witnessing a child endure pain and suffering—physical or psychic. He or she often identifies with the parents of the child. This reaction intensifies when the caregiver is also a parent, especially if his or her healthy child is the same age as the patient. For the caregiver who does not yet have children, the specter of a fatally ill child may loom threateningly. In surveys, medical and nursing staff often cite the personal pain of losing a child as the most difficult experience in their work with dying children. Special attention should be paid to the

grief experienced by trainees with little previous experience with death and dying. Interns are in special need of emotional support following a patient's death. Reviewing each death on the next morning's rounds provides the needed debriefing and shows respect for the patient who has died. When possible and it feels appropriate, clinicians can write a card or attend the funeral or memorial service, which may facilitate closure.

For all these reasons, the professionals who engage in this extraordinarily rich and demanding work articulate significant needs for support themselves. Otherwise, the toll of cumulative unresolved grief exacts a heavy toll in their personal and professional lives. A cohesive team and/or the opportunity for individual and group consultation are crucial for those who are intimately engaged in repeated cycles of attachment.

CONCLUSION AND FUTURE DIRECTIONS

Patients with hematologic malignancies and their families face unique challenges compared with patients with solid tumors. These challenges include: the need to undergo high-risk treatments with significant symptom burden and prolonged hospitalization to achieve cure; significant prognostic uncertainty; difficult decisions about the benefits and burdens of life-sustaining transfusions of blood products when the prognosis of the cancer is weeks to months; increased likelihood of receiving more aggressive care in the last month of life; and more deaths in the hospital.[5,22,27]

There is growing evidence that integration of palliative care into the care of patients with hematologic malignancies is achievable and can improve patient and family outcomes.[29] Appropriate triggers for members of the hematologic oncology team to request a palliative care consultation could include patients with high risk of refractory symptoms (e.g., severe graft-versus-host disease) or high mortality risk (e.g., relapse after bone marrow transplant, or hospitalized patients with end-stage disease). Research is needed to characterize and alleviate the symptom burden of patients with hematologic malignancy at all points in their illness trajectories,[30] and measure the effectiveness of specialty-level palliative care interventions to relieve patients' and families' suffering.[14]

REFERENCES

1. Institute of Medicine: *When children die: Improving palliative and end-of-life care for children and their families*, Washington, DC, 2003, National Academy Press.

2. IOM (Institute of Medicine): *Dying in America: Improving quality and honoring individual preferences near the end of life*, Washington, DC, 2014, The National Academies Press.

3. Quill TE, Abernethy AP: Generalist plus Specialist Palliative Care—Creating a More Sustainable Model. *N Engl J Med* 368:1173–1175, 2013.

4. Feudtner C, Womer J, Augustin R, et al: Pediatric Palliative Care Programs in Children's Hospitals: A Cross-Sectional National Survey. *Pediatrics* 132(6):1063–1070, 2013. doi: 10.1542/peds.2013-1286. published ahead of print November 4, 2013.

5. Hui D, Didwaniya N, Vidal M, et al: Quality of end-of-life care in patients with hematologic malignancies: a retrospective cohort study. *Cancer* 120(10):1572–1578, 2014.

6. Levy MH, Smith T, Alvarez-Perez A, et al: Palliative care, Version 1. 2014. Featured updates to the NCCN Guidelines. *J Natl Compr Canc Netw* 12(10):1379–1388, 2014. <http://www.nccn.org/professionals/physician_gls/f_guidelines.asp#palliative>.

7. Sourkes B: *Armfuls of time: The psychological experience of the child with a life-threatening illness*, Pittsburgh, 1995, University of Pittsburgh Press, p 11, 31, 114, 156, 167.

8. Waldman E, Wolfe J: Palliative care for children with cancer. *Nat Rev Clin Oncol* 10(2):100–107, 2013.

9. Ullrich C, Duncan J, Joselow M, et al: Pediatric palliative care. In Kliegman RM, Behrman RE, Stanton BF, et al, editors: *Nelson textbook of pediatrics*, ed 19, Philadelphia, 2011, Elsevier.

10. de Vos MA, Bos AP, Plötz FB, et al: Talking With Parents About End-of-Life Decisions for Their Children. *Pediatrics* 135(2):e465–e476, 2015.

11. Goldman RE, Sullivan A, Back AL, et al: Patients' reflections on communication in the second-opinion hematology-oncology consultation. *Patient Educ Couns* 76(1):44–50, 2009.

12. Abrahm, Janet L: *A Physician's Guide to Pain and Symptom Management in Cancer Patients*, ed 3, Baltimore, 2014, Johns Hopkins University Press.

13. Mack JW, Wolfe J, Grier HE, et al: Communication about prognosis between parents and physicians of children with cancer: Parent preferences and the impact of prognostic information. *J Clin Oncol* 24:5265, 2006.

14. LeBlanc TW: Palliative care and hematologic malignancies: old dog, new tricks? *J Oncol Pract* 10(6):e404–e407, 2014.

15. Odejide OO, Salas Coronado DY, Watts CD, et al: End-of-life care for blood cancers: a series of focus groups with hematologic oncologists. *J Oncol Pract* 10(6):e396–e403, 2014.

16. Alexande SC, Sullivan AM, Back AL, et al: Information giving and receiving in hematological malignancy consultations. *Psychooncology* 21:297, 2012.

17. Jackson VA, Jacobsen J, Greer JA, et al: The cultivation of prognostic awareness through the provision of early palliative care in the ambulatory setting: a communication guide. *J Palliat Med* 16(8):894–900, 2013.

18. Bona K, London WB, Guo D, et al: Prevalence and Impact of Financial Hardship among New England Pediatric Stem Cell Transplantation Families. *Biol Blood Marrow Transplant* 21(2):312–318, 2015.

19. Wolfe J, Grier H, Klar N, et al: Symptoms and suffering at the end of life in children with cancer. *N Engl J Med* 342:326, 2000.

20. Dussel V, Joffe SJ, Hilden JM, et al: Considerations about hastening death among parents of children who die of cancer. *Arch Pediatr Adolesc Med* 164:1, 2010.

21. Wolfe J, Orellana L, Ullrich C, et al: Symptoms and Distress in Children With Advanced Cancer: Prospective Patient-Reported Outcomes From the PediQUEST Study. *J Clin Oncol* 2015. pii: JCO.2014.59.1222. [Epub ahead of print] PubMed PMID 25918277.

22. Manitta V, Zordan R, Cole-Sinclair M, et al: The symptom burden of patients with hematological malignancy: a cross-sectional observational study. *J Pain Symptom Manage* 42(3):432–442, 2011.

23. Balboni TA, Paulk ME, Balboni MJ, et al: Provision of spiritual care to patients with advanced cancer: Associations with medical care and quality of life near death. *J Clin Oncol* 28:445, 2010.

24. Block SD: Psychological issues in end-of-life care. *J Palliat Med* 9:751, 2006.

25. Miovic M, Block S: Psychiatric disorders in advanced cancer. *Cancer* 110:1665, 2007.

26. Friedrichsdorf SJ, Postier A, Dreyfus J, et al: Improved quality of life at end of life related to home-based palliative care in children with cancer. *J Palliat Med* 18(2):143–150, 2015.

27. LeBlanc TW, Abernethy AP, Casarett DJ: What is different about patients with hematologic malignancies? A retrospective cohort study of cancer patients referred to a hospice research network. *J Pain Symptom Manage* 49(3):505–512, 2015.

28. Rosenberg AR, Postier A, Osenga K, et al: Long-term psychosocial outcomes among bereaved siblings of children with cancer. *J Pain Symptom Manage* 49(1):55–65, 2015.

29. Selvaggi KJ, Vick JB, Jessell SA, et al: Bridging the gap: a palliative care consultation service in a hematological malignancy-bone marrow transplant unit. *J Community Support Oncol* 12(2):50–55, 2014.

30. Cleeland CS, Williams LA: Symptom burden in hematologic malignancies. *Blood* 123(24):3686–3687, 2014.

LATE COMPLICATIONS OF HEMATOLOGIC DISEASES AND THEIR THERAPIES

Wendy Landier and Smita Bhatia

The past three decades have seen a marked improvement in survival for patients with hematologic malignancies. The 5-year survival is as follows: leukemia, 58%; Hodgkin lymphoma (HL), 87%; non-Hodgkin lymphoma (NHL), 71%; and multiple myeloma, 43%.[1] As a consequence, the population of long-term cancer survivors continues to grow. As of January 1, 2014, there were 316,210 leukemia survivors living in the United States, 197,850 HL survivors, and 569,820 NHL survivors.[2]

Attendant with this success is an increasing awareness of the occurrence of long-term morbidity and mortality associated with the very treatments responsible for the improvement in survival. The subject of long-term morbidity suffered by cancer survivors has been the topic of numerous reports.[3–12] These reports demonstrate that survivors are at risk for developing adverse outcomes, including premature death, subsequent neoplasms, organ dysfunction (e.g., cardiac, pulmonary, gonadal), reduced growth, decreased fertility, impaired intellectual function, difficulties obtaining employment and insurance, and overall reduced quality of life.

Hematopoietic cell transplantation (HCT) is the treatment of choice for patients with hematologic malignancies experiencing disease recurrence after conventional regimens and for those with disease characteristics associated with poor prognosis if treated with conventional chemotherapy and radiation regimens. Complications observed after HCT often have a multifactorial origin encompassing issues related to prior cancer therapy, intensity of the preparative regimen, graft-versus-host disease (GVHD), and other posttransplantation complications.[13–22]

This chapter summarizes select adverse outcomes among individuals treated for hematologic malignancies with conventional therapy alone or with HCT. Recommendations for providing ongoing follow-up care to this population of survivors are also reviewed.

CARDIOVASCULAR DISEASE

One of the more serious adverse events encountered in survivors of hematologic malignancies is the development of late-occurring cardiovascular events, which include coronary artery disease (CAD) (myocardial infarction, atherosclerotic heart disease, and angina pectoris) and cardiac disease (cardiomyopathy and congestive heart failure [CHF], valvular disease, conductive abnormalities, and constrictive pericarditis). These complications are more common than expected,[23,24] and often occur earlier than would be expected for the general population.[13,25,26]

Cardiac Disease

The anthracycline class of drugs is a well-known cause of late-onset cardiomyopathy. Anthracyclines are directly toxic to the myocardium through a variety of mechanisms, including free radical-mediated oxidative damage and induction of cellular apoptosis. Compared with the general population, survivors of childhood cancer are at a 15-fold increased risk of developing CHF[6] and at a sevenfold increased risk of premature death due to cardiac causes.[27] There is a strong dose-dependent relationship between anthracycline exposure and risk of CHF. Among childhood cancer survivors, the incidence of CHF is less than 5% with cumulative anthracycline exposure of less than 250 mg/m^2, approaches 10% at doses between 250 mg/m^2 and 600 mg/m^2, and exceeds 30% for doses higher than 600 mg/m^2.[28–30] However, cumulative anthracycline exposure as low as 101–150 mg/m^2 may be associated with a 3.9-fold increased risk for cardiomyopathy when compared with those unexposed to anthracyclines.[31]

Among survivors of adult-onset cancer, the incidence of CHF has been estimated at 7.5% to 26% with a dosage of 550 mg/m^2.[32] However, this cumulative anthracycline exposure has considerably higher dosages than the 300 mg/m^2 typically used for patients treated with six cycles of doxorubicin (Adriamycin), bleomycin, vinblastine, and dacarbazine (ABVD) or rituximab, cyclophosphamide, doxorubicin, vincristine, and prednisone (R-CHOP); the cardiac effects of moderate-dose doxorubicin, given as part of ABVD or R-CHOP to young adults, are less clear. Small case series either show no cardiac toxicity[33,34] or significant deterioration in several echocardiographic measures of ventricular function with 6 months of exposure.[35] In addition, 5-year cumulative risks of significant cardiac events and CHF were 19% and 10%, respectively.[36] Among survivors older than 65 years of age, the risk of late-onset CHF was 29% higher among those exposed to doxorubicin, compared with those not treated with doxorubicin, and an increase in the number of cycles of doxorubicin-containing chemotherapy was significantly associated with increasing risk of CHF.[37] In a clinical trial designed to evaluate cardiac toxicity after R-CHOP for diffuse large B-cell lymphoma (DLBCL) (median age at treatment: 68 years), 6% of the patients developed CHF after six to eight cycles.[38]

Among HCT recipients, the risk of CHF is highest after autologous HCT, approaching 10% at 15 years after HCT.[24] Autologous HCT survivors are at a nearly fivefold risk of CHF when compared with age-matched and sex-matched individuals from the general population. Outcome after post-HCT CHF is poor, with less than 50% of patients surviving 5 years after a diagnosis of CHF.[39] The risk of late-occurring CHF is primarily due to pre-HCT exposure to anthracyclines.[24,39] A recent study found that a doxorubicin dose ≥300 mg/m^2 and a cardiac radiation therapy (RT) dose greater than 30 Gy were independent risk factors for left ventricular systolic dysfunction.[40]

Modifying Factors for Cardiac Disease

Young age at exposure is a significant modifier of anthracycline-related cardiotoxicity.[41,42] Females treated in childhood are at greater risk of developing doxorubicin-induced ventricular dysfunction than are males.[28] The combined use of doxorubicin and chest radiation has been associated with a greater risk of late cardiac toxicity than either treatment given alone. For men treated for HL at age 40 years, the estimated 15-year rate of cardiac-related hospitalization was 9.8% (standardized incidence ratio [SIR]: 1.92) following mantle RT (median dose: 35 Gy) and 16.5% following combined doxorubicin with mediastinal RT (SIR: 2.80).[33,34] Another study found that the addition of anthracyclines to mediastinal RT significantly increased the risk of CHF (relative risk [RR]: 2.81) vs mediastinal RT alone.[33]

The presence of one or more conventional cardiac risk factors (diabetes, dyslipidemia, smoking, and hypertension) has a significant effect on the incidence of heart disease among both HL survivors and older patients with DLBCL.[33,37] The risk of post-HCT anthracycline-related cardiotoxicity also increases significantly among individuals with one or more conventional cardiac risk factors.[23,24,43,44]

Arterial Disease

Radiation to the chest produces late-onset intimal thickening of the coronary arteries and microvascular damage that causes reduced myocardial perfusion. Several cohort studies have shown that patients who received mediastinal irradiation for HL had an increased risk of CAD compared with the respective general populations.[45–51] The risk of radiation-related CAD is generally higher among men and among younger patients. A large, retrospective cohort study reported the risk of deaths related to myocardial infarction to be 2.5-fold higher among HL patients when compared with an age-matched and sex-matched general population. While the RR declined with increasing age of the HL cohort, the absolute excess risks of death from myocardial infarction increased with older age up to age 65 years at first treatment. The statistically significantly increased risk of myocardial infarction mortality persisted through to 25 years after first treatment. Risks were increased statistically significantly for patients treated with supradiaphragmatic radiation, anthracyclines, or vincristine. Patients treated with the doxorubicin, bleomycin, vinblastine, and dacarbazine regimen were at a 9.5-fold increased risk of mortality due to myocardial infarction. Among those exposed to supradiaphragmatic radiation and vincristine and followed for 20 or more years after first treatment, the risk was 14.8-fold that of the general population.[52]

Arterial disease in the transplant setting is related to an accelerated atherosclerosis, attributed to pre-HCT and conditioning-related radiotherapy, and is compounded by the development of cardiovascular risk factors (hypertension, diabetes, and dyslipidemia) in the early post-HCT period.[43,53] The cumulative incidence of arterial events such as clinically overt CAD or stroke among allogeneic HCT recipients is 10% at 15 years and the risk exceeds 20% at 20 years.[25,26] In this population, the median age at first myocardial infarction is as low as 53 years (range: 35–66 years),[44,54] which is earlier than would be expected for the general population (67 years)[55] or that reported for survivors of autologous HCT (61 years).[44,54]

Cardiovascular Risk Factors

The risk of developing cardiovascular risk factors such as hypertension, diabetes, and dyslipidemia is especially high in allogeneic HCT recipients when compared with autologous HCT recipients, as well as age-matched and sex-matched individuals in the general population.[44,56] The 10-year cumulative incidence of hypertension, diabetes, and dyslipidemia in allogeneic HCT recipients was 37.7%, 18.1%, and 46.7%, respectively; the risk for multiple (>2) cardiovascular risk factors approached 40% (compared with 26% in survivors of autologous HCT).

Conditioning with total body irradiation (TBI) has been associated with an increased risk of dyslipidemia and diabetes in pediatric[57,58] and adult[56] survivors of HCT. Abdominal radiotherapy possibly contributes to insulin resistance and/or metabolic syndrome, suggesting a role for radiation-induced pancreatic or hepatic injury.[59,60] The increased risk of diabetes and dyslipidemia among HCT survivors with prior exposure to TBI could potentially be due to the combined effects of abdominal radiotherapy and post-HCT gonadal dysfunction.[61]

Prevention of Cardiotoxicity

Given the known cardiac complications of cancer therapy, prevention of cardiotoxicity is a focus of active investigation. There is strong evidence for dexrazoxane as a cardioprotectant. Dexrazoxane decreases oxygen free radicals through intracellular iron chelation.[62] In two metaanalyses, dexrazoxane was associated with 60% to 80% fewer clinical and subclinical cardiac events during and after anthracycline-based therapy.[63,64] Overall, toxicity and measures of tumor response were similar between patients exposed and unexposed to dexrazoxane.[63] Currently, the Food and Drug Administration approves dexrazoxane for women with metastatic breast cancer who have received 300 mg/m² of doxorubicin and who need additional anthracycline-based therapy. The American Society of Clinical Oncology also recommends considering dexrazoxane for adults with any history of cancer who have already received 300 mg/m² of doxorubicin-based therapy.[65]

Intermediate or surrogate endpoints in randomized clinical trials show that dexrazoxane reduces cardiotoxicity in children exposed to anthracyclines.[66,67] Among 206 children with acute lymphoblastic leukemia (ALL), those receiving dexrazoxane had fewer episodes of elevated cardiac troponin T (cTnT) concentrations after anthracycline treatment (21% vs. 50%, $p < .001$)[67] Longer term follow-up data demonstrate that various echocardiographic indices of left ventricular (LV) structure and function are worse in those not receiving dexrazoxane.[66] Girls benefit from dexrazoxane more than boys, particularly with respect to changes in the LV end-diastolic thickness-to-dimension ratio, a marker of pathologic LV remodeling. Dexrazoxane was also found to demonstrate cardioprotection in children treated with doxorubicin for T-cell ALL and lymphoma.[68] A recent report demonstrates no impact on late mortality among HL patients randomized to dexrazoxane.[69] However, comprehensive longer term follow-up is required to document that dexrazoxane does indeed have a cardioprotective effect while maintaining comparable event-free survival.[70,71]

Previous reports have suggested that doxorubicin-induced cardiotoxicity can be prevented by continuous infusion of the drug.[72–74] Lipshultz et al[75] compared cardiac outcomes in children with leukemia receiving bolus or continuous infusion doxorubicin and reported that continuous doxorubicin infusion over 48 hours did not offer a cardioprotective advantage over bolus infusion. Both regimens were associated with progressive subclinical cardiotoxicity. Several other studies have reported no statistically significant difference in echocardiographic characteristics of children with cancer 5–7 years after treatment with either continuous infusion (over 6–24 hours) or bolus infusion of anthracyclines.[76,77]

Liposome-encapsulated anthracyclines have been explored for their propensity to result in a lower incidence of cardiotoxicity. The premise behind this theory is as follows: liposome-encapsulated anthracyclines escape the capillaries with wide endothelial gaps in the tumor, thus reaching high concentrations in the interstitial fluid of the tumor bed, but are less likely to escape the tight capillary junctions of the heart. Biopsy results have confirmed the relative safety in clinical use.[78,79] Data on the potential cardioprotection associated with liposomal formulations of anthracyclines is limited. A phase I study of liposomal daunorubicin in 48 children reported no cardioprotection.[80]

Specific recommendations for monitoring, based on age and therapeutic exposure, are delineated within the Children's Oncology Group Long-Term Follow-Up Guidelines[81] (COG LTFU guidelines) available at http://www.survivorshipguidelines.org.[82] According to these guidelines, patients exposed to anthracyclines need ongoing monitoring for late-onset cardiomyopathy using serial noninvasive testing (echocardiogram) and physical examination. The frequency of echocardiograms can range from yearly to every 5 years, depending on cumulative anthracycline dose, age at exposure, and treatment with mediastinal radiation. Pregnant women previously treated with anthracyclines should be closely monitored, because changes in volume during the third trimester could add significant stress to a potentially compromised myocardium. In addition to monitoring for cardiomyopathy, survivors who received radiation involving the heart field also need monitoring for potential early-onset atherosclerosis. Heart-healthy lifestyles should be encouraged for all survivors, including implementation of a regular exercise program, dietary recommendations, and screening for dyslipidemia. Joint recommendations for monitoring long-term survivors of HCT by the European Group for Blood and Marrow Transplantation (EBMT)/Center for International Blood and Marrow Transplant Research CIBMTR)/ American Society for Blood and Marrow Transplantation (ASBMT) suggest that at a minimum, cholesterol and high-density lipoprotein-cholesterol (HDL-C) should be checked at least every 5 years for men starting by age 35 years and women starting at 45 years of age. It is suggested that screening for dyslipidemia should start at 20 years of age for smokers, patients with diabetes, or patients with a family history of heart disease. Abnormalities (total cholesterol >200 mg/dL or HDL-C <40 mg/dL) should be followed up with a full fasting lipoprotein profile.[83]

PULMONARY EFFECTS

Compromise of pulmonary function among survivors of hematologic malignancies has been reported after conventional therapy.[13,14,84–86] Impairments evident by pulmonary function testing include reductions in total lung capacity (TLC), forced vital capacity (FVC), forced expiratory volume in the first second of expiration (FEV$_1$), and gas transfer (diffusing capacity of lung for carbon monoxide [DLCO]), suggesting obstructive and restrictive defects. Risk factors include exposure to certain chemotherapeutic agents (particularly bleomycin), radiation to the chest, underlying lung disease, female sex, and a younger age at exposure to the pulmonary-toxic therapeutic agents. In a recent study, Armenian et al[87] demonstrated an elevated risk of pulmonary compromise among childhood cancer survivors when compared with healthy controls and identified populations at increased risk for pulmonary toxicity. Compared with healthy controls, childhood cancer survivors were 6.5-fold more likely to develop restrictive defects and 5.2-fold more likely to develop diffusion abnormalities. Among childhood cancer survivors, higher radiation dose (>20 Gy) and younger age at exposure (<16 years) was associated with restrictive disease. Female sex and higher chest radiation dose were associated with diffusion abnormalities. Importantly, over a period of 5 years, diffusion capacity declined among females and those exposed to high doses of chest radiation.

Pulmonary complications, both infectious and noninfectious, are common after HCT. Multiple factors are thought to contribute to pulmonary complications, including the type and duration of immunological defects produced by the underlying disease and treatment, the development of GVHD, and the conditioning regimens employed. These complications are classified as early or late, depending on whether they occur before or after 100 days from transplantation. Early noninfectious pulmonary complications typically include pulmonary edema, upper airway complications, diffuse alveolar hemorrhage, and pleural effusion. Bronchiolitis obliterans, venoocclusive disease, and secondary malignancies occur late after HCT. Idiopathic pneumonia syndrome, GVHD, and radiation-induced lung injury can occur in early or late periods after HCT (reviewed in Khurshid and Anderson).[88]

The following pulmonary function tests are noted to decline after HCT: FEV$_1$/FVC, forced mid-expiratory flow, TLC, DLCO, residual volume (RV), functional residual capacity, and RV/TLC. Older age at the time of allogeneic HCT is associated with lower FEV$_1$/FVC and DLCO, and higher RV/TLC. Bronchiolitis obliterans syndrome is a progressive, insidious lung disease occurring after allogeneic HCT and results in progressive circumferential fibrosis and ultimate cicatrization of the small terminal airways, manifesting as new fixed airflow obstruction (reviewed in Williams et al).[89] Bronchiolitis obliterans has been shown to have a strong correlation with chronic GVHD and has been reported in up to 6% of HCT recipients. Most patients present when the degree of airflow is severe, causing significant dyspnea on exertion and a persistent nonproductive cough. Lung biopsy findings demonstrating damage to the bronchiolar epithelium, obliteration of bronchiolar lumens, inflammation between the epithelium and the smooth muscle, and pulmonary fibrosis are characteristic. The National Institutes of Health definition of bronchiolitis

obliterans requires the following: (1) absence of active infection, (2) decreased FEV$_1$ (<75% of predicted value), (3) evidence of airway obstruction with a ratio of FEV$_1$ to FVC of less than 0.7, (4) elevated RV of air (>120% of predicted normal), or (5) an expiratory chest computed tomographic (CT) scan or lung biopsy results that reveals air trapping or bronchiectasis. Recommended therapy includes high-dose systemic steroids for a protracted course, with or without the addition of other immunosuppressants. Leukotriene inhibitors have emerged as a potential therapy because of the elevated levels of leukotrienes implicated in bronchiolitis obliterans.

The COG LTFU guidelines recommend monitoring for pulmonary dysfunction in childhood cancer survivors that includes assessment of symptoms such as chronic cough or dyspnea on annual follow-up. Risks of smoking and exposure to second-hand smoke should be discussed with all patients. The best approach to chronic pulmonary toxicity of anticancer therapy is preventive and includes respecting cumulative dosage restrictions of bleomycin and alkylators, limiting radiation dosage and port sizes, and avoidance of primary or second-hand smoke. Pulmonary function tests are recommended as a baseline upon entry into long-term follow-up for patients at risk, repeated as clinically indicated in symptomatic patients and in those with subclinical abnormalities identified on screening evaluation. Repeat evaluation should also be considered for at-risk patients before general anesthesia. Influenza and pneumococcal vaccines are encouraged in survivors at risk for pulmonary compromise.[82] Joint recommendations for monitoring long-term survivors of HCT by the EBMT/CIBMTR/ASBMT suggest: (1) routine clinical assessment at 6 months, 1 year, and annually thereafter, (2) institution of active smoking cessation programs, and (3) pulmonary function tests and focused radiologic assessment at 1 year after allogeneic HCT for patients with signs or symptoms of lung compromise or earlier as clinically indicated. Annual testing is recommended thereafter for patients with recognized defects or appropriate clinical circumstances. For autologous HCT recipients, pulmonary function testing should be performed for those with known deficits before HCT or with those exposed to radiation or other pulmonary toxic agents during or after transplantation. Chest radiographic studies are indicated based on symptoms or abnormal pulmonary function test results.[83]

ENDOCRINOLOGIC EFFECTS

Thyroid

Patients with hematologic malignancies treated with cranial, craniospinal, or mantle irradiation are at increased risk for thyroid complications. Among survivors of HL, and to a lesser extent leukemia, abnormalities of the thyroid gland, including hypothyroidism, hyperthyroidism, and thyroid neoplasms, have been reported to occur at rates significantly higher than those found in the general population.[73–75] Hypothyroidism is the most common nonmalignant late effect involving the thyroid gland.[90] After exposure to radiation at doses above 15 Gy, laboratory evidence of primary hypothyroidism is evident in 40% to 90% of patients with HL and NHL[91–93]; risk increases with radiation dose.[94]

In an analysis of 1791 5-year survivors of pediatric HL (median age at follow-up: 30 years), Sklar et al[95] reported the occurrence of at least one thyroid abnormality in 34% of subjects. The risk for hypothyroidism was increased 17-fold compared with sibling controls; increasing dose of radiation, older age at diagnosis of HL, and female sex were identified to be significant independent predictors of increased risk. The actuarial risk for hypothyroidism for subjects treated with 45 Gy or more was 50% at 20 years after diagnosis of HL. Hyperthyroidism was reported to occur in only 5%. In a seminal study of 1677 patients with HL treated at Stanford University Hospital between 1961 and 1989 with irradiation involving the thyroid (mean age at diagnosis: 28 years; mean duration of follow-up: 9.9 years), the actuarial risk for developing thyroid disease was 52% at 20 years and 67% at 26 years after treatment. In this population, the actuarial risk for developing overt or subclinical hypothyroidism was 44% by 25 years after therapy; the risk for developing thyroid cancer was 1.7% (15.6 times the expected risk).[91] Most cases of overt hypothyroidism after HCT result from primary hypothyroidism caused by radiation injury. The incidence of hypothyroidism after HCT depends on the type of myeloablative conditioning regimen, ranging from 10% to over 50% after fractionated TBI, to as high as 90% after exposure to single-dose TBI.[16,96]

Thyroid nodules are common in patients treated with neck radiation for HL, but the majority of these do not undergo malignant transformation.[97,98] In a study of 647 children treated for HL, 67 developed thyroid nodules during or after therapy (median time between diagnosis of HL and thyroid nodule was 10.5 years, with a range of 0.2–24.8 years). All but one of these patients had received neck radiation as part of their therapy, with a median dose to the thyroid of 35 Gy. Seven (10%) of the 67 nodules were malignant.[97]

Monitoring for survivors at risk for thyroid complications should include yearly thyroid examination as well as yearly measurement of free thyroxine and thyroid-stimulating hormone.[82]

Growth

Poor linear growth and short adult stature are common complications after successful treatment of hematologic malignancies in childhood. The adverse impact of central nervous system (CNS) irradiation on adult final height among childhood leukemia patients has been well documented, with final heights below the fifth percentile in 10% to 15% of survivors.[99–102] The effects of cranial irradiation appear to be related to age and sex, with females and children younger than 8 years at the time of therapy being more susceptible.[103,104] The precise mechanisms by which cranial irradiation induces short stature are not clear. Disturbances in growth hormone production have not been found to correlate well with observed growth patterns in these patients.[105,106] The phenomenon of early onset of puberty in girls receiving cranial irradiation may play some role in the reduction of final height.[107,108] In childhood leukemia survivors not treated with cranial irradiation, there are conflicting results regarding the impact of chemotherapy on final height.[100,109]

Impaired linear growth after HCT is likely due to an interaction of multiple factors, including host characteristics (young age), treatment exposures (prior cranial irradiation, TBI), and post-HCT complications, such as chronic GVHD.[96] Findings suggest that final height is unaffected in children who receive busulfan or cyclophosphamide as pretransplant conditioning.[110]

Survivors should be monitored using standardized growth curves until final height is achieved. An endocrine consultation should be obtained for children who received cranial radiation in doses ≥30 Gy and for those whose height is less than the third percentile, or who have poor growth for age or pubertal stage.[82,104]

Obesity

An increased prevalence of obesity has been reported among survivors of childhood ALL.[111–113] In an analysis from the Childhood Cancer Survivor Study, Oeffinger et al[114] compared the distribution of the body mass index (BMI) of 1765 adult survivors of childhood ALL with that of 2565 adult siblings of childhood cancer survivors. Survivors were significantly more likely to be overweight (BMI of 25 to <30) or obese (BMI ≥30). Risk factors for obesity were cranial irradiation, female sex, and age 0–4 years at diagnosis of leukemia. Females diagnosed under the age of 4 years who received a cranial radiation dose of more than 20 Gy were found to have a 3.8-fold increased risk for obesity. In a recent report of survivors of standard-risk childhood ALL treated without cranial radiation, there was no increased risk of overweight or obesity compared with general population health data.[115] Obesity has the potential to adversely impact the overall health status in survivors and is associated with insulin resistance, diabetes mellitus, hypertension, and dyslipidemia. The prevalence of growth hormone deficiency related to cranial radiation in

childhood ranges from 29% to 39%,[116] with increased risk at higher doses and longer time from treatment,[116] and may predispose adult survivors of childhood ALL, particularly females, to abdominal obesity[117] and metabolic syndrome.[118] Yearly monitoring of BMI is recommended for all survivors.

Gonadal Dysfunction

Treatment-related gonadal dysfunction has been well documented in male and female patients after therapy for hematologic malignancies and there is a reasonable body of research that provides a basis for counseling patients regarding the long-term gonadal effects of radiation and chemotherapy.

Radiation effects on the ovary are age and dose dependent. It has been estimated that there is a 50% depletion in oocytes after exposure of the ovaries to 2 Gy.[119] Amenorrhea develops in approximately 68% of prepubescent females treated for HL with ovarian doses of 12–15 Gy, whereas 100% of adult females older than 40 years of age will sustain irreversible ovarian failure after doses of 4–7 Gy.[120] Spinal irradiation for the treatment of childhood leukemia appears to result in clinically significant ovarian damage in some survivors,[121] and cranial irradiation in young girls is associated with an increased risk for premature puberty.[122]

The effects of radiation on testicular function, including germ cell number and Leydig cell function, have been investigated. Reduced sperm production has been observed after testicular doses of 1–6 Gy and follows a dose-dependent pattern.[123] Azoospermia has been reported among HL patients with calculated testicular irradiation exposures ranging from 1–3 Gy.[124] Testicular doses between 4–6 Gy have been associated with prolonged azoospermia and decreased testicular volume.[125] Spermatogenesis is impaired in 75% to 100% of male childhood HL survivors in whom radiation and chemotherapy were combined.[90] Leydig cells, although also affected by radiation in a dose-dependent fashion, require higher exposure levels to sustain damage than those seen for the germ cells.[126] Testicular doses of 24 Gy among prepubertal males have been reported to be associated with delayed pubertal development and abnormal testosterone and gonadotropin levels.[127–129]

Ovarian and testicular damage can also result from chemotherapeutic agents, with alkylating agents showing the strongest association. Effects of chemotherapy on gonadal function are typically sex, age, and dose dependent. While older studies have suggested that the ovaries tend to be less sensitive to the effects of alkylating agent exposure compared with the testes,[130] this may have been due to a lack of reliable markers for measuring ovarian function.[90] Ovarian dysfunction has been well documented in HL patients treated with alkylating agents, singly or in combination (e.g., MOPP regimen consisting of mechlorethamine, vincristine [Oncovin], procarbazine, and prednisolone, or a COPP regimen consisting of cyclophosphamide, vincristine [Oncovin], procarbazine, and prednisolone)[130–133] MOPP and COPP regimens have been reported to result in azoospermia in more than 90% of exposed males,[134] with a negative correlation seen between cumulative doses of alkylating agents and sperm concentration.[135] Even with a reduction in the dose of cyclophosphamide in the hybrid COPP/adriamycin, bleomycin, and vinblastine (ABV) regimen for HL, the majority of young males are infertile, likely due to the procarbazine component in this regimen.[136] In a study of 6224 male survivors of childhood cancer between 15 and 44 years of age, those with a diagnosis of hematologic malignancy were significantly less likely to sire a pregnancy compared with sibling controls; those with a diagnosis of HL were least likely to sire a pregnancy (RR of fertility: 0.34; 95% confidence interval [CI]: 0.28–0.41), followed by NHL (RR: 0.60; 95% CI: 0.48–0.74), and leukemia (RR: 0.70; 95% CI: 0.59–0.84); $p < .001$ for all comparisons.[137]

Young boys and adolescent males with aplastic anemia who receive standard-dose cyclophosphamide alone (200 mg/kg) as the pretransplant conditioning regimen appear to retain normal Leydig cell function, as do males who receive busulfan and cyclophosphamide, with normal plasma concentrations of luteinizing hormone and testosterone, and normal progression through puberty.[96] Evidence of germ cell damage can occur and is more likely among patients treated after puberty.[138] Semen analyses have been normal in approximately two-thirds of men after high-dose cyclophosphamide and several men have fathered normal children. Men treated with TBI-based regimens who have not received prior testicular irradiation generally retain normal Leydig cell function, regardless of their age at treatment.[138] Germ cell dysfunction occurs in all men treated with TBI-based regimens and azoospermia is the rule; however, some younger males (age <25 years at HCT) without chronic GVHD have showed some degree of spermatogenesis following standard-dose TBI.[139]

Female patients treated with high-dose cyclophosphamide alone retain normal ovarian function regardless of age at exposure, although these subjects may be at an increased risk for early menopause as they reach the third decade of life.[140] These individuals can sustain a normal pregnancy resulting in normal offspring. Females treated with busulfan and cyclophosphamide are at very high risk for ovarian failure and premature menopause.[141] The outcome of ovarian function after TBI appears to be determined by the age at exposure. Approximately 50% of prepubertal girls receiving fractionated TBI enter puberty spontaneously and premature ovarian failure is seen in all patients who are older than 10 years of age when treated with TBI.[96] Pregnancies among survivors of TBI are at an increased risk for spontaneous abortion, premature labor, and low-birthweight offspring.[142]

Assessment for gonadal dysfunction includes a thorough history and physical examination; additionally, a morning serum testosterone level in males and serum estradiol, follicle-stimulating hormone level, and luteinizing hormone level in females, should be obtained during early adolescence and as clinically indicated in patients with delayed or arrested puberty or who have symptoms of gonadal dysfunction. Semen analysis may be obtained in sexually mature males desiring to know their fertility status.[82,143,144]

PREGNANCY OUTCOMES

Offspring of survivors of childhood hematologic malignancies do not appear to be at increased risks for cancer or congenital malformations.[145,146] In a study of 593 adult survivors of childhood ALL, 15.7% (93 out of 593) of survivors (mean age: 22.6 years) had given birth to or fathered a total of 140 live-born offspring, compared with 29.8% (122 out of 409) of sibling controls (mean age: 25.2 years). There was no significant difference in the rate of birth defects between offspring of survivors (3.6% [5 out of 140]) versus sibling controls (3.5% [8 out of 228]; RR: 1.02; 95% CI: 0.34–3.05).[147] In a review of pregnancy outcomes of participants in the Childhood Cancer Survivor Study,[133] the offspring of survivors were more likely to be premature (born before 37 weeks' gestation) compared with the survivors' female siblings (odds ratio [OR]: 1.9; 95% CI: 1.4–2.4; $p < .001$); and the offspring of women who received uterine radiation at a dose of more than 5 Gy were more likely to be small for gestational age (OR: 4.0; 95% CI: 1.6–9.8; $p = .003$). The frequency of premature birth was not related to prior maternal exposure to alkylating agents, but prior exposure to doxorubicin or daunorubicin increased the risk for low birthweight independent of pelvic irradiation history.[133] There were no significantly increased rates of congenital anomalies[146] or genetic diseases[148] in the offspring of survivors who received potentially mutagenic therapy (i.e., radiation or alkylating agents).

MUSCULOSKELETAL EFFECTS

Osteonecrosis is a painful and debilitating condition that develops when the blood supply to the bone is disrupted, usually in areas of terminal circulation. The condition is believed to be the result of vascular compromise with resultant death of bone and cell tissues or disruption of bone-repair mechanisms.[149,150] Osteonecrosis has been reported after conventional therapy for hematologic malignancies,

particularly after exposure to dexamethasone between the ages of 10 and 20 years. This complication usually develops during or shortly after completion of therapy but may progress over time.[151–153] Mattano et al[151] described the magnitude of risk and associated risk factors for development of osteonecrosis in children with ALL treated on Children's Oncology Group therapeutic protocols. The cumulative incidence was 9.3% at 3 years; the incidence was higher in older patients (14.2% for patients ≥10 years of age vs. 0.9% for patients <10 years of age) and higher among whites than African Americans. Furthermore, the incidence was higher among patients randomized to receive two 21-day dexamethasone courses versus one course.

Osteonecrosis is increasingly being reported among HCT recipients.[154–157] Campbell et al[158] conducted a retrospective cohort study and described the cumulative incidence of osteonecrosis to be 2.9% among autologous HCT recipients, 5.4% among allogeneic HCT recipients, and 15% among unrelated donor HCT recipients. Among allogeneic HCT recipients, male sex, presence of chronic GVHD, and exposure to cyclosporine, tacrolimus, prednisone, and mycophenolate mofetil rendered patients at increased risk, in particular among patients with a history of exposure to three or more drugs. The mean latency period was 18 months. The hip joint was the most commonly involved joint (80%); however, the knee, wrist, and ankle joints were also affected. The cumulative incidence of surgery (mainly arthroplasty) approached 31% at 1 year from osteonecrosis diagnosis. Li et al[157] conducted a case-control study of children who underwent allogeneic HCT and found that children at highest risk included those who underwent transplant during the period of rapid pubertal growth and those who received myeloablative conditioning and immunosuppression for treatment of GVHD.

Osteopenia (bone density 1–2.5 standard deviations below mean) or osteoporosis (bone density >2.5 standard deviations below mean) is commonly seen in survivors of hematologic malignancies.[159–161] Risk factors include therapy with corticosteroids, methotrexate (at higher doses), and cranial irradiation with resultant pituitary insufficiency or gonadal dysfunction. Survivors of HCT are also at increased risk for reduced bone mineral density; identified risk factors in these patients include treatment with corticosteroids for chronic GVHD, prior cranial irradiation (resulting in growth hormone deficiency), and gonadal failure.[96] Lifestyle factors that increase the risk for osteopenia include lack of regular weight-bearing exercise, inadequate calcium and vitamin D intake, smoking, and excessive alcohol consumption.[162,163]

Detection and diagnosis of musculoskeletal sequelae depend largely on anticipating these issues in vulnerable hosts, on taking a careful history, and on performing a thorough physical examination. Pain or a history of fractures may be the only indication of osteonecrosis or osteoporosis. Because of progress with various interventions (including the use of calcium supplementation, calcitonin, bisphosphonates, and hormone replacement in patients with gonadal failure), the COG LTFU guidelines recommend a baseline dual-energy x-ray absorptiometry or quantitative CT scan for survivors a minimum of 2 years following completion of treatment, with repeat studies as clinically indicated.[82] Joint recommendations for monitoring long-term survivors of HCT by the EBMT/CIBMTR/ASBMT suggest a screening dual-photon densitometry performed at 1 year after transplantation in adult women or for any patient who has received prolonged treatment with corticosteroids or calcineurin inhibitors.[83] Screening for osteonecrosis is not recommended[82,83]; however, clinicians should maintain a high level of suspicion for patients with exposure to irradiation or prolonged corticosteroids.

NEUROCOGNITIVE EFFECTS

Childhood cancer survivors are at increased risk for neurocognitive impairment. Cranial radiation has long been associated with neurocognitive late effects,[164–166] typically a dose of 24 Gy is associated with cognitive deficits,[167] although antimetabolite chemotherapy and corticosteroids have also been implicated as potential contributors to neurocognitive impairment.[168–171] Additional risk factors include increased treatment intensity, younger age at treatment exposure, and female sex.[169,172–176] Neurocognitive deficits usually become evident within 1–2 years following cranial radiation and are progressive in nature. The decline over time is typically reflective of the child's failure to acquire new abilities or information at a rate similar to peers, rather than because of a progressive loss of skills and knowledge. Survivors of childhood ALL are at risk for neurocognitive problems, generally characterized by reduced attention, processing speed, executive function, and global intellectual function.[174] Affected children with information-processing deficits exhibit academic difficulties and are prone to problems with receptive and expressive language, attention span, and visual and perceptual motor skills. The deficits observed after chemotherapy alone are restricted to attention, executive function, and complex fine-motor functioning; global intellectual function is relatively preserved. Neurocognitive function in long-term survivors of childhood cancer appears particularly vulnerable to the effects of fatigue and sleep disruption.[177] The neurocognitive impairment observed in survivors of childhood ALL persists into adulthood; this impairment is associated with reduced educational attainment and unemployment,[178] independent living, and health care use.[179]

A spectrum of neuropathological syndromes related to leukoencephalopathy[180] may occur in survivors of childhood hematologic malignancies, including radionecrosis, necrotizing leukoencephalopathy, mineralizing microangiopathy and dystrophic calcification, cerebellar sclerosis, and spinal cord dysfunction, manifesting clinically as ataxia, spasticity, dysarthria, hemiparesis, or seizures. Imaging abnormalities may or may not be evident in these patients. Leukoencephalopathy has been primarily associated with methotrexate-induced injury of white matter. However, cranial irradiation may play an additive role through disruption of the blood–brain barrier, allowing greater exposure of the brain to systemic therapy. Although some abnormalities have been detected by diagnostic imaging studies, the abnormalities observed have not been well demonstrated to correlate with clinical findings and neurocognitive status. In a recent study, brain grey and white matter volume and diffusion tensor imaging was compared between survivors treated with and without radiation and healthy controls. ALL survivors had a lower ratio of white matter to intracranial volume in frontal and temporal lobes compared with control subjects. ALL survivors treated with chemotherapy alone performed worse in processing speed, verbal selective reminding, and academics compared with population norms but performed better than survivors treated with cranial RT on verbal selective reminding, processing speed, and memory span. There were significant associations between neurocognitive performance and brain imaging, particularly for frontal and temporal white and grey matter volume. ALL survivors treated with chemotherapy alone demonstrated significant long-term differences in neurocognitive function and altered neuroanatomical integrity.[181]

Long-term survivors of childhood HL may also be at risk for neurocognitive impairment. This is associated with radiologic indices suggestive of reduced brain integrity and occurs in the presence of symptoms of cardiopulmonary dysfunction.[182]

Many survivors of adult-onset hematologic malignancies also experience impairments of neurocognitive function, including memory loss, distractibility, and difficulty performing multiple tasks. These patients may also concurrently suffer from mood disturbances and symptoms that compromise their ability to function adequately, including fatigue and pain.[183]

HCT survivors are also at risk for neurocognitive late effects. Prospective, longitudinal evaluations of intellectual and adaptive functioning of children receiving a transplant have revealed declines in intellectual function, particularly among those less than 6 years of age at transplantation.[184] Among the adult populations, a prospective longitudinal study design was used to describe neurocognitive function over 5 years after allogeneic HCT for cancer survivors and compared with matched controls.[185] Survivors recovered significant cognitive function from posttransplantation (80 days) to 5 years in all tests except verbal recall. Between 1 and 5 years, verbal fluency improved, as did executive function, but motor dexterity did not, remaining significantly below population norms. Over 40% of the survivors had mild or greater deficits, a proportion that was significantly higher than that among the controls (17.5%). Neurocognitive sequelae among adults undergoing HCT include slowed reaction time, reduced attention and concentration, and difficulties in reasoning and problem solving, memory impairment, problems with executive functioning and processing speed, and cognitive impairment.[186–189] Reduced memory function is associated with older age, longer interval since HCT, chronic GVHD, and long-term cyclosporine use.[190] Other predictors include fatigue and poor physical functioning. Lower education level and poorer social functioning appear to impact cognitive performance. It is therefore prudent to query post-HCT patients regarding perceived deficits in neuropsychological functioning and to refer patients with these problems to a neuropsychologist who is experienced in the follow-up care of HCT patients.

The COG LTFU guidelines recommend a baseline neuropsychological evaluation for patients who received therapy that may affect neurocognitive function. This should be repeated as clinically indicated and at key transition points (e.g., transitioning from grade school to middle/high school); an annual assessment of their vocational or educational progress should also be monitored.[82] Joint recommendations for monitoring long-term survivors of HCT by the EBMT/CIBMTR/ASBMT suggest that all recipients of HCT should undergo clinical evaluation for symptoms or signs of neurologic dysfunction at 1 year after HCT. Additional tests such as neuropsychologic testing may be warranted for those with symptoms or signs.[83]

OTHER TOXICITIES

Ocular Effects

Survivors of hematologic malignancies are at risk for the development of cataracts as a consequence of therapy with corticosteroids, cranial irradiation,[191,192] TBI,[193] or busulfan.[194] In a cohort of childhood ALL survivors who were treated with chemotherapy with or without cranial radiation and received a mean cumulative prednisone equivalent dose of 5.2 gm/m^2, cumulative incidence of cataracts was 26 ± 8.1% at 25 years; cranial radiation was the only significant risk factor.[195] Belkacemi et al[196] studied 1063 patients who underwent HCT for acute leukemia; the overall 10-year incidence of cataracts in this group of patients was 50%. Single-dose TBI was associated with a 60% incidence of cataracts, fractionated TBI was associated with a 43% incidence for those receiving six or fewer fractions, and a 7% incidence was reported for those receiving more than six fractions. Factors independently associated with an increased risk for cataract formation in this cohort were older age (>23 years), allogeneic bone marrow transplantation, higher dose rate (>0.04 Gy/min), and steroid administration for longer than 100 days. Xerophthalmia may also occur as a late complication because of decreased lacrimation resulting from damage to the lacrimal gland during radiation or, in HCT patients, from chronic GVHD.[197] Westeneng et al[198] followed 101 adults up to 24 months after allogeneic HCT and reported ocular GVHD in 54% of patients, manifesting mainly as xerophthalmia and conjunctivitis; blepharitis and uveitis were encountered less often. Tabbara et al[199] reported major ocular complications in 13% of 620 patients (age range: 9–65 years) after allogeneic HCT; complications included chronic ocular GVHD, corneal ulcers, cataracts, glaucoma, cytomegalovirus retinitis, fungal endophthalmitis, and the acquisition of allergic conjunctivitis from atopic donors.

Audiologic Effects

Survivors of hematologic malignancies who received platinum chemotherapy, those who had cranial irradiation at a young age (especially during infancy),[200] and those who required supportive therapy with aminoglycoside antibiotics[201] are at risk for therapy-related hearing loss. Hearing loss associated with ototoxic agents is generally sensorineural in origin and is usually irreversible. Although a low incidence of hearing loss has been reported in survivors of HCT performed in childhood, the risk is elevated threefold to fourfold over that in the general population.[193] Data are beginning to emerge regarding genetic polymorphisms associated with increased susceptibility to platinum-related hearing loss; these data may prove useful in identifying future patients who are at increased risk for hearing loss as a consequence of platinum-based chemotherapy.[202]

Dental Effects

Children whose teeth have not completely developed at the time of cancer treatment are most vulnerable to dental complications and treatment with chemotherapy during early childhood may result in qualitative problems with enamel and root development.[203] However, patients of all ages who received RT involving the head or neck (including cranial irradiation and TBI) are susceptible to dental complications, most often manifesting as increased susceptibility to dental caries and gingivitis as a result of diminished salivary gland function. Patients who have undergone HCT are at increased risks for dental caries, gum disease, and xerostomia[204]; abnormalities of tooth development are seen in survivors who underwent HCT during childhood.[205] Younger age at transplantation (especially under 6 years) and TBI doses above 10 Gy are associated with the greatest risk.[205]

Hepatic Effects

Although acute hepatic dysfunction may be seen with certain chemotherapeutic agents, including antimetabolites and anthracyclines, there has generally been a low reported incidence of delayed hepatotoxicity in patients receiving these agents.[206] However, reports of chronic hepatotoxicity and portal hypertension have emerged in survivors of childhood ALL who received 6-thioguanine–based maintenance therapy,[207–210] and these survivors require long-term surveillance for this complication.[82,211] Chronic viral hepatitis, resulting from transfusion of contaminated blood or serum products, should be considered in the differential diagnosis of all survivors with persistently elevated alanine aminotransferase levels. Hepatitis C is the most prevalent type of hepatitis seen in survivors transfused before universal screening of the blood supply for this infection (implemented in the United States in July 1992).[212,213] Cirrhosis and hepatocellular carcinoma are potential sequelae of untreated chronic viral hepatitis and potential causes of morbidity and mortality in this population. In addition, iron overload associated with HCT for hematopoietic malignancies may also be a contributing factor to hepatotoxicity in survivors.[214,215]

Second and Subsequent Malignancies

Second or subsequent malignancies are defined as histologically distinct cancers developing after the occurrence of a first cancer. Subsequent malignancies are conventionally categorized into two major types: therapy-related myelodysplastic syndrome/acute myeloid leukemia (t-MDS/AML) and solid tumors. The latency between diagnosis and treatment of the primary cancer and the development of t-MDS/AML is generally short, whereas nonhematopoietic malignancies or solid tumors seem to have a longer latency, and the risk continues to rise for three or more decades. A wide variety of factors influence the risk for subsequent malignancies.

Several large epidemiologic studies have attempted to determine the magnitude of the burden of subsequent malignancies after adult-onset primary cancer. For example, 470,000 cancer patients registered between 1953 and 1991 in Finland were followed for the development of a second cancer.[216] Overall, the cohort was not at an increased risk for developing a second cancer when compared with the risk for cancer in an age-matched and sex-matched healthy population. However, patients less than 50 years of age at the diagnosis of their primary cancer were at a 1.7-fold increased risk for developing a second cancer. Another cohort of 633,964 cancer patients diagnosed between 1958 and 1996 in Sweden and followed for the development of subsequent cancers revealed a modestly increased risk (less than twofold), when compared with the general population.[217] The Swedish family-cancer database was used to analyze site-specific risk of second primary malignancies following 53,159 hematologic malignancies diagnosed between 1958 and 1996. Among 18,960 patients with NHL, there was a 1.2-fold significant increase in risk of subsequent malignancies. Among the 5353 patients with HL, there was a 1.7-fold significant increase in subsequent malignancies. Among the 8098 patients with ALL, there was a 1.3-fold increased risk of subsequent malignancies.[218]

However, when we examine the risk of subsequent neoplasms among childhood cancer survivors, a somewhat different picture emerges. The cumulative incidence of subsequent malignant neoplasms (SMNs) exceeds 20% at 30 years after diagnosis of the primary cancer.[219] The cumulative incidence is 9% for nonmelanoma skin cancer (NMSC) and 3% for meningioma. The cumulative incidence is 8% for SMNs excluding NMSC; this represents a sixfold increased risk of SMNs among cancer survivors compared with the general population. HL survivors demonstrate the highest risk of subsequent malignancies (8.7-fold compared with the general population). Treatment with RT and specific chemotherapeutic agents is associated with increased risk of subsequent malignancies; female sex, older age at diagnosis, and earlier treatment era modify that association. Breast cancer is the most common subsequent malignancy, followed by thyroid cancer.[219] Subsequent malignancies are the leading cause of nonrelapse late mortality.[220] The risk of subsequent malignancies remains elevated for more than 20 years from diagnosis of the primary cancer. Multiple subsequent neoplasms are common among aging survivors of childhood cancer. Cumulative incidence of a second subsequent malignancy was reported as 47% at 20 years after the first SMN. A first SMN of NMSC identifies a population at high risk for a subsequent invasive SMN.[221]

The magnitude of risk for subsequent malignant neoplasms after HCT ranges from fourfold to 11-fold that of the general population. Several host and clinical factors are associated with an increased risk for subsequent malignant neoplasms after HCT. These include age at HCT, pre-HCT exposure to chemotherapy and radiation, exposure to TBI as part of conditioning, infection with oncogenic viruses (Epstein-Barr virus and hepatitis B and C viruses), prolonged immunosuppression after HCT, autologous versus allogeneic HCT, and original cancer.

The cumulative incidence of solid tumors after allogeneic HCT ranges from 7% to 11% at 15 years posttransplantation.[222–225] The magnitude of risk of solid tumors exceeds twofold that of an age-matched and sex-matched general population; the risk reaches threefold among patients followed for 15 or more years after HCT. Solid tumors are unequivocally related to the RT used to treat the primary cancer, typically have a long latency, and the risk is high among those exposed to irradiation at a young age. Thus among patients exposed to radiation at an age less than 30 years, the risk is ninefold that of the general population, whereas for those older than 30 years it approaches that of the general population. Solid tumors commonly seen after HCT include melanoma, cancers of the oral cavity and salivary glands, brain, liver, cervix, thyroid, breast, bone, and connective tissue.

t-MDS/AML is the major cause of nonrelapse mortality in patients undergoing autologous HCT for patients with a primary diagnosis of HL or NHL.[226,227] The cumulative probability of t-MDS/AML ranges from 1.1% at 20 months to 24.3% at 43 months after autologous HCT, with a median latency of 12–24 months after HCT (range: 4 months to 6 years). Using the World Health Organization classification, two types of t-MDS/AML are recognized, related closely to the therapeutic exposure: alkylating agent/radiation and topoisomerase II inhibitor.[228] The alkylating agent-related t-MDS/AML typically develops 4–7 years after exposure. Cytopenias are common. Roughly 65% of the patients present with myelodysplasia; the remaining present with AML but carry myelodysplastic features.

Abnormalities involving chromosomes 5 (-5/del[5q]) and 7 (-7/del[7q]) are frequently seen. AML secondary to topoisomerase II inhibitors presents as overt leukemia, without a preceding myelodysplastic phase. The latency is brief, ranging from 6 months to 5 years, and is associated with balanced translocations involving chromosome bands 11q23 or 21q22.

Subsequent Malignancies Among Survivors of Acute Lymphoblastic Leukemia

Evaluation of large cohorts of patients with childhood ALL entered on Children's Oncology Group therapeutic trials have shown that the cumulative incidence of second and subsequent malignancies approaches 4% at 15 years from diagnosis of ALL.[229–231] CNS tumors, the most common subsequent malignancy observed among survivors of childhood ALL, are predominantly associated with exposure to cranial irradiation.[232] Histologically, radiation-related late-occurring neoplasms include high-grade gliomas (glioblastomas and malignant astrocytomas), peripheral neuroectodermal tumors, ependymomas and meningiomas, and basal cell carcinomas (BCCs).[229,230,233,234] Other commonly reported subsequent malignancies among ALL survivors include thyroid cancer and t-MDS/AML. Secondary thyroid malignancies are generally associated with radiation exposure to the thyroid gland as part of CNS irradiation, either prophylactic or for treatment of CNS leukemia. Thyroid malignancy has been reported to represent between 6% and 17% of secondary cancers among large cohorts of ALL survivors[229,230,232] and typically develops 10 or more years from treatment. The risk of t-MDS/AML after therapy for ALL is generally low, except among those patients treated with epipodophyllotoxin therapy, where a cumulative risk of 3.8% at 6 years has been reported.[235] Therapy-related AML associated with topoisomerase II inhibitors is characterized typically by a shorter latency period (3–5 years from therapeutic exposure) than that seen for t-MDS/AML after alkylating agents, lack of a myelodysplastic phase, and the presence of 11q23 rearrangements with mutations in the mixed-lineage leukemia (*MLL*) gene. Epipodophyllotoxin-associated secondary AML depends more on the schedule of drug administration than total cumulative dose.[236]

Subsequent Malignancies Among Survivors of Hodgkin Lymphoma

Survivors of HL demonstrate the highest risk for subsequent malignancies. This is particularly true for patients treated in the earlier eras with predominantly radiation-based therapies; these patients are at 10-fold increased risk when compared with the general population.[237] A number of studies, with cohorts ranging from 499 to 5925 HL patients, have reported the cumulative incidence of second malignancies to range from 7.6% at 20 years to 18.0% at 30 years.[232,238–242] The sex difference in a 30-year cumulative incidence of any SMN of 10.9% among males and 26.1% in females (*p* < .001) is driven by the incidence of invasive breast cancer.[242]

Early studies of HL identified the increased risk for t-MDS/AML among patients treated with MOPP-based therapy, which included mechlorethamine and cyclophosphamide.[243,244] These alkylating agent-associated t-MDS/AMLs are characterized by a relatively short latency period, presence of chromosomal abnormalities involving chromosomes 5 and/or 7, and are often preceded by a phase of myelodysplasia. The risk for t-MDS/AML usually does not extend beyond the first 10–15 years after therapeutic exposure. Extended follow-up studies of early cohorts have already reported excess risks for lung and gastrointestinal cancers.[237,245–248] More recent studies, with longer follow-up of cohorts, demonstrate that the most frequently observed solid second malignancies include breast cancer, thyroid cancer, and bone/soft tissue sarcomas.[237,248–250] Compared with the general US population, SIRs are highest for bone cancer 22.3 (95% CI: 10.0–49.6), thyroid cancer 17.6, and breast cancer 17.0 per 10,000 person-years, respectively. Cumulative incidence of

invasive breast SMN at 30 years after diagnosis is 18.3%, with no apparent plateau in incidence within the cohort at this time.[242]

With extended follow-up of cohorts of young HL survivors, increased risks for common adult carcinomas, including colorectal, lung, and stomach, have emerged, and these cancers are being diagnosed at younger ages than observed in the general population.[237] In a large population-based study of solid tumor risk among 18,862 5-year survivors reported to 13 registries, breast, lung, and gastrointestinal cancers accounted for almost two-thirds of the estimated excess number of cases.[251]

Subsequent Breast Cancer

Breast cancer is the most common solid SMN after HL, largely due to chest radiation for treatment of HL. The risk of radiation-related breast cancer among female HL survivors ranges from 25-fold to 55-fold that of the general population.* For female HL patients treated with chest radiation at less than 16 years of age, the cumulative incidence of breast cancer approaches 20% by age 45 years.[237,242]

The latency after chest radiation ranges from 7 to 10 years, and the risk of breast cancer increases in a linear fashion with radiation dose, with an estimated RR of 6.4 at a dose of 20 Gy and 11.8 at a dose of 40 Gy.[242,258] Moreover, 40% of identified cases were found to have developed contralateral disease. Among women treated for childhood cancer with chest RT, those treated with whole-lung irradiation have a greater risk of breast cancer than previously recognized, demonstrating the importance of radiation volume.[259] There appears to be a protective effect of early menopause either because of alkylating agents or radiation dose above 5 Gy to the ovaries, suggesting that ovarian hormones play an important role in promoting tumorigenesis once an initiating event has been produced by radiation.[257,258,260] The 25-year cumulative incidence of breast cancer is reported to be 11% after allogeneic HCT.[261] Allogeneic HCT survivors are at a 2.2-fold increased risk for developing breast cancer when compared with an age and sex-matched general population. The median latency from HCT to diagnosis of breast cancer is 12.5 years. The incidence is higher among those exposed to TBI (17%) than among those who did not receive TBI (3%). The risk is increased among those exposed to TBI at a younger age. The substantially increased RRs of breast cancer observed at 10–20 years postdiagnosis are not sustained into ages at which the risk of breast cancer in the general population becomes substantial; among women who survived to an age of at least 50 years, there is currently no evidence of an increased risk of breast cancer compared with the general population.[262] Importantly, mortality associated with breast cancer after childhood cancer is substantial; breast cancer–specific mortality at 5 and 10 years was 12% and 19%, respectively.[259]

Travis et al[263] developed estimates of cumulative absolute risk for use in counseling patients. For example, the cumulative absolute risks for an HL survivor who was treated at age 25 years with a chest radiation dose of 40 Gy or more without alkylating agents were estimated to be 1.4% after 10 years, 11% after 20 years, and 29% after 30 years.

Subsequent Thyroid Cancer

Thyroid cancer is observed after neck radiation for HL, ALL, and brain tumors, and after TBI for HCT.[219,232,264] The risk of thyroid cancer has been reported to be 18-fold that of the general population.[95] RT at a young age is the major risk factor for the development of thyroid cancer. A linear dose–response relationship between thyroid cancer and radiation is observed up to 20 Gy, with a decline in the OR at higher doses, demonstrating evidence for a cell kill effect.[265,266] Female sex, younger age at exposure, and longer time since exposure are significant modifiers of the radiation-related risk

---

*References 219, 232, 237, 238, 248, 249, 252–257.

of thyroid cancer.[267] Thyroid cancer develops after a latency of 8.5 years and is associated with an excellent outcome.

Subsequent Central Nervous System Tumors

Meningiomas and gliomas develop after cranial radiation for management of CNS disease among ALL or NHL patients. Gliomas occurred a median of 9 years from the original diagnosis; for meningiomas, the latency is 17 years. For gliomas, the excess RR per Gy was highest among children exposed at less than 5 years of age. The overall SIR was 8.7 for the gliomas, and the excess absolute risk was 1.9 per 1000 person-years.[219,230,232,268–272] The risk for second brain tumors demonstrates a linear relation with radiation dose; the dose–response appears weaker for gliomas than for meningiomas.[268,269,273] Possible effects of chemotherapy on the risk of second brain tumors have also been described by some.[269] Increased exposure to intrathecal methotrexate significantly increases risk of meningioma.[273]

Therapy-Related Myelodysplastic Syndrome/Acute Myeloid Leukemia

Several studies have described an increased risk for t-MDS/AML after autologous HCT, particularly for HL or NHL; pretransplantation therapy with alkylating agents, topoisomerase II inhibitors, and RT; use of peripheral blood hematopoietic cells; stem cell mobilization with etoposide; difficult stem cell harvests; conditioning with TBI; number of CD34+ cells infused; and a history of multiple transplants.[224,226] Thus t-MDS/AML after autologous HCT is the result of cumulative toxicity that includes pre-HCT chemotherapy (alkylators and topoisomerase II inhibitors), topoisomerase II inhibitors used for stem cell mobilization, and transplantation-related conditioning. The diagnosis of t-MDS/AML after autologous HCT confers a uniformly poor prognosis, with a median survival of 6 months in patients treated with conventional chemotherapy.

Subsequent Skin Cancer

Among allogeneic HCT recipients, the incidence of BCCs is 6.5% at 20 years, whereas the incidence for squamous cell carcinoma (SCC) is 3.4%.[274] TBI increases the risk for BCC, especially in younger patients. SCC risk is increased among patients with acute GVHD, whereas chronic GVHD is associated with both BCC and SCC.[275] Immunologic alterations predispose patients to SCC of the buccal cavity particularly, hence the association with chronic GVHD.[274] In patients with prolonged immunosuppression, oncogenic viruses such as human papillomavirus contribute to SCC of the skin and buccal mucosa.[274] BCC is one of the most frequent SMNs in childhood cancer survivors.[219,276] Childhood cancer survivors are at a fivefold increased risk of NMSC compared with the general population.[277] Ninety percent of patients have previously received RT; 90% of tumors occur within the radiation field. Radiation is associated with a sixfold increase in risk.[278]

Recommendations for Screening and Follow-Up

The elevated risk of breast cancer noted among survivors of childhood and adolescent cancers supports the importance of evidence-based screening guidelines for this high-risk group.[252] Because outcome after breast cancer is closely linked to stage at diagnosis, close surveillance resulting in early diagnosis should confer survival advantage. Mammography, the most widely accepted screening tool for breast cancer in the general population, may not be the ideal screening tool by itself for radiation-related breast cancers, occurring in relatively young women with dense breasts, hence the American Cancer Society recommends including adjunct screening with magnetic resonance imaging.[279] Thus the following are recommendations

for females who received radiation with potential impact to the breast (i.e., radiation doses of 20 Gy or higher to the mantle, mediastinal, whole lung, and axillary fields): monthly breast self-examination beginning at puberty; annual clinical breast examinations beginning at puberty until age 25 years; and a clinical breast examination every 6 months, with annual mammograms and magnetic resonance images beginning 8 years after radiation or at age 25 years (whichever occurs later). Females who received TBI or cumulative chest radiation doses of 10–19 Gy should be counseled regarding the benefits and risks/harms of screening; if a decision is made to screen, the same recommendations apply as for those women who received radiation doses of 20 Gy or higher.[82] Screening of those at risk for early-onset colorectal cancer (i.e., radiation doses of ≥30 Gy to the abdomen, pelvis, or spine) should include colonoscopy every 5 years beginning at age 35 years or 10 years following radiation (whichever occurs last).[82] Joint recommendations for monitoring long-term survivors of HCT by the EBMT/CIBMTR/ASBMT suggest that all recipients of HCT should be advised of the risks for subsequent malignancies and encouraged to perform screening self-examinations, such as breast and skin examinations. All patients should be advised to avoid high-risk behaviors, including avoidance of tobacco or excessive unprotected exposure of skin to ultraviolet light.[83]

Late Mortality

Childhood cancer survivors remain at risk for disease-associated and treatment-associated late mortality, and the excess mortality persists long after diagnosis.[220,280,281] Overall mortality among survivors has been described to be eightfold that of the general population. Recurrent disease is the most common cause of premature death. Increases in cause-specific mortality are seen for deaths due to SMNs, cardiac, and pulmonary causes. Extended follow-up of these cohorts demonstrates changing patterns of cancer-specific mortality with increasing time from diagnosis.[27,280] Thus excess risk for deaths from recurrence declines with time, while the excess risk for deaths from SMNs and cardiovascular causes increases; subsequent to 45 years from diagnosis, recurrence accounted for only 7% of the excess number of deaths while SMNs and cardiovascular causes accounted for 51% and 26% of the excess number of deaths respectively.[280] Childhood cancer survivors are at a 15-fold increased risk of SMN-related deaths, 8.8-fold increased risk of pulmonary deaths, and 7-fold increased risk of death due to cardiac causes when compared with the general population.[220] The high burden of morbidity carried by HCT recipients can result in premature death. Mortality rates are fourfold to ninefold higher than in the expected population for at least 30 years following HCT, producing an estimated lower life expectancy of 30% compared with the general population, regardless of current age.[282] Relapse of primary disease and chronic GVHD are the main causes of premature death. Nonrelapse-related mortality is greater among patients who are over 18 years of age when undergoing HCT, as well as among those with chronic GVHD. Compared with the general population, allogeneic HCT recipients are 3.6 times more likely to die of SMNs, 15.1 times more likely to die of pulmonary complications, and 2.3 times more likely to die of a cardiac compromise. However, the conditional survival probability at 10–20 years after allogeneic HCT exceeds 80% for those individuals who were alive and disease free 2–5 years after HCT.[283,284] On the other hand, autologous HCT recipients demonstrate a conditional 5-year survival that approaches 75% among those who have survived 2 or more years and approaches 90% among those who have survived 10 years after HCT. Among those who survive the first 10 years, nonrelapse-related mortality exceeds relapse-related mortality.[285] Primary disease and subsequent malignancies are the most common cause of death.[227]

Psychosocial Effects

Survivors of hematopoietic malignancies are at risk for adverse psychosocial outcomes that may affect their overall quality of life, including anxiety, depression, posttraumatic stress disorder, and barriers to accessing the healthcare system because of problems obtaining health insurance coverage. The impact of cancer therapy on psychosocial functioning is dependent on many variables, including intensity and duration of therapy, treatment-related complications, family functioning, developmental processes, and treatment-specific sequelae such as altered cognitive or physical functioning.[286]

Results from an analysis of 5736 long-term survivors of childhood leukemia and lymphoma demonstrated that although a relatively low proportion reported symptoms indicative of depression (4.6%) and somatic distress (10.8%), they were significantly more likely to report these symptoms when compared with sibling controls.[287] In a study of 6542 childhood cancer survivors (55% of whom were survivors of leukemia/lymphoma), the risk for posttraumatic stress disorder was increased by 4.6-fold, 4.1-fold, and 3.8-fold for survivors of HL, NHL, and leukemia respectively, compared with sibling controls; increased risk was associated with lower educational level (high school or less), lower income (<$20,000 annually), being unmarried, being unemployed, and having had more intensive treatment.[288] Long-term survivors of adult-onset HL report poorer health-related quality of life, primarily in physical health, when compared with a healthy general population.[289] Survivors of HL also appear to be at increased risk for psychosocial distress when compared with acute leukemia survivors; areas of greatest impact for these patients include impaired family and sexual functioning.[290] There is growing interest in the reported occurrences of fatigue and sleep disturbances among cancer survivors, particularly those with HL,[291-293] which may contribute to depression.

Fatigue, psychological distress, psychiatric symptoms, mood disturbances, and sexual difficulties are commonly reported by HCT survivors.[294] Risk factors for impaired health-related quality of life include older age, advanced disease at transplantation, presence of chronic GVHD, and lower level of education. Fatigue and sleep disturbances have been reported in up to 65% of the patient cohorts studied,[295] and sexual disturbances are prevalent in 25% of HCT survivors[296] (see box on Evaluating Survivors for Potential Late Effects).

POTENTIAL LATE EFFECTS BY DIAGNOSIS

Therapeutic approaches to hematologic malignancies vary widely depending on the patient's age at diagnosis, biologic subtype and staging of disease, year (era) of diagnosis, initial response to therapy, and physician/institutional preference. Even though two patients may share an identical diagnosis, their risks for late effects may differ

---

Evaluating Survivors for Potential Late Effects

To diminish the incidence and severity of untoward late effects and to improve the quality of survival for patients with hematopoietic malignancies, systematic evaluation of outcomes with subsequent modification of current and future therapies is required. To decrease late morbidity and mortality rates and to meet the specialized healthcare needs of this group of patients, ongoing comprehensive follow-up care with attention to early detection and intervention for late effects are essential.

Patients are generally eligible to enter formal long-term follow-up care when the risk for relapse of their primary disease is minimal. For most hematologic malignancies, this occurs when a patient is at least 2 years off therapy. When a patient enters long-term follow-up, the focus of care shifts from vigilant surveillance for disease recurrence to a survivorship model of health maintenance or promotion and management of treatment-related late effects. Effective management of these late effects requires ongoing surveillance, early intervention, and when possible, prevention.

The long-term complications of treatment for which an individual survivor is at risk are determined by several factors, including the patient's diagnosis, age at treatment, specific chemotherapeutic agents received (including cumulative doses), specific radiation fields and doses, therapy-related complications, degree of psychosocial support received, genetic predisposition, and current health-related behaviors (e.g., diet, physical activity, tobacco, and alcohol use).

---

significantly because of differences in therapy, age at exposure to therapy, or pharmacogenetics. General associations of late effects with conventional treatment for common hematologic malignancies are reviewed in Tables 93.1–93.3. The risk for specific late effects in survivors who have undergone HCT depends on the conditioning regimen, donor source, complications experienced during the transplantation process, presence or absence of GVHD, and prior cancer therapy. Transplantation-related sequelae have been reviewed throughout the text of this chapter.

Acute Lymphoblastic Leukemia

ALL is a heterogeneous disease. Therapy for ALL ranges from a relatively innocuous, antimetabolite-based approach for low-risk childhood ALL[297] to marrow-ablative therapy followed by HCT for very high-risk disease in all age groups.[298,299] The risk for long-term complications for individual survivors varies widely and is dependent on the specific therapy received as well as the patient's age at time of treatment.[300,301] Potential late effects that may occur as a consequence of conventional therapy for ALL are listed in Table 93.1.

Acute Myeloid Leukemia

Therapy for AML is generally more intense and of shorter duration than that used for treatment of ALL. Higher doses of anthracycline chemotherapy are often employed, as is consolidation therapy

---

TABLE 93.1	Late Effects Associated With Conventional Therapy for Acute Lymphoblastic Leukemia and Non-Hodgkin Lymphoma
Common Therapeutic Exposures	**Potential Late Effects**
Vincristine	Peripheral neuropathy, Raynaud phenomenon
Corticosteroids	Cataracts, osteopenia, osteoporosis, avascular necrosis
Asparaginase	No known late effects
Mercaptopurine	Hepatic dysfunction (rare)
Thioguanine	Portal hypertension, hepatotoxicity (when used continuously in maintenance therapy)
Methotrexate (systemic)	Osteopenia, osteoporosis, osteonecrosis, renal dysfunction (rare), hepatic dysfunction (rare)
Methotrexate (intrathecal, high dose), or cytarabine (high dose)	Neurocognitive deficits, clinical leukoencephalopathy
Cranial or craniospinal irradiation	Neurocognitive deficits, clinical leukoencephalopathy, cataracts, hypothyroidism, second malignant neoplasm in radiation field (e.g., skin, thyroid, brain), short stature, scoliosis or kyphosis, obesity
Anthracyclines	Cardiomyopathy, arrhythmias, subclinical left ventricular dysfunction, secondary AML
Cyclophosphamide	Hypogonadism, hemorrhagic cystitis, dysfunctional voiding, bladder malignancy, secondary AML or MDS
Blood products	Chronic viral hepatitis, HIV

AML, Acute myeloid leukemia; HIV, human immunodeficiency virus; MDS, myelodysplastic syndrome.

TABLE 93.2   Late Effects Associated With Conventional Therapy for Acute Myeloid Leukemia

Common Therapeutic Exposures	Potential Late Effects
Anthracyclines	Cardiomyopathy, arrhythmias, subclinical left ventricular dysfunction, secondary acute myeloid leukemia
Corticosteroids	Cataracts, osteopenia, osteoporosis, avascular necrosis
Asparaginase	No known late effects
Cytarabine (high dose)	Neurocognitive deficits, clinical leukoencephalopathy
Blood products	Chronic viral hepatitis, human immunodeficiency virus infection

TABLE 93.3   Late Effects Associated With Conventional Therapy for Hodgkin Lymphoma

Common Therapeutic Exposures	Potential Late Effects
Anthracyclines	Cardiomyopathy, arrhythmias, subclinical left ventricular dysfunction, secondary AML or MDS
Corticosteroids	Cataracts, osteopenia, osteoporosis, avascular necrosis
Bleomycin	Pulmonary dysfunction
Vincristine, vinblastine	Peripheral neuropathy, Raynaud phenomenon
Procarbazine, mechlorethamine, dacarbazine	Hypogonadism, infertility, secondary AML or MDS
Cyclophosphamide	Hypogonadism, infertility, hemorrhagic cystitis, dysfunctional voiding, bladder malignancy, secondary AML or MDS
Mantle irradiation	Hypothyroidism, premature cardiovascular disease, cardiac valvular disease, cardiomyopathy, arrhythmias, carotid artery disease, scoliosis or kyphosis, second malignant neoplasm in radiation field (e.g., thyroid, breast), pulmonary dysfunction
Inverted Y irradiation	Hypogonadism, infertility, adverse pregnancy outcome, second malignant neoplasm in radiation field (e.g., gastrointestinal)
Splenectomy	Acute life-threatening infections
Blood products	Chronic viral hepatitis, HIV

AML, Acute myeloid leukemia; HIV, human immunodeficiency virus; MDS, myelodysplastic syndrome.

with HCT.[301,302] Typically patients with AML receive less CNS-directed therapy than those with ALL. Examples of potential late effects associated with conventional therapy for AML are listed in Table 93.2.

Hodgkin Lymphoma

Therapy for HL relies on the use of alkylating agents, antitumor antibiotics (including anthracyclines and bleomycin), corticosteroids, and RT. Some patients may be aplenic as a consequence of the staging procedures performed in the earlier era.[303] Examples of potential late effects associated with conventional therapy for HL are listed in Table 93.3.

Late Effects Research: What Is Needed

Medical Issues Faced by This Population
- Premature death.
- Second malignancies.
- Organ dysfunction (e.g., cardiac, pulmonary, gonadal).
- Impaired growth and development.
- Decreased fertility.
- Neurocognitive impairment.
- Difficulties obtaining employment and insurance.
- Overall reduced quality of life.

Issues to Be Considered by Physicians Providing Care to This Population
- Providing long-term follow-up care for cancer survivors.
- Models of care delivery.
- Guidelines for ongoing screening and management.

Major Clinical and Research Challenges
- Cancer survivorship research continually changing because of new;
    - Therapeutic agents or combinations of agents (including targeted therapies).
    - Radiation oncology techniques.
    - Surgical procedures.
    - Supportive care techniques.

Future Directions
- Research is needed to;
    - More clearly define survivors at greatest risk for specific outcomes.
    - Identify genetic predispositions to certain key outcomes and the role of gene–environment interactions.
    - Identify the role of lifestyle choices (e.g., alcohol, tobacco, diet, exercise) in modification of risks for late adverse outcomes.
    - Understand the potential long-term impact of cancer therapy in order to effectively counsel survivors.
    - Develop effective intervention strategies to prevent or minimize the impact of adverse late effects.
    - Develop scientifically valid, evidence-based recommendations for clinical follow-up of survivors, which should include screening for potential late effects and application of proven approaches for health promotion.
- Much of the current information available relates to outcomes within the first decade after treatment, and only minimal data address the longer term outcomes that may subsequently occur. Large sample sizes within the context of well-characterized cohorts with complete long-term follow-up remain the greatest challenge to sound survivorship research.

Non-Hodgkin Lymphoma

The potential late effects after therapy for NHL are therapy specific and similar to those experienced by survivors of ALL (see Table 93.1).[303] Those patients whose treatment included HCT are also at risk for transplantation-related sequelae.

Chronic Myeloid Leukemia

Long-term survivors of CML have usually either undergone HCT or are receiving tyrosine kinase inhibitors long term. Among HCT recipients, there is a significant risk for late effects as a result of the transplantation-conditioning regimen, as well as treatment for and sequelae of GVHD.[17] With the transition in the early 2000s to tyrosine kinase inhibitor therapy for CML as the predominant treatment modality, the long-term effects of these agents will need to be studied in detail in the growing cohort of CML survivors[304] (see box on Late Effects Research: What Is Needed and the section Providing Clinical Care to Survivors).

PROVIDING CLINICAL CARE TO SURVIVORS

A summary of cancer treatment and a survivorship care plan are critical components of care provision for survivors of hematologic malignancies (see box on Survivorship Care Plans). Guidelines for long-term follow-up of survivors of hematologic malignancies and those who underwent HCT in childhood, adolescence, or young adulthood have been developed by the Children's Oncology Group[82] and are available at http://www.survivorshipguidelines.org; HCT long-term follow-up guidelines have also been developed by an international group of transplant experts.[83] In order to provide risk-based guideline-directed follow-up care, a comprehensive treatment summary is needed (Table 93.4) and a copy should be given to each survivor with instructions to share this information with all healthcare providers. Survivors should undergo annual comprehensive, multi-disciplinary health evaluations (Fig. 93.1) with special attention to the detection of potential late effects specific to the patient's diagnosis and treatment history (Table 93.5). Because certain late effects have prolonged asymptomatic intervals before becoming clinically evident (e.g., late-onset CHF as a result of anthracycline-induced cardiomy-opathy), ongoing evaluation is important to identify and provide early intervention for these potential complications. Health education regarding potential health risks and risk-reduction measures should be provided to each survivor. Targeted health education materials related to potential late complications of therapy during childhood, adolescence, or young adulthood have been developed by the Children's Oncology Group[305] and are available at http://www.survivorshipguidelines.org. After completion of each annual evaluation, identified late effects should be systematically recorded, and recommendations for any additional testing and for health maintenance and promotion should be shared with the patient and his or her primary healthcare provider. To optimize future follow-up care for all survivors, patients should be invited to participate in any relevant research studies for which they are eligible (see box on Late Effects Research: What Is Needed).

FUTURE DIRECTIONS

Better understanding of treatment-related toxicity has not only guided the design of less toxic therapies, but also the development of

---

Survivorship Care Plans

Survivorship care plans have been identified by the Institute of Medicine[309,310] as an important tool to facilitate follow-up care. Survivorship care plans should include both a summary of cancer treatment and a follow-up plan that can be used to enhance communication between care providers, coordinate care, and encourage health monitoring and promotion.[306] Specific elements of the survivorship care plan should include:

- Diagnosis, including histologic subtype and stage if relevant.
- Contact information for all cancer care providers and institutions where care was received.
- Surgical procedure(s) with dates.
- Chemo/biotherapy drugs received and completion dates for each.
- Radiation treatment dates with anatomical area(s) treated.
- Ongoing toxicities or treatment side effects.
- Genetic/hereditary risk factors or predisposing conditions, if relevant, including genetic testing results if performed.
- List of potential late and/or long-term effects.
- List of possible symptoms of cancer recurrence and surveillance testing schedule.
- Follow-up visit schedule, including who will provide care, and schedule of recommended screening/testing as indicated.
- Recommendations regarding general health maintenance/promotion.
- Information regarding common survivorship issues (e.g., emotional, financial, work/employment).

TABLE 93.4	Comprehensive Treatment Summary
Topic	**Specific Information to Include**
Demographics	Name
	Record number or patient identification number
	Date of birth
	Sex
	Race or ethnicity
Diagnosis	Date or age at diagnosis
	Referring physician or institution
	Treating physician or institution
	Presenting symptoms
	Past medical history
	Family history (including cancer in first- or second-degree relatives)
	Physical examination findings at presentation
	Initial diagnostics (complete blood cell count, chemistry panel, radiographic studies)
	Diagnostic procedures (biopsies, cytologic studies)
	Pathology (morphology, histology, cytochemistry, flow cytometry)
	Cytogenetics
	Central nervous system status (if applicable)
	Stage (if applicable)
	Metastatic sites (if applicable)
	Initial response to therapy (e.g., RER, SER, date first complete remission achieved)
	Relapse(s) dates, age at relapse(s), relapse site(s)
Treatment	Date of initial treatment (initiated and completed)
	Date(s) for treatment of relapse (initiated and completed)
	Final off-therapy date
	Chemotherapy agents received, including route of administration (list all)
	Cumulative doses (in mg/m^2) and age at treatment for all alkylators, anthracyclines, and heavy metals
	Dose ranges for cytarabine and methotrexate (e.g., standard dose vs. high dose >1000 mg/m^2)
	Radiation fields, doses, shielding, age at treatment
	Surgical procedure(s)
	Transfusion(s), including all blood or serum products
	Stem cell transplantation(s), including donor source, preparative regimen, GVHD prophylaxis or treatment
Acute complications	Significant therapy-related complications (e.g., tumor lysis, septic shock, typhlitis, acute GVHD)
	Significant treatment required for complications (e.g., hemodialysis, amphotericin, aminoglycosides)
Complications after therapy	Significant complications after completion of therapy (e.g., herpes zoster, acute life-threatening infection after splenectomy)

GVHD, Graft-versus-host disease; RER, rapid early response; SER, slow early response.
Modified from Children's Oncology Group Summary of Cancer Treatment, 2013. http://www.survivorshipguidelines.org

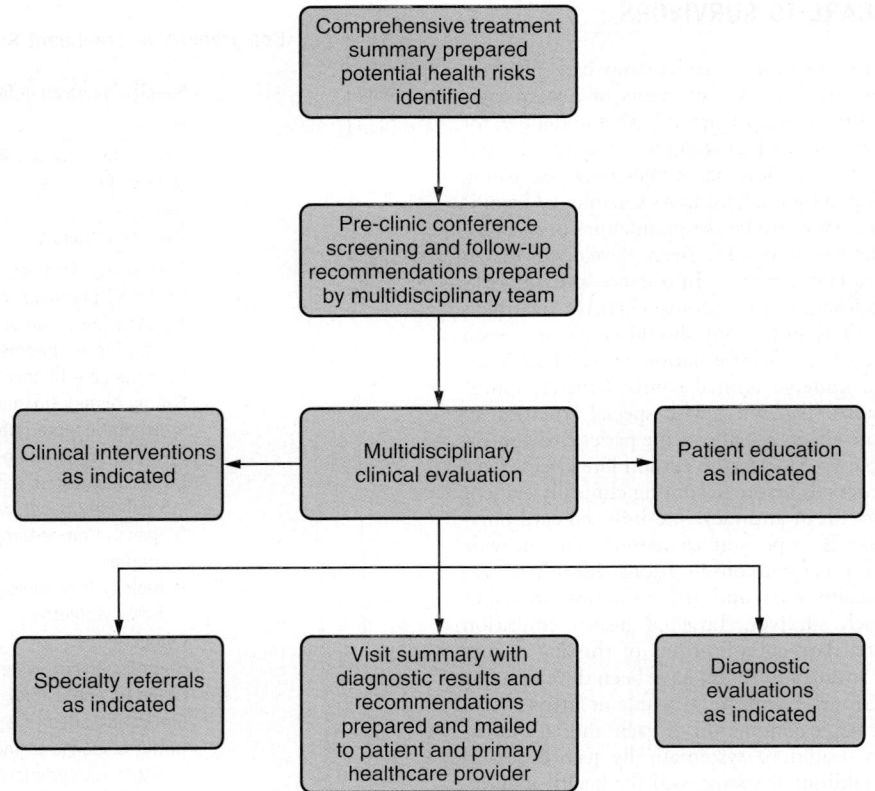

Fig. 93.1 ANNUAL COMPREHENSIVE MULTIDISCIPLINARY HEALTH EVALUATION FOR THE CANCER SURVIVOR.

TABLE 93.5	Monitoring for Potential Late Effects		
Potential Late Effects	**Therapeutic Exposure**	**Recommended Monitoring**	**Suggested Interventions**
Adverse psychosocial effects (e.g., depression, anxiety, posttraumatic stress disorder, limitations in healthcare access, risky behaviors, psychosocial disability due to pain, fatigue)	Diagnosis and treatment for hematologic malignancy	Clinical interview: yearly	Psychologic or social work consultation if indicated
Dental abnormalities (abnormal tooth development, increased susceptibility to caries and gum disease)	Chemotherapy Cranial irradiation TBI	Dental examination: every 6 months	Professional dental cleaning every 6 months; use of fluoridated toothpaste; topical fluoride applications as indicated; Panorex radiograph before orthodontic or dental procedures for patients treated before completion of tooth development
Peripheral neuropathy Raynaud phenomenon	Vincristine Vinblastine	Neurologic examination if symptomatic	Physical therapy if indicated; advise patient to protect against precipitating factors (e.g., cold environment)
Neurocognitive deficits	Methotrexate (intrathecal, high-dose systemic) Cytarabine (high-dose systemic) Cranial irradiation TBI	Formal neuropsychologic testing: baseline on entry to long-term follow-up; repeat as clinically indicated if evidence of impaired performance Clinical interview yearly, including assessment of educational and vocational progress	Referral for specialized educational services, curricular modifications, or vocational training programs if indicated

TABLE 93.5 **Monitoring for Potential Late Effects—cont'd**

Potential Late Effects	Therapeutic Exposure	Recommended Monitoring	Suggested Interventions
Clinical leukoencephalopathy	Methotrexate (intrathecal, high-dose systemic) Cytarabine (high-dose systemic) Cranial irradiation	Clinical evaluation: yearly Brain MRI or CT if clinically indicated	Neurology consultation if clinically indicated
Cataracts	Corticosteroids Busulfan Cranial irradiation TBI	Funduscopic examination and visual acuity evaluation: yearly Ophthalmologic examination: yearly for patients who received TBI or cranial radiation ≥30 Gy; every 3 years for cranial radiation <30 Gy	Ophthalmology consultation if abnormalities detected
Xerophthalmia	Chronic GVHD related to HCT	History and eye examination yearly	Artificial tears, ophthalmology consultation if indicated
Xerostomia	Cranial irradiation Chronic GVHD related to HCT	Dental evaluation: every 6 months	Meticulous oral hygiene Artificial saliva products if indicated
Hearing loss	Platinum chemotherapy Aminoglycoside antibiotics Cranial irradiation	History and physical examination: yearly Audiogram: baseline at entry into long-term follow-up, then as clinically indicated; every 5 years if cranial radiation dose ≥30 Gy	Audiology consultation if indicated
Hypothyroidism Thyroid nodules Thyroid malignancy	Cranial, cervical, spinal, mantle, or mediastinal irradiation; TBI	Free T_4, TSH, thyroid examination: yearly	Endocrine or surgical referral as indicated
Cardiomyopathy Arrhythmias Subclinical left ventricular dysfunction	Anthracyclines Chest or thoracic irradiation (e.g., mantle, mediastinal)	Detailed history of exertional tolerance (e.g., dyspnea on exertion, chest pain): yearly ECG (for evaluation of QT interval): baseline on entry into long-term follow-up; ECHO: baseline on entry into long-term follow-up, then every 1–5 years as indicated based on age at therapy and total anthracycline or radiation dose	Cardiology consultation if indicated; additional cardiology evaluation of patients who are pregnant or planning to become pregnant if patient received ≥300 mg/m² of an anthracycline, radiation dose ≥30 Gy, or any dose of anthracycline combined with irradiation
Pericarditis Pericardial fibrosis Valvular disease Premature atherosclerotic heart disease	Chest or thoracic irradiation (e.g., mantle, mediastinal)	Consider cardiology consultation 5–10 years after irradiation to evaluate risk for coronary artery disease in patients who received doses ≥40 Gy Fasting glucose or hemoglobin A1c and lipid profiles: every 2 years	Cardiology consultation if indicated; additional cardiology evaluation in patients who are pregnant or planning to become pregnant if patient received anthracycline combined with radiation, ≥300 mg/m² anthracycline, or radiation dose ≥30 Gy
Pulmonary dysfunction (fibrosis, interstitial pneumonitis)	Bleomycin Busulfan Chest/thoracic irradiation TBI Chronic GVHD related to HCT	Pulmonary function testing: baseline at entry into long-term follow-up and as clinically indicated for patients with progressive dysfunction	Pulmonary consultation for symptomatic patients; influenza and pneumococcal vaccine; counsel patients to avoid smoking and avoid scuba diving
Thrombosis Vascular insufficiency Infection of retained cuff or line tract	Central venous catheter	History and physical examination: yearly as clinically indicated	Surgical referral as indicated
Hepatic dysfunction	Mercaptopurine, thioguanine, methotrexate (systemic), HCT	ALT, AST, bilirubin: baseline on entry into long-term follow-up; repeat if clinically indicated	If abnormal results for baseline studies, obtain prothrombin time (to assess hepatic synthetic function) and viral hepatitis screening
Chronic viral hepatitis	Blood products	Hepatitis C antibody and HCV RNA by PCR: once if transfused before universal screening of blood supply (1992 in the United States) Hepatitis B surface antigen and core antibody: once if transfused before universal screening of blood supply (1972 in the United States)	Gastroenterology or hepatology consultation and annual AFP for patients with chronic hepatitis; hepatitis A and B immunizations in patients lacking immunity

Continued

TABLE 93.5   Monitoring for Potential Late Effects—cont'd

Potential Late Effects	Therapeutic Exposure	Recommended Monitoring	Suggested Interventions
HIV infection	Blood products	HIV-1 and HIV-2 antibodies: once if transfused before universal screening of blood supply (1985 in the United States)	Infectious disease consultation for patients with confirmed infection
Life-threatening infection	Splenectomy Splenic radiation ≥40 Gy Chronic active GVHD	Physical examination at time of febrile illness to evaluate degree of illness and for potential source of infection	Counsel patients regarding risk of life-threatening infections and indication for medical alert bracelet Administer parenteral antibiotics and continue close medical observation in patients with temperature ≥38.3°C (101°F) or other signs of serious infection; immunize with pneumococcal, meningococcal, and HIB vaccines
Iron overload	HCT (and patients requiring multiple red blood cell transfusions)	Serum ferritin: at entry into long-term follow-up	If abnormal, consider chelation, or repeat as clinically indicated until within normal limits
Bowel obstruction Chronic enterocolitis Fistulas and strictures	Abdominal surgery Abdominal or pelvic irradiation Chronic GVHD related to HCT (esophageal strictures, vaginal stenosis)	History and physical examination: yearly and as clinically indicated Serum protein and albumin levels: yearly in patients with chronic diarrhea or fistula	Surgical and gastroenterology consultations as clinically indicated
Renal insufficiency	TBI Abdominal or splenic irradiation Ifosfamide Platinum chemotherapy Methotrexate	Blood pressure: yearly Urinalysis: yearly BUN, creatinine, electrolytes, calcium, magnesium, phosphorus baseline and repeat as clinically indicated	Nephrology consultation for proteinuria, hypertension, progressive renal insufficiency
Hemorrhagic cystitis Bladder fibrosis Dysfunctional voiding Bladder malignancy	Cyclophosphamide Ifosfamide Irradiation of abdomen, pelvis, iliac, inguinal sites	Voiding history: yearly	Urinalysis and urology consultation as clinically indicated for incontinence, dysfunctional voiding, macroscopic hematuria (culture negative)
Growth hormone deficiency	Cranial irradiation TBI	Height, weight: every 6 months during puberty until growth is complete Obtain bone age in poorly growing children	Endocrine referral for patients failing to follow normal growth curve
Overweight/obesity	Cranial irradiation	BP, growth percentile, BMI: yearly	Endocrine referral as indicated
Dyslipidemia	TBI	Lipid profile every 2 years	
Hypogonadism Infertility	Alkylating agents Cranial irradiation Abdominal or pelvic irradiation Testicular irradiation Spinal irradiation >25 Gy TBI	Menstrual history, sexual function, height, weight: yearly Pubertal history, Tanner stage: yearly until maturity FSH, LH, estradiol: baseline at age 13 (females); Testosterone: baseline at age 14 (males); or at entry into long-term follow-up and for clinical symptoms of estrogen or testosterone deficiency Semen analysis: as indicated or requested by patient	Endocrine referral for hypogonadal patients (for hormone-replacement therapy); reproductive endocrinology referral for patients desiring evaluation of fertility options
Precocious puberty	Cranial irradiation	Physical examination, height, weight, Tanner stage: yearly until maturity LH, FSH, estradiol, or testosterone: as clinically indicated in patients with accelerated pubertal progression Obtain bone age in rapidly growing prepubertal children	Endocrine referral as indicated
Adverse pregnancy outcomes (e.g., spontaneous abortion, premature delivery, low-birthweight infant)	Irradiation of abdomen, pelvis, iliac, inguinal, paraaortic sites TBI	History: yearly and as clinically indicated	High-risk obstetric care

TABLE 93.5 **Monitoring for Potential Late Effects—cont'd**

Potential Late Effects	Therapeutic Exposure	Recommended Monitoring	Suggested Interventions
Osteopenia, osteoporosis	Corticosteroids Methotrexate (high-dose systemic) HCT	Bone-density study (DEXA scan or quantitative CT scan): baseline at entry into long-term follow-up, repeat as clinically indicated	Calcium and vitamin D supplementation; weight-bearing exercise; treatment of exacerbating conditions (e.g., hypogonadism); consider pharmacologic intervention (e.g., bisphosphonates)
Avascular necrosis	Corticosteroids Methotrexate (systemic) HCT	History: yearly; MRI if clinically indicated	Orthopedic consultation if indicated
Scoliosis/kyphosis	Irradiation of trunk (e.g., mantle, spine, abdomen, pelvis)	Physical examination of spine: yearly (every 6 months during pubertal growth spurt) Radiologic imaging of the spine if clinical evidence of scoliosis or kyphosis	Orthopedic referral
Joint contractures	Chronic GVHD related to HCT	Physical examination yearly	Orthopedic referral if indicated
Chronic infection	Chronic GVHD related to HCT	History: yearly	Prophylactic antiinfective agents; infectious disease consultation if indicated
Vitiligo Scleroderma Joint contractures Nail dysplasia Dysplastic nevi Skin cancer Secondary benign or malignant neoplasms in radiation field	Chronic GVHD related to HCT Irradiation (any field)	Physical examination: yearly Careful physical examination, inspection and palpation of irradiated skin and soft tissues: yearly	Dermatology or rehabilitation consultation if clinically indicated Dermatology or surgical referral and radiographs if indicated for any suspicious lesions
Bone malignancies Brain tumor	Cranial irradiation	History and physical examination: yearly Brain MRI: baseline at maturity for all patients and as clinically indicated	Neurosurgical consultation as indicated
Breast cancer	Chest or thorax irradiation ≥20 Gy (mantle radiation field) TBI or chest or thorax irradiation 10–19 Gy (mantle radiation field)	Clinical breast examination: yearly until age 25, then every 6 months Mammogram and breast MRI: yearly beginning at age 25 or 8 years after irradiation (whichever comes last) Discuss benefits and risks/harms of screening; if decision is made to screen, follow above recommendations	Teach breast self-examination; instruct patient to perform monthly self-examination and report changes immediately; surgical consultation if clinically indicated
Gastrointestinal malignancy	Abdominal, pelvic, spinal irradiation ≥30 Gy	Colonoscopy every 5 years beginning 10 years after radiation or at age 35, whichever comes last; or more frequently as clinically indicated	Surgical consultation if indicated
AML (preceding myelodysplastic phase associated with alkylating agents)	Anthracyclines Epipodophyllotoxins Alkylating agents Stem cell priming with etoposide Autologous transplantation for NHL or Hodgkin lymphoma	Physical examination: yearly for 10 years after therapy CBC and differential and bone marrow evaluation if clinically indicated	Counsel patient to report fatigue, bruising, bleeding, bone pain

AFP, α-Fetoprotein; ALT, alanine aminotransferase; AML, acute myeloid leukemia; AST, aspartate aminotransferase; BMI, body mass index; BP, blood pressure; BUN, blood urea nitrogen; CBC, complete blood cell count; CT, computed tomography; DEXA, dual-energy x-ray absorptiometry; ECG, electrocardiogram; ECHO, echocardiogram; FSH, follicle-stimulating hormone; GFR, glomerular filtration rate; GVHD, graft-versus-host disease; HCT, hematopoietic cell transplantation; HCV, hepatitis C virus; hemoglobin A1c, glycosylated hemoglobin; HIB, *Haemophilus influenzae* type B; HIV, human immunodeficiency virus; LH, luteinizing hormone; MRI, magnetic resonance imaging; NHL, non-Hodgkin lymphoma; PCR, polymerase chain reaction; RNA, ribonucleic acid; T_4, thyroxine; TBI, total body irradiation; TSH, thyroid-stimulating protein.

Modified from Children's Oncology Group: *Long-term follow-up guidelines for survivors of childhood, adolescent, and young adult cancers*, version 4.0, 2013, Children's Oncology Group. http://www.survivorshipguidelines.org

treatment summaries,[82] survivorship plans,[306] and efforts to harmonize survivorship guidelines worldwide[307] that serve as a model for the survivorship care of adult patients with cancer. It is important that more recent cohorts of cancer survivors continue to be followed to determine how therapy modifications impact the prevalence and spectrum of late effects. It is important to apply known interventions

that can reduce the impact of cancer and treatment-related late effects on quality of life, morbidity, and mortality, as well as to develop and test new interventions. For example, survivors of HL who are treated with chest radiation have an increased risk of developing lung cancer, and tobacco use increases this risk 20-fold. Successful smoking prevention and cessation strategies among survivors can decrease the risk of this prevalent and highly morbid cancer of adulthood, while also decreasing the development and progression of atherosclerosis and other SMNs. Screening of young women at increased risk of breast cancer due to chest radiation has already been mentioned. Survivors of childhood cancer, particularly those who received radiation to the hypothalamic–pituitary axis, are also at risk of obesity. Obesity can, in turn, exacerbate the increased risks of cardiovascular disease associated with anthracycline chemotherapy and RT to the chest. Modifiable cardiovascular risk factors, such as hypertension, can potentiate the risk of major cardiac events and both behavioral and medical interventions can potentially reduce these risks. Research to define optimal intervention strategies and well-integrated survivorship care models are needed. Execution of these intervention strategies in the setting of clinical trials would permit evaluation of interventions in early detection, leading to a reduction in morbidity and mortality and, ultimately, improvement in the overall quality of life of cancer survivors.

The advantages of studying outcomes in cancer survivors, including detailed knowledge of the therapeutic exposures coupled with close follow-up after these exposures, enables researchers to study testable hypotheses and determine the effects of host and therapy-related factors in the development of adverse outcomes ranging from carcinogenesis and organ dysfunction to psychosocial consequences. Opportunities also exist to explore gene and environment interactions that may modify susceptibility to develop adverse outcomes, thus providing insights into the identification of high-risk populations.

The growing population of cancer survivors carries a significant burden of morbidity, necessitating comprehensive long-term follow-up of these survivors.[308] This follow-up should ideally begin at the completion of active therapy, with a documented summarization of therapeutic exposures and recommendations for follow-up, thus ensuring standardization of care received by the survivors.[306,309,310] However, many barriers prevent effective follow-up, the most fundamental being the lack of knowledge regarding survivorship issues demonstrated by both the long-term survivors and the primary care physicians caring for them. Shortcomings of the healthcare system also pose potential barriers, and include logistical issues such as a lack of capacity within centers, training and educational deficiencies, inadequate communication between pediatric oncologists, and primary care physicians that subsequently provide the large bulk of follow-up. Finally, a major obstacle faced by cancer survivors in the United States has been the difficulty in obtaining affordable health insurance, especially for young adults, which has made it difficult for survivors to seek and obtain appropriate long-term follow-up care. The enactment of the Patient Protection and Affordable Care Act (ACA) in the United States in 2010 included several provisions designed to broaden coverage and potentially transform patterns of health care for previously uninsured survivors; the impact of this change on healthcare received by the cancer survivors is beginning to emerge.[311]

Despite these unique opportunities, conduct of survivorship research faces several challenges. Cancer survivorship research can be expected to evolve during the next several years as better treatment options, new agents, and combinations of agents are developed for the cancer patients who do not now survive. Targeted therapies will contribute to increased survivorship. Evaluation of their late effects will need to keep in step with their increased usage. Refinements in RT and minimally invasive surgeries are intended to minimize late effects. Evidence-based research will need to determine whether they will live up to this expectation. Advances in supportive care, including transfusions and hematopoietic growth factors, also require ongoing surveillance for identification of late effects. Furthermore, the influence of genetic profiles on susceptibility to late effects, as well as their interaction with lifestyle exposures such as tobacco, alcohol, and diet, is of growing interest and has not been fully explored. However, the

multifactorial etiology of the adverse effects, coupled with the heterogeneous nature of the patient population, necessitates large sample sizes within the context of well-characterized cohorts with complete long-term follow-up, and this remains the greatest challenge to sound survivorship research.

SUGGESTED READINGS

Armenian SH, Meadows AT, Bhatia S: Late effects of childhood cancer and its treatment. In Pizzo PA, Poplack DG, editors: *Principles and practice of pediatric oncology*, Philadelphia, 2011, Lippincott Raven, pp 1431–1462.

Baker KS, Ness KK, Weisdorf D, et al: Late effects in survivors of acute leukemia treated with hematopoietic cell transplantation: a report from the Bone Marrow Transplant Survivor Study. *Leukemia* 24:2039, 2010.

Bhatia S: Caring for the long-term survivor after allogeneic stem cell transplantation. *Hematology Am Soc Hematol Educ Program* 2014(1):495–503, 2014.

Children's Oncology Group: *Children's Oncology Group Long-Term Follow-Up Guidelines for Survivors of Childhood, Adolescent, and Young Adult Cancers, Version 4.0.* Monrovia, CA: Children's Oncology Group, <http://www.survivorshipguidelines.org>, 2013.

de Moor JS, Mariotto AB, Parry C, et al: Cancer survivors in the United States: prevalence across the survivorship trajectory and implications for care. *Cancer Epidemiol Biomarkers Prev* 22:561–570, 2013.

Guy GP, Jr, Ekwueme DU, Yabroff KR, et al: Economic burden of cancer survivorship among adults in the United States. *J Clin Oncol* 31(30):3749–3757, 2013.

Hewitt ME, Greenfield DM, Stovall E, editors: *From cancer patient to cancer survivor: lost in transition*, Washington, D.C., 2006, The National Academies Press.

Hewitt ME, Weiner SL, Simone JV, editors: *Childhood cancer survivorship: improving care and quality of life*, Washington, D.C., 2003, The National Academies Press.

Hudson MM, Oeffinger KC, Jones K, et al: Age-dependent changes in health status in the Childhood Cancer Survivor cohort. *J Clin Oncol* 33(5):479–491, 2015.

Landier W, Armenian S, Bhatia S: Late effects of childhood cancer and its treatment. *Pediatr Clin North Am* 62(1):275–300, 2015.

Majhail NS, Rizzo JD, Lee SJ, et al: Recommended screening and preventive practices for long-term survivors after hematopoietic cell transplantation. *Biol Blood Marrow Transplant* 18(3):348–371, 2012.

Mayer DK, Nekhlyudov L, Snyder CF, et al: American Society of Clinical Oncology clinical expert statement on cancer survivorship care planning. *J Oncol Pract* 10(6):345–351, 2014.

Oeffinger KC, Mertens AC, Sklar CA, et al: Chronic health conditions in adult survivors of childhood cancer. *N Engl J Med* 355(15):1572–1582, 2006.

Phillips SM, Padgett LS, Leisenring WM, et al: Survivors of childhood cancer in the United States: prevalence and burden of morbidity. *Cancer Epidemiol Biomarkers Prev* 24(4):653–663, 2015.

Rowland JH, Hewitt M, Ganz PA: Cancer survivorship: a new challenge in delivering quality cancer care. *J Clin Oncol* 24(32):5101–5104, 2006.

Sun CL, Kersey JH, Francisco L, et al: Burden of morbidity in 10+ year survivors of hematopoietic cell transplantation: report from the bone marrow transplantation survivor study. *Biol Blood Marrow Transplant* 19(7):1073–1080, 2013.

Vanderwalde AM, Sun CL, Laddaran L, et al: Conditional survival and cause-specific mortality after autologous hematopoietic cell transplantation for hematological malignancies. *Leukemia* 27(5):1139–1145, 2013.

REFERENCES

For the complete list of references, log on to www.expertconsult.com.

CELL-BASED THERAPIES

OVERVIEW AND HISTORICAL PERSPECTIVE OF CURRENT CELL-BASED THERAPIES

Leslie E. Silberstein and Helen E. Heslop

The discovery in 1900 by Karl Landsteiner of the ABO blood group system paved the way for transfusion therapy, that is, the ability to safely infuse living blood cells as a therapeutic modality (see Chapters 95–109). Thus, the discipline began with the collection by venipuncture of whole blood, which required anticoagulation and storage at refrigerated temperatures. These procedures were optimized when it became possible to isolate different cell populations, such as red blood cells, platelets, and granulocytes. The term *blood banking* refers to collection and storage of blood products, both of which are highly regulated by the United States Food and Drug Administration (FDA).

The pioneering work by E. Donnall Thomas and others between 1950 and 1970, demonstrating the feasibility of transfusing bone marrow cells (i.e., bone marrow transplantation) as a treatment modality marked the next significant development of cellular therapies (see Chapters 103–109).[1] The success of bone marrow engraftment is related to the presence of hematopoietic stem and progenitor cells in the bone marrow; immune cells in the graft, including T cells and natural killer cells, mediate graft-versus-tumor effects in patients transplanted for hematologic malignancy. Hematopoietic stem cell populations, currently used for therapy of malignant and nonmalignant disease, can be isolated from bone marrow, from (mobilized) peripheral blood, and from umbilical cord blood (see Chapter 95). An exciting new development in hematopoietic stem cell transplantation is the genetic manipulation/transduction of the hematopoietic stem cell to correct hereditary disorders such as the congenital immunodeficiencies and hemoglobinopathies (see Chapter 98).[2,3] More recently, the ability to isolate and expand cell populations in culture has led to the evaluation of a number of cell therapy strategies. Only one approach, a dendritic cell vaccine, has so far been approved by the FDA in the United States,[4] but several CD19 CAR products have obtained breakthrough designation and will likely be approved soon.[5] Infusions of other cells expanded ex vivo or significantly manipulated are conducted as experimental procedures through the FDA's Investigational New Drug application process. Many such studies use autologous cells, which do not have a risk for transferring communicable disease, but (because they are patient-specific products) make late-stage clinical trials more challenging. The use of allogeneic cells requires careful assessment of donor eligibility because of the risk for infectious disease transmission or transfer of immune reactivity (Table 94.1).[6] Allogeneic cells may also be used to produce a patient-specific product in some clinical settings, such as treatment of relapse postallogeneic transplant in which full HLA matching is required. In other applications, however, third-party cells may have benefits, including the advantage of broad applicability since a larger number of patients can receive a product generated from a single donor.

A broad range of cell types are currently being evaluated in clinical trials (see Chapters 97–101). Immune cell populations with distinct biologic properties are being infused to treat cancer and infectious diseases, and some approaches have progressed to late-phase testing (see Chapters 100 and 101). Nonhematopoietic stromal cells from bone marrow have attracted considerable interest recently for use in tissue repair and immunomodulation, largely because of their multilineage differentiation potential and their secretion of cytokines and chemokines (see Chapter 99). Their use, while experimental, is promising. Thus, significant experience in cell-based therapies

involving hematopoietic/bone marrow-derived cells has evolved, similar to blood banking and transfusion medicine, into a highly regulated discipline with oversight by several regulatory agencies, including the FDA and the National Institutes of Health Recombinant DNA Advisory Board (see Chapters 96 and 97).

TABLE 94.1	Evaluation of Allogeneic Donor for Eligibility to Provide Cell Therapy Product	
Evaluation/Test[a]	**Rationale/Purpose**
Complete history and physical	To review the donor's medical and social history for risk factors for communicable disease agents and diseases. To review for clinical evidence of risk factors or diseases.
Donor questionnaire	To evaluate risk factors for communicable disease (using uniform donor questionnaire[b] drafted by an international task force).
CBC, platelets, differential	To evaluate for evidence of hematologic abnormalities.
Electrolytes, BUN, creatinine, glucose, total protein, albumin, total bilirubin, alkaline phosphatase, ALT, AST, LDH	To evaluate for evidence of liver or electrolyte abnormalities.
ABO typing	To confirm identity.
HLA typing	To conduct HLA matching for some indications. To confirm identity.
HIV-1 antibody, HIV-2 antibody, HIV NAT, HTLV-1/2 antibodies, HBs antigen, HBc antibody, HCV NAT, CMV antibody, serologic test for syphilis, West Nile virus NAT, Chagas disease (if indicated by region)	To exclude communicable disease agents. Must be collected at the time of recovery of the cells or tissue from the donor; or up to 7 days before or after recovery. For donors of peripheral blood stem/progenitor cells, oocytes and bone marrow may be collected for testing up to 30 days.

[a]The donor eligibility rule requires human cell and tissue products establishments to screen and test cell and tissue donors for risk factors for, and clinical evidence of, relevant communicable disease agents or diseases. Additional Investigational New Drug-specific tests may also be mandated. All facilities need to use United States Food and Drug Administration-approved testing.
[b]Foundation for the Accreditation of Cellular Therapy (FACT) Standards: HPC Donor History Questionnaire http://www.factwebsite.org/Inner.aspx?id=163
ALT, Alanine aminotransferase; AST, aspartate aminotransferase; BUN, blood urea nitrogen; CBC, complete blood cell count; CMV, cytomegalovirus; HBc, hemoglobin C; HBs, hemoglobin S; HCV, hepatitis C virus; HIV, human immunodeficiency virus; HLA, human leukocyte antigen; HTLV-1/2, human T-lymphotropic virus-1/2; LDH, lactate dehydrogenase; NAT, nucleic acid testing.

The next frontier of cellular therapies is being driven by the discovery and ability to culture stem cell populations from various other adult tissues (retina, cornea, heart, lung, etc.), embryonic stem cells, and inducible pluripotent stem cells. The therapeutic application of these cell populations, although intensely investigated worldwide, is regarded as preliminary at present and guidelines have been published for clinical development.[7] Similarly, gene editing is also being used to modify hematopoietic stem cells and immune effector cells in preclinical studies, but there are ethical considerations with transfer to the clinic.[8]

REFERENCES

1. Weiden PL, Flournoy N, Thomas ED, et al: Antileukemic effect of graft-versus-host disease in human recipients of allogeneic-marrow grafts. *N Engl J Med* 300:1068–1073, 1979.

2. Fischer A, Hacein-Bey Abina S, Touzot F, et al: Gene therapy for primary immunodeficiencies. *Clin Genet* 88(6):507–515, 2015.

3. Naldini L: Gene therapy returns to centre stage. *Nature* 526(7573):351–360, 2015.

4. Cheever MA, Higano CS: PROVENGE (Sipuleucel-T) in prostate cancer: the first FDA-approved therapeutic cancer vaccine. *Clin Cancer Res* 17(11):3520–3526, 2011.

5. June CH, Riddell SR, Schumacher TN: Adoptive cellular therapy: a race to the finish line. *Sci Transl Med* 7(280):280ps7, 2015.

6. Horowitz MM, Confer DL: Evaluation of hematopoietic stem cell donors. *Hematology Am Soc Hematol Educ Program* 469–475, 2005.

7. Kimmelman J, Hyun I, Benvenisty N, et al: Policy: Global standards for stem-cell research. *Nature* 533(7603):311–313, 2016.

8. Kohn DB, Porteus MH, Scharenberg AM: Ethical and regulatory aspects of genome editing. *Blood* 127(21):2553–2560, 2016.

PRACTICAL ASPECTS OF HEMATOLOGIC STEM CELL HARVESTING AND MOBILIZATION

Scott D. Rowley and Michele L. Donato

Hematopoietic stem cell (HSC) products for autologous or allogeneic transplantation are available from bone marrow, peripheral blood, or umbilical cord blood (UCB) sources. Bone marrow was the original source of cells for transplantation because of the ease and reliability of collecting adequate numbers of cells for transplantation, and it remains the standard with which other sources of HSCs are compared.

Peripheral blood stem cell (PBSC) products have virtually replaced bone marrow as the HSC component for autologous transplantation and are frequently used for allogeneic transplantation. Virtually all patients undergoing autologous HSC transplantation will have PBSCs as the source of HSCs, based on the advantages of ease of scheduling of collections, greater quantities of HSCs resulting in faster hematologic recovery and shorter and less costly hospital stays,[1–6] and potentially lower risks for tumor cell contamination of the graft. The rapid engraftment kinetics of PBSCs compared with bone marrow is widely recognized. Median times to achieve an absolute neutrophil count greater than 500/μL and platelet transfusion independence after PBSC transplantation typically are approximately 11 to 14 days. The allogeneic donor has a wide range of options, including marrow, PBSC, or UCB products from human leukocyte antigen (HLA)-compatible or partially compatible related or unrelated donors. The availability of HLA-matched related or unrelated donors is the primary consideration in the selection of a donor, but donor health or donation preferences may restrict what products will be available to the recipient. The patient's physician may select a stem cell source based on the expected transplant outcomes. PBSC products, for example, have the greatest quantity of HSCs and will result in faster hematologic recovery compared with marrow or UCB transplants. Bone marrow transplantation has a higher risk of graft failure, resulting in a twofold higher probability of second harvest request compared with PBSC donation.[7] In some reports, PBSC transplantation also results in a survival advantage. However, PBSC transplantation is associated with a higher risk for difficult-to-control chronic graft-versus-host disease (GVHD) and may not be appropriate for use in patients who would not benefit from a robust graft-versus-leukemia effect, such as those treated for nonmalignant diseases. The transplant recipient may request a source of cells, but the donor has the right to decide about the method of donation. Although GVHD prophylaxis with posttransplant methotrexate will slow engraftment, the kinetics of engraftment for the allogeneic PBSC recipient is similar to that experienced by the autologous PBSC recipient. A number of phase III studies involving either autologous or allogeneic HSC transplantation confirmed the more rapid engraftment kinetics for recipients of PBSCs,[8–11] and this effect is not limited to HSCs collected from the peripheral blood, because cytokine administration to the patient or donor before marrow harvesting will also increase the number of HSCs collected and result in quicker hematologic recovery.[12–14] The disadvantages to use of PBSC components compared with bone marrow or UCB for autologous or allogeneic transplantation include the possible need for multiple days of collection (especially for autologous transplantation), the inability to collect adequate components from all patients and donors, and a possibly higher risk for chronic GVHD or the occurrence of chronic GVHD that is more difficult to control[15] (see box on Choice of Hematologic Stem Cell Product for Transplantation).

UCB from public banks has the advantage of being immediately available, reducing the time to transplantation. Targeting collection of UCB products from ethnic populations not well represented in donor registries will facilitate treatment of ethnic minority patients. The relative immunologic naïveté of the cord blood donor allows use of HLA-mismatched products without an undue increase in GVHD risk.[16] The much smaller quantity of HSCs in the cord blood product results in slower hematologic recovery and a higher risk for primary engraftment failure, which may be partially offset by infusion of multiple products, and the older adult patient, in particular, may also be at greater risk for posttransplant infections because of the relative immature immune system of the donor.

SELECTION AND EVALUATION OF THE STEM CELL DONOR

Selection of the Stem Cell Donor

The primary selection criterion for the patient undergoing autologous HSC collection and transplantation is the diagnosis of an illness amenable to treatment with a dose-intense regimen requiring HSC support. Extensive prior treatments, especially with marrow-toxic chemotherapy regimens or with radiotherapy, may prohibit collection of adequate quantities of autologous HSCs, which would exclude a patient from this treatment option. Proper management of patients with a disease amenable to dose-intensive therapy should include provisions for HSC collection before extensive marrow-toxic agents are administered. In general, however, any serious comorbid illnesses that would preclude either marrow or PBSC collection would also disqualify the patient from treatment with dose-intensive regimens used in preparation for autologous HSC transplantation.

The selection of the allogeneic HSC donor is more complex. The HLA major histocompatibility complex is the primary consideration in selection of a donor for allogeneic HSC transplantation, since its loci contribute significantly to host-versus-graft (leading to immunologic rejection of donor HSCs) and to graft-versus-host (leading to GVHD and graft-versus-leukemia) reactions.[17,18] Donor age, gender, and parity are secondary considerations in the selection of an allogeneic HSC donor.[18,19] Mismatching for killer-cell immunoglobulin-like receptor ligands may reduce the risk for posttransplant relapse of disease.[20] More than 30% of allogeneic HSC transplants from related or unrelated donors will involve ABO-disparate donors and recipients, and donor and recipient pairs may also differ for other red blood cell antigens, with no clear evidence of deleterious effect on engraftment, survival, or GVHD.[21] Cancer, autoimmune disorders, and genetic diseases such as the hemoglobinopathies can be transmitted to the allograft recipient; thus, donor health is an important consideration in donor selection and determination of donor eligibility.

Evaluation of Hematopoietic Stem Cell Donor Suitability and Eligibility

The immediate precollection evaluation of a patient or donor is intended to address the risks of the collection procedure to the donor

Virtually all patients undergoing autologous hematopoietic stem cell (HSC) transplantation will have peripheral blood stem cells (PBSCs) as the source of HSC, based on the following advantages: ease of collection, greater quantities of HSCs (resulting in faster hematologic recovery and shorter and less costly hospital stays), and potentially lower risks for tumor cell contamination of the graft.

The allogeneic donor has a wider range of options, including marrow, PBSCs, or umbilical cord blood (UCB) products from human leukocyte antigen-compatible or partially compatible related or unrelated donors. The transplant recipient may request a source of cells, but the donor has the right to decide about the method of donation. PBSC products have the greatest quantity of HSCs and will result in faster hematologic recovery compared with marrow or UCB transplants. In some reports, PBSC transplantation resulted in a survival advantage. However, PBSC transplantation is also associated with a higher risk for difficult-to-control chronic graft-versus-host disease (GVHD) and may not be appropriate for use in patients who would not benefit from a robust graft-versus-leukemia effect, such as those treated for nonmalignant disease. UCB has the advantage of being immediately available, reducing the time to transplantation. Targeted collection of UCB products from ethnic populations not well represented in the various donor registries will facilitate treatment of ethnic minority patients. The relative immature immunity of the cord blood donors allows the use of human leukocyte antigen-mismatched products without an undue increase in GVHD risk. Infusion of two cord blood units may achieve a greater graft-versus-tumor effect (this concept has not been proven), even though one unit will be rejected. The much smaller quantity of HSCs in the cord blood product results in slower hematologic recovery, and the adult patient, in particular, may be at greater risk for posttransplant infection because of the relative immature immune system of the donor.

Hematopoietic stem cell (HSC) transplantation involves the infusion of a "blood product", and allogeneic and syngeneic donors must be evaluated for risks for disease transmission as per the current criteria for blood or tissue donation ("donor eligibility"). Exemptions from criteria that specifically address the risk for disease transmission are permissible, if the risks of excluding an otherwise appropriate donor outweigh the risks for disease transmission to the transplant recipient, who may not have an alternate donor. Informed consent must be obtained for the evaluation and collection procedures. Informed consent also must be specifically obtained for the release of protected donor health information to the transplant recipient, allowing proper informed consent for the transplant to be obtained. Minors and donors not competent to provide consent must be represented by a third party not involved in the care of the recipient. Ideally, similar courtesy will be provided to the adult competent donor.

Donors must also be evaluated for health issues that would increase the risks resulting from the collection procedures ("donor suitability"). For marrow donors, this includes the risks of anesthesia and harvesting in the prone position; for PBSC donors, evaluation should include the risks of mobilization medications and apheresis, including the need for venous catheter placement.

The donor collection facility's standard operating procedures for evaluation of HSC donors must meet the Foundation for the Accreditation of Cellular Therapy/Joint Accreditation Committee or AABB standards and United States Food and Drug Administration (or other regulatory agency) regulations, and include policies and procedures for the following:

- Education of donor, including education regarding procedures, risks and alternatives, and possible request for future donations;
- Medical history, including special attention to history of autoimmune disorders, arthritis, cardiac and vascular disease, and history of cancer;
- History of high-risk behaviors, such as recent tattoos, body piercing, sexual practices, and travel;
- Physical examination, including vein assessment (PBSC donors) and oral examination (marrow donors undergoing inhalational anesthesia);
- Laboratory studies, including verification human leukocyte antigen typing, ABO typing, complete blood count, chemistry panel, infectious disease panel, urinalysis, ECG, CXR;
- Consent for the collection procedures and the release of protected health information to the stem cell recipient;
- Documentation of both donor eligibility and suitability before initiation of the transplant conditioning regimen.

("donor suitability") and the risks for transmission of disease from the donor to the recipient ("donor eligibility"). The same general health criteria apply to both bone marrow and PBSC donors. Patients undergoing autologous HSC collection and transplantation are not at risk for transmitting disease to themselves, and determination of donor eligibility is not medically required or economically justifiable, but these patients must be evaluated for their suitability for the collection procedures. All allogeneic and syngeneic HSC donors must be evaluated for donor eligibility, as well as suitability, using the same criteria currently applied to blood or other tissue donors, including a targeted history regarding behaviors exposing the donor to infection, recent or concurrent illnesses, and medication use.[22–26] This evaluation of the allogeneic donor suitability and eligibility must be clearly documented in the donor medical record, with appropriate additional documentation of donor eligibility placed in the intended recipient's medical record before initiation of the transplant conditioning regimen. Older donors have a greater probability of comorbid medical conditions, which will increase the risks of the collection procedures, and the risks to the allogeneic donor with underlying health problems must be fully considered before subjecting the donor to HSC collection. Published standards describe evaluation of the donor for the risk of the donation process, as well as the risk for transmission of disease to the recipient.[22–24,26] Evaluation by appropriate consultants may be required before autologous or allogeneic donor approval is finalized. Procedures involving donors with acute infectious illnesses should be delayed, if at all possible, because of the risk for disease transmission. Genetic disorders, such as hemoglobinopathies, will be transmitted to the recipient as a direct consequence of stem cell engraftment. Cancer can be transmitted, as illustrated by the transmission of donor leukemia not detected during initial evaluation of the donor,[27] and donors previously treated for cancer should be evaluated for the probability of recurrent disease that could be transferred to the immunocompromised recipient.[28] Collection of PBSCs is generally an outpatient procedure conducted in the clinic setting. In contrast, marrow harvesting has the luxury of the intensive support capability of the operating room. PBSC collection, therefore, should never be viewed as a safer alternative to marrow harvesting for the donor with

underlying health problems. Pediatric donors present different challenges, based on the smaller size and varying ages (and ability to cooperate) of the donors (see box on Evaluation of the Allogeneic or Syngeneic Marrow or Peripheral Blood Stem Cell Donor).

Use of a donor who does not meet eligibility criteria and who poses a risk for transmission of disease requires appropriate informed consent both from the donor (for disclosure of this confidential health information to the recipient and for counseling of the recipient) and from the recipient (for use of the stem cell product). The potential conflict of interest between protecting donor confidentiality and patient needs must be recognized by the personnel caring for each person, and preferably, the donor and patient should be represented by different physicians.[29]

Determination of Suitability for Bone Marrow Donation

Anesthesia and blood loss present the greatest risks for serious complications to the bone marrow donor. Most marrow harvesting is performed under general anesthesia, which requires intubation for control of the airway for a surgical procedure being performed on a prone patient. Regional (spinal or epidural) anesthesia may not be effectively established, so patients and donors who express a preference for this form of anesthesia must be counseled about the potential need for general anesthesia. The health assessment must include questioning about a history of joint disease of the cervical spine and mandible, and examination of the mouth if general anesthesia requiring intubation is chosen. Patients and donors with comorbid conditions, such as aortic stenosis sensitive to changes in blood volume and blood pressure, may require anesthesia consultation and plans for invasive monitoring during the surgical procedure. A history of marrow fibrosis, pelvic irradiation, or pelvic tumor involvement may exclude a patient from marrow harvesting, although unilateral harvesting from the posterior and iliac crests and aspiration of the sternum may achieve adequate quantities of cells for transplantation.

Determination of Suitability for Peripheral Blood Stem Cell Donation

The PBSC donor is exposed to the risks of cytokine (and chemokine) administration and the risks related to the apheresis procedure, including the risks of central venous catheter insertion and use. No long-term health consequences have been associated with G-CSF administration, and the specific toxicities with these agents are described later. G-CSF may lead to a flare of autoimmune disorders and may increase the risk for blood clots, particularly for donors who are sedentary or who may be traveling shortly after the donation procedures.[30] The PBSC donor must be assessed for venous access before the patient receives conditioning, and consent for use of a central venous catheter must be obtained if the venous access is deemed inadequate for the apheresis procedure.

Suitability and Eligibility for Umbilical Cord Blood Donation

Evaluation of the donor for UCB donation begins with a history of maternal and paternal illnesses and exposures to infectious diseases. Although linkage between the infant and the product is currently maintained, an update of infant health is not obtained at the time of transplantation, which may be several years after collection. Therefore, parental medical history includes specific questions addressing the risks for transmission of hereditary or acquired blood-borne diseases. A comprehensive genetic and family history should be obtained. Testing for infectious diseases is obtained from the mother at the time of collection to minimize loss of product through such testing.

Public UCB banks set criteria for the storage of units in order to avoid the collection and storage of UCB units that would not be acceptable for transplantation.[31] Exclusion criteria for potential donors in one multicenter study, for example, included the following: multiple gestation; premature delivery; active chorioamnionitis or sepsis; mother being the recipient of an organ transplant; mother with history of cancer; mother with high-risk behaviors or previously diagnosed with HIV, hepatitis, or syphilis; and mother having an active venereal disease such as vaginal herpes simplex and delivering vaginally.

COLLECTION OF BONE MARROW FOR TRANSPLANTATION

Bone Marrow-Collection Techniques

Bone marrow is typically harvested from the posterior iliac crests using virtually the same techniques used to obtain diagnostic samples in the clinic. The primary differences between obtaining diagnostic specimens and cell quantities adequate for transplantation are the volume of blood and marrow removed, which requires attention to fluid and blood component replacement during the procedure, and the need for appropriate anesthesia. Bone marrow harvesting from healthy donors presents little risk for serious morbidity, permitting

the ethical recruitment of allogeneic and syngeneic donors, including pediatric bone marrow donors and donors not related to the recipient.[22-25] Multiple aspirations are performed with collection of approximately 5 mL of marrow from each puncture site. If properly spaced, no more than two or three skin-puncture sites per side usually are required. Other harvest sites, such as the anterior iliac crests or sternum, can be used, but at increased risk for complications from accidental laceration or perforation of contiguous anatomic structures. For patients with a history of radiation or tumor involvement of one pelvic crest, adequate cells can be harvested from the anterior and posterior crests of the other side.

The prescription for marrow collection will define the desired quantity of nucleated cells per kg recipient weight to be collected. Ideally, this quantity of cells will be collected in a minimal total volume and procedure duration. Although transplant registries may require physicians to be experienced in marrow harvesting, defined as the number of procedures performed, few published studies report a correlation between such experience and harvest yields or donor complications.[32] The nucleated cell yield (cells per volume aspirated) appears greater for needles with side aspiration ports.[33] Smaller quantities aspirated per "pull" also improves cell yield.[34] Warming of the donor may improve cell yield.[35] Quality-assurance management should review for each harvest team the nucleated cell yield per volume of marrow, total volume aspirated, use of blood replacement, and duration of anesthesia.

Marrow is collected in the day surgery suite using either general or regional anesthesia. With proper fluid and blood replacement, overnight hospitalization should not be required. Bone marrow harvesting necessitates placing the donor into the prone position, which has specific considerations to avoid complications directly resulting from this positioning.[36] Donors must be supported, at a minimum, by positioning on chest rolls. For the healthy donor, the risks for serious complications from either general or regional anesthesia are minimal, although a multivariate analysis of adverse events performed by the National Marrow Donor Program for unrelated donors reported a higher risk for serious adverse events for donors receiving regional anesthesia.[37,38] Use of spinal or epidural anesthesia avoids the nausea that may occur with general anesthesia, especially for younger women, but hypotension from loss of vascular tone in the lower extremities often occurs as the volume of marrow is collected. General anesthesia is preferable for the donor with comorbid disorders such as cardiovascular or cerebral vascular disease because of the better control of donor airway and lower risk for hypotension during the harvest procedures. Local anesthesia is acceptable only if a very limited harvest is being performed, because local anesthesia does not achieve anesthesia of the marrow space and because large quantities of lidocaine, for example, are cardiotoxic.

Both heparin and acid-citrate-dextran-A (ACD-A) can be used for anticoagulation of bone marrow products. ACD-A decreases the accumulation of lactic acid and may be preferable, especially for products that will be transported or stored for longer periods before infusion or cryopreservation.[39]

Toxicity of Bone Marrow Collection

Anesthesia complications present the major health risk to the donor; marrow aspiration is generally well tolerated, although postharvest discomfort is experienced to some extent by all donors.[40] Complications include hemorrhage and infections at skin-puncture sites. Severe hematomas and neuralgias rarely occur, and training regarding pelvic anatomy is required to decrease the risk for damage to vessels and nerves lying under or adjacent to the iliac crest harvest sites. Irritation of the sacral nerves may result from needle penetration through the pelvic bone or from blood tracking into the nerve roots, and requires several months of convalescence. Localized pain is common, may last for several days, and may require a brief period of opioid medication. In a survey of over 9000 donors for unrelated bone marrow transplantation, 82% reported collection site pain, with a median time to recovery of 3 weeks (see Figs. 95.1 and 95.2).[38] Pain associated with

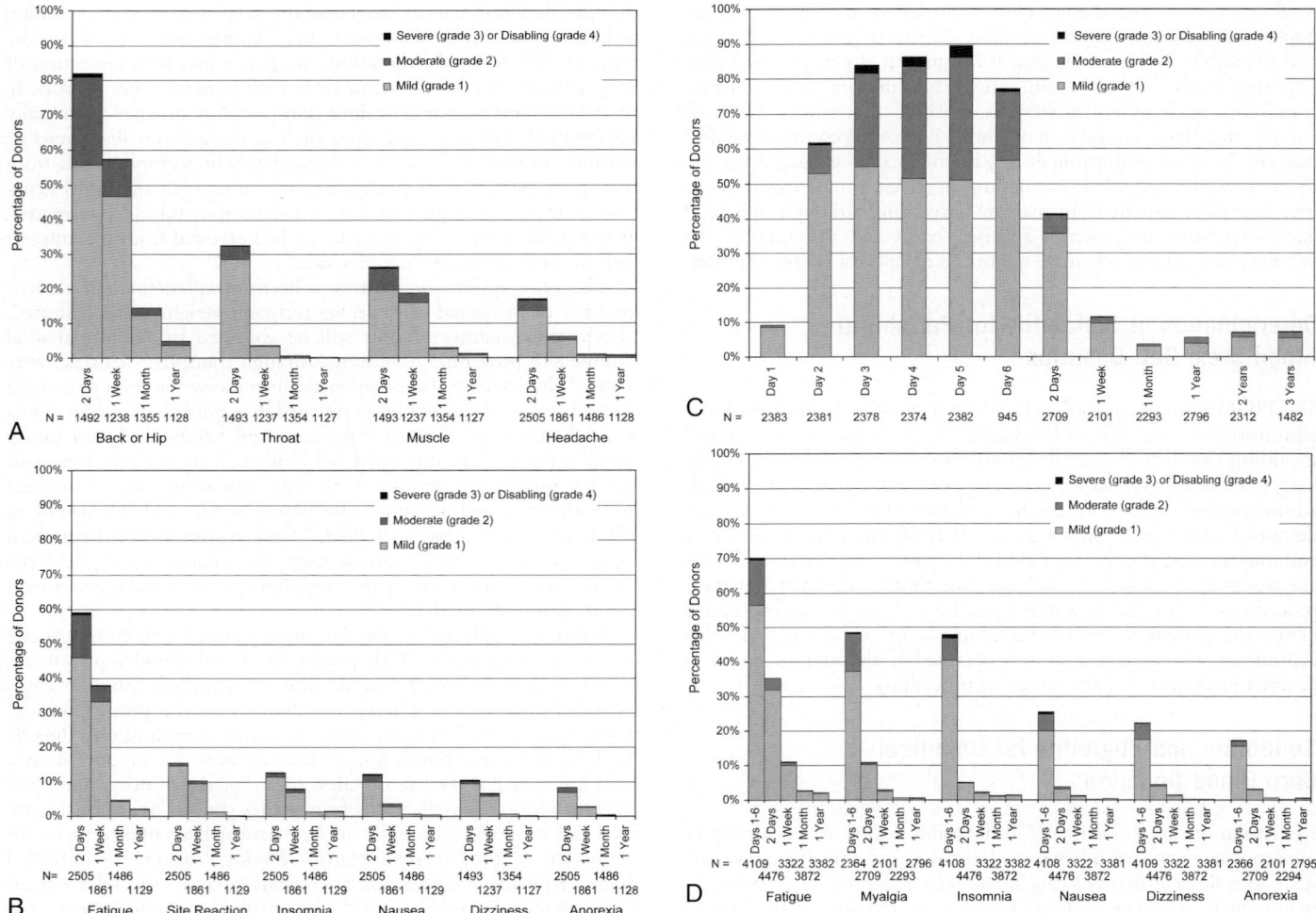

Fig. 95.1 (A) Percentage of BM donors reporting pain at selected sites over time. Reports of pain and pain severity were collected at the indicated time points post-donation. Throat pain is largely restricted to donors receiving general anesthesia, whereas headache is more common in donors receiving regional anesthesia, for example, epidural. (B) Six most frequently reported body symptoms experienced by BM donors at the indicated time points post-donation. (C) Percentage of PBSC donors reporting bone pain over time. Reports of bone pain and severity of pain were collected at the indicated time points during mobilization, collection, and post-donation. Day 1 is the first day of filgrastim administration; day 5 is the first day of apheresis. Bone pain represents pain in at least one of the following sites: general bone pain, back, head, limb, joint, hip, and neck. The severity of bone pain is defined as the maximum grade among these pain sites. (D) Six most frequently reported body symptoms experienced by PBSC donors during mobilization and collection, and at the indicated time points post-donation. The percentages for day 1 to day 6 represent the frequencies of the highest grade of symptoms during mobilization and collection. *(From* Biol Blood Marrow Transplant. *14(9 Suppl):29–36, 2008, doi: 10.1016/j.bbmt.2008.05.018.)*

the anesthesia procedures (throat pain, 33%; postanesthesia headache, 17%) was reported by a large proportion of the donors. Fatigue was reported by 59% of donors. Serious adverse effects were reported for 125 donors (1.35%), with 116 donors reporting serious complications considered to be a consequence of the collection procedures. Most of the serious complications ($n = 69$) were mechanical injury to tissue, bone, or nerve; and a smaller number ($n = 45$) were related to anesthesia. Infection and grand mal seizure were reported for one donor each. A retrospective survey of donor events reported by the European Group for Blood and Marrow Transplantation described almost 28,000 bone marrow donors, with one death from pulmonary embolism.[41] An additional 12 donors experienced severe adverse events, including four cardiac arrests (three during anesthesia), two episodes of severe hypertension, one pulmonary embolism from heparin-induced thrombocytopenia, one episode of pulmonary edema, one donor with a subdural hematoma, and three events not otherwise specified. This retrospective survey did not include all donors and may have underreported adverse events. This report,

furthermore, did not report the experiences of related and unrelated donors separately. The adverse events reported by unrelated donor registries will underestimate the risks faced by donors for related recipients, who may undergo collection despite comorbid illnesses that would preclude participation in an unrelated donor registry.[26,42] Most donors are able to return to routine activities 1 to 2 days after harvesting. The total recovery time for the 67 donors reporting serious mechanical injury was a median of 10 months (range: 1–96 months).[37] Toxicity was more likely to occur for less experienced harvest teams,[32] and harvest teams must address training and maintenance of harvest skills in their quality-assurance plans. Any team associated with a second severe mechanical injury should specifically be evaluated, in light of the very low probability of these events.

The usual volume harvested from healthy donors is approximately 10–15 mL of marrow per kilogram of recipient bodyweight to achieve the desired nucleated cell and CD34$^+$ cell doses. This results in a blood loss of 800–1000 mL for donors providing marrow for an average-sized adult recipient. The quantity of marrow harvested from

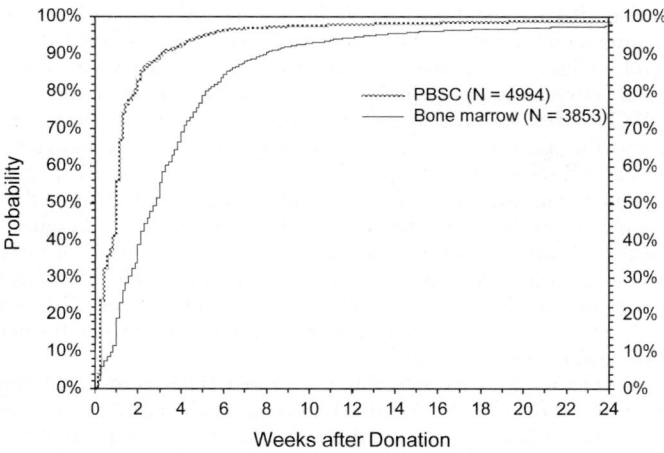

Fig. 95.2 Kaplan-Meier plots of time to recovery from stem cell donation (first donations performed from November 2001 through March 2006). *(From* Biol Blood Marrow Transplant. *14[9 Suppl]:29–36, 2008, doi: 10.1016/j. bbmt.2008.05.018.)*

autologous patients may be greater, reflecting previous chemotherapy given to these patients causing decreased marrow cellularity. Donors for pediatric recipients will lose proportionately less blood. Most patients and donors receive blood transfusions to alleviate symptoms of volume depletion. With proper preharvest autologous blood storage, use of homologous blood for healthy first-time allogeneic donors should be extremely rare. For a blood loss of less than 10 mL/ kg of donor weight, salt solutions are acceptable for volume replacement. Colloid solutions, such as hydroxyethyl starch, can be used to avoid homologous blood transfusion for blood losses between 10 and 20 mL/kg donor weight. Blood transfusion will be required for larger blood losses (>20 mL/kg) or for patients with comorbid illnesses. Homologous blood transfusions must be irradiated to prevent transfusion-associated GVHD in the transplant recipient caused by "passenger lymphocytes" from the third-party blood donor. Donors undergoing a second harvest shortly after the first harvest are more likely to require homologous blood.[24] Oral iron supplements should be considered for healthy donors, particularly for female donors or donors from whom a proportionately large blood volume is to be harvested.

COLLECTION OF UMBILICAL CORD BLOOD STEM CELLS FOR TRANSPLANTATION

Cord Blood Collection Techniques

Advantages of this source of HSCs include the ability of public cord blood banks to target collections from ethnic-minority populations not well represented in the various unrelated donor registries and the relative immaturity of the donor immune system allowing transplantation of HLA-mismatched units without overwhelming GVHD. The primary obstacle to the widespread use of cord blood cells is the limited quantity of HSCs collected, and one public UCB bank predicted that from less than 5% to less than 38% (depending on the cell dose criterion for transplantation) of the units stored in that bank would be acceptable for transplantation of an 80-kg adult patient.[43] The speed and success of engraftment are predicted by the total nucleated cell dose and, more important, by the quantity of CD34+ cells or infused colony-forming units (CFUs).[44]

UCB is collected from the placental vein after delivery of the infant and transection of the cord, either before delivery of the placenta by the obstetrician or by laboratory personnel after delivery of the placenta.[43] Published reports conflict regarding the volume of UCB collected and the likelihood of obtaining a product inadequate

for storage with either in utero or ex utero collection techniques. The timing of cord clamping after delivery of the infant is associated with the volume of cord blood collected, and greater volumes are collected with earlier clamping. Greater cell quantities were found for infants with greater birth weight, but no difference was found based on gender or gestational age. Ethnic background appears to predict the cell quantities, with smaller quantities of cells collected from ethnic minorities compared with whites.[45] UCB is usually collected by cannulation of the umbilical cord veins with aspiration of the blood into a collection bag. Collection of cord blood into open containers results in an unacceptable rate of bacterial contamination. Perfusion of the placenta with salt solutions may increase the cell number collected, but this technique has not been widely adopted. Many cord blood banks reduce the volume of the product by red cell and plasma depletion to minimize storage space and to reduce possible infusion-related toxicities from mature blood cells contained in unfractionated cord blood units.[46] Bacterial contamination of UCB products is of concern, especially in the collection of products for related donor transplantation by obstetricians with limited or no experience in HSC collection and processing.[47] The identification and evaluation of the donor and the collection techniques used should be viewed as the first steps in a manufacturing process with adequately validated procedures, personnel training, quality control, and performance improvement oversight.

COLLECTION OF PERIPHERAL BLOOD STEM CELLS FOR TRANSPLANTATION

Background

The presence of HSCs in the peripheral circulation was suggested by animal studies as early as 1951.[48] Although the nature of the survival agent was not recognized at that time, parabiosis experiments demonstrated that some factor in the blood of a healthy animal was able to rescue another animal from the effects of lethal irradiation. Subsequently, a number of animal models demonstrated the presence of HSCs in the peripheral blood and the successful use of these cells to rescue animals from the marrow-lethal effects of radiation. The concentration of HSCs in the peripheral blood is normally very low, requiring the processing of large quantities of blood to collect the quantity of HSCs equivalent to what could be collected in a bone marrow harvest. For this reason, PBSC transplantation was initially used by a few transplant programs that explored this source of HSCs for patients who otherwise were ineligible for marrow harvesting, collecting cells during steady-state hematopoiesis or during the transient increase in circulating HSCs that occurred during recovery from marrow hypoplasia-producing chemotherapy.[49–53] These early reports noted that engraftment could be achieved sooner after infusion of PBSC components compared with marrow cell transplantation. However, because of the occasionally limited quantity of HSCs that was collected from the peripheral blood, the kinetics of engraftment for some patients was considerably slower. The effective mobilization of HSCs achieved by cytokine or chemokine administration,[54–56] and the reliability of same-day flow cytometric analysis in assessing the quality of the collection, are the direct bases for the rapid and widespread adoption of PBSCs as a source of HSCs for transplantation (see box on Mobilization and Collection of Peripheral Blood Stem Cell for Autologous Transplantation).

Mobilization of Hematopoietic Stem Cells Into Peripheral Blood

The self-renewal and differentiation of HSCs is controlled by the surrounding microenvironment of the stem cell niche(s) in which the HSC reside.[57] These niches are composed of a complex three-dimensional architecture of a variety of cell types including sinusoidal endothelial cells, sympathetic nerve fibers, cells of the osteoblastic

---

Mobilization and Collection of Peripheral Blood Stem Cells for Autologous PBSC Transplantation

Five important considerations when prescribing a mobilization regimen for collection of peripheral blood stem cells (PBSCs) for autologous transplantation are as follows: (1) A regimen of chemotherapy followed by granulocyte colony-stimulating factor (G-CSF) results in higher numbers of circulating CD34⁺ cells than will be found with G-CSF alone. (2) The choice of chemotherapy (or cytokine alone mobilization) should be appropriate to the disease and stage of disease for the patient. (3) Each cycle of prior chemotherapy and any previous treatment with radiotherapy will decrease the response to mobilization therapy. (4) Tumor infiltration of the marrow will increase the probability of circulating tumor cells and will decrease the response to mobilization therapy. (5) Some patients will benefit from tandem cycles of dose-intense therapy, and the prescription should target adequate quantities of CD34⁺ cells for these patients. With these considerations in mind, elective collection of PBSCs either before extensive treatment or after a limited number of cycles of debulking chemotherapy should be considered. Additional cycles of chemotherapy can be given after PBSC collection is completed, for those patients who require further tumor reduction before proceeding to transplantation. The timing of apheresis after chemotherapy and G-CSF mobilization is best guided by measurement of the level of peripheral blood CD34⁺ cells. Daily or every-other-day quantification of these cells can be initiated after the white blood cell count reaches 1000/μL. Patients with poor mobilization of CD34⁺ cells should be considered for large-volume apheresis or addition of a chemokine such as plerixafor to reduce the costs associated with daily doses of G-CSF, laboratory testing, apheresis procedures, and cryopreservation. Patients who fail to mobilize may have successful collections if given a short drug "holiday" before undergoing mobilization with high-dose G-CSF with plerixafor.

---

lineage, macrophages, and mesenchymal stem cells that are responsible for controlling the balance between HSC quiescence, self-renewal, and differentiation. A number of pathways with mutually recognized cellular adhesion molecules and their respective ligands responsible for the spontaneous migration of HSCs from the stem cell niche, as well as the multistep process of homing back into the niche, have been identified.[58] The mechanisms by which granulocyte colony-stimulating factor (G-CSF) and other cytokines promote mobilization of HSCs are being elucidated and appear to be an indirect effect (HSCs do not express receptors for G-CSF) on the CXC-chemokine receptor 4 (CXCR4)/stromal cell–derived factor-1 (SDF-1) axis mediated by monocytes and the sympathetic nervous system.[57] The mechanisms of mobilization by chemotherapy and CXCR4 antagonists such as plerixafor are also being determined, and the elucidation of the mechanisms of mobilization and homing may result in more effective harvesting and transplantation techniques.[59]

Cytokine Mobilization

The ability of recombinant hematopoietic cytokines to increase the level of myeloid progenitor cells in the blood, as well as mature blood cells, was reported in 1988 by different groups for both G-CSF and granulocyte-macrophage colony-stimulating factor (GM-CSF).[60,61] Subsequently, a number of different investigators reported the collection of PBSCs from patients using a variety of mobilization regimens, including cytokines alone, cytokine combinations, and combinations of chemotherapy with cytokines. Various other recombinant human hematopoietic cytokines, including erythropoietin and fusion molecules, increase the quantity of CD34⁺ cells in the peripheral blood but have not been developed for clinical transplantation.

Granulocyte Colony-Stimulating Factors Including Biosimilars

G-CSF is the cytokine most commonly used because of its efficacy compared with other cytokines and its relatively benign toxicity

profile. Recombinant methionyl human G-CSF (filgrastim) and recombinant human G-CSF (lenograstim) were the two forms of this cytokine initially available for clinical use.[62] There are slight differences between these two similar cytokines in their ability to mobilize PBSCs. Watts and colleagues[63] studied 20 healthy volunteers and found that peak levels of colony-forming unit–granulocyte-macrophages (CFU-GMs) in the peripheral blood were 28% higher after treatment with the glycosylated molecule (lenograstim), attributed to the higher specific activity of this form. De Arriba and colleagues[64] treated 30 women with breast cancer in a randomized study of these two drugs, using dosages containing bioequivalent units of activity and found no difference in mobilization of CD34⁺ cells. The two forms have otherwise similar biologic activity and are not further distinguished in this discussion.

Regulatory agencies including the United States Food and Drug Administration (US FDA), the European Medicines Agency, and others established regulatory pathways leading to approval of biologic medicines that are highly similar to an already-approved biologic product ("biosimilar").[65,66] In the US, The Biologics Price Competition and Innovation Act of 2009 created an abbreviated licensure pathway for biological products shown to be "biosimilar" to or "interchangeable" with an FDA-licensed biologic product, known as the "reference product." This abbreviated licensure pathway permits reliance on existing scientific knowledge about the safety and effectiveness of the reference product, and enables a biosimilar biologic product to be licensed based on less than a full complement of product-specific preclinical and clinical data usually required before marketing of a new drug. The biosimilar must show it has no clinically meaningful differences in terms of safety and effectiveness from the reference product. Only minor differences in clinically inactive components are allowable. Filgrastim-sndz is the first biosimilar drug approved by the US FDA, and is marketed with the same indication for use as filgrastim. Tbo-filgrastim, however, was licensed under a different mechanism, and does not have US FDA approval for use in PBPC collection. The use of a biosimilar G-CSF in mobilization of PBPCs must be extrapolated from laboratory data such as mobilization of CD34⁺ cells, and it is conceivable, although considered very unlikely, that differences in the mobilization of stem and other cells, as well as in toxicity to the donor, may occur.[67,68] Clinical experience describing similar mobilization results are now being reported for these drugs.[69]

Mobilization of Hematopoietic Stem Cells Using Granulocyte Colony-Stimulating Factor

G-CSF is the most potent cytokine currently available for mobilization of HSCs. In a randomized study of healthy volunteers comparing G-CSF, GM-CSF, and the combination of both, Lane and colleagues[70] reported an average 0.99% CD34⁺ cells in the peripheral blood of healthy donors treated with 10 μg/kg per day of G-CSF compared with 0.25% for donors treated with the same dose of GM-CSF. The quantity of CD34⁺ cells in the peripheral blood before treatment averaged 1.6/μL. After GM-CSF treatment, the level increased to 3/μL, but with G-CSF, the level increased to 61/μL. Each group underwent one leukapheresis on the 5th day of treatment, and the collections from donors treated with G-CSF averaged 119 × 10⁶ CD34⁺ cells compared with 12.6 × 10⁶ for the donors treated with GM-CSF.

The appearance of CD34⁺ cells during administration of G-CSF follows a distinct time course, with the maximal level of CD34⁺ cells occurring on day 5 after daily G-CSF administration.[71] Smaller numbers of CD34⁺ are present on days 4 and 6, and the level falls rapidly on subsequent days despite a continual rise in white blood cell (WBC) count.

The number of CD34⁺ cells collected after G-CSF treatment is proportional to the number of these cells in the peripheral blood before initiation of the cytokine.[18] Although doses as low as 5 mcg/kg/day have been used, there is a dose response to G-CSF, with higher average levels of CD34⁺ cells achieved with 10 mcg/kg/day compared with 5 mcg/kg/day.[72] With appropriate dosing of allogeneic donors, adequate numbers of CD34[+] cells can be collected in one procedure for transplantation of most patients. A similar dose response is observed in autologous patients and may extend to doses as high as 40 mcg/kg/day.[72] An advantage to twice-daily dosing of G-CSF has been suggested but not confirmed. Anderlini and colleagues[73] compared administration of 6 mcg/kg given twice daily with 12 mcg/kg given once daily and found no differences in CD34[+] cells per liter of blood processed during the apheresis procedure or the total yield of CD34[+] cells per kilogram collected. In contrast, a second trial enrolling primarily pediatric patients noted better results with the twice-daily schedule.[74] Patients, especially those previously treated with chemotherapy or radiotherapy, will generally have lower quantities of CD34[+] cells mobilized.[59]

Toxicity and Complications of Granulocyte Colony-Stimulating Factor

The toxicity of G-CSF has been most clearly defined in studies of allogeneic donors.[30,75,76] The autologous patient will experience a similar toxicity profile, but with the added complications of the underlying malignancy and its treatment.

Almost all recipients of G-CSF will develop somatic complaints, of which skeletal pain is most prominent (see Fig. 95.1), but also including fatigue, insomnia, and nausea.[30,37,38,41,75-77] The somatic complaints are generally tolerable, and few donors will require reduction in dose or discontinuation of the medicine. At present, there appear to be minimal, if any, long-term health risks for the donor. Few serious complications of the mobilization regimen and donation process have been reported.[77] G-CSF increases spleen size, with a rare patient or donor experiencing splenic rupture. G-CSF may induce a hypercoagulable state, which is of concern for donors (and patients) requiring central venous catheter placement or for those who may have other risk factors for the development of deep venous thrombosis (such as air travel immediately after the collection procedures). Patients with autoimmune disorders may experience a flare-up of their disease during administration of G-CSF, and a variety of case reports of ophthalmologic and other adverse events have been reported for healthy donors or patients treated with G-CSF.

Of concern is the possibility that cytokine administration will increase the risk for marrow dysplasia or malignancy. Although this is a theoretical concern in that these cytokines are known to stimulate growth of leukemia cells, no clinical evidence from large registry reviews of healthy donor experiences indicates that these agents will induce abnormalities in the hematopoietic stem cell.[77,78]

G-CSF administration results in a number of changes in blood counts and chemistries in addition to the coagulation factor changes. Alanine aminotransferase, lactate dehydrogenase, and alkaline phosphatase levels increase, and the levels of blood urea nitrogen and bilirubin may decrease.[76] The elevation in alkaline phosphatase level is primarily of bone origin; γ-glutamyl transferase levels remain normal. These abnormalities of serum chemistries resolve within 2 weeks after discontinuation of the medication. G-CSF administration also will result in a decrease in platelet count, especially if the cytokine is administered over 5 to 10 days.[76] WBC counts fall rapidly after discontinuation of G-CSF. In approximately 10% of donors, the WBC count may fall to abnormal levels (but generally still remain above 1000/μL), reaching a nadir 10 to 14 days after discontinuation of the cytokine before stabilizing at normal levels.

Granulocyte-Macrophage Colony-Stimulating Factor

Much of the early experience with the use of hematopoietic cytokines for mobilization of HSCs involved GM-CSF and chemotherapy.[61,79] GM-CSF is not as potent as G-CSF,[70,79] although as with G-CSF, there is a dose response in mobilization of PBSCs with GM-CSF over a range from 0.3 to 30 mcg/kg/day, without a plateau.[80] In this dose-ranging study, however, the average increase in CFU-GM in the blood at this highest dose level again was only 8.4-fold. In a randomized study comparing GM-CSF with G-CSF, or both drugs used in sequence after chemotherapy administration, patients had faster recovery of counts, required less supportive care including transfusions, and achieved greater collections of CD34+ cells if given one of the G-CSF–containing regimens.[79]

Administration of GM-CSF results in somatic complaints and hepatic function abnormalities similar to those reported after G-CSF administration. In addition, 44% to 80% of patients experience fever, sometimes after each dose, as well as generalized or local skin reactions. Doses greater than 20 mcg/kg/day are poorly tolerated because of fluid retention, pleural and pericardial inflammation, and venous thrombosis. A "first-dose reaction", characterized by hypoxia and hypotension occurring within 3 hours of administration, has been described for some recipients, especially after intravenous administration.

Other Hematopoietic Cytokines

Recognition of the mobilization potential of G-CSF led many investigators to study other hematopoietic cytokines, including erythropoietin, monocyte–colony-stimulating factor, interleukin (IL)-3, PIXY 321 (a fusion molecule), and stem cell factor (SCF) for their capacity to mobilize HSCS into the peripheral blood. Used as single agents, these cytokines resulted in only an approximately 5- to 10-fold increase in circulating CFU-GM or CD34[+] cells.

Chemotherapy Plus Cytokine Mobilization

The number of HSCs in the peripheral blood is moderately increased during the early hematologic recovery phase after marrow hypoplasia-producing chemotherapy. Chemotherapy plus cytokine generally mobilizes greater numbers of PBSCs than either agent alone. This finding was confirmed in a randomized study comparing cyclophosphamide followed by G-CSF versus G-CSF alone, in which higher numbers of CD34 cells were found for the patients treated with the chemotherapy-based regimen.[81] However, no differences in the degree of tumor cell contamination of PBSC components, speed of hematological recovery after transplantation, or survival probability were found. A wide variety of different chemotherapy regimens has been used successfully for mobilization of HSCs into the blood, with cyclophosphamide- or ifosfamide-based regimens being most commonly used. The primary consideration is that the choice of chemotherapy used for mobilization must also meet the treatment needs of the patient. Demirer and colleagues[82] studied the effect of different chemotherapy regimens for mobilization of HSCs for patients with breast cancer. Four regimens were used, all involving cyclophosphamide (CY), but including etoposide with or without cisplatin, or paclitaxel. All patients also received G-CSF. The median quantity of CD34[+] cells collected on the first day of apheresis after cyclophosphamide mobilization was 0.9×10^6 per kilogram of patient weight. The addition of etoposide and then of etoposide and cisplatin increased the first-day yield to 8.1×10^6 and 3.5×10^6 CD34[+] cells/kg, respectively, in separate cohorts of patients. The median number of CD34[+] cells harvested on the first day of apheresis after cyclophosphamide plus paclitaxel was 11.1×10^6/kg, and more than 50% of the women mobilized with this last regimen achieved the target dose of CD34[+] cells in one apheresis procedure. Of the 100 women studied, 94 achieved the target dose of greater than 5×10^6 CD34[+] cells/kg. Only four patients failed to reach a lower but acceptable dose of 2.5×10^6 CD34[+] cells/kg.

Chemokines

Chemokines (chemoattractant cytokines) are a family of approximately 40 related small proteins that influence leukocyte (and malignant cell) migration and function.[83] Chemokines with varying effects on different WBC populations have been identified, as have a number of chemokine receptors. The roles of chemokines and chemokine receptors in the trafficking of HSCs into and from the bone marrow compartment are under active investigation.[84]

In a preclinical study, administration to both mice and rhesus monkeys of a modified CXC chemokine growth-related oncogene-β after 4 days of G-CSF resulted in a fivefold increase in the number of circulating stem and progenitor cells compared with G-CSF alone, with also a much shorter time course of release, measured in hours.[85] Furthermore, more rapid recovery of hematopoietic function was observed for animals given similar quantities of cells collected after administration of the chemokine and cytokine combination. IL-8, a related ligand for the CXCR2, mobilizes stem cells within 15 to 30 minutes of injection into mice,[86] which appears to involve increased matrix metalloproteinase-9 activity detectable immediately before the appearance of HSCs in the peripheral circulation. Murine studies demonstrate a mobilizing effect of the chemokine SDF-1 and its receptor CXCR4 that can be blocked by neutralizing antibodies to either.[86] The bicyclam molecule plerixafor disrupts SDF-1/CXCR4 binding and has been shown to result in mobilization of HSC in murine, canine, and nonhuman transplant models.

Similar signaling pathways are used for mobilization and homing of normal and malignant hematopoietic cells.[87] Although PBSC products collected after G-CSF mobilization generally contain fewer detectable tumor cells than does bone marrow harvested from the same patient, the effects of chemokine treatment on the degree of PBSC contamination and on disease relapse after autologous transplantation remain to be elucidated. For example, acute myelogenous leukemia cells express CXCR4 in varying levels and homing of primary human acute myeloid leukemia cells into nonobese diabetic/severe combined immunodeficiency mice is CXCR4 dependent, similar to normal human stem cells. Similar studies of chemokine control on tumor cell growth, migration, and metastasis are being reported from a number of laboratories. There are now reports of a possibly increased risk of posttransplant myelodysplasia or acute leukemia after transplantation using plerixafor-mobilized cells,[88] although others have reported that poor mobilizers (who are more likely to receive this chemokine) have a higher risk of posttransplant myelodysplasia,[89] complicating determination of causation of this complication of transplantation.

Plerixafor

Plerixafor (AMD3100) is a small-molecule inhibitor of CXCR4. Clinical studies of HSC mobilization using plerixafor with or without G-CSF priming are being reported in both healthy donors and patients undergoing autologous or allogeneic HSC transplantation. In a study involving normal volunteers, a single dose of plerixafor was equal in mobilization of CD34$^+$ cells to administration of a standard 5-day course of G-CSF.[90] However, a single dose of plerixafor given on day 5 of a daily course of G-CSF administration resulted in a further 3.8-fold increase in circulating CD34$^+$ cells (as well as B and T cells, which may be important in allogeneic transplantation). Randomized phase III studies conducted in patients undergoing autologous PBSC transplantation in the treatment of multiple myeloma or non-Hodgkin lymphoma demonstrated a clear increase in CD34$^+$ cells collected by the addition of plerixafor to filgrastim.[91,92] Plerixafor was also effective in remobilization attempts for patients who failed initial collection goals.[93] Plerixafor clearance is proportional to the degree of renal function in patients with renal failure.[94] Minor gastrointestinal symptoms appear to be the most common toxicities of this medication.

Strategies for the Patient Who Is Difficult to Mobilize

Most patients achieve the targeted dose of CD34$^+$ cells after processing 20 to 30 L of blood in one to three apheresis procedures. However, approximately 5% to as many as 30% of patients in various series have inadequate collections because only small numbers of HSCs are present in the peripheral blood despite the administration of hematopoietic cytokines. Of note, the number of days of apheresis also predicts the kinetics of neutrophil engraftment independent of the CD34$^+$ cell dose infused, indicating an undefined measurement of graft quality, probably a reflection of the various quantities of CD34$^+$ cell subsets and CD34$^-$ stem cells, as well as the characteristics of the stem cell niche.[95] Patient-specific factors predictive of poor mobilization include older age, marrow disease, prior radiotherapy, and prior chemotherapy.[59] Approximately 50% of patients who fail to achieve the targeted dose of CD34$^+$ cells will achieve this goal on a second attempt. High-dose (15 mg/kg twice daily) G-CSF after a 2- to 4-week drug holiday to allow marrow recovery is one strategy. Combination cytokine therapy is also of potential value in this situation, and the combination of SCF with G-CSF may be effective for patients who reside in countries where SCF is available. The addition of GM-CSF to G-CSF is not of proven value. The addition of plerixafor will often be effective when used in combination with G-CSF for collection of PBSCs from patients who failed a prior mobilization attempt.[93] Treatment with the use of cyclophosphamide- or ifosfamide-based mobilizing chemotherapy plus a cytokine regimen also will be effective, but will be associated with increased toxicity.[96] Bone marrow collection is very unlikely to achieve an acceptable product in that the poor mobilization of PBSCs predicts for a poor marrow harvest. Patients who fail initial collection attempts will frequently fail subsequent attempts, and transplantation of these patients with a lower dose of CD34$^+$ cells (as low as 1×10^6 CD34$^+$ cells/kg) may be an option.

It is, therefore, strongly preferable to avoid collection failure. Consideration should be given to the prophylactic collection of PBSCs early in the course of treatment for patients who later may be candidates for autologous HSC transplantation but who are advised to receive multiple courses of therapy or therapy involving alkylating agents or radiation therapy. HSCs can be collected and cryopreserved before extensive therapy while the patient has good marrow function and stored for years without obvious progressive loss of engraftment potential.

Timing of Apheresis

A major problem with chemotherapy-based mobilization regimens is the difficulty in determining the optimal time to commence HSC collection. Apheresis devices can collect only those CD34$^+$ cells actually being released into and circulating in the peripheral blood. It is possible to estimate the quantity of CD34$^+$ cells that will be collected during apheresis by multiplying the quantity of CD34$^+$ cells in the blood by the total volume of blood processed during the apheresis procedure and by the efficiency of the apheresis device in collecting these cells. If the device has an efficiency of 50% and the patient undergoes a 10-L exchange, approximately 5×10^7 CD34$^+$ cells will be collected for a peripheral blood level of 10 CD34$^+$ cells/μL and 5×10^8 CD34$^+$ cells for a blood level of CD34$^+$ cells that is 10-fold higher. Although many protocols call for initiation of apheresis after chemotherapy mobilization when the WBC count has recovered to greater than 1000/μL, there is a poor, if any, correlation between the peripheral blood white cell or mononuclear cell counts and the CD34$^+$ cells in the peripheral blood. Characteristics that suggest a higher CD34$^+$ cell level are a rapidly rising WBC count, shift in differential to immature myeloid cells, circulating nucleated red cells, and platelet transfusion independence. However, it is much more cost effective to obtain an actual measurement of CD34$^+$ cells in the blood and to time the apheresis collection when these cells are present in adequate numbers. Fig. 95.3 shows such a relationship for patients with lower concentrations of CD34$^+$ cells in the peripheral blood and illustrates the very poor collections obtained when the peripheral blood CD34$^+$ count is less than 10/μL. Although there is considerable error in the enumeration of CD34$^+$ cells at levels less than 5/μL, this error is not clinically relevant because even a doubling of the CD34$^+$ cells in this low range still results in a very poor apheresis yield.

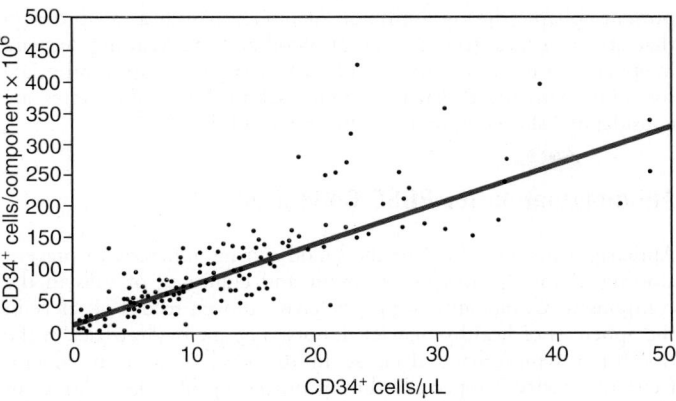

Fig. 95.3 RELATIONSHIP BETWEEN QUANTITY OF CD34+ CELLS IN THE PERIPHERAL BLOOD AND NUMBER COLLECTED BY APHERESIS USING APHERESIS AND FLOW CYTOMETRIC TECHNIQUES. Data shown are limited to peripheral blood CD34+ cell numbers <50.0/μL ($n = 157$, $r = 0.82$, $p < .001$).

Physician Prescription for Apheresis and Peripheral Blood Stem Cell Processing

The attending physician should be aware of apheresis and laboratory procedures in order to maximize the value of peripheral blood stem cell (PBSC) products. The choices of venous access, anticoagulant(s), blood volume processed, target dose of CD34+ cells, and cryopreservation volumes can be individualized. Apheresis unit staff may ask for guidance regarding pain medications, concurrent medications, and blood transfusions (although it is advisable to avoid transfusion during the apheresis procedure because of citrate or other reactions, and because changes in the hematocrit may affect the efficiency of the collection). Adequate numbers of CD34+ cells can be collected for more than one cycle of chemotherapy. It is important to communicate with the cryopreservation facility if PBSC components will be used to support more than one cycle of chemotherapy or if dimethyl sulfoxide toxicity is of concern, in order to facilitate appropriate packaging of each product. Current cytometric techniques for quantification of CD34+ cells require at least 1 hour of processing, so it may not be practical to prescribe the number of CD34+ cells to be frozen in each bag. However, it is possible to divide the component into the number of bags equaling the number of anticipated infusions so that equal numbers of CD34+ cells will be available for each.

The level of CD34+ cells in the peripheral blood at which to start apheresis is a clinical decision. Although levels in the range of 50–100/μL or greater will reduce the number of apheresis procedures necessary to achieve a target goal of CD34+ cells, each day's delay in initiating apheresis incurs the costs of additional cytokine administration and blood testing. In some patients who previously have undergone extensive treatment and who may show a slowly rising WBC count, multiple apheresis procedures may be necessary to achieve the target goal. No patient should undergo apheresis if the peripheral blood CD34+ cell count is less than 5/μL (see Fig. 95.3). For patients with CD34+ cell counts in the range of 10–20/μL, it is possible to process more blood per day using large-volume leukapheresis (LVL) techniques, thereby reducing the numbers of days the patients are required to return to the apheresis unit. Most patients mobilized with chemotherapy have a rising CD34+ cell count in the peripheral blood, so starting apheresis the day after the patient has achieved a desirable CD34+ level generally is feasible.[97]

The timing of apheresis after G-CSF mobilization differs from the timing after chemotherapy and cytokine mobilization. For both patients and healthy donors, the peak concentration of CD34+ cells occurs on day 5 of G-CSF administration (after 4 daily doses).[71] Lower levels are present on day 4, and the concentration continues to fall after day 6, even if cytokine administration is continued and despite a possible continued rise in WBC count. Thus, PBSC collection should be initiated on day 4 or 5 of G-CSF administration. The kinetics of CD34+ cells in the peripheral blood for patients and donors mobilized with G-CSF alone are so reliable that monitoring of peripheral blood levels is not necessary unless there is concern that the patient has failed to mobilize cells and it is practical to obtain the cell count rapidly enough to initiate apheresis on the same day.

Timing of Apheresis Using Plerixafor

Plerixafor administration results in a rapid mobilization of HSCs into the peripheral blood, with peak CD34+ cell and CFU-GM concentrations occurring about 6 to 10 hours but with a wide range of activity extending to over 24 hours after administration of a dose of 240 mcg/kg.[98–100] The initial phase III studies demonstrating the efficacy of this agent in patients failing to mobilize adequate cells with G-CSF alone required administration of plerixafor about 10 hours before apheresis, and then daily administration of plerixafor on the same schedule until completion of collections. The broad duration of activity may allow alternate timing schedules and, conceivably, two apheresis procedures after one dose of plerixafor (particularly for patients with renal impairment[94]). Although rigorous clinical studies

addressing alternate timing schedules have not been performed, small studies have demonstrated the ability to collect PBSCs with alternate schedules.[101,102] In a study of 11 patients who failed two previous attempts to collect PBSCs using G-CSF alone, Lefrere et al[102] found an early rise in circulating CD34+ cells, as early as 3 hours, with a fall in circulating CD34+ cells occurring after 8–12 hours.

Collection of PBSCs by Apheresis

A number of apheresis devices are available for separating HSCs from the peripheral blood. The devices may be classified as continuous flow (e.g., Fenwal CS3000, COBE Spectra, Spectra Optia, Fenwal Amicus) or discontinuous flow (e.g., Haemonetics family of equipment). Discontinuous-flow devices have the advantage of requiring only a single venous access. Continuous-flow devices require two access lines for aspiration and return of blood, but they process much larger volumes of blood in a shorter period of time. All apheresis devices collect HSCs. Continuous-flow devices are more efficient in the collection of PBSCs and are, accordingly, preferred over discontinuous-flow devices (see box on Physician Prescription for Apheresis and Peripheral Blood Stem Cell Processing). The ideal apheresis device will have: a high efficiency of CD34+ cell collection with minimal contamination of the product by mature blood cells such as granulocytes, which complicate subsequent processing and can increase infusion toxicity; rapid blood processing with minimal anticoagulant use reducing toxicity to the donor; and minimal depletion of platelets. The various apheresis devices, in general, have similar efficacies in collecting CD34+ cells from the peripheral blood, but may vary in processing time, and in final product volume and mature blood cell contamination.[103]

Apheresis Technology

Apheresis technology is widely used for collection of platelets and other blood products from healthy donors and is considered to be without major risk to the donor. The important safety considerations for PBSC collection are the same as for platelet collection and include the venous access to be used for the procedure, the extracorporeal volume of blood during the procedure, and the solutions administered to the donor. Of note, however, PBSC collection for autologous transplantation involves patients with underlying medical conditions who may require considerable nursing care during the procedure. In a prospective evaluation of 2408 healthy unrelated volunteer donors, apheresis-associated adverse events were reported by 20% of female donors ($n = 964$) and 7% of male donors ($n = 1444$) on the first day of apheresis, falling to 10% and 4%, respectively, on the second day of collection (if performed).[77] Most (51%) of reported adverse events were related to citrate infusion. A smaller proportion of donors (22%) reported problems with venous access. Rare (1–6% of events) adverse events included hypertension or hypotension, allergic reactions, fatigue, and syncope. The placement of a central venous catheter was required by 17% of female donors and 4% of male donors. Also, larger-volume and repetitive exchanges will result in platelet depletion.[76] The platelet count may reach its nadir several days after completion of the apheresis collections and discontinuation of G-CSF, and donors should be counseled in this regard.

Important caveats are that the donors in this analysis from the unrelated donor registry met strictly defined health criteria and were between 18 and 69 years of age. A higher probability of adverse events may be expected in patients and in donors of older (or younger) age. For example, in an older retrospective publication, Goldberg and colleagues[104] studied the complications occurring during 554 PBSC collections from 75 consecutive patients. Patient diagnoses and the mobilization treatment regimens were varied. All but one patient had subclavian or jugular venous system catheters placed for apheresis. A median of nine collections per patient were performed using a discontinuous-flow apheresis device. The most common problems were related to the venous catheters: 50% of patients developed at least one occlusion. Hypocalcemia occurred in 14.6% of patients and hypotension in 13.3%. Sixteen percent of patients experienced infectious complications during the PBSC collection period.

Staffing of the apheresis unit should be appropriate for the medical condition of the patients undergoing apheresis. Staffing must include nurses familiar with the care of the oncologic patient who may be recovering from marrow hypoplasia complicated by neutropenic fever requiring multiple medications and the care of a central venous catheter. Collection of PBSCs by apheresis in the outpatient setting should be performed only after careful review of the medical support requirements for the individual patient or donor, and it should never be assumed to be a safer alternative for the donor or patient with a serious comorbid illness than marrow harvesting conducted in the intensive care setting of the operating room.

Venous Access

Adequate venous access is required for optimal apheresis technique. Continuous-flow apheresis devices require two-lumen access with a stable blood flow capacity generally greater than 20 mL/min. Single-lumen access may be used with discontinuous-flow apheresis devices, although at a much slower rate of blood processing. The great majority ($\approx$95%) of adult male allogeneic PBSC donors have adequate arm veins for the procedure to be conducted "vein to vein," with female donors more likely to require alternate venous access.[77] Some donors, especially those with small veins and undergoing several daily procedures, may require placement of a temporary venous catheter. Venous access for the patient undergoing collection for autologous PBSC transplantation is much more heterogeneous. Vein-to-vein procedures can be performed, even on several consecutive days, with proper phlebotomy technique and postcollection care of the phlebotomy site. Most patients received previous chemotherapy or are proceeding directly to transplantation, conditions for which tunneled access is commonly placed. Ideally, this venous access should be appropriate both for the apheresis procedures and the subsequent transplant. Length, lumen size, and wall stiffness all affect the blood flow that can be achieved through a catheter. For this reason, the commonly used dual-lumen Hickman or Broviac catheters are usually unsuitable for apheresis, as are all subcutaneously placed ports. Most triple-lumen catheters are inadequate because of the small lumen size. If such access is already in place, consideration can be given to replacement with a shorter, stiffer tunneled catheter or to placement of a temporary percutaneous dialysis/apheresis catheter. The catheters designed for dialysis and apheresis have adequate wall thickness to

prevent collapse during aspiration of blood, as well as a tip design that decreases local recirculation of blood and the resulting decrease in apheresis efficiency. Catheters of 10 F or larger size are appropriate for adult patients. Pediatric patients, whose blood flow rates are considerably slower, may use catheter sizes of 5–7 F.[105]

Anticoagulation for PBSC Collection

Anticoagulants are added to the blood during apheresis to prevent clotting of the extracorporeal circuit and clumping of cells in the component. Citrate anticoagulants have a proven record of safety in the apheresis of healthy platelet donors. The major drawback is the risk for a symptomatic decrease in the level of ionized calcium ("citrate toxicity"), especially during processing of large volumes of blood. Citrate ions chelate calcium ions (and other divalent cations such as magnesium), making them unavailable for Ca^{2+}-dependent metabolic reactions. ACD-A contains 10.67 g of citrate per 500-mL volume in the form of trisodium citrate and citric acid. Citrate is diffused throughout the extravascular space, and this diffusion is the first defense against citrate toxicity. The body size and difference in muscle mass between men and women results in an increased risk for citrate toxicity for women in particular and smaller donors in general. Metabolism by liver, kidney, and muscle also reduces the concentration of citrate. Metabolism of citrate becomes an important clinical consideration during processing of larger blood volumes or at higher rates of blood flow. The initial signs of citrate toxicity include circumoral or acral paresthesias and may progress to nausea, vomiting, loss of consciousness, tetany, and seizures. Because pediatric patients may not be able to relate the initial symptoms of the condition, citrate toxicity should be considered as the cause of any change of behavior, such as crying, during the apheresis procedure. Citrate toxicity is prevented by limiting the quantity of citrate infused either by decreasing the blood flow rate through the apheresis device or changing the blood-to-citrate ratio. The processing of blood from patients experiencing the initial symptoms of citrate toxicity should be temporarily halted until the symptoms abate and then resumed at a slower rate. The benefit of oral calcium supplements for these patients is not proven and may cause abdominal discomfort. Heparin can be used as a replacement for some or all of the citrate, although additional citrate should be added to the component bag to prevent clumping of platelets. Some centers that use citrate anticoagulants also administer intermittent or continuous infusions of calcium gluconate during the procedure, especially if large volumes of blood are being processed. However, excessive calcium replacement can induce cardiac dysfunction.

Large-Volume Leukapheresis

The apheresis device has a uniform and fairly reproducible efficiency of collection. Thus, for a consistent quantity of blood processed through the machine, the quantity of CD34+ cells collected is directly related to the number present in the peripheral blood. Greater quantities of CD34+ cells can be collected by increasing the number of these cells in the peripheral circulation or by increasing the volume of blood processed in each procedure (LVL). For patients with lower CD34+ cell levels, multiple apheresis procedures will be required to achieve the target dose of CD34+ cells needed for transplantation. An alternate approach is to process the same total quantity of blood but in fewer, longer procedures. LVL is not standardly defined, but in general usage it refers to processing of more than two or three times the patient's blood volume. Typically, the quantity of blood processed is six or more times the patient's blood volume, often 25–36 L of blood. The advantage of LVL is that it reduces the number of days of cytokine administration and apheresis, with associated reduced costs of laboratory processing and testing. The apheresis techniques are the same as those used for processing of smaller volumes of blood, although blood flow rates may be increased to reduce the time required. The risks of LVL are the increased time required and the

TABLE 95.1	Replenishment of CD34+ Cells During Large-Volume Leukapheresis[a]				
			CD34+ Cells		
UPN	Blood (per µL)	Blood (Total)	Harvested (Total)	Released (Total)	Released (per min)
10,605	6.5	34.9	123.5	88.6	0.3
10,698	15.6	603.3	1438.1	540.8	2.1
10,849	30.7	109.7	211.1	62.6	0.3
10,920	37.9	214.2	952.8	57.0	1.6
11,128	66.1	280.6	1010.8	532.7	1.9

[a]Shown are numbers of CD34+ cells in the peripheral blood or apheresis component for five patients with acute myelogenous leukemia or multiple myeloma undergoing large-volume leukapheresis after granulocyte colony-stimulating factor (G-CSF) or chemotherapy plus G-CSF mobilization treatment. Blood volumes processed were six times the calculated blood volume of the patient. Peripheral blood stem cell collection was performed on the COBE Spectra. The total number of CD34+ cells in the blood (third column) was calculated from the level of CD34+ cells in the blood and the estimated blood volume of the patient. The total number of CD34+ cells released (fifth column) was calculated from the total number in the apheresis component and the number in the peripheral blood after collection minus the total number in the peripheral blood at the start of the collection procedure. All CD34+ cell quantities (except blood levels reported per µL) are × 10^6.
Full data are given in Rowley SD, Yu J, Heimfeld S, et al: Trafficking of CD34+ cells into the peripheral circulation during collection of peripheral blood stem cells by apheresis. *Bone Marrow Transplant* 28:649, 2001.

higher risk for citrate (or other anticoagulant) toxicity. Patients will also incur a proportional drop in platelet counts and may become profoundly thrombocytopenic.

Most reports of LVL describe the collection of more CD34+ cells than are calculated to be present in the peripheral blood at the initiation of the apheresis procedure. This results from the ongoing release of cells from the marrow replacing those cells removed by apheresis (or returning to the marrow space).[106] Apheresis of CD34+ cells is a three-compartment system consisting of the extracorporeal circuit of the apheresis device (including the collection bag), the peripheral blood, and the marrow. It is not obvious that the apheresis technique itself "mobilizes" CD34+ cells. Apheresis-induced mobilization, if it occurs, may be related to a decrease in divalent cations resulting from the citrate anticoagulant, possibly affecting cell adhesion forces.

Studies at the Fred Hutchinson Cancer Research Center demonstrated a continuous release of CD34+ cells from the marrow (and, presumably, return to the marrow space).[106] Patients having higher levels of CD34+ cells in the peripheral blood appeared to have a greater number of these cells circulating between the marrow and peripheral blood compartments (Table 95.1). In this model the apheresis device merely serves as a siphon, removing these cells from the blood as they are released from the marrow. If this description of CD34+ cell kinetics is accurate, it may be possible to deplete these cells from the blood and marrow by prolonged processing, but probably only if limited numbers of them are present in the marrow compartment. Also, the model suggests that higher blood flow rates used to shorten the apheresis procedure may be counterproductive for patients with low CD34+ cell levels in the blood because of the slower rate of release of CD34+ cells in these patients.

Pediatric Donors and Patients

PBSCs can be collected from pediatric patients, including infants. The special challenges of the pediatric patient arise from the fixed extracorporeal blood volume of the apheresis device, the need for venous catheters for blood access, and the management of a patient who may be unwilling or unable to rest quietly for the period of apheresis. It is especially important in management of the pediatric patient that timing of apheresis be optimal to minimize the number of procedures required to achieve the desired quantity of PBSCs.

Given these considerations, a number of centers have reported successful collection of PBSCs from pediatric patients and donors.

Almost all pediatric patients undergo insertion of a venous catheter adequate for the flow rates expected, although older patients (>12 years) may tolerate vein-to-vein procedures. The whole blood flow rate for the pediatric patient is much reduced compared with that of adult patients, and catheters as small as 5 F may be adequate.

Appropriate management of fluid balance during the apheresis procedure is critical for the smaller patient. The volume of red blood cells contained in the extracorporeal circuit of the continuous-flow apheresis device could represent 30% to 50% of the red cell mass of a pediatric donor. Although discontinuous-flow devices are appealing because of the feasibility of performing apheresis with a single-lumen venous access, they may result in even higher extracorporeal volumes and should be avoided in the smallest patients. The obvious solution to this problem is to prime the apheresis device with ABO-compatible, irradiated red blood cells (leukocyte-depleted and cytomegalovirus-negative blood is also desirable) when the blood in the extracorporeal circuit is expected to exceed 15% of the patient's blood volume. Packed red blood cell units can be diluted with saline or albumin (to reduce the loss of plasma protein that may occur). The red cells remaining in the extracorporeal circuit at the completion of the run need not be returned ("rinse-back"), although if performed slowly with monitoring of vital signs, rinse-back may actually increase the hematocrit after the procedure and otherwise reduce the need for red cell transfusions for these patients. For the intermediate-size pediatric patient (weight 25–50 kg), the apheresis device can be primed with a 5% albumin solution. This step will reduce the albumin loss that otherwise would occur. However, clotting proteins and other proteins not contained in this solution may decrease with repetitive apheresis.

The pediatric patient may not exhibit or relate the prodromal symptoms associated with citrate toxicity. Continuous calcium gluconate infusion can be incorporated into the procedure, or heparin can be added to the citrate anticoagulant solution or used as the sole anticoagulant. Sedation of the pediatric patient is usually not necessary and hinders the ability to recognize the symptoms of citrate toxicity. (Some patients may require antihistamine premedication if the apheresis device is primed with red blood cells.) Centers routinely performing pediatric PBSC collection should design an environment conducive to the management of pediatric patients and develop support procedures that recognize the unique physical and cognitive features of pediatric patients.

The range in blood volumes for pediatric donors of differing ages is greater than the range for adult donors. Therefore, most centers set a goal for volume processed based on the individual's blood volume instead of a set volume (e.g., two blood volumes vs. 6 L of blood) for all patients. The pediatric patient may undergo LVL to achieve the target goal of HSCs with fewer procedures. Blood flow rates for pediatric patients are slower than for adults to minimize the risk for citrate reaction. As with adults, the timing of apheresis can be optimized by monitoring the quantity of CD34+ cells in the peripheral blood.

QUALITY CONTROL OF HSC PRODUCTS

Quantity of Bone Marrow Cells for Transplantation

Cell dose is normally used as a surrogate for the stem cell content of the marrow product because the definition of adequate HSC products predated the availability of flow cytometric analysis of HSC content, and nucleated cell counting is the only quality-control measure easily performed during the collection procedure. For autologous transplantation, cell doses of 1×10^8 nucleated cells/kg are adequate. Based on early reports that smaller quantities increased the risk for engraftment failure, most centers target 3×10^8 nucleated cells/kg of recipient weight for allogeneic transplantation. However, those early reports were of patients being treated for aplastic anemia, in which engraftment failure is a more common event. A review of unrelated donor transplantation found that recipients of higher marrow cell doses experienced faster neutrophil and platelet engraftment, as well as better leukemia-free survival.[107] Pretreatment of the marrow donor with either GM-CSF or G-CSF may increase the number of myeloid progenitor cells harvested and decrease the period of posttransplant aplasia to that achievable by PBSC transplantation. CD34+ cell dose is now being correlated with transplant outcomes—with more rapid engraftment kinetics, possibly lower transplant-related mortality, and better overall survival, for example, in recipients of allogeneic bone marrow products containing higher quantities of CD34+ cells.[108] This assay should be a routine component of bone marrow product quality control.[108]

Definition of Adequate PBSC Component(s)

The quantity of CD34+ cells in a PBSC component varies greatly and is dependent on the number in the peripheral blood at the time of apheresis, the volume of blood processed, and the efficiency of the apheresis device. Therefore, any definition of an adequate component cannot include a set number of CD34+ cells to be contained in any single apheresis component. Instead, one or more components will be collected to meet the appropriate dose of these cells for transplantation. The dose of CD34+ cells required for infusion depends on the intended treatment regimen. For marrow-ablative regimens, increasingly higher CD34+ doses results in greater likelihood of rapid engraftment (Figs. 95.4 and 95.5).[109] Lower doses of CD34+ cells appear satisfactory for nonablative regimens.

Patients who receive a dose of CD34+ cells above a certain threshold will engraft. At lower doses of CD34+ cells, considerable heterogeneity occurs in engraftment speed, especially for platelet engraftment. Why this heterogeneity exists is not known, but it may reflect a weakness in the correlation between CD34+ cells and the cells responsible for engraftment, a greater heterogeneity of CD34+ subsets collected, or perhaps simply a greater degree of error in the measurement of CD34+ cells at the lower cell concentrations. As the dose of CD34+ cells increases, the engraftment kinetics becomes both more rapid and more consistent for the population studied.[109]

Subset analysis of CD34+ cells may improve the accuracy of predicting neutrophil and platelet engraftment kinetics but does not appear to predict engraftment failure enough to be of clinical utility. Pecora and colleagues[110] reported that the quantity of CD34+CD33− cells infused was identified as an independent factor predictive of engraftment kinetics. Dercksen and colleagues[111] reported better correlation between the number of CD34+CD33− cells and time to granulocyte engraftment, and between the number of CD34+CD41+

cells and time to platelet engraftment than found with the overall number of CD34+ cells. Coexpression of adhesion molecules is also predictive of hematopoietic recovery, with the same pathways important for both mobilization and homing of HSCs.[112] Given the limited range in recovery times when adequate numbers of CD34+ cells are collected and infused, however, this additional information is currently of limited clinical value.

CD34+ cell dose is also predictive of outcome of allogeneic PBSC (and marrow) transplantation.[108,113] Higher CD34+ cell doses result in better neutrophil and platelet engraftments after either related or unrelated donor transplantation and may correlate with better survival after bone marrow transplantation, but may also be associated with the development of more chronic GVHD.

Tumor Cell Contamination

The probability that tumor cell contamination of HSC product could contribute to relapse was demonstrated by Brenner and colleagues[114] in studies involving the autologous transplantation of genetically marked marrow cells, as well as in individual case reports describing the transmission of malignancy to allogeneic recipients from donors with occult disease at time of harvesting.[27,28] Sensitive immunocytostaining techniques, clonal assays, flow cytometric analysis, and polymerase chain reaction amplification of malignant genetic material detect tumor cells in the autologous PBSC components of many patients with a variety of malignancies.[115] In general, the incidence of contamination (number of patients with positive components) and the level of contamination (number of tumor cells per number of normal cells) is much less for PBSCs than for marrow products.

The presence of tumor cells at the time of collection or persisting after ex vivo processing may correlate with the extent of systemic disease or the chemotherapy sensitivity of disease at the time of cell collection. Whether patients transplanted with autologous PBSCs have a lower relapse rate compared with patients receiving bone marrow is not well defined, and appropriate phase III studies of this question will be difficult to design and enroll with patients in light of the other well-defined advantages of PBSC transplantation. In a retrospective study, Sharp and colleagues[116] demonstrated similar probabilities of relapse-free survival in recipients of PBSCs or marrow components if the components were free of lymphoma cells. In that study, patients with marrow involvement by lymphoma were assigned to transplantation with PBSCs. The authors concluded that PBSC transplantation is a sensible approach to the patient with overt marrow involvement. However, Brugger and colleagues[117] demonstrated that patients with breast cancer involvement of the marrow

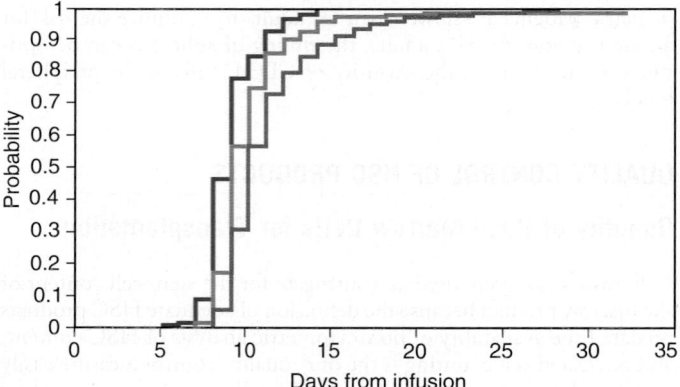

Fig. 95.4 Kaplan–Meier probability of achieving ≥0.5 × 10⁹ neutrophils/L for <5.0 × 10⁶ *(red)*, >5.0–10.0 × 10⁶ *(blue)*, and >10 × 10⁶ *(green)* CD34+ cells per kilogram *(p = .0001)*. *PBSC,* Peripheral blood stem cell. *(From Weaver CH, Hazelton B, Birch R, et al: An analysis of engraftment kinetics as a function of the CD34 content of peripheral blood progenitor cell collections in 692 patients after the administration of myeloablative chemotherapy. Blood 86:3961, 1995.)*

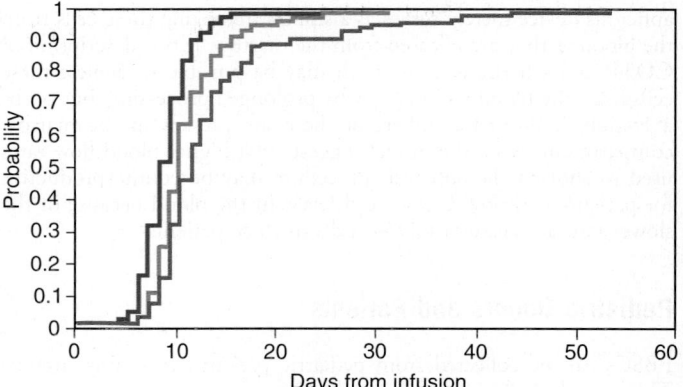

Fig. 95.5 Kaplan–Meier probability of achieving ≥20.0 × 10⁹ platelets/L for <5.0 × 10⁶ *(red)*, >5.0–10.0 × 10⁶ *(blue)*, and >10 × 10⁶ *(green)* CD34+ cells/kg *(p = .0001)*. *(From Weaver CH, Hazelton B, Birch R, et al: An analysis of engraftment kinetics as a function of the CD34 content of peripheral blood progenitor cell collections in 692 patients after the administration of myeloablative chemotherapy. Blood 86:3961, 1995.)*

at the time of chemotherapy mobilization were likely to mobilize tumor cells into the blood. The most disturbing finding of this study is that the tumor cells were detected in the peripheral blood at the same time as CD34[+] cells.[117] Similarly, Pecora and colleagues[118] found a relationship between the ability to detect tumors in PBSC components and in bone marrow samples, but they also found a higher incidence of positive PBSC components for patients who required greater numbers of apheresis procedures to achieve the target dose of CD34[+] cells. Investigators at The Johns Hopkins Oncology Center found no difference in the incidence of tumor contamination of PBSC components between patients treated with chemotherapy and cytokines and those treated with cytokines alone.[119] Ex vivo purging of tumor cells from PBPC products has not been shown to reduce the risk for relapse after autologous transplantation, either because the techniques are not adequate in depleting minimal residual disease or because patients relapse primarily from endogenous disease surviving the pretransplant conditioning regimen. Patients with marrow involvement may benefit from several cycles of debulking (in vivo purging) chemotherapy before collection of HSCs, with the caveat that extensive chemotherapy will also decrease the subsequent yield of PBSCs. Tumor cells in the HSC inoculum likely will not benefit the patient, but until further data demonstrating a deleterious effect on transplant outcomes are available, it is advisable that reports of tumor contamination in the collections for individual patients be interpreted with caution.

Microbial Contamination of Hematopoietic Stem Cell Components

Bacterial culture is an essential quality-control component in HSC collection and transplantation used to identify errors and breakdowns in manufacturing technique. Skin flora are the bacteria usually isolated, and infusion of culture-positive HSC products is generally without clinical sequelae, although serious infections have occurred after infusion of HSC products contaminated during processing.[47] Culture-positive products need not be automatically destroyed. Any decision regarding the disposition of a culture-positive HSC product must be made by the patient's transplant physician after considering the type of contamination, the anticipated risks from use of the component, and the ability to replace the culture-positive product(s) in a timely manner.

The incidence of culture-positive PBSC components is considerably less than that for marrow. The actual incidence of contamination for all HSC products is likely several times higher than reported, however, because most laboratories will culture only a very small volume of product (≈1 mL). In a retrospective review of 2935 HSC products processed and transplanted at one center, positive microbial products were reported for 1.3% of bone marrow products, 0.7% of PBSC products, and 2.0% of UCB products.[47] Coagulase-negative *Staphylococcus* and *Bacillus* species accounted for 23 of the 38 positive cultures, but *Escherichia coli*, *Klebsiella pneumonia*, and *Pseudomonas cepacia* were cultured from one product each. The recipient of the *Pseudomonas*-contaminated product subsequently died of complications of *Pseudomonas* sepsis, but no adverse sequelae could be documented for any of the other 34 recipients of culture-positive products. The highest rate of contamination occurred in the UCB products collected for related donor transplantation (5 out of 18, 27.8%), likely a reflection of the collection techniques in place at the time, and illustrating the need for strict quality control in the collection and processing of HSC products.

Quantitation of CD34[+] Cells

Quantification of CD34 antigen-positive cells by flow cytometry has become the standard of care for management of the PBSC donor because it provides a rapid and clinically relevant assessment of HSC content in the peripheral blood or in the PBSC product. This antigen is found on HSCs (including a variety of subpopulations) and limited

populations of other blood cells,[120] and can be identified using a variety of commercially available antibodies. If antibodies directly conjugated with dyes are used, the technique requires only about 1 hour of preparation time. Cell viability using propidium iodide or 7-aminoactinomycin D exclusion can simultaneously be determined if the cells are analyzed while still fresh, or the cells can be fixed after staining for analysis at a later date. Other antibodies can be added for analysis of CD34 subsets if desired (and if the flow cytometer has proper detectors to detect the different emission wavelengths of the fluorochromes used). A strong correlation exists between the numbers of CD34[+] cells and CFU-GM in the sample, but with ratios of about 5:1 to 20:1.[121] Thus, CD34 analysis will provide data similar to that obtainable with cell cultures, except that the latter demonstrates the functional viability of the progenitor cells. Mobilized PBPC products contain a heterogeneous mixture of cells including CD34[+] cells belonging to different cell subsets. Subset analysis of CD34[+] cells will provide additional information regarding early and sustained engraftment after autologous PBPC transplantation but does not appear to be clinically useful for the patient who easily meets the PBSC collection goal.

The major difficulty with analysis of CD34[+] cells is the low frequency of these cells. Clinical decisions to initiate apheresis are being made for CD34[+] cell levels as low as $10/\mu L$. This may represent a cell frequency that is 0.01% or less of the nucleated cells in the specimen. This enumeration is possible because of multidimensional measurements obtained by flow cytometry. Most cytometers can measure at least five characteristics of each cell, including size, granularity, and the presence of up to three different fluorochromes. Thus, the cells of interest can be separated in five-dimensional space, achieving discrimination of cells as rare as 1:10,000. The difficulties arise from developing an adequate technique that makes optimal use of the cytometer to measure these rare cells. Sources of errors include (A) sampling of the HSC product, (B) cell counting, (C) cytometer calibration and operation, (D) choice of antibody and fluorochrome, (E) lysis technique, and (F) gating strategy. Moreover, cytometry provides a proportion of cells that must be multiplied by the cell count to obtain an absolute number. The steps involved in preparing a specimen for cytometry may alter the proportion of cells in the sample, and this error will be translated into an error in the absolute number. Clinically, this imprecision may explain some of the range in engraftment kinetics observed for patients receiving low doses of CD34[+] cells.

SUGGESTED READINGS

Barker JN, Byam C, Scaradavou A: How I treat: the selection and acquisition of unrelated cord blood grafts. *Blood* 117(8):2332–2339, 2011.

Bosi A, Bartolozzi B: Safety of bone marrow stem cell donation: a review. *Transplant Proc* 42(6):2192–2194, 2010.

Boulais PE, Frenette PS: Making sense of hematopoietic stem cell niches. *Blood* 125(17):2621–2629, 2015.

Broxmeyer HE: Chemokines in hematopoiesis. *Curr Opin Hematol* 15(1):49–58, 2008.

Buell JF, Beebe TM, Trofe J, et al: Donor transmitted malignancies. *Ann Transplant* 9(1):53–56, 2004.

Confer DL, Shaw BE, Pamphilon DH: WMDA guidelines for subsequent donations following initial BM or PBSCs. *Bone Marrow Transplant* 46(11):1409–1412, 2011.

Dettke M, Buchta C, Wiesinger H, et al: Anticoagulation in large-volume leukapheresis: comparison between citrate versus heparin-based anticoagulation on safety and CD34+ cell collection efficiency. *Cytotherapy* 14(3):350–358, 2012.

DiPersio JF, Micallef IN, Stiff PJ, et al: Phase III prospective randomized double-blind placebo-controlled trial of plerixafor plus granulocyte colony-stimulating factor compared with placebo plus granulocyte colony-stimulating factor for autologous stem-cell mobilization and transplantation for patients with non-Hodgkin's lymphoma. *J Clin Oncol* 27(28):4767–4773, 2009.

Duong HK, Savani BN, Copelan E, et al: Peripheral blood progenitor cell mobilization for autologous and allogeneic hematopoietic cell transplantation: guidelines from the American Society for Blood and Marrow Transplantation. *Biol Blood Marrow Transplant* 20(9):1262–1273, 2014.

Giralt S, Costa L, Schriber J, et al: Optimizing autologous stem cell mobilization strategies to improve patient outcomes: consensus guidelines and recommendations. *Biol Blood Marrow Transplant* 20(3):295–308, 2014.

Heimfeld S: HLA-identical stem cell transplantation: is there an optimal CD34 cell dose? *Bone Marrow Transplant* 31(10):839–845, 2003.

Horowitz MM, Confer DL: Evaluation of hematopoietic stem cell donors. *Hematology Am Soc Hematol Educ Program* 469–475, 2005.

Kao GS, Kim HT, Daley H, et al: Validation of short-term handling and storage conditions for marrow and peripheral blood stem cell products. *Transfusion* 51(1):137–147, 2011.

Kurtzberg J, Cairo MS, Fraser JK, et al: Results of the Cord Blood Transplantation (COBLT) Study unrelated donor banking program. *Transfusion* 45(6):842–855, 2005.

Malik S, Bolwell B, Rybicki L, et al: Apheresis days required for harvesting CD34+ cells predicts hematopoietic recovery and survival following autologous transplantation. *Bone Marrow Transplant* 46(12):1519–1525, 2011.

Miller JP, Perry EH, Price TH, et al: Recovery and safety profiles of marrow and PBSC donors: experience of the National Marrow Donor Program. *Biol Blood Marrow Transplant* 14(9 Suppl):29–36, 2008.

Morrison SJ, Scadden DT: The bone marrow niche for haematopoietic stem cells. *Nature* 505(7483):327–334, 2014.

Pulsipher MA, Chitphakdithai P, Logan BR, et al: Acute toxicities of unrelated bone marrow versus peripheral blood stem cell donation: results of a prospective trial from the National Marrow Donor Program. *Blood* 121(1):197–206, 2013.

Rowley SD, Yu J, Heimfeld S, et al: Trafficking of CD34+ cells into the peripheral circulation during collection of peripheral blood stem cells by apheresis. *Bone Marrow Transplant* 28(7):649–656, 2001.

Sacchi N, Costeas P, Hartwell L, et al: Haematopoietic stem cell donor registries: World Marrow Donor Association recommendations for evaluation of donor health. *Bone Marrow Transplant* 42(1):9–14, 2008.

Sharma M, Afrin F, Satija N, et al: Stromal-derived factor-1/CXCR4 signaling: indispensable role in homing and engraftment of hematopoietic stem cells in bone marrow. *Stem Cells Dev* 20(6):933–946, 2011.

Solves P, Mirabet V, Perales A, et al: Banking strategies for improving the hematopoietic stem cell content of umbilical cord blood units for transplantation. *Curr Stem Cell Res Ther* 3(2):79–84, 2008.

Thomas ED, Storb R: Technique for human marrow grafting. *Blood* 36(4):507–515, 1970.

To LB, Levesque J-P, Herbert KE: How I treat patients who mobilize hematopoietic stem cells poorly. *Blood* 118(17):4530–4540, 2011.

Weaver CH, Hazelton B, Birch R, et al: An analysis of engraftment kinetics as a function of the CD34 content of peripheral blood progenitor cell collections in 692 patients after the administration of myeloablative chemotherapy. *Blood* 86(10):3961–3969, 1995.

Worel N, Buser A, Greinix HT, et al: Suitability criteria for adult related donors: a consensus statement from the Worldwide Network for Blood and Marrow Transplantation (WBMT) Standing Committee on Donor Issues. *Biol Blood Marrow Transplant* 2015. [Epub ahead of print].

REFERENCES

For the complete list of references, log on to www.expertconsult.com.

INVESTIGATIONAL NEW DRUG–ENABLING PROCESSES FOR CELL-BASED THERAPIES

Robert Lindblad, Traci Heath Mondoro, Deborah Wood, and Gillian Armstrong

The use of donated human cells as more than replacement therapy has become a reality over the course of the last several years. While basic and clinical scientists are developing many new and promising strategies to improve immune reconstitution and transplant outcome at the manufacturing and individual patient level, they are dependent on many others to implement these new therapies on a larger scale. Ultimately, implementation of procedures that were successful in the laboratory can be expensive and difficult to scale up to a process that will produce the required dosage while maintaining the consistent cellular product quality needed for clinical trials. To cope with these issues, many institutions have established specialized cell-processing centers; however, a specialized cell-processing laboratory and specially trained laboratory staff do not resolve all the problems associated with scaling a new procedure for a clinical trial. In some cases, equivalent reagents and processes suitable for use in large-scale clinical trials are not available.

In addition to the technical challenges of producing clinical grade cells in larger quantities, all of this work involving more than minimally manipulated cell therapy products must be performed under the Investigational New Drug (IND) process through the US Food and Drug Administration (FDA). The use of any cell product that is more than minimally manipulated and is for a nonhomologous indication in humans requires an IND, and even if the cellular therapy has been approved, a new IND may be needed if the agent is being tested in new populations or a situation where the risks to the patient are unknown (Table 96.1). An IND-enabling pre-clinical program is geared toward generating and collecting critical safety/toxicology/pharmacology data required to allow first-in-human studies. Appropriately designed pre-clinical studies are essential to the successful development and characterization of clinical scale manufacturing processes that will enable the filing of a well-supported IND with the FDA for a clinical trial. After IND filing, the FDA will review the procedures in place for the procurement, storage, and processing of the cells, as well as the proposed clinical trial design. A clinical study that is not likely to yield interpretable results is considered an unethical study because it places participants at risk without the prospect of either direct or generalizable benefit.

As the field of cellular therapy moved beyond transfusion of blood components and bone marrow transplantation, it became apparent that the processing and preparation of the cellular product was becoming a science unto itself. The isolation and identification of the desired cell population could take months, and the optimization of this process could take years. This did not include the development and validation of potency assays. All of this work is expensive, labor intensive, and requires staff qualified to perform at the highest technical level. Even though these tasks are vital to the production process, they are not hypothesis driven, so this type of work does not meet the requirements for National Institutes of Health (NIH) research project grants. One of the review criteria for NIH grant applications and contract proposals is innovation. Work required to develop and validate scale-up procedures and potency assays is not considered innovative and therefore is not eligible for discovery research that is typically funded through NIH grants. Many investigators perform this translational work by piecing

together funding from institutional or philanthropic sources. The National Heart, Lung, and Blood Institute (NHLBI) will accept grant applications for cell therapy studies that include manufacturing and translational studies. The National Institute of Biomedical Imaging and Bioengineering (NIBIB) funds hypothesis-driven research related to technologies, and some investigators have been able to utilize services provided by NIH Clinical and Translational Sciences Awards (CTSA) programs. Regardless of the source of funding, this chapter will provide general information about requirements during the IND-enabling phase of the development of a cellular therapy before it is tested for safety in a clinical trial. Critical elements involved in the stages of cell therapy product development are outlined in Fig. 96.1.

OVERVIEW OF THE CELL THERAPY PRODUCT

Novel cell-based therapy offers great potential for treating a number of currently untreatable disorders and diseases including immune reconstitution, tissue repair and regeneration, and metabolic support. Cell-based therapies can be derived from a variety of human autologous, allogeneic, or xenogeneic tissue sources such as blood, bone marrow, adipose, umbilical cord blood, fetal, embryonic stem cell lines, and induced pluripotent cells. Cellular engineering techniques such as selection, depletion, expansion, and genetic modification can be applied to alter or modify a cell to achieve a desired therapeutic effect. With these novel cell therapies, however, come development, manufacturing, characterization, and testing challenges in consistently generating a safe and effective cell therapy product.

Challenges for Cell Therapy Product and Manufacturing Development

Current good manufacturing practices (cGMPs) govern manufacturing processes to ensure consistent manufacture of safe, pure, and potent products.[1] Current good tissue practices (cGTPs) govern the methods used in, and the facilities used for, the manufacture of human cells, tissues, and cellular and tissue-based products (HCT/Ps). cGTPs focus on the prevention of the introduction, transmission, and spread of communicable diseases or other adverse events while preserving product function and integrity.[2]

Biological Variability

Living biological products present unique challenges. With cell-based therapy there is inherent patient-to-patient biological variability and cellular heterogeneity. Cell therapy products are derived from tissue sources that contain multiple cell types. In addition to known "active components," there are known and unknown cell subpopulations that may be considered "contaminants" or "inactive components," or could be critical to the biologic function of the product. Viability alone is a poor marker of cell function. Evolving characterization and

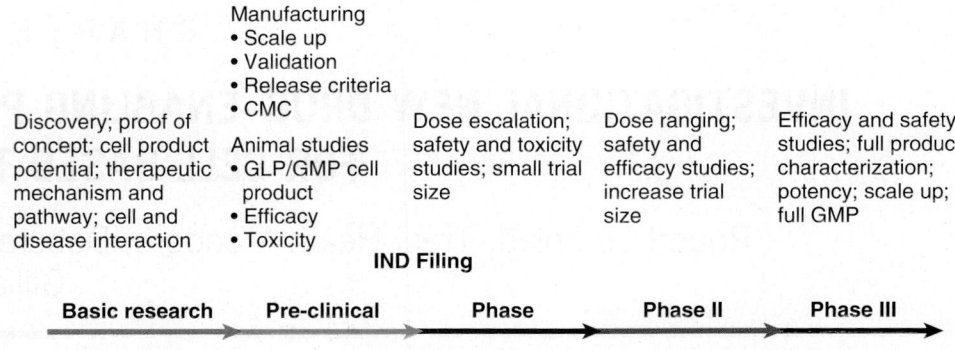

Fig. 96.1 CELL THERAPY PRODUCT DEVELOPMENT. *CMC,* chemistry, manufacturing and controls; *GLP,* good laboratory practices; *GMP,* good manufacturing practices; *IND,* investigational new drug.

TABLE 96.1 Regulation of Human Cells, Tissues, and Cellular and Tissue-Based Products	
HCT/Ps Regulated Under 351 of the PHS Act	**HCT/Ps Regulated Under 361 of the PHS Act**
Require IND submission and premarket approval; do not meet the definition of exempt products described for 361 products; 21 CFR 1271	No IND required/no premarket approval requirement
More than minimally manipulated	• Minimally manipulated, and • For homologous use, and • Not a combination product, *AND either* • has no cellular or systemic effect *or* • if it is active on a cellular or systemic basis is used in an autologous setting, in an allogeneic setting in first- or second-degree blood relatives, or is for reproductive use
Not intended for homologous use	
Associated with a device or scaffold[a]	
Cellular or systemic effect or dependent of metabolic activity of the cells for its primary function	

[a]Cell therapies that also have a device or scaffold associated with them can be regulated by the Center for Devices and Radiological Health (CDRH) as a consultant to the Center for Biologics Evaluation and Research (CBER) or as the lead center if the scaffold is the primary mode of action.

rigorous process control are therefore critical to counter the intrinsic heterogeneity and variability of cell therapy products.[3]

Characterization

Cell therapy products are difficult to fully characterize. Critical decisions need to be made in the product-development stage and the establishment of a desired characterization profile should occur early in the process to drive development. Successful product development demonstrates that a cell therapy product can be consistently manufactured which is safe, pure, potent, effective, and stable. Of these five elements, developing a potency assay for cell therapy products is most challenging. Potency measures the product's relevant biological function and therefore is a critical aspect of both safety and efficacy. Potency requires understanding a mechanism of action that is relevant to the use of the product in humans. Biological products are inherently complex, variable, and often heterogeneous, with complex and/or poorly defined mechanisms of action(s). Despite complex cell-engineering processes, the final product may contain both therapeutic and nontherapeutic cells; however, it can be difficult to ascertain if the combination of "active" and "inactive" components contribute to biological function. Because cells and cell lines are genetically diverse, they may behave differently during manufacturing than they did under experimental conditions. Cell-characterization testing, particularly with respect to potency, will evolve and change significantly during pre-clinical testing and clinical product development.[4]

Raw Materials

Many types of raw materials are used in cell therapy manufacturing. Such materials include culture media, sera, growth factors, cytokines, and "feeder cells," which are used to support cell growth. They may be simple or complex and may remain in the final therapeutic product as active substances, excipients, or as impurities, and, as such, their levels should be measured, controlled, and justified. They may also be used in the manufacturing process as ancillary products. A qualification program for raw materials that includes microbial testing (sterility, pyrogenicity [endotoxin], mycoplasma, and other adventitious agents) needs to be implemented to ensure the consistency and quality of raw materials and be designed to address identification and selection of the material, suitability of materials for use in manufacturing, characterization of materials, justification for use of animal-derived materials (i.e., fetal bovine serum), and quality assurance (QA) for all materials.[5]

Adventitious Agents

Adventitious agents (e.g., viruses, endotoxin mycoplasma, bacteria, parasites, fungi) may originate from the source (e.g., infected animals, tissues), during cell culture manipulation (e.g., repeated passages and manipulation in the laboratory), or by using contaminated biological reagents. Unidentified diseases may exist in the use of xenogeneic cells. The range of infectious agents that produce little or no effect in animals may have severe consequences in humans. With xenogeneic materials rigorous qualification of source animals and primary cell substrates is critical. Also, complex cell engineering procedures may extend over months, and can result in increased risk of contamination and other adverse effects. A risk-based assessment of the quality control (QC) aspects of the manufacturing process is necessary as poor controls of production processes can lead to the introduction of adventitious agents or other contaminants, or to inadvertent changes in the safety, potency, purity, or stability of the biological product that may not be detectable in final product testing, which is a keystone of the final product release.[6]

Aseptic Processing

As living functional cells are the product, terminal sterilization is not an option, therefore aseptic processing is required, with the use of closed manufacturing systems to the extent possible. This is considered a critical aspect of the manufacturing process and should be defined and validated as such, particularly as the risk of delivering a contaminated product is increased not only because of the inability to sterilize the product, but also because the timelines involved with cell products and product administration may occur before final sterility testing has been completed. The nature of the starting material and processes that involve open or closed manipulations determine the level of a controlled environment to be implemented.

Target Cell Population

Cells of therapeutic interest are often found in small numbers. Therefore an important first step of cell processing can be the initial isolation or enrichment of a cell population of interest from the tissue source. Several commercial fully automated closed systems are already in use and include the CliniMACS Prodigy system (Miltenyi Biotec), the Sepax 2 system (Biosafe SA), and the Elutra system (Terumo BCT). Cell-culturing processes can be specific to a given cell type; for example, cells such as T cells can be grown in nonadherent suspension culture where large-scale bioreactors, such as bag-based and traditional stirred-tank vessels, are used. This culturing system requires a small surface area and can produce high cell yield. There is a growing interest in ex vivo expansion of adherent cells for a variety of clinical applications. Mesenchymal stromal cells are grown adherently on tissue culture-treated surfaces but require a large surface area to be produced on a large scale. Miltenyi Biotec culture bags offer a closed-system process along with the CLINImacs (MABio). Multilayered flasks have been developed (CellCube and CellSTACK, Corning) to address surface area. Bioreactors (G-Rex, Wilson Wolf Manufacturing and WAVE, GE Healthcare Life Sciences) and microcarrier-based culturing systems (SoloHill Engineering) are designed to support cell growth at a variety of scales.[7]

Autologous Versus Allogeneic Products

Given their unique donor specificity, autologous products are attractive because of their decreased risk of immunologic reactions, bioincompatibility, and communicable disease transmission. However, they are inherently more limited and more variable owing to individual patient characteristics and/or disease state. Use of allogeneic donors is associated with greater risk than autologous donation because of the risk of infectious disease transmission from the donor to the recipient, overall risk of an immune response, and donor-to-donor variability. However, allogeneic cells have the potential to treat hundreds of patients from a single manufactured lot of cells and can be an "off-the-shelf" product.

Methods used in the production of cell products for clinical therapies depend on the nature of the final product and their targeted population. Autologous products are patient-specific and are manufactured using a "scaled out" approach. Cells are manufactured in small-volume batches and each patient constitutes their own "lot" of product. Allogeneic product manufacturing can use a scaled-up approach with a bulk manufacturing strategy to produce larger-volume batches to treat multiple patients.

In summary, cell therapy products are being used in a variety of therapeutic indications and their development for and use in other indications is progressing into the clinic. However, the clinical administration of living biologics carries elements of risk. Rigid control processes to minimize risk need to be implemented. Characterization, although a predictor of efficacy, is not a predictor of safety or quality. As full characterization is unlikely, it is imperative that manufacturing and aseptic processes be designed and validated to produce a safe, reliable product. If manufacturing methods change, as is often the case, essentially a new product is created, and recharacterization and repeat testing will be required to assess the impact of those changes on the product.

THE REGULATION OF CELL THERAPY PRODUCTS

The Center for Biologics Evaluation and Research (CBER) currently regulates cell therapy products considered as HCT/Ps under two sections of the Public Health Service (PHS) Act.[8,9] Section 361 includes products that require no IND be filed prior to the initiation of clinical studies and are consistent with products defined in 21 CFR 1271.10,[10] i.e., minimally manipulated, homologous use, not a combination product, and either has no cellular or systemic effect, or, if it is active on a cellular or systemic basis, is used in an autologous setting, in an allogeneic setting in first- or second-degree blood relatives, or is for reproductive use. Section 351 of the PHS Act[10,11] includes products that require clinical data be collected under an IND application, and do not meet the definition of exempt products described above for Section 361 products. Cell therapies that also have a device or scaffold associated with them can be regulated by the Center for Devices and Radiological Health (CDRH) as a consultant to CBER or as the lead center if the scaffold is the primary mode of action. Table 96.1 summarizes regulation of HCT/Ps as Section 351 and 361 products.

THE INVESTIGATIONAL NEW DRUG PROCESS

Presented below is a summary of the basic procedures to file an IND with the FDA. The regulatory pathway to conduct a clinical trial using a cell therapy product will involve an IND if the product does not meet the major criteria defining minimally manipulated products.

IND Sponsor/Investigator

The *Sponsor* of an IND trial is the individual or organization that takes legal responsibility for and initiates the clinical investigation. This may be an individual, an academic institution, the government (the NIH), or a pharmaceutical company. In contrast, the *Investigator* is the individual who actually conducts the clinical trial and under whose direction the investigational product is administered. In many small cell-therapy clinical trials, the sponsor may in fact also be the investigator, so that the trial is conducted under a single individual who is designated as a *Sponsor/Investigator*.[12]

Requesting a Meeting

Product regulatory development almost always begins with meetings between the sponsor and the FDA. Even with the availability of various Guidance Documents, sponsors are rarely in a position to submit a successful IND application with a cellular therapeutic product without direct FDA interactions in order to agree on submission details. The agency has designated meeting types to create a consistent level of support for products under development. A meeting request is submitted to the FDA stating the type of meeting requested with draft questions and suggested dates for the meeting.

Type A meetings are used to discuss products stalled in the development pathway and products that have been placed on clinical hold after a clinical trial is already underway. Type B meetings (the most common) include several specified time points in the development of a product. These include a pre-IND, end of phase I, end of phase II/pre–phase III, pre–biological license application (BLA), product license application (PLA), establishment license application (ELA), and new drug application (NDA) meetings. Type C meetings are any other meetings not covered under type A or B.[13,14] Under the performance goals set for the FDA, type A meetings should occur within 30 calendar days from receiving the request, type B meetings within 60 days, and type C meetings within 75 days.

Background information, sufficient to allow the FDA to answer the questions posed, should be submitted to the agency with the type A meeting request and 30 days prior to the scheduled meeting for type B and C meetings.[14]

Pre-IND Meeting

For cell therapy products the most critical meeting is the pre-IND meeting. The content of a pre-IND package that the sponsor sends to the FDA 30 days prior to the meeting will be driven by the questions the investigator wants to pose to the FDA, but generally includes a synopsis of the proposed clinical protocol, pre-clinical information (pharmacology and toxicology), any existing clinical information, a manufacturing section presenting proposed manufacturing methods and specifications, and copies of pertinent references. A list of questions that the sponsor would like the FDA to address and focus the discussion is critical to the success of the meeting. The FDA will specifically address these questions and provide a formal response prior to the meeting, which becomes part of the meeting minutes, allowing the meeting to be further focused on outstanding issues. Questions should include issues related to the pre-clinical testing data, chemistry, manufacturing, and controls (CMC) information, and the clinical protocol (safety assessments, inclusion/exclusion criteria).

The sponsor, the principal investigator, the individual responsible for the pre-clinical work, and the cell manufacturer should attend the pre-IND meeting. The FDA will be represented by reviewers to match these areas. After the pre-IND meeting, FDA reviewers in general make themselves available for further discussion and clarification, or can review a new manufacturing technique or a pre-clinical study to ensure that the sponsor and the FDA are in agreement regarding the next steps. This is a collaborative process with the goal of moving the process into the clinical arena as quickly and as safely as possible. Engaging the FDA early on in the IND submission process is recommended to facilitate the overall success of the IND. Within CBER, pre-pre IND meetings are available that are nonbinding, informal scientific discussions between CBER reviewers (pharmacology/toxicology) and the sponsor to initiate dialogue at an early stage in the process to facilitate design of expensive pre-clinical studies and allow data to be collected and presented at a type B, pre-IND meeting. This structure reflects the willingness of the CBER to engage the cell therapy community early in the development process and helps avoid delays because of lack of communication.

IND Submission

The submission of the IND will follow the pre-IND meeting and must fully address the issues raised at the pre-IND meeting in order to move forward. Once the IND is submitted, the FDA has 30 days to respond. The clinical study may proceed unless the FDA reviewers provide comments, or place the IND on hold within that 30-day time limit. Typically the FDA will have comments and will contact the IND sponsor prior to the 30-day deadline, requesting clarifications or updates to key documents. The IND submission will be organized in a similar fashion to the pre-IND package noted earlier. Several key sections in the IND are the clinical protocol with appropriate eligibility, endpoints, stopping rules and dosing justification, the CMC section, and the pre-clinical section.[12]

Chemistry, Manufacturing, and Control Section

Unlike chemical manufacturers that may produce a single large lot of drug to treat multiple individuals, cell therapies can be a single lot to treat a single individual or a small number of patients. The CMC section of a cellular therapy IND is crucial to the success of an IND submission.[15] From the regulations in 21 CFR 312.23,[16] sufficient information is required to assure the proper identification, safety, quality, and purity of the cell product. The *drug substance* is the starting material(s) including the procurement, process description, and test methods used to determine identity, strength, quality, and purity. The *drug product* is the end product, and its composition, manufacturing methods and packaging, and stability data should be included. Setting appropriate specifications with acceptable criteria for the drug product is crucial. Components used in the manufacturing of the IND—active, inactive compendial, and noncompendial excipients—should be listed. If available, Certificates of Analysis for reagents not FDA approved should be submitted. The IND/GMP Sliding Scale was developed with the recognition that manufacturing under cGMP is a challenge for early-stage cell therapy research. Perceived deviations from standard cGMP can be acceptable with scientific justification and an alternative approach proposed. The FDA will not direct the development of the product but will respond to the data-driven suggestions put forward by the sponsor in an IND application.

The format of the information that is included in the CMC section of an IND is described in CFR 312.23.[16] Typical problems encountered with submission of CMC sections include:

- Poor organization and key elements missing from the submission
- Incomplete descriptions of materials and reagents used in the manufacturing process
- Insufficient facility information
- Insufficient details regarding release criteria and tests employed
- Insufficient standard operating procedures (SOPs)

Pharmacology/Toxicology Section

The pharmacology/toxicology section must support the planned clinical trial. Pharmacology information should describe the pharmacologic effects and mechanism of action in the animal model and provide information on the absorption, distribution, metabolism, and excretion of the product. In cellular therapies much of this information is not readily measurable, but cell survival posttransplantation, cell migration, and tissue integration can be explored in pre-clinical studies, and therefore an attempt to organize the pre-clinical data to address these areas should be made. If this information is not known, it should be stated. Toxicology studies, however, are critical to the initiation of clinical trials in humans.

Pre-clinical animal studies in general will be conducted in two species under good laboratory practices (GLP) conditions including a developed protocol and complete data record keeping. An adequate number of animals, typically of both sexes, and adequate sampling time points for pharmacokinetic analysis are required. The appropriate studies include a proof-of-concept demonstration in a relevant animal model of the disease/injury and healthy animal toxicology studies. One study must include the same route of administration, the same cell manufacturing technique, and the same product as will be proposed in the clinical study. Deviations from this ideal should be clearly explained and justified scientifically. The pre-pre IND meeting is the time to come to an agreement with the FDA regarding the acceptable animal models in which to conduct these studies prior to embarking on time-consuming, expensive pathways that do not adequately answer the questions to advance the development process.

Cross-Referencing

The FDA permits one IND to cross-reference information that is already on file at the agency; for example, in another IND or a drug master file. Written authorization must be obtained from the sponsor of the submission that is being cross-referenced and be included in the new IND. Specific details including the submission and volume number, the heading, and page numbers should be provided to identify what material is being cross-referenced. This allows FDA reviewers to quickly locate the referenced materials, facilitating the review process.

An IND Hold

Once the IND is filed, the FDA has 30 days to respond with comments prior to the IND automatically becoming active. If there are safety concerns, the FDA applies a clinical hold to stop the clinical investigation from proceeding until identified issues are adequately addressed.[17] For new INDs, this represents a failure of the pre-IND process. If the sponsor in the pre-IND meeting presents sufficient detail and asks appropriate questions, then potential hold issues will be addressed prior to the IND submission. The FDA will put a clinical trial on hold for predefined reasons that include:

- Exposure to unreasonable risk for significant illness or injury
- Clinical investigators are not qualified
- The investigator brochure is misleading, erroneous or incomplete (multicenter studies)
- The IND does not contain sufficient information to assess risk
- Gender exclusion for a condition that occurs in both men and women

In practice, a clinical hold on cell therapy INDs is applied for several reasons, which include:

- The clinical trial does not provide adequate safety protection, which includes appropriate dosing, based on the preliminary clinical or pre-clinical data, appropriate dose escalation, and appropriate stopping rules for the trial
- The pre-clinical data do not support the clinical trial based on product manufacturing or route of delivery
- The manufacturing section has inadequate characterization of the product, inadequate controls over manufacturing and insufficient details

These issues should all be addressed in the pre-IND process.

IND Maintenance

When an IND becomes active, future communication with the FDA outside of specific meeting requests occur through the submission of IND amendments. Each submission is sequentially numbered and adds to the overall content of the IND. Amendments are submitted to the IND on a rolling basis and include protocol revisions, expedited safety reports, changes to the manufacturing technique or to the facility, key personnel changes, and any other significant changes to the clinical or manufacturing portions of the IND. Additionally, each IND sponsor is required to submit an annual report, summarizing the clinical study conducted over the past year. In some cases, the FDA may require more frequent progress reports. Each annual progress report is an opportunity to submit other details regarding the INDs that were not submitted during the year. The annual report is due within 60 days of the anniversary date of the IND becoming active.

WHEN IS A CELL THERAPY PRODUCT READY TO BE TESTED IN A CLINICAL TRIAL?

The ultimate test of the cellular therapy is its performance in human trials. This is the last step of an incredibly complex journey. The cell population has been identified along with a manufacturing method and assays to characterize the consistency and key properties of the product. The manufactured product has been tested in animal models for both proof-of-concept data including the route of administration, dosing schemes, and toxicology. The best way to make the transition from animals to humans smoothly is, if possible, to continue working with the same cell-processing facility and staff that have been preparing the product throughout the pre-clinical study stage. Good communication among the investigator, the cell-processing staff, and the FDA is key for the success of the clinical trial. When this occurs, it is then easier to solve inevitable operational difficulties, attribute adverse events, and solve recruitment problems that may occur during the course of the trial.

Trial Design Considerations

Initial clinical studies are safety based, typically at a single center, and expose a small number of patients to the new therapy while carefully monitoring for adverse effects and collecting preliminary efficacy data. As development continues, clinical trial design can be broken down into two broad areas: scientific and operational. The scientific area includes the clinical questions to be answered and the statistical methods used to answer them. The investigator and the cell-processing staff should meet early with statistical staff to determine how to phrase the clinical questions such that they can be answered with appropriate clinical endpoints. If a surrogate endpoint is proposed, this should be discussed with FDA staff to ensure it is acceptable from a regulatory standpoint. The method of endpoint measurement must be determined. Is there an existing validated assay to measure the endpoint? Is the assay commercially available and is it FDA approved for clinical use, or is it a "research-based" assay? The statisticians will calculate the appropriate sample size that is required to answer the questions with sufficient statistical power. Once the sample size is derived, the investigators must determine if the trial can be conducted at one center or if a multicenter study is needed.

Operational Issues

These are addressed using experience gained from prior clinical trials, or may need to be solved through pilot studies or "dry runs" by the manufacturing and clinical staff, including the use of any device needed to deliver the cell therapy product. The first operational details to be worked out are those involving the timing of manufacture and the delivery to the patient. If the trial must be conducted at multiple sites, will there be a central manufacturing site or will processing staff need to be trained at each recruitment site?

Shipping and Administration of Cellular Products

Shipping is considered an extension of storage conditions. Selecting the right vendor is essential to shipping a stable product. The shipping containers purchased must be validated by the laboratory prior to their use. Transport documentation is a cGTP requirement for traceability of donor to final product purposes [1271.290(e)].[18] The US Department of Transportation has guidance on classifying biological materials in accordance with 49 CFR 171.[19]

Depending on the type of product, certain postshipment release testing may be indicated prior to product use in the clinic. This requires cell therapy expertise at the receiving site or significant training. Shipping-validation procedures can be conducted to determine which tests are required for certain products. Establishing postshipment acceptance criteria is critical for the use of many cell therapy products.[20] Practice runs are recommended for shipment of the product, especially if the timing of the administration is crucial. For example, if a product is to be administered during a surgical procedure, it will be important to know the product viability if there are delays in shipment or postshipment testing, or during the surgical procedure.

In addition to a product meeting the appropriate release criteria, the product administration process needs to be monitored. Patient baseline and postadministration evaluations are conducted, adverse events are documented, and any deviations from the product administration procedures/processes are recorded. Such documentation can allow the cell-processing laboratory to evaluate common elements across different products as well as observe any product-specific trending.

Quality Control/Quality Assurance

A parallel process to the manufacturing process and pre-clinical studies is QC and QA. QA begins before the manufacture of the cellular therapeutic begins. It is based on the manufacturing process and confirms that each step from raw material procurement to product release can be performed in a consistent and regulation-compliant manner. QC is product based and confirms whether or not the final cell therapy product satisfies the preestablished specifications for final release. Managers and third-party auditors are responsible for QA through the development of process documentation, establishing SOPs, conducting audits, and training. Inspectors and area supervisors perform QC by performing and receiving inspection reports at all points throughout the manufacturing process.

Data and Adverse Event Monitoring

In addition to the QC/QA of the cellular therapeutic, there is also the QC of data collection. Case report forms must be tailored to the study and need to be linked to the source data collected during the manufacture and delivery of the cells, and throughout the clinical trial. The forms should be tested for ease of completion so that data coming in from the clinical sites will be easy to collect and interpret. Data coordinators and/or research nurses should be given rigorous training on the completion of these forms and should know how long each form takes to complete so they will be able to give a reasonable estimate of how many subjects they can follow within a given time period.[21]

Single-center trials are often monitored by an institutional safety monitoring committee (SMC), whereas multicenter trials typically have a centralized independent data safety monitoring board (DSMB) that is often convened by the sponsor (NIH or a pharmaceutical company). A monitoring plan must be developed for the collection and reporting of adverse events to the SMC/DSMB and the FDA. This is another step where good communication is essential. The trial investigator and the cell-processing facility must meet regularly to discuss any adverse events and events that occur during product administration to determine if they are attributable to the cellular product or the subject's underlying disease. The FDA and the SMC/DSMB must be informed of these events to determine if a prespecified stopping boundary has been crossed.

CONCLUSIONS

The development of novel cellular therapeutics is a long and complex process requiring an IND. There are many translational steps to be completed before exposure to humans is feasible. These steps range from practical issues such as the shipment of cells to the complicated issues of setting acceptable product specifications and conducting pre-clinical studies in animal models to predict product safety profile. Investigators need to develop good working relationships with the cell-processing facility staff and statistical staff in order to conduct a technical and scientifically robust clinical trial. The key to a successful IND is early and frequent communication with the FDA.

SUGGESTED READINGS

Gee A, editor: *Cell therapy cGMP facilities and manufacturing*, New York, 2009, Springer-Verlag.

Gee AP, Sumstad D, Stanson J, et al: A multicenter comparison study between the Endosafe® PTS™ rapid-release testing system and traditional methods for detecting endotoxin in cell-therapy products. *Cytotherapy* 10:427, 2008.

Guidance for Industry: Eligibility Determination for Donors of Human Cells, Tissues, and Cellular and Tissue-Based Products (HCT/P's) Final Guidance, August 2007.

Guidance for Industry: Guidance for Human Somatic Cell Therapy and Gene Therapy, March 1998.

Preti RA: Bringing safe and effective cell therapies to the bedside. *Nature Biotechnol* 23:801, 2005.

REFERENCES

For the complete list of references, log on to www.expertconsult.com.

CHAPTER 97

GRAFT ENGINEERING AND CELL PROCESSING

Adrian P. Gee

Hematopoietic stem cell transplantation (HSCT) originated using bone marrow (BM) cells from allogeneic donors. Sources of cells have subsequently increased to include autologous marrow, growth factor-mobilized peripheral blood, umbilical cord blood, and placenta. In this chapter, the ex vivo processing of these cells and other cells used in the context of HSCT is reviewed. Processing may range from simple depletion of ABO-incompatible red blood cells (RBCs) or plasma, to more complex procedures designed to engineer the graft components to enhance engraftment, prevent graft-versus-host disease (GVHD), or to introduce genetic modifications into the cells. Facilities performing these procedures are often involved in other types of cellular therapies. These include provision of cells for adjuvant therapies in the post-HSCT setting and to support clinical trials in regenerative medicine. The dramatic growth in these new applications has attracted the interest of regulatory agencies, which have worked hard to develop an appropriate strategy to address a complex new area of medicine. An understanding of the regulations is therefore essential because they are based on the type of cellular therapy product.

REGULATORY ISSUES WITH CELL PROCESSING

Regulation of a fast-moving field, such as cellular therapies, has posed a challenge to the United States Food and Drug Administration (FDA) and other national regulatory authorities. However, in the past few years, a risk-based structure has emerged in the United States of America that has clarified the strategy. In brief, manufacturers of cellular therapy products need to determine whether they fall under Investigational New Drug (IND) regulations, which require manufacturing of the product under good manufacturing practices (GMP); whether they fall under Part 1271 of Title 21 of the Code of Federal Regulations (21CFR) Human Cells, Tissues, and Cellular and Tissue-Based Products (HCT/Ps), which require manufacturing of the product under good tissue practices (GTP); or whether they are exempt from both of these regulations.

GTP regulations, which came into effect in May 2005, were established nominally to prevent the introduction, transmission, and spread of communicable diseases by HCT/Ps. This was based on the presumption that most posttransplant infections and admissions to intensive care units were attributable to administration of contaminated products. The validity of this assumption is open to question. GTP regulations provide a framework for screening, performing ex vivo processing, storing, and distributing HCT/Ps, and provide the FDA with an overview of current activities by requiring an annual registration of collection and processing facilities. The Part 1271 regulations effectively filled a gap in the law that left unregulated HCT/Ps that were minimally manipulated (e.g., were not cultured ex vivo, genetically modified, or activated ex vivo), were intended for homologous use, or were not combined with another article (e.g., a matrix or scaffold) for administration. Minimally manipulated HCT/Ps should not exert a systemic effect and should not be dependent on the metabolic activity of living cells for their function. If this were not the case, then the cells should be for autologous use only, for use in a first- or second-degree blood relative, or for reproductive use. Cellular products that fall into this classification are referred to as *Type 361 products*. The Part 1271 regulations do not apply to vascularized organs for transplantation; whole blood or blood components;

and, important for this discussion, minimally manipulated BM for homologous use and not combined with another article. This therefore means that traditional HSCTs do not fall under FDA regulations, and that these procedures are currently considered practice of medicine.

With the exceptions noted, most other cellular therapy and HSCT products fall under IND regulations and are referred to as *Type 351 products*. These are cells that have been cultured ex vivo and transduced or activated ex vivo, and therefore are more than minimally manipulated. The facility processing these cells is required to operate under GMP. These regulations were originally developed for the pharmaceutical industry to ensure that drugs are manufactured under a controlled and auditable process that ensures their safety, purity, and potency. The FDA has indicated that the application of GMP to cellular therapy products follows a continuum, such that products that are manufactured for a phase I/II clinical trial under an IND are not expected to be prepared under full GMP. As the trial proceeds the expectation is that the application of GMP will become more rigorous, such that a phase III product would be extensively characterized and manufactured using a fully validated process.

Implementation of Part 1271 regulations has had an impact on the "routine" laboratory that prepares cells primarily for HSCT. Laboratories that use cells other than BM must now register annually with the FDA; ensure that donors meet eligibility requirements (or document why noneligible donors are used); and manufacture, store, and distribute the cells under GTP. If a laboratory has previous experience manufacturing products under GMP conditions, it already will be familiar with most of the features of GTP. In general, these cover personnel, procedures, facilities, environmental control and monitoring, equipment, supplies and reagents, recovery, processing and process controls, process changes, process validation, labeling controls, storage, receipt, predistribution shipment and distribution, records, tracking, and complaints. Implementation of the components of GMP and/or GTP operations is a time-consuming process that requires development, implementation, and maintenance of numerous components and generates a considerable volume of documentation. Professional societies, such as the Foundation for the Accreditation of Cellular Therapy (FACT) and AABB (formerly the American Association of Blood Banks), have developed standards and an accreditation process that takes into account GTP/GMP regulations and provides a framework around which compliance can be built (see Professional Standards section).

An exception from the products described earlier is cord blood. In the United States, cord blood is a licensed product and facilities that prepare and bank cord blood are required to obtain a Biologics License. This allows the manufacturer to introduce, or deliver for introduction, a biologic product into interstate commerce (21 CFR 601.2).

Central to both GMP and GTP regulations is the establishment and maintenance of a quality program. This must ensure that the appropriate regulations are being followed on an ongoing basis; that mechanisms are in place for detecting, reviewing, and remediating errors and deviations from regulations, policies, and procedures; and that an audit program will be developed, implemented, and maintained. Activities performed by the quality program must be documented, and the program should be staffed by individuals who are not involved in hands-on manufacturing of the products.

Holders of INDs must provide the agency with an annual report on the protocol and include a listing of the products administered and those that have been prepared but not used. In addition, cell-processing facilities should be prepared to assist the IND sponsor by providing information on products that have been associated with severe adverse reactions in the recipients, and whether these were attributable to product quality. For Type 361 products, the facility must report, as Biological Product Deviations, any contaminated products that have been administered to a patient.

PROFESSIONAL STANDARDS

The two major accrediting organizations in the United States for cellular therapies are FACT and AABB. Whereas FACT offers accreditation of collection, processing, and clinical use of cellular therapy products, the AABB focuses on collection and laboratory processing. Both organizations inspect based on standards that are published every 18 months to 3 years. In the case of FACT, the standards are published in collaboration with the Joint Committee on Accreditation in Europe. FACT also publishes separate standards in collaboration with NetCord that cover cord blood banking. Both organizations have worked to harmonize their standards with American, Canadian, Australasian, and European regulatory agencies; therefore, accreditation by either organization is of great assistance on the pathway to regulatory compliance. A number of other professional organizations accredit particular aspects of operations within the cell-processing facility. These include the College of American Pathologists, which accredits general laboratories, and hematology and flow cytometry facilities; the American Society for Histocompatibility and Immunogenetics; and the European Federation for Immunogenetics, which accredits histocompatibility-testing laboratories. Some organizations, such as the College of American Pathologists and StemCell Technologies, also provide proficiency testing services for laboratory staff.

MANIPULATION OF HEMATOPOIETIC STEM CELL TRANSPLANTATION PRODUCTS

Manipulation of a product for hematopoietic rescue is intended to remove a component that is unwanted or may cause adverse effects or to enrich a desired population, such as CD34+ cells. As discussed previously, the degree of manipulation may determine the regulations under which the product is manufactured and handled. The FDA defines minimal manipulation as processing that does not alter the relevant biologic characteristics of the cells or tissues. This includes procedures such as RBC and plasma depletion, and cell selection using an approved device. By contrast, more than minimal manipulation would include activities such as culture ex vivo, genetic modification, and ex vivo activation.

Routine Minimal Manipulation for Volume Reduction or ABO Incompatibility

The most widely used form of manipulation in the hematopoietic progenitor cell (HPC)-processing facility is probably removal of erythrocytes and/or plasma to overcome incompatibility between donor and recipient (Table 97.1). This process is performed largely using techniques that were developed by the blood banking industry.

Plasma depletion to remove donor antibodies that may react with recipient cells is achieved by centrifugation of the graft, usually in a transfer pack, at approximately 2000 g for 10 minutes at ambient temperature. The pack then is placed in a plasma expresser, which compresses the product bag so that plasma can be forced out and into a separate collection bag. Plasma depletion can also be used to reduce the volume of ABO-compatible grafts when the donor is large and the recipient small.

| TABLE 97.1 | Processing Performed to Address ABO Incompatibilities Between Hematopoietic Stem Cell Donors and Recipients |

Recipient ABO Type	Donor ABO Type	Type of Processing
ABO identical	ABO identical	No special processing required
A or B	AB	RBC depletion
O	A/B/AB	RBC depletion
A	B	RBC + plasma depletion
B	A	RBC + plasma depletion
Antibody to RBCs	N/A	RBC depletion
A/B/AB	O	Plasma depletion
AB	A or B	Plasma depletion

N/A, Not applicable; RBC, red blood cell.

RBC depletion removes incompatible donor erythrocytes that would stimulate a reaction by the donor upon administration. Most facilities establish a maximum volume of incompatible RBCs that can be infused with HPCs; exceeding this limit can result in hemolysis and a transfusion reaction. Depletion of erythrocytes can be achieved most simply by centrifugation. The product is centrifuged at approximately 3000 g for approximately 10 minutes at ambient temperature, and the leukocyte-rich buffy coat is collected at the interface between the plasma layer and the RBCs.

RBC depletion can also be achieved by sedimenting erythrocytes using hydroxyethyl starch (hetastarch). This promotes RBC sedimentation by formation of erythrocyte rouleaux. The hematocrit of the product is first adjusted to approximately 25% by addition of normal saline, and 6% hetastarch (Hespan) is added at a volume:volume ratio of 1:6 to 1:7. Sedimentation can be performed under gravity or may be accelerated by centrifugation.

The most rigorous erythrocyte depletion is achieved by centrifugation of the collection on a Ficoll-Hypaque density gradient. This process enriches mononuclear cells at the interface between the gradient and the layered cells after centrifugation and depletes erythrocytes, platelets, and granulocytes. As a result of enrichment for mononuclear cells, the overall nucleated cell recovery is lower than with other techniques in which granulocytes are retained.

Automated devices are available for preparing buffy coats and density gradient-enriched cells. For larger volumes, the COBE 2991 Cell Processor from Terumo can be used. This requires a minimum volume of 150 mL RBCs for operation and may therefore not be suitable for pediatric processing. It is capable of preparing buffy coats and density-separated cell preparations using a functionally closed disposable set.

The COBE Spectra from Terumo is in common use to collect peripheral blood progenitor cells by apheresis. The device is also less widely used in the processing facility to enrich mononuclear cells from BM.

For smaller starting volumes, the Sepax device from Biosafe can be used (Fig. 97.1). It has found widespread application in cord blood banks for buffy coat preparation (with or without addition of hydroxyethyl starch) and has also been used for volume reduction of peripheral blood progenitor cell collections, density gradient separation of BM, and for cell washing. The device has a small footprint, uses functionally closed disposables, and provides a print-out of operations.

Xpress devices for cord blood and marrow processing are available from Thermogenesis. The AXP AutoXpress is designed for enriching mononuclear cells from cord blood that is transferred to the processing set, which is then placed into the AXP device. This fits into a centrifuge bucket, and during spinning the red and mononuclear cells are collected into separate bags and the plasma is retained in the processing set. The MarrowXpress performs a similar procedure on marrow harvests. Both devices provide closed sterile systems, and the

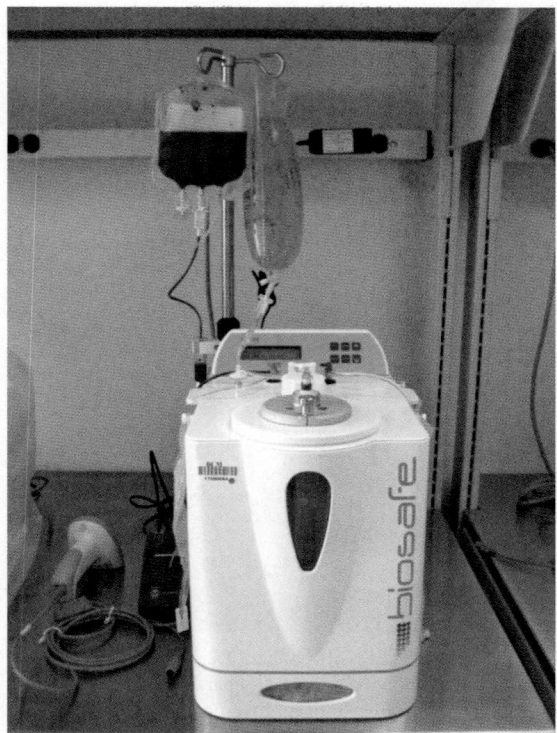

Fig. 97.1 THE BIOSAFE SEPAX DEVICE. Used for automated processing of hematopoietic cells. A newer version of this device provides additional good manufacturing practice features.

XpressTRAK software enables data tracking to assist with regulatory compliance.

Purging of Autologous Grafts

Autologous HPCs can be used for recipients lacking a human leukocyte antigen (HLA)-matched related or unrelated donor. It has been proposed that occult viable tumor cells collected with the graft and returned to the patient could act as a source for disease relapse. Gene-marking studies have supported this hypothesis. As a result, much effort has been exerted to develop methods for the ex vivo detection and removal of tumor cells from autologous grafts. Techniques have included incubation with chemotherapeutic drugs, such as 4-hydroperoxycyclophosphamide, photosensitizing agents, and antisense oligonucleotides. Alternatively, tumor-directed monoclonal antibodies (MAbs) can be used to identify the cells and effect their removal. The MAb-coated tumor cells can be eliminated by addition of serum complement, or by capturing them on a solid phase, such as a column matrix, a plastic sheet, or magnetic particles. These particles may be large (5 μm diameter) so they can be collected, with the attached tumor cells, in a standard magnetic field. The matrix material may be much smaller, such as nanoparticles or ferrofluids, which coat the cells. These are then collected on a metal matrix placed in a field generated by permanent magnets. Such systems are capable of depleting 4–6 logs of tumor cells from a graft. However, even at such high efficiencies, and given the limits of our ability to detect residual tumor cells, the clinical value of purging autologous grafts is debatable. There has also been a decline in interest in purging techniques because of the potential benefits of a graft-versus-tumor (GVT) effect detected in recipients of allogeneic grafts.

T-Cell Depletion of Allogeneic Products

T cells in HPC grafts have the potential to cause severe or lethal GVHD or potentially to exert a beneficial GVT effect (discussed in Chapter 108). Considerable work has been done to determine whether these opposing effects are produced by distinct subpopulations of T lymphocytes. This would allow ex vivo manipulation of allogeneic grafts to remove differentially the GVHD-producing T cells while sparing those that mediate GVT responses. Various subpopulations of T cells have been identified as candidate effector subpopulations; however, there is no widespread consensus as to which subsets should be targeted.

Methods are available for eliminating T cells from grafts using approaches similar to those used for purging tumor cells. Early techniques included use of soybean agglutinin to aggregate the majority of nonprogenitor cells and rosetting of sheep erythrocytes with T cells to facilitate their removal. Although successful, these techniques are not "FDA friendly" and do not offer the specificity that likely is required to engineer T-cell subpopulations in allogeneic grafts. This is made possible by the use of MAbs directed toward the antigens that are currently used to identify T-lymphocyte subpopulations. The target population then can be removed with high efficiency using immunomagnetic separation, as described previously for purging autologous grafts. The challenge remains to identify the appropriate target T-cell populations and to source clinical grade MAbs for these procedures. A number of potential target antigens have been identified and separation techniques implemented. They range from pan–T-cell depletions using antibodies to CD3 and CD2, to depletions of helper and cytotoxic T cells using MAbs against CD4 and CD8, to stimulation and removal of alloreactive populations by targeting activation antigens.

Efforts have recently focused on depletion of αβ-positive T cells from the graft. This spares the donor-derived alloreactive natural killer (NK) and γδ T cells, which may provide a tumor-directed response. Promising early clinical results have been obtained using this approach. An alternative approach is to administer regulatory T cells (Tregs) posttransplant to prevent and treat GVHD. A first-in-man clinical study was performed using in vitro-expanded Tregs from partially HLA-matched third party umbilical cord blood units that were administered to 23 patients receiving double-cord blood transplants. Results were compared with 108 historical controls. No Treg acute toxicities were seen, and there was a reduced incidence of grades II–IV acute GVHD, but since this was a phase I study it was not designed to demonstrate efficacy. Later studies support the finding that donor Treg infusions can prevent GVHD after allogeneic transplantation. Evidence that Tregs can be used to treat GVHD is still under evaluation

Methods that eliminate or physically remove either T cells or tumor cells from grafts are referred to as *negative selection techniques*. They are affected by variables such as target antigen expression, sensitivity of detection technologies for quantitating separation efficiency, and other technical hurdles. These may be difficult to control in order to achieve the ideal composition of the graft and the target level of residual T cells, or T-cell subsets, remains to be established. A dose of 10^5 T cells/kg is generally regarded as the goal to minimize the risk of GVHD while facilitating engraftment. There are also no approved devices for negative selection, so these types of procedures must be performed under an IND.

For many years, the goal was to replace negative selection with a procedure in which HPC populations could be specifically enriched by positive selection. This would effectively deplete T cells or tumor cells from allogeneic and autologous grafts, respectively. The problem was the lack of a method for identifying the target HPCs until the CD34 antigen was identified on a small population of progenitor cells, including the pluripotent cells required for hematopoietic transplantation. The subsequent availability of MAbs directed against this antigen made possible the development of techniques for enrichment of these cells. Immobilization of the antibodies on a matrix (e.g., plastic sheets) and cellulose and magnetic particles was used as the primary approach, and a number of devices were commercially developed. The first to achieve FDA approval for use with apheresis products was the Baxter Isolex 300i, which uses Dynal 5-μm magnetic beads as the separation modality and releases

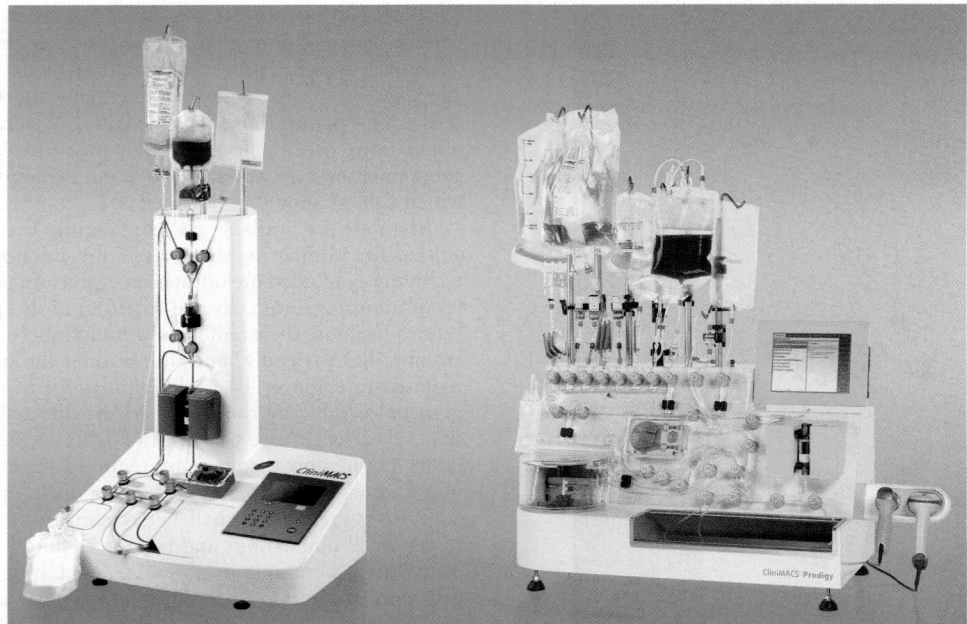

Fig. 97.2 MILTENYI CLINIMACS CELL SEPARATOR AND PRODIGY CELL PROCESSOR. The Prodigy (right side) is a self-contained cell separation and processing device. CliniMACS is a cell separation system using magnetic nanoparticles conjugated with monoclonal antibody to the target antigen. Investigators should determine the status of regulatory approval of these devices before clinical use. *(Copyright 2015 Miltenyi Biotec GmbH. All rights reserved.)*

CD34$^+$ cells from the beads using a competitive binding peptide. This device was recently withdrawn from the market for this application and is currently under evaluation for use in regenerative medicine protocols.

An alternative is the CliniMACS system (Miltenyi Biotec; Fig. 97.2), which currently has regulatory approval in Europe but still requires an IND for use in the United States for other than one specific indication. This uses anti-CD34 nanoparticles to effect separation. The labeling with and removal of unbound CD34 reagent is performed manually. The CD34 reagent-treated cells are then processed on the device, where they are retained on a column located in a high-gradient magnetic field. Nonlabeled cells flow through the column and are collected in the negative fraction. The labeled cells are recovered from the column after several automated separation and washing cycles by removing the magnetic field. The nanoparticles remain on the CD34$^+$ cells; however, they are biocompatible and may be infused into the recipient. The device normally achieves purities in excess of 90% with yields of approximately 60%. This results in passive depletion of 4–6 logs of T cells. The device may be used with a variety of MAbs directed against antigens expressed by various types (T, B, and NK cells), potentially allowing it to be used as a platform for multiple types of graft engineering. Recently, Miltenyi Biotec has introduced a new device (the Prodigy; see Fig. 97.2), which can automatically perform many of the steps requiring manual intervention on the CliniMACs. Additional features provide the potential ability to fully automate the preparation of a variety of cellular therapy products in a functionally closed system. The regulatory status of these devices should be discussed with the FDA before clinical use.

Positive selection techniques may, however, passively deplete from the graft certain cells that could be of potential benefit to the recipient. These include some stromal elements, GVT-mediating T cells, and other populations that may facilitate engraftment. As our understanding of the identity of these populations improves, it may be possible to recover them from the normally discarded negative fraction and add them back to the CD34$^+$ cells, or to administer them in the posttransplant period as donor leukocyte infusions (see later discussion).

TABLE 97.2	**Methods Used for T-Cell Depletion of Hematopoietic Grafts**
Destruction in Situ	**Physical Separation**
Monoclonal antibody-based	Monoclonal antibody-based
Antibody + complement	Immunomagnetic separation
Immunotoxins (e.g., ricin)	Negative selection (T-cell removal)
Panning and immunoaffinity columns	Positive selection (CD34 selection) CliniMACs device
Cytotoxic drugs (e.g., 4-HC)	Rosetting with sheep erythrocytes
Photopheresis	Lectins (e.g., soybean agglutinin) Centrifugal elutriation

4-HC, 4-Hydroperoxycyclophosphamide.

Table 97.2 lists various methods of direct T-lymphocyte depletion and indirect depletion by HPC enrichment.

EVALUATION OF MANIPULATED GRAFTS

Most allograft engineering has focused on T-lymphocyte depletion and has emphasized quantitative versus qualitative removal. The majority of allografts are infused immediately after preparation rather than after cryopreservation and storage. This restricts the types of assays that can be used to evaluate graft composition to those that have a rapid turnaround, and the implications of infusing large numbers of T lymphocytes can be severe or lethal. Therefore, it is important to have available methods that can rapidly enumerate the numbers of T lymphocytes within the graft. Although early methods used detection of E-rosette–forming cells or manual immunofluorescence after staining with pan–T-lymphocyte–directed MAbs, most laboratories currently rely on flow cytometry. This technology is widely used in routine clinical laboratories; however, some precautions must be taken when it is used for T-depleted allografts.

Flow Cytometry

Accurate enumeration of very small numbers of target cells by cytometry requires rare event analysis. In this technique, large numbers of events must be accumulated and carefully analyzed if reliable data are to be obtained. This approach has been widely adopted for counting CD34$^+$ cells in unfractionated grafts but is often neglected when enumerating T lymphocytes in depleted grafts. The choice of MAb for detection of the T-lymphocyte population also is critical when a MAb-mediated depletion technology is used. The same MAb should not be used for both depletion and analysis because cells that became coated with the antibody during the depletion phase, but were not effectively removed, will be blocked from detection. However, they can be detected by adding an antiimmunoglobulin antibody conjugated to a fluorochrome different from the one conjugated to the T-lymphocyte–directed MAb. The most sensitive detection is achieved by using panels of non–cross-blocking anti–T-lymphocyte antibodies directed against a variety of epitopes.

It is important to include a viability stain in the analysis panel. Although this is less crucial when T-lymphocyte depletion is achieved by physical removal of target cells, it is extremely important when in situ elimination methods are used. In these cases, the depleted allograft may contain dead or dying T lymphocytes that will be detected by flow cytometry but may not contribute to postinfusion events. Suitable viability stains include propidium iodide and 7-aminoactinomycin. Analysis of cell viability after ex vivo depletion is not straightforward. Cell death may not be expressed immediately but develops in the hours or days after processing and infusion. Under such circumstances, the analysis of apoptotic cells by a combination of Annexin-V staining with 7-aminoactinomycin may provide a more accurate estimate of cell damage. This approach can be used in combination with simultaneous staining for T-cell surface markers to provide additional information. In some cases, incubating the cells for a period before analysis is advisable (e.g., in the case of depletion by immunotoxins, cells require time to divide to manifest the toxic

effects). Stimulation of cells with interleukin-2 (IL-2) and ex vivo culture also has been used to detect functional residual T lymphocytes. In some cases, this method has shown a correlation between the numbers of T lymphocytes in the cultured sample and the development of clinical GVHD in the graft recipient.

Tetramer Analysis

Enumeration of T cells bearing receptors for specific antigens can be achieved using tetramer analysis (Fig. 97.3). In this procedure, soluble versions of heavy chain of major histocompatibility complex molecules are synthesized and adopt the appropriate conformation when a synthetic peptide representing the epitope is recognized by the T-cell receptor and β2-microglobulin is added. The carboxyl-terminus of the MHC molecule is biotinylated, and four of these peptide/MHC–biotin complexes assemble into a tetramer when streptavidin is added. The streptavidin is tagged with a fluorochrome; therefore, T cells reactive with the chosen peptide–MHC complex become fluorescently stained and can be detected by flow cytometry.

Functional Assays

Flow cytometry detects residual cells by their ability to bind MAbs. Routine flow does not provide information on the functional capacity of these cells, which may be important when assessing the graft for its potential to mediate GVHD or GVT. For this purpose, a number of assays have been developed. These are not suitable for use as release tests because of their turnaround time, but they can provide retrospective information that may correlate with clinical outcome. They include limiting dilution analysis, in which a range of dilutions of the graft are plated out and assessed for the ability of T cells to form colonies in response to the addition of stimulants, such as phytohemagglutinin and IL-2. Based on the proportion of colony-forming

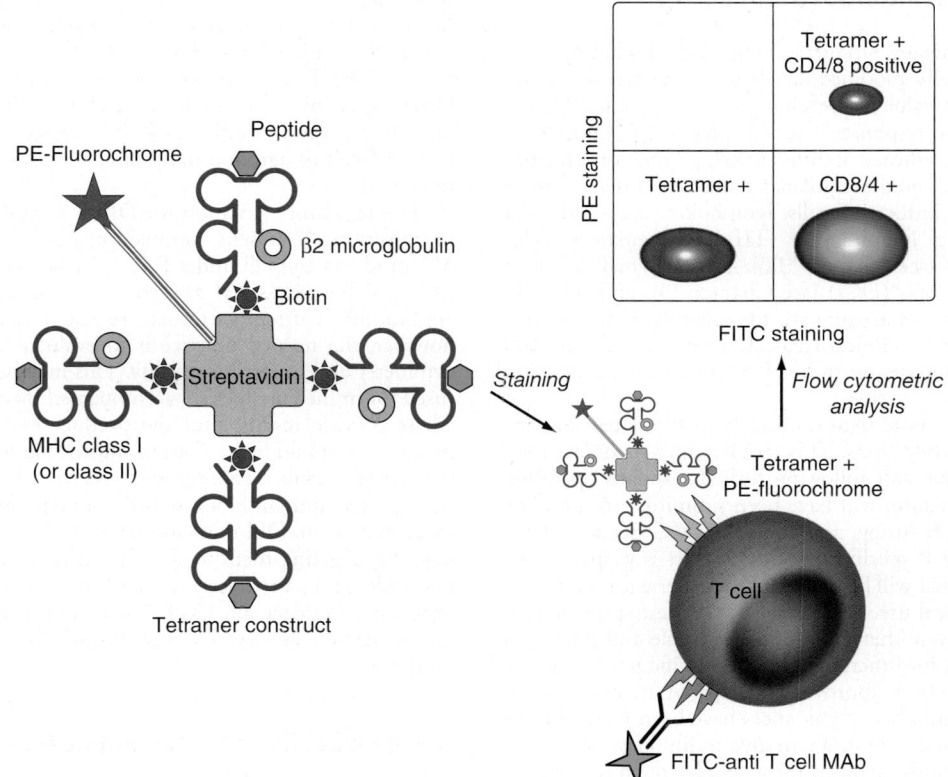

Fig. 97.3 TETRAMER STAINING TO DETECT ANTIGEN-SPECIFIC T CELLS. See text for details. *FITC*, Fluorescein isothiocyanate; *MAb*, monoclonal antibody; *MHC*, major histocompatibility complex; *PE*, phycoerythrin.

TABLE 97.3	Immunotherapeutic Cells Frequently Used in HSCT Recipients
Cell Type	**Clinical Use**
T regulatory cells	Prevention/treatment GVHD
Mesenchymal stromal cells	Immunosuppressive effect (GVHD) Regenerative applications
NK cells, TIL cells, LAK cells, NKT	Anticancer response
CAR-T cells	Anticancer response
Dendritic cells	Anticancer vaccines Antigen-presenting cells

CAR, Chimeric antigen receptor; GVHD, graft-versus-host disease; LAK, lymphokine activated; NK, natural killer; NKT, natural killer T cells; TIL, tumor-infiltrating lymphocyte.

wells at the various dilutions, it is possible to determine by Poisson distribution the number of T cells present in the original graft.

Another approach is use of an enzyme-linked immunosorbent spot (ELISpot) assay in which cells are stimulated to produce an analyte that is characteristic of their normal function. The cells are plated onto a surface that has been coated with an antibody directed against that analyte and incubated for a fixed period. The secreted analyte binds to this antibody, and the cells and any other unbound material are washed away. The surface is incubated with a biotinylated antibody directed against the analyte and washed and incubated with alkaline phosphatase linked to streptavidin. After washing, the plate is incubated with a substrate solution. A blue-black precipitate will appear at sites were the analyte was produced, with each spot representing an analyte-secreting cell. The spots can be enumerated manually or by using an ELISpot reader.

CELLULAR THERAPY PRODUCTS

A number of cellular therapy products (Table 97.3), including some that have been genetically modified, are being evaluated in clinical trials to determine their value in preventing or treating GVHD, and for potential antitumor responses (see Chapter 108). These have examined the safety and efficacy of different cell populations, including, but not limited to, nonmanipulated leukocyte infusions from HPC donors, cytokine-induced T cells, lymphokine-activated killer cells, tumor-infiltrating lymphocytes (TILs), T-regulatory cells, antigen-specific T cells (see Chapter 100), mesenchymal cells (see Chapter 99), dendritic cells (DCs) (see Chapter 23), and NK cells (see Chapter 101). Detailed accounts of the scientific basis for such studies as well as results of clinical trials are given in Chapters 100 and 101. This section focuses on processing and product evaluation issues.

Cells that have been more than minimally manipulated must be prepared under GMP conditions. This requires that manufacturing be performed by trained staff following formal standard operating procedures. These procedures will have been submitted to the FDA in the chemistry, manufacturing, and control (CMC) section of the IND application and will specify how the product is prepared, the reagents and materials that will be used, and the criteria for the release of the product for clinical use. Release criteria are test specifications that are designed to ensure that the product is sterile and pure, and they may include assays for functionality. The specific tests for sterility and purity that have been approved by the FDA are described in 21CFR 610.12, and a number of guidances have been issued by the FDA on the use and validation of alternative techniques.

In the normal release mechanism for a cellular therapy product, the quality unit reviews the production records and issues a certificate of analysis (Fig. 97.4). This document details the testing that was performed together with test method, the testing laboratory, the specification required by the FDA, and the actual results obtained. Routine testing required for most cellular therapy products consists of aerobic, anaerobic, and fungal sterility; endotoxin levels (by Limulus amebocyte method, e.g., Endosafe from Charles River); mycoplasma for ex vivo expanded cells (assayed by the culture method or by a validated polymerase chain reaction based method); identity and purity (by flow cytometry and, in some cases, HLA typing); and, for products in later stages of evaluation, functionality (e.g., cytotoxic activity toward target cells or secretion of specific bioactive products). Products that have been transduced with a retroviral vector will also require testing for replication-competent virus. Use of non–FDA-approved test methods should be cleared with the FDA at the IND application stage. Regulatory agencies also like to see some form of stability testing program that evaluates the stability of the cellular product over time in storage in the frozen state and when thawed for administration.

Phase I studies are designed to evaluate the safety of the product and should include assessment of reactions to infusion, risks for contamination during preparation, and delayed effects after administration. Clinical efficacy is evaluated during phase II/III. At this time, progress should be made toward the development of an in vitro assay for potency that correlates with clinical efficacy. This can be problematic because most in vitro assays currently used are unreliable as predictors of the clinical value of the product, and some form of surrogate marker has been substituted.

Donor Leukocyte Infusions

The ability of infusions of donor leukocytes (DLI) to mediate antitumor responses was originally described in patients with chronic myeloid leukemia in hematologic relapse after allogeneic stem cell transplantation, but lymphomas and Hodgkin disease also are sensitive to the effects of DLI. Remission rates of up to 80% have been reported in chronic myeloid leukemia patients who relapse after transplant. Up to 90% responses have been described in patients with Epstein-Barr virus (EBV)-associated lymphoproliferative disease. Moderate success has been achieved with use of DLI after relapse in other malignancies such as acute myeloid leukemia (15%–40%), low-grade lymphomas (≤60%), and metastatic multiple myeloma (40%–60%). Fewer than 5% of patients with relapsed acute lymphoblastic leukemia respond to DLI alone. Although the etiology is unclear, the reason could be lack of antigenic expression, downregulation of T-cell recognition molecules, or tumor burden at the time of treatment.

The regulatory situation for DLI is complicated and is probably in transition. At present, nonmanipulated DLI are classified as Type 361 products and fall under Part 1271 of 21CFR. It is possible that they will be reclassified as Type 351 products requiring an IND application. Currently, formal release criteria are not required; however, the normal practice is to evaluate T-cell content by flow cytometry and to test for sterility. This may be done by a gram stain (used for immediate release) accompanied by culture-based methods. These provide results after the product has been infused. Formal procedures should be in place to inform the recipient's physician if a positive test result is subsequently received. The contaminant should be speciated and antibiotic sensitivities obtained and communicated to the physician. DLI that have been manipulated ex vivo in any way (e.g., by targeting them to specific antigens or by transduction with a suicide gene, as described later) will be classified as Type 351 products requiring an IND. These products will require formal release testing as described previously for other cellular therapy products.

Nonspecifically Activated Autologous T Cells

T cells can be expanded ex vivo through polyclonal activation using phytohemagglutinin, anti-CD3 antibody, or a combination of anti-CD3 and anti-CD28 antibodies. Several groups have evaluated

CAGT GMP — Center for Cell & Gene Therapy — Good Manufacturing Practices Facility

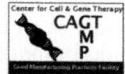

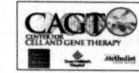

CERTIFICATE OF ANALYSIS

GMP Facility, Center for Cell & Gene Therapy
Baylor College of Medicine
Caution: New Drug-Limited by Federal Law to Investigational Use
Properly identify intended recipient and component
For Autologous Use Only

CAGT — Center for Cell and Gene Therapy

T Cells Whole Blood: VZV-Specific T-Lymphocytes Transduced with the SFG.iCasp9.2A.CAR-GD2.CD28.OX40ζ [VEGAS Protocol]

Patient Name:	**DOE, John**
CAGT #	**P9999**
Hospital #:	**MRN 1234567**
Component #	**C6688.41.21**
Vector Lot #:	**RV1202.C**
Date frozen	**06/30/15 Store below -150°C**

TEST	LABORATORY	SPECIFICATION	RESULT
Viability by dye exclusion	CAGT GMP Facility Houston, Texas	>70% viable	93.8% viable 06/30/15
Endotoxin (LAL – Endosafe) (Cell supernatant)	CAGT QC Laboratory, Houston, Texas	<5.0 EU/ml	<2.0 EU/ml 07/09/15
Mycoplasma (MycoAlert)	CAGT QC Laboratory, Houston, Texas	Negative	Negative 07/02/15
Sterility Bactec Bacterial Sterility (Cells) Bactec Anaerobic Sterility (Cells) Bactec Fungal (Supernatant)	Houston Adult Hospital Laboratory Services	Negative @ 7 days	Negative @ 14 days 07/15/15 Negative @ 14 days 07/15/15 Negative @ 14 days 07/14/15
Immunophenotyping	CAGT 17th Floor Translational Lab. Houston, Texas CAGT GMP Flow Facility, Houston, Texas	≥20% expression of GD2 CAR by FACS analysis <0.1% (CD3/CD16/CD56)^{neg} (CD83/32)^{pos}	88.9% expression of GD2 CAR by FACS analysis 06/29/15 0.01% (CD3/CD16/CD56)^{neg} (CD83/32)^{pos} 07/06/15
Cytotoxic Activity (^{51}Cr Release)	CAGT 17th Floor Translational Lab. Houston, Texas	Killing of GD2$^+$ targets ≥ 20% in cytotoxicity assay @ 20:1 Effector:Target ratio	Killing of GD2$^+$ targets 86.8% in cytotoxicity assay @ 20:1 Effector:Target ratio 06/29/15
Antigen specificity by γ-IFN Elispot assay	CAGT 17th Floor Translational Lab. Houston, Texas	>20 spot-forming cells above background in response to VZV pepmixes	229 spot-forming cells above background in response to VZV pepmixes 07/01/15
HLA Typing	**Donor & CTLs** Houston Adult Hospital Histocompatibility Laboratories	HLA Identity between CTLs and Donor **Donor** A*11,*32; B*15,*38 Cw* DRB1*04,*13; DQB1*03,*06; DRB3*01; DRB4*01 DRB5* 05/28/15	**CTLs** A*11,*32; B*15,*38 Cw* DRB1*04,*13; DQB1*03,*06; DRB3*01; DRB4*01 DRB5* 07/08/15
Replication-Competent Retrovirus	CAGT QC Laboratory	Sample sent for testing	Sample sent for testing 06/30/15

Approved for Release for Autologous Use Only by:

_______________________________ 07/17/15
John Smith
Director, Quality Assurance

_______________________________ 07/17/15
Helen Johns
Laboratory Medical Director

Valid Certificate consists of 1 signed page — Page 1 of 1

Fig. 97.4 SAMPLE CERTIFICATE OF ANALYSIS USED FOR THE RELEASE OF CELLULAR PRODUCTS MANUFACTURED UNDER AN INVESTIGATIONAL NEW DRUG.

whether such expanded T cells have antitumor activity. Faster recovery of lymphocyte counts with improved outcome after autologous transplant observed in non-Hodgkin and Hodgkin lymphoma led to a phase I study evaluating the infusion of autologous CD3/CD28-activated cells after a CD34-selected stem cell transplantation.

Cells prepared for these types of studies are Type 351 products because they are cultured ex vivo and may have undergone some form of activation. Manufacturing must be carried out under GMP, and the clinical studies must be performed under an IND. The IND application must describe in the CMC the procedure for manufacturing the cells and the criteria that will be used to determine whether they can be released for clinical use. Many manufacturing procedures use reagents and materials that are not approved for human use, and the application should include information about these materials and what testing will be performed before they can be used for manufacturing the clinical product. Justification should be provided for the use of nonapproved media and supplements and any potentially undesirable ancillary products, such as antibiotics. Evidence should be provided on the efficacy of their removal before administration of the product.

The release criteria for autologous T-cell products are similar to those described for generic Type 351 products. They include tests for sterility, endotoxin, mycoplasma, and identity and purity (i.e., by flow cytometry); some test of potency is recommended, but is not usually required for phase I studies. A draft of the certificate of analysis, which will be used for release, should be included in the IND submission.

Tumor-Infiltrating Lymphocytes

TILs are cells harvested from tumor sites and are expanded ex vivo with IL-2. As the cells are being expanded, increased tumor specificity is achieved by pulsing the cells with tumor-specific peptides or transducing them with a retrovirus encoding a tumor-specific T-cell receptor. A major limitation is that patients must have preexisting lymphocytes that can both respond to tumor and be expanded ex vivo. Transfer of these cells has led to tumor regression in 50% of lymphodepleted patients with metastatic melanoma.

A number of methods have been developed for isolation of TILs from tumors. They include mechanical disruption, enzymatic treatment, differential centrifugation approaches, and positive immunomagnetic selection. The method of choice depends on the type of tissue from which the cells are to be extracted and the availability of reagents, such as MAbs, to enrich the T-cell population of interest. As with T-cell depletion of allogeneic grafts, the predominant effector TIL cell population is not fully characterized, and the availability of this information should facilitate the design of more effective separation techniques. A number of approved enzymes and centrifugation media are available, and several companies have suitable MAbs that have been prepared under GMP conditions but have not been submitted for FDA approval.

The extracted cells are expanded ex vivo, usually starting in semiopen systems such as cluster plates. The initial populations may be tested in a cytotoxicity assay in an attempt to identify the effector population, which can then be selected for expansion. The expansion phase usually progresses through a number of types of cultures as cell numbers increase. These may progress from plates to T flasks and gas-permeable bags to hollow fiber and culture bag bioreactors. The culture medium contains IL-2 as the primary cytokine, although other agents alone and in combination may be used to promote outgrowth of specific cell subpopulations.

Some investigators have used irradiated tumor cells to restimulate TILs during culture; others have performed selective separations to enrich the effector cells during expansion. Highly characterized tissue culture media, such as the serum-free lymphocyte medium AIM V (Thermo Fisher Scientific), have been used for expansion. The goal is to use the simplest medium with the fewest additives that will support growth of functional cells. When possible, the media should be free of animal serum and proteins to simplify the regulatory issues. However, the FDA is aware that complex media and serum combinations may be required to support growth of some cell types and is willing to consider them, particularly if the cells can be washed into an approved excipient for administration.

Initiation of a phase I study using TILs or TIL subpopulations will not require complete characterization of the effector cell population, but some preliminary information should be available that allows quantification of the putative effectors for dosing purposes. In most cases, flow cytometric analysis will be used, and the target antigens may be pan–T-cell markers or specific combinations of T

subset markers. When other constituents of the product may adversely affect the activity of effector cells, it may be necessary to set an upper limit for contamination by these cells in the clinical product. Most facilities perform some type of functional assay as a part of the release process, which in the case of TILs may be cytokine release or cytotoxic activity toward tumor cells of the appropriate histologic type.

Allodepleted Cells

The major drawback of DLI is the significant risk of GVHD, which is the most important source of treatment-related mortality. Given that the frequency of tumor or viral antigen-specific T cells in most cases is considerably lower than that of alloreactive T cells, it is necessary to expand antigen-specific T cells ex vivo not only to enhance antitumor activity, but also to try to separate GVHD from GVT effect. An alternative method for separating GVHD from GVT effect is to selectively deplete alloreactive donor T cells ex vivo. Selective allodepletion is performed by removing donor T cells that express activation markers after coculture with nonleukemic recipient cells. Activation markers investigated include CD25 and CD69 and the increased sensitivity of activated T cells to photosensitizing dyes. A number of phase I/II studies using immunotoxin directed against CD25 have demonstrated the feasibility of this approach, with accelerated reconstitution of virus-specific and total T-cell numbers and low rates of severe GVHD. Relapse rates remained high in this study, which probably reflects the high-risk nature of the patient population.

Potential recipients of allodepleted cells often receive a CD34-selected HPC graft. As a part of the CD34 selection process, a negatively selected population of cells that includes T cells becomes available. However, this fraction usually is not used as the source of cells for allodepletion. These cells usually have been obtained from donors who received granulocyte-macrophage colony-stimulating factor for mobilization of peripheral blood progenitor cells, and during processing for CD34 selection they were exposed to anti-CD34 MAbs. Therefore, it is preferable to obtain cells for allodepletion from a peripheral blood draw of the donor before administration of growth factor for mobilization. The T-cell–enriched fraction is usually obtained by centrifugation on a Ficoll-Hypaque density cushion. The cells are washed and coincubated with irradiated recipient mononuclear cells, which act as stimulators. A convenient source for stimulator cells is obtained by generation of a cell line from the donor by infection of his or her peripheral blood mononuclear cells with a laboratory strain of EBV. The coincubation step produces stimulation of alloreactive donor T cells with resulting expression of activation markers, which can then be targeted to remove the alloreactive population. Methods for elimination include cytotoxic drugs (e.g., methotrexate), anti-CD25 MAbs conjugated to the toxin ricin, and immunomagnetic selection. All of the regulatory issues associated with the manufacturing and release of Type 351 products apply to allodepleted T-cell products. Release criteria include routine assays for sterility and purity. HLA typing may be included as a confirmation that the cells in the product are of donor origin. Functional assays may include demonstration that the allodepleted cells fail to proliferate when cultured in a primary mixed lymphocyte reaction (MLR). If a suicide gene has been introduced (see next section), testing will include demonstration that it can be efficiently activated.

Suicide Gene-Transduced Lymphocytes

Although treatment with DLI has led to remission in patients with disease after HSC transplantation, unmanipulated cells also contain alloreactive T cells and can induce GVHD. The incidence of GVHD ranges from 55% to 90% and is associated with a treatment-related mortality rate of about 20%. Approaches that maintain the GVT effect while decreasing the incidence of GVHD have been evaluated and include transduction of donor T cells with a "suicide gene."

Genes can be introduced into DLI or alloreactive-depleted cells to express the herpes simplex virus-1 thymidine kinase (HSV-tk). If GVHD develops, Ganciclovir is administered to the recipient, resulting in suicide of the transduced donor leukocytes.

Alternative suicide genes based on the dimerization of Fas or Caspase-9 in the apoptotic pathway have been developed to circumvent the problem of immunogenicity of HSV-tk. The inducible Caspase construct also encodes a selection marker, such as CD19, that can be used to enrich the transduced population. In the event that GVHD develops after administration of the Caspase-transduced cells, the suicide activation drug can be administered to the recipient to eradicate the transduced T cells by dimerization of Caspase 9 and activation of the apoptosis pathway.

Antigen-Specific Cytotoxic T Lymphocytes

Two major prerequisites for generating antigen-specific cytotoxic T lymphocytes (CTLs) are the identification of appropriate viral (in the case of EBV-associated lymphomas) or tumor target antigens and the availability of suitable antigen-presenting cells (APCs). After being identified, CTL lines can be generated by coculturing T cells with APCs that express the target antigen. The lines are then expanded by restimulation with the antigen of choice and the addition of cytokines such as IL-2.

To generate antigen-specific CTLs, it is necessary to have a good source of APCs and a source of antigen to present to T cells. A variety of APCs have been evaluated, including fibroblasts, monocytes, and DCs, using different sources of antigen, including virus lysate or lysate of antigen-positive cells, peptides, or transduction of the APC, such as lymphoblastoid cells (LCLs) and DCs with an immunodominant antigen. Use of lysates as the antigen source can be problematic because they are likely to be variable and difficult to standardize. Alternatively, many processing laboratories may not be experienced in handling virus and virus-infected cells.

LCLs prepared using laboratory strains of EBV make excellent APCs for use in manufacturing EBV-specific T cells. They present EBV antigens efficiently, and they express high levels of costimulatory molecules. The normal procedure for generating the LCL is coincubation with EBV derived from the tamarin B95-8 cell line. This line has undergone extensive testing and has been approved for use as a source of "clinical" EBV. The resulting LCLs are cultured in media containing acyclovir to eliminate any residual EBV. The LCLs are used to repeatedly stimulate T cells (as a mononuclear cell fraction of peripheral blood leukocytes), resulting in a population that is directed toward the immunodominant EBV antigens. These CTLs can be frozen while release testing is performed. They are delivered frozen to the bedside, where they are thawed and administered intravenously. Release testing consists of the routine tests described earlier for Type 351 products. For allogeneic CTLs, functionality is usually assessed by cytotoxicity assays, which must demonstrate less than 10% killing of autologous blasts.

One limitation of this approach is that expansion of virus-specific T cells to achieve adequate dose levels is extremely time consuming. All of these procedures require several weeks to generate APCs. More recently accelerated methods of production have been developed. These include the use of direct T-cell stimulation using mixtures of peptides for overlapping regions of the target antigen(s) (PepMix, JPT) and the use of disposable bioreactors that provide improved gas exchange, thereby markedly improving rates of T-cell expansion.

An alternative strategy is to manufacture and bank third-party allogeneic EBV-specific CTLs with a range of HLA types so that an "off-the-shelf" product is available. Clinical responses have been described for patients who received partially matched allogeneic CTLs. The generation of banks of CTLs requires careful donor screening and HLA typing to allow at least partial matching with the intended recipient.

The use of T cells transduced to express chimeric antigen receptors directed against tumor antigens has produced very promising results in early-phase clinical trials in CD19+ leukemias. The chimeric antigen receptor often incorporates other moieties that are designed to dampen inhibitory signals from the cancer or to amplify a beneficial immune response. Manufacture of these cells requires preparation of an appropriate construct and delivery system (viral or nonviral vector) that is used to modify the expanded T-cell population. Release testing is similar to that required for other gene-modified cellular therapeutics (see Fig. 97.4).

Natural Killer Cells

NK cells are effectors from the innate immune system that also mediate antiviral and antitumor immunity. Studies have shown that haploidentical NK cells infused after lymphodepleting chemotherapy can have antitumor effects. Most facilities use a simple positive selection with clinical scale immunomagnetic methods involving CD56 selection or CD3 depletion for such products. These procedures must be done under an IND because of lack of commercially available devices and reagents for this indication. Recent evidence has suggested that cryopreserved NK cells have impaired functionality on recipients, in contrast to cells that are infused fresh. This poses an additional challenge to the manufacturer, who must coordinate testing and possible shipment of the fresh product. It is not clear whether the same finding may apply to other cell therapy products.

When preparing an IND application for NK cell enrichment, care should be taken to ensure that the MAbs used for the selection or depletion are of the highest quality available. A certificate of analysis for these reagents should be submitted with the IND application, and the agency will probably require detailed information on their manufacturing (i.e., to ensure that the process includes robust procedures for virus inactivation or removal). The same type of information may be required for any ancillary reagents (e.g., buffers and protein sources used to supplement buffers). Preclinical data demonstrating that the enrichment technique is effective should be provided and accompanied by data from clinical scale validation enrichments, providing evidence that the NK cells can be separated with acceptable viability, purity, and yield for the proposed study. The CMC section of the IND application should include information on the methods used to store, label, and administer the cells. Engineered APCs, such as the K562-mb15-41BBL cell line, if used to stimulate NK cells, should initially have been grown and tested as a Master Cell Bank, from which a Working Cell Bank is generated and tested for routine use.

Dendritic Cells

DCs are powerful APCs that can be used in vitro or in vivo to elicit immune response to the antigen they are presenting. A number of studies have evaluated tumor antigen-primed DCs for treatment of hematologic malignancies and solid tumors. Antigen-primed DCs are used to target T cells in vitro toward specific antigens. These cells then can be used therapeutically to eliminate viruses or tumor cells bearing that antigen. DCs can be derived from BM or cord blood and mobilized, and resting peripheral blood obtained from normal donors and patients. The normal procedure consists of enriching monocytes from the source material, which has been accomplished by plastic adherence or CD14-based immunomagnetic selection (or by depletion of CD19+ B cells and CD2+ T cells). An alternative approach is use of elutriation to collect an enriched monocyte fraction from the donor. A purpose-built elutriation system for collection of monocytes is available (the Elutra, Terumo BCT). This method has also been used successfully to enrich monocytes from cryopreserved mobilized apheresis collections.

The monocyte fraction can be cultured in polystyrene tissue culture flasks or gas-permeable bags in culture medium containing IL-4 and granulocyte-macrophage colony-stimulating factor to induce DC differentiation. This is followed by culture in medium containing proinflammatory mediators to accelerate maturation. A number of supplements have been used during this phase, including CD40 ligand or poly(I:C), interferon-α, tumor necrosis factor-α, IL-6, IL-1α, and prostaglandin E$_2$. Some protocols add proinflammatory mediators at the initiation of the cultures rather than after induction of differentiation. One issue for manufacturers is finding clinical or GMP-grade cytokines and growth factors. Some sources now are available, and many manufacturers assist investigators by providing information on test procedures and stability information. Attempts have been made to expand DCs in serum-free medium with varying degrees of success; improved growth and maturation have generally been obtained in the presence of human AB or autologous serum. Of note, minor changes in composition of the culture medium and even in the type of vessel used for culture have been reported to affect the yield, phenotype, and functional activity of the resulting DCs. Cultured DCs have been effectively transfected using native tumor DNA or lentiviral or adenoviral vectors. The cells can be cryopreserved for later administration or use.

Assessment of DC product usually involves immunophenotyping (CD1a$^+$, CD80$^+$, CD83$^+$) and some type of functional assay (ability to generate an allogeneic T-cell response or response to a recall antigen as measured by proliferation assay) in addition to the standard release assays.

Mesenchymal Stromal Cells

Mesenchymal stromal cells (MSCs) are cells with multilineage potential that have shown efficacy in promoting engraftment and suppressing GVHD. They are also widely used in regenerative medicine applications, where their mode of action is not well understood. In vitro MSCs are capable of differentiating into bone, cartilage, cardiac and skeletal muscle, neuronal cells, adipose and connective tissue, and tendons. The cells are not inherently immunogenic and do not appear to be recognized by allogeneic T cells or NK cells. They express very low levels of MHC class II and intermediate levels of class I antigens. They appear to be able to suppress T-cell proliferation and function of both memory T and naive T cells in vitro, as well as inhibit the development of monocyte-derived DCs in vitro.

A number of technical variables affect MSC culture and expansion ex vivo. They include culture medium, passaging density, serum type and concentration, population selection, culture vessel, and use of growth factors. To reduce some of this variability and decrease the cost of preclinical testing, the FDA often encourages investigators to adopt a manufacturing process that is in current clinical trials. The following is a basic procedure. MSCs are usually isolated from BM collected from the iliac crest. The cells are diluted, and the mononuclear fraction is isolated using a Ficoll-Hypaque density cushion (GE Healthcare Life Sciences). This fraction is plated into culture flasks to enrich for adherent cells. The nonadherent population is removed after approximately 7 days of incubation. The adherent cells are washed and detached by incubation with trypsin/ethylenediaminetetraacetic acid (alternatively, TrypZean [Sigma-Aldrich], a recombinant form of trypsin, can be substituted) and then cultured and passaged at weekly intervals. In a study designed to optimize culture conditions, the best results were obtained when cells were cultured in low-glucose Dulbecco's modified Eagle medium-based media containing 10% fetal bovine serum (human platelet lysate is now frequently substituted) and GlutaMAX (Thermo Fisher) instead of L-glutamine. The cells also proliferated better when plated at low cell densities (5000–10,000 cells/cm^2) in Falcon flasks. Use of basic fibroblast growth factor as a growth supplement was found to be effective; however, it caused HLA-DR induction and upregulated HLA class I expression. This did not affect the immunosuppressive capabilities of the cells. An increase in osteogenic and adipogenic potential was noted, but neurogenesis and engraftment support for CD34$^+$ cells were slightly suppressed. A number of media specifically designed for culture of MSCs are commercially available (e.g., PRIME-XV from Irvine Scientific, STEMPRO MSC SFM, a serum-free formulation from Invitrogen, and MesenCult, a basal culture medium from StemCell Technologies). Various investigators have

reported success growing MSCs in serum-free media or using platelet lysate, autologous serum, or human AB serum as alternatives to fetal bovine serum. The traditional method for producing MSCs in tissue culture flasks is laborious and involves many open procedures that could result in product contamination. An alternative method is to use a functionally closed, hollow-fiber bioreactor, such as the Quantum from Terumo. In this system whole marrow is loaded into the reactor and the adherent cells attach to the fibers. Nonadherent cells are flushed from the fibers, which are perfused with the culture medium. Growth is monitored by glucose consumption and/or lactate production, and the flow rate of medium is increased based on these readings. The cells are removed from the fibers by routine enzymatic treatment.

Mesenchymal stromal cells can be characterized by their expression of CD105, CD73, and CD90 and their lack of expression of CD45, CD34, CD14 or CD11b, CD79a or CD19, and HLA-DR. They must be plastic adherent under standard culture conditions and must be capable of differentiating into osteoblasts, adipocytes, and chondroblasts in vitro. Differentiation assays involve growing MSCs under conditions that promote differentiation along the specific pathway. For neurogenic differentiation, the medium contains linoleic acid, platelet-derived growth factor, and epidermal growth factor. Neural cells are identified by immunostaining with antibodies against tubulin BIII, synaptophysin, galactocerebroside, neurofilament M, and neuronal nuclei. To assess adipogenic potential, the medium contains dexamethasone, isobutylmethylxanthine, and indomethacin. The lipid droplets in the generated adipocytes are visualized by staining with Sudan Black IV. Osteogenic differentiation is measured by culturing the cells in medium containing dexamethasone, β-glycerophosphate, and L-ascorbic acid 2-phosphate. Calcium accumulation and alkaline phosphatase activity in the resulting cells is visualized by alkaline phosphatase/Von Kossa staining, and the osteogenic differentiation is measured as the percentage of mineralized area in the total cultured area.

The ability of MSCs to suppress an MLR is used as an indication of their immunosuppressive activity. A traditional MLR assay is used; however, in the test wells, the MLR is performed on a layer of MSCs seeded the day before. The response is traditionally measured by uptake of tritiated thymidine. Numerous animal assays for MSCs are available but are predominantly used in preclinical studies and are not useful as release assays. Release criteria consist of the usual assays for sterility, endotoxin, and mycoplasma, with immunophenotyping for the MSC population. Depending on the intended use of the MSC, the release process may require an assay showing potential for differentiation into a specific lineage or ability to suppress an immune response such as an MLR assay.

Genetically Modified Cell Therapy Products

Many cell therapy approaches involve genetic modification of either APCs or effector cells (see earlier discussion). This therapy requires a source of vector that has been manufactured to meet regulatory requirements. Viral vector specifications changed markedly after the death of a gene therapy patient in Philadelphia, and they continue to evolve. Manufacturers must maintain close contact with the FDA to ensure that their products meet current specifications. Manufacturing and testing of viral vectors is extremely expensive, and use of genetically modified products requires additional monitoring of recipients. Use of vectors to transduce or transfect cellular therapy products ex vivo usually requires additional testing of the product, which may include detection of replication-competent virus and checking the functionality of the introduced vector (by detecting expression of the gene product).

Gene-Modified Tumor Vaccines

Tumor vaccines as an approach to inducing or stimulating immunity have been evaluated. Various techniques have been tested, including the use of DCs pulsed with a tumor-associated antigen preparation and the use of the entire tumor cells as an immunogen, either unmodified or transduced with immunostimulatory genes, aimed at eliciting a broad-based, robust immune response.

From the manufacturing perspective, the autologous product is much more of a challenge because a stable tumor cell line must be isolated from each patient. This can be an extremely difficult process. Many isolated lines do not expand well in culture, or they change phenotype over time. In some patients, the line cannot be generated; other patients progress clinically before the vaccine is available and are excluded from the study. As a result, the autologous approach has a relatively high "failure rate". The allogeneic cell line approach is technically easier because a line is selected before the study and can be used as the generic immunogen. This line must be tested extensively for infectious agents and should pass the FDA testing criteria for Master and Working Cell Banks. Currently, testing of this type costs $100,000–200,000 for each line. Scientifically, the drawback is that the selected line may not adequately express the antigen or range of antigens present on each patient's tumor. In addition, the choice of immunostimulatory molecules that are expressed or enhanced by transduction of the cell line may not be those that would most effectively evoke an immune response. These products are relatively expensive to produce, involving not only the costs of testing the tumor cell line, but also the expense of manufacturing and testing the vectors used for transduction. However, these are one-time costs because the same vaccine is used for all patients in the study.

Release testing involves testing for sterility, endotoxin, and mycoplasma, with immunophenotyping of the cells and some form of test demonstrating that the line has been effectively transduced (e.g., flow cytometry for CD40 ligand and IL-2 production in the examples described earlier). Because the product will be stored cryopreserved over the course of the study and thawed for administration to each patient, the requirement for an ongoing stability study should be anticipated.

FUTURE DIRECTIONS

The science and practice of hematopoietic transplantation has expanded dramatically over the past 10 years and has stimulated entirely new areas of medicine. New sources of stem cells have been discovered that have expanded the availability of grafts and provided new insights into stem cell biology. An improved understanding of the immunology of transplantation and immune responses to malignancies has led to more sophisticated methods to manipulate the hematopoietic graft and the immune system in the recipient to produce more favorable outcomes. The ability to target T cells to residual disease by genetic modification of the cells to express chimeric antigen receptors has produced promising results that have reinvigorated prospects for effective immunotherapy of cancer.

In parallel, the regulatory situation has become clearer and we are starting to see widespread development of commercial reagents and devices that facilitate easier compliance when manufacturing cell products.

These advances in knowledge coupled to development in technology promise a bright future for engineering specific cell populations to provide targeted therapies.

SUGGESTED READINGS

PROFESSIONAL STANDARDS FOR CELLULAR THERAPY

AABB Standards for Cellular Therapy Services, AABB, Bethesda, MD.
FACT Common Standards for Cellular Therapy. Foundation for Accreditation of Cellular Therapy, Omaha, NE.

FACT-JACIE International Standards for Cellular Therapy Product Collection: Processing and Administration. Foundation for Accreditation of Cellular Therapy, Omaha, NE.
NetCord-FACT International Standards for Cord Blood Collection, Processing, and Release for Administration, Omaha, NE.

FDA REGULATIONS: CGMP AND CGTP

cGMP in Manufacturing, Processing, Packing, or Holding of Drugs and Finished Pharmaceuticals. Code of Federal Regulations Title 21, Parts 210 and 211.
Human Cells, Tissues, and Cellular and Tissue Based Products. Code of Federal Regulations Title 21, Part 1271.

FDA GUIDANCES ON CELLULAR AND GENE THERAPY

Guidance for FDA Reviewers and Sponsors: Content and Review of Chemistry, Manufacturing, and Control (CMC) Information for Human Somatic Cell Therapy Investigational New Drug Applications (INDs). U.S. Department of Health and Human Services, Food and Drug Administration, Center for Biologics Evaluation and Research, April 2008.
Guidance for Industry: CGMP for Phase 1 Investigational Drugs. U.S. Department of Health and Human Services, Food and Drug Administration, Center for Biologics Evaluation and Research, July 2008.
Guidance for Industry: Considerations for the Design of Early-Phase Clinical Trials of Cellular and Gene Therapy Products. U.S. Department of Health and Human Services, Food and Drug Administration, Center for Biologics Evaluation and Research, June 2015.

GMP FACILITIES AND PRODUCT MANUFACTURING

Cell therapy – cGMP facilities and manufacturing. Gee AP, editor: New York, NY, 2009, Springer.
Cellular therapy: principles, methods, and regulations. Areman E, editor: Bethesda, MD, 2009, AABB.

SPECIFIC CELL TYPES: CURRENT REVIEWS

OVERVIEW

June CH, Riddell SR, Schumacher TN: Adoptive cellular therapy: a race to the finish line. Sci Transl Med 7(280):280ps7, 2015.
Kongtim P, Lee DA, Cooper LJ, et al: Haploidentical Hematopoietic Stem Cell Transplantation as a Platform for Post-Transplantation Cellular Therapy. Biol Blood Marrow Transplant 21(10):1714–1720, 2015.
Melero I, Berman DM, Aznar MA, et al: Evolving synergisitic combinations of targeted immunotherapies to combat cancer. Nat Rev Cancer 15:457, 2015.
Themeli M, Riviere I, Sadelain M: New cell sources for T cell engineering and adoptive immunotherapy. Cell Stem Cell 16(4):357–3566, 2015.

MESENCHYMAL STROMAL CELLS

Luk F, de Witte SF, Bramer WM, et al: Efficacy of Immunotherapy with mesenchymal stem cells in man: a systematic review. Expert Rev Clin Immunol 11:617, 2015.

DENDRITIC CELLS

Atta J, Berk E, Cintolo JA, et al: Rationale for a multimodality strategy to enhance the efficacy of cell based cancer immunotherapy. Front Immunol 2:271, 2015.

NATURAL KILLER CELLS

Cichocki F, Verneris MR, Cooley S, et al: The Past, Present, and Future of NK Cells in Hematopoietic Cell Transplantation and Adoptive Transfer. *Curr Top Microbiol Immunol* 2015 Jun 3.

TUMOR-INFILTRATING LYMPHOCYTE CELLS

Hinrichs CS, Rosenberg SA: Exploiting the curative potential of adoptive T cell therapy for cancer. *Immunol Rev* 257:56, 2014.

T AND CAR-T CELLS

Brenner MK: Will T cell therapy for cancer ever be a standard of care? *Cancer Gene Ther* 19:818, 2012.

Gill S, June CH: Going viral: chimeric antigen receptor T cell therapy for hematological malignancies. *Immunol Rev* 263:68, 2015.

Leen AM, Heslop HE, Brenner MK: Antiviral T-cell therapy. *Immunol Rev* 258(1):12–29, 2014.

TUMOR VACCINES

Kissick HT, Sanda MG: The role of active vaccination in cancer immunotherapy: lessons from clinical trials. *Curr Opin Immunol* 35:15, 2015.

REGULATORY T CELLS

Attridge K, Walker LS: Homeostasis and function of regulatory T cells (Tregs) in vivo: lessons learned from TCR transgenic Tregs. *Immunol Rev* 259:23, 2014.

Michael M, Shimoni A, Nagler A: Regulatory T cells in allogeneic stem cell transplantation. *Clin Dev Immunol* 2013:608951, 2013. [Epub].

Monty M, Gaugler B: A bit of sweetness for GVHD prevention. *Blood* 125:1364, 2015.

CHAPTER 98

PRINCIPLES OF CELL-BASED GENETIC THERAPIES

David A. Williams

The use of gene transfer to treat human diseases has now been demonstrated to be efficacious in a limited number of instances. Proof-of-principle successes in several monogenic diseases—both hematologic and nonhematologic—have been published and widely publicized in the past decade. The previous occurrence of serious adverse events in some trials related to insertional mutagenesis has stimulated rapid development of safer vector systems. This chapter discusses the basic biology of vector systems applicable to blood diseases, the details of the application of gene therapy to blood diseases using specific trials as examples of this technology, and the modifications in vector systems driven by clinical experience that predict future trials. The chapter also discusses the evolving field of somatic cell reprogramming and genome editing that may impact clinical applications in the future.

HEMATOLOGIC DISEASES, CELLULAR TARGETS, AND THE BASIS FOR GENETIC THERAPIES

Gene therapy is defined as the introduction of new genetic material into the cells of an organism for therapeutic purposes. Broadly speaking, two types of gene therapy can be envisioned. The introduction of genetic material into germ cells such that the new DNA can be expected to be passed into the gene pool. This is termed *germline gene therapy* and is currently banned in the United States and around the world. The potential for newer methods of genome engineering to be utilized in clinical applications (discussed later) has led to more recent calls for extending this restriction. In contrast, introduction of new genetic material into specialized cells of the body with no risk of the new genetic material being passed onto subsequent generations is termed *somatic gene therapy*. The ultimate goal of gene therapy is to correct the targeted genetic disease by *replacement* of the defective gene in situ. Such gene replacement could be envisioned via a process termed *homologous recombination*. Homologous recombination in mammalian cells is widely practiced in laboratories but up to now has been relatively inefficient, although newer technology may overcome some of the previous limitations to efficient genome editing. Advantages of this approach would include a reduction in the risk of inadvertent disruption or dysregulation of expression of a critical gene sequence and regulated (appropriate level and distribution) expression of the normal (replaced) gene. However, the frequency of homologous recombination (in contrast to random chromosomal integration) in mammalian cells and primary tissues makes therapeutic use of homologous recombination somewhat impractical at this point. Methods to effect homologous recombination have improved in the past 5 years and may make this goal attainable in the future.

The requirements for successful application of our current gene transfer technology for treatment of human diseases include knowledge of the abnormal gene sequence responsible for the disease phenotype and the availability of the corresponding normal gene sequence that can be packaged into current vector backbones for efficient recombinant virus production. In addition, the cells responsible for the disease phenotype must be identified and accessible for genetic manipulation. Finally, a means of introducing and expressing the correct gene sequence in cells such that the disease phenotype can be reversed is needed. Although effectively accomplished nearly three decades ago in murine studies, this latter requirement encompassing both in vivo administration of DNA sequences and ex vivo cell manipulation has been the most difficult to consistently meet in human applications using current gene transfer technology.

Since the early development of virus vectors, blood-forming cells have been used as one optimal target for ex vivo gene transfer studies. For this purpose, hematopoietic stem and progenitor cells (HPSCs) are isolated, manipulated in the laboratory, and administered back to the patient. The advantages of these cells as targets of gene transfer are multiple. First, all blood cells are derived from a common progenitor cell, the hematopoietic stem cell (HSC), which is both long lived in vivo and capable of significant self-renewal. The latter capacity and the pluripotency of HSCs is exploited to amplify the genetically manipulated cells into large cell numbers of multiple blood lineages derived from the genetically altered cells in vivo. There is a long and successful experience in obtaining these stem cells from the bone marrow (BM) and peripheral and umbilical cord blood. There is extensive experience in the use of HSCs in the clinical setting for transplantation, and there is experience in purification of these cells and limited knowledge of the requirements for ex vivo manipulation of the cells. In addition, the experience of HSC transplantation (HSCT) has defined a variety of genetic diseases in which the phenotype can be altered by the successful engraftment of normal allogeneic donor cells. Finally, the blood system is involved as a major dose-limiting organ in cancer therapies and both a target and an effector organ in immune reactions, providing a large group of diseases that could theoretically be approached using gene transfer technology. As noted earlier, there are already a large number of monogenic diseases of the blood extensively characterized, with more being defined at the molecular level on a regular basis as whole-exome and whole-genome sequencing is being applied to rare disease phenotypes. In addition to HSC targets, another application of gene transfer technology exploits the experience in adoptive T-cell immunotherapy. In this application, T cells (and less well developed to this point, other immune effector cells) are modified ex vivo in an attempt to enhance potency and specificity. This application of gene transfer technology will not be reviewed here.

The field of gene therapy is rapidly evolving. Successes of "proof-of-principle" small trials have demonstrated the utility of gene transfer approach in a sizable number of patients but in a limited number of diseases. The technology itself is quickly evolving in response to new understanding of viruses, the regulation of gene expression, and gene editing. The application of gene transfer technology to HSC gene therapy has been made possible by exploitation of viruses that have evolved the capacity to efficiently and precisely insert viral genomes into cellular chromosomes of infected cells. The field has taken more than 30 years to evolve to its current state of clinical application. Although this might be viewed as a slow pace, in reality, this time frame parallels the development of many other novel therapies. This developmental phase also reflects the complexities of the biologic systems involved and the caution required in moving forward in the face of serious adverse events seen in early safety trials. It is indeed an exciting time with respect to the clinical application of gene transfer technology in human diseases.

VECTOR SYSTEMS

The initial impetus to develop gene transfer for human studies derived from the exploitation of oncoretroviruses, mainly murine γ-retroviruses, as vectors for gene delivery in the early 1980s. However, since these early studies, a multitude of virus vectors have been developed. All vector systems exploit the virus life cycle to increase the frequency and fidelity of gene transfer. Although many vector systems have been developed, retrovirus and lentivirus vectors have become the most used platforms for human gene therapy trials involving HSCs, and this review will focus primarily on these vector systems and the closely related foamy virus and avian virus vectors (reviewed by Touw and Erkeland[1]). As noted, the majority of trials registered with the Recombinant DNA Advisory Committee of the National Institutes of Health use retroviruses, with nonintegrating adenovirus vectors, adeno-associated virus, and nonvirus (liposomes and plasmids) systems making up the second- and third-largest groups. The latter are primarily focused on immune stimulation trials in cancer and have limited relevance to the use of HPSCs for the treatment of genetic blood diseases.

Retrovirus Vectors

The use of γ-retroviruses as gene transfer vectors takes advantage of the normal virus life cycle. The virus, a membrane-bound particle enclosing a dimer of genomic RNA, Gag, and reverse-transcriptase proteins, interacts with specific cell surface receptors on the target cell. After entry into the cytoplasm, the virus is uncoated, and the genomic messenger (m)RNA is reverse transcribed into DNA. Subsequent polymerase activity yields a double-stranded (DS) DNA provirus molecule. For γ-retroviruses, transport into the nucleus depends on the loss of the nuclear membrane, which accompanies cell division (see later discussion). Integration of the DS provirus in the chromosome is semi-random. The occurrence of insertional activation of oncogenes in several human trials and the subsequent scrutiny of insertion sites in HSC-derived progeny in both murine and human cells using deep sequencing methods have provided a more detailed understanding of the subtle but biologically relevant preferences for insertions of these vectors (see later discussion). After being integrated, the provirus can give rise to mRNA, leading to encoded protein products. Full-length (genomic) mRNA can also be used as the genomic nucleic acid in newly formed virus particles, which are budded nonlytically from the cell surface after assembly in the cytoplasm of the infected cell. The use of retroviruses for gene delivery depends on the capacity to replace viral genes with other heterologous gene sequences and to provide necessary viral proteins in trans in specialized cell lines, called *packaging cells*. The advanced generation of packaging cells appears to be capable of generating pure stocks of recombinant virus without contaminating wild-type helper virus, an important safety consideration. Indeed, to date in human trials, there have been no reports of inadvertent generation of infectious virus. Thus, the infection with replication-incompetent (i.e., helper-free) retrovirus vectors would be predicted to yield integration into the targeted cell population but no further spread of virus in the body of the treated patient. The proteins provided in trans for γ-retroviruses are generally Gag, reverse transcriptase, and envelope proteins, the latter defining the host range of infection. In summary, the advantages of retrovirus vectors include the high efficiency of stable transfer of intact DNA sequences, the broad range of host cells susceptible to infection by retroviruses, and the ability to generate helper-free recombinant virus via stable packaging cell lines.

Despite these advantages, the application of retrovirus vectors for treatment of human blood diseases in early trials was disappointing. In multiple studies, transduction of long-lived and transplantable HSCs has been extremely low. In most studies, the frequency of circulating marked blood cells was too low to effect phenotypic correction of any disease, usually less than 0.1%. The biologic parameters contributing to the poor results in human trials are varied. The major impediments appear to include the low levels of viral receptors on the surface of human HSCs, reducing the efficiency of interaction of virus particles with these target cells, and the quiescent nature of the majority of HSCs, which hinders the transport of the provirus into the nucleus and thus reduces integration frequency. Practical issues, including the difficulty in obtaining high-titer virus in large-scale preparations required for human trials, have also been noted.

These difficulties have led to various strategies and the development of entirely new vector systems, which seek to improve gene transfer methods in human HSCs. These strategies include attempts to increase virus–cell interactions or methods to enhance the chances of successful DNA integration. Different viral envelopes were used to pseudotype recombinant particles to more efficiently target CD34 cells. The use of various cell surface markers, such as CD34, to purify the target cell population can also increase the multiplicity of infection at a given virus titer and has been used in clinical transplantation protocols. Thus, the development of antibody-based enrichment of the CD34+ HPSC compartment from human hematopoietic tissues using magnetic column purification provides a rapid, clinically applicable method to further enhance retroviral transduction by increasing the vector-to-target cell ratio. Methods to increase physical interactions between vector particles and target cells include colocalization on fibronectin and centrifugation methods. Where polycations such as polybrene had previously been used to enhance transduction frequencies by negating electrostatic charge repulsion between target cells and viral particles, the characterization of the recombinant CH296 fibronectin fragment (Retronectin) as a matrix upon which one could colocalize HSCs and viral particles was a significant advance in the quest to improve CD34+ transduction frequencies. Other efforts to increase the chances of DNA integration have focused on attempts to increase the number of HSCs that are undergoing cell division (primarily the use of cytokines that effect stem cell proliferation). The development of improved in vitro growth media formulations incorporating novel cytokine cocktails achieved the dual aim of promoting HSC division, which is required for transduction with γ-retroviral vectors while minimizing stem cell loss via apoptosis or differentiation. Finally, the use of new virus systems that do not require nuclear membrane disruption (and, therefore, cell division) for entry of the provirus DNA into the nucleus, including primarily lentivirus vectors but potentially also vectors based on foamy viruses, appears to be the most significant development in the field in the past decade. These newer vector systems will be discussed later.

In addition to advancing stem cell transduction methodology, additional work has focused on developing retroviral vectors that would express transgene cassettes at levels that would be high enough to elicit a therapeutic benefit and be resistant to gene silencing. Advances in vector design such as the optimization of long-terminal repeat (LTR) enhancer and promoter elements and viral leader sequences resulted in recombinant vectors that were able to mediate high-level transgene expression in both primitive and mature hematopoietic cells. As discussed in detail later, although these powerful promoter and enhancer elements provided robust expression of transgenes, they also appear to be capable of long-range activation of endogenous regulatory sequences as a form of insertional mutagenesis, which can have significant deleterious effects. Taken together, these technologic advances served as the platform for the first successful gene therapy trial in humans.

The use of pharmacologic in vivo selection in combination with gene transfer, both in the setting of cancer trials and in genetic diseases, remains a potentially important method to enhance the reconstitution of human recipients with gene-modified blood cells, but it has not yet gained widespread usage. General considerations include the need for a particular drug to effect damage to BM stem or progenitor cells. A gene or genes encoding resistance to this agent would need to be identified and resistance in vivo to the agent would need to be demonstrated after overexpression of this gene in BM cells. For applications in cancer therapies, dose intensification of drugs used within chemotherapeutic regimens should improve antitumor efficacy. Work is ongoing to use transgenic expression of O^6-methylguanine methyltransferase (MGMT), which generates resistance to bis-chloroethylnitrosourea, temazolamide, and 1-(2-chloroethyl)-3-cyclohexyl-1-nitrosourea and cytidine deaminase, which generates resistance to cytosine arabinoside, gemcitabine, decitobine, and azacytodine for applications in cancer. For noncancer applications (for coselection of a nonselectable therapeutic gene in a genetic disease application), the mutagenic potential of the chemotherapy agent must be considered as a risk in relation to the overall benefit of the gene therapy procedure. Several chemoresistance genes and chemotherapy drug combinations are currently under investigation for this application, and encouraging preclinical studies have led to a limited number of early-phase human studies in cancer patients. In a recently reported human trial in which *MGMT* gene transfer was utilized, patients receiving temazolamide for treatment of brain tumors tolerated significantly more chemotherapy compared with historical controls, with transient increases in gene-modified cells in the peripheral blood in a few patients.[2]

Lentivirus Vectors

One of the key advances in the gene therapy field in the past decade has been the development of recombinant vectors based on lentiviruses, including human immunodeficiency virus (HIV). These vectors were originally developed after the observation that targets of HIV included more differentiated cells, such as macrophages, that are often also postmitotic, suggesting this group of retroviruses has evolved a method of circumventing the block in infection of γ-retroviruses seen in nondividing cells. Investigators demonstrated lentivirus vectors derived from HIV were capable of infecting nondividing neurons after direct injection into the brain. Subsequently, Naldini and colleagues showed efficient infection of growth-arrested cells. As with γ-retroviruses, lentivirus vectors use key viral gene products in trans to generate replication-defective infectious particles carrying the transgene of interest. To date, most lentivirus vectors use vesicular stomatitis virus as envelope sequence, which provides a very broad range of target cells susceptible to lentivirus vector transduction. In the case of lentivirus vectors, viral Gag and Pol, as well as Tat and Rev protein expression are required in trans for efficient virus production along with the envelope proteins. These proteins are usually supplied from separate plasmids, and recombinant lentivirus production is today generally created using "four-plasmid" systems encompassing all the necessary viral proteins on three plasmids and the transfer vector sequences on the fourth plasmid. In addition to *gag* and *pol*, the transfer vector contains all the virus regulatory sequences required in cis for packaging an infectious particle, including the *psi* packaging sequence, integrase, and reverse transcriptase. Thus, generation of high-titer recombinant virus is more complicated than γ-retroviruses and remains a significant issue for large-scale, clinical grade production for use in human trials.

To reduce the chances of generation of replication-competent retroviruses (RCRs), a major safety concern with HIV, most of the nonessential viral sequences have been removed from currently utilized vectors. This included *viv*, *vpu*, *vpr*, and *nef* genes, and subsequently *tat*, an important regulator of viral transcription. Recombinant vectors generated without these sequences were demonstrated to efficiently infect a variety of cells. RCR testing is based on sensitive assays to detect Gag protein by p24 immunoassays or polymerase chain reaction. In addition, lentivirus vectors have traditionally been produced using the "self-inactivating design" (SIN) for added safety because of reduced risk of recombination with and subsequent mobilization of endogenous HIV viruses. The transfer vector thus contains a deletion of the 5′ LTR U3 region and is devoid of viral enhancer and promoter sequences. During reverse transcription, the 5′ LTR is replicated, and the integrated provirus is thus devoid of both 5′ and 3′ U3 regions. In SIN constructs, the transgene of interest is thus expressed from an internal promoter that can be chosen with varying strengths. This added safety feature ultimately has also proven important to reduce the risk of insertional mutagenesis (see later), by which integration near cellular genes are inadvertently activated by the LTR enhancer sequences of vectors.

Lentivirus vectors were originally developed for use in a wide range of tissues in which cells are largely nondividing. Early work focused on brain, retinal cells, liver, pancreatic islets, airway epithelium, and muscle. However, it was subsequently appreciated that the requirement of stimulating HSCs into division with various cytokines to effect efficient transduction with γ-retrovirus vectors may have negative effects on engraftment, or that a large fraction of HSCs remain quiescent and therefore resistant to transduction during clinical transduction protocols. After several groups reported successful transduction of primitive HSC populations in protocols in which these cells remained resistant to transduction by γ-retroviruses, the adaption of lentivirus vectors has now included several recent human trials, and initial results are encouraging. In a trial for childhood cerebral adrenoleukodystrophy (CCALD),[3] long-term "marking" in the myeloid compartment appears to be 10% to 20%, a level that is about 100-fold higher than the marking in the myeloid compartment seen in previous trials in immunodeficiency conditions that used γ-retrovirus vectors. In addition to the safety advantage of SIN vector design used in all lentivirus vectors, there is an additional theoretical advantage of the preference of lentiviruses for integration away from transcription start sites (TSS) of genes in contrast to γ-retroviruses. However, the recent experience with a lentivirus vector used in a single patient with thalassemia,[4] in which abnormal splicing resulted in clonal expansion in the erythroid compartment, suggests that insertion within genes including intronic and noncoding regions of genes may also have potential adverse effects on endogenous sequences. These trials are described in more detail later. Thus, the long-term safety of lentiviruses in human trials remains to be determined, and important aspects of insertional mutagenesis are described in more detail later.

Foamy Virus Vectors

Foamy viruses possess several features that have been exploited to yield vectors for the purpose of transducing HSCs. Foamy viruses are members of the spumaretroviruses family. They have been shown to be endemic retroviruses in a wide range of animals but are not found in humans. These vectors are the largest of the retroviruses (≈14 kb) and thus yield vectors with a capacity to efficiently package large amounts of genetic sequences. The virus has a DNA genome that is reversed transcribed within the virion particle, forming a stable preintegration complex within the transduced cell. As with γ-retrovirus vectors, the virus packaging signals have been successfully exploited to allow production of high-titer, replication-free vector stocks. Based on accidental exposure of a limited number of animal care workers, it has been reported that infection of humans with wild-type foamy virus has no pathologic effects. Foamy virus vectors have been used to successfully transduce mouse and human hematopoietic cells. Proof-of-principle work by Hickstein's group has demonstrated correction of canine leukocyte adhesion deficiency using a foamy virus vector expressing CD18 after transduction and infusion of CD34+ cells after submyeloablative conditioning. No human trials have been opened to date using this vector system, but several are planned for the future.

Alpharetroviruses

Retrovirus vectors derived from Rous sarcoma virus, which is a member of the alpharetrovirus family, have been described. Although these vectors maintain genomic integration as part of the viral life cycle, they have attracted recent attention because of their propensity to integrate in a relatively neutral fashion with respect to promoter regions and TSS of genes. In large animal studies, alpharetrovirus-transduced HSC-derived progeny demonstrated integrations that were not clustered in gene-rich CpG or TSS regions of the genome. The development of a self-inactivating alpharetrovirus with a split-packaging design by Schambach and colleagues[5] has provided proof-of-principle with respect to the capacity to generate high-titer, replication-free vector stocks from stable producer cell lines that use internal promoters to express transgenes in a potentially safer fashion than γ-retrovirus vectors. Such vectors have been demonstrated to efficiently infect murine and human hematopoietic cells, including T lymphocytes, at low multiplicity of infection.[5]

EXPERIENCE IN HEMATOLOGIC CLINICAL TRIALS TO DATE

X-Linked Severe Combined Immunodeficiency

Severe combined immunodeficiency (SCID) comprises a number of rare monogenic diseases, with common features including a block in T-cell differentiation and impaired B-cell and natural killer (NK) cell immunity. Studies of pattern of inheritance, immune function, and genotypes have led to the identification of at least 11 distinct SCID conditions. The most common variant of SCID results from the deficiency in expression or function of the common cytokine receptor γ chain, which is shared by the receptors for interleukin (IL)-2, IL-4, IL-7, IL-9, IL-15, and IL-21. This condition is inherited in a sex-linked fashion (X-linked SCID or SCID-X1) and accounts for 40% to 50% of all SCID cases. SCID-X1 is characterized by abnormal development or function of T, B, and NK cells, although B cells are usually present in humans (so-called T-minus, B-plus SCID). Survival depends on the reconstitution of T-cell development and function by allogeneic BM transplantation (BMT). If a genotypically matched family donor is available, HSCT confers greater than 80% chance of long-term survival. The absence of T and NK cells in the patient allows for the engraftment of donor cells without preparative chemotherapy conditioning; thus, this is the treatment of choice with minimal toxicity. When a genotypically matched family member is not available, haploidentical donors (e.g., a parent) or closely matched unrelated donors are used, with varying preference center to center, and a survival rate of 64% to 78% has been reported. These inferior outcomes may be attributed to the increased risk of graft rejection or graft-versus-host disease (GVHD), as well as the effects of T-cell depletion, immune suppression causing slower immune reconstitution, or conditioning with increased risk of infection. Haploidentical transplants rigorously depleted of T cells, similar to genotypically related transplant, are performed in some institutions without preparative chemotherapy conditioning; however, B-cell reconstitution is poor, and the majority of patients require intravenous immunoglobulin (IVIG) replacement for life. Interestingly, spontaneous partial correction of severe T-cell immunodeficiencies, including SCID, has previously been reported, suggesting a selective advantage of wild-type T cells over defective T cells.

Three independent gene therapy trials aimed at correcting the immunologic defect of SCID-X1 patients who lack a genotypically matched BM donor have been reported.[6] In the initially reported trials, a total of 20 patients have been treated.[7,8] Despite minor technical differences in the two protocols, the basic design of both gene therapy trials is quite similar: the complete coding region of the human γ-chain was cloned into a "first-generation" γ-retroviral vector regulated by the murine leukemia virus (MLV) LTR sequences, which was used to infect BM-derived CD34+ cells in vitro. The transduction occurred in the presence of early acting cytokines (stem cell factor, thrombopoietin, IL-3, and FMS-like tyrosine kinase 3 ligand) and the CH296 human fragment of fibronectin described earlier. Cells were subsequently infused without prior conditioning or cytoreductive treatment. Minor differences between the two protocols included the uses of a threefold higher concentration of IL-3 and 4% fetal cell serum in the French trial. Additionally, the French investigators used the amphotropic envelope pseudotype compared with the use of gibbon ape leukemia virus envelope in the British trial. Results in both trials have been extremely encouraging.

In the French trial, 10 children younger than the age of 1 year were enrolled between 1999 and 2002. Nine out of 10 infants developed normal numbers of T and NK cells, with good immune function. In seven of the nine patients who developed T cells, T-cell counts reached normal levels within 3 months and have remained normal at the time of the last published follow-up. Protective levels of antibodies, including antibody production after immunization, were achieved, and the prophylactic administration of IVIG was discontinued. At almost more than 10 years after gene therapy, these patients continued to retain a functional immune system, enabling them to live normally.

However, serious adverse events related to gene therapy have been reported in four patients in the French trial, occurring 31 to 68 months after gene therapy, and in one patient in the British trial. In these patients, untoward effects of viral integration into the genome resulted in T-cell leukemia, leading to the death of one of the four affected patients. Much research has subsequently been directed at elucidating the mechanism responsible for these adverse events. Retroviral integration in the proximity of proto-oncogenes, particularly the LIM domain only 2 (LMO2) promoter, was involved in leukemogenesis in three French patients and one British patient. An integration of the unaltered γ-chain–encoding viral vector on chromosome 11q13, near the first exon of the LMO2 gene, led to the unregulated transcription of LMO2, giving rise to a T-cell acute lymphoblastic leukemia (T-ALL)–like lymphoproliferation in the initial two patients. In the patient in the British trial, the integration of the vector 35 kb upstream of the LMO2 locus cooperated with secondary genetic aberrations, including a gain-of-function mutation of NOTCH1, a deletion at the CDKN2A tumor-suppressor gene locus, and a translocation of the T-cell receptor β region, to give rise to T-ALL. LMO2 is a master regulator of human hematopoiesis that is involved in stem cell growth and is not normally expressed in T cells. However, LMO2 activation has been implicated in some cases of human T-cell leukemia. In addition, LMO2 transgenic mice have been shown to develop T-ALL within 10 months. It is increasingly clear that retroviral vectors may "turn on" cellular proto-oncogenes adjacent to their integration site in the genome. The strong promoter or enhancer activity of the retroviral LTR element shows particular propensity to the upregulation of genes neighboring the integration site. Multiple studies now indicate that γ-retroviral vectors, such as the vectors used in the two SCID-X1 trials, preferentially integrate into the 5′ end of genes near the TSS. In addition, γ-retroviral vectors have been shown to integrate in or near a number of proto-oncogenes that are actively expressed in human CD34+ cells. When human CD34+ cells were transduced with retroviral vectors ex vivo, 21% of retroviral integrations occurred at recurrent insertion sites ("hot spots"), which were highly enriched for proto-oncogenes and growth-controlling genes. A series of papers investigating the vector integration sites in both SCID-X1 trials and a trial treating adenosine deaminase (ADA) deficiency, the ADA-SCID trial (see later), observed a greater-than-random frequency of vector integrations near the TSS of genes that are active in HSCs. Interestingly, in the SCID-X1 trial, a skewing of vector integration site distribution in vivo was noted. Compared with retroviral integration sites (RIS) recovered from transduced CD34+ cells, RIS recovered from T cells in vivo 9 to 30 months after transplantation showed an overrepresentation of RIS within or near genes encoding proteins with kinase activity, transferase activity, or proteins involved in phosphorous metabolism. This skewing of RIS in vivo suggests a selection of T cells as a result of viral integration in certain growth- and survival-promoting genes. A more recent trial in X-SCID utilizing a SIN γ-retrovirus design reports early follow-up on nine patients,[6] although the trial is still accruing patients (NCT01129544). The virus design is noteworthy in that it is more directly comparable to a lentivirus, since the viral enhancer elements are deleted and expression of the IL-2 γ-chain is from an "internally positioned" cellular promoter. The initial results reported efficacy similar to the previous SCID-X1 trials—no leukemias and integration analysis that appears safer than those seen in the previous two trials. In the eight evaluable patients treated in this trial, six demonstrated correction of T-cell reconstitution. One patient died prior to full engraftment of gene-modified cells of preexisting viral infection that did not resolve after gene therapy. The two failures correlated with lower vector copy number in the transduced product as a result of inadequate gene transfer. This study is particularly noteworthy as the only human study in which a γ-retrovirus vector deleted of enhancer elements has been utilized. It thus provides a platform for more direct comparison with previous γ-retrovirus and lentivirus trials with respect to safety and efficacy.

Strikingly, in contrast to five cases of insertional mutagenesis in the two SCID-X1 trials, no adverse events have been reported in the 10 patients treated in the ADA-SCID trial, despite a similar RIS pattern observed in this patient group. There have been no leukemias reported in more than 40 patients treated worldwide (including in London, Los Angeles, and at the NIH) and most of these have benefited from gene therapy. The observation of the difference in leukemia in these trials has led to the proposal of a "disease effect" contributing to oncogenesis of γ-chain gene therapy. Woods and colleagues demonstrated lentiviral transduction of γc$^{-/-}$ mice with vectors containing the human common γ-chain (cγ) or an inert control gene at very high viral doses.[8a] They observed the induction of T-cell malignancies in one-third of the animals receiving cγ-transduced cells but not in the control groups. The merit of this very limited study was subsequently challenged, primarily on the basis of a viral dose much higher than that used in clinical scenarios and incomplete data on the pathogenesis of the malignancies, particularly as they relate to the downstream activation level of a key signaling target of the common γ-chain, Janus kinase 3, in the tumors. In addition, the lentiviral vector used in this study incorporated a hybrid promoter or enhancer element that is extremely powerful and likely to possess a greater transactivating potential than promoter or enhancer elements that would be considered for clinical gene therapy use. More recent occurrence of leukemia in another trial for Wiskott-Aldrich syndrome (WAS; see later) using the same vector backbone further challenges the presence of SCID-X1 disease or transgene effects in these leukemias.

In summary, thus far, 5 out of 20 patients treated with gene therapy for SCID-X1 have encountered a life-threatening severe adverse event, thought to be triggered by retroviral activation of LMO2 in 4 patients. Four patients were salvaged with chemotherapy, and one patient succumbed to the disease after an unsuccessful allogeneic BMT. At this point, the use of MLV-based retroviral vectors with LTR promoter enhancer elements intact is viewed as contraindicated in this disease by most investigators in the field. The continued development of safety-enhanced vectors and the validation of these vectors in clinically relevant systems have emerged as a major priority in the field, and, as noted above, an international trial has recently been reported using a γ-retrovirus that is deleted of LTR enhancer elements. Transgene expression is mediated by a weak cellular promoter in this vector. Data suggest that early efficacy is maintained despite lower expression of the cγ-chain and that the deletion of the γ-retrovirus enhancer is a key to improved safety.[6]

Adenosine Deaminase Deficiency

ADA is a housekeeping enzyme of the purine metabolic pathway that is expressed in all tissues of the body. Deficiency of this enzyme leads to a buildup of toxic metabolites with detrimental systemic effects, including neurodevelopmental deficiencies, sensorineuronal deafness, and skeletal abnormalities. Importantly, ADA deficiency causes abnormal T-, B-, and NK-cell development, resulting in the SCID phenotype. As is the case with the more common SCID-X1, untreated patients generally succumb to severe opportunistic infections in the first year of life. Treatment strategies used to manage affected patients include allogeneic HSCT, enzyme-replacement therapy, and, more recently, gene therapy. Allogeneic HSCT from a human leukocyte antigen-matched family donor offers good immunologic and biochemical correction with 73% survival. However, outcomes after mismatched and haploidentical transplants are less impressive. Likewise, the exogenous replacement of ADA, administered in a polyethylene glycol (PEG) conjugate by intramuscular injection on a weekly or twice-weekly schedule, results in systemic detoxification and immune reconstitution. In the long term, however, about half of the patients receiving PEG-ADA replacement continue to require IVIG infusions, and some patients show a decline in T-cell numbers over time.

A number of gene therapy trials for ADA deficiency were initiated in the early 1990s, targeting retroviral gene transfer into various cell types, including peripheral blood lymphocytes, umbilical cord blood, BM, and CD34$^+$ selected stem cells. These early studies failed to produce clear efficacy. By contrast, more recent studies introduced key modifications to the gene therapy protocol, including the use of a reduced-intensity myelosuppressive conditioning regimen and the withdrawal of concurrent PEG-ADA replacement. The Milan-based group of Aiuti and colleagues have reported on their initial experience with 10 children.[11] Patients were conditioned with 4 mg/kg of busulfan before the infusion of transduced cells. The mean age at the time of gene therapy was 2.2 years. All children on this trial are healthy and thriving, with the longest published follow-up time now more than 64 months. Gene therapy has resulted in a substantial increase of lymphocyte counts and normalization of T-cell function. A recent update on this trial,[9] published in abstract form, reports that 18 patients have been treated and are alive and, of these, 15 do not require replacement enzyme treatment.

Similarly, four patients have been treated in London.[10] One patient that has been reported in detail had been treated with PEG-ADA for 3 years but showed a gradual decline in T-cell numbers despite effective metabolic correction. Because a matched BM donor was not available, the patient was enrolled on the ADA-SCID gene therapy trial. PEG-ADA replacement was stopped 1 month before gene therapy, and the patient was conditioned with a single dose of 140 mg/m2 of melphalan before infusion of the transduced BM CD34$^+$ cells. At the time of the last published follow-up, the patient was 2 years from gene therapy, clinically well, and off prophylactic antibiotic therapy.[10a] An increase in T-cell numbers and normalization of the proliferative response have been noted. Importantly, no adverse events have occurred thus far in the patients treated for ADA-SCID at these two centers.

Aiuti and colleagues recently published a comprehensive genome-wide analysis of RIS of five patients treated in Milan. This paper analyzed the RIS patterns in CD34$^+$ cells before infusion as well as RIS in vivo up to 47 months after gene therapy. As anticipated, a nonrandom proviral integration pattern, favoring TSS and gene-dense regions, was observed in the pretransplant cells. RIS observed in vivo in T cells were additionally enriched for TSS, suggesting the occurrence of in vivo selection. More recently, Aiuti and colleagues[11] have demonstrated that cellular genes in the proximity of the proviral integration site are subject to moderate dysregulation in gene modified T-cell clones isolated from patients. However, in contrast to the SCID-X1 trial, no in vivo skewing toward RIS in genes affecting survival, cell cycling, signal transduction, or proliferation were observed, making a clonal dominance effect appear less likely. Interestingly, only one RIS was detected at the *MDS-EVI1* locus and became undetectable at later time points. This is in contrast to the clonal dominance of *MDS-EVI1* integration sites observed in the X-linked Chronic Granulomatous Disease trial (see later). Additionally, an overrepresentation of RIS was noted in the proximity of the *CCND2* and *LMO2* genes, with a total of 5 out of 523 RIS recovered in vivo. Notably, the *CCND2* insertions were detected only in the first 2 years of follow-up and not subsequently. *LMO2* insertions were also overrepresented in the pretransplant CD34$^+$ samples, highlighting the fact that the *LMO2* gene is a hotspot for retroviral integration in human CD34$^+$ cells. The lack of in vivo expansion of clones carrying *LMO2* RIS indicates that this integration site may not be sufficient to mediate clonal dominance and leukemic transformation. Rather, additional cooperating mutations or insertions are required for malignant transformation. The lack of malignant transformation in two ADA-SCID trials may point to the role of the genetic background or the role of the therapeutic transgene introduced into human CD34$^+$ cells. However, the patient cohort remains relatively small, and follow-up is still short term. As noted previously, over 40 patients have now been treated worldwide, with no leukemias reported in any trial in this disease to date.[12] An ongoing new multicenter trial utilizes a lentivirus platform (NCT01279720). Overall, the genotoxicity profile in the ADA-SCID trials has been sufficiently favorable to continue to recommend this experimental therapy to patients and families lacking a perfectly matched sibling donor. Indeed, this vector and treatment portfolio has been licensed in 2011 to a major pharmaceutical company for clinical development.

Chronic Granulomatous Disease

Chronic granulomatous disease (CGD) is an inherited disorder of phagocyte dysfunction characterized by often life-threatening invasive fungal and bacterial infections and by granuloma formation in vital organs. CGD results from a mutation in one of four subunits of the reduced form of nicotinamide adenine dinucleotide phosphate oxidase of phagocytes. The inability to form microbiocidal oxygen species renders the phagocytes unable to fight invasive infections. Almost 70% of CGD cases result from defects in the X-linked gene encoding gp91^{phox} (X-CGD). With conventional therapy, including lifelong antimicrobial prophylaxis and interferon-γ therapy, the yearly mortality rate of X-CGD remains at 5%. HSCT is curative for patients with a perfectly matched sibling donor but remains risky in patients with active infections. Unrelated donor transplantations are not routinely recommended. Thus, the development of a gene therapy approach that uses autologous HSC provides an important therapeutic advance for this patient group. In previous clinical gene therapy trials conducted without myeloreductive conditioning, the engraftment level of gene-modified cells remained low.

In 2002, the German group of Grez and colleagues in Frankfurt, Germany, initiated a gene therapy trial of X-CGD.[12a] The initial patients received a mild immunosuppressive preparative regimen and failed to engraft significant numbers of gene-modified cells. However, 2 years later, low-dose busulfan—modeled on the successful gene therapy trial for ADA-SCID—was incorporated into the preparative regimen, and additional patients were treated. This group of patients has been followed with unprecedented sophistication by the prospective monitoring of integration sites that marks each hematopoietic cell before transplantation and then allows the tracking of these cells in vivo. The initial two patients treated were 26 and 25 years old. Both patients carried the diagnosis of X-CGD and had failed to clear invasive infections, including a *Staphylococcus aureus* liver abscess and pulmonary aspergillosis with medical treatment. Thus, autologous peripheral blood CD34$^+$ cells were mobilized with granulocyte colony-stimulating factor and collected. Gene transfer was performed using a γ-retroviral vector SF71gp91^{phox}. This vector, containing the spleen focus-forming virus LTR elements (in contrast to the Moloney MLV LTR in the two SCID trials) was chosen for its ability to achieve high expression levels in transduced HSCs. The in vitro transduction rates in the two patients were 45% and 39.5%, respectively, with a proviral copy number of 2.6 and 1.5 per transduced cell. Proviral integration occurred preferentially in gene-coding regions (47–52%) and was highly skewed toward the 5-kb sequence surrounding TSS. Moreover, the clonal distribution pattern was not stable over time. Rather, starting 5 months after therapy, a less diverse integration pattern emerged, indicating the appearance of dominant clones.

Clinically, following a period of cytopenia after conditioning and cell infusion, the initial engraftment rates detected in the peripheral blood were 12% to 13%. Significant improvement in the previously refractory infections was noted 50 to 60 days after therapy. Surprisingly, a gradual increase in the number of gene-corrected cells up to 50% to 60% of all peripheral blood cells was observed, starting around day 150 after transplant. This coincided with increased oxidase activity and occurred in the absence of altered blood counts. These events were accompanied by a selective outgrowth of progenitors carrying vector insertions that activated one of three oncogenes: *PRDM16*, *SETBP1*, and most notably *MDS-EVI1*. Although all three genes are well-known cancer-associated genes, most clonal outgrowths were exhausted after a few months with the exception of *MDS-EVI1*, which increased to 67% to 90% in both patients approximately 1 year after cell infusion. Of note, the dominant *MDS-EVI1* clones initially did not transgress the boundaries of the normal myeloid pool because these cells remained cytokine dependent

in vitro and failed to engraft in immunocompromised mice, suggesting their benign nature. Thus, the expansion of gp91^{phox+} cells, although clearly providing therapeutic benefit during the initial phase, was viewed with mixed feelings by the investigators and the general gene therapy community.

More recent follow-up on these two study patients has been provided.[13,14] Indeed, although gene marking remained high in both patients, downregulation of gene expression was noted as a result of CpG methylation in the viral LTR promoter. As a consequence, gp91phox expression was suppressed, but the capacity of the LTR-encoded enhancer to transactivate nearby genes remained intact. One patient died 2.5 years after therapy of severe sepsis. The second patient developed monosomy 7 and myelodysplastic syndrome (MDS) and died after an unsuccessful unrelated donor BMT.[13] Of note, the EVI1 locus has previously been identified as a common target of retroviral oncogenesis. EVI1, which is not detected in normal hematopoietic cells, has been associated with myeloid leukemia and MDS. The constitutive overexpression of EvI1 in mouse BM cells has been shown to induce MDS in mice and data from the CGD trial suggest that dysregulated expression is associated with genomic instability, presumably contributing to the acquisition of additional somatic mutations. Despite these molecular events, the infusion of gene-corrected CD34$^+$ cells was highly effective with regard to clearing refractory pyogenic infections, raising the possibility of using gene therapy to bridge patients with refractory pyogenic infections into eligibility for allogeneic HSCT. A multiinstitutional international trial has recently opened in which the GP91^{phox} gene is expressed in a lentivirus backbone via a chimeric myeloid internal promoter (NCT01855685).

Wiskott-Aldrich Syndrome

WAS is an X-linked immunodeficiency caused by inactivating mutations in the WAS protein (WASP). WASP plays a regulatory role in cell signaling and cytoskeletal reorganization in hematopoietic cells. The disease is fatal and is characterized by severe combined immunodeficiency, thrombocytopenia, elevated frequency of tumor formation, eczema, and other autoimmune manifestations. The only currently available curative therapy for WAS is BM transplant, but as with the other primary immunodeficiencies, the availability of suitably matched donors is limiting. A clinical trial for the genetic correction of WAS via retroviral delivery of the WASP cDNA into autologous CD34$^+$ cells was recently reported.[15] A combination of a relatively high cell dose (7–8 × 10^6 CD34$^+$/kg body weight) and good transduction efficiency led to gene marking across both myeloid and lymphoid lineages. A marked clinical benefit from gene therapy has been reported in one of the patients.[15] Of particular note is the fact that the architecture of the vector backbone used in this trial is similar to that used in both the CGD and the SCID trials described earlier. That is, the γ-retroviral vector has an intact LTR that contains the enhancer and promoter from the spleen focus-forming virus.[16] Recent reports describe T-cell leukemia from insertional mutagenesis in 7 of the 10 patients in this trial.[17] Thus, a common molecular etiology in this trial strongly suggests that the initial vector design (intact strong viral LTRs containing enhancer elements that can transactivate promoters over long distances) are unsafe. In addition, the occurrence of T-cell leukemia in a disease other than SCID weakens the argument that the leukemias in X-SCID was related either to the transgene or some unknown disease-specific characteristic. In any regard, use of the "first-generation" MLV backbone in human trials may now be ended. More recently, several new clinical trials have opened that utilize a SIN lentivirus vector for treatment of WAS (NCT02333760, NCT01410825, and NCT01347346). These trials utilize the same vector backbone. In a total of 10 patients studied, 9 were reported alive and showed clinical benefit with reduced autoimmunity, including improvement in eczema and reduced platelet transfusion dependence with no serious bleeding. One patient died from preexisting viral infection that did not resolve after gene therapy. In one study it was noted that the degree of myeloid engraftment and platelet reconstitution in this disease treatment correlated with the dosage of gene-corrected cells.

Childhood Cerebral X-Linked Adrenoleukodystrophy

Childhood cerebral X-linked CCALD is a fatal neurodegenerative disease that results from progressive neural demyelination within the brain. The defective gene that is responsible for the phenotype, adenosine triphosphate-binding cassette D1 (ABCD1), encodes a transmembrane transport protein that is responsible for the shuttling of fatty acids into peroxisomes, where they are subsequently degraded. ALD is characterized by an accumulation of very long-chain fatty acids, although the exact pathophysiology of the disease is unknown. Cerebral demyelination is associated with inflammation evident on gadolinium magnetic resonance imaging studies. Most patients progress from no symptoms to a vegetative state and death within 8 years of diagnosis. Allogeneic BM transplant has been found to be therapeutic for cerebral demyelination, presumably because of the infiltration of donor-derived microglia cells into the brain. However, because of the very rapidly progressive nature of the demyelination and the time required to generate mature microglia from transplanted HSCs, BM transplant is most effective when administered as soon after the development of demyelination evident by imaging methods as possible. In cases in which CCALD is successfully treated with HSCT, continued progression of the disease occurs for 18 months to 2 years before disease arrest. Myelin inflammation resolves, but lost neurologic function is not regained in successfully treated patients. Because of the time constraints imposed upon finding a suitable human leukocyte antigen-matched donor and the occurrence of GVHD, the genetic correction of autologous BM CD34$^+$ cells is an attractive experimental therapeutic option.

A phase I gene therapy trial using a recombinant HIV-1–based lentiviral vector to deliver the ABCD1 cDNA into CD34$^+$ cells has been reported from Paris.[3] In the three patients who have been enrolled to date, a transduction efficiency of 30% to 50% in CD34$^+$ cells was achieved, with mean vector copy numbers of 0.6 to 0.7 per cell. Patients were preconditioned with cyclophosphamide and busulfan, and between 9% and 23% multilineage gene-marked chimerism has been reported in a follow-up period that extends up to 16 months. In the two patients who had been followed for 16 months after transplant, HSC gene therapy resulted in arrests of neurologic functional loss and resolution of central nervous system inflammation that are similar to those achieved with allogeneic transplant. This trial is particularly noteworthy in that it is the first trial to report reconstitution of BM cells that have been transduced with a recombinant lentiviral vector. Molecular characterization of lentiviral integration sites in engrafting cells indicated that reconstitution was polyclonal, but detailed analysis of genomic loci targeted by this vector has yet to be reported. A multisite, biotechnology-sponsored phase II/III registration trial is currently accruing patients in several countries using a similar lentivirus vector in this disease (NCT01896102).

β-Thalassemia

Patients treated in a clinical trial that used a lentiviral vector for the correction of β-thalassemia have recently been reported[4] and subsequent updates are in abstract form.[18,19] Two patients treated have become transfusion independent and a third patient has shown increasing levels of gene-modified red blood cells expressing transgenic hemoglobin. Thalassemias result from mutations that attenuate the expression of either the α- or β-globin chains that compromise hemoglobin synthesis and thus cause ineffective erythropoiesis. Because adult hemoglobin consists of a tetramer of two α- and two β-chains, inherited mutations at the β-globin locus cause a mismatch in the ratio of these two chains, thus preventing the correct assembly of the hemoglobin molecule. Clinically, this may result in transfusion-dependent anemia, which in turn can promote the serious side effect of iron overload. In general, disease severity correlates with the degree

to which inactivation mutations inhibit β-globin expression. However, other genetic loci can modulate the disease phenotype, for example, by inducing adult expression of the fetal γ-globin gene, which can be efficiently incorporated into functional hemoglobin in place of the β-globin chain. In particular, Orkin's group has recently demonstrated that the transcription factor BCL11A plays a major role in switching γ-globin off and β-globin expression on during the transition from fetal to adult life.[19a] Gene therapy of β-thalassemia is complicated by the requirement for an exact stoichiometry of α- and β-globin chains to facilitate efficient assembly of hemoglobin. Thus, an effective gene therapy vector must be able to facilitate high level expression of β-globin in the range of that mediated by the normal endogenous gene in an erythroid-specific context. Lineage-specific expression of the β-globin chain is particularly important in the context of genetic modification of HSC to prevent high-level expression of β-globin in nonerythroid hematopoietic lineages.

The lentiviral vector used in the trial mentioned earlier comprises a SIN configuration with elements from the β-globin locus control region driving expression of the β-globin cDNA that has been mutated to enhance β-globin chain stability. Additionally, the vector's expression cassette is flanked by chromatin insulator elements that function to both prevent silencing of the transgene expression cassette by inhibitory chromatin structure surrounding the integration site and to prevent the vector-encoded enhancer from modulating expression of endogenous genes near to the insertion site. An interim report on the findings of the clinical trial describes that, in 2007, a single patient with severe transfusion-dependent β-thalassemia major received CD34$^+$ cells transduced with the lentiviral vector described earlier.[4] There was a clear demonstration of clinical efficacy because the patient has been transfusion independent for 15 months. Of note, posttransplant molecular analysis revealed a clonal skewing of peripheral blood cells. The clone, which harbors a proviral integration within the high-mobility group A2 proteins (HMGA2) gene locus, is reported to be stable. Insertion of the provirus into this locus resulted in the production of a 3′ truncated mRNA resulting from the introduction of a cryptic splice acceptor, present in the vector insulator element, into intron 3 of the gene. This truncated mRNA, comprising exons 1–3, was expressed at elevated levels because of a loss of negative posttranscriptional regulation by Let-7 miRNAs because the miRNA target sequence in exon 5 was lost. HMGA2 has been found to be mutated in chromosomal translocations, primarily in benign tumors and less often in malignant tumors. Although the clinical implications of this clonal outgrowth are unclear, this event clearly demonstrates that lentiviral vectors can contribute to insertional mutagenesis, albeit in this case via modulation of posttranscriptional regulation of gene expression. Indeed, the propensity to insert in coding sequences may lead to an abundance of abnormal mRNA splicing variants.

Several additional trials are planned using a similar approach to express either a sickle-resistant mutated β-globin protein or to increase expression of protective fetal hemoglobin, or to reverse the so-called *fetal to adult globin switch* based on recent data showing "cure" of humanized sickle mice by genetic deletion of BCL11A expressing short hairpin RNA against this transcription factor or by gene-edited deletion of the BCL11A gene in HSCs.[20] These trials represent important extensions of the technology from very rare diseases to a disease with a much larger patient population.

INSERTIONAL MUTAGENESIS

From an early stage in the development of retroviral vectors for gene therapy applications, there has been a concern that recombinant vectors could elicit cellular transformation by altering expression of either cellular proto-oncogenes or tumor suppressor genes that are proximal to the genomic integration site. This phenomenon, referred to as *insertional mutagenesis*, was characterized as a property of wild-type γ-retroviruses. Having greatly reduced the likelihood that retroviral gene therapy vectors could generate replication-competent virus, the risk of a recombinant vector being able to transform a cell via insertional mutagenesis was initially perceived by many investigators to be very low. The lack of efficacy in preclinical models using human hematopoietic stem and progenitor (CD34⁺) cells also shifted emphasis away from the risks of insertional mutagenesis. However, soon after the publication detailing the efficacy of the Paris-based SCID-X1 trial, work emerged from the group of Baum and colleagues that would reestablish the importance of insertional mutagenesis as a significant risk factor in the retroviral-mediated genetic correction of hematopoietic cells and that ultimately predicted the appearance of leukemia in the SCID, CGD, and WAS gene therapy trials described earlier. Baum demonstrated for the first time that a replication-incompetent retroviral vector backbone designed for gene therapy applications could cause cellular transformation via insertional mutagenesis in the context of a transplant model of transduced murine HSCs. In this and a subsequent study, it was found that a single retroviral insertion in the vicinity of the ecotropic viral integration site 1 (*Evi1*) gene or the related PR domain-containing 16 (*PRDM16*) gene resulted in their overexpression, likely because of the influence of the LTR viral enhancer element, and was sufficient to initiate a cascade of events resulting in leukemic transformation in vivo. Furthermore, a high copy number infection of murine BM with recombinant retroviral vectors was able to facilitate combinatorial hits, which caused leukemogenesis. The pattern of cellular genes that combine to promote cellular transformation demonstrated a significant overlap with those that are deregulated in experiments that used RCR vectors to provoke the development of leukemia. Although murine HSCs likely represent a more readily transformed target than their human counterparts, these studies formally established the mutagenic potential of recombinant retroviral vectors intended for gene therapy applications.

Baum's group then made the seminal observation that at low copy numbers, retroviral-transduced murine HSCs are selectively expanded during transplant dependent upon proviral insertion sites. These nonmalignant dominant clones are enriched for proviral integration sites in the locale of genes encoding signal transduction molecules and growth-promoting genes. Analysis of mRNA expression levels in these clones revealed that the proviral insertion did indeed alter transcriptional regulation of genes proximal to the integration site and led to the hypothesis that this was a powerful method to identify proengraftment genes through positive selection. These observations were found to have direct translational relevance in the gene therapy trial for CGD where the nonmalignant expansion of dominant retroviral transduced clones in two patients was found to correlate with insertional upregulation of growth-promoting genes. Subsequent experience with γ-retroviruses used in the clinical trial for WAS confirmed that insertional leukemogenesis in the SCID-X1 trial was not a disease-specific side effect. Multiple children in the WAS trial have developed T-cell leukemia.[17] Thus far, leukemias associated with replication-incompetent retrovirus vectors are associated with insertional activation of known proto-oncogenes by viral promoter and enhancer sequences (reviewed by Kohn et al[21]).

Wild-type and recombinant retroviral vectors (including α, γ, spuma, and lenti) integrate into the host genome in a semi-random manner and demonstrate insertion site biases that are dependent on the accessibility of the insertion site in the target cell and variations in the viral integrase enzyme that depend on retroviral genus. γ-retroviruses such as MLV have been shown to exert a clear preference for integration in the region immediately surrounding the TSS of actively transcribed genes. Although lentiviral vectors also demonstrate a preference to integrate within the loci of actively transcribed genes, their integration profile favors sites that are downstream of the TSS within the body of the primary transcript.

Using viral chimeras, it has been shown that incorporation of MLV integrase into an HIV-1–based vector alters the integration pattern of the lentivirus to more closely resemble that associated with a γ-retroviral vector. It is possible that this phenomenon results from the binding of the MLV integrase with cell type-specific transcription factors, resulting in the recruitment of the preintegration complex to the promoter and enhancer region of actively transcribed genes. This work clearly demonstrates that γ-retroviral and lentiviral vectors have

developed distinct mechanisms of integrase-dependent integration that may have an impact on the mutagenic potential of recombinant retroviral vectors. If one considers the possibility of integrating vectors upregulating oncogene expression via either read-through transcription or enhancer effects on the endogenous promoter, then γ-retroviral vectors could be considered as potentially more mutagenic than lentiviral vectors in this context because of their preference for integration near the TSS. Conversely, preferential integration within the body of the primary transcript may result in lentiviral vectors having a higher probability of interrupting, for example, tumor suppressor gene expression, or as noted earlier in the treatment of one patient with thalassemia in altering normal gene splicing. Progress has been made in the development of model systems to functionally evaluate the relative mutagenic potential of different vector systems. However, the model systems developed to date have a clear preference to detect mutagenesis mediated via upregulation of oncogene transcription. It is not clear whether this is a reflection of tumor suppressor gene inactivation being inconsequential as a mechanism of insertional mutagenesis or is a result of bias within the model system. Clearly, the preliminary results from the β-thalassemia trial described earlier demonstrate that lentiviral vectors may mediate insertional mutagenesis via alternate mechanisms.

As noted earlier, other related retroviral vector systems have also been shown to have an integration pattern that is distinct from γ-retroviral vectors, and as such may represent a safer vector configuration. Recombinant foamy virus vectors do not preferentially integrate within genes, and their integration pattern does not significantly correlate with actively transcribed genes. Likewise, avian sarcoma leukosis (α-retrovirus) vectors do not favor gene-rich regions or TSS as preferred integration sites. However, these novel vectors systems have not been as well characterized as γ-retroviral or lentiviral vectors with regards to safety and efficacy, and have not yet been translated to clinical use in the near future.

RECENT MODIFICATIONS OF VECTOR SYSTEMS BASED ON CLINICAL EXPERIENCE

New Cell Targets in Genetic Engineering

Despite recent advances in improving ex vivo manipulation of HSCs for the purpose of gene transfer, an ongoing limitation of this technology is the loss of engraftment potential of manipulated cells. This is dramatically emphasized in genetic diseases such as Fanconi anemia, in which the disease process itself leads to a marked reduction in HSC targets and, in addition, in HSCs, which appear to have increased susceptibility to in vitro stress. An exciting area of recent research advances that may in the future address this issue and also allow prescreening at the molecular level of insertions to determine safety is the use of embryonic stem (ES) or induced pluripotent stem (iPS; next paragraph) cells. These cells offer exciting possibilities for studying mechanisms of pluripotency; establishing models for disease-specific investigations; and enabling future applications in genetic and cellular therapies, including tissue engineering for regenerative medicine. ES cells can be propagated and expanded in vitro, making them amenable to manipulations, including the genetic correction of molecular defects. ES cells can be differentiated into a number of cells resembling mature cell types in vitro. In theory, cell therapy using donor cells of the same genetic constitution as the recipient may avoid the issues related to the immune barrier of allogeneic transplantation. One of the key ethical and practical barriers to applying ES cell research to human diseases is the need for obtaining human oocytes or embryos for the in vitro generation of ES cell lines.

A key recent finding with potential applications in cell and gene therapy has been the observation that many somatic tissues can be "reprogrammed" into pluripotent stem cells with characteristics of ES cells, termed *iPS cells*, and direct reprogramming of differentiated somatic cells by gene transfer of a small number of defined transcription factors has been shown to yield cells that are indistinguishable from inner cell mass-derived ES cells. Takahashi et al reasoned that forcing the expression of ES cell-specific genes, particularly transcription factors in somatic cells, might induce (reprogram) somatic cells to take on the properties of ES cells, much like factors present in oocytes can reprogram somatic nuclei in mammals.[21a] By systematic screening experiments, four factors, including some known to be involved in the process of self-renewal (Oct3/4, Sox2), and others associated with transformation and maintenance of ES cell pluripotency (c-Myc, Klf 4), were identified as sufficient to achieve reprogramming. The resultant cells, termed *iPS cells*, exhibited key features of ES cells, including the fulfillment of stringent pluripotency requirements. This work was subsequently confirmed and expanded upon by other groups describing the application of this technology to human cells. Proof-of-concept for the utility of iPS cells in regenerative medicine of inherited blood disorders was recently provided when iPS cells were generated from tail tip fibroblasts in a humanized sickle cell anemia mouse model. The genetic sickle hemoglobin defect of the iPS cells was corrected in vitro via homologous recombination. Using established protocols for the differentiation of hematopoietic progenitors from ES cells, hematopoietic cells capable of reconstituting lethally irradiated recipient mice were generated.

Transplantation of these cells into irradiated recipients resulted in robust engraftment and amelioration of the sickle cell phenotype in transplant recipients. Reprogramming of a panel of disease-specific human iPS cells, including patients with blood diseases, has been demonstrated. Human iPS cell lines shared defining features with human ES cells, including morphology, proliferation, feeder dependence, surface markers, gene expression, promoter and telomerase activities, in vivo differentiation, and teratoma formation. In analogy to the murine system, the reprogramming viruses are strongly silenced in human iPS cells, indicating that the maintenance of pluripotency does not depend on continuous transgene expression. Enforced transgene expression appears to initiate a sequence of stochastic events over several days that eventually induces a small fraction of cells (0.001–0.5% of cells) to acquire a stable pluripotent state. During direct reprogramming, gradual changes lead to a stable epigenetic state that is indistinguishable from inner cell mass-derived ES cells. For example, the Dnmt3a and Dnmt3b methyltransferases become activated and silence the viral transgenes as endogenous pluripotency factors are transcriptionally reactivated. Human iPS cell lines thus represent a novel stem cell population that can be studied with regard to normal and pathologic tissue formation in vitro, enabling disease investigation, drug development, and a platform for producing autologous cell therapies that avoid immune rejection. Moreover, the creation of iPS cells allows the correction of genetic defects and exhaustive molecular characterization at the clonal level before tissue reconstruction. While genetic transduction with exogenous genes, particularly oncogenes such as *c-MYC* and *KLF4*, and the use of integrating retroviral delivery systems are clear handicaps of this technology with regard to future clinical translation, newer methods have utilized nonintegrating vectors and even mRNA transduction to generate iPS. However, to date, robust reconstitution of murine hematopoiesis has not been consistently demonstrated, and there are no successful reports of in vivo reconstitution of human hematopoiesis in model systems. These all represent significant barriers to the translation of this powerful technology into human therapies.

One utility of targeting iPS cells for genetic therapies is that these cells can be cloned and expanded, allowing analysis of vector insertion sites before clinical use. In addition, reprogramming has now been accomplished, albeit at lower efficiencies using both nonintegrating vectors and protein transduction. Reprogramming has also now been accomplished with the expression of fewer transcription factors, most notably without c-Myc. Several laboratories have demonstrated that targeting specific loci is associated with limited or no adverse effects on expression of neighboring genes (reviewed by Sadelain et al[22]). For example, targeting of the *AAVS1* locus located on chromosome 19 has been well characterized. This locus encodes the *PPP1R1C* gene that is ubiquitously expressed. Insertion at this site appears to provide a "safe harbor" with respect to genotoxicity and allows stable and long-term expression of transgenes in human embryonic stem cells.

Finally, Naldini and colleagues have demonstrated that targeted insertion into two genomic sites (*IL2RG* and *CCR5*) using zinc-finger technology leads to no detectable alteration in the expression of nearby genes and sustained expression of the transgene cargo.[23] The frequency of directed site-specific integration in primary fibroblasts was as high as 10%.[23] In addition, elegant work by Sadelain and colleagues has demonstrated the feasibility of screening large numbers of iPS-derived clones for both integration in operationally defined safe harbors and for clinically relevant transgene expression using vectors that express globin genes.[24] Thus, this approach offers exciting future applications in treating a variety of human diseases.

Site-Directed Homologous Recombination to Correct Gene Mutations

A long-standing but unrealized goal of genetic therapy has been homologous recombination to affect replacement of abnormal disease-causing gene mutations. Although human ES cells theoretically provide an ideal target for such correction, gene targeting in these cells has proven difficult. Zinc-finger nuclease (ZFN)-mediated DS breaks allow high-efficiency site-specific homologous recombination and has been used to target a number of genes in human cells. ZFNs are generated by fusing the FokI nuclease domain to a DNA recognition domain composed of engineered C_2H_2 zinc finger motifs that specify the genomic DNA binding site for the chimeric protein. Compared with standard homologous recombination vectors, one advantage of ZFN is the relatively short stretch of homology needed (500 bp vs. 10–12 kb) to mediate genomic targeting. Binding of two fusion proteins to cognate DNA allows dimerization of the nuclease, leading to generation of a DS DNA break. When donor DNA with homology to sequence flanking the DS break is present, repair occurs with incorporation of the incoming DNA sequence. This system has been successfully used to target genes in multiple species and has recently been demonstrated in both human ES cells and iPS cells to effectively target both expressed and nonexpressed genes with a frequency of 1% to 20% and has been termed *genome editing*. Because the development of a DNA DS break is a prerequisite to ZFN-mediated gene editing and such breaks induce both p53 and HDR, this approach, although attractive, could also have significant "off-target" effects. In addition, as efficiency improves, direct targeting in HSCs is possible and a trial is currently under development to utilize ZFN-mediated deletion of *BCL11A*, which repressed fetal hemoglobin expression for the treatment of β-thalassemia.[25]

Other systems that seek to target specific genetic loci have also been described and are at different levels of development. As with ZFN nucleases, these approaches use cellular DNA repair mechanisms to introduce exogenous DNA sequences into the chromosome. Thus, methods to increase the efficiency of targeting by introducing DNA DS breaks as well as several other methods have exploited endonucleases that target rare DNA sequences to establish these DS breaks. Alternative methods in development include meganucleases and transcription activator-like effector nucleases.[26] Even more recently, bacterial immunity-related clustered regularly interspaced short palindromic repeats have shown higher efficiencies of genome editing by expressing the Cas9 protein and guide RNAs to target the mammalian genome at specific locations. Challenges of all of these approaches include efficiency of targeting in primary cells and potential off-target effects on the genome, and will likely also depend on technologic advances that allow ex vivo HSC cloning and large-scale expansion. At present, the use of ES or iPS cells is clearly amendable to this approach, but as noted earlier, use of these cells to derive transplantable HSCs is a major impediment to clinical utilization.

FUTURE DIRECTIONS

The use of gene transfer to treat human diseases has now been successful in several diseases. Compared with allogeneic BMT, ex vivo gene therapy using autologous cells obviates the need to search for an appropriate donor, eliminates the risk of GVHD, and in some cases reduces the intensity of preparative regimen required before transplant, which also reduces toxicity. Thus, in some diseases, this therapeutic approach can now be considered an alternative to standard therapy. Insertional mutagenesis, which has resulted in serious adverse events in several trials, has stimulated rapid development of putative safer vector systems that are being tested in human trials but remains a challenge. Rapid progress in molecular technology, such as high-throughput sequencing and the development of new sources of expandable stem cell sources, offers significant potential for ongoing development of gene transfer in regenerative biology for a wide range of human conditions.

ACKNOWLEDGEMENTS

Funding from NIH DK062757, CA113969, AI097628, DK090913, and the NHLBI Gene Therapy Resource Program. I would like to thank members of my laboratory and members of the Transatlantic Gene Therapy Consortium for productive collaborations.

SUGGESTED READINGS

Aiuti A, Cassani B, Andolfi G, et al: Multilineage hematopoietic reconstitution without clonal selection in ADA-SCID patients treated with stem cell gene therapy. *J Clin Invest* 117:2233–2240, 2007.

Aiuti A, Slavin S, Aker M, et al: Correction of ADA-SCID by stem cell gene therapy combined with nonmyeloablative conditioning. *Science* 296:2410–2413, 2002.

Bauer TR, Jr, Allen JM, Hai M, et al: Successful treatment of canine leukocyte adhesion deficiency by foamy virus vectors. *Nat Med* 14:93–97, 2008.

Cartier N, Hacein-Bey-Abina S, Bartholomae CC, et al: Hematopoietic stem cell gene therapy with a lentiviral vector in X-linked adrenoleukodystrophy. *Science* 326:818–823, 2009.

Cavazzana-Calvo M, Hacein-Bey S, de Saint Basile G, et al: Gene therapy of human severe combined immunodeficiency (SCID)-X1 disease. *Science* 288:669–672, 2000.

Cavazzana-Calvo M, Payen E, Negre O, et al: Transfusion independence and HMGA2 activation after gene therapy of human beta-thalassaemia. *Nature* 467:318–322, 2010.

Gaspar HB, Parsley KL, Howe S, et al: Gene therapy of X-linked severe combined immunodeficiency by use of a pseudotyped gammaretroviral vector. *Lancet* 364:2181–2187, 2004.

Hacein-Bey-Abina S, Le Deist F, Carlier F, et al: Sustained correction of X-linked severe combined immunodeficiency by ex vivo gene therapy. *N Engl J Med* 346:1185–1193, 2002.

Hacein-Bey-Abina S, Von Kalle C, Schmidt M, et al: LMO2-associated clonal T cell proliferation in two patients after gene therapy for SCID-X1. *Science* 302:415–419, 2003.

Hanna J, Wernig M, Markoulaki S, et al: Treatment of sickle cell anemia mouse model with iPS cells generated from autologous skin. *Science* 318:1920–1923, 2007.

Hirschhorn R, Yang DR, Puck JM, et al: Spontaneous *in vivo* reversion to normal of an inherited mutation in a patient with adenosine deaminase deficiency. *Nat Genet* 13:290–295, 1996.

Howe SJ, Mansour MR, Schwarzwaelder K, et al: Insertional mutagenesis combined with acquired somatic mutations causes leukemogenesis following gene therapy of SCID-X1 patients. *J Clin Invest* 118:3143–3150, 2008.

Laufs S, Nagy KZ, Giordano FA, et al: Insertion of retroviral vectors in NOD/SCID repopulating human peripheral blood progenitor cells occurs preferentially in the vicinity of transcription start regions and in introns. *Mol Ther* 10:874–881, 2004.

Li Z, Dullmann J, Schiedlmeier B, et al: Murine leukemia induced by retroviral gene marking. *Science* 296:497, 2002.

Milsom M, Schambach A, Williams DA, et al: Chemoprotective gene delivery. In Harington KJ, Vile RG, Pandha H, editors: *Viral therapy of cancer*, Indianapolis, IN, 2008, Wiley Press, pp 376–391.

Miyoshi H, Smith KA, Mosier DE, et al: Transduction of human CD34(+) cells that mediate long-term engraftment of NOD/SCID mice by HIV vectors. *Science* 283:682–686, 1999.

Moritz T, Patel VP, Williams DA: Bone marrow extracellular matrix molecules improve gene transfer into human hematopoietic cells via retroviral vectors. *J Clin Invest* 93:1451–1457, 1994.

Naldini L, Blomer U, Gallay P, et al: In vivo gene delivery and stable transduction of nondividing cells by a lentiviral vector. *Science* 272:263–267, 1996.

Ott MG, Stein S, Schultze-Strasser S, et al: Phase I/II gene therapy study for Chronic Granulomatous Disease: results, lessons and perspectives. *Blood (ASH Annual Meeting Abstracts)* 110:503, 2007.

Pai S, Notarangelo L, Harris C, et al: Somatic gene therapy for X-linked severe combined immunodeficiency using a self-inactivating modified gammaretroviral vector results in an improved preclinical safety profile and early clinical efficacy in a human patient. *Blood (ASH Annual Meeting Abstracts)* 118:164, 2011.

Park IH, Zhao R, West JA, et al: Reprogramming of human somatic cells to pluripotency with defined factors. *Nature* 451:141–146, 2008.

Porteus MH, Carroll D: Gene targeting using zinc finger nucleases. *Nat Biotechnol* 23:967–973, 2005.

Sadelain M, Papapetrou EP, Bushman FD: Safe harbours for the integration of new DNA in the human genome. *Nat Rev Cancer* 12:51–58, 2012.

Sankaran VG, Menne TF, Xu J, et al: Human fetal hemoglobin expression is regulated by the developmental stage-specific repressor BCL11A. *Science* 322:1839–1842, 2008.

Stein S, Ott MG, Schultze-Strasser S, et al: Genomic instability and myelodysplasia with monosomy 7 consequent to EVI1 activation after gene therapy for chronic granulomatous disease. *Nat Med* 16:198–204, 2010.

Takahashi K, Tanabe K, Ohnuki M, et al: Induction of pluripotent stem cells from adult human fibroblasts by defined factors. *Cell* 131:861–872, 2007.

Thrasher AJ, Gaspar HB, Baum C, et al: Gene therapy: X-SCID transgene leukaemogenicity. *Nature* 443:E5–E6, discussion E6-E7, 2006.

Urnov FD, Miller JC, Lee YL, et al: Highly efficient endogenous human gene correction using designed zinc-finger nucleases. *Nature* 435:646–651, 2005.

Williams DA, Thrasher AJ: Concise review: lessons learned from clinical trials of gene therapy in monogenic immunodeficiency diseases. *Stem Cells Transl Med* 3:636–642, 2014.

Xu J, Peng C, Sankaran VG, et al: Correction of sickle cell disease in adult mice by interference with fetal hemoglobin silencing. *Science* 334:993–996, 2011.

Yu J, Vodyanik MA, Smuga-Otto K, et al: Induced pluripotent stem cell lines derived from human somatic cells. *Science* 318:1917–1920, 2007.

REFERENCES

For the complete list of references, log on to www.expertconsult.com.

Alexander Friedenstein first described, in 1974, fibroblast-like colony-forming units (CFU-F) isolated from the bone marrow (BM) by plastic adherence in tissue culture plates that could support hematopoiesis in vitro.[1] The culture-expanded progeny derived from CFU-F could proliferate robustly and differentiate into mesenchymal lineages. In 1991, Arnold Caplan from Case Western Reserve University introduced the term *mesenchymal stem cells* (hereafter MSCs) to name this unique cell population, referring to their mesenchymal plasticity and potential use in bone repair.[2] He and others then proceeded to demonstrate that these cells could differentiate into several mesenchymal lineages, such as bone, cartilage, muscle, and fat, and serve as progenitor cells for nonhematopoietic tissues.[3] The intrinsic mesenchymal plasticity deployed by culture-expanded MSCs informed the notion that they could be used in regenerative medicine for the treatment of congenital mesenchymal disorders such as *osteogenesis imperfecta* (OI). Based on the ability of MSCs to migrate to the bone and differentiate into osteoblasts, Edwin Horwitz et al hypothesized that the infusion of whole BM containing mesenchymal progenitors could attenuate if not cure OI. In 1999 the first clinical study was conducted on three infants with severe deforming OI[4] infused with unmanipulated BM graft from human leukocyte antigen (HLA)–identical or single antigen-mismatched siblings following a myeloablative regimen. All patients presented hematopoietic engraftment, and new bone formation could be seen in bone biopsies performed 3 months after implantation. Total body bone mineralization and growth were increased, while fracture incidence was reduced in the first 6 months following BM transplantation. Encouraged by these results, this group conducted a second clinical trial published in 2002, in which OI infants were not only given BM transplant, but were also infused with in vitro expanded allogeneic MSCs.[5] Of the six infants treated, five presented MSC engraftment in BM—albeit at a very low frequency—accompanied by a net increase in growth. However, only one child had a substantial increase in total body mineralization. Since no changes were observed in the only patient in whom injected MSCs did not engraft, the beneficial effects seen in the other infants can presumably be attributed to the infused MSCs and their paracrine effect. Contemporaneous to the OI studies, a first-in-human clinical use of culture-expanded autologous marrow MSCs by Hillard Lazarus was conducted in 1995 as adoptive cell therapy for support of hematopoiesis in the setting of autologous peripheral blood stem cell transplantation (SCT).[6] In addition to their trophic effects on hematopoiesis, intravenous transfusion of MSCs were later shown to deploy robust immune suppressive properties in a nonhuman primate model of skin allotransplantation, which augured a 2004 case report from the Karolinska Institute by Katarina LeBlanc describing the anecdotal yet substantial effect of haploidentical MSCs on steroid-resistant grade IV acute graft-versus-host disease (GVHD) in a 9-year-old boy (Fig. 99.1).[7] This report was followed by a series of phase II studies of allogeneic MSCs in prevention and treatment of acute, steroid-refractory GVHD.[8] However, a phase III clinical trial of an industrial random donor MSC product in steroid-resistant acute GVHD reported in 2009 that it failed to meet its primary endpoint of durable GVHD remission.[9] Notwithstanding, culture-expanded MSC-like cells derived from marrow, adipose tissue, or umbilical cord are under intense clinical study for ailments falling roughly into three categories: adjunct to hematopoietic stem cell (HSC) transplantation, autoimmune and inflammatory disease, and tissue repair. See box titled "Considerations in Development of MSC-like Cells as a Cellular Pharmaceutical for GVHD".

ENDOGENOUS MESENCHYMAL STEM CELLS

The estimated frequency of CFU-F progenitors relative to total nucleated cells in marrow is approximately 1:100,000 to 1:240,000. Despite their relative rarity, endogenous marrow MSCs are active components of the BM hematopoietic niche.[10] They are mainly localized in the endosteum of the bone where they give rise to pericytes, myofibroblasts, osteocytes, and endothelial cells, as well as all functional elements of the BM stroma supporting HSCs and progenitor cells development. MSCs have also been identified in vivo as perivascular cells expressing the STRO1, CD146 and 3G5 antigens. Despite a close relationship between these two cell types in terms of surface phenotype and qualitative in vitro assays, MSCs in general lack the contractility of pericytes and may show marked differences in gene expression. In addition, some have described a neuroectodermal origin of MSCs through either Sox1[+] neuroepithelial cells or Nestin[+] precursors. MSCs also express fibronectin, laminin, collagen, and proteoglycans, which are part of the extracellular matrix of the BM stroma. Importantly, MSCs directly interact with hematopoietic cells via an array of surface markers and cytokines, which regulate different aspects of HSC development: quiescence, proliferation, and differentiation. Cell–cell contact between MSCs and hematopoietic cells is mediated by several adhesion molecules such as intercellular adhesion molecule (ICAM)-1, ICAM-2, ICAM-3, vascular cell adhesion molecule (VCAM)-1, leukocyte function–associated antigen (LFA)-3, CD44, and CD72. Among factors secreted, MSCs were shown to express hematopoietic growth factors such as bone morphologic protein 4 (BMP4), Flt-3, leukemia inhibitory factor (LIF), oncostatin M (OSM), stem cell factor (SCF), stromal cell-derived factor-1 (SDF-1), and transforming growth factor-β (TGF-β), and interleukins such as interleukin (IL)-1, IL-6, IL-7, IL-8, IL-11, IL-14, and IL-15. CFU-F–forming cells from BM can be obtained through the prospective isolation of CD45[−] MSCs with anti-STRO1, anti-CD271, or anti-CD146 antibodies, or selection for nestin-expressing cells. Nevertheless, not enough data concerning purified MSCs are available to assume that endogenous MSC progenitors possess the same immune regulatory properties of ex vivo expanded culture-adapted MSCs.[11] Therefore, almost the entire amount of data concerning the immunological properties of MSCs refers to adherent expanded, culture-adapted MSCs.

BONE MARROW MESENCHYMAL STEM CELL MANUFACTURE AND PHENOTYPE

The manufacture of MSCs in large numbers requires collection and processing of marrow followed by ex vivo culture expansion in serum-containing growth media. Typical processing protocols involve Ficoll enrichment of mononuclear cells from liquid BM aspirates and subsequent plating of unfractionated nucleated cells onto plastic tissue culture plates maintained within humidified incubators set at 37°C and 5% CO_2. Within a week or so, plastic adherent CFU-F arise, and subsequent passaging depletes nonadherent myelolymphoid cells and gives rise to a homogenous polyclonal population of

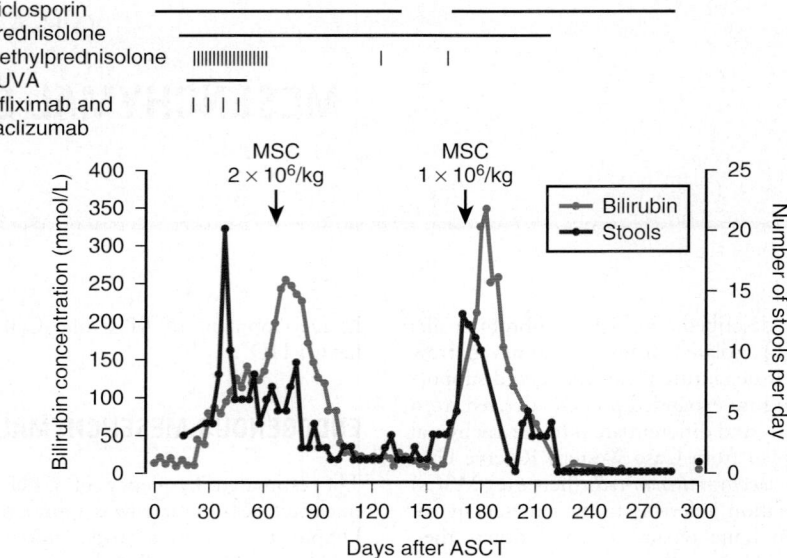

Ciclosporin
Prednisolone
Methylprednisolone
PUVA
Infliximab and
daclizumab

Fig. 99.1 CLINICAL COURSE AND IMMUNOSUPPRESSION OF THE FIRST GRAFT VERSUS-HOST DISEASE PATIENT TO BE TREATED WITH MESENCHYMAL STEM CELLS. Pharmacologic immune suppression is indicated *(top)*; arrows indicate the time of MSC infusions. *ASCT*, Allogeneic stem cell transplantation; *MSC*, mesenchymal stem cell; *PUVA*, psoralen and ultraviolet light A. *(With permission from Le Blanc K, Rasmusson I, Sundberg B, et al: Treatment of severe acute graft-versus-host disease with third party haploidentical mesenchymal stem cells.* Lancet *363:1439, 2004.)*

plate-adherent MSCs with a doubling time of roughly 24–72 hours. Serial passaging allows for continued expansion for up to more than 50 cell doublings. Under microscopic observation, human MSCs appear morphologically heterogeneous and contain fast-replicating spindle- or round-shaped cells and slow-replicating large cells. The International Society of Cellular Therapy (ISCT) arrived at the conclusion that although the cell culture may contain stem cells, most culture-expanded progeny do not meet the criteria attributed to stem cells (self-renewal and mesenchymal pluripotency). Therefore they proposed the name multipotent *mesenchymal stromal cells*, since MSCs are consistently found to be part of the stroma independent of the tissue from which they arise.[12] Indeed, cell populations with multipotent mesenchymal plasticity and self-renewing potential are found in various tissue such as adipose tissue, umbilical cord blood (CB), and placenta, to name a few. As the field of MSC research matured, different isolation methods, tissue origins and characterization criteria were developed. In order to standardize the elements defining MSCs, the ISCT proposed a list of criteria published in 2006.[12] It was proposed that first, MSC populations must be plastic adherent; second, although many isolation methods based on surface cell markers have been established, the only markers recognized for MSCs are CD105+, CD73+, CD90+, and negative hematopoietic cell markers CD45, CD34, CD14 or CD11b, CD79a or CD19, and human leukocyte antigen, antigen D related (HLA-DR); third, cells should be shown to differentiate into osteoblasts, adipocytes, and chondroblasts in vitro (Fig. 99.2); and finally, the origin of the cells should always be clearly stated, such as "bone marrow–derived" or "adipose-derived MSC." Subsequent guidance from the ISCT[13] and the International Federation for Adipose Therapeutics and Science (IFATS)[14] regarding phenotypic characteristics of adipose-derived MSCs and cytokine-activated cells provides an evolving understanding of phenotype and function (Table 99.1). See box titled "MSC Phenotype: Does Form Predict Function?".

IMMUNE PROFILE OF MESENCHYMAL STEM CELLS

MSCs are typically identified by their coexpression of CD73, CD90, and CD105. Although these markers provide identity to MSCs, the

TABLE 99.1   Phenotypic Profile of Culture Expanded MSCs From Adipose Tissue, Marrow and Following IFN-γ Priming

	ASC[a]	BM-MSC[a]	IFN-γ-activated MSCs[b]
CD13	++	++	++
CD44	++	++	++
CD73	++	++	++
CD90	++	++	++
CD105	++	++	++
CD10	++	±	
MHC class I	+	+	++
CD106	–	+	++
CD36	+	–	
CD34	±	–	–
CD45	–	–	–
CD14 or CD11b	–	–	–
CD19 or CD79α	–	–	–
HLA-DR	–	–	++
IDO	–	–	+++
PD-L1	–	–	+++
CD80	–	–	–
CD86	–	–	–

[a]Adapted from International Federation for Adipose Therapeutics and Science and the International Society of Cellular Therapy (ISCT) Position Statement on Adipose Stromal Cells.[12,14]
[b]Adapted from the ISCT Working Proposal on Immunological Characterization of Mesenchymal Stem Cells.[13]
ASC, Adipose Stromal cell; BM, bone marrow; HLA-DR, human leukocyte antigen, antigen D related; IDO, indoleamine dioxygenase; IFN-γ, interferon-γ; MHC, major histocompatibility complex; MSC, mesenchymal stromal cell; PD-L1, programmed death-ligand 1.

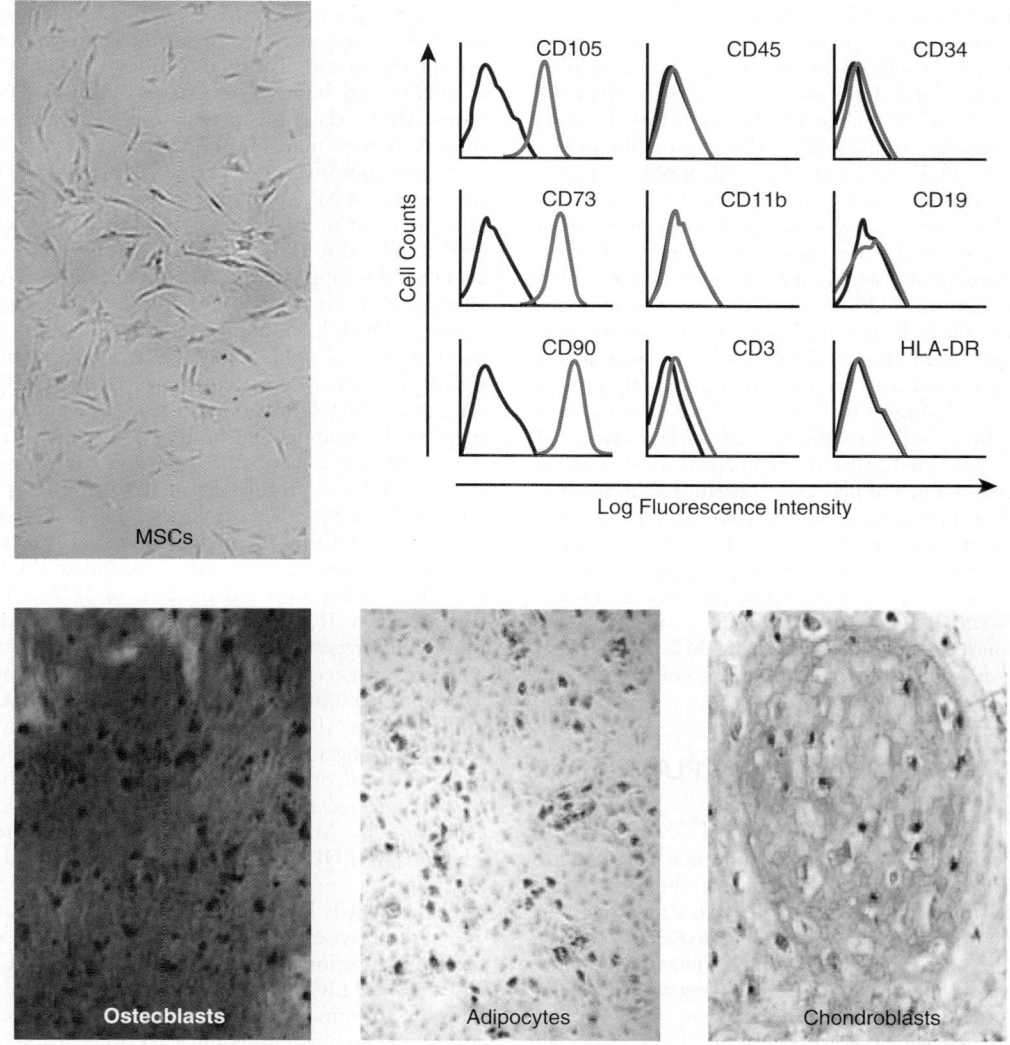

Fig. 99.2 A PANEL OF DATA DEMONSTRATING THE DEFINING CHARACTERISTICS OF MESENCHYMAL STROMAL CELLS: ADHERENCE, IMMUNOPHENOTYPE, AND IN VITRO DIFFERENTIATION. *Top left,* photomicrograph of undifferentiated MSCs showing the characteristic spindle shape and adherent properties of the cells. Original magnification, ×40. *Top right,* flow cytometry histograms demonstrating the typical expression pattern of surface antigens *(blue line)* and isotype control *(red line),* as indicated. *Bottom,* immunocytochemical staining demonstrating the differentiation of MSCs into osteoblasts (Alizarin Red stain), adipocytes (Oil Red O stain), and chondroblasts (Alcian Blue stain). *MSC,* Mesenchymal stem cell. *(With permission from Martinez C, Hofmann TJ, Marino R, et al: Human bone marrow mesenchymal stromal cells express the neural ganglioside GD2: A novel surface marker for the identification of MSCs.* Blood *109:4245, 2007.)*

role of these molecules in MSCs has not been established. However, CD73, an ectoenzyme that catalyzes the dephosphorylation of adenosine monophosphates into adenosine, is known to suppress adaptive immune responses. MSCs constitutively express major histocompatibility complex (MHC) class I molecules and are able to present MHC class I-restricted epitopes from transfected tumor antigens or virally introduced antigens to CD8+ T lymphocytes. It has been demonstrated that human MSCs are capable of cross-presentation of soluble antigens and effective antigenic presentation to naive CD8+ T cells. Expression of CD80, CD86, CD28, ICOSL, and 41BBL co-stimulatory molecules are not observed on MSCs; however, they express low levels of CD54/ICAM-1 or CD106/VCAM-1, both of which could play a role in T-cell co-stimulation. MSCs have been shown to produce basal levels of biologically active chemokines, cytokines, and inflammatory mediators, in particular CXC-chemokine ligand 12 (CXCL-12)/SDF-1, IL-6, prostaglandin E2 (PGE$_2$), and TGF-β. CXCL-12 is a small chemotactic cytokine that is often found in inflammatory sites and is an important

chemoattractant for a variety of cells, in particular hematopoietic stem/progenitor cells. It supports the function of MSCs in HSC niches and tissue regeneration. The role of CXCL-12 in the immune properties of MSC has not been fully investigated; however, while this cytokine has been described to mediate attraction and proliferation of lymphocytes, it may also favor the establishment of immune tolerance in vivo. IL-6 is a well-characterized cytokine that functions in inflammation, lymphocyte proliferation, and B-cell maturation. Compared with primary blood macrophages, basal production of IL-6 and PGE$_2$ is substantial in MSCs. For instance, primary unstimulated human macrophages produce less than 1 ng/48 h/10^6 cells of IL-6, while human MSCs produce 5–30 ng/48 h/10^6 cells of IL-6, and production of PGE$_2$ and IL-6 by MSCs is increased upon exposure to inflammatory products, such as tumor necrosis factor-α (TNF-α) or Toll-like receptor (TLR) ligands. Accordingly, inhibition of IL-6 produced by MSCs results in enhanced suppression of proliferation of activated lymphocytes in vitro. IL-6 was shown to be responsible for neutrophil protection from apoptosis in cultures with low numbers of human MSCs and has been suggested to play a role in the blocking of monocyte differentiation into DCs. MSC-derived TGF-β was shown to play a role in the inhibition of natural killer (NK) cells in vitro and is the dominant cytokine that drives the polarization of FoxP3⁻ CD4⁺ T cells to FoxP3⁺ regulatory T (Treg) cells. Accordingly, production of TGF-β by MSCs favors the induction of Treg cells in vivo. PGE$_2$ is a metabolic product of arachidonic acid conversion by the enzyme COX-1 and COX-2. MSCs constitutively express COX-2 and secrete low levels of PGE$_2$. Expression of COX-2 and secretion of PGE$_2$ are considerably increased when encountering an inflammatory signal such as interferon (IFN)-γ, TNF-α, or lipopolysaccharide (LPS). In addition to its role in the inflammatory reaction, PGE$_2$ is described as an important pathway in T-cell immunosuppression mediated by MSCs. Human MSCs have also been shown to express an array of other potential immune suppressive effectors, including LIF, HLA-G, TNF-α–stimulated gene/protein 6 (TSG-6), as well as soluble and cell surface-associated galectins, in particular galectin-1, galectin -3, and galectin -8. Expression of several molecules known to play an important role in fetomaternal tolerance such as indoleamine dioxygenase (IDO) occurs in human MSCs and these appear to be central in the suppressor functionality of human culture-expanded MSCs. Exposure of MSCs to IFN-γ increases the expression of these factors that mediate inhibitory action on T, B, and NK cell activities. MSCs can also affect differentiation of monocytes to IL-10-producing M2 macrophages and dendritic cells, as well as their maturation, migration, and functions.[15]

MESENCHYMAL STROMAL CELL IMMUNE PLASTICITY IN RESPONSE TO INFLAMMATORY CUES

In a resting state, cultured MSCs display immune homeostatic features biased toward suppression and are further highly responsive to environmental inflammatory cues.[16] In vivo experiments in rodents and nonhuman primates have demonstrated that although a large portion of MSCs are trapped in the lung following systemic intravenous administration, infused MSCs can migrate to several organs such as the liver, spleen, BM, and kidneys. Their migratory potential is associated with the expression of VCAM-1, which allows them to interact with endothelial cells. In addition, MSCs can express chemokine receptors (CCR1, CCR7, CCR9, CXCR4, CXCR5, and CXCR6) that promote their migration to specific sites, such as the BM via SDF-1, or to inflamed tissue via other CC and CXC chemokines. MSCs express multiple receptors for inflammatory signals, such as receptors for chemokines, type I and II IFNs, IL-1, and TNF-α, as well as TLRs that bind to pathogen-associated conserved motifs. These mediators are produced by fully activated immune cells and upregulate the expression of immunosuppressive factors by MSCs, which in turn dampens the immune and/or inflammatory response. IFN-γ is a well-studied immunomodulatory cytokine that robustly modulates the immunobiology of MSCs, and the in vivo suppressive properties of MSCs are likely dependent on activation by IFN-γ secreted by activated lymphoid effector cells. The importance of IFN-γ for augmentation of the veto properties of MSCs has been demonstrated in multiple key seminal observations: anti-IFN-γ receptor antibodies abrogate the suppressive properties of MSCs; IFN-γ receptor knock out of MSCs does not inhibit T cells[17]; and, IFN-γ licensing is crucial for MSCs to suppress T-cell effector functions. Accordingly, in vivo experiments in murine GVHD models demonstrated that MSCs were not effective at controlling GVHD if mice were transplanted with T cells defective for IFN-γ production, and MSCs pretreated with IFN-γ were more potent than nontreated MSCs at inhibiting GVHD. The downstream effects of IFN-γ activation on MSCs are protean. IFN-γ–primed MSCs robustly upregulate markers such as MHC I and II molecules, immune modulatory molecules (CD200, CD274/PD-L1/B7-H1), cytokine/chemokine receptors (CXCR3, CXCR4, CXCR5, CCR7, CD119/IFN-γ receptor), adhesion molecules (CD54, CD106), DNAM ligands (CD112, CD155), NKG2D ligands (macrophage

inflammatory complex [MIC] A/B, UL binding protein 1, 2, 3), and Notch receptors (Jagged-1). Intriguingly, human MSCs do not upregulate co-stimulatory molecules (CD80, CD86) in response to IFN-γ, and immune modulators such as TGF-β can markedly blunt MHC class II upregulation in response to inflammatory stimuli. IFN-γ–inducible IDO expression plays a major role in the immunosuppressive properties of MSCs and defines an important component of MSC immune plasticity. IDO catabolizes conversion of tryptophan to kynurenine, which is an inhibitor of T-cell proliferation. Blocking IDO catabolic activity with 1-methyl tryptophan abolishes the suppressive activity of MSCs on T-cell proliferation in vitro. Another tryptophan-degrading enzyme, tryptophan 2,3 dioxygenase (TDO), has a homeostatic housekeeping role predominantly in the liver, and unlike IDO it does not respond to immunoactive signals. Human MSCs were shown to express TDO in the resting stage and IFN-γ stimulation does not upregulate its expression. This suggests the leading role of IFN-γ–inducible IDO in modulating the tryptophan catabolic pathway and subsequent immunosuppression by MSCs. Upregulation of IDO by IFN-γ can be augmented synergistically by other cytokines such as TNF-α, which are poor inducers of IDO by themselves alone. TLR activators such as LPS and polyI:C have been shown to upregulate IDO through autocrine IFN-β signaling loop independent of IFN-γ. Interestingly, MSCs with defective IFN-γ receptor 1 can still suppress T-cell proliferation. This suggests that other immunosuppressive mechanisms are operative in synergy with IFN-γ–induced effects on MSCs to regulate T-cell proliferation, such as: HLA-G5, PGE2, galectins, insulin-like growth factor (IGF)-binding proteins, and TSG-6. The breadth and effectiveness of an ongoing immune response are determined by both T-cell proliferation and their effector function, as defined by cytokine secretion and degranulation, respectively. Thus, IDO expression by MSCs targets the proliferative response of T cells while PDL1/PDL2-PD-1 interaction likely regulates memory T-cell function.

Whereas it is known that most somatic cells express one or two TLRs, the exact expression profile of TLRs in MSCs is controversial. Protein expression of TLR1, TLR2, TLR3, TLR4, TLR5, TLR6, TLR7, and TLR9 has been reported in human and mouse MSCs; however, in humans only TLR3 and TLR4 were expressed at levels comparable to blood mononuclear cells. The response to TLR ligands in MSCs appears quite different compared with macrophages. When activated, both cell types secrete chemokines, PGE$_2$, and IL-6; however, only macrophages produce IL-10, TNF-α, and, following IFN-γ priming, IL-12. In addition, factors secreted by TLR-activated MSCs, in particular PGE$_2$, act in vitro and in vivo on surrounding macrophages, resulting in increased production of IL-10. It has been shown that MSCs can reduce mortality in a mouse model of peritonitis associated with septicemia and release of bacterial toxins in the circulation.[18] In this study, MSCs injected in the systemic circulation of septic mice localized in the lung, where they were found surrounded by macrophages. These macrophages were shown to produce increased levels of the antiinflammatory cytokine IL-10 both in vivo and ex vivo in response to bacterial LPS compared with untreated septic mice. In vitro assays suggested that the suppressive effect of MSCs on the macrophage inflammatory response to LPS was dependent on the expression of the LPS receptor TLR4 by both cell types. Results suggested that LPS or TNF-α–mediated activation of MSCs upregulated the expression of cyclooxygenase 2 and PGE2 by MSCs, which in turn bind to the EP2 and EP4 receptors on macrophages, stimulating the production of IL-10.

A fundamental discrepancy between the immune cell physiology of MSCs from different species is the relative importance of nitric oxide (NO) and IDO in murine and human MSCs.[19] After inflammatory priming, human MSCs express extremely high levels of IDO and low levels of inducible nitric oxide synthase (iNOS), which is opposite to that seen with mouse MSCs. The in vitro functional relevance of IDO bioactivity in human MSCs can be readily shown by use of the specific inhibitor L-1 methyltryptophan (L-1MT), which completely abolishes the inhibition of T-cell proliferation, whereas mouse MSCs are unaffected by L-1MT. Inhibition of NO production in mouse MSCs abolishes their ability to suppress T-cell proliferation, a phenomenon not observed in human MSCs. In addition to IDO, other human-specific tolerance molecules such as HLA-G are upregulated by IFN-γ in human MSCs but not in the murine system. These important differences between the mechanisms of priming and action of immunosuppression by mouse versus human MSCs highlight some of the limitations of in vivo studies assessing the immunosuppressive mechanism of action properties of murine MSCs in animal models of disease.

MESENCHYMAL STROMAL CELL IMMUNE PRIVILEGE: A CONTROVERSIAL ISSUE

Based on the extensive results demonstrating the immunosuppressive effect of MSCs in vitro, it was suggested that MSCs could use their immunosuppressive mechanisms to evade the immune system and therefore be used as an immune-privileged "off the shelf" allogeneic donor product for clinical applications. Several studies have suggested that allogeneic MSCs are ignored by the immune system and/or are weakly immunogenic. For instance, the persistence of fetal MSCs in the bone marrow of the mothers was reported decades after pregnancies. Baboons that received allogeneic MSCs injected at high doses (5×10^6 MSCs/kg), first intravenously and then intramuscularly developed alloantigen-specific antibodies but had reduced alloantigen-induced PBMC proliferation compared with naive controls, and persistence of donor MSCs could be observed 4 weeks later. In contrast, other studies have suggested that MSCs can be fully recognized by the immune system and/or support immune cell activation in an antigen-independent fashion, challenging the notion of immune privilege.[20] In mice and pigs, allogeneic MSCs injected subcutaneously induced both alloantigen-specific T- and B-cell responses. In a rat model of transplantation, allogeneic heart transplants were rejected earlier if recipients were previously sensitized to donor MSCs. In human MSCs, detailed analyses showed that in certain experimental conditions MSCs can support in vitro allogeneic T-cell proliferation, LPS- or antigen-induced IgG secretion by spleen B cells, or suppress neutrophil apoptosis. These events could be initiated through direct antigenic recognition of MSCs and soluble factors produced by MSCs, in particular IL-6. Paradoxically, IFN-γ stimulation of MSCs enables them to acquire antigen-presenting cell-like features. Human and mouse MSCs activated by IFN-γ upregulate MHC class I molecule expression and MHC class I-mediated antigen presentation of endogenously expressed viral proteins to cytotoxic T lymphocyte lines. Expression of MHC class II molecules and antigenic presentation to CD4$^+$ T cells was observed to be induced by IFN-γ, and depended in vitro on IFN-γ concentration. Antigenic presentation by mouse or human MSCs to CD8$^+$ or CD4$^+$ T lymphocytes induced IFN-γ and IL-2 production by T lymphocytes and T lymphocyte proliferation. Antigen processing was not affected by sole treatment with TNF-α, or TLR3 or TLR4 ligands. In addition, MSCs can present extracellular soluble proteins to CD8$^+$ T cells through their MHC class I molecules. This function, a hallmark of professional antigen-presenting cells, is known as *cross-presentation* and is critical for the mounting of a T-cell immune response targeted at extracellular pathogens or tumor antigens. Although MSCs do not express the classical B7 co-stimulatory molecules CD80 and CD86, they express other surface molecules (ICAM and LFA-3) and cytokines (IL-6 and IL-7), which can deliver co-stimulatory signals necessary for T-cell activation.

MESENCHYMAL STROMAL CELLS FOR THE PREVENTION AND TREATMENT OF STEROID-REFRACTORY ACUTE GRAFT-VERSUS HOST DISEASE

Based upon their dual role in supporting hematopoiesis and modulating immunity, MSCs have been studied as a companion transfusion product for HSC transplantation (SCT), and can be categorized into two broad categories: prevention and treatment of GVHD, and adjuvant to HSC engraftment. Much has been done since the first described successful treatment of a 9-year-old boy suffering from acute steroid-resistant GVHD with MSCs. Several phase I/II clinical and multiinstitutional trials have been published with encouraging results in adult or pediatric patients. In most studies, MSCs were infused intravenously at a dose of $1-8 \times 10^6$ MSCs/kg in subjects with GVHD. The intravenous route allowed the injection of several doses of MSCs, and the number of MSC infusions was often increased in patients with partial responses. MSCs were from HLA-identical siblings or HLA-matched or -mismatched donors; however, the response rate to MSC infusion was not related to the degree of HLA matching. The largest academic, multicenter phase II experimental study was described in 2008, in which 55 adult and pediatric patients with steroid-resistant acute GVHD were treated with steroids and MSC infusions. Thirty patients had a complete response, 53% of whom were alive 2 years later. Although similar results were obtained in other studies, some failed to reach a positive outcome. An industry-sponsored phase III randomized, placebo-controlled clinical trial for steroid-refractory acute GVHD in adults and children was completed in 2009 and the results presented in February 2010 at the BMT Tandem Meetings. Six infusions of industrial MSCs (Prochymal, Osiris Therapeutics) were administered at a dose of 2×10^6 MSCs/kg twice a week for 3–4 consecutive weeks, in addition to standard glucocorticoid therapy. The results that have been released to date demonstrate that in adults there was no statistical difference between MSCs and placebo on the overall response rate (35% vs. 30%; $n = 244$). Nevertheless, in a post-hoc analysis MSCs improved liver GVHD (day 100 response rates of 76% vs. 47%) or gastrointestinal GVHD (day 100 response rates of 82% vs. 68%). In pediatric patients, Prochymal showed a trend of improvement in durable CR rates (64% vs. 43%; $n = 28$), allowing for conditional approval of by Canadian and New Zealand authorities for use in children.[21]

Although numerous clinical studies using MSCs for the treatment of GVHD have been conducted, the mechanisms by which MSCs mediate their immunosuppressive effect against GVHD in humans is still unknown. It was described that acute GVHD is accompanied by a burst in cytokine production by activated donor immune cells, including IFN-γ and TNF-α. In a mouse model of GVHD using MSCs from iNOS-knock out mice, it was demonstrated that NO produced by MSCs in response to the presence of high levels of IFN-γ was principally responsible for the immunosuppressive effect observed. It was also shown that IFN-γ stimulation of MSCs is the key element promoting the immunosuppressive effect of MSCs. The latter study suggested that the effectiveness of MSC infusions to treat mice undergoing allogeneic BM transplant varied with the phase of the disease and the level of circulating IFN-γ. Co-transplantation of MSCs with HSCs did not prevent the appearance of GVHD, whereas MSC infusion 20 days post-HSC transplantation (when levels of IFN-γ are high) or implantation of prestimulated MSCs with IFN-γ resulted in enhanced survival. Additional studies hinted that the timing of MSC administration relative to HSC transplant may dramatically influence the outcome of both the graft-versus-leukemia (GVL) response and GVHD. Ning et al. reported results from a clinical trial in which patients with hematological malignancy underwent haploidentical peripheral blood stem cell (PBSC) transplantation in combination with MSCs or not, where they observed a reduction of GVHD in MSC-injected patients but also a 60% tumor relapse compared with a 20% relapse in the non-MSC group.[22]

MESENCHYMAL STROMAL CELLS TO PROMOTE HEMATOPOIETIC STEM CELL ENGRAFTMENT IN PRECLINICAL MODELS OF STEM CELL TRANSPLANTATION

Engraftment of HSCs is a considerable barrier to successful transplant, particularly in allogeneic SCT for nonmalignant diseases. Graft failure is predominantly immune mediated, where recipient T cells play a dominant role in rejecting donor hematopoietic cells. The risk of graft failure therefore increases with the degree of human leukocyte antigen mismatch, the intensity of pretransplant conditioning, and ex vivo graft T-cell depletion. The majority of preclinical murine studies examining the use of human MSCs have utilized immune-defective nonobese diabetic (NOD)/severe combined immunodeficiency (SCID) mice that have received sublethal doses of radiation prior to human HSC transplantation. MSCs isolated from human fetal lung, fetal BM, adult BM, and placenta enhance engraftment of single human CD34+ CB, although results were not statistically significant using placental MSCs. Both placental and BM MSCs enhance double-CB engraftment in the NOD/SCID mouse model. Third-party human BM MSCs also increase the engraftment of double CB compared with single CB. Both human placental and BM MSCs also significantly decrease single-cord dominance in this model. In an effort to identify MSC subsets that may show enhanced ability to support HSC engraftment, MSCs expressing markers that enrich for CFU-F activity such as the low-affinity nerve growth factor receptor (LNGFR, CD271) and STRO-1 have been examined. The infusion of selected human CD271+ marrow-derived MSCs has been compared with the infusion of standard MSCs for engraftment of human CD133+ peripheral blood cells into NOD/SCID mice. In this study, CD271+ MSCs displayed full MSC CFU-F activity (with none in the CD271− fraction) and demonstrated one- to threefold higher proliferation compared with standard MSCs. While both MSC subsets increased engraftment, CD271+ MSCs resulted in greater CD45+ donor cell engraftment. Similarly, both STRO-1+ and STRO-1− MSCs have been shown to increase BM, peripheral blood, and spleen engraftment of human CB cells in this model, although STRO-1− MSCs are superior in this effect. The MSC donor source may also impact the effect of MSCs on engraftment. In murine models, syngeneic murine BM-derived MSCs significantly increase donor murine HSC engraftment, whereas donor-derived MSCs significantly decrease engraftment, and third-party MSCs have no effect.[23] In contrast, in a NOD/SCID model, autologous or allogeneic MSCs comparably increase myeloid engraftment of human CD45+ cells. This suggests that, at least in a murine model of SCT, MSCs are not immunologically inert, and that the donor source of MSCs can lead to profound differences in engraftment depending on the transplant model. MSCs had no effect in two canine models of SCT using different MSC and HSC donor sources. Third-party MSCs (either from primary culture or an immortalized clonal population) had no impact on the engraftment of canine haploidentical BM cells following total-body irradiation when compared with BM cells alone, with half of the animals rejecting grafts and half developing fatal acute GVHD. Donor-derived BM MSCs also had no impact on engraftment in a canine leukocyte antigen-identical transplant model using nonmyeloablative conditioning (1 Gray), a model in which costimulation (CTLA4) blockade or anti-CD154 has been successful. Failure of MSCs in these canine models may be attributed to numerous reasons, including the source of MSCs, intensity of conditioning, absence of posttransplant immunosuppression, and/or the dosing schedule of MSCs. Finally, MSCs have been studied in a nonhuman primate model of autologous CD34+ intra-BM transplant in which autologous BM MSCs increased the percentage of donor CFUs found in recipient BM, although the primates were not followed long term.

CLINICAL TRIALS OF MESENCHYMAL STROMAL CELLS TO PROMOTE HEMATOPOIETIC STEM CELL ENGRAFTMENT

A number of clinical trials have been published demonstrating the use of MSCs to promote allogeneic HSC engraftment. Several clinical trials have evaluated the use of MSCs following CB transplantation using third-party or haploidentical MSCs. Following infusion of haploidentical MSCs, pediatric patients with high-risk acute leukemia had engraftment and rates of GVHD comparable to historical controls; all eight patients engrafted with a low rate of acute GVHD. A similar study utilized haploidentical MSCs in pediatric patients with hematologic malignancies and hemophagocytic lymphohistiocytosis. Compared with a historical control group, there were comparable rates of engraftment, although patients receiving MSCs had significantly less grade III–IV acute GVHD. Interestingly, no patients in either of these studies developed chronic GVHD. Finally, a study of adult patients with high-risk hematologic malignancies found comparable rates of CB engraftment in patients receiving donor-derived (mostly haploidentical) MSCs to that of a concurrent control group. All patients receiving MSCs had rapid donor engraftment with a low incidence of chronic GVHD and no grade III–IV acute GVHD.

In addition to being given early in SCT to support HSC engraftment, MSCs have been employed to promote ex vivo expansion of HSCs. In an elegant study by de Lima et al,[24] adult patients with hematologic malignancies receiving double-CB transplant had the smaller CB expanded in ex vivo coculture with third-party MSCs, then infused on day 0 following receipt of the unmanipulated larger CB unit. Patients had significantly more rapid neutrophil and platelet engraftment and higher cumulative incidence of neutrophil and platelet engraftment when compared to a matched historical control group. The expanded cord predominated early post-SCT, while the unmanipulated cord predominated long term. The authors attribute this observation to coculture increasing progenitor cells committed to megakaryocyte and myeloid lineages, and depleting cells important in long-term repopulation. Interestingly, several other clinical trials in which MSCs were coinfused with allogenic BM also demonstrated that, despite successful donor HSC engraftment, donor MSCs cannot be recovered from the marrow compartment posttransplant. This observation suggests that allogeneic MSCs do not meaningfully engraft into the host BM, but rather likely support the newly engrafted donor HSCs through the transient expression of hematopoietic cytokines and immune modulation.

SAFETY PROFILE OF ADOPTIVELY TRANSFERRED MESENCHYMAL STROMAL CELLS

Numerous studies on a variety of conditions have thus far documented safety following infusion of MSCs, and a recent metaanalysis of 36 studies (including 11 SCT studies) demonstrated no association with acute infusion toxicity, organ toxicity, malignancy, infection, or death, with a significant association only seen with transient fever.[25] The genomic stability of cultured adult stem cells and MSCs in particular is robust and not as significant a source of concern.[26] Based upon the immunosuppressive properties of MSCs, downstream effects on malignant cells and infections have been of particular concern in SCT patients. The study by Ning et al[22] is the only published study reporting an increase in relapse rates following MSC infusion, although the study did not report statistical analyses and did not preserve the randomization. The inverse relationship found between GVHD and relapse in this study, however, does fit with numerous other studies documenting the same effect (likely due to decreased GVL) and warrants continued long-term monitoring in patients receiving MSCs in the malignant setting. Increased rates of infectious complications have been reported in several small nonrandomized trials, but as previously stated no association was found in a recent meta-analysis.[25] Cytomegalovirus (CMV) viral loads and the rate of CMV disease were higher than expected in 31 patients receiving MSCs as treatment for GVHD or hemorrhagic cystitis. All cases of CMV disease, however, occurred in a GVHD-affected organ and most were described as mild.[27] Furthermore, this study was single arm without even a historical comparison group reported, so it is difficult to ascribe a causative effect. A cohort of pediatric patients receiving MSCs as treatment for steroid-refractory GVHD had comparable rates of CMV, Epstein-Barr virus, and adenovirus when compared to historical controls, although adenoviral infection resulted in decreased survival, particularly when it occurred following MSC infusion.

While an effect on adenovirus-specific T cells was found in vitro, no in vivo effect was found, and the authors note significantly higher rates of HLA-mismatched grafts in the MSC group. A retrospective analysis of 1021 patients transplanted at the Karolinska University Hospital found MSC infusion to be a significant predictor of post-transplant lymphoproliferative disease on multivariate analysis, a finding that has not been previously reported. As none of these studies were randomized trials, they serve as further reminders that long-term monitoring in patients receiving MSCs is necessary, particularly in future randomized trials.

REGULATORY OVERSIGHT OF MESENCHYMAL STROMAL CELLS DEVELOPMENT AND MARKETING APPROVAL

The clinical evidence-based development of HSC transplantation as a therapeutic modality has historically been performed as "practice of medicine", akin to organ transplantation and transfusion medicine. In this particular setting, the cellular product is considered minimally manipulated and is therefore recognized as a 361 product by the US Food and Drug Administration (FDA). In contrast, any cellular product that requires some adulteration, nonhomologous use, or more-than-minimal manipulation is considered a 351 product and regulated by the FDA as a drug.[28] In order to evaluate these products on humans in the United States, the academic investigator or company will need to develop a manufacturing process and controls that meet the requirements of the FDA. The FDA's requirements for manufacturing investigational cell therapy products include adherence to the following regulations: 21 CFR 210/211 Current Good Manufacturing Practice (cGMP), 21 CFR 600 and 610 Biological Products General and Biological Products Standards, and 21 CFR 1271 Human Cells, Tissues, and Cellular and Tissue-Based Products (HCT/Ps). These regulations require the establishment of systems for the design, monitoring, and controls of the manufacturing process and facility. For an academic researcher or a startup company, establishing systems and facilities that are compliant with these regulations requires a considerable amount of resources and time. Consequently, manufacturing stands as a major hurdle to overcome for the clinical translation of cell therapy technologies—particularly for individuals, companies, or academic health centers with limited resources. MSC-like cells that have undergone ex vivo culture expansion fall under this regulatory oversight, and an FDA Center for Biologics Evaluation and Research (CBER) Investigational New Drug (IND) application is mandatorily required to engage in human clinical trials.[29] Clinical trials demonstrating an impact on clinical outcomes are required to eventually secure FDA marketing approval and Biologics License Application (BLA) for reimbursement and deployment. Herein lies a substantive distinction in traditional evidence-based clinical science and the pathway to widespread adoption of progress in clinical centers and the regulatory requirements imposed upon more-than-minimal manipulated cell products for the same end. Whereas any accredited clinical center can readily adopt practice of medicine cell therapy technologies without licensing requirements, the same is not true for adoption of more-than-minimally manipulated (e.g., 351) cell therapies. This regulation of cells as drugs favors a development model driven by industry where mass-produced universal product amenable to batch manufacture and release testing is compatible with a sustainable business model consistent with drug cell manufacture and deployment. In contrast, personalized cell medicine, as exemplified by autologous PBSC transplantation, is typically provided as a medical service within accredited medical centers. Providing such services within medical centers with the additional encumbrance of BLA requirement is a challenge for which no clear pathway has been defined. Although industrial models based on manufacture of personalized cell therapies have been feasible, the business sustainability of such has been a challenge, as exemplified by the bankruptcy of Dendreon Corporation (WA, USA), which obtained the first ever FDA marketing approval for an industrial manufactured autologous cell-based vaccine pharmaceutical. The added requirements for regulatory science and innovative reimbursement models in traditional medical center service-based care delivery will likely have a substantial impact on deployment of MSC-based technologies. See box titled "Cryobiology and Fitness of Thawed MSC Cellular Pharmaceuticals."

FUTURE DIRECTIONS

The number of clinical trials examining the use of MSCs for treatment of acute, steroid-resistant GVHD and other immune ailments is growing exponentially. Subtle differences in donor source, culture methods, and expansion levels make head-to-head comparisons of the different MSC products challenging when interrogating their utility. The European experience in exploiting random donor MSCs to treat GVHD is wide in its breadth and robustness. Although solely phase II studies, as an aggregate their cumulative experience and the very meaningful differences in MSC cell preparation when compared to their industrial counterpart, in particular the use of early passage cells, point toward key remedies that may be buttressed by mechanistic interrogation. Virtually all human clinical trials carried out to date involve the use of culture-expanded MSCs maintained in their default setting. Preclinical animal data strongly support the notion that the use of augmented MSCs prior to infusion, either by the use of cytokine activation, genetic engineering, or reprogramming robustly, enhances their pharmaceutical potency.[30] Therein lies the path for MSC v2.0. In closing, understanding this mechanism and how it relates to clinical utility remains the only rational path to the successful development of MSCs to their full clinical potential.

Considerations in Development of MSC-like Cells as a Cellular Pharmaceutical for GVHD.

The use of allogeneic mesenchymal stromal cells (MSCs) for the treatment of steroid-resistant graft-versus-host disease (GVHD) builds upon encouraging phase II clinical trial data published by European academic collaborative groups in the past few years. However, a large multicenter phase III clinical trial (NCT00366145) conducted in the USA examining the use of an industrial marrow-derived MSC product (Prochymal) reported in 2009 that it failed to meet its primary clinical endpoint of achieving a significant increase of complete response of steroid-resistant GVHD lasting at least 28 days. This pivotal phase III study does not support the use of Prochymal in this clinical indication and has not gained FDA marketing approval. The field of MSC cell therapy is faced with a paradox regarding the clinical utility of MSCs for GVHD, with opposite clinical outcomes when testing industrial and locally sourced MSCs. MSC cell biology informs us that there may well be meaningful distinctions between the functionality of industrial MSCs and those manufactured by academic centers. Most typically, a polyclonal pool of culture-expanded random donor MSCs is manufactured, and here lies a major difference: academic centers seldom manufacture more than 5–10 MSC doses from a single volunteer donor, whereas up to 10,000 doses are manufactured per donor for Prochymal lots. From a cell biology perspective, genetic reprogramming will inexorably occur when progenitor cells are continuously culture expanded to achieve large lots of qualified pharmaceutical. Although MSC cultures are polyclonal at onset, expansion pressure leads to clonal impoverishment with time. Culture-expanded human MSCs have been shown to undergo telomere shortening and other alterations of phenotype, which may play a role in modifying their regenerative and immunosuppressive properties or triggering an immune response, limiting their survival and function in vivo. Among these acquired alterations is the gradual entry into senescence of MSCs as they approach replicative exhaustion. Although senescent MSCs have a virtually indistinguishable marker phenotype from nonsenescent MSCs, their functional properties, immune in particular, may be significantly altered. Clinical data from the Karolinska Institute suggest that late-passage MSCs are less effective than comparable early-passage MSCs with regard to survival outcomes in GVHD patients. The MSC manufacture protocols utilized by academic collaborative groups would predictably minimize meaningful epigenetic reprogramming of MSCs when compared to industrialized expansion scale, and therein lies a plausible shortcoming to industrial-scale culture expansion of MSCs and their effectiveness in human trials.

Cryobiology and Fitness of Thawed MSC Cellular Pharmaceuticals

Mesenchymal stromal cells (MSCs) from either a marrow or adipose source, autologous, or of random donor origin are being investigated in a large number of clinical trials as a cellular pharmaceutical for treatment of immune disorders such as Crohn disease, systemic lupus erythematous, multiple sclerosis, graft-versus-host disease, and others. Most typically, a polyclonal pool of ex vivo culture-expanded cells is cryopreserved and banked for later use. Human subjects subsequently receive an intravenous transfusion of thawed MSCs that were retrieved directly from cryostorage no more than a few hours beforehand. It is assumed that viable, immediate post-thaw MSCs deploy the same bio-chemical, homing, and immunomodulatory features as their pre-freeze counterparts. This assumption may be erroneous and may provide, in part, an explanation for the discrepancy between preclinical animal models of MSC effectiveness and negative outcomes of prospective randomized clinical trials. In contrast to what is done in human trials, virtually all published preclinical work in mice reports the effect of live, metabolically fit MSCs. It has been shown that MSCs deploy a heat shock response immediately post-thaw, as well as trigger an instant blood-mediated inflammatory reaction (IBMIR). These acquired MSC pysiologic anomalies are associated with a profound alteration of their in vivo distribution and fate post-intravenous transfusion, markedly blunts their ability to exert immunomodulatory effects, and renders them susceptible to complement-mediated lysis. This fundamental discrepancy in the handling of MSCs at time of adoptive transfer to animal models and human subjects provides an explanation for the apparent paradox of MSC utility for mice but not in men. A funda-mental truism applicable to most cell-based therapies may be that metabolically fit, undamaged cells are distinct than a thawed product as a cellular pharmaceutical.

MSC Phenotype: Does Form Predict Function?

Mesenchymal stromal cells (MSCs) are a cellular product that is ex vivo culture expanded using established, clinically applicable methods. According to the International Society of Cell Therapy guidelines, MSCs must be plastic adherent when maintained in standard culture condi-tions, express major histocompatibility complex class I molecules as well as surface CD105, CD90, CD73, and CD44; lack expression of hematopoietic markers CD45, CD34, CD11b, and CD19; and retain the ability to differentiate to osteoblasts, adipocytes, and chondroblasts in vitro (Table 99.1). Although useful in confirming identity, these markers have virtually no utility in predicting function or immunosuppressive potency. Indeed, these markers are remarkably uniform in their expres-sion among different individual donors, and the assumption is that marrow MSCs are equipotent independent of donor fitness, age, or biology. This assumption may be flawed, especially when interrogating the immune plasticity of MSCs derived from otherwise indistinguish-able donor source. It is now well established that cytokine licensing of human MSCs with interferon-γ (IFN-γ) markedly potentiates their immunosuppressive properties in vitro, and murine data support the theory that in vivo IFN-γ responsiveness is mandatory for their suppres-sion function. Utilizing IFN-γ-induced IDO upregulation as a surrogate marker of suppressor function, it has been shown that there are substantial differences in the magnitude of IDO responsiveness arising from IFN-γ activation of otherwise indistinguishable MSC preparations from normal human donors and that the magnitude of IDO response among individual donors correlates with MSC veto function. This observation strongly suggests that IFN-γ responsiveness is not uniform among human subjects and that MSCs derived from low IDO inducers may be substantially less potent than cells derived from high inducers. Clinical studies exploiting mass-produced MSCs on an industrial scale where thousands of doses derived from a few donors are used to treat a multiplicity of subjects, which may lead to an unfavorable potency bias. For example, if many patients receive MSCs derived from a normal volunteer who happens to be a low IFN-γ responder, the outcome may be not as good as if patients had received cells from a high IFN-γ responder donor. Mechanistically-defined MSC potency profiling may provide scientific rationale for selection of volunteer donors whose MSC deploys the greatest veto function and avoid the pitfalls of less potent MSC products in subjects participating in pivotal clinical trials.

REFERENCES

1. Friedenstein AJ, Chailakhyan RK, Latsinik NV, et al: Stromal cells responsible for transferring the microenvironment of the hemopoietic tissues. Cloning in vitro and retransplantation in vivo. *Transplantation* 17:331, 1974. PMID 4150881. 414.
2. Caplan AI: Mesenchymal stem cells. *J Orthop Res* 9:641–650, 1991. PMID 1870029. 412.
3. Prockop DJ: Marrow stromal cells as stem cells for nonhematopoietic tissues. *Science* 276:71–74, 1997. PMID 9082988. 415.
4. Horwitz EM, Prockop DJ, Fitzpatrick LA, et al: Transplantability and therapeutic effects of bone marrow-derived mesenchymal cells in chil-dren with osteogenesis imperfecta. *Nat Med* 5:309–313, 1999. PMID 10086387. 423.
5. Horwitz EM, Gordon PL, Koo WK, et al: Isolated allogeneic bone marrow-derived mesenchymal cells engraft and stimulate growth in children with osteogenesis imperfecta: Implications for cell therapy of bone. *Proc Natl Acad Sci USA* 99:8932–8937, 2002. PMID 12084934. 424124401.
6. Lazarus HM, Haynesworth SE, Gerson SL, et al: Ex vivo expansion and subsequent infusion of human bone marrow-derived stromal progenitor cells (mesenchymal progenitor cells): implications for thera-peutic use. *Bone Marrow Transplant* 16:557–564, 1995. PMID 8528172. 410.
7. Le Blanc K, Rasmusson I, Sundberg B, et al: Treatment of severe acute graft-versus-host disease with third party haploidentical mesenchymal stem cells. *Lancet* 363:1439–1441, 2004. PMID 15121408. 134.
8. Baron F, Storb R: Mesenchymal stromal cells: a new tool against graft-versus-host disease? *Biol Blood Marrow Transplant* 18:822–840, 2012. PMID 21963621. 4293310956.
9. Galipeau J: The mesenchymal stromal cells dilemma–does a negative phase III trial of random donor mesenchymal stromal cells in steroid-resistant graft-versus-host disease represent a death knell or a bump in the road? *Cytotherapy* 15:2–8, 2013. PMID 23260081. 220.
10. Kfoury Y, Scadden DT: Mesenchymal cell contributions to the stem cell niche. *Cell Stem Cell* 16:239–253, 2015. PMID 25748931. 437.
11. Bianco P, Cao X, Frenette PS, et al: The meaning, the sense and the significance: translating the science of mesenchymal stem cells into medicine. *Nat Med* 19:35–42, 2013. PMID 23296015. 4313998103.
12. Dominici M, Le Blanc K, Mueller I, et al: Minimal criteria for defining multipotent mesenchymal stromal cells. The International Society for Cellular Therapy position statement. *Cytotherapy* 8:315–317, 2006. PMID 16923606. 150.
13. Krampera M, Galipeau J, Shi Y, et al: Immunological characterization of multipotent mesenchymal stromal cells–The International Society for Cellular Therapy (ISCT) working proposal. *Cytotherapy* 15:1054–1061, 2013. PMID 23602578. 250.
14. Bourin P, Bunnell BA, Casteilla L, et al: Stromal cells from the adipose tissue-derived stromal vascular fraction and culture expanded adipose tissue-derived stromal/stem cells: a joint statement of the International Federation for Adipose Therapeutics and Science (IFATS) and the Inter-national Society for Cellular Therapy (ISCT). *Cytotherapy* 15:641–648, 2013. PMID 23570660. 4273979435.
15. Bernardo ME, Fibbe WE: Mesenchymal stromal cells: sensors and switchers of inflammation. *Cell Stem Cell* 13:392–402, 2013. PMID 24094322. 242.
16. Le Blanc K, Mougiakakos D: Multipotent mesenchymal stromal cells and the innate immune system. *Nat Rev Immunol* 12:383–396, 2012. PMID 22531326. 128.
17. Ren G, Zhang L, Zhao X, et al: Mesenchymal stem cell-mediated immunosuppression occurs via concerted action of chemokines and nitric oxide. *Cell Stem Cell* 2:141–150, 2008. PMID 18371435. 153.
18. Nemeth K, Leelahavanichkul A, Yuen PS, et al: Bone marrow stromal cells attenuate sepsis via prostaglandin E(2)-dependent reprogramming of host macrophages to increase their interleukin-10 production. *Nat Med* 15:42–49, 2009. PMID 19098906. 4352706487.
19. Ren G, Su J, Zhang L, et al: Species variation in the mechanisms of mesenchymal stem cell-mediated immunosuppression. *Stem Cells* 27:1954–1962, 2009. PMID 19544427. 152.

20. Ankrum JA, Ong JF, Karp JM: Mesenchymal stem cells: immune evasive, not immune privileged. *Nat Biotechnol* 32:252–260, 2014. PMID 24561556. 4284320647.

21. Trounson A, McDonald C: Stem Cell Therapies in Clinical Trials: Progress and Challenges. *Cell Stem Cell* 17:11–22, 2015. PMID 26140604. 438.

22. Ning H, Yang F, Jiang M, et al: The correlation between co-transplantation of mesenchymal stem cells and higher recurrence rate in hematologic malignancy patients: outcome of a pilot clinical study. *Leukemia* 22:593–599, 2008. PMID 18185520. 433.

23. Nauta AJ, Westerhuis G, Kruisselbrink AB, et al: Donor-derived mesenchymal stem cells are immunogenic in an allogeneic host and stimulate donor graft rejection in a nonmyeloablative setting. *Blood* 108:2114–2120, 2006. PMID 16690970. 1431895546.

24. de Lima M, McNiece I, Robinson SN, et al: Cord-blood engraftment with ex vivo mesenchymal-cell coculture. *N Engl J Med* 367:2305–2315, 2012. PMID 23234514. 205.

25. Lalu MM, McIntyre L, Pugliese C, et al: Safety of cell therapy with mesenchymal stromal cells (SafeCell): a systematic review and meta-analysis of clinical trials. *PLoS ONE* 7:e47559, 2012. PMID 23133515. 4063485008.

26. Sensebe L, Tarte K, Galipeau J, et al: Limited acquisition of chromosomal aberrations in human adult mesenchymal stromal cells. *Cell Stem Cell* 10:9–10, author reply -1, 2012. PMID 22226349. 8.

27. von Bahr L, Sundberg B, Lonnies L, et al: Long-term complications, immunologic effects, and role of passage for outcome in mesenchymal stromal cell therapy. *Biol Blood Marrow Transplant* 18:557–564, 2012. PMID 21820393. 130.

28. Sipp D, Turner L: Stem cells. U.S. regulation of stem cells as medical products. *Science* 338:1296–1297, 2012. PMID 23224541. 436.

29. Mendicino M, Bailey AM, Wonnacott K, et al: MSC-based product characterization for clinical trials: an FDA perspective. *Cell Stem Cell* 14:141–145, 2014. PMID 24506881. 439.

30. Dimmeler S, Ding S, Rando TA, et al: Translational strategies and challenges in regenerative medicine. *Nat Med* 20:814–821, 2014. PMID 25100527. 434.

CHAPTER 100

T-CELL THERAPY OF HEMATOLOGIC DISEASES

Gianpietro Dotti and Malcolm K. Brenner

INTRODUCTION

Conventional modalities for treating cancer remain unsatisfactory. Despite the introduction of small molecules that target specific molecular lesions or pathways within the cancer cells, cure rates for many common tumors remain low, while adverse events are still distressingly high. Cancer immunotherapy represents a promising extension of highly targeted cancer therapy with a favorable toxicity profile and excellent pharmacoeconomics. Until recently, most attention has been on the development of conventional monoclonal antibodies that target specific tumor-expressed antigens. Over the past few years, the focus of monoclonal antibody therapy has shifted to agents that recruit innate or adaptive immune responses against the tumor, either by blocking immune regulation by tumors or by simultaneously engaging tumor cells and effector lymphocytes (bispecific antibodies).[1,2] More recently, however, strikingly beneficial results with direct (adoptive) transfer of immune system cells are now being reported.[3] Although to date, these have primarily been obtained in patients with leukemia, lymphoma, melanoma, or neuroblastoma, methodologies are being developed to allow us to extend the tumor range.

Many human tumors express tumor-specific antigens (TSAs) or tumor-associated antigens (TAAs) that can be recognized by the host immune system and induce antitumor cell-mediated and humoral immune responses. Although these responses may be transient and are not always associated with clinical responses, they provide evidence for the existence of tumor-directed immunity in humans that may also have antitumor activity. Several barriers block the development of more effective antitumor immunity in people with cancer. First, many human tumors express few major histocompatibility complex (MHC) molecules or have poor processing of their potential tumor antigens. Even when TAA/TSA are processed and presented, most tumors lack the costimulatory molecules necessary to implement a long-lived and effective immune response. In addition to these passive defenses against immunity, many tumors can "edit" the immune system to their advantage, secreting cytokines such as TGFβ or by expressing molecules such as programmed death-ligand 1 (PD-L1) that act as inhibitory or check point signals to cytotoxic effector T-cell growth, function and survival, or that favor expansion of Th2/regulatory T cells rather than effector T cells. Finally, intensive chemotherapy and radiotherapy can themselves severely reduce immune function by destroying antigen presenting cells and dividing T lymphocytes.

As our understanding of the molecular basis of tumor immune escape has increased, it has been possible to derive countermeasures that may allow us to induce more potent antitumor immune responses, and that will soon allow us to extend effective therapies to a broad range of common tumors.

TYPES OF CELLULAR IMMUNOTHERAPY

Cellular immunotherapy may be *active,* using cell-based vaccines derived from tumor cells themselves or antigen-presenting cells expressing TAA/TSA from proteins or peptides, or *passive,* by direct adoptive transfer of viable immune cells. The former approach relies on the intact afferent and efferent immune system of the host responding to the stimulus with an effective antitumor response, while the latter is the cellular equivalent of antibody serotherapy, in which the transferred immune cells are expected to attack the tumor cells directly, albeit with a phase of in vivo expansion, and to subsequently establish a pool of memory cells to provide long-term protection against resurgent disease. Several cell subsets are currently being studied in adoptive transfer protocols, including activated T lymphocytes (ATL), tumor infiltrating T lymphocytes, antigen-specific cytotoxic T lymphocytes (CTL), natural killer (NK) cells, γδ T cells and natural killer T (NKT) cells. In this chapter, we discuss adoptive transfer of ATL and CTL.

Adoptive Cell Therapy With T Lymphocytes

In principle, lymphocytes have the ability to traffic through multiple tissue planes and to be self-renewing. These assets, coupled with their ability to destroy tumor or viral infected target cells through a range of mechanisms makes them an appealing resource for adoptive transfer, and a multiplicity of clinical studies using this approach have now been described. Adoptive lymphocyte therapies may use allogeneic or autologous cells, which may be of tightly defined specificity (e.g., T-cell clones) or broad phenotype and activity (e.g., tumor infiltrating lymphocytes). As we have learned more about the molecular basis of immune recognition and immune regulation, it has become possible to genetically modify the infused lymphocytes to alter their specificity or behavior. In this section, we describe examples of each type of T-cell adoptive transfer and discuss the relative merits and limitations of each.

Donor Lymphocyte Infusion

It has long been apparent that the curative effects of allogeneic hematopoietic stem cell transplants (HSCT) for many hematologic malignancies can be attributed to a graft-versus-leukemia (GVL) effect largely mediated by the incoming T cells within the donor graft. Thus, patients with chronic graft-versus-host disease (GVHD) were well recognized as having a lower probability of relapse than individuals without this unpleasant complication. Similarly, recipients of syngeneic grafts have the lowest rate of GVHD and the highest risk of relapse. In 1990, Kolb and colleagues took advantage of this observation and deliberately infused donor lymphocytes in an attempt to eliminate recurrent disease in patients with chronic myeloid leukemia (CML). Their positive results have been confirmed in multiple studies worldwide, and remission can be induced in more than 50% of CML patients who relapse after transplantation by stopping immunosuppressive treatment or infusing donor lymphocytes. Unfortunately, donor lymphocyte infusion (DLI) is much less effective at treating other types of relapsed leukemias after transplantation, with a 29% remission rate for acute myeloid leukemia and only 5% for acute lymphoblastic leukemia (ALL). It is not clear why these differences occur, since all these leukemias present the minor histocompatibility antigens (mHags) that are likely the targets of this GVL effect, although many mHags have yet to be defined. DLI therapy may also produce severe adverse effects, since the frequency of broadly alloreactive effector cells is usually much higher than the frequency of lymphocytes targeted exclusively to the relapsed malignancy. As a consequence, patients receiving DLI often develop GVHD. This complication of DLI usually increases in frequency and severity if donor and recipient are unrelated or human leukocyte antigen (HLA) haploidentical. Strategies aimed at retaining the benefits of GVL whilst preventing GVHD have included the depletion of alloreactive T cells in the donor lymphocyte product and the incorporation of suicide genes into the infused donor T cells so that they may be killed if the GVHD activity exceeds the benefits from GVL.[4,5] Recently, the manipulation of the stem cell graft to deplete only the αβ T-cell receptor (TCR)+ T lymphocytes whilst retaining the γδTCR+ T-cell compartment may reduce GVHD without compromising stem cell engraftment and retain some protection against opportunistic infections.[6] Ultimately, investigators may wish to identify tumor-restricted target antigens on the malignant cells and infuse antigen specific T cells directed to them. It has proved feasible to prepare donor-derived T lymphocytes specific for mHags and to show both the feasibility and potential efficacy of the approach, although scalability remains challenging.[7]

Infusion of Activated T Lymphocytes

When T cells are polyclonally stimulated, for example by simultaneously cross-linking their CD3 and CD28 receptors by CD3/CD28 monoclonal antibodies on beads, then the cells proliferate. They also secrete tumoricidal cytokines such as TNFα and can mediate MHC-unrestricted cytotoxicity towards a range of tumor target cells. Efforts have been made to harness these effects by producing large numbers of CD3/CD28-activated T cells for cancer patients and infusing them. Although infusion of CD3/CD28-ATL after autologous stem cell transplant may improve patients T-cell reconstitution, as yet there is no evidence to suggest improved antitumor activity.[8] ATL that are additionally primed with interferon gamma (IFN-γ) and interleukin (IL)-2 (so called cytokine-induced killer cells or CIK) may have superior clinical potential for hematologic malignancies and early phase clinical trials may be showing clinical benefits.[9]

Adoptive Immunotherapy With Virus-Specific Cytotoxic T Lymphocytes

Viral infections are one of the most common causes of morbidity and mortality after allogeneic HSCT, and are more prevalent as the degree of antigen mismatching between donor and recipient is increased. Cord blood transplantation in particular, is associated with often-intractable virus infections that are becoming recognized as a major limitation of the approach. The most common problematic viral infections after allogeneic HSCT are reactivated herpes viruses, including cytomegalovirus (CMV) which typically causes pneumonitis and hepatitis and the gamma herpes virus Epstein-Barr Virus (EBV), which may cause a rapidly fatal lymphoproliferative disease (LPD). In children and recipients of cord blood transplants, adenoviral disease is also common. Adoptive transfer of virus-specific T cells (VSTs) appears to effectively prevent and treat these infections after transplant. Infusion of even small numbers of specific cells (10^6 or less) may be sufficient for benefit, since the lymphodepletion of the immediate posttransplant period is associated with the release of homeostatic cytokines such as IL-7 and IL-15 which augment the expansion of virus specific T cells when they encounter their antigen.

The feasibility of adoptive transfer of VSTs after HSCT has greatly increased over the past decade because of the simplification of the procedures required to isolate or expand these cells ex vivo. The pioneering approach developed at Fred Hutchinson Cancer Research Center and St. Jude Children's Research Hospital aimed at generating ex vivo CMV-specific CD8+ T-cell clones and polyclonal EBV-VSTs were effective in controlling CMV and EBV-reactivation after allogeneic HSCT, respectively. However, the broad application of these therapeutic approaches was significantly limited by the laborious process required to generate VSTs with sufficient specificity and in sufficient number for adoptive transfer. The recent introduction of long-peptide libraries (pepmixes) as a source of viral antigens, allowed

significant reduction of the time necessary for the generation of clinical grade VSTs (<10 days), without compromising their specificity or increasing the risk of GVHD.[10] Another important change has been the creation of banks in which VSTs from donors with common HLA polymorphisms can be manufactured in advance and stored for immediate administration to partially HLA matched transplant recipients with active virus infections. Crawford and colleagues previously demonstrated that such a "third party" bank of polyclonal EBV-VSTs could be safely infused based on the best available HLA match and had a high success rate in patients who developed EBV-lymphoproliferation after solid organ transplantation (SOT). In a phase-II multicenter trial, 33 patients with EBV-LPD had an overall response rate of 64% at 5 weeks and 52% at 6 months. These impressive results in SOT recipients led us to develop a similar multicenter study to evaluate whether "best matched" VSTs may have similar activity against EBV, CMV, and adenovirus after allogeneic HSCT. We observed a circa 75% response rate to all three viruses, comparable to the reported response rates obtained by infusing VSTs generated from the stem cell donor.[11] This approach may be suited for further scale up and broader application. An alternative approach is to eliminate ex vivo expansion of VSTs by selecting such cells directly from leukapheresis products. This can be accomplished by using HLA-multimers to bind the relevant cells, or by overnight exposure to viral peptides to stimulate γ-IFN production followed by bead selection of γ-IFN+ cells. These selected VSTs are then infused into the recipients without any ex vivo expansion, and their use is being explored for the prevention and treatment of CMV and other viral infections after HSCT.

Adoptive Immunotherapy of Virus-Associated Malignancies

The encouraging results of adoptive immunotherapy with EBV-VSTs in the immunocompromised host led us to extend this strategy to other EBV-associated tumors (lymphoma and nasopharyngeal cancer) that develop in the immunocompetent patient. Unlike EBV-LPD, which expresses the highly immunogenic viral latency antigens EBNA1, EBNA2, and EBNA3, these other EBV tumors express a limited number of poorly processed (EBNA1) or weakly stimulatory (latent membrane protein [LMP]1 and LMP2) EBV-derived antigens. We have therefore used VSTs specific for these EBV antigens, beginning with the cells directed to LMP2. Initially, the VSTs were generated from patients with Hodgkin lymphoma or non-Hodgkin lymphoma by using dendritic cells that are engineered to overexpress LMP2. The infusion of polyclonal LMP2-specific T cells containing both CD4+ and CD8+ T cells increased LMP2-specific T-cell responses, and lead to sustained complete tumor regression in 56% of patients with relapsed/resistant EBV+ lymphoma.[12] Complete responses have also been obtained in EBV-associated nasopharyngeal carcinoma (NPC), a tumor which originates from the epithelial cells of the nasopharynx, and a promising increase in overall survival has been obtained in phase II studies. Like EBV-associated lymphomas, NPC express the same restricted set of weakly immunogenic viral antigens including EBNA1, LMP1, and LMP2. As for the VSTs infused after allogeneic HSCT, simplification of manufacture has been accomplished by using peptide libraries as a source of viral antigens. VSTs so generated retain their specificity and may have increased longevity in vivo based on their less differentiated phenotype. The development of this simplified therapeutic strategy has allowed the implementation of larger scale commercialization.

Infection with human papilloma virus (HPV; particularly serotypes 16 and 18) has been associated with orogenital epithelial cancers. T lymphocytes directed to the persisting viral antigens (such as E5 and E6) may be effective treatment for these tumors, and a recent study using T cells genetically manipulated to express an anti-HPV E6 TCR induced sustained tumor regression in two patients with advanced metastatic cervical cancer (Hinrichs et al, unpublished data). A number of groups are now exploring the value of the approach.

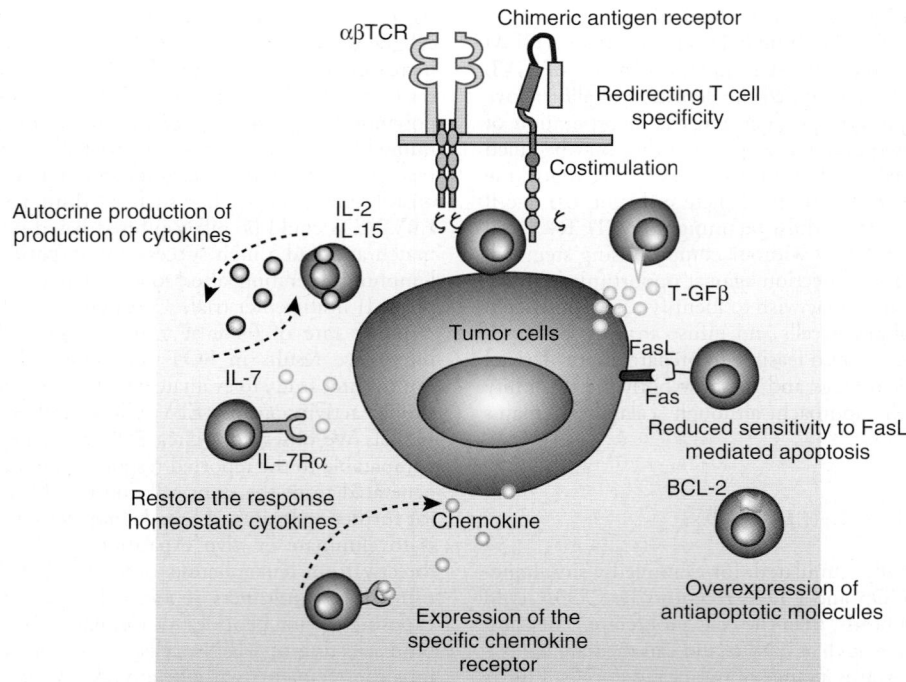

Fig. 100.1 GENETIC MODIFICATIONS OF T LYMPHOCYTES FOR ADOPTIVE T-CELL THERAPY. *TCR,* T-cell receptor.

Adoptive Immunotherapy of Virus Independent Malignancies

The majority of human malignancies are not evidently associated with viral infection and thus alternative antigens must be targeted by T cells to achieve antitumor responses. Many different types of tumor-associated or TSAs have been described and several attempts have been implemented to target these antigens, either by stimulating T cells in vivo through vaccination with the antigens, or ex vivo through isolation of specific CTLs. Unfortunately, multiple, physiologic and pathologic factors significantly limit the success of these approaches. Physiologically, the great majority of T cells with high affinity for self-antigens have been deleted during T-cell development. Thus, in cancer patients, T cells specific for self-antigens that can potentially recognize tumor cells have suboptimal affinity for the target antigen and are also frequently functionally anergic because of the highly immunosuppressive tumor environment (Fig. 100.1). Indeed, recent evidence suggests that effective antitumor responses in patients infused with ex vivo expanded tumor infiltrating lymphocytes are preferentially directed against neoantigens from mutated genes in tumor cells rather than to the unmutated self-antigens, even if these are more highly expressed on the tumor cells than by normal tissues.[13] The importance of such neoantigens is supported by recent clinical studies using monoclonal antibodies to molecules such as PD-1, PD-L1, or cytotoxic T lymphocyte antigen 4 (CTLA-4), which block T-cell inhibitory pathways. In these studies, clinical responses are preferentially observed in patients affected by highly mutated tumors.[14] For all these reasons, the production of effector T cells with the ability to target solid tumors effectively, while resisting their immune evasion strategies will likely require extensive engineering of the effector cells, by genetic modification or other means.

GENETIC MODIFICATION OF T CELLS

Early clinical studies using genetic modification only attempted to "mark" the T-cell infused to follow their fate in the peripheral blood or other tissues. More recently, efforts have been devoted to "redirecting" the antigen-specificity of T lymphocytes and thus providing them with robust antitumor activity. To overcome the low affinity of tumor-specific CTLs detected in vivo, investigators have cloned T-cell receptor α and β chains (αβTCR) of high affinity.[15] Alternatively, tumor-specificity has been generated by the construction of chimeric antigen receptors (CARs)[16] which are most commonly composed of the binding domains of a monoclonal antibody and the ξ signaling domain of the CD3αβ TCR as well as components of costimulatory molecules to ensure signaling and T-cell activation once the CAR has been engaged (see Fig. 100.1). Finally, interest in genetic modification of T cells has also arisen as a means of incorporating countermeasures to the multiplicity of immune evasion strategies used by potentially immunogenic tumor cells or to enhance the "survival' of T cells in vivo (see Fig. 100.1). Because T lymphocytes can be long-lived cells and may proliferate extensively in vivo, most gene transfer studies have used integrating vectors such as gamma-retroviral vectors, lentiviral vectors or transposon/ transposase integrating plasmids to ensure long-term expression of the therapeutic transgene.[16]

Artificial αβT-Cell Receptors

The large-scale culture of T lymphocytes to enrich the scanty precursors specific for weak TAAs is often unsuccessful and always tedious. This process can be bypassed by introducing additional T-cell receptor genes with predetermined specificity and high affinity for the weak tumor antigen into a polyclonal population of T cells. Technical improvements in retroviral transduction mean that >30% of polyclonal T lymphocytes can now be induced to express a transgenic TCR with high affinity for TAAs including MART-1, melanoma antigen (MAGE)-3, MDM2, WT1, NY-ISO, survivin, and for mHags such as HA1 and infectious agents such as human immunodeficiency virus (HIV)-1 and EBV.[17,18]

Polyclonal T cells expressing transgenic MART-1 specific αβTCRs have been infused in patients with metastatic melanoma after lymphodepleting chemoradiotherapy.[15] Up to 30% of these patients had objective regression of metastatic disease. Similar results have been obtained in patients with metastatic synovial cell sarcomas and melanoma who were given T cells expressing an NY-ESO-1 specific αβTCR.[17] Although most of these patients had no severe adverse events, toxicity was observed in normal tissues containing melanocytes such as skin and uvea in melanoma patients infused with MART-1 T cells.[15] Colitis was also reported in patients with metastatic colon carcinoma who received T cells expressing a TCR directed to the carcinoembryonic antigen that is also expressed at low level in normal epithelia cells of the gut.[19] Thus T cells with high-affinity transgenic TCR may produce "on target" but "off organ" toxicities to normal tissues that physiologically express the target antigen at low level. The first TCR gene therapy trial for patients with acute leukemia targeting WT1 is currently recruiting patients.

The major problem of TCR gene transfer in polyclonal T lymphocytes harboring their own native αβTCR was hypothesized to be the "cross-pairing" between transgenic α or β receptor chains and the reciprocal endogenous TCR α- and β-chains, that could create loss of function or—and potentially worse—gain of function receptors that may produce autoimmune disease, an adverse effect clearly demonstrable in mouse models.[20] These events have not been reported in clinical trials so far, but unfortunately other unexpected toxicities have been observed. Patients with myeloma or melanoma were given T cells modified to express a TCR specific for MAGE-A3 that had been synthetically affinity-enhanced. Two of the recipients rapidly developed lethal cardiotoxicity caused by an unanticipated cross-reactivity of the transgenic TCR against peptide epitopes derived from Titin, which were expressed only by cardiac myocytes.[21] In a second study, the infusion of T cells expressing a transgenic high affinity MAGE-A3 TCR caused lethal neurotoxicity possibly caused by the simultaneous cross-reactivity of a MAGE-A12-derived peptide expressed in human brain.[22] These results strongly indicate that T cells engineered with high-affinity TCR can be effective, but can also reveal unexpected and lethal cross-reactivity with other peptide epitopes that would not be recognized by TCR with more physiologic binding affinity.[18,21] While such unanticipated toxicities may be avoided by ever more extensive preclinical evaluation, reliance on "superaffinity" TCR may be intrinsically hazardous.

Chimeric Antigen Receptors

The cytotoxic activity of T cells through their native or transgenic TCR is MHC-restricted so that multiple distinct transgenic αβTCR would be required to recognize tumor antigens associated with the multiple MHC polymorphisms in a human population, precluding a "universal" receptor. In addition, tumor cells can downregulate MHC molecules and avoid immune recognition by conventional TCRs. In an attempt to overcome this limitation, MHC unrestricted CARs have been generated.[16] CARs are most commonly prepared by joining the light and heavy chain variable regions of a monoclonal antibody expressed as a single-chain Fv (scFv) molecule to the cytoplasmic signaling domains derived from CD3ζ cytoplasmic and intracytoplasmic endodomains derived from costimulatory molecules such as CD28, 4-1BB and OX40.[16] Thus when CARs are expressed by polyclonal T lymphocytes or VSTs, they can combine the antigen specificity of an antibody with the cytotoxic properties of T cells, together with the costimulatory signals provided by professional antigen presenting cells that allow survival and proliferation of activated T lymphocytes. Since CARs bind to target antigens in an HLA-unrestricted manner, they are resistant to many of the tumor immune evasion mechanisms, such as downregulation of HLA class I molecules or failure to process or present proteins, used by tumor cells to escape immune attack. Adoptive transfer of polyclonal activated T cells expressing a second generation CD19-specific CAR caused impressive clinical responses in patients with ALL and lymphomas with >75% complete response rates in relapsed/refractory ALL patients in several phase I clinical trials (Table 100.1). The small size and significant heterogeneity of these studies precludes definitive conclusions, but the data suggest that adoptive transfer of CAR-T cells is more effective in patients with B-ALL than in other B-cell malignancies. The effects also seem greatest when lymphopenia is

induced before infusion of the CAR-T cells. It is not yet known how the composition of the CAR affects the outcome, but patients can achieve remission regardless the type of CAR costimulation (CD28 or 4-1BB) used, although only 4-1BB costimulation appears to be associated with prolonged CAR–T-cell engraftment. Because the CD19 target molecule is also expressed by normal B cells, the eradication of B-cell leukemia is also associated with B-cell aplasia, which was sustained during the period of robust CAR–T-cell engraftment. CD19-specific CAR-T cells have been successfully used in both autologous and allogeneic (after HSCT) settings.

Despite their remarkable success, administration of CD19–CAR-T cells is also associated with potentially lethal acute toxicity caused by a profound perturbation of the immune system, often termed the systemic inflammatory response syndrome, which is manifest by hyperpyrexia, hypotension, and respiratory distress with high levels of circulating proinflammatory cytokines. Although investigators can usually control this unwanted outcome, larger scale clinical studies will be essential to assess the feasibility of safely introducing the approach into more generalized clinical practice.

CAR–T-cell therapies for other hematologic malignancies such as myeloid leukemia and multiple myeloma are also in preclinical stages or in phase I clinical trials. While targeting several candidate antigens such as B-cell maturation antigen (BCMA) or CS1 could be effective in controlling the proliferation of the malignant plasma cells of multiple myeloma without causing "on target" toxicities, the selection of antigens that can selectively control myeloblasts without causing myelosuppression remains more challenging.[16] Recent clinical experience using CD33-specific CAR–T-cells in a single patient with acute myeloid leukemia suggests that the only potential clinical application of CARs targeting shared myeloid antigen is the induction of remission in preparation for hematopoietic stem cell transplantation.[26]

Optimizing T-Cell Trafficking and Overcoming Tumor Immune Evasion

The expression of transgenic TCRs or CARs in T lymphocytes confers potent cytotoxic activity and potential long-term persistence to these cells. However, other functional T-cell properties may need to be addressed to maximize their antitumor effects. Table 100.2 and Fig. 100.1 summarize some of the T-cell modifications that may optimize the antitumor activity of T lymphocytes. For example, CD19-specific CAR-T cells may be more effective for the treatment of ALL than of lymphoma in part because they more efficiently eliminate tumor cells from the circulation and bone marrow than the lymph nodes. Many lymphomas are characterized by a particular chemokine milieu to which engineered T cells can be adapted. For example, Hodgkin lymphomas may produce high levels of TARC, and T cells coexpressing a CAR specific for the Hodgkin disease–associated CD30 antigen and a transgenic chemokine receptor CCR4 have significantly enhanced traffic to the tumor and consequently better antitumor activity in animal models.[16] Even when tumor-specific T cells efficiently reach the tumor-environment, other tumor-associated factors may hamper T-cell survival and function. For example, many tumors, including hematologic malignancies, and their tumor-associated stroma produce transforming growth factor (TGF)-β, which favors the development of immune tolerance and T-cell anergy, inducing T effector cell growth arrest with induction of regulatory T cells. Transfection of a dominant negative form of TGF-β RII (dnTGF-β RII) confers resistance to the antiproliferative effects of TGF-β and improves the persistence of T cells and antitumor effects in preclinical models,[16] and such approach is currently being studied in patients with EBV-associated lymphomas.

Achievement of sustained clinical responses upon T-cell transfer is strongly dependent on in vivo T-cell expansion and persistence, which in turn requires the infused T cells to contain a population with a stemness/memory signature and the availability of cytokines that sustain T-cell replication and survival. We do not yet know the optimal means by which stem/memory T cells can be preserved before adoptive transfer.[27,28] Nonetheless it is clear that infusion of

TABLE 100.1	Clinical Trials Using CD19-Targeted CAR-Modified T Cells With Published Results							
Reference	CD19-Positive Targeted Diseases	N	T-Cell Origin	Auxiliary Therapy	Cell Dose Range ($\times 10^6$)	Persistence	Outcomes	Best Response Duration
[a]Savoldo[23]	DLBCL, transformed FL	6	Autologous	None	40–400/m^2	Up to 6 wk	2 SD, 4 NR	SD × 6 wk
[a]Kalos[23]	CLL	3	Autologous	Lymphodepletion (BEN or CTX/PTS)	0.15–16/kg	Up to 26 wk	2 CR, 1 PR	CR × 48+ wk
[a]Brentjens[23]	CLL, ALL	9	Autologous	None or lymphodepletion (CTX)	2–30/kg	Up to 6 wk	1 PR, 2 SD, 1 cCR, 4 NR, 1 death	PR × 12 wk
[a]Kochenderfer[23]	FL, CLL, SMZL	8	Autologous	Lymphodepletion (CTX/FLU) and IL-2	5–55/kg	Up to 26 wk	1 CR, 5 PR, 1 SD, 1 NE	CR × 60+ wk
[a]Brentjens[23]	ALL	5	Autologous	Lymphodepletion (CTX)	1.5–3/kg	Up to 8 wk	4 CR, 1 cCR	CR × 13 wk
[a]Cruz[23]	ALL, CLL, transformed CLL	8	Allogeneic	Allo-HSCT preparative regimen; none immediately before T-cell infusion	19–110/m^2	Up to 12 wk	1 CR, 1 PR, 1 SD, 2 cCR, 3 NR	CR × 12 wk
[a]Kochenderfer[23]	CLL, DLBCL, MCL	10	Allogeneic	Allo-HSCT preparative regimen, DLI; none immediately before T-cell infusion	1–10/kg	Up to 4 wk	1 CR, 1 PR, 6 SD, 2 NR	CR × 39+ wk
[a]Davila[23]	ALL	16	Autologous	Lymphodepletion (CTX)	0.5–3/kg	Up to 12 wk	12 CR, 2 cCR, 2 NR	CR × 13 wk
Maude[3]	ALL	30	Autologous	Lymphodepletion (Flu/CTX or others)	0.76–20/kg	Up to 6 mo	27 CR	CR × 24+ mo
Lee[24]	ALL/NHL	21	Autologous	Lymphodepletion (Flu/CTX)	1–3/kg	4 wk	14 CR	NA
Kochenderfer[25]	NHL	15	Autologous	Lymphodepletion (Flu/CTX)	1–5/kg	Up to 8 wk	8 CR	CR × 9+ mo

[a]Ref 23 refers to a review article that summarizes these clinical trials.
–, none; ALL, acute lymphoblastic leukemia; Allo-HSCT, allogeneic hematopoietic stem cell transplantation; BEN, bendamustine; cCR, continued complete response (i.e., patient had no evidence of disease before and after infusion); CLL, chronic lymphocytic leukemia; CR, complete response; CTX, cyclophosphamide; DLBCL, diffuse large B-cell lymphoma; DLI, donor lymphocyte infusion; FL, follicular lymphoma; Flu, fludarabine; NA, not applicable since patients in CR underwent allogeneic stem cell transplant; NE, not evaluable; NHL, non-Hodgkin lymphoma; NR, no response; PR, partial response; PTS, pentostatin; SD, stable disease; SMZL, splenic marginal zone lymphoma.

tumor-specific T cells in a lymphodepleted host benefits T-cell expansion, likely because the infused T cells can exploit the favorable homeostatic cytokine milieu (including production of IL-7 and IL-15) and the transient depletion of regulatory T cells. Exogenous cytokines, such as recombinant IL-2 can also be infused, but may cause significant toxicity and concomitant expansion of regulatory T cells. Recombinant IL-15 infusions were anticipated to be more effective and better tolerated than IL-2, but toxicity remains problematic.[29] Thus investigators have developed T-cell engineering strategies that make tumor-directed T cells which produce their own cytokines or express receptors for specific cytokines.[16] While these approaches are effective in preclinical models, we do not know if they can replace or augment the use of lymphodepleting agents before adoptive transfer.

The molecular pathways responsible for the regulation and contraction of the T-cell immune response (immune check-points) have become a major focus of effective immunotherapies, and as described earlier ("Adoptive Immunotherapy of Virus Independent Malignancies") monoclonal antibodies that interrupt pathways such as the CD28/CTLA-4 and the PD-1/PD-L1 axes have emerged as potent new agents for the treatment of cancer, inducing sustained clinical responses in tumors likely mediated by the functional release of suppressed tumor-specific T cells recognizing neoantigens.[14,30] Many investigators therefore believe that the adoptive transfer of tumor-specific T cells generated ex vivo will synergize with infusion of checkpoint antibodies, and this is an active area of clinical research.

T Lymphocytes and Transfer of Safety Genes

A major problem of any successful cell therapy is that adverse events produced by the infused cells may persist and worsen if the cells survive and proliferate. A classic example is the GVHD that occurs when allogeneic donor T cells are transferred with the hematopoietic graft. It is also clear, however, that even nonalloreactive T cells may cause serious and even lethal toxicities, particularly if they are genetically modified to target highly expressed self-antigens present both on tumors and normal tissues (see "Adoptive Immunotherapy of Virus Independent Malignancies" and "Chimeric Antigen Receptors" mentioned earlier).

Similarly, efforts to enhance the survival and expansion of T cells may lead to uncontrolled expansion of the manipulated T cells, an event that may even occur as a result of retroviral genotoxicity alone. While malignant transformation has so far only been observed in clinical studies of hematopoietic stem cells transduced by murine oncoretroviral vectors, there is understandable concern that it can potentially occur after the transfer of gene-modified T cells. For all these reasons, therefore, there has been increasing interest in the incorporation of safety switches or suicide genes in any T cell that is adoptively transferred to humans.

Safety or suicide genes have been best studied in the recipients of DLI in patients with hematologic malignancies relapsed after allogeneic HSC transplantation to prevent the occurrence of GVHD. Adequate doses of donor T cells can only be safely given if there is some means by which unwanted alloreactivity can be abrogated in

TABLE 100.2	Causes of Immunosuppression in Cancer Patients

Immunosuppression Induced by Tumors

Release of chemokine by tumor cells that attract immunosuppressive T lymphocytes

Antigen-specific CD4+/CD8+ T-cell tolerance

Defective proximal TCR signaling (decreased expressions of CD3δ chain, p56^{lck}, p59^{fyn} tyrosine kinases)

Impairment of antigen-processing machinery (TAP, LMP2, LMP7) or downregulation of MHC molecules and costimulatory molecules

Activation of negative costimulatory signals (CTLA-4, PD-1, B7-H4, BTLA)

Tumor-derived immunosuppressive cytokines (TGF-β, IL-10, VEGF, PGE$_2$)

Expression of immunomodulatory or proapoptotic molecules by tumor (tryptophan-depleting enzyme IDO, galectin-1, FasL, TRAIL)

Recruitment and expansion of immunosuppressive cell populations (regulatory T cells, myeloid/plasmocytoid dendritic cells)

Immunosuppression Induced by Therapy

Neutropenia, depletion and functional impairment of monocytes

Hypogammaglobulinemia (decreased levels of IgA and IgM)

Defective T cell-mediated immune response

BTLA, B- and T-lymphocyte attenuator; CTLA, cytotoxic T lymphocyte antigen; FasL, Fas-Fas ligand; Ig, immunoglobulin; IL, interleukin; LMP7, latent membrane protein 7; MHC, major histocompatibility complex; PD-1, programmed death-1; PGE2, prostaglandin E$_2$; TAP, transporter associated with antigen processing; TCR, T-cell receptor; TGF-β, transforming growth factor-β; TRAIL, tumor necrosis factor–related apoptosis-inducing ligand; VEGF, vascular endothelial growth factor.

vivo. Over the past 10 years, efforts have been made to achieve this aim by genetically modifying T cells through the introduction of suicide genes, of which the herpes simplex thymidine kinase (HSVtk) is the most popular and advanced in term of clinical development, as it is currently being tested in a phase III clinical trial.[4] HSVtk phosphorylates specific nucleoside analogues, including gancyclovir (GCV), to nucleoside monophosphates. These compounds block effective DNA synthesis and kill dividing cells. In several clinical trials, this gene has been transferred to donor T lymphocytes, which have then been given to the allogeneic stem cell transplant recipient to prevent or treat relapse.

The approach has had some success. HSVtk gene modified–T cells persist in the circulation in most of the patients, and are removed after the administration of GCV, often with an improvement in GVHD.[4] However, several problems remain. HSVtk is a viral protein and in some patients, a cell-mediated immune response against HSVtk is detected, causing undesired premature elimination of transgenic cells. Other drawbacks of HSVtk include the unintended elimination of gene-modified cells when GCV is used for treatment of CMV reactivation, GCV resistance that may occur from truncated HSVtk generated from cryptic splice donor and acceptor sites, and slow elimination of transgenic cells as HSVtk requires DNA synthesis to be active; such delayed activity may be undesirable if T cells are acutely toxic.

Investigators attempted to overcome some of these limitations by developing new suicide genes based on human molecules that are potentially less immunogenic. In particular, suicide genes based on chimeric molecules derived from human proteins that are involved in the apoptotic pathway and modified to be activated by a small molecule have been generated (inducible Fas and inducible Caspase9). Two clinical studies have used the *iCaspase9* (*iC9*) gene which consists of the sequence of the human FK506-binding protein with an F36V mutation, connected to human caspase-9 deleted for its endogenous activation and caspase-activating recruitment domain. FKBP12-F36V binds with high affinity an otherwise bioinert small molecule

dimerizing agent (AP1903). In the presence of the drug, the iCasp9 promolecule dimerizes and activates the intrinsic apoptotic pathway leading to cell death. The study infused donor-derived iCaspase9-T cells after haploidentical stem cell transplant and if patients developed GVHD, administered a single dose of the dimerizing drug. There was rapid destruction of >95% of the cells with prompt resolution of GVHD and faster immune reconstitution that allowed robust protection against opportunistic infection.[5] These promising results prompted the design of multicenter studies to reach the Food and Drug Administration approval and commercialization.

FUTURE APPLICATIONS AND IMPLEMENTATION OF CELL THERAPIES FOR CANCER

With the approval of the first cell therapeutics for cancer (ProVenge; Dendreon), and the publication of increasing numbers of reports of complete tumor responses after cellular immunotherapy, there is increasing hope that this methodology will finally take its place in cancer therapeutics. T-cell therapies with engineered T cells for B-cell lymphoid malignancies are currently a clinical reality, but much remains to be done to ensure the effectiveness and safety of these therapies. Equally important, and as illustrated by the fate of the Dendreon cancer vaccine, much remains to be learned about development of a sustainable economic model for their affordable and broad clinical application. Nonetheless the integration of cellular therapies with other biologic agents and small molecules continues to offer the prospect of truly transformative therapies for the treatment of hematologic and other malignancies.

REFERENCES

1. Topalian SL, Hodi FS, Brahmer JR, et al: Safety, activity, and immune correlates of anti-PD-1 antibody in cancer. *N Engl J Med* 366:2443–2454, 2012.
2. Bargou R, Leo E, Zugmaier G, et al: Tumor regression in cancer patients by very low doses of a T cell-engaging antibody. *Science* 321:974–977, 2008.
3. Maude SL, Frey N, Shaw PA, et al: Chimeric antigen receptor T cells for sustained remissions in leukemia. *N Engl J Med* 371:1507–1517, 2014.
4. Ciceri F, Bonini C, Stanghellini MT, et al: Infusion of suicide-gene-engineered donor lymphocytes after family haploidentical haemopoietic stem-cell transplantation for leukaemia (the TK007 trial): a non-randomised phase I-II study. *Lancet Oncol* 10:489–500, 2009.
5. Di Stasi A, Tey SK, Dotti G, et al: Inducible apoptosis as a safety switch for adoptive cell therapy. *N Engl J Med* 365:1673–1683, 2011.
6. Bertaina A, Merli P, Rutella S, et al: HLA-haploidentical stem cell transplantation after removal of alphabeta+ T and B cells in children with nonmalignant disorders. *Blood* 124:822–826, 2014.
7. Warren EH, Fujii N, Akatsuka Y, et al: Therapy of relapsed leukemia after allogeneic hematopoietic cell transplantation with T cells specific for minor histocompatibility antigens. *Blood* 115:3869–3878, 2010.
8. Rapoport AP, Aqui NA, Stadtmauer EA, et al: Combination immunotherapy using adoptive T-cell transfer and tumor antigen vaccination on the basis of hTERT and survivin after ASCT for myeloma. *Blood* 117:788–797, 2011.
9. Hontscha C, Borck Y, Zhou H, et al: Clinical trials on CIK cells: first report of the international registry on CIK cells (IRCC). *J Cancer Res Clin Oncol* 137:305–310, 2011.
10. Papadopoulou A, Gerdemann U, Katari UL, et al: Activity of broad-spectrum T cells as treatment for AdV, EBV, CMV, BKV, and HHV6 infections after HSCT. *Sci Transl Med* 6:242ra83, 2014.
11. Leen AM, Bollard CM, Mendizabal AM, et al: Multicenter study of banked third-party virus-specific T cells to treat severe viral infections after hematopoietic stem cell transplantation. *Blood* 121:5113–5123, 2013.
12. Bollard CM, Gottschalk S, Torrano V, et al: Sustained complete responses in patients with lymphoma receiving autologous cytotoxic

T lymphocytes targeting Epstein-Barr virus latent membrane proteins. *J Clin Oncol* 32:798–808, 2014.

13. Robbins PF, Lu YC, El-Gamil M, et al: Mining exomic sequencing data to identify mutated antigens recognized by adoptively transferred tumor-reactive T cells. *Nat Med* 19:747–752, 2013.

14. Rizvi NA, Hellmann MD, Snyder A, et al: Mutational landscape determines sensitivity to PD-1 blockade in non-small cell lung cancer. *Science* 2015.

15. Morgan RA, Dudley ME, Wunderlich JR, et al: Cancer regression in patients after transfer of genetically engineered lymphocytes. *Science* 314:126–129, 2006.

16. Dotti G, Gottschalk S, Savoldo B, et al: Design and development of therapies using chimeric antigen receptor-expressing T cells. *Immunol Rev* 257:107–126, 2014.

17. Robbins PF, Morgan RA, Feldman SA, et al: Tumor regression in patients with metastatic synovial cell sarcoma and melanoma using genetically engineered lymphocytes reactive with NY-ESO-1. *J Clin Oncol* 29:917–924, 2011.

18. Arber C, Feng X, Abhyankar H, et al: Survivin-specific T cell receptor targets tumor but not T cells. *J Clin Invest* 125:157–168, 2015.

19. Parkhurst MR, Yang JC, Langan RC, et al: T cells targeting carcinoembryonic antigen can mediate regression of metastatic colorectal cancer but induce severe transient colitis. *Mol Ther* 19:620–626, 2011.

20. Bendle GM, Linnemann C, Hooijkaas AI, et al: Lethal graft-versus-host disease in mouse models of T cell receptor gene therapy. *Nat Med* 16:565–570, 1p, 2010.

21. Linette GP, Stadtmauer EA, Maus MV, et al: Cardiovascular toxicity and titin cross-reactivity of affinity-enhanced T cells in myeloma and melanoma. *Blood* 122:863–871, 2013.

22. Morgan RA, Chinnasamy N, bate-Daga D, et al: Cancer regression and neurological toxicity following anti-MAGE-A3 TCR gene therapy. *J Immunother* 36:133–151, 2013.

23. Ramos CA, Savoldo B, Dotti G: CD19-CAR trials. *Cancer J* 20:112–118, 2014.

24. Lee DW, Kochenderfer JN, Stetler-Stevenson M, et al: T cells expressing CD19 chimeric antigen receptors for acute lymphoblastic leukaemia in children and young adults: a phase 1 dose-escalation trial. *Lancet* 385:517–528, 2015.

25. Kochenderfer JN, Dudley ME, Kassim SH, et al: Chemotherapy-Refractory Diffuse Large B-Cell Lymphoma and Indolent B-Cell Malignancies Can Be Effectively Treated With Autologous T Cells Expressing an Anti-CD19 Chimeric Antigen Receptor. *J Clin Oncol* 33:540–549, 2015.

26. Wang QS, Wang Y, Lv HY, et al: Treatment of CD33-directed chimeric antigen receptor-modified T cells in one patient with relapsed and refractory acute myeloid leukemia. *Mol Ther* 23:184–191, 2015.

27. Gattinoni L, Lugli E, Ji Y, et al: A human memory T cell subset with stem cell-like properties. *Nat Med* 17:1290–1297, 2011.

28. Xu Y, Zhang M, Ramos CA, et al: Closely related T-memory stem cells correlate with in vivo expansion of CAR.CD19-T cells and are preserved by IL-7 and IL-15. *Blood* 123:3750–3759, 2014.

29. Conlon KC, Lugli E, Welles HC, et al: Redistribution, hyperproliferation, activation of natural killer cells and CD8 T cells, and cytokine production during first-in-human clinical trial of recombinant human interleukin-15 in patients with cancer. *J Clin Oncol* 33:74–82, 2015.

30. Topalian SL, Hodi FS, Brahmer JR, et al: Safety, activity, and immune correlates of anti-PD-1 antibody in cancer. *N Engl J Med* 366:2443–2454, 2012.

CHAPTER 101

NATURAL KILLER CELL–BASED THERAPIES

Sarah Cooley, Michael R. Verneris, and Jeffrey S. Miller

INTRODUCTION

The antitumor effect of allogeneic hematopoietic cell transplantation (allo-HCT) is mediated through both high-dose chemotherapy and immune reactions. Although relapse rates remain high, reduced intensity regimens do provide protection from relapse, demonstrating that allogeneic immune cells can eradicate leukemia and lymphoma. Exactly which cell populations contribute to the graft-versus-leukemia effect is not entirely established, and may vary among individuals and diseases. Immune cell populations can be mechanistically divided into two broad categories; the innate (natural killer [NK] cells and antigen presenting cells [APC]) and adaptive (T cell and B cells) arms of the immune system. It is commonly believed that mature innate immune cells are able to perform their biologic functions without prior activation, while in contrast adaptive immune cells require antigen presentation, activation, and expansion before they can act. These paradigms are changing. It is becoming increasingly clear that human cytomegalovirus (CMV) induces profound changes in the NK-cell repertoire promoting NK-cell populations that are capable of immunologic memory. These populations have been termed "adaptive NK cells." Likewise, under certain conditions, T cells can mediate major histocompatibility complex (MHC)-unrestricted killing, typically considered a quality of the innate system. Importantly, cells from all components of the immune system are regulated in concert to achieve a balance between immune response and tolerance. Because the antitumor efficacy of conventional cytotoxic agents is limited by off target toxicity and resistance, targeted immune cell–based therapies provide an attractive alternative. Progress in cytokine biology and improvements in techniques to separate, expand, and target cells through immune engagers or chimeric antigen receptors (CARs) have transformed the concept of NK cell–based therapy. This chapter examines characteristics of NK cells and discusses how they may be manipulated to treat malignancy and combat infection, both in HCT and non-HCT settings.

NATURAL KILLER CELL BIOLOGY

NK cells were first described functionally in 1975 for their ability to lyse virally infected cells and tumor targets without prior sensitization. NK cells comprise 10% to 15% of the peripheral blood (PB) lymphocyte pool in normal humans, but they are also found in the bone marrow, spleen, liver, lymph nodes, lungs, and pregnant uterus (Fig. 101.1). Defined by the expression of CD56 or NKp46 and by the lack of a CD3/T-cell receptor complex, they develop from marrow-derived progenitors via distinct developmental stages in secondary lymphoid tissue.[1] Mature NK cells can be functionally distinguished by CD56 density. The CD56[dim] subset exhibits natural cytotoxicity (killing of class I–negative targets) and displays Fc receptors (CD16) that facilitate the recognition of immunoglobulin-coated targets, a process called antibody-dependent cellular cytotoxicity (ADCC). CD56[dim] cells also produce cytokines in response to the above stimuli. In contrast, CD56[bright] NK cells are more proliferative and are less cytotoxic. CD56[bright] cells respond to monocyte-derived cytokines (interleukin [IL]-12, IL-15, and IL-18) to rapidly produce large amounts of interferon gamma (IFN-γ). NK cells also proliferate and become activated in response to IL-2, IL-15,

and IL-21. IL-15 is of particular importance for NK cell development and homeostasis. Trans presentation of IL-15 by IL-15Rα on APCs appears to be the physiologic source of cytokine leading to NK activation.[2] These cytokines enhance the expression of CD56 on activated cells, producing a population that should not be confused with steady-state CD56[bright] cells, which have different functional properties.

Natural Killer Cell Functions

NK cells provide a link between the innate and adaptive immune systems[3] and play an important role in immune surveillance, pregnancy outcomes, and response to infections (see Fig. 101.1). NK cell function can be divided into several separate activities that include interaction with APCs, activation, expansion, homing to malignant or virally infected targets, direct cell–cell killing, and cytokine production. These responses may differ based on the stimulus and the NK cell subset studied. Activated NK cells produce cytokines and chemokines, including IFN-γ, tumor necrosis factor, granulocyte macrophage colony-stimulating factor, and transforming growth factor beta. NK cells also express β2 integrins such as leukocyte function–associated antigen-1 (LFA-1) and CD2, which bind to molecules such as intracellular adhesion molecule-1 and LFA-3 on APCs and other cells. If the balance of activating and inhibitor receptor signaling favors activation (see later), target-cell apoptosis occurs via membrane bound death receptors (Fas ligand [FasL] and tumor necrosis factor-related apoptosis inducing ligand [TRAIL]) or by releasing cytotoxic molecules (perforin and granzyme) into a small area between the NK cell and the target cells (called the immune synapse). These activated NK cells then produce cytokines. It is believed that the activating signal threshold required for IFN-γ production is higher than that needed for CD107a degranulation or cytotoxicity after target cell exposure. It is not known whether cytokine production or direct cell killing is physiologically most important for a therapeutic NK cell response, and it is likely that both are required for efficacy.

Natural Killer Cell Receptors

Unlike T cells or B cells that express a single, unique, rearranged antigen receptor, NK cells express a variety of different receptors that trigger either inhibition or activation. Many of the inhibitory receptors are MHC class I–specific, such that engagement of self results in a *reduction* in NK cell function. Thus recognition of MHC class I, which is ubiquitously expressed by healthy tissues, leads to NK cell tolerance. In contrast, the loss of MHC class I, which occurs during the process of viral infection and malignant transformation, leads to the *lack* of engagement of these inhibitory receptors and, in turn, permits activation of the NK cell via other receptor–ligand interactions. The activating receptors often recognize ligands that are induced by cell stress, such as MHC I–related chain A and B, the unique long (UL) 16-binding proteins (ULBPs), nectin-2, and CD48.[4] The net balance of activating and inhibitory signals determines the NK cell response to a target, favoring elimination of infected, transformed, or stressed cells.

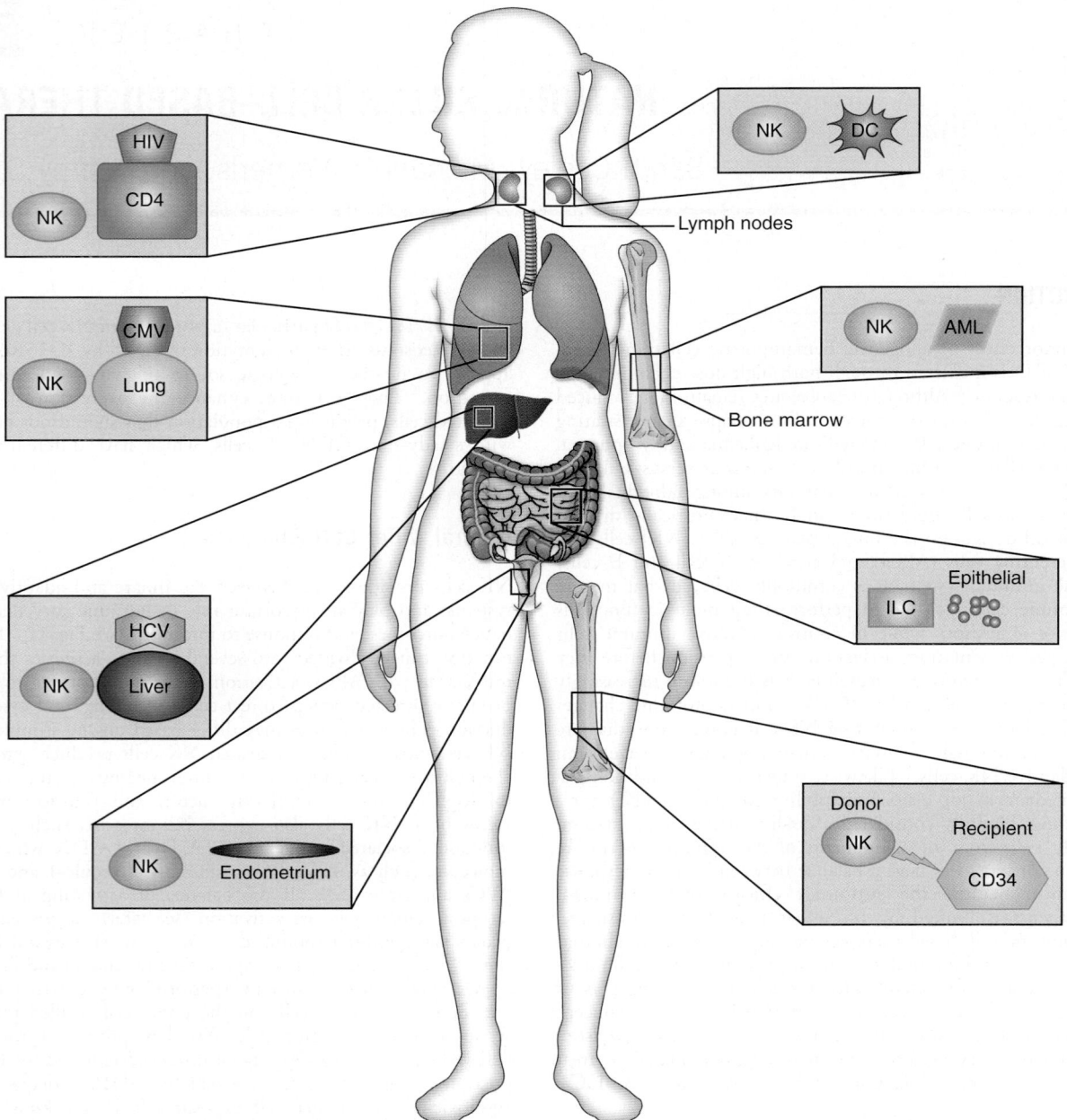

Fig. 101.1 ROLES OF NATURAL KILLER CELLS IN CANCER AND HEALTH. The expanding roles of NK cells in both health and cancer are depicted. NK cells play a critical role in initiation of immune responses by interacting with dendritic cells (DCs), resulting in reciprocal activation of both cell types (i.e., NK cells activate DCs and vice versa). NK-induced DC activation likely also results in the initiation of adaptive immune responses by inducing DCs to present antigens to T cells. Activated NK cells can go on to destroy malignant tissues including leukemia. In the setting of allogeneic transplantation, NK cells can eradicate recipient stem cells, thereby facilitating allogeneic stem-cell engraftment. Emerging data shows that a subpopulation of NK cells or similar cells (known as innate lymphoid cells) produce IL-22 and interact with lymph node stroma to mediate mucosal immunity and may accelerate immune responses after transplantation. A unique population of uterine NK cells is responsible for the maintenance of pregnancy. Still other roles for NK cells include the surveillance for and response to infectious organisms including hepatitis C virus, cytomegalovirus, and human immunodeficiency virus. *AML,* Acute myeloid leukemia; *CMV,* cytomegalovirus; *DC,* dendritic cell; *HCV,* hepatitis C virus; *HIV,* human immunodeficiency virus; *ILC,* innate lymphoid cell; *NK,* natural killer.

Killer Immunoglobulin-Like Receptors

The killer immunoglobulin-like receptor *(KIR)* gene cluster, located on chromosome 19q13.4, encodes 15 different molecules in the immunoglobulin (Ig) superfamily. *KIR* genes contain either two or three extracellular domains (2D or 3D), a transmembrane region, and an intracellular domain that is either long (containing inhibitory motifs) or short (containing docking sites for activating molecules). In addition, there are two pseudogenes (*KIR2DP1* and *KIR3DP1*). Individuals carry two KIR haplotypes, which can be defined as A or B, based on their *KIR* gene content. All haplotypes include three framework genes bounded by *KIR3DL3* at the centromeric (Cen) end, *KIR3DL2* at the telomeric end and *KIR2DL4* in the middle. The A KIR haplotype contains a fixed content of genes that also includes the inhibitory receptors KIR2DL1, KIR2DL3, and KIR3DL1 along with a single activating receptor (KIR2DS4). In contrast, B KIR haplotypes contain a variable number of activating (*KIR2DS1, KIR2DS2, KIR2DS3, KIR2DS5, KIR3DS1*) and inhibitory (*KIR2DL5A/B, KIR2DL2*) genes. *KIR2DL2/3* and *KIR3DL1/S1* are genes whose alleles determine whether they define KIR A (KIR2DL2 and 3DL1) or KIR B (KIR2DL3 or KIR3DS1) haplotypes.

Inhibitory KIR recognizes self-class I human leukocyte antigen (HLA) molecules on potential target cells. This interaction suppresses the NK cell effector responses. Inhibitory KIR recognizes polymorphisms of HLA-C and B in a biallelic manner (i.e., C1 versus C2 and Bw4 versus Bw6). KIR2DL1, KIR2DL2/KIR2DL3 and KIR3DL1 bind HLA class I C2, C1, and Bw4 alleles, respectively. These inhibitory receptor–ligand interactions are complex, as the mere expression of the receptors does not predict the cellular response. Rather, the affinity of a given KIR seems to depend on allelic polymorphisms both of KIR and its MHC class I ligand. In addition, the receptor–ligand binding rules are not absolute, as KIR2DL2 can bind both HLA-C1 and HLA-C2 alleles. KIR also binds to HLA-A alleles (A3 and A11) that contain the Bw4 epitope, and KIR3DL2 binds some HLA-A alleles in the context of certain peptides. Our understanding of the KIR system is further complicated by the fact that the natural ligands for activating KIR remain largely unknown. Although some bind MHC molecules at low affinity, it is not known whether MHC proteins function as the natural ligands in vivo. Although KIR2DS1 has been shown to bind HLA-C2, KIR2DS2 does not bind HLA-C1 but recently has been shown to recognize threonine 80 of HLA-A11, which can be modified by peptide.[5]

Additional Natural Killer Cell Receptors

Several other families of activating and inhibitory receptors influence NK cell function, some of which bind HLA molecules. The NKG2 family of C-type lectin receptors that heterodimerize with CD94 may be either inhibitory (NKG2A) or activating (NKG2C), and can recognize nonclassic HLA-E. NKG2D does not heterodimerize with CD94 and recognizes stress-induced molecules such as MHC class I polypeptide-related sequence A/B (MICA and MICB) or viral-derived proteins like the CMV-related UL binding proteins (ULBP1-6). Additional receptors include the natural cytotoxicity receptors NKp30, NKp46, and NKp44, DNAM-1, and Nectin-2 (CD122), 2B4, Ig-like receptors, and leukocyte-associated immunoglobulin-like receptor-1. These activating receptors are believed to play a role in communication between NK cells and dendritic cells as well as determining whether an NK cell can recognize a target.

Natural Killer Cell Education—The Acquisition of Function, Self-Tolerance, and Alloreactivity

A mechanistic explanation for the phenomenon of "hybrid resistance" and "missing self" is derived from the characterization of NK cell inhibitory receptors that recognize self-MHC class I. In both instances, because they fail to engage inhibitory receptors, target cells lacking self-MHC class I expression are sensitive to NK-mediated killing. Thus NK cells detect either allogeneic cells or disease-associated downregulation/loss of MHC class I on virally infected or tumor cells.[6] The process of inhibitory receptor signaling that leads to the acquisition of cytotoxicity and cytokine production has been referred to as "NK cell education" or "NK licensing."[7,8] NK cells lacking both KIR and NKG2A are hyporesponsive and cannot be educated until inhibitory receptors are expressed. Relevant to the field of allo-HCT, NK cell education may not be fixed. For instance, adoptive transfer of hypofunctional NK cells from β2-microglobulin knockout mice (that lack MHC class I) into wild-type mice leads to their education

and gain of function. Conversely, adoptive transfer of fully functional NK cells from wild-type mice into β2-microglobulin knockout hosts results in NK hyporesponsiveness.[9,10] Collectively, these data support the model of NK cell education as a dynamic, inherently plastic process where low level, tonic inhibitory signals are required to maintain cytotoxic capacity. It has also been demonstrated that the cumulative strength of inhibitory receptor signaling correlates with functional thresholds. This model, aptly compared to a "rheostat," permits self-tolerance in the normal state and allows for enhanced sensitivity to damage to healthy cells through class I downregulation.[11] Importantly, it must be emphasized that not all acquisition of NK cell function is through NK cell education. NK cells can overcome rules of NK cell education in the presence of high concentrations of cytokines, in settings such as in vitro activation where exogenous cytokines are applied or during inflammatory conditions where high levels of cytokines are present. In the mouse, the importance of inflammation-induced cytokine production leading to enhanced NK function is clearly demonstrated by the ability of NK cells from β2-microglobulin knockout mice, which are hyporesponsive in vitro, to clear murine CMV. In summary, NK education determines the function of NK cells at steady state, but other factors may overcome or even dominate, especially when cytokines are administered to patients or used to stimulate NK cells that are adoptively transferred.

Natural Killer Cell Recognition of Tumors

Although the antitumor efficacy of NK cells has been most evident for myeloid malignancies, a wide variety of solid tumors including breast, ovarian, hepatocellular, colon, neuroblastoma, Ewing sarcoma, rhabdomyosarcoma, and melanoma can be sensitive to NK cell lysis. The relative resistance of some tumors may be caused by a higher expression of class I HLA, which inversely correlates with the susceptibility of primary pre–B cell acute lymphoblastic leukemia (ALL) blasts to NK cell lysis.[12] Successful destruction of a target requires coengagement of NK cell receptors by both inhibitory and activating signals. Accordingly, activating receptors such as NKG2D play an important role in immune surveillance and killing of acute myeloid leukemia (AML) stem cells. Other tumor ligands that correlate with responsiveness to NK cell-mediated killing include DNAM-1 on myelodysplastic syndrome blasts, CD137 ligand on AML targets, and B7-H3, which protects neuroblastoma from NK lysis. When considering therapeutic uses of NK cells and interventions such as the use of anti-KIR or anti-NKG2A antibodies to promote tumor lysis, it is important to remember that many NK cells circulating in steady-state peripheral blood variably express KIR and NKG2A. Therefore maximum killing of targets such as leukemia blasts may require blockade of multiple inhibitory receptor interactions.

Innate Lymphoid Cells

Until recently, NK cells were the only known lymphocyte population that could be considered "innate lymphoid cells." However, more recently, it has been appreciated that there are a variety of different innate lymphoid cell (ILC) populations, known as ILC1, ILC2, and ILC3 cells. Similar to the T-cell paradigm, ILCs have been categorized by key transcription factor expression, which drives unique cytokine production in response to activation.[13] More specifically, ILC1 cells (including NK cells) are characterized by T-bet expression and produce IFN-γ in response to the monocyte-derived cytokines IL-12 and IL-18. ILC2 cells express GATA-3 and produce IL-5 and IL-13 following stimulation with IL-25 and IL-33, and ILC3 cells express the transcription factor ROR-γt and produce IL-22 in response to IL-1 and IL-23 stimulation. The physiologic role for these cells, both in health and pathology is still emerging, but recent studies suggest that ILC1 cells play a role in anticancer responses and ILC2 and ILC3 cells may assist in response to pulmonary and intestinal pathogens and may also have a role in preventing graft-versus-host disease (GVHD).

CLINICAL APPLICATIONS OF NATURAL KILLER CELLS

Determination of Donor Natural Killer Cell Alloreactivity

It is widely accepted that the ability of NK cells to contribute to protection from relapse and infection requires that they be functionally competent and present in sufficient numbers. As described earlier, NK cells are alloreactive against targets that lack self-HLA ligands for the inhibitory receptors that contributed to their education or licensing. Recent studies have suggested that the diversity of the NK cell repertoire is massive (6000–30,000 phenotypically distinct individual clones in an individual),[14] allowing NK cell education to occur through multiple receptor–ligand interactions. Several models have been developed to predict NK cell alloreactivity, but the aforementioned diversity suggests that the in vivo response is more complicated than the existing models. Donor and recipient HLA typing can be used to determine KIR–ligand mismatch or incompatibility, as defined by the Perugia group,[15] which predicts that donor-derived NK cells will be alloreactive in the graft-versus-host direction when recipients lack C2, C1, or Bw4 alleles that are present in the donor. Alternatively, in the KIR–ligand absence model, alloreactive potential is based entirely on the number of KIR ligands (HLA molecules) a recipient lacks. The receptor–ligand model of alloreactivity requires knowledge of the inhibitory KIR expression in the donor (based on assessment of the donor KIR genotype or phenotype). Because *KIR* genes have multiple alleles with variable levels of expression and functional activity, alloreactivity may be best determined by evaluating the donor KIR genotype with functional assessments of their KIR phenotype.

The Role of Natural Killer Cells in Hematopoietic Cell Transplantation

NK cells are the first lymphocyte population to reconstitute after HCT. Engrafted alloreactive NK cells may mediate: (1) decreased rates of GVHD by targeting of host APC; (2) improved engraftment by secretion of stem cell trophic cytokines and elimination of host immune barriers; (3) targeting minimal residual leukemia and reduce relapse; and (4) decreased infectious complications. An early report published by the Perugia Group in 2002 demonstrated a beneficial effect of alloreactive NK cells and showed that donor KIR–ligand mismatched NK cells in the GVHD direction play a key role in achieving durable remission after CD34+ selected (T-cell deplete) haploidentical transplantation for AML, but not ALL. KIR–ligand mismatched donors were associated with improved engraftment, decreased relapse, and decreased GVHD.[15] However, in a long-term follow up of 112 patients, only decreased relapse in patients transplanted while in complete remission and improved disease-free survival were maintained. Subsequent analyses of the role of KIR–ligand mismatching and KIR–ligand absence in different settings have produced mixed results. In umbilical cord blood (UCB) transplantation, the effect of KIR–ligand mismatching on outcomes appears to depend on either the intensity of the preparative regimen or the drugs used (i.e., ATG or not).[16,17] In a 2009 study of 169 children treated with autologous HCT for neuroblastoma, KIR–ligand absence was strongly associated with improved survival and decreased risk of disease progression.[18] Inconsistent effects of KIR–ligand mismatch and KIR–ligand absence strategies are likely caused by differences in the stem cell source, conditioning, degree of T-cell depletion, and post-HCT immunosuppression used, all of which can affect NK cell development, education, and function. Despite this confusion, NK cell effects continue to emerge, implicating them as having a key role in protecting against relapse in myeloid malignancies. Similar promise

has been demonstrated in pediatric, but not adult ALL, suggesting that unique interactions between NK cells and targets might account for these differences.

Natural Killer Cell Function After Hematopoietic Cell Transplantation

Despite their high numbers early after HCT, engrafting NK cells are not fully functional. This has been demonstrated by several investigators.[19,20] Foley et al studied simultaneous NK cell functions in response to target cell exposure.[21] They reported that degranulation stimulated by class I–negative targets recovered early after transplant, suggesting that NK cells could be educated through either NKG2A or KIR. NK cells from double umbilical cord grafts exhibited CD107a hyperfunction compared to adult unrelated donors, which may explain the enhanced relapse protection seen in this setting. In marked contrast, IFN-γ production was severely diminished for at least 6 months post-HCT, especially in settings of T-cell depleted grafts (even without posttransplant immune suppression) or grafts containing naive T cells (UCB), suggesting that NK cells require T cells for optimal education. This defect could be rapidly reversed by short-term exposure to IL-15. In addition, and in contrast to CD107a degranulation, IFN-γ production could only be educated through self-KIR (NK cells expressing KIR that encounter their cognate ligand [MHC class I] in the recipient), suggesting a hierarchy of thresholds for different NK effector functions. Lastly, different conditioning regimens may have varied effects on the tempo of NK and T-cell reconstitution after transplantation and may therefore affect function and impact on clinical outcomes.

Donor Selection Based on Killer Immunoglobulin-Like Receptor Genotype

Another approach to capitalize on the beneficial effects of NK cells after HCT is to consider the full KIR genotype of potential donors. In a study of 448 patients undergoing myeloablative HLA-matched or -mismatched unrelated donor (URD) HCT for AML, the 3-year overall survival was significantly higher after transplantation from a KIR B/x genotype donor (containing at least 1 B haplotype), irrespective of recipient KIR genotype, with a 30% improvement in relative risk of relapse-free survival.[22] A subsequent analysis of 1409 URD transplant recipients confirmed these findings and refined the beneficial effect of *KIR B* genes to AML patients. Similar effects were not seen in ALL. In addition, this later study showed that the most benefit from donor KIR B genotype was localized to genes present in the centromeric part of the *KIR* locus. The greatest protection from relapse and best disease-free survival, in both HLA matched and mismatched transplants, was associated with donors homozygous for this region. Donors could be stratified by KIR into those with Best (Cen-B homozygous present in 11% of the population), Better (≥2 B defining domains as seen in 20% of the population), or Neutral donor KIR genotypes. A publicly available calculator to determine this stratification is available online (http://www.ebi.ac.uk/ipd/kir/donor_b_content.html). KIR genotyping as few as three of the best HLA matched donor candidates should substantially increase the frequency of URD transplants from donors with favorable *KIR* gene content (from 31% to 79%) AML.[23] New studies suggest that the benefit of Better/Best donors is further enhanced in HLA-C1 but not HLA-C2 recipients, which may inhibit KIR2DS1+ NK cells by downtuning NK cell educations in the context of HLA-C2.[24,25] Several prospective trials using different graft sources designed to select donors for relapse protection are underway. The benefit of donor KIR B/x has been verified in other studies, and all *KIR B* genes contribute the clinical benefit. The B-haplotype *KIR* genes *2DL5A*, *2DS1*, and *3DS1* were associated with an AML-specific fourfold reduction in relapse in a study of 246 T-cell depleted HLA-matched sibling transplants, and KIR B haplotypes were associated with improved survival and reduced TRM in association with less CMV reactivation in otherwise similar patients. In conclusion, in addition to HLA matching, donor selection for *KIR* genes is a promising strategy to improve outcome after HCT, but benefit may not be seen in all settings. While the benefits of NK cells can be realized in AML, the HLA-matched setting,[26] in the autologous setting,[27] and new studies in pediatric ALL,[28,29] the benefit of a *KIR B/x* donor may be lessened when reduced intensity conditioning is used for transplantation by unknown mechanisms.

Making Natural Killer Cells Antigen Specific

Despite their ability to recognize malignant transformation or viral infection, NK cells are limited by their lack of antigen specificity. Bispecific or Trispecific killer engagers (termed BiKEs or TriKEs) have been developed to overcome this limitation. These novel drugs use the single chain antigen binding regions of antibodies (scFv) to redirect NK cells to targets. For instance, scFvs directed against CD16 on NK cells can be combined with an scFv against a tumor-associated antigen (i.e., CD33). They promote the formation of an immunologic synapse that is both antigen specific and leads to the engagement of other receptor/ligand pairs between NK cells and their targets. For example, CD16x33 BiKEs have been designed to target AML, and have the additional benefit of recognizing and killing CD33+ myeloid-derived suppressor cells.[30] The activation induced by BiKEs and TriKEs is potent enough to overcome inhibitory signaling through class I recognizing NK cell receptors. This platform is flexible and modular (for example, CD19 could be easily substituted for CD33), making it an exportable therapeutic approach without the need for gene therapy. The CD16x19x22 TriKE construct targets two tumor-associated antigens (CD19 and CD22) via CD16, or alternatively via the agonistic 41BB-ligand. An alternative approach being explored by some groups is the introduction of CARs into NK cells, but difficulties in lentiviral gene transduction may make other approaches such as the introduction of CARs into induced pluripotent stem cell (iPS)-derived NK cells or NK cell lines a more realistic approach because of their off-the-shelf renewal properties.

Control of Viral Infection

Perhaps the greatest advance in NK cell biology over the past 5 years derives from studies of the impact of murine CMV on NK cells. It had been recognized that murine CMV infection leads to expansion of a population of Ly49H+ NK cells that recognize the murine CMV protein M157. Following repeat challenges with CMV, these cells expand and attenuate CMV disease. Moreover, Ly49H+ cells can be adoptively transferred and protect mice from CMV-induced lethality. In 2004, Lopez-Botet and colleagues[30a] found a unique population of NKG2C+ NK cells in CMV-seropositive but not CMV-seronegative humans. These cells were not induced by other herpes viruses such as herpes simplex virus or Epstein-Barr virus (EBV). NKG2C+ NK cells were also enriched in vitro when cultured with human CMV infected fibroblasts. Definitive data now shows that NKG2C+ and NKG2C+/CD57+ NK cells expand in vivo when immunosuppressed patients reactivate CMV after solid organ or hematopoietic cell transplantation.[31,32] These NKG2C+ NK cells are long-lived and exhibit a high frequency of self-KIR expressing NK cells capable of enhanced target cell killing and IFN-γ production compared to NK cells lacking NKG2C. These findings suggest that NKG2C+ NK cells represent a unique NK cell population primed by human CMV. Although Ly49 recognizes murine CMV, it is not clear that NKG2C directly recognizes human CMV. The NKG2C+ population was also found to expand in victims of a hantavirus outbreak in Sweden and a chikungunya virus outbreak in Africa, suggesting that these NK cells may be involved in the response to multiple viral infections. However, both of these populations also had prior exposure to CMV, so at present it is unclear whether these viruses also induce NKG2C+ NK cells or whether they lead to concurrent CMV reactivation. It is interesting that NKG2C/CD94 and NKG2A/CD94 both recognize

HLA-E, often expressed on cancer cells. One simple explanation for how CMV influences NK cell function is by the conversion of HLA-E recognition on CMV-exposed NK cells from inhibition through NKG2A to activation through NKG2C as NK cells usually express one or the other receptor but not both. Recently, Lee et al[33] and Schlums et al[34] refined our understanding of subsets of NKG2C+ NK cells by precisely defining them by the additional loss of their adaptor or signaling proteins spleen tyrosine kinase, EAT-2 and FcεRγ. They refer to these CMV-induced, long-lived cells as "adaptive NK cells" drawing parallels between these cells and the T-cell arms of the (adaptive) immune system. In support of this, CMV induced a unique NK-cell methylation signature resembling CD8+ T cells that was distinctly different from conventional/canonic NK cells. In summary, data suggest that CMV exposure, latent CMV, and CMV reactivation has a profound effect on the NK cell repertoire with induction of adaptive NK cells. This is important in transplantation because 25% to 50% of seropositive patients will reactivate CMV. It has recently been discovered in the post-gancyclovir era that CMV reactivation protects against transplant relapse and prolongs disease-free survival[35,36] suggesting that adaptive NK cells may play a role as antitumor effectors that merits further study. Recently, IL-12/IL-18 in addition to IL-15 has been shown to induce a population of primed NK cells that are long lived, and these cells are in clinical trials.[37] How these cells compare to CMV-induced adaptive NK cells is under study.

Adoptive Transfer of Natural Killer Cells

Although methods to exploit the beneficial effects of NK cells engrafting after allo-HCT are increasing, it should be recognized that NK cells are also well suited for adoptive cellular therapies. Many groups tested methods to induce autologous NK cell activity, such as treatment with prolonged, low-dose IL-2 subcutaneously, higher dose IL-2 intravenously, and infusions of ex vivo IL-2–activated NK cells. While these approaches induced in vivo NK cell expansion and function, they were shown by several investigational teams to have only limited clinical efficacy; therefore, the Minnesota Group pioneered the use of haploidentical NK cell infusions.[37a] This approach was based on the likelihood that haploidentical NK cells, educated in the donor, would mediate stronger graft-versus-leukemia reactions because they are not exposed to immune suppressive mechanisms seen in cancer patients. It was further hypothesized that this would result in a higher frequency of alloreactive NK cells (NK cells with inhibitory receptors functionally educated through a different inhibitory receptor that will not be inhibited by class I expressed by the tumor). The safety and success of NK cell infusions was established in a trial using haplotype mismatched, related-donor NK cell products followed by subcutaneous IL-2 to induce in vivo NK survival and expansion.[38] Successful expansion was achieved only after a lymphodepleting regimen of high dose cyclophosphamide and fludarabine. Interestingly, complete remissions in AML correlated with in vivo NK expansion and higher proportions of circulating (and functional) NK cells. The importance of the high-dose chemotherapy regimen delivered before NK cell transfer cannot be overstated. Chemotherapy not only creates space for the NK cells to expand, but also results in a surge of endogenous IL-15 and IL-7 and transiently prevents recipient T cells from rejecting allogeneic NK cells. This platform allows in vivo expanded NK cells to partially overcome the rules of NK cell education and tolerance, potentially obviating the need to select specific alloreactive NK cell donors. This assumption requires formal clinical testing. Other modifications have shown that elimination of regulatory T cells with IL-2 diphtheria toxin fusion protein can enhance the clinical activity of NK cell infusions.[39] Adoptive transfer of haploidentical NK cells has been tested in other settings. In a pediatric cohort, recovery of functional donor-derived CD56+/CD16+ NK cells that lysed K562 targets mediated strong ADCC activity against neuroblastoma and leukemic blasts by day +14 after the infusion. The use of NK cell–based therapies to target minimal residual disease is being tested. This preemptive approach is

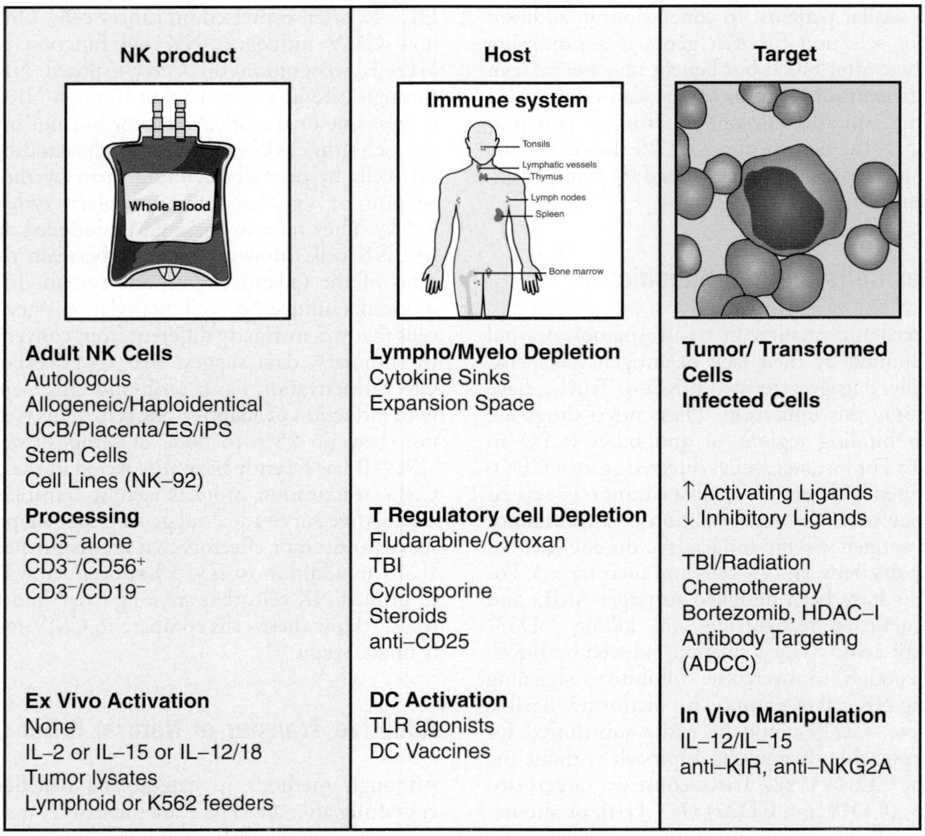

Fig. 101.2 MANIPULATIONS TO INCREASE THE EFFECTIVENESS OF ADOPTIVE NATURAL KILLER CELL THERAPIES. Current approaches to improve the effectiveness of adoptive transfer of NK cells involve a balance between factors from the NK cell product, the host, and the tumor target. The NK cell product can be derived from adult blood and can be autologous (although there is greater concern for "self" MHC inhibition through inhibitory receptors), allogeneic, derived from primitive progenitors, or even NK cell lines, all of which may be more amenable to gene therapy. The optimal product may be the one that gives rise to longer in vivo persistence and survival, which needs formal testing. Use of donor NK cells infused across allogeneic barriers involves variable degrees of purity, and clinical trials have been published using each of these manipulations. At a minimum, a T-cell depleted product is needed to prevent GVHD. Contaminating B cells have also been shown to contribute to complications such as EBV-induced lymphoproliferative disease and autoimmune hemolytic anemia as part of a passenger lymphocyte syndrome. It is still unclear whether NK cell products should be administered without activation (fresh or frozen), with IL-2 or IL-15, or using activation through other mechanisms (such as CMV reactivation or tumor cell lysates). Several investigators are exploring ex vivo expansion, a process that requires lymphoblastoid cell line or membrane bound IL-15 or IL-21 and 41BB-ligand transduced K562 feeders. The success of adoptive transfer is absolutely dependent on host factors that determine whether the recipient is permissive to adoptive transfer. Success depends on lymphodepletion allowing for transient removal of cytokines sinks to free up cytokines such as endogenous IL-15 as well as added myelodepletion that provides space for adoptively transferred cells. Immune barriers to adoptive transfer include an increase in regulatory T cells, especially when IL-2 is administered to the patient, and methods to blunt this inhibitory response may be effective if they do not dampen NK cell function. As NK cells and DC coactivate each other, use of DC vaccines or TLR-7 or TLR-9 agonists that work through DC may be synergistic. Lastly, there are a number of manipulations that involve the target itself to enhance sensitivity to NK cell adoptive transfer. These manipulations are intended to promote interactions between NK cells and their targets based on known biology to enhance activation interactions, decrease inhibition, or to prolong NK cell survival. It is anticipated that a combination of these variables will ultimately be needed for clinical efficacy, and these strategies may need to be tailored to different tumor types. *ADCC,* antibody-dependent cell-mediated cytotoxicity; *CMV,* cytomegalovirus; *DC,* dendritic cell, *EBV,* Epstein-Barr virus; *ES,* embryonic stem cells; *GVHD,* graft-versus-host disease; *HDAC-1,* histone deacetylase 1; *IL,* interleukin; *iPS,* induced pluripotent stem cells, *KIR,* killer immunoglobulin-like receptor; *MHC,* major histocompatibility complex; *NK,* natural killer; *TBI,* total body irradiation; *TLR,* toll-like receptor; *UCB,* umbilical cord blood.

being tested by use of NK cell donor lymphocyte infusions after haploidentical HCT in adults with AML. A published study in pediatric patients used NK cells as consolidation therapy to maintain remissions in a nontransplant setting. This platform is being adapted for testing in elderly AML patients. Additional studies to explore applications in multiple myeloma, lymphoma, and solid tumors are being developed.

FUTURE DIRECTIONS

Several promising strategies to exploit NK cell alloreactivity to treat cancer are in development. These include various approaches to develop in vivo or ex vivo expanded products, manipulations of the host immune system, and strategies to modify the tumor targets to enhance their sensitivity to NK cell–mediated killing (Fig. 101.2). Unlike T cells, haplotype mismatched or completely HLA-mismatched NK cells can be given without risk of GVHD, although a recent report cautions that conclusion when using highly expanded NK cells ex vivo using membrane bound IL-15 and 41BB-ligand K562 feeders, because some patients developed a syndrome that histologically and clinically was indistinguishable from GVHD.[40] Adoptive transfer is limited by the cell dose attained from a single leukopheresis and the current requirement for high dose lymphodepleting chemotherapy. In vivo expansion, while detectable, is transient and appears to require the use of exogenous cytokines such as IL-2, which is associated with induction of suppressive regulatory T cells. The use of IL-15 (or IL-15/IL-15Rα complexes to trans present IL-15), the true homeostatic factor for NK cells, is now being tested in patients receiving adoptively transferred NK cells to treat their AML or posttransplant relapse. A major advantage of IL-15 is that unlike IL-2, it does not stimulate regulatory T cells. Various methods to enrich the NK cell fraction in haploidentical apheresis products are being tested, including depletion of T (CD3) and B (CD19) cells, or positive selection for CD56+ NK cells. Several investigators are also exploring ex vivo NK expansion using EBV-transformed or modified K562 feeder cells to increase the infused NK cell dose, potentially circumventing the need for in vivo expansion. The use of "off-the-shelf" NK cell lines, such as NK-92, may provide a large supply of highly cytotoxic NK cells that could be used for repeated infusions. Other approaches using NK cell products derived from UCB or placental progenitors, embryonic stem cells, or induced iPS cell sources are also being developed. UCB stem cell–derived ILC that produce IL-22 may enhance tissue integrity and improve immune reconstitution after HCT. Alternative forms of activation, such as combining NK cells with either toll-like receptor agonists and/or dendritic cell vaccines, are also being explored. Other possibilities are being aimed at sensitizing the target cells using chemotherapy (bortezomib or histone deacetylase inhibitors), or irradiation. Lastly, if cytokines such as IL-15 can safely and efficiently expand autologous NK cells in vivo, it may be possible to mimic an allogeneic approach by in vivo or ex vivo expansion of NK cells. Combining these with antibodies (anti-KIR and anti-NKG2A) that block inhibitory receptors or BiKEs that deliver potent activation signals that overcome inhibition through class I MHC receptors may be incredibly powerful.

CONCLUSION

The therapeutic use of NK cells is a promising strategy to treat cancer in both transplant and nontransplant settings. NK cells have the potential to induce graft-versus-tumor effects without inducing GVHD. To date, the majority of data supporting the antileukemic effect of NK cells has emerged from the allo-HCT literature. However, the complexities of allo-HCT, including variations in preparative regimens, stem cell sources, graft products, posttransplant immune suppression, and disease specific differences all complicate our understanding of the underlying biologic mechanisms. This limits the design of effective therapies exploiting NK cell alloreactivity. Investigators developing strategies using adoptive transfer of NK cells are

working to establish proof of concept and to develop exportable techniques. Development of platforms that support robust in vivo or ex vivo NK cell expansion and education, selection of NK donors based on their NK cell receptor genes, manipulation of tumor NK cell receptor ligand expression, and coordination of NK cell interactions with other immune cells are underway at many institutions. Ultimately, combination therapy using several strategies will likely prove most successful. In particular, cytokines such as IL-15, antibodies to block inhibitory receptors, methods to induce adaptive NK cells with properties of immune memory, and the use of BiKEs or TriKEs to make NK cells antigen-specific hold great promise.

REFERENCES

1. Freud AG, Yokohama A, Becknell B, et al: Evidence for discrete stages of human natural killer cell differentiation in vivo. *J Exp Med* 203:1033, 2006.
2. Huntington ND, Legrand N, Alves NL, et al: IL-15 trans-presentation promotes human NK cell development and differentiation in vivo. *J Exp Med* 206:25–34, 2009.
3. Walzer T, Dalod M, Robbins SH, et al: Natural-killer cells and dendritic cells: "l'union fait la force". *Blood* 106:2252–2258, 2005.
4. Lopez-Botet M, Angulo A, Guma M: Natural killer cell receptors for major histocompatibility complex class I and related molecules in cytomegalovirus infection. *Tissue Antigens* 63:195–203, 2004.
5. Liu J, Xiao Z, Ko HL, et al: Activating killer cell immunoglobulin-like receptor 2DS2 binds to HLA-A*11. *Proc Natl Acad Sci USA* 111:2662–2667, 2014.
6. Kim S, Poursine-Laurent J, Truscott SM, et al: Licensing of natural killer cells by host major histocompatibility complex class I molecules. *Nature* 436:709–713, 2005.
7. Raulet DH: Missing self recognition and self tolerance of natural killer (NK) cells. *Semin Immunol* 18:145–150, 2006.
8. Parham P: Taking license with natural killer cell maturation and repertoire development. *Immunol Rev* 214:155–160, 2006.
9. Joncker NT, Shifrin N, Delebecque F, et al: Mature natural killer cells reset their responsiveness when exposed to an altered MHC environment. *J Exp Med* 207:2065–2072, 2010.
10. Elliott JM, Wahle JA, Yokoyama WM: MHC class I-deficient natural killer cells acquire a licensed phenotype after transfer into an MHC class I-sufficient environment. *J Exp Med* 207:2073–2079, 2010.
11. Brodin P, Karre K, Hoglund P: NK cell education: not an on-off switch but a tunable rheostat. *Trends Immunol* 30:143–149, 2009.
12. Feuchtinger T, Pfeiffer M, Pfaffle A, et al: Cytolytic activity of NK cell clones against acute childhood precursor-B-cell leukaemia is influenced by HLA class I expression on blasts and the differential KIR phenotype of NK clones. *Bone Marrow Transplant* 43:875–881, 2009.
13. Di Santo JP: Staying innate: transcription factor maintenance of innate lymphoid cell identity. *Immunol Rev* 261:169–176, 2014.
14. Horowitz A, Strauss-Albee DM, Leipold M, et al: Genetic and environmental determinants of human NK cell diversity revealed by mass cytometry. *Sci Transl Med* 5:208ra145, 2013.
15. Ruggeri L, Mancusi A, Burchielli E, et al: Effectiveness of donor natural killer cell alloreactivity in mismatched hematopoietic transplants. *Science* 295:2097–2100, 2002.
16. Brunstein CG, Wagner JE, Weisdorf DJ, et al: Negative effect of KIR alloreactivity in recipients of umbilical cord blood transplant depends on transplantation conditioning intensity. *Blood* 113:5628–5634, 2009.
17. Willemze R, Rodrigues CA, Labopin M, et al: KIR-ligand incompatibility in the graft-versus-host direction improves outcomes after umbilical cord blood transplantation for acute leukemia. *Leukemia* 23:492–500, 2009.
18. Venstrom JM, Zheng J, Noor N, et al: KIR and HLA genotypes are associated with disease progression and survival following autologous hematopoietic stem cell transplantation for high-risk neuroblastoma. *Clin Cancer Res* 15:7330–7334, 2009.
19. Yu J, Venstrom JM, Liu XR, et al: Breaking tolerance to self, circulating natural killer cells expressing inhibitory KIR for non-self HLA exhibit

effector function after T cell-depleted allogeneic hematopoietic cell transplantation. *Blood* 113:3875–3884, 2009.

20. Fauriat C, Ivarsson MA, Ljunggren HG, et al: Education of human natural killer cells by activating killer cell immunoglobulin-like receptors. *Blood* 115:1166–1174, 2010.

21. Foley B, Cooley S, Verneris MR, et al: NK cell education after allogeneic transplantation: dissociation between recovery of cytokine-producing and cytotoxic functions. *Blood* 118:2784–2792, 2011.

22. Cooley S, Trachtenberg E, Bergemann TL, et al: Donors with group B KIR haplotypes improve relapse-free survival after unrelated hematopoietic cell transplantation for acute myelogenous leukemia. *Blood* 113:726–732, 2009.

23. Cooley S, Weisdorf DJ, Guethlein LA, et al: Donor selection for natural killer cell receptor genes leads to superior survival after unrelated transplantation for acute myelogenous leukemia. *Blood* 116:2411–2419, 2010.

24. Cooley S, Weisdorf DJ, Guethlein LA, et al: Donor Killer Cell Ig-like Receptor B Haplotypes, Recipient HLA-C1, and HLA-C Mismatch Enhance the Clinical Benefit of Unrelated Transplantation for Acute Myelogenous Leukemia. *J Immunol* 192:4592–4600, 2014.

25. Venstrom JM, Pittari G, Gooley TA, et al: HLA-C-dependent prevention of leukemia relapse by donor activating KIR2DS1. *N Engl J Med* 367:805–816, 2012.

26. Impola U, Turpeinen H, Alakulppi N, et al: Donor Haplotype B of NK KIR Receptor Reduces the Relapse Risk in HLA-Identical Sibling Hematopoietic Stem Cell Transplantation of AML Patients. *Front Immunol* 5:405, 2014.

27. Delgado DC, Hank JA, Kolesar J, et al: Genotypes of NK cell KIR receptors, their ligands, and Fcgamma receptors in the response of neuroblastoma patients to Hu14.18-IL2 immunotherapy. *Cancer Res* 70:9554–9561, 2010.

28. Oevermann L, Michaelis SU, Mezger M, et al: KIR B haplotype donors confer a reduced risk of relapse after haploidentical transplantation in children with acute lymphoblastic leukemia. *Blood* 124:2744–2747, 2014.

29. Verneris MR, Miller JS: KIR B or not to be? … that is the question for ALL. *Blood* 124:2623–2624, 2014.

30. Gleason MK, Ross JA, Warlick ED, et al: CD16xCD33 bispecific killer cell engager (BiKE) activates NK cells against primary MDS and MDSC CD33+ targets. *Blood* 123:3016–3026, 2014.

30a. Gumá M, Angulo A, Vilches C, et al: Imprint of human cytomegalovirus infection on the NK cell receptor repertoire. *Blood* 104(12):3664–3671, 2004.

31. Foley B, Cooley S, Verneris MR, et al: Cytomegalovirus reactivation after allogeneic transplantation promotes a lasting increase in educated NKG2C+ natural killer cells with potent function. *Blood* 119:2665–2674, 2012.

32. Lopez-Verges S, Milush JM, Schwartz BS, et al: Expansion of a unique CD57(+)NKG2Chi natural killer cell subset during acute human cytomegalovirus infection. *Proc Natl Acad Sci USA* 108:14725–14732, 2011.

33. Lee J, Zhang T, Hwang I, et al: Epigenetic Modification and Antibody-Dependent Expansion of Memory-like NK Cells in Human Cytomegalovirus-Infected Individuals. *Immunity* 42:431–442, 2015.

34. Schlums H, Cichocki F, Tesi B, et al: Cytomegalovirus infection drives adaptive epigenetic diversification of NK cells with altered signaling and effector function. *Immunity* 42:443–456, 2015.

35. Elmaagacli AH, Steckel NK, Koldehoff M, et al: Early human cytomegalovirus replication after transplantation is associated with a decreased relapse risk: evidence for a putative virus-versus-leukemia effect in acute myeloid leukemia patients. *Blood* 118:1402–1412, 2011.

36. Green ML, Leisenring WM, Xie H, et al: CMV reactivation after allogeneic HCT and relapse risk: evidence for early protection in acute myeloid leukemia. *Blood* 122:1316–1324, 2013.

37. Romee R, Schneider SE, Leong JW, et al: Cytokine activation induces human memory-like NK cells. *Blood* 120:4751–4760, 2012.

37a. Miller JS, Soignier Y, Panoskaltsis-Mortari A, et al: Successful adoptive transfer and in vivo expansion of human haploidentical NK cells in patients with cancer. *Blood* 105(8):3051–3057, 2005.

38. Miller JS, Soignier Y, Panoskaltsis-Mortari A, et al: Successful adoptive transfer and in vivo expansion of human haploidentical NK cells in patients with cancer. *Blood* 105:3051–3057, 2005.

39. Bachanova V, Cooley S, Defor TE, et al: Clearance of acute myeloid leukemia by haploidentical natural killer cells is improved using IL-2 diphtheria toxin fusion protein. *Blood* 123:3855–3863, 2014.

40. Shah NN, Baird K, Delbrook CP, et al: Acute GVHD in patients receiving IL-15/4-1BBL activated NK cells following T-cell-depleted stem cell transplantation. *Blood* 125:784–792, 2015.

IMMUNE CHECKPOINT BLOCKADE IN HEMATOLOGIC MALIGNANCIES

Reid Merryman and Philippe Armand

INTRODUCTION

The acquisition of a malignant phenotype by a cell is accompanied by many genetic and epigenetic changes. These changes result in the generation of distinct antigens ("tumor neoantigens"), which can be potentially recognized by T-cell receptors (TCRs) and targeted by a cell-mediated immune response. T-cell activation is a complex and carefully regulated process governed by stimulatory and inhibitory signals from antigen presenting cells (APCs) and other cells in the surrounding microenvironment. Many inhibitory and costimulatory receptors, termed "immune checkpoints," have now been identified. Tumor cells are known to interfere with the normal operation of these pathways, providing a critical mechanism by which they can evade immune destruction. Our understanding of both the normal regulation of T-cell function and its dysregulation by malignant cells has accelerated greatly in recent years, allowing therapeutic intervention at the level of the immune synapse. The clinical development of immune checkpoint-blocking monoclonal antibodies (mAbs) now allows the therapeutic modulation of those pathways in vivo and the restoration of antitumor immune activity in patients. Already, antibodies for two targets—cytotoxic T lymphocyte-associated antigen 4 (CTLA-4) and the programmed cell death protein 1 (PD-1) pathway—have shown impressive efficacy in clinical trials. Several other targets are under investigation with promising preclinical and early clinical results (Fig. 102.1). Checkpoint blockade therapies (CBT) have been more extensively studied in solid malignancies, but a small number of early phase studies have generated exciting results in hematologic malignancies (HMs), particularly in Hodgkin lymphoma (HL). Given those early results, and the well-known susceptibility of many HMs to immunotherapy, illustrated by the success of allogeneic hematopoietic stem cell transplant (HSCT) across many HM subtypes, there is today a real hope that CBT could profoundly influence the treatment paradigms in HMs.

CYTOTOXIC T LYMPHOCYTE-ASSOCIATED ANTIGEN 4

CTLA-4, an inhibitory receptor expressed on T cells, was the first immune checkpoint receptor to be targeted for immunotherapy. Upon T-cell activation, CTLA-4 is generally upregulated, which results in the dampening of T-cell function through several mechanisms. First, CTLA-4 counteracts the costimulatory receptor CD28 by binding to their shared ligands CD80 and CD86 with greater affinity.[1] It triggers multiple inhibitory cell signaling pathways leading to T-cell anergy.[2,3] Finally, it downregulates the function of T-helper cells and enhances the action of regulatory T cells (Tregs) through mechanisms that are not yet fully understood.[1] The multifactorial actions of CTLA-4 underpin its importance in maintaining immune tolerance, which is demonstrated by the immune hyperactivation phenotype of the lethal CTLA-4 knockout mouse.[4]

Given its fundamental role in immune tolerance, CTLA-4 was a natural target for testing the concept of immune checkpoint blockade; however, the prospect of blocking CTLA-4 in humans also raised the specter of significant autoimmune toxicity. In fact, clinical trials of CTLA-4 blockade using the mAb ipilimumab (Bristol-Myers Squibb, Princeton, NJ, USA) in patients with melanoma showed not only a manageable safety profile but also an unprecedented overall survival benefit with significant rates of long-term survival.[5] Beyond melanoma, ipilimumab has also shown therapeutic benefit in prostate, pancreatic, and nonsmall-cell lung cancer cancers.[6–8] These results sparked interest in using CTLA-4 blockade in the treatment of HMs. In 2009, the first reported study, a phase 1 trial of ipilimumab in relapsed or refractory (R/R) non-Hodgkin lymphoma (NHL), demonstrated an 11% objective response rate (ORR). The response rate was less notable than the duration of the two clinical responses—a complete response (CR) in a patient with diffuse large B-cell lymphoma (DLBCL) lasting 31 months and a partial response (PR) in a patient with follicular lymphoma (FL) lasting 14 months.[9] Such durable responses with single agent therapy spurred interest in CTLA-4 blockade specifically and CBT in general within HMs. There are ongoing trials of ipilimumab in myeloid and lymphoid malignancies (NCT01757639, NCT01896999, NCT01729806). In addition, ipilimumab has shown promise for the postallogeneic transplant relapse setting, where it may augment the graft-versus-tumor (GVT) effect, as discussed later.

Importantly, early clinical results in HMs suggested that immune-related adverse events (irAEs) with ipilimumab are similar to those seen in solid malignancies. Continued observation and reporting will be necessary to ensure that rates of pneumonitis, colitis, dermatitis, endocrinopathies, and other immune side effects are generally manageable in HMs, as they appear to be in solid malignancies.

PROGRAMMED CELL DEATH PROTEIN 1

PD-1 is an inhibitory immune checkpoint receptor expressed on T cells and other lymphocytes. Like CTLA-4, PD-1 is upregulated upon T-cell activation. When bound to one of its two ligands (PD-L1 or PD-L2), it inhibits T-cell activation via phosphatase activity in a mechanism that appears to be distinct from that of CTLA-4.[2] In addition to CD8+ effector T cells, PD-1 is expressed on Tregs where it promotes their proliferation and downregulation of immune responses.[10] PD-1 is expressed on tumor-infiltrating lymphocytes across many different types of tumors, and its ligands PD-L1 and PD-L2 are upregulated in many different tumors.[10–12] In contrast to CTLA-4, which regulates early phases of T-cell activation, the PD-1 pathway appears to be most important during the effector phase of T-cell activation that occurs within the tumor microenvironment.[10] It was therefore hoped that PD-1 blockade would provide a more targeted immune-enhancing approach at a later stage of T-cell activation and therefore result in lower rates of irAEs compared with CTLA-4 blockade.

Like CTLA-4, PD-1 blockade showed important therapeutic activity in melanoma, where phase III studies have shown benefit in heavily pretreated patients.[13] Trials of PD-1 and PD-L1 blockade have also demonstrated benefit in nonsmall-cell lung cancer, RCC, and other solid malignancies.[14–16] Multiple mAbs against PD-1 and PD-L1 have been developed and are in different stages of investigation. At this time, three PD-1 inhibitors—nivolumab (Bristol-Myers Squibb, Princeton, NJ, USA), pembrolizumab (Merck, Kenilworth, NJ, USA), and pidilizumab (CureTech, Yavne, Israel)—have been studied in published trials in HMs, with preliminary

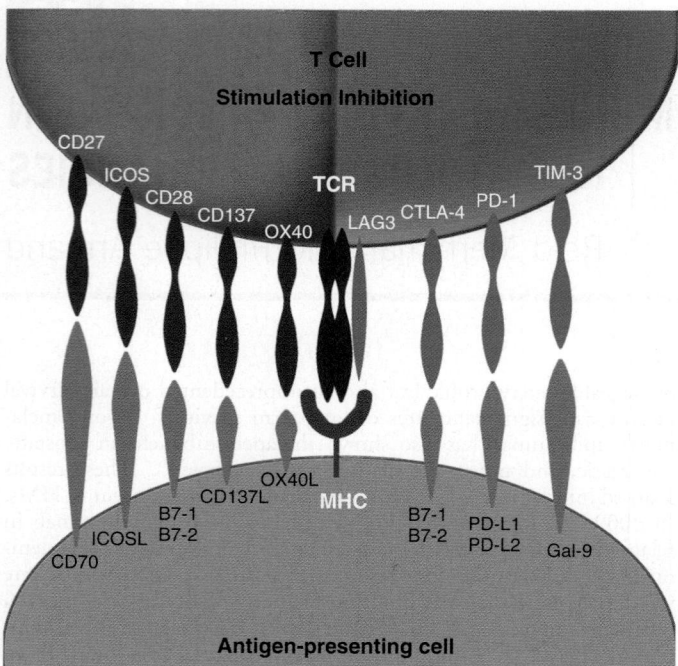

Fig. 102.1 COSTIMULATORY AND INHIBITORY RECEPTORS. A partial list of stimulatory and inhibitory T-cell coreceptors currently in clinical development with their cognate ligands. *MHC,* Major histocompatibility complex; *TCR,* T-cell receptor.

results hinting at the potential therapeutic effectiveness of this approach.

Hodgkin Lymphoma

Among all HMs, there was particular interest in using PD-1 blockade in HL. HL is unique among lymphomas for its tissue architecture, which is composed of relatively rare Reed-Sternberg (RS) tumor cells surrounded by a much larger population of immune infiltrating cells that appear unable to generate an anti-RS cell activity. Genetic analyses of HL demonstrated frequent 9p24.1 amplification, driving increased expression of both PD-L1 and PD-L2, as well as increased activity of the Janus activated kinase/signal transducer and activator of transcription (JAK/STAT) pathway, which itself leads to increased expression of PD-L1.[17] Epstein-Barr virus (EBV) infection, which occurs relatively commonly in HL, is also associated with increased PD-L1 expression.[18] These mechanisms explain the high rates of PD-L1 and PD-L2 expression seen in HL and, additionally, suggest that this upregulation may be more fixed than in other tumors.

Based on these observations, patients with HL were included in independent expansion cohorts in two phase 1 trials examining PD-1 blockade with nivolumab (NCT01592370) and pembrolizumab (NCT01953692) within a mixed group of patients with R/R HMs. HL patients in both studies were heavily pretreated, with the majority having relapsed or progressed after brentuximab and autologous stem cell transplantation. Despite this, CR rates of 17% and 21% and ORRs of 87% and 65% were seen with nivolumab and pembrolizumab, respectively. The durability of responses with single-agent therapy have also been impressive with ongoing responses for greater than 1 year in many patients. Importantly, the mAbs in both trials showed an acceptable safety profile in HL with limited irAEs and no drug-related grade 4 or 5 toxicities.[19,20] While these trials were small and merit confirmation, they have generated hope that PD-1 blockade could bring about a fundamental shift in the treatment of R/R HL. As more clinical data accumulate, PD-1 blockade will likely move to earlier stages of treatment. Additional studies are planned and ongoing within HL.

Non-Hodgkin Lymphoma

While PD-1 blockade has shown the most promise in HL, clinical activity has also been seen in multiple types of NHL including FL, DLBCL, and T-cell lymphoma. Interest in CBT in NHL has been driven by the durable responses seen with ipilimumab,[9] as well as by an early study of pidilizumab in patients with R/R HMs that demonstrated an isolated CR in a patient with FL.[21] Based on these results, a phase II trial examined combination therapy with pidilizumab and rituximab in patients with rituximab-sensitive relapsed FL. Among 32 patients, the ORR was 66%, with a 52% CR rate.[22] While it is difficult to assess the activity of this combination without a monotherapy control arm, these rates compare favorably with historic controls treated with rituximab alone. In addition, immunohistochemical analysis showed that PD-1 expression was significantly higher on T cells of responders, mechanistically supporting the role of PD-1 activity in the combination.[22] Preliminary results from the previously mentioned phase 1 nivolumab trial (NCT01592370) also demonstrated activity in FL and DLBCL with OR rates of 40% and 36%, respectively.[23] The underlying biology of PD-1 blockade in these malignancies is less well understood. In general, FL is considered to be one of the more immune sensitive HMs based on occasionally witnessed spontaneous regressions and responsiveness to nonspecific immune activators like bacillus Calmette-Guérin and interleukin-2.[22] Because of this, it is an attractive target for PD-1 blockade and immune checkpoint blockade in general. Within DLBCL, PD-L1 expression appears to be restricted to a subset of tumors, as discussed later, which could explain the activity seen with nivolumab. Larger phase II studies in FL and DLBCL are ongoing. Lastly, the phase 1 nivolumab trial also demonstrated a 17% ORR in a mixed population of T-cell NHLs.[23] The significance of these findings is not yet clear, but this represents an exciting new area of investigation for an otherwise difficult to treat, chemorefractory group of malignancies.

Multiple Myeloma

Multiple myeloma (MM) has been included in trials of PD-1 blockade based on preclinical data showing PD-L1 expression on MM cells and PD-1 upregulation on immune cells in the MM microenvironment.[24,25] Despite these observations, early data obtained with PD-1 blockade has been disappointing. In the phase 1 nivolumab trial, no CRs or PRs were observed in 27 patients with MM; however, 18 of 27 (67%) had stable disease lasting several months.[23] CBT experience in solid tumors suggests that such stable disease may reflect antitumor activity and provide sustained periods of disease control; more investigation is needed in MM to determine if there is indeed a true clinical benefit from CBT. Based on these early results, PD-1 blockade is being investigated in early phase trials as part of combination therapy with lenalidomide, pomalidomide, and a novel Bruton tyrosine kinase inhibitor (NCT02077959, NCT02289222, NCT02362035).

Safety

In the limited experience with PD-1 blockade in HMs, the safety profile of the drugs appears to be comparable with the more extensive experience in solid malignancies. IrAEs with PD-1 therapy appear to be less common than with CTLA-4 blockade, specifically with lower rates of colitis and endocrinopathies. Within the phase 1 nivolumab, the largest trial published thus far in HM, the rate of pneumonitis was around 10%, which is only slightly higher than that seen in solid malignancies, despite high rates of prior treatment with potentially pneumotoxic regimens (including radiation therapy and brentuximab).[23] Additional studies are clearly needed, but these results suggest that PD-1 blockade is generally tolerable for patients with HM.

CHECKPOINT BLOCKADE THERAPIES AFTER HEMATOPOIETIC STEM CELL TRANSPLANTATION

HSCT, using autologous or allogeneic grafts, is an important part of the treatment of many HMs, and may provide a fruitful setting for CBT. In the case of autologous HSCT, the minimal disease burden and presence of a remodeled immune system with a relative preponderance in the early post-HSCT period of immune cells that are targets of CBT, like natural killer (NK) cells and T-effector cells,[26] may allow the effective leveraging of CBT. PD-1 blockade has already been studied after autologous transplant in DLBCL. In an international phase 2 study, 72 patients with DLBCL received three doses of pidilizumab beginning 1–3 months after autologous stem cell transplant. Progression-free survival at 18 months after HSCT was 72%, higher than the 52% rate observed in a similar historic control cohort. Notably, the rate of progression-free survival among the higher risk group of patients with positron emission tomography (PET)-positive disease before transplant was 70%. In addition, among the 35 patients with measurable disease after transplant, the overall response rate after pidilizumab was 51% (CR, 34%). Importantly, pidilizumab was well tolerated without significant irAEs.[27] Together, these findings suggest that PD-1 blockade may have direct antitumor activity and important clinical activity in the postautologous transplant setting, warranting additional studies. Based on these promising early results, there are now several ongoing trials of PD-1 blockade after autologous transplant in HL, DLBCL, and MM (NCT02362997, NCT02181738, NCT02038933, and NCT02331368).

Allogeneic HSCT also represents an attractive, if challenging, field in which to deploy CBT. This form of transplantation is an important part of treatment for many HMs, as the attendant GVT effect may be salutary in patients who are not curable with conventional chemotherapy or autologous HSCT. Yet failure to develop an effective GVT occurs frequently, manifesting as postallogeneic HSCT relapse, and the outcomes for those patients are usually dismal. The postallogeneic transplant setting is attractive for CBT because the treatment strategy is already based on immune manipulation. CBT was studied in this context in a phase 1 study of ipilimumab in patients with recurrent or progressive disease after allogeneic transplant. Remarkably, ipilimumab did not induce significant graft-versus-host disease (GVHD) and the rate of irAEs did not differ greatly from that seen outside of the transplant setting. In addition, objective responses were seen in three patients including two sustained CRs in patients with HL.[28] In a follow-up study investigating repeated dosing of ipilimumab in the posttransplant relapse setting, 6 of 27 patients have achieved formal responses including 4 CRs in acute myeloid leukemia and 2 PRs in patients with MM and HL. These responses are notable given that these patients had been highly pretreated including some who had received prior donor lymphocyte infusion after posttransplant relapse. They suggest an important potential role for CBT after allogeneic transplant. With repeated dosing, ipilimumab did result in increased irAEs, including two patients with grade 4 pneumonitis, three cases of GVHD, and one treatment-related death.[29] In most cases, however, AEs were manageable and did not prevent continued treatment with ipilimumab; however, safety of CBT in this setting will need to be carefully monitored.

LESSONS FROM CTLA-4 AND PD-1 BLOCKADE

Selection of Tumors and Patients

Unlike CTLA-4, the expression of PD-1 and its ligands varies widely across tumor types and patients. Differences in expression have been helpful in predicting the responses to PD-1 blockade in solid tumors, and those lessons may be instructive for the development of CBT in

HM and for targeting of other immune checkpoints. Initial studies in solid malignancies suggested that tumors with demonstrable PD-L1 expression on the tumor cell surface had higher response rates to PD-1 blockade[30,31]; at first look, this pattern seems to also hold in HMs, as response rates have been highest in HL where PD-L1 expression is very frequent.[32] However, in solid tumors, patients whose tumors did not demonstrate PD-L1 expression have also had meaningful responses, suggesting that PD-L1 expression should not yet be used to exclude patients from clinical trials.

Indeed, variation in tumor cell surface expression of PD-L1 is unlikely to entirely explain the apparent differences in clinical response to PD-1 blockade among HL, various NHLs, and MM. PD-L1 expression is a highly dynamic process that varies with time and environment and is likely poorly captured by isolated in vitro tumor biopsy analyses. Tumor-cell ligand expression also ignores the important role of immune cells in the tumor microenvironment whose expression of PD-1 and its ligands may affect response to therapy. While its role is less clearly delineated, PD-L2 may also be an important predictive marker for response to PD-1 blockade. PD-L2 amplification is uncommon in solid malignancies, but it is overexpressed in HL, primary mediastinal large B-cell lymphoma (PMBL), and some T-cell lymphomas.[12,23] Lastly, the impressive response rates in HL also suggest that the *mechanism* of PD-L1 overexpression may be important; in the case of HL, constitutive overexpression of PD-L1/2 driven by EBV infection or genetic amplification events may result in a unique dependence on the PD-1 signaling pathway for survival, which could underlie HL's high vulnerability to PD-1 blockade. This phenomenon occurs in a few other HMs: there are virally-driven DLBCL and T-cell NHL subtypes, which appear to also show very frequent PD-L1 surface expression; and a specific NHL subtype, PMBL, which also harbors frequent 9p24.1 amplification and concomitant PD-L1 and PD-L2 expression.[12,32] Those tumor subtypes are very attractive targets for PD-1 blockade, as is being explored in ongoing trials.

Treatment Setting

Clinical experience with CBT in HMs thus far has been limited to the R/R setting; however, treatment will likely move to earlier stages of diseases in the coming years, at least in HL. This transition has several important implications. Published trials have used CBT to augment the immune response of patients who have received numerous rounds of cytotoxic therapy. In newly diagnosed patients who have relatively normal immune function, responses may be significantly different. For this reason, earlier treatment with CBT may result in a more robust antitumor immune response. At the same time, it may also increase the incidence and severity of irAEs. Continued investigation is critical to determine how the setting of treatment will alter its efficacy and tolerability.

At this time, there is limited but exciting experience with CBT after HSCT. Yet if continued investigations confirm the early results, post-HSCT CBT may become an important part of transplantation, and may affect both the efficacy of HSCT and its place in the treatment course of patients with HMs.

Endpoint Definition

Early trials in CBT in solid malignancies showed that patients occasionally had evidence of progression before a response, longer times to CR than with traditional treatments, and long-term disease stability despite meeting traditional criteria for progressive disease.[30] As a result, new response criteria, the immune-related response criteria, were proposed for solid malignancies to account for different radiographic responses to therapy and to prevent early withdrawal of treatment from patients who might eventually show a response.[33] Hints of a similar pattern of delayed radiographic responses and disease stability have been seen in HMs. For example, 21% of patients had a delayed response (4 months or more after initiation of therapy) in a trial of pidilizumab in FL.[22] With the rapid growth of CBT trials in HM, there may soon be enough data to establish patterns of response by computed tomography (CT) and PET imaging, which can be used to revise response criteria for treatment with CBT.

FUTURE DIRECTIONS

Beyond CTLA-4 and PD-1

The interaction between T cells and tumor cells is complex, and our understanding of the inhibitory and costimulatory receptors that govern T-cell response is rapidly growing. With the success of CTLA-4 and PD-1 blockade, there is great interest in many of the other checkpoint receptors that regulate T-cell activation. For some of these receptors, mAbs have been developed and are in early stages of clinical development. Killer immunoglobulin-like receptor (KIR) is an inhibitory receptor found on NK cells. Similar to PD-1 and CTLA-4 on effector T cells, KIR is believed to facilitate evasion from NK cell-mediated immune destruction. Phase 1 trials of the Anti-KIR monoclonal antibody, lirilumab (Bristol-Myers Squibb, Princeton, NJ, USA), in MM and acute myeloid leukemia have demonstrated satisfactory tolerability and safety,[34,35] and additional studies are underway (NCT 01248455, NCT01687387). Lymphocyte activation gene 3 (LAG-3), an inhibitory immune checkpoint receptor, is currently being targeted in a phase 1 trial in R/R HMs (NCT02061761). Another inhibitory receptor, CD27, is being targeted by the mAb varlilumab (Celldex Therapeutics, Hampton, NJ, USA) in a phase 1 trial in HMs with a documented PR in a patient with HL (NCT01460134). Multiple costimulatory receptors have also been targeted and are in early trials. Urelumab (Bristol-Myers Squibb, Princeton, NJ, USA), an anti-CD137 monoclonal antibody, is under investigation in a phase I trial with rituximab in patients with R/R B-cell malignancies (NCT01775631). In addition, an anti-Ox40L mAb is currently being studied in combination with PD-1 or CTLA-4 blockade in HMs in a phase 1 trial (NCT02205333). As our understanding of immune checkpoint blockade expands, it is likely that additional targeted therapies will reach the clinic in the coming years.

Concepts in Combination Therapy

With early trials demonstrating safety and efficacy for CBT, checkpoint-blocking antibodies are being combined together and with other antitumor therapies including cytotoxic drugs, targeted therapies, radiation therapy, and other forms of immunotherapy. This approach may lead to responses across a broader group of HMs than is possible with single-agent therapy.

Cytotoxic and targeted therapies may have a synergistic effect with checkpoint-blocking antibodies by increasing tumor antigen presentation and thereby stimulating immune destruction. On the other hand, there is uncertainty regarding how cytotoxic and targeted therapies, many of which deplete lymphocyte populations, will affect CBT, as the latter depends on intact effector T-cell function for its antitumor effect. For this reason, the timing of combination therapy may be important to maximize benefits. Combination therapy in FL with pidilizumab and rituximab was well tolerated with suggestion of increased clinical efficacy,[22] but experience with combination therapy in both solid and HMs is very limited. Again, ongoing trials in HMs may provide an early answer, as several trials are currently combining checkpoint-blocking antibodies with other agents including anti-CD19 and anti-CD20 in NHL (NCT02271945, NCT02220842), lenalidomide, and a novel Bruton tyrosine kinase inhibitor in MM (NCT02077959, NCT02362035), brentuximab in HL (NCT01896999), and dasatinib in chronic myeloid leukemia (NCT02011945).

Local radiation therapy likely also increases tumor antigen presentation through tumor cell destruction and may have less systemic immunosuppressive effects. A retrospective series in melanoma reported an abscopal effect, whereby local radiation therapy in combination with CBT resulted in significant improvement in systemic disease control.[36] Combination therapy with local radiation therapy and ipilimumab in low-grade B-cell lymphomas is currently being investigated in a phase 1 trial (NCT02254772).

Another combination strategy is dual blockade with two immune checkpoint-blocking antibodies to further augment antitumor immune function. As discussed previously, T-cell activation is governed by numerous receptors and while CTLA-4 and PD-1 are critical actors, changes in expression of other checkpoint receptors may be sufficient to overcome single receptor blockade. The mechanism of immune evasion for patients failing CBT is not yet well understood, but could involve upregulation of alternative checkpoint receptors. Supporting this theory, a recent study in melanoma revealed that mice treated with CTLA-4 blockade and radiotherapy increased expression of PD-L1 in an apparent escape pathway from CTLA-4 blockade.[37] Additional knowledge of the pattern and frequency of these escape pathways will be useful in planning combination therapy.

Dual therapy with PD-1 and CTLA-4 blockade has shown tolerability and clinical benefit in a phase 1 study in melanoma.[38] Several phase 1 trials are underway in HMs including combination therapy with nivolumab and urelumab in NHL (NCT02253992) an anti-Ox40L mAb and a PD-L1 inhibitor in aggressive B-cell lymphomas (NCT02205333), and nivolumab plus ipilimumab or lirilumab in R/R HMs (NCT01592370). Results from those studies are eagerly anticipated to chart the future course of combination CBT.

Finally, CBT could be combined with other types of immunotherapies including tumor vaccines, oncolytic viral therapies, bispecific antibodies, and chimeric antigen receptor T cells. While there are very few results of this strategy at present, a murine study combining tumor vaccine and pidilizumab in MM,[39] and early results from a clinical trial in humans suggest that future efforts are worth pursuing.[40]

CONCLUSION

Immune checkpoint blockade therapy targeting CTLA-4 and PD-1 has shown impressive results in early trials in several types of HMs. The dramatic response rates seen with PD-1 blockade in HL may not be easily replicated in other HMs. However, with judicious selection of tumor targets, of treatment setting, of combination partner(s), with appropriate endpoint assessment, and with diligently and collaboratively pursued correlative studies, there is hope that CBT-based therapy may in the near future, fundamentally alter the treatment paradigm for many HMs.

REFERENCES

1. Pardoll DM: The blockade of immune checkpoints in cancer immunotherapy. *Nat Rev Cancer* 12(4):252–264, 2012.
2. Parry RV, et al: CTLA-4 and PD-1 receptors inhibit T-cell activation by distinct mechanisms. *Mol Cell Biol* 25(21):9543–9553, 2005.
3. Schneider H, et al: Reversal of the TCR stop signal by CTLA-4. *Science* 313(5795):1972–1975, 2006.
4. Tivol EA, et al: Loss of CTLA-4 leads to massive lymphoproliferation and fatal multiorgan tissue destruction, revealing a critical negative regulatory role of CTLA-4. *Immunity* 3(5):541–547, 1995.
5. Hodi FS, et al: Improved survival with ipilimumab in patients with metastatic melanoma. *N Engl J Med* 363(8):711–723, 2010.
6. Kwon ED, et al: Ipilimumab versus placebo after radiotherapy in patients with metastatic castration-resistant prostate cancer that had progressed after docetaxel chemotherapy (CA184-043): a multicentre, randomised, double-blind, phase 3 trial. *Lancet Oncol* 15(7):700–712, 2014.
7. Le DT, et al: Evaluation of ipilimumab in combination with allogeneic pancreatic tumor cells transfected with a GM-CSF gene in previously treated pancreatic cancer. *J Immunother* 36(7):382–389, 2013.
8. Lynch TJ, et al: Ipilimumab in combination with paclitaxel and carboplatin as first-line treatment in stage IIIB/IV non-small-cell lung cancer:

results from a randomized, double-blind, multicenter phase II study. *J Clin Oncol* 30(17):2046–2054, 2012.

9. Ansell SM, et al: Phase I study of ipilimumab, an anti-CTLA-4 monoclonal antibody, in patients with relapsed and refractory B-cell non-Hodgkin lymphoma. *Clin Cancer Res* 15(20):6446–6453, 2009.

10. Dong H, et al: Tumor-associated B7-H1 promotes T-cell apoptosis: a potential mechanism of immune evasion. *Nat Med* 8(8):793–800, 2002.

11. Ahmadzadeh M, et al: Tumor antigen-specific CD8 T cells infiltrating the tumor express high levels of PD-1 and are functionally impaired. *Blood* 114(8):1537–1544, 2009.

12. Rosenwald A, et al: Molecular diagnosis of primary mediastinal B cell lymphoma identifies a clinically favorable subgroup of diffuse large B cell lymphoma related to Hodgkin lymphoma. *J Exp Med* 198(6):851–862, 2003.

13. Weber JS, D'Angelo SP, Minor D, et al: Nivolumab versus chemotherapy in patients with advanced melanoma who progressed after anti-CTLA-4 treatment (CheckMate 037): a randomized, controlled, open-label, phase 3 trial. *Lancet Oncol* 4:375–384, 2015.

14. Topalian SL, et al: Safety, activity, and immune correlates of anti-PD-1 antibody in cancer. *N Engl J Med* 366(26):2443–2454, 2012.

15. Powles T, et al: MPDL3280A (anti-PD-L1) treatment leads to clinical activity in metastatic bladder cancer. *Nature* 515(7528):558–562, 2014.

16. Brahmer JR, et al: Safety and activity of anti-PD-L1 antibody in patients with advanced cancer. *N Engl J Med* 366(26):2455–2465, 2012.

17. Green MR, et al: Integrative analysis reveals selective 9p24.1 amplification, increased PD-1 ligand expression, and further induction via JAK2 in nodular sclerosing Hodgkin lymphoma and primary mediastinal large B-cell lymphoma. *Blood* 116(17):3268–3277, 2010.

18. Green MR, et al: Constitutive AP-1 activity and EBV infection induce PD-L1 in Hodgkin lymphomas and posttransplant lymphoproliferative disorders: implications for targeted therapy. *Clin Cancer Res* 18(6):1611–1618, 2012.

19. Ansell SM, et al: PD-1 blockade with nivolumab in relapsed or refractory Hodgkin's lymphoma. *N Engl J Med* 372(4):311–319, 2015.

20. Moskowitz CH, Ribrag V, Michot J-M, et al: PD-1 Blockade with the Monoclonal Antibody Pembrolizumab (MK-3475) in Patients with Classical Hodgkin Lymphoma after Brentuximab Vedotin Failure: Preliminary Results from a Phase 1b Study (KEYNOTE-013). *Blood* 124:290, 2014.

21. Berger R, et al: Phase I safety and pharmacokinetic study of CT-011, a humanized antibody interacting with PD-1, in patients with advanced hematologic malignancies. *Clin Cancer Res* 14(10):3044–3051, 2008.

22. Westin JR, et al: Safety and activity of PD1 blockade by pidilizumab in combination with rituximab in patients with relapsed follicular lymphoma: a single group, open-label, phase 2 trial. *Lancet Oncol* 15(1):69–77, 2014.

23. Lesokhin AM, Ansell SM, Armand P, et al: Preliminary Results of a Phase I Study of Nivolumab (BMS-936558) in Patients with Relapsed or Refractory Lymphoid Malignancies. *Blood* (ASH Annual Meeting Meeting Abstracts) 124:291, 2014.

24. Liu J, et al: Plasma cells from multiple myeloma patients express B7-H1 (PD-L1) and increase expression after stimulation with IFN-{gamma}

and TLR ligands via a MyD88-, TRAF6-, and MEK-dependent pathway. *Blood* 110(1):296–304, 2007.

25. Yousef S, et al: Immunomodulatory molecule PD-L1 is expressed on malignant plasma cells and myeloma-propagating pre-plasma cells in the bone marrow of multiple myeloma patients. *Blood Cancer J* 5:e285, 2015.

26. Porrata LF, Litzow MR, Markovic SN: Immune reconstitution after autologous hematopoietic stem cell transplantation. *Mayo Clin Proc* 76(4):407–412, 2001.

27. Armand P, et al: Disabling immune tolerance by programmed death-1 blockade with pidilizumab after autologous hematopoietic stem-cell transplantation for diffuse large B-cell lymphoma: results of an international phase II trial. *J Clin Oncol* 31(33):4199–4206, 2013.

28. Bashey A, et al: CTLA4 blockade with ipilimumab to treat relapse of malignancy after allogeneic hematopoietic cell transplantation. *Blood* 113(7):1581–1588, 2009.

29. Davids MS, Kim HT, Costello C, et al: A Multicenter Phase I Study of CTLA4 Blockade with Ipilimumab for Relapsed Hematologic Malignancies after Allogeneic Hematopoietic Cell Transplantation. *Blood* 214:3964, 2014.

30. Postow MA, Callahan MK, Wolchok JD: Immune Checkpoint Blockade in Cancer Therapy. *J Clin Oncol* 2015.

31. Taube JM, et al: Association of PD-1, PD-1 ligands, and other features of the tumor immune microenvironment with response to anti-PD-1 therapy. *Clin Cancer Res* 20(19):5064–5074, 2014.

32. Chen BJ, et al: PD-L1 expression is characteristic of a subset of aggressive B-cell lymphomas and virus-associated malignancies. *Clin Cancer Res* 19(13):3462–3473, 2013.

33. Wolchok JD, et al: Guidelines for the evaluation of immune therapy activity in solid tumors: immune-related response criteria. *Clin Cancer Res* 15(23):7412–7420, 2009.

34. Benson DM, Jr, et al: A phase 1 trial of the anti-KIR antibody IPH2101 in patients with relapsed/refractory multiple myeloma. *Blood* 120(22):4324–4333, 2012.

35. Vey N, et al: A phase 1 trial of the anti-inhibitory KIR mAb IPH2101 for AML in complete remission. *Blood* 120(22):4317–4323, 2012.

36. Grimaldi AM, et al: Abscopal effects of radiotherapy on advanced melanoma patients who progressed after ipilimumab immunotherapy. *Oncoimmunology* 3:e28780, 2014.

37. Twyman-Saint Victor C, et al: Radiation and dual checkpoint blockade activate non-redundant immune mechanisms in cancer. *Nature* 2015.

38. Wolchok JD, et al: Nivolumab plus ipilimumab in advanced melanoma. *N Engl J Med* 369(2):122–133, 2013.

39. Rosenblatt J, et al: PD-1 blockade by CT-011, anti-PD-1 antibody, enhances ex vivo T-cell responses to autologous dendritic cell/myeloma fusion vaccine. *J Immunother* 34(5):409–418, 2011.

40. Rosenblatt J, Avivi I, Vasir D, et al: Blockade of PD-1 in Combination with Dendritic Cell/Myeloma Fusion Cell Vaccination Following Autologous Stem Cell Transplantation. *Biol Blood Marrow Transplant* 19:2013.

PART

X

TRANSPLANTATION

OVERVIEW AND CHOICE OF DONOR OF HEMATOPOIETIC STEM CELL TRANSPLANTATION

Helen E. Heslop

Since the first hematopoietic stem cell transplants (HSCTs) were performed more than 50 years ago, this modality has become a well-established therapeutic option for many hematologic malignancies as well as for bone marrow (BM) failure states, immune deficiencies, and inborn errors of metabolism (Table 103.1).[1,2] The wider application of allogeneic transplantation has been possible because of increased knowledge of the genetic basis of histocompatibility and advances in molecular methodology to more accurately type donors and recipients. In addition, the development of large donor registries and cord blood banks has expanded access to transplant as well as increasing the likelihood that a recipient will find a well-matched donor.[3]

Over the last 20 years, there has also been identification of additional sources of stem cells so that BM, peripheral blood (PB), and umbilical cord blood (UCB) are all widely used in clinical practice to provide long-term hematopoietic reconstitution. The increasing use of reduced-intensity conditioning regimens has made transplant an option for older patients and patients with comorbidities. Finally, there have been improvements in graft-versus-host disease (GVHD) prophylaxis and supportive care during the period of hematopoietic and immune suppression after transplant. Allogeneic HSCT should therefore be considered for patients in whom this procedure is likely to result in superior long-term disease-free survival (DFS) compared with other therapeutic modalities. Potential candidates must also have a suitable source of hematopoietic stem cells (HSCs) available at an appropriate time in the course of the disease.

This chapter provides an overview of HSCT procedures, including conditioning regimens, selection of donor and HSC source, and common early and late posttransplant complications. These topics are discussed in depth in Chapters 104 to 109, and the disease specific indications are discussed in the relevant disease chapters (see Table 103.1 for details). Technical aspects of transplant, including HSC harvesting and cell processing, are discussed in Chapters 95 and 97.

ALLOGENEIC TRANSPLANTATION

Allogeneic transplant is a potential treatment for patients with relapsed or high-risk hematologic malignancy as well as for patients with inherited and acquired disorders of the hemopoietic and immune systems. The goal is to replace the recipient's hemopoietic and immune systems with normal HSCs from a closely matched donor whose hematopoietic stem and progenitor cells obtained from donor BM or other sources can home to the recipient's hematopoietic microenvironment and engraft. The major criteria for choosing an allogeneic donor is the degree of histocompatibility between the donor and recipient because the risks of both graft rejection and of GVHD increase with the degree of genetic disparity. The most important determinant of alloreactivity is matching at loci in the major histocompatibility complex (MHC) that includes human leukocyte antigens (HLA), encoded by class I (*HLA-A*, *HLA-B*, and *HLA-C*) and class II (*HLA-DR*, *HLA-DQ*, and *HLA-DP*) genes. HLA molecules were originally defined by serology, but molecular testing is now routine because gene sequencing has revealed multiple alleles for most serologically defined specificities (see Chapter 105).[4]

Other determinants include minor histocompatibility antigens, which are naturally processed peptides derived from normal cellular proteins that can stimulate an MHC-restricted response when different polymorphisms are present in donor and recipient. Natural killer (NK) cells may also contribute to alloreactivity, particularly in the setting of haploidentical transplantation (Chapter 101).[5] There is also increasing evidence that genetic loci outside of the MHC may influence the risk of transplant complications such as infection or regimen-related mortality, and several groups have undertaken genome-wide association assays to define genetic variants that might predict these complications.[6]

Donor Choice

The choice of donor for an allogeneic HSCT depends on several factors, including donor choices, the urgency of the transplant, and the patient's disease status. The optimal donor is a matched sibling sharing HLA class I and HLA class II alleles, but because each child inherits one set of paternal and one set of maternal HLA antigens, the likelihood of any sibling matching is only 25%. For patients who lack such donors, other options include a closely matched unrelated or cord donor or a haploidentical family member. Development of high-resolution molecular tissue typing methods and establishment of large donor registries have facilitated transplants from closely HLA-matched unrelated donors. These volunteer donors are healthy individuals between 18 and 60 years of age who fulfill eligibility requirements similar to those applied to blood donors. With increasing registry size, the chance of finding a donor has increased, so that more than 70% of Caucasian patients can identify an HLA-A, B, C, and DRB1 allele-matched unrelated donor.[7] The likelihood of finding a donor matching at these eight loci (or 10 loci if matching at DQB1 is also included) varies for different ethnic groups and is less for groups with more polymorphism of HLA antigens.[3] The initial results of transplantation from unrelated donors were inferior to those seen after matched sibling transplantation because of increased incidences of graft rejection and of GVHD caused by the greater genetic disparity. Over the past decade, though, results have gradually improved in both single-center and multicenter registry studies, reflecting better donor–recipient matching and advances in GVHD prophylaxis and supportive care.[7] A recent study has examined donor characteristics that predict outcome and found that after adjustment for patient disease and comorbidities when the donor was a 10/10 match, there was a significantly improved survival if the donor was young (aged 18–32 years).[8] Indeed for every 10-year increment in donor age, there was a 5.5% increase in the hazard ratio for overall mortality.[8] Overall donor age is the most important factor after donor–recipient HLA match when selecting an unrelated donor.

For a patient who lacks a matched sibling or 10/10 matched unrelated donor, the options are a mismatched unrelated donor, a haploidentical donor, or a cord, and each choice has benefits and disadvantages (Table 103.2).[9] One limitation of unrelated donor transplant is the time required to identify and screen an unrelated donor, which can be up to 3–6 months. Cord units by contrast can be obtained within 1 week of identifying a suitable matched unit while almost everyone has a haploidentical donor who is usually highly motivated and available for additional products. This source also has the potential for more graft-versus-tumor effects because of increased alloreactivity and the potential for a beneficial killer-cell immunoglobulin-like receptor mismatch. A haploidentical donor also has a lower "cost of goods" for procurement of the product. Several studies have compared outcomes of mismatched unrelated,

cord, and haploidentical donor transplants, but they do not show a definitive advantage for either source of HSCs.[9,10] Most transplant units have therefore developed algorithms for donor selection based on local experience and patient characteristics such as size and disease.

Autologous Transplantation

In autologous transplantation the recipient's own HSCs are collected then reinfused after high-dose chemotherapy to produce hemopoietic reconstitution. This approach allows dose intensification in settings where there is a correlation between dose and tumor response rate and hematopoietic toxicity is a limiting factor for dose intensification. HSCs are harvested and cryopreserved and then reinfused after doses of chemotherapy and radiotherapy that would otherwise be lethal or require a prolonged period of recovery. In general, autologous transplant is well tolerated, and data from the Center for International Bone Marrow Transplant Research (CIBMTR) show that the 100-day mortality rate is less than 5%.[8] The major cause of failure after autologous transplant is relapse of the primary disease. One longer-term concern is that recipients of autologous transplant have an increased risk of secondary therapy-related myeloid leukemia or myelodysplastic syndromes (t-MDS/acute myeloid leukemia [AML]) although this may also reflect effects of previous treatment. Indeed, a study that identified a pattern of altered gene expression in patients who developed t-MDS/AML after transplant for lymphoma found that the genetic programs associated with t-MDS/AML are perturbed pre transplant.[11]

The most common indications for autologous transplant are currently myeloma, non-Hodgkin lymphoma, and Hodgkin lymphoma, in which it has been shown in randomized trials or concluded in evidence-based reviews that dose intensification and hemopoietic rescue result in improved DFS.[12,13] Patients with newly diagnosed myeloma who are considered potential candidates for autologous transplant autologous stem cell transplantation are usually treated with two to four cycles of therapy that usually includes an immuno-modulatory agent and a proteasome inhibitor before proceeding to autograft.[14] High- or intermediate-dose melphalan is the most widely used conditioning regimen with patients who are younger than the age of 65 years and do not have significant comorbidities receiving high-dose regimens (200 mg/m^2); older patients or those with comorbidities receive a reduced dose regimen (usually 140 mg/m^2).[14] The optimal postautograft therapy is under investigation. A multicenter randomized trial showed no advantage for performing nonmyeloablative allogeneic HSCT compared with tandem autologous HSCT for patients with standard-risk multiple myeloma,[15] while lenalidomide maintenance therapy, initiated at day 100 after hematopoietic stem-cell transplantation, was associated with a significantly longer time to disease progression and significantly improved overall survival among patients with myeloma.[16] Current studies are evaluating vaccines

TABLE 103.1   Hematologic Disorders Treated by Hematopoietic Stem Cell Transplantation

Hematologic Malignancies	Chapters
Acute lymphoblastic leukemia	65 (pediatric), 66, 104 (adult)
Acute myeloid leukemia	61, 104 (adult), 62 (pediatric)
Myelodysplasia	61, 104 (adult), 63 (pediatric)
Myeloproliferative disorders	63 (pediatric), 70 (myelofibrosis)
Chronic lymphocytic leukemia	77, 104
Chronic myeloid leukemia	63 (pediatric), 67 (adult)
Multiple myeloma	86, 104
Hodgkin lymphoma	75, 104 (adult), 84 (pediatric)
Non-Hodgkin lymphoma	80 (follicular), 81 (mantle cell), 82 (diffuse large B cell), 84 (pediatric), 104 (all types)
Nonmalignant Disorders	
Hemoglobinopathies	
Sickle cell disease	42
Thalassemia	40
Immune deficiencies	
SCID	51
Wiskott–Aldrich syndrome	51
Bone marrow failure syndromes	
Aplastic anemia	30
Paroxysmal nocturnal hemoglobulinuria	31
Fanconi anemia and other inherited bone marrow failure syndromes	29
Neutrophil disorders	
Chronic granulomatous disease	50
Histiocytic disorders	
Hemophagocytic lymphohistiocytosis	52
Lysosomal storage diseases	53

SCID, Severe combined immunodeficiency.

TABLE 103.2   Donor Choice

	Mismatched Unrelated Donor	Haploidentical Donor	Cord
Availability	Over 80%	Over 95%	Over 80%
Time to procure	1–4 months	Immediate	2–5 days
Engraftment	Over 95%	Over 95%	Over 90% with slower engraftment
GVHD	Moderate	More genetic disparity but moderate with most modern regimens	Moderate—may be less acute but chronic similar
Availability donor for posttransplant immune therapy	Usually, but takes 2–4 weeks	Yes	No
Relative cost	Moderate	Low if unmanipulated product. Moderate if ex vivo selection	Moderate (1 unit) or high (2 units)
Risk of relapse	Moderate	Higher with regimens that are effective in preventing GVHD	Moderate

and immune effector cells posttransplant to reduce the risk of relapse.

Both American Society for Blood and Marrow Transplantation and National Comprehensive Cancer Network guidelines recommend autologous transplantation in patients with relapsed or refractory diffuse large B-cell lymphoma as well as selected patients with follicular lymphoma. Several large studies have also showed benefit from consolidating with an autograft after initial therapy in patients with mantle-cell lymphoma. A number of different myeloablative conditioning regimens are used in patients with non-Hodgkin lymphoma with the most common being BCNU, etoposide, cytosine arabinoside, and melphalan (BEAM), often in combination with rituximab.

SOURCE OF HEMATOPOIETIC STEM CELLS

The major sources of stem cells for transplant are BM, mobilized PB, and cord blood.

Autologous Donors

In autologous transplantation, the source of HSCs is mobilized PB in almost all adults and more than 90% of pediatric patients. Cytokine-mobilized PB stem cells (PBSCs) can be harvested either after treatment with recombinant human granulocyte colony-stimulating factor (G-CSF) alone or with G-CSF given after chemotherapy. In patients who are heavily pretreated and difficult to mobilize, plerixifor, an antagonist of CXCR4 that interferes with adhesion of hematopoietic progenitors in the microenvironment thereby promoting their circulation in the PB, can be used to increase the mobilization of CD34+ stem cells when given in combination with standard G-CSF therapy.

The success of HSC mobilization is related to the amount of previous chemotherapy with some drugs such as alkylating agents having a particularly adverse effect on the success of HSC mobilization. The International Myeloma Working Group has therefore recommended early mobilization of stem cells, preferably within the first four cycles of initial therapy.[17]

Allogeneic Donors

BM was the historic source of HSCs for transplant and remains the most widely used source in children. Marrow can be harvested from the posterior iliac crests of allogeneic donors in amounts up to 10–20 mL per kilogram of recipient weight to obtain sufficient HSCs for engraftment. Cytokine-mobilized allogeneic PBSC harvest has become an alternative to marrow as a source of HSCs and is now the most widely used source in adults receiving allogeneic transplants. In both single-center randomized studies and CIBMTR registry studies, use of this source of stem cells from matched sibling donors resulted in more rapid engraftment with no increase in acute GVHD. However, there was a higher incidence of chronic GVHD associated with a lower risk of relapse, which translated to improved DFS in patients transplanted for advanced hematologic malignancies. However, this survival benefit was not seen in patients with early stage disease. A large, prospective, randomized trial in recipients of unrelated HSCs who were randomized to receive BM-versus-PB grafts for hematologic malignancies shows no difference in overall survival at 2 years but a higher incidence of chronic GVHD in the recipients who received PB.[18] Longer follow up is needed to determine if this more frequent development of chronic GVHD will be associated with higher late mortality.

Umbilical Cord Blood

Another alternative source of stem cells is cord blood. There are several large cord banks where cord blood is collected, cryopreserved,

and tested for infectious agents in accordance with standards developed by governmental and specialty oversight organizations. This worldwide network for UCB cell procurement, typing, and storage has collected a large inventory of cords and has facilitated more than 20,000 unrelated donor UCB transplants. A major advantage of cord transplant is the immediate availability of cryopreserved units. Cord transplants have slower engraftment, but they also may also induce less GVHD because of the relative naivety of cord T cells. One limitation is the cell count, which can be limiting for individuals weighing more than 50 kg. However, several studies show that double cord blood transplant, with each unit sharing at least 4/6 HLA antigens with the recipient, can overcome this problem and extend the use of cord transplant to larger adult recipients (see Chapter 107).

CONDITIONING REGIMENS

The conditioning regimen has different roles in autologous and allogeneic transplant. In autologous transplant, the aim of the conditioning regimen is to intensify doses of chemotherapy agents that would be limited by hematopoietic toxicity. In allogeneic transplant, the goal of conditioning is to achieve immunosuppression of the recipient sufficient to prevent rejection of the donor BM cells and to destroy residual malignant cells (see Chapter 104). Historically, patients transplanted for malignancy have received intensive fully ablative regimens in which hematopoietic reconstitution would not occur without HSC support. Conditioning regimens are discussed in more detail in Chapter 104, but the most commonly used allogeneic regimens use total-body irradiation and cyclophosphamide or chemotherapy alone with combinations such as busulfan and cyclophosphamide. Biologic agents, such as antithymocyte globulin and monoclonal antibodies, may also be included in some regimens to increase immunosuppression. Reduced-intensity conditioning regimens were developed in the late 1990s and are primarily immunosuppressive, relying on graft-versus-leukemia mechanisms to eradicate malignancy. Reduced-intensity conditioning is often used in older patients or patients with comorbidities in whom the toxicity associated with ablative conditioning would be unacceptable. A variety of regimens based on low-dose total-body irradiation or fludarabine have been used.

COMPLICATIONS AFTER STEM CELL TRANSPLANTATION

Patients who receive transplants are at risk of a number of short- and long-term complications and require long-term follow up. Guidelines for screening and monitoring long-term survivors have been published,[19] and there is increasing interest in research to define the quality of life in long-term transplant survivors. Recipients of both allogeneic and autologous transplant have risks of infection during the period of hematopoietic and immune reconstitution and short- and long-term complications from toxicities from the conditioning regimen. Allograft recipients are also at risk of graft failure and GVHD because of the genetic disparity between donor and recipient.

Acute Graft-Versus-Host Disease

GVHD is the most important cause of mortality, morbidity, and diminished quality of life after allogeneic HCT and results from alloreactivity between donor and recipient. The process is initiated by donor T lymphocytes that recognize antigenic disparities between donor and recipient. In the initial phase, chemotherapy or radiation given as part of the conditioning regimen results in production of inflammatory cytokines secreted by damaged host cells.[20] The release of microbial products that are produced by intestinal flora, as well as the release of cytokines by damaged host tissues, lead to the activation of innate immune cells by pathogen recognition receptors such as Toll-like receptors. After infusion of the HSC product, donor T cells become activated by exposure to host antigens and further activate other immune effectors, resulting in secretion of cytokines and clinical manifestations of GVHD. Chronic GVHD is defined as GVHD occurring after day 100 after transplant, although this definition is somewhat arbitrary. Chronic GVHD often occurs in a patient who has had preceding acute GVHD, although it may arise de novo. It targets the skin, liver, and gastrointestinal tract but may also target other organs and shares features with autoimmune diseases such as scleroderma.

Graft Failure

Graft failure results when recipient immune system cells that survive the conditioning regimen are able to eliminate the incoming donor BM. It is uncommon after fully ablative allogeneic HSCT for hematologic malignancies, but higher incidences are seen after reduced-intensity conditioning and when cord blood is the source of HSCs. Other risk factors include the degree of mismatch between donor and recipient, a low nucleated cell dose, and T-cell depletion of the donor product. Patients who experience graft failure may be retransplanted after additional immunosuppressive conditioning, but mortality from infection caused by prolonged neutropenia is significant.

Infections

After engraftment of the donor HSCs, donor-derived cells reconstitute the recipient's immune system. This is usually a rapid process after autologous transplant but is more prolonged after allogeneic transplant and may be further delayed in a recipient who develops GVHD and requires additional immunosuppression. During the early period after HSC infusion, neutropenic patients are at risk for bacterial infection, fungal infection, and infection with respiratory viruses (see Chapter 89). After engraftment, allogeneic recipients are at risk for viral infection, particularly reactivation of herpes viruses such as cytomegalovirus. Late infectious complications are mainly seen in allogeneic recipients, in whom a major risk factor is chronic GVHD. International consensus guidelines on the management of infections posttransplant have been published.[21]

Regimen-Related Toxicity

A number of early and late posttransplant complications are related to the conditioning regimen as well as previous therapies and pretransplant comorbidities. These include pneumonitis, sinusoidal obstruction syndrome, hemorrhagic cystitis, growth impairment, and endocrine abnormalities and are described in Chapter 109.

Secondary Malignancies

After HSCT, recipients have a twofold to sevenfold increased risk of developing a secondary neoplasm, with the most frequently seen malignancies being Epstein-Barr virus-related posttransplant lymphoproliferative disease (EBV-PTLD), therapy-related AML and myelodysplasia, and a variety of solid tumors.[22] As discussed earlier, autologous transplant recipients are at risk of developing therapy-related MDS and AML because of previous therapy as well as transplant conditioning. Recipients of allogeneic transplant have an increased incidence of both PTLD and solid cancers.

Treatment of Relapse

Relapse remains a major cause of treatment failure after HSCT for hematologic malignancies, and present treatment options are inadequate. Maneuvers that are commonly used are withdrawal of immune suppression, donor lymphocyte infusions, chemotherapy,

and second transplants. Chemotherapy may induce some responses but rarely results in long-term disease control. Increasing knowledge of the molecular basis of graft-versus-tumor responses has stimulated interest in the use of immunotherapy to treat relapse. Infusion of unmanipulated donor lymphocytes can result in significant clinical responses in patients with relapsed CML, but responses are less frequent in other hematologic malignancies.[23] More recently, T cells genetically modified with chimeric antigen receptors have shown very encouraging response rates when treating relapse of CD19+ve malignancies after autologous or allogeneic transplant, but longer follow up is needed.[24–26] Other current research is focusing on targeting lineage-specific antigens, such as Wilms Tumor 1, preferentially expressed antigen of melanoma, or proteinase 3 or mutation specific antigens.[27] Additional immunotherapy approaches under investigation include the administration of antitumor vaccines or NK cells.[28]

FUTURE DIRECTIONS

An ongoing challenge is to delineate the indications for transplant as new drugs are incorporated in primary therapies for many hematologic malignancies and as risk factors continue to be redefined by new information from genetic sequencing and proteomics studies. The wider use of reduced-intensity transplant offers the prospect of using such transplants as a platform for immunotherapy, and transplant will likely be integrated more closely with other cell therapies such as infusions of NK cells, cytotoxic T cells, and regulatory T cells. The question of optimal stem cell source for patients who lack a matched sibling or 10/10 matched unrelated donor is an open issue as novel regimens to improve outcomes are being evaluated for cord and haploidentical transplants. Finally, there is a need for comparative effectiveness studies that include quality of life measures to compare transplant with other therapeutic options.

REFERENCES

1. Appelbaum FR: Hematopoietic-cell transplantation at 50. *N Engl J Med* 357(15):1472–1475, 2007.
2. Jenq RR, van den Brink MR: Allogeneic haematopoietic stem cell transplantation: individualized stem cell and immune therapy of cancer. *Nat Rev Cancer* 10(3):213–221, 2010.
3. Anasetti C: Use of alternative donors for allogeneic stem cell transplantation. *Hematology Am Soc Hematol Educ Program* 2015:220–224, 2015.
4. Nunes E, Heslop H, Fernandez-Vina M, et al: Definitions of histocompatibility typing terms. *Blood* 118(23):e180–e183, 2011.
5. Venstrom JM, Pittari G, Gooley TA, et al: HLA-C-dependent prevention of leukemia relapse by donor activating KIR2DS1. *N Engl J Med* 367(9):805–816, 2012.
6. Warren EH, Zhang XC, Li S, et al: Effect of MHC and non-MHC donor/recipient genetic disparity on the outcome of allogeneic HCT. *Blood* 120(14):2796–2806, 2012.
7. Gratwohl A, Pasquini MC, Aljurf M, et al: One million haemopoietic stem-cell transplants: a retrospective observational study. *Lancet Haematol* 2(3):e91–e100, 2015.
8. Kollman C, Spellman SR, Zhang MJ, et al: The effect of donor characteristics on survival after unrelated donor transplantation for hematologic malignancy. *Blood* 127(2):260–267, 2016.
9. Kekre N, Antin JH: Hematopoietic stem cell transplantation donor sources in the 21st century: choosing the ideal donor when a perfect match does not exist. *Blood* 124(3):334–343, 2014.
10. Brunstein CG, Fuchs EJ, Carter SL, et al: Alternative donor transplantation after reduced intensity conditioning: results of parallel phase 2 trials using partially HLA-mismatched related bone marrow or unrelated double umbilical cord blood grafts. *Blood* 118(2):282–288, 2011.
11. Li L, Li M, Sun C, et al: Altered hematopoietic cell gene expression precedes development of therapy-related myelodysplasia/acute myeloid leukemia and identifies patients at risk. *Cancer Cell* 20(5):591–605, 2011.

12. Oliansky DM, Czuczman M, Fisher RI, et al: The role of cytotoxic therapy with hematopoietic stem cell transplantation in the treatment of diffuse large B cell lymphoma: update of the 2001 evidence-based review. *Biol Blood Marrow Transplant* 17(1):20–47 e30, 2011.

13. Oliansky DM, Gordon LI, King J, et al: The role of cytotoxic therapy with hematopoietic stem cell transplantation in the treatment of follicular lymphoma: an evidence-based review. *Biol Blood Marrow Transplant* 16(4):443–468, 2010.

14. Palumbo A, Anderson K: Multiple myeloma. *N Engl J Med* 364(11):1046–1060, 2011.

15. Krishnan A, Pasquini MC, Logan B, et al: Autologous haemopoietic stem-cell transplantation followed by allogeneic or autologous haemopoietic stem-cell transplantation in patients with multiple myeloma (BMT CTN 0102): a phase 3 biological assignment trial. *Lancet Oncol* 12(13):1195–1203, 2011.

16. McCarthy PL, Owzar K, Hofmeister CC, et al: Lenalidomide after stem-cell transplantation for multiple myeloma. *N Engl J Med* 366(19):1770–1781, 2012.

17. Kumar S, Giralt S, Stadtmauer EA, et al: Mobilization in myeloma revisited: IMWG consensus perspectives on stem cell collection following initial therapy with thalidomide-, lenalidomide-, or bortezomib-containing regimens. *Blood* 114(9):1729–1735, 2009.

18. Anasetti C, Logan BR, Lee SJ, et al: Peripheral-blood stem cells versus bone marrow from unrelated donors. *N Engl J Med* 367(16):1487–1496, 2012.

19. Majhail NS, Rizzo JD, Lee SJ, et al: Recommended screening and preventive practices for long-term survivors after hematopoietic cell transplantation. *Biol Blood Marrow Transplant* 18(3):348–371, 2012.

20. Blazar BR, Murphy WJ, Abedi M: Advances in graft-versus-host disease biology and therapy. *Nat Rev Immunol* 12(6):443–458, 2012.

21. Tomblyn M, Chiller T, Einsele H, et al: Guidelines for preventing infectious complications among hematopoietic cell transplantation recipients: a global perspective. *Biol Blood Marrow Transplant* 15(10):1143–1238, 2009.

22. Rizzo JD, Curtis RE, Socie G, et al: Solid cancers after allogeneic hematopoietic cell transplantation. *Blood* 113(5):1175–1183, 2009.

23. Kolb HJ: Graft-versus-leukemia effects of transplantation and donor lymphocytes. *Blood* 112(12):4371–4383, 2008.

24. Kochenderfer JN, Dudley ME, Carpenter RO, et al: Donor-derived CD19-targeted T cells cause regression of malignancy persisting after allogeneic hematopoietic stem cell transplantation. *Blood* 122(25):4129–4139, 2013.

25. Davila ML, Riviere I, Wang X, et al: Efficacy and toxicity management of 19-28z CAR T cell therapy in B cell acute lymphoblastic leukemia. *Sci Transl Med* 6(224):224ra225, 2014.

26. Maude SL, Frey N, Shaw PA, et al: Chimeric antigen receptor T cells for sustained remissions in leukemia. *N Engl J Med* 371(16):1507–1517, 2014.

27. Rooney CM, Leen AM, Vera JF, et al: T lymphocytes targeting native receptors. *Immunol Rev* 257(1):39–55, 2014.

28. Rosenblatt J, Avivi I, Vasir B, et al: Vaccination with dendritic cell/tumor fusions following autologous stem cell transplant induces immunologic and clinical responses in multiple myeloma patients. *Clin Cancer Res* 19(13):3640–3648, 2013.

INDICATIONS AND OUTCOMES OF ALLOGENEIC HEMATOPOIETIC CELL TRANSPLANTATION FOR HEMATOLOGIC MALIGNANCIES IN ADULTS

Mehdi Hamadani and Parameswaran N. Hari

BACKGROUND

Thomas et al[1] first reported long-term leukemia-free survival following human leukocyte antigen (HLA) identical sibling hematopoietic cell transplantation (HCT) in patients with refractory acute leukemia in the 1970s. Since then, allogeneic HCT has evolved to become a frequently used and effective therapy for many hematologic malignancies. Changes in both HCT and nontransplant therapies have modified the indications and applicability of HCT over time. In chronic myelogenous leukemia (CML), HCT (once the mainstay for cure), is now largely supplanted by molecularly targeted therapy. In recent years, and especially after the advent of reduced intensity conditioning (RIC) in the late 1990s, allogeneic HCT is increasingly used in older patients and as a salvage strategy for lymphoma or myeloma not responding to chemotherapy or autologous HCT. Transplant-related mortality (TRM), while steadily declining, still remains a challenge. General principles, indications and optimal timing of allogeneic HCT for hematologic malignancies and long-term outcomes following HCT are discussed in this chapter.

Allogeneic HCT involves administration of a conditioning (or preparative) regimen of chemotherapy (with or without radiation) and immune suppressive medications, followed by infusion of donor hematopoietic progenitor cells. Most patients then receive prolonged (several months) therapy with immune suppressive agents to prevent or treat graft-versus-host disease (GVHD). The purpose of the conditioning regimen is generally twofold: to eradicate malignant cells and to eliminate host immune cells (capable of rejecting even HLA-identical sibling donor cells). The ability to restore hematopoiesis with donor hematopoietic progenitor cells permits the administration of substantially higher (myeloablative) doses of cytotoxic therapy, than is otherwise possible. Although originally regarded primarily as a way of rescuing patients from therapy-induced marrow aplasia, it is now accepted that graft-versus-malignancy (GVM) effects conferred by alloreactive donor cells contribute substantially to cancer eradication and longer-term relapse prevention.

PATIENT POPULATION

Accompanying the growth of HCT, a coordinated, international effort evolved to collect and analyze data on transplant outcomes through the International Bone Marrow Transplant Registry (IBMTR), established in 1972. The IBMTR affiliated with the United States (US) National Marrow Donor Program (NMDP) in 2004 to become the Center for International Blood and Marrow Transplant Research (CIBMTR). The CIBMTR currently collects data on HCT outcomes from more than 400 transplant centers worldwide and on all allogeneic transplants in the US. In 2013, approximately 9600 allogeneic transplants were performed in adults (age >18 years) in the US. These data show that hematologic malignancies (and premalignant conditions) remain the most common indications for allogeneic HCT. Acute myeloid leukemia (AML), myelodysplastic syndrome/myeloproliferative disorders (MDS/

MPD) and acute lymphoblastic leukemia (ALL) currently constitute the three most common indication of allogeneic transplantation (Fig. 104.1).

Improved immunosuppression and supportive care and the use of RIC have led to an increase in allogeneic HCT for older adults in recent years. Only 4% of allogeneic HCT recipients in 1987–1992 were older than 50 years. In 2013, 34% were older than 55 years and 10% were 65 years or older. Allogeneic transplantation in patients without HLA-identical siblings was facilitated by establishment of large unrelated donor registries. In 1987–1992, <10% of HCTs for hematologic malignancies used unrelated donors; in 2013, this figure was >50%. More transplantation in older adults and increasing use of unrelated donors were the main reasons for the steady growth in allogeneic HCT over the last decade. Similarly, the use of haploidentical related donor HCT is on the rise. In 2001, less than 50 related donor haploidentical transplants were reported to the CIBMTR, compared with nearly 500 transplants in 2013.

CONDITIONING REGIMENS

Historically, conditioning regimens included myeloablative doses of cytotoxic drugs with or without radiation, intended not only to provide disease control, but also host immunosuppression (to prevent graft rejection). Myeloablative regimens for hematologic malignancies often involve a combination of cyclophosphamide (commonly 60 mg/kg/day for 2 days) and total-body irradiation (TBI) (5–15 Gy, single or fractionated doses). Many regimens substitute busulfan (typically 3.2 mg/kg/day intravenously for 4 days or pharmacokinetic guided similar dose) in place of TBI. Posttransplant survival rates with cyclophosphamide and TBI and with cyclophosphamide and busulfan (BuCy) are similar though recent prospective data suggest an advantage for BuCy in myeloid malignancies (AML/MDS/CML). Other drugs such as etoposide, melphalan and thiotepa, are sometimes added to or substituted for cyclophosphamide and/or busulfan in a variety of regimens in efforts to provide better, generally disease-specific, antineoplastic activity. Large prospective trials comparing efficacy of these regimens are lacking. A CIBMTR study suggested better outcomes in ALL in second complete remission (CR2) with either higher doses of TBI or substitution of cyclophosphamide by etoposide in a standard dose TBI regimen.

Myeloablative conditioning regimens are associated with significant risk of regimen-related toxicity. Toxicity can be minimized and efficacy improved with careful pharmacokinetic monitoring of certain drugs, e.g., busulfan. Another strategy for lowering treatment related mortality is by reducing the dose-intensity of the conditioning regimen. This approach uses lower doses of cytotoxic drugs and/or radiation to facilitate donor cell engraftment and relies more on GVM effects to eradicate malignant cells. The lower doses of cytotoxic agents produce less host tissue damage and less inflammatory cytokine secretion resulting in lower rates of regimen-related morbidity and mortality. Use of RIC regimens has greatly increased the applicability of allogeneic HCT in patients ineligible for traditional myeloablative regimens because of age or comorbidities. The development of these

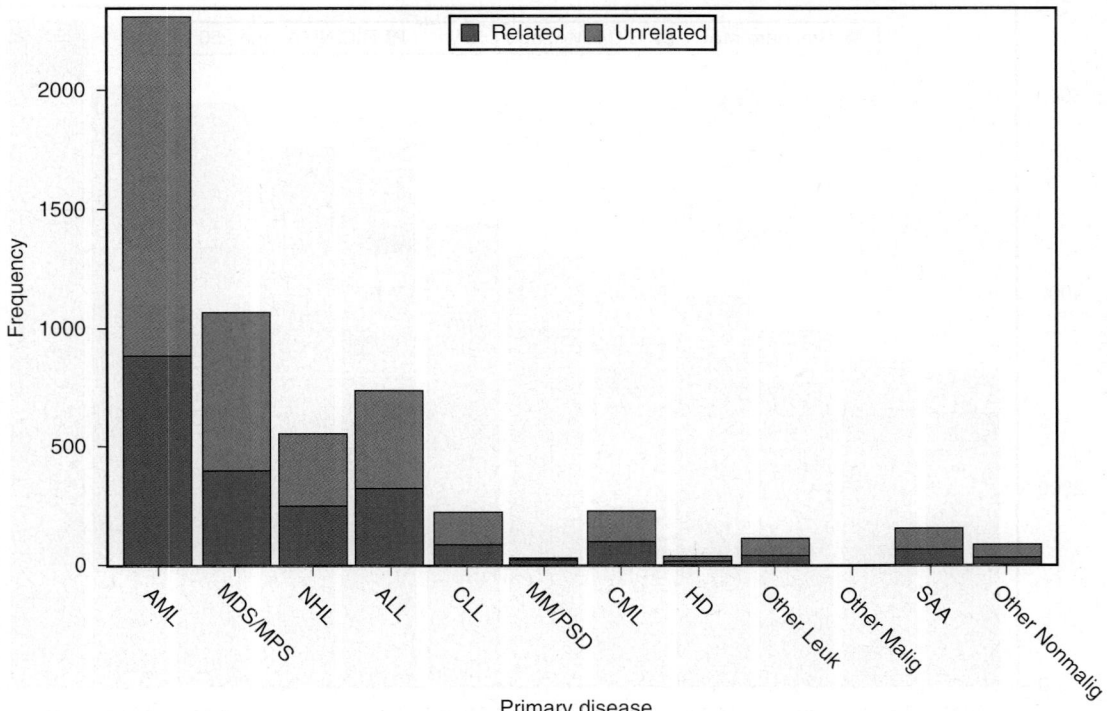

Fig. 104.1 INDICATIONS FOR ALLOGENEIC HEMATOPOIETIC STEM CELL TRANSPLANTA-TION IN ADULTS (US DATA), 2013. *ALL,* acute lymphoblastic leukemia; *AML,* acute myeloid leukemia; *CLL,* chronic lymphocytic leukemia; *CML,* chronic myeloid leukemia; *HD,* Hodgkin disease; *Leuk,* leukemia; *Malig,* malignancy; *MDS,* myelodysplastic syndrome; *MM,* multiple myeloma; *MPS,* myeloproliferative syndrome; *NHL,* non-Hodgkin lymphoma; *PSD,* plasma cell dyscrasia; *SAA,* severe aplastic anemia.

novel conditioning regimens produced a major change in practice in the past decade (Fig. 104.2).

Consensus criteria have been developed by the CIBMTR and the European Society for Blood and Marrow transplantation (EBMT) to distinguish between myeloablative, reduced intensity and nonmyeloablative regimens based on the likelihood of the regimen to produce toxicity to the recipient marrow (Table 104.1).[2] Myeloablative regimens produce profound pancytopenia and are usually fatal in the absence of stem cell rescue. Nonmyeloablative regimens cause brief and often less severe pancytopenia and in the absence of donor stem cell rescue, autologous hematopoietic recovery is likely to occur. RIC regimens are an intermediate category not fitting well in either of the above, since they produce pancytopenia that may recover without stem cell rescue but which is prolonged and, in clinical practice, requires stem cell support.

RIC regimens induce less immune compromise in the immediate post-HCT setting as the duration and depth of neutropenia is reduced and host-derived immunocompetent cells are not immediately eliminated. In addition, the reduced risk of organ toxicity makes RIC regimens attractive for patients ineligible for conventional high-dose regimens.[3] Whether these benefits outweigh the risks of potentially reduced antitumor effects in patients fit for myeloablative conditioning regimens, remains controversial.

It is generally accepted that reduced intensity regimens allow HCT to be done in some patients who will not be offered HCT with myeloablative conditioning. For example, in the US, the proportion of transplantations done in patients older than 60 years increased from <5% before 2000 to ~22% in 2013. Two-thirds of the latter patients received RIC regimens. The Seattle consortium described the outcomes of 372 "older" patients (aged 60–75 years) receiving non-myeloablative regimens.[3] Increasing age was not associated with increase in organ toxicity or GVHD and 5-year survival of the entire

cohort was 35%. However, RIC regimens are increasingly used in patients of all ages receiving both related and unrelated donor transplants, as is shown in Fig. 104.2.

Despite the growing popularity of RIC regimens, large retrospective database studies from the EBMT and CIBMTR (summarized in Table 104.2) have generally failed to show a definite survival advantage resulting from the use of such conditioning regimens. Although RIC regimens allow a potent graft-versus-leukemia response to occur with lower toxicity, there are concerns about a higher risk of disease relapse following RIC regimens. Since the distribution of conditioning regimens in registry studies reflects physician choice or patient selection bias, retrospective data are of limited use. Randomized trials have been performed to gauge the true impact of regimen intensity. The US prospective trial Bone Marrow Transplant-Clinical Trial Network (BMT-CTN 0901) randomized patients with myeloid malignancies eligible for myeloablative conditioning to RIC-versus-myeloablative regimens. This trial was suspended after enrolling 272 out of the planned 356 patients when early results indicated better outcomes for myeloablative regimens (National Heart, Lung and Blood Institute clinical advisory and personal communication—Mary Horowitz). Detailed results are not available yet and RIC transplants remain the standard of care for those not eligible for myeloablative conditioning. A recently concluded prospective European trial (RICMAC) showed similar 2-year relapse-free and overall survival for busulfan based RIC versus myeloablative regimens in patients with MDS and secondary AML.[4]

GRAFT SOURCES

The sources of hematopoietic cells for transplantation, historically donor bone marrow, now also include peripheral blood hematopoietic

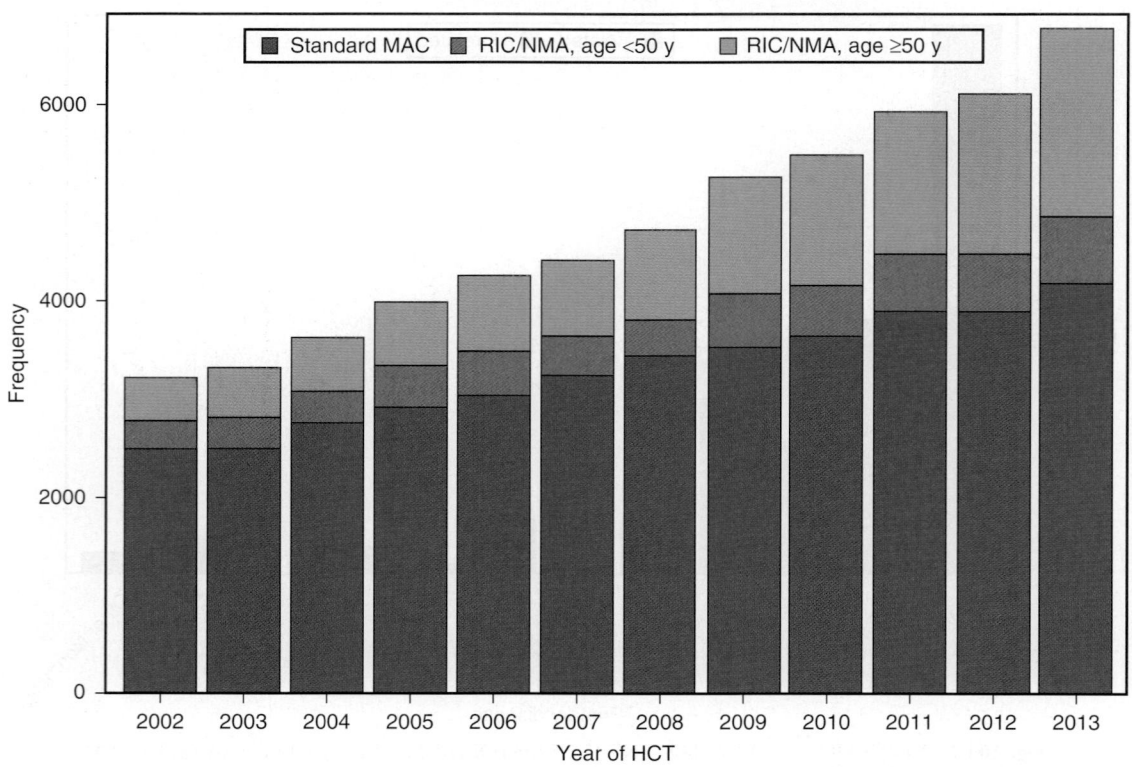

Allogeneic Transplants Registered with the CIBMTR in the United States, 2002–2013, by Conditioning Regimen Intensity & Patient Age

Fig. 104.2 CONDITIONING REGIMEN INTENSITY AND PATIENT AGE: CHANGING TREND OVER TIME (2002–2013). *MAC,* myeloablative conditioning; *NMA,* nonmyeloablative; *RIC,* reduced intensity conditioning.

TABLE 104.1	Consensus Definition of Conditioning Regimen Intensity

Myeloablative Conditioning
Profound Cytopenia, Not Likely to Recover Without Hematopoietic Cell Rescue

Total body irradiation >5 Gy single dose or >8 Gy fractionated
Busulfan >8 mg/kg orally or intravenous equivalent

Nonmyeloablative
Minimal Cytopenia, Autologous Recovery of Hematopoiesis Likely Even Without Transplant

Total body irradiation <2 Gy + purine nucleoside analogue
Fludarabine + cyclophosphamide + antithymocyte globulin
Fludarabine + cytarabine + idarubicin
Cladribine + cytarabine
Total lymphoid irradiation + antithymocyte globulin

Reduced Intensity Conditioning

Regimens that are intermediate between the above categories

cells collected by leukapheresis and umbilical cord blood. The composition of grafts from bone marrow, peripheral blood and cord blood varies in terms of the proportion of pluripotent stem cells to lineage-committed late progenitor cells and in the characteristics of immune reactive cells. Bone marrow is the primary source of allogeneic donor cells for transplantation in children and peripheral blood the main source in adults (Fig. 104.3). Among all allografts, umbilical cord blood is used for nearly 30% of transplants in children (younger than 20 years). The proportion of transplants in adults using cord blood grafts increased from about 2% in 2004 to 4.5% in 2013.

Several randomized trials have compared matched sibling bone marrow-versus-peripheral blood grafts in patients with hematologic malignancy following myeloablative conditioning regimens. These studies in general, showed no difference in the rates of acute GVHD between the two graft sources and a higher risk of chronic GVHD with peripheral blood grafts. While survival outcomes were similar in most studies, the US and Canadian randomized studies reported a disease-free and overall survival advantage respectively favoring peripheral blood grafts.[5,6] A metaanalysis using individual patient-level data from nine randomized trials of related donor peripheral blood-versus-bone marrow transplants suggested that patients receiving peripheral blood grafts had faster hematopoietic recovery,[6] a lower relapse rate if transplanted for hematologic malignancy and higher overall and disease-free survival if transplanted for advanced-stage disease. However, peripheral blood was also associated with a significantly increased risk of extensive chronic GVHD. Prospective data evaluating graft sources for unrelated donor transplantation are sparse. The BMT-CTN 0201 is the only randomized trial (*n* = 551) comparing unrelated donor marrow versus peripheral blood grafts for hematologic malignancies. This study showed a higher risk of chronic GVHD in patients receiving peripheral blood grafts (53% versus 41% for marrow grafts). Notably, survival and the incidence of relapse and acute GVHD were similar, while graft failure was more common among recipients of marrow grafts.[7] The relative importance of graft sources in patients receiving lower-intensity conditioning is not known, but a recent CIBMTR study comparing unrelated bone marrow versus peripheral blood grafts following RIC, showed no difference between the two sources in terms of rates of acute or chronic GVHD, relapse risk and survival outcomes.[8]

ALTERNATIVE DONOR TRANSPLANTS—CORD BLOOD AND HAPLOIDENTICAL GRAFTS

A major obstacle to allogeneic HCT is donor availability for the majority (70%) of adult patients without an HLA-identical sibling.

TABLE 104.2   Retrospective Registry-Based Comparisons of NMA/RIC versus Myeloablative Allogeneic HCT

Group	Disease	Donor	RIC vs. MAC (N)	TRM RIC vs. MAC	Relapse	Comments
EBMT[33]	MDS or sAML >50	MUD 39%	315 vs. 407	32% vs. 44% at 4 years	41% vs. 33% at 4 years	Survival 31% at 4 years. RIC predicted for greater relapse but lower TRM in multivariate model. Wide variety of different conditioning regimens used.
EBMT[34]	MM	MUD 12%	320 vs. 196	24% vs. 37% at 2 years	27% vs. 54%	TRM lower after RIC but relapse risk is double
EBMT[35]	AML	Sibling	215 vs. 621	22% vs. 32% at 3 years	45% vs. 27% at 3 years	Relapse rate higher and TRM lower in RIC but OS similar (41% vs. 45%) in both groups.
EBMT[36]	CLL	MUD 22%	73 vs. 82	19% vs. 26%	28% vs. 11%	Similar TRM but higher relapse risk after RIC
EBMT[37]	HL	MUD 13%	89 vs. 79	23% vs. 46% at 1 year	57% vs. 30%	Relapse rate higher and TRM lower in RIC but OS similar
CIBMTR[38]	Follicular NHL	Sibling	88 vs. 120	23% in both at 1 year	17% vs. 8%	RIC associated with higher risk of relapse but similar TRM while lower KPS impacted on TRM. OS was similar.
EBMT[39]	ALL	Sibling	127 vs. 449	21% vs. 29%	32% vs. 38%	TRM lower after RIC but higher relapse rate. Leukemia-free survival similar to MAC
CIBMTR[40]	AML/MDS	MUD/Sibling	1448 vs. 3731	3-year TRM similar	Lower risk of relapse in Myeloablative	Overall and disease-free survival was highest for myeloablative group

ALL, Acute lymphoblastic leukemia; AML, acute myeloid leukemia; CIBMTR, Center for International Blood and Marrow Transplant Research; CLL, chronic lymphocytic leukemia; EBMT, European Society for Blood and Marrow transplantation; HCT, hematopoietic cell transplantation; HL, Hodgkin lymphoma; KPS, Karnofsky performance score; MAC, myeloablative conditioning; MDS, myelodysplastic syndrome; MM, multiple myeloma; MUD, matched unrelated donor; NHL, Non-Hodgkin lymphoma; NMA, nonmyeloablative; OS, overall survival; RIC, reduced intensity conditioning; TRM, transplant-related mortality; sAML, secondary acute myeloid leukemia.

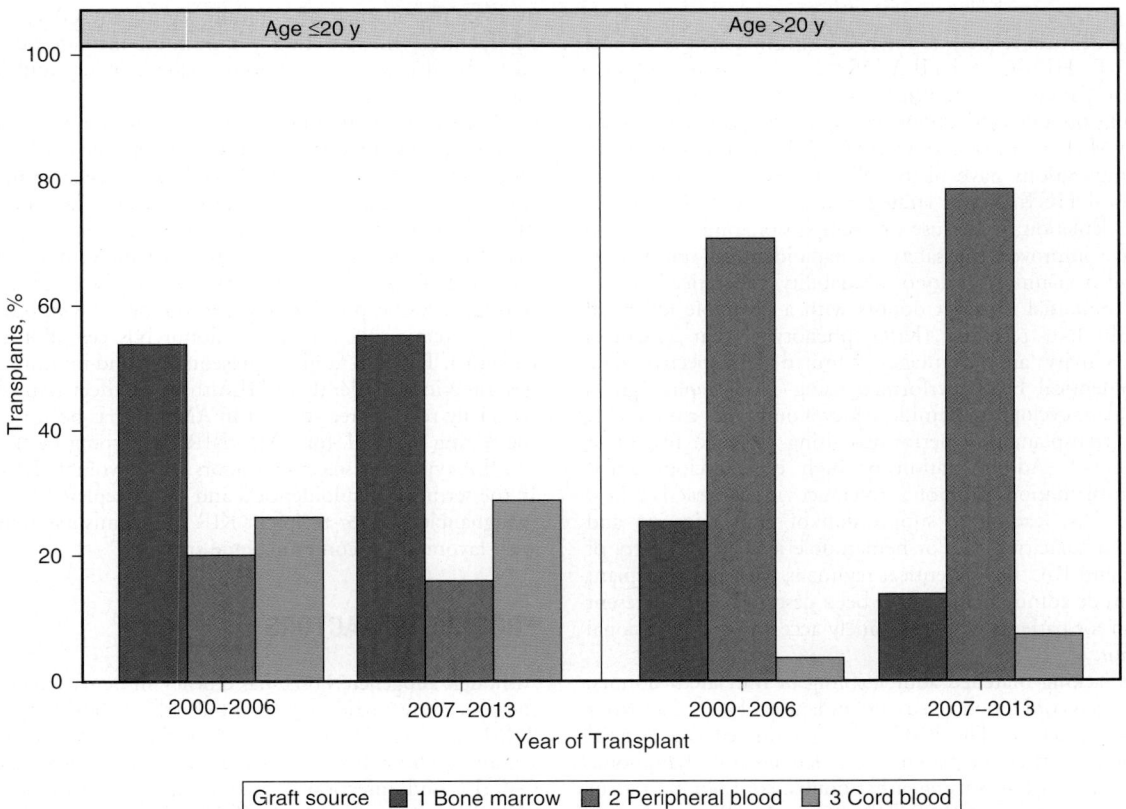

Fig. 104.3 ALLOGENEIC STEM CELL SOURCES, BY DONOR TYPE VERSUS DONOR AGE, 2000–2013.

The likelihood of finding an optimal adult unrelated donor (i.e., a donor matched at high resolution at HLA-A, HLA-B, HLA-C, and -DRB1) varies among racial and ethnic groups depending on the size and composition of unrelated donor registries. Within the US population, the highest likelihood for finding an optimal donor is for whites of European descent, at 75%, and the lowest among blacks of South or Central American descent, at 16%.[9] The unrelated donor search process can be time-consuming, raising the risk of disease progression before transplantation can be performed. As a source of hematopoietic stem cells for unrelated donor transplantation, umbilical cord blood offers several advantages. It is readily available and entails no risk to the donor. Current data also indicate that HLA-matching criteria for cord blood transplantation need not be as stringent as for adult donor transplantation. Hence cord-blood units mismatched at one or two HLA loci are available for almost all patients <20 years of age and for more than 80% of patients ≥20 years of age, regardless of racial and ethnic background.[9] Drawbacks of cord blood transplants include procurement costs, often limited number of hematopoietic cells in each cord blood unit and relatively high rates of TRM.

The numbers of cord blood transplants have increased steadily, especially in children but also in adults. Comparative data on cord blood versus adult donor transplantation in adults come from registry studies and consistently suggests slower hematopoietic recovery but lower rates of GVHD with cord blood grafts. A CIBMTR comparison of adult leukemia patients receiving cord blood versus matched or mismatched unrelated marrow grafts indicated that rates of relapse, TRM, treatment failure and overall mortality were not significantly different between recipients of cord blood or mismatched marrow transplants.[10] Based on current data, a one or two HLA-antigen mismatched cord blood graft of appropriate cell dose is an acceptable alternative for patients with hematologic malignancies who need HCT but do not have a readily available HLA-identical adult (sibling or unrelated) donor. Patients without a single cord unit of adequate cell dose may receive two units to facilitate engraftment.[11] Other approaches to facilitate engraftment with limited cord blood cell doses, including ex vivo cell expansion techniques are in clinical trials.

HLA haploidentical related-donor HCT (mismatched at ≥2 loci HLA-A, HLA-B, HLA-C and HLA-DR; usually parents, siblings, or children of patients) is another option for patients without matched sibling or unrelated donors. Despite the potential benefit of a strong GVM effect, the risk of severe GVHD, graft rejection and infectious complications have historically limited the applicability of haploidentical HCT. Newer strategies using intense ex vivo or in vivo T-cell depletion or the use of cyclophosphamide posttransplantation have improved the safety of haploidentical transplants. Immediate and near-universal donor availability, theoretically lower costs and the potential to select donors with a favorable killer-cell immunoglobulin-like receptor (KIR) phenotype that enhances antileukemia activity are advantages. Limited retrospective data suggest haploidentical HCT performed using T-cell–replete grafts and posttransplant cyclophosphamide achieves outcomes comparable with those of transplantation performed using matched related or unrelated donors.[12] Administration of high dose cyclophosphamide posttransplantation promotes tolerance in alloreactive host and donor T cells, leading to suppression of graft rejection and GVHD without toxicity to donor hematopoietic cells. A variety of myeloablative and RIC haploidentical regimens with posttransplant cyclophosphamide administration have been described and represent another option for patients who lack timely access to a conventional unrelated donor.

In patients lacking matched adult (sibling or unrelated) donors, the choice between cord blood versus haploidentical HCT is a matter of much ongoing debate. The BMT-CTN conducted two parallel multicenter phase 2 trials in patients with leukemia or lymphoma and no suitable adult donors using either double cord blood units or haploidentical marrow grafts (BMT-CTN 0603) after RIC.[13] Survival at 1 year was similar: 54% after cord blood HCT and 62% after haploidentical marrow grafts. The incidence of TRM and relapse after cord blood grafts were 24% and 31%, respectively; corresponding incidences after haploidentical marrow grafts were 7% and 45%. The ongoing BMT-CTN 1101 study comparing umbilical cord blood versus haploidentical marrow grafts will hopefully inform clinical decision making about the relative risks/benefits of these two alternative donor sources.

GRAFT VERSUS MALIGNANCY EFFECTS

Donor derived alloreactive cells are capable of mounting a potent anticancer immune response. Barnes and Loutit[13a] studied leukemic mice treated with high-dose TBI and compared those receiving syngeneic and allogeneic bone marrow infusions. Mice receiving syngeneic marrow died quickly of leukemia whereas those receiving allogeneic cells survived longer but eventually developed fatal GVHD. Importantly, the allografted mice had no evidence of leukemia at death. Several canine and murine experiments reproduced these results.[14] Antitumor effects of allogeneic cells could be specific, i.e., after sensitization of the donor or the donor's cells to antigens present on malignant cells, or nonspecific, i.e., associated with GVHD, an immune reaction of donor lymphocytes against normal and malignant host cells presumably triggered by differences in histocompatibility antigens.[15] The term graft-versus-leukemia was coined by Bortin and coworkers[14] to indicate the adoptive immunotherapeutic effect of transplanted donor cells against the recipient's leukemia cells. Clinical evidence for the importance of GVM effects in eradicating tumor includes: 1) lower incidence of disease relapse in allograft recipients with acute and/or chronic GVHD than in those without GVHD[15]; 2) higher relapse rates after syngeneic versus allogeneic HCT[15]; 3) higher relapse rates after T-cell depleted transplants[15]; 4) durable remissions induced after posttransplant relapse by infusion of donor lymphocytes without other antileukemia therapy; and 5) durable remissions achieved after very low doses of conditioning agents (e.g., 2 Gy TBI) and allogeneic HCT.[3] GVM effects are associated with GVHD and measures that prevent or suppress GVHD may allow more relapse but significant anticancer effects are demonstrable even in the absence of clinically significant GVHD, especially in AML and CML. The efficacy of immune-mediated antitumor effects varies by disease; they are most evident in myeloid leukemias and indolent lymphomas.

The role of natural killer (NK) cells in the posttransplant setting is of increasing interest. After HCT, donor-derived NK cells promote engraftment, reduce the risk of GVHD, enhance immune reconstitution and also decrease the risk of relapse especially in AML.[16] In the physiologic state, NK cells can engage and kill target cells lacking major histocompatibility (HLA) class I molecules. This function is regulated by signaling through the KIR family. In the allogeneic HCT setting; lack of expression of the inhibitory KIR ligand on the recipient's leukemic cells can trigger donor NK cell alloreactivity against leukemia. The KIR family represents a second immunogenetic system inherited independently of HLA that can affect transplant outcomes especially relapse-free survival in AML. It has been proposed that in the setting of HCT for AML, KIR genotyping be used in addition to HLA typing by selecting donors with favorable KIR haplotypes.[17] In the setting of haploidentical and T-cell depleted HCT for myeloid malignancies, donor-recipient KIR ligand mismatching is associated with favorable outcomes in some studies.

PROGNOSTIC FACTORS

Although allogeneic HCT has efficacy in hematologic malignancies, the procedure carries a substantial risk of morbidity and mortality. TRM may result from toxicity of the pretransplant conditioning regimen to lung, liver, and other organs, complications of cytopenia, GVHD, and infection related to delayed immune reconstitution especially in the setting of GVHD or its treatment. The risk of TRM may be 30% or higher in adults receiving unrelated or alternative donor transplantation. In addition, many patients have recurrence of

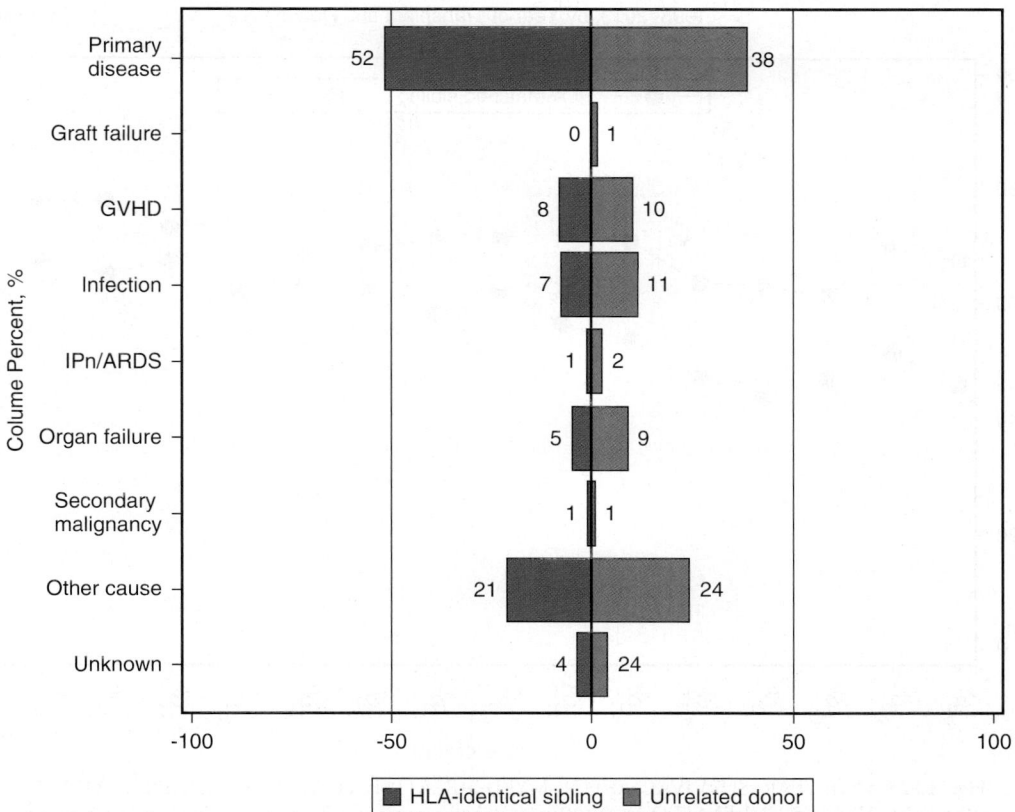

Fig. 104.4 CAUSES OF DEATH AFTER TRANSPLANTATION, 2008–2013. *ARDS,* adult respiratory distress syndrome; *GVHD,* graft-versus-host disease; *HLA,* human leukocyte antigen; *IPn,* idiopathic pneumonia syndrome.

their malignancy despite intensive conditioning and GVM effects. Primary causes of death after allogeneic transplantation for hematologic malignancy are shown in (Fig. 104.4). The prognosis of transplant recipients is influenced by several factors associated with risk of TRM and/or cancer recurrence or progression.

Donor Factors

TRM rates are generally lower after HLA-identical sibling than after unrelated donor or alternative donor transplants because of less graft failure, faster immune reconstitution and less GVHD. However, considerable progress has been made in reducing TRM rates after both HLA-identical sibling and alternative donor HCT. For matched sibling donor HCT in AML in CR1, the incidence of TRM decreased from 29% from 1985–1989 to about 15% from 2000–2004 and 14% from 2005–2009. For unrelated donor HCT, the incidence of TRM from 1990–1994 was 39%, which decreased to 31% by 2000–2004 and 21% from 2005–2009.[18] Among alternative donor transplants, those from more closely HLA-matched donors tend to have lower risks of GVHD and TRM. Donor-recipient HLA mismatching is associated with increased risk of posttransplant complications including graft rejection, acute and chronic GVHD and mortality; risks increase progressively with multiple HLA mismatches. With modern molecular HLA typing techniques (allowing selection of more closely HLA-matched donors) and current GVHD prevention strategies, the difference in outcomes between HLA-matched sibling and unrelated donor transplantation has narrowed (Fig. 104.5).

Adoption of molecularly-defined HLA matching techniques, calcineurin inhibitor–based GVHD prophylaxis, fungal prophylaxis with azoles, leukocyte reduction of blood products, newer assays for viral reactivation, pharmacokinetic testing of conditioning agents and posttransplant cyclophosphamide for induction of allogeneic tolerance are some of the major innovations that have impacted TRM.

Timing of Transplantation

In general, HCT outcomes are better when transplantation is done earlier in the disease course. Transplantation for advanced disease is associated with higher risks of both relapse and TRM. High TRM in the setting of advanced disease likely reflects patients' poorer clinical status and the cumulative effects of more extensive prior treatment. Since some hematologic malignancies have excellent prognosis with nontransplant therapy, e.g., children with standard risk ALL or adults with acute promyelocytic leukemia, appropriate timing of transplantation requires consideration of likely outcomes with transplant and nontransplant therapies. However, even when not used early, transplantation should not be inordinately delayed, since patients with refractory disease or severe complications from extensive prior therapy are unlikely to benefit. For patients with diseases potentially curable by allografting, appropriate timing of transplantation should be considered early in planning management strategies. This includes determining the availability of suitable related or unrelated donors. The American Society for Blood and Marrow Transplantation (ASBMT) developed evidence-based guidelines (see Pink Box 104.1) based upon current clinical practice and available literature (available online at http://www.asbmt.org/?page=GuidelineStatements)

Patient- and Disease-Related Factors

TRM is lower and, consequently, survival is higher, in patients who are young, cytomegalovirus antibody screen-negative, and have good

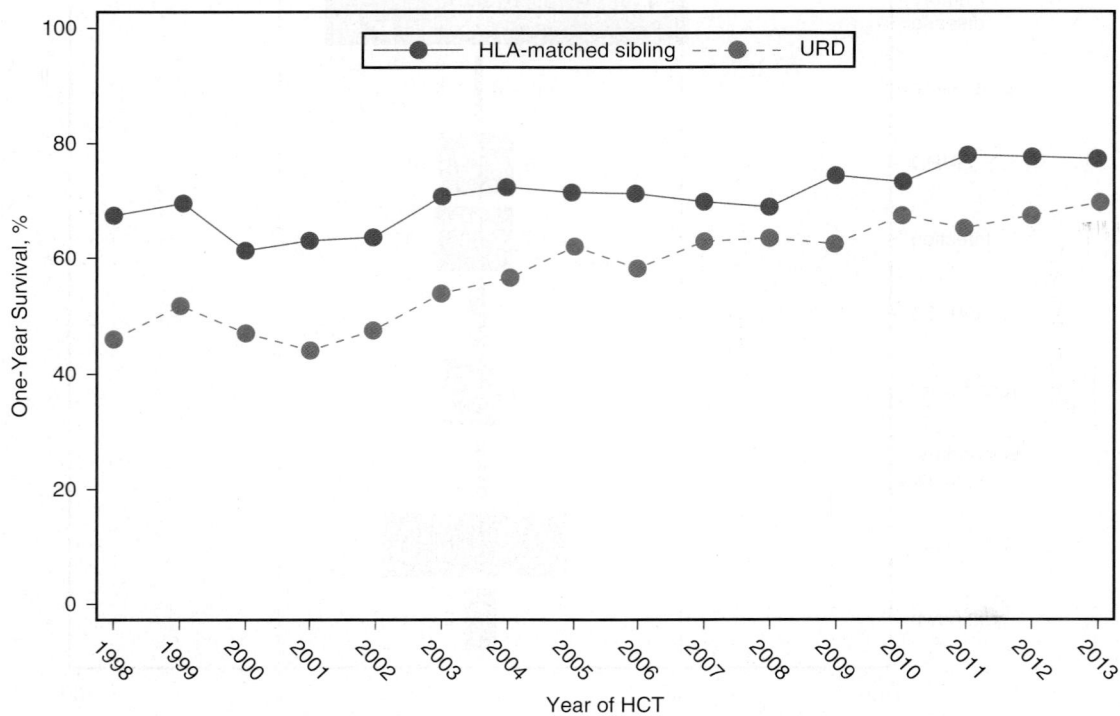

One-Year Survival after a Myelablative Conditioning Regimen for Acute
Leukemias in any Remission, CML or MDS, Age <50 yrs, in the United States,
1998–2013, by Year of Transplant and Donor Type

Fig. 104.5 ONE-YEAR SURVIVAL AFTER MYELOABLATIVE HCT IN YOUNGER PATIENTS (RELATED VERSUS UNRELATED DONOR). *HCT,* hematopoietic cell transplantation; *URD,* unrelated donors.

BOX 104.1	ASBMT Consensus Policy for Allogeneic Transplantation
Disease State	**Policy Regarding: Allogeneic Transplantation**
AML in adults	1. Survival advantage is established for allogeneic HCT vs. chemotherapy for patients under age 55 years with high risk cytogenetics. 2. Insufficient evidence to routinely recommend allogeneic HCT for patients with intermediate risk cytogenetics. 3. No survival advantage for allogeneic HCT in patients under age 55 years with low-risk cytogenetics. 4. Insufficient data to make a recommendation for the use of myeloablative regimens for patients over age 55 years. 5. Insufficient data to make a recommendation for RIC followed by HCT vs. chemotherapy. 6. For patients in second complete remission, allogeneic HCT is recommended if there is an available donor. *Details available at:* http://c.ymcdn.com/sites/www.asbmt.org/resource/resmgr/Docs/AdultAML_PositionStatement.pdf
ALL in adults	1. In first CR, allogeneic HCT as first-choice therapy is appropriate for all risk groups. In younger patients (<35 years), with standard risk, Ph-negative ALL, HCT results in superior survival compared with chemotherapy. In older (>35 years) patients, with standard risk Ph-negative ALL, higher TRM diminishes survival benefits of HCT. 2. In second CR, allogeneic HCT is recommended over chemotherapy. 3. There is similar survival after related and unrelated donor HCT for ALL. 4. RIC may produce similar outcomes to myeloablative but available data are limited. RIC is appropriate only for patients with ALL in remission and unsuited for myeloablative conditioning. *Details available at:* http://c.ymcdn.com/sites/www.asbmt.org/resource/resmgr/Docs/Adult_ALL_PositionStatement.pdf
Diffuse Large B-cell Lymphoma	1. Survival outcomes are equivalent for autologous and allogeneic HCT; neither option is recommended over the other. Comparison between the two techniques is biased by different patient selection criteria. 2. Based on limited data, RIC is an acceptable alternative for selected patients who cannot tolerate a myeloablative regimen. *Details available at:* http://c.ymcdn.com/sites/www.asbmt.org/resource/resmgr/Docs/DLBCL_PositionStatement.pdf
Follicular Lymphoma	1. Autologous versus allogeneic HCT: there are insufficient data to recommend one option over the other as comparison between the two techniques is biased by different patient selection criteria. 2. Based on limited data and expert opinion, RIC is an acceptable alternative approach to myeloablative conditioning. 3. Based on expert opinion, matched unrelated donor transplants are considered as effective as matched related donor transplants. *Details available at:* http://c.ymcdn.com/sites/www.asbmt.org/resource/resmgr/Docs/FollicularLymphoma_PositionS.pdf
Myeloma	1. Autologous transplant is preferred over allogeneic HCT based on current evidence. Studies are ongoing to further evaluate the role of allogeneic HCT. *Details available at:* http://c.ymcdn.com/sites/www.asbmt.org/resource/resmgr/Docs/MultipleMyeloma_PositionStat.pdf

ALL, Acute lymphoblastic leukemia; AML, acute myeloid leukemia; ASBMT, American Society for Blood and Marrow Transplantation; CR, complete remission; HCT, hematopoietic cell transplantation; Ph, Philadelphia chromosome; RIC, reduced intensity conditioning, TRM, transplant-related mortality.

BOX 104.2   Hematopoietic Cell Transplantation-Specific Comorbidity Index (HCT-CI)

Comorbidity	Explanation	HCT-CI score
Arrhythmia	Atrial fibrillation or flutter, sick sinus syndrome, or ventricular arrhythmias	1
Cardiac	Coronary artery disease, congestive heart failure, myocardial infarction, or ejection fraction ≤50%	1
Inflammatory bowel disease	Crohn disease or ulcerative colitis	1
Diabetes	Requiring treatment with insulin or oral hypoglycemics	1
Cerebrovascular disease	Transient ischemic attack or cerebrovascular accident	1
Psychiatric disturbance	Depression or anxiety requiring psychiatric consult or treatment	1
Hepatic, mild	Chronic hepatitis, bilirubin > ULN to 1.5 × ULN, or AST/ALT > ULN to 2.5 × ULN	1
Obesity	Patients with a body mass index >35 kg/m⁺	1
Infection	Requiring treatment after day 0	1
Rheumatologic	SLE, rheumatoid arthritis, polymyositis, mixed connective tissue disease, or polymyalgia rheumatica	2
Peptic ulcer	Requiring treatment	2
Moderate/severe renal	Serum creatinine >2 mg/dL, on dialysis, or prior renal transplantation	2
Moderate pulmonary	DLCO and/or FEV₁ 66% to 80% or dyspnea on slight activity	2
Prior solid tumor	Treated at any time point in the patient's past history, excluding nonmelanoma skin cancer	3
Heart valve disease	Except mitral valve prolapse	3
Severe pulmonary	DLCO and/or FEV₁ ≤65% or dyspnea at rest or requiring oxygen	3
Moderate/severe hepatic	Liver cirrhosis, bilirubin > 1.5 × ULN, or AST/ALT > 2.5 × ULN	3

HCT-CI of 0 predicts 2 year TRM of 14%
HCT-CI of 1-2 predicts 2 year TRM of 21%
HCT-CI of ≥3 predicts 2 year TRM of 41%

ALT, Alanine aminotransferase; AST, aspartate aminotransferase; CI, confidence interval; DLCO, diffusing capacity of the lungs for carbon monoxide; FEV₁, forced expiratory volume in the first second of expiration; HCT, hematopoietic cell transplantation; SLE, systemic lupus erythematosus; ULN, upper limit of normal.

BOX 104.3   Refined Disease Risk Index (DRI)

Refined DRI Category	Definition of Refined DRI category	2-Year Overall Survival
Low	• Hodgkin lymphoma, mantle cell lymphoma, indolent non-Hodgkin lymphoma (NHL), chronic lymphocytic leukemia (CLL) or favorable-cytogenetics acute myeloid leukemia (AML) in complete remission (CR) • CLL or indolent NHL in partial remission (PR) • First or second chronic phase chronic myelogenous leukemia (CML).	66%
Intermediate	• CML advance phase • Mantle cell lymphoma, T-cell NHL, Hodgkin lymphoma, or aggressive NHL in PR • CLL or indolent NHL with stable or progressive disease • Acute lymphoblastic leukemia (ALL) in first CR • Intermediate-cytogenetics AML or aggressive NHL in CR • Myeloproliferative neoplasm • Low-risk myelodysplastic syndrome (MDS) with adverse-cytogenetic or high-risk MDS with intermediate-cytogenetics • Multiple myeloma in CR/very good PR/PR	51%
High	• T-cell NHL, Hodgkin lymphoma, mantle cell lymphoma, myeloma with stable or progressive disease • Burkitt lymphoma in CR • ALL in second or third CR • Adverse-cytogenetics AML in CR • Intermediate-cytogenetic AML with induction failure or active relapse • High-risk MDS with intermediate cytogenetics and advanced disease • Any-risk MDS with adverse cytogenetics and advanced disease	33%
Very High	• CML blast phase • Burkitt lymphoma in PR • Adverse-cytogenetic AML or ALL with induction failure or active relapse • Aggressive NHL with stable or progressive disease	23%

performance scores and no active infection. While age is still a significant barrier to successful allogeneic HCT, the presence and extent of medical comorbid conditions rather than an arbitrary chronologic age cutoff, is increasingly recognized as a major determinant of TRM. Box 104.2 depicts the commonly used HCT-Comorbidity Index (HCT-CI), for estimating risk of TRM posttransplantation.[19]

Although many factors influence the outcome of allogeneic HCT, disease type and disease status at the time of transplantation are the strongest determinants of post-HCT survival. The CIBMTR recently reported a Refined Disease Risk Index (R-DRI) (see Box 104.3), as a useful prognostic tool to predict overall survival postallogeneic HCT, based on patient's disease type and remission status.[20] Both

HCT-CI and R-DRI are increasingly used in clinical decision making to determine patient eligibility and optimal conditioning intensity pre-HCT.

CLINICAL RESEARCH IN ALLOGENEIC TRANSPLANTATION

The number of HCTs performed in the US is increasing at a rate of approximately 5% per year. Only a minority of patients have their transplants performed on clinical trials. Challenges unique to the field of HCT such as small numbers treated at individual centers, the wide variety of indications and multiple competing risks in the peritransplant period, make it difficult to perform single center studies. To overcome these challenges, in the US, a national multicenter transplant study network (BMT-CTN) has been established. The BMT-CTN has thus far launched 36 multicenter trials and accrued more than 7000 patients.

While clinical trials focus on short- and intermediate-term outcomes, there is also a need for long-term follow up of transplant recipients. Outcomes registries, such as those maintained by the CIBMTR and EBMT, are important in facilitating additional clinical research. The CIBMTR maintains a large database of clinical information on the outcome of HCTs performed in 500 transplant centers in nearly 50 countries. The database includes information on more than 370,000 transplant recipients. Data quality and consecutive registration are ensured through extensive computer checks and on-site audits. Data collection is through a web-based data entry program. Some important questions, such as results of HCT in specific patient groups and rare diseases, analysis of prognostic factors, evaluation of new transplant regimens, comparison of HCT with nontransplant therapy, defining intercenter variability in practice and outcome are difficult to address in randomized trials and can be studied using registry data. Analysis of outcomes after transplantation needs an understanding of statistic methodologies such as multistate modeling. Such models involve competing risks problems such as the study of relapse versus death in remission or the complex interrelationship between engraftment, transplant complications (such as infection or GVHD), and primary events such as death or relapse.[21] Outcomes registries also provide a platform to analyze the availability, access, disparities, and economics of HCT. A biospecimen repository maintained by the NMDP and associated with the CIBMTR database allows the linkage of clinical and immunologic data for analysis and has led to important insights into transplant immunobiology.

LONG-TERM SURVIVAL AFTER ALLOGENEIC TRANSPLANTATION

Most deaths related to HCT occur within the first 2 years. However, an analysis of 2 year survivors found that, compared with age and nationality matched death rates among the general population, subsequent survival was still inferior for HCT recipients.[22] Overall, 85% of 2-year survivors were still alive at 10 years post-HCT. Late relapse was the major cause of late deaths and was associated with advanced disease at HCT. Older age and GVHD were the other major predictors of late mortality.

The number of long-term HCT survivors is growing. Most 5-year survivors are well, off all immune suppression and leading normal lives. However, transplant recipients remain at risk for late complications including late infections, cataracts, abnormalities of growth and development, thyroid disorders, chronic lung disease and avascular necrosis. There is also an increased incidence of leukemias, myelodysplasia, and solid tumors in transplant recipients compared with the general population. Lifelong surveillance is necessary, as is increased awareness of late complications among the many nontransplant physicians who will care for these patients. Recommended long-term follow up of HCT recipients is summarized in Box 104.4.

DISEASE-SPECIFIC INDICATIONS FOR ALLOGENEIC TRANSPLANTATION

Acute Myeloid Leukemia

There is general agreement that most patients under the age of about 60 years who fail conventional therapy and who have good performance status are best treated with allogeneic transplantation if an appropriate related or unrelated donor is available. HCT is not recommended for those with favorable risk cytogenetics in first complete remission (CR1).

The National Comprehensive Cancer Network (NCCN) guidelines, widely used to guide cancer therapy in the US, distinguishes between patients ≤60 versus those >60 years. Among younger patients, the panel recommended a postremission strategy based on factors such as the expected relapse rates with high dose cytarabine therapy alone, salvage treatment options at relapse and patient-specific comorbidities that predict for TRM. The guidelines uniformly endorsed allogeneic HCT, from related or unrelated donors including cord blood HCT, in first CR for patients with unfavorable cytogenetic or molecular abnormalities, therapy-related AML or prior myelodysplasia. Among those older than 60 years, the recommendation was to consider HCT as an early option in those achieving a CR and as treatment for induction failure only in patients with low volume residual disease. For relapsed AML, HCT was recommended irrespective of age but only after a second CR was achieved or in the context of a clinical trial. For patients with acute promyelocytic leukemia, the recommendation was to reserve allogeneic HCT for relapsed patients with persistent disease despite salvage therapy.

The ASBMT evidence-based policy for allogeneic HCT in AML recommends HCT in the relapse setting (after achievement of CR2) and in patients with poor-risk cytogenetics in first remission. The ASBMT guidelines did not routinely recommend: allogeneic HCT for patients with intermediate risk cytogenetics; or the routine use of myeloablative conditioning for patients over age 55 years. The European Leukemia-Net guidelines are mostly in line with the ASBMT evidence-based policy, but provide greater detail about allogeneic HCT in cytogenetically normal (CN) AML.[23] These guidelines recommend considering HCT for patients with CN-AML and unfavorable molecular markers, that is, those who lack the favorable genotypes of mutated nucleophosmin 1 (NPM1) without FMS-related tyrosine kinase 3-internal tandems duplication (FLT3-ITD) or mutated CCAAT/enhancer binding protein alpha (CEBPA). In addition, allogeneic HCT was endorsed for FLT3-ITD + AML.

A systematic review of various national guidelines found the following[24]:

a. Consistent recommendations that patients with relapsed or refractory disease or high-risk cytogenetics be considered for HCT early;
b. Consistent recommendations that patients with good prognosis cytogenetics receive HCT only after failure of nontransplant therapy;
c. Inconsistent recommendations for patients with intermediate risk disease or without a family donor regarding transplantation in first remission;
d. Lack of consensus regarding the efficacy of reduced-intensity conditioning;
e. Most national guidelines recommend a risk-based approach to guide selection of chemotherapy versus transplant approaches using factors such as patient age, comorbid conditions, disease phenotype at diagnosis and the number of cycles of therapy before remission.

Acute Lymphoblastic Leukemia

Allogeneic HCT in first remission from related or unrelated donors is generally accepted as the most effective available therapy for

BOX 104.4	Recommended Practices for Allogeneic Transplant Recipients in Long-term Follow-up			
	6 mo	12 mo	Annual	Comments ([a])
Liver:				
Liver Function Tests	√	√	a	Annual check only if previously abnormal or new signs/symptoms
Serum Ferritin		√	a	
Respiratory:				
Clinical Assessment	√	√	√	
Smoking/Tobacco Avoidance	√	√	√	
Formal Pulmonary Function Tests		√	a	Annual study/Imaging as needed in follow up of prior/new abnormalities
Chest X-Ray	a	a	a	
Bone Density Screening		√	a	Consider repeat testing in ones with recognized defects, ongoing risk factors or for response assessment
Kidney:				
Blood Pressure Screen	√	√	√	
Proteinuria Screen	√	√	a	As needed annually
BUN/Creatinine level	√	√	√	
Nervous System:				
Clinical Assessment		√	a	Annually as needed
Endocrine:				
Thyroid Function		√	a	Annually as needed
Gonadal Function in postpubertal women		√	√	
Cardiac/Vascular:				
Cardiovascular Risk Factor Screen		√	√	
Immune System/Infection Risk:				
Encapsulated organism Prophylaxis	a	a	a	If on immune suppression or with ongoing GVHD
Pneumocystis prophylaxis	√	a	a	
CMV test	√	√		
Immunizations		√	√	
Endocarditis prophylaxis		a	a	Follow AHA guidelines
Antifungal/Antiherpes viral prophylaxis	a	a	a	If on immune suppression or with GVHD; if not, no consensus
Second Cancer Risk:				
Cancer Risk Assessment and Education		√	√	
Pap Smear		√	√	
Mammogram (women over 40 years)		√	√	
Breast/Skin/Testes self-examination		√	√	
Clinical Screen for second cancers		√	√	
Psychosocial:				
Clinical psychosocial and QOL screen	√	√	√	
Sexual function screen	√	√	√	
Dental Assessment	√	√	√	
Ocular:				
Clinical Evaluation	√	√	√	
Fundus Exam		√	a	As needed annually
Schirmer test	a	a		If with ongoing GVHD or on immune suppression

AHA, American Heart Association; BUN, blood urea nitrogen; CMV, cytomegalovirus; GVHD, graft-versus-host disease; QOL, quality of life.

patients with Philadelphia chromosome (Ph)-positive ALL. For adults with Ph-negative ALL, the appropriate timing of HCT is more controversial despite the largest prospective study (Medical Research Council/Eastern Cooperative Oncology Group [MRC/ECOG]) and a metaanalysis suggesting a survival advantage for those assigned to transplant in CR1.[25,26] Allogeneic transplantation is currently considered by NCCN expert consensus as the best curative therapy for adult patients with high-risk features such Ph+ ALL or those with a poor response to initial induction therapy and among adults with t(4;11) ALL. Evidence-based policy statement from the ASBMT recommended allogeneic HCT for standard-risk, young (<35 years) adults in first CR and for ALL in second or higher remission. Related and unrelated donor HCT were recommended as being similar in outcomes.[27] For those without suitable matched adult donors, cord blood grafts should be considered.

Chronic Myelogenous Leukemia

In general, HCT is indicated for patients whose initial presentation is in blast phase and should be considered for those with a suboptimal response or relapse while on tyrosine kinase inhibitors (TKIs). HCT

is also a consideration for patients who have BCR-ABL mutations that predict for TKI nonresponse (e.g., T325I mutation). It is important to establish a monitoring plan for early signs of progression and for mutation screening since outcomes are significantly better if HCT is performed before transformation to advanced disease. Definitions of suboptimal response and failure with TKIs and guidelines for monitoring have been developed.[28] European Leukemia-Net guidelines recently addressed timing of allogeneic HCT in CML.[28] Allogeneic HCT was recommended in all CML patients presenting in blast phase, and for the accelerated phase patients who do not achieve an optimal response. HCT transplantation was also recommended for TKI-treated chronic phase patients subsequently progressing to accelerated or blast phase, after achieving optimal disease control. For patients in chronic phase, recommendation was to reserve allogeneic HCT for those who are resistant or intolerant to at least one second-generation TKI, and in patients developing T315I mutation.

Chronic Lymphocytic Leukemia

Current NCCN guidelines recommend allogeneic HCT in chronic lymphocytic leukemia (CLL) for those of younger age with high-risk disease (TP53 deletion, 11q deletion) in the frontline setting and for those with CLL relapsing shortly after initial response (<2 years) irrespective of cytogenetics. The EBMT consensus group has recommended allogeneic HCT as a reasonable treatment option for younger patients with nonresponse, or relapse (within 12 months) after purine analogue therapy.[29] Patients who relapse within 24 months after having a response to purine analogue-based combinations and patients with TP53 abnormalities and those with Richter transformation requiring treatment are also considered candidates for transplant evaluation. The role and timing of allogeneic HCT in the era of Bruton Tyrosine Kinase inhibitors will need to be redefined.

Diffuse Large B-Cell Lymphoma

The ASBMT panel recommends autologous transplantation as the treatment of choice for relapsed or refractory chemosensitive diffuse large B-cell lymphoma. Allogeneic HCT is a consideration in the context of clinical trials and in select situations such as autologous mobilization failure, persistent bone marrow disease, and after a failed autologous transplant.[30]

Follicular Lymphoma

A systematic review by the ASBMT noted the lack of high-quality evidence regarding indications for allogeneic HCT in follicular lymphoma.[31] The consensus panel recommended autologous HCT for relapsed disease or transformed follicular lymphoma. In the allogeneic setting, RIC was considered an acceptable alternative to myeloablative regimens. The panel found no differences in outcomes between HLA identical sibling donors and matched unrelated donors. Given the efficacy of rituximab-based salvage treatments and autologous HCT for follicular lymphoma, allogeneic HCT is generally used for patients who have failed, are likely to fail, or are unable to proceed to salvage autologous HCT. However, late application of allogeneic HCT may be less effective especially for chemotherapy refractory disease. The NCCN guideline panel recommended autologous transplantation in second or third remission as a standard consolidative strategy for relapsed follicular lymphoma.[32] Allogeneic HCT was a consideration for highly selected patients and those with histologic transformation to a higher grade (especially in the context of a clinical trial).

Mantle Cell Lymphoma

NCCN guidelines recommend autologous transplantation as an adjunct to initial therapy in eligible patients.[32] Expert opinion is that allogeneic HCT has a limited role as upfront consolidation in chemotherapy-sensitive disease. Given the poor prognosis of recurrent mantle cell lymphoma and the curative potential of allogeneic HCT, it is a reasonable option for patients relapsing after upfront autologous transplantation or those with chemotherapy refractory disease.

T-Cell Lymphoma

NCCN guidelines recommend consideration of allogeneic HCT in the relapsed or refractory setting in T-cell lymphoma.[32] In cutaneous T-cell lymphoma, allogeneic HCT is considered in the setting of progressive or refractory stage IIB–IV disease after failure of biologic agents and at least one line of chemotherapy.

Hodgkin Lymphoma

NCCN guidelines currently consider allogeneic HCT in progressive or relapsed Hodgkin lymphoma as a category 3 recommendation (major disagreement) and recommend that this treatment should therefore ideally be performed as part of a clinical trial.

Multiple Myeloma

The NCCN guidelines consider allogeneic HCT with myeloablative conditioning as an accepted option in the setting of a clinical trial, in those responding to primary therapy or with primary progressive disease. The guidelines did not recommend allogeneic HCT with nonmyeloablative conditioning alone as an option. RIC with allogeneic HCT following autologous HCT was considered a category 2A recommendation (reflecting uniform NCCN consensus, based on lower-level evidence including clinical experience, that the recommendation is appropriate). Allogeneic HCT in the relapsed setting after a prior autograft was considered a grade III recommendation reflecting major disagreement.

REFERENCES

1. Thomas E, Storb R, Clift RA, et al: Bone-marrow transplantation (first of two parts). *N Engl J Med* 292(16):832–843, 1975.
2. Bacigalupo A, Ballen K, Rizzo D, et al: Defining the intensity of conditioning regimens: working definitions. *Biol Blood Marrow Transplant* 15(12):1628–1633, 2009.
3. Sorror ML, Sandmaier BM, Storer BE, et al: Long-term outcomes among older patients following nonmyeloablative conditioning and allogeneic hematopoietic cell transplantation for advanced hematologic malignancies. *JAMA* 306(17):1874–1883, 2011.
4. Kröger N, Brand R, Niederwieser D, et al: Reduced intensity vs. standard conditioning followed by allogeneic stem cell transplantation for patients with MDS or secondary AML: a prospective, randomized phase III study of the chronic malignancies working party of the EBMT (RICMAC-Trial). *Blood* 124(21):320, 2014.
5. Mielcarek M, Storer B, Martin PJ, et al: Long-term outcomes after transplantation of HLA-identical related G-CSF-mobilized peripheral blood mononuclear cells versus bone marrow. *Blood* 119(11):2675–2678, 2012.
6. Couban S, Simpson DR, Barnett MJ, et al: A randomized multicenter comparison of bone marrow and peripheral blood in recipients of matched sibling allogeneic transplants for myeloid malignancies. *Blood* 100(5):1525–1531, 2002.
7. Anasetti C, Logan BR, Lee SJ, et al: Peripheral-blood stem cells versus bone marrow from unrelated donors. *N Engl J Med* 367(16):1487–1496, 2012.
8. Eapen M, Logan BR, Horowitz MM, et al: Bone marrow or peripheral blood for reduced-intensity conditioning unrelated donor transplantation. *J Clin Oncol* 2014.
9. Gragert L, Eapen M, Williams E, et al: HLA match likelihoods for hematopoietic stem-cell grafts in the U.S. registry. *N Engl J Med* 371(4):339–348, 2014.
10. Laughlin MJ, Eapen M, Rubinstein P, et al: Outcomes after transplantation of cord blood or bone marrow from unrelated donors in adults with leukemia. *N Engl J Med* 351(22):2265–2275, 2004.
11. Wagner JE, Jr, Eapen M, Carter S, et al: One-unit versus two-unit cord-blood transplantation for hematologic cancers. *N Engl J Med* 371(18):1685–1694, 2014.
12. Bashey A, Zhang X, Sizemore CA, et al: T-cell-replete HLA-haploidentical hematopoietic transplantation for hematologic malignancies using post-transplantation cyclophosphamide results in outcomes equivalent to those of contemporaneous HLA-matched related and unrelated donor transplantation. *J Clin Oncol* 31(10):1310–1316, 2013.
13. Brunstein CG, Fuchs EJ, Carter SL, et al: Alternative donor transplantation after reduced intensity conditioning: results of parallel phase 2 trials using partially HLA-mismatched related bone marrow or unrelated double umbilical cord blood grafts. *Blood* 118(2):282–288, 2011.
13a. Barnes DW, Loutit JF, Micklem HS: "Secondary disease" of radiation chimeras: a syndrome due to lymphoid aplasia. *Ann N Y Acad Sci* 99:374–385, 1962.

14. Bortin MM, Truitt RL, Rimm AA, et al: Graft-versus-leukaemia reactivity induced by alloimmunisation without augmentation of graft-versus-host reactivity. *Nature* 281(5731):490–491. 1979.

15. Horowitz MM, Gale RP, Sondel PM, et al: Graft-versus-leukemia reactions after bone marrow transplantation. *Blood* 75(3):555–562, 1990.

16. Leung W, Iyengar R, Turner V, et al: Determinants of antileukemia effects of allogeneic NK cells. *J Immunol* 172(1):644–650, 2004.

17. Cooley S, Weisdorf DJ, Guethlein LA, et al: Donor selection for natural killer cell receptor genes leads to superior survival after unrelated transplantation for acute myelogenous leukemia. *Blood* 116(14):2411–2419, 2010.

18. Horan JT, Logan BR, Agovi-Johnson MA, et al: Reducing the risk for transplantation-related mortality after allogeneic hematopoietic cell transplantation: how much progress has been made? *J Clin Oncol* 29(7):805–813, 2011.

19. Sorror ML, Maris MB, Storb R, et al: Hematopoietic cell transplantation (HCT)-specific comorbidity index: a new tool for risk assessment before allogeneic HCT. *Blood* 106(8):2912–2919, 2005.

20. Armand P, Kim HT, Logan BR, et al: Validation and refinement of the Disease Risk Index for allogeneic stem cell transplantation. *Blood* 123(23):3664–3671, 2014.

21. Eapen M, Rocha V: Principles and analysis of hematopoietic stem cell transplantation outcomes: the physician's perspective. *Lifetime Data Anal* 14(4):379–388, 2008.

22. Socie G, Stone JV, Wingard JR, et al: Long-term survival and late deaths after allogeneic bone marrow transplantation. Late Effects Working Committee of the International Bone Marrow Transplant Registry. *N Engl J Med* 341(1):14–21, 1999.

23. Dohner H, Estey EH, Amadori S, et al: Diagnosis and management of acute myeloid leukemia in adults: recommendations from an international expert panel, on behalf of the European LeukemiaNet. *Blood* 115(3):453–474, 2010.

24. Hubel K, Weingart O, Naumann F, et al: Allogeneic stem cell transplant in adult patients with acute myelogenous leukemia: a systematic analysis of international guidelines and recommendations. *Leuk Lymphoma* 52(3):444–457, 2011.

25. Goldstone AH, Richards SM, Lazarus HM, et al: In adults with standard-risk acute lymphoblastic leukemia, the greatest benefit is achieved from a matched sibling allogeneic transplantation in first complete remission, and an autologous transplantation is less effective than conventional consolidation/maintenance chemotherapy in all patients: final results of the International ALL Trial (MRC UKALL XII/ECOG E2993). *Blood* 111(4):1827–1833, 2008.

26. Pidala J, Djulbegovic B, Anasetti C, et al: Allogeneic hematopoietic cell transplantation for adult acute lymphoblastic leukemia (ALL) in first complete remission. *Cochrane Database Syst Rev* (10):CD008818, 2011. doi(10):CD008818.

27. Oliansky DM, Larson RA, Weisdorf D, et al: The role of cytotoxic therapy with hematopoietic stem cell transplantation in the treatment of adult acute lymphoblastic leukemia: update of the 2006 evidence-based review. *Biol Blood Marrow Transplant* 18(1):16–17, 2012.

28. Baccarani M, Deininger MW, Rosti G, et al: European LeukemiaNet recommendations for the management of chronic myeloid leukemia: 2013. *Blood* 122(6):872–884, 2013.

29. Dreger P, Corradini P, Kimby E, et al: Indications for allogeneic stem cell transplantation in chronic lymphocytic leukemia: the EBMT transplant consensus. *Leukemia* 21(1):12–17, 2007.

30. Oliansky DM, Czuczman M, Fisher RI, et al: The role of cytotoxic therapy with hematopoietic stem cell transplantation in the treatment of diffuse large B cell lymphoma: update of the 2001 evidence-based review. *Biol Blood Marrow Transplant* 17(1):20–47.e30, 2011.

31. Oliansky DM, Gordon LI, King J, et al: The role of cytotoxic therapy with hematopoietic stem cell transplantation in the treatment of follicular lymphoma: an evidence-based review. *Biol Blood Marrow Transplant* 16(4):443–468, 2010.

32. Zelenetz AD, Wierda WG, Abramson JS, et al: Non-Hodgkin's lymphomas, version 1.2013. *J Natl Compr Canc Netw* 11(3):257–272, quiz 273, 2013.

33. Lim Z, Brand R, Martino R, et al: Allogeneic hematopoietic stem-cell transplantation for patients 50 years or older with myelodysplastic syndromes or secondary acute myeloid leukemia. *J Clin Oncol* 28(3):405–411, 2010.

34. Crawley C, Iacobelli S, Björkstrand B, et al: Reduced-intensity conditioning for myeloma: lower nonrelapse mortality but higher relapse rates compared with myeloablative conditioning. *Blood* 109:3588–3594, 2007.

35. Martino R, Iacobelli S, Brand R, et al: Retrospective comparison of reduced-intensity conditioning and conventional high-dose conditioning for allogeneic hematopoietic stem cell transplantation using HLA-identical sibling donors in myelodysplastic syndromes. *Blood* 108:836–846, 2006.

36. Dreger P, Brand R, Milligan D, et al: Reduced-intensity conditioning lowers treatment-related mortality of allogeneic stem cell transplantation for chronic lymphocytic leukemia: a population-matched analysis. *Leukemia* 19:1029–1033, 2005.

37. Sureda A, Robinson S, Canals C, et al: Reduced-intensity conditioning compared with conventional allogeneic stem-cell transplantation in relapsed or refractory Hodgkin's lymphoma: An analysis from the Lymphoma Working Party of the European Group for Blood and Marrow Transplantation. *J Clin Oncol* 26:455–462, 2008.

38. Hari P, Carreras J, Zhang MJ, et al: Allogeneic transplants in follicular lymphoma: higher risk of disease progression after reduced-intensity compared to myeloablative conditioning. *Biol Blood Marrow Transplant* 14:236–245, 2008.

39. Mohty M, Labopin M, Volin L, et al: Reduced-intensity versus conventional myeloablative conditioning allogeneic stem cell transplantation for patients with acute lymphoblastic leukemia: A retrospective study from the European Group for Blood and Marrow Transplantation. *Blood* 116:4439–4443, 2010.

40. Luger SM, Ringdén O, Zhang MJ, et al: Similar outcomes using myeloablative vs. reduced-intensity allogeneic transplant preparative regimens for AML or MDS. *Bone Marrow Transplant* 47:203, 2012.

CHAPTER 105

UNRELATED DONOR HEMATOPOIETIC CELL TRANSPLANTATION

Effie W. Petersdorf and Claudio Anasetti

The outcomes of unrelated donor hematopoietic cell transplantation (HCT) have greatly improved as a result of better understanding of the diversity of genes that give rise to host-versus-graft (HVG) and graft-versus-host (GVH) allorecognition. Development of robust typing methods that define functional variation of human leukocyte antigen (HLA) genes have greatly accelerated understanding of gene–gene interactions that lead to graft failure, graft-versus-host disease (GVHD), and graft-versus-leukemia (GVL). Continued growth of registries of volunteer donors worldwide now provides the potential for identifying suitable donors for up to 75% of white patients in need of a transplant. The major challenges are to increase the safety and efficacy of unrelated donor HCT therapy through improved prevention and treatment of GVHD while leveraging control of leukemia through GVL effects. For unrelated HCT to be more widely applied to patients of diverse ethnic and racial backgrounds, more information on permissible HLA mismatches is needed so that mismatched donors can be safely used when matched donors are not available. This chapter chronicles genotyping methods used for donor selection and the clinical results of unrelated donor HCT in the era of DNA typing for *HLA* genes.

DONOR IDENTIFICATION AND LIKELIHOOD OF TRANSPLANTATION

The field of unrelated donor HCT has witnessed a rapid growth over the past 25 years. Data from the Center for International Bone Marrow Transplant Research (CIBMTR) show that among all allogeneic transplantations performed in the United States, the number of transplants from unrelated donors has exceeded that from related donors since 2006 (http://www.CIBMTR.org). Similar statistics from the European Group for Blood and Marrow Transplantation show that 52% of all allogeneic transplants are performed with unrelated donors (http://www.ebmt.org). The primary indications for unrelated donor HCT are acute myeloid leukemia, myelodysplastic syndrome/myeloproliferative disorders, acute lymphoblastic leukemia, non-Hodgkin lymphoma, and other nonmalignant disorders. Between 2002 and 2006, patients older than 60 years of age comprised the fastest growing group of transplant recipients as a result of the introduction of nonmyeloablative and reduced-intensity conditioning regimens (http://www.CIBMTR.org).

Unrelated HCT has been made feasible by the establishment of registries of volunteer donors worldwide. The Anthony Nolan Appeal was the first effort to demonstrate the feasibility of donor recruitment. Now known as the Anthony Nolan Research Institute, this registry was the first to promote access to HLA-matched bone marrow (BM) donors for patients around the world. In the United States, early efforts for donor recruitment were spearheaded by individual centers. Growing interest in unrelated donor HCT led the US Congress to authorize the creation of a national registry comprising a network of donor centers, transplant centers, and a national coordinating center through the Transplant Act of 1984. Two years later, a federal contract to establish a national registry was awarded to the National Marrow Donor Program (NMDP). In the Netherlands, Professor Jon J. van Rood led the Europdonor Foundation in the collection of HLA data from donor registries around the world and in the formation of a database of HLA phenotypes known as Bone Marrow Donors Worldwide (http://www.bmdw.org). Continued

growth in registry size worldwide has increased the chances that well-matched donors can be identified. The NMDP registers 52,000 new donors each month (http://www.bethematch.org). Today, more than 10.5 million donors are available through the NMDP, and more than 25 million donors are available through international cooperative agreements with registries around the world (http://www.worldmarrow.org).[1] With this database of 25 million donors, North American white patients have a 75% chance of identifying an unrelated donor matched at HLA-A, HLA-B, HLA-C, and HLA-DRB1 (HLA "8/8").[2] This number increases to 97% if the donor selection criteria are relaxed to accommodate one HLA mismatch (HLA "7/8"). The situation is not as favorable for patients of non-European white background. For African Americans, the likelihood of finding an HLA 8/8–matched donor is only 19% but improves to 76% with HLA 7/8 donors. These statistics emphasize that although the total number of donors is climbing, the challenges for the future remain achieving the ideal optimal registry size and composition to improve the odds that every patient in need of a transplant has at least one suitable donor.

The availability of HLA-matched donors is only one potential barrier to transplantation for patients. In a single center study of 531 patients who initiated a search for an unrelated donor,[3] an 8/8 HLA-A, HLA-B, HLA-C, HLA-DRB1–matched donor was available for 54% of these patients; a further 30% had a donor with a single HLA mismatch, and 16% had no suitable donor. Factors that increased the chances of a patient undergoing unrelated donor transplantation included race (white patients are more likely; $p = .03$), younger age ($p = .01$), lower disease risk ($p = .005$), and availability of an HLA 8/8–matched donor ($p = .005$; Box 105.1). The reasons for patients not pursuing transplant can be varied, but most often are caused by disease progression, alternative treatment plan choices, and medical ineligibility. Having a suitable donor not only allowed patients to reach transplantation but also improved the overall survival of patients with good performance status, compared with not having a suitable donor.[3]

DONOR EVALUATION AND SELECTION

Selection of unrelated donors includes consideration for the level of the HLA tissue-type match with the recipient and the presence of recipient antidonor HLA antibodies, which place the patient at high risk for nonengraftment in the setting of HLA mismatching.[4] One of the earliest studies to highlight the importance of anti-HLA antibodies in nonengraftment found an over twofold higher risk of graft failure after haploidentical related donor transplantation when the patient possessed antidonor lymphocytotoxic antibodies.[5] More recently, anti–HLA-DP antibodies were associated with graft failure after transplantation from otherwise HLA-A, HLA-B, HLA-C, HLA-DR, HLA-DQ–matched unrelated donors.[6] The increased utilization of cord blood sources for stem cells in transplantation has prompted evaluation of the role of anti-HLA antibodies in cord blood, and the experience has paralleled that of unrelated donor transplantation.[7-11] Collectively, this experience has led to the formulation of strategies for antibody screening before allogeneic transplantation.[12]

Evaluation of unrelated donors includes a screening medical history, physical examination, and laboratory testing for risks

TABLE 105.1 | **Common Definitions in Human Leukocyte Antigen Genetics**

Term	Definition	Example
Allele	Unique sequence of an *HLA* gene defined by molecular methods	DRB1*04:01 allele is a unique sequence defined as DR4 by serologic methods
Antigen	Antibody-defined protein	DR4 antigen is a serologically-defined protein product of an *HLA* gene
Haplotype	*HLA* genes inherited as a chromosomal unit	HLA-A1, HLA-B8, HLA-DR3 is a common haplotype among white populations
Genotype	Molecularly-defined HLA allele or sequence	Genotypically-matched donor and recipient are identical for the HLA alleles at a given *HLA* gene (e.g., HLA-DRB1*04:01)
Phenotype	Serologically-defined HLA protein or antigen	Phenotypically-matched donor and recipient share the same HLA antigen (e.g., HLA-DR4)

HLA, Human leukocyte antigen.

TABLE 105.2 | **Polymorphism of Human Leukocyte Antigen Genes**

	Antigens	Alleles
HLA-A	24	3285
HLA-B	50	4077
HLA-C	9	2801
HLA-DRB1	15	1825
HLA-DQB1	9	876
HLA-DPB1	6	587

HLA, Human leukocyte antigen.
Available at http://www.ebi.ac.uk/ipd/imgt/hla/stats.html.

associated with transmissible elements akin to blood transfusion donors. Special focus is placed on risks of transmission of hepatitis, human immunodeficiency virus (HIV), malaria, West Nile virus, transmissible spongiform encephalitis (Creutzfeldt-Jacob disease), and Chagas disease. Donor screening includes blood tests for HIV 1 and 2, hepatitis B virus, hepatitis C virus, *Treponema pallidum*, human T-cell lymphotrophic virus I and II, and cytomegalovirus.

Increased awareness for the health and safety of the unrelated donor has led to the establishment of standards for donation.[13,14] These standards include donor recruitment, confidentiality, health assessment and eligibility, donors as research participants, and adverse events following donation. With the use of peripheral-blood stem cells as a primary source of progenitor cells for transplantation,[15] a comprehensive review of the long-term effects of granulocyte colony-stimulating factor has not revealed increased incidence of hematologic malignancies among volunteer donors.[16]

PROCESS OF IDENTIFYING A SUITABLE UNRELATED DONOR

Human Leukocyte Antigen Typing and Donor Matching in the DNA Era: Genetics of the Human Leukocyte Antigen Complex

The advent of molecular techniques has made possible the definition of unique sequence variants (alleles) that encode each HLA molecule that is recognized by an antibody (antigen; Table 105.1). Polymorphism ensures that a large array of foreign peptides can be presented to the immune system by HLA molecules. As of October 2015, more than 3285 HLA-A, 4077 HLA-B, 2801 HLA-C, 1825 HLA-DRB1, 876 HLA-DQB1, and 587 HLA-DPB1 alleles have been defined in diverse human populations (http://www.ebi.ac.uk/ipd/imgt/hla/stats.html; Table 105.2). HLA nomenclature accommodates the steady discovery of new human variants. The HLA prefix is followed by a hyphen and the gene name (e.g., HLA-A). The gene is listed followed by an asterisk to separate the gene from the unique sequence (HLA-A*). The unique sequence name embodies up to four kinds of information, each delimited by a colon. The first set of numbers after the asterisk and before the first colon correspond to the serologic antigen equivalent (e.g., HLA-A*02 refers to sequences of the

HLA-A2 antigen family). The second set of numbers provides the unique protein that correspond to the subtype (HLA-A*02:101). The third set of numbers indicate synonymous substitutions (HLA-A*02:101:01). The last series of numbers give information on non-coding variation often denoting expression (HLA-A*02:101:01:02 N). Letter suffixes are used to denote alleles that are not expressed (also known as "null"; N), low cell surface expression (L), a soluble secreted molecule not present on the surface of the cell (S), a cytoplasmic product not expressed on the cell surface (C), a protein with aberrant expression (A), and a sequence of questionable expression (Q). This new nomenclature has no limits on the number of digits for each of the four categories and in this way, obviates the need for constant renumbering.

DNA genotyping was adopted as the standard technique for selection of HLA-matched unrelated donors because unrelated individuals who are matched for HLA antigens may not necessarily share the same HLA sequences. If HLA alleles can be expressed in any combination and if inheritance of alleles were random, then the total estimated number of possible five-locus HLA-A, HLA-B, HLA-C, HLA-DRB1, and HLA-DQB1 genotypes would be exceedingly high, and the chances of identifying a fully matched donor would be very low. Clinical experience demonstrates that donor identification is successful, and is caused by the underlying genetic hallmark of the major histocompatibility complex known as linkage disequilibrium (LD). LD refers to the observation that HLA alleles are found in association with each other at an observed frequency that exceeds their expected frequency. The probability of identifying a matched donor for a given patient is higher when the patient and donor share a similar ethnic background. Linked *HLA* genes are inherited from each parent as a haplotype in classic Mendelian fashion (see Assessment of Human Leukocyte Antigen Haplotypes later). *HLA* gene and haplotype frequencies provide important data for estimating optimal registry size and composition (http://www.allelefrequencies.net). Given the polymorphism of allele sequences that encompass variants of a single serologically defined antigen, it is not surprising that antigen-matched donor and patient pairs may differ for their alleles (Table 105.3).

HUMAN LEUKOCYTE ANTIGEN TYPING METHODS

HLA antigens important in transplantation were historically characterized using serologic typing methods. Typing by serology entails reacting alloantisera containing antibodies against cells in a complement-dependent microcytotoxicity assay. The development of standardized tissue typing reagents and methods of nomenclature for *HLA* genes have been facilitated by a series of 16 international histocompatibility workshops (Table 105.4). The advent of polymerase chain reaction (PCR) in the 1980s revolutionized donor typing and matching and has greatly accelerated understanding of the HLA barrier in transplantation. Guidelines for typing volunteer donors using DNA-based methods are available. To transition from

TABLE 105.3   Definition of Matching for Alleles and Antigens

Match Status	Donor	Recipient
Antigen[a]-matched	HLA-B*44	HLA-B*44
Antigen-matched and allele[b]-matched	HLA-B*44:02	HLA-B*44:02
Antigen-matched but allele-mismatched	HLA-B*44:03	HLA-B*44:02
Antigen-mismatched	HLA-B*44	HLA-B*27

Human leukocyte antigen (HLA) alleles and antigens are designated according to the World Health Organization Nomenclature for Factors of the HLA System.
[a]Defined by serology.
[b]Defined by DNA sequencing.

TABLE 105.4   International Histocompatibility Workshops and Conferences

Workshop	Year	Chairman	Venue	Advances	
First	1964	D.B. Amos	Durham, NC, USA	Definition of "Hu-L," "LA," and "Four" antigen specificities	
Second	1965	J.J. Van Rood	Leiden, The Netherlands	MLC testing	
Third	1967	R. Ceppellini	Turin, Italy	Family studies HLA in renal transplantation	
Fourth	1970	P. Terasaki	Los Angeles, CA, USA	Definition of 27 HLA-A, HLA-B, and HLA-C specificities	
Fifth	1972	J. Dausset	Evian, France	Worldwide typing of 49 populations	
Sixth	1975	F. Kissmeyer	Aarhus, Denmark	Description of Dw specificities, Nielsen	
Seventh	1977	W. Bodmer	Oxford, England	Definition of DR1-7 specificities HTC testing	
Eighth	1980	P. Terasaki	Los Angeles, CA, USA	Definition of HLA-MB (DQ) MT (DR52/53) HLA in renal transplantation and disease association	
Ninth	1984	E. Albert W. Mayr	Munich, Germany Vienna, Austria	New class I and II specificities HLA class II in renal transplantation	
10th	1987	B. Dupont	Scanticon, NJ, USA New York, NY, USA	Establishment of RFLP/T cell clones and HTC methods Creation of panel of homozygous cell lines	
11th	1991	T. Sasazuki K. Tsuji	Yokohama, Japan	HLA class I PCR typing anthropology	
12th	1996	D. Charron	Saint-Malo, France Paris, France	Sequencing Class I DNA typing/HLA in medicine	
13th	2002	J. Hansen	Seattle, WA, USA Victoria, British Columbia, Canada	Virtual DNA analysis Identification of SNP markers HLA in anthropology, disease association, HCT	http://www.ihwg.org
14th	2005	J. McCluskey	Melbourne, Australia	MHC and anthropology, disease, infection, HCT, cancer nonclassical genes, NK-KIR, cytokine genes	http://www.ihwg.org
15th	2008	M. Gerbase and M-E Moraes	Buzios, Brazil	Brazil Population Studies, Bioinformatics Tools	
16th	2012	S.G.E. Marsh and D. Middleton	Liverpool, UK	Population-based alleles and haplotypes; next generation sequencing tools	
17th	2017	M. Fernandez-Vina	Stanford, CA, USA	Next generation sequencing	

HCT, Hematopoietic cell transplantation; HLA, human leukocyte antigen; HTC, homozygous typing cells; KIR, killer-cell immunoglobulin-like receptor; MHC, major histocompatibility complex; MLC, mixed lymphocyte culture; NK, natural killer; PCR, polymerase chain reaction; RFLP, restriction fragment length polymorphism; SNP, single nucleotide polymorphism.

serologic to DNA-based methods, development of dictionaries of HLA alleles and antigen equivalents has become a necessity because many donors in the registries have been typed only by serologic assays. Interpretation and use of molecular typing data for donor search and selection has required the development of informatics programs.

Low-resolution DNA-based typing methods can define groups of alleles that are serologic equivalent (e.g., HLA-A*02 is DNA-defined and is equivalent to HLA-A2 that is serologically-defined). Intermediate-resolution DNA typing methods provide additional information but not to the level of the complete DNA sequence that distinguishes one allele from another (e.g., the information is sufficient to delineate one group of alleles that include HLA-A*02:01 and another that include HLA*02:05 but cannot definitely assign the allele). High-resolution typing defines the unique DNA sequence of an allele (e.g., HLA-A*02:01). The term "6/6" matched refers to recipients and donors who share the same low-resolution–defined HLA-A, HLA-B, and HLA-DR genes. The term "8/8" refers to high-resolution matching at the four loci HLA-A, HLA-B, HLA-C, and HLA-DRB1. When HLA-DQB1 is added, "10/10" refers to high-resolution matching at the five loci. When HLA-DPB1 is added, "12/12" refers to donor–recipient pairs that are allele matched at all six genetic loci.

Several PCR-based HLA typing approaches are widely used by clinical tissue typing laboratories in support of unrelated HCT programs. The sequence-specific primer method uses a panel of primers to amplify the *HLA* locus or alleles. The PCR products are electrophoresed on a gel, and assignment of an HLA type is made by examining the composite pattern of positive and negative PCR reaction methods.

The sequence-specific oligonucleotide probe hybridization (SSOPH) method uses a solid phase support to immobilize PCR-amplified products. Nonradioactive-labeled oligonucleotide probes are allowed to hybridize to the support. Whereas probes with sequences complementary to the target DNA will hybridize, probes with as few as one nucleotide difference will fail to hybridize. Alternatively, SSOPH methods can use probes that are immobilized to the solid phase support and allow PCR-amplified target DNA to hybridize to the support.

A variation of the SSOPH method is oligonucleotide array technology. Arrays can simultaneously query multiple regions of polymorphisms in many *HLA* genes. Oligonucleotide probes can be designed to all four potential nucleotides, thereby enabling detection of new sequence polymorphisms with the same sensitivity and specificity as sequencing-based typing. Redundancy of probe sequences allows combinations of alleles to be distinguished in heterozygous individuals. Commercial platforms are now available and provide quality-controlled reagents for high throughput genotyping.[17,18]

In addition to probe-based assays, Sanger sequencing of *HLA* genes has been an established method for high-resolution typing.[19] Newer sequencing approaches include "next generation sequencing" (NGS) platforms that provide not only high resolution of HLA alleles but also have the advantage of short-range phasing of exons 2, 3, and 4 of class I genes, and of exons 2 and 3 of class II genes.[20,21] The capability of linking sequences across exons substantially reduces the number of theoretical ambiguities of allele combinations. NGS approaches for HLA typing are supported by software for automated assignment of HLA alleles.[22] Because many samples may be tested simultaneously, NGS is a cost-effective typing method for typing donors recruited into registries.[23,24]

ASSESSMENT OF THE VECTOR OF MISMATCHING

The "vector" or "direction" of HLA compatibility between a donor and a recipient has biologic relevance in defining the risks of graft failure and GVHD. The concept of the vector was first demonstrated in cases of haploidentical related mismatched transplantation and defines HVG and GVH alloreactivity.[25] Patients homozygous for the mismatched *HLA* locus had lower rates of severe acute GVHD but

TABLE 105.5	Vector of Mismatch		
		Examples	
Vector	**Definition**	**Donor**	**Recipient**
HVG	Presence of donor alleles not present in the recipient	DRB1*01:01,04:01[a] DRB1*01:01,04:01[b]	DRB1*01:01,04:10 DRB1*01:01,01:01
GVH	Presence of recipient alleles not present in the donor	DRB1*01:01,04:01[a] DRB1*01:01,01:01[b]	DRB1*01:01,04:10 DRB1*01:01,04:10

[a]These combinations contain bidirectional (both HVG and GVHD) mismatch vectors.
[b]Unidirectional mismatches.
GVH, Graft-versus-host; HVG, host-versus-graft.

higher rates of graft failure than heterozygous patients. These clinical observations led to the establishment of the "vector of HLA incompatibility" in allogeneic transplantation: whereas the presence of donor alleles not shared by the recipient determines HVG allorecognition, the presence of recipient alleles not shared by the donor provides the immunologic basis for GVH allorecognition (Table 105.5). "Bidirectional" mismatching refers to the situation in which both HVG and GVH vectors are present at a given *HLA* locus. "Unidirectional" mismatching describes the situation in which either the donor or the recipient is homozygous for the same allele at the mismatched locus. A unidirectional GVH vector mismatch occurs when the donor is homozygous and the recipient is heterozygous and shares one allele with the donor (e.g., patient DRB1*01:01, *04:10 versus donor DRB1*01:01, *01:01). A unidirectional HVG vector mismatch occurs when the patient is homozygous and the donor is heterozygous and shares one allele with the patient (e.g., patient DRB1*01:01, *01:01 versus donor DRB1*01:01, *04:01).

Clinical outcomes analyses that evaluate the association between HLA disparity and risk of graft failure or GVHD should specify the vector of incompatibility that is used to define the comparison groups. In a recent evaluation of unrelated donor transplants performed through the NMDP and CIBMTR,[26] unidirectional GVH vector mismatching among patients and HLA 7/8–matched donors was associated with similar risk as bidirectional HLA mismatches among HLA 7/8 transplant pairs. Patients who were homozygous at an *HLA* locus, receiving a transplant from a donor heterozygous at that locus (HLA 7/8 HVG vector mismatch) had lower risk of GVHD than patients receiving an HLA 7/8 transplant involving a GVH vector mismatch. These observations are consistent with the early haploidentical transplant experience and demonstrate the importance of the HLA vector of incompatibility in defining risks of GVHD and graft failure.

ASSESSMENT OF HUMAN LEUKOCYTE ANTIGEN HAPLOTYPES

Patients who are candidates for allogeneic transplantation undergo a pedigree analysis to determine the availability of potential HLA genotypically identical siblings who could serve as a donor (Box 105.2). The family study, which includes typing of the propositus' mother, father, and all full siblings, provides an internal verification of the patient's HLA haplotypes. Because *HLA* genes segregate in classic Mendelian fashion, the probability that a sibling inherits the same parental haplotypes is 25% (genotypically identical). The probability that a sibling inherits one identical paternal or maternal haplotype plus one nonshared haplotype is 50% (haploidentical). The probability of inheriting neither of the same haplotypes is 25% (complete mismatch).

When no related donor is available or suitable, a search for an unrelated donor is initiated. A search of all available international registries today includes consideration of more than 25 million donors worldwide (http://www.nmdp.org; http://www.worldmarrow.org). In the assessment of every unrelated donor, matching for each *HLA* genetic locus allele is considered. However, gene-by-gene identity for HLA-A, HLA-B, HLA-C, HLA-DR, and HLA-DQ between two unrelated individuals does not necessarily signify that the HLA alleles are linked on the same chromosomal haplotype. Hence it is possible for two unrelated individuals who share the same HLA genotype to have different HLA haplotypes. The clinical significance of haplotype matching is described in the section entitled Beyond Classic HLA: Major Histocompatibility Complex Resident Variation.

CLINICAL IMPORTANCE OF DONOR HLA MATCHING IN CASES OF UNRELATED DONOR HCT

The first successful human allogeneic BM transplantations were performed in 1968. Early clinical experience in allogeneic transplantation identified both HLA and non-HLA factors as important in defining posttransplantation complications. Donor HLA mismatching was identified as a risk factor for graft failure after HCT from relatives. Non-HLA factors associated with an increased risk of graft failure included transplantation of a lower BM cell dose, use of T cell–depleted BM, and transplantation of BM from a cross-match–positive donor (presence of antidonor lymphocyte antibodies in the patient's serum pretransplant). HLA mismatching was also shown to increase the incidence and severity of acute GVHD.

Use of HLA-matched unrelated donors as the source of BM was first applied in the case of a patient with severe aplastic anemia. Durable engraftment and immunologic reconstitution were early barriers to successful unrelated donor HCT. As clinical experience matured and tissue typing methods became more robust, unrelated donor HCT was established as a therapeutic approach for treatment of hematologic disorders when an HLA-identical sibling is not available. DNA-based methods have become established as the gold standard for HLA testing because serologically identical recipients and potential unrelated donors can be mismatched for one or more alleles that are identified by DNA testing methods.

The collective worldwide experience demonstrates that patients have superior outcome after HLA-matched unrelated HCT than after HLA-mismatched transplantation (Table 105.6). The general recommendations for donor selection are: (1) If the patient has many potential 8/8 donors, additional matching for HLA-DQB1 (HLA 10/10) and HLA-DPB1 (HLA 12/12) may further enhance patient outcomes. (2) When an HLA 8/8– or 10/10–matched donor cannot be identified, use of a donor mismatched for a single allele can be considered (see Table 105.6). A mismatch for HLA-DQB1 alone seems forgiving (HLA 9/10), but mismatch for HLA-DQB1 plus another locus appears to increase mortality. Among HLA-A, HLA-B, HLA-C, HLA-DRB1, HLA-DQB1 10/10–matched donors, criteria for the selection of donors with one HLA-DPB1 (HLA 11/12) mismatch have recently become available, and provide additional means to optimize overall transplant outcomes. (3) Multiple mismatches are less well tolerated and should be limited. (4) When HLA-DRB1–mismatched donors are identified, assessment of HLA-DRB3, HLA-DRB4, or HLA-DRB5 may help to uncover coincident mismatching at these loci; cumulative mismatching at multiple *HLA-DRB* genes increases risks after transplantation. (5) Permissible HLA

BOX 105.2	Principles of Patient-Donor Human Leukocyte Antigen Matching and Selection

Establish the Patient's Haplotypes

When an allogeneic transplant is being considered a part of the treatment regimen for a patient, HLA typing of the patient and first degree relatives is performed early in the planning process to identify suitable related donors. Typing of family members provides two key pieces of information: (1) the availability of an HLA genotypically-matched sibling or a suitable haploidentical related donor, and (2) confirmation of the patient's HLA tissue type. When both parents of the patient are available for tissue typing, the family study allows confirmation of the paternal and maternal HLA haplotypes, and this information is invaluable for predicting the probability of finding unrelated donors. In the absence of parents, tissue typing of available siblings might yield sufficient information for the four parental haplotypes.

Characterize Human Leukocyte Antigens at High Resolution

DNA-based methods are the mainstay for tissue typing. Molecular methods provide information of allelic variants at HLA-A, HLA-B, HLA-C, HLA-DRB1, HLA-DQB1, and HLA-DPB1 that have been shown to have biologic implications in graft-versus-host and host-versus-graft allorecognition. When a search for an unrelated donor yields potential registry donors that lack high-resolution typing, often knowledge of the patient's haplotypes may help to direct typing of donors that have the highest probability of matching the patient's alleles.

Determine the Presence of Antidonor Antibodies Against Mismatched Human Leukocyte Antigen Mismatches

The risk of graft failure is significantly increased when the patient has mounted an anti-HLA response against donor-mismatched antigens. Screening donors with patient sera, especially when the donor has known HLA mismatches, is an essential step of donor selection. When no HLA-matched donors are available, avoiding the use of donors whose HLA mismatches are the same specificity as the anti-HLA antibodies in the patient may reduce the risk of graft failure.

Identify Backup Donors

Efficiency of the unrelated donor search process is highly dependent on the racial and ethnic background of the recipient and on the composition of the donor registries. The availability of unrelated donors must also factor into the planning of the transplant, including the identification of a primary donor and backup donors.

TABLE 105.6	Impact of Specific Single-Locus HLA Mismatches on Risks After Unrelated Donor Transplantation

Mismatched Locus	Graft Failure	GVHD	GVL Effect	Survival	Notes
HLA-A	↑ 27,28	↑ 29,30		↓ 29,31	Allele and antigen mismatches are similarly risky; in some reports, antigen mismatches are riskier than allele mismatches.
HLA-B	↑ 28	↑ 29,30		↓ 31	Insufficient data on allele versus antigen mismatches.
HLA-C	↑ 28,32	↑ 29,30,33,34	Yes 31	↓ 31,33	Antigen mismatches much riskier than allele mismatches. C*03:03,03:04 mismatch is low risk. GVL effect present.
HLA-DRB1		↑↓ 29,30		↓ 31	Insufficient data on allele versus antigen mismatches. Global trend for lower survival.
HLA-DQB1		↓ 29			Only when DQB1 is the only mismatched locus (HLA 9/10).
HLA-DPB1	↑ 35–38		Yes31	↓ 31	GVL effect present.

HLA, Human leukocyte antigen; GVHD, graft-versus-host disease; GVL, graft-versus-leukemia.

mismatches have been proposed as defined by polymorphism for selected HLA class I residues that participate in selecting the peptide repertoire or direct contact with the T-cell receptor. (6) Polymorphisms outside of the classic *HLA* loci may be clinically significant.

HUMAN LEUKOCYTE ANTIGEN–MATCHED UNRELATED DONOR HEMATOPOIETIC CELL TRANSPLANTATION

The impact of more complete and precise donor HLA matching is dramatic. Overall survival after transplantation for the treatment of acute myeloid leukemia, myelodysplastic syndrome, acute lymphoblastic leukemia, and CML from an HLA 8/8-matched unrelated donor can approach the results observed after HLA-identical sibling transplantation (http://www.marrow.org). For all modalities, the underlying disease diagnosis and stage of disease at transplantation remain the most important prognostic features that affect disease-free survival. The general rules for donor HLA matching are applicable to different graft sources (BM or peripheral blood stem cells) and to different intensities of the conditioning regimen (ablative, reduced intensity, nonmyeloablative) in which HLA matching is globally associated with better outcome than HLA mismatching.[39,40]

SINGLE-LOCUS MISMATCHED UNRELATED HEMATOPOIETIC CELL TRANSPLANTATION

Early studies of patients receiving HLA antigen-matched, MLC-compatible unrelated donor HCT uniformly reported a relatively high incidence of acute GVHD and transplant-related mortality (TRM) compared with transplantations from HLA-identical siblings. The possibility that undetected donor–recipient mismatching for HLA allele variants could be responsible for increased complications in cases of unrelated donor HCT suggested that the safety and success of unrelated donor transplantations could be improved by further advances in HLA typing and donor matching and prompted close examination of serologically identical unrelated transplant pairs using DNA typing methods.

The importance of high-resolution matching of unrelated donors for HLA-A, HLA-B, HLA-C and HLA-DRB1 was confirmed by several large analyses (see Table 105.6). In summary, when an HLA-matched donor is not available, distinguishing allele mismatches and antigen mismatches at HLA-A, HLA-B, and HLA-C provides an algorithm for the prioritization of mismatched donors; in general, avoidance of antigen mismatches is preferred.

The importance of the HLA-DP locus has been demonstrated in several recent analyses in which the role of specific HLA-DPβ epitopes as well as level of HLA-DP expression have been shown to have clinical relevance, as described later. Population studies have shown that HLA-DP is unique among other *HLA* genes because of very weak LD between HLA-DP and HLA-A, HLA-B, HLA-C, HLA-DR, and HLA-DQ. As a result, fewer than 20% of HLA-A, HLA-B, HLA-C, HLA-DRB1, and HLA-DQB1–matched unrelated donor pairs are also matched for HLA-DP. Retrospective examination of HLA-DP has required very large transplant populations so that sufficient numbers of HLA-DP–matched pairs could be compared with mismatched pairs. Furthermore, the measured effects attributed to single loci in early studies likely measured additive effects of HLA-DP with HLA-A, HLA-B, and HLA-DR. HLA-DP does function as a classic transplantation antigen with respect to GVHD. Mismatching for two DPB1 allele increases the risk of acute GVHD compared with one or no HLA-DP mismatch. Analysis of the structural basis of HLA alloreactivity sheds light on specific epitopes encoded by HLA-DP exon 2 that are responsible for increased GVHD risk.[41]

New information from the Japan Marrow Donor Program (JMDP) suggests that the beneficial graft-versus-leukemia (GVL) effect is not equally apparent for every HLA mismatch.[42] In a retrospective analysis of 7898 Japanese patients transplanted with T-cell replete marrow from Japanese unrelated donors, only HLA-C and HLA-DPB1 mismatching were associated with lower risk of relapse.

These novel observations suggest that the underlying mechanisms leading to GVL may involve T- and/or NK-mediated effects of these two loci.

Beyond *HLA-A, HLA-B, HLA-C, HLA-DR,* and *HLA-DQ* genes, a series of class II genes known as *HLA-DRB3, DRB4,* and *DRB5* exist on certain HLA-DRB1 haplotypes and have recently been shown to contribute to clinical outcome.[43] HLA-DRB3 is linked to HLA-DR3, DR5, and DR6 haplotypes; DRB4 to HLA-DR4, DR7, and DR9 haplotypes, and DRB5 to DR2 haplotypes. When a patient and donor are mismatched HLA-DRB1, the probability of additional mismatching at DRB3/4/5 is increased on these specific HLA-DR haplotypes. The cumulative impact of multiloci mismatching inclusive of DRB3/4/5 on mortality was significant, particularly when three or more mismatches are present. These data suggest that when an HLA-DRB1–mismatched donor is identified, additional characterization of HLA-DRB3/4/5 on relevant HLA-DR haplotypes, is warranted.

Selection of Mismatched Donors: Emerging Concepts for Permissible Mismatches

Given that many patients have only HLA-mismatched unrelated donors,[2] research efforts have been focused on identifying properties of HLA mismatches that do not increase risks to patients, also known as "permissible HLA mismatches" (Box 105.3). Three major

---

BOX 105.3	**Research in Progress: New Immunogenetic Factors for Consideration in Transplantation**

Permissible HLA Mismatches

When an HLA-matched donor is not available, criteria for the selection of mismatched donors is needed. There are currently four concepts for evaluating HLA-mismatched donors. Extensive registry and transplant center data suggest that where possible, limiting the total number of HLA mismatches is associated with lower posttransplant complications.

Second, defining a given patient–donor mismatch as "allele" (detectable by high-resolution DNA methods, for example HLA-A*02:01) or "antigen" (equivalent to the serologic phenotype of the antigen, for example HLA-A2) has utility in lower risks, particularly for the *HLA-C* locus where HLA-C allele mismatches have less associated risk of mortality than HLA-C antigen mismatches.

A third area of active research is the definition of residues of class I and II molecules and their amino acid substitutions that are associated with transplant risks. Hypervariable positions having direct influence on the peptide-binding region of the molecule have been most commonly studied and show that some amino acid substitutions at certain positions are more detrimental than others. The most noteworthy residues identified to date include residues 99 and 116 of HLA-C and residue 9 of HLA-B. The ability of T cells to recognize these epitopes lends functional support to this model.

A fourth new concept is the role of the level of HLA expression. Mismatched patient HLA-C antigens that are expressed at lower levels on the cell surface are associated with lower risk of graft-versus-host disease than patient antigens expressed at higher levels. Mismatching between low-expression donor HLA-DP and high-expression patient HLA-DP alleles is associated with high risks of clinically significant GVHD.

Haplotypes

The Japanese transplant experience strongly suggests a role for highly conserved HLA haplotypes and transplant outcome.

Novel Markers

Surveys of the major histocompatibility complex with the aid of single nucleotide polymorphism markers have uncovered undetected variation that is associated with transplant outcome. These data suggest that HLA haplotype encode additional genes that have clinical relevance. Future research into the identification of the causative genes will shed light on the pathways involved in graft-versus-host allorecognition.

GVHD, Graft-versus-host disease; HLA, human leukocyte antigen.

approaches have been taken including understanding whether there are differences in risks associated with patient–donor mismatching for (1) DNA-defined alleles ("high-resolution mismatches") compared with antigens ("low-resolution mismatches"); (2) specific amino acid positions, or groups of alleles defined by T-cell reactivity ("T-cell epitope" or TCE mismatches), and (3) low- or high-expression HLA allotypes.

Alleles and Antigens

With the availability of molecular methods for defining the HLA alleles of transplant recipients and donors, it now is possible to evaluate the impact of the location and number of mismatched amino acid residues as potential factors defining the permissibility of a mismatch. In a single-center study of graft failure after myeloablative unrelated HCT, donor–recipient mismatching for HLA-A, HLA-B, or HLA-C antigens conferred greater risk for graft failure than did single allele mismatches at these loci.[44] The allele and antigen mismatches represented in this study population differed in the number of nonsynonymous substitutions (a change in amino acids) and in the location of the mismatch in the α_1 and α_2 domains of the molecule, suggesting that multiple mismatches for residues that affect peptide binding and T-cell receptor contact might have been instrumental in evoking T-cell responses that led to graft failure in these patients.

Single-center and registry-based studies have examined allele and antigen mismatches and the risks conferred by each kind of mismatch on TRM and survival (see Table 105.6). In an early CIMBTR analysis, each HLA-A, HLA-B, HLA-C, or HLA-DRB1 mismatch was found to confer a 9% to 10% lower overall survival compared with a baseline of 8/8 allele matches.[4] A follow-up registry analysis of patients receiving growth factor mobilized peripheral blood stem cell transplants confirms the high-risk nature of HLA-C antigen mismatches, more so than HLA-C allele mismatches.[39] Among HLA-C allele mismatches, the high frequency mismatch between C*03:03 and C*03:04 appears to be associated with risks comparable with HLA-C–matching, described in detail later in the section entitled The Level of HLA Expression. These data are consistent with the graft failure study discussed earlier in which a predominance of HLA-C mismatches and allele disparities did not contribute to increased risk. These studies demonstrate that avoidance of HLA-A, HLA-B, HLA-C, and HLA-DRB1 allele mismatches lowers the risks of posttransplant complications.

Mismatching at Amino Acid Residues and T-Cell Epitopes

The hypothesis that donor–recipient mismatching at certain amino acid substitutions in the class I HLA molecule may be associated with higher posttransplant risks compared with mismatching at other residues was first tested by Ferrara et al.[45] Amino acid mismatching at residue 116 was found to be associated with significantly increased risks of acute GVHD and TRM compared with matching at this residue. Following these intriguing findings, the JMDP evaluated 5210 Japanese recipients of unrelated donor transplants to identify mismatched residues of HLA-A, HLA-B, HLA-C, HLA-DRB1, HLA-DQB1, or HLA-DPB1 molecules that correlate with clinical outcome.[46] Analysis of each allele-defined mismatch yielded four HLA-A, one HLA-B, seven HLA-C, two HLA-DR/DQ, and two HLA-DP mismatch combinations to be significantly associated with increased posttransplant complications. Each allele was subsequently defined by its putative amino acid sequence, and all polymorphic donor–recipient mismatched positions at each locus were individually analyzed for associations. Donor–recipient mismatching for Tyr9–Phe9 of HLA-A and for Tyr9–Ser9, Asn77–Ser77, Lys80–Asn80, Tyr99–Phe99, Leu116–Ser116, and Arg156–Leu156 of HLA-C were identified to be clinically significant. When the study group was restricted to pairs matched at HLA-C for positions 77 and 80 that

define killer-cell immunoglobulin-like receptor (KIR) ligands, donor–recipient mismatching at positions 9, 99, 156, and 163 were found to correlate strongly with GVHD risk. This study demonstrates that mismatching for positions of HLA-A or HLA-C that participate in peptide binding is functional and provides a basis for defining nonpermissive HLA allele mismatches. Of the 10 mismatch combinations associated with GVHD risk, the JMDP explored whether the same mismatch combinations were involved in both GVHD and relapse (GVL effects) or only one.[47] In a population of 4643 transplants, 10 mismatch combinations (4 for HLA-C and 6 for HLA-DPB1) were statistically significantly associated with lowered relapse; however, only a subset were also involved in GVHD.

A recent CIBMTR analysis of HLA-matched and HLA-mismatched unrelated donor transplants performed in the United States has identified three critical amino acid substitutions of class I and their role in GVHD.[48] Patient–donor mismatching at residue 116 of HLA-C is associated with severe acute GVHD, and mismatching at residue 99 with increased transplant-related mortality. Residue 9 of HLA-B was identified as a susceptibility position, associated with increased risk of chronic GVHD. These results suggest that HLA mismatches do not confer equivalent risks to GVHD and relapse and that approaches for separating GVH from GVL may be possible through selected HLA combinations. Statistic models have been developed to predict peptide binding of HLA molecules as an approach to predict HLA alleles that lead to diverse binding of peptide and that may consequently affect T-cell recognition of HLA and its minors.

Initial observations suggested a role for HLA-DPB1 mismatching in graft failure.[41] The importance of T-cell epitope (TCE) recognition of HLA-DPB1 mismatches in GVHD, relapse, and mortality was subsequently elucidated in a large population of unrelated donor transplants. In this retrospective analysis of 8539 transplants performed worldwide, HLA-DPB1 TCE groups were assigned according to alloreactive T-cell cross-reactivity patterns established in a patient with graft failure after transplantation for thalassemia.[49,50] Compared with permissive HLA-DPB1 mismatches (i.e., outcomes similar for mismatches compared with matches), nonpermissive HLA-DPB1 mismatches (i.e., outcomes associated with mismatches were worse than those associated with other mismatches or matches) were associated with significantly higher risks of severe acute GVHD, nonrelapse morality, and overall mortality. The TCE concept that mismatching at certain amino acid positions of HLA class I and II molecules may affect transplant outcomes differently than mismatching at other amino acid positions, has recently been validated by the NMDP/CIBMTR.[51] In this large US study of 8003 transplants, nonpermissive HLA-DPB1 mismatching was associated with higher transplant-related mortality compared with permissive mismatches or HLA-DPB1 matches.

THE LEVEL OF HLA EXPRESSION

HLA expression has recently emerged as a key feature of alloimmunity in infections and autoimmune diseases including HIV-AIDS and Crohn disease.[52] The level of expression of HLA-C and HLA-DP allotypes has recently been found to be an important feature of the permissivity of donor–recipient mismatching at these two loci. Whereas high expression of HLA-C is associated with low viral set-point in HIV-AIDS, high expression of HLA-C is associated with increased risk of Crohn disease. In a recent analysis of unrelated donor transplants mismatched for only a single HLA-C determinant, the level of HLA-C expression was found to be informative for permissive and nonpermissive HLA-C mismatches.[53] As the level of expression of the patient's mismatched HLA-C allotype increased, the risks of acute GVHD and nonrelapse mortality also increased. When mismatches were examined for C*03 and 07 (allotypes expressed at the lowest levels) and C*01 and 14 (allotypes expressed at the highest levels), mismatching for high-expression mismatches was associated with increased risk when the HLA-C mismatch was also mismatched at residue 116 and for natural KIR ligands. Residue 116 and KIR ligand mismatches that were low-expression had similar risks as HLA-C matches.

The 3′ untranslated region of the *HLA-DPB1* locus is resident to a single nucleotide polymorphism that affects the level of expression of HLA-DP allotypes, and the ability of hepatitis B–infected individuals to control infection from this virus. In unrelated donor transplantation, an HLA-DPB1 mismatch between a low-expression HLA-DPB1 donor allele and a high-expression HLA-DPB1 recipient allele was recently identified as a risk factor for severe acute GVHD. These data demonstrate that polymorphisms that reside within regulatory regions of *HLA* genes have clinical significance, and underscore a need for a more complete understanding of HLA expression in defining permissible HLA mismatches. Taken together, the results offer a new approach for understanding HLA-mediated immune responses in transplantation, infectious diseases, and autoimmune disorders.

BEYOND CLASSIC HLA: MAJOR HISTOCOMPATIBILITY COMPLEX RESIDENT VARIATION

Currently, gene-by-gene matching between recipients and unrelated donors is performed to approximate the haplotype matching that is feasible between genotypically identical sibling pairs. However, HLA-matched unrelated donors and recipients are not related to one another; therefore they are described as identical by state. This opens the possibility that genes other than classic HLA may be clinically relevant. The major histocompatibility complex (MHC) is the most diverse region in the human genome known to date. More than 300 loci have been verified within the extended 7.6-megabase (Mb) MHC region have immune function.[54] Hence, current donor matching is performed for less than 5% of the total gene content of the MHC.

In addition to the classic *HLA* loci, the MHC is residence to the nonclassic *HLA-E, HLA-F, HLA-G, MICA,* and *MICB* genes. Data suggest a role for HLA-E in transplant outcome.[55] Increased risk for bacterial infections and corresponding TRM at day 180 posttransplant were found in recipients transplanted from HLA-E*01:01,01:01 homozygous unrelated donors. HLA-E*01:03,01:03 homozygosity among HLA-identical siblings conferred protection against acute GVHD and TRM, leading to increased overall survival. These data point to the potential involvement of the innate immune system in GVHD. New information on *MICA* in transplantation has become available.[56] In a retrospective study of 236 patients transplanted from HLA-matched and HLA-mismatched unrelated donors, 8.4% were mismatched for *MICA*. The presence of *MICA* disparity was associated with higher risk of overall grades II–IV acute GVHD and higher gastrointestinal GVHD independent of HLA mismatching. Because the gastrointestinal epithelium is the sole organ where *MICA* is expressed, the data suggest that MICA serves as a classic transplantation antigen.

Mapping with microsatellite (Msat) markers was among the earliest approaches for discovering disease-causing variation in many model systems, including autoimmunity and cancer. Msats provide indirect information because Msats themselves are not functional. Their LD with putative functional genes, however, provides the basis for its application in estimating optimal donor registry size and composition and for donor selection. Studies have used Msats to query the MHC region for novel determinants. Tumor necrosis factor variation within the class III region of the HLA complex has recently been identified as a risk factor for transplant outcomes.[57] These studies provide key evidence that variation outside of the classic *HLA* genetic loci both exist and are potentially functional in transplantation.

More recently, with the availability of a complete sequence of the MHC, mapping with the use of single-nucleotide polymorphisms (SNPs) has provided investigators with a robust tool for disease mapping.[58] The MHC is characterized by LD of discrete segments or blocks of sequences that reside between *HLA* genes. Although the specific content of these blocks is under investigation, donor–recipient matching for these regions is associated with superior clinical

outcome. The map of the MHC continues to be refined for both simple variation such as that represented by SNPs to more complex variation, including insertions and deletions (http://www.sanger.ac.uk/HGP/Chr6?MHC). The content of several common HLA haplotypes, including HLA-A1, B8, DR3 and HLA-A2, B DR15, showcases the extreme levels of sequence conservation over long stretches of the MHC, upward of 4 Mb in some haplotypes.[58] This work importantly shows the need for similarly dense sequence information on common as well as rare haplotypes in all ethnicities and racial populations to understand how such variation may be clinically relevant.

How can knowledge of haplotype content facilitate the discovery of new transplantation determinants? The available sequence alignments demonstrate that the classic *HLA* loci serve as robust markers for the undetected linked variation on the haplotype. To test the hypothesis that the HLA haplotype serves as a tool for querying such areas outside of classic loci, a novel long-range phasing technique has been developed.[59] By physically linking *HLA-A* with *HLA-B* with *HLA-DR* on the same strand of DNA, this technique has been applied to test the hypothesis that HLA-identical unrelated donors and recipients encode different HLA haplotypes, and furthermore, haplotype mismatching is associated with increased posttransplant risks conferred by variation that is linked to the different haplotypes.[60] In this study, a homogeneous population of HLA-A, HLA-B, HLA-C, HLA-DRB1, HLA-DQB1 allele-matched unrelated transplants were characterized using the phasing method. Of these pairs, 20% were found to have different physical linkage of HLA-A, HLA-B, and HLA-DR. Haplotype mismatching was associated with a significantly increased risk of grade III–IV acute GVHD. The increased risk of GVHD was offset by lower relapse, leading to similar overall survival. This study demonstrates that variation linked to the haplotype is functional and that the HLA haplotype can be used as a surrogate marker for GVHD risk.

Fine mapping will entail comprehensive analysis of both simple and complex MHC variation. In this way, comparative sequences analysis of common and rare haplotypes continues to be an important research area.[61] The JMDP carried out an extensive analysis of three commonly observed HLA haplotypes in their transplant population.[62] This work has provided invaluable information on the degree of conservation within and across haplotypes of the Japanese population and provides insight into the possible genetic basis for differences in GVHD risk among Japanese patients compared with white patients. In North American populations, SNPs, the most common and simplest form of human genetic variation, have been used to identify candidate regions within the MHC that may harbor novel variants that have functional consequences in unrelated donor transplantation.[63,64] This work has shown, in HLA-A, HLA-B, HLA-C, HLA-DRB1, HLA-DQB1–matched transplantation, two novel markers have been validated as determinants of survival and acute GVHD.[63] In single-locus mismatched unrelated donor transplantation, candidate markers have been identified and validation is underway.[64] The data in HLA-mismatched transplantation provides new information on susceptibility genes but also sheds light on the risks associated with mismatching for classic *HLA* genes. When the effects of SNP genotype or mismatching are accounted, comparison of mismatching at HLA-A, HLA-B, HLA-DRB1, and HLA-DQB1 relative to HLA-C demonstrates the deleterious nature of HLA-A, and HLA-C mismatching, but also highlights the permissive nature of HLA-DQB1 mismatches. These data point towards new understanding of the alloimmunogenecity of HLA in unrelated donor transplantation.

FUTURE DIRECTIONS

The HLA genetic system regulates the transplantation barrier. Clinical outcome after unrelated donor transplantation can be achieved with donor matching for the highly polymorphic *HLA* loci. When HLA disparity cannot be avoided, judicious selection of a donor with the fewest HLA mismatches and avoidance of certain loci may provide patients with the opportunity for lifesaving transplantation.

Disease stage remains a strong predictor of overall transplant outcome, and expediency in timing of transplantation for patients with high-risk disease is paramount. New research avenues include identification of novel MHC resident genetic variation that may contribute to risks of GVHD and TRM and the precise role of HLA region variation in preventing transplant complications and disease relapse.

SUGGESTED READINGS

Anasetti C, Logan BR, Lee SL, et al: Peripheral-blood stem cells versus bone marrow from unrelated donors. *N Engl J Med* 367:1487–1496, 2012.

Fernandez-Vina MA, Klein JP, Haagenson M, et al: Multiple mismatches at the low expression HLA loci DP, DQ, and DRB3/4/5 associate with adverse outcomes in hematopoietic stem cell transplantation. *Blood* 121:4603–4610, 2013.

Fleischhauer K, Shaw BE, Gooley T, et al: Effect of T-cell-epitope matching at HLA-DPB1 in recipients of unrelated-donor haemopoietic-cell transplantation: a retrospective study. [Erratum appears in Lancet Oncol. 2012 Apr;13(4):e134-5]. *Lancet Oncol* 13:366–374, 2012.

Foeken LM, Green A, Hurley CK, et al: Monitoring the international use of unrelated donors for transplantation: the WMDA annual reports. *Bone Marrow Transplant* 45:811, 2010.

Gragert L, Eapen M, Williams E, et al: HLA match likelihoods for hematopoietic stem-cell grafts in the US registry. *N Engl J Med* 371:339–348, 2014.

Hurley CK, Woolfrey A, Wang T, et al: The impact of HLA unidirectional mismatches on the outcome of myeloablative hematopoietic stem cell transplantation with unrelated donors. *Blood* 121:4800–4806, 2013.

Kawase T, Matsuo K, Kashiwase K, et al: HLA mismatch combinations associated with decreased risk of relapse: implications for the molecular mechanism. *Blood* 113:2851, 2009.

Lee SJ, Klein J, Haagenson M, et al: High-resolution donor-recipient HLA matching contributes to the success of unrelated donor marrow transplantation. *Blood* 110:4576, 2007.

Morishima S, Ogawa S, Matsubara A, et al: Impact of highly conserved HLA haplotype on acute graft-versus-host disease. *Blood* 115:4664, 2010.

Morishima Y, Yabe T, Matsuo K, et al: Effects of HLA allele and killer immunoglobulin-like receptor ligand matching on clinical outcome in leukemia patients undergoing transplantation with T-cell-replete marrow from an unrelated donor. *Biol Blood Marrow Transplant* 13:315, 2007.

Petersdorf E, Gooley TA, Malkki M, et al: HLA-C expression levels define permissible mismatches in hematopoietic cell transplantation. *Blood* 124:3996–4003, 2014.

Petersdorf EW, Malkki M, Gooley TA, et al: MHC haplotype matching for unrelated hematopoietic cell transplantation. *PLoS Med* 4:e8, 2007.

Petersdorf EW, Malkki M, Horowitz MM, et al: Mapping MHC haplotype effects in unrelated donor hematopoietic cell transplantation. *Blood* 121:1896–1905, 2013.

Petersdorf EW, Malkki M, O'hUigin C, et al: High HLA-DP expression and graft-versus-host disease. *N Engl J Med* 373:599–609, 2015.

Pidala J, Kim J, Schell M, et al: Race/ethnicity affects the probability of finding an HLA-A,B,C, and DRB1 allele-matched unrelated donor and likelihood of subsequent transplant utilization. *Bone Marrow Transplant* 48:346–350, 2013.

Pidala J, Sarwal M, Roedder S, et al: Biologic markers of chronic GVHD. *Bone Marrow Transplant* 2013. [Epub ahead of print].

Woolfrey A, Klein JP, Haagenson M, et al: HLA-C antigen mismatch is associated with worse outcome in unrelated donor peripheral blood stem cell transplantation. *Biol Blood Marrow Transplant* 17:885, 2011.

REFERENCES

For the complete list of references, log on to www.expertconsult.com.

CHAPTER 106

HAPLOIDENTICAL HEMATOPOIETIC CELL TRANSPLANTATION

Ephraim Fuchs

Allogeneic hematopoietic stem cell transplant (alloHSCT) is a potentially effective treatment for a wide range of hematologic malignancies and nonmalignant hematologic or immunologic disorders. Sources of donor stem cells for alloHSCT include human leukocyte antigen (HLA)-matched siblings, suitably HLA-matched unrelated adult donors, partially HLA-mismatched unrelated donors, related or unrelated donor umbilical cord blood, or partially HLA-mismatched related (HLA-haploidentical ["haplo"]) donors. Historically, the paramount consideration in choosing between graft sources has been the degree of HLA match between donor and recipient. A fully HLA-matched sibling has been the preferred donor for alloHSCT because transplants from HLA-matched siblings have been associated with the lowest incidence of graft failure, graft-versus-host disease (GVHD), and nonrelapse mortality (NRM), as well as with the highest overall survival (OS) and event-free survival. Unfortunately, only 30% of patients referred for alloHSCT have an HLA-matched sibling, and the availability of closely matched unrelated donors varies significantly by patient ethnicity, being as low as 19% for African Americans or as high as 80% for white people of Northern European origin.[1] HLA mismatching between donor and recipient is associated with increased alloreactivity of donor and recipient T cells, leading to higher risks of GVHD and NRM, as well as to worse outcomes. In the past two decades, techniques have been developed to mitigate alloreactivity to the point that outcomes of HLA-haploidentical stem cell transplant (SCT) rival those of umbilical cord blood and unrelated donor (URD) transplants. This chapter starts by defining what is an HLA-haploidentical donor and presents the immunobiology of the immune response to allogeneic HLA molecules. A history of HLA-haploidentical hematopoietic cell transplantation (HCT) is provided, culminating in a presentation of modern approaches and results. Finally, considerations that are unique to or enabled by HLA-haploidentical HCT are discussed.

DEFINITIONS: WHAT IS AN HLA HAPLOTYPE, AND WHO IS AN HLA-HAPLOIDENTICAL DONOR?

A haplotype is a set of genes that are arranged closely together on a chromosome and are inherited as a biologic unit. The HLA locus on chromosome 6p13.2 comprises a set of tightly linked genes encoding molecules that present peptide antigens to T cells. The HLA locus contains three regions:

1. The class I region encodes the "classical" class I genes HLA-A, HLA-B, and HLA-C, which present antigens to CD8[+] T cells, as well as nonclassical HLA-E, HLA-F, and HLA-G molecules.
2. The class II region encodes HLA-DRB1, HLA-DQB1, and HLA-DPB1, which present antigens to CD4[+] T cells, as well as nonclassical class II molecules HLA-DM and HLA-DO.
3. The class III region encodes molecules not known to be involved in histocompatibility reactions.

An HLA haplotype is defined as the set of histocompatibility genes that are on the same chromosome 6 and so are inherited together. Each individual has two HLA haplotypes, one on the chromosome 6 inherited from the individual's mother and the other on the chromosome 6 inherited from the individual's father.

An HLA-haploidentical donor is a related donor who shares, by common inheritance, exactly one HLA haplotype with the transplant recipient and differs by a number of HLA genes on the unshared HLA haplotype. When typing is performed for three HLA class I genes, HLA-A, HLA-B, and HLA-C, and three class II genes, HLA-DRB1, HLA-DQB1, and HLA-DPB1, HLA disparity between the HLA-haploidentical donor and recipient ranges from 0 to 6 alleles or antigens. By definition, a parent and a child are HLA haploidentical to each other, and each biological sibling or half-sibling of a patient has a 50% chance of being HLA haploidentical to each other. Other potential haplo donors include aunts, uncles, nieces, and nephews, who each have a 50% chance of being HLA haploidentical, and cousins, who have a 25% chance of being HLA haploidentical.

Mismatching of HLA alleles or antigens can occur in the graft-versus-host (GVH) direction only, the host-versus-graft (HVG) direction only, or bidirectionally. When the donor is homozygous for an HLA allele but the recipient is heterozygous at the same genetic locus, there is a mismatch in the GVH direction only. Conversely, when the recipient is homozygous for an HLA allele but the donor is heterozygous, there is a mismatch in the HVG direction only. HLA mismatches in the GVH direction stimulate GVHD, whereas HLA mismatches in the HVG direction stimulate rejection of the hematopoietic stem cell (HSC) graft by host T cells. The number of HLA mismatches between an HLA-haploidentical donor and recipient should be expressed as the number of mismatches in the GVH direction as well as the number of mismatches in the HVG direction. For example, the patient in Fig. 106.1 differs from sibling 2 by four antigens (and alleles) in the GVH direction and by five antigens (and alleles) in the HVG direction, and from sibling 3 by three antigens (versus four alleles) in the GVH direction and by three antigens (versus five alleles) in the HVG direction.

WHY HLA-HAPLOIDENTICAL BONE MARROW TRANSPLANT? (see Box 106.1)

Advantages and Limitations of Haploidentical Donors

The major advantages of the HLA-haploidentical donor option over the other donor types include:

1. *Near-universal availability of highly motivated donors:* Patients have an average of 2.7 potential HLA-haploidentical donors among first-degree relatives. By comparison, only approximately 30% of patients have an HLA-matched sibling, and availability of a URD genotypically matched at eight of eight alleles (HLA-A, HLA-B, HLA-C, and HLA-DRB1) ranges from 19% to 80%, depending on the recipient's ethnic background.[1]
2. *Rapid availability:* The time to identify and mobilize an adult URD can be longer than 3 months for up to 25% of patients. An HLA-haploidentical donor can be identified and mobilized within 2 weeks to 1 month.
3. *Adequate doses of HSCs:* HLA-haploidentical grafts have sufficient doses of HSCs for transplant of adult recipients and of memory T cells for immune reconstitution. In contrast, the total dose of nucleated cells in a single umbilical cord blood unit may be suboptimal for engraftment in larger adults, leading to delayed immune reconstitution.
4. *Low cost of graft acquisition:* The costs of acquiring grafts from adult URDs and especially from umbilical cord blood banks can be substantially higher than acquiring them from related donors.

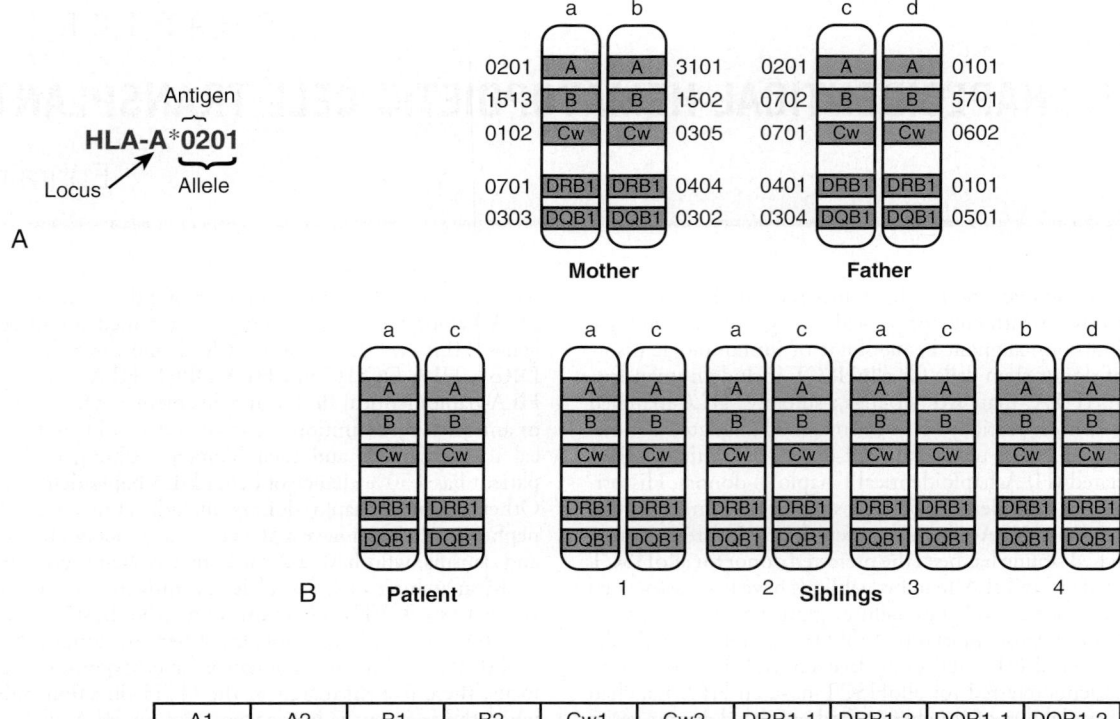

Fig. 106.1 HIGH-RESOLUTION HUMAN LEUKOCYTE ANTIGEN TYPING IN A REPRESENTA-TIVE FAMILY. (A) Nomenclature employed for high-resolution typing. The human leukocyte antigen (HLA) genetic locus is identified by the capital letter after the hyphen. The first two digits after the asterisk are the antigen designation, which facilitates comparisons of results of low- or intermediate-resolution versus high-resolution HLA typing. The four-digit code designates allele level type by high-resolution methods, such as sequence-based typing or a combination of sequence-specific priming and sequence-specific oligonucleotide probes. (B) Family study. Results of high-resolution HLA typing are shown for the parents. Based upon HLA typing of the children, membership of individual HLA alleles in haplotypes, designated "a," "b," "c," and "d," are assigned. The allele composition of the haplotypes is then used to assign haplotype inheritance in the children. The patient is genotypically HLA matched to sibling 1 and is completely mismatched for both HLA haplotypes with sibling 4. Siblings 2 and 3 are partially HLA mismatched, or HLA haploidentical, to the patient, and would be considered potential donors for allogeneic stem cell transplant only if sibling 1 is not a suitable or willing donor. (C) High-resolution HLA typing of the patient is aligned with typing of the HLA-haploidentical siblings to facilitate analysis of the degree of mismatching in both the rejection (host-versus-graft) and graft-versus-host directions. Alleles of the shared haplotype are aligned in columns A1, B1, Cw1, DRB1-1, and DQB1-1. Alleles that are mismatched in the graft-versus-host direction are in *blue boxes*, whereas alleles that are mismatched in the host-versus-graft direction are outlined in *red boxes*.

5. *Availability of the donor for repeated donations of HSCs to treat graft failure or lymphocytes to treat relapse:* Umbilical cord blood is a nonrecurring source of cells. If a patient has a relapse of the underlying hematologic malignancy after umbilical cord blood transplant (UCBT), donor lymphocytes to treat the relapse will not be available.
6. *Graft-versus-leukemia (GVL) effect:* For patients with high-risk acute leukemia, HLA-haploidentical HCT may be associated with a stronger GVL effect than HLA-matched sibling HCT, resulting in a lower cumulative incidence of relapse[2] and an improved OS.[3]

The major challenge of HLA-haploidentical HCT is the high frequency of host and donor T cells reactive to HLA alloantigens,[4] resulting in intense bidirectional alloreactivity and, in the absence of effective prophylactic measures, high incidence of fatal graft rejection or severe or fatal GVHD.

The problems associated with bidirectional alloreactivity were exemplified by an analysis of over 2000 allogeneic HCTs performed between 1985 and 1991 and reported to the International Bone Marrow Transplant Registry.[5] Compared with HLA-matched sibling HCTs, two HLA antigen-mismatched related donor transplants resulted in higher rates of transplant-related mortality (55% vs. 21% at 3 years after transplant among leukemia patients), graft failure (16% vs. 1%), moderate-severe acute GVHD (56% vs. 29%), and chronic GVHD (60% vs. 42%). T-cell depletion (TCD) of the donor graft reduced the incidence of acute GVHD, but at the cost of increased incidence of graft rejection, and it did not improve leukemia-free survival (LFS).[6] Several advances in graft engineering beginning in the 1990s, as well as in pharmacologic modulation of alloreactivity beginning in the 2000s, have reduced the incidence of GVHD and NRM, improved OS and progression-free survival (PFS), and made this graft source an acceptable alternative for

The number of human leukocyte antigen (HLA)-haploidentical stem cell transplant procedures performed is increasing on a global scale. China is the leader in HLA-haploidentical ("haplo") stem cell transplants (SCTs) on a per-country basis, perhaps because the one-child policy there nullifies the availability of an HLA-matched sibling for many patients. In the past 5 years, the number of haplo transplants performed in Europe and the United States has more than doubled. Reports of successful haplo SCTs are appearing in the published literature from countries with more limited economic resources, such as Brazil, India, and Romania.

There are clinical, practical, and economic reasons for the increasing popularity of HLA-haploidentical SCT. Clinically, results of the procedure have improved dramatically over the past 10 to 15 years, to the point that the outcomes of haplo SCT approach or equal those of HLA-matched sibling or unrelated donor transplantation (see "Integrating HLA-Haploidentical SCT into Clinical Practice: Comparison of Outcomes With Other Graft Sources"). Absent these improvements, all other advantages of haplo donors would be meaningless. A major practical advantage of the haplo option is donor availability. A haplo donor can be found for nearly every patient referred for allogeneic SCT, because every biologic child or parent of a patient is HLA haploidentical, and each sibling or half-sibling has a 50% chance of being HLA haploidentical. The likelihood of finding a haplo donor increases further if one is willing to consider second-degree relatives, such as aunts, uncles, nieces, nephews, or cousins, as donors. The wide availability of haplo donors is especially important for members of ethnic minority groups that are underrepresented in registries of volunteer unrelated donors. Relatives, especially parents and children, tend to be highly motivated to donate and can do so more than once if needed to treat graft failure or relapse. The treating center has greater control over the timing of transplants when haplo donors than when unrelated donors are used. Clinical trials and advances in adoptive cellular therapy of cancer may be easier using related donors, because unrelated donor lymphocytes for infusion are regulated by the U.S. Food and Drug Administration as a biologic. Thus an investigational new drug application must be filed for any clinical trial employing the infusion of lymphocytes from unrelated donors, but not for minimally manipulated lymphocytes from related donors.

Finally, haplo stem cells are inexpensive compared with stem cells from unrelated adult volunteers or from umbilical cord blood. This, combined with the growing availability of inexpensive methods of graft-versus-host disease prophylaxis for haplo SCT (especially posttransplant cyclophosphamide), makes the haplo option increasingly attractive in countries with limited economic resources. In many countries, the government allocates a fixed budget for allogeneic stem cell transplantation. By lowering the total cost of the transplant for each patient, the haplo option permits more patients to receive this potentially lifesaving procedure.

patients lacking an HLA-matched sibling or URD (see Modern Approaches to HLA-Haploidentical SCT section later).

IMMUNOLOGIC CONSIDERATIONS IN HLA-HAPLOIDENTICAL HSCT

The HLA class I and class II molecules play a central role in the human immune response to infection and to transplanted tissues. The HLA class I molecules HLA-A, HLA-B, and HLA-C present peptide antigens, generally 8–11 amino acids in length, for recognition by $CD8^+$ T cells. These molecules can also deliver stimulatory or inhibitory signals to natural killer (NK) cells. The HLA class II molecules HLA-DRB1, HLA-DQB1, and HLA-DPB1 present peptide antigens, generally 14–18 amino acids in length, for recognition by $CD4^+$ T cells.

The biologic mechanisms underlying the high incidence of graft rejection and severe GVHD when crossing the HLA barrier remain to be elucidated, but two fundamental characteristics of T-cell alloreactivity are likely responsible. The first is the high frequency of T

cells reactive against allogeneic HLA molecules. T cells recognize a complex determinant comprising specific amino acid residues of the HLA molecule as well as amino acid residues of the bound peptide. It has been estimated that there are 50,000 to 100,000 copies of each HLA molecule on a cell surface, with as many as 5000 different peptides being presented. Thus each allogeneic HLA molecule provides as many as 5000 distinct recognition units corresponding to 5000 distinct alloreactive T cells. In contrast, a non-HLA or "minor" histocompatibility antigen consists of a single allelic peptide presented by a single species of HLA molecule. Thus whereas the frequency of T cells reactive to a single minor histocompatibility antigen is on the order of 1 in 50,000, the frequency of anti-HLA alloreactive T cells has been estimated to be on the order of 5% to 10%.[4] The higher frequency of T cells reactive to allogeneic HLA molecules than to minor histocompatibility antigens corresponds to a higher incidence of graft rejection and GVHD after HLA-haploidentical SCT than after HLA-matched SCT. The second property of alloreactive T cells that contributes to a high incidence of graft failure and GVHD after haploSCT is a significant proportion of HLA-alloreactive memory T cells,[7] even in donors and recipients who have not been exposed to allogeneic HLA molecules through pregnancy or blood transfusions. T cells that are immunized against environmental antigens, especially viruses, can cross-react against allogeneic major histocompatibility complex (MHC) molecules.[8,9] The phenomenon in which viral infection triggers cross-reactive memory against allogeneic HLA molecules is termed *heterologous immunity* and may be a formidable barrier to the establishment of donor hematopoietic cell chimerism[10] or the induction of tolerance to transplanted organs.[11] Unlike naive T cells, which are sensitive to chemotherapy-induced apoptosis and to immunologic tolerance induction by antigen without costimulation,[12] memory T cells are more resistant to chemotherapy-induced death, can induce costimulatory signals on antigen-presenting cells that they encounter,[13] and are resistant to tolerance induction by regulatory T cells (Tregs)[14,15] or to T cell–depleting antibodies.[16–18] The presence and substantial number of memory T cells reactive to allogeneic HLA molecules make control of graft rejection and GVHD more challenging after HLA-haploidentical SCT than after HLA-matched SCT.

B cells and NK cells also participate in the immune response to HLA-mismatched tissues. Allogeneic HLA molecules can elicit the formation of alloantibodies. Preexisting donor-specific antibodies (DSA) against HLA molecules are a major risk factor for graft failure after HLA-haploidentical SCT. Pregnancy and blood transfusions are sensitizing events that can lead to the formation of antibodies against HLA molecules. The prevalence of antidonor HLA antibodies in parous women has been reported to be as high as 42%[19]; such sensitization is directed against unshared HLA molecules expressed by their children. DSA can be detected by flow cytometric crossmatch tests using beads coated with a single HLA or by complement-dependent cytotoxicity (CDC) testing, in which the patient's serum is mixed with donor lymphocytes in the presence of complement. In one study, a positive crossmatch for antidonor lymphocytotoxic antibody was associated with a 2.3-fold increased risk of graft failure.[20] A positive crossmatch by CDC assay should be considered a contraindication to the use of the donor against whom the antibodies are directed. Patients with DSA detectable by flow cytometric crossmatch assay but not by CDC assay may be considered for a desensitization protocol to reduce the level of antibody in the serum so as to allow engraftment of the transplanted cells, as discussed later.

NK Cell Alloreactions After Allo-SCT

NK cells may play a significant role in inducing GVL effects after haploidentical SCT in humans. NK cells belong to the family of innate lymphoid cells. Unlike T and B cells, they do not express rearranging receptors for antigen, but like $CD8^+$ T cells, they express receptors for HLA class I molecules, including HLA-B and HLA-C. Moreover, like $CD8^+$ T cells, they secrete interferon-γ and kill target cells via granzyme- and perforin-mediated cytotoxicity.

A current consensus, the "missing self" hypothesis,[21,22] is that NK cells have evolved to detect and rapidly eliminate virally infected or tumor cells that have downregulated cell surface expression of MHC class I molecules to evade the $CD8^+$ T-cell arm of the immune response.

The molecular basis of NK cell alloreactivity is incompletely understood, but it involves a dynamic balance of signals through activating as well as inhibitory receptors on the NK cell. The killer immunoglobulin-like receptors (KIRs) are encoded by a set of linked genes called the leukocyte receptor complex (LRC) on human chromosome 19q13.4.[23] KIRs contain two or three extracellular Ig-like domains and either a short (S) or a long (L) cytoplasmic tail, which mediates activating or inhibitory signals, respectively. The LRC is marked by significant interindividual variation in KIR gene content as well as significant allelic variation in individual KIR genes.[24] As a consequence, the KIR locus is second only to the HLA locus in the number of polymorphisms, and unrelated individuals are unlikely to share KIR genotypes.

Distinct HLA class I molecules comprise the ligands for specific inhibitory KIRs (iKIRs). An organizing principle of NK cell biology is that NK cell self-tolerance is mediated by inhibitory signals delivered by self HLA class I molecules through iKIRs. The ontogeny of receptor expression on individual NK cells is poorly understood, but it is currently thought that each NK cell expresses at least one inhibitory receptor for a self HLA class I molecule.[25] There are four distinct categories of HLA ligands for iKIRs (Fig. 106.2). The C1 group of HLA ligands is characterized by the presence of an asparagine residue at position 80 of the HLA-C molecule and is recognized by either KIR2DL2 or KIR2DL3. The complementary C2 group of HLA ligands is distinguished by a lysine residue at position 80 of the HLA-C molecule and is recognized by KIR2DL1. The Bw4 serologic group is recognized by KIR3DL1. Finally, KIR3DL2 recognizes HLA-3 and HLA-11 molecules. Developing NK cells undergo a host MHC class I–dependent functional maturation process, termed *licensing*[26,27] or, more recently, *education*.[28] Education endows an NK cell with the ability to kill MHC class I–deficient targets but also provides a mechanism for self-tolerance because the same MHC class I ligand that licenses the developing NK cell also inhibits the activity of the mature NK cell. Licensing is not an all-or-none phenomenon, and there are degrees of licensing depending upon the affinity of an iKIR for its HLA ligand. Further, there is evidence that transplanted NK cells can attune themselves to the new HLA environment, indicating that NK cell alloreactivity is a complex and dynamic phenomenon.[29] Because the genes comprising the LRC and the HLA locus are on chromosomes 19 and 6, respectively, KIR and HLA molecules are inherited independently, so individuals can inherit an iKIR but not its ligand, resulting in an NK cell that cannot be licensed during development. Unlicensed NK cells would be predicted to be poorly functional; unexpectedly, however, they dominate the early response to cytomegalovirus (CMV) infection in mice,[30] and they also may be potent mediators of antibody-dependent cellular cytotoxicity.[31] DNA damage resulting from transplant conditioning or inflammatory conditions such as viral infection may be sufficient to induce stress ligands of NK cell activation receptors,[32] break tolerance in unlicensed NK cells, and generate autoreactivity,[33–35] including tumor regression. In contrast to HLA-matched transplants, where donors and recipients express the same ligands for iKIRs, in HLA-haploidentical SCTs, the recipient may lack the HLA ligand for the iKIR on a licensed donor NK cell, releasing the cell from inhibition and resulting in donor NK cell alloreactivity. Unlicensed donor NK cells may also be activated by a dominance of stimulatory NK cell ligands in the inflammatory milieu of a conditioned recipient, but this scenario is not unique to HLA-haploidentical SCT and may also occur after HLA-matched SCT as long as the recipient lacks HLA ligands for iKIR molecules. Although the mechanisms of NK cell alloreactivity remain to be fully elucidated, there is great interest in harnessing their activity for preventing or controlling relapse of hematologic malignancy after HLA-haploidentical SCT.

Models of NK Cell Reactivity After SCT

The KIR ligand incompatibility model was first formulated by Ruggeri et al[36–38] to account for NK alloreactivity after rigorously T cell–depleted, stem cell–enriched, HLA-haploidentical SCT.[39,40] The model predicts NK cell alloreactivity when the donor expresses, but the recipient lacks, an HLA ligand (HLA group C1, C2, or Bw4) for an iKIR. In this situation, the donor is predicted to contain NK cells that have been licensed by, and are self-tolerant of, an HLA molecule that is present in the donor, but after HLA-haploidentical SCT, these NK cells are activated by recipient cells lacking expression of that HLA molecule. Support for the ligand incompatibility model was

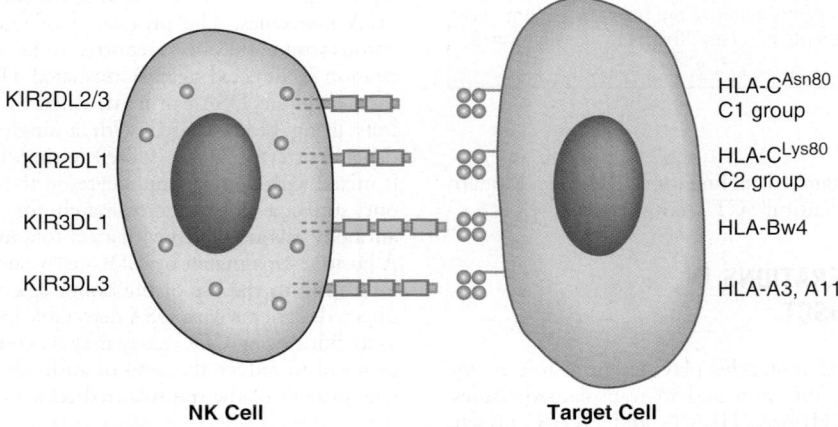

Fig. 106.2 INTERACTIONS BETWEEN INHIBITORY KILLER IMMUNOGLOBULIN-LIKE RECEPTORS AND THEIR HUMAN LEUKOCYTE ANTIGEN LIGANDS OF RELEVANCE TO NATURAL KILLER CELL ALLOREACTIVITY AFTER ALLOGENEIC STEM CELL TRANSPLANT. For convenience, a single natural killer (NK) cell expressing four distinct inhibitory killer immunoglobulin-like receptors (iKIRs) is shown. Each NK cell need express only one molecular species of iKIR for functional maturation to occur. Individual members of the HLA-C1, HLA-C2, and HLA-Bw4 groups are listed in Table 106.1. High-resolution HLA typing is required to determine whether specific alleles of HLA-B and HLA-Cw are ligands of specific iKIRs. High-resolution typing of HLA-B and HLA-Cw loci are incorporated into the ligand incompatibility, receptor ligand, and missing ligand models of NK cell alloreactivity (see Fig. 106.3). Interactions between KIR3DL2 and HLA-A3 or HLA-A11 are generally not considered in these models.

provided by the ability to generate donor alloreactive NK clones in all 51 ligand incompatible donor–recipient pairs but in none of the 61 donors who were KIR ligand matched with their recipients.[38] NK alloreactivity in the GVH direction was predicted to have three functional consequences[37]: (1) a GVL effect arising from donor NK cytotoxicity against leukemia cells; (2) a decreased rate of graft rejection arising from donor NK cell killing of host T cells; and (3) a decreased rate of GVHD arising from donor NK cell elimination of host antigen-presenting cells such as dendritic cells, which are required to initiate GVH reactions.[41] Clinical trials performed by Ruggeri et al (hereinafter the Perugia group) have consistently demonstrated a strong antitumor effect of KIR ligand incompatibility in acute myeloid leukemia (AML) but not in acute lymphoblastic leukemia (ALL).

The missing ligand model predicts NK-mediated GVH reactions when the transplant recipient is missing at least one of the three major classes of HLA ligands for iKIR. The missing ligand model differs from the ligand incompatibility model only in that it does not require the presence on donor cells of the HLA ligand that is missing in the recipient. Consequently, donors who are predicted by the ligand incompatibility model to contain alloreactive NK cells against their recipients are a subset of the donors who are predicted by the missing ligand model to contain antirecipient alloreactive NK cells.

The KIR ligand incompatibility and missing KIR ligand models were compared for their ability to predict relapse after T cell–replete (TCR), URD SCT for hematologic malignancies.[42] Among recipients of HLA-mismatched transplants, recipient homozygosity for HLA-B or HLA-C KIR epitopes was used to define "missing" KIR ligands and was associated with a decreased hazard of relapse (hazard ratio [HR], 0.61; 95% confidence interval [CI], 0.43–0.85; $p = .004$). The effect was observed in patients with AML, chronic myeloid leukemia, or ALL. The same effect was not observed in HLA-identical unrelated transplants. KIR ligand incompatibility was not associated with a decreased risk of relapse in recipients of either HLA-mismatched or HLA-matched grafts.

COMPLICATIONS OF HLA-HAPLOIDENTICAL SCT

Regardless of the immunologic disparity between donor and recipient, all patients undergoing allogeneic SCT are at risk for the same complications, namely conditioning regimen toxicity, graft failure, GVHD, infection, and relapse. Intense bidirectional alloreactivity after HLA-haploidentical SCT results in higher risks of both graft failure and acute GVHD than HLA-matched sibling SCT. Strategies employed to reduce the risk of one complication of haploidentical SCT have, to much frustration, resulted in an increased incidence of another serious complication. For example, TCD of the donor graft reduces the risk of GVHD but increases the risk of fatal graft failure.[6,43] Consequently, in early studies, TCD did not improve the outcome of HLA-haploidentical SCT.[6] Increased conditioning regimen intensity reduces the risk of graft failure but increases the risk of regimen-related toxicity[44] and also may increase the risk of GVHD.[45,46] Finally, low rates of graft rejection and GVHD can be achieved by giving rigorously T cell–depleted grafts to intensively conditioned recipients, but immune reconstitution is significantly delayed, and NRM approaches or exceeds 40%,[39,40,47,48] much of it due to infection. The following section describes transplant complications whose incidence and/or severity may be affected by the immunologic disparity between donor and recipient.

Graft Failure

Graft failure is a serious complication of allogeneic SCT and is nearly always fatal after myeloablative conditioning.[49] Graft failure may be primary, marked by the lack of initial engraftment (neutrophils >500/μL) and absence of donor hematopoietic chimerism, or it may be secondary, manifested as initial hematologic recovery followed by neutropenia and loss of donor chimerism. The primary cause

of graft failure is immunologic rejection mediated by radioresistant host T and/or NK cells.[50,51] Among patients receiving myeloablative conditioning, the incidence of either primary or secondary (late) graft failure was 2.0% in recipients of HLA-matched sibling marrow, but it was 12.3% in recipients of marrow from HLA-haploidentical related donors ($p < .0001$).[20] The incidence of graft failure correlated with the degree of HLA incompatibility, occurring in 3 (7%) of 43 patients receiving haploidentical grafts mismatched for 0 HLA antigens (HLA phenotypically matched grafts from a parent or child), 11 (9%) of 121 recipients of 1 HLA antigen-mismatched graft, 18 (21%) of 86 recipients of 2 HLA antigen-mismatched grafts, and 1 of 19 recipients of 3 HLA antigen-mismatched grafts ($p = .028$). The effect of increasing HLA disparity on the risk of graft rejection after myeloablative SCT was also confirmed in an analysis performed by the Center for International Blood and Marrow Transplant Research (CIBMTR) consortium.[6] In this study, the risk of graft rejection among recipients of grafts mismatched for two or three HLA antigens was approximately six to eight times greater than among recipients of grafts from HLA-matched siblings. TCD of the donor graft increased the risk of graft failure after HLA-mismatched as well as HLA-matched SCT. In another study, the risk of graft failure was increased in patients mismatched with the donor for both HLA-B and HLA-DR antigens, as well as in patients with a positive lymphocytotoxic crossmatch against donor cells.[20] The presence of a positive crossmatch predicts both graft failure[52–54] and poor OS for patients receiving HLA-mismatched grafts.[55] Crossmatching, either by lymphocytotoxic or by solid-phase immunoassay (SPI) (the "virtual crossmatch"),[56] is strongly recommended as a step in determining donor eligibility before HLA-mismatched SCT. If the crossmatch is positive, further testing is recommended to assess for the presence in the patient of antidonor HLA antibodies. In cases where the flow cytometric crossmatch is positive but the cytotoxic crossmatch is negative or predicted to be negative by virtual crossmatching, plasmapheresis or immunoadsorption can be used to clear antidonor HLA antibodies and permit engraftment after HLA-haploidentical SCT.[19,57] If the cytotoxic crossmatch is or is predicted to be positive, then a search for a different donor is recommended.

In addition to the degree of HLA disparity between donor and recipient, several other factors influence the risk of graft rejection after HLA-haploidentical bone marrow transplant (BMT), including characteristics of the patient, the graft, the conditioning regimen, and posttransplant immunoprophylaxis.[58] A competent host immune system is clearly required for allogeneic graft rejection, because the barrier to engraftment is lower in patients with severe combined immunodeficiency than in patients with hematologic malignancies.[59] Conversely, sensitization of immunocompetent recipients, for instance by blood transfusions, increases the risk of graft rejection following allogeneic SCT. The dose of donor T cells and stem cells also has a powerful influence on donor cell engraftment after haploidentical SCT. Early studies clearly established that depletion of T cells from the graft significantly increases the risk of graft failure following HLA-haploidentical SCT.[6] In some series, the risk of graft failure following TCD approached 50%.[59] However, the detrimental effects of TCD on donor cell engraftment can be overcome by augmenting recipient immunosuppression and escalating the dose of transplanted stem cells.[60,61] These studies ultimately led to the concept and practice of using "megadoses" of haploidentical CD34$^+$ stem cells (>10^7/kg of recipient body weight) obtained from granulocyte colony-stimulating factor (G-CSF)–mobilized peripheral blood collections.[62,63] Studies in mice suggest that megadoses of mismatched stem cells induce tolerance by the "veto" mechanism,[64–66] in which the cytotoxicity of alloreactive donor cells is inhibited by recipient cells expressing the alloantigen.[67,68] Transplant of megadoses of stem cells into intensively conditioned recipients enables TCD of haploidentical grafts to decrease the risk of acute GVHD without increasing the risk of fatal graft failure.[39,40]

Increasing the intensity of transplant conditioning also lowers the risk of graft failure after HLA-haploidentical SCT. For example, increased intensity of total body irradiation (TBI) was inversely correlated with the rate of graft failure among patients with leukemia receiving transplants from HLA-haploidentical donors.[20] Finally, posttransplant pharmacologic immunosuppression is likely to decrease the risk of graft failure following mismatched SCT. Although this has not been studied intensively in the HLA-haploidentical setting, the risk of graft failure after HLA-matched sibling BMT was significantly lower among patients receiving posttransplant prophylaxis with methotrexate (MTX), cyclosporine (CsA), or both than among patients receiving no GVHD prophylaxis.[43]

GVHD

Severe acute GVHD was a major complication of early trials of TCR, HLA-haploidentical SCT.[69] These early studies examined the relationship of serologic HLA incompatibility to the incidence and severity of GVHD. Among patients receiving MTX as sole posttransplant prophylaxis, the cumulative incidence of acute GVHD by day 100 was 34% among recipients of phenotypically HLA-matched grafts and 84% among recipients of three-loci-incompatible marrow.[70] The vector of incompatibility has been found to influence the risk of GVHD. In a study conducted at the Fred Hutchinson Cancer Research Center, recipients of grafts with one HLA antigen mismatch were categorized according to the vector of incompatibility. The cumulative incidence of acute GVHD by day 100 was 18% when the incompatibility was solely in the HVG direction (homozygous recipient of a heterozygous graft [$n = 17$]), but it was greater than 50% when there was incompatibility in the GVH direction (heterozygous recipients of a homozygous or heterozygous graft [$n = 87$]; $p = .03$).[69] There was no significant difference in the incidence of acute GVHD between recipients of grafts mismatched for a single HLA class I antigen versus a single HLA class II antigen. In a CIBMTR study,[6] recipients of bone marrow mismatched for two or three HLA antigens had a three- to fivefold higher risk of GVHD compared with recipients of HLA-matched sibling grafts. TCD of the graft significantly reduced the risk of GVHD after HLA-mismatched as well as HLA-matched sibling BMT.

The adverse effect of HLA mismatch on the incidence of acute GVHD was confirmed in a subsequent analysis by the CIBMTR.[5] The incidence of grades II–IV acute GVHD was 29% among 1176 recipients of HLA-matched sibling marrow, 44% among 223 recipients of one HLA antigen–mismatched related marrow ($p < .001$), and 56% among 86 recipients of 2 HLA antigen-mismatched marrow ($p < .001$). The incidence of grades III–IV acute GVHD also differed significantly according to degree of incompatibility: 13% for HLA-matched siblings, 27% for two antigen–mismatched donors ($p < .001$), and 36% for two antigen–mismatched relatives ($p < .001$). Among patients surviving at least 90 days with evidence of donor engraftment, the incidence of chronic GVHD by 2 years was 42% for recipients of HLA-matched sibling marrow, 52% for recipients of one HLA antigen–mismatched marrow ($p < .001$), and 60% for recipients of two HLA antigen–mismatched marrow ($p = .02$).

An analysis of the outcomes of allogeneic SCTs performed in Japan between 1991 and 2000 identified serologic HLA mismatch, higher age, and high-risk disease as independent risk factors for both short survival and the development of grades III–IV acute GVHD.[2] Importantly, the correlation between HLA mismatch and the risk of acute GVHD was preserved when the data were analyzed according to the degree of HLA allele mismatch, as determined by molecular typing methods. There was no significant difference in the risk of acute GVHD between patients mismatched for a single HLA class I allele versus a single HLA class II allele. The risk of grades III–IV acute GVHD was significantly higher after one HLA antigen–mismatched SCT than after HLA-matched URD BMT (30% vs. 16%; $p = .0013$). These data demonstrate that recipients of one HLA antigen–mismatched related grafts have a higher risk of severe acute GVHD than recipients of HLA-matched sibling or unrelated grafts.

The increased risk of acute GVHD with increasing HLA mismatch between donor and recipient has also been confirmed among recipients of HLA-haploidentical stem cells after reduced-intensity conditioning (RIC).[71] The cumulative incidence of acute GVHD in

this study was 39% (95% CI, 33% to 45%) in recipients with HLA-matched donors, 44% (95% CI, 30% to 57%) in those with one-locus-mismatched donors, and 50% (95% CI, 29% to 68%) in those with two- or three-loci-mismatched donors. In a multivariable analysis, patients who received a graft from a one-locus-mismatched donor and a two- or three-loci-mismatched donor had an HR for acute GVHD of 1.83 (95% CI, 1.04–3.22; $p = .035$) or 2.44 (95% CI, 1.14–5.21; $p = .021$), respectively, compared with those from an HLA-matched donor. There was no increased risk of chronic GVHD among recipients of partially HLA-mismatched grafts after RIC as compared with recipients of HLA-matched sibling SCTs.

Hyperacute GVHD is defined in the literature as GVHD occurring within the first 14 days after allogeneic SCT.[72] Hyperacute GVHD may be accompanied by high fever (>40°C) and may involve a more extensive skin rash and lower response to therapy than GVHD diagnosed after transplant day 14. HLA mismatch is associated with hyperacute GVHD: HLA-haploidentical donors carry a 4.1-fold higher relative risk of developing the syndrome compared with recipients of grafts from HLA-matched siblings.

In the past decade, novel methods of preventing GVHD after HLA-haploidentical SCT have been developed, and these methods appear to have reduced or eliminated the detrimental impact of HLA mismatch on GVHD, NRM, and OS. These methods and their clinical effects are discussed later in the Modern Approaches to HLA-Haploidentical SCT section.

Impaired Immune Reconstitution and Infection

Rapid reconstitution of innate and adaptive immunity is critical for resistance to opportunistic infections after allogeneic SCT. Patients who undergo HLA-haploidentical SCT have had significantly impaired immune reconstitution as measured by delayed recovery of CD4$^+$ T cells compared with recipients of HLA-matched sibling grafts.[73] A number of factors contribute to impaired immune reconstitution after HLA-haploidentical SCT. Damage to lymphoid tissues resulting from conditioning may interfere with T-cell homing and the generation of immunologic memory. The rigorous TCD necessary to prevent GVHD in the haploidentical setting results in profound posttransplant immunodeficiency.[74,75] Finally, acute and chronic GVHD both interfere with immune reconstitution,[76] in part through inhibition of thymopoiesis.[77] The result of delayed immune reconstitution after T cell–depleted haploidentical SCT is an increased incidence of morbidity and NRM secondary to opportunistic infection. For example, among 101 patients receiving intensive conditioning and megadoses of rigorously T cell–depleted grafts in Perugia, Italy, 27 died as a result of opportunistic infection.[40] Infection was the cause of death in 7 of 29 patients with hematologic malignancies receiving RIC and haploidentical grafts depleted of CD3$^+$ and CD19$^+$ cells by magnetic cell sorting.[78] Infectious complications remain high even in the context of strategies designed to selectively deplete alloreactive T cells while sparing immunity to pathogens. In a study done at the Dana-Farber Cancer Institute, haploidentical donor grafts were exposed to recipient cells in the presence of T-costimulatory blockade, either CTLA4-Ig ($n = 19$) or a combination of antibodies to B7-1 and B7-2 ($n = 5$), to induce selective tolerance in alloreactive T cells before their transplant into lethally conditioned recipients. Despite this maneuver, 12 of the 24 patients died as a result of treatment-related causes, 6 as a result of infection with or without GVHD.[79] Conditioning agents that deplete host and donor T cells, such as antithymocyte globulin (ATG) or alemtuzumab (a monoclonal antibody against CD52 expressed on both B and T cells), may also increase the incidence of opportunistic infection after haploidentical SCT. Among 49 patients receiving haploidentical SCT after a non-myeloablative conditioning regimen containing alemtuzumab, the rate of CMV reactivation was 86%, and 11 patients (22%) died as a result of opportunistic infections.[80] These results illustrate the general observation that strategies employed to reduce graft rejection and/or GVHD tend to increase the incidence and severity of opportunistic infections after haploidentical SCT.

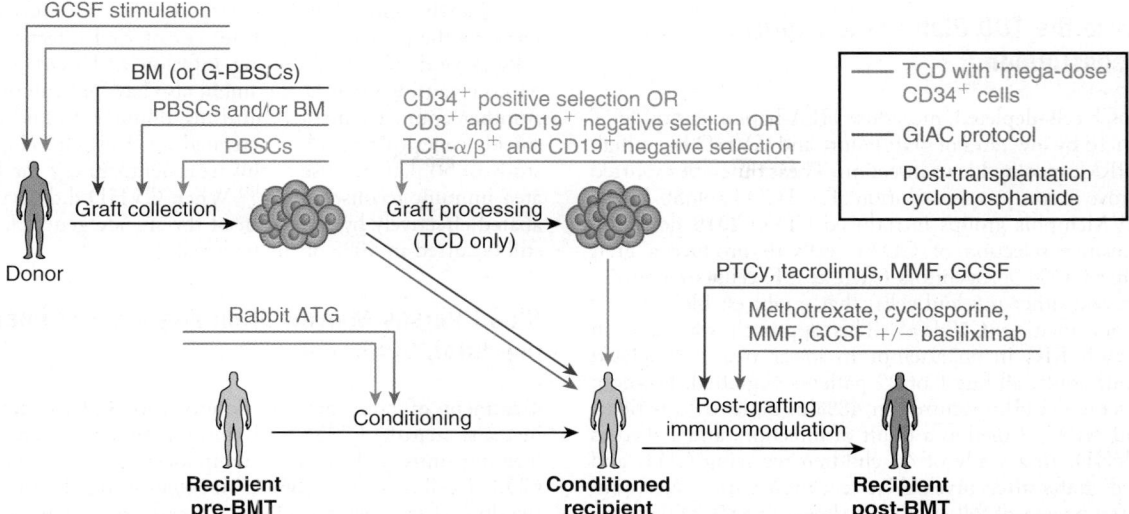

Fig. 106.3 COMPONENTS OF EACH TRANSPLANTATION PLATFORM. Interventions on the donor or the recipient for each transplantation platform are shown at each stage of the transplant procedure. *ATG,* Antithymocyte globulin; *BM,* bone marrow; *BMT,* blood or bone marrow transplant; *GCSF,* granulocyte colony-stimulating factor; *GIAC,* granulocyte colony-stimulating factor stimulation of the donor; intensified immunosuppression including cyclosporine A, mycophenolate mofetil, and methotrexate; antithymocyte globulin; and combination of peripheral blood and bone marrow allografts; *G-PBSCs,* granulocyte colony-stimulating factor-mobilized peripheral blood stem cells; *MMF,* mycophenolate mofetil; *PBSCs,* peripheral blood stem cells; *PTCy,* posttransplant cyclophosphamide; *TCD,* T-cell depletion; *TCR,* T-cell receptor.

MODERN APPROACHES TO HLA-HAPLOIDENTICAL SCT

"Megadose" T Cell–Depleted Stem Cell Grafts

A turning point for haploidentical, T cell–depleted BMT came in 1993[62] with the clinical application of an extensively T cell–depleted megadose of stem cells, a concept pioneered in animal models by Reisner in the late 1980s.[60,63] "Megadose" SCTs (Fig. 106.3), piloted by Aversa and colleagues, initially consisted of G-CSF–mobilized peripheral blood stem cells (PBSCs) and bone marrow cells, both depleted of T cells ex vivo by soybean agglutination and erythrocyte rosetting[62] and a conditioning regimen including TBI, cyclophosphamide, thiotepa, and ATG, with no additional pharmacologic immunosuppression after transplant. The Perugia group subsequently modified this regimen extensively, with fludarabine replacing cyclophosphamide in the TBI-based conditioning regimen after the observation in the mouse model that fludarabine and TBI provided equivalent immunosuppressive effect.[81] The substitution of fludarabine for cyclophosphamide represented an attempt to reduce the conditioning regimen toxicity without jeopardizing its immunosuppressive effect. In addition, the total lung dose of radiation was decreased from 6 to 4 Gy. Other advances included implementation of a CD34+ selection device that provided a 4.5-log TCD, as well as not treating the recipient with filgrastim (G-CSF) after transplant, which may impair dendritic cell production of interleukin (IL)-12, leading to abnormalities in antigen-presenting function and T-cell reactivity.[82,83] Over the past two decades, the Perugia group has demonstrated that full HLA haplotype–mismatched transplants can be successful in patients with acute leukemia in first or second complete remission (CR1 or CR2, respectively) when a megadose of stem cells is infused after an immunoablative and myeloablative conditioning regimen.[84] Among 104 patients who underwent transplants for acute leukemia, acute GVHD occurred in only 8 of 101 assessable patients, and chronic GVHD developed in 5 of 70 evaluable patients.[40] However, the megadose SCT regimen is associated with an increased rate of infectious morbidity and mortality, secondary to a prolonged time to immune reconstitution. Early results showed a transplant-related mortality risk of approximately 40%,[39] with infection being the leading cause of death. Somewhat improved immune reconstitution and fewer deaths secondary to infection occurred when G-CSF was discontinued.

Those who have reported other approaches using myeloablative conditioning and high-dose CD34+ cell–selected grafts described similarly favorable engraftment and GVHD rates, but, unfortunately, recurrent malignancy and problems with infection-related deaths were encountered. In a Canadian multicenter study, all 11 study patients engrafted without GVHD, but 10 of 11 patients died as a result of leukemic relapse or infection.[47] Waller et al reported a 93% mortality rate in patients who received T cell–depleted, CD34+ enriched, HLA-haploidentical SCT after an ATG-based regimen, with most deaths being a result of infection or relapse.[85] In a retrospective analysis done in Japan, severe infections occurred in 20 of 32 patients receiving CD34+-selected PBSCs from two or three HLA antigen–mismatched related donors.[86] Seventeen (53%) of 32 patients died as a result of treatment-related causes, including 10 (31%) caused by infection, and 9 patients died as a result of complications of progressive disease. These results suggest that transplant of highly purified CD34+ PBSCs from haploidentical donors is associated with a low incidence of GVHD but an increased risk of disease progression or fatal infection.

The Acute Leukemia Working Party of the European Blood and Marrow Transplant Group Registry has reported outcomes of 266 patients with acute leukemia receiving myeloablative conditioning and CD34+-selected, "megadose" PBSC grafts from HLA-haploidentical related donors.[87] For the 119 patients who were not in remission at the time of transplant, the cumulative incidence of transplant-related mortality was 66% for AML and 44% for ALL, and the cumulative incidence of relapse was 32% and 49%, respectively. Only five patients were alive between 5 and 56 months after transplant. Eighty-six patients with AML and 61 patients with ALL underwent transplant in remission. Grade II–IV acute GVHD was observed in 4 patients with AML (5%) and 11 patients with ALL (18%). Among patients who survived more than 100 days, chronic GVHD was observed in 6 (10%) of 56 patients with AML and 7 (19%) of 39 patients with ALL. The cumulative incidence of NRM for patients with AML who underwent transplant in CR1 (n = 25) or CR>2 (n = 61) was 36% or 54%, respectively, and for patients with ALL, the corresponding incidence rates were 61% (n = 24) and 44% (n = 37) for patients in CR1 and CR≥2, respectively.

Refinements to the TCD Platform to Improve Immune Reconstitution

Early studies of T cell–depleted, megadose HLA-haploidentical SCT were characterized by low rates of graft failure and GVHD but a high incidence of NRM, mostly due to infection. These outcomes spurred efforts to improve immune reconstitution after TCD haploSCT. The Tübingen and Memphis groups introduced CD3/CD19 depletion rather than positive selection of CD34+ cells to produce a graft containing other CD34− progenitors (such as NK cells, monocytes, dendritic cells, and other myeloid cells) that might enable immune recovery without inciting GVHD.[88] This approach was used in combination with RIC in an attempt to lower treatment-related toxicity.[78] In one study, all but 1 of 29 patients engrafted; however, grades II–IV acute GVHD occurred in 48% of patients, 8 patients (28%) still had NRM, 7 died as a result of infection, and 1 died as a result of GVHD. In a study of 46 children receiving CD3- and CD19-depleted grafts after myeloablative conditioning, successful engraftment after 5 years of follow-up was shown in 88% of patients, and grades II–IV acute GVHD occurred in 20%, grades III–IV acute GVHD in 7%, chronic GVHD in 21%, and NRM in 20%.[88] In this latter study, relapse occurred in 63% of patients after 2 years of follow-up, although 43% of patients undergoing transplant had active disease at the time of treatment. Overall, the use of CD3/CD19 depletion may reduce NRM, but at the cost of a higher risk of GVHD compared with CD34+ selection.

The increased risk of infection seen after TCD haploSCT may be due to the depletion from the adult donor graft of pathogen-specific memory T cells that provide protection from infection until new donor T cells differentiate from hematopoietic precursors in the recipient thymus. Research has been focused on infusing grafts containing selected populations of T cells to enhance immune reconstitution without substantially increasing the risk of GVHD. Adding back low numbers of T cells that have been depleted of alloreactive cells or that have been anergized by IL-10 is a straightforward and promising approach to improving immune reconstitution without exacerbating GVHD.[89,90]

A second approach is focused on depleting only T cells expressing the αβ T-cell receptor (TcRαβ). TcRγδ (γδ+) T cells have been found to mediate virus-specific responses to both CMV and Epstein-Barr virus,[91–93] both of which cause substantial posttransplant morbidity and mortality. Furthermore, γδ+ T cells have antitumor activity[91,92,94] while potentially also posing a lower risk for initiating GVHD than αβ+ T cells.[95,96] Following successful clinical scale depletion of αβ+ but not γδ+ T cells,[97] results of a small study of 23 pediatric patients with nonmalignant disorders were published in 2014.[98] The researchers in this study used combined depletion of αβ+ T cells and B cells and detected GVHD rates similar to those seen in patients who received CD34+-selected TCD haploBMT, but with an encouragingly low NRM of 9.3%.[98]

Another approach, reported by the Perugia group, involves infusing immunomagnetically selected Tregs 4 days before transplant and infusing conventional T cells on the same day as the TCD allograft.[99,100] In the first study of 28 patients, 26 successfully engrafted.[99] Only two patients developed grades II–IV acute GVHD, and both received the highest T-cell doses in the study cohort; no chronic GVHD was observed. T-cell reconstitution was markedly improved, including expanded T-cell repertoires and improved pathogen-specific responses. No patients developed CMV-associated disease. Unfortunately, NRM still occurred in 13 patients (50%), 8 of whom died following infection. An updated report of an expanded cohort of patients showed similar results and suggested that, in both mouse and human models, the infusion of Tregs did not seem to affect graft-versus-tumor immunity.[100] Indeed, relapse rates in patients treated in this study, using add-back of low numbers of Tregs and conventional T cells, were strikingly lower than those in historical control subjects. Still, NRM remained high, particularly death as a result of infection, despite laboratory evidence of improved immune reconstitution.

A fourth approach involves infusing virus-specific cytotoxic T-cell lines for the prevention or treatment of viral infections.[101] These T cells expand in vivo following infusion and exert antiviral effects without causing GVHD and might also have antitumor activity.[101,102] Another approach involves infusing donor lymphocytes expressing suicide genes that could be activated if GVHD developed.[103,104] In a study of 50 patients, use of this treatment strategy markedly accelerated immune reconstitution.[103] When GVHD did occur, it could be abated effectively by induction of the suicide gene. However, NRM still occurred in 40% of the patients.

Blood Versus Marrow From Filgrastim-Primed Donors: the "GIAC" Protocol

Treatment of bone marrow donors with G-CSF before donation increases marrow CD34+ cells and granulocyte-macrophage colony-forming units, reduces total lymphocytes, and reverses the CD4+/CD8+ T-cell ratio (Fig. 106.3). To enhance engraftment by increasing the dose of transplanted HSCs, 15 patients with high-risk leukemia received myeloablative conditioning with cytarabine; cyclophosphamide; and 1000-cGy TBI; G-CSF–primed bone marrow from haploidentical donors; and GVHD prophylaxis with rabbit ATG (5 mg/kg/day on days −4 through −1), CsA, MTX, and mycophenolate mofetil (MMF).[105] At the time of reporting, all 15 patients had prompt trilineage hematopoietic engraftment; the cumulative incidence of GVHD was 33%; and 9 of 15 patients were alive at a median follow-up of 22 months (range, 13–35 months). On the basis of these results, Lu et al compared the outcomes of 293 patients with leukemia receiving HLA-matched sibling (n = 158) or HLA-haploidentical related grafts (n = 135) from G-CSF–primed donors.[106] Patients undergoing haploidentical SCT were conditioned with cytarabine, oral busulfan, cyclophosphamide, and methyl-CCNU (1-[2-chloroethyl]-3-[4-methylcyclohexyl]-1-nitrosourea); received G-CSF primed bone marrow on day 0 (n = 134) and/or G-CSF–primed peripheral blood on day 1 (n = 131); and received GVHD prophylaxis with ATG 2.5 mg/kg/day on days −4 through −1, CsA, MTX, and MMF. This protocol is now termed the GIAC protocol: (1) G-CSF stimulation of the donor; (2) intensified immunosuppression, including CsA, MMF, and MTX; (3) antithymocyte globulin; and (4) combination of peripheral blood and bone marrow allografts. All but two haploidentical SCT patients on the GIAC protocol had sustained engraftment of donor neutrophils. The cumulative incidence of acute grades II–IV, grades III–IV, and chronic GVHD in recipients of matched versus mismatched SCT were 32% versus 40% (p = .13), 11% versus 16% (no p value provided), and 56% versus 55% (p = .90). Mismatched patients had a higher incidence of CMV antigenemia (65% vs. 39%; p < .001) and hemorrhagic cystitis (35% vs. 13%; p < .001) but not of CMV disease. Two-year rates of relapse and NRM were 13% versus 18% (p = .40) and 14% versus 22% (p = .10) for recipients of matched versus mismatched transplants, respectively. The 2-year probability of LFS was 71% versus 64% and that of OS was 72% versus 71% (p = .72) in the matched and mismatched cohorts, respectively. In a follow-up report of 157 consecutive recipients of G-CSF–primed bone marrow plus peripheral blood from haploidentical related donors, recipients of CD3+ T-cell doses higher than the median (1.77 × 10^8/kg) had a significantly lower NRM, better LFS, and better OS.[107] The Beijing results are extremely encouraging. Novel aspects of the regimen that may contribute to the low rates of graft failure and GVHD may be the use of low-dose rabbit ATG[108]; the use of G-CSF–mobilized bone marrow plus peripheral blood[82,109]; and the combination of CSP, MTX, and MMF.

Two other Chinese research groups reported very similar results of retrospective studies comparing outcomes of patients who received haploBMT with those of patients who received HLA-matched sibling or HLA-matched unrelated alloBMT.[110,111] Researchers in a prospective, multicenter study of haploBMT (n = 231) versus HLA-matched sibling (n = 219) alloBMT using biologic randomization based on donor availability confirmed similar outcomes between the two groups.[112]

Several groups have attempted to reduce the incidence of GVHD seen with use of the GIAC protocol. In a Korean study, researchers used a modification of this platform with RIC and only G-CSF-PBSC allografts, and their results showed lower rates of grades II–IV acute (20%) and chronic (34%) GVHD.[113] The Air Force General Hospital group modified its protocol, which used TBI-based conditioning and only GCSF-primed bone marrow, by adding basiliximab for further GVHD prophylaxis.[114,115] This approach resulted in a markedly lower rate of grades II–IV acute GVHD of 11%; although chronic GVHD was still seen in most patients, it was mostly limited in severity. The Rome Transplant Network employed this same GVHD prophylaxis approach in 97 patients and had encouraging results in terms of GVHD (grades II–IV and grades III–IV acute GVHD of 31% and 9%, respectively, and extensive chronic GVHD of 12%), but 1-year NRM was 32%.[116]

Survival outcomes of patients with acute leukemia who received haploBMT using the GIAC protocol have been particularly encouraging. In fact, results of one study suggested that even patients treated for very high-risk acute leukemia with haploBMT had better outcomes than patients receiving HLA-matched sibling alloBMT, owing primarily to a much lower incidence of relapse in the haploBMT group (26% vs. 49%; p = .008).[3] In 2009, the Peking University research group reported the results of a study of 250 consecutive patients with acute leukemia, 108 of whom had AML and 142 of whom had ALL.[117] Survival outcomes of patients with AML were particularly favorable, with 3-year OS outcomes of 73% and 56% reported for standard-risk and high-risk groups, respectively. Similarly excellent outcomes were seen in a second study of adult patients with AML in CR1.[112] However, outcomes of patients with high-risk ALL appear poor because of very high rates of NRM (51% after 3 years of follow-up) and relapse (49% after 3 years of follow-up).[117] Patients with standard-risk ALL, however, had an encouraging 3-year OS of 60%.[117] Two other studies have confirmed excellent survival of patients with ALL in CR1 treated with haploBMT using the GIAC protocol.[112,118] Researchers in another study retrospectively investigated adult patients with ALL who had high-risk disease and were in CR1 but lacked an HLA-matched sibling or HLA-matched URD.[119] Consolidation with either 2 years of chemotherapy (n = 104) or haploBMT (n = 79) was chosen by the patients; those who received haploBMT had markedly better 3-year disease-free survival (DFS) (64% vs. 21%), OS (72% vs. 27%), and cumulative incidence of relapse (19% vs. 61%) than chemotherapy-treated patients.[119] In multivariate analyses, treatment with haploBMT was the only factor associated with less relapse and better OS.

In these studies of haploBMT using the GIAC protocol, the extent of HLA disparity did not affect OS.[110,120,121] Although findings of a later study suggested that HLA-B mismatching was associated with higher acute GVHD and NRM as well as worse DFS and OS,[122] the Peking University group's latest analysis did not confirm this finding.[121] In an analysis of the effects of donor characteristics on patient outcomes, the lowest NRM and highest OS were seen when using younger, male donors.[121] Less acute GVHD was seen when the donor was the patient's child or an HLA-haploidentical relative who was mismatched for noninherited maternal HLA antigens (NIMA); however, neither of these donor types was associated with improved survival. By contrast, use of maternal donors was associated with higher acute and chronic GVHD and worse survival. Overall, the authors suggested that a NIMA-mismatched male child was the best possible donor for haploBMT using the GIAC protocol, whereas use of older mothers and noninherited paternal antigen-mismatched donors should probably be avoided.[121]

Posttransplant Cyclophosphamide

The effects of cyclophosphamide, one of the oldest chemotherapeutic agents, on immunologic tolerance have been studied since the early 1960s.[123] High-dose cyclophosphamide was found to be effective in prolonging the survival of MHC-mismatched mouse skin allografts only when the drug was given shortly after allograft placement or up to the fourth posttransplant day, with the optimal effectiveness of this treatment being at 2 days posttransplant.[124] This work was continued by a number of other investigators, but it was most fully explored by a Kyushu University group whose results were published in a series of 13 related reports from 1984 to 1987, with related mechanistic studies continuing into the mid-1990s.[125,126] By administering donor spleen cells followed 48–72 hours later by cyclophosphamide, long-lasting tolerance to MHC-compatible, but not MHC-incompatible, skin allografts was established. Three primary mechanisms of posttransplant cyclophosphamide (PTCy)-induced tolerance were delineated in this model: (1) direct elimination of host T cells responding to donor antigens in the periphery, (2) intrathymic clonal deletion of donor-reactive host T cells, and (3) generation of tolerogen-specific host suppressor T cells.[127] Suppressor T cells were found to inhibit responses to both major and minor histocompatibility antigens through active suppression but not clonal deletion of alloreactive T cells.[128] Induction of tolerance by PTCy was disrupted by the administration of CsA or corticosteroids before adoptive cell transfer and cyclophosphamide treatment,[129,130] but it was not affected by the administration of G-CSF starting the day after PTCy treatment.[131]

Subsequently, the PTCy approach was extended to alloBMT. In MHC-mismatched mouse models, treatment with PTCy reduced the dose of radiation required to induce reliable engraftment[132] and also prevented GVHD and prolonged survival.[133] Graft failure could be further reduced by the use of antilymphocyte globulin,[134] and radiation in the conditioning regimen could be replaced entirely by fludarabine, although high levels of donor chimerism required at least 100 cGy of TBI.[135] The resultant mixed chimeras were tolerant to both donor and host but maintained reactivity against third-party alloantigens in mixed lymphocyte culture.[132–134] This tolerogenic effect allowed skin and heart allografts from the MHC-mismatched donor strain to survive, whereas MHC-disparate third-party grafts were rejected.[132,135]

Parallel to the effects seen on host T cells in skin allograft models, in mouse alloBMT models treatment with PTCy inhibited GVHD through elimination of alloreactive donor T cells.[136] Donor T cells exposed to antigen on day 0 were largely depleted by PTCy, whereas nonalloreactive donor T cells, which divided more slowly in a lymphopenic environment, were relatively spared (Fig. 106.4).[136] However, destruction of alloreactive donor T cells was necessary but not sufficient for PTCy-induced tolerance. The role of Tregs in inducing, as opposed to maintaining, tolerance is controversial. In mouse models of MHC-matched alloBMT in which donor CD4+ T cells promote GVHD, donor Tregs were necessary to prevent lethal GVHD after PTCy treatment,[137,138] an effect consistent with the results from skin allograft models. In these mouse and human studies, donor Tregs were resistant to PTCy-induced cytotoxicity, owing to increased expression of aldehyde dehydrogenase, the enzyme primarily responsible for in vivo detoxification of cyclophosphamide,[139] upon allogeneic stimulation in a lymphopenic environment.[137,138] In contrast, PTCy can induce tolerance in alloreactive CD8+ T cells in the absence of CD4+ T cells, including CD4+ Tregs.[137] Other studies have shown that Tregs are not required for cyclophosphamide-induced tolerance of tumor-reactive T cells[140] or for transplant tolerance induced by bendamustine.[141]

PTCy is the most commonly employed approach to selective alloreactive TCD, although ex vivo approaches also have been explored. These strategies include using mixed lymphocyte cultures to eliminate alloactivated cells that either express the activation marker CD25 or retain a dye that becomes highly cytotoxic upon activation with visible light.[142–144] This latter photodepletion approach also spares Tregs and has reportedly shown promise in ongoing clinical studies.[145,146]

Clinical Outcomes of HaploSCT With PTCy

In a phase I study of 13 patients at the John Hopkins Hospital (JHH), patients received PTCy 50 mg/kg 3 days after receiving TCR haploBMT using RIC with fludarabine and low-dose (200 cGy) TBI

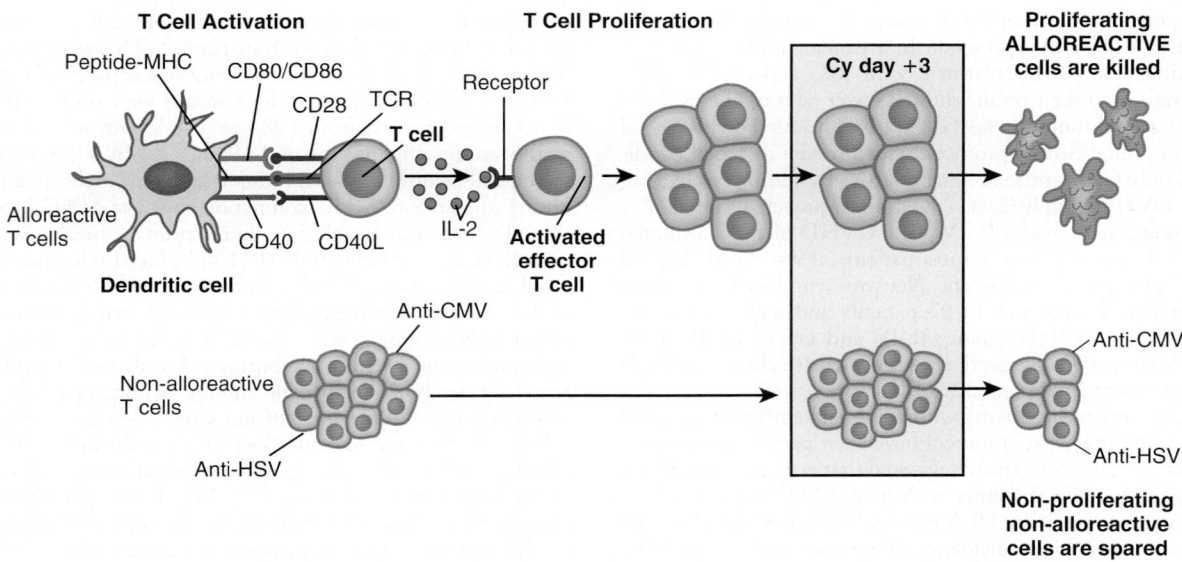

Fig. 106.4 CYCLOPHOSPHAMIDE-INDUCED TOLERANCE TO HISTOCOMPATIBILITY ANTI-GENS. On the day of transplant, alloreactive donor and host T cells encounter alloantigen on the surface of host and donor antigen-presenting cells, which also provide costimulatory ligands for T-cell activation *(top left)*. The alloreactive T cells secrete cytokines such as interleukin (IL)-2 and proliferate. Because cyclophosphamide is more toxic to proliferating than to resting cells, the drug induces substantial killing of the alloreactive population while relatively sparing the resting, nonalloreactive T cells, including cells responsible for immunity to pathogens *(bottom)*. Thus this protocol provides for selective allodepletion while permitting rapid immune reconstitution. *CMV,* Cytomegalovirus; *HSV,* herpes simplex virus; *MHC,* major histocompatibility complex; *TCR,* T-cell receptor.

with (*n* = 10) or without (*n* = 3) cyclophosphamide.[147] For additional GVHD prophylaxis, MMF and tacrolimus were administered the day after patients received PTCy (posttransplant day 4) and continued for at least 30 days. Among the 10 patients in the second cohort, 8 successfully engrafted and 6 had grades II–IV acute GVHD. Six of these ten patients, five of whom had active disease at haploBMT, were alive at a median follow-up of 284 days.

Researchers in a phase I/II study of 68 patients at two institutions sought to improve upon this regimen by further reducing the incidence of GVHD and graft failure.[148] Twenty-eight patients were treated at the Fred Hutchinson Cancer Research Center in Seattle and received TCR haploBMT in line with the protocol described previously, except that tacrolimus was continued until 180 days posttransplant. Forty patients treated at JHH also received a second dose of PTCy on the fourth posttransplant day. Twelve (13%) of sixty-eight patients had graft failure; however, owing to the low-intensity conditioning used, all but one experienced rapid autologous neutrophil recovery at a median of 15 days posttransplant. Engrafted patients achieved complete or near-complete donor chimerism by 1–2 months post-transplant. Grades II–IV and grades III–IV acute GVHD occurred in 34% and 6% of patients, respectively. The incidence of extensive chronic GVHD was low in both cohorts, but it was significantly lower in patients receiving two doses of PTCy (5% vs. 25%). NRM was 15% after 1 year of follow-up. Consistent with preclinical data suggesting sparing of nonalloreactive T cells,[136,149] no patient had CMV disease; only two died as a result of fungal infections (one had graft failure). Longer follow-up of an expanded cohort of 210 patients treated in line with the JHH protocol confirmed low rates of NRM, acute GVHD, and chronic GVHD.[150] The extent of HLA disparity had no negative effects on acute GVHD or PFS.[151] The relatively high rate of relapse (55%) in part reflected the advanced disease state of patients who received transplants; a disease risk–stratified analysis of 372 patients showed that survival outcomes were comparable with those of patients receiving HLA-matched alloBMT.[152]

Nevertheless, in an effort to reduce relapse rates, the impact of intensifying the conditioning of the PTCy haploBMT protocol was investigated. In two studies, myeloablative conditioning was associated with similar rates of acute GVHD and slightly higher, but still favorable, rates of chronic GVHD (26% and 35%, respectively), similar rates of NRM (18% and 10%, respectively), and lower rates of relapse (22% and 40%, respectively).[153,154] The first of these two studies also spaced the PTCy to be administered on posttransplant days 3 and 5 and started MMF and CsA treatment before PTCy.[153] Unlike in preclinical studies,[129] tolerance was not abrogated by starting CsA before PTCy, as evidenced by low rates of grades II–IV acute GVHD (12%) and chronic GVHD. Researchers in another study used TBI-based ablative conditioning with PBSCs for haploBMT and showed excellent survival (78%) with low rates of NRM (3%) and relapse (24% for all patients and 0% for patients with low to intermediate disease risk) after 2 years of follow-up, albeit with higher rates of acute (23% grades III–IV) and chronic (56% overall and 22% moderate/severe disease) GVHD.[155] An alternative two-step approach to myeloablative PTCy haploBMT separates the induction of tolerance to donor cells (step 1) from hematopoietic rescue (step 2). Thus patients lethally conditioned with total body irradiation (TBI) are given peripheral blood cells containing a fixed dose of T cells on pretransplantation day −6 and cyclophosphamide 60 mg/kg/day on days −3 and −2 for tolerance induction (step 1), and then receive a CD34-selected PBSC graft from the same donor on day 0.[156,157] This procedure mimicked the timing of the standard PTCy platform, except that stem cells were spared exposure to cyclophosphamide. Results for patients who were in remission at the time of haploBMT have been quite encouraging: Grades III–IV acute (4%) and chronic (21%) GVHD rates were low, NRM was only 3.6%, and relapse-related mortality was 19%, leading to 2-year DFS and OS of 74% and 77%, respectively.

Several groups have explored the use of PBSCs for PTCy haploBMT in an attempt to further improve engraftment and reduce relapse.[154,155,158,159] However, the effects of this substitution are currently unclear, particularly because heterogeneity between studies makes a definitive assessment of the impact on relapse challenging. Graft failure appears to be similar to that of, or at most only slightly improved by, the use of PBSCs. The substitution of PBSCs for bone marrow would be expected to produce higher rates of chronic GVHD,[160] although it is not obvious if this is indeed true for PTCy. Three studies investigating the replacement of bone marrow with PBSCs have shown higher but still favorable rates of chronic GVHD,[154,155,157] whereas two others have demonstrated rates of chronic GVHD similar to those seen using haploBMT plus PTCy.[158,159] In these studies, the rates of grades III–IV acute GVHD and NRM were not consistently higher than previously seen in patients who received bone marrow. A matched pairs analysis found no significant increase in the incidence of acute or chronic GVHD or NRM, but relapse incidence was significantly lower and event-free survival was significantly improved with HLA-haploidentical PBSC grafts as compared with bone marrow.[161]

HaploBMT with PTCy has generally been well tolerated, although a few potential complications are of particular note. Fever characteristically occurs within the first few days posttransplant, particularly when using PBSCs.[154,156,162] These fevers can become quite severe, are generally culture negative, and are thought to be cytokine mediated and related to uncontrolled alloreactivity; therefore they tend to abate within hours to days of cyclophosphamide administration. Severe cytokine release syndrome has been reported in patients receiving HLA-haploidentical PBSCs and posttransplant cyclophosphamide, and it is associated with increased NRM.[163] In these cases, the syndrome is associated with elevated serum levels of IL-6, and symptoms of cytokine release syndrome can be abated by the administration of tocilizumab, a humanized antibody against IL-6. Hemorrhagic cystitis occurs not infrequently after haploBMT with PTCy, but it generally is of limited severity and is regularly attributable to polyomavirus (predominantly BK virus) infection.[154,164-166] Graft rejection remains a potential complication of haploBMT using either PTCy or TCD and can be related to DSA present pretransplant in the recipient.[19,52] In patients with detectable DSA to all potential HLA-haploidentical donors, desensitization procedures can reduce DSA titers such that haploBMT can be performed successfully.[19,167,168] Notably, Epstein-Barr virus–related posttransplant lymphoproliferative disease within the first year posttransplant was not seen among 785 patients treated with PTCy,[169] and no increase in donor-derived malignancies was detected.[170]

PTCy in Other Transplant Settings

PTCy has shown promise in facilitating solid-organ transplant. One group reported an approach to combined kidney transplant/BMT in which fludarabine/cyclophosphamide conditioning was administered before renal transplant and column-selected PBSCs were given the day after renal transplant.[171-173] MMF and tacrolimus were started 2 days before kidney transplant and PTCy was given at 50 mg/kg 3 days posttransplant. According to the latest report, 12 of 19 patients[173] achieved functional tolerance as demonstrated by successful cessation of all immunosuppression without graft rejection; tolerance induction appeared to be dependent on achieving sustained donor chimerism.[172]

Studies Comparing Modern Haploidentical Transplant Platforms

There are only two published studies comparing different HLA-haploidentical transplant platforms. In both of them, data were analyzed retrospectively. In a retrospective study of 65 adult patients receiving haploBMT using either PTCy or megadose T cell–depleted stem cells for GVHD prophylaxis, survival was significantly better after PTCy.[174] Disease progression was similar between the patient groups; therefore this difference was largely a result of markedly lower NRM after PTCy (16% vs. 42% at 1 year) with a lower risk of viral (twofold lower) and fungal (fivefold lower) infections. Following PTCy, T-cell reconstitution was more rapid, and the incidence of chronic GVHD was lower (7% vs. 18%).

Posttransplant cyclophosphamide has also been compared with ATG as GVHD prophylaxis after HLA-haploidentical SCT for patients with AML.[174a] Patients in the PTCy group (n = 193) had significantly less severe (grades III–IV) acute GVHD than the 115 patients in the ATG group (5% vs. 12%, respectively; p = .01); the incidence of chronic GVHD was not significantly different. Recipients of PTCy had a significantly lower incidence of NRM (22% vs. 30%; p = .02), with no difference in relapse incidence. Compared with patients in the ATG group, patients receiving PTCy had improved LFS (HR, 1.48; 95% CI, 1.03–2.12; p = .03) and a trend for higher OS (HR, 1.43; 95% CI, 0.98–2.09; p = .06). Taken together, these results suggest that TCR haploBMT with PTCy may be associated with a lower incidence of NRM, a similar incidence of disease relapse, and improved LFS compared with haploSCT using either megadose T cell–depleted grafts or TCR grafts with ATG-based prophylaxis.

Integrating HLA-Haploidentical SCT Into Clinical Practice: Comparison of Outcomes With Other Graft Sources

A long-standing dogma in the field of allogeneic SCT has been that (1) HLA-matched sibling donors are associated with the best outcomes; (2) if an HLA-matched sibling donor is not available, the next best donor is a well-matched (10/10 allele match at HLA-A, HLA-B, HLA-Cw, HLA-DRB1, and HLA-DQB1) URD; and (3) in the absence of a well-matched sibling or URD, the choices boil down to partially HLA-mismatched adult URDs, URD umbilical cord blood, and HLA-haploidentical first-degree relatives (Table 106.1). It is worth noting that no prospective, randomized trials comparing different graft sources have been published, so the dogma is based upon retrospective, registry-based studies. Several recent studies, albeit nonrandomized, call into question the positioning of HLA-haploidentical SCT at or near the bottom of the list of preferred donors.

HLA-Haploidentical BMT Versus UCBT

The Acute Leukemia Working Party of the European Blood and Marrow Transplant Organization compared outcomes after UCBT and haplo-SCT in adults with de novo AML (n = 918, comprising 360 haploSCT, 558 UCBT) and ALL (n = 528, comprising 158 haploSCT, 370 UCBT).[175] Conditioning regimens were a mixture of myeloablative conditioning and RIC, and GVHD prophylaxis for recipients of haplo transplants included PTCy in 163, ATG in 244, and neither ATG nor PTCy in 111. UCBT was associated with delayed engraftment and a higher incidence of graft failure, but a lower incidence of chronic GVHD, for both AML and ALL patients. There were no significant differences between graft sources in the incidence of NRM or relapse or in LFS. The authors concluded that both haplo and UCBT grafts are acceptable approaches for patients with acute leukemia lacking an HLA-matched donor.

The Blood and Marrow Transplant Clinical Trials Network (BMT CTN) in the United States conducted two parallel trials of RIC followed by either double-UCBT (dUCBT) (BMT CTN 0604) or HLA-haploidentical BMT with posttransplant cyclophosphamide for patients with acute leukemia or lymphoma.[176,177] The 100-day cumulative incidence of grades II–IV acute GVHD was 40% after dUCBT and 32% after haploBMT. The 1-year cumulative incidence rates of NRM and relapse after dUCBT transplant were 24% and 31%, respectively, with corresponding results of 7% and 45% after haploBMT. OS and PFS were 39% (95% CI, 26%–53%) and 36% (95% CI, 23%–49%), respectively, after dUCBT and 54% (95% CI, 39%–67%) and 35% (95% CI, 21%–48%), respectively, after haploBMT. The similar PFS seen in these two trials provided equipoise for the current phase III, prospective randomized BMT CTN trial (ClinicalTrials.gov identifier NCT01597778) comparing these two different graft sources after RIC.

TABLE 106.1   Selected Studies Comparing Transplant Outcomes Using Human Leukocyte Antigen–Haploidentical Versus Other Graft Sources

Author, Year	Study Type	Disease(s)	Donor (n)	Graft-Versus-Host Disease (%)			NRM (%)	Relapse (%)	Overall Survival (%)	Event-Free Survival (%)
				Grades II–IV Acute	Grades III–IV Acute	Chronic				
Studies Employing GIAC Protocol for HLA-Haploidentical SCT										
Lu, 2006	Retrospective	AML, ALL, CML, MDS	Haplo (135)	40	–	55	22[a]	18[a]	71[a]	64[a]
			MSD (158)	32	–	56	14	13	72	71
Wang, 2015	Prospective	AML	Haplo (231)	36	–	42	13	15	79[b]	74[b]
			MSD (219)	13	–	15	8	15	82	78
Wang, 2016	Biologically randomized	Ph⁻ ALL	Haplo (121)	28[b]	6	38[b]	13[b]	18[b]	75[b]	68[b]
			MSD (89)	13	2	25	11	24	69	64
Mo, 2016	Retrospective	ALL	Haplo (65)	62[d]	34	64[a]	13[a]	16[a]	82[a]	71[a,c]
			Single Cord (65)	28	15[c]	6[d]	19	24	70	57
Studies Employing HLA-Haploidentical SCT With High-Dose, Posttransplant Cyclophosphamide										
Bashey,[185] 2016	Retrospective	Many	Haplo (116)	41	–	31[a]	17[a]	29[a]	57[a]	54[a]
			MUD (178)	48	–	47[d]	16	34	59	50
			MSD (181)	28[d]	–	44[c]	14	30	72[c]	56
Ciurea, 2015	Retrospective	AML	Haplo (MA; 104)	16	7	30	14[b]	44[b]	45[b]	42[b]
			MUD (MA; 1245)	33[d]	13[c]	53[d]	20	39	50	41
Kanate, 2015	Retrospective	Lymphoma	Haplo (185)	27	8	13[e]	17[b]	36	60	47
			MUD with ATG (241)	49[c]	17	33[d]	26[c]	36	50	38[c]
			MUD without ATG (491)	40	12	51[d]	22	28	62	49
Ghosh,[187] 2016	Retrospective	Lymphoma	Haplo (180)	27	8	12[e]	15[b]	37[b]	61[b]	48[b]
			MSD (807)	25	8	45[d]	13	40	62	48

[a]Outcome at 2 years after transplant.
[b]Outcome at 3 years after transplant.
[c].01 < p < .05 compared with haplo.
[d]p < .01 compared with haplo.
[e]Outcome at 1 year after transplant.

ALL, Acute lymphocytic leukemia; AML, acute myeloid leukemia; ATG, antithymocyte globulin; CML, chronic myeloid leukemia; GIAC, granulocyte colony-stimulating factor stimulation of the donor; intensified immunosuppression including cyclosporine A, mycophenolate mofetil, and methotrexate; Haplo, human leukocyte antigen haploidentical; HLA, Human leukocyte antigen; MA, myeloablative conditioning; MDS, myelodysplastic syndrome; MSD, human leukocyte antigen–matched sibling donor; MUD, human leukocyte antigen–matched unrelated donor; NRM, nonrelapse mortality; Ph, Philadelphia chromosome; SCT, stem cell transplant.

HLA-Haploidentical Versus HLA-Matched URD SCT

GIAC Protocol

The Beijing group and the European Society for Blood and Marrow Transplantation conducted a retrospective comparison of patients with AML and intermediate-risk cytogenetics receiving haploidentical transplants using the GIAC protocol ($n = 87$) versus control subjects receiving fully matched (10/10) URD transplants ($n = 87$).[178] Cases and control subjects were matched for age ±5 years, interval from CR1 to transplant, and the number of induction courses required to achieve CR1. Outcomes were similar in both groups: The 5-year LFS was 60.3% in the URD group versus 73.5% in the haplo group ($p = .15$), OS was 63.6% versus 78.2% ($p = .15$), relapse incidence was 24% versus 12.7% ($p = .08$), and NRM was 15.7% versus 13.8% ($p = .96$).

Posttransplant Cyclophosphamide

The CIBMTR has compared outcomes of URD BMT with those of haploBMT plus PTCy for patients with AML[179] as well as for patients with lymphoma.[180] For patients with AML, neutrophil recovery by day 30 was lower after haploidentical compared with matched unrelated donor (MUD) transplants (90% vs. 97%; $p = .02$), but 3-month acute GVHD grades II–IV (16 vs. 33%; $p < .0001$) and 3-year chronic GVHD (30% vs. 53%; $p < .0001$) incidence favored the haploidentical group. Similar differences in GVHD were also seen after nonmyeloablative conditioning. Three-year probability of OS after myeloablative conditioning was 45% after haplo transplants versus 50% after MUD transplants ($p = .38$). Corresponding rates after RIC were 46% for haplo and 44% for MUD transplants ($p = .71$)

The study of patients with lymphoma was restricted to those receiving RIC only and compared three groups: haploidentical transplants with PTCy versus URD transplants, with or without ATG. The 1-year cumulative incidence rates of chronic GVHD were 13%, 51%, and 33% among patients receiving haploBMT with PTCy, URD BMT without ATG, and URD BMT with ATG, respectively ($p < .001$). In multivariate analysis, grades III–IV acute GVHD was higher in URD without ATG ($p = .001$), as well as URD with ATG ($p = .01$), relative to haploidentical transplants. Cumulative incidence rates of relapse/progression at 3 years were 36%, 28%, and 36% in the haploidentical, URD without ATG, and URD with ATG groups, respectively ($p = .07$). Corresponding 3-year OS rates were 60%, 62%, and 50%, respectively, in the three groups, with multivariate analysis showing no survival difference between URD without ATG ($p = .21$) or URD with ATG ($p = .16$) relative to haploidentical transplants. The data demonstrate that, for patients with lymphoma, haploidentical transplants with PTCy produce survival outcomes as good as those seen after transplants using URDs, but with less chronic GVHD.

HLA-Haploidentical Versus HLA-Matched Sibling Donors

GIAC Protocol

Single-center, nonrandomized studies suggested that survival after HLA-haploidentical SCT using the GIAC protocol or after HLA-matched sibling SCT was similar.[106,181] These studies motivated a prospective, multicenter trial in which patients with AML in CR1 were assigned to receive a transplant after myeloablative conditioning from an HLA-matched sibling ($n = 219$) or, if a matched sibling was not available, an HLA-haploidentical donor ($n = 231$) with treatment to the GIAC protocol.[182] Patients assigned to the haplo arm were significantly younger (median age, 28 years) than patients receiving matched sibling grafts (median age, 40 years). Patients receiving haplo grafts had significantly higher incidence of grades II–IV acute

GVHD (36% vs. 13%; $p < .001$), grades III–IV acute GVHD (10% vs. 3%; $p = .004$), and chronic GVHD (42% vs. 15%; $p < .001$) than patients receiving grafts from matched siblings. However, there were no significant differences between recipients of haplo versus matched sibling transplants in the 3-year incidence of relapse (15% vs. 15%; $p = .98$) or NRM (13% vs. 8%; $p = .13$) or for 3-year DFS (74% vs. 78%; $p = .34$) or 3-year OS (79% vs. 82%; $p = .36$).

Posttransplant Cyclophosphamide

A variety of reports from single centers have retrospectively analyzed the outcomes of transplants from either matched siblings or haploidentical first-degree relatives.[183–186] Bashey et al[185] reported that patients treated with haploBMT plus PTCy experienced a higher incidence of acute GVHD (41% vs. 21%; $p = .005$) and significantly worse survival (58% vs. 72%; $p = .02$). The other studies did not show significantly worse survival after haploidentical BMT, and two[185,186] showed a significantly lower incidence of chronic GVHD without a corresponding increase in relapse.

The CIBMTR recently compared outcomes of patients with lymphoma undergoing RIC followed by either HLA-matched sibling SCT ($n = 807$) or HLA-haploidentical BMT with PTCy as part of GVHD prophylaxis ($n = 180$).[187] Although platelet recovery was delayed among those treated with haploBMT plus PTCy, the cumulative incidence of chronic GVHD was significantly lower after haploBMT (12% vs. 45%; $p < .001$), and there were no significant differences between haploBMT and HLA-matched sibling BMT in 3-year rates of NRM (15% vs. 13%; $p = .41$), relapse/progression (37% vs. 40%; $p = .51$), PFS (48% vs. 48%; $p = .96$), or OS (61% vs. 62%; $p = .82$).

PRACTICAL CONSIDERATIONS IN HLA-HAPLOIDENTICAL STEM CELL TRANSPLANT

The following sections provide management recommendations for clinical situations that are frequently encountered and for which the donor relationship and immunologic disparity require unique consideration.

Selection of the HLA-Haploidentical Donor (see Box 106.2)

Potential HLA-haploidentical donors include parents, children, siblings, half-siblings, cousins, nieces, nephews, and grandchildren. In our experience, each patient has, on average, two or three potential HLA-haploidentical first-degree relatives who are willing and medically able to donate. Several patient and donor characteristics influence the choice of donor, including medical and psychologic suitability of the donor, donor age, sex, and parity, presence of antidonor HLA antibodies in the patient's serum, donor-recipient HLA mismatch, red blood cell ABO group compatibility, and donor and recipient CMV serology. Regardless of transplant platform, there are two absolute contraindications to donation: (1) the donor is medically or psychologically unfit to donate, or (2) the recipient has antibodies against donor HLA molecules at a level that would produce a positive result in a CDC assay (see Management of the Patient with Antidonor HLA Antibodies section later).

The transplant platform used may also influence donor choice. In a study of 118 patients receiving megadose T cell–depleted transplants, 5-year event-free survival was better in patients who received transplants from the mother than from the father (50.6% ± 7.6% vs. 11.1% ± 4.2%; $p < .001$), with better survival resulting from both a reduced incidence of relapse and transplant-related mortality. The 5-year event-free survival was 27.0% ± 6% and 25.5% ± 9% for patients who received transplants from an HLA haploidentical sister ($n = 30$) or brother ($n = 49$), respectively ($p = .63$). On the basis of these results, the authors suggested that the mother of the patient

A 58-year-old woman is found to have acute myeloid leukemia (AML) harboring the FLT3 internal tandem duplication. She achieves complete remission with induction chemotherapy. Human leukocyte antigen (HLA) typing reveals that her 65-year-old brother is an HLA-matched sibling. On evaluation, he appears to be healthy but is found to have a white blood cell count of 3200/μL and a platelet count of 140,000/μl. The patient also has three children: a 32-year-old son and two daughters, ages 30 and 27 years. All three children are healthy and have normal blood counts. The patient is mismatched with the son bidirectionally at HLA-A, HLA-B, HLA-C, HLA-DRB1, and HLA-DQB1, whereas she is mismatched to the daughters, who are HLA matched to each other, bidirectionally at HLA-A, and bidirectionally at HLA-DRB1. Solid-phase immunoassays demonstrate antibodies against HLA-DRB1*1501, present in the daughters, with a mean fluorescence intensity of 15,000, and a weaker antibody against HLA-DQB1*0501, present in the son, with a mean fluorescence intensity of 1000. The patient and both daughters are blood type A+ and cytomegalovirus (CMV) seropositive, but her son is blood type O– and CMV seropositive.

This case presents a number of considerations for selection of the appropriate donor. Remissions in patients with AML and the FLT3 tend to be brief, so there may not be time to search, identify, and mobilize an unrelated donor. Ordinarily, an HLA-matched sibling would be the first choice of donor, but the patient's 65-year-old brother has abnormal blood counts, raising the possibility of an underlying clonal hematopoietic disorder. Caution should be exercised in using this donor, even if examination of his bone marrow and an AML mutation panel are both normal. The strength of the antibody against HLA-DRB1, a high-expression HLA molecule, is consistent with a positive crossmatch result on a complement-dependent cytotoxicity (CDC) assay. Antidonor HLA antibodies resulting in a positive CDC assay are an absolute contraindication to donation, so the daughters are ruled out. In contrast, the patient's antibody against HLA-DQB1*0501 would not rule out her son as a donor. It is a weak antibody that would not result in a positive flow cytometric or CDC assay. Low-level antibodies against the low-expression HLA molecules, such as HLA-DQB1 or HLA-DRB3, HLA-DRB4, or HLA-DRB5, are generally not a contraindication to the use of a donor. However, the bone marrow transplant physician should always consult closely with the immunogenetics laboratory in cases where antidonor antibodies are present.

Although the son has a minor ABO incompatibility and is heavily HLA mismatched with the mother, neither is a contraindication to transplant, and modern approaches to HLA-haploidentical stem cell transplant have reduced if not eliminated the detrimental impact of HLA mismatching on outcome. He is therefore an appropriate donor for transplant for his mother. Umbilical cord blood is another potential source of stem cells for this patient. At present, there are no clinical data that would mandate the choice of an HLA-haploidentical donor over umbilical cord blood, or vice versa.

is the preferred HLA-haploidentical donor for megadose, T cell–depleted HSCT. Wang et al studied outcomes of 1210 patients treated with the GIAC protocol. With this platform, younger donors and male donors were found to be associated with less NRM and better survival. Less acute GVHD was seen when using the patient's child or an HLA-haploidentical relative who was mismatched for NIMA as the donor; however, use of either of these donor types was not associated with any significant improvement in patient survival outcomes. By contrast, use of maternal donors was associated with higher acute and chronic GVHD and worse survival. Overall, the authors suggested that a NIMA-mismatched male child was the best possible donor for haploBMT using the GIAC protocol, whereas use of older mother donors and noninherited paternal antigen-mismatched donors should be avoided.[188]

Management of the Patient With Antidonor HLA Antibodies

HLA-mismatch was also historically associated with graft failure, with rates of 12% and 2% after HLA-mismatched and HLA-matched

related donor allografting, respectively.[15] The same study showed that the presence of antidonor lymphocytotoxic antibodies on crossmatch was associated with a 39% graft failure rate, compared with 10% in patients with a negative crossmatch. In haploBMT with PTCy, Ciurea et al found that graft failure occurred in 75% of recipients with DSA compared with 5% of recipients without DSA ($p = .008$) and that antibodies to HLA-DRB1 were most frequent.[16] In subsequent analyses by Ciurea et al, the overall incidence of DSA in haploBMT assessments was 18%, 86% of whom were women.[53] Thirty-two percent of patients with DSA experienced graft rejection. The mean fluorescence intensity (MFI) of antidonor HLA antibody was 10,055 for patients who experienced rejection versus 2065 for those with engraftment. Graft failure was associated with a complement assay that detects C1q-binding DSA, with only one C1q-negative patient (who had an MFI of 6265) without engraftment. Patients with C1q-binding DSA also had a higher median MFI than C1q-negative patients (15,279 vs. 2471). All male patients were C1q negative, and their median MFI levels were much lower. Pregnancy was associated with a much higher risk of developing DSA than transfusion of blood products.

DSA can be quantified by SPI using fluorescent beads coated with a single phenotype and single HLA antigens. SPI results can be correlated with crossmatching by flow cytometry or CDC assays to generate a "virtual crossmatch."[18] Gladstone et al found that HLA-directed DSA occurred in 14.5% of all patients and 42% of women undergoing haplotransplant evaluation.[19] In patients without alternative available donors, plasmapheresis combined with anti-CMV intravenous immunoglobulin, tacrolimus, and MMF starting 1 to 2 weeks before conditioning, depending on the level of DSA, was associated with a 64.4% mean reduction in DSA levels.[19,167] Fifteen patients received this treatment, and the fourteen patients who achieved DSA reduction to negative or weak levels underwent transplant and engrafted. Ciurea et al proposed an alternative desensitization method of plasma exchange, rituximab, and intravenous immunoglobulin, which they found to be only partially effective.[53] However, combining that regimen with the infusion of donor HLA antigens via a buffy coat 24 hours before SCT was highly effective. They also reported that clearing of DSA may be unnecessary, with reduction to non-complement-binding levels sufficient to achieve engraftment.

The management of a patient with antidonor HLA antibodies depends to a great extent upon the strength of the antibodies and upon the availability of other donors. All other factors being equal, preference should be given to donors against whom the patient does not have antibodies. Not all antibody specificities are equal. For example, antibodies against low-expression HLA molecules such as HLA-DQB1 or HLA-DRB3, HLA-DRB4, or HLA-DRB5 may not carry as high a risk of graft rejection as antibodies against the high-expression HLA molecules, HLA-A, HLA-B, HLA-Cw, and HLA-DRB1. We quantify antibody strengths using SPI with single HLA antigen–coated beads. The SPI reports antibody strength as MFI. An antibody with an MFI of 1000 to 3000 is considered a weak antibody, one with an MFI of 3000 to 15,000 is considered a moderate antibody, and one with an MFI greater than 15,000 is considered a strong antibody. Antibodies with an MFI greater than 10,000 are generally associated with a positive CDC crossmatch. It is critically important to consult with an immunogeneticist with experience in the management of patients with DSA. As a general rule, we never use a donor if the MFI of antidonor HLA antibody is greater than 10,000. For patients with antibodies associated with a positive flow cytometric crossmatch but a negative CDC crossmatch (MFI 3000 to 10,000), strategies to reduce the risk of graft rejection by lowering the concentration of antidonor HLA antibody have been developed. One such method of desensitizing patients includes plasma exchange and intravenous immunoglobulin every other day combined with tacrolimus and MMF,[19,168] which was followed by sustained engraftment of HLA-haploidentical stem cells in 14 of 15 treated patients.[167] Other methods to desensitize patients with antidonor HLA antibodies include treatment with bortezomib, transfusion of platelets expressing the targeted HLA antigens, or the combination of rituximab and plasma exchange, with[53] or without[189] intravenous immunoglobulin.

In summary, the presence of antidonor HLA antibodies that produces a positive result on a CDC assay, or an MFI greater than 10,000 determined by SPI, is an absolute contraindication to the use of a donor who expresses the targeted HLA molecule. Antibodies of intermediate strength, corresponding to a positive flow cytometric crossmatch test or an antibody against a high-expression HLA molecule with MFI of 3000 to 10,000, may be reduced by a desensitization protocol to allow the use of a donor expressing the targeted HLA molecules. Antidonor HLA antibodies with an MFI less than 3000 measured by SPI may not require desensitization. Management of the patient with antidonor HLA antibodies must involve a close collaboration of the transplant physician and the immunogenetics laboratory.

Management of Suspected Graft Failure

Graft failure occurs when donor HSCs are unable to support long-term hematopoiesis in the recipient, resulting in loss of donor hematopoietic chimerism. Potential causes of graft failure include a poor-quality graft containing a low number of CD34+ cells; viral infection in the recipient (such as CMV, human herpesvirus 6, adenovirus, or parvovirus); or immunologic rejection by antidonor HLA antibodies, alloreactive recipient T cells, or both. Immunologic rejection of the donor graft almost certainly accounts for the higher incidence of graft failure after HLA-haploidentical as compared with HLA-matched SCTs.

The definition of graft failure depends upon the intensity of the conditioning regimen employed. Chimerism studies are required to make a diagnosis of graft failure. Management of graft failure depends to some extent on the perceived risk of irreversible pancytopenia and upon the risk of disease relapse. Graft failure after myeloablative conditioning is likely to be fatal unless the patient is effectively salvaged by a second stem cell graft, whereas autologous hematopoiesis often returns in the event of graft failure after nonmyeloablative conditioning.

PBSCs from HLA-haploidentical donors have been used successfully to salvage graft failure after myeloablative conditioning and HCT from partially HLA-mismatched URDs, from URD umbilical cord blood,[190,191] or from HLA-haploidentical donors.[192,193] When salvaging graft failure after HLA-haploidentical SCT, the question arises whether to use the same donor or switch to a different donor for the second transplant. It is important to test the patient for the presence of antibodies against the mismatched HLA molecules of the original donor because a positive test would demonstrate immunity against this donor's cells and a strong risk of rejection if the same donor is used. Preclinical studies demonstrate that graft rejection after nonmyeloablative conditioning can induce cellular immunity against donor cells without detectable antidonor antibody.[194] Thus lack of antidonor antibody does not mean lack of sensitization against a failed HLA-haploidentical allograft. If it is possible to switch to an HLA-haploidentical donor who does not share the same mismatched HLA haplotype as the original donor, then a new donor is preferred.

Treatment of Relapsed Hematologic Malignancy After HLA-Haploidentical SCT

Relapse remains a significant complication of allogeneic SCT, including HLA-haploidentical SCT. There is substantial controversy regarding whether HLA disparity between donor and recipient reduces relapse through a more intense GVH reaction. Most studies have not shown decreased relapse rates after HLA-haploidentical as compared with HLA-matched SCT,[180,187,195] though such studies may be confounded by significant differences between donor types in the GVHD prophylaxis regimens employed. Other studies have shown a decreased risk of relapse associated with HLA mismatching,[196] especially for patients with poor-risk hematologic malignancies.[2] Approximately one-third of leukemic relapses after

HLA-haploidentical SCT are associated with loss of the mismatched HLA locus via acquired uniparental disomy, a process in which the unshared HLA haplotype on chromosome 6 is replaced by the shared HLA haplotype.[197,198] HLA-alloreactive T cells must be providing the selective pressure that results in the emergence of these variants, because relapse is never associated with loss of the shared HLA haplotype, and HLA loss by uniparental disomy has not been described after HLA-matched SCT. Clinically, relapses of AML associated with loss of mismatched HLA tend to occur later than relapses with preserved HLA expression (307 days vs. 88 days; $p < .001$),[199] but they tend to carry a similar poor prognosis. Donor lymphocyte infusion (DLI) may not be effective in light of the loss of the major targets of alloreactive T cells. OS at 6 months after relapse was 28.5% for patients with HLA loss and 27.4% for patients with "classical" relapse. Survival may be improved by performing a second transplant, especially from a different donor, though NRM is high (7 of 17 patients).

DLIs have been administered to patients with relapsed hematologic malignancy after HLA-haploidentical SCT plus PTCy. In one study, DLI was administered as a series of escalating infusions (ranging from 10^3 to 10^7 T cells/kg), with or without preceding chemotherapy, to patients with acute leukemia in molecular ($n = 20$) or hematologic ($n = 12$) relapse, or to patients with Hodgkin lymphoma ($n = 10$).[200] The incidence rates of acute GVHD after DLI in these groups were 15%, 17%, and 10%, respectively, and the response rates were 45%, 33%, and 70%. Two-year actuarial survival rates were 43%, 19%, and 80%, respectively. In a second report, 40 patients, including 16 with AML and 11 with lymphoma, received DLI starting at a dose of 10^5 CD3+ T cells/kg with subsequent dose escalation.[201] The most commonly used first dose was 10^6 CD3+ T cells/kg. Acute GVHD developed in 10 patients, 6 patients had grades III–IV, and 3 developed chronic GVHD. Twelve patients (30%) achieved a complete response with a median duration of 11.8 months. Eight patients were alive in complete response at the time of reporting, six for more than 1 year.

The Beijing group developed a modified DLI approach in which patients with relapsed leukemia after haploBMT received chemotherapy and peripheral blood leukocytes from filgrastim-treated donors followed by an immunosuppressive drug (CsA or MTX) for 2 to 8 weeks after DLI.[202] One hundred twenty-four patients in relapse after haploBMT received chemotherapy followed by modified DLI containing a median of 4×10^7 CD3+ T cells/kg of recipient weight. The cumulative incidence of DLI-associated acute GVHD was 53.2% for grades II–IV and 28.4% for grades III–IV. The duration of GVHD prophylaxis after DLI was the only risk factor for DLI-associated grades III–IV acute GVHD ($p < .05$). The 2-year OS, NRM, and cumulative incidence of relapse after DLI were 47.2%, 34.1%, and 34.6%, respectively. A subsequent study compared the antileukemic effects of chemotherapy alone ($n = 32$) versus chemotherapy followed by modified DLI ($n = 50$), with immunosuppression given for 4 to 8 weeks after DLI, in patients with relapsed acute leukemia after haploBMT.[203] In patients receiving chemotherapy followed by modified DLI, the CR rate was significantly higher (64.0% vs. 12.5%; $p = .000$), the incidence of relapse was significantly lower (50.0% vs. 100.0%; $p = .000$) and DFS was significantly improved (36.0% vs. 0.0%; $p = .000$) compared with patients receiving chemotherapy alone. Multivariate analysis demonstrated that patients with chronic GVHD after intervention ($p = .000$) and patients receiving chemotherapy followed by modified DLI ($p = .037$) were associated with a lower relapse rate.

In summary, hematologic malignancies in relapse after HLA-haploidentical SCT can be treated with DLIs. Patients with relapse of acute leukemia in the first 6 months after transplant generally have a poor prognosis. For patients with relapse of leukemia after 6 months, HLA typing of the leukemia blasts is recommended. If mismatched HLA expression is preserved, DLI with or without preceding chemotherapy may be used. For patients in overt hematologic relapse, a starting dose of 10^6 CD3+ T cells/kg may be used. If mismatched HLA alleles have been lost, a second transplant procedure from a different donor may provide the best outcome.

CONCLUSIONS

HLA-haploidentical donors are a rapid and near universally available source of HSCs for transplant into patients with poor-risk hematologic malignancies. HLA mismatch between donor and recipient stimulates not only alloreactive T cells but also NK and B cells, which generates unique biologic and clinical considerations. The major drawback of HLA-haploidentical SCT is intense bidirectional alloreactivity resulting in higher incidences of graft failure, GVHD, and NRM. Three modern approaches to haploSCT have mitigated these complications substantially: (1) megadose T cell–depleted SCTs; (2) the GIAC protocol involving administration of ATG, filgrastim-mobilized marrow plus PBSCs, and intensive posttransplant immunosuppression; and (3) high-dose, posttransplant cyclophosphamide as part of GVHD prophylaxis. Outcomes of haploSCT for hematologic malignancies using these strategies now approach those seen after HLA-matched SCT. Prospective randomized trials comparing different graft sources will be needed to determine the donor priority for patients referred for allogeneic SCT. Priorities for future research include improving immune reconstitution and preventing or treating relapsed malignancy.

SUGGESTED READINGS

Abboud R, Keller J, Slade M, et al: Severe cytokine-release syndrome after T cell-replete peripheral blood haploidentical donor transplantation is associated with poor survival and anti-IL-6 therapy is safe and well tolerated. *Biol Blood Marrow Transplant* 22:2016, 1851.

Aboul Nour H, Patil N, Chewning JH, et al: Safety of repeated un-manipulated peripheral blood stem cell haploidentical transplant for graft failure. *Bone Marrow Transplant* 52:157, 2017.

Al-Homsi AS, Cole K, Bogema M, et al: Short course of post-transplantation cyclophosphamide and bortezomib for graft-versus-host disease prevention after allogeneic peripheral blood stem cell transplantation is feasible and yields favorable results: a phase I study. *Biol Blood Marrow Transplant* 21:1315, 2015.

Arcese W, Picardi A, Santarone S, et al: Haploidentical, G-CSF-primed, unmanipulated bone marrow transplantation for patients with high-risk hematological malignancies: an update. *Bone Marrow Transplant* 50(Suppl 2):S24, 2015.

Bramanti S, Nocco A, Mauro E, et al: Desensitization with plasma exchange in a patient with human leukocyte antigen donor-specific antibodies before T-cell–replete haploidentical transplantation. *Transfusion* 56(5):1096–1100, 2016.

Chen H, Liu KY, Xu LP, et al: Haploidentical hematopoietic stem cell transplantation without in vitro T cell depletion for the treatment of Philadelphia chromosome–positive acute lymphoblastic leukemia. *Biol Blood Marrow Transplant* 21:1110, 2015.

Ciurea SO, Thall PF, Milton DR, et al: Complement-binding donor-specific anti-HLA antibodies and risk of primary graft failure in hematopoietic stem cell transplantation. *Biol Blood Marrow Transplant* 21(8):1392–1398, 2015.

Ciurea SO, Zhang MJ, Bacigalupo AA, et al: Haploidentical transplant with posttransplant cyclophosphamide vs matched unrelated donor transplant for acute myeloid leukemia. *Blood* 126(8):1033–1040, 2015.

Crocchiolo R, Bramanti S, Vai A, et al: Infections after T-replete haploidentical transplantation and high-dose cyclophosphamide as graft-versus-host disease prophylaxis. *Transpl Infect Dis* 17:242, 2015.

Crucitti L, Crocchiolo R, Toffalori C, et al: Incidence, risk factors and clinical outcome of leukemia relapses with loss of the mismatched HLA after partially incompatible hematopoietic stem cell transplantation. *Leukemia* 29(5):1143–1152, 2015.

Epperla N, Pasquini M, Pierce K, et al: Salvage haploidentical hematopoietic cell transplantation for graft rejection following a prior haploidentical allograft. *Bone Marrow Transplant* 52:147, 2017.

Ghosh N, Karmali R, Rocha V, et al: Reduced-intensity transplantation for lymphomas using haploidentical related donors versus HLA-matched sibling donors: a Center for International Blood and Marrow Transplant Research analysis. *J Clin Oncol* 34:3141, 2016.

Kanate AS, Mussetti A, Kharfan-Dabaja MA, et al: Reduced-intensity transplantation for lymphomas using haploidentical related donors vs HLA-matched unrelated donors. *Blood* 127(7):938–947, 2016.

Leffell MS, Jones RJ, Gladstone DE: Donor HLA-specific Abs: to BMT or not to BMT? *Bone Marrow Transplant* 50:751, 2015.

Leventhal JR, Elliott MJ, Yolcu ES, et al: Immune reconstitution/immunocompetence in recipients of kidney plus hematopoietic stem/facilitating cell transplants. *Transplantation* 99(2):288–298, 2015.

McCurdy SR, Kanakry JA, Showel MM, et al: Risk-stratified outcomes of nonmyeloablative, HLA-haploidentical BMT with high-dose posttransplantation cyclophosphamide. *Blood* 125:3024, 2015.

O'Donnell PV, Eapen M, Horowitz MM, et al: Comparable outcomes with marrow or peripheral blood as stem cell sources for hematopoietic cell transplantation from haploidentical donors after non-ablative conditioning: a matched-pair analysis. *Bone Marrow Transplant* 51:2016, 1599.

O'Donnell P, Raj K, Pagliuca A: High fever occurring 4 to 5 days posttransplant of haploidentical bone marrow or peripheral blood stem cells after reduced-intensity conditioning associated with the use of posttransplant cyclophosphamide as prophylaxis for graft-versus-host disease. *Biol Blood Marrow Transplant* 21(1):197–198, 2015.

Or-Geva N, Reisner Y: The evolution of T-cell depletion in haploidentical stem-cell transplantation. *Br J Haematol* 172(5):667–684, 2016.

Rimondo A, Crocchiolo R, El-Cheikh J, et al: The calcineurin inhibitor and the intensity of the conditioning regimen may affect the occurrence of polyomavirus-associated hemorrhagic cystitis after haploidentical hematopoietic stem cell transplantation with post-transplant cyclophosphamide. *Bone Marrow Transplant* 52:135, 2017.

Ringdén O, Labopin M, Ciceri F, et al: Is there a stronger graft-versus-leukemia effect using HLA-haploidentical donors than with HLA-identical siblings? *Leukemia* 30:447, 2016.

Ruggeri A, Labopin M, Sanz G, et al: Comparison of outcomes after unrelated cord blood and unmanipulated haploidentical stem cell transplantation in adults with acute leukemia. *Leukemia* 29(9):1891–1900, 2015.

Ruggeri A, Roth-Guepin G, Battipaglia G, et al: Incidence and risk factors for hemorrhagic cystitis in unmanipulated haploidentical transplant recipients. *Transpl Infect Dis* 17:822, 2015.

Solomon SR, Sizemore CA, Sanacore M, et al: Total body irradiation-based myeloablative haploidentical stem cell transplantation is a safe and effective alternative to unrelated donor transplantation in patients without matched sibling donors. *Biol Blood Marrow Transplant* 21:1299, 2015.

Stokes J, Hoffman EA, Zeng Y, et al: Post-transplant bendamustine reduces GvHD while preserving GvL in experimental haploidentical bone marrow transplantation. *Br J Haematol* 174(1):102–116, 2016.

Tang BL, Zhu XY, Zheng CC, et al: Successful early unmanipulated haploidentical transplantation with reduced-intensity conditioning for primary graft failure after cord blood transplantation in hematologic malignancy patients. *Bone Marrow Transplant* 50(2):248–252, 2015.

Wang Y, Liu QF, Xu LP, et al: Haploidentical vs identical-sibling transplant for AML in remission: a multicenter, prospective study. *Blood* 125(25):3956–3962, 2015.

REFERENCES

For the complete list of references, log on to www.expertconsult.com.

UNRELATED DONOR CORD BLOOD TRANSPLANTATION FOR HEMATOLOGIC MALIGNANCIES

Rohtesh S. Mehta, Amanda Olson, Doris M. Ponce, and Elizabeth J. Shpall

Cord blood (CB) is now routinely used as an alternative stem cell source for patients without a matched related or unrelated peripheral blood (PB) or bone marrow (BM) graft. In the late 1980s, Broxmeyer and colleagues[1] reported that CB is a rich source of hematopoietic stem cells (HSCs) and progenitors, setting the stage for the first related donor CB transplantation (CBT) in 1988.[2] Subsequently, placental blood banking programs were initiated in 1992 to 1993 in New York, Milan, Dusseldorf, and Paris.[3,4] The first unrelated donor CBT was performed in 1993, and the first unrelated donor CBT series were published in 1996.[5,6] Public CB banks have since grown in number with an estimated 600,000 public CB units banked globally.[7] Furthermore, the number of CBT continues to increase.[8] In 2010–2011, CBT accounted for more than one-fourth of all allogeneic stem cell transplants (SCT) in patients younger than 20 years, but less than 10% among patients older than 20 years.[8]

The use of CB stem cells has several unique benefits. Given it is a cryopreserved product, it has rapid accessibility, does not carry the risk of donor unavailability, minimizes the risk of infection transmission, has less stringent human leukocyte antigen (HLA) match requirements because of the naive neonatal immune system, and is associated with lower than expected rates of graft-versus-host disease (GVHD). Barker et al[9] reported that recipients of CB grafts were transplanted a median of 25 days earlier than unrelated donor transplant recipients. This is particularly advantageous for patients in need of an urgent transplant. Further, CB has facilitated the extension of transplant access especially to racial and ethnic minorities. Although there are more than 11 million potential marrow donors in the National Marrow Donor Program (NMDP) registry, only 27% are from racial and ethnic minority groups compared with CB units where 45% belong to the minority group.[10] A recent NMDP registry analysis showed that the likelihood of finding an optimal (8/8 or 7/8 HLA-matched) adult donor is 75% for whites of European decent, but it is less than 20% for American blacks and varies from 27% to 52% for other ethnicities. By contrast, a suitable CB graft can be obtained for 80% to 96% of adult patients across all races and almost universally for younger patients.[11] (Fig. 107.1)

SINGLE UNIT CORD BLOOD TRANSPLANTATION

Engraftment

Unrelated donor CBT was initiated using single-unit grafts. Studies have demonstrated that higher cell dose and better donor–recipient HLA match are independent factors associated with improved neutrophil engraftment.[12–19] The 1997 Eurocord analysis was the first large series reporting on 143 related and unrelated donor CBT recipients. In unrelated donor CBT recipients, improved neutrophil and platelet engraftment were both associated with a higher total nucleated cell (TNC) dose above the median of 3.7×10^7/kg and donor–recipient HLA match.[15] In 1998, Rubinstein et al[18] confirmed these findings in an analysis of 562 CBT facilitated by the New York Blood Center (NYBC) as did an updated analysis by Gluckman and Rocha[20] in 2004. In 2002, Wagner et al[19] reported that infused

$CD34^+$ cell dose was superior to infused TNC dose in determining the success of neutrophil and platelet engraftment in an analysis of 102 CBT (median age, 7.4 years) with recipients of units with less than 1.7×10^5 $CD34^+$ cells/kg having a significantly lower neutrophil engraftment incidence of 72% at a median of 34 days compared with higher cell doses ($p < .01$).

These analyses have the limitation that cell dose and HLA match are analyzed separately and yet these graft characteristics must be considered together in the selection of individual units. In 2009, Rocha and Gluckman[21] reported on 925 recipients of single-unit CBT transplanted for malignant disease and found that neutrophil engraftment was related to the number of cells infused ($p < .0001$) and HLA match with a significant difference between zero and one (81%), two (75%), and three and four (63%) HLA disparities ($p = .037$). The role of HLA match was partially abrogated by an increase in cell dose except for recipients of highly mismatched grafts. In 2010, Barker et al[12] analyzed the combined effect of TNC dose and donor–recipient HLA match in 1061 single-unit CBT recipients transplanted for hematologic malignancies after myeloablative conditioning. The best neutrophil engraftment was associated with a fully HLA-A, HLA-B antigen, and HLA-DRB1 matched unit or a cryopreserved TNC greater than 10.0×10^7/kg with one or two mismatches. The worst was with a unit with three mismatches or a cryopreserved TNC below 2.5×10^7/kg with one or two mismatches (Fig. 107.2). There was no difference in neutrophil engraftment in recipients of one versus two mismatched units, and in this setting, the TNC dose determined neutrophil engraftment.

Graft-Versus-Host Disease

Single-unit CBT is associated with a lower than expected incidence of GVHD for the degree of donor–recipient HLA mismatch, which allows use of units with a less stringent HLA match (i.e., only a 4-6/6 HLA-A, HLA-B antigen, HLA-DRB1 allele match). Incidences of grade II–IV acute GVHD have been reported between 10% and 50% and likely vary according to the GVHD prophylaxis used and the inclusion of antithymocyte or antilymphocyte globulin (ATG/ALG) in the conditioning.[12,15,22–26] As with transplantation of adult donors, the major graft determinant of acute GVHD is the HLA match, although with CB, the permissible mismatch is considerably greater than can be tolerated with HSC transplantation from adult donors.

Although an effect of HLA mismatch could not be demonstrated in early series of unrelated donor CBT,[14,15,18,19] a later large NYBC retrospective analysis of 1061 single-unit CBT recipients demonstrated that recipients of matched CB units had significantly less grade III–IV acute GVHD and that increasing mismatch was associated with a progressively increased risk of severe acute GVHD.[12] There was also an association between the degree of mismatch and chronic GVHD, although this only reached significance in recipients of units with three mismatches.[12]

The influence of deeper HLA-matching using allele-level high resolution typing as well as the impact of HLA-C matching have also been explored in single-unit CBTs. In the Cord Blood

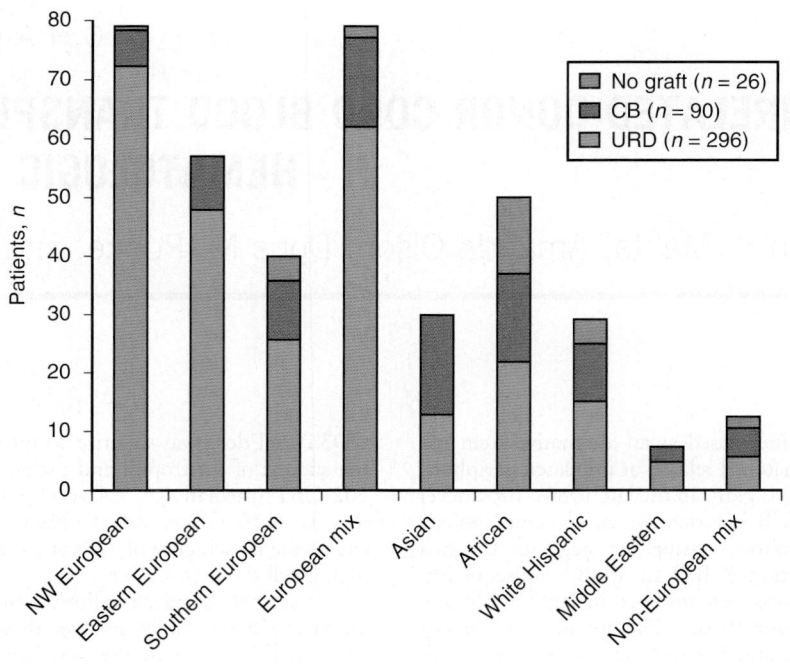

Fig. 107.1 COMPARISON OF PATIENT ANCESTRY IN RECIPIENTS OF UNRELATED VOLUNTEER DONOR (URD) OR CORD BLOOD (CB) TRANSPLANTATION, OR THOSE WHO LACKED A SUITABLE GRAFT. *(From Barker JN, Byam CE, Kernan NA, et al: Availability of cord blood extends allogeneic hematopoietic stem cell transplant access to racial and ethnic minorities.* Biol Blood Marrow Transplant *16:1541, 2010.)*

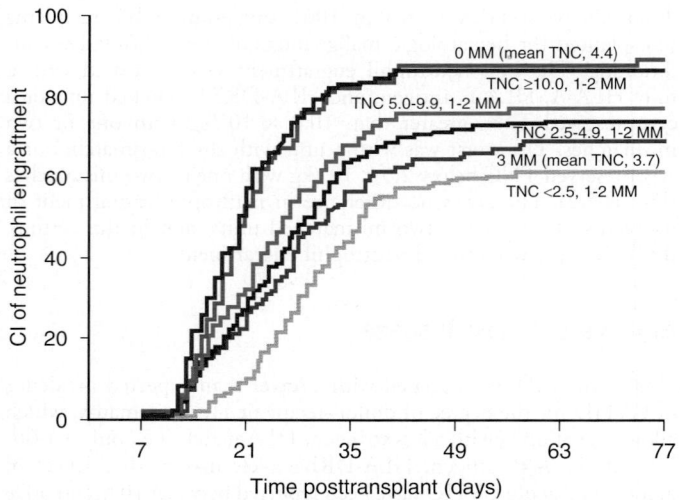

Fig. 107.2 NEUTROPHIL ENGRAFTMENT AFTER MYELOABLATIVE SINGLE-UNIT CORD BLOOD TRANSPLANTATION FACILITATED BY THE NEW YORK BLOOD CENTER ACCORDING TO CRYOPRESERVED TOTAL NUCLEATED CELL (TNC) DOSE AND HUMAN LEUKOCYTE ANTIGEN MATCH. *CI,* Cumulative incidence; *MM,* mismatched. *(From Barker JN, Scaradavou A, Stevens CE: Combined effect of total nucleated cell dose and HLA match on transplantation outcome in 1061 cord blood recipients with hematologic malignancies.* Blood *115:1843, 2010.)*

Transplantation Study involving 191 children (median age 7.7 years), Kurtzberg et al[23] showed that high-resolution matching at HLA-A, HLA-B, and HLA-DRB1 alleles was protective against GVHD. There was a significantly higher incidence of grade II–IV ($p = .02$) and grade III–IV ($p = .02$) acute GVHD in recipients of units with less than 5/6 allele match. A later study by Eapen et al[27] in 803 recipients of single CB units examined the effect of match at HLA-A, HLA-B, HLA-C at intermediate resolution and HLA-DRB1 at allele resolution. The authors did not find a significant effect of HLA-match on grade II–IV acute GVHD, but high-resolution matching was not examined at HLA class I. A recent study by Eapen et al[28] analyzed the effect of allele-level matching at HLA-A, HLA-B, HLA-C, and HLA-DRB1 in 1568 children with single-unit CBT. The risk of grade II–IV acute GVHD was higher with three or four mismatches, but not with one, two or five mismatches, compared with matched CBT. There was no difference in the risk of chronic GVHD between matched or any mismatched CBT. Also, there was no impact of mismatching at a specific *HLA* loci on any of the outcomes. Of note, allele level typing was not available for 50% of the patients, which was then estimated using the *Haplogic III* developed by the NMDP based on the available low/intermediate level testing.

Relapse

During the early years of CBT, there was concern that the neonatal immune system would not adequately protect against relapse. However, multiple series have demonstrated a strong protection against relapse after CBT with the major determinant of relapse being the recipients' disease status.[19,22,23,29] The NYBC series of 1061 single-unit CBT recipients showed no association between HLA match and the incidence of relapse. Subgroup analysis in only relapsed patients, only remission patients, and only those who engrafted also failed to demonstrate any association.[12] However, the 2011 analysis of Eapen et al[27] ($n = 803$) showed a lower relapse incidence after CBT mismatched at more than one loci compared with recipients of units matched at HLA-A, HLA-B, HLA-C, and HLA-DRB1, although the number of mismatched loci had no effect. Moreover, in the recent study by Eapen et al[28] assessing allele level matching at HLA-A, HLA-B, HLA-C, and HLA-DRB1, reduced relapse was noted only for units mismatched at four alleles (but not <3 or 5 alleles) compared with matched units (hazard ratio [HR] 0.50; $p = .001$). The reason for disparity in the findings of these studies is not known, and this area requires further investigation before definitive conclusions can be drawn.

Transplant-Related Mortality and Survival

Early series of single-unit CBT demonstrated high transplant-related mortality (TRM) and consequently poor survival after single-unit CBT. This likely related to the high-risk nature of the patient population and standards of supportive care as well as the characteristics of the transplanted units. Factors such as disease status and recipient cytomegalovirus (CMV) positivity are strong determinants of survival after single-unit CBT.[23] From the standpoint of the graft, both TNC dose and HLA-match influence TRM and survival. In addition to low TNC dose being associated with increased TRM and decreased survival,[12,15,18,19] the 68 adult patient analysis of Laughlin et al[16] and the Wagner et al[19] 102 patient analysis demonstrated a higher CD34+ cell dose (>1.2 and 1.7, respectively) were associated with significantly improved disease-free survival (DFS). Also, increasing HLA-mismatch is significantly associated with increased TRM and lower survival.[12,19,27] The 2010 NYBC analysis of combined TNC dose and HLA match showed that recipients of 6/6 HLA-matched units had the lowest TRM and best survival regardless of the dose at least within the dose range tested (Fig. 107.3).[12] Recipients of units with one HLA-mismatch and a TNC dose 2.5 to 4.9×10^7/kg had a similar TRM as those receiving units with two mismatches and a TNC greater than 5.0×10^7/kg despite the higher cell dose in the latter group (see Fig. 107.3). Recipients of single units with one or two mismatches and a TNC below 2.5×10^7/kg had very high TRM and poor survival.

In the 2011 Eapen series evaluating the contribution of HLA-C matching after single unit CBT, patients matched at HLA-A, HLA-B, and HLA-DRB1 had a higher TRM if mismatched at HLA-C ($n = 23$; HR 3.97; $p = .018$) as compared with those matched at all four loci ($n = 69$).[27] TRM was also higher in 5/6 but 6/8 matched CBT recipients mismatched at one of HLA-A, HLA-B, or HLA-DRB1 plus HLA-C ($n = 234$; HR 1.70; $p = .029$) compared with those who were 5/6 and 7/8 matched (i.e., when there was a single HLA mismatch at HLA-A, HLA-B, or HLA-DRB1 but a match at HLA-C; $n = 127$). This study suggests that HLA-C matching is an important determinant of survival and should be considered in unit selection algorithms. In a recent study by Eapen et al[28] using allele level matching, significantly higher nonrelapse mortality (NRM) was noted with units mismatched at any number of alleles (HLA-A, HLA-B, HLA-C, or HLA-DRB1) compared with HLA-matched

units (HR ranging from 2.8 to 4.6 for 1 to 5 allele mismatches).[28] The author recommended avoiding CB units with greater than three allele mismatches. Of note, only 7% of the units in their study were complete allele matched and 90% of the 4/6 matched patients by current standard were reported to have greater than or equal to three allele-level mismatches. Therefore, if greater than three allele mismatches are to be avoided, that would require massive addition of high-quality CB units to the global inventory.[30] Therefore, the application of the study results, which are highly informative, is impractical for current clinical practice.

Comparison of Single-Unit Cord Blood Transplantation and Adult Donor Allografts

Although the use of CBT as an alternative HSC source has increased substantially, no randomized studies evaluating survival after CBT versus adult donor allografts have yet been reported. Retrospective comparisons have demonstrated varying results depending on whether the series evaluated children or adults and if matched versus mismatched unrelated volunteer donors were included. Selected series are summarized in Table 107.1. In 2007, Eapen and colleagues[26] compared the outcomes of pediatric single-unit CBT with those of unrelated volunteer BM recipients who were transplanted for the treatment of acute leukemia. Compared with the recipients of 8/8 allele-matched unrelated donor BM transplantation (BMT), the 5-year LFS in recipients of one or two HLA-mismatched CBT was similar. Notably, however, a significantly higher LFS was observed in recipients of 6/6 HLA-matched units. Interestingly, TRM was similar in 6/6 HLA-matched and 5/6 HLA-matched high cell dose compared with that of allele-matched unrelated donor recipients' transplant ($p = .0659$ and .1332, respectively). By contrast, TRM was higher in recipients of one antigen HLA-mismatched low cell dose and two antigen HLA-mismatched of any cell dose compared with allele-matched unrelated donor recipients ($p = .0455$ and .0003, respectively).

A similar analysis done in adult patients with acute leukemia demonstrated that single-unit CBT recipients had a higher TRM compared with recipients of 8/8 HLA-matched unrelated donor transplants but a similar TRM to that of 7/8 HLA-mismatched unrelated donor transplant recipients.[22] The Japanese group of Takahashi et al[25] compared CBT recipients with unrelated donor BM or PB HSC transplantation for the treatment of hematologic malignancies. They demonstrated a slower neutrophil recovery in CBT recipients but a similar rate of neutrophil engraftment. The incidences of grade III–IV acute GVHD and extensive chronic GVHD were higher after unrelated donor transplantation. No differences were demonstrated in TRM, relapse, or DFS between the groups. Atsuta et al[31] conducted a disease-specific analysis comparing CBT to unrelated donor BMT in patients with acute leukemia. The patients had similar age distribution, and all received myeloablative conditioning. In the acute myeloid leukemia group, there was a similar relapse rate but higher TRM in CBT recipients, resulting in lower survival, but similar relapse and survival rates were seen in the acute lymphoblastic leukemia (ALL) group. The risk of developing extensive chronic GVHD was lower in CBT recipients.

DOUBLE-UNIT CORD BLOOD TRANSPLANTATION

The transplantation of HSC from more than one donor is an approach that was originally reported by Mathé et al,[32] who infused multiple aliquots of BM from different donors. In 1972, Ende and Ende[33] published the first case of allogeneic CBT using multiple small CB units. Subsequently, double-unit CBT (DCBT) was formally investigated by the University of Minnesota as a method to augment graft cell dose. These investigators demonstrated the safety and feasibility of this approach.[33] Barker et al[34] reported two series of DCBT after myeloablative and reduced-intensity conditioning (RIC) conditioning in patients with high-risk hematologic malignancies.[35] The myeloablative series evaluated 23 patients (median age 24 years) and

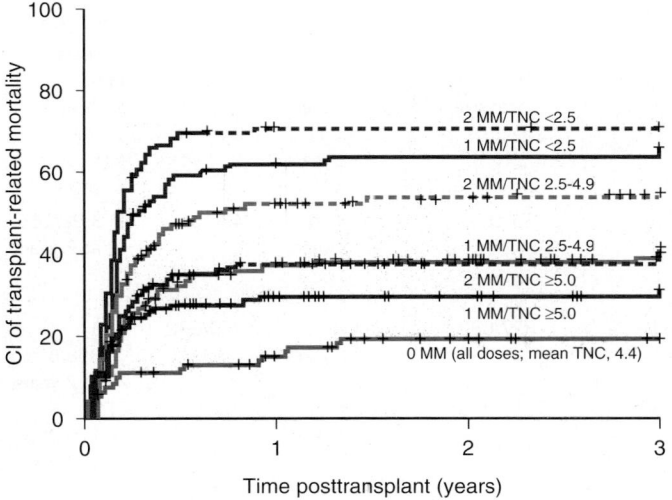

Fig. 107.3 CUMULATIVE INCIDENCE (CI) OF TRANSPLANT-RELATED MORTALITY (TRM) ACCORDING TO THE COMBINED TOTAL NUCLEATED CELL (TNC) DOSE AND HUMAN LEUKOCYTE ANTIGEN MISMATCH AFTER SINGLE-UNIT MYELOABLATIVE CORD BLOOD TRANSPLANTATION. *MM,* Mismatched. *(From Barker JN, Scaradavou A, Stevens CE: Combined effect of total nucleated cell dose and HLA match on transplantation outcome in 1061 cord blood recipients with hematologic malignancies.* Blood 115:1843, 2010.)

TABLE 107.1

Comparison of Single-Unit Cord Blood Transplantation With Adult Donor Hematopoietic Stem Cell Transplantation

Reference	Graft (Patients n)	Age Median (range), in years	Conditioning (Patients n)	CI (%) of Neutrophil Engraftment / Days to Neutrophil Engraftment, Median (range)	II–IV Acute GVHD	III–IV Acute GVHD	Chronic GVHD	NRM/TRM	Relapse	Survival
Eapen et al[26]	503 CBT 35 matched	Unknown (<1 to <16)	TBI 69% Non-TBI 31%	25 (9–90) days 85% at day +42	8/34	3/34	10/33	2/35	11/35	5-year LFS 60%
	1-Ag MM 157 high dose		TBI 68% Non-TBI 30%	80% at day +42	62/149	29/149	27/147	45/157	46/157	5-year LFS 45%
	44 low dose		TBI 82% Non-TBI 14%	59% at day +42	16/44	9/44	7/39	19/44	9/44	5-year LFS 36%
	2-Ag MM 267		TBI 78% Non-TBI 20%	76% at day +42	107/259	69/259	38/247	124/267	52/267	5-year LFS 33%
	282 BM Matched 116		TBI 84% Non-TBI 16%	19 (9–33) days 97% at day +42	53/116	21/116	37/116	24/116	45/116	5-year LFS 38%
	MM 166		TBI 92% Non-TBI 8%	97% at day +42	100/166	54/166	66/166	51/166	51/166	5-yr LFS 37%
Takahashi et al[25]	100 CBT	38 (16–55)	TBI-based	91% at day +60 22 (16–46) days	51%	6%	Overall 73% Extensive 23%	8% at day 100 9% at 1 year	17% at 3-years	DFS 70% at 3 years
	71 RD 55 BM/16 PBSC	40 (16–58)	TBI-based	96% at day +60 17 (10–35) days	36%	13%	Overall 49% Extensive 30%	4% at day 100 13% at 1 year	26% at 3 years	DFS 60% at 3 years
Atsuta et al[31]	CBT 173 AML	38 (16–69)	TBI-based (89%) Bu-Cy (10%)	77% at day +100	32%	–	Overall 28% Extensive 8%	30% at 1 year 33% at 2 years	27% at 1 year 31% at 2 years	LFS 43% at 1 year 36% at 2 years
	UD-BMT 311 AML	38 (16–60)	TBI-based (82%) Bu-Cy (18%)	94% at day +100	35%	–	Overall 32% Extensive 20%	19% at 1 year 22% at 2 years	20% at 1 year 24% at 2 years	LFS 62% at 1 year 54% at 2 years
	CBT 114 ALL	34 (16–58)	TBI-based (97%) Bu-Cy (3%)	80% at day +100	28%	–	Overall 27% Extensive 10%	21% at 1 year 24% at 2 years	27% at 1 year 19% at 2 years	LFS 52% at 1 year 45% at 2 years
	UD-BMT 222 ALL	32 (16–59)	TBI-based (91%) Bu-Cy (5%)	97% at day +100	42%	–	Overall 30% Extensive 17%	23% at 1 year 25% at 2 years	31% at 1 year 24% at 2 years	LFS 58% at 1 year 51% at 2 years
Eapen et[22]	165 CB	28 (16 to >50)	TBI (55%) ATG (72%)	24 (12–68) days 80% at day +42	49/162	–	39/161	37% at 2 years	43/165	LFS 98/165 at 2 years
	888 URD PBSC 632 matched	33 (16 to >50)	TBI (66%) ATG (18%)	14 (5–28) days 96% at day +42	303/630	–	327/632	24% at 2 years	209/632	LFS 358/632 at 2 years
	265 1-Ag MM				134/256	–	113/256	38% at 2 years	77/256	LFS 170/256 at 2 years
	472 URD BM 332 matched	39 (16 to >50)	TBI (68%) ATG (28%)	19 (6–41) days 93% at day +42	129/332	–	132/332	22% at 2 years	112/332	LFS 188/332 at 2 years
	140 1-Ag MM				64/139	–	51/140	34% at 2 years	42/140	DFS 80/140

Ag, Antigen; ALL, acute lymphoid leukemia; AML, acute myeloid leukemia; BM, bone marrow; CBT, cord blood transplantation; DFS, disease-free survival; GVHD, graft-versus-host disease; LFS, leukemia-free survival; MM, mismatched; NRM, nonrelapse mortality; PBSC, peripheral blood stem cell; RD, related donor; TBI, total-body irradiation; TRM, transplant-related mortality; URD, unrelated donor.

demonstrated that all evaluable patients achieved donor-derived neutrophil engraftment at a median of 23 days. The striking finding of this report was the high level of engraftment despite sustained hematopoiesis being mediated by a single donor in nearly all patients and the high 1-year overall survival (OS) of 72%. The RIC series demonstrated that it was possible to engraft CB after conditioning with cyclophosphamide 50 mg/kg, fludarabine 200 mg/m2, and 200 cGy of total body irradiation. In 2007, Brunstein et al[36] updated the RIC experience in 110 adults (17 single-unit CBT and 93 DCBT) and demonstrated neutrophil engraftment in 92% but a higher probability of 3-year event-free survival of 39% in DCBT recipients compared with 24% in single-unit recipients ($p = .05$). The high incidences of donor-derived neutrophil engraftment have been subsequently replicated at other centers.[37–41]

Determinants of Unit Dominance

After DCBT single cord provides long-term engraftment while the second unit is lost in a majority of cases usually within 30–60 days and evidently within 1 year.[34,36,38,40,42,43] Myeloablative conditioning regimens lead to an early dominance of single unit,[34] while nonmyeloablative conditioning regimens are associated delayed emergence of single dominant unit.[36] Less than 5% of patients may have evidence of stable persistent mixed-unit chimerism,[41,44–49] defined as detection of both CB units at varying proportions for at least 1 year posttransplantation.[50] This is more common after nonmyeloablative conditioning regimens and if two CB units are closely HLA-matched to each other.[36] Moreover, a review of studies with persistent mixed-unit chimerism suggests that HLA-C matching between the cords may be associated with a higher likelihood of mixed-unit chimerism through intercord tolerance induction.[50] The determinants of DCBT unit dominance remain to be fully elucidated. Better HLA match, ABO group, and higher infused TNC or

CD34+ cell doses have not predicted which unit will win. Current evidence suggests that unit dominance is predominantly immune-mediated, although unit hematopoietic potential can also play a role (Table 107.2).

Host Factors as Determinants of Unit Dominance

Based on earlier studies using DCBT murine models and correlating findings that the dominant unit in mice correlated clinically in 18 of 21 patients, it was suggested that unit dominance is not related to host-versus-graft factors.[51] Later studies showed that there was no effect of donor-specific anti-HLA antibodies in on the speed of engraftment or unit dominance in recipients of DCBT,[52] providing further evidence that host factors do not play a major role in unit dominance.

Hematopoietic Potency as a Determinant of Unit Dominance

Although the infused CD34+ cell or colony-forming unit dose has not been associated with unit dominance, studies suggest that high CD34+ cell viability, which correlates with colony-forming unit potential, predicts unit dominance.[41,53,59,60] Thus, damage to the unit as reflected by a low percentage of viable CD34+ cells likely impairs engraftment potential.

Immune Factors as Determinants of Unit Dominance

The role of graft T-cells in predicting unit dominance is supported by the studies showing that higher infused CD3+ cell dose correlates with the engrafting unit.[41,61] Murine models have also suggested

TABLE 107.2	Potential Determinants of Unit Dominance After Double-Unit Cord Blood Transplantation			
Potential Mechanism	**Reference**	**Finding**		**Implications**
Host factors	Eldjerou et al[51]	Unit dominance in mice correlated with clinical engraftment.		Host factors do not influence unit dominance.
	Brunstein et al[52]	Donor specific anti-HLA antibodies had no influence on unit dominance.		
Unit factors Hematopoietic potential	Scaradavou et al[53]	Infused TNC/kg, CD34+/kg, and CFU doses were not associated with unit engraftment. However, units with low CD34+ viability were very unlikely to engraft.		Infused CD34+ cell dose and CFU, CFC, or CAFC content do not directly influence unit dominance, but poor-quality units are very unlikely to engraft in humans.
	Eldjerou et al[51]	In vitro CFC and CAFC content did not correlate with unit dominance.		
Immune factors	Barker et al[34] Scaradavou et al[53] Avery et al[41]	Higher infused CD3+ cell dose is associated with unit dominance.		Graft-versus-graft interactions dictate unit dominance.
	Kim et al[54]	DCBT with MNC associated with unit dominance whereas coengraftment achieved with lineage depletion or MSC infusion.		
	Yahata et al[55]	Mixed chimerism achieved by CD34+ selection.		
	Eldjerou et al[51]	Loss of unit dominance with CD34+ DCBT restored with addition of CD34- cells.		
	Delaney et al[56]	Unmanipulated unit is dominant when coinfused with T-cell depleted expanded CB.		
	Gutman et al[57]	Dominant unit CD8+ T cells directed against the nondominant unit detected in patients with single unit dominance.		
	Avery et al[41]	High level of unit–unit match associated with increased likelihood of coengraftment.		
	Brunstein et al[58]	Higher prevalence of dual chimerism after Treg infusion.		

CAFC, 5 Cobblestone area-forming cell; CB, cord blood; CFC, colony forming cell; CFU, colony forming unit; DCBT, double-unit cord blood transplantation; HLA, human leukocyte antigen; MNC, mononuclear cell; MSC, mesenchymal stromal cell; TNC, total nucleated cell dose; Treg, regulatory T cell.

that an immune mechanism accounts for unit dominance. Studies in nonobese diabetic severe combined immunodeficient interleukin-2 receptor gamma null (NOD/SCID/IL-2R-γ^{null}) mice demonstrated that despite each unit engrafting alone, coinfusion of mononuclear cells as a double-unit graft was associated with predominance of one CB unit.[54,55] Further, unit dominance could be mitigated (and engraftment of both units achieved) with either lineage depletion of the units or cotransplantation of third-party BM-derived mesenchymal stromal cells and mixed chimerism could be generated by CD34$^+$ cell selection.[54,55] It was also shown that the unit dominance was T-cell–mediated and involved both CD4$^+$ and CD8$^+$ cells. Furthermore, it can be hypothesized that the failure of sustained engraftment of ex vivo expanded CB units in clinical trials of DCBT in which one of two units is expanded is not attributable to failure to expand or maintain sufficient progenitors in the manipulated unit but because the expanded unit is T-cell depleted and therefore cannot compete with a T-cell replete unmanipulated unit.[56]

Graft-versus-graft interactions also play a role in determining unit dominance. This is suggested from NOD/SCID/IL2R-γ^{null} murine study showing that DCBT using CD34$^+$ cells was associated with loss of both unit dominance, and addition of CD34$^-$ cells from only one of the two units restored unit dominance, with engraftment being mediated by the origin of the CD34$^-$ cells.[51] Moreover, Brunstein et al[58] evaluated the safety of ex vivo expanded regulatory T cells (Tregs) in DBCT recipients and found an increased prevalence of coengraftment of both units (dual donor chimerism), suggesting that graft-versus-graft interactions could be ameliorated by suppressing T-cell responses.

Additional evidence in favor of an immune basis for unit dominance comes from the study by Gutman et al,[57] who identified CD8$^+$ T cells derived from the dominant unit that recognized the

nondominant unit were present in the PB 28 days after transplantation in 9 of 10 DCBT recipients engrafting with single units regardless of the conditioning regimen. Interestingly, the three patients who had persistent mixed chimerism also did not develop an alloreactive CD8$^+$ T-cell response.

Clinical data from Avery et al[41] have demonstrated a role of HLA-match in unit dominance. Interestingly, in this analysis of 84 DCBT recipients, the dominant units were not necessarily better HLA-matched to the recipient compared with the nondominant unit of a double-unit pair (Fig. 107.4). However, the unit–unit HLA match influenced the length of time the ultimately nonengrafting unit was able to be detected. Specifically, recipients of double-unit grafts in whom the unit–unit HLA match was 7/10 or greater HLA-allele matched were significantly more likely to have initial coengraftment and transient persistence of the ultimately nonengrafting unit with one patient having sustained engraftment of both units long term. By contrast, recipients of units highly mismatched (<6/10) to each other were more likely to have engraftment with only a single unit. This is likely because of an enhanced unit-versus-unit immune response, whereas closely HLA-matched units are more likely to be relatively tolerant of each other, and in this setting, at least transient coengraftment is possible.

Taken together, these findings suggest that unit dominance likely involves a complex interplay of hematopoietic potential as suggested by the role of CD34$^+$ cell viability as well as immune factors that are likely T-cell–mediated because no role for natural killer (NK) cells has been identified to date.[62] Future studies need to elucidate the specific cell population mediating the graft-versus-graft effect in the setting of the transplantation of two units with adequate engraftment potential. This will enhance our CB unit selection process for infusion and for novel graft manipulation techniques elaborated later.

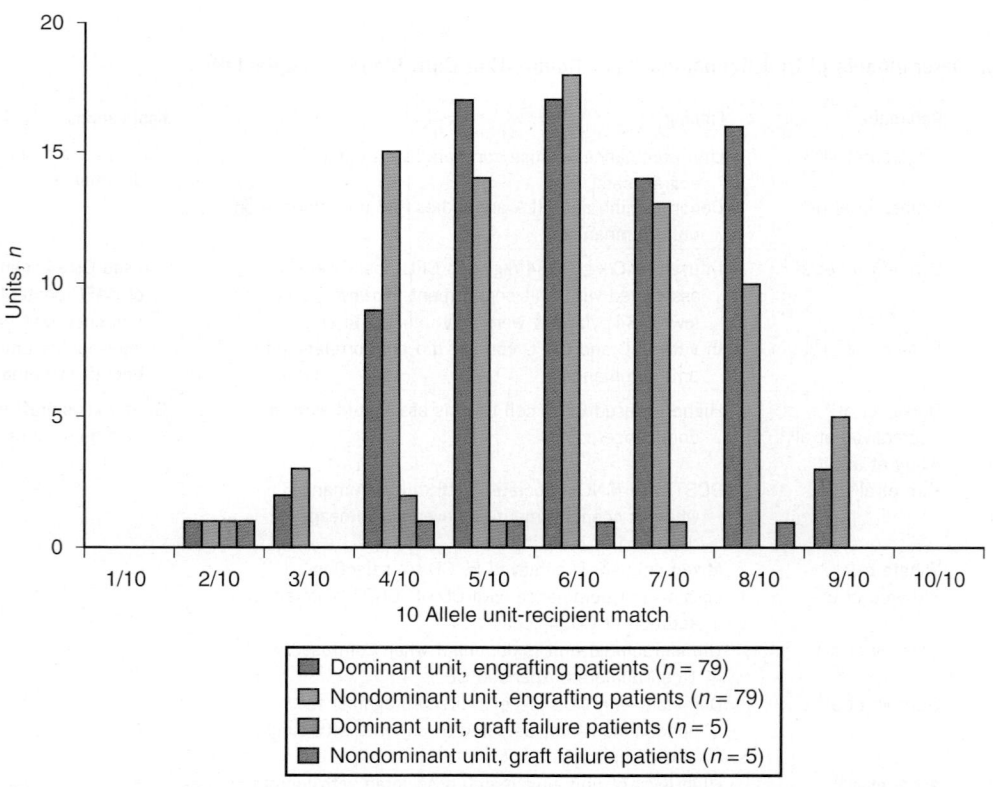

Fig. 107.4 INFLUENCE OF HIGH RESOLUTION UNIT-RECIPIENT HUMAN LEUKOCYTE ANTIGEN MATCH ON SUSTAINED DONOR ENGRAFTMENT AFTER DOUBLE-UNIT D BLOOD TRANSPLANTATION ($n = 84$). The engrafting units were not better matched to the recipient. *(From Avery S, Shi W, Lubin M, et al: Influence of infused cell dose and HLA match on engraftment after double-unit cord blood allografts.* Blood *117:3277, 2011.)*

CORD BLOOD UNIT SELECTION

Efficient search and selection of CB units requires decision making as to what banks to consider and what factors to prioritize in unit selection. The unit selection algorithm currently used at the Memorial Sloan-Kettering Cancer Center (MSKCC) is shown in Fig. 107.5.[63] The M.D. Anderson Cancer Center (MDACC) uses a similar approach. Primary unit selection criteria are based on the prethaw cryopreserved TNC/kg, the unit-recipient HLA match (4-6/6 of HLA-A, HLA-B antigen, and HLA-DRB1 allele), and the bank of origin based on the authors' experience with the bank and their accreditation. Other factors such as the availability of confirmatory HLA typing on an attached segment and the completeness of maternal infectious disease marker and hemoglobinopathy testing are also taken into account.

The exact threshold for acceptable TNC/kg has yet to be established and varies with HLA match. For example, the 2010 NYBC analysis of single-unit CBT demonstrated that recipients of units with a 6/6 HLA match had the best transplantation outcomes regardless of the cryopreserved TNC dose. By contrast, recipients of 4/6 units required a TNC dose of 5.0×10^7/kg or greater to achieve similar TRM and DFS to that of recipients of 5/6 units with TNC of $2.5-4.9 \times 10^7$/kg.[12] Although the numbers of DCBT recipients available do not yet permit such analysis, it is likely that similar principles will be found associated with the engrafting unit in DBCT recipients. Indeed, Avery et al[41] have reported that a higher infused TNC and CD34+ cell dose in the engrafting unit of a double-unit pair was strongly associated with the speed and success of neutrophil engraftment. However, because it is not currently possible to predict which unit will predominate at the time of

double-unit graft selection, a minimum threshold for each unit of a double-unit graft is needed. Based on the analysis by Avery et al[41] a minimum TNC dose threshold of at least 2.0×10^7/kg is currently recommended in DCBT. The age of cryopreserved CB units should not be criteria when selecting CB units. A study showed that units cryopreserved for up to 11 years before transplantation had no impact on postthaw TNC recovery or neutrophil or platelet engraftment in 288 single CBT recipients.[64]

Recent analyses have highlighted new factors to be considered in unit selection. The 2009 NYBC analysis evaluated the impact of fetal exposure to noninherited maternal antigens (NIMAs) on the outcome of CBT.[65] The 79 single-unit CBT recipients that had an HLA-mismatched antigen that was identical to a donor NIMA engrafted earlier and had lower TRM and overall mortality. There was also a lower tendency toward relapse among patients with myeloid malignancies. Subsequently, in 2011, the NYBC analyzed the effect of HLA-mismatch vector in 1202 single-unit CBT recipients.[66] They identified 98 donor–recipient pairs with only unidirectional mismatches (58 in the graft-versus-host direction and 40 in the rejection direction). The graft-versus-host vector group had faster engraftment and decreased TRM and overall mortality compared with the one-bidirectional mismatch reference group, but recipients of rejection only mismatched units had slower engraftment, a higher incidence of graft failure, and higher relapse rates. Also in 2011, Eapen et al[27] reported that HLA-C matching is important in addition to HLA-A, HLA-B, and HLA-DRB1, although how to balance this against TNC dose needs to be further investigated. Finally, the potential importance of antigens in the patients that are shared with inherited paternal antigens in the CB donor that could be a target for maternal T cells has recently been reported as a potential mechanism of reduced relapse after CBT.[67]

The findings concerning the importance of HLA-mismatch vector and HLA-C can be immediately incorporated into CB unit selection algorithms, but incorporation of NIMA and inherited paternal antigen will require banks to provide maternal typing. In addition, although the best available CB unit or units are selected as the graft, it is important to identify and reserve at least one backup unit in the event of problems with unit shipment, mislabeling, problems with thaw, or graft failure.[68-70] At both MSKCC and MDACC, the authors select one domestic unit as backup to ensure the timely infusion of an optimal CB product.

It is unclear if recipients should be assessed pretransplant for anti-HLA antibodies possessing specific alloreactivity against CB units (donor specific antibodies, DSAs), as these may have an impact on post-DCBT outcomes although the data are rather conflicting. Cutler et al[71] analyzed the outcomes of 73 DCBT recipients after either myeloablative or RIC regimens. DSAs were detected in 24% of the patients, of which about 60% were directed against one CB unit and the rest targeted both units. Rate of graft failure was drastically higher in patients with DSAs directed against both units (57%) compared with those with DSAs against single unit (18%) or those with no DSAs (5.5%). Also, time to neutrophil engraftment was prolonged (29 days versus 21 days; $p = .004$) and day 100 mortality or relapse was increased in patients with any DSA. Noteworthy, more than 70% of patients received RIC regimens that included ATG. Another study using RIC regimens in 294 CBT recipients found DSAs in 14 patients (4.7%), half of whom received single CBT.[72] As seen in the Cutler study,[71] patients with DSAs had significantly worse neutrophil engraftment (44% versus 81%, $p = .006$), 1-year TRM (46% versus 32% $p = .06$) and a trend towards poor OS (42% versus 29%; $p = .07$) compared with those without DSAs. On the contrary, Brunstein et al[52] found no impact of DSAs in their study of 126 DCBT recipients. Overall, DSAs were present in about 15% of the patients, of which two-thirds were directed against one CB unit and one-third against both units. The cumulative incidence of neutrophil engraftment was similar in patients with DSAs against at least one CB unit (78%; median, 24.5 days) compared with patients with irrelevant anti-HLA antibodies (84%; median, 24 days) and those with no antibody (86%; median, 19 days), $p = .54$. Overall, 35% of entire study cohort received myeloablative conditioning, but the type

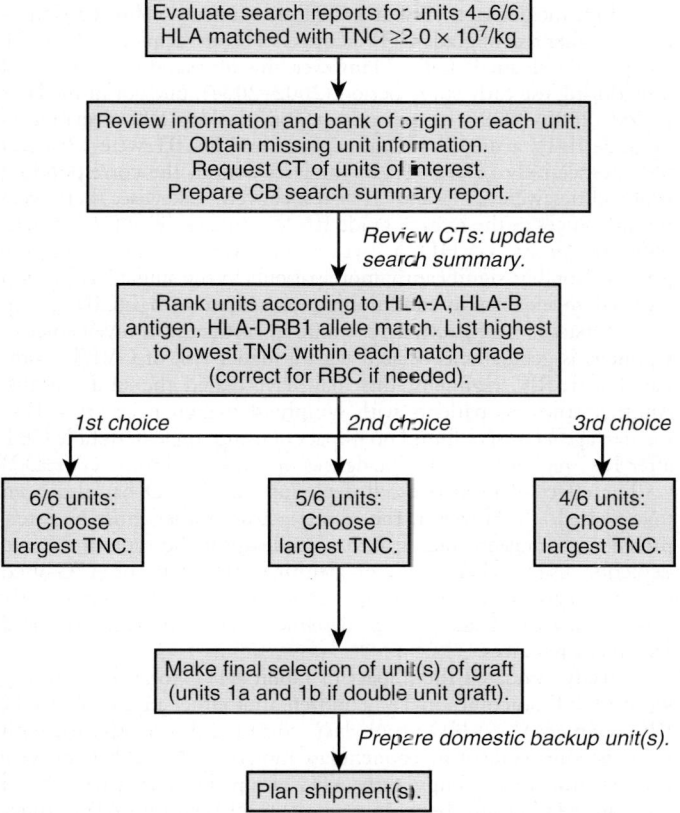

Fig. 107.5 CURRENT MEMORIAL SLOAN-KETTERING CANCER CENTER AND M.D. ANDERSON CANCER CENTER SCHEMA OF HOW TO SELECT CORD BLOOD (CB) UNITS. *CT,* Confirmatory typing; *HLA,* human leukocyte antigen; *RBC,* red blood cell; *TNC,* total nucleated cell. *(From Barker JN, Byam C, Scaradavou A: How I treat: the selection and acquisition of unrelated cord blood grafts.* Blood *117:2332, 2011.)*

of conditioning specifically used in patients with DSAs was not reported. Similar to these findings, more recently Dahi et al[73] also showed no impact of DSAs on engraftment in 82 DCBT recipients who were transplanted with either myeloablative (82%) or nonmyeloablative (18%) conditioning. DSAs were present in about 15% of patients, half of which targeted both CB units. There was no difference in cumulative incidence of engraftment at day 42 in patients with DSAs (92%), without DSAs (95%), or those with nonspecific HLA-antibodies (100%). Intriguingly, half of the patients with DSAs against one CB unit actually engrafted with that unit. Of note, all patients with DSAs in this study received myeloablative conditioning. Therefore, it is possible that the use of DCBT and myeloablative conditioning may overcome any potential adverse effect of DSAs. Some of the differences in these studies could be explained by differences in underlying patient population, type of conditioning regimen, GVHD prophylaxis, use of ATG or not, assay used to detect DSAs, threshold for labeling DSAs as positive and the median fluorescence intensity of DSAs. Although virtual cross-match techniques may be used to screen for DSAs,[74] it is debatable if their presence should be assessed in all patients being considered for CBT. It certainly adds to health care costs and may delay search for an "appropriate" unit.

DOUBLE-UNIT VERSUS SINGLE-UNIT CORD BLOOD TRANSPLANTATION

Engraftment

The use of double-unit CB grafts is now a standard approach to augment cell dose, although DCBT does not improve or hasten engraftment compared with adequately dosed single-unit CBT.[75-77] A recent phase III, multicenter, randomized trial conducted by the Blood and Marrow Transplant Clinical Trials Network (BMTCTN) in collaboration with Children's Oncology Group (BMTCTN-0501 trial), involving children (median age 9.9 years) with hematologic malignancies compared the use of single ($n = 112$) with double ($n = 108$) CBT after myeloablative conditioning.[77] The study found no difference in the incidence of neutrophil recovery (88% versus 89%), or the time to neutrophil engraftment between the groups (23 versus 21 days respectively). On the contrary, the recipients of single CBT had significantly faster platelet engraftment compared with DCBT recipients (median 58 versus 84 days, respectively).

In the absence of a randomized controlled trial in adults, data from retrospective series and a small prospective study suggest similar rapidity and cumulative incidence of engraftment between single or double CBT recipients. A retrospective analysis of the CIBMTR and the NYBC registries compared single ($n = 106$) with double ($n = 303$) CBT after myeloablative ($n = 216$) or RIC regimens ($n = 193$) in adults with acute leukemia.[76] The median time to neutrophil engraftment (20 days in both groups) and the probability of neutrophil engraftment by day 42 were identical in both groups (81% after single CBT versus 78% after DCBT, $p = .83$).

A prospective study in adults (median age 53.5 years) compared single CBT ($n = 27$) with DCBT ($n = 23$) after RIC regimens.[75] Patients underwent single CBT if cryopreserved TNC dose in one unit was $>2.5 \times 10^7$/kg recipient weight. Once again, there were no differences in the median time to neutrophil engraftment among single CBT (25 days) or DCBT (23 days), or the cumulative incidence of neutrophil engraftment at day 100 posttransplantation (88.4% versus 91.3% respectively, $p = .99$).

Graft-Versus-Host Disease

GVHD is a major cause of morbidity and one of the leading causes of mortality after DCBT.[22,26,38,78-81] Also, DCBT may be associated with an increased incidence of acute GVHD compared with single CBT in a specific subset of patients, especially if transplantation is performed without the use of ATG or ALG.[78,82] The results across studies are variable because of heterogeneity in study population,

transplant procedures and study designs. The following section highlights some of these differences.

In the BMTCTN-0501 randomized trial,[77] a higher incidence of grade III–IV acute GVHD was noted in children receiving double-unit than those receiving single-unit CBT (23% versus 13%, $p = .02$). Similarly, the incidence of chronic extensive GVHD was higher in the DCBT group at 1 year after transplantation (15% versus 9%, $p = .05$). A retrospective study conducted by the Eurocord and Acute Leukemia Working Party of European Blood and Marrow Transplant (EBMT) group[81] in adults with acute leukemia ($n = 239$) receiving myeloablative conditioning found higher risk of grade II–IV acute GVHD after DCBT compared with single CBT (43% versus 26%, $p = .005$); however, two-thirds of these events were grade II acute GVHD. Age less than 35 years (HR 0.55, 95% CI, 0.34–0.88, $p = .01$) and the use of single CBT (HR 0.84, 95% CI, 0.41–0.96, $p = .02$) were independently associated with lower risk of acute GVHD.

In a retrospective analysis by MacMillan et al[82] comparing single-unit ($n = 80$) and double-unit ($n = 185$) CBT, the incidence of grade II–IV acute GVHD was noted to be significantly higher in recipients of DCBT (58% versus 39%, $p < .01$). However, the increased risk was predominantly accounted by grade II skin acute GVHD, and the overall incidence of grade III–IV acute GVHD was similar among the groups (19% versus 18%). Of note, differential use of ATG, differences in age, year of transplant, conditioning regimens and GVHD prophylaxis between the groups are some of the important biases in the study. For instance, the single CBT group was younger (median age 23 years) and ATG was used in more than half of them. In contrast, the median age of patients in the double-CBT group was 45 years and only about a quarter received ATG. Younger age and higher use of ATG may explain lower incidence of acute GVHD seen after single CBT.

On the other hand, the CIBMTR-NYBC registry analysis of adequately dosed single ($n = 106$, median age 33 years) or double ($n = 303$, median age 43 years) CBT in adults also showed significantly higher risk of grade II–IV acute GVHD in recipients of DCBT compared with single CBT.[76] However, this increased risk was noted only during the early study period (2002–2004), but not in the later period (2005–2009). In the early period, the day 100 probabilities of grade II–IV acute GVHD after single and DCBT were 18% and 58% respectively ($p < .001$). In the later period, the corresponding probabilities were 27% and 31% respectively. Likewise, there were no differences in the rates of grade III–IV acute GVHD (14% versus 18%) or chronic GVHD at 2-years (24% versus 31%) among the groups. Notably, significantly more patients in the single CBT group received myeloablative conditioning compared with DCBT group (72% versus 45% respectively, $p < .0001$). As the use of myeloablative regimens is generally associated with a higher risk of GVHD compared with RIC regimens, this may have biased the study results. Another study in patients with lymphoid malignancies ($n = 104$, median age 41 years), found no impact of using single or double CBT after RIC regimens on the incidences of acute or chronic GVHD.[83]

The effect of in vivo T-cell depletion on GVHD has also been investigated.[84-87] However, the results across studies must be interpreted with caution, taking into consideration the type of in vivo depletion used (ATG, ALG, or alemtuzumab), type of ATG used (rabbit versus horse), dose (high versus low) and the timing (early versus delayed) in addition to baseline patient characteristics and transplant practices.

A study evaluated the impact of rabbit ATG (total dose 10 mg/kg) on CBT outcomes in 127 children after either myeloablative or RIC regimens.[84] GVHD prophylaxis consisted of cyclosporine with either prednisolone or mycophenolate mofetil (MMF). Patients were divided into three groups: early ATG group (between days −9 and −5), late ATG group (between days −5 and 0), and no-ATG group. The study found an increased risk of acute GVHD and lower rates of viral infections and infection related deaths in the group that did not receive ATG compared with the groups that did. Further, the risk of acute GVHD was significantly higher in the no-ATG group (HR 8.2, $p < .001$) and early-ATG group (odds ratio [OR] 3.9, $p = .005$) compared with the late-ATG group. However, there were no differences in chronic GVHD or other outcomes including neutrophil engraftment, NRM, relapse and OS between the groups. Although patients in the early-ATG group had significantly faster CD3+, CD4+, and CD4+-naive T-cell immune reconstitution at 1 and 2 months post-CBT compared with patients in the late-ATG group, yet, there were no differences in viral reactivation episodes in early and late-ATG groups. This is likely related to attainment of similar immune reconstitution by 3 months post-CBT in both groups. Therefore, the early use of ATG does not offer any clinical advantage over not using ATG at all.

Series of DCBT in adults incorporating ATG have demonstrated lower rates of GVHD than what is typically seen after CBT without the use of ATG. For example, Cutler et al[85] reported an overall incidence of grade II–IV acute GVHD of 9.4% and chronic GVHD of 12.5% in adults (n = 32, median age 53 years) after RIC using rabbit ATG (days –7, –5, –3, –1; total dose 6.0 mg/kg) and GVHD prophylaxis with sirolimus plus tacrolimus. Unsurprisingly, immune reconstitution was remarkably prolonged; the CD4+CD45RA+, CD4+CD45RO+, and CD4+CD25+ T-cell subsets did not reach the pretransplantation levels even at 2-years posttransplantation. Consequently, five patients developed Epstein Barr virus (EBV) reactivation leading to fatal posttransplant lymphoproliferative disorder and five additional patients died of sepsis (4 caused by human herpesvirus-6 and EBV-related meningoencephalitis). The NRM at 2-years was 34.4%, which is considerably higher than what is reported by other RIC CBT series.[78,86,88–94] Another study included 42 adults RIC DCBT patients (median age 49 years) who received rabbit ATG and tacrolimus/sirolimus (69%) or cyclosporine based (31%) GVHD prophylaxis.[86] The dose and timing of ATG were not mentioned. Although there were low incidence of grade II–IV acute GVHD (21%) and chronic GVHD (24%), but as expected, T-cell immune reconstitution was substantially prolonged. The median number of CD4+ T cells did not reach >200 cells/mL even 9 months posttransplant leading to high rate of early infection (59%) within the first 100 days after transplantation. Similarly, Brunstein et al[87] showed an increased risk of EBV–related complications with the use of high dose equine ATG (15 mg/kg given every 12 hours for 6 doses, days –5, –4, and –3) after Fludarabine/Cytaradine/total body irradiation (TBI) RIC regimen but not after myeloablative regimens. The incidence of EBV–related complications was 3.3% in patients with myeloablative CBT, but in patients with RIC CBT the incidence was 21% if ATG was used and 2% if was omitted, $p < .01$.

Although the use of ATG is associated with a higher risk of serious infections, including fatal EBV–related complications,[85,87,95] delayed immune reconstitution,[85,86,96] increased risk of TRM,[36,83] and possibly increased risk of relapse,[97] the exclusion of ATG on the other hand is associated with an increased incidence of acute GVHD. Series of studies from MSKCC omitted the use of ATG in DCBT recipients after either myeloablative (70%, median age 24 years) or RIC (30%, median age 10 years).[78,98,99] GVHD prophylaxis consisted of a calcineurin inhibitor and MMF. The omission of ATG led to rapid T-cell immune reconstitution (median CD4+ T-cell count >200 cells/μL by day 120 post-CBT) with resultant low incidence of serious infections or deaths caused by infections. Consequently, cumulative incidence of 2-year TRM was low (21% at day +100 and 25% at 2-years), but cumulative incidences of grade II–IV acute GVHD were high (43%).

Thus, better understanding of the pathophysiology of GVHD after DCBT is needed to incorporate effective prevention and treatment strategies balancing the risks of GVHD and infections.

Relapse and Disease-Free Survival

Disease relapse is the most common cause of mortality after CBT, contributing to 30% to 60% of deaths. In general, various DCBT studies reported an average relapse risk of approximately 10% to 35% and DFS of about 30% to 55% at 2–5 years depending upon underlying patient characteristics, disease risk and type, type of conditioning regimen and transplant practices.[38,76,79,81,100–103] A few retrospective series suggest that DCBT is associated with a lower risk of relapse compared with single CBT in certain patients,[36,42,83] while other studies did not find a similar association.[76,81]

The Eurocord-Netcord investigators showed that the use of DCBT with either myeloablative conditioning or RIC was associated with a significantly lower risk of relapse or progression at 2-years compared with single CBT (13% versus 38%; $p = .009$) in adults with lymphoid malignancies, but without any difference in DFS.[83] Verneris et al[42] analyzed the risk of acute leukemia relapse in 177 recipients of myeloablative CBT and found that for patients in first or second complete remission, the risk of relapse was markedly reduced in DCBT recipients compared with single CBT recipients (19% versus 34%, $p = .03$). Again, no differences in leukemia-free survival (LFS) were noted between the groups (55% in single and 58% in DCBT group at 1-year, $p = .35$). However, the single CBT group included pediatric patients (n = 84, median age 8 years) while the DCBT arm included mostly adults (n = 93, median age 24 years). Another study in 110 adults with various hematologic malignancies noted a trend towards lower relapse after DCBT with nonmyeloablative conditioning (30% versus 41%, $p = .07$) and significantly improved 3-year DFS after DCBT (39% versus 24%, $p = .05$) compared with single CBT.[36] Another large registry study (n = 239) by the Eurocord and the EBMT group in adults with acute leukemia in first complete remission receiving myeloablative conditioning found significantly improved 2-year DFS in DCBT group (48%) and single CBT patients who received thiotepa/busulfan/fludarabine conditioning (48%), compared with single CBT performed with either busulfan- or TBI-based conditioning (30%), $p = .003$. No difference in the risk of relapse at 2-years (20% versus 19%, $p = .72$) was noted in single or double CBT recipients respectively.[81] Of note, DCBT recipients were younger, received higher cell dose, and ATG was used less frequently than other groups.

Contrarily, the CIBMTR-NYBC registry study of adult leukemia patients did not find any difference in 2-year probabilities of relapse (32% versus 36%) or DFS (30% versus 32%) after single or double CBT, respectively. Correspondingly, the BMTCTN-0501 phase III randomized study in pediatric patients found similar rates of 1-year relapse (12% versus 14%, $p = .12$) and DFS (70% versus 64%, $p = .11$) among single-unit or DCBT recipients respectively.[77] Therefore, it is likely that the dissimilarities in relapse or DFS risk noted across studies are reflections of differences in patients, disease type, risk and remission status, and transplant characteristics.

Nonrelapse Mortality and Overall Survival

In general, the use of myeloablative conditioning is associated with lower risk of relapse at the expense of higher toxicity and NRM. On the other hand, RIC regimens are well tolerated and result in lower TRM but are associated with higher risk of relapse, thus resulting in similar OS as seen after myeloablative conditioning.[104,105] The use of double-unit graft does not add to NRM compared with the use of single CBT.[42,76,77,81] The average 2–3 year cumulative incidence of NRM reported by various DCBT studies is about 20% to 45% and OS is in the range of 35% to 65%, which are comparable with those observed after single CBT.

The BMTCTN-0501 randomized trial in pediatric patients reported similar 1-year OS (65% versus 73%; $p = .17$) and 1-year TRM (19% versus 22%; $p = .43$) among single-unit or DCBT recipients respectively.[77] In adults, the Eurocord and the EBMT registry study found similar 2-year NRM after myeloablative single or double CBT (38% versus 34%, $p = .95$).[81] Similarly, the CIBMTR-NYBC registry analysis found a trend toward lower 6-month probability of TRM after DCBT compared with single CBT (21% versus 31%, $p = .06$) in adult patients with acute leukemia, without any difference in 2-year OS (35% versus 33%, $p = .66$).[76]

Studies also imply that DCBT recipients who survive early posttransplant period are very unlikely to die of delayed transplant-related causes. In the MSKCC series of DCBT recipients of either myeloablative (n = 53; 71%) or nonmyeloablative (n = 22; 29%) conditioning, 2-year TRM of 25% was almost entirely accounted for by patients dying in the first 6 months after transplant.[78] In another study, the median time to TRM was 3 months; few deaths occurred after 1-year posttransplantation which resulted in 1- and 3-year OS rates of 57% and 52% respectively.[38] Steady immune recovery observed after 6 months of transplantation likely contributes to this protection against late mortality.[38]

Comparison of Double-Unit Cord Blood Transplantation With Adult Donor Allografts

A number of retrospective studies have shown comparable outcomes after DCBT and adult donor transplantation, supporting the use of double-unit grafts as an alternative stem cell source (Table 107.3). However, DCBT is associated with significantly prolonged engraftment of neutrophils and platelets, and increased NRM compared with other types of allografts.[22,26,94,100,102,106–109]

After **myeloablative** conditioning DCBT, the median time to neutrophil engraftment is 3 weeks and that to platelet engraftment is 5 weeks approximately.[22,26,102,106–109] The risks of acute GVHD, especially grade III–IV (5–25%), and chronic GVHD (20–40% at 3 years), especially extensive, are significantly lower after DCBT compared with other graft sources.[102,107,109] The risk of NRM at 2–5 year is typically higher after CBT (about 35–40%) than after other types of transplants (15–35%).[107,109] One of the most important factors contributing to high NRM is delayed neutrophil engraftment. As shown by Brunstein et al,[107] 5-year NRM was 41% in DCBT patients who engrafted beyond 26 days compared with 16% in patients who achieved neutrophil engraftment within 26 days, which was similar to NRM seen with other donor types. The risk of relapse at 3–5 years is about 12% to 22% after DCBT. Various studies comparing DCBT with other types of transplants showed inconsistent findings. A study by Gutman et al[106] in 31 CBT patients (87% DCBT) showed significantly lower cumulative incidence of relapse at 2-years after CBT (3.2%) compared with matched unrelated donors (MUD; 23%) and mismatched unrelated donors (MMUD; 26%). A subsequent larger study by Brunstein et al[107] similarly showed marked reduction in relapse risk at 5-year after DCBT (15%) compared with matched related donors (MRD; 43%), MUD (37%) and MMUD (35%), p < .01. However, a few recent studies involving patients with either single or double CBT did not find a similar advantage of relapse prevention after CBT.[102,108,109] However, these studies have some notable differences between CBT group and their comparative arms. In the study by Liu et al,[109] there were appreciably more high-risk patients in the CBT group (87%) compared with the MRD recipients (47%). Also, conditioning regimens differed significantly between the groups. Another study included ALL patients in complete remission (CR)1 and CR2, and ATG was used more commonly in the CBT group compared with other allografts (31% versus 21%).[102] A third study by Konuma et al[108] included high-risk patients (65%) older than 45 years of age who received CBT with methotrexate-based GVHD prophylaxis compared with MMF-based regimen used in

TABLE 107.3   Comparison of Double-Unit Cord Blood Transplantation With Adult Donor HSC Transplantation

Reference	Graft (Patients n)	Age Median (range), in years	Conditioning (Patients n)	CI (%) of Neutrophil Engraftment — Days to Neutrophil Engraftment, Median (range)	II–IV Acute GVHD	III–IV Acute GVHD	Chronic GVHD	TRM	Relapse	Survival
Myeloablative Regimens										
Gutman et al[106]	31 CBT (27 DCBT)	22 (0.6–42)	CY/TBI/FLU		80.6%	29.0%		20.6% at 2 years	3.2% at 2 years	PFS 76.2% at 2 years OS 74.5% at 2 years
	31 MMUD	25 (1–48)	CY/TBI (21) BU/CY (10)		87.1%	35.5%		29.2% at 2 years	23% at 2 years	PFS 47.8% at 2 years OS 50% at 2 years
	31 MUD	25 (0.9–41)	CY/TBI (24) BU/CY (5)		67.7%	12.9%		17% at 2 years	25.8% at 2 years	PFS 57.1% at 2 years OS 59.7% at 2 years
Brunstein et al[107]	128 DCBT	25 (10–46)	Flu/Cy/TBI	26 (13–45)	60%	22%	26% at 2 years	34% (5 years)	15% (5 years)	LFS 51% (5 years)
	204 MRD (92% PB)	40 (12–67)	Flu/Cy/TBI	16 (11–39)	65%	13%	47% at 2 years	24% (5 years)	43% (5 years)	LFS 33% (5 years)
	152 MUD (58% PB)	31 (10–57)		19 (11–39)	80%	14%	43% at 2 years	14% (5 years)	37% (5 years)	LFS 48% (5 years)
	52 MMUD (65% PB)	31 (10–51)		18.5 (8–33)	85%	37%	48% at 2 years	27% (5 years)	35% (5 years)	LFS 38% (5 years)
Konuma et al[108]	66 CBT	49 (45–55)	MA (TBI-based)	22 (18–34) days, 93.9% at day 60	– (HR 0.90; p = .76)	9.2%	Extensive: 27/58	3% day +100 16% at 5 years	22% at 5 years	5-year OS: 67.4%
	31 RD BMT/ PBSCT	48 (45–58)	MA (TBI-based)	18 (11–40) days, 96.8% at day 60		16%	Extensive: 13/27	6.5% day +100 32.7% at 5 years	16.7% at 5 years	5-year OS: 55.2%

TABLE 107.3 Comparison of Double-Unit Cord Blood Transplantation With Adult Donor HSC Transplantation—cont'd

Reference	Graft (Patients *n*)	Age Median (range), in years	Conditioning (Patients *n*)	CI (%) of Neutrophil Engraftment / Days to Neutrophil Engraftment, Median (range)	II–IV Acute GVHD	III–IV Acute GVHD	Chronic GVHD	TRM	Relapse	Survival
Liu et al[109]	70 CBT	23 (16–46)	MA TBI-based (93%) Bu-based (7%)	19 (13–32)	40%	4%	Overall 20.7% Extensive 3.4%	34.2% at 6 months 35.7% at 2 years	11.9% at 3 years	DFS 55% at 3 years
	115 MRD (59% PB, 50% PB + BM, 6% BM)	32 (16–58)	MA TBI-based (26%) Bu-based (74%)	12 (10–18)	15%	10%	Overall 42.2% Extensive 14.6%	8.7% at 6 months 25.3% at 2 years	16.2% at 3 years	DFS 60% at 3 years
Marks et al[102]	116 CBT	25 (16–59)	MA TBI-based (94%) Bu-based (4%)	25 days 57% at day +28 91% at day +60	27%	9%	39% at 3 years	TRM 42% at 3 years	22% at 3 years	OS: 44% at 3 years
	546 8/8 matched (33.3% BM, 66.6% PB)	32 (16–59)	MA TBI-based (89%) Bu-based (11%)	95% at day +28 97% at day +60	47%	16%	42% at 3 years	31% at 3 years	25% at 3 years	OS: 44% at 3 years
	140 7/8 matched (40% BM, 60% PB)	33 (16–59)	MA TBI-based (89%) Bu-based (10%)	96% at day +28 97% at day +60	41%	24%	45% at 3 years	39% at 3 years	28% at 3 years	OS: 43% at 3 years
Reduced Intensity Regimens										
Majhail et al[88]	43 CBT	59 (55–69)	Flu/Cy/TBI (84%) ATG (40%)	89% at day +42	49%		17% at 1 year	28% at day +180		PFS 34% at 3 years OS: 34% at 3 years
	47 MRD	58 (55–70)	Flu/Cy/TBI (70%) ATG (13%)	100% at day +42	42%		40% at 1 year (*p* = .02)	23% at day +180		PFS: 30% at 3 years OS: 43% at 3 years
Brunstein et al[89]	50 CBT	58 (16–69)	Flu/Cy/TBI	15 days (4–47) 94% at day +56	40%	21%	25% at 1 year	24% at 1 year	31% at 1 year	OS: 54% at 1 year PFS: 46% at 1 year
	50 Haplo-BM	48 (7–70)	Flu/Cy/TBI	16 days (12–83) 96% at day +56	32%	0%	13% at 1 year	7% at 1 year	45% at 1 year	OS: 62% at 1 year PFS: 48% at 1 year
Ponce et al[78]	75 DCBT	37 (<1–66)	53 MA 22 NMA No T-depletion	93% MA (24 days) NMA (10 days)	43%		28%	25% (2 years)	20% at 2 years	55% (2 years)
	108 RD	47 (<1–71)	89 MA 19 NMA 66% T-depletion	100% MA (11 days) NMA (11 days)	Unmodified 27%, TCD 8%		Unmodified 31%, TCD 12%	15% at 2 years	19% (unmodified) and 19% (TCD) at 2 years	66%
	184 URD	48 (1–71)	156 MA 28 NMA 68% T-depletion	97% MA (11 days) NMA (10 days)	Unmodified 31%, TCD 12%		Unmodified 44%, TCD 19%	27% at 2 years	9% (unmodified) and 24% (TCD) at 2 years	55%

Continued

TABLE 107.3   Comparison of Double-Unit Cord Blood Transplantation With Adult Donor HSC Transplantation—cont'd

Reference	Graft (Patients n)	Age Median (range), in years	Conditioning (Patients n)	CI (%) of Neutrophil Engraftment — Days to Neutrophil Engraftment, Median (range)	II–IV Acute GVHD	III–IV Acute GVHD	Chronic GVHD	TRM	Relapse	Survival
Brunstein et al[90]	121 CBT	55 (23–68)	Flu/Cy/TBI	9 days 83% at day +28 93% at day +42	50%	17%	34% at 2 years	19% at 2 years	49% at 2 years	2-year LFS: 31% 2-year OS: 37%
	40 CBT	48 (21–67)	Other	20 days 83% at day +28 92% at day +42	33%	18%	36% at 2 years	52% at 2 years	35% at 2 years	2-year LFS: 15% 2-year OS: 19%
	313 8/8-PBPC	59 (23–69)	Other	13 days 93% at day +28 98% at day +42	33%	14%	56% at 2 years	21% at 2 years	44% at 2 years	2-year LFS: 35% 2-year OS: 44%
	111 7/8-PBPC	58 (21–69)	Other	12 days 92% at day +28 96% at day +42	40%	23%	54% at 2 years	28% at 2 years	44% at 2 years	2-year LFS: 29% 2-year OS: 37%
Chen et al[91]	64 CBT	53 (19–67)	RIC ATG 99%	21.5 (13–70) days 85.9% by day +50	14.1%	3.1%	21.9% at 2-years	26.9% at 2 years	42.7% at 3 years	OS: 46% at 3 years PFS: 30% at 3 years
	221 URD (97% PB)	58 (19–73)	RIC ATG 0%	13 (2–181) days 98.6% by day +50	20.3%	6.8%	53.9% at 2-years	10.4% at 2-years	49.8% at 3 years	OS: 50% at 3 years PFS: 40% at 3 years
Jacobson et al[86]	42 CBT	49 (20–67)	Flu/Mel based ATG (100%)	21.5 (13–107)	21%		24%	11% at 2 years	40% at 2 years	PFS: 49% at 2 years OS: 66% at 2 years
	102 PB–MUD	56 (20–73)	Bu/Flu based ATG 0%		12%		54%	11% at 2 years	32% at 2 years	PFS: 57% at 2 years PFS: 68% at 2 years
Robin et al[92]	129 CBT	57 (20–72)	RIC In-vivo T-depletion (40%)	20 (6–72) days 78%	31%		23% at 2 years	42% at 2 years	30%	PFS: 28% at 2 years OS: 30% at 2 years
	502 PB–MUD	60 (20–76)	RIC In vivo T-depletion (83%)	16 (3–60) days 98%	29%	–	41% at 2 years	31% at 2 years	25%	PFS: 44% at 2 years OS: 49% at 2 years
	379 10/10 PB	60 (24–76)	RIC In vivo T-depletion (82%)	–	–	–	35% at 2 years	32% at 2 years	23%	PFS: 50% at 2 years OS: 45% at 2 years
	107 9/10 PB	61 (20–74)	RIC In vivo T-depletion (87%)	–	–	–	44% at 2 years	36% at 2 years	28%	PFS: 36% at 2 years OS: 43% at 2 years
Rodrigues et al[93]	104 CBT	48 (18–67)	RIC ATG/ALG/ Alemtuzumab (21%)	81% at day +60	29% at 3 years		26% at 3 years	29% at 3 years	41% at 3 years	OS: 56% at 3 years
	541 MUD	50 (18–70)	RIC ATG/ALG/ Alemtuzumab (73%)	95% at day +60	32% at 3 years		52% at 3 years	28% at 3 years	36% at 3 years	OS: 49% at 3 years

TABLE 107.3   Comparison of Double-Unit Cord Blood Transplantation With Adult Donor HSC Transplantation—cont'd

Reference	Graft (Patients n)	Age Median (range), in years	Conditioning (Patients n)	Days to Neutrophil Engraftment, Median (range)	II–IV Acute GVHD	III–IV Acute GVHD	Chronic GVHD	TRM	Relapse	Survival
Weisdorf et al[100]	205 CBT (60% DCBT)	59 (50–71)	MA 21% RIC 79% In vivo T-depletion (32%)	69% at day +28	35%		28% at 3 years	35% at 3 years	35% at 3 years	OS: 30% at 3 years
	441 8/8 URD (86% PB)	58 (50–75)	MA 46% RIC 54% In vivo T-depletion (39%)	97% at day +28	36%		53% at 3 years	27% at 3 years	35% at 3 years	OS: 43% at 3 years
	94 7/8 URD (85% PB)	58 (50–72)	MA 50% RIC 50% In vivo T-depletion (50%)	91% at day +28	44%		59% at 3 years	41% at 3 years	26% at 3 years	OS: 37% at 3 years
Warlick et al[94]	151 CBT	18–74	MA 36% RIC 64% ATG 15%	16 days 96% at day +50		24%		20% at 1 year	36% at 2 years	OS: 36% at 6 years DFS: 34% at 6 years
	187 MRD	18–74	MA 60% RIC 40% ATG 11%			9%		20% at 1 year	26% at 2 years	OS: 47% at 6 years DFS: 44% at 6 years
	55 MUD	18–74	MA 65% RIC 35% ATG 45%			15%		25% at 1 year	20% at 2 years	OS: 54% at 6 years DFS: 50% at 6 years
	21 MMUD	18–74	MA 90% RIC 10% ATG 48%			24%		14% at 1 years	33% at 2 years	OS: 51% at 6 years DFS: 39% at 6 years

ATG, Antilymphocyte globulin; Bu/Flu, busulfan/fludarabine; CBT, cord blood transplantation; CI, confidence interval; DCBT, double-unit CBT; DFS, disease-free survival; GVHD, graft-versus-host disease; LFS, leukemia-free survival; MA, myeloablative; MMUD, mismatched unrelated donor; MRD, matched related donor; MUD, matched unrelated donor; NMA, nonmyeloablative; OS, overall survival; PB, peripheral blood; PBSCT, peripheral blood stem cell transplantation; PFS, progression-free survival; RD, related donor; RIC, reduced-intensity conditioning; TBI, total body irradiation; TCD, T-cell depleted; TRM, transplant-related mortality; URD, unrelated donor.

other studies. Also, the authors do no mention if the patients received single or double CB grafts.

Other long-term outcomes such as DFS and OS are similar after DCBT and other types of transplants.[22,26,102,106–109] Therefore, DCBT with myeloablative conditioning is an appealing alternative as it offers a substantial advantage of lower risk of GVHD without jeopardizing graft-versus-tumor effect.

The introduction of **RIC** regimens extends the application of DCBT in older (>45–50 years) and infirm individuals who are otherwise not candidates for myeloablative conditioning. Multiples studies showed encouraging results after RIC DCBT compared with other graft sources.[86,88–92,94,100,101] Time to neutrophil engraftment is faster after RIC (average 15 ± 5 days) compared with myeloablative CBT; however it is still slower than what is achieved with other types of transplants.[86,88–92,94,100,101] The risk of chronic GVHD at 1–3 years is lower after CBT (15–30%), while other outcomes such as grade II–IV acute GVHD (15–50%), 1–3 years relapse (30–45%), DFS (30–60%), and OS (35–60%) are comparable with other transplants types.[86,88–92,94,100,101] As seen with myeloablative DCBT, a few studies using RIC regimens also showed an increased risk of TRM after DCBT (10–30% at 0.5–3 years).[91,100] Most of the TRM and other

complications seen after CBT are encountered during the early posttransplantation period. These are related to delayed time to hematopoietic recovery and immune reconstitution compared with the transplantation of related and unrelated donor PB HSCs. This leads to prolonged hospitalization, higher rates of early infectious complications, and increased early TRM. Thus, strategies to enhance engraftment are of immense interest.

NOVEL STRATEGIES TO ENHANCE ENGRAFTMENT

Studies investigating the infusion of multiple small CB units have not enhanced engraftment.[110] Results of direct intra-BM injection of CB have been mixed,[111,112] with a study at the University of Minnesota being abandoned for futility. New approaches focusing on enhancing engraftment are summarized in Table 107.4.

The Spanish group of Fernandez et al[125] evaluated the coinfusion of CD34+ cells from a related haploidentical donor with a single-unit CBT as a "bridge" strategy to shorten the period of posttransplant neutropenia. Subsequently, these investigators updated their experience using mobilized PB HSCs from either a haploidentical or an

TABLE
107.4   **Potential Strategies to Enhance Cord Blood Engraftment**

Strategy	Reference	Protocol	Patients (*n*)	Median Age (year)	Neutrophil Engraftment	Platelet Engraftment (≥20,000/mm³)	Outcomes
Coinfusion of HSC	Bautista et al[113]	Single CB units + coinfusion of TCD HSC from haploidentical or third-party donors	55	34	96%; median ANC, 10 days (9–36 days)	78%; median time, 32 days (13–98 days)	DFS 47% and OS 56% at 5 years
	Liu et al[114]	Single CB units + coinfusion of TCD HSC from haploidentical related donors	45	50	95%; median ANC 11 days (9–15 days)	83%; median time, 19 days (15–33 days)	PFS 42% and OS 55% at 1 year
Stem cell expansion	de Lima et al[115]	CB ex vivo expansion with copper chelator TEPA	10	21	Median ANC, 30 days (16–46 days); 9/10 patients engrafted	Median, 48 days (35–105 days) in 6/10 patients	30% survival at 25 months
	Stiff et al[116]	CB ex vivo expansion with copper chelator TEPA	101	37	21 days	54 days	Improved survival at day 100 compared with controls
	Delaney et al[56]	Notch-mediated expansion of CD34⁺ cells	10	27	Median ANC, 16 days (7–34 days); 1 patient had primary graft rejection	Unknown	7/10 alive
	de Lima et al[117]	CB ex vivo expansion with MSC	32	35	97%; median ANC, 15 days (9–42 days)	Median, 40 days (13–62 days)	OS 40% at 5 years
	Horwitz et al[118]	Nicotinamide	11	45	Median ANC, 13 days	Median, 33 days	OS 82% PFS 73%
	Wagner et al[119]	SR1					
Stem cell homing	Campbell et al[120] Christopherson et al[121,122]	CD26 inhibition	N/A (mice)	N/A	Significant increase in engraftment	Unknown	N/A
	Cutler et al[123]	CB treated with PGE₂ Cohort 1	9	43	Median ANC, 24 days in 7/9	Median, 72.5 days	2 graft failures
		CB treated with PGE₂ Cohort 2	12	57.5	Median ANC, 17.5 days (14–31 days)	Median, 43 days (20–60 days)	No graft failure
	Popat et al[124]	Fucosylation of CB CD34⁺ cells	22	42	Median ANC, 17 days (12–34 days)	Median, 35 days (18–100 days)	1 patient died from sepsis on day 23; 1 had secondary graft failure.

ANC, Absolute neutrophil count; CB, cord blood; DFS, disease-free survival; HSC, hematopoietic stem cell; MSC, mesenchymal stem cell; N/A, not applicable; OS, overall survival; PGE₂, prostaglandin E₂; PFS, progression-free survival; TCD, T cell depleted; TEPA, tetraethylenepentamine.

unmatched third-party donor to support single-unit CBT.[113] This series included 55 patients with high-risk hematologic malignancies. The median time to neutrophil recovery was 10 days, and the maximum cumulative incidence of neutrophil engraftment was 96%; the median time to platelets greater than 20,000/mm³ was 32 days with an incidence of 78%. The cumulative incidence of full CB chimerism was 91% and took a median of 44 days. Grade II–IV acute GVHD developed in 10 patients and grade III–IV acute GVHD in 6 patients. Twenty-two patients died (3 relapses, 6 organ failures, 4 GVHD, 8 infections, 1 graft failure). The 5-year OS and DFS were 56% and 47%, respectively. The van Besien group recently reported similar findings that included 45 patients with hematologic malignancies (47% had refractory or untreated relapse) who received RIC followed by transplantation of a single CB unit and CD34⁺ cells from a haploidentical donor.[114] Rapid engraftment was obtained with cumulative incidences for neutrophil and platelet (>20,000/mm³) engraftment of 95% at day 50 and 83% at day 100, respectively, with a median time to recovery of 11 days for neutrophils and 19 days for platelets. However, the percentage of host-derived hematopoiesis was 5% by day 180, and four patients had graft failure (2 primary and 2 secondary). The cumulative incidence of grade II–IV acute GVHD was 25%, and the 1-year OS and progression-free survival (PFS) rates were 55% and 42%, respectively.

A recent study from the MSKCC assessed the use of DCBT combined with haploidentical CD34+ cells in 39 patients (median 48 years) after myeloablative (*n* = 2) or RIC (*n* = 37).[126] The median infused TNC dose of CB units was 2.30 × 10⁷/kg and 1.86 × 10⁷/kg and the median infused CD34+ cell dose from haploidentical donors was 3.1 × 10⁶/kg. One patient with DSAs to the haploidential and both CB units had graft rejection. In the remaining evaluable patients, the median time to neutrophil engraftment was 13 days (range 11–38), one of which had graft rejection at a later time. All of the remaining 36 patients had sustained CB engraftment and rejected the haploidentical graft at some point. In these patients, haploidentical graft contributed to either bridge engraftment without transient neutropenia (*n* = 20), bridge engraftment with transient neutropenia (*n* = 5), or no engraftment (*n* = 11). One of the significant complications noted in the study was occurrence of preengraftment syndrome in 76% of patients, which was severe in 8%, but responded to steroids in all cases.[126]

Ex vivo CB expansion is another approach to enhance neutrophil recovery. Given that cellular copper has been implicated in the regulation and differentiation of HSCs, Peled et al[127,128] cultured CD34⁺38⁻ CB HSCs with a copper chelator tetraethylenepentamide (TEPA). A group of investigators at the MDACC conducted a phase I/II clinical trial in which CD133+ selected CB hematopoietic progenitors from a portion of a single CB unit were cultured with TEPA and cytokines for 21 days and coinfused with the unmanipulated portion in 10 patients.[115] Although this technique led to an average expansion of 219-fold for TNC and sixfold for CD34+ cells, yet the time to hematopoietic recovery was not improved. The median time to neutrophil recovery was 30 days and median time to platelets engraftment was 48 days. Of note, this study used tacrolimus and methotrexate as GVHD prophylaxis, which may have contributed to delayed engraftment. Subsequently, Stiff et al[116] reported a prospective multicenter trial using this technique in patients undergoing single CBT with myeloablative conditioning, but replacing methotrexate with MMF. A portion of CB unit was expanded ex vivo and infused with the unmanipulated fraction of the same CB unit in 101 patients (median age 37 years). In contrast to the MDACC study, this group attained an average expansion of 400-fold for TNC and 77-fold for CD34+ cells. Compared with DCBT controls from the CIBMTR and the Eurocord registries, the times to neutrophil engraftment (21 versus 28 days, $p < .0001$) and platelet engraftment (54 versus 105 days, $p = .008$) were significantly faster in the study group. There were no differences in the rates of acute (19.4%) or chronic (18.4%) GVHD and 100-day survival was significantly improved compared with the controls.

Delaney et al[56] studied a double-unit CB strategy in which CD34+ selected CB progenitors were transduced with an engineered Notch ligand (Delta1$^{ext-IgG}$) and cultured for 16 days with cytokines. This led to an average expansion of 562-fold for TNC and 164-fold for CD34+ cells. A phase I study is ongoing in leukemia patients receiving myeloablative DCBT, in which an entire expanded unit is infused after the infusion of an unmanipulated unit. In the preliminary analysis ($n = 10$), the median time to neutrophil engraftment was 16 days. No infusional toxicities were noted but primary graft rejection occurred in one patient. All evaluable patients developed grade II acute GVHD, except one who had grade III acute GVHD. There was no extensive chronic GVHD, while limited chronic GVHD was noted in three patients. Two patients had long-term persistence of the expanded cells, until day 180 and day 240, but not beyond one year, after which the unexpanded CB unit completely contributed to engraftment.

The MDACC group explored another approach to expand CB CD34+ cells by coculturing with mesenchymal stromal cells derived from either haploidentical family member BM or "off-the-shelf" universal donors.[117] This approach was tested in a clinical trial in 31 patients (median age 31 years) after myeloablative DCBT and low dose rabbit ATG (1.25 mg/kg on day –4 and 1.75 mg/kg on day –3). After 14 days of coculture, they achieved median 40-fold expansion of CD34+ cells and 14-fold for TNC. The expanded unit was infused following the infusion of the unmanipulated unit. This resulted in significantly improved engraftment compared with the CIBMTR controls. The cumulative incidence of engraftment at day 42 was 96% (compared with 78% in the controls, $p < .001$), with faster neutrophil recovery (median 15 days versus 24 days, $p < .001$) and platelet recovery (42 days versus 49 days, $p = .03$). The cumulative incidences of grade II–IV (42%) and III–IV acute GVHD (13%) and chronic GVHD (45%) were similar to the controls. In the 28 evaluable patients, 54% had hematopoiesis derived solely from unmanipulated cord, while the rest had hematopoiesis derived from both units by day 30. At 6 months post-CBT, the expanded CB was detected in 13% of the patients.

Horwitz et al[118] reported results of a phase I clinical trial using CB expansion with nicotinamide, which inhibits differentiation and enhances functionality of hematopoietic stem and progenitor cells. In this study, 11 patients (median age 45 years) received TBI-based myeloablative conditioning DCBT, where the CD133+ selected fraction of one CB unit was expanded ex vivo for 3 weeks with nicotinamide and then infused along with its CD133-fraction and a second unmanipulated cord. This led to significantly improved median times to neutrophil (13 days) and platelet (33 days) engraftment compared with their institutional controls. One patient had primary graft failure. Five patients developed grade II–IV acute GVHD and there was no cases of grade III–IV acute GVHD. One-year OS was 82% and PFS was 73%.

Preclinical data with aryl hydrocarbon receptor antagonists[129] and novel cytokines[130,131] with enhanced HSC expansion capacity are promising approaches that are currently under investigation. The University of Minnesota group presented the results of a phase I/II study using StemReginin1 (SR1), an aryl hydrocarbon receptor antagonist.[119] This technique led to 328-fold expansion of CD34+cells resulting in 100% neutrophil engraftment in 17 DCBT patients after myeloablative conditioning. The median time to neutrophil engraftment was shorter in 11 patients in whom the SR1-expanded cord predominated (11 days) compared with patients in whom the unmanipulated cord predominated (23 days). This group are now evaluating the safety and feasibility of infusing a single cord expanded with SR1.

A different approach to improving engraftment is to enhance stem cell homing to the BM niche. The Broxmeyer group reported that endogenous CD26 expression negatively regulates the homing and engraftment of stem cells.[120,121] Campbell et al[120] evaluated pretreated purified CD34+ human CB cells with a CD26 peptidase inhibitor (Ditropin A) and found a significant enhanced engraftment in NOD/SCID mice. Christopherson et al[122] demonstrated that transplantation of either CD34+ or lineage depleted human CB cells in NOD/SCID/B2m-^{null} mice after treatment with a CD26 inhibitor was associated with a significant improvement in the engraftment of long-term repopulating.

Cutler et al[123] investigated the safety and efficacy of ex vivo treatment of one of the CB units with a prostaglandin E_2 (PGE$_2$) derivative (dmPGE2) as a method to enhance engraftment by improved homing. The trial included 21 patients undergoing DCBT with fludarabine, melphalan, and ATG (4 mg/kg) conditioning. During their initial study period, the smaller CB unit was thawed on the day of transplantation and treated with dmPGE$_2$ for 60 minutes at 4°C, but as the authors found two graft failures without any engraftment improvement in this set of patients, they decided to treat the larger of the units at 37°C for 120 minutes. The treated CB unit was then infused within 4 hours of the untreated unit. The median time to neutrophil engraftment was 24 days and 17.5 days in the two cohorts respectively. The corresponding times for platelet engraftments were 72.5 and 43 days. In the second cohort, 10 of 12 patients had 100% hematopoiesis from the dmPGE$_2$ treated CB unit which was sustained for up to 27 months post-CBT.

Hidalgo et al[132] found that the defect in CB homing was associated with a reduced α-1,3-fucosyltransferase expression and activity in CB CD34+ cells, decreasing their ability to bind to P- and E-selectins expressed by the BM vasculature. Subsequently, investigators at the MDACC[133] demonstrated that human CD34+ CB cells fucosylated using a recombinant fucosyl transferase in a murine model exhibited improved engraftment. The group reported results of their phase I clinical trial using this approach in 22 adults undergoing myeloablative or RIC DCBT and rabbit ATG (total dose 3 mg/kg infused over 2 days), where one CB unit was infused unmanipulated while the other unit was ex vivo fucosylated for 30 minutes at room temperature before infusion.[124] The cumulative incidence of neutrophil engraftment was 95.5% and all evaluable patients had 100% donor chimerism by day +30 posttransplantation. The median times to neutrophil engraftment (17 days versus 26 days, $p = .0023$) and platelet engraftment (35 days versus 45 days, $p = .0520$) were significantly improved compared with the institutional historical controls. There were no differences in the cumulative incidences of acute grade II–IV GVHD (41%), acute grade III–IV GVHD (9%), or chronic GVHD (5%) compared with the controls. This approach is especially attractive as it is quick and does not require prolonged ex vivo culture or a Good Manufacturing Practice (GMP) laboratory, thus making it universally adoptable across centers. The multicenter phase III study has been approved by the FDA and is expected to open to accrual soon.

Although these novel techniques have led to significant improvement in the rapidity of hematopoietic recovery, the impact of these strategies on immune reconstitution is still unclear. This is of interest because disease relapse is the leading cause of mortality and viral infections (especially CMV, EBV, adenovirus, and BK virus) contribute to significant morbidity and mortality in the post-CBT period.

Further, in addition to delayed quantitative immune reconstitution after DCBT,[86,134,135] there are delays in functional recovery of viral-specific T-cells for the first year posttransplantation.[136] Therefore, strategies to enhance immune recovery after CBT are critically needed.

ADOPTIVE IMMUNOTHERAPY

Adoptive immunotherapy is an attractive strategy not only to enhance antitumor responses but also to prevent GVHD and treat viral infections.[137] (Table 107.5). Sun et al[138] have reported the generation of CD4+ EBV-specific cytotoxic lymphocytes from CB, and Park et al[139] have generated CMV pp65-specific T cells from CB. The O'Reilly group at MSKCC has investigated the alternative approach of using third-party EBV-specific cytotoxic T lymphocytes (CTLs) to successfully treat EBV-associated posttransplant lymphoma in two CBT recipients who failed tapering of immunosuppression and rituximab therapy.[140] A group of investigators at the Baylor College of Medicine has generated multivirus-specific T cells from CB lymphocytes to prevent and treat CMV, EBV, and adenovirus.[141,142] The preliminary results of a phase I trial evaluating the efficacy of this approach in eight patients showed it to be safe. No patient developed GVHD from infusion of these cells. More strikingly, the CTLs were able to clear CMV reactivation within weeks of infusion in most of the patients without the use of conventional treatment. Similarly, all patients with high EBV loads and almost every patient with adenovirus infection were able to clear the viruses.[143] Furthermore, the same group generated genetically modified CD19-chimeric receptor antigen T-cells that not only possess an antitumor activity against B-cell ALL cells but are also active against EBV, CMV, and adenovirus.[144] This is a fascinating approach to treating viruses and disease relapse with a single infused product.

The use of donor lymphocyte infusion to prevent or treat disease relapse, which has been successfully used after PB or BM transplants, has been historically limited in the setting of CBT because of limitation of cell dose. However, the advent of ex vivo expansion techniques has now made this feasible and has created opportunities to develop tumor specific CB CTLs.[146] Ex vivo expanded CB NK cells have demonstrated in vitro and in vivo antitumor effects.[145,147] Several early phase clinical trials are evaluating the safety and efficacy of prophylactic CB NK infusion in the setting of CBT for patients with chronic

lymphocytic leukemia [ClinicalTrials.gov: NCT01619761, NCT02280525] and other high-risk myeloid malignancies [ClinicalTrials.gov: NCT01823198], and in conjunction with autologous SCT for patients with multiple myeloma [ClinicalTrials.gov: NCT01729091].

Adoptive immunotherapy using ex vivo expanded Tregs is another area of investigation to prevent or treat GVHD. Brunstein et al[58] reported the results of a phase I clinical trial of CB derived ex vivo expanded Tregs from a third CB unit, which were infused in addition to a double-unit CB grafts in 23 patients (median age 52 years) using Flu/Cy/TBI RIC regimen. The incidence of grade II–IV acute GVHD was significantly lower in the group that received Tregs compared with historical controls (43% versus 61%, $p = .05$), but there were no differences in grade III–IV acute GVHD between the groups (17% versus 23%). The cumulative incidence of viral and fungal infections by day +100 in Treg treated patients (39%) was similar to controls (53%). Further, there were no differences in the risks of relapse or mortality between the groups. Of note, the infused Tregs persisted in circulation for 2 weeks. The MDACC group recently demonstrated enhanced in vivo persistence of fucosylated CB derived Tregs in a xenogenic GVHD mouse model.[148] Moreover, the infusion of fucosylated Tregs was associated with improved clinical GVHD score as well as OS at day 30 compared with mice that received nonfucosylated Tregs (70% versus 23%, $p < .0001$). The clinical impact of this novel GVHD prophylaxis approach in CBT recipients is of interest.

FUTURE DIRECTIONS

CB is a promising alternative HSC source for use in the transplantation of patients with high-risk hematologic malignancies. CBT extends transplant access to patients from ethnic and racial minorities and those in need of urgent transplantation. Furthermore, survival after CBT has greatly improved because of larger CB inventory; possibly better unit quality; and improved conditioning regimens, grafts, and supportive care. Single-unit CBT has been shown to be comparable with unrelated donor transplantation in children,[26] and DCBT has had DFS comparable with the transplantation of adult donor HSC.[22,26,102,106–109] CBT should be considered as an immediate alternative in patients with high-risk hematologic malignancies who are candidates for allogeneic HSC transplantation but lack a suitable related donor.

SUGGESTED READINGS

Avery S, Shi W, Lubin M, et al: Influence of infused cell dose and HLA-match on engraftment after double-unit cord blood allografts. *Blood* 117:3277, 2011.

Ballen KK, Gluckman E, Broxmeyer HE: Umbilical cord blood transplantation: the first 25 years and beyond. *Blood* 122(4):491–498, 2013.

Barker JN, Byam CE, Kernan NA, et al: Availability of cord blood extends allogeneic hematopoietic stem cell transplant access to racial and ethnic minorities. *Biol Blood Marrow Transplant* 16:1541, 2010.

Barker JN, Byam C, Scaradavou A: How I treat: the selection and acquisition of unrelated cord blood grafts. *Blood* 117:2332, 2011.

Barker JN, Doubrovina E, Sauter C, et al: Successful treatment of EBV-associated posttransplantation lymphoma after cord blood transplantation using third-party EBV-specific cytotoxic T lymphocytes. *Blood* 116:5045, 2010.

Barker JN, Scaradavou A, Stevens CE: Combined effect of total nucleated cell dose and HLA match on transplantation outcome in 1061 cord blood recipients with hematologic malignancies. *Blood* 115:1843, 2010.

Barker JN, Weisdorf DJ, DeFor TE, et al: Transplantation of two partially HLA-matched umbilical cord blood units to enhance engraftment in adults with hematologic malignancy. *Blood* 105:1343, 2005.

Bautista G, Cabrera JR, Regidor C, et al: Cord blood transplants supported by co-infusion of mobilized hematopoietic stem cells from a third-party donor. *Bone Marrow Transplant* 43:365, 2009.

TABLE 107.5	Cellular Therapeutic Strategies to Mitigate Viral Infections, Relapse, and Graft-Versus-Host Disease After Cord Blood Transplantation	
Target	**Strategy**	**Results**
Antiviral	Multivirus specific CTLs (CMV, EBV, adenovirus)[142]	Lysed antigen-pulsed and virus infected targets
	Third-party EBV-specific CTLs[140]	2 EBV PTLD patients achieved durable CR
Antitumor	IL-2 expansion of CB NK cells[145]	Cytolytic effect in vitro and in vivo against leukemia cells
Antitumor and antiviral	CB-derived CTLs against CD19 and viruses (CMV, EBV, adenovirus)[144]	In vitro antileukemic and antiviral effect
GVHD prevention	Infusion of ex vivo expanded CB Treg[58]	23 patients accrued; aGVHD incidence decreased without increase in relapse

aGVHD, Acute graft-versus-host disease; CB, cord blood; CMV, cytomegalovirus; CR, complete remission; CTL, cytotoxic T-cell lymphocyte; EBV, Epstein-Barr virus; GVHD, graft-versus-host disease; IL-2, interleukin-2; NK, natural killer; PTLD, posttransplant lymphoproliferative disease; Treg, regulatory T cell.

Brunstein C, Barker JN, Weisdorf DJ, et al: Umbilical cord blood transplantation after non-myeloablative conditioning: impact on transplant outcomes in 110 adults with hematological disease. *Blood* 110:3064, 2007.

Brunstein CG, Fuchs EJ, Carter SL, et al: Alternative donor transplantation: results of parallel phase II trials using HLA-mismatched related bone marrow or unrelated umbilical cord blood grafts. *Blood* 118:282, 2011.

Brunstein CG, Gutman JA, Weisdorf DJ, et al: Allogeneic hematopoietic cell transplantation for hematological malignancy: relative risks and benefits of double umbilical cord blood. *Blood* 116:4693, 2010.

Christopherson KW, 2nd, Hangoc G, Mantel CR, et al: Modulation of hematopoietic stem cell homing and engraftment by CD26. *Science* 305:1000, 2004.

Delaney C, Heimfeld S, Brashem-Stein C, et al: Notch-mediated expansion of human cord blood progenitor cells capable of rapid myeloid reconstitution. *Nat Med* 16:232, 2010.

de Lima M, McNiece I, Robinson SN, et al: Cord-blood engraftment with ex vivo mesenchymal-cell coculture. *N Engl J Med* 367(24):2305–2315, 2012.

Eapen M, Klein JP, Sanz GF, et al: Effect of donor-recipient HLA matching at HLA A, B, C, and DRB1 on outcomes after umbilical-cord blood transplantation for leukaemia and myelodysplastic syndrome: a retrospective analysis. *Lancet Oncol* 11:653, 2010.

Eapen M, Rocha V, Sanz G, et al: Effect of graft source on unrelated donor haemopoietic stem-cell transplantation in adults with acute leukaemia: a retrospective analysis. *Lancet Oncol* 11:653, 2010.

Eapen M, Rubinstein P, Zhang MJ, et al: Comparison of outcomes after transplantation of unrelated donor umbilical cord blood and bone marrow in children with acute leukemia. *Lancet* 369:1947, 2007.

Eldjerou LK, Chaudhury S, Baisre-de Leon A, et al: An *in vivo* model of double unit cord blood transplantation that correlates with clinical engraftment. *Blood* 116:3999, 2010.

Gutman JA, Turtle CJ, Manley TJ, et al: Single-unit dominance after double-unit umbilical cord blood transplantation coincides with a specific CD8+ T-cell response against the nonengrafted unit. *Blood* 115:757, 2010.

Hanley PJ, Cruz CR, Savoldo B, et al: Functionally active virus-specific T cells that target CMV, adenovirus, and EBV can be expanded from naive T-cell populations in cord blood and will target a range of viral epitopes. *Blood* 114:2009, 1958.

Kurtzberg J, Prasad VK, Carter SL, et al: Results of the Cord Blood Transplantation Study (COBLT): clinical outcomes of unrelated donor umbilical cord blood transplantation in pediatric patients with hematologic malignancies. *Blood* 112:4318, 2008.

Liu H, Rich ES, Godley L, et al: Reduced-intensity conditioning with combined haploidentical and cord blood transplantation results in rapid engraftment, low GVHD, and durable remissions. *Blood* 118:6438, 2011.

MacMillan ML, Weisdorf DJ, Brunstein CG, et al: Acute graft-versus-host disease after unrelated donor umbilical cord blood transplantation: analysis of risk factors. *Blood* 113:2410, 2009.

Micklethwaite KP, Savoldo B, Hanley PJ, et al: Derivation of human T lymphocytes from cord blood and peripheral blood with antiviral and antileukemic specificity from a single culture as protection against infection and relapse after stem cell transplantation. *Blood* 115:2695, 2010.

Ponce DM, Zheng J, Gonzales AM, et al: Reduced late mortality risk contributes to similar survival after double-unit cord blood transplantation compared with related and unrelated donor hematopoietic stem cell transplantation. *Biol Blood Marrow Transplant* 17:1316, 2011.

Purtill D, Smith K, Devlin S, et al: Dominant unit CD34+ cell dose predicts engraftment after double-unit cord blood transplantation and is influenced by bank practice. *Blood* 124(19):2905–2912, 2014.

Rocha V, Gluckman E: Improving outcomes of cord blood transplantation: HLA matching, cell dose and other graft- and transplantation-related factors. *Br J Haematol* 147:262, 2009.

Scaradavou A, Smith KM, Hawke R, et al: Cord blood units with low CD34+ cell viability have a low probability of engraftment after double unit transplantation. *Biol Blood Marrow Transplant* 16:500, 2010.

Stevens CE, Carrier C, Carpenter C, et al: HLA mismatch direction in cord blood transplantation: impact on outcome and implications for cord blood unit selection. *Blood* 118:3969, 2011.

van Rood JJ, Stevens CE, Smits J, et al: Reexposure of cord blood to non-inherited maternal HLA antigens improves transplant outcome in hematological malignancies. *Proc Natl Acad Sci USA* 106:19952, 2009.

Verneris MR, Brunstein CG, Barker J, et al: Relapse risk after umbilical cord blood transplantation: enhanced graft-versus-leukemia effect in recipients of 2 units. *Blood* 114:4293, 2009.

Wagner JE, Barker JN, DeFor TE, et al: Transplantation of unrelated donor umbilical cord blood in 102 patients with malignant and nonmalignant diseases: influence of CD34 cell dose and HLA disparity on treatment-related mortality and survival. *Blood* 100:1611, 2002.

Wagner JE, Jr, Eapen M, Carter S, et al: One-unit versus two-unit cord-blood transplantation for hematologic cancers. *N Engl J Med* 371(18):1685–1694, 2014.

REFERENCES

For the complete list of references, log on to www.expertconsult.com.

CHAPTER 108

GRAFT-VERSUS-HOST DISEASE AND GRAFT-VERSUS-LEUKEMIA RESPONSES

Pavan Reddy and James L.M. Ferrara

The ability of allogeneic hematopoietic cell transplantation (HCT) to cure certain hematologic malignancies is widely recognized. An important therapeutic aspect of HCT in eradicating malignant cells is the graft-versus-leukemia (GVL) effect. The importance of the GVL effect in allogeneic HCT has been recognized since the earliest experiments in stem cell transplantation. Forty years ago, Barnes and colleagues noted that leukemic mice treated with a subtherapeutic dose of radiation and a syngeneic (identical twin) graft transplant were more likely to relapse than mice given an allogeneic stem cell transplant.[1,2] They hypothesized that the allogeneic graft contained cells with immune reactivity necessary for eradicating residual leukemia cells. They also noted that recipients of allogeneic grafts, though less likely to relapse, died of a "wasting syndrome" now recognized as graft-versus-host disease (GVHD). Thus in addition to describing GVL, these experiments highlighted for the first time the intricate relationship between GVL and GVHD. Since these early experiments, both GVHD and the GVL effect have been studied extensively.[3] This chapter reviews the pathophysiology, clinical features, and treatment of GVHD and summarizes current understanding of the relationships between GVHD and the GVL effect.

GRAFT-VERSUS-HOST DISEASE: CLINICAL AND PATHOLOGIC ASPECTS

Ten years after the work of Barnes and Loutit, Billingham formulated the requirements for the development of GVHD: the graft must contain immunologically competent cells, the recipient must express tissue antigens that are not present in the transplant donor, and the recipient must be incapable of mounting an effective response to destroy the transplanted cells.[4] According to these criteria, GVHD can develop in various clinical settings when tissues containing immunocompetent cells (blood products, bone marrow, and some solid organs) are transferred between persons. The most common setting for the development of GVHD is following allogeneic HCT; without prophylactic immunosuppression, most allogeneic HCTs will be complicated by GVHD. GVHD is induced by mismatches between histocompatibility antigens between the donor and recipient. Matching of the major histocompatibility complex (MHC) antigens hastens engraftment and reduces the severity of GVHD.[5] In humans, the MHC region lies on the short arm of chromosome 6 and is called the HLA (human leukocyte antigen) region.[6] The HLA region is divided into two classes, class I and class II, each containing numerous gene loci that encode a large number of polymorphic alleles. MHC class I molecules are involved in the presentation of peptides to $CD8^+$ T cells, and class II molecules present peptides to $CD4^+$ T cells.[6,7] The determination of HLA types has become much more accurate with molecular techniques that replace earlier serologic or cellular methods. In patients whose ancestry involves extensive interracial mixing, the chances of identifying an HLA identical donor are diminished.[8]

Despite HLA identity between a patient and donor, substantial numbers of patients still develop GVHD because of differences in minor histocompatibility antigens (MiHAs) that lie outside the HLA loci. Most minor antigens are expressed on the cell surface as degraded peptides bound to specific HLA molecules, but the precise elucidation of many human minor antigens is yet to be accomplished.[9] In the United States, the average patient has a 25% chance of having an HLA match within his or her immediate family.[8] Patients who lack an HLA-identical family member donor must seek unrelated donor volunteers or cord blood donations.

Acute Graft-Versus-Host Disease

Acute GVHD can occur within days (in recipients who are not HLA-matched with the donor or in patients not given any prophylaxis) or as late as 6 months after transplantation. The incidence ranges from less than 10% to more than 80%, depending on the degree of histoincompatibility between donor and recipient, the number of T cells in the graft, the patient's age, and the GVHD prophylactic regimen.[10] The principal target organs include the immune system, skin, liver, and intestine. GVHD occurs first and most commonly in the skin as a pruritic maculopapular rash, often involving the palms, soles, and ears; it can progress to total-body erythroderma, with bullae formation, rupture along the epidermal-dermal border, and desquamation in severe cases.[10] Gastrointestinal (GI) and liver manifestations often appear later and rarely represent the first and only findings. Intestinal symptoms include anorexia, nausea, diarrhea (sometimes bloody), abdominal pain, and paralytic ileus.[10] Liver dysfunction includes hyperbilirubinemia and increased serum alkaline phosphatase and aminotransferase values. Coagulation studies may become abnormal, and hepatic failure with ascites and encephalopathy may develop in severe cases.[10–12] Hepatic GVHD can be distinguished from hepatic venoocclusive disease by weight gain or pain in the right upper quadrant in the latter.[12] Acute GVHD also results in the delayed recovery of immunocompetence.[10] The clinical result is profound immunodeficiency and susceptibility to infections, often further accentuated by the immunosuppressive agents used to treat GVHD.[10]

Pathologically, the sine qua non of acute GVHD is selective epithelial damage of target organs.[13,14] The epidermis and hair follicles are damaged and sometimes destroyed. Small bile ducts are profoundly affected, with segmental disruption. The destruction of intestinal crypts results in mucosal ulcerations that may be either patchy or diffuse. Other epithelial surfaces, such as the conjunctivae, vagina, and esophagus, are less commonly involved. A peculiarity of GVHD histology is the early paucity of mononuclear cell infiltrates; however, as the disease progresses, the inflammatory component may be substantial. Studies that identified inflammatory cytokines as soluble mediators of GVHD have suggested that direct contact between target cells and lymphocytes is not always required (see following sections). GVHD lesions are not evenly distributed: in the skin, damage is prominent at the tip of rete ridges; in the intestine, at the base of the crypts; and in the liver, in the periductular epithelium. These areas all contain a high proportion of stem cells, giving rise to the idea that GVHD targets may be undifferentiated epithelial cells with primitive surface antigens.[15]

The histologic severity of GVHD is at best semiquantitative, and consequently pathologic scores are not used to grade GVHD. Because it is often difficult to obtain an adequate tissue biopsy, and because it can be very difficult to distinguish GVHD from other post-HCT complications such as drug eruptions or infectious complications, the physician is left to use clinical judgment.

An independent committee of a multicenter phase III trial that assessed the presence and severity of GVHD was unable to confirm a high incidence of GVHD.[16,17] Standard grading systems generally include clinical changes in the skin, GI tract, liver, and performance status (Table 108.1).[18] Although the severity of GVHD is often difficult to quantify, the overall maximal grade correlates with disease outcome: mild GVHD (grade I or II) is associated with little mortality, whereas higher grades are associated with significantly decreased survival.[18,19] Recent advances in the use of biomarkers at the onset of disease may soon be sufficiently accurate to guide therapy.[19]

Clinical Features of Acute Graft-Versus-Host Disease

The clinical features, staging, and grading of acute GVHD are summarized in Tables 108.1 and 108.2. In a comprehensive review of patients receiving therapy for acute GVHD, Martin and colleagues[20] found that 81% had skin involvement, 54% had GI involvement, and 50% had liver involvement at the initiation of therapy. After high-intensity (myeloablative) conditioning, acute GVHD generally occurs within 14–35 days of stem cell infusion. The time of onset may depend on the degree of histocompatibility, the number of donor T cells infused, and the prophylactic regimen for GVHD. A

rapid and severe form of GVHD may occur in patients with severe HLA mismatches and in patients who receive T-cell replete transplants without or with inadequate in vivo GVHD prophylaxis.[21] Although such GVHD is sometimes called "hyperacute," this term is misleading because it is pathophysiologically distinct from hyperacute rejection after solid organ allografting, which is caused by preformed antibodies. This form of GVHD, which is manifested by fever, generalized erythroderma and desquamation, and often edema, typically occurs about 1 week after stem cell infusion and may be rapidly fatal. In patients receiving standard (in vivo) GVHD prophylaxis such as a combination of cyclosporine and methotrexate, the median onset of GVHD is typically 21–25 days after transplantation; however, after in vitro T-cell depletion of the graft, the onset of GVHD symptoms may be much later.[21] Thus the findings of rash and diarrhea by 1 week after transplantation would very likely be because of ineffective prophylaxis and would be very unlikely with the use of calcineurin inhibitors or in vitro T-cell depletion of the stem cell inoculum. A less ominous syndrome of fever, rash, and fluid retention occurring in the first 1–2 weeks after stem cell infusion is the "engraftment syndrome." These manifestations may be seen with either allogeneic or autologous transplantation. Although this syndrome's pathophysiology is poorly understood, it is thought to be caused by a wave of cytokine production as the graft starts to recover. These symptoms are related to, but distinct from, the "cytokine storm"[22] of acute GVHD because there is no concomitant T-cell–mediated attack. This syndrome responds immediately to steroids in most patients, and it typically presents earlier than acute GVHD.[15]

Skin is the most commonly affected organ (Fig. 108.1). In patients receiving transplants after myeloablative conditioning, the skin is usually the first organ involved, and GVHD often coincides with engraftment. However, the presentation of GVHD is more varied following nonmyeloablative transplants or donor lymphocyte infusions.[23] The characteristic maculopapular rash can spread throughout

TABLE 108.1	Clinical Manifestations and Staging of Acute Graft-Versus-Host Disease	
Organ	**Clinical Manifestations**	**Staging**
Skin	Erythematous, maculopapular rash involving palms and soles; may become confluent Severe disease: bullae	Stage 1: <25% rash Stage 2: 25%–50% rash Stage 3: generalized erythroderma Stage 4: bullae
Liver	Painless jaundice with conjugated hyperbilirubinemia and increased alkaline phosphatase	Stage 1: bili 2–3 mg/dL Stage 2: bili 3.1–6 mg/dL Stage 3: bili 6.1–15 mg/dL Stage 4: bili >15 mg/dL
Gastrointestinal tract	Upper: nausea, vomiting, anorexia Lower: diarrhea, abdominal cramps, distension, ileus, bleeding	Stage 1: diarrhea >500 mL/day Stage 2: diarrhea >1000 mL/day Stage 3: diarrhea >1500 mL/day Stage 4: ileus, bleeding

TABLE 108.2	Glucksberg Criteria for Staging of Acute Graft-Versus-Host Disease[a]			
Overall Grade	**Skin**	**Liver**		**Gut**
I	1–2	0		0
II	1–3	1	and/or	1
III	2–3	2–4	and/or	2–3
IV	2–4	2–4	and/or	2–4

[a]See Table 108.1 for individual organ staging. Traditionally, individual organs are staged without regard to attribution. The overall grade of graft-versus-host disease, however, reflects the actual extent of graft-versus-host disease. To achieve each overall grade, skin disease, liver and/or gut involvement are required.

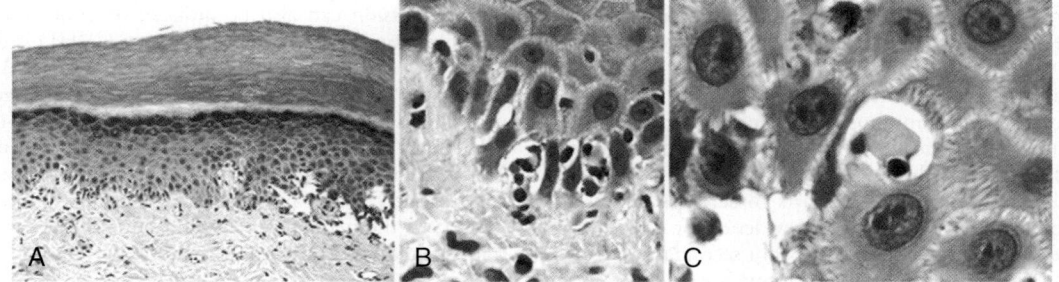

Fig. 108.1 GRAFT-VERSUS-HOST DISEASE, SKIN BIOPSY. This 40-year-old man with a history of relapsed Hodgkin lymphoma was status-postallogeneic stem cell transplant with donor lymphocyte infusion. He developed painful oral ulcers and a macular-papular rash on the arms, hand, and chest. The skin biopsy is from the palmar surface of the hand (A). It shows a scant lymphoid infiltrate in the dermis with a developing subepithelial blister *(right)*. There is basal vacuolar change with single lymphocytes in the epithelium, as well as apoptotic keratinocytes accompanied by lymphocytes (B, and detail, C). *(Courtesy Vesna Petronic-Rosic and Mark Racz, University of Chicago.)*

the rest of the body but usually spares the scalp; it is often described as feeling like a sunburn, tight or pruritic. In severe cases the skin may blister and ulcerate.[24] Histologic confirmation is critical to rule out drug reactions, viral infections, etc. Apoptosis at the base of dermal crypts is characteristic. Other features include dyskeratosis, exocytosis of lymphocytes, satellite lymphocytes adjacent to dyskeratotic epidermal keratinocytes, and dermal perivascular lymphocytic infiltration.[25]

GI tract involvement of GVHD may present as nausea, vomiting, anorexia, diarrhea, and/or abdominal pain.[26] It is a panintestinal process, often with differences in severity between the upper and lower GI tracts. Gastric involvement gives rise to postprandial vomiting that is not always preceded by nausea. Although gastroparesis is seen after bone marrow transplant, it is usually not associated with GVHD. The diarrhea of GVHD is secretory; significant GI blood loss may occur as a result of mucosal ulceration and is associated with a poor prognosis.[27] In advanced disease, diffuse, severe abdominal pain, and distension is accompanied by voluminous diarrhea (>2 liters/day).[19,28]

Radiologic findings of the GI tract include luminal dilatation with thickening of the wall of the small bowel and air/fluid levels suggestive of an ileus on abdominal flat plates or small bowel series. Abdominal computed tomography may show the "ribbon" sign of diffuse thickening of the small bowel wall.[24] Little correlation exists between the extent of disease and the appearance of mucosa on endoscopy, but mucosal sloughing is pathognomonic for severe disease.[29] Nevertheless, some studies have shown that antral biopsies correlate well with the severity of GVHD in the duodenum and in the colon even when the presenting symptom is diarrhea.[29] Histologic analysis of tissue is imperative to establish the diagnosis. The histologic features of GI GVHD are the presence of apoptotic bodies in the base of crypts, crypt abscesses, crypt loss, loss of Paneth cells, and flattening of the surface epithelium.[28,30,31]

Liver function test abnormalities are common after bone marrow transplant and occur secondary to venoocclusive disease, drug toxicity, viral infection, sepsis, iron overload, and other causes of extrahepatic biliary obstruction.[12] The exact incidence of hepatic GVHD is unknown because many patients do not undergo liver biopsies. The development of jaundice or an increase in the alkaline phosphatase and bilirubin may be the initial features of acute GVHD of the liver. The histologic features of hepatic GVHD are endothelialitis, lymphocytic infiltration of the portal areas, pericholangitis, and bile duct destruction and loss.[19,32]

Other Organs

Whether GVHD affects organs other than the classic triad of skin, liver, and gut has remained a matter of debate, although numerous reports suggest additional organ manifestations. The most likely candidate is the lung. Lung toxicity, including interstitial pneumonitis and diffuse alveolar hemorrhage, may occur in 20% to 60% of allogeneic transplant recipients but in fewer autologous transplant recipients. Causes of pulmonary damage other than GVHD include engraftment syndrome (see earlier), infection, radiation pneumonitis, and chemotherapy-related toxicity (e.g., methotrexate, busulfan).[21,33] One retrospective analysis failed to link severe pulmonary complications to clinical acute GVHD per se.[34] The mortality caused by pneumonia increases with the severity of GVHD, but this association may be related to increased immunosuppressive therapy.[21] A histopathologic signature of lymphocytic bronchitis has been associated with GVHD,[33] although not always.

Despite the ability of kidneys and hearts to serve as targets of transplant rejection, there is no convincing evidence for direct renal or cardiac damage from acute GVHD that is not secondary to drugs or infection. Similarly, neurologic complications are also common after transplantation but most can be attributed to drug toxicity, infection, or vascular insults.

Differential Diagnosis

Acute GVHD ought to be distinguished from any process that causes a constellation of fever, erythematous skin rash, and pulmonary edema that may occur during neutrophil recovery and has been termed engraftment or capillary leak syndrome.[35,36] In allogeneic transplant recipients distinction from acute GVHD is difficult. Engraftment syndrome is thought to reflect cellular and cytokine activities during early recovery of (donor-derived) blood cell counts and/or homeostatic proliferation of lymphocytes, but a precise delineation of the activated cells and mechanisms has not been demonstrated. Engraftment syndrome may be associated with increased mortality, primarily but not exclusively from pulmonary failure. Corticosteroid therapy may be effective particularly for the treatment of pulmonary manifestations.[37] Skin rashes may reflect delayed reactions to the conditioning regimen, antibiotics, or infections; furthermore, histopathologic skin changes consistent with acute GVHD can be mimicked by chemoradiotherapy and drug reactions.[21,38] Diarrhea can be a consequence of total-body irradiation (TBI), viral infection (especially with cytomegalovirus and other herpes viruses), parasitic infection, *Clostridium difficile* infection, nonspecific gastritis, narcotic withdrawal, and drug reactions: all of which mimic GVHD of the gut. Liver dysfunction can be caused by parenteral nutrition, venoocclusive disease, and viral or drug-induced hepatitis.

Genetic Basis of Graft-Versus-Host Disease

The graft-versus-host (GVH) reaction was first noted when irradiated mice were infused with allogeneic marrow and spleen cells.[39] Although mice recovered from radiation-induced injury and marrow aplasia, they subsequently died with "secondary disease,"[39] a phenomenon subsequently recognized as acute GVHD. Three requirements for the development of GVHD were formulated by Billingham.[4] First, the graft must contain immunologically competent cells, now recognized as mature T cells. In both experimental and clinical allogeneic HCT, the severity of GVHD correlates with the number of donor T cells transfused.[40,41] The precise nature of these cells and the mechanisms they use are now understood in greater detail (see later). Second, the recipient must be incapable of rejecting the transplanted cells (i.e., immunocompromised). After allogeneic HCT, the recipient is typically immunosuppressed by chemotherapy and/or radiotherapy before the hematopoietic cell infusion.[42] Third, the recipient must express tissue antigens that are not present in the transplant donor. Thus Billingham's third postulate stipulates that the GVH reaction occurs when donor immune cells recognize disparate host antigens.[4] These differences are governed by the genetic polymorphisms.[42]

HLA Matching

Recognition of alloantigens depends on the match with the presenting major histocompatibility molecule.[43–45] In humans, the MHC is governed by the HLA antigens that are encoded by the MHC gene complex on the short arm of chromosome 6 and can be categorized as class I, II, and III. Class I antigens (HLA-A, HLA-B, and HLA-C) are expressed on almost all cells of the body.[46] Class II antigens (DR, DQ, and DP) are primarily expressed on hematopoietic cells, although their expression can also be induced on other cell types following inflammation.[46] The incidence of acute GVHD is directly related to the degree of MHC mismatch.[42] The role of HLA mismatching of cord blood (CB) donors is more difficult to analyze compared with unrelated donor HCT, because allele typing of CB units for HLA-A, HLA-B, HLA-C, DRB1, and DQB1 is not routinely performed.[47] Nonetheless, the total number of HLA disparities between the recipient and the CB unit has been shown to correlate with risk for acute GVHD as the frequency of severe acute GVHD is lower in patients transplanted with HLA-matched (6/6) CB units.[47–49]

Minor Histocompatibility Antigens

In most clinical allogeneic transplants where MHC of donor and recipient are matched, donor T cells recognize MHC-bound peptides derived from the protein products of polymorphic genes (MiHAs) that are present in the host but not in the donor.[9,50–55] Substantial numbers (50%) of patients will develop acute GVHD despite receiving HLA-identical grafts as well as optimal postgrafting immune suppression.[9,42,56] MiHAs are widely but variably expressed in different tissue,[51,56] which is one possible explanation for the unique target organ distribution in GVHD. Many MiHAs such as HA-1 and HA-2 are expressed on hematopoietic cells, which may be one reason for the host immune system to be a primary target for the GVH response, and helps explain the critical role of direct presentation by professional recipient antigen-presenting cells (APCs) in the GVH response.[57] By contrast, other MiHAs such as H-Y and HA-3 are expressed ubiquitously.[56] MiHAs do not all equally induce lethal GVHD but show hierarchic immunodominance.[58,59] Furthermore, the difference in a single immunodominant MiHA is insufficient to elicit GVHD in murine models, even though a single MiHA can elicit T-cell–mediated damage in a skin explant model.[60,61] However, the role of specific MiHAs that are able to induce clinical GVHD has not been systematically evaluated in large groups of patients.[62]

Other Non-HLA Genes

Genetic polymorphisms in several non-HLA genes such as in killer-cell immunoglobulin-like receptors (KIRs), cytokines, and nucleotide-binding oligomerization domain containing 2 (NOD2) genes have recently been shown to modulate the severity and incidence of GVHD.

KIRs on natural killer (NK) cells that bind to the HLA class I gene products are encoded on chromosome 19. Polymorphisms in the transmembrane and cytoplasmic domains of KIRs govern whether the receptor has inhibitory (such as KIR2DL1, 2DL2, 2DL3, and 3DL1) or activating potential. Two competing models have been proposed for HLA-KIR allorecognition by donor NK cells following allogeneic HCT: the "mismatched ligand" and the "missing ligand" models.[5,63-66] Both models are supported by several clinical observations, albeit in patients receiving very different transplant and immunosuppressive regimens (see Chapters 20 and 102).[64,67-69]

Proinflammatory cytokines involved in the classic cytokine storm of GVHD cause pathologic damage to target organs, such as the skin, liver, and GI tract (see later).[22] Several cytokine gene polymorphisms in both recipients and donors have been implicated. Specifically, tumor necrosis factor (TNF) polymorphisms (TNFd3/d3 in the recipient, TNF863 and TNF857 in donors and/or recipients and TNFd4, TNF-α-1031C, and tumor necrosis factor receptor (TNFR) II-196R in the donors) have been associated with an increased risk for acute GVHD and transplant-related mortality (TRM).[70,71] The three common haplotypes of the interleukin (IL)-10 gene promoter region in recipients, representing high, intermediate, and low production of IL-10, have been associated with severity of acute GVHD following HLA-matched sibling donor allogeneic HCT.[72] By contrast, smaller studies have found neither IL-10 nor TNF-α polymorphisms to be associated with GVHD following HLA-mismatched cord blood transplantation.[71,73] Interferon-gamma (IFN-γ) polymorphisms of the 2/2 genotype (high IFN-γ production) and 3/3 genotype (low IFN-γ production) have been associated with decreased or increased acute GVHD, respectively.[71,74]

NOD2/caspase-activating recruitment domain 15 (CARD15) gene polymorphisms in both the donors and recipients were recently shown to have a striking association between GI GVHD and overall mortality following related and unrelated donor allogeneic HCT.[75] Several of the associations with non-HLA polymorphisms will need to be confirmed in larger and more diverse populations. Furthermore, it is likely that the importance of non-HLA gene polymorphisms in GVHD will differ depending on the donor source (related versus unrelated), HLA disparity (matched versus mismatched), graft source (CB versus bone marrow [BM] versus peripheral blood stem cells), and the intensity of the conditioning.

PATHOPHYSIOLOGY OF ACUTE GRAFT-VERSUS-HOST DISEASE

It is helpful to remember two important principles when considering the pathophysiology of acute GVHD. First, acute GVHD represents exaggerated but normal inflammatory responses against foreign antigens (alloantigens) that are ubiquitously expressed in a setting where they are undesirable. The donor lymphocytes that have been infused into the recipient function appropriately, given the foreign environment they encounter. Second, donor lymphocytes encounter tissues in the recipient that have been often profoundly damaged. The effects of the underlying disease, prior infections, and the intensity of conditioning regimen all result in substantial changes not only in the immune cells but also in the endothelial and epithelial cells. Thus the allogeneic donor cells rapidly encounter not simply a foreign environment, but one that has been altered to promote the activation and proliferation of inflammatory cells. Therefore the pathophysiology of acute GVHD may be considered a distortion of the normal inflammatory cellular responses that, in addition to the absolute requirement of donor T cells, involves multiple other innate and adaptive cells and mediators.[76] The development and evolution of acute GVHD can be conceptualized in three sequential phases (Fig. 108.2) to provide a unified perspective on the complex cellular interactions and inflammatory cascades that lead to acute GVHD: (1) activation of the APCs; (2) donor T-cell activation, differentiation, and migration; and (3) effector phase.[76] It is important to note that this three-phase description permits a unified perspective on GVHD biology but it is not meant to suggest that all three phases are of equal importance or that GVHD occurs in a stepwise and sequential manner. The spatiotemporal relationships among these biologic processes, depending on the context, are likely to vary and their relevance to the induction, severity, and maintenance of GVHD may depend on the factors cited earlier.

Phase 1: Activation of Antigen-Presenting Cells

The earliest phase of acute GVHD is initiated by the profound damage caused by the underlying disease and infections and further exacerbated by bone marrow transplantation (BMT) conditioning regimens (which include TBI and chemotherapy) that are administered even before the infusion of donor cells.[77-81] This first step results in activation of the APCs.[7] Specifically, damaged host tissues respond with multiple changes, including the secretion of proinflammatory cytokines, such as TNF-α, IL-1 and IL-6 described as the cytokine storm.[79,80,82,83]

Such changes increase expression of adhesion molecules, costimulatory molecules, MHC antigens, and chemokine gradients that alert the residual host and the infused donor immune cells.[80] These "danger signals" activate host APCs.[84,85] Damage to the GI tract from the conditioning is particularly important in this process because it allows for systemic translocation of immunostimulatory microbial products such as lipopolysaccharide (LPS) that further enhance the activation of host APCs, and the secondary lymphoid tissue in the GI tract is likely the initial site of interaction between activated APCs and donor T cells.[80,86,87] This scenario accords with the observation that an increased risk for GVHD is associated with intensive conditioning regimens that cause extensive injury to epithelial and endothelial surfaces with a subsequent release of inflammatory cytokines and increases in expression of cell surface adhesion molecules.[80,81] The relationship among conditioning intensity, inflammatory cytokine, and GVHD severity has been supported by elegant murine studies.[82] Furthermore, the observations from these experimental studies have led to two recent clinical innovations to reduce clinical acute GVHD: (1) reduced intensity conditioning to decrease the damage to host tissues and thus limit activation of host APC and (2) KIR mismatches between donor and recipients to eliminate the host APCs by the alloreactive NK cells.[65,88]

Host-type APCs that are present and have been primed by conditioning are critical for the induction of this phase; recent evidence suggests that donor-type APCs exacerbate GVHD, but in certain experimental models, donor-type APC chimeras also induce GVHD.[85,89-91] In clinical situations, if donor-type APCs are present in sufficient quantity and have been appropriately primed, they too might play a role in the initiation and exacerbation of GVHD.[92-94] Among the cells with antigen-presenting capability, dendritic cells

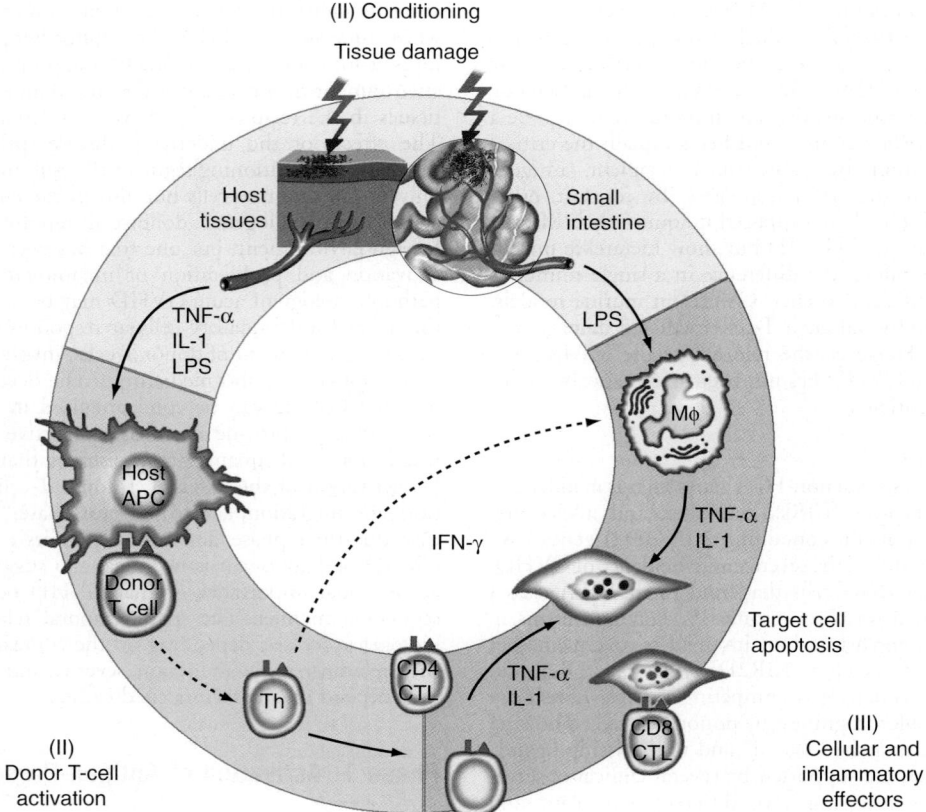

Fig. 108.2 PATHOPHYSIOLOGY OF GRAFT-VERSUS-HOST DISEASE. During step 1, irradiation and chemotherapy both damage and activate host tissues, including intestinal mucosa, liver, and the skin. Activated cell hosts then secrete inflammatory cytokines (e.g., TNF-α and IL-1), which can be measured in the systemic circulation. The cytokine release has important effects on APCs of the host, including increased expression of adhesion molecules (e.g., ICAM-1, VCAM-1) and of MHC class II antigens. These changes in the APCs enhance the recognition of host MHC and/or minor H antigens by mature donor T cells. During step 2, donor T-cell activation is characterized by proliferation of GVHD T cells and secretion of the Th1 cytokines IL-2 and IFN-γ. Both of these cytokines play central roles in clonal T-cell expansion, induction of CTL and NK cell responses, and the priming of mononuclear phagocytes. In step 3, mononuclear phagocytes primed by IFN-γ are triggered by a second signal such as endotoxin LPS to secrete cytopathic amounts of IL-I and TNF-α. LPS can leak through the intestinal mucosa damaged by the conditioning regimen to stimulate gut-associated lymphoid tissue or Kupffer cells in the liver; LPS that penetrates the epidermis may stimulate keratinocytes, dermal fibroblasts, and macrophages to produce similar cytokines in the skin. This mechanism results in the amplification of local tissue injury and further production of inflammatory effectors such as nitric oxide, which, together with CTL and NK effectors, leads to the observed target tissue destruction in the stem cell transplant host. CTL effectors use Fas/FasL, perforin/granzyme B, and membrane-bound cytokines to lyse target cells. *APC,* Antigen-presenting cell; *CTL,* cytotoxic T lymphocyte; *GVHD,* graft-versus-host disease; *ICAM,* intercellular adhesion molecule; *IFN,* interferon; *IL,* interleukin; *LPS,* lipopolysaccharide; *MHC,* major histocompatibility complex; *NK,* natural killer; *TNF,* tumor necrosis factor; *VCAM,* vascular cell adhesion molecule.

(DCs) are the most potent and play an important role in the induction of GVHD.[95] Experimental data suggest that GVHD can be regulated by qualitatively or quantitatively modulating distinct DC subsets.[96–101] Langerhans cells were also shown to be sufficient for the induction of GVHD when all other APCs were unable to prime donor T cells, although the role for Langerhans cells when all APCs are intact is dispensable.[102,103] Studies have yet to define roles for other DC subsets. In one clinical study persistence of host DC after day 100 correlated with the severity of acute GVHD, whereas elimination of host DCs was associated with reduced severity of acute GVHD.[93] The allostimulatory capacity of mature monocyte-derived DCs (mDCs) after reduced-intensity transplants was lower for up to 6 months compared with the mDCs from myeloablative transplant recipients, thus suggesting a role for host DCs and the reduction in danger signals secondary to less intense conditioning in acute

GVHD.[104] Nonetheless, this concept of enhanced host APC activation explains a number of clinical observations such as increased risks for acute GVHD associated with advanced-stage malignancy, conditioning intensity, and histories of viral infections. However, recent data suggest that even in the absence of all host hematopoietic derived APCs, GVHD can still be initiated by host nonhematopoietic cells.[105] The exact nature of the host nonhematopoietic cells that can initiate GVHD and the context under which they may play a more dominant role remains to be understood. Moreover when all of host CD11c⁺ DCs are eliminated, the severity of GVHD was found to be enhanced demonstrating a role for host DCs in mitigating GVHD severity.[106,107] Furthermore, a specific subset of host DCs, the CD8⁺ DCs might mitigate GVHD severity.[108,109] By contrast donor-derived DCs, specifically, CD103⁺CD11b⁻ DCs migrate from the colon and markedly enhance alloantigen presentation within the mesenteric lymph nodes (mLNs).[110] Critically, alloantigen presentation in the mLNs imprints gut-homing integrin signatures on donor T cells, leading to their emigration into the GI tract where they mediate fulminant disease. Thus anatomically distinct, donor DC subsets amplify GVHD. GVHD once initiated by host hematopoietic and/ or nonhematopoietic recipient APCs, generates a profound, localized, and lethal feed-forward cascade of donor DC-mediated indirect alloantigen presentation and cytokine secretion within the GI tract and aggravates its severity.

Other professional APCs such as monocytes/macrophages or semiprofessional APCs might also play a role in this phase.[7] For example, recent data suggest that host-type B cells might play a regulatory role under certain contexts,[111] whereas in other contexts, they were dispensable for GVHD induction. Similarly, host basophils have been shown not to affect the induction or severity of acute GVHD.[112,113] A small subset of radioresistant host-derived neutrophils infiltrate intestines after allo-HCT and the infiltration levels are dependent on the local microbial flora while such infiltration is not seen in germ-free conditions. Depletion of these neutrophils has been shown to reduce GVHD mortality.[114] Data suggest that radiosensitive hematopoietic-derived APCs may not be obligatory for induction of APCs. Also, host or donor-type nonhematopoietic stem cells (such as endothelial cells, epithelial cells, or stromal cells) can function as APCs in the context of inflammation.[105] The role of these cells in the presence and absence of professional hematopoietic-derived APCs remains to be elucidated.

Alloantigen presentation by the host APCs has been shown to be modulated by the local microflora and by the release of PAMPs and also by the release of damage associated molecular patterns (DAMP) molecules from condition-mediated damage. Classically, tissue damage releases exogenous and endogenous damage/pathogen-associated molecules termed DAMPs/PAMPs that are detected by pattern recognition receptors. Examples of pattern recognition receptors include Toll-like receptors (TLR) and NOD-like receptors that result in the activation of APCs.[115] The purine nucleoside adenosine triphosphate (ATP) is one DAMP whose release has been implicated as an early danger signal following tissue damage after allogeneic HCT. Elevated levels of ATP are found in peritoneal fluids of humans and mice following GVHD or irradiation. ATP interaction with the purinergic receptor $P2X_7$ on host APCs resulted in increased expression of costimulatory molecules CD80/CD86 and production of inflammatory cytokines. Interrupting this interaction reduced GVHD in experimental models.[116] More recently, a multiprotein complex termed the Nlrp3 inflammasome was shown to respond to DAMPs/PAMPs such as uric acid.[117] Mice deficient in critical components of Nlrp3 or adaptor protein for caspase-1 cleavage demonstrated less severe GVHD. Emerging data have demonstrated a role for negative regulators of DAMP responses in controlling the severity of GVHD. Siglecs are a family of sialic acid binding Ig-like lectins, which function as counter regulators to immune activation and Siglec-G$^{-/-}$ animals have increased GVHD, an effect confined to radiosensitive host APCs. In contrast, the enhanced Siglec-G signaling with CD24 in wild-type animals was protective.[118] Likewise inhibition of endogenous DAMPs such as heparan sulfate by endogenous protease inhibitors such as alpha-1 antitrypsin also mitigated GVHD in mice.[119,120] These and other data suggest that DAMPs such as ATP, heparin sulfate, and uric acid may have nonredundant roles in the aggravation of GVHD.

In addition to the role of LPS, recent observations have brought back renewed interest in the role of the quantitative and qualitative contributions of microbiota-driven inflammatory signals on GVHD. These signals are influenced by the variety and pathogenicity of organisms present, and have been demonstrated to affect the severity of GVHD.[121–123] It is apparent that GVHD mediates a loss of Paneth cell-derived antimicrobial peptides that play an important role in shaping the diversity of microbiota, in addition to the use of pharmaceutic antimicrobials, nonetheless our mechanistic understanding of the changes in microflora is currently limited. Understanding these mechanisms may offer manipulable targets to alter this primary, inflammation-mediated, initiation phase of GVHD.

Phase 2: Donor T-Cell Activation, Differentiation, and Migration

The infused donor T cells interact with the primed APCs leading to the initiation of the second phase of acute GVHD. This phase includes antigen presentation by primed APCs and the subsequent activation, proliferation, differentiation, and migration of alloreactive donor T cells. After allogeneic hematopoietic stem cell transplants, both host and donor-derived APCs are present in secondary lymphoid organs.[124,125] The T-cell receptor (TCR) of the donor T cells can recognize alloantigens either on host APCs (direct presentation) or donor APCs (indirect presentation).[126,127] In direct presentation, donor T cells recognize either the peptide bound to allogeneic MHC molecules or allogeneic MHC molecules without peptide.[127,128] During indirect presentation, T cells respond to the peptide generated by degradation of the allogeneic MHC molecules presented on self-MHC.[128] Experimental studies demonstrated that APCs derived from the host, rather than from the donor, are critical in inducing GVHD across MiHA mismatch.[7,126] Recent data suggest that presentation of distinct target antigens by the host-type and donor-type APCs might play a differential role in mediating target organ damage.[7,129,130] In humans, most cases of acute GVHD developed when both host DCs and donor DCs were present in peripheral blood after BMT.[93]

Costimulation

The interaction of donor lymphocyte TCR with the host allopeptide presented on the MHC of APCs alone is insufficient to induce T-cell activation.[7,131] Both TCR ligation and costimulation via a "second" signal through interaction between the T-cell costimulatory molecules and their ligands on APCs are required to achieve T-cell proliferation, differentiation, and survival.[132] The danger signals generated in phase 1 augment these interactions and significant progress has been made on the nature and impact of these second signals.[133,134] Costimulatory pathways are now known to deliver both positive and negative signals and molecules from two major families: the B7 family and the TNF receptor (TNFR) family play pivotal roles in GVHD.[135] Interruption of the second signal by the blockade of various positive costimulatory molecules (CD28, ICOS, CD40, CD30, 4-1BB, and OX40) reduces acute GVHD in several murine models, whereas antagonism of the inhibitory signals (programmed death (PD)-1 and cytotoxic T lymphocyte antigen (CTLA)-4) exacerbates the severity of acute GVHD.[136–142] The role of adhesion molecule DNAX accessory molecule-1 (DNAM-1) was recently explored in GVHD.[143,144] Splenocytes deficient in DNAM-1 and prophylactic treatment with anti–DNAM-1 antibody prevented and treated GVHD. The various T-cell and APC costimulatory molecules and the impact on acute GVHD are summarized in Table 108.3. The specific context and the hierarchy in which each of these signals plays a dominant role in the modulation of GVHD remain to be determined.

T-Cell Subsets

T cells consist of several subsets whose responses differ based on antigenic stimuli, activation thresholds, and effector functions. The alloantigen composition of the host determines which donor T-cell subsets proliferate and differentiate.

CD4$^+$, CD8$^+$ Cells and Naive/Memory T-Cell Subsets

CD4 and CD8 proteins are coreceptors for constant portions of MHC class II and class I molecules, respectively.[145] Therefore MHC class I (HLA-A, HLA-B, HLA-C) differences stimulate CD8$^+$ T cells and MHC class II (HLA-DR HLA-DP, HLA-DQ) differences stimulate CD4$^+$ T cells.[145–148] In the majority of HLA-identical BMT, acute GVHD can be induced by either or both CD4$^+$ and CD8$^+$ subsets in response to MiHAs.[149]

Several independent groups have found that although the naive (CD62L$^+$) T cells were alloreactive and caused acute GVHD, this was

TABLE
108.3

TABLE 108.3 T Cell–Antigen-Presenting Cell Interactions

T Cell	APC
Adhesion	
ICAMs	LFA-1
LFA-1	ICAMs
CD2 (LFA-2)	LFA-3
CD 226 (DNAM-1)	CD155, CD112
Recognition	
TCR/CD4	MHC II
TCR/CD8	MHC I
Costimulation	
CD28	CD80/86
CD152 (CTLA-4)	CD80/86
ICOS	B7H/B7RP-1
PD-1	PD-L1, PD-L2
Unknown	B7-H3
CD154 (CD40L)	CD40
CD134 (OX 40)	CD134L (OX40L)
CD137 (4-1BB)	CD137L (4-1BBL)
HVEM	LIGHT

APC, Antigen-presenting cell; CTLA-4, cytotoxic T lymphocyte antigen 4; DNAM-1, DNAX accessory molecule-1; HVEM, HSV glycoprotein D for herpesvirus entry mediator; ICAM, intercellular adhesion molecule; L, ligand; LFA, leukocyte function–associated antigen; LIGHT, homologous to lymphotoxins, shows inducible expression, and competes with HVEM, a receptor expressed by T lymphocytes; MHC, major histocompatibility complex; PD, programmed death; TCR, T-cell receptor.

not the case for the memory (CD62L⁻) T cells across different donor/recipient strain combinations.[150–153] Furthermore, expression of naive T-cell marker CD62L was also found to be critical for regulation of GVHD by donor natural regulatory T cells.[154] By contrast, another recent study demonstrated that alloreactive memory T cells and their precursor cells (memory stem cells) caused robust GVHD.[155,156]

Regulatory T Cells

Recent advances indicate that distinct subsets of regulatory CD4⁺CD25⁺, CD4⁺CD25⁻IL10⁺ Tr cells, γδT cells, DN⁻ T cells, NKT cells, and regulatory DCs control immune responses by induction of anergy or active suppression of alloreactive T cells.[97,98,157–165] Several studies have demonstrated a critical role for the natural donor CD4⁺CD25⁺ Foxp3⁺ regulatory T cells (Treg), obtained from naive animals or generated ex vivo, in the outcome of acute GVHD. Some studies have demonstrated that donor CD4⁺CD25⁺ T cells suppressed the early expansion of alloreactive donor T cells and their capacity to induce acute GVHD without abrogating GVL effector functions, while others have shown that depending on the tumors used and the context, GVL may be reduced as well.[166–168] The mechanisms by which donor Tregs suppress GVHD are being better understood. The presence of signal transducer and activation of transcription (STAT)1 signaling has been shown to enhance Treg-mediated suppression of GVHD.[169] A key role for host APCs in the induction of GVHD protection, and for donor APCs in the sustenance of the protection by the infused mature Tregs has been demonstrated.[170] Several small clinical trials that either include expanding Tregs in vivo with IL-2, or by epigenetic targeting of histone acetylation at the *Foxp3* locus, or by preferential expansion of Tregs by cyclophosphamide have shown clinical benefit in early phase II trials.[171–174] Direct infusion of ex vivo expanded donor Tregs has also demonstrated potential clinical benefit in small early phase trials and several clinical trials are underway in the United States and Europe with attempts to substantially expand these cells ex vivo and use for prevention of GVHD.[175,176]

Host NK1.1⁺ T cells are another T-cell subset that has been shown to suppress acute GVHD in an IL-4 dependent manner.[164,165,177] By contrast, donor NKT cells were found to reduce GVHD and enhance perforin-mediated GVL in an IFN-γ dependent manner.[178–180] Recent clinical data suggest that enhancing recipient NKT cells by repeated TLI conditioning promoted Th2 polarization and dramatically reduced GVHD.[165] Experimental data also show that activated donor NK cells can reduce GVHD through the elimination of host APCs or by secretion of transforming growth factor-β (TGF-β).[179] A murine BMT study using mice lacking SH2-containing inositol phosphatase, in which the NK compartment is dominated by cells that express two inhibitory receptors capable of binding either self or allogeneic MHC ligands, suggests that host NK cells may play a role in the initiation of GVHD.[181]

T-Cell Apoptosis and Signaling

Deletional mechanisms of tolerance fall into two categories: (1) central (thymic) deletion and (2) peripheral deletion.[182] Central deletion is an effective way to eliminate continued thymic production of alloreactive T cells. To this end, lymphoablative treatments have been used as a condition to create a mixed hematopoietic chimeric state in murine BMT models.[183] In this strategy, donor cells seed the thymus and maturing donor-reactive T-cell clones are deleted through intrathymic apoptosis.[184,185] The pathways of T-cell apoptosis by which peripheral deletion occurs can be broadly categorized into activation-induced cell death (AICD) and passive cell death (PCD).[186] An important mediator of AICD in T cells is the Fas receptor.[187] Activated T cells expressing the Fas molecule undergo apoptotic cell death when brought into contact with cells expressing Fas ligand. A critical role for Fas-mediated AICD has been clearly demonstrated in attenuation of acute GVHD by several type 1 T helper (Th1) cytokines.[42] PCD, or "death by neglect," illustrates the exquisite dependence of activated T cells on growth factors (e.g., IL-2, IL-4, IL-7, and/or IL-15) for survival; apoptotic cell death in this instance is largely because of rapid downregulation of B-cell lymphoma 2.[188–190] Transplantation of B-cell lymphoma-extra large T cells into nonirradiated recipients significantly exacerbates GVHD; however, no difference in GVHD mortality is observed in animals that have been lethally irradiated.[191] Selective elimination of donor T cells in vivo after BMT using transgenic T cells in which a thymidine kinase (TK) suicide gene is targeted to T cells has also been shown to attenuate the severity of acute GVHD.[191–194] Another recent approach to prevent GVHD is the selective depletion of alloantigen-specific donor T cells by a photodynamic cell-purging process, wherein donor T cells are treated with photoactive 4,5-dibromorhodamine 123 and subsequently exposed to visible light.[195] Targeting alloreactive T-cell bioenergetics has emerged as a newer strategy to mitigate GVHD in mice.[196,197] Thus several deletional mechanisms have been shown to reduce acute GVHD but the conditions under which one or another of these deletional mechanisms predominate remain to be determined.

APC and T-cell activation results in rapid intracellular biochemical signaling cascades that activate or negatively regulate alloreactive donor T-cell responses. The calcineurin-nuclear factor of activated T cell (NFAT) pathway has been shown to be an effective target for mitigating GVHD and forms the bedrock of clinical care. Specifically, the calcineurin inhibitors cyclosporine and tacrolimus. Cyclosporine binds to the cytosolic protein peptidyl prolyl cis-trans isomerase A (also known as cyclophilin), whereas tacrolimus binds to the peptidyl-prolyl cis-trans isomerase FK506-binding protein (FKBP)12, and these complexes (cyclosporine–cyclophilin or tacrolimus–FKBP12) inhibit calcineurin, thereby blocking the dephosphorylation of NFAT and its nuclear translocation.[198] These events prevent NFAT from exerting its transcriptional function, resulting in the inhibition of transcription of IL-2 and of other cytokines and ultimately leading to a reduced function of T-cells and mitigation of GVHD. Merging data have identified several key T-cell signaling pathways, many of which are being targeted in the clinic. Notably, the mammalian target of rapamycin (mTOR) pathway has been shown to be critical for blocking IL-2–mediated signal transduction and prevents cell-cycle progression in naive T cells.[199] Inhibition of mTOR with sirolimus is being used clinically to prevent and treat GVHD. Several additional signaling pathways that regulate alloreactive T-cell responses have recently been identified, such as Notch, protein kinase C (PKC) θ, spleen tyrosine kinase (syk), Janus-activated kinase (JAK)2, signal transducer and activator of transcription (STAT)3 and nuclear factor kappa-B (NFκB).[115] Emerging data are further defining a role for regulation T-cell proliferation/apoptosis epigenetic regulation through posttranslational modification by ubiquitination[200,201] or acetylation,[202] or by microRNAs (miRNAs). Specifically miRNAs such as miRNA 412 and miRNA 155 modulate alloimmunity by regulation of T-cell cycling and thus mitigate GVHD.[203,204]

Cytokines and T-Cell Differentiation

Classically the Th1 cytokines (IFN-γ, IL-2), TNF-α and IL-6 have been implicated in the cytokine storm that occurs early after BMT and have been shown to be critical for the pathophysiology of acute GVHD.[83,205–208] In addition to IL-2, several other common γ-chain cytokines (IL-21, IL-7, and IL-15) have been shown to play critical and potentially nonredundant roles in GVHD pathogenesis.[209] Type 1 or Tc1/Th1 maturation is recognized as the dominant pattern in acute GVHD.[210,211] Increased quantities of Th1-associated cytokines, TNF and IFN-γ, in acute GVHD are associated with earlier onset and more severe disease in preclinical models and clinical BMT. Although the dominance of Th1 subsets is well established, Th2 and Th17 subsets are also involved in pathology, and the balance between subsets determines acute GVHD severity, in addition to organ specificity, and the pathogenic or protective effects of any subset cannot be viewed in isolation.[212,213] Specifically, Th2 differentiation is often seen as opposing Th1 differentiation; however, this subset is also recognized as causing acute GVHD but with predominant pathology in pulmonary, hepatic, and cutaneous tissues,[214] in contrast to the strong GI association with Th1. Cutaneous pathology also may be generated by Th17 cells; although they are more commonly associated with chronic GVHD, they also have been associated with acute pathology.[215,216] Recent data have shown that blockade of L-33 binding with the Th2 ST2 receptor during allogeneic-hematopoietic cell transplantation by exogenous ST2-Fc infusions had a marked reduction in GVHD lethality, indicating a role for ST2 as a decoy receptor modulating GVHD.[217] Th17 differentiation is initiated by IL-6,[218] and RORγt is the defining transcription factor, whereas maintenance and amplification relies on IL-23 and IL-21, respectively. The use of RORC-deficient donor T cells results in attenuated acute GVHD severity and lethality.[219] Further studies are needed to better define the role of this subset in late acute GVHD versus early chronic GVHD, as well as the relative contribution of IL-17 from CD4 and CD8 T cells to end-organ pathology.

Leukocyte Migration

Donor T cells migrate to lymphoid tissues, recognize alloantigens on either host or donor APCs, and become activated. They then exit the lymphoid tissues and traffic to the target organs and cause tissue damage.[220] The molecular interactions necessary for T-cell migration and the role of lymphoid organs during acute GVHD have recently become the focus of a growing body of research. Chemokines play a critical role in the migration of immune cells to secondary lymphoid organs and target tissues.[221] T-lymphocyte production of macrophage inflammatory protein-1-alpha is critical to the recruitment of CD8+ but not CD4+ T cells to the liver, lung, and spleen during acute GVHD.[222] Several chemokines such as CCL2-5, CXC-chemokine ligand (CXCL)2, CXCL9-11, CCL17, and CCL27 are overexpressed and might play a critical role in the migration of leukocyte subsets to target organs liver, spleen, skin, and lungs during acute GVHD.[220,223] CXC-chemokine receptor (CXCR)3+ T and CCR5+ T cells cause acute GVHD in the liver and intestine.[220,224–226] CCR5 expression has also been found to be critical for Treg migration in GVHD.[227] Recent

clinical data from an early phase trial suggests that this may be a viable clinical strategy.[228] In addition to chemokines and their receptors, expression of selectins and integrins and their ligands also regulate the migration of inflammatory cells to target organs.[221] For example, interaction between α4β7 integrin and its ligand MadCAM-1 are important for homing of donor T cells to Peyer patches and in the initiation of intestinal GVHD.[86,229] αLβ2/intercellular adhesion molecule 1(ICAM1), ICAM2, ICAM3, and α4β1/vascular cell adhesion molecule (VCAM)2 interactions are important for homing to the lung and liver after experimental HCT.[220] The expression of CD62L on donor Tregs is critical for their regulation of acute GVHD, suggesting that their migration in secondary tissues is critical for their regulatory effects.[125] The migratory requirement of donor T cells to specific lymph nodes (e.g., Peyer patches) for the induction of GVHD might depend on other factors such as the conditioning regimen, inflammatory milieu, etc.[86,230] Furthermore, FTY720, a pharmacologic sphingosine-1-phosphate receptor agonist, inhibited GVHD in murine but not in canine models of HCT.[231,232] Thus significant species differences may also factor in the ability of these molecules to regulate GVHD.

Phase 3: Effector Phase

The effector phase that leads to the GVHD target organ damage is a complex cascade of multiple cellular and inflammatory effectors that further modulate each other's responses either simultaneously or successively. Effector mechanisms of acute GVHD can be grouped into cellular and inflammatory effectors. Inflammatory chemokines expressed in inflamed tissues upon stimulation by proinflammatory effectors, such as cytokines, are specialized for the recruitment of effector cells, such as cytotoxic T lymphocytes (CTLs).[233] Furthermore, the spatiotemporal expression of the cytochemokine gradients might determine not only the severity but also the unusual cluster of GVHD target organs (skin, gut, and liver).[220,234]

Cellular Effectors

CTLs are the major cellular effectors of GVHD.[235,236] The principle CTL effector pathways that have been evaluated after allogeneic BMT are the Fas-Fas ligand (FasL), the perforin-granzyme (or granule exocytosis), and the TNFR-like death receptors (DR), such as TNF-related apoptosis-inducing ligand (TRAIL: DR4, 5 ligand) and TNF-like weak inducers of apoptosis (TWEAK: DR3 ligand).[236–241] The involvement of each of these molecules in GVHD has been tested by using donor cells that are unable to mediate each pathway. Perforin is stored in cytotoxic granules of CTLs and NK cells, together with granzymes and other proteins. Although the exact mechanisms remain unclear, following the recognition of a target cell through the TCR-MHC interaction, perforin is secreted and inserted into the cell-membrane, forming "perforin pores" that allow granzymes to enter the target cells and induce apoptosis through various downstream effector pathways such as caspases.[242]

Transplantation of perforin-deficient T cells results in a marked delay in the onset of GVHD in transplants across MiHA disparities only, both MHC and MiHA disparities, and across isolated MHC I or II disparities.[236,243–247] However, mortality and clinical and histologic signs of GVHD were still induced even in the absence of perforin-dependent killing in these studies, demonstrating that the perforin-granzyme pathway plays little role in target organ damage. A role for the perforin-granzyme pathway for GVHD induction is also evident in studies using donor T-cell subsets. Perforin-deficient or granzyme B-deficient CD8+ T cells caused less mortality than wild-type T cells in experimental transplants across a single MHC class I mismatch. This pathway, however, seems to be less important compared with the Fas/FasL pathway in CD4-mediated GVHD.[246–248] Thus it seems that CD4+ CTLs preferentially use the Fas-FasL pathway, whereas CD8+ CTLs primarily use the perforin-granzyme pathway.

Fas, a TNF-receptor family member, is expressed by many tissues, including GVHD target organs.[249] Its expression can be upregulated by inflammatory cytokines such as IFN-γ and TNF-α during GVHD, and the expression of FasL is also increased on donor T cells, indicating that FasL-mediated cytotoxicity may be a particularly important effector pathway in GVHD.[236,250] FasL-defective T cells cause less GVHD in the liver, skin, and lymphoid organs.[245,248,250] The Fas-FasL pathway is particularly important in hepatic GVHD, consistent with the keen sensitivity of hepatocytes to Fas-mediated cytotoxicity in experimental models of murine hepatitis.[236] Fas-deficient recipients are protected from hepatic GVHD, but not from other organ GVHD, and administration of anti-FasL (but not anti-TNF) monoclonal antibodies (MAbs) significantly blocked hepatic GVHD damage occurring in murine models.[236,251,252] Although the use of FasL-deficient donor T cells or the administration of neutralizing FasL MAbs had no effect on the development of intestinal GVHD in several studies, the Fas-FasL pathway may play a role in this target organ, because intestinal epithelial lymphocytes exhibit increased FasL-mediated killing potential.[253] Elevated serum levels of soluble FasL and Fas have also been observed in at least some patients with acute GVHD.[254,255]

The use of a perforin-granzyme and FasL cytotoxic double-deficient (cdd) T cells, showed that they were unable to induce lethal GVHD across MHC class I and class II disparities after sublethal irradiation.[244] However, when recipients were conditioned with a lethal dose of irradiation, cdd CD4+ T cells produced similar mortality to wild-type CD4+ T cells.[240] These results were confirmed by a recent study demonstrating that GVHD target damage can occur in mice that lack alloantigen expression on the epithelium, preventing direct interaction between CTLs and target cells.[241]

Recently, several additional TNF family apoptosis-inducing receptors/ligands have been identified, including TWEAK, TRAIL, and LTβ/LIGHT, all of which have been proposed to play a role in GVHD and GVL responses.[136,256-262] However, whether these distinct pathways play a more specific role for GVHD mediated by distinct T-cell subsets in certain situations remains unknown. Taken together, experimental data suggest some distinction between the use of different lytic pathways for the specific GVHD target organs and GVL, but the clinical applicability of these observations is as yet largely unknown.

Inflammatory Effectors

Inflammatory cytokines synergize with CTLs resulting in the amplification of local tissue injury and further promotion of an inflammation, which ultimately leads to the observed target tissue destruction in the transplant recipient.[263]

The cytokines TNF-α, IL-6, and IL-1 are produced by an abundance of cell types during processes of both innate and adaptive immunity; they often have synergistic, pleiotropic, and redundant effects on both activation and effector phases of GVHD.[207,219] A critical role for TNF-α in the pathophysiology of acute GVHD was first suggested over 20 years ago because mice transplanted with mixtures of allogeneic BM and T cells developed severe skin, gut, and lung lesions that were associated with high levels of TNF-α messenger RNA (mRNA) in these tissues.[264] Target organ damage could be inhibited by infusion of anti–TNF-α MAbs, and mortality could be reduced from 100% to 50% by the administration of the soluble form of the TNF-α receptor (sTNFR), an antagonist of TNF-α.[79,82,265] TNF-TNF1 interactions on donor T cells promote alloreactive T-cell responses and TNF-TNFR2 interactions are critical for intestinal GVHD.[211,259,266] TNF-α also seems to be an important effector molecule in GVHD in skin and lymphoid tissue.[264,267] In addition, TNF-α might also be involved in hepatic GVHD, probably by enhancing effector cell migration to the liver via the induction of inflammatory chemokines.[268] The second major proinflammatory cytokine that appears to play an important role in the effector phase of acute GVHD is IL-1.[42,263] Secretion of IL-1 appears to occur predominantly during the effector phase of GVHD of the spleen and skin, two major GVHD target organs.[269] A similar increase in mononuclear cell IL-1 mRNA has been shown during clinical acute GVHD. Mice receiving IL-1 displayed a wasting syndrome and increased mortality that appeared to be an accelerated form of disease. By contrast, intraperitoneal administration of IL-1 receptor antagonist (IL-1RA) was able to reverse the development of GVHD in the majority of animals, providing a significant survival advantage to treated animals.[270] However, the attempt to use IL-1RA to prevent acute GVHD in a randomized trial was not successful.[271]

As a result of activation during GVHD, macrophages also produce nitric oxide (NO), which contributes to the deleterious effects on GVHD target tissues, particularly immunosuppression.[272] NO also inhibits the repair mechanisms of target tissue destruction by inhibiting proliferation of epithelial stem cells in the gut and skin.[273] In humans and rats, the development of GVHD is preceded by an increase in serum levels of NO oxidation products.[274-276]

IL-6 has also been identified as a critical cytokine that promotes a proinflammatory response during GVHD. Recent data suggest that IL-6 might in fact be the most critical cytokine that increases GVHD severity. It has direct cytopathic effects on the GI tract following allogeneic BMT and likely inhibits the reconstitution of Tregs.[208,277] It plays a dominant role in mitigating lung injury after allo-BMT.[278] Recent clinical trial demonstrated that targeting IL-6 early after transplant, particularly following high-intensity conditioning could mitigate GVHD.

BIOMARKERS OF ACUTE GRAFT-VERSUS-HOST DISEASE

Emerging data from large datasets have identified and validated plasma biomarkers with important prognostic value at the onset of symptoms of acute GVHD. Markers of systemic GVHD include IL-2Rα, TNFR1, IL-8, and hepatocyte growth factor.[1,279] Elafin has been identified as a biomarker specific for skin GVHD, and regenerating islet-derived 3-alpha (REG3α) as a biomarker of gastrointestinal GVHD, and ST2 or the soluble IL-33 receptor as a maker of resistance to therapy.[2-4,280-282]

Recently, the concentrations of three of these plasma biomarkers (TNFR1, ST2, and Reg3α) were used in the creation of an algorithm that computed the probability of nonrelapse mortality (NRM) for individual patients.[5,283] The algorithm was developed in a multicenter training set of 328 patients, and two separate multicenter validation sets of 164 and 300 patients, respectively. The investigators identified thresholds that created three distinct Ann Arbor GVHD scores. In all three datasets (training, test, and validation), the cumulative incidence of 6-month NRM significantly increased as the Ann Arbor GVHD score increased: 8% for score 1, 27% for score 2, and 46% for score 3 (P <.0001). Conversely, the response to primary GVHD treatment decreased as the GVHD score increased: 86% for score 1, 67% for score 2, and 46% for score 3, P <.0001). These findings suggest that biomarker-based scores can be used to guide risk-adapted therapy at the onset of acute GVHD. High-risk patients with a score of 3 are candidates for intensive primary therapy, while low-risk patients with a score of 1 are candidates for rapid tapers of systemic steroid therapy.

Recently the number of Paneth cells in duodenal biopsies for GVHD has been shown to correlate with response to treatment and with long-term survival.[6,31] The plasma concentration of REG3α, the clinical severity of GVHD, and the histologic severity at GVHD diagnosis independently predicted lack of response to GVHD therapy 4 weeks following treatment and TRM. Patients who had all three risk factors experienced significantly greater NRM than those with any two of the risk factors (86% versus 66%, P <.001). The integration of clinical stage, histologic grade, and biomarkers into a single grading system may permit better risk stratification and rapid identification of patients for whom standard treatment is likely to be insufficient.[3,281]

These biomarkers may also provide new insights into the biology of GVHD. For example, the IL-22-Reg3 axis protects the epithelial barrier function of the intestinal mucosa. Intestinal stem cells (ISCs) are principal cellular targets of GVHD in the GI tract, where intestinal flora are critical for amplification of GVHD damage. ISCs are protected by antibacterial proteins such as REG3α secreted by neighboring Paneth cells. Mucosal barrier disruption caused by stem cell dropout and subsequent lack of mucosal regeneration may preferentially allow Paneth cell proteins, including REG3α, to traverse into the bloodstream. Thus the plasma levels of REG3α may serve as a "liquid biopsy" and surrogate marker for the cumulative area of these breaches to GI mucosal barrier integrity, a parameter impossible to measure by individual tissue biopsies.

Prevention of Acute Graft-Versus-Host Disease

Elimination of T cells with monoclonal antibodies, immunotoxins, lectins, CD34 columns, or physical techniques are effective at reducing GVHD. A typical unmanipulated marrow transplant entails the infusion of approximately 10^7 T cells per kg of recipient weight. A T-cell dose less than or equal to 10^5 per kg has been associated with complete control of GVHD.[41] More recently, the combination of very high stem cell numbers and less than 3×10^4 CD3 cells per kg allowed haploidentical transplantation without GVHD.[284] Presumably host immune cells that survive the initial conditioning are responsible for graft rejection. When the stem cell source contains large numbers of T cells, the GVH reaction further reduces the residual population capable of alloreactivity, thus decreasing graft rejection. To some degree, the higher graft failure rates may be controlled by increasing the intensity of the immunosuppression of the conditioning regimen,[285,286] or adding back T cells.[287] Overall there has been no improvement in survival that can be definitively attributed to T-cell depletion.

Treatment of established GVHD with specific T-cell antibodies has produced mixed results. Although antithymocyte globulin has definite activity in established GVHD, the nonspecific clearance of T cells may result in increased opportunistic infections and no improvement in survival. More specific therapy with the humanized anti–IL-2 receptor antibody, daclizumab[288,289] or the humanized anti-CD3 antibody, visilizumab[290,291] are promising, since they offer the potential of selectively removing the activated T cells. However, an increased risk for infection may still be observed.[292]

The first generally prescribed GVHD preventive regimen was the administration of intermittent low-dose methotrexate as developed in a dog model by Thomas and Storb.[293] The principle of this approach was to administer a cell cycle–specific chemotherapeutic agent immediately after the transplant, when the T cells have started to divide after exposure to allogeneic antigens. Subsequently, the addition of antithymocyte globulin, prednisone, or both resulted in incremental improvement in the GVHD rate but no improvement in survival.[294,295] Ultimately, the course of methotrexate was abbreviated and combined with a T-cell activation inhibitor, such as cyclosporine or tacrolimus. The introduction of cyclosporine in the late 1970s was a significant advance in GVHD prevention. A similar agent, tacrolimus, has been shown to provide similar control of GVHD.[296] As a single agent, cyclosporine was about as effective as methotrexate.[297] However, in combination with methotrexate, there was a significant reduction in the incidence of GVHD and an improvement in survival.[298] Subsequent trials of tacrolimus and methotrexate compared with cyclosporine and methotrexate showed no advantage for either combination.[296] The addition of prednisone to the conventional two-drug regimen resulted in similar rates of GVHD and no improvement in survival.[299]

Sirolimus (rapamycin) is a macrocyclic lactone immunosuppressant that is similar in structure to tacrolimus and cyclosporine. All three drugs bind to immunophilins; however, sirolimus complexed with FKBP12 inhibits T-cell proliferation by interfering with signal transduction and cell-cycle progression and can prevent GVHD.[300] Because Sirolimus acts through a separate mechanism from the tacrolimus-FKBP complex (and cyclosporine-cyclophilin complex), it may be synergistic with both tacrolimus and cyclosporine. More recently, mycophenolate mofetil (MMF) has been studied. It is the prodrug of mycophenolic acid (MPA), a selective inhibitor of inosine monophosphate dehydrogenase, an enzyme critical to the de novo synthesis of guanosine nucleotide. Since T lymphocytes are more dependent on such synthesis than myeloid or mucosal cells, MPA preferentially inhibits proliferative responses of T cells.[301]

One hypothesis that flows from the three-step model of GVHD posits that reduction of intestinal colonization with bacteria could prevent GVHD. Animal studies in germ-free environments support this notion; GVHD was not observed until mice were colonized with gram-negative organisms.[302] Later, gut decontamination and use of a laminar air flow environment was associated with less GVHD and better survival in patients with severe aplastic anemia.[303] Similarly, studies of intestinal decontamination in patients with malignancies have shown less GVHD in some,[304,305] but not all studies.[306] Finally, another recent approach to GVHD prevention has been the use of nonmyeloablative conditioning transplants. Administration of vorinostat in combination with standard GVHD prophylaxis after related-donor reduced-intensity conditioning hemopoietic stem-cell transplantation reduced cumulative incidence of grade II–IV acute GVHD by day 100 to 22%, lower than the expected incidence of severe acute GVHD.[172] A less intensive preparative regimen decreases the tissue toxicity and subsequent release of cytokines in animal models.[79,82] Patients generally experience mild toxicity in the initial peritransplant period and develop little or no GVHD, although many develop GVHD later, especially after donor lymphocyte infusions. In fact, the rates of GVHD are often higher than with conventional transplants, and GVHD is associated with a significant portion of the GVL effect.[307–309]

A recent study has shown that addition of one dose of a humanized anti–IL-6 monoclonal antibody (tocilizumab) in addition to standard cyclosporine methotrexate prophylaxis resulted in only 12% Grade II–IV acute GVHD in 48 patients.[310,311] An important role for TNF-α in clinical acute GVHD has been suggested by studies demonstrating elevated levels of TNF-α in the serum of patients with acute GVHD and other endothelial complications such as venoocclusive disease.[312–315] Therapy of GVHD with humanized anti-TNF-α (infliximab)[316,317] or a dimeric fusion protein consisting of the extracellular ligand-binding portion of the human TNF-α receptor (TNFR) linked to the Fc portion of human immunoglobulin G1 (etanercept)[318] have shown some promise.[319,320] The second major proinflammatory cytokine that appears to play an important role in the effector phase of acute GVHD is IL-1. Secretion of IL-1 appears to occur predominantly during the effector phase of GVHD in the spleen and skin, two major GVHD target organs.[269] IL-1RA is a naturally occurring pure competitive inhibitor of IL-1 that is produced by monocytes/macrophages and keratinocytes. Of note, the IL-1RA gene is polymorphic, and the presence in the donor of the allele that is linked to higher secretion of IL-1RA was associated with less acute GVHD.[321] Two-phase I/II trials showed promising data that specific inhibition of IL-1 with either the soluble receptor or IL-1RA could result in remissions in 50% to 60% of patients with steroid-resistant GVHD.[322,323] However, a subsequent randomized trial of the addition of IL-1RA or placebo to cyclosporine and methotrexate beginning at the time of conditioning and continuing through day 14 after stem cell infusion did not show any protective effect of the drug, despite the attainment of very high plasma levels.[271,324] Therefore, at least as administered in this study, IL-1 inhibition was insufficient to prevent GVHD in humans. IL-11 was also able to protect the GI tract in animal models and prevent GVHD, but it did not prevent clinical GVHD.[324] Thus not all preclinical strategies successfully translate to new therapies.

Therapy for Acute Graft-Versus-Host Disease

Glucocorticoid steroids are the initial therapy for acute GVHD. The mechanisms by which steroids work are multifactorial; they act as lympholytic agents and inhibit the release of inflammatory cytokines such as IL-1, IL-2, IL-6, gamma interferon, and TNF-α. Because of its intravenous availability, methylprednisolone is the steroid most commonly given for acute GVHD. Various dosing regimens have been used, none of which is clearly superior. High-bolus doses (10–20 mg/kg or 500 mg/m²) have higher initial response rates, but flares on tapering and opportunistic infections are common. Both the Seattle and Minnesota transplant groups have found that treatment with steroids was as effective as, or more effective than, other therapies or combination of therapies, with 20% to 40% of patients having durable long-term responses.[325,326] Long-term salvage rates for patients who did not respond to steroids were 20% or less; most patients eventually died from infection, acute GVHD, and/or chronic GVHD. More recently, a randomized trial demonstrated that topical therapy with oral budesonide can have prednisone sparing effects and is efficacious in treatment of GI GVHD.[327] Clinically, two types of failure of corticosteroid treatment of acute GVHD can be distinguished: true steroid resistance (i.e., progression of GVHD symptoms and manifestations while patients are receiving full-dose corticosteroid treatment) and steroid dependence (i.e., reoccurrence [or flare] of GVHD during or after tapering of steroid treatment).[328] In general, the prognosis with true steroid-resistant GVHD is worse than the prognosis of steroid-dependent patients.[328] A comparison of trials dealing with steroid-resistant GVHD is hampered by variable inclusion of both patient groups in many of these trials. A number of agents have been tested, including chemical immunosuppressants such as MMF, antithymocyte globulin (ATG), anti-CD3, anti-T-cell antibodies, and more specific agents directed against activation or adhesion molecules anti-CD25, anti-CD147, or cytokines or extracorporeal photopheresis.[328,329] To date, there are no randomized trials testing one agent versus the other in this clinical situation. Recent data suggested a role for TNF inhibition when added to steroids in treating GVHD, although a randomized trial failed to demonstrate any difference when compared with the addition of pentostatin or anti-IL2 to steroids and was inferior to the addition of MMF.[319,330]

Targeted elimination of alloreactive T cells has recently been demonstrated to be a safe and efficacious method to mitigate GVHD. Fusion of human caspase 9 to a modified human FK-binding protein that allowed for dimerization when exposed to a synthetic dimerizing drug led to the rapid death of 90% of alloreactive T cells expressing this construct and mitigated acute GVHD in a pilot trial of five patients following haploidentical BMT.[331]

Other Supportive Approaches

Infections are the main cause of death in patients with steroid-refractory acute GVHD, and careful surveillance and control of infections is mandatory in patients with acute GVHD. Fungal infections, especially aspergillosis, are the leading complication. Prophylaxis and early aggressive treatment should be facilitated by the introduction of new azoles (voriconazole, posiconazole) or echinocandins (caspofungin, micafungin), which broaden therapeutic efficacy with acceptable toxicity. Other supplementary approaches have been suggested, such as the use of octreotide[332] and oral beclomethasone (or budesonide) to control large volumes of diarrhea.[327]

CHRONIC GRAFT-VERSUS-HOST DISEASE

Chronic GVHD was initially defined as a GVHD syndrome presenting more than 100 days after transplantation; its onset occurred either as an extension of acute GVHD (progressive), after a disease-free interval (quiescent), or with no precedent (de novo).[333,334] Chronic GVHD may be limited or extensive (see Table 108.3). Any grade of acute GVHD increases the probability of chronic GVHD, although no singular pathologic feature of the former predicts the development of the latter. Its incidence ranges from 30% to 60% after transplantation with the bone marrow, although it may be higher after peripheral blood progenitor transplants.[335]

As with acute GVHD, the immune system appears to be affected in all patients, who are highly susceptible to bacterial, viral, fungal, and opportunistic infections. Specific abnormalities of cellular immunity include decreases in the production of antibodies against specific antigens, defects in the number and function of CD4⁺ T cells, and increases in the number of nonspecific suppressor cells, which further diminish lymphocyte responses. Skin changes resembling widespread lichen planus with papulosquamous dermatitis, plaques, desquamation, dyspigmentation, and vitiligo occur in 80% of patients.[309,336] Destruction of dermal appendages leads to alopecia and onychodysplasia. Severe chronic GVHD of the skin can resemble scleroderma, with induration, joint contractures, atrophy, and chronic skin ulcers. Chronic cholestatic liver disease occurs in 80% of patients and often resembles acute GVHD; it rarely progresses to cirrhosis. Severe mucositis of the mouth and esophagus can result in weight loss and malnutrition. Intestinal involvement, however, is infrequent.[309,336] Chronic GVHD also produces a sicca syndrome, with atrophy and dryness of mucosal surfaces caused by lymphocytic destruction of exocrine glands, usually affecting the eyes, mouth, airways, skin, and esophagus.[24,336,337] The hematopoietic system may also be affected, and thrombocytopenia is an unfavorable prognostic factor in patients with chronic GVHD.[309] Important predictors of unfavorable outcome are progressive onset, lichenoid skin changes, elevated serum bilirubin level, continued thrombocytopenia, and failure to respond to 9 months of therapy.[309,338–340] Among patients with none of these risk factors, 70% are expected to survive, compared with less than 20% with two or more of these risk factors.[340]

Histologic examination of the immune system reveals involution of thymic epithelium, disappearance of Hassall corpuscles, depletion of lymphocytes, and absence of secondary germinal centers in lymph nodes.[337] Pathologic skin findings include epidermal atrophy with changes characteristic of lichen planus and striking inflammation around eccrine units. Sclerosis of the dermis and fibrosis of the hypodermis subsequently develop. GI lesions include localized inflammation of the mucosa and stricture formation in the esophagus and small intestine.[336] Histologic findings in the liver are often similar to those that occur in acute GVHD but are more intense, with chronic changes such as fibrosis and hyalinization of portal triads, obliteration of bile ducts, and hepatocellular cholestasis.[309] The endocrine glands of the eyes, mouth, esophagus, and bronchi show destruction focused on centrally draining ducts, with secondary involvement of alveolar components.[337] Findings of bronchiolitis obliterans, similar to those that occur in rejection of lung transplants, are now generally considered a pulmonary manifestation of chronic GVHD, although the pathogenesis of this process remains unclear.[337]

Clinical Manifestations of Chronic Graft-Versus-Host Disease

Chronic GVHD can present with a plethora of clinical manifestations. Because of its unpredictable pattern and the late onset, when patients are no longer receiving care at their transplant center, the diagnosis is often delayed or not recognized. The staging of chronic GVHD is summarized in Table 108.4. However, consensus criteria recently developed by the National Institutes of Health (NIH) might soon become the standard for diagnosing and evaluating responses for chronic GVHD.[341,342]

Dermatologic

Skin involvement in chronic GVHD presents with varied features. Lichenoid chronic GVHD presents as an erythematous, papular rash that resembles lichen planus with no typical distribution pattern.[24] Sclerodermatous GVHD may involve the dermis and/or the muscular fascia and clinically resembles systemic sclerosis. The skin is thickened, tight, and fragile, with very poor wound healing. Either hypo or hyperpigmentation may occur. In severe cases the skin may become blistered and ulcerate. Hair changes can include increased brittleness, premature graying, and alopecia. Fingernails and toenails may also be

TABLE 108.4	Commonly Administered Drugs for Graft-Versus-Host Disease Prophylaxis and Treatment	
Drug	**Mechanism**	**Adverse Effects**
Corticosteroids	Direct lymphocyte toxicity; suppress proinflammatory cytokines such as TNF-α	Hyperglycemia, acute psychosis, severe myopathy, neuropathy, osteoporosis, cataract development
Methotrexate (MTX)	Antimetabolite: inhibit T-cell proliferation	Significant renal, hepatic, and gastrointestinal toxicities
Cyclosporine A (CSA)	IL-2 suppressor; blocks Ca²⁺-dependent signal transduction distal to TCR engagement	Renal and hepatic insufficiency, hypertension, hyperglycemia, headache, nausea and vomiting, hirsutism, gum hypertrophy, seizure with severe toxicity
Tacrolimus (FK506)	IL-2 receptor; blocks Ca²⁺-dependent signal transduction distal to TCR engagement	Similar to CSA
Mycophenolate mofetil (MMF)	Inhibits de novo purine synthesis	Body aches, abdominal pain, nausea and vomiting, diarrhea, neutropenia
Sirolimus	mTOR inhibitor	Thrombocytopenia, hyperlipidemia, TTP
Antithymocyte globulin (ATG)	Polyclonal immunoglobulin	Anaphylaxis, serum sickness

IL-2, Interleukin-2; mTOR, mammalian target of rapamycin; TCR, T-cell receptor; TNF-α, tumor necrosis factor-α; TTP, thrombotic thrombocytopenic purpura.

affected by chronic GVHD. Destruction of sweat glands can cause hyperthermia.[343]

Ocular

Ocular GVHD usually presents with xerophthalmia or dry eyes. Irreversible destruction of the lacrimal glands results in dryness, photophobia, and burning. Local therapy with preservative-free tears and ointment or the placement of punctal plugs by an ophthalmologist might be required. Conjunctival GVHD, a rare manifestation of severe chronic GVHD, has a poor prognosis.[24,343]

Oral

Oral GVHD causes xerostomia and/or food sensitivity.[343] More advanced disease may cause odynophagia caused by esophageal damage and strictures, although esophageal involvement occurs rarely without oral disease. Physical examination may reveal only erythema with a few white plaques, prompting a misdiagnosis of thrush or herpetic infections. Lichenoid changes in advanced disease can cause extensive plaque formation.[24]

Gastrointestinal

Patients with chronic GVHD have GI complaints that mimic other disease states, including acute GVHD, infection, dysmotility, lactose intolerance, pancreatic insufficiency, and drug-related side effects. In one retrospective review of the intestinal biopsies of patients with chronic GVHD and persistent GI symptoms, a majority of patients had evidence of both acute and chronic GVHD, and only 7% of the patients had isolated chronic GVHD.[24,336] Thus although chronic GVHD may involve the GI tract alone, it may be difficult to diagnose in those circumstances without concurrent acute GVHD.

Hepatic

Hepatic disease typically presents as cholestasis with elevated serum levels of alkaline phosphatase and bilirubin. Isolated hepatic chronic GVHD has become more common with the increasing use of donor lymphocyte infusions.[11] Liver biopsy is required to confirm the diagnosis of chronic hepatic GVHD in patients with no other target organ involvement.

Pulmonary

Bronchiolitis obliterans is a late and serious manifestation of chronic GVHD. Patients typically present with a cough or dyspnea.[343] Severe sclerotic disease of the chest wall may also give rise to similar symptoms with no intrinsic pulmonary disease. Pulmonary function tests demonstrate obstructive physiology and a reduction in DLCO. Chest computed tomography results may be normal or may show hyperinflation with a ground-glass appearance. Overall, patients with bronchiolitis obliterans have minimal response to therapy and a very poor prognosis. Patients with chronic GVHD are also at risk for chronic sinopulmonary infections, but symptoms may be minimal.[24]

Hematopoietic

Cytopenias in chronic GVHD are common. This may be a result of stromal damage, but autoimmune neutropenia, anemia, and/or thrombocytopenia are also seen. Thrombocytopenia at the time of chronic GVHD diagnosis is associated with poor prognosis. However, thrombocytopenia posttransplant is a poor prognostic factor regardless of GVHD, and eosinophilia is occasionally seen with chronic GVHD.

Immunologic

Chronic GVHD is inherently immunosuppressive. Functional asplenia with an increased susceptibility to encapsulated bacteria is common, and circulating Howell-Jolly bodies can be seen on peripheral blood smear. Patients are also at risk for invasive fungal infections and *Pneumocystis carinii* pneumonia. Hypoglobulinemia is common, and patients with levels below 500 mg/dL should be supplemented with intravenous immunoglobulin.

Musculoskeletal

Fascial involvement in sclerodermatous GVHD is usually associated with skin changes. Fasciitis in joint areas can cause severe restriction of range of motion. Muscle cramps are a common complaint in patients with chronic GVHD, but myositis with elevated muscle enzymes is rare. Many patients with chronic GVHD are on steroid therapy and have low levels of sex hormone posttransplant. Thus avascular necrosis, osteopenia, and osteoporosis are frequent complications.

Although several cases have been described, it is yet to be determined in large studies whether kidneys, which are primary targets in some animal models of chronic GVHD, are also involved.[344] Among the myriad clinical features of chronic GVHD, three definitive signs appear to be risk factors for increased mortality: (1) extensive skin GVHD involving greater than 50% of the body surface area, (2) platelet count of less than 100,000/μL, and (3) progressive onset and acute GVHD that continues uninterrupted beyond day 100.[345] However, chronic GVHD remains, except in cases with obvious features, a difficult diagnosis; response to therapy is even more difficult to assess. Recent criteria established by the NIH consensus conference might prove to be beneficial in establishing uniform guidelines for diagnosis, treatment, and response.[342] The NIH consensus criteria are currently being evaluated.

Differential Diagnosis

The distinction between chronic and acute GVHD has been traditionally based on the time of onset. However, with the advent of low-intensity HCT, that distinction has become less relevant. The NIH working group has, in addition to the two main categories of GVHD, added two subcategories. The broad category of acute GVHD includes (1) classic acute GVHD (maculopapular rash, nausea, vomiting, anorexia, profuse diarrhea, ileus, or cholestatic hepatitis), occurring within 100 days after transplantation or donor leukocyte infusion (DLI), (without diagnostic or distinctive signs of chronic GVHD), and (2) persistent, recurrent, or late acute GVHD: features of classic acute GVHD without diagnostic or distinctive manifestations of chronic GVHD occurring beyond 100 days of transplantation or DLI (often seen after withdrawal of immune suppression). The broad category of chronic GVHD includes (1) classic chronic GVHD without features characteristic of acute GVHD and (2) an overlap syndrome in which features of chronic and acute GVHD appear together. In the absence of histologic or clinical signs or symptoms of chronic GVHD, the persistence, recurrence, or new onset of characteristic skin, GI tract, or liver abnormalities should be classified as acute GVHD regardless of the time after transplantation. With appropriate stratification, patients with persistent, recurrent, or late acute GVHD or overlap syndrome can be included in clinical trials with patients who have chronic GVHD.

CHRONIC GRAFT-VERSUS-HOST DISEASE: PATHOPHYSIOLOGY

The pathophysiology of chronic GVHD is generally much less well understood than that of acute GVHD and has undergone less intensive experimental modeling.[24] It is important to recognize that chronic GVHD was originally defined as a temporal rather than a clinical or pathophysiologic entity. The initial clinical reports of chronic GVHD described abnormalities that occurred at least 150 days after stem cell infusion.[346,347] By convention, day 100 after stem cell infusion is used as an arbitrary divider between acute and chronic GVHD. But some manifestations of acute GVHD occur after day 100, and some manifestations of chronic GVHD may occur before day 100. Thus it is preferable to consider the clinical symptoms and signs per se rather than their timing of onset.

Relatively little is known about the pathophysiology of chronic GVHD. This is in part because of the absence of appropriate animal models that can capture the kinetics and the protean manifestation of chronic GVHD.[348] However, recent studies using multiple models that collectively mimic many of the chronic GVHD manifestations have begun to shed light on the complex biology.

T cells: Based on certain clinical features chronic GVHD has been considered to be an autoimmune disease, with some experimental data suggesting that chronic GVHD results from defective central negative selection, which leads to the generation of autoreactive clones that escape tolerogenic mechanisms operating in the periphery.[349,350] The autoreactive cells of chronic GVHD are associated with a damaged thymus, which can be injured by several mechanisms,

including acute GVHD, the conditioning regimen, or age-related involution and atrophy. In chronic GVHD the ability of the thymus to delete autoreactive T cells (negative selection) and to induce tolerance is impaired.[24,351,352] Chronic GVHD could also be a product of T cells that have undergone relatively chronic antigen stimulation as a result of the presence of inexhaustible and ubiquitous MiHA antigens. Allo-T cells under circumstances of chronic MiHA antigen stimulation can induce syndromes resembling those induced by the chronic antigen stimulation in autoimmune diseases. This concept is also consistent with the proposal of acute GVHD as a risk factor for chronic GVHD. The antigens targeted in chronic GVHD could be the same dominant ones targeted in acute GVHD, but the reactive T cells could be different; for example, they may secrete TGF-β. Recent data have shown that the balance between Treg and conventional T-cells is critical for chronic GVHD.[171]

Cytokines: TGF-β has been implicated in the development of fibrosis and chronic GVHD.[180] IL-17 and subsequent T-cell differentiation along the Th17 pathway have recently been strongly associated with cGVHD. IL-17 was shown more recently to result in colony stimulating factor (CSF)1-dependent macrophage accumulation in skin and lung, which drives tissue fibrosis.[353] Systemic IL-17 levels increase late after clinical BMT, at a time when chronic GVHD develops.[311] Inhibition of Th17 differentiation and CSF1 appear to be relevant to the development of chronic GVHD.

IL-2 is critical for Treg homeostasis. Recent data have shown that Treg:conventional T-cell balance is critical for chronic GVHD.[171] In addition, inhibition of terminal cytokines involved in fibrosis, such as TGF-β and IL-13, represent additional targets; however, TGF-β inhibition may be problematic given its important role in Treg homeostasis.

B cells: In some patient subsets, responses to rituximab, presence of MiHA-specific antibodies, and the presence of chronic GVHD after T-cell depletion (TCD) allo-BMT would indicate that in addition to donor T cells, donor B cells might be a direct effector or might have a role in priming T cells as APCs.[354,355] Murine models demonstrated a pathogenic role for donor B cells and alloantibody production in causing experimental chronic GVHD. It is also clear that T follicular helper (T_{FH}) cells and IL-21 play important roles in the development of chronic GVHD via the stimulation of germinal center B cells and alloantibody generation.[356] Two tyrosine kinases expressed in the hepatocellular carcinoma (TEC) family of kinases, IL-2–inducible kinase (ITK) and Bruton tyrosine kinase (BTK), share close homology and play critical roles in both T-cell and B-cell function. ITK helps to drive T-cell activation and differentiation while BTK is essential for B-cell receptor signaling. In mouse studies treatment with ibrutinib, an ITK and BTK inhibitor, reversed lung pathology and pulmonary dysfunction in mice with established chronic GVHD in a model dependent on cooperation between T_{FH} and germinal center B cells; additionally, ibrutinib reduced the progression of sclerodermatous chronic GVHD in mice.[357] Targeting syk in B cells has been shown to mitigate chronic GVHD in several models. Syk deletion in vivo was effective in treating established chronic GVHD, as was a small-molecule inhibitor of Syk, fostamatinib, which normalized germinal center formation and decreased activated CD80/86(+) dendritic cells.[358] In multiple distinct models of sclerodermatous chronic GVHD, clinical and pathologic disease manifestations were not eliminated when mice were therapeutically treated with fostamatinib, though both clinical and immunologic effects could be observed in one of these scleroderma models.

BIOMARKERS OF ACUTE GRAFT-VERSUS-HOST DISEASE

Less progress has been made with biomarkers for chronic GVHD than for acute GVHD; nevertheless, several are beginning to emerge. CXCL9 has been identified and validated in several hundred patients from at least two HCT centers.[7,359] Other biomarkers with potential utility include soluble B-cell activation factor (sBAFF), anti-dsDNA antibody, soluble IL-2 receptor alpha (sIL-2Rα), and soluble CD13 (sCD13); sBAFF and anti-dsDNA also may be elevated in patients with late-onset chronic GVHD, but these biomarkers need to be validated in much larger cohorts before definitive conclusions can be drawn.

THERAPY FOR CHRONIC GRAFT-VERSUS-HOST DISEASE

Chronic GVHD has a major impact on both quality of life and survival, frequently involves multiple organs, and necessitates prolonged immunosuppressive therapy.[360] One report noted that 15% of cancer-free patients were still receiving immunosuppressive therapy after 7 years.[361] The more severe forms of chronic GVHD are clearly associated with a lower disease-free survival. Thus the potential benefit of a GVL effect is shadowed by significant treatment-related mortality.[361]

Current therapies for chronic GVHD are of limited efficacy, and there is no long-term satisfactory regimen for patients who do not respond to front-line steroid-based therapy. Indeed, no medication has been approved by the Food and Drug Administration for use in chronic GVHD. The lack of standardized response criteria to measure therapeutic efficacy poses a major obstacle to pursuing therapeutic trials in chronic GVHD. Overall survival and/or discontinuation of systemic immunosuppression are accepted long-term endpoints in chronic GVHD trials. The recent NIH-sponsored consensus project provided, for the first time, a set of standardized measures and definitions to use as response criteria in chronic GVHD.[341,342] Nonetheless, these recommendations are yet to be tested and validated in prospective studies. The NIH consensus conference has defined response measures that are classified in two main groups: clinician-assessed and patient-reported (Table 108.5).[348]

The prevention of acute GVHD has not consistently resulted in a lower incidence of chronic GVHD. A clear example is the use of reduced-intensity transplants, consistently associated with a lower incidence of acute GVHD but with no major impact on chronic GVHD.[362,363] The extended use of GVHD prophylaxis with cyclosporine, or variations in the cyclosporine dosage used, showed no beneficial effects on the incidence of chronic GVHD.[360,364] The addition of thalidomide to cyclosporine and methotrexate prophylaxis, the administration of intravenous immunoglobulin, and early treatment based on biopsy findings of subclinical GVHD in an attempt to preemptively treat chronic GVHD were unsuccessful.[360] A randomized placebo- controlled study in Europe showed that the addition of ATG Fresenius resulted in a significant reduction in the severity and incidence of chronic GVHD.[8,365]

The most commonly used therapies to treat chronic GVHD are cyclosporine A (CSA) and prednisone. Sullivan and colleagues[366] reported that prednisone alone is superior to prednisone plus azathioprine for primary treatment of patients with chronic GVHD.

However, in patients classified as high-risk on the basis of platelet counts below 100,000/μL, treatment with prednisone alone resulted in only 26% 5-year survival. When a similar group of patients was treated with alternating-day CSA and prednisone, 5-year survival exceeded 50%.[367] A randomized study of patients with extensive GVHD found no difference when prednisone alone was compared with prednisone plus CSA.[24] For chronic GVHD that recurs or fails to respond to initial therapy, there is no standard treatment. A small recent study has shown that an 8 week administration of low dose, subcutaneous IL-2 ameliorated several manifestations of chronic GVHD that was resistant to steroids, particularly in the skin.[9,368] This improvement was associated with an increase in Tregs. This increase was caused by enhanced, proliferation, thymic export and resistance to apoptosis.[10,171] Randomized clinical trials of this approach are currently being conducted. Other experimental therapies include psoralen plus ultraviolet light A, MMF, thalidomide, total lymphoid irradiation, Plaquenil, extracorporeal photopheresis, pentostatin, and acetretin.[338] (see Table 108.4, for list of the commonly used GVHD drugs and their side effects.)

Transfusion-Associated Graft-Versus-Host Disease

Most blood products administered to immunocompromised patients are now irradiated or at least leukocyte-depleted to avoid the transfusion of viable alloreactive T cells. With most homologous blood products, the MHC incompatibility between donor and recipient results in rapid clearance of transfused T cells by the recipient's immune system. However, occasionally, transfusions from donors who are homozygous for one of the recipient's MHC haplotypes are not recognized as foreign by the recipient.[369–371] These cells can survive, "engraft," and mount an immunologic attack against the unshared haplotype in the patient, resulting in transfusion-induced GVHD.[371] Transfusion-associated GVHD differs from GVHD occurring after transplantation in terms of kinetics and manifestations (i.e., with transfusion-associated GVHD, the recipient marrow is a major target).[370] Since the number of stem cells in the offending blood product is inadequate, there is no hemopoietic recovery from donor cells. This syndrome is generally fatal as a result of refractory pancytopenia and/or other organ involvement.

GRAFT-VERSUS-LEUKEMIA RESPONSES

The GVL response after allogeneic HCT results from the immunologic attack of the host tissue and, by extension, the leukemia (i.e., the tumor). This response represents a potent form of immunotherapy that circumvents some of the "immunoediting" mechanisms used by tumor cells to develop in the hosts. The power of the alloimmune response to eliminate malignancy was first reported more than 50 years ago in experimental models by Barnes et al.[1] However, GVL as its own entity and its close association with GVHD were not established until another 15 years later.[372] GVL responses demonstrate the clearest and arguably to date, the most potent demonstration of the power to harness the immune system to eradicate malignant diseases. The critical and direct evidence of GVL effect in clinical transplantation has been provided by the use of DLI to treat relapses after allogeneic HCT.[373–375] Kolb and colleagues first reported three patients with relapsed chronic myeloid leukemia (CML) who achieved complete cytogenetic remission after treatment with IFN-α and DLI from the original donors.[376] Subsequently, these findings have been confirmed in several reports.[377–379]

The most recent and dramatic effect of the GVL effect has been demonstrated using genetic engineering to create tumor antigen-specific T cells (CAR T-cell therapy). Most discussion below is geared towards biology of GVL responses after allo-BMT. The mechanisms of GVL responses after CAR T-cell therapy while seemingly evident (antigen-specific T cells eliminating leukemia and other cells expressing the antigen), the mechanisms for failure and complications are just being explored.

	National Institutes of Health Chronic Graft-Versus-Host Disease Measures	
TABLE 108.5		

Measure	Clinician-Assessed	Patient-Reported
Chronic GVHD Specific Core Measures		
Signs	Organ-specific measures	Not applicable
Symptoms	Clinician-assessed symptoms	Patient-reported symptoms
Global rating	Mild, moderate, or severe	Mild, moderate, or severe
	0–10 severity scale	0–10 severity scale
	7-point change scale	7-point change scale
Chronic GVHD Nonspecific Ancillary Measures		
Function	Grip strength	Patient-reported function
	2-minute walk time	
Quality of life	—	Patient-reported health-related quality of life

GVHD, Graft-versus-host disease.

Clinical Features of Graft-Versus-Leukemia

Clinical evidence that the donor graft mediates an important anti-leukemic effect comes from higher relapse rates for recipients of syngeneic stem cells than for recipients of HLA-matched sibling grafts.[380] These findings have also been confirmed in a multicenter analysis of HCT recipients with acute myelogenous leukemia (AML) in first remission and subsequent retrospective analyses by the International Bone Marrow Transplant Registry (IBMTR).[381–383] The second IBMTR analysis also showed that the magnitude of this GVL effect is greater for patients with CML and AML and not statistically significant for patients with acute lymphoblastic leukemia (ALL) in first remission.[384,385]

Several case reports of patients with relapse of leukemia after allogeneic HCT noted remissions of the malignancy either after abrupt withdrawal of immunosuppression or during a flare of acute GVHD.[386–389] Patients who develop GVHD after allogeneic HCT experience relapse less frequently than similar patients who do not develop clinical disease. GVHD is protective against relapse both for HCT recipients with advanced leukemia[390–392] and for patients who receive transplants in earlier stages of malignancy.[393] Additional analyses also suggest that the magnitude of the GVL effect appears to be disease and stage-specific.[392–394] Initial reports suggested that chronic GVHD was most protective against relapse,[392] but other analyses demonstrate that acute GVHD is also protective.[393] Based on these reports, newer trials of immunotherapy are designed to include cessation of immunosuppressive therapy (without taper) to induce a GVL reaction for patients whose malignancy has relapsed after HCT. Furthermore, Childs and colleagues demonstrated that the graft-versus-tumor (GVT) effect also plays an important role in inducing remissions from a nonhematologic malignancy, renal cell carcinoma.[395]

Another line of clinical evidence regarding the GVL effect of allogeneic HCT and its tight linkage to GVHD comes from the studies using T-cell depletion of the donor graft. Donor T cells included in the stem cell graft are critical for acute GVHD, and T-cell depletion by various strategies is one of the most successful means of reducing the incidence and severity of GVHD after allogeneic HCT.[26,396–401] Unfortunately, although T-cell depletion results in less treatment-related morbidity and mortality, improved overall survival rates have not been reliably demonstrated. This failure is caused in large part by a reciprocal increase in the subsequent relapse rate after T-cell depletion, as well as to graft failure and other complications.[394,402,403] T-cell depletion increases relapse rates particularly in CML.[393,394,404] This observation provides further strong, albeit indirect, evidence that allogeneic donor T cells are important mediators not only of GVHD, but also of the GVL properties of the allogeneic stem cell graft. Finally, the most compelling evidence of donor T cells in mediating GVL comes from the observations made from donor lymphocyte infusions (discussed later). The induction of GVL is a complex process.

Genetic Basis

The immunotherapeutic effect that occurs in the allo-BMT setting is primarily mediated by allogeneic donor T or NK cells directed against the alloantigens shared by the recipient tumor and target tissues and/or tumor-specific antigens (TSAs) that have the advantage of not being subjected to tolerance mechanisms by the host tumor.[56,405,406] Understanding of the exquisite specificity of T-cell responses led to attempts to identify specific antigens that are responsible for the GVL effect. Much of the focus has been on the identification of (1) certain oncogenic viral proteins (because these are absent in normal cells but expressed by transformed tumor cells [certain Epstein-Barr virus peptides such as Epstein-Barr virus nuclear antigen-1, latent membrane protein {LMP}-1, LMP, LCL]), (2) antigens that are expressed in a tissue-specific fashion (melanoma specific proteins), and (3) proteins that are overexpressed in tumors (WT1, proteinase 3, survivin, telomerase reverse transcriptase, CYPB1, and human epidermal growth factor receptor 2/neu).[53,56]

Although these antigens are specific, most T-cell responses to these antigens are limited because of the poor immunogenicity of these proteins, expression on normal cells, defects in the processing or presentation of tumor antigens, or production of factors that disable T-cell responses. Thus clinical attempts to obtain high specificity of T-cell responses have been offset with difficulties in obtaining enough sensitivity and vice versa. Furthermore, given the current concepts of stem cell origins of leukemia and cancers, identification of the immunogenic proteins that are specifically expressed in the malignant stem cells and harnessing T-cell responses to those antigens will be needed for the optimal GVL effect to cure malignancy.[407,408]

In contrast to the TSAs or tumor-associated antigens (TAAs) discussed earlier, alloantigens are not subjected to tolerance mechanisms. Vaccination strategies with autologous T cells using TAAs or TSAs have yielded disappointing clinical antitumor responses.[409] By contrast, allogeneic HCT has met with remarkable GVL responses perhaps owing to recognition of minor alloantigens in addition to the TAAs.[410] This concept has been demonstrated by recent murine studies, which showed that alloantigen on the tumor cells is required for GVL responses and that the principal targets of GVL are the immunodominant allogeneic MiHAs rather than the TAAs.[60,91] Thus T cells specific for MiHA antigens could provide for a potent GVL effect. Significant progress has been made in the identification of MiHAs that are specifically expressed in the host hematopoietic tissues and therefore might allow for a GVL response without causing GVHD.[53] Together, these results suggest that in addition to tumor-specific proteins, expression of alloantigens and cognate interactions between donor T cells and the tumor tissues are required for the effective induction of the majority of GVL responses. However, T cells specific for some MiHAs are also responsible for GVHD, and a means of consistently separating the beneficial GVL effect from GVHD has not yet been clinically achieved.

Killer-Cell Immunoglobulin-Like Receptor Polymorphisms

The two competing models described earlier, the "mismatched ligand" and the "missing ligand" models for HLA-KIR allorecognition, have been supported by clinical observations of GVL responses in different patient and transplant populations.[65,66] The former model has been shown to separate GVL and GVHD responses in the context of TCD haploidentical HCT for AML.[46,67] Even though this model is supported by elegant laboratory studies, it was found to be invalid for ALL and also for AML after unrelated donor HCT with immunosuppression.[67] Recent retrospective clinical data suggest that GVHD and GVL can be separated by the "missing ligand" model in CML/AML and myelodysplastic syndrome patients after TCD HLA identical sibling HCT.[46,66,69] Further validation of either models by clinical prospective studies and a better understanding of the balance between the inhibitory and activating receptor-ligand interaction of the NK cells are needed to adequately exploit the interface between HLA-KIR genetics to separate GVHD from GVL (see Chapter 102).[64,411]

Chimeric Antigen Receptor T Cells and Cytokine Release Syndrome

Infusion of unselected CD19 specific CAR T cells is associated with a massive cytokine storm that causes severe toxicity, known as cytokine release syndrome (CRS). CRS is a nonantigen-specific toxicity that occurs as a result of high-level immune activation.[412,413] The magnitude of immune activation typically required to mediate clinical benefit using modern immunotherapies exceeds the levels of immune activation that occur in more natural settings. The symptomatology and severity associated with CRS varies greatly and many features of CRS mimic infection. Thus fever is a hallmark, at times temperatures exceeding 40.0°C. Other features, some potentially life threatening, include adult respiratory distress syndrome, fluid retention, neurologic toxicity, cardiac, renal and/or hepatic failure, and disseminated intravascular coagulation. Some of these, particularly lung and cardiac dysfunction, can be rapid onset and severe, but are typically reversible. Neurologic symptoms occurring in the context of CRS are varied and may occur coincident with other symptoms of CRS or may arise when the other symptoms of CRS are resolving.[414] Magnetic resonance imaging often reveals no abnormalities. IL-6 appears to be the most relevant cytokine in CRS, although likely not the only cytokine involved. CRS may also be associated with findings of macrophage activation syndrome/hemophagocytic lymphohistiocytosis.[414] In addition, rapid turnover of underlying leukemia/tumor might lead to tumor lysis syndrome that may coincide or contribute to the severity of CRS. Appropriate supportive care, steroids, and anti–IL-6, tociluzimab remain the current mainstay for management of CRS. Furthermore, whether CRS severity is dependent on the type of T cell being engineered (central versus effector versus naive versus bulk),or the type of vector and/or antigen being targeted remains unknown.

Immunobiology of Graft-Versus-Leukemia Responses

Given the tight association of clinical GVHD and GVL, as well as the common biologic principles governing these responses after allogeneic HCT, it is important to discuss the similarities and distinctions between them in the context of the three cellular phases of GVHD.[415]

Phase 1: Activation of Antigen-Presenting Cells

The concept that tumor eradication after allogeneic HCT might not require toxic chemoradiotherapy and could be achieved primarily by the immunotherapeutic effect from the GVL responses has led to the clinical development of nonmyeloablative HCT for hematologic and nonhematologic malignancies.[416] Phase 1 is characterized by the development of the cytokine storm-generated danger signals from the conditioning regimen and the subsequent activation of APCs.[415] Experimental data suggested that the reduction in conditioning would attenuate the cytokine storm, lead to the development of mixed donor-host chimerism, and confine the GVH response primarily to secondary lymphoid organs, thus cause less severe GVHD without impairing GVL responses.[417–419] However, nonmyeloablative HCT has delayed the kinetics but did not reduce the overall incidence of GVHD and a significant number of patients either failed to respond or relapsed.[21] Furthermore, recent murine and human studies have suggested that homeostatic expansion of T cells in a lymphopenic environment induced by conditioning (as opposed to mere immunosuppression) improves the antitumor efficacy of adoptively transferred syngeneic or autologous T cells by increasing the availability of space, enhancing the memory responses, and reducing the competition for homeostatic cytokines (such as IL-7 and IL-15) for transferred T cells while eliminating regulatory T cells.[420–422] Thus low-intensity HCT clearly demonstrates the principle of the GVL effect, but the roles of the cytokine storm and homeostatic expansion of allogeneic T cells in shaping the intensity of GVL responses are not known.

Host and donor APCs are critical for the induction and severity of GVHD.[7] Activation of APCs is the key step in phase 1 of GVHD.[415] Significant progress has been made in understanding the role of APCs in GVL. Recent experimental evidence has demonstrated a crucial role for professional host APCs in the induction of GVL responses mediated by donor T cells, even when the tumor cells showed some features of APCs.[91,423] Tumors that merely express costimulatory molecules may still be unable to stimulate an effective immune response because of their various "immunoediting" processes that cause ineffective antigen presentation.[424] However, when the tumor cell itself functions as a professional APC, as with CML, it can generate an effective GVL response.[425,426] By contrast, cancers such as acute leukemias that seldom differentiate into APCs generate poor GVL

responses. Data also demonstrated that given sufficient time and a low tumor burden, cross-presentation of TAAs and/or alloantigens by professional donor APCs can occur and may promote or sustain GVL responses by maintaining or expanding alloreactive T cells after initial priming on host APCs.[91,426] This concept is consistent with clinical GVL responses in CML in which the final stage of a GVL response to CML may be the result of donor T cells responding not directly to the small number of CML stem cells or progenitors (which would be undifferentiated and therefore poor APCs) but to tumor antigens cross-presented on professional donor APCs. Emerging data suggest that enhancing such cross-presentation is sufficient to elicit effective GVL responses against acute or advanced leukemia. These data, however, suggest that GVL responses generated after low-intensity conditioning may not be as robust as those after full intensity HCT and highlight the need for a clearer understanding of the effects of the cytokine storm and lymphopenia generated danger signals on the activation of APCs in mediating GVL.

Recent data showed that APC subsets could potentially be modulated to enhance the GVL effect without aggravating GVHD. Host-derived CD8α[+]DCs were shown to be required for the induction of optimal GVT responses when Batf3 deficient mice were used as recipients in experimental allo-HCT.[109] TLR3 stimulation via poly I:C in host CD8α[+]DCs, enhanced GVL responses without exacerbating GVHD. However, cellular processes of regulating GVL responses in host APCs still remain unclear. The molecular mechanisms underpinning the role of host APC subsets in GVL are just now being deciphered. It has been observed that absence of Ikaros in host hematopoietic APCs exacerbates GVHD, but without concomitantly enhancing GVT responses in multiple models.[427] The role of donor-derived DCs in mediating GVL is also being explored. Initial reports regarding this association demonstrated that donor APCs are not required for GVL responses, but play an indispensable role in GVHD in a MHC-matched, MiHA-mismatched BMT model. In order to present host TSAs, via donor APCs, to donor CD8[+]T cells, donor APCs must have the capacity for cross-presentation as they do not express both endogenous alloantigens and TSAs.[428] Furthermore, additional studies are needed to determine which specific subsets of donor APCs play a critical role in enhancing GVT responses. Reports suggest that donor CD11b[−] APCs within the BM grafts consist mostly of pDC progenitors (pre-pDCs) and enhance the GVL activity of donor T cells by promoting differentiation into Th1/type 1 CTLs. Pre-pDCs also regulate GVH and GVT responses altering the balance between donor Tregs and inflammatory T cells by inducing indoleamine 2,3-dioxygenase synthesis.[428]

Phase 2: Donor T-Cell Activation

The core of GVL responses, as with GVHD, is also dependent on the activation of appropriate numbers of T cells. The "second" signals from professional APCs (or certain tumor cells that function as effective APCs) are critical for generating an effective GVL response.[230] Several of the costimulatory pathways that modulate GVHD have also been evaluated in mediating GVL responses. Blockade of CD28 costimulation preserved GVL responses but reduced GVHD in murine studies.[429] However, when the tumor cells also expressed B7 molecules, such blockade reduced the GVL responses.[425] Ex vivo blockade of CD40-CD40L interaction has been shown to reduce GVHD by generating Tregs but still preserve GVL. By contrast, blockade of the 4-1BB pathway reduced both GVHD and GVL.[140] The other costimulatory molecules (OX40 and ICOS) and the inhibitory molecules (CTLA-4 and PD-1) also modulate antitumor responses.[141,142] A better understanding of the context (i.e., low intensity or DLI) and the hierarchy of timing, duration, and extent of costimulatory requirements of donor T-cell subsets might allow for balancing the intensity of GVL and GVHD responses. Clinical and experimental evidence suggest that donor T-cell numbers correlate with the severity of GVHD and GVL responses. TCD grafts had reduced GVHD but increased disease relapse, suggesting a role for

T-cell numbers in GVL responses as well.[430] Clinical attempts to separate GVHD and GVL by regulating allogeneic T-cell dose have met with limited success. For example, administration of 1×10^5 T cells/kg after HLA-matched sibling transplantation did not mediate GVL effects and yet was associated with a measurable incidence of GVHD. Thus infusion of the correct numbers of donor T-cell effectors is crucial for GVL responses.[430] This has been demonstrated by durable responses that are observed in CML and other malignancies after DLI (see later), despite the experimental evidence that host APCs stimulate a stronger GVL response than do donor APCs.[91,426] This could be because, clinically, DLI is almost always given without immunosuppression to an individual who has not developed GVHD either from the chemical immunosuppression or physical removal of donor T cells from the allograft. This lack of immunosuppression after DLI increases the likelihood of a GVH response, and DLI is almost always associated with clinical GVHD. The delivery of additional allogeneic effector cells in DLI also increases the effector:target ratio compared with the time of initial HCT. The latter is also clinically demonstrated by a more effective GVL response to DLI against minimal residual disease (BCR-ABL positivity by PCR) compared with the response against high leukemic burden (e.g., blast crisis) in CML patients.[426] Thus DLI provides the proof, in principle, for the concepts that sufficient T-cell numbers and appropriate antigen presentation are required for both GVHD and an effective GVL response.

T-Cell Subsets

Most experimental studies have implicated donor CD8+ T cells as the primary mediators of GVL, but there are no clinical data for CD8+-mediated GVL responses in the absence of CD4 T cells.[56,236,426] Moreover, some clinical data suggest a role for greater CD4-mediated GVL responses without an increase in GVHD after allogeneic HCT and DLI.[423,431-434] But it is unclear whether CD4+ T-cell initiated GVL responses occur in the absence of generation of MiHA specific CD8+ T cells. Given the critical requirement of alloantigens for most GVL responses, the specific requirement of CD4 and/or CD8 T cells for GVL and GVHD is likely to be determined by the expression of the relevant immunodominant MiHAs and/or TAAs. Therefore it is unlikely that GVHD and GVL responses can be separated under all circumstances merely by depletion of either subset of alloreactive T cells. However, experimental data suggest it might be possible to separate GVHD and GVL when certain donor T-cell subsets are either depleted or infused (DLI) at an appropriate interval after transplant.[423] But the optimal time interval, if any, after clinical HCT is yet to be determined.

Because of recent identification and understanding of the role of various T-cell subsets in mediating immune responses, depletion of specific T-cell subsets to separate GVHD and GVL remains an area of active investigation. For example, recent experimental data suggest that CD62L expressing naive T cells home to secondary lymph nodes and are critical for initiating GVHD.[151] By contrast, CD62L-negative effector memory T cells with enhanced reactivity to recall antigens mediated GVL responses with minimal GVHD.[151] An important caveat to these data is the fact that the lack of a priori knowledge of the repertoire of human memory T cells would make it difficult to predict whether these cells might cross-react only with TAAs or with the recipient's alloantigens. Using CD62L status alone as a determinant of GVHD potential can also have other unintended consequences; recent studies have demonstrated that its expression is critical for the regulation of GVHD by Tregs (see later). Moreover, it is not known whether the behavior of human memory T cells parallels that of murine memory T cells in their migratory, functional, and cytolytic capabilities. Although Tregs reduce antitumor immunity in murine models and in human subjects, experimental data suggest that administration of donor-type Tregs, either at the time of HCT or when delayed, reduced GVHD but preserved CD8+-mediated perforin-dependent GVL responses.[435,436] Similar preservation of experimental GVL was also observed by harnessing donor NKT cell function with granulocyte colony stimulating factor analogues.[178,179] However, it remains unclear whether these observations are valid after

clinical HCT when the GVL responses might not be entirely dependent on CD8 T cells.

T-Cell Migration

It is conceivable that manipulation of these interactions to focus the alloimmune response to lymphohematopoietic tissues would enhance GVL responses but not GVHD. For example, blockade of the CCR9 ligand TECK or CCR5 and CCL17 may prevent the migration of donor T cells to GI tract and skin respectively, but preserve GVL.[220] Pharmacologic manipulation with the immunosuppressive agent FTY720 has recently provided the proof in principle for this approach.[231] Given the redundancy, strategies to modulate the chemokine biology for separation of GVHD and GVL will require greater understanding of these networks in modulating the migration not only of specific T-cell subsets but also of the other immune cells in the context of different conditioning regimens.

Phase 3: Effector Phase of Graft-Versus-Leukemia

The effector arm of GVL is also characterized primarily by the antigen-specific cellular components and less by the inflammatory components of alloresponse. Experimental data demonstrate that neutralization of IL-1α reduced GVHD but preserved GVL.[269] By contrast, donor TNF-α secretion contributes to both GVHD and GVL effects, and in some cases, antagonism of TNF-α reduced GVHD and GVL responses.[437-439] Nonetheless, antagonism of nonspecific inflammatory effectors (such as either IL-1 or TNF-α) appears to regulate GVHD to a greater extent than GVL responses after experimental allogeneic HCT.[439]

Several lines of experimental and clinical data demonstrate that antigen-specific donor T-cell subsets and NK cells are the key effectors of GVL.[56] The cytotoxic pathways that are operative in the NK and T cell–mediated antitumor responses have been well characterized.[56] Fas ligand-mediated CTL of tumor targets is used by both NK and T (mostly Th1) cells, but most murine experiments with FasL-deficient donor T cells suggested that FasL is a key effector molecule for causing GVHD but not GVL.[236] However, one study found that FasL is required for CD4+-mediated GVL against myeloid leukemia.[440,441] By contrast, even though perforin-mediated CTL pathways are also used by T (mostly Th2) and NK cells, experimental data with perforin-deficient donor T cells demonstrated a loss of GVL with a diminution in the severity of GVHD.[236] In some other experimental models, perforin was required only for GVL but not for GVHD.[236] Recent data showed that TRAIL-mediated CTL had no effect on GVHD severity but was required for optimal GVL.[257] Therefore strategies that increase donor T cell TRAIL expression or enhance the susceptibility of tumors to TRAIL-mediated CTL (such as histone deacetylase inhibitors) may promote a robust GVL effect without exacerbating GVHD.[442-444] Thus significant progress has been made in recent understanding of the CTL pathways used by donor T cells for GVL responses, but the role and context of use of these pathways by donor NK and NKT cells after allogeneic HCT are not known.

It is likely that effector cells responsible for the GVL and GVHD effects of HCT will similarly be responsible for the GVL effect associated with DLI, although this assumption has not been formally proven. The administration of select subsets of donor mononuclear cell fractions is the ideal setting in which to dissect the cellular mechanisms responsible for GVL induction and strategies that delay the infusion of these various cellular subsets will help define the mechanisms and enhance the efficacy of DLI.

Immunobiology of Cytokine Release Syndrome After Chimeric Antigen Receptor T-Cell Therapy

CRS has been typically reported with mAb infusions, such as anti-CD3 (OKT3), and the CD28 superagonist etc.[445,446] In recent years it has been increasingly appreciated as the major acute toxicity from infusion of CAR T cells and bispecific antibodies for leukemia.[447,448]

It is characterized by an acute (days, depending on the inducing agent) and intense inflammatory response wherein the majority of the infused CAR T cells along with other immune cells such as NK cells, monocyte-macrophages, and dendritic cells become activated and release inflammatory cytokines.[449,450] Much remains to be understood about the biology of CRS following CAR T-cell therapy. However, it appears that the incidence and severity of the syndrome is greater in patients with large tumor burdens, presumably because of higher levels of T-cell expansion and activation.[414] However, as yet, no clear relationship between the cell infusion dose and the incidence/severity of CRS has been observed. It is associated with a massive proinflammatory cytokine storm with elevated IFN-γ, IL-6, TNF-α, IL-2, granulocyte-macrophage colony-stimulating factor and IL-5.[414] Amongst these cytokines, it appears that in many instances IL-6 may be the most critical cytokine and its effects are likely from trans-signaling. The source of IL-6 and mechanisms remain unknown. The biology behind the incidence of neurotoxicities remains unclear. It is also unknown whether CRS is required for eventual clinical response and/or if mitigating it blunts response rates. Furthermore, whether CRS is reduced when selected T cells (central memory subset) are engineered with CARs instead of using bulk T cells remains an open question. The relationship of CRS with the type of vectors or other methodologic aspects also remains unknown.

Several other critical mechanisms for enhancing the efficacy of CAR T cells or for mitigating their toxicities remain to be understood. The data on whether other targets (instead of CD19) can be as effective remain to be explored. The role of costimulatory domains in promoting efficacy, toxicity or exhaustion remains largely unknown. Recent experimental observations suggest that CARs against non-CD19 targets may be more susceptible to exhaustion and in these cells CD28 costimulation augments, whereas 4-1BB costimulation reduces, exhaustion induced by persistent CAR signaling.[451] Thus much remains to be understood with regards to the immunobiology of CRS, and CAR T-cell therapy.

FUTURE DIRECTIONS

Complications of HCT, particularly GVHD, remain major barriers to the wider application of allogeneic HCT for a variety of diseases. Recent advances in the biology of genetic polymorphisms, the chemocytokine networks, several novel cellular subsets including regulatory T cells, and the direct mediators of cellular cytotoxicity have led to improved understanding of this complex disease process. Animal studies show that modulation of several mediators of the complex GVHD cascade may be able to reduce the undesirable inflammatory aspects of GVHD while preserving the benefits of GVL. However, most of the laboratory observations remain to be studied in well-controlled clinical trials. Multiple cellular effectors may be involved in GVL, although donor T-cell recognition of host antigens is an important element of this process. Cellular immunotherapy such as DLI offers a strategy for separating GVHD and the GVL effect. Both experimental and clinical data suggest that posttransplantation cellular immunotherapy can be performed relatively safely and effectively, and optimization of patient selection, cell dose, and timing of administration may all serve to limit toxicity and enhance the potential GVL effects.

SUGGESTED READINGS

Alousi AM, Weisdorf DJ, Logan BR, et al: Etanercept, mycophenolate, denileukin or pentostatin plus corticosteroids for acute graft vs. host disease: a randomized phase II trial from the BMT CTN. *Blood* 114:511, 2009.

Anasetti C, Beatty PG, Storb R, et al: Effect of HLA incompatibility on graft-versus-host disease, relapse, and survival after marrow transplantation for patients with leukemia or lymphoma. *Hum Immunol* 29:79, 1990.

Billingham RE: The biology of graft-versus-host reactions. *Harvey Lect* 62:21, 1966-67.

Blazar BR, Murphy WJ, Abedi M: Advances in graft-versus-host disease biology and therapy. *Nat Rev Immunol* 12(6):443, 2012.

Choi SW, Braun T, Chang L, et al: Vorinostat plus tacrolimus and mycophenolate to prevent graft-versus-host disease after related-donor reduced-intensity conditioning allogeneic haemopoietic stem-cell transplantation: a phase 1/2 trial. *Lancet Oncol* 15(1):87, 2014.

Den Haan JM, Sherman NE, Blokland E, et al: Identification of a graft versus host disease-associated human minor histocompatibility antigen. *Science* 268:1476, 1995.

Dickinson AM, Middleton PG, Rocha V, et al: Genetic polymorphisms predicting the outcome of bone marrow transplants. *Br J Haematol* 127:479, 2004.

Edinger M, Hoffmann P, Ermann J, et al: CD4+CD25+ regulatory T cells preserve graft-versus-tumor activity while inhibiting graft-versus-host disease after bone marrow transplantation. *Nat Med* 9:1144, 2003.

Glucksberg H, Storb R, Fefer A, et al: Clinical manifestations of graft-versus-host disease in human recipients of marrow from HL-A-matched sibling donors. *Transplantation* 18:295, 1974.

Goulmy E, Schipper R, Pool J, et al: Mismatches of minor histocompatibility antigens between HLA-identical donors and recipients and the development of graft-versus-host disease after bone marrow transplantation. *N Engl J Med* 334:281, 1996.

Henden AS, Hill GR: Cytokines in Graft-Versus-Host Disease. *J Immunol* 194:4604, 2015.

Kolb H, Mittermuller J, Clemm C, et al: Donor leukocyte transfusions for treatment of recurrent chronic myelogenous leukemia in marrow transplant patients. *Blood* 76:2462, 1990.

Korngold R, Sprent J: Negative selection of T cells causing lethal graft-versus-host disease across minor histocompatibility barriers. Role of the H-2 complex. *J Exp Med* 151:1114, 1980.

Levine JE, Braun TM, Harris AC, et al: A prognostic score for acute graft-versus-host disease based on biomarkers: a multicentre study. *Lancet Haematol* 2:e21–e29, 2015.

Lindemans CA, Calafiore M, Mertelsmann AM, et al: Interleukin-22 promotes intestinal-stem-cell-mediated epithelial regeneration. *Nature* 528(7583):560–564, 2015.

Lowsky R, Takahashi T, Liu YP, et al: Protective conditioning for acute graft-versus-host disease. *N Engl J Med* 353:1321, 2005.

Martin PJ, Weisdorf D, Przepiorka D, et al: National Institutes of Health Consensus Development Project on Criteria for Clinical Trials in Chronic Graft-versus-Host Disease: VI. Design of Clinical Trials Working Group report. *Biol Blood Marrow Transplant* 12:491, 2006.

Mathewson ND, Jenq R, Mathew AV, et al: Gut microbiome-derived metabolites modulate intestinal epithelial cell damage and mitigate graft-versus-host disease. *Nat Immunol* 17(5):505–513, 2016.

Petersdorf EW, Hansen JA, Martin PJ, et al: Major-histocompatibility-complex class I alleles and antigens in hematopoietic-cell transplantation. *N Engl J Med* 345:1794, 2001.

Ratanatharathorn V, Nash RA, Przepiorka D, et al: Phase III study comparing methotrexate and tacrolimus (prograf, FK506) with methotrexate and cyclosporine for graft-versus-host disease prophylaxis after HLA-identical sibling bone marrow transplantation. *Blood* 92:2303, 1998.

Reddy P, Maeda Y, Liu C, et al: A crucial role for antigen-presenting cells and alloantigen expression in graft-versus-leukemia responses. *Nat Med* 11:1244, 2005.

Shlomchik WD, Couzens MS, Tang CB, et al: Prevention of graft versus host disease by inactivation of host antigen-presenting cells. *Science* 285:412, 1999.

Shulman HM, Sharma P, Amos D, et al: A coded histologic study of hepatic graft-versus-host disease after human bone marrow transplantation. *Hepatology* 8:463, 1988.

Storb R, Deeg HJ, Whitehead J, et al: Methotrexate and cyclosporine compared with cyclosporine alone for prophylaxis of acute graft versus host disease after marrow transplantation for leukemia. *N Engl J Med* 314:729, 1986.

van Bekkum DW, Roodenburg J, Heidt PJ, et al: Mitigation of secondary disease of allogeneic mouse radiation chimeras by modification of the intestinal microflora. *J Natl Cancer Inst* 52:401, 1974.

Vander Lugt MT, Braun TM, Hanash S, et al: ST2 as a marker for risk of therapy-resistant graft-versus-host disease and death. *N Engl J Med* 369(6):529–539, 2013.

Weiden PL, Flournoy N, Thomas ED, et al: Antileukemic effect of graft-versus-host disease in human recipients of allogeneic-marrow grafts. *N Engl J Med* 300:1068, 1979.

Wekerle T, Kurtz J, Ito H, et al: Allogeneic bone marrow transplantation with co-stimulatory blockade induces macrochimerism and tolerance without cytoreductive host treatment. *Nat Med* 6:464, 2000.

Zeiser R, Blazar BR: Preclinical models of acute and chronic graft-versus-host disease: how predictive are they for a successful clinical translation? *Blood* 127:3117–3126, 2016.

REFERENCES

For the complete list of references, log on to www.expertconsult.com.

CHAPTER 109

COMPLICATIONS AFTER HEMATOPOIETIC CELL TRANSPLANTATION

Shernan G. Holtan, Navneet S. Majhail, and Daniel J. Weisdorf

The high-dose therapy used in hematopoietic cell transplantation (HCT) results in toxicities induced directly by the treatment and secondarily by the prolonged immunodeficiency and extended recovery process. Identification of risk factors for particular complications allows the design of risk-specific supportive care regimens that may reduce the morbidity and mortality accompanying transplantation. HCT-related complications can be broadly classified into infections, early noninfectious complications (within 3 months of HCT), late noninfectious complications (after 3 months of HCT), and graft-versus-host disease (GVHD) (Table 109.1).

INFECTIONS

Infections are among the most frequent causes of nonrelapse mortality in HCT recipients and cause significant morbidity, both in the early and late transplant period (Table 109.2). Immune defects occurring in the posttransplant period can be divided into predictable phases based on time from engraftment (sustained absolute neutrophil count >500/μL), with characteristic infections in each phase (Fig. 109.1). Antimicrobial prophylaxis regimens tailored to address the risk of specific infections during these time periods are effective in limiting the incidence of posttransplant opportunistic infections (Table 109.3). Evidence-based guidelines for preventing infectious complications in HCT recipients have been published and can be used as a reference for determining infection risk and assigning antimicrobial prophylaxis for individual patients.[1]

Engraftment generally occurs within 7–14 days in autologous and 10–28 days in allogeneic HCT recipients. Recipients of grafts from unrelated donors (URD) or umbilical cord blood (UCB) tend to engraft later compared with sibling donors; marrow grafts recover a bit more slowly than filgrastim-mobilized peripheral blood stem cell (PBSC) grafts. Importantly, up to 5% of URDs (or potentially greater if human leukocyte antigen [HLA]-mismatched) and approximately 10% of UCB grafts may fail to engraft leading to prolonged neutropenia and extended transfusion dependence. In addition to neutropenia, the main risk factors for infection during this preengraftment phase are disruption of mucocutaneous barriers and indwelling venous catheters. Bacterial infections can occur in up to 30% of transplant recipients during this initial period and usually arise from normal flora of the skin (coagulase-negative *Staphylococcus*), oropharynx, and gastrointestinal tract (*Streptococcus viridans*, *Enterococcus* spp. and enteric gram-negative bacilli). Colonizing yeasts or inhaled airborne molds also invade because of neutropenia and disruption of normal host flora and can lead to systemic mycotic infections (most often candida or aspergillus spp.) in 10% to 15% of patients. Reactivation of latent herpes viruses (herpes simplex, cytomegalovirus [CMV] or human herpesvirus [HHV]-6 can occur, but may be contained by antiviral prophylaxis.

The predominant immunologic defects seen in the early and late postengraftment period are impairments of cellular and humoral immune systems. This underlying severe immune dysfunction is enhanced and prolonged by acute and chronic GVHD and by corticosteroids and the immunosuppressive agents used for GVHD prevention and treatment. The incidence of late opportunistic infections is much lower in autologous HCT recipients because of faster immune reconstitution and the lack of immunosuppressive drug therapy. Immune reconstitution can take up to 2 years to fully recover in allogeneic HCT recipients and may be incomplete because of ongoing GVHD. Patients with chronic GVHD can be functionally asplenic and be at risk for infections by encapsulated bacteria including pneumococcus or *H. influenza*. In addition, chronic GVHD patients on long-term immunosuppression remain susceptible to fungi (*Aspergillus* spp., *Candida* spp. and *Pneumocystis jiroveci*) and viruses including CMV and varicella zoster virus (VZV). Additional factors that can delay immune reconstitution include donor-recipient HLA disparity, with depletion of T cells either through ex vivo graft manipulation or in vivo with antithymocyte globulin (ATG) or alemtuzumab. URDs and possibly UCB as a graft source may also augment infection risks.[2,3] Antimicrobial prophylaxis should continue beyond the initial posttransplant period, typically for at least 3–6 months after cessation of all immunosuppression, especially in patients being treated for chronic GVHD. Some centers use total T cell (CD3+) and particularly CD4 cell levels as surrogate markers of T-cell recovery and to guide decisions regarding the intensity and duration of infection surveillance and antimicrobial prophylaxis. Supplemental intravenous immunoglobulin (IVIg) has been considered for patients with persistent hypogammaglobulinemia (immunoglobulin G [IgG] levels <400 mg/dL), but its prophylactic use is costly, does not prolong survival or prevent late infections, and may impair humoral immune reconstitution. Patients with GVHD and those with indwelling venous access undergoing endoscopy or dental procedures should receive antibiotics for endocarditis prophylaxis. Published guidelines are available for immunization of HCT survivors (Table 109.4).[1]

Based on the type and dose of conditioning chemotherapy and radiation, recipients of nonmyeloablative or reduced-intensity conditioning (NMA/RIC) regimens can exhibit varying degrees of myelosuppression.[4] The incidence of bacterial infections is lower in NMA/RIC recipients because of the shorter duration of posttransplant neutropenia. However, the degree of lymphodepletion tends to be comparable with that seen with myeloablative regimens and the risks of invasive aspergillosis and CMV reactivation remain unchanged.

Among UCB HCT recipients, neutrophil engraftment and immune reconstitution can be delayed and a higher incidence of bacterial and viral infections in the early posttransplant period has been reported. Overall, the risk of serious infections among children receiving UCB grafts is comparable with that of URD marrow and is lower than that of a T-cell depleted graft source.[2] Among adult UCB HCT recipients, the incidence of infections is higher in the early posttransplant period; however, infections do not compromise the risks of overall and nonrelapse mortality compared with URD HCT.[2]

The approach to managing posttransplant infections is generally similar to that for infections in patients with cancer, especially acute leukemia (Chapter 89). However, certain infections, particularly caused by viruses and fungi, are more common in the HCT population and are discussed in further detail here.

Febrile Neutropenia

A large proportion of patients develop fever in the early posttransplantation period though an infectious pathogen is identified in only

TABLE 109.1	Major Complications of Hematopoietic Cell Transplantation	
	Complication	**Incidence (%)**
Infections	Bacterial infections	
	Gram-positive bacteremia	20–30
	Gram-negative bacteremia	5–10
	Viral infections	
	Cytomegalovirus	5–40 in high risk patients[a]
	Herpes simplex virus	5–10 in seropositive patients
	Varicella-zoster virus	10–50 in seropositive patients
	Respiratory viruses	10–20
	Fungal infections	
	Candida	5–10
	Aspergillus and other molds	5–15
	Pneumocystis jirovecii	<1
	Other infections	
	Toxoplasma gondii	2–7 in seropositive patients
Early noninfectious	Regimen-related toxicity	
Complications	Mucositis	60–75
(0–3 months)	Hemorrhagic cystitis	5–10
	Venoocclusive disease	5–40
	Pneumonitis	10–20
	Alveolar hemorrhage	5–10
	Graft failure	2–10
	Adverse drug reactions	Common
Late noninfectious	Organ specific late effects	
Complications	Cataracts	25–40
(>3 months)	Hypothyroidism	30–50
	Sterility/hypogonadism	50–90
	Growth disturbances	30–50 in prepubertal children
	Osteoporosis/avascular necrosis	5–20
	Malignant relapse	Variable
	Second cancers	2–12
Graft-versus-host disease	Acute	20–50 with related, 40–90 with unrelated donors, 20–50 with UCB
	Chronic	20–40 with related, 40–70 with unrelated donors, 20–40 with UCB

[a]CMV-seropositive HCT recipients or CMV-seronegative recipients with a CMV-seropositive donor.
UCB, umbilical cord blood.

50% of patients. Fever may also be caused by tissue inflammation (oropharyngeal or enteric mucositis), transfusions, amphotericin (now used infrequently in the era of mold-active azoles), or other drug fever. Bacterial infections caused by aerobic bacteria such as coagulase-negative *Staphylococci*, *Viridans streptococci* and enteric gram-negative bacilli are the primary concern during this neutropenic phase, although there is also an ongoing risk of infections with yeasts.

Prophylactic strategies can include suppressive antimicrobials, directed against aerobic, particularly enteric bacteria and fungi.

Empiric therapy with broad spectrum antibiotics is usually started at fever onset along with appropriate clinical and microbiologic evaluation. The choice of antibiotics depends on prior and current antibiotic usage modified by local resistance patterns and can be based on recommendations available for the treatment of febrile neutropenia in cancer patients.[5] Among patients with persistent febrile neutropenia, that is fever without an identified focus that continues despite 3–5 days of appropriate broad-spectrum antibiotics, invasive fungal infections should be considered.[6] Initiating empiric antifungal therapy with mold-active agents such as voriconazole, an echinocandin or amphotericin is generally recommended at this stage. The choice of agent is dependent on prior exposure to antimold agents for prophylaxis where resistant species (e.g., zygomycetes) may emerge. Empiric mold specific therapy can be started earlier in patients who have experienced prolonged periods of neutropenia pre-HCT (e.g., patients with myelodysplastic syndromes [MDSs]). Repeated vigorous investigation to identify sources of infection (e.g., with computed tomography [CT] scan of the chest and sinuses), even for fever recurring after initial defervescence, is essential. Although administration of myeloid growth factors (granulocyte colony-stimulating factor [G-CSF] or granulocyte-macrophage CSF [GM-CSF]) reduces the duration of neutropenia and accelerates engraftment, they have not been demonstrated to reduce mortality from early posttransplant infections. Granulocyte infusions are applied rarely for life-threatening infections during the preengraftment phase. Novel cellular therapies, such as third-party expanded myeloid progenitor cells are currently being studied for their role in providing protection from severe infections before engraftment.

Cytomegalovirus Infection

Epidemiology and Risk Factors

Despite the introduction of effective antiviral therapies, CMV infection continues to be a major cause of infection-related morbidity and mortality in HCT recipients.[7] The risk of CMV reactivation spans both the early and late transplant period, especially in patients with GVHD on prolonged immunosuppression. Although the incidence of early CMV disease with organ involvement has declined to 3% to 6% with the use of empiric antiviral drug therapy directed by routine surveillance with CMV DNA polymerase chain reaction (PCR) or antigenemia testing, late onset CMV infection is still seen in up to 20% to 40% of patients.[7]

Seropositivity of the recipient is the most important risk factor for CMV infection in HCT recipients, and reactivation of latent virus is the most important mechanism resulting in CMV disease. Nearly all CMV infections (<5%) in seronegative recipients are the result of exogenous exposure (primary CMV infection), either from a seropositive stem cell donor or from cellular blood products collected from CMV seropositive donors. The possibility of false negative serology pre-HCT should also be considered in patients with early CMV reactivation. CMV infection and especially end-organ CMV disease is also more frequent following allogeneic HCT, with CMV infections occurring in less than 5% of autograft recipients. However, autologous HCT recipients who have previously received T-cell suppressive therapies (e.g., fludarabine, alemtuzumab) can be at high-risk for CMV infection. Among patients undergoing allogeneic transplantation, the risk may be greater with URD compared with related donors. Although the prevalence of donor seropositivity is nearly zero in UCB grafts, the risk of posttransplant CMV infection may be similar as recipient CMV status is still the predominant risk factor for infection although the CMV naive UCB graft confers no latent protective immunity against CMV.[8] Other factors that delay immune reconstitution may also increase the risk for CMV infection, including older recipient age, greater donor-recipient HLA mismatch, acute and chronic GVHD, and need for prolonged immunosuppression, especially with high-dose corticosteroids. CMV

TABLE 109.2 Common Infections in Hematopoietic Cell Transplant Recipients

Pathogen	Risk Period After HCT	Risk Factors	Common Clinical Syndromes	Treatment
Gram-positive cocci	1–4 wk	Neutropenia Mucositis Central venous catheters Skin breakdown	Bacteremia	Antibiotics based on susceptibility testing
Enterobacteriaceae spp.	1–4 wk	Neutropenia Skin breakdown GI mucosal breakdown	Bacteremia	Antibiotics based on susceptibility testing
Clostridium difficile	1–8 wk	Antibiotics	Colitis	Metronidazole Oral vancomycin
Encapsulated bacteria[a]	>12 wk	Chronic GVHD Chronic immunosuppression	Sinusitis Pneumonia	Antibiotics based on susceptibility testing
Candida spp.	1–4 wk	Neutropenia Skin breakdown GI mucosal breakdown	Candidemia Mucocutaneous Hepatosplenic	Azoles Echinocandins Amphotericin
Aspergillus spp.	1–4 wk >8 wk	HLA-disparity CMV infection Acute or chronic GVHD Chronic immunosuppression High-dose corticosteroids	Sinusitis Pulmonary nodules or infiltrates	Mold-specific azoles Echinocandins Amphotericin
Pneumocystis jirovecii	>4 wk	Chronic GVHD Chronic immunosuppression	Pneumonia	TMP-SMX Dapsone Pentamidine
CMV	>4 wk	Recipient or donor seropositivity HLA-disparity Acute or chronic GVHD Chronic immunosuppression	Viremia Enteritis Interstitial pneumonitis	Ganciclovir Valganciclovir Foscarnet Cidofovir or Brindcidofovir
HSV	1–4 wk	Recipient seropositivity	Oropharyngeal Esophagitis	Acyclovir Valacyclovir Foscarnet
VZV	>4 wk	Recipient seropositivity History of chicken pox HLA disparity Acute or chronic GVHD Chronic immunosuppression	Cutaneous Interstitial pneumonitis Hepatitis	Acyclovir Valacyclovir Foscarnet
EBV	>4 wk	HLA disparity T-cell depletion	Viremia PTLD	Rituximab Reduce immunosuppression Virus-specific T cells Cytotoxic chemotherapy

[a]Includes *S. pneumoniae, H. influenzae,* and *N. meningitidis.*
CMV, cytomegalovirus; EBV, Epstein-Barr virus; GI, gastrointestinal tract; GVHD, graft-versus-host disease; HCT, hematopoietic cell transplantation; HLA, human leukocyte antigen; HSV, herpes simplex virus; PTLD, posttransplant lymphoproliferative disorder; TMP-SMX, trimethoprim-sulfamethoxazole; VZV, varicella-zoster virus.

TABLE 109.3 Recommended Antimicrobial Prophylaxis Against Common Infections

Pathogen	Preventing Early Disease (0–100 days after HCT)	Preventing Late Disease (>100 days after HCT)
Bacterial infections	No specific recommendations[a]	Antibiotics (based on local resistance patterns) to prevent infections caused by encapsulated bacteria (*S. pneumoniae, H. influenzae,* and *N. meningitidis*) in patients on chronic immunosuppression
CMV	Prophylaxis or preemptive treatment with ganciclovir or valganciclovir in high risk patients[b]	Preemptive treatment with ganciclovir or valganciclovir in high-risk patients[b]
HSV	Acyclovir in seropositive patients	Acyclovir in patients with recurrent HSV infections
Yeast infections	Fluconazole	Fluconazole in patients on chronic immunosuppression
Mold infections	No specific recommendations[c]	No specific recommendations[a]
Pneumocystis jirovecii	Trimethoprim-sulfamethoxazole (preferred) or dapsone or pentamidine	Trimethoprim-sulfamethoxazole (preferred) or dapsone or pentamidine in patients on chronic immunosuppression
Respiratory viruses	Isolation; masks; hand-washing Vaccination of household contacts	Vaccination of patient and household contacts

[a]Limited data exist favoring fluoroquinolones such as levofloxacin. No impact on infection-related mortality.
[b]CMV-seropositive HCT recipients or CMV-seronegative recipients with a CMV-seropositive donor.
[c]Limited data available. Prospective testing of voriconazole and posaconazole suggests possible benefit as prophylaxis. No impact on mold-related mortality.
CMV, cytomegalovirus; HCT, hematopoietic cell transplantation; HSV, herpes simplex virus.

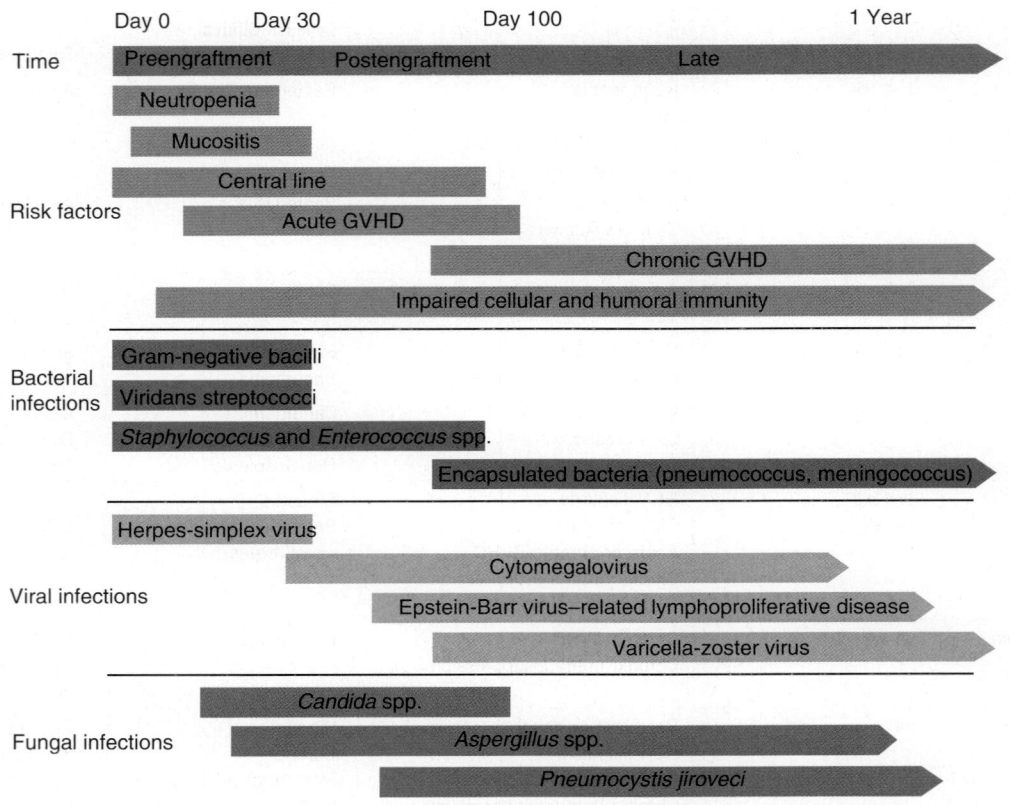

Fig. 109.1 COMMON INFECTIONS IN HCT RECIPIENTS. *GVHD*, Graft-versus-host disease.

TABLE 109.4	Recommended Vaccinations for Hematopoietic Cell Transplant Recipients	
Vaccine[a]	Time Post-HCT to Initiate Vaccine (months)	No. of Doses[b]
Pneumococcal conjugate (PCV)	3–6	2–3[c]
Tetanus, diphtheria, acellular pertussis[d]	6–12	3
Haemophilus influenzae conjugate	6–12	3
Inactivated polio	6–12	3
Recombinant hepatitis B	6–12	3
Inactivated influenza	4–6	1–2 yearly[e]
Measles-mumps-rubella (live)	24	1–2[f]
Varicella zoster	24	1[f]

[a]Vaccinations are deferred in patients with chronic GVHD until discontinuation of immunosuppression
[b]A minimum of 1 month interval between doses is suggested
[c]Following the primary series of three PCV doses, a dose of the 23-valent polysaccharide pneumococcal vaccine (PPSV23) to broaden the immune response might be given. For patients with chronic GVHD who are likely to respond poorly to PPSV23, a fourth dose of the PCV should be considered instead of PPSV23.
[d]Diphtheria tetanus pertussis vaccine (DTaP) is preferred, however, Tdap can be used if DTaP is not available.
[e]For children <9 years of age, two doses are recommended yearly between transplant and 9 years of age.
[f]Not recommended <24 months post-HCT, in patients with active GVHD and in patients on immune suppression. In children, two doses of MMR are favored. Lower viral dose vaccines (varicella vaccine, live [varivax], not zoster vaccine, live [zostavax]) may be preferred as potentially safer.
GVHD, Graft-versus-host disease; MMR, major molecular response; PPSV23, 23-valent; pneumococcal polysaccharide vaccine; Tdap, tetanus toxoid, reduced diphtheria toxoid, and acellular pertussis vaccine.

reactivation posttransplantation has been recently associated with natural killer (NK) cell maturation toward an innate memory-cell phenotype that may contribute to both infection control and possibly to reduced cancer relapse after allogeneic HCT.[9]

Clinical Presentation and Diagnosis

The most common manifestation of CMV infection is asymptomatic reactivation noted by screening antigenemia or DNA PCR testing. CMV organ infection and disease are most often pneumonia and enteritis. CMV is the most common specific cause of interstitial pneumonitis and is responsible for up to 50% of all cases. Infection at other sites such as retinitis, hepatitis and central nervous system disease are less common and are usually seen in late-onset or persisting CMV infection. Indirect effects of CMV infection may include increased risks of graft rejection plus bacterial and fungal superinfection. The presence of posttransplant CMV viremia is a strong predictor of subsequent clinical CMV disease. CMV pneumonia develops in 60% of patients with untreated asymptomatic viremia, and treatment of viremia can reduce the incidence of CMV pneumonia to less than 5%. Although autologous HCT recipients have a lower risk of developing CMV infection, the severity of infection (e.g., pneumonia), if it develops, is similar to that observed in recipients of allogeneic HCT.

The diagnosis of CMV can be made either by demonstration of characteristic cytology or cytopathic effects in tissue culture or by the use of more sensitive molecular methods that detect viral proteins or DNA. Commonly used molecular assays include CMV DNA detection methods, and the pp65 antigenemia assay. Detection of the CMV pp65 antigen in leukocytes has been the commonly used method for CMV surveillance after HCT, but is ineffective during early post-HCT leukopenia. However, direct detection of CMV DNA either by PCR or DNA hybrid capture assay is the most sensitive method to detect CMV. Furthermore, plasma CMV DNA PCR, though not as sensitive as whole blood PCR, can be a valuable tool to monitor CMV during periods of neutropenia when CMV antigenemia testing is unreliable. In addition, quantitative real-time PCR assays allow estimation of viral load which can assist in determining need for therapy and risk of disease progression and in monitoring response among patients receiving anti-CMV treatment. Viral cultures of urine, saliva, blood or bronchioalveolar lavage (BAL), using either rapid shell-vial or routine culture techniques, have limited clinical utility since they are less sensitive than antigen or DNA detection techniques and take much longer to report. Shell-vial cultures of CMV from BAL fluid are less specific for CMV pneumonia and can be positive in asymptomatic seropositive patients without pneumonia who are shedding CMV in oral or respiratory secretions. Despite this lack of specificity, even in asymptomatic patients, finding CMV in BAL fluid is a strong predictor for the development of subsequent CMV pneumonia, and treatment should be initiated.

Prevention and Treatment

For seronegative recipients, the use of seronegative donors and CMV-safe blood products is the mainstay of prevention of CMV disease (Box 109.1). For high-risk patients (seropositive recipients or seropositive donors for seronegative recipients), two general strategies can be used, both of which have been effective in reducing early CMV infection rates to less than 10%.[7] The first is the "preemptive" approach, which involves prompt treatment of early CMV viremia with ganciclovir, valganciclovir, or foscarnet before it can lead to clinical disease. The second is the "general prophylaxis" approach, in which all at-risk patients are treated with antiviral prophylaxis. The former approach requires availability and frequent scheduled application of reliable and rapid early diagnostic tests. The latter approach can reduce the rate of early CMV infection, but does not impact mortality or the risk for late CMV infection and is associated with a higher incidence of ganciclovir-induced myelosuppression. Both approaches require aggressive surveillance to allow prompt detection of infection. High-dose acyclovir or valacyclovir, although not as effective as ganciclovir, also reduces the incidence of CMV viremia, but continued surveillance for CMV is still required with prompt initiation of preemptive therapy with ganciclovir or foscarnet when viremia develops. Unlike ganciclovir, which has to be administered intravenously, its prodrug valganciclovir, has excellent oral bioavailability and is often used for prophylaxis and preemptive therapy of CMV infection among HCT recipients. Since autologous HCT recipients have a lower risk of CMV disease, the preemptive approach to preventing CMV infection is usually sufficient. Surveillance for CMV is continued weekly until at least day 100 posttransplant for high-risk patients and is continued longer in patients with chronic GVHD on high-dose immunosuppression.

CMV disease, especially pneumonia, must be diagnosed and treated promptly as it remains associated with very high rates of mortality. The combined use of ganciclovir and IVIg has been the most successful treatment for CMV pneumonia, with resolution in 50% to 75% of nonventilator dependent patients. Prolonged therapy (>2 months) with the combination is indicated because shorter treatment regimens have been associated with recurrence of CMV pneumonia. Foscarnet can be effective in clinical settings in which ganciclovir fails or is associated with excess toxicity, usually myelosuppression. Although treatment is generally similar, with ganciclovir or foscarnet plus immunoglobulin, CMV enteritis, hepatitis, and retinitis are variably responsive. Valganciclovir may be considered for treatment of mild to moderate CMV organ disease, although more prolonged administration may be required.[10] Adoptive cellular therapies (using approaches to enhance NK or infuse CMV-specific T cells) are also being explored. Although rare, CMV antiviral resistance can occur and ganciclovir or foscarnet can be used as alternative drugs for second-line therapy. Cidofovir can be considered when disease progresses despite treatment with ganciclovir and foscarnet and a

| BOX 109.1 | Approach to Prevention and Treatment of Cytomegalovirus Infection |

Prevention

1. Seronegative recipient with seronegative donor (allogeneic and autologous): Transfuse only cytomegalovirus (CMV) safe blood products. Leukocyte depletion by filtration and blood from CMV-seronegative donors are clinically equivalent alternatives.
2. Seronegative recipient with seropositive donor (allogeneic): Deliver only CMV-safe blood products (seronegative or leukocyte depleted), but administer chemoprophylaxis as well to prevent reactivation of donor-derived and transmitted latent virus.
3. Seropositive recipients: Prophylaxis with acyclovir appears to be somewhat useful. Use of immunoglobulin may be beneficial. There is no proven role for seronegative blood products. Ganciclovir is highly effective when given prophylactically, but is myelosuppressive. Patients who must interrupt the course of ganciclovir because of leukopenia are at risk for development of CMV reactivation and disease. Ganciclovir (or valganciclovir) is the current best prophylaxis in high-risk patients, but is not indicated for autologous recipients. Intensive surveillance and early preemptive therapy may be equivalently effective.
4. All patients need periodic (weekly) monitoring for CMV antigenemia or CMV DNA polymerase chain reaction for 8–12 weeks posttransplantation. Longer duration (beyond 12 weeks) surveillance is appropriate for allograft recipients, especially those with graft-versus-host disease.

Treatment

1. Asymptomatic infections (allogeneic and autologous): Ganciclovir or valganciclovir treatment of asymptomatic infection detected in blood or bronchioalveolar lavage (BAL), by either molecular detection or antigenic methods, is recommended to prevent the development of CMV pneumonia. Intensive induction treatment (2 weeks) followed by a maintenance phase of 5+ days/week therapy for an additional 4–8 weeks is necessary.
2. CMV pneumonia: Ganciclovir in combination with immunoglobulin is recommended. This should be instituted promptly. Once the disease has progressed to cause respiratory failure and ventilator dependence, survival is limited.

No Treatment

1. Empiric CMV therapy for interstitial pneumonitis is not indicated in seronegative recipients with seronegative graft and blood donors. Diagnostic evidence of CMV infection should be obtained.
2. Empiric CMV therapy for interstitial pneumonitis is also not indicated in patients whose BAL is negative for CMV by direct staining and molecular testing. However, BAL CMV studies have a small (<5%) false-negative rate, and close follow up and monitoring is still required.
3. Asymptomatic CMV viruria does not require therapy, but does need close follow up and serial blood viral testing for surveillance of systemic disease.

liposomal formulation of cidofovir with good oral bioavailability (CMX-001, brincidofovir) is being studied in prophylaxis and treatment of CMV infections in HCT.

Other Latent Viral Infections

Primary and reactivation infections of other herpesviruses can occur after transplantation. Herpes simplex virus (HSV) infection is uncommon with the use of acyclovir or valacyclovir prophylaxis in seropositive patients. Acyclovir-resistant HSV infection can occur in patients given low-dose prophylaxis or intermittent treatment and in recipients of T-cell depleted grafts. Foscarnet is the drug of choice for resistant disease with cidofovir reserved as an alternative agent. VZV reactivation can occur in 30% to 50% of HCT recipients with previous exposure to VZV, and can be effectively delayed and possibly prevented by acyclovir prophylaxis. Acyclovir prophylaxis has been suggested for the 6–12 months after transplantation for VZV seropositive autologous and allogeneic HCT recipients; patients with chronic GVHD need to continue prophylaxis for the duration of their immunosuppression.[1]

Human polyomavirus type I, also known as BK virus, can cause hemorrhagic cystitis in the early posttransplant period. Urine PCR can identify BK virus and distinguish it from hemorrhagic cystitis caused by other infections (e.g., adenovirus) and urotoxic agents (e.g., cyclophosphamide). Quinolone antibiotics suppress BK virus replication in vivo and in vitro and may have a role as prophylaxis in patients at high risk for hemorrhagic cystitis.[1] Along with bladder irrigation or forced polyuria intravesical or intravenous cidofovir has been used for the treatment of BK virus hemorrhagic cystitis.[1] Rarely, BK virus encephalitis has been described postallogeneic HCT. Another polyoma virus, John Cunningham virus, can reactivate in immunocompromised HCT recipients and lead progressive multifocal leukoencephalopathy, a fatal demyelinating disease of the central nervous system. Severe immune deficiency is the primary risk factor for these opportunistic infections, and treatment is primarily supportive and aimed at an improving immune function, if possible.

HHV-6 can also reactivate from latency post-HCT, with incidence ranging from 20% in recipients of grafts from matched sibling donors, 46% in URDs, and 69% of recipients of UCB grafts, at a median of 23 days after HCT.[11] Although reactivation is common, routine surveillance is not necessary. Rather, preemptive treatment of a high viral load (>25,000 copies) with ganciclovir or foscarnet, in the presence of symptoms (headache, mental status changes, unexplained fever and/or rash, delayed engraftment or marrow suppression) should be considered. Reactivation of HHV-6 is common and is rarely associated with poor post-HCT outcomes.

Acquired Viral Infections

HCT recipients can be prone to community-acquired respiratory viral (CRV) infections with influenza, parainfluenza, and respiratory syncytial virus (RSV). As upper respiratory infections can progress to more serious lower respiratory infections and certain CRVs can be treated, appropriate diagnostic testing (e.g., nasopharyngeal swabs) should be considered to identify the virus if possible. Zanamivir or oseltamivir can be used for chemoprophylaxis and prompt treatment of influenza. Aerosolized and possibly oral ribavarin can be considered in patients with RSV infection, especially if they are early posttransplantation or have lower respiratory tract involvement.

Adenovirus infections can occasionally occur after allogeneic HCT, especially among recipients of T-cell depleted or mismatched grafts and in patients with GVHD. Novel antivirals are needed to treat respiratory viral infections in HCT recipients. An inhaled antiviral, DAS181, cleaves sialic acid-containing receptors on the surface of host respiratory epithelial cells, thus preventing influenza and parainfluenza attachment to and infection of respiratory cells, is currently undergoing clinical study.[12]

Fungal Infections

Invasive fungal infections are among the leading causes of mortality in HCT recipients. The vast majority of fungal infections in this setting are caused by yeasts (*Candida* spp.) or molds (*Aspergillus* spp.).

Candida Infections

Candida albicans has been the leading cause of yeast infections in HCT recipients, but the current widespread use of azole prophylaxis in the early transplant period has reduced the overall incidence, but led to the emergence of a variety of non-*albicans* species, such as *Candida tropicalis, Candida krusei* and *Candida glabrata*, as important pathogens.[13] These yeasts are normal inhabitants of the skin, oral and gastrointestinal mucosa which overgrow as normal commensal flora are disrupted by broad-spectrum antibacterials. Breakdown of these mucosal surfaces caused by radiation and chemotherapy, compounded by neutropenia in the preengraftment period, can greatly increase the risk of invasion and systemic yeast infections. Presence of indwelling central venous catheters and alteration of normal surface flora arising from antibiotics are additional risk factors for *Candida* infections.[1]

Clinical manifestations can range from localized mucocutaneous to disseminated deep-tissue infection. A high index of suspicion is needed for the diagnosis of *Candida* infections, especially in patients with persistent febrile neutropenia, since blood cultures are usually not very sensitive for isolation and identification of *Candida* spp. Oral and esophageal candidiasis frequently occurs in the early posttransplant period and should be treated aggressively as these can serve as portals for subsequent systemic infection. Venous catheter infections can be difficult to eradicate with antifungal agents alone and necessitate removal of the central line. Patients with candidemia are also at risk for endovascular infections such as endocarditis, thrombophlebitis or endophthalmitis. Hepatosplenic candidiasis is the most common manifestation of disseminated candidiasis, although it is increasingly rare with widespread use of effective anticandida azoles and echinocandins. Specific signs or symptoms related to organ involvement may be absent and the diagnosis frequently has to be made by abdominal CT scan imaging.

Prophylaxis with fluconazole is recommended in the preengraftment and early postengraftment periods, especially among allogeneic HCT recipients.[1,14,15] In patients who are at high-risk for mold infections, caspofungin, micafungin, voriconazole, or posaconazole can be considered as they have antimold activity. *Candida krusei* and *Candida glabrata* are intrinsically resistant to fluconazole and other agents (e.g., posaconazole, voriconazole, or micafungin) should be preferred for prophylaxis in patients colonized with fluconazole-resistant *Candida* species. Itraconazole is another active agent, but its use is limited by its tolerability, absorption, and toxicities. Cross-resistance to azoles can occur among *Candida* species. Antifungal agents for treatment of suspected or known invasive candidiasis include voriconazole or posaconazole, echinocandins or an amphotericin formulation, especially when infection occurs in the setting of ongoing fluconazole prophylaxis.[15]

Aspergillus Infections

Most mold infections in HCT recipients are caused by *Aspergillus fumigatus, Aspergillus flavus,* and *Aspergillus niger,* which gain entry through breakdown of mucosal surfaces in the nasal passages, sinuses, and the lower respiratory tract. *Aspergillus* infections can occur early after HCT (during the neutropenic phase) or later, especially complicating the immunosuppression associated with acute or chronic GVHD. Risk factors for *Aspergillus* infections include allogeneic (more than autologous) HCT, prolonged neutropenia, and GVHD.[16] Transplantation for diseases that cause extended neutropenia or neutrophil dysfunction pretransplantation (e.g., aplastic anemia and MDS, Fanconi anemia, or chronic granulomatous disease) also increases the risk. Prior history of *Aspergillus* infection has also been observed to be a risk factor for recrudescence after HCT.

Aspergillus occurring in the posttransplant setting can be difficult to diagnose premortem. Hence, a high index of suspicion and an aggressive approach is required to establish its diagnosis and initiate therapy. Since the nasal passages and tracheobronchial tree are the most common portals of entry for *Aspergillus* spp., these two sites are also the most common sites of infection. Sinusitis is frequently symptomatic and more advanced disease can be associated with erosion, vascular invasion and necrosis of surrounding structures. Pulmonary manifestations typically include nodular infiltrates, usually distributed along the lung periphery, with pleuritic pain or cough as an initial symptom. Frank consolidation (with a halo sign on CT scan) or cavitary lesions can be seen in more advanced stages of pulmonary involvement. *Aspergillus* has angioinvasive properties and can present with hemoptysis or with intravascular dissemination to the skin or brain.

Blood cultures have a very low sensitivity in detecting *Aspergillus* and diagnosis has to rely on demonstration of typical fungal morphology on culture or histopathology or on tests to detect fungal components or nucleic acids. Nasal and bronchial washings for *Aspergillus* also may not be sensitive and lung biopsy may be required to obtain a definitive diagnosis. The galactomannan assay is an enzyme-linked immunosorbent assay to detect the *Aspergillus* cell wall glycoprotein; it has a high specificity, but low sensitivity for diagnosing invasive aspergillosis and has not been reproducible in well-designed trials. Similarly, testing for β-D-glucan has modest clinical utility, but low sensitivity. Molecular methods for diagnosis, including PCR for *Aspergillus* DNA, are also undergoing development. More invasive evaluations (e.g., fine needle aspiration or biopsy) are often needed to confirm the presence of *Aspergillus* in suspicious lesions identified on clinical exam or imaging studies.

The use of high-efficiency air filters has reduced the nosocomial acquisition of *Aspergillus*, at least during the early neutropenic phase when isolation measures are used. The optimal pharmacologic strategy for primary prophylaxis against aspergillosis in HCT recipients is not well defined. Posaconazole has been shown to be effective for prophylaxis in HCT recipients with GVHD. A large randomized trial showed no difference in fungal-free survival between voriconazole and fluconazole in HCT recipients at low risk for disease progression or early HCT mortality, although there was a trend towards fewer *Aspergillus* infections and less empiric antifungal use in voriconazole recipients.[17] Inhaled or low dose intravenous amphotericin has not been effective for primary prophylaxis. In patients with a previous history of invasive aspergillosis, secondary prophylaxis with a mold-specific azole (e.g., oral voriconazole or posaconazole) or parenteral echinocandins or an amphotericin preparation is recommended, possibly for the duration of intensive immunosuppression. Therapy with a mold-specific azole, an echinocandin, or an amphotericin preparation should be initiated in patients with invasive aspergillosis or in high-risk patients with persistent febrile neutropenia.[18] Azoles and echinocandins have a more favorable side effect profile compared with amphotericin formulations. Patients with disease progressing on a single antimold drug might need combination therapy with two antimold agents. The role of adjunctive measures such as cytokine growth factors, immunoglobulin infusion, or granulocyte transfusion remains undefined.

Other molds including fusarium, alternaria or the zygomycetes may present similarly and might be difficult to distinguish on tissue biopsy.[19] Aggressive antifungal therapy is required for their management and may require multidrug therapy. Granulocyte transfusions may be an important adjunct for treatment of invasive fungal infections during neutropenia, but formal studies have not demonstrated improvements in survival.[20,21]

EARLY NONINFECTIOUS COMPLICATIONS

High-dose chemotherapy and radiation regimens are used before transplantation for their antineoplastic and immunosuppressive effects. However, these treatments can damage host tissue, resulting in significant morbidity. Early HCT-associated complications can frequently simulate infections or be compounded by concurrent infections. In addition, because epithelial tissue repair may be delayed by ongoing neutropenia and local microinvasive infection, delay in hematopoietic engraftment can exaggerate and prolong these toxicities.

Graft Failure

Failure to establish hematologic engraftment (primary graft failure) and loss of an established graft (late graft failure) are serious, though uncommon complications of both autologous and allogeneic HCT. Delayed or poor graft function can exaggerate and prolong the risks of infection and can increase the risk of peritransplant mortality. Graft failure can occur if insufficient hematopoietic progenitors are infused. A minimum of approximately 2×10^4 colony-forming cells from marrow per kilogram (kg) recipient weight are needed to

establish autologous engraftment. This is accomplished by infusing approximately 1×10^8 autologous marrow mononuclear cells/kg. Most investigators recommend infusion of a minimum of at least 2×10^8 marrow mononuclear cells/kg to ensure establishment of an allogeneic graft. UCB derived hematopoietic grafts can engraft with a lower number of cells. Stem cells and progenitors can be damaged by cryopreservation or by ex vivo purging, and additional cells are required if intensive purging, especially with alkylators, is performed though currently this approach to autograft preparation is uncommon. Selection of CD34+ cells as a technique for tumor cell depletion does not compromise engraftment, unless the quantitative cell losses through selection are excessive.

The use of hematopoietic stem cells and progenitors harvested from the blood by apheresis instead of the bone marrow has become widely prevalent, both for autologous and allogeneic HCT. Autologous peripheral blood hematopoietic cell grafts (PBSC) are collected after mobilization of marrow-derived progenitors into the blood by cytokine (G-CSF or GM-CSF) therapy or during recovery from myelosuppressive chemotherapy, often in combination with growth factors (Chapter 97). Progenitor content of blood or marrow grafts is assayed by quantitation of mononuclear cells expressing the hematopoietic progenitor-associated surface marker CD34. Peripheral graft mobilization can be further enriched by the use of plerixafor, an inhibitor of CXC-chemokine receptor 4 that releases cells from the marrow. Allogeneic grafts are mobilized from healthy donors using growth factors alone, nearly exclusively using G-CSF though clinical trials with plerixafor are ongoing.

Graft failure is uncommon if $>2 \times 10^6$ CD34+ cells/kg or more are collected, cryopreserved, and later infused as an autologous graft though guidelines often target $>5 \times 10^6$/kg for prompt neutrophil and platelet recovery. The minimum CD34 content for an allogeneic graft is less well defined, but more than 5×10^6 CD34+ cells/kg is frequently cited as a target collection for an allogeneic donor allograft. Mobilized PBSC grafts yield satisfactory and more rapid trilineage hematopoietic recovery than grafts from marrow-derived cells. Similar to marrow grafting, late graft failure is possible, but unlikely (<5%) after transplantation using PBSC. Infusion of a sufficient graft cell dose (nucleated or CD34+ cells) may be the most important controllable factor to limit the risk of graft failure.

Recipient myelofibrosis or splenomegaly can interfere with engraftment. Splenomegaly can delay hematologic recovery, presumably because both progenitors and mature blood cells are sequestered in the spleen and may particularly prolong dependence on platelet transfusions. The presence of moderate severe myelofibrosis also delays engraftment, perhaps because of faulty homing of stem cells in the marrow microenvironment.

Posttransplantation therapy can jeopardize engraftment. Graft failure or poor graft function has been associated with use of methotrexate, ATG, acyclovir, ganciclovir, trimethoprim-sulfamethoxazole (TMP-SMX), and mycophenolate mofetil (MMF). Posttransplant complications such as CMV, HHV-6 or fungal infections, and acute and chronic GVHD can also compromise successful engraftment.

Allogeneic HCT, especially using unrelated or mismatched donors, poses unique engraftment problems. Transplants between siblings completely matched at *HLA-A, HLA-B,* and *HLA-DR* loci are rarely (1%–3%) associated with graft failure; however, the probability of graft failure in the related-donor transplantation setting increases to near 10% with greater degrees of donor-recipient HLA incompatibility. This may be overcome by the promising use of post-HCT cyclophosphamide to deplete alloreactive host and particularly donor cells.[22] The problem is more frequently observed, although still <5% in the volunteer adult URD setting, where primary or secondary graft failure may occur even after transplantation from donors well matched at the *HLA-A, HLA-B, HLA-C,* and *HLA-DR* loci. In some cases, failure of URD stem cells to engraft may result from reactivity against other important histocompatibility determinants, including HLA-C or donor-specific antibodies against HLA class I or class II molecules.[23] Early failure of an allogeneic graft can be accompanied by emergence of cytotoxic T-lymphocytes of host origin, presumably representing immune-mediated graft rejection. This may be blunted by effective host immunosuppression by the conditioning regimen and peritransplant immunoprophylaxis. T-lymphocyte depletion of donor marrow performed as GVHD prophylaxis can also adversely affect engraftment, even from matched sibling donors. Ex vivo marrow manipulation can deplete stem cells. T-cell depletion can also render the graft immunoincompetent and functionally less capable of preventing graft rejection.

Compared with related or URD allografts, time to neutrophil recovery is significantly delayed in patients receiving UCB grafts. In addition, the overall incidence of graft failure is somewhat greater, currently 5% to 15% with present selection strategies. The most critical determinants of engraftment following UCB transplantation are both HLA matching and cell dose, and units with a total nucleated cell dose of at least 2.5×10^7 cells/kg or more have a greater probability of successful engraftment. Since each UCB unit has a limited number of hematopoietic stem and progenitor cells, methods to overcome this limitation of cell dose are being investigated. These include transplantation using multiple UCB units, ex vivo expansion to increase the number of progenitor cells, and approaches to improve homing including intrabone marrow injection of the graft or preincubation with prostaglandins. Increasing overall cell dose and the added antihost immunologic response with transplantation of two UCB units has increased the chances of successful engraftment, especially in adults.

The use of recombinant G-CSF or GM-CSF, which stimulate myelopoiesis, has improved the treatment of graft failure. Improvement in myelopoiesis can be seen in 50% to 60% patients with poor graft function within 14–21 days after initiation of growth factor therapy. Myeloid growth factor therapy can increase peripheral blood leukocyte recovery, but has little effect on platelet reconstitution. Recombinant human thrombopoietin receptor agonists are now available, although their efficacy and safety profile in HCT recipients is currently being studied. Limited experience suggests the value of recombinant erythropoietin in reducing red blood cell transfusion needs.

A second stem cell infusion can be useful if graft failure occurs. In the case of a failed autograft, infusion of previously harvested and frozen marrow or blood cells frequently reestablishes functional hematopoiesis and hematologic improvement. In the case of graft failure after related-donor transplantation, a second infusion of donor marrow or cytokine-mobilized PBSC may allow successful engraftment. Sometimes, because of the presumption of immune-mediated rejection, reconditioning with reduced doses of cytotoxic agents or further immunosuppression with ATG, corticosteroids, or cyclosporine is used to prepare the recipient for a second infusion.

The treatment of graft failure after URD transplantation poses special problems. URDs may not be available for a second marrow harvest or blood stem cell apheresis. In experimental settings where graft failure risks are high, it may be prudent to store autologous stem cells from patients undergoing URD transplantation, although this is rarely done. The original donor is not available in recipients of unrelated UCB grafts and the only treatment option for graft failure in this setting is a second transplant using cells from a different UCB or volunteer adult donor (related or unrelated) second allograft, or reinfusion of autologous backup cells, if available. Because of variability in the circumstances and donor options available, there are few clear data on the outcomes of second allografts in these situations.[24]

Sinusoidal Obstruction Syndrome

Sinusoidal obstruction syndrome (SOS), also known as hepatic venoocclusive disease, is a serious liver disorder characterized by jaundice, ascites, fluid retention, and hepatomegaly that complicates up to 5% to 50% of HCT's.[25] The varying reported incidence is based upon stringency of the definition of the clinical diagnosis (Box 109.2). The primary initiating event is thought to be portal hypertension caused by inflammatory and edematous obstruction of hepatic sinusoids and venules, which secondarily leads to damage to surrounding centrilobular hepatocytes. Chemotherapy and total body irradiation

---

BOX 109.2 Sinusoidal Obstruction Syndrome

Diagnostic Criteria for Sinusoidal Obstruction Syndrome (SOS)

Bilirubin ≥2 mg/dL before day 21 post-HCT and at least two of the following: (1) hepatomegaly or right upper quadrant pain, (2) ascites, or (3) weight gain >5% over baseline.

SOS is a clinical diagnosis; liver ultrasound with Doppler studies or liver biopsy can support or confirm the diagnosis.

Risk Factors

Pretransplant Factors

Prior hepatic inflammatory disease (e.g., chronic hepatitis B or C, nonalcoholic steatohepatitis, alcoholic hepatitis)
Prior hepatic fibrotic disease (e.g., cirrhosis)
Extensive pre-HCT chemotherapy
Prior exposure to gemtuzumab ozogamicin
Prior liver irradiation

Transplant-Related Factors

Conditioning regimen (e.g., myeloablative total body irradiation or busulfan-based regimens)
Exposure to other agents (e.g., sirolimus, itraconazole)

Prognostic Factors

Adverse prognostic factors include: development of multiorgan failure, rapid increase in weight, rapid increase in bilirubin.

Treatment

For >70% of patients, SOS will recover spontaneously with supportive care. However, mortality rates are >80% for patients with severe SOS. Treatment options, especially for patients with more severe SOS, includes:

Pharmacologic

Ursodeoxycholic acid (prophylaxis)
Defibrotide (investigational—prophylaxis and treatment)
Low-dose heparin and low-molecular-weight heparin (prophylaxis)
Tissue plasminogen activator (investigational – prophylaxis and treatment)
Antithrombin III (investigational—prophylaxis and treatment)

Nonpharmacologic

Supportive care with management of multiorgan failure
Transjugular intrahepatic portosystemic shunt
Liver transplantation

(TBI) used in pretransplant conditioning regimens produce sinusoidal endothelial injury. Subsequent deposition of fibronectin and factor VIII/von Willebrand factor at the site of damaged endothelium can lead to activation of the coagulation system and subsequent sinusoidal obstruction. Such changes are often associated with depressed plasma protein C levels and other signs of procoagulant activity, including lower antithrombin III levels and elevated factor VIII and fibrinogen levels. Cytokines such as tumor necrosis factor (TNF)-α and alterations in the levels of nitric oxide and matrix metalloproteinases may also have a role in its pathogenesis.

Risk factors associated with the development of SOS include history of pretransplant hepatitis or liver injury, intensive preparative regimens, increased TBI dose and dose rate and increased busulfan dose. SOS may also be more frequent after mismatched related or URD transplantation. Prior therapy with gemtuzumab ozogamicin also increases the risk of posttransplant SOS. Sirolimus has also been shown to increase the risks of SOS after myeloablative allogeneic HCT, particularly using busulfan-based regimens.

Signs of SOS usually occur within 2–4 weeks after hematopoietic graft infusion, but may be recognized much sooner, even during administration of an intensive preparative regimen. Clinical evidence of venoocclusive disease includes hyperbilirubinemia, tender hepatomegaly, ascites, and weight gain.[25] More advanced stages can be associated with encephalopathy along with renal, pulmonary, and multiorgan failure. The diagnosis of SOS is primarily based on clinical criteria that include presence of jaundice, plus either hepatomegaly, weight gain, and/or ascites within 2–3 weeks of stem cell infusion. However, other causes of hyperbilirubinemia and weight gain early after transplantation (e.g., drugs, hepatitis, capillary leak, cardiac failure, volume overload) can complicate the differential diagnosis, particularly for milder or less abrupt presentations of these symptoms. Percutaneous or transabdominal needle biopsy of the liver is hazardous in severely thrombocytopenic transplant recipients and should be avoided. Transvenous biopsies may provide sufficient histologic material for diagnosis and may allow determination of hepatic wedge pressure product (greater than 10 mm is associated with SOS), but may be associated with hemorrhagic complications as well. Ultrasonographic Doppler flow studies demonstrating reversal of portal flow or a higher portal vein resistive index have been suggested as a noninvasive means of confirming the diagnosis, but their validity has recently been questioned. SOS can be graded from mild to severe depending on the degree of hyperbilirubinemia and weight gain. Severe SOS is almost universally fatal within several weeks of onset.

Effective methods for prevention and treatment of SOS have not been defined. Limited understanding of the cellular and microvascular pathophysiology of SOS has confounded development of more rational approaches to its prevention and treatment. Possible approaches include preventive therapy with low-dose heparin, prostaglandin E, pentoxifylline (a TNF-α blocking agent), although none has proved effective in carefully performed prospective trials. Post-HCT hepatic injury including SOS has become less frequent with widespread and prolonged administration of ursodiol as a choleretic and hepatic protectant. Recombinant tissue plasminogen factor has been used successfully to treat established SOS, however, thrombolytics are associated with substantially increased risk of hemorrhage. Transjugular intrahepatic portosystemic shunts have also been used with some success. Early experience with defibrotide, a single-stranded polyribonucleotide with fibrinolytic, antithrombotic, and antiischemic properties, has been favorable with 30% to 40% of patients with severe SOS achieving complete resolution and improvement in survival.[26] Its efficacy in the prophylaxis and management of severe SOS is currently being investigated in larger clinical trials.

Interstitial Pneumonitis

Interstitial pneumonitis is a common and frequently fatal complication, affecting up to 35% of allogeneic transplant recipients, although recent advances in supportive care have substantially reduced this risk. Interstitial pneumonitis is notably less common after autografting. It is characterized by diffuse, interstitial inflammation accompanied by hypoxemia, dyspnea, and nonproductive cough, sometimes with fever. Risk factors associated with the development of interstitial pneumonitis include use of methotrexate for GVHD prophylaxis, older age at transplant, severe GVHD, interval from diagnosis of hematologic disease to HCT of 6 months or greater, poor pretransplant performance status and use of higher TBI dose rate (>4 cGy/min). Remarkably, in one study, the reported risk of interstitial pneumonitis was 8% when none of these risk factors were present, compared with 94% when all six factors were present. It has been hypothesized that URD transplantation is more immunosuppressive and thus associated with more severe opportunistic infections and greater risk of interstitial pneumonitis, but this has not been rigorously investigated.

The course of interstitial pneumonitis is often catastrophic, manifesting with rapidly progressive tachypnea, hypoxemia, and hemodynamic compromise. Therefore, therapeutic intervention most frequently occurs before the return of definitive results of diagnostic tests and must be initiated based on the assessment of clinical risk factors and the underlying clinical setting (Box 109.3).

BOX 109.3   Approach to Interstitial Pneumonitis

The presentation of interstitial pneumonitis after hematopoietic cell transplantation (HCT) should be considered an urgent medical situation and empiric broad-spectrum therapy must be initiated early. The choice of therapy is influenced by the following:

1. Timing: Within the first 3 weeks after HCT, interstitial pneumonitis is more likely to be idiopathic (including diffuse alveolar hemorrhage) or fungal than caused by cytomegalovirus (CMV) infection. Beyond 6 weeks, idiopathic pneumonitis is unusual and the cause is more likely infectious. *Pneumocystis jirovecii* pneumonia is rare beyond 1 year after transplantation except in patients with ongoing chronic graft-versus-host disease. Respiratory syncytial virus (RSV) infections are seasonal (fall and winter), and community outbreaks can be prevalent. Influenza is also seasonal, whereas parainfluenza can occur year round.

2. CMV serology and prophylaxis: If a seronegative recipient has received a seronegative graft and noninfective (seronegative or leukocyte-depleted) blood, CMV pneumonia is unusual. Seropositive recipients are at higher risk, although with ganciclovir or other antiviral prophylaxis, the risk is markedly reduced. Other prophylactic regimens for CMV, such as acyclovir or intravenous immunoglobulin, have still been associated with significant risk for serious CMV infection in the seropositive recipient. Serial negative testing for CMV antigenemia or DNA-polymerase chain reaction makes CMV pneumonitis less likely.

3. Prolonged neutropenia: This factor is associated with infectious causes, particularly with fungal pneumonias.

4. Type of transplant: Diffuse alveolar hemorrhage is less frequently seen in patients undergoing autologous HCT. CMV pneumonia is unusual (2%–3%) in autologous recipients, but it still has a high case fatality rate. All infectious causes are more common after allogeneic HCT. More intensive conditioning regimens (e.g., higher total body irradiation, carmustine) are associated with greater risks of pneumonitis.

5. Compliance and prophylaxis: A thorough assessment of what prophylaxis the patient has actually been receiving (e.g., trimethoprim-sulfamethoxazole, penicillin, CMV prophylaxis, transfusions outside the transplant center) is critical to assess risk.

6. Chest radiograph: The pattern and distribution of the infiltrate may narrow the differential diagnosis. Cardiac enlargement or pleural effusions may suggest pulmonary edema. A chest computed tomography scan is useful, especially if nodularity, pleural involvement, or cavitary lesions (possibly fungal) are suspected.

7. Epidemiology: Identification of the causes of other recent cases can be most helpful with infections that are horizontally transmitted (e.g., RSV) or have common environmental risk factors (e.g., *Aspergillus* infection associated with construction).

8. Bronchoalveolar lavage (BAL): This can be extremely useful to establish a specific diagnosis or to exclude others. CMV rarely causes pneumonia without positive BAL findings (either direct staining of CMV-associated antigens in BAL cells or DNA-PCR). BAL also usually detects RSV, *Pneumocystis jirovecii* and other respiratory viruses, though not as rapidly, but is required to identify alveolar hemorrhage. It is less sensitive for diagnosis of fungal pneumonias. Galactomannan or β-D-glucan studies of serum or BAL may indicate fungal pneumonia, but are insensitive.

9. Lung biopsy: Although this is the gold standard for definitive diagnosis of most of the possible causes of interstitial pneumonitis, it can often be avoided through the use of clinical diagnostic measures listed. It may be necessary for the definitive diagnosis of fungal pneumonias, pulmonary changes associated with chronic graft-versus-host disease (bronchiolitis obliterans), or idiopathic interstitial pneumonitis. Either bronchoscopic(transbronchial), open surgical or video-assisted thoracoscopic can be used. Transbronchial biopsies are insufficient for other than very diffuse processes and carry risks of bleeding and/or pneumothorax. The surgical approaches are more invasive, but more often definitive.

10. Ventilator therapy: Progressive respiratory failure after HCT is rarely reversible, especially in adults. Although aggressive diagnostic and therapeutic measures are essential, some centers offer patients and their families the option of foregoing mechanical ventilatory support if survival is not expected. Preliminary discussion of this possible complication in pretransplant patient counseling can facilitate decision-making if respiratory failure does occur.

Infectious Causes of Interstitial Pneumonitis

Infections are the most common cause of interstitial pneumonitis in HCT recipients. CMV and *Aspergillus* are the most common infections associated with interstitial pneumonitis and have been discussed earlier. Other important, though relatively uncommon infections to consider are *Pneumocystis jirovecii*, RSV and similar respiratory viruses.

Pneumonitis caused by *Pneumocystis* has a typical bilateral distribution with a 'butterfly' pattern on chest radiograph and prominent hypoxemia, and rarely causes pleural effusions. The previously reported 5% to 15% risk of *Pneumocystis* pneumonia has been largely eliminated by routine use of prophylaxis with TMP-SMX (first choice), dapsone, atovaquone, or inhaled pentamidine. Prophylaxis with TMP-SMX virtually eliminates *Pneumocystis* pneumonia from the differential diagnosis, but only if patient compliance with therapy is certain. Diagnosis requires cytologic evaluation of silver-stained preparations of BAL cells or sputum, although transbronchial lung biopsy may slightly increase the diagnostic yield of a bronchoscopic examination. *Pneumocystis* pneumonia is effectively treated with high dose TMP-SMX or parenteral pentamidine. Prophylaxis against *Pneumocystis* pneumonia should be continued through the period of immunosuppression (6 months to 1 year posttransplantation) and for the duration of any therapy for chronic GVHD.

RSV is a potentially fatal cause of interstitial pneumonitis and typically occurs in the fall and winter months. RSV should be suspected if the patient presents a history of rhinorrhea and if RSV has been frequently recognized in the community or in the hospital. Diagnosis can be made by rapid antigen or PCR testing on nasal washings or BAL specimens. Because of the possibility of horizontal transmission, patients with RSV should be isolated. Inhaled and sometimes oral ribavarin is used for treatment of RSV-associated pneumonia. Other community acquired viruses, such as parainfluenza or influenza can also cause interstitial pneumonitis in the transplant recipient. Their presentation is clinically indistinguishable from RSV though parainfluenza pneumonitis is not seasonal and may be seen year round. Yearly influenza vaccination for HCT recipients and especially their household contacts may be effective in reducing risks of this infection.

Noninfectious Causes of Interstitial Pneumonitis

Idiopathic Interstitial Pneumonitis

Idiopathic interstitial pneumonitis is a diagnosis of exclusion based on typical findings and ruling out infectious causes. Its timing is somewhat earlier than other causes of interstitial pneumonitis, typically occurring within the first 2–7 weeks after HCT. The recognized risk factors for idiopathic interstitial pneumonitis include older age at transplant, extensive pretransplant chemotherapy, high-dose cyclophosphamide, TBI (higher total dose and dose rate), blood transfusions, administration of methotrexate and GVHD.[27]

The observation that idiopathic interstitial pneumonitis is as frequent among syngeneic as among allogeneic recipients and has an equally high incidence in T-cell depleted grafts, suggests that immunosuppression is less of a risk factor for idiopathic interstitial pneumonitis than it is for infectious interstitial pneumonitis. Clinical observations support a toxic cause for idiopathic interstitial pneumonitis, and radiation-induced lung damage appears to be the major contributor, especially the use of high-dose TBI. Effective therapy has not been established, although high-dose corticosteroids are often administered. Inflammatory cytokines, including interleukin (IL)-1 and TNF-α, have been implicated in lung injury. Etanercept, a TNF-α binding protein has been reported to improve lung function in patients with idiopathic interstitial pneumonitis, particularly if administered before the need for mechanic ventilation. Its use was not confirmed to be better than placebo when used in combination with corticosteroids in a recent, though small, multicenter trial.[28,29]

Diffuse Alveolar Hemorrhage

Alveolar hemorrhage is a clinical syndrome of acute onset of pulmonary infiltrates and hypoxemia with a progressively bloodier BAL on bronchoscopy.[30] Alveolar hemorrhage arising from noninfectious causes has been called diffuse alveolar hemorrhage, but it is often difficult to distinguish it from infection-associated pulmonary hemorrhage, especially in the early posttransplant period.[30] The reported incidence of diffuse alveolar hemorrhage ranges from 2% to 5% in autologous and 5% to 10% in allogeneic HCT recipients. Its pathogenesis is not known, but it most likely develops as result of a complex interaction of a variety of factors, including alveolar injury from radiation and chemotherapy, inflammatory damage caused by neutrophils and cytokines, and underlying infections. Older age at transplant, use of an allogeneic donor source, and GVHD are risk factors for this syndrome. The risk is similar with NMA and myeloablative conditioning regimens.[31] Onset typically occurs within the first 3 months of transplantation with dyspnea, hypoxia, and cough, although late-onset alveolar hemorrhage is also possible. Hemoptysis is usually absent and bronchoscopy with BAL is required to confirm the diagnosis and to exclude infectious etiologies. This syndrome is very serious and the majority of patients develop respiratory failure with mortality rates of more than 70%. Hemorrhage occurring in the periengraftment period is associated with a better outcome compared with later-onset hemorrhage. Treatment includes correction of any coagulopathy and aggressive ventilatory support. High-dose corticosteroids have been used for its management, but their efficacy has not been clearly proven. Small case series have reported the successful use of recombinant factor VIIa and aminocaproic acid, but their efficacy needs to be confirmed in clinical trials. Cytokine antagonists (e.g., etanercept) might have a therapeutic role that is being investigated in clinical trials.

LATE NONINFECTIOUS COMPLICATIONS

Improvements in transplantation techniques and supportive care have led to an increasing number of long-term HCT survivors. Among HCT recipients who remain disease-free through 2–5 years posttransplantation, the probability of survival over the following 10–20 years is more than 80%.[32,33] These survivors remain at risk for late transplant associated complications, which can include specific organ dysfunction, second cancers, infections because of ongoing immunodeficiency, functional impairments, and compromise in the quality of life (QOL; Table 109.5).[34] Guidelines for screening and prevention of late effects in HCT survivors have been published.[4,35] In addition, following general population guidelines for screening and prevention of cancers and chronic diseases and promoting a generally healthy lifestyle is recommended for all HCT survivors.

Organ-Specific Late Effects

A multitude of pre-, peri-, and post-HCT factors determine a patient's overall risk for developing specific late complications. Risk factors include age at the time of HCT, gender, and lifestyle factors such as tobacco and alcohol use. In addition, patients may have preexisting comorbidities such as chronic renal insufficiency or cardiovascular disease that can be exacerbated by chemotherapy, radiation, and other medications they receive to treat their malignancy and during HCT. Exposure to chemotherapy and radiation as part of initial treatment of underlying hematologic disorder or as part of the conditioning regimen given before HCT also can contribute to organ-specific complications. Allogeneic HCT recipients who develop chronic GVHD may require long-term treatment with glucocorticoids, calcineurin inhibitors (e.g., cyclosporine or tacrolimus), or other immunosuppressive agents and can be prone to developing medication-related side effects, infections

TABLE 109.5	**Selected Late Complications of Hematopoietic Cell Transplantation**	
Complication	**Risk Factors**	**Monitoring and Prevention**
Endocrine		
Hypothyroidism	TBI/radiation	Periodic assessment of thyroid and gonadal function
Hypogonadism	Chronic GVHD	
Growth retardation	Chemotherapy	
Ocular		
Cataracts	TBI/radiation	Periodic eye exam
Keratoconjunctivitis sicca	Corticosteroids	
	Chronic GVHD	
Oral		
Dental caries	TBI/radiation	Periodic dental assessment
Dry mouth	Chronic GVHD	
Cardiovascular		
Coronary artery disease	TBI/radiation	Periodic clinical evaluation
Cerebrovascular disease	Chemotherapy	Modification of risk factors
Respiratory		
Bronchiolitis obliterans	TBI/radiation	Periodic clinical evaluation
Interstitial pneumonitis	Chronic GVHD	Smoking cessation
	Infections	
Hepatic		
Cirrhosis	Hepatitis B or C	Periodic liver function tests
Iron overload	Transfusions	Serum ferritin level
Renal		
Nephropathy	TBI/radiation	Periodic serum creatinine and urinalysis
	Chemotherapy	Control hypertension
	Cyclosporine	
Skeletal		
Osteoporosis	TBI/radiation	Periodic bone densitometry
Avascular necrosis	Corticosteroids	
Second cancers	TBI/radiation	Periodic cancer screening
	Chemotherapy	
	Chronic GVHD	

GVHD, Graft-versus-host disease; TBI, total body irradiation.

and second malignancies, especially those associated with chronic immunodeficiency.

Although any organ system can be involved, certain organs have a greater predilection for late-onset problems post-HCT. Cataracts develop in more than one-third of patients by 5-years posttransplantation and often require surgical therapy. Hypothyroidism can be seen in up to 50% and hypogonadism in up to 90% of HCT survivors. The majority of HCT survivors become permanently sterile, although HCT without TBI can be fertility-sparing in nearly one-third of men and women. Prepubertal children may retain fertility, although secondary sexual development may be delayed. Up to 50% of children undergoing HCT also develop growth retardation. Musculoskeletal complications including osteoporosis and avascular necrosis of weight-bearing joints can be particularly debilitating. An increased incidence of cardiovascular events and diabetes has also been reported. The risk for most organ-specific late complications continues to

increase with time and continued surveillance for these problems indicated in all HCT survivors.

Second Cancers

Secondary cancers are a rare, but devastating complication of HCT. They account for 5% to 10% of deaths among greater than 2 year survivors. These malignancies can be broadly categorized as post-transplant lymphoproliferative disorders (PTLD), hematologic malignancies, and solid cancers.[36,37]

PTLD comprise a heterogeneous group of lymphoid proliferations, primarily involving B-lymphocytes that develop as a result of uncontrolled Epstein-Barr virus (EBV) infection. (Chapter 54) They occur almost exclusively in allogeneic HCT recipients, with an overall incidence of 1% to 2%. They typically manifest soon after transplantation with more than 80% of cases diagnosed within the first year. Since T cells play an important role in preventing proliferation of EBV-infected lymphocytes, removal of T cells from the hematopoietic graft or anti–T-cell serotherapy with ATG or alemtuzumab are strong risk factors for PTLD. A greater degree of immunosuppression, such as that resulting from GVHD and use of grafts from unrelated or HLA-mismatched donors, also increases the risk for PTLD. Treatment of PTLD is often challenging, and available treatments are not very effective. Withdrawal of immunosuppression is usually attempted first, but can be difficult in patients with active GVHD. Treatment options include anti-CD20 monoclonal antibody rituximab, antiviral therapy with acyclovir or ganciclovir, multiagent chemotherapy, or infusion of EBV-specific cytotoxic T lymphocytes. Since PTLD is associated with high mortality rates, active surveillance for EBV reactivation in high-risk settings and initiation of preemptive therapy, often with rituximab, is important.

Secondary MDS and acute myeloid leukemia (AML) can be seen in 5% to 15% of autologous HCT recipients, but is extremely rare among allogeneic HCT recipients. They usually occur following a latency period of 2–5 years.[36] Bone marrow evaluation can show cytogenetic abnormalities characteristic of other treatment-induced AML/MDS (e.g., balanced translocations to 11q23, monosomy of 5q and 7q or multiple, complex chromosomal aberrations). Risk factors for secondary MDS/AML include older age at transplant, the type, intensity and duration of pre-HCT chemotherapy (especially alkylating agents), and use of TBI. Outcomes are very poor and long-term survival rates are less than 20%, sometimes following a second allograft for this new malignancy.

Secondary solid cancers have a latency period of 3–5 years following HCT. Subsequently, their incidence continues to rise with time and is higher than what may be expected in age- and gender-matched general populations. Their cumulative incidence ranges from 1% to 2% at five years, 2% to 6% at 10 years, and 4% to 15% at 15 years posttransplantation.[36] Younger age at transplantation, use of TBI and chronic GVHD are important risk factors for solid cancers. Solid cancers at variety of sites have been reported, including cancers of the head and neck, liver, brain and nervous system, thyroid, and bone and connective tissue. Since there is no plateau in the incidence of secondary solid cancers after HCT, their overall risk has not been completely realized, and longer follow up than what is currently available is needed before the true magnitude of risk will become apparent. Lifelong cancer screening is recommended for all HCT survivors according to established guidelines (Table 109.6).[4,35]

Quality of Life After Transplantation

Despite the early morbidity associated with HCT, the majority of transplant survivors attain high levels of physical and psychologic QOL and return to full-time employment by 3–5 years posttransplant. However, up to 20% to 40% of long-term survivors continue to have functional, psychological, and cognitive impairments years after HCT.[38,39] The major risk factors for compromised QOL are older age and advanced disease at transplantation, chronic GVHD

TABLE 109.6	Screening Guidelines for Common Cancers After Hematopoietic Cell Transplantation
Site	**Screening Recommendations**
Breast	Mammogram annually starting at age 40 years; in women who have received ≥20 Gy to the chest region begin at age 25 years or 8 years after radiation, whichever is later
Cervix	Pap smear every year (for regular Pap test) or every 2 years (for liquid-based Pap test); may screen every 2–3 years after 30 years of age if patient has three consecutive normal tests
Colorectal	Beginning at age 50 years, fecal occult blood annually and/or flexible sigmoidoscopy every 5 years, or double contrast barium enema every 5 years, or colonoscopy every 10 years; certain high-risk groups (e.g., patients with inflammatory bowel disease) may need earlier initiation and more frequent screening
Lung	Yearly pulmonary exam with imaging as appropriate
Oral	Yearly oral cavity exam
Thyroid	Yearly thyroid exam
Skin	Yearly skin exam

Pap, Papanicolaou.

and presence of medical late effects. Although chronic GVHD is a strong predictor of poor QOL, the overall health and functional status improves with resolution of GVHD and eventually reaches a level comparable with that seen in patients with no history of chronic GVHD. Gender specific differences in QOL have also been observed with females more likely to report impairments in psychologic and sexual domains. Cognitive deficits, particularly involving executive function, memory and motor skills, have been reported in 30% to 60% of HCT survivors. The risk of developing these neuropsychological sequelae is increased in patients receiving transplantation at an older age, although a recent prospective study did not identify any association of cognitive deficit with intensity of conditioning, cyclosporine, length of inpatient stay, or the development of GVHD.[40]

GRAFT-VERSUS-HOST DISEASE

GVHD is a clinicopathologic syndrome initiated by T cell–mediated alloreactivity that commonly occurs as a complication of allogeneic HCT and leads to significant morbidity and mortality (also see Chapter 108). It is usually classified as acute GVHD or chronic GVHD. Acute GVHD may be further characterized as classic acute GVHD (onset ≤100 days) and persistent, recurrent or late-onset acute GVHD (onset >100 days). In the absence of clinical features characteristic of acute GVHD, chronic GVHD is called classic chronic GVHD. When features of both acute and chronic GVHD appear together, it is classified as overlap syndrome, based upon a consensus conference proposed definition. Recent revisions lend lesser support for maintaining this overlap syndrome as an independent category.[41]

Current understanding of the pathogenesis of GVHD suggests that alloreactive donor T-lymphocytes recognize histocompatibility antigens on host cells and initiate secondary inflammatory injury, leading to the clinical symptoms of GVHD.[42] This alloreactive response can be initiated or accelerated by conditioning regimen-induced tissue injury with release of proinflammatory cytokines, primarily IL-1 and TNF-α. GVHD is more frequent and more severe in recipients of partially matched transplants, suggesting that major histocompatibility complex encoded molecules may be the prime antigenic targets initiating the alloreactive T-cell response. Minor histocompatibility antigens also play an important role in its pathogenesis, especially in HLA-identical sibling donor grafts. Activated donor-derived T-cells produce IL-2 and interferon-γ, expand and differentiate into effector cells and recruit mononuclear phagocytes and neutrophils and possibly NK cells which ultimately yield host tissue destruction, primarily through apoptosis. T-cell depletion of the graft reduces the risk of acute and chronic GVHD, albeit at the cost of increasing risks of disease relapse caused by blunting of the graft-versus-tumor response. Alternative mechanisms may also be involved in the pathogenesis of chronic GVHD including autoreactivity, loss of self-tolerance and B-cell dysregulation.[42]

Acute Graft-Versus-Host Disease

Risk Factors and Clinical Features

Up to 50% of patients receiving HLA-identical sibling-donor and up to 90% of patients receiving URD HCT develop acute GVHD. Donor-recipient HLA disparity is the most important risk factor for acute GVHD. Additional risk factors include increasing recipient and donor age, use of alloimmunized donors such as parous women, and HCT from unrelated instead of sibling donors. Among recipients of UCB, acute GVHD occurs in 20% to 60% of patients; incidence of acute GVHD, though of only moderate severity, may be higher among recipients of double UCB transplantation.[43]

Skin, liver, and gastrointestinal tract are the most common sites of GVHD. Acute GVHD of the skin is characterized by a maculo-papular rash that, when severe, can lead to bullae or even resemble toxic epidermal necrolysis. Hepatic involvement manifests as cholestatic hepatitis with marked elevation of serum bilirubin and alkaline phosphatase, but usually only mild transaminase alterations. In the intestine, upper gastrointestinal tract GVHD can produce nausea, vomiting and anorexia, whereas small bowel and colon GVHD produces large volume secretory diarrhea. The diagnosis is clinical but frequently requires histologic confirmation to distinguish it from other frequent toxicities in the early posttransplantation period (e.g., hypersensitivity drug rash, drug-induced cholestasis, SOS, or infectious enteritis). The histologic hallmark of acute GVHD is apoptosis of the proliferative and regenerative cell layer of the epidermis, intestinal or biliary epithelium.

Acute GVHD is graded according to organs involved (skin, liver or gastrointestinal tract) and the extent (stage) of each organ involvement. Mild to moderate (grade I or II) GVHD is characterized by limited organ involvement and carries an excellent prognosis. Severe (grade III or IV) GVHD has extensive multiorgan involvement with significant morbidity and poor survival, commonly evolves to chronic GVHD and is associated with an increased risk of secondary opportunistic infections.

Prophylaxis of Graft-Versus-Host Disease

The most effective techniques for GVHD prevention have involved ex vivo depletion of donor T-lymphocytes, most often coupling immunologic recognition (monoclonal anti–T-cell antibodies) with depletion techniques (immunomagnetic beads, complement cytotoxicity or toxin immunoconjugates). Immunomagnetic selection of CD34+ cells from the graft (negatively selecting out T cells) has been used more widely in recent years.[44] Although vigorous T-cell depletion prevents acute GVHD, it also may increase the risks of graft failure and neoplastic relapse after transplantation.

Pharmacologic immunosuppression administered in the first several months after transplantation can prevent or blunt the initiating T-cell recognition and proliferative response that triggers GVHD and can allow development of immune system tolerance and complete lymphohematopoietic chimerism. Methotrexate, corticosteroids, ATG, cyclosporine, tacrolimus, MMF and sirolimus have been used for prophylaxis of GVHD and have successfully reduced both the frequency and the severity of clinical GVHD.[45] Despite the potential role of inflammatory cytokines in initiation and amplification of GVHD, clinical blockade of IL-1, IL-2, or TNF-α has not been effective in GVHD prophylaxis. Current therapies being tested in addition to the backbone of calcineurin inhibitors in multicenter trials include posttransplant cyclophosphamide (to lyse proliferating alloreactive donor T cells), bortezomib, and maraviroc (inhibits lymphocyte chemotaxis, but not function).

Treatment of Acute Graft-Versus-Host Disease

Therapy for acute GVHD requires both immunosuppression to blunt the T-cell–induced tissue injury and appropriate supportive care. Corticosteroids are the mainstay of initial therapy for acute GVHD. GVHD involving limited areas of the skin can be treated with topical corticosteroids alone. Oral beclomethasone can be used to treat early stage GVHD of the upper gastrointestinal tract. Corticosteroids (2 mg/kg per day prednisone) are initial therapy for more advanced GVHD and yield response rates of approximately 50%. No regimen has shown a consistent increase in response rates or improvement in survival compared with corticosteroids alone. In a recent large randomized phase II trial comparing corticosteroids with MMF, pentostatin, etanercept or denileukin diftitox, efficacy and toxicity data suggested the combination of MMF and corticosteroids to be most promising.[46] This combination was not superior to corticosteroids alone in the follow-up randomized phase III trial, however.[47] Other investigational therapies include inhibitors of lymphocyte homing to intestinal tissues and infusion of mesenchymal stem cells. Prognosis is poor for patients with steroid-resistant disease, which is GVHD that does not respond to initial therapy with corticosteroids. Up to 10% to 40% of patients will respond to salvage therapy with ATG or other drugs such as sirolimus, tacrolimus, MMF, pentostatin or cyclosporine, either as single agents or in combination. Monoclonal antibodies and immunotoxins directed against T-cells or inflammatory cytokines have been investigated, although their effectiveness has not been demonstrated outside of small case series. Specific agents with reported activity in steroid-refractory acute GVHD include pentostatin, etanercept and infliximab (TNF-α receptor blockers), dacluzimab and denileukin diftitox (IL-2 receptor inhibitors), and visilizumab (anti-CD3 antibody). Extracorporeal photochemotherapy has also been reported to have some efficacy in steroid-refractory acute GVHD. In addition to effective immunosuppression, successful management of acute GVHD involves attention to supportive care, particularly skin care, nutrition and limitation of polypharmacy-associated drug interactions. Infections are a leading cause of death in patients with GVHD and attention should be paid to infection surveillance and prophylaxis.

Chronic Graft-Versus-Host Disease

Risk Factors and Clinical Features

Chronic GVHD is a complex syndrome in recipients of allogeneic HCT that occurs later, typically between 3–7 months posttransplant, although it can also begin before 3 months and even beyond 2 years. Its incidence ranges from 30% to 50% in HLA-matched sibling donor transplants to 50% to 70% in HLA-matched URD transplants and it is the leading cause of nonrelapse late mortality in allogeneic HCT survivors. Recipients of UCB grafts have lower risks compared with matched adult URD HCT and comparable or even lower than matched related donor HCT recipients. Chronic GVHD occurs most frequently in patients with preceding acute GVHD, but can also manifest de novo without any preceding acute GVHD. The distinction between classic chronic GVHD and overlap syndrome requires attention to clinical symptoms and signs which are characteristic and thus diagnostic of chronic GVHD.

Acute GVHD is the most important risk factor for development of subsequent chronic GVHD. Use of mismatched or URDs and transplantation using peripheral blood derived hematopoietic stem cells instead of bone marrow also increases its risk. Other reported risk factors for chronic GVHD include older recipient age, use of a female donor, CMV seropositivity, high graft CD34+ cell count, and

TABLE 109.7	Common Clinical Manifestations of Chronic Graft-Versus-Host Disease
Organ System	**Clinical Manifestations**
Cutaneous	Poikiloderma, lichen planus, dermal sclerosis, morphea-like features, hypopigmentation or hyperpigmentation, ichthyosis, nail dystrophy, onycholysis
Ocular	Keratoconjunctivitis sicca, conjunctivitis, corneal ulcerations
Oral	Lichen planus, hyperkeratotic plaques, xerostomia, mucosal atrophy, ulcers, restriction of mouth opening from sclerosis
Pulmonary	Bronchiolitis obliterans, bronchiolitis obliterans-organizing pneumonia
Gastrointestinal	Esophageal web and strictures, malabsorption syndrome, exocrine pancreatic insufficiency
Hepatic	Cholestasis
Genitourinary	Vaginal stenosis or scarring, lichen planus
Musculoskeletal	Fasciitis, joint contractures from sclerosis, myositis or polymyositis, arthritis
Hematopoietic	Thrombocytopenia, eosinophilia, lymphopenia, hemolytic anemia, hypogammaglobulinemia

treatment with donor lymphocyte infusion. Similar to acute GVHD, in vitro or in vivo T-cell depletion of the graft can reduce the incidence of chronic GVHD.

Chronic GVHD can affect any organ system; however, certain pathognomonic clinical signs and symptoms have to be present to establish the diagnosis (Table 109.7).[48] Other clinical manifestations, though not diagnostic of chronic GVHD, can be characteristic, though may be seen in acute GVHD as well. Additional investigations including biopsies might be needed to verify the diagnosis and to rule out other etiologies, such as infections, drug effects and malignancies. The skin, mouth, eyes, and liver are the most commonly involved sites of chronic GVHD. The cutaneous manifestations resemble autoimmune disease and can include poikiloderma, lichen planus-like eruptions or scleroderma (sclerosis). An inflammatory dermatitis can progress to severe dermal and periarticular fibrosis with loss of skin appendages (hair and sweat glands) as well as significant skin tightness, fasciitis and loss of joint flexibility. Additional manifestations include dry eyes and dry mouth, which can resemble Sjögren syndrome clinically and histologically; enteritis with anorexia, early satiety, malabsorption, weight loss and failure to thrive, or esophageal dysmotility or stricture; and cholestatic (or sometimes hepatitic) jaundice. Pulmonary involvement in the form of bronchiolitis obliterans is an uncommon manifestation, but can be particularly debilitating and dangerous. In addition, the profound immune dysfunction associated with chronic GVHD because of hypogammaglobulinemia, impaired cellular immunity and functional asplenia, greatly increases the risk of secondary infections from bacteria, viruses and fungi. After the onset of chronic GVHD, 25% to 40% of patients die within 2 years, often of infections.

Chronic GVHD can be classified as mild, moderate, or severe depending on the number of organs involved and the degree of individual organ involvement. In general, factors associated with an adverse prognosis include thrombocytopenia, progressive onset from acute GVHD, poor performance status, lack of response to initial therapy and extensive skin or lung involvement.

Treatment of Chronic Graft-Versus-Host Disease

Although acute GVHD is one of the strongest predictors for chronic GVHD, strategies to limit acute GVHD such as prolonging or intensifying initial immunosuppression have not been consistently effective in preventing subsequent chronic GVHD. As with acute GVHD, the specific immunosuppressive therapy for chronic GVHD is most often corticosteroids, usually in combination with cyclosporine. The ongoing and long lasting nature of the syndrome demands that reduced doses and, if possible, alternate day steroid therapy be used to minimize chronic complications of prolonged corticosteroid therapy. Typical corticosteroid regimens start with daily prednisone 1 mg/kg per day and responding patients are tapered down to 0.5–1 mg/kg every other day and continued on this dose for 6–9 months beyond any active GVHD symptoms, followed by a slow withdrawal of immunosuppression. Longer therapy may be required for some patients, and early withdrawal of therapy has been frequently accompanied by flares of chronic GVHD. Salvage therapies including high-dose corticosteroids, sirolimus, tacrolimus, MMF, thalidomide, azathioprine, and hydroxychloroquine have been tried with limited response rates. Newer approaches currently being investigated as potential therapies for chronic GVHD include modulation of T-cell function, B-cell depletion, induction of immune tolerance and cytokine blockade. Small uncontrolled studies have reported the use of pentostatin, alemtuzumab and ATG to inhibit T-cell function and rituximab to eliminate B-cells with response rates of 30% to 50%. T-cell immunomodulation using extracorporeal photopheresis has been shown to have some activity, especially in sclerotic cutaneous chronic GVHD. Preliminary studies using daclizumab, etanercept, and infliximab for blockade of the cytokine-mediated inflammatory response have also shown short-term responses. The treatment of chronic GVHD demands particular attention to prophylaxis and aggressive therapy of secondary opportunistic infections. Most successful strategies for treating chronic GVHD incorporate long-term reduced-dose immunosuppressive therapy, aggressive antimicrobial prophylaxis and supportive care. Strategies favoring development of donor-derived regulatory T cells which may facilitate the development of immunologic tolerance including avoidance of calcineurin inhibitors (cyclosporine or tacrolimus) or photopheresis are being studied.

FUTURE DIRECTIONS

Complications of HCT are one of the major barriers to the wider application of transplantation for a variety of diseases. Currently, only one in four adult HCT recipients survives to 1 year post-HCT without experiencing a major complication.[49] The impact of newer transplantation modalities, including the use of NMA or RIC regimens, alternative donor transplantation with UCB, and incorporation of immune-based therapies within transplantation regimens, on early and late complications are areas of current investigation. Better tools to predict the risk of post-HCT complications and nonrelapse mortality are needed as well. Genomic and proteomic approaches to HCT complications are being investigated to monitor and predict complications. Although they are some years from use in clinical practice, these approaches could have many potential applications in transplantation, including prediction of risk for complications and GVHD, refining donor selection, and utilization of pharmacogenomic data to individualize conditioning regimens and immunosuppression. Each of these facets represent areas of ongoing vigorous research to improve the safety and effectiveness of HCT.

SUGGESTED READINGS

Alousi AM, Weisdorf DJ, Logan BR, et al: Etanercept, mycophenolate, denileukin, or pentostatin plus corticosteroids for acute graft-versus-host disease: a randomized phase 2 trial from the Blood and Marrow Transplant Clinical Trials Network. *Blood* 114:511, 2009.

Armenian SH, Sun CL, Kawashima T, et al: Long-term health-related outcomes in survivors of childhood cancer treated with HSCT versus conventional therapy: a report from the Bone Marrow Transplant Survivor Study (BMTSS) and Childhood Cancer Survivor Study (CCSS). *Blood* 118(5):1413–1420, 2011.

Betts BC, Young JA, Ustun C, et al: Human herpesvirus 6 infection after hematopoietic cell transplantation: is routine surveillance necessary? *Biol Blood Marrow Transplant* 17(10):1562–1568, 2011.

Boeckh M, Ljungman P: How we treat cytomegalovirus in hematopoietic cell transplant recipients. *Blood* 113(23):5711–5719, 2009.

Bolanos-Meade J, Logan BR, Alousi AM, et al: Phase 3 clinical trial of steroids/mycophenolate mofetil vs steroids/placebo as therapy for acute GVHD: BMT CTN 0802. *Blood* 124(22):3221–3227, 2014; quiz 3335.

Ciurea SO, Thall PF, Wang X, et al: Donor-specific anti-HLA Abs and graft failure in matched unrelated donor hematopoietic stem cell transplantation. *Blood* 118(22):5957–5964, 2011.

Ferrara JL, Levine JE, Reddy P, et al: Graft-versus-host disease. *Lancet* 373(9674):1550–1561, 2009.

Filipovich AH, Weisdorf D, Pavletic S, et al: National Institutes of Health consensus development project on criteria for clinical trials in chronic graft-versus-host disease: I. Diagnosis and staging working group report. *Biol Blood Marrow Transplant* 11(12):945–956, 2005.

Foley B, Cooley S, Verneris MR, et al: Cytomegalovirus reactivation after allogeneic transplantation promotes a lasting increase in educated NKG2C+ natural killer cells with potent function. *Blood* 119(11):2665–2674, 2012.

Freifeld AG, Bow EJ, Sepkowitz KA, et al: Clinical practice guideline for the use of antimicrobial agents in neutropenic patients with cancer: 2010 Update by the Infectious Diseases Society of America. *Clin Infect Dis* 52(4):427–431, 2011.

Gooley TA, Chien JW, Pergam SA, et al: Reduced mortality after allogeneic hematopoietic-cell transplantation. *N Engl J Med* 363(22):2091–2101, 2010.

Holtan SG, DeFor T, Lazaryan A, et al: Composite end point of graft-versus-host disease-free, relapse-free survival after allogeneic hematopoietic cell transplantation. *Blood* 125(8):1333–1338, 2015.

MacMillan ML, Weisdorf DJ, Brunstein CG, et al: Acute graft-versus-host disease after unrelated donor umbilical cord blood transplantation: analysis of risk factors. *Blood* 113(11):2410–2415, 2009.

Majhail NS, Parks K, DeFor TE, et al: Diffuse alveolar hemorrhage and infection-associated alveolar hemorrhage following hematopoietic stem cell transplantation: related and high-risk clinical syndromes. *Biol Blood Marrow Transplant* 12(10):1038–1046, 2006.

Majhail NS, Rizzo JD, Lee SJ, et al: Recommended screening and preventive practices for long-term survivors after hematopoietic cell transplantation. *Bone Marrow Transplant* 47(3):337–341, 2012.

Majhail NS: Secondary cancers following allogeneic haematopoietic cell transplantation in adults. *Br J Haematol* 154(3):301–310, 2011.

McDonald GB: Hepatobiliary complications of hematopoietic cell transplantation, 40 years on. *Hepatology* 51(4):1450–1460, 2010.

Panoskaltsis-Mortari A, Griese M, Madtes DK, et al: An official American Thoracic Society research statement: noninfectious lung injury after hematopoietic stem cell transplantation: idiopathic pneumonia syndrome. *Am J Respir Crit Care Med* 183(9):1262–1279, 2011.

Rizzo JD, Wingard JR, Tichelli A, et al: Recommended screening and preventive practices for long-term survivors after hematopoietic cell transplantation: joint recommendations of the European Group for Blood and Marrow Transplantation, the Center for International Blood and Marrow Transplant Research, and the American Society of Blood and Marrow Transplantation. *Biol Blood Marrow Transplant* 12(2):138–151, 2006.

Rizzo JD, Curtis RE, Socie G, et al: Solid cancers after allogeneic hematopoietic cell transplantation. *Blood* 113(5):1175–1183, 2009.

Sun CL, Francisco L, Baker KS, et al: Adverse psychological outcomes in long-term survivors of hematopoietic cell transplantation: a report from the Bone Marrow Transplant Survivor Study (BMTSS). *Blood* 118(17):4723–4731, 2011.

Sun CL, Francisco L, Kawashima T, et al: Prevalence and predictors of chronic health conditions after hematopoietic cell transplantation: a report from the Bone Marrow Transplant Survivor Study. *Blood* 116(17):3129–3139, 2010; quiz 3377.

Tomblyn M, Chiller T, Einsele H, et al: Guidelines for preventing infectious complications among hematopoietic cell transplantation recipients: a global perspective. *Biol Blood Marrow Transplant* 15(10):1143–1238, 2009.

Weisdorf D: GVHD the nuts and bolts. *Hematology Am Soc Hematol Educ Program* 62–67, 2007.

Wingard JR, et al: Long-term survival and late deaths after allogeneic hematopoietic cell transplantation. *J Clin Oncol* 29(16):2230–2239, 2011.

Wingard JR, Majhail NS, Brazauskas R, et al: Randomized, double-blind trial of fluconazole versus voriconazole for prevention of invasive fungal infection after allogeneic hematopoietic cell transplantation. *Blood* 116(24):5111–5118, 2010.

Yanik GA, Horowitz MM, Weisdorf DJ, et al: Randomized, double-blind, placebo-controlled trial of soluble tumor necrosis factor receptor: Enbrel (etanercept) for the treatment of idiopathic pneumonia syndrome after allogeneic stem cell transplantation: blood and marrow transplant clinical trials network protocol. *Biol Blood Marrow Transplant* 20(6):858–864, 2014.

REFERENCES

For the complete list of references, log on to www.expertconsult.com.

PART XI

TRANSFUSION MEDICINE

CHAPTER 110

HUMAN BLOOD GROUP ANTIGENS AND ANTIBODIES

Connie M. Westhoff, Jill R. Storry, and Beth H. Shaz

Pretransfusion testing includes ABO and Rhesus (Rh) type and antibody screening to determine whether a patient has an unexpected red blood cell (RBC) antibody. If the antibody screen is positive, an identification panel is performed to identify the specificity of the antibody. Unexpected antibodies can be clinically significant causing hemolysis (i.e., acute or delayed hemolytic reaction) after transfusion of RBCs carrying the reciprocal antigen, or can be insignificant. The clinical significance of an antibody is assessed by correlating the serologic information with clinical experiences reported in the literature and with the patient's medical history. Notably, the majority of clinically significant antibodies (outside the ABO system) are in response to RBC antigen exposure either through transfusion or pregnancy. Other antibody characteristics that are used to predict clinical significance include immunoglobulin (Ig) class and in vitro characteristics such as strength of reactivity and titer; however, no foolproof method exists to predict the clinical significance. For antibodies with well-known clinical significance, antigen-negative blood is selected for transfusion. Predicting clinical significance is more difficult when a patient has an antibody to a novel or rare high-prevalence antigen and requires a transfusion but antigen-negative blood is not available.

ERYTHROCYTE BLOOD GROUP ANTIGENS

Erythrocyte blood group antigens are polymorphic, inherited, carbohydrate, or protein structures located on the surface of the RBC membrane. There are more than 300 blood group antigens, most of which are included in 36 different blood group systems (Table 110.1). The protein antigens are primarily located on integral transmembrane proteins, but a few are on glycosylphosphatidylinositol (GPI)–linked proteins (Fig. 110.1). Some antigens are carbohydrates attached to proteins or lipids, some require a combination of a specific portion of protein and carbohydrate, and a few antigens are carried on proteins that are adsorbed from the plasma. Many of the proteins carrying blood group antigens reside in the erythrocyte membrane as complexes with other proteins.

Recognition of a new blood group antigen begins with discovery of an antibody. When an individual whose RBCs lack an antigen is exposed to RBCs that possess the antigen, he or she may mount an immune response and produce antibodies that react with the antigen. Depending on the characteristics of the antibody and the number and topology of antigens in the RBC membrane, the interaction in vivo between antibody and antigen may result in removal of antibody-coated RBCs by the reticuloendothelial system or in hemolysis if complement is activated.

In blood group testing, most assays are designed to detect antibody-antigen binding with clumping of the RBCs ("agglutination") as the detectable endpoint. The ability to detect and identify blood group antigens and antibodies has contributed significantly to current safe supportive blood transfusion practice, to the appropriate management of pregnancies at risk for hemolytic disease of the fetus and newborn (HDFN), and to management of hematopoietic progenitor cell and solid organ transplantation.

Terminology

Some blood group systems bear the family surname in which the antibody was first discovered (Kell, Kidd, Duffy, etc.), with abbreviations to indicate antigens (K/k, Jk^a/Jk^b, Fy^a/Fy^b, etc.). Others have been given letter designations (A, B, D, M, N, etc.). A committee for terminology of RBC surface antigens and alleles, organized by the International Society of Blood Transfusion (ISBT), works to standardize terminology of new blood group antigens and the coding alleles.

DNA-Based Typing for Blood Group Antigens

The majority of genes encoding blood group antigens have been identified and cloned, and the molecular basis of most blood group antigens has been determined.[1,2] Details concerning the alleles associated with blood group antigens are found on the ISBT nomenclature and the Blood Group Antigen Gene Mutation Database (BGMUT) websites (www.ncbi.nlm.nih.gov/gv/mhc/xslcgi.cgi?cmd=bgmut/home; www.isbtweb.org/working-parties/red-cell-immunogenetics-and-blood-group-terminology/). Knowledge of the genes has advanced understanding of the structure and function of the components carrying antigens and resulted in an appreciation of diseases associated with loss of expression of some blood groups, for example, null phenotypes (Table 110.1). Of importance, knowledge of the gene has made it possible to perform DNA analyses to predict the serologic phenotype, to determine gene dosage (zygosity), to perform noninvasive fetal typing, and to type for numerous blood group antigens in a single assay.

Although the simple hemagglutination test remains the principal assay for RBC antigen typing for ABO and Rh, antibody screen, and compatibility testing; genotyping for minor blood group antigens has become commonplace in several clinical situations (Table 110.2). These include determination of the extended blood group phenotype in patients who are multiply transfused, which avoids false typing because of contaminating donor RBCs and aids determination of antibody specificity. This approach is also preferred in patients with strongly direct antiglobulin test (DAT)-positive RBCs, as well as for typing for antigens when no serologic reagents are available and for fetal typing from amniocytes or from free DNA present in the maternal plasma. In these instances[2a] and others (Table 110.2), hemagglutination is not helpful and genomic analysis is a useful adjunct to routine testing. More recently, genotyping is useful in patients treated with daratumumab (anti-CD38) because treatment results in panreactivity on antibody screening (all cells being reactive). High-throughput genotyping systems have enabled blood centers to screen donors for a large number of antigens in a single assay.

Blood Group Antibodies

The common causes of immunization against blood group antigens are transfusion, pregnancy, transplantation, or occasionally, practices such as sharing needles. "Naturally occurring" antibodies are not a result of RBC exposure; rather, a response to microbes encountered by way of the digestive tract and other mucosal surfaces regularly (e.g., anti-A, anti-B,) or sometimes (e.g., anti-M, -P, $-P^k$, -P1, $-Le^a$, $-Le^b$, -I, -IH) which result in production of antibodies with these specificities. These are the most common antibodies present in children and nontransfused male patients, and are primarily IgM. These multivalent IgM antibodies directed to carbohydrate antigens optimally bind and directly agglutinate to RBCs at temperatures below 37°C. Most are not clinically significant (outside of ABO).

TABLE 110.1   Blood Group Systems, Antigens, Expression, and Disease Associations

ISBT System Name (Number)	Gene Name	Predicted Topology (Number of Amino Acids [AA])	Component Name	Principal Associated Blood Group Antigens (null phenotype)	Present in Other Tissue	Disease Association	Function
ABO (001)	ABO	Glycosyl-transferases Type II (354 AA)	Carbohydrate	A, B, AB, A1 (group O)	Secretions, platelets, broad tissue distribution	Altered in some hematologic disorders, leukemia	Glycosylation
MNS (002)	GYPA (MN) GYPB (Ss)	Type I (131 AA) Type I (72 AA)	GPA GPB	M, N, S, s, U, Vw; M^k M^k lack GPA and GPB; En(a−) lack GPA; S−s−U− lack GPB	Renal endothelium and epithelium	Decreased Plasmodium falciparum invasion; May be receptor for Escherichia coli	Negative charge on sialic acid; receptor for microbes
P (003)	A4GALT	Galactosyl-transferase Type II (353 AA)	Carbohydrate	P1, Pk (P1−, PP1Pk−)	Lymphocytes, granulocytes, monocytes, platelets	Receptor E. coli and Parvovirus-B19; Miscarriage	Glycosylation
Rh (004)	RHD RHCE	Multipass—12 spans (417 AA)	RhD RhCE	D, C, E, c, e, G, V/VS (Rh_{null} syndrome)	RBC-specific	Hemolytic anemia; stomatocytosis; Reduced expression and mosaicism in hematologic malignancies	Structural link to underlying cytoskeleton
Lutheran (005)	LU	Type I IgSF (597 AA) (557 AA)	Lutheran glycoprotein B-CAM	Lu^a, Lu^b, Lu3, Au^a, Au^b (recessive Lu(a−b−))	Broad tissue distribution; Not on lymphocytes, granulocytes, monocytes or platelets	Increased expression possibly involved in vasocclusion in sickle cell disease	Possibly adhesion; may mediate intracellular signaling; Binds to laminin
Kell (006)	KEL	Type II (732 AA)	Kell glycoprotein	K, k, Kp^a, Kp^b, Ku, Js^a, Js^b (K_o or K_{null})	Broad tissue distribution; Bone marrow, fetal liver, testes, brain, heart, skeletal muscle	Depressed in McLeod syndrome (see XK)	Cleaves big endothelin 3 to ET-3 (a potent vasoconstrictor)
Lewis (007)	FUT3 (LE)	Not endogenous to RBCs Type II (361 AA)	Carbohydrate Adsorbed from plasma	Le^a, Le^b, Le^{ab}, Le^{bh}, ALe^b, BLe^b (Le(a−b−))	Saliva and body fluids; Blood cells, GI, skeletal muscle, kidney, adrenal	Increased expression in fucosidosis	Fucosyl transferase
Duffy (008)	ACKR1 (FY)	Multipass—7 spans (338 AA)	Fy glycoprotein	Fy^a, Fy^b, Fy3, Fy6 (Fy(a−b−))	Broad tissue distribution; Endothelial and epithelial cells, Purkinje cells, colon, lung, spleen, thyroid, thymus, kidney	Plasmodium vivax receptor; RBC null-resistant to P. vivax	Chemokine receptor
Kidd (009)	SLC14A1 (JK)	Multipass—10 spans (389 AA)	Kidd glycoprotein	Jk^a, Jk^b, Jk3 (Jk(a−b−) or Jk_{null})	Kidney: vasa recta endothelium; Renal medulla	Urine concentrating defect	Urea transport
Diego (010)	SLC4A1 (DI)	Multipass—14 spans (911 AA)	Band 3, AE1	Di^a, Di^b, Wr^a, Wr^b, (1 reported—transfusion dependent; predicted to be incompatible with life)	Kidney: intercalated cells of distal and collecting tubules	Southeast Asian ovalocytosis, hereditary spherocytosis, renal tubular acidosis	Anion transport CO_2/HCO_3^- exchange
Yt (011)	ACHE (YT)	GPI-linked (557 AA)	Acetyl-cholinesterase	Yt^a, Yt^b	Brain, muscle, nerves	Absent from PNH III RBCs	Enzymatic
Xg (012)	MIC2 (XG1)	Type I (180 AA) (163 AA)	Xg^a glycoprotein	Xg^a	The antigen may be restricted to RBC, but CD99 has broad tissue distribution		Adhesion molecule

System	Gene (symbol)	Protein/Component	Molecular structure	Antigens	Tissue distribution	Disease/clinical association	Function
Scianna (013)	ERMAP (SC)	ERMAP	Type I (475 AA)	Sc1, Sc2, Sc3, Rd (Sc -1, -2, -3)			Possible adhesion
Dombrock (014)	ART4 (DO)	Do glycoprotein; ART 4	GPI-linked (314 AA)	Do^a, Do^b, Gy^a, Hy, Jo^a (Gy(a-))	Lymphocytes, spleen, lymph nodes, GI, ovary, testes, heart, liver	Absent from PNH III RBCs	Enzymatic
Colton (015)	AQP1 (CO)	Aquaporin	Multipass—6 spans (269 AA)	Co^a, Co^b, Co3 (Co(a-b-))	Broad tissue distribution Kidney, liver, gallbladder, eye, capillary endothelium	Monosomy 7, congenital dyserythropoietic anemia	Water transport
Landsteiner-Wiener (016)	ICAM4 (LW)	LW glycoprotein ICAM-4	Type I IgSF (241 AA)	LW^a, LW^b, LW^{ab} (LW(a-b-))		Depressed in some malignant diseases; decreased in Rh_{null} syndrome	Ligand for integrins
Chido/ Rodgers (017)	C4A, C4B (CH/RG)	C4A; C4B	Not endogenous to RBC (1191 AA)	Ch1, Ch2, Rg1	Adsorbed from plasma	Certain phenotypes increased susceptibility to autoimmune conditions and infections C4-deficient predisposes for SLE	Part of the complement cascade
H (018)	FUT1(H)	Carbohydrate	Fucosyl-transferase Type II (365 AA)	H (Bombay O_h)	Broad distribution Soluble—all fluids except CSF in secretors	Decreased in some tumor cells Increased in hematopoietic stress	Glycosylation
Kx (019)	XK (XK)	XK glycoprotein	Multipass—10 spans (444 AA)	Kx (McLeod)	Fetal liver, adult skeletal muscle, brain, pancreas, heart	X-linked midlife onset neuropathy, elevated CPK, muscular dystrophy, acanthocytosis; sometimes associated with CGD	Transport; possible neuro-transmitter
Gerbich (020)	GYPC (GE)	GPC GPD	Type I (128 AA) (107 AA)	Ge2, Ge3, Ge4 (Leach phenotype)	Fetal liver, renal endothelium	Hereditary elliptocytosis, hemolytic anemia, receptor P. falciparum	Structural Interacts with protein 4.1 and p55
Cromer (021)	CD55 (CROM)	DAF	GPI-linked (347 AA)	Cr^a, Tc^a, Tc^b, Tc^c, Dr^a, Es^a, IFC (Inab)	Vascular endothelium Epithelial GI, GU, CNS Soluble form in plasma and urine	Absent from PNH III RBCs Dr^a is receptor for uropathogenic E. coli	Complement regulation; binds C3b; disassembles C3/C5 convertase
Knops (022)	CR1 (KN)	CR1	Type I (1998 AA)	Kn^a, Kn^b, McC^a, Sl^a, Yk^a, KCAM (no nulls reported)	Blood cells, glomerular podocytes, follicular dendritic cells	Antigens depressed in certain autoimmune and malignant conditions	Complement regulation; binds C3b and C4b; mediates phagocytosis
Indian (023)	CD44 (IN)	Hermes antigen	Type I (341 AA)	In^a, In^b	Wide tissue distribution	1 case—congenital dyserythropoietic anemia	Binds hyaluronic acid; mediates adhesion of leukocytes
Ok (024)	BSG (OK)	Basigin	Type I IgSF (248 AA)	Ok^a	All cells tested	Receptor P. falciparum	Possible adhesion
RAPH (025)	MER2	CD151	Multipass—4 spans (253 AA)	MER2 (Raph-)	Fibroblasts	Absence associated with renal disease and kidney failure	

Continued

TABLE 110.1 Blood Group Systems, Antigens, Expression, and Disease Associations—cont'd

ISBT System Name (Number)	Gene Name	Predicted Topology (Number of Amino Acids [AA])	Component Name	Principal Associated Blood Group Antigens (null phenotype)	Present in Other Tissue	Disease Association	Function
JMH (026)	SEMA-L (JMH)	GPI-linked (656 AA)	Semaphorin 7A	JMH		Absent from PNHIII RBCs	Adhesion molecule
I (027)	GCNT2	N-acetyl-glucosaminyl-transferase type II (400 AA)	Carbohydrate	I (I– or i adult)	Broad tissue distribution	Cataracts in Asians	Glycosylation
Globoside (028)	B3GALT1	N-acetyl-galactosaminyl-transferase type II (331 AA)	Carbohydrate (Gb$_4$, globoside)	P (P–) P^k and p	Broad tissue distribution Placenta (trophoblasts and interstitial cells)	Receptor E. coli and Parvovirus-B19 Spontaneous abortion	Glycosylation
GIL (029)	AQP3 (GIL)	Multipass—6 spans (292 AA)	AQP3	GIL (GIL–)	Board tissue distribution Kidney, prostate, GI tract, spleen, skin, eye		Glycerol/ water/ urea transport
RHAG (030)	RHAG	Multipass—12 spans (409 AA)	Rh-associated glycoprotein	RHAG1 or Duclos, RHAG2 or Ol^a, RHAG3 or DL, RHAG4 (Rh$_{null}$ regulator)	RBC-specific but homologs RhBG, RhCG in kidney, liver, skin, GI tract	Hereditary overhydrated stomatocytosis	Ammonia transport
FORS (031)	GBGT1	Type II (347 AA)	Carbohydrate	FORS1	Broad tissue distribution		Glycosyltransferase
JR (032)	ABCG2	Type III – 6 spans (655 AA)	ATP-binding cassette sub-family G member 2	Jr^a (Jr(a–))	Broad tissue distribution. High in placenta, seminal vesicles.	Gout; multidrug resistance in cancer	Urate exporter; porphyrin hemostasis
LAN (033)	ABCB6	Type III – 6 spans (842 AA)	ATP-binding cassette sub-family B member 6, mitochondrial	Lan (Lan–)	Broad tissue distribution	Dyschromatosis universalis hereditaria; Microphthalmia	Binds heme and porphyrins. Important in heme synthesis
VEL (034)	SMIM1	Type 1 (78 AA)	SMIM1	Vel (Vel–)	RBCs, salivary glands, testis		Not known
CD59 (035)	CD59	GPI-linked (128 AA)	CD59 glycoprotein	CD59.1 (CD59.1–)	Broad tissue distribution; Soluble form in plasma	Hemolytic anemia, with or without polyneuropathy	Complement regulation; inhibits MAC complex
AUG	SLC29A1	Type III – 11 spans (456 AA)	Equilibrative nucleoside transporter 1	At^a (At(a–))	Broad tissue distribution	Pseudo gout in the null phenotype	Nucleoside transmembrane transporter

^{a}Type I, protein with a single pass through the RBC lipid bilayer with its amino terminus to the outside of the cell; type II, protein with a single pass through the RBC lipid bilayer with its amino terminus to the inside of the cell. AEI, Anion exchanger 1; AQP, aquaporin; C4, fourth component of complement; CGD, chronic granulomatous disease; CR1, complement receptor 1; CSF, colony-stimulating factor; CNS, central nervous system; DAF, decay-accelerating factor; ERMAP, erythrocyte membrane-associated protein; GPA, glycophorin A; GPB, glycophorin B; GPC, glycophorin C; GPD, glycophorin D; GI, gastrointestinal; GPI, glycosylphosphatidylinositol; GU, genitourinary; ICAM4, intercellular adhesion molecule 4; IgSF, immunoglobulin super family; ISBT, International Society of Blood Transfusion; PNH, paroxysmal nocturnal hemoglobinuria; RBC, red blood cell; SLE, systemic lupus erythematosus.

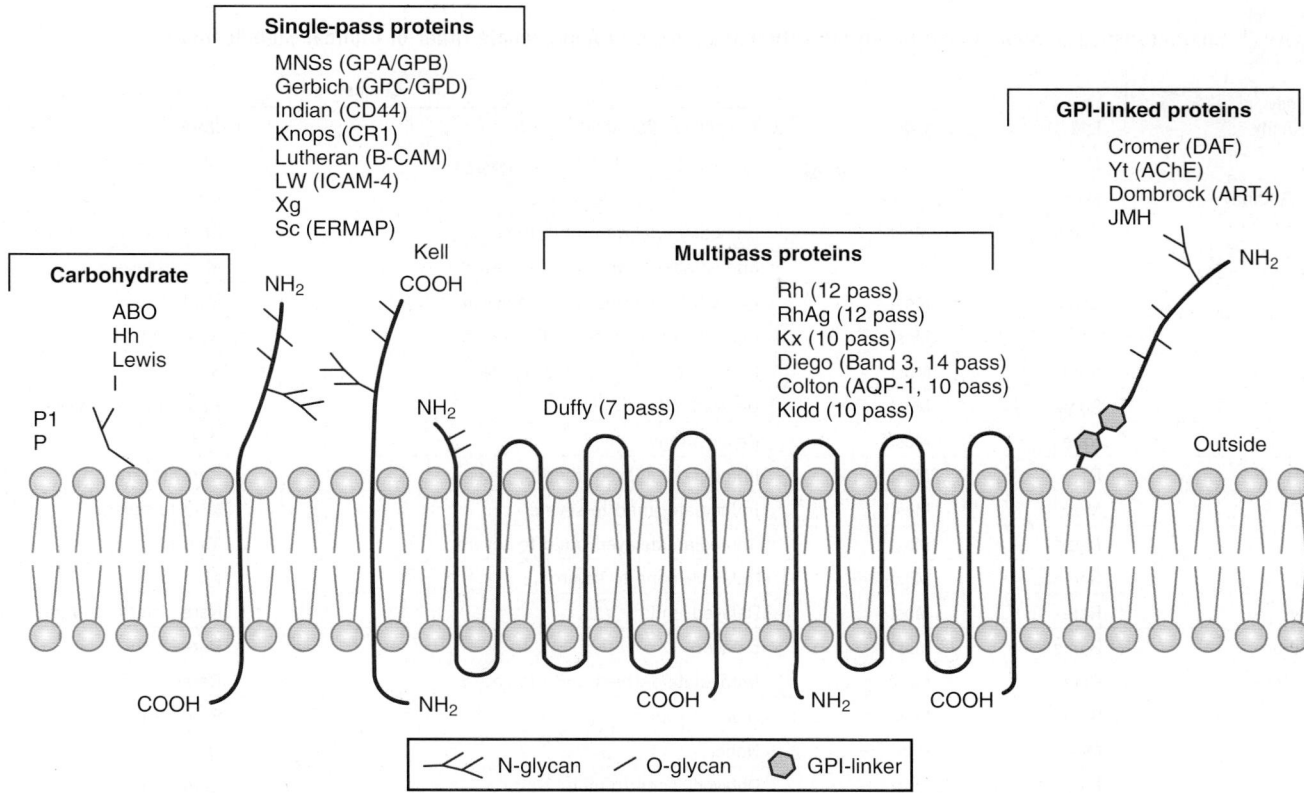

Fig. 110.1 MODEL OF BLOOD GROUP PROTEINS IN THE RED BLOOD CELL MEMBRANE. Schematic representation of the red blood cell (RBC) molecules that carry blood group antigens and the predicted structure. These include carbohydrates, single and multipass proteins, and GPI-linked proteins in the RBC membrane. AQP-1 (aquaporin-1), COOH (carboxyl group), CR1 (complement receptor 1), DAF (decay-accelerating factor), ERMAP (erythrocyte membrane-associated protein), GPA (Glycophorin A), GPB (glycophorin B), GPC (glycophorin C), GPD (glycophorin D), GPI (glycosylphosphatidylinositol), ICAM-4 (intercellular adhesion molecule 1), LW (landsteiner-wiener), Rh (rhesus), RhAG (Rh-associated glycoprotein).

TABLE 110.2	**Uses of DNA-Based Genotyping Assays for Transfusion Medicine**

Type patients who have been recently transfused

Type patients who are being treated with monoclonal antibody therapy, for example anti-CD38

Type RBCs coated with immunoglobulin

Type patients with AIHA (to select antigen-negative RBCs for transfusion and absorption of autoantibodies when searching for underlying alloantibodies)

Type RBCs when commercial antisera are not available

Type for numerous blood group antigens in a single assay

Identify weak D and partial D (to determine candidate for Rh immune globulin or avoid use of limited Rh-negative donor supply)

Resolve blood group typing discrepancies

Determine paternal zygosity for *RHD* and HPA

Type fetus to determine risk for HDFN or NAIT

AIHA, Autoimmune hemolytic anemia; HDFN, hemolytic disease of the fetus and newborn; HPA, human platelet antigen; NAIT, neonatal alloimmune thrombocytopenia; RBC, red blood cell.

Exceptions occur if the antibody is reactive at 37°C and/or has an IgG component. Antibodies that are considered not to be clinically significant unless the antibody reacts in tests performed at 37°C include those to A1, P1, M, N, Lu^a, Le^a, Le^b, I, IH, and Sd^a antigens.

In contrast, antibodies occurring following immunization to protein antigens such as those in the Rh, Kell, Kidd, and Duffy blood group systems are primarily of the IgG isotype that react at 37°C and are detected by the indirect antiglobulin test (IAT). These bivalent antibodies optimally bind to, but do not directly agglutinate, RBCs at 37°C. The addition of an antiglobulin reagent (i.e., antihuman IgG (AHG), also known as Coombs serum) is required to induce RBC agglutination. Most of these are clinically significant antibodies, with the exception of antibodies to Knops (Kn), Chido/Rodgers (Ch/Rg) and JMH systems (Table 110.3 summarizes the Ig class and clinical significance associated with alloantibodies; see also box on Indirect Antiglobulin Test and Direct Antiglobulin Test).

Antibodies recognizing antigens in the ABO system are by far the most clinically significant and are present in nearly all individuals who lack the antigen (they typically appear by 4 months of age). Other clinically significant antibodies occur in the following approximate order, from the most to the least commonly encountered in transfusion practice: anti-D, anti-K, anti-E, anti-c, anti-Fy^a, anti-C, anti-Jk^a, anti-S, and anti-Jk^b. Clinically significant antibodies occur in approximately 3% of transfused patients[3] but have a higher incidence of 35% to 55% in patients undergoing chronic transfusion.[4-8] The frequency of antibody production depends on the antigen immunogenicity and prevalence of the antigen in a population.

Compatibility Procedures and Location of Antigen-Negative Blood

Manual tube, solid phase, or gel-column methods based on agglutination of RBCs are the most common serologic assays performed in transfusion medicine laboratories.

TABLE 110.3   Characteristics of Some Blood Group Alloantibodies (Listed in Approximate Order of Clinical Significance)

Antibody Specificity	IgM	IgG	Clinical Transfusion Reaction	HDFN
ABO	Most	Some	Immediate; mild to severe	Common; mild to moderate
H in Bombay	Most	Some	Immediate; mild to severe	Rare; mild
Rh	Some	Most	Immediate/delayed; mild to severe	Common; mild to severe
RhAG	Rare	Most	Immediate/delayed; mild to severe	Mild to severe
Kell	Some	Most	Immediate/delayed; mild to severe	Mild to severe
Kidd	Few	Most	Immediate/delayed; mild to severe	Rare; mild
Duffy	Rare	Most	Immediate/delayed; mild to severe	Rare; mild
S	Some	Most	Delayed/mild	Rare; mild to severe
s	Rare	Most	Delayed/mild	Rare; mild to severe
U	Rare	Most	Immediate/delayed; mild to severe	Rare; severe
PP1P[k]	Most[a]	Most[a]	Immediate; mild to severe	Mild to severe[b]
Vel	Most[a]	Most[a]	Immediate/delayed; mild to severe	Mild to severe
Diego	Some	Most	Delayed; none to severe	Mild to severe
Colton	Rare	Most	Delayed; mild	Rare; mild to severe
Lutheran	Some	Most	Delayed	Rare; mild
Dombrock	Rare	Most	Immediate/delayed; mild to severe	Rare; mild
M	Some	Most	Delayed (rare)	Rare; mild to severe
N	Most	Rare	None	None
LW[a]	Rare	Most	Delayed; none to mild	Rare; mild
Yt[a]	Rare	Most	Delayed (rare); none to mild	None
Ch/Rg	Rare	Most	Anaphylactic (rare)	None
JMH	Rare	Most	Delayed (rare in genetic variants); none to mild	None
P1	Most	Rare	None (rare)	None
Le[a]	Most	Few	Immediate (rare)	None
Le[b]	Most	Few	None	None
I	Most	Rare	None None to mild in I adults	None
Knops	Rare	Most	None	None
Xg[a]	Rare	Most	None	None

[a]Most examples of these antibodies are both IgM and IgG.
[b]Seldom hemolysis of fetal cells but high incidence of recurrent spontaneous abortions.
IgG, Immunoglobulin G; IgM, immunoglobulin M; HDFN, Hemolytic disease of the fetus and newborn; Rh, rhesus; RhAG, Rh-associated glycoprotein.

ABO

Commercially available mouse monoclonal anti-A and anti-B are used to determine ABO type, and these reagents directly agglutinate RBCs at room temperature. To confirm the RBC ABO reactivity, the plasma is tested for the presence of the corresponding agglutinins by testing with commercially available group A1 and group B RBCs. In both tests, agglutination is macroscopically visible.

Rhesus

Patient and donor RBCs are routinely tested for the presence of the D antigen in the Rh system. Reagents containing monoclonal anti-D that directly agglutinate D-positive (Rh-positive) RBCs suspended in saline at room temperature are commonly used for testing. Testing by a method that detects expression of a weak D antigen on RBCs is required for donors, but additional testing for weak D is optional when testing patient samples. Exceptions include typing the RBCs of a newborn when the mother is D-negative to determine whether she is a candidate for Rh immune globulin (RhIG) (see box on Rh Immune Globulin).

Antibody Screening

Patient plasma is incubated at 37°C with commercially available reagent RBCs of known antigen type. After incubation, unbound antibodies are removed by washing with saline, and an antiglobulin reagent containing either AHG, or a mixture of AHG and antihuman complement is added. Column agglutination technology is now widely used and eliminates the requirement to wash unbound IgG. If the antibody screen is positive, the specificity of the antibody is determined by testing the plasma against a panel of different group O reagent RBCs (usually 10) varying in antigen phenotype (termed antibody identification).

Compatibility Testing

Once a patient is actively immunized to an RBC antigen and produces a clinically significant alloantibody, the patient is considered immunized for life and should be transfused with antigen-negative RBCs, even if the antibody is no longer detectable. Patients with passively acquired antibody (e.g., neonates with maternal antibody; recipients of plasma and platelet products or RhIG) need to be

Indirect Antiglobulin Test and Direct Antiglobulin Test

The indirect antiglobulin test (IAT) is used to detect alloantibodies in patient sera in vitro following incubation at 37°C and includes antibody screening and identification and crossmatching with donor red blood cells (RBCs). IAT is also sometimes used for antigen typing to detect RBCs coated with antibody following incubation with reagent antisera. After incubation, unbound antibodies are removed by washing with saline and an antiglobulin reagent containing either antihuman IgG (AHG) or a mixture of AHG and monoclonal antihuman complement is added. Differential agglutination suggests the presence of antibodies to one or more specific RBC antigens while agglutination of all cells suggests the presence of an antibody to a high-prevalence antigen or the presence of an autoantibody.

The direct antiglobulin test (DAT) is used to detect the presence of antibody or complement (or both) on the surface of RBCs in vivo such as autoantibodies coating the patient's cells in warm autoimmune hemolytic anemia, cold hemagglutinin disease, or alloantibodies coating the patient's cells in immediate or delayed transfusion reactions, or hemolytic disease of the fetus and newborn. Patient RBCs obtained in ethylenediaminetetraacetic acid, to prevent in vitro complement deposition on the RBCs, are washed with saline and then incubated with a commercial antiglobulin reagent containing AHG or antihuman complement or a mixture of the two. Antiglobulin reagents containing anti-IgM or anti-IgA are available in specialized centers to detect coating of RBCs by antibodies of these isotypes.

Rh Immune Globulin

Rh immune globulin (RhIG) is a human plasma-derived hyperimmunoglobulin product consisting of IgG antibodies to D antigen that is administered to D-negative pregnant women who are at risk for D sensitization. RhIG is administered (1) at 28 weeks gestational age, (2) when there is a risk for fetal maternal hemorrhage through amniocentesis, trauma, or other procedures, and (3) postpartum in the case of a known or potential D-positive newborn or fetus. If the Rh(D) typing of a pregnant woman is discrepant with prior results, or typing reactions are weaker than expected, or if variable reactivity is seen, RHD genotyping should be considered to guide RhIG prophylaxis and selection of blood for transfusion.

RhIG is sometimes administered outside of pregnancy to D-negative patients who receive D-positive blood products, most commonly whole blood derived platelet products. This is primarily considered for females of childbearing potential when the formation of anti-D has serious consequences. Because the risk for D alloimmunization from whole blood derived platelet transfusion is less than 4%, and even less for apheresis platelets, the majority of D-incompatible platelets are given without RhIG administration. RhIG in significantly higher doses is used to treat immune thrombocytopenic purpura (ITP) in patients who are D-positive and have not been splenectomized.

For prevention of D-sensitization in the United States, 300 μg are routinely administered, but dosing is increased if there is evidence of large fetal-maternal hemorrhage (300 μg for every 15 mL of RBC exposure or 30 mL of whole blood exposure). The dose is calculated based on the estimated volume of D-positive fetal RBCs from Kleihauer-Betke or flow cytometry, which is more precise. RhIG dosing calculators are available. RhIG should be given within 72 hours, which was the time period for the original studies, but should not be withheld if not administered within this time period. Adverse events to low doses used to prevent D immunization include fever, chills, and pain at the injection site. Rarely, hypersensitivity reactions are noted. RhIG doses used to treat ITP are substantial: 50 μg/kg for hemoglobin values ≥10 g/dL and 25–40 μg/kg when hemoglobin is 8–10 g/dL. Adverse events include possible anemia, hemolysis, disseminated intravascular coagulopathy, and rarely, death (Chapter 131).

TABLE 110.4 Approaches to Supplying Red Blood Cell Products to Prevent Alloimmunization in Patients With Sickle Cell Disease or Other Transfusion-Dependent Anemia

Phenotype or genotype for clinically significant antigens before transfusion
Provide antigen-matched blood for C, E, and K prophylactically
Provide blood negative for the major antigens that the patient lacks after the patient makes an antibody

antigen-negative blood will to some extent depend on the prevalence of the target antigen(s) in the donor population. Transfusion service staff are vital for communication between the patient's physician and/or consultant transfusion medicine specialist to determine the immediate and ongoing transfusion needs of the patient and to ensure that antigen-negative blood is available. Understanding the risks and benefits of transfusion are important, as well as understanding the potential clinical significance of the antibody and the urgency of transfusion. When a patient's antibody is directed at a high-prevalence antigen, it is important to test siblings in the quest for compatible blood and to urge the patient to donate blood for long-term storage when clinical status permits. In hemolytic anemia because of warm-reactive autoantibodies, compatibility may be difficult to demonstrate. In this scenario, the important issue is to be sure that there are no clinically significant alloantibodies underlying the warm reactive autoantibodies. Donor RBCs antigen-matched with the patient for clinically significant blood group antigens should be considered in lieu of transfusion with "least incompatible" blood to minimize alloimmunization.

Prevention of Alloimmunization

Transfusion management of patients who require chronic transfusion therapy, in particular patients with sickle cell disease can be challenging.[9–11] Many programs attempt to reduce or prevent alloimmunization by transfusion of RBCs that are prophylactically antigen-matched, typically for C, E, and K,[12] and some match for additional antigens. Some centers match for extended antigens once the patient makes an antibody (Table 110.4). The goal is to prevent hemolytic or delayed transfusion reactions, which are known to be underreported because they can manifest as a sickle cell crisis and may result in decreasing the transfusion interval.

Blood Group Disease Association

The absence of some blood group antigens and their carrier molecules can result in disease. For example, an absence of the Rh and Rh-associated glycoprotein (RhAG) proteins causes stomatocytosis[13] and anemia, termed *Rh_null syndrome*. The absence of Xk protein is associated with the *McLeod syndrome*, which is associated with myopathy and neurodegeneration. RBCs and white blood cells from patients with leukocyte adhesion deficiency II (also known as *congenital disorder of glycosylation type II*) lack antigens that are dependent on fucose. The RBCs have the Le(a–b–) Bombay phenotype and the white blood cells lack sialyl-Le^x, which explains the high white blood cell count and infections in these patients. Hemagglutination is a simple test that can be used to diagnose these syndromes. In patients with paroxysmal nocturnal hemoglobinuria, a proportion of the RBCs will lack antigens carried on GPI-linked proteins. Other associations between blood group antigens and diseases are summarized in Table 110.1.

Diseases associated with antibodies to blood group antigens include hemolytic disease of the newborn, warm autoimmune hemolytic anemia, cold hemagglutinin disease, and paroxysmal cold hemoglobinuria. Hemagglutination is a valuable aid in diagnosis of these conditions.

transfused with antigen-negative RBCs only while the passive antibody is present. Selection of blood for transfusion to patients with alloantibodies requires typing of donor units for the corresponding antigen to identify antigen-negative units and crossmatch of the selected units with the patient's plasma. Antigen-negative units are provided by, or can be located by, most donor centers. Provision of

Blood Group Systems

Presented here is a brief description of the most clinically relevant blood group systems in approximate order of clinical significance. For further information and prevalence of blood group antigens in different populations, refer to specialized texts such as *Human Blood Groups, The Blood Group Antigen Facts Book,* and the AABB *Technical Manual.*[2,3,14]

Carbohydrate Blood Groups

ABO and H

The ABO blood group system is by far the most clinically significant, because of the presence of naturally occurring IgM antibodies (and sometimes IgG). The original observation by Landsteiner that certain human erythrocyte suspensions were agglutinated by other human sera led to the recognition of ABO polymorphism.[14a] This initial observation is still the cornerstone of modern transfusion practice more than a century later.

Antigens and Their Synthesis

ABH antigens occur on glycoproteins and glycolipids and are synthesized in a stepwise fashion by glycosyltransferases that sequentially add specific monosaccharides in specific linkages to a growing oligosaccharide precursor chain (reviewed in Clausen and Hakomori[15]). The terminal sugar determines antigen specificity (Fig. 110.2). Group O individuals have H antigen only, the terminal sugar of which is fucose, and this is the precursor substrate for A and B antigens. Group O individuals have defective A or B transferases. The A and B transferase enzymes differ only by the nature of the monosaccharide added to the chain. *N*-acetyl-D-galactosamine is added by A-transferase, and D-galactose is added by B-transferase. In clinical practice, four ABO phenotypes (A, B, O, and AB) are discriminated. In addition, two common variations of group A (A_1 and A_2) can be distinguished. The differences between A_1 and A_2 phenotypes are quantitative and qualitative. Not only is the A_1 transferase more efficient in converting H to A antigen (approximately five times more A sites per RBC on A_1 RBCs than on A_2 RBCs), it also has the capacity to make A_1 antigen on the repetitive A epitope. Quantitatively normal ABH expression also requires the branching of carbohydrate chains, which is performed by the blood group I enzyme. Some H antigen precursor remains on A and B RBCs in this order: $A_2 > B > A_2B > A_1 > A_1B$.

Inherited and Acquired ABH Variation In addition to the main ABO types, there are many other inherited phenotypes with a weaker expression of the specified antigen, for example, A_3, A_x, A_{el}, B_3, B(A), and cis-AB. This can cause problems in determining the ABO blood group, but for patients needing immediate transfusion, the selection

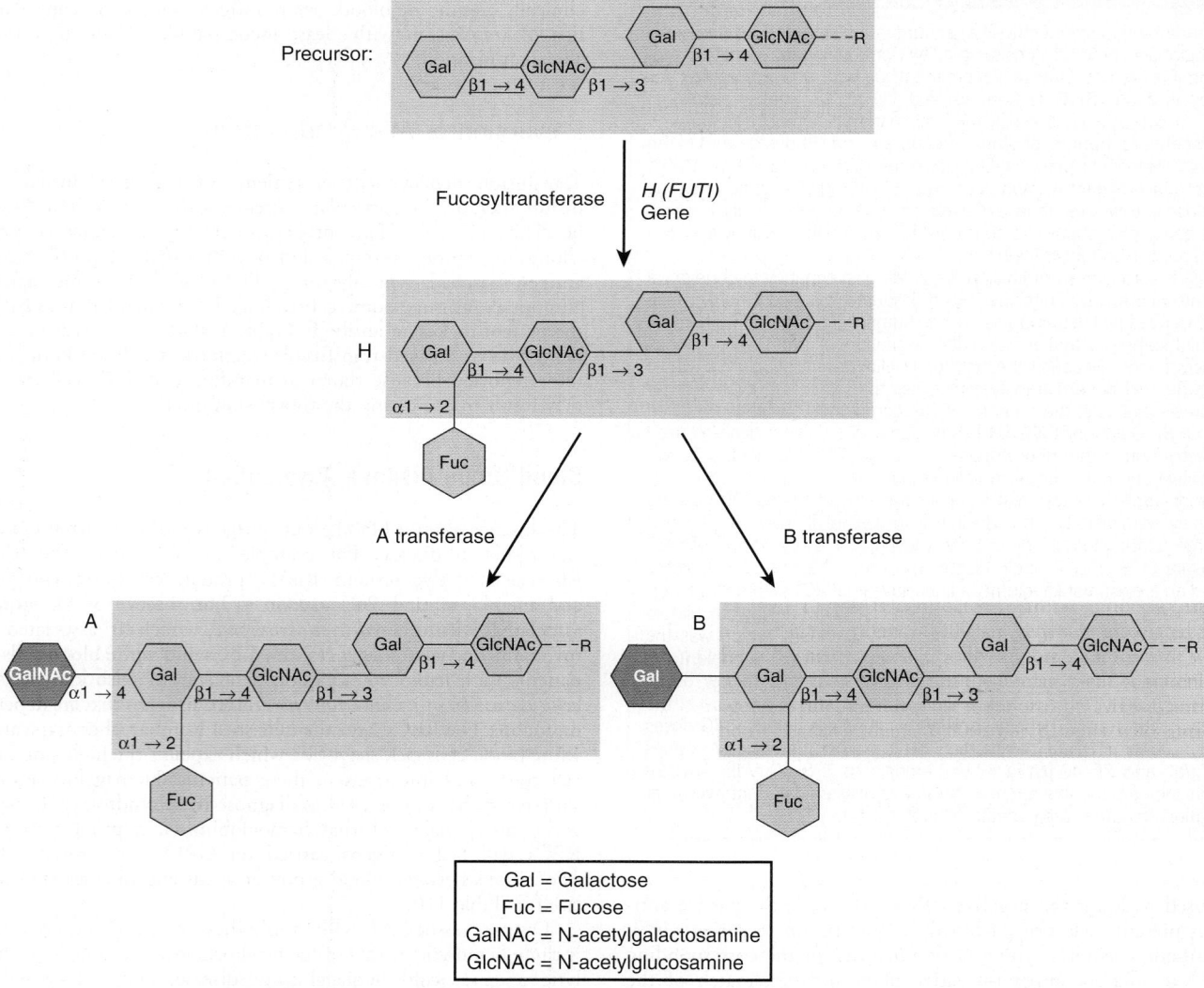

Fig. 110.2 BIOCHEMICAL STRUCTURES OF ABH ANTIGENS. Schematic representation of the terminal portions of the carbohydrate structures carrying the H, A, and B antigens on red blood cells.

of group O red cells and AB plasma products is an option. In blood donors, if very weak expression of A or B antigens on the RBCs is not detected, the major risk is that they may be transfused to a patient whose antibodies may cause accelerated destruction of the transfused cells.

Rare Bombay (O_h) phenotype RBCs, first reported in Bombay (Mumbai), India, lack H antigen and, consequently, A and B antigens. Other variants with weak H expression on RBCs, with or without H in secretions, also occur (para-Bombay) and have been reviewed.[16] Of clinical relevance, potent anti-H with the same hemolytic potential as anti-A and anti-B can be produced by Bombay individuals. Anti-H is often found in para-Bombay individuals but is generally not a potent antibody. HDFN caused by anti-H has not been reported.

Acquired B antigen is a rare phenomenon that results from the action of bacterial deacetylase, an enzyme that can remove an acetyl group from the A-terminal sugar, *N*-acetylgalactosamine. Galactosamine is similar to galactose, the B-specific terminal residue, and anti-B reagents can cross-react with the deacetylated structure. Acquired B can occur in individuals suffering from gram-negative infections of gastrointestinal origin or carcinoma and can be clinically significant if a patient's blood group is misinterpreted and group AB blood is transfused. Other polyagglutinable states (e.g., T, Tn, Tk) are detected by naturally occurring antibodies found in the serum of most people; these can be identified by a panel of lectins.

A or B antigen expression can weaken in patients with acute leukemia or stress hematopoiesis or, occasionally, during pregnancy. Chromosomal deletions or lesions that involve the *ABO* locus can result in the loss of transferase expression in the leukemic cell population. A decrease in A or B antigen expression, when found without a hematologic disorder, can be prognostic of a preleukemic state.

Genes and Enzymes The ABO gene was cloned in 1990 following purification of A transferase; since then, over 200 different alleles have been described.[17] There are only four amino acid differences between A and B transferases in the catalytic domain, two of which (Leu-266Met and Gly268Ala) are primarily responsible for the substrate specificity. The group O phenotype results from mutations in ABO that cause a loss of glycosyltransferase activity. The most common group O allele *(ABO*O1)* results from a single nucleotide deletion near the 5′ end of the gene that causes a frameshift and early termination with no active enzyme production. The rare B(A) and cis-AB phenotypes have both A and B enzyme activity from a single allele caused by variant glycosyltransferases that have a combination of A-specific and B-specific residues.

The fucosyltransferases required for H synthesis are encoded by two closely linked genes on chromosome 19, *FUT1* (or H) and *FUT2* (or *Se* for secretor), which have different substrate specificity and expression in tissues. Homozygosity for defective *FUT2* alleles is responsible for the common nonsecretor phenotype in which A, B, and/or H antigen are not present in secretions. Individuals homozygous for null alleles at both the *FUT1* and *FUT2* loci have the Bombay phenotype (see earlier section).

ABO and Transplantation As tissue antigens, ABO antigens are important in solid organ transplantation. Recipient antibodies will react with antigens on the transplanted organ and complement activation at the surface of endothelial cells can result in rapid destruction and hyperacute rejection. However, successful transplantation across ABO barriers is possible, particularly with blood group A_2 to O and with current immunosuppressive and pretreatment regiments including removal of ABO antibodies.[18] Allogeneic hematopoietic stem cell transplantations are routinely performed regardless of ABO compatibility, but occasionally initial hemolysis or pure red cell anemia because of persisting anti-A or anti-B titers in the recipient can result.

Antibodies Anti-A and anti-B are found in the sera of individuals who lack the corresponding antigens. They are produced in response to environmental stimulants, such as bacteria. These antibodies are produced after birth, reaching a peak at 5–10 years of age, and declining with increasing age. The antibodies are mostly IgM and can activate complement, which in conjunction with the high density of ABO antigen sites on RBCs, are responsible for the severe, life-threatening transfusion reactions that may result following ABO-incompatible transfusions. In contrast, HDFN caused by ABO antibodies is usually mild because (1) placental transfer is limited to the fraction of IgG anti-A and anti-B found in maternal serum, (2) ABH antigens are not fully developed on fetal RBCs because of a lack of fully branched carbohydrate chains, and (3) tissue ABH antigens provide additional targets for the antibodies.

Platelets have intrinsic A, B, and H antigens; thus ABO incompatibility can decrease the posttransfusion platelet increment, but this is often not of clinical significance.[19] However, platelets from donors with an A_2 phenotype lack both A and H antigens. Approximately 20% of group A platelets would be from A_2 donors and would be appropriate for "universal" use. Platelets from A_2 donors may also be a superior product for patients undergoing A/O major mismatch allogeneic progenitor cell transplantation.[20]

Potent anti-H (along with anti-A and anti-B) found in O_h (Bombay) individuals will destroy transfused RBCs of any ABO group, so these individuals must be transfused only with H− RBCs. In contrast, anti-H identified in individuals with low expression of H antigen, notably A_1B and A_1, is usually IgM, reacts only at lower temperatures, and is thus clinically insignificant.

Other Carbohydrate Blood Group Systems

As for all glycoconjugate structures, sequential enzymatic action is required to build other carbohydrate antigenic epitopes, and the genetic background of all these involves different glycosyltransferase loci.

The null p phenotype, P_2^k and P_1^k, are of clinical interest because of potent naturally occurring antibodies that are present in plasma of individuals whose RBCs lack the glycolipid-based antigens P1/P/P^k, P1/P/PX2, or P/PX2, respectively. In analogy with the ABO blood group system, antibodies of IgM and IgG class (anti-PP1P^k, anti-P1PPX2, or anti-PPX2) are made against the missing antigens. Although the incidence of the null phenotypes is only 5–10 per million, they have attracted considerable interest because of their relationship to disease and as receptors for pathogens. Women with p and P^k phenotypes suffer a high incidence of spontaneous abortion, a phenomenon most likely caused by destruction of the placenta by anti-P. In addition, anti-P and anti-P^k cause hemolytic transfusion reactions if antigen-positive RBCs are transfused. Transient autoanti-P, produced following a viral infection, causes paroxysmal cold hemoglobinuria and lysis of autologous P-positive RBC. P antigen (also known as *globoside*) is the cellular receptor for the parvo-B19 virus that causes erythema infectiosum (fifth disease) in children, sometimes complicated by severe aplastic anemia because of lysis of early erythroid precursors. P-fimbriated *Escherichia coli* expresses both P-binding and P^k-binding molecules at the tips of their pili, a finding with implications for uropathogenicity. Individuals lacking P, or P^k and P, appear to be naturally resistant to these bacterial and viral infections. In contrast to anti-P and anti-P^k, it should be noted that anti-P1 is a cold-reactive agglutinin that seldom has clinical importance. The clinical importance of anti-PX2 made by P^k individuals is unclear.

Lewis antigens are fucosylated glycolipids that are synthesized by nonerythroid cells, circulate in plasma, and are passively adsorbed onto RBC. Antibodies to Lewis can be made by individuals with the Le(a−b−) phenotype. These antibodies are of IgM class and seldom cause any clinical problems. Lewis antibodies are commonly found in pregnant women.

The i and I antigens are nonterminal epitopes on linear and branched carbohydrate structures, respectively, carrying ABH antigens at their terminal ends. During the first years of life, linear chains are modified into branched chains, resulting in the appearance of I antigens. The i phenotype is very rare among adults, but it is the normal state on RBCs from fetuses and infants. The gene encoding the I-branching β-1,6-*N*-acetylglucosaminyltransferase (*GCNT2*) has three alternative forms of exon 1 with common exons 2 and 3. Mutations in exon 2 or exon 3 silence *GCNT2* and give rise to the form of the i phenotype that is associated with cataracts in Asians. Mutations in exon 1C silence the gene in erythrocytes (but not in other tissues) and lead to the i phenotype without cataracts.

Alloanti-I made by a person with the rare i adult phenotype can be clinically significant and cause destruction of transfused I-positive RBCs. However, the sera of all I-positive individuals contain autoanti-I that is clinically benign and reactive only at or below room temperature. In contrast, cold hemagglutinin disease is characterized by a high titer of complement-fixing monoclonal anti-I, which causes in vivo hemolysis and hemolytic anemia. The titer and thermal range of autoanti-I is often increased following infection with *Mycoplasma pneumoniae*. If transfusion cannot be avoided, donor RBCs should be transfused through a blood warmer.

The FORS1 blood group antigen is a rare low prevalence antigen that is A-like in that it is defined by a terminal *N*-acetylgalactosamine and was first recognized as a weak A subgroup. The antigen has been defined as Forssman antigen, commonly found on the RBCs of nonprimate mammals, and arises from a gain-of-function mutation in the *GBGT1* pseudogene. The clinical relevance of anti-FORS1 found naturally occurring in the plasma of most individuals is not known.

Protein Blood Groups

Rhe, Rhe-associated glycoprotein, and LW Blood Group Systems

The Rh system is second only to the ABO system in importance in transfusion medicine. Rh antigens, especially D, are highly immunogenic; thus in most countries, blood for transfusion is tested and labeled with the D antigen type (Rh-positive or Rh-negative) and D–recipients are transfused with D–RBC products.

Three systems for naming Rh antigens have been used. Two are shown in Table 110.5, which indicates the incidence of the common Rh haplotypes present in different ethnic groups. The Fisher-Race nomenclature was based on the premise that there were three closely linked genes (D, C/c, and E/e), whereas the Wiener nomenclature (Rh-Hr) was based on the belief that a single gene encoded multiple factors (antigens). Although it is now well established that two genes, *RHD* and *RHCE*, encode the Rh proteins, the Fisher-Race (D, C/c, and E/e) terminology is often preferred for written communication; for spoken communication, a modified version of the Wiener nomenclature is preferred. Uppercase *R* indicates that D antigen is present and use of a lowercase *r* (or "little r") indicates that it is absent. The

C or c and E or e antigens carried with D are represented by subscripts: 1 for Ce (R_1), 2 for cE (R_2), 0 for ce (R_0), and Z for CE (R_z). The presence of these antigens without D is represented by a superscript: prime for Ce (r′), double-prime for cE (r″), and y for CE (r^y). This terminology allows one to convey the common Rh antigens (the phenotype) with a single term. The third system of numeric designations is not widely used in the laboratory, with a few exceptions (Rh17, Rh32, Rh33).

Genes, Proteins, Antigens, and Phenotypes The Rh proteins are designated RhD (encoded by *RHD*), which carries the D antigen, and RhCE (encoded by *RHCE*), which carries the CE antigens (either ce, cE, Ce, or CE). RhD differs from the various forms of RhCE by 32–35 amino acids. RhD and RhCE are not glycosylated but form a complex in the RBC membrane with RhAG (Rh-associated glycoprotein). Other proteins present in the Rh-complex are CD47 (an integrin-associated protein), LW, and glycophorin B. The Rh-complex also associates with band 3 (the anion exchanger) as a macrocomplex in the membrane.

The D-negative (Rh-negative) phenotype is prevalent in whites (15%–17%), less common in African blacks (3%–5%), and rare in Asians (<0.1%). The absence of D in Europeans is primarily caused by a deletion of the *RHD* gene. African blacks and rare D-negative whites and Asians carry a *RHD* gene that is silenced by a variety of molecular events.[3]

RBCs with weak D have D antigen but at lower levels than normal because of one or more amino acid changes that are often predicted to be in the intracellular or transmembrane regions of RhD. The RBCs do not lack, or have altered, epitopes of D. Many individuals with a serologic weak D phenotype have weak D types 1, 2, and 3 by *RHD* genotyping, and individuals with these genotypes can safely receive D-positive blood and do not make clinically significant anti-D.[21,22]

Partial D antigens (previously called *D categories* or *D mosaics*) are caused either by point mutations in *RHD* that encode amino acid changes that alter D epitopes, or by replacement of *RHD* nucleotides or exons by the equivalent part of *RHCE* that result in loss of D epitopes. RBCs with a partial D antigen may have strong or weak reactivity with anti-D. Because patients with partial D antigens can make anti-D directed to the D epitopes that are altered or absent, they ideally should receive D-negative blood and women of childbearing potential are candidates for Rh immune globulin. In practice, many type as D-positive and are recognized only after they make anti-D. However, in the United States monoclonal D typing reagents licensed by the Food and Drugs Administration for patient testing classify partial DVI phenotypes as D-negative in direct testing, and as D-positive by IAT. *RHD* genotyping is very useful to distinguish weak D phenotypes from partial D to guide selection of blood for transfusion and prevent D alloimmunization and to avoid unnecessary Rh immune globulin injection (see box on Weak or Variable D Typing).

TABLE 110.5	Prevalence of the Principal Rhesus Haplotypes			
Fisher-Race Haplotype	**Modified Weiner Haplotype**	**Incidence (%)**		
		White	**African Black**	**Asian**
Rh-Positive				
DCe	R_1	42	17	70
DcE	R_2	14	11	21
Dce	R_0	4	44	3
DCE	R_z	<0.01	<0.01	1
Rh-Negative				
ce	r	37	26	3
Ce	r′	2	2	2
cE	r″	1	<0.01	<0.01
CE	r^y	<0.01	<0.01	<0.01

Weak or Variable D-Typing

Clinically significant D-sensitization potentially results in a pregnancy with a fetus at risk for hemolytic disease of the fetus and newborn and hemolytic transfusion reactions if transfused with D-positive red blood cells (RBCs). Individuals with RBCs that express a partial D antigen are at risk for D-sensitization, whereas those with weak D antigen are usually not at risk. These cannot be distinguished by serologic reactivity, because either may present as weak or moderately positive or give variable results with anti-D reagents. Particularly in the prenatal setting, *RHD* genotyping should be done to distinguish weak D from partial D. Women with weak D expression, particularly weak D types 1, 2, and 3, are not at risk for clinically significant D-sensitization and therefore are not candidates for RhIG prophylaxis. In contrast, individuals with partial D, lack D epitopes and have produced clinically significant anti-D and should receive RhIG prophylaxis. *RHD* genotyping avoids unnecessary treatment with RhIG and excess use of Rh-negative blood in patients with weak D antigen.

Several phenotypes, including D– –, Dc–, and DC^w–, have an enhanced expression of D antigen and no, or variant, CE antigens. They are caused by replacement of portions of *RHCE* by *RHD*. The RhD sequences in RhCE, along with a normal RhD, explain the enhanced D and account for the lack, or reduced expression, of CE antigens. Immunized individuals with these CE-depleted phenotypes can make antibodies to high-prevalence Rh antigens.

C and c antigens differ by four amino acids, but only residue Ser103Pro is predicted to be extracellular. E and e differ by one amino acid, Pro226Ala. The RhD and various combinations of RhCE proteins (ce, Ce, cE, and CE) are typical for the majority of white transfusion recipients. However, Rh proteins in other ethnic groups often carry additional polymorphisms, particularly in individuals of African descent, and this fact often complicates transfusion in patients with sickle cell disease. For example, the RBCs of more than 30% of blacks are VS+ because of a Leu245Val substitution in Rhce, and expression of this antigen is associated with variant expression of e antigen. Many other amino acid changes in Rhce, as well as in RhD, are associated with production of Rh antibodies in patients with sickle cell disease. RH genotyping by DNA methods allows enhanced Rh antigen matching of patients and donors and is particularly important in patients who present with Rh antibodies reacting with all, or the majority, of cells tested.

The Rh_null phenotype is very rare and occurs on two genetic backgrounds: the "regulator" type, caused by mutations in *RHAG*, which encodes an Rh-associated glycoprotein, and the "amorph" type, caused by mutations in *RHCE* on a D– (deleted *RHD*) background. Rh_null RBCs are stomatocytic, fragile, and associated with anemia. RhAG is involved in maintenance of cation balance in RBCs.[13]

Antibodies Most Rh antibodies are IgG and do not activate complement. As a result, primarily extravascular hemolysis, rather than intravascular hemolysis, occurs in transfusion reactions involving Rh antibodies. The antibodies are almost always caused by RBC immunization from pregnancy or transfusion and usually persist for years. Anti-D can cause severe hemolytic transfusion reactions and HDFN, but the incidence of anti-D has decreased with the prophylactic use of Rh immune globulin. Most Rh antibodies should be considered as having the potential to be clinically significant for HDFN and hemolytic transfusion reactions. If serum antibody levels fall below detectable levels, subsequent exposure to the antigen characteristically produces a rapid secondary immune response. Autoantibodies in the sera of patients with warm autoimmune hemolytic anemia, as well as in some cases of drug-induced autoimmune hemolytic anemia, appear to demonstrate relative specificity to high-prevalence Rh antigens, although specificity for other members of the Rh complex have not been ruled out (see box on Transfusion Management of Patients With Warm Autoimmune Hemolytic Anemia).

RHAG Blood Group System

RhAG glycoprotein, encoded by *RHAG*, is highly similar to the RhD and RhCE proteins. It carries four blood group antigens: two of high prevalence (RHAG1 and 3) and two of low prevalence (RHAG 2 and 4). Antibodies to RHAG4 cause HDFN. RhAG is important for erythrocyte ion balance in RBCs and is required for the expression of RhD and RhCE proteins forming the core of the Rh-complex.

LW Blood Group System

Rh and LW are independent blood group systems but have a phenotypic relationship. In adults, D-positive RBCs have a stronger expression of LW antigen than D-negative RBCs, and anti-LW can be confused with anti-D. Transient loss of LW antigens from RBCs has been described in pregnancy and in patients with diseases, particularly Hodgkin disease, lymphoma, leukemia, sarcoma, and other forms of malignancy. Loss of LW antigens is usually associated with the production of antibodies that appear to be alloanti-LW.

Kell and Kx Systems

The Kell glycoprotein is highly folded through multiple intrachain disulfide bonds and is covalently linked to the XK protein in the RBC

Transfusion Management of Patients With Warm Autoimmune Hemolytic Anemia

Patients with warm autoimmune hemolytic anemia may present with jaundice, fatigue, and anemia, or they may show no overt clinical manifestations. The antibody screen and antibody identification panel will show all red blood cells (RBCs) positive (panagglutinin) with anti-IgG in the indirect antiglobulin test. The autocontrol (patient's own plasma and RBCs) will also be positive.

History: A transfusion history should be obtained to differentiate these results from a hemolytic transfusion reaction or hemolysis because of an alloantibody.

DAT: A direct antiglobulin test should be performed with anti-IgG and anti-C3. In clinically significant hemolysis, the DAT is usually strongly positive.

Eluate: If patient has been recently transfused (3–4 months), an eluate should be prepared from the patient cells to remove the antibody(ies); the eluate should be tested to determine specificity. The eluate is usually reactive with all cells when tested by the IAT with anti-IgG.

Phenotype or genotype: Type the patient's RBCs for minor blood group antigens (Cc, Ee, K, Jka/b, Fya/b, Ss) if the patient has not been recently transfused. When possible, IgM typing reagents are used because the patient's own antibody-coated RBCs may result in false-positive typing. Some laboratories are able to remove the IgG from the RBCs and perform a phenotype, but alternatively, genotyping for minor blood group antigens including Do^a/b antigens (there is no serologic reagent) can be performed.

Adsorption: Adsorb the serum autoantibody onto the patient's own RBCs to test for underlying alloantibody if the patient has not been recently transfused (3–4 months). If the patient has been recently transfused or if the low hematocrit results in insufficient autologous RBCs, perform alloadsorption with well-characterized RBCs (usually three with known antigen profiles). Test the adsorbed serum for underlying alloantibodies.

Crossmatch: Perform with neat and with adsorbed plasma. Crossmatch performed with neat plasma will usually be incompatible.

Communication: Inform ordering physician of reactivity and of delay in receiving crossmatched RBCs. Provide emergency-release RBCs if patient's clinical situation warrants. Inform the physician that the patient may hemolyze transfused RBCs similar to hemolysis of his or her own RBCs.

Transfusion: Consider providing RBC units negative for minor antigens that the patient also lacks. Consider matching for Cc, Ee, K, Jka/b, Fya/b, Ss (and Doa/b if possible). This potentially enables RBC units to be available before completion of the antibody identification testing. Transfusion with antigen-matched units potentially allows continued transfusion without need for autoadsorption or alloadsorption unless signs and symptoms of RBC destruction occur or there is a change in reactivity in antibody screening or the DAT.

membrane. Kell is highly polymorphic because of single amino acid substitutions in the glycoprotein that account for 35 of 36 antigens described to date. The K antigen is remarkably immunogenic eventhough it differs from wild-type (k, small k) by only one amino acid, and it appears that loss of an *N*-glycan exposes the peptide, thereby rendering it immunogenic.

Inherited weak expression of Kell antigens, termed K_mod phenotype, occurs with amino acid changes in the protein, with Kp^a in cis, and in the McLeod phenotype.[23] Transient depression of Kell system antigens may also occur in autoimmune hemolytic anemia, in microbial infections, and was reported in two cases of idiopathic thrombocytopenia purpura. The lack of Kell antigens (the K_0 or K_null phenotype) is caused by multiple different gene defects.

HDFN caused by anti-K can result in severe neonatal anemia, and unlike anti-D, maternal antibody titers and amniotic bilirubin levels are not good predictors of the severity of the disease. Kell antigens are expressed very early during erythropoiesis, and anti-K has been shown to suppress erythropoiesis in vitro. This may explain the low level of bilirubin observed in cases of neonatal anemia; thus Doppler screening of the fetal middle cerebral artery peak systolic velocity is used to monitor anemia. Other unusual consequences of Kell antibodies include risk for fetal thrombocytopenia and neutropenia.

McLeod Syndrome This uncommon syndrome is associated with the loss of expression of Kx protein caused by mutations and deletions in the *XK* gene.[23] The syndrome, which is X-linked and manifests only in males, may be underdiagnosed. The physical characteristics, which often develop only after the fourth decade of life, include muscular and neurologic problems. A minority of patients with chronic granulomatous disease also have the McLeod phenotype as a result of X-chromosome deletions encompassing both genes. Carrier females have two populations of RBCs (one of the McLeod phenotype and one of normal phenotype).

Duffy Blood Group System

The Duffy (*FY*), previously known as *DARC* now designated *ACKR1* for atypical chemokine receptor, glycoprotein is a promiscuous chemokine receptor found on RBCs and on endothelial cells in the kidney and brain that binds a family of chemotactic and proinflammatory peptides from the CXC (IL-8, MGSA) and the CC (RANTES, MCP-1, MIP-1) classes. The physiologic role of FY is clear, but on RBCs the receptor may allow RBCs to act as scavengers for excess chemokines. FY is also a receptor to which *Plasmodium vivax* merozoites can bind to invade RBC and cause malaria.

Antigens The Fy^a and Fy^b antigens differ by a single amino acid (Gly42Asp) located on the N-terminal extracellular domain of the FY glycoprotein and is responsible for the common Fy(a+b−), Fy(a−b+), and Fy(a+b+) phenotypes. The null Fy(a−b−) phenotype is rare in most ethnic groups, but it is common in people of African and Arabian origins. The null phenotype most often results from a mutation in the promoter region of FY that disrupts a binding site for the erythroid transcription factor GATA-1 and results in loss of FY on RBCs.[24] Because the erythroid promoter controls expression only in erythroid cells, FY expression in other tissues is unaffected. All individuals of African origin with a mutated GATA box to date have been shown to carry FYB and therefore Fy^b is expressed on nonerythroid tissues. This explains why Fy(a−b−) individuals make anti-Fy^a but not anti-Fy^b. Fy(a−b−) caused by a mutated GATA box on an FYA allele has been found in Papua New Guinea, another malaria-endemic region.

Antibodies FY antigens are much less immunogenic than Rh and K. Anti-Fy^b is less common than anti-Fy^a, and both antibodies can cause delayed hemolytic transfusion reaction (DHTR) and rarely HDFN. Anti-Fy3 is made by Fy(a−b−) individuals who are exceptions to above, and it is speculated they may lack FY protein on all cells.

Kidd Blood Group System

The Kidd (JK) blood group protein was implicated in urea transport when RBCs lacking the antigens were shown to resist lysis in 2 M urea. The protein is present in RBCs and kidney medulla and is a constitutive urea transporter, but failure to express Kidd does not result in an overt clinical syndrome; the only observed manifestation is a reduced capacity to concentrate urine.[25]

Antigens The Jk^a and Jk^b antigens differ by a single amino acid (Asp280Asn) and are responsible for the common Jk(a+b−), Jk(a−b+), and Jk(a+b+) phenotypes. The Jk(a−b−) or Jk$_{null}$ phenotype is uncommon and occurs with greater incidence in Polynesians, Asians, and Finns. Many different molecular changes in both JKA and JKB alleles have been shown to abolish expression of the Kidd blood group protein. Weakly expressed variants of Jk^a and Jk^b antigens are also not uncommon.

Antibodies JK antibodies are responsible for at least one-third of cases of DHTR. The antibodies often drop to undetectable levels or react only with cells that are homozygous for the antigen and escape

detection in the sensitized patient's serum before transfusion. JK antibodies only rarely cause HDFN, and if they do, it is typically not severe. Anti-Jk3, sometimes referred to as anti-Jk^{ab}, is produced by Jk(a−b−) individuals, and rare donors must be located for transfusion.

MNS System

M and N antigens are carried on alternative forms of glycophorin A (GPA), whereas S and s antigens are carried on alternative forms of glycophorin B (GPB). M/N and S/s are homologous proteins encoded by adjacent genes and consequently show linkage disequilibrium in inheritance of the antigens. The MNS system is highly polymorphic and most of the 49 antigens are the result of amino acid substitutions or rearrangements between *GYPA* and *GYPB*. Persons who are S−s− are usually of African origin. They either also lack the high-prevalence U antigen arising from a deletion of *GYPB* or express variant weak U antigen as a result of an altered form of *GYPB*.

Antibodies Anti-S, anti-s, and anti-U are usually IgG and can be clinically significant antibodies. Anti-M and anti-N can be naturally occurring, may be reactive at room temperature or below, and are often clinically insignificant.

Other Protein Antigens

Antibodies to antigens in the following systems are less common than those described earlier in this chapter, and information regarding their general clinical significance is summarized in Table 110.3.

Lutheran System

Lutheran (Lu), along with Secretor, provided the first example of autosomal linkage in humans, the first example of autosomal crossing over, and the first indication that crossing over in humans is more common in females than in males. The Lu system consists of four antithetical pairs of antigens and 16 independent high-prevalence antigens. The Lu(a−b−) phenotype is rare, but in the majority of individuals, it is caused by heterozygosity for silencing mutations in the *EKLF/KLF1* gene.[26] KLF1 is a transcription factor that regulates many erythroid-specific genes, and the expression of antigens in other blood group systems (e.g., Kn, In) is also affected. In one family, heterozygosity for a mutation in the *GATA1* gene was shown to be responsible for the Lu(a−b−) phenotype.

Antibodies Antibodies in this system are rarely encountered because the antigens are not highly immunogenic. They are usually IgG and give characteristic agglutinates surrounded by unagglutinated RBCs. They can cause mild transfusion reactions, but do not typically cause HDFN. Anti-Lu3 is found in the serum of immunized people of the rare recessive Lu(a−b−) phenotype, and the antibody is usually IgG and may cause DHTR or HDFN. Blood with the Lu(a−b−) phenotype should be used for transfusion of patients with these antibodies.

Diego System

The Diego (Di) blood group antigens are on Band 3 anion transport protein (AE1), one of the most abundant erythrocyte glycoproteins. AE1 forms complexes with many other proteins in the cell membrane and is important for RBC stability. The Diego blood group system contains three antithetical pairs of antigens and 16 low-prevalence antigens. Di^b antigen has a prevalence of greater than 99.9%, but Di^a is rare in most populations. Exceptions include South American Indians (Di^a occurs in 54% of this population) and North American Indians, approximately 12% of whom are Di(a+).

Antibodies Di antibodies are usually IgG and do not bind complement. These antibodies have caused DHTR (usually delayed) and HDFN. Autoantibodies to band 3 are common in patients with warm autoimmune hemolytic anemia.

Yt Blood Group System

The Yt system was named in 1956 when an antibody was found in the serum of patient whose last name was Cartwright. Yt^a occurs with a prevalence of more than 99% in random blood samples, and Yt^b is found with a prevalence of approximately 8%, except in Israelis, in whom it has a prevalence of 20% or higher.

Antibodies Yt antibodies usually are IgG and do not bind complement. These antibodies have caused DHTR but not HDFN.

Scianna Blood Group System

The Scianna (Sc) antigens are expressed by the RBC adhesion protein, erythrocyte membrane-associated protein. Sc1 is a high-prevalence antigen (prevalence ≈99.9%), and Sc2 is a low-prevalence antigen (1%); there are five other Scianna antigens.

Antibodies Sc antibodies are usually IgG, and some bind complement. These antibodies have not caused DHTR, and although they have caused a positive DAT in cord RBCs, they have not caused HDFN. Several examples of autoanti-Sc1 have been reported, some reactive in tests using patient serum but not plasma. Autoanti-Sc3–like antibodies have been described in one patient with lymphoma and in one patient with Hodgkin disease whose RBCs had suppressed Sc antigens.[2]

Dombrock Blood Group System

Dombrock (Do) antigens are carried on a GPI-linked glycoprotein that is a member of the mono-ADP-ribosyltransferase family, although Do has no demonstrable enzyme activity on the RBC. The Do blood group system consists of two antithetical antigens, Do^a and Do^b, and eight other antigens of high prevalence. The null phenotype is Gy(a–).

Antibodies Do^a and Do^b antigens are poor immunogens, and anti-Do^a and anti-Do^b are rarely found as single specificities. Antibodies in the Do system are usually IgG and do not bind complement. These antibodies have caused DHTR and a positive DAT but no clinical HDFN.

Colton Blood Group System

The Colton (Co) antigens are carried on aquaporin-1 (AQP-1), the first water channel protein characterized in mammals, and are also found in the kidney. The function of AQP-1 in RBCs may be to rehydrate rapidly after shrinking in the hypertonic environment of the renal medulla. Co^a has a prevalence of 99.9%, its antithetical antigen Co^b has a prevalence of 10%, and Co3 and Co4 are present on all RBCs except those of the very rare Co(a–b–) null phenotype. Co4 is a high prevalence antigen, the absence of which has been seen in three families only. Apparently healthy propositi with the Co(a–b–) phenotype and AQP-1 deficiency have RBCs with an 80% reduction in the ability to transport water. The residual water transport in these RBCs may be through another member of the water channel protein family, AQP-3, which transports water, glycerol, and urea, and carries the blood group antigen GIL.

Antibodies Antibodies in the Co system are usually IgG and some bind complement. The antibodies have caused DHTR and HDFN.

Gerbich Blood Group System

The Gerbich system antigens are carried on glycophorin C (GPC) and glycophorin D (GPD). There are six high-prevalence antigens and five low-prevalence antigens. The two glycoproteins are products of the *GYPC* gene. The gene consists of four exons, and the smaller GPD is generated by the use of an alternative translation initiation site.

Antibodies The antibodies may be immune or naturally occurring. Most are IgG and some of these bind complement. Some antibodies may be IgM. Although some antibodies have caused DHTR, others

have been benign. Anti-Ge3 has caused HDFN, and similar to Kell antibodies, the disease is associated with severe anemia. Clinical HDFN associated with anti-Ge2 has not been reported, but the antibodies have been eluted from DAT-positive cord RBCs.

Cromer Blood Group System

The Cromer (Cr) antigens are carried on decay-accelerating factor (DAF, CD55), a complement control protein attached to the RBC membrane through GPI-linkage. Cr is a system of two sets of antithetical antigens ($Tc^a/Tc^b/Tc^c$ and WES^a/WES^b), 16 high-prevalence antigens, and three low-prevalence antigens. The Cr(a–) phenotype is the least rare of the negative phenotypes, and with the exception of one Spanish-American woman, all people with Cr(a–) RBCs are black. Most of the other phenotypes are exceedingly rare.

Antibodies Antibodies in the Cr system are usually IgG and do not bind complement. The antibodies have caused mild DHTR but not HDFN.

Knops Blood Group System

The Kn blood group antigens are carried on complement receptor 1 (CR1). Kn^a, Sl^a, and McC^a antigens are fairly common and have a similar prevalence (>90%) in different populations; however, Sl^a is present on RBCs of 98% of whites, but on only 60% of African Americans. Typing for Kn system antigens can be challenging because the low level of expression on the RBCs in some disease processes gives false-negative results. RBC CR1 is important in the processing of immune complexes, binding them for transport to the liver and spleen for removal from the circulation. The CR1 copy number per RBC (and thus antigen strength) is reduced in SLE, cold agglutinin disease, paroxysmal nocturnal hemoglobinuria (PNH), hemolytic anemia, insulin-dependent diabetes mellitus, acquired immunodeficiency syndrome, some malignant tumors, and any condition associated with increased clearance of immune complexes. CR1 (the Sl^a antigen in particular) may act as a receptor for the malarial parasite *Plasmodium falciparum*; thus the Sl(a–) phenotype may provide selective advantage.

Antibodies Antibodies in the Kn system are usually IgG, and they do not bind complement. The antibodies do not cause DHTR or HDFN, and once identified, they can usually be ignored for clinical purposes. Identification may be complicated by the fluctuation of antigen expression on RBCs. In the Kn system, anti-Kn^a is the most common antibody in whites, and anti-Sl^a is the most common in African Americans.

Indian Blood Group System

The antigens of the In system are carried on CD44. CD44 has a diverse range of biologic functions involving cell-cell and cell-matrix interactions in cells other than RBCs. It is an adhesion molecule in lymphocytes, monocytes, and some tumor cells. CD44 binds to hyaluronate and other components of the extracellular matrix and is also involved in immune stimulation, as well as signaling between cells. In^b is a common antigen, and In^a is rare in white persons but has a prevalence of 4% in Indians, 10% in Iranians, and nearly 12% in Arabs.

Antibodies Antibodies in the Indian system are usually IgG and do not bind complement. Some antibodies may directly agglutinate RBCs, but the reactivity is greatly enhanced by the IAT. These antibodies have caused decreased RBC survival and a positive DAT in the neonate but not HDFN. A severe DHTR caused by anti-In^b has been reported.

Chido/Rodgers Blood Group System

Although the Ch and Rg antigens are readily detected on RBCs, they are located on the fourth component of complement (C4), which becomes bound to RBCs from the plasma. In complement activation through the classic pathway, C4 becomes bound to the RBC membrane and undergoes further cleavage; ultimately, a tryptic fragment,

C4d, remains on the RBC. This C4d glycoprotein carries the Ch/Rg blood group antigens. The antigens are stable in stored serum or plasma, and the phenotypes of this system are most accurately defined in plasma by agglutination inhibition tests.

Antibodies Antibodies in the Ch/Rg system are usually IgG, do not activate complement, and are considered benign. Considerable variation may be common in the reaction strength obtained with different RBC samples. Although these antibodies do not generally cause DHTR, they have caused anaphylactic reactions. The antibodies have not caused HDFN.

JR Blood Group System

The Jr^a antigen is carried on ABCG2, a member of the ATP-binding cassette family of multipass membrane proteins. The protein is broadly distributed and is a high-affinity urate transporter. It is also involved in porphyrin transport and in multidrug resistance in some cancers. The Jr(a−) phenotype is the null phenotype and Jr(a−) individuals lack the protein. Many different mutations have been identified for this phenotype although it is more common among the Japanese (where it is associated with gout) and the Roma population in Europe.

Antibodies Anti-Jr^a are usually IgG, do not activate complement and do not generally cause DHTR or HDFN, however two cases of severe HDFN have been reported.

Lan Blood Group System

Lan too, is carried by an ATP-binding cassette protein, in this case ABCB6, a protein that is widely expressed. It is highly expressed in fetal liver and upregulated during erythropoiesis. ABCB6 is important in heme synthesis and transports heme and porphyrins into the mitochondria. The Lan− phenotype is the null phenotype and it arises from many different molecular backgrounds but is not associated with a disease phenotype. Lan antigen expression is variable on erythrocytes.

Antibodies Anti-Lan are generally IgG and do not bind complement but have caused mild to severe DHTR and mild HDFN.

Vel Blood Group System

The Vel blood group antigen is dependent on the SMIM1 protein for expression and a 17-bp mutation in the *SMIM1* gene accounts for the vast majority of Vel− individuals and absence of SMIM1. The protein is widely expressed but more highly expressed on erythrocytes, salivary glands, and testes, although its function is unknown. Vel antigen expression is variable on RBCs.

Antibodies Anti-Vel are often a mixture of IgM and IgG and readily bind complement. While HDFN caused by anti-Vel is rare, the antibodies can cause severe hemolytic transfusion reactions.

CD59 Blood Group System

An antibody in the plasma of a young patient with CD59 deficiency qualified CD59 as a blood group antigen. CD59 is a GPI-linked protein on the erythrocyte and is important in complement regulation. It inhibits the formation of the membrane attack complex (MAC) by specifically binding to C8 and C9. Like other GPI-linked proteins, it is absent from the erythrocytes of PNH patients and its absence is the underlying cause of hemolysis.

Antibodies Only one example of the antibody has been reported. It was clinically benign although a positive DAT was observed following one of the transfusions.

Augustine Blood Group System

The blood group system Augustine (symbol AUG; number 036) was recently assigned to the equilibrative nucleoside transporter 1 protein (SLC29A1; ENT1) after it was identified as the carrier of the At^a antigen. The At(a−) phenotype in individuals of African origin is defined by an amino acid polymorphism on SLC29A1 (p.Glu391Lys), while the At(a−) members of a rare family affected by bone malformation lacked the protein due to an inactivating mutation in the *SLC29A1* gene: c.589+1G>C. The antigen defined by the antibody produced by the null phenotype was named AUG1, and the antigen defined by the amino acid Glu391 (At^a) was named AUG2.[27]

Antibodies. Anti-At^a are mostly IgG although may contain IgM. While HDFN due to anti-At^a is rare, the antibodies can cause severe hemolytic transfusion reactions.

REFERENCES

1. Reid ME, Lomas-Francis C, Olsson ML: *Blood group antigen facts book*, ed 3, San Diego, 2012, Academic Press.
2. Daniels G: *Human blood groups*, ed 3, Oxford, 2013, Wiley-Blackwell.
2a. Association Bulletin #16-02: *Mitigating the anti-CD38 interference with serologic testing*, 2016, AABB. <https://www.aabb.org/programs/publications/bulletins/Documents/ab16->.
3. Heddle NM, Soutar RL, O'Hoski PL, et al: A prospective study to determine the frequency and clinical significance of alloimmunization post-transfusion. *Br J Haematol* 91:1000, 1995.
4. Rosse WF, Gallagher D, Kinney TR, et al: Transfusion and alloimmunization in sickle cell disease. *Blood* 76:1431, 1990.
5. Aygun B, Padmanabhan S, Paley C, et al: Clinical significance of RBC alloantibodies and autoantibodies in sickle cell patients who received transfusions. *Transfusion* 42:37, 2002.
6. Vichinsky EP, Earles A, Johnson RA, et al: Alloimmunization in sickle cell anemia and transfusion of racially unmatched blood. *N Engl J Med* 322:1617, 1990.
7. Cox JV, Steane E, Cunningham G, et al: Risk of alloimmunization and delayed hemolytic transfusion reactions in patients with sickle cell disease. *Arch Intern Med* 148:2485, 1988.
8. Chou ST, Jackson T, Vege S, et al: High prevalence of red blood cell alloimmunization in sickle cell disease despite transfusion from Rh-matched minority donors. *Blood* 122:1062, 2013.
9. Chou ST, Westhoff CM: The role of molecular immunohematology in sickle cell disease. *Transfus Apher Sci* 44:73, 2011.
10. Yazdanbakhsh K, Ware RE, Noizat-Pirenne F: Red blood cell alloimmunization in sickle cell disease: pathophysiology, risk factors, and transfusion management. *Blood* 120:528, 2012.
11. Matteocci A, Pierelli L: Red blood cell alloimmunization in sickle cell disease and in thalassaemia: current status, future perspectives and potential role of molecular typing. *Vox Sang* 106:197, 2014.
12. Osby M, Shulman IA: Phenotype matching of donor red blood cell units for nonalloimmunized sickle cell disease patients: a survey of 1182 North American laboratories. *Arch Path Lab Med* 129:190, 2005.
13. Bruce LJ, Guizouarn H, Burton NM, et al: The monovalent cation leak in overhydrated stomatocytic red blood cells results from amino acid substitutions in the Rh-associated glycoprotein. *Blood* 113:1350, 2009.
14. Fung MK, Grossman BJ, Westhoff CM, et al, editors: *Technical manual*, ed 18, Bethesda, Md, 2014, American Association of Blood Banks.
14a. Schwarz HP, Dorner F: Karl Landsteiner and his major contributions to haematology. *Br J Haematol* 121:556–565, 2003.
15. Clausen H, Hakomori S: ABH and related histo-blood group antigens; immunochemical differences in carrier isotypes and their distribution. *Vox Sang* 56:1, 1989.
16. Oriol R, Candelier JJ, Mollicone R: Molecular genetics of H. *Vox Sang* 78:105, 2000.
17. Storry JR, Olsson ML: The ABO blood group system revisited: A review and update. *Immunohematology* 25:48, 2009.
18. Rydberg L: ABO-incompatibility in solid organ transplantation. *Transfus Med* 11:325, 2001.
19. Curtis BR, Edwards JT, Hessner MJ, et al: Blood group A and B antigens are strongly expressed on platelets of some individuals. *Blood* 96:1574, 2000.
20. Cooling LL, Kelly K, Barton J, et al: Determinants of ABH expression on human blood platelets. *Blood* 105:3356, 2005.

21. Flegel WA: Homing in on D antigen immunogenicity. *Transfusion* 45:466, 2005.

22. Sandler SG, Flegel WA, Westhoff CM, et al: It's time to phase in RHD genotyping for patients with a serologic weak D phenotype. *Transfusion* 55:680, 2015.

23. Danek A, Rubio JP, Rampoldi L, et al: McLeod neuroacanthocytosis: Genotype and phenotype. *Ann Neurol* 50:755, 2001.

24. Tournamille C, Colin Y, Cartron JP, et al: Disruption of a GATA motif in the *Duffy* gene promoter abolishes erythroid gene expression in Duffy-negative individuals. *Nat Genet* 10:224, 1995.

25. Sands JM, Gargus JJ, Frohlich O, et al: Urinary concentrating ability in patients with Jk(a-b-) blood type who lack carrier-mediated urea transport. *J Am Soc Nephrol* 2:1689, 1992.

26. Singleton BK, Burton NM, Green C, et al: Mutations in EKLF/KLF1 form the molecular basis of the rare blood group In(Lu) phenotype. *Blood* 112:2081, 2008.

27. Daniels G, Ballif BA, Helias V, et al: Lack of the nucleoside transporter ENT1 results in the Augustine-null blood type and ectopic mineralization. *Blood* 125:3651–3654, 2015.

CHAPTER 111

PRINCIPLES OF RED BLOOD CELL TRANSFUSION

Yen-Michael S. Hsu, Paul M. Ness, and Melissa M. Cushing

The clinical practice of transfusion medicine has evolved substantially since the discovery of the ABO system around 1900. Two technologic advances set the stage for clinical practice through blood component therapy. First, the introduction of a safe and effective anticoagulant-preservative solution (suggested by Loutit and Mollison) allowed for the preservation of blood products. Second, in the mid-1960s, the introduction of plastic blood bags by Walter and Murphy, combined with the ability to store blood for extended periods, created opportunities to use transfusions in varied clinical settings. With these discoveries, the era of modern component therapy began. In 2011, approximately 13.8 million units of whole blood/red blood cells (RBC) were transfused in the United States; whole blood transfusions accounted for only 0.15% of total transfusions. This chapter reviews appropriate RBC transfusion practice in a variety of clinical settings, the clinical implications of RBC storage, the pathogenesis of red cell alloimmunization, and existing and emerging alternatives to allogeneic RBC transfusions.

RED BLOOD CELL COMPONENTS

Modern transfusion medicine practice aims to provide the specific component of the blood required, rather than whole blood: red cells for oxygen-carrying capacity, plasma for coagulation proteins, and platelets for microvascular bleeding. The component therapy approach allows for optimal use of a limited community resource (Table 111.1). Today, the clinician wishing to increase the patient's oxygen-carrying capacity is more likely to use an RBC concentrate than whole blood, although there may still be situations in which whole blood, if available, is appropriate. For particular clinical applications, several modifications can be made to RBC products to render them leukocyte or plasma depleted. RBCs can also be frozen for long-term storage.

Whole Blood

A unit of whole blood is collected in citrate phosphate dextrose adenine (CPDA)-1 anticoagulant, giving it a shelf-life of 35 days and a volume of approximately 510 mL (450 mL of blood plus 63 mL of CPDA-1). Within 24 hours of collection, the granulocytes are dysfunctional, and several plasma coagulation factors including factors V and VIII have fallen. Although clinicians have been taught that whole blood stored at 4°C has no functional platelets, evolving studies have demonstrated in vitro that platelet quantities and function are maintained for 10–14 days after collection, leading to new interest in the use of whole blood for resuscitation.

Whole blood has the advantage of correcting simultaneous deficits in oxygen-carrying capacity and blood volume. Therefore, whole blood is useful in the management of trauma or in surgical cases involving extensive blood loss. In this setting, whole blood has two distinct advantages: (a) it provides colloid osmotic pressure and coagulation factors not supplied by crystalloid solutions and (b) it does not expose the recipient to RBCs and plasma from different donors.

The goal of using whole blood for all cases of concomitant RBC and volume deficit is difficult to achieve in practice. Most indications for whole blood transfusion are now well managed exclusively with blood component therapy, but the use of fresh whole blood has persisted in military settings. In the civilian setting, the simultaneous need for volume and oxygen-carrying capacity can usually be met by combining red cells with crystalloid or colloid solutions. In massive transfusions, however, this clinical axiom is being questioned, and current approaches are designed to minimize crystalloid exposure. In some cases of trauma and cardiovascular surgery, platelet transfusion may be indicated to combat microvascular bleeding from dilutional thrombocytopenia or bypass-associated platelet dysfunction. The transfusion of platelets usually supplies the equivalent of several units of relatively fresh plasma so that there is often no reason for further donor exposure by the administration of thawed plasma.

There has been recent renewed interest in fresh whole blood for patients with severe coagulopathy and shock. Few prospective trials have compared fresh whole blood with component therapy. The potential advantages for fresh whole blood are a relative increase in hemoglobin (Hb) concentration, coagulation factors, and platelets compared with component therapy. In addition, fresh products avoid some of the negative effects of storage and processing. A Food and Drug Administration (FDA) approved platelet-sparing leukocyte reduction filter is available for fresh whole blood. However, the use of fresh whole blood is limited due to the lack of published randomized controlled studies on specific indications and the demonstration of significant clinical benefits. The methods to achieve adequate pathogen removal and the determination of optimal storage conditions for whole blood products are the subjects of active investigations.

Increasingly studies in trauma patients have demonstrated a benefit to the early use of increased ratios of plasma and platelets to RBCs, including the PROPPR study that found there was a significant reduction in the time to hemostasis and a reduction in death by exsanguination within 24 hours for patients receiving a 1:1:1 ratio of RBC:plasma:platelets versus a 2:1:1 ratio. Whole blood transfusion is also being looked at as an alternate approach to provide trauma patients with early plasma and platelets.

Red Blood Cells

RBCs (also referred to as *packed RBCs* or *RBC concentrates*) are obtained from anticoagulated whole blood after removal of most of the platelet-rich plasma for the production of frozen plasma or platelets, or both. At most blood centers, the RBCs are then mixed with 100 mL of an additive nutrient solution that extends the storage period to 42 days and results in flow properties similar to those of whole blood.

RBCs are the product of choice for the correction of an isolated defect in oxygen-carrying capacity, as in cases of chronic anemia. In addition, RBCs rather than whole blood are used for the emergent transfusion of patients of unknown ABO type. The use of concentrated group O RBCs without plasma containing anti-A and anti-B can minimize potential hemolysis of the recipient's red cells.

Leukocyte-Reduced Red Blood Cells

Leukocyte-reduced RBCs (LRRCs) can be prepared by a variety of methods, resulting in differing degrees of white blood cell (WBC)

TABLE 111.1	Red Blood Cell (RBC) Components: Characteristics and Indications	
Component	**Characteristics**	**Indications**
Whole blood	High volume; good flow	Combined red cell/volume deficit (massive hemorrhage; exchange transfusion)
RBCs	Lower volume Higher hematocrit	Red cell deficit
Leukocyte-reduced RBCs	Good flow in AS-1	Prevention of febrile reactions Reduction of alloimmunization Reduction of immunomodulatory effects
Washed RBCs	Plasma depletion	Prevention of severe allergic reactions
	Must use within 24 hours	Prevention of anaphylaxis in IgA deficiency
Frozen RBCs	Long-term storage Plasma and leukocyte depletion	Rare donor unit storage Autologous storage for postponed surgery
	Must use within 24 hours of thawing	

Ig, Immunoglobulin.

removal. Currently, the most widely used method of leukoreduction is filtration that can be performed either in the laboratory or at the bedside. The various filters on the market result in greater than 99% leukocyte reduction while depleting less than 10% of the red cells. Blood bags with in-line filters allow prestorage leukoreduction.

The major indication for the use of LRRCs is the prevention of the febrile nonhemolytic transfusion reaction, the most common adverse effect of transfusion, particularly in multiply transfused patients or multiparous females. These reactions are believed to be mediated by antibodies directed against leukocyte antigens (human leukocyte antigen, HLA, or granulocyte-specific antigens). Depletion of leukocytes to less than 5×10^6 has been shown to prevent, or at least ameliorate, such reactions in most patients. Increasing evidence suggests that cytokines play a role in causing these reactions. Because cytokines may be released from leukocytes during storage, prestorage leukoreduction procedures are the preferred mode of leukoreduction.

A second important indication for LRRCs is the mitigation of alloimmunization to HLA antigens that can adversely affect post transfusion platelet increments and the search for HLA-compatible donors for stem cell and solid organ transplantations. This approach will be effective only if leukoreduced platelets are also used. According to current AABB standards, the total leukocyte number must be less than 5×10^6 when intended for this purpose. With the introduction of third-generation leukoreduction filters for both RBCs and platelets, this goal is achievable. A multicenter study known as TRAP showed that the use of leukoreduction filters for platelet products significantly decreased the rate of alloimmunization, but did not completely eliminate the problem.

A third indication for the use of LRRCs is to prevent transfusion-transmitted cytomegalovirus (CMV). CMV is found in low copy numbers outside of cells, and leukoreduced blood components are considered CMV safe. RBCs that are either leukoreduced or from CMV seronegative donors are associated with 1% to 1.5% CMV-transmission failure rates, and thus some institutions use the "belt and suspenders" approach of providing leukoreduced RBCs from a CMV seronegative in their vulnerable populations.

A final indication for the use of LRRCs is to prevent Transfusion Related Immunomodulation (TRIM), which is of particular concern in the postoperative period. A large metaanalysis previously demonstrated that patients who receive a blood transfusion are more likely to experience a postoperative infection than patients not transfused.

This effect has been found to be dose-dependent and is thought to be mediated by suppressing the patient's immune function. The mechanism of TRIM has yet to be defined, but multiple theories have been proposed. It has been suggested that immunologically active WBCs or soluble biologic response modifiers released from WBCs during storage down regulate the recipient's immune function. Alternative theories suggest that soluble mediators circulating in allogeneic plasma may have an immune modulatory effect. Universal leukoreduction has been found by some studies, but not by others, to mitigate the immunomodulatory effect of allogeneic transfusions.

Washed Red Blood Cells

RBCs are washed using isotonic saline solutions by either automated or manual techniques. Automated techniques are more efficient, but there is always some degree of RBC loss with each wash cycle. When the washing is performed in an open system, the resulting product must be transfused within 24 hours because of concerns over potential bacterial contamination.

The primary aim of washing is to remove plasma proteins, although some leukocytes and platelets are removed simultaneously. The major indication for washed RBCs is the prevention of severe allergic transfusion reactions, most likely mediated by recipient IgE antibodies against donor plasma proteins. Washing is recommended when reactions are severe and refractory to steroid and antihistamine administration. In IgA-deficient patients who have preformed antibody to IgA, the exposure to IgA-containing plasma can cause anaphylaxis. Therefore, high volume cell washes may be required to prepare cellular components for transfusion in IgA-deficient patients.

Irradiated Red Blood Cells

RBCs are irradiated with either gamma-ray or x-ray technology with a minimum dose of 25 Gy not exceeding 50 Gy. Red cells expire 28 days after irradiation or on the original expiration date, whichever is sooner. A method is used to ensure that irradiation has occurred with each batch. The primary aim of irradiation is to prevent the rare, but often fatal risk of transfusion-associated graft-versus-host disease (TA-GVHD) by the abrogation of the proliferative potential of donor T lymphocytes. GVDH can occur after the transfusion of immunologically competent donor lymphocytes, usually to an immuno-incompetent recipient. Ultraviolet light activated nucleic acid cross-linking techniques have also been shown to effectively inactivate T lymphocytes; however, currently, the FDA has not approved it as an acceptable alternative to gamma or x-ray irradiation to prevent TA-GVHD. Some patient populations with indications for irradiated products include neonates, patients with hematologic malignancies, stem cell transplant recipients, and patients with congenital immune deficiencies. There is still much debate among experts regarding which additional patient populations may be at risk for TA-GVHD. It has been suggested that a policy of universal blood component irradiation could prevent TA-GVHD in patients with currently unsuspected risks, including advanced age, unrecognized immune deficiencies in the recipient, or unsuspected donor-recipient immune similarities. Pathogen reduction is a term that refers to one of several methods to reduce the risk of blood-borne pathogens. If efficacious systems to apply pathogen reduction to red cell components by induction of DNA/RNA cross-linking become approved, another advantage would be the inactivation of white cells, which would eliminate the need for gamma irradiation to prevent TA-GVHD

Frozen Red Blood Cells

RBCs can be frozen (with glycerol used as a cryoprotective agent) and stored in liquid nitrogen or mechanical freezers. The required concentration of glycerol depends on the rate and the temperature of freezing. The freezing process destroys other blood constituents, except for a small percentage of immunocompetent lymphocytes. RBCs are prepared for transfusion by thawing and washing away the glycerol using a series of progressively less hypertonic crystalloid solutions, allowing glycerol to diffuse gradually from the cells to prevent hemolysis. The cells are resuspended in an isotonic saline solution containing glucose. The extensive washing removes approximately 99.9% of the plasma as well as cellular debris.

RBCs can be stored in the frozen state up to 10 years with good viability. After thawing and washing, storage is typically limited to 24 hours because of the open system. Frozen cells have been shown to maintain prefreezing adenosine triphosphate (ATP) and 2,3-diphosphoglycerate (DPG) levels. To maintain these factors at high levels, the standard is to freeze within 6 days of collection. When it is necessary to freeze older units, rejuvenation with a solution containing pyruvate, glucose, phosphate, and adenine has provided excellent results. The major indication for frozen RBCs is the stockpiling of rare donor units for patients who have developed alloantibodies. Some patients with rare phenotypes can make autologous donations that can be frozen for later use. Cells from autologous donors can be frozen if more units are required than can be collected in the 42-day liquid storage period or if surgery is postponed. Because of the high cost and cumbersome nature of freeze-thaw procedures, other uses of frozen RBCs are somewhat difficult to justify.

APPROPRIATE TRANSFUSION PRACTICE IN VARIOUS CLINICAL SETTINGS

The response to RBC transfusion varies from patient to patient. In the absence of increased red cell destruction or sequestration, one unit of RBCs can be expected to increase the Hb level by 1 g/dL or the hematocrit level by approximately 3%. This rise is usually not fully realized until approximately 24 hours after transfusion, when the plasma volume has had time to return to normal. On the basis of a half-life of approximately 57.7 days for donor red cells, Mollison and associates calculated that an average-sized adult requires 24 mL of RBCs per day to maintain a given hematocrit level, assuming no red cell production. Patients with red cell aplasia require approximately 2 units of RBCs every 2 weeks.

Several factors can adversely affect the survival of transfused red cells. Hemolysis, caused by either immune-mediated red cell damage or mechanical trauma, shortens the survival of transfused cells, much as it shortens the survival of the patient's own cells. Hypersplenism can lead to initial sequestration as well as increased destruction of red cells. Continued blood loss is another obvious cause of suboptimal response to transfusion. It should also be emphasized that transfusion suppresses erythropoiesis, so that the net result of transfusion may be less than expected if transfusions are administered on a chronic basis.

Chronic Anemia

As a rule, signs and symptoms attributable to anemia are unlikely to develop at a Hb level of greater than 7 or 8 g/dL. When the anemia is of gradual onset, the body's compensatory mechanisms for maintaining oxygen delivery to the tissues come into play. Both cardiac output and intracellular 2,3-DPG increase, and thus, oxygen unloads at a lower oxygen saturation of Hb. When chronic anemia is due to red cell destruction, the healthy bone marrow responds by increasing erythropoiesis up to sixfold.

RBC transfusion more commonly provides symptomatic support rather than definitive therapy for anemia. Transfusion should be used only when there is no definitive treatment for the underlying cause, or when the severity of the anemia and the clinical manifestations in the patient make it impossible to wait for the effects of the treatment to be realized.

Generalizations about RBC transfusion indications and practices are difficult to make and are usually inappropriate. The clinical impact of anemia varies depending on its pathogenesis, rate of onset, the presence or absence of accompanying hypovolemia, and, most importantly, the individual patient. The Hb level at which a given individual manifests the signs and symptoms of anemia relates, in part, to underlying health status, cardiorespiratory reserve, and tissue oxygen demand.

Perioperative Period

Many generalizations have been made about the appropriate transfusion management of acute blood loss, often with little hard data to support the arguments. One rule of thumb is that blood loss of 10% or less of total blood volume requires no replacement therapy at all; loss of up to 20% can be replaced exclusively with crystalloid solutions; and loss of greater than 25% generally requires RBC transfusion to restore oxygen-carrying capacity, along with crystalloid and sometimes colloid solutions to restore intravascular oncotic pressure to achieve adequate perfusion. For years, the threshold of 10 g/dL of Hb had been used as the gold standard for the RBC transfusion trigger during the perioperative period, but 7 g/dL is now more commonly used. Each case must be evaluated individually on the basis of clinical signs and symptoms, rather than on the basis of laboratory values. If the cardiovascular system is healthy and the degree of hypoperfusion is not significant, good tissue oxygenation can be maintained at much lower Hb levels. A National Institutes of Health consensus conference suggested that many surgical patients do not need transfusion unless the Hb level falls to less than 7 g/dL. Given that RBC transfusion should be tailored to individual needs, the question arises as to whether there is any readily available, objective measurement that can be used to determine how low the Hb level can safely be allowed to fall before RBC transfusion is initiated.

Global hemodynamic parameters do not always correlate with microvascular perfusion. Assessment of tissue oxygenation at the microvascular level would help evaluate the effectiveness of a red cell transfusion, evaluate the effect of red cell storage on end-organ perfusion, and provide data about when to transfuse. Several general methods are available to evaluate the microcirculation and include direct assessment using image techniques and indirect methods of assessment, such as measures of microvascular oxygen availability and function. Direct assessment can be performed using laser Doppler flowmetry, imaging of the microcirculation, intravital microscopy, orthogonal polarization spectral imaging, and sidestream dark-field imaging. Assessments of oxygen availability include oxygen electrodes, reflectance spectrophotometry, and near-infrared spectroscopy. The techniques described are currently considered research tools and are not available in routine clinical practice. Many have yet to prove reliable and reproducible in the clinical setting. Further, some are only useful in specific organ systems and do not reflect the global oxygenation of the patient. To be useful at the bedside, a technique must be technically simple, rapid and noninvasive without large interoperator variation. Such a device has yet to become available.

The Society of Thoracic Surgeons and the Society of Cardiovascular Anesthesiologists published clinical practice guidelines that identified six variables that increased a patient's risk of postoperative blood transfusion: advanced age, low preoperative red cell volume, preoperative antiplatelet or antithrombotic drugs, reoperative or complex procedures, emergency operations, and noncardiac patient comorbidities. The report recommended developing institution-specific protocols to screen for high risk patients and apply blood conservation interventions, such as erythropoietin or antifibrinolytic administration, intraoperative blood salvage or normovolemic hemodilution, and institution-specific blood transfusion algorithms supplemented with point-of-care testing. In 2015, the American Society of Anesthesiologists published a practice guideline for perioperative blood management that emphasizes the preoperative patient assessment and encourages greater utilization of pharmacologic agents and point of care testing-directed transfusion algorithms to minimize blood transfusion.

Randomized clinical trials have evaluated the effects of different transfusion thresholds in distinct clinical settings; however the thresholds used in the studies differ widely. Many of the studies found no difference in outcome. Most studies were not powered to adequately evaluate clinically important outcomes. Few studies included more than 100 patients. The Transfusion Requirements in Critical Care trial included 838 intensive care unit (ICU) patients who were randomized to a restrictive transfusion strategy (transfused at Hb 7 g/dL) or liberal strategy (transfused at 10 g/dL). The 30-day mortality was slightly lower in the restrictive group (18.7% versus 23.3%), but not significantly lower. The FOCUS trial, a 2600 patient, multicenter randomized trial designed to determine whether patients with cardiovascular disease or risk factors undergoing surgical repair of the hip benefit from a lower (<8 g/dL) or liberal transfusion trigger (transfused at 10 g/dL), has recently been completed. The results showed that liberal transfusion did not reduce mortality or in-hospital morbidity in this patient cohort. Other studies have now been published in the ICU, in sepsis, and in upper gastrointestinal (GI) bleeding that support the use of conservative transfusion triggers. On the other hand, there is a need for studies of transfusion triggers in patients with cardiac ischemia or in neurosurgery where clinicians have been reluctant to adopt conservative red cell triggers.

Red Blood Cell Transfusion in Neonates

In neonates it is convenient to consider periodic, small-volume transfusion separately from massive transfusion situations. The trigger for transfusion and the optimal type of component are very different in these two settings. The potential adverse effects may be quite distinct.

Low-volume RBC transfusion is rarely indicated in full-term infants unless acute blood loss has occurred at birth or an intrauterine situation has led to prenatal anemia. In contrast, premature infants are frequent recipients of transfusions. In the intensive care setting, the premature infant is subjected to frequent blood sampling, and iatrogenic anemia may necessitate transfusion. Anemia of prematurity is also a well-recognized entity; premature infants have a slightly lower Hb value at birth. In addition, the postnatal decline in Hb occurs earlier and is more pronounced in premature infants. The mechanism for anemia of prematurity appears to involve a relatively lower output of erythropoietin in response to a given degree of anemia. This phenomenon is attributed in part to the fact that the liver, rather than the kidney, is the major site of erythropoietin production in these infants. Although some practitioners have considered this degree of anemia to be physiologic, the benign nature of this condition remains controversial.

Another debate among neonatologists concerns the triggers for RBC transfusion, as in what clinical signs and symptoms are valid reflections of poor tissue oxygenation. Congestive heart failure and severe pulmonary disease are generally accepted indications for transfusion, but recurrent apnea, tachypnea, tachycardia, and failure to thrive are also used as transfusion triggers. In recent times, the rate of transfusion and the donor exposure rate of premature infants have consistently declined. These changes, however, reflect improvements in patient care (e.g., microtesting methods resulting in less iatrogenic blood loss; the use of surfactant resulting in decreased respiratory distress and the use of a single unit to supply one infant over a longer period) rather than being attributable to changes in the transfusion trigger. The prolonged use of single units has become possible with the advent of the sterile docking technology that preserves the full shelf-life of the unit of RBCs, as well as with the accumulating evidence that fresh blood is not necessary for low-volume transfusions in neonates because supernatant potassium and decreased pH are not of concern in this setting. Two recent studies have provided additional information about the relative risks and benefits of using restrictive rather than more liberal criteria for very low birth weight infants. One study showed that a liberal transfusion practice resulted in more infants receiving transfusion but conferred little evidence of

benefit. The other study showed a lower risk of apnea and major brain injury for the liberal transfusion arm of the study. Therefore, the safest transfusion trigger in the preterm infant still remains unclear, and further studies are indicated. Most institutions assess the clinical situation and consider the postnatal age and whether a neonate has oxygen requirements when determining the need for a RBC transfusion.

The dose of a RBC transfusion in a neonate can vary by institution between 5 and 20 mL/kg. Few studies have assessed the optimal dose in this patient population and further studies are needed. Paul et al compared 10 and 20 mL/kg and found that the larger volume did not cause impaired pulmonary function. Wong et al demonstrated extra transfusion episodes could be avoided with 20 mL/kg versus 15 mL/kg, without any additional risk to the patient. Many transfusion services now routinely use RBCs stored in additive solutions for low volume RBC transfusion and thus prefer a dose of 20 mL/kg to account for the lower hematocrit of an additive unit.

Finally, several trials of erythropoietin therapy in premature infants have been undertaken. The administration of relatively high-dose erythropoietin has been shown to raise Hb levels and reticulocyte counts in healthy premature infants, but the effect in sicker neonates is unclear. Although transfusion exposure was decreased, the significance of this observation is diminished, given the promise of new strategies for limiting transfusions and donor exposure. The high cost and the increased risk of retinopathy associated with erythropoietin treatment does not justify its use in this patient population.

In the case of massive transfusion, the situation differs. There have been marked increases in massive transfusion in recent years in full-term as well as premature infants. Hemolytic disease of the newborn remains a prominent indication for exchange transfusion; however, the recent use of intravenous immune globulin to decrease red cell antibody levels in newborns has decreased the necessity of this procedure. The two triggers for exchange are (a) rapidly rising levels of unconjugated bilirubin that may lead to kernicterus and permanent central nervous system damage and (b) congestive heart failure secondary to severe anemia. Whole blood exchange transfusion is especially beneficial in cases of hemolytic disease of the newborn because it clears the bilirubin, the offending antibody, and the antibody-coated red cells before lysis, while providing a source of red cells lacking the offending antigen. A two-blood-volume exchange is commonly performed by using a fresh unit of blood concentrated to a final hematocrit level of approximately 50%. In cases of hyperbilirubinemia resulting from other causes (e.g., that associated with liver immaturity in premature infants), phototherapy is the treatment of choice because its effects are usually more sustained, and exchange transfusion is used only for cases of marked elevations. Extracorporeal membrane oxygenation and open-heart surgery are two other situations that the neonate may be exposed to large volumes of allogeneic RBCs. The extracorporeal membrane oxygenation circuit requires a prime with RBCs, as do many of the types of extracorporeal circuits used for cardiopulmonary bypass.

Although accumulating evidence supports the safety of using RBC units of any age and with any preservative solution for low-volume transfusions in neonates, the same transfusion policies may not apply to massive transfusion. Newborn physiology is unique in several ways that may have implications for massive transfusion therapy. The newborn does not handle metabolites in a mature fashion. Renal immaturity may lead to problems in clearing potassium or acid from stored RBCs, and the immature liver may not catabolize citrate efficiently. These problems are accentuated and protracted in the premature infant. To address the concern about potassium load, fresh (<7 days old) or washed RBCs are often used, although the necessity of this practice is actively debated. Fresh blood may also be preferred because of its higher 2,3-DPG levels and better red cell integrity. The citrate problem is probably best handled by using slow infusion rates, because the use of bicarbonate or calcium replacement to counteract the acid load or calcium-chelating effects of citrate is controversial. Finally, the use of RBCs stored in the newer preservative solutions (CPDA-1, Adsol, Nutricel, Optisol) is avoided by some authorities because of the risk of renal damage and renal stones due to adenine metabolites. If CPD RBCs are not available, the additive solution can be removed and the cells washed. RBCs preserved in additive solutions also have a lower hematocrit level that must be taken into account in making calculations for exchange transfusion.

The humoral and cellular immune systems of the neonate are immature, especially in the premature infant. There is a small but real risk of transfusion-induced GVHD in premature infants receiving RBC transfusions and in the fetus undergoing intrauterine transfusion. Irradiation of RBCs should be performed in both settings. Another risk of transfusion in low birth weight (<1500 g) premature infants is the development of clinical CMV infection in infants of CMV-seronegative mothers. CMV safe blood, either CMV seronegative or leukoreduced, should be provided to these infants. Some retrospective studies have suggested that other rare RBC transfusion-associated complications in this particularly vulnerable patient group include necrotizing enterocolitis and intraventricular hemorrhage. However, a causal relationship has yet to be established through clinical studies.

Novel ideas to prevent anemia and decrease donor exposure in premature infants and other neonates include delayed cord clamping, cord milking, umbilical vein blood sampling from the delivered placenta, and autologous cord blood transfusion. One review of 10 delayed cord clamping studies, and demonstrated lower transfusion requirements in the delayed versus early clamped group. However, a randomized controlled trial by Strauss et al found no difference in transfusion needs between delayed and early clamped groups. A few studies have looked at autologous cord blood transfusions in neonates. One study found that the amount of blood harvested was insufficient to cover all transfusions in low birth weight infants. In addition, studies have demonstrated that blood processing problems, bacterial contamination, and costs are all barriers to the routine collection and autotransfusion of cord blood.

Red Blood Cell Transfusion in the Allogeneic Hematopoietic Stem Cell Transplantation Recipient

Red cell engraftment is usually the last phase of hematopoietic recovery after stem cell transplantation; therefore, RBC transfusion is common during the posttransplantation period. As hematopoietic stem cells and progenitor cells lack ABO antigens, the transplantation outcome is not significantly affected by the red cell antigen/antibody incompatibility between the donor and the recipient. However RBC transfusion requirements and blood product selection can vary significantly depending on the type of ABO incompatibility. The phenotyping of non-ABO/Rh red cell antigens from the donor and recipient is not required in the absence of a positive red cell antibody screen in the recipient. Patients with an autologous stem cell transplant have less RBC transfusion requirements when compared with patients receiving allogeneic stem cell transplantation.

In the setting of allogeneic stem cell transplantation, there are four major categories of ABO antigen matching: full compatibility, minor incompatibility, major incompatibility, and bidirectional incompatibility. In addition, Rh type must be taken into consideration. Rh positive recipients with Rh negative donors should receive Rh negative RBCs, but Rh negative recipients with Rh positive donors may receive Rh positive RBCs. Apheresis platelets and plasma may be given without regard to Rh. The blood product selection algorithm is shown in (Table 111.2). Minor incompatibility is defined as the presence of blood group antibodies in donor plasma (e.g., group O donor to group A recipient). In minor incompatible stem cell transplantation, the incompatible plasma in the donor stem cell product may result in some hemolysis of the recipient's endogenous RBCs during the early phase of the posttransplantation period. Minor incompatibility is occasionally complicated by passenger lymphocyte syndrome, where transient hemolysis may occur if donor-derived lymphocytes in the stem cell graft remain viable and form blood group–specific antibodies, which are incompatible with the recipient's

TABLE 111.2	Transfusion After ABO Incompatible Hematopoietic Stem Cell Transplantation			
ABO Group			**Product Selection**	
Donor	**Recipient**	**Type of Mismatch**	**RBC**	**Plasma/Platelets**
A	O	Major	O	A
A	B	Bi-directional	O	AB
A	AB	Minor	A	AB
B	O	Major	O	B
B	A	Bi-directional	O	AB
B	AB	Minor	B	AB
O	A	Minor	O	A
O	B	Minor	O	B
O	AB	Minor	O	AB
AB	A	Major	A	AB
AB	B	Major	B	AB
AB	O	Major	O	AB

RBC, Red blood cell.

red cells. Typically, passenger lymphocyte syndrome involves ABO incompatibility, but hemolysis resulting from serologic incompatibility in other blood group systems has been reported. If hemolysis increases a few days after transplantation, passenger lymphocyte syndrome should be considered. Once the donor is engrafted and incompatible recipient red cells are removed, donor red cells will have normal survival in the recipient. Major incompatibility is defined by the presence of blood group antibodies in recipient plasma (e.g., group A donor to a group O recipient). Major ABO incompatible transplantation may result in pure red cell aplasia (PRCA) due to persisting incompatible ABO antibody targeting the donor's engrafting erythropoietic precursors expressing ABO antigens. Although there may be no evident hemolysis, the donor red cell engraftment could be further delayed and result in prolonged RBC transfusion support. Finally, bidirectional incompatibility is defined as the presence of incompatible ABO antigens and antibodies contributed by both donor and recipient (e.g., group A donor to group B recipient). Bidirectional incompatible transplants may cause the problems associated with both minor and major ABO incompatible transplants. To predict the severity of these complications and provide management, an ABO antibody titer can be performed on either the stem cell product or the recipient. However, titers do not correlate perfectly with the clinical outcomes. When a high titer incompatible ABO antibody is discovered in a minor incompatibility, the stem cell product can be plasma-reduced to avoid an immediate hemolytic reaction. Occasionally, in major incompatibilities, plasma exchange can be considered if the recipient has a high level of incompatible ABO antibody to prevent hemolysis at the time of transplant or PRCA.

RED BLOOD CELL PRESERVATION AND STORAGE

The first key to the storage of blood is a stable, minimally toxic anticoagulant with preservative properties. During the early 1900s, it was recognized that citrate met these criteria. Citrate is slightly more toxic than heparin, especially when given rapidly and in large amounts, but citrate has preservative action that heparin lacks. Citrate has the added advantage of not causing systemic anticoagulation in the recipient.

The other factor essential for long-term storage is a mechanism to maintain cell viability and function. Freshly transfused RBCs have a good survival rate in the recipient's circulation, with a destruction rate approximately equal to that of the recipient's own cells: 1% per day.

Discoveries during the past two decades have raised clinical concern regarding the efficacy and risk of RBC transfusion. Changes within the RBC and its supernatant during RBC storage have been associated with reduced tissue oxygenation and other adverse effects in patients receiving RBC components stored for extended periods. The biochemical, structural, and functional changes are collectively termed the red cell storage lesion. The alterations found with the storage lesion along with the clinical implications will be discussed in this section.

BIOCHEMICAL CHANGES ASSOCIATED WITH RED BLOOD CELL STORAGE

Adenosine Triphosphate Levels

ATP levels appear to be a major determinant of red cell viability. The drop in cellular ATP levels during storage has been correlated with increased cell rigidity and with loss of membrane lipid, leading to decreased red cell life span. For this reason, most efforts to extend RBC storage have focused on ways to maintain intracellular ATP levels. First, dextrose was introduced into the citrate solution (citrate-phosphate-dextrose [CPD]: 21 day shelf life), and then adenine was added (CPDA-1: 35 day shelf life). Three additive solutions containing additional dextrose and adenine (Nutricel, or AS-3) or dextrose and adenine plus mannitol (Adsol, or AS-1) and (Optisol, or AS-5) allow extension of the maximum storage time to 42 days (Table 111.3). The majority of today's RBC supply is stored in an additive solution.

2,3-Diphosphoglycerate Levels

Stored RBCs must also maintain their capacity to deliver oxygen. It was not until 1967 that the central role of 2,3-DPG in releasing oxygen from oxyhemoglobin was recognized. Attention was then focused on ways to maintain high levels of 2,3-DPG in stored RBCs. The first anticoagulant introduced on a large scale, acid citrate-dextrose, was ineffective because of its low initial pH; however, the subsequently developed CPD, with its higher initial pH and slower fall in pH, was superior. CPDA-1 and additive solutions have not further improved 2,3-DPG maintenance. Although 2,3-DPG depletion of stored RBCs is known to decrease oxygen delivery, the clinical significance of this finding is unclear. 2,3-DPG levels in stored RBCs are rapidly regenerated in vivo, rising to greater than 50% of normal within several hours and to normal within 24 hours of transfusion. Although a patient with normal cardiac status should be able to compensate by increasing cardiac output to maintain normal oxygen delivery until 2,3-DPG levels are regenerated, an improvement in 2,3-DPG preservation in stored RBCs is still desirable.

TABLE 111.3	Biochemical Changes in Stored Red Blood Cells			
Variable	CPDA-1	CPDA-1	Adsol	
		CPDA-1 Fresh	35 Days	35 Days
In vivo survival (at 24 hours) (%)	100	<71.0	<88.0	
pH		<7.5	<6.7	<6.7
ATP (% initial)	100	<45.0	<76.0	
2,3-DPG (% initial)	100	<10.0	<10.0	
Plasma K⁺ (mEq/L)	5.1	<78.5	<49.0	

CPDA-1, Citrate phosphate dextrose adenine-1; DPG, 2,3-diphosphoglycerate. Data from Zuck TF, Bensinger TA, Peck CC, et al: The in vivo survival of red cells stored in modified CPD with adenine: Report of a multi-institutional cooperative effort. *Transfusion* 17:34, 1977; and Moore GL, Peck CC, Sohmer RR, Zuck TF: Some properties of blood stored in anticoagulant CPDA-1 solution: A brief summary. *Transfusion* 21:135, 1981.

Citrate

Infusion of large volumes of blood with citrate anticoagulant over a short period may cause plasma citrate levels to reach the toxic range. The primary concern is the cardiovascular effects of hypocalcemia caused by chelation of calcium by citrate. The risk of citrate toxicity is exacerbated by liver dysfunction or liver immaturity. Despite these theoretical considerations, there is little documented evidence of clinical citrate toxicity, which can usually be prevented by slower infusion. If large amounts of blood have to be infused over a very short period, administration of calcium gluconate can be considered, but whether the benefits justify the risk is controversial.

Potassium

Another issue with prolonged storage is the excess potassium in the RBC supernatant that could potentially cause cardiac arrhythmias. At a storage temperature of 4°C, the red cell sodium-potassium pump is essentially nonfunctional, and intracellular and extracellular levels gradually equilibrate. In addition, hemolysis results in increased potassium in the supernatant. However, because the total volume of plasma in RBC concentrates is low (approximately 70 mL), the total potassium burden is only approximately 5.5 mEq at product expiration. Practically speaking, the potassium load is rarely a clinical problem except in the setting of preexisting hyperkalemia and renal failure in adults. In children with rapid or massive transfusions, hyperkalemic cardiac arrest is more commonly recognized. In these situations, fresher units of RBCs or washed RBCs can be used.

Di(2-ethylhexyl)phthalate

Since their introduction in the 1960s, plastic blood bags used for storing RBCs have been made from polyvinylchloride containing the lipophilic plasticizer di(2-ethylhexyl)phthalate (DEHP), which confers pliability. The safety of DEHP has been questioned for years owing to its tendency to leach from the bag and to be present at levels of 50–70 mg/L in stored RBCs. The storage of RBCs in bags made of polyvinyl chloride plasticized with DEHP has caused more recent concern because of the reported association between DEHP exposure and impaired development of the male genital tract. One of the benefits of using DEHP for RBC storage is the prevention of hemolysis. DEHP leaches out from the plastic bag and intercalates and stabilizes the red cell membrane. Shorter storage lessens the load of DEHP delivered to the recipient. Although there are potential replacement plasticizers, DEHP is most commonly used since the exposure to DEHP through transfusion is generally felt to be less than other environmental exposures.

Storage Length of Red Blood Cells

Current Status

The current expiration time of an RBC unit stored in an additive solution is 42 days. The allowable storage time is regulated by the FDA and requires: 1) the recovery of at least 75% of red cells transfused twenty-four hours after infusion, and 2) less than 1% hemolysis, both at the end of the storage limit. There is no criterion based on the clinical ability of transfused red cells to oxygenate tissue. The 2011 National Blood Collection and Utilization Survey reported that the mean age of RBC units at transfusion was 17.9 days.

Many variables affect the age of a specific RBC unit at transfusion. The blood group of the unit will impact the length of storage. Group O units tend to be issued quickly due to their universal compatibility; as a result, Group O units are often issued with a shorter age. Group B and AB tend to be stored the longest. Transfusion service policies will also affect the overall age of RBC units at the time of transfusion. Busy tertiary care hospitals tend to transfuse some of the oldest units since they may receive units returned from smaller community centers who did not expect to use them before their outdate. Hospitals that have blood refrigerators outside the blood bank tend to age units in the refrigerators because it is cumbersome to rotate the units out frequently. Hospitals with high crossmatched to transfused ratios also tend to have older units on their shelves.

Red Blood Cell Storage Lesion

The RBC storage lesion includes all the changes that occur to blood components during blood bank storage. The lesion includes biochemical and structural changes to the red cell, as well as changes that occur in the storage supernatant. The structural changes include red cell membrane loss that leads to the reversible evolution of the shape of the red cell from a biconcave disc to a spheroechinocyte. After this stage, further red cell membrane loss becomes irreversible, and microvesicles are produced. Red cell vesicles are quickly cleared by macrophages due to exposed negatively charged lipids. The infusion of a large amount of red cell vesicles during a RBC transfusion may overwhelm the reticuloendothelial system and cause a proinflammatory and prothrombotic response. The shape changes are also associated with a rheologic effect, including increased viscosity and reduced flow within the capillaries, leading to decreased tissue perfusion. Many of the biochemical and structural changes, aside from vesiculation, are reversible when the RBCs enter human circulation where pH, ATP levels, and 2,3 DPG levels are normal.

Older red cells become more susceptible to oxidative damage, although this change generally occurs at a lower rate during in vitro conditions than in vivo due to the lower storage temperature. However, during a transfusion the human circulation is confronted by a bolus of equally damaged RBCs that may overwhelm the reticuloendothelial system. The work of Hod and Spitalnik emphasized that up to 25% of transfused RBCs with prolonged storage are cleared within 24 hours. The rate of delivery of heme-iron to the reticuloendothelial system may abruptly increase as much as 60-fold after transfusion of even a single unit of RBCs. This can surpass the rate of uptake by transferrin and produce circulating nontransferrin bound iron that may in turn lead to the myriad of problems associated with iron overload.

Irradiated cells are exposed to additional oxidative stress that can damage red cell protein and lipid. WBCs in the component also break down during storage and release proteases and lipases. Lysophospholipids and glycosidases are produced. Glycosidases may remove sialic acid and other sugars from the red cell membrane and can cause increased binding of stored red cells to endothelial cells and potentially contribute to endothelial inflammation. Increased lysophospholipids, such as platelet activating factor, have been found in units that have caused TRALI.

Clinical Relevance of the Red Cell Storage Lesion

Retrospective or prospective observational studies in many diverse patient populations have suggested numerous adverse events that may be associated with prolonged RBC storage, including increased risk for mortality, postoperative infection, multiorgan failure, deep venous thrombosis, or increased length of stay in the ICU or hospital. The observational studies on this topic have a number of significant limitations. First, larger volumes of RBC transfusion predict worse outcomes. Patients who are transfused larger volumes are statistically more likely to receive older RBCs. Second, confounding factors may not be recognized and, as a result, are discounted in nonrandomized studies. Third, individual methodologies in the presently available studies have varied markedly. Some studies have looked at the effect of mean storage age of all units transfused on outcome and some have broken storage time into categorical groups (i.e., is storage less than 14 days safer than storage beyond 14 days). In addition, studies have not used a single definition for "older" units; some have defined older units as greater than 14 days, greater than 21 days, or greater than

28 days. The definitions of age have not been based on either clinical or microcirculatory relevance or related to the feasibility and practicality of blood collection. Most studies have been designed for convenience and feasibility; a red cell storage age study with a definition of an older RBC unit as greater than 14 days of storage is achievable given current hospital inventories. Fourteen days is close to the average age of RBCs stored in a blood bank, but from a blood collection and inventory management perspective, an expiration time of 14 days would be disastrous for both hospitals and blood collection facilities. Authorities have argued that studies should be designed to measure storage age differences between lengths of storage that would actually be achievable given current inventory levels and difficulties in donor recruiting.

Published studies have focused on three patient groups that consume large numbers of RBC components: cardiac surgery, trauma, and critical care patients. A publication on the effect of RBC storage age on hematopoietic transplant recipients has also been recently published.

The Age of RBCs in Premature Infants study, a double-blinded study evaluating the effectiveness of RBCs stored no longer than seven days versus standard-issue RBCs in 377 neonates requiring transfusions has been published. The primary outcome revealed that using fresh blood of less than 7 days old did not improve the clinical outcome of these vulnerable premature infants. Recently, the Red Cell Storage Duration Study evaluated 1098 patients undergoing complex cardiac surgical procedures who were likely to require RBC transfusion. Patients were randomized to receive RBC units stored for either 10 or fewer days or 21 or more days. The median storage times of the transfused RBCs were 7 days versus 28 days for the two groups. RBC storage duration was not associated with a change in the Multiple Organ Dysfunction Score (MODS) or the 28-day mortality. Adverse events did not differ between the groups, except that hyperbilirubinemia was more common in the older storage age group.

The Age of Blood Evaluation study investigated the effect of leukoreduced RBCs stored 7 days or less versus leukoreduced standard-issue RBCs on 90-day all-cause mortality. Investigators enrolled 2430 adult participants receiving their first RBC unit in an intensive care unit. The study found that fresh versus standard-issue red cells did not decrease 90-day mortality among critically ill adults. Most recently, the Age of Blood in Children in Pediatric Intensive Care Units trial has been initiated to examine the effect of transfusing less than 7-day old blood (versus standard-issue age) in over 1500 pediatric ICU patients requiring transfusion. The primary outcome is new or progressive MODS.

Although the randomized prospective trial seems to be the only option to determine the clinical consequences of the RBC storage lesion, conducting a well-designed trial is not an easy task. Limited blood bank inventories to supply the longer and shorter storage duration arms, difficulty in consenting patients, and difficulty in selecting outcome measures to study have made creating the ideal study a formidable challenge.

The published studies evaluating whether adverse clinical consequences are associated with prolonged RBC storage have yet to satisfactorily answer this important question in all patient populations. The current RBC inventory almost always meets hospital needs with a 42 day RBC expiration period but is not currently equipped to meet the needs of a less than 7 day inventory, or even a less than 21 day inventory. Although it is logical to expect that there is a limit to RBC storage, beyond which the risks of transfusion outweigh the benefits of transfusion, none of the randomized studies described above is designed to determine this limit.

Animal studies have been able to provide additional information about the safety of RBCs stored for longer amounts of time than the clinical trials in humans. Natanson et al found that older blood (42 days of storage) increases the risk of transfusion (survival and multiple organ injury) in canine subjects with infection. In addition, in critically ill dogs with infection, they showed a favorable risk-to-benefit ratio for washing older blood. However, fresh blood (7 days of storage) was superior to older blood, whether washed or not.

RED CELL ALLOIMMUNIZATION

Overview

RBCs have over 300 blood group antigens that are capable of mounting humoral responses in antigen-naive transfused recipients. Direct exposure to nonself red cells from allogeneic blood transfusion, circulating fetal red cells in pregnant females, or even occasionally stem cell/organ transplantation can cause red cell alloimmunization. In addition, recent studies have shown that indirect immune modulation mediated via proinflammatory factors in stored RBCs, a proinflammatory state in the host (e.g., endothelial damage or higher turnover rate of red cells in patients with chronic transfusion), and passive transfer of WBC antibodies (anti-HLA and anti-HNA) are associated with a higher risk of RBC alloimmunization. Matzinger's Danger Theory/Model further proposes that nonself antigen exposure with local danger signals from injured cells can synergize immune responses. Therefore, red cell alloimmunization represents an intricate yet complex interplay between transfused allogeneic RBCs and host immunity.

The humoral response can be categorized into two phases. The primary response occurs immediately when foreign antigen activates B lymphocytes leading to the high-affinity mutation selection process. This process allows the activated B cells to proliferate and differentiate into memory/plasma B cells that produce a specific antibody against the antigen. Although, the initially generated antibody may not lead to significant hemolysis of sensitized red cells. Upon reexposure to the same antigen (e.g., transfusing an individual who had preformed antibody but at an undetectable level), the second phase of the immune response (anamnestic response) can lead to rapid and robust antibody production from the pregenerated antigen-specific memory/plasma B cells. This response often causes clinically significant hemolysis that may even lead to a fatality in these transfused individuals. In the blood bank, a process is in place to prevent clinically significant hemolysis in transfused patients with preformed red cell alloantibody. There are two isotypes of red cell antibodies that are routinely evaluated in the blood bank. Immunoglobulin M (IgM) is a pentavalent antibody that appears during the early phase of antibody generation. It is primarily restricted to the intravascular compartment, can fix complement on the transfused red cells with cognate antigens, and could result in intravascular hemolysis. On the contrary, IgG antibody is produced mostly by memory/plasma B cells that can migrate to the extravascular compartment (e.g., amniotic fluid, tissues, etc.). Due to its capacity to move between compartments, it is commonly associated with extravascular hemolysis and fetal hemolysis.

Individuals at Risk

Both the immunogenicity and quantity of foreign red cell antigens are critical determinants of alloimmunization. Therefore, frequent transfusion exposure and transfusion across different ethnic groups are the most common factors associated with alloimmunization. This issue is of great concern in patients with transfusion dependent hemoglobinopathies [e.g., sickle cell disease (SCD) and thalassemia] and PRCA (e.g., Diamond-Blackfan anemia). In particular, SCD is associated with rapid sequestration of defective red cells and endothelial damage. The discrepancy in the prevalence of certain red cell antigens, such as in the Rh system (DCcEe) and Kell (K1), between blood donors (mostly Whites) and SCD patients (mostly African descent) significantly contributes to the increase in red cell alloimmunization rate compared with the general population. Interestingly, by molecular genotyping, it was found that SCD patients have a high frequency of polymorphisms that can result in red cell alloimmunization even when serologically matched red cells are transfused. In addition, the endothelial damage and chronic inflammatory state associated with SCD have been hypothesized to cause synergy in red cell alloimmunization. Genetic factors predisposing SCD patients to red cell alloimmunization have been studied, and patients with HLA-B35 have a sixfold higher likelihood of making red cell alloantibodies compared

with SCD patients lacking HLA-B35. GWAS studies currently being pursued may clarify the role of genetic factors. Interestingly, the rate of alloimmunization was not proportionally observed in patients receiving massive transfusion with uncrossmatched RBCs. This observation may be due to transient immunosuppression in the setting of severe physiologic stress or by immune modulation due to the overwhelming amount of foreign RBCs transfused. This phenomenon was also shown in pediatric SCD patients receiving RBC exchange. On rare occasions, solid organ transplant can also be a source of red cell alloimmunization as it may expose the recipient to residual donor red cells with foreign antigens, despite immediate saline perfusion to rinse the organ of blood. Clinical hemolysis may be observed, but severe hemolytic complications are more likely a result of passenger lymphocytes that are capable of mounting an anamnestic response to antigen-positive recipient red cells (Passenger Lymphocyte Syndrome). From knowledge gained through observational studies, the risk of red cell alloimmunization seems to be associated with both red cell exposure and host immune responses. However, the complete pathophysiology still remains to be determined.

Molecular Pathophysiology

The exact cause of human RBC alloimmunization under myriad clinical circumstances is multifactorial and difficult to accurately identify. Thus, reductionist animal model based studies will be needed to investigate the mechanisms and identify the specific etiologies of this clinical entity. Given the well-defined genetic background, ready availability of a large number of participants, ability to adapt to many genetic manipulations, and largely conserved lineage-specific genes in the mouse immune system, mouse models are ideal to investigate this complex clinical entity. For example, transgenic human Rh, Kell, and Duffy antigen-expressing mice have been generated to study the interaction with their cognate alloantibodies. In addition, human hemolytic disease of the fetus and newborn (HDFN) associated with alloantibody against the Kell antigen has been closely recapitulated in pregnant transgenic Kell mice. Unlike the HDFN associated with alloantibody against the RhD antigen that can be prevented with administration of Rh immune globulin, HDFN associated with alloantibody against the Kell antigen still lacks effective prevention. Therefore, this anti-Kell mouse model will be useful in revealing the mechanism of alloimmunization against the Kell antigen.

There is a high red cell alloimmunization rate in SCD patients. The transgenic murine model of SCD revealed that the sickle cell genetic mutation alone was not sufficient to independently cause RBC alloimmunization. This study further suggests the critical roles of environmental factors involved in this immune response. Indeed, other mouse model studies have found that viral analog-induced inflammation (e.g., polyinosinic polycytidylic acid, or poly:IC) can independently enhance RBC alloimmunization. Furthermore, experimental mice transfused in the absence of inflammation developed immune tolerance against the transfused foreign red cell antigens as compared with control mice in the presence of poly:IC. This observation is supported by the fact that most transfused individuals without infections do not make alloantibodies to nonself red cell antigens. Also, exogenous inflammatory factors accumulated during RBC storage (storage lesion) were found to enhance sensitization to foreign RBCs leading to a more than 10-fold increase in alloantibody production. This concept has not yet been tested in prospective controlled clinical trials.

While animal models are able to provide the reductionist view of red cell alloimmunization and can serve as a platform to study the mechanism of red cell alloimmunization, the study conclusions may have limited general applicability. For example, the transgenic SCD mouse model has inherent differences in disease manifestations (e.g., massive splenomegaly, large vessel vasculopathy, etc.) that are not observed in human SCD patients. In addition to the interspecies genetic variation, the homogeneous nature of the experimental mouse's genetic background may not fully capture the true pathophysiology of red cell alloimmunization in the human population.

Nevertheless, mouse models provide a molecular view of the disease pathogenesis and generate many new hypotheses to further elucidate the mechanism of red cell alloimmunization.

Red Blood Cell Alloimmunization Mitigation Strategies

Blood transfusion is one of the most common therapies provided in a hospital, and millions of blood products are transfused every year worldwide. Therefore, a carefully planned strategy to prevent red cell alloimmunization is urgently needed. Reducing red cell alloimmunization can occur in three areas: blood collection/manufacturing, hospital transfusion services, and through patient care. At the blood center, prestorage leukoreduction can effectively remove more than 99.99% of the original WBCs. This process minimizes the inflammatory or "danger" signals infused into recipients at the time of foreign red cell antigen exposure and thus may reduce subsequent alloimmunization. Some blood centers have also begun to provide non-ABO red cell antigen typing on RBC units to minimize transfusing RBCs with mismatched red cell antigens. Clinical interventions have also been proposed to reduce red cell alloimmunization risk. Surgical splenectomy was shown in mouse models and observed in transfusion-dependent patients (e.g., thalassemia) to reduce the alloimmunization rate; however, this procedure is not as effective if the initial antigen exposure occurred prior to spleen removal. Since sickle cell patients develop asplenia at early ages, this finding may also not be relevant to the high incidence of alloimmunization in sickle cell anemia. Immunosuppression can also theoretically retard the red cell alloimmunization rate. However, one must consider the adverse clinical impact of these drugs. More studies on drug types and dosages are needed to refine this strategy. Finally, blood bank practice plays a daily pivotal role in preventing red cell alloimmunization in hospital patients. Molecular/genetic typing can permit red cell antigen matching at a higher resolution and precision than traditional serologic red cell antigen typing. This additional testing is particularly helpful in patients with hemoglobinopathies or high titer warm autoantibodies, who are especially vulnerable to red cell alloantibody formation. In the current climate of medical care, patients often do not receive care at the same institution; therefore blood bank results may not fully and accurately transfer between hospitals. Recently, the National Patient Antibody Registry was developed to address this issue. By integrating patient test results from hospital blood banks and blood centers within a region or across the nation, this shared database not only reduces blood issuing time, but can also facilitate the selection of antigen-matched RBCs to prevent or mitigate alloimmunization. Collectively, the approaches described above to reduce alloimmunization were derived from clinical trials, observational studies, and studies using mouse-models. As many of these approaches incur additional cost and effort, a validated cost-effective strategy is needed to further improve patient care and reduce red cell alloimmunization. In view of the high costs of finding antigen negative blood and the fact that many patients with sickle cell anemia do not become alloimmunized, another strategy that remains reasonable until antigen negative blood becomes more cost effective is to monitor patients carefully and switch to antigen matching after the first detection of a red cell antibody

ALTERNATIVES TO ALLOGENEIC RED CELL TRANSFUSIONS

There are many alternatives to standard allogeneic red cell transfusions for a patient requiring elective surgery (Table 111.4). Potential alternatives include banking autologous units before the surgery, acute normovolemic hemodilution, pharmacologic therapies (i.e., erythropoietin or fibrinolysis inhibitors), perioperative salvage, virally inactivated donor red cells, or blood substitutes. All current options have their own unique benefits and drawbacks, and some of these alternatives are not yet available. In cases where an emergency transfusion is needed, the first three options would not be possible as they

TABLE 111.4	Alternatives to Standard Allogeneic Transfusions
Hemodilution	
Intraoperative autologous transfusion	
Perioperative blood salvage	
Lower transfusion trigger	
Pharmacologic therapies	
Pathogen inactivation	
Red Cell Substitutes	
Stem cell derived RBCs	

all require significant planning. Only virally inactivated components and red cell substitutes (both of which are still works in progress) would be available for unanticipated transfusion needs.

Autologous Blood Transfusion

Advantages of Autologous Blood Transfusion

The substitution of autologous blood components for those collected from other (allogeneic) donors eliminates transfusion-transmitted diseases such as viral hepatitis and acquired immunodeficiency syndrome. Immunologic complications related to the transfusion of foreign cells, including hemolysis and febrile reactions to WBCs, are also prevented. Other advantages, though possible, are less clearly established. For example, erythropoiesis may be sufficiently stimulated in the repeatedly bled autologous donor to hasten recovery from postoperative anemia. Intraoperatively salvaged red cells are spared the acquired membrane defects ("storage lesion") and 2,3-DPG deficiencies of refrigerated red cells.

An important drawback to these techniques is their increased expense in contrast to the simpler allogeneic transfusions they replace. In addition, the availability of autologous components may result in their use in situations where transfusion might not have otherwise been considered. Patients with suboptimal compensatory erythropoiesis and donation-induced anemia at the time of surgery are also more likely to be given transfusions. Based upon the current level of viral safety in blood components in the developed world, the use of autologous blood has dropped significantly from times when viral testing was not available or reliable.

Preoperative Autologous Blood Collection

The typical volunteer allogeneic blood donor is allowed to give one unit of blood no more than once every 8 weeks, to prevent iron deficiency. However, provided that bone marrow erythropoiesis can be stimulated and satisfactory iron supplies maintained, blood can be collected as frequently as once a week from an autologous donor. Although the shelf-life of refrigerated RBCs is limited to 42 days, frozen storage for up to 10 years is possible at less than 65°C using glycerol as a cryopreservative.

From a cardiovascular standpoint, phlebotomy is well tolerated by a variety of seemingly high-risk donors, including the elderly, children, pregnant women, and patients with coronary artery disease. By contrast, anemia frequently develops during the donation interval and limits the number of autologous units that can be collected. In addition to marginal iron stores, erythropoietin levels often do not increase during the donation interval, probably because the hematocrit level of most donors is not allowed to fall to less than 30%. This situation may be improved by the administration of the recombinant growth hormone erythropoietin to autologous donors. The use of preoperatively donated autologous blood has also been reported for a variety of surgical procedures, including radical prostatectomy; hysterectomies and other gynecologic procedures; colorectal, biliary, and gastric surgery; orthopedic surgery, and neurosurgery. Since many of these procedures are now performed using laparoscopy or other techniques to limit blood loss, the demand for predeposit autologous transfusion support has fallen in recent years.

Autologous blood has been safely collected from women during pregnancy for use during childbirth. Nevertheless, the transfusion rate at delivery is quite low (<2.5% in many institutions) and most autologous donations are unused. Long-term (frozen) storage of autologous RBCs in the absence of a planned transfusion episode is largely ineffective and expensive.

Intraoperative Blood Salvage

Cell salvage occurs in three phases: collection, washing, and reinfusion. RBCs are collected from the operative field using a dedicated double lumen suction device. One lumen suctions blood from the operative field and the other lumen adds heparinized saline to the salvaged blood. The anticoagulated blood then passes through a filter and is collected in a reservoir. If less than 1 L of blood is collected, further processing is foregone and the collected blood is discarded.

In most circumstances the contents in the bag can be washed to remove free Hb, surgical irrigation solutions, and other debris. Instruments are available that include both a reservoir for collecting salvaged blood and a centrifugal washer. Large aliquots (>500 mL) can be fully washed in as little as 3 minutes. As a result of this speed, autologous blood salvage has become practical in situations in which blood loss may be extremely rapid, such as trauma or liver transplantation.

The hematocrit level of unwashed blood is typically low because of dilution from irrigating surgical fluids and some degree of mechanical hemolysis. Free Hb levels are sometimes greater than 1000 mg in unwashed blood, and hemoglobinemia and hemoglobinuria may occur after the transfusion, although renal sequelae are surprisingly low. Despite this evidence of red cell injury, the survival rate of ^{51}Cr-labeled salvaged cells is normal in most patients studied.

There are many potential complications associated with cell salvage, such as nonimmune hemolysis, air embolus, febrile nonhemolytic transfusion reactions, mistransfusion, coagulopathy, and contamination with drugs. Transfusion of salvaged blood has resulted in coagulation abnormalities, including hypofibrinogenemia, prolonged prothrombin time and partial thromboplastin time, elevated fibrin degradation products, and thrombocytopenia. These coagulation abnormalities most likely reflect the characteristics of the salvaged blood itself, which, after exposure to serosal surfaces, becomes deficient in coagulation factors and platelets and, in the case of unwashed blood, has high levels of fibrin degradation products (Table 111.5).

Fat, fibrin, bone fragments, and microaggregates often contaminate salvaged autologous blood. However, infusion of unwashed blood has not been proved harmful in either animals or humans, possibly because routine blood filters remove most particulate material. Other contaminants, such as heparin, topical antibiotics, hemostatic agents, and biologic substances such as tissue enzymes, can be at least partially removed by washing. Complete removal of bacteria is also not possible, even when the salvaged blood is washed with antibiotics. Thus, collection of blood from a contaminated site (e.g., with intestinal contents) is usually considered to be contraindicated;

in fact, manufacturers contraindicate the use of cell salvage in cases where there is potential contamination of salvaged blood with enteric contents. However, in recent years this viewpoint has been reconsidered as studies have found that autotransfusion of microbiologically contaminated salvaged blood have demonstrated no adverse outcomes or increase in postoperative infectious complications. Tumor cells have been found in blood salvaged during cancer operations, and thus many practitioners consider cancer another contraindication. Others believe that filtration would remove salvaged tumor cells.

Approximately one-half the blood lost during surgery can be salvaged. The rest is usually irretrievably absorbed in drapes and sponges or damaged during collection. The use of salvaged autologous blood has been associated with a 50% reduction in allogeneic blood use in orthopedic procedures such as spinal surgery and hip replacement, and is also effective in vascular surgical procedures such as aortic reconstruction. Autologous salvage has been a useful adjunct in the treatment of some Jehovah's Witnesses whose literal acceptance of the Bible includes abstention from routine allogeneic blood transfusions.

Both the canister systems and RBC processors used to collect intraoperative autologous blood can also be used to collect postoperative blood drainage, such as that from the mediastinum after open heart surgery, from the knee or hip after orthopedic procedures, or from the peritoneal cavity after hepatic injury. Because blood salvaged from a serosal cavity has little residual fibrinogen and platelets, clotting is not a problem, and the addition of anticoagulants is usually unnecessary. Shed mediastinal blood after open-heart surgery contains high levels of cardiac muscle enzymes, especially creatine kinase, as well as lactate dehydrogenase from hemolyzed RBCs. Therefore, reinfusion of shed blood results in elevated levels of both enzymes that can confound the diagnosis of myocardial infarction (MI) in the postoperative period. Reinfusion of shed mediastinal blood has been shown to reduce the need for allogeneic transfusions.

Hemodilution

The collection of autologous blood during surgery for later reinfusion at the end of the procedure was first suggested in open-heart operations, in which it was hoped that a supply of platelets undamaged by exposure to the membrane oxygenator might reduce the incidence of coagulopathies. Hemodilution itself reduces RBC loss: a patient with a hematocrit level of 45% and 2 L blood loss during surgery loses roughly 900 mL of RBCs, but one with a hematocrit level of 20% from hemodilution loses only 400 mL of RBCs. Hemodilution is less expensive to accomplish than preoperative autologous blood donation and may be the only option available when surgery is performed in other than elective settings. Proponents claim that the induced anemia may even be beneficial to the patient, in that oxygen delivery at a hematocrit level of 30% is enhanced by an increased cardiac output resulting from the decreased blood viscosity. Other advantages of hemodilution over predeposit autologous transfusion are the provision of fresh red cells along with plasma and platelets that may be important in maintaining hemostasis.

Reductions in allogeneic blood needs have been reported after marked intraoperative hemodilution (after the hematocrit is lowered

TABLE 111.5	Autologous Blood Salvage Systems[a]: Characteristics of Collected Blood						
System	Hardware	Software	Hematocrit	Free Hemoglobin	Platelet Count	Coagulation Factors	Fibrin Degradation Products
Collection without washing	Rigid plastic container	Plastic bag	Low (25%)	Very high (200 mg%)	Low (100,000/mm³)	Low (35–75%)	High (300 mg%)
Collection followed by washing	Integral or separate blood cell processor	Disposable plastic bowl and tubing	High (60%)	Low (<50 mg%)	Very low (10,000/mm³)	Absent (0%)	Absent (0%)

[a]Typical results of laboratory tests are shown. Transfusion of large volumes of salvaged blood results in similar alterations in these tests in the recipient.
Data from Noon GP: Intraoperative autotransfusion. *Surgery* 84:719, 1978; and Silva R, Moore EE, Bar-Or D, et al: The risk: benefit ratio of autotransfusion-comparison to banked blood in a canine model. *J Trauma* 24:557, 1984.

by 50%). More modest hemodilution (e.g., removal of 2 units of blood at the beginning of surgery) is also beneficial, according to some investigators but the amount of red cells saved is small. Furthermore, one group has provided evidence that hemodilution may jeopardize patients at risk of ischemic myocardial injury. More research is needed to establish the safety, efficacy, and ideal protocols for this form of blood conservation. The availability of blood substitutes may facilitate augmented hemodilution for some patients who are expected to have large volumes of blood loss or who refuse blood transfusions.

BLOOD SUBSTITUTES

The search for blood substitutes began when our early scientific ancestors tested alternatives to human blood, including animal blood, milk, and wine. Modern research into the use of animal blood includes the work by Amberson et al, who reported the successful use of a bovine hemosylate for exchange transfusions in cats and dogs. Further work revealed that human and bovine hemosylates caused renal dysfunction in human recipients. The suspected cause of this nephrotoxicity was the stromal lipid component of the RBC membrane. The logical next step in the search for the ideal substitute was the development of stroma-free Hb (Hb tetramer). Unfortunately, in 1978 Savitsky et al demonstrated renal dysfunction, hypertension, and abdominal pain using stroma-free Hb in healthy volunteers. It was hypothesized that these adverse events were due to the instability of the Hb tetramer. Since then, efforts have been made to produce stabilized products with desirable oxygen off-loading characteristics and extended intravascular retention times.

Today, the United States blood supply is increasingly safe and has sufficient capacity to meet most patient needs. There is room for considerable improvement, however, in supply levels and risk reduction. The shrinking donor pool (owing to lack of willingness and/or ability) and the increasing transfusion requirements of an aging population may lead to shortage of blood products. The threat of new and emerging infections results in the vulnerability of human-derived oxygen carriers. The continuous battle against emerging infectious diseases underscore the risk of a tainted blood supply and depletion of transfusion resources. Theoretically, the ideal red cell substitute would solve both of these issues (Table 111.6). There have been many attempts to develop red cell substitutes in the past, but no product has been able to fulfil all of the above criteria or meet the Food and Drug Administration's requirements of purity, potency, and safety. There is no licensed red cell substitute available.

RED BLOOD CELL SUBSTITUTES

It is important to differentiate between "blood substitutes" and red cell substitutes. Red cell substitutes are oxygen carriers and do not replace all components and functions of blood, for example,

TABLE 111.6	The Ideal Red Cell Substitute

Delivers oxygen (and maybe enhances delivery)
Does not transmit disease
Does not have immunosuppressive effects
Available in abundant supply
Universally compatible (no need to type and crossmatch)
Prolonged shelf-life and stable at a range of temperatures
Similar in vivo half-life to the RBC
Available at a reasonable cost
Easy to administer
Able to access all areas of the human body (including ischemic tissue)
Effective on room air or ambient conditions

RBC, Red blood cell.

coagulation factors and WBCs. There are two main categories of oxygen carriers that show promise as RBC substitutes: perfluorocarbons (PFCs) and Hb-based oxygen carriers (HBOC).

Perfluorocarbons

PFCs are chemically and biologically inert artificial fluorinated organic fluids that are immiscible in water and have a high solubility for oxygen. The amount of dissolved oxygen in PFC is linearly related to the ambient oxygen tension, unlike Hb; gas molecules are not chemically bound to PFCs but are absorbed and released by simple diffusion. Products require oxygen inhalation by the patient, as the oxygen delivery capacity is less than 30% of normal blood. PFC has been shown to reduce the need for RBC transfusion, but has been associated with an increase in stroke rates. Although some PFCs are still being investigated, there are no major trials ongoing and no licensed products in the United States.

Hemoglobin-Based Oxygen Carriers

As RBCs age and degrade, the stroma and unmodified Hb released can lead to various adverse effects in the transfused recipients. Therefore, the HBOC that were most recently in clinical development were stroma-free and engineered to produce desirable oxygen dissociation characteristics as well as an adequate in vivo half-life with minimal toxicities. Stroma-free Hb has a very high oxygen affinity compared with native Hb in a RBC because of a lack of 2,3-DPG. Furthermore, the Hb tetramer is such a small molecule that the kidney rapidly removes it.

Four different methods have been suggested to avoid toxicities: stabilization, polymerization, conjugation, and Hb vesicles. HBOC can be prepared from different Hb sources (e.g., bovine RBCs or recombinant Hb harvested from bacteria/yeasts). However, the safety concerns of using Hb from nonhuman sources, such as the potential for transmitting diseases, immunogenicity, and toxicities have not been fully addressed. While one of the commercially available HBOCs (e.g., Bovine-derived Oxyglobin, HBOC-301) is approved for veterinary use, there is no HBOC product approved for clinical use although several products are in clinical development phases. All faced significant challenges in proving their safety and efficacy in early and late phase clinical trials. A large metaanalysis by Natanson et al identified 16 randomized controlled trials in which adult patients received HBOCs therapeutically. The analysis reviewed the association between HBOCs and the risk of MI and mortality in clinical trials. The study included five different HBOCs in the analysis and reported a 30% increase in risk of death and threefold increase in risk of MI when all HBOC trials were pooled. The metaanalysis has been criticized for including trials of varying methodologies performed on heterogeneous patient populations in different settings with different controls. The authors of the metaanalysis criticized the United States government oversight, as well as the transparency and timeliness in reporting the results of the HBOC clinical trials. The editorial that accompanied the publication in the Journal of the American Medical Association made a recommendation that further phase III trials of HBOCs should not be conducted until the mechanisms and potential toxicities are better understood. The effects may be due to the interaction of Hb and nitric oxide, a concern not fully appreciated in the early days of blood substitute research, but potentially addressed by the expansion of knowledge about NO and mitigating its effects. Although some HBOCs are still being investigated, there are no major trials ongoing and no licensed products in the United States.

Potential Clinical Applications

RBC substitutes have many potential applications. One of the most compelling needs would be the use for rapid resuscitation during military and civilian traumas. In developing a specific plan to avoid the consequences of blood unavailability after national disasters involving large-scale injuries, blood substitutes could play a key role as an immediate treatment option. In addition to these acute emergency situations, there is a wide range of less urgent applications where oxygen carriers might provide a viable solution to difficult situations, including supporting solid organ perfusion during transport/storage, augmenting perioperative hemodilution, transfusion of patients who refuse human blood components because of religious beliefs (e.g., Jehovah's Witnesses), transfusion of patients with rare blood types or antibodies to high incidence antigens, organ preservation for transplant surgery, transfusion in patients with autoimmune hemolytic anemia in whom it is difficult to detect underlying antibodies, and reducing alloimmunization risk in patients receiving frequent transfusions. Since blood transfusion therapy is not available to handle some of these indications, there remains an unmet medical need for a safe and efficacious RBC substitute.

Red Blood Cells Derived From Stem Cells

Due to the threat of future blood shortages, the possible shortening of RBC storage, and unlikely availability of RBC substitutes in clinical use, a new source of RBCs is needed. Blood substitutes will not answer this need in the near future. The generation of RBCs derived from stem cells could meet this need, and this method is currently under intense development by researchers worldwide.

Umbilical cord blood is an accessible source of stem cells with proliferative capacity; however, the proliferation is not infinite, requiring a system of production in batches. Neildez-Nguyen et al first reported the possibility of converting umbilical cord stem cells into erythroid progenitors that can continue to mature into terminally differentiated RBCs in vivo. Giarratana et al subsequently demonstrated that adult mobilized hematopoietic stem progenitor cells can also be differentiated into RBCs and found that the survival of the cultured RBCs was similar to that of native RBCs. Under optimized expansion and differentiation conditions, Giarratana et al reported that they were able to generate 4 to 30 million RBCs from one hematopoietic stem progenitor cell obtained from apheresis donors. While this expansion scheme could be adequate to generate clinically useful transfusable RBCs, it may not justify the donor risks (e.g., G-CSF–mobilized apheresis collection) for the sole purpose of RBC production. Stem cells cultured from umbilical cords would necessitate the use of cord blood banks and would still be dependent on human donation. Alternatively, embryonic stem cells and induced pluripotent stem cells (iPSCs) can be obtained, generated, then maintained indefinitely in culture, thus providing an unlimited source of cells. Like embryonic stem cells, iPSCs are capable of in vitro self-renewal and differentiation into cell types from all germ layers. However, they possess an advantage over embryonic cells in that they pose no ethical dilemma and can be selected based on known phenotypes. Researchers have been able to demonstrate that iPSCs can differentiate into terminally mature and fully functional red cells.

A number of challenges must be overcome before we have an unlimited supply of clinical grade RBCs. The ideal choice for the initial cell type (e.g., hematopoietic stem cell, erythroblast, etc.) remains to be determined. The method of reprogramming the cells must be established to avoid the risk of potential mutation and tumor development (although this is less of an issue for red cells as they are enucleate and can be safely irradiated) while still ensuring the functionality of the end product. Finally, the use of GMP conditions for mass production within a reasonable amount of time and at a reasonable cost seems to be the greatest hurdle to date. The current challenges in utilizing iPSCs to generate RBCs are the inefficiency in erythroid commitment and the suboptimal cellular amplification. A number of strategies are under development to solve this crucial problem. Until mass amplification is possible, the iPSCs could be developed, not as an unlimited supply, but as a source of cells expressing a rare blood group used to treat alloimmunized patients with rare blood types. Currently, the available methods for ex vivo manufacturing of RBCs for clinical use are expensive and unrealistic.

SUGGESTED READINGS

Amberson WR, Mulder AG, Steggerda FR, et al: Mammalian life without red blood corpuscles. *Science* 78(2014):106–107, 1933.

American Society of Anesthesiologists Task Force on Perioperative Blood Management: Practice guidelines for perioperative blood management: an updated report by the American Society of Anesthesiologists Task Force on Perioperative Blood Management. *Anesthesiology* 122(2):241–275, 2015.

Ashworth A, Klein AA: Cell Salvage as part of a blood conservation strategy in anesthesia. *Br J Anaeth* 105(4):401–416, 2010.

Bell EF, Strauss RG, Widness JA, et al: Randomized trial of liberal versus restrictive guidelines for red blood cell transfusion in preterm infants. *Pediatrics* 115(6):1685–1691, 2005.

Vamvakas EC, Blajchman MA: Transfusion-related immunomodulation (TRIM): an update. *Blood Rev* 21(6):327–348, 2007.

Chou S, Jackson T, Vege S, et al: High prevalence of red blood cell alloimmunization in sickle cell disease despite transfusion from Rh-matched minority donors. *Blood* 122(6):1062–1071, 2013.

Dzik WH, Anderson JK, O'Neill EM, et al: A prospective, randomized clinical trial of universal WBC reduction. *Transfusion* 42(9):1114–1122, 2002.

Fergusson DA, Hebert P, Hogan DL, et al: Effect of fresh red blood cell transfusion on clinical outcomes in premature, very low-birth-weight infants: the ARIPI randomized trial. *JAMA* 308(14):1443–1451, 2012.

Giarratana MC, Rouard H, Dumont A, et al: Proof of principle for transfusion of in vitro-generated red blood cells. *Blood* 118(19):5071–5079, 2011.

Goodnough LT, Rudnick S, Price TH, et al: Increased preoperative collection of autologous blood with recombinant human erythropoietin: a controlled trial. *N Engl J Med* 321(17):1163–1168, 1989.

Hebert PC, Wells G, Blajchman MA, et al: A multicenter, randomized controlled clinical trial of transfusion requirements in critical care. *N Engl J Med* 340(6):409–417, 1999.

Hendrickson JE, Tormey CA, Shaz BH: Red blood cell alloimmunization mitigation strategies. *Transfus Med Rev* 28(3):137–144, 2014.

Hod EA, Brittenham GM, Billote GB, et al: Transfusion of human volunteers with older, stored red blood cells produces extravascular hemolysis and circulating non-transferrin bound iron. *Blood* 118(25):6675–6682, 2011.

Hod EA, Zhang N, Sokol SA, et al: Transfusion of red blood cells after prolonged storage produces harmful effects that are mediated by iron and inflammation. *Blood* 115(21):4284–4292, 2010.

Holcomb JB, Tilley BC, Baraniuk S, et al: Transfusion of plasma, platelets, and red blood cells in a 1:1:1 vs a 1:1:2 ratio and mortality in patients with severe trauma: the PROPPR randomized clinical trial. *JAMA* 313(5):471–482, 2015.

King KE, Ness PM: Treatment of Autoimmune Hemolytic Anemia. *Semin Hematol* 42(3):131–136, 2005.

Kirpalani H, Whyte RK, Andersen C, et al: The premature infants in need of tranfusion (PINT) study: a randomized, controlled trial of a restrictive (low) versus liberal (high) transfusion threshold for extremely low birth weight infants. *J Pediatr* 149(3):301–307, 2006.

Klein HG: Transfusion-associated graft-versus-host disease: less fresh blood and more gray (Gy) for an aging population. *Transfusion* 46(6):878–880, 2006.

Klein HG, Anstee DJ: *Mollison's Blood Transfusion in Clinical Medicine*, ed 11, Malden, MA, 2005, Blackwell Publishing, p 389.

Lee AC, Reduque LL, Luban NLC, et al: Transfusion-associated hyperkalemic cardiac arrest in pediatric patients receiving massive transfusions. *Transfusion* 54(1):244–254, 2014.

Mazurier C, Douay L, Lapillonne H: Red blood cells from induced pluripotent stem cells: hurdles and developments. *Curr Opin Hematol* 18(4):249–253, 2011.

Meryman HT, Hornblower M: A method for freezing and washing red blood cells using high glycerol concentration. *Transfusion* 12(3):145–156, 1972.

Natanson C, Kern SJ, Lurie P, et al: Cell-free Hb-based blood substitutes and risk of myocardial infarction and death, a meta-analysis. *JAMA* 299(19):2304–2312, 2008.

Neildez-Nguyen TM, Wajcman H, Marden MC, et al: Human erythroid cells produced ex vivo at large scale differentiate into red blood cells in vivo. *Nat Biotechnol* 20(5):467–472, 2002.

Ness PM, Bourke DL, Walsh PC: A randomized trial of perioperative hemo-dilution versus transfusion of preoperatively deposited autologous blood in elective surgery. *Transfusion* 32(3):226–230, 1992.

NIH Consensus Conference: Perioperative red blood cell transfusion. *JAMA* 260(18):2700–2703, 1988.

Ness PM, Cushing MM: Oxygen therapeutics. Pursuit of an alternative to the donor red blood cell. *Arch Pathol Lab Med* 131(5):734–741, 2007.

Paglino JC, Pomper GJ, Fisch GS, et al: Reduction of febrile but not allergic reactions to RBCs and platelets after conversion to universal prestorage leukoreduction. *Transfusion* 44(1):16–24, 2004.

Paul DA, Leef KH, Locke RG, et al: Transfusion volume in infants with very low birth weight: a randomized trial of 10 versus 20 mL/kg. *J Pediatr Hematol Oncol* 24(1):43–46, 2002.

Peyrard T, Bardiaux L, Krause C, et al: Banking of pluripotent adult stem cells as an unlimited source for red blood cell production: potential applications for alloimmunized patients and rare blood challenges. *Transfus Med Rev* 25(3):206–216, 2011.

Report of the US Department of Health and Human Services: *The 2011 national blood collection and utilization survey report*, Washington, DC, 2011, US Department of Health and Human Services, Office of the Assistant Secretary for Health.

Ryder AB, Zimring JC, Hendrickson JE: Factors influencing RBC alloim-munization: lessons learned from murine models. *Transfus Med Hemother* 41(6):406–419, 2014.

Savitsky JP, Doczi J, Black J, et al: A clinical safety trial of stroma-free hemoglobin. *Clin Pharmacol Ther* 23(1):73–80, 1978.

Sehgal LR, Sebala LP, Takagi I, et al: Evaluation of oxygen extraction ratio as a physiologic transfusion trigger in coronary artery bypass graft surgery patients. *Transfusion* 41(5):591–595, 2001.

Steiner ME, Ness PM, Assmann SF, et al: Effects of red-cell storage duration on patients undergoing cardiac surgery. *N Engl J Med* 372(15):1419–1429, 2015.

Strauss RG, Mock DM, Johnson KJ, et al: A randomized clinical trial comparing immediate versus delayed clamping of the umbilical cord in preterm infants: short-term clinical and laboratory endpoints. *Transfusion* 48(4):658–665, 2008.

Tinmouth A, Fergusson D, Yee IC, et al: Clinical consequences of red cell storage in the critically ill. *Transfusion* 46(11):2014–2024, 2006.

TRAP Study Group: Leukocytic reduction and ultraviolet B irradiation of platelets to prevent alloimmunization and refractoriness to platelet transfusions. *N Engl J Med* 337(26):1861–1869, 1997.

Von Lindern JS, Brand A: The use of blood products in perinatal medicine. *Semin Fetal Neonatal Med* 13(4):272–281, 2008.

Wang D, Cortés-Puch I, Sun J, et al: Transfusion of older stored blood worsens outcomes in canines depending on the presence and severity of pneumonia. *Transfusion* 54(7):1712–1724, 2014.

Wong H, Connelly R, Day A, et al: A comparison of high and standard blood transfusion volumes in premature infants. *Acta Paediatr* 94(5):624–625, 2005.

CLINICAL CONSIDERATIONS IN PLATELET TRANSFUSION THERAPY

Richard M. Kaufman

PLATELET COLLECTION AND MANUFACTURING

Platelet components are either prepared from whole blood donations (platelet concentrates) or, more commonly, are collected by apheresis (single donor platelets). In the United States, whole blood-derived platelet concentrates are made using the platelet-rich plasma (PRP) method. First, a whole blood unit is separated by gentle centrifugation (slow spin) into red blood cells (RBCs) and PRP. The PRP is then centrifuged a second time (hard spin) to isolate one platelet concentrate plus one unit of plasma. Each platelet concentrate contains approximately 5.5×10^{10} platelets suspended in a plasma volume of approximately 50 mL. In Europe and Canada, the alternate buffy coat method is used to produce platelet concentrates. Platelets are stored at room temperature under continuous gentle agitation for up to 5 days. To prepare an adult dose of platelets for transfusion, four to six platelet concentrates are pooled together.

Apheresis platelet units are collected from a single platelet donor by continuous flow centrifugation using an automated device. A high volume of whole blood is processed through the machine, and the platelets are retained in a sterile collection bag. According to AABB (formerly, the American Association of Blood Banks) standards, an apheresis platelet unit should contain a minimum of 3×10^{11} platelets,[1] a dose that is approximately equivalent to five pooled platelet concentrates. Current devices allow many different combinations of blood products to be collected during a single apheresis donation, such as 1 unit of platelets plus 1 unit of RBCs. Apheresis platelet units generally contain less than 1×10^6 white blood cells (WBCs) per unit; thus, they meet the current AABB definition for leukoreduced blood products ($<5 \times 10^6$ WBCs/unit).[1] Although apheresis platelets cost more to produce than whole blood-derived platelet concentrates, they have become increasingly popular. In the United States in 2011, approximately 2 million therapeutic doses of platelets were provided as apheresis platelets, and only 200,000 equivalent doses were administered as whole blood-derived platelet concentrates.[2]

Apheresis platelets provide limited advantages over whole blood-derived platelet concentrates. Radiolabeling studies indicate that apheresis platelets circulate longer in vivo than pooled concentrates, most likely reflecting gentler handling and less platelet activation during collection. Recipients of apheresis platelets are exposed to fewer donors per transfusion (1 donor versus 4–6 as with a pool of platelet concentrates), so in principle, apheresis platelets should pose a lower risk of viral transmission than whole blood-derived platelets. However, given that the per-unit transfusion-transmission risks for HIV and hepatitis C virus have been reduced to less than 1 per 1,000,000,[3] the viral safety advantage of apheresis platelets over whole blood-derived platelets is marginal. Data from surveillance culture studies suggest that apheresis platelets may be less likely than platelet concentrates to become contaminated with bacteria. At one time, it was predicted that apheresis platelets would be less likely than pooled concentrates to provoke platelet alloimmunization by virtue of exposing recipients to fewer unique donor human leukocyte antigens (HLAs). This hypothesis was not confirmed empirically, however. Although they express surface HLA class I antigens, platelets appear to be rather poor immunogens. HLA alloimmunization to platelets primarily appears to be triggered by contaminating WBCs within a platelet unit. Thus, alloimmunization is not platelet dose dependent, and simply providing leukoreduced platelet units prevents most cases of immune-mediated platelet refractoriness.[4] When platelet refractoriness does occur, it is often in multiparous women, who were initially sensitized to foreign (paternal) HLA antigens in previous pregnancies.[5]

PROPHYLACTIC PLATELET TRANSFUSION

Most platelet units are transfused to prevent bleeding in nonbleeding patients, rather than to treat active bleeding. Before 1960, platelet transfusions were not widely available, and death from hemorrhage was common among patients with leukemia who received chemotherapy. In 1962, Gaydos and colleagues[6] published a seminal study demonstrating a relationship between platelet count and likelihood of bleeding. After this study was published, prophylactic platelet transfusion rapidly became standard practice. Notably, based on their data, no specific platelet transfusion trigger was suggested by the authors. Regardless, a platelet count of 20,000/μL was widely adopted at the time as the standard prophylactic platelet transfusion trigger.

Later studies suggested that a lower transfusion trigger would be as effective as a trigger of 20,000/μL. Slichter and Harker,[7] for instance, performed RBC radiolabeling studies in thrombocytopenic patients who were not receiving platelet transfusions. They demonstrated that only patients with platelet counts below 5000/μL had significantly elevated fecal RBC loss.[7] Years later, several clinical studies directly challenged the 20,000/μL trigger. Platelet transfusion triggers of 10,000/μL versus 20,000/μL were compared directly in three randomized prospective studies of patients with acute leukemia.[8–10] These studies, as well as a nonrandomized prospective trial,[11] did not show an increased incidence of bleeding when a trigger of 10,000/μL is used. Most recently, the Platelet Dosing (PLADO) trial demonstrated that the risk of bleeding among patients with hypoproliferative thrombocytopenia only increased at platelet counts below 6000/μL.[12] As shown in Fig. 112.1, the risk of spontaneous bleeding was equivalent between platelet counts of 6000/μL and 80,000/μL.

Severe hemorrhage in the setting of therapy-related hypoproliferative thrombocytopenia is now quite rare. Given the substantial changes in both chemotherapy and the supportive care of patients with hematologic malignancy that have occurred over the past several decades, two randomized controlled trials recently examined whether routine platelet prophylaxis still provides a clinical benefit. In the study by Wandt and colleagues,[13] patients receiving chemotherapy or undergoing autologous hematopoietic stem cell transplantation (HSCT) were randomly assigned to receive platelet transfusions only when bleeding occurred, or standard prophylactic platelet transfusions for a morning platelet count at or below 10,000/μL. Grade 2 or higher bleeding occurred in 42% of patients receiving therapeutic platelet transfusions only, versus 19% in patients receiving platelet prophylaxis ($p < .001$). There were significantly more intracerebral hemorrhages in the no-prophylaxis group (7% versus 2%, $p = .01$), and there were two deaths due to bleeding in the no-prophylaxis group compared with zero in the prophylaxis group. In the Trial of Prophylactic Platelets,[14] a similar population of patients

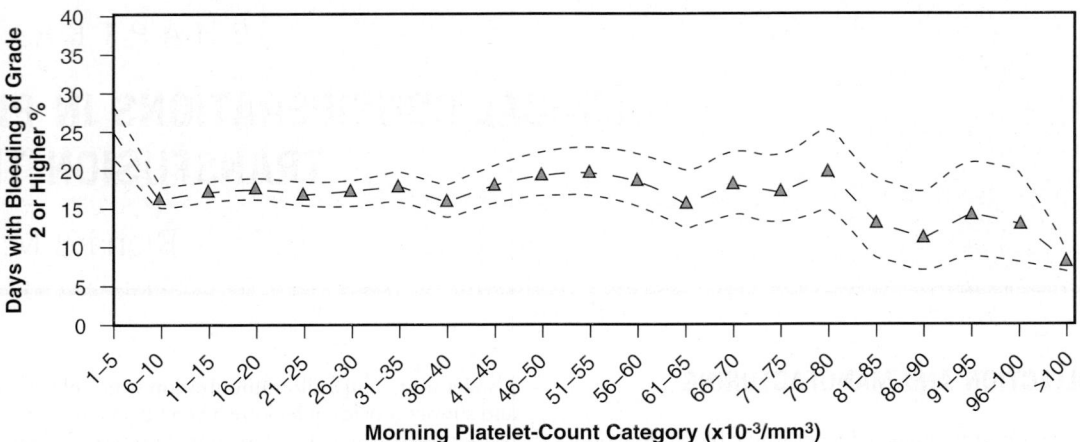

Fig. 112.1 RELATIONSHIP BETWEEN PLATELET COUNT AND SPONTANEOUS BLEEDING AMONG PATIENTS WITH THERAPY-INDUCED HYPOPROLIFERATIVE THROMBOCYTOPE- NIA. The percentage of days that adult or pediatric patients with hematologic malignancy enrolled in the PLADO trial had grade 2 or higher bleeding is shown as a function of morning platelet count. The 95% confidence intervals are shown as dashed lines. The bleeding risk was equivalent for platelet counts between 6000 and 80,000/μL.[12]

was randomized to no prophylactic platelet transfusions or routine prophylaxis. Grade 2 or higher bleeding occurred in 50% of patients in the no-prophylaxis group versus 43% in the prophylaxis group (*p* = .06 for noninferiority.) There were no deaths due to bleeding in this study. In both trials, bleeding occurred more frequently among patients being treated for acute leukemia versus autologous stem cell transplant recipients. Overall, the results of these trials support the continued use of prophylactic platelet transfusions for patients with hematologic malignancy and therapy-induced hypoproliferative thrombocytopenia.[15]

Prophylactic Platelet Dosing

There are currently thought to be two distinct clearance mechanisms for platelets. Most platelets undergo senescence after circulating in the peripheral blood for 8 to 10 days. But there is also evidence for a second clearance route in which there is a fixed daily loss of platelets that occurs independent of platelet age. Platelets exiting the circula- tion via this second route are postulated to function in maintaining vascular integrity. In principle, a low dose of platelets could be used to meet this daily requirement. This hypothesis was tested directly by the 2010 PLADO trial. A total of 1272 patients undergoing HSCor chemotherapy were randomly assigned to receive low-, medium-, or high-dose platelets for a morning count of 10,000/μL or lower. The risk of spontaneous bleeding was not increased until patient platelet counts fell to 5000/μL or lower. No differences were observed in bleeding rates among the three treatment groups, supporting the concept that few platelets are required to maintain hemostasis. Although significantly fewer total platelets were transfused to patients in the low-dose group, platelet transfusions were required more frequently.[12]

Prophylactic Platelets for Invasive Bedside Procedures

To date, there have been no large randomized trials evaluating the need for platelet prophylaxis before invasive bedside procedures such as lumbar puncture. However, retrospective data provide reassurance that moderate thrombocytopenia does not pose a serious risk for performing such procedures. Howard et al[16] reviewed the records of 956 consecutive pediatric patients with newly diagnosed acute

lymphoblastic leukemia who underwent lumbar puncture. No serious hemorrhagic complications were observed after 5223 lumbar punc- tures, including 170 procedures that were done when the platelet count was 11,000 to 20,000/μL. The authors concluded that pro- phylactic platelet transfusion was unnecessary in patients with platelet counts above 10,000/μL. Lumbar punctures were performed in only 29 patients with platelet counts of 10,000/μL or less, making it difficult to assess the risk of bleeding in patients with very low platelet counts. A similar, albeit much smaller, retrospective study examined the same issue in adult patients with acute leukemia.[17] No hemor- rhagic complications were observed after 195 lumbar punctures, including 35 that were done with platelet counts of 20,000 to 30,000/μL. With very limited data published data available on severely thrombocytopenic adults, AABB has suggested 50,000/μL as a minimum safe platelet count for lumbar puncture in adult patients. For central venous catheter placements, AABB has suggested 20,000/μL as a minimum safe platelet count, based on multiple observational studies.[15] Relatively few studies have been published to date addressing the question of a safety minimum platelet count for other types of bedside procedures (thoracentesis, paracentesis, etc.)

Prophylactic Platelets for Major Surgical Procedures

There are currently no data from randomized trials addressing the question of what constitutes an adequate platelet count before surgery. Retrospective studies, though, suggest that patients with platelet counts of 50,000/μL or higher are not at excess bleeding risk during surgery. Bishop and colleagues[18] reported a series of 95 patients with acute leukemia who underwent 130 surgical procedures with platelet counts of less than 50,000/μL. Intraoperative blood loss exceeded 500 mL in only 7% of cases. No relationship was seen between the preoperative platelet count and surgical blood loss. These data suggest that prophylactic platelet transfusions need not be administered before surgery when the preoperative platelet count is at least 50,000/μL. This rule of thumb is thought to apply to most types of surgery (cardiac, orthopedic, and so on). For a few types of surgeries, however, requiring a higher platelet count (70,000–100,000/μL) is traditional, although no published data currently exist either to support or refute this approach. These settings include neurosurgery, retinal surgeries, and other procedures in which the risk is not that the patient may exsanguinate but rather that even a minor bleed might cause clinically significant damage in a vulnerable vital structure such as the brain.

ADVERSE EFFECTS OF PLATELET TRANSFUSION

Infectious Risks

Platelets are associated with essentially the same range of infectious pathogens as other blood components, but septic transfusion reactions caused by bacterially contaminated units comprise a unique risk of platelet transfusion. Over time, improvements in donor screening virtually eliminated the risk of transfusion transmission of hepatitis B virus, hepatitis C virus, and HIV. The risk of septic transfusion reactions remained fairly constant over this same time period, so eventually, platelet bacterial contamination became, by default, the most frequent infectious risk of transfusion. Unlike other blood components, which are stored either refrigerated or frozen, platelets are stored at room temperature. The reason is that if platelets are refrigerated before transfusion, they are cleared rapidly from the recipient's circulation.[19] Although room temperature storage allows transfused platelets to circulate in vivo, it has the downside of promoting bacterial growth. Because of this risk, platelet storage is ordinarily limited to only 5 days, making platelet inventory management extremely challenging.

In the 1990s, numerous studies demonstrated that contaminating bacteria, usually representing skin flora from the donor, could be cultured out of approximately 1 of 3000 platelet units. Clinically apparent septic transfusion reactions were thought to occur after approximately 1 of 25,000 platelet transfusions, although there is considerable uncertainty around this point estimate. In response to the issue, AABB developed the following standard:

> *5.1.5.1 The blood bank or transfusion service shall have methods to limit and detect or inactivate bacteria in all platelet components. Standard 5.6.2 applies [skin disinfection].*[1]

How this standard is being met varies by facility. Many blood collection centers have begun routinely culturing platelet units using an automated culture system. The BacT/ALERT system (BioMerieux), used by many centers, works by continuously monitoring for bacterial production of CO_2 within culture bottles. Platelet units are sampled on the day after collection. The samples are cultured for a period of time, typically 24 hours, and if the cultures fail to produce abnormal levels of CO_2, the product is released into inventory. Overall, culture-based bacterial screening appears to have decreased, but not eliminated, the risk of septic reactions.[20] Rapid, point-of-issue tests that can be used to test the sterility of a platelet unit just before issue have also been developed, but are not widely used due to issues of logistics and cost. Reducing the bacterial risk further may ultimately require alternative approaches, such as pathogen reduction.[21] Pathogen inactivation systems, using photoactivated reagents such as amotosalen or riboflavin plus ultraviolet (UV) light, can provide up to 6 logs of killing of spiked virus or bacteria within 1 unit of platelets. Such systems have been used in Europe and elsewhere, and in 2015, a pathogen reduction system for platelets and plasma was licensed for use in the U.S.[22]

Allergic and Febrile Nonhemolytic Transfusion Reactions

The typical RBC unit contains approximately 20 mL of plasma. Platelet units contain far more plasma, approximately 200 mL on average. There are multiple potential adverse effects associated with this large plasma content. Indeed, in the PLADO trial, higher platelet doses were associated with significantly increased risk of transfusion-related adverse events.[23] Febrile nonhemolytic reactions, defined as an increase in temperature of more than 1°C, are the most common reactions seen after platelet transfusion. In a classic study, Heddle and colleagues[24] demonstrated that the plasma component of platelet units, rather than the cellular component, causes most reactions. Cytokines that accumulate during product storage have been implicated. Allergic transfusion reactions are the second most-common type of adverse event associated with platelet transfusion.[23] Allergic reactions to blood products occur when the recipient has a preexisting allergy to a plasma protein component. Allergic reactions range from mild, uncomplicated urticarial reactions (most common) to full-blown anaphylaxis. Platelet Additive Solution (PAS) platelet units are those in which a preservative solution replaces most of the residual plasma. Using PAS platelets has been shown to reduce the risk of allergic reactions.[25]

ABO and Hemolytic Reactions to Platelets

Whenever possible, platelet units are assigned so as to match the donor plasma with recipient RBC type. For example, a type A patient would ordinarily receive type A or AB platelets, which do not contain anti-A antibody. When platelet inventories are constrained, however, it is common for blood banks to issue ABO-incompatible platelets. For example, a type A patient might receive type O platelets, containing anti-A. The passive transfusion of donor anti-A or anti-B to a patient usually does not cause adverse sequelae. Rarely, however, hemolysis may be observed. Most often, this occurs with units from type O donors, who occasionally have high titer anti-A, anti-B, or anti-A,B antibody. In a typical type O adult, the titer of circulating anti-A is on the order of 128 to 256. Some donors, however, have anti-A titers of 10,000 or higher. Recipients of products from donors with high-titer anti-A (and less frequently, anti-B) rarely do have clinically apparent hemolysis, and a small number of fatalities have been reported.[26] This is considered to be a low-risk event, but it may be on the rise in the United States because of the increased number of single-donor apheresis platelet units used. One strategy to deal with this issue is to measure the anti-A/B titer on all platelet donors; components exceeding a threshold titer are assigned to type-specific recipients. An alternate strategy is to reduce the load of plasma in a platelet unit before transfusing the unit to a non–ABO-identical recipient, either by washing or concentrating the unit, or by using a PAS unit (above.)

Transfusion-Related Acute Lung Injury

Transfusion-related acute lung injury (TRALI) is an acute respiratory distress syndrome associated with the transfusion of any plasma-containing blood component, including platelets.[27] Most cases of TRALI appear to be precipitated by the passive transfusion of donor anti-HLA or (less commonly) anti-neutrophil antibody. It is believed that products containing higher volumes of plasma such as fresh-frozen plasma (FFP) and apheresis platelets carry a higher risk of TRALI. Approximately one-third of female blood donors have circulating anti-HLA antibody because of prior sensitization during pregnancy. To help mitigate against the risk of TRALI, many countries, including the United States, now produce FFP from the blood of male donors only. Although this strategy has been relatively easy to apply to FFP production, female platelet donors are still needed to ensure an adequate platelet supply. A variety of strategies are being implemented to screen female platelet donors for anti-HLA antibody and to defer women who are antibody positive.

D Sensitization

The Rh(D) antigen is the most immunogenic RBC protein antigen. More than 80% of individuals who are D-negative will form anti-D after a single D-positive RBC transfusion. Anti-D is associated with both hemolytic transfusion reactions and hemolytic disease of the fetus and newborn. For this reason, it is standard practice to provide D-negative individuals exclusively with D-negative RBC units.

Platelet units contain a small number of contaminating RBCs. In the case of whole blood-derived platelet concentrates, approximately 0.3 to 0.5 mL RBCs may be present. In contrast, current apheresis platelets contain far fewer RBCs (≈0.0002 to 0.0007 mL per unit). When possible, D-negative platelet units are given to D-negative recipients. However, inventory constraints often force blood banks to issue D-positive platelet products to D-negative recipients. Transfusion of such units is associated with a low but nonzero risk of sensitization and formation of anti-D. D sensitization can be prevented by administering Rh immune globulin, as is done to prevent fetomaternal Rh sensitization in D-negative mothers of D-positive children. The risk of sensitization is very low among D-negative immunocompromised patients transfused with D-positive platelets (e.g., HSCT patients).[28] In this setting, the value of Rh immune globulin (RhIG) prophylaxis appears to be low.

PLATELET REFRACTORINESS

Causes of Refractoriness to Platelet Transfusion

Platelet refractoriness is defined as an inappropriately low platelet increment after repeated platelet transfusions. It can be caused by nonimmune or immune factors (Table 112.1). The most commonly reported nonimmune causes of platelet refractoriness include fever, sepsis, bleeding, splenomegaly, and disseminated intravascular coagulation. In a small subset of cases, platelet refractoriness is immune mediated. Platelets express HLA class I antigens, ABO antigens, and several platelet-specific antigens. Any of these molecules may potentially serve as an immune stimulus in a transfusion recipient. Whereas antibodies directed against HLA molecules are responsible for most cases of immune-mediated platelet refractoriness, antibodies to the human platelet antigens (anti-HPA) are less frequently implicated.

Diagnosis of Platelet Refractoriness

Because fewer than half of all platelet-refractory patients have demonstrable anti-HLA or antiplatelet antibodies, evaluation of both an immediate response to platelet transfusion and an 18- to 24-hour posttransfusion platelet survival is needed to help establish the cause of platelet refractoriness. Platelet counts obtained from 10 minutes to 1 hour after transfusion that repeatedly fail to demonstrate a corrected count increment of more than 5000/μL usually indicate immune-mediated platelet refractoriness. If the 10-minute to 1-hour posttransfusion platelet count shows a reasonable increment but the platelet count falls back to baseline by 18 to 24 hours, a nonimmune mechanism of refractoriness may be presumed (see Table 112.1). In cases of suspected immune-mediated refractoriness, HLA antibody screening (panel reactive antibody [PRA]) provides valuable supporting evidence that allosensitization has occurred.[29] A patient with a PRA greater than 70% may be considered to be "severely immunized" and a good candidate for HLA-matched platelets (below).

Detection of Anti-Human Leukocyte Antigen Antibodies

Several assays are available to detect the presence of anti-HLA class I antibodies in the serum of alloimmunized patients. Years ago, the most commonly used test was the lymphocytotoxicity assay (LCA). The results of the LCA correlate well with the response to platelet transfusion. However, this assay does not detect anti-HLA antibodies that do not activate complement. The anti-HLA antibodies can also be detected using an HLA-specific solid-phase enzyme-linked immunosorbent assay, glycoprotein-specific monoclonal antibody-specific immobilization of platelet antigens, or flow cytometric detection of antibody binding to beads coated with purified HLA antigens. The flow cytometry-based methodology has significantly improved sensitivity over LCA and, similar to solid-phase assays, it can detect both complement-fixing and noncomplement-fixing antibodies.

TABLE 112.1	Causes of Refractoriness to Platelet Transfusion
Nonimmune	
Fever	
Sepsis	
Drug associated	
Active bleeding	
Splenomegaly	
Disseminated intravascular coagulation	
Venoocclusive disease	
Immune	
Anti-HLA antibodies	
Anti-HPA antibodies	
ABO mismatch	
Drug-dependent antibodies	

HLA, Human leukocyte antigen; HPA, human platelet antigen.

Detection of Antiplatelet Antibodies

The most commonly used methods for detection of anti-HPA antibodies are solid-phase assays using purified platelet antigens for detection of antibody specificity. However, testing for anti-HPA antibodies is not typically performed in the workup of platelet refractory patients, mainly because the importance of these antibodies in causing clinical refractoriness is not well established.

Prevention of Alloimmunization

Although they express HLA class I antigens, platelets themselves are fairly weak immunogens. It has been shown that contaminating leukocytes in platelet products are primarily responsible for stimulating HLA antibody formation in platelet transfusion recipients. Thus removing WBCs from blood products (leukoreduction) is an essential means of preventing alloimmunization and subsequent platelet refractoriness. The definitive study showing this was the Trial to Reduce Alloimmunization to Platelets (TRAP study)[5] that compared alloimmunization rates in 530 newly diagnosed patients with acute myeloid leukemia randomized to receive unmodified, pooled platelet concentrates (control); filtered, pooled platelet concentrates (F-PC); filtered single-donor apheresis platelets (F-AP); or UV-B-irradiated pooled platelet concentrates (UVB-PC). Anti-HLA antibodies were detected in 45% of control participants compared with 17% to 21% of patients receiving modified platelets. A total of 13% of control group patients became platelet refractory versus only 3% in the F-PC group, 4% in the F-AP group, and 5% in the UVB-PC group.

Management of Platelet-Refractory Patients

When platelet refractoriness has been demonstrated, several strategies may facilitate achieving therapeutic platelet increments in vivo (Table 112.2). A trial of ABO-matched, fresh (1–2 days old) platelets may be helpful. In cases of immune-mediated refractoriness, a trial of HLA-matched platelets, antigen-negative platelets, or cross-matched platelets should be considered. The basic principles for selection of HLA-matched platelets are outlined in Table 112.3. In most cases, alloimmune refractory patients will show some degree of response to HLA-matched platelets. Because of the high degree of polymorphism of the HLA loci, it is often not possible to find perfect HLA-A and HLA-B locus matches, leading to the use of platelets mismatched at one or more loci (Table 112.4). In general, transfusion of grade A- or BU-matched platelets can result in an increase in platelet count that is superior to platelet increment obtained using either cross matched platelets or platelets with different degrees of HLA mismatching (BX, C, or D). An additional step that may help in finding compatible

TABLE 112.2   Management of the Platelet-Refractory Patient

Obtain 10-minute to 1-hour posttransfusion platelet count on two occasions.

If there is an appropriate increment in platelet count after a single platelet transfusion, continue to transfuse random platelets and treat nonimmune factors associated with decreased platelet survival such as sepsis and DIC, discontinue offending drugs, and so on.

If the 10-minute to 1-hour posttransfusion platelet counts demonstrate no platelet increment (or only a marginal increment), obtain the patient's HLA type and screen the patient for the presence of anti-HLA antibodies (panel reactive antibody test).

While awaiting HLA antigen typing and antibody screening results, consider transfusion of "fresh" (<3 days old) ABO-matched platelets.

If PRA shows less than 20% reactivity, continue with "fresh" ABO-matched random platelets.

If PRA shows more than 20% reactivity, obtain anti-HLA antibody specificity. Use the recipient's HLA typing information to locate grade A or B matched platelet units for transfusion. Avoid transfusion of platelets containing antigens against which the recipient has antibodies. Consider recruiting recipient's family for platelet donation.

Transfusion of cross match-compatible platelets is an option if there is a poor response to grade A- or B-matched platelets or if the recipient has antibodies to platelet-specific antigens.

All HLA-matched or cross-matched platelet units must be irradiated before transfusion to prevent transfusion-associated GVHD.

DIC, Disseminated intravascular coagulation; GVHD, graft-versus-host disease; HLA, human leukocyte antigen; PRA, panel reactive antibody.

TABLE 112.3   Traditional Platelet Selection Guidelines for Refractoriness Caused by Alloimmunization

ABO antigens are expressed on platelets. Consider transfusion of ABO-matched platelets while awaiting the recipient's HLA type and antibody specificity

Platelet matching for the recipient's HLA-A and HLA-B antigens is important.

Platelet matching for the recipient's HLA-C antigens is not essential.

Determine the antigen specificity of recipient's antiplatelet antibodies and try to transfuse antigen negative platelets.

Some HLA antigens may be weakly expressed on platelets. Consider giving platelets mismatched for those antigens (e.g., HLA-B12 and its splits B44, B45)

If HLA-matched platelets are unavailable, consider transfusion of platelets mismatched for HLA antigens that are serologically cross-reactive with the recipient's HLA antigens.

If platelets mismatched for serologically cross-reactive antigens are not effective, matching for HLA-associated antigen systems such as Bw4/Bw6 may be helpful.

HLA, Human leukocyte antigen.

TABLE 112.4   Grades of Human Leukocyte Antigen–Matched Platelets

Match Grade	Description
A	4-antigen match (donor and recipient match at both HLA-A and HLA-B loci)
B1U	1 antigen unknown or blank (e.g., donor is: A2, –; B5, 27)
B1X	1 cross-reactive group[a]
B2UX	1 antigen blank and 1 cross-reactive[a]
C	1 mismatched antigen present
D	≥2 mismatched antigens present
R	Random

[a]The clusters of human leukocyte antigen (HLA) that share antigenic epitopes can be classified into cross-reactive antigen groups. Antibodies recognizing one HLA molecule within the group cross-react with other members of the same group.

Adapted from Brecher ME, editor: *Technical manual*, ed 15, Bethesda, MD, 2005, American Association of Blood Banks.

The most challenging cases are the rare instances involving immune-refractory patients who are actively bleeding and HLA-matched platelets or cross matched platelets are either ineffective or unavailable. In such cases, patients are typically transfused with repeated doses of random HLA-incompatible platelets during hemorrhagic episodes. The efficacy of this practice is unclear.

REFERENCES

1. Levitt J: *Standards for blood banks and transfusion services*, 29 ed, Bethesda, 2012, AABB.
2. Whitaker BI: *The 2011 national blood collection and utilization survey report*, Washington, DC, 2013, U.S. Department of Health and Human Services.
3. Zou S, Stramer SL, Dodd RY: Donor Testing and Risk: Current Prevalence, Incidence, and Residual Risk of Transfusion-Transmissible Agents in US Allogeneic Donations. *Transfus Med Rev* 26(2):119–128, 2012.
4. Slichter SJ: Leukocyte reduction and ultraviolet B irradiation of platelets to prevent alloimmunization and refractoriness to platelet transfusions. The Trial to Reduce Alloimmunization to Platelets Study Group. *N Engl J Med* 337(26):1861–1869, 1997.
5. Slichter SJ: Factors affecting posttransfusion platelet increments, platelet refractoriness, and platelet transfusion intervals in thrombocytopenic patients. *Blood* 105(10):4106–4114, 2005.
6. Gaydos LA, Freireich EJ, Mantel N: The quantitative relation between platelet count and hemorrhage in patients with acute leukemia. *N Engl J Med* 266(18):905–909, 1962.
7. Slichter SJ, Harker LA: Thrombocytopenia: Mechanisms and management of defects in platelet production. *Clin Haematol* 7:523, 1978.
8. Heckman KD, Weiner GJ, Davis CS, et al: Randomized study of prophylactic platelet transfusion threshold during induction therapy for adult acute leukemia: 10,000/microL versus 20,000/microL. *J Clin Oncol* 15(3):1143–1149, 1997.
9. Rebulla P, Finazzi G, Marangoni F, et al: The threshold for prophylactic platelet transfusions in adults with acute myeloid leukemia. Gruppo Italiano Malattie Ematologiche Maligne dell'Adulto. *N Engl J Med* 337(26):1870–1875, 1997.
10. Zumberg MS, del Rosario MLU, Nejame CF, et al: A prospective randomized trial of prophylactic platelet transfusion and bleeding incidence in hematopoietic stem cell transplant recipients: 10,000/L versus 20,000/microL trigger. *Biol Blood Marrow Transplant* 8(10):569–576, 2002.
11. Gmür J, Burger J, Schanz U, et al: Safety of stringent prophylactic platelet transfusion policy for patients with acute leukaemia. *Lancet* 338(8777):1223–1226, 1991.

platelets is flow cytometric detection of anti-HLA antibody specificity using single HLA antigen-coated beads. This information can be used to find donors that may be HLA mismatched with the recipient, but whose platelets lack the antigens to which the patient has specific antibodies. Furthermore, family members may be considered as platelet donors in addition to the available pool of HLA-matched volunteer donors. As an alternative to HLA antigen matching, patients may benefit from receiving donor platelets that are cross match compatible with the patient's serum. The major benefit of cross matching is a potentially larger pool of donors that would have been excluded by strict HLA antigen matching. Also, platelet cross matching may be helpful in cases of refractoriness caused by antibodies directed against platelet-specific antigens.[30]

12. Slichter SJ, Kaufman RM, Assmann SF, et al: Dose of prophylactic platelet transfusions and prevention of hemorrhage. *N Engl J Med* 362(7):600–613, 2010.

13. Wandt H, Schaefer-Eckart K, Wendelin K, et al: Therapeutic platelet transfusion versus routine prophylactic transfusion in patients with haematological malignancies: an open-label, multicentre, randomised study. *The Lancet.* 380(9850):1309–1316, 2012.

14. Stanworth SJ, Estcourt LJ, Powter G, et al: A no-prophylaxis platelet-transfusion strategy for hematologic cancers. *N Engl J Med* 368(19):1771–1780, 2013.

15. Kaufman RM, Djulbegovic B, Gernsheimer T, et al: Platelet Transfusion: A Clinical Practice Guideline From the AABB. *Ann Intern Med* 162(3):205–213, 2015.

16. Howard SC, Gajjar A, Ribeiro RC, et al: Safety of lumbar puncture for children with acute lymphoblastic leukemia and thrombocytopenia. *JAMA* 284(17):2222–2224, 2000.

17. Vavricka SR, Walter RB, Irani S, et al: Safety of lumbar puncture for adults with acute leukemia and restrictive prophylactic platelet transfusion. *Ann Hematol* 82(9):570–573, 2003.

18. Bishop JF, Schiffer CA, Aisner J, et al: Surgery in acute leukemia: a review of 167 operations in thrombocytopenic patients. *Am J Hematol* 26(2):147–155, 1987.

19. Murphy S, Gardner FH: Effect of storage temperature on maintenance of platelet viability–deleterious effect of refrigerated storage. *N Engl J Med* 280(20):1094–1098, 1969.

20. Eder AF, Kennedy JM, Dy BA, et al: Bacterial screening of apheresis platelets and the residual risk of septic transfusion reactions: the American Red Cross experience (2004–2006). *Transfusion* 47(7):1134–1142, 2007.

21. Seltsam A, Müller TH: Update on the use of pathogen-reduced human plasma and platelet concentrates. *Br J Haematol* 162(4):442–454, 2013.

22. McCullough J: Therapeutic efficacy and safety of platelets treated with a photochemical process for pathogen inactivation: the SPRINT Trial. *Blood* 104(5):1534–1541, 2004.

23. Kaufman RM, Assmann SF, Triulzi DJ, et al: Transfusion-related adverse events in the Platelet Dose study. *Transfusion* 2014. doi: 10.1111/trf.12791. n/a–n/a.

24. Heddle NM, Klama L, Meyer R, et al: A randomized controlled trial comparing plasma removal with white cell reduction to prevent reactions to platelets. *Transfusion* 39(3):231–238, 1999.

25. Tobian AAR, Fuller AK, Uglik K, et al: The impact of platelet additive solution apheresis platelets on allergic transfusion reactions and corrected count increment (CME). *Transfusion* 54(6):1523–1529, 2013.

26. Josephson CD, Castillejo M-I, Grima K, et al: ABO-mismatched platelet transfusions: Strategies to mitigate patient exposure to naturally occurring hemolytic antibodies. *Transfus Apher Sci* 42(1):83–88, 2010.

27. Toy P, Gajic O, Bacchetti P, et al: Transfusion related acute lung injury: incidence and risk factors. *Blood* 119(7):1757–1767, 2012.

28. Cid J, Lozano M, Fernández-Avilés F, et al: Anti-D alloimmunization after D-mismatched allogeneic hematopoietic stem cell transplantation in patients with hematologic diseases. *Transfusion* 46(2):169–173, 2006.

29. Dzik S: How I do it: platelet support for refractory patients. *Transfusion* 47(3):374–378, 2007.

30. Vassallo RR, Fung M, Rebulla P, et al: Utility of cross-matched platelet transfusions in patients with hypoproliferative thrombocytopenia: a systematic review. *Transfusion* 54(4):1180–1191, 2013.

HUMAN LEUKOCYTE ANTIGEN AND HUMAN NEUTROPHIL ANTIGEN SYSTEMS

Ena Wang, Sharon Adams, David F. Stroncek, and Francesco M. Marincola

This chapter reviews human leukocyte antigen (HLA) and human neutrophil antigen (HNA) systems. A general background of the structure, function, and nomenclature of both systems and their relevance in clinical hematology is presented. Analysis of HLA gene products is applied in clinical settings (1) to select compatible donor-recipient pairs for transplantation, (2) to select HLA-compatible single-donor platelet products for thrombocytopenic patients refractory to standard transfusion of random pooled platelets, (3) to screen for genetic factors that may contribute to the prevalence of diseases, and (4) for forensic purposes in which the identity of individuals may contribute to solving legal disputes or criminal investigations. In addition, we discuss new applications that have broadened the relevance of HLA in the area of immune pathology. HLA phenotypes determine the suitability of patients for epitope-specific immunization. Tetrameric HLA/epitope complexes (tHLA) allow enumeration of antigen-specific T-cell responses. Furthermore, molecular identification of T-cell epitopes associated with distinct diseases and characterization of the communication between immune effector cells through HLA–HLA ligand interactions extend the relevance of HLA to biologic fields. These biologic fields encompass natural killer (NK) and cytotoxic T-cell function, antigen recognition in the context of infection, autoimmunity, graft-versus-neoplasia (GVN) effect, and autologous cancer rejection. Finally, the recognition that polymorphism extends to other protein families relevant to immune pathology including cytokines, their receptors, and killer cell-inhibitory receptors has broadened the significance of immunogenetics beyond HLA. Thus this chapter emphasizes the importance of viewing human pathologic conditions through the kaleidoscopic complexity of human polymorphism.

GENETICS, STRUCTURE, AND FUNCTION OF HUMAN LEUKOCYTE ANTIGEN MOLECULES

HLAs embrace a family of genes clustered in the short arm of chromosome 6 as the human version of the major histocompatibility complex (MHC), initially identified in mice as responsible for graft rejection between genetically unrelated strains (transplantation antigens).[1] Credit for the description of the human MHC goes to three individuals. In 1952, Jean Dausset observed that serum of individuals who had received several transfusions contained hemagglutinins (HAs) specific to the donors' leukocytes. In 1958, Rose Payne noted that the only requirement for the development of HAs against leukocytes was a history of previous transfusion or pregnancy and concluded that these antibodies were directed against antigens on the surface of circulating leukocytes. This conclusion was concomitantly and independently confirmed by Jon van Rood, who observed that multiple pregnancies immunize mothers against leukocytes leaked from the fetus into the mother's circulation. Based on these discoveries, the term *human leukocyte antigen* was subsequently adopted.[2] It should be clarified, however, that this historical name is misleading. HLA molecule expression is neither limited to leukocytes nor do they display, in natural conditions, antigenic behavior. In fact, several are expressed by most somatic cells and, rather than being antigens, chaperone protein bioproducts to the cell surface for recognition by T cells. There is, however, some substance to the name, because HLAs, by virtue of being densely packed on the cell surface, are exposed to recognition in a foreign environment such as allotransplantation or xenoinfusion performed to induce anti-HLA antibodies as diagnostic reagents.

ORGANIZATION OF THE HUMAN LEUKOCYTE ANTIGEN GENES

HLA genes constitute a string of coding sequences that regulate the expression of molecules with similar but not identical function. Residing in a region that spans approximately 4000 kilobases of the short arm of chromosome 6 (Fig. 113.1),[3] HLA contains several genes and pseudogenes characterized by sequence homology and functional similarity. Of them, 47 are officially recognized by the World Health Organization (WHO) nomenclature committee and include classic HLA class I and class II genes associated with antigen processing such as proteasomal units PSMB8 and PSMB9, or peptide transport TAP1 and TAP2.[4] Both HLA and HLA-associated genes can be physically grouped into three subregions according to chromosomal location. In centromeric to telomeric direction, the first is HLA class II region comprising the α-and β-chains of HLA-DR, HLA-DQ, HLA-DP, HLA-DM, and HLA-DO as well as TAP and PSMB. Sandwiched between the class II and class I region, class III region encodes for functionally unrelated genes such as complement components, heat shock proteins, and tumor necrosis factor. The reason for their genetic link to the HLA complex is unknown, but their immunologic function seems more than coincidental. The class I region is mostly telomeric and includes HLA-A, HLA-B, and HLA-C loci; the non-classic HLA-E, HLA-F, and HLA-G loci; and several pseudogenes.

General terminology separates HLA genes into classic and non-classic. Classic HLA genes have been well characterized and are clearly associated with presentation of antigen to immune cells. They are further subdivided into class I (HLA-A, HLA-B, HLA-C) and class II (HLA-DR, HLA-DQ, and HLA-DP). In general, HLA class I and II genes have very similar structure and function.[5,6] They contain six to eight exons coding for functionally distinct domains (Fig. 113.2). The first exon encodes a leader sequence; the following exons (exons 2 to 4) are highly polymorphic and encode extracellular domains responsible for peptide binding and T cell-antigen receptor (TCR) engagement. Because they are exposed on the cell surface, these domains are also responsible for alloreactivity. The last exons encode a conserved transmembrane and small intracellular domains whose functions are unclear.

Only the heavy chain of HLA class I is encoded in the MHC region. Genes encoding HLA-A, HLA-B, and HLA-C contain three exons coding for α_1, α_2, and α_3 extracytoplasmic domains, one transmembrane, and three cytoplasmic domains (Fig. 113.3). The associated class I light chain, β_2-microglobulin, is encoded on chromosome 15.[7] By contrast, the HLA class II molecule is composed of a heterodimer of an α-chain and β-chain encoded in the MHC region. Although the genetics are different, the protein product is structurally similar to HLA class I, with two helices resulting in the antigen-presenting part of the molecule (Fig. 113.4).

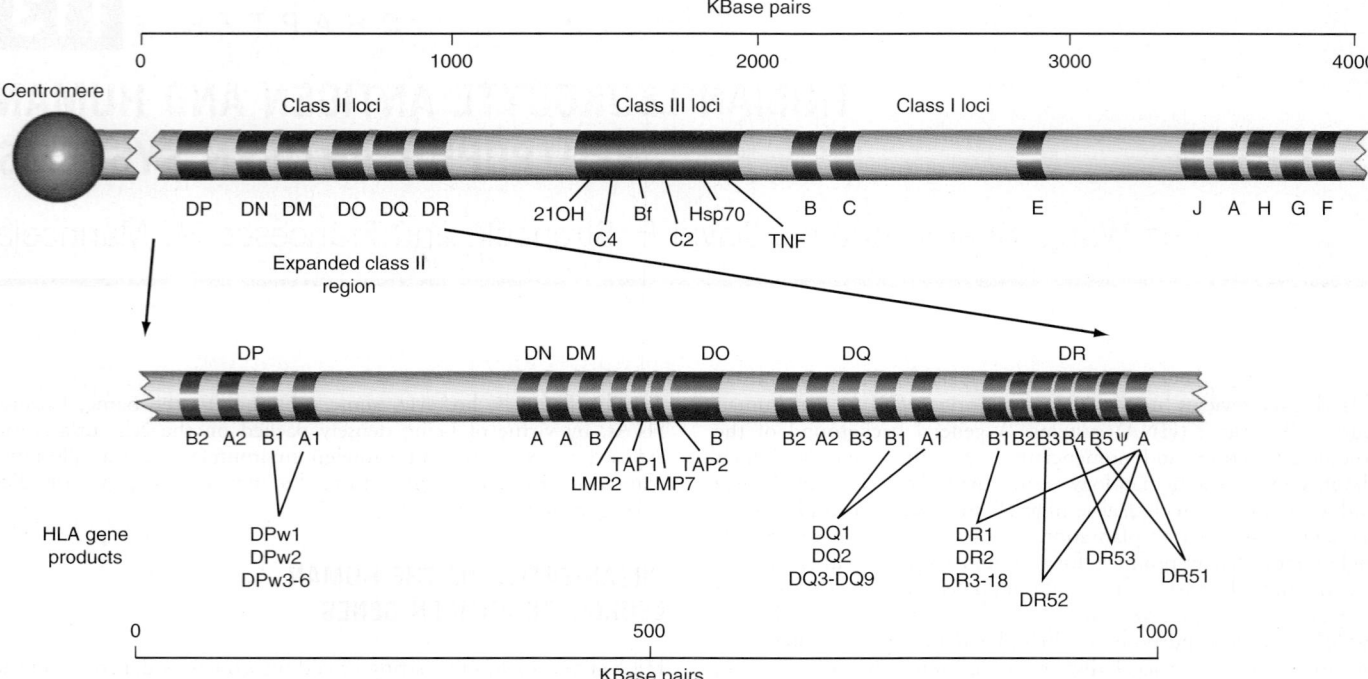

Fig. 113.1 PHYSICAL MAP OF THE HUMAN LEUKOCYTE ANTIGEN (HLA) GENETIC COMPLEX, ILLUSTRATING THE CLUSTERS OF GENES ACCORDING TO THE CLASS OF ENCODED GENE PRODUCTS. The symbol ψ represents four DRB pseudogenes, designated 7, 8, and 9. Other pseudogenes are shown in *gray*.

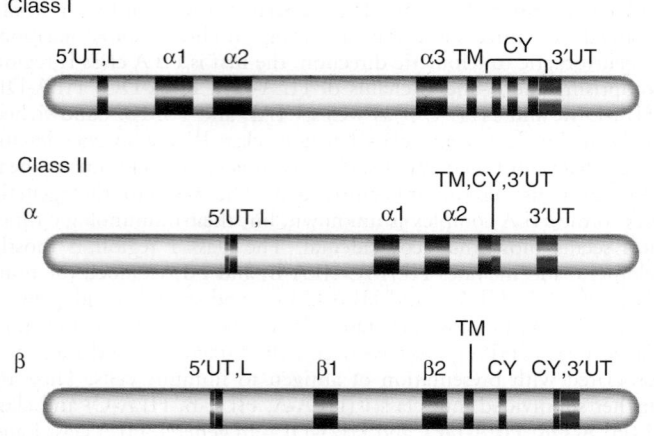

Fig. 113.2 ORGANIZATION OF CLASS I AND II MAJOR HISTO-COMPATIBILITY COMPLEX (MHC) GENES. *5′UT* and *3′UT*, Untranslated regions in the 5′ and 3′ ends of the gene; *α, β,* exons encoding extracellular domains. *CY,* Exon encoding cytoplasmic tail; *L,* leader sequence; *TM,* transmembrane exon. *(From Germain RN, Malissen B: Analysis of the expression and function of class-II major histocompatibility complex-encoded molecules by DNA-mediated gene transfer.* Annu Rev Immunol *4:281, 1986.)*

All DR molecules use DRA for α-chains but can use alleles coded by DRB1, DRB3, DRB4, or DRB5 for β-chains. DP, DQ, DM, and DO molecules are the product of DPA1 and DPB1, DQA1 and DQB1, DMA and DMB, and DOA and DOB genes, respectively. HLA DRB1 locus is expressed in all HLA haplotypes (the set of HLA alleles derived from the same parental chromosome and therefore genetically linked). However, only one other HLA DR locus is present in each individual chromosome. Thus each haplotype can have either DRB5 (DR1 haplotype); DRB3, DRB4, or DRB5 loci (DR2 haplotype); DRB4 locus (DR4 and DR7 haplotype); or none (DR8 and DR10 haplotype).[3]

INHERITANCE AND LINKAGE DISEQUILIBRIUM

Because of their proximity within a short chromosomal distance, HLA genes are inherited en bloc from each parent unless a recombinant event occurs. Thus each HLA haplotype behaves as a unit and is transmitted through generations according to mendelian principles. Because there are four possible genotypes (two from each parent), the probability of genotypic identity between two siblings is 25%. Most HLA phenotypically identical siblings are also HLA genotypically identical, because the genetic pool of derivation is restricted to the parents. In 2% of cases, recombinant HLA haplotypes (a set of genes derived partially from two chromosomes through recombination) deviate from this rule.

The occurrence of HLA haplotypes within a population with a frequency higher than expected from the prevalence of individual alleles is called *linkage disequilibrium.* In large populations, gene frequencies achieve equilibrium within a few generations unless selective pressure influences individuals' survival and mating capacity (Hardy-Weinberg principle). In equilibrium, gene prevalence is maintained based solely on its frequency. Thus, assuming that there were 18, 36, and 8 alleles for the HLA-A, HLA-B, and HLA-C loci, respectively (number of alleles known when this example was described[2]), theoretically 18 × 36 × 8 = 5184 HLA class I allelic combinations or haplotypes would be possible. Adding HLA class II genes to the calculation yields an astronomical number, making the identification of two HLA-matched individuals unlikely. However, individual alleles occur with different frequency, and an allele that occurs with high frequency is predominant in a given population, such as HLA-A2 in whites and A24 or A11 in Asians.[8] Because predominant alleles come with the related haplotype, most theoretical permutations never occur, and the chances of identifying matched individuals are much higher than theoretically possible.

STRUCTURE OF THE HUMAN LEUKOCYTE ANTIGEN CLASS I AND II

The structure of HLA molecules and their relationship with their natural ligand, the TCR, has been well characterized by crystallography.[9–11] HLA molecules are heterodimer glycoproteins belonging to the immunoglobulin superfamily with common features (Fig. 113.4). This includes two α-helical domains protruding toward the extracellular milieu. Between them lies a flat surface formed by β-sheet structures that contributes to the formation of a groove accommodating peptides generated from intracellular (HLA class I) or extracellular proteins (HLA class II) (Fig. 113.5). The helices/peptide complex is exposed for TCR recognition. Because HLA polymorphism is clustered within the α-helixes and β-sheets domains, peptides display variable affinity for distinct HLA alleles.[12,13] It has been proposed that a given peptide can bind to closely related alleles, and HLA superfamilies with similar binding characteristics have been described.[14–16] However, peptide binding to related but distinct HLA alleles is associated with conformational dissimilarity caused by differential interaction with variant residues in the binding groove.[17] The TCR interaction with HLA required for productive engagement spans a surface including the peptide and portions of the α- and β-helix.[11,18–20] This double requirement of interaction between TCR and HLA/peptide complex represents the structural basis for HLA restriction. Degenerate and promiscuous TCR recognition of peptides presented by distinct HLA alleles within the same superfamily has also been described.[21] Although this concept holds in general, several exceptions can be expected because single amino acid variants in the HLA molecule may disallow binding of a peptide or may not be permissive to TCR engagement.[22–24]

The binding affinity of a given peptide for an HLA allele can be predicted through algorithms that compile available information to identify amino acid residues that fit distinct pockets of the HLA groove.[13,25] Several algorithms implement this information with experimental testing based on the refolding capability of HLA heavy chains exposed to known peptide sequences in the presence of β₂-microglobulin and/or their dissociation rates (see www.bimas.dcrt.nih.gov or www.uni-tuebingen.de/uni/kxi). This is based on the principle that the affinity of a peptide for a given HLA promotes that stability of the noncovalent assembly of heavy chain with β₂-microglobulin.[13,26] Finally, peptide binding can be shown by direct elutriation from purified HLA heavy chains.[12,27]

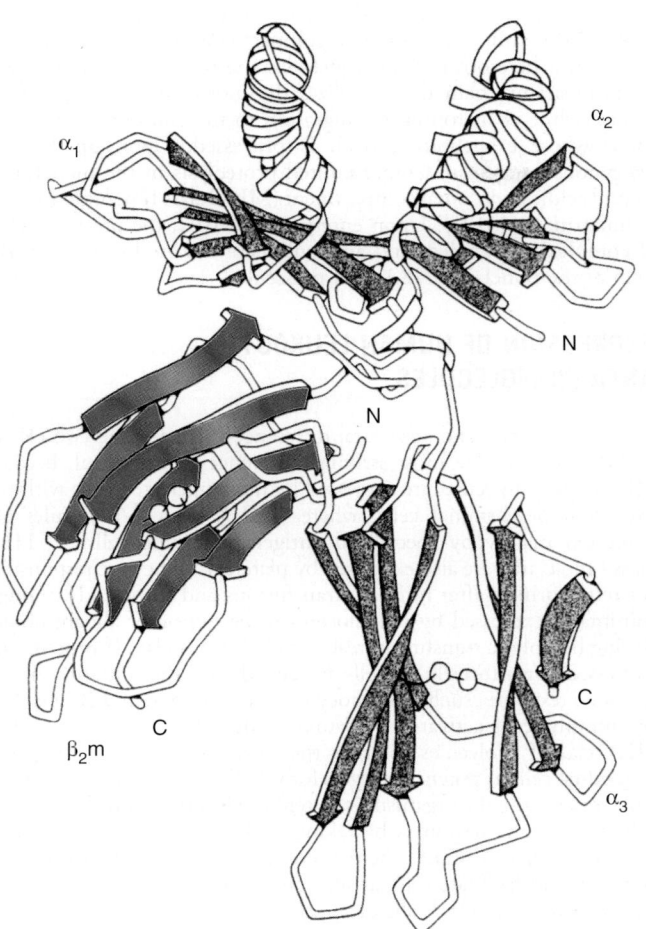

Fig. 113.3 THREE-DIMENSIONAL CONFIGURATION OF HLA-A2, MODELED FROM X-RAY CRYSTALLOGRAPHIC STUDIES. *HLA, Human leukocyte antigen. (From Bjorkman PJ, Saper MA, Samraoui B, et al: Structure of the human class I histocompatibility antigen, HLA-A2. Nature 329:506, 1987.)*

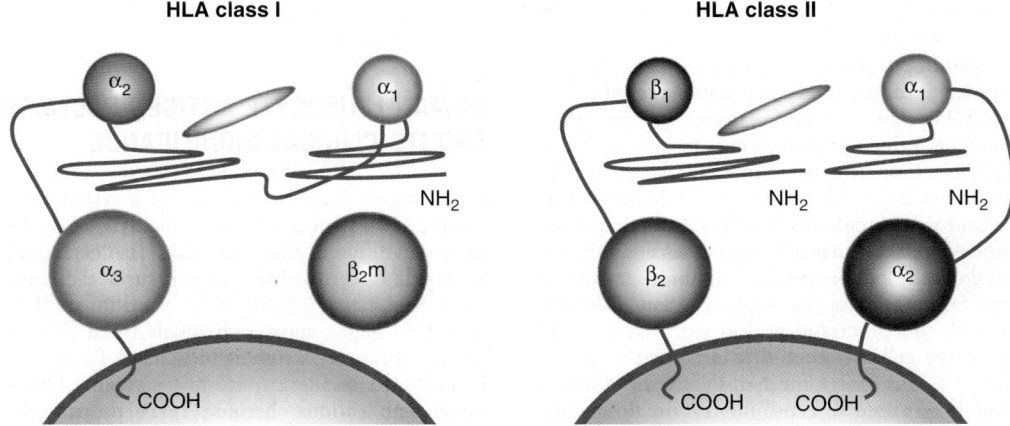

Fig. 113.4 SCHEMATIC DIAGRAM OF HUMAN LEUKOCYTE ANTIGEN (HLA) CLASS I AND CLASS II MOLECULES POINTING TO THEIR STRUCTURAL SIMILARITY. In both HLA classes, two immunoglobulin-type domains reside close to the cell membrane (α₃ and β₂m for class I and α₂ and β₂ for class II). The other two domains project toward the extracellular milieu with α-helices (α₁ and α₂ for class I and α₁ and β₁ for class II) and a platform of parallel β-sheets that form a peptide-binding groove.

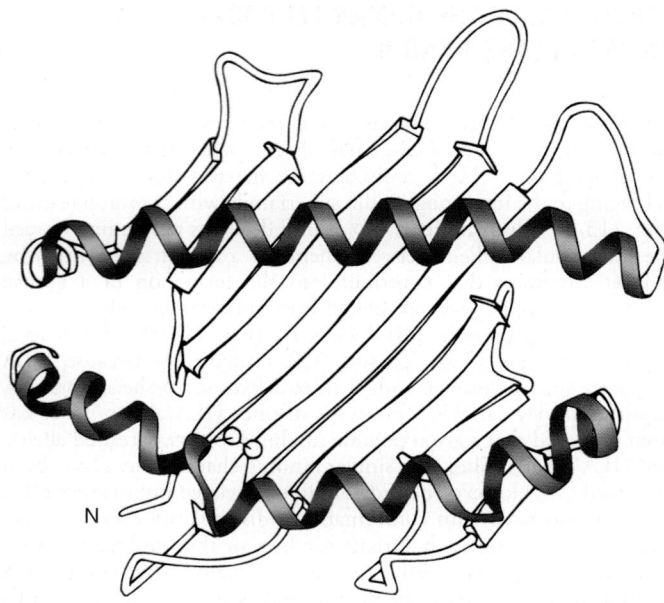

N

Fig. 113.5 SCHEME OF THE PEPTIDE GROOVE OF A HUMAN LEUKOCYTE ANTIGEN (HLA) CLASS I MOLECULE, FORMED BY THE α_1 AND α_2 DOMAINS AT THE SIDE AND THE β-SHEETS AT THE BOTTOM. The view is looking down on the vertically oriented molecule: the T-cell receptor point of view. *(From Bjorkman PJ, Saper MA, Samraoui B, et al: Structure of the human class I histocompatibility antigen, HLA-A2.* Nature *329:506, 1987.)*

Beyond the interactive component of the HLA molecule with TCR, other domains act as coreceptors for the TCR. CD8$^+$ cytotoxic T cells bind to the α_3-domain of HLA class I through CD8, whereas CD4$^+$ T cells interact with HLA class II-specific domains. Although the coreceptor-TCR interaction is not an absolute requirement in most cases, it determines HLA class I or II restriction of individual T cells.[28] Specific to HLA class I is the assembly with β_2-microglobulin on stabilization in the presence of high-affinity peptides derived from the cleavage of intracellular proteins (endogenous pathway of antigen presentation).[29] Most peptides derive from degradation of self-protein in the cytosol by proteasomes (PSMB) and other proteases.[30] Soluble peptides (9 to 10 amino acids long) are then chaperoned into the endosomal compartment by transporter molecules associated with antigen processing (TAP1 and TAP2). Within this compartment, they bind to heavy chains according to each individual's HLA phenotype. The binding and stability of the HLA-peptide complex depends on the affinity of each peptide for a particular allele. If the stability is sufficient, the peptide-loaded HLA migrates to the cell surface. Intracellular pathogens produce proteins that are also degraded by proteasomes into peptides that compete with self-peptides for binding to HLA class I molecules. Thus the function of the endogenous pathway of antigen presentation is to provide information to the extracellular compartment of intracellular events. In physiologic conditions, only self-peptides are presented, and therefore minimal interactions occur with circulating T cells. During infection, pathogen-derived peptides signal cellular infection to T cells, whereas antibodies that cannot cross the cell membrane remain insensitive to intracellular pathogens. Several pathogens, such as cytomegalovirus (CMV), can interfere with this process as well as with reduction of HLA/peptide density on the cell surface and, consequently, diminished T-cell recognition.[31,32] This escape mechanism can be counteracted by the host through increased susceptibility of virally infected cells to NK cell-mediated cytolysis.[33] Reciprocally, viruses can evade NK cells and escape recognition by modulating HLA expression.[34–36]

HLA class II molecules bind to longer peptides derived from the metabolism of molecules endocytosed from the extracellular compartment (exogenous pathway of antigen presentation).[29] This is a specialized process used by professional antigen-presenting cells such

as macrophages and dendritic cells. HLA class II molecules are assembled within the endosomal compartment where they are composed of a heterotrimer. This includes the α- and β-chains plus a short invariant chain that stabilizes the molecule by occupying its groove while chaperoning its migration to the endosomal compartment where exogenous antigen is processed. Upon uptake, the exogenous antigen undergoes limited proteolysis in the membrane-bound acidic endosomal compartment (MHC class II peptide-loading compartment, MIIC). Upon entering the MIIC, the pre-HLA class II complex is degraded, and antigenic peptides are loaded with the help of the nonclassic HLA-DM molecule.[37]

EXPRESSION OF HUMAN LEUKOCYTE ANTIGEN MOLECULES

There are genetic and structural differences between the two classes of HLA alleles. The most striking difference is functional, because HLA class I molecules are expressed by most nucleated cells with the exception of germinal cells, whereas HLA class II molecules are expressed mainly by specialized antigen-presenting cells.[38,39] HLA class I molecules are also expressed by platelets.[40] They are responsible for refractoriness after multiple transfusions and sufficiently, though minimally, expressed by reticulocytes to be targets of alloantibodies during hemolytic transfusion reactions.[41–45] HLA class II proteins are expressed constitutively by cells associated with the initiation of the immune response, such as monocytes, macrophages, and B cells,[46] or by immune cells activated by cytokines during inflammation. Thus HLA class I molecules instruct the host about the condition of individual cells as potential targets for CD8$^+$ cytotoxic T cells responsible for clearing the organisms of altered cells. HLA class II molecules initiate immune responses by taking up pathogen components and presenting them to CD4$^+$ helper T cells, which can in turn initiate humoral and facilitate cellular immune responses.

Expression of HLA alleles is sensitive to environmental conditions and can be modulated by cytokines among which interferons play a major role.[47] This is particularly important for HLA-B and HLA-C normally expressed at a lower density than HLA-A, but are more sensitive to cytokine induction.[48,49] In addition, HLA class II molecules can be expressed by most cells following cytokine stimulation.[50,51] Thus the ability of cells to present antigen in association with HLA is strongly influenced by the surrounding environment. This might explain why chronic inflammation induced by alloreactions during graft-versus-host disease (GVHD) may facilitate the presentation of tumor-specific antigens by tumor cells with consequent development of GVN effect. In addition, it might explain how systemic administration of proinflammatory cytokines such as interleukin (IL)-2 may stimulate immune responses by increasing the antigen-presenting ability of cells within the tumor microenvironment.[52]

HUMAN LEUKOCYTE ANTIGEN POLYMORPHISM AND ITS CLINICAL SIGNIFICANCE

A striking characteristic of the HLA system is its extreme polymorphism.[53] By chance, most individuals are heterozygote and therefore carry two different alleles for each HLA gene that, being codominant, are equally expressed on the cell surface. Because everybody carries three HLA class I (-A,-B, and -C) and three HLA class II (-DR, -DQ, and -DP) genes, most individuals (with the exception of homozygotes) express six different HLA class I and six different HLA class II molecules on the surface of their cells. This has important functional implications, because HLA polymorphism is clustered in domains of the HLA molecule associated with peptide binding and interaction with the TCR. Thus most individuals have a broad repertoire of molecules capable of presenting different pathogen components to immune cells leading to the belief that HLA polymorphism improves the chances of a given species of surviving infection.[54] This paradigm is difficult to demonstrate in human pathologic conditions in which the natural history of infectious diseases rarely correlates with HLA phenotype. An exception is the strong association between HLA-B*5701 and lack of progression to acquired immunodeficiency syndrome of individuals infected with human immunodeficiency virus (HIV).[55] Associations have been observed between HLA phenotype and predisposition for nasopharyngeal carcinoma.[56,57] This is of particular interest because nasopharyngeal carcinoma is a virally induced cancer against which T cells can mediate immune surveillance. HLA associations have also been described with less consistency than other virally driven tumors, such as cervical carcinoma,[58] or immunogenic tumors, such as melanoma.[59,60]

The difficulty in demonstrating conclusive associations between infectious disease and HLA in humans could be caused by the successful implementation of antigen presentation through a broad repertoire of HLA genes that could compensate for each other in limitations in antigen presentation. Chickens carry a single MHC locus, and their susceptibility to infection appears to be clearly related to MHC. For instance, Kaufman et al[54] have shown that chickens carrying a particular Bf (the only MHC class I gene in chickens) allele are fully protected from Rous virus-induced sarcomas, because this allele (B-f12) can bind several antigenic peptides from its proteins. On the contrary, chickens homozygous for B-f4 are killed by the same infection, because this allele cannot bind peptides from sarcoma virus proteins.[54]

HLA polymorphism is the basis of alloimmunization because most individuals are likely to have different HLA molecules on the surface of their cells. Hundreds of HLA alleles have been identified through high-resolution typing, making the chances of two individuals having identical HLA phenotypes extremely low. Thus partial mismatches are commonly accepted in transplantation cases and are at the root of hyperacute, acute, and chronic rejections. Hyperacute rejection is caused by preformed antibodies against donor HLA alleles in patients presensitized by multiple transfusions.[61] Acute and chronic rejection result from a combination of humoral and cellular immune reactivity toward HLA alleles of the donor.[62,63] In addition to allosensitization, HLA alleles can mediate GVHD whereby hematopoietic cells derived from the grafted tissue recognize and reject the host tissues. They do this by identifying polymorphisms of intracellular proteins of the host [minor histocompatibility antigens (mHags)] presented in association with donor-recipient matched HLA alleles.

NONCLASSIC MHC AND MHC CLASS I CHAIN-RELATED MOLECULES

Besides the three ubiquitously expressed highly polymorphic classic HLA class I molecules, humans encode three relatively conserved nonclassic, selectively expressed (HLA-E, HLA-F, and HLA-G) MHC class I genes (also known as MHC-Ib). These evolved at different rates in primates reflecting differential involvement in the modulation of immune responses.[4,64,65] In addition, these molecules are characterized by unique patterns of transcription, protein structure, and immunologic function.[66]

The MHC class I-related chain genes (MICA and MICB) are located within the MHC region and are characterized by high polymorphism (more than 50 alleles so far identified).[67] The molecules encoded by these genes do not appear to bind peptides or associate with β_2-microglobulin. Their polymorphic variants are not concentrated around the peptide-binding groove, yet they seem to have functional significance, because most mutations are nonsynonymous, suggesting selective pressure as a driving force. Their tissue distribution is restricted to epithelial and endothelial cells and fibroblasts. It appears that MIC genes modulate the function of NK and CD8+ T cells by binding the NKG2D stimulating receptor.[68] Also, MIC genes have been implicated in transplant rejection because alloantibodies against them are often found in transplant recipients that may exert complement-mediated cytotoxicity against endothelial cells from the graft.

Other unusual MHC-like molecules are present in the genome and have disparate functions, including presentation of lipid antigens (CD1), transport of immunoglobulins (Fc receptor), and regulation of iron metabolism (hemochromatosis gene product).[69] Contrary to classic MHC class I genes that are constitutively expressed, nonclassic MHC and MIC gene expression is dependent on stimulation by proinflammatory cytokines.[70] In addition, two nonclassic MHC class II proteins (HLA-DM and HLA-DO) have been described as mediators of peptide exchange by stabilizing empty MHC class II molecules.[37] Finally, it is possible that several nonclassic MHC molecules whose function is to present peptides to lymphocytes may be present throughout the genome. Because of their limited polymorphism, however, these genes may have evolved to serve specialized presentation functions.[71]

Characterized by low polymorphism, the regulation of HLA-G expression follows a nonclassic behavior. Aberrant cytokine-responsive regulatory sequences may be responsible for its predominant expression by trophoblasts that do not express other HLA proteins.[72-75] It may also account for its low levels in a variety of human tissues.[76] Lack of responsiveness to common immunostimulatory pathways (NF-κB, interferon-γ, or CIITA) is most pronounced in HLA-G cells and is shared by other nonclassic MHC such as HLA-E.[77] Also, HLA-G is expressed in a variety of cancers.[72] It is hard to know what the relevance of HLA-G expression is, because it can occur in various membrane-bound or soluble isoforms with distinct functional characteristics.[72] Functional isoforms that include the α-1 and α-2 domains bind and present peptides from cytoplasmic proteins.[78] Because of the minimal polymorphism, however, the repertoire of peptides presented is likely to be limited, suggesting that peptide binding is necessary to stabilize the molecule rather than being involved in antigen presentation.

Functionally, HLA-G is thought to modulate the function of NK cells through interactions with their inhibitory receptors.[79] In addition, the HLA-G leader sequence contains a peptide that can bind and stabilize the expression of HLA-E, which, in turn, inhibits NK cells.[80] Because the HLA-G–derived leader peptide has the strongest affinity for HLA-E (among all HLA class I molecules), it is likely that HLA-G is a powerful direct and indirect inhibitor of NK cells, reducing the risk for cardiac rejection or inducing immune escape of cancer cells.[72,81] Although much has been published about the immunoregulatory role of HLA-G, its true function remains unknown, principally because of discordant findings reported by various groups.[74] With the goal of achieving consensus, a workshop was recently organized to standardize methods of analysis of HLA-G.[66]

HLA-E is minimally polymorphic,[4] binds hydrophobic peptides from other HLA class I leader sequences, and interacts with CD94/NKG2 lectin-like receptors present predominately on NK and partially on CD8+ T cells.[82-85] The peptide binding is highly specific and stabilizes the HLA-E protein, allowing its migration to the cell surface. Thus surface density of HLA-E is an indirect reflection of the number of HLA class I alleles expressed by a cell.[86] The interaction of HLA-E with CD94/NKG2 protects HLA-E–expressing cells from killing. Cells damaged by viral infection or neoplastic degeneration may lose HLA class I expression. As a backup mechanism of protection, reduced HLA class I expression results in decreased expression of HLA-E, leading to vulnerability to NK cells.[87] Some viruses express mimic peptides that bind and stabilize HLA-E so that, although classic MHC molecules are downregulated, HLA-E expression is maintained, allowing the pathogen to simultaneously escape CD8+ T- and NK-cell killing.[88]

The function of HLA-F remains enigmatic. Its transcriptional regulation is closest to classic HLA molecules in that it can be induced by NF-κB, interferon regulatory factor-1, and class II trans-activator.[89] However, contrary to classic HLA molecules, HLA-F is predominantly empty, mostly intracellular, with a restricted pattern of expression.[90] Its tissue distribution appears to be limited to B cells, therefore it is mostly found in lymphatic organs.[90] Structural studies suggest that HLA-F is a peptide-binding molecule and may reach the cell surface under favorable conditions when a suitable peptide is present.[91] Once on the cell surface, HLA-F may interact with the effector-cell receptors IL-T2 and IL-T4, as suggested by HLA-F tetrameric complexes-binding studies.[91] Thus it is possible that in specific yet unknown conditions, HLA-F may modulate the function of immune effector cells similarly to HLA-E and HLA-G.

NON-HUMAN LEUKOCYTE ANTIGEN POLYMORPHISM AND ITS CLINICAL SIGNIFICANCE

Although this chapter is dedicated to HLA, it would be incomplete without mentioning the increasingly recognized polymorphisms of other immune modulators. The significance of non-HLA polymorphism is evidenced by the development of GVHD in the presence of HLA identical matching among relatives. As recently summarized,[92] three general areas of polymorphism are being investigated: NK cell-receptor genes, mHags, and cytokines. Over the last decade, much progress has been made in identifying the mechanisms of action of NK cells. A major breakthrough was made in the discovery of HLA class I-specific inhibitory receptors and in the role they play in the regulation of NK function with consequent effects on the eradication of hematologic malignancies, prevention of graft rejection, or induction of GVHD.[93] NK cells recognize HLA molecules via killer immunoglobulin-like receptors (KIRs). The regulation of NK cell function by KIRs is further discussed in Chapter 22. KIRs are glycoproteins encoded by at least 17 different genes located on chromosome 19q13.4.[94] All human KIR genes derive from a gene encoding three immunoglobulin (Ig)-like domains (D0, D1, and D2) and a long cytoplasmic tail. However, the KIRs genes are diverse and may encode either two or three Ig-like domains and either a long or short cytoplasmic tail (Table 113.1). The long cytoplasmic tails contain one or two immunoreceptor tyrosine-based inhibition motifs.[95] Although KIR molecules with long cytoplasmic tails inhibit NK cytotoxicity, those with short tails do not. The names given to KIR genes are based on the molecule that they encode. The first digit corresponds to the number of Ig-like domains in the molecule and a *D* denotes domain. The D is followed by either an *L* for long cytoplasmic tail or *S* for short cytoplasmic tail or *p* for a pseudogene. The last digit indicates the number of the KIR gene.[96]

Expression of KIR in individual NK cells is complex because NK cells may express several members of the KIR family. The number of KIR genes in each haplotype varies among individuals. The most common haplotype is known as group A, and is made up of six genes (2DL1, 2DL2 or 2DL3, 3DL1, 3DL2, 2DS4, and 2DL4). Various KIR genes can recognize different HLA-A, HLA-B, and HLA-C molecules. HLA-C antigens can be divided into two groups based on polymorphisms at amino acid positions 77 and 80 of their class I heavy chains. One group has asparagine (Asn) at position 77 and lysine (Lys) at 80 and the other has serine (Ser) at 77 and Asn at 80. Some KIRs recognize HLA-C antigens with Asn 77 and Lys 80, whereas other KIRs recognize HLA-C antigens with Ser 77 and Lys 80. The polymorphism at position 80 is most important. Another group of KIR reacts with HLA-B antigens that carry specific combinations of amino acids at positions 77 and 83 of the heavy chain that

forms HLA-Bw4. Because a single KIR can interact with multiple HLA class I alleles, KIR recognition of HLA class I molecules is degenerate. Another NK inhibitory receptor (CD94-NKG2A) recognizes the nonclassic HLA-E molecule. In addition, each of the KIR genes is extensively polymorphic.

Because the genes for KIR, HLA, and CD94-NKG2A are located in separate chromosomes, they segregate independently and consequently individuals can carry genes for KIR for which there is no correspondent HLA ligand.[97] As HLA-E is expressed in all individuals, NK cells that bear the CD94-NKG2A receptor are not alloreactive. Because the specificity of KIR for their ligands is broad and each individual carries several KIRs, it is likely that in most cases all NK cells of a given person express at least one KIR that is specific for a self-HLA class I allele. Thus in autologous settings, NK cells kill only aberrant cells that have lost HLA class I expression. By contrast, NK cells can kill allogeneic cells that do not express HLA class I alleles recognized by their KIR. Thus, by knowing the KIR repertoire of a given transplant recipient and the HLA type of the donor, it would theoretically be possible to predict the likelihood of an NK-mediated alloreaction. Importantly, it appears that alloreactive NK cells undergo proliferation on exposure to the stimulatory cells and therefore can preferentially expand in the presence of allogeneic tissue. NK cells also express activating receptors that are responsible for their lytic activity. Although the identity of the ligands for these receptors has not been identified, it is possible that they are expressed primarily by activated or proliferating cells. It is therefore possible that during the inflammatory process induced in allogeneic conditions, normal cells can become activated by cytokines and express ligands, which are responsible for NK activation in the absence of HLA class I molecules reactive with the inhibitory receptors.[93] The relevance of KIR in transplantation has been well studied in the context of haploidentical hematopoietic transplantation. In this case, several combinations are possible: NK cells from the graft express KIRs that do not interact with the donor's HLA (graft-versus-host alloreactivity). It seems that the presence of graft-versus-host reactive NK cells associated with incompatibilities between donor and recipient (especially HLA-C families) has favorable effects on the outcome of acute myeloid leukemia.[98] Alternatively, a good match may be present between graft NK and host HLA as well as between host NK and graft HLA. In such a case, no alloreactivity occurs. Finally, the graft's HLA type may be unsuitable for the host's NK repertoire, and the host's reactivity may lead to graft rejection. Alloreactive grafted NK cells seem to prevent GVHD while inducing GVN.[93]

Like HLA, KIR genes are polymorphic, and their variability is clustered in positions likely to affect the overall structure of the molecule. The relevance of KIR gene polymorphism in the outcome of hematopoietic stem cell transplantation (HSCT) is unclear. It appears that the risk for GVHD is highest in the context of unrelated HSCT when the recipient KIR genotype is included in the donor KIR genotype.[99] These results show that compatibility between KIR genotypes themselves may influence the outcome of HSCT.

The mHags are represented by polymorphic molecules whose peptides containing variant sequences are presented by HLA alleles. They have been shown to be targets of cytotoxic T cells, which can lyse leukemia cells.[98,100] In addition, some mHags are selectively expressed by neoplastic cells.[101] At present, little is known about the identity of mHag epitopes in the context of various HLA types and their significance in the development of GVHD and GVN.

Cytokines are another large family of molecules associated with antigen recognition, graft rejection, and GVHD. Their polymorphism is becoming an important area of investigation in the context of transplantation, autoimmunity, and cancer.[102] Polymorphic sites reside in regulatory regions so that genetic variants are associated with high or low production of a given cytokine rather than differences in its function. A Web site compiles information about cytokine polymorphism (www.bris.ac.uk/Depts/PathAndMicro/services/GAI/cytokine4.htm). Although no consensus has been achieved yet, several studies have shown associations between various cytokine genotypes and propensity toward disease and transplant outcome. These studies have been summarized elsewhere.[92,103] A strong

TABLE 113.1	HLA Class I Alleles Recognized by Different Killer Immunoglobulin-Like Receptors	
KIR	**HLA Class I Allele**	**Amino Acid Sequence Motif**
P58.1 (KIR2DL1)	HLA-C2, HLA-C4, HLA-C5, HLA-C6	Asn 77, Lys 80
P58.2 (KIR2DL2/3)	HLA-C1, HLA-C3, HLA-C7, HLA-C8	Ser 77, Asn 80
P70 (KIR3DL1)	HLA-Bw4 public specificity	Aa 77-83
P140 (KIR3DL2)	HLA-A3, HLA-A11	
(KIR2DL4)	HLA-G	

Aa, Amino acid; Asn, asparagine; HLA, human leukocyte antigen; KIR, killer immunoglobulin-like receptor; Lys, lysine; Ser, serine.

association was recently noted between a low IL-10 producer genotype and a tendency to develop melanoma and prostate cancer.[104,105]

HUMAN LEUKOCYTE ANTIGEN NOMENCLATURE

The history of the HLA system nomenclature was summarized by Sir Walter Bodmer who, together with Ruggero Ceppellini, was primarily involved in its development.[106] It began as HL-A, for *human leukocyte locus A*. With the recognition that HLA molecules are encoded by more than one locus, the A came to stand for *antigen* and a locus designation was added after HLA (i.e., HLA-A, HLA-B, HLA-C, HLA-D, etc.).[2] From then on, the WHO has updated nomenclature on a quarterly basis. The most recent update was assigned in January 2015, as seen in Table 113.2.[4] At present, two systems are used. An immunologically defined nomenclature is based on the identification of HLA antigens on the surface of leukocytes. Therefore HLA phenotypes described by immunologic methods are

conventionally called *HLA antigens*.[107] The second system is based on the molecular identification of nucleotide sequences in genomic deoxyribonucleic acid (DNA), and results are conventionally referred to as *HLA alleles*. Because molecular typing has higher resolution, it has gained increasing popularity.

IMMUNOLOGICALLY DEFINED HUMAN LEUKOCYTE ANTIGEN NOMENCLATURE

Immunologically defined nomenclature follows this rule: HLA separated by a hyphen from a capital letter identifying the locus encoding distinct HLA class I (-A, -B, -C) or class II (-DR, -DQ, -DP) antigens. The letter is followed by a number that identifies a serologic family of alleles sharing epitopes recognized by alloantibodies or alloreactive cytotoxic T cells. With improved understanding of the molecular genetics of the HLA region, various appendages have been removed from the HLA nomenclature. For instance, the letter *w* was used to

TABLE 113.2	Name of Genes in the HLA Region Considered by the WHO Nomenclature Committee		
Name	**Previous Equivalents**	**Molecular Characteristics**	**No. of Alleles January (2015)**
HLA-A	–	Class I α-chain	3107
HLA-B	–	Class I α-chain	3887
HLA-C	–	Class I α-chain	2623
HLA-E	E, "6.2"	Associated with class I 6.2-kBa Hind III fragment	17
HLA-F	F, "5.4"	Associated with class I 5.4-kBa Hind III fragment	22
HLA-G	G, "6.0"	Associated with class I 6.0-kBa Hind III fragment	50
HLA-H	H, AR, "12.4", HLA-54	Pseudogene association with class I 5.4-kBa Hind III fragment	12
HLA-J	cda 12, HLA-59	Pseudogene association with class I 5.9-kBa Hind III fragment	9
HLA-K	HLA-70	Pseudogene association with class I 7.0-kBa Hind III fragment	6
HLA-L	HLA-92	Pseudogene association with class I 9.2-kBa Hind III fragment	5
HLA-X	–	Class I gene fragment	0
HLA-DRA	DRα	DR α-chain	7
HLA-DRB1	DRβI, DR1B	DR β₁ determining specificity for DR1, DR2, DR3, etc.	1726
HLA-DRB2	DRβII2	Pseudogene with DRβ-like sequence	1
HLA-DRB3	DRβIII, DR3B	DR β3 determining DR52, Dw24, w25, -26 specificity	59
HLA-DRB4	DRβIV, DR4B	DR β4 determining DR53 specificity	15
HLA-DRB5	DRβV, DR5B	DR β5 determining DR52, Dw24, w25, -26 specificity	21
HLA-DRB6	DRBX, DRBσ	Pseudogene found in DR1, DR2, and DR10 haplotypes	3
HLA-DRB7	DRBψ1	Pseudogene found in DR4, DR7, and DR9 haplotypes	2
HLA-DRB8	DRBψ2	Pseudogene found in DR4, DR7, and DR9 haplotypes	1
HLA-DRB9	M 4.2 β exon	Pseudogene isolated fragment	1
HLA-DQA1	DQα1, DQ1A	DQ α-chain as expressed	54
HLA-DQB1	DQβ1, DQ1B	DQ β-chain as expressed	780
HLA-DOA	DNA, DZα, DOα	DO α-chain	12
HLA-DOB	DOβ	DO β-chain	13
HLA-DMA	RING 6	DM α-chain	7
HLA-DMB	RING 7	DM β-chain	13
HLA-DPA1	DPα1, DP1A	DP α-chain as expressed	33
HLA-DPB1	DPβ1, DP1B	DP β-chain as expressed	520
TAP1	ABCB2, RING4	ABC (ATP-binding cassette) transporter	12
TAP2	ABCB3, RING 11	ABC (ATP-binding cassette) transporter	12
MICA	PERB 11.1	Class I chain-related gene	101
MICB	PERB 11.2	Class I chain-related gene 18	41

ATP, Adenosine triphosphate; HLA, human leukocyte antigen; WHO, World Health Organization.
Data from Marsh SGE, Albert AD, Bodmer WF, et al: Nomenclature for factors of the HLA system, 2010. *Tissue Antigens* 75:291, 2010.

indicate a provisional assignment, and this has been discontinued, but it is occasionally added to HLA-C antigen nomenclature to distinguish it from complement genes; DP and DW also maintained this letter to reinforce the dependency of their immune identification predominantly through cellular techniques. Finally, HLA-Bw4 and HLA-Bw6 retain the *w* to emphasize that the public epitopes are shared by several HLA-B and some HLA-A antigens. More recently, a bridge between immunologic and molecular nomenclature has been proposed whereby HLA antigens that encompass a single gene product can be assigned a two-digit numeric extension corresponding to the molecular nomenclature for that allele.[108]

SEQUENCE-DEFINED ALLELIC NOMENCLATURE

The 10th International Histocompatibility Workshop recommended in 1987 a sequence-based nomenclature to describe alleles not distinguishable by immunologic methods.[108] Since then, the number of HLA alleles has rapidly increased. As of January 2015, a total of 13,023 alleles for HLA exist. This is a drastic increase from the original numbers established in 2003. Other designations are summarized in Table 113.2. HLA designates molecules belonging to the human MHC followed by the locus (-A, -B, etc.). Alleles are then identified after an asterisk (*). Each HLA allele name has a unique number corresponding to up to four sets of digits separated by colons. The length of the allele designation is dependent on the sequence of the allele and that of its nearest relative. All alleles receive at least a four digit name that corresponds to the first two sets of digits, longer names are only assigned when necessary. The digits before the first colon describe the type, which often corresponds to the serologic antigen carried by an allotype. The next set of digits are used to list the subtypes, numbers being assigned in the order that the DNA sequences have been determined. Alleles whose numbers differ in the two sets of digits must differ in one or more nucleotide substitutions that change the amino acid sequence of the encoded protein. Alleles that differ only by synonymous nucleotide substitutions (also called silent or noncoding substitutions) within the coding sequence are distinguished by the use of the third set of digits. Alleles that only differ by sequence polymorphisms in the introns or in the 5′ or 3′ untranslated regions that flank the exons and introns are distinguished by the use of the fourth set of digits.[109] A four-digit number is used when the first two digits refer to the original serologic family (e.g., HLA-A2 serologically would be HLA-A*02). Often numbers are missing because an original assignment was revoked (e.g., this is why there is no HLA-A*24:01). When silent mutations are identified (variation in nucleotide sequence that does not translate into changes in amino acid sequence), the name of the allele remains identical, but another two digits are added to designate a variant that has no functional significance. New sequences are submitted to European Molecular Biology Laboratory (EMBL; www.ebi.ac.uk/Submissions/index.html), GenBank (www.ncbi.nlm.nih.gov/Genbank/index.html), or DNA Data Bank of Japan (DDBJ; http://www.ddbj.nig.ac.jp/submission-e.html).

Requirements for new allele naming were described by Marsh et al.[4] The WHO committee also made recommendations about naming alleles with aberrant expression such as HLA-G isoforms and KIR. Some alleles are identifiable at the genomic level but are not translated into protein (pseudogenes). These are indicated by the addition of an *N* (for null) following the numerical designation of the allele. Mutations inducing a reduction of expression are marked by *L* (low expression). An *S* denotes alleles expressed as soluble secreted molecules, such as HLA-B*44:02:01:02S characterized by an intronic variant that disallows the expression of the transmembrane domain of the HLA molecule and is therefore only in soluble form. Differential splicing of HLA-G leads to production of membrane-bound and soluble forms, which are respectively denoted by a lowercase *m* or *s* before HLA. Limited cytoplasmic expression is denoted by *C* and aberrant expression by *A*. Finally, KIR polymorphism will be classified by a new system that is in preparation.[4,97,110] A nomenclature system for cytokine polymorphism has not yet been developed.[111]

HUMAN LEUKOCYTE ANTIGEN TYPING IN CLINICAL HEMATOLOGY AND DETERMINATION OF COMPATIBILITY HLA TYPING

Originally HLA typing was done primarily in support of transplantation or transfusion needs with the purpose of identifying histocompatibility through the best match between donor and recipient. Allosensitization of recipients previously exposed to heterologous cell products is tested by identifying alloreactive antibodies in serum, and crossmatch procedures are performed to grade compatibility of candidate donor-recipient pairs. In addition, HLA testing has been applied to identify links between a given disease and the genetic makeup of its carriers.[112] Strong associations are exemplified by birdshot uveitis (a disease occurring exclusively in HLA-A29 individuals),[113] type 1 diabetes and other autoimmune diseases,[114–116] or long-term survival of HIV-infected individuals.[55] These studies evaluated the role that genetic background may have contributed over environmental factors.[112,117] HLA associations are thought to be caused by the differential ability of distinct alleles to present immunogenic epitopes[113,115] or by the close linkage to the HLA class III region where potent immunomodulators such as tumor necrosis factor-α are located.[118] It has also been suggested that HLA associations may be predictors of immune responsiveness of cancer to immune therapy.[60] However, such associations have remained quite difficult to reproduce.[119] HLA typing is requested for enrollment of patients into and interpretation of immunization protocols,[24] because specific HLA-epitope combinations require high-resolution typing.[22,120]

Serologic testing takes advantage of fetomaternal sensitization. In mammals, the progeny carries a full haplotype of paternal origin, and pregnant women may develop antibodies against the paternal haplotype. Maternal serum samples are collected at term and characterized by testing their ability to kill HLA-bearing repository cell lines of known phenotype in the presence of complement (complement-dependent cytotoxicity [CDC]).[121] CDC is used for HLA typing by exposing circulating cells expressing HLA class I (most cells) and class II (predominantly B cells) antigens from the individual (to be typed to previously characterized sera or monoclonal antibodies).[122] Conversely, already typed repository cell lines are used in CDC to identify alloantibodies in sera of sensitized individuals. The fraction of cell lines killed by the sera roughly grades the intensity of allosensitization or panel reactive antibody (PRA) reactivity. Some antibodies activate complement and kill with poor efficiency, known as the *cytotoxicity-negative absorption-positive (CYNAP) phenomenon*.[123] As judged by cytotoxicity testing, CYNAP may underestimate allosensitization. By modifying CDC with the addition of antihuman antibodies suitable for complement activation, CYNAP can be circumvented (augmented CDC). In this case, however, relatively innocuous antibodies can cause overestimation of clinically relevant allosensitization.[124]

Other methods identify alloantibodies, including immobilization of HLA molecules on solid surface to capture soluble antibodies and flow cytometry using a spectrum of microbeads loaded with known HLA alleles.[125–129] An interlaboratory comparison of serum screening for HLA-antibody determination suggested that enzyme-linked immunosorbent assay and flow cytometry yield higher PRA activity values compared with CDC or augmented CDC.[125,127] However, the study suggested a lack of consistency among participant laboratories, leaving the question of which method most accurately defines clinically relevant allosensitization unsolved, and a panel of various methods may be most informative.[72]

CDC is declining in interest in the United States because most laboratories are switching to easier-to-handle and higher-resolution molecular methods. However, immunologic methods remain valuable to characterize functional aspects of HLA because molecular methods cannot define whether an HLA allele is expressed nor, at least until recently,[130] grade allosensitization. Thus it is likely that immunologic methods will continue to complement molecular methods in the future.[130]

The usefulness of conventional serologic typing of HLA antigens has been limited by the availability of allele-specific sera. Most important, because antibodies identify structural differences on the surface of HLA molecules, variants caused by nucleotide polymorphism in nonexposed areas such as the peptide-binding groove of the HLA heavy chain are not detectable. However, these differences are of functional significance because they determine the specificity and affinity of peptide binding and T-cell recognition of self and allogeneic target cells.[23,131-133] DNA-based typing directly determines the sequence,[134] and its resolution is limited only by the number of allele-specific probes used to identify an ever-growing number of alleles (see www.anthonynolan.com/HIG/index.htm). Various polymerase chain reaction (PCR)-based methods have been described, among which sequence-specific primer and sequence-specific oligonucleotide probe-based methods are the most universally used.[134-137] The rich nature of HLA has led to proportionally increasing complexity of the assays used to cover all possible alleles. As a consequence, accurate HLA typing for donor and recipient matching in transplantation has become increasingly complex and burdensome. In addition, because of the important role that HLA molecules play in antigen presentation and the stringency of the relationship between epitope and associated HLA allele, high-resolution typing is increasingly requested for appropriate enrollment of patients into immunization protocols aimed at the enhancement of T-cell responses.[138] Therefore high-resolution HLA typing is increasingly in demand in clinical and experimental settings.

Although oligonucleotide-based methods could theoretically discriminate any known polymorphic site, they have two major limitations. First, they require a specific PCR reaction for each allele investigated. Because each individual has only two alleles for each locus, a disproportionately large number of PCR reactions must be performed to cover all possible polymorphisms to identify the two borne by the individual tested. Because both methods are based on specific interactions with known oligonucleotide sequences unique to a particular allele, they cannot identify unknown polymorphisms unless the variation occurs within the region spanned by one of the oligonucleotides used in the assay. Because of these limitations, interest is growing for definitive typing methods that yield conclusive information about the identity of the alleles typed. The most comprehensive method is sequence-based typing. Unfortunately, its use has been limited by the cost of equipment and reagents and by the high level of expertise and time required for the interpretation of each typing. More recently, high-throughput, robotic, sequence-based typing has been developed that allows sequencing of hundreds of genomic fragments each day.[139-141] However, even sequence-based typing has some technical limitations. Some combinations of HLA class I and class II

alleles result in ambiguous allele combinations that require additional testing for resolution.[142] Finally, new methods based on high-density array technology are being developed that may allow extensive typing of known and unknown polymorphisms on microchips.[143,144]

High-resolution methods yield high-resolution information of an individual's HLA type. However, the wealth of information is counterbalanced by increased difficulty in identifying suitable HLA alleles during donor-recipient pairing or accrual into immunization protocols restricted to specific HLA-epitope combinations. Thus, at present, clinicians are faced with the daunting task of applying high-resolution typing results of unclear relevance to clinical settings.[145]

TESTING FOR ALLOSENSITIZATION AND DETERMINATION OF COMPATIBLE RECIPIENT-DONOR PAIRS

Any cell-containing product transfused or transplanted between different individuals should be compatible in an ideal situation. Yet, in most cases, histocompatibility is not prospectively sought. Thus patients with multiple exposures to blood products often become reactive to various antigens, including HLA. Transplant candidates often develop prior alloreactivity following transfusion of platelet concentrates contaminated with leukocytes, even though the incidence of allosensitization is much less because of leukodepletion of blood products. Alloreactivity must be documented before transplantation, because alloreactive patients can still undergo transplantation, provided that the donor has no mismatched HLA antigens reacting with the patient's antibodies. Patients who have received repeated platelet transfusions may become allosensitized and consequently refractory to further transfusions unless HLA-compatible platelets are used. Obviously the best compatibility consists of identical matching. It is often impossible to identify a perfectly matched unrelated donor, particularly in the case of rare HLA types. Thus other strategies are adopted to identify the best possible match or compatible mismatch. Selection of unrelated donor-recipient pairs is carried out through typing with serologic, cellular, and molecular methods.[146] The chances of identifying compatible donors based on full or partial HLA matching have become increasingly low with the increasing resolution of the typing methods.[145] To broaden compatibility, matching criteria of donor-recipient pairs are based on shared public epitopes assigned to cross-reactive groups (CREGs)[147] or shared amino acid polymorphisms defined through sequence information (Table 113.3).[148] The

TABLE 113.3	Population Frequencies of Major Cross Reactive or Determinants Present on HLA-A and HLA-B Gene Products		
Major Cross-Reactive Group	Public Epitope	Associated Private Epitopes	Approximate Epitope Frequency (%)[a]
1C	1p	A1, 3, 9 (23, 24), 11, 29, 30, 31, 36, 80	79
	10p	A10 (25, 26, 34, 43, 66), 11, 28 (68, 69), 32, 33, 74	
2C	28p	A2, 28 (68, 69), 9, 17	70
	9p	A2, 28 (68, 69), 9 (23, 24)	
	17p	A2, B17 (57, 58)	
5C	5p	B5 (51, 52), 18, 35, 53, 78	50
	21p	B5 (51, 52), 15 (62, 63, 75, 76, 77), 17 (57, 58), 21 (49, 50), 35, 53, 70 (71, 72), 73, 74, 78	
7C	7p	B7, 8, 41, 42, 48, 81	54
	22p	B7, 22 (54, 55, 56), 27, 42, 46	
	27p	B7, 13, 27, 40 (60, 61), 47	
8C	8p	B8, 14 (64, 65), 16 (38, 39), 18	38
12C	12p	B12 (44, 45), 13, 21 (49, 50), 40 (60, 61), 41	44
Bw4	Bw4	B13, 27, 37, 38, 47, 49, 51, 52, 53, 57, 58, 59, 63, 77, A24, 25, 32	79
Bw6	Bw6	B7, 8, 18, 35, 39, 41, 42, 45, 46, 48, 50, 54, 55, 56, 60, 61, 62, 64, 65, 67, 71, 72, 73, 75, 76, 78, 81	87

[a]North American white populations of European origin.

preexistence of alloantibodies restricts the identification of compatible donors even further. Highly sensitized recipients with PRA activity exceeding 85% of tested specificities (generally between 30% and 60%) represent a particularly challenging group.[149] An alternative approach to the exclusion of alloreactive determinants is the inclusion of acceptable antigen mismatches expressed in a panel of cells that give negative reactions with the recipient sera,[150] which extends the repertoire of possible donors. All these are fundamental tools for the identification of nonrelated, not fully matched donor-recipient pairs. Unfortunately, even these compromises often fail to identify a suitable match.

Duquesnoy[149] described a molecularly based algorithm to identify histocompatible pairs called *HLAMatchmaker*. This method focuses on the structural basis of HLA class I polymorphism so that compatible HLA mismatches can be identified without extensive serum screening. This algorithm is based on the principle that short amino acid sequences (triplets) characterizing polymorphic sites of the HLA molecules are critical components of allosensitizing epitopes. Such amino acids reside in the α-helices and β-loops of the heavy chain. Because each HLA molecule expresses a characteristic string of these determinants, it is possible to characterize each molecule according to the linear sequence of amino acid triplets present on its surface. Based on the reasonable assumption that none of the triplets present in the HLA repertoire of the recipient is self-immunogenic, it is possible through a process of electronic recombination to identify donors with HLA alleles different from the recipient's but containing exclusively shared triplets. These HLA alleles will be compatible, because they do not contain any epitope absent in the recipient.

In theory, a large number of triplets could occur if polymorphisms were randomly distributed. However, most HLA molecules span conserved domains, and only a total of 142 different polymorphic triplets designate serologically defined HLA-A, HLA-B, and HLA-C antigens.[149] Triplet polymorphism can occur in 30 locations on HLA-A, 27 in HLA-B, and 19 in HLA-C chains. Because the HLAMatchmaker algorithm includes interlocus comparison, it is possible to accumulate the information into a single database. Among the 142 polymorphic triplets, 29 are polymorphic for one class I locus but monomorphic for another class I locus. Such polymorphic triplets cannot be immunogenic because they are always present on the patient's own HLA antigens, whereas the remaining 113 triplets have immunogenic potential. With this algorithm, it is possible to significantly broaden the number of molecularly matched HLA alleles and significantly increase the chances of identifying a compatible donor, particularly in those cases in which the recipient has a rare HLA phenotype. In addition, HLAMatchmaker considers triplets that are present in the panel cells that give negative reactions with the recipient's serum. These negative panel cells can be expected to share antigens with the patient's, but other HLA antigens may be present and contain mismatched triplets apparently not immunogenic for that patient. Such triplets are therefore acceptable and can be added to the algorithm for the identification of possible donors. Thus HLAMatchmaker assesses HLA compatibility at a molecular level by determining whether or not a triplet in a given position of a mismatched HLA antigen is also found in the same position in any of the recipient's own HLA-A, HLA-B, and HLA-C molecules. A shared triplet in the same position on a mismatched HLA antigen cannot elicit a specific antibody response in that patient. Preliminary verification of the algorithm in a series of high-PRA renal patients suggested that this is a proper strategy at least in highly sensitized renal transplantation candidates waiting for unrelated donors.[150,151] HLAMatchmaker is also effective at selecting an optimal HLA-typed platelet component for alloimmunized thrombocytopenic patients.[152]

A new version of HLAMatchmaker considers so-called *eplets* and is based on the structural definitions of functional epitopes on well-characterized protein antigens that have been complexed with an antibody.[153] Eplets represent amino acid residue configurations within a 3- to 3.5-Å radius of each polymorphic residue on the HLA molecular surface. Many eplets correspond to triplets, but eplets represents a more complete repertoire of structurally defined epitopes.

THE HUMAN LEUKOCYTE ANTIGEN MOLECULES AS ANTIGENS AND HLA ALLOIMMUNIZATION

By no means are HLA molecules antigenic in physiologic condition (with the exception of maternofetal alloimmunization). However, because of their high density on the surface of cells, they can become highly immunogenic in the nonphysiologic event in which cells from different individuals are exposed to another person's immune system. The mechanism or mechanisms leading to allosensitization are believed to follow two pathways. The first pathway mimics the one followed during most immune reactions in which antigen is up-taken by antigen-presenting cells and presented to autologous lymphocytes (indirect pathway). In this case the donor's HLA molecules are processed into peptides through the exogenous pathway of antigen presentation and presented to autologous T cells as linear peptides.[154,155] This pathway is believed to be responsible for the development of alloantibodies as well as T-helper cell responses, but its role in the development of cytotoxic T-cell responses remains unclear. Because this pathway depends on the presentation of donor HLA molecules by recipient HLA alleles, it may explain why the humoral response to HLA class I allodeterminants correlates with the HLA phenotype of the responder.[156] The indirect pathway of HLA allorecognition has been associated with allograft rejection.[157] Because the function of HLA molecules is to present antigenic determinants to T cells, it could be easily envisioned how minor changes in their structure could be misinterpreted as antigenic epitopes. Intact HLA molecules residing on the surface of donor cells are a perfect target for T cell-mediated allorecognition (direct pathway) either through the direct cytotoxic effect of T cells against target cells or by the activation of helper T cells through HLA class II engagement, leading to stimulation of antibody-mediated immune responses.[158]

Humoral responses mediated most frequently by IgM are predominant in the sensitization to infrequent allogeneic exposure because they require smaller amounts of antigenic material. T-cell responses become more manifest in the context of transplantation in which the persistence of the allogeneic stimulus allows the expansion and sustenance of alloreactive cytotoxic T cells. Antibodies and TCR have different requirements for their engagement, which means epitopes recognized by T cells and antibodies are different. Antibodies require interaction with a small structure, including a limited number of amino acids; thus any sequence combination on the surface of an HLA allele not present in the individual exposed to the alloreaction may represent an epitope. T cells have much lower binding affinity for their ligand and require a complete interaction with the peptide as well as the α- and β-helices of the HLA class I heavy chain.[11] Although several B-cell epitopes recognized by antibodies can be identified in a given HLA molecule, generally the whole HLA molecule is necessary for T cell-dependent allorecognition. Definition and topographic mapping of epitopes defined by serologic or cellular methods has revealed distinct regions of hypervariability in the α-1 and α-2 domains of the class I heavy chains and in the α-1 and β-1 domains of class II molecules.[159] Two types of antibody-defined epitopes can be identified according to their frequency among HLA alleles. Private epitopes are almost, but not totally unique for a single serologically defined HLA antigen and are used for typing. These epitopes are generally shared by all molecular alleles present in that given family, and fine differences among alleles within a general family cannot be distinguished by antibodies. Public epitopes are more widely distributed and cluster distinct serologic families into groups. These epitopes bear an immunodominant character. Immune sera that identify public epitopes have been considered predictive of major CREGs with the idea that alloreactivity among patients belonging to the same CREG may be less likely (Table 113.3). The predictive value of CREGs in transplant outcome or platelet transfusion results, however, remains to be demonstrated.

Not all patients who have been exposed to alloantigens develop alloantibodies, and in fact, exposure to low doses of donor-specific HLA antigens through donor transfusion may have a beneficial effect on graft survival.[160] Obviously, the degree of compatibility in the context of allosensitization may vary according to the degree of mismatch between donor and recipient. In addition, alloantibodies are one aspect of alloreaction that does not take into account cellular responses. These have been more difficult to document, although they are likely to play an important role in the context of acute transplant rejection. Several hypotheses have been discussed about the reason or reasons for the capriciousness of allosensitization, including the presence of regulatory immune responses or cytokine-mediated immunosuppression. Currently the mechanism modulating the quality and quantity of alloimmunity remains elusive, and different aspects of this algorithm are discussed ad hoc in this chapter, with particular attention to molecularly defined algorithms for the prediction of histocompatibility.[130,149,161,162]

Clearly, HLA matching is beneficial in patients undergoing renal transplantation. An analysis of more than 150,000 recipients receiving transplants in different centers participating in the Collaborative Transplant Study showed that a complete mismatch (6 HLA-A+B+DR) had a 17% lower survival expectation than no mismatch ($p < .0001$).[163] Matching was particularly beneficial in patients with highly reactive preformed alloantibodies. The same study suggested that high-resolution matching based on molecular typing improved graft survival. Similar results were observed in cases of cardiac transplantation in which HLA matching yielded significantly better results ($p < .0001$). This is particularly important because donor hearts are currently not allocated according to HLA match in most centers. In cases of liver transplantation, HLA matching was not beneficial.[164]

Donor-specific hyporesponsiveness has been particularly well documented in the context of renal allotransplantation and may limit the need for immunosuppression. A recent randomized study suggested that pretransplant donor transfusions improved the survival of cadaver kidney grafts in patients receiving modern immunosuppressive regimens, but the mechanism remains unclear.[165,166] Although most centers currently do not implement deliberate blood transfusions, the usefulness of this approach needs to be investigated further.

Approximately 5% to 10% of platelet transfusions are given to patients who have been previously exposed to HLA class I-expressing heterologous cells and are reactive to HLA antigens. Such patients are refractory to random-donor platelets and must be given HLA-matched or semi-matched platelet apheresis components.[41–44] However, a provision of HLA-matched platelets does not always improve platelet recovery and survival. Possibly, the ineffective platelet transfusion is in part caused by unrecognized HLA mismatches between the donor and recipient resulting from the low-resolution methods used for typing, thus higher resolution methods have been advocated. It is currently controversial whether or not molecularly based HLA typing confers an advantage over serologic typing, and this principle was recently questioned in the context of hematopoietic cell transplantation.[167,168]

HUMAN LEUKOCYTE ANTIGEN AS A FUNCTIONAL MEDIATOR OF GRAFT-VERSUS-HOST DISEASE AND/OR GRAFT-VERSUS-NEOPLASIA EFFECT

Allogeneic or syngeneic HSCT is used predominately for the treatment of hematologic malignancies[169–171] and other hematologic disorders such as aplastic anemia,[172] thalassemia,[173] or myelodysplastic syndrome.[174] This strategy can induce long-term disease-free survival in chronic myelogenous leukemia patients.[169,171] The objective of HSCT in cases of malignancy is to cure the patient by eradication of the neoplastic cells with myeloablative chemotherapy followed by restoration of hematopoiesis through the transplantation of normal hematopoietic stem cells derived from HLA-compatible normal donors. This strategy is characterized by the insurgence of an immune reaction toward the host's normal cells (GVHD) that is often associated and preferentially targets neoplastic cells (GVN

effect).[175–185] Both the GVHD and the GVN effect occur in the presence of a full HLA match; thus the HLA molecules are not targets of allosensitization themselves, but present polymorphic molecules expressed by the recipient's cells recognized by the grafted immune cells.

GRAFT-VERSUS-HOST DISEASE

GVHD represents the alloimmune reaction of donor lymphocytes against normal cells of the recipient. GVHD occurs predominantly in association with HSCT compared with other types of transplants because the hematopoietic transplant is enriched with immune cells. Myeloablative therapy is generally administered before transplantation and, as a consequence, in most cases prevents graft rejection. GVHD is a major complication of HSCT, and a fine balance between GVHD and graft rejection is maintained by modulating the level of posttransplantation immunosuppression.[179] In addition, other major disturbances associated with HSCT, such as overwhelming infection, leukemia, or tumor relapse, and other regimen-related morbidities are strongly influenced by the treatment of GVHD. With the advent of nonmyeloablative HSCT for the treatment of nonhematologic diseases such as solid tumors, GVHD has reached a predominant role because of its close association with GVN effect.

T-cell depletion has been advocated for the prevention of GVHD by decreasing the probability of cellular and humoral alloresponses.[186,187] This strategy decreases the occurrence of GVHD but is associated with an increased risk for graft rejection and tumor or leukemia relapse.[179] In fact, Weiden et al[188] observed that survivors of severe acute GVHD had a significantly lower incidence of tumor relapse compared with patients who did not experience GVHD. This association appeared mandatory, and it was believed that the beneficial GVN reaction was inseparable from GVHD.

The risk for GVHD increases with genetic distancing between donor and recipient. Thus recipients of transplants from HLA-identical twins have a lesser chance of developing GVHD than recipients of transplants from HLA-unrelated donors and from donors with only a partial HLA match.[189,190] Interestingly, although the genetic closeness between donor and recipient appears to decrease the risk for GVHD, it also decreases the therapeutic benefit, with increased chances of tumor relapse.

GRAFT-VERSUS-NEOPLASIA EFFECT

It was originally observed that a beneficial collateral effect of GVHD was the rejection of neoplastic cells by the donor immune system in the context of hematologic malignancies (graft-versus-leukemia effect).[183] It was rapidly recognized that the graft-versus-leukemia effect could play a powerful therapeutic role in the treatment of refractory malignant disorders, including some solid tumors (graft-versus-tumor effect).[180] Because the biology and clinical principles underlining the two effects are likely similar, for simplicity, in this chapter we coin a unifying term: *graft-versus-neoplasia effect*. Indeed, there is a perception that the GVN reaction is the most potent form of tumor immunotherapy currently in clinical use. Its mechanism of action is still poorly understood. T cells definitely play a fundamental role in the initiation and maintenance of the alloreaction toward neoplastic cells.[191] A sevenfold increase in the chance of relapse was noted in patients with chronic myelogenous leukemia who received a T cell-depleted HSCT as compared with a subset of patients who had received a T cell-depleted HSCT but did not develop GVHD.[186,187] This result suggested that GVHD is a biologic entity different from the GVN effect. In addition, on leukemia relapse, administration of donor lymphocyte infusion could reinduce clinical remission.[192] Finally, leukemia-specific CD8+ T cells have been identified in circulating lymphocytes at the time of leukemia regression.[193] NK cells play an additional role in mediating this phenomenon, and clinical data suggests that mismatch of NK receptor and ligands during allogeneic HSCT can be used to enhance the GVN effect.[93,194] Appreciation of the GVN effect has led to the development of nonmyeloablative stem cell transplants designed to immunosuppress the host to a level sufficient to permit engraftment of the donor immune cells to generate GVN without inducing the serious complications associated with myeloablation.[179] The GVN effect has gained popularity in the last decade to the point that allogeneic-based immunotherapeutic approaches have been advocated for several nonhematologic malignancies.[179] The rationale is largely based on the assumption that the immune cell repertoire capable of recognizing cancer cells in the allogeneic context is broader than in the autologous system. Donor T cells can target not only tumor-specific antigens but also allelic variants of these antigens; mHag; and, in the case of HLA-mismatched transplants, HLA antigens disparate from the donor expressed by the tumor cells.[195–197] Although there are several theories about how the GVN effect occurs, it remains unclear why allo-T cells have a better chance of targeting tumor cells in an allogeneic context as compared with the natural insurgence of antitumor immunity described for several solid tumors.

HUMAN LEUKOCYTE ANTIGEN AND T CELL-DIRECTED IMMUNIZATION

The last decade has witnessed remarkable progress in the identification and mapping of T-cell epitopes for various infectious diseases and cancer. In particular, progress was made in mapping HLA-associated epitopes for HIV, CMV, and Epstein-Barr virus.[198–201] In addition, the molecular identification of tumor-associated antigens has yielded a large number of epitopes that could be used to immunize against neoplasia.[202] A comprehensive discussion of these topics is beyond the scope of this chapter, but we address a few points framing the relevance of HLA in the context of T cell-directed immunization (viral specific T cells).

The identification of T-cell epitopes led to two major areas of clinical investigation. The first is active-specific immunization to prevent or treat ongoing infections or cancer. The second is the harvest and in vitro expansion of immunization-induced T cells for adoptive transfer. In general, active immunization has proved successful in inducing epitope-specific T cells easily detectable among circulating lymphocytes.[120,203–205] However, often the immunization-induced enhancement of T-cell function is not associated with clinical improvement. Although the reason for the clinical ineffectiveness of immunization-induced T cells is unclear, it has been postulated that they may be quantitatively or qualitatively inadequate for eradicating disease.[203,206] Therefore a second strategy is being pursued whereby the number of antigen-specific T cells is amplified in vitro for autologous or donor-derived adoptive transfer. This second strategy has met some promising success in the context of ganciclovir-resistant CMV infection,[207] Epstein-Barr virus–induced posttransplantation lymphoproliferative disorders,[208] and metastatic melanoma.[209]

Whether delivered as a primary form of therapy or to prime in vivo T cells for further ex vivo expansion, epitope-specific vaccination encounters the major limitation of a stringent requirement for HLA allelic association. Although super families of HLA alleles may share epitopes,[14,16] in practical terms, clinically relevant HLA-epitope associations are restricted to few peptide-allele combinations for a given protein.[22] Patients considered for enrollment in immunization protocols are best served by high-resolution HLA typing to exclude subtypes with unproven immunogenic potential for a given epitope. To bypass the stringent HLA requirements demanded by epitope-specific vaccination, whole-antigen delivery is suggested. This is based on the assumption that the epitope repertoire of a protein can be adjusted to distinct HLA phenotypes by a cellular process of self-selection naturally coupling peptides to HLA according to binding affinity. Although theoretically indisputable, in practice, the truth of this assumption depends on the efficiency with which individual molecules are processed and presented in association with distinct HLA alleles. Even in these settings, high-resolution typing is desirable

because it allows accurate interpretation of immunization results by allowing a comparison between the detailed genetic makeup of the individual receiving the vaccine and his or her antigen-specific immune response. It is likely that in the future HLA laboratories will receive increasing demands for high-resolution, definitive typing for appropriate patient enrollment and for subsequent interpretation of immune responses.

MONITORING IMMUNE RESPONSES WITH TETRAMERIC HUMAN LEUKOCYTE ANTIGEN-PEPTIDE COMPLEXES

A growing understanding of the molecular immunology of T-cell interactions with HLA/epitope complexes in the context of infectious disease, virally induced malignancies, and spontaneous tumors as well as interest in their treatment with T cell-directed vaccines has generated more attention to the issue of using accurate methods to quantify ex vivo the extent of antigen-specific immune responses.[210] The most commonly used assays available for the enumeration of antigen-specific T cells include tHLA; intracellular fluorescence-activated cell sorter staining for cytokine expression on cognate stimulation; detection of cytokine release by enzyme-linked immunospot assay; and quantitative real-time PCR, recently reviewed by Keilholz et al.[211] tHLAs are complexes of four HLA molecules combined with a specific peptide and bound to a fluorochrome (Fig. 113.6). These complexes bind to complementary TCR and identify antigen-specific T cells,[212] measuring cellular responses against specific epitopes with sensitivity as low as 1 in 5000 CD8+ T cells. To synthesize tHLA molecules, soluble HLA heavy chains containing a biotinylation site and recombinant β2-microglobulin are synthesized and purified. They are then refolded in the presence of the specific epitope, and the monomer is isolated by gel filtration and is biotinylated. Fluorescent streptavidin is added to induce tetramerization. An aliquot of tetramers is added to the peripheral blood mononuclear cells together with other antibodies for a more detailed characterization of antigen-specific T cells.[206] Analysis is performed using a flow cytometer. Because of the specificity of vaccines, the patient's HLA type and specific peptide must be identified and synthesized to provide the adequate tetramer. Pentameric HLA/peptide complexes have recently become available and in some laboratories have replaced the use of tHLA.

Analysis of tHLA offers many potential advantages over other T-cell assays. This method is quantitative and enables an estimation of the avidity between TCR and peptide-loaded HLA class I molecules. tHLA staining does not kill the labeled cells, allowing sorting of subpopulations by flow cytometry for additional analysis or expansion for adoptive transfer. With tHLA, specific T cells can be analyzed from blood samples without the prerequisite of in vitro culture, and all specific cytotoxic T lymphocytes are detected, regardless of their functional status.[203,206,213]

HUMAN LEUKOCYTE ANTIGEN SUMMARY

The relevance of HLA in clinical pathology has broadened from its role as a predictor of allosensitization to a mediator of GVHD and GVN. The understanding of action mechanisms in various nonclassic HLA genes as well as KIR has opened a new field. The study examining the function of the innate immune response in the context of transplantation and other immunopathologies is a result of this. Together with HLA, immunogenetics is rapidly growing, driven by the realization that polymorphism is the hallmark of human immunopathology as its spans mHag, KIR, cytokines, and their receptors. Each of these is interwoven in an intricate array of interdependent functions that cannot be discounted. Modern methods should be able to adopt high-throughput systems for the parallel assessment of all these variables when addressing the genetic makeup of an individual in correlation with the natural or therapeutic history of his or her disease. The comparison of donor and recipient protein profiling and cytokine polymorphism may offer insights

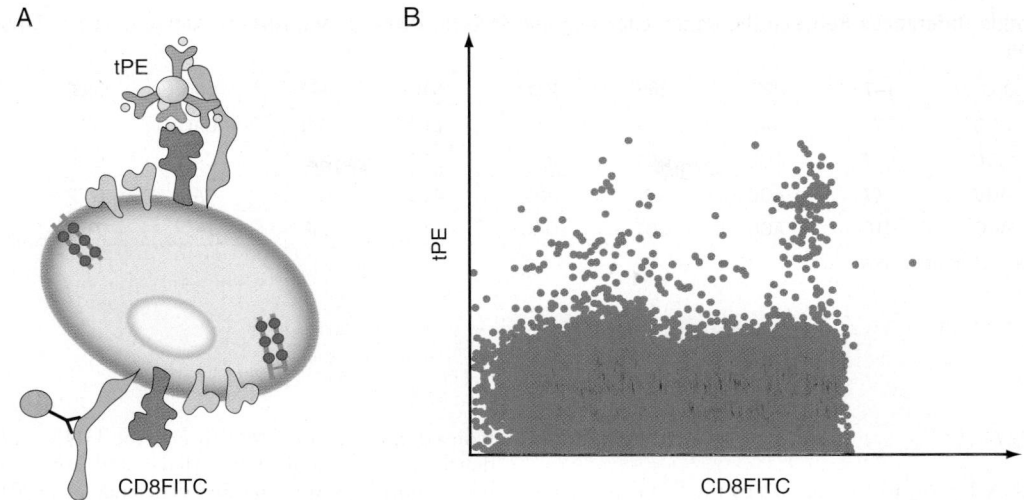

Fig. 113.6 SCHEMATIC REPRESENTATION OF THE MECHANISM OF BINDING OF TETRA-MERIC PEPTIDE/HUMAN LEUKOCYTE ANTIGEN COMPLEXES (THLA) TO ANTIGEN-SPECIFIC T CELLS. (A) Binding of tHLA to T-cell receptor. The tHLA consists of four HLA/peptide complexes identical to the ones recognized by the T cell on the surface of live cells. Each HLA molecule is modified to contain one biotin molecule that serves as a bridge for binding to tetravalent streptavidin molecules fluorescently labeled. (B) Actual fluorescence-activated cell sorter analysis result of CD8+, tHLA-positive T cells. *(Modified from Monsurro V, Nargosen D: Immunotracking of specific cancer vaccine CD8 lymphocytes. ASHI Q 26:100, 2003.)*

into the rejection mechanism when matched-donor grafts are used. Finally, the increased use of T cell-directed immunization is driving renewed interest in high-resolution typing of HLA molecules to allow a more accurate interpretation of clinical and immunologic results. In the coming years, there will be an abundance of data generated from various methods for next generation sequencing. Utilization of this data will have a tremendous impact on understanding the clinical and immunologic implications in regards to HLA. This data will require an enormous effort with bioinformatics at the forefront.

HUMAN NEUTROPHIL ANTIGENS AND THEIR CLINICAL SIGNIFICANCE

Lalezari et al described the first granulocyte antigens.[214,215] These antigens were designated *N* for neutrophil. Each antigen system was described alphabetically, and each allele was described numerically in order of discovery. They identified NA1 in 1966 and its allele, NA2, in 1972.[214,215] Reports of several other granulocyte antigens followed.

A new nomenclature was established in 1998 by the International Society of Blood Transfusion Working Party (Table 113.4).[216] In this nomenclature, antigen systems are referred to as *human neutrophil antigens,* or HNA. The antigen systems—that is, the polymorphic forms of the immunogenic proteins—are indicated by integers, and specific antigens within each system are designated alphabetically by date of publication. Alleles of the coding genes are named according to the Guidelines for Human Gene Nomenclature. Neutrophil antigens NA1 and NA2 became HNA-1a and HNA-1b, respectively, and NB1 became HNA-2. The serology, biochemistry, molecular biology, and clinical significance of these antigens are reviewed here.

THE HNA-1 ANTIGEN SYSTEM

Expression of HNA-1 Antigens

HNA-1 antigens are expressed only on neutrophils. HNA-1 antigens are located on the low-affinity Fc-γ receptor IIIb (FcγRIIIb), CD16.[217-220] FcγRIIIb, HNA-1a, HNA-1b, HNA-1c, and HNA-1d

TABLE 113.4	International Society of Blood Transfusion Nomenclature			
Antigen System	Antigens	Location	Former Name	Alleles
HNA-1	HNA-1a	FcγRIIIb, CD16	NA1	FCGR3B*01
	HNA-1b	FcγRIIIb, CD16	NA2	FCGR3B*02
	HNA-1c	FcγRIIIb, CD16	SH	FCGR3B*03
	HNA-1d	FcγRIIIb, CD16		FCGR3B*02
HNA-2	HNA-2	CD177 (NB1 gp)	NB1	CD177
HNA-3	HNA-3a	CTL-2	5b	SLC44A2*01
HNA-4	HNA-4a	CD11b (CR3)	Mart(a)	ITGAM*01
HNA-5	HNA-5a	CD11a (LFA-1)	Ond(a)	ITGAL*01

CR3, C3bi receptor; gp, glycoprotein; HNA, human neutrophil antigen; LFA-1, leukocyte function–associated antigen-1.

antigens are expressed on all segmented neutrophils, approximately one-half of neutrophilic metamyelocytes, and approximately 10% of neutrophilic myelocytes.[221] Neutrophil expression of FcγRIIIb and HNA-1 antigens are diminished by the treatment of neutrophils with stimulants such as complement component C5a and chemotaxin F-met-leu-phe or granulocyte colony-stimulating factor (G-CSF). Soluble FcγRIIIb is present in plasma, and it has the same HNA-1 polymorphisms found on neutrophils. FcγRIIIb released from granulocytes is the source of the soluble FcγRIIIb and HNA-1 antigens.[222]

Biochemistry

FcγRIIIb is a glycoprotein with 233 amino acids and is glycosylphosphatidylinositol (GPI) anchored.[217-220] Its molecular weight is 50 to 80 kDa, and the glycoprotein has *N*-linked carbohydrate side chains. The HNA-1a form of FcγRIIIb is 50 to 65 kDa, while the HNA-1b form of FcγRIIIb is 65 to 80 kDa, and the heterozygous form is 50 to 80 kDa. Differences in *N*-glycosylation account for the differences in molecular mass.

TABLE 113.5 Nucleotide Differences Between the Genes Encoding the HNA-1a, HNA-1b, and HNA-1c Antigens of Fcγ RIIIb Base Pair Position

Gene	141	147	227	266	277	349	473	505	559	641	733
FCGR3B*01	AGG	CTC	A**A**C	GCT	GAC	**G**TC	GAC	CAC	GTT	TCT	TGA[a]
FCGR3B*02	AG**C**	CT**T**	AGC	GCT	**A**AC	ATC	GAC	CAC	GTT	TCT	TGA[a]
FCGR3B*03	AG**C**	CT**T**	AGC	G**A**T	**A**AC	ATC	GAC	CAC	GTT	TCT	TGA[a]
FCGR3A	AGG	CTC	AGC	GCT	GAC	ATC	G**G**C	T**A**C	T**T**T	T**T**T	**C**GA

Note: Differences among genes are in bold.
*N-Glycosylation site.
[a]Stop codon.
HNA, Human neutrophil antigen.

Molecular Biology

FcγRIIIb and the HNA-1 antigens are encoded by the FCGR3B gene located on chromosome 1q23-24 within a cluster of two families of Fc γ R genes, FCGR2, and FCGR3. The FCGR3 family is made up of FCGR3A and FCGR3B. FCGR3B is highly homologous to FCGR3A, which encodes FcγRIIIa. Only four nucleotides differ between FCGR3B and FCGR3A (Table 113.5). The most important difference between the two genes is a C to T change at 733 in FCGR3B that creates a stop codon. As a result, FCGR3A has 21 more amino acids than FCGR3B, and FCGR3A is a transmembrane rather than GPI-anchored glycoprotein. FcγRIIIa is not recognized by antibodies specific to HNA-1 antigens, but the similarities between FCGR3A and FCGR3B complicate genotyping of HNA-1 alleles.

HNA-1a, HNA-1b, HNA-1c, and HNA-1d Polymorphisms

The neutrophil-specific HNA-1 antigen system is made up of four alleles, HNA-1a, HNA-1b, HNA-1c, and HNA-1d.[223] (Table 113.4). The gene frequencies of the alleles vary widely among different racial groups. Among whites, the frequency of the gene encoding HNA-1a, FCGR3B*01, is between 0.30 and 0.37, and the frequency of the gene encoding HNA-1b, FCGR3B*02, is from 0.63 to 0.70.[224–228] In Japanese and Chinese populations, the FCGR3B*01 gene frequency is from 0.60 to 0.66, and the FCGR3B*02 gene frequency is from 0.30 to 0.33.[217,218,221,225–228] The frequency of the gene encoding HNA-1c, FCGR3B*03, also varies among racial groups. FCGR3B*03 is expressed by neutrophils in 4% to 5% of whites and 25% to 38% of African Americans.[229]

The FCGR3B*01 gene differs from the FCGR3B*02 gene by only five nucleotides in the coding region, at positions 141, 147, 227, 277, and 349 (Table 113.5).[217–220] Four of the nucleotide changes result in changes in amino acid sequence between the HNA-1a and HNA-1b forms of the glycoprotein. The fifth polymorphism at 147 is silent. The glycosylation pattern of the protein differs between the two antigens because of two nucleotide changes at bases 227 and 277. The HNA-1b form has six N-linked glycosylation sites, while the HNA-1a form has four glycosylation sites.

The gene encoding the HNA-1c form of FcγRIIIb, FCGR3B*03, is identical to FCGR3B*02 except for a C to A substitution at nucleotide 266 resulting in an alanine to aspartate change at amino acid 78 of FcγRIIIb (Table 113.5).[223] In many cases, FCGR3B*03 exists on the same chromosome with a second or duplicate FCGR3B gene.[223,230]

Antibodies to HNA-1d have recently been described in two cases of neonatal immune neutropenia. The antigen HNA-1d is also encoded by FCGRB*02.[231]

FcγRIIIB Deficiency

Blood cells from patients with paroxysmal nocturnal hemoglobinuria lack the GPI-linked glycoproteins, and their granulocytes express reduced amounts of FcγRIIIb and the HNA-1 antigens.[220] Genetic deficiencies of granulocyte FcγRIIIb and HNA-1 antigens have also been reported. With inherited deficiency of FcγRIIIb, the FCGR3B gene is deleted along with an adjacent gene, FCGR2C.[224,232] Among white patients the incidence of individuals homozygous for FCGR3B deletion is about 0.1%.[233,234] However, among Africans and African Americans the incidence is much higher; in one study, 3 of 126 Africans were found to be FCGR3B deficient,[229] and, in another, 1 of 53 was found to be FCGR3B deficient.[227]

Function of HNA-1 Antigens

The low-affinity Fc-γ receptors link humoral immunity to cellular immune function; specifically, Fc γ Rs on effector cells recognize cytotoxic IgG molecules and immune complexes containing IgG molecules. Polymorphisms in FcγRIIIb affect neutrophil function. Neutrophils that are homozygous for HNA-1b have a lower affinity for IgG3 than granulocytes homozygous for HNA-1a.[235] Neutrophils from people who are homozygous for HNA-1b phagocytize erythrocytes sensitized with IgG1 and IgG3 anti-Rh monoclonal antibodies and bacteria opsonized with IgG1 at a lower level than granulocytes homozygous for HNA-1a.[236,237]

Clinical Relevance of FCγRIIIB Deficiency

Despite the important role of FcγRIIIb in neutrophil function, deletion of the entire FcγRIIIB gene does not cause major clinical problems, and most people with FcγRIIIb deficiency are healthy. However, too few patients have been studied to identify a slight increase in susceptibility to infection or autoimmune disease due to FcγRIIIb deficiency.

THE HNA-2 ANTIGEN SYSTEM

HNA-2 is an isoantigen without allelic variation. It was first described in 1971 by Lalezari et al and was known as NB1.[238] Monoclonal antibodies specific to HNA-2 have been clustered as CD177.

Expression of HNA-2

HNA-2 is expressed only in neutrophils, neutrophilic metamyelocytes, and myelocytes.[221,239] HNA-2 is unique in that it is expressed in subpopulations of neutrophils. The mean size of the HNA-2–positive subpopulation of neutrophils is 45% to 65%.[240–242] The expression of HNA-2 is greater on neutrophils from women than men.[241,243] The size of the HNA-2–positive subpopulation of neutrophils from women is approximately 60%, compared with approximately 50% for men. Neutrophil expression of HNA-2 is greater in pregnant women than in healthy female blood donors.[243] The surface expression of HNA-2 is slightly upregulated by treatment with the chemotactic peptide F-met-leu-phe.[240] The administration of G-CSF to healthy patients for several days increases the proportion of neutrophils expressing HNA-2 to near 90%.[244]

CD177 Glycoprotein Biochemistry

The glycoprotein carrying HNA-2a, CD177, was previously known as the NB1 glycoprotein. It is located on neutrophil plasma membranes and secondary granules[240,245] and is linked to the plasma membrane via a GPI anchor.[240] Although some GPI-anchored proteins are shed by F-met-leu-phe–treated neutrophils, CD177 is not, nor is soluble CD177 glycoprotein present in plasma.[240] The molecular weight of CD177 is 58 to 64 kDa, and it contains *N*-linked carbohydrate side chains.[240,245]

Molecular Biology

The gene encoding CD177 is located on chromosome 19q13.31, and its coding region consists of 1311 base pairs that code for a protein of 416 and a signal peptide of 21 amino acids.[246,247] The predicted protein has two cysteine-rich domains, three potential *N*-linked glycosylation sites, and a potential ω-site for attachment of the GPI anchor.[247] This gene belongs to the Ly-6 snake toxin superfamily. Other genes in this family include urokinase-type plasminogen activator receptor (uPAR; CD87) and decay-accelerating factor (CD59).

Polymorphisms

HNA-2 is expressed in neutrophils by approximately 97% of whites, 95% of African Americans, and 89% to 99% of Japanese.[241,248–250] HNA-2–negative neutrophil phenotype is caused by a CD177 transcription defect.[251] HNA-2 genes from two women with HNA-2–negative neutrophils who produced HNA-2a–specific alloantibodies have been studied, and CD177 complementary DNA (cDNA) sequences were present in both women.[251] The HNA-2–negative phenotype was the result of different off-frame insertions at the RNA level, resulting in CD177 glycoprotein deficiency in neutrophils.[251]

Clinical Relevance of HNA-2 Antigens

The rare women who produce HNA-2–specific alloantibodies and who lack NB1 glycoprotein are healthy. The expression of HNA-2 is reduced in neutrophils from people with paroxysmal nocturnal hemoglobinuria and chronic myelogenous leukemia,[239] but it is unknown whether this has any clinical significance. CD177 mRNA is overexpressed by neutrophils from patients with polycythemia rubra vera and essential thrombocytosis.[252,253] The role of CD177 in neutrophil function is unknown. In some studies HNA-2 may have a role in the adhesion of neutrophils to endothelial cells.[254]

HNA-3 ANTIGEN SYSTEMS

The HNA-3 antigen system has one antigen, HNA-3a, which was previously known as 5b. HNA-3a is expressed by neutrophils, lymphocytes, platelets, endothelial cells, kidney, spleen, and placental cells. HNA-3a has a gene frequency of 0.66.[255] HNA-3a is located on the Choline Transporter-like protein-2 (CTL-2) and is encoded by SLC44A2. The HNA-3a phenotype is due to a nucleotide polymorphism that results in an arginine rather than a glutamine at position 154 of CTL-2.[256,257] Several cases of transfusion-related acute lung injury (TRALI) have been associated with transfusion of plasma containing anti-HNA-3a.[258,259]

HNA-4 AND HNA-5 ANTIGEN SYSTEMS

HNA-4 and HNA-5 antigens are located in the β_2-integrins. Each antigen system contains only a single antigen, HNA-4a and HNA-5a, respectively. HNA-4a antigen was previously known as Mart(a). HNA-4a has a phenotype frequency of 99.1% in white patients. HNA-4a has been located on the αM chain (CD11b) of the C3bi receptor (CR3) and is caused by a single nucleotide substitution of G to A at position 302 of the gene ITGAM.[260] The substitution is predicted to result in an arginine to histidine polymorphism at amino acid 61.

A second polymorphism of the β_2-integrins, HNA-5a, was first described as Ond(a). HNA-5a was found to be expressed on the αL integrin unit, leukocyte function-associated antigen-1 (LFA-1) (CD11a), and is caused by a G to C single nucleotide substitution at position 2446 of the gene ITGAL. This change predicts an amino acid change of arginine to threonine at amino acid 766.[260]

CLINICAL SIGNIFICANCE OF ANTIBODIES TO NEUTROPHIL ANTIGENS

Alloimmune Neonatal Neutropenia

During pregnancy, mothers can become alloimmunized to neutrophil antigens. Maternal IgG directed to neutrophils can cross the placenta and destroy the neonate's neutrophils. Maternal alloimmunization to neutrophil antigens can occur in utero and affect the first child. Most neonates experience isolated neutropenia, but the cytopenias are self-limiting and resolve as the antibody is cleared. The alloimmunized mothers produce and carry the antibodies; but the antibodies do not react with the mother's blood cells or tissues, and they have normal neutrophil counts. Antibodies to neutrophil-specific antigens HNA-1a, HNA-1b, and HNA-2 most commonly cause neonatal alloimmune neutropenia (Table 113.6).[255,261] Antibodies to HNA-1c and HNA-3a rarely cause alloimmune neonatal neutropenia. Mothers with FcγRIIIb deficiency have produced FcγRIIIb-specific antibodies that caused neonatal neutropenia.[233,255,261]

Newborns with alloimmune neutropenia are usually asymptomatic. Most often, the neutropenia is detected in the first week of life when the neonate becomes febrile or develops an infection and a neutrophil count is performed. Typically the counts are 0.100 to 0.200×10^9/L. Some neonates have normal neutrophil counts the first day of life, but they become neutropenic on their second day.[261] White blood cell count, platelet count, and hemoglobin level are usually normal; but eosinophilia or monocytosis may be present. If a bone marrow biopsy is performed, it often shows normal numbers of erythroid progenitors and megakaryocytes with hyperplasia of myeloid progenitors.

TABLE 113.6	Specificities of Antibodies in Alloimmune Neonatal Neutropenia	
Antigen	**N = 18[211] (%)**	**N = 48[253] (%)**
HNA-1a	28	10
HNA-1b	22	8
FcγRIIIb	0	8
HNA-2a	11	2
HNA-3a	0	2
Unknown	0	15
HLA class I[251]	11	54
Negative	28	38

HLA, Human leukocyte antigen; HNA, human neutrophil antigen.

The clinical course is quite variable. An occasional infant is asymptomatic, but almost all affected children have an infection. The most common infections are umbilicus infections, skin infections, abscesses, and respiratory tract infections. Less commonly, infants experience otitis media, urinary tract infections (UTIs), and gastroenteritis. Serious infections such as sepsis, pneumonia, and meningitis can occur. The duration of the neutropenia may be as short as a few days or as long as 28 weeks.[261] The mean duration of neutropenia is about 11 weeks.[261]

For an asymptomatic child, no immediate treatment may be required. Prompt and aggressive antibiotic treatment of children with fevers or other signs of infections is indicated. Intravenous immunoglobulin has a limited role in the treatment of neonatal alloimmune neutropenia. Approximately half the patients treated have a transient increase in count lasting only a few days. The use of G-CSF to treat alloimmune neutropenia has also had mixed results. The administration of G-CSF elevates the neutrophil count in some but not all neonates.[261]

AUTOIMMUNE NEUTROPENIA OF CHILDHOOD

Autoimmune neutropenia has been well described in children.[262-265] Typically the onset of the autoimmune neutropenia of children begins at 8 months of age, but children between 1 and 36 months of age can be affected. Most studies found that neutrophil counts recover spontaneously by the age of 5 years, with a median of 13 to 20 months of neutropenia.[262-265]

In most cases, children presented with severe neutropenia, having neutrophil counts less than 0.5×10^9/L. Monocytosis has been reported to occur in up to 38% of patients. Results of bone marrow biopsies in affected patients usually show normal to hypercellular marrow with a decreased number of mature granulocytes. Febrile episodes and infections, including bacterial skin infections, otitis media, respiratory tract infections, and UTIs, are common. Life-threatening complications are rare.

Antibodies to neutrophils can be detected in up to 98% of affected patients. If antibody specificity is identified, the antibodies are almost always specific to epitopes located on FcγRIIIb. The antibodies are directed to HNA-1a in 10% to 46% of patients, to HNA-1b in 2% to 3% of patients, and rarely to FcγRIIIb epitopes expressed by granulocytes from all donors.[262,265]

Autoimmune neutropenia has been treated with corticosteroids, intravenous immunoglobulin, and G-CSF. Approximately half the patients responded to intravenous immunoglobulin, but neutrophil counts remained elevated for only 1 week.[262] Almost all the patients responded to G-CSF and 75% to corticosteroids, and neutrophil counts remained elevated as long as the drugs were given.

TRANSFUSION REACTIONS

Antibodies to neutrophil and HLA antigens can cause febrile nonhemolytic transfusion reactions and TRALI. Before the widespread transfusion of leukocyte-reduced blood components, approximately 0.5% of transfusions were associated with febrile nonhemolytic transfusion reactions, and leukocyte antibodies are a common cause of these reactions. These febrile reactions are caused by the interaction of leukocyte antibodies in the transfusion recipient with leukocytes contained in the transfused blood components. These reactions can be prevented by the use of components that have been filtered to remove leukocytes.

A more serious type of transfusion reaction associated with leukocyte antibodies is the acute noncardiac pulmonary edema, or TRALI. This entity is characterized by acute respiratory distress that usually occurs within 4 hours after a transfusion. These reactions are characterized by dyspnea, hypoxia, and bilateral pulmonary infiltrates on chest radiograph without cardiomegaly or pulmonary vascular congestion. The mortality rate associated with TRALI is approximately 5%.[266] Of patients with TRALI, 80%

have rapid resolution of pulmonary infiltrates and return of arterial blood gas values to normal within 96 hours after the initial respiratory insult. However, pulmonary infiltrates have persisted for at least 7 days after the transfusion reaction in 17% of TRALI patients.

TRALI has been associated with both neutrophil and HLA antibodies. Antibodies reported in these reactions include HNA-1a, HNA-1b, HNA-2, HNA-3a, and HLA class I and II antibodies. Most of these cases involve the passive transfusion of the offending antibody in donor plasma, as contrasted with the reactivity of the recipient's antibody with donor leukocytes to cause febrile nonhemolytic reactions. Retrospective studies involving antibodies to HNA-3a have implicated blood components from single donors with anti-HNA-3a in several TRALI cases.[258]

NEUTROPHIL ANTIGENS SUMMARY

Five neutrophil antigen systems, HNA-1, HNA-2, HNA-3, HNA-4 and HNA-5 have been well described. HNA-1 antigens are located on FcγRIIIb, and antibodies to these antigens are frequently implicated in autoimmune and alloimmune neutropenia. HNA-2 is located on CD177 glycoprotein, and antibodies to HNA-2 are found in patients with alloimmune and autoimmune neutropenia. Antibodies to HNA-3a are rare; but relative to other neutrophil antibodies, may be more frequently associated with cases of TRALI. The significance, if any, of HNA-4a and HNA-5a antibodies is uncertain.

REFERENCES

For the complete list of references, log on to www.expertconsult.com.

SUGGESTED READINGS

Braun WE: Update in kidney transplantation: Increasing clinical success, expanding waiting lists. *Cleve Clin J Med* 69:501, 2002.

Bux J, Behrens G, Jaeger G, et al: Diagnosis and clinical course of autoimmune neutropenia in infancy: Analysis of 240 cases. *Blood* 91:181, 1998.

Bux J, Jung KD, Kauth T, et al: Serological and clinical aspects of granulocyte antibodies leading to alloimmune neonatal neutropenia. *Transfus Med* 2:143, 1992.

Childs R, Srinivasan R: Advances in allogeneic stem cell transplantation: Directing graft-versus-leukemia at solid tumors. *Cancer J Sci Am* 8:2, 2002.

Daser A, Michinson H, Michinson A, et al: Non-classical-MHC genetics of immunological disease in man and mouse: The key role of proinflammatory cytokine genes. *Cytokine* 8:593, 1996.

Dawkins RL, Degli-Esposti MP, Abraham LJ, et al: Conservation versus polymorphism of the MHC in relation to transplantation, immune responses and autoimmune disease. In Klein J, Klein D, editors: *Molecular evolution of the major histocompatibility complex*, Berlin, 1991, Springer-Verlag, p 391.

De Haas M, Kleijer M, van Zwieten R, et al: Neutrophil FcγRIIIb deficiency, nature, and clinical consequences: A study of 21 individuals from 14 families. *Blood* 86:2403, 1995.

Duquesnoy RJ, Marrari M: HLAMatchmaker: A molecularly based algorithm for histocompatibility determination. II. Verification of the algorithm and determination of the relative immunogenicity of amino acid triplet-defined epitopes. *Hum Immunol* 63:353, 2002.

Hennecke J, Wiley DC: T cell-receptor-MHC interactions up close. *Cell* 104:1, 2001.

Kim CJ, Parkinson DR, Marincola FM: Immunodominance across the HLA polymorphism: Implications for cancer immunotherapy. *J Immunother* 21:1, 1997.

Kissel K, Santoso S, Hofmann C, et al: Molecular basis of the neutrophil glycoprotein NB1 (CD177) involved in the pathogenesis of immune neutropenias and transfusion reactions. *Eur J Immunol* 31:1301, 2001.

Matzinger P: An innate sense of danger. *Semin Immunol* 10:399, 1998.

Opelz G, Vanrenterghem Y, Kirste G, et al: Prospective evaluation of pretransplant blood transfusion in cadaver kidney recipients. *Transplantation* 63:964, 1997.

Opelz G, Wujciak T, Dohler B, et al: HLA compatibility and organ transplant survival: Collaborative transplant study. *Rev Immunogenet* 1:334, 1999.

Parker KC, Bednarek MA, Coligan JE: Scheme for ranking potential HLA-A2 binding peptides based on independent binding of individual peptide side-chains. *J Immunol* 152:163, 1994.

Petersdorf EW, Hansen JA, Martin PJ, et al: Major-histocompatibility-complex class I alleles and antigens in hematopoietic-cell transplantation. *N Engl J Med* 345:2001, 1794.

Petz LD, Garratty G, Calhoun L, et al: Selecting donors of platelets for refractory patients on the basis of HLA antibody specificity. *Transfusion* 40:1446, 2000.

Stroncek DF, Skubitz KM, McCullough J: Biochemical nature of the neutrophil-specific antigen NB1. *Blood* 75:744, 1990.

Velardi A, Ruggeri L, Moretta A, et al: NK cells: A lesson from mismatched hematopoietic transplantation. *Trends Immunol* 23:438, 2002.

CHAPTER 114

PRINCIPLES OF NEUTROPHIL (GRANULOCYTE) TRANSFUSIONS

Ronald G. Strauss

Current leukapheresis technology and donor management/stimulation permit collection of large numbers of several types of blood leukocytes (e.g., neutrophils, hematopoietic progenitors/stem cells, and lymphocytes) from either healthy donors (allogeneic use) or patients (autologous use)—who often are stimulated with recombinant cytokines such as granulocyte colony-stimulating factor (G-CSF)—to be used for transfusion and transplantation or for further processing (e.g., ex vivo expansion and genetic manipulation). Polymorphonuclear neutrophils (PMNs) are granulocytic leukocytes that are collected from healthy donors and issued as a standard blood component (granulocytes, pheresis). This chapter analyzes the use of neutrophil (i.e., granulocyte) transfusions (GTX) as an adjunct to antimicrobial drugs in the treatment and prevention of progressive infections in patients with severe neutropenia or PMN dysfunction.

Life-threatening infections with bacteria, yeast, or other fungi continue to be a consequence of severe neutropenia ($<0.5 \times 10^9$/L blood PMNs), most commonly occurring after intense chemotherapy or hematopoietic progenitor cell (HPC) transplantation, and disorders of PMN dysfunction such as chronic granulomatous disease. The most frequent clinical situation today is neutropenic fever and infection following intense chemotherapy or HPC transplantation given to treat hematologic malignancies. Neutropenic infections cause considerable morbidity, occasionally are fatal, and add considerable cost to the management of these patients. However, because of improved antifungal prophylaxis and therapy immediately following HPC transplantation, severe fungal infections often occur later after neutrophil engraftment (i.e., due primarily to long-standing immunodeficiency, not to severe neutropenia), and neutrophil transfusions (GTX), of course, are not warranted during this later time in the posttransplant period. Thus the number of patients with severe fungal infections, for whom GTX previously were considered, has decreased, further questioning the need in some physicians' opinions for GTX therapy.

Previous attempts to prevent infections in severely neutropenic patients by transfusing PMN concentrates (i.e., prophylactic GTX) achieved only questionable success. Although rates of certain infections were significantly reduced by prophylactic GTX, many adverse effects, such as pulmonary infiltrates and cytomegalovirus infections, were reported, and GTX were expensive. Thus prophylactic GTX have gained little support over the years. Similarly, use of therapeutic GTX to resolve existing infections has not gained lasting acceptance, despite many reports, including randomized clinical trials, documenting significant benefit for some patients. This lack of enthusiasm for GTX can be explained by the continuing development of new and very effective antimicrobial drugs to prevent and treat infections and by the availability of recombinant hematopoietic growth factors and peripheral blood hematopoietic progenitor cell (PBHPC) transfusions—both of which hasten patient recovery from myelotoxic therapy and, thereby, shorten the period of severe neutropenia and consequent risk of neutropenic infections.

Historically, PMN concentrates were collected for transfusion from unstimulated donors or those stimulated only with corticosteroids, and contained woefully inadequate numbers of PMNs. Currently, very large numbers of PMNs can be collected from normal donors using G-CSF plus corticosteroid (i.e., dexamethasone) marrow stimulation followed by large-volume leukapheresis, during which several liters (e.g., 7 L) of donor blood are processed. In this chapter the historical and modern experiences with GTX are reviewed, and the current technology of PMN collection is discussed.

THERAPEUTIC GTX FOR NEUTROPENIC INFECTIONS: HISTORICAL EXPERIENCE

The historical experience with GTX will be critically reviewed because it provides the underpinnings for continued interest in this mode of therapy, despite its lack of universal acceptance over the 40 or so years since publication of the first controlled trials. In the third edition of this book, 34 papers were reviewed that reported the therapeutic use of GTX—collected before the advent of G-CSF donor stimulation—in severely neutropenic patients ($<5 \times 10^9$/L blood PMNs), and only a summary of their findings will be presented here to lay the basis for modern GTX therapy.

Results of the historical studies were tabulated (Table 114.1) according to the index infection that prompted GTX therapy. Patients were counted only once (e.g., patients with septicemia were listed only in the septicemia group, even if they had another infection, such as pneumonia). As an exception, all patients with invasive fungal infections were counted together because it was impossible to accurately separate sepsis, pneumonia, sinusitis, and so forth into distinct categories. All patients given GTX for a designated type of infection were enumerated in the "Treated" column. The treated patients, those for whom the actual course and mortality of the index infection could be clearly documented, were enumerated again in the "Evaluable" column. GTX therapy was considered successful if so stated by the authors. Combining data from multiple reports of varying experimental design, admittedly, is of limited value for drawing firm conclusions, and it was done simply to document the surprising breadth of historical reported experience.

To obtain more definitive information regarding efficacy of historical GTX (i.e., collected without G-CSF), the seven controlled studies were analyzed in more detail.[1-7] In these seven studies, the response of infected neutropenic patients to treatment with GTX plus antibiotics (study group) was compared with that of comparable patients given antibiotics alone and evaluated concurrently (control group). The design, size, and results of these seven studies are presented in Tables 114.2 and 114.3. Despite the limited donor stimulation and somewhat primitive leukapheresis technology, three of the seven studies reported a significant overall benefit for GTX.[4-6] In two additional studies,[1,3] overall success was not demonstrated for GTX, but certain subgroups of patients were found to benefit significantly. Thus some measure of success for GTX was evident in five of the seven controlled studies. However, this success was counterbalanced by four studies that were negative in some respect—two totally[2,7] and two partially negative.[1,3]

An explanation of these inconsistent results is evident on critical analysis of the adequacy of GTX support (see Table 114.3). Patients in the three successful trials received relatively high doses of PMNs (generally $\geq 1.7 \times 10^{10}$/day).[4-6] Donors were selected to be both erythrocyte and leukocyte compatible. By contrast, the four controlled studies yielding negative results can legitimately be criticized. Two of the four studies with negative conclusions used PMNs collected by filtration leukapheresis for some patients.[1,3] It is now known that such PMNs are defective, and they are no longer transfused. In the negative studies using PMNs collected by centrifugation

TABLE 114.1	Infectious Problems in Neutropenic Patients Treated With Historical Granulocyte Transfusions in 34 Studies		
Type of Infection	Treated	Evaluable	Success Rate (%)
Bacterial septicemia	298	206	127/206 (62)
Sepsis organism unspecified	132	39	18/39 (46)
Invasive yeast or other fungus	83	77	28/77 (36)
Pneumonia	120	11	7/11 (64)
Localized infections	143	47	39/47 (83)
Fever etiology unknown	184	85	64/85 (75)

TABLE 114.2	Results of Seven Controlled Studies Evaluating Historical Therapeutic Granulocyte Transfusions in Neutropenic Patients					
			Study Group		Control Group	
Investigators	Success	n	Survival (%)	n	Survival (%)
Higby et al[5]	Yes	17	76	19	26
Vogler and Winton[6]	Yes	17	59	13	15
Herzig et al[4]	Yes	13	75	14	36
Alavi et al[1]	Partial	12	82	19	62
Graw et al[3]	Partial	39	46	37	30
Winston et al[7]	No	48	63	47	72
Fortuny et al[2]	No	17	78	22	80

TABLE 114.3	Design of Seven Controlled Studies Evaluating Historical Therapeutic Granulocyte Transfusions in Neutropenic Patients					
Investigators	Randomized?	Collection Method	Dose ($\times 10^{10}$)	Schedule	HLA[a]	WBC[a]
Higby et al[5]	Yes	Filtration	2.2	Daily	No	Yes
Vogler and Winton[6]	Yes	Centrifugation	2.7	Daily	Yes	Yes
Herzig et al[4]	Yes	Filtration	1.7	Daily	No	Yes
		Centrifugation	0.4	Daily	No	Yes
Alavi et al[1]	Yes	Filtration	5.9	Daily	No	No
Graw et al[3]	No	Filtration	2.0	Daily	No	Yes
		Centrifugation	0.6	Daily	No	Yes
Winston et al[7]	Yes	Centrifugation	0.5	Daily	No	No
Fortuny et al[2]	No	Centrifugation	0.4	Daily	No	Yes

[a]Donors selected to be compatible with recipient either by HLA typing (A and B loci matched, at least in part) or by leukocyte crossmatching.
HLA, Human leukocyte antigen; WBC, white blood cell.

leukapheresis,[2,3,7] the dose was extremely low (0.41 to 0.56 $\times 10^{10}$ per concentrate). As another factor, investigators in two of the four negative studies[1,7] made no provision for the possibility of leukocyte alloimmunization, because donors were selected solely on the basis of erythrocyte compatibility. Finally, control subjects responded reasonably well to antibiotics alone in three of the four negative studies,[1,3,7] suggesting that some patients fared so well with conventional treatment that they had no apparent need for additional therapeutic modalities.

These impressions from the seven controlled GTX trials have been analyzed by formal meta-analysis,[8] with conclusions that the dose of PMNs transfused and the survival rate of the nontransfused control subjects were primarily responsible for the differing success rates of the historical studies. In clinical settings in which the survival rate of nontransfused control subjects was low, study subjects benefited from receiving adequate doses of GTX, prompting the authors to suggest that severely neutropenic patients with life-threatening infections should be considered to receive GTX given in adequate doses.[8]

THERAPEUTIC GTX FOR NEUTROPENIC INFECTIONS: MODERN EXPERIENCE

Bacterial, yeast, and other fungal infections occur frequently in patients with severe neutropenia or PMN dysfunction, and when these infections fail to promptly respond to antimicrobial drugs, they pose a major challenge for which modern therapeutic GTX offer a possible answer. Recipients of HPC transplants—particularly marrow transplant patients—often become severely neutropenic and exhibit PMN dysfunction shortly after transplant. Importantly, they manifest defective cellular and humoral immunity for months after transplantation. Altered immunity is particularly profound when the HPC

graft is T-lymphocyte depleted to diminish graft-versus-host disease. Hence all types of infection pose a threat, with yeast and other fungal infections being major problems. In a series of 1186 marrow transplant patients, 10% developed a noncandidal fungal infection, with only 17% of infected patients surviving. When the marrow graft is depleted of T lymphocytes, the rate of infection is increased twofold to sevenfold above that occurring with standard bone marrow transplantation.

Data are insufficient to determine the proper role of GTX in treating yeast or other fungal infections (which are the most difficult to treat). Historical case reports, experimental studies in animals, and experience in treating patients with chronic granulomatous disease have supported the efficacy of GTX in fungal infections. In contrast, a large historical clinical study reported that GTX collected without G-CSF donor stimulation were of no benefit in treating yeast or other fungal infections in 87 bone marrow transplant patients, 50 of whom received GTX. Although this study was a retrospective review with several shortcomings, it is supported by the disappointing finding of the poor response of invasive/tissue fungal infections in neutropenic patients to even modern GTX in some reports.

At this time, two randomized clinical trials of therapeutic GTX collected after G-CSF donor stimulation have been reported, but fail to clearly establish the efficacy or potential toxicity of modern GTX. Their shortcomings will be discussed. Because the randomized trials fail to provide definitive information, five case reports (Table 114.4) and six uncontrolled studies of multiple patients (Table 114.5) will be reviewed to provide as much information as possible for making clinical decisions.[9–19]

Clarke et al[9] and Catalano et al[11] each reported single patients (see Table 114.4) with aplastic anemia undergoing HPC transplantation and with fungal infections that responded favorably to strikingly different doses of PMNs. Similarly, Ozsahin et al[12] and Bielorai et

TABLE 114.4   Case Reports of Modern Therapeutic Granulocyte Transfusions Using Neutrophils Collected From Granulocyte Colony-Stimulating Factor–Stimulated Donors in Neutropenic Patients

Investigators	PMNs × 10¹⁰ per Each GTX	Stimulation	Leukapheresis	Outcomes
Clarke et al[9]	5.3[a]	G-CSF 5–10 µg/kg	Dextran 10 L processed	One patient with fungus recovered
Catalano et al[11]	1.9	G-CSF 300 µg/dose	Not described	One patient with fungus recovered
Ozsahin et al[12]	3.1	G-CSF 5 µg/kg	Hetastarch 5–7 L processed	One patient with fungus recovered
Bielorai et al[13]	7.0[a]	G-CSF 5 µg/kg	Not described	One patient with fungus recovered
Bielorai et al[14]	4.8-6.8	Not described	Not described	One patient with vancomycin-resistant *Enterococcus* recovered

[a]Assumptions made because PMN dose expressed × 10¹⁰ unclear in these reports. Dose calculated that would be given to a 70-kg recipient for Clarke et al and Bielorai et al.
G-CSF, Granulocyte colony-stimulating factor; GTX, granulocyte transfusions; PMN, neutrophil.

TABLE 114.5   Groups of Neutropenic Patients Treated With Modern Therapeutic Granulocyte Transfusions Using Neutrophils Collected From Granulocyte Colony-Stimulating Factor–Stimulated Donors

Investigators	PMNs × 10¹⁰ per Each GTX	Stimulation	Leukapheresis	Outcomes
Hester et al[10]	4.1	G-CSF 5 µg/kg	Pentastarch 7 L processed	60% (9 of 15) success with yeast (4 patients) and other fungus (11 patients)
Grigg et al[15]	5.9[a]	G-CSF 10 µg/kg	Dextran 10 L processed	100% (3 of 3) success with bacterial infection 0% (0 of 5) success with progressive fungus 67% (2 of 3) success with stable fungus
Peters et al[16]	3.5a	G-CSF 5 µg/kg or Prednisolone	Hetastarch 6.4 L processed	82% (14 of 17) success with bacterial infection 54% (7 of 13) success with fungal infection
Price et al[17]	8.2	G-CSF 600 µg/kg plus Dexamethasone 8 mg	Hetastarch 10 L processed	100% (4 of 4) success with bacterial infection 0% (0 of 8) success with invasive fungus 57% (4 of 7) success with yeast infection
Lee et al[18]	5.1-10.6	G-CSF 5 µg/kg and/or Dexamethasone 3 mg/m²	Pentastarch 6–10 L processed	40% (10 of 25) success with multiple-organism infections
Hubel et al[19]	4.6-8.1	G-CSF 600 mg/kg with or without Dexamethasone 8 mg	Hetastarch or pentastarch 10 L processed	55% (unrelated donor) success with bacterial infection 75% (family donor) success with bacterial infection 0% (unrelated donor) success with yeast infection 40% (family donor) success with yeast infection 15% (unrelated donor) success with fungal infection 25% (family donor) success with fungal infection

[a]Assumptions made because PMN dose expressed × 10¹⁰ unclear in these reports. PMN dose calculated using values for range of leukocytes collected, percentage of collected cells being myeloid, and volume of units collected (Grigg et al). Dose calculated that would be given to a 70-kg recipient for Peters et al.
G-CSF, Granulocyte colony-stimulating factor; GTX, granulocyte transfusions; PMN, neutrophil.

al[13] each reported single patients (see Table 114.4) with chronic granulomatous disease and fungal infections that responded favorably to GTX during the transplantation period. Bielorai et al[14] reported a single patient with acute leukemia and sepsis with progressive, antibiotic-resistant bacteria whose infection cleared slowly with GTX.

Hester et al[10] transfused 15 patients with hematologic malignancies and infections (see Table 114.5). PMNs were collected from donors stimulated only with G-CSF and selected without regard for leukocyte compatibility. Although GTX were successful in most patients, it was not possible to distinguish responses of yeast versus other fungal infections. Lee et al[18] transfused 25 patients with hematologic malignancies, many of whom were infected with multiple organisms. PMNs were collected from donors stimulated with G-CSF alone (67% of donors), G-CSF plus dexamethasone (25% of donors), or dexamethasone alone (8% of donors). Of patients with sepsis, 50% (2 of 4) responded favorably, and 38% (8 of 21) of patients with progressive localized infections responded favorably. Grigg et al[15] transfused 11 patients (see Table 114.5). Eight patients had hematologic malignancies and progressive infections, five of the eight

undergoing progenitor cell transplantation and three receiving chemotherapy. Three additional patients who were undergoing progenitor cell transplantation had stable fungal infections. PMNs were collected from donors stimulated only with G-CSF and selected without regard for leukocyte compatibility. Success was excellent for bacterial and stable fungal infections but was quite poor for progressive fungal infections with organ dysfunction, a troubling pattern reported by others.[17]

Peters et al[16] transfused 30 patients (see Table 114.5) with hematologic disorders—18 undergoing HPC transplantation. PMNs were collected from donors stimulated with G-CSF or prednisolone and selected without regard for leukocyte compatibility. The exact PMN dose transfused is uncertain because values from 0.9×10^{10} to 14.4×10^{10} can be calculated from data reported, and it was impossible to distinguish the success of GTX from G-CSF–stimulated versus prednisolone-stimulated donors. However, the outcome of bacterial infections appeared to be superior to that of fungal infections.

Price et al[17] transfused 19 patients (see Table 114.5) with hematologic malignancies, 16 who had received HPC transplants and three who were pretransplantation recipients. PMNs were collected from donors stimulated with G-CSF and dexamethasone. Although donors were selected without regard for leukocyte compatibility, recipients were documented not to exhibit evidence of leukocyte alloimmunization at study entry. Bacterial infections responded well, and yeast infections responded modestly. Despite very high PMN doses, success for other invasive fungal infections was dismal.

Hubel et al[19] expanded the study of Price et al[17] to a total of 74 patients (see Table 114.5) with HPC transplants. Controls were 74 historical patients not given GTX. Donors were either family members or unrelated individuals stimulated with G-CSF with or without dexamethasone. Comparative favorable responses varied with family versus unrelated donors but were approximately 70% for bacterial, 50% for yeast, and 20% for other fungal infections, values similar to the historical control patients not given GTX.

The report of Safdar et al[20] did not lend itself to presentation in Table 114.5 because many aspects of the patients and their infections are quite heterogeneous. The study was a case-control retrospective analysis of 491 cancer patients with candidemia—29 given GTX and 462 not. Donors were stimulated with G-CSF plus dexamethasone, and GTX were given either daily or on alternate days. Not all patients were evaluable, but unexpectedly only 35% of patients given GTX resolved their infections versus 67% of those not given GTX ($p <$ .001).

No firm conclusions can be drawn from these somewhat anecdotal and very heterogeneous reports of modern therapeutic GTX, but on the basis of these preliminary findings, bacterial infections appeared to respond well to modern GTX, relatively mild yeast and other fungal infections responded modestly well, whereas, serious and/or invasive fungal infections with tissue damage often resisted even the large doses of PMNs transfused with modern GTX.[15–17] Accordingly the precise role of modern therapeutic GTX, collected from donors stimulated with G-CSF plus corticosteroids, was addressed by two randomized clinical trials.

As background for judging the quality and recognizing the shortcomings of the randomized trials, modern therapeutic GTX is defined as PMNs collected from donors stimulated with G-CSF, preferably combined with dexamethasone, by means of centrifugation leukapheresis using an erythrocyte-sedimenting agent, while processing large volumes of donor blood. An ideal PMN collection should include: (1) 300–480 μg G-CSF given subcutaneously plus 8 mg dexamethasone given orally to the donor approximately 12 hours before leukapheresis begins; (2) hetastarch plus concentrated citrate infused throughout the entire leukapheresis procedure at a ratio of 1 part hetastarch to 12 to 14 parts donor blood; and (3) processing of 8 to 10 L of donor blood. The goal should be to transfuse 6 to 8 $\times$ 10^{10} neutrophils per GTX, with a lower limit of 4 $\times$ 10^{10}.

Two randomized clinical trials have been reported, but both have shortcomings or flaws that preclude firm guidelines for clinical practice. The first published randomized clinical trial of modern GTX provided no definitive guidelines for transfusion practices[21] because of problems including: (1) lack of completion due to poor enrollment; (2) donors stimulated only with G-CSF and not dexamethasone resulting in relatively low PMN doses for individual GTX; and (3) GTX were given every other day, not daily, resulting in low PMN doses for the overall course of GTX. Thus the trial failed to test efficacy of modern "high-dose" GTX.[21]

The second and most recent randomized clinical trial (RING),[22] like the first trial, was stopped before completion due to slow enrollment and, accordingly, failed to provide definitive guidelines for clinical practice. RING is a multicenter (14 clinical sites in the United States) randomized clinical trial in which 114 infected neutropenic (<500 neutrophils/μL blood) patients were randomly allocated to treatment either with daily GTX collected from donors stimulated with G-CSF plus dexamethasone plus antibiotics ($n = 56$) or with antibiotics alone ($n = 58$). The primary endpoint was composite, consisting of survival at 42 days after randomization plus a favorable microbial response determined by a blinded adjudication panel.

Results by intention-to-treat analysis (i.e., all subjects enrolled into the two arms, regardless of whether or not they received the therapy

dictated for each arm) were nearly identical ($p >$ .99) with 42% in the GTX arm versus 43% of controls having a favorable response. Similarly, by per-protocol analysis (i.e., only patients actually treated as intended), results were not different ($p =$ .64), with 49% favorable in the GTX arm versus 41% of controls. No differences in success rates were noted when subsets of subjects were analyzed per specific type of infection (i.e., bacteremia, fungemia, invasive/tissue bacterial infections, or invasive/tissue fungal infections).

Although results appeared to be "negative" (i.e., no advantage for GTX), 32% of patients in the GTX arm received less than the intended dose of PMNs/granulocytes. When patients actually given the intended "high-dose" GTX were compared with those given the unintended lower doses of GTX, the "high-dose" GTX patients had significantly higher success rates ($p =$ .01). Specifically the success rate was 58% for 26 patients given at least three GTX with an average dose per transfusion of at least 5 $\times$ 10^{10} compared with 11% success for 9 patients receiving lower leukocyte doses.

The reasons for the poor PMN/granulocyte doses given in the RING trial could not be determined, but the findings suggest that the potential benefits of high-dose GTX still remain a possibility, provided high-dose GTX (at least 4 $\times$ 10^{10} neutrophils per transfusion) are actually given.[22] The findings also demonstrate that the collection of quality neutrophil/granulocyte concentrates requires expertise and careful quality assessment to consistently provide a product with any hope of benefit.

As a case in point, in a retrospective review of patients with invasive *Fusarium* infections, 11 patients with severe neutropenia and failure to respond to antifungal drugs received a median of seven GTX containing a mean of 6.84 $\times$ 10^{10} granulocytes per GTX.[23] Ten of eleven patients (91%) had a favorable response, compared with an expected response of <50% when antifungal drugs are given without GTX. Over 98% of donors were unrelated community donors who were given 480 μg G-CSF subcutaneously plus 8 mg dexamethasone orally, 12–18 hours and 12 hours before leukapheresis, respectively. Seven liters of donor blood were processed by continuous-flow leukapheresis using 500 mL of 6% hetastarch and anticoagulated with 30 mL of 46.7% trisodium citrate at a hetastarch to donor blood ratio of 1:12 throughout the procedure.

Conclusions regarding the role of modern therapeutic GTX at this time are as follows. The use of G-CSF plus dexamethasone to stimulate PMN donors has brought GTX therapy into a new era, as it is now possible to collect relatively large numbers of PMNs (granulocytes) (>4 $\times$ 10^{10}). However, definitive quality data to provide firm guidelines for clinical practice remain elusive. Randomized clinical trials have proven extremely difficult to complete because of poor and/or slow patient enrollment and the lack of dependable neutrophil/granulocyte leukapheresis products. There are strong hints that transfusing >4 $\times$ 10^{10} neutrophils/granulocytes daily to severely neutropenic infected patients may be beneficial and, despite lack of definitive proof of efficacy, should be considered in clinical settings where severely neutropenic patients suffer significant morbidity and/or mortality from infections.

THERAPEUTIC GTX IN INFANTS AND CHILDREN

Children with severe neutropenia due to marrow failure during chemotherapy or HPC transplantation suffer infections similar to those of adult patients, and the principles for therapeutic GTX are comparable to those discussed in the previous section. Accordingly, they will not be reiterated other than to note that GTX, generally, are transfused infrequently with doses of PMNs/granulocytes decreased commensurate with smaller body size. Alternatively, it may be wise to transfuse an entire standard leukapheresis collection to provide very high doses of PMNs, assuming the overall condition of the patient permits the large volume of the GTX.

An indication for GTX is severe infection occurring in children with congenital disorders of PMN dysfunction, who have adequate numbers of blood PMNs, but are susceptible to serious infection because their PMNs fail to kill pathogenic microorganisms. Patients with severe forms of PMN dysfunction are relatively rare, and no randomized clinical trials have been reported to establish the efficacy of therapeutic GTX in their management. Firm recommendations about the use of GTX to treat patients cannot be made. However, several patients with chronic granulomatous disease, complicated by progressive life-threatening fungal infections, have been reported to benefit. Because of the possibility of alloimmunization to leukocyte and red blood cell antigens plus the other risks of allogeneic transfusions, such as pulmonary reactions and transfusion-transmitted infections, therapeutic GTX are recommended only for progressive infections that cannot be controlled with antimicrobial drugs. Because of lifelong problems with infections, prophylactic GTX are impractical.

Neonates (infants within the first month of life) are another group of patients who may suffer life-threatening bacterial infections caused, at least in part, by PMN dysfunction and neutropenia—absolute or relative (i.e., normal neonates exhibit a physiologic neutrophilia compared with normal PMN counts in older children and adults)—consequently, absolute blood PMN counts as high as 3.0×10^9/L might prompt consideration of GTX in neonates.[23] Although four of six controlled trials assessing the efficacy of therapeutic GTX in neonatal sepsis found a significant benefit for GTX, this form of therapy is rarely used today. Accordingly, they will not be discussed further.

PROPHYLACTIC GRANULOCYTE TRANSFUSIONS IN NEUTROPENIC PATIENTS

Based on historical reports, prophylactic GTX were of marginal value. In 12 reports, benefits were few, whereas risks and expenses were substantial. However, some measure of success was found in 7 of 12 studies; the remaining 5 studies failed to show a benefit for prophylactic GTX. In none of these 5 negative studies were large numbers of PMNs obtained from matched donors and transfused daily. In a situation analogous to that for the negative therapeutic GTX trials, the failure of prophylactic GTX might be explained, at least in part, by inadequate transfusions.

The role of modern prophylactic GTX (i.e., from G-CSF–stimulated donors) has not been established by definitive clinical trials. However, two factors suggest possible success: (1) because of the rapid recovery from myeloablation, hastened by peripheral blood HPC transplantation plus treatment of patients with recombinant growth factors such as G-CSF, the period of severe neutropenia may be as short as 1 week; and (2) this relatively brief period of severe neutropenia might literally be eliminated by transfusing large doses of PMNs collected from donors stimulated with G-CSF plus corticosteroids. A few studies have begun to explore this possibility (Table 114.6).

Adkins et al[24] transfused 10 allogeneic marrow recipients with PMNs collected from their human leukocyte antigen (HLA)-matched sibling marrow donors (see Table 114.6). Leukapheresis was performed on days 1, 3, and 5 posttransplant, and GTX were infused.

Recipients were given 7.5 µg/kg G-CSF every 12 hours until blood PMNs were greater than or equal to 1.5×10^9/L. Recipient blood PMNs were maintained at greater than 1.5×10^9/L throughout the 5 days of posttransplant GTX. By comparison, a historical group of control recipients treated with G-CSF, but no GTX, exhibited lower mean blood PMN counts of less than 0.5×10^9/L posttransplant. Prophylactic GTX seemed promising in this setting and perhaps would have been even more effective (i.e., higher recipient blood PMN counts and fewer infections) if given daily.

In another study, Adkins et al[25] transfused 23 autologous peripheral HPC recipients with PMNs collected from first-degree relative donors (see Table 114.6). Leukapheresis was performed on posttransplant days 2, 4, 6, and 8, and GTX were infused. Recipients were given 5 µg/kg G-CSF daily until the blood PMN count was greater than or equal to 1.5×10^9/L. Recipients were studied for the effects of lymphocytotoxic antibodies (i.e., leukocyte alloimmunization) on GTX effectiveness. The 15 recipients who did not exhibit lymphocytotoxic antibodies during the 10-day study period experienced a mean of 4.1 febrile days and required 7.3 days of antibiotics. Values for the eight recipients with lymphocytotoxic antibodies were less desirable—6.3 febrile days and 10.5 days of antibiotics. Rates of documented infections were not reported.

No firm conclusions can be drawn from these reports of modern prophylactic GTX because (1) no nontransfused control subjects were included, (2) few patients were studied, and (3) most patients were given GTX every other day, rather than daily—possibly providing a lower-than-optimal dose of PMNs. Modern prophylactic GTX appear promising, but their efficacy, potential adverse effects, and economic analysis await definition by randomized clinical trials.

ALTERNATIVE OR ADDITIVE MEASURES TO GRANULOCYTE TRANSFUSIONS

Patients with severe neutropenia, particularly those undergoing intense chemotherapy or HPC transplantation, exhibit a variety of abnormalities in multiple body defense mechanisms, most of which cannot be corrected by GTX. Consequently infections that occur in these patients often occur after the period of severe neutropenia and accordingly do not respond to GTX. To bolster body defenses, a number of additional therapies have been evaluated, two of which are the use of recombinant myeloid growth factors (i.e., cytokines) and intravenous immunoglobulin (IVIg). A critical analysis of the biology and clinical use of these agents is beyond the scope of this chapter.

AUTHOR'S APPROACH TO THERAPEUTIC GTX

1. Consider for severe bacterial, yeast, or other fungal infection in a neutropenic patient ($<0.5 \times 10^9$ PMNs/µL blood) when the infection progresses despite optimal antimicrobial therapy.

TABLE 114.6	Modern Prophylactic Granulocyte Transfusion Studies Using Neutrophils Collected From Granulocyte Colony-Stimulating Factor–Stimulated Donors in Hematopoietic Progenitor Cell Transplant Recipients			
Investigator	PMNs × 10^{10} per Each GTX	Stimulation	Leukapheresis	Outcomes
Adkins et al[24]	4.1 (day 1) 5.1 (day 3) 6.1 (day 5)	G-CSF 5 µg/kg × 5 Days posttransplant	Hetastarch 7 L processed Days 1, 3, and 5	60% (6 of 10) afebrile 40% (4 of 10) febrile 3 culture positive
Adkins et al[25]	5.6 (day 2) 7.0 (day 4) 8.5 (day 6) 9.9 (day 8)	G-CSF 10 µg/kg	Hetastarch 7 L processed Days 2, 4, 6, and 8	Reduction of fever and antibiotics if no leukocyte antibodies

G-CSF, Granulocyte colony-stimulating factor; GTX, granulocyte transfusions; PMN, neutrophil.

2. Collect PMNs (4 to 8 × 10^{10}) from allogeneic blood donors, as follows:
   a. Stimulate neutrophilia by giving the donor 300 to 480 µg G-CSF subcutaneously plus 8 mg dexamethasone orally 12 hours (±4 hours) before beginning leukapheresis;
   b. Process 10 L of donor blood using a continuous-flow blood separator with citrated hydroxyethyl starch solution infused throughout the entire collection.
3. Transfuse one granulocyte concentrate (4 to 8 × 10^{10} PMNs) daily until bone marrow recovery (blood PMNs >1.0 × 10^9/L without granulocyte transfusion) or clinical resolution of infection.

REFERENCES

1. Alavi JB, Root RK, Djerassi I, et al: A randomized clinical trial of granulocyte transfusions for infection in acute leukemia. *N Engl J Med* 296:706, 1977.
2. Fortuny IE, Bloomfield CD, Hadlock DC, et al: Granulocyte transfusion: A controlled study in patients with acute non-lymphocytic leukemia. *Transfusion* 15:548, 1975.
3. Graw RG, Jr, Herzig G, Perry S, et al: Normal granulocyte transfusion therapy. *N Engl J Med* 287:367, 1972.
4. Herzig RH, Herzig GP, Graw RG, Jr, et al: Successful granulocyte transfusion therapy for gram-negative septicemia. *N Engl J Med* 396:702, 1977.
5. Higby DJ, Yates JW, Henderson ES, et al: Filtration leukapheresis for granulocytic transfusion therapy. *N Engl J Med* 292:761, 1975.
6. Vogler WR, Winton EF: A controlled study of the efficacy of granulocyte transfusions in patients with neutropenia. *Am J Med* 63:548, 1977.
7. Winston DJ, Ho WG, Gale RP: Therapeutic granulocyte transfusions for documented infections: A controlled trial in 95 infectious granulocytopenic episodes. *Ann Intern Med* 97:509, 1982.
8. Vamvakas EC, Pineda AA: Meta-analysis of clinical studies of the efficacy of granulocyte transfusions in the treatment of bacterial sepsis. *J Clin Apher* 11:1, 1996.
9. Clarke K, Szer J, Shelton M, et al: Multiple granulocyte transfusions facilitating unrelated bone marrow transplantation in a patient with very severe aplastic anemia complicated by suspected fungal infection. *Bone Marrow Transplant* 16:723, 1995.
10. Hester JP, Dignani MC, Anaissie EJ, et al: Collection and transfusion of granulocyte concentrates from donors primed with granulocyte stimulating factor and response of myelosuppressed patients with established infection. *J Clin Apher* 10:188, 1995.
11. Catalano L, Fontana R, Scarpato N, et al: Combined treatment with amphotericin-B and granulocyte transfusion from G-CSF-stimulated donors in an aplastic patient with invasive aspergillosis undergoing bone marrow transplantation. *Haematologica* 82:71, 1997.
12. Ozsahin H, von Planta M, Muller I, et al: Successful treatment of invasive aspergillosis in chronic granulomatous disease by bone marrow transplantation, granulocyte colony-stimulating factor-mobilized granulocytes, and liposomal amphotericin-B. *Blood* 92:2719, 1998.
13. Bielorai B, Toren A, Wolach B, et al: Successful treatment of invasive aspergillosis in chronic granulomatous disease by granulocyte transfusions followed by peripheral blood stem cell transplantation. *Bone Marrow Transplant* 26:1025, 2000.
14. Bielorai B, Neumann Y, Avigad I, et al: Successful treatment of vancomycin-resistant *Enterococcus* sepsis in a neutropenic patient with G-CSF-mobilized granulocyte transfusions. *Med Pediatr Oncol* 34:221, 2000.
15. Grigg A, Vecchi L, Bardy P, et al: G-CSF stimulated donor granulocyte collections for prophylaxis and therapy of neutropenic sepsis. *Aust N Z J Med* 26:813, 1996.
16. Peters C, Minkov M, Matthes-Martin S, et al: Leucocyte transfusions from rhG-CSF or prednisolone stimulated donors for treatment of severe infections in immunocompromised neutropenic patients. *Br J Haematol* 106:689, 1999.
17. Price TH, Bowden RA, Boeckh M, et al: Phase I/II trial of neutrophil transfusions from donors stimulated with G-CSF and dexamethasone for treatment of patients with infections in hematopoietic stem cell transplantation. *Blood* 95:3302, 2000.
18. Lee J-J, Chung I-J, Park M-R, et al: Clinical efficacy of granulocyte transfusion therapy in patients with neutropenia-related infections. *Leukemia* 15:203, 2001.
19. Hubel K, Carter RA, Liles WC, et al: Granulocyte transfusion therapy for infections in candidates and recipients of HPC transplantation: A comparative analysis of feasibility and outcome for community versus related donors. *Transfusion* 42:1414, 2002.
20. Safdar A, Hanna HA, Boktour M, et al: Impact of high-dose granulocyte transfusions in patients with cancer with candidemia. *Cancer* 101:2859, 2004.
21. Seidel MG, Peters C, Wacker A, et al: Randomized phase III study of granulocyte transfusions in neutropenic patients. *Bone Marrow Transplant* 42:679, 2008.
22. Price TH, Boeckh M, Harrison RW, et al: *Efficacy of transfusion with granulocytes from G-CSF/dexamethasone treated donors in neutropenic patients with infection.* Blood First Edition Paper, prepublished online Sept 2, 2015; doi: 10.1182/blood-2015-05-645986.
23. Strauss RG: Current status of granulocyte transfusions to treat neonatal sepsis. *J Clin Apher* 5:25, 1989.
24. Adkins D, Spitzer G, Johnston M, et al: Transfusions of granulocyte-colony-stimulating factor-mobilized granulocyte components to allogeneic transplant recipients: Analysis of kinetics and factors determining posttransfusion neutrophil and platelet counts. *Transplantation* 37:737, 1997.
25. Adkins DR, Goodnough LT, Shenoy S, et al: Effect of leukocyte compatibility on neutrophil increment after transfusion of granulocyte colony-stimulating factor-mobilized prophylactic granulocyte transfusions and on clinical outcomes after stem cell transplantation. *Blood* 95:3605, 2000.

CHAPTER 115

TRANSFUSION OF PLASMA AND PLASMA DERIVATIVES: PLASMA, CRYOPRECIPITATE, ALBUMIN, AND IMMUNOGLOBULINS

Matthew S. Karafin, Christopher D. Hillyer, and Beth H. Shaz

Plasma and its derivatives are well-established clinical resources, but cost risk of infectious disease transmission, although rare, and other adverse effects mandate their appropriate use. Even to this day however, much still remains to be clarified regarding the appropriate clinical use of plasma products. The 2015 National Institute of Health-National Heart Lung and Blood Institute State of the Science Symposium revealed that significant and fundamental gaps in our knowledge regarding the most predictive clinical hemostatic tests (i.e., viscoelastic versus traditional coagulation tests), best products (i.e., frozen versus liquid plasma), new products (i.e., freeze dried plasma), and appropriate clinical indications/protocols for plasma product use remain. Plasma can be separated from red blood cells (RBCs) through centrifugation of whole blood at the time of collection, or can be collected by apheresis as a single product or as a by-product of platelet or RBC apheresis. Plasma can be processed into derivatives through cold ethanol fractionation (method of Cohn). In this chapter, the features and uses of plasma products, which include fresh frozen plasma (FFP), plasma frozen within 24 hours of phlebotomy (FP24), thawed plasma, liquid plasma, solvent detergent treated plasma (SD-plasma), pathogen-reduced/ inactivated plasma as well as plasma derivate, including cryoprecipitate-reduced plasma, cryoprecipitate, albumin, intravenous immunoglobulin (IVIg) and intramuscular immunoglobulin (Ig) are discussed. The use of plasma-derived clotting factor concentrates as well as coagulation factor concentrates that are genetically engineered as therapy for specific clotting factor deficiencies are discussed in Chapter 120.

PLASMA PRODUCTS

Plasma is the acellular, fluid compartment of blood and it consists of 90% water, 7% protein and colloids, and 2% to 3% nutrients, crystalloids, hormones, and vitamins. The protein fraction contains the soluble clotting factors: fibrinogen, factor XIII, von Willebrand Factor (vWF), factor VIII primarily bound to its carrier protein vWF, and the vitamin K-dependent coagulation factors II, VII, IX, and X. Clotting proteins are the constituents for which transfusion of plasma is required. Plasma products include FFP, FP24, thawed plasma, SD-plasma, and pathogen reduced/inactivated plasma which can be used interchangeably. Notably, FFP and FP24 are both termed FFP in some countries outside of the United States.

FFP and FP24

Plasma frozen at −18°C or colder within 8 hours of donation (6 hours with the use of some storage bags after apheresis collection) can be labelled as FFP. This product may be stored up to 1 year before use, at which time it is thawed at 37°C over 20 to 30 minutes. A second type of frozen plasma, the most commonly used in the United States, is FP24 plasma. FP24 is frozen at −18°C or colder within 24 hours of collection. The difference between FFP and FP24, using historic data, is a reduction in the following factors: fibrinogen 12%, factor V 15%, factor VIII 23%, and factor XI 7%. More recently, a direct comparison between FFP and FP24 mean factor activity immediately postthaw revealed the following changes in activity levels: factor II

0%, factor V +1%, factor VII −16%, factor VIII −15%, factor IX +6%, factor X 0%, vWF antigen activity +34%, vWF:ristocetin cofactor activity +22%, fibrinogen +29 mg/dL, antithrombin 0%, protein C −19%, and protein S −5%. A disintegrin and metalloproteinase with a thrombospondin type 1 motif, member 13 (ADAMTS13) activity level is also equivalent in FFP, FP24, and cryoprecipitate-reduced plasma (discussed later). All of the factors evaluated in this study reveal that FP24 immediately postthaw had activities above the minimum activity required for safe surgical hemostasis (factor II 97%, factor V 86%, factor VII 89%, factor VIII 66%, factor IX 88%, factor X 94%, vWF:Ristocetin cofactor activity 123%, fibrinogen 309 mg/dL). Therefore, studies support that FFP and FP24 can be used interchangeably.

Thawed Plasma

Coagulation factors are also well maintained in thawed FFP and FP24 stored at 1°C to 6°C for up to 5 days, termed thawed plasma. Studies show that during 5 days of storage, most clotting factors, including ADAMTS13, remain stable. However, there is evidence that activity levels fall significantly for factors V, VII, and VIII. A review by Eder and Sebock revealed that at day 5, factor V, VII, and VIII activity levels fell from day 1 on average by 16%, 20%, and 41%, respectively, if the FFP was derived from whole blood, and 9%, 4%, and 14%, respectively, if the FFP was derived via apheresis. Although some recent evidence suggests that thrombin generation may be slower in 5-day-old thawed plasma, the decrease in clotting factor activity for both FFP and FP24 is generally not considered to be of clinical significance, as the mean factor activity levels for 5-day-old thawed plasma remain above the minimum activity required for safe surgical hemostasis (on average, FFP: factor V 67%, factor VII 70%, factor VIII 43%; FP24: factor V 59%, factor VII 77%, factor VIII 48%). Stored thawed plasma improves patient care and is more cost-effective than frozen plasma because there is no preparation time required. This difference consequently results in a decreased turn-around time, and a substantially reduced wastage rate.

Liquid Plasma

Liquid plasma is produced from whole blood within 5 days of the whole blood expiration date. Liquid plasma is maintained at 1°C to 6°C and stored for up to 26 days. It is deficient in labile clotting factors (i.e., factor V, VIII). It is used primarily for immediate treatment of acutely bleeding patients, especially where reversal of the effects of warfarin is required, as the vitamin K−dependent factors FII, FVII, F IX, and FX are relatively stable under these storage conditions. Liquid plasma remains rarely used in the United States, but studies in Europe demonstrate at least comparable efficacy to FFP in urgent situations.

Freeze-Dried Plasma (Lyophilized Plasma)

Freeze-dried plasma is produced and pooled from 10 or fewer apheresis plasma donors. The plasma undergoes a cryodessication process to form a 215 g powder in a sterile bottle. The plasma is then rehydrated for use via 200 mL of sterile water with soft agitation. While not in use yet in the United States (but used in Europe), the product is being actively investigated for use in military situations. Early studies suggest that the product is safe and efficacious for treatment of war injuries.

Cryoprecipitate-Reduced Plasma

Cryoprecipitate-reduced plasma, also known as cryosupernatant or cryoreduced-plasma, is the remaining supernatant after the removal of cryoprecipitate from FFP, which is subsequently refrozen. This product is deficient in factor VIII, factor XIII, vWF, fibrinogen, and fibronectin. Cryoprecipitate reduced plasma is only indicated in the treatment of patients with thrombotic thrombocytopenic purpura (TTP), and thus cannot be used interchangeably with thawed plasma, FFP, or FP24. It can be thawed and stored for up to 5 days at 1°C to 6°C termed, thawed plasma cryoprecipitate reduced.

Solvent-Detergent Plasma (SD-Plasma)

SD-plasma is a product manufactured from ≤2500 pooled plasma products that has been treated with solvent (tri-η-butyl phosphate)/detergent (triton X-100) to inactivate lipid-enveloped viruses (HIV, hepatitis B, hepatitis C). The product is distributed in 200 mL containers, frozen at −18°C with a shelf life of 1 year. The coagulation factor levels are comparable to FFP and FP24, and SD-plasma has less viability between units. SD-plasma was recently approved by the U.S. Food and Drug Administration (FDA), and has the added advantage of a substantially reduced risk of transfusion-related acute lung injury (TRALI) and has a lower rate of allergic reactions.

Pathogen-Reduced/Inactivated Plasma

Other pathogen-reduction methods have been developed including amotosalen photochemical treatment with ultraviolet (UVA) light, which has recently been FDA approved. Riboflavin-treated plasma with UVA light and methylene blue-treated plasma have also been developed, but these have not yet been FDA approved, but are approved in Europe. Studies in Europe show that these methods are also quite effective at reducing the risk of viral contamination, but are deficient in some clotting factors, such as fibrinogen and factor VIII (approximately 80% retention in comparison with control plasma).

Recovered and Source Plasma (Plasma for Manufacture)

There are plasma products that are not used for transfusion, but are used for further manufacturing into plasma derivatives. These products include recovered plasma (liquid plasma and "plasma") that are derived from whole blood and are sent to a manufacturer from a collection facility through a "short supply agreement". Liquid plasma, as noted previously, is defined as plasma that is separated from whole blood at any time during storage at 1°C to 6°C, up to 5 days after the whole blood expiration date. "Plasma" is defined as liquid plasma that is frozen at −18°C or colder with a frozen shelf life of 5 years. Source plasma, a FDA licensed product, is collected by apheresis which is intended for further manufacturing. The Plasma Protein Therapeutics Association promotes safe collection and manufacturing practices of plasma derivatives. Source plasma can be collected more frequently under special donor programs; the donors can be compensated for their time, and can be collected in an open or closed system. Source plasma is frozen immediately in the United States and within 24 to 72 hours in Europe.

Indications

Most guidelines consistently support plasma transfusions for correcting multiple acquired coagulation factor deficiencies, as seen in liver failure or disseminated intravascular coagulopathy (DIC), massive transfusion, reversal of warfarin effect, and certain indications as a replacement fluid in therapeutic plasma exchange (Table 115.1). However, according to one recent metaanalysis, there are no published or ongoing trials regarding the optimal transfusion strategy for these indications. As there are currently no evidence-based laboratory value "triggers" for plasma administration, any recommendation needs to be carefully weighed against the patient's presence, or risk, of bleeding.

Plasma is typically indicated when prothrombin time (PT) and/or partial thromboplastin time (PTT) are greater than 1.5 to 1.7 times normal paired with the presence of bleeding or anticipated bleeding. The justification for these current recommendations is that there is compelling evidence that plasma transfusions are ineffective in correcting mild to moderate abnormalities of coagulation screening tests. One study demonstrated that fewer than 15% of patients with a pretransfusion PT between 13.1 and 17.0 seconds had some correction after plasma transfusion, and less than 1% completely normalized. Another study found that minimally prolonged international normalized ratios (INRs) decreased with treatment of the underlying disease alone, and that the addition of plasma did not statistically change the INR over time. On the other hand, marked reductions in substantially elevated coagulation studies can occur with relatively modest plasma transfusion volumes. This variable response to plasma can be largely explained because of the nonlinear, exponential relationship between clotting factors activity levels and coagulation test results (Fig. 115.1).

Audits of recent transfusion practices have consistently demonstrated that plasma product use is inappropriately high. Recent estimates suggest up to 83% (reported range: 10–83%) of plasma transfusions are not administered according to published guidelines. The most commonly cited reason for plasma administration is a preprocedural elevation in coagulation studies. This indication is not evidence-based, especially when the coagulation abnormality is mild-moderate. Moreover, plasma should not be used as a volume expander or as a source of nutrients. Clinical situations where plasma transfusions may be beneficial are further defined in the following sections.

Liver Failure

Patients with liver failure may develop low levels of the vitamin K-dependent clotting factors (factors II, VII, IX, and X). These

---

TABLE 115.1	Indications for Plasma Product Transfusion Indicated

Disseminated intravascular coagulation
Liver failure
Massive transfusion
Multiple acquired coagulation factor deficiency
Plasma infusion or exchange for thrombotic thrombocytic purpura and other thrombotic microangiopathies, diffuse alveolar hemorrhage, and catastrophic antiphospholipid syndrome
Rapid reversal of warfarin effect when prothrombin complex concentrate is not available
Replacement of an inherited single plasma factor deficiency for which no coagulation factor concentrate exists

Not Indicated

Burns
Immunodeficiency
Source of nutrients
Volume expansion
Wound healing

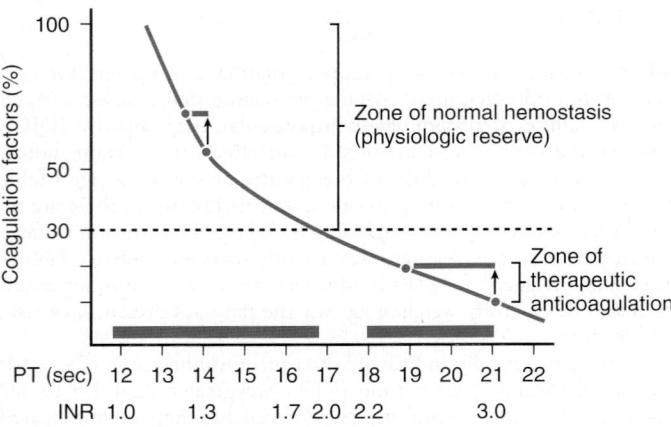

Fig. 115.1 RELATIONSHIP BETWEEN FACTOR ACTIVITY LEVELS AND COAGULATION STUDIES. The general relationship between the concentration of coagulation factors and the result of PT and INR studies. The normalization of modest elevations in the INR required much larger volumes of plasma than would be expected and modest doses of plasma can result in marked changes in the INR when markedly elevated. The cause of this phenomenon can be explained by the nonlinear, exponential, relationship between coagulation factor concentration and standard coagulation test results. As shown earlier, small increases of coagulation factors correlate with marked changes in coagulation studies when coagulation factors are depleted. The opposite is true when the coagulation factors are at higher concentrations. *INR*, International normalized ratio; *PT*, prothrombin time. *(Adapted from Levi M, Toh CH, Thachil J, Watson HG: Guidelines for the diagnosis and management of disseminated intravascular coagulation. Br J Haematol 145:24–33, 2009.)*

patients develop a prolonged PT/INR, PTT, and thrombin time. Fibrin split products may also be elevated in these patients, and in later stages, the fibrinogen level may be decreased. Prolongation of the PT and PTT has been correlated with both an increased risk of bleeding and mortality in these patients. Moreover, hemorrhage, most often secondary to an anatomic lesion, may be complicated by the coagulopathy resulting from these abnormalities. Patients with orthotopic liver transplantation complicated by preexisting severe liver disease and liver disease with DIC are two such examples that may require large plasma volumes.

While elevations in coagulation tests are correlated with the incidence of bleeding in these patients, growing evidence now suggests that the PT and PTT are, in themselves, poor predictors of surgical bleeding. The reason for this lack of association may be twofold. First, PT and PTT values do not correlate well with plasma factor activity levels. One study identified that up to 50% of patients with abnormal coagulation tests had coagulation activity levels considered sufficient for adequate thrombus formation. Moreover, studies demonstrate that mild abnormalities in these coagulation tests do not correct—even with infusion of large quantities of plasma, because of the mathematical difficulty of infusing normal levels of factors into mildly deficient blood to get enough plasma to decrease the PT/PTT (see Fig. 115.1). Second, the lack of increased/excessive bleeding noted in some patients with liver disease and elevated coagulation tests may be caused by a parallel reduction in anticoagulant proteins, such as proteins C and S. Therefore, patients with liver disease may not bleed as much as expected because they retain a homeostatic balance between coagulant and anticoagulant proteins.

A growing body of evidence suggests that the use of plasma in the context of severe liver disease and perioperatively during liver transplant does not significantly improve outcome. One study demonstrated that appropriate plasma transfusions did not significantly alter thrombin generation in cirrhotic liver patients. Another study demonstrated in 293 patients who received plasma transfusions during hepatectomy that there was no significant difference in complication

rate or postoperative liver function tests between those who received plasma from those who did not. Two other studies showed a poor correlation between number of plasma transfusions, PT and PTT values, and number of RBCs transfusions needed during liver transplantation. Lastly, a randomized control trial revealed that intranasal desmopressin was both less expensive and as effective as plasma transfusions for liver disease patients with an INR between 2.0 and 3.0 undergoing minor surgery.

As a result of these studies, authorities now suggest that the use of plasma be more limited in liver disease and hepatectomy patients. The transfusion of plasma in these patients should be guided by a combination of clinical assessment, the evidence and degree of bleeding, and by coagulation test results. Plasma products are currently not recommended prophylactically before a surgical challenge or liver biopsy in these patients. However, as noted previously, plasma transfusions may be considered when the PT/PTT is greater than 1.5 to 1.7 times normal, or if the INR is 2.0 or greater when the risk of bleeding is considered high.

Massive Transfusion

Massive transfusion is generally defined as receiving 10 or more units of RBCs within 24 hours (or one blood volume). Trauma patients may arrive at the hospital with a prolonged PT (termed acute trauma induced coagulopathy, early trauma induced coagulopathy, or acute coagulopathy of trauma). Early trauma induced coagulopathy is associated with increased mortality and increased use of blood products. Trauma patients can also develop a secondary coagulopathy, termed the lethal triad, secondary to dilutional coagulopathy, acidosis and hypothermia. The dilutional coagulopathy is secondary to the administration of crystalloid and RBCs without coagulation factor support. Studies have shown that the early use of plasma and platelets in trauma patients undergoing massive transfusion appears to decrease the incidence of secondary coagulopathy (lethal triad) and improve survival in these patients. In addition, the early administration of tranexamic acid has been shown to reduce mortality in bleeding patients.

Some experts have previously argued that plasma should be used only in the context of abnormal coagulation studies in a massively bleeding patient. However, recent studies have shown that this may not be the most effective approach. Because of the rapidity required to treat severely bleeding patients, standardized hospital-based massive transfusion protocols providing predetermined transfusions of RBCs, plasma, cryoprecipitate, and platelets are in use and have been associated with improved survival. Further, massive transfusion protocols identify who is responsible for different aspects of the patient's care, what laboratory tests should be ordered and when, and what blood products should be prepared and at what intervals. Some protocols are laboratory based while others have preset blood product volumes and ratios, and lastly, some integrate both. Importantly, hospitals develop these protocols using a multidisciplinary team, defining quality measures with periodic review to adjust the protocol based on new evidence and data.

The optimal ratio of RBCs and plasma in the context of massive transfusion is under active investigation. Multiple studies in both the military and civilian literature have shown a reduction in morbidity and mortality with a transfusion ratio of 1 unit of plasma for every 1 to 3 RBC units transfused in the context of severe posttraumatic bleeding. The Prospective Observational Multicenter Major Trauma Transfusion (PROMMTT) study demonstrated that clinicians generally are transfusing patients with a blood product ratio of 1:1:1 or 1:1:2 (plasma:platelet:RBC) and that early transfusion of plasma (within minutes of arrival to a trauma center) was associated with improved 6-hour survival after admission. The recently published Pragmatic, Randomized Optimal Platelet and Plasma Ratios trial was designed to compare the effectiveness and safety of a 1:1:1 transfusion ratio with a 1:1:2 transfusion ratio in patients with trauma who were predicted to receive a massive transfusion. This randomized clinical trial found no overall difference in survival based on transfusion ratio, but did find that those who were randomized to receive more plasma (1 : 1 : 1 ratio) achieved hemostasis more frequently. Consequently, data support no advantage of 1 : 1 : 1 versus 1 : 1 : 2, and further study comparing 1 : 1 : 2 versus 1 : 1 : 3 is needed.

Questions regarding best practice still remain. One European group has suggested that the use of prothrombin complex concentrate (PCC) and fibrinogen concentrates, instead of plasma, provide a safer alternative for massive transfusion patients. The increased use of whole blood, as an alternative to using the 1 : 1 : 1 component ratio, is being studied and has been shown to have similar efficacy in pilot trials. Other studies are investigating the early use of cryoprecipitate and the use of concentrated and/or lyophilized plasma. The optimal blood type for emergency plasma transfusions is also under active investigation. During the initial resuscitation phase of these patients, the patient's blood type is often unknown. Emergency release plasma, traditionally group AB, is used until blood typing has been completed, and the plasma used can be switched to the patient's identified ABO type. The theoretic advantage in using group AB plasma is its lack of anti-A and anti-B antibodies, thus theoretically avoiding the risk of acute hemolytic transfusion reactions. However, since AB plasma is the least common type of plasma, there is a possibility of shortages. Studies now support the use of group A plasma in massive support situations as the universal product, and have so far shown no increased risk to the recipient and no substantial effect on clinical outcomes. Some provide low titer, typically defined as less than 1 : 100, group A plasma while other do not titer group A plasma. Since patients typically receive group O RBCs and about 80% of the population is group O or group A, the risk of hemolysis is low.

In the recent past, trauma patients would be provided primarily crystalloid and albumin, followed by component transfusion therapy based on specific transfusion "triggers." A hemoglobin less than 8 g/dL for RBCs, a PT greater than 1.5 times normal for plasma, a platelet count less than 50,000/μL for platelet transfusions, and a fibrinogen less than 100 g/dL for cryoprecipitate were often used. These "triggers" have now been incorporated as part of some massive transfusion protocols as algorithms to guide therapy. In these protocols, component therapy is guided by rapid and regular laboratory value correlation. To improve the speed by which one can address coagulation abnormalities, some protocols now use thromboelastography (TEG) or other point-of-care tests. TEG technology provides a dynamic and global assessment of the coagulation process, and can provide rapid assessments of the patient's platelet function, coagulation cascade, and fibrinolysis. The mechanism underlying TEG technology and the interpretation of TEG data are beyond the scope of this chapter. Currently, sufficient data are lacking to universally recommend the use of TEG in massive transfusion protocols.

Massive transfusion in other conditions, such as liver, cardiac, or orthopedic surgery and obstetric hemorrhage, likely have a different pathophysiology and thus transfusion management of these patients may be different than trauma patients. Studies exploring the use of massive transfusion protocols in these situations are lacking, but institutions should have policies in place for rapid availability of blood products and laboratory testing.

Disseminated Intravascular Coagulation

DIC may be secondary to sepsis, liver disease, hypotension, surgery-associated hypoperfusion, trauma, obstetric complications, leukemia (usually promyelocytic), or underlying malignancy. Successful treatment of the underlying cause is paramount. Recent guidelines suggest, based on low quality evidence, that plasma therapy should not be initiated based on abnormal laboratory results alone. Rather, patients with DIC and bleeding, those requiring an invasive procedure, and those at risk for bleeding complications should be given plasma in amounts sufficient to correct or ameliorate the coagulopathy or hemorrhagic diathesis. Large volumes of plasma are often necessary to correct the coagulation defect in these patients. However, in patients with severe liver disease, bleeding, and DIC, plasma infusions often fail to normalize the PT and PTT.

Rapid Reversal of Warfarin Effect

Warfarin inhibits the hepatic synthesis of vitamin K-dependent clotting factors (factors II, VII, IX, and X) by blocking the recovery of the form of vitamin K that is active in the carboxylation of these proteins. Warfarin therapy induces functional deficiencies of these factors, which correct within 48 hours after the discontinuation of warfarin if diet and vitamin K absorption are normal.

The use of plasma in the context of warfarin anticoagulation is well established, but is becoming less relevant because of the availability of four factor PCC. Recent randomized control trials comparing PCC with plasma have demonstrated a similar clinical efficacy between the two products, but superior rate of INR normalization for those who receive PCC. Plasma is generally not indicated for warfarin reversal when the patient is not bleeding and when the patient has an INR <9, as vitamin K administration corrects the coagulopathy in 12 to 18 hours. In patients anticoagulated with warfarin who have active bleeding, require emergency surgery, or have serious trauma, however, the deficient clotting factors can be immediately provided by PCC, or plasma transfusions Plasma use may not be optimal in all situations of warfarin-induced bleeding, though, as large volumes of plasma might be required for adequate warfarin reversal, and lengthy infusion times, especially in those who are volume sensitive, might delay needed surgical intervention.

Consequently, four factor PCC, which was approved for use by the FDA in April 2013, should be chosen as the first-line therapy for rapid reversal of life or limb threatening warfarin anticoagulation. For nonemergent or nonthreatening reversal, vitamin K can be administered. Studies have shown that PCC can reverse a warfarin-induced coagulopathy faster with lower mortality and less volume overload than plasma or vitamin K alone. Also, INR levels need to be closely followed to ensure warfarin reversal is sustained.

Thrombotic Thrombocytopenic Purpura and Other Thrombotic Microangiopathies

In patients with TTP, plasma exchange (TPE) with plasma as the replacement fluid is life-saving. Plasma infusion or exchange is also critical in the treatment of individuals who have congenital TTP. TPE has decreased the mortality of TTP from over 90% to less than 10% (see Chapter 134). Six randomized control trials have demonstrated that TPE is most effective in patients who have an autoantibody to ADAMTS13. This is caused by both the removal of a patient's plasma containing the inhibitor coupled with the addition of donor plasma containing the functional vWF-cleaving protease. The FDA has also approved the use of cryoprecipitate-reduced plasma for refractory TTP, defined as those who are unresponsive to plasma exchange with FFP. Some authorities advocate the use of cryoprecipitate-reduced plasma as a first-line therapy for TTP, as these products have a lower level of vWF than FFP, a comparable ADAMTS13 activity, and lower amounts of ADAMTS13–larger vWF multimer complexes. However, the most recent multicenter prospective randomized trial comparing exchange transfusion with plasma and cryoprecipitate reduced plasma for the initial treatment of TTP demonstrated equal efficacy between plasma and cryoprecipitate-reduced plasma for the initial therapy in TTP.

Standard therapy involves daily TPE with plasma replacing 1.0 to 1.5 plasma volumes until the platelet count is above 150×10^9/L, and lactate dehydrogenase is near normal for 2 to 3 consecutive days. Treatment should be initiated immediately or at least within 24 hours of diagnosis, and if TPE is not available to initiate treatment, plasma infusions can be used until TPE is available. The total number of treatments required is variable and is based on each individual's clinical response, but studies have shown that the median number of TPEs needed to establish hematologic recovery is about 7 to 8.

TPE is not indicated in the treatment of individuals with diarrhea associated hemolytic uremic syndrome (HUS) (also termed thrombotic microangiopathy, Shiga toxin mediated) unless there are severe neurological symptoms. Seven randomized control trials were performed evaluating the efficacy of TPE for typical cases of HUS. These trials found that the use of plasma was not superior to supportive therapies alone. TPE with plasma replacement fluid, however, is currently indicated in diarrhea-negative (atypical) HUS (aHUS), which is caused by a number of inherited and sporadic conditions that lead to the uncontrolled activation of the alternative complement system (i.e., deficiency or autoantibody to complement factor H). A complete discussion of aHUS is beyond the scope of this chapter. Typically, all patients diagnosed with aHUS are empirically treated with TPE or plasma transfusions until underlying disease or mutation is further defined, which then determines treatment. TPE has been theoretically proposed to effectively remove the potentially causative autoantibody or mutated circulating complement regulator, while replacing absent or defective complement regulators. The reported clinical response varies depending on the underlying cause, however. For some causes of aHUS, plasma infusion can be initiated. Recently, Eculizumab, a humanized monoclonal antibody against C5, has been shown to be an effective alternative treatment for some causes of aHUS (see Chapter 134).

TPE with plasma replacement may also be indicated in other thrombotic microangiopathies. Some medications cause thrombotic microangiopathies that require plasma exchange. Current examples include ticlopidine and clopidogrel, and potentially cyclosporine or tacrolimus. Lastly, TPE with plasma may also be used in the treatment of thrombotic microangiopathy associated with stem cell transplantation.

Plasma as replacement fluid, either partially or completely, for TPE is used in other diseases with risk of hemorrhage caused by the resulting coagulopathy, such as diffuse alveolar hemorrhage, liver failure, and perioperatively.

Prophylactic Use of Plasma

Studies have shown that prophylactic administration of plasma to nonbleeding recipients with abnormal coagulation studies (i.e., PT, aPTT, INR) is unlikely to produce a clinical benefit and unnecessarily exposes the patient to the risks of plasma transfusion. Moreover, systematic reviews of whether a prolonged PT or aPTT even predicts bleeding found no significant difference in the risk of bleeding between patients with a prolonged PT or aPTT and those with normal clotting parameters in the setting of bronchoscopy, central vein cannulation, angiography, or liver biopsy. Despite this ambiguity, a number of randomized control trials and metaanalyses have evaluated the efficacy of the prophylactic use of plasma products to reduce the risk of bleeding. One trial, the Northern Neonatal Nursing Initiative Group Trial, randomized 776 neonates, and evaluated whether plasma transfusion prophylaxis could prevent intraventricular hemorrhage in comparison with volume expanders (gelofusine or dextrose-saline). In a second large randomized clinical trial, 275 patients were randomized to see whether plasma transfusions could prophylactically prevent bleeding in acute pancreatitis patients. Neither large study showed clinical benefit of prophylactic plasma use. In one systematic review, 55 other randomized clinical trials were reviewed and evaluated. Only 17 of these 55 involved a control group that did not receive plasma. Overall, like the two largest studies, the results of these randomized control trials failed to show evidence for the efficacy of prophylactic plasma use across multiple clinical and laboratory outcomes. Similarly, a second metaanalysis evaluated 25 independent studies of minor surgical procedures and found that there was no significant difference in bleeding risk between those who did and did not have a coagulopathy. Despite this evidence, current recommendations still recommend that a pretransfusion INR of ≥1.5 to 1.7 be used as a transfusion trigger, as the prophylactic use of plasma is theoretically justified when the clinical risk of bleeding is greater than potential harms of using plasma.

Dosage

One unit of plasma derived from a unit of whole blood contains 200 to 280 mL. When plasma is collected by apheresis, as much as 800 mL can be obtained from one individual ("jumbo" plasma units), but the majority of units clinically used have a volume around 250 mL. On average, there is 0.7 to 1 unit/mL of activity of each coagulation factor per milliliter of plasma and 1 to 2 mg/mL of fibrinogen. The appropriate dose of plasma may be estimated from the plasma volume, the desired increment of factor activity, and the expected half-life of the factor being replaced (i.e., factor VII has a half-life of only 4–6 hours, and thus plasma doses should be repeated every few hours if replacing factor VII in a patient with factor VII deficiency). Alternatively, the plasma dosage may be estimated as 10 to 15 mL/kg, and ideally should be ordered as the number of milliliters to be infused. The frequency of administration depends on the clinical response to the infusion and correction of laboratory parameters. Moreover, plasma infusions should be given as close to the time as it is needed to allow for its maximum hemostatic effect if given preprocedure. A recent one-year evaluation of 10 U.S. hospitals revealed that the current median dose of plasma was 2.0 units with 15.2% receiving only 1 unit. The median weight-adjusted plasma dose was only 7.3 mL/kg with only 29% of doses being at least 10 mL/kg and 15.5% being 15 mL/kg. Based on these findings, a large proportion of patients in the United States are likely being underdosed.

Compatibility

Plasma is screened for unexpected RBC antibodies during product testing and should be ABO-type compatible for transfusion (see later). Notably, group AB plasma is universally compatible with all patients and group O plasma is only compatible with patients with group O RBCs.

	Plasma Product ABO Type			
Patient ABO type	O	A	B	AB
O	Yes	Yes	Yes	Yes
A	No	Yes	No	Yes
B	No	No	Yes	Yes
AB	No	No	No	Yes

Yes = compatible blood types
No = incompatible blood types

Adverse Events

Plasma transfusion is associated with a number of infectious and noninfectious adverse events. Transfusion transmitted diseases traditionally include HIV, hepatitis B, and hepatitis C (Chapter 120), which are currently rare. Noninfectious risks include allergic reactions, TRALI, transfusion-associated circulatory overload (TACO), and hemolytic reactions (Chapter 119).

Transfusion-Related Acute Lung Injury

TRALI is noncardiogenic pulmonary edema associated with the transfusion of blood products. TRALI is usually caused by neutrophil and pulmonary endothelial activation, usually caused by transfused donor white cell antibodies, including human leukocyte antigen (HLA) antibodies and human neutrophil antigen (HNA) antibodies. These donor antibodies react with the recipient's white cells in the pulmonary vasculature causing leukoagglutination, activation of the complement cascade, cytokine release, and pulmonary edema. Approximately 5% of TRALI is caused by the opposite mechanisms, which are recipient white cell antibodies against transfused donor white cells. Nonimmune mechanisms are also postulated to mediate TRALI, including bioactive lipids and CD40 ligand.

TRALI is the most common cause of transfusion-associated mortality in the United States and is usually associated with transfusion of blood products containing large volumes of plasma containing white blood cell antibodies. Patients at higher risk include those with shock, chronic alcohol abuse, positive fluid balance, higher peak airway pressure, and current smoker. Signs and symptoms appear within 2 to 6 hours of transfusion and include respiratory distress with dyspnea, tachypnea, hypoxia, fever, tachycardia, and hypotension. Bilateral pulmonary infiltrates on chest x-ray may be seen with no evidence of left atrial hypertension. In cases of suspected TRALI, the transfusion should be discontinued. Medical management is primarily supportive, commonly with supplemental oxygen and endotracheal intubation, if needed. Diuresis is not indicated, and the role of steroids is unclear. The majority of patients improve within 2 days, although TRALI has a 5% to 25% mortality rate.

Multiple strategies have been implemented to reduce the risk of TRALI and have resulted in a substantial decline in its incidence. First, donors implicated in prior TRALI reactions are deferred from further blood donation. Second, multiparous female donors can be tested for HLA and HNA antibodies, and blood products with high volume plasma (i.e., plasma and apheresis platelets) are not made from those with high-titer antibodies. Third, plasma supplied to hospitals for transfusion can be only from male donors while the female plasma is diverted for fractionation. Currently, these strategies have reduced the risk of TRALI from 1:4000 to 1:12,000 without significantly reducing blood product availability.

Allergic Reactions

Allergic transfusion reactions occur when preformed recipient antibodies bind to transfused allergens. Allergic transfusion reactions occur in approximately 1% to 3% of plasma transfusions. Anaphylactic reactions occur in approximately 1 in 20,000 to 1 in 50,000 transfusions. The majority of allergic transfusion reactions are mild. Mild reactions consist of urticaria with or without generalized pruritus or flushing. More severe symptoms include hoarseness, stridor, wheezing, dyspnea, hypotension, gastrointestinal symptoms, and shock. Mild reactions can be treated with antihistamines, while more severe reactions can be treated with epinephrine, H1-receptor antagonists, and steroids.

Anaphylactic reactions may be secondary to anti-IgA, usually found in rare patients with IgA deficiency (0.13% of the population). Patients who have severe allergic reactions should be tested for IgA deficiency and the presence of anti-IgA. If anti-IgA is identified, the patient should receive plasma products from IgA-deficient donors or washed RBC and platelets products.

Premedication with antihistamine is used to mitigate allergic transfusion reactions and is indicated in patients who have multiple prior or moderate allergic reactions. Unlike platelet products, however, which can be washed or concentrated before administration, there are currently no other preventative measures, other than premedication, to diminish the risk or severity of allergic reactions in plasma transfusion recipients. Consequently, oral premedication with antihistamines can be given 30 to 60 minutes before a transfusion, while intravenous premedication can be given 10 minutes before a transfusion in patients with a history of allergic reactions to plasma products.

Transfusion-Associated Circulatory Overload

TACO results from vascular fluid volume overload following the transfusion of blood products, and is most common in very young or elderly patients with cardiac dysfunction or positive fluid balance.

TACO is also likely underdiagnosed and underreported. Studies show that the mean age of patients who develop TACO range from about 70 to 85 years. Additional known risk factors for TACO include larger volumes of transfusion, greater plasma transfusion volume, and a faster transfusion rate. The incidence of TACO is unknown, but it is increasingly recognized clinically. Studies have reported the incidence to range from 1 in 356 to 1 in 10,000 blood products transfused or 1% to 8% of transfusion recipients, depending on the study population and data collection methodology, and are currently associated with a mortality rate of 5% to 15% in the United States.

Symptoms include dyspnea, orthopnea, cough, chest tightness, cyanosis, hypertension, and headache. Symptoms usually present at the end of transfusion but may occur up to 6 hours posttransfusion. Diagnosis is based on the presence of cardiogenic pulmonary edema. Management includes discontinuing transfusion, diuretic therapy, oxygen supplementation, and sitting the patient upright. Avoiding rapid transfusion can prevent TACO, unless clinically indicated. Transfusions should be administered slowly, usually 1 mL/kg/h, particularly in patients at risk for TACO.

CRYOPRECIPITATE

Cryoprecipitate is prepared from 1 unit of FFP thawed at 4°C. The precipitate is then refrozen and stored at −18°C or colder for 1 year. Cryoprecipitate, volume of 10 to 15 mL, contains 80 to 100 units of factor VIII, 100 to 250 mg of fibrinogen, and 50 to 60 mg of fibronectin as well as vWF and factor XIII.

Cryoprecipitate takes 10 to 15 minutes to thaw at 30°C to 37°C, and then requires pooling before infusion. Prepooled (pooled before storage) cryoprecipitate products are now available, easing the burden of preparation on the transfusion services. Once pooled and thawed, cryoprecipitate is maintained at 20°C to 24°C and outdates in 4 hours (6 hours if unpooled or pooled in a closed system).

Indications

Cryoprecipitate is used predominantly to treat bleeding associated with fibrinogen deficiency (Table 115.2). Cryoprecipitate should not be used to treat factor XIII, vWF, and factor VIII deficiencies, as virally inactivated factor concentrates are available. Human fibrinogen concentrate is also available and FDA approved, which is primarily used for congenital fibrinogen factor deficiency in the United States and broader indications in Europe. Like plasma, recent studies also indicate that actual administered doses of cryoprecipitate vary widely, suggesting inconsistent practice and uncertainty over the evidence informing optimal use. One large audit, for instance, demonstrated that across 25 Canadian hospitals and 4370 units of cryoprecipitate transfusions, only 24% of transfusions were considered clinically appropriate, and 34% of cryoprecipitate transfusions were deemed inappropriate according to published national guidelines (i.e.,

TABLE 115.2	Administration of Cryoprecipitate
Indicated	
Congenital afibrinogenemia if fibrinogen concentrate unavailable	
Dysfibrinogenemia	
Factor XIII deficiency	
Fibrinogen deficiency	
Massive transfusion	
Reversal of thrombolytic therapy	
Possibly Indicated	
Amniotic fluid embolism (used as last resort to replace depleted fibronectin)	
Snake bites	
Uremic bleeding	

Transfusion Medicine Advisory Group of British Columbia, Canada Guidelines for cryoprecipitate transfusion).

Fibrinogen Deficiency

Fibrinogen deficiency is the primary indication for cryoprecipitate transfusion. The deficiency may be caused by congenital afibrinogenemia or dysfibrinogenemia, severe liver disease, DIC, or massive transfusion. Patients with the later indications often have concomitant decreases in clotting factor levels and require the coadministration of plasma products. It is important to obtain fibrinogen measurements because levels less than 100 mg/dL cause prolongation of the PT and PTT, despite adequate clotting factor replacement. Very low levels of fibrinogen occur during liver transplantation (<100 mg/dL), where transfusion support with cryoprecipitate is vital.

A specific purified human fibrinogen concentrate is now available, and may represent a safer alternative for direct fibrinogen replacement in isolated fibrinogen deficiencies, such as inherited hypofibrinogenemia. Fibrinogen concentrates undergo viral inactivation and have a standardized fibrinogen content; these are used preferentially over cryoprecipitate in some countries, but studies have not demonstrated a clinical benefit over cryoprecipitate. In the United States, fibrinogen concentrate is FDA approved for treatment of bleeding in patients with congenital fibrinogen deficiency.

Fibrin Glue/Sealant

Fibrin glue/sealant results from the mixture of a fibrinogen source (from plasma, platelet-rich plasma, or allogeneic/autologous cryoprecipitate) with a thrombin source (bovine, human, or recombinant). The enhanced local hemostasis achieved by the sealant product is through the action of thrombin on fibrinogen. "Fibrin glue" is a non–FDA-approved thrombin/preparation, and it has been widely used in Europe many years. Fibrin and thrombin sealants are FDA-approved alternatives to fibrin glue and are advantageous over locally made fibrin glues, because of standard dosing. Fibrin and thrombin containing glues/sealants can be used for multiple surgical purposes, including as a topical hemostat (creating a blood clot to halt bleeding), as a sealant (agents to prevent leakage of potentially nonclotting fluids, i.e., cerebrospinal fluid), or as an adhesive (bonds different tissues together). Multiple fibrin or thrombin containing products are now FDA approved for use.

The safety profile of each product differs depending on the product components and source. Bovine thrombin has been reported to cause anaphylaxis (because of bovine allergies), coagulopathy through formation of antibodies to factor V or II, and rarely death caused by severe systemic hypotensive reactions. Consequently, bovine products have an FDA mandated black-box warning on their package inserts. Pooled human plasma sources have the potential risk of viral or prion disease transmission. Reports indicate that hepatitis A and parvovirus B19 are particularly difficult to remove from these products despite current cleansing and filtration methods, and it is recommended that patients be counselled about this risk. Recombinant products, while eliminating the risk of infectious transmission or antibody formation, may also cause allergic reactions because of the hamster or snake proteins used to manufacture the product. Lastly, autologous fibrin clot preparations have been used, although the infectious risks (e.g., HIV and hepatitis) associated with the use of heterologous fibrin glue are eliminated by replacement with the autologous source, but are resource intensive. Given the current safety of the blood supply, the infectious risks are extremely low, particularly for pathogen inactivated products.

Alternatively, albumin mixed with glutaraldehyde has been used to form both an effective sealant and adhesive. The FDA has currently approved an albumin-based product to seal large blood vessel anastomoses and to reattach layers of the aorta in the context of an aortic dissection. Other successful reported uses include as

a sealant in breast cancer surgery, and to reduce air leaks in lung volume reduction procedures. Side effects of this compound can be significant, however, and include nerve and muscle necrosis, sinoatrial node damage, calcium metabolism abnormalities, mucosal and skin irritation, adhesive emboli, limitation of aortic growth, and pseudoaneurysms.

Uremic Bleeding

Abnormal bleeding is a common complication of uremia and is primarily caused by platelet dysfunction and defective interaction with endothelium. Use of cryoprecipitate as a source of vWF has been speculated to correct the platelet dysfunction. However, cryoprecipitate has been shown not to affect platelet aggregation in vitro, but does shorten the bleeding time. In 1980, a single study published in the *New England Journal of Medicine* led to the widespread, but temporary, use of cryoprecipitate for the treatment of uremic bleeding. Since that time, variable response reports have been published. Numerous alternative strategies are currently available for the prevention and treatment of uremic type bleeding including dialysis, erythropoietin, RBC transfusion, desmopressin, and conjugated estrogens, and, as such, cryoprecipitate is now rarely used in the prevention or treatment or uremic bleeding.

Massive Transfusion

While most studies regarding massive transfusion evaluate the use of platelets and plasma, some studies suggest that regular doses of cryoprecipitate may also help improve survival. In general, the current use of cryoprecipitate in massive support is not standardized and the use is based on theoretic efficacy. According to the recently published PROMMTT study, there are wide differences (7–82%) in the use of cryoprecipitate at U.S. level 1 trauma centers, and inclusion of cryoprecipitate in massive transfusion protocols vary significantly. Specifically, some PROMMTT sites used cryoprecipitate after a certain number of RBC units infused, while others used fibrinogen triggers, such as 100 mg/dL. While the PROMMTT study found no significant differences in mortality between those that did and did not receive cryoprecipitate, other studies have shown benefit. One study found that a high transfusion ratio involving cryoprecipitate in 214 massive transfusion patients resulted in improved 30-day survival (66% versus 41%). Another key study found that maintaining a ≥0.2 g fibrinogen/RBC (10 units of cryoprecipitate used for every 10 units of RBCs) unit ratio resulted in significantly higher survival rates (76% versus 48%). Lastly, military trauma patients in the MATTERs II study who received a combination of cryoprecipitate and Tranexamic acid had the lowest observed mortality despite high injury severity scores (odds ratio, 0.34). While a small randomized feasibility study has been performed (CRYOSTAT trial), and demonstrated that cryoprecipitate can be prepared early during trauma resuscitation, larger randomized prospective clinical trials are still needed. Consequently, while still under investigation, current data tentatively support the use of cryoprecipitate in the context of massive transfusion protocols, however cryoprecipitate remains indicated in the treatment of hypofibrinogenemia. See box "Severe Maternal Hemorrhage."

Dosage

The dosage of cryoprecipitate is calculated on the basis of the amount of fibrinogen present in 1 unit of cryoprecipitate, the plasma volume, and the desired increment. The difficulty in determining the correct amount to administer is primarily caused by variability in the fibrinogen content of cryoprecipitate, secondary by variability in donors and component processing and preparation. The goal of therapy should be to maintain the measured fibrinogen at greater than 100 mL/dL, although increasing studies and some consensus recommendations

Severe Maternal Hemorrhage

Major obstetric hemorrhage is a leading cause of maternal morbidity and mortality, and is preventable and/or treatable. Significant obstetric hemorrhage is defined as active bleeding >1000 mL within the 24 hours following birth that continues despite the use of initial measures including first-line uterotonic agents and uterine massage. Early assessment and aggressive treatment of postpartum hemorrhage (PPH) are important for reducing morbidity and mortality rates. A critical first step in managing PPH is rapid recognition that clinically significant bleeding has occurred, with effective communication of the situation to the appropriate team members, both clinical and laboratory staff. Subsequent measures include immediate resuscitation with definitive action to arrest the bleeding (obstetric, surgical, and/or hematologic) and ongoing assessment and monitoring of the response to treatment. In these cases, blood ordering protocols specific to obstetric patients may be helpful. A massive transfusion protocol, similar to that seen in acute trauma patients ensures sustained availability of blood products while the bleeding remains uncontrolled. Unique to maternal hemorrhage, hypofibrinogenemia is an important predictor for the later development of severe bleeding. Consequently, point-of-care technologies, such as thromboelastography and rotational thromboelastometry, in addition to fibrinogen levels can identify decreased fibrin clot quality during PPH, which correlate with low fibrinogen levels and can assist in transfusion management. Early administration of 1 to 2 g tranexamic acid is also recommended, followed by an additional dose in cases of ongoing bleeding. Early fibrinogen replacement using an appropriate dose of cryoprecipitate may also be beneficial in these cases.

---

have revised target levels to at least 150 to 200 mg/dL, or a TEG Maximum clot firmness (MCF) reading of 6 to 8 mm. It is estimated that a dose of 8 to 10 units of cryoprecipitate will increase the fibrinogen in a 70 kg adult by 50 to 70 mg/dL, but how this dose affects a TEG is unclear. Dosing frequency should be determined based on clinical and laboratory responses, as factor XIII and fibrinogen are very stable proteins. Specifically, the half-life of fibrinogen is 4 days, and factor XIII has a half-life of 9 days.

Compatibility

Cryoprecipitate can contain minimal anti-A and/or anti-B antibodies and, as such, ABO and D compatibility is not necessary for most adult and pediatric patients.

Adverse Events

Cryoprecipitate has similar adverse event risk as other blood products, including transfusion-transmitted diseases, hemolytic reactions and allergic reactions. Since it contains less plasma and no leukocytes, febrile and allergic reactions are less likely to occur.

ALBUMIN

Albumin, an important plasma protein, contributes primarily to the maintenance of plasma colloid oncotic pressure; it is also involved in the transport of numerous substances, such as unconjugated bilirubin, various hormones, and drugs. Albumin also has an established role in acid-base function, free radical scavenging, is antiapoptotic, antithrombotic, and has positive and negative effects on vascular integrity. The human body content of albumin is 4 to 5 g/kg, and is responsible for 80% of the osmotic pressure of human plasma. Albumin is clinically available in four forms: 5% solution in saline; 25% solution in distilled water; albumin conjugated with polyethylene glycol; and purified protein fraction, which is 5% total protein (88% albumin and 12% globulins). These products are heat-treated and albumin has not been documented to transmit infectious diseases (single outbreak occurred with albumin transfusion-associated hepatitis B with purified protein fraction in 1973).

TABLE 115.3	Administration of Albumin

Indicated
After large-volume paracentesis
Nephrotic syndrome resistant to potent diuretics
Ovarian hyperstimulation syndrome
Volume/fluid replacement in plasmapheresis

Possibly Indicated
Adult respiratory distress syndrome
Cardiopulmonary bypass pump priming
Fluid resuscitation in shock/sepsis/burns
Neonatal kernicterus/hyperbilirubinemia
To reduce enteral feeding intolerance

Not Indicated
Correction of measured hypoalbuminemia or hypoproteinemia
Nutritional deficiency, total parenteral nutrition
Preeclampsia
Red blood cell suspension
Simple volume expansion (surgery, burns)
Wound healing

Investigational
Cadaveric renal transplantation
Cerebral ischemia
Stroke

Common Usages
Cardiopulmonary bypass, pump priming
Extensive burns
Hypotension
Intraoperative fluid requirement exceeding 5–6 L in adults
Labile pulmonary, cardiovascular status
Liver disease, hypoalbuminemia, diuresis
Nephrotic syndrome, proteinuria, and hypoalbuminemia
Plasma exchange
Premature infant undergoing major surgery
Protein-losing enteropathy, hypoalbuminemia
Resuscitation
Serum albumin <20 g/dL

Indications

A decrease in measured plasma albumin is found in many situations, including chronic liver disease, chronic renal failure, sepsis, malignancy, burns, critical illness, severe head trauma, and hemorrhage, and is often, in itself, not a clinically significant concern. Mild edema arising from hypoalbuminemia does not require albumin therapy. However, inadequate synthesis, as seen in severe liver disease and severe malnutrition, or excessive loss, as seen in nephrotic syndrome and protein-losing enteropathy, can lead to significant hypoalbuminemia with intravascular volume depletion, anasarca, ascites, and pleural effusions. Hypoalbuminemia is associated with poor clinical outcome in some studies, yet correction of low serum albumin levels in critically ill patients does not improve outcome measures such as mortality, duration of intensive care unit (ICU) and hospital stay, or mechanic ventilation. Historically, albumin had a broader use (i.e., nutritional support, correction of hypoalbuminemia, volume replacement), but recent studies support its benefit in fewer situations, including nephrotic syndrome resistant to potent diuretic therapy, after large-volume paracentesis, and in ovarian hyperstimulation syndrome (OHSS) (Table 115.3).

Intravascular Volume Expansion

As noted, albumin provides the majority of plasma colloid oncotic pressure. Infused albumin provides colloid oncotic pressure; however, 50% of the infused protein is lost to the extravascular fluid compartment within 4 hours. Crystalloid may also provide volume expansion and is more quickly redistributed into total body fluids. Studies investigating the use of albumin in various situations including volume expansion during and after surgery, as priming solution in cardiopulmonary bypass, or in maintaining colloid oncotic pressure, found no clinical benefit compared with controls. In 1998, the Cochrane Injuries Group performed a systematic review of randomized control trials in albumin treatment of critically ill patients and concluded that there was no evidence that albumin use for volume expansion reduces mortality in patients. They also suggested that albumin increases mortality, but this conclusion was not confirmed in later randomized control trials or subsequent metaanalyses. The SAFE trial found in 6997 patients across 16 ICUs that there was no difference in survival between those ICU patients who received albumin versus normal saline. In another randomized study, the SAFE trial investigators found that albumin use was associated with a trend toward better outcomes in patients with severe sepsis 2-year postrandomization. A smaller prospective study further revealed that albumin was at least equivalent to plasma in clinical endpoints (perioperative/postoperative RBC transfusions, postoperative blood loss, duration of ICU stay, major complications) as a plasma expander in the context of pediatric craniofacial surgeries. One conclusion from these prospective randomized trials is, contrary to previous reports, the use of albumin is at least clinically equivalent to saline or plasma for intravascular volume resuscitation in some clinical settings. Moreover, the Italian Society of Transfusion Medicine and Immunohematology recently recommended that albumin may be useful for hypovolemia in some patients with hemorrhagic shock, patients undergoing major surgery, such as cardiac surgery, patients with severe burns, and patients postliver transplant when crystalloids and other colloids did not provide adequate clinical benefit.

Hypoalbuminemia

Low serum albumin is an independent predictor of morbidity and mortality in many clinical settings. However, correction of low serum albumin levels in ill patients does not improve outcome measures such as mortality. However, two randomized controlled studies showed that correction of hypoalbuminemia did improve respiratory, cardiovascular, and central nervous system function. Current guidelines support the use of albumin to correct hypoalbuminemia for patients with ascites, large volume paracentesis, hepatorenal syndrome, and spontaneous bacterial peritonitis. Recent studies with albumin infusions have also been done in end-stage liver disease patients for hypoalbuminemia. However, results are less encouraging, with studies indicating no additional benefits or reduction in morbidity.

Cirrhosis

The use of albumin in cirrhotic patients dates to before 1950. In this setting, albumin was recommended for temporary improvement in hyponatremia, spontaneous bacterial peritonitis, or prevention of the complications associated with paracentesis, including volume shifts and hyponatremia, as noted earlier. Several studies demonstrated that after large-volume paracentesis (>5 L), hyponatremia and renal insufficiency were improved with albumin infusion compared with other volume-expanding agents. Moreover, a single randomized control trial of albumin use in cirrhotic patients with spontaneous bacterial peritonitis revealed that albumin administration with antibiotics resulted in reduced mortality and a reduced risk of renal failure in comparison with antibiotic use alone.

Nephrotic Syndrome

Albumin has been used to increase colloid oncotic pressure with the intention of increasing diuresis via increasing vascular pressure at the level of the glomerulus. Several studies have shown that albumin use

in this context have resulted in no clinical benefit. However, other studies have suggested that albumin use is associated with increased hypertension, respiratory distress, and electrolyte abnormalities. Consequently, the current recommended use of albumin for nephrotic syndrome patients is limited to patients in whom diuretic therapy is poorly tolerated or ineffective or in those with massive ascites or anasarca.

Ovarian Hyperstimulation Syndrome

OHSS is usually a result of iatrogenic administration of human chorionic gonadotrophin (hCG) to induce ovulation. OHSS is typified by enlarged ovaries which release vascular endothelial growth factor that can result in increased capillary permeability. This, in turn, leads to a fluid shift out of the intravascular compartment to the abdominal/pleural spaces resulting in ascites and hypovolemia. In the most severe form, the patient can develop tense ascites, oliguria, dyspnea, hemodynamic instability, and thromboembolism. Treatment includes fluid restriction, analgesics, and close monitoring; occasionally hospitalization may be necessary.

Mild OHSS occurs in approximately one-third and moderate-severe in approximately 5% of women receiving exogenous hCG. Increased risk of OHSS includes young age, low body weight, polycystic ovarian syndrome, high dose hCG, high or rapid rise in estradiol level, and previous history of OHSS. In addition, the risk is proportional to the number of developing follicles and number of oocytes retrieved. Moderate-severe OHSS can be mitigated by closely monitoring women during treatment and subsequently withholding or reducing hCG administration when there is a large number of intermediate size developing follicles present or when estradiol levels are elevated.

In 2011, the Cochrane collaboration systematically reviewed eight randomized clinical trials of albumin administration in OHSS, and concluded that there is only a borderline statistically significant decrease in the incidence and severity of OHSS when albumin was administered during oocyte retrieval in high-risk women. In contrast, the metaanalysis further revealed that the use of hydroxyethyl starch (HES) resulted in a markedly decreased incidence of severe OHSS. In addition, Bellver et al. published a large randomized trial that demonstrated no difference in moderate-severe OHSS when 40 g of albumin was administered after the retrieval of 20 or more oocytes. Only one (nonrandomized) study to date has compared human albumin and 6% HES. This study concluded in 16 patients with severe OHSS that patients who received HES had a higher urine output, needed less abdominal paracentesis and drainage of pleural effusions, and had a shortened hospital stay than patients who received albumin. Therefore, while still clinically used, albumin may be inferior to other therapies in the prevention of OHSS.

Therapeutic Apheresis

Albumin is the replacement fluid of choice for many apheresis indications. Albumin reduces the risk of adverse events during apheresis procedures by reducing the risk of viral transmission, allergic reactions, and TRALI in comparison to plasma use (see plasma section). Albumin can also be used in combination with saline during apheresis procedures, but excessive use of saline results in hypotensive reactions. Albumin is also indicated if large (>15% of the total blood volume) blood volumes are removed to prevent hypotensive reactions in other therapeutic apheresis procedures (leukapheresis, plateletpheresis).

While albumin is generally well tolerated in therapeutic apheresis patients, albumin use can result in significant hypotension, bradycardia, and flushing in patients receiving angiotensin converting enzyme inhibitor (ACE) therapy. ACE inhibitors prevent the patient's ability to metabolize bradykinins that are present in the albumin and activated during the apheresis procedure. In patients taking ACE inhibitors, symptoms can be prevented by using plasma, or halting ACE inhibitor use and delaying the start of apheresis therapy.

Emerging Indications

Serum albumin has been shown to be a free radical scavenger. Because of this function, some have recommended albumin as an adjuvant therapy in patients with sepsis. There are no confirmed data on the benefits of albumin therapy in this patient population, however. In other conditions associated with systemic inflammation such as acute lung injury or acute respiratory distress syndrome, albumin therapy use was found to improve oxygenation and hemodynamic status.

Dose

The volume and speed of administration should be determined by the patient's volume status, condition, and response to the product. In an adult, the total daily dose should not exceed the theoretical amount present in normal plasma (2g/kg/day), in the absence of acute hemorrhage. In the pediatric population, albumin dose again depends on the patient's condition, but 0.5 to 1.0 g/kg/dose with a maximum dose of 6 g/kg/day could be used as a general guideline. Albumin 5% is oncotically equivalent to normal human plasma. Albumin 25% provides less infusion volume per amount of albumin and is usually administered to patients with fluid or sodium intake restriction. Albumin 25% expands the blood volume by 3.5 times by drawing fluid into the intravascular space.

Adverse Effects

Albumin is a plasma derivative used widely and associated with rare adverse reactions. Allergic reactions, including urticaria, may be encountered. Changes in vital signs (heart rate, blood pressure, respiration rate), nausea, emesis, and fever/chills have also been rarely reported. Volume overload and dilutional anemia as well as hypocalcemia may occur. Albumin has not been associated with transfusion-transmitted diseases.

INTRAVENOUS IMMUNOGLOBULIN

IVIg is prepared by fractionation of large pools of human plasma. There are numerous preparations available in the United States and throughout the world. Subcutaneous preparations of Ig are also now available. Each preparation is slightly different and has theoretic advantages and disadvantages and specific licensed indications. Ideally, IVIg should contain each IgG subclass; retain Fc receptor activity; have a normal half-life; demonstrate virus neutralization, opsonization, and intracellular killing; and have antibacterial capsular polysaccharide antibody. Furthermore, vasoactive impurities should be absent, and no transmissible infectious agents should be present. The uses of IVIg have been extensively reviewed and the number of theoretical and accepted uses for IVIg is rapidly expanding.

Indications

IVIg is indicated for replacement of Igs or for its immunomodulatory effects. Currently, there are six FDA approved indications for IVIg treatment: primary immunodeficiency, pediatric HIV infections, secondary immunodeficiency in chronic lymphocytic leukemia (CLL), idiopathic thrombocytopenic purpura (ITP), Kawasaki disease, and allogeneic stem cell transplantation in patients older than 20 years of age. Some of the FDA indications are no longer applicable, such as in patients with CLL and HIV, given better medications. IVIg is also considered first-line therapy for multiple other conditions, such as Guillain-Barré syndrome, chronic inflammatory demyelinating polyradiculoneuropathy (CIDP), neonatal alloimmune thrombocytopenia (NAIT), posttransfusion purpura (PTP), myasthenia gravis and stiff-person syndrome (Table 115.4). An exhaustive review of all the known established and investigational uses for IVIg cannot be

reasonably summarized in this chapter. For further information, some excellent reviews are cited in the reference section. A brief summary of some of the more well-established uses of IVIg are presented in the following section.

Primary Immunodeficiency Syndromes

Primary congenital immunodeficiency syndromes have been treated with intramuscular Ig for the past 30 years. The use of intramuscular Ig has certain disadvantages: delayed absorption, delivery of inadequate amounts because of small muscle mass, and pain at the injection site. IVIg overcomes these disadvantages, and used prophylactically in patients with primary immunodeficiency has been demonstrated to reduce the number of febrile and infectious episodes as well as improve survival rate. IVIg use in IgG subclass deficiencies is also beneficial.

Chronic Lymphocytic Leukemia

CLL may be associated with hypogammaglobulinemia and complications of repeated bacterial infections. IVIg decreases the incidence and severity of bacterial infections in CLL patients with hypogammaglobulinemia and has become accepted prophylactic therapy.

Bone Marrow Transplantation

The use of prophylactic IVIg or cytomegalovirus (CMV)–IVIg in CMV-negative bone marrow transplant recipients during the first 100 days posttransplant has been demonstrated to reduce the incidence of symptomatic CMV-associated disease, including CMV interstitial pneumonia, in some trials. Because of the high cost of this treatment and the increasing use of prophylactic ganciclovir, IVIg is currently not indicated for the prophylaxis of CMV infections in bone marrow transplant recipients. In established CMV-interstitial pneumonia, IVIg in combination with ganciclovir has been shown to reduce the mortality rate and has become the recommended treatment modality. Its role in preventing severe graft-versus-host disease is unclear. Prolonged IVIg therapy during graft-versus-host disease prevention may suppress humoral immunity recovery.

Pediatric Human Immunodeficiency Virus Infection

The defects in humoral and cellular immunity observed in children with HIV infection predispose them to life-threatening bacterial infections. Studies previously demonstrated that the administration of IVIg to HIV-infected children could reduce the incidence and severity of bacterial infections as well as the frequency of hospitalization. More recently, studies have now shown that IVIg does not improve outcome, likely because of improved medications for HIV and HIV-associated infections.

Idiopathic Thrombocytopenic Purpura

IVIg and Rh immune globulin are routinely and effectively used in the treatment of acute and chronic ITP. IVIg significantly raises the platelet count within 5 days in adults with chronic ITP and in children with acute ITP. The mechanism of action of IVIg in ITP is unknown; one postulation is Fc receptor blockade decreases the removal of antibody-coated platelets. Other proposed mechanisms include suppressed antiplatelet antibody synthesis, increased antiviral immunity, and blockage by antiidiotypic antibodies. In general, IVIg induces responses in most patients within 1 to 2 days. Responses are of variable duration and are rarely sustained, although maintenance therapy may be of some value. IVIg may be effective in chronic ITP refractory to corticosteroids or splenectomy; and may show greater efficacy in conjunction with corticosteroids.

TABLE 115.4   Administration of Intravenous Immunoglobulins

Indicated

Ataxia-telangiectasia
Chronic inflammatory demyelinating polyneuropathy
Chronic lymphocytic leukemia
Common variable immunodeficiency
Cytomegalovirus-interstitial pneumonia after bone marrow transplantation
Guillain–Barré syndrome
Graft-versus-host disease after bone marrow transplantation
Hemolytic disease of the fetus and newborn
Idiopathic thrombocytopenic purpura
Immunoglobulin G subclass deficiency
Inflammatory myopathies (refractory dermatomyositis and polymyositis)
Myasthenia gravis
Mucocutaneous lymph node syndrome (Kawasaki disease)
Neonatal alloimmune thrombocytopenia
Parvovirus infection
Pediatric human immunodeficiency virus infection
Persistent deficit in antibody production after bone marrow transplantation
Posttransfusion purpura
Primary immunodeficiency syndromes
Secondary hypogammaglobulinemia
Severe combined immunodeficiency
Stiff-person syndrome
Wiskott-Aldrich syndrome
X-linked agammaglobulinemia

Possibly Indicated

Antiphospholipid syndrome in pregnancy
Autoimmune hemolytic anemia (warm type unresponsive to prednisone)
Factor VIII inhibitors (refractory)
Graves ophthalmopathy
Immune neutropenia
Multiple myeloma (stable disease, high risk for infections)
Pemphigus

Solid organ transplantation (kidney)
Systemic lupus erythematosus (refractory, severe, active)
Thrombocytopenia refractory to platelet transfusion
Vasculitis (refractory to standard therapy)

Investigational

Acquired von Willebrand disease
Amyotrophic lateral sclerosis
Burn patients
Chronic fatigue syndrome
Chronic human parvovirus B19 infection
Chronic idiopathic pericarditis
Chronic pain syndromes
Congestive heart failure
Dilated cardiomyopathy
Graft-versus-host disease
Human immunodeficiency virus infection
Immune-mediated aplastic anemia
Inflammatory bowel disease
Intractable childhood epilepsy
Multiple sclerosis
Myocarditis
Necrotizing fasciitis
Neonatal sepsis
Neonatal hemochromatosis
Postpartum cardiomyopathy
Prevention of nosocomial postoperative infections
Prophylaxis in transplant recipients against cytomegalovirus infection
Recurrent unexplained spontaneous abortions
Rheumatoid arthritis
Sepsis and septic shock
Toxic epidermal necrolysis/Stevens-Johnson syndrome
Toxic shock syndrome

Although IVIg has shown equal efficacy with corticosteroids in pediatric acute ITP and in 75% of adults with chronic ITP, because of the transient responses and high cost, its use is justified only in clinical situations requiring rapid elevation of platelet count or if standard therapy has failed. IVIg is, therefore, indicated in acute bleeding episodes or before urgent surgery, including splenectomy; in patients at high risk of intracranial hemorrhage; and in those in whom corticosteroids are contraindicated or ineffective. IVIg has also been used to treat ITP during pregnancy, postinfectious thrombocytopenia, ITP associated with HIV infection, and neonatal thrombocytopenia. Intravenous anti-D immune globulin (also known as Rh immune globulin) has demonstrated efficacy in Rh-positive, nonsplenecto-mized individuals with ITP. It has been suggested that the mechanism of action may involve a shift in the immune-mediated destruction from platelets to the antibody-coated RBCs (Chapter 131).

Kawasaki Disease

The mucocutaneous lymph node syndrome (Kawasaki disease) has been treated with aspirin with or without concomitant IVIg admin-istration. Coronary artery aneurysm, a serious complication of this disease, was significantly reduced in the IVIg-treated group. However, in a multicenter retrospective survey of all children treated with Kawasaki disease, persistent or recrudescent fever after their first course of IVIg was associated with a statistically significant risk of treatment failure. Furthermore, IVIg retreatment in those patients with persistent fever after IVIg treatment failure was approximately 60%. Current randomized trials are now being done to compare the efficacy of newer, and perhaps better, therapies, such as infliximab (anti-tumor necrosis factor α). To date, these randomized control

studies show that infliximab is at least as safe and as efficacious as IVIg in these refractory patients. One retrospective review has even suggested that infliximab might result in faster resolution of fever and fewer days of hospitalization in comparison with IVIg. While studies are still ongoing, IVIg may soon be replaced by alternative therapies in this refractory patient population.

With regard to the pathogenesis of Kawasaki disease, decreased peripheral blood lymphocyte apoptosis has been demonstrated. Therefore, the effect of IVIg in Kawasaki disease has been postulated to partially reverse inhibited lymphocyte apoptosis.

Solid Organ Transplantation

The presence of high-titer reactive antibodies against incompatible graft HLA or ABO antigens increases the risk of early solid organ, antibody-mediated, graft rejection and mortality, especially in kidney and cardiac transplants. For some patients who have HLA antibodies to undergo transplantation, these antibodies must be removed or decreased. While morbidity and mortality can be reduced by selecting an adequately cross-matched donor, IVIg with or without plasma exchange has also been shown to decrease sensitization of incompat-ible antigens in patients awaiting renal and cardiac transplantations. In addition, IVIg with or without plasma exchange is used in the treatment of biopsy-proven antibody-mediated rejection. One review discussed three randomized control trials which investigated the use of IVIg for renal transplantation and revealed a trend in improvement in desensitization rates and a statistically significant decrease in time to transplant for patients treated with IVIg, superior graft survival rate in kidney transplant patients desensitized with IVIg, and a lower rate of recurrent acute rejection with IVIg in comparison to OKT3 (murine monoclonal antibody to CD3 antigen of human T cells). Consequently, current consensus renal transplant guidelines indicate IVIg is a useful treatment modality for desensitization of patients with HLA antibodies and in patients with acute rejection.

Randomized trials have not yet been performed for ABO incompatible kidney transplants, heart, liver, or lung transplants. Moreover, there is a paucity of data for transplant outcomes, and current studies have small numbers without data on donor specific antibody levels. Current guidelines assert that there is insufficient evidence to make a recommendation for or against the routine use of IVIg for desensitization in these transplants.

Aplastic Anemia Secondary to Parvovirus

Parvovirus B19 infection can result in severe anemia and reticulocytopenia, especially in immunocompromised individuals or individuals with sickle cell disease or thalassemia, and the use of IVIg is considered first-line therapy in the treatment of these patients (typical dose 0.5 g/kg weekly for 4 weeks).

Chronic Inflammatory Demyelinating Polyradiculoneuropathy

CIDP is a chronic disorder resulting in demyelination of peripheral nerves that result in weakness and sensory changes. Equivalent outcomes have been observed in the treatment of CIDP with IVIg (reported dose 400 mg/kg/day for 5 days, once each month, or 1 g/kg/day for 2 days, once each month), TPE, or glucocorticosteroids. The decision as to which treatment to use is made on an individual basis balancing the risks and benefits of each treatment modality.

Dermatomyositis

Dermatomyositis is a chronic inflammatory disorder that results in progressive weakness and rash. IVIg (typical dose 2.0 g/kg per month administered over 2–5 days) results in improved muscle strength and neuromuscular symptoms.

Guillain-Barré Syndrome (Acute Inflammatory Demyelinating Polyneuropathy)

Guillain-Barré syndrome is an acute demyelinating peripheral neuropathy affecting both motor and sensory nerves. IVIg (typical dose 400 mg/kg/day for 5 days or 1.0 g/kg/day for 2 days or 2.0 g/kg as a single dose) is likely equivalent to TPE in improving disability and shortening the time to improvement.

Hypogammaglobulinemia Associated With Multiple Myeloma

Multiple myeloma is a monoclonal B-cell (plasma cell) disorder with clinical symptoms arising as a result of plasma cell infiltration of the bone marrow, monoclonal Ig in the blood and urine, and immunosuppression. IVIg has shown to be beneficial in preventing serious infections in plateau-phase multiple myeloma or other hematologic malignancy, where the patients have hypogammaglobinemia, at doses of 0.4 g/kg every 4 weeks, with subsequent dosing adjusted based on trough levels.

IgM Paraproteinemic Demyelinating Neuropathy

Paraproteinemic demyelinating neuropathy is a chronic disorder resulting in decreased sensory and motor function, similar to CIDP,

in association with monoclonal Igs. One placebo-controlled trial demonstrated that IVIg may improve short-term morbidity, but the remainder of the available evidence is mixed. The use of IVIg for this condition has recently fallen out of favor with current consensus groups.

Inclusion Body Myositis

Inclusion body myositis is an inflammatory myopathy resulting in chronic muscular weakness. Randomized trials using IVIg appear to result in short-term improvement in strength scores and improved swallowing in patients with inclusion body myositis, and are equivalent to treatment with glucocorticosteroids in one small clinical study. The use of IVIg for this condition has also recently fallen out of favor with current consensus groups because of the lack of known sustained benefit for patients with this condition.

Lambert-Eaton Myasthenic Syndrome

Lambert-Eaton myasthenic syndrome results from antibodies to the neuromuscular junction, leading to autonomic dysfunction. One randomized control trial reveals that IVIg significantly improves generalized central and peripheral muscle strength and decreases serum calcium channel antibody titers. A total dose of 2.0 g/kg given over 2 to 5 days is a recommended initial treatment.

Multifocal Motor Neuropathy

Multifocal motor neuropathy is a chronic progressive disorder resulting in primarily hand weakness. IVIg is now considered a first-line treatment for this condition, and improved strength can be seen at a dose of 2.0 g/kg over 2 to 5 days.

Multiple Sclerosis

Multiple sclerosis is a chronic progressive or relapsing and remitting disorder characterized by brain white mater demyelination. There are two published metaanalyses, and several randomized controlled clinical trials in patients with relapsing-remitting multiple sclerosis using a wide range of IVIg doses that demonstrate the success of IVIg in reducing the number of exacerbations and disability in patients with relapsing-remitting multiple sclerosis in comparison with placebo. However, no studies to date have compared IVIg with standard therapies, and one clinical trial (PRIVIG trial) has raised doubt that IVIg is effective as a routine treatment. Consequently, IVIg is considered a viable second-line option for those patients who fail, decline, or are unable to tolerate standard immunomodulatory therapies such as β-interferon and glatiramer acetate.

Myasthenia Gravis

Myasthenia gravis is a chronic neurologic autoimmune disorder characterized by weakness and fatigue upon repetitive skeletal muscle use, which improves with rest. IVIg has been used successfully as a short-term measure for acute severe exacerbations of myasthenia gravis at a dose of 2.0 g/kg given over 2 to 5 days, and appears comparable with TPE. A definitive randomized control trial comparing the two treatment modalities has not been done, however.

Neonatal Alloimmune Thrombocytopenia

NAIT is a rare condition that results from maternal platelet alloantibodies against the fetal/neonatal platelets resulting in neonatal/fetal thrombocytopenia. Studies evaluating the use of IVIg for NAIT are limited, but unlikely to improve because of the rarity of the condition. The treatment of NAIT during pregnancy is maternal administration of 1.0 g/kg IVIg weekly as a first-line therapy beginning at 20 weeks of gestational age with the use of glucocorticosteroids, or 2.0 g/kg weekly if steroids are not used. Once at 32 weeks of gestation, the IVIg dose is increased to 2.0 g/kg weekly with corticosteroids. Moreover, the neonate may need to receive IVIg and platelet transfusions after delivery to increase fetal platelet counts to prevent intracerebral hemorrhage at a dose of 1.0 g/kg (Chapter 131).

Hemolytic Disease of the Fetus and Newborn

Hemolytic Disease of the Fetus and Newborn (HDFN) results from maternal RBC alloantibodies binding to fetal/neonatal RBCs and may result in hemolysis, leading to anemia or hydrops fetalis and death depending on the severity. Two metaanalyses reveal that IVIg significantly reduces the need for exchange transfusions in patients with HDFN. IVIg is now consequently recommended at a dose of 0.5 to 1.0 g/kg to treat newborns with HDFN if there is established jaundice and a rising total serum bilirubin despite phototherapy. In addition, maternal IVIg infusion (with or without therapeutic plasma exchange) has been used in severe cases of HDFN where treatment must occur before the ability to perform intrauterine transfusions.

Posttransfusion Purpura

PTP is a rare complication of transfusion resulting in acute, profound thrombocytopenia, secondary to platelet antibodies that destroy both transfused and autologous platelets. While the evidence evaluating the effect of IVIg in these patients is limited to multiple case reports, the available evidence suggests that IVIg should be a first-line therapy for this condition. PTP treatment with IVIg at a dose of 2 g/kg over 2 days or 0.4–0.5 g/kg daily for 5 days can result in a rapid increase in platelet count.

Sepsis and Septic Shock in Adults

The use of IVIg in adult patients with bacterial sepsis or septic shock is potentially beneficial. One randomized control trial reveled that in ICU patients with intraabdominal sepsis and shock, IVIg with antibiotics was superior to antibiotics with albumin in improving patient survival. Encouraging results have also been identified in patients receiving IVIg for streptococcal toxic shock syndrome, but further studies are currently needed.

Stiff-Person Syndrome

Stiff-person syndrome is a neurologic disorder associated with truncal and limb rigidity and heightened sensitivity. One small randomized control trial suggests that IVIg could play a positive role in improving stiffness and sensitivity symptoms. Currently, IVIg is considered a second-line therapy for those who fail or cannot tolerate GABA (glutamic acid decarboxylase)-ergic medications. A dose of 2.0 g/kg given over 2 to 5 days is the current recommended starting dose.

Dosage

The dosage and frequency for IVIg varies significantly depending on the age of the patient and the clinical indication. Many typical dosages were described in the preceding section. In general, patients require 200 to 800 mg/kg intravenously every 3 to 4 weeks to achieve adequate IgG levels if immunodeficient (usually 500 mg/dL) and

needing protection against infection. Initially, serial IgG level determination may allow the physician to individualize the dose and schedule. These are affected by the recovery, half-life, redistribution, and catabolism of IVIg, which vary from product to product and patient to patient. Patients with ITP are usually initially treated with 400 to 1000 mg/kg daily for 2 to 5 consecutive days with a maximum dose of 2.0 g/kg. Maintenance doses of 400 to 1000 mg/kg/dose every 3 to 6 weeks is recommended in some patients (particularly children) based on clinical response and platelet count. Kawasaki disease is treated with 2.0 g/kg as a single dose in combination with aspirin. Currently, direct comparisons between different IVIg formulations or brands are lacking, and so evidence-based recommendations cannot be made along these lines.

Adverse Effects

Infusions of IVIg should be started slowly and patients should be closely monitored. If the initial rate (0.5 mL/kg/h) is well tolerated, the rate can be increased gradually, but not more than eightfold. That said, initial and maximum infusion rates vary by IVIg product, and product inserts should be consulted prior to selecting an appropriate infusion rate. Fever, headache, nausea, vomiting, fatigue, backache, leg cramps, urticaria, flushing, elevation of blood pressure, and thrombophlebitis may be seen. Adverse events have been reported in 2% to 10% of infusions. IgA-deficient patients may have IgG anti-IgA antibodies, which can cause anaphylactic reactions. This complication is rare and may be avoided by using products with a lower concentration of IgA. Aggregated IgG may produce chills, nausea, flushing, chest tightness, and wheezing. Rarely, IVIg preparations contain RBC antibodies that can produce hemolysis or interfere with serologic evaluations, including RBC compatibility testing. IVIg treatment will produce a false positive direct antiglobulin test, and sometimes positive hepatitis and CMV serologies. Serum sickness can also occur. Lastly, high-dose IVIg therapy has been associated with thrombosis, reversible acute renal failure, TRALI, and aseptic meningitis. Improved manufacturing processes currently in place render IVIg free of enveloped and nonenveloped viruses.

HYPERIMMUNE IMMUNOGLOBULIN PRODUCTS

Hyperimmune globulins are concentrated immune globulins with specificity for an antigen, or group of antigens. These products are manufactured in a similar manner to that used for IVIg product production. However, donors for these specific products are unique in that they have high titers for the Ig specificity of interest. The donor high titers can be achieved via natural immunity, prophylactic immunization, or target immunization, depending on the antibody of interest. These products are generally used to provide passive immunity for a variety of conditions that are described in more detail in the following sections (Table 115.5).

TABLE 115.5	Hyperimmune and Intramuscular Immunoglobulins

Antithymocyte globulin
Botulism immunoglobulin
Cytomegalovirus immunoglobulin
Hepatitis A immunoglobulin
Hepatitis B immunoglobulin
Rabies immunoglobulin
Respiratory syncytial virus immunoglobulin
Rh(D) immunoglobulin
Tetanus immunoglobulin
Vaccinia immunoglobulin
Varicella-zoster immunoglobulin
Western equine encephalitis immunoglobulin

Antithymocyte Globulin

Antithymocyte globulin is a purified concentrated globulin made from hyperimmune serum of horses immunized with human T lymphocytes. Antithymocyte globulin is used in renal transplant patients as an adjunct therapy in the treatment of graft rejection. It is also used in patients with aplastic anemia who are not candidates for bone marrow transplantation.

Hyperimmune Immunoglobulin

Hyperimmune globulin is used to prevent the development of specific clinical disease or alter its symptomatology. Hepatitis B Ig is used to provide passive immunity to hepatitis B virus associated with needle stick exposure or sexual contact with hepatitis B surface antigen-positive individuals, postliver transplantation for prevention of recurrence, and prevention of hepatitis B vertical transmission. Other hyperimmunoglobulins include botulism, CMV, hepatitis A, rabies, respiratory syncytial virus, tetanus, vaccinia, and varicella-zoster virus Igs.

Rh Immunoglobulin

Rh Ig has two primary indications: prevention of D antigen alloimmunization and treatment of ITP. Rh Ig is given to D-negative mothers after potential exposure to fetal D-positive RBCs, such as after abortion or amniocentesis, as well as at 28-weeks gestational age, and postpartum if the child proves to be D positive. The therapeutic effect is thought to be caused by antibody feedback with T-cell suppression of the B-cell clone responsible for the formation of anti-D antibody. Rh Ig can also be given to prevent immunization in D-negative individuals given D-positive blood products, such as platelets.

Rh Ig is dosed to adequately prevent D immunization. In the United States, 300 µg are administered after event resulting in maternal-fetal hemorrhage, 28 weeks and postpartum. Doses are increased for evidence of large maternal-fetal hemorrhage (300 µg for every 15 mL of RBC exposure). This dosing is also used in the prevention of D alloimmunization after receipt of RBC containing blood product. Rh Ig should be given within 72 hours after RBC exposure. Adverse events to low doses, such as those used to prevent D immunization include fever, chills, and pain at the injection site. Rarely, hypersensitivity reactions are noted. See box "Weak, Partial D, and Rh Ig Use" for more information.

Weak, Partial D, and Rh Ig Use

Clinically significant D sensitization potentially results in a pregnancy with a fetus at risk for hemolytic disease of the fetus and newborn and hemolytic transfusion reactions if transfused with D-positive red blood cells. In rare cases, as a result of a mutation in the *D* gene, a person may have amino acid substitutions affecting a part of the normal D protein that changes the antigen on the external aspect of the red cell. These patients are described as having "partial D." When someone with partial D is exposed to blood from someone with a normal form of D, they may make an antibody against the portions of the D antigen that they lack. Individuals with red blood cells that express a partial D antigen are thus at risk for D-sensitization and may benefit from Rh Ig administration to prevent D sensitization. Mutations which result in fewer "normal" D antigens on a red cell are known as having a "weak" D. Those with weak D antigens are usually not at risk for D sensitization because they have a normal D protein, and thus do not require Rh Ig administration. Partial and weak D antigens cannot be distinguished by serologic reactivity, because either may present as weak, moderately, or strongly positive or give variable results with anti-D reagents. Particularly in the prenatal setting, RhD genotyping can be done to distinguish weak D from partial D to help determine need for Rh Ig administration.

Rh Ig doses are substantially higher for the treatment of ITP: 50 µg/kg for hemoglobin ≥10 L/dL and 25 to 40 µg/kg when hemoglobin is 8 to 10 g/dL. Rh Ig use in ITP is indicated in D-positive patients with intact spleen. Adverse events at high doses of Rh Ig include hemolysis, DIC, and rarely death (Chapter 131).

SUGGESTED READINGS

AABB: Information piece: alternatives to transfusable single-donor plasma components. <http://www.aabb.org/programs/clinical/Documents/Alternatives-to-Transfusable-Single-Donor-Plasma-Components.pdf>, 2014.

AABB: *Standards for blood banks and transfusion services*, ed 29, Bethesda (MD), 2014, AABB.

Bellver J, Muñoz EA, Ballesteros A, et al: Intravenous albumin does not prevent moderate-severe ovarian hyperstimulation syndrome in high-risk IVF patients: a randomized controlled study. *Hum Reprod* 18:2283–2288, 2003.

Callum JL, Karkouti K, Lin Y: Cryoprecipitate: The current state of knowledge. *Transfus Med Rev* 23:177–188, 2009.

Cardigan R, Lawrie AS, Mackie IJ, et al: The quality of fresh-frozen plasma produced from whole blood stored at 4°C overnight. *Transfusion* 45:1342, 2005.

Eder AF, Sebok MA: Plasma components: FFP, FP24, and thawed plasma. *Immunohematology* 23:150–157, 2007.

Shaz BH, Hillyer CD, Roshal M, et al: *Transfusion Medicine and Hemostasis: Clinical and Laboratory Aspects*, ed 2, 2013, Elsevier.

Holcomb JB, del Junco DJ, Fox EE, et al; PROMMTT Study Group: The Prospective, Observational, Multicenter, Major Trauma Transfusion (PROMMTT) study: comparative effectiveness of a time-varying treatment with competing risks. *JAMA Surg* 148(2):127–136, 2013.

Holcomb JB, Tilley BC, Baraniuk S, et al; PROPPR Study Group: Transfusion of plasma, platelets, and red blood cells in a 1:1:1 vs a 1:1:2 ratio and mortality in patients with severe trauma: the PROPPR randomized clinical trial. *JAMA* 313(5):471–482, 2015.

Holland LL, Brooks JP: Toward rational fresh frozen plasma transfusion: The effect of plasma transfusion on coagulation test results. *Am J Clin Pathol* 126:133–139, 2006.

Ketchem L, Hess JR, Hiippala S: Indications for early fresh frozen plasma, cryoprecipitate, and platelet transfusion in trauma. *J Trauma* 60:S51, 2006.

Kor DJ, Stubbs JR, Gajic O: Perioperative coagulation management-fresh frozen plasma. *Best Prac Res Clinical Anaesthesiol* 24:51–64, 2010.

Levi M, Toh CH, Thachil J, et al: Guidelines for the diagnosis and management of disseminated intravascular coagulation. *Br J Haematol* 145:24–33, 2009.

Levy JH, Goodnough LT: How I use fibrinogen replacement therapy in acquired bleeding. *Blood* 125(9):1387–1393, 2015.

Levy JH, Welsby I, Goodnough LT: Fibrinogen as a therapeutic target for bleeding: a review of critical levels and replacement therapy. *Transfusion* 54(5):1389–1405, 2014.

Liumbruno G, Bennardello F, Lattanzio A, et al: Recommendations for the use of albumin and immunoglobulins. *Blood Transfus* 7:216–234, 2009.

Pandey S, Vyas GN: Adverse effects of plasma transfusion. *Transfusion* 52(Suppl 1):65S–79S, 2012.

Pantanowitz L, Kruskall M, Uhl L: Cryoprecipitate patterns of use. *Am J Clin Pathol* 119:874, 2003.

Roback JD, Caldwell S, Carson J, et al. American Association for the Study of Liver; American Academy of Pediatrics; United States Army; American Society of Anesthesiology; American Society of Hematology: Evidence-based practice guidelines for plasma transfusion. *Transfusion* 50:1227–1239, 2010.

Robinson P, Anderson D, Brouwers M, et al: IVIG Hematology and Neurology Expert Panels. Evidence-based guidelines on the use of IVIG for hematologic and neurologic conditions. *Transfus Med Rev* 21:S3–S8, 2007.

SAFE study investigators: A comparison of albumin and saline for fluid resuscitation in the ICU. *N Engl J Med* 350:2247–2256, 2004.

SAFE study investigators: Saline or albumin for fluid resuscitation in patients with traumatic brain injury. *N Engl J Med* 357:874–884, 2007.

Sandler SG: The status of pathogen-reduced plasma. *Transfus Apher Sci* 43:393–399, 2010.

Scott E, Puca K, Heraly J, et al: Evaluation and comparison of coagulation factor activity is fresh-frozen plasma and 24-hour plasma at thaw and after 120 hours of 1 to 6°C storage. *Transfusion* 49:1584–1591, 2009.

Shaz BH, Stowell SR, Hillyer CD: Transfusion-related acute lung injury: from bedside to bench and back. *Blood* 117:1463–1471, 2011.

Shehata N, Palda VA, Meyer RM, et al: The use of immunoglobulin therapy for patients undergoing solid organ transplantation: An evidence based practice guideline. *Transfus Med Rev* 24:S7–S27, 2010.

Spotnitz WD, Burks S: Hemostats, sealants, and adhesives II: Update as well as how and when to use the components of the surgical toolbox. *Clin Appl Thromb Hemost* 16:497, 2010.

Stanworth SJ: The evidence-based use of FFP and cryoprecipitate for abnormalities of coagulation tests and clinical coagulopathy. *Hematology* 179–186, 2007.

Stanworth SJ, Brunskill S, Hyde CJ, et al: What is the evidence base for the clinical use of FFP: a systematic review of randomized controlled trials. *Br J Haematol* 126:139–152, 2004.

Schwartz J, Padmanbhan A, Aqui N, et al: Guidelines on the use of therapeutic apheresis in clinical practice—evidence-based approach from the writing committee of the American Society for Apheresis: the Seventh Special Issue. *J Clin Apher* 31:149–162, 2016.

Theusinger OM, Goslings D, Studt JD, et al: Quarantine versus pathogen-reduced plasma-coagulation factor content and rotational thromboelastometry coagulation. *Transfusion* 2016 Epub.

Triulzi D, Gottschall J, Murphy E, et al; NHLBI Recipient Epidemiology and Donor Evaluation Study-III (REDS-III): A multicenter study of plasma use in the United States. *Transfusion* 2014. doi:10.1111/trf.12970. [Epub ahead of print].

Zielinski MD, Johnson PM, Jenkins D, et al: Emergency use of prethawed Group A plasma in trauma patients. *J Trauma Acute Care Surg* 74(1):69–74, 2013.

CHAPTER 116

PREPARATION OF PLASMA-DERIVED AND RECOMBINANT HUMAN PLASMA PROTEINS

David B. Clark

The development of large-scale methods for the preparation of human plasma proteins began more than 70 years ago, soon after the outbreak of World War II. The US Armed Forces issued an urgent request to the medical community for 300,000 units of human whole blood or plasma, which appeared to be an impossibly large amount at the time. Thinking that albumin could be used instead of plasma, Dr. Edwin J. Cohn of Harvard Medical School drew together a task force of investigators who developed methods for the fractionation of plasma based on differential precipitation of various proteins with ethanol. Although albumin was the only product distributed during the war, the remaining plasma fractions were carefully preserved, and other preparations, including fibrinogen and immunoglobulins, were soon developed. This was the beginning of the plasma fractionation industry.

PLASMA FRACTIONATION

Beginning in the post-World War II era and continuing to the present, major improvements have occurred in the preparation of human plasma protein products. Most large-scale manufacture of plasma-derived products is still based on modifications of the original method developed by Cohn's group supplemented by more selective purification techniques to produce a wide variety of products. In addition, genetic engineering technology has allowed recombinant human plasma proteins to be produced in cell culture systems and transgenic animals. This chapter describes current methods and future directions for the preparation of plasma-derived and recombinant human plasma proteins for clinical use, primarily for products available in the United States.

Plasma is estimated to contain approximately 10,000 different proteins, most of which have yet to be identified. One of the unique features of plasma fractionation is the ability to produce multiple products from a single raw material. Plasma for fractionation is derived from two sources, either directly by plasmapheresis, termed *source plasma*, or as a byproduct of whole blood donation, termed *recovered plasma*. The plasma is usually shipped frozen as individual units from local blood or plasma collection centers to a central processing plant.

At the plant, sufficient units to produce typically 2000–3000-L pools are thawed slowly at 1° to 5°C to produce cryoprecipitate, a cold-insoluble fraction that contains significant amounts of factor VIII, von Willebrand factor (vWF), fibrinogen, fibronectin, and factor XIII, along with a number of other proteins present in smaller quantities. The cryoprecipitate is usually recovered by centrifugation. The cryo-supernatant or cryo-poor plasma may be treated with a chromatographic media to capture the factor IX complex or anti-thrombin (AT) before it enters the Cohn process. There it goes through a series of precipitations as the ethanol concentration is increased in steps from 8% to 40% at specific combinations of pH, ionic strength, protein concentration, and cold temperature. The precipitates and supernatants are separated either by the traditional continuous-flow centrifugation or in large-scale filter presses. The method provides both relatively pure fractions containing albumin and immunoglobulins, which need minimal additional processing, as well as fractions enriched in other proteins, which are used as the starting materials for further purification. Fig. 116.1 shows a schematic of the ethanol process.

The first precipitate, fraction I at 8% alcohol, contains factor VIII, fibrinogen, and other poorly soluble proteins. Fractions II and III are precipitated together and contain the immunoglobulins, which are separated in a subsequent series of precipitations to produce fraction II, essentially pure immunoglobulins. Because many of the fraction I proteins are removed in the cryoprecipitate, some manufacturers do not produce a separate fraction I. Instead they collect a combined fraction I + II + III. Fraction IV, produced from the supernatant of fraction (I +) II + III, is sometimes produced in two subfractions. Fraction IV-1 contains the vitamin K–dependent (VKD) clotting factors, AT and α_1-proteinase inhibitor (API), whereas fraction IV-4 contains transferrin, haptoglobin, and some of the albumin. Fraction V is almost pure albumin.

PRODUCT SAFETY

Ensuring the safety of plasma products depends on a complex system that starts with donor selection and carries all the way through to the patient receiving the product. The system is highly redundant so that a failure in one area may be compensated for by another.

Donor Selection, Screening, and Testing

Gone are the days when anyone could be a donor, with prisons and mental hospitals providing much of the country's plasma. Plasma collection centers screen their potential donors rigorously, both for medical history and any social behaviors that might put them at risk of infection. Plasma products licensed in the United States are only produced from plasma collected from US donors in US Food and Drug Administration (FDA)–licensed establishments.

Every donation is tested for a number of different viral diseases by a battery of tests, again with redundancy. Sensitive antigen and antibody tests are followed by NAT testing (nuclear amplification or nucleic acid testing, a form of polymerase chain reaction), which can detect extremely small numbers of virus particles. Because of the "window period" between the time a donor is infected and the time antibodies or viruses can be detected in his or her plasma, most manufacturers also hold donations for at least 60 days until a donor has returned for a repeat donation. If the repeat donation still tests negative, there is a high likelihood that the first donation is safe. In addition to FDA oversight, many manufacturers and collection agencies belong to the Plasma Protein Therapeutic Association (PPTA), which has strict quality regulations to help ensure the safety of donated plasma.

Viral Inactivation and Removal Processes

Maximizing the safety of the incoming plasma is only the first step. Viral inactivation and removal methods are now incorporated into all purification processes. One of the early methods, still used today, is pasteurization of albumin; otherwise, except for donor screening

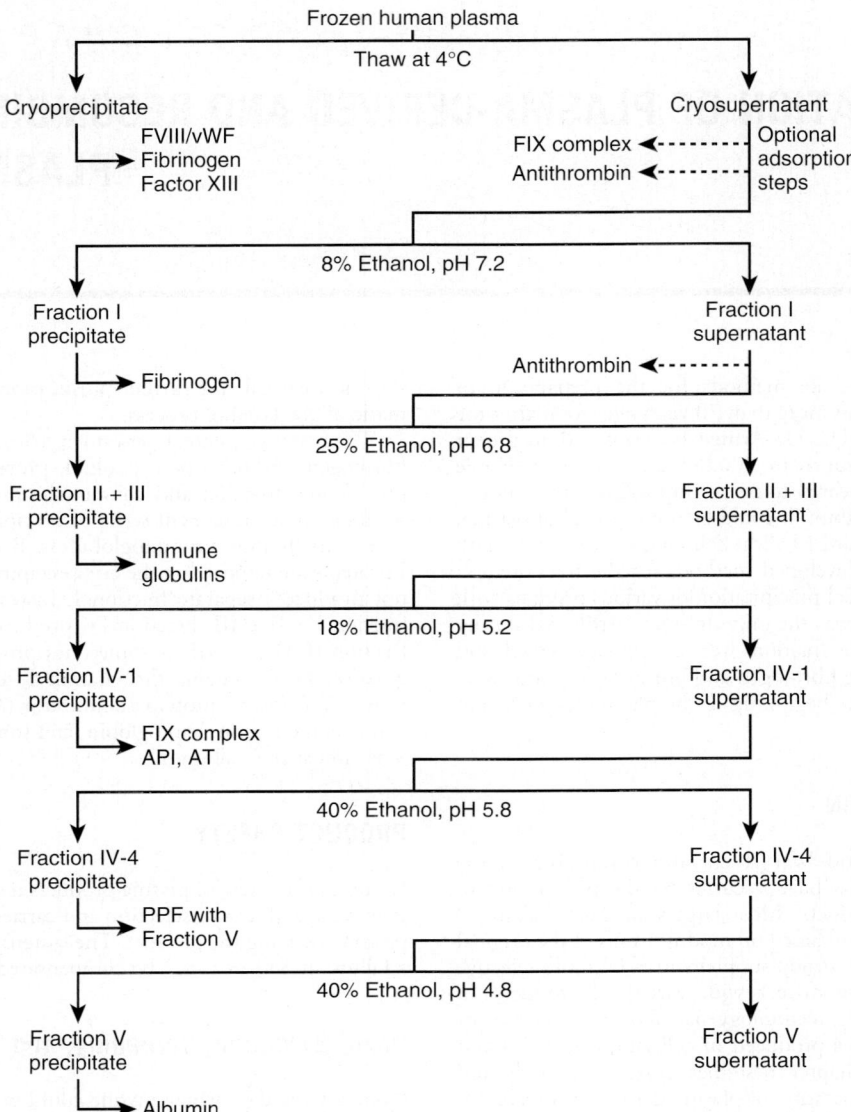

Fig. 116.1 SCHEMATIC OF A TYPICAL PLASMA FRACTIONATION PROCESS. The *dashed lines* show optional steps. *API*, α₁-Proteinase inhibitor; *AT*, antithrombin; *FIX*, factor IX; *FVIII*, factor VIII; *PPF*, plasma protein fraction; *vWF*, von Willebrand factor.

and testing, most other early products had no antiviral treatment. That all changed with the AIDS crisis in the early 1980s, when many in the hemophilia community became infected with HIV from clotting factor concentrates.

Since then, many viral inactivation and removal methods have been developed, including various types of heat treatment, solvent and detergent treatment, and nanofiltration. Manufacturers have also realized that many of their purification methods remove viruses, which works well as long as they take steps to protect the processed products from recontamination. Many of those steps also remove prions, the agents of the transmissible spongiform encephalopathies.

The bottom line is that modern plasma-derived products are extremely safe, as shown both theoretically and by actual experience over the past 30 years. Still, many patients and physicians prefer recombinant products because of their perceived greater safety in terms of the future unknown, emergent virus.

PLASMA PRODUCTS

The following sections provide information about the plasma-derived and recombinant plasma protein products available in the United

States in 2015. Additional details, including manufacturing and viral reduction methods, are listed in the tables for most products. The manufacturing methods were taken from the prescribing information sheets provided with each product and from the published literature. However, most manufacturers consider their processes proprietary, so some descriptions are not very detailed.

Fresh-Frozen Plasma

Whole plasma is still used to treat various conditions, including as a source of coagulation proteins that are not available in purified form and for replacement of significant blood loss. Plasma from a single donor that has been separated from the red blood cells, placed in a freezer within 8 hours after phlebotomy, and stored at −18°C or less is labeled as fresh-frozen plasma. *Fresh-frozen plasma* undergoes essentially the same donor screening and donation testing as plasma for fractionation and has a low risk of infectious disease transmission. In addition, INTERCEPT plasma was recently licensed by FDA as a viral-inactivated plasma for treatment of thrombotic thrombocytopenic purpura. The INTERCEPT process uses a psoralen, amotosalen, and ultraviolet light to inactivate viruses.

Albumin and Plasma Protein Fraction

Albumin remains one of the major products of human plasma fractionation. Literally tons of albumin have been isolated and millions of units have been infused. Albumin, recovered in very pure form in fraction V, is pasteurized in the final vial for 10 hours at 60°C with sodium acetyltryptophanate and sodium caprylate added as stabilizers.

Albumin is a commodity product, with little to distinguish one manufacturer's product from another's. There are small differences in purity, but those are only clinically relevant in rare cases. Three albumin products are manufactured in the United States: *albumin (human) 25% solution, albumin (human) 5% solution*, and *plasma protein fraction (human)* or PPF. In albumin (human), more than 96% of the protein content must be albumin. PPF, obtained by coprecipitating fraction IV-4 with fraction V, has a lower purity of greater than 83% albumin. PPF is more economical to produce than albumin, but the rapid infusion of PPF has been associated with hypotensive episodes.

Immune Globulins and Hyperimmune Globulins

Since the early 1950s, immune globulin products have been prepared from Cohn fraction II + III by the method developed by Oncley, a collaborator of Cohn. The Oncley process uses additional ethanol precipitations to remove lipoproteins, immunoglobulins A and M (IgA and IgM), and other plasma proteins, leaving fraction II, which contains purified immunoglobulin G (IgG). Whereas immune globulin is prepared from the plasma of unselected normal donors, hyperimmune globulins are prepared from the plasma of donors with high antibody titers against specific antigens [e.g., rho(D), hepatitis B, rabies, and tetanus]. These donors may be identified during convalescent periods after infection or transfusion, or they may be specifically immunized to produce the desired antibodies. The immune globulin products are listed in Tables 116.1 and 116.2.

Intravenous Immune Globulin Concentrates

The original immune globulin concentrates, initially termed *immune serum globulin* and currently *immune globulin (human)*, were administered by the intramuscular route, with the associated problems of limited injectable volume, poor bioavailability, and discomfort at the injection site. Intravenous (IV) injection of immune globulin (human) causes serious clinical reactions, which are attributed to complement-activating aggregates in these products.

To overcome these limitations, *immune globulin intravenous (human)* (IGIV) products were developed using a variety of methods to remove or inactivate anticomplementary aggregates. Today most intramuscular immune globulin usage is limited to hyperimmune products. Although immune globulin products tend to be self-protecting from viral transmission because of the large pools of antibodies they contain, infections have occurred, and as a result all manufacturers have incorporated viral inactivation or removal steps in their production processes.

The development of IGIV has permitted the administration of much higher doses, with a subsequent expansion in immunoglobulin therapy. Although immune globulin products were originally also considered commodity products, the increased usage has led manufacturers to distinguish their products in various ways. As shown in the tables, products are available in both lyophilized and liquid forms, with various strengths and purities. IgA content and product formulation are also distinguishing factors.

Subcutaneous Immune Globulin Concentrates

The first patient treated for primary immune deficiency was actually given subcutaneous injections of immunoglobulins, but as described above, intramuscular and later IV injection became the preferred methods. Recently, however, two immune globulin concentrates for subcutaneous injection have been marketed, Hizentra and HyQvia. HyQvia is also formulated with recombinant hyaluronidase to improve dispersion and absorption of the immune globulins in subcutaneous infusion. These products are intended for patients who have problems with IV infusion.

COAGULATION FACTOR CONCENTRATES

Transfusion of whole blood was shown in the mid-1800s to curtail bleeding in patients with hemophilia, and by 1940, bleeding episodes were being routinely treated with plasma. However, large amounts of plasma were needed, and this method of therapy could not provide normal levels of coagulation factors without producing hypervolemia. The development of more highly purified plasma-derived coagulation factor concentrates and more recently of recombinant concentrates has resulted in dramatic increases in the quality of life and life expectancy for patients with hemophilia. Hemophilia treatment is a large market, and the development of improved coagulation factor concentrates continues to be a major focus of research.

Factor VIII Concentrates

Factor VIII is the protein that is missing or defective in patients with hemophilia A. Factor VIII concentrates, generically termed *antihemophilic factor (human)* or AHF, for the treatment of hemophilia A have evolved from cryoprecipitates to very high-purity plasma-derived products to recombinant products. The various AHF concentrates available in the United States are listed in Table 116.3.

Cryoprecipitate

In a landmark discovery for hemophilia A treatment, cryoprecipitate was discovered in the mid-1950s to contain much of the factor VIII activity of the original plasma. By 1965, single-donor cryoprecipitate with factor VIII concentrations five to 30 times that of plasma became widely available for use in the treatment of patients with hemophilia A. Single-donor cryoprecipitate is still available from many blood banks but does carry a risk of viral transmission.

Intermediate- and High-Purity Antihemophilic Factor Concentrates

The development of AHF concentrates purified approximately 3000-fold over plasma was the next significant advance in the treatment of hemophilia A. Cryoprecipitate was used as the starting material, and a variety of methods were developed to remove fibrinogen, immunoglobulins, and other contaminating proteins. These were the mainstay of hemophilia A treatment for many years and are still available, their chief advantage being lower cost. Some of these products are also indicated as a source of vWF, which circulates in a complex with factor VIII. Products purified 5000-20,000–fold over plasma were subsequently developed using various chromatographic methods, but they have primarily been supplanted by immunoaffinity-purified products in the United States.

Immunoaffinity-Purified Concentrates

The next major advance in the preparation of AHF concentrates was the use of murine monoclonal antibodies (mAbs) immobilized on a chromatographic column for the purification of factor VIII. Factor VIII concentrates partially purified by conventional means are applied to an immunoaffinity column that binds either factor VIII directly or the factor VIII/vWF complex. The columns are washed extensively to remove unwanted proteins and then eluted with a solution that

TABLE 116.1 Immune Globulin Products[a]

Generic Name	Manufacturer or Distributor	Brand Name (Product Form)	Purity IgA Content	Production Methods (Formulation)[b]	Virus Inactivation or Removal Methods
Immune globulin (human)	Grifols Therapeutics	GamaSTAN S/D (15%–18% solution)	≥96% GG IgA: N/A	CEF (glycine)	PS, S/D, TSE
Immune globulin intravenous (human)	Baxter Healthcare	Gammagard S/D (lyophilized)	≥90% GG IgA <2.2 µg/mL	CEF, IEC (albumin, glycine, glucose, and PEG)	PS, S/D
		Gammagard S/D, IgA <1 µg/mL in a 5% solution (lyophilized)	≥90% GG IgA <1 µg/mL	CEF, IEC (albumin, glycine, glucose, and PEG)	PS, S/D
	Bio Products Laboratory	Gammaplex (5% solution)	>95% GG IgA <10 µg/mL	CEF, IEC (D-sorbitol, glycine, sodium acetate, and P80)	S/D, NF, low pH
	Biotest Pharmaceuticals	Bivigam (10% solution)	≥96% GG IgA <200 µg/mL	CEF (glycine, P80)	PS, low pH, S/D, NF
	CSL Behring	Carimune NF, Nanofiltered (lyophilized)	≥96% GG IgA: N/A	CEF, pH 4/pepsin treatment (sucrose)	PS, NF, low pH, DF, TSE
		Privigen (10% solution)	≥98% GG IgA ≤25 µg/mL	CEF, FAF, IEC (L-proline)	NF, low pH, DF, TSE
	Grifols Biologicals	Flebogamma 5% DIF (5% solution)	≥97% GG IgA ≤50 µg/mL	CEF, PEG PPTN, IEC (D-sorbitol and PEG)	PS, low pH, PST, S/D, NF, TSE
		Flebogamma 10% DIF (10% solution)	≥97% GG IgA ≤100 µg/mL	CEF, PEG PPTN, IEC (D-sorbitol and PEG)	PS, low pH, PST, S/D, NF, TSE
	Octapharma USA	Octagam, 5% (5% solution)	≥96% GG IgA ≤200 µg/mL	CEF, CHR (maltose)	PS, low pH, S/D
		Octagam, 10% (10% solution)	≥96% GG IgA ≤200 µg/mL	CEF, CHR (maltose)	PS, low pH, S/D
Immune globulin infusion (human)	Baxter Healthcare	Gammagard Liquid (10% solution)	≥98% GG IgA ~37 µg/mL	CEF, IEC (glycine)	S/D, NF, low pH
Immune globulin infusion (human), 10% with recombinant human hyaluronidase	Baxter Healthcare	HyQvia (10% solution)	≥98% GG IgA ~37 µg/mL	CEF, IEC (hyaluronidase, glycine)	S/D, NF, low pH
Immune globulin injection (human), 10% caprylate/ chromatography purified	Grifols Therapeutics	Gamunex-C (10% solution) Also distributed as Gammaked by Kedrion Biopharma	≥98% GG IgA ~46 µg/mL	CEF, OAF, IEC (glycine)	PS, DF, low pH, TSE
Immune globulin subcutaneous (human)	CSL Behring	Hizentra (20% solution)	≥98% GG IgA ≤50 µg/mL	CEF, OAF, IEC (L-proline and P80)	Low pH, DF, NF, TSE

Various forms of filtration and ultrafiltration are common in plasma fractionation, so those steps are not listed.

[a]These products were marketed in the United States in 2015. Data were obtained from manufacturers, distributors, and available literature.

[b]Not including NaCl.

CHR, Chromatography (specific method not available); CEF, cold ethanol fractionation; DF, depth filtration; FAF, fatty acid fractionation; GG, gamma globulin; IEC, ion-exchange chromatography; IgA, immunoglobulin A; N/A, not available; NF, nanofiltration; OAF, octanoic acid fractionation; P80, polysorbate 80; PEG, polyethylene glycol; PPTN, precipitation; PS, purification steps; PST, pasteurization (heat treatment in solution); S/D, solvent/detergent; TSE, validated for removal of transmissible spongiform encephalopathies.

disrupts the antibody binding. A final chromatography step removes the harsh elution solutions as well as any mAb that might have leached off the column to produce a factor VIII concentrate that is essentially pure before the addition of albumin as a stabilizer.

Recombinant Antihemophilic Factor Concentrates

One of the remarkable early accomplishments of molecular biology was the elucidation of the structure of factor VIII, its molecular cloning, and the successful production of two recombinant human factor VIII products, Recombinate and Kogenate. Additional recombinant factor VIII products have followed. Because proper posttranslational processing is essential for factor VIII functionality, the products are produced in mammalian cells, either baby hamster kidney (BHK) cells or Chinese hamster ovary (CHO) cells. A newer product, Eloctate, is produced in human embryonic kidney (HEK) cells. Recombinant factor VIII is purified by various types of chromatography.

One of the major driving forces for development of recombinant products is viral safety; they are seen as inherently safer because they are not produced from plasma. However, the first generation of recombinant products used animal-derived proteins and sera in their cell culture media and in the production of the mAbs used for purification, plus human albumin to stabilize the products in the final vial, all potential sources of viral contamination. With this in

TABLE 116.2 Hyperimmune Globulin Products[a]

Generic Name	Manufacturer or Distributor	Brand Name (Product Form)	Potency Purity IgA Content	Production Methods (Formulation)[b]	Virus Inactivation or Removal Methods
Botulism immune globulin intravenous (human)	California Department of Public Health FFF Enterprises	BabyBIG (lyophilized)	Antibotulism type A toxin ≥15 IU/mL Antibotulism type B toxin ≥4.0 IU/mL % GG: N/A IgA: N/A	CEF, HIC (sucrose and albumin)	PS, S/D, NF
Cytomegalovirus immune globulin intravenous (human)	CSL Behring	Cytogam (5% solution)	Anti-CMV: N/A % GG: N/A IgA: N/A	CEF (sucrose and albumin)	S/D
Hepatitis B immune globulin (human)	Biotest Pharmaceuticals	Nabi-HB (5% solution)	Anti-HBs >312 IU/mL % GG: N/A IgA ≤40 µg/mL	CEF (glycine and P80)	PS, S/D, NF
	Grifols Therapeutics	HyperHEP B S/D (15%–18% solution)	Anti-HBs ≥220 IU/mL % GG: N/A IgA: N/A	CEF, PPTN (glycine)	PS, S/D, TSE
Hepatitis B immune globulin intravenous (human)	Emergent Biosolutions	HepaGam B (5% solution)	Anti-HBs >312 IU/mL % GG: N/A IgA <40 µg/mL	IEC (maltose and P80)	PS, S/D, NF
Rabies immune globulin (human)	Grifols Therapeutics	HyperRAB S/D (15%–18% solution)	Anti-rabies ~150 IU/mL % GG: N/A IgA: N/A	CEF, PPTN (glycine)	PS, S/D, TSE
	Sanofi Pasteur	Imogam Rabies-HT (10%–18% solution)	Anti-rabies ≥150 IU/mL % GG: N/A IgA: N/A	CEF (glycine)	PS, PST
Rh$_o$(D) immune globulin (human)	Grifols Therapeutics	HyperRHO S/D Full Dose (15%–18% solution)	Anti-D ≥1500 IU/dose % GG: N/A IgA: N/A	CEF, PPTN (glycine)	PS, S/D, TSE
		HyperRHO S/D Mini Dose (15%–18% solution)	Anti-D ≥250 IU/dose % GG: N/A IgA: N/A	CEF, PPTN (glycine)	PS, S/D, TSE
	Kedrion Biopharma	RhoGAM Ultra-Filtered PLUS (300 µg; 1500 IU; 5% solution, prefilled syringe)	Anti-D: 1500 IU/dose ≥98% GG IgA <15 µg/dose	CEF (glycine and P80)	PS, S/D, NF
		MICRhoGAM Ultra-Filtered PLUS (50 µg; 250 IU; 5% solution, prefilled syringe)	Anti-D: 250 IU/dose ≥98% GG IgA <15 µg/dose	CEF (glycine and P80)	PS, S/D, NF
Rh$_o$(D) immune globulin intravenous (human)	CSL Behring	Rhophylac (3% solution, prefilled syringe)	Anti-D: 750 IU/mL ≥95% GG IgA <5 µg/mL	IEC, AH (albumin and glycine)	PS, S/D, NF
	Emergent Biosolutions	WinRho SDF (liquid)	Anti-D ~1150 IU/mL % GG: N/A IgA ~5 µg/mL	IEC (maltose and P80)	PS, S/D, NF
Tetanus immune globulin (human)	Grifols Therapeutics	HyperTET S/D (15%–18% solution, prefilled syringe)	Tetanus antitoxin ≥250 units/vial % GG: N/A IgA: N/A	CEF, PPTN (glycine)	PS, S/D, TSE
Vaccinia immune globulin intravenous (human)	Emergent Biosolutions	VIGIV (4%–7% solution)	Anti-vaccinia ≥3300 units/mL % GG: N/A IgA <40 µg/mL	IEC (maltose and P80)	PS, S/D, NF
Varicella zoster immune globulin (human)	Emergent Biosolutions	VariZIG (lyophilized)	Anti-VZV: 125 IU/vial % GG: N/A IgA: N/A	IEC (glycine and P80)	PS, S/D, NF

Various forms of filtration and ultrafiltration are common in plasma fractionation, so those steps are not listed.

[a]These products were marketed in the United States in 2015. Data were obtained from manufacturers, distributors, and available literature.

[b]Not including NaCl.

AH, Aluminum hydroxide adsorption; CMV, cytomegalovirus; CEF, cold ethanol fractionation; GG, gamma globulin; HBs, hepatitis B surface antigen; HIC, hydrophobic interaction chromatography; IEC, ion-exchange chromatography; IgA, immunoglobulin A; IU, international unit; N/A, not available; NF, nanofiltration; P80, polysorbate 80; PPTN, precipitation; PS, purification steps; PST, pasteurization (heat treatment in solution); S/D, solvent/detergent; TSE, validated for removal of transmissible spongiform encephalopathies; VZV, varicella zoster virus.

TABLE 116.3   Antihemophilic Factor and von Willebrand Factor Concentrates[a]

Generic Name	Manufacturer or Distributor	Brand Name	Specific Activity[b]	Production Methods	Virus Inactivation or Removal Methods
Antihemophilic factor (human)	Baxter Healthcare	HEMOFIL M	2–22 ~2000[c]	CP, CAP, IAC, IEC	PS, S/D, NF
	CSL Behring	Monoclate-P	4–10 >3000[c]	CP, CAP, AH, IAC, AC	PS, PST
	Kedrion Biopharma	Koāte-DVI	9–22 ~50[c]	CP, AH, PEG PPTN, glycine PPTN, SEC	PS, S/D, HT
Antihemophilic factor/von Willebrand factor complex (human)	CSL Behring	Humate-P	1–2 ~40[c] vWF/FVIII = 2.4	CP, AH, glycine PPTN, NaCl PPTN	PS, PST
	Grifols Biologicals	Alphanate	≥5 ~150[c] vWF/FVIII ≥0.4	CP, PEG PPTN, AC, NaCl PPTN,	PS, S/D, HT, Lyo, TSE
von Willebrand factor/coagulation factor VIII complex (human)	Octapharma USA	Wilate	≥60[d] vWF/FVIII = 1.0	CP, AH, IEC, SEC	PS, S/D, HT
Antihemophilic factor (recombinant)	Baxter Healthcare	Recombinate	2–20 >4000[c]	CHO, IAC, IEC	PS
		Advate	4000–10,000	CHO, IAC, IEC	S/D
	Bayer Healthcare	Kogenate FS (also distributed as Helixate FS by CSL Behring)	2600–6800	BHK, IEC, IAC, IMAC	PS, S/D, TSE
	Novo Nordisk	Novoeight	8340	CHO, IAC, CHR	Det, NF
	Pfizer	ReFacto	9110–13,700	CHO, CHR	None
		Xyntha	5900–9900	CHO, IEC, AC, SEC	PS, S/D, NF
Antihemophilic factor (recombinant), Fc fusion protein	Biogen Idec	Eloctate	N/A	HEK, IAC, CHR	Det, NF
Antihemophilic factor (recombinant), porcine sequence	Baxter Healthcare	Obizur	11,000–18,000	BHK, CHR	S/D, NF

Various forms of filtration and ultrafiltration are common in production processes, so those steps are not listed.
[a]These products were marketed in the United States in 2015. Data were obtained from manufacturers, distributors and available literature. All products are lyophilized.
[b]IU-factor VIII/mg of total protein.
[c]Before addition of human albumin.
[d]Specific activity of both vWF and FVIII in IU/mg of total protein.
AC, Affinity chromatography; AH, aluminum hydroxide adsorption; BHK, baby hamster kidney cell culture; CAP, cold acid precipitation; CHO, Chinese hamster ovary cell culture; CHR, chromatography (specific method not available); CP, cryoprecipitation; Det, detergent; FVIII, factor VIII; HEK, human embryonic kidney cell culture; HT, dry heat treatment; IAC, immunoaffinity chromatography; IEC, ion-exchange chromatography; IMAC, immobilized metal affinity chromatography; IU, international units; Lyo, lyophilization; N/A, not available; NF, nanofiltration; PEG, polyethylene glycol; PPTN, precipitation; PS, purification steps; PST, pasteurization (heat treatment in solution); S/D, solvent/detergent; SEC, size exclusion chromatography; TSE, validated for removal of transmissible spongiform encephalopathies; vWF, von Willebrand factor.

mind, manufacturers went still further to develop recombinant products completely free of human- and animal-derived proteins, both in their production processes and in their formulations. Most current production methods for recombinant products also incorporate viral inactivation or removal procedures for an added measure of safety.

One of the potential benefits of recombinant technology is the ability to design completely new proteins that do not occur in nature, ones that potentially perform better or are easier to produce than their natural counterparts. The factor VIII molecule is a multidomain complex consisting of a heavy chain with A1, A2, and B domains and a light chain consisting of A3, C1, and C2 domains. Previous research had shown that the B domain is not necessary for coagulant activity, so a B domain-deleted product, ReFacto, was developed. Eliminating the B domain, which is highly glycosylated, increased the expression of the molecule as much as 20-fold over full-length factor VIII. Xyntha was later introduced as an updated version of ReFacto with an improved manufacturing process.

Many hemophilia A patients are on prophylactic treatment regimens that require infusions every other day to maintain an increased factor VIII level in the bloodstream. To reduce the frequency of

infusions, a number of manufacturers are developing factor VIII molecules that have longer lifetimes in circulation. They are all taking the approach of connecting factor VIII to another molecule that has a longer half-life such as albumin or an immunoglobulin fragment. The first product to reach the market is Eloctate, which is a recombinant fusion protein of factor VIII and the Fc fragment of an immunoglobulin molecule. Eloctate reduces the frequency of infusions from every other day to once every 3–5 days.

Another new product, Obizur, is a recombinant porcine factor VIII that is indicated for patients with acquired hemophilia A. Antibodies against human factor VIII often do not react to porcine factor VIII, but the porcine molecule is active in the human coagulation process.

Factor IX Concentrates

Factor IX is the protein that is missing or defective in patients with hemophilia B. Two types of plasma-derived factor IX concentrates are available today: factor IX complex, which contains significant amounts of the other VKD clotting factors, and coagulation factor

TABLE 116.4	Factor IX and Other Coagulation Factor and Anticoagulant Concentrates[a]				
Generic Name	Manufacture or Distributor	Brand Name	Specific Activity[b]	Production Methods	Virus Inactivation or Removal Methods
Factor IX complex	Baxter Healthcare	Bebulin	2	CP, IEC	PS, VHT, NF
	Grifols Biologicals	Profilnine	4	CP, IEC	PS, S/D, NF
Prothrombin complex concentrate (human)	CSL Behring	Kcentra	N/A	CP, IEC, AS, CPA	PS, PST, NF
Coagulation factor IX (human)	CSL Behring	Mononine	≥190	CP, IEC, IAC, HIC	PS, CT, NF
	Grifols Biologicals	AlphaNine SD	≥150	CP, IEC, BCA, AC	PS, S/D, NF
Coagulation factor IX (recombinant)	Pfizer	BeneFIX	≥200	CHO, IEC, AC, IMAC	NF
	Baxter Healthcare	Rixubis	≥200	CHO, CHR	S/D, NF
Coagulation Factor IX (recombinant), Fc fusion protein	Biogen Idec	Alprolix	N/A	HEK, PAC, IEC	PS, NF
Anti-inhibitor coagulant complex	Baxter Healthcare	FEIBA	N/A	CP, CEF, IEC, SA	PS, VHT, NF
Coagulation factor VIIa (recombinant)	Novo Nordisk	NovoSeven RT	N/A	BHK, AA, IEC, IAC	PS
Antithrombin III (human)	Grifols Therapeutics	Thrombate III	N/A	CP, CEF, AC	PST, NF, TSE
Antithrombin III (recombinant)	rEVO Biologics	ATryn	>99% AT	TGM, AC, IEC, HIC	PS, HT, NF
Factor XIII concentrate (human)	CSL Behring	Corifact	N/A	CP, CEF, AH, IEC	PS, PST, NF
Coagulation factor XIII A-subunit (recombinant)	Novo Nordisk	Tretten	N/A	YST, HIC, IEC	None
Fibrinogen concentrate (human)	CSL Behring	RiaSTAP	N/A	CP, AH, glycine PPTN	PS, PST
Protein C concentrate (human)	Baxter Healthcare	Ceprotin	N/A	CP, CEF, IAC, IEC	PS, P80, VHT

Various forms of filtration and ultrafiltration are common in production processes, so those steps are not listed.

[a]These products were marketed in the United States in 2015. Data were obtained from manufacturers, distributors, and available literature.

[b]IU-factor IX/mg of total protein.

AA, Autocatalytic activation; AC, affinity chromatography; AH, aluminum hydroxide adsorption; AS, ammonium sulfate precipitation; AT, antithrombin; BCA, barium citrate adsorption; BHK, baby hamster kidney cell culture; CHO, Chinese hamster ovary cell culture; CHR, chromatography (specific method not available); CP, cryoprecipitation; CPA, calcium phosphate adsorption; CEF, cold ethanol fractionation; CT, chemical treatment; HEK, human embryonic kidney cell culture; HIC, hydrophobic interaction chromatography; HT, heat treatment; IAC, immunoaffinity chromatography; IEC, ion-exchange chromatography; IMAC, immobilized metal affinity chromatography; IU, international units; N/A, not available or not applicable; NF, nanofiltration; P80, polysorbate 80 treatment; PAC, Protein A chromatography; PPTN, precipitation; PS, purification steps; PST, pasteurization (heat treatment in solution); SA, surface activation; S/D, solvent/detergent; TGM, transgenic goat milk; TSE, validated for removal of transmissible spongiform encephalopathies; VHT, vapor heat treatment; YST, yeast cell culture.

IX (human), a preparation substantially free of these other proteins. Recombinant factor IX products are also available. The factor IX concentrates available in the United States are listed in Table 116.4.

Factor IX Complex Concentrates

The VKD proteins are serine proteases that include clotting factors II, VII, IX, and X and the anticoagulants protein C and protein S. Because of their similar structures, they tend to co-purify by most of the methods used to isolate them from plasma. Thus, the original factor IX products for treatment of hemophilia B were mixtures of the VKD proteins called *factor IX complex*. Because the protein in highest concentration in these products is prothrombin (factor II), they have also been identified as *prothrombin complex concentrates* (PCCs).

The VKD proteins were originally adsorbed from either cryo-poor plasma or fraction IV-4 using tricalcium phosphate. Later, ion exchange chromatography resins were used with cryo-poor plasma with the advantage that the supernatant plasma can then be further fractionated by the Cohn method for the production of immune globulins, albumin, and other products with little loss in yield.

Coagulation Factor IX Concentrates

With the widespread use of factor IX complex, it became apparent that serious thromboembolic episodes and acute myocardial infarction were major complications of its infusion, especially when used in large quantities for extended periods, such as for surgical procedures and in patients with liver disease. The cause of the thrombogenicity has not been conclusively determined, but the problem led to the development of more highly purified concentrates that are essentially free of the other VKD clotting factors. These products are designated *coagulation factor IX (human)*. Of the two products available in the United States, Mononine is prepared by immunoaffinity chromatography using a mAb to factor IX, and AlphaNine SD is purified by heparin affinity chromatography. These preparations have proven to be largely nonthrombogenic in clinical use.

Recombinant Factor IX Concentrates

Recombinant coagulation factor IX products have also been developed. They are produced in cell culture by mammalian cells and are purified using several chromatography steps. As with the latest generation AHF products, they are produced without human or animal proteins and include viral inactivation/removal steps to eliminate any viruses that might be present.

Manufacturers are also developing factor IX products with longer half-lives in circulation. The first to be marketed, Alprolix, is a recombinant fusion protein of factor IX bound to the Fc portion of an immunoglobulin molecule. The longer half-life reduces the frequency of prophylactic infusions from about once every third day to once a week or longer.

OTHER COAGULATION AND ANTICOAGULANT CONCENTRATES

Now that the risk of infection has essentially been eliminated, the major complication in hemophilia treatment is the development of inhibitors, neutralizing antibodies directed against factor VIII or factor IX. There are two primary means of treating bleeding in inhibitor patients, both based on administration of activated clotting factors.

Factor IX complex was known to be somewhat effective in preventing bleeding in inhibitor patients, possibly because it contains small amounts of activated clotting factors. Based on that information, two activated factor IX complex products were developed, one of which, FEIBA, is still available. FEIBA, which is named for factor eight inhibitor bypassing activity, is generically named *anti-inhibitor coagulant complex* and is indicated for inhibitor treatment in both hemophilia A and B.

The hypothesis that administration of activated clotting factors can bypass inhibitors also led to the development of NovoSeven, a recombinant activated factor VII concentrate. NovoSeven has been extensively studied and is currently the most widely used option for inhibitor treatment, especially for patients who have never been exposed to plasma-derived products. However, both FEIBA and NovoSeven do carry a risk of thromboembolic complications. FEIBA and NovoSeven are listed in Table 116.4.

von Willebrand disease (vWD), caused by missing or abnormal vWF, is actually the most common inherited coagulation disorder. vWF is a large protein that circulates in a complex with factor VIII. It stabilizes factor VIII in the bloodstream but also has coagulation functions of its own. Several intermediate-purity viral-inactivated AHF concentrates that contain significant amounts of vWF are also indicated for replacement therapy for vWD. These vWF/AHF concentrates are listed in Table 116.3.

Fibrinogen is the final protein in the coagulation cascade. It is cleaved by thrombin to form fibrin, a protein that naturally self-associates to form a clot. RiaSTAP is a plasma-derived concentrate for replacement therapy in fibrinogen-deficient patients that is made from the concentrated fibrinogen in cryoprecipitate. Interestingly, fibrinogen was also one of the first plasma products developed, but it was soon taken off the market because it almost universally transmitted viral infections. RiaSTAP is pasteurized (heat treated) in solution for 20 hours at 60°C, twice as long as the typical treatment for pasteurized plasma products. Significant viral removal has also been demonstrated for its purification process, and the resulting product is considered safe. RiaSTAP is listed in Table 116.4.

Factor XIII does not participate directly in the coagulation cascade but instead stabilizes the final clot by cross-linking the fibrin molecules. Factor XIII deficiency is rare and is characterized by weak clots prone to rebleeding. Before the availability of factor XIII concentrates, patients were usually treated with plasma or cryoprecipitate, both of which carry a risk of viral infection. Plasma-derived Corifact is purified from cryoprecipitate and employs a unique process step using Vitacel, a wheat-based vegetable fiber, to remove fibrinogen, after which the factor XIII is further purified by ion-exchange chromatography. Tretten is a recombinant version of the A subunit of factor XIII, a deficiency of which is the usual cause of factor XIII deficiency. Tretten is produced in yeast and purified by chromatography. Tretten and Corifact are listed in Table 116.4.

Anticoagulant Concentrates

Antithrombin III, now generally just called AT, is an anticoagulant. As its name suggests, it inhibits thrombin (activated factor II), but it also inhibits the activated forms of factors IX, X, XI, and XII. It belongs to the serpin family named for their activity as serine protease inhibitors. Heparin is a cofactor that increases the native activity of AT significantly, from 500- to 1000-fold for factor Xa inhibition up to 1 million-fold for factor IXa inhibition. The affinity of AT for heparin is also used to purify the protein by affinity chromatography on an immobilized heparin column. Thrombate III, the only plasma-derived product currently on the US market, is purified by heparin affinity chromatography from Cohn fraction IV-1. ATryn, a recombinant AT, was the first recombinant human plasma protein produced in transgenic animals to be approved anywhere. It is made in the milk of transgenic goats and also purified by heparin affinity chromatography. The two available AT concentrates are listed in Table 116.4.

Protein C is a serine protease with a structure similar to clotting factors II, VII, IX, and X, but it is an anticoagulant that cleaves activated factors V and VIII. Patients deficient in protein C are susceptible to thrombosis. One plasma-derived protein C concentrate, Ceprotin, is available. Ceprotin is listed in Table 116.4.

Fibrin Sealant and Thrombin

Fibrinogen and thrombin are also used as topical hemostatic agents, together as fibrin sealant, and as standalone thrombin concentrates. The fibrin sealant and thrombin products available in the United States are listed in Table 116.5.

Fibrin sealant uses the clot-forming reaction of thrombin and fibrinogen to form a physiologic glue or sealant that has become widely used in surgical procedures. All three fibrin sealant products on the US market are made from human plasma-derived fibrinogen and thrombin. Fibrinogen is purified directly from cryoprecipitate followed by further purification steps. ARTISS and TISSEEL contain a plasmin inhibitor, synthetic aprotinin, which is used to delay clot lysis. EVICEL contains a more highly purified fibrinogen component that has minimal plasmin activity and therefore does not contain a clot lysis inhibitor. Both fibrinogen preparations contain residual factor XIII for clot stabilization, and additional factor XIII is recruited from the patient's bloodstream during use. Fibrin sealant is also the basis of two patches or bandages that are used to promote clotting.

Thrombin is produced from prothrombin (factor II) purified from the factor IX complex captured by ion exchange from cryosupernatant plasma. Prothrombin is autocatalytically activated to thrombin in the presence of calcium. Both the fibrinogen and thrombin components are also treated for viral inactivation and removal. Three standalone thrombin products are also available for use in promoting topical hemostasis. For years, bovine thrombin was the standard of care for such use; however, research has suggested that it may have been responsible for postsurgical hemostatic problems in some patients. The cause was apparently contamination with bovine factor V, against which some patients developed antibodies that cross-reacted with their own human factor V. Most bovine thrombin products were taken off the market, but Thrombin-JMI, the sole remaining bovine product, was instead further purified to reduce bovine factor V to undetectable levels. A plasma-derived human thrombin product, EVITHROM, was also developed, which is the same thrombin used in EVICEL fibrin sealant.

The recombinant human thrombin product, RECOTHROM, is another example of a bioengineered protein. The VKD clotting factors contain a domain called the Gla region that is rich in a unique amino acid, γ-carboxyglutamic acid (Gla). The posttranslational modifications required to produce the Gla residues are a rate-limiting step in the production of all of the VKD proteins in cell culture. Presence of the Gla region is absolutely necessary for the function of most of the clotting factors but not for thrombin. Therefore, the Gla-less molecule prethrombin-1 is produced in CHO cells, with a significant increase in production rate. Prethrombin-1 is activated to thrombin using a proprietary enzyme system. RECOTHROM behaves similarly to human and bovine thrombin in clinical use.

PLASMA PROTEINASE INHIBITORS

The proteinase inhibitors that are present in human plasma play critical roles in the regulation of the coagulation, fibrinolytic, complement, and kinin cascade systems. Most of these inhibitors have similar amino acid and structural properties and are members of the serpin superfamily of proteins. AT, an anticoagulant, was discussed earlier. Two other proteinase inhibitors, API and C1 esterase inhibitor, are also available for treatment of deficient patients. These concentrates are listed in Table 116.6.

TABLE 116.5	Fibrin Sealants and Thrombin Concentrates[a]			
Generic Name	Manufacturer/Distributor	Brand Name (Product Format)	Production Methods	Virus Inactivation or Removal Methods
Fibrin sealant (human)	Baxter Healthcare	Artiss (frozen solutions in prefilled syringe)	FC: CP, OS TC: IEC, CA	FC and TC: PS, VHT, S/D
	Omrix/Ethicon	Evicel (frozen solutions)	FC: CP, AH, HIC, AC TC: CP, IEC, CA	FC: S/D, PST TC: S/D, NF
Fibrin sealant (Tisseel)	Baxter Healthcare	Tisseel (lyophilized or frozen solutions)	FC: CP, OS TC: IEC, CA	FC and TC: PS, VHT, S/D
Fibrin sealant patch	Omrix/Ethicon	Evarrest (lyophilized absorbable patch)	FC: CP, AH, HIC, AC TC: CP, IEC, CA	FC: S/D, PST TC: S/D, NF
	Takeda/Baxter Healthcare	TachoSil (lyophilized absorbable patch)	FC: CP, glycine PPTN, AH, HIC, AC TC: CP, CHR, AS, CTA	FC and TC: PS Final product: GI
Thrombin, topical (bovine)	GenTrac/Pfizer	Thrombin-JMI (lyophilized)	Thrombin: BP, IEC, TA, NF Bovine thromboplastin: GBL, MHA, AS	PS, NF, TSE
Thrombin topical (human)	Omrix /Ethicon	Evithrom (frozen solution)	CP, IEC, CA	S/D, NF
Thrombin, topical (recombinant)	The Medicines Company	Recothrom (lyophilized)	CHO, EA, AC, IEC	S/D, NF

Various forms of filtration and ultrafiltration are common in production processes, so those steps are not listed.
[a]These products were marketed in the United States in 2015. Data were obtained from manufacturers, distributors, and available literature.
AC, Affinity chromatography; AH, aluminum hydroxide adsorption; AS, ammonium sulfate precipitation; BP, bovine plasma; CA, calcium activation; CHO, Chinese hamster ovary cell culture; CHR, chromatography (specific method not available); CP, cryoprecipitation; CTA, citrate activation; EA, enzymatic activation; FC, fibrinogen component; GBL, ground bovine lung tissue; GI, gamma irradiation; HIC, hydrophobic interaction chromatography; IEC, ion-exchange chromatography; MHA, magnesium hydroxide gel adsorption; NF, nanofiltration; OS, other steps, not specified; PPTN, precipitation; PS, purification steps; PST, pasteurization (heat treatment in solution); S/D, solvent/detergent; TA, thromboplastin activation; TC, thrombin component; TSE, validated for removal of transmissible spongiform encephalopathies; VHT, vapor heat treatment.

α_1-Proteinase Inhibitor

α_1-Proteinase inhibitor (human), also known as α_1-antitrypsin, was the first of the serpins to be isolated and characterized. Although the protein was originally named for its antitrypsin activity, its primary physiologic function appears to be the inhibition of neutrophil elastase in the lung. API replacement therapy is indicated for chronic treatment of individuals with hereditary deficiency. However, even with four products available, the supply is tight because of the limited amount ultimately available from plasma. One issue is the poor efficiency of IV administration. It is estimated that only approximately 2% of the infused API ends up in the lung. Studies have suggested that aerosol delivery of API directly into the lungs by inhalation would be efficacious and could replace IV administration because of its lower cost and greater convenience. API is also a good candidate for recombinant production.

C1 Esterase Inhibitor

C1 esterase inhibitor (human) acts as a regulator in the complement and fibrinolytic systems and as an inhibitor of factor XIIa and kallikrein. Its name comes from its inhibition of the complement proteins C1r and C1s. Patients deficient in C1 esterase inhibitor are at risk for attacks of hereditary angioedema. Two plasma-derived C1 esterase inhibitor concentrates are licensed in the United States. RUCONEST, a recombinant product produced in transgenic rabbits, was also licensed recently. The products are listed in Table 116.6.

FUTURE DIRECTIONS

New Plasma-Derived Concentrates

With licensure of a number of new products in the past few years, including protein C, vWF, factor XIII and C1 esterase inhibitor, the United States is catching up with Europe and other parts of the world. Concentrates of factor VII and factor XI are also available elsewhere. Several other proteins in plasma would be potentially useful as therapeutic products, including butyrylcholinesterase for reversal of succinylcholine-induced apnea and treatment of cocaine overdose and other coagulation factors and inhibitors, such as factors X and XII and protein S. However, the prevalence of deficiency disorders of these proteins is small, so they would be true orphan drugs with limited markets. There are also potential improvements that can be made to current plasma-derived and recombinant concentrates. In addition to enhanced purification and viral clearance methods, products can be made more user friendly.

Alternate delivery systems could also potentially improve the utility of many products. Delivery of clotting factors by inhalation, ingestion, and subcutaneous injection has been explored. As mentioned earlier, several studies have looked at aerosol delivery of API. Production of fibrin sealant in a powder form that could be sprinkled on a wound has also been studied.

Recombinant Plasma Protein Concentrates

Almost all plasma proteins licensed for human use have been cloned and expressed in biologically active forms in animal cells in the laboratory, and several have been developed into licensed products, as described earlier. The main advantages of recombinantly produced proteins include freedom from human viruses and a potentially unlimited supply. AT and C1 esterase inhibitor have already been produced in the milk of transgenic animals, and others such as API, which are required in relatively large amounts, are also candidates. Transgenic cows, goats, pigs, and sheep can produce large quantities of human proteins, typically 1–10 g/L in milk. In contrast, the animal cell culture systems routinely used for production of the types of plasma proteins described here produce substantially less protein, typically 0.01–0.1 g/L.

Recombinant proteins can also be produced in modified forms that may give them advantageous new properties such as increased

TABLE 116.6 α_1-Proteinase Inhibitor and C1 Esterase Inhibitor Concentrates[a]

Generic Name	Manufacturer/Distributor	Brand Name (Product Format)	Potency Specific Activity[b]	Production Methods	Virus Inactivation or Removal Methods
Alpha$_1$-proteinase inhibitor (human)	Baxter Healthcare	Aralast NP (lyophilized)	≥16 ≥0.55	CEF, PEG PPTN, ZnCl$_2$ PPTN, IEC	PS, S/D, NF
	CSL Behring	Zemaira (lyophilized)	~50 ≥0.7	CEF, EXTN, DST, IEC, HIC	PST, NF
	Grifols Therapeutics	Prolastin-C (lyophilized)	~50 ≥0.7	CEF, PEG PPTN, IEC	PS, S/D, NF, TSE
	Kamada/Baxter Healthcare	Glassia (liquid)	20 ≥0.7	CEF, CHR	S/D, NF
C1 esterase inhibitor (human)	CSL Behring	Berinert (lyophilized)	50 SA: N/A	HIC, IEC, AS	PS, PST, NF
	Sanquin Blood Supply Foundation/ ViroPharma Biologics	Cinryze (lyophilized)	62.5 4.0–9.0	CHR, PEG PPTN	PS, PST, NF
C1 esterase inhibitor (recombinant)	Pharming Group/Santaris	Ruconest (lyophilized)	150 SA: N/A	TRM, IEC, ZCC	PS, PST, NF

Various forms of filtration and ultrafiltration are common in production processes, so those steps are not listed.
[a]These products were marketed in the United States in 2015. Data were obtained from manufacturers, distributors, and available literature.
[b]For α_1-proteinase inhibitor products, potency is in mg-API/mL-solution and specific activity is in mg-active API/mg-total protein. For C1 esterase inhibitor products, potency is in units/mL-solution and specific activity is in units/mg-total protein.
API, α_1-Proteinase inhibitor; AS, ammonium sulfate precipitation; CEF, cold ethanol fractionation; CHR, chromatography (specific method not available); DST, dithiothreitol and silicon dioxide treatment; EXTN, extraction (specific details not available); HIC, hydrophobic interaction chromatography; IEC, ion-exchange chromatography; N/A, not available; NF, nanofiltration; PEG, polyethylene glycol; PPTN, precipitation; PS, purification steps; PST, pasteurization (heat treatment in solution); SA, specific activity; S/D, solvent/detergent; TRM, transgenic rabbit milk; TSE, validated for removal of transmissible spongiform encephalopathies; ZCC, zinc-chelating chromatography.

potency, longer half-lives, or varied specificity. Examples include the longer acting factor VIII and IX products being developed. Another product already available is B domain-deleted factor VIII described earlier.

SUGGESTED READINGS

GENERAL OVERVIEWS OF PLASMA PRODUCTS AND PRODUCTION METHODS

Burnouf T: Modern plasma fractionation. *Transfus Med Rev* 21:101, 2007.
Farrugia A, Evers T, et al: Plasma fractionation issues. *Biologicals* 37:88, 2009.
Farrugia A, Quinti I: Manufacture of immunoglobulin products for patients with primary antibody deficiencies - the effect of processing conditions on product safety and efficacy. *Front Immunol* 5:665, 2014.
Ofosu FA, Freedman J, Semple JW: Plasma-derived biological medicines used to promote haemostasis. *Thromb Haemost* 99:851, 2008.
Radosevich M, Burnouf T: Intravenous immunoglobulin G: trends in production methods, quality control and quality assurance. *Vox Sang* 98:12, 2010.

RECOMBINANT PLASMA PRODUCTS

Burnouf T: Recombinant plasma proteins. *Vox Sang* 100:68, 2011.
Grillberger L, Kreil TR, et al: Emerging trends in plasma-free manufacturing of recombinant protein therapeutics expressed in mammalian cells. *Biotechnol J* 4:186, 2009.
Maksimenko OG, Deykin AV, et al: Use of transgenic animals in biotechnology: prospects and problems. *Acta Naturae* 5:33, 2013.
Oldenburg J, Albert T: Novel products for haemostasis - current status. *Haemophilia* 20(Suppl 4):23, 2014.

Peyvandi F, Garagiola I, Seregni S: Future of coagulation factor replacement therapy. *J Thromb Haemost* 11(Suppl 1):84, 2013.
Pipe SW: The hope and reality of long-acting hemophilia products. *Am J Hematol* 87(Suppl 1):S33, 2012.

SAFETY OF PLASMA PRODUCTS

Cai K, Groner A, et al: Prion removal capacity of plasma protein manufacturing processes: a data collection from PPTA member companies. *Transfusion* 53:1894, 2013.
Dichtelmuller HO, Biesert L, et al: Contribution to safety of immunoglobulin and albumin from virus partitioning and inactivation by cold ethanol fractionation: a data collection from Plasma Protein Therapeutics Association member companies. *Transfusion* 51:1412, 2011.
Klamroth R, Groner A, Simon TL: Pathogen inactivation and removal methods for plasma-derived clotting factor concentrates. *Transfusion* 54:1406, 2014.
Velthove KJ, Over J, et al: Viral safety of human plasma-derived medicinal products: impact of regulation requirements. *Transfus Med Rev* 27:179, 2013.

HISTORY OF PLASMA PRODUCT PRODUCTION

Cohn EJ, Strong LE, et al: Preparation and properties of serum and plasma proteins. IV. A system for the separation into fractions of the protein and lipoprotein components of biological tissues and fluids. *J Am Chem Soc* 68:459, 1946.
Palmer JW: The evolution of large-scale human plasma fractionation in the United States. In Sgouris JR, Rene A, editors: *Proceedings of the workshop on albumin*, Washington, DC, 1976, DHEW Publication No. (NIH) 76-925, US Government Printing Office.

TRANSFUSION THERAPY FOR COAGULATION FACTOR DEFICIENCIES

Elizabeth Roman, Peter J. Larson, and Catherine S. Manno

This chapter reviews products available to treat deficiencies of plasma coagulation proteins. The development of blood component therapy and subsequently protein concentrates that are enriched in particular coagulation factors and other proteins made possible the effective treatment of bleeding episodes in patients with hemophilia and other diatheses. In the 1940s, a collaborative effort funded by the US government was undertaken among protein scientists with the goal of rapidly developing a method to isolate albumin from human plasma to provide a lyophilized intravascular volume expander for use in the military. As part of this effort, Dr. Edwin Cohn developed an ethanol fractionation procedure that was amenable to large-scale manufacture.[1] Building on the foundation of the Cohn fractionation procedure (see Chapter 116), the first coagulation factor concentrates were developed in the mid-1960s and provided a safer and more effective treatment for patients with the X-linked coagulation deficiencies, hemophilia A and B. Given the limited human plasma resource as a raw material for production of all but a few coagulation protein concentrates, manufacturers of human plasma–based products attempt to derive the maximum yield from each pool of plasma. Manufacturers of plasma-derived products strive to maximize the therapeutic potential of pooled human plasma by deriving more products from these processes.

Development of recombinant products was fueled by infectious disease transmission through human plasma–derived products. Currently licensed products are produced in mammalian cell culture to optimize necessary posttranslational modifications required for biologic activity. These recombinant expression processes are complicated and expensive. Transgenic recombinant technology has been explored as a way to decrease or eliminate reliance on the human plasma resource and the technically rigorous production of recombinant proteins using mammalian cell culture methods.

Recombinant technology has made significant progress recently in the evolution of long-acting factor VIII and IX preparations, which are effective in preventing as well as treating bleeding episodes; however, the progress has been more significant in the extension of the factor IX half-life. By conjugation to fusion protein (immunoglobulin Fc) the half-lives of these coagulation proteins have been extended. This has had a great impact on the daily life of patients with hemophilia who use factor concentrate as prophylaxis, as extending the factor half-life has reduced the burden of numerous weekly infusions, while maintaining factor efficacy.

In addition, this new era holds vast promise in gene therapy for factor IX deficiency. Enhancing a patient's ability to produce even a modest increase in factor levels could transform the individual from a severe to moderate hemophilia patient, eliminating the need for routine prophylactic therapy and reducing the number of spontaneous or trauma-related bleeding episodes.

HEMOPHILIA A AND B

The hemophilias are X-linked disorders caused by deficiencies of either factor VIII (hemophilia A, or classic hemophilia) or factor IX (hemophilia B, or Christmas disease). The genes for these coagulation factors are located in close proximity on the long arm of the X chromosome. Whereas hemophilia A affects 1:5000 males,

hemophilia B affects 1:30,000. This difference in incidence is roughly correlated with the size of the genes, and more than 30% of cases arise from spontaneous mutations.

The major morbidity of the severe hemophilias A and B is arthropathy, a result of recurrent joint bleeding developing over the course of years in those with inhibitors or those who are untreated or undertreated. The major cause of hemorrhagic mortality is bleeding into critical closed spaces (e.g., intracranial).[2] Central nervous system (CNS) bleeding occurs in 3% to 14% of patients, and mortality from CNS hemorrhage ranges from 20% to 50%[3–5] with neurologic sequelae (including seizures, motor impairment, or mental retardation) observed in 40% to 50% of survivors.[3] CNS bleeding episodes occur predominantly in patients with severe disease (<1% factor level).[3] A more detailed discussion of the hemophilias and the molecular biology of factors VIII and IX can be found in Chapter 135.

TRANSFUSION THERAPY FOR HEMOPHILIA A AND B

History of Transfusion for Hemophilia

Transfusion was first proposed by Schönlein and his student Hopf in 1832 as a treatment for "bleeders" who were suffering from exsanguinating hemorrhage, and these two were likely the first to have used the term *Haemophilie* to describe the disease.[6,7] The first effective transfusion-based intervention for hemophilia is credited to Samuel Lane who, in 1840, infused 10–12 ounces of fresh human blood into a 12-year-old boy with postoperative hemorrhage after eye surgery for correction of a squint.[8] Subsequently, a variety of interventions, using the infusion of human and animal blood and blood derivatives, were used in the therapy of hemorrhage in patients with congenital bleeding diatheses (Table 117.1). Citrated plasma was first used in 1923 for the treatment of hemophilia by Feissly in a father-to-son transfusion.[9] Development of modern blood banking in the 1930s and expansion of transfusion during and after World War II allowed for more widespread use of whole blood and subsequently frozen plasma in the treatment of hemophilia. Because of limited availability, the use of whole blood and components of whole blood for the treatment of hemophilia and other diseases was initially confined to larger metropolitan areas. In addition, volume constraints associated with the quantity of whole blood or plasma needed to achieve therapeutic levels of coagulation limited their usefulness.[10]

The advent of modern transfusion therapy for hemophilia came with the observation that the cold-insoluble precipitate remaining after thawing of frozen plasma at 4°C contains high concentrations of factor VIII.[32] Application of this procedure to the separation of components of whole blood[19] allowed for the production of a reduced-volume blood product known as *cryoprecipitate*. Cryoprecipitate derived from a single whole blood collection contains approximately 125 units of factor VIII and quickly replaced frozen plasma as the therapy of choice for the treatment of bleeding episodes in hemophilia A in the 1960s. The availability of cryoprecipitate made the treatment of bleeding episodes by patients in their homes, rather than at a hospital, a reality. In addition, the development of quantitative assays for factor VIII[15] and for factor IX[14] meant that the

TABLE 117.1	Development of Transfusion Therapy for Hemophilia
1832	Schönlein proposes transfusion for exsanguination[7]
1840	Lane transfuses whole blood to stop postoperative bleeding in hemophilia[8]
1905	Weil reports use of human serum to treat hemophilia[11]
1911	Addis fractionates plasma by acid method[12]
1923	Feissly uses citrated plasma in ABO-mismatched father-to-son transfusion for hemophilia[9]
1930s–1940s	Development of modern blood banking. Availability of whole blood and frozen plasma for therapy (allows levels of approximately 5%)
1946	Cohn develops ethanol fractionation of plasma[1]
1949	Graham uses FFP in canine hemophilia model[13]
1945–1960	Fractionation of plasmas with AHF activity
1952	Biggs distinguishes hemophilia B from hemophilia A[14]
1953	Graham, Langdell, and Brinkhous develop quantitative assays to measure AHF[15,16]
1958	Barium precipitation of plasma to enrich for factor IX[17,18]
1963	Wagner uses glycine precipitation to partially purify factor VIII
1964	Pool develops clinically useful cryoprecipitate for factor VIII deficiency (allows levels of >20%)[19]
1966	Johnson uses PEG to partially purify factor VIII[20]
1967	Brinkhous develops glycine and PEG method to produce large-scale high potency factor VIII product (allows levels of 100%)[21]
1965–1970	Home infusion therapy
1969	Hoag produces large-scale prothrombin complex concentrate for factor IX deficiency[22]
1970s	HBsAg assay is developed
1978–1985	HIV contaminates blood supply and factor concentrates
1979–1986	Heat treatment of factor concentrates reduces transmission of hepatitis B and HIV[23,24]
1985	Assay for HIV is licensed
1982	Immunoaffinity method of purification for factor VIII[25,26]
1986	S/D method of treating infusible protein solutions to inactivate enveloped viruses[27,28]
1992–1993	First recombinant factor VIII concentrates are licensed[29,30]
1998	Recombinant factor IX concentrate is licensed[31]
1999	Nucleic acid amplification testing of blood donors
1999	Recombinant factor VIIa approved for hemophilia A and B with inhibitor
2007	Recombinant factor VIIa approved for acquired hemophilia
2011	First plasma-derived factor XIII product approved by the FDA
2011	Successful report of AAV mediated gene therapy for factor IX deficiency

AHF, Human antihemophilic factor; FDA, Food and Drug Administration; FFP, fresh-frozen plasma; HBsAg, hepatitis B surface antigen; PEG, polyethylene glycol; S/D, solvent/detergent.

two diseases could now be distinguished and effects of transfusion therapy on circulating levels of factors could be more accurately assessed.

Before the discovery of plasma cryoprecipitate, significant advances had been made in the fractionation of plasma using ethanol,[1] glycine,[33] polyethylene glycol,[20] a combination of glycine and polyethylene glycol,[21] and calcium or barium[17,22,34] to precipitate plasma proteins. These techniques, in conjunction with cold precipitation of frozen plasma, laid the groundwork that resulted in the production of the first factor VIII and factor IX concentrates for clinical use.[21,22] These concentrates could be lyophilized and stored at temperatures up to 4°C with extended stability. Infusion of factor concentrates resulted in high circulating levels of factor VIII and factor IX without the complication of volume overload and paved the way for intensive infusion therapy for serious and life-threatening bleeding complications such as intracranial, retroperitoneal, and retropharyngeal hemorrhages and major surgery. Because they were produced from large pools of single plasma donations (>1000), initial concentrates were nearly universally contaminated with viral pathogens such as hepatitis B and non-A, non-B hepatitis (hepatitis C).[35] Initial attempts to attenuate viral transmission using pasteurization and dry heat, instituted by manufacturers in the late 1970s and early 1980s,[23,36] were found to limit the transmission of hepatitis B. Eventually, these techniques were found to inactivate the human immunodeficiency virus (HIV).[24,37,38] Before the widespread application of these techniques, however, the majority of patients with severe hemophilia treated with concentrates between 1978 and 1985 were infected with HIV and hepatitis C virus. This tragic consequence of infusion therapy helped fuel the development of modern strategies to reduce the risk of viral transmission by products derived from human plasma. These strategies include (1) careful screening of potential donors for risk factors leading to infection with transfusion-transmissible infections, (2) more vigilant surveillance of the blood donor base for the appearance of new pathogens, (3) development and implementation of testing specific for markers of infectious agents, (4) purification strategies that reduce viral load in final products, and (5) physical and chemical viral inactivation methods to treat infusible products. Finally, development and refinement in techniques of molecular biology in the 1970s and 1980s resulted in the cloning of the genes for many plasma proteins, including factor VIII and factor IX.[39–41] Within the next decade, the production and licensure of biologically active recombinant factor VIII and factor IX products had become a reality.[29,42–44] Concentrates of these recombinant products have been shown to be effective and have not been associated with the transmission of pathogens. Further development of recombinant products centered on the removal of all human and animal proteins in the production and formulation of products to further reduce the risk of their inadvertent contamination with emerging pathogens, such as variant prions,[45,46] and newly discovered agents, such as hepatitis G virus and other transfusion transmitted viruses.[47,48] In addition, episodic supply constraints incurred in the manufacture of recombinant proteins in mammalian cell culture systems resulting in supply shortages of recombinant factor VIII[49] have led to greater interest in transgenic production of human plasma proteins compared with mammalian cell culture. With transgenic systems, raw material from which the protein of interest is purified (milk, plant tissue) can be produced in abundance.

Attenuation of Pathogens in Blood-Derived and Other Biologic Products

The development of factor VIII and factor IX concentrates in the 1960s improved the life expectancy of patients with hemophilia from approximately 11 years (before effective transfusion therapy) to nearly normal.[50] Experience with these first-generation concentrates, however, showed that they invariably transmitted the viral agents responsible for hepatitis B and hepatitis C,[35] which are associated with chronic hepatitis with attendant morbidity and mortality, including cirrhosis and hepatocellular carcinoma. Although efforts

TABLE 117.2 Viruses Implicated in Transfusion of Plasma-Derived Products

Virus	Nucleic Acid Human Disease	Human Disease	Known Transmission by Blood	Lipid Enveloped	Size (nm)	Reduction/Inactivation
HIV	RNA	Yes (AIDS)	Yes	Yes	100–120	S/D
HBV	DNA	Yes (acute and chronic hepatitis)	Yes	Yes	40–45	S/D
HCV	RNA	Yes (acute and chronic hepatitis)	Yes	Yes	40–60	S/D
Parvovirus B19	DNA	Yes (fifth disease, transient erythroblastopenia of childhood, chronic anemia in immunocompromised patients)	Yes	No	18–20	Incompletely by heat; nanofiltration
HAV	RNA	Yes	Yes	No	25–30	Incompletely by heat
Hepatitis G	RNA	No	Yes	Yes		?S/D
TTV	DNA	No	Yes	No		?S/D
HHV-8	DNA	Kaposi sarcoma	Unknown			
SEN V	DNA			No		
TSE (prion)	Peptide	Yes (CJD)	Unknown	N/A	250 kDa	Unknown

CJD, Creutzfeldt-Jakob disease; HAV, hepatitis A virus; HHV-8, human herpesvirus 8; N/A, not applicable; S/D, solvent/detergent; SEN V, SEN virus; TSE, transmissible spongiform encephalopathy; TTV, torque teneo virus.
Data from Teitel J: Transmissible agents and the safety of coagulation factor concentrates. World Federation of Hemophilia. *Facts and Figures* 7:1,118 1999; and Allain JP: Emerging viruses in blood transfusion. *Vox Sang* 78:243, 2000.

were being directed at methods to attenuate these known hepatitis viruses during the late 1970s and early 1980s,[23,36] HIV contaminated the human blood supply. More than 70% of patients in many countries and 30% to 40% of hemophilia patients worldwide were infected with HIV.[51–54] More recently, concern about the prion agents responsible for transmissible spongiform encephalopathies such as Creutzfeldt-Jakob disease (CJD), variant CJD, and bovine spongiform encephalopathy, as well as newly identified viral agents in the blood supply,[47,48] have reinforced the need for continued surveillance and further refinements in the production of products for the treatment of hemophilia. This attention has also been focused on recombinant products because some currently licensed products use added human or animal protein in fermentation or as stabilizers during purification or formulation. Table 117.2 lists agents that are potential contaminants of human plasma. Other viruses such as cytomegalovirus and human T-lymphotropic virus type I are transmissible primarily by cellular blood products.

Although ideal, the absolute removal of infectious agents in transfusable products may be unattainable and in fact may be unnecessary because the primary goal is to make them noninfectious. Practically, this can be accomplished by reducing the levels of the contaminating agent below the level of infectivity. The most relevant agents, viruses and prions, are small and therefore difficult to separate from protein components of plasma. Some pathogens are resistant to currently used methods of inactivation. In addition, as exemplified by HIV and prions, new agents may periodically emerge in the human population by crossing species barriers. Unless detected rapidly, newly emerging agents have the potential for global dissemination, especially if they are transmitted by transfusion of contaminated blood products. Despite these limitations, the safety of infusible products derived from human or animal sources (which includes cultured mammalian cells expressing recombinant protein) can be optimized by reducing the initial viral load in the source material (human plasma, culture medium, or transgenic material). With human plasma, this is accomplished by screening to limit potentially infected donors, by removal and inactivation of infectious agents, and by prospective surveillance of all products and recipients of products that potentially may become contaminated. Progress continues in technology to reduce virus transmission; nanofiltration, an example of this, allows for more than 4–6 log reduction of viruses through size exclusion by filtering the solution through membranes with extremely small poor size (15–40 nm) and without denaturing

plasma proteins.[55] Nonenveloped viruses such as hepatitis A and parvovirus B19, both smaller than 30 nm, can be effectively removed by nanofiltration. Benefix (Pfizer) undergoes nanofiltration.

Current discussions in the medical, health economic, and patient communities center around achieving an appropriate balance between safety and costs given that plasma-derived products on the market today are extremely safe with regard to pathogen transmission.[56]

Infusion Regimens and Dosing for Hemophilia

The mainstay of therapy for hemophilia involves the treatment of bleeding episodes with the infusion of products capable of replacing the missing factor VIII or IX. This so-called on-demand therapy is effective in staunching hemorrhage but not before tissue damage has occurred. Bleeding is especially destructive in the synovium, where a vicious cycle develops in which the initial bleed results in a proliferative inflammatory response and hypertrophy of synovial tissues that then become more susceptible to further trauma and bleeding. The result in the short term is repeated bleeds into the same joint, resulting in what is referred to as a "target joint," and eventually chronic joint destruction or hemophilic arthropathy. Patients with chronic arthropathy often require surgical intervention, including synovectomy, debridement, joint replacement, or even joint fusion.

With the availability of factor concentrates that allowed for the attainment of high plasma levels of factor VIII or IX, prophylactic therapy became possible. This approach was pioneered by Swedish treaters who have demonstrated that the use of prophylactic regimens,[57] wherein trough factor levels are maintained at greater than 1% of normal, reduces the incidence of arthropathy and CNS hemorrhage.[56] Greater availability of virally safe factor concentrates has allowed for the initiation of prophylactic regimens in early childhood. This "primary" form of prophylaxis has become the standard of care in developed countries. For prophylaxis, the National Hemophilia Foundation Medical and Scientific Advisory Council recommends infusion of factor VIII 25–50 U/kg 3 times a week or every other day for hemophilia A and factor IX 40–100 U/kg 2 or 3 times a week for hemophilia B.[58] Prophylaxis is not universally practiced, however, owing to the high cost of factor concentrates, the requirement for frequent intravenous (IV) infusion, and the need for placement of central venous catheters in some patients, especially small children, to obtain IV access. The cost of factor makes primary prophylaxis

TABLE 117.3	Dosing Regimens for Bleeding and Prophylaxis in Hemophilia				
Site	Factor Level (%)	Dose Hemophilia A (U/kg)	Dose Hemophilia B (U/kg)	Duration of Treatment	Comments
Joint	30–70	15–35	30–70	1–3 d	Splinting, temporary splinting, no weight bearing
Life threatening (e.g., intracranial, retropharyngeal, retroperitoneal)	80–100	40–50	80–100	1–14 d	Antifibrinolytic therapy with retropharyngeal bleeds
Soft tissue	30–50	15–25	30–50	2–5 d	Higher levels can be used for compartment syndrome
Surgery	80–100	40–50	80–100	10–14 d (or shorter for minor procedures)	Significant blood loss can occur into large muscles of the lower extremity and the iliopsoas
Oral	20–50	10–25	20–50	1–2 d	Antifibrinolytic therapy
Gastrointestinal[a]	30–100	15–50	30–100	2–3 d	Should be evaluated for source
Genitourinary[b]	30–50	15–25	30–50	1–2 d	Avoid antifibrinolytic therapy
Prophylaxis[c]	50	25	50	qod or 3×/wk	Steroids may be useful

[a]Depending on severity.
[b]Painless spontaneous hematuria often requires no treatment other than fluid intake. Persistence requires treatment and evaluation.
[c]Use of a schedule of 25 U/kg qod and a dose of 40 U/kg with an interval of 2 days between the next dose may increase compliance by decreasing infusions to three per week.
qod, Every other day.
Data from DiMichele D: Hemophilia 1996. New approach to an old disease. *Pediatr Clin North Am* 43:709, 1996; Mannucci PM: Haemophilia treatment protocols around the world: Towards a consensus. *Haemophilia* 4:421, 1998; and Lusher J: *Treatment of congenital coagulopathies*, 1999, AABB Press.

and even on-demand treatment prohibitive to more than 60% of the hemophilia patients in the world.[59]

To understand how prophylaxis is currently being instituted in the United States, a survey of hemophilia treatment centers was conducted: 62 centers responded, and 32% (or 20 centers) initiated prophylaxis on a once-weekly schedule, 21% (13 centers) on a twice-weekly schedule, and 47% on a thrice-weekly schedule.[60] This survey demonstrated the diversity in practice and deviation from the recommendation from the National Hemophilia Foundation. Alternative schedules for prophylaxis have been investigated. For example, the Canadian Hemophilia Primary Prophylaxis Study, a small, prospective, multicenter study, evaluated a tailored prophylaxis regimen in 25 patients with severe hemophilia A; patients were started at 50 U/kg once a week and were escalated to 30 U/kg twice weekly and then 25 U/kg on alternate days if one of the three situations occurred: development of a target joint, four bleeds in 3 months, or five or more bleeds occurred into any one joint. This seemed to be well tolerated, resulting in 1.2 bleeds per year while maintaining good joint function; long-term follow-up of tailored prophylaxis is needed, but it may be a cost-effective and central line-sparing option.[61]

Dosing regimens for the treatment of bleeding episodes in hemophilia have also evolved paralleling the availability of high-concentration pathogen-safe replacement products. Although no universal regimen for "on-demand" treatment has been established, certain trends prevail. In general, for nonlife-threatening bleeding episodes, the goal of therapy is to achieve a plasma factor VIII or IX level of between 30% and 100%. For life-threatening bleeds or prophylaxis for surgical procedures, the goal is a level of 100% to be maintained by repeated bolus infusions or continuous infusion for a duration of 10–14 days or longer, depending on the severity of the bleed or surgical intervention.

The majority of prophylaxis regimens aim at achieving a trough factor level of approximately 1%. Primary prophylaxis, instituted in young children, is aimed at preventing any joint bleeding episodes that would eventually result in chronic arthropathy. Secondary prophylaxis refers to limited or prolonged periods of prophylactic therapy, instituted after a serious bleed or the development of repeated bleeding into a single joint (target joint); tertiary prophylaxis entails initiation of prophylaxis subsequent to the onset of joint disease. A prospective randomized trial evaluating the safety and efficacy of a preemptive approach using once-weekly dosing before the first bleed to reduce inhibitor formation is currently in the planning stages.[62]

To prevent the development of a target joint and chronic arthropathy, many hemophilia treatment centers have recently adopted a regimen of two, three, or more infusions after a hemarthrosis (aggressive on-demand treatment). Specific dosing regimens for bleeding episodes have been developed by treaters and treatment centers. Although slight variations in indications and target plasma levels of factor VIII and factor IX among treatment centers exist, representative dosing regimens are similar and are presented in Table 117.3.[63-65]

Venous Access in Hemophilia Patients

Parents of young hemophilia patients are taught how to administer factor preparations through a butterfly needle until the patient is old enough to be taught to self-infuse. Alternatively, visiting nurse services obtain peripheral access for some patients. Factor administration via peripheral veins can be very challenging in infants and in patients who require frequent IV therapies, such as those with inhibitors; therefore, more permanent venous access is required in some patients. Options for venous access include externally tunneled or fully implantable catheters or arteriovenous fistulas (AVFs).[66] Hemophilia practitioners differ in their approach to venous access; one survey indicated that central venous access devices are widely used in 89%

of centers and avoided in 11%.[60] Complications such as infections and thrombosis limit the life of a device and add to the morbidity of the patient. From a metaanalysis of 48 studies, the incidence of infection was 0.66 per 1000 catheter-days. A multivariate analysis of these data showed that the presence of an inhibitor was associated with an increased risk of infection; additionally, they demonstrated that the risk of infection with a fully implantable device was one-third that of an external device.[67] In one prospective study of catheter-related deep venous thrombosis (DVT) in boys with hemophilia, 69% of children had a DVT when screened and 81% at the 2-year rescreening.[68] One study of 38 hemophilia patients confirmed that AVF is feasible, with complications in 34% of the patients; this group suggests that in patients with inhibitors, AVF should be considered the first line for venous access because they frequently require long-term, daily administration of factor.[69] In deciding on which approach to IV access for a patient, practitioners should address the risks and benefits of each type of device on an individual basis. Use of central catheters is attended by the risks of catheter-induced septic and thrombotic complications.[70] With longer acting products becoming available and the potential for more convenient modes of administration (subcutaneous), the need for semi-permanent vascular access devices will decrease over time.

TREATMENT OF HEMOPHILIA

Products Available for Treatment of Factor VIII Deficiency

Products available for the treatment of bleeding episodes or prophylaxis against bleeding in patients with mild or moderate hemophilia A include DDAVP (1-deamino 8-D arginine vasopressin), a vasoactive peptide that stimulates release of stored factor VIII, and infusible products containing exogenous factor VIII protein. These may be blood components, concentrates purified from blood plasma, or concentrates containing recombinant factor VIII protein.

DDAVP

The preferred product for treatment of patients with mild or moderate hemophilia A is the synthetic octapeptide DDAVP, a vasopressin analog. DDAVP causes a release of factor VIII (and von Willebrand factor [vWF]) from endothelial cells, raising plasma factor VIII by approximately threefold (range, 2–12-fold) in patients with hemophilia in whom the disease is caused by decreased production or secretion of a functional protein or a protein that has decreased activity. To be effective, DDAVP relies on a partial quantitative deficiency of factor VIII; thus, patients with severe hemophilia will not benefit from its use if the causative mutation results in no synthesis, secretion, or a nonfunctional protein. In a retrospective study assessing response to a DDAVP challenge in mild or moderate hemophilia, 57% of patients with mild hemophilia had a positive response, and several who failed the initial challenge had a response after a mean of 6 years, increasing the response rate to 71% in the mild group.[71] The response to DDAVP in an individual patient is typically reproducible, and an effective response must be documented before its routine use or as prophylaxis for bleeding in surgical procedures (see box on 1-Deamino 8-D Arginine Vasopressin Trial). IV and intranasal preparations are available. The IV product has been used in a subcutaneous route of administration. The intranasal preparation more easily allows a patient to administer the compound on an as-needed basis in a home therapy regimen. The phenomenon of tachyphylaxis, the decreased effectiveness of repeated doses of the same compound, occurs after several, typically three, consecutive doses.

Injectable DDAVP (Sanofi Aventis) is available in 4 μg/mL. The recommended dose is 0.3 μg/kg, mixed in 30 mL normal saline (for children <10 kg, 10 mL normal saline), infused IV slowly over 30 minutes. This dose can be repeated after 12–24 hours. DDAVP nasal

---

1-Deamino 8-D Arginine Vasopressin Trial

1. Collect citrated plasma from the patient immediately before DDAVP infusion for testing with the postinfusion blood specimen.
2. Administer DDAVP IV (0.3 μg/1 kg) in 25–50 mL normal saline.
3. Wait approximately 30 minutes after the infusion, carefully observing the patient for possible adverse side effects (increased blood pressure, facial flushing, signs or symptoms of hyponatremia).
4. Collect post-DDAVP infusion specimen in sodium citrate at 60, 120, and 240 minutes.
5. Compare the pre- and post-DDAVP factor VIII and vWF:Ag levels to confirm a therapeutic response, threefold increase from baseline (for mild or moderate hemophilia, response is defined as twofold increase in factor VIII: C levels or an absolute level above 0.31 U/mL at 1 hour).[71]

---

spray Stimate (CSL Behring) is available in a metered-dose pump that delivers 0.1 mL (150 μg) per activation (spray). The dose is one activation for patients weighing less than 50 kg and two activations in separate nostrils for those weighing more than 50 kg. In general, only three consecutive doses of DDAVP should be used unless otherwise advised by an experienced hemophilia treater. Because DDAVP is a vasopressin analog, there is a risk of fluid retention with its use. Changes in fluid balance can result in hyponatremia and seizures, especially when DDAVP is used in individuals on nonfluid-restricted or salt-restricted diets (e.g., elderly or very young patients or surgical patients undergoing fluid replacement with solutions with concentrations <0.9% sodium). For this reason, DDAVP is not recommended for children younger than 2 years of age. Caution is advised with the use of DDAVP in patients at risk for arterial thrombosis because there have been reports of myocardial infarction and cerebral thrombosis with its use.[72]

Factor VIII Concentrates

In developed countries, the current standard of care for the treatment and prevention of bleeding episodes in patients with severe hemophilia A and in patients with mild or moderate disease who do not respond to DDAVP is the infusion of recombinant human factor VIII. Recovery of recombinant factor VIII ranges from 1.5% to 2.5%/ IU/kg so that dosing assumes a rise in plasma factor VIII activity of 2% for every 1 IU/kg infused. Available concentrates are optimized to enhance viral clearance during purification and undergo one or more viral inactivation steps during manufacture. Plasma-derived factor VIII concentrates, treated with multiple purification and viral inactivation steps, are also available and have an excellent recent record of safety.

Intermediate- and High-Purity Plasma-Derived Concentrates

Intermediate-purity plasma-derived concentrates are prepared from cryoprecipitated plasma or fresh-frozen plasma (FFP), from which factor VIII is further purified using precipitation, gel permeation, ion exchange, or affinity chromatography, often in combination. Specific factor VIII coagulant activity in these products ranges from 2 to more than 100 IU/mg of protein, and many of the methods used also copurify significant amounts of vWF, making them useful for the treatment of some patients with von Willebrand disease (vWD; see later discussion on treatment of vWD). More highly purified plasma-derived concentrates are produced using heparin ligand or immuno-affinity purification methods and have specific activities ranging from 140 to greater than 3000 IU/mg. To stabilize the factor VIII molecule, the majority of these products are formulated by adding human albumin before lyophilization.

Recombinant Factor VIII Products

Highly purified recombinant factor VIII concentrates have been licensed in North America, Europe, and Japan since the early 1990s. These are either full-length or B domain–deleted molecules (the B domain is not required for activity in coagulation) that are expressed in mammalian cell culture (Chinese hamster ovary or baby hamster kidney cell lines) and are purified using immunoaffinity techniques. The development of these recombinant products was fueled primarily by concerns regarding safety of the human blood donor pool and the viral epidemics that occurred within the hemophilia population with the use of early plasma-derived products. As with highly purified plasma-derived factor VIII concentrates, the first-generation recombinant products are formulated with added albumin as a stabilizer. "Second generation" products (Kogenate FS, Bayer, Refacto, Pfizer) have been developed that stabilize the factor VIII molecule with nonprotein excipients.[73–75] Third-generation products (Advate, Baxter, Xyntha, Pfizer) do not have human proteins or other additives in the cell culture or as a stabilizer. Recombinant production methods that do not rely on the human plasma resource theoretically should provide for unlimited supply.

The first long-acting recombinant factor VIII product, Eloctate, Biogen Idec, synthesized in a human embryonic kidney cell line, was US Food and Drugs Administration (FDA) approved in June 2014. It is a B domain–deleted factor VIII covalently linked to human immunoglobulin G1; this Fc fusion protein has extended the half-life of factor VIII: in adults, almost 20 hours, 12–17 years old almost 16.5 hours, 6–11 years old about 14.5 hours and 2–5 years old, 12 hours.[76] Almost all of the patients (99%) receiving Eloctate for 6 months have been able to use the product every 3 days or longer to maintain a factor VIII level 1% to 3%.[76] Eloctate, Biogen Idec, has been used on demand, for prophylaxis and in the perioperative setting. For prophylaxis, Biogen Idec recommends 50 IU/kg every 4 days and suggests personalizing the dose based on response, 25–65 IU/kg at 3–5 day intervals.[76] The package insert also indicates that children less than 6 years old, may require more frequent or higher doses (up to 80 IU/kg).[76] For minor and moderate bleeds, Eloctate 20–30 IU/kg can be given every 24–48 hours; however in children less than 6 years old, Eloctate should be given every 12–24 hours.[76] For major bleeding episodes, Eloctate 40–50 IU/kg should be given every 12–24 hours and in children less than 6 years old, Eloctate should be given every 8–24 hours.[76] Many other long-acting factor VIII products are currently under investigation.

Novel Direction for Factor VIII Deficiency

In a phase I, dose escalating study, ACE910, Roche, a humanized bispecific antibody which binds both IXa and X, essentially mimicking how factor VIII functions, was given to patients with severe hemophilia with ($n = 11$) and without inhibitors ($n = 7$); this unique agent was given subcutaneously weekly and was well tolerated.[77] Further testing is needed but the possibility of a weekly subcutaneous injection would be life altering for patients with factor VIII deficiency, both with and without inhibitors.

Gene Therapy for Factor IX Deficiency

A landmark paper was published in December 2011 describing a phase 1 trial of the first six patients with severe factor IX deficiency who received one peripheral IV injection of an adeno-associated virus (AAV) expressing a factor IX gene, at three different doses. This vector was selected as it does not intercalate into the host genome and a capsid of AAV serotype 8 was added to avoid immunogenicity. Another advantage of using this serotype is the propensity for it to home to the liver. Sixty-seven percent of the patients in the trial no longer needed prophylaxis and the other 33% needed less factor. Patients who received the highest dose experienced a transient elevation of the alanine aminotransferase, between week 7 and 10, which resolved with prednisolone; this effect correlates with finding AAV8-capsid specific T cells in the peripheral blood.[78] These authors recently published an update on the long-term outcome of 10 men (22–64 years old) treated with gene therapy using the AAV8 construct; the additional four patients received the high dose of the vector and had on average 5% factor IX levels, with a decrease in bleeding episodes, sustained over 4 years.[79]

Plasma/Cryoprecipitate

In communities where virally inactivated factor VIII concentrates are not available, cryoprecipitate provides an effective alternative to therapy with concentrates for hemophilia A and vWD patients. Cryoprecipitate is a small-volume product (10–15 mL) enriched in factor VIII, vWF, fibrinogen, fibronectin, and factor XIII. Dosing can be calculated assuming approximately 80–150 IU of factor VIII per bag of cryoprecipitate (derived from a 450-mL single whole blood donor collection unit). Thus, a typical 1750-IU dose (50% correction for a 70-kg patient) would require between 10 and 21 bags or units. The limitations of cryoprecipitate therapy are (1) lack of a viral inactivation step in manufacture of the component and (2) lack of convenience, because multiple units must be pooled into a large volume ($\approx$70–100 mL) for infusion. FFP and whole blood provide less desirable alternatives because adequate therapy with both of these products suffers from the limitations described for cryoprecipitate, and their use often results in intravascular volume overload. Solvent/detergent (S/D)–treated FFP product is available in some countries. ABO group–specific S/D plasma is prepared by S/D treatment (TNBP and Triton ×100) of a pool of up to 2500 donors. After removal of the solvent and detergent components, 200-mL aliquots are refrozen for infusion.

Products Available for Treatment of Factor IX Deficiency

Factor IX Concentrates

As with replacement therapy for factor VIII deficiency, intermediate- and high-purity products derived from plasma for the treatment of factor IX deficiency are available, as well as a single recombinant factor IX product. All of these concentrates also undergo at least one viral inactivation or exclusion step in manufacture. The volume of distribution of factor IX is approximately twice the plasma volume. This can be explained in part by the affinity of factor IX for type IV collagen present in the extracellular matrix.[80] Recovery of factor IX after infusion is therefore approximately 1%/IU/kg. The recovery observed with recombinant factor IX is approximately 20% lower than that observed with plasma-derived factor IX.[81] This is likely caused by differences in posttranslational modifications between recombinant factor IX and plasma-derived factor IX.

Intermediate-purity factor IX products are generally purified from plasma using anion-exchange chromatography or calcium or barium precipitate adsorption. These methods select for proteins that contain highly negatively charged epitopes. The vitamin K–dependent (VKD) coagulation factors, by virtue of their gamma-carboxyglutamic acid–rich domains, are such proteins; thus, these techniques copurify varying amounts of the other VKD coagulation factors, factor VII, factor X, and prothrombin with factor IX. Hence, the products are referred to as *prothrombin complex concentrates* (PCCs). The levels of vitamin K proteins in these products vary and can be obtained from the manufacturer. In addition, the PCCs are contaminated with trace amounts of activated forms of VKD factors. The presence of these activated factors is the likely explanation for thromboses that have occurred with the use of these intermediate-purity products, typically in the setting of postoperative immobility or hepatic dysfunction.[82] To minimize the risk of thrombosis with the use of PCCs, it is advisable to achieve a peak factor IX level no higher than 50%.[83] Some clinicians add small amounts of heparin to infusions of these products to prevent thrombosis, and some manufacturers have formulated PCCs with heparin or antithrombin III.

High-purity factor IX products are produced from plasma using techniques of ligand affinity or immunoaffinity chromatography and typically have specific activities greater than 150 IU/mg. Three single high-purity recombinant factor IX products have been licensed in the United States (Alphanine, Grifols; Mononine, CSL Behring; and BeneFIX, Wyeth). Because specific products have different recovery results, consulting the package insert and performing recovery studies are recommended; for example, 1 IU BeneFIX/kg will increase the circulating activity of factor IX by 0.8 ± 0.2 and 0.7 ± 0.3 IU/dL in adults and pediatric (younger than 15 years old) patients, respectively.[84] Also, the initial dose of BeneFIX should be given under direct medical supervision because the potential for an allergic reaction is significant.[77] Thrombotic complications have not been reported with these high-purity products; some thrombotic events have been associated with continuous administration, which is not an approved method.[77] In patients with a history of allergy and inhibitors, an irreversible nephrotic syndrome has been reported during immune tolerance induction.[85]

In communities where factor IX concentrates are not available, plasma may provide a means of replacing factor IX in hemophilia B patients during bleeding episodes. Each unit of FFP derived from a 450-mL whole blood collection contains approximately 200 IU of factor IX. Replacement to therapeutic levels of factor IX with FFP is difficult because of the complication of volume overload. In some areas, S/D plasma provides a virally inactivated alternative to FFP.

The first long-acting recombinant factor IX product, Alprolix, Biogen Idec, synthesized in a human embryonic kidney cell line and purified by nanofiltration was FDA approved in March 2014. This factor IX is covalently linked to human immunoglobulin G1; this Fc fusion protein has extended the half-life of factor IX: in adults, almost 86.5 hours, 12–17-years old about 83.5 hours, 6–11 years old about 72 hours and 2–5 years old almost 66.5 hours.[86] Some patients with factor IX deficiency may only need factor IX three times a month with this product. It should be noted that kaolin-based assays may underestimate the factor IX level.[86]

Other Useful Adjuncts for Treatment of Bleeding in Hemophilia A and B

The antifibrinolytic agents tranexamic acid and ε-aminocaproic acid (EACA) (Amicar, Xanodyne Pharmaceuticals) are sometimes used in conjunction with clotting factor replacement therapy or DDAVP in the treatment of bleeding that occurs with hemophilia and other bleeding disorders. These agents interact with the lysine-binding site of plasminogen and enhance its activation. The more important effect of lysine analogs is that their occupancy of this site inhibits binding of the zymogen, plasminogen, to fibrin, which is necessary for full fibrinolytic activity. Antifibrinolytics are useful in the setting of mucosal bleeding and may substantially reduce the need for clotting factor concentrates in the setting of oral mucosal bleeding with tooth extractions. These agents are administered preoperatively and continued postoperatively until wound healing occurs. Although tranexamic acid is more potent, it is less readily absorbed when given orally. Tranexamic acid is administered at 25 mg/kg orally or 10 mg/kg IV preoperatively, and therapy can be continued postoperatively using oral rinses with a 5% solution. EACA is used at a dose of 100 mg/kg preoperatively followed by 100 mg/kg every 6 hours either orally or IV (maximum dose, 24 g/day). Dosing of EACA should be reduced in patients with renal insufficiency.

INHIBITORS OF FACTOR VIII AND FACTOR IX

A major complication in the treatment of patients with hemophilia is the development of inhibitory antibodies against the infused factors that interfere with factor activity. Rarely, antibodies may develop that do not affect activity but increase clearance of factor VIII or factor IX. The incidence of factor VIII inhibitors is approximately 30%, and inhibitors typically develop within the first 20 exposures to replacement therapy.[87,88] Well-designed prospective studies of the use of recombinant factor VIII in previously untreated patients revealed

that many of these inhibitors are low titer and transient in nature.[42,43] Patients with low-titer, transient inhibitors can be managed with increased doses of factor VIII. Inhibitors to factor IX occur less frequently; with an estimated incidence of approximately 1% to 3%.[89] Patients with factor IX antibodies may have anaphylactic reactions when treated with high-purity products.[90,91]

Patients with high-titer inhibitors to either factor VIII or factor IX do not usually achieve hemostasis after factor replacement and thus present a treatment challenge. Treatment of patients who develop inhibitors involves two approaches: (1) acute treatment of bleeding episodes and (2) immune tolerance induction therapy, whereby the patient is treated frequently (often daily) with factor VIII or factor IX in an effort to suppress the production of inhibitors by the immune system (similar to allergic desensitization therapy).

Treatment of acute bleeding episodes can be accomplished by two methods. For patients with low-titer inhibitors (<5 Bethesda units [BU], a laboratory measurement of inhibitor activity), hemostasis can be accomplished with large doses of factor VIII or factor IX (e.g., as high as 200 IU/kg given at frequent intervals) in an effort to neutralize or "override" the circulating inhibitor. A neutralization approach is usually ineffective for patients with high-titer inhibitors (>5–10 BU) and is expensive because of the large amounts of factor required. These patients and patients with low-titer inhibitors who fail to respond to override therapy can be treated using products that act to "bypass" the inhibitor. The only current bypass agents include activated prothrombin complex concentrates (FEIBA, Baxter Bioscience) (aPCC), which contain factors VII, X, and prothrombin in addition to factor IX that enhance production of thrombin generation by activating the coagulation pathway at points further down than the factor VIIIa/factor IXa step. FEIBA is used as first-line treatment of bleeding episodes in patients with inhibitors by some treaters even though the concentrate is derived from human plasma.

Recombinant activated factor VII (rFVIIa) (NovoSeven, Novo Nordisk) product was licensed in Europe and the United States with an indication for use as a bypass agent in the treatment of inhibitors in patients with hemophilia A and hemophilia B, as well as for bleeding and perioperative management in Glanzmann thrombasthenia, who are refractory to platelet transfusion. Another recombinant VII product, AryoSeven (Aryogen), which is biosimilar to NovoSeven is available and was shown to be as effective in the management of acute bleeding episodes.[92] The dose of rFVIIa is 90 μg/kg. Recombinant activated factor VIIa is administered every 2 hours compared with every 8–12 hours for PCCs or aPCCs. Thrombosis has also been reported with the use of rFVIIa[93,94] and PCCs.[95]

Despite the success achieved with immune tolerance induction regimens (80%–90%),[96] "bypass" agents are still needed in patients undergoing tolerization because an interval potentially as long as 2–3 years exists between the time that induction is initiated and the inhibitor is suppressed. Bleeding episodes that occur before achievement of tolerance usually require treatment with one or other of the bypassing agents.

Recently, Leissinger et al[97] demonstrated in hemophilia A patients with high-titer inhibitors the superiority of prophylactic thrice-weekly FEIBA (Baxter) at 85 U/kg over on-demand therapy. In a prospective, randomized, crossover study with a 3-month washout between the two arms, which were each 6 months, the prophylaxis regimen prevented progression of joint disease in high-titer inhibitor patients; and is now recommended for prophylaxis in high-titer inhibitor patients (see box Treatment of Life-Threatening Bleeding Episodes in Patients With Inhibitors Against Factor VIII or Factor IX).

Treatment of life-threatening bleeds in the context of a high-titer inhibitor represents a significant challenge. The effect of nonfactor VIII concentrates (bypass agents), when the inhibitor titer is greater than 10 BU (precluding the use of factor VIII), is difficult to monitor in the laboratory because plasma factor levels do not reflect hemostasis. Adjunctive therapies are frequently used in this setting to lower the titer of the antibody to allow for treatment of the patient with factor VIII concentrates. Aggressive regimens are used in which circulating antibodies are depleted using plasmapheresis or staphylococcal protein A immunoadsorption, and reduction of antibody

---

Treatment of Life-Threatening Bleeding Episodes in Patients With Inhibitors Against Factor VIII or Factor IX

Concentrates

1. Factor VIII containing concentrates in high doses (as high as 150–200 IU/kg) if inhibitor titer is low (<5–10 BU). High-dose continuous infusion of factor VIII (≈10 IU/kg/hour) after a high-dose bolus may be useful.
2. Recombinant factor VIIa. Dose is 90 μg/kg (or a dose up to 320 μg/kg) administered every 2 hours. Risk of thrombosis exists with this product.
3. Activated PCCs at a dose of 50–75 IU/kg every 8–12 hours. Risk of thrombosis exists with this product.

Immunomodulation

1. Antibody depletion
   a. Plasmapheresis
   b. Extracorporeal immunoadsorption of plasma (staphylococcal protein A column therapy and other methods)
2. Suppression of antibody production
   a. High-dose steroids (equivalent of prednisone 80 mg/day)
   b. Cyclophosphamide (10–15 mg/kg load and 2–3 mg/kg/day)
   c. Intravenous immunoglobulin (1 g/kg daily for 2 days)
   d. More aggressive regimens that may include vincristine, azathioprine, cyclosporine, or interferon-γ

Conservative Measures

1. Immobilization
2. Compression
3. Local application of hemostatic agents
4. Antifibrinolytics
5. Avoid venipunctures, intramuscular injections, arterial puncture, and lumbar punctures
6. Avoid use of medications that inhibit platelet function (ASA, NSAIDs)
7. DDAVP may be effective in some patients with low-titer inhibitors

ASA, aspirin; BU, Bethesda unit; NSAIDs, nonsteroidal antiinflammatory drugs; PCC, prothrombin complex concentrate.

---

production is attempted using immunomodulatory agents such as steroids, cyclophosphamide, and IV infusion of immunoglobulin G (IgG).[98–101] These strategies for acutely reducing antibody titers are also used by some hemophilia treaters at the outset of immune tolerance induction. In a phase II trial, Leissinger et al evaluated the safety and efficacy of rituximab, without concurrent immune tolerance induction (ITI), to reduce high-titer inhibitor levels in hemophilia A patients,[102] although the study was designed to enroll 43 patients, only 23 were enrolled and the Data Safety Monitoring Board closed the study because of poor accrual over 4 years. Three of 16 (18.8%) had a major response (inhibitor titer <5 BU) and one with a minor response (initial inhibitor titer <5 BU but increased after factor VIII exposure).[103] Several case reports or series of patients with severe hemophilia have demonstrated a greater advantage from rituximab when used in conjunction with ITI.[104,105] In a recent review of inhibitor eradication with rituximab, Franchini and Mannucci concluded that the combination of ITI with rituximab in mild to moderate hemophilia is likely to be more beneficial[106] than when used without simultaneous factor VIII. Also, rituximab has been used successfully in the setting of acquired hemophilia A, mostly with concurrent immunosuppression.[105]

VON WILLEBRAND DISEASE

vWD is an autosomal dominant bleeding disorder first described by Erik von Willebrand in 1926, who named this bleeding diathesis *pseudohemophilia*. vWD is relatively common, with a prevalence of up to 2% of the general population.[107] The penetrance and severity of the disease vary depending on the type of vWD (type 1, 2, or 3); the specific mutation; the number of affected genes; the patient's blood type; and numerous drug, hormonal, and stress-related

parameters. These factors, particularly the subtype of vWD and the patient's response to DDAVP, influence the recommended treatment for acute bleeding episodes or for prophylaxis against bleeding.

Although the disease had been described in the 1920s, the primary defect had earlier been attributed to either platelets or the vessel wall. An understanding of the missing protein in vWD and its relationship to factor VIII was not appreciated until the 1950s. Correction of the defect with transfusion of plasma, but not with platelet concentrates alone, defined the disease as one involving a missing plasma protein factor (vWF), not a platelet or vessel wall defect.[108] A correlation between vWD and factor VIII activity had previously been observed—the observation that a plasma fraction from patients lacking factor VIII (hemophilia A) could correct the defect in vWD in addition to the autosomal inheritance pattern, which helped further differentiate hemophilia A from vWD.[108] A more detailed discussion of clinical features and pathophysiology of vWD and the molecular biology of vWF can be found in Chapter 138.

Transfusion Therapy for von Willebrand Disease

The specific treatment for vWD varies with the bleeding symptoms and signs and with the individual diagnostic subtype of vWD (see Chapter 138). Treatment is guided further by laboratory results indicating the potential success of increasing vWF with DDAVP and the clinical experience with a particular patient and his or her natural biologic family members who have vWD. When possible, attempts should be made to treat the patient without exposing him or her to plasma-derived products.

Nonprotein-Based Treatment

DDAVP is a synthetic octapeptide homolog of vasopressin that results in the release of stored vWF from Weibel Palade bodies of the endothelium (see section on treatment of hemophilia A). DDAVP is often effective for type 1 disease and may be useful in certain patients with type 2 disease. It is not appropriate for use in patients with type 3 disease in whom no stores of vWF exist. Before the use of DDAVP, a DDAVP trial should be conducted to document its efficacy in an individual patient. The trial is performed as described for hemophilia A. The phenomenon of tachyphylaxis is also observed when DDAVP is used to treat vWD. For bleeding that does not respond to DDAVP or in patients in whom a poor response is observed with DDAVP, other modalities (typically protein based) must be used.

As described for hemophilia A, the antifibrinolytic agent EACA or tranexamic acid are often administered in the setting of dental surgery to inhibit fibrinolysis. Care should be taken when these agents are administered in patients with a predisposition to thrombosis.

Estrogens upregulate vWF synthesis and may be useful especially in women. Therapy with estrogens should also help ameliorate menorrhagia in affected symptomatic patients.

Plasma-Protein–Based Therapy

Factor VIII Concentrates

Some intermediate-purity factor VIII concentrates are manufactured from plasma using methods that copurify significant amounts of vWF. Many of the products listed in Table 117.4 contain vWF. Humate-P (ZLB Behring), Alphanate (Grifols USA), and Wilate (Octapharma), which is 1:1 vWF:RCo/factor VIII, are currently licensed for the treatment of vWD. Others, including Koate-DVI (Talecris Biotherapeutics), have been tested in vitro and in vivo for their potential use in therapy for vWD.[109–111] The multimeric pattern of VWF in these concentrates varies, and no product has the pattern of multimers that is present in normal plasma.[110] Because many of these products are effective clinically, the importance of these differences in multimer pattern remains to be determined. In addition,

TABLE 117.4   Other Coagulation Deficiencies

Factor	Incidence	Inheritance	Chromosome	Half-Life	Target Plasma Level	Treatment Product[a]
I (fibrinogen)	1–2/10⁶		4	2–4 days	50–100 mg/dL	Concentrates
Afibrinogen		AR				Cryoprecipitate
Hypofibrinogen		AR or AD				
Dysfibrinogen		AR or AD				
II (prothrombin)	<1/10⁶	AD	11	3 days	30%	PCCs Plasma
V	1/10⁶	AR	1	36 hours	25%	Plasma
VII	2/10⁶	AR	13	3–6 hours	25%	rFVIIa Concentrates PCCs Plasma
X	2/10⁶	AR	13	40 hours	10%–25%	PCCs Plasma
XI		AR or AD	4	80 hours	20%–40%	Concentrates Plasma
XIII	<1/10⁶	AR	1.6	9 days	5%	Concentrates Cryoprecipitate Plasma

[a]Products are listed in order of viral safety.
AD, Autosomal dominant; AR, autosomal recessive; PCC, prothrombin complex concentrates.
Data from Cohen AJ and Kessler: Treatment of inherited coagulation disorders. *Am J Med* 99:675, 1995.

when using multiple doses of these products, factor VIII and vWF:RCo should be monitored because there is an increased risk of thrombotic events with the accumulation of factor VIII.

von Willebrand Factor Concentrates (Plasma Derived and Recombinant)

Several chromatography-purified plasma-derived concentrates enriched in vWF have been studied by manufacturers in Europe.[112,113] Preliminary reports suggest that these are amenable to viral inactivation steps and may be effective both in vitro and in vivo.[110] To date, none of these have been developed as widely licensed products. Recombinant vWF (BAX 111, Baxter) which is albumin- and plasma-free and synthesized in Chinese hamster ovaries has been developed. In patients with severe vWD, a phase 3 multicenter trial of recombinant vWF (BAX 111, Baxter), given alone or with Advate, Baxter was effective in treating all 22 patients with bleeding episodes; no thrombosis or inhibitors occurred during the study.[114] A biologic license application was submitted to the FDA for BAX111.

Cryoprecipitate

Cryoprecipitate was the mainstay of plasma-based therapy for bleeding in patients with vWD until the availability of virally inactivated intermediate-purity factor VIII concentrates with preserved functional vWF protein. These factor VIII concentrates are the products of choice for the treatment of bleeding in patients with types 1 and 2 vWD who are unresponsive to DDAVP and for bleeding in patients with type 3 vWD. Owing to the small potential for viral contamination of cryoprecipitate, manufacture of which does not include steps to inactivate viral pathogens, cryoprecipitate is currently indicated only when virally safe concentrates containing vWF are unavailable.

ACQUIRED FACTOR VIII AND VON WILLEBRAND FACTOR DEFICIENCY

Antibodies that inhibit the activity of factor VIII can develop in previously normal patients. Most of these patients have no underlying disease; however, factor VIII antibodies can arise in the setting of autoimmune disorders or in the postpartum period. Although approximately one-third of inhibitors disappear spontaneously, the mortality rate among affected patients is significant.

In adults, acquired vWD is a rare autoimmune disorder that can occur in association with other autoimmune disorders or lymphoproliferative disease. Antibody may interact with the epitopes on

vWF required for its normal activity or result in increased clearance of antibody–vWF complexes.

In children, acquired vWD is extremely rare but has been reported in the context of Wilms tumor, hypothyroidism, and congenital heart disease and some medications; with treatment of the underlying disorder, vWF normalizes.

Treatment

Therapy for those patients with relatively high inhibitor titers (>5 BU) includes bypassing agents (FEIBA or rFVIIa) to stop bleeding and immunosuppression to reduce inhibitor levels. Plasmapheresis or immunoadsorption can be used to reduce the circulating levels of inhibitors. Immunosuppressive agents and IV IgG are useful adjuncts to abrogate production of the autoantibody. DDAVP can also be effective in some patients with low-titer inhibitors. Unlike inhibitors that develop with hemophilia A, exposure to factor VIII usually does not result in increased antibody titers.[115] Conservative measures to control hemorrhage should also be used in conjunction with the above, including immobilization and compression, topical or local hemostatic agents, and antifibrinolytic therapy. The use of venipunctures, intramuscular injections, and drugs with platelet inhibitory activity should be minimized or avoided.

OTHER COAGULATION PROTEIN DEFICIENCIES

Approximately 15% of inherited bleeding disorders are caused by deficiencies of coagulation factors other than factor VIII, factor IX, or vWF. Inherited deficiencies of fibrinogen and factors II, V, VII, X, XI, and XIII may result in bleeding, requiring treatment. The genes for these factors are not located on the X chromosome; thus two gene defects are typically required for symptomatic disease. Consanguinity is frequent in affected kindreds. The characteristics of these deficiencies are presented in Table 117.4. Hereditary deficiencies of factor XII, prekallikrein, and high-molecular-weight kininogen have not been described to result in bleeding diatheses.

The mainstays of therapy for these disorders are cryoprecipitate (for fibrinogen deficiency) and plasma. In some countries, concentrates enriched in the missing protein have been available. An S/D-treated pooled plasma product is also available in some regions. Pooled S/D-treated plasma has the advantage over FFP in that it is virally inactivated but has the drawback of exposing the patient to a large number of donors (2500) with each dose.

Fibrinogen Deficiency

Bleeding disorders can result from low to absent levels of fibrinogen (hypofibrinogenemia or afibrinogenemia) or a protein with abnormal function (dysfibrinogenemia). The inheritance pattern for the former is autosomal recessive and for the latter is autosomal dominant. Dysfibrinogenemias can result in bleeding or hypercoagulability. The gene for fibrinogen is located on chromosome 4. Because fibrinogen is required for the formation of a fibrin clot, it is surprising that afibrinogenemic patients survive gestation and birth. Diagnosis is made when patients present with bleeding from the umbilical stump, intracranial hemorrhage, or mucosal bleeding. Hemarthroses can occur but are less common than observed with the hemophilias. Wound healing may be delayed. Increased incidence of fetal wastage in patients with afibrinogenemia and hypofibrinogenemia is observed, and term gestation is rarely achieved without replacement of fibrinogen.[116-118] Because the substrate for clot formation, fibrinogen, is missing or deficient, the prothrombin time (PT), activated partial thromboplastin time (aPTT), thrombin clotting time (TCT), and coagulation assays that have fibrin formation as their end points are all prolonged. Replacement of fibrinogen is accomplished with cryoprecipitate with a goal of achieving a plasma level between 50 and 100 mg/dL and at least 60 mg/dL for maintenance of pregnancy.[118] Each bag of cryoprecipitate contains approximately 200 to 300 mg of fibrinogen. The biologic half-life of fibrinogen is between 2 and 4 days. Virally inactivated, highly purified fibrinogen concentrates are available in Europe, China, and Japan (Japan Green Cross, Aventis, LFB) and in the United States, RiaSTAP, CSL Behring is available. These fibrinogen concentrates offer many advantages over cryoprecipitate, including: viral inactivation, standardized fibrinogen content, smaller infusion volume and expedited time to treat the patient as reconstitution is swift, since it is stored as a lyophilized powder, and there is no need for cross-matching.[119] Adverse reactions to treatment include the development of fibrinogen antibodies; allergic reactions; and, paradoxically, thrombosis.

Prothrombin Deficiency

Congenital prothrombin deficiency is a rare autosomal recessive disorder estimated to be present at a rate of 0.5 cases per million. Disease has been described with both homozygous and heterozygous defects (including compound heterozygotes). No reports of a prothrombinemia appear in the literature, suggesting that complete lack of the protein is incompatible with normal development. Hemorrhagic symptoms include bruising; hemarthroses; intracranial, mucosal, and deep tissue bleeding; and menorrhagia.[120] Correlation between bleeding and prothrombin levels is poor. Both the PT and the aPTT are prolonged, and the thrombin time is normal. Treatment of prothrombin deficiency includes plasma at a dose of 15–25 mL/kg followed by 3 mL/kg every 12–24 hours to achieve levels of approximately 30%. The half-life of prothrombin is approximately 3 days. PCCs contain prothrombin and other VKD factors and can be used to treat prothrombin-deficient patients who are undergoing major surgery or life-threatening bleeds. Caution should be exercised because these have been associated with thrombosis.

Factor V Deficiency

Inherited deficiency of factor V occurs in fewer than 1:1,000,000 people with an autosomal recessive inheritance pattern (homozygous or compound heterozygous), resulting in factor V levels less than 20%. Symptoms include bleeding from the umbilical stump and mucous membranes, ecchymoses, menorrhagia, postpartum bleeding, and intracranial hemorrhage. Hemarthroses can occur but are

less common than with severe hemophilia. Correlation between bleeding and factor V levels is poor. No factor V–enriched plasma concentrates are available. Because factor V is in the common pathway of coagulation, in deficiency states, both the PT and the aPTT are prolonged. Treatment of bleeding involves the infusion of plasma at 15–20 mL/kg with a goal of achieving levels of 20%. The half-life of factor V is approximately 36 hours. Because platelets contain stored factor V,[121] they have been used to treat bleeding. Platelet infusion may result in the production of platelet-specific antibodies.

Factor VII Deficiency

Factor VII deficiency occurs in approximately 1:500,000 people; it is autosomal recessive and of the rare inherited coagulation disorders, factor VII deficiency is the most common. Severe bleeding occurs with levels below 1%, and symptoms in severely affected patients are similar to those observed with severe hemophilia. Intracranial hemorrhage may occur in up to 16% of cases and in neonates after vaginal delivery. The PT is prolonged, but the aPTT and thrombin time are normal. PCCs contain factor VII and may provide a benefit over plasma because they are virally inactivated. As with the use of these products for factor VIII and factor IX inhibitors, thrombosis has been reported. Several plasma-derived factor VII concentrates (LFB, Baxter and PFL) have been developed and have been used to treat congenital deficiency. Recombinant activated factor VII concentrate is effective in the treatment of bleeding with a congenital factor VII deficiency.[122-125] This can be used at a dose of 10–40 µg/kg every 4–6 hours.[126] Inhibitors to factor VIIa have developed in patients with congenital factor VII deficiency.[122]

Factor X Deficiency

Congenital deficiency of factor X is a rare condition resulting from homozygous or compound heterozygous defects in the autosomal genes for factor X located on chromosome 13. Bleeding is correlated with factor X levels, and symptoms include epistaxis, menorrhagia, hemarthrosis, intracranial or gastrointestinal hemorrhage, hematuria, and umbilical cord bleeding. Because factor X is a component of prothrombinase (the first step in the common pathway), diagnosis is suggested by both a prolonged PT and a prolonged aPTT but a normal TCT. Treatment is with plasma products (FFP or S/D-treated plasma) at approximately 15–25 mL/kg followed by 5 mL/kg every 24 hours with a goal of plasma factor X activity levels of 20%. PCCs can be used; however, they contain variable amounts of factor X. As with the use of PCCs for other indications, the risk of thrombosis is increased. Currently, a Phase III, multicenter study to investigate the pharmacokinetics, safety, and efficacy of a high purity factor X (Bio Products Laboratory) in patients with moderate to severe factor X deficiency was completed and results are not yet available.[127]

Factor XI Deficiency

Congenital factor XI deficiency (sometimes called hemophilia C) is an autosomal disorder with a recessive pattern of inheritance and is particularly common in Ashkenazi Jews in whom two specific mutations account for the approximately 8% prevalence of an abnormal factor XI gene.[123,124] The factor XI gene is located on chromosome 4. Bleeding symptoms are variable and include postsurgical or traumatic bleeding or heavy menses in women. Spontaneous hemorrhage and musculoskeletal bleeding are not typical of the disorder, and these characteristics distinguish this disorder from hemophilia A and B. Plasma levels of factor XI do not correlate with bleeding symptoms unlike the factor levels in hemophilia A and B. The aPTT is prolonged with factor XI deficiency; PT and thrombin time are normal. Patients with factor XI deficiency are usually treated before surgical procedures with a goal of factor XI levels between 30 and 45 U/dL.[123] Plasma (FFP and S/D-treated plasma) provides the mainstay of

CHAPTER 118

HEMAPHERESIS

Sandhya R. Panch and Harvey G. Klein

Therapeutic bloodletting is an ancient therapy, fashionable, albeit unproved, and practiced well into the 19th century. About the time that scientific skepticism began to temper the widespread use of therapeutic phlebotomy, a new technique for blood removal, apheresis, appeared in the research laboratory.[1] The term *apheresis*, derived from a Greek verb meaning "to take away or withdraw," was coined to describe removal of one component of blood with return of the remaining components to the donor. Like phlebotomy, apheresis was used first to treat patients but later became more important for collecting blood components for transfusion. Increasingly, apheresis techniques are used to collect cell populations from the peripheral blood of healthy donors and patients for purposes of hematopoietic stem/progenitor cell (HPC) transplantation and immune cell therapies. Annually in the United States, about 1.9 million units of red blood cells (RBCs), 2.5 million units of platelets, and 2500 granulocyte doses are collected by apheresis and more than 50,000 units of peripheral blood-hematopoietic stem and progenitor cells (PB-HSPC) and therapeutic cellular therapy products are collected at hospital and blood center apheresis facilities.[2]

PRINCIPLES OF APHERESIS

The principal objective of apheresis is efficient removal of some circulating blood component, either cells (cytapheresis) or some plasma solute (plasmapheresis). For most disorders the treatment goal is to deplete the circulating cell or substance directly responsible for the disease process. Apheresis can also mobilize cells and plasma components from tissue depots. For example, lymphocytes may be mobilized from the spleen and lymph nodes of some patients with chronic lymphocytic leukemia (CLL), and low-density lipoproteins (LDLs) can be removed from tissue stores in patients with familial hypercholesterolemia. The apheresis procedure itself mobilizes $CD34^+$ cells from extravascular depots in peripheral blood-hematopoietic stem and progenitor cells (PB-HSPC) donors, resulting in collection of more than twice as many $CD34^+$ cells than estimated based on preapheresis peripheral blood cell counts (Fig. 118.1). Apheresis may have other, less obvious effects. Lymphocyte depletion may modify immune responsiveness in some disease states, possibly by disturbing the control mechanisms of cellular immune regulation. Plasmapheresis enhances splenic clearance of immune complexes in certain autoimmune disorders. When therapeutic effect is judged by clinical improvement rather than by efficiency of solute removal, apheresis is more often a helpful adjunct than a form of first-line therapy.

Several mathematical models formulated for different clinical conditions describe the kinetics of apheresis. Removal of most blood constituents follows a logarithmic curve (Fig. 118.2). This model assumes that the substance removed is neither synthesized nor degraded substantially during the procedure, remains within the intravascular compartment, and mixes instantaneously and completely with any plasma replacement solution. When the goal of plasmapheresis is to supply a deficient substance, for example, the cleavase ADAMTS13 in the treatment of thrombotic thrombocytopenic purpura (TTP), replacement follows logarithmic kinetics similar to those developed for solute removal. From Fig. 118.2, it is evident that removal of 1.5–2.0 volumes will reduce an intravascular substance by approximately 80% and that processing larger volumes results in little additional gain. Specific cell removal with centrifugal automated cell separators depends on the number of cells available, the volume of blood processed, the efficiency of the particular instrument, and the separation characteristics of the different cells. Most commercially available instruments remove platelets and lymphocytes extremely efficiently. Granulocytes and other mononuclear cells, including HPCs from peripheral blood, cannot be cleanly separated from other cells by standard centrifugal apheresis equipment (Fig. 118.3). Optimal harvesting of these cells requires special techniques such as stimulating the donor with corticosteroids or cytokines and adding sedimenting agents to enhance cell separation.

Whereas this model accurately estimates removal of cells and large proteins such as fibrinogen and immunoglobulin (Ig) M, removal of smaller solutes such as IgG and albumin-bound drugs is less efficient. Transfer of these moieties from the extravascular to the intravascular compartment depends both on diffusion along a concentration gradient and on active transport. The rate of clearance can be calculated using diffusion coefficients, sieving coefficients, and lymphatic flow rate, although in practice this degree of accuracy is rarely necessary.

TECHNOLOGY AND TECHNIQUES

The plasmapheresis technique that originated in the animal laboratory required manual resuspension of RBCs and posed a substantial risk of microbial contamination of the components being reinfused. With the introduction of sterile, disposable, interconnected plastic blood bags, plasmapheresis became relatively safe and easy. However, manual apheresis proved too inefficient and labor intensive for collecting large component volumes and raised concerns that the separated units of RBCs might be reinfused accidentally into the wrong donor or patient. The introduction of automated online blood cell separators solved these problems. Automated apheresis instruments use microprocessor technology to draw and anticoagulate blood, separate components either by centrifugation or by filtration, collect the desired component, and recombine the remaining components for return to the patient or donor. The equipment contains disposable plastic software in the blood path and uses anticoagulants containing citrate or combinations of citrate and heparin that do not result in clinical anticoagulation of the patient or donor. Most instruments function well at blood flow rates of 30–80 mL/min and can operate from peripheral venous access or from a variety of multilumen central venous catheters. Newer therapeutic apheresis devices are smaller and more automated, allowing for implementation of more safety functions and improved portability.

Because the ideal method for treating disorders mediated by abnormal plasma components is to remove the offending substance selectively, a variety of online filtration and column adsorption techniques have been introduced or proposed. Ligands bound to a column matrix may be relatively nonspecific chemical sorbents, such as charcoal or heparin, or specific ligands, such as monoclonal antibodies and recombinant protein antigens. Two such columns are commercially available: one using staphylococcal protein A and the other using negatively charged dextran sulfate cellulose beads. Staphylococcal protein A has high affinity for the Fc portion of IgG1, IgG2, and IgG4 and for immune complexes containing these IgG subtypes. This column is approved for use in therapeutic apheresis procedures for patients with chronic immune thrombocytopenia and selected adult patients with rheumatoid arthritis. The dextran sulfate cellulose

Cell type	Blood concentration			Cell content			Apparent volume of distribution	
	Initial	End	% change[a]	Blood[b]	Product[c]	Fraction[d]	Liters	No. of blood volumes
CD34 Cells								
25 L	0.077	0.045	−45	3.8	7.9	2.3	25.9	5.3
15 L ×2	0.078	0.039	−50	3.9	8.1	2.3	22.2	5.1

[a] Percentage change, end vs. initial

[b] Estimated initial content in peripheral blood

[c] Total product content

[d] Total product content divided by estimated initial content in peripheral blood. L, liters. CD34 cell concentration in 10^9/L, CD34 cell content x 10^8 cells.

Fig. 118.1 TWENTY HEALTHY MOBILIZED DONORS UNDERWENT EITHER A SINGLE LARGE VOLUME LEUKAPHERESIS PROCEDURE OF 25 L OR TWO CONSECUTIVE-DAY SMALLER VOLUME PROCEDURES OF 15 L EACH. In both study groups, more than twice as many CD34 cells were collected than the estimated total content of these cells in the peripheral blood before apheresis, providing evidence for the existence of a large extravascular pool of peripheral blood stem cells, which becomes accessible to collection by leukapheresis. *(Modified from Bolan CD, Carter CS, Wesley RA, et al: Prospective evaluation of cell kinetics, yields and donor experiences during a single large-volume apheresis versus two smaller volume consecutive day collections of allogeneic peripheral blood stem cells.* Br J Hematol *120:801, 2003, by permission of the authors.)*

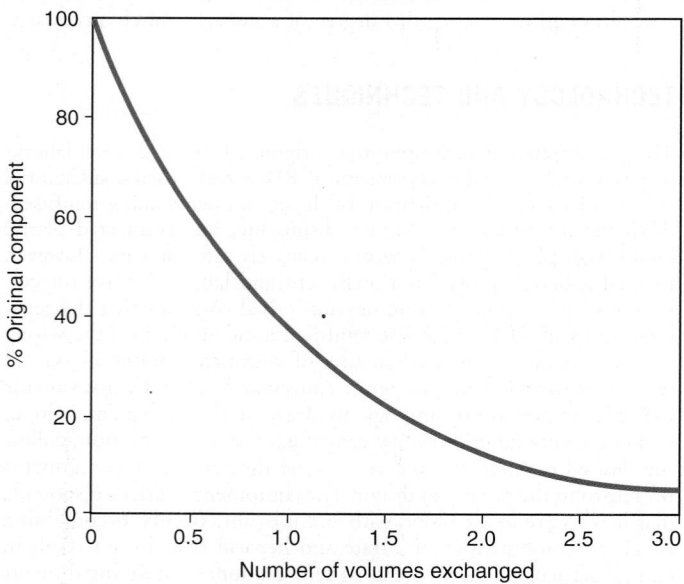

Fig. 118.2 RELATIONSHIP BETWEEN VOLUMES REMOVED BY APHERESIS AND PERCENTAGE OF THE TARGET COMPONENT REMAINING. The relation is valid for blood volumes during red blood cell exchange or for plasma volumes during plasmapheresis if the target solute remains primarily within the intravascular compartment.

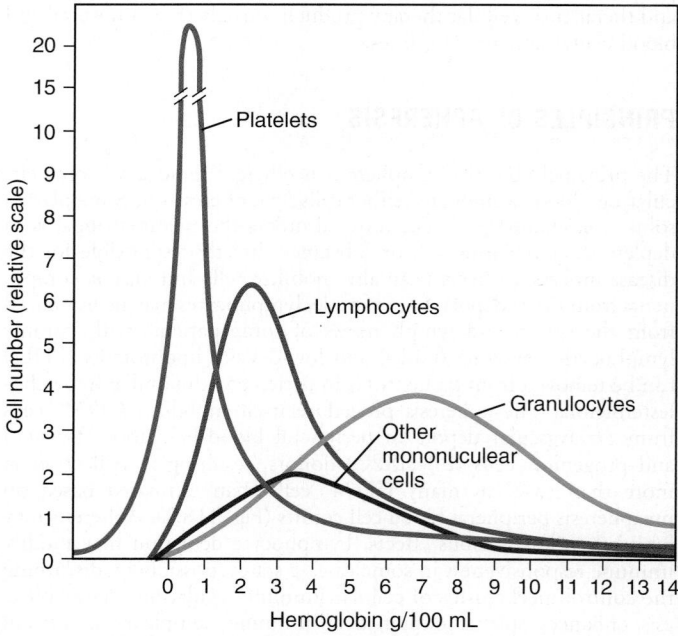

Fig. 118.3 SCHEMATIC DISTRIBUTION OF CELLS AT THE COLLECTION PORT OF A CENTRIFUGAL CELL SEPARATOR. The number and percentage of each cell type collected can be varied by adjusting the site of collection along the interface or by changing centrifugal force, blood flow rate, or rate of cell removal.

columns selectively remove LDL, very-low-density lipoprotein, and lipoprotein, and have proved effective in managing patients with homozygous hypercholesterolemia who have not responded to diet and cholesterol-lowering drug therapy (Fig. 118.4). A similar technique, heparin-induced extracorporeal lipoprotein precipitation, uses low pH and negatively charged heparin to precipitate lipoproteins and remove the precipitate by filtration online (H.E.L.P. Plasmat Futura, Braun Medical). Apheresis technology has also been adapted for extracorporeal phototherapy of patient leukocytes (photopheresis) to treat cutaneous T-cell lymphoma and to modulate the pathologic immune response in graft-versus-host disease (GVHD), solid organ transplant, and autoimmune diseases (see later discussion).

Therapeutic Cytapheresis

Common indications for therapeutic cell removal are listed in Table 118.1. Most of these procedures entail simple apheresis of the patient's peripheral blood with diversion for discarding the affected RBC, white blood cell (WBC), or platelet fraction. Special apheresis technologies have been approved, such as photopheresis devices, that divert a cell fraction that is photochemically treated in the extracorporeal circuit and returned to the patient's circulation, and

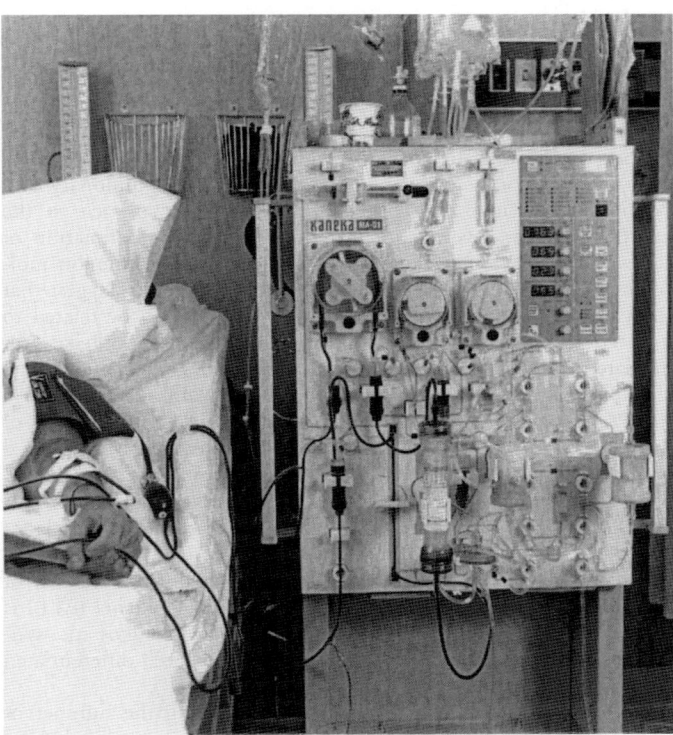

Fig. 118.4 TWO-STAGE THERAPEUTIC PLASMAPHERESIS. Plasma is separated from cells by filtration and then passed through parallel adsorption columns to remove low-density lipoproteins from a patient with homozygous familial hypercholesterolemia.

TABLE 118.1	Common Indications for Therapeutic Cytapheresis

Erythrocytapheresis
Acute complications of sickle cell disease
Prophylaxis for recurrent stroke
Frequent severe pain crises
Hyperparasitemia (malaria, babesiosis)
Hemochromatosis

Leukapheresis
Leukemia with hyperleukocytosis syndrome
Cutaneous T-cell lymphoma (photopheresis)
Peripheral blood stem cell collection

Plateletpheresis
Symptomatic thrombocytosis

apheresis immunoabsorption columns, which selectively remove immunoglobulins in the plasma by binding to a solid matrix.

Erythrocytapheresis

RBC exchange (erythrocytapheresis) is used most often to manage or prevent the acute vasoocclusive complications of sickle cell disease. Compared with manual exchange transfusion, mechanical cell separators offer the advantages of speed and ease and reduce the risks of rapid blood volume alteration and increased blood viscosity that may occur with simple transfusion. Automated procedures can be performed with all centrifugal instruments, and programmed procedures allow accurate prediction of target hemoglobin (Hb) concentration and percent HbA at the conclusion of the procedure. A single volume exchange will remove about two-thirds of the circulating cells.

Sickle cell anemia occurs in individuals who are homozygous for a single mutation in codon 6 of the *β-globin* gene, resulting in

substitution of a single amino acid. Although the defect appears simple, the pathophysiology of the vasoocclusive crises is complex, involving Hb polymerization, change in cell shape, adhesion to endothelial cells, dysregulated nitric oxide homeostasis, and release of free Hb and inflammatory cytokines.[3] Clinical manifestations vary from patient to patient. The rationale behind exchange transfusion involves improving tissue oxygenation, reducing hemolysis, and preventing microvascular sickling by diluting the patient's abnormal RBCs, simultaneously correcting anemia and favorably altering whole blood viscosity and rheology. No clinical data support a single optimal level of HbA; however, as few as 30% of transfused cells markedly decrease blood viscosity. At mixtures of 50% or greater, resistance to membrane filterability approaches normal. In nonemergency situations, such levels can often be achieved with a simple transfusion regimen. For simple and exchange transfusions, raising the level of HbA to between 60% and 70% while lowering the level of HbS to 30% is generally efficacious, although even higher levels of HbA are often used to treat an ongoing crisis. Clinical indications for exchange transfusion in patients with sickle cell anemia remain controversial, with limited controlled study data available. Simple transfusion has been shown to improve renal concentrating ability and splenic function in young sickle cell patients; exchange transfusion improves exercise tolerance and reverses the periodic oscillations in cutaneous blood flow associated with this disease. Such observations have encouraged the use of exchange transfusion for acute complications of sickle cell disease such as acute chest syndrome, priapism, cerebrovascular accident, and hepatic and retinal infarction. Exchange transfusion for sickle cell patients has also been used for prophylaxis during pregnancy and before surgery, although prophylactic transfusion in these settings remains controversial. The only randomized trial of transfusion during pregnancy has shown that prophylactic transfusion sufficient to reduce the incidence of painful crises did not reduce other maternal morbidity or perinatal mortality. The risk of intrauterine growth restriction may be reduced by prophylactic exchange transfusion; however, the study is limited by the retrospective observational nature of the data. In a randomized study of patients with sickle cell disease undergoing surgery, a conservative simple transfusion regimen (to increase the Hb level to 10 g/dL) was as effective as an aggressive regimen (to lower the HbS level to <30%) with respect to perioperative complications not related to transfusion. The patients in the aggressive regimen group received twice as many units of blood, had a proportionally increased RBC alloimmunization rate, and had more hemolytic transfusion reactions. A subsequent trial has confirmed that preoperative transfusion is associated with decreased perioperative complications in patients with sickle cell disease who are scheduled to undergo low-risk and medium-risk surgeries.[4]

Transfusion prophylaxis is now clearly indicated for children at high risk for stroke. A randomized controlled study demonstrated a risk reduction of 90% in the patients who were maintained at levels of 30% or less HbS by simple or exchange transfusion. This result confirms earlier experience and indicates that in this group of children with sickle cell anemia, transfusion therapy should begin before the first event and continue indefinitely. A second trial addressed whether transfusion could be safely discontinued to avoid the cumulative long-term risks of iron overload and RBC alloimmunization. After 10 months of randomization, half of the patients who discontinued transfusion had developed central nervous system abnormalities, including reversion to abnormal transcranial Doppler findings and a small number of strokes, necessitating early termination of the trial. For chronic management, repeated erythrocytapheresis may be preferable to simple transfusion for patients at high risk for stroke who have developed iron overload to levels associated with organ damage. Exchange transfusion, although relatively safe and convenient, carries all the complications of RBC transfusion. Patients are exposed to a large number of donors and are at a small but significant risk of contracting hepatitis and other blood-borne infections. As many as 33% of all patients develop alloantibodies, and life-threatening delayed hemolytic transfusion reactions have been reported. In addition, an immunohematologic study of multiply transfused sickle cell patients shows that 85% of heavily transfused patients are alloimmunized to human leukocyte antigens (HLAs), platelet-specific antigens, or both. Most centers avoid inducing nonhemolytic transfusion reactions and HLA alloimmunization by using leukocyte-depleted RBCs. Extended RBC phenotyping at diagnosis and provision of phenotypically matched blood, when practical, can reduce the risk of RBC alloimmunization and associated hemolytic transfusion reactions. Despite the removal of RBCs during exchange, most patients remain in positive iron balance, although iron accumulation is slow and chelation is rarely required to prevent transfusional hemosiderosis.

Other indications for RBC exchange are rare. The procedure has been used for patients with overwhelming RBC parasitic infections, such as severe and complicated malaria and babesiosis. In malaria, exchange transfusion may have at least three beneficial effects. An automated exchange rapidly decreases the concentration of circulating parasites while improving the rheologic properties of the blood by replacing the infected RBCs. The exchange may also reduce levels of proinflammatory cytokines and may help sustain life until conventional therapy and natural immunity take effect. Although the efficacy of this therapy has not been evaluated by controlled trials, prospective studies and review of published cases suggest the use of erythrocytapheresis for parasitemia greater than 10% to 15% or even less in selected patients such as those with cerebral malaria or pulmonary edema. Case reports document RBC exchange in such diverse conditions as carbon monoxide poisoning and glucose-6-phosphate dehydrogenase (G6PD)–deficient hemolysis.

Automated RBC removal with volume replacement (isovolemic hemodilution) can be performed rapidly and safely in polycythemic subjects. This maneuver should be reserved for polycythemic patients with an urgent clinical indication to lower the hematocrit (e.g., evolving thrombotic stroke) for which standard single-unit manual phlebotomy might be inadvisably slow. Automated double RBC apheresis technology has more recently been used to treat individuals with hereditary hemochromatosis. This procedure removes excess iron more rapidly than manual phlebotomy and is well received by patients because it lowers the frequency of clinic visits (Fig. 118.5).[5]

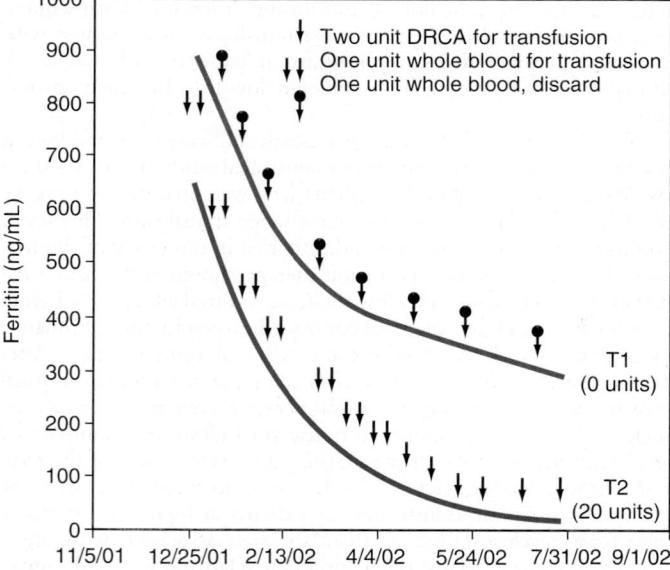

Fig. 118.5 ONE TWIN WAS TREATED WITH MANUAL PHLEBOTOMY (T1) AND THE OTHER WITH DOUBLE RED BLOOD CELL APHERESIS (T2). In the same time period, ferritin levels declined more rapidly and to lower levels in the twin treated with double red blood cell apheresis. *DRCA*, Double red blood cell apheresis. (Unpublished data from Bolan CD, Leitman SF, with permission of the authors.)

Leukapheresis

Therapeutic leukapheresis has been used most successfully to help manage patients with acute leukemia and extremely high WBC numbers, so-called acute hyperleukocytic leukemia (AHL). When the fractional volume of leukocytes (leukocrit) exceeds 20%, blood viscosity increases and leukocytes can interfere with pulmonary and cerebral blood flow and compete with tissue for oxygen in the microcirculation. Investigations of the expression and function of adhesion receptors in leukemic cells and the role of adhesion molecules in leukocyte-induced acute lung injury in sepsis suggest that the pathophysiology of leukostasis in AHL may also be related to interactions between leukemic blasts, platelets, and endothelial cells mediated by locally released adhesion molecules. A single-volume leukapheresis procedure generally reduces the WBC count by 20% to 50%, depending on the differing sedimentation characteristics of the specific blast cell population. Ordinarily, leukapheresis is initiated in a patient with acute myeloid leukemia (AML) or in the accelerated phases of chronic myeloid leukemia (CML) when the blast count exceeds 100,000/mm³ or when rapidly rising blast counts are higher than 50,000/mm³, especially when evidence of central nervous system or pulmonary symptoms appears. The threshold for initiation of leukapheresis in patients with acute lymphocytic leukemia (ALL) is generally higher (WBC count >200,000/mm³). Leukostatic syndromes do not occur when concentrations of well-differentiated lymphocytes exceed even several million/mm³.

Although leukapheresis is effective in reducing the number of circulating blasts, the evidence for clinical benefit is anecdotal. Case reports and small series describe dramatic improvement of patients with evolving strokes and respiratory insufficiency, but the absence of a randomized controlled trial necessitates reliance on retrospective studies. Leukapheresis may reduce early death (ED) rates but does not improve the overall survival of patients with AML.[6] Trials reporting reduction in ED should be interpreted with caution. Because one retrospective cohort study associated leukapheresis with a poorer outcome attributed to a delay in commencing chemotherapy,[7] it seems imprudent to delay other immediate measures for treatment of patients with AHL (infusion of intravenous [IV] fluids, administration of hydroxyurea, and uricosuric medication, urinary alkalization, correction of coagulopathy and thrombocytopenia) while awaiting leukapheresis.

Mechanical cytoreduction for managing other leukemic processes has limited value. Although repeated leukapheresis has adequately reduced the WBC count in a series of patients with CML, the median patient survival rate was not significantly different from that of similar patients treated with conventional chemotherapy. Chronic leukapheresis can provide acceptable control of the peripheral WBC count in clinical situations such as pregnancy, when cytotoxic agents may best be avoided, but cytoreduction alone does not appear to alter the course of CML. In a small series of gravid patients leukapheresis in combination with interferon has successfully controlled the disease until therapy with tyrosine kinase inhibitors could be initiated after delivery.[8] Early studies of patients with CLL suggested short-term clinical benefit of leukapheresis, but long-term support of patients when the disease is refractory to chemotherapy does not appear to prolong life.

Lymphocyte removal by apheresis has also been used to modify immune responsiveness in patients with autoimmune diseases and to enhance solid organ allograft survival and reverse solid organ graft rejection. Evidence of clinical efficacy in these situations is sparse. Removal of large numbers of lymphocytes over a period of a few weeks can suppress peripheral lymphocyte counts in patients with rheumatoid arthritis for up to 1 year and can alter skin test reactivity and lymphocyte mitogen responsiveness to a variety of stimulants. Selected patients experience a modest but significant reduction in disease activity; however, the subset of patients who may derive substantial benefit from this therapy is difficult to identify. Because leukocytes are a major source of inflammatory cytokines implicated in the pathogenesis of inflammatory bowel diseases (IBD), nonpharmacologic methods for selective leukoreduction have been developed to treat these chronic, relapsing, lifelong disorders. Although IBD respond to a variety of drug regimens, leukapheresis may have a role as a "steroid-sparing" intervention for patients who develop toxicity from long-term steroid use. Cellsorba removes leukocytes by extracorporeal filtration. Granulocyte-monocyte apheresis (Adacolumn) selectively adsorbs cells through columns filled with cellulose beads.[9] Clinical trials using Adacolumn technology have promising results in the treatment of ulcerative colitis, with remission rates in excess of 70% compared with conventional medical therapy. These studies should be interpreted with caution given their high risk of bias and the inclusion of predominantly Japanese patients, which may limit how the results apply to populations with different genetic and environmental factors.[10] The optimum course of therapy is yet to be defined. Recent trials have investigated the safety and efficacy of procedures varying from weekly to a daily basis.[11]

Extracorporeal Photopheresis

Photopheresis, although not strictly a "cell removal" procedure, is considered "apheresis" as it involves automated extracorporeal photochemotherapy (ECP) treatment that includes leukapheresis, extracorporeal photoactivation with 8-methoxypsoralen (8-MOP), a light-sensitizing agent, and ex vivo ultraviolet A irradiation. The treated leukocyte fraction (Fig. 118.6) delivering the light-sensitizing agent directly to the extracorporeal leukocyte fraction avoids any potential toxicity from oral administration of 8-MOP. The mechanism of action of photopheresis is unproved, but may involve induction of apoptosis of pathogenic T lymphocytes and induction of a dendritic cell-mediated cytotoxic T-cell response. This therapy has minimal toxicity and is highly effective in the treatment of patients with advanced cutaneous T-cell lymphoma. Patients who present with the erythrodermic disease form and circulating malignant cells have the best clinical response. Photopheresis is typically performed once or twice a month. Symptomatic patients with a higher circulating tumor burden benefit from a more intense regimen.[12] More recently, the major use of this technology involves modulation of immune rejection of transplanted organs and management of GVHD after stem cell transplantation in patients who do not respond to standard immunosuppressive therapy. In steroid-refractory acute GVHD, ECP is thought to enhance regulatory T-cell activity, likely inhibiting the cytotoxic T-cells implicated in the pathogenesis of this condition. Response rates in steroid refractory acute GVHD in pediatric and adult patients range from 52% to 100%. Based on these promising results, trials evaluating the utility of ECP as a GVHD preventive strategy are currently underway. Patients with chronic extensive GVHD have also been treated, with responses observed in approximately two-thirds of the steroid-dependent patients, with cutaneous, oral, and ocular forms of the disease. Treatment which is more aggressive than the traditional bimonthly schedule may be required. A response may facilitate a reduction in immunosuppression ("steroid sparing") with continued photopheresis based on results from a randomized phase II trial.[13] In chronic visceral GVHD, where a clear benefit is yet to be established, consideration for treatment should include the logistic challenges of frequent hospital visits and the prolonged need for central venous catheter care and/or transfusion support.

Acute rejection in cardiac transplantation occurs in 25% of recipients in the first year. In 30% to 50% of cases, acute rejection is T-cell mediated. Prospective studies have shown benefit of photopheresis in prevention of rejection. In the case of lung transplant, chronic rejection is manifest as bronchiolitis obliterans syndrome (BOS), presenting as progressive dyspnea and airflow limitation. In a recent prospective nonrandomized study, the rate of decline in lung function stabilized within 6 months of starting ECP therapy compared with rates of FEV_1 (forced expiratory volume in the first second of expiration) which were worsening at baseline. Rates of retransplantation were lower and survival was higher among patients who received ECP treatment. Patients with cystic fibrosis and those with longer interval to BOS development since transplant were less likely

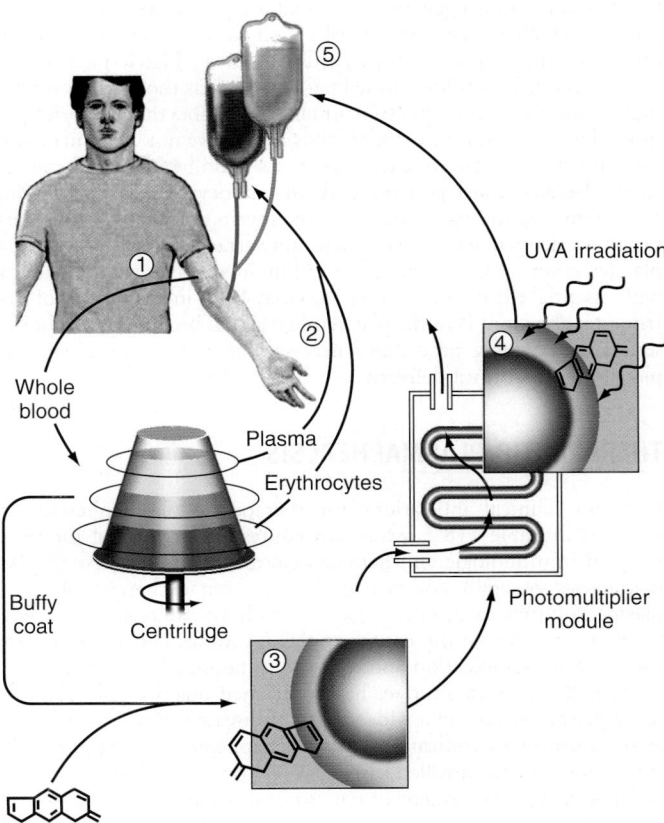

Fig. 118.6 OVERVIEW OF A PHOTOPHERESIS PROCEDURE. (1) Vascular access is achieved by placement of a peripheral intravenous line or through a temporary central venous catheter. Whole blood is withdrawn from the patient, mixed with an anticoagulant solution, and pumped to a centrifuge, where it is separated into plasma, red blood cell, and mononuclear cell (buffy coat) fractions by elutriation. (2) After the collection of each mononuclear cell fraction, the uncollected red blood cells and plasma are pumped from the plasma/return bag through a blood filter and returned to the patient. (3) The mononuclear cell fractions are mixed with 8-methoxypsoralen and then (4) pumped through a sterile cassette surrounded by ultraviolet A (UVA) bulbs, resulting in a controlled rate and amount of UVA exposure. (5) The treated cell fraction is filtered and returned to the patient.

to respond to therapy.[14] Of the substantial number of autoimmune disorders for which ECP therapy has been studied, data from small randomized trials have shown benefit in systemic sclerosis (improvement is skin and joint disease severity), and in Crohn disease (steroid-sparing effect). No significant benefit was demonstrated in type I diabetes or in multiple sclerosis (MS).[15] The acute adverse effects of photopheresis include photosensitivity, low-grade fever, and transient hypotension. Anemia and iron deficiency caused by incomplete reinfusion of RBCs may occur in patients undergoing repeated photopheresis. In patients with inadequate peripheral venous access requiring central venous catheter placement, infection, bleeding, and recurrent clotting are risk factors.

Plateletpheresis

Therapeutic plateletpheresis is generally reserved for patients with myeloproliferative disorders and hemorrhage or thrombosis associated with an increase in circulating platelets. Many centers consider using plateletpheresis when the patient's peripheral platelet count is greater than $10^6/mm^3$, although no consistent relationship between the level of platelet elevation and the occurrence of symptoms has been found, and no generally accepted assay of platelet dysfunction predicts which patients are at risk. A single cytapheresis procedure can lower the platelet count by 30% to 50%. Plateletpheresis can have dramatic effects for selected patients such as those with evolving digital gangrene. Attempts to maintain thrombocythemic patients at normal platelet counts by cytapheresis alone have not been successful; more practical long-term chemotherapy should be instituted concurrently. Because most patients with thrombocytosis do not develop symptoms, including patients with myeloproliferative disorders, prophylactic plateletpheresis seems unwarranted regardless of the platelet count. One possible exception involves pregnant patients with essential thrombocythemia who may be at increased risk of first trimester abortion; Periodic plateletpheresis has been used in a limited series, with weekly procedures necessary to reduce the circulating platelet number until delivery.

THERAPEUTIC PLASMAPHERESIS

Common clinical indications for therapeutic plasmapheresis are outlined in Table 118.2. Most procedures are performed for treatment of immunologic and hematologic disorders. A course of plasmapheresis generally consists of five to seven exchanges of 1–1.5 plasma volumes each, either daily or with an interval of 1–2 days between procedures; the course of therapy varies depending on the specific disease indication and rate and duration of response.

Several expert committees have published practice guidelines for using plasmapheresis in a wide variety of disease states.[16] Some of the least controversial indications for plasmapheresis are supported by small series of uncontrolled cases that rely on some objective clinical or laboratory measurement of patient improvement.

Hematologic Indications

Two of the most common indications for plasmapheresis are treatment of TTP and treatment of clinical syndromes associated with paraproteinemias. Plasma exchange with fresh-frozen plasma (FFP) replacement has been estimated to improve survival rates of patients with TTP from 10% to more than 75%. Comprehensive reviews of the clinical and laboratory evaluation and treatment of patients with suspected TTP, including management with plasma exchange therapy, have been published.[17] Treatment usually involves daily single-volume plasma exchange with both frequency and duration of treatment

TABLE 118.2	Common Indications for Therapeutic Plasmapheresis

Hematologic Diseases (Including Blood Cell–Specific Autoimmune Diseases)

Thrombotic thrombocytopenic purpura
Idiopathic thrombocytopenic purpura (immunoabsorption)
Hyperviscosity
Posttransfusion purpura
Cold agglutinin syndrome
ABO-mismatched marrow transplant (recipient)

Autoimmune Diseases

Cryoglobulinemia
Rheumatoid arthritis (immunoadsorption, lymphoplasmapheresis)
Myasthenia gravis
Goodpasture syndrome
Guillain-Barré syndrome
Chronic inflammatory demyelinating polyneuropathy

Metabolic Diseases

Homozygous familial hypercholesterolemia (selective adsorption)
Refsum disease

Other

Drug overdose and poisoning

guided by clinical response and continued until the platelet count is above 150,000/μL and lactate dehydrogenase is near normal for 2–3 consecutive days. The persistence of schistocytes on the peripheral blood smear does not preclude weaning or discontinuation of treatment. Typically, patients should respond within 2 or 3 days of beginning treatment. In desperately ill and deteriorating patients, escalating the intensity of plasma exchange to twice daily may be necessary.[18] Despite initial reports of improved response rates in certain patients, recent experience suggests that the use of cryoprecipitate-poor plasma may not be more effective than the use of standard FFP as a specific replacement fluid for plasma exchange in patients with TTP. The effectiveness of plasma exchange in this setting may derive from removal of antibody to or replacement of the von Willebrand factor–cleaving zinc metalloprotease, ADAMTS13. However, patients with clinical features of TTP and only moderate ADAMTS13 deficiency or even normal activity may respond to plasma exchange. Plasma exchange for hematopoietic progenitor cell transplant recipients exhibiting clinical features of TTP, now generally referred to as transplantation-associated thrombotic microangiopathy (TAM), has proved far less efficacious. This syndrome likely differs in pathogenesis from classic TTP in many aspects, including the absence of severe ADAMTS13 deficiency, the spectrum of clinical symptoms, and the lack of evidence of systemic microthrombus formation. Furthermore, plasma exchange has been unsuccessful in reversing most cases of TAM. Finally, atypical hemolytic uremic syndrome (aHUS), a rare form of thrombotic microangiopathy with high mortality, may be difficult to distinguish clinically from TTP in adults. aHUS results from uncontrolled complement activation, does not respond at all to plasma therapies, and is instead treated with eculizamab to block the terminal complement complex.

Small, uncontrolled studies and extensive clinical experience support the use of plasmapheresis as an adjunctive therapy for patients with paraproteinemia and hyperviscosity syndrome and with some paraproteinemias in the absence of hyperviscosity. Waldenström macroglobulinemia manifests as a lymphoplasmacytic lymphoma with a monoclonal IgM protein in the plasma. Because IgM is a large molecule and resides predominantly in the intravascular space, as little as one apheresis procedure will result in improvement in symptoms. Recurrence of symptoms and rising plasma viscosity will determine the need and frequency of repeated exchanges. Comprehensive reviews describing the rationale and treatment schedules for plasmapheresis in patients with a variety of paraproteinemias, including cryoglobulinemia and Waldenström macroglobulinemia have been published.

Low-Density Lipoprotein Apheresis and Other Metabolic Disease Indications

Evidence that cutaneous lesions and vascular lesions regress in individuals with familial hypercholesterolemia as LDL levels are controlled by plasmapheresis has encouraged the use of apheresis column absorption procedures in patients with homozygous disease and in poorly controlled heterozygous patients. LDL apheresis removes apolipoprotein B–containing lipoproteins from the blood by a variety of techniques, including dextran sulfate cellulose adsorption, immunoadsorption, and heparin-induced extracorporeal precipitation. Short-term safety and efficacy have been demonstrated. Patients have now been treated successfully for several years; however, additional experience with this therapy will be required to prove long-term benefit for refractory hypercholesterolemia and coronary artery disease for heterozygotes in particular.[19] In 36 homozygous children in two studies, 20% to 22% developed new aortocoronary lesions or showed progression of existing lesions while on apheresis despite impressive reductions in mean LDL cholesterol.[20,21] Side effects such as malaise, shivering, and pain at the phlebotomy site are common but mild, and the treatments are generally well tolerated. Patients with severe hypertriglyceridemia are at risk of developing acute pancreatitis. Plasma exchange appears to reduce recurrent episodes by an average 67% but requires continuation of medical therapy.

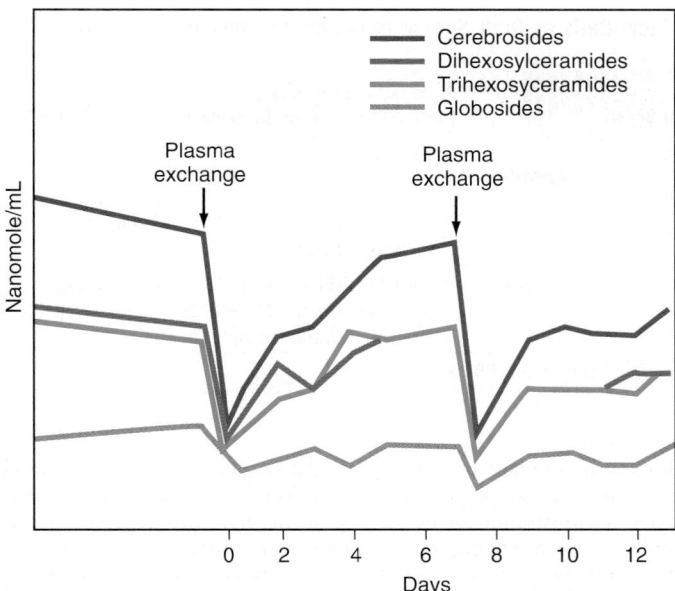

Fig. 118.7 PLASMA EXCHANGE TO REMOVE PLASMA NEUTRAL GLYCOLIPIDS IN A PATIENT WITH FABRY DISEASE. The plasma lipid recovery curve appears to be biphasic, reflecting initial reequilibration from tissue stores and subsequent new synthesis of that glycolipid.

Simple plasma exchange may be used in patients with other inherited metabolic diseases, such as Refsum disease. The frequency of exchange depends primarily on total body burden, rate of synthesis, and plasma concentration of the solute to be removed (Fig. 118.7). Less evidence exists to support a role for repeated treatments in these diseases.

Immune Disease Indications and Immunoadsorption Therapies

Plasma exchange appears to have at least a temporary adjunctive role in managing some rheumatic diseases and other immune disorders characterized by circulating autoantibodies. Early success was reported in patients with Goodpasture syndrome, a disorder characterized by a specific pathogenic autoantibody directed against the renal glomerular and pulmonary alveolar basement membrane. Plasmapheresis has demonstrated similar success in myasthenia gravis, pemphigus, and Eaton-Lambert syndrome. Although nonselective plasma exchange has been used in a variety of other rheumatic diseases such as systemic lupus erythematosus (SLE) and rheumatoid vasculitis, with the exception of treatment of patients with Goodpasture syndrome (in which plasma exchange is considered first-line adjuvant therapy), such use remains unproved and should be reserved for circumstances in which a vital organ or life itself is endangered. Selective leukapheresis by Adacolumn technology in a series of patients with SLE has shown clinical benefit, but trial interpretation is limited by the uncontrolled nature and small size.

In some immune disorders, such as immune thrombocytopenic purpura (ITP) and immune inhibitors to coagulation proteins, plasma exchange may be helpful during a catastrophic event, but in general, benefit of nonselective plasma exchange therapy is not established.

Plasma exchange appears to be a useful therapeutic option in renal transplant patients threatened with refractory humoral rejection and is now widely used to overcome ABO and HLA incompatibilities between renal transplant patients and their only available donors. Several studies have shown successful reversal of acute humoral rejection mediated by HLA-specific donor antibody using a combination of plasmapheresis and IV immune globulin (IVIg), which is superior to high dose IVIg alone.[22] A conditioning regimen consisting of pretransplant plasmapheresis, immunosuppressive medications, and low-dose cytomegalovirus immune globulin effectively reduces donor-specific antibody and isoagglutinin titers with and without posttransplant splenectomy and anti-CD20 treatment. The strength of donor-specific antibodies is also important and can be determined by titration, but greater sensitivity and specificity may be obtained using Luminex flow-bead technology. Patients with strong HLA antibodies have increased mean bead fluorescence and were more likely to have acute rejection; however, the introduction of peritransplantation apheresis reduced acute rejection from 66% to 7%.[23]

Plasma exchange has also been used to treat patients with focal segmental glomerulosclerosis, both for primary disease refractory to standard immunosuppressive therapy and for treatment of patients with recurrent disease after renal transplantation.

Two immunoadsorption columns have been approved in the United States for removal of autoantibodies to factor VIII or factor IX (Immunosorba staphylococcal protein A–agarose column) and treatment of ITP and rheumatoid arthritis (Prosorba staphylococcal protein A–silica column). Several case series describe the use of immunoadsorption for patients with immune inhibitors to factor VIII or factor IX. A phase III, multicenter, sham-controlled randomized study of staphylococcal protein A column immunoadsorption shows a significant increase in clinical response in adult patients with longstanding rheumatoid arthritis. Sparse published evidence exists to support the use of immunoadsorption therapy in patients with chronic ITP refractory to standard medical management.

Plasmapheresis is effective first- or second-line therapy in selected patients with certain neurologic disorders. Controlled clinical trials of plasmapheresis have demonstrated efficacy in at least two of the polyradiculoneuropathies. In Guillain-Barré syndrome, plasmapheresis should be considered when patients are unable to walk independently or require mechanic ventilation. However, IVIg alone may be equally effective and is more readily available.[16] Periodic plasmapheresis may be necessary in patients with a chronic inflammatory demyelinating neuropathy. Because the long-term prognosis varies, plasmapheresis may be used in conjunction with steroids and IVIg. Rapid deterioration may occur upon discontinuation.

MS is a relapsing and progressive disorder with demyelination of the central nervous system white matter. Patients who present with acute fulminant demyelination may benefit from early plasma exchange, particularly when they fail to respond to high-dose corticosteroids.[24] The majority of patients have a relapsing-remitting form of the disease, and plasmapheresis may be of benefit. Unfortunately, for chronic progressive forms of MS, plasma exchange has consistently been shown to be ineffective.

REPLACEMENT FLUIDS FOR PLASMA EXCHANGE

The success of therapeutic apheresis procedures seldom depends on the composition of the replacement solution that is used; the single exception is TTP (discussed in the previous section). With therapeutic plasmapheresis for most other disorders, the primary function of the replacement solution is to maintain intravascular volume. Additional requirements include restoration of important plasma proteins, maintenance of colloid osmotic pressure, maintenance of electrolyte balance, and preservation of trace elements lost during a prolonged course of plasmapheresis procedures. In moderately well-nourished patients, homeostatic mechanisms normally obviate the need for precise plasma replacement, and 5% albumin in normal saline or combinations of albumin and crystalloid are usually sufficient. Commonly used is 60% to 80% replacement by colloid, with the crystalloid component consisting of a combination of normal saline and an anticoagulant. Patients with clinical conditions such as hypotension, hypoalbuminemia, or preexisting coagulopathies should receive solutions prepared specifically to meet their individual requirements. Routine supplementation with calcium, potassium, or immunoglobulins is unnecessary. However, for large-volume apheresis procedures to collect PB-HSPC, IV calcium supplementation is beneficial (discussed in the following section). Because less than 500 mL is removed

TABLE 118.3	Bone Marrow Versus Cytokine Stimulated Peripheral Blood Stem Cells as Graft Source of Choice for Hematopoietic Stem Cell Transplantation			
Disease Category	Recipient Age Group	Type of Donor	Preferred Graft Source (Unstimulated BM vs. Cytokine Stimulated PB HSPC)	
Nonmalignant (e.g., severe aplastic anemia)	All ages	Sibling	BM HSPCs	
Malignant	Pediatric	Sibling	BM HSPCs	
Malignant	Adult	Sibling	PB or BM HSPCs (PB HSPCs preferred in high-risk leukemia)	
Malignant	Adult	Matched unrelated donor	PB or BM HSPCs (PB HSPCs preferred if high graft failure risk; BM HSPCs if high cGVHD risk, prior immunosuppression)	

BM, Bone marrow; cGVHD, chronic graft-versus-host disease; HSPC, hematopoietic stem and progenitor cell; PB, peripheral blood.

during most cell collection procedures and therapeutic cell depletions, no volume replacement beyond the anticoagulant and saline priming solution is required. Problems of decreased availability and high cost of albumin have led some centers to develop protocols for alternatives to plasma-derived volume expanders, such as hydroxyethyl starch (HES), for full- or partial-volume replacement with plasma exchange. One center has used a combination of 3% HES and 5% albumin mixture successfully, but patients did experience mild adverse events more frequently than did historical control subjects.[25] Although such solutions are generally well tolerated, extensive replacement with HES in patients undergoing longer courses of plasmapheresis, especially those with impaired renal function, can result in diffuse tissue accumulation of the larger starch molecules (acquired lysosomal storage).

HEMATOPOEITIC STEM CELL COLLECTION

Blood cell separators developed for hemapheresis are used to collect peripheral blood cells for cellular therapy. The most common application of apheresis technology for cell therapy indications is the collection of HPCs from peripheral blood after administration of recombinant hematopoietic growth factor or chemotherapy, or both, to "mobilize" large numbers of HPCs into the circulation. The collected mononuclear cell fraction contains a subset of progenitor cells that, on infusion, can home to and reconstitute the bone marrow in patients who receive ablative radiation or chemotherapy, or both. Similarly, donor leukocytes obtained from leukapheresis procedures may be used for donor lymphocyte infusion or subject to further processing for immunotherapy.

Peripheral Blood Hematopoietic Stem and Progenitor Cells

Pluripotent HPCs, and quite possibly primordial hematopoietic stem cells capable of reconstituting the bone marrow and the immune system, have long been known to circulate in the peripheral blood. Numerous studies have confirmed the potential for rapid and durable engraftment of peripheral blood hematopoietic stem and progenitor cells (PB HSPCs) mobilized into the circulation by hematopoietic growth factors harvested by large-volume leukapheresis procedures and subsequently administered to patients with marrow aplasia after high-dose chemotherapy. The concentration of hematopoietic stem and progenitor cells in the peripheral blood can be increased by the administration of cytokines such as granulocyte colony-stimulating factor (G-CSF) and granulocyte-macrophage colony-stimulating factor (GM-CSF) and by the administration of chemotherapy. CD34$^+$ hematopoietic cell numbers in the peripheral blood generally rise 20- to 40-fold (from 1–3 cells/μL to 40–70 cells/μL) after administration of G-CSF alone, and they increase 100- to 1000-fold when chemotherapy rebound is enhanced by administration of G-CSF. Efforts to define optimal collection conditions have been

limited by the lack of a standardized assay; however, time and level of increase of donor peripheral blood WBC and CD34$^+$ cell counts after administration of mobilizing agents have proved to be useful indicators. Despite ongoing problems with interlaboratory standardization, flow cytometric analysis of cells labeled with a fluorochrome-conjugated CD34 antibody are used for "real-time" decision making about the timing and adequacy of PB HSPC collections. Several prestimulation donor variables are important. Increasing age, white ethnicity, and female gender are associated with significantly lower post–G-CSF CD34$^+$ cell counts, which would favor younger males as donors when high cell doses are required.[26]

Several clinical scale devices for CD34$^+$ cell enrichment of leukapheresis collections by immunoabsorption or immunomagnetic techniques are available. This "positive selection" of CD34$^+$ hematopoietic cells also results in reduced numbers of cells that do not express the CD34 antigen, such as T lymphocytes. T-cell–reduced products may confer a lower risk of GVHD, and the ability to produce apheresis products enriched for CD34$^+$ cells facilitates graft manipulations for experimental cell therapies such as ex vivo expansion of CD34$^+$ cells. However, some studies suggest a higher incidence of engraftment failure and possibly delayed immune reconstitution in certain patient populations when transplants are performed with highly purified CD34-selected, T-cell–depleted products.

Over the last decade, PB HSPCs have surpassed bone marrow HSPCs as the predominant graft source in the clinical setting for various hematopoietic stem cell transplants. PB HSPCs are the graft of choice in 99% of conditions where autologous transplants are indicated. For allogeneic transplants, especially which use stem cells from matched unrelated donors or in pediatric transplants, bone marrow stem cells still remain the popular graft source. PB HSPC transplants result in higher rates of clinically significant chronic GVHD in these situations. Table 118.3 provides a summary of comparisons of bone marrow versus PB HSPCs in different types of allogeneic stem cell transplants.

From a donor perspective, the discomfort and inconvenience of multiple-day cytokine administration may be a significant deterrent. Most donors experience some degree of malaise and bone pain, and some donors require hospitalization for more serious adverse reactions to G-CSF administration. However, a large prospective trial of the National Marrow Donor Program found intensity and duration of pain in the pericollection period (during G-CSF administration before apheresis among PB HSPC donors and following bone marrow biopsy procedure in bone marrow HSPC donors) was similar for persons undergoing HSPC collection by either apheresis or bone marrow biopsy. Further, 3% of bone marrow donors reported ongoing low-grade site pain after 6 months of completing the procedure whereas recovery was complete for PB HSPC donors by this time. Risk factors for worse toxicities, including older age, female gender, and obesity were similar among bone marrow and PB HSPC donors.[27] While concerns remain regarding the hypothetic long-term effects of exposure of healthy donors to growth factors, another recent prospective study with more than 20,000 donor-years of follow-up, showed no evidence of increased risk for cancer, autoimmune illness, and stroke in donors receiving G-CSF.[28] Splenic enlargement occurs commonly, and several instances of splenic rupture have been reported. Citrate toxicity is a common complication of PB-HSPC collections; although usually mild and transient, it may be severe and even life-threatening in some individuals (see previous section). Venous access requires large-bore multilumen catheters, and these appear particularly susceptible to clotting, especially when patients receive recombinant cytokine stimulation. Hemorrhage, especially in thrombocytopenic patients, is another potentially severe complication of central venous catheter placement.

Some patients who have received multiple prior cycles of chemotherapy and a small proportion of normal healthy donors, referred to as "poor mobilizers," fail to respond adequately to mobilization regimens. In this circumstance, Plerixafor, a reversible CXCR4 antagonist that can block the adhesion of HPCs to the bone marrow stroma can enhance collections by releasing these cells into the circulation. In a randomized controlled trial, the combination of G-CSF and Plerixafor resulted in a significantly higher proportion of patients with non-Hodgkin lymphoma achieving their target cell dose in fewer apheresis days.[29] Similar success is achieved with multiple myeloma patients achieving a 4.8-fold increase peripheral blood CD34 cell count compared with 1.7-fold with G-CSF alone. Emerging evidence indicates that Plerixafor may be administered "just-in-time" to rescue collections for patients who mobilize poorly with G-CSF alone. While the optimum circumstances and timing for administration have not yet been determined, some guidelines recommend addition of Plerixafor for circulating CD34$^+$ cell counts fewer than 20×10^6/L on two consecutive days accompanied by increasing WBCs.[30]

COMPLICATIONS OF THERAPEUTIC APHERESIS

Automated apheresis is a minimal-risk procedure for normal healthy blood and plasma donors. The current generation of blood cell separators is remarkably reliable and equipped with sensitive detection and alarm systems to alert the operator to potential problems. Nevertheless, serious morbidity and rare deaths have been associated with therapeutic procedures. In most reports, deaths are related to either complications associated with the use of central venous access catheters or to cardiac and respiratory problems in patients who were critically ill before apheresis; in the latter, the contributory role of the apheresis procedure is often questionable. The most common adverse effects of therapeutic apheresis are citrate-induced hypocalcemia, allergic reactions (usually to donor plasma or other blood components), vasovagal reactions, and hypovolemia. If transient paresthesia and mild vasovagal events are excluded, approximately 5% of all therapeutic apheresis procedures have medical complications. The frequency of adverse reactions is influenced by the experience of the operator and the nature of the patient population being treated. Expected and predictable effects of therapeutic apheresis include alterations in laboratory parameters caused by removal and dilution by replacement fluids. A 5% to 15% decrease in Hb and hematocrit, a 20% to 30% decrease in platelet count, and mild transient increase in leukocyte count are commonly observed. Significantly but transiently abnormal coagulation test results are often observed (recovery generally occurs within 48 hours after a single-volume exchange procedure), as well as clinically insignificant decreased levels of other plasma proteins after serial plasma exchange procedures. The most common adverse effect of both donor and therapeutic apheresis procedures is symptomatic hypocalcemia caused by infusion of calcium-chelating citrate ions in the anticoagulant, and if used as replacement fluid, anticoagulant donor plasma. Hypocalcemia is usually manifested by mild perioral or acral paresthesia, or both, requiring no intervention other than slowing the reinfusion rate. The benefit of oral calcium supplements in this setting is questionable, although the practice is widespread. Hyperventilation may exacerbate the symptoms of hypocalcemia. More severe citrate toxicity is uncommon; signs may range from involuntary carpopedal spasm, nausea, and vomiting to frank tetany with spasm in other muscle groups, including life-threatening laryngospasm and grand mal seizure.

Severe toxicity is most commonly experienced by small patients, particularly women, when the blood flow rate is rapid and the procedure is prolonged beyond a few hours. Symptoms correlate inversely with the level of ionized calcium. Extremely low concentrations of ionized calcium are encountered routinely in therapeutic procedures that process more than 15 L of blood. Acute severe hypocalcemia leading to fatal cardiac arrhythmia has been reported in patients who have undergone apheresis. Controlled infusions of 10% calcium gluconate or calcium chloride are effective in the management of these complications. Because metabolism of citrate occurs predominantly in the liver and kidney, patients with conditions affecting these organs are at increased risk for severe citrate reactions. Studies of therapeutic plasma exchange procedures and of PB-HSPC donations performed with and without calcium gluconate or calcium chloride infusion show the effectiveness of continuous calcium infusion for the prevention of mild to moderate citrate toxicity (Fig. 118.8). A study of plateletpheresis donors documented sustained effects of citrate infusion on bone metabolism demonstrated by changes in alkaline phosphatase, osteocalcin, parathyroid hormone, and 1,25-dihydroxyvitamin D levels, suggesting the potential for long-term effects on bone metabolism in these donors. Magnesium, another divalent cation, is also bound by citrate. Despite decreases in serum ionized magnesium levels to 39% below baseline, clinical effects are not typically observed even during large-volume leukapheresis procedures. The most severe allergic complications occur when plasma is used as the replacement solution, and this risk increases with repeated exposure. Allergic reactions to ethylene oxide, an agent used in the sterilization of plastic disposable equipment, have been reported. IV diphenhydramine is usually effective in managing allergic reactions; premedication with steroids and precautions against anaphylaxis may be necessary for sensitized individuals. Atypical (hypotension and flushing) and anaphylactic reactions have been reported in patients receiving angiotensin-converting enzyme inhibitors undergoing different apheresis procedures, including immunoadsorption with staphylococcal protein A columns. These medications should be discontinued for at least 24 hours before apheresis. Unlike

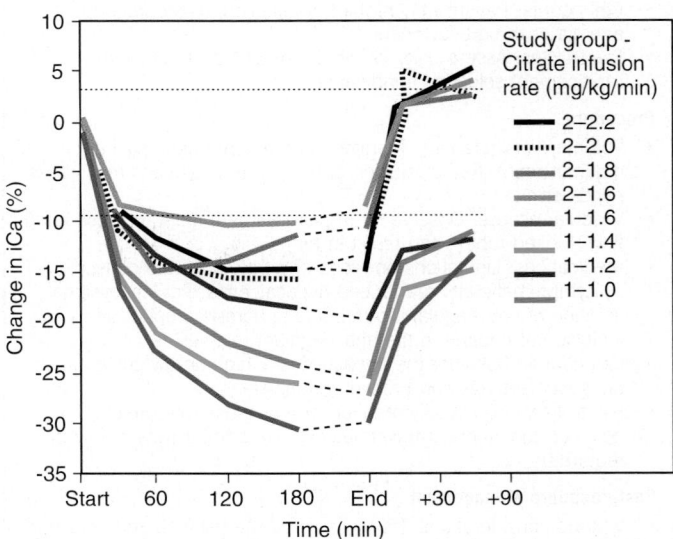

Fig. 118.8 LEVELS OF IONIZED CALCIUM ARE MARKEDLY LOWER IN PROCEDURES PERFORMED WITHOUT PROPHYLACTIC CALCIUM INFUSION AND REMAIN BELOW THE REFERENCE RANGE 90 MINUTES AFTER COMPLETION OF APHERESIS. *Dotted lines* indicate upper and lower limits of the reference range. *Open symbols* represent procedures without prophylactic calcium; *solid symbols* represent those with calcium infusion. *Dashed lines* between 180 minutes and end-procedural values (End) reflect varying procedure duration. *iCa*, Ionized calcium. *(From Bolan CD, Cecco SA, Wesley RA, et al: Controlled study of citrate effects and response to i.v. calcium administration during allogeneic peripheral blood progenitor cell donation.* Transfusion *42:935, 2002, used by permission).*

donors undergoing apheresis for donation of RBCs, platelets, or plasma, donors undergoing apheresis for collection of therapeutic granulocytes are stimulated with steroids and G-CSF before donation. The well-known association of long-term steroid treatment and posterior subcapsular cataracts is likely irrelevant in the context of short-term steroid stimulation for donor granulocyte mobilization. However, an increased number posterior subcapsular cataracts has been detected in three separate studies including an analysis of 100 granulocyte donors compared with age-matched plateletpheresis donors, suggesting that granulocyte donors may be at increased risk for cataract formation. Repeated steroid stimulation for granulocyte collection warrants regular ophthalmologic examination and close follow up.[31] Serious complications indirectly associated with therapeutic apheresis include adverse consequences of large-needle vascular access; namely, retroperitoneal or pericardial hemorrhage, phlebotomy site aneurysm formation, pneumo- or hemothorax, thrombosis, nerve damage, and infection. A retrospective review of 381 therapeutic plasma exchange procedures at one institution reported an approximately 1% incidence of severe complications, all of them related to central venous catheters (see box on Patient Management Issues for Therapeutic Apheresis).

Patient Management Issues for Therapeutic Apheresis

Important issues to consider when preparing a patient for therapeutic apheresis, for monitoring the patient during the procedure, and for managing the patient after removal from the apheresis device include:

Preparation

- Volume considerations: Calculate volume to be processed or exchanged; order replacement solutions; assess patient volume status. A blood prime may be necessary for children who weigh less than 25 kg.
- Vascular access: Assess need for apheresis line placement. Note that not all large catheters are suitable for apheresis procedures.
- Medications: Evaluate impact of medications (Coumadin, platelet inhibitory agents, angiotensin-converting enzyme inhibitors) and indications to suspend certain medications. Albumin-bound medications may be depleted by apheresis.
- Cell counts: Patient may require transfusion for preprocedure anemia or thrombocytopenia.
- Electrolytes: Assess risks for citrate toxicity; order calcium replacement solutions if indicated.

Procedure

- Volume considerations: Monitor replacement fluids (saline-to-albumin ratio). Rapid infusion of refrigerated solutions may cause hypothermia.
- Vascular access: Observe for impaired, intermittent, or obstructed flow. Kinked tubing can result in hemolysis.
- Medications: Limitations on blood or citrate flow rate caused by symptomatic citrate-induced hypocalcemia may necessitate addition of anticoagulant to the final apheresis product or inclusion of heparin in the anticoagulant regimen.
- Cell counts: Consider the impact of very high or low cell counts on device settings and procedure efficiency.
- Electrolytes: Continually monitor for adverse citrate effects; bolus or continuous intravenous calcium administration may be required.

Postprocedure Management

- Volume considerations: Review net volume balance and consider additional infusion or administration of diuretic if needed.
- Vascular access: The decision to remove the apheresis catheter should include the possibility of additional apheresis or procedures; monitor for complications associated with maintenance or removal of venous catheter.
- Medications: Determine when to restart medications; consider the impact of transiently reduced coagulation factor levels.
- Cell counts: The patient may require transfusion for postprocedure thrombocytopenia; monitor cumulative red blood cell and platelet loss after repeated procedures.
- Electrolytes: Assess for imbalance postprocedure with attention to ionized calcium and magnesium as indicated by symptoms.

PEDIATRIC HEMAPHERESIS

Therapeutic apheresis in pediatrics poses a particular challenge. The indications for apheresis in children are limited by a lack of clinical trial data. Therefore the evidence for therapy in many diseases is extrapolated from trials in adults despite differing patient physiology and an age-dependent presentation and natural history of the disease. For example, hemolytic uremic syndrome is more common in children and responds to supportive care; at the other end of the spectrum of this disease, TTP is more common in adults and necessitates plasma exchange.

Similarly the mechanics of apheresis were developed for adults and therefore designed for their larger circulating blood volume. Therefore depending on the size of the child, modifications to the apheresis procedure may be necessary. Central venous catheters are required in most circumstances because the caliber of peripheral venous access is too small to permit adequate blood flow.

Technical Aspects

In pediatric apheresis, maintenance of isovolemia is essential to prevent circulatory compromise, particularly in an acutely ill child who may have some degree of cardiac or renal impairment. The beginning and end of the apheresis procedure involves negative and positive intravascular fluid shifts, respectively. Typically, this has negligible impact on an adult's circulation but can represent a substantial proportion of the total blood volume (TBV) of an infant. The volume of the patient's blood required to fill the apheresis circuit at the start of the procedure is the extracorporeal volume (ECV). Symptomatic hypovolemia becomes increasingly likely as ECV exceeds 15% of TBV. An ECV of 400 mL represents 8% of the TBV of a 70-kg patient but may be as much as 35% for a 15-kg infant. Modification of the apheresis procedure is necessary for safe management in infants and small children.

In adults, the apheresis circuit is primed with saline, which is then diverted to the collection or waste bag. One option permits return of saline prime to the patient, which may be useful for larger children. For children who weigh less than 25 kg, a prime with RBCs is often necessary to prevent intravascular volume depletion and severe anemia. Upon completion, fluids remaining in the apheresis circuit, typically returned to the adult patient, are not returned in pediatrics to avoid a positive fluid shift causing fluid overload.

PEDIATRIC APHERESIS

Pediatric therapeutic apheresis accounts for about 10% of all apheresis procedures performed. The majority of apheresis procedures in children are erythrocytapheresis for patients with sickle cell disease and mononuclear cell collections for HPCs to be used in conjunction with high-dose chemotherapy. Leukapheresis is performed in symptomatic leukostasis in acute leukemias, but may not be beneficial as prophylaxis in hyperleukocytosis. Indications for ECP and LDL-apheresis follow guidelines discussed earlier. In solid organ rejection, both ECP and therapeutic plasma exchange (TPE) have been used as adjunct treatment modalities with sparse data thus far. As in adults, TPE is shown to be efficacious in acute and chronic demyelinating neuropathies and in severe refractory myasthenia gravis. TPE may also benefit children with rare neurologic disorders; pediatric autoimmune neuropsychiatric disorders associated with streptococcal infection and Sydenham chorea (SC) are autoimmune neuropsychiatric disorders that occur rarely after infection with group A β-hemolytic streptococcal infections. Circulating immune factors may contribute to the pathogenesis of these diseases. These conditions respond to IVIg and plasmapheresis. In a small randomized study, 50% of patients with SC also responded to plasmapheresis, and although superior to corticosteroids, treatment with IVIg had the best response, with 72% of patients having a reduction in symptoms of chorea. Small pediatric studies have demonstrated benefit of

TPE specifically in recurrent focal segmental glomerulosclerosis, especially when it occurs post renal transplantation. It has been attempted with marginal success in severe refractory vasculitides such as Henoch-Schönlein purpura, Kawasaki disease and ANCA-associated vasculitides.[32]

REFERENCES

1. Abel JJ, Rowntree LG, Turner BB: Plasma removal with return of corpuscles (plasmaphaeresis). The Journal of Pharmacology and experimental therapeutics Vol. V. No. 6, July, 1914. *Transfus Sci* 11(166):1990.

2. Whitaker BL, Henry RA: *The 2011 National Blood Collection and Utilization Survey Report*, Washington DC, 2011, US Department of Health and Human Services.

3. Kato GJ, Gladwin MT, Steinberg MH: Deconstructing sickle cell disease: reappraisal of the role of hemolysis in the development of clinical subphenotypes. *Blood Rev* 21(1):37–47, 2007.

4. Howard J, Malfroy M, Llewelyn C, et al: The Transfusion Alternatives Preoperatively in Sickle Cell Disease (TAPS) study: a randomised, controlled, multicentre clinical trial. *Lancet* 381(9870):930–938, 2013.

5. Rombout-Sestrienkova E, Nieman FH, Essers BA, et al: Erythrocytapheresis versus phlebotomy in the initial treatment of HFE hemochromatosis patients: results from a randomized trial. *Transfusion* 52(3):470–477, 2012.

6. De Santis GC, de Oliveira LC, Romano LG, et al: Therapeutic leukapheresis in patients with leukostasis secondary to acute myelogenous leukemia. *J Clin Apher* 26(4):181–185, 2011.

7. Chang MC, Chen TY, Tang JL, et al: Leukapheresis and cranial irradiation in patients with hyperleukocytic acute myeloid leukemia: no impact on early mortality and intracranial hemorrhage. *Am J Hematol* 82(11):976–980, 2007.

8. Klamova H, Markova M, Moravcova J, et al: Response to treatment in women with chronic myeloid leukemia during pregnancy and after delivery. *Leuk Res* 33(11):1567–1569, 2009.

9. Vernia P, D'Ovidio V, Meo D: Leukocytapheresis in the treatment of inflammatory bowel disease: Current position and perspectives. *Transfus Apher Sci* 43(2):227–229, 2010.

10. Thanaraj S, Hamlin PJ, Ford AC: Systematic review: granulocyte/monocyte adsorptive apheresis for ulcerative colitis. *Aliment Pharmacol Ther* 32(11–12):1297–1306, 2010.

11. Yamamoto T, Umegae S, Matsumoto K: Daily granulocyte and monocyte adsorptive apheresis in patients with active ulcerative colitis: a prospective safety and feasibility study. *J Gastroenterol* 46(8):1003–1009, 2011.

12. Knobler R, Berlin G, Calzavara-Pinton P, et al: Guidelines on the use of extracorporeal photopheresis. *J Eur Acad Dermatol Venereol* 28(Suppl 1):1–37, 2014.

13. Flowers ME, Apperley JF, van Besien K, et al: A multicenter prospective phase 2 randomized study of extracorporeal photopheresis for treatment of chronic graft-versus-host disease. *Blood* 112(7):2667–2674, 2008.

14. Jaksch P, Knobler R: ECP and solid organ transplantation. *Transfus Apher Sci* 50(3):358–362, 2014.

15. Kuzmina Z, Stroncek D, Pavletic SZ: Extracorporeal photopheresis as a therapy for autoimmune diseases. *J Clin Apher* 30:224–237, 2015.

16. Schwartz J, Winters JL, Padmanabhan A, et al: Guidelines on the use of therapeutic apheresis in clinical practice-evidence-based approach from the Writing Committee of the American Society for Apheresis: the sixth special issue. *J Clin Apher* 28(3):145–284, 2013.

17. George JN, Nester CM: Syndromes of thrombotic microangiopathy. *N Engl J Med* 371:654–666, 2014.

18. Nguyen L, Li X, Duvall D, et al: Twice-daily plasma exchange for patients with refractory thrombotic thrombocytopenic purpura: the experience of the Oklahoma Registry, 1989 through 2006. *Transfusion* 48(2):349–357, 2008.

19. Bruckert E: Recommendations for the management of patients with homozygous familial hypercholesterolaemia: overview of a new European Atherosclerosis Society consensus statement. *Atheroscler Suppl* 15(2):26–32, 2014.

20. Hudgins LC, Kleinman B, Scheuer A, et al: Long-term safety and efficacy of low-density lipoprotein apheresis in childhood for homozygous familial hypercholesterolemia. *Am J Cardiol* 102(9):1199–1204, 2008.

21. Kolansky DM, Cuchel M, Clark BJ, et al: Longitudinal evaluation and assessment of cardiovascular disease in patients with homozygous familial hypercholesterolemia. *Am J Cardiol* 102(11):1438–1443, 2008.

22. Lefaucheur C, Nochy D, Andrade J, et al: Comparison of combination Plasmapheresis/IVIg/anti-CD20 versus high-dose IVIg in the treatment of antibody-mediated rejection. *Am J Transplant* 9(5):1099–1107, 2009.

23. Akalin E, Dinavahi R, Friedlander R, et al: Addition of plasmapheresis decreases the incidence of acute antibody-mediated rejection in sensitized patients with strong donor-specific antibodies. *Clin J Am Soc Nephrol* 3(4):1160–1167, 2008.

24. Llufriu S, Castillo J, Blanco Y, et al: Plasma exchange for acute attacks of CNS demyelination: Predictors of improvement at 6 months. *Neurology* 73(12):949–953, 2009.

25. Agreda-Vasquez GP, Espinosa-Poblano I, Sanchez-Guerrero SA, et al: Starch and albumin mixture as replacement fluid in therapeutic plasma exchange is safe and effective. *J Clin Apher* 23(5):163–167, 2008.

26. Vasu S, Leitman SF, Tisdale JF, et al: Donor demographic and laboratory predictors of allogeneic peripheral blood stem cell mobilization in an ethnically diverse population. *Blood* 112(5):2092–2100, 2008.

27. Pulsipher MA, Chitphakdithai P, Logan BR, et al: Acute toxicities of unrelated bone marrow versus peripheral blood stem cell donation: results of a prospective trial from the National Marrow Donor Program. *Blood* 121(1):197–206, 2013.

28. Pulsipher MA, Chitphakdithai P, Logan BR, et al: Lower risk for serious adverse events and no increased risk for cancer after PBSC vs BM donation. *Blood* 123(23):3655–3663, 2014.

29. DiPersio JF, Micallef IN, Stiff PJ, et al: Phase III prospective randomized double-blind placebo-controlled trial of plerixafor plus granulocyte colony-stimulating factor compared with placebo plus granulocyte colony-stimulating factor for autologous stem-cell mobilization and transplantation for patients with non-Hodgkin's lymphoma. *J Clin Oncol* 27(28):4767–4773, 2009.

30. Bilgin YM, Visser O, Beckers EA, et al: Evaluation of Dutch guideline for just-in-time addition of plerixafor to stem cell mobilization in patients who fail with granulocyte-colony-stimulating factor. *Transfusion* 2014.

31. Clayton JA, Vitale S, Kim J, et al: Prevalence of posterior subcapsular cataracts in volunteer cytapheresis donors. *Transfusion* 51(5):921–928, 2011.

32. Kim YA, Sloan SR: Pediatric therapeutic apheresis: rationale and indications for plasmapheresis, cytapheresis, extracorporeal photopheresis, and LDL apheresis. *Pediatr Clin North Am* 60:1569–1580, 2013.

TRANSFUSION REACTIONS TO BLOOD AND CELL THERAPY PRODUCTS

William Savage

A *transfusion reaction* can be defined broadly as any untoward clinical event that is the consequence of infusing a blood or cell therapy product. Transfusion reactions are classified by how close to transfusion they occur (timing), how much morbidity is caused (severity), how strong the causal association of the event is with transfusion (imputability), and how closely the reactions fit a consensus definition of a transfusion reaction type. Every year, approximately 40 fatalities attributable to transfusion are reported to the US Food and Drugs Administration (FDA).

It is important to recognize that many transfusion reactions can mimic pathology unrelated to transfusion. The differential diagnosis of any untoward clinical event should always consider adverse sequelae of transfusion, even when transfusion occurred weeks earlier. This chapter will review the presentation, mechanisms, and management of transfusion reactions (Table 119.1). Approximate risks of selected transfusion reactions are shown in Fig. 119.1.

HEMOLYTIC TRANSFUSION REACTIONS

Hemolytic transfusion reactions are caused by the immune-mediated clearance of transfused red blood cells (RBCs). Immune-mediated hemolysis can be classified clinically according to the timing of the reaction (acute or delayed) and mechanistically by site of hemolysis (intravascular with terminal complement activation or extravascular with phagocytosis in liver and spleen, Table 119.2).[1,2] Although hemolytic transfusion reactions are mechanistically considered immune-mediated in most cases, thermal, osmotic, infectious, and mechanical destruction of RBCs also can lead to acute hemolysis.

ACUTE INTRAVASCULAR HEMOLYTIC TRANSFUSION REACTIONS

Acute hemolytic reactions are those that occur typically during or immediately after incompatible RBCs are transfused into a patient who already possesses the corresponding antibody. ABO-incompatible RBC transfusion is the prototypical example of an acute, intravascular hemolytic transfusion reaction. ABO antibodies are spontaneously occurring immunoglobulin (Ig) M and IgG antibodies to foreign A and B blood group antigens. IgM antibodies efficiently fix complement after binding to ABO-incompatible RBCs and are responsible for initiating the hemolytic and inflammatory cascades that cause a clinically significant acute intravascular hemolytic transfusion reaction. Such a reaction could occur, for example, after transfusion of A RBCs into an O recipient who has significant amounts of circulating anti-A (see box titled "Acute Hemolytic Transfusion Reaction"). Acute hemolytic reactions can also occur with incompatible plasma transfusion. Because of limited platelet inventories, platelet components with incompatible plasma to the recipient are frequently transfused, for example an O platelet with anti-A transfused into an A recipient. This plasma incompatibility (i.e., minor incompatibility) can occasionally result in acute, ABO-incompatible hemolytic reactions.

Factors that determine the severity of hemolysis include the antibody titer, antibody avidity, antibody subtype, antigen density on the RBC membrane, and volume and rate of incompatible blood

transfused. Transfusing as little as 30 cm³ of incompatible blood can be fatal, and there is a direct relationship between increasing volumes of incompatible blood transfused and mortality.

In IgM-mediated ABO-incompatible transfusion reactions, activation of the complement cascade generates anaphylatoxins C3a and C5a, which lead to capillary leak, hypotension, and phagocyte and mast cell activation. Furthermore, the deposition of C3b on the RBC membrane increases extravascular hemolysis. Excessive terminal complement activation results in C5b-9 membrane attack complexes overwhelming complement regulatory factors on the RBC membrane leading to osmotic lysis. Plasma heme also induces renal vasoconstriction through nitric oxide scavenging.

In addition to complement components, cytokines also play a role in the clinical syndrome, including fever. For example, interleukin (IL)-1β, IL-6, and tumor necrosis factor (TNF)-α have pyrogenic activity; IL-8 is a neutrophil chemotactic and activating factor. These four cytokines have been generated in various in vitro models of intravascular hemolysis and IgG-mediated RBC incompatibility. TNF-α induces tissue factor expression on endothelium while decreasing thrombomodulin, which contributes to disseminated intravascular coagulation (DIC). TNF-α also promotes endothelin production, which promotes renal vasoconstriction. The clinical variability of hemolytic transfusion reactions is explained in part by the relative balance of cytokine production in the transfusion recipient. Factors that increase the circulating levels of proinflammatory cytokines and chemokines often result in more severe reactions.

An acute intravascular hemolytic transfusion reaction is a medical emergency. Initial clinical symptoms can include fever and chills, shortness of breath, chest pain, dizziness, and back or flank pain. Some patients report feeling anxiety or pain or warmth ascending from the site of infusion. Often the first sign of an immediate hemolytic transfusion reaction is fever. Therefore RBC transfusions must be stopped and evaluated by blood bank testing when fever develops (≥1°C). The transfused incompatible RBCs undergo complement-mediated osmotic lysis, producing hemoglobinemia and hemoglobinuria. Cardinal signs of an acute intravascular hemolytic transfusion reaction are the presence of red plasma (hemoglobinemia) and red/dark urine (hemoglobinuria). Acute transfusion reactions can quickly progress to shock and acute renal failure. Many patients, curiously even anephric patients, often complain of lower back pain. It is speculated that this symptom is caused by ischemic muscle pain or vasospasm, rather than by kidney pain from developing renal failure.

Laboratory tests for hemolysis can be useful if there is clinical ambiguity about the type of reaction and useful for guiding ongoing management of severe hemolytic reactions. Because most ABO-incompatible transfusion reactions are caused by errors in safety systems, an important initial evaluation is confirmation of blood incompatibility and determination of where an error occurred. There may be a systemic error that could put other patients at risk. Laboratory findings include hemoglobinuria, hemoglobinemia, and a haptoglobin level that is low to undetectable. During the hemolytic episode, the bilirubin (especially indirect bilirubin) usually increases only modestly (2–3 mg/dL) if the patient has normal liver function. Because of the lysis of RBCs, levels of lactate dehydrogenase (LDH) may rise markedly. If the patient shows no signs of cardiovascular instability and if hemostatic and renal function is unchanged at least

24 hours after the incompatible transfusion, the episode can be considered to be over, with serious sequelae unlikely. The direct antiglobulin test (DAT) becomes positive in an immune hemolytic reaction (if tested before all the incompatible RBCs are destroyed). Preparation of an antibody eluate is often necessary to identify the presence of an offending IgG antibody. An elution is a procedure that chemically separates the bound antibody from the RBCs and concentrates it so that it may be identified.

Initial therapy consists of immediately stopping the transfusion, administering intravenous fluids, cardiorespiratory support, and ensuring a brisk diuresis. Increasing renal blood flow is the best way to prevent acute oliguric renal failure. Usually, 0.9% NaCl is infused to maintain a urine output of 100 mL/hour for approximately 24 hours. Diuresis can be achieved with loop diuretics or mannitol. Mannitol, if chosen, must be used with caution; if acute tubular necrosis (ATN) occurs before mannitol infusion, pulmonary edema may occur as a result of the acute increase in intravascular volume secondary to fluid expansion. Maintaining hydration and diuresis can be complicated in the setting of heart failure and underlying renal disease. The mechanisms responsible for the beneficial effect of increased renal blood flow likely include increased clearance of free hemoglobin and a return of more physiologic control of renal vasodilation. Creatinine and blood urea nitrogen (BUN) should be monitored; dialysis may be necessary for treatment of oliguric acute renal failure. Support of blood pressure and respiration may require the use of vasopressors, bronchodilators, or intubation. DIC can occur in severe cases. The prothrombin time, activated partial thromboplastin time, and fibrinogen level should be monitored (see box on Workup of an Acute Intravascular Hemolytic Transfusion Reaction).

Hyperhemolysis is a specific type of acute intravascular hemolysis of bystander RBCs that do not express the antigen to which an immune-mediated hemolysis is directed. Hyperhemolysis occurs in

Acute Hemolytic Transfusion Reaction

A 15-year-old blood group O male with sickle cell disease presents for routine simple transfusion for primary prevention of stroke. He has no history of red blood cell (RBC) alloimmunization and his pretransfusion compatibility testing shows a negative screen for RBC alloantibodies. Seven minutes into the transfusion, the patient reports not feeling well. He quickly develops chills, abdominal pain, flank pain, and pain at the infusion site. The transfusion is stopped. Vital signs show a 15-mm Hg drop in systolic blood pressure from baseline value, pulse of 130, and a temperature increase from afebrile pretransfusion to 38.9°C. Gross hematuria is seen in a subsequent urine sample. Reinspection of the blood unit shows that it is group A and labeled with the name of the child receiving blood in the infusion chair next to him. The patient is transferred to the emergency room where he is evaluated for renal failure and DIC.

Recognition of the signs and symptoms at an acute hemolytic transfusion reaction are paramount for transfusion safety. Stopping transfusion at the first sign of incompatibility, usually fever, is critical for preventing severe sequelae. Although almost all febrile reactions to blood transfusion are not caused by blood incompatibility, it is impossible to exclude this possibility at the bedside. All transfusion reactions need to be reported to the blood bank to exclude incompatibility.

TABLE 119.1   Types of Acute Transfusion Reactions

Reaction Type	Presenting Signs and Symptoms
Acute hemolytic	Fever, chills, dyspnea, vomiting, hypotension, tachycardia, infusion site pain, back pain, hemoglobinuria, hemoglobinemia, indirect hyperbilirubinemia, renal failure, DIC
Febrile reaction	Fever, chills, rigors
Allergic	Urticaria, pruritus, flushing, angioedema, dyspnea, bronchospasm stridor, hypotension, tachycardia, abdominal cramping
Hypervolemic	Dyspnea, tachycardia, hypertension, headache, jugular venous distention
Septic	Fever, chills, hypotension, tachycardia, vomiting
Transfusion-related acute lung injury	Dyspnea, hypoxemia, fever, hypotension

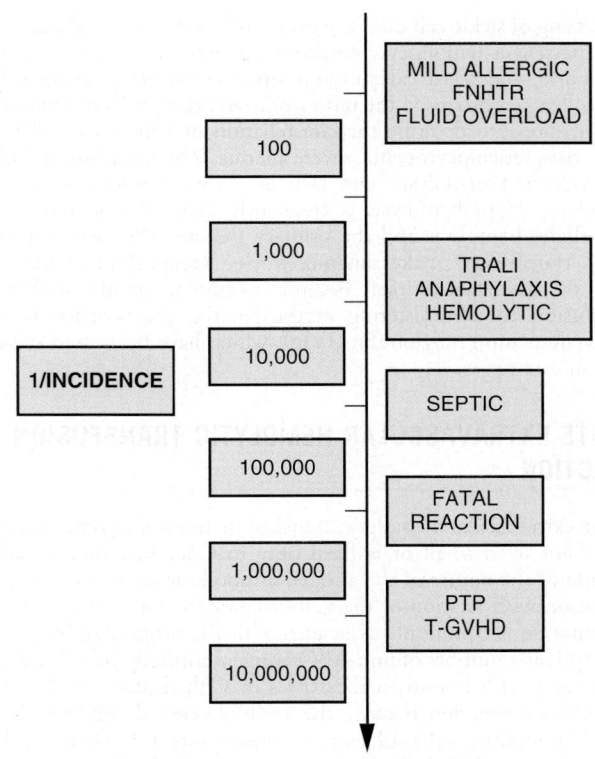

Fig. 119.1 APPROXIMATE RISK OF VARIOUS TRANSFUSION COMPLICATIONS. *FNHTR*, Febrile nonhemolytic transfusion reaction; *PTP*, posttransfusion purpura; *t-GVHD*, transfusion-associated graft-versus-host disease; *TRALI*, transfusion-related acute lung injury.

TABLE 119.2   Hemolytic Transfusion Reactions: Serologic Presentation

Type	Antibody Detectable Initially	Primary Antibody Type	Degree of Complement Binding	Example
Acute intravascular	Yes	IgM	Full (C1-9)	ABO system
Acute extravascular	Yes	IgG	None/partial	Rh system
Delayed intravascular	No	IgG	Full (C1-9)	Kidd system
Delayed extravascular	No	IgG	None/partial	Duffy system

the setting of sickle cell disease with transfusion, acute malarial infection, passenger lymphocyte syndrome, paroxysmal nocturnal hemoglobinuria, and select cases of autoimmune hemolytic anemia. Petz and colleagues proposed the term *sickle cell hemolytic transfusion reaction syndrome* to describe the constellation of hemolysis, sickle cell pain crisis, reticulocytopenia, severe anemia, RBC transfusion leading to accelerated hemolysis, and lack of a clear serologic reason for hemolysis. Hyperhemolysis is frequently fatal because transfusion exacerbates hemolysis and the primary treatment for severe anemia (RBC transfusion) makes anemia worse. Recognition of this syndrome is therefore critical because treatment should shift from transfusion to administering erythropoietin, glucocorticoids, and intravenous immunoglobulin (IVIg), which have been used successfully in case series.

ACUTE EXTRAVASCULAR HEMOLYTIC TRANSFUSION REACTION

In an extravascular hemolytic transfusion reaction, complement is either not fixed at all or is fixed only to C3b. In either situation, because of the nature of the antigen-antibody reaction, complement activation with fixation of the C5b-9 complex does not occur. This presentation is commonly associated with Rh antibodies, but can be seen with any number of non-ABO antigen-antibody complexes. The presence of IgG bound to the RBCs or C3b fixation results in an extravascular reaction because the antibody-coated cells are cleared by IgG receptors in the spleen or C3b receptors in the liver. In these circumstances, RBC lysis does not occur in the intravascular space. Because of the lack of generation of C3a or C5a, an extravascular hemolytic transfusion reaction does not usually present as a clinical emergency. It is characterized by a positive DAT caused by recipient RBC alloantibodies binding to the incompatible circulating donor RBCs. Moreover, an increase in indirect bilirubin, an increase in LDH, a decrease in hematocrit, a decrease in haptoglobin, and an increase in colorless urine urobilinogen can occur, but hemoglobinuria and hemoglobinemia are rarely present. The patient typically remains clinically stable. Renal failure, shock, and hemostatic abnormalities, such as DIC, are rarely seen unless the amount of incompatible blood infused is excessive. However, patients often have a low-grade fever.

When an extravascular hemolytic transfusion reaction is suspected, the diagnostic test of choice is a DAT with an eluate. The eluate is performed to identify the antibody coating the RBCs. The positive DAT result reflects the patient's antibody (or antibodies) coating the

incompatible donor RBCs. Because this is not an autoantibody, the patient's own RBCs are not involved in the reaction.

Typically an acute extravascular hemolytic transfusion reaction requires no special therapeutic intervention if the volume of incompatible blood transfused is relatively low. The patient characteristically recovers in a few days as the incompatible donor RBCs are cleared from the circulation. If the volume of incompatible blood transfused was high, hemolysis can quickly lead to a severe anemia. Communication with the blood bank is key to identifying how many units of incompatible units were transfused.

Extravascular acute reactions may occur if the patient's preexisting alloantibody was missed by the blood bank during the antibody screening process, if a wrongly labeled sample was used, if the unit of blood was labeled for the wrong patient, or if the unit was hung on the wrong patient.

DELAYED HEMOLYTIC REACTIONS

The pathogenesis of a delayed hemolytic transfusion reactions (DHTR) is similar to that described for acute hemolytic reactions. However, in DHTRs, the patient develops hemolysis 3–10 days after the transfusion as an anamnestic antibody response to a blood antigen previously known to the patient's immune system through transfusion, pregnancy, or hematopoietic stem cell transplantation (HSCT). Delayed hemolytic reactions occur more slowly than acute reactions and are less likely to present as a clinical emergency. Hemoglobinuria and hemoglobinemia can occur but are less pronounced than with an acute intravascular reaction. This is probably because of the gradual increase in antibody, as well as the fact that most DHTRs are caused by antibodies not efficient at activating complement. The need for intervention is much less likely than with an acute hemolytic transfusion reaction, but hematologic and renal monitoring are prudent.

DHTRs are the most common presentation of transfusion-associated immune hemolysis. DHTRs often involve the Rh system. Patients present with a fever, a falling hematocrit, and the development of a positive DAT with an eluate demonstrating a new RBC alloantibody. Because these reactions are typically mild in nature, they are usually addressed with supportive care only. In patients with sickle cell disease, DHTRs can precipitate vasoocclusive crises, autoantibody production, or hyperhemolysis. It is prudent to take a transfusion history in people with sickle cell disease who present with new complications.

One final note regarding the serologic evaluation of a transfusion reaction: posttransfusion testing may be complicated and difficult to interpret because of the possibility of autoantibodies or the involvement of medications. In such circumstances, referral to the pretransfusion specimen is often helpful. In cases of more complex evaluations, consultation with an expert serologist is recommended to detect and identify new alloantibodies in the patient's plasma, which may be responsible for a hemolytic transfusion reaction.

FEBRILE NONHEMOLYTIC TRANSFUSION REACTIONS

A febrile nonhemolytic transfusion reaction (FNHTR) is suspected when a transient temperature rise of 1°C to over 38°C or more occurs during or after transfusion and when no other cause for the fever can be identified.[3] In addition to fever, FNHTRs are often associated with rigors and chills. In fact, rigors and chills can also manifest without a concomitant fever, an atypical or "afebrile" FNHTR. In these cases, temperature increases may be masked by antipyretic premedication.

Evidence supports two mechanisms of FNHTR: antileukocyte antibodies and a storage lesion of released cytokines. Cytotoxic or agglutinating antibodies having human leukocyte antigen (HLA) specificity, neutrophil specificity, or platelet specificity may be present in the recipient's plasma and react against antigens present on transfused donor lymphocytes, granulocytes, or platelets. Conversely, donor plasma may contain the offending antibody that can react with the corresponding cellular antigens in the recipient's blood. Leukocyte-derived cytokines IL-8, IL-1β, and IL-6 accumulate in platelet products in particular and induce fever. IL-1, through prostaglandin PGE$_2$ synthesis, is thought to stimulate the thermoregulatory center of the hypothalamus to produce fever. Other mediators such as macrophage inflammatory proteins (e.g., MIP-1) may also participate in the febrile response, but this reaction is not mediated through prostaglandin synthesis. CD154 (CD40 ligand) derived from platelets is also involved in febrile reactions by inducing cyclooxygenase-2 and PGE$_2$. Leukoreduction is less effective at preventing FNHTRs to platelets than to red cell components because of platelet-derived biologic response modifiers. Nevertheless, studies show that generation of cytokines during storage is directly proportional to the leukocyte count of the unit and the duration of storage.

The frequency of febrile reactions for a nonleukoreduced unit has been estimated to be 6.8 per 100 units RBCs transfused and 2.2 per 100 units platelet transfused. With the advent of prestorage leukoreduction, these risks have been decreased to about 0.09–1.1 per 100 units RBCs transfused and 0.04–1.56 per 100 units platelet transfused. Reactions are most commonly seen in recipients who have been exposed to multiple white cell or platelet antigens. Patients with bone marrow failure (primary or chemotherapy-induced) are at risk as a result of frequent transfusions, as are multiparous women who may have received multiple exposures during pregnancy and childbirth. These groups of patients can form multiple HLA-, granulocyte-, or platelet-specific antibodies that will react with white cells or platelets upon subsequent exposure.

The workup of a febrile reaction must be undertaken promptly, because fever may also be the first sign of other, more severe reactions, including acute hemolysis or sepsis. A hemolytic transfusion reaction may be ruled out by reconfirming the ABO and Rh type of the patient and the donor unit, repeating crossmatching to confirm patient-donor compatibility, evaluating the results of the pretransfusion and posttransfusion DATs, evaluating the serum for hemolysis, and rechecking the accuracy of paperwork. The posttransfusion DAT should yield negative findings, because FNHTRs do not involve RBC alloantibodies.

As laboratory testing is being completed, the workup should include bedside patient evaluation. Fever and chills may be attributable to drugs or underlying diseases, or they may be associated with infection or inflammation. Neutropenic fever often complicates the clinical picture in patients undergoing myeloablative chemotherapy, a population of patients likely to undergo repeated RBC or platelet transfusions. Blood cultures of the patient and the blood product should be considered, especially if the patient has high fever or shows signs of sepsis (see later text and box for a more in-depth discussion of septic transfusion reactions). The difficulty lies in knowing when to order blood cultures, because there is a false-positive incidence as a result of contamination during culturing. It is not routine to identify the specificities of HLA, platelet, or granulocyte antibodies that could cause FNHTRs. Accordingly the diagnosis of an FNHTR is usually made as a diagnosis of exclusion without isolating an identifiable antibody.

Fever from an FNHTR usually responds to antipyretics, including aspirin, nonsteroidal antiinflammatory drugs (NSAIDs), and acetaminophen. Aspirin and NSAIDs should be avoided in thrombocytopenic patients because of their inhibitory effects on platelet cyclooxygenase, including inhibition of transfused platelets. Diphenhydramine is not indicated for treatment or prevention of febrile reactions.

For patients with no history of febrile reactions, routine premedication is unnecessary. Most patients do not experience subsequent FNHTRs. Those with a history of clinically significant FNHTRs may be premedicated with acetaminophen or an NSAID. Those patients with severe reactions despite premedication may require more intensive pharmacotherapy, including corticosteroids 1–2 hours before transfusion. Patients with severe rigors can be treated with meperidine. Febrile reactions after granulocyte transfusions and, less frequently, after platelet transfusions can be so severe that hypotension may occur.

Septic Transfusion Reaction

A 29-year-old women in week 38 of pregnancy received a unit of apheresis platelets prophylactically in clinic for a chronic bone marrow failure syndrome of unclear etiology. During the infusion, she developed flank pain and coughing. The transfusion was stopped and the patient was admitted. She became febrile to 39.3°C 90 minutes after transfusion. Blood cultures from the patient and bag grew *Staphylococcus aureus* within 12 hours.

Blood transfusion is common in people with bone marrow failure, either primary or secondary to myeloablative chemotherapy. These patients are also often neutropenic, have central venous catheters, and/or are taking immunosuppressive medications. Despite these underlying risk factors, transfusion should always be considered a potential source of bacteremia. It is critical to always consider blood components as a source of infection. There are usually other components manufactured from the same collection, and the blood bank must quarantine them before release to another patient. It is only when the blood bank is notified of a suspected septic reaction that this is possible. Yomtovian and colleagues prospectively cultured all platelets issued from a large hospital blood bank and found contaminated units similar to other reported rates (~1:2000). When they relied on passive reporting of septic reactions from clinicians, the incidence fell to zero, only to increase back to baseline once active culturing of platelets resumed.

Prevention of febrile reactions also relies on the use of leukocyte-depleted blood components. Several leukocyte depletion techniques are available. Prestorage leukocyte depletion filters are the most common method used for preventing febrile reactions. They remove up to 4 logs (99.99%) of leukocytes, often lowering the level of white cells in a unit of blood from 10^9 to 10^5. They also are useful for preventing or delaying the onset of HLA alloimmunization and preventing cytomegalovirus transmission. For these reasons, leukoreduction is universal in many centers. Cell washing or use of frozen deglycerolized RBCs can remove up to 95% of contaminating white cells. Individuals with a history of recurrent, severe febrile reactions should have notations made in their blood bank record to ensure future use of leukocyte-reduced components.

ALLERGIC TRANSFUSION REACTIONS

Allergic transfusion reactions complicate up to 3% of all transfusions. The allergic manifestations occur on a spectrum of severity. They can include flushing, urticaria, pruritus, angioedema, hypotension, bronchospasm, stridor, abdominal pain, and emesis. Anaphylaxis is a systemic immediate hypersensitivity reaction, which can be defined as allergic signs and symptoms in skin/mucosa and at least one other organ system (cardiovascular, respiratory, gastrointestinal). Shock is the most ominous manifestation of anaphylaxis, but bronchospasm and upper airway angioedema are more common manifestations (see box titled "Management and Prevention of Allergic Transfusion Reaction).

Allergic transfusion reactions manifest as other IgE-mediated, immediate hypersensitivity reactions. The incidence is associated with the plasma content of the product, so it is thought that a plasma protein is responsible for many reactions. Examples of IgG or IgE with specificity to IgA, haptoglobin, and C4 have been described. There are several reports of allergic transfusion reactions to autologous transfusion, suggesting that a storage lesion may be responsible for some reactions. Passive transfer of IgE with allergen exposure in the recipient is a mechanism that has been described for food and antibiotic-mediated allergic transfusion reactions, but these are uncommon.

Mast cells are the primary allergic effector cells for immediate hypersensitivity reactions; basophils may play a secondary role. Mast cells and basophils can be activated by cross-linking cell surface high-affinity IgE receptors or via IgE-independent mechanisms, such as complement receptor binding by C5a. Upon activation, histamine is released immediately, as it is stored preformed in granules. Platelet activating factor, a potent arachidonic acid derivative that mediates anaphylactic shock, is produced rapidly, along with a variety of other eicosanoids, for example, leukotrienes.

Over 90% of allergic transfusion reactions occur during infusion. When allergic symptoms develop, transfusion should be stopped and the patient given 25–50 mg of diphenhydramine. The transfusion may resume, but only if the symptoms resolve and the patient feels well. A mild allergic reaction (urticaria and pruritus) during a blood transfusion usually does not progress to a more severe anaphylactic reaction after infusion of additional blood from the same unit. The severity of allergic transfusion reactions is not directly related to volume infused or infusion rate.

Most patients never experience an allergic transfusion reaction, and for those who have one, it is usually isolated. Even among the minority of patients with recurrent reactions, most transfusions are tolerated well. Patients who have had more than one mild allergic reaction may continue to receive routine units. Washed RBCs or plasma-reduced platelets can be used to prevent severe, recurrent reactions; however, washing cellular products compromises component quality. Washing RBCs leads to accelerated in vitro hemolysis. Washing platelets increases platelet activation and lowers posttransfusion platelet count increments. Platelets collected in platelet additive solution and pooled, solvent detergent plasma are relatively new products that have been shown to reduce the incidence of allergic transfusion reactions. Leukocyte depletion or microaggregate filters are of no value.

There is no evidence that antihistamine premedication prevents allergic transfusion reactions, although antihistamines do mitigate symptoms when they occur. Studies in healthy volunteers support a synergistic role for treating histamine-mediated reactions with both H1 and H2 receptor antagonists, for example, diphenhydramine and ranitidine, respectively. Corticosteroids, provided in advance of a transfusion, also may be useful in patients with serious recurrent reactions.

Most anaphylactic transfusion reactions are idiopathic. Case reports describe moderate or severe anaphylactic reactions in patients who are severely IgA deficient (<0.05 mg/dL) and have anti-IgA antibodies. The generalizability of this mechanism is low. Most cases of fatal anaphylaxis are not related to IgA deficiency, and most severely IgA-deficient people tolerate transfusions well. Thus, patients with incidental IgA deficiency may receive routine blood components, and IgA/anti-IgA testing should be reserved for patients with anaphylactic reactions. Quantitative haptoglobin can also be considered as a screening test, as rare cases of haptoglobin deficiency are associated with anaphylactic reactions.

HYPOTENSIVE TRANSFUSION REACTION

A less recognized, but severe acute transfusion reaction is isolated hypotension during or immediately following a blood product infusion. For adults, the definition includes a drop in systolic blood pressure greater than 30 mmHg to below 80 mmHg, and it is most likely when hypotension occurs within minutes of the start of the transfusion and resolves quickly after the transfusion is stopped. This type of transfusion reaction was initially reported after transfusion of platelets administered through some types of bedside leukoreduction filters. Later it was also reported in other types of blood products including plasma and RBCs. The pathogenesis of this syndrome appears to be related to the activation of the contact pathway (prekallikrein converting to kallikrein) induced in plasma by the negatively charged surface of some leukoreduction filters. Kallikrein activation stimulates the conversion of high-molecular-weight kininogen to bradykinin. Notably these reactions have also been reported in cases where leukoreduction filters were used before storage, indicating that bradykinin generation may occur via pathways other than via bedside filtration. The syndrome is often more severe in patients already taking angiotensin-converting enzyme (ACE) inhibitors. ACE is identical to kininase II, which is responsible for degrading bradykinin. Blockage of the kininase II degradation of bradykinin by ACE inhibitors results in a prolonged bradykinin half-life and a reaction that can be very severe. Two surgical settings that may pose increased risk of hypotensive reactions include (1) procedures involving the prostate, because another kallikrein gene family member, *hK2*, can generate bradykinin, and (2) cardiac bypass surgery because the pulmonary vasculature is an important site for kinin metabolism.

INFECTIOUS COMPLICATIONS OF TRANSFUSION

Transfusion-transmitted diseases are discussed in detail in Chapter 120. A focus on the clinical presentation of acute reactions is presented here.

Bacterial contamination of stored blood can pose grave risks to the recipient. Bacteria can enter the blood collection bag during venipuncture as a result of inadequate skin preparation, during component preparation, or through the collection of blood from a donor with an occult infection or asymptomatic bacteremia. Platelet concentrates, stored at room temperature, have the highest risk of bacterial contamination. Many reports describe fatal septic transfusion reactions caused by platelet components containing a variety of species, including *Pseudomonas, Salmonella,* and *Staphylococcus.* Bacteria that grow well at refrigerated blood bank temperatures (1°C to 6°C), including *Pseudomonas, Yersinia, Enterobacter,* and *Flavobacterium,* are organisms commonly associated with a contaminated unit of RBCs. Units of blood that are contaminated need not be obviously discolored, malodorous, or clotted; it is extremely difficult to determine by simple visual inspection whether a unit is contaminated.

Patients who receive a unit of contaminated blood may develop fever, rigors, skin flushing, abdominal cramps, myalgias, DIC, renal failure, hypotension, and cardiac arrest. These reactions may be immediate, or there may be a delay of several hours before the symptoms become apparent. Especially for gram-positive bacteria, a reaction to infusion of a contaminated unit may not be distinguishable from an FNHTR. Shock in a septic transfusion reaction is attributable to endotoxin produced by gram-negative bacteria. Septic transfusions differ from acute hemolytic reactions most notably by the absence of characteristic hemoglobinuria and hemoglobinemia.

For a patient who appeared well and suddenly develops rigors, fever, and/or shock during an infusion, an infected component should be considered. Blood infusion should be stopped the moment any transfusion reaction is suspected, and appropriate samples should be sent to the blood bank for a DAT, hemolysis check, and bacterial culture. Broad-spectrum antibiotics should be started immediately if infusion of contaminated blood is suspected and continued until the culture results are reported. It is also important to consider a bacterially contaminated blood component when a patient presents with signs of bacteremia several hours after a transfusion is completed. Gram-positive bacteria, which are the most common bacterial contaminants in platelet components, are less likely to cause shock, and presentation of signs and symptoms of infection may be delayed by several hours.

Because of the decrease in viral transmission by blood transfusion, septic transfusion reactions now account for a significant portion of the transfusion-related infections in the United States. Data from the Bacterial Contamination of Blood study showed that from 1998 to 2000, the rate of transfusion-transmitted bacteremia was 9.98 per million single-donor platelets, 10.64 per million pooled platelets, and 0.21 per million RBC units; the rate of fatal reactions was 1.94 per million single-donor platelets, 2.22 per million pooled platelets, and 0.13 per million RBC units, respectively. To decrease the likelihood of a septic unit of platelets being transfused, the expiration date of units of platelet concentrate has been limited to a 5-day outdate. To further reduce the risk for bacterial transmission through platelet transfusion, platelet concentrates must be tested for bacterial contamination. There are two bacterial detection systems approved by the FDA for screening of blood components. Since the implementation of the mandatory bacterial testing for platelets, FDA data indicate that the mortality associated with septic transfusion reactions in the United States has decreased, although the risks for septic transfusion reaction have not been eradicated.

Viral and parasitic transmission through transfusion does not lead to acute reactions. Rather, subacute infectious syndromes present days to months after transfusion. As with bacteremia, it is important to always consider transfusion as an infectious source. A full description of the infectious agents transmissible through transfusion are surveyed in the following chapter.

TRANSFUSION-RELATED ACUTE LUNG INJURY

Transfusion-related acute lung injury (TRALI), is the leading cause of transfusion-related death reported to the FDA. For the period of 2009–2013, 38% (72 of 190) of reported fatalities to the FDA were caused by TRALI. Symptoms of TRALI range from mild dyspnea to severe noncardiogenic pulmonary edema, with symptoms and signs that include dyspnea, oxygen desaturation, respiratory failure, chills, fever, and hypotension. Most patients require oxygen support, and many require mechanical ventilation. TRALI, by definition, develops within 6 hours of starting a transfusion, but typically reactions occur within 2 hours. Because the pulmonary edema is noncardiogenic, there is no elevation in cardiopulmonary pressures. The chest radiograph may reveal pulmonary edema pattern (bilateral infiltrates), but should not show vascular congestion. Copious amounts of fluid are produced in the lungs, as is characteristic of hypervolemia; however, the noncardiogenic reaction usually follows infusion of volumes of blood too small to produce fluid overload. It is often postulated that TRALI consists of a "two-hit" event, the first "hit" being an underlying clinical condition that leads to the sequestration and priming of neutrophils in the lung tissue, and the second being the transfusion of blood products containing anti-HLA or anti-HNA (human neutrophil antigen) antibodies

that activate the neutrophils in the lung parenchyma, leading to edema. Complement and monocyte activation with aggregation of white blood cells also may occur when leukoagglutinins present in the recipient react with leukocytes contained in the infused donor blood. As a result of the leukocyte antigen-antibody reaction, the activated leukocytes express adhesive molecules on their surface (CD11/CD18), which then permit leukocytes to attach to pulmonary endothelial cells and migrate to the interstitial space between the pulmonary capillaries and the alveolar epithelium. Once in the interstitial space, neutrophils degranulate and through enzymatic digestion produce capillary dehiscence that results in fluid filling the alveolar sacs. Pulmonary leukostasis with pulmonary edema thus occurs as a result of microvascular occlusion and capillary leakage. Complement-activated granulocytes also produce oxygen radicals that damage pulmonary endothelial cells, resulting in a further increase in pulmonary vascular permeability and additional passage of fluid into alveolar spaces. It has been reported that aged blood products may accumulate bioactive lipids and soluble mediators, such as CD40L, that hamper the chemokine scavenging ability of erythrocytes as a result of reduction in the expression of the Duffy antigens, and this may represent a second hit in the two-hit model. Rodent model systems for TRALI have also been described, and some of these models suggest a role for platelets in TRALI. Work is ongoing to elucidate the different mechanisms leading to this syndrome, which may be a final common pathway from a variety of initiating insults.

Because TRALI is hard to distinguish from fluid overload without central cardiovascular pressure measurements, it is often not straightforward to diagnose. When a patient shows signs of noncardiogenic pulmonary edema, the infusion should be immediately stopped, as it should be with all other reactions. These HLA/neutrophil antigen-antibody reactions are usually donor-specific and should not recur with a unit from a different donor.

Treatment is supportive (Table 119.3). Donors who are implicated in TRALI reactions should be permanently deferred from blood donation. Hence reporting of these reactions to the blood bank is important so that implicated donors can be identified and tested. Antileukocyte antibodies are most likely present in blood donors who are multiparous women. The exclusion of these donors has proven to be effective. Using male-only plasma started in the 2000s and led to a reduction in TRALI fatalities by more than half.

TABLE 119.3	Transfusion-Related Acute Lung Injury
Onset	Within 6 hours of start of transfusion, usually within 2 hours
Frequency	1:10,000 transfusions
Signs and symptoms	Hypoxemia, fever, hypotension, tachypnea, dyspnea, diffuse pulmonary edema,
Pathogenesis	HLA/granulocyte-specific antibodies (usually of donor origin) reacting with recipient leukocytes or directly with endothelium. Lysophosphotidylcholines that accumulate during component storage can activate neutrophils in an antibody-independent manner.
Diagnosis	Chest radiograph; blood gases; post/pretransfusion NT-BNP ratio <1.5; blood for HLA or antineutrophil antibodies
Differential diagnosis	Fluid overload; septic transfusion; anaphylaxis; unrelated acute lung injury
Treatment	Stop transfusion. Provide respiratory support (administer O_2, intubation may be needed), support blood pressure, no evidence supporting glucocorticoids or diuretics.

HLA, Human leukocyte antigen; NT-BNP, N-terminal brain-natriuretic peptide.

TRANSFUSION-ASSOCIATED CIRCULATORY OVERLOAD

Transfusion-associated circulatory overload (TACO) results from hydrostatic transudate accumulation in the lungs and should be considered in patients who, during a blood infusion, develop sudden onset of dyspnea, jugular venous distention, tachycardia, congestive heart failure, or other signs of fluid overload. Unless there is severe hemorrhage or life-threatening shock, blood should not be infused rapidly, because the acute expansion of a patient's intravascular volume may exceed the capacity of the cardiovascular and renal systems to compensate, resulting in fluid overload. Likewise, rapidly transfusing an anemic patient who is euvolemic may cause harm. This caveat applies to transfusion of any blood component. Patients with compromised cardiopulmonary status may not tolerate acute blood volume expansion and may develop right- or left-sided heart failure. This is especially true for infants, the elderly, and people with renal failure.

If TACO is suspected, the transfusion should be stopped and the patient's blood volume reduced by diuretics. If there is a concern that the patient may not tolerate infusion of a full unit of blood or component within the 4-hour period allotted for infusion of blood components, the blood bank often can divide the product into smaller portions, which can be transfused in aliquots. As a general guide, infusions in nonbleeding adults should occur at less than 2–3 mL/kg/hour. The rate should be lowered to 1 mL/kg/hour for patients at risk for fluid overload. For a blood component of 300 mL with a typical 4-hour expiration, a 75-kg adult would receive the component at 1 mL/kg/hour if transfused over 4 hours. Diuretics may be given to patients with compromised cardiopulmonary status before transfusion. Diagnostically, if the patient improves with diuretics, it is suggestive of TACO.

The initial stages of transfusion-induced hypervolemia may be difficult to distinguish from hemolytic transfusion reaction, FNHTR, allergic reaction, or TRALI. The absence of hemoglobinuria and hemoglobinemia and the absence of a positive posttransfusion DAT result distinguish the reaction from one caused by immune hemolysis. Likewise, the absence of fever, chills, or urticaria should help distinguish TACO from the febrile or allergic types of reactions. The clinical use of laboratory testing such as N-terminal probrain natriuretic peptide (NT-proBNP) may aid in the diagnosis; when NT-proBNP is at least 50% higher posttransfusion than pretransfusion levels, NT-proBNP is sensitive and specific for TACO and makes other diagnoses in the differential less likely. TRALI is less likely when NT-proBNP is elevated.

Transfusion-Associated Graft-Versus-Host Disease

Transfusion-associated graft-versus-host disease (t-GVHD) occurs when immunologically competent lymphocytes are introduced into a host who cannot destroy the donor lymphocytes. The immunocompetent donor lymphocytes engraft, host HLA antigen is presented to donor lymphocytes, and the activated lymphocytes attack host tissues. t-GVHD occurs after transfusion of nonirradiated cellular blood components, especially when the blood donor and recipient share HLA antigens. t-GVHD has a much higher fatality rate than HSCT-related GVHD because the donor lymphocytes produce recipient bone marrow aplasia in addition to typical liver, gut, and skin manifestations of acute GVHD. In GVHD after bone marrow transplantation, the bone marrow is of donor origin, and bone marrow aplasia does not occur.

Posttransfusion GVHD is fatal in more than 90% of cases, primarily because of aplasia of the recipient's bone marrow. It often occurs 8–10 days after transfusion with marked pancytopenia, as well as gut, skin, and liver GVHD. The signs and symptoms include nausea, vomiting, anorexia, fever, diarrhea, liver dysfunction, and erythroderma. Patients often die of infection and hemorrhage within 3–4 weeks. There is no effective treatment, with the possible exception of bone marrow transplantation, if posttransfusion GVHD is recognized early and a suitable donor can be found in a short time.

Risk Groups for Transfusion-Associated Graft-Versus-Host Disease[a]
Congenital T-cell defects (known or suspected)
Immunologic immaturity (fetus or premature infant)
Intrauterine transfusion
Neonates undergoing intrauterine exchange transfusion or extracorporeal membrane oxygenation
Solid organ and hematopoietic stem cell transplant
Lymphoma and hematologic malignancy
Solid tumors
Fludarabine
Haplotype sharing between donor and recipient
Transfusions from blood relatives
Human leukocyte antigen-matched platelets
Granulocyte transfusions

[a]Risks not identified for human immunodeficiency virus infection/acquired immunodeficiency syndrome or aplastic anemia (except in setting of bone marrow transplantation or immunosuppressive therapy).

Reports have shown that haploidentical directed donor units of blood may produce fatal posttransfusion GVHD even in immunocompetent recipients. The use of irradiated blood (2500 cGy) is thus recommended in clinical situations in which posttransfusion GVHD is considered possible, such as when patients receive directed blood transfusions from their relatives. Leukocyte-reduction filters should not be used as prophylaxis against GVHD, because the number of leukocytes needed to produce the disease is not known. Case reports of fatal GVHD in patients who received leukoreduced, but not irradiated, blood have been published. GVHD continues to be a rare, but extremely serious, complication of blood transfusion. From 2009 to 2013, two fatalities from transfusion-associated GVHD were reported to the FDA. There is no clear evidence that prophylactic irradiation is indicated for patients with human immunodeficiency virus infection (see box on Risk Groups for Transfusion-Associated Graft-Versus-Host Disease). Of note, irradiation of RBCs causes membrane damage, permitting slow leakage of potassium and hemoglobin extracellularly. Nevertheless, rather than track which patients need irradiated blood, many centers provide universal irradiation of RBC components without adverse sequelae.

Posttransfusion Purpura

Posttransfusion purpura (PTP) is a rare and self-limiting thrombocytopenia occurring 5–10 days posttransfusion in patients lacking a specific platelet antigen, usually HPA-1a (also called PLA1, GPIIIa, CD61). These patients often have a history of sensitization with prior transfusions or pregnancies. Indeed, about 85% of cases occur in women. After resensitization by transfusion, patients can develop potent antibodies against the platelet-specific antigen that they are lacking but which is present on donor platelets. These platelet antibodies often have a high titer and can fix complement. As a result, the transfused platelets and the patient's own platelets are also destroyed through the adsorption of the antigen or immune complexes on their own platelets. A concurrent autoimmune process may also involve destruction of the recipient's own platelets, as shown in one case report of a positive antibody against the patient's own platelets. The thrombocytopenia can be marked with a platelet count falling below 10,000/μL. The onset is sudden, although self-limited, and usually resolves in 2 weeks. This severe thrombocytopenia can help distinguish PTP from heparin-induced thrombocytopenia, which can also be considered in the differential diagnosis when thrombocytopenia develops 5–10 days after combined heparin exposure and blood transfusion, for example, major surgery. In patients who already have thrombocytopenia, diagnosing PTP can be difficult, especially when the patient already has immune-mediated platelet destruction. PTP can be considered if platelet refractoriness continues despite transfusion of HLA-matched platelets. IVIg appears to be an effective treatment, although plasma exchange, steroids, and splenectomy may also be useful. Patients with acute bleeding and needing platelet support should receive platelets without the platelet-specific antigen, if possible. If random donor platelets are given, patients can develop severe reactions, including allergic reactions. Recurrence of PTP is rare.

Hypothermia

Hypothermia can occur with rapid infusion of large quantities of refrigerated (1–6°C) blood, such as in cases of rapid and massive transfusions. Rapid infusion of blood (1 unit every 5 minutes) may lower the temperature of the sinoatrial node to less than 30°C, at which point ventricular fibrillation may occur. Hypothermia also induces coagulopathy, possibly attributed to inefficient enzymatic activity below physiologic temperatures. Use of warming devices may reduce the incidence of coagulopathies associated with major trauma and also help to overcome cardiac complications. Most transfusions need not be given this rapidly. For routine transfusion, blood does not have to be warmed. Indeed, overwarming a unit of blood can cause RBC thermal injury and produce hemolysis, DIC, or shock.

If blood is to be warmed, the temperature must be monitored and kept below a level that could cause hemolysis. Usually, this is less than 42°C. Heating blood under running hot tap water or heating in a microwave device is unacceptable.

Electrolyte Toxicity

Citrate, a component of the preservative solution used in blood storage, functions as an anticoagulant by chelating calcium and interfering with the coagulation cascade. Rapid transfusion of citrated blood is associated with a drop in ionized calcium levels. Citrate-containing blood products, however, are routinely infused without any problem because the citrate is rapidly metabolized to bicarbonate. In patients with normal liver function, citrate infusion is unlikely to produce reactions. Mild to severe citrate toxicity can be seen, however, in individuals undergoing therapeutic apheresis when citrate is infused to anticoagulate blood flowing through the instrument and large volumes of citrated RBCs or plasma are simultaneously reinfused.

The effects of hypocalcemia range from mild circumoral paresthesias to frank tetany. However, severe citrate toxicity, even with massive transfusion, is rare. More commonly, the reaction is mild and self-limiting and can be treated by merely slowing the rate of reinfusion. If prolonged QT intervals or signs of tetany are seen, calcium can be administered. Calcium need not be infused routinely, even after large-volume blood transfusions. However, it is prudent to monitor calcium status in patients undergoing massive transfusion and patients at risk for hypocalcemia arising from citrate toxicity. Under no circumstances should calcium be added to a unit of blood or a line used for blood infusion because it would recalcify the unit and cause clots to form. In addition to the effects on calcium, the metabolism of citrate also can result in a metabolic alkalosis because of the generation of large amounts of bicarbonate.

Citrate also chelates magnesium, so correction of the hypocalcemia may require infusion of magnesium, as well. Actual clinical complications of transfusion-induced hypomagnesemia, however, have not been well documented other than in cases of apheresis.

Hyperkalemia caused by infusion of stored blood is a rare occurrence. Although hyperkalemia is often thought to be a problem in massive transfusion, development of hypokalemia is of greater concern. With storage, leakage of potassium from RBCs to the extracellular fluid occurs. However, after infusion the RBCs reverse the biochemical storage lesion by restoring the Na-K ATP membrane pump, and intracellular potassium levels are restored. As the citrate is metabolized to bicarbonate, the blood becomes alkalotic, contributing to hypokalemia. In massive transfusion, it is not uncommon for this to result in the need for administration of potassium. Depending on the storage solution, the potassium content in the supernatant of an RBC unit can reach 7 mEq at the end of storage. Neonates and children can receive transfusions of up to 20 mL/kg RBC for routine transfusions over 3–4 hours without concern for hyperkalemia. For large volume transfusions or transfusion in the setting of hyperkalemia, fresher or washed RBC components can be requested. As there is increased potassium leakage from RBCs after exposure to 25 Gy of radiation to prevent posttransfusion GVHD, a maximum 28-day shelf life from the day of irradiation is imposed on this blood component.

Iron Overload

Iron loading from RBC transfusion is not categorized as a transfusion reaction, but it is a common adverse consequence of chronic RBC transfusion. One milliliter of RBCs at a hematocrit of a typical RBC unit contains approximately 0.75 mg of iron. A unit of blood with 300 mL of RBCs thus contains approximately 225 mg of iron, and 4 units of blood contain ~1 g of iron, roughly the amount stored in the bone marrow. Men and nonmenstruating women lose only approximately 1 mg of iron each day. Continued use of transfusion therapy in individuals with a hemolytic anemia, such as those with thalassemia or sickle cell disease, in which iron is not lost from the body but is recycled, can thus result in the accumulation of excessive tissue stores of iron. Over long periods, the iron that is stored in parenchymal cells results in oxidative injury and organ failure, particularly in the heart, liver, and endocrine organs. Iron chelation therapy is now widely used to mitigate positive iron balance. The availability of oral iron chelators such as deferasirox and deferiprone provides expanded access to iron chelation therapy.

Air Emboli

Since the replacement of evacuated glass bottles by plastic blood bags, the risk for air embolism from phlebotomy or transfusion has virtually disappeared from transfusion practice. Air, however, still may be infused into patients by the roller pumps contained in various transfusion devices, especially apheresis machines and intraoperative salvage machines. All such devices currently manufactured, however, contain air-in-line sensors. However, any operators using this equipment must be well trained and remain alert to the potential risk for air embolization at all times while the patient is being treated. Patients who receive air intravenously experience acute cardiopulmonary insufficiency. The air tends to lodge in the right ventricle, preventing blood from entering the pulmonary circulation. Acute cyanosis, pain, cough, shock, and arrhythmia may occur, and death may result unless immediate action is taken. The patient should be placed head-down on the left side; this may displace the air bubble from the pulmonary valve. Use and removal of central lines may also pose a risk for air embolism.

Complications Associated With Massive Transfusion

Massive transfusion is variably defined as the transfusion of one whole blood volume within 24 hours, 4 units of RBCs in 1 hour with anticipation of more blood needed, or transfusion of 50% of total blood volume in 3 hours. Common problems associated with massive transfusion include coagulopathy, hypothermia, and metabolic abnormalities.

Coagulopathy of massive transfusion is multifactorial and can have devastating consequences. Classically the coagulopathy associated with massive transfusion was thought to be attributable solely to consumption of factors owing to ongoing hemorrhage and/or dilution owing to the large volume of fluids and RBCs typically infused. However, the understanding of hemostasis in massive transfusion now includes a form of coagulopathy that occurs *before* coagulation factors and platelets are consumed. Early coagulopathy, described primarily in the setting of trauma, is driven by tissue hypoperfusion and increased fibrinolysis. Early coagulopathy is not

TABLE 119.4	Common Hematopoietic Stem Cell Infusion Reactions	
Types	**Presentations**	**Treatment and Prevention**
DMSO toxicity	Halitosis, nausea, vomiting, flushing, coughing, chest tightness, dyspnea, abdominal pain, hypotension, hypertension, cardiac toxicity (such as bradycardia and other arrhythmias), and rarely neurologic toxicity, such as syncope and transient encephalopathy	Antihistamine Antiemetics Limiting DMSO infusion volume
Minor ABO mismatch	Delayed hemolysis (1–2 weeks post HSC infusion)	Plasma depletion of HSC product RBC transfusion support compatible with donor and recipient Monitor for hemolysis RBC exchange with donor- and recipient-compatible blood if massive hemolysis
Major ABO mismatch	Hemolysis at the time of infusion Delayed RBC engraftment	Limiting the infusion of incompatible RBC Hydration Monitor for RBC engraftment Modify immunosuppression Plasmapheresis to remove isohemagglutinins if significant RBC engraftment delay

DMSO, Dimethyl sulfoxide; HSC, hematopoietic stem cell; RBC, red blood cell.

likely to respond to traditional transfusion therapy and may only be resolved with restoration of circulatory capacity and inhibition of fibrinolysis.

Despite enhancements in understanding of early coagulopathy, platelet/coagulation factor dilution and consumption still remain outstanding problems in the setting of massive transfusion. Patients undergoing large-scale transfusion must be regularly monitored for hematocrit, platelet count, prothrombin time, activated partial thromboplastin time, and fibrinogen. Reasonable goals to promote hemostasis in the setting of massive transfusion are to maintain (1) hematocrit >25%, (2) platelets >50,000/µL, (3) international normalized ratio (INR) <1.7, and (4) fibrinogen ≥100–150 mg/dL. Therefore it is imperative that clinicians provide more than just RBCs to massively bleeding patients. To ensure a more appropriate provision of plasma and platelet products, many facilities have developed protocols consisting of preset numbers of RBC, fresh frozen plasma (FFP), and platelet units that are immediately issued upon requests for massive transfusion. Such protocols, developed in conjunction with surgical and trauma services, can drastically improve the efficiency of blood product provision in the setting of massive transfusion. Although massive transfusion protocols are useful tools to combat coagulopathy, controversy remains regarding the numbers of plasma and platelet products that should be provided to patients transfused with large volumes of RBCs. Trials and reports from military trauma centers have promoted use of protocols based around a 1:1:1 ratio of RBC/plasma/platelets units. Data from combat theaters suggest that such ratios are successful in avoiding the coagulopathy of massive transfusion and ultimately lead to improved survival. Despite these data, it is unclear whether such approaches are relevant to noncombat, civilian hospitals, which frequently issue massive transfusions for wide-ranging indications such as surgical complications, large gastrointestinal or retroperitoneal hemorrhages, or blunt trauma. A 2015 randomized controlled trial (PROPPR Trial) compared 1:1:1 and 2:1:1 RBC/plasma/platelet transfusion protocols in civilian trauma patients. Results showed an absolute difference of 4% lower 24-hour and 30-day mortality in the 1:1:1 group, but the difference was not statistically significant.

Complications Associated With Hematopoietic Stem Cell Infusion

Hematopoietic stem cells (HSCs), the most widely used cell therapy products, may be derived from bone marrow, peripheral blood, and cord blood. As with blood transfusions, the infusion of HSCs carries the risk of the same types of transfusion reactions. However, additional risks are associated with HSC infusion, such as those related to cryopreservatives. In general, infusions of cryopreserved cells are more likely to cause reactions, as they contain higher concentrations of lysed RBCs and granulocytes than other blood products. For most reactions, it is difficult to identify the causative agent. Moreover, because of the irreplaceable nature of HSC products, higher risks may be tolerated. Only those reactions that are unique or more problematic for HSC infusions are discussed in this section. A summary of the reactions is given in Table 119.4.

Dimethyl Sulfoxide Toxicity

The most common reactions to HSC have been attributed to dimethyl sulfoxide (DMSO), the most widely used cryopreservative. A variety of symptoms are associated with DMSO infusion and are generally dose-dependent. A garlic odor commonly accompanies DMSO infusion, and nausea and vomiting are often reported. Additional DMSO-related symptoms include flushing, coughing, chest tightness, dyspnea, abdominal pain, hypotension, hypertension, cardiac toxicity (such as bradycardia and other arrhythmias), and rarely, neurologic toxicity (such as syncope and transient encephalopathy). Some cases of DMSO toxicity are thought to arise from the release of histamine. Agents such as diphenhydramine have been used for the treatment and prevention of DMSO-related toxicity. Antiemetic agents such as prochlorperazine have been useful for ameliorating nausea and vomiting. Most clinical services have protocols in place to limit the volume of DMSO that can be infused, such as setting an upper infusion limit of 1 g/kg/day, dividing HSC infusion doses, or washing HSC products to remove DMSO (this, however, may result in cellular loss).

Red Blood Cell Engraftment and Hemolysis

Although mismatched ABO and non-ABO blood groups do not prevent successful HSCT, these antigens (and their corresponding antibodies) can create problems during the transplant period. When considering incompatibilities within the ABO system, three scenarios are possible: (1) antibodies present in the recipient interact with incompatible cells present in the graft (major incompatibility), (2) antibodies present in the plasma portion of the graft mediate hemolysis of recipient RBCs (minor incompatibility), or (3) antibodies present in both the recipient and the donor interact with incompatible RBCs (bidirectional, or two-way, incompatibility). It has been shown that both major and bidirectional ABO incompatibility can delay stem cell engraftment. In such cases, anti-A and/or B antibodies suppress RBC precursors expressing these antigens, leading to reticulocytopenia and prolonged anemia. In the most severe form of this process, HSC recipients can develop pure RBC aplasia, a condition wherein bone marrow shows a virtual absence of immature erythroid elements more than 3 months posttransplantation. In cases of either delayed engraftment or pure RBC aplasia, patients are dependent on RBC transfusions for prolonged periods of time.

Another risk factor associated with HSC infusion is the possibility for RBC hemolysis. Both ABO and non-ABO antibodies are capable of mediating RBC lysis. In such conditions, preformed antibodies in either the recipient or HSC plasma can cause accelerated clearance of incompatible RBCs by either intra- or extravascular mechanisms. Presentation of hemolytic transfusion reactions immediately after HSC infusion is no different from that of typical transfusion reaction. Policies and protocols should be in place to prevent postinfusion HSC-related hemolysis—for example, plasma depletion of HSC products (in cases of minor mismatch and bidirectional ABO incompatibility), limiting the infusion of incompatible RBCs (in cases of major mismatch and bidirectional ABO), hydration of patients, and prospective monitoring for hemolysis.

Although delayed hemolysis is rarely clinically significant in major ABO-mismatched HSC transplant, clinically significant delayed hemolysis is commonly reported in minor and bidirectional ABO-incompatible HSC transplants. As a result of donor lymphocyte engraftment, typically occurring 1–2 weeks after HSC infusion, donor ABO antibodies can cause hemolysis of residual recipient RBCs. This delayed hemolysis is typically clinically evident with decreased hemoglobin, increased indirect bilirubin, increased LDH, and decreased haptoglobin, and patients often require RBC transfusion. Sometimes the hemolysis can be acute and massive and result in multiorgan failure and death. Thus it is important to monitor patients closely for anemia and hemolysis after minor and bidirectional ABO-incompatible HSC infusion, especially in the first two weeks post-HSC infusion. Timely support and treatments such as RBC exchange with donor type blood can be provided for massive hemolysis.

Infectious Complications

As a result of an underlying bacteremia during collection, or contamination through collection, processing, storage, thawing, and sampling, some HSC products may harbor microbial organisms capable of mediating septic reactions during or immediately after HSC infusion. Such reactions may manifest with fever, tachycardia, hypotension, nausea, or vomiting. Patients experiencing such symptoms should be treated with broad-spectrum antibiotics to cover both gram-positive and gram-negative organisms. Bone marrow collections have a higher contamination rate than apheresis HSC collections, although typically with coagulase negative *Staphylococcus aureus* and *Propionibacterium acnes* that grow only with extended culture.

Fortunately, bacterial contamination of an HSC unit is often known well in advance of an actual HSC infusion because HSC products are typically cultured at the time of collection and processing. As such, clinical teams can be prepared for such reactions. In such circumstances, preventative measures include provision of pre-infusion antibiotics to cover the documented organism(s) and close patient surveillance during and after infusion. One additional option would be to avoid infusion of a contaminated unit altogether. This is possible if a patient has multiple, separate HSC products available for infusion. Clinical and transplant teams can preferentially infuse noncontaminated HSC units first, saving the contaminated unit as a "last resort" should the graft fail.

Other Infusion Complications Related to Hematopoietic Stem Cell Products

In addition to the problems related to DMSO and ABO mismatches, other adverse reactions sometimes occur with the use of HSC products. Nausea and vomiting are frequently reported with infusion of freshly collected HSC products such as fresh marrow. Fever and chills are commonly seen with cryopreserved HSC; these have been speculated to be caused by the cellular debris and cytokines contained in HSC products. Antipyretics and steroid premedication may be used for prevention. Severe adverse reactions to HSC infusion (such as cardiac arrest and neurologic symptoms, including loss of consciousness and seizure) have been linked to high granulocyte counts in HSC products.

Respiratory problems are increasingly being recognized as an important cause of morbidity and mortality in the setting of HSC infusion. Although many of these are late-onset problems (e.g., infectious complications associated with immunosuppression occurring days or weeks after transplantation), some pulmonary issues will arise acutely during HSC infusion. The National Marrow Donor Program (NMDP) issued a report in 2010 regarding seven patients who experienced hypertension, chest pain, and decreased oxygen saturation after infusion of cord blood. Even though no clear-cut cause-effect relationship was established, some recommendations were made, including minimizing thaw to infusion time, filtering HSC products with standard 150–250-μm blood filters, avoiding very high infusion rate, and others. In addition, the classic pulmonary complications encountered during HSC infusion may resemble TRALI in that they are associated with dyspnea, hypoxemia, a low-grade fever, and bilateral pulmonary infiltrates, all occurring within a short time after initiation or completion of infusion. Some authors have attributed these problems to a noncardiogenic capillary leak syndrome that appears to be independent of cardiac function, similar to the proposed pathophysiology of TRALI.

Patients demonstrating signs or symptoms of respiratory distress during HSC infusion must be treated aggressively. The first response should be to stop the HSC infusion and provide immediate respiratory support. The provision of corticosteroids or other immunosuppressive agents is not likely to be of benefit for such reactions. It may also be prudent to investigate whether the patient's symptoms are related to circulatory overload rather than arising from noncardiogenic pulmonary edema. This distinction may be assisted by measuring plasma levels of brain-natriuretic peptide (BNP). If BNP is elevated, then the patient's symptoms may be attributable, in part, to volume overload.

National Healthcare Safety Network

The National Healthcare Safety Network (NHSN) is a national program of combined governmental and private sector agencies designed to evaluate and track transfusion reactions and other adverse effects associated with infusion of blood products and derivatives. Similar programs exist in other countries, including the United Kingdom (Serious Hazards of Transfusion, SHOT), the Netherlands (Transfusion and Transplantation Related Incidents in Patients, TRIP), and Canada (Transfusion Transmitted Injuries Surveillance System, TTISS). Hemovigilance systems in other countries have established efficacy of safety interventions, for example, reduction in TRALI using male-only plasma donors, and they can identify emerging threats to transfusion safety, especially when events are uncommon and are detectable only when large numbers of outcomes are evaluated in aggregate.

The Hemovigilance Module, the first protocol release of the Biovigilance Component of NHSN, was developed through a public-private partnership between the Centers for Disease Control and Prevention (CDC) and subject-matter experts convened by AABB. The Hemovigilance Module is designed for transfusion services staff in health care facilities to monitor recipient adverse reactions and quality-control incidents related to blood transfusion.

The Hemovigilance Module provides standard criteria and definitions to participating facilities to report adverse events related to blood transfusion that will result in aggregate data suitable for trend analyses and benchmarking. Participating facilities can analyze their data independently within NHSN and will be able to compare their data with national aggregate rates through NHSN in the future.

The following transfusion reaction categories are used to identify types of adverse events related to blood transfusion:

- Allergic
- Acute hemolytic
- Delayed hemolytic
- Delayed serologic
- Febrile nonhemolytic
- Hypotensive
- Posttransfusion purpura
- Transfusion-associated circulatory overload (TACO)
- Transfusion-associated dyspnea
- Transfusion-associated graft-versus-host disease
- Transfusion-related acute lung injury (TRALI)
- Transfusion-transmitted infection

Transfusion reactions are further classified by their severity and imputability—that is, the likelihood that the reaction is attributable to infusion of the blood product being investigated. Protocols, forms, and enrollment information are available online (http://www.cdc.gov/nhsn/PDFs/Biovigilance/BV-HV-protocol-current.pdf).

SUGGESTED READINGS

Alessandrino P, Bernasconi P, Caldera D, et al: Adverse events occurring during bone marrow or peripheral blood progenitor cell infusion: analysis of 126 cases. *Bone Marrow Transplant* 23:533, 1999.

Benumof J: Minimizing venous air embolism from reinfusion bags [comment]. *Anesthesiology* 91:1999, 1962.

Gilliss B, Looney M: Experimental models of transfusion-related acute lung injury. *Transfus Med Rev* 25:1, 2011.

Hardy J, de Moerloose P, Samama C: The coagulopathy of massive transfusion. *Vox Sang* 89:123, 2005.

Heddle NM, Blajchman MA, Meyer RM, et al: A randomized controlled trial comparing the frequency of acute reactions to plasma-removed platelets and prestorage WBC-reduced platelets. *Transfusion* 42:556, 2002.

Holcomb JB, Tilley BC, Baraniuk S, et al: Transfusion of plasma, platelets, and red blood cells in a 1:1:1 vs a 1:1:2 ratio and mortality in patients with severe trauma: the PROPPR randomized clinical trial. *JAMA* 313:471, 2015.

Kelly M, Roy DC, Labbe AC, et al: What is the clinical significance of infusing hematopoietic cell grafts contaminated with bacteria? *Bone Marrow Transplant* 38:183, 2006.

Kuehnert M, Roth VR, Haley NR, et al: Transfusion-transmitted bacterial infection in the United States, 1998 through 2000. *Transfusion* 41:1493, 2001.

Popovsky MA: *Transfusion reactions*, Bethesda, MD, 2012, AABB Press.

Sachs UJ, Wasel W, Bayat B, et al: Mechanism of transfusion-related acute lung injury induced by HLA class II antibodies. *Blood* 117:669, 2011.

Sandler SG, Eder AF, Goldman M, et al: The entity of immunoglobulin A-related anaphylactic transfusion reactions is not evidence based. *Transfusion* 55:199, 2015.

Savage WJ, Hamilton RG, Tobian AR, et al: Defining risk factors and presentations of allergic transfusion reactions. *J Allerg Clin Imm* 133:1772, 2014.

Shimada E, Tadokoro K, Watanabe Y, et al: Anaphylactic transfusion reactions in haptoglobin-deficient patients with IgE and IgG haptoglobin antibodies. *Transfusion* 42:766, 2002.

Sihler K, Napolitano L: Complications of massive transfusion. *Chest* 137:209, 2010.

Stowell SR, Winkler AM, Maier CL, et al: Initiation and regulation of complement during hemolytic transfusion reactions. *Clin Dev Immunol* 2012:307093, 2012.

Tobian A, Sokoll LJ, Tisch DJ, et al: N-terminal pro-brain natriuretic peptide is a useful diagnostic marker for transfusion-associated circulatory overload. *Transfusion* 48:1143, 2008.

Toy P, Gajic O, Bacchetti P, et al: Transfusion-related acute lung injury: incidence and risk factors. *Blood* 119:2002, 1757.

U.S. Food and Drug Administration: *Vaccines, Blood & Biologics: Fatalities reported to FDA following blood collection and transfusion*: Annual summary for fiscal Year 2013. <http://www.fda.gov/BiologicsBloodVaccines/SafetyAvailability/ReportaProblem/TransfusionDonationFatalities/ucm391574.htm>.

Uchida S, Tadokoro K, Takahashi M, et al: Analysis of 66 patients definitive with transfusion-associated graft-versus-host disease and the effect of universal irradiation of blood. *Transfusion Med* 23:416, 2013.

Vlaar A, Hofstra JJ, Determann RM, et al: The incidence, risk factors, and outcome of transfusion-related acute lung injury in a cohort of cardiac surgery patients: a prospective nested case-control study. *Blood* 117:4218, 2011.

Wiersum-Osselton J, Middleburg RA, Beckers EA, et al: Male-only fresh-frozen plasma for transfusion-related acute lung injury prevention: before-and-after comparative cohort study. *Transfusion* 51:1278, 2011.

Worel N, Greinix HT, Keil F, et al: Severe immune hemolysis after minor ABO-mismatched allogeneic peripheral blood progenitor cell transplantation occurs more frequently after nonmyeloablative than myeloablative conditioning. *Transfusion* 42:1293, 2002.

Yomtovian RA, Palavecino EL, Dysktra AH, et al: Evolution of surveillance methods for detection of bacterial contamination of platelets in a university hospital, 1991 through 2004. *Transfusion* 46:719–730, 2006.

CHAPTER 120

TRANSFUSION-TRANSMITTED DISEASES

Susan L. Stramer and Roger Y. Dodd

Adverse reactions following blood transfusion reflect immunologic, pathophysiologic, and microbiologic events. This chapter presents information about transfusion-associated viral, bacterial, parasitic, and prion infections and discusses a number of emerging agents. Transfusion-transmitted infection risk mitigation through blood donor screening and blood testing strategies are presented.[1] The boxed discussions provide insights into interventions aimed at reducing risk from known and emerging threats and new technologies for reducing or eliminating microbial contamination. Red cell, platelet, and plasma transfusion represent important therapeutic modalities for appropriately selected patients. Awareness of the hazards of transfusion and the rate at which these events occur should enable physicians to better determine the benefit/risk ratios when prescribing transfusions.

HEPATITIS VIRUSES

The hepatitis viruses can be classified according to their predominant modes of transmission, parenteral and enteric, with the parenterally transmitted agents, hepatitis B virus (HBV) and hepatitis C virus (HCV) dominating concerns about transfusion transmission because many individuals unknowingly infected with these agents become asymptomatic chronic carriers and may make blood donations.

Parenterally-Transmitted Hepatitides

Hepatitis B

HBV is a deoxyribonucleic acid (DNA) virus in the family *Hepadnaviridae*. The infectious virion is occasionally referred to as the Dane particle and has surface and core components, surface antigen (HBsAg), and core antigen (HBcAg), respectively. Epitopes on the viral surface provide a basis for epidemiologic studies and consist of the HBsAg "a," d/y, and w/r determinants. However, this approach is being replaced by genotyping and DNA sequencing methods. Recombinant vaccines containing the "a" determinant confer protective immunity to a high proportion of vaccinees and are dramatically altering the incidence and prevalence of HBV infection in the general population where they are in wide use and consequently also impact the frequency of HBV infection in the donor population.

The average incubation period (the time from infection to liver enzyme elevation and symptomatic hepatitis) is 59 days (range, 5 to 12 weeks) but may be as long as 6 months. Symptoms, which occur in 30% to 50% of infected persons age 5 years and older, include fatigue, anorexia, nausea, vomiting, jaundice, dark urine, light stools, arthralgias, rashes, vasculitis, and glomerulonephritis. The risk for progression to chronic infection is inversely related to age at infection. HBV infection becomes chronic in more than 90% of infants, 25% to 50% of children 1 to 5 years of age, and fewer than 5% of older children and adults. Approximately 5% of the US population has serologic evidence of prior HBV infection (antibodies against HBcAg [anti-HBc] reactive). From the mid-1980s through 2013, with increasing immunization in early childhood, the incidence of acute HBV infection has decreased. In 2013 41 states reported HBV infections to the US Centers for Disease Control and Prevention (CDC) of which approximately 3000 were acute cases, or 1 case per 100,000

population, and an additional 12,400 were chronic hepatitis (www.cdc.gov/hepatitis/statistics, Viral Hepatitis–Statistics and Surveillance). It is estimated in the United States that approximately 12 million persons are infected, with 5000 deaths each year resulting from hepatitis B and its complications.

Based largely on data from parenteral exposures of health care workers, HBV is 100 times more infectious than human immunodeficiency virus (HIV) and 10 times more infectious than HCV. The predominant mode of transmission to adults and adolescents is through sexual contact. Forty percent have infected partners, 15% are males having sex with other males, injecting drug users account for 14% of cases, and one-third have no identifiable risk. A recent study of risk factors in blood donors found to be infected with HBV found that of 292 infected donors surveyed, the characteristics most frequently associated with infection were living abroad or having immigrated to the United States (51% vs. controls at 6%), a family member infected with hepatitis (15% vs. 2%), having been in a jail or detention for 3 nights or more (19% vs. 5%) and having taken illegal drugs (20% vs. 12%).[2]

HBsAg is detectable in blood approximately 4 weeks (30 to 60 days) after infection. Subsequently, immunoglobulin M (IgM) anti-HBc antibodies appear coincident with symptom onset. High viral titers (10^{10} genomes/mL) present at that time decline subsequently. HBsAg persists transiently in acute infections for up to 4 months (average 63 days). More recent data using extremely sensitive HBsAg assays for blood donation screening show the mean period of HBsAg duration to be 43 days.[3] Antibodies against HBsAg (anti-HBs) develop subsequently and are generally thought to protect against reinfection although recent studies on blood donors have identified a few breakthrough cases of infection. These cases were mainly caused by HBV genotypes differing from that of the vaccine strain and were mild and self-limited.[4] Such donations were not detected by HBsAg blood donation screening but required more sensitive HBV DNA screening.

Some anti-HBc–positive and HBsAg-negative individuals have circulating HBV DNA, and this pattern defines so-called occult HBV infection (OBI). In rare cases, OBI may be accompanied by anti-HBs, usually at levels below 200 mIU per mL. Donors with OBI may transmit HBV via blood transfusion, but the frequency of such infection is low, and seems to be absent if anti-HBs is present.[5] Although anti-HBs usually confers immunity to reinfection, sufficient virus remains in the liver to transmit HBV following liver transplant from anti-HBs–positive donors through reactivation under intense immunosuppression.

Blood donors in the United States are currently queried for a history of hepatitis and risks associated with hepatitis and screened for HBsAg, anti-HBc and HBV DNA. It should, however, be noted that the FDA has eliminated the requirement to ask about a history of viral hepatitis, effective May 2016.[6] The detection of HBV DNA is performed by nucleic acid testing (NAT) in minipools of 6–16 donations each as now required per Food and Drug Administration (FDA) Guidance, Use of Nucleic Acid Tests on Pooled and Individual Samples from Donors of Whole Blood and Blood Components, including Source Plasma, to Reduce the Risk of Transmission of Hepatitis B Virus (www.fda.gov/BiologicsBloodVaccines/GuidanceComplianceRegulatoryInformation/Guidances/default.htm, October 2013) and made final in updates to the Code of Federal Regulations.[6] The risk for HBV transmission per unit in the United States has

TABLE 120.1	Risk for Transfusion-Transmitted Diseases in the United States
Pathogenic Agent or Disease	**Average Estimated Risk Per Unit**
Hepatitis A	Rare
Hepatitis B	1 per 765,000–1,006,000
Hepatitis C	1 per 1,149,000
Human immunodeficiency virus	1 per 1,467,000
Human T-lymphotropic viruses 1, 2	1 per 4,364,000
Cytomegalovirus	Infrequent
Parvovirus B19	Rare
West Nile virus	Rare
Malaria	0–3 cases per year
Babesiosis	1 per 18,000 in highly endemic regions; 1 per 100,000 endemic regions overall
Chagas disease	20 transfusion-associated cases reported
Creutzfeldt-Jakob disease	4 vCJD transfusion-associated cases reported
Bacterial contamination:	
Red cells	1 per 30,000
Septic reactions	1 per 500,000–1 per 10,000,000
Platelets	1 per 3000–1 per 8000
Septic reaction	1 per 100,000
Emerging infections: Arboviruses including dengue viruses, chikungunya and Zika viruses Pandemic influenza viruses (H5N1, H1N1)	Risk unknown

vCJD, Variant Creutzfeldt-Jakob disease.

recently decreased substantially as a result of very sensitive HBsAg testing, the implementation of NAT, and a recent decline in the incidence of HBV infection among donors undoubtedly because of universal vaccination (Table 120.1).[3,4,7] Before NAT implementation, most contemporary HBV transfusion-transmitted infections were attributable to blood donations from asymptomatic donors during acute infection preceding the development of detectable HBsAg. Early in infection, HBV replicates relatively slowly with a doubling time of approximately 2.6 days. The current window period between infection and the detection of HBV DNA by NAT ranges from 30 to 38 days depending on the infectious dose, which, early in infection, is estimated to be between 1 and 10 copies per mL.[8] Since the implementation of HBV NAT in the United States, there have been no documented cases of breakthrough HBV transfusion transmissions. The per unit residual risk is estimated to be 1 per 843,000 to 1 per 1,208,000, depending on which infectious dose is used for this calculation.[7]

There is evidence that some HBsAg assays will not detect all HBsAg and HBc gene variants of HBV. Because all blood donations are screened by HBV NAT, HBsAg, and anti-HBc, it is unlikely that any mutant strain of HBV would go undetected in the United States. Among 12.8 million blood donors to the American Red Cross during 2009–11, 1 per 9337 were infected with HBV. Of these, 1090 were positive for HBsAg, with or without HBV DNA (1 per 11,736), and only 5 were identified solely by NAT in minipools (1 per 2.55 million).[7] However, more recent data, also from the American Red Cross, demonstrate the HBV DNA detection rate of

seronegative donations by NAT to be 1 per 600,000 donations. NAT on individual donation aliquots has the potential to reduce the risk for transfusion-transmitted HBV further by detecting newly infected donors slightly earlier than the HBsAg tests licensed for blood donor screening, but the additional cost of individual donation-NAT in the United States would be high with very little to no demonstrable clinical benefit.

Hepatitis D

Hepatitis D virus (HDV) was originally called the delta agent. It is a defective ribonucleic acid (RNA)–containing passenger virus that requires active synthesis of HBsAg to act as a "helper" for assembly of HDV virions. As many as 10% of HBV infections are accompanied by HDV worldwide. Its prevalence is very low in the United States but higher in injection drug users. HDV superinfection of chronic HBV carriers is associated with worsened chronic sequelae and with fulminant hepatitis. Screening for HBV acts synergistically to prevent transfusion-associated HDV cases by identifying donors that are co-infected with HBV and HDV. There has never been a HBV-HDV–related transfusion transmission reported.

Hepatitis C

HCV is an RNA virus in the family *Flaviviridae*, genus *Hepacivirus*. There are six genotypes that share similar epidemiology, pathogenesis, and natural histories. In the United States, genotypes 1, 2, and 3 cause 75%, 10%, and 10% of infections, respectively. Genotype 1 responds relatively poorly to traditional treatment regimens using pegylated interferon combined with oral doses of ribavirin compared with genotypes 2 and 3; the overall cure rate for all genotypes using this regimen was no better than 40% to 50%. Recently approved HCV protease inhibitors are materially improving these rates. Two new oral regimens of Harvoni and Viekira Pac are now the standard of care in the United States, and result in a sustained virologic response of greater than 90% (www.cdc.gov/hepatitis/statistics, Viral Hepatitis–Statistics and Surveillance).

HCV is distinguished by a low rate of recognized acute infection and by a high rate of chronic infection, with substantial morbidity and mortality over long periods of observation as a result. In the United States there are an estimated 3.2 million chronic infections.

The most common source of HCV acquisition is injection drug use. The prevalence of HCV in US adults (20 to 59 years old) with any history of illegal injection drug use is greater than 45%. Other risks include blood transfusion before donor serologic screening began in 1990, a high lifetime number of sex partners, exposure in health care settings, including through dialysis, among infants born to HCV-infected mothers, and tattoos in unregulated settings. In a large series, 15% to 30% of patients report no risk factors. Vertical transmission occurs to 3% to 7% of infants of mothers with active infections. In contrast to HBV, sexual transmission is an inefficient route of infection and much less often reported, but was found to be the most likely mode of transmission of HCV among HIV-infected men who have sex with men (MSM) in New York City. In 2012 CDC recommended that individuals born during 1945–1965 have one-time HCV screening since among all persons living with HCV infection, about 75% were born during this time. Such individuals have a 3% prevalence, which is five times higher than the prevalence seen in adults born in other years. Among blood donors, 0.03% have confirmed-positive HCV test results. There have been studies on risk factors among HCV-infected blood donors, and despite policies requiring deferral of injection drug users, such use is the most common risk factor.[2,9] Of 316 blood donors followed who were HCV-confirmed positive, risks identified via a retrospective questionnaire revealed risks versus control donors of illegal drug use (37% vs. <1% for controls), followed by jail or detention (57% vs. 5%), history of a blood transfusion before screening (18% vs. 7%), and living in a household with someone having hepatitis (15% vs. 2%).

At most 20% to 30% of newly infected persons develop recognizable symptoms during acute HCV infection. Some 20% of infected individuals clear their infection over a relatively short initial period, remaining antibody positive but RNA negative. Chronic infection develops in 75% to 85% of persons infected after 45 years of age and in 50% to 60% of those infected as children or young adults. Chronic HCV infection progresses to cirrhosis in 15% to 30% over 30 years of observation. Hepatocellular carcinoma occurs in 1% to 4% per year in those with cirrhosis. HCV is among the most prevalent causes of chronic hepatitis, cirrhosis, and primary liver cancer in the developed world and is the most common indication for liver transplantation in the United States, resulting in around 2400 procedures annually.

A single positive anti-HCV result cannot distinguish between acute and chronic HCV infection or between current or cleared infection. In 2012 laboratory criteria for the confirmation of anti-HCV reactivity were modified to add one specific assay including RNA detection, using a supplemental anti-HCV assay (as available) or a single value above a specific threshold on the screening test.[10] The risk for posttransfusion HCV infection declined progressively with the introduction of surrogate markers for non-A, non-B hepatitis in the 1980s (alanine aminotransferase [ALT] and anti-HBc) and of serologic testing for HCV antibodies in May 1990, followed sequentially by improved serologic testing and NAT. The seronegative-window period for the first-generation HCV antibody test extended to 6 months from infection, but was reduced to 82 and 70 days with second- and third-generation assays, respectively. NAT further reduced the window period to approximately 7 days. The risk per unit declined from an estimated 1 per 276,000 units to 1 per 1,935,000 units.[11]

Like HBV, in the United States, testing for HCV RNA has used NAT in small minipools combining aliquots from 16 to 24 donations (currently 6 to 16). Loss of test sensitivity because of sample pooling was tolerable given the rapid increase or burst of HCV viremia before antibody seroconversion (estimated doubling time of 10.8 hours in that period during the 40–50-day window period) and the high titer of viremia that remains preceding antibody seroconversion. However, the rest of the world (except the United States, Canada, the United Kingdom and most of Germany) has implemented NAT for screening individual donation samples intended for transfusion. The HCV RNA yield by NAT in seronegative donations using data from the American Red Cross is 1 per 225,000 donations.

As an alternative to NAT assays, enzyme immunoassays (EIAs) have been developed that detect HCV HBcAg in serum or plasma, either as an individual analyte in parallel with antibody assays or as HCV antigen-antibody combination assays. These tests reduce the preseroconversion-window period and were adopted in some developing countries. They are less sensitive than HCV NAT and are not approved for blood donor screening in the United States.[12] Since the implementation of NAT, reports of transfusion-transmitted HCV are virtually nonexistent.

The high seroprevalence of HCV at the onset of serology screening in the early 1990s, the prolonged interval between infection and clinical manifestations, and the relatively high rate of HCV clinical sequelae prompted blood collection facilities and hospitals to conduct "look-back" notification of previous recipients of blood given by donors found on subsequent donations to be HCV infected. Look-back was subsequently made mandatory in companion rules from FDA and the Centers for Medicare and Medicaid Services. In general, HCV look-back programs found half or fewer of targeted transfused individuals alive, but were able to find both seropositive and RNA-positive recipients who were unaware of their status.

Enterically Transmitted Hepatitides

Hepatitis A

The hepatitis A virus (HAV), a nonenveloped picornavirus, genus *Hepatovirus*, is transmitted predominantly by the fecal-oral route,

with an average incubation period of 28 days (range, 15 to 50 days) with signs or symptoms persisting for less than 2 months. The incidence of HAV infection in the United States fell by 76% between 1997 and 2003 after the recommendation for targeted immunization of members in high-risk communities. Populations at risk include those in areas where extended community outbreaks occur and children living in states that have high and intermediate rates of disease, staff and residents of closed communities, close personal contacts of cases, the staff and parents of children in day-care centers, and those with common-source exposure to infected food or water. For many sporadic cases there is no recognized source. HAV is self-limited with no chronic carrier state, but approximately 10% to 15% of infected individuals develop a more prolonged or relapsing illness. It is the most frequent cause of hepatitis among children under 11 years of age.

Transfusion-related transmission, although rare, is caused by a blood donation from a recently infected, asymptomatic, viremic individual. The peak viremia occurs 2 weeks before onset of jaundice or elevation of hepatocellular enzymes and persists for a median period of 42 days (range, up to 59 days). The virus is quite resistant to many inactivation procedures, including the pathogen-reduction procedures being developed for cellular blood components (e.g., licensed psoralens or investigational riboflavin, both with ultraviolet [UV] irradiation) and fresh-frozen plasma (solvent/detergent and methylene blue). Transmission by clotting-factor concentrates treated with the solvent/detergent pathogen-reduction process occurred in the 1990s, but not thereafter. Plasma for further manufacture is routinely screened for HAV RNA by pooled NAT.

An indefinite deferral for a clinical history of viral hepatitis after age 11 years has been required in the United States (regardless of the specific viral agent). Because most viral hepatitis in the United States before 11 years is HAV, with its relatively brief and self-limited viremia, individuals with a history of hepatitis before the age of 11 are allowed to donate on the assumption they had HAV. As pointed out previously, the FDA has now issued new rules for donor suitability that do not require questioning for a history of viral hepatitis.[6] A 120-day deferral is recommended after exposure to HAV during community outbreaks to prevent transfusion transmission. Screening for HAV is not done for donation of blood for transfusion.

Hepatitis E

The hepatitis E virus (HEV) is a small, nonenveloped single-stranded RNA virus in the *Hepeviridae* family. HEV was first recognized in the 1980s in Afghanistan among soldiers with unexplained hepatitis. There is a single serotype but at least four genotypes with differing geographic distributions and epidemiologic patterns. Genotypes 1 and 2 are generally associated with large, water-borne (fecal-orally transmitted) outbreaks in less developed tropical countries. Illness is usually self-limited but can be lethal in pregnant women, their fetuses, and patients with chronic liver disease. Genotypes 3 and 4 appear to be animal viruses that result in zoonotic infection of humans, most often through consumption of inadequately cooked pork products. Genotype 3 seems to be widely distributed and is present in developed countries, whereas genotype 4 seems to be more comment in certain Asian countries. Transfusion-related transmission, mostly of serotype 3, has been well-documented in Japan, France, England, the Netherlands, and Spain.[13]

Recent studies suggest a wide range of seroprevalence rates, but some of the variability may be attributable to the differences in performance characteristics of the tests used and some to dietary habits. Most studies indicate a cohort effect, with prevalence rates increasing with age. Transfusion infectivity is logically associated with the presence of detectable viral RNA in the plasma and the frequency of this finding varies between 1 in 1000 to 1 in 10,000 donations.

In a large study in England,[14] 225,000 donations were tested and 79, or 1 in 2848, were found to be positive when tested for HEV RNA. For 43 of these, recipient tracing was possible and 18 (42%) showed evidence of transfusion-transmitted infection. In contrast, in a smaller, blinded study in the United States, 7.7% of donors were anti-HEV positive and only two of approximately 19,000 were RNA positive: recipient follow-up was not possible.[15] A current broader concern is the finding that highly immunosuppressed patients (such as solid-organ transplant recipients) do develop chronic HEV infections with long-term clinical sequelae, although these have not been specifically linked to infection via transfusion.

Non–A-E Hepatitis

Cases of posttransfusion hepatitis only rarely if ever occur but there remains speculation that undiscovered hepatitis agents exist. A small but consistent percentage of community-acquired hepatitis cases test negative for known hepatitis viruses, some cirrhosis is classified as "cryptogenic," an etiologic agent for hepatitis-associated aplastic anemia eludes description, and the cause of some cases of acute liver failure remains elusive. Several candidate agents have been proposed as non–A-E hepatitis viruses. None of these agents have been shown to be pathogenic and are instead likely commensal and nonpathogenic.

GBV-C (initially called hepatitis G virus) is a flavivirus with no confirmed disease association that is transmitted parenterally, including frequently from transfusion. Of interest, GBV-C infection may delay progression of disease in those co-infected with HIV, which has led to studies of the interactions of these viruses.[16]

From 1% to 4% of US blood donors are viremic compared with 15% to 20% of injection drug users who have detectable GBV-C RNA. Infection occurs frequently among those infected with HCV and HIV. More people have antibodies against the E2 envelope protein, in the absence of RNA, suggesting viral clearance. GBV-C has not been shown to cause liver disease or other morbidity, and hence there is no consideration of donor screening at this time. GBV-C is now referred to as a human pegivirus. A second human pegivirus has recently been described associated with HCV likely as a result of an acute parenteral co-infection event, but again, has not been associated with hepatitis or any pathology. This virus was identified by next generation sequencing.[17] Likely other such commensal agents will continue to be identified by use of sophisticated molecular techniques.

The torque teno virus (TTV) complex is a genetically diverse group of nonenveloped DNA viruses in the family *Circoviridae*, which was discovered in 1997. They cause viremia, and they are transmitted by transfusion, but they cause no recognized liver disease or other clinical illness.

SEN virus (SENV), another member of the *Circoviridae*, was described using degenerate polymerase chain reaction (PCR) primers while working with TTV. After an initial report associating SENV variants in two patients with transfusion-associated non–A-E hepatitis, subsequent epidemiologic studies have failed to link SENV with clinical hepatitis.

RETROVIRAL INFECTION

Human Immunodeficiency Virus

The HIVs type 1 and type 2 (HIV-1 and HIV-2) are retroviruses of the family *Retroviridae*, genus *Lentivirus*, and the etiologic agents of the acquired immunodeficiency syndrome (AIDS). They are enveloped viruses with two linear, positive-sense RNA molecules, 9.2 kb in length. The predominant transmission mechanisms are sexual, perinatal, and parenteral. An acute retroviral syndrome may be seen around 21 days after infection, although this period may range from 5 to 70 days and may involve fever, lymphadenopathy, and rash. If untreated, the incubation period for full-blown AIDS is measured in years. Molecular characterization divides HIV-1 into three groups: group M (main), group O (outliers), and group N (non-M/O). Group M subtype B infections predominate in the United States; only 3% of HIV-positive blood donors have non-B strains. Very rare

group O infections have been detected in the United States among patients who were born, lived, or had sexual contact in endemic regions of West and Central Africa. HIV-2 infected persons in the United States are rare (less than 1% of HIV cases diagnosed annually) and have, for the most part, been infected after heterosexual transmission from West African emigrants or residents. HIV-2 disease requires a longer time to evolve and is less severe than that from HIV-1 There have been five confirmed cases of HIV-2 infection among blood donors in the United States.

In 2010 CDC estimated a total of 1.2 million people in the United States 13 years or older are living with HIV infection, or 1 per 300 Americans, with over 10% of those unaware of their infection. The highest number of new infections occurs in those 25 to 34 years old with about 50,000 new infections per year and about half of those in African-American males, most of whom are MSM. MSM continue to bear the greatest burden of HIV infection among all race and ethnic groups. Although MSM represent 4% of the US population, in 2010 MSM accounted for nearly 80% of all new HIV infections in males and over 60% of all new HIV infections. Antiretroviral therapy for HIV treatment has improved dramatically since the advent of combination therapy in 1996, even against multidrug resistant viruses. HIV-associated morbidity and mortality have significantly been reduced so that HIV treatment has converted HIV infection to a chronic, versus a fatal disease.

Antibody testing of blood donors detects both HIV-1 and its variants and HIV-2.[18] Antibody testing for HIV-1 began in 1985, with the addition of HIV-2 in 1992 (although HIV-1 tests before that time detected most HIV-2 infections arising from over 60% sequence homology between the two viruses) and for HIV-1 group O in 2006.

Both serologic testing and NAT are performed on every blood donation. First-generation antibody tests had a window period (time between infection and detection) of 45 days on average, but has decreased significantly as tests became more sensitive leading to less than a 20-day window period. HIV-1 NAT, implemented in 1999 (in duplex tests with HCV performed in pools of 6–16 donations) detects RNA at a minimum concentration of approximately 5 copies per milliliter (50% lower limit of detection) leaving about a 9-day window period of risk in which an infected donor could donate and not be detected by any test in current use. Rare genetic variants of HIV may escape NAT detection when nucleotide sequence changes affect NAT primer or probe binding sites, but the vast majority of these infections will be detected serologically. Further, tests are now designed to detect two or more separate sequences representing different viral regions. Currently, the frequency of confirmed-positive test results for antibodies to HIV is 0.26 per 10,000 donations. Almost all of these are also RNA-positive as the finding of an infected donor with low-level RNA levels is very rare (on the order of 2%). One donation per 900,000 is confirmed positive for RNA in the absence of antibody (NAT yield).[11]

To interdict donations in the window period between exposure and test positivity, each blood donor is asked at each donation about exposure risks using questions developed in the early to mid-1980s, subsequent to the first reports of AIDS in hemophiliacs and transfusion recipients. These initial interventions targeted blood donations from homosexually active men and injection drug users, substantially reducing the transmission risk between 1983 and 1985. Five clusters of transfusion transmissions have been documented subsequent to the introduction of NAT, three before 2002 and one in 2008.[8,19] It is of interest to note that in two cases, although the transfused plasma component transmitted HIV, the corresponding red cell component did not. Modeling suggests a residual risk for HIV transmission persists at approximately one transmission per 1.5 million donations, because NAT cannot detect HIV infection during the immunosilent 9-day eclipse phase between infection and test reactivity. Processing and quarantine procedural errors do not now appear to be a risk for transmission of HIV via transfusion. Fourth-generation tests combine HIV-1/2 antibody and HIV antigen detection and detect almost 90% of infections detected by NAT. Their role is expanding worldwide even in countries that use HIV-1 NAT. In 2014 the CDC published revised guidelines for laboratory diagnosis of HIV infection (http://dx.doi.org/10.15620/cdc.23447).[20]

Recent studies have shown that the predominant risk factors for HIV infection among 149 male infected blood donors surveyed retrospectively continues to be a history of MSM behavior (62% in cases vs. 2% in controls) or of a male having sex with an HIV-positive individual (26% in cases and none in controls). Of note, 50% of MSM activity occurred within the last 12 months. Although in the past, injection drug use was also a prominent risk factor, this has decreased in prominence (24% in cases vs. 5% in controls).[2]

In 2015 the US FDA formally reconsidered the original policy of permanent lifetime deferral of MSM even once since 1977 and have now issued Guidance permitting donation by those who have not engaged in MSM in the prior year, thus reducing the deferral period to 1 year, in common with a number of other countries, including Australia[21] and the United Kingdom (www.fda.gov/BiologicsBloodVaccines/GuidanceComplianceRegulatoryInformation/Guidances/default.htm, Revised Recommendations for Reducing the Risk of Human Immunodeficiency Virus Transmission by Blood and Blood Products, Dec 2015).

Most consider the blood supply in the developed world to be at its highest historical safety level. This reflects incremental improvements in donor selection and history screening, blood testing, and process control that span four decades. For years, blood collection professionals and government regulators formulated blood safety policy decisions in an apparent aim to achieve zero-risk blood supply. In part, this reflects the perceived delayed response of the transfusion medicine community in the early 1980s to the emergence of human immunodeficiency virus (HIV) in the blood supply and the recognition of the scope and severity of post-transfusion non-A, non-B hepatitis (subsequently hepatitis C [HCV]) following that. It reflects also the "dread fear" associated with transfusion-associated HIV. This reaction is seen when devastating, unpredictable, and stigmatizing events threaten potential victims who have little ability to escape the risk. This fear was validated by numerous transfusion-related HIV cases. It was amplified by widely publicized lawsuits, indictments, and criminal convictions of health ministers and policy makers in the 1980s and 1990s (*l'affaire du sang contaminé* in France addressing HIV and Canada's Royal Commission of Inquiry on the Blood System into blood collection agencies' response to non-A, non-B hepatitis risk) (Fig. 120.1). (See box on Blood Safety Decision Making.)

Human T-Lymphotropic Virus-1 and Virus-2

Human T-lymphotropic virus-1 (HTLV-1) and HTLV-2 are closely related deltaretroviruses with 60% to 70% sequence homology and shared tropism for T-lymphocytes. In contrast to HIV, HTLV is rarely present in cell-free plasma and shows little active replication in infected humans. HTLV-1 is distributed worldwide, with endemic foci in southern Japan, the Caribbean, certain parts of South America, Africa, the Middle East, and Melanesia. HTLV-2 is endemic among Amerindians in both North and South America and African Pygmies. An epidemic of HTLV-2 infections has occurred over the past 40 to

---

Blood Safety Decision Making

Not surprisingly, from the 1980s until now, donor deferrals and blood-testing interventions have been rapidly, successively, and additively implemented for emerging and theoretical risks. Collection facilities introduced antibody testing to the HBcAg of HBV (anti-HBc) and ALT testing as surrogates for non-A, non-B hepatitis, HIV-1 p24 antigen testing, then NAT for hepatitis C and HIV and subsequently HBV, extensive deferrals for the risks attending transmissible spongiform encephalopathies (TSEs,) NAT for West Nile virus (WNV), and antibody testing for *Trypanosoma cruzi*. The cost-benefit estimates for some of these interventions exceeded by orders of magnitude generally accepted thresholds but did not deter their adoption. In general, the implementation of these measures was undertaken by the blood providers, but at the time of writing, it is unlikely that this reactive approach can be sustained in the current health care–reform environment and in the face of declining funding for blood providers, at least in the United States.

Application, after HIV entered the blood supply, of a stringent form of the precautionary principle (originally promulgated for environmental protection, not transfusion safety) pushed decision making toward avoidance of all risks. The precautionary principle promotes implementation of measures to mitigate risk even if evidence of a risk is incomplete. It is supposed to be tempered by proportionality; that is, any measures adopted are to be proportional to the risk and with those used in similar circumstances, but some have argued that this has not been the case with blood safety measures, at least by the metric of cost-benefit. Nevertheless, although in potential conflict with evidence-based decision making, this approach resonated with policy advocates charged with transfusion safety. In contrast, when the risk for transfusion transmission of variant Creutzfeldt Jakob (vCJD) disease (the human form of bovine spongiform encephalopathy, BSE) emerged as theoretical, modeling was used to balance the perceived risk against the impact of extensive donor deferrals on the adequacy of the blood supply and to arrive at a policy decision. Some argue that the magnitude of risk does not justify the stringency of the donor deferral policy given the small risk in a country that was not BSE endemic or lacked any BSE-contaminated materials in their food supply, but the process was the first to attempt to balance risk with adequacy. Subsequently, vCJD was shown to be transfusion transmissible.[22]

Hemovigilance programs, such as the Serious Hazards of Transfusion (SHOT) in the United Kingdom and others in Canada, France, and a smaller program in the United States, have emerged, supplying evidence about a much broader range of transfusion hazards than just infections. For example, a data-driven decision to minimize plasma transfusions from potentially alloimmunized female donors resulted in a dramatic reduction in transfusion-related acute lung injury (TRALI) in the United Kingdom, and studies in the United States have reproduced this finding.

These systems provide an opportunity for monitoring the risks and benefits of new initiatives, (e.g., proactive pathogen reduction). Pathogen-reduction processes (see box on Pathogen Reduction) offer the opportunity to abrogate most of the residual risk for all of the historically important transfusion-transmitted viral infections, bacterial contamination of platelets, babesiosis and malaria contaminated red cells, WNV infections, and Chagas disease. Pathogen reduction could eliminate the often lengthy, reactive, iterative paradigm of emergence of a new pathogen in the population, recognition of a material threat to transfusion recipients, development of donor-deferral strategies followed by development and refinement of test systems that has characterized our historical approach. Critically, broadly active pathogen-reduction processes offer a layer of protection against unsuspected emergence of new agents.[23] If already in use, they would need only to be validated as active against a new agent or appropriate model agents. The challenge with this approach is broad-based availability (all components) and wide-scale acceptance, the impact on product quality, and the potential long-term toxicities that may not be apparent in premarketing clinical trials or implementation to date.[24-26]

More recently, as cost pressures for health care increase, transfusion professionals are questioning whether the zero-risk paradigm remains relevant. A consensus conference held in Toronto in October 2010 addressed concerns about "safety at any cost" and inconsistent decision-making practices affecting the blood supply. This initiative has led to a definitive effort to establish a framework for risk-based decision-making under the direction of the Alliance of Blood Operators (www.allianceofbloodoperators.org/abo-resources/risk-based-decision-making/rbdm-framework.aspx). The process involves risk identification, risk assessment, risk management, and risk communication, along with an assessment of risk tolerance, in the context of full and open communication with stakeholders.[27] Risk will never be zero, and there is now a realization that cost considerations,[28] politics, ideology, and public opinion cannot be ignored.

Pathogen Reduction

Pathogen-reduction technology (PRT) offers a proactive strategy to address new threats; these technologies involve physical, chemical, and photochemical treatments of blood components to inactivate or decrease viral, bacterial, and parasite infectivity.[23,25]

Beginning in the 1980s, heat treatment, nanofiltration, and solvent/detergent treatment eliminated or reduced viral transmission in products derived from large-scale plasma fractionation such as albumin, immunoglobulin, and hemostatic factor concentrates.

In the past two decades, attention turned to whole blood–derived components: frozen plasma, platelets, and red cells. For these, PRT utilizes solvent-detergent, ultraviolet (UV) and methylene blue and visible light treatment for plasma; amotosalen (psoralen) and UVA light, and riboflavin (vitamin B₂) and UVB and UVA light for plasma and platelets; and riboflavin/UV light and S303 (a labile alkylating compound) for whole blood or red cells. Many European countries use PRT for platelets and plasma. Amotosalen/UVA-treated plasma and platelets (Intercept, Cerus Corporation) and solvent-detergent plasma (OctaPlas, OctaPharma) are FDA-approved and available in the United States. Because solvent-detergent does not inactivate nonenveloped viruses, OctaPharma screens all incoming units in pools to prevent the introduction of HAV, HEV and B19. Breakthough HEV infections have been described with Intercept-treated plasma in France.

Amotosalen/UVA (Intercept, Cerus) and riboflavin/UV (TerumoBCT) have advanced furthest in investigation in North America. They provide significant antiviral activity against all agents for which tests are performed currently, human immunodeficiency virus (HIV), hepatitis B and C viruses (HBV and HCV), human T-lymphotropic virus (HTLV), West Nile virus (WNV), the parasite, *Trypanosoma cruzi,* and cytomegalovirus, but the two methods appear to differ in their inactivation capacity. PRT also inactivates agents causing bacterial contamination of platelets; inactivates white blood cells to prevent transfusion-associated graft-versus-host disease; decreases formation and release of cytokines during storage, reducing febrile, nonhemolytic transfusion reactions; and abrogates white blood cell–induced alloantibody (e.g., human leukocyte antigen [HLA] antibody) formation mitigating alloimmune platelet refractoriness. Intercept-treated plasma (as mentioned) and platelets are FDA approved and available in the United States; clinical studies on pathogen-inactivated red cells (Cerus) and whole blood (TerumoBCT) are ongoing.

Methylene blue and visible light inactivate pathogens in plasma by targeting nucleic acids. However, this alters fibrinogen structure. Because it damages cell membranes, methylene blue is not used for platelets or red cells. It is not effective against hepatitis A or parvovirus and is not recommend for use in the treatment of thrombotic thrombocytopenic purpura.

Amotosalen/UVA targets nucleic acids. Platelets treated with these technologies have somewhat lower 1-hour post-transfusion corrected-count counts.[26] In clinical trials, mild and moderate bleeding frequency is increased, but not severe bleeding complications; the time between transfusions and the total number of platelet transfusions have not generally been different. Pulmonary toxicity similar to transfusion-related acute lung injury (TRALI) has been reported in clinical trials and in animal model experiments in which UV light has been implicated. Previous clinical trials in red blood cells (RBCs) were halted because of asymptomatic immunoreactivity against the red cell neoantigens believed to be the result of treatment, and are being resumed with a reformulated process. Preliminary reports suggest riboflavin/UV causes functional impairment in red cells stored nearest the 42-day expiration Although, there have been discussions about the potential for adverse reactions to treated products, extensive reviews of European data do not support the additional concern. Nevertheless, initial implementation of the Intercept platelet technology will be accompanied by Phase 4 studies in the United States.

Interest in PRT remains high because it reduces sepsis-related platelet transfusion complications and will eliminate the need for complex testing procedures to reduce bacterial risk related to contaminated platelets; inactivates parasites such as *Babesia microti,* and *Plasmodium falciparum;* mitigates risks associated with recognized emerging pathogens such as dengue, chikungunya, and Zika viruses; and proactively decreases threats from unknown, emerging pathogens. It should be noted that inactivation capabilities differ greatly between the various technologies, and each must be evaluated for its intended use.

50 years among intravenous drug users in the United States, Brazil, and Europe. Transmission of both HTLV-1 and HTLV-2 occurs by parenteral exposures, sexual contact, and by vertical transmission from mother to child during pregnancy and breastfeeding.

Diseases associated with HTLV-1 infection include adult T-cell leukemia/lymphoma (ATL), HTLV-associated myelopathy/tropical spastic paraparesis (HAM/TSP), lymphocytic pneumonitis, uveitis, polymyositis, and arthritis. HTLV-2 does not appear to cause hematologic malignancy but has been associated with HAM/TSP and linked to a higher rate of common infections such as acute bronchitis, pneumonia, and urinary tract infections, suggesting a subtle immunomodulatory effect of the virus.[29]

ATL occurs in only 1% to 5% of infected persons following a latent period of decades. The illness is characterized by malignant lymphocytosis and leukemia, lymphadenopathy, hepatomegaly, abnormal liver function test results, splenomegaly, skin lesions, bone lesions, and hypercalcemia. HAM/TSP occurs in approximately 2% of individuals infected with HTLV-1 and HTLV-2. Patients with transfusion-associated HAM/TSP develop neurologic symptoms rather more rapidly, at a median of 3.3 years after transfusion. This illness is characterized by slowly progressive chronic spastic paraparesis, lower limb weakness, urinary incontinence, impotence, sensory disturbances, low back pain, hyperreflexia, and impaired vibration sense.

Blood donor screening for HTLV-1 antibodies began in 1988, and more sensitive combination HTLV-1/2 assays that detect close to 100% of HTLV-2 infections were introduced in 1998. The prevalence of HTLV confirmed-positive donors decreased approximately 10-fold during the 1990s to the current value of 0.004%. The rate is threefold higher in female compared with male donors. Incident infections are rare in repeat donors, an observation that has led to one-time testing of donors in some European countries, but an incidence of 3 per million donor years of follow up is felt by some to be too high for adoption of this strategy in the United States. Cell-free components such as plasma and cryoprecipitate do not transmit HTLV, and less than 30% of infected cellular components transmit. The residual risk for transfusion-associated HTLV infection using contemporary serologic testing is approximately 1 per 2.4 million donations, but since the initiation of testing using these contemporary tests, there has not been a breakthrough HTLV infection by transfusion. The contribution of blood-donor serologic testing to this low residual risk is confounded by the effect of effective leukoreduction that reduces HTLV-1 copy numbers in red blood cell (RBC) concentrates by up to 6 logs, to below the infectious dose of 10^7 to 10^8 infected cells per unit (one of a number of arguments used in support of universal leukoreduction of blood components).

The deferral, notification, and counseling of healthy blood donors after a repeatedly reactive screening test for HTLVs has been problematic, and tens of thousands have been affected since screening started. The vast majority of such tests are false positive, a licensed confirmatory test is now available and will greatly improve this situation.

HUMAN HERPESVIRUS INFECTIONS

Human herpesviruses (HHVs) are enveloped, structurally complex double-stranded DNA viruses that cause common infectious diseases. Primary infection is followed by lifelong carrier states and the possibility of reactivation. They are classified in three subfamilies, *Alphaherpesvirinae, Betaherpesvirinae,* and *Gammaherpesvirinae,* of which the latter two contain the herpesviruses that are of greatest concern from a transfusion medicine standpoint. Members of the *Alphaherpesvirinae* subfamily, herpes simplex viruses (HSVs) and varicella-zoster virus (VZV), are rarely, if ever, associated with transfusion-transmitted infections. Transfusion-transmitted cytomegalovirus (CMV) is well recognized. Transmissions of Epstein-Barr virus (EBV) and HHVs 6–8 by blood are virtually nonexistent in the United States because of the use of primarily leukocyte-depleted (leukoreduced) blood products.

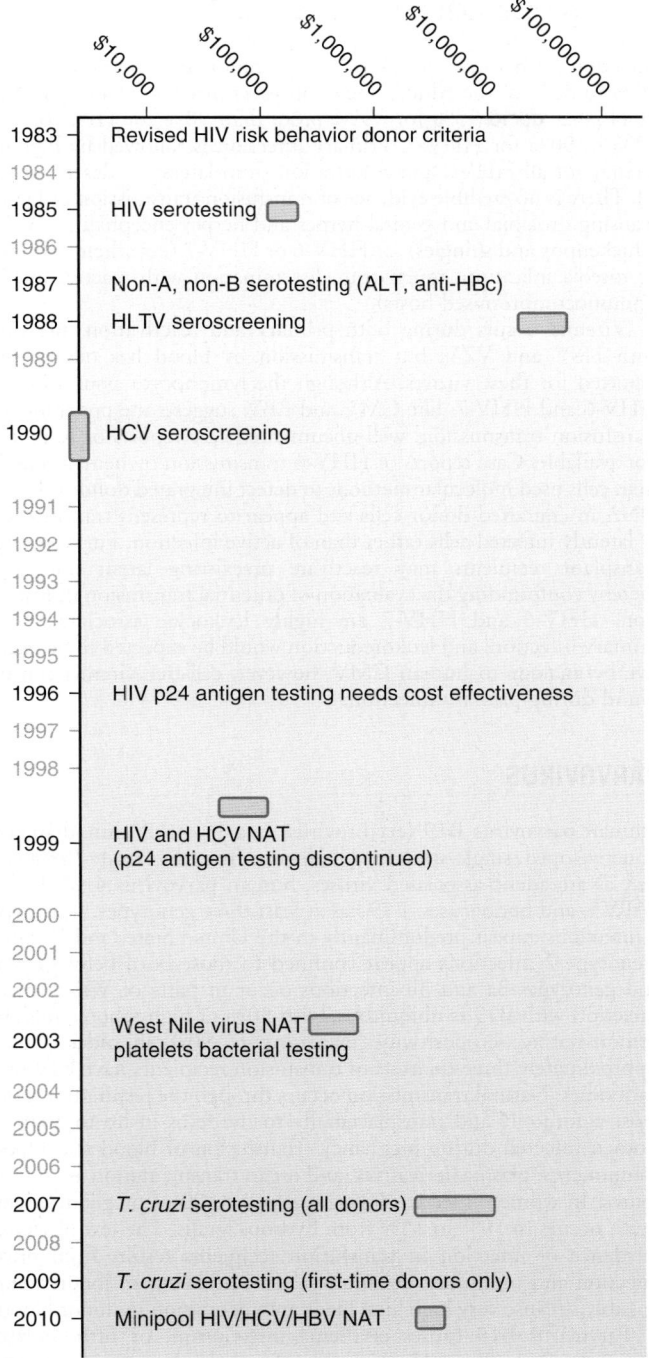

DOLLARS PER QUALITY-ADJUSTED LIFE-YEAR (QALY)

$10,000 $100,000 $1,000,000 $10,000,000 $100,000,000

1983 — Revised HIV risk behavior donor criteria
1984
1985 — HIV serotesting
1986
1987 — Non-A, non-B serotesting (ALT, anti-HBc)
1988 — HLTV seroscreening
1989
1990 — HCV seroscreening
1991
1992
1993
1994
1995
1996 — HIV p24 antigen testing needs cost effectiveness
1997
1998
1999 — HIV and HCV NAT (p24 antigen testing discontinued)
2000
2001
2002
2003 — West Nile virus NAT platelets bacterial testing
2004
2005
2006
2007 — T. cruzi serotesting (all donors)
2008
2009 — T. cruzi serotesting (first-time donors only)
2010 — Minipool HIV/HCV/HBV NAT

Fig. 120.1 VARIOUS SAFETY MEASURES INTRODUCED DURING THE PAST THREE DECADES OF ENHANCED TRANSFUSION SAFETY. The x-axis displays costs associated with these advances per quality-adjusted life-year. Hepatitis C virus seroscreening saves costs. Estimates for platelet bacterial culturing and human immunodeficiency virus p24 antigen testing are not available. *ALT,* Alanine aminotransferase; *anti-HBc,* antibodies against HBcAg; *HBV,* hepatitis B virus; *HCV,* hepatitis C virus; *HIV,* human immunodeficiency virus; *HLTV,* human T-lymphotropic virus; *NAT,* nucleic acid testing; *QALY,* quality-adjusted life-year; *T. cruzi, Trypanosoma cruzi.*

TABLE 120.2	Patients Benefiting From Cytomegalovirus Risk–Reduced Blood Components[a]

Infants <1200 g with CMV-seronegative mothers
Seronegative autologous and allogeneic (CMV-seronegative donors) stem cell transplant recipients
Seronegative stem cell transplant candidates
Seronegative recipients of seronegative solid organ transplants
Seronegative pregnant women
Fetuses receiving intrauterine transfusions
Immunosuppressed patients receiving granulocyte transfusions
HIV-seropositive/CMV-seronegative patients

[a]CMV risk–reduced components include CMV-seronegative and leukocyte-reduced components.
CMV, Cytomegalovirus; HIV, human immunodeficiency virus.

Cytomegalovirus

CMV, a betaherpesvirus, infects a wide range of cell types, including leukocytes of the monocyte-macrophage lineage and their progenitors. In the United States, in the population-based National Health and Nutrition Examination Survey (NHANES) III study, 58.9% of individuals more than 5 years old were seropositive, indicating prior CMV infection. Prevalence increases with age and is dependent on race/ethnicity and other demographic factors. The prevention of transfusion-transmitted CMV infection has depended on the use of "CMV safe" blood including a combination of leukoreduced and CMV-seronegative blood. There is, however, some evidence that acute infection may result in plasma viremia and thus the potential for transfusion infectivity.

Primary CMV infection in immunocompetent individuals is usually community acquired, often asymptomatic or associated with a mild, self-limited infectious mononucleosis syndrome. After virtually all infections, latent virus persists permanently in cellular reservoirs, allowing lifelong reactivation, and in the setting of transfusion or transplantation, the potential for viral transmission via nonleukoreduced cellular blood products, and allografts.

In immunosuppressed patients, CMV infection can cause severe morbidity and mortality from pneumonitis, hepatitis, gastroenteritis, retinitis, and other inflammatory conditions. CMV infection in low-birth-weight infants is associated with sepsis-like syndromes, respiratory distress, and liver and bone marrow dysfunction. Their infections can be acquired in utero, from breast milk, or from transfusion. Reported infant morbidity varies considerably but can approach 50% of seronegative low-birth-weight infants receiving unscreened, non-leukoreduced blood. CMV-seronegative marrow transplant patients are also susceptible to CMV infection; but the adoption of routine monitoring for CMV antigen or nucleic acid in transplant recipients and of preemptive antiviral therapy have decreased this risk. Seronegative solid organ transplant recipients are also susceptible to symptomatic transfusion-transmitted CMV infections. CMV-seronegative, HIV-infected patients are another group at risk for transfusion-transmitted primary CMV infection. The historical risk for CMV infection in immunosuppressed recipients receiving CMV-unscreened, nonleukoreduced blood components varies from 13.5% to 53.3%. The residual risk for CMV infection in seronegative, immunocompetent patients who receive nonleukoreduced cellular blood components unscreened for presence of CMV antibodies is approximately 1%. CMV transmission strictly attributable to blood is rare to nonexistent with the combination of leukoreduction and CMV antibody screening. CMV antibody screening will be replaced by pathogen reduction methods in the future.

Current practice in the United States is diverse. In a meta-analysis of 11 controlled trials in allogeneic marrow transplantation, 12 of 829 recipients of seronegative units versus 24 of 878 receiving leukoreduced but unscreened units developed CMV infections.[30] Pooling of data from three studies of seronegative or leukoreduced components, in comparison with CMV unscreened components, demonstrated statistically identical 93.1% and 92.3% reduced risks of CMV infection, respectively. Thus most clinicians consider leukoreduction and CMV seronegative blood to be equivalent; however, clinicians caring for neonates are more likely to require serologic screening. American Association of Blood Banks (AABB) recommends that each institution review its internal policies for blood use in patients vulnerable to CMV infection. Table 120.2 lists patient populations for whom use of "CMV risk–reduced" components, that is, CMV seronegative, leukoreduced, or both, are thought to be beneficial. The failure of clinicians to recognize recipients requiring CMV-safe transfusion and to request such components is an argument that has been advanced in support of universal prestorage (versus bedside) leukoreduction.

CMV DNA blood donation screening by NAT may be considered an additional risk reduction measure for donors with seronegative window-period infections. However, current NAT assays would be expected to be equivalent to serologic screening in detecting latently infected blood donors. Any consideration of additional testing is complicated by the absence of randomized studies using contemporary leukoreduction methods and by our lack of understanding of the clinical impact of transfusion-transmitted CMV in an era of CMV monitoring and treatment. But with the advent of pathogen reduction measures the need for any CMV donor screening will become obsolete.

EPSTEIN-BARR VIRUS (HHV-4)

EBV, a gammaherpesvirus, is the causative agent of heterophile antibody-positive infectious mononucleosis and is etiologically associated with Burkitt lymphoma, nasopharyngeal carcinoma, and posttransplant lymphoproliferative disease. Transfusion transmission of the virus is unusual because more than 90% of the adult population is infected, and second infection is prevented by host virus-specific cytotoxic T-lymphocytes, capable of lysing EBV-infected B lymphocytes when viral peptides are expressed on the lymphocyte surface. Rare cases of transfusion-transmitted EBV presenting as infectious mononucleosis have been described in immunocompetent recipients and in immunosuppressed patients following solid organ transplantation. Aggressive EBV-associated lymphoproliferative disorders have been observed in patients with immune injury after cord blood stem cell transplantation but have not been documented following transfusion. B lymphocytes are the likely source of transfusion-transmitted EBV infection, so leukoreduction is an attractive strategy to prevent infection in transfusion recipients. Nonclinical studies suggest that leukoreduction is capable of removing detectable EBV DNA from platelet concentrates and RBCs.

Kaposi Sarcoma Herpesvirus (HHV-8)

HHV-8 is a gammaherpes virus causally linked to Kaposi sarcoma, primary effusion lymphoma, and multicentric Castleman disease. It is highly cell-associated with lymphocytes and monocyte-macrophages. Although generally spread person to person, including sexually, it has been shown to be transmitted by transplantation. There is convincing evidence of HHV-8 transmission by transfusion in sub-Saharan Africa, where the seroprevalence of HHV-8 among blood donors is 40%, and fresh, nonleukoreduced blood transfusions are commonly used. The seroprevalence of HHV-8 among US blood donors has been reported to be as high as 20% to 25%, but a multicenter study using well-characterized antibody tests on donations from five representative US regions estimated a seroprevalence of only 3.5% and showed no evidence of viremia by PCR. The possibility has been raised that transfusions in the United States have transmitted HHV-8, but subsequently reported studies comparing transfused patients with untransfused controls are not suggestive. Similar to what has been established for CMV infection, it is assumed that widespread leukoreduction in the United States mitigates the risk for HHV-8 transmission by transfusion, but this has not been proven.

Other Herpesviruses (Herpes Simplex, Varicella-Zoster Virus, Human Herpesviruses 6 and 7)

Infection with these viruses is very common to ubiquitous. From 50% to 80% of the adult population is seroreactive to HSV-1 and/or HSV-2, up to 95% for VZV, more than 90% for HHV-6, and 70% to 90% for HHV-7. Primary infection is followed by lifelong latency for all HHVs, and reactivation from latency is described for all. There is no credible evidence of transfusion transmission of HSVs (causing orolabial and genital herpes and herpes encephalitis), VZV (chickenpox and shingles), or HHV-6 or HHV-7 (exanthem subitum or roseola infantum, multiorgan dissemination with reactivation in immunocompromised hosts).

Viremia occurs during both primary and reactivation infection with HSV and VZV, but transmission by blood has never been reported for these viruses. Although the lymphocyte association of HHV-6 and HHV-7, like CMV and EBV, suggests the possibility of transfusion transmission, well-documented case reports or series are not available. Case reports of HHV-6 transmission by hematopoietic stem cells used molecular methods to detect integrated donor HHV-6 DNA in engrafted donor cells and appear to represent transmission of latently infected cells rather than active infection. Furthermore, transplant recipients may reactivate preexisting latent infection, thereby confounding the evaluation of potential transfusion transmission. HHV-6 and HHV-7 are highly leukocyte associated after primary infection, and leukoreduction would be expected to be effective by analogy to human CMV; however, cell-free viremia can be found during primary infection.

PARVOVIRUS

Human parvovirus B19 (erythrovirus) is a 19- to 23-nm–diameter nonenveloped, single-stranded DNA virus from the family *Parvoviridae*, as are adeno-associated viruses, human parvovirus 4 (PARV4), PARV5, and bocaviruses. B19 has at least three genotypes. Genotype 1 infections appear predominantly in the United States and Europe. Genotype 2 infections appear confined to those born before 1973, and genotypes 3a and 3b infections occur in parts of West Africa. Infection with B19 is ubiquitous, with 50% of high school children demonstrating seropositivity, increasing to 90% in older adults. Approximately three-quarters of transfusion recipients have B19 IgG antibodies. Natural transmission occurs through the respiratory route most commonly and transplacentally to the fetus in up to 30% of women infected during pregnancy. Transfusion of blood and blood components, plasma derivatives, and organ transplantation are minor routes. In women infected during weeks 9 to 20 of pregnancy, fetal death occurs in 10% to 15% from hydrops fetalis. The low observed incidence of infection in transfusion recipients results from prior infection and immunity, co-infusion of neutralizing antibodies, and possibly because very high viral loads are uncommon in donor blood.

Parvovirus B19 causes erythema infectiosum, or fifth disease, oligoarthritis, and neurologic and myocardial infections. Following acute infection, viral replication leads to extremely high-titer viremia that declines at the time of IgM seroconversion approximately 9 days following infection. B19 may persist in bone marrow, liver, tonsils, and skin of healthy persons with no recognized clinical significance, and low levels of B19 DNA have been amplified from the blood of healthy people for several years after primary infection. The virus is highly tropic for erythroid progenitor cells using the P-blood group antigen, or globoside, as its receptor, causing aplastic crises in patients with sickle cell anemia, other inherited hemolytic diseases, and conditions associated with decreased RBC survival, malaria, and HIV/AIDS. Acute infection impairs erythropoiesis for 7 to 10 days, with complete cessation for 3 to 7 days, resulting in hemoglobin decreases. Persistent infection, causing red cell aplasia, occurs in those who fail to develop neutralizing antibodies to the viral capsid protein 1. In these patients, the virus continues to circulate at high titer, greater than 10^{12} International Units (IU) or equivalent genome copies per mL. Patients at risk for persistent infection include those receiving chemotherapy and immunosuppression, organ transplant recipients, and those with HIV. Infection in these groups tends to respond favorably to intravenous immunoglobulin infusions.

B19 virus–impaired erythropoiesis appears to be multifactorial. B19 viral nonstructural protein 1 (NS1) mediates apoptosis via an 11-kDa protein that perturbs signal transduction and induces apoptosis. B19 viral DNA activates Toll-like receptor 9 inhibiting cell growth and is toxic for infected cells.

Blood and plasma-derivative transmission involves donations during the transient 1- to 2-week high-titer viremic period. The prevalence of B19 viremia has been reported as 0.003% to 0.84% in blood and plasma donors. In a study involving more than 12,100 B19 DNA–tested blood donations, given to surgical patients with a 78% pretransfusion B19 IgG seroprevalence, no B19 transmissions occurred from transfusions containing less than 10^6 IU per mL.[31] Hence most blood transfusion recipients are believed to be at low risk for an infectious exposure. However, careful studies in Japan have demonstrated some transmissions from components with comparatively low viral loads of around 10^5 IU per mL).[32,33]

By contrast, recipients of plasma-derived products made from manufacturing pools of thousands of donations have a significant risk because the virus survives partitioning, ethanol fractionation, and other antiinfective measures applied to derivatives, and a single high-titer viremic donation can overcome the neutralizing activity of antibody in the pool. Recipients of coagulation concentrates are at highest risk, whereas those of intravenous immunoglobulin and albumin are less so based on cohort studies of prevalence. In one report, 14% of viremic plasma donors had titers between 10^4 and 10^7 IU per mL, and one in 13,000 had titers greater than 10^7. In observational studies, seroconversion occurred among recipients of plasma derivatives with high titers, $10^{7.5}$ to $10^{8.5}$ IU per mL, treated with the solvent/detergent pathogen-reduction technique, suggesting that the protective effect of neutralizing anti-B19 antibodies is exceeded in the presence of high viral loads (see box on Pathogen Reduction). Since B19 is a nonenveloped virus, solvent/detergent pathogen-reduction treatment is ineffective in preventing B19 transmission in hemophilia patients receiving factor concentrates. Freeze-drying and dry-heat treatment (80°C [176°F] for 72 hours) inactivate more than 4.7 logs B19, but this is not always sufficient to prevent transmission. Currently, plasma derivative manufacturers use "in-process" NAT to identify and remove source (from paid and volunteer donors) and recovered (from volunteer whole blood donors) plasma units with the objective to assure that manufacturing pools have parvovirus B19 DNA titers no greater than 10^4 IU per mL. Approximately 1 per 10,000 plasma units is withheld from further processing. For volunteer whole blood donors, 1 per 6000 to 1 per 16,000 have titers greater than 10^6 IU per mL. Because individual whole-blood donations rarely cause recognized parvovirus infection, testing of single red cell units, platelets, or plasma for transfusion for B19 DNA is not currently required, although some advocate use of B19-tested blood components for those potentially at risk, including pregnant women, neonates, those with reduced RBC survival, and immunocompromised patients.

Of note, PARV4 and PARV5 have been detected in pooled plasma derivative samples, but the clinical significance is not known; limited clinical disease associations have been described.[34]

WEST NILE VIRUS

WNV is a mosquito-borne lipid-enveloped RNA virus in the Japanese encephalitis complex of the family *Flaviviridae*. Transmitted bird-to-bird primarily by culicine mosquito vectors, human infections occur incidentally. The first cases were identified in the West Nile district of Uganda in 1937. Subsequently, outbreaks occurred in the Middle East, South Africa, and Europe. The first North American cases appeared in New York City in 1999. Starting in July 2000, WNV cases spread to the Mid-Atlantic States. This was followed in the next 3 years by transcontinental dissemination. During the summer of 2002, a model suggesting a significant risk for WNV infection in blood donors was published,[35] and then four recipients of organ allografts from a single donor developed neuroinvasive WNV infection. Infection of the organ donor was traced to donor blood transfused before death from trauma. Transfusion transmission was documented in 23 recipients in 2002[36] against a background of 2946 cases of WNV-meningoencephalitis (WNME). These events provoked a multidisciplinary effort, successfully engaging the blood community, the manufacturers of blood donor–screening NAT platforms, and public health officials and regulators to develop and deploy, under an investigational new drug (IND) exemption, high-throughput screening tests in the 10 months before the 2003 transmission season began. WNV test implementation represents the benchmark for responsiveness to a serious emerging transfusion-transmitted infection in the United States.[37,38]

In 2003 2946 WNME were reported and 714 healthy blood donors tested WNV RNA positive. In 2004 case reports declined in the Northeast but extended westward into Arizona and Southern California. In 2005 more than 1300 WNME cases were reported, with approximately 25% occurring in California, relatively high activity in South Dakota, Nebraska, Louisiana, and Illinois, and low activity in the Northeast. In 2006 over 400 WNV RNA-positive blood donors were identified. Subsequently WNV activity was reported in Washington State for the first time, and high rates of infection were noted in Idaho, California, Nebraska, Illinois, Louisiana, and the Dakotas. By 2011 fewer than 150 blood donors tested positive with the highest frequencies in New York, Texas, Arizona, and California. The frequency of both WNME cases and RNA-positive blood donors continues to vary by year and remain unpredictable. In total from 2002–2014, nearly 19,000 cases of WNME have been recorded with 4355 RNA-positive blood donors identified, which are related in magnitude by year.[39]

WNV RNA is believed to appear 1 to 3 days after a bite of an infected mosquito. In contrast to HIV and HCV, peak WNV levels are low (maximum observed 720,000 copies/mL, median 3500 copies/mL compared with 10^5 to 10^7 copies for HIV and HCV). In cohort studies of blood donors with positive WNV RNA tests, only 29% to 61% (retrospectively) describe any symptoms before or after donation consistent with WNV infection, compared with 3% to 20% of those not infected, demonstrating that the donor history is neither sensitive nor specific enough to prevent transfusion transmission.[40] Testing for antibodies also will not prevent transmission because IgM antibodies appear a median of 14 days and IgG antibodies a median of 17 days after infection and infectivity disappears rapidly with the development of antibody. These data explain the selection of WNV NAT for the testing strategy. To maximize efficiency, donation samples are tested in minipools containing aliquots from 6 to 16 donors, as is done for HCV, HBV, and HIV.

Despite minipool NAT, six transfusion-associated WNV cases occurred during 2003. The implicated donors were antibody-negative and had low-level RNA that escaped detection in the minipool (i.e., diluted) samples. At the end of 2003 an observation was made, even before the documentation of these transfusion transmissions, that the viral load in some donor samples is too low for detection by minipool NAT. Consequently, strategies have been developed to switch from minipool-NAT to NAT on individual donation aliquots in areas experiencing high WNV activity.[41] In total, following the 23 cases of transfusion-transmitted WNV documented before the initiation of donation NAT screening, an additional 14 have been reported, most related to donations having only low-levels of RNA; the last was in 2016. All implicated donations, except one in 2002, have been IgM negative. Blood centers must remain vigilant for appropriate conversion to individual donation-NAT for this strategy to be effective.

DENGUE VIRUSES

This mosquito-borne infection is of great interest as an emerging pathogen with the potential to spread by transfusion. Forty percent of the world's population lives in areas with risk for dengue, including many areas visited by US travelers. It has spread rapidly in Latin America and the Caribbean since the 1980s. Dengue is endemic in Puerto Rico, the US Virgin Islands, and American Samoa, and there have been outbreaks in Hawaii, Texas, and Florida during the last 10 years. Dengue is caused by four related flaviviruses spread person to person by *Aedes aegypti* and *Aedes albopictus,* which are present in 16 and 35 US states, respectively. Over 2.3 million dengue clinical cases occurred in the Americas during 2015.

Most infections are asymptomatic, but illness ranges from undifferentiated fever to classic break-bone fever and severe dengue (dengue hemorrhagic fever and dengue shock syndrome). An approximately 7-day viremia is a feature of both asymptomatic and symptomatic infection, and asymptomatic blood donors from Hong Kong, Singapore, Brazil, and Puerto Rico have transmitted dengue to blood recipients in seven clusters. Although such reports are limited, compared with the high rates of vector-borne infection, there is no systematic surveillance for transfusion-transmitted dengue and its recognition in the face of widespread outbreaks is problematic.[42] RNA-positive, asymptomatic donors have been identified in Brazil, Central America, and Puerto Rico using NAT and antigen detection tests. Rates of donor RNA positivity in Puerto Rico are comparable to those found in US donors during the most active WNV seasons.[43,44] A recent study in Brazil documented transfusion transmission; however, when patient charts of those donors who received an RNA-positive unit and were shown to be infected were compared with control recipients who did not receive an RNA-positive unit, there was no reported increase in clinical illness.[45] This further illustrates the difficulty in identifying transfusion-transmitted dengue among severely ill patients who are frequently transfused.[44]

In the absence of significant outbreaks of locally-transmitted dengue in the continental United States, transfusion risk relates mainly to return of infected, asymptomatic or presymptomatic travelers to the United States from endemic areas A 3- to 14-day incubation period precedes symptom onset. Deferral for travel to malarious areas (1 year for a US resident) offers some protection, but a large proportion of dengue-affected areas frequently visited from the United States are malaria-free and donor-travelers to those areas could potentially introduce the virus into the community and the blood supply. Careful surveillance and a high index of suspicion when sustained febrile illness occurs following transfusion are required to recognize transfusion-related dengue. Preliminary data on travelers from the United States to dengue-endemic destinations that are malaria-free suggest that 2- to 4-week deferral for travel to dengue-affected areas may have a greater adverse impact on blood donation than current malaria deferrals. To date, however, there are no instances of transfusion-transmitted dengue in the continental United States that are attributable to donor exposure through travel. The conditions for sustained spread of dengue exist in large areas of the United States: a source of infection from travelers and immigrants; a susceptible population; and competent vectors. Whether the recently identified outbreaks in the United States will continue or increase, and whether sustained transmission will begin is unknown. Transfusion-transmitted dengue has been identified by one group as one of the three highest-priority emerging infections posing a potential threat to transfusion recipients in the United States and Canada and has been the subject of discussions at the FDA's Blood Products Advisory Committee (see box on Emerging Infections).

CHIKUNGUNYA VIRUS

Chikungunya virus is another tropical arbovirus transmitted by *Aedes* spp. mosquitoes. It is a togavirus of the alphavirus group and, although first recognized in Africa has been notably responsible for explosive outbreaks in the islands of the Indian Ocean and has most recently spread to the Caribbean, where more than 1.7 million clinical cases were reported from the end of 2013 to the middle of 2015, including RNA positivity in blood donors.[51] Although there have been no reported cases of transmission by transfusion, the similarity of early infection to that of dengue has resulted in significant concern.

Emerging Infections

The experiences with human immunodeficiency virus (HIV), new variant Creutzfeldt-Jakob disease (vCJD), and West Nile virus (WNV) have made it clear that planning for the emergence of new pathogens that may threaten the blood supply is critical in order to shorten the interval from emergence to mitigation. To that end, the characteristics of pathogens likely to enter the blood supply must be understood. These include the ability of the agent to establish an asymptomatic blood-borne phase, to survive under contemporary processing and storage conditions, to establish infection by the intravenous route, and to cause significant morbidity in a transfusion recipient.

Using these characteristics and a review of contemporary literature, the Transfusion Transmitted Diseases Committee of the American Association of Blood Banks (AABB), from 2005 to 2009 produced a compendium of infectious agents that might become relevant to transfusion medicine and attempted to prioritize those that were identified.[46] A series of 68 fact sheets was developed. The fact sheets provide transfusion medicine professionals and clinicians with an overview of the agents' phylogeny, epidemiology, clinical characteristics, and interventions that might be useful to protect the safety of the blood supply. Three agents were included in the highest priority stratum: *Babesia* sp., dengue viruses, and the vCJD prion; a section on each is included in this chapter. The fact sheets are freely available online, cover many of the agents discussed in this chapter, and have been updated when required (www.aabb.org/tm/eid/Pages/eidpostpub.aspx).

Since the original publication, several new monographs have been added, reflecting an ongoing "horizon-scanning" initiative designed to alert the medical community to potential threats. These include yellow fever and the yellow fever vaccine viruses after the latter was transmitted to blood recipients when recent vaccine recipients failed to divulge that information during blood donation. Other fact sheets have been updated and rereleased to capture relevant new information (see box on Xenotropic Murine Leukemia Virus-Related Virus). The availability of these materials to the transfusion medicine and general medical communities is meant to increase awareness that unexpected infections in transfusion recipients should trigger consideration of that source and to provide background allowing the rational consideration of approaches to avert and minimize their spread.[47]

Xenotropic Murine Leukemia Virus–Related Virus

The alleged association of the gammaretrovirus xenotropic murine leukemia virus–related virus (XMRV) with chronic fatigue syndrome/myalgic encephalomyelitis (CFS/ME) is paradigmatic of the difficulties inherent in the real-time assessment of potential and emerging transfusion-transmissible infections. A group of CFS/ME patients and controls were evaluated using polymerase chain reaction (PCR), virus isolation, serology, and immunohistochemistry.[48] Evidence of the virus's presence was strongly associated with the clinical diagnosis, culturable virus was found in plasma, and the issue of transfusion transmission was appropriately raised.

Multiple subsequent studies from other groups over the ensuing 2 years failed to confirm the presence of XMRV in a variety of populations. Several publications suggested that PCR contamination underlies some positive results; however, data now indicate that XMRV arose as a recombinant of two murine leukemia viruses during passages in nude mice, leading to the conclusion that the initial findings were an artifact.[49] With these findings, the original publication was retracted. The absence of transfusion transmission and of the agent were also demonstrated in studies on the donor pool.[50] The amount of research and resulting publications on this recombinant laboratory-generated virus were simply another lesson in caution that is required prior to claims of a viral agent being a human pathogen, or in this case, being the result of recombinant contamination.

Notably, French authorities responded to the outbreak in La Réunion by halting local collection of red cells (providing for the island's needs by supplying blood from the French mainland) and by implementation of limited NAT and the use of pathogen reduction for platelets.[52] Other precautions that have been used have been to strengthen requirements of postdonation information from donors (a process that is enhanced by the high [50%–80%] frequency of symptoms among infected subjects), along with deferrals for residence in affected areas. Chikungunya symptoms are similar to those of dengue, but without the impact upon the circulatory system. Arthralgia is, however, a prominent symptom and may be prolonged. Routine testing is not currently available.

ZIKA VIRUS

Zika virus is another tropical arbovirus of the flavivirus group. Again, first recognized in Africa, it has been circulating in the Pacific islands at relatively modest levels. In 2007 the first human outbreak was recognized on the island of Yap in Micronesia with subsequent spread in 2013 to French Polynesia.[53] Testing performed in Polynesia showed 2.8% of presenting donors to have Zika virus RNA. Within 2015 Zika virus and associated disease emerged in Brazil and has now spread to beyond other South and Central American countries, Mexico, and the Caribbean including travel-associated cases in the United States.[54] A particular concern is that the infection seems to be associated with an unexpectedly high and troubling incidence of microcephaly, a neurologic developmental abnormality.[55,56] Increases have been noted, particularly in Brazil, where it is believed that the increase is a consequence of maternal infection and transmission to the developing fetus. In addition, during the outbreak in Polynesia, a 20-fold increase in the number of reported Guillain-Barré syndrome cases were reported; a similar increase is also being noted in Brazil. Other than mosquito transmission, like dengue, transfusion transmission has been reported. Unlike the other mosquito-borne viruses, Zika appears to be sexually transmitted (and can be recovered from urine and semen).[57] The World Health Organization has called a public health emergency of international concern to increase surveillance and vector control and to expedite the development of diagnostics, treatment, and vaccine development. Given the similarity to and relationship with dengue, there are concerns about the spread of Zika virus and local transmission in the continental United States. Most recently (August 2016), the implementation of universal, individual donation NAT for Zika virus RNA has been required for all blood collected in the United States.

PANDEMIC INFLUENZA A

There was interest in the transfusion safety implications of influenza A even before the swine origin A-H1N1 pandemic of 2009–2010.[58] Viremia in donors, and the potential for infection of recipients were discussed during meetings of an AABB pandemic influenza planning task force as early as 2008, based on old literature demonstrating the virus in the blood of experimentally infected volunteers and case reports of viral dissemination during human infection with highly pathogenic avian A-H5N1 virus. Subsequent studies have failed to identify influenza viruses in donors drawn in US communities during periods of high seasonal influenza activity or in donors with the onset of influenza-like illness immediately following donations.[59] The current consensus is that pandemic influenza is not likely a threat to blood recipients, but that disruption of the blood supply in a severe pandemic is a more important possibility, requiring careful advance planning.

BACTERIAL CONTAMINATION

Bacterial contamination of red cell and platelet components occurs primarily as a result of the inability to achieve complete skin disinfection at the donor phlebotomy site, where bacterial populations survive in skin appendages below the accessible surface and contaminate skin plugs made by the phlebotomy needle and enter the blood bag. Transient asymptomatic bacteremia at the time of blood donation, a break in technique during pooling the contents of or sealing blood containers, disruption of blood bag integrity or its contamination during manufacturing are other rare sources. Bacterial

proliferation occurs more rapidly in platelet concentrates stored at room temperature than in red cells maintained at 4°C (39.2°F).

The rate of bacterial contamination in allogeneic platelets was estimated at 1 per 1000 to 3000 units with life-threatening septic reactions occurring in one per 15,000 to 100,000 recipients before routine implementation of culture-based tests to detect bacteria in apheresis platelets in 2004. These tests reduced contamination rates to approximately 1 per 5000 to 8500 platelet units. Clinical septic reactions occur in approximately 30% of recipients receiving contaminated platelets. Bacterial contamination was responsible for 33 of 267 (12%) of transfusion-related deaths reported to the FDA from 2005 to 2009.[60] In subsequent reporting periods (2008–2012 and 2010–2014) bacterial contamination of platelets (primarily *Staphylococcus aureus* and *Serratia marcescens*) were responsible for 13 of 198 (7%) and 11 of 176 (6%) recipient fatalities (www.fda.gov/BiologicsBloodVaccines/SafetyAvailability/ReportaProblem/TransfusionDonationFatalities/). The downward trend is undoubtedly caused by interventions that have been put into place (increased attention to arm scrub, improved antiseptic solutions used, sample diversion of the first 40 mL or so containing the skin plug and bacterial testing). Only acute hemolytic reactions and TRALI are responsible for more fatalities in the referenced reporting periods. However, there is consensus that these reactions are badly underrecognized and underreported. Culturing fails to detect 50% to 75% of contaminated units. This undetected contamination occurs largely because minimal bacterial levels, present when cultures are obtained, yield culture aliquots without bacteria. Subsequently the few bacteria remaining in the blood bag can grow out during storage, producing transfusions with significant bacterial levels. To minimize this, collection facilities generally hold apheresis platelets for approximately 24 hours after collection before sampling for culture to allow low bacterial inocula to proliferate, improving the sensitivity of culture. As mentioned, improved skin antisepsis and diversion for laboratory testing of the first 40 mL of blood, which contains the skin plug, provide further reduction of contamination rates, transfusion reactions, and fatality rates by lowering the bacterial load that otherwise would enter the final component container.

Septic transfusion reactions should be suspected when one or more of the following occur within 1 to 4 hours of transfusion: temperature elevations greater than 1–2°C (1.8–3.6°F), chills and rigors, tachycardia more than 120 beats per minute or an increase of 40 beats per minute, or an increase or fall in systolic blood pressure of greater than 30 mmHg. Additional signs and symptoms can include nausea, vomiting, diarrhea, bleeding, oliguria, or septic shock. Septic transfusion reactions may be confused with hemolytic transfusion reactions, febrile, nonhemolytic transfusion reactions, or TRALI.

Platelet concentrates contaminated with *Staphylococcus aureus*, *Serratia marcescens*, *Staphylococcus epidermidis*, *Escherichia coli*, and *Streptococcus* species account for most of clinically recognizable reactions. *Propionibacterium acnes* is a frequent culture isolate from platelets during storage when an anaerobic culture is also performed but is not believed to be responsible for a significant number of reactions. A clinically relevant case of *Clostridium perfringens*, another anaerobe, has been reported.[61] The bacterial dose in platelet concentrates and species virulence correlate with the clinical outcome. Bacterial concentrations greater than 10^5 colony-forming units (CFU)/mL are more likely to result in severe reactions or fatalities. Alternatively, low concentrations, 10^4 or fewer CFU/mL of skin organisms, frequently elicit no reaction. Endotoxin elaboration by gram-negative organisms is associated with the most severe reactions, but the vast majority of gram-negative organisms are easily detected by bacterial culture.

In addition, bacteria grow at variable rates. *S. epidermidis* grows slowly, and *P. acnes* requires on average 3 days for detection. Because collection agencies continue bacterial culturing until the platelet unit expiration date or detection of growth, there is further opportunity to intercept released platelets that have not been transfused and to alert physicians about the potential risk for bacterial contamination in cases where the units have been administered. However, the vast majority of septic reactions are associated with false-negative culture tests because of sampling insufficiency as noted earlier. The overall rate of bacterial contaminated apheresis platelets is 1 per 5000 and for septic transfusion reactions is 1 per 107,000 distributed components.[61]

Before the mid-1980s, platelet concentrates were stored for 7 days. Following reports of septic reactions, the shelf life was reduced to 5 days to decrease the interval during which bacteria could proliferate. In the United States, blood suppliers distributed platelets from 2005 to 2008 with a 7-day shelf life following enrollment in an FDA-mandated postmarket surveillance study (Post Approval Surveillance Study of Platelet Outcomes, Release Tested [PASSPORT]) that included testing for bacterial contamination by a sensitive culture method. Initial experience suggested that extended platelet storage coupled with bacterial testing substantially decreased platelet loss from outdating. However, the PASSPORT study found 1 per 4329 tested platelet products with negative bacterial cultures had bacterial growth when tested at the end of storage, 7 days later.[62] Septic transfusion reactions occurred in approximately 1 per 25,000 platelet transfusions; some following infusion of 3-day stored platelets, most with those stored 4 days or longer, leading to reinstatement of the 5-day platelet shelf life.

Alternative methods for detecting bacterial contamination include point-of-release testing in the hospital transfusion service. Considered a supplement to culture-based testing, this assay can be used shortly before issuing platelets for transfusion to detect units missed by early culture. This rapid qualitative immunoassay tests for the presence of conserved bacterial antigens (gram-negative lipopolysaccharide and gram-positive lipoteichoic acid). In one report using this test, 1 per 3000 platelet doses contained gram-positive organisms when issued 3 or more days after collection.[63] Other methods, under development for mitigating septic platelet events, include microcolorimetry, bacterial spore biosensors, real-time PCR, flow cytometry, and detection of other bacterial cell wall constituents. Pathogen-reduction technology using licensed psoralens (Intercept) or riboflavin plus UV light provides an opportunity for inactivating multiple pathogens before they can proliferate. Again, however, not all technologies inactivate different bacterial isolates with the same efficiency.

RBC bacterial contamination rates approximate 1 per 30,000 units with adverse clinical outcomes occurring in 1 per 500,000 transfusions and fatalities occurring at a rate of 1 per 10 million. Most septic reactions occur in units stored for 4 weeks or longer, reflecting the delayed growth of bacteria at 4°C (39.2°F).

Bacteria isolated from contaminated red cell units include *S. marcescens*, *E. coli*, *Pseudomonas* species (especially *Pseudomonas fluorescens*), and *Yersinia enterocolitica*. The latter two are psychrophilic and known to proliferate in the cold. Gram-positive skin saprophytes account for most of the organism-contaminating platelet concentrates, with the remaining attributed to gram-negative organisms associated with occult bacteremia.

Immediate recognition of a platelet or red cell septic reaction and immediate discontinuation of the transfusion, supportive care, and antibiotic administration are the mainstays of therapy. Prevention relies on careful donor selection and scrupulous adherence to aseptic techniques and precautions from component collection, processing, transport, and storage to transfusion at the bedside. The Gram stain reveals bacteria in platelet concentrates contaminated with more than 10^5 to 10^6 CFU/mL.

A proportion of donors of platelet units contaminated with *Streptococcus bovis* or *Streptococcus infantarius* have been found to have colonic polyps or colon cancer.

SPIROCHETE INFECTIONS

Syphilis

US blood banks first screened donors with a serologic test for syphilis in 1938, and screening has been a regulatory requirement since 1958. It was the first test mandated for US donors and stood alone before

the discovery of the Australia antigen almost two decades later. More than 100 transfusion syphilis cases were published before World War II, and many more certainly occurred. The last alleged case of transfusion-transmitted syphilis in the United States, however, was in 1966. Since then, hundreds of millions of components have been transfused in this country without another recognized case. There are multiple explanations for the disappearance of transfusion-transmitted syphilis in addition to improvements in testing: (1) the dramatic decline in the incidence of early syphilis in the United States over the decades, more than an order of magnitude, reducing the reservoir of donors able to transmit; (2) the end of direct donor-to-recipient transfusion combined with the loss of viability of *Treponema pallidum* in stored blood—the latter attributed to poor survival in refrigerated RBCs and to the high oxygen tension in platelets stored at higher temperatures; (3) the ubiquitous administration of antibiotics for trivial to serious viral, bacterial, and noninfectious clinical syndromes, especially to those sick enough to be transfused; (4) donor deferral for behavioral correlates of syphilis risk (e.g., male sex with males, occurrence of recent sexually transmitted infection in donors, exchange of drugs or money for sex, injection drug use); (5) passive surveillance for transfusion-transmitted syphilis compounded by the failure of recognition by physicians (who may have never seen syphilis, venereal or otherwise); and (6) donor illness during spirochetemia severe enough to prevent their presentation to donate blood or causing deferral. The relative contributions of each of these factors are unquantified.

Most blood collection facilities screen donors with an automated test for detecting treponemal antibodies (e.g., *T. pallidum* hemagglutination assay and *T. pallidum* particle agglutination assay; treponemal antibody confirmatory test usually follows using a variety of methods such as enzyme-linked immunosorbent assay (ELISA) or fluorescent treponemal antibody, absorbed (FTA-abs) test; most blood centers further test donors with treponemal antibody reactivity using a nontreponemal test (e.g., rapid plasma reagin [RPR]) to stage the reactivity as recent or past. Approximately 50% of donors with confirmed positive treponemal test results have evidence of a treated syphilis infection. Donations with reactive syphilis tests are generally discarded. Blood centers defer donors with positive treponemal confirmatory tests; donors may be reentered (regardless of their nontreponemal test results) 12 months after completion of treatment for syphilis. Treponemal and nontreponemal false positivity occurs in healthy donors caused by cross-reactivity with a wide variety of infectious diseases other than syphilis, in those with high-titer human leukocyte antigen (HLA) antibodies, after some immunizations, with autoimmune disease and other chronic inflammatory disease, and have increasing prevalence with increasing age.

Most true treponemal antibody positives are the "serologic scar" of remote (often treated) infection and pose no risk to blood recipients. A recommendation to discontinue donor screening for syphilis was made in 1985 but not acted upon initially because of the perception that testing might be functioning as a surrogate for HIV or other transfusion-transmissible viruses.[64] This hypothesis has been rejected, but, because the role of syphilis testing in the elimination of transfusion syphilis is unclear, syphilis testing continues even though it has no apparent value. Although small PCR studies of reactive donors have been universally negative, rabbit inoculation studies using samples from confirmed reactive donors will likely be required to eliminate syphilis testing, and it seems unlikely the resources will be found to do a study of the required size.

Lyme Disease

Borrelia burgdorferi is the spirochete that causes Lyme disease, the most frequent tick-borne infection in North America and Europe. The agent was discovered in 1977 during investigations of an arthritis cluster in Connecticut children. Cases reported in the United States doubled between 1992 and 2006 to almost 20,000. Geographic distribution of cases is highly focused, with the majority of reported cases occurring in 10 northeast and north central states. *Ixodes scapularis*, the black-legged tick, transmits *B. burgdorferi* in those areas, and *Ixodes pacificus*, the western black-legged tick, transmits the infection along the Pacific coast. The ticks feed predominantly in late spring and early summer during the nymph stage. Emergence has been associated with environmental changes that increase deer and rodent reservoir populations and changing residential patterns putting humans in more intimate contact with the tick vectors. Rodents are the reservoir. Although deer are not infected, they transport and maintain the ticks. Birds may also play a role in transporting the vector ticks.

The characteristic erythema chronicum migrans ("bull's-eye") rash is present in 70% to 80% of cases within 30 days of infection. The wide variety of clinical findings includes malaise, fatigue, headache, myalgias, large joint arthralgias and arthritis, and neurologic and cardiac signs and symptoms. These may not immediately suggest Lyme disease in the absence of a typical rash or known tick exposure. Serologic testing supports the clinical diagnosis. Unfortunately, poor specificity is recognized with many screening methods, and a two-step approach using a sensitive EIA or immunofluorescence assay (IFA) followed by a confirmatory, more specific, immunoblot is recommended by the CDC.

B. burgdorferi spirochetemia occurs in 44% of patients with clinical Lyme disease and peaks 7 to 10 days after tick bite. The spirochete can survive in red cells, platelets, and frozen plasma for at least the duration of their routine storage. Transfusion transmission of *B. burgdorferi* has been demonstrated in a murine model. Despite these observations, no human transfusion-associated cases have been reported. This may reflect the relatively short spirochetemic phase and low levels of organisms, as well as deferral of donors with nonspecific illness or signs and symptoms of Lyme borreliosis. Although there are no official standards or guidance, it would be prudent for individuals with a history of Lyme disease to be deferred until well and treatment has been completed.

Other Tick-Borne Bacteria

The rickettsia that cause human monocytic ehrlichiosis (HME) and human granulocytic anaplasmosis (HGA; formerly human granulocytic ehrlichiosis) are intracellular bacteria that survive in stored blood. *Ehrlichia chaffeensis* causes HME and is transmitted to humans by Lone Star tick (*Amblyomma americanum*) bites. Most cases occur in the south central and southeastern United States. *Anaplasma phagocytophilum* causes HGA and occurs predominantly in the northeastern and upper midwestern areas of the United States. *I. scapularis* and *I. pacificus* (the Lyme borreliosis vector) transmit the organism. Signs and symptoms include fever, chills, and headache, often associated with thrombocytopenia, leukopenia, and increased liver enzyme levels. Intracellular aggregates of microcolonies of bacteria referred to as morulae appear in monocytes in the HME, and inclusions appear in granulocytes in HGA. Seroprevalence studies in blood donors in Wisconsin and Connecticut report 0.5% to 3.5% seropositivity for *A. phagocytophilum* antibodies. At least nine cases of transfusion-transmitted HGA from asymptomatic donors have been recognized after nonleukoreduced RBC transfusion; however, cases have occurred as well following leukoreduction including one from apheresis platelets.[65] Both *Ehrlichia* and *Anaplasma* spp. are white blood cell–associated, and it has been suggested that leukoreduction may mitigate their impact. The infectivity of *Orientia tsutsugamushi*, the rickettsial agent of scrub typhus, is reduced by up to 10^5 by filtration leukoreduction, but infectious *E. chaffeensis* survived in refrigerated red cells and could be isolated from the packed RBCs after filtration.

In a study of heavily tick-exposed military recruits in Arkansas, which included a look back to 10 blood recipients of units from soldiers infected with *E. chaffeensis* and *Rickettsia rickettsii* (the agent of Rocky Mountain spotted fever [RMSF]), no clinical illness occurred in recipients. One possible RMSF seroconversion was reported. There is a single case report of transfusion-associated RMSF

that involved a donor developing symptoms 3 days postdonation. The recipient developed symptoms 6 days posttransfusion.

PARASITIC INFECTIONS

Malaria

Five *Plasmodium* species (*Plasmodium falciparum*, *Plasmodium vivax*, *Plasmodium ovale*, *Plasmodium malariae*, and *Plasmodium knowlesi*) and occasionally others cause the protozoan disease malaria. In 2008 243 million cases occurred worldwide, with most in sub-Saharan Africa. Other endemic areas include parts of Asia and South America and more limited areas in Mexico, Central America, and the Caribbean. Of 1478 imported cases in the United States in 2009, 735 were acquired in Africa, 142 in Asia/Western Pacific, and 103 in the Americas.[66] West Africa accounted for most cases associated with Africa, and Honduras, Haiti, and Guyana for most of the cases from the Americas. During 2009 only two cases were acquired in Mexico, both *P. vivax*. In 2003 eight autochthonous infections occurred in Palm Beach, Florida; but none subsequently. Vectorial transmission, overwhelmingly the most common route, is by the bite of an infected female *Anopheles* mosquito. *Anopheles* mosquitoes generally feed between dusk and dawn, thereby limiting the risk to tourists who usually visit malaria areas during daylight hours. Almost three-quarters of those who acquired malaria were visiting friends or relatives in endemic areas. Missionaries and business travelers represent fewer than 20% of infected US citizens. Leisure travelers make up the small remainder.

P. falciparum accounts for 40% to 46% of US cases detected recently, *P. vivax* 11% to 20%, and *P. malariae* and *P. ovale* approximately 2% each. For the remainder, most are undetermined with a few mixed-species infections. *P. knowlesi* has not yet been reported.

Seventy percent of imported cases in the United States occur among returning travelers who were visiting friends or relatives, ethnically and racially distinct from the majority population of the United States (where malaria is not endemic), who return to their homelands (countries where malaria is endemic) to visit friends or relatives. The region of origin is very relevant to measures designed to prevent malaria transmission by transfusion because many of these individuals are semiimmune and therefore can be parasitemic while asymptomatic. In contrast, donors without malarial immunity who travel to endemic areas and become infected are nearly always symptomatic when they are parasitemic and would not be accepted as blood donors. Malaria symptoms occurred within 1 month of arrival in the United States in 84% of those infected with *P. falciparum* and 56% of those with *P. vivax* in 2009. The latter represents almost all cases of relapsing malaria. No acute onsets involving the four most frequent *Plasmodium* species occurred at an interval greater than 1 year.

One hundred transfusion cases have been recognized and reported in the United States since 1963. Since 1999 there have been 19 (0 to 3 per year) including one in 2007, none in 2008, two in 2009 and one each in 2010 and 2011; from 2012–2015, no cases have yet to be reported. In the majority of the 100, the case would have been prevented had the extant donor deferral criteria been appropriately applied.

The incubation period for transfusion-associated malaria ranges from 8 to 90 days. *P. falciparum* has the shortest time, mean 17 days (range, 8 to 36 days) and *P. malariae* the longest, mean 50 days (range, 8 to 90 days). Most cases involved RBC or whole-blood transfusion, although a few transmissions from platelet transfusions have occurred, presumably related to RBC contamination. Transmission from frozen plasma has not been reported.

Current strategies for reducing the low risk for transfusion transmission in the United States involve deferral of residents of nonendemic areas who have traveled to malaria-endemic regions during the previous 12 months, those with residence in endemic areas for 3 years since their last potential exposure in such regions, and those with a history of malaria for 3 years after resolution. Apart from incomplete elicitation of malaria risk history, residual risk remains because transfusion transmissions of *P. falciparum*, *P. vivax*, and *P. ovale* have been reported 13, 27, and 7 years, respectively, after departure from malarious areas. Because *P. malariae* infection can persist for more than 70 years without symptoms, elimination of transfusion-induced malaria is a practical impossibility. At this time, licensed in vitro screening for at-risk donors using antibody tests, antigen detection, or NAT are unavailable in the United States. It is not clear that the limited commercial potential of assays to be used on a relatively small fraction of donors will justify the investment required to pass the stringent regulatory requirements of a blood donor screening assay. Donor deferral guidelines have been modified in 2014 to reduce the loss of more than 60,000 potential donors with travel to areas of Mexico where the malaria risk is minimal.[67]

Babesiosis

Babesia species that infect humans include *Babesia microti*, *Babesia duncani* (previously WA1 type), *Babesia divergens* (limited primarily to Europe), *B. divergens*–like (MO1 and EU1), and *Babesia venatorum*. *B. microti*, an intraerythrocytic protozoan, causes most human infections. The white-footed mouse, *Peromyscus leucopus,* serves as the reservoir and the deer or black-legged tick, *I. scapularis* (also the vector of Lyme borreliosis and HGA), as the vector. Transmission follows bites from infected ticks, primarily nymphs, from May through early September. The defined transmission period has less relevance for transfusion transmission because asymptomatic blood donors can be infected chronically.[68] Most cases occur in Massachusetts and its coastal islands, Rhode Island, Connecticut, New York, New Jersey, Wisconsin, and Minnesota; these states are considered the seven endemic states. This geographic range has expanded recently, attributed to expansion of white-tailed deer, *Odocoileus virginianus,* populations. Although not a competent host, deer provide a blood meal and transportation for adult ticks to new areas.

The vast majority of both vectorial and transfusion-associated *Babesia* cases involve *B. microti*. *B. duncani* infections include those previously designated WA1. *B. divergens* cases occur predominantly in Europe. The incubation period varies from 1 to 9 weeks. The severity of illness associated with *Babesia* infections relates more to the infected individual's immune status than the *Babesia* species. The very young, older adults, persons who have had a splenectomy, and those with hereditary hemolytic disorders are at greatest risk for morbidity and mortality. Approximately one-third of infected subjects remain asymptomatic, and parasitemia may persist for more than 2 years. Typical symptoms resemble malaria and include fever, headache, chills, sweats, and arthralgia, myalgia, malaise, nausea, diarrhea, and hemolytic anemia. Parasitemia levels vary from 1% to 2% in otherwise healthy hosts to 85% in immunocompromised and asplenic patients. Case fatality rates approximate 5%.

Case reports of transfusion-associated *Babesia* infections include red cell units stored for up to 42 days. *Babesia* transmission has been reported following transfusion of cryopreserved red cells, and four cases involve whole blood–derived platelet transfusions presumably contaminated with red cells. At least 159 transfusion-associated *B. microti* cases have occurred, primarily in endemic regions, but cases in nonendemic states reflect the interstate movement of both blood components and blood donors and highlight the high index of suspicion required to recognize cases.[69] More than three-quarters of the reports occurred during the past decade. The all-cause mortality rate approaches 19%. Babesia represented the highest number of reported transfusion-related fatalities to the FDA from any single microbial infection in the periods of 2008–2012 and again in 2010–2014 including 8 of 21 (38%) and 4 of 15 (27%), respectively. The total number of transfusion-related fatalities in these periods was 198 and 176, respectively (www.fda.gov/BiologicsBloodVaccines/SafetyAvailability/ReportaProblem/TransfusionDonationFatalities/). There are three reports of transfusion-transmission involving *B. duncani,* and single cases have been reported from Japan (*B. microti*–like) and Germany.

Babesiosis has been made a nationally notifiable infection in 2011 and included in the nascent biovigilance network of the National Healthcare Safety Network, so more accurate measurements of transfusion risk may become available in the future. In 2011–2013 up to 29 states reported a total of 3857 cases nationally of which 95% occurred in seven states in New England and the upper Midwest and increased to 98.5% in nine states (adding New Hampshire and Maine) (http://www.cdc.gov/mmwr/preview/mmwrhtml/mm6127a2.htm). Transfusion-transmission risk estimates in endemic states have occurred with the advent of investigational testing and are about 1 per 18,000 red cell units transfused in the highly endemic states of New England to an overall risk of approximately 1 per 100,000 units throughout the all nine endemic states mentioned (including New Hampshire and Maine, where an increasing number of transfusion-related cases have been reported).

Febrile patients must be queried for a transfusion history and babesiosis considered when transfusion has occurred. Diagnostic laboratory evaluation includes blood smear examination, which requires differentiation of *Babesia* sp. from *Plasmodium* infections. Tetrad or "Maltese cross" forms are diagnostic for *Babesia* but occur infrequently. Diagnostic testing most frequently involves indirect IFA testing for identifying persons with low-level parasitemia such as patients with chronic infections but remains positive for up to 5 years after resolution or cure of babesiosis. PCR testing is more sensitive for detecting acute infections before seroconversion.

In the absence of an FDA-licensed test, mitigation of transfusion transmission involves deferral of potential donors with a history of *Babesia* infection. Questioning donors about tick exposure or tick bite has no predictive value as a donor-screening question. Investigational testing most widely uses IFA and PCR to screen donations. One US blood center's screening program screens red cell units intended for immunosuppressed patients considered at highest risk for *Babesia* infection complications such as neonates, pediatric patients with sickle cell disease, and pediatric oncology patients. However, when cases of transfusion-transmitted babesiosis are carefully studied, such groups only represent about half of those who have developed transfusion-transmitted babesiosis. The same investigational assays (IFA and PCR) are being used together by another system in highly endemic regions for screening of red cells units. Retrospective studies have demonstrated the feasibility and suitable performance characteristics of the combination of these tests, yielding a combined specificity of 99.8%[70] and demonstrating an absence of transfusion transmission by screened units. Donor prevalence in endemic areas is 0.3%. Currently this program only screens enough units to supply those hospitals requesting babesia-screened blood. An attractive alternative to testing is the eventual development of red cell or whole blood pathogen-reduction technologies.

Leishmaniasis

Phlebotomine (Old World) and *Lutzomyia* (New World) sand-fly bites transmit *Leishmania* infections to humans in most of the tropical and subtropical world. *Trypanosomatidae* of various species cause visceral infection also known as kala-azar (*L. donovani, L. infantum,* and others). Additional species are involved in cutaneous and mucocutaneous infections (*L. tropica, L. major, L. mexicana, L. braziliensis,* and others given a variety of local names). In addition, transplacental, sexual, and transfusion transmissions occur.[71] The promastigote form of the parasite resides in the gastrointestinal tract of sand flies and is inoculated into humans through a skin bite. In humans, promastigotes are phagocytosed by monocytes, where they transform into amastigotes that reproduce and reside in macrophages and the reticuloendothelial system. Organisms in monocytes and free amastigotes are released during refrigerated storage, transform back into extracellular promastigotes, and mediate transfusion transmission. *L. tropica* also survives in monocytes contained in frozen red cell preparations and in platelet concentrates stored at room temperature. At least 10 cases of transfusion-associated leishmaniasis attributed to *L donovani* have been reported in endemic areas, mostly in young children or neonates. A probable case of platelet transfusion–transmitted *L. donovani* was reported in India. A presumed case of transfusion-transmitted *L. mexicana* in a renal transplant recipient was mistakenly diagnosed as Chagas disease because of serologic cross-reactivity between *Trypanosoma cruzi* and *Leishmania*. *L. infantum* DNA was amplified from 6% of peripheral blood mononuclear cells of blood donors with *Leishmania* antibodies in the Balearic Islands. Several animal model studies also demonstrate transmission by blood transfusion.

Asymptomatic infections occur frequently in healthy donors exposed in endemic areas, and the organisms may circulate in peripheral blood more than 1 year following exposure. Foxhounds infected with *Leishmania* species have been found in 18 US states and two Canadian provinces, but transmission has not extended to humans.

Following reports of *L. tropica*–related viscerotropic leishmaniasis in veterans of Operation Desert Storm, between August 1990 and December 1992, those serving in that theater of operations were deferred from blood donation for 1 year. The deferral period reflected the development of fever, malaise, abdominal pain, and intermittent diarrhea up to 7 months after return to the United States. *L. tropica* was found in the bone marrow of seven patients and in the lymph nodes in one. When intracellular amastigotes were seen in the peripheral blood of the one patient in whom this was studied following reports of cutaneous and visceral leishmaniasis among troops involved in the Afghanistan and Iraq wars, a similar 1-year deferral following departure from Iraq and Afghanistan was implemented. The military continues to enforce lifetime deferral for any clinical history of *Leishmania* infection.

The possibility of transmission to humans during military deployment and travel and the large number of military personnel returning from Iraq and Afghanistan raise concerns about future transfusion transmission. To date, there are no cases of transfusion-transmitted leishmaniasis in the United States. The widespread use of leukoreduction filters likely has a beneficial role because these filters reduce both intracellular and extracellular parasite concentrations by 3 to 4 logs.

Toxoplasmosis

Toxoplasmosis is caused by the obligate intracellular protozoan parasite *Toxoplasma gondii*, whose usual host is the domestic cat. The parasite is transmitted by exposure to cat feces, by eating raw or undercooked pork, goat, lamb, beef, or wild game, and congenitally. In the NHANES from 1999–2004, 24.8% of foreign-born US residents age 12 to 49 years of age, compared with 8.2% of US–born residents, had serologic evidence of infection; approximately 50% of those with antibody harbor parasites in tissue. Transfusion-associated disease has been described in immunocompromised patients receiving granulocyte concentrates from donors with chronic myelocytic leukemia who would not qualify as blood donors currently. One possible transfusion-related case involves a platelet transfusion. Red cells and frozen plasma transmission have not been reported.

Chagas Disease

The protozoan parasite *Trypanosoma cruzi* causes Chagas disease. The infection is widespread in Latin America; approximately 8 to 10 million people are affected. Humans become infected when bitten by *Trypanosoma cruzi*–infected insects of the Reduviidae family (triatomine, assassin, kissing, or chinch bugs). Congenital transmission from mother to fetus, organ transplantation, blood transfusion, and ingestion are recognized routes as well. Once infection occurs, low-level, intermittently detectable parasitemia usually persists for life. Treatment with benznidazole or nifurtimox can reduce the risk for chronic sequelae, but neither of these drugs is FDA approved and access to only one of these is through an IND with the CDC. Treatment is most effective during the acute stage of infection. At least 18 mammalian species in the United States serve as reservoirs, including armadillos, opossums, and raccoons, and vectors are present in the lower two-thirds of the country, but autochthonous vector transmission is rare but has been increasingly reported especially in rural areas of Texas. CDC estimates at least 20 states have had isolation of the insect vector and 17 states with the mammalian reservoir. An estimated 300,000 people in the United States and Canada are estimated to be infected with *T. cruzi*; most are immigrants from Latin America. *T. cruzi* organisms remain viable in whole blood stored at refrigerator temperatures for 18 days, for longer than 8 months in citrated blood samples stored at room temperature, and following freezing and thawing. In South America, early data suggested that approximately 13% to 49% of recipients of fresh whole blood from parasitemic donors become infected. There has been concern that additional transfusion-associated Chagas disease cases will occur as immigration increases to the United States from Central and South America.

American trypanosomiasis, or Chagas disease, consists of an acute phase that varies from asymptomatic to manifestations that include fever, skin rash, and conjunctivitis with edema around the eyelids, lymphadenopathy, and hepatosplenomegaly. The acute phase usually resolves in 4 to 8 weeks unless severe myocarditis or meningoencephalitis intervenes. The latter is associated with fatal outcomes. Intracellular *T. cruzi* amastigotes remain in cardiac and skeletal muscle following the acute phase. Following an indeterminate stage of undetermined duration, chronic disease occurs in 20% to 30% of infected patients, manifesting as cardiac disease (initially conduction and left ventricular wall abnormalities), megacolon, or achalasia. Diagnosis is made on clinical and serologic grounds most often. Xenodiagnosis, hemoculture, and nucleic acid amplification tests are also available.

Risk factors for transfusion-transmitted *T. cruzi* infection include birth or residence in endemic regions such as Central America, South America, or Southeastern Mexico; living in dwellings with palm leaf–thatched roofs or mud walls, where vector insects reside; oral intake of contaminated foodstuffs; and receipt of unscreened blood transfusions in Latin America. Among donors who lived in poor housing or received a blood transfusion in endemic areas, 3% to 4% had *T. cruzi* antibodies. One study, conducted in California in the 1990s, found that 1 per 340 blood donors had a risk factor for Chagas disease. A large survey conducted from 1994 to 1998 in Los Angeles and Miami among immigrant blood donors from endemic areas found *T. cruzi* seroprevalence rates of 1 per 7500 and 1 per 9000, respectively. However, none of the 18 recipients in this survey who received blood from a seropositive donor, and who were available for testing, had evidence of infection.

A look-back study involving blood donations in Mexico made before determining the donors were *T. cruzi*–seropositive, found four of nine recipients of subsequently determined seropositive whole blood or platelets to be seropositive.

Since 1987, 30 years before testing started in the United States and Canada, seven cases of transfusion-associated Chagas disease were reported in those countries; symptoms developed 2 to 3 months after transfusion. In six cases, platelets were the implicated component; and the unit in the seventh case was not identified. In each of the six cases, the implicated donor emigrated from a *T. cruzi*–endemic region (Bolivia, Mexico, Paraguay, and Chile) between 16 and 33 years before the implicated donation. *T. cruzi* may separate with platelets, or room-temperature storage may favor parasite survival. In addition, acute Chagas disease has been reported in organ transplant recipients. More recently, two transfusion-related infections were identified in the United States as a result of recipient tracing (look-back) studies (but these represented fewer than 1% of all studied individuals exposed to transfusion of blood from infected donors; see later). Additional transfusion-associated cases have been reported from Spain, all derived from donors who had emigrated from South America for a total of 20 cases ever documented when combining all reported transfusion-associated cases from the United States, Canada and Spain, the countries with the highest immigration rates from Latin America.[72]

The assumed increasing prevalence of *T. cruzi*–infected blood donors with immigration into the United States from Latin America, the reports of transfusion-associated cases, and some autochthonous infections triggered efforts to mitigate the risk for transfusion-transmitted Chagas disease in the United States. Questioning donors about region of birth or extended stay and transfusion in Chagas-endemic areas could interdict 75% of infected donors but would result in deferral of large numbers of noninfected donors. Leukoreduction decreases *T. cruzi* transmission in a mouse model by 50% to 70%, consistent with *Leishmania* and the rickettsia *Anaplasma*. Pathogen-reduction techniques successfully decrease *T. cruzi* viability in plasma and cellular products.

Serologic screening, used for many years in Latin America, was chosen as the preferred strategy for the United States. The first serologic test for screening blood donors, based on a *T. cruzi* whole-parasite lysate, achieved FDA licensure in December 2006, and voluntary screening commenced in early 2007. Approximately 1 per 30,000 donations showed confirmed reactive serologic results, a lower prevalence than estimated. In 2010 the FDA licensed a second assay that uses chimeric recombinant antigens and in 2011, a licensed supplemental test using the same antigen constructs was FDA licensed. Seropositive donors are overwhelmingly immigrants from *T. cruzi*–endemic countries with asymptomatic chronic infections, although a small number of seropositive donors may have acquired the infection in the United States via vertical transmission from infected immigrant mothers, or very rarely by autochthonous vectorial transmission. From the investigation of antibody-positive donors lacking any immigration or maternal risk factors, autochthonous transmission has been estimated to occur at the rate of 1 per 354,000 donors.[73]

Look-back studies involving recipients of prior donations from those found positive for *T. cruzi* antibodies on a subsequent donation showed rates of transfusion transmission much lower than predicted. Only two occurred (0.8%), both from the same apheresis platelet donor born in Argentina, among 253 recipients tested. In light of these findings, testing donors is now required only once rather that at each donation.[74] Concern that those tested once might contract *T. cruzi* during travel or within the United States seems unfounded in that no seroconversions have been observed in more than 4 million blood donors during 6 million person-years of follow up. The unexpectedly low rate of transmission may relate to differences in blood component processing and storage in the United States compared with Latin America (absence of the transfusion of fresh whole blood), some underrepresentation of platelet donors in the look backs completed to date, or other biases. Although all donors are asked a question about having a history of Chagas disease, with the advent of sensitive testing, the question has no residual value and has been removed from the donor history questionnaire according to FDA rules.[75]

TRANSMISSIBLE SPONGIFORM ENCEPHALOPATHIES

The transmissible TSEs (prion diseases) are rare, lethal neurodegenerative diseases generally accepted to be caused by nucleic acid–free proteins called PrP^TSE, as distinguished from the normal cellular protein, PrP^C. The existence of additional factors has not been excluded, but current consensus supports the involvement of infectious proteins. PrP^TSE is an abnormal conformation of PrP^C that induces transformation (recruitment) of additional PrP^C to PrP^TSE, resulting in deposits of insoluble aggregates in central nervous system tissue followed by progressive dementia and other characteristic neurologic findings. Classic Creutzfeldt-Jakob disease (CJD) is diagnosed at a rate of approximately one case per million population per year worldwide. It occurs as sporadic CJD, vertically transmitted familial diseases caused by germline mutations in the human *PRNP* gene (e.g., fatal familial insomnia and Gerstmann-Sträussler-Scheinker syndrome), iatrogenically transmitted infection (e.g., from dura mater implantation, contaminated surgical equipment, injection of human pituitary-derived growth hormone, or corneal transplant) and can be spread horizontally (Kuru associated with consumption of human brain during ritual cannibalism is of historical interest).

There are no documented cases of transfusion transmission of sporadic CJD, the familial or iatrogenic forms, and cohort studies of intensively transfused patient groups have failed to establish any epidemiologic association in both the United Kingdom and the United States.[22,76] In an ongoing look-back effort, no cases of CJD have been observed among 461 recipients (of whom 85 were still alive as of December 31, 2008) of blood components from 40 donors subsequently diagnosed with CJD. A case-control study of CJD patients, compared with control patients with CJD ruled out, found a fivefold increased risk for CJD with a history of transfusion more than 10 years before TSE onset, but the authors recognized critical sources of bias in their methods and their findings are unconfirmed. Nevertheless, as a result of the iatrogenic transmissions and long incubation period of the disease (as demonstrated in growth hormone transmissions), concern arose in the mid-1990s that CJD transmission could occur from asymptomatic donors to transfusion or derivative recipients. This theoretical risk resulted in lifetime donor deferral requirements for iatrogenic exposure to or a family history of classic CJD.

Like classic CJD, vCJD is a fatal, degenerative neurologic disease. It occurs in younger patients than classic CJD and has distinctive clinical, radiographic, histopathologic, and biochemical features. The first reports of vCJD from the United Kingdom were published in 1996. The etiologic agent is the same prion that causes BSE or "mad cow disease." Transmission of the BSE prion to humans occurred by consumption of beef and other bovine products containing infectious neural or reticuloendothelial tissue. In the United Kingdom the vCJD epidemic followed a massive epidemic of BSE in the 1980s and 1990s. The latter was traced to the recycling of material from dead sheep and cattle (offal) into feed for cattle. This practice was banned in 1988, and the vCJD outbreak subsided after a peak of 28 cases in 2000. The number of new vCJD diagnoses in the United Kingdom rose steadily in the first few years after 1995 from 3 in 1995 to 28 in 2000, but decreased since then to 5, 5, 5, 1, 3, 3, and 2 from 2005 to July 2011, by which time 175 (172 deaths, 3 living) definite or probable cases of vCJD had been reported in the United Kingdom. An additional 49 cases have been diagnosed elsewhere, mostly in France and several other European countries. A few cases have been identified outside Europe, including 3 cases in the United States (2 associated with exposure in the United Kingdom and 1 in Saudi Arabia), 2 from Canada, and 1 each from Japan, Taiwan, and Saudi Arabia. Most but not all of the patients with non-European cases had more than 6 months' exposure in the United Kingdom during the BSE epidemic. Although it appears that the vCJD outbreak is waning (and is much smaller than initially feared), concern persists that there could be a second wave of the epidemic caused by delayed onset of the disease in infected individuals. This is based in part on observations of abnormal prion protein accumulation in random surgical tissue samples in the United Kingdom, which may represent preclinical vCJD disease. In one retrospective study, 3 of 12,674 appendectomy and tonsillectomy specimens from persons 20 to 29 years of age were positive. Furthermore, a critical polymorphism at codon 129 of the PrP^C gene coding for methionine or valine leads to variation in the susceptibility to and incubation period of human TSEs. All of the clinical cases reported to date are methionine homozygotes. Because only 37% of the general British population is homozygous for methionine, and are maximally susceptible to vCJD, a larger population (52%) of heterozygotes and valine homozygotes (11%) may be at risk for asymptomatic infection in a prolonged incubation period.

Four transfusion-transmitted infections with the vCJD prion have been reported in the United Kingdom. Although they may have developed vCJD independent of transfusion, this possibility is regarded highly unlikely based on epidemiologic and statistic considerations. Three of the four cases were diagnosed with clinical vCJD 6.5, 7.8, and 9 years after receiving nonleukocyte reduced RBCs or a blood component from two different donors who developed clinical symptoms of vCJD 40 and 21 months after donating. These three with symptomatic disease were homozygous for methionine at codon 129. The fourth case was heterozygous (methionine/valine) and had no clinical signs or symptoms of vCJD at death from unrelated causes, but had abnormal prion protein aggregates in lymphoid (but not neural) tissues at autopsy and was considered to have preclinical infection. Five years before death the recipient received nonleukocyte reduced RBCs from a donor who developed clinical vCJD 18 months after donating. These four cases represent 6% of the 67 UK recipients who received blood components from 18 different donors subsequently diagnosed with vCJD (and an estimated 23% of exposed methionine homozygotes). In light of these cases and animal transfusion experiments, TSE transmission and disease from transfusion is no longer regarded as a theoretical event.[22] A single case reports a potential epidemiologic link between exposure to plasma derivatives and transmission of the agent to a recipient.

Prion-removal strategies (e.g., affinity filters) remain under evaluation, especially in the United Kingdom, but none is expected to be suitable for consideration for use in the United States in the immediate future. There are currently no blood donor–screening tests for vCJD, leaving risk mitigation dependent on removal of donors that could have asymptomatic infection. Initially, primarily on the basis of the prominent distribution of vCJD prion in reticuloendothelial tissue compared with classic prion protein (PrP^C,), on subsequent reports of animal and human infection by transfusion, and then on the early observation that nearly all cases of vCJD were associated with potential exposure in the United Kingdom or to UK bovine products, the FDA adopted and has modified donor-deferral policies sequentially since 1999.[77] The first called for indefinite deferral of donors who had spent more than 6 months in the United Kingdom from 1980 to 1996, before control of the food chain and of recipients of bovine insulin from the UK. Models predicted that this would remove approximately 90% of the risk at a "cost" of deferring approximately 5% of otherwise eligible donors. These were subsequently expanded to include US military personnel and their dependents who spent certain durations on bases in the European Union where UK beef was imported during the BSE epidemic and recipients of transfusions in the United Kingdom and France during the peak risk periods of their BSE epidemics. Experience at US blood centers has largely confirmed the donor loss predictions of the FDA models.

Chronic wasting disease (CWD) of deer and elk is prevalent at rates as high as 15% in cervid populations in multiple areas of the United States and Canada. Concern has been expressed that, given the popularity of hunting, there may be risk for exposure to and infection with the CWD prion during handling or consumption of infected animals. Apparent clusters of classic CJD in hunters have been alleged, but on full evaluation have not been shown to have a relationship to the CWD agent. There is currently no plan to intervene for this theoretical risk in hunters who donate blood beyond hygienic measures when handling cervids or their tissues.

FUTURE DIRECTIONS

The residual risk for transmitting HIV, HBV, and HCV is less than 1 per million units transfused, an extremely low rate. In contrast, platelet septic events are reported at a frequency of 1 per 100,000 units. Transmission of known, emerging infectious agents such as dengue, Zika virus, *B. microti*, and those currently unrecognized remain problematic. Continued safety of the blood supply requires constant vigilance, early detection, reporting of untoward events, and excellent communication and cooperation between those providing blood components and those prescribing them.

SUGGESTED READINGS

Aubuchon JP, Prowse CV, editors: *Pathogen inactivation: the penultimate paradigm shift*, Bethesda MD, 2010. AABB Press.

Bennett JL, Blajchman MA, Delage G, et al: Proceedings of a consensus conference: risk-based decision making for blood safety. *Transfus Med Rev* 25:267, 2011.

Berg MG, Lee D, Coller K, et al: Discovery of a novel human pegivirus in blood associated with hepatitis C virus co-infection. *PLoS Pathog* 11:e1005325, 2015.

Brennan CA, Yamaguchi J, Devare SG, et al: Expanded evaluation of blood donors in the United States for human immunodeficiency virus type 1 non-B subtypes and antiretroviral drug-resistant strains: 2005 through 2007. *Transfusion* 50:2707, 2010.

Busch MP: Cooley Award Lecture. Transfusion-transmitted viral infections: building bridges to transfusion medicine to reduce risks and understand epidemiology and pathogenesis. *Transfusion* 46:1624, 2006.

Centers for Disease Control and Prevention and Association of Public Health Laboratories: *Laboratory Testing for the Diagnosis of HIV Infection: Updated Recommendations*. Available at http://dx.doi.org/10.15620/cdc.23447. Published June 27, 2014. Accessed 31.01.16.

Centers for Disease Control and Prevention: HIV transmission through transfusion—Missouri and Colorado, 2008. *MMWR* 59:1335, 2010.

Custer B, Kessler D, Vahidnia F, et al: For the NHLBI Retrovirus Epidemiology Donor Study-II (REDS-II) Risk factors for retrovirus and hepatitis virus infections in accepted blood donors. *Transfusion* 55:1098–1107, 2014.

FDA Final Rule: Docket No FDA-2006N-0040. *Fed Regist* 80(99):29842–29906, 2015.

Hewitt PE, Ijaz S, Brailsford SR, et al: Hepatitis E virus in blood components: a prevalence and transmission study in southeast England. *Lancet* 384:1766–1773, 2014.

Jackson BR, Busch MP, Stramer SL, et al: The cost-effectiveness of NAT for HIV, HCV, and HBV in whole-blood donations. *Transfusion* 43:721, 2003.

Kleinman SH, Lelie N, Busch MP: Infectivity of human immunodeficiency virus-1, hepatitis C virus, and hepatitis B virus and risk of transmission by transfusion. *Transfusion* 49:2454–2489, 2009.

Kleinman Steven, Cameron C, Custer B, et al: Modeling the risk of an emerging pathogen entering the Canadian blood supply. *Transfusion* 50:2592, 2010.

Laperche S, Nübling CM, Stramer SL, et al: Sensitivity of hepatitis C virus core antigen and antibody combination assays in a global panel of window period samples. *Transfusion* 55:2489–2498, 2015.

Murphy EL, Glynn SA, Fridey J, et al: Increased prevalence of infectious diseases and other adverse outcomes in human T lymphotropic virus types I- and II-infected blood donors. Retrovirus Epidemiology Donor Study (REDS) Study Group. *J Infect Dis* 176:1468, 1997.

Orton SL, Stramer SL, Dodd RY, et al: Risk factors for HCV infection among blood donors confirmed to be positive for the presence of HCV RNA and not reactive for the presence of anti-HCV. *Transfusion* 44:275–281, 2004.

Petrik J, Lozano M, Seed CR, et al: Hepatitis E. *Vox Sang* 110:93–103, 2016.

Seed CR, Kiely P, Law M, et al: No evidence of a significantly increased risk of transfusion-transmitted human immunodeficiency virus infection in Australia subsequent to implementing a 12-month deferral for men who have had sex with men. *Transfusion* 50:2722, 2010.

Seghatchian J, Hervig T, Putter JS: Effect of pathogen inactivation on the storage lesion in red cells and platelet concentrates. *Transfus Apher Sci* 45:75, 2011.

Snyder EL, Stramer SL, Benjamin RJ: The safety of the blood supply – time to raise the bar. *N Engl J Med* 372:1882–1885, 2015.

Stramer SL, Dodd RY, Brodsky JP: The value of screening signal-to-cutoff ratios for hepatitis C virus antibody confirmation. *Transfusion* 53:1497–1500, 2013.

Stramer SL, Moritz ED, Foster GA, et al: Hepatitis E virus: seroprevalence and frequency of viral RNA detection among U.S. blood donors. *Transfusion* 56:481–488, 2016.

Stramer SL, Notari EP, Krysztof DE, et al: Hepatitis B virus testing by minipool nucleic acid testing: does it improve blood safety? *Transfusion* 53:2449–2458, 2013.

Stramer SL, Wend U, Candotti D, et al: Nucleic acid testing to detect HBV infection in blood donors. *N Engl J Med* 364:236–247, 2011.

Taira R, Satake M, Momose S, et al: Residual risk of transfusion-transmitted hepatitis B virus (HBV) infection caused by blood components derived from donors with occult HBV infection in Japan. *Transfusion* 1393–1404, 2013.

Urwin PJM, Mackenzie JM, Llewelyn CA, et al: Creutzfeldt–Jakob disease and blood transfusion: updated results of the UK Transfusion Medicine Epidemiology Review Study. *Vox Sang* 110:310–316, 2016.

Vamvakas EC: Is white blood cell reduction equivalent to antibody screening in preventing transmission of cytomegalovirus by transfusion? A review of the literature and meta-analysis. *Transfus Med Rev* 19:181, 2005.

Xiang J, Wunschmann S, Diekema DJ, et al: Effect of coinfection with GB virus C on survival among patients with HIV infection. *N Engl J Med* 345:704, 2001.

Zou S, Dorsey KA, Notari EP, et al: Prevalence, incidence, and residual risk of human immunodeficiency virus and hepatitis C virus infections among United States blood donors since the introduction of nucleic acid testing. *Transfusion* 50:1495–1504, 2010.

Zou S, Stramer SL, Notari EP, et al: Current incidence and residual risk of hepatitis B infection among blood donors in the United States. *Transfusion* 49:1609–1620, 2009.

REFERENCES

For the complete list of references, log on to www.expertconsult.com.

CHAPTER 121

PEDIATRIC TRANSFUSION MEDICINE

Cassandra D. Josephson and Steven R. Sloan

A variety of neonatal and pediatric patients require blood component transfusions. This chapter focuses on aspects of blood-bank laboratory testing, blood products and components, transfusion indications, and potential adverse events that are specifically relevant to neonates and children.

PEDIATRIC BLOOD BANKING

Blood and Blood Components

Several different blood components, including whole blood, reconstituted whole blood, red blood cells (RBCs), platelets, plasma, and cryoprecipitated antihemophilic factor (CRYO) may be available from a blood bank for transfusion. Recently, additional components have become available in the United States. They are photochemically-treated INTERCEPT platelets and plasma, and solvent detergent–treated plasma, Octaplas. The availability of specific component types varies between blood suppliers.

- Whole blood is infrequently used and may not be available from a particular blood bank or blood supplier, but it may be available on request and is used by some pediatric cardiac surgery services. Whole blood contains all RBCs, plasma, platelets, and an anticoagulant preservative solution containing citrate, phosphate, dextrose, and possibly adenine.
- RBC units mostly contain RBCs but also contain some plasma and a preservative solution. Most RBC units contain an additive preservative solution that includes some combination of adenine, dextrose, and mannitol. Additive solutions are safe for relatively small ($\leq$20 mL/kg) transfusions. There are concerns over the safety of these additives given in large transfusions to neonates, and their safety in this setting has never been proven in a randomized clinical trial. In view of this concern, some hospital blood banks provide nonadditive RBC units or wash additive units intended for large transfusions to neonates. Because many blood centers provide only additive RBC units to hospital blood banks and washing an RBC unit takes approximately 1 hour, blood banks have been unable to supply RBC units without additives in many situations. Thus many institutions now have significant experience transfusing large volumes of additive RBC units to neonates and have not noticed any problems.
- Two general types of platelet units are available in the United States, although any one blood bank or hospital may stock only one of these types. These two types, whole blood–derived platelets (platelets) and platelets collected by apheresis (pheresis platelets), differ in their size. A platelet unit contains approximately 5.5 to 10×10^{10} platelets in about 50 mL, whereas a pheresis platelet unit contains at least 3×10^{11} platelets in about 200 mL. It is often easier to use platelet units for small children because pheresis platelets usually need to be aliquoted to provide the correct dose. However, many blood centers exclusively provide only one type of platelet component. Recently, two modifications of platelet components were approved in the United States, although these had been in use in other countries for several years.
  - Platelets that have undergone pathogen inactivation using the INTERCEPT Blood System (Cerus Corporation, Concord, CA) which mixes amotosalen HCl, a synthetic psoralen

compound that intercalates with nucleic acid and, on activation with ultraviolet (UV) light, cross-links pathogen and white blood cell DNA, inhibiting replication.[1] Almost all of the amotosalen, a potential carcinogen, is removed during processing. However, INTERCEPT platelets are contraindicated for neonatal patients treated with phototherapy devices emitting wavelengths <425 nm due to potential erythema from interaction between UV light and amotosalen.
  - Platelets stored in a Platelet Additive Solution (PAS). PAS platelets contain very little plasma, which reduces the risk of allergic reactions and transfusion-related acute lung injury (TRALI), but also lowers the dose of coagulation factors contained in the platelet component.
- Plasma is frozen to retain functional plasma proteins including clotting factors. Depending on the timing of freezing and thawing, the component may be called fresh frozen plasma (FFP) or another name. However, all of these plasma components contain all the necessary clotting factors. Two pathogen-inactivated plasma products, that had been available in several countries, are now available in the United States:
  - INTERCEPT(Cerus Corporation, Concord, CA) treated plasma using the same system as described above.
  - Octaplas (Octapharma, Hoboken, NJ) is a filtered pooled plasma product that is subjected to solvent/detergent treatment to inactivate lipid-enveloped viruses.[2] Its safety and efficacy in pediatric patients has not been evaluated which would be important in neonates whose coagulation system regulation differs from adults. Specifically, Octaplas contains low concentrations of protein S and α2-antiplasmin, two inhibitors of the coagulation system that are present in low concentrations in neonates.[3,4]
- Cryoprecipitate is prepared from plasma and contains high concentrations of fibrinogen.
- Because pediatric patients require smaller doses of blood components, they often require only a portion of a component.
- RBCs are stored refrigerated and hence can be prepared in aliquots as needed if the blood bank has the necessary equipment. Alternatively the blood center can collect RBC units into a collection system in which additional bags are attached for dispensing aliquots. Whole blood is also stored refrigerated, but its use is very limited and it is almost never prepared in aliquots.
- All platelet components are stored at room temperature under constant agitation and can be prepared in aliquots when needed in the blood bank if the blood bank has the necessary equipment and supplies. However, 1 unit of whole blood–derived platelets does not contain many doses, even for infants, and most blood banks do not aliquot them.
- All plasma products are stored frozen, and are not generally aliquoted after thawing. However, many blood centers will prepare plasma aliquots before freezing.
- Because even small infants rarely require less than 1 unit of cryoprecipitate, this component is rarely prepared in aliquots.

Directed Donations

Families often prefer to donate blood for their children using a process known as directed donations, and some blood banks permit this. If this is done without medical reason, it offers no benefit and there are potential risks. Although directed donors need to go through the same screening and infectious disease testing process as all allogeneic blood donors, some studies suggest that directed donors have a slightly higher risk for infectious disease transmission.

In addition, directed donors may be a poor choice for immunologic reasons. For example, if a neonate has alloimmune thrombocytopenia or anemia, the pathologic antibody is a passively acquired maternal antibody directed against inherited paternal antigens. In this case, blood donated by the father would be recognized by the antibody in the baby's circulation and cleared just as the neonate's own platelets or erythrocytes are cleared. Another example in which immune concerns make directed donors a poor choice involves transplants. Some patients may require a future tissue or bone marrow transplant, and blood relatives often serve as the best donors for such transplants. However, prior transfusions from relatives may sensitize the patient's immune system to antigens present on the tissues of blood relatives, complicating those potential tissue or bone marrow transplants.

TECHNICAL CONSIDERATIONS/MECHANICAL DEVICES

Smaller pediatric patients require small transfusions administered at slow rates. Aliquots of components often need to be prepared. This can be performed by collecting blood into collection bags interconnected with sterile tubes or by attaching additional containers to a standard blood component by using a sterile docking device that produces a sterile weld between two separate tubing sets.

Blood components must be filtered to remove microaggregates before transfusion. For an adult patient, this is normally accomplished by transfusing the component through a filter contained within the blood administration set. These standard blood administration sets are not ideal for transfusing small patients because 20 to 40 mL of the component is lost in the dead space of the administration set. Pediatric microaggregate filters with much smaller dead space are available.

For nonbleeding patients, blood components are generally transfused at a rate of no more than 5 mL/kg/h. For infants, this corresponds to a lower rate than can be regulated by most standard infusion pumps. Hence these transfusions are usually performed using syringe pumps, with the blood component aliquot being transferred to a syringe for the transfusion. Often the blood bank prepares aliquots of a blood component through a pediatric microaggregate filter directly into a syringe, eliminating the need for bedside microaggregate filtration.

TRANSFUSION MEDICINE: GENERAL INDICATIONS AND DOSING

Indications for RBC Transfusion in Neonates, Children, and Adolescents

Neonates Less Than 4 Months Old

RBC transfusions are more commonly administered to hospitalized neonates than any other pediatric patient age-group, and RBCs are the component most often transfused in this population. Symptomatic anemia is the major indication for simple transfusion and an RBC transfusion should be considered when the venous hemoglobin is less than 13 g/dL in the first 24 hours of life or when a neonate has lost approximately 10% of his/her blood volume. A transfusion dose of 10–15 mL/kg of RBCs should yield an increase in the neonate of 2–3 g/dL of hemoglobin after transfusion.

Two randomized clinical trials of premature infants in neonatal intensive care units, examining restrictive versus liberal RBC transfusion practices, had conflicting results.[5,6] Therefore most guidelines

TABLE 121.1	Guidelines for Transfusion of Red Blood Cells in Infants Less Than 4 Months of Age

1. Hematocrit <20% with low reticulocyte count and symptomatic anemia (tachycardia, tachypnea, poor feeding)
2. Hematocrit <30% and
   a. On <35% oxygen hood, or
   b. On oxygen by nasal cannula, or
   c. On continuous positive airway pressure and/or intermittent mandatory ventilation on mechanical ventilation with mean airway pressure <6 cm of water, or
   d. With significant tachycardia or tachypnea (heart rate >180 beats per minute for 24 hours or respiratory rate >80 breaths per minute for 24 hours)
   e. With significant apnea or bradycardia (more than six episodes in 12 hours or two episodes in 24 hours requiring bag and mask ventilation while receiving therapeutic doses of methylxanthines), or
   f. With slow weight gain (<10 g/day observed over 4 days while receiving >100 kcal/kg/day)
3. Hematocrit <35% and
   a. On >35% oxygen hood, or
   b. On continuous positive airway pressure/intermittent mandatory ventilation with mean airway pressure >6–8 cm of water
4. Hematocrit <45% and
   a. On extracorporeal membrane oxygenation (ECMO), or
   b. With congenital cyanotic heart disease

RBC, Red blood cell.

are based on experience rather than evidence-based medicine (Table 121.1). An ongoing study (http://clinicaltrials.gov/01702805) has the promise of providing definitive evidence to inform RBC transfusion practice in this population.[7] One prospective randomized clinical trial found equivalent clinical outcomes in neonates transfused with fresh RBCs stored for less than 7 days as those transfused with standard-issue RBCs with a mean age of 14.6 days, although some have criticized the generalizability of the study results.[8,9]

Older Infants, Children, and Adolescents

RBC transfusion indications for infants older than 4 months and for young children are similar to those of adults. However, there are several noteworthy differences between children and adults: total blood volume, ability to tolerate blood loss, and age-specific hemoglobin levels (Table 121.2). In infants, RBC transfusions are primarily given for surgical losses, anemia of chronic diseases, and malignancies. Infants inherently have lower hemoglobin levels than adults and remain asymptomatic at lower hemoglobin concentrations, especially if the anemia occurs gradually. Even with these physiologic differences, general transfusion-trigger guidelines for pediatric intensive care unit patients are similar to those for adults, with a transfusion trigger of 7 g/dL of hemoglobin for hemodynamically stable patients being shown to be safe for these patients.[10] This threshold has also been found to be safe for hematopoietic progenitor cell (HPC) transplant patients.[11] The usual dose of RBCs is 10 to 15 mL/kg. There is no evidence that pediatric patients benefit from transfusion of RBCs of a particular age, although it is currently the subject of a multicenter study (http://clinicaltrials.gov/01977547).

Platelets

Platelet transfusion support in pediatric patients is usually intended as a prophylactic strategy to prevent bleeding (Table 121.3). The prophylactic platelet transfusion thresholds in premature infants are

TABLE 121.2	Guidelines for Transfusion of Red Blood Cells in Patients More Than 4 Months of Age

1. Emergency surgical procedure in patient with significant postoperative anemia
2. Preoperative anemia when other corrective therapy is not available
3. Intraoperative blood loss ≥15% total blood volume
4. Hematocrit <2–24%
   a. In perioperative period, with signs and symptoms of anemia
   b. While on chemotherapy/radiotherapy
   c. Chronic congenital or acquired symptomatic anemia
5. Hematocrit <21%, hemodynamically stable patients >3 days old in the pediatric intensive care unit
6. Acute blood loss with hypovolemia not responsive to other therapy
7. Hematocrit <40% and
   a. With severe pulmonary disease
   b. On ECMO
8. Sickle cell disease and
   a. Cerebrovascular accident
   b. Acute chest syndrome
   c. Splenic sequestration
   d. Aplastic crisis
   e. Recurrent priapism
   f. Preoperatively when general anesthesia is planned (target hemoglobin 10 mg/dL)
9. Chronic transfusion programs for disorders of RBC production (e.g., β-thalassemia major and Diamond-Blackfan syndrome unresponsive to therapy)

ECMO, Extracorporeal membrane oxygenation; RBC, red blood cell.

TABLE 121.3	Guidelines for Transfusion of Platelets in Neonates and Older Children

Platelet Count <150,000/μL

1. Platelet count 5000–10,000/μL with failure of platelet production
2. Platelet count <30,000/μL in neonate with failure of platelet production
3. Platelet count <50,000/μL in stable premature infant
   a. With active bleeding, or
   b. Before an invasive procedure with failure of platelet production
4. Platelet count <100,000/μL in sick premature infant
   a. With active bleeding, or
   b. Before an invasive procedure in patient with DIC

Without Thrombocytopenia

1. Active bleeding with qualitative platelet defect
2. Unexplained excessive bleeding during cardiopulmonary bypass
3. Patient receiving ECMO with
   a. Platelet count <100,000/μL
   b. Higher platelet counts and bleeding

DIC, Disseminated intravascular coagulation; ECMO, extracorporeal membrane oxygenation.
Modified from Roseff SD, Luban NLC, Manno CS. Guidelines for assessing appropriateness of pediatric transfusion. *Transfusion* 42:1398, 2002 and Wong CC, Luban NLC: Intrauterine, neonatal, and pediatric transfusion. In: Mintz PD, editor: *Transfusion therapy: Clinical principles and practice,* ed 2. Bethesda, MD, 2005, AABB Press, p 159.

TABLE 121.4	Guidelines for Transfusion of Frozen Plasma and Cryoprecipitate in Neonates and Older Children

Frozen Plasma

1. Support during treatment of DIC
2. Replacement therapy
   a. When specific factor concentrates are not available, including but not limited to, antithrombin, protein C or S deficiency, and factor II, factor V, factor X, and factor XI deficiencies
   b. During therapeutic plasma exchange when FFP is indicated (cryoprecipitate-poor plasma, plasma from which the cryoprecipitate has been removed)
3. Reversal of warfarin in an emergency situation, such as before an invasive procedure with active bleeding
   Note: Frozen plasma is not indicated for volume expansion or enhancement of wound healing

Cryoprecipitate

1. Hypofibrinogenemia or dysfibrinogenemia with active bleeding
2. Hypofibrinogenemia or dysfibrinogenemia, undergoing an invasive procedure
3. Factor XIII deficiency with active bleeding or undergoing an invasive procedure in the absence of factor XIII concentrate
4. Limited directed-donor cryoprecipitate for bleeding episodes in small children with hemophilia A (when recombinant and plasma-derived factor VIII products are not available)
5. In the preparation of fibrin sealant
6. von Willebrand disease with active bleeding: Cryoprecipitate is used in von Willebrand disease only when both of the following are true:
   a. 1-Deamino-8-D-arginine vasopressin is contraindicated, not available, or does not elicit response
   b. Virus-inactivated plasma-derived factor VIII concentrate (which contains von Willebrand factor) is not available

DIC, Disseminated intravascular coagulation; FFP, fresh frozen plasma.

quite controversial and based primarily on expert consensus rather than evidence-based medicine. In sharp contrast to adults, who rarely develop spontaneous severe bleeding until their platelet counts fall below 10,000/μL, preterm infants with other complicating illnesses may bleed at higher platelet counts. The increased risk may be secondary to (1) lower levels of plasma coagulation factors, (2) natural anticoagulants that potentiate thrombin inhibition, (3) intrinsic or extrinsic platelet dysfunction, and (4) increased vascular fragility. Platelet counts and function in older children are similar to those of adults, and the indications for platelet transfusions do not differ from the indications for adults.

Frozen Plasma and Cryoprecipitate

Frozen plasma is used in preterm and term infants most commonly to treat multiple factor deficiencies or vitamin K deficiency, a condition that can occur in infants not prophylactically given vitamin K after birth, especially if the mother ingested certain drugs during pregnancy such as warfarin, cephalosporins, or some anticonvulsants (Table 121.4). Dosing for all pediatric patients is 10 to 15 mL/kg. This should result in an increase in all factor activity of 15% to 20% unless there is a marked consumptive coagulopathy. As mentioned previously, solvent detergent–treated plasma, Octaplas, may not be safe for neonates as it has low concentrations of protein S and α2-antiplasmin.

Cryoprecipitate is used primarily to treat disorders resulting from a decrease in or dysfunction of fibrinogen or factor XIII deficiency. These indications are similar to those for adults. Children should receive 1 to 2 units of CRYO/10 kg patient weight. One unit or less of cryoprecipitate is usually sufficient to achieve hemostatic levels in infants and premature infants. The expected rise in fibrinogen should be 60 to 100 mg/dL.

Granulocytes

Granulocytes, whose efficacy, especially at low doses, is unproven, may be indicated for neutropenic children with infections unresponsive to standard antimicrobial therapy.[12] In addition, children with granulocyte dysfunction (e.g., chronic granulomatous disease [CGD]) severe infections may also benefit from granulocyte transfusions.

However, patients with CGD are at significant risk for developing anti-HLA antibodies from granulocyte transfusions, which can render granulocyte transfusions ineffective and can complicate possible future hematopoietic cell transplants.[13]

TRANSFUSION MEDICINE: INDICATIONS IN UNIQUE PEDIATRIC POPULATIONS

Hemolytic Disease of the Fetus and Newborn

Hemolytic disease of the fetus and newborn (HDFN) occurs when the mother's immune system recognizes a foreign, paternally inherited antigen on fetal erythrocytes. The incidence of HDFN dramatically declined after the introduction of Rh immune globulin to prevent sensitization of the mother to RhD. Although introduction of Rh immune globulin has prevented most cases of HDFN due to RhD sensitization, it has not totally eliminated HDFN due to RhD or reduced HDFN due to other antibodies.

Most significant cases of HDFN are due to antibodies recognizing antigens other than ABO system antigens. These antibodies should be detected in the blood-bank antibody screen of the blood specimen of the pregnant or postpartum woman. Also necessary for diagnosis, the corresponding antigens would be present on fetal or newborn erythrocytes, or predicted to be present on fetal erythrocytes based on molecular testing of fetal DNA. The direct antiglobulin test (DAT) of the fetal or newborn's erythrocytes is usually positive, although it can be negative in transfused patients. Although antibody titers can be used to help predict the severity of the disease during pregnancy, they are generally not useful in the newborn. After birth, the severity of the anemia and the resulting hyperbilirubinemia serve as markers for the severity of HDFN. Rates of rise in bilirubin level are most helpful in determining whether an exchange transfusion will be necessary, with increases of 8 to 13 μmol/L/h despite phototherapy indicating that exchange transfusion will likely be necessary.[14]

RBCs transfused in utero to the fetus need to be compatible with the ABO type of the fetus and mother and hence are usually blood group O. They need to lack the antigen(s) to which the mother has made antibodies, and they need to be crossmatch compatible with her serum. The RBCs should be irradiated to prevent transfusion-associated graft-versus-host disease (TA-GVHD), and cytomegalovirus (CMV) safe to minimize the risk for transfusion-transmitted CMV. Relatively fresh RBCs also are usually chosen for these transfusions.

Reconstituted whole blood is usually used for neonatal exchange transfusions. The blood is prepared by removing most of the preservative solution from an RBC unit and adding plasma, usually so that the final hematocrit is 40% to 45%.

Neonatal Alloimmune Thrombocytopenia

The pathophysiology of neonatal alloimmune thrombocytopenia (NAIT) is similar to that of HDFN in that both involve immune-mediated attack and destruction of fetal and neonatal blood cells by the mother's immune system. Unlike HDFN, NAIT often affects a woman's first pregnancy. In addition, the antigens involved are due to polymorphisms on platelet-specific proteins. Although a variety of antigens can be implicated, the human platelet antigen-1 (HPA-1) protein is most frequently implicated in whites, with approximately 70% to 80% of cases being due to women who lack the HPA-1a antigen making antibodies against HPA-1a that is expressed on fetal platelets.[15] When NAIT is suspected, maternal serum can be tested for antibodies to platelet antigens, and the parent's or patient's platelet antigens can be determined by molecular means in which their platelet antigens are indirectly determined from their DNA. An affected infant or fetus may require platelet transfusions. Although random platelets may be of some transient benefit, antigen-negative units are best. Maternal platelets lack the antigen, but because the plasma contains the pathogenic antibody, the platelet unit should be washed before transfusion. Alternatively, antigen-negative units may be available. Indeed, major blood centers usually have HPA-1a-negative units available.

TABLE 121.5 Indications for Extracorporeal Membrane Oxygenation for Neonates and Pediatric Patients

Neonatal
Meconium aspiration
Respiratory distress syndrome
Persistent pulmonary hypertension
Congenital diaphragmatic hernia
Sepsis

Pediatric
Bacterial pneumonia
Viral pneumonia
Acute respiratory distress syndrome
Burns
Inhalation injuries
Near drowning
Sepsis

Extracorporeal Membrane Oxygenation

Extracorporeal membrane oxygenation (ECMO) is an intervention in which whole blood is removed from the patient's venous circulation and circulated through a machine to remove carbon dioxide and replenish oxygen before being returned to the patient. This prolonged intervention is reserved for patients with more than 80% mortality risk and those who have been unresponsive to conventional ventilator support and medical treatment but still potentially can recover. In neonates and children, ECMO has become a lifesaving therapy in the treatment of multiple disorders; Table 121.5[16] lists indications for ECMO support in neonates and children. Standardized guidelines for transfusion practice have not been established, resulting in individualized centers establishing their own criteria. In order to prevent thrombosis and platelet activation in the extracorporeal circuit which is comprised of extensive tubing, patients are anticoagulated, usually with heparin, resulting in a significant risk of bleeding.[17] Bleeding during ECMO is a common complication and may be caused by any of the following factors necessary for operating the ECMO circuit or resulting from the thrombogenic surface of the circuit: (1) systemic heparinization, (2) platelet dysfunction, (3) thrombocytopenia, (4) other coagulation defects, and (5) nonendothelial cell surface lining the circuitry. It is recommended that hospital transfusion services and ECMO staff be in close communication to agree on local protocols to ensure safe, efficient, and consistent care (Table 121.6 provides an example protocol from one institution).[16] Blood products for ECMO are typically ABO and Rh specific and crossmatch compatible for priming. The RBC units for priming circuits are typically relatively fresh, irradiated, and CMV seronegative and/or leukoreduced.

Trauma

Hemorrhagic shock requiring massive transfusion can occur in children. Prothrombin time (PT), activated partial thromboplastin time (aPTT), and platelet count abnormalities upon emergency room admission are strongly associated with mortality.[18] Transfusion management of a pediatric trauma patient often must be guided by the patient's estimated blood loss and associated signs and symptoms, such as hypotension or tachycardia, and bleeding. A prospective study found that a ratio of 1:1:1 of RBC to plasma to platelet units transfused did not decrease overall mortality but decreased hemorrhagic deaths in trauma patients.[19] The use of such a massive transfusion strategy has not been rigorously tested in pediatric patients.

TABLE 121.6	Blood Product Protocols for Extracorporeal Membrane Oxygenation				
Clinical Scenario	Urgency	Products	Blood Groups	Storage
Cardiac arrest	5–10 min	2 units RBCs	O-negative RBCs	<14 days, AS
ECMO circuit disruption	5–10 min	2 units RBCs	O-negative RBCs	<14 days, AS
Progressive septic shock, nonneonate	30 min	2 units RBCs	O-negative RBCs or type specific	<10 days, any preservative
Neonate transferred for ECMO	1–2 hr	2 units RBCs 1 unit FFP 1 unit platelets	O-negative RBCs AB plasma	<10 days, CPD or CPDA-1
Cardiac ICU	30–60 min	2 units RBCs	Type specific	<7 days, AS
Gradual respiratory or cardiac failure on conventional support	Hours-days	2 units RBCs	Type specific	<10 days, CPD

AS, Additive solution unit is acceptable; CPD, citrate phosphate dextrose; CPDA-1, citrate phosphate dextrose adenine; ECMO, extracorporeal membrane oxygenation; FFP, fresh frozen plasma; ICU, intensive care unit; RBC, red blood cell.
Modified from protocols developed at The Children's Hospital of Philadelphia. Friedman DF, Montenegro LM: Extracorporeal membrane oxygenation and cardiopulmonary bypass. In: Hillyer CD, Strauss RG, Luban NLC, editors: *Handbook of pediatric transfusion medicine*, London, 2004, Elsevier Academic Press, p 181.

Although some have advocated adopting similar protocols for pediatric trauma centers, this has occurred in only a few places, most likely because there are little data on transfusions in pediatric trauma patients.[20]

Hemoglobinopathies

In patients with sickle cell disease (SCD), chronic transfusion therapy has been shown to reduce the risk for both primary and secondary stroke, by decreasing the hemoglobin S content of the patient's blood, as well as achieving a reduction in sickling, suppression of erythropoiesis, and preventing an increase in blood viscosity.[21,22] The risk for recurrent stroke has been reduced to less than 10% if hemoglobin levels are maintained between 8 and 9 g/dL and hemoglobin S levels below 30%. Simple or partial-exchange transfusion therapy can achieve this goal when performed approximately every 3 to 4 weeks. Chronic erythrocytapheresis has also been used for this therapy with an added mission to mitigate iron overload complications. Chronic transfusion treatment for stroke most times is an indefinite therapy, that is, once the patient is placed on it, cessation is not possible because it has been shown to lead to recurrent stroke.[21] Table 121.2 describes other indications for patients with SCD needing either simple or chronic RBC transfusion therapy. Products for patients with SCD should be screened at a minimum for hemoglobin S and should be leukocyte reduced to reduce the risk for febrile nonhemolytic transfusion reactions and to reduce the risk for human leukocyte antigen (HLA) alloimmunization resulting in platelet refractoriness that can complicate possible stem cell transplantation.

In children with SCD, it also is useful to prevent alloimmunization to minor RBC antibodies because in most children with severe SCD, RBC transfusion is the only therapy available to treat the multiple manifestations of SCD. Overall the SCD patient has higher rates of alloimmunization than other chronically transfused patient groups. The antibodies most frequently produced are against common Rh, Kell, Duffy, and Kidd system antigens. Some sickle cell treatment centers perform thorough phenotype analysis of a patient's red cells before initiating transfusion therapy. This testing helps to reduce the rate of alloimmunization by allowing preferential selection of phenotypically similar units.[23] However, particularly for patients who are not yet alloimmunized, this process remains controversial because phenotypically compatible units may be difficult to obtain and expensive.[24] One common protocol followed for nonalloimmunized patients is pretransfusion phenotypic matching for C, E, and K antigens to reduce the incidence of alloimmunization. Once a patient has developed a red cell antibody, some centers extend matching to additional red cell antigens (Fy, Jk, S) to prevent further alloimmunization. However, care must be taken with some of these strategies as recent studies have found no benefit in alloimmunization rates by providing Rh-matched RBC units from minority donors.[25] The benefits of RBC transfusion therapy in SCD disease must constantly be weighed against the costs (e.g., iron overload, RBC alloimmunization, and increased donor exposure risks). As a result of these issues, some clinicians have proposed that a clinically successful course of transfusions that maintains the hemoglobin S below 30% could, after several years, be transitioned to a strategy of more limited transfusions with a hemoglobin S target of 40% to 50% to reduce the risks for iron overload.[21] Patients with SCD may also be at risk for delayed hemolytic transfusion reactions, the development of autoantibodies, and "hyperhemolytic" syndrome, a phenomenon in which a patient hemolyzes both the native and transfused erythrocytes following RBC transfusion. The mechanism is not well characterized.

Thalassemia

Thalassemia with severe anemia is usually treated with chronic transfusion therapy to improve tissue oxygenation and suppress extramedullary erythropoiesis in the liver, spleen, and bone marrow. This approach mitigates many of the complications caused by the ineffective erythropoiesis. In contrast to chronic transfusion regimens used to treat SCD, most β-thalassemia major patients requiring chronic transfusion therapy start at a very young age. The treatment goals in this population are characterized by (1) increasing oxygen-carrying capacity by anemia correction, (2) preventing progressive hypersplenism, (3) suppression of endogenous erythropoiesis, and (4) reduction of gastrointestinal absorption of iron.[26] The target hemoglobin levels are usually 8 to 9 g/dL, where normal growth and development can occur in these patients. Supertransfusion protocols aim for higher target hemoglobin levels (11 to 12 g/dL) to reduce organomegaly from extramedullary hematopoiesis. Iron overload is a complication of this RBC transfusion protocol that cannot be prevented and must be treated with chelation therapy beginning early in childhood. In a recent report from the Centers for Disease Control and Prevention on transfusion complications in thalassemia patients in the thalassemia network in the United States from 2004–2012, iron-induced multi-organ dysfunction from transfusion was common despite chelation. Transfusion-transmitted disease pathogens were found in almost one-quarter of those patients monitored and almost 50% of patients experienced transfusion reactions including allergic, febrile nonhemolytic, and hemolytic. RBC alloimmunization was found in 19% of all patients with the most common antigens being E, Kell, and C. Years of transfusion was found to be the strongest predictor of alloantibody formation.[27] Phenotypic-matching protocols are used in some locations to prevent RBC alloimmunization, but data supporting or refuting this practice are scant and further research is needed.

Autoimmune Hemolytic Anemia

Autoimmune hemolytic anemia in children occurs predominantly in young children, with a median age of 3.8 years, and 53% are associated with other immunologic diseases, according to one study in which 74% of the cases had both immunoglobulin G (IgG) and C3d on their surface.[28] Like adult cases, most cases of autoimmune hemolytic anemia in children have antibody reactivity to all RBCs from all donors.

Children also may develop autoimmune hemolytic anemia associated with a Donath-Landsteiner antibody, which is rarely seen in adults. Classically the Donath-Landsteiner antibody is associated with paroxysmal cold hemoglobinuria, a disease in which patients developed paroxysms of hemoglobinuria following exposure to cold temperatures.[29] However, some children with a Donath-Landsteiner antibody develop symptoms of anemia that are not obviously associated with exposure to cold. The syndrome often develops following an infection such as a respiratory infection.

The Donath-Landsteiner antibody is an IgG antibody that binds erythrocytes, usually recognizing the P antigen, at cold temperatures (<20°C [68°F]) and fixes early components of complement. The fixed complement does not cause significant hemolysis at cold temperatures, but upon warming, the entire complement complex binds and lyses the erythrocytes. Initial testing in the blood bank may be entirely normal or may reveal a positive DAT for C3. The Donath-Landsteiner antibody can be detected only by special testing in which the patient's plasma is incubated with erythrocytes in cold temperatures followed by warm temperatures.

Hematopoietic Cellular Transplant Patients

Transfusion support for HPC transplant patients is similar to that for adult patients, although there are few published studies on transfusion of pediatric HPC transplant patients. RBC transfusions are often not needed in these patients whose hemoglobin level is at least 7 g/dL.[11] No studies in the modern era have been published on platelet transfusions in these patients, but use of a transfusion trigger of 10,000 platelets/μL, like that used for adults, seems reasonable for those patients without a significant bleeding risk other than thrombocytopenia.

Apheresis

Pediatric apheresis is used for many of the same indications as for adults. However, additional aspects need to be considered in treating pediatric patients. Many children require vascular access through a central vein because the peripheral veins of many children are too small. In addition, peripheral access requires patients to remain seated or reclining with limited arm movement for the procedure duration, and younger patients are often unable to comply with this given that procedures usually last at least 2 hours. During the procedures, children are susceptible to symptomatic hypocalcemia from citrate anticoagulation. For this reason, some pediatric centers use heparin to anticoagulate patients, although prophylactic cation replacement can successfully prevent most symptoms in pediatric apheresis patients.[30] Apheresis procedures subject the patient to volume shifts, which are usually a loss of less than 200 mL of fluid during the procedure and a gain of up to 300 mL at the end of the procedure. The actual fluid shifts depend on the machine, the procedure, and the parameters for that procedure. In some cases, the volume shifts may be too large to be safe for the patient. In these cases, most machines can be primed with 5% albumin, an RBC unit, or reconstituted whole blood. Using a prime solution, it is possible to minimize fluid shifts so that the patient is effectively volume neutral for the

entire procedure. Procedures to accomplish this are usually only available at centers that perform apheresis on relatively large numbers of pediatric patients.

Special Processing and Prevention of Adverse Events in Pediatric Patients

Special processing of blood products is performed more frequently for children than for adults. This is especially true for the preterm infant population, specifically in very low-birth-weight (VLBW) infants weighing less than 1500 g and extremely low-birth-weight infants weighing less than 1000 g.

Leukocyte-Reduced Blood Components

Leukoreduced cellular blood products are used in greater than 80% of blood components transfused to children in the United States. The rationale behind the use in pediatric patients has primarily been extrapolated from adult studies. In general, leukoreduction reduces transmission of CMV,[31] decreases HLA alloimmunization,[32] and decreases the frequency of febrile nonhemolytic transfusion reactions. The benefits of leukoreduction for neonates differ from the benefits for older patients. While neonates younger than 4 months of age rarely develop transfusion reactions and rarely become HLA alloimmunized, some neonates, especially premature infants, are at risk for transfusion-transmitted CMV.[31] Additionally, one study of premature infants found that implementation of universal leukoreduction was associated with decreased incidences of retinopathy, prematurity, and bronchopulmonary dysplasia, and decreased length of hospitalization.[33]

Cytomegalovirus-Seronegative Blood Components

Some immunosuppressed pediatric patients, including premature infants, are at risk of significant disease from CMV infection. Transfusion-transmitted CMV can occur because many healthy blood donors have been infected at some point and their leukocytes harbor the virus. Approaches to reduce the risk of transfusion transmission of CMV include transfusion of blood components that test negative for antibodies to CMV (CMV seronegative), are leukoreduced, or both. Although each of these approaches is highly effective, none of these approaches provides zero risk of transfusion-transmitted CMV since blood from donors who were recently infected can lack antibodies to CMV and can contain cell-free virions that are not removed by leukoreduction. The risk of transfusion-transmitted CMV in VLBW infants (<1500 g) is less than 1% when the units are leukoreduced and CMV seronegative.[34] This approach has not been directly compared to using only CMV seronegative or using only leukoreduced units. However, results from older studies found that the residual risk for transfusion-transmitted CMV in adults from CMV seronegative blood components to be between 1% and 3% but current risks are likely lower, and one study found no infants acquiring transfusion-transmitted CMV from transfusion of CMV seronegative blood components.[35] Leukoreduction is also very effective, reducing the rate of transfusion-transmitted CMV to less than 1% in immunosuppressed patients of all ages.[36] Some have recommended the combined approach of using leukoreduced CMV seronegative units for prevention of transfusion-transmitted CMV for some of the most at-risk patients.[37] Despite confidence in the safety of using CMV seronegative units, it may not be practical and cost effective to rely on CMV seronegative donors as they often constitute less than or equal to one-half of the blood donor pool.

Irradiation

Mortality rates associated with TA-GVHD are as high as 80% to 90%, with no effective treatments. As a result, identifying neonates and children who are immunosuppressed is paramount, so irradiation of cellular components can be performed to prevent this noninfectious serious hazard of transfusion. There are differing expert opinions and practices, and local protocols based on patient populations, available equipment, and best practices at each institution should be followed. The following patients should receive irradiated cellular blood components: (1) premature infants with birth weight less than 1200 g, (2) any child with known or suspected cellular immune deficiency (e.g., severe combined immunodeficiency), (3) any child with significant immunosuppression due to chemotherapy or radiation treatment, (4) any child who receives blood components from blood relatives, and (5) any child who receives HLA-matched or crossmatched platelet components.

Washing

Washing removes the supernatant from RBC or platelet units and is usually performed to reduce the risk of allergic reactions related to plasma. For very young children, washing may also be performed to reduce the concentration of extracellular potassium or to remove anticoagulant-preservative solutions. Washing can also be used to remove pathologic antibodies from a donor unit. Most donor units lack such antibodies. However, if maternal RBC or platelet units are used to treat her newborn with HDFN or neonatal alloimmune thrombocytopenic purpura, respectively, then her plasma would contain the pathogenic antibodies and the units should be washed prior to transfusion. Indeed, because maternal blood contains pathologic antibodies in these settings, its use for these patients is not generally recommended. However, a maternal component may be used because it may be the only component available that lacks the antigen recognized by her antibodies

Volume Reduction

Volume reduction, involving removal of plasma, is primarily used for patients who cannot tolerate the volume of a blood component transfusion, such as some infants with compromised cardiac function. However, it may also be employed for infants and children who receive ABO-mismatched platelet transfusions, because several deaths have been reported in the literature of children who have received out-of-group platelets (e.g., O platelet pheresis to A recipient).[38] Not all blood banks volume-reduce such platelets.

Reconstitution of RBCs for Neonatal Exchange Transfusion

During a neonatal exchange, the infant's whole blood is replaced with reconstituted whole blood prepared from type-compatible RBCs and plasma. Typically, RBCs less than 5 to 7 days old are used to minimize the concentration of extracellular potassium and, theoretically, provide transfused RBCs that will have maximal in vivo benefit, although this has never been demonstrated. Because of theoretical concerns associated with large volumes of RBC additives transfused to premature infants, nonadditive units are sometimes selected or additives are removed from the RBCs prior to reconstitution. Most blood banks also provide RBC units that are negative for sickle hemoglobin to avoid the rare potential of intravascular sickling. RBC units should be leukoreduced, CMV seronegative, or both to reduce the incidence of transfusion- transmitted CMV. The RBC unit should also be irradiated to prevent TA-GVHD if the infant is considered at risk of this by local criteria. If irradiated, the RBC or reconstituted whole blood should be irradiated just before the exchange to minimize liberation of potassium from intracellular stores. Alternatively the RBC unit can be irradiated prior to volume reduction or washing. The glucose load during an exchange transfusion can be high due to the fact that banked plasma contains added dextrose and because glucose is added to RBC preservative solutions.

Hence glucose levels should be monitored during the first few hours of the exchange.

The goal of most exchanges is to exchange twice the blood volume of the neonate. The volume needed can be calculated based on the fact that the blood volume of a neonate ranges from 100 mL/kg for the most premature to 85 mL/kg for term infants. Usually, one RBC unit is sufficient for a two-volume exchange. The reconstituted whole blood should have a hematocrit of approximately 40% to 50% and must be adequately mixed to maintain the intended hematocrit throughout the exchange transfusion.

The reconstituted whole blood should be transfused through a standard filter and an inline blood warmer. In general, no more than 5 mL/kg of body weight or 5% of the infant's blood volume is to be removed and replaced during a 2–5 minute cycle. The exchange should be performed at a slow pace, so as to not cause sudden hemodynamic changes that can result in cerebral blood flow shifts in intracranial pressure, precipitating an intraventricular hemorrhage.[39] A double-volume exchange transfusion typically takes 1.5 to 2 hours.

REFERENCES

1. FDA. *INTERCEPT® Blood System for Platelets–Small Volume (SV) Processing Set.* 2014: Intercept Package Insert.
2. Beeck H, Hellstern P: In vitro characterization of solvent/detergent-treated human plasma and of quarantine fresh frozen plasma. *Vox Sang* 74(Suppl 1):219–223, 1998.
3. Albisetti M: The fibrinolytic system in children. *Semin Thromb Hemost* 29:339, 2003.
4. El Beshlawy A, Alaraby I, Abou Hussein H, et al: Study of protein C, protein S, and antithrombin III in newborns with sepsis. *Pediatr Crit Care Med* 11(1):52–59, 2010.
5. Bell EF, Strauss RG, Widness JA, et al: Randomized trial of liberal versus restrictive guidelines for red blood cell transfusion in preterm infants. *Pediatrics* 115(6):1685–1691, 2005.
6. Kirpalani H, Whyte RK, Andersen C, et al: The Premature Infants in Need of Transfusion (PINT) study: a randomized, controlled trial of a restrictive (low) versus liberal (high) transfusion threshold for extremely low birth weight infants. *J Pediatr* 149(3):301–307, 2006.
7. Nickel RS, Josephson CD: Neonatal Transfusion Medicine: Five Major Unanswered Research Questions for the Twenty-First Century. *Clin Perinatol* 42(3):499–513, 2015.
8. Fergusson DA, Hebert P, Hogan DL, et al: Effect of fresh red blood cell transfusions on clinical outcomes in premature, very-low-birth-weight infants: the ARIPI randomized trial. *JAMA* 308(14):1443–1451, 2012.
9. Patel RM, Josephson CD: Storage age of red blood cells for transfusion of premature infants. *JAMA* 309(6):544–545, 2013.
10. Lacroix J, Hebert PC, Hutchison JS, et al: Transfusion strategies for patients in pediatric intensive care units. *N Engl J Med* 356(16):1609–1619, 2007.
11. Lightdale JR, Randolph AG, Tran CM, et al: Impact of a Conservative Red Blood Cell Transfusion Strategy in Children Undergoing Hematopoietic Stem Cell Transplantation. *Biol Blood Marrow Transplant* 2011.
12. Price TH, Boeckh M, Harrison RW, et al: Efficacy of transfusion with granulocytes from G-CSF/dexamethasone treated donors in neutropenic patients with infection. *Blood* 2015.
13. Heim KF, Fleisher TA, Stroncek DF, et al: The relationship between alloimmunization and posttransfusion granulocyte survival: experience in a chronic granulomatous disease cohort. *Transfusion* 51(6):1154–1162, 2011.
14. Wennberg RP, Depp R, Heinrichs WL: Indications for early exchange transfusion in patients with erythroblastosis fetalis. *J Pediatr* 92(5):789–792, 1978.
15. Davoren A, Curtis BR, Aster RH, et al: Human platelet antigen-specific alloantibodies implicated in 1162 cases of neonatal alloimmune thrombocytopenia. *Transfusion* 44(8):1220–1225, 2004.
16. Friedman DF, Montenegro LM: Extracorporeal Membrane Oxygenation and Cardiopulmonary Bypass. In Hillyer CD, Strauss RG, Luban NLC,

editors: *Handbook of Pediatric Transfusion Medicine*, London, 2004, Elsevier Academic Press, pp 181–189.

17. Meliones JN, Hansell DR: Extracorporeal membrane oxygenation: The role of blood components. In Chambers LA, Isssitt LA, editors: *Supporting the pediatric transfusion recipient*, Bethesda, MD, 1994, AABB, pp 87–107.

18. Hendrickson JE, Shaz BH, Pereira G, et al: Coagulopathy is prevalent and associated with adverse outcomes in transfused pediatric trauma patients. *J Pediatr* 160(2):204–209 e3, 2012.

19. Holcomb JB, Tilley BC, Baraniuk S, et al: Transfusion of plasma, platelets, and red blood cells in a 1:1:1 vs a 1:1:2 ratio and mortality in patients with severe trauma: the PROPPR randomized clinical trial. *JAMA* 313(5):471–482, 2015.

20. Dehmer JJ, Adamson WT: Massive transfusion and blood product use in the pediatric trauma patient. *Semin Pediatr Surg* 19(4):286–291, 2010.

21. Adams RJ, Brambilla D: Discontinuing prophylactic transfusions used to prevent stroke in sickle cell disease. *N Engl J Med* 353(26):2769–2778, 2005.

22. Adams RJ, McKie VC, Hsu L, et al: Prevention of a first stroke by transfusions in children with sickle cell anemia and abnormal results on transcranial Doppler ultrasonography. *N Engl J Med* 339(1):5–11, 1998.

23. Vichinsky EP, Luban NL, Wright E, et al: Prospective RBC phenotype matching in a stroke-prevention trial in sickle cell anemia: a multicenter transfusion trial. *Transfusion* 41(9):1086–1092, 2001.

24. Castro O, Sandler SG, Houston-Yu P, et al: Predicting the effect of transfusing only phenotype-matched RBCs to patients with sickle cell disease: theoretical and practical implications. *Transfusion* 42(6):684–690, 2002.

25. Chou ST, Jackson T, Vege S, et al: High prevalence of red blood cell alloimmunization in sickle cell disease despite transfusion from Rh-matched minority donors. *Blood* 122(6):1062–1071, 2013.

26. Olivieri NF: The beta-thalassemias. *N Engl J Med* 341(2):99–109, 1999.

27. Vichinsky E, Neumayr L, Trimble S, et al: Transfusion complications in thalassemia patients: a report from the Centers for Disease Control and Prevention (CME). *Transfusion* 54(4):972–981, quiz 1, 2014.

28. Aladjidi N, Leverger G, Leblanc T, et al: New insights into childhood autoimmune hemolytic anemia: a French national observational study of 265 children. *Haematologica* 96(5):655–663, 2011.

29. Eder AF: Review: acute Donath-Landsteiner hemolytic anemia. *Immunohematology* 21(2):56–62, 2005.

30. Bolan CD, Yau YY, Cullis HC, et al: Pediatric large-volume leukapheresis: a single institution experience with heparin versus citrate-based anticoagulant regimens. *Transfusion* 44(2):229–238, 2004.

31. Gilbert GL, Hayes K, Hudson IL, et al: Prevention of transfusion-acquired cytomegalovirus infection in infants by blood filtration to remove leucocytes. Neonatal Cytomegalovirus Infection Study Group. *Lancet* 1(8649):1228–1231, 1989.

32. Leukocyte reduction and ultraviolet B irradiation of platelets to prevent alloimmunization and refractoriness to platelet transfusions. The Trial to Reduce Alloimmunization to Platelets Study Group. *N Engl J Med* 337(26):1861–1869, 1997.

33. Fergusson D, Hebert PC, Lee SK, et al: Clinical outcomes following institution of universal leukoreduction of blood transfusions for premature infants. *JAMA* 289(15):1950–1956, 2003.

34. Josephson CD, Caliendo AM, Easley KA, et al: Blood transfusion and breast milk transmission of cytomegalovirus in very low-birth-weight infants: a prospective cohort study. *JAMA Pediatr* 168(11):1054–1062, 2014.

35. Yeager AS, Grumet FC, Hafleigh EB, et al: Prevention of transfusion-acquired cytomegalovirus infections in newborn infants. *J Pediatr* 98(2):281–287, 1981.

36. Vamvakas EC: Is white blood cell reduction equivalent to antibody screening in preventing transmission of cytomegalovirus by transfusion? A review of the literature and meta-analysis. *Transfus Med Rev* 19(3):181–199, 2005.

37. Laupacis A, Brown J, Costello B, et al: Prevention of posttransfusion CMV in the era of universal WBC reduction: a consensus statement. *Transfusion* 41(4):560–569, 2001.

38. Josephson CD, Castillejo MI, Grima K, et al: ABO-mismatched platelet transfusions: strategies to mitigate patient exposure to naturally occurring hemolytic antibodies. *Transfus Apher Sci* 42(1):83–88, 2010.

39. Bada HS, Chua C, Salmon JH, et al: Changes in intracranial pressure during exchange transfusion. *J Pediatr* 94(1):129–132, 1979.

HEMOSTASIS AND THROMBOSIS

CHAPTER 122

OVERVIEW OF HEMOSTASIS AND THROMBOSIS

James C. Fredenburgh and Jeffrey I. Weitz

Hemostasis preserves vascular integrity by balancing the physiologic processes that maintain blood in a fluid state under normal circumstances and prevent excessive bleeding after vascular injury. Preservation of blood fluidity depends on an intact vascular endothelium and a complex series of regulatory pathways that maintain platelets in a quiescent state and keep the coagulation system in check. In contrast, arrest of bleeding requires rapid formation of hemostatic plugs at sites of vascular injury to prevent exsanguination. Perturbation of hemostasis can lead to bleeding or thrombosis. Bleeding will occur if there is failure to seal vascular leaks either because of defective hemostatic plug formation or because of premature breakdown of the plugs. In contrast, thrombosis may occur if prothrombotic stimuli are unregulated.

Thrombosis can occur in arteries or veins and is a major cause of morbidity and mortality. Arterial thrombosis is the most common cause of acute coronary syndromes, ischemic stroke, and limb gangrene, whereas thrombosis in the deep veins of the leg leads to postthrombotic syndrome and pulmonary embolism, which can be fatal.

Most arterial thrombi form on top of disrupted atherosclerotic plaques, because plaque rupture exposes thrombogenic material in the plaque core to the blood.[1] This material then triggers platelet aggregation and fibrin formation, which results in the generation of a platelet-rich thrombus that temporarily or permanently occludes blood flow. Temporary occlusion of blood flow in coronary arteries may trigger unstable angina, whereas persistent obstruction causes myocardial infarction. The same processes can occur in the cerebral circulation, where temporary arterial occlusion may manifest as a transient ischemic attack, and persistent occlusion can lead to a stroke. Likewise, critical limb ischemia can occur if there is superimposed thrombosis on ruptured atherosclerotic plaques in the major arteries supplying blood to the lower extremities.

In contrast to arterial thrombi, venous thrombi rarely form at sites of obvious vascular disruption. Although they can develop after surgical trauma to veins, or secondary to indwelling venous catheters, they usually originate in the valve cusps of the deep veins of the calf or in the muscular sinuses, where there is stasis.[2] Sluggish blood flow in these veins reduces the oxygen supply to the avascular valve cusps. Hypoxemia induces endothelial cells lining the valve cusps to become activated and express adhesion molecules onto their surfaces. Tissue factor–bearing leukocytes and microparticles adhere to these activated cells and induce coagulation. Impaired blood flow exacerbates local thrombus formation by reducing clearance of activated clotting factors. These responses constitute the three axes of the Virchow triad associated with development of thrombosis: stasis, hypercoagulability of the blood, and activation or disruption of the endothelium. Calf vein thrombi that extend into the proximal veins of the leg can dislodge and travel to the lungs to produce pulmonary embolism.[3]

Arterial and venous thrombi contain platelets and fibrin, but the proportions differ. Arterial thrombi are rich in platelets because of the high shear on this side of the circulatory system. In contrast, venous thrombi, which form under low shear conditions, contain relatively few platelets and consist mostly of fibrin and trapped red blood cells. Because of the predominance of platelets, arterial thrombi appear white, whereas venous thrombi appear red.

The antithrombotic drugs used for prevention and treatment of thrombosis target components of thrombi and include antiplatelet drugs, which inhibit platelets; anticoagulants, which attenuate coagulation; and fibrinolytic agents that induce fibrin degradation (see Chapter 149). With the predominance of platelets in arterial thrombi, strategies to inhibit or treat arterial thrombosis focus mainly on antiplatelet agents, although in the acute setting, strategies often include anticoagulants and fibrinolytic agents. When arterial thrombi are occlusive and rapid restoration of blood flow is imperative, mechanical and pharmacologic methods enable thrombus extraction, compression, or degradation. Although rarely used for this indication, anticoagulants can also prevent recurrent ischemic events after acute myocardial infarction. Anticoagulants are the mainstay for prevention and treatment of venous thromboembolism because fibrin is the predominant component of venous thrombi (see Chapter 142). Antiplatelet drugs are less effective than anticoagulants because of the limited platelet content of venous thrombi. Selected patients with venous thromboembolism benefit from fibrinolytic therapy—for example, patients with massive or submassive pulmonary embolism achieve more rapid restoration of pulmonary blood flow with systemic or catheter-directed fibrinolytic therapy than with anticoagulant therapy alone. Certain patients with extensive deep vein thrombosis in the iliac and/or femoral veins may also have a better outcome with catheter-directed fibrinolytic therapy and/or mechanical thrombus extraction in addition to anticoagulants (see Chapter 143).

This chapter provides an overview of hemostasis and thrombosis by highlighting the processes involved in platelet activation and aggregation, blood coagulation, and fibrinolysis.

HEMOSTATIC SYSTEM

The major components of the hemostatic system are the vascular endothelium, platelets, and the coagulation and fibrinolytic systems.

Vascular Endothelium

A monolayer of endothelial cells lines the intimal surface of the circulatory tree and separates the blood from the prothrombotic subendothelial components of the vessel wall (see Chapter 123). As such, the vascular endothelium encompasses about 10^{13} cells and covers a vast surface area. Rather than serving as a static barrier, the healthy vascular endothelium is a dynamic organ (Fig. 122.1) that actively regulates hemostasis by inhibiting platelets, suppressing coagulation, promoting fibrinolysis, and modulating vascular tone and permeability.[4] Defective vascular function can lead to bleeding if the endothelium becomes more permeable to blood cells, if vasoconstriction does not occur, or if premature degradation of hemostatic plugs reopens repaired vasculature.

Platelet Inhibition

Endothelial cells synthesize prostacyclin and nitric oxide and release them into the blood.[4] These agents not only serve as potent vasodilators but also inhibit platelet activation and subsequent aggregation by stimulating adenylate cyclase and increasing intracellular levels of cyclic adenosine monophosphahte (cAMP). In addition, endothelial cells express CD39 on their surfaces, a membrane-associated ecto-adenosine diphosphatase (ADPase). By degrading adenosine

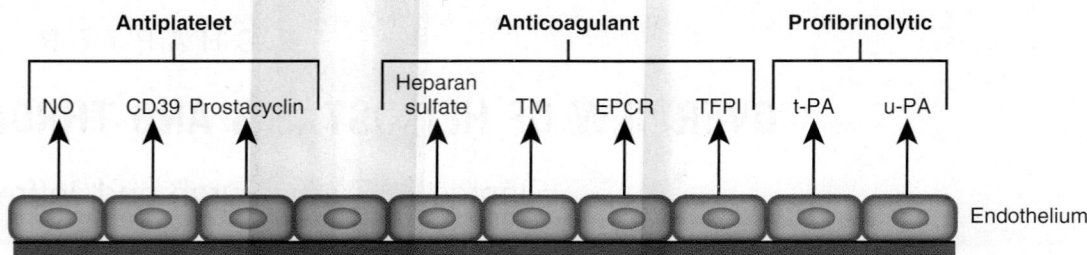

Fig. 122.1 THE ANTITHROMBOTIC FUNCTIONS OF THE ENDOTHELIUM. The healthy endothelium has (a) antiplatelet activity because of synthesis and release of prostacyclin and nitric oxide (NO) and expression of CD39, a membrane-associated ectoADPase; (b) anticoagulant activity because of heparan sulfate proteoglycan-mediated activation of antithrombin and expression of thrombomodulin (TM) and endothelial protein C receptor (EPCR), which are involved in protein C activation, and surface-bound tissue factor pathway inhibitor (TFPI); and (c) profibrinolytic activity because of release of tissue and urokinase-type plasminogen activator (t-PA and u-PA, respectively).

diphosphate (ADP), which is a platelet agonist, CD39 attenuates platelet activation.

Anticoagulant Activity

Intact endothelial cells play an essential part in the regulation of thrombin generation through a variety of mechanisms. Endothelial cells produce heparan sulfate proteoglycans, which bind circulating antithrombin and accelerate the rate at which it inhibits thrombin and other coagulation enzymes. Tissue factor pathway inhibitor (TFPI), a naturally occurring inhibitor of coagulation, binds heparan sulfate on the endothelial cell surface.[5] Administration of heparin or low-molecular-weight heparin (LMWH) displaces glycosaminoglycan-bound TFPI from the vascular endothelium, and released TFPI may contribute to the antithrombotic activity of these drugs.

Endothelial cells regulate thrombin generation by expressing thrombomodulin and endothelial cell protein C receptor (EPCR) on their surfaces. Thrombomodulin binds thrombin and alters this enzyme's substrate specificity such that it no longer acts as a procoagulant but becomes a potent activator of protein C (see Chapter 127). Activated protein C serves as an anticoagulant by degrading and inactivating activated factor V and factor VIII (factor Va and VIIIa, respectively), key cofactors involved in thrombin generation. Protein S acts as a cofactor in this reaction, and EPCR enhances this pathway by binding protein C and presenting it to the thrombin–thrombomodulin complex for activation. In addition to its role as an anticoagulant, activated protein C also regulates inflammation and preserves the barrier function of the endothelium.[6]

Fibrinolytic Activity

The vascular endothelium promotes fibrinolysis by synthesizing and releasing tissue-type and urokinase-type plasminogen activator (t-PA and u-PA, respectively), which initiate fibrinolysis by converting plasminogen to plasmin (see Chapter 126). Endothelial cells in most vascular beds synthesize t-PA constitutively and release it in response to stimuli such as thrombin or bradykinin. In contrast, perturbed endothelial cells produce u-PA in the settings of inflammation and wound repair.

Endothelial cells also produce type 1 plasminogen activator inhibitor (PAI-1), the major regulator of both t-PA and u-PA. Therefore net fibrinolytic activity depends on the dynamic balance between the release of plasminogen activators and PAI-1. Fibrinolysis localizes to the endothelial cell surface because these cells express annexin II, a coreceptor for plasminogen and t-PA that promotes their interaction. Therefore healthy vessels actively resist thrombosis and help maintain platelets in a quiescent state.

Vascular Tone and Permeability

In addition to synthesizing potent vasodilators, such as prostacyclin and nitric oxide, endothelial cells also produce a group of counterregulatory peptides known as endothelins that induce vasoconstriction. Endothelial cell permeability is influenced by the connections that join endothelial cells to their neighbors. Macromolecules traverse the endothelium via patent intercellular junctions, by endocytosis, or through transendothelial pores. Vasodilatation, severe thrombocytopenia, and high doses of heparin can increase endothelial permeability, which may contribute to bleeding. Activated protein C may also contribute to the barrier function of the endothelium.

Platelets

Platelets are anucleate cellular particles released into the circulation after programmed fragmentation of bone marrow megakaryocytes (see Chapter 124). Because they are anucleate, platelets have limited capacity to synthesize proteins. Consequently, platelet protein composition is determined by the parent cell as well as by those factors endocytosed from the circulation. Thrombopoietin, a glycoprotein synthesized in the liver and kidneys, regulates megakaryocytic proliferation and maturation as well as platelet production. Once they enter the circulation, platelets have a life span of 7 to 10 days.

Damage to the intimal lining of the vessel exposes the underlying subendothelial matrix. Platelets home to sites of vascular disruption and adhere to the exposed matrix proteins (see Chapter 125). Adherent platelets undergo activation and not only release substances that recruit additional platelets to the site of injury, but also promote thrombin generation and subsequent fibrin formation (Fig. 122.2). A potent platelet agonist, thrombin amplifies platelet recruitment and activation. Activated platelets then aggregate to form a plug that seals the leak in the vasculature.[7] An understanding of the steps in these highly integrated processes helps pinpoint the sites of action of antiplatelet drugs and rationalizes the utility of anticoagulants for the treatment of arterial thrombosis and venous thrombosis.

Adhesion

Platelets adhere to exposed von Willebrand factor (vWF) and collagen, originating from endothelial cells and the subendothelium, respectively. The platelet monolayer promotes thrombin generation and subsequent fibrin formation. These events depend on constitutively expressed receptors on the platelet surface, $\alpha_2\beta_1$ and glycoprotein (GP) VI, which bind collagen, and GPIbα and GPIIb/IIIa ($\alpha_{IIb}\beta_3$), which bind vWF. The platelet surface is crowded with receptors, but those involved in adhesion are the most abundant: every

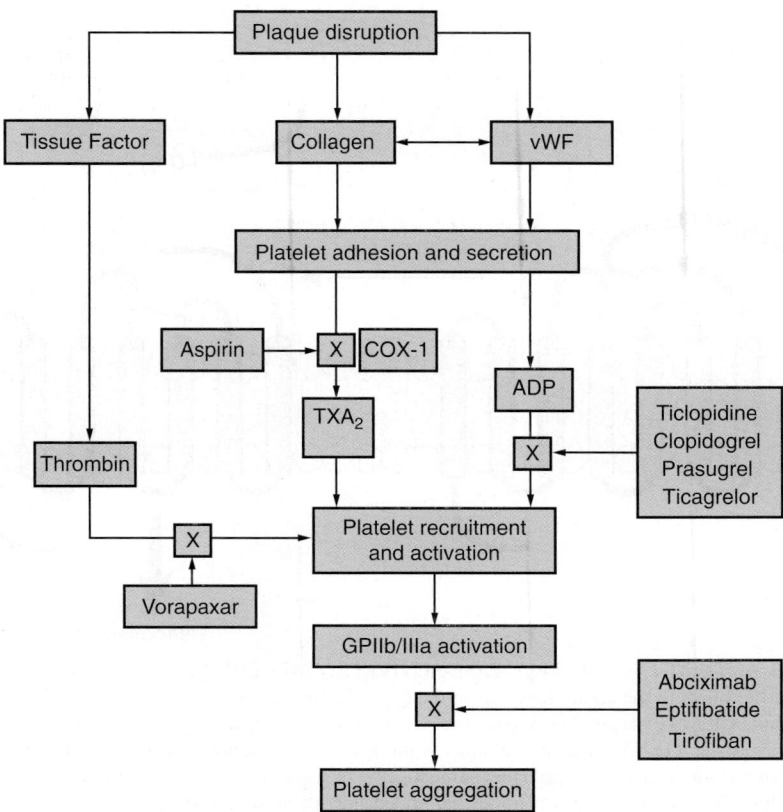

Fig. 122.2 SITES OF ACTION OF ANTIPLATELET DRUGS. Aspirin inhibits thromboxane A_2 (TXA_2) synthesis by irreversibly acetylating cyclooxygenase-1 (COX-1). Reduced TXA_2 release attenuates platelet activation and recruitment to the site of vascular injury. Ticlopidine, clopidogrel, and prasugrel irreversibly block $P2Y_{12}$, a key ADP receptor on the platelet surface; whereas ticagrelor is a reversible inhibitor of $P2Y_{12}$. Abciximab, eptifibatide, and tirofiban inhibit the final common pathway of platelet aggregation by blocking fibrinogen and von Willebrand factor (vWF) binding to activated glycoprotein (GP) IIb/IIIa. Vorapaxar inhibits thrombin-mediated platelet activation by targeting protease activated receptor-1 (PAR-1), the major thrombin receptor on platelets.

platelet has about 40,000 to 80,000 copies of GPIIb/IIIa and 25,000 copies of GPIbα. Receptors cluster in cholesterol-enriched subdomains, which render them more mobile, thereby increasing the efficiency of platelet adhesion and subsequent activation (see Chapter 125).

Under low shear conditions, such as in the venous circulation, collagen can capture and activate platelets on its own. Captured platelets undergo cytoskeletal reorganization that causes them to flatten and adhere more closely to the damaged vessel wall. Under high shear conditions in the arterial system, however, collagen and vWF must act in concert to support optimal platelet adhesion and activation. vWF synthesized by endothelial cells and megakaryocytes assembles into multimers that range from 550 to over 10,000 kDa. When released from storage in the Weibel-Palade bodies of endothelial cells or the α-granules of platelets, most of the vWF enters the circulation, but the vWF released from the abluminal surface of endothelial cells accumulates in the subendothelial matrix, where it binds collagen via its A3 domain. This surface-immobilized vWF can simultaneously bind platelets via its A1 domain. In contrast, circulating vWF does not react with unstimulated platelets. This difference in reactivity likely reflects vWF conformation; circulating vWF is in a coiled conformation that prevents access of its platelet-binding domain to vWF receptors on the platelet surface, whereas immobilized vWF assumes an elongated shape that exposes its A1 domain. Shear forces at sites of vascular injury also unfold vWF, thus contributing to the abundance of platelets in arterial thrombi. In this extended conformation, large vWF multimers serve as the molecular glue that tethers platelets to the damaged vessel wall with sufficient strength to withstand higher shear forces.[8] Large vWF multimers

provide additional binding sites for collagen and heighten platelet adhesion because platelets have more vWF receptors than collagen receptors. Adhesion to collagen or vWF results in platelet activation, the next step in platelet plug formation.

Activation and Secretion

Adhesion to collagen and vWF initiates signaling pathways that result in platelet activation. These pathways induce cyclooxygenase-1 (COX-1)–dependent synthesis and release of thromboxane A_2, and trigger the release of ADP from storage granules. Thromboxane A_2 is a potent vasoconstrictor, and like ADP, locally activates ambient platelets and recruits them to the site of injury. This process results in expansion of the platelet plug. To activate platelets, thromboxane A_2 and ADP must bind to their respective receptors on the platelet membrane. The thromboxane receptor (TP) is a G protein coupled–receptor that is found on platelets and on the endothelium, which explains why thromboxane A_2 induces vasoconstriction as well as platelet activation.[9] ADP interacts with a family of G protein–coupled receptors on the platelet membrane. Most important of these is $P2Y_{12}$, which is the target of the thienopyridines, but $P2Y_1$ also contributes to ADP-induced platelet activation, and maximal ADP-induced platelet activation requires activation of both receptors. A third ADP receptor, $P2X_1$, is an adenosine triphosphate (ATP)–gated calcium channel. Platelet storage granules contain ATP as well as ADP; ATP released during the platelet activation process may contribute to the platelet recruitment process in a $P2X_1$-dependent fashion.

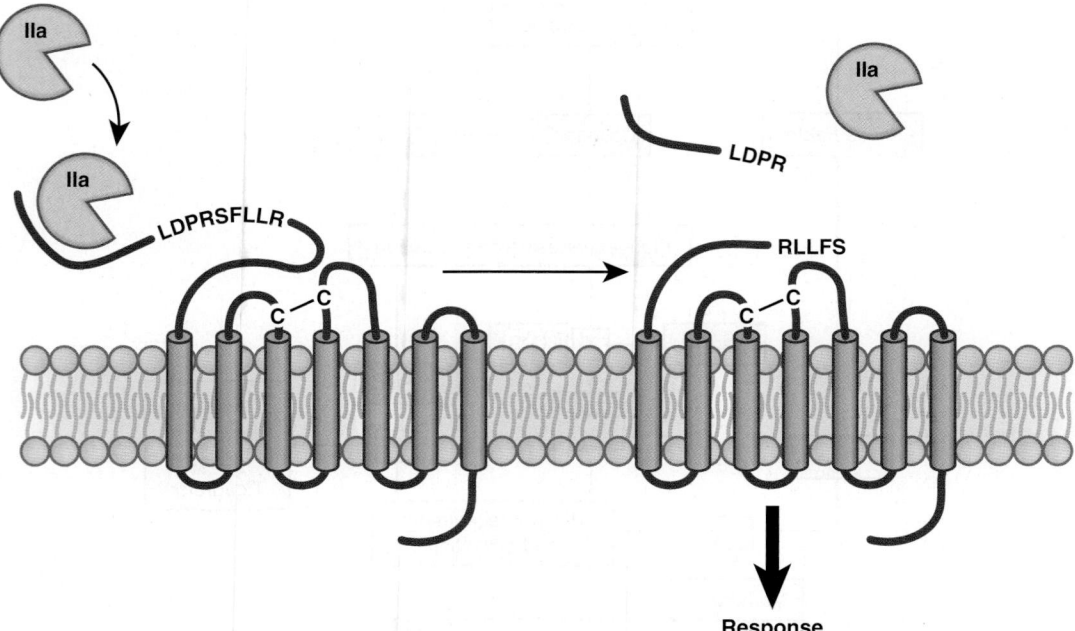

Fig. 122.3 ACTIVATION OF PROTEASE-ACTIVATED RECEPTOR (PAR)-1 BY THROMBIN. Thrombin (IIa) binds to the amino terminus of the extracellular domain of PAR-1 where it cleaves a specific peptide bond. Cleavage of this bond generates a new amino-terminal sequence of Ser-Phe-Leu-Leu-Arg (SFLLR) that acts as a tethered ligand and binds to the body of the receptor, thereby activating it. Thrombin then dissociates from the receptor. Analogues of the first five or six amino acids of the tethered ligand sequences, known as thrombin receptor agonist peptides, can independently activate PAR-1.

Although TP and the various ADP receptors signal through different pathways, they all trigger an increase in the intracellular calcium concentration in platelets. This in turn induces shape change via cytoskeletal rearrangement, granule mobilization and release, and subsequent platelet aggregation. Activated platelets promote coagulation by cycling phosphatidylserine from the inner membrane bilayer to the outer layer. Surface exposure of this anionic phospholipid is essential for assembly of coagulation factor complexes (see Chapter 126). Once assembled, these clotting factor complexes trigger a burst of thrombin generation and subsequent fibrin formation. In addition to converting fibrinogen to fibrin, thrombin amplifies platelet recruitment and activation, thus promoting expansion of the platelet plug. Thrombin binds to protease-activated receptors types 1 and 4 (PAR1 and PAR4, respectively) on the platelet surface and cleaves their extended amino-termini, thereby generating new amino-termini that serve as tethered ligands that bind internally and activate the receptors (Fig. 122.3). Whereas low concentrations of thrombin cleave PAR1, PAR4 cleavage requires higher thrombin concentrations.[10] Cleavage of either receptor triggers platelet activation.

In addition to providing a surface on which clotting factors assemble, activated platelets also promote fibrin formation and subsequent stabilization by releasing factor V, factor XI, fibrinogen, and factor XIII (see Chapter 125). Thus there is coordinated activation of platelets and coagulation, and the fibrin network that results from thrombin action helps anchor the platelet aggregates at the site of injury. Activated platelets also release adhesive proteins, such as vWF, thrombospondin, and fibronectin, which augment platelet adhesion at sites of injury, as well as growth factors, such as platelet-derived growth factor (PDGF) and transforming growth factor-beta (TGF-β), which promote wound healing. Platelet aggregation is the final step in the formation of the platelet plug.

Aggregation

GPIIb/IIIa mediates platelet-to-platelet linkages that result in the formation of clumps of platelets. On nonactivated platelets, GPIIb/

IIIa exhibits minimal affinity for its ligands. Upon platelet activation, GPIIb/IIIa undergoes a conformational transformation, which reflects transmission of inside-out signals from its cytoplasmic domain to its extracellular domain.[11] This transformation enhances the affinity of GPIIb/IIIa for its ligands, fibrinogen, and, under high shear conditions, vWF (see Chapter 125). Cryptic Arg-Gly-Asp (RGD) peptide sequences located in fibrinogen and vWF, as well as a platelet-binding Lys-Gly-Asp (KGD) sequence in fibrinogen, mediate their interaction with GPIIb/IIIa. When subjected to high shear, circulating vWF elongates and exposes its platelet-binding domain, which enables its interaction with the conformationally activated GPIIb/IIIa. Similarly, initial binding to GPIIb/IIIa leads to a conformational change in fibrinogen that unmasks additional binding sites. Divalent fibrinogen and multivalent vWF molecules serve as bridges and bind adjacent platelets together. Once bound to GPIIb/IIIa, fibrinogen and vWF induce outside–inside signals that augment platelet activation and result in the activation of additional GPIIb/IIIa receptors, creating a positive feedback loop. Because GPIIb/IIIa acts as the final effector in platelet aggregation, it is a logical target for potent antiplatelet drugs (see Chapters 130 and 149). Fibrin, the ultimate product of the coagulation system, tethers the platelet aggregates together and anchors them to the site of injury.

Coagulation

Coagulation results in the generation of thrombin, which converts soluble fibrinogen to fibrin. Coagulation occurs through a series of concerted activation steps, wherein a nascent protease activates an inactive enzyme precursor (zymogen); a process that is repeated in a cascade-like fashion. The principal enzyme complexes are composed of a vitamin K–dependent enzyme and a non-enzyme cofactor assembled on anionic phospholipid membranes in a calcium-dependent fashion (see Chapter 126). Because each enzyme complex activates a substrate that becomes the enzyme component of the subsequent complex, a small stimulus can produce a robust response. Initially the small amount of thrombin generated activates

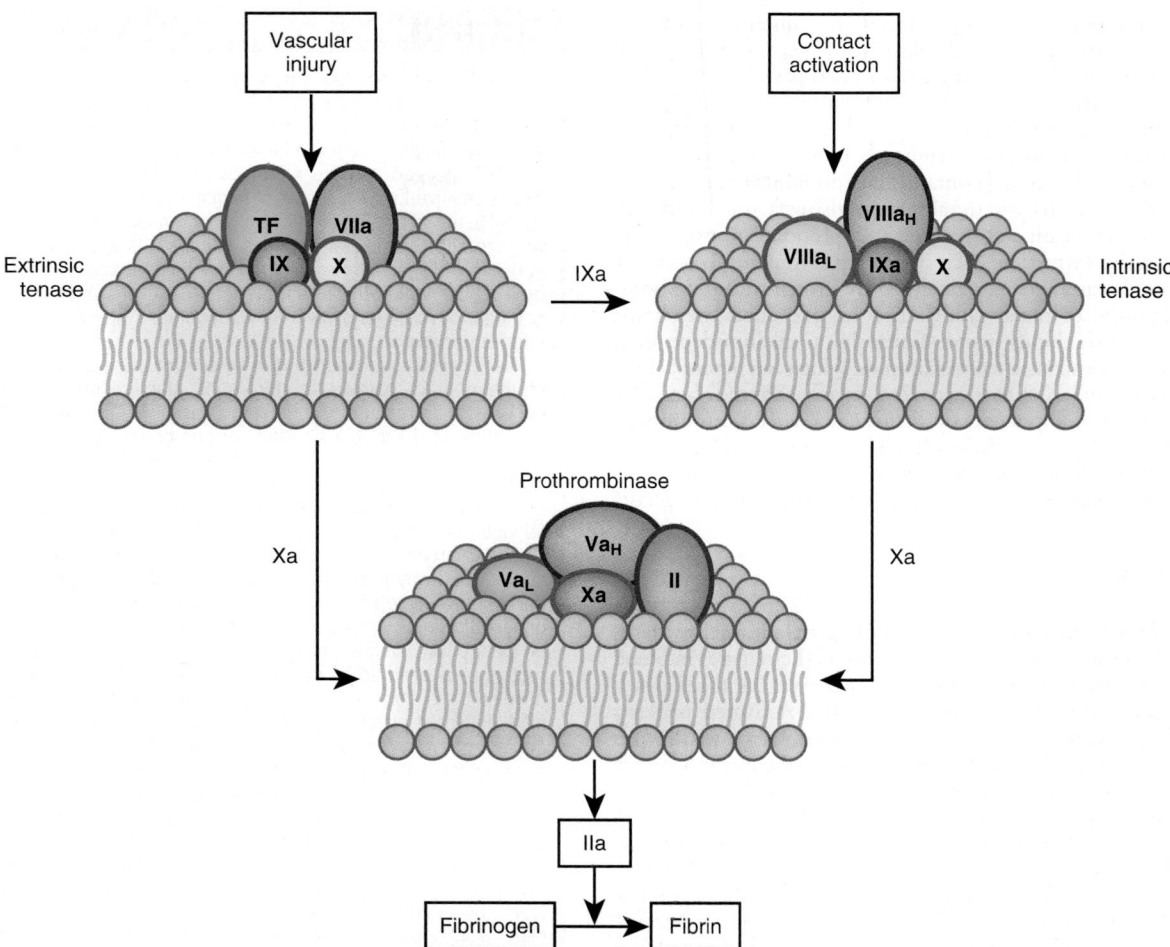

Fig. 122.4 COAGULATION SYSTEM. Coagulation occurs through the action of discrete enzyme complexes, which are composed of a vitamin K–dependent enzyme and a non-enzyme cofactor. These complexes assemble on anionic phospholipid membranes in a calcium-dependent fashion. Vascular injury exposes tissue factor (TF), which binds factor VIIa to form extrinsic tenase. Extrinsic tenase activates factors IX and X. Factor IXa binds to factor VIIIa to form intrinsic tenase, which activates factor X. The contact system also leads to activation of factor IX in response to exposure of anionic surfaces. Factor Xa binds to factor Va to form prothrombinase, which converts prothrombin (II) to thrombin (IIa). Thrombin then converts soluble fibrinogen into insoluble fibrin.

non-enzyme cofactors and platelets. The activated platelets then provide an anionic surface on which the coagulation complexes assemble to promote rapid thrombin generation. The three predominant enzyme complexes involved in thrombin generation are extrinsic tenase, intrinsic tenase, and prothrombinase, named for their substrates, factor X and prothrombin (Fig. 122.4).

Coagulation can be divided into three phases: initiation, propagation, and termination.[12,13] These phases reflect the exquisite control over thrombin activity necessary to effect hemostasis. The initiation phase, which is predominantly mediated by extrinsic tenase, is responsible for generating the initial burst of thrombin required for platelet and coagulation factor activation. The propagation phase is largely mediated by intrinsic tenase and is responsible for the explosive thrombin generation necessary to sustain the coagulant response. The termination phase, which is mediated by numerous protease inhibitors, ensures that thrombin generation is localized and finite. Each of the activation complexes exhibits similar composition, assembly, and regulation.

Because initiation and propagation reactions require a membrane surface for assembly of factors, cells play a key role in coagulation. Tissue factor exposure on monocytes and extravascular cells and platelet membrane capacitation are recognized key steps. However, other cells also make important contributions. For example, damaged endothelium appears to support coagulation because mice deficient in PAR4, the major thrombin receptor on mouse platelets, still exhibit significant thrombus formation after laser injury. Red blood cells also bind to damaged endothelium and express procoagulant phospholipids on their surface, thereby providing additional sites for assembly of coagulation complexes. In addition, activated neutrophils extrude web-like structures known as neutrophil extracellular traps (NETs). Composed of nuclear DNA, histones, and metalloproteases, NETs promote coagulation by binding and activating platelets, trapping red blood cells, and activating the contact pathway. Thus cells contribute to coagulation at numerous sites in the cascade.

Extrinsic Tenase

This complex forms upon exposure of tissue factor–expressing cells to the blood.[14] Tissue factor exposure occurs after atherosclerotic plaque rupture because the core of the plaque is rich in macrophages and other cells that express tissue factor. Denuding injury to the vessel wall also exposes tissue factor constitutively expressed by subendothelial fibroblasts and smooth muscle cells. In addition to cells in the vessel wall, circulating monocytes and monocyte-derived microparticles (small membrane fragments) also provide a source of tissue factor. When tissue factor–bearing monocytes or microparticles bind to platelets or other leukocytes and their plasma membranes fuse, tissue factor transfer occurs. By binding to adhesion molecules expressed on activated endothelial cells or to P-selectin on activated platelets, these tissue factor–bearing cells or microparticles can initiate or augment coagulation. This phenomenon likely explains how venous thrombi develop in the absence of obvious vessel wall injury.

Tissue factor is an integral membrane protein that serves as a receptor for factor VIIa. Blood contains trace amounts of factor VIIa, which has negligible activity in the absence of tissue factor.[14] Although tissue factor is present on cell surfaces, it is proposed to exist in an encrypted, inactive form. The decryption step is thought to occur by a disulfide bond rearrangement catalyzed by protein-disulfide isomerase and exposure of phosphatidylserine on the outer membrane surface. Factor VIIa binds tissue factor in a calcium-dependent fashion to form the extrinsic tenase complex, which is a potent activator of factors IX and X. Once activated, factor IXa and factor Xa serve as the enzyme components of intrinsic tenase and prothrombinase, respectively. Because sufficient levels of factor Xa and thrombin are formed in response to exposure of tissue factor, the extrinsic tenase complex is considered the essential mediator of the initiation phase.

Intrinsic Tenase

Factor IXa binds to factor VIIIa on anionic platelet or cell surfaces to form the intrinsic tenase complex.[15] Factor VIII circulates in blood in complex with vWF. Thrombin cleaves factor VIII and releases it from vWF, converting it to its activated form. Activated platelets express binding sites for factor VIIIa. Once bound, factor VIIIa binds factor IXa in a calcium-dependent fashion to form the intrinsic tenase complex, which then activates factor X. The loss in catalytic efficiency of intrinsic tenase that occurs with a deficiency of factors VIII or IX in hemophilia A and B, respectively, highlights their importance. Absence of the membrane or factor VIIIa almost completely abolishes enzymatic activity, and the catalytic efficiency of the complete complex is 10^6-fold greater than that of factor IXa alone.[15] Because intrinsic tenase activates factor X at a rate 50- to 100-fold faster than extrinsic tenase, it plays a critical role in the amplification of factor Xa and subsequent thrombin generation. Thus intrinsic tenase is crucial to the propagation phase of coagulation.

Contact Pathway

The contact pathway is so named because initial identification of its constituents (factors XII, XI, IX, and kallikrein), required contact with artificial agents such as ellagic acid or silica for activation. For this reason, the contact pathway lost prominence when the physiologic tissue factor pathway was identified. Current thinking is that tissue factor exposure represents the sole pathway for activation of coagulation and thus the contact system is unimportant for hemostasis because patients deficient in factor XII, prekallikrein, and high-molecular-weight kininogen do not have bleeding problems (see Chapter 126). Although patients with severe deficiency of factor XI can bleed after trauma or surgery, spontaneous bleeding is uncommon, and the plasma level of factor XI does not reliably predict the propensity for bleeding (see Chapter 137). The capacity of thrombin to feedback and activate platelet-bound factor XI may help to explain this phenomenon. It also is possible that platelet-derived factor XI may be more important for hemostasis than circulating factor XI.

We cannot ignore the contact pathway, however, because catheters and other blood-contacting medical devices, such as stents or mechanical valves, likely trigger clotting through this mechanism. Factor XII bound to charged or artificial surfaces undergoes a conformational change that results in its activation. Factor XIIa converts prekallikrein to kallikrein in a reaction accelerated by high-molecular-weight kininogen, and factor XIIa and kallikrein both feed back to activate additional factor XII. Factor XIIa propagates coagulation by activating factor XI and generating factor XIa, the predominant activator of factor IX (Fig. 122.5). (See box on Emerging Role of the Contact Pathway)

Emerging Role of the Contact Pathway

The contact pathway has emerged as an important player in thrombosis. It has long been recognized that the contact pathway is dispensable for hemostasis because of the lack of a bleeding diathesis in patients with hereditary deficiency of factor XII, prekallikrein, or high-molecular-weight kininogen and the mild bleeding diathesis with factor XI deficiency relative to deficiencies of factor VIII or factor IX. However, until recently, the role of the contact pathway remained elusive. The pathway was ignored for several decades because its activators were mainly nonphysiologic substances such as kaolin or ellagic acid, compounded by the observation that thrombin could activate factor XI, providing a potential physiologic bypass for the contact system as the activator of intrinsic tenase.

The renaissance in our understanding of the important contribution of the contact pathway to thrombus stabilization and propagation occurred as a result of the identification of new physiologic activators, the attenuated thrombosis after venous or arterial injury observed in mice deficient in factor XII or XI, and the development of contact pathway–specific inhibitors. Reports that factor XI-deficient mice were protected from arterial injury–induced thrombosis to the same extent as factor IX-deficient mice, but did not experience bleeding, provide a clear demarcation between hemostasis and thrombosis. The role of the contact pathway in thrombosis gained credibility with the observation that mice lacking factor XII were also resistant to clot formation at sites of vascular injury. However, the physiologic mechanism for activation of the pathway remained unclear until studies showed that nuclear material released from neutrophils in the form of neutrophil extracellular traps, nucleic acids, and inorganic polyphosphates released from activated platelets or microorganisms, activated coagulation in a contact pathway–dependent fashion. With a valid association between the contact pathway and physiologic activators, investigation into the role of the contact pathway in thrombosis exploded.

Renewed interest in the contact pathway has spurred investigation of factors XI and XII as targets for new antithrombotic drugs. Agents targeting factors XI and XII include biological inhibitors, antibodies, small molecule inhibitors, and aptamers. Another approach is to reduce factor levels by inhibiting protein expression through the use of antisense oligonucleotides (ASO). This approach has been successfully applied to factor XI, where administration of an ASO reduced postoperative thrombosis in patients undergoing total knee arthroplasty, without an increase in bleeding. Similar interest in targeting the contact pathway is directed at device-related thrombosis. Thrombosis is a major cause of failure of blood-contacting medical devices, a problem that can lead to life-threatening complications including pulmonary embolism, coronary occlusion, and stroke. and activation of the contact pathway by the artificial surface is thought to be the primary cause. Therefore the contact pathway has emerged as an attractive target for development of agents that reduce thrombosis with little impact on hemostasis.

In addition to its role in device-related thrombosis, the contact pathway may also contribute to the stability of arterial and venous thrombi.[16] NETs, and DNA and RNA released from damaged cells in atherosclerotic plaques, activate factor XII, and mice given DNA- or RNA-degrading enzymes exhibit attenuated thrombosis at sites of arterial injury. Polyphosphates released from activated platelets also activate factor XII, and may provide another stimulus for contact pathway activation. Mice deficient in factor XII or factor XI form small unstable thrombi at sites of arterial or venous damage, suggesting that factor XII and factor XI contribute to thrombogenesis (see Chapter 137). There is mounting evidence that the same is true in humans. Thus patients with unstable angina have increased plasma levels of factor XIa which could reflect activation by factor XIIa, although activation by thrombin remains a possibility. The best evidence for the importance of the contact system comes from the results of a phase II study that demonstrated that knock down of factor XI with an antisense oligonucleotide in patients undergoing elective knee arthroplasty reduced the risk of postoperative venous thromboembolism to a greater extent than enoxaparin. Furthermore, the thrombi that did form in patients with low levels of factor XI were very small in size, consistent with the role of factor XI in thrombus growth. Therefore the contact system is not only an important driver

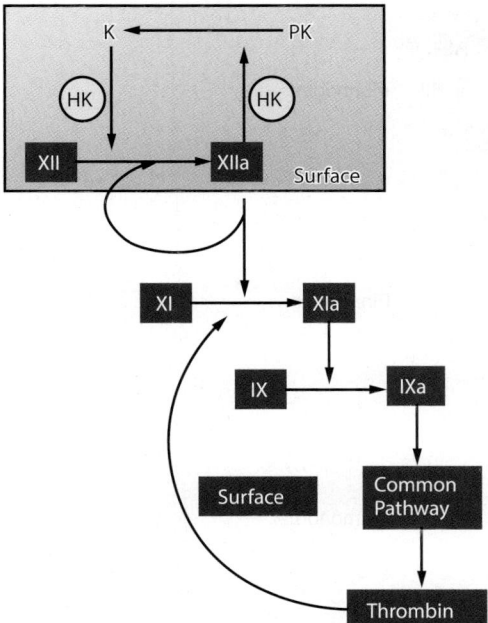

Fig. 122.5 CONTACT SYSTEM. Factor XII (XII) is activated by contact with negatively charged surfaces. XIIa converts prekallikrein (PK) to kallikrein (K), which can feed back to activate more XII. Likewise, XIIa also can feed back to amplify its own generation. About 75% of circulating PK is bound to high-molecular-weight kininogen (HK), which localizes it to anionic surfaces and promotes PK activation. XIIa propagates clotting by activating XI, which then activates IX. The resultant IXa assembles into the intrinsic tenase complex, which activates X to initiate the common pathway of coagulation. Thrombin can feedback activate factor XI to further propagate coagulation.

of thrombosis in blood-contacting medical devices but may also contribute to thrombus propagation in situations where tissue factor initiates coagulation, such as after major surgery.

Prothrombinase

Being the only physiologic producer of thrombin, the prothrombinase complex is essential for hemostasis. Factor Xa binds to factor Va, its activated cofactor, on anionic phospholipid membrane surfaces to form the prothrombinase complex. Activated platelets release factor V from their α-granules, and this platelet-derived factor V may play a more important role in hemostasis than its plasma counterpart.[17] Whereas plasma factor V requires thrombin activation to exert its cofactor activity, the partially activated factor V released from platelets already exhibits substantial cofactor activity. Activated platelets express specific factor Va binding sites on their surface, and bound factor Va serves as a receptor for factor Xa. The catalytic efficiency of factor Xa activation of prothrombin increases by 10^5-fold when factor Xa incorporates into the prothrombinase complex.[13] Prothrombin binds to the prothrombinase complex, where it undergoes conversion to thrombin in a reaction that releases prothrombin fragment 1.2 (F1.2). Plasma levels of F1.2, therefore, provide a marker of prothrombin activation. Prothrombin is the most abundant coagulation factor, and the efficiency of activation generates high local levels of thrombin.

Termination

Because thrombin clots fibrinogen, activates cells and platelets, and mediates anticoagulant and antifibrinolytic processes, it is imperative to regulate its activity and location. Thus the termination phase plays a critical role in balancing the procoagulant forces. Two principal

inhibitors modulate coagulation: TFPI and antithrombin. TFPI, which is located on platelets and microvascular endothelial cells, inhibits factor VIIa in a factor Xa-dependent manner. TFPI effectively halts tissue factor-mediated initiation of coagulation, but not before sufficient factor Xa is generated to propagate clotting. The high levels of thrombin produced during the amplification phase are controlled by antithrombin. This serine protease inhibitor (serpin) also inactivates other coagulation proteases, including factors VIIa, IXa, Xa, and XIa. Although antithrombin is abundant, it exhibits only moderate inhibitory activity, except in the presence of cell-associated glycosaminoglycans, such as heparan sulfate. This is the biochemical basis for use of heparin as an anticoagulant (see Chapter 149). Further regulation of thrombin generation is mediated by the protein C anticoagulant pathway which is catalyzed by thrombin. These processes ensure that thrombin generation is localized and limited. Sufficient thrombin is produced, however, to ensure that coagulation occurs.

Fibrin Formation

Thrombin converts soluble fibrinogen into insoluble fibrin. Fibrinogen is a dimeric molecule, each half of which is composed of three polypeptide chains, the Aα, Bβ, and γ chains. Numerous disulfide bonds covalently link the chains together and join the two halves of the fibrinogen molecule (Fig. 122.6). Electron micrographic studies of fibrinogen reveal a trinodular structure with a central E domain flanked by two D domains. Crystal structures show symmetry of design with the central E domain, which contains the amino termini of the fibrinogen chains, joined to the lateral D domains by coiled-coil regions.

Fibrinogen circulates in a soluble form. Thrombin binds to the amino termini of the Aα and Bβ chains of fibrinogen, where it cleaves specific peptide bonds to release fibrinopeptide A and fibrinopeptide B and generates fibrin monomer (Fig. 122.6). Because they are products of thrombin action on fibrinogen, plasma levels of these fibrinopeptides provide an index of thrombin activity. Fibrinopeptide release creates new amino termini that extend as knobs from the E domain of one fibrin monomer and insert into preformed holes in the D domains of other fibrin monomers. This creates long strands known as protofibrils, consisting of fibrin monomers noncovalently linked together in a half-staggered, overlapping fashion.[18]

Noncovalently linked fibrin protofibrils lack tensile strength.[18] The stability of the fibrin network is enhanced by platelets and procoagulant cells.[19] Platelets not only bind fibrin via GPIIb/IIIa and promote formation of a dense fibrin network, but they also release factor XIII. By covalently cross-linking α and γ chains of adjacent fibrin monomers, factor XIIIa stabilizes the fibrin in a calcium-dependent fashion and renders it relatively resistant to physical strain and degradation. Factor XIII circulates in blood as a heterodimer consisting of pairs of A and B subunits. The active and calcium binding sites on factor XIII are localized to the A subunit. Platelets contain large amounts of factor XIII in their cytoplasm, but platelet-derived factor XIII consists only of the A subunits (see Chapter 125). Both plasma and platelet factor XIII are activated by thrombin.

Hemostasis depends on the dynamic balance between the formation of fibrin and its degradation. The fibrinolytic system mediates fibrin breakdown.

Fibrinolytic System

Fibrinolysis initiates when plasminogen activators convert plasminogen to plasmin, which then degrades fibrin into soluble fragments. Blood contains two immunologically and functionally distinct plasminogen activators, t-PA and u-PA. t-PA mediates intravascular fibrin degradation, whereas u-PA binds to a specific u-PA receptor (u-PAR) on the surface of cells, where it activates cell-bound plasminogen. Consequently, pericellular proteolysis during cell migration and tissue remodeling and repair are the major functions of u-PA.[20]

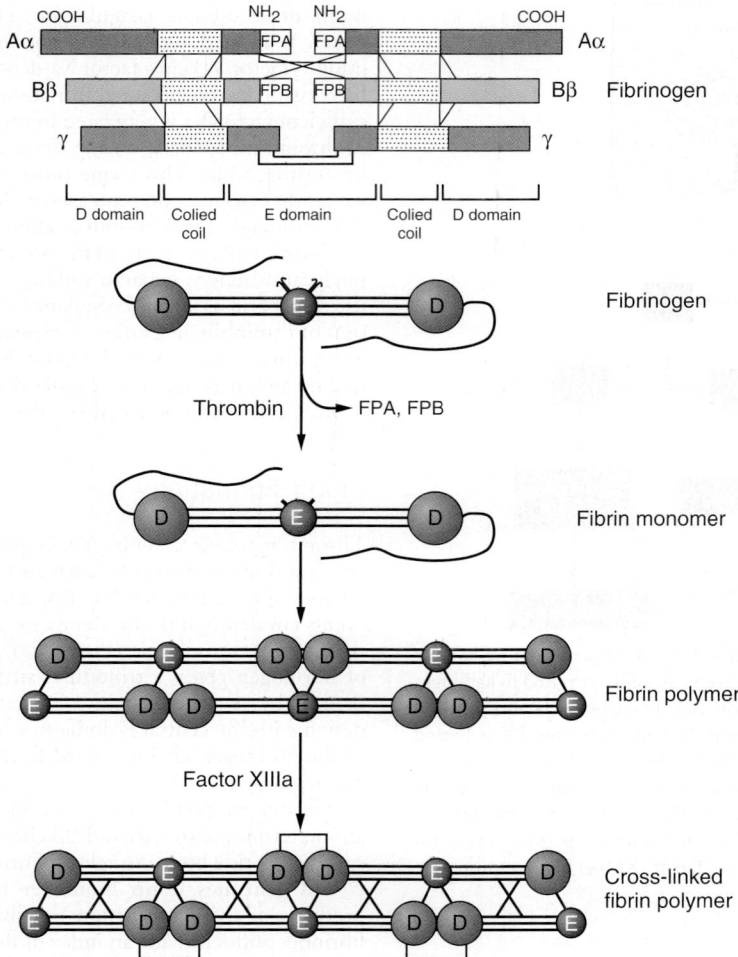

Fig. 122.6 FIBRINOGEN STRUCTURE AND CONVERSION OF FIBRINOGEN TO FIBRIN. A dimeric molecule, each half of fibrinogen is composed of three polypeptide chains, Aα, Bβ, and γ. Numerous disulfide bonds *(lines)* covalently link the chains together and join the two halves of the fibrinogen molecule to yield a trinodular structure with a central E domain linked via the coiled-coil regions to two lateral D domains. To convert fibrinogen to fibrin, thrombin cleaves specific peptide bonds at the amino (NH₂) termini of the Aα and Bβ chains of fibrinogen to release fibrinopeptide A (FPA) and fibrinopeptide B (FPB), thereby generating fibrin monomer. Fibrin monomers polymerize to generate protofibrils arranged in a half-staggered overlapping fashion. By covalently cross-linking α and γ chains of adjacent fibrin monomers, factor XIIIa stabilizes the fibrin network and renders it resistant to degradation.

Regulation of fibrinolysis occurs on a number of levels (see Chapter 127). The substrate of the fibrinolytic system, fibrin, serves a transient but essential stimulatory role that subsides as it degrades. The serpins, PAI-1, and to a lesser extent, PAI-2, inhibit the plasminogen activators, whereas α₂-antiplasmin inhibits plasmin. Endothelial cells synthesize PAI-1, which inhibits both t-PA and u-PA, whereas monocytes and the placenta synthesize PAI-2, which specifically inhibits u-PA. Thrombin-activatable fibrinolysis inhibitor (TAFI) also modulates fibrinolysis and provides a link between fibrinolysis and coagulation.[21] Thrombosis can occur if there is impaired activation of the fibrinolytic system, whereas excessive activation leads to bleeding. Therefore a review of the mechanisms of action of t-PA, u-PA, and TAFI is worthwhile.

Mechanism of Action of Tissue-Type Plasminogen Activator

t-PA, a serine protease, contains five discrete domains: a fibronectin-like finger domain, an epidermal growth factor (EGF) domain, two kringle domains, and a protease domain. Synthesized as a single-chain polypeptide, t-PA is converted into a two-chain form by plasmin.

Single- and two-chain forms of t-PA convert plasminogen to plasmin. Native Glu-plasminogen is a single-chain polypeptide with a Glu residue at its amino-terminus. Plasmin cleavage near the amino-terminus generates Lys-plasminogen, a truncated form with a Lys residue at its new amino terminus.[20] t-PA cleaves a single peptide bond to convert single-chain Glu- or Lys-plasminogen into two-chain plasmin, composed of a heavy chain containing five kringle domains and a light chain containing the catalytic domain. Because its open conformation exposes the t-PA cleavage site, Lys-plasminogen is a better substrate than Glu-plasminogen, which assumes a circular closed conformation that renders this bond less accessible.

t-PA has little enzymatic activity in the absence of fibrin, but its activity increases by at least three orders of magnitude when fibrin is present. This increase in activity reflects the capacity of fibrin to serve as a template that binds t-PA and plasminogen and promotes their interaction. t-PA binds to fibrin via its finger and second kringle domains, whereas plasminogen binds fibrin via its kringle domains. Kringle domains are triple loop-like structures that bind Lys residues on fibrin and other proteins. As fibrin undergoes degradation, more Lys residues are exposed, which provide additional binding sites for t-PA and plasminogen. Consequently, degraded fibrin stimulates t-PA activation of plasminogen more than intact fibrin.

α$_2$-Antiplasmin, another serpin, rapidly inhibits circulating plasmin by docking to its first kringle domain and then inhibiting the active site.[20] Because plasmin binds to fibrin via its kringle domains, plasmin generated on the fibrin surface resists inhibition by α$_2$-antiplasmin. This phenomenon endows fibrin-bound plasmin with the capacity to degrade fibrin. Factor XIIIa cross-links small amounts of α$_2$-antiplasmin onto fibrin, which prevents premature fibrinolysis.[19]

Like fibrin, endothelial cells bind t-PA and plasminogen and markedly promote activation by colocalization of enzyme and substrate. Cell-surface binding is mediated by receptors such as annexin II, gangliosides, and α-enolase, as well as an orphan transmembrane protein expressed with a carboxy-terminal lysine residue. Plasminogen binds to exposed lysine residues on these receptors via its kringle domains. Lipoprotein a, which also possesses kringle domains, impairs cell-based fibrinolysis by competing with plasminogen for cell-surface binding. This phenomenon may explain the association between elevated lipoprotein a levels and atherosclerosis.

Mechanism of Action of Urokinase-Type Plasminogen Activator

Synthesized as a single-chain polypeptide, single-chain u-PA (scu-PA) has minimal enzymatic activity. Plasmin converts scu-PA into a two-chain form that is enzymatically active and capable of binding u-PAR, the u-PA receptor on cell surfaces. Further cleavage at the amino-terminus of two-chain u-PA yields a truncated, lower-molecular-weight form that lacks the u-PAR binding domain.

Two-chain forms of u-PA readily convert plasminogen to plasmin in the absence or presence of fibrin.[20] In contrast, scu-PA does not activate plasminogen in the absence of fibrin, but it can activate fibrin-bound plasminogen, because plasminogen adopts the readily activatable open conformation. Like the higher-molecular-weight form of two-chain u-PA, scu-PA binds to cell surface u-PAR, where plasmin can activate it. Many tumor cells elaborate u-PA and express u-PAR on their surface. As with fibrin and plasminogen receptors, colocalization of the reactants greatly promotes activation. Plasmin generated on these cancer cells endows them with the capacity for metastasis because plasmin readily degrades components of the extracellular matrix and activates growth factors and other degradative proteases.

Mechanism of Action of TAFI

TAFI, a procarboxypeptidase B–like molecule synthesized in the liver, circulates in blood in a latent form where thrombin bound to thrombomodulin can activate it to TAFIa (see Chapters 126 and 127). Unless bound to thrombomodulin, thrombin activates TAFI inefficiently.[21] TAFIa attenuates fibrinolysis by cleaving Lys residues from the carboxy termini of chains of degrading fibrin, thereby removing binding sites for plasminogen, plasmin, and t-PA, attenuating activation, and promoting inhibition. TAFI links fibrinolysis to coagulation because the thrombin–thrombomodulin complex not only activates TAFI, which attenuates fibrinolysis, but also activates protein C, which mutes thrombin generation.

TAFIa has a short half-life in plasma because the enzyme is unstable.[21] Genetic polymorphisms can result in synthesis of more stable forms of TAFIa. Persistent attenuation of fibrinolysis by these variant forms of TAFIa may render patients susceptible to thrombosis.

DISORDERS OF HEMOSTASIS OR THROMBOSIS

A physiologic host defense mechanism, hemostasis focuses on arrest of bleeding by forming hemostatic plugs composed of platelets and fibrin at sites of vessel injury. In contrast, thrombosis reflects a pathologic process associated with intravascular thrombi that fill the lumens of arteries or veins.

TABLE 122.1	Comparison of the Features of Disorders of Primary, Secondary, or Tertiary Hemostasis		
Features	Primary	Secondary	Tertiary
Components involved	Platelets, vWF, and vessel wall	Coagulation	Fibrinolysis factors
Site of bleeding	Skin and mucocutaneous and soft tissues	Muscles, joints, and deep tissues	Wounds and genitourinary tract
Physical findings	Petechiae and ecchymoses	Hematomas and hemarthroses	Hematuria and menorrhagia
Timing of bleeding	Immediate	Delayed	Delayed
Inheritance	Autosomal dominant	Autosomal or X-linked recessive	Autosomal recessive

vWF, von Willebrand factor.

TABLE 122.2	Disorders of Primary Hemostasis	
Components Affected	Causes
Platelets	Quantitative or qualitative platelet disorders
vWF	Inherited or acquired deficiency or dysfunction of vWF
Vessel wall	Vasculitis or abnormalities of connective tissue supporting the vasculature

vWF, von Willebrand factor.

Hemostatic Disorders

Bleeding can occur if there is abnormal platelet plug formation and/or reduced thrombin generation and subsequent fibrin clot formation at the site of vascular injury; disorders of primary and secondary hemostasis, respectively. Bleeding also can occur if the platelet/fibrin clot is prematurely degraded because of excessive fibrinolysis; a disorder of tertiary hemostasis. The features distinguishing disorders of primary, secondary, and tertiary hemostasis are outlined in Table 122.1. Hemorrhagic disorders can be inherited or acquired, and the clinical and laboratory evaluation of such disorders is detailed in Chapters 128 and 129, respectively.

Disorders of Primary Hemostasis

Platelet plug formation, the first step in the arrest of bleeding at sites of injury, requires three key components (a) an adequate number of functional platelets, (b) vWF, the molecular glue that mediates platelet adhesion to the damaged vessel wall even in the face of high shear, and (c) a normal blood vessel that constricts in response to injury (Table 122.2). Because the platelet plug provides the first line of defense against bleeding, patients with disorders of primary hemostasis often present with immediate bleeding after injury, and petechiae (pinpoint hemorrhages) may be noted. In addition to skin bleeding, mucocutaneous bleeding, which may manifest as epistaxis, bleeding gums, or hematochezia, is common as is excessive menstrual bleeding in women (see Chapter 128).

Disorders of primary hemostasis may be inherited or acquired.[22] Thrombocytopenia or congenital or acquired disorders of platelet function are common causes of bleeding. Thrombocytopenia can be the result of decreased production, which can occur because of failure, infiltration, or fibrosis of the bone marrow (see Chapters 29 and 30), increased platelet destruction, or abnormal distribution because of platelet pooling in the spleen (see Chapter 132). Increased destruction of platelets can occur via immune mechanisms, such as immune thrombocytopenic purpura (ITP), alloimmune thrombocytopenia, posttransfusion purpura, and drug-induced thrombocytopenia (see Chapter 131), or nonimmune mechanisms, which include microangiopathic disorders, such as thrombotic thrombocytopenic purpura and hemolytic uremic syndrome (see Chapter 134), as well as consumption because of activation of coagulation, such as occurs with disseminated intravascular coagulation (see Chapter 139).

Platelet function disorders include disorders of platelet (a) adhesion, such as von Willebrand disease (see Chapter 138) and Bernard-Soulier syndrome (see Chapter 125); (b) thromboxane synthesis; (c) secretion, such as alpha or dense granule deficiency or aspirin-like secretion defects; (d) aggregation, such as Glanzmann thrombasthenia (see Chapter 125); or (e) procoagulant activity (Scott syndrome) where the platelets fail to support clotting factor complex assembly (see Chapter 126). Acquired disorders of platelet function can occur in patients taking drugs that impair platelet function, such as aspirin or nonsteroidal antiinflammatory drugs, or in patients with uremia, paraproteins or myelodysplastic or myeloproliferative disorders (see Chapter 130).

Bleeding can also occur with inflammation or malformations of the blood vessels or abnormalities of the connective tissue supporting the blood vessels. Inflammatory disorders include Henoch-Schonlein purpura (see Chapter 152) and the vasculitis that occurs with paraproteins or cryoglobulins or in patients with systemic lupus erythematosis or other immune disorders.[23] Hereditary hemorrhagic telangiectasia is an inherited disorder associated with malformations of the capillaries. Telangiectatic vessels can often be seen in the oral and nasal cavities of patients with this disorder and bleeding episodes, primarily from the nose and gastrointestinal tract, are common. Abnormalities of the connective tissue matrix supporting the blood vessels include Marfan syndrome, Ehlers-Danlos syndrome, and pseudoxanthoma elasticum.[24] Patients with these disorders frequently report easy bruising.

Disorders of Secondary Hemostasis

Secondary hemostasis depends on rapid generation of sufficient amounts of thrombin to generate a fibrin mesh that not only consolidates the platelet aggregates that form at sites of vascular injury, but also is stable enough to provide a barrier that prevents leakage of blood from the damaged blood vessel.[19] Secondary hemostasis can be compromised by (a) impaired thrombin generation because of congenital or acquired deficiencies of coagulation factors or cofactors or intake of drugs that inhibit one or more steps in the coagulation pathways, (b) congenital or acquired fibrinogen deficiency or dysfunction, and/or (c) impaired cross-linking of fibrinogen because of congenital or acquired deficiency of factor XIII (Table 122.3).

Examples of inherited deficiencies of coagulation factors include hemophilia A and B, deficiencies of factor VIII and factor IX, respectively (see Chapter 135). Because of redundancy in the coagulation system, only patients with a factor VIII or factor IX level less than 1% have severe disease characterized by spontaneous bleeding or

bleeding with minimal trauma. Those with factor levels between 1% and 5% have an intermediate phenotype, whereas patients with factor VIII or IX levels above 5% usually have mild disease and bleed only with trauma or surgery. The frequency of bleeding episodes in patients with severe hemophilia can be reduced with prophylactic administration of the appropriate factor concentrate; such treatment is also administered to hemophiliacs with overt bleeding, or in preparation for surgery or other major interventions. Long-lasting factor VIII and IX molecules have been developed to reduce the frequency of factor replacement. The half-lives of these recombinant full-length or truncated proteins have been prolonged by conjugating them to hydrophilic polymers such as polyethylene glycol or by fusing them with albumin or the Fc fragment of IgG_1. Conjugation to polyethylene glycol protects the proteins from proteolytic degradation, whereas fusion technology creates new recycling pathways that diminish natural protein breakdown (see Chapter 136). Management of hemophilia becomes more complicated if patients develop inhibitory antibodies that attenuate or abolish the activity of the infused factor.

Congenital deficiencies of prothrombin (factor II), factors V, VII, X, or XI (hemophilia C), or fibrinogen are less common causes of bleeding (see Chapter 137). In contrast, deficiencies of components of the contact pathway—factor XII, high-molecular-weight kininogen, and prekallikrein—are not associated with bleeding. The clinical and laboratory evaluation of such patients is detailed in Chapters 128 and 129, respectively, whereas their treatment is outlined in Chapter 115.

Acquired deficiencies of coagulation factors can result from decreased synthesis due to severe liver disease, vitamin K deficiency or intake of drugs that interfere with vitamin K metabolism, consumption because of excessive activation of coagulation (e.g., disseminated intravascular coagulation; see Chapter 139), or accelerated clearance due to adsorption by paraproteins or amyloid (see Chapters 86 and 87) or to autoantibodies that shorten the half-life or attenuate or abolish clotting factor activity.

Congenital disorders of fibrinogen include absence or low levels of fibrinogen (afibrinogenemia and hypofibrinogenemia, respectively) or synthesis of a dysfunctional protein (dysfibrinogenemia). Acquired disorders of fibrinogen include decreased synthesis or production of an abnormal fibrinogen, increased fibrinogen consumption or the presence of inhibitors that interfere with fibrin polymerization, such as paraproteins, autoantibodies, particularly in patients with systemic lupus erythematosis or other immune disorders or elevated levels of fibrin(ogen) degradation products.

Stabilization of fibrin requires cross-linking of the α and γ chains of adjacent fibrin monomers to yield a polymer that is resistant to premature breakdown. Factor XIIIa, a transglutaminase, performs this function by catalyzing the condensation of lysine residues on one chain with glutamic acid residues on another chain.[25] Congenital or acquired deficiency of factor XIII can impair cross-linking, resulting in bleeding. The hallmarks of severe factor XIII deficiency include umbilical stump bleeding in the neonatal period (see Chapter 150), intracranial hemorrhage with little or no trauma, recurrent soft tissue hemorrhages, and, in females, recurrent spontaneous miscarriages.

Disorders of Tertiary Hemostasis

Tertiary hemostasis depends on the generation of plasmin, which degrades fibrin and restores blood flow in damaged vessels. Premature lysis of fibrin in hemostatic plugs can lead to bleeding; this can occur systemically or can be localized (Table 122.4). Systemic fibrinolysis that occurs in the absence of activation of coagulation, so-called primary hyperfibrinolysis, is rare but can occur with inherited deficiency of PAI-1 or α_2-antiplasmin, the inhibitors of the plasminogen activators and plasmin, respectively, advanced liver disease, and some snake bites. More commonly, systemic hyperfibrinolysis is secondary to activation of coagulation by procoagulants such as tissue factor (e.g., in patients with metastatic cancer) or artificial surfaces (e.g., in cardiopulmonary bypass surgery or with cardiac assist devices). Examples of localized hyperfibrinolysis include menorrhagia or hematuria after prostatectomy triggered by excessive plasmin generation

TABLE 122.3	Disorders of Secondary Hemostasis
Components Affected	Causes
Coagulation factors	Congenital deficiency, autoantibodies, increased consumption, or drugs that attenuate thrombin generation or thrombin activity
Fibrinogen	Decreased production; increased consumption or synthesis of an abnormal protein
	Impaired fibrin polymerization because of fibrin(ogen) degradation products or paraproteins
Fibrin cross-linking	Congenital or acquired factor XIII deficiency

TABLE 122.4	Disorders of Tertiary Hemostasis
Component Affected	**Causes**
Plasminogen activators	Increased t-PA or u-PA release in the GU tract or other tissues
Plasmin	Deficiency of PAI-1 or α_2-antiplasmin, resulting in an increased plasmin concentration
Plasminogen activation	Enhanced plasminogen activation secondary to activation of coagulation by procoagulants, such as cancer cells, artificial surfaces, or snake venoms

GU, Genitourinary; PAI-1, plasminogen activator inhibitor 1; t-PA, tissue plasminogen activator; u-PA, urokinase-type plasminogen activator.

induced by the high concentrations of t-PA and u-PA in the uterus and genitourinary tract, respectively.

Thrombotic Disorders

Thrombosis may occur in arteries, in the chambers of the heart, or in the veins. Factors contributing to thrombosis in these sites include endothelial injury or activation, reduced blood flow, and hypercoagulability of the blood, the so-called Virchow triad.

Arterial Thrombosis

Most arterial thrombi occur on top of disrupted atherosclerotic plaques. Plaques with a thin fibrous cap and a lipid-rich core are most prone to disruption. Erosion or rupture of the fibrous cap exposes thrombogenic material in the lipid-rich core to the blood and triggers platelet activation and thrombin generation. The extent of plaque disruption and the content of thrombogenic material in the plaque determine the consequences of the event, regardless of whether it occurs in the cerebral circulation (see Chapter 145), the coronary circulation (see Chapter 146), or the major arteries of the legs (see Chapter 148), but host factors also contribute. Breakdown of regulatory mechanisms that limit platelet activation and inhibit coagulation can augment thrombosis at sites of plaque disruption.

Decreased production of nitric oxide and prostacyclin by diseased endothelial cells can trigger vasoconstriction and platelet activation. Proinflammatory cytokines lower thrombomodulin expression by endothelial cells, which promotes thrombin generation, and they stimulate PAI-1 expression which inhibits fibrinolysis.

Products of blood coagulation contribute to atherogenesis, as well as to its complications (see Chapter 144). Microscopic erosions in the vessel wall trigger the formation of tiny platelet-rich thrombi.[26] Activated platelets release PDGF and TGF-β, which promote a fibrotic response. Thrombin generated at the site of injury not only activates platelets and converts fibrinogen to fibrin, but also activates PAR-1 on smooth muscle cells and induces their proliferation, migration, and elaboration of extracellular matrix. Incorporation of thrombi into plaques promotes plaque growth, and decreased endothelial cell production of heparan sulfate—which normally limits smooth muscle proliferation—contributes to plaque expansion.[26] The multiple links between atherosclerosis and thrombosis have prompted the term atherothrombosis (see Chapter 144).

Intracardiac Thrombosis

Thrombi can form in the left ventricle after transmural myocardial infarction or with an aneurysm or dyskinetic ventricle, or in the left atrial appendage, particularly in patients with atrial fibrillation (see Chapter 147). Damage to the endothelium after myocardial infarction and abnormal blood flow are the major triggers for left ventricular thrombus formation. With rapid atrial fibrillation, there also is stasis and turbulent blood flow in the left atrial appendage, which is a long, blind-ended trabeculated pouch.[27] This may lead to localized activation of endothelial cells and subsequent loss of their anticoagulant phenotype, a process amplified by adhesion of leukocytes and subsequent elaboration of proinflammatory cytokines. The generation of thrombin creates a local hypercoagulable state that likely promotes thrombus formation on the abnormal endothelium. Embolization of these thrombi to the brain is a common cause of ischemic stroke and the major cause of mortality and morbidity in patients with atrial fibrillation.

Venous Thrombosis

The causes of venous thrombosis include those associated with hypercoagulability, which can be genetic or acquired, and the mainly acquired risk factors, such as advanced age, obesity, or cancer, which are associated with immobility (see Chapters 140 and 142). Inherited hypercoagulable states and these acquired risk factors combine to establish the intrinsic risk of thrombosis for each individual.[2] Superimposed triggering factors, such as surgery, pregnancy, or hormonal therapy, modify this risk, and thrombosis occurs when the combination of genetic, acquired, and triggering forces exceed a critical threshold.[28]

Some acquired or triggering factors entail a higher risk than others. For example, major orthopedic surgery, neurosurgery, multiple trauma, and metastatic cancer (particularly adenocarcinoma) are associated with the highest risk; prolonged bed rest, antiphospholipid antibodies (see Chapter 141), and the puerperium are associated with an intermediate risk; whereas pregnancy, obesity, long-distance travel, or the use of oral contraceptives or hormonal replacement therapy are mild risk factors. Up to half of patients who present with venous thromboembolism before the age of 45 have inherited hypercoagulable disorders—so-called thrombophilia (see Chapter 140)—particularly those whose event occurred in the absence of risk factors or with minimal provocation, such as after minor trauma or a long-haul flight or with estrogen use.[29]

TREATMENT OF DISORDERS OF HEMOSTASIS AND THROMBOSIS

By the midpoint of the 20th century, two major anticoagulant drugs had been discovered, characterized, and given to humans for prevention or treatment of thrombotic disorders. Heparin and vitamin K antagonists, such as warfarin, dominated treatment regimens for decades. In the same era, determination of their mechanisms of action and dosing was aided by the discovery of the main players of the coagulation system, resulting from the development of sensitive functional assays to monitor their activity. Heparin and warfarin still represent effective members of the anticoagulant armamentarium; however, detailed understanding of the biochemistry and cell biology of hemostasis has directly contributed to the development of new therapies. Heparin derivatives with more predictable pharmacokinetics have improved therapy and reduced complications (see Chapter 149). Small molecule, direct inhibitors of thrombin and factor Xa have been developed as non–vitamin K antagonist (or direct) oral anticoagulants, such as dabigatran, rivaroxaban, apixaban, and edoxaban, that are replacing conventional therapies (see Chapter 149). The resurgence of interest in the contact system as a potential mediator of thrombosis has led to the investigation of factors IX, XI, and XII as new targets for therapy. Likewise new antiplatelet agents that antagonize activation or aggregation steps are being used in conjunction with aspirin to prevent and treat arterial thrombosis (see Chapter 146). On the hemostasis side, regimens to treat bleeding disorders include administration of factors VIIa, VIII, or IX, and prothrombin complex concentrates (see Chapters 135, 136, and 137). The new agents and treatment regimens highlight the therapeutic benefit that has resulted from our detailed understanding of hemostasis and thrombosis.

REFERENCES

1. Lippi G, Franchini M, Targher G: Arterial thrombus formation in cardiovascular disease. *Nat Rev Cardiol* 8:502, 2011.
2. Reitsma PH, Versteeg HH, Middledorp S: Mechanistic view of risk factors for venous thromboembolism. *Arterioscler Thromb Vasc Biol* 32(3):563–568, 2012.
3. Morris TA: Natural history of venous thromboembolism. *Crit Care Clin* 27(4):869–884, 2011.
4. van Hinsbergh VW: Endothelium – role in regulation and coagulation and inflammation. *Semin Immunopathol* 34(1):93–106, 2012.
5. Wood JP, Ellery PE, Maroney SA, et al: Biology of tissue factor pathway inhibitor. *Blood* 123(19):2934–2943, 2014.
6. Esmon CT: Protein C anticoagulant system–anti-inflammatory effects. *Semin Immunopathol* 34(1):127–132, 2012.
7. Nieswandt B, Pleines I, Bender M: Platelet adhesion and activation mechanisms in arterial thrombosis and ischaemic stroke. *J Thromb Haemost* 9(Suppl 1):92–104, 2011.
8. Di Stasio E, De Cristofaro R: The effect of shear stress on protein conformation: physical forces operating on biochemical systems: the case of von Willebrand factor. *Biophys Chem* 153(1):1–8, 2010.
9. Hechler B, Gachet C: P2 receptors and platelet function. *Purinergic Signal* 7(3):293–303, 2011.
10. Alberelli MA, De Candia E: Functional role of protease activated receptors in vascular biology. *Vascul Pharmacol* 62(2):72–81, 2014.
11. Bennett JS, Moore DT: Regulation of platelet beta 3 integrins. *Haematologica* 95(7):1049–1051, 2010.
12. Versteeg HH, Heemskerk JW, Levi M, et al: New fundamentals in hemostasis. *Physiol Rev* 93(1):327–358, 2013.
13. Mann KG: Thrombin generation in hemorrhage control and vascular occlusion. *Circulation* 124(2):225–235, 2011.
14. Rao LV, Pendurthi UR: Regulation of tissue factor coagulant activity on cell surfaces. *J Thromb Haemost* 10(11):2242–2253, 2012.
15. Ahmad SS, London FS, Walsh PN: The assembly of the factor X-activating complex on activated human platelets. *J Thromb Haemost* 1(1):48–59, 2003.
16. Woodruff RS, Sullenger B, Becker RC: The many faces of the contact pathway and their role in thrombosis. *J Thromb Thrombolysis* 32(1):9–20, 2011.
17. Fager AM, Wood JP, Bouchard BA, et al: Properties of procoagulant platelets: defining and characterizing the subpopulation binding a functional prothrombinase. *Arterioscler Thromb Vasc Biol* 30(12):2400–2407, 2010.
18. Lord ST: Molecular mechanisms affecting fibrin structure and stability. *Arterioscler Thromb Vasc Biol* 31(3):494–499, 2011.
19. Wolberg AS: Plasma and cellular contributions to fibrin network formation, structure and stability. *Haemophilia* 16(Suppl 3):7–12, 2010.
20. Schaller J, Gerber SS: The plasmin-antiplasmin system: structural and functional aspects. *Cell Mol Life Sci* 68(5):785–801, 2011.
21. Heylen E, Willemse J, Hendriks D: An update on the role of carboxypeptidase U (TAFIa) in fibrinolysis. *Front Biosci* 17:2427–2450, 2011.
22. Broos K, Feys HB, DeMeyer SF, et al: Platelets at work in primary hemostasis. *Blood Rev* 25(4):155–167, 2011.
23. Eby C: Pathogenesis and management of bleeding and thrombosis in plasma cell dyscrasias. *Br J Haematol* 145(2):151–163, 2009.
24. Malfait F, DePaepe A: Bleeding in the heritable connective tissue disorders: mechanisms, diagnosis and treatment. *Blood Rev* 23(5):191–197, 2009.
25. Komaromi I, Bagoly Z, Muszbek L: Factor XIII: novel structural and functional aspects. *J Thromb Haemost* 9(1):9–20, 2011.
26. Borissoff JI, Spronk HM, ten Cate H: The hemostatic system as a modulator of atherosclerosis. *N Engl J Med* 364(18):1746–1760, 2011.
27. Watson T, Shantsila E, Lip GY: Mechanisms of thrombogenesis in atrial fibrillation: Virchow's triad revisited. *Lancet* 373(9658):155–166, 2009.
28. Tchaikovski SN, Rosing J: Mechanisms of estrogen-induced venous thromboembolism. *Thromb Res* 126(1):5–11, 2010.
29. Anderson JA, Weitz JI: Hypercoagulable states. *Crit Care Clin* 27(4):933–952, 2011.

The vasculature plays a major role in conveying and distributing hematopoietic cells, nutrients, gases, metabolites, and various chemical mediators.[1] The interior of the vessel wall is lined by the endothelium, comprising more than 1012 endothelial cells, covering a surface of approximately 500 m[2] and weighing approximately 1 kg in total.[2,3] The endothelium forms a continuous monolayer at the interface between blood and tissue. Thus it contributes significantly to sensing and transducing of signals between blood and tissue, trafficking of hematopoietic cells, and maintenance of a nonthrombogenic surface permitting flow of blood. Normally quiescent with cell turnover measured on the order of years, endothelial cells have a remarkable capacity to proliferate and vascularize tissues in physiologic (menstrual cycle) and pathologic (tumorigenesis, diabetic retinopathy) situations.[4] The endothelium is critical for initiating and potentiating the inflammatory response. The pathogenesis of several disorders, such as atherosclerosis, hypertension, diabetic angiopathy, and microangiopathic hemolytic anemias, involves dysfunction of the endothelial lining. The complexity and the vast array of its functional responses have led to the description of the endothelium as a distributed organ.[5] This chapter provides a conceptual framework of the structure and development of the vessel wall and the physiologic functions of the endothelium as it relates to the hematopoietic system.

STRUCTURE OF THE VESSEL WALL

The circulatory system has traditionally been divided into the macrovasculature (vessels >100 μm in diameter) and the microvasculature.[6] The arterial system transports blood to tissues, resists changes in blood pressure proximally, and regulates blood flow distally. Veins return blood to the heart and act as capacitance vessels because they contain approximately 70% of the total blood volume. Venules with luminal diameters less than 50 μm are structurally similar to capillaries.[6] Capillaries and microvessels in general are particularly important in the exchange of gases, macromolecules, and cells between blood and tissue. Although large vessels play an important role in maintaining vascular tone, a significant proportion of peripheral resistance arises from the capillaries.[7] Capillary endothelial cells also have a metabolic role, as in the conversion of angiotensin and hydrolysis of lipoproteins. Finally, sprouting of new vessels is initiated in the microvasculature.

Macrovasculature

Large vessels are composed of three layers: intima, media, and adventitia.[6,8] The intima comprises the endothelium and the subendothelium. The endothelial cells of large vessels contain a distinct rod-shaped organelle, measuring approximately 3 μm × 0.1 μm, called the Weibel-Palade body.[9] Ultrastructural studies indicate the presence of a single membrane around the Weibel-Palade body with tubular structures within. This organelle contains von Willebrand factor (vWF), and P-selectin has been reported to be present on the surrounding membrane.[10–12] The abluminal face of the endothelium rests on a basement membrane, which supports the endothelial cell and can act as a secondary barrier against the extravasation of blood.[2] The subendothelial matrix contains occasional smooth muscle cells and scattered macrophages. Both smooth muscle cells and endothelial cells contribute to the extracellular matrix (ECM) of the intima, along with ECM components including elastin and collagen.[13,14] In large vessels, the media is separated from the intima by a layer of elastin, the internal elastic lamina. Diseases associated with mutations in elastin include supravalvular aortic stenosis,[15,16] Williams syndrome,[17] and autosomal dominant cutis laxa.[18] The medial layer is composed primarily of concentric layers of smooth muscle cells and their secreted matrix, which is a complex mix of glycoproteins and proteoglycans. This layer is responsible for the structural integrity of the wall and for maintaining vascular tone. Mutations of the fibrillin-1 gene, a microfilament protein in elastic fibers, result in disruption of the media in Marfan syndrome.[12] Defects of type III collagen can cause aortic rupture in patients with Ehlers-Danlos syndrome type IV.[14] An attenuated band of elastic fibers, the external elastic lamina, separates the adventitia from the media. The adventitia is composed of loose connective tissue, and the outer portion of the media contains an ECM scaffold containing fibroblasts, small nerves, progenitor cells, lymphatic vessels, and nutritive blood vessels, the vasa vasorum. The adventitia has been recognized as a dynamic environment, important in the growth, disease, and repair of the artery. The external limit of the adventitial layer is loosely defined and becomes continuous with the surrounding connective tissue of the organ.[6,8]

Microvasculature

Capillaries and postcapillary venules are composed of two cell types: endothelial cells and pericytes.[19] Pericytes and endothelial cells are invested with a basement membrane and, depending on the vascular bed, variable amounts of matrix separate the two cell types. Both cell types contribute to secretion of basement membrane proteins, demonstrating that pericyte–endothelial interaction plays a key role in basement membrane formation, maintenance, and remodeling. Long pericyte processes extend over the abluminal surface of the endothelial cell,[20] and reciprocal extensions of the endothelial cell make contact with the pericyte. At distinct points in the basement membrane, pericytes and endothelial cells form specialized junctions with each other. Adherens junctions connect the cytoskeleton of pericytes and endothelial cells, mediating contact inhibition through contractile forces. Gap junctions between the cytoplasms of pericytes and endothelial cells enable communication through the passage of metabolites and ionic currents.[21] A variety of functions have been ascribed to the pericyte, including[19,22,23] (1) a contractile function, which regulates blood flow; (2) multipotential capabilities resulting in differentiation to adipocytes, osteoblasts, phagocytes, and smooth muscle cells; and (3) regulation of capillary growth. The best evidence probably exists for the last function. In animal models[24,25] and human disease (diabetic microangiopathy, hemangiomata),[26] a lack of pericytes is associated with microaneurysms and disordered microvasculature. In addition, there is a temporal correlation between pericyte contact and cessation of vessel growth in wound healing,[27] and pericyte contact suppresses endothelial cell migration and proliferation in vitro.[19]

Endothelial Structure and Function

In contrast to circulating blood cells and vascular smooth muscle cells but similar to epithelial cells, the endothelium exhibits polarity manifested by the asymmetric distribution of cell surface glycoproteins and by the unidirectional secretion of some ECM proteins and chemical mediators.[28,29] Although in cultured endothelial cells an apical–basal polarity is established before confluence, intercellular junctions may have a role in maintaining the asymmetry in vivo.[28,30]

Four types of intercellular junctions between adjacent endothelial cells have been described[30,31]: tight junctions, gap junctions, adherens junctions, and syndesmos. Their distribution varies along the vascular tree, with tight junctions occurring more frequently in the larger arteries and brain vasculature, correlating with a more stringent requirement for permeability control. The molecular structure of endothelial tight junctions is similar to that of epithelial cells, consisting of a network of fibrils, with the integral membrane components composed of occludin, claudin-5, and junctional adhesion molecules (JAMs), which associate with various structural and signaling proteins on the cytoplasmic face.[32] The distribution of gap junctions tends to follow that of tight junctions. Connexin 37, connexin 40, and connexin 43 are gap junction proteins that have been detected in endothelial cells. Gap junctions mediate communication between adjacent endothelial cells, and between endothelial cells and pericytes or smooth muscle cells; they also contribute to the endothelial barrier and vascular integrity. Adherens junctions are formed by transmembrane glycoproteins called cadherins, which make the link between cell-to-cell contacts and the cytoskeleton. Several different types of cadherins are expressed in endothelial cells. The endothelial-specific cadherin vascular endothelial cadherin (VE-cadherin [cadherin-5]) is expressed on virtually all types of endothelium.[31] Similar to other cadherins, VE-cadherin forms homotypic contacts with VE-cadherin on adjacent cells. Within the cell, VE-cadherin complexes with catenins, which, through other proteins, contact the actin cytoskeleton. Homotypic engagement of VE-cadherin results in density-dependent inhibition of endothelial proliferation, which appears to be mediated by association of vascular endothelial growth factor receptor 2 (VEGFR-2) with VE-cadherin, thereby sequestering VEGFR-2 at the membrane and preventing its internalization into signaling compartments.[33] The structure of the fourth type of junction, the syndesmos, is not well elucidated.

Other membrane proteins that are located at interendothelial junctions include platelet endothelial cell adhesion molecule 1 (PECAM-1), which may be important in directing the formation of junctions, nectins, JAMs, endothelial cell-selective adhesion molecule (ESAM), and the integrins (particularly $\alpha2\beta1$ and $\alpha5\beta1$).[34,35] In addition to the functions listed previously, intercellular contacts are important in maintaining cell survival.[36]

On the luminal side, endothelium is exposed to blood elements and, under pathologic conditions, to circulating molecules such as cytokines and bacterial products. Engagement of endothelial receptors by these humoral factors activates a well-described series of responses, including the recruitment and transmigration of leukocytes and changes in endothelial cell coagulant activity (see The Endothelium as a Nonthrombogenic Surface section). Biomechanical forces resulting from pulsatile blood flow have been shown to mediate striking changes in endothelial morphology and metabolism. Vessels must withstand three types of physical forces: radial distension (tension), longitudinal stretch, and tangential shear stress. In response to flow (shear stress), endothelial cells reorganize their cytoskeletal architecture, rearrange focal contacts at the basal surface, and align in the direction of flow.[37–39] Some endothelial cell responses following exposure to physical forces occur within seconds, such as activation of potassium channels and increased release of nitric oxide (NO), resulting in vasodilation. Other endothelial cell responses to flow are related to changes in gene expression and occur after a delay of a few hours. Elements in the promoters of various adhesion molecule and growth factor genes have been shown to contain sequences that respond to shear stress (in a positive or negative fashion) and have been referred to as the *shear stress response element*.[37–39]

Endothelial cells vectorially secrete certain ECM proteins to the abluminal face. The matrix molecules that are secreted by endothelium include several types of collagen, elastin, fibronectin, laminins, and proteoglycans (e.g., heparan sulfate and dermatan sulfate). The exact composition of the subendothelium varies with location in the vascular tree, age, and disease states.[2,14,40] Endothelial cells bind to the ECM via heterodimeric cell surface glycoproteins—the integrins—which link and integrate matrix proteins to the cytoskeleton at sites referred to as *focal contacts*.[41] The integrins detected in resting endothelium include $\alpha6\beta1$, $\alpha5\beta1$, $\alpha2\beta1$, and $\alpha v\beta3$.[42] Interestingly, endothelial cells express integrins on luminal as well as abluminal surfaces.[42] The ECM serves several important functions: (1) it serves as a barrier to macromolecules in the event of disruption of the endothelium; (2) it sequesters growth factors and mediates their high-affinity binding to endothelial cells (e.g., heparan sulfate binds to fibroblast growth factor [FGF]); and (3) it acts as a counterstructure for the binding of endothelial cell integrins.[14,40,43] This binding of endothelial cells to the ECM serves at least four purposes: (1) Whereas certain matrix molecules provide a physical scaffold, others act as haptotactic agents, inducing endothelial cells to migrate.[14] (2) Clustering of integrins at focal adhesion contacts by certain matrix molecules can transduce survival or differentiation signals by causing phosphorylation of various proteins and lipids.[43] Whereas fibronectin and vitronectin provide survival signals, laminins appear to signal differentiation.[44–46] (3) By maintaining cell shape, integrin-mediated cell spreading provides an antiapoptotic signal independent of direct integrin-initiated signal transduction.[47] (4) By anchoring the cell, the matrix provides a mechanism whereby blood flow at the luminal surface of the endothelium creates shear stress, which also transmits signals to cells.[37]

Endothelial Heterogeneity

Despite their common features, quiescent endothelial cells in vivo represent a widely heterogeneous population, with their phenotype depending on vessel caliber and location. Exposure to different physical forces (e.g., arteries vs. veins) and the different functions served by vessels of different caliber are reflected in different endothelial phenotypes.[48] However, study of the molecular basis of the heterogeneity of these different populations is just beginning. Experiments using serial analysis of gene expression and in vivo delivery of phage display peptide libraries have revealed organ- and tumor vasculature–specific molecules that will help to elucidate the molecular basis of endothelial heterogeneity.[49–51] Within the microvasculature is a structural heterogeneity of capillaries, depending on the organ supplied. Even within a single organ, endothelial cells exhibit different phenotypes, depending on their functional role. When microvessels from different organs are harvested and cultured in vitro, they lose some of their distinctive characteristics with progressive passaging. Some specialization of the different endothelial cells can be retained if they are cocultured with cells or matrix from the organ from which they are derived. Thus matrix proteins, soluble factors from the organ, or heterotypic contacts with parenchymal cells or pericyte or smooth muscle cells are believed to be important factors in specifying endothelial cell phenotype.[52] Conversely, emerging evidence indicates that endothelial cells in turn provide instructive morphogenic cues during organogenesis and in adults.[53] Specific examples of microvessels found in hematopoietic tissues are discussed in the following sections. Endothelial cells from veins and arteries and from capillaries of different organs demonstrate heterogeneity at structural, functional, and molecular levels.[54] Intriguingly, phenotypic heterogeneity also exists between neighboring endothelial cells exposed to the same extracellular environment. In the case of endothelial-restricted vWF expression, heterogeneity denoted by mosaic vWF expression proved dynamically regulated by bistable transitions in the DNA methylation status of the vWF promoter, suggesting novel stochastic phenotype switching potentials in endothelial microenvironments.[55]

High Endothelial Venules

Lymphocyte migration into secondary lymphoid sites, such as lymph nodes, Peyer patches, and chronically inflamed nonlymphoid tissues, occurs at specialized postcapillary venules called *high endothelial venules* (HEVs).[56] The endothelial cells of these venules (HEV-ECs) exhibit a plump or cuboidal morphology (hence the name high endothelial venule), display intense biosynthetic activity, and are encircled by a continuous thick basal lamina formed from ECM components produced by surrounding pericyte-like cells called *fibroblastic reticular cells*. HEV-ECs are composed of free ribosomes, multivesicular bodies, well-developed Golgi apparatus, tissue-specific adhesion molecules, and chemokines.[57] They secrete a thick glycocalyx, of which a proportion is glycosylation-dependent cell adhesion molecule 1, a ligand for L-selectin.[58] CD34 is another HEV "addressin" on peripheral lymph node endothelial cells. Endothelium of mesenteric lymph nodes and Peyer patches express mucosal addressin cellular adhesion molecule 1 (MAdCAM-1) as a ligand for L-selectin and $\alpha4\beta7$ integrin. HEV-EC express additional L-selectin ligands grouped together as peripheral node addressins (PNAd) including glycosylation-dependent cellular adhesion molecule 1 (GlyCAM-1),[59] endomucin,[60] and nepmucin.[61] Expression of these different addressins may recruit specific subpopulations of lymphocytes to different lymphoid tissues (i.e., they facilitate the "homing" of lymphocytes). Several other proteins, including the chemokine receptor DARC (Duffy antigen receptor for chemokines) and the antiadhesive matrix protein Hevin, have been identified as being preferentially expressed by the high endothelial venule.[62] Tight junctions are present at intermittent spots, and extensive overlap between the membranes of adjacent cells prevents macromolecules from interendothelial transit. However, when lymphoid cells transit to the high endothelial venule, there is a temporary breach in the barrier.[58] Evidence suggests that the high endothelial venule not only plays a critical role in homing and recruitment of immune cells, but also can influence the outcome of the immune response.[63]

Bone Marrow Sinuses

Much less is known about the bone marrow (BM) sinuses than about the high endothelial venule. The BM sinus endothelial cell is flat, in contrast to that of the high endothelial venule, with loose interdigitated junctions and the basal lamina is discontinuous. It has been suggested that hematopoietic cells traverse pores present at attenuated areas of the endothelium rather than move by an interendothelial route.[64] Clearly, the BM sinus endothelial cell is specialized given the regulated egress of cells from the BM. For example, if a red blood cell (RBC) that still is nucleated begins to enter the circulation, the body of the cell is allowed to cross and is released as a reticulocyte, while the nucleus is retained extravascularly. The adventitial reticular cell (similar to a pericyte) is also thought to play an important role in controlling hematopoietic cell egress.[65] Stromal cell–derived factor 1 (SDF-1; also called CXC-chemokine ligand [CXCL]12) and chemokine receptor CXC-chemokine receptor (CXCR)4 interactions are essential for stem cell homing, mobilization, and transendothelial migration into the BM.[66,67] SDF-1 activates the integrins lymphocyte function-associated antigen 1 (LFA-1 [$\alpha L\beta2$]), very late antigen 4 (VLA-4 [$\alpha4\beta1$]), and very late antigen 5 (VLA-5 [$\alpha5\beta1$]). Whereas vascular cell adhesion molecule 1 (VCAM-1), which is expressed on BM endothelial cells (and spleen endothelial cells in the mouse), appears to be the major BM addressin for hematopoietic progenitor cells expressing VLA-4, intercellular adhesion molecule 1 (ICAM-1) binds LFA-1.[67,68] Endothelial selectins also have been implicated in promoting hematopoietic stem and progenitor cell homing to the BM.[69] Factors such as CD44, cytoskeletal rearrangement, and matrix metalloproteinases (MMPs) are other key players in the homing process related to the endothelium.[67] The BM endothelium is also involved in regulating hematopoiesis (see Relationship Between Vascular Development and Hematopoiesis section).

VASCULAR DEVELOPMENT AND DIFFERENTIATION

The human embryo develops a vascular system by the third week, when its nutritional needs are no longer met by diffusion.[70] Vascular development proceeds in several ways. Vasculogenesis is the process whereby blood vessels form de novo from the differentiation of mesodermal precursors. Angiogenesis is the outgrowth of new capillaries from preexisting vessels and is thought to be the major mode of new vessel development in the adult. Arteriogenesis, or collateral development, is the rapid enlargement of preexisting collateral arterioles after occlusion of a supply artery. Lymphangiogenesis is the development of lymphatic vessels, which are required for transportation of extravasated lymph and lymphoid cells. Finally, in some neoplasms, tumor cells rather than endothelial cells form vascular channels or a portion of some vessels, a process termed *vasculogenic mimicry*.[71] A similar nonendothelial cell lining of vascular channels can be created by placental cytotrophoblasts forming hybrid fetal–maternal vessels in the endometrium.[71]

Vasculogenesis

Vasculogenesis in the yolk sac proceeds initially by the differentiation of mesodermal cells into angioblasts.[72] Angioblasts are vascular cells that express some, but not all, endothelial markers. These cells arise from mesodermal cells resting on the endoderm (splanchnopleuric mesoderm) but not from the mesoderm adjacent to the ectoderm (somatopleuric mesoderm). Thus it is believed that whereas the endoderm positively regulates vascular development, the ectoderm negatively regulates vasculogenesis. Organs that are primarily of ectodermal origin (e.g., brain and kidney) are vascularized by angiogenesis and not by vasculogenesis. The mesodermal cells migrating outward from the endoderm form primitive structures termed *blood islands*. Whereas the cells at the center of the blood island are hematopoietic precursors, those arranged peripherally are angioblastic precursors. Vasculogenesis within the embryo begins shortly after that in the yolk sac, again in close association with endoderm.[73] However, except for a region on the ventral aspect of the embryonic aorta, intraembryonic vascular development occurs in solitary angioblasts rather than blood islands. Angioblasts differentiate in situ and form primary capillary plexuses with lumens, or they migrate and fuse with other angioblasts or capillaries. Fusion of angioblasts or blood islands results in the formation of a capillary plexus that undergoes extensive remodeling over the developmental period.[72]

Vasculogenesis in the Adult

Although initially said to occur primarily in the embryo, vasculogenesis may also play a role in promoting vascular development in adults. The identification of circulating BM-derived vascular precursors and the demonstration that these precursors can integrate into the vasculature at sites of angiogenesis describe an adult form of de novo vessel development.[74] Two distinct BM-derived precursors with the ability to differentiate into vascular cells have been identified: (1) accumulating evidence points to a single precursor, the hemangioblast, which can differentiate into either hematopoietic or endothelial cells,[75] and (2) a multipotent nonhematopoietic adult progenitor cell, which is thought to represent a BM mesenchymal stem cell (BM-MSC). When injected intravenously into adult mice, these MSCs differentiate into vascular cells, hematopoietic cells, and several epithelial cell types.[76,77] Once seeded on a synthetic graft, BM-MSCs differentiate into both smooth muscle and endothelial cells in vivo.[78] Both types of multipotential precursor populations express CD133, a cell surface marker that is lost upon further maturation.[79] However, only the hemangioblast expresses CD34. Whether MSCs are able to circulate and thus contribute to neovascularization outside the BM remains to be shown. Various stresses, including neoplasia, sepsis, burns, and trauma, have been suggested to induce mobilization of BM-derived endothelial precursors, which express CD133, CD34, and VEGFR-2.[79] Cytokines that reportedly induce mobilization of BM-derived endothelial precursors include VEGF-A and granulocyte macrophage colony-stimulating factor (GM-CSF),[79] as well as SDF-1, which stimulates mobilization of CXCR4+ BM cells, including hematopoietic stem cells (HSCs) and EPCs.[80,81] Recent data have implicated IL-8 as a regulator in mobilizing EPCs into the peripheral circulation by binding both CXCR1 and CXCR2.[82] The contribution of BM-derived vascular precursors to angiogenic vessels in tumors is highly variable, depending on the study, the model used, and the tumor cell type used.[83] The degree of endothelial precursor incorporation into the angiogenic vasculature is highly controversial; several groups suggest negligible, if any, involvement by distant precursors.[83] The problem arises in part from the poor definition of a circulating endothelial precursor cell. Many, if not all, of the markers used to define this rare cell population are shared with hematopoietic stem or progenitor cells, and the distinction between the endothelial and hematopoietic precursor has not been rigorously addressed in the majority of studies. More recent work has suggested that BM-derived, perivascular CD11b+ hematopoietic cells secreting angiogenic cytokines have been misidentified as endothelial precursor cells.[84,85]

Angiogenesis

In a normal adult, angiogenesis occurs primarily in the female reproductive system. However, angiogenesis is a process that has a major impact in several pathologic situations. Probably the best known and studied example of pathologic neovascularization occurs during tumor progression. Angiogenesis also is important in chronic inflammation, ischemia, and wound healing.

Capillary sprouts from the existing microvasculature form secondary to an inciting stimulus that results in increased vascular permeability, accumulation of extravascular fibrin, and local proteolytic degradation of the basement membrane.[86-88] Endothelial cells overlying the disrupted region become "activated," change shape, and extend elongated processes into the surrounding tissue. Filopodia extending from the specialized endothelial cells at the tip of the vascular sprout guide the migration of the nascent vessel.[89] Directed migration toward the angiogenic stimulation results in the formation of a column of endothelial cells. Just proximal to the migrating tip of the column is a region of proliferating endothelial cells. These proliferating cells cause an increase in the length of the sprout. In the region of proliferation, up to 20% of endothelial cells may enter the cell cycle. This is in marked contrast to quiescent endothelium, of which less than 0.01% of cells are cycling. Proximal to the proliferative zone, the endothelial cells undergo another shape change, adhere tightly to each other, and begin to form a lumen. Evidence suggests that endothelial lumina arise through the formation and fusion of intracellular vacuoles.[90] Secondary sprouting from the migrating tip results in a capillary plexus, and fusion of individual sprouts at their tips closes the loop and circulates blood into the vascularized area. Activated macrophages and platelets, by secreting growth factors, cytokines, proteases, and protease inhibitors, can influence all phases of the angiogenic process.[91]

The morphologic features described are characteristic of sprouting angiogenesis. Another mechanism of angiogenesis, "intussusceptive microvascular growth," refers to vascular network formation by insertion of interstitial tissue columns, called *tissue pillars* or *posts*, into existing vascular lumen and subsequent growth of these columns, resulting in partitioning of the vessel lumen. Periendothelial cells, including pericytes and myofibroblasts, which invade the pillar core stabilize the structure in association with collagen fibrils. The mechanisms of intussusceptive angiogenesis are less well described, but hemodynamic factors appear to be involved.[92]

Recruitment of Periendothelial Cells

Whether formed by vasculogenesis or angiogenesis, maturation of new vessels requires recruitment of smooth muscle cells or pericytes to reestablish vessel integrity. Periendothelial cells provide structural support, assist in production of the ECM, provide contractile function so as to modulate vessel caliber, and maintain the cells in a quiescent state. Genetically altered mice that fail to invest their vessels with pericytes develop microaneurysms.[24] In embryos, periendothelial cells are thought to be derived from locally available mesenchymal cells as endothelial cells invade organ rudiments. Local derivation of periendothelial cells may be one mechanism that allows for tissue-specific phenotype of the vasculature.[19] Evidence suggests that embryonic endothelial cells may transdifferentiate into vascular smooth muscle cells.[93] Evidence also indicates that some periendothelial cells are derived from the neural crest during embryogenesis and from BM-derived precursors in adults.[94-97] Although some studies have shown pericytes to be potential antivascular targets for tumor therapy,[96,98] other work has suggested that pericytes act to limit tumor metastasis.[99]

Extracellular Matrix

It is thought that whereas interstitial collagens (e.g., collagen I) and provisional plasma-derived fibronectin–fibrin matrices stimulate endothelial tubular morphogenic events, laminin-rich matrices lead to endothelial differentiation and stabilization events.[91] Mice deficient in fibronectin die during embryogenesis and show vascular defects. Type I collagen-deficient mice die of circulatory failure just before birth. Although most tumor vessels are covered by basement membrane, this layer has multiple structural abnormalities consistent with ongoing vascular activation in tumors.[100] ECM proteins or their proteolytic fragments have been shown to inhibit angiogenesis.

Dissolution of the underlying matrix by MMPs and heparanases allows endothelial cells to migrate at the initiation of angiogenesis.[101,102] Matrix-bound growth factors are also released as a consequence of ECM degradation. The balance between positive and negative regulators is the basis of tight control in this process. Tissue plasminogen activator (t-PA) and urokinase plasminogen activator (u-PA), by generating plasmin, can activate collagenases and other MMPs. Plasminogen activator inhibitors (PAIs) may block angiogenesis at this step. Action of the MMPs is required for angiogenesis, and the tissue inhibitors of MMPs regulate their function.[103]

Cell Adhesion Molecules

Of the various classes of cell adhesion molecules involved in angiogenesis, the integrins have been the most studied.[14,104,105] Although it is universally accepted that integrins and integrin ligands function in angiogenesis, their exact actions remain unclear. In particular, substantial controversy surrounds the role of $\alpha v \beta 3$ integrin.[14,104,106] Immunohistochemical studies localize this integrin to the tips of sprouting vessels. Neutralizing antibodies abrogate angiogenesis and induce vascular cell apoptosis in vivo, and inhibitory peptides or peptidomimetics blocking adhesive functions of integrin $\alpha v \beta 3$ inhibit angiogenesis in a variety of animal models.[107] However, mice lacking αv show extensive angiogenesis, and mice and humans (Glanzmann thrombasthenia) lacking $\beta 3$ integrin also show normal angiogenesis. Notwithstanding the discrepancies outlined, preclinical studies have validated $\alpha v \beta 3$ and potentially other integrins ($\alpha v \beta 5$, $\alpha 1 \beta 1$, $\alpha 2 \beta 1$, $\alpha 5 \beta 1$, $\alpha 6 \beta 4$) as therapeutic antiangiogenic targets, and clinical trials with combination therapy are currently in progress.[108] One of the integrin receptors for fibronectin, $\alpha 5 \beta 1$, has been shown to be necessary for vascular development, and $\alpha 2 \beta 1$ seems important for the formation of tubes by endothelial cells in vitro. However, there likely is a dynamic regulation of $\beta 1$ integrins during angiogenesis because constitutive activation of this integrin inhibits endothelial sprouting in vitro and angiogenesis in vivo.[109] The junctional proteins VE-cadherin and PECAM-1, and possibly JAM-1, are expressed early in development and have a role in assembling the vasculature.[33,110,111]

Guidance Molecules

Similar to the nervous system, the vascular system forms a highly ordered, branching network. The ordering of this patterned network is dependent on multiple attractive and repulsive cues, many of which are common to both the nervous and vascular systems.[112,113] Tip cells express a distinctive profile of genes with substantially higher expression compared with stalk cells of molecular markers including platelet-derived growth factor (PDGF)-B, VEGFR-2, uncoordinated (Unc)5b, Delta-like (Dll)4, and VEGFR-3. Whereas VEGF165 acts as an attractive cue to the tip cell of the endothelial sprout, Netrin-1 signals to Unc5b on the vasculature act as a repulsive cue. Netrin-4 can also bind Neogenin, which in turn recruits and activates Unc5b to mediate repulsion. Other guidance pathways implicated in vascular patterning and angiogenesis are ephrinB2–EphB4, plexinD1–semaphorin, and Slit–Robo interactions, as well as the neuropilins. Patterning and specification of small arteries along peripheral nerves in the skin of the embryonic limb involves nerve-derived VEGF; in other situations, neuronal patterning is dependent on the vasculature.[114,115] Thus the congruent patterning of the neural and vascular systems likely is caused by use of common signals and may require cross-talk between the two systems.

Remodeling, Regression, and Apoptosis

Even though the vasculature is laid down before circulation begins, hemodynamic forces are important for maintenance and remodeling. Most of the vessels laid down during vasculogenesis regress or are remodeled. After neovascularization (e.g., during wound healing), the vessels regress when no longer needed. A chronic decrease in blood flow results in narrowing of the vessel lumen. This change in vessel caliber is dependent on an intact and functional endothelium.[116] Remodeling, which involves loss of some vessels as well as changes in lumen diameter and wall thickness, requires both cell death and proliferation (as well as remodeling of the ECM). In addition to survival signals transmitted by integrins, shear stress is important for endothelial survival and vessel healing after injury.[117–119] Oxygen tension is important in vascular maintenance. Hypoxia increases levels of VEGF, which provides signals for vessel maintenance and neovascularization.[120] Hyperoxia, on the other hand, inhibits VEGF expression, which leads to regression and death of retinal vessels.[121] In some models, regression of vessels occurs by apoptosis of vascular cells.[122,123] Endothelial cells express several antiapoptotic molecules to maintain viability when quiescent and when stressed.[124,125] Most likely, an intricate balance between cell death and proliferation is maintained by activators and inhibitors of both processes.

Role of Ligand–Receptor Interactions

Numerous factors regulate vascular development and differentiation in a positive or negative fashion. Some of the key molecules and their receptors are discussed here. A model for vascular development is shown in Fig. 123.1.

Inducers of Angiogenesis

Fibroblast Growth Factors

The role of FGFs in vascular development remains murky.[126–128] Because of possible functional redundancy in the numerous family members, assigning specific roles to the various members of the FGF family has been difficult. Evidence suggests that FGF receptors signal

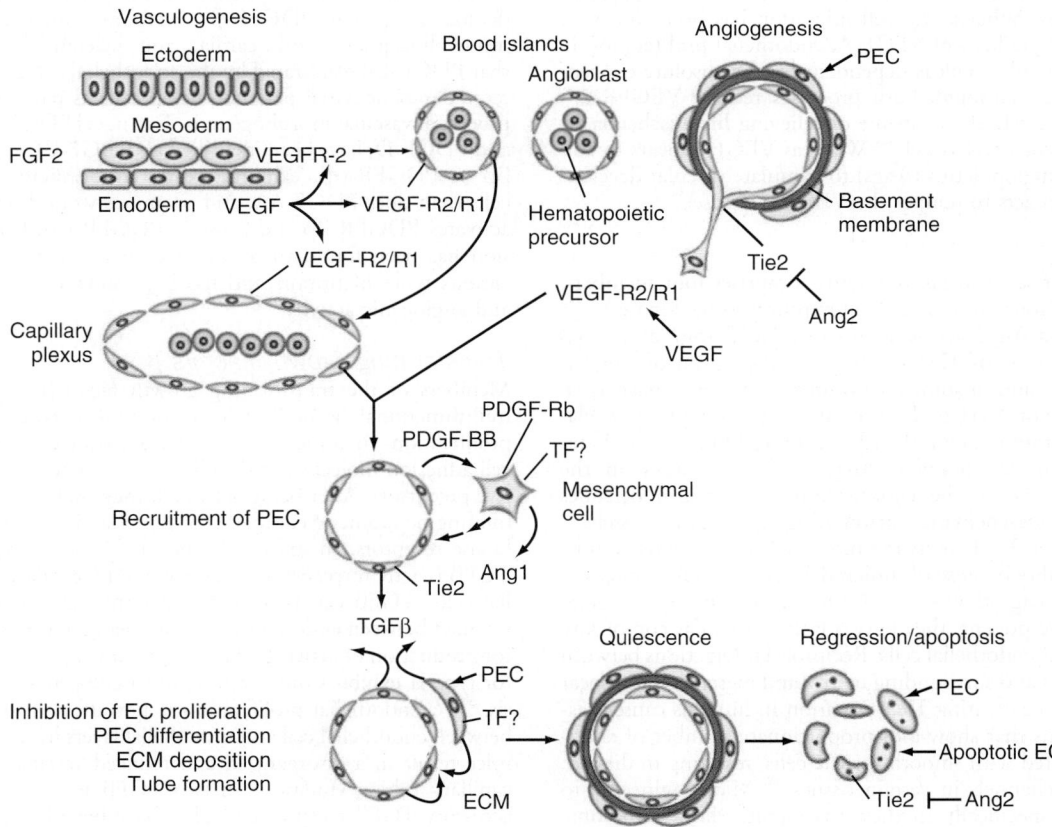

Fig. 123.1 MODEL FOR VASCULAR DEVELOPMENT. The role of secreted proteins and membrane receptors in vascular development is highlighted, but other factors such as cell adhesion molecules and extracellular matrix components also contribute significantly. *Ang,* Angiopoietin; *EC,* extracellular; *ECM,* extracellular matrix; *FGF2,* fibroblast growth factor 2; *PDGF,* platelet-derived growth factor; *PEC,* periendothelial cell (smooth muscle cell, pericyte); *TF,* tissue factor; *TGFβ,* transforming growth factor-β; *VEGF,* vascular endothelial cell growth factor; *VEGFR,* vascular endothelial cell growth factor receptor.

an inductive pathway by upregulating VEGFR-2 in differentiating mesoderm before vascular morphogenesis.[128–130] FGF2 may induce neovascularization in adults indirectly through activation of the VEGF–VEGFR pathway.[131]

Vascular Endothelial Growth Factors

Eight members of the VEGF family have been identified[86,126,128,132–137]: VEGF-A (also called vascular permeability factor), VEGF-B, VEGF-C, VEGF-D, VEGF-E (a viral ortholog), VEGF-F, VEGF-b, and placental growth factor. Three members of the receptor tyrosine kinase family[126,135,136]—VEGFR-1 (flt-1), VEGFR-2 (flk-1/KDR), and VEGFR-3 (flt-4)—respond differentially to individual members of the VEGF family. In addition, the coreceptors for VEGF, neuropilin 1 and neuropilin 2, have been identified on arterial and venous endothelial cells, respectively. Neuropilin 1 is a coreceptor for VEGFR-2 that enhances binding of the VEGF-A isoform VEGF165 to VEGFR-2.[135] VEGF-A functions as a homodimer. However, it also heterodimerizes with VEGF-B and placental growth factor, and it has a crucial dose-dependent effect on vasculogenesis.[86,126,128,135,136] Whereas VEGF-A binds VEGFR-1 and VEGFR-2, VEGF-C binds VEGFR-2 and VEGFR-3. Whereas placental growth factor specifically activates VEGFR-1, VEGF-E binds only VEGFR-2.[128,135,136] Lack of VEGFR-2 prevents the development of endothelial cells and a hematopoietic system because cells lacking VEGFR-2 do not reach the correct location to form blood islands.[138] Mice that have been rendered deficient for VEGFR-1 have normal hematopoietic progenitors and abundant endothelial cells, but they do not form capillary tubes or functional vessels.[139] Both VEGFR-2– and VEGFR-1–deficient mice die at an early embryonic stage, as do neuropilin 1– and neuropilin 2–deficient mice. In von Hippel-Lindau disease, development of hemangioblastomas may be caused by stabilization of VEGF mRNA.[140] VEGF is also believed to play a key role in propagating tumor angiogenesis. Whereas tip cell migration has been shown to be dependent on a gradient of VEGF-A, endothelial proliferation in the lengthening vascular stalk is dependent on the absolute concentration of VEGF-A, although both processes require VEGFR-2.[89] Finally, injection of VEGF is capable of relieving limb ischemia by the generation of collateral vessels.[88] Whereas VEGF appears to collaborate with the angiopoietins (Angs) to stimulate vascular development, VE-cadherin acts to temper the VEGF response.[33]

Angiopoietins

The Ang family of secreted glycoproteins comprises four members: Ang1 to Ang4. All four bind to Tie2, a receptor tyrosine kinase.[141–144] Whereas Ang1 and Ang4 act as agonists of Tie2, Ang2 and Ang3 function as antagonists of Tie2.[144] However, the action of Ang2 is context dependent, and in some environments, it may behave as an agonist.[144] Binding of Ang1 to Tie2 results in tyrosine phosphorylation of Tie2 and promotes endothelial cell survival but not proliferation.[141,144] Early in development, Ang1 is found mainly in the myocardium surrounding the endocardium, but it also becomes expressed in the mesenchyme surrounding developing vessels.[141] Disruption of either Ang1 or its receptor Tie2 in the mouse results in embryonic lethality because of similar defects.[142,145] These mice die at a slightly later stage than do VEGFR-deficient mice. Although endothelial cells are present, they have a lack of vascular complexity and a scarcity of periendothelial cells. Reciprocal interactions between the endothelial cells and surrounding matrix and mesenchyme appear to be disrupted. An activating Tie2 mutation in humans causes vascular malformations that show a disproportionate number of endothelial cells compared with smooth muscle cells, resulting in dilated, tortuous vascular channels in certain tissues.[146] Mice engineered to overexpress Ang2 specifically in their vasculature show embryonic lethality and vascular defects that are reminiscent of those seen in Ang1- or Tie2-null embryos.[143] In one proposed model, Ang1–Tie2 coupling mediates vascular maturation by sustaining endothelial cell–periendothelial cell–matrix interactions and may be involved in maintaining endothelial cell quiescence. Because Ang2 is found only at sites of vascular remodeling, Ang2 loosens matrix contacts, thus allowing access and responsiveness to angiogenic factors such as

VEGF.[143,144] In the absence of growth factors, disruption of the vessel architecture by Ang2 may result in vascular cell apoptosis and vessel regression. However, Ang2-deficient mice are born alive, and the major defect appears to be lymphatic development.[144] Thus despite major advances, the data are conflicting. The response of endothelial cells to the angiopoietins likely is context dependent and endothelial cell type specific.[144]

Tie1 is a receptor tyrosine kinase that exhibits structural similarities to Tie2. A ligand for Tie1 has not yet been identified.[126,147] Disruption of the Tie1 gene in mice results in lethality at a much later point in development; Tie1-null mice may survive up to birth.[145,148] Tie1$^{-/-}$ mice die of hemorrhage and edema, implicating Tie1 in signaling the control of fluid exchange across capillaries and in maintenance of vessel integrity under hemodynamic stress. Chimeric mice that express Tie1$^{-/-}$ and Tie1$^{+/-}$ endothelial cells show underrepresentation of Tie1$^{-/-}$ cells in vessels primarily derived by angiogenesis but not in embryonic vessels derived by vasculogenesis, suggesting a differential function for Tie1 in angiogenesis.[149] Evidence also implicates a role for Tie1 in combination with Ang1 in establishing vascular polarity.[150]

Platelet-Derived Growth Factors

The PDGF family is composed of four chains. PDGF-A and PDGF-B can associate in a homodimeric or heterodimeric fashion.[151] Similarly, the receptors α and β are receptor tyrosine kinases that can form homodimers or heterodimers. PDGF-BB can bind the receptors PDGFR-ββ or PDGFR-αβ, but PDGFR-ββ binds only PDGF-BB and not PDGF-AA or PDGF-AB.[126] Mice that are null for PDGF-B die perinatally of renal, hematologic, and cardiovascular abnormalities.[152] The large vessels and heart of these mice are dilated, and microvessels exhibit microaneurysms because of a lack of pericytes.[24,152] PDGFR-β knock-out mice do not show an overtly abnormal cardiovascular phenotype, but generation of chimeric mice demonstrates that PDGFR-β$^{-/-}$ cells are underrepresented in all muscle lineages (smooth, cardiac, and skeletal).[153,154] Thus it appears that PDGF-BB elaborated by the endothelial cell provides a signal to recruit mesenchymal periendothelial cells as part of the maturation process of vascular morphogenesis. Two novel PDGF chains, PDGF-C and PDGF-D, have been identified.[155] PDGF-CC can bind PDGFR-ββ or PDGFR-αβ, exhibits greater mitogenicity of mesenchymal cells than does PDGF-AA, and promotes wound repair. PDGF-DD activates PDGFR-ββ and possibly PDGFR-αβ. PDGF-DD expression has been found to be elevated in the serum of patients with various types of tumors and has been shown to have transforming and angiogenic activity.[155]

Transforming Growth Factors β

Members of the transforming growth factor-β (TGFβ) family are multifunctional homodimeric peptides with diverse effects on cell proliferation, migration, differentiation, adhesion, and expression of cell adhesion molecules and ECM.[126,156,157] They are secreted as inactive precursors. After being activated, they transmit signals to cells by binding heteromeric complexes of type I and type II serine/threonine kinase receptors. In most cell types, the type I receptor engaged by TGFβ is activin receptor-like kinase 5 (ALK5). However, in endothelial cells, TGFβ can bind and signal through ALK5 and ALK1.[158] Contact between endothelial cells and periendothelial cells is required for production of active TGFβ.[19] Mice lacking TGFβ or TGFβ receptor type II exhibit similar defects in vasculogenesis and hematopoiesis.[156,157] Endothelial proliferation is not affected, but poor contacts between endothelial cell and mesothelial layers in embryos of TGFβ$^{-/-}$ mice result in a disorganized and reduced vascular network lacking capillary tubes. Mutations in two TGFβ receptors, ALK1 and the accessory TGFβ receptor endoglin, have been linked to the vascular disorder hereditary hemorrhagic telangiectasia.[158] Disruption of TGFβ signaling likely plays a role in the telangiectasia seen in this disorder.

Notch

The Notch family is composed of four receptors (Notch1 through Notch4) and five ligands (Jagged1 and Jagged2 and Delta-like 1 [Dll1], Dll3, and Dll4). Ligand engagement results in a series of proteolytic clips that release the Notch intracellular domain, which then translocates to the nucleus where it effects transcriptional activation via the DNA-binding protein CSL (also called *RBP-Jκ* or *CBF1*).[159] Gene targeting studies have revealed a critical role for Notch1, Dll1, Dll4, and Jagged1 in vascular development and remodeling.[159] Dll4–Notch1 signaling between endothelial cells within the angiogenic sprout serves to restrict tip cell formation in response to VEGF.[160–162] Consequently, inhibition of Dll4 in adult mice results in increased endothelial proliferation, sprouting, and branching and increased tumor vascularity.[163,164] However, the vasculature is disorganized and poorly perfused; thus Dll4 blockade inhibits tumor growth in several models.[163,164]

Coagulation Factors

Tissue factor (TF) is a member of the cytokine receptor superfamily. In addition to its role in initiating coagulation as a cofactor for factor VII, TF may be involved in intracellular signaling. TF knock-out mice have abnormalities of their large vessels and microvasculature secondary to defects in mesenchymal cell and periendothelial cell accumulation and function.[25] Elevated TF expression in various tumors and the associated angiogenic endothelium has been reported.[165] Expression of mutant oncogenes (K-*ras*, *EGFR*) or tumor suppressor genes (*PTEN*, *p53*) leads to increased TF expression and activity, and this may link tumor angiogenesis and the hypercoagulable states manifested in cancer.[165] Abnormal development of the vasculature also affects 50% of mice that are deficient in factor V. The affected mice die in utero, and the 50% embryonic lethality is similar to that observed in thrombin receptor–deficient mice that die without obvious coagulation defects.[166] Factor V–dependent generation of thrombin may be important for early vascular development by signaling through the thrombin receptor.[167] Thrombin can promote angiogenesis through a mechanism that is independent of fibrin formation.[167,168] Studies have suggested that thrombin can stimulate release of angiogenic factors (e.g., VEGF-A) from tumor cells and platelets, as well as induce VEGFR-2 on endothelial cells.[168] In addition, APC and protein C inhibitor have been shown to contribute not only to the regulation of hemostasis but also to cell inflammation, proliferation, apoptosis, tumor biology, and angiogenesis.[169] Regarding angiogenesis, APC increases proliferation of vascular endothelial cells and angiogenesis by APC receptor–mediated activation of mitogen-activated protein kinase, phosphatidylinositol 3-kinase, and endothelial nitric oxide synthase (eNOS) pathways.[170]

Clinical trials have revealed that treatment with low-molecular–weight heparins improves the survival time of cancer patients receiving chemotherapy, an effect that appears to be independent of the anticoagulant properties of the low-molecular-weight heparins.[171,172] Although antiangiogenic effects of specific heparanase-generated fragments of unfractionated heparins have been demonstrated in vitro, the mechanism of the antitumor effect remains to be defined.

The potential involvement of fibrinolytic factors in angiogenesis has been mentioned. Interestingly, fragments 1 and 2 of prothrombin have been reported to inhibit angiogenesis, and various other fragments of coagulation and fibrinolytic proteins also may inhibit angiogenesis.[173]

Other Factors

Various other families of ligand–receptor pairs play a role in angiogenesis. They include ephrin–Eph, Wnt–frizzled, neuropilin–semaphorin, slit–Robo, and sonic hedgehog–patched/smoothened. Various chemokines have been shown to modulate angiogenesis in either a positive or negative fashion.

Inhibitors of Angiogenesis

As with the angiogenesis inducers, multiple factors have been reported to negatively regulate vascular morphogenesis.[88,173] Of interest is a class of endogenous angiogenesis inhibitors that are fragments of larger proteins that have little or no angiogenesis-related activity in their intact form. They include fragments of ECM proteins such as fibronectin, collagen type IV α3 chain (tumstatin), and collagen type XIII (endostatin), as well as coagulation protein fragments such as plasminogen (angiostatin) and antithrombin.[173] The mechanism of action of these protein fragments depends on the particular polypeptide, but the functional effect usually is inhibition of endothelial proliferation or induction of apoptosis.[173–175] Other endogenous inhibitors include interferons, chemokines, and interleukin-12 (IL-12).

More than 100 compounds are in clinical trials attempting to cause regression of tumors by inhibiting angiogenesis.[176] These compounds can be broadly divided into those that act directly by targeting the angiogenic endothelial cell and those that act indirectly by targeting activators of angiogenesis. The latter category includes targeting of oncogenes (e.g., mutant EGFR or Her2) because many aberrantly activated oncogenes have been shown to induce expression of angiogenic factors. The first clear-cut evidence of efficacy in clinical trials of an angiogenic inhibitor for tumor therapy came from regimens directed against the VEGF pathway (e.g., bevacizumab).[177,178] Because of the short improvement in overall and progression-free survival with the addition of VEGF inhibitors over standard chemotherapy, it is likely that heterogeneity and inherent instability of tumor cell populations result in the selection of malignant cells that feed their vasculature through factors other than VEGF. In this regard, use of indirect angiogenic inhibitors still suffers from the likelihood of tumors becoming resistant to the therapy.

Whether the mechanism of action of these inhibitors is truly caused by the abrogation of a functional vascular supply is an open question. VEGF inhibitors "normalize" the aberrant, leaky tumor vasculature. Other than in renal cancer, VEGF inhibitors have shown effect only when used in combination chemotherapy regimens, which has led to the proposal that VEGF pathway inhibition improves vessel functionality and perfusion, thus facilitating delivery of chemotherapeutic agents.[177,178] VEGF–VEGFR signaling also acts in an autocrine fashion within some tumor cell populations, raising the possibility that positive outcomes may have as much to do with direct tumor kill as with an antiangiogenic effect. Finally, as with organogenesis, the vasculature may provide a juxtacrine or paracrine role in supporting tumor viability and proliferation independent of the provision of a circulatory system for delivery of nutrients and oxygen.[53]

Some of the more common side effects observed with use of VEGF-A inhibitors were not predicted a priori but may be understandable in retrospect. For instance, hypertension and arterial thrombosis are common side effects. Two possible reasons may explain the hypertensive side effect. One is that VEGF directly activates eNOS and thus may be responsible in part for basal production of NO.[179] Another potential explanation is that podocyte-derived VEGF is required for proper glomerular function throughout life.[53] Heterozygous loss of podocyte VEGF results in hypertension and proteinuria in adult mice.[53] Given that proteinuria is also commonly seen in patients treated with VEGF inhibitors, the latter explanation would tie two of the side effects seen. The reasons for arterial thrombosis are less obvious. Because arterial circulation is more dependent on VEGF, it is possible that arterial endothelial apoptosis serves as a nidus for localized activation of coagulation and platelet aggregation. Apoptotic endothelial cells have been shown to increase thrombin-generating capacity and bind to unactivated platelets and leukocytes.[180–182]

More recently, the use of PDGF inhibitors to target pericytes has been shown to be a potentially effective antiangiogenic strategy, particularly in combination with antiendothelial (anti-VEGF) molecules.[96,98] "Metronomic" or low-dose, frequent scheduling of traditional cytotoxic agents also is reported to have an antiangiogenic effect and has proven efficacious in animal studies.[183] Antivasculogenic therapy directed against recruitment of BM-derived vascular precursors may have a role in future cancer therapeutic regimens, but thus far the evidence is weak at best.[79]

Arteriogenesis

Arteriogenesis is a term coined to distinguish the development of collateral vessels in adults from the process of angiogenesis.[184,185]

Remodeling of a preexisting collateral arteriole is thought to be caused by flow-induced changes secondary to occlusion of a supply artery. The consequent increase in shear stress through the collateral arteriole activates endothelial cells, resulting in monocyte recruitment and infiltration into the media. Elaboration of various cytokines, growth factors, and proteases from monocytes and endothelial cells causes matrix degradation, smooth muscle cell proliferation, and rapid enlargement of the preexisting arteriole. Factors thought to promote arteriogenesis include FGF-2, placental growth factor, PDGF-BB, TGFβ1, monocyte chemoattractant protein 1, and GM-CSF.[185,186]

Lymphangiogenesis

The lymphatics comprise a low-flow, low-pressure system that collects extravasated fluid from the tissues and transfers it back to the venous system via the thoracic duct. Lymphatic vessels also serve an immune function by transporting lymphoid and antigen-presenting cells to lymphoid organs.[187] Lymphatic vessels share features with blood vessels, but they also exhibit differences. Lymphatic vessels develop shortly after blood vessels and may arise de novo from precursor mesenchymal cells (lymphangioblasts) in a process akin to vasculogenesis.[188] Alternatively, other studies suggest that specific venous endothelial cells differentiate to lymphatic endothelium in response to signals that have yet to be determined.[189] VEGF-C and VEGF-D, by activating VEGFR-3 and Ang2 potentially through Tie2 activation, are growth factors necessary for lymphatic vessels.[190] The α9β1 integrin and matrix interacting protein CCBE1 are necessary for proper lymphatic development, and the homeobox transcription factor Prox1 appears to induce transdifferentiation of venous to lymphatic endothelial cells.[189–191] The earliest described regulator of early lymphatic endothelial cell specification is Sox18 (sex determining Region Y Box 18), a transcriptional regulator of Prox1expression. Lymphedema can be caused by congenital defects, parasitic (filariasis) or neoplastic obstruction, or surgical resection. Congenital lymphedema (Milroy disease) is linked to inactivating mutations of VEGFR-3.[187] Whether lymphatic vessel density in human tumors correlates with disease progression is not clear, but in animal models, induction of lymphangiogenesis by VEGF-C or VEGF-D promotes lymph node metastasis.[187]

Relationship Between Vascular Development and Hematopoiesis

Hematopoietic cells and endothelial cells are intertwined in several ways. First, there is the likely existence of a common precursor (see Vasculogenesis section earlier). Second, the endothelium is intimately involved in hematopoiesis, having a supportive role structurally and nutritionally. Finally, the endothelium organizes the controlled egress and ingress of hematopoietic cells in hematopoietic and other tissues. The last issue is covered in the Interaction of Blood Cells With the Vessel Wall section.

BM stromal cells secrete cytokines, produce ECM, and are in direct cellular contact with hematopoietic cells, thereby providing a microenvironment suitable for hematopoietic proliferation, differentiation, and self-renewal.[192] Many studies demonstrate the supportive role of endothelium in hematopoiesis.[193–195] The physical proximity of endothelium and hematopoietic precursors within the BM and the requirement of blood cells to transit BM endothelium to reach the circulation is presumptive evidence of an important role for endothelium. BM endothelial cells constitutively express high levels of IL-6, stem cell factor, granulocyte colony-stimulating factor (G-CSF), and granulocyte macrophage colony-stimulating factor (GM-CSF).[193] Both yolk sac and BM endothelial cells support long-term proliferation and differentiation of hematopoietic cells in vitro.[193] BM endothelial cell expression of notch ligand jagged supports long-term notch-dependent HSC proliferation and renewal.[196] However, endothelial cells also have been reported to inhibit hematopoiesis.[197]

Significant evidence now indicates that hematopoietic stem and progenitor cells are not randomly distributed in the BM, but rather are spatially and possibly physically associated with the endosteum and the blood vessels.[195] Functional differences between the osteoblastic and vascular niches have been described. It has been suggested that whereas the osteoblastic niche maintains quiescence of HSCs, stem and progenitor cells that are activated for differentiation and mobilization reside at the vascular niche.[194] Translocation of megakaryocyte progenitors to the vicinity of the BM sinuses is sufficient to induce megakaryocyte maturation and platelet production.[195] However, a study has identified CXCL12 (SDF-1)–abundant reticular cells that are located in close proximity to the sinusoidal endothelium as well as the endosteum.[198] The authors confirmed that the CXCL12–CXCR4 signaling axis is required for maintenance of HSCs in the BM, and these findings raise the possibility that the vascular and osteoblastic niches may not be that different.[198] In all likelihood, endothelial cells and osteoblasts, in concert with other stromal cells, provide a finely tuned system to modulate hematopoiesis in the BM such that differentiation, proliferation, and self-renewal occur in a regulated fashion.

Human endothelial cells have been reported to express receptors for IL-3, stem cell factor, erythropoietin, and thrombopoietin, and show functional responses to IL-3 and erythropoietin.[199–201] The shared responses to growth factors, combined with the importance of macrophages in angiogenesis and the production of cytokines by monocytes and macrophages, suggest that hematopoietic cells play a reciprocal role in maintaining the endothelium.

PHYSIOLOGIC FUNCTIONS OF THE ENDOTHELIUM

The Endothelium as a Barrier

The microvessels (capillaries and postcapillary venules) act as the exchange vessels of the circulation. However, as with other endothelial functions, vessel permeability is dependent on the type of vessel and its location. Movement of lipophilic and low-molecular-weight hydrophilic substances between blood and tissue is virtually unimpeded, but the vessels are selectively permeable to macromolecules. This semiselective barrier is necessary to maintain the fluid balance between intravascular and extravascular compartments, yet antibodies, hormones, cytokines, and other molecules must have access to the interstitial space for the initiation and potentiation of various processes, including inflammation, immune response, and wound repair.

Movement of macromolecules across the vessel wall is governed by (1) hydrostatic and oncotic pressure gradients; (2) physicochemical properties of the molecule, such as size, shape, and charge; and (3) properties of the barrier. The barrier of the vessel wall is formed by the cellular components, endothelial cells, and pericytes, as well as by the charge and compactness of the matrix components, glycocalyx, and basement membrane. Macromolecules can pass either directly through the endothelial cell (transcellular path) or between adjacent endothelial cells (paracellular path). Surprisingly, the mechanisms of macromolecular movement remain controversial, and data generated by physiologists, morphologists, and cell biologists have not been consolidated into a model that satisfies the findings of the different groups.[202]

To explain cellular transport in endothelium, physiologists have proposed the existence of two sets of "pores" based on experiments measuring the movement of dextran and other macromolecules: a small pore of radius 3–5 nm for transport of water and small hydrophilic molecules, and a large pore of radius 25–60 nm for macromolecular transport.[202–204] Although water mainly moves across the continuous endothelium via the paracellular route, a significant proportion (≤40%) can traverse the endothelium via the transcellular route by water-transporting membrane channels, the aquaporins.[205] Macromolecular transport into cells can proceed by receptor-mediated systems, such as clathrin-coated pits, in which the molecules usually are targeted to the lysosome, but may be transported through

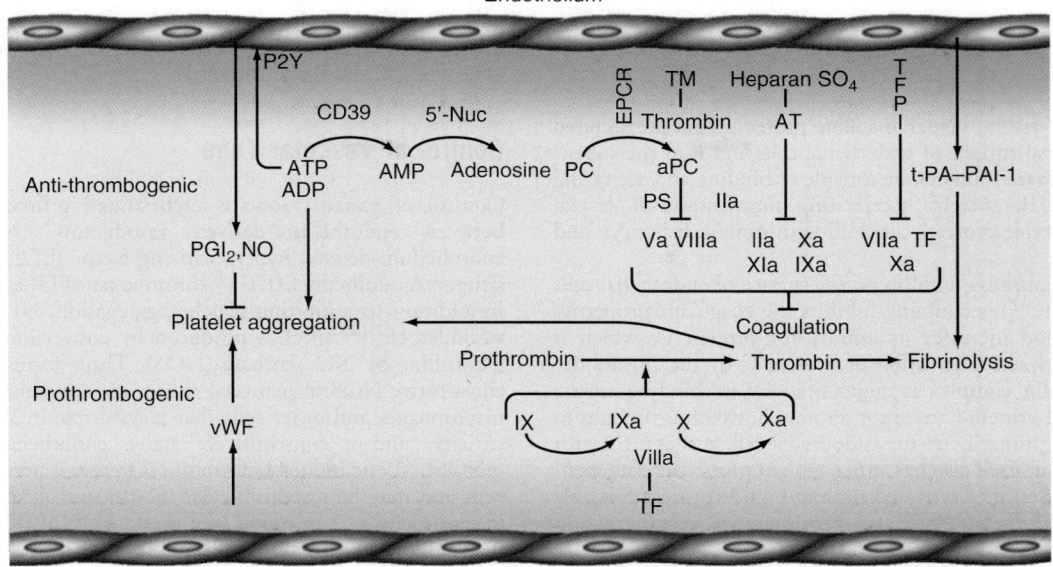

Fig. 123.2 OVERVIEW OF ENDOTHELIAL FUNCTION IN COAGULATION. *ADP*, Adenosine diphosphate; *AMP*, adenosine monophosphate; *AT*, antithrombin; *ATP*, adenosine triphosphate; *EPCR*, endothelial protein C receptor; *5'-Nuc*, ecto-5'-nucleotidase; *NO*, nitric oxide; *P2Y*, purinergic receptor 1; *PAI-1*, plasminogen activator inhibitor 1; *PC*, protein C; *PGI₂*, prostaglandin I2 (prostacyclin); *PS*, protein S; *TF*, tissue factor; *TFPI*, tissue factor pathway inhibitor; *TM*, thrombomodulin; *t-PA*, tissue plasminogen activator; *vWF*, von Willebrand factor.

the cell. Alternatively, molecules can be moved across the cell by plasmalemmal vesicles or caveolae, which are abundant in capillary endothelial cells. Caveolae are 50–100-nm membrane invaginations that can participate in transcytosis as well as in the translocation of glycosylphosphatidylinositol-linked proteins into the cytoplasm and in transmembrane signaling.[206] Because of the known leakiness of tumor microvasculature, investigators have studied these microvessels and identified a structure designated the vesiculovacuolar organelle.[207] These organelles are grape-like clusters of interconnecting uncoated vesicles and vacuoles that span the entire thickness of vascular endothelium, thereby providing a potential transendothelial connection between the vascular lumen and the extravascular space.[207] Interestingly, their function is enhanced by injection into normal skin of VEGF, which is known to increase the permeability of vessels.[207] Localization of caveolin to vesiculovacuolar organelles suggests that this structure is a fusion of caveolae.[207]

During inflammation, binding of neutrophils to the endothelium results in the generation of oxidants that can mediate endothelial cell injury and increase permeability.[208] Upon adhesion of neutrophils to the endothelium, leukocyte CD18 (β2 integrin)-mediated signals trigger the release of the neutrophil cationic protein called *heparin-binding protein/CAP37/azurocidin*, which in turn induces formation of gaps between endothelial cells and macromolecular efflux.[209] Thrombin, an inflammatory mediator, can increase endothelial permeability by several mechanisms resulting from activation of its receptor on endothelial cells.[210–212] First is an increase in transcellular vesicular permeability. Second is increased paracellular permeability that results from phosphorylation of endothelial cell nonmyosin light chains and contractile activity generated by movement of actin and myosin filaments past each other. The contraction and retraction of endothelial cells are accompanied by "loosening" of intercellular junctions and focal integrin contacts with the ECM. Finally, thrombin may alter the repulsive effect of the negatively charged glycocalyx. An increase in paracellular permeability may result from alteration of cell–cell contacts present at tight junctions and adherens junctions secondary to posttranslational modification of components of these junctions such as claudins and VE-cadherin.[202] Pericyte contractility also has been hypoth-

esized as a mechanism for increasing permeability in inflammatory states.[212]

The Endothelium as a Nonthrombogenic Surface

The molecular mechanisms of hemostasis and thrombosis are addressed in Chapters 115 and 116 and 118–120. This section places the endothelium in the appropriate context in these processes. An overview of endothelial cell contributions to the anticoagulant and procoagulant states is shown in Fig. 123.2. Normal unperturbed endothelium presents a nonthrombogenic surface to the circulation by inhibiting platelet aggregation, preventing the activation and propagation of coagulation and enhancing fibrinolysis.[213–217] These activities are accomplished by both passive and active processes. Conversely, when injured or under inflammatory conditions, the endothelium may become procoagulant.

When in close proximity to endothelial cells, platelets become unresponsive to agonists. This inhibition of platelet aggregation is accomplished by secretion of prostacyclin (prostaglandin I2 [PGI₂]) and NO, and by surface expression of an ecto-adenosine phosphatase (ADPase)/CD39/nucleoside triphosphate diphosphohydrolase (NTPDase-1).[216,218] Prostacyclin is synthesized mainly by vascular endothelial and smooth muscle cells as a product of arachidonic acid metabolism. It inhibits platelet activation, secretion, and aggregation, as well as monocyte interactions with endothelial cells. It also causes vascular smooth muscle cell relaxation. NO similarly has a wide range of functions, including inhibition of platelet adhesion, activation, and aggregation. Most of the NO released from endothelial cells is elaborated abluminally, where it acts on the smooth muscle cell to cause vasodilation. However, some NO may enter the lumen and thereby diffuse into platelets. Prostacyclin and NO can act synergistically to reverse platelet aggregation.[216] The released platelet agonist, ADP, can be inactivated by endothelial membrane-associated CD39.[218] Metabolism of ATP and ADP to adenosine monophosphate (AMP) by CD39 eliminates platelet recruitment and returns platelets to their resting state. Adenosine, which is generated by hydrolysis of AMP by ecto-5'-nucleotidase, acts to inhibit platelet aggregation and cause vasodilation. ATP/ADP can stimulate purinoreceptors on endothelial cells, resulting in synthesis and release of PGI$_2$ and NO.[219]

Endothelial cells use three main pathways to inhibit thrombin generation and limit coagulation[213,215,220,221]:

1. Antithrombin system: Heparan sulfate proteoglycans are secreted onto the luminal surface of endothelial cells and into the subendothelium. Heparan sulfates are capable of binding and activating antithrombin III, thereby accelerating inactivation of several procoagulant serine proteases, including thrombin, factor Xa, and factor IXa.
2. Protein C[222]: Thrombomodulin on the surface of endothelial cells binds thrombin. This coupling inhibits the coagulant properties of thrombin and increases its affinity for protein C, which it cleaves and activates. Activation of protein C by the thrombin–thrombomodulin complex is augmented by its binding to the endothelial cell protein C receptor. Protein S, which is thought to be synthesized primarily by the endothelial cell, acts as a cofactor for protein C but itself also has anticoagulant properties. Independent of the presence of activated protein C, free protein S is able to inhibit the prothrombinase and intrinsic tenase complexes and interact directly with factors Va and VIIIa.
3. Tissue factor pathway inhibitor (TFPI)[223]: TFPI is a Kunitz-type serine protease inhibitor that modulates TF-initiated coagulation. TFPI binds to and directly inhibits the TF–factor VIIa–factor Xa complex. It is mainly produced by and bound to endothelial cells, likely to surface glycosaminoglycans. There is also a plasma pool bound to low-density lipoprotein.

If coagulation occurs despite the many anticoagulant mechanisms, endothelial cells also provide proteins to promote fibrinolysis.[215] Endothelium is a major source of t-PA.[224,225] Approximately 40% of t-PA is bound to its inhibitor, PAI-1, which is also secreted by endothelial cells. Stresses such as exercise, acidosis, hypoxia, shear forces, increased venous pressure, and thrombin cause release of t-PA,[224,225] and presumably activate plasminogen. Receptors for plasminogen and t-PA are present on the endothelial cell surface, allowing for effective localized production of fibrinolytic activity.

Although intact endothelium is necessary to maintain blood in a fluid state and inhibit coagulation under normal conditions, injured endothelium can rapidly downregulate its anticoagulant functions and become procoagulant even without overt vascular damage as occurs with trauma or surgery. Further tissue injury or vascular pathology also leads to exposure of the underlying matrix, which is procoagulant by virtue of its binding to and activation of platelets. Endothelial cells that have been induced to undergo apoptosis in vitro become procoagulant. Apoptotic endothelial cells expose phosphatidylserine on their surface and downregulate their anticoagulant properties. Apoptotic endothelial cells and vascular smooth muscle cells also increase thrombin formation in recalcified citrated plasma, and apoptotic endothelial cells show increased adhesion to unactivated platelets.[180,181,226] Thrombosis resulting from procoagulant changes induced by endothelial apoptosis could contribute to the pathogenesis of diverse diseases.[227]

Even without endothelial death, perturbation of the vascular lining by inflammatory mediators could tip the balance such that the endothelium converts from a nonthrombogenic to a procoagulant surface because of downregulation of anticoagulant properties as well as induction of procoagulant properties. For example, the setting of acute inflammation is associated with increased release of vWF, platelet-activating factor, and fibronectin, all of which may potentiate thrombus formation. Tumor necrosis factor (TNF), IL-1, and lipopolysaccharide can increase the expression of PAI-1 in endothelial cells with downregulation or no change in t-PA levels, thereby impairing fibrinolysis. TNF, IL-1, and lipopolysaccharide also have been shown to downregulate thrombomodulin as well as to induce expression of TF on cultured endothelial cells. However, whether endothelial cells express TF on their luminal surfaces in vivo is controversial.[228] More recently, circulating microparticles generated by leukocytes and vascular cells have been shown to be a source of blood-borne TF and

to contribute to coagulation.[229] Although most microparticles probably are derived from platelets and monocytes, endothelial-derived microparticles may be an important source of circulating TF under conditions of drastic activation.[229,230]

Control of Vascular Tone

Control of vascular tone is orchestrated primarily by a balance between endothelium-derived vasodilators (NO, PGI$_2$, and endothelium-derived hyperpolarizing factor [EDHF]) and vasoconstrictors (endothelin-1 [ET-1], thromboxane (TXA$_2$) and superoxide). In addition to inhibiting platelet aggregation, NO and PGI$_2$ act as vasodilators.[231,232] NO is produced by conversion of L-arginine to L-citrulline by NO synthase (NOS). Three forms of NOS exist: a constitutive NOS in neuronal tissue; an inducible enzyme found in macrophages and other cells that plays a role in NO-induced cytotoxicity; and a constitutively active endothelial form, NOSIII (eNOS).[233] The inducible form of NOS also is present in endothelial cells and may be responsible for the uncontrolled vasodilation seen in septic shock.[233] Injection into the forearm of L-arginine analogues that inhibit NOS causes substantial vasoconstriction. Conversely, eNOS-deficient mice are hypertensive, suggesting that NO release is crucial for maintaining basal vasodilation.[231,232] The major physiologic stimulus for continuous production of NO in vivo is shear stress. The action of NO on platelets (antiaggregatory), endothelial cells, and smooth muscle cells (relaxation) is caused by activation of guanylyl cyclase and formation of cyclic guanosine 3′,5′-cyclic monophosphate. Whereas NO is quite unstable, the formation of S-nitrosothiols in the presence of oxygen and thiols provides a stable reservoir of NO.[234] Hemoglobin is an avid scavenger of NO, which may account for the vasoconstriction observed with administration of cell-free, hemoglobin-based RBC substitute.[235] Physiologically, however, S-nitrosohemoglobin acts as a regulator of blood flow. Deoxygenation is accompanied by an allosteric change in S-nitrosohemoglobin that releases the NO group, relaxing blood vessels to bring blood flow in line with local oxygen requirements.[236]

Prostacyclin (PGI$_2$), on the other hand, does not appear to have as global a role in vasodilation as does NO. PGI$_2$ is synthesized mainly by endothelial cells and acts locally at sites of injury. It may counterbalance the vasoconstriction induced by the platelet-produced arachidonic acid metabolite thromboxane A$_2$ (TXA$_2$). Most PGI$_2$ is released luminally, where it has an antiplatelet effect. Whereas PGI$_2$ transduces a cellular signal by increasing the levels of cyclic AMP (cAMP), TXA$_2$ signals via the phosphoinositol pathway and lowering of cAMP levels. Synthesis of prostaglandins is catalyzed by the action of cyclooxygenases (COX-1 and COX-2) on arachidonic acid. Aspirin inhibits COX irreversibly in both platelets and endothelial cells. However, the clinical effect is seen primarily in platelets for two reasons.[232,233] One reason is that platelets, being nonnucleated, cannot synthesize new COX, but endothelial cells can. Therefore TXA$_2$ synthesis recovers only when new platelets enter the circulation, but COX production by endothelial cells restores PGI$_2$ levels within a few hours. The second reason is that platelets encounter orally administered aspirin before it is deacetylated by the liver and diluted by the venous circulation. The important balance in the activity of PGI$_2$ and TXA$_2$ to homeostasis in the healthy vessel becomes evident when using selective COX-2 inhibitors to reduce inflammation, which decreases the production of PGI$_2$ without affecting the production of TXA$_2$ resulting in vasoconstriction and platelet aggregation unopposed by PGI$_2$, and increased risk for cardiac events.

Early experimental evidence suggested that endothelial cells release other relaxing factors (i.e., EDHF), which act by increasing the membrane potential of smooth muscle cells. Hyperpolarization of isolated coronary arteries occurs in the presence of an arginine analogue, a NOS inhibitor, and indomethacin, a COX inhibitor, suggesting that EDHF, NO, and prostanoids contribute differentially to relaxation in human coronary arteries.[237] The nature of EDHF is unclear, but it encompasses different biologic mechanisms. These mechanisms involve an increase in intracellular calcium concentration, the opening of calcium-activated potassium channels, and the hyperpolarization of endothelial cells, resulting in an endothelium-dependent hyperpolarization of smooth muscle cells.[238] Smooth muscle cell hyperpolarization may occur through direct myoendothelial electrical coupling or through accumulation of potassium ions in the intercellular space. Findings suggest that EDHF represents cytochrome P450-linked arachidonate metabolites in some blood vessels but also lipoxygenase derivatives and hydrogen peroxide.[238]

ET-1 is a 21-amino acid peptide, released preferentially at the abluminal surface of endothelial cells, that exhibits potent vasoconstrictor activity.[239,240] Of the three known ETs, only ET-1 is produced by endothelial cells. At least two receptors (ET-A and ET-B) bind to all three ETs. Whereas ET-A is abundantly expressed on smooth muscle cells, ET-B is predominantly expressed on endothelial cells. The vasoconstrictor activity of ET-1 is preferentially mediated by ET-A receptors on smooth muscle cells. Engagement of ET-B on endothelial cells by ET-3 may paradoxically cause a transient vasodilation. Little evidence indicates that ET-1 plays a role in essential hypertension, but it might contribute to pregnancy-induced hypertension and may play a role in reperfusion injury after ischemia.[240] ET-1 does appear to play a role in pulmonary arterial hypertension, and the dual ET receptor antagonist bosentan and ET-A antagonist ambrisentan have been approved for treatment of this disease.[241,242]

Another seemingly important regulator of vascular tone is the superoxide anion.[231,243] The source of this free radical may be the endothelium itself or inflammatory cells that have been recruited to sites of injury or inflammation. Interaction of superoxide radicals and NO produces peroxynitrite and reduces the concentration of NO. Peroxynitrite can oxidize low-density lipoprotein (LDL) and deleteriously modify other proteins, thereby causing endothelial dysfunction. Increased production of superoxide inhibits synthesis of PGI_2 but not that of TXA_2.[243]

The endothelium expresses angiotensin-converting enzyme at its surface; this enzyme converts angiotensin I to angiotensin II, a potent vasoconstrictor. The interaction among ET, angiotensin II, and α-adrenergic agonists in the pathogenesis of hypertension is complex.[244] An altered balance of the vasoactive substances described in this section has been proposed to cause endothelial dysfunction and the attendant vascular pathology observed in atherosclerosis, hypertension, and diabetes mellitus. Alteration of vascular function in these diseases then may perpetuate endothelial dysfunction and, consequently, worsen disease.

Interaction of Blood Cells With the Vessel Wall

Leukocytes

In the absence of any inflammatory stimulus, neutrophils circulate freely and do not interact significantly with the endothelium. This contrasts with continuous, low-level physiologic traffic of monocytes and lymphocytes across the vessel wall. Monocytes emigrate from the bloodstream to develop into tissue macrophages that may exhibit tissue- or organ-specific functions. To maintain immune surveillance of tissue, lymphocytes recirculate between blood and lymphatics, gaining entrance to the latter at the high endothelial venule of postcapillary venules in lymphoid tissue.

Intravital microscopic studies have established a sequence of events involved in leukocyte emigration at extravascular sites of inflammation. Under conditions of flow, leukocytes first tether to and then roll along the endothelium of postcapillary venules adjacent to the site of inflammation. Some of the rolling leukocytes are activated and adhere firmly. The adherent leukocytes migrate along the endothelial surface and diapedese between endothelial junctions to enter the extravascular tissue. These steps in emigration tethering, rolling, activation, firm adhesion, and diapedesis also are involved in lymphocyte emigration at high endothelial venules. They result from the interaction of distinct leukocyte and endothelial receptors in an adhesion cascade (Fig. 123.3; see Chapter 16).[245,246] Rolling is observed only under flow conditions and is the consequence of shear forces acting on the leukocyte and adhesive interactions between selectin receptors and their glycoconjugate counterstructures.[247] It is initiated primarily by activation of the endothelium by extravascular stimuli such as bacterial-derived products or by endogenous mediators produced by the endothelium or cells in tissue. Early on, rolling is mediated by endothelial P-selectin, which is rapidly translocated from Weibel-Palade bodies to the luminal surface, and L-selectin on leukocyte microvilli. E-selectin is involved only at later time points because it is not constitutively expressed by endothelium but rather is induced over hours by de novo synthesis.

For leukocytes to circulate freely, their integrin receptors must be minimally adhesive, but they also must be able to increase binding rapidly at sites of inflammation. After being tethered to endothelium by selectin interactions, leukocyte integrin receptors are activated by endothelial membrane-expressed platelet-activating factor, endothelial membrane-bound chemokines, or locally secreted chemoattractants. Activation of leukocyte integrins involves changes in receptor affinity or affinity-independent receptor clustering,[248] which promotes firm adhesion to endothelial ligands, which are members of the immunoglobulin gene superfamily (IgSF). These IgSF ligands are constitutively expressed (ICAM-1, ICAM-2), further upregulated (ICAM-1), or induced (VCAM-1) by inflammatory mediators (Table 123.1). Although these activation-dependent increases in leukocyte integrin binding to endothelial IgSF ligands are necessary for shear-resistant firm adhesion, subsequent leukocyte migration over the endothelium requires reversible adhesion caused by cyclic modulation of receptor avidity.[249]

There are several caveats regarding the current multistep model of initial selectin-mediated rolling and subsequent integrin-mediated firm adhesion.[250] First, selectin-mediated rolling is not a prerequisite for emigration under conditions of reduced flow, as might occur at sites of inflammation.[251] Second, the model was developed from observations in the systemic microcirculation, where leukocyte emigration occurs in postcapillary venules under relatively low shear forces. However, selectins do not appear to play a major role in neutrophil emigration in the pulmonary microcirculation, where emigration occurs predominantly in capillaries,[252] or in the liver microvasculature, where leukocytes emigrate primarily in sinusoids.[253] Third, under some conditions leukocytes are able to tether and roll via receptors other than selectins and α4 integrins (e.g., CD44[254] or VAP-1[255]). Finally, several other adhesion pathways have been implicated in leukocyte adhesion to endothelium in vitro, and their roles in the adhesion cascade in vivo remain to be defined.[250]

When adherent, leukocytes migrate upon the endothelial luminal surface. Upon encountering an intercellular junction, some leukocytes diapedese between endothelial cells (paracellular pathway), enter extravascular tissue, and then migrate to the site of inflammatory or immune reaction.[256,257] This process of transendothelial migration uses leukocyte integrin interactions with endothelial IgSF ligands[258] and several junctional proteins, including PECAM-1 (CD31),[259] JAM-1,[260] CD99,[261] CD99L2,[262] ESAM,[263] PVR,[264] and CD47.[265] Diapedesis involves signaling by the leukocyte to the endothelial cell that triggers opening of endothelial cell junctions.[266] Although leukocyte migration is primarily paracellular (i.e., through endothelial cell–cell junctions), under certain circumstances, leukocytes may emigrate directly through the body of an endothelial cell (transcellular pathway).[267]

Leukocyte recruitment is terminated by several mechanisms. Whereas E-selectin and P-selectin are removed from the endothelial cell surface by endocytosis,[268] L-selectin is cleaved from leukocytes by a membrane protease.[269] Decay of cytokine, chemokine, or chemoattractant generation leads to gradual resolution of endothelial adhesion molecule expression and integrin activation. Locally expressed mediators, such as NO,[270] TGFβ,[271] and Fas ligand,[272] also inhibit further leukocyte adhesion to endothelium.

The adhesion molecules involved in leukocyte trafficking from bloodstream to tissue have emerged as important therapeutic targets. Extensive preclinical studies showed that blockade of leukocyte or endothelial adhesion molecules was efficacious in diverse disease models,[273] prompting the development of adhesion antagonists for

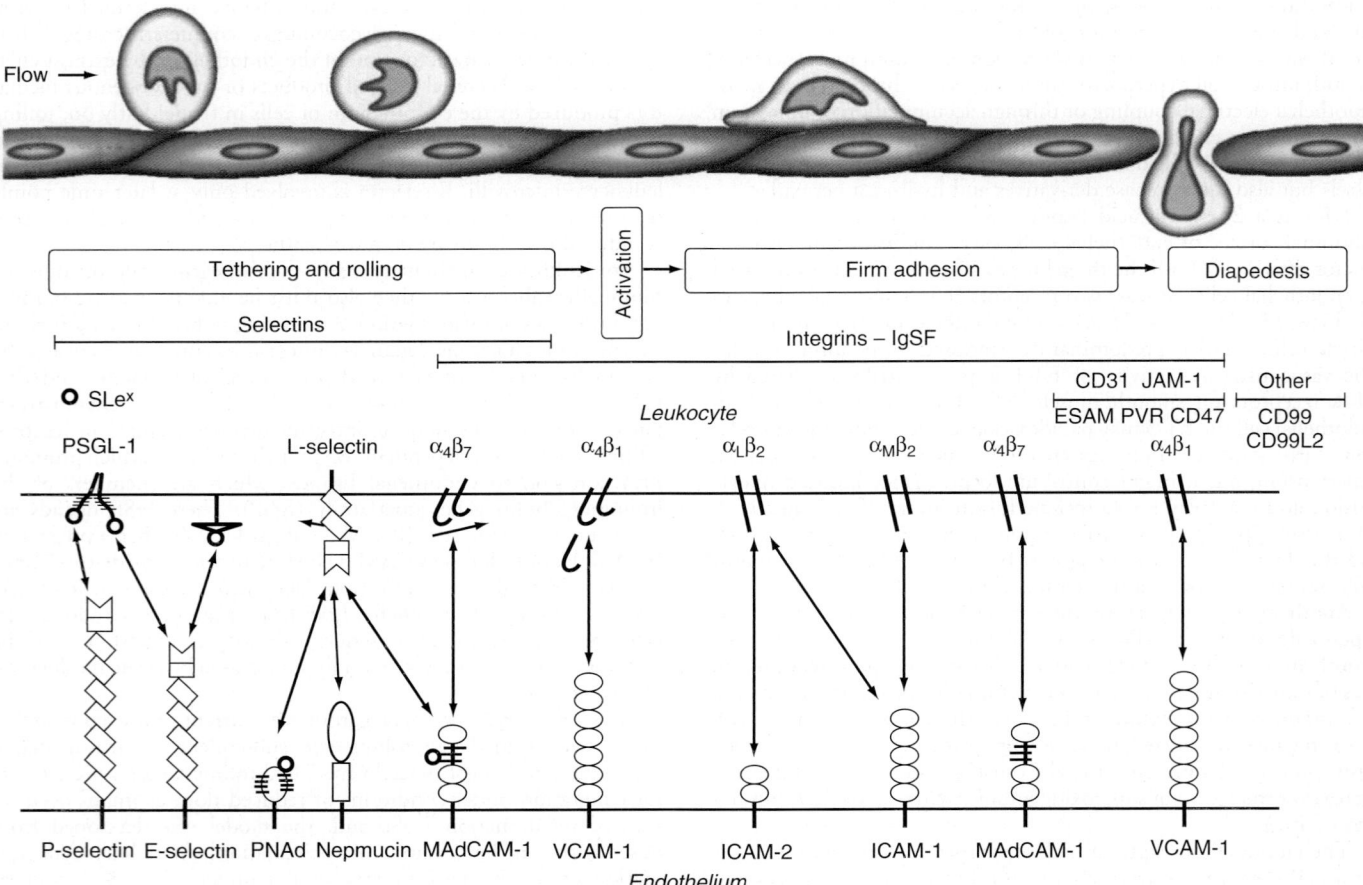

Fig. 123.3 ADHESION CASCADE. Under conditions of flow, leukocytes first tether to endothelial ligands and then roll along the vessel wall. Tethering is mediated predominantly by interaction of P-selectin and L-selectin with their cognate glycoconjugate ligands. P-selectin binds to SLe^x and sulfate residues expressed on PSGL-1. L-selectin binds to an uncharacterized ligand(s) on inflamed endothelium and to sulfated SLe^x-like moieties on PNAd and MAdCAM-1 and sialomucin nepmucin on high endothelial venules. E-selectin, $\alpha_4\beta_1$ (very late antigen 4 [VLA-4]), and $\alpha_4\beta_7$ stabilize rolling initiated by P-selectin and L-selectin. E-selectin recognizes SLe^x on PSGL-1 and other glycoproteins or glycolipids. After tethering and rolling, leukocyte integrin receptors are activated, most often by chemoattractants (e.g., chemokines) via G protein–coupled receptors. After activation, integrin receptors engage endothelial immunoglobulin gene superfamily ligands to promote firm adhesion. Leukocyte $\alpha_L\beta_2$ (leukocyte function antigen 1 [LFA-1]) binds to ICAM-1 and ICAM-2, $\alpha_M\beta_2$ (macrophage 1 [Mac-1]) to ICAM-1, $\alpha_4\beta_1$ (VLA-4) to VCAM-1, and $\alpha_4\beta_7$ to MAdCAM-1. The adherent leukocyte then migrates across endothelium to interendothelial junctions, where it diapedeses between endothelial cells via leukocyte integrin receptors and their endothelial immunoglobulin gene superfamily ligands as well as endothelial junctional proteins such as CD31 (PECAM-1), CD99, CD99L2, ESAM, and JAM-1. *ESAM*, endothelial cell-selective adhesion molecule; *ICAM*, intercellular adhesion molecule; *IgSF*, immunoglobulin gene superfamily; *JAM-1*, junctional adhesion molecule 1; *MAdCAM*, mucosal addressin cell adhesion molecule; *PNAd*, peripheral node addressin; *PSGL*, P-selectin glycoprotein ligand; *PVR*, poliovirus receptor; *SLe^x*, sialyl Lewis X; *VCAM*, vascular cell adhesion molecule 1.

clinical trials in a variety of diseases. However, results were disappointing overall, with many unsuccessful clinical trials of various adhesion antagonists in multiple disease indications.[274,275] Moreover, the report of progressive multifocal leukoencephalopathy, a rare viral infection of the CNS, in several patients treated with the α4-integrin antagonist natalizumab[276] highlights the risks of targeting molecules that are pivotal in host defense and repair as well as in disease. Nevertheless, the potential of antiadhesion therapy is demonstrated by the approval of two integrin antagonists: efalizumab for treatment of psoriasis[277] and natalizumab for treatment of multiple sclerosis.[278]

Platelets

Similar to neutrophils, unactivated platelets do not interact with unperturbed endothelium. After a vascular injury that produces endothelial denudation or retraction, platelets rapidly adhere to the exposed subendothelium. As discussed in greater detail in Chapters 115 and 116, at high shear rates this initial adhesion does not require platelet activation and involves platelet glycoprotein Ib/V/IX (GPIb–V–IX) binding to vWF in the subendothelial matrix and platelet GPVI binding to collagen in the injured arterial wall. Platelet activation occurs after adhesion, leading to platelet spreading mediated by integrin receptors binding to matrix components and aggregation mediated by fibrinogen binding to GPIIb/IIIa (αIIbβ3). Evidence indicates that platelets can bind directly to activated endothelium in vivo via endothelial P-selectin[279] and PECAM-1[280], and to roll on venular endothelium via interaction of platelet GPIbα and endothelial P-selectin.[281] Platelets have been shown to bind to high endothelial venules in vivo via platelet P-selectin.[282] In vitro platelets can adhere to intact endothelium via a platelet GPIIb/IIIa-dependent bridging mechanism involving platelet-bound adhesive

TABLE 123.1 Endothelial Cell Activation[a]

Agonist	Response
Thrombin	Secretion of vWF, P-selectin, TFPI, and PDGF Synthesis of PAF, IL-8, IL-6, and E-selectin
IL-1β, TNF-α, LPS	Synthesis of adhesion molecules (ICAM-1, VCAM-1, E-selectin), chemokines (IL-8, MCP-1), cytokines (IL-6, CD40), procoagulant proteins (TF, PAI-1, t-PA, u-PA), and cytoprotective molecules (A1, IAP) Downregulation of anticoagulant proteins (TM)
Reduced/disturbed shear stress	Increased expression of proinflammatory genes (e.g., VCAM-1, ICAM-1, MCP-1)
VEGF	Decreased eNOS activity Increased expression of cytoprotective genes (A1, MnSOD), Ang2, COX-2

[a]Selected agonists and responses. Many other stimuli (e.g., lipoproteins, hypoxia, microbes, and microbial products) have been reported to upregulate or downregulate various endothelial responses.
Ang, Angiopoietin; A1, Bcl-2 homologue; COX-2, cyclooxygenase 2; eNOS, endothelial nitric oxide synthase; IAP, inhibitor of apoptosis protein; ICAM, intercellular adhesion molecule; IL, interleukin; LPS, lipopolysaccharide; MCP, monocyte chemoattractant protein; MnSOD, manganese superoxide dismutase; PAF, platelet-activating factor; PAI, plasminogen activator inhibitor; PDGF, platelet-derived growth factor; TF, tissue factor; TFPI, tissue factor pathway inhibitor; TM, thrombomodulin; TNF, tumor necrosis factor; t-PA, tissue plasminogen activator; u-PA, urokinase-type plasminogen activator; VCAM, vascular cell adhesion molecule; VEGF, vascular endothelial growth factor; vWF, von Willebrand factor.

proteins and the endothelial cell receptors ICAM-1, αVβ3 integrin, and GPIbα.[283] Platelet adhesion to intact endothelium via these various pathways may contribute to thrombus formation in the circulation and may provide a link between thrombosis and inflammation in diseases such as atherosclerosis.[284] Platelet–endothelial interactions also may contribute to the pathogenesis of thrombotic thrombocytopenic purpura. Normally, ultra-large vWF remains attached to endothelium via P-selectin until it is cleaved by the plasma metalloproteinase a disintegrin and metalloproteinase with thrombospondin (ADAMTS-13). Failure of this mechanism in thrombotic thrombocytopenic purpura because of a deficiency of ADAMTS-13 may lead to spontaneous platelet adhesion to endothelium and microvascular thrombosis.[285]

Red Blood Cells

Plasmodium falciparum–infected and sickled RBCs interact significantly with endothelium, and these adhesive interactions are thought to play an important role in the pathogenesis of human diseases.

Among the human malarial parasites, only *P. falciparum* modifies the surface of the parasitized RBCs so that asexual parasites and gametocytes are able to adhere to the vascular endothelium.[286,287] Binding of trophozoite- and schizont-infected RBCs to endothelium not only allows the parasite to escape destruction in the spleen, but also may contribute to the pathogenesis of cerebral malaria.[287,288] Multiple endothelial adhesion receptors have been implicated in mediating cytoadherence of infected RBCs, including P-selectin, ICAM-1, VCAM-1, and CD36.[289]

Binding of young sickled RBCs to postcapillary endothelium with secondary trapping of poorly deformable, often irreversibly sickled cells is thought to be an important pathogenic factor in vasoocclusive events.[290] Several interactions between sickle RBC receptors and endothelial ligands have been described, including α4β1/VCAM-1;[291] α4β1/Lutheran blood group (basal cell adhesion molecule)[292]; and ICAM-4/αVβ3.[293] The adhesive proteins thrombospondin and vWF promote adhesion by serving as bridging factors between various sickle RBC and endothelial adhesion molecules. In addition to direct

adhesion to endothelium, sickle RBC binding to adherent leukocytes has been proposed as a mechanism for sickle cell vascular occlusion.[294] As with leukocyte adhesion to endothelium in inflammatory and immune disease, drugs targeting sickle RBC adhesive interactions with endothelial cells or leukocytes may prove useful in preventing or treating vasoocclusive crises.

Endothelial Cell Activation and Dysfunction

Although once viewed as a passive barrier between blood and tissue, the endothelium now is evident to be a dynamic and heterogeneous organ that responds to diverse stimuli, ranging from coagulation proteins and cytokines to hemodynamic forces and growth factors. Activation of endothelial cells induces a complex proinflammatory and prothrombotic phenotype as well as expression of certain cytoprotective genes (see Table 123.1).[295,296] Multiple transcription factors, particularly nuclear factor-κB[297] and early growth response 1,[298] regulate these responses.[295] Endothelial activation undoubtedly is an important event in host defense and repair, but it also may contribute to the pathogenesis of diverse diseases, ranging from sepsis[299] to atherosclerosis.[300]

Endothelial dysfunction is characterized by a reduction in the bioavailability of vasodilators, particularly NO, leading to impairment of endothelium-dependent vasodilation, or by an increase in endothelium-derived contracting factors.[301] Endothelial dysfunction is prominent in atherosclerosis but also has been described in diabetes, preeclampsia, hypertension, uremia, and other diseases. In a broader sense, endothelial dysfunction encompasses proinflammatory and procoagulant changes as well as apoptotic cell death.[227,302,303]

A number of noninvasive approaches for assessing endothelial function in vascular diseases have been developed. Endothelial vasodilatory responses can be evaluated by high-resolution ultrasound measurement of flow-mediated vasodilation or by plethysmography of changes in forearm blood flow during reactive hyperemia.[304] Endothelial activation can be assessed in plasma by circulating markers such as soluble endothelial adhesion molecules (e.g., sVCAM-1, sICAM-1, sE-selectin) and endothelial coagulation proteins (e.g., vWF and thrombomodulin)[305] or endothelial microparticles.[306] Circulating endothelial cells reflect significant vascular damage or cell death.[307]

SUGGESTED READINGS

Aird WC: Spatial and temporal dynamics of the endothelium. *J Thromb Haemost* 3:1392, 2005.

Aird WC: Phenotypic heterogeneity of the endothelium: I. Structure, function, and mechanisms. *Circ Res* 100:158, 2007.

Bazzoni G, Dejana E: Endothelial cell-to-cell junctions: molecular organization and role in vascular homeostasis. *Physiol Rev* 84:869, 2004.

Butler JM, Nolan DJ, Vertes EL, et al: Endothelial cells are essential for the self-renewal and repopulation of notch-dependent hematopoietic stem cells. *Cell Stem Cell* 6:251, 2010.

Carmeliet P: Blood vessels and nerves: common signals, pathways and diseases. *Nat Rev Genet* 4:710, 2003.

Conway EM, Collen D, Carmeliet P: Molecular mechanisms of blood vessel growth. *Cardiovasc Res* 49:507, 2001.

Coultas L, Chawengsaksophak K, Rossant J: Endothelial cells and VEGF in vascular development. *Nature* 438:937, 2005.

De Palma M, Naldini L: Role of haematopoietic cells and endothelial progenitors in tumour angiogenesis. *Biochim Biophys Acta* 1766:159, 2006.

Gerhardt H, Betsholtz C: Endothelial-pericyte interactions in angiogenesis. *Cell Tissue Res* 22:15, 2003.

Harrison DG, Widder J, Grumbach I, et al: Endothelial mechanotransduction, nitric oxide and vascular inflammation. *J Intern Med* 259:351, 2006.

Hebbel RP, Yamada O, Moldow CF, et al: Abnormal adherence of sickle erythrocytes to cultured vascular endothelium: Possible mechanism for microvascular occlusion in sickle cell disease. *J Clin Invest* 65:154, 1980.

Kerbel R, Folkman J: Clinical translation of angiogenesis inhibitors. *Nat Rev Cancer* 2:727, 2002.

Lapidot T, Dar A, Kollet O: How do stem cells find their way home? *Blood* 106:1901, 2005.

Luster AD, Alon R, von Andrian UH: Immune cell migration in inflammation: present and future therapeutic targets. *Nat Immunol* 6:1182, 2005.

Miyasaka M, Tanaka T: Lymphocyte trafficking across high endothelial venules: dogmas and enigmas. *Nat Rev Immunol* 4:360, 2004.

Mehta D, Malik AB: Signaling mechanisms regulating endothelial permeability. *Physiol Rev* 86:279, 2006.

Minami T, Aird WC: Endothelial cell gene regulation. *Trends Cardiovasc Med* 15:174, 2005.

Petri B, Bixel MG: Molecular events during leukocyte diapedesis. *FEBS J* 273:4399, 2006.

Pober JS, Min W: Endothelial cell dysfunction, injury and death. *Handb Exp Pharmacol* 135:2006.

Rafii S, Lyden D, Benezra R, et al: Vascular and haematopoietic stem cells: Novel targets for anti-angiogenesis therapy? *Nat Rev Cancer* 2:826, 2002.

Rak J, Milsom C, May L, et al: Tissue factor in cancer and angiogenesis: The molecular link between genetic tumor progression, tumor neovascularization, and cancer coagulopathy. *Semin Thromb Hemost* 32:54, 2006.

Schofield L, Grau GE: Immunological processes in malaria pathogenesis. *Nat Rev Immunol* 5:722, 2005.

Shih T, Lindley C: Bevacizumab: an angiogenesis inhibitor for the treatment of solid malignancies. *Clin Ther* 28:1779, 2006.

Yin T, Li L: The stem cell niches in bone. *J Clin Invest* 116:1195, 2006.

Yonekawa K, Harlan JM: Targeting leukocyte integrins in human diseases. *J Leukoc Biol* 77:129, 2005.

REFERENCES

For the complete list of references, log on to www.expertconsult.com.

MEGAKARYOCYTE AND PLATELET STRUCTURE

Joseph E. Italiano, Jr. and John H. Hartwig

Platelets are small anucleate fragments that are formed from the cytoplasm of megakaryocytes and have a characteristic discoid shape. To assemble and release platelets, megakaryocytes become polyploid by endomitosis and follow a maturation program that results in the conversion of the bulk of their cytoplasm into multiple long processes called *proplatelets*. To produce its quota of 1000–2000 platelets, a megakaryocyte may protrude as many as 10–20 proplatelets, each of which begins as a blunt protrusion that over time thins and branches repeatedly. Platelets form selectively at the ends of proplatelets. As platelets develop, their content of granules and organelles is delivered to them in a stream of individual particles moving from the megakaryocyte cell body to the nascent platelet buds at the proplatelet tips. Platelet formation can be arbitrarily divided into two phases. The first phase takes days to complete and requires megakaryocyte-specific growth factors. Massive nuclear proliferation to 16–32N and enlargement of the megakaryocyte cytoplasm occur as the platelet is filled with cytoskeletal proteins, platelet-specific granules, and sufficient membrane to complete the platelet assembly process. The second phase is relatively rapid and can be completed in hours. During this phase, megakaryocytes generate platelets by remodeling their cytoplasm first into proplatelets, then preplatelets, which undergo fission to generate discoid platelets.

MEGAKARYOCYTE DEVELOPMENT

Endomitosis

Hematopoietic stem cells, which are endowed with the genetic capacity to differentiate into multiple lineages, are induced down the pathway to become megakaryocytes by their exposure to certain growth factors.[1] Megakaryocytes become polyploid (i.e., 4N, 16N, 32N, 64N) through repeated cycles of DNA replication without cell division.[2–5] Normally ploidy ranges from 4 to 64 times the haploid DNA complement, but the majority of cells fall within three ploidy classes (8N, 16N, and 32N), with 16N being dominant (Fig. 124.1).[6,7] Ploidy number appears to be a predetermined event, possibly signifying genetic diversity among megakaryocyte populations. Megakaryocyte polyploidization results in a functional gene amplification whose likely function is an increase in protein synthesis.[8] This process, called *endomitosis*, is a shortened mitosis caused by a block in late anaphase.[9,10]

Whereas cells undergoing diploid mitoses proceed through cytokinesis and complete abscission division, megakaryocytes exhibit regression of the cleavage furrow and reenter G_1 as polyploid cells.[1] During polyploidization of megakaryocytes, the nuclear envelope breaks down, and an abnormal spherical mitotic spindle forms. The spindle has attached chromosomes that align from a position equidistant from the spindle poles. Sister chromatids segregate and move toward their respective poles (anaphase A). However, the spindle poles fail to move apart and do not undergo the microtubule-driven separation typically observed during anaphase B. Individual chromatids are not moved to the poles, and subsequently a single nuclear envelope encapsulates the entire set of sister chromatids.[9,10] In most cell types, checkpoints and feedback controls ensure that DNA replication and cell division are tightly coupled. Megakaryocytes appear to be an exception to this rule, indicating they have managed to deregulate this process. Proposed mechanisms for regulating endomitosis include a reduction in mitosis-promoting factor[11,12] or decreased

expression of cyclin B.[12–15] Cyclins appear to play a critical role in directing endomitosis. Cyclin D3 is overexpressed in the G_1 phase of maturing megakaryocytes,[16] but a triple knockout of cyclins D1, D2, and D3 in mice does not appear to affect megakaryocyte development.[17] In contrast, cyclin E-deficient mice exhibit a profound defect in megakaryocyte development.[18] The molecular programming involved in endomitosis is characterized by the mislocalization or absence of at least two critical regulators of mitosis: the chromosomal passenger proteins Aurora-B/AIM-1 and survivin. AIM-1, a serine/threonine kinase in the Aurora family that is implicated in mitosis, is downregulated as megakaryocyte polyploidization occurs, suggesting its loss may lead to the abortive mitosis and polyploidization.[19,20] However, while Aurora kinase A is required for hematopoiesis, it is dispensable for mouse megakaryocyte endomitosis and differentiation.[21] Whereas deletion of the APC/C cofactor Cdc20 causes mitotic arrest and severe thrombocytopenia, lack of the kinases Aurora-B, Cdk1, or Cdk2 does not affect endomitosis of megakaryocytes or platelet counts. Deletion of Cdk1 forces a change to endocycles without mitosis, whereas polyploidization in the absence of cdk1 and cdk2 occurs in the presence of aberrant replication events. Notably, ablation of these kinases rescues defects in Cdc20 null megakaryocytes. The observations suggest that endomitosis can be functionally replaced by alternative polyploidization mechanisms in vivo. One explanation for endomitosis could be inhibition of microtubule-based forces in anaphase B. Spindle pole separation during anaphase B is believed to be powered by the sliding of antiparallel interdigitating microtubules past each other[22] mediated by the mitotic kinesin-like protein 1. This protein localizes at regions of overlapping microtubules during anaphase B and studies in vitro indicate that it can slide microtubules past each other.[23] Therefore lack of spindle pole separation during endomitosis may result from failure of megakaryocytes to undergo normal spindle orientation and/or the absence of signals that localize or activate a kinesin motor molecule that provides force for sliding.

Cytoplasmic Maturation

Megakaryocytes, the largest of the hematopoietic cells, undergo a pronounced cytoplasmic maturation to attain their large volumes (15,000 fL). Cytoplasmic maturation begins during endomitosis and increases considerably after all DNA amplification has ended (Fig. 124.2). Megakaryocytes enlarge dramatically as they mature, reaching sizes of 100–150 μm in diameter in culture and in bone marrow. During this process, the megakaryocyte cytoplasm rapidly fills with platelet-specific proteins, organelles, and membrane systems that ultimately are subdivided and packaged into platelets (Fig. 124.3). Their cytoplasmic space expands and, except for the most cortical regions, becomes densely filled with internal membranes that subsequently serve as the repository for the plasma membrane to be regurgitated for coating proplatelets as they extend.[24] This internal membrane system, which is one of the most striking features of mature megakaryocytes, has been referred to as the *demarcation membrane system* (DMS). The DMS, first described by Yamada in 1957, consists of an extensive, tortuous, branching network of membrane channels composed of flattened cisternae and tubules. Initially, the DMS was proposed to play an essential role in platelet formation by defining preformed "platelet territories" or "platelet fields" within the megakaryocyte cytoplasm.[26,27] Release of individual

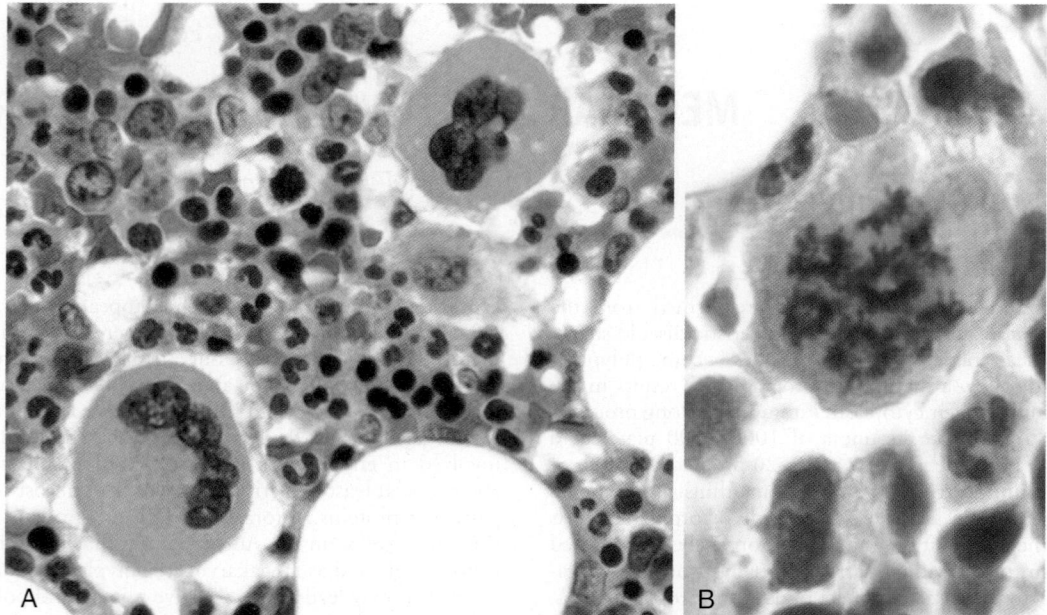

Fig. 124.1 POLYPLOID MEGAKARYOCYTES IN THE BONE MARROW. Large polyploid megakaryo-cytes are seen in the bone marrow on a typical hematoxylin- and eosin-stained slide and are recognized by their abundant pink cytoplasm and large nuclei (A). The degree of polyploidization is difficult to determine. Rarely, megakaryocytes can be seen in mitosis (B), and when chromosomes are aligned in metaphase plates, the high ploidy level become quite apparent. In the mitotic figure illustrated, the megakaryocyte is a 16N form with eight 2N metaphase plates.

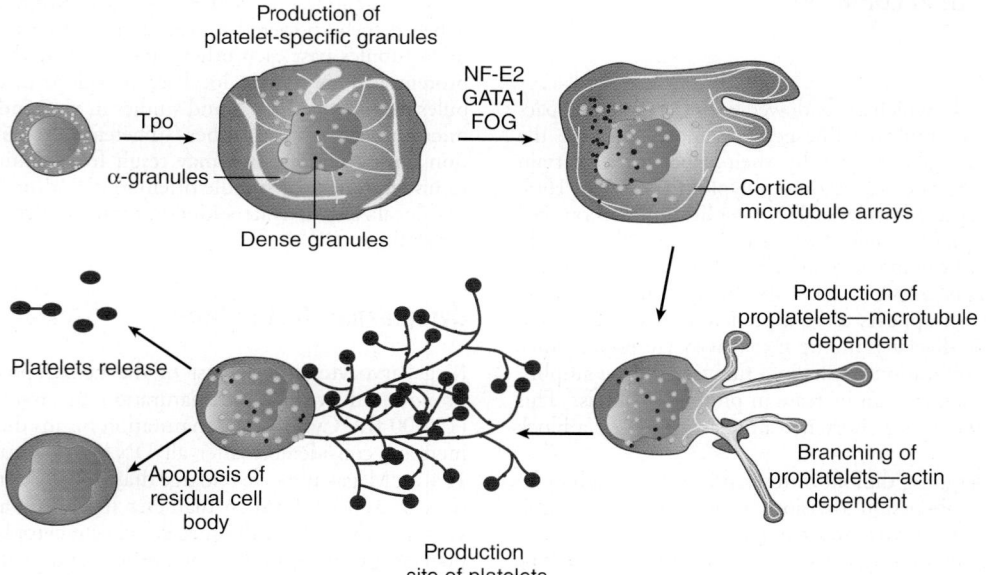

Fig. 124.2 SUMMARY OF THE MAJOR EVENTS THAT LEAD TO PLATELET FORMATION AND RELEASE FROM MEGAKARYOCYTES. Hematopoietic stem cells are converted into megakaryocytes by exposure to the specific growth factor TPO. TPO initiates a maturation program that amplifies the mega-karyocyte DNA and leads to synthesis of platelet-specific proteins. In particular, cytoskeletal elements, membrane systems, and receptor proteins are made in bulk, and the megakaryocyte becomes filled with platelet-specific granules. Platelet production begins when microtubules aggregate in the cell cortex, and one pole of the megakaryocyte spontaneously elaborates pseudopodia. These begin as large blunt pseudopodia, which subsequently thin and branch into proplatelets. The branching reaction is dependent on a localized assembly of actin and is inhibited by drugs that disrupt actin filaments. Platelets are assembled primarily at the ends of the proplatelets. Intracellular organelles are delivered to the platelet buds along microtubule tracks in the shafts. Platelets are released from the ends of proplatelets. *FOG*, Friend of *GATA1*; *GATA1*, GATA binding protein 1; *TPO*, thrombopoietin.

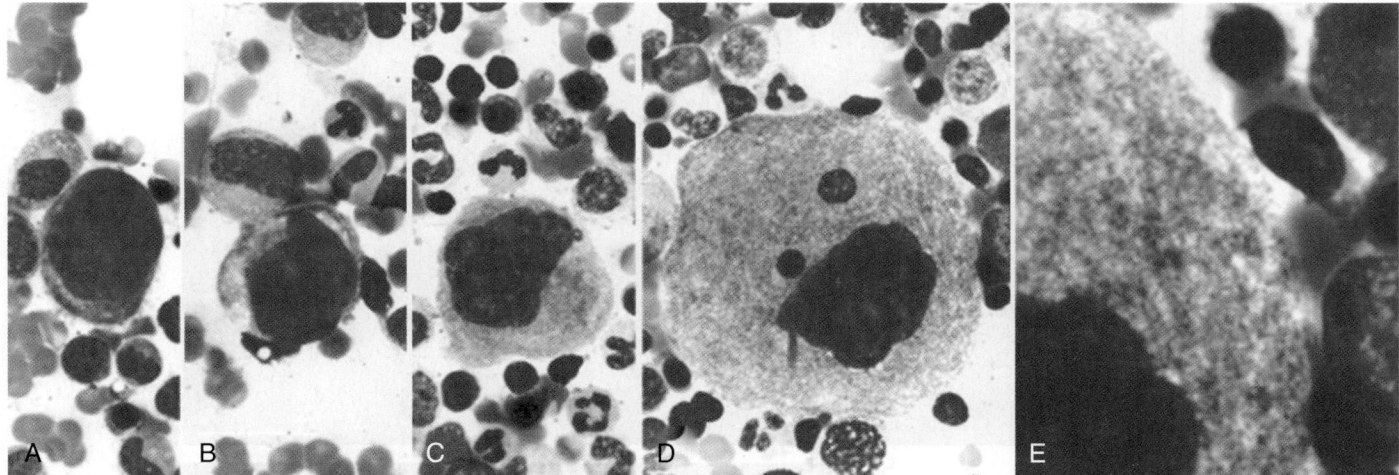

Fig. 124.3 PLATELET PRODUCTION IN THE MEGAKARYOCYTE. (A) Immature polyploid mega-karyoblast with little differentiation. (B) Megakaryocyte with early Golgi zone. (C) Early platelet production in cytoplasm. (D) Late-stage megakaryocyte with abundant internal membranes, organelles, and platelet-specific proteins. (E) Early formation of demarcation membranes.

platelets was postulated to occur by massive fragmentation of the megakaryocyte cytoplasm along DMS fracture lines between these fields. However, studies demonstrating that platelets are primarily assembled and released from proplatelet ends (see Platelet Formation later in this chapter) are inconsistent with this notion and indicate instead that the DMS functions predominantly as a membrane reserve for proplatelet formation.[24] Direct visualization of mature DMSs containing phosphatidylinositol 4,5-bisphosphate suggests that it is the source of proplatelet membranes.[2] Studies by Eckly et al[28] have begun to provide insights into how the DMS forms and matures. To develop the DMS, the megakaryocyte plasma membrane enfolds at specific sites to generate a perinuclear pre-DMS. Next, the pre-DMS is expanded into its mature form by material added from Golgi-derived vesicles and by endoplasmic reticulum-mediated lipid transfer. This structural description is in line with studies on platelet glycosyltransferases, which arrive early in the forming DMS and eventually make their way to the megakaryocyte and platelet surface.[29] Thus far only a handful of proteins have been identified to participate in DMS formation based on alteration in its structure in certain knockout mouse models. Membrane-deforming proteins that use F-BAR domains to curve membranes or use GTP as an energy source to bud vesicles from membranes appear to be necessary for normal megakaryocyte maturation and platelet release. Gross disruptions in DMS structure are found in megakaryocytes isolated from either filamin A knockout, pascin2 knockout, dynamin 2 knockout, or Cdc42 interacting protein 4 (CIP4) knockout mice. CIP4 is an F-BAR protein that induces membrane tubulation and localizes to membrane lipids via its BAR domain and interacts with the Wiskott-Aldrich syndrome protein (WASp).[30] CIP4$^{-/-}$ mice have mild thrombocytopenia with a 25% decrease in platelet counts. While megakaryocyte numbers and ploidy are normal in CIP4$^{-/-}$ knockout mice, megakaryocytes isolated from these mice are less effective in producing proplatelets in vitro.

Dynamins are highly conserved large mechanochemical GTPases involved in endocytosis and vesicle transport, and mutations in dynamin 2 have been associated with thrombocytopenia in humans. Dynamin-2–dependent endocytosis is required for megakaryocyte development in mice.[31] Filamin connects αGPIbα to the actin cytoskeleton and binds pacsin2, a molecule that deforms membranes. Pacsin 2 has an F-BAR and SH3 domain that binds dynamin and N-WASp. Pacsin2 plays an important role in organizing internal membranes during megakaryocyte development and platelet production.

Maturing megakaryocytes, like other granulated cells, contain an abundance of ribosomes and rough endoplasmic reticulum, where protein synthesis occurs. During this phase of megakaryocyte development, the cytoplasm fills with cytoskeletal proteins, platelet-specific receptors and secretory granules, and normal cellular organelles such as mitochondria and lysosomes.

One of the hallmark features of the mature megakaryocyte is its abundance of platelet-specific secretory granules. The two specific granules destined for platelets are α-granules and dense granules. α-Granules, the more abundant and larger of the two (200–500 nm in diameter), contain proteins that enhance platelet adhesion, promote cell-cell interactions, regulate angiogenesis, and stimulate vascular repair. α-Granules store matrix proteins and contain glyco-protein receptors in their membranes (Fig. 124.4A). The bulk of cellular P-selectin and a portion of $\alpha_{IIb}\beta_3$ and the glycoprotein Ib/IX/V complex, a receptor for von Willebrand factor (vWF), are expressed in the membranes of α-granules. Adhesion molecules within the granules include vWF, fibrinogen, fibronectin, vitronectin, and thrombospondin. α-Granule proteins can be derived from different sources. Some proteins, such as α-thromboglobulin and vWF, are synthesized by megakaryocytes. However, fibrinogen, also a major component of α-granules, is not synthesized by megakaryocytes and is taken up from plasma by an endocytic mechanism requiring fibrinogen binding to $\alpha_{IIb}\beta_3$. Although little is known about the intracellular trafficking of proteins in megakaryocytes, experiments using cryosectioning and immunoelectron microscopy suggest that multivesicular bodies are an essential intermediate stage in the formation of platelet α-granules. During megakaryocyte development, large (≈0.5 μm) multivesicular bodies undergo a gradual transition from granules containing 30–70-nm internal vesicles to granules containing secretion concentrates.

The second and smaller type of platelet granule is the dense granule. Platelets contain relatively few dense granules, which are approximately 150 nm in diameter. Dense granules have electron opaque cores and function primarily to recruit additional platelets to sites of vascular injury. Dense granules contain soluble activating agents, such as serotonin and ADP, as well as divalent cations. When the megakaryocyte reaches a certain point of maturation, proplatelet production begins, and granules are sent into the proplatelets destined for platelets.

REGULATION OF MEGAKARYOCYTE DEVELOPMENT

The development of megakaryocytes and the process of platelet biogenesis occur within a complex bone marrow environment where both cytokines and adhesive interactions play an essential role.

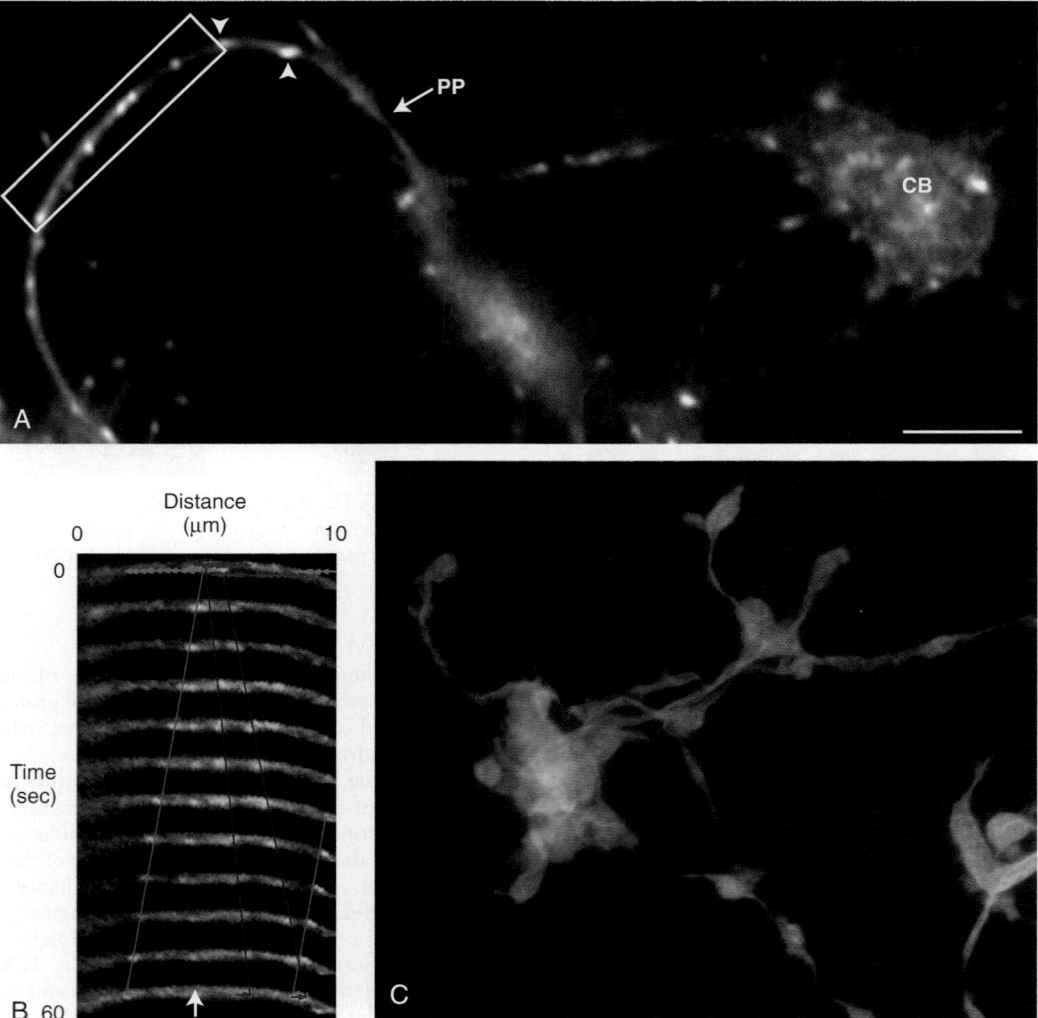

Fig. 124.4 MICROTUBULE DYNAMICS DURING PROPLATELET FORMATION. (A) Visualization of plus-end microtubule assembly in living megakaryocytes expressing end-binding protein 3 (EB3)-green fluorescent protein (GFP). First frame from the time-lapse sequence (B) of a living megakaryocyte that was retrovirally directed to express EB3-GFP. The cell body (CB) is at the right of the micrograph, and proplatelets (PP) extend to the left. EB3-GFP labels growing microtubule plus ends in a characteristic "comet" staining pattern that has a bright front and a dim tail. (B) The kymograph shows movement over time. Images are every 5 seconds. EB3-GFP comets undergo bidirectional movements in PP, demonstrating that microtubules are organized as bipolar arrays. Some EB3-GFP comets move toward the tip and are highlighted in *green*; others that move toward the cell body are highlighted in *red*. (C) Distribution of α-granules in megakaryocytes and PP projections visualized by fluorescence microscopy. α-Granules are stained with Alexa 568 *(red)*–labeled anti–von Willebrand factor antibodies. The proplatelets have been co-stained with Alexa 488 *(green)* antitubulin antibodies to highlight the microtubules.

Megakaryocytes are imprisoned within the subendothelial layer of the bone marrow sinuses where development and platelet biogenesis are regulated at multiple levels by several cytokines. Thrombopoietin (TPO), which is synthesized in bone marrow and the liver, is the principal regulator of thrombopoiesis. TPO also plays a central role in hematopoietic stem cell survival and proliferation. Circulating levels of TPO induce proliferation and maturation of megakaryocyte progenitors by binding to the c-Mpl receptor and signaling induction. TPO regulates all stages of megakaryocyte development, from the hematopoietic stem cell stage through cytoplasmic maturation. TPO increases platelet production by increasing both the number and size of individual megakaryocytes. c-Mpl activation is regulated by a complex array of signaling molecules that turn on specific transcription factors (see Transcriptional Regulation of Platelet Formation later in this chapter) to drive megakaryocyte proliferation and maturation. Although TPO appears to function as the main regulator of megakaryocyte development, it is not exclusive in this action. The cytokine stem cell factor, granulocyte-macrophage colony-stimulating factor, FLT ligand, interleukin (IL)-3, IL-6, IL-11, and erythropoietin also can regulate megakaryocyte development but appear to function mainly in concert with TPO. Mice that lack TPO or its receptor c-Mpl have approximately 15% of the normal platelet count. The discovery of TPO in 1994 and the development of primary megakaryocyte or mouse embryonic stem cell cultures that can be induced to faithfully reconstitute platelet formation has provided systems for studying megakaryocytes in the act of making platelets in vitro. Megakaryocytes isolated from mouse fetal liver and incubated with TPO for 4–5 days mature into huge polyploid cells that are capable of generating and releasing large numbers of platelets. In a similar fashion, mouse embryonic stem cells can be induced to mature into large polyploid megakaryocytes in the presence of stromal cells and TPO, IL-6, and IL-11. This process requires 10–12 days, during which the conversion of embryonic stem cells into hematopoietic stem cells very likely occurs in the first half of the time period and the maturation of hematopoietic stem cells into proplatelet-producing megakaryocytes in the second half. Human embryonic stem cells can be coaxed to differentiate into mature megakaryocytes,[3] although the process takes several more days in culture. Recently, platelets have been generated from induced human pluripotent stem cells in culture using a doxycycline-controlled c-MYC expression vector.[4]

PLATELET FORMATION

Proplatelets and the Cytoskeletal Mechanics of Platelet Formation

The discovery of TPO and the development of megakaryocyte cultures that reconstitute platelet formation in vitro have allowed visualization of megakaryocytes in the act of forming platelets.[5] The actual mechanical process of platelet production begins when mature megakaryocytes start to elaborate proplatelets (see Fig. 124.2 and Fig. 124.5). This process is distinguished by the erosion of one pole of the megakaryocyte cytoplasm (see Fig. 124.5). Multiple thick pseudopodia are extended and subsequently elongate to yield thin tubules. As these slender tubules grow, they branch repeatedly and develop periodic densities along their length that impart a beaded appearance.[5,6] The first insight into the cytoskeletal mechanics of platelet formation dates from the work of Tablin and colleagues, who showed that proplatelet formation is dependent on microtubules; that is, proplatelet elaboration is inhibited by microtubule poisons. Microtubule poisons are effective because the extension of proplatelets from the megakaryocyte is mediated by the assembly of microtubules and their reorganization into cortical bundles. Cortical bundles align in the shafts of proplatelets, and proplatelet elongation is driven by sliding movements between overlapping microtubules composed of these bundles.[7] The microtubule bundles form loops at the end of each proplatelet, and ultimately a single microtubule is rolled into a coil at the proplatelet end to define the platelet territory. Cytoplasmic tubulin in solution is an $\alpha\beta$ dimer that reversibly polymerizes into microtubules, which are long, hollow cylinders with an outer diameter of 25 nm. Several studies reveal an essential role in platelet biogenesis for β_1 tubulin, a divergent and lineage-specific β tubulin that is a major component of the megakaryocyte proplatelet cytoskeleton and marginal microtubule coil of the platelet. β_1 Tubulin, which is expressed exclusively in platelets and megakaryocytes during the late stages of megakaryocyte development, is essential for the production of normal numbers of platelets, as well as for the discoid shape of platelets. The evidence supporting the role of β_1 tubulin in these processes comes from several sources. First, mRNA subtraction between wild-type and NF-E2–deficient megakaryocytes identifies β_1

tubulin as a downstream effector of the megakaryocyte transcription factor NF-E2 that is absent in NF-E2–deficient megakaryocytes. Second, genetic elimination of the β_1-tubulin gene in mice results in thrombocytopenia.[6] Third, megakaryocytes isolated from β_1-tubulin knockout mice fail to form proplatelets in vitro and instead extend only a small number of blunt protrusions.

The first event that signals proplatelet production is the consolidation of microtubules into large bundles at the megakaryocyte cortex that subsequently are reorganized into parallel bundles in the shafts of the proplatelets (Fig. 124.6).[8] Microtubule bundles are thick near the body of the megakaryocyte as they enter the proplatelet shaft but become progressively thinner along the shaft, such that only 5–10 microtubules remain at the end of the proplatelet. Of note, the microtubule bundles that run down the proplatelet shaft make characteristic U turns in the tips and reenter the shaft, forming teardrop-shaped structures (Fig. 124.7). This creates a bipolar orientation of bundles near the proplatelet tip, a geometry required to explain the bidirectional granule and organelle traffic observed in proplatelets. The looped arrangement of microtubules in proplatelet tips also constrains the elongation mechanism used to grow proplatelets because of an insufficient number of free microtubule ends to nucleate this reaction.

Direct visualization of microtubule dynamics in living megakaryocytes using green fluorescent protein (GFP) technology has provided insights into how microtubules orient to power proplatelet elongation (see Fig. 124.4A,B). End-binding protein 3 (EB3), a microtubule plus end-binding protein associated only with growing microtubules, fused to GFP was retrovirally expressed in murine megakaryocytes and used as a marker to localize microtubule plus ends and to follow plus end dynamics.[7] Immature megakaryocytes without proplatelets use a centrosomal-coupled microtubule nucleation/assembly reaction, which appears as a prominent starburst pattern when visualized with EB3-GFP. Microtubules assemble only from the centrosome and grow outward into the cell cortex, where they turn and run parallel to the cell edges. Just before proplatelet production begins, however, centrosomal assembly ends and microtubules release and consolidate into the cortex as bundles. Fluorescence time-lapse microscopy of living, proplatelet-producing megakaryocytes expressing EB3-GFP reveals that as proplatelets elongate, microtubules assemble continuously throughout the entire proplatelet. EB3-GFP studies also reveal that microtubules polymerize in both directions in proplatelets—that is, toward both the tips and cell body—demonstrating that microtubules composing the bundles have a mixed polarity. The cytoplasmic Ran-binding protein, RanBP10, is a β_1-tubulin–binding protein that appears to regulate the assembly of proplatelet microtubules.[9] Even though microtubules are continuously assembling at their plus ends in proplatelets, polymerization per se does not provide the force for proplatelet elongation. First, the rates of microtubule polymerization

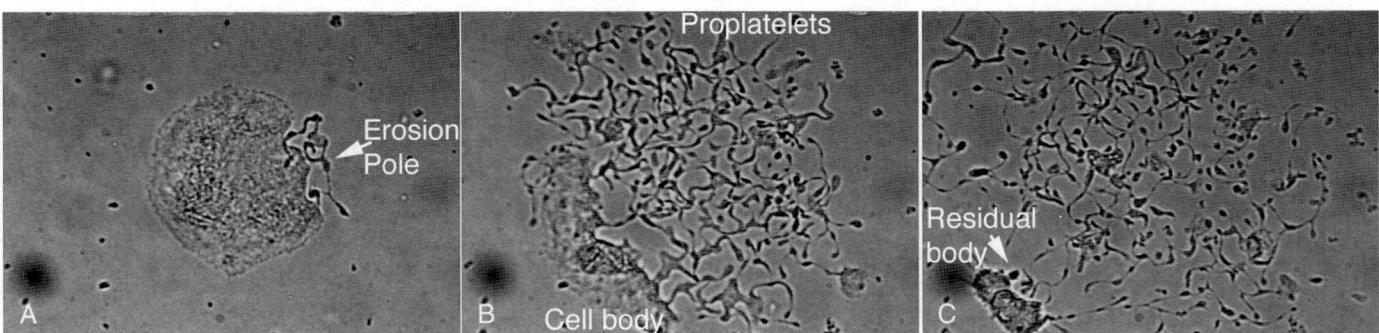

Fig. 124.5 FORMATION OF PROPLATELETS BY A MOUSE MEGAKARYOCYTE. Time-lapse sequence of a maturing megakaryocyte showing the events that lead to elaboration of proplatelets in vitro. (A) Platelet production begins when the megakaryocyte cytoplasm starts to erode at one pole (*arrow*). (B) The bulk of the megakaryocyte cytoplasm has been converted into multiple proplatelet processes that continue to lengthen and form swellings along their length. These processes are highly dynamic and undergo bending and branching. (C) Once the bulk of the megakaryocyte cytoplasm has been converted into proplatelets, the entire process ends in a rapid retraction that separates the released proplatelets from the residual cell body.

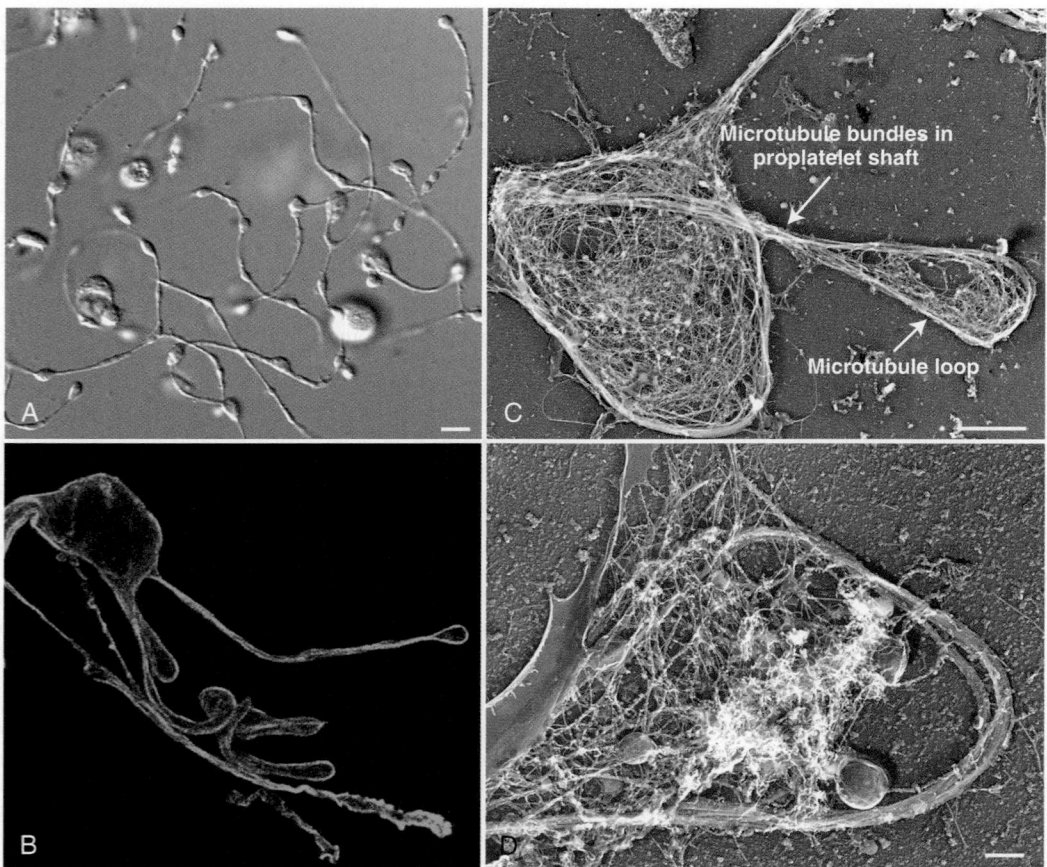

Fig. 124.6 STRUCTURE OF PROPLATELETS. (A) Differential interference contrast image of proplatelets elaborated by mouse megakaryocytes in culture (bar = 5 μm). (B) Staining of proplatelets with Alexa 488 antitubulin immunoglobulin G reveals that the microtubules line the shaft of the proplatelet and form loops at the proplatelet tips (bar = 5 μm). (C, D) Organization of microtubules in the tips of proplatelets. (C) Microtubules form bundles in the proplatelet shafts (bar = 2 μm). (D) Microtubules loop in the proplatelet ends and reenter the proplatelet shafts (bar = 0.2 μm).

(average 10.2 μm/min) are approximately 10-fold faster than the proplatelet elongation rate. Second, proplatelet elongation continues when microtubule polymerization is blocked with drugs that inhibit net assembly, suggesting an alternative mechanism for proplatelet elongation. Third, proplatelets possess an inherent microtubule sliding mechanism. Cytoplasmic dynein, a minus-end microtubule molecular motor protein, localizes along the microtubules of the proplatelet and appears to directly contribute to microtubule sliding because inhibition of dynein through disassembly of the dynactin complex prevents proplatelet formation. Microtubule sliding can be reactivated in detergent-permeabilized proplatelets. Adenosine triphosphate, which is known to support the enzymatic activity of microtubule-based molecular motors, activates elongation in permeabilized proplatelets that contain dynein and its regulatory complex dynactin. More recent analysis has indicated six types of behaviors that characterize the elaboration of proplatelets: elongation, branching, pausing, fusions, fragmentations, and retractions. While the average elongation rate for proplatelets over time is 1 μm/min, extension normally occurs in bursts and pauses. Burst rates greatly exceed the average rates, and under flow rates of less than 30 μm/min have been observed. These rates correlate well with the sliding rates of microtubules within the bundles. Fluorescence recovery after photobleaching studies have demonstrated that microtubule sliding drives proplatelet elongation and is dependent on cytoplasmic dynein.[32] Thus dynein-facilitated microtubule sliding appears to be the key event driving proplatelet elongation.

Nascent platelets assemble at the bulbous ends of proplatelets, as defined by the rolling of a single microtubule into a coil having the same diameter as the coil found in the mature platelet. Given that maturation of the platelet is limited to these sites; efficient platelet production requires a large number of proplatelet ends. Megakaryocytes use a unique mechanical process to repeatedly bifurcate the shafts of the proplatelet, thereby amplifying the number of ends. To accomplish this task, the shaft of elongating proplatelets is bent on itself and a new proplatelet grows out of the bend; a process that results in bifurcation of the shaft. Whereas proplatelet elongation is mediated by microtubules, actin mediates the bending and branching of proplatelet shafts. Actin filament assemblies decorate branch points, and agents that disrupt actin assembly, such as the cytochalasins, abolish proplatelet branching. One possibility is that proplatelet bending and branching are regulated by the actin-based molecular motor myosin. Myosin II is an ATPase motor that makes up 2%–5% of the total platelet protein. Myosin II binds to actin filaments and generates force for contraction. Each myosin has two heads and a long, rod-like tail whose function is to permit the molecules to assemble into bipolar filaments. Of interest, a mutation in the tail domain of the nonmuscle myosin heavy chain A gene in humans results in several disorders, including May-Hegglin anomaly, Sebastian syndrome, and Fechtner syndrome. These rare autosomal platelet disorders are characterized by thrombocytopenia with giant platelets. Recent findings have implicated myosin IIA in restricting proplatelet production until megakaryocytes attain full maturity. The loss of myosin IIA function through targeted gene disruption in mice, through dominant inhibitory mutations in humans, or by manipulation of cultured megakaryocytes appears to accelerate proplatelet production. Consequently, platelet production is inefficient and

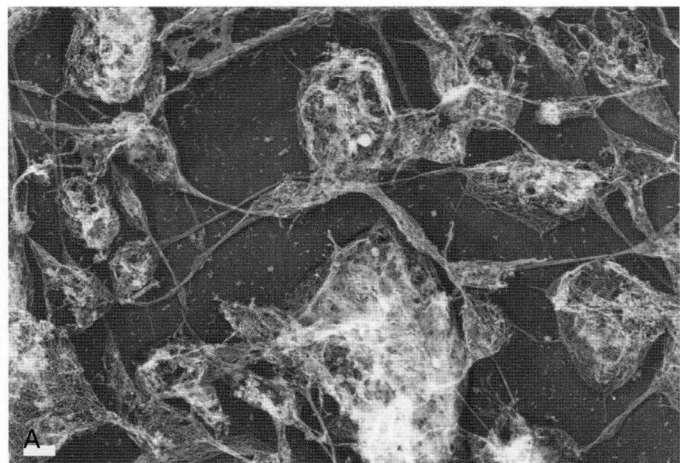

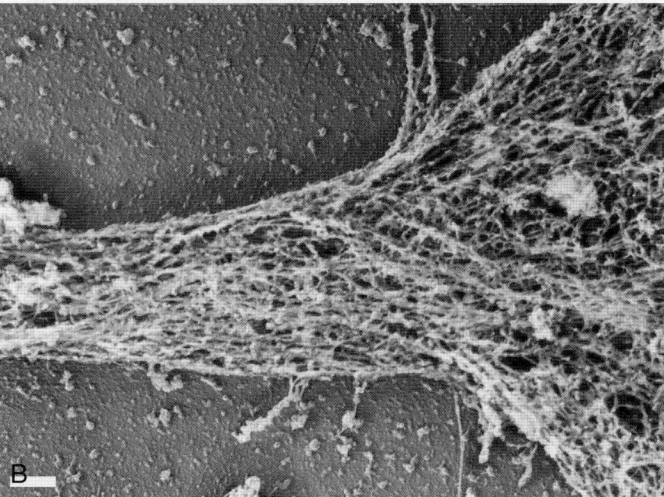

Fig. 124.7 MEMBRANE SKELETON OF THE PROPLATELET. Representative electron micrographs of the detergent-insoluble proplatelet cytoskeleton. Proplatelets were permeabilized with 0.75% Triton X-100, 5 μM phallacidin, and 0.1% glutaraldehyde. Examination through electron microscopy reveals that the plasma membrane of the proplatelet tube is supported by a fibrous membrane skeleton that is similar in structure to the membrane skeleton of mature platelets. (A) This low-magnification field shows that an intact membrane skeleton laminates the underside and extends along the entire length of proplatelets (bar = 1 μm). (B) High-magnification, three-dimensional electron micrograph of the proplatelet membrane skeleton reveals a lattice-like network of elongated filamentous strands, similar in nature to the spectrin-based network in red blood cells and platelets. The membrane skeleton continuously laminates the underside of the proplatelet. A cytoplasmic bridge is shown *(left)* linking to a swelling *(right)* (bar = 200 nm).

produces platelets that vary extensively in shape, content, and diameter. These findings also suggest that the Rho-ROCK-myosin light chain pathway regulates myosin IIA.

Because proplatelets elongate, but do not branch in the presence of the actin-disrupting drug cytochalasin B, it is unexpected that the deletion of certain actin-associated proteins from the megakaryocyte lineage leads to macrothrombocytopenia. It seems likely that removal of actin-modulating proteins alters and/or increases filamentous actin and that the cytoskeletal structure appears to have a dominant inhibitory effect on proplatelet production and release. The absence of the cytoplasmic actin crosslinking protein Filamin A in conditional knockout mice whose megakaryocyte lineage lacks Filamin A results in macrothrombocytopenia in which platelet counts are reduced by 80%–90%.[33] Conditional knockout mice lacking the actin turnover protein cofilin-1 in the megakaryocyte lineage also contain giant platelets with a platelet count reduced by 60%–80% of normal. In

contrast, mice lacking the actin turnover protein ADF have normal platelet counts and morphology.[34] On the other hand, when ADF[−/−] mice are crossed with cofilin-1 knockout mice, platelet production is severely reduced and morphologies of platelets are highly variable. Mice that contain megakaryocytes that specifically lack profilin 1, a small protein that promotes actin filament assembly, have macrothrombocytopenia with reduced platelet counts.[35] Profilin-null platelets have a thickened microtubule coil with hyperacetylated microtubules, and in some ways, the profilin 1 knockout phenotype is similar to the behavior of platelets in Wiskott-Aldrich syndrome, or in WASp knockout mice. Defective proplatelet production has also been observed in mice in which the small regulatory GTPases Rho, Cdc42, and Rac have been deleted in the megakaryocyte lineage.[36,37]

In addition to playing an essential role in proplatelet elongation, the microtubules lining the shafts of proplatelets serve a secondary function: transport of membrane, organelles, and granules into proplatelets and assembling platelets at proplatelet ends (see Fig. 124.4C). Organelles are sent individually from the cell body into the proplatelets, where they move bidirectionally until they are captured at proplatelet tips.[14] Immunofluorescence and electron microscopic studies indicate that organelles are intimately associated with microtubules, and actin poisons do not diminish organelle motion. Thus movement appears to involve microtubule-based forces. Bidirectional organelle movement is conveyed in part by the bipolar arrangement of microtubules within the proplatelet because kinesin-coated latex beads move in both directions over the microtubule arrays of permeabilized proplatelets. Of the two major microtubule motors, kinesin and cytoplasmic dynein, only the plus end-directed kinesin is localized in a pattern similar to organelles and granules, and is likely responsible for transporting these elements along microtubules. It appears that two mechanisms of organelle and granule movement are involved in platelet assembly: first, organelles and granules travel along microtubules, and second, the microtubules themselves slide bidirectionally in relation to other motile filaments, indirectly moving organelles along proplatelets in a piggyback manner.

Although the roles of microtubules and actin filaments in proplatelet development have been extensively studied, our understanding of the function of the membrane skeleton has only recently been established. High-resolution electron microscopy reveals that proplatelets have a dense spectrin-based membrane skeleton similar in structure to that of mature blood platelets. Nonerythroid spectrin subunits, alpha-II and beta-II spectrin, are predominately expressed in mouse megakaryocytes, proplatelets, and platelets, but erythroid alpha-I and beta-I spectrin isoforms are also expressed (see Fig. 124.6).[15] Assembly of spectrin tetramers is required for development of the DMS and proplatelet elaboration because expression of a spectrin tetramer–disrupting construct in megakaryocytes inhibits both processes. Furthermore, integration of this spectrin-disrupting construct into a permeabilized proplatelet system quickly destabilizes proplatelets, resulting in massive blebbing and swelling. Spectrin tetramers also stabilize the barbell-like shapes found in the penultimate stage in platelet production (see later). Taken together, these studies suggest a role for spectrin in different steps of megakaryocyte development through its participation in the formation of demarcation membranes and in the maintenance of proplatelet structure.

Platelet Maturation at the Proplatelet Tip

Platelet maturation at proplatelet tips ends when a single microtubule detaches from the microtubule bundle and is rolled into a coil. To complete construction of mature platelets, once the fundamental cytoskeletal components have been delivered to and assembled in the platelet buds, the buds must fill with their organelle and granule content.

Granules are sent to nascent platelets on the microtubule tracks of the proplatelets. The concentration of this cargo in the platelet occurs by an end-trapping mechanism as granules and organelles, which enter the nascent platelet, continue to move in the tip but do not return to the proplatelet shaft.

Release of Mature Platelets

Details of how mature platelets release from the proplatelet tips are beginning to come into focus. In vitro, maturation of proplatelets ends in a rapid retraction that separates a variable portion of the proplatelets from the residual cell body, leaving behind a naked, denuded nucleus (see Fig. 124.5C). Activation of apoptotic pathways in the cell body has been shown to be coincident with this event. Junt and colleagues have used intravital fluorescence microscopy to visualize proplatelet production in the opened cranial marrow cavity of living mice.[16] Yellow fluorescent protein (YFP)–labeled megakaryocytes were seen to protrude proplatelets and release megakaryocyte fragments into the marrow sinusoids of living mice. Notably, these anucleate fragments typically exceed platelet dimensions, suggesting that platelet morphogenesis continues in the circulation. In line with these observations, we have recently identified a previously unrecognized intermediate stage in platelet formation and release, which we termed the *preplatelet*.[17] Preplatelets are defined as discoid cells (3–10 μm) that retain the capacity to convert into barbell-shaped proplatelets and undergo fission into platelets. The conversion of preplatelets to barbell proplatelets is powered by microtubule-based forces. It is likely that the microtubule motors that drive proplatelet extension are involved in aspects of platelet release, as well as in the process of microtubule coiling. Sliding of an uncoiled portion of the microtubule relative to the rigid microtubule bundle in the proplatelet tip would provide a simple mechanism to effect platelet release and would explain the variable morphology of the small but reproducible percentage (<5%) of dumbbell-shaped platelets that are present in blood. Recently, it was demonstrated that individual human platelets have the innate capacity to duplicate and form new cell bodies that undergo fission into platelets.[18] The morphologic similarities between platelets that form new cell bodies and preplatelets are striking. Whether or not newly released platelets exhibit a preplatelet phenotype, which allows them to form barbell-shapes and divide again, is not clear.

Location of Platelet Release

Megakaryocytes are produced in the bone marrow, and some undergo fragmentation into platelets in this location. It has been suggested that, by extending into the bone marrow sinusoids, proplatelets provide a mechanism for extension into the bone, allowing release of platelets directly into the circulation.[19,20] Megakaryocytes have been identified in intravascular sites within the lung, leading to a theory that some platelets are formed from their parent cell in the pulmonary circulation.

Transcriptional Regulation of Platelet Formation

Megakaryocyte development and platelet formation are controlled by the coordinated action of transcription factors that specifically turn on the genes of megakaryocyte precursors or suppress the expression of genes that support other cell types.[22] Gene-targeting studies in mice have identified several genes that are crucial for megakaryocyte development and platelet formation. Leading the list of transcription factors that play an essential role in megakaryocyte maturation and platelet biogenesis is the basic leucine zipper heterodimer NF-E2. NF-E2 is a protein composed of a ubiquitously expressed 18–20-kDa small-Maf subunit and a p45 subunit that is restricted to erythroid and megakaryocytic lineages. Although NF-E2 was postulated to be a transcription factor that specifically drove the expression of genes essential for erythropoiesis, mice lacking p45 NF-E2 do not exhibit defects in erythropoiesis. Instead, mice deficient in the p45 subunit or two of the small-Maf subunits die of hemorrhage shortly after birth because of a complete lack of circulating platelets. Although megakaryocytes undergo normal endomitosis and proliferate in response to TPO, mice deficient in p45 NF-E2 produce increased numbers of megakaryocytes that are larger than normal, contain fewer granules,

exhibit a highly disorganized DMS, and fail to generate proplatelets in vitro, a phenotype indicative of a late block in megakaryocyte maturation. Therefore NF-E2 appears to control the transcription of a limited number of genes involved in cytoplasmic maturation and platelet formation. Shivdasani and colleagues generated a subtracted cDNA library enriched in transcripts downregulated in NF-E2 knockout megakaryocytes. Using this approach, these investigators have started to identify the downstream targets of NF-E2 and to analyze their role in the terminal stages of megakaryocyte differentiation. Putative transcriptional targets of NF-E2 include β_1 tubulin, thromboxane synthase, and proteins that regulate inside-out signaling via $\alpha_{IIb}\beta_3$ integrin. The zinc finger protein GATA1 is also a transcription factor that plays a critical role in driving the expression of genes essential for megakaryocyte maturation. However, unlike NF-E2, which appears to drive the later stage of megakaryocyte development, *GATA1* functions at multiple stages of development. Initially, GATA proteins were thought to regulate red blood cell maturation because genetic disruption of the *GATA1* gene in mice results in embryonic lethality secondary to a block in erythropoiesis. However, several more recent observations also implicate *GATA1* as a regulator of megakaryocyte differentiation. First, forced expression of *GATA1* in the early myeloid cell line 416b induces megakaryocyte differentiation. Second, Shivdasani and colleagues used targeted mutagenesis of regulatory elements within the *GATA1* locus to generate mice with a selective loss of *GATA1* in the megakaryocyte lineage. These knockdown mice expressed sufficient levels of *GATA1* in erythroid cells to circumvent the embryonic lethality caused by anemia. *GATA1* deficiency in megakaryocytes leads to severe thrombocytopenia. Platelet counts are reduced to approximately 15% of normal, and the small numbers of circulating platelets are round and larger than normal. These mice have increased numbers of small megakaryocytes that exhibit an accelerated rate of proliferation. The small cytoplasmic volume of *GATA1*-deficient megakaryocytes typically contains an excess of rough endoplasmic reticulum, very few platelet-specific granules, and an underdeveloped or disorganized DMS, suggesting that maturation of megakaryocytes is arrested in GATA1-deficient megakaryocytes.

A family with X-linked dyserythropoietic anemia and thrombocytopenia due to a mutation in *GATA1* has been described. A single-nucleotide substitution in the N-terminal zinc finger of *GATA1* inhibits the interaction of *GATA1* with its essential cofactor, friend of *GATA1* (FOG). Although megakaryocytes in affected family members are abundant, they are unusually small and exhibit several abnormal features, including an abundance of smooth endoplasmic reticulum, an underdeveloped DMS, and a lack of granules. These observations suggest an essential role for the *FOG1-GATA1* interaction in thrombopoiesis. Genetic elimination of FOG in mice unexpectedly resulted in specific ablation of the megakaryocyte lineage, suggesting a *GATA1*-independent role for FOG in the early stages of megakaryocyte development; therefore *GATA1* and FOG are required for megakaryocyte generation from a common bipotential progenitor.

Several knockout mice also indicate a role for additional transcription factors in megakaryocyte development. Mice carrying a null mutation in *Fli-1*, a member of the ETS family of winged helix-turn-helix transcription factors that bind purine-rich sequences in gene promoters, exhibit defects in megakaryocyte development. Megakaryocytes cultured from mice lacking *Fli-1* contain reduced numbers of α-granules, disorganization of the demarcation membranes, and a reduction in size. Mice lacking the hematopoietic zinc finger (Hzf) protein, a transcription factor that is predominantly expressed in megakaryocytes, have reduced numbers of α-granules in megakaryocytes and platelets. Therefore Hzf may regulate the transcription of genes involved in the synthesis of α-granule components and/or their packaging into α-granules. SCL, a basic helix-loop-helix transcription factor initially identified in a subset of human T-cell leukemia with multilineage characteristics, also appears to be critical for megakaryopoiesis. Results of deletion of SCL in mice indicate that this transcription factor is required for proper erythroid and megakaryocyte development.

PLATELETS

Structure of the Resting Platelet

Megakaryocyte development culminates in the release of mature discoid platelets having dimensions of approximately 3.0 × 0.5 μm and a cytoplasmic volume of 7 fL.[23] The evolutionary explanation for the discoid shape of the platelet is unknown. Discoid shape may permit more efficient flow or dispersion of clot-promoting elements or may simply reflect the microtubule-based mechanism by which platelets are produced. In humans, platelets, once released from the ends of proplatelets, normally circulate for 7–10 days. Given that nearly 1 trillion platelets circulate in an adult human, each day an adult produces approximately 100 billion platelets.

The precise morphology of newly released platelets is unknown. However, when released into the circulation or maintained in culture, platelets have a very reproducible structure. Although they are heterogeneous in size, presumably because of changes in size as they age, platelets have discoid shapes with flat, featureless surfaces (Fig. 124.8A and Fig. 124.9A) that are interrupted only by pit-like openings into the open canalicular system (OCS). The OCS is an extensive system of internal membrane conduits that serves as a passageway to the outside world into which granular contents are released. It also is a reservoir of plasma membrane, membrane receptors, and proteins. For example, approximately 30% of the thrombin receptors are localized in the OCS of the resting platelet, awaiting movement to the surface when the cells are activated. Although contiguous with the plasma membrane, not all proteins on the cell surface can enter the OCS. Factors controlling movement into the OCS remain to be defined but likely depend on the actin cytoskeleton. Entry restriction, however, occurs at the necks of OCS infoldings. The third function of the OCS is to serve as a source of redundant plasma membrane for cell spreading. OCS membrane initially is disgorged to the surface following cell activation. When cells are activated in solution, much of this membrane is subsequently reabsorbed into the remnants of the OCS.

A small thin zone of cytoplasm separates the plasma membrane of the resting platelet from a marginal microtubule coil and the general intracellular space, which contains all inclusion bodies and the internal cytoskeleton of the cell. This zone is filled with the spectrin-based membrane skeleton (see Fig. 124.9A). Beneath this zone sits a microtubule coil. Then follows the cytoplasmic space, which is filled with filaments of actin that embed granules, organelles, the OCS, and other specialized membrane systems such as smooth endoplasmic reticulum.

Platelets actively recruit other blood-borne cells to areas of vascular damage by releasing mediators packaged in intracellular granules (described earlier in Cytoplasmic Maturation) that initiate secondary homeostatic interactions and that express a "sticky" apical surface after the platelets adhere. In the resting platelet, granules

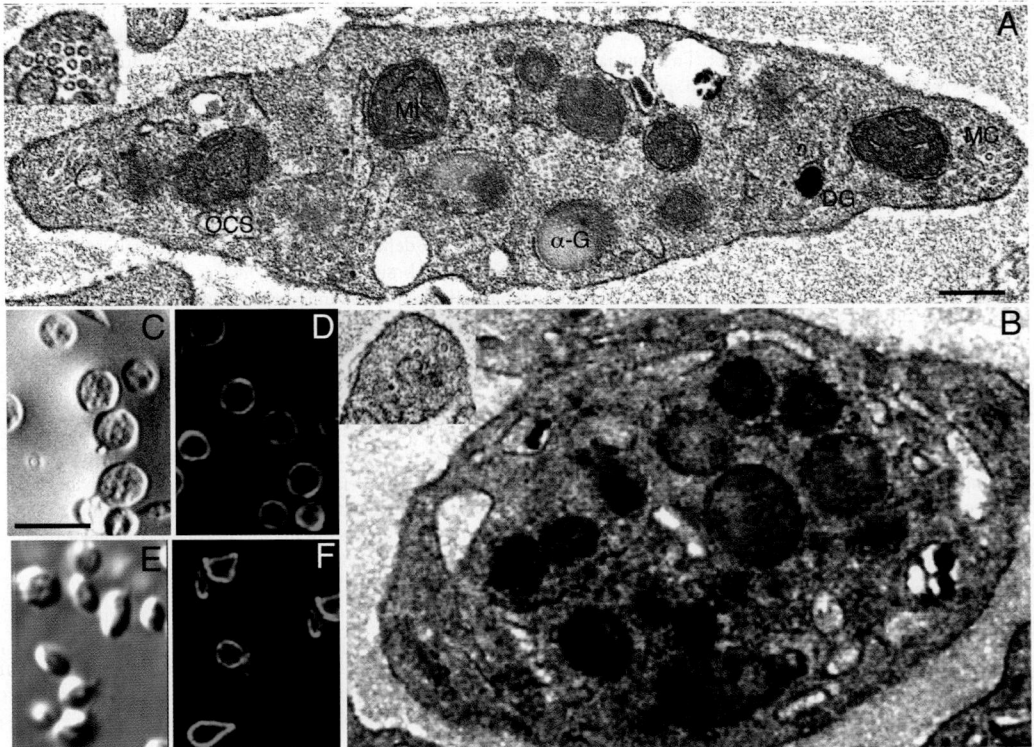

Fig. 124.8 COMPARISON OF THE STRUCTURE OF NORMAL MOUSE PLATELETS (A, C, D) WITH THOSE LACKING β_1 TUBULIN (B, E, F). (A) Electron micrograph of a resting mouse platelet sectioned through its thin axis. The cut plane reveals the microtubule coil (MC) at the cell periphery. The *inset* shows a high-magnification cross-section through the MC of the resting platelet. The microtubule is wound 11 times in this platelet, forming the coil. The cytoplasmic space embeds mitochondria (MT), α-granules (α-G), and dense granules (DG). Spaces created by the open canalicular system (OCS) are apparent. (B) Electron micrograph of a thin section through a platelet isolated from a mouse lacking β_1 tubulin (bar = 0.2 μm). Platelets from these animals are spherical (E) and have only a rudimentary microtubule coil *(inset)*. In this platelet the microtubule is twisted twice. (C) Differential interference contrast image of resting platelets shows them to be flat discs. (D) MC of the resting mouse platelet. Staining of fixed mouse platelets with Alexa 488 antitubulin immunoglobulin G (IgG) reveals the MC. This coil resides at the periphery of the platelet. (E) Differential interference contrast image of platelets lacking β_1 tubulin. (F) Staining of fixed mouse β_1-tubulin–deficient platelets with Alexa 488 antitubulin IgG reveals the coil is defective and bent in a number of places throughout the platelets. (C–F are the same magnification; bar = 5 μm.)

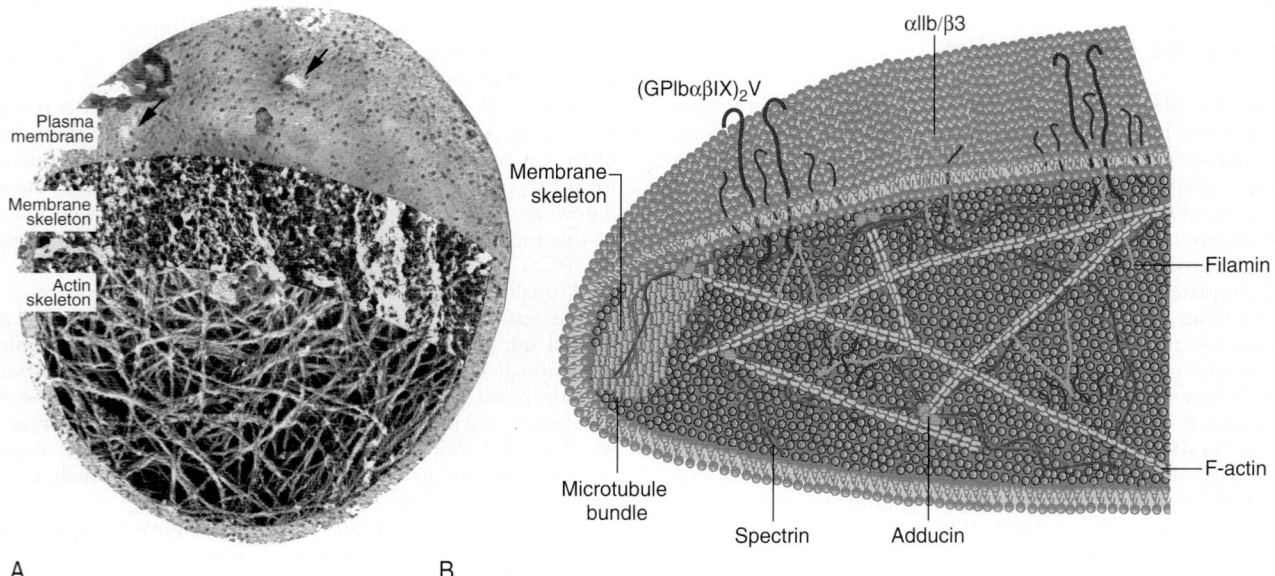

Fig. 124.9 STRUCTURE OF THE RESTING HUMAN BLOOD PLATELET AND ITS ACTIN-BASED CYTOSKELETON. (A) Composite illustrating the major actin cytoskeletal layers of the resting platelet. *Plasma membrane*: The plasma membrane of the resting cell is flat and featureless, except for periodic invaginations that lead into the open canalicular system (OCS) *(arrows)*. *Membrane skeleton*: The plasma membrane of the platelet is supported by a submembranous spectrin-based skeleton. This network is composed primarily of spectrin molecules, which are tetramers with actin binding sites at the ends. Actin filament ends dock on spectrin to complete the network. The association between spectrin and F actin is promoted by adducin. *Actin cytoskeleton*: As discussed earlier, the spectrin network is both directly and indirectly attached to the underlying actin filaments. Filament ends interconnect spectrin molecules, whereas the filamin links run from the filament sides to the plasma membrane receptor (GPIbαβIX)$_2$V. The cytoplasmic space has a dense filling of actin filaments. Actin filaments from the cell center radiate outward. As the filaments approach the plasma membrane, they turn and run in parallel with it. The actin filaments have been decorated using myosin subfragment 1 (S1), which gives them a twisted cable-like appearance in frozen samples. Myosin S1 labeling reveals the polarity of the actin filament. "Pointed" and "barbed" ends are definable. The ends of actin filaments are bound by the ends of spectrin molecules on the edges of the membrane network *(arrowhead)*. A microtubule coil composed of a single long microtubule resides just beneath the plasma membrane at the periphery of the thin axis of the platelet (not shown) (bar = 0.5 μm). (B) Schematic showing the structural features of the resting blood platelet cytoskeleton. Resting cells have discoid shapes. Structural elements that support this shape are (1) a marginal microtubule coil, (2) a spectrin-based membrane skeleton, and (3) a rigid network of cross-linked cytoplasmic actin filaments (only a small number of the actin filaments have been added to this illustration so that they will not obscure the rest of the structures in the cell). Platelets have a specialized membrane skeleton composed of spectrin, actin, and many associated proteins. Spectrin tetramers (200 nm long and 5 nm wide) have actin filament-binding sites at each molecular end. The membrane skeleton is held in compression between the plasma membrane and the cytoplasmic actin by filamin connections from the sides of actin filaments to the cytoplasmic tails of GPIbα subunit of the membrane glycoprotein complex that binds to von Willebrand factor (GPIbαβIX)$_2$V complex. Greater than 98% of the barbed ends of actin filaments are capped by adducin and capZ in the resting platelet.

are juxtaposed together and are in intimate association with the membranes of the OCS. The release reaction of platelet granules differs from that of other cells. Granules rarely fuse with the plasma membrane; instead they exocytose into the OCS. Platelets also contain lysosomes and a few mitochondria, which are easily identified under the electron microscope by their internal system of membrane cristae.

Cytoskeleton of the Resting Platelet

Although both microtubule- and actin-based forces have been considered in the elaboration and branching of proplatelets, respectively, it is the integration of the microtubule and actin cytoskeletal elements that uniquely defines the shape of the mature platelet. One of the most distinguishing features of the resting platelet is its marginal microtubule coil (see Fig. 124.8). αβ-Tubulin dimers assemble into microtubule polymers under physiologic conditions. In resting platelets, tubulin is equally divided between dimer and polymer fractions. In many cell types, αβ-tubulin subunits are in a dynamic equilibrium with microtubules such that reversible cycles of assembly-disassembly of microtubules are observed. Microtubules are long, hollow polymers (24 nm in diameter) that are responsible for many types of cellular movements, such as segregation of chromosomes during mitosis and transport of organelles across the cell. The microtubule ring of the resting platelet, initially characterized in the late 1960s by White and Krivit, was described as a single microtubule approximately 100 μm long and is coiled 8–12 times inside the periphery of the platelet. However, recent work suggests that the marginal band is highly dynamic and consists of multiple microtubules with mixed polarity that undergo constant assembly and disassembly.[24] This may accommodate the shrinkage of microtubule coil diameters that occurs with aging of platelets. Antagonistic microtubule motors appear to keep the marginal microtubule coil in its resting state.[38] The primary function of the microtubule coil is to maintain the discoid shape of the resting platelet. Disassembly of platelet microtubules with drugs such as vincristine, colchicine, or nocodazole causes platelets to become round and to lose their discoid shape. Cooling the platelets also causes disassembly of the microtubule coil and loss of the discoid shape. Mice lacking β_1 tubulin, the major hematopoietic β-tubulin isoform, produce platelets that lack their characteristic discoid shapes and have defective marginal bands. Genetic elimination of β_1 tubulin in mice results in thrombocytopenia with circulating platelet counts below 50% of normal. β_1-Tubulin–deficient platelets are spherical in shape, apparently due to shortened marginal bands with fewer coilings. Whereas normal platelets possess a marginal band that consists of 8–12 coils, β_1-tubulin knockout platelets contain only 2–3 coils. A human β_1-tubulin functional substitution (AG→CC) inducing both structural and functional platelet alterations has been described. Of note, the Q43P β_1-tubulin variant was found in 10.6% of the general population and in 24.2% of 33 unrelated patients with undefined congenital macrothrombocytopenia. Electron microscopy revealed enlarged spherocytic platelets with a disrupted marginal band and structural alterations. Platelets with the Q43P β_1-tubulin variant showed mild platelet dysfunction with reduced ATP secretion, attenuated thrombin receptor-activating peptide (TRAP)–induced aggregation, and impaired adhesion to collagen under flow conditions.[25] A more-than-doubled prevalence of the β_1-tubulin variant was observed in healthy subjects not undergoing ischemic events, raising the possibility that the variant confers an evolutionary advantage and a protective cardiovascular role.

Actin is the most abundant of all the platelet proteins, with 2 million molecules expressed per platelet. Of these molecules, 800,000 assemble to form the 2000–5000 linear actin polymers that exist in the resting cell (see Fig. 124.9A). The remainder of the actin is maintained in storage as a 1:1 complex with β_4 thymosin, which can be converted to filaments during platelet activation to drive cell spreading. All evidence indicates that the filaments of the resting platelet are interconnected at various points into a rigid cytoplasmic network because platelets express high concentrations of actin cross-linking proteins, including filamin and α-actinin.[7] Both filamin and α-actinin are homodimers in solution. Three filamin genes are located on chromosomes 3, 7, and X. Filamin A (X) and filamin B (3) are expressed in platelets. Filamin A is expressed at levels more than 10-fold higher than that of filamin B. Filamin subunits are elongated strands composed primarily of 24 repeats, each approximately 100 amino acids in length and folded into immunoglobulin G-like β-barrels. Each strand has an N-terminus actin-binding site that shares homology with other actin-binding proteins, two rod domains that are end-to-end assemblies of the repeat units, interrupted by two hinge domains between repeats 15 and 16, and 23 and 24, and a C-terminus self-association site (Fig. 124.10B). Subunits assemble to form V-shaped bipolar molecules—that is, the self-association site is the vertex of the V, and the actin-binding sites are on the free ends. Inclusion of the first hinge in filamin depends on alternative RNA splicing. Filamin now is recognized to be a prototype "scaffolding

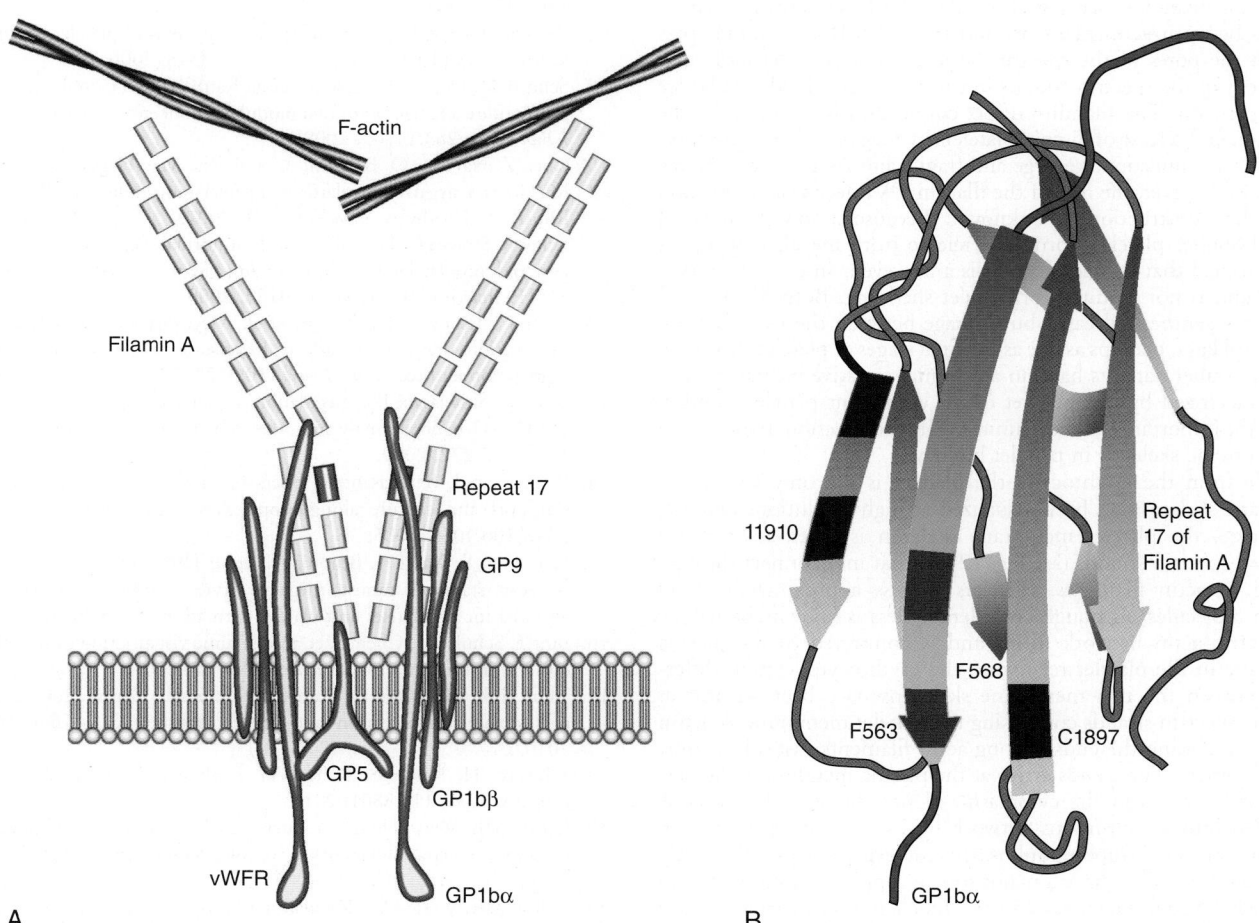

Fig. 124.10 INTERACTION OF FILAMIN A WITH THE VON WILLEBRAND FACTOR RECEPTOR. (A) Model showing the orientation of filamin A when interacting with the GPIbα chain of the vWFR and cytoplasmic actin filaments. For tight binding of filamin A to vWFR, both GPIbα chains of the receptor must be engaged by a single filamin A molecule. (B) Ribbon diagram showing the interface between filamin A repeat 17 and the filamin A binding region of the GPIbα tail (residues 556–577). Critical residues that provide the lock-and-key interaction between the two domains are indicated. *GPIbα*, glycoprotein Ibα; *vWFR*, von Willebrand factor receptor.

molecule" that collects binding partners and localizes them adjacent to the plasma membrane. Partners bound by filamin members include the small GTPases, RalA, Rac, Rho, and Cdc42, with RalA binding in a GTP-dependent manner; the exchange factors Trio and Toll; kinases such as PAK1; phosphatases; and transmembrane proteins. Most partner proteins are bound within the C-terminus portion of filamin.

Central to the structural organization of the resting platelet is an interaction between filamin and the cytoplasmic tail of the GPIbα subunit of the GPIb-IX-V complex.[27] The second rod domain (repeat 17) of filamin has a binding site for the cytoplasmic tail of GPIbα. The interaction between filamin A and GPIbα occurs at the atomic level. Repeat 17 of filamin A has a groove between certain β-sheet strands that forms a pocket for the GPIbα tail (see Fig. 124.10). Binding between filamin A and GPIbα is driven by entropic forces, and the alignment and specificity are provided by large residues that create a lock-and-key fit between the two molecules. Whereas the interaction between one filamin A subunit and GPIbα has an affinity of approximately 10 μM, high-affinity binding (10 nM) occurs when each filamin A subunit in a molecule and both GPIbα chains in a vWF receptor are engaged. Studies have shown that the bulk of platelet filamin (>90%) is in complex with GPIbα. This interaction has three consequences. First, it positions filamin's self-association domain and associated partner proteins at the plasma membrane while dangling filamin's actin binding sites into the cytoplasm. Second, because a large fraction of filamin is bound to actin, it aligns the GPIb-IX-V complexes on the surface of the platelet over the underlying filaments (see Fig. 124.9B). Third, because the filamin linkages between actin filaments and the GPIb-IX-V complex pass through the pores of the spectrin lattice, it restrains the molecular movement of the spectrin strands in this lattice and holds the lattice in compression. The filamin-GPIbα connection is essential for the formation and release of discoid platelets by megakaryocytes; platelets lacking this connection are large and fragile and are produced in low numbers. However, the role of the filamin-vWF receptor connection in platelet construction is unknown. Because a low number of Bernard-Soulier platelets form and release from megakaryocytes, it can be argued that this connection is a late event in the maturation process and is not required for platelet shedding. Both filamin and GPIbα are synthesized early, but linkage between the two may not occur until later, perhaps as late as the final stages of platelet shedding. Bernard-Soulier patients have an autosomal recessive bleeding disorder characterized by low platelet count with giant platelets, underscoring the importance of the filamin-GPIbα connection in stabilizing the membrane skeleton in platelet biology.

Aside from the erythrocyte, the platelet is the only cell whose membrane skeleton has been visualized at high resolution. Like the erythrocyte, the platelet membrane skeleton is a self-assembly of elongated spectrin strands (see Fig. 124.9) that interconnect through binding to actin filaments. Platelets express approximately 2000 spectrin molecules. Although considerably less is known about how the spectrin-actin network forms and is connected to the plasma membrane in the platelet relative to the erythrocyte, certain differences between the two membrane skeletons have been identified. First, the spectrin strands composing the platelet membrane skeleton interconnect using the ends of long actin filaments instead of short actin oligomers. These ends arrive at the plasma membrane originating from filaments in the cytoplasm. Hence the spectrin lattice is assembled into a continuous network by its association with actin filaments. Second, tropomodulins are not expressed at sufficiently high levels, if at all, to have a major role in capping the pointed ends of the platelet actin filaments. Instead, biochemical experiments have revealed that a substantial number (≈2000) of these ends are free in the resting platelet. Third, although little tropomodulin protein is expressed, α adducin and γ adducin are abundantly expressed and appear to cap many of the barbed ends of the filaments composing the resting actin cytoskeleton. Adducin is a key component of the membrane skeleton, forming a triad complex with spectrin and actin. Capping of barbed filament ends by adducin also serves the function of targeting them to the spectrin-based membrane skeleton because

the affinity of spectrin for adducin-actin complexes is greater than for either actin or adducin alone. Platelet glycoproteins involved in attaching spectrin to the membrane remain to be defined.

REFERENCES

1. Bluteau D, Lordier L, Di Stefano A, et al: Regulation of megakaryocyte maturation and platelet formation. *J Thromb Haemost* 7:227, 2009.
2. Schulze H, Korpal M, Hurov J, et al: Characterization of the megakaryocyte demarcation membrane system and its role in thrombopoiesis. *Blood* 107:3868, 2006.
3. Lu SJ, Li F, Yin H, et al: Platelets generated from human embryonic stem cells are functional in vitro and in the microcirculation of living mice. *Cell Res* 2011.
4. Takayama N, Nishimura S, Nakamura S, et al: Transient activation of c-MYC expression is critical for efficient platelet generation from human induced pluripotent stem cells. *J Exp Med* 207:2817, 2010.
5. Italiano JE, Jr, Lecine P, Shivdasani RA, et al: Blood platelets are assembled principally at the ends of proplatelet processes produced by differentiated megakaryocytes. *J Cell Biol* 147:1299, 1999.
6. Schwer H, Lecine P, Tiwari S, et al: A lineage-restricted and divergent b tubulin isoform is essential for the biogenesis, structure and function of mammalian blood platelets. *Curr Biol* 11:579, 2001.
7. Patel S, Richardson J, Schulze H, et al: Differential roles of microtubule assembly and sliding in proplatelet formation by megakaryocytes. *Blood* 106:4076, 2005.
8. Patel S, Hartwig J, Italiano J, Jr: The biogenesis of platelets from megakaryocyte proplatelets. *J Clin Invest* 115:3348, 2006.
9. Schulze H, Dose M, Korpal M, et al: RanBP10 is a cytoplasmic guanine nucleotide exchange factor that modulates noncentrosomal microtubules. *J Biol Chem* 283:14109, 2008.
10. Chen Z, Naveiras O, Balduini A, et al: The May-Hegglin anomaly gene MYH9 is a negative regulator of platelet biogenesis modulated by the Rho-ROCK pathway. *Blood* 110:171, 2007.
11. Eckly A, Strassel C, Freund M, et al: Abnormal megakaryocyte morphology and proplatelet formation in mice with megakaryocyte-restricted MYH9 inactivation. *Blood* 113:3182, 2009.
12. Leon C, Eckly A, Hechler B, et al: Megakaryocyte-restricted MYH9 inactivation dramatically affects hemostasis while preserving platelet aggregation and secretion. *Blood* 110:3183, 2007.
13. Chen Z, Shivdasani RA: Regulation of platelet biogenesis: insights from the May-Hegglin anomaly and other MYH9-related disorders. *J Thromb Haemost* 7:272, 2009.
14. Richardson J, Shivdasani R, Boers C, et al: Mechanisms of organelle transport and capture along proplatelets during platelet production. *Blood* 106:4066, 2005.
15. Patel-Hett S, Wang H, Begonja AJ, et al: The spectrin-based membrane skeleton stabilizes mouse megakaryocyte membrane systems and is essential for proplatelet and platelet formation. *Blood* 2011.
16. Junt T, Schulze H, Chen Z, et al: Dynamic visualization of thrombopoiesis within bone marrow. *Science* 317:1767, 2007.
17. Thon JN, Montalvo A, Patel-Hett S, et al: Cytoskeletal mechanics of proplatelet maturation and platelet release. *J Cell Biol* 191:861, 2010.
18. Schwertz H, Koster S, Kahr WH, et al: Anucleate platelets generate progeny. *Blood* 115:3801, 2010.
19. Larson MK, Watson SP: A product of their environment: do megakaryocytes rely on extracellular cues for proplatelet formation? *Platelets* 17:435, 2006.
20. Larson MK, Watson SP: Regulation of proplatelet formation and platelet release by integrin alpha IIb beta3. *Blood* 108:1509, 2006.
21. Goldenson B, Kirsammer G, Stankiewicz MJ, et al: Aurora kinase A is required for hematopoiesis, but is dispensable for murine megakaryocyte endomitosis and differentiation. *Blood* 125:2141, 2015.
22. Dore LC, Crispino JD: Transcription factor networks in erythroid cell and megakaryocyte development. *Blood* 2011.
23. Hartwig JH: The platelet: form and function. *Semin Hematol* 43:S94, 2006.

24. Patel-Hett S, Richardson JL, Schulze H, et al: Visualization of microtubule growth in living platelets reveals a dynamic marginal band with multiple microtubules. *Blood* 111:4605, 2008.

25. Freson K, De Vos R, Wittevrognel C, et al: The β1-tubulin Q43P functional polymorphism reduces the risk of cardiovascular disease in men by modulating platelet function and structure. *Blood* 106:2356, 2005.

26. Nakamura F, Stossel TP, Hartwig JH: The filamins: organizers of cell structure and function. *Cell Adh Migr* 5:160, 2011.

27. Nakamura F, Pudas R, Heikkinen O, et al: The structure of the GP1b-filamin A complex. *Blood* 107:1925, 2005.

28. Eckly A, Heijnen H, Pertuy F, et al: Biogenesis of the demarcation membrane system (DMS) in megakaryocytes. *Blood* 123:921, 2014.

29. Wandall HH, Rumjantseva V, Sørensen AL, et al: The origin and function of platelet glycosyltransferases. *Blood* 120:626, 2012.

30. Chen Y, Aardema J, Kale S, et al: Loss of the F-BAR protein CIP4 reduces platelet production by impairing membrane-cytoskeleton remodeling. *Blood* 22:1695, 2013.

31. Bender M, Giannini S, Grozovsky R, et al: Dynamin 2-dependent endocytosis is required for normal megakaryocyte development in mice. *Blood* 125:1014, 2015.

32. Bender M, Thon JN, Ehrlicher AJ, et al: Microtubule sliding drives proplatelet elongation and is dependent on cytoplasmic dynein. *Blood* 125:860, 2015.

33. Begonja A, Hoffmeister KM, Hartwig JH, et al: FlnA-null megakaryocytes prematurely release large and fragile platelets that circulate poorly. *Blood* 118:2285, 2011.

34. Bender M, Eckly A, Hartwig JH: ADF/n-cofilin-dependent actin turnover determines platelet formation and sizing. *Blood* 116:1767, 2010.

35. Bender M, Stritt S, Nurden P, et al: Megakaryocyte-specific Profilin1-deficiency alters microtubule stability and causes a Wiskott-Aldrich syndrome-like platelet defect. *Nat Commun* 5:4746, 2014.

36. Pleines I, Dütting S, Cherpokova D, et al: Defective tubulin organization and proplatelet formation in murine megakaryocytes lacking Rac1 and Cdc42. *Blood* 122:3178, 2013.

37. Pleines I, Hagedorn I, Gupta S: Megakaryocyte-specific RhoA deficiency causes macrothrombocytopenia and defective platelet activation in hemostasis and thrombosis. *Blood* 119:1054, 2012.

38. Diagouraga B, Grichine A, Fertin A, et al: Motor-driven marginal band coiling promotes cell shape change during platelet activation. *J Cell Biol* 204:177, 2014.

CHAPTER 125

MOLECULAR BASIS OF PLATELET FUNCTION

Margaret L. Rand and Sara J. Israels

The primary physiological role of platelets is to support hemostasis at sites of vascular injury by forming a plug that arrests blood loss (Fig. 125.1). Normally, disc-shaped platelets circulate in the bloodstream without adhering to the endothelium of the vessel wall. When the endothelium is damaged, platelets adhere to the exposed subendothelial collagen and, at high shear, to collagen-immobilized von Willebrand factor (VWF). Platelet adhesion at the site of vessel wall damage initiates activation events via intracellular signaling pathways that trigger (1) reorganization of the actin cytoskeleton that results in a shape change from discs to irregular spheres with filopodia, and enables platelet spreading to increase surface contact; (2) secretion of dense granule and α granule contents, including ADP from the dense granules; (3) formation and release of second messengers including thromboxane A_2 (TxA_2); and (4) exposure of phosphatidylserine (PS) on the platelet surface, thereby creating a procoagulant activated platelet surface for assembly of coagulation factor complexes that accelerate the generation of thrombin. Platelet agonists, including ADP, TxA_2, and thrombin, bind to their specific membrane receptors, initiating signaling pathways that convert integrin αIIbβ3 from a low-affinity resting state to a high-affinity activated state capable of binding its ligands. Divalent fibrinogen and multivalent VWF function as bridges between αIIbβ3 on adjacent activated platelets, resulting in aggregation and plug formation. This series of platelet responses is essential for the hemostatic function of platelets, and when impaired by congenital or acquired defects, bleeding can occur. However, if these same events take place on a ruptured atherosclerotic plaque, they can lead to the formation of a platelet-rich thrombus that can occlude the arterial lumen and lead to ischemia.

This chapter addresses the molecular basis of platelet activation and primary hemostatic plug formation. Significant progress has been made in defining the molecular mechanisms that govern platelet responses, facilitated by the study of patients with congenital defects of platelet function and/or number, and by the study of genetically modified animals. Recently, the field of platelet biology has expanded to encompass the platelet's role in inflammation, host defense and tumor progression.[1–3] What we have learned about the molecular mechanisms of platelets in the setting of hemostasis and thrombosis is now being applied in new areas to address new questions.

MOLECULAR BASIS OF PLATELET ADHESION

Substrates for Platelet Attachment and Spreading

Platelet plug formation is initiated by contact of circulating platelets with proteins in the subendothelial extracellular matrix (ECM). Normal endothelium maintains an effective barrier that prevents circulating platelets from contact with these ECM proteins. In addition to the physical barrier, endothelial cells actively inhibit platelet activation by release of nitric oxide, prostacyclin, and enzymes (CD39/CD73) involved in the metabolism of ADP.[4] At sites of vascular injury, where endothelium is lost or damaged and the ECM becomes exposed to flowing blood, platelets come into close contact with ECM adhesive proteins that promote initial attachment and subsequent activation.

The subendothelial matrix can be viewed as a dynamic and mutable interface that provides multiple substrates to support platelet adhesion (Table 125.1). These substrates include collagens,[5] immobilized VWF,[6] fibronectin,[7] laminin,[8] and thrombospondin-1.[9] Plasma proteins fibrinogen,[10] vitronectin,[11] and circulating VWF also interact with platelets after binding to matrix components. The roles of collagen and VWF are well defined, while the contributions of other adhesive proteins to the initial attachment of platelets are less well established. Studies of mice deficient in individual matrix proteins have been useful in determining the contribution of these proteins to the integrated function of the ECM in the formation, growth, and stabilization of the platelet plug.

Shear rates in flowing blood, which vary depending on vessel caliber, influence the contribution of specific matrix proteins. At low shear, platelets can be captured by collagens, but at higher shear rates (>1000 s^{-1}), VWF becomes critical in ensuring efficient platelet attachment via the receptor glycoprotein (GP)Ibα (Fig. 125.2A) (see section on Platelet Adhesion Receptors). VWF, secreted from endothelial cells and recruited from plasma, binds to type VI collagen in the vascular matrix via the VWF A1 domain, and to types I and III collagen in both superficial and deeper layers of the matrix via the VWF A3 domain.[12]

Collagen types I, III, and VI exposed at sites of vascular injury are key substrates for direct platelet adhesion. Collagen is a fibrillar protein made up of tropocollagen monomers packed into units of five to generate microfibrils.[13] Collagens have motifs that are not only recognized by VWF, but also by the platelet collagen receptors α2β1 and GPVI[5,14] (see section on Platelet Adhesion Receptors). At low shear, collagen can function independently of VWF to capture platelets at the matrix surface. However, under high shear, collagen and VWF, with their respective receptors, function in concert.[12,15]

Platelet adhesion is supported by other substrates in the matrix, and by plasma proteins that interact with the matrix. It is likely that these proteins fine-tune the primary hemostatic response depending on the site or severity of the injury. Plasma proteins including fibronectin,[7,16] vitronectin,[11] and fibrinogen (and its polymerized product fibrin), matrix protein laminin[8] and platelet α granule protein thrombospondin-1[9] all support platelet adhesion in experimental systems. It is likely that most of these proteins play an ancillary role in vivo via mechanisms that include enhancing VWF immobilization in the matrix (laminin), protecting large VWF multimers from degradation (thrombospondin-1), or bridging between platelet receptors and matrix collagen (fibronectin).

Platelet Adhesion Receptors

Nomenclature

The individual adhesive proteins serve as ligands for specific receptors on the platelet surface (Table 125.1). Several nomenclature systems have been used to identify the membrane glycoproteins of the platelet, such that the same receptor may have multiple designations. The original and still widely used system designates the membrane glycoproteins according to their electrophoretic mobility upon sodium dodecyl sulfate polyacrylamide gel electrophoresis; protein separation is on the basis of molecular weight, with higher molecular-weight proteins migrating more slowly. Glycoproteins were designated as GPI, II, III, and so on, with GPI having the highest molecular weight. With greater resolution techniques, additional glycoproteins were

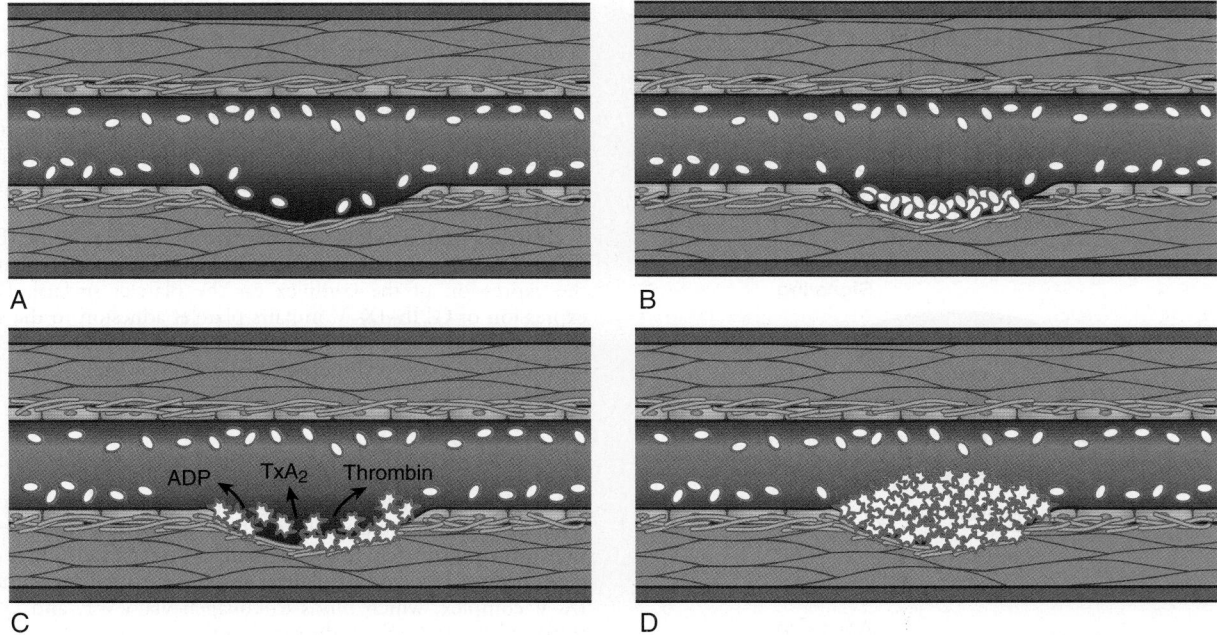

Fig. 125.1 HEMOSTATIC RESPONSE OF PLATELETS TO VESSEL WALL INJURY. (A) Disruption of the endothelial cell lining of the blood vessel exposes constituents of the subendothelial extracellular matrix. (B) Platelets adhere to and spread on matrix constituents. (C) Activated platelets secrete ADP, synthesize and release TxA_2, and promote the generation of thrombin. (D) ADP, TxA_2, and thrombin activate additional platelets that aggregate to form a platelet plug. *TxA₂*, Thromboxane A₂.

TABLE 125.1	Subendothelial Matrix Adhesive Proteins and Their Platelet Receptors
Adhesive Protein	**Receptor(s)**
Collagen	GPIa–IIa ($\alpha 2\beta 1$)[a] GPVI
von Willebrand factor	GPIb–IX–V GPIIb–IIIa ($\alpha IIb\beta 3$)
Fibronectin	GPIc–IIa ($\alpha 5\beta 1$) GPIIb–IIIa ($\alpha IIb\beta 3$)
Thrombospondin-1	$\alpha v\beta 3$
Vitronectin	$\alpha v\beta 3$ GPIIb–IIIa ($\alpha IIb\beta 3$)
Laminin	$\alpha 6\beta 1$

[a]Alternative name for receptor is given in brackets.

identified, hence the subdivision designations, e.g., GPIa, GPIb, GPIc; GPIIa, GPIIb. Many of the membrane glycoproteins on the platelet surface exist as noncovalent complexes, e.g., GPIa–IIa, GPIb–IX–V, GPIIb–IIIa.

In addition to the GP nomenclature system, the $\alpha\beta$ integrin nomenclature system is used. Several of the platelet membrane glycoproteins are members of the integrin family of adhesion receptors (see later), e.g., GPIa–IIa is $\alpha 2\beta 1$, GPIIb–IIIa is $\alpha IIb\beta 3$. Some glycoproteins also have cluster of differentiation (CD) designations, e.g., CD41 for GPIIb and CD61 for GPIIIa. Finally, some receptors have been named based on their function (e.g., the fibrinogen, fibronectin, and vitronectin receptors). Although functional designations can be appropriate from a descriptive standpoint, at least two different membrane glycoproteins on platelets serve as receptors for vitronectin and fibronectin (see Table 125.1), and several are receptors for collagen (see later). Beyond creating nomenclature complexity, redundancy of platelet receptors endows the platelet with the capacity to form multiple contacts with a single matrix constituent. Thus, a single ligand may initiate several distinct functional responses by engaging different receptors.

The Integrin Family of Adhesion Receptors

Integrins are members of a superfamily of broadly distributed adhesion receptors that mediate cell-matrix and cell-cell interactions. They are composed of noncovalently associated α and β transmembrane polypeptide subunits with large extracellular domains and short cytoplasmic tails. Of the 18 known α subunits, platelets express five, and of the eight known β subunits, platelets express two, with a total of five different platelet integrins. It is estimated that half of the surface area of an activated platelet is occupied by integrin receptors. Many of the glycoprotein receptors on platelets that mediate cell-matrix adhesion are members of the integrin family (Table 125.1). $\alpha 2\beta 1$ is a receptor for subendothelial collagen (see later); $\alpha 5\beta 1$ for fibronectin; $\alpha 6\beta 1$ for laminin; $\alpha IIb\beta 3$ for fibrinogen, VWF, and fibronectin; and $\alpha v\beta 3$ for vitronectin. Of the integrins expressed on blood cells, $\alpha IIb\beta 3$ is the most narrowly distributed and is restricted predominantly to platelets and megakaryocytes. It not only plays a prominent role in cell-cell adhesion, i.e., platelet aggregation (see section on Molecular Basis of Platelet Aggregation), but in many other platelet responses, including the association of platelets with tumor cells, an interaction involved in tumor metastasis.

Role of GPIb–IX–V in Platelet Adhesion

GPIb–IX–V is a notable example of a major cell surface molecule involved in platelet adhesion that is not a member of the integrin family. GPIb is composed of an α (heavy) chain and two β (light) chains; the α and β chains both span the platelet membrane and are linked by disulfide bonds.[17] GPIX and GPV are smaller single-chain transmembrane polypeptides that are noncovalently associated with GPIb, and all three subunits (members of the leucine-rich repeat protein superfamily) are necessary for the expression of the complex on the platelet surface. The GPIbα-GPIbβ–IX–V complex has a

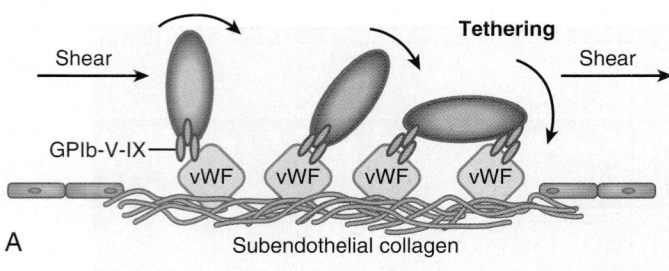

Tethering

Shear →   ← Shear

GPIb-V-IX

vWF vWF vWF vWF

A   Subendothelial collagen

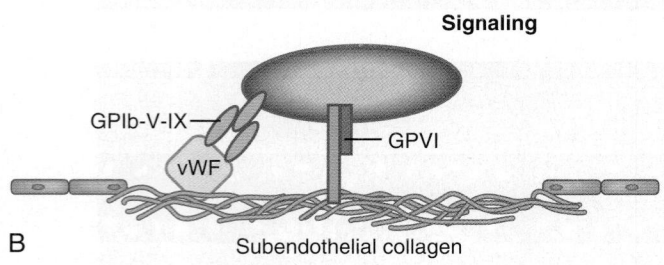

Signaling

GPIb-V-IX

vWF   GPVI

B   Subendothelial collagen

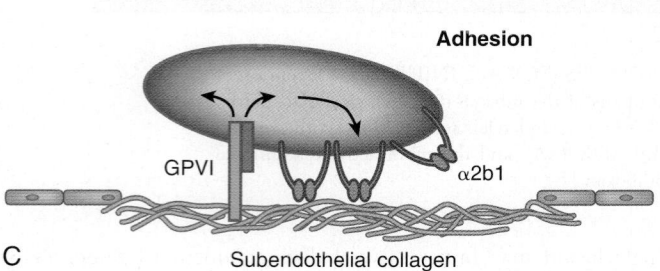

Adhesion

GPVI   α2b1

C   Subendothelial collagen

Fig. 125.2 ADHESION TO THE SUBENDOTHELIUM IS A MULTI-STEP PROCESS. (A) Collagen-bound VWF in the subendothelium undergoes a conformational change when exposed to arterial shear rates such that GPIbα of the GPIb–IX–V complex binds to the VWF A1 domain. These rapidly formed bonds are quickly broken and reestablished, causing platelet translocation, or rolling, along the subendothelium. (B) The translocation process slows platelet transit, allowing the signaling receptor GPVI to bind directly to collagen. (C) GPVI-mediated signal transduction pathways activate the integrin α2β1, enabling it to bind strongly to collagen. This final association between the platelet and collagen is stable and allows the platelet to adhere firmly to the subendothelium. *GP*, Glycoprotein; *VWF*, von Willebrand factor.

stoichiometry of 2:4:2:1 and exists in high copy number on the platelet surface (approximately 25,000 molecules per platelet) with the N-terminus of GPIbα being the major ligand-binding subunit of the complex. Platelet activation and aging are associated with shedding of glycocalicin, a large proteolytic N-terminal fragment of GPIbα that is cleaved by ADAM17 or other sheddases. The cytoplasmic tail of GPIbα binds to a number of proteins, including the signaling molecule 14-3-3ζ and the cytoskeletal protein filamin A (an actin-binding protein)[18] (see section on the Platelet Cytoskeleton).

GPIb–IX–V plays a major role in hemostasis and thrombosis as a receptor for immobilized VWF in the subendothelium. Plasma VWF does not interact with platelet GPIb–IX–V, but at the high shear rates that occur in the arterial microcirculation, a conformational change in VWF bound to subendothelial collagen exposes a GPIbα binding site in the A1 domain. Thus, GPIb–IX–V binds to subendothelial VWF; this interaction is reversible with fast on and off rates, which allows for translocation (rolling) of platelets on the surface (Fig. 125.2A).[12,15] A polymorphism in the GPIbα gene leads to variable numbers of tandem repeats in the macroglycopeptide region of the protein between the ligand-binding region and the plasma membrane. The length of this region, which is determined by the number of

tandem 13 amino acid repeats (one to four), may have a role in regulating platelet adhesion to VWF.

In addition to serving as a receptor for VWF in the subendothelium, GPIb–IX–V is also a receptor for the soluble agonist thrombin (see section on Soluble Agonist Receptors). Other adhesive ligands for GPIb–IX–V include the counter-receptors P-selectin (CD62P), expressed on activated platelets and endothelial cells, and leukocyte integrin Mac-1 (αMβ2), which is involved in the formation of platelet-leukocyte conjugates.[18]

Platelets from patients with Bernard-Soulier syndrome (BSS) lack GPIb–IX–V as a result of mutations in GPIb or GPIX that prevent the expression of the complex on the platelet surface. Decreased expression of GPIb–IX–V impairs platelet adhesion to the subendothelium and can result in a significant bleeding diathesis (see section on Molecular Basis of Inherited Platelet Disorders).

Collagen Receptors

Subendothelial collagen has long been recognized as an important initiator of platelet responses, serving as a substrate for platelet adhesion, which ultimately results in platelet aggregation. Three different receptors are involved in platelet responses to collagen: the GPIb–IX–V complex, which binds to collagen via VWF, and GPVI and α2β1 (GPIa–IIa), which directly bind to collagen.

GPVI, with approximately 4000–6000 copies per platelet, is a transmembrane protein member of the immunoglobulin superfamily and has two extracellular immunoglobulin domains. As an immunoreceptor tyrosine-based activation motif (ITAM)-coupled receptor, its cytoplasmic domain contains a proline-rich sequence that binds to tyrosine kinases involved in platelet signaling[12,19] (see section on Activation Pathways). GPVI is noncovalently associated with the Fc receptor γ chain (FcRγ) dimer, which is required for GPVI surface expression. There is in vitro and in vivo evidence of shedding of GPVI from the surface of activated platelets by the action of ADAM17 and during platelet aging in the circulation. Deficiencies of GPVI can be associated with a mild bleeding diathesis (see section on Genetic Basis of Inherited Platelet Function Disorders).

α2β1, with approximately 2000 copies per platelet, is the major collagen-binding integrin on the platelet surface.[12,20] It undergoes a conformational change to a high-affinity state to allow it to bind to collagen. Silent polymorphisms in the α2 gene control its expression level, with higher plasma membrane levels associated with enhanced adhesion to collagen in vitro and an increased risk of cardiovascular disease.

The adhesion of platelets to collagen is a complex, multistep process. An initial interaction of GPIb–IX–V with VWF in the subendothelium (see earlier) facilitates a direct, low-affinity interaction of GPVI with collagen (Fig. 125.2B). Binding of GPVI to collagen is a potent stimulus to intracellular signaling pathways (see section on Activation Pathways). As a result of this signaling cascade, α2β1 is activated to bind to collagen with high affinity (Fig. 125.2C), thereby forming a stable interaction. Alternatively, or in addition, low levels of constitutively activated α2β1 can initiate direct binding of platelets to collagen, thereby assisting GPVI to bind and to initiate activation signaling. At high shear, GPVI plays the major role in mediating stable adhesion, while at lower shear, α2β1 is more important.[19,21]

CLEC2 Adhesion Receptor

CLEC2 is a transmembrane C-type lectin that was originally described as the receptor responsible for platelet activation by the snake venom rhodocytin, inducing signaling events similar to those initiated by GPVI (see section on Activation Pathways). CLEC2 contributes to thrombosis in mouse models,[22] even though it does not have a ligand in the ECM. CLEC2 has now been recognized as the receptor responsible for platelet activation upon binding to the membrane glycoprotein podoplanin on lymphatic endothelial cells; this binding

Platelet G Protein-Coupled Receptors, Their Associated G Proteins (A), and Their Effectors (B)

(A)

Agonist	GPCR	G Protein
Thrombin	PAR1	G_q, G_i, $G_{12/13}$
	PAR4	G_q, $G_{12/13}$
ADP	P2Y1	G_q, $G_{12/13}$
	P2Y12	G_i
TxA_2	TP	G_q, $G_{12/13}$
PGI_2	IP	G_s

(B)

G Protein Subunit(s)	Effector	Function
$G\alpha_q$	PLC-β	$\uparrow IP_3$/DAG
$G\beta\gamma_i$	PLC-β	$\uparrow IP_3$/DAG
	PI3K-γ	$\uparrow$3-PPIs
$G\alpha_{12/13}$	p115-RhoGEF	Actin cytoskeleton reorganization
$G\alpha_s$	Adenylate cyclase	$\uparrow$cAMP
$G\alpha_i$	Adenylate cyclase	$\downarrow$cAMP

ADP, Adenosine 5′-diphosphate; cAMP, cyclic adenosine monophosphate; DAG, diacylglycerol; GPCR; G protein-coupled receptor; IP, prostaglandin I_2 (prostacyclin) receptor; IP_3, inositol-1,4,5-trisphosphate; PAR, protease-activated receptor; PGI_2, prostaglandin I_2 (prostacyclin); PI, phosphoinositide; PLC, phospholipase C; 3-PPIs, 3-phosphorylated phosphoinositides; TP, thromboxane/prostanoid; TxA_2, thromboxane A_2.
Adapted from Brass LF, Newman DK, Wannermacher KM, et al: Signal transduction during platelet plug formation. In: Michelson AD, editor. Platelets, 3rd edition. San Diego: Academic Press; p. 367-398, 2013, with permission.

and subsequent intracellular signaling regulates blood and lymphatic vascular separation during fetal development.[23]

MOLECULAR BASIS OF PLATELET ACTIVATION

Soluble Agonist Receptors

The majority of agonist receptors on platelets are members of the superfamily of trimeric G protein–coupled receptors (GPCRs) that contain seven transmembrane spanning α-helices, four extracellular loops and domains, and four intracellular loops and domains. Upon binding of their ligands, intracellular signaling is initiated via G proteins (GTP-binding proteins) associated with the GPCRs at the inner plasma membrane, leading to diverse downstream responses (see section on Activation Pathways). The platelet GPCRs include receptors for thrombin, ADP, the arachidonate metabolite TxA_2, and epinephrine (Table 125.2).[24] Deficiencies or dysfunction of these GPCRs can result in bleeding diatheses ranging from mild to severe (see section on Molecular Basis of Inherited Platelet Disorders).

Thrombin Receptors

Thrombin receptors on platelets belong to the protease-activated receptor (PAR) family, GPCRs with a unique activation mechanism that involves cleavage of the N-terminal extracellular domain, thereby creating a new N-terminus that acts as a tethered ligand for the receptor. PAR1 and PAR4 are present on human platelets (PAR3 and PAR4 on mouse platelets); PAR1 is the high-affinity thrombin receptor (~2500 copies per platelet), responding to thrombin at nanomolar concentrations, and PAR4 is a lower affinity receptor.[25] After thrombin cleavage of the N-terminus of PAR1, the tethered ligand (peptide sequence: Ser-Phe-Leu-Leu-Arg-Asn; SFLLRN) undergoes a conformational change and forms an intramolecular complex with a region also on the N-terminal extracellular domain of the receptor, referred to as ligand binding site-1. This triggers the G protein cycle of PAR1's associated G proteins. PAR4 is nonhomologous with PAR1 in both the peptide sequence of the tethered ligand (Gly-Tyr-Pro-Gly-Lys-Phe; GYPGKF) and its binding characteristics. Although PAR4 requires a higher concentration of thrombin for cleavage, once cleaved, it produces a more sustained signal than PAR1. GPIb–IX–V also possesses a high-affinity binding site for thrombin on GPIbα that facilitates PAR1 cleavage by thrombin.

ADP and ATP Receptors

ADP is an important primary platelet agonist and also amplifies other primary responses following its secretion from platelet dense granules. Platelets have two ADP receptors: P2Y1 and P2Y12, which are GPCRs that are coupled to different G proteins. ADP binding to P2Y1 (~150 copies per platelet), which is coupled to the α subunits of G_q and $G_{12/13}$, mediates a transient rise in intracellular calcium, and induces platelet shape change and rapidly reversible aggregation. ADP binding to P2Y12 (~600 copies per platelet), which is coupled to the α subunit of G_i, results in inhibition of adenylyl cyclase, decreased levels of cyclic AMP (cAMP) and enhancement of the aggregation and secretion responses produced by other agonists. Full aggregation responses to ADP in vitro require concurrent activation of both receptor pathways.[26]

ATP is an antagonist of P2Y1 and P2Y12, but an activator of P2X1, a ligand-gated ion channel, that causes rapid influx of Ca^{2+} from the external milieu through the ion channel and amplifies responses to other agonists. The effects of ADP and ATP are modulated in vivo by CD39, a nucleoside triphosphate diphosphohydrolase (NTPDase-1) expressed by endothelial and vascular smooth muscle cells that hydrolyzes both ATP and ADP, thereby maintaining homeostasis and preventing inappropriate platelet activation.[4]

Thromboxane A_2 Receptor

In humans, the TxA_2 thromboxane/prostanoid (TP) receptor exists in two isoforms, the result of alternative splicing (TPα and TPβ). TPα is the dominant form expressed on platelets, with approximately 1000 copies per platelet.[27]

Epinephrine Receptor

Epinephrine is a relatively weak agonist but plays a role in potentiating platelet activation by other agonists, manifested through its ability to inhibit cAMP formation. In humans, the epinephrine receptor is the α_{2A}-adrenergic receptor (~300 copies per platelet).

Activation Pathways

Once a subendothelial or soluble agonist binds to its receptor on the platelet surface, intracellular signaling pathways (detailed in Fig. 125.1) are set into motion. These signaling pathways result in reorganization of the cytoskeleton and platelet shape change, storage granule exocytosis, TxA_2 synthesis, PS surface exposure, and $\alpha IIb\beta 3$ activation.

The signaling pathways, initiated by collagen binding to GPVI, and by thrombin, ADP, TxA_2, and epinephrine binding to their specific GPCRs, comprise a "molecular toolkit"[28] of signaling molecules, which will be considered briefly. The monomeric G proteins, also known as small (low molecular weight) GTPases, which regulate integrin activation and cytoskeletal reorganization, are described later in the sections Molecular Mechanisms of Aggregation and Cytoskeletal Reorganization, respectively. Much has been learned about the signaling pathways from genetically modified mice. The reader is referred to comprehensive reviews of platelet signaling for more detail.[28–35]

Heterotrimeric G Proteins Are Early Response Elements for Most Soluble Platelet Agonists[24,28]

The GPCRs for soluble platelet agonists are constitutively associated at the inner plasma membrane with specific heterotrimeric G proteins (consisting of α, β, and γ subunits) of the families G_q, $G_{12/13}$, and G_i (Table 125.2A). The receptor for the potent platelet inhibitory molecule, prostaglandin I_2 (PGI_2; prostacyclin) is also a GPCR and is coupled to G_s.

In the basal, resting state, GDP is bound to the α subunit of the G protein. Upon ligand binding, a GPCR acts as a guanine nucleotide exchange factor, promoting exchange of GDP for GTP on different classes of the α subunit. Sites on the α and $\beta\gamma$ subunits are thereby exposed, allowing for activation of effector molecules including the β isoform of phospholipase C (PLC-β), the γ isoform of phosphatidylinositol 3-kinase (PI3K), and a Rho-specific guanine nucleotide exchange factor, p115-RhoGEF (Table 125.2B). Adenylate cyclase is activated via G_s and inhibited by G_i. Intrinsic GTPase activity of the α subunit hydrolyzes the bound GTP to GDP, thus restoring the G protein to its resting conformation.

Protein Tyrosine Kinases Modulate Enzyme Activity and Allow for the Formation of Signaling Complexes[28–30]

GPVI is the most potent signaling collagen receptor. Clustering of GPVI upon binding to collagen results in phosphorylation of its constitutively-associated FcRγ by tyrosine kinases of the Src family (Fyn and Lyn) that are associated with the cytoplasmic domain of GPVI. Phosphorylation of tandem ITAM motifs enables binding of Syk via Src homology 2 (SH2) domains. Activation of the tyrosine kinase Syk leads to the phosphorylation of the adaptor protein LAT, which serves as the platform for the assembly of a signalosome—a complex of multiple signaling enzymes and adaptor molecules (e.g., SLP 76, Btk, Gads, Gab1) within membrane lipid rafts. The signalosome serves as a membrane scaffold for phosphorylation/activation of effectors including phospholipase C-γ (PLC-γ) and the α, β, and δ isoforms of PI3K.

The platelet receptor platelet-endothelial cell adhesion molecule (PECAM)1 negatively regulates GPVI signaling by recruiting the tyrosine phosphatase SHP2, and reducing LAT signalosome assembly.

The signaling pathway initiated by binding of GPIb–IX–V to VWF is similar to that of GPVI in that both involve activation of PLC-γ via FcRγ, Fyn and Lyn, and Syk. Binding of platelets to podoplanin via CLEC2 also induces signaling events similar to those initiated through GPVI. However, rather than (tandem) ITAM phosphorylation, it involves hemi-ITAM phosphorylation.[29]

Phospholipase C Is Responsible for the Hydrolysis of Membrane PI-4,5P$_2$[28]

Activation of PLC, either the β-isoform (by thrombin, ADP, or TxA_2 via G_q) or the γ-isoform (by collagen, protein tyrosine kinases, and scaffold molecules) results in the hydrolysis of the minor inner plasma membrane leaflet phospholipid phosphatidylinositol-4,5-bisphosphate (PI-4,5P$_2$). The two second messengers that are formed, soluble inositol-1,4,5-trisphosphate (IP_3) and membrane-associated diacylglycerol (DAG), lead, respectively, to increased cytosolic Ca^{2+} concentrations and activation of protein kinase C (PKC), a serine/threonine kinase.

Phosphatidylinositol 3-Kinase Forms 3-Phosphorylated Phosphoinositides[28,32]

Activation of PI3K isoforms, either the γ (via G_i) or the α, β, and δ (via the collagen signaling pathway), results in phosphorylation of

PI-4P and PI-4,5P$_2$ to yield PI-3,4P$_2$ and PI-3,4,5P$_3$, respectively. Inner membrane leaflet PIP_3 functions in signaling by interacting with Akt via binding motifs termed pleckstrin homology domains (PH), thereby activating Akt to function as a serine/threonine kinase.

Serine/Threonine Kinases Regulate the Activity of Other Proteins and Enable the Development of Signaling Complexes[31,33]

PKC is a central protein kinase in the PLC signaling pathway that, upon activation by DAG and Ca^{2+}, phosphorylates the serine and threonine residues of many platelet proteins, including pleckstrin. The serine/threonine kinase Akt is an effector of PI3K, activating Rap1B. PKC is important in platelet secretion and both PKC and Akt are involved in αIIbβ3 activation, resulting in aggregation.

Cytosolic Ca^{2+}[28,34]

An increase in the intracellular Ca^{2+} concentration ($[Ca^{2+}]_i$) is a key event that triggers platelet activation and aggregation; Ca^{2+}-dependent responses include shape change, secretion, procoagulant surface exposure, TxA_2 formation, and αIIbβ3 activation. The basal $[Ca^{2+}]_i$ is maintained at approximately 0.1 μM and can increase to greater than 1 μM with strong stimulation. The initial increase results from IP_3-mediated release of Ca^{2+} from the dense tubular system (DTS). Upon depletion of this Ca^{2+} pool, store-operated Ca^{2+} (SOC) influx occurs from the platelet exterior. Stromal interaction molecule 1 (STIM1), a protein in the DTS membrane, undergoes a conformational change when DTS Ca^{2+} is depleted, allowing it to bind and activate Orai1, the major SOC Ca^{2+}-selective release-activated Ca^{2+} (CRAC) channel in the platelet plasma membrane.

Phospholipase A$_2$ Is Responsible for the Synthesis of TxA$_2$[28]

An increase in $[Ca^{2+}]_i$ is one of the main triggers for activation of cytosolic phospholipase A_2 (cPLA2), resulting in the formation of the proaggregatory prostanoid TxA_2. cPLA2 hydrolyzes the polyunsaturated fatty acid arachidonate from the C2 position of inner plasma membrane leaflet phospholipids, and arachidonate is converted to the cyclic endoperoxide intermediates prostaglandin (PG)G_2 and PGH_2 by cyclooxygenase (COX)-1. Thromboxane synthase in the platelet cytosol metabolizes PGH_2 to TxA_2, which diffuses out of the platelet and is available to activate additional platelets via the TP receptor.

cAMP[28]

Activation of adenylate cyclase via G_s increases the intracellular level of cAMP, which activates protein kinase A (PKA). This serine/threonine kinase is responsible for phosphorylating proteins including GPIbβ, filamin, myosin light chain (MLC), and Rap1B. Elevated levels of cAMP result in sequestration of intracellular Ca^{2+} in the DTS, and inhibition of cytoskeletal rearrangement, granule secretion, and aggregation. Inhibition of adenylate cyclase via G_i is important in facilitating activation of platelets by lowering cAMP concentrations that are raised above basal levels by PGI_2 produced by the endothelium.

Reorganization of the Actin Cytoskeleton

Platelet plug formation requires platelets to undergo a rapid change from their resting discoid shape to active forms spread over the damaged subendothelium that then recruit additional platelets by providing an enlarged surface area for platelet-platelet or platelet-leukocyte interactions. The discoid shape of the circulating platelet is maintained by an internal cytoskeleton composed of polymers of actin and tubulin and their associated proteins (see also Chapter 124). Shape change requires the remodeling of the resting cytoskeleton and the assembly of new cytoskeletal fibers to transform the platelet into its activated configuration.

The Resting Platelet Cytoskeleton

The resting platelet cytoskeleton maintains cell shape and integrity as the platelet encounters the high shear forces of blood flow in small vessels. The spectrin-based membrane skeleton (similar but not identical to that of erythrocytes) forms a contiguous network with actin filaments to support platelet ultrastructure. Actin is the single most abundant platelet protein (2 million copies per platelet), forming 2000–5000 linear actin polymer filaments that are cross-linked to form a rigid cytoplasmic network. Cross-linking proteins include filamin A and B, and α-actinin. The interaction between filamin A/B and the cytoplasmic tail of the VWF receptor GPIbα provides structural stability and the major link between the plasma membrane and the actin cytoskeleton. Loss of this linkage in platelets deficient in either GPIbα (BSS) or filamin A results in loss of restraint of the spectrin lattice, swelling of the membrane skeleton, and large fragile platelets that are subject to rapid clearance from the circulation.[15]

Platelets contain a long microtubule wound 8–12 times into a coil that sits just beneath the plasma membrane, maintaining the discoid shape of the resting platelet. Microtubules are rigid polymers made up of $\alpha\beta$-tubulin heterodimeric subunits. β1-tubulin deficient mice have platelets that are spherical and fail to develop a discoid shape due to aberrant microtubule assembly.[36] A heterozygous human variant in β1-tubulin, which may be present in as many as 10% of the general population, results in decreased levels of β1-tubulin and a subset of spherocytic platelets.[37]

Cytoskeletal Reorganization During Platelet Activation

The assembly and disassembly of the actin cytoskeleton allows platelets to spread. Following platelet activation, the platelet makes contact with the ECM, initially changing shape from disc to sphere and developing filopodia, followed by flattening and spreading of broad lamellae. Granules and organelles are relocated to the center of the cell. The filopodia are filled with long actin filaments originating in the center of the cell. Increases in $[Ca^{2+}]_i$ initiated by signaling through G_q result in activation of gelsolin, a multidomain protein with binding sites for Ca^{2+}, actin, and phospholipid. Ca^{2+} binding alters the conformation of gelsolin such that it binds and cleaves actin filaments, leading to disassembly of the resting actin cytoskeleton and allowing the platelet to change shape. Signaling via $G_{12/13}$ and p115-RhoGEF activates the small, monomeric G protein RhoA that is also involved in regulating actin filament formation and myosin contraction. For example, actin filaments are stabilized by the activation of Rho-activated kinase (p160ROCK) and LIM-kinase.

Assembly of the activated platelet cytoskeleton doubles the actin filament content of the platelet by exposing nucleation ends on existing actin filaments (the result of severing of filaments by gelsolin) or creating new nucleation sites (by the Arp 2/3 complex). The Arp2/3 complex is enriched in the periphery of the activated platelet where actin assembly is occurring, and the complex is activated by proteins associated with cell adhesion sites and by the Wiskott-Aldrich syndrome protein (WASp) family members.[38]

Platelets are also the force-generating component of clot retraction. αIIbβ3 is tethered to underlying actin filaments in association with cytoplasmic proteins talin, filamin, paxillin, zyxin, α-actinin, and vinculin. Association of cytoplasmic myosin with actin provides the motor for the contractile force. Platelets contain nonmuscle myosin IIA and IIB; myosin II is a hexamer made up of two heavy chains and four light chains. Assembly into bipolar filaments is the result of Ca^{2+}-activated phosphorylation of the 20-kDa MLCs by MLC kinase, enhanced by blocking MLC dephosphorylation through Rho kinase. *MYH9*-related disease is the result of mutations in the gene for nonmuscle myosin heavy chain IIA (NMMHC-IIA)[39] (see section on Molecular Basis of Inherited Platelet Disorders).

Secretion of Granules

Platelet activation leads to the release of a diverse list of molecules that stimulate or inhibit platelets or other blood and vascular cells, covalently modify the thrombus to affect its mechanical properties, regulate coagulation, contribute to cell adhesive events, and modulate wound healing, inflammation, and angiogenesis.

Most of the substances that are actively and selectively secreted from platelets are packaged in storage granules formed in megakaryocytes. Platelets contain three types of granules: dense (δ) granules, α granules, and lysosomal granules (Fig. 125.3A).

Dense Granules

Dense granules belong to the family of lysosome-related organelles (LROs) that also includes melanosomes, cytotoxic T-cell granules, and neutrophil azurophilic granules. Platelets contain three to eight dense granules, storing high concentrations of cations (Ca^{2+}, Mg^{2+}, K^+), polyphosphate, nucleotides (ADP, ATP, GTP), and bioactive amines (serotonin and histamine). These granules are innately dense when viewed by electron microscopy due to their Ca^{2+} content. Biogenesis of LRO complexes (BLOCs) are protein complexes that are critical in vesicle trafficking and dense granule formation.[40] Mutations in specific protein members of BLOCs 1, 2, and 3, or in the adaptor protein complex 3 (AP3) result in dense granule deficiency and associated LRO abnormalities in mice and in Hermansky-Pudlak syndrome (HPS) 1–9 in humans, characterized by mucocutaneous bleeding and oculocutaneous albinism[41] (see section on Molecular Basis of Inherited Platelet Function Disorders).

α Granules

α Granules are unique to platelets and are the most abundant granule type: 50–80 granules per platelet, taking up 10% of the platelet volume. They contain a large number of proteins that are either synthesized by megakaryocytes or taken up from plasma by endocytosis. Genetic defects in *NBEAL2* and *VPS33B*, genes involved in α granule synthesis, result in α granule deficiency syndromes[42–46] (see section on Molecular Basis of Inherited Platelet Disorders). Proteomic studies have demonstrated that there are more than 300 unique proteins released by α granules.[47] These proteins have diverse functions and can be classified as coagulants and anticoagulants (e.g., factors V and XI, antithrombin, protein S, plasminogen activator inhibitor-1); adhesion proteins (e.g., fibrinogen, VWF, thrombospondin-1); chemokines (e.g., CXC-chemokine ligand 4 [CXCL4; platelet factor 4], CXCL7 [β-thromboglobulin]); growth factors (e.g., epidermal growth factor, transforming growth factor-β); angiogenic factors (e.g., vascular endothelial growth factor, platelet-derived growth factor, angiostatin); and immune mediators (e.g., precursors of complement factors C3 and C4)[48] (Fig. 125.3A). There appears to be heterogeneity in the cargo protein content of subsets of α granules, with pro- and antiangiogenic proteins stored in distinct subsets and differentially released.[49] Membrane-bound proteins in α granules include integrins, immunoglobulin family receptors, leucine-rich repeat family receptors and tetraspanins. Most of these are also present on the resting platelet plasma membrane, but some, such as P-selectin (CD62P), are only expressed on the plasma membrane following granule exocytosis.[46]

Lysosomal Granules

Platelets have small numbers of primary and secondary lysosomes that contain enzymes involved in degradation of proteins, carbohydrates, and lipids. These enzymes include cathepsins, elastase, collagenases, galactosidase, glucuronidase, and acid phosphatase.

Mechanism of Granule Secretion

The secretion of platelet granule contents occurs through mechanisms analogous to those required for the exocytosis of granules from neurons and mast cells. Platelet secretion is triggered by a variety of strong agonists such as thrombin. Induction of secretion by weak agonists (e.g., ADP) occurs when the cells are brought into close contact, such as during aggregation,[50] and is dependent on TxA_2 to amplify the effect of the primary agonist.

In most cells, exocytosis occurs when vesicles fuse with the plasma membrane and release their contents into the extracellular milieu. In platelets, granules clustered centrally by platelet shape change also fuse with one another and with the open canalicular system (OCS), a system of invaginations of the plasma membrane extending into the interior of the platelet; the granule contents diffuse to the external environment. Membrane fusion is driven by the soluble *N*-ethylmaleimide–sensitive factor (NSF) attachment protein receptors (SNAREs). Platelets have the three basic components of SNARE machinery: tSNAREs (target receptors associated with open canalicular system and plasma membrane), vSNAREs (vesicle-associated receptors associated with the granule membranes), and soluble regulators (including NSF and NSF-attachment proteins).[48,51] vSNAREs including vesicle-associated membrane proteins (VAMPs) interact with syntaxin isoforms and synaptosomal-associated protein (SNAP)-23 on the target membranes to form four helix bundles

that bring the vesicular and target membranes into close proximity (Fig. 125.3B). SNARE function is tightly regulated by chaperone proteins. NSF regulates membrane interaction by disassembling SNARE complexes on the same membrane so that they are available to form complexes with proteins on opposing membranes. The Sec1/Munc proteins (Munc18a, b, and c, and Munc13-4) and Rab GTPases regulate granule docking,[51] a preliminary step to granule membrane fusion (Fig. 125.3B).

Activation pathways involving intracellular Ca^{2+}, Rab GTPase, and PKC isoforms regulate the SNARE complex interactions. PKC isoforms phosphorylate several of the SNARE proteins and their regulators including Munc18c, syntaxin 4, and SNAP-23. The PKC substrate pleckstrin is also a critical mediator of granule exocytosis: pleckstrin-deficient mice show markedly impaired platelet secretion.[52]

The important role of granule releasates in hemostasis is underlined by the bleeding diathesis in people with granule deficiencies or defects of granule exocytosis. α Granules secrete fibrinogen and VWF, which mediate platelet-platelet and platelet-ECM interactions. Of the total VWF, 20% is contained in α granules, which are enriched in the most potent high-molecular-weight VWF multimers. ADP released from dense granules is essential for recruitment of additional platelets to the primary plug. Other mediators released from α granules play key roles in additional functions including wound repair, angiogenesis, and host defense. However, these modulators can also be pathogenic, contributing to the inflammatory response and atherosclerosis (Fig. 125.3A).

Procoagulant Surface Exposure and Microparticles

The phospholipids of the plasma membrane of resting platelets are asymmetrically distributed between the leaflets of the membrane bilayer, with choline-containing phospholipids predominating in the

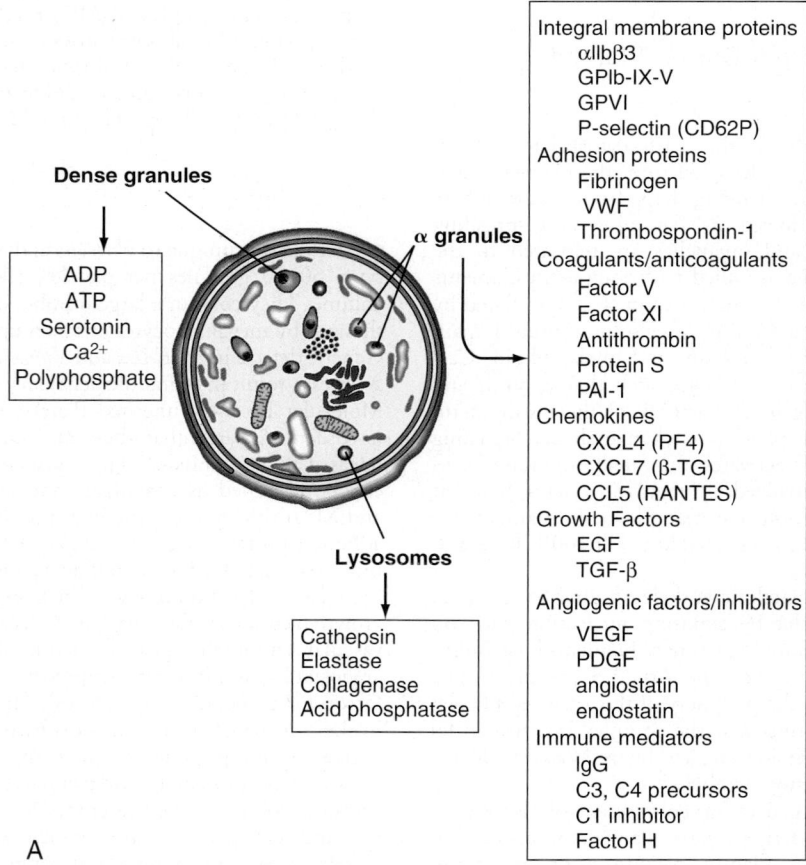

Fig. 125.3 (A) PLATELET GRANULE CONTENTS RELEASED BY SECRETION. Examples of bioactive substances stored in platelet dense granules, α granules, and lysosomes.

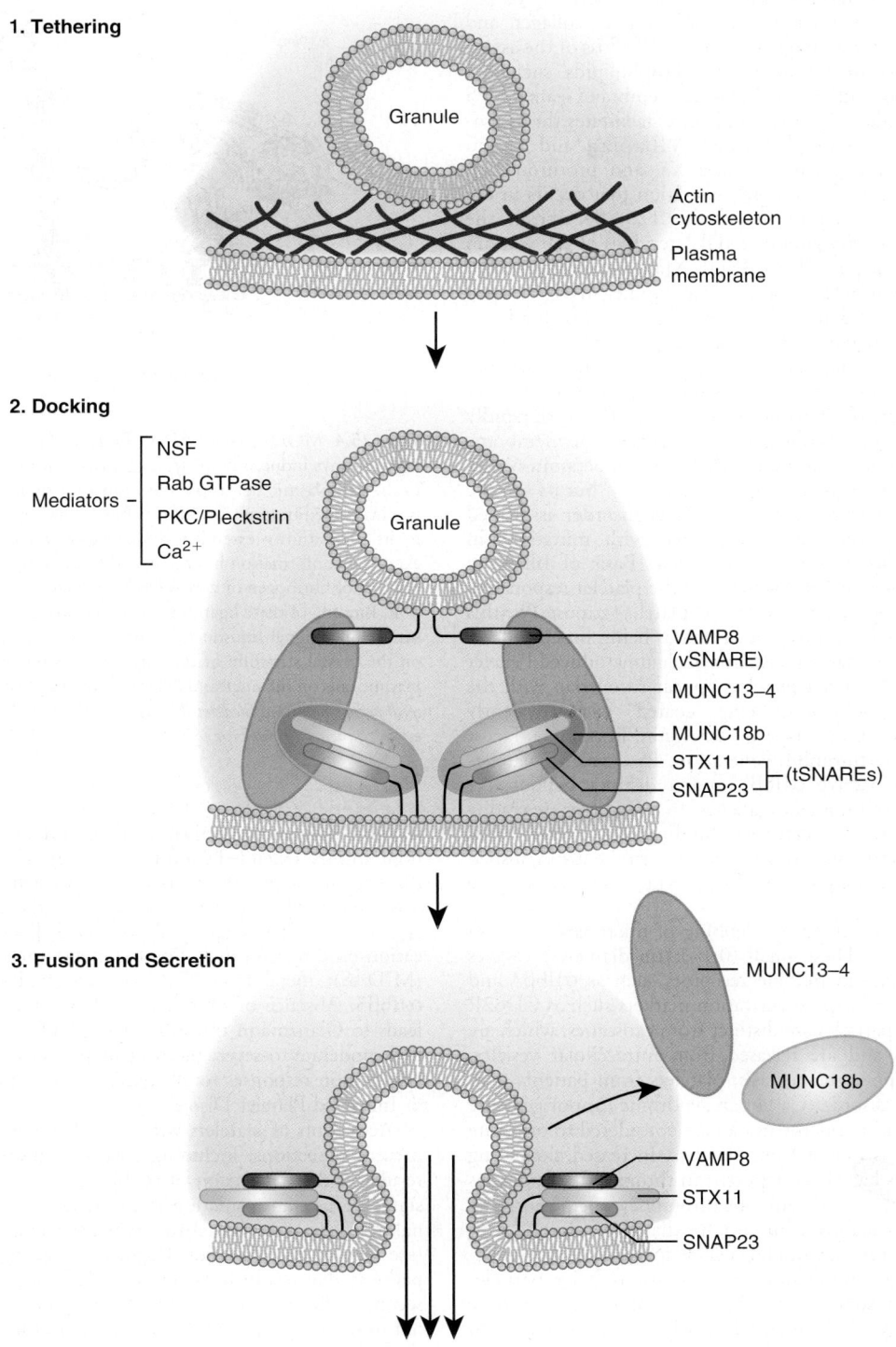

1. Tethering

Granule

Actin cytoskeleton

Plasma membrane

2. Docking

Mediators –
- NSF
- Rab GTPase
- PKC/Pleckstrin
- Ca^{2+}

Granule

VAMP8 (vSNARE)

MUNC13–4

MUNC18b

STX11 ⎤
SNAP23 ⎦ (tSNAREs)

3. Fusion and Secretion

MUNC13–4

MUNC18b

VAMP8

STX11

SNAP23

B   Granule contents

Fig. 125.3, cont'd (B) MOLECULAR CONTROL OF GRANULE SECRETION. This is a schematic diagram of steps in granule secretion. (1) Tethering: attachment of granules to the membrane cytoskeleton. (2) Docking: the engagement of vSNAREs on the granule membrane and tSNAREs on the target membrane to form a prefusion complex. In platelets, these docking proteins are VAMP8 on α granule and dense granule membranes, STX11/SNAP-23 complex on the plasma membrane and accessory proteins Munc13-4 and Munc18b/Munc18-2. (3) Fusion/secretion: involves the zippering of opposing SNAREs, applying force to fuse the granule and plasma membranes, resulting in release of the granule contents. Additional mediators of this active process include Rab GTPases, PKC, pleckstrin, Ca^{2+}, and NSF. *β-TG*, β-Thromboglobulin; *CXCL*, CXC-chemokine ligand; *EGF*, epidermal growth factor; *GP*, glycoprotein; *IgG*, immunoglobulin G; *NSF*, N-ethylmaleimide-sensitive factor; *PAI-1*, plasminogen activator inhibitor-1; *PDGF*, platelet-derived growth factor; *PF4*, platelet factor 4; *PKC*, protein kinase C; *RANTES*, regulated upon activation, normal T-cell expressed, and secreted; *SNAP-23*, synaptosomal-associated protein-23; *SNARE*, soluble N-ethylmaleimide–sensitive factor attachment protein receptor; *STX11*, syntaxin 11; *TGF-β*, transforming growth factor-β; *tSNARE*, target SNARE; *VAMP8*, vesicle-associated membrane protein 8; *VEGF*, vascular endothelial growth factor; *vSNARE*, vesicle-associated SNARE; *VWF*, von Willebrand factor.

outer cytoplasmic leaflet, and the minor anionic aminophospholipid PS predominating in the inner. Platelet adhesion to collagen and stimulation with thrombin synergistically result in a loss of the asymmetry, or "scrambling," of the membrane phospholipids, such that PS becomes exposed on the external plasma membrane leaflet.[53] PS translocated to the surface of activated platelets facilitates the assembly of the intrinsic tenase complex (factors VIIIa, IXa, and X) and prothrombinase complex (factors Va and Xa, and prothrombin), contributing to the burst of thrombin generation that occurs in the propagation phase of coagulation (see Chapter 126). Specifically, the negatively charged γ-carboxyglutamate (Gla) residues of the vitamin K-dependent factors, factors VII(a), IX(a), X(a), and prothrombin, mediate Ca^{2+}-dependent binding of the factors to negatively-charged PS. There is recent evidence that plasminogen also binds to PS-exposing platelets, thereby linking coagulation and fibrinolysis.[54]

Exposure of PS on the platelet surface requires sustained increases in $[Ca^{2+}]_i$ via influx across the plasma membrane, and activation of phospholipid scramblase (see Chapter 130, Fig. 130.1), which rapidly and nonspecifically transports phospholipids between the membrane leaflets. The transmembrane protein TMEM16F (anoctamin 6) has recently been shown to be essential for PS exposure,[55] but its specific role is not yet clear. Scott syndrome, a platelet disorder associated with a defect in PS exposure, is associated with mutations in *TMEM16F* (*ANO6*; see section on Molecular Basis of Inherited Platelet Disorders). There is heterogeneity in the platelet response to stimulation: only a proportion of activated platelets expose PS (this population of platelets is variously described as being procoagulant, superactivated, coated, or having Sustained Calcium-Induced Platelet [SCIP] morphology).[56] Coated platelets appear to overlap with the PS-exposing platelet population, being "coated" with covalently linked platelet secretion products (e.g., serotonin, fibrinogen, factor Va). Besides supporting thrombin generation, PS-exposing platelets are characterized by inactive αIIbβ3 and a distinct balloon-like morphology with loss of internal organelles. In vitro, they are readily identified by annexin A5 or lactadherin binding. The pathway that leads to rapid PS exposure on activated platelets can be distinguished from a slower intrinsic apoptotic pathway, which involves caspase activation.[57]

PS exposure is accompanied by blebbing of microparticles from the plasma membrane.[58] These small (0.1–1 μm diameter) vesicles not only express platelet membrane receptors such as αIIbβ3 and GPIb–IX–V, but can also express activation markers such as CD62P. Platelet-derived microparticles are distinct from exosomes, which are smaller (40–100 nm) and are released from intracellular vesicles. Microparticles can support hemostasis; platelets from patients with the very rare bleeding disorder Castaman syndrome cannot generate microparticles. Circulating microparticles are considered to originate from megakaryocytes as well as from platelets. Increased circulating levels of microparticles have been reported in thrombotic conditions such as myocardial infarction, thrombotic thrombocytopenic purpura, sickle cell disease, and diabetes, immune-mediated conditions such as immune thrombocytopenia and heparin-induced thrombocytopenia, and in malignancy and inflammatory conditions. Microparticles formed by platelets activated via GPVI have been shown to contribute to the pathophysiology of rheumatoid arthritis, delivering IL-1 to synovial fibroblasts,[59] an example of how microparticles may play a role in platelet-cell communication by delivering bioactive molecules to target cells.

MOLECULAR BASIS OF PLATELET AGGREGATION

αIIbβ3 and Molecular Mechanisms of Aggregation

Integrin αIIbβ3 is the most abundant membrane protein on the platelet surface, with 40,000–80,000 copies per resting platelet, a very high receptor density for such a small cell. Platelet activation can produce an additional 10% increase in this number as a result of expression from internal pools, i.e., α-granule membranes. On resting platelets, αIIbβ3 is in a low-affinity bent conformation that is unable

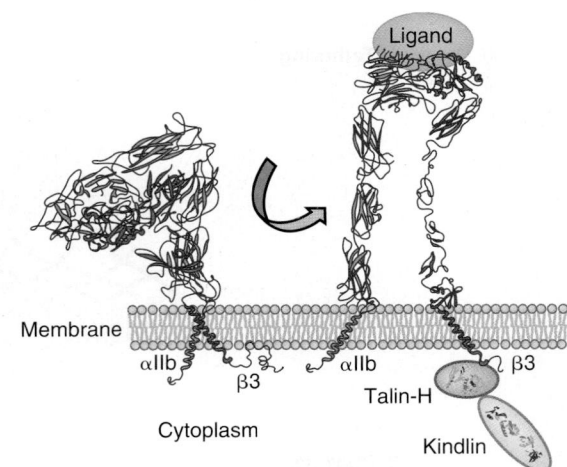

Fig. 125.4 MODEL SHOWING THE ACTIVATION OF αIIbβ3. Signaling pathways induced by platelet agonists result in talin and kindlin binding to the cytoplasmic tail of β3 and inside-out signaling such that the integrin is transformed from its low-affinity bent conformation on the resting platelet to its high-affinity extended conformation on the activated platelet. The extended conformation has the ligand binding site exposed, allowing for the binding of fibrinogen or von Willebrand factor, and thus for platelet aggregation. Binding of these ligands initiates outside-in signaling, triggering further intracellular signal transduction and platelet responses. This model is based on the crystal structure of the extracellular domain of αvβ3, and the cytoplasmic tails on the nuclear magnetic resonance structure of αIIbβ3. *(Adapted, with permission, from Bledzka K, Smyth SS, Plow EF. Integrin αIIbβ3. From discovery to efficacious therapeutic target. Circ Res 112:1189, 2013.)*

to bind its ligands. Activation of αIIbβ3 results in a change to a high-affinity, extended conformation (Fig. 125.4), allowing it to bind divalent fibrinogen or multivalent VWF which can bridge to other activated αIIbβ3 molecules on adjacent platelets, mediating platelet aggregation. The N-terminal portion of β3 contains three divalent cation-binding sites including the metal-ion dependent adhesion site (MIDAS); metal ions (Ca^{2+}) are required for ligand binding to αIIbβ3. Absence or dysfunction of αIIbβ3 on the platelet surface leads to Glanzmann thrombasthenia (GT), a disorder characterized by a moderate-to-severe bleeding diathesis and absent in vitro platelet aggregation responses to all agonists (see section on Molecular Basis of Inherited Platelet Disorders).

Activation of platelets with any of the agonists described in the preceding sections, including collagen, thrombin, ADP, and TxA$_2$, results in the conversion of αIIbβ3 from its resting to its activated state.[60] This transformation is a consequence of the intracellular signaling pathways set in motion when the agonist binds to its receptor (see section on Activation Pathways), leading to the final common pathway that results in aggregation; it occurs rapidly, on the order of seconds, after platelet exposure to an agonist. The signal is transmitted to the cytoplasmic tails of αIIbβ3 and from the cytoplasmic tail through the transmembrane helices, ultimately inducing a change in the extracellular domain to render αIIbβ3 competent to bind its ligands. The signaling process responsible for this transformation is referred to as "inside-out" signaling through αIIbβ3.

Specifically, it is the agonist-induced increase in $[Ca^{2+}]_i$ and DAG formation that result in the final common pathway of integrin activation.[61] Via the Ca^{2+}- and DAG-regulated guanine nucleotide exchange factor (CalDAG-GEFI), the small monomeric G protein (GTPase) Rap1 is activated and binds to Rap1-GTP-interacting adaptor molecule (RIAM); RIAM promotes binding of the cytoskeletal protein talin to the cytoplasmic domain of β3. Talin cooperates with kindlin-3, which also binds to the cytoplasmic domain of β3, to unclasp the complex between the αIIb and β3 cytoplasmic tails. This leads to a dissociation of the transmembrane complex of the αIIb and β3 subunits, inducing a conformational change in the extracellular domains. The bent conformation of αIIbβ3 is transitioned through intermediaries to an extended conformation that exposes the ligand-binding site (see Fig. 125.4) for fibrinogen and VWF.

Both fibrinogen and VWF bind to activated αIIbβ3 via Arg-Gly-Asp (RGD) sequences. Fibrinogen contains two such sequences, RGD-Ser and RGD-Phe, in its Aα chains, and VWF contains one in its C1 domain. The RGD sequence is a broadly used recognition code in cellular adhesive reactions; it is found on a variety of proteins, and it is recognized by several other integrin receptors. Fibrinogen has a second binding sequence for activated αIIbβ3, -X-X-Lys-Gln-Ala-Gly-Asp-Val (XXKQAGDV), in the C-terminus of its γ-chains; evidence indicates that this sequence is the primary one by which fibrinogen binds to activated αIIbβ3.[61] While fibrinogen binding mediates platelet aggregation at low shear, it is VWF binding that mediates aggregation at high shear.[62]

In turn, ligand binding induces conformational changes to activated αIIbβ3, resulting in exposure of binding sites on the cytoplasmic tails of the integrin for cytoskeletal and signaling proteins, and activation of protein kinases and phosphatases. This "outside-in" signaling is important in platelet responses such as full platelet spreading, irreversible aggregation, and clot stability and retraction.[28,61]

Upon aggregation, the close platelet-platelet contact facilitates binding of additional cell surface ligands on one platelet to cell surface receptors on adjacent platelets. Such binding can affect platelet activation and thrombus stability via initiation of intracellular signaling or formation of additional contacts between platelets. These ligand/receptor pairs include: ephrin/Eph kinase; semaphorin4D/CD72 (in humans) and a member of the plexin B family (in humans and mice); and growth-arrest specific gene 6 (Gas-6)/receptor tyrosine kinases Tyro3, Axl, and Mer.[28,62]

Laboratory Evaluation of Aggregation

The in vitro aggregation response of platelets is most commonly assessed using aggregometry, considered to be the gold standard of platelet function testing.[63] In the aggregometer, platelet responses are measured in suspension, bypassing the initial adhesion response of platelets to the subendothelial ECM that occurs in vivo (see section on Platelet Adhesion). Optical or turbidometric aggregometry, now more often referred to as *light transmission aggregometry (LTA)*, was developed in the 1960s; in LTA, light transmission through a rapidly stirred suspension of platelets is recorded upon addition of a soluble agonist (Table 125.3). With all agonists except epinephrine, there is an initial, transient, small decrease in light transmission from baseline due to actin cytoskeleton reorganization and platelet shape change from discs to more rounded forms with extended filipodia. This is followed by a larger increase in light transmission as the platelets aggregate. Depending on the agonist and its concentration, platelets may deaggregate, indicated by a subsequent decrease in light transmission (Fig. 125.5).

In clinical laboratories, platelet-rich plasma (PRP), obtained by low-speed centrifugation of a whole blood specimen anticoagulated with citrate, is routinely used in LTA assessment of platelet function. Citrate lowers the plasma concentration of Ca^{2+} to the micromolar range, which is still sufficient for aggregation to occur. In research laboratories, LTA of platelets isolated from plasma and suspended in balanced salt solutions (e.g., Tyrode's solution) is often used. In this case, Ca^{2+} must be added to the suspending medium to allow aggregation to occur. LTA measures platelet aggregation under conditions of low shear, in which aggregation is dependent on fibrinogen binding to activated αIIbβ3. This is in contrast with tests such as the Platelet Function Analyzer (PFA-100/200) (see Chapter 129), which measures aggregation under conditions of high shear ($5000-6000$ s^{-1}), in which aggregation is mediated by VWF binding to activated αIIbβ3.

Some of the commonly used platelet agonists are listed in Table 125.3. Of particular physiological relevance are the platelet-derived aggregating agents—ADP, and the arachidonate metabolite TxA₂—that provide a mechanism for stimulated platelets to recruit additional

TABLE 125.3 Agonists Used in the Laboratory Evaluation of Aggregation

Agonist	In vivo/In vitro Mechanism of Action
Thrombin receptor-activating peptide (TRAP)[a]	SFLLRN (Ser-Phe-Leu-Leu-Arg-Asn), the peptide sequence of the new N-terminus of PAR-1 after thrombin cleavage (binds to uncleaved PAR-1 in vitro)
ADP	Released from platelet dense granules; acts synergistically with many other agonists (binds to P2Y1 and P2Y12)
Arachidonate	Is metabolized by the cyclooxygenase pathway to TxA₂ which is released from stimulated platelets and is rapidly metabolized in plasma (TxA₂ binds to TP)
U46619	Stable TxA₂ mimetic (binds to TP)
Collagen	In subendothelial extracellular matrix (binds to GPVI and α2β1)
Epinephrine[b]	A weak agonist that is not associated with platelet shape change and that potentiates other agonists; may allow for hormonal regulation of hemostasis (binds to α₂ₐ-adrenergic receptor)
Ca²⁺-ionophore	Directly mobilizes intracellular Ca²⁺ (does not bind to a receptor)
Ristocetin[c]	An antibiotic that changes the conformation of VWF, exposing the binding site for GPIbα of the GPIb–IX–V complex, allowing platelet agglutination by VWF

[a]TRAP is used as a substitute for thrombin. Thrombin binds to GPIb–IX–V and cleaves PAR-1 and PAR-4, but is not often used in the assessment of platelet aggregation in citrated platelet-rich plasma as it causes fibrin clot formation.
[b]Reduced response to epinephrine occurs in a proportion of healthy individuals due to natural variation in receptor density, and is not necessarily indicative of a platelet function disorder.
[c]In contrast with the other agonists that stimulate aggregation, an energy-requiring process, ristocetin induces platelet agglutination via VWF, a process that does not require platelets to be metabolically active.
ADP, Adenosine 5′-diphosphate; GP, glycoprotein; PAR, protease-activating receptor; TP, thromboxane/prostanoid; TxA₂, thromboxane A₂; VWF, von Willebrand factor.

platelets to an aggregate in vivo. As described earlier, these agonists activate platelets by binding to specific receptors and triggering intracellular signaling pathways that ultimately converge to a set of common steps that permit the platelets to aggregate. Platelet aggregation, mediated by ligand binding to activated αIIbβ3, is energy dependent, and can be distinguished on this basis from platelet agglutination induced by ristocetin (Table 125.3), mediated by VWF binding to GPIbα of the GPIb–IX–V complex, which does not require platelets to be metabolically active. Many preanalytical and analytical variables affect the results obtained by LTA and recommendations for clinical laboratory standardization have been published recently.[64,65]

Platelet aggregation can also be measured by whole-blood aggregometry. This test measures platelet aggregation in diluted, anticoagulated whole blood as the change in impedance or resistance between two electrodes when platelets adhere to the electrodes and aggregate in response to soluble agonists (see earlier and Table 125.3). Whole-blood aggregometry has the advantages over LTA of requiring smaller blood volumes and less sample manipulation. Certain light transmission/whole-blood aggregometers also provide simultaneous measurements of dense granule secretion, specifically ATP release (using lumi-aggregometry).

The information gained from aggregometry has been extremely useful in the diagnosis of platelet function disorders, whether inherited or acquired.[64] However, aggregation as measured in vitro does

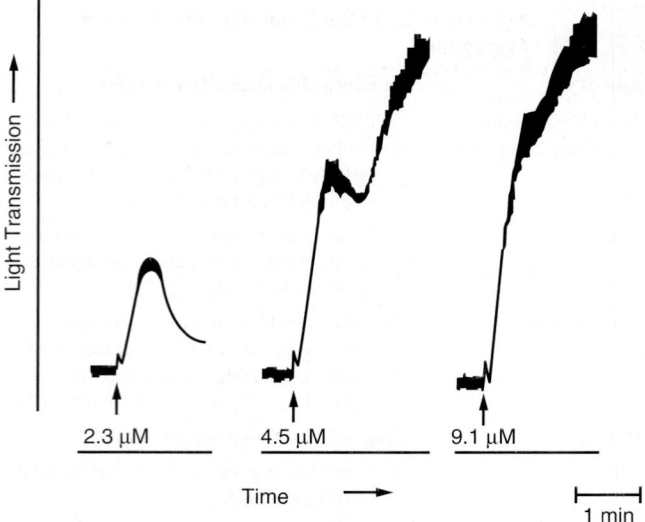

Fig. 125.5 AGGREGATION RESPONSES OF PLATELETS IN CITRATED PLATELET-RICH PLASMA STIMULATED WITH ADP. (Note that the micromolar concentration of Ca^{2+} in citrated platelet-rich plasma is sufficient to allow aggregation to occur.) The *arrows* indicate the addition of increasing concentrations of ADP from left to right. Following addition of the agonist, platelet shape change is observed as a slight decrease in light transmission, followed by an increase in light transmission as the platelets aggregate. The lowest concentration of ADP (2.3 μM; left) induces primary aggregation followed by deaggregation, as indicated by the subsequent decrease in light transmission. The intermediate concentration of ADP (4.5 μM; middle) induces primary aggregation followed by a secondary wave of aggregation; the secondary wave occurs due to thromboxane A_2 formation by the stimulated platelets and subsequent granule content exocytosis, including ADP. At the highest concentration of ADP (9.1 μM; right), there is fusion of the two phases of aggregation so that only a single wave of aggregation is apparent. *(Adapted, with permission, from Rand ML, Leung R, Packham MA: Platelet function assays.* Transfus Apher Sci *28:307, 2003.)*

not always reflect platelet function in vivo; clinical bleeding and the aggregation response of platelets do not necessarily coincide. This disparity reflects, in part, the importance of platelet adhesion under flow conditions in hemostatic plug/arterial thrombus formation, an effect that is not detected by aggregometry.[62] Tests that allow for measurement of adhesion of platelets to multiple surfaces under flow conditions at variable shear rates, and for measurement of multiple outcomes to characterize platelet responses will, in the future, provide additional information about platelet function.[66]

MOLECULAR BASIS OF INHERITED PLATELET DISORDERS

Inherited platelet disorders are a heterogeneous group of bleeding disorders involving defects in platelet function and/or number (usually thrombocytopenia). The bleeding symptoms experienced by patients are primarily mucocutaneous, such as epistaxis, bruising, bleeding from the oropharynx or gastrointestinal tract, menorrhagia, and postpartum and surgical (including dental) bleeding; these symptoms can range from very mild to life threatening, depending on the disorder (severity may vary among individuals with the same disorder). The prevalence of these disorders is unknown, as there are no population-based data. While severe disorders such as GT and BSS are relatively easy to diagnose, rare, milder disorders are more difficult to characterize and it is likely that they are more common than previously appreciated.[67] Much has been learned about platelet development, structure and function, and the underlying

Platelet Aggregation Testing for the Diagnosis of Platelet Disorders

Platelet aggregometry is the mainstay in the work-up of platelet function disorders (PFDs). Abnormalities in aggregation tracings can point towards specific diagnoses and direct further testing.

Glanzmann Thrombasthenia

In this severe PFD in which there are quantitative or qualitative defects in integrin αIIbβ3 (GPIIb–IIIa), the receptor to which fibrinogen/von Willebrand factor (VWF) binds on activated platelets, there is absent aggregation response to all agonists. However, agglutination in response to a high concentration of ristocetin occurs, as it is independent of αIIbβ3.

Bernard-Soulier Syndrome

This disorder with defective surface expression of the adhesive VWF receptor GPIb–IX–V is characterized by a lack of agglutination to a high concentration of ristocetin. Note that in von Willebrand disease (VWD) there is an absent agglutination response to a high concentration of ristocetin because of deficient VWF.

Defects in Agonist/Adhesion Receptors

P2Y12: a defect in this ADP receptor results in decreased and reversible aggregation responses to ADP. TPα: thromboxane A_2 (TxA₂) receptor defects show decreased aggregation responses to arachidonic acid, collagen and the stable TxA₂ mimetic U46619. GPVI: a defect in this collagen receptor is characterized by a decreased aggregation response to collagen.

Storage Granule Deficiencies/Secretion Defects

In these disorders, secondary aggregation responses to ADP, collagen, epinephrine, and arachidonic acid can be reduced, but it should be noted that secretion defects may be present with a normal aggregation profile. In dense granule disorders, secretion as measured by lumiaggregometry is decreased.

Platelet Type VWD/Type 2B VWD

These gain-of-function disorders in the VWF binding site of GPIbα or in the GPIbα binding site of VWF, respectively, are characterized by an abnormally increased agglutination response to a low concentration of ristocetin.

Effects of Antiplatelet Medications

Aggregation responses will also be affected by antiplatelet medications. For example, individuals taking aspirin or other nonsteroidal antiinflammatory drugs will have decreased responses to arachidonic acid, but not to U46619. Patients taking P2Y12 receptor blockers, i.e., clopidogrel, prasugrel, ticagrelor, or cangrelor, will have decreased and reversible responses to ADP, depending on the extent of inhibition of the receptor.

genetic basis of specific disorders from the investigation of patients; indeed, the molecular defects in many of the disorders have now been identified (Fig. 125.6). Important insights have also been provided by characterization of mouse models in which platelet proteins have been altered genetically.[68] The reader is referred to comprehensive reviews of inherited disorders of platelets for more details.[69–72]

Inherited Platelet Function Disorders

Inherited platelet function disorders encompass defects in: platelet adhesion, with deficiencies or dysfunction of receptors for subendothelial VWF or collagen; platelet activation, including deficiencies or dysfunction of receptors for soluble agonists, of cytoskeletal proteins, of signaling pathways, of dense and α granules, and of PS exposure; and platelet aggregation, with deficiencies or dysfunction of integrin αIIbβ3. Most of the disorders described later have an autosomal recessive pattern of inheritance, and thus affected individuals have homozygous or compound heterozygous gene mutations. The disorders vary significantly in their severity, and some present with associated thrombocytopenia.

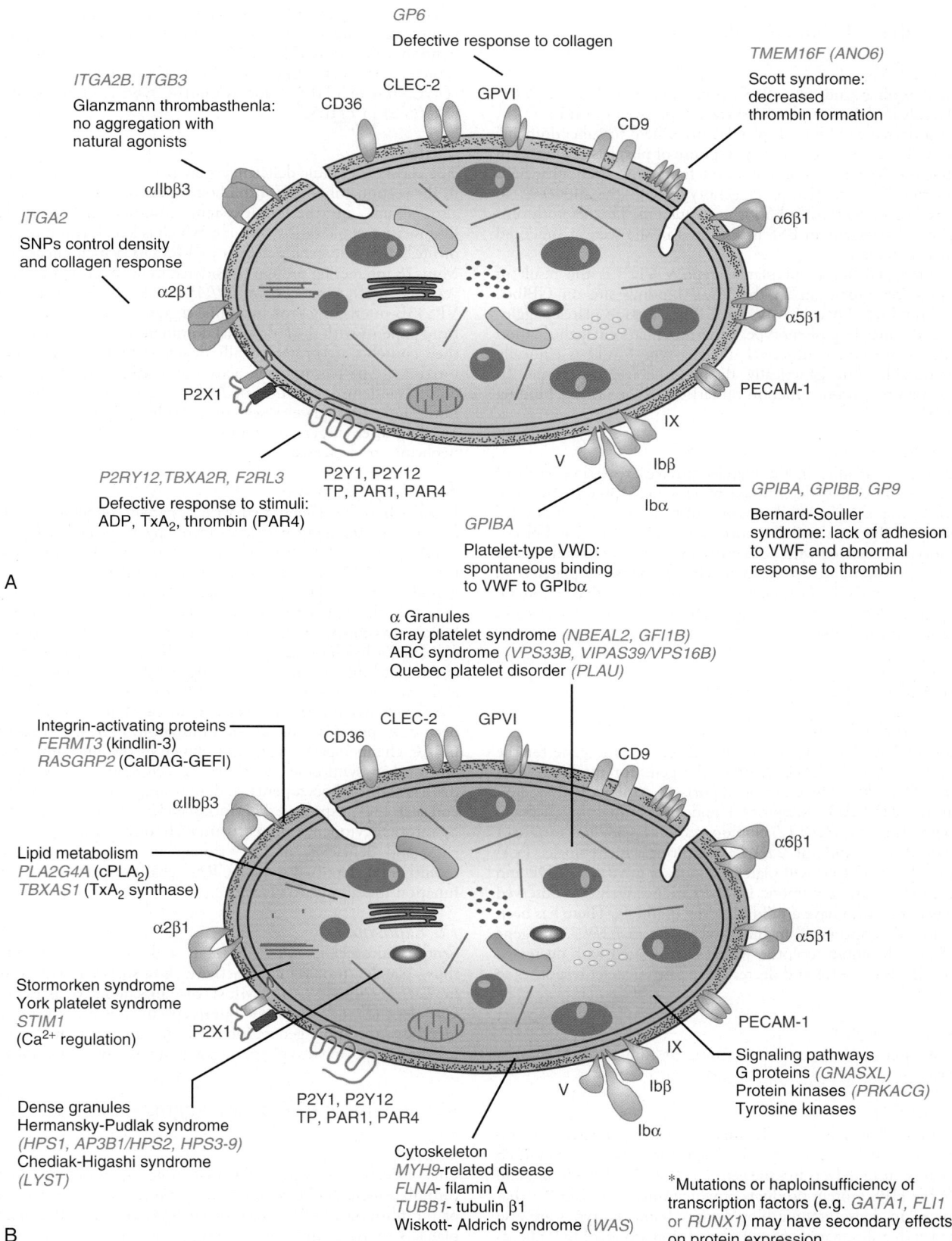

Fig. 125.6 GENETIC CAUSES OF INHERITED PLATELET DISORDERS. (A) Surface membrane receptor defects and (B) granule and intracellular protein defects. *ARC,* Arthrogryposis-renal dysfunction-cholestasis; *cPLA₂,* cytosolic phospholipase A₂; *CalDAG-GEF,* Ca^{2+} and diacylglycerol-regulated guanine nucleotide exchange factor; *GP,* glycoprotein; *PAR,* protease-activated receptor; *PECAM,* platelet-endothelial cell adhesion molecule; *SNP,* single-nucleotide polymorphism; *TxA₂,* thromboxane A₂; *VWD,* von Willebrand disease; *VWF,* von Willebrand factor. *(Adapted, with permission, from Nurden AT, Nurden P: Inherited disorders of platelet function.* J Thromb Haemost *13(Suppl 1):S2, 2015.)*

Abnormalities of Platelet Adhesion

GPIb–IX–V[73]

In Bernard-Soulier syndrome (BSS), mutations in *GP1BA*, *GP1BB*, or *GP9* result in defective platelet surface expression of GPIb–IX–V, and thus a decreased ability of platelets to adhere to subendothelial VWF, as well as a decreased in vitro response of platelets to thrombin and ristocetin. Missense, nonsense, and frameshift alterations have been described[69,74]; correlation of genotype with the moderate to severe bleeding phenotype in BSS is not apparent. The macrothrombocytopenia that occurs in BSS is discussed in the section Inherited Thrombocytopenias.

The autosomal dominant platelet-type VWD[75] is the result of gain-of-function mutations in the VWF binding site on GPIbα. Enhanced binding of plasma VWF to GPIbα leads to platelet agglutination and a bleeding phenotype. In vitro, enhanced agglutination to low-dose ristocetin is observed. Platelet-type VWD is clinically indistinguishable, but genetically distinguishable, from type 2B VWD, caused by gain-of-function mutations in the GPIbα binding site of VWF.

Collagen Receptors

There is wide variability in the platelet surface expression levels of GPVI and α2β1 that is determined by specific haplotypes in *GP6* and *ITGA2*, respectively. While absence of α2β1 expression has not been observed, there are several reports of patients with a mild bleeding phenotype associated with *GP6* mutations, leading to deficiencies in GPVI expression and decreased in vitro response of platelets to collagen.[69] Acquired GPVI deficiency can also occur, with ectodomain shedding (i.e., cleavage) of the receptor from the platelet surface in response to autoantibodies.

Abnormalities of Platelet Activation

Soluble Agonist Receptors

Rare patients have been described with defects in the gene for the ADP receptor P2Y12 (*P2RY12*) or in the gene for the TxA$_2$ TPα receptor (*TBXA2R*). (There are no reports of patients with a deficiency in the P2Y1 ADP receptor.) The defects mimic the effects of antiplatelet drugs: for *P2RY12*, clopidogrel, prasugrel, and ticagrelor that block P2Y12; and for *TBXA2R*, aspirin, which blocks TxA$_2$ formation. As such, decreased platelet responses in vitro to ADP and the stable thromboxane mimetic U46619, respectively, are observed in these patients, who have a mild bleeding diathesis. There has been a recent first description of an inherited defect in *F2RL3*, the gene for the PAR4 thrombin receptor, which is associated with decreased expression levels of PAR4 and decreased in vitro platelet responses to thrombin.[76]

Cytoskeletal Defects

These are discussed later in the section on Inherited Thrombocytopenias.

Dense Granules[77]

Hermansky-Pudlak syndrome is characterized by oculocutaneous albinism and platelet-dense granule deficiency.[78] The distinct HPS subtypes arise from defects in nine genes, *HPS1*, *AP3B1* (*HPS2*), and *HPS3-9*, the HPS protein products of which interact in BLOCs that are involved in dense granule biogenesis.[41] Some subtypes are also associated with pulmonary fibrosis and granulomatous colitis. Patients with Chediak-Higashi syndrome have severe immunological defects in addition to oculocutaneous albinism and dense granule deficiency; they have mutations in the *LYST* gene, the product of which is a vesicular transport protein. These syndromic dense granule deficiencies are associated with mild-to-moderate bleeding; in vitro secretion responses as measured by lumiaggregometry are reduced.

Normal numbers of granules with decreased secretion responses are indicative of defective granule secretion processes. For example, in vitro evidence of dense and α granule secretion defects with normal granule cargo are observed in some forms of familial hemophagocytic lymphohistiocytosis (FHL). Mutations for genes encoding SNARE proteins or their regulators have been identified: Munc13-4 (*UNC13D*) in FHL3,[79] and Munc18b/syntaxin binding protein 2 (*STXBP2*) in FHL5.[80]

α Granules

The classic α granule deficiency, gray platelet syndrome, is discussed in the section Inherited Thrombocytopenias. Platelet α granules are also absent in the multisystem disorder arthrogryposis-renal dysfunction-cholestasis syndrome, which is lethal within the first year of life. Here, the gene defect is in *VPS33B*, which encodes a Sec1/Munc18 interacting protein considered to be involved in intracellular vesicular trafficking, or in *VIPAS39* (*VPS16B*), which encodes VPS33B-interacting protein. While α granules are present in platelets from patients with the autosomal dominant Quebec platelet disorder, their contents are proteolytically degraded by plasmin generated by urokinase-type plasminogen activator (u-PA), abnormally expressed due to tandem duplication of *PLAU*, the u-PA gene. Inappropriate fibrinolysis after platelet secretion results in symptoms of delayed bleeding after surgery or trauma; in vitro platelet responses to epinephrine are decreased.

Signaling Pathways

Patients have been identified with apparent congenital disorders in a variety of signaling pathways involving G proteins (G$_q$, G$_s$, G$_i$), cPLA$_2$, and PLC, PKC-θ, Ca^{2+} mobilization, TxA$_2$ formation (including COX-1 and thromboxane synthase deficiencies), and granule secretion. However, for the most part, the underlying genetic defects in these patients, who experience mild-to-moderate bleeding, remain unknown. An insertion mutation in the extra-large Gα$_s$ gene (*GNASXL*) has been associated with Gα$_s$ hyperfunction in platelets and a bleeding phenotype, neurological problems, and mild skeletal abnormalities. Mutations in *PLA2G4A* encoding cPLA2 and in *TBXAS1* encoding thromboxane synthase (Ghosal syndrome) have been described. Gain-of-function mutations in *STIM1* resulting in a CRAC channelopathy have been shown in the autosomal dominant Stormorken syndrome, which is characterized by a mild bleeding diathesis, thrombocytopenia, and, in resting platelets, elevated [Ca^{2+}]$_i$ and surface PS exposure. The York platelet syndrome,[81] characterized by thrombocytopenia, ultrastructural abnormalities in platelet organelles, and deficiency of Ca^{2+} storage in dense granules, has also recently been reported to be a CRAC channelopathy due to gain-of-function mutations in *STIM1*.

PS Exposure

Scott syndrome, in which there is a defect in PS exposure and thus, platelet procoagulant activity, is associated with mutations in *TMEM16F* (*ANO6*); TMEM16F (anoctamin 6) is essential for Ca^{2+}-dependent PS exposure, but its specific role is not yet clarified.[82] Decreased thrombin generation results in a moderate-to-severe bleeding phenotype; in vitro platelet aggregation responses are not affected.

Abnormalities of Platelet Aggregation

αIIbβ3[83]

One of the best characterized platelet function disorders, Glanzmann thrombasthenia (GT), results from quantitative or qualitative defects of the fibrinogen/VWF receptor αIIbβ3, and thus the inability of platelets to aggregate. The bleeding phenotype ranges from mild to life-threatening hemorrhage, and in vitro there are absent aggregation responses to all agonists, while ristocetin-induced agglutination is intact. Type I GT is defined as <5% surface-expressed αIIbβ3; type II, as 5%–25%; and variant, as normal expression levels of a αIIbβ3 complex that is nonfunctional. Approximately 200 mutations have been described in the *ITGA2B* and *ITGB3* genes, most commonly missense and nonsense mutations, and those involving splice mutations and small deletions and insertions with frame shifts; genotype does not necessarily correlate with phenotype.[84] Rare mutations result in macrothrombocytopenia (see section on Inherited Thrombocytopenias).

Defects in the gene for kindlin-3 (*FERMT3*) or CalDAG-GEFI (*RASGRP2*) have been reported that prevent activation of αIIbβ3, with subsequent absence of platelet aggregation. Deficiency in kindlin-3 is the basis for leukocyte deficiency-III syndrome, a severe disorder that encompasses defective integrin β2 function in leukocytes and associated susceptibility to infections and poor wound healing, as well as severe bleeding.

Inherited Thrombocytopenias

Inherited thrombocytopenias vary significantly in their severity, platelet morphology, and presence or absence of associated platelet dysfunction. There are approximately 20 human gene defects known to be associated with inherited thrombocytopenias. In terms of molecular mechanism, these can best be understood in the context of megakaryocyte differentiation, maturation, proplatelet formation, and platelet release (Fig. 125.6; see also Chapter 124).[85,86]

Abnormalities of Megakaryocyte Differentiation

Defects in megakaryocyte maturation result in deficiency or absence of bone marrow megakaryocytes. Known defects include:

Congenital Amegakaryocytic Thrombocytopenia (CAMT)
This is an autosomal recessive disease caused by mutations in *MPL*, the gene for the thrombopoietin (TPO) receptor. Binding of TPO to its receptor activates multiple signaling pathways including JAK2/STAT, Ras/MAPK, and PI3K. TPO is essential for commitment and differentiation in megakaryocytes but also in the erythroid and granulocytes lineages, as patients with CAMT, although thrombocytopenic at birth, develop trilineage bone marrow hypoplasia in the first few years of life.[87]

Thrombocytopenia with Absent Radii (TAR)
This is an autosomal recessive disorder characterized by absent radii and isolated thrombocytopenia, also present at birth. In contrast to CAMT, platelet counts improve with age and other cell lines are unaffected. The cause is a compound inheritance of a low-frequency single-nucleotide polymorphism and a rare null allele in *RBM8A*, a gene encoding the exon-junction complex subunit member Y14. This complex is involved in RNA processing and nuclear export. It is still unknown how this defect affects megakaryocyte maturation, although it may affect TPO signaling through its receptor.[88]

Amegakaryocytic Thrombocytopenia with Radio-Ulnar Synostosis (ATRUS)
This is the result of heterozygous defects in *HOXA11*, a member of the *HOX* gene family of transcription factors involved in embryonic development. These patients have thrombocytopenia from birth that does not improve with time, associated with fusion of the proximal radius and ulna.[87]

Abnormalities of Megakaryocyte Maturation

Defects in differentiation are associated with mutations in specific transcription factors. Some of these mutations are associated with an increased risk of myeloid malignancies and some are associated with additional functional platelet defects. They are characterized by immature or dysplastic bone marrow megakaryocytes.

Familial Platelet Disorder With Predisposition to Acute Myeloid Leukemia
Familial platelet disorder with predisposition to acute myeloid leukemia (FPD/AML) is the result of heterozygous mutations in

RUNX1 (also called *AML1* or *CBFA2*) that encodes the alpha subunit of the core-binding factor transcription complex. This complex regulates expression of genes involved in stem cell proliferation versus differentiation in hematopoiesis. The loss of this regulation predisposes to the development of myelodysplastic syndrome and AML in approximately 40% of individuals with germ-line *RUNX1* mutations. In some pedigrees, the thrombocytopenia is accompanied by abnormalities of granule structure or defects in granule secretion.[89]

Paris-Trousseau Thrombocytopenia and Jacobsen Syndrome
Paris-Trousseau thrombocytopenia and Jacobsen syndrome are disorders caused by deletions in chromosome 11q23-ter, the severity of the syndrome, which includes cardiac and facial defects, depending on the size of the deletion. The loss of one copy of the transcription factor gene *FLI1* results in macrothrombocytopenia, and platelets with abnormal α granules and internal membrane structure (see Chapter 124).[89]

GATA-1–Related Thrombocytopenias
These are X-linked diseases associated with anemia, indicating this transcription factor's involvement in both megakaryocytic and erythroid maturation (see Chapter 124). Mutations in *GATA-1* that interfere with binding to its cofactor FOG1 result in dyserythropoietic anemia with thrombocytopenia and defects in α granule maturation.[69]

ANKRD26-Related Thrombocytopenia
This is the result of point mutations in the 5′-UTR of *ANKRD26*, leading to gene overexpression, dysmegakaryopoiesis, and an increased risk of myeloid malignancies. Some affected individuals also have evidence of dysregulation of erythroid and myeloid maturation.[90]

Gray Platelet Syndrome
Gray platelet syndrome (GPS) is the result of homozygous mutations in *NBEAL2*, a regulator of membrane dynamics and vesicle trafficking, affecting α granule development. The disorder is characterized by macrothrombocytopenia, absent platelet α granules, splenomegaly, and progressive bone marrow fibrosis.[42–44] The *Nbeal2*[−/−] mouse also shows evidence of abnormal megakaryocyte maturation.[91] Recently, mutations in *GFI1B*, encoding a transcription factor involved in megakaryopoeisis and erythropoiesis, have been identified in association a phenotype similar to GPS. Affected individuals have macrothrombocytopenia and α granule deficiency, and some have erythrocyte abnormalities.[92]

Abnormalities of Proplatelet Formation and Platelet Release

The central role of platelet cytoskeletal components and their interaction with surface membrane receptors in proplatelet formation and platelet production have been clarified by the identification of inherited defects in these molecules that are associated with thrombocytopenias.

MYH9-Related Disease
Previously referred to as the May-Hegglin, Sebastian, and Fechtner syndromes and Epstein anomaly, *MYH9*-related disease is the result of autosomal dominant mutations in *MYH9*, the gene that encodes NMMHC-IIA. NMM is involved in the generation of energy-driven skeletal forces involved in cytokinesis, cell motility, and shape change. Affected individuals have macrothrombocytopenia from birth, the result of branching defects in proplatelets. Branching increases the number of free proplatelet ends and the number of platelets released. There also appear to be defects in the timing of platelet release. Some *MYH9* mutations are also associated with leukocyte inclusions and the development of progressive renal dysfunction, sensorineural hearing loss, and cataracts.[39]

ACTN1- and FLNA-Related Thrombocytopenias

These result from mutations in the genes that encode α-actinin or filamin A, both functioning as cross-linking proteins in the actin-based cytoskeleton. Filamin A is also critical in binding the cytoplasmic tail of GPIbα to the filamentous actin network. Monoallelic mutations in either gene result in abnormalities of proplatelet formation and variable degrees of macrothrombocytopenia.[86]

Wiskott-Aldrich Syndrome and X-linked Thrombocytopenia

Wiskott-Aldrich syndrome (WAS) and X-linked thrombocytopenia (XLT) are caused by mutations in the *WAS* gene. Mutations that result in nonexpression of WASp cause WAS that manifests as severe immune dysregulation, in addition to thrombocytopenia. XLT is caused by mutations that decrease expression of the normal protein. These syndromes have the unique characteristic of microthrombocytopenia. WASp is involved in regulation of actin polymerization; the defect in platelet production may be the result of ectopic platelet shedding by megakaryocytes.[85,93]

Bernard-Soulier Syndrome

In addition to the functional adhesive defect (described in the section on Abnormalities of Platelet Adhesion), patients have thrombocytopenia and giant platelets. Abnormalities in proplatelet formation resemble those seen in mutations of cytoskeletal proteins, suggesting that the anchoring of the actin filament network by GPIbα to the plasma membrane is a required part of this process, disrupted by deficiency of the GPIb–IX–V transmembrane protein complex.[15,86] Most heterozygotes do not have macrothrombocytopenia, but there are exceptions where specific mutations (e.g., p.A156V, the Bolzano mutation) or monoallelic BSS (e.g., Velo-Cardio-Facial syndrome) cause mild macrothrombocytopenia.

ITGA2B/ITGB3-Related Thrombocytopenias

These are rare macrothrombocytopenias with functional defects associated with specific monoallelic mutations in *ITGA2B* or *ITGB3* that are distinct from the mutations that cause GT, described previously. These mutations result in constitutive activation of αIIbβ3 and downstream effectors, defects in actin-myosin reorganization, and abnormalities of proplatelet formation.[94]

TUBB1-Related Thrombocytopenia

This is caused by mutations in the gene for β1-tubulin and is associated with platelets that are spherical rather than discoid, the result of abnormalities of the microtubule coil[95] (see also Chapter 124).

PRKACG-Related Macrothrombocytopenia

This is the result of a germ-line mutation in the gene encoding the γ-catalytic subunit of the cAMP-dependent protein kinase (PK), PKA. There is a defect in proplatelet formation and a low level of filamin A in megakaryocytes.[96]

SUGGESTED READINGS

Bertozzi CC, Schmaier AA, Mericko P, et al: Platelets regulate lymphatic vascular development through CLEC-2-SLP-76 signaling. *Blood* 116(4):661–670, 2010.

Blair P, Flaumenhaft R: Platelet alpha-granules: basic biology and clinical correlates. *Blood Rev* 23(4):177–189, 2009.

Bledzka K, Smyth SS, Plow EF: Integrin alphaIIbbeta3: from discovery to efficacious therapeutic target. *Circ Res* 112(8):1189–1200, 2013.

Boilard E, Nigrovic PA, Larabee K, et al: Platelets amplify inflammation in arthritis via collagen-dependent microparticle production. *Science* 327(5965):580–583, 2010.

Brass LF, Newman DK, Wannermacher KM, et al: Signal transduction during platelet plug formation. In Michelson AD, editor: *Platelets*, ed 3, San Diego, 2013, Academic Press, pp 367–398.

Bryckaert M, Rosa JP, Denis CV, et al: Of von Willebrand factor and platelets. *Cell Mol Life Sci* 72(2):307–326, 2015.

Franco AT, Corken A, Ware J: Platelets at the interface of thrombosis, inflammation, and cancer. *Blood* 126(5):582–588, 2015.

Freson K, Wijgaerts A, van Geet C: Update on the causes of platelet disorders and functional consequences. *Int J Lab Hematol* 36(3):313–325, 2014.

Harrison P, Lordkipanidze M: Testing platelet function. *Hematol Oncol Clin North Am* 27(3):411–441, 2013.

Harrison P, Mackie I, Mumford A, et al: Guidelines for the laboratory investigation of heritable disorders of platelet function. *Br J Haematol* 155(1):30–44, 2011.

Heemskerk JW, Mattheij NJ, Cosemans JM: Platelet-based coagulation: different populations, different functions. *J Thromb Haemost* 11(1):2–16, 2013.

Huizing M, Helip-Wooley A, Westbroek W, et al: Disorders of lysosome-related organelle biogenesis: clinical and molecular genetics. *Annu Rev Genomics Hum Genet* 9:359–386, 2008.

Italiano JE, Jr, Richardson JL, Patel-Hett S, et al: Angiogenesis is regulated by a novel mechanism: pro- and antiangiogenic proteins are organized into separate platelet alpha granules and differentially released. *Blood* 111(3):1227–1233, 2008.

Kunishima S, Saito H: Advances in the understanding of MYH9 disorders. *Curr Opin Hematol* 17(5):405–410, 2010.

Li R, Emsley J: The organizing principle of the platelet glycoprotein Ib-IX-V complex. *J Thromb Haemost* 11(4):605–614, 2013.

McFadyen JD, Kaplan ZS: Platelets are not just for clots. *Transfus Med Rev* 29(2):110–119, 2015.

Nieuwland R, van der Pol E, Gardiner C, et al: Platelet-derived microparticles. In Michelson AD, editor: *Platelets*, ed 3, San Diego, 2013, Academic Press, pp 453–467.

Notarangelo LD, Ochs HD: Wiskott-Aldrich Syndrome: a model for defective actin reorganization, cell trafficking and synapse formation. *Curr Opin Immunol* 15(5):585–591, 2003.

Nurden AT, Nurden P: Congenital platelet disorders and understanding of platelet function. *Br J Haematol* 165(2):165–178, 2014.

Nurden AT, Nurden P: Inherited disorders of platelet function: selected updates. *J Thromb Haemost* 13(Suppl 1):S2–S9, 2015.

Nurden AT, Pillois X, Fiore M, et al: Glanzmann thrombasthenia-like syndromes associated with Macrothrombocytopenias and mutations in the genes encoding the alphaIIbbeta3 integrin. *Semin Thromb Hemost* 37(6):698–706, 2011.

Pecci A, Balduini CL: Lessons in platelet production from inherited thrombocytopenias. *Br J Haematol* 165(2):179–192, 2014.

Ruggeri ZM: Platelet adhesion under flow. *Microcirculation* 16(1):58–83, 2009.

Senis YA, Mazharian A, Mori J: Src family kinases: at the forefront of platelet activation. *Blood* 124(13):2013–2024, 2014.

Seward SL, Jr, Gahl WA: Hermansky-Pudlak syndrome: health care throughout life. *Pediatrics* 132(1):153–160, 2013.

Tijssen MR, Ghevaert C: Transcription factors in late megakaryopoiesis and related platelet disorders. *J Thromb Haemost* 11(4):593–604, 2013.

Varga-Szabo D, Braun A, Nieswandt B: STIM and Orai in platelet function. *Cell Calcium* 50(3):270–278, 2011.

Versteeg HH, Heemskerk JW, Levi M, et al: New fundamentals in hemostasis. *Physiol Rev* 93(1):327–358, 2013.

Watson SP, Farndale RW, Moroi M, et al: Platelet collagen receptors. In Marder VJ, Aird WC, Bennett JS, et al, editors: *Hemostasis and thrombosis. Basic principles and clinical practice*, ed 6, Philadelphia, 2013, Lippincott Williams & Wilkins, pp 420–430.

Wei AH, Schoenwaelder SM, Andrews RK, et al: New insights into the haemostatic function of platelets. *Br J Haematol* 147(4):415–430, 2009.

REFERENCES

For the complete list of references, log on to www.expertconsult.com.

CHAPTER 126

MOLECULAR BASIS OF BLOOD COAGULATION

Kathleen Brummel-Ziedins and Kenneth G. Mann

Blood is the principal vehicle delivering oxygen and nutrients to the various tissues and organs of the body. Blood flow and the integrity of the vasculature are essential to life itself. The hemostatic process has evolved to provide damage recognition and protection from blood loss after perforation of the vasculature while at the same time preventing the systemic activation of the clotting system. However, pathologic occlusions are associated with dysregulation of the intravascular system, resulting in venous or arterial thrombosis. The fine line between vascular occlusion and hemostasis is defined by the complex interplay between pro- and anticoagulant materials provided by the blood, the vasculature, and subvascular elements. The appropriate functions occur as a consequence of intense focal development and regulation of enzymatic activity at sites of vascular injury.

The development of the inventory of components involved in plasma clotting were initially based on the most abundant procoagulant plasma proteins, notably prothrombin and fibrinogen, and extended during the past century with the identification of genetic abnormalities that led to bleeding and deviations in laboratory tests that evolved as the inventory of congenital defects expanded. In some instances, laboratory test results indicating a defect in the procoagulant system were not mirrored by hemostatic pathology. In a similar fashion, the congenital defects associated with thrombosis led to the discovery of anticoagulant proteins in blood and vascular counterparts associated with their presentation and activation.

The functional connections between procoagulant "factors" were developed by mixing and matching plasmas associated with different hemostatic disorders. This inventory and its connectivity were ratified and expanded by experiments performed with transgenically mutated mice.

The dynamics of the plasma coagulation process as expressed are a consequence of the molar concentrations of the pro- and anticoagulant components in blood and the vasculature, and the kinetic processes associated with the dynamics of both the activation and functions of the various proteins associated with the process.

The initial result of the activation of the procoagulant hemostatic process is the formation of a fibrin–platelet plug that forms the temporary seal of the vascular perforation in hemostasis. The generation of an occlusive fibrin–platelet plug blocking further flow through an element of the vasculature is thrombosis. In both instances, the fibrin–platelet scaffold is ultimately removed and substituted by vascular repair, new cells, and connective tissue. In thrombosis, the platelet–fibrin plug is removed mechanically or by biochemical intervention to restore flow to the flow-starved vascular bed.

The elements of clotted fibrinogen–platelet plug are dissolved by the fibrinolytic system, a tightly regulated dynamic system involving enzyme activation, feedback regulation, and blockade by a potent series of inhibitors. Just as there is an interplay between the pro- and anticoagulant components that brings about a blood clot in hemostasis, similar mechanisms occur when blood clots are dissolved via the fibrinolytic process, which is essential for tissue repair. This chapter describes the components of the pro- and anticoagulant system and the pro- and antifibrinolytic system, and the interplay between these systems. The common feature of both systems is the focal presentation of activity that is dependent on the presentation of surface-bound enzymatic complexes that can cleave their respective substrates.

Blood coagulation can best be understood if viewed as a choreographed system that starts from an inventory of the key players, the relationship or connectivity of these players, and the dynamic catalytic processes. These processes together keep blood in a fluid state but primed to react to vascular injury in an explosive manner. Therefore following sections describe the process of blood coagulation in terms of the inventory, the connectivity, and then the dynamics.

INVENTORY: PROCOAGULANT, ANTICOAGULANT, AND FIBRINOLYTIC PROTEINS, INHIBITORS AND RECEPTORS

Putting together an inventory of the blood coagulation components is still ongoing, but what we currently know to date began from initial observations that were made in the fifth century and recorded in the Babylonian Talmud. It was noted that if two male children died of bleeding after circumcision, the third should not be circumcised.[1] Over the centuries, many more hypotheses were made regarding what happens to blood when it escapes from the body.[2,3] The realization that clots stem blood loss only occurred in the 18th century.[2,3] The existence of thrombin, the key enzyme in blood coagulation, was recognized in the 19th century.[2,4]

In 1905, Paul Morawitz proposed the classic theory of coagulation.[5] He hypothesized that in the presence of calcium and thromboplastin, prothrombin was converted to thrombin, which in turn converted fibrinogen to the fibrin clot. These clotting factors were subsequently assigned Roman numerals, factor I (fibrinogen), factor II (prothrombin), factor III (thromboplastin; tissue factor membrane), and factor IV (calcium).[6] As more coagulation factors were introduced, they were assigned consecutive Roman numerals. The activated forms are distinguished by a lower case "a" after their Roman numeral designation. Therefore the activated form of factor V becomes factor Va.

More complex descriptions of the coagulation system were as a "cascade" or "waterfall." Macfarlane[7] and Davie and Ratnoff[8] proposed that in an intrinsic pathway, involving only plasma, blood coagulated by a sequence of events in which the reactions occurred in a defined series leading to fibrin clot formation. Over the past six decades, the Morawitz/Davie and Macfarlane pathways have been significantly expanded (Fig. 126.1). Each reaction shares a similar mechanism in which an inactive zymogen protein is converted to an active enzyme and each "enzyme" is a surface-bound multiprotein complex consisting of a surface, divalent calcium ions (Ca^{2+}), a protease, and a cofactor. Although some facets of these initial descriptions are still valid, the emerging concept of coagulation and fibrinolysis centers on a complex network of highly interwoven concurrent processes. Procoagulant and fibrinolytic events occur simultaneously with many positive- and negative-feedback loops regulating the processes.

To fully understand the multiple simultaneous processes that occur to effect a hemostatic response, we will first inventory the key procoagulant, anticoagulant, and fibrinolytic participants. The inventory sections discuss vitamin K–dependent protein family, cofactor proteins, the intrinsic accessory pathway proteins, endothelium, platelets, proteinase inhibitors, clot proteins, and fibrinolysis proteins.

The Vitamin K–Dependent Protein Family

Vitamin K–dependent proteins, synthesized in the liver, play a central role in blood coagulation through either procoagulant or anticoagulant mechanisms. The vitamin K–dependent protein family includes

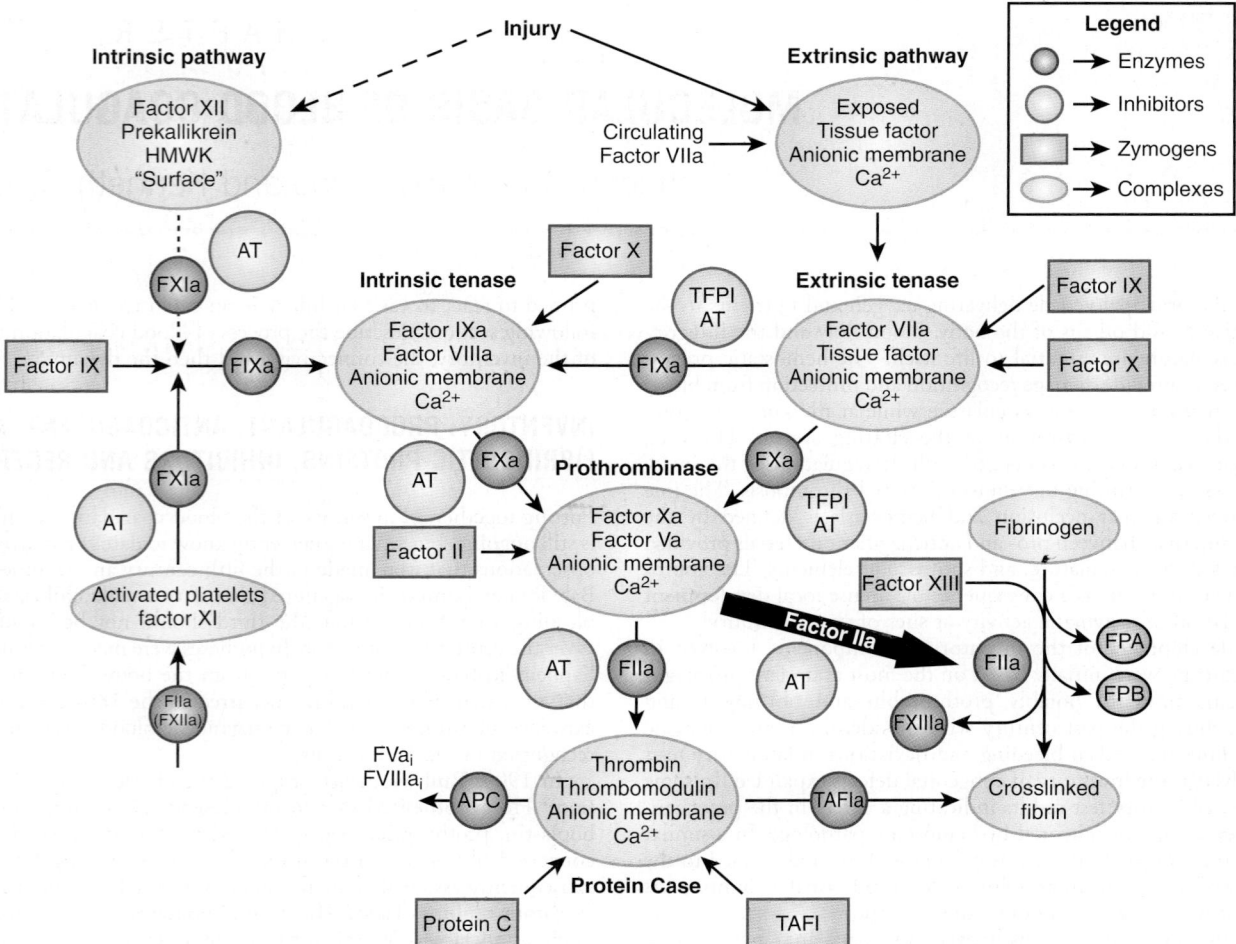

Fig. 126.1 OVERVIEW OF HEMOSTASIS. Coagulation is initiated via two pathways, the primary extrinsic pathway *(right)* and the accessory (historically called the *contact* or *intrinsic pathway*) *(left)*. An illustration of the multistep processes are as follows: enzymes *(small circles)*, inhibitors *(large circles)*, zymogens *(boxes)*, or complexes *(ovals)*. The accessory pathway has no known bleeding etiology associated with it; thus this path is considered accessory to hemostasis. Upon injury to the vessel wall, tissue factor, the cofactor for the extrinsic tenase complex, is exposed to circulating factor VIIa and forms the vitamin K–dependent complex extrinsic tenase. Factor IX and factor X are converted to the serine proteases FIXa and FXa, which then form the intrinsic tenase and prothrombinase complexes, respectively. The combined actions of intrinsic and extrinsic tenase and the prothrombinase complexes lead to an explosive burst of thrombin (IIa). Thrombin not only functions as a procoagulant but also acts as an anticoagulant when complexed with the cofactor thrombomodulin in the protein Case complex. The product of the protein Case reaction, APC, inactivates the cofactors factors Va and VIIIa. The cleaved species, FVa$_i$ and FVIIIa$_i$, no longer support the respective procoagulant activities of the prothrombinase and intrinsic tenase complexes. When thrombin is generated through procoagulant mechanisms, thrombin cleaves fibrinogen, releasing FPA and FPB, and activates factor XIII to form a cross-linked fibrin clot. Thrombin–thrombomodulin also activates TAFI, which delays fibrin degradation by plasmin. The procoagulant response is downregulated by the stoichiometric inhibitors TFPI and AT. TFPI serves to attenuate the activity of extrinsic tenase, the trigger of coagulation. AT directly inhibits thrombin, FIXa, and factor Xa. The accessory pathway provides an alternate route for the generation of factor IXa. Thrombin has also been shown to activate factor XI. *APC,* Activated protein C; *AT,* antithrombin; *FIXa,* factor IXa; *FPA,* fibrinopeptide A; *FPB,* fibrinopeptide B; *FVa$_i$,* factor Va$_i$; *FVIIIa$_i$,* factor VIIIa$_i$; *FXa,* factor Xa; *HMWK,* high-molecular-weight kininogen; *TAFI,* thrombin-activatable fibrinolysis inhibitor; *TFPI,* tissue factor pathway inhibitor.

the zymogen procoagulant factors VII, IX, X, and prothrombin, and the anticoagulants protein C, protein S, and protein Z (Fig. 126.2 and Table 126.1). Except for protein S and protein Z, after cleavage to their active forms these proteins are serine proteases related to the trypsin and chymotrypsin superfamily. Peptide bond cleavage at specific sites converts the vitamin K–dependent zymogens to their active serine protease forms. All share nroncatalytic domains, each of which is characterized by highly conserved regions that fold, independently from the rest of the molecule, into a characteristic

three-dimensional shape. The domains of the vitamin K–dependent proteins are illustrated in Fig. 126.2. Several reviews have been written on vitamin K–dependent proteins.[9–11]

Vitamin K is essential for the biosynthesis of these clotting factors by participating in the cyclic oxidation and reduction of the enzyme that converts 9–13 N-terminal glutamate residues to γ-carboxy glutamate (Gla; Fig. 126.2; see reviews listed in the References[9,12–14]). This posttranslational modification to form Gla residues adds a net negative charge to the molecules that enables the vitamin K–dependent

TABLE 126.1 Procoagulant, Anticoagulant, and Fibrinolytic Proteins, Inhibitors, and Receptors

Protein	Molecular Weight (kD)	Plasma Concentration (nmol/L)	Plasma Concentration (µg/mL)	Plasma $t_{1/2}$ (Days)	Clinical Phenotype Associated with Deficiency	Functional Classification
Procoagulant Proteins and Receptors						
Factor XII	80	500	40	2-3	None	Protease zymogen
HMW kininogen	120	670	80		None	Cofactor
LMW kininogen	66	1300	90			Cofactor
Prekallikrein	85/88	486	42			Protease zymogen
Factor XI	160	30	4.8	2.5-3.3	Sometimes bleeding	Protease zymogen
Tissue factor	44			N/A		Cell-associated cofactor
Factor VII	50	10	0.5	0.25	Bleeding (Occasionally thrombotic)	VKD protease zymogen
Factor X	59	170	10	1.5	Bleeding	VKD protease zymogen
Factor IX	55	90	5	1	Bleeding	VKD protease zymogen
Factor V	330	20	6.6	0.5	Bleeding[a]	Soluble procofactor
Factor VIII	285	1.1-1.5	0.3-0.4	0.3-0.5	Bleeding	Soluble procofactor
vWF	255	Varies	10		Bleeding	Carrier for factor VIII
Factor II	72	1400	100	2.5	Bleeding[b]	VKD protease zymogen
Fibrinogen	340	7400	2500	3-5	Bleeding[c]	Structural clot protein
Factor XIII	320	94	30	9-10	Bleeding	Transglutaminase zymogen
Anticoagulant Proteins, Inhibitors, and Receptors						
Protein C	62	65	4	0.33	Thrombotic	Proteinase zymogen
Protein S	69	300	20	1.75	Thrombotic	Inhibitory cofactor
Protein Z	62	47	2.9	2.5	Sometimes thrombotic	Inhibitory cofactor
Thrombomodulin	100	N/A	N/A	N/A		Cofactor/modulator
Tissue factor pathway inhibitor	40	1-4	0.1	minutes		Proteinase inhibitor
Antithrombin	58	2400	140	2.5-3	Thrombotic	Proteinase inhibitor
Heparin cofactor II	66	500-1400	33-90	2.5	Often thrombotic	Proteinase inhibitor
α_2-Macroglobulin	735	2700-4000	2-3000	<1 hour		Proteinase inhibitor
α_1-Proteinase inhibitor	53	28,000-65,000	1500-3500	6		Proteinase inhibitor
Endothelial protein C receptor						Receptor
Fibrinolytic Proteins, Inhibitors, and Receptors						
Plasminogen	88	2300	210	2.2		Proteinase zymogen
t-PA	70	0.07	0.005	<5 min		Proteinase zymogen
u-PA	54	0.04	0.002	5 min		Proteinase zymogen
TAFI	58	75	4.5	10 min	Thrombotic	Carboxypeptidase
FSAP	64	190	12			Fibrinolytic zymogen
PAI-1	52	0.2	0.01	<10 min	Bleeding	Proteinase inhibitor
PAI-2	47/60	<0.070	<0.005	–		Proteinase inhibitor
α-Antiplasmin	70	500	70	2.6	Bleeding	Proteinase inhibitor

[a]Factor V Leiden mutatation associated with thrombosis.
[b]Prothrombin 20210A mutation associated with thrombosis.
[c]Some fibrinogen mutations associated with thrombosis.
HMW, High-molecular-weight; LMW, low-molecular-weight; VKD, vitamin K–dependent; vWF, von Willebrand factor. FSAP, Factor VII–activating protease; PAI, plasminogen activator inhibitor; TAFI, thrombin-activatable fibrinolysis inhibitor; t-PA, tissue plasminogen activator; u-PA, urinary plasminogen activator (urokinase); u-PAR, urokinase-type plasminogen activator receptor.

proteins to interact with Ca^{2+} and a membrane surface.[15,16] Blocking the formation of the Gla residues is the basis for anticoagulant therapy with coumarin (warfarin) derivatives, which are chemically similar in structure to vitamin K (Fig. 126.3). The Ca^{2+} binding association with this modification is also the basis for the anticoagulant activity of sodium citrate, a calcium chelator, found in the blue-top vacuum tubes used for clinical laboratory testing of clotting activity. The level of inhibition achieved with the same dose of warfarin varies among patients. Increased sensitivity to warfarin has been identified in patients when started after surgery.[17,18] Factors affecting the level of anticoagulation include dietary intake of vitamin K; liver function; concomitant medications that either reduce or enhance the warfarin effect[19]; common polymorphisms in the vitamin K epoxide reductase complex subunit 1 (VKORC1), which is responsible for vitamin K reduction; and polymorphisms in CYP2C9, which affect warfarin metabolism (see reviews listed in the References[20,21]). Therefore genotyping may be helpful to personalize starting doses of warfarin. Ultimately, proper monitoring of warfarin therapy is essential. This is done using the prothrombin time (PT) with the assay sensitivity corrected using the international normalized ratio (INR).[22,23]

The NH_2-terminal Gla domains are followed by either a kringle domain in factor II or an epidermal growth factor–like domain (EGF) in factor VII, factor IX, factor X, protein C, protein S, and protein Z (see Fig. 126.2). Protein S is not a serine protease precursor and instead contains a thrombin-sensitive region before the EGF domain and a sex hormone–binding globulin–like domain (SHBG) in the COOH-terminus.[24] Protein Z contains a "pseudo catalytic domain" in the COOH-terminus and does not function as a serine protease enzyme.[25]

Vitamin K–dependent protein complexes are essential for establishing hemostatic balance (Fig. 126.4). Each complex is composed of a serine protease enzyme, a cofactor that functions as a surface receptor or enhancer for the enzyme Ca^{2+}, and a negatively charged membrane surface provided by activated or damaged cells (e.g., endothelial cells, monocytes, and platelets). There are four vitamin K–dependent complexes: the extrinsic tenase complex (factor

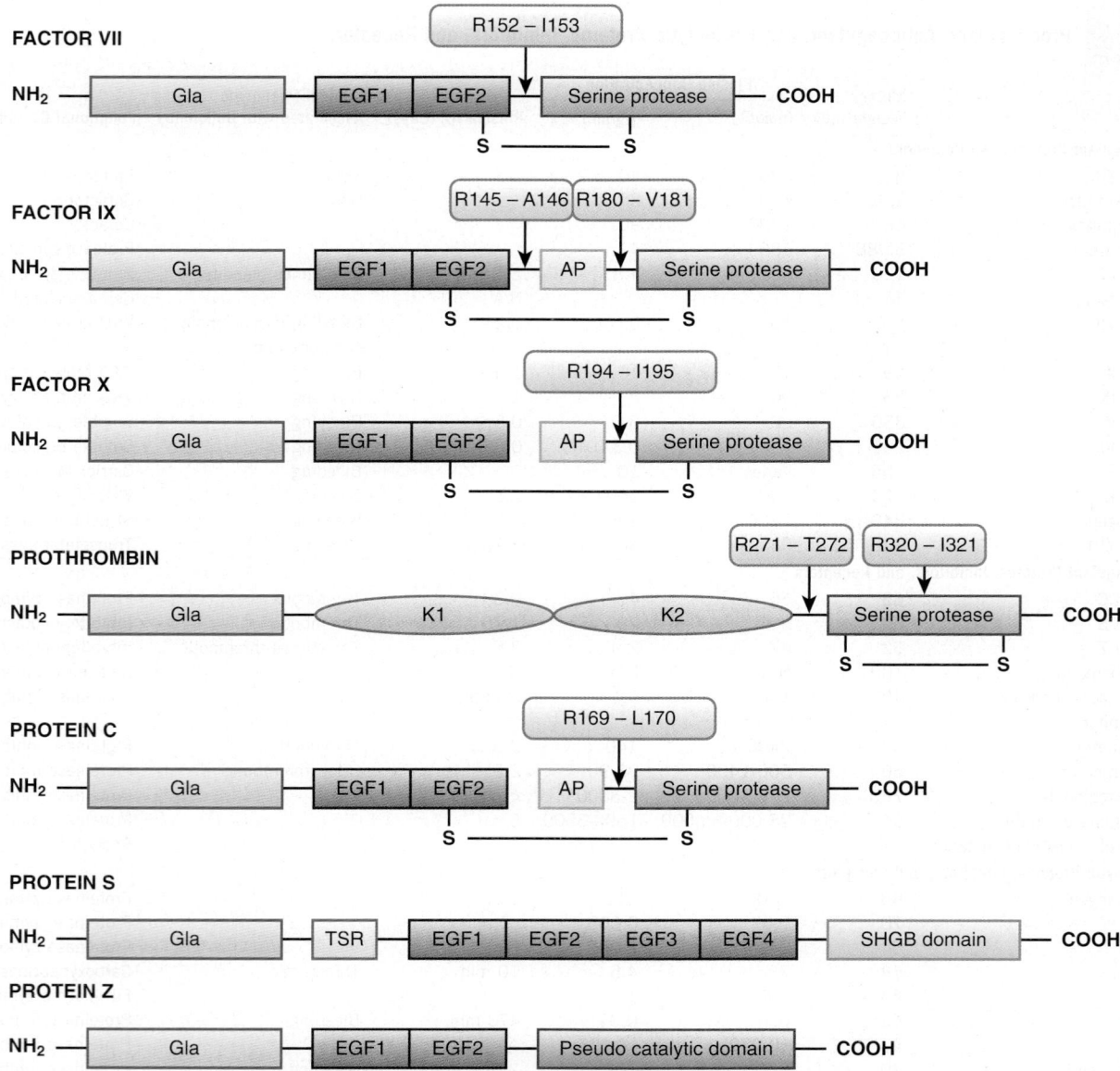

Fig. 126.2 SCHEMATIC REPRESENTATION OF THE VITAMIN K–DEPENDENT PROTEINS. The vitamin K–dependent proteins can be divided into two classes, procoagulant (factors II, VII, IX, and X) and anticoagulant (protein C, protein S, and protein Z). The building blocks for these proteins include an NH$_2$-terminal Gla domain, consisting of nine to 13 Gla residues, followed by either an EGF–like domain in factor VII, factor IX, factor X, protein C, protein S, and protein Z, or a K domain in prothrombin. In protein S, a TSR precedes the EGF domain. Active sites are contained within the serine protease domain. Cleavage sites for the conversion of zymogens to their active forms are designated by *arrows*; activating proteases are placed in *boxes* above the *arrows*. Factor IX, factor X, and protein C are activated by proteolytic removal of an AP. Protein S, which is not a serine protease precursor, contains an SHGB at the COOH-terminus. Protein Z also contains a "pseudo catalytic domain" in the COOH-terminus and does not function as a serine protease. Disulfide bonds (-S-S-) critical to the integrity of the two-chain zymogens or active forms are presented. *AP*, Activation peptide; *EGF*, epidermal growth factor; *K*, kringle; *SHGB*, sex hormone–binding globulin–like domain; *TSR*, thrombin-sensitive region.

VIIa–tissue factor), the intrinsic tenase complex (factor IXa–factor VIIIa), the prothrombinase complex (factor Xa–factor Va), and the anticoagulant protein Case complex (thrombin–thrombomodulin).

When the serine protease is associated with its respective cofactor on an appropriate membrane surface with Ca^{2+}, the specific reactions occur at a rate that is 10^4–10^9-fold faster than that of protease–substrate combination alone.[26] One way to visualize the importance of the assembly of these macromolecular complexes in the formation of the hemostatic plug is to note that if a healthy person takes 4 minutes for his or her blood to clot, then in the absence of membrane and cofactor, blood clot formation would take approximately 3.8 years.

Cofactor Proteins

There are two categories of procoagulant cofactor proteins; the cell-bound cofactors (tissue factor and thrombomodulin) and the soluble plasma-derived procoagulant procofactors (factor V and factor VIII with its circulating carrier von Willebrand factor [vWF]).

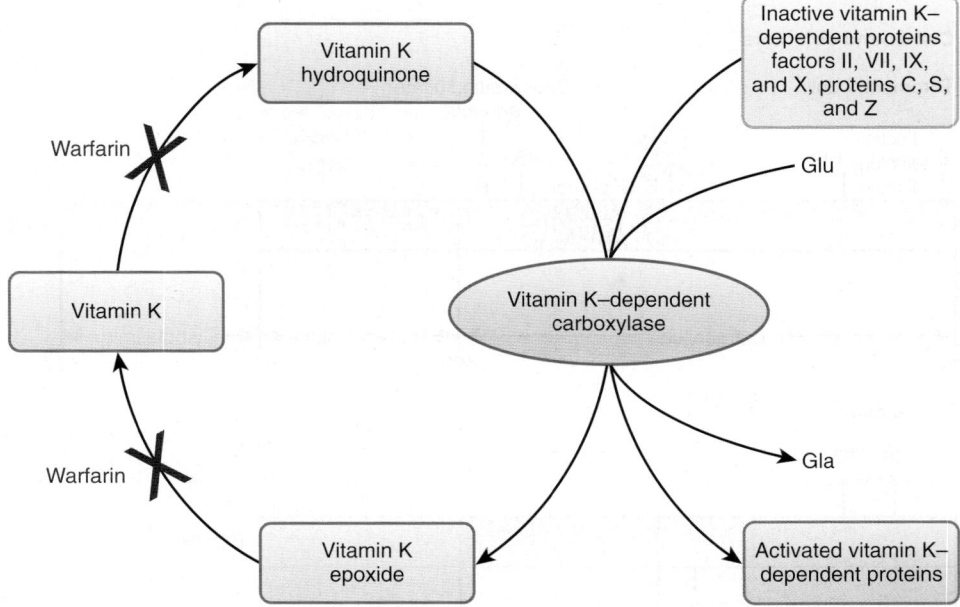

Fig. 126.3 VITAMIN K–DEPENDENT PROCESS AND WARFARIN EFFECT. Schematic representation of the mechanism of γ-carboxy glutamate generation by a vitamin K–dependent reaction cycle to produce an active protein is illustrated. The regeneration of vitamin K hydroquinone by the vitamin K–dependent reductases is inhibited by warfarin.

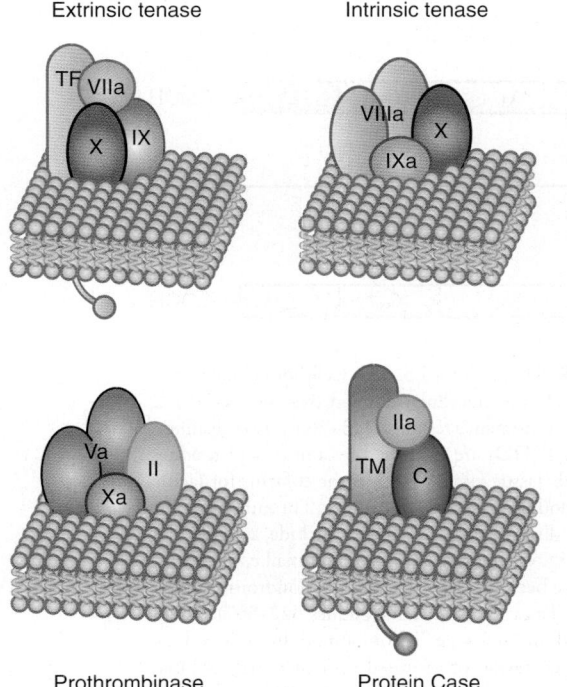

Fig. 126.4 VITAMIN K–DEPENDENT COMPLEXES. Three procoagulant complexes (extrinsic tenase, intrinsic tenase, and prothrombinase) and one anticoagulant complex (protein Case) are illustrated. Each membrane complex consists of a vitamin K–dependent serine protease (factor VIIa [VIIa], factor IXa [IXa], factor Xa [Xa], or thrombin [IIa]) and a soluble or cell surface–associated cofactor (factor VIIIa [heavy and light chain VIII$_H$ and VIII$_L$], factor Va [heavy and light chain V$_H$ and V$_L$], tissue factor [TF], or thrombomodulin [TM]). Each serine protease is shown in association with the appropriate cofactor protein and zymogen substrate(s) on the membrane surface. The membrane serves as a scaffold for the coagulation reactants, enhancing the reaction rates by 10^4–10^9-fold.

Cell-Bound Cofactors

Tissue Factor

Tissue factor is a transmembrane protein that functions as a nonenzymatic cofactor for factor VIIa in the extrinsic tenase complex[27] (see reviews listed in the References[28,29]; Fig. 126.5A). In the absence of injury or inflammatory stimuli, tissue factor is not expressed on cellular surfaces in direct contact with circulating blood (see the review listed in the References[30]). Presentation of tissue factor to the circulation is the event that triggers the primary procoagulant pathway of coagulation[31–33] (see Fig. 126.1). There are no known mutations or deficiencies of human tissue factor, and tissue factor deletion in mice is lethal during embryonic development,[34] leading to the speculation that tissue factor is essential for life.

Tissue factor activity is primarily regulated by controlling its presentation. The commonly accepted sources of functional tissue factor are the subendothelium exposed upon vascular damage or monocytes stimulated by cytokines. However, there is controversy regarding the source and presentation of active tissue factor and whether functional tissue factor circulates in blood in healthy and pathologic states.[35–40] Microparticle sources of blood-borne tissue factor are generally defined as submicron-sized cell-derived membrane fragments produced in response to activation or apoptosis. Their role in hemostasis is still debated.[28,35,41,42]

Thrombomodulin

Thrombomodulin is a type 1 transmembrane protein constitutively expressed on the surface of vascular endothelial cells (see Fig. 126.5A). Thrombomodulin is a high-affinity receptor for all thrombin forms and acts as a cofactor for the thrombin-dependent activation of protein C.[43] The endothelial cell protein C receptor (EPCR) provides cell-specific binding sites for both protein C and activated protein C (APC).[44–47] When bound to thrombomodulin, thrombin's procoagulant activities (e.g., its capacity to generate fibrin and activate factor V, factor VIII, factor XI, and platelets) are neutralized, and the rate of inactivation of thrombin by antithrombin is increased.[48–50] The generation of APC by the thrombin–thrombomodulin complex leads to inactivation of the procoagulant cofactors factor Va and factor VIIIa, thus suppressing thrombin formation.[51,52] Thrombin–thrombomodulin, or the "protein Case" (see Fig. 126.4) complex,

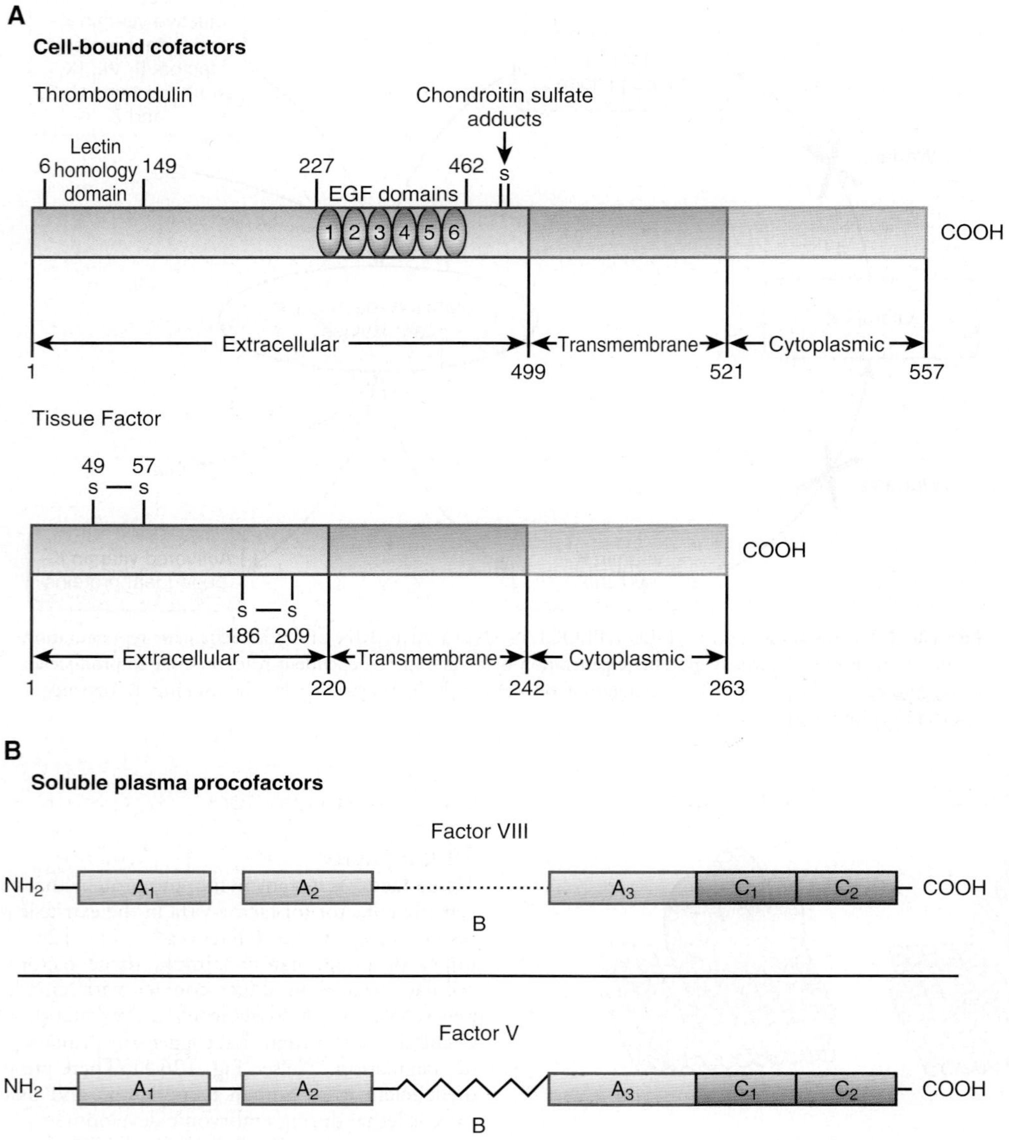

A

Cell-bound cofactors

Thrombomodulin

Chondroitin sulfate
adducts

Lectin
6 homology 149   227   462 S
domain   EGF domains

1 2 3 4 5 6   COOH

Extracellular →← Transmembrane →← Cytoplasmic →

1   499   521   557

Tissue Factor

49 57
S — S

COOH

S — S
186 209

Extracellular →← Transmembrane →← Cytoplasmic →

1   220   242   263

B

Soluble plasma procofactors

Factor VIII

NH₂ — A₁ — A₂ ········· A₃ C₁ C₂ — COOH

B

Factor V

NH₂ — A₁ — A₂ ⋀⋁⋀ A₃ C₁ C₂ — COOH

B

Fig. 126.5 CELL-BOUND AND SOLUBLE COFACTOR STRUCTURES. (A) Cell-bound cofactors: tissue factor and thrombomodulin. Tissue factor is composed of an extracellular domain (residues 1–219), a transmembrane domain (residues 220–242), and a cytoplasmic domain (residues 243–263). Two disulfide bonds (-S-S-) and the sites of the three carbohydrate moieties (CHO) are identified by amino acid residue. One cysteine (C^{245}) contains a thiol ester linkage to a fatty acid. Tissue factor, which is the cofactor for factor VIIa in the extrinsic tenase complex, is exposed on the subendothelial surface after injury. Thrombomodulin is an endothelial cell-surface glycoprotein composed of five distinct domains. These include a lectin-like domain (residues 6–149), a domain containing six EGF–like regions (residues 227–462), a small extracellular domain rich in threonine and serine residues (S^{472} and S^{474} have been identified as sites of chondroitin sulfate adducts), a membrane-spanning region (residues 499–521), and a cytoplasmic tail (residues 522–557). There are nine known glycosylation sites (CHO) on the thrombomodulin molecule. Thrombomodulin functions as the cofactor in the protein Case complex and assists in the generation of activated protein C. (B) Soluble plasma procofactors: factor VIII and factor V. The linear domain structures (A1–A2–A3–C1–C2) are illustrated with *horizontal arrows* bracketed by the beginning and ending amino acid number. Thrombin (IIa) and activated protein C cleavage sites are shown with *vertical arrows*. The B regions (factor V, residues 709–1545; factor VIII, residues 740–1689) are represented by the *crosshatched regions*. *EGF,* Epidermal growth factor.

also has an antifibrinolytic role via activation of the fibrinolysis inhibitor, thrombin-activatable fibrinolysis inhibitor (TAFI; see reviews listed in the References[53–56]).

Thrombomodulin activity on the surface of endothelial cells is decreased by inflammatory cytokines,[57,58] and this decrease may contribute to the hypercoagulation characteristic of inflammatory states.

Soluble Plasma Procofactors

Factor V

Factor V is a large single-chain glycoprotein (GP) that circulates in human plasma (see Table 126.1 and Fig. 126.5B) and is also contained in the α-granules of human platelets, with approximately 18%–25% of the total factor V found in platelets.[59] The procofactor

factor V is proteolyzed by α-thrombin to the active cofactor factor Va.[60] Factor Va functions both as a factor Xa receptor and positive modulator of factor Xa catalytic potential in the prothrombinase complex (see Fig. 126.4).[61] Factor Va is proteolytically inactivated by APC.[62,63] The importance of this regulatory mechanism is demonstrated by the "APC resistance" syndrome associated with factor V^{Leiden}.[64,65] Individuals with factor V^{Leiden} have a G to A substitution at nucleotide 1691 in the factor V gene that results in an Arg^{506}→Gln mutation at the protein level.[66] Factor Va^{Leiden} has normal cofactor activity as part of the prothrombinase complex. However, unlike normal factor Va, factor Va^{Leiden} is more slowly inactivated by APC. The Arg^{506}→Gln mutation hinders the first step in the series of inactivating cleavages by APC. Cleaved factor Va^{Leiden} retains limited cofactor activity and continues to promote thrombin generation. The identification, role in coagulation, and overall importance of factor V in hemostasis have been described in numerous reviews.[61,67]

Factor VIII

The soluble procofactor factor VIII, or antihemophilic factor (see Fig. 126.5B), circulates in plasma in complex with the large multimeric protein vWF.[68] vWF acts to regulate the plasma concentration of factor VIII. Factor VIII interaction with vWF requires the NH$_2$- and COOH-termini of the factor VIII light chain (A3, C1, and C2 domains), although a specific vWF binding site has been identified at residues 1673–1684 on the light chain.[68–71] Factor VIII is activated by thrombin cleavage at three sites (Arg^{372}, Arg^{740}, Arg^{1689}) to generate the heterotrimeric cofactor factor VIIIa.[72] The vWF binding site is removed from the factor VIII protein by thrombin cleavage at Arg^{1689}. After forming, vWF–free factor VIIIa forms a complex with the serine protease factor IXa, Ca^{2+}, and a membrane (provided by platelets), resulting in the intrinsic tenase (see Fig. 126.4). Factor VIIIa function is downregulated by the relatively rapid dissociation of the noncovalently associated A2 subunit, which is produced by the cleavages required for activation. Factor VIII is homologous (40% identity) to the procofactor factor V.[73]

Deficiency of factor VIII, or hemophilia A, is a well-characterized bleeding disorder linked to the X chromosome.[74] Hemophilia A therefore occurs almost exclusively in males at a frequency of 1 in 5000 to 1 in 10,000 individuals.[75]

von Willebrand Factor

vWF has several key roles in coagulation. It is synthesized in endothelial cells and also contained in the α-granules of human platelets.[76] vWF is a large adhesive GP that circulates in plasma as a heterogeneous mixture of disulfide-linked multimers that range in size from dimers (M$_r$ = 600,000) to extremely large multimers of more than 20 million kDa. vWF has binding sites for factor VIII, heparin, collagen, platelet GPIb, and platelet GPIIb–IIIa.[77–90] vWF acts as the bridge between platelets to promote platelet aggregation. The primary platelet binding site for vWF is the GPIb–IX–V receptor complex. GPIb–IX–V is an active receptor on unstimulated platelets and serves to promote platelet aggregation and adhesion to vWF in the absence of platelet activation.[91]

vWF is a structural protein and is part of the subendothelial matrix. Endothelial cells secrete vWF multimers, which are larger than those found circulating in plasma.[92] The function of these large multimeric forms of vWF is to bind to and agglutinate blood platelets under high shear conditions. These large multimers of vWF are degraded by a specific metalloprotease called a disintegrin and metalloproteinase with a thrombospondin type 1 motif, member 13 (ADAMTS)-13.[93–95] In familial and acquired thrombotic thrombocytopenic purpura, ultra-large vWF multimers are correlated with defective ADAMTS-13 activity.[96]

ABO blood type has a significant influence on vWF levels, with individuals of types A, B, or AB blood having much higher levels of vWF than those with type O blood.[97,98] vWF is also known for its role in ristocetin-induced platelet agglutination,[99,100] which is the basis of clinical assays for von Willebrand disease, a fairly common disorder that is estimated to occur in 1%–2% of the general population (see Chapter 138).[101–104] vWF is also an acute-phase reactant,

and vWF levels are elevated as a result of stress, pregnancy, or surgical trauma.[105–108]

The Intrinsic Accessory Pathway Proteins

The designation "intrinsic accessory pathway" emerged as the relationship between genetic deficiencies and bleeding phenotypes was established (see Fig. 126.1). Deficiencies of proteins associated with the intrinsic or accessory pathway (factor XII, prekallikrein, and high-molecular-weight kininogen [HMWK]) are not ordinarily associated with excessive bleeding, even after surgical challenge.[109–111] In contrast, deficiencies of the protein components of the extrinsic or primary pathway (prothrombin and factors V, VII, VIII, IX, and X) can lead to severe bleeding diatheses.[112–116] The physiologic role of the accessory pathway is therefore not clearly understood.[117]

Although the intrinsic pathway proteins have no defined role in normal hemostasis, these accessory pathway factors are thought to play a key role in disseminated intravascular coagulation associated with the systemic inflammatory response syndrome[118,119] and in the promotion of thrombus stability,[117,120,121] and may be a new target to control pathologic coagulation.[122] Also, the accessory pathway is important in cardiopulmonary bypass because of contact between blood components and synthetic surfaces.[119] Recent evidence suggests that biologic activation of the contact pathway system may be accomplished through assembly of these proteins on endothelial cell membranes and that prekallikrein is activated by an endothelial cell membrane cysteine protease rather than by factor XII.[123,124] Extracellular RNA derived from damaged or necrotic cells has also been found to participate in the activation of proteases of the contact pathway by providing a procoagulant cofactor template for factor XII- or XI-induced contact activation.[125] Polyphosphates, linear inorganic polymers of 60–100 phosphate residues, released from platelets have also been shown to activate fXII.[126]

In principle, factor XI represents an intersection point for the two pathways. Individuals with factor XI deficiency (hemophilia C) have a variable bleeding phenotype upon surgical challenge,[127,128] therefore establishing an essential role for factor XI in hemostasis. During the coagulation process, factor XIa formation appears to be catalyzed by thrombin as part of a positive-feedback loop stemming from thrombin generation.[129] Factor XIa then functions in the propagation phase of thrombin generation in association with the primary pathway by activation of factor IX.[130]

Three proteins, factor XII, prekallikrein, and HMWK, are required for activity of the intrinsic or accessory pathway. Factor XII and prekallikrein are zymogens that are activated to generate serine proteases, and HMWK is a nonenzymatic procofactor (Fig. 126.6). The activation of this pathway in vitro is accomplished when factor XII autoactivates to factor XIIa upon exposure to foreign surfaces, including kaolin, dextran sulfate, and sulfatides.[131–133] The substrates for factor XIIa, prekallikrein, and factor XI exist in noncovalent complex with HMWK and become activated to kallikrein and factor XIa, respectively.[134] Positive-feedback loops exist in which kallikrein cleaves HMWK, thereby releasing bradykinin and allowing more prekallikrein and factor XI to associate and activate.[135] This pathway is also negatively regulated by the cleavage of HMWK by factor XIa.[136]

Proteinase Inhibitors

Proteinases, enzymes that hydrolyze peptide bonds, are found in a wide array of biologic systems, including the blood coagulation process (clot formation and fibrinolysis), digestive system, apoptotic cascades, and the immune system. To keep these systems in balance between activation and inhibition, a complex system of proteinase inhibitors has evolved. In blood, proteinase inhibitors constitute a significant percentage of circulating proteins. In general, proteinases that activate the coagulation and fibrinolytic cascades have highly defined substrate specificities. Coagulation is kept in check through

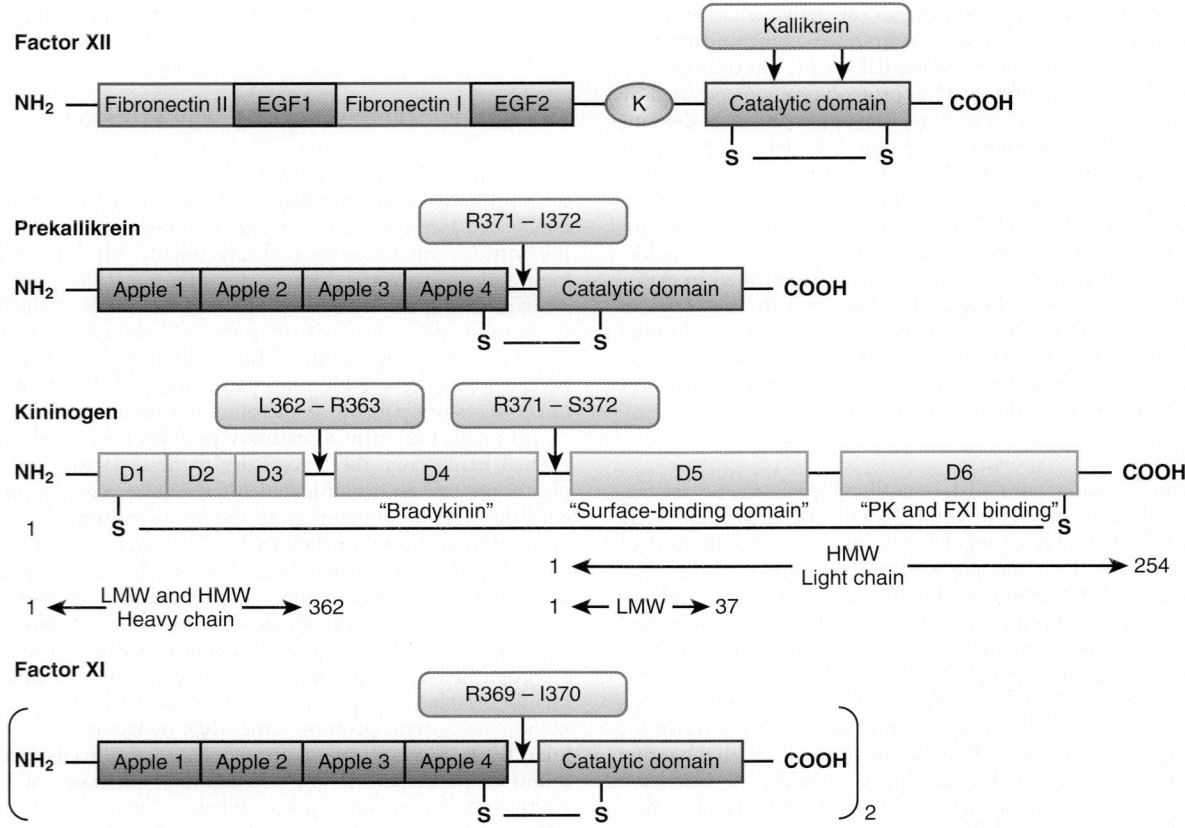

Fig. 126.6 SCHEMATIC REPRESENTATION OF THE ACCESSORY PATHWAY (INTRINSIC) PROTEINS. Factor XII, prekallikrein, kininogen, and factor XI are shown with their various domains depicted. Cleavage sites for activation are identified with an *arrow*, and with the specific amino acid residues of the site shown. Key interchain disulfide bonds (-S-S-) are included. For the kininogens, *horizontal arrows* indicate the amino acid residues defining heavy and light chain regions of the activated forms of the cofactors. Factor XI is illustrated as a monomer. *EGF*, Epidermal growth factor; *FXI*, factor XI; *HMW*, high molecular weight; *LMW*, low molecular weight; *PK*, prekallikrein.

the action of several specific and broad-spectrum proteinase inhibitors. Specific clot formation inhibitors are antithrombin, tissue factor pathway inhibitor (TFPI), heparin cofactor II, and protein C inhibitor. Together specific and broad-spectrum inhibitors function to localize, limit, and control hemostasis (see Chapter 127).

Antithrombin

Antithrombin is a member of the serpin proteinase inhibitory family and circulates in blood as a single-chain GP[137] (see Table 126.1; Fig. 126.7). Congenital antithrombin deficiency exhibits an autosomal dominant pattern of inheritance, with an incidence of 1 in 2000 to 1 in 5000.[138] Individuals with this deficiency have partial expression of antithrombin and are prone to venous thromboembolic disease.[139] The complete absence of antithrombin is lethal.

Antithrombin has a broad spectrum of inhibitory activity, with most of its target proteases participating in the coagulation cascade (see Fig. 126.1). It is primarily an inhibitor of the serine proteases thrombin, factor Xa, factor IXa, factor VIIa–tissue factor, factor XIa, factor XIIa, kallikrein, and HMWK.[140–142] Heparin and heparan sulfate potentiate these reactions, and heparin is used for the prevention and treatment of thrombosis. When antithrombin is complexed with heparin, its rate of inhibition of several coagulation proteases is accelerated by up to 10,000-fold. The general mechanism of inhibition involves reaction of the active site of the enzyme with a peptide loop structure (the reactive center loop) of antithrombin, forming a tight, equimolar (1:1) complex. Inactivation proceeds through covalent bond formation between antithrombin and the protease followed by inactivating structural rearrangements of both antithrombin and the protease.

Antithrombin also displays antiproliferative and antiinflammatory properties that primarily derive from its ability to inhibit thrombin. In addition, latent or cleaved forms of antithrombin have antiangiogenic activities.[143]

Tissue Factor Pathway Inhibitor

TFPI, formerly called *extrinsic pathway inhibitor* or *lipoprotein-associated coagulation inhibitor*, is a multivalent Kunitz-type plasma proteinase inhibitor. It circulates in plasma as a heterogeneous collection of partially proteolyzed forms[144–147] (see Table 126.1 and Fig. 126.7). Up to 90% of circulating TFPI is found associated with lipoproteins, primarily low-density lipoprotein.[144,148,149] Parenteral TFPI is cleared from the circulation mainly by the liver and has an unusually short half-life (minutes) compared with other proteinase inhibitors.

Many reviews of TFPI have been published.[150–160] The importance of TFPI in blood coagulation is best illustrated through transgenic mice with complete TFPI deficiency; the deficiency is embryonic lethal.[154] However, this lethality in mice can be rescued by heterozygous or homozygous factor VII deficiency.[161] This implies that diminishing the level of factor VII lessens the need for TFPI-mediated inhibition of the factor VIIa–tissue factor coagulation pathway during embryogenesis.[161] Similarly, the combination of low normal TFPI with factor V Leiden is lethal.[162,163] Mice with combined heterozygous TFPI deficiency and homozygous apolipoprotein E deficiency develop more extensive atherosclerosis burden,[164] raising the possibility that TFPI contributes to protection from atherosclerosis, as well as serving as a regulator of thrombosis.

TFPI is the principal stoichiometric inhibitor of the extrinsic factor tenase complex (factor VIIa–tissue factor).[165] Effective TFPI

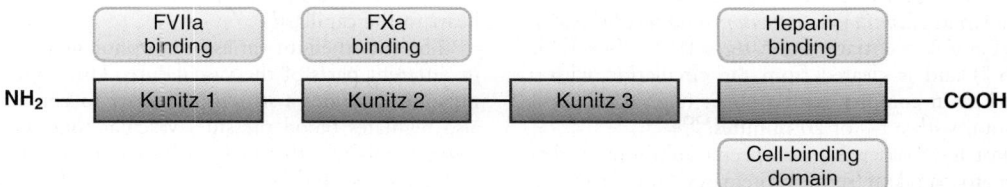

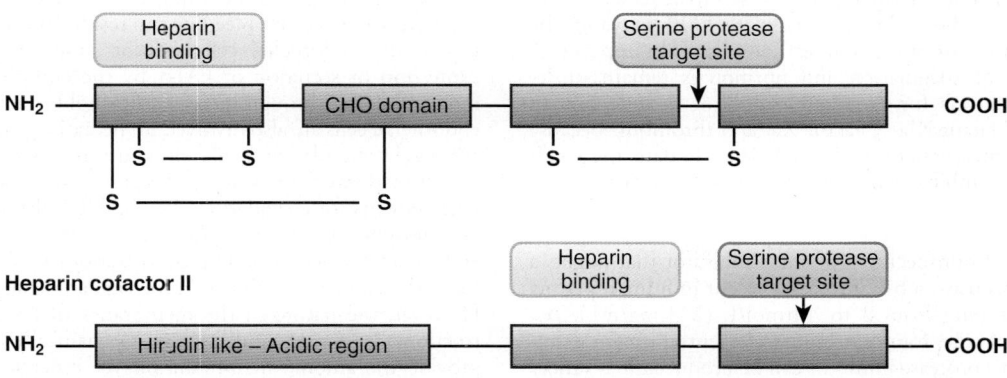

Protein C inhibitor

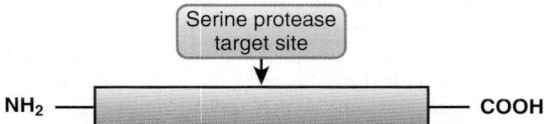

Fig. 126.7 SCHEMATIC REPRESENTATION OF SEVERAL PROTEINASE INHIBITORS. Tissue factor pathway inhibitor (TFPI) contains three Kunitz domains. TFPI inhibits the serine proteases FVIIa and FXa, shutting down the extrinsic pathway of coagulation. Kunitz 1 domain binds FVIIa, and Kunitz 2 domain binds FXa. The COOH-terminus of TFPI contains a basic region, the cell-binding domain, which binds to heparin. Antithrombin (AT) contains two intrachain disulfide bonds (-S-S-) in its NH$_2$-terminus and one in its COOH-terminus with a carbohydrate-rich domain (CHO) in between. The region of interaction between the active sites of target proteases and AT is illustrated (reactive center loop). Heparin binding occurs in the NH$_2$-terminus and enhances the rate of inhibition of serine proteases. Heparin cofactor II inhibits thrombin. Structurally, the inhibitor contains an NH$_2$-terminus hirudin-like region, a heparin or dermatan sulfate binding region, and a reactive center loop. The reactive site is shown at Leu[444]. Protein C inhibitor is a serine protease inhibitor that inhibits several proteases, including activated protein C, thrombin, and FXa. It is also a potent inhibitor of the thrombin–thrombomodulin complex. The reactive bond (Arg[354]) in the reactive center loop is shown. *FVIIa*, Factor VIIa; *FXa*, factor Xa.

inhibition of the factor VIIa–tissue factor complex depends on the presence of factor Xa. Thus inhibition of the extrinsic factor tenase by TFPI occurs only after significant factor IXa and factor Xa formation. Inhibition by TFPI is achieved by formation of the stable quaternary, by tissue factor–factor VIIa–TFPI–factor Xa complex, and by formation of the factor Xa–TFPI complex directly.

Heparin Cofactor II

Heparin cofactor II is a member of the serpin family (see Fig. 126.7). The plasma concentration of heparin cofactor II is 0.5–1.4 μmol/L[166,167] (see Table 126.1). Its plasma half-life is approximately 2.5 days. Similar to antithrombin, heparin cofactor II inhibits thrombin in a reaction that is accelerated more than 1000-fold by heparin.[168] However, unlike antithrombin, the only coagulation enzyme inhibited by heparin cofactor II is thrombin.[169] The rate of thrombin inhibition by heparin cofactor II in the absence or presence of heparin or heparin-like molecules is significantly slower than by antithrombin under similar conditions. Considering that the plasma concentration of heparin cofactor II is 25%–50% that of antithrombin and that low levels of heparin cofactor II are not strongly associated with

thrombosis,[170] the physiologic role of heparin cofactor II as a systemic thrombin inhibitor has been questioned.

In vitro, heparin cofactor II inhibition of thrombin is accelerated by dermatan sulfate proteoglycans synthesized by fibroblasts and vascular smooth muscle cells.[171] Thus heparin cofactor II may be uniquely suited to regulate extravascular thrombin in areas of vascular endothelium disruption in which heparin cofactor II would be exclusively stimulated by dermatan sulfate in the subendothelium. In addition, heparin cofactor II may participate in regulation of acute inflammation and wound healing by harboring a peptide chemotactic for neutrophils and monocytes that is released by leukocyte proteolysis.[172]

Heparin cofactor II may also have a role in protection from thrombosis during pregnancy. Increased levels of dermatan sulfate in the maternal and fetal circulation[173] along with increased levels of heparin cofactor II in pregnant women have been reported.[174,175] Low levels of thrombin–heparin cofactor II complexes are detected in normal plasma samples; elevated levels were detected in patients with disseminated intravascular coagulation.[176] Although inherited deficiency of heparin cofactor II has been associated with thrombosis, this is not always the case.[177–179]

Protein C Inhibitor

Protein C inhibitor is a member of the serine proteinase inhibitor family and is also known as *plasminogen activator inhibitor-3* (PAI-3). It circulates in blood at a concentration of 5 µg/mL[180,181] (see Table 126.1 and Fig. 126.7) and is cleared from the circulation with a half-life of 1 day. When in complex with a target (e.g., APC), it is cleared from circulation with a $t_{1/2}$ of 20 minutes.[182]

Protein C inhibitor is considered a nonspecific inhibitor in that its targets range from procoagulant (serine proteinases), anticoagulant, and fibrinolytic enzymes to plasma and tissue kallikreins, the sperm protease acrosin, and prostate-specific antigen.[183,184] The major target of protein C inhibitor, as its name suggests, appears to be APC.[182,185,186] Protein C inhibitor has been shown to regulate TAFI activation by inhibiting the thrombin–thrombomodulin complex.[187] Its importance as a dual regulator of coagulation and fibrinolysis remains unresolved.[188,189] Other targets for protein C inhibitor include human plasma kallikrein,[190] factor XIa,[190] factor Xa, and thrombin. Because there are no documented patients with a deficiency to date, the actual function of protein C inhibitor in vivo has yet to be elucidated.

α₂-Macroglobulin

α₂-Macroglobulin is a nonspecific proteinase inhibitor that targets a broad spectrum of protease substrates. It is present in human plasma at concentrations ranging from 2 to 4 µmol/L (2–3 mg/mL). α₂-Macroglobulin can also be found in higher concentrations in extravascular fluids.[191] This protease inhibitor can be produced in a variety of cells, including hepatocytes, fibroblasts, and macrophages.[192,193] Human α₂-macroglobulin circulates in plasma as a tetramer.[191–198] α₂-Macroglobulin has a unique mechanism of action, which accounts for its broad specificity. The initial step involves the "bait region" of α₂-macroglobulin.[199] After proteolysis in this bait region, α₂-macroglobulin undergoes conformational changes that trap the proteinase inside the molecule.[199] Consequently, α₂-macroglobulin inhibits a broad range of proteinases. It is distinctive in its capacity to inhibit members from each of four mechanistic classes of proteinases (serine, cysteine, and aspartic proteinases, and metalloproteinases). α₂-Macroglobulin functions as a secondary inhibitor of serine proteinases in plasma by inhibiting thrombin, kallikrein, and plasmin.[200,201] It may also be important in preventing thromboembolic events when there is a congenital deficiency of antithrombin or acquired deficiency in sepsis.[202,203] α₂-Macroglobulin also inhibits various growth factors and cytokines, including transforming growth factor-α (TGF-α),[204] interleukin (IL)-1β,[205] IL-6,[206] acidic fibroblast growth factor,[207] basic fibroblast growth factor,[207] tumor necrosis factor-α (TNF-α),[208] and IL-2.[209] Polymorphisms identified in α₂-macroglobulin have been thought to play a role in Alzheimer disease.[210–212] Overall, the biologic role of α₂-macroglobulin in vivo is still being elucidated.

Reduced levels of α₂-macroglobulin in humans have been observed in individuals with chronic obstructive lung disease[213] and metastatic cancer.[214] Complete deficiency has not been reported, suggesting that absence of α₂-macroglobulin is incompatible with survival. Inactivation of the α₂-macroglobulin gene in mice has no obvious phenotype, but the mice are resistant to endotoxin challenge.[215] It has been suggested that α₂-macroglobulin serves as a neutralizer of TGF-α and an inducer of nitric oxide synthesis in mice.[216]

Endothelium

Blood cells and the vasculature are crucial to normal hemostasis. Multiple processes involving components of the vessel wall, circulating platelets, and plasma protein moieties interact to maintain blood fluidity. These must be precisely choreographed to allow the vasculature to perform its myriad complex physiologic activities (Fig. 126.8). The endothelium, the thin layer of cells that lines the interior of blood and lymphatic vessels, plays a key role because of its strategic interface among organs, tissues, and circulating blood. The cells that form the endothelium are called *endothelial cells*, those in direct contact with blood are called *vascular endothelial cells*, and those in direct contact with lymph are known as *lymphatic endothelial cells*. Vascular endothelial cells line the entire circulatory system (from the heart to the capillaries).

The endothelium varies in morphology and physiologic function in different parts of the vasculature. This complex cellular network not only provides a structural barrier to contain flowing blood but also regulates blood pressure, vascular tone, permeability, and processes involving other cells such as smooth muscle cells, leukocytes, and platelets, and deposits an intricate basement membrane and extracellular matrix.[217] In addition, the endothelium is involved in inflammatory and immune responses and angiogenesis.[218] Defects in vascular endothelium function, therefore, have profound physiologic implications. Excessive bleeding can result from structural abnormalities of the endothelial cell layer or supporting matrix. Impaired expression or secretion of PAI-1 by the endothelium likewise promotes bleeding through increased fibrinolytic activity.[219] Conversely, endothelial cells are also involved in mediating processes that promote atherosclerotic plaque formation and thrombotic pathologies.[220]

The early work of Ware and Seegers[221] identified the phospholipid requirements for coagulation. The biologic elements contributing to the phospholipid include damaged vascular tissue-activated platelets and inflammatory cells. The contributions of the membrane to the formation and expression of procoagulant complexes are essential. However, the nature of the membranes that support procoagulant reactions is poorly understood. Mechanically damaged cells can provide the anionic membrane bilayer inner leaflet phospholipids, which can support general procoagulant complex formation; however, more subtle cellular activation events also generate selective complex-forming sites on intact cells. Activated platelet membranes express individual binding sites for the factor IXa–factor VIIIa and factor Xa–factor Va complexes. Hemorrhagic pathology is therefore associated with thrombocytopenia and is also displayed in a rare disease, Scott syndrome, which appears to result from the improper presentation of these platelet binding sites.[222] Binding sites have also been reported on a number of peripheral blood cells, especially activated monocytes. The vascular endothelium itself can provide binding sites after stimulation by cytokine growth factors.[223] The endothelium also provides the anticoagulant thrombomodulin, TFPI and heparan sulfate. The EPCR provides cell-specific binding sites for both protein C and APC.[44,224] EPCR is downregulated by TNF-α.[44] Monocytes appear to express specific binding sites for APC that are distinct from the endothelial cell protein C receptor.[225] The cell-expressed binding sites may be important in the antiinflammatory properties of APC.[46]

A further consequence of damage to the endothelium is the release of pathologic quantities of vWF, which promote platelet aggregation and adhesion to the subendothelium, and thus the formation of potentially fatal thrombi. Endothelial dysfunction is also linked with hypertension, diabetes, obesity, and hyperlipidemia.

Platelets

Platelets, or thrombocytes, are vital to procoagulant events and contribute to the fibrinolytic process as well. They are small, irregularly shaped clear cell fragments, which are derived from megakaryocytes. The average lifespan of a platelet is approximately 5–9 days. Platelets are at the balance of bleeding or clotting events: when platelet numbers are low (thrombocytopenia), excessive bleeding can occur, and when platelet numbers are high (thrombocytosis), thrombosis can occur. Disorders that reduce the number of platelets but typically cause thrombosis instead of bleeding are heparin-induced thrombocytopenia and thrombotic thrombocytopenic purpura.

Similar to the endothelium, the undisturbed platelet presents a nonthrombogenic surface. Important components of platelet physiology are surface adhesion protein complexes and the platelet secretory granules: α-granules, lysosomes, and dense granules. Contents of the α-granules include procoagulant and adhesive proteins such as fibrinogen, fibronectin, thrombospondin, vWF, P-selectin, HMWK, platelet factor 4, osteonectin, factor V,[59] and factor XI.[226] Other α-granule contents, α₁-antitrypsin, protein S, TFPI, and platelet

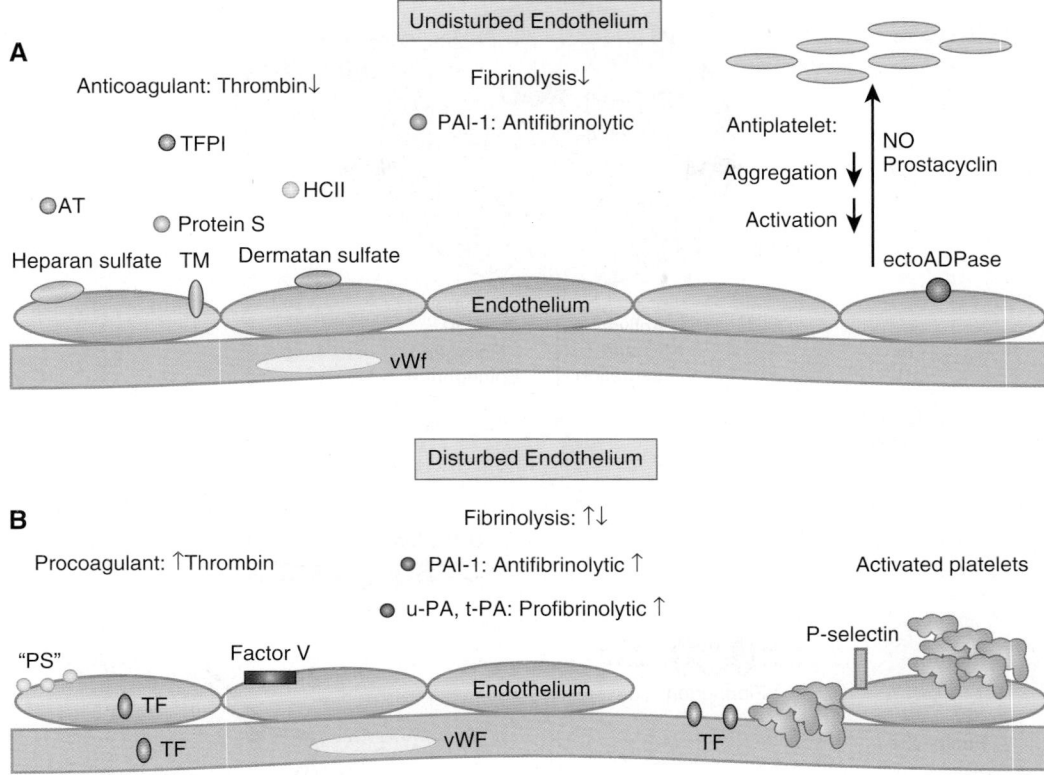

Fig. 126.8 SCHEMATIC OF THE CHANGES THAT OCCUR TO THE ENDOTHELIUM UPON INJURY. Under normal conditions in the absence of injury or chemical stimulus (A), *the undisturbed endothelium* actively downregulates thrombin generation through production of TFPI, AT, protein S, heparan sulfate, TM, and dermatan sulfate. The undisturbed endothelium is also antifibrinolytic and secretes PAI-1. In the absence of a stimulus, the endothelium likewise prevents platelet activation, secretion, and aggregation through production of NO, prostacyclin, and the membrane-associated protein ectoADPase. When the *endothelium is disturbed* (B), the endothelium becomes procoagulant and accelerates thrombin formation by exposing or expressing anionic phospholipid ("PS"), TF, and factor V. The fibrinolytic response is modulated by the release of both antifibrinolytic and profibrinolytic molecules. u-PA and t-PA are profibrinolytic and serve to activate plasminogen; PAI-1 inhibits both enzymes and is antifibrinolytic. Platelet activation, secretion, and aggregation are also promoted under conditions in which the endothelium is disrupted. vWF in the subendothelial matrix is exposed, allowing platelets to attach to the surface of the vessel. P-selectin likewise promotes platelet attachment. *AT*, Antithrombin; *NO*, nitric oxide; *PAI-1*, plasminogen activator inhibitor-1; *TFPI*, tissue factor pathway inhibitor; *TF*, tissue factor; *TM*, thrombomodulin; *t-PA*, tissue plasminogen activator; *u-PA*, urokinase plasminogen activator; *vWF*, von Willebrand factor.

inhibitor of factor XI, are involved in anticoagulant activities.[227-229] The α-granule also contains proteins that mediate both pro- and antifibrinolytic processes. These proteins include plasminogen, α2-antiplasmin, factor XIII, and PAI-1.[230-234] In the unstimulated platelet, the granule contents remain internalized and anionic phospholipid is sequestered in the inner leaflet of the plasma membrane. Prostaglandin I2 (prostacyclin) and nitric oxide released from endothelial cells, the presence of CD39, and the inability of normal plasma vWF to bind spontaneously to the platelet surface are the inhibitory mechanisms that keep platelets unactivated.[235]

When the vascular system is perturbed, platelet plug formation occurs in stages. During the first stage, platelets adhere and are activated by exposure to collagen and vWF and other matrix components (Fig. 126.9). The cytoskeleton spreads and platelet–fibrinogen aggregates are formed and the contents of the granules are secreted.[236-238] The activated platelets adhere to each other, endothelial cells, leukocytes, and components of the subendothelial matrix.[239] The phosphatidyl serine–rich internal face of cell membranes are exposed and present a highly procoagulant surface to the circulation.[240] In addition, activated platelets express specific receptors or binding sites for the assembly of the procoagulant multiprotein complexes (Fig. 126.10). There are approximately 3000 factor Va binding sites on the activated platelet

membrane.[241] Factor Va forms part of the receptor for factor Xa. Factor Xa is also reported to bind to effector cell protease receptor-1 (EPR-1) molecules expressed on activated platelets.[241-244]

In the extension phase of platelet plug formation, where activated platelets accumulate on top of the initial monolayer of platelets bound to collagen, the presence of receptors on the platelet surface allows agonists such as thrombin, adenosine diphosphate, and thromboxane A2 to recruit additional circulating platelets into the growing hemostatic plug (see Fig. 126.10). Subsequently, during the platelet plug formation perpetuation phase, close contacts between platelets promote the growth and stabilization of the hemostatic plug, in part through contact-dependent signaling mechanisms.[235]

Clot Proteins

A central event in blood coagulation is the conversion of soluble fibrinogen (factor I) to insoluble fibrin (see Fig. 126.1; see reviews listed in the References[245,246]). Fibrinogen functions in hemostasis to stem blood loss. It serves as a molecular bridge to support interplatelet aggregation, and it is the precursor of fibrin, which is the main component of the protein scaffolding of the forming hemostatic plug.

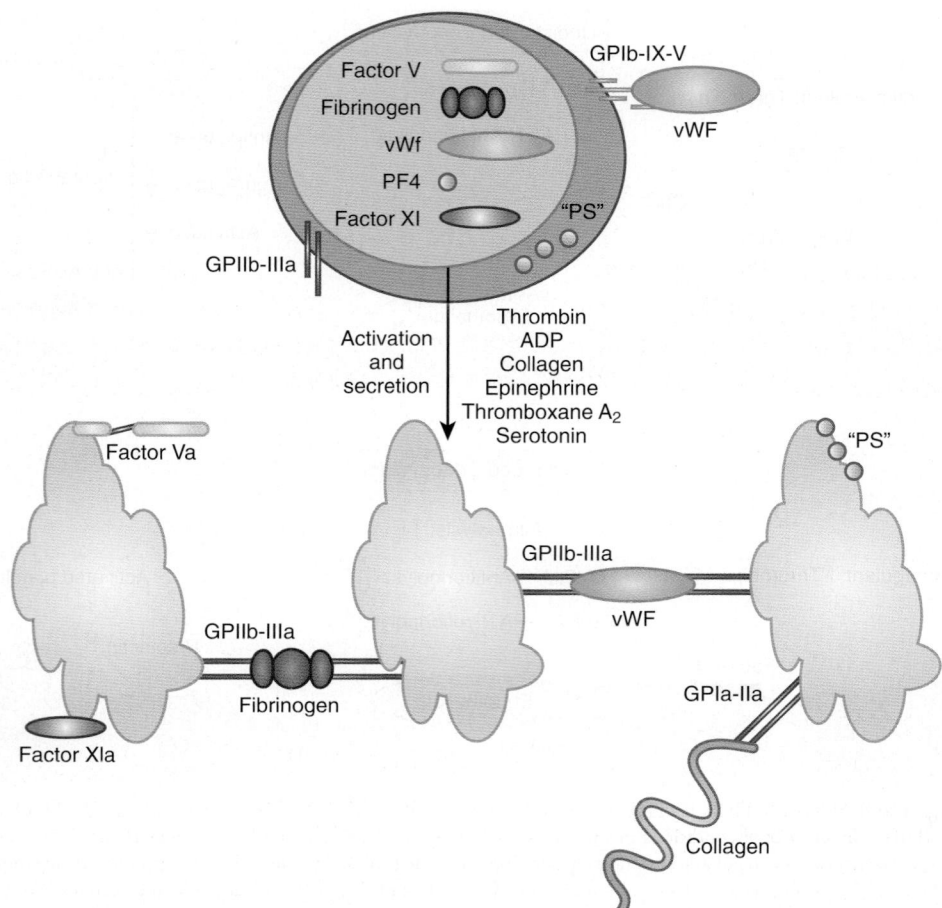

Fig. 126.9 SCHEMATIC OF PLATELET ACTIVATION, SECRETION, AND AGGREGATION. Platelets have multiple functions in hemostasis. They serve as reservoirs of factor V, fibrinogen, vWF, PF4, and factor XI. Platelets also contribute a significant portion of the anionic phospholipid ("PS") necessary for membrane-dependent complex formation and function. In the unstimulated state, proteins and other molecules are sequestered in the platelet granules. Anionic phospholipid is found only in the inner leaflet of the platelet membrane and is not exposed to flowing blood. The GPIb–IX–V complex, which recognizes vWF, is an active receptor, but the GPIIb–IIIa receptor, which recognizes a variety of molecules, including fibrinogen and vWF, is not active. The GP Ib–IX–V receptor likely allows unstimulated platelets to attach to exposed subendothelial vWF, thereby promoting procoagulant events before platelet activation. Upon activation by a variety of agonists, platelets secrete granule contents, become activated and bind factor V/Va and factor XI/XIa, and expose anionic phospholipid. The GPII—IIIa receptor serves to link platelets to each other and the vessel wall. Collagen receptors, such as GPIa–IIa, promote both platelet activation and aggregation. *ADP*, Adenosine diphosphate; *GP*, glycoprotein; *PF4*, platelet factor 4; *vWF*, von Willebrand factor.

Platelet aggregation critically depends on fibrinogen binding to activated platelets via the platelet fibrinogen receptor GPIIb/IIIa as well as fibrin adhesion (see Fig. 126.10). Fibrinogen/fibrin also regulates thrombin activity by interactions that include the proteolytic cleavage by thrombin of fibrinopeptides[247,248] to form a fibrin clot and thrombin exosite binding to fibrin, which potentially limits the diffusion of thrombin, thereby regulating clot propagation. The structure, stability, and duration of insoluble fibrin are controlled by an interplay between fibrin formation and fibrinolysis, which includes other molecular and cellular components.

The description of fibrinogen activation and fibrin assembly has been based on studies using citrated plasmas or purified proteins. The three main players in fibrinogen to fibrin conversion are the enzyme thrombin, the substrates fibrinogen, and the cross-linking tranglutaminase factor XIII. Fibrinogen is composed of six polypeptide chains (two Aα, two Bβ, and two γ chains) that form two symmetrical half molecules (three chains each) with the NH2-termini cross-linked to each other. The outside two domains of fibrinogen are composed of the Bβ and γ chains, and designated as the D domain. The central domain that contains the NH2-termini of all the chains

is designated as the E domain. From x-ray crystallographic data, fibrinogen has a trinodular structure aligned as D–E–D domains (Fig. 126.11).

The kinetics of fibrinogen cleavage by thrombin results in the hydrolysis of Arg–Gly bonds removing small, polar N-terminal fragments (fibrinopeptides [FPs]) from the NH2-terminal of the Aα and Bβ chains Fig. 126.11.[249,250] Cleavage at the Arg–Gly bond of the Aα chain releases FPA and forms fibrin I. The release of two FPA peptides exposes a site in the E domain that interacts with a site in the D domain to form overlapping fibrils. Subsequent cleavage of the Arg–Gly bond on the Bβ chain releases FPB to form fibrin II, presumably increasing lateral aggregation of the protofibrils.[251]

An important enzyme for the structure and stability of the fibrin clot is transglutaminase factor XIIIa.[252–254] Its function is to cross-link fibrin and other adhesive proteins, including integrin receptors, providing a stable network. Only the Aα chain and the γ chain, which have donor (Gln) and acceptor (Lys) sites, participate in cross-linking of adjacent glutamyl and lysyl residues by factor XIIIa.[251,255–257]

Fibrinogen is also required for competent inflammatory reactions. Fibrinogen is an acute-phase reactant whose levels increase during

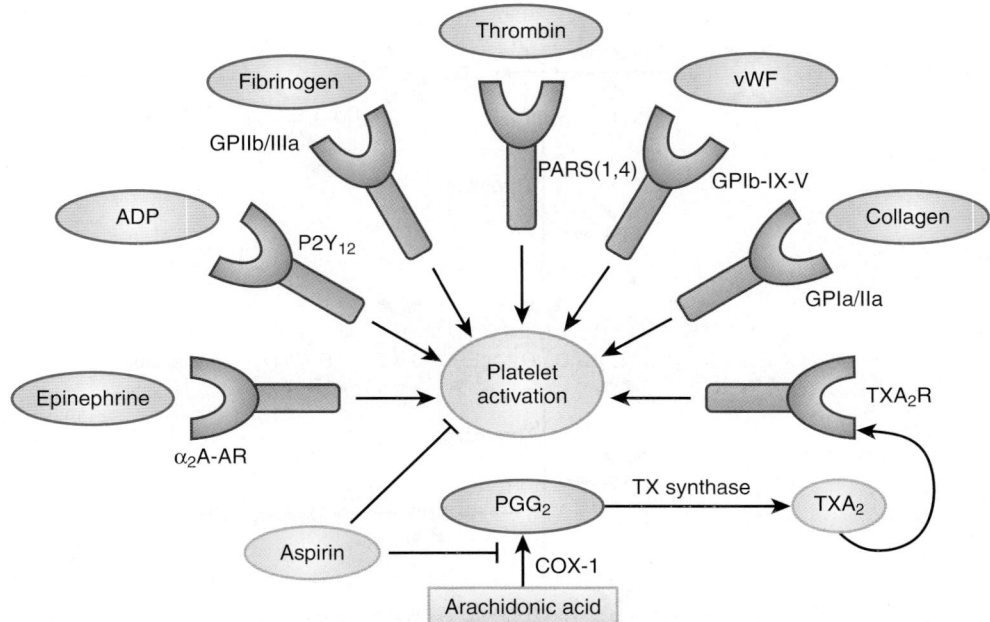

Fig. 126.10 SELECTED PLATELET RECEPTOR TARGETS AND THEIR RESPECTIVE INHIBITORY AGENTS. When a platelet encounters a break in the endothelium, it encounters molecules that trigger its activation, such as collagen, TXA_2, ADP, and thrombin. The ability of platelets to adhere, aggregate, respond to agonists, aid in coagulation, and bind fibrin are all processes mediated by the plasma membrane glycoproteins of the platelet. The platelet GPIbIX–V constitutes the receptor for vWF. GPIa/IIa mediates platelet–collagen interactions. GPIIb/IIIa is a receptor for fibrinogen. $P2Y_{12}$ is a chemoreceptor for ADP. The α_2A-AR is expressed on platelets and binds the naturally occurring ligand epinephrine. COX-1 is responsible for the formation of prostaglandins and thromboxane. COX-1 converts arachidonic acid to PGG_2. Aspirin irreversibly inhibits COX-1. *α_2A-AR*, α_2A-adrenergic receptor; *COX-1*, cyclooxygenase-1; *GP*, glycoprotein; *PGG_2*, prostaglandin G_2; *TX*, thromboxane; *TXA_2*, thromboxane A_2; *TXA_2R*, thromboxane A_2 receptor; *vWF*, von Willebrand factor.

inflammation.[258,259] In these situations, fibrinogen functions as a bridging molecule in cell–cell interactions.[260,261] Fibrin and fibrinogen constitute a matrix that modulates cellular responses in a variety of cell types, including endothelial cells, epithelial cells, leukocytes, platelets, and fibroblasts. Cellular receptors that bind fibrinogen and fibrin include the integrins $\alpha_{IIb}\beta_3$, $\alpha_V\beta_3$, and $\alpha_5\beta_1$, and the cellular adhesion molecules intercellular adhesion molecule-1 and vascular endothelial cadherin.[262–265]

Fibrin clot-based assays have been extensively used in the clinical diagnosis of bleeding disorders. Two in vitro plasma tests, the PT[266,267] and the activated partial thromboplastin time (aPTT),[268] segregate the coagulation process into tissue factor–initiated or surface contact processes, respectively. The aPTT, which initiates coagulation by the introduction of a foreign surface, only examines the biologic constituents intrinsic to plasma. This assay is sensitive to isolated or combined deficiencies of factor XII, HMWK, prekallikrein, factor XI, factor VIII, factor IX, factor X, factor V, prothrombin, and fibrinogen. The PT assay is based on initiating coagulation via an extrinsic source of tissue factor (thromboplastin). The PT assay is sensitive to isolated or combined deficiencies of factor VII, factor X, factor V, prothrombin, and fibrinogen. Although these in vitro clotting assays help establish a basis for hemostasis, abnormal test results are not always mirrored by human pathology associated with bleeding or thrombosis.

Fibrinolysis Proteins

Clot formation is integrated with clot dissolution (fibrinolysis). Fibrinolysis, the elimination of blood clots, has two types, primary fibrinolysis and secondary fibrinolysis. Whereas primary fibrinolysis is a normal body process, secondary fibrinolysis is the breakdown of clots caused by a medicine, a medical disorder, or some other cause.

The biochemical mechanisms of clot dissolution center on fibrin-specific activation of plasminogen to plasmin. The key proteins involved are plasminogen, the plasminogen activators tissue plasminogen activator (t-PA) and urokinase plasminogen activator (u-PA), and the inhibitors (PAI-1, α_2-antiplasmin, and TAFIa). Plasminogen is the inactive precursor of the enzyme plasmin, which is the primary catalyst of fibrin degradation (Fig. 126.12).[269] The process of plasminogen activation can occur through three distinct pathways: (1) the intrinsic activator system (analogous to the contact system of blood coagulation), (2) the extrinsic activators (t-PA and u-PA), and (3) an exogenous activator system involving pharmacologic agents (fibrinolytic drugs). The primary pathway used in vivo appears to be the extrinsic pathway. However, both the intrinsic as well as exogenous activator systems can play important roles in human disease.

t-PA and u-PA, secreted by the endothelium, have unique structures and properties that affect the specificity and rate of plasmin generation (see Fig. 126.12).[270] After being generated, plasmin digests fibrin in a pattern that produces a collection of degradation products, including fragment X, fragment Y, and the core fragments, fragments D and E. The first step in degrading fibrin is the removal of the α chains, thus exposing the coiled coils. As these coils are cleaved, different sized fragments are released.[271] Fibrinogen is represented as a trinodular structure (D–E–D domains) with each E domain and D domain separated by a coiled coil domain. Upon formation of fibrin cross-links occur between alternating molecules of fibrin at the D domain (D=D). Plasmin degrades fibrin, releasing various sized fragments, the smallest of which is the D=D or D-dimer ($M_r = 180,000$). The largest of these fragments is XXD, X=D–E–D, with a mass of 595,000.[272,273] Elevated levels of D-dimer are found in the blood of patients with various thrombotic and thrombolytic disorders.[274]

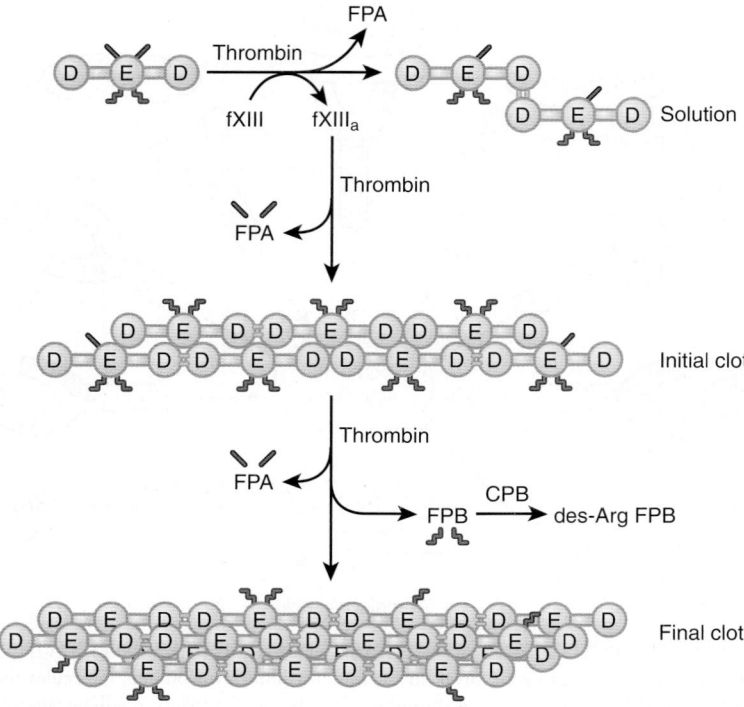

Fig. 126.11 SCHEMATIC REPRESENTATION OF WHOLE-BLOOD FIBRIN FORMATION. At the start of clot formation, thrombin simultaneously acts on fibrinogen (D-E-D) and FXIII. A portion (≈40%) of FPA is released from fibrinogen, and an initial clot is formed from the complementary overlap of the exposed sites between the E and D domains of adjacent fibrin molecules. fXIIIa simultaneously cross-links adjacent D domains (D=D). Thus the initial soluble fibrin clot is composed of fibrinogen, fibrin, and γ-γ dimers with FPB still attached. The initial clot is continuously acted on by thrombin, releasing the remaining FPA and some of the FPB to yield a final clot with the majority of FPB still attached. The released FPB is selectively acted on by a CPB (potentially thrombin-activatable fibrinolysis inhibitor a), which cleaves the C-terminal arginine to produce des-Arg FPB. The significance of this cleavage is still unclear. *CBP,* Carboxypeptidase B–like enzyme; *FPA,* fibrinopeptide A; *FPB,* fibrinopeptide B; *FXIII,* factor XIII; *FXIIIa,* activated factor XIIIa. *(From Brummel KE, Butenas S, Mann KG: An integrated study of fibrinogen during blood coagulation.* J Biol Chem *274:22862, 1999, with permission.)*

These circulating fragments are cleared by other proteases or by the kidney and liver.

Inhibitors of the Fibrinolytic System

Plasminogen activation in blood is primarily inhibited by PAI-1, which targets u-PA and t-PA. PAI-1 also has a role in tissue remodeling by interfering with vitronectin-dependent processes of cell adhesion and migration.[275] Congenital deficiency of PAI-1 is rare, with homozygous individuals displaying abnormal bleeding in response to trauma.[276] Platelets contribute to the fibrinolytic process by binding t-PA and plasminogen, and supporting plasmin generation. Increased levels of plasma PAI-1 delay fibrin removal by shortening the functional lifetime of plasminogen activators, thereby shifting hemostasis to a more thrombotic state.[277]

TAFI is a plasma zymogen with homology to procarboxypeptidases A and B (see Fig. 126.12).[55,278–280] Activation of TAFI yields the exopeptidase (TAFIa) with carboxypeptidase B–like substrate specificity. TAFIa catalyzes the removal of basic amino acids (arginine, lysine) from the COOH-termini of polypeptides. The activation of many of the cofactors and zymogens of the coagulation and fibrinolytic cascades results in the generation of functional proteins with COOH-terminus arginine or lysine residues. COOH-terminus lysine residues that appear in fibrin fragments degraded with plasmin have been identified as the major substrates for TAFIa. The physiologic activator of TAFIa is the thrombin–thrombomodulin complex, thus defining TAFIa as a coagulation-dependent activity.[281] Because TAFIa functions as an attenuator of fibrinolysis,[53] an adequate rate of TAFIa

generation appears critical for the stabilization of the blood clot. Plasmas with specific deficiencies in the coagulation pathway exhibit reduced rates of thrombin production, decreased levels of TAFIa, and premature clot lysis.[257,282,283]

Fibrinolytic drugs are often given after a myocardial infarct or ischemic stroke to dissolve the fibrin clot blocking the coronary or cerebral artery. Fibrinolytic drugs are also used in massive pulmonary embolism. Antifibrinolytics, such as aminocaproic acid (ε-aminocaproic acid) and tranexamic acid, are used as inhibitors of fibrinolysis.

CONNECTIVITY AND DYNAMICS IN HEMOSTASIS

In the healthy state, the hemostatic system is relatively quiescent, with the vascular endothelial cells, the blood, and the extravascular tissue functioning to maintain fluidity. Blood platelets remain in a quiescent state because of the endothelial cell lining of the blood vessel being an active anticoagulant that secretes small molecules and enzymes. The endothelium also provides constituent anticoagulant proteins, which inhibit the blood coagulation system. These vascular anticoagulant systems are both passive and dynamic in nature, and function in cooperation with plasma components. The blood supplies pro- and anticoagulant proteins in the plasma and platelets, which contribute to the coagulation reaction. If the endothelium becomes damaged, the pro- and anticoagulant levels become imbalanced, and cells that should remain in the blood can leak through blood vessels into adjacent body tissue, which triggers a response. The dimensions of the response are relevant to the injury. The extravascular compartment and blood interact to rapidly produce a vigorous local

Plasminogen

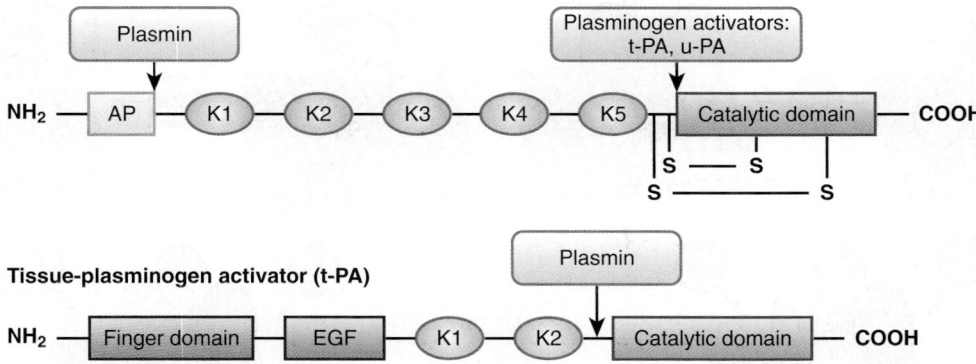

Tissue-plasminogen activator (t-PA)

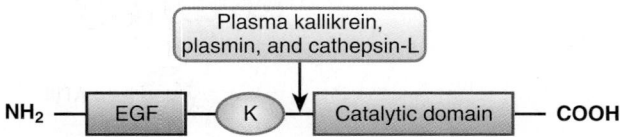

Single chain-urokinase plasminogen activator (sc-uPA)

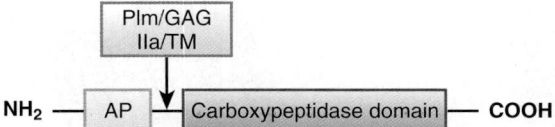

Thrombin activatable fibrinolysis inhibitor (TAFI)

Fig. 126.12 SCHEMATIC OF FIBRINOLYTIC PROTEINS. *Plasminogen* is the inactive precursor of the enzyme plasmin, which is the primary catalyst of fibrin degradation. The domain structure of human plasminogen is represented by Kringle domains (K1–K5), a catalytic domain, and the *arrows* indicate the sites of proteolytic cleavage by plasmin, elastase, and plasminogen activators (t-PA and u-PA). Disulfide bonds are illustrated by -S-S-. The t-PA molecule is a serine proteinase and consists of an A and B chain. The A chain consists of a fibronectin finger–like domain, an EGF–like domain, and two kringle domains. The K2 domain and the finger domain of t-PA are involved in the binding of t-PA to fibrin. The B-chain of t-PA contains the active site catalytic triad. Single-chain t-PA is an efficient plasminogen activator in the presence of fibrin and is converted to the two-chain form by cleavage of the peptide bond between R^{275} and I^{276}. This cleavage is performed primarily by the action of plasmin during fibrinolysis. *Single-chain u-PA* (sc-uPA) is a serine protease and is an ineffective catalyst. Plasmin or plasma kallikrein can hydrolyze the K^{158}–I^{159} peptide bond, converting sc-uPA into the fully active two-chain form (two-chain urokinase-type plasminogen activator). u-PA is composed of an EGF domain (EGF), a single kringle domain, a connecting peptide region, and the serine protease-type catalytic domain. *Thrombin-activatable fibrinolysis inhibitor* (TAFI): Activation of TAFI (TAFIa) yields an exopeptidase with carboxypeptidase B–like substrate specificity. TAFIa delays fibrinolysis by cleaving COOH-terminus Arg (R) or Lys (K) residues made available as a consequence of partial plasmin digestion of the fibrin clot. Removing these residues attenuates the self-amplifying mechanism of fibrin-based plasmin formation wherein partial plasmin proteolysis of fibrin increases the number of binding sites (COOH-terminal lysines) available for efficient plasminogen activation. TAFI contains an activation peptide region and a carboxypeptidase domain. It is activated by the thrombin–thrombomodulin complexes (IIa/TM) and plasmin–glycosaminoglycan complexes (Plm/GAG) by hydrolysis of the R^{92}–A^{93} bond. EGF, Epidermal growth factor; *sc-uPA*, Single-chain u-PA; *t-PA*, tissue plasminogen activator; *u-PA*, urokinase plasminogen activator.

coagulation response, which attenuates blood loss and initiates the vascular repair process in four phases: initiation, propagation, termination, and elimination and fibrinolysis.[284–286]

Initiation

If vascular injury occurs, a measured response is triggered in that the extent of damage regulates platelet and fibrin deposition. Activated platelets provide the membrane surfaces upon which coagulation enzymes can be anchored, assembled, and expressed. Therefore the activated platelet membrane provides both an initiating and limiting component to the extent of a coagulation reaction.[287] More vascular damage produces more anchored activated platelets, and more membrane allows the assembly of more coagulation enzymes, which ultimately results in increased fibrin formation.

When the vascular system is perturbed, the initial stages of the hemostatic response are triggered. The initial principal player is the extrinsic tenase complex (tissue factor–factor VIIa), which is composed of a cell membrane; tissue factor exposed by vascular damage or cytokine stimulation; Ca^{2+}; and the serine protease plasma factor VIIa, which is already present in its active form at 1%–2% of the factor VII zymogen concentration[53,288] (Fig. 126.13). Before binding to tissue factor, the plasma serine protease factor VIIa is essentially

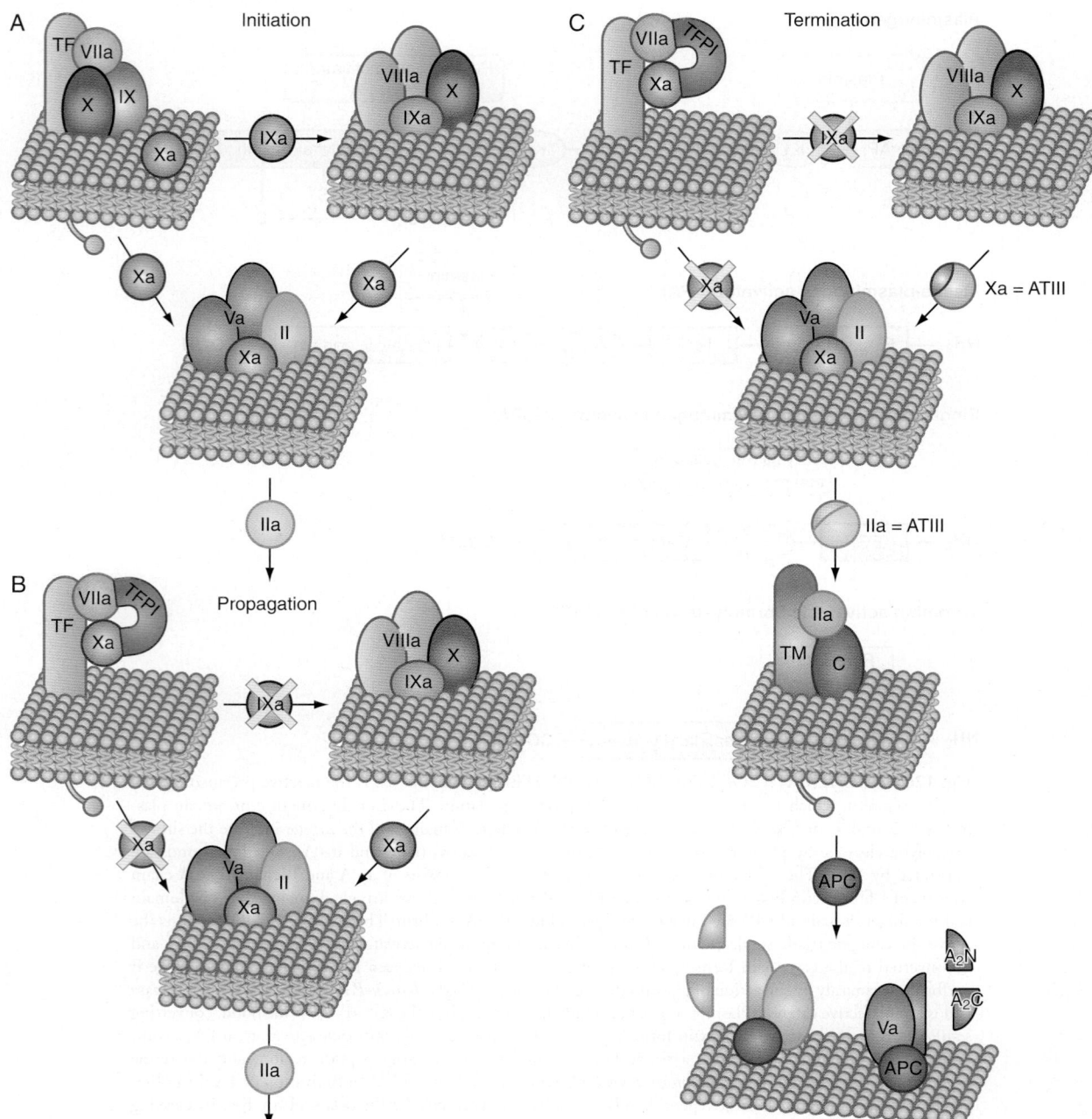

Fig. 126.13 REGULATION OF THE DYNAMIC PROCOAGULANT RESPONSE. Initiation (A), propagation (B), and termination (C) of thrombin generation and the procoagulant response are illustrated. Four vitamin K–dependent complexes are shown: extrinsic tenase, intrinsic tenase, prothrombinase, and protein Case. The procoagulant response is regulated by the stoichiometric inhibitors AT and TFPI. AT inhibits thrombin, factor Xa, and factor IXa that are free in solution. TFPI inhibits both factor Xa and the factor VIIa–TF–factor Xa complex. APC generated from the protein Case complex (TM–thrombin [IIa]) inactivates factor Va and factor VIIIa by proteolysis of their heavy chains. Low levels of thrombin are required to initiate clot formation (initiation phase) and trigger the coagulation cascade response (propagation phase). The enzymes, cofactors, and inhibitors act together to generate a hemostatic response that can be divided into an initiation phase and a propagation and termination phase. During the initiation phase, factors X and IX are converted to their respective serine proteases factor Xa and factor IXa; low levels of thrombin are subsequently generated by factor Xa. This thrombin then can activate platelets and the procofactors factors V and VIII, which stimulate further thrombin generation during the propagation phase. Thrombin generation is attenuated by shutting down the initiation phase by means of the stoichiometric inhibitor of the extrinsic tenase complex, TFPI, followed by AT, which directly inhibits thrombin and factors Xa and IXa. *APC*, Activated protein C; *AT*, antithrombin; *C*, protein Case; *TF*, tissue factor; *TFPI*, tissue factor pathway inhibitor; *TM*, thrombomodulin. *(From Mann KG: Coagulation explosion, Burlington, Vermont, 1997, Vermont Business Graphics, with permission.)*

inert from the catalytic perspective and thus impervious to the abundant protease inhibitors in plasma.[289] Factor VII also competes with factor VIIa for tissue factor binding, thus serving as a negative regulator that buffers the overall reaction.[290,291] Factor VII–activating protease (FSAP) has also been shown to activate factor VII in the absence of tissue factor.[292–294] The physiologic function of FSAP still is unclear, but most recently has been suggested to be involved in inflammation (see the review listed in the References[295]). The extrinsic tenase complex (tissue factor–factor VIIa) activates low levels of the zymogens factor X and factor IX to their respective serine protease enzymes factor Xa (≈10 pM) and factor IXa (≈1 pM).[296,297] Factor X is the more efficient and abundant substrate.[298,299]

The extrinsic tenase complex is under tight supervision by TFPI, which can bind both the complex and the product factor Xa (see Fig. 126.13).[300,301] TFPI, present in low abundance in blood, is released from the vasculature by heparin.[302] If the initiating procoagulant stimulus is sufficient to overcome the level of this anticoagulant response, a threshold is exceeded and downstream complexes can be formed.

The limited amounts of factor Xa that escapes inhibition by TFPI and antithrombin bind to available membrane sites and can activate tiny amounts of prothrombin to thrombin (see Fig. 126.13).[303] The time period in which factor Xa directly generates picomolar amounts of thrombin[304] is referred to as the *initiation phase* of blood coagulation (Fig. 126.14). During the initiation phase, circulating blood cells

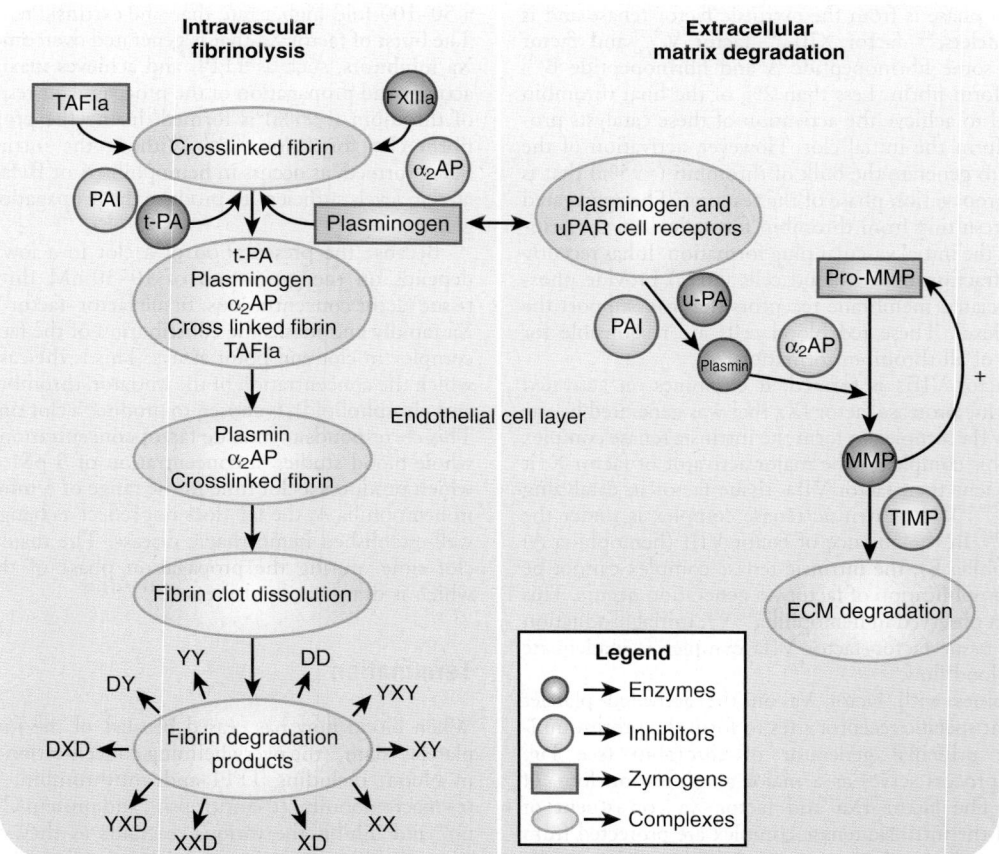

Fig. 126.14 SCHEMATIC OF THE DYNAMIC INTERACTION BETWEEN THE PROTEINS AND INHIBITORS OF FIBRINOLYSIS. Cross-linked fibrin formation is integrated with fibrin clot dissolution and degradation of its products. Two pathways are shown, intravascular fibrinolysis and extracellular matrix, separated by an endothelial cell layer. The enzymes *(red circles)*, inhibitors *(blue circles)*, zymogens *(green boxes)*, and complexes *(large yellow ovals)* are illustrated in a simplified form to show this multicomponent process. The key proteins of the fibrinolytic system *(left panel)* are plasminogen, the plasminogen activator t-PA, PAIs, α₂-AP and TAFI, and the transglutaminase FXIIIa. t-PA and plasminogen both bind to the fibrin surface, cross-linked by FXIIIa, where t-PA is an effective catalyst of plasminogen conversion to plasmin. Initially, plasmin proteolysis of fibrin generates new COOH-terminus lysine residues, which function as higher affinity binding sites for plasminogen, setting up an amplifying loop of plasminogen activation. Formation of activated TAFIa results in removal of the plasmin-generated COOH-terminus lysine residues, thus suppressing the rate of fibrin lysis. Opposing these events are antifibrinolytic mechanisms. Soluble and cross-linked α₂-AP complexes with plasmin, rendering it inactive. PAI rapidly reacts with t-PA, thus reducing the concentration of the plasminogen activator. Fibrin degradation occurs by plasmin cleavage at the D-E-D domains of fibrin polymers to yield a variety of polymers as illustrated (for a definition of the D-E-D domain, see Fig. 126.11). Plasminogen can cross the endothelial cell layer and become converted to plasmin by the u-PA *(right panel)*. Plasmin can convert latent MMPs (pro-MMPs) to their active form (MMPs). MMPs themselves can act in a positive-feedback mechanism to convert pro-MMPs to more MMPs, which ultimately degrade the extracellular matrix. Plasmin-mediated effects are inhibited by PAI and α₂-AP. MMP-mediated effects are inhibited by TIMPs. *α₂-AP,* α₂-Antiplasmin; *ECM,* extracellular matrix; *FXIIIa,* activated factor XIII; *MMP,* matrix metalloproteinase; *PAI,* plasminogen activator inhibitor; *t-PA,* tissue plasminogen activator; *TAFI,* thrombin-activatable fibrinolysis inhibitor; *TIMP,* tissue inhibitors of metalloproteinases; *u-PA,* urokinase plasminogen activator.

and procoagulant proteins are activated,[305] the procoagulant elements necessary for the full procoagulant response are generated, and a preliminary fibrin network is formed.[306] Although this process is inefficient, this initial thrombin is essential for the acceleration of the process by serving as the activator of platelets through cleavage of protease–activated receptors (PAR1 and PAR4)[307] and the activation of the procofactors factor V and factor VIII.[129] Thrombin also activates factor XI to factor XIa,[130] initiating the accessory pathway that enhances factor IX activation.[308]

In analyses of tissue factor–induced activation of the coagulation process in whole blood, the initial period of thrombin generation (based on levels of thrombin–antithrombin complexes) illustrates that most catalyst formation occurs before fibrin clot formation (see Fig. 126.14).[305] The small amount of thrombin that is generated during the initiation phase is from the extrinsic factor tenase and is able to activate platelets,[309] factor XIII,[310] factor V,[311] and factor VIII[312], and release some fibrinopeptide A and fibrinopeptide B[263] from fibrinogen to form fibrin. Less than 2% of the final thrombin produced is required to achieve the activation of these catalysts produced in blood to form the initial clot. However, activation of the catalysts is essential to generate the bulk of thrombin (≈95%) that is formed during the propagation phase of the reaction. The aggregated platelets and fibrin resulting from thrombin formation are the principal components of the initial vascular plug formation. It has recently been shown that a fraction of red blood cells (≤1%) provide phosphatidyl serine–associated membrane receptors that can support the procoagulant complexes. These red blood cells are responsible for approximately 30% of all thrombin formation.[313]

After cofactor factor VIIIa is formed, it combines on activated platelets with the serine protease factor IXa that was generated by the tissue factor–factor VIIa complex to form the intrinsic tenase complex (see Fig. 126.13). This complex is the major activator of factor X; it is 50-fold more efficient than factor VIIa–tissue factor in catalyzing factor X activation.[299,314] The extrinsic tenase complex is under the control of TFPI.[315,316] In the absence of factor VIII (hemophilia A) or factor IX (hemophilia B), the intrinsic tenase complex cannot be assembled; thus no amplification of factor Xa generation occurs. This is the principal defect observed in hemophilia[317,318]: initial production of factor Xa by the tissue factor–factor VIIa complex is inadequate to efficiently stem blood flow.

Factor Xa combines with factor Va on the activated platelet membrane surfaces at specific receptor sites to form the prothrombinase complex; the principal generator of thrombin (see Fig. 126.13).[319,320] This process serves as a major amplification loop of blood coagulation. The factor IXa and factor Xa constituent of prothrombinase and the intrinsic tenase complex are protected from inhibition by antithrombin and other plasma inhibitors when in the complexed form.

Propagation

When a sufficient stimulus is provided to overcome the antagonist–inhibitor threshold, the accumulating mass of activated platelets will support increasing intrinsic tenase and prothrombinase complex formation on their surfaces through specific platelet receptors, and the local inhibitor concentrations are overwhelmed (see Fig. 126.13). These platelet-bound catalysts execute the propagation phase of the reaction, during which massive amounts of thrombin are produced.[321] This phase of thrombin generation continues independent of the initially presented tissue factor as long as there is a continuous supply of blood to deliver new plasma procoagulant reactants, platelets, and fibrinogen to the site of perforation in the vascular endothelium.

Essential to the formation of the prothrombinase complex is the generation of factor Xa. Factor Xa is a unique regulatory enzyme in that it is formed through both the intrinsic tenase and the extrinsic tenase complexes. Under normal conditions, the concentration of factor Xa is the rate-limiting component of the prothrombinase complex. The other components of the complex, platelets (membrane

surface–binding sites), and the cofactor (factor Va) are activated rapidly to produce a surplus that is ready for action.[319] The coagulation mechanism can become sensitive to factor V or platelets when confronted with congenital deficiencies, thrombocytopenia, platelet pathology, or pharmacologic interventions.[322,323]

The initial factor Xa is generated via the tissue factor–factor VIIa complex during the initiation phase. Additional factor Xa is then generated by the intrinsic tenase complex (factor IXa–factor VIIIa–membrane–Ca²⁺). Initially, the concentration of the factor VIIa–tissue factor complex is higher than the concentration of the factor VIIIa–factor IXa complex, which requires activation and assembly. As time progresses, the contribution of the intrinsic tenase complex to factor Xa generation exceeds that of the extrinsic tenase.[324] The intrinsic tenase complex is kinetically more efficient and activates factor X at a 50–100-fold higher rate than the extrinsic tenase complex.[299,325,326] The burst of factor Xa that is generated overcomes the levels of factor Xa inhibitors, such as TFPI, and achieves maximal prothrombinase activity and propagation of the procoagulant response.[162,315] The bulk of thrombin (≈95%) is formed during the propagation phase after fibrin clot formation.[305,327] Without the intrinsic tenase complex being formed, as occurs in hemophilia A or B, factor Xa is not generated in levels sufficient to produce the propagation phase of thrombin generation.[317,328]

Because the presentation of a clot in a low tissue factor model depends on the generation of 10–30 nM thrombin,[305,327] at high tissue factor concentrations, tissue factor–factor VIIa generates factor Xa rapidly and masks the contribution of the factor VIIIa–factor IXa complex in clot end point assays. This is the case for the PT[266,267] in which the concentration of the initiator, thromboplastin (tissue factor and phospholipid), is chosen to produce a clot time of 11–15 seconds. This corresponds to a tissue factor concentration over 20 nM. In our whole-blood studies, a concentration of 5 pM tissue factor is used, which produces a clot time in the range of 5 minutes.[305,327] Therefore in hemophilia A, the PT does not reflect a change in clot time in this well-established hemorrhagic disease. The major defect occurs after clot time, during the propagation phase of thrombin generation, which is dramatically decreased.[317,321,329]

Termination

When blood flow has ceased because of the formation of a fibrin–platelet "dam," the overwhelming concentration of inhibitors present in blood, including TFPI and antithrombin, heparin cofactor II, α_2-macroglobulin, α_1-antitrypsin, and protein C inhibitor, can "catch up" and inhibit the various reactants as they dissociate from their respective complexes (see Fig. 126.13).[150,315,330–332]

In the intact vasculature surrounding the growing thrombus, procoagulant enzymes and cofactors escaping the wound site are rapidly quenched under normal circumstances by the stoichiometric and dynamic inhibitory systems of blood in cooperation with elements of the vascular endothelium. The free serine proteases (thrombin, factor IXa, and factor Xa) of the coagulation system in the plasma environment are rapidly inhibited by the surplus of antithrombin molecules. The reaction is accelerated by the interaction of antithrombin with heparan sulfate proteoglycans presented constitutively on the surface of vascular endothelial cells.[333]

Any thrombin escaping from the wound site may bind resident thrombomodulin molecules constitutively expressed by vascular endothelial cells. Thrombomodulin-bound thrombin is converted from a procoagulant enzyme to an anticoagulant enzyme.[334,335] The thrombin–thrombomodulin complex (protein Case) activates protein C, which in turn downregulates the intrinsic factor tenase and prothrombinase procoagulants by cleaving factor VIIIa and factor Va, respectively. The rates of APC inactivation of factors Va and VIIIa are enhanced by protein S. TAFI is also activated by protein Case and serves to delay clot lysis (see reviews listed in the References[53,336]). Cleavage of factor Va by APC and inhibition of thrombin generation also reduces thrombin–thrombomodulin–mediated TAFI activation.[337]

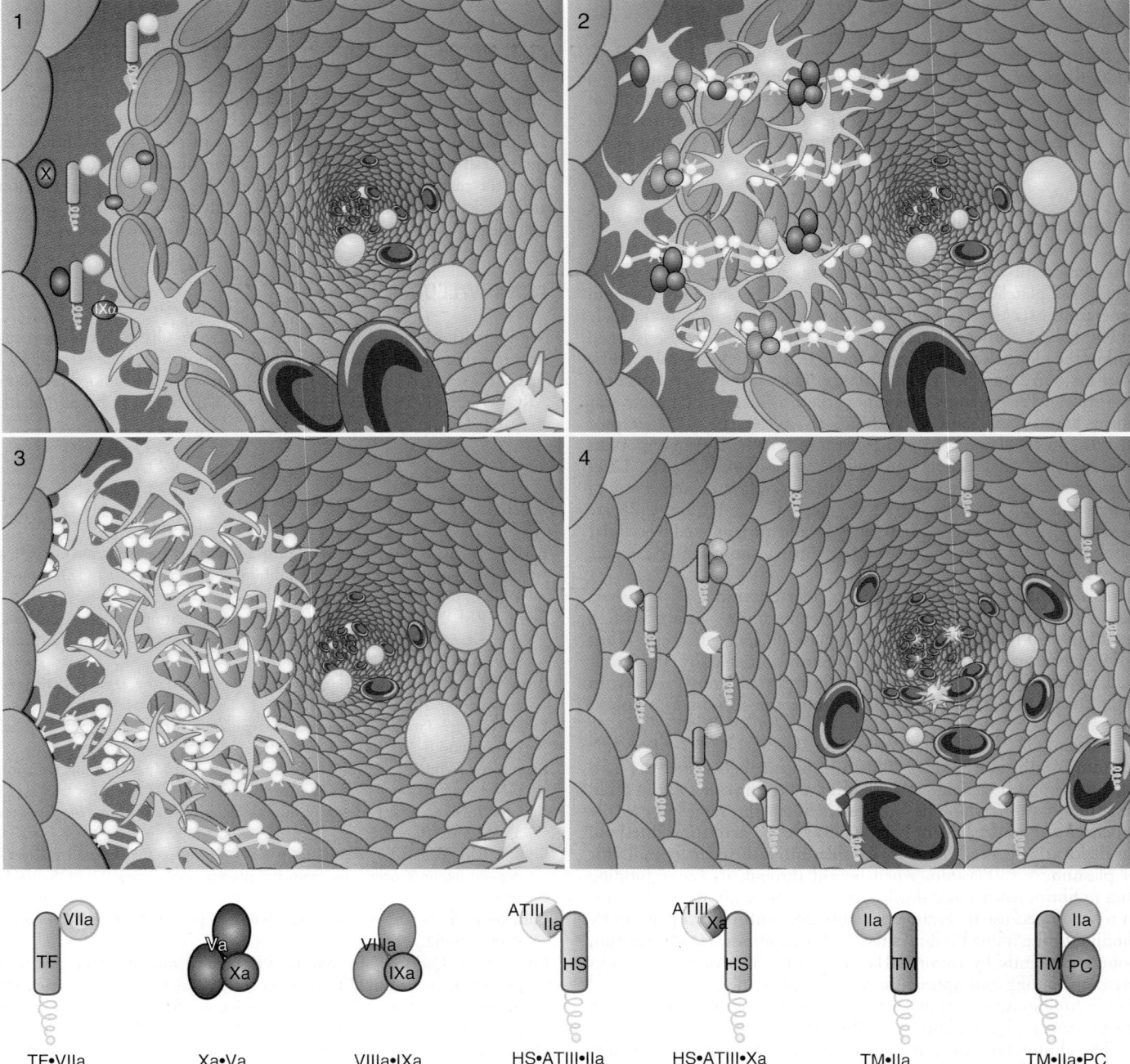

Fig. 126.15 SCHEMATIC OF THE DYNAMIC EVENTS DURING TISSUE FACTOR–INITIATED BLOOD COAGULATION. A cross-section of a blood vessel showing the luminal space, endothelial cell layer, and extravascular region is presented at the site of a perforation. The blood coagulation process in response is depicted in four stages. *Extrinsic tenase* complex, TF•VIIa; *prothrombinase* complex, Xa•Va; *intrinsic tenase*, VIIIa•IXa; AT–endothelial cell HS proteoglycan complex bound to thrombin or FXa, HS•AT•(IIa or Xa); protein C bound to TM–thrombin, TM•IIa•PC. *Stage 1.* Perforation results in delivery of blood, and with it circulating factor VIIa and platelets, to an extravascular space rich in membrane-bound TF. Platelets adhere to collagen and von Willebrand factor associated with the extravascular tissue, and TF binds factor VIIa, initiating the process of factor IX and factor X activation. Factor Xa activates small amounts of prothrombin to thrombin, which activates more platelets and converts factor V and factor VIII to factor Va and factor VIIIa. *Stage 2.* The reaction is propagated by platelet-bound intrinsic tenase and prothrombinase, with the former being the principal factor Xa generator. Initial clotting occurs and fibrin begins to fill in the void in cooperation with activated platelets. *Stage 3.* A barrier composed of activated platelets ladened with procoagulant complexes and enmeshed in fibrin scaffolding is formed. The reaction in the now filled perforation is terminated by reagent consumption, attenuating further thrombin generation, but functional procoagulant enzyme complexes persist because they are protected from the dynamic inhibitory processes found on the intravascular face. *Stage 4.* View downstream of the perforation. Enzymes escaping from the plugged perforation are captured by antithrombin–heparan complexes, and the protein C system is activated by residual thrombin binding to endothelial cell TM, initiating the dynamic anticoagulant system. These intravascular processes work against occlusion of the vessel despite the continuous resupply of reactants across the intravascular face of the thrombus. *AT,* Antithrombin; *PC,* protein C; *HS,* heparan sulfate; *TF,* tissue factor; *TM,* thrombomodulin. *(From Orfeo T, Butenas S, Brummel-Ziedins KE, Mann KG: The tissue factor requirement in blood coagulation. J Biol Chem 280:42887, 2005, with permission.)*

When operating properly, this system of blood leakage attenuation displays the appropriate level of procoagulant required to obstruct blood loss but is precluded from systemic activation of the coagulation system. The converse to hemostasis occurs when the damaging insult for the vasculature is internal to the vessel lumen.[338]

Elimination and Fibrinolysis

The hemostatic or pathologic thrombus is structurally composed of aggregated platelets and cross-linked fibrin. The steps in thrombin generation of a cross-linked fibrin clot are shown diagrammatically in Fig. 126.11. Other plasma proteins and blood cells are also trapped within the clot. Clot formation is integrated with clot dissolution by plasmin to maintain hemostatic balance. The plasminogen system has two roles: t-PA generates plasmin at the fibrin surface and governs fibrin homeostasis, and u-PA binds to a cellular u-PA receptor (u-PAR) and generates pericellular plasmin, which plays an important role in tissue remodeling and cellular migration.[339,340] The latter function is, to a great extent, mediated by plasmin activation of matrix metalloproteinases, which degrade ECM. t-PA and u-PA are secreted by vascular endothelial cells[341,342] and are regulated by cellular cytokines and components produced during the clotting cascade, including thrombin.

In the absence of fibrin, t-PA is a poor enzyme.[343-345] However, both t-PA and plasminogen bind to the fibrin surface with a resulting 100-fold enhancement in plasminogen activation. Thus t-PA activation of fibrinolysis is primarily initiated by and localized to fibrin.[343,345] The digestion of fibrin by plasmin[346] is seen in Fig. 126.14 and further described under the section Fibrinolysis Proteins.[274,346-349]

Fibrinolysis is regulated primarily by PAI-1,[350,351] PAI-2,[352] α_2-antiplasmin, and TAFI.[353] The antagonism between PAI-1 and the plasminogen activators u-PA and t-PA provides a threshold response of the fibrinolytic process in much the same way as the procoagulant–anticoagulant balance provides an activation threshold for the clotting process.[354-357] α_2-Antiplasmin is the primary inhibitor of plasmin.[358-360] Plasmin, when bound through its lysine binding sites to fibrin, reacts more slowly with α_2-antiplasmin than when free in solution because α_2-antiplasmin interacts with plasma plasmin by binding to the lysine binding sites.[358-362] In contrast, α_2-antiplasmin, bound covalently by factor XIIIa to the Aα chain of fibrin, blocks plasmin binding and appears to decrease plasminogen activation.[363] TAFIa functions in vitro as an antifibrinolytic factor by suppressing the positive-feedback pathway of fibrinolysis.[255,256,337]

The elimination phase begins the process of tissue repair by dissolving the fibrin–platelet clot generated in the earlier phases of hemostasis. The damaged vascular tissue not only requires plasmin to clear the fibrin clot, but also to initiate removal of damaged tissue to allow for cell migration into the injured area.[364,365] Plasmin activates a variety of matrix metalloproteinases that degrade subendothelial matrix components and extricate the damaged tissue.[365,366] These processes mark the beginnings of the final stages of the hemostatic response, repair, and regeneration.

The importance of the tight regulation of these processes is perhaps best illustrated by malfunctions of the hemostatic response. An inappropriate response can lead to one of two opposing but equally undesirable outcomes. Failure to form a sufficient hemostatic plug to arrest blood flow subsequent to vascular injury can result in pathologic hemorrhage. Excessive clot formation or failure to efficiently lyse a clot may result in thrombosis with consequent vascular obstruction. Under normal circumstances, the vascular endothelium together with the aforementioned positive- and negative-feedback loops within the procoagulant pathways prevent these negative outcomes by actively controlling the coagulation process until a triggering stimulus of sufficient magnitude threatens vascular integrity (Fig. 126.15). Initiation of the procoagulant response also initiates the fibrinolytic response simultaneously with repair and regeneration processes.

FUTURE DIRECTIONS

This chapter describes the process of blood coagulation (extrinsic and intrinsic pathway) by dividing it into sections based on procoagulant, anticoagulant, and fibrinolytic enzymes, cofactors, and inhibitors in the overall process of fibrin formation and fibrin dissolution. When all of the players are present, the overall process of blood coagulation and fibrinolysis is best described as a dynamic threshold-limited, complex, intertwined process that together promotes hemostasis.

ACKNOWLEDGEMENTS

We the authors would like to thank Matthew Gissel in the preparation of this chapter. The authors were supported by the NIH-DOD TACTIC study 1-UM-1-HL120877-2, the Systems Biology program ARO-W911NF-10-1-0376, and by the United States Naval Health Research Center contract W911QY-15-C-0027.

SUGGESTED READINGS

Bajzar L, Manuel R, Nesheim ME: Purification and characterization of TAFI, a thrombin-activable fibrinolysis inhibitor. *J Biol Chem* 270:14477–14484, 1995.

Bertina RM, Koeleman BP, Koster T, et al: Mutation in blood coagulation factor V associated with resistance to activated protein C. *Nature* 369:64–67, 1994.

Broze GJ, Jr: Tissue factor pathway inhibitor and the revised theory of coagulation. *Annu Rev Med* 46:103–112, 1995.

Broze GJ, Jr: Protein Z–dependent regulation of coagulation. *Thromb Haemost* 86:8–13, 2001.

Brummel KE, Butenas S, Mann KG: An integrated study of fibrinogen during blood coagulation. *J Biol Chem* 274:22862–22870, 1999.

Butenas S, Mann KG: Kinetics of human factor VII activation. *Biochemistry* 35:1904–1910, 1996.

Camire RM, Pollak ES, Kaushansky K, et al: Sec-retable human platelet–derived factor V originates from the plasma pool. *Blood* 92:3035–3041, 1998.

Castellino FJ: Human protein C and activated protein C. *Trends Cardiovasc Med* 5:55–62, 1995.

Dahlback B, Carlsson M, Svensson PJ: Familial thrombophilia due to a previously unrecognized mechanism characterized by poor anticoagulant response to activated protein C: prediction of a cofactor to activated protein C. *Proc Natl Acad Sci USA* 90:1004–1008, 1993.

Davie EW, Ratnoff OD: Waterfall sequence for intrinsic blood clotting. *Science* 145:1310–1312, 1964.

Fukudome K, Esmon CT: Identification, cloning, and regulation of a novel endothelial cell protein C/activated protein C receptor. *J Biol Chem* 269:26486–26491, 1994.

Gailani D, Broze GJ, Jr: Factor XI activation in a revised model of blood coagulation. *Science* 253:909–912, 1991.

Healy AM, Rayburn HB, Rosenberg RD, et al: Absence of the blood-clotting regulator thrombomodulin causes embryonic lethality in mice before development of a functional cardiovascular system. *Proc Natl Acad Sci USA* 92:850–854, 1995.

Kahn ML, Zheng YW, Huang W, et al: A dual thrombin receptor system for platelet activation. *Nature* 394:690–694, 1998.

Kalafatis M, Mann KG: The role of the membrane in the inactivation of factor Va by plasmin. Amino acid region 307-348 of factor V plays a critical role in factor Va cofactor function. *J Biol Chem* 276:18614–18623, 2001.

Kalafatis M, Rand MD, Mann KG: The mechanism of inactivation of human factor V and human factor Va by activated protein C. *J Biol Chem* 269:31869–31880, 1994.

Koedam JA, Meijers JC, Sixma JJ, et al: Inactivation of human factor VIII by activated protein C. Cofactor activity of protein S and protective effect of von Willebrand factor. *J Clin Invest* 82:1236–1243, 1988.

Lord ST: Fibrinogen and fibrin: scaffold proteins in hemostasis. *Curr Opin Hematol* 14:236–241, 2007.

Lu D, Kalafatis M, Mann KG, et al: Comparison of activated protein C/protein S–mediated inactivation of human factor VIII and factor V. *Blood* 87:4708–4717, 1996.

Mann KG, Jenny RJ, Krishnaswamy S: Cofactor proteins in the assembly and expression of blood clotting enzyme complexes. *Annu Rev Biochem* 57:915–956, 1988.

Mann KG, Kalafatis M: Factor V: a combination of Dr Jekyll and Mr Hyde. *Blood* 101:20–30, 2003.

Mann KG, Nesheim ME, Church WR, et al: Surface-dependent reactions of the vitamin K–dependent enzyme complexes. *Blood* 76:1–16, 1990.

Parker KA, Tollefsen DM: The protease specificity of heparin cofactor II. Inhibition of thrombin generated during coagulation. *J Biol Chem* 260:3501–3505, 1985.

Patthy L: Evolution of the proteases of blood coagulation and fibrinolysis by assembly from modules. *Cell* 41:657–663, 1985.

Pittman DD, Tomkinson KN, Kaufman RJ: Post-translational requirements for functional factor V and factor VIII secretion in mammalian cells. *J Biol Chem* 269:17329–17337, 1994.

Saenko EL, Scandella D: The acidic region of the factor VIII light chain and the C2 domain together form the high affinity binding site for von Willebrand factor. *J Biol Chem* 272:18007–18014, 1997.

Stafford DW: The vitamin K cycle. *J Thromb Haemost* 3:1873–1878, 2005.

Stenflo J, Ferlund P, Egan W, et al: Vitamin K dependent modifications of glutamic acid residues in prothrombin. *Proc Natl Acad Sci USA* 71:2730–2733, 1974.

van't Veer C, Mann KG: Regulation of tissue factor initiated thrombin generation by the stoichiometric inhibitors tissue factor pathway inhibitor, antithrombin-III, and heparin cofactor-II. *J Biol Chem* 272:4367–4377, 1997.

Weiler-Guettler H, Christie PD, Beeler DL, et al: A targeted point mutation in thrombomodulin generates viable mice with a prethrombotic state. *J Clin Invest* 101:1983–1991, 1998.

REFERENCES

For the complete list of references, log on to www.expertconsult.com.

CHAPTER 127

REGULATORY MECHANISMS IN HEMOSTASIS

James A. Huntington and Trevor P. Baglin

MAIN POINTS

- Hemostasis and thrombosis result from the localized production of thrombin.
- Thrombin is the final protease generated in the coagulation cascade of zymogen activation events.
- The regulation of hemostasis relies on maintaining the lumen of blood vessels (intravascular space) as an anticoagulant environment and the extravascular space as a procoagulant environment.
- The principal drivers of coagulation in the extravascular space are tissue factor (TF) and collagen.
- The procoagulant activity of von Willebrand factor (vWF) is controlled through limited proteolysis by ADAMTS13.
- Tissue factor pathway inhibitor (TFPI) limits the initiation of the coagulation cascade.
- The protein C pathway regulates propagation of the thrombin explosion.
- Antithrombin (AT) is a serpin (serine protease inhibitor) that neutralizes coagulation proteases in the absence and presence of heparin-like molecules.
- Hemostasis reflects the dynamic balance between coagulation and fibrinolysis; excessive fibrinolytic activity relative to thrombin generation may compromise hemostasis.

KEY EVENTS IN BLOOD COAGULATION

It is essential that blood remains fluid within the circulation, but that it clots rapidly when there is loss of vascular integrity. Hemostasis refers to the formation of a blood clot to limit blood loss into the extravascular space or hemorrhage outside the tissues. The term thrombosis refers to pathologic clot formation within the lumen of a blood vessel that impedes blood flow.

Blood coagulation is the result of a biologic amplification system in which plasma zymogens of serine proteases are converted into active enzymes (Fig. 127.1).[1,2] Enzyme activation occurs in a sequential manner and is dependent on the assembly of enzyme–cofactor complexes on phospholipid membranes, principally on the surface of activated platelets (Fig. 127.2).[3] The final event in the amplification process is the formation of the effector enzyme, thrombin. At each step in this process, specific protease inhibitors control the amount of enzyme generated while simultaneous regulatory mechanisms control the availability of phospholipid and the cofactor-dependent assembly of enzymatic complexes on the membrane of activated platelets.

Hemostasis is triggered by the exposure of extravascular tissue to certain protein and cellular components of blood. Nonendothelial cells express TF on their surface and collagen is present in the extracellular space. TF binds factor VIIa to initiate the coagulation cascade, and collagen binds platelets and initiates their activation. These events contribute synergistically to produce a large amount of thrombin from a small trigger.[5] Thrombin ultimately converts soluble fibrinogen into an insoluble fibrin clot to form an impermeable platelet–fibrin barrier. This barrier is rapidly stabilized by platelet-dependent clot retraction and thrombin-mediated fibrin crosslinking

(through activation of factor XIII) and suppression of the fibrinolytic system (through activation of thrombin-activatable fibrinolysis inhibitor [TAFI]).

Both hemostasis and thrombosis are dependent on the action of thrombin. In order to maintain blood in a fluid state in the circulation but permit rapid coagulation when a blood vessel is ruptured it is necessary to regulate thrombin formation so that it occurs rapidly and is limited to sites of vascular injury. The regulation of thrombin generation is both spatial (compartmentalization) and temporal (kinetic). The traditional paradigm of blood coagulation is that hemostasis and thrombosis are inseparable, primarily due to their shared dependence on thrombin. There is now emerging evidence of dissociation between hemostasis and thrombosis, potentially due to subtle differences in the triggering or propagation of thrombin generation.[6,7] However, the most important consideration is that hemostasis and thrombosis are distinct from a spatial perspective (extravascular versus lumenal). Consequently, regulation of hemostasis relies principally on maintaining the lumen of blood vessels (intravascular space) as an anticoagulant environment and the extravascular space as a procoagulant environment.

THE ANTICOAGULANT INTRAVASCULAR SPACE

Blood Flow

The importance of blood flow as a regulatory mechanism is apparent from observations of arterial and venous thrombosis. The arterial system is a high-pressure, high-flow system and thrombosis typically occurs only in the presence of endothelial injury, for example atherosclerosis with plaque rupture or vasculitis. In contrast the venous system is a low-pressure, low-flow system, and venous thrombosis usually occurs in the absence of endothelial damage. Sluggish flow resulting from immobility or pooling of venous blood in valve pockets is an important contributory factor to venous thrombosis. Similarly, thrombus formation is common in atrial fibrillation where lack of coordinated contraction of the atria results in irregular blood flow (stasis) in the left atrial appendage.

Blood Components

Although the potential to convert from a liquid to a solid gel is an inherent property of blood, the components responsible for the phase change circulate in inactive states. The platelets are plate-like and inactive, with a membrane unable to bind clotting proteins and with receptors in inactive conformations. The proteases are all in inactive zymogen states, requiring cleavage of an activation peptide and the subsequent zymogen-to-protease conformational change typical of the chymotrypsin family of serine proteases.[8,9] A possible exception to this is the small fraction of factor VII that circulates as factor VIIa; however, factor VIIa is still zymogen-like until it binds to TF to complete its activating conformational change.[10] Clotting proteases that escape from the site of a clot into the blood are inhibited by a reservoir of inhibitory activity provided by a high (2.3 µM) concentration of the serpin, AT.[11]

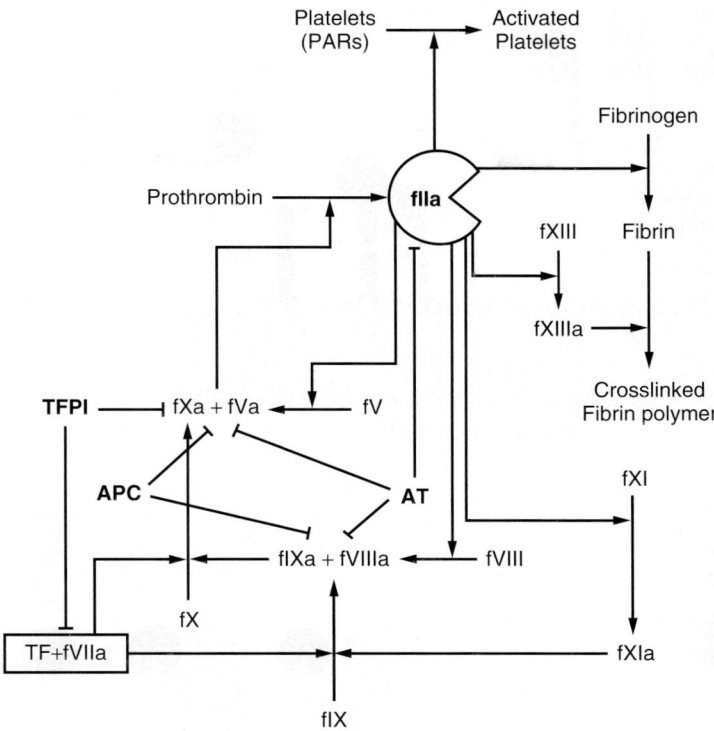

Fig. 127.1 THE HEMOSTATIC NETWORK OF ACTIVATION AND INHIBITION EVENTS. Clotting is initiated by the exposure of the subendothelial space containing tissue factor (TF)–expressing cells and collagen. TF binds to factor (f)VIIa *(boxed)* to form the extrinsic Xase complex. The fXa that is generated binds to fVa to form the prothrombinase complex, which then converts prothrombin to thrombin (fIIa). fIIa activates platelets through cleavage of PARs, converts fibrinogen to fibrin, activates fXIII, which cross-links the fibrin, and stimulates its own formation through activation of fV, fVIII and fXI. Inhibitors of coagulation include tissue factor pathway inhibitor (TFPI), antithrombin (AT) and activated protein C (APC) *(bold)*.

Endothelium

Tight junctions between endothelial cells prevent exposure of blood components to the extravascular space, and their lumenal surfaces are carpeted with negatively charged glycoproteins and proteoglycans that repel circulating platelets and keep them inert.[12] Other important regulators of platelet activation are secreted by endothelial cells: nitric oxide (NO) or endothelium-derived relaxing factor, prostacyclin (PgI$_2$), and the ectonucleotidase, NTPDase-1 (CD39). NO and PgI$_2$ are constitutively expressed, but secretion is stimulated by mechanical stimuli such as cyclic stretch and shear stress. These molecules regulate platelet activation by stimulation of inhibitory signaling pathways within platelets. NTPDase-1 suppresses platelet activation by hydrolyzing the platelet agonist ADP. Endothelial cells also express potent inhibitors of the clotting proteases, including TFPI, thrombomodulin, and glycosaminoglycans (GAGs), such as heparan sulfate and dermatan sulfate. TFPI directly inhibits the initiating complex of TF–factor VIIa–factor Xa; thrombomodulin binds to thrombin and converts it from a procoagulant into an efficient activator of the protein C pathway; and GAGs bind to and activate endogenous protease inhibitors (serpins), AT, protease nexin-1 (PN-1), and heparin cofactor II (HCII). GAG-associated AT inhibits factor IXa, factor Xa and thrombin, whereas PN-1 and HCII are specific for thrombin.

THE PROCOAGULANT EXTRAVASCULAR SPACE

Tissue Factor and Collagen

The principal drivers of coagulation in the extravascular space are TF and collagen.[13–15] TF binds and allosterically activates factor VIIa to

generate sufficient factor Xa for a small amount of thrombin to be formed (Fig. 127.1). This thrombin can activate platelets by binding to GpIbα and cleaving protease-activated receptor (PAR) 1, thereby exposing phosphatidylserine on the platelet surface and setting the stage for the thrombin explosion.[16] The principal procoagulant activity of collagen is to bind to platelet receptors, thereby tethering and accumulating platelets at the site of vascular damage. Exposed collagen also binds vWF (via its A3 domain) inducing a conformational change in the vWF A1 domain that enhances its affinity for GpIbα and leads to platelet adhesion and activation. The platelets contribute to hemostasis first by forming a platelet plug, through adhesion and aggregation, and then by contributing to coagulation by providing a catalytic surface that enhances thrombin generation. This catalytic activity, known as the platelet procoagulant response, results from exposure of negatively charged phospholipid (phosphatidylserine) on the platelet surface during the platelet activation process. These activated platelets are the structural foundation for the assembly of the macromolecular intrinsic tenase (factor VIIIa–factor IXa) and prothrombinase (factor Va–factor Xa) complexes (Fig. 127.2). These homologous enzymatic complexes are the "engines" of blood coagulation and are required for generating sufficient quantities of factor Xa and thrombin to form a stable thrombus. The anionic membrane helps to capture, orient and approximate the enzymes, cofactors and substrates involved in the biological amplification process of thrombin generation. The activation of factor X by the intrinsic tenase complex is 10^9-fold faster than that by factor IXa alone, whereas the conversion of prothrombin to thrombin by the prothrombinase complex is 10^6-fold faster than that by factor Xa alone (in the absence of membranes).[17] The structure of the prothrombinase complex from the venom of the Australian eastern brown snake (*Pseudonaja textilis*) was recently published, allowing the generation of a detailed model

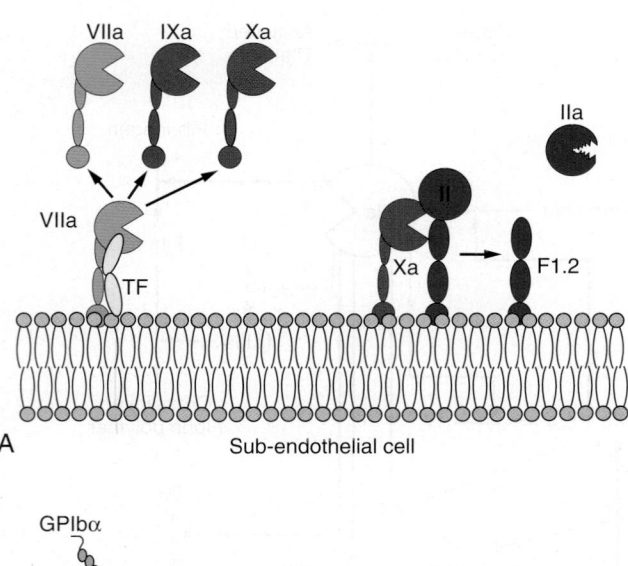

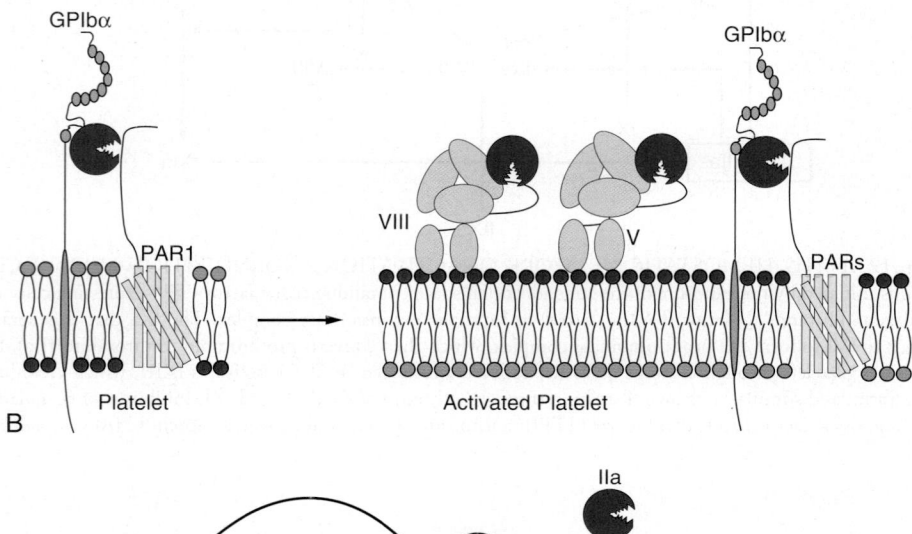

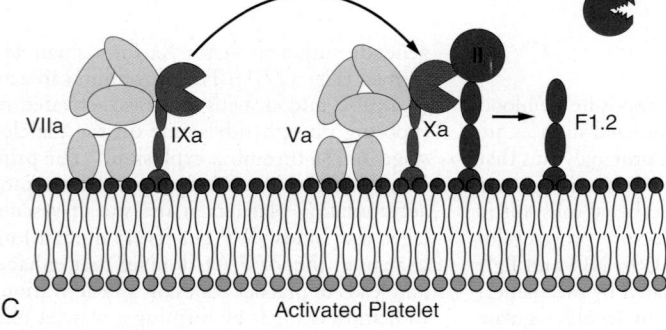

Fig. 127.2 ASSEMBLY OF THE CRITICAL HEMOSTATIC COMPLEXES OCCURS ON THE SURFACE OF SUBENDOTHELIAL CELLS AND PLATELETS. (A) All extravascular cell types express tissue factor (TF) on their surfaces so that clotting is initiated when they come into contact with blood. The factor VIIa–TF complex can activate factor VII, factor IX and factor X. The factor Xa created at this stage is thought to activate a small amount of thrombin (IIa) from prothrombin (II). (B) Thrombin can then bind to the platelets via the receptor GPIbα and cleave protease-activated receptor (PAR) 1 to scramble the membrane bilayer and expose phosphatidylserine *(red surface)*. The phosphatidylserine-rich surface of the activated platelet binds the circulating procofactors, factor VIII and factor V with high affinity. Thrombin activates these cofactors and continues to cleave PARs. (C) Activated platelets now serve as the template for the formation of the two "engines" of hemostasis, the intrinsic Xase complex (factor VIIIa and factor IXa) and the prothrombinase complex (factor Va and factor Xa), leading to the thrombin explosion. *(Adapted from Huntington J: Structural insights into the life history of thrombin. In Tanaka K, Davie E, Ikeda Y, et al, editors: Recent advances in thrombosis and hemostasis, Japan, 2008, Springer, p 80–106,*[4] *with permission.)*

of the human orthologue.[18,19] The components of the tenase and prothrombinase complexes are similar in sequence and structure, and it has always been assumed that they assemble in an analogous manner. However, how the very different substrates of factor X and prothrombin bind to their respective complexes has yet to be resolved.

THE REGULATORS OF COAGULATION

ADAMTS13

Platelet adhesion is an early event in hemostasis and is initiated primarily through vWF, which acts as a molecular bridge between exposed collagen and the GPIb/IX/V receptor on the platelet membrane.[20] vWF, a multidomain protein that forms large disulfide-linked multimers, is secreted from endothelial cells in a latent form that is unable to bind platelets. Binding to exposed collagen via the A3 domain in environments with high shear stress causes vWF to partially unfold, exposing the binding site for platelet glycoprotein receptor GPIbα, which is located in the A1 domain (Fig. 127.3A).[21] The ease of unfolding, and therefore the procoagulant activity, is related to the size of the multimers, and this in turn is regulated by the multidomain metalloprotease ADAMTS13 (vWF-cleaving protease). Although ADAMTS13 circulates in a constitutively active state, its ability to cleave vWF is dependent on the unfolding of the A2 domain that harbors the scissile bond, Tyr^{1605}–Met^{1606}. Cleavage of ultralarge multimers of vWF by ADAMTS13 reduces the capacity of vWF to initiate platelet adhesion and spontaneous platelet aggregation. The importance of this regulatory mechanism is highlighted by the microvascular thrombosis that characterizes thrombotic thrombocytopenic purpura (TTP), a disorder associated with deficiency of ADAMTS13.[22]

Tissue Factor Pathway Inhibitor

TFPI is an endogenous inhibitor of the extrinsic Xase complex.[23] It is expressed by endothelial cells in α and β isoforms generated by alternative splicing of its premessenger RNA (Fig. 127.3B). The α form is composed of three Kunitz domains (K1, K2, K3) followed by an unstructured basic C-terminal region. The first and second Kunitz domains inhibit factor VIIa and factor Xa, respectively. Inhibition is thought to be a two-step process with binding of factor Xa to K2 followed by binding of K1 to factor VIIa-TF. The third Kunitz domain does not possess inhibitory activity but binds to protein S, and the basic C-terminus binds to cell surface GAGs. The β-isoform consists of the first and second Kunitz domains and a glycophosphatidylinositol (GPI)-anchor on the C-terminus that tethers it to the surface of the endothelial cell that produced it. Endothelial cells secrete both α- and β-isoforms, but platelets only produce the soluble α isoform. The basic C-terminal tail of the α isoform has been shown to bind to an acidic stretch on factor Va that has been activated by factor Xa and on the partially activated factor V that is released from platelets.[24] However, that acidic stretch is missing in thrombin-activated factor Va, so the relevance of this interaction in normal clotting is unclear. Protein S binding to the K3 domain helps to localize TFPIα to cell surfaces and thus effects a cofactor activity, enhancing the rate of inhibition of factor Xa by 90-fold.[25]

Serpins

The principal inhibitor of the coagulation proteases is the serpin, AT, also known as SERPINC1 and previously as ATIII.[11] Like all other members of the serpin family of protease inhibitors, AT utilizes a mousetrap-like mechanism whereby the protease (mouse) takes a bite of the reactive center loop (cheese), and before the protease can disengage, the serpin (trap) releases its stored energy through

a conformational change (snap) that crushes the protease.[26] AT circulates at about 2.3 μM and acts to mop up lumenal thrombin and factor Xa. A fraction of AT is associated with heparan sulfate on vascular endothelial cells, where it helps to confer an anticoagulant environment to intact vessels. Heparan sulfate binding also activates AT roughly 1000-fold toward its main targets, thrombin, factor Xa, and factor IXa. This is indeed how the structurally related GAG heparin asserts its therapeutic anticoagulant effect. About one-third of the chains of medicinal heparin (much less for heparan sulfate) contain a pentasaccharide sequence that binds AT with high affinity and induces a conformational change in AT. Low-molecular-weight heparins, including the synthetic pentasaccharide fondaparinux, accelerate inhibition of factor IXa and factor Xa, but have almost no effect on thrombin inhibition. This is because thrombin is insensitive to the conformational change in AT conferred by heparin binding, and instead requires long chains composed of at least 18 saccharide units to "bridge" AT to thrombin.[27] Factors IXa and Xa can also be bridged, but this is a secondary effect to the allosteric activation by heparins, and requires longer heparin chains than those needed for thrombin (36 or more saccharide units in length).[28] Other serpins play relatively minor roles in regulating clotting proteases, including heparin cofactor II (HCII or SERPIND1), which inhibits thrombin and is activated by dermatan sulfate and heparin; protease nexin-1 (PN-1 or SERPINE2), which is a specific thrombin inhibitor and is only found on cell surfaces bound to GAGs; and protein C inhibitor (PCI or SERPINA5), which is a promiscuous inhibitor of coagulation proteases and can be activated by GAGs to inhibit thrombin, factor Xa, factor XIa and the TF–factor VIIa complex.[29] The structures of most of these recognition complexes have been solved by x-ray crystallography.

Protein C Pathway

Protein C is activated by thrombin bound to thrombomodulin on the surface of endothelial cells.[30] Activation is more efficient when protein C binds to the endothelial cell protein C receptor (EPCR) via its Gla domain.[31] Activated protein C (APC) is a physiologic anticoagulant that down-regulates thrombin generation by cleaving and inactivating factor Va and factor VIIIa, the cofactors of the prothrombinase and intrinsic Xase complexes, respectively; protein S acts as a cofactor for APC-mediated inactivation of factor Va and factor VIIIa by helping target APC to the negatively charged surface of activated platelets.[32] Deficiency in protein C results in thrombophilia and its complete absence is associated with purpura fulminans.[33] The most common thrombophilic mutation is the Leiden mutation in factor V that reduces the rate of factor Va inactivation by APC.[34] Conversely, excessive APC activity is associated with bleeding.[35]

Fibrinolysis

Fibrin is a key component of the hemostatic clot and is the primary target for plasmin, the effector protease of the fibrinolytic system. During healing of an injured vessel, the thrombus is lysed by plasmin. Plasmin is generated by plasminogen activators, principally tissue plasminogen activator (tPA). It is essential that tPA and plasmin activity are regulated to prevent hyperfibrinolysis.[36] The principle inhibitors of these enzymes are the serpins plasminogen activator inhibitor 1 (PAI-1) and antiplasmin. In addition, during hemostasis thrombin down-regulates fibrinolytic activity through activation of TAFI. However, hyperfibrinolysis may occur if there is excessive tPA or plasmin. Dysregulation and consequent hyperfibrinolysis occur in disseminated intravascular coagulation (DIC), liver disease, nephrotic syndrome and with some metastatic tumors. Very rarely, heritable deficiencies of PAI-1 or antiplasmin produce hyperfibrinolysis and a bleeding tendency. In addition, normal fibrinolysis may contribute to bleeding when there is inadequate thrombin generation, as in hemophilia.[36]

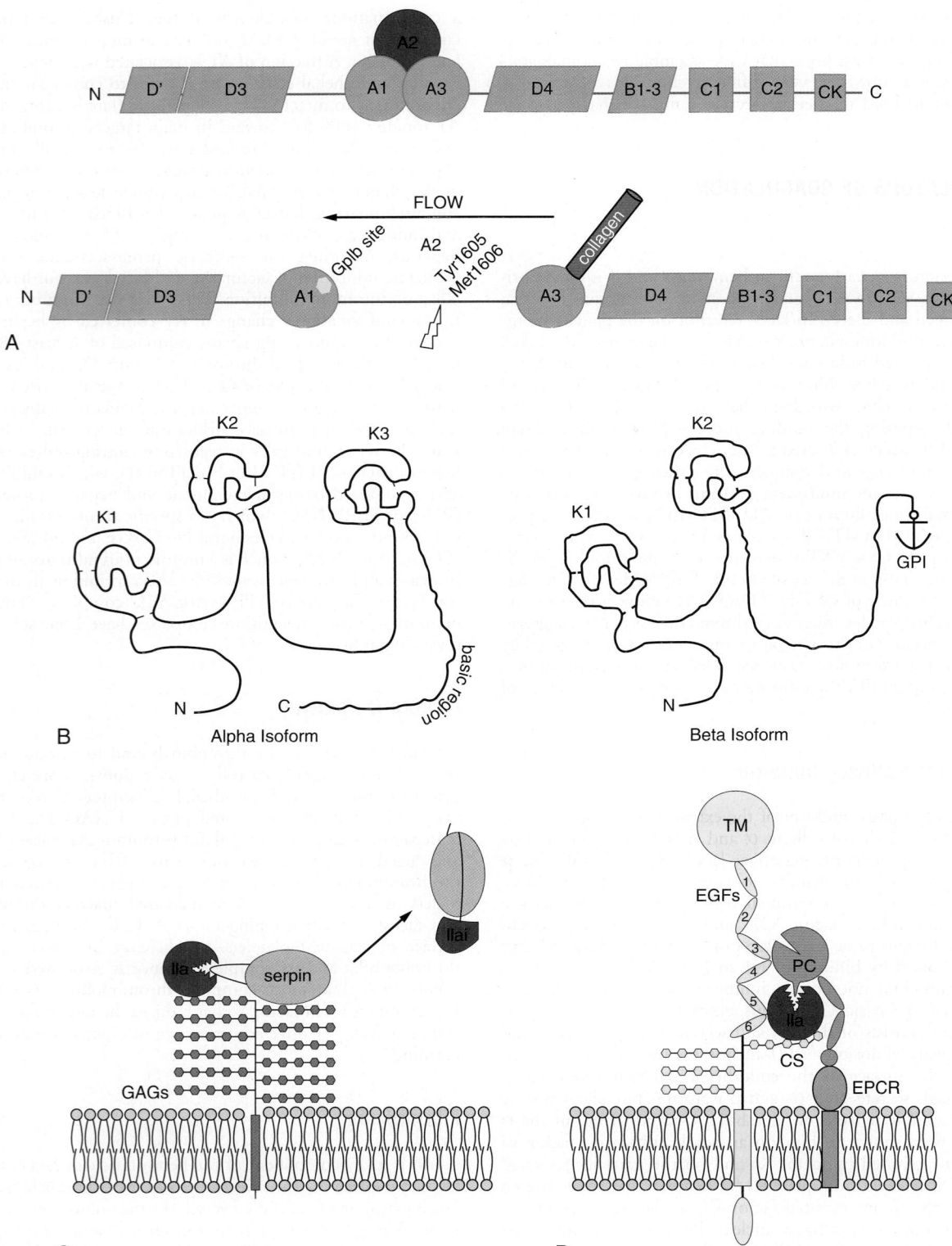

Fig. 127.3 PRINCIPAL REGULATORS OF HEMOSTASIS. (A) von Willebrand factor (vWF) is a multidomain protein that circulates as large disulfide-linked multimers. A schematic of the monomer is shown in its latent state *(top)*, where the platelet receptor binding site (GpIb) on the A1 domain and the ADAMTS13 cleavage site in the A2 domain are obscured. Binding of the A3 domain to collagen *(green cylinder)* in a high shear environment *(flow)* unfolds the A2 domain *(red)* exposing both cryptic sites: GpIb site *(yellow)* and ADAMTS13 cleavage site *(lightning bolt)*. (B) The alpha and beta isoforms of tissue factor pathway inhibitor (TFPI) are shown *(schematics)*. The alpha form is the predominant circulating form, and is composed of three Kunitz domains (K1, K2, and K3) and a basic C-terminus. K1 inhibits factor VIIa and K2 inhibits factor Xa. The beta isoform is devoid of the noninhibitory K3 domain and basic region, and ends with a C-terminal glycophosphatidylinositol (GPI)-anchor *(anchor)*. This form is exclusively found on cell surfaces. (C) Serpins inhibit thrombin (IIa) and other serine proteases, often accelerated by the presence of endothelial cell glycosaminoglycans (GAGs). Inhibition leads to conformational changes in both the serpin and the protease, and in the case of AT and thrombin, results in release from GAGs for receptor-mediated clearance. (D) Endothelial cells also express the transmembrane protein thrombomodulin (TM), composed of six epidermal growth factor-like (EGF) domains. EGF domains 5 and 6 bind thrombin and support activation of protein C (PC). EPCR binding to the Gla domain of PC accelerates the reaction, and the presence of a chondroitin sulfate (CS) moiety on thrombomodulin increases its binding affinity for thrombin. *(Panels C and D were adapted from Huntington J: Structural insights into the life history of thrombin. In Tanaka K, Davie E, Ikeda Y, et al, editors: Recent advances in thrombosis and hemostasis, Japan, 2008, Springer, p 80–106,[4] with permission.)*

REFERENCES

1. Macfarlane RG: An Enzyme Cascade in the Blood Clotting Mechanism, and Its Function as a Biochemical Amplifier. *Nature* 202:498–499, 1964.

2. Davie EW, Ratnoff OD: Waterfall Sequence for Intrinsic Blood Clotting. *Science* 145:1310–1312, 1964.

3. Hoffman M, Monroe DM, Roberts HR: Cellular interactions in hemostasis. *Haemostasis* 26(Suppl 1):12–16, 1996.

4. Huntington J: Structural Insights into the Life History of Thrombin. In Tanaka K, Davie E, Ikeda Y, et al, editors: *Recent Advances in Thrombosis and Hemostasis 2008*, Japan, 2008, Springer, pp 80–106.

5. Mann KG, Brummel K, Butenas S: What is all that thrombin for? *J Thromb Haemost* 1(7):1504–1514, 2003.

6. Buller HR, Gailani D, Weitz JI: Factor XI antisense oligonucleotide for venous thrombosis. *N Engl J Med* 372(17):1672, 2015.

7. Kenne E, Renne T: Factor XII: a drug target for safe interference with thrombosis and inflammation. *Drug Discov Today* 19(9):1459–1464, 2014.

8. Fehlhammer H, Bode W, Huber R: Crystal structure of bovine trypsinogen at 1-8 A resolution. II. Crystallographic refinement, refined crystal structure and comparison with bovine trypsin. *J Mol Biol* 111(4):415–438, 1977.

9. Huntington JA: Slow thrombin is zymogen-like. *J Thromb Haemost* 7(Suppl 1):159–164, 2009.

10. Eigenbrot C, Kirchhofer D: New insight into how tissue factor allosterically regulates factor VIIa. *Trends Cardiovasc Med* 12(1):19–26, 2002.

11. Bjork I, Olson ST: Antithrombin. A bloody important serpin. *Adv Exp Med Biol* 425:17–33, 1997.

12. Verhamme P, Hoylaerts MF: The pivotal role of the endothelium in haemostasis and thrombosis. *Acta Clin Belg* 61(5):213–219, 2006.

13. Butenas S: Tissue factor structure and function. *Scientifica.* 2012:964862, 2012.

14. Gardiner EE, Andrews RK: Structure and function of platelet receptors initiating blood clotting. *Adv Exp Med Biol* 844:263–275, 2014.

15. Nuyttens BP, Thijs T, Deckmyn H, et al: Platelet adhesion to collagen. *Thromb Res* 127(Suppl 2):S26–S29, 2011.

16. De Candia E: Mechanisms of platelet activation by thrombin: a short history. *Thromb Res* 129(3):250–256, 2012.

17. Kane WH, Davie EW: Blood coagulation factors V and VIII: structural and functional similarities and their relationship to hemorrhagic and thrombotic disorders. *Blood* 71(3):539–555, 1988.

18. Lechtenberg BC, Murray-Rust TA, Johnson DJ, et al: Crystal structure of the prothrombinase complex from the venom of Pseudonaja textilis. *Blood* 122(16):2777–2783, 2013.

19. Pomowski A, Ustok FI, Huntington JA: Homology model of human prothrombinase based on the crystal structure of Pseutarin C. *Biol Chem* 395(10):1233–1241, 2014.

20. Lenting PJ, Casari C, Christophe OD, et al: von Willebrand factor: the old, the new and the unknown. *J Thromb Haemost* 10(12):2428–2437, 2012.

21. Crawley JT, de Groot R, Xiang Y, et al: Unraveling the scissile bond: how ADAMTS13 recognizes and cleaves von Willebrand factor. *Blood* 118(12):3212–3221, 2011.

22. Sadler JE: Von Willebrand factor, ADAMTS13, and thrombotic thrombocytopenic purpura. *Blood* 112(1):11–18, 2008.

23. Wood JP, Ellery PE, Maroney SA, et al: Biology of tissue factor pathway inhibitor. *Blood* 123(19):2934–2943, 2014.

24. Wood JP, Bunce MW, Maroney SA, et al: Tissue factor pathway inhibitor-alpha inhibits prothrombinase during the initiation of blood coagulation. *Proc Natl Acad Sci USA* 110(44):17838–17843, 2013.

25. Wood JP, Ellery PE, Maroney SA, et al: Protein S is a cofactor for platelet and endothelial tissue factor pathway inhibitor-alpha but not for cell surface-associated tissue factor pathway inhibitor. *Arterioscler Thromb Vasc Biol* 34(1):169–176, 2014.

26. Huntington JA, Read RJ, Carrell RW: Structure of a serpin-protease complex shows inhibition by deformation. *Nature* 407(6806):923–926, 2000.

27. Bray B, Lane DA, Freyssinet JM, et al: Anti-thrombin activities of heparin. Effect of saccharide chain length on thrombin inhibition by heparin cofactor II and by antithrombin. *Biochem J* 262(1):225–232, 1989.

28. Rezaie AR, Olson ST: Calcium enhances heparin catalysis of the antithrombin-factor Xa reaction by promoting the assembly of an intermediate heparin-antithrombin-factor Xa bridging complex. Demonstration by rapid kinetics studies. *Biochemistry* 39(39):12083–12090, 2000.

29. Rau JC, Beaulieu LM, Huntington JA, et al: Serpins in thrombosis, hemostasis and fibrinolysis. *J Thromb Haemost* 5(Suppl 1):102–115, 2007.

30. Esmon CT, Owen WG: Identification of an endothelial cell cofactor for thrombin-catalyzed activation of protein C. *Proc Natl Acad Sci USA* 78(4):2249–2252, 1981.

31. Mohan Rao LV, Esmon CT, Pendurthi UR: Endothelial cell protein C receptor: a multiliganded and multifunctional receptor. *Blood* 124(10):1553–1562, 2014.

32. Esmon CT: The protein C pathway. *Chest* 124(3 Suppl):26S–32S, 2003.

33. Reitsma PH: Protein C deficiency: from gene defects to disease. *Thromb Haemost* 78(1):344–350, 1997.

34. Griffin JH, Heeb MJ, Kojima Y, et al: Activated protein C resistance: molecular mechanisms. *Thromb Haemost* 74(1):444–448, 1995.

35. Langdown J, Luddington RJ, Huntington JA, et al: A hereditary bleeding disorder resulting from a premature stop codon in thrombomodulin (p.Cys537Stop). *Blood* 124(12):1951–1956, 2014.

36. Chapin JC, Hajjar KA: Fibrinolysis and the control of blood coagulation. *Blood Rev* 29(1):17–24, 2015.

CHAPTER 128

CLINICAL APPROACH TO THE PATIENT WITH BLEEDING OR BRUISING

Catherine P.M. Hayward

Bruising and bleeding problems are common reasons for a hematology referral.[1] The management of an acute bleed (e.g., life-threatening hemorrhage from an acquired factor VIII inhibitor, an anticoagulant drug, or a postpartum hemorrhage) should be the first priority because diagnostic test results are often not immediately available. However, most assessments of bruising and bleeding symptoms are not urgent.

The assessment of bleeding or bruising can be challenging because some individuals without bleeding problems often experience bleeding symptoms (e.g., bruising with trauma, nosebleeds).[1-3] Furthermore, most individuals referred for assessment of bleeding or bruising will have experienced some bleeding symptoms that may or may not reflect an underlying bleeding disorder.[3] Because many individuals referred to a hematologist for an evaluation for a bleeding disorder will be diagnosed with a bleeding disorder, there is a high pretest probability for a bleeding disorder among such patients.[3]

Some referrals for bleeding disorder assessment are for asymptomatic problems (e.g., abnormal coagulation tests caused by vitamin K deficiency, evaluation of a familial bleeding problem after diagnosis of other relatives). Mild bleeding symptoms (e.g., bruising, nosebleeds, possible abnormal bleeding with prior surgery) are more common than severe symptoms (e.g., severe bleed from anticoagulant therapy, life-threatening postpartum hemorrhage, joint bleed) among referred individuals. Sometimes the bleeding symptoms reflect an underlying bone marrow disorder (e.g., bleeding associated with thrombocytopenia caused by leukemia, or a platelet function defect induced by a myelodysplastic or myeloproliferative syndrome), which can develop as a complication of some inherited bleeding disorders (e.g., inherited thrombocytopenia caused by a RUNX1, ANKRD or FLI1 mutation). Some causes of bleeding, such as vitamin C deficiency (scurvy), are rare in developed countries. When considering possible causes of bleeding or bruising, it is important to identify symptoms that are of concern to the patient and/or the referring physician and to determine the extent of bleeding that the person has experienced.[1,3] The next step is to formulate a differential diagnosis and plan for bleeding symptom management (e.g., control of menorrhagia), including strategies to minimize future bleeding risks from exposure to surgery and other invasive procedures.[3]

Fig. 128.1 provides a general guide to the steps involved in clinical assessment. Bleeding-history assessment tools provide a detailed framework to evaluate the medical history and to determine which symptoms should be considered more suspicious of an underlying bleeding problem.[4-8] Bleeding-history assessment tools have been used to standardize and quantify bleeding for research purposes, and some have a reasonable utility for ruling out a bleeding disorder when performing an initial assessment for bleeding problems[5] (see box on Influences on Presenting Problems). While a very high bleeding score is consistent with a bleeding problem,[4-8] there is overlap of scores for individuals with and without bleeding problems.[4,5,7,8] These tools provide evidence that some bleeding symptoms are uncommon unless there is a bleeding disorder (e.g., joint bleeds, bruises that are as large or larger than an orange or that track downward).[2,4,5,7,8] Nonetheless, further research is needed to determine the accuracy of recommended bleeding assessment tools for detecting a bleeding disorder at the time of bleeding disorder assessment (see box on Case 1: Illustration of a Mild, Inherited Bleeding Problem).

Some bleeding symptoms, such as menorrhagia or nosebleeds, are not specific to any particular type of bleeding problem.[1,3,7] Bleeding can be triggered or exacerbated by therapies for atherosclerotic disease (e.g., aspirin and/or P2Y12 inhibitors), venous thromboembolic disease (prophylaxis or treatment with anticoagulants), inflammatory states (e.g., treatment with prednisone or other glucocorticoids) and pain (prescription or nonprescription use of nonsteroidal antiinflammatory drugs).[1-3] Bruising can also reflect systemic or topical corticosteroid use and the effects of age- or sun-exposure related changes in the skin (i.e., senile purpura).[1,3]

Without treatment, severe bleeding disorders typically cause abnormal bleeding with all major hemostatic challenges. On the other hand, bleeding may not occur with every challenge in persons with mild defects and lower bleeding risk (e.g., those with a 5- to 10-fold increased risk for bleeding). Age influences the bleeding history by increasing the likelihood of exposures to hemostatic challenges and the development of sequelae such as arthropathy in patients with severe hemophilia.[6,7] A severe unexplained bleed with surgery may be considered suspicious of a bleeding problem. However, if the person reports that prior challenges did not result in bleeding, this narrows down the possibilities to a mild inherited bleeding disorder, an acquired bleeding disorder, an iatrogenic condition (e.g., bleeding while on anticoagulant therapy or a technical problem during surgery that caused bleeding) or a problem that is not related to a congenital or acquired bleeding disorder (e.g., a postpartum hemorrhage after a Caesarian section from uterine atony or retained products of conception). A bleeding disorder assessment needs to consider both familial and personal bleeding symptoms (see box on Case 2: Illustration of The Importance of Assessing Both Personal and Familial Bleeding Problems).

The timing of bleeding with challenges is evaluated to determine whether the bleeding problem reflects a common bleeding disorder, such as von Willebrand disease, a platelet function disorder, an undefined mucocutaneous bleeding problem, or a rarer cause, such as a defect or deficiency in a coagulation factor or fibrinolytic protein[1,3] (see box on Case 3: Illustration of the Importance of Assessing Bleeding Problems Over Time; see also boxes on Cases 1 and 2). Although patients will often know whether bleeding began on the day of a challenge, their recall of timing details is often better when procedures were done without general anesthesia (e.g., dental extractions, biopsies).[1,3,7] Bleeding within a few hours or on the same day of a challenge (e.g., surgery or dental extraction) is most suggestive of a defect involving von Willebrand factor or platelets.[1,3,7] Delayed bleeding (beginning 1 or more days after a challenge) is most suggestive of a coagulation or fibrinolytic defect (see boxes on Cases 1 and 2).[1,3,7] However, the onset of some bleeding, such as postpartum hemorrhage, can be delayed in persons with von Willebrand disease or platelet function disorders.[1,3,9-13] Postpartum bleeding may be absent or inconsistent in women with mild bleeding disorders because pregnancy increases the levels of some hemostatic proteins, including fibrinogen and von Willebrand factor. Bleeding during pregnancy after implantation is uncommon with most bleeding disorders, although it can be severe in individuals with bleeding disorders who develop placental abruption (e.g., from an untreated fibrinogen disorder or factor XIII deficiency). Intracranial bleeding in a child may suggest a severe defect or deficiency of factor XIII, a coagulation factor deficiency, or a fibrinolytic inhibitor, but other conditions should be considered if the diagnostic tests for these conditions are negative.

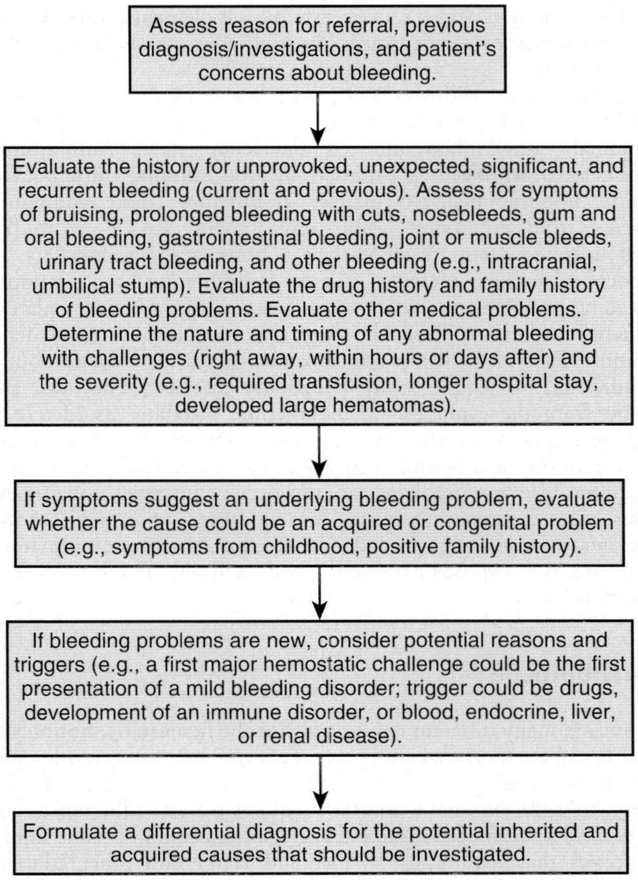

Assess reason for referral, previous diagnosis/investigations, and patient's concerns about bleeding.

↓

Evaluate the history for unprovoked, unexpected, significant, and recurrent bleeding (current and previous). Assess for symptoms of bruising, prolonged bleeding with cuts, nosebleeds, gum and oral bleeding, gastrointestinal bleeding, joint or muscle bleeds, urinary tract bleeding, and other bleeding (e.g., intracranial, umbilical stump). Evaluate the drug history and family history of bleeding problems. Evaluate other medical problems. Determine the nature and timing of any abnormal bleeding with challenges (right away, within hours or days after) and the severity (e.g., required transfusion, longer hospital stay, developed large hematomas).

↓

If symptoms suggest an underlying bleeding problem, evaluate whether the cause could be an acquired or congenital problem (e.g., symptoms from childhood, positive family history).

↓

If bleeding problems are new, consider potential reasons and triggers (e.g., a first major hemostatic challenge could be the first presentation of a mild bleeding disorder; trigger could be drugs, development of an immune disorder, or blood, endocrine, liver, or renal disease).

↓

Formulate a differential diagnosis for the potential inherited and acquired causes that should be investigated.

Fig. 128.1 STEPS TO EVALUATE BLEEDING AND BRUISING PROBLEMS.

Influences on Presenting Problems

When evaluating a bleeding history, it is important to recognize that the presenting problems are influenced by the following factors:
1. The nature and severity of the defect, and the presence of single or multiple risk factors for bleeding
2. Whether the bleeding problem is congenital or acquired
3. Antecedent exposure to hemostatic challenges (such as surgery, dental extraction, menses, and childbirth) and the risk for bleeding with each of these challenges
4. The presence of other medical problems (e.g., renal, hepatic, or thyroid disease), including anemia
5. Variability in the bleeding symptoms experienced by individuals without bleeding disorders (e.g., nosebleeds, bruising) and by individuals with known bleeding disorders, even within families with the same defect
6. Local factors (e.g., sun-damage to the skin, vascular lesions, diverticular disease, or cancerous lesions in the gastrointestinal tract) and the possibility of nonaccidental trauma
7. Treatments that increase the risk for bleeding (e.g., antiplatelet drugs, such as aspirin and nonsteroidal antiinflammatory drug used for pain control, anticoagulant therapy, etc.)
8. Whether treatments were used to prevent or control bleeding
9. Whether treatments prescribed for other reasons may have reduced bleeding (e.g., reduced menstrual bleeding while on oral contraceptives to prevent pregnancy)

EPIDEMIOLOGY

An understanding of the epidemiology of bleeding problems requires distinction between symptoms that rarely represent a pathologic condition and do not require investigation or therapy (e.g., isolated "easy bruising", brief nosebleeds) and those that are

Case 1: Illustration of a Mild, Inherited Bleeding Problem

A 77-year-old man who is starting treatment for multiple myeloma was discovered to have a prolonged activated partial thromboplastin time. Review of his records indicated that the abnormality was present on a previous admission for spinal cord compression, which was treated with surgery. He required 4 units of packed red blood cells several days after this surgery because of delayed postoperative bleeding. There was no other bleeding history. He was found to have mild factor IX deficiency, unrelated to the myeloma, and his daughter proved to be a carrier of this defect.

Case 2: Illustration of the Importance of Assessing Both Personal and Familial Bleeding Problems

A 22-year-old woman was referred for evaluation of a possible platelet disorder. She had a history of menorrhagia (4 days out of 7 days of menstrual flow were heavy when not on treatment), prolonged nosebleeds in childhood, and hematuria with urinary tract infections. She did not have thrombocytopenia, and she had no exposure to major hemostatic challenges. Her father, uncle, and grandfather had a striking bleeding history, and two of them had thrombocytopenia. The bleeding in her relatives included joint bleeds with trauma and severe, delayed-onset bleeding after trauma and surgery (usually more than a day later), which continued for weeks despite platelet transfusions. One of these relatives reported no bleeding when he had a tooth extracted while receiving fibrinolytic inhibitor therapy. Although menorrhagia is not specific to any one type of bleeding disorder, the delayed bleeding in affected relatives suggests a possible autosomal dominant disorder and either a fibrinolytic defect or a factor defect or deficiency (e.g., dysfibrinogenemia; the latter had been excluded in previous tests of the affected relatives). Because of the family history of thrombocytopenia, joint bleeds, and delayed bleeding, which did not respond well to platelet transfusions, testing was done for the Quebec platelet disorder. Genetic testing for duplication mutation of the urokinase plasminogen activator gene confirmed this diagnosis in the patient and her relatives. This case illustrates the importance of evaluating both the personal and family bleeding history and highlights the fact that bleeding-symptom severity can vary among affected family members, in part because of their different exposures to challenges and treatments.

Case 3: Illustration of the Importance of Assessing Bleeding Problems Over Time

A 72-year-old man was referred for evaluation of a severe bleed after receiving a single dose of low-molecular-weight heparin for unconfirmed deep vein thrombosis. He had a history of a similar bleeding episode several years previously while on warfarin treatment for atrial fibrillation. There was no other bleeding history, and the patient subsequently developed a spontaneous iliopsoas bleed. He had undergone numerous surgeries earlier in life without any bleeding problems, and there was no family history of bleeding. The bleeding history suggested the possibility of an acquired bleeding problem, possibly acquired von Willebrand disease or an acquired factor deficiency. Diagnostic testing indicated that he had acquired factor XIII deficiency. This case illustrates the fact that there may be more than one risk factor for bleeding: in this case, several exposures to anticoagulants triggered bleeding in a patient with an acquired factor deficiency. On initial treatment of his iliopsoas bleed with factor XIII concentrate, there was partial neutralization of the infused factor followed by accelerated clearance, consistent with acquired factor XIII deficiency secondary to an autoantibody.

more suspicious, require treatment, and/or are highly predictive of a bleeding problem.[1-3] Some individuals have multiple risk factors for bleeding (e.g., low von Willebrand factor levels, exposure to drugs that inhibit platelet function after a surgical procedure associated with a high risk for bleeding).[3] Although some symptoms, such as nosebleeds, easy bruising, and menorrhagia, are quite prevalent in the general population (10% or more report these symptoms), these problems are more frequent and more severe in individuals with bleeding disorders.[1-5,7,9,14-18] Menorrhagia requiring treatment is common among women, and it can sometimes be life-threatening in those with severe bleeding disorders.[10,12,14,16,17] With moderate or severe disorders, there is less uncertainty about the disease prevalence than there is for milder disorders (e.g., type 1 von Willebrand disease) where there is ongoing debate about the diagnostic criteria that define a pathologic abnormality.[9] There is less information on the prevalence of disorders that require complex tests for diagnosis and have many potential causes (e.g., platelet function disorders). Undefined disorders (definite bleeding problems despite normal or nondiagnostic test findings) have emerged as a common cause of mucocutaneous bleeding.[18,19]

The process of referral for bleeding makes it likely that the person has had some bleeding symptoms that may or may not reflect an underlying congenital or acquired bleeding problem.[1,3] Because of this referral bias, the prevalence of bleeding disorders in tertiary referral clinics is much higher than in the general population. The prevalence of inherited bleeding disorders in the general population is quite low (from 0.00023% to over 1% for von Willebrand disease, with much lower estimates based on studies of bleeding disorder–clinic cases compared with those derived from population screening studies that used higher cutoffs to define quantitative deficiencies; 0.005% to 0.01% for hemophilia; and much lower for other coagulation factor deficiencies). Consequently, unselected screening is not recommended.[1,3,9,20] Founder effects in populations can alter the prevalence of both common and rare inherited bleeding disorders.

A person with a first-degree relative with an autosomal dominant bleeding problem (e.g., Case 2), or a sibling with a recessively inherited disorder, has a higher pretest probability of an inherited bleeding disorder.[7,9] When assessing the relative of someone with a positive family history of a bleeding problem, it is important to realize that the person may have the same condition, with or without additional defects, or a different bleeding problem.[7] Furthermore, it is common for affected family members to show some variability in the severity of their bleeding symptoms (e.g., Case 2).[7,9] Index cases typically have more severe bleeding symptoms.[1,4] Accordingly, laboratory investigations are often used to assess family members at high risk, even in the absence of a remarkable personal bleeding history.

Common bleeding disorders that are inherited as autosomal dominant traits include von Willebrand disease, many common platelet function disorders (including many secretion defects, MYH9-related disorders, gain-of-function disorders such as platelet-type von Willebrand disease and Quebec platelet disorder), and dysfibrinogenemia.[1,3,9,15] Because the diagnostic criteria for mild von Willebrand disease have changed,[9] a positive personal or family history often requires reevaluation over time.

X-linked bleeding disorders include hemophilia A, hemophilia B, and X-linked congenital platelet disorders (e.g., Wiskott-Aldrich syndrome or thrombocytopenia caused by GATA1 mutations).[1,3,15] X-linked disorders typically affect males but can affect women with skewed X-chromosome inactivation or Turner syndrome. Recessively inherited bleeding disorders are the rarest, and their prevalence is highest in populations in which consanguinity is culturally accepted.[21]

Acquired bleeding problems are common, and the most frequent cause is a drug-induced defect.[1,3] Drugs that alter hemostasis may cause bleeding on their own or they may unmask or worsen symptoms from a mild or moderate underlying bleeding disorder.[1,3,9,22] Drug-induced problems to consider include the following: (1) use of prescription or nonprescription nonsteroidal antiinflammatory drugs (NSAIDs) that transiently inhibit platelet cyclooxygenase-1 (patients may not recall taking these drugs if they received them after a surgical procedure[2,3,22]); (2) aspirin or $P2Y_{12}$ or $\alpha_{IIb}\beta_3$ inhibitors used for acute or chronic prevention or treatment of cardiovascular disorders; (3) anticoagulants prescribed for the prevention or treatment of venous thromboembolic disease, atrial fibrillation, or acute management of atherosclerotic disease; (4) antidepressant medications (e.g., serotonin reuptake inhibitors), which may cause bruising; and (5) glucocorticoid therapy.[1,19,23,24] Some dietary practices affect platelet function (e.g., use of fish oil supplements, ingestion of herbal supplements with aspirin-like properties), as can acute alcohol intoxication.[3,15]

Among adults with von Willebrand disease, factor VIII deficiency, and factor XIII deficiency, about 10% of the cases result from an acquired, autoantibody-induced deficiency state. Autoimmune causes of other bleeding disorders include immune thrombocytopenia, immune-mediated platelet dysfunction (more commonly arising from antibodies against glycoprotein IbIXV or $\alpha_{IIb}\beta_3$), and acquired factor V deficiency.[1,3] Bone marrow disorders are associated with an increased risk for autoimmune or nonimmune bleeding problems, including thrombocytopenia, secondary platelet function defects of diverse etiology (e.g., acquired forms of dense granule deficiency, Glanzmann thrombasthenia, or Bernard-Soulier syndrome), or acquired von Willebrand disease.[15] They can also result from the evolution of an inherited bleeding disorder (e.g., the development of acute myelogenous leukemia or myelodysplastic syndrome in a person with a RUNX1 or ANKRD mutation). Acquired bleeding problems can also occur with renal impairment, liver disease, hypothyroidism, or Cushing syndrome.[1,3] Some patients present with acquired skin bleeding that, on examination, is restricted to exposed parts of the body and reflects sun damage to the skin.

PATHOBIOLOGY

There are many different components of the hemostatic, fibrinolytic and vascular response to injury that are important for prevention and control of bleeding (see Chapters 122, 123, 125–127, 130, 131, 135, 137 and 138). Normal hemostasis requires platelet adhesion to collagen and platelet activation and aggregation at sites of tissue injury, processes that require von Willebrand factor and other adhesive proteins; the initiation of coagulation by tissue factor; followed by amplification and propagation of coagulation to generate thrombin and convert fibrinogen to fibrin. It also requires stabilization of fibrin through the cross-linking actions of activated factor XIII. The activation of fibrinolysis (which is important for wound healing) is part of the normal response to tissue injury and repair. Fibrinolysis is retarded by platelets (which release large quantities of stored plasminogen activator inhibitor 1 [PAI-1]) and accelerated by deficiencies or defects in PAI-1 or α_2-antiplasmin, gain-of-function defects in plasminogen activators, and pathologic states that increase fibrinolysis. The interdependence of hemostatic mechanisms explains why a failure of platelet adhesive mechanisms (e.g., from defects in platelet number or function or von Willebrand disease) may cause persistent, delayed, and/or recurrent bleeding from a wound site, particularly if initial hemostasis was inadequately managed or controlled. That activation of fibrinolysis occurring during hemostasis explains why fibrinolytic inhibitors are often effective for treating diverse bleeding problems (e.g., menorrhagia and bleeding from oral/nasal surgical or dental procedures) in patients with conditions ranging from von Willebrand disease and platelet disorders to factor deficiencies and fibrinolytic defects. Some individuals with severe nosebleeds or gastrointestinal bleeds from platelet function disorders (e.g., Glanzmann thrombasthenia) that are refractory to platelet transfusions (because of development of antibodies) may respond to treatment with recombinant factor VIIa.

Hemostasis is also influenced by other factors, such as anemia. The red cell number in blood influences platelet margination, which facilitates platelet adhesion to the injured vessel wall. Accordingly, anemia can worsen bleeding and increase bleeding risk. Some disorders of hemostasis reflect defects in the vessel wall. For example, hereditary hemorrhagic telangiectasia (HHT), which is often (but not always) associated with telangiectasia on the nose, lips and oral cavity,[25] can cause troublesome bleeding from vascular malformations. HHT can cause epistaxis (present in about 95% of persons with this disorder), gastrointestinal bleeding, and less commonly, intracranial or pulmonary hemorrhage, typically without excessive bleeding with surgical procedures or menorrhagia.[1,3,25]

CLINICAL MANIFESTATIONS

Age of Presentation and Extent of Symptoms

Inherited bleeding disorders can present at any age, but if severe, a bleeding disorder typically presents at a younger age.[1,3,6,7,26] Milder disorders can present at any age and may require a significant hemostatic challenge to come to medical attention, often a major surgical procedure or a dental extraction.[1,3,6,7,26] Women with mild, moderate, or severe inherited bleeding disorders may present with troublesome bleeding at the onset of menses or with childbirth-related bleeding.[1,3,7,26] When the bleeding risk is only mildly increased (e.g., low von Willebrand factor levels without other defects, mild inherited platelet secretion defects), there may be a history of bleeding with some, but not all, hemostatic challenges.[1,3,9]

The severity of the bleeding disorder affects the number, severity, and type of manifestations. Numerical scores, derived from standardized bleeding-history assessment tools, show considerable overlap among subjects with different disease severities.[4,5] Although use of a standardized tool to quantify bleeding symptoms has been recommended by the International Society on Thrombosis and Haemostasis,[6] the tool requires further prospective validation before it is used in routine clinical practice.

Family History and Syndromic Disorders

It is important to consider that the family history of an inherited bleeding disorder is influenced by the disorder severity, the mode of inheritance, and whether there is more than one bleeding disorder in the family. The family history is often negative in the case of an acquired problem, such as iatrogenic bleeding from anticoagulant therapy or a technical problem complicating a surgical or dental procedure.[1] The family history is typically positive when the disorder is autosomal dominant and has high penetrance.[3,7,9] The family history is negative in individuals with novel mutations and in those with recessive disorders unless there are affected siblings or many affected relatives from consanguinity or founder effects. Individuals with mild disorders who have never had a hemostatic challenge may be referred after another family member is identified to have a bleeding problem or if the person has bleeding after a significant hemostatic challenge.[1,3] Early identification of a bleeding disorder may alter the natural history, particularly if treatment is given before hemostatic challenges.[7]

Some patients have other clinical problems that suggest the possibility of a syndromic disorder (e.g., albinism or a history of delayed pigmentation, hearing loss, nephritis, absent radii) or an alternative diagnosis (e.g., hyperextensibility of the joints because of Ehlers-Danlos syndrome). An evaluation for symptoms and signs of joint hypermobility (affecting the spine, elbows, knees, and/or metacarpophalangeal joints) can help assess for collagen disorders amongst individuals referred for bleeding symptom assessment.[27]

Bruising, Petechiae, and Other Skin Changes

Bruising (which reflects bleeding into the skin) is a commonly reported bleeding symptom.[2–4,7,9,15] Bruising is reported more frequently by women than men.[2] Some bruising symptoms are more suggestive of a bleeding problem than others. For example, bruises from bleeding disorders often occur after minimal or no recalled trauma.[3,4,7,9,15] Bruises that are unusually large (e.g., as big or bigger than an orange) or lumpy or that migrate (i.e., track downward to the feet over time) are consistent with more extensive bleeding into cutaneous or subcutaneous tissues and are more specific, but not highly sensitive, for bleeding disorders.[4,7,9] When bruises are large or multiple, patients may hide them (by wearing pants and long-sleeved shirts) to avoid being questioned. Severe bruising symptoms may lead to lifestyle changes (e.g., avoidance of sports or other activities that increase the risk for bruising).[7] When there is significant swelling with

a bruise, imaging (e.g., with ultrasound) may be necessary to exclude bleeding into deeper tissues.

Bruising symptoms (that are normal or abnormal) can fluctuate over time, depending on activity levels and exposure to drugs or trauma that increase the risk of bruising (e.g., increased bruising when moving house, traveling, or engaging in physical sports; bruising in a toddler who just started walking; worsened bruising after initiating antidepressant therapy). Like normal bruising, bruising from bleeding disorders usually occurs at sites that are commonly exposed to trauma (e.g., lower limbs, outer hips, arms). However, bruising with acquired hemophilia A may be extensive and involve other regions (e.g., the trunk). This type of bruising is most often autoantibody related because it does not occur in congenital hemophilia, even if there is an inhibitor.

Skin examination sometimes reveals bruising associated with skin pigmentation changes from iron deposition. This is typical of repeated bleeds in persons with severe platelet function disorders or moderate to severe forms of von Willebrand disease. These pigment changes are typically localized to sites of recurrent trauma (e.g., anterior shins), and the distribution (which can be spotty) helps to distinguish the finding from the pigmentation associated with venous stasis.

Petechiae and/or oral blood blisters are typical of severe thrombocytopenia and are less commonly seen in other conditions, including severe platelet function disorders. Scurvy can cause perifollicular hemorrhage (often on the shins), bruising, and gum bleeding, typically with associated swelling and redness. Schamberg disease is a pigmented purpuric dermatitis that does not represent a bleeding problem and can be mistaken for petechiae. Early lesions of purpura fulminans, from congenital deficiency of protein C or protein S, may be mistaken for bruises, but the age of the patient and the distribution of the lesions help to establish the diagnosis. Skin bleeding from minor lesions (e.g., skin cancers) can be unusually troublesome for patients with severe bleeding disorders.

Epistaxis

Epistaxis is a commonly reported bleeding symptom that does not always reflect a bleeding disorder, even when the bleeding is frequent and/or requires medical interventions.[2–5,7] Although nosebleeds can be caused by mucocutaneous bleeding disorders (e.g., platelet or von Willebrand factor problems), they can also result from severe deficiencies of common pathway coagulation factors (e.g., congenital deficiency of factor V, factor X, or prothrombin), fibrinolytic defects (PAI-1 or α_2-antiplasmin deficiency, increased platelet urokinase plasminogen activator from Quebec platelet disorder) or HHT.[1,3,7,9,15,21] Nosebleeds from bleeding disorders or other causes are often worse in childhood.

When the volume of bleeding from the nose is large, the patient may experience passage of clots from the nose or may present with melena. Although nosebleeds are not specific to bleeding disorders, it is important to ask about them because severe nosebleeds can be disabling for some individuals with bleeding disorders, such as von Willebrand disease.[3,9]

Gum Bleeding and Bleeding With Loss of Primary Teeth

Gum bleeding can be problematic with inherited or acquired bleeding disorders that affect platelets or von Willebrand factor, although it more frequently reflects gum disease.[1,3,9,21] Severe bleeding with the loss of primary teeth is also suspicious of an underlying bleeding disorder.[1,3,7,9]

Gastrointestinal Bleeding

Gastrointestinal bleeding can complicate a bleeding disorder, but it is rarely the presenting problem, and it requires investigation to determine the source of the bleeding.[1,3,4,9] Gastrointestinal bleeding can be severe with HHT.[25]

Challenge-Related Bleeding

The assessment of challenge-related bleeding is an important part of taking a bleeding history. Bleeding related to accidental trauma may be more difficult to evaluate than bleeding associated with surgery or dental procedures because accidental trauma often causes bleeding, and it is difficult to determine whether the extent of bleeding was excessive.[7] In addition, large wounds may continue to bleed until sutured.

A history of bleeding with surgical or dental procedures can include being told that there was excessive bleeding by a dentist, physician, or other health care worker and/or experiencing excessive oozing or drainage from an incision or extraction sites; wound hematomas; delayed wound healing; bleeding requiring repeated surgery, suturing of an extraction site, an admission to hospital, a longer hospital stay, and/or transfer to the intensive care unit; and receiving blood transfusions, drugs, and/or factor replacement for hemorrhage control.[1,3,7] Patients may not spontaneously report some symptoms, such as extensive bruising around surgical incisions. Occasionally an operative report or other medical document provides important confirmation that there was abnormal bleeding with surgery (e.g., an operative note that documents generalized oozing during a procedure and greater-than-expected total blood loss).[1,3] Iatrogenic reasons (e.g., oozing vessels that were not cauterized or ligated) should be considered when there is a history of an isolated bleeding episode.

Many individuals undergo dental extractions at some point in their life. Bleeding that persists beyond the first day, or that becomes problematic one or more days after a dental extraction, should be considered suggestive of a bleeding disorder.[1,3] Severe bleeding with dental cleaning should be considered suggestive of a congenital or an acquired bleeding disorder (e.g., von Willebrand disease or a platelet function disorder).

In individuals with a moderate-to-severe bleeding problem, bleeding after surgery, dental procedures, or a severe throat infection can lead to airway compromise, whereas bleeding from a surgical or traumatic limb injury can lead to compartment syndrome.[1,3,28]

Bleeding Symptoms Restricted to Women

Women with bleeding disorders experience more bleeding than men because of the hemostatic challenges associated with menses and childbirth.[16,29] Such women are also at increased risk for developing endometriosis and hemorrhage from ovarian cysts.[16,29] They may also report troublesome bruising or bleeding with sexual activity.

Menorrhagia is a fairly common manifestation of bleeding disorders, and the hemostatic cause can be von Willebrand disease, a platelet disorder, or a defect in coagulation or fibrinolysis.[7,15,16,29] However, menorrhagia can arise from other causes, such as fibroids.[3,17,29] Menorrhagia from inherited bleeding disorders is often long standing, but it can be influenced by treatments. Accordingly, it is important to ask about menses when on, and not on, treatment. Menorrhagia can develop as a manifestation of an acquired bleeding problem (e.g., from acquired von Willebrand disease or anticoagulant therapy for deep vein thrombosis).

In general, it is more helpful to ask women quantitative or categorical questions about menses, rather than qualitative questions (e.g., are/were your menstrual periods heavy?). Questions to consider include the following: How many days of bleeding do you have with your typical menstrual periods? How many days of this bleeding were heavy flow? On your heavy days of flow, did you soak through sanitary products in an hour or less? What treatments have you taken for heavy periods? When you were not on treatment, how many days of bleeding (and how many days of heavy flow) did you have with a typical menstrual period? Were your periods like this

when they first began, or did the heavy-flow problems start later in your life?

Menses up to 7 days in total duration, with 2–3 days of heavy flow, can be considered normal.[4,5,7,16,29] Although influenced by the absorbency of the products used, soaking through sanitary products in less than an hour is suspicious of menorrhagia, as is doubling up on products because of heavy flow and gushing and flooding accidents. Dysmenorrhea is common among women with bleeding disorders, and the passage of large blood clots (which reflect increased flow), which is typically painful, suggests the possibility of a bleeding disorder.[5] Pictorial bleeding-assessment tools (which are not applicable to an initial consultation visit) can be helpful to document menorrhagia and responses to treatment.[11,29]

Postpartum hemorrhage is rarely caused by an underlying bleeding problem, and it can be complicated by a profound acquired coagulopathy, typically with severe fibrinogen depletion.[11–13] On the other hand, excessive or prolonged bleeding after childbirth or pregnancy loss can be problematic for some women with bleeding problems.[9,11] In addition, severe fibrinogen disorders and factor XIII deficiency compromise carrying a pregnancy to term and need to be excluded if the patient has unexplained pregnancy losses that are associated with hemorrhagic placental abruption[3] (see box on Case 4: Evaluation of an Isolated Symptom—Recurrent Pregnancy Loss With Bleeding).

During the first week after childbirth, the bleeding (lochia) is typically characterized by brighter red flow than a normal period. Afterward, the flow usually lightens and continues for up to 6 weeks postpartum. Flow can be heavier, or persist longer, in women with bleeding disorders.[9,11]

Anemia Related to Bleeding

A history of anemia and/or prior treatment with iron replacement is frequently reported by women with bleeding disorders.[3,16] Pallor of the palms is often observed when the hemoglobin is below 10 g/dL. Anemia is uncommon in individuals with bleeding disorders unless there is acute bleeding or chronic persistent bleeding leading to iron deficiency that compromises red cell production. Many women with bleeding disorders and menorrhagia have low iron stores, but not anemia. Low iron stores may also reflect ongoing gastrointestinal bleeding (overt or occult), which if present, requires investigation even if there is a known congenital or acquired bleeding problem. Some bleeding disorders (e.g., platelet disorders from GATA1 mutations) are associated with anemia and thrombocytopenia.

Joint Bleeds and Muscle Bleeds

Joint bleeds and bleeding into muscles (e.g., iliopsoas bleeds), which are uncommon bleeding symptoms, suggest a severe coagulation

---

Case 4: Evaluation of an Isolated Symptom—Recurrent Pregnancy Loss With Bleeding

A 32-year-old woman was referred for evaluation of a low fibrinogen level in the setting of acute placental abruption, resulting in a third pregnancy loss (this time in the third trimester). She had no prior bleeding history apart from having suffered three placental abruptions associated with severe bleeding that required transfusion. The family history was negative for bleeding problems. She had previously been investigated for thrombophilia but had not been tested for a bleeding disorder. The low fibrinogen level persisted over many months (levels of approximately 90 mg/dL), suggesting that the defect was inherited. She received fibrinogen concentrate for two subsequent pregnancies, which she carried to term and delivered without bleeding problems. This case illustrates the need to consider inherited disorders when the bleeding symptoms are unusual and severe, even if there is only one bleeding symptom. It also illustrates that prognosis is dependent on diagnosis and treatment.

defect or a fibrinolytic disorder.[1,3-7] However, bleeding into a joint after an injury or an orthopedic (e.g., arthroscopic) procedure can be experienced by persons with other types of bleeding disorders.[1,3-7] In patients with severe factor deficiencies, the clinical assessment should evaluate for symptoms and signs of arthropathy and muscle wasting and if relevant, neurologic sequelae complicating compartment syndrome bleeds.

Subdural and Intracranial Hemorrhage

A newborn or child presenting with spontaneous intracranial hemorrhage or a large cephalohematoma should be investigated for severe underlying bleeding disorders, such as thrombocytopenia, hemophilia, factor XIII deficiency, other coagulation factor deficiencies, or a severe defect in platelets or von Willebrand factor.[1,3-5] Trauma-related subdural or intracranial hemorrhages can also be manifestations of a severe bleeding disorder.[1,3-5] In adults, ischemic strokes are more frequent than hemorrhagic strokes, although hemorrhagic strokes appear to predominate with some bleeding disorders (e.g., Quebec platelet disorder[7]), and they can be complications of antithrombotic drug treatment.

Hematuria

Urinary tract bleeding with an infection is a commonly reported symptom, whereas spontaneous (or unexplained) hematuria can complicate hemophilia and other bleeding disorders, such as Quebec platelet disorder.[3,7,28]

Bleeding at Birth, Age-Related Changes in Bleeding, and Very Rare Bleeding Symptoms

Many individuals cannot answer questions about bleeding at the time that they were born. Nonetheless, bleeding from the umbilical stump or a cephalohematoma at birth can be symptoms of a bleeding disorder.[4,5,7] Menarche can be associated with a marked increase in bleeding in women with inherited or acquired bleeding problems. Some individuals with inherited bleeding disorders report a reduction in their bleeding symptoms as they age, which could reflect lifestyle adaptation and age-related increases in hemostatic protein levels (e.g., von Willebrand factor or fibrinogen) and thrombin generation. Increases in bleeding with aging can suggest an acquired problem (see box on Case 5: Illustration of Changes in Bleeding Problems Over Time).

Some types of bleeds are quite rare among individuals with bleeding disorders, including spontaneous hemorrhage into the spleen, which can lead to rupture (see box on Signs of Active or Recent Bleeding).

LABORATORY MANIFESTATIONS

The general investigations that are appropriate for most assessments of bleeding problems include (1) a complete blood count (to establish if there is thrombocytopenia or anemia), (2) an assessment for a low ferritin level to evaluate for iron deficiency (less commonly associated with microcytosis or anemia; iron deficiency should be corrected if bleeding risks are increased), (3) a blood group and antibody screen, particularly for individuals with prior pregnancies or transfusions and upcoming surgery or major dental procedures, and (4) tests of renal function (creatinine) if antifibrinolytic therapy will be considered because the dosage is dependent on renal function or if an MYH9-related disorder is suspected (see box on The Laboratory Manifestations of Bleeding Disorders). The bleeding time test is no longer recommended, because of its technical limitations and poor sensitivity to common bleeding disorders.[3,15,30] Electrolyte levels merit monitoring when repeated doses of desmopressin therapy are given

Case 5: Illustration of Changes in Bleeding Problems Over Time
A 65-year-old woman presents for urgent evaluation of a bleeding problem, requiring treatment for a symptomatic, expanding subdural hematoma. She had been previously diagnosed with type 1 von Willebrand disease but indicated that she had no bleeding problems (despite many challenges) until she reached 30 years of age, when she began to experience increasing problems with bruising, menorrhagia, and challenge-related bleeding, including severe gum bleeds with routine dental cleaning. An activated partial thromboplastin time (aPTT) had been performed and was elevated. Testing confirmed a low level of factor VIII (14%) and a low level of ristocetin cofactor activity (less than 10%). The patient was given emergency treatment with plasma-derived von Willebrand factor concentrate containing factor VIII. Intravenous γ-globulin was given because she had a very poor response to replacement, suggesting rapid clearance of von Willebrand factor and factor VIII. Within 24 hours of the intravenous γ-globulin administration, her von Willebrand factor and factor VIII levels increased above normal, consistent with acquired von Willebrand syndrome. Additional tests indicated that she had an immunoglobulin (Ig) G paraprotein without evidence of myeloma. Several features of her presentation suggested that her von Willebrand factor abnormalities were probably acquired and not because of type 1 von Willebrand disease (which is more common): her increasing bleeding symptoms over time and lack of bleeding problems during childhood or early adulthood, her very low level of factor VIII (because of its clearance with von Willebrand factor), the IgG paraprotein, her poor response to von Willebrand factor replacement, and her excellent response to intravenous γ-globulin. She has since been managed with intermittent intravenous γ-globulin treatment.

Signs of Active or Recent Bleeding and Conditions Associated With Bleeding
Although findings from the physical examination in bleeding disorders are often normal, it is important to look for signs of active or recent bleeding, including the following:
1. Petechiae, perifollicular hemorrhages (typical of scurvy)
2. Oral blood blisters, particularly if the patient has thrombocytopenia
3. Ecchymoses, hematomas, and skin pigmentation changes because of recurrent bleeds
4. Signs of active bleeding from a site of trauma or an incision, including excessive blood loss into drains
5. Sequelae of previous bleeds in individuals known or suspected to have a severe bleeding disorder, such as muscle wasting and arthropathy, neurologic abnormalities from prior intracranial or compartment syndrome bleeds
6. Pallor arising from anemia: the palms are usually notably pale when the hemoglobin is less than 10 g/dL
7. Signs of an underlying hematologic disorder, such as lymphadenopathy and/or splenomegaly
8. Signs of acute or chronic liver disease, such as jaundice, hepatomegaly, spider nevi, palmar erythema, or Dupuytren contractures
9. Signs of an endocrine disorder, such as hypothyroidism or Cushing syndrome
10. Vascular lesions such as telangiectasia on the face, lips, tongue, buccal mucosa, or fingers which can suggest hereditary hemorrhagic telangiectasia
11. Hyperextensibility if the bleeding history suggests a collagen disorder as a potential diagnosis
12. Signs suggestive of a syndromic bleeding disorder (albinism, hearing impairment, absent radii)

and/or if the fluid balance is difficult to assess. Tests of liver function are warranted if the person has risks for transfusion-acquired, chronic liver disease. Tests for liver and thyroid disease (particularly hypothyroidism) can be helpful if the history suggests an acquired bleeding problem of unknown etiology. Screening for Cushing syndrome (24-hour urine test for free cortisol) should be restricted

TABLE 128.1 Differential Diagnosis of Bleeding Problems

Major Categories	Comments
No bleeding disorder	Symptoms do not reflect a bleeding disorder and have another explanation (e.g., a surgical bleed, not caused by a bleeding disorder).
Possible bleeding disorder	The laboratory findings are nondiagnostic, and the bleeding history is considered equivocal (e.g., unexplained serious bleed with one surgical procedure; unexplained menorrhagia without other bleeding problems).
Definite bleeding disorder, undefined or indeterminate type	The bleeding history is consistent with a bleeding disorder; however, the laboratory findings are nondiagnostic. Commonly the bleeding history resembles mild to moderate defects in platelet function or von Willebrand factor. The diagnosis should only be made once an adequate evaluation for common bleeding disorders (e.g., for von Willebrand disease and platelet aggregation and release defects) is completed. If testing is not complete, the classification should indicate the types of conditions excluded or not excluded, for example: mild mucocutaneous bleeding problem, von Willebrand disease excluded, mild mucocutaneous bleeding problem, platelet release defects not yet excluded.
Definite bleeding disorder with a defined cause	The symptoms and laboratory findings are considered diagnostic of a bleeding disorder. Tables 128.2 and 128.3 summarize many of the potential inherited and acquired causes.

to patients with acquired bleeding problems that suggest this possibility (e.g., bleeding associated with obesity, the development of type 2 diabetes, hypertension, striae, and/or changes in physical appearance).

The investigations for a bleeding problem typically also include screening tests (prothrombin time, aPTT, thrombin clotting time, and fibrinogen level), which are inexpensive tests, that detect acquired coagulopathies much more commonly than they detect inherited bleeding disorders because of differences in prevalence. These investigations are useful as a baseline for individuals at risk for developing a dilutional coagulopathy from bleeding and as initial investigations of a possible inherited or acquired coagulation disorder. Abnormalities, if detected, require further evaluation to determine if the cause is a fibrinogen disorder or a deficiency of one or more coagulation factors. Screening tests for von Willebrand disease are warranted for individuals with a personal or familial history of mucocutaneous bleeding.[9] Platelet function disorders should be evaluated by aggregation tests and tests for dense granule release, if available, because these tests are useful for assessing common bleeding disorders.[15,19,30] Chapter 129 provides more detail on the specific diagnostic tests that are appropriate for a laboratory workup of bleeding problems.

DIFFERENTIAL DIAGNOSIS OF BRUISING AND BLEEDING

The initial differential diagnosis should focus on three major categories (Table 128.1): deciding whether there is (1) no bleeding disorder, (2) a possible bleeding disorder (equivocal bleeding history and nondiagnostic laboratory findings), or (3) a definite bleeding disorder.

There are many potential inherited and acquired causes of definite bleeding problems (summarized in Tables 128.2 and 128.3). The history should be evaluated to determine if the problems suggest a defect in the initial control of bleeding (e.g., defects in platelet adhesion from von Willebrand disease or a platelet problem) or if there are delayed bleeding problems that suggest a defect in a coagulation factor or a fibrinolytic protein. Laboratory findings are important for distinguishing undefined bleeding problems from von Willebrand disease and platelet function disorders, because their symptoms are quite similar.[1,3,18,30]

Acquired bleeding problems arising from drugs are often diagnosed solely on the basis of the medical history (i.e., acquired bleeding problems that occurred while taking a medication that inhibits coagulation or platelet function), although laboratory testing can be useful to rule out other causes. The subject's medical history and laboratory findings are helpful for determining if there is a possibility of acquired bleeding problems from a bone marrow disorder, liver disease, renal failure, or an endocrine disorder (e.g., hypothyroidism or, less commonly, Cushing syndrome).

PROGNOSIS

The prognosis for bleeding problems depends on the severity and nature of the hemostatic defect, exacerbating factors, and whether these problems can be readily corrected (e.g., vitamin K to correct a deficiency, discontinuing aspirin) or if they require hemostatic therapies, such as factor concentrates and/or drugs (e.g., desmopressin, tranexamic acid, or aminocaproic acid). Life expectancy is generally normal unless there is a severe bleeding disorder (e.g., severe hemophilia) or a complication (e.g., transfusion-acquired chronic hepatitis or human immunodeficiency virus). The prognosis for some rare disorders significantly improves after puberty (e.g., factor IX Leyden). A few show progressive worsening over time (e.g., development of aplasia from congenital amegakaryocytic thrombocytopenia, transformation of thrombocytopenia from an inherited RUNX1 mutation into myelodysplasia or acute myeloid leukemia). Other disorders (e.g., acquired hemophilia) may go into complete remission after immunosuppressive treatment with risk for later relapses.

Mild platelet function disorders, mild type 1 von Willebrand disease, and many common undefined conditions that cause mucocutaneous bleeding usually respond well to prophylactic desmopressin therapy, which is given to prevent bleeding with major surgical and dental procedures or bleeding with childbirth. Nonetheless, it is important to have a specific diagnosis to manage situations in which desmopressin therapy alone is insufficient to control bleeding.

Women with bleeding disorders have a similar prognosis to men, although they often have a greater burden of symptoms because of menorrhagia and childbirth-related bleeding.[1,3] Their outcomes with pregnancy and childbirth are often similar to individuals without bleeding disorders provided that they receive treatment to control bleeding with delivery.[1,3] However, some disorders have sufficiently

TABLE 128.2	Differential Diagnosis of Congenital Bleeding Disorders

Disorder	Comments
Fibrinogen deficiency or dysfunction	Deficiencies can be mild-moderate hypofibrinogenemia or severe afibrinogenemia. Fibrinogen function is abnormal in dysfibrinogenemias, which can present with bleeding, thrombosis, or both. Fibrinogen levels can be reduced in some dysfibrinogenemias.
X-linked coagulation factor deficiencies—hemophilia	Presentation is influenced by the degree of deficiency. Factor VIII deficiency is more common than factor IX deficiency. If factor VIII is low, von Willebrand disease needs to be excluded as the cause.
Rarer, coagulation factor deficiencies	Deficiencies can affect factors XI, V, II, VII, or X, and the presentation is dependent on the severity of the deficiency. Hereditary deficiencies of multiple coagulation factors are rare (e.g., of factors V and VIII, or multiple vitamin K–dependent coagulation factors for congenital defects impairing γ-carboxylation) and can easily be excluded by measuring multiple factors.
Fibrinolytic defects	Causes include disorders caused by loss of function, such as α_2-antiplasmin or PAI-1 deficiency, and by gain-of-function defects, such as Quebec platelet disorder (overexpression of urokinase plasminogen activator in megakaryocytes).
von Willebrand disease	Causes include quantitative (partial type 1 to severe type 3) and qualitative defects (loss of function in type 2M and 2A, gain of function in type 2B and platelet-type). Type 1 von Willebrand disease can be confused with low von Willebrand factor levels (e.g., because of blood group O).
Platelet disorders	These conditions can affect platelet number, function, or both. The most common type of platelet function disorder is a platelet secretion defect, which may or may not also impair aggregation responses. Disorders of platelet function are commonly subclassified by the nature of the defect, such as the following: 1. Defects of membrane receptors for adhesive proteins (e.g., Glanzmann thrombasthenia and Bernard-Soulier syndrome) or agonists (e.g., $P2Y_{12}$ deficiency) 2. Defects of signaling or secretion (the largest subcategory) 3. Cytoskeletal defects (e.g., MYH9-related disorders) 4. Storage pool disorders (e.g., gray platelet syndrome, dense granule deficiency, $\alpha\gamma$-storage pool deficiency, Quebec platelet disorder) 5. Defects of procoagulant function (e.g., Scott syndrome)
Vascular disorders	Congenital vascular malformation, including hereditary hemorrhagic telangiectasia, Ehlers-Danlos syndrome

PAI-1, Plasminogen activator inhibitor 1.

good outcomes with childbirth that treatment for uncomplicated childbirth is not required (e.g., for Quebec platelet disorder).[7,28] Childbirth plans for women with bleeding disorders requires consideration of the options for pain management and avoidance of procedures, such as spinal or epidural anesthesia, to limit bleeding risks unless the defect can be readily corrected.

THERAPY

An individual's bleeding history is an important consideration whenever formulating therapeutic plans to control and minimize bleeding risks. Some symptoms do not warrant therapy (e.g., bruising), whereas treatment is important for controlling menorrhagia and for preventing and limiting challenge-related bleeding (e.g., from major or minor surgery and dental procedures, and traumas). For severe disorders, prophylactic treatment is warranted to prevent spontaneous bleeding and to limit challenge-related bleeding, which can be severe. The focus of therapy for some acquired conditions (e.g., acquired hemophilia) is immunosuppressive therapy to achieve a remission while managing any acute bleeding that warrants therapy. For individuals with mild bleeding disorders, who have undergone multiple prior surgical procedures without bleeding, it may be appropriate to have treatment available (e.g., desmopressin on "standby") that is to be administered if and when abnormal bleeding occurs, provided that the procedural-related risks of bleeding are small and readily managed (e.g., biopsy under local anesthetic) while waiting for the medication to have an effect.

For women with bleeding disorders, there are general treatments that can be considered for symptomatic management regardless of the type of bleeding disorder. For example, options for menorrhagia management include oral contraceptives, antifibrinolytic drugs, and hormone-releasing intrauterine devices. When menorrhagia limits lifestyle and further pregnancies are not desired, surgical options

(endometrial ablation, hysterectomy) may be preferred options, particularly when menopause is not imminent.

General management of bleeding often includes supportive care, correction and prevention of anemia (e.g., iron replacement for iron deficiency), and immunization against viruses that may be acquired by blood transfusion (e.g., hepatitis A and B) (see box on Case 6: Illustration of Changes in Bleeding Outcomes With Treatment). If the patient is immobilized or is undergoing a procedure with significant risks for thrombosis, there should be plans for thromboprophylaxis if the defect can be corrected during this treatment (e.g., by factor replacement therapy for hemophilia or von Willebrand disease, fibrinolytic inhibitor therapy for Quebec platelet disorder) or for alternative thromboprophylaxis if this is not possible (e.g., use of venous compression devices without anticoagulant drugs if the treatment will provide only brief hemostatic correction [e.g., desmopressin, platelet transfusions]). Other measures to limit bleeding risks from bleeding disorders, with surgery, include the avoidance of intramuscular injections, spinal and epidural anesthesia, and NSAIDs for pain management. In older individuals with bleeding disorders and symptomatic atherosclerotic disease (e.g., angina), aspirin therapy may be appropriate, with increased vigilance for signs and symptoms of significant bleeding.

FUTURE DIRECTIONS

The development of a bleeding-assessment tool with sufficient utility to distinguish persons with bleeding disorders from those without significant bleeding problems could improve the clinical assessment of bleeding disorders. There is a need for more information on the genetic causes of common disorders (e.g., type 1 von Willebrand disease, common platelet function disorders such as secretion defects) to further understand bleeding disorder pathogenesis and bleeding risks.

TABLE 128.3	Differential Diagnosis of Acquired Bleeding Problems
Disorder	**Comments**
Drug induced	Aspirin, NSAIDs, other platelet function inhibitors (e.g., $P2Y_{12}$ and $\alpha_{IIb}\beta_3$ inhibitors), anticoagulants, fibrinolytic drugs, and antidepressants are common causes
Acquired factor deficiencies	The causes can be immune (e.g., acquired factor VIII deficiency, acquired factor V deficiency) or nonimmune. Reductions in multiple factors can result from vitamin K deficiency, treatment with vitamin K antagonists, liver disease, hemodilution, and rarely snakebites. Severe acquired hypofibrinogenemia is commonly caused by a postpartum coagulopathy or severe liver disease. Prothrombin deficiency occurs with some lupus anticoagulants. Amyloidosis can cause an acquired factor X deficiency, which may be associated with reductions in other coagulation factors synthesized in the liver if the liver is involved.
Disseminated intravascular coagulation	The manifestations can include thrombocytopenia, consumption of coagulation factors, including fibrinogen, and impairment of hemostatic mechanisms from the fibrin/fibrinogen degradation products. Causes are wide ranging and include postpartum consumptive states, prostate and other cancers, and snakebites.
Acquired von Willebrand disease	The cause can be immune (often in association with an IgG paraprotein) or nonimmune (e.g., increased proteolysis of von Willebrand factor with stenotic aortic valvular disease).
Immune thrombocytopenia	Bleeding is usually influenced by the extent of the thrombocytopenia. Some autoantibodies interfere with platelet membrane receptor function, causing bleeding disproportionate to the thrombocytopenia.
Non–drug induced, acquired platelet function disorders	The cause can be immune (see earlier) or nonimmune, typically from bone marrow disorders, although secretion defects can be secondary to Cushing syndrome or hypothyroidism.
Liver disease	Liver disease can cause thrombocytopenia, deficiencies of coagulation factors, hypofibrinogenemia and dysfibrinogenemia, and increased fibrinolysis. In mild liver disease, factor VII and sometimes factors XI and XII are low. Fibrinogen is often increased in early liver disease, and if low, the finding suggests severe liver disease.
Renal disease	Anemia is an important predictor of uremic bleeding. Uremic bleeding is typically associated with severe renal impairment.
Hypothyroidism	Hypothyroidism can cause an acquired von Willebrand disease and acquired defects in platelet function.
Cushing syndrome	This syndrome should be suspected when there are symptoms and findings suggestive of Cushing syndrome or treatment with systemic or topical glucocorticoids.
Surgical bleeding	This is often a diagnosis of exclusion, although the procedural notes sometimes document that a technical problem was encountered that led to abnormal bleeding.
Vitamin K deficiency	Newborns are at risk, as are individuals with malabsorption and/or receiving broad-spectrum antibiotics that reduce vitamin K production by reducing gut bacteria. Older adults are also at greater risk for developing vitamin K deficiency, because of reduced stores from poorer intake of vitamin K. If the patient does not respond to parenteral vitamin K, other causes should be considered.
Vitamin C deficiency (scurvy)	This diagnosis should be considered when there is lethargy with skin and gum bleeding (perifollicular hemorrhages, gum bleeding with swelling). The condition is rare in developed countries. The cause is usually a very poor diet or malabsorption.

IgG, Immunoglobulin G; NSAID, nonsteroidal antiinflammatory drug.

Case 6: Illustration of Changes in Bleeding Outcomes With Treatment

A 38-year-old woman was evaluated for a bleeding disorder. Her family physician had already excluded the possibility of von Willebrand disease. The patient had a long-standing history of massive bruises, often without recollection of trauma, prolonged nosebleeds requiring medical attention since early childhood, prolonged bleeding from minor cuts, and severe bleeding requiring blood transfusions with many surgical procedures. She had a history of recurrent iron-deficiency anemia, menorrhagia requiring medical therapies, and immediate postpartum bleeding. Her father had a history of bleeding problems, but the cause of the bleeding problem in the family was unknown. The history suggested an inherited disorder, possibly a platelet function disorder or a form of von Willebrand disease. The testing indicated that she had a platelet secretion defect with multiple aggregation abnormalities, with no evidence of von Willebrand disease. She underwent additional surgical procedures, using desmopressin treatment to reduce her bleeding risks, with no abnormal bleeding. Her menorrhagia was controlled with tranexamic treatment. She self-administered desmopressin treatment to control nosebleeds, with good effect. This case illustrates that treatment affects bleeding outcomes and the importance of evaluating for common defects in hemostasis.

For more information on therapies for specific disorders, see the chapters on hemophilia (Chapters 135 and 136), rare coagulation factor deficiencies (Chapter 137), von Willebrand factor (Chapter 138), and platelet disorders (Chapters 125 and 130–132).

REFERENCES

1. Greaves M, Watson HG: Approach to the diagnosis and management of mild bleeding disorders. *J Thromb Haemost* 5:167, 2007.
2. Mauer AC, Khazanov NA, Levenkova N, et al: Impact of sex, age, race, ethnicity and aspirin use on bleeding symptoms in healthy adults. *J Thromb Haemost* 9:100, 2011.
3. Hayward CP: Diagnosis and management of mild bleeding disorders. *Hematology Am Soc Hematol Educ Program* 423, 2005.
4. O'Brien SH: Bleeding scores: are they really useful. *Hematology Am Soc Hematol Educ Program* 152:2012, 2012.
5. Rydz N, James PD: The evolution and value of bleeding assessment tools. *J Thromb Haemost* 10:2223, 2012.
6. Rodeghiero F, Tosetto A, Abshire T, et al: ISTH/SSC bleeding assessment tool: a standardized questionnaire and a proposal for a new bleeding score for inherited bleeding disorders. *J Thromb Haemost* 8:2063, 2010.
7. McKay H, Derome F, Haq MA, et al: Bleeding risks associated with inheritance of the Quebec platelet disorder. *Blood* 104:159, 2004.

8. Mauer AC, Barbour EM, Khazanov NA, et al: Creating an ontology-based human phenotyping system: The Rockefeller University bleeding history experience. *Clin Transl Sci* 2:382, 2009.

9. Nichols WL, Hultin MB, James AH, et al: von Willebrand disease (VWD): evidence-based diagnosis and management guidelines, the National Heart, Lung, and Blood Institute (NHLBI) Expert Panel report (USA). *Haemophilia* 14:171, 2008.

10. James AH: Women and bleeding disorders. *Haemophilia* 16:160, 2010.

11. Chi C, Bapir M, Lee CA, et al: Puerperal loss (lochia) in women with or without inherited bleeding disorders. *Am J Obstet Gynecol* 203:56, 2010.

12. Siboni SM, Spreafico M, Calo L, et al: Gynaecological and obstetrical problems in women with different bleeding disorders. *Haemophilia* 15:1291, 2009.

13. Kadir RA, Kingman CE, Chi C, et al: Is primary postpartum haemorrhage a good predictor of inherited bleeding disorders? *Haemophilia* 13:178, 2007.

14. Philipp CS, Faiz A, Heit JA, et al: Evaluation of a screening tool for bleeding disorders in a U.S. multisite cohort of women with menorrhagia. *Am J Obstet Gynecol* 204:209, 2011.

15. Hayward CP: Diagnostic evaluation of platelet function disorders. *Blood Rev* 25:169, 2011.

16. James AH, Kouides PA, Abdul-Kadir R, et al: Evaluation and management of acute menorrhagia in women with and without underlying bleeding disorders: consensus from an international expert panel. *Eur J Obstet Gynecol Reprod Biol* 158:124, 2011.

17. Kouides PA: Bleeding symptom assessment and hemostasis evaluation of menorrhagia. *Curr Opin Hematol* 15:465, 2008.

18. Quiroga T, Mezzano D: Is my patient a bleeder? A diagnostic framework for mild bleeding disorders. *Hematology Am Soc Hematol Educ Program* 466:2012, 2012.

19. Hayward CP, Pai M, Liu Y, et al: Diagnostic utility of light transmission platelet aggregometry: results from a prospective study of individuals referred for bleeding disorder assessments. *J Thromb Haemost* 7:676, 2009.

20. McHugh J, Holt C, O'Keeffe D: An assessment of the utility of unselected coagulation screening in general hospital practice. *Blood Coagul Fibrinolysis* 22:106, 2011.

21. Borhany M, Pahore Z, Ul Qadr Z, et al: Bleeding disorders in the tribe: result of consanguineous in breeding. *Orphanet J Rare Dis* 5:23, 2010.

22. Masso Gonzalez EL, Patrignani P, Tacconelli S, et al: Variability among nonsteroidal antiinflammatory drugs in risk of upper gastrointestinal bleeding. *Arthritis Rheum* 62:2010, 1592.

23. Loewen P, Dahri K: Risk of bleeding with oral anticoagulants: an updated systematic review and performance analysis of clinical prediction rules. *Ann Hematol* 90:1191, 2011.

24. Chen WT, White CM, Phung OJ, et al: Association between CHADS$_2$ risk factors and anticoagulation-related bleeding: a systematic literature review. *Mayo Clin Proc* 86:509, 2011.

25. McDonald J, Bayrak-Toydemir P, Pyeritz RE: Hereditary hemorrhagic telangiectasia: An overview of diagnosis, management, and pathogenesis. *Genet Med* 13:607, 2011.

26. Mikhail S, Kouides P: von Willebrand disease in the pediatric and adolescent population. *J Pediatr Adolesc Gynecol* 23:S3, 2010.

27. Jackson SC, Odiaman L, Card RT, et al: Suspected collagen disorders in the bleeding disorder clinic: a case-control study. *Hemophilia* 19:246, 2013.

28. Hayward CP, Rivard GE: Quebec platelet disorder. *Expert Rev Hematol* 4:137, 2011.

29. Peyvandi F, Garagiola I, Menegatti M: Gynecological and obstetrical manifestations of inherited bleeding disorders in women. *J Thromb Haemost* 9:236, 2011.

30. Gresele P: Subcommittee on Platelet Physiology. Diagnosis of inherited platelet function disorders: guidance from the SSC of the ISTH. *J Thromb Haemost* 13:314, 2015.

CHAPTER 129

LABORATORY EVALUATION OF HEMOSTATIC AND THROMBOTIC DISORDERS

Menaka Pai

This chapter provides a practical approach to the laboratory evaluation of hemostatic and thrombotic disorders. Any assessment of hemostatic or thrombotic disorders must start with a thorough history and physical exam. These can provide clues to guide subsequent laboratory testing, diagnosis and management.

Physiologic hemostasis is a complex interplay of cellular or plasma elements: the adhesion of platelets to damaged endothelium, the aggregation of platelets to form a temporary plug, the successive activation of coagulation factors to form a stabilizing fibrin clot, clot retraction to repair endothelial damage, and finally clot breakdown through fibrinolysis (Fig. 129.1). Commonly available laboratory tests focus on the individual components of hemostasis by testing coagulation proteins, platelets, and fibrinolytic proteins; this chapter is organized into similar components, to provide a structured laboratory approach to the patient with a hemostatic or thrombotic problem. Yet the clinician must be mindful that in the body, the components of hemostasis work together to form a product that is more than the sum of its parts.

LABORATORY EVALUATION OF COAGULATION PROTEINS

The Physiology Underlying Laboratory Evaluation of Coagulation Proteins

For over half a century, the process of fibrin clot formation has been conceptualized as a "coagulation cascade." This is based on the waterfall hypothesis of Davie, Ratnoff, and MacFarlane, who almost simultaneously reported a sequence of proteolytic reactions starting with factor XII (Hageman factor) activation by surface contact and ending with thrombin's proteolysis of fibrinogen to form fibrin.[1,2] However, upon its introduction, this hypothesis of successive necessary proteolytic reactions already appeared to be too simplistic. Nearly a decade earlier, Ratnoff had identified that deficiencies of factor XII were not associated with bleeding; others soon established that deficiency of factor XII's cofactors (prekallikrein and high-molecular-weight kininogen) did not result in a bleeding phenotype either. In 1977, Osterud and Rappaport recognized that the factor VIIa/tissue factor complex can activate factor IX to factor IXa.[3] Broze later recognized that this complex cannot directly activate factor X, because of the presence of tissue factor pathway inhibitor (TFPI); factor IX activation is a prerequisite. Though deficiency of factor XII and its antecedents is not associated with bleeding, factor XI deficiency is. In 1991, Gailani and Broze explained this by proposing that factor XI can be activated independent of factor XII, as formed thrombin cycles back to activate factor XI and thus amplifies its own formation.[4] Factor XII, long considered to have no role in coagulation in vivo, has been found to play a role in thrombus formation and angiogenesis.[5] Our understanding of hemostasis has advanced still further in recent years, as blood coagulation research is increasingly performed under flow conditions with cellular elements in vitro, and in live animals in vivo.

The physiologic "coagulation cascade" now appears to be an intricate system with built-in shortcuts and feedback loops. It is triggered by factor VIIa and tissue factor, and results in the activation

of zymogens that become serine proteases. This system functions in concert with platelet activation and fibrinolysis (Fig. 129.2). However, clinical laboratory testing of coagulation proteins is not based on this current understanding—it follows the original Ratnoff-Davie-MacFarlane surface-activated coagulation cascade hypothesis.[1,2] These tests attempt to mimic in vivo processes by carrying them out in vitro, and thus do not capture the true complexity of physiologic hemostasis. They are still useful in diagnosing coagulation protein deficiencies and important bleeding disorders. However, they can be misleading, as they can also detect abnormalities of questionable clinical significance. The clinician must therefore understand the distinction between the complexity of physiologic hemostasis and the simplistic picture presented by laboratory tests.

As we proceed in reviewing tests for coagulation proteins, we can place them into three technical categories:

1. **Immunologic tests**, which include enzyme-linked immunosorbent assays (ELISA), immunoelectrophoresis, and immunoturbidimetric (latex agglutination) tests. These tests are quantitative, and detect specific proteins with polyclonal or monoclonal antibodies. Their sensitivity and specificity depend on the antibody used (polyclonal versus monoclonal) and the presence of interfering substances (e.g., rheumatoid factor, other autoantibodies).
2. **Chromogenic or amidolytic assays**, which measure the activity of the serine proteases of the coagulation system as they react with synthetic peptides. The reaction (and thus the activity of serine protease) can be measured as the synthetic peptide releases a colored dye. Chromogenic assays are affected by the specificity of the peptide substrate. A disadvantage of these assays is that their fairly narrow measure of an enzyme's activity may not correlate with its biologic activity in vivo or its activity in clot-based assays.
3. **Clot-based or coagulation assays** that are functional, and compare the clotting potential of a patient's plasma with standard plasma that has a known clotting potential. These tests are more difficult and time-consuming to perform than the others, and are susceptible to interference from other factors. However, they most closely approximate in vivo hemostasis.

SCREENING FOR COAGULATION PROTEIN DEFECTS: ACTIVATED PARTIAL THROMBOPLASTIN TIME, PROTHROMBIN TIME AND THROMBIN CLOTTING TIME

The three assays most commonly used to screen for coagulation protein defects are: (1) the activated partial thromboplastin time (APTT), induced in vitro by surface-activation of factor XII; (2) the prothrombin time (PT), induced in vitro by the addition of excess tissue factor; and (3) the thrombin clotting time (TCT), a test of fibrinogen integrity and thrombin inhibition. The PT, APTT, and TCT are clot-based assays that measure the rate of clot formation, and are based on the waterfall hypothesis of coagulation. They trigger a sequence of proteolytic reactions in the intrinsic, extrinsic, and common pathways (Fig. 129.3). The reactions culminate in the proteolysis of fibrinogen to form a fibrin clot, which causes soluble

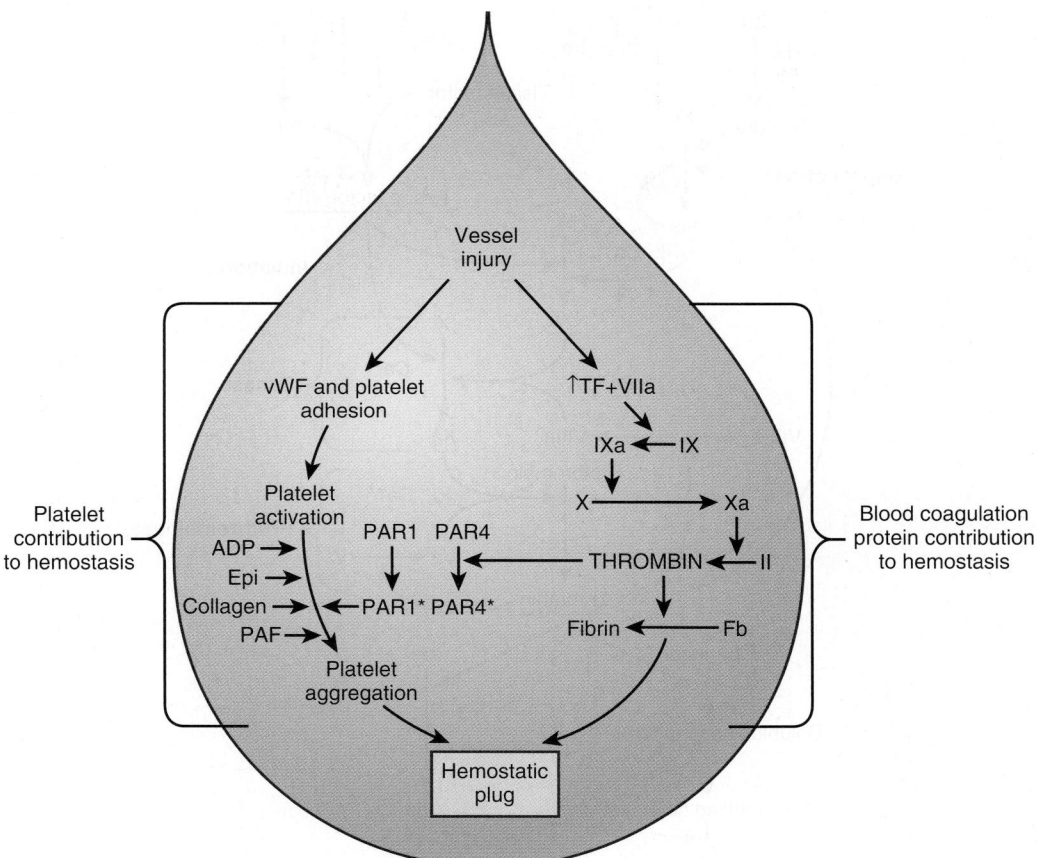

Fig. 129.1 SCHEMATIC DIAGRAM OF HEMOSTASIS. Two equally important arms of activity contribute to physiologic hemostasis. The platelet contribution to hemostasis is as follows. When a vessel is injured, exposing collagen, platelets adhere to the injury site via von Willebrand factor and, in high-shear areas, glycoprotein VI (not shown in figure). Upon adherence, the platelets are activated and release their granule contents. Released ADP and other granule contents recruit more platelets to the injury site. Simultaneously at the site of injury, subendothelial cell tissue factor is upregulated and with activated factor VII (VIIa) activates factor IX to activated factor IX (IXa) and, sequentially, factor X to activated factor X (Xa), and prothrombin (II) to thrombin. Exposed collagen also allows for factor XII autoactivation and generation of additional thrombin in the milieu of activating platelets (not shown in figure). Thrombin stimulates more platelets, enhancing the platelet plug. Thrombin also proteolyzes fibrinogen to form fibrin monomer, which then polymerizes into a fibrin clot. These events occur on or about the activated platelet surface. *Epi*, Epinephrine; *Fb*, fibrinogen; *PAF*, platelet-activating factor; *PAR*, protease-activated receptor, *TF*, tissue factor; *vWF*, von Willebrand factor.

proteins to precipitate in the patient's plasma sample. These soluble proteins can be detected by either increased electric impedance or decreased optical clarity, based on the instrumentation used to measure the result.

Any defect in one of the coagulation proteins along the pathway to clot formation will give an abnormal result (i.e., a delayed time to clot formation), (see Fig. 129.3). For example, a factor XI deficiency will lead to a prolonged APTT. Furthermore, because clot formation depends on a series of reactions, any substance (e.g., inhibitory antibodies, anticoagulants) that interferes with the assay *downstream* from a specific coagulation protein will lead to an abnormal result. For example, a profound fibrinogen deficiency will lead to a prolonged APTT and PT, even when the levels and function of all the upstream coagulation proteins are normal.

In the APTT assay, activation of the blood coagulation system occurs when factor XII comes in contact with a negatively charged surface such as kaolin, celite, silica, or elagic acid (hence the intrinsic pathway's alias as the "contact pathway"). This causes the protein to change shape, allowing its autoactivation and subsequent initiation of the cascade of proteolytic reactions seen in the coagulation system. The APTT measures many proteins that are critical to physiologic hemostasis, including factor VIII and factor IX. However, it also

measures proteins like factor XII, prekallikrein, and high-molecular-weight kininogen that are not necessary for physiologic hemostasis. To perform the APTT assay, equal parts of a negatively charged surface and phospholipid mixture are incubated with patient plasma for a predetermined time. Calcium chloride is added to recalcify the citrated plasma, and the time to clot formation is measured. The APTT assay measures all the proteins of the intrinsic system (factor XII, prekallikrein, high-molecular-weight kininogen, factor XI, factor IX, and factor VIII) and the proteins of the common pathway (factors X, V, II, and fibrinogen). These proteins have different threshold levels to which they must fall before the APTT shows an abnormality. For example, most commercial APTT reagents detect a decrease in factor VIII when the protein level decreases to 35% to 45% of normal (i.e., 0.35–0.45 U/mL). Alternatively, factor XII and high-molecular-weight kininogen levels must fall to 10% to 15% of normal before the APTT becomes abnormal. The sensitivity of the screening tests for detection of specific abnormalities varies with the factor being tested, the commercial reagent used in the assay, and the equipment platform for measurement. Each clinical laboratory should know the level of decrease for each coagulation factor that produces an abnormal APTT with their current equipment and reagents.

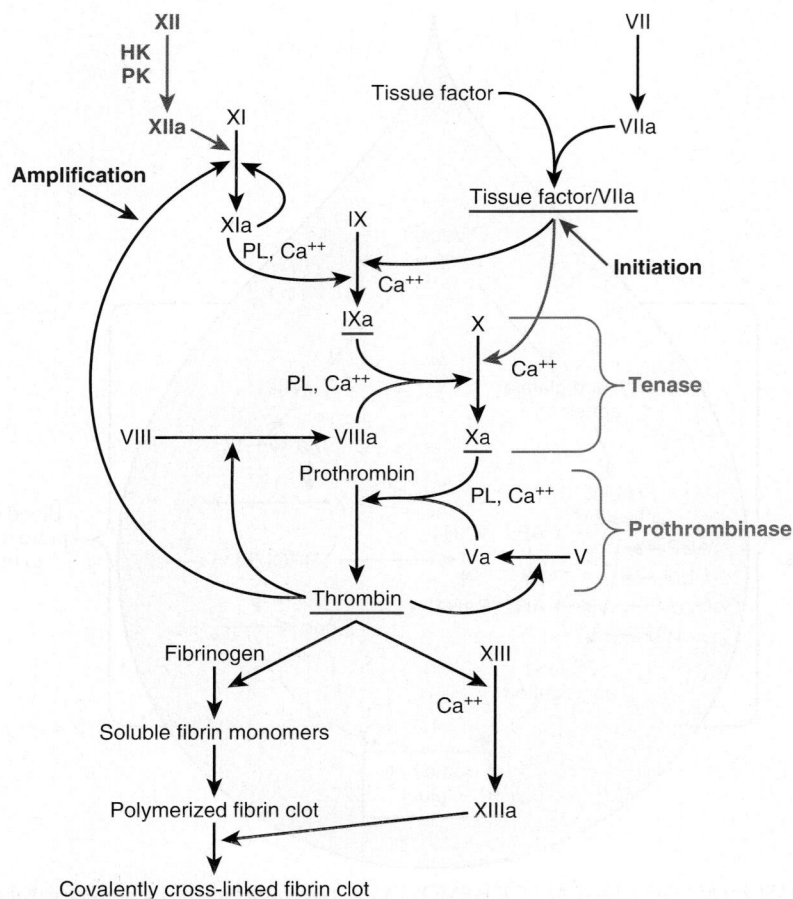

Fig. 129.2 SCHEMATIC DIAGRAM OF PHYSIOLOGIC HEMOSTASIS. Formation of the tissue factor–activated factor VII complex (TF/VIIa) results in factor IX activation to activated factor IX (IXa). TF/VIIa does *not* normally activate factor X directly *(brown line)*. Activated factor IX activates factor X to activated factor X (Xa) in the presence of activated factor VIII (VIIIa), which must have been formed from some prior thrombin activation of factor VIII (tenase). Activated factor X in the presence of activated factor V activates prothrombin to thrombin (IIa) (prothrombinase). Thrombin proteolyzes fibrinogen to form a fibrin clot. If more thrombin is needed, thrombin can activate factor XI to activated factor XI (XIa), which then activates more factor IX to factor IXa, which makes more activated factor X and thrombin. If more thrombin-induced clot formation is needed, thrombin also activates carboxypeptidase U to form a thrombin-activatable fibrinolysis inhibitor that inhibits fibrinolysis (pathway not shown). Factor XI also can be activated by activated factor XII, which is formed secondarily by the constitutive activation of prekallikrein in the presence of high-molecular-weight kininogen by contact activation in collagen-exposed injured vessels. These latter mechanisms are *not* constitutive for physiologic hemostasis. However, in nonphysiologic states, such as sepsis, clot formation in the intravascular compartment, or cardiopulmonary bypass, activated factor XII can activate factor XI to initiate hemostasis with thrombin formation. This latter mechanism is the basis of the activated partial thromboplastin time, a major screening test for hemostatic disorders. *HK,* High-molecular-weight kininogen; *PK,* prekallikrein; *PL,* Phospholipid; *TF,* tissue factor; *Va,* activated factor V. *(Modified from Schmaier AH, Miller J: Coagulation and fibrinolysis. In McPherson RA, Pincus MR, editors:* Henry's clinical diagnosis and management by laboratory methods, *ed 22, Philadelphia, 2011, Elsevier, p 785).*

In the PT assay, addition of excess tissue factor creates a nonphysiologic change in the normal stoichiometric relationship of coagulation factors, allowing factor VIIa to overcome the inhibitory effect of TFPI; the factor VIIa/tissue factor complex then activates factor X to factor Xa (this bypasses the usual physiologic requirement for this process to occur through factor IX activation). To perform the PT assay, one part patient plasma and two parts tissue thromboplastin (tissue-derived or recombinant human tissue factor) and phospholipid are incubated for a predetermined time. The plasma is then recalcified by the addition of calcium chloride, and the time required to clot formation is measured. The PT assay measures the extrinsic pathway of coagulation, which consists of factor VII and the proteins of the common pathway (factors X, V, II, and fibrinogen). Like the APTT, the PT becomes abnormal at different threshold levels for different factors, depending on the commercial reagent and the

equipment platform. For example, factor VII levels must generally fall below 35% to 40% before the PT becomes abnormal.

The PT can also be used to monitor warfarin therapy if the test reporting is modified so it can be interpreted universally. Because of the plethora of commercially available PT reagents and coagulation instruments, it is impossible to know the normal range for the PT from any given laboratory. The international normalized ratio (INR) was thus developed to standardize the reporting of the PT, and create a universal benchmark for monitoring warfarin therapy. INR = (patient PT/mean laboratory PT)^{ISI}, where the ISI (international sensitivity index) for a given thromboplastin reagent is a measure of its responsiveness to reduction of the vitamin K–dependent coagulation factors, factors II, VII, IX, and X. The ISI (provided by each reagent's manufacturer, but ideally locally validated) is based on the degree of variation of the thromboplastin reagent from the World

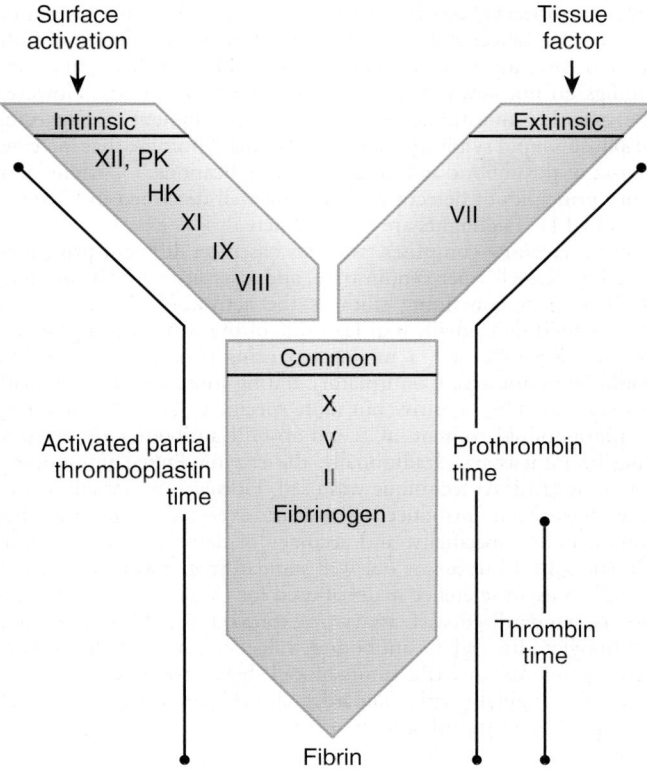

Fig. 129.3 ORGANIZATION OF THE COAGULATION SYSTEM BASED ON CURRENT SCREENING ASSAYS. The intrinsic coagulation system consists of the protein factors XII, XI, IX, and VIII and prekallikrein and high-molecular-weight kininogen. The extrinsic coagulation system consists of tissue factor and factor VII. The common pathway of the coagulation system consists of factors X, V, and II and fibrinogen (I). The activated partial thromboplastin time requires the presence of every protein except tissue factor and factor VII. The prothrombin time requires factors VII, X, V, and II, and fibrinogen. The thrombin clotting time only tests the integrity of fibrinogen. *(Modified from Schmaier AH: Approach to the bleeding patient. In Schmaier AH, Petruzzelli LM, editors: Hematology for the medical student, Philadelphia, 2003, Lippincott Williams & Wilkins, p 79).*

Health Organization (WHO) reference thromboplastin. This reference has an arbitrarily assigned value of 1. INR derivation can be performed by developing a calibration line for any given thromboplastin, using orthogonal regression or linear regression and incorporating the PT determined with the WHO standard.[6] Determination of the ISI requires samples from a minimum of 20 normal donors and 60 patients on stable warfarin therapy with INRs from 1.5 to 5.0.[7] The higher the ISI, the less sensitive the thromboplastin. In practice, changes in the INR are considered interchangeable with changes in the PT. However, the INR is correctly used only to characterize the degree of PT prolongation of a plasma sample from a patient on warfarin.

In the TCT assay, exogenous thrombin is added to examine the integrity of its major substrate, fibrinogen. To perform this assay, purified thrombin is added to plasma, and the time to clot formation is measured. The TCT is thus a direct measure of the conversion of fibrinogen to fibrin (see Fig. 129.3). When performing this assay, it is essential to use the minimal amount of α-thrombin (3000 U/mg specific activity) that will reproducibly "clot" fibrinogen, usually 2–6 U/mL, aiming for approximately 20 seconds with pooled normal plasma to achieve maximal sensitivity for a clinically useful assay. This assay is distinguishable from the clottable fibrinogen assay (Clauss assay) by the amount of thrombin used. The clottable fibrinogen assay uses far more thrombin (100 U/mL) and calculates the amount of functional fibrinogen in patient plasma compared with known levels of functional fibrinogen in calibration plasma.[8] A prolonged

TCT, as indicated by values outside the 95% confidence interval for the time to clot of a population of 20 or more normal donors, suggests reduced fibrinogen levels (usually <100 mg/dL), abnormal fibrinogen function, or the presence of an inhibitor of the exogenous thrombin (e.g., heparin or a direct thrombin inhibitor). The TCT can also be elevated if there is interference with fibrin polymerization, which can be caused by elevated levels of fibrinogen degradation products or the presence of a paraprotein. Some drugs, such as valproic acid, also cause elevation of the TCT.[9]

EVALUATION OF SPECIFIC COAGULATION PROTEIN DEFECTS

When the APTT, PT, or TCT indicate a coagulation protein defect, the plasma concentration of the coagulation factors should be evaluated. Factor assays determine the nature and severity of coagulation protein defects, and can also be used to monitor factor replacement therapy. Coagulation protein defects can take three forms: a true protein deficiency; an abnormal protein that cannot participate in its physiologic function(s); or an inhibitor that targets the active site of the protein or enhances its clearance. Inherited protein deficiencies and abnormalities can be caused by deletions, insertions, and missense/nonsense mutations in individual genes. Inhibitors are generally immunoglobulins, although abnormally produced endogenous heparin, fibronectin, or cryoglobulins can also serve as acquired inhibitors to coagulation proteins.

If a coagulation protein defect is suspected, clinical laboratory testing can be done with immunologic, chromogenic or clot-based assays. Clot-based assays for coagulation proteins are functional: they will be abnormal with both true deficiencies and dysfunctional proteins. These take the form of one-stage assays that use the APTT (for factor XII, prekallikrein, high-molecular-weight kininogen, factors XI, IX, and VIII) or the PT (for factors VII, X, V, and II) as the platform. Specific factor–deficient plasma is the key to clot-based factor assays. These assays are based on the principle that when plasma (either from a reference standard or from a patient) containing the factor is added to plasma completely deficient in that factor, it can "correct" (i.e., shorten) the prolonged clotting time. For example, a factor VIII assay requires reference plasma, factor VIII–deficient plasma (which has <1 U/dL of factor VIII and normal levels of all other factors), and patient plasma. A number of different dilutions of the reference plasma are set up, creating a range of known concentrations of factor VIII. Factor VIII–deficient plasma is added to each dilution, and after incubation for a predetermined time, APTTs are performed according to laboratory protocol. A calibration curve can then be set up by plotting the known concentration of factor VIII present (x-axis) against the time to clot in seconds (y-axis). This process is repeated, substituting patient plasma for reference plasma. If the patient plasma has decreased levels of factor VIII, it cannot compensate for the absence of factor VIII in the factor VIII–deficient plasma; the time to clot formation is prolonged when compared to a similar dilution of reference plasma. By comparing the time to clot of the patient's plasma to the calibration curve, the level of factor VIII in the patient's plasma can be quantitated.

Immunologic assays can be used to establish the quantity (as opposed to the quality) of coagulation proteins. When used together with clot-based tests, these assays can detect a protein with reduced function, but normal production. For example, an abnormal fibrinogen (dysfibrinogenemia) can be detected by measuring clottable fibrinogen and fibrinogen antigen on the same sample. If fibrinogen clottability is less than 90% of the amount of fibrinogen antigen, the protein produced is likely functionally abnormal.

Evaluation of Specific Inhibitors of Coagulation Proteins

An inhibitor is generally suspected when a prolonged clot-based assay does not correct after mixing patient plasma in equal quantities with normal plasma (i.e., in a 1:1 mix), or if an apparent factor deficiency is not consistent with the patient's clinical history. Screening for inhibitors is accomplished by using a 1:1 mix in a clot-based assay. If coagulation factor–deficient plasma is mixed with normal plasma, clotting will not be impaired, as the normal plasma will compensate for the deficient plasma and "correct" its prolonged clotting time. However, if inhibitor-containing plasma is mixed with normal plasma, clotting will be impaired, as the inhibitor will decrease the activity of coagulation factors in the normal plasma as well. Specific inhibitors of coagulation proteins are generally time-dependent, that is, clotting may not be impaired immediately after the 1:1 mix is performed. However, if it is incubated for 2 hours, the clotting time will be prolonged.

Inhibitors of specific coagulation proteins increase a patient's risk for bleeding. The most common acquired inhibitor is an antibody to factor VIII (see Chapters 135 and 136). It can occur as an alloantibody in persons with hemophilia, or as an autoantibody in those with previously normal hemostasis.[10] Patients with an autoantibody-type acquired factor VIII inhibitor present with a prolonged APTT and hemophilia-like bleeding. Both males and females can develop this type of inhibitor. It is characteristically seen in older adult patients, patients with B-cell malignancies, patients with connective tissue disorders such as systemic lupus erythematosus, and in the postpartum period. Management decisions in these patients are influenced by the severity of bleeding and the titer of the inhibitor.[10,11] Quantitative measurement of factor VIII inhibitors is performed using the Bethesda method. This method is based on the observation that if a coagulation factor is incubated with plasma containing its specific inhibitor, the factor will be progressively neutralized. If the amount of factor added and the duration of incubation are standardized, the inhibitor strength can be measured according to how much of the factor is inhibited. One Bethesda unit is defined as the amount of factor VIII inhibitor that will neutralize 50% of 1 unit of factor VIII in normal plasma after 2 hours of incubation at 37°C. Normal plasma pool is considered to represent 1 unit of factor VIII. The Bethesda assay is performed by incubating patient plasma with normal plasma for 2 hours at 37°C At the end of the incubation period, the residual factor VIII is assayed and plotted against a standard graph of Bethesda units versus residual factor VIII activity. The factor VIII percentage nearest to 50% (between 30% and 60%) is chosen for calculating the strength of inhibitor. At 50% inhibition, the test plasma contains, by definition, 1 Bethesda inhibitor unit per mL. The Nijmegen modification allows for more accurate determination of inhibitor titers at low levels of factor VIII inhibition. Increases in pH and decreases in protein concentrations can lead to increased inactivation of factor VIII, potentially leading to false-positive results using the standard Bethesda assay. The Nijmegen modification buffers normal plasma with 0.1 M imidazole buffer, and uses immunodepleted factor VIII–deficient plasma in the control mixture.

Inhibitors directed against other coagulation factors are rare. Autoantibodies against von Willebrand disease (vWD) can develop in the context of a paraproteinemia, whereas autoantibodies against prothrombin are a rare complication of systemic lupus erythematosus. Inhibitors to other factors can be measured with modifications of the Bethesda method.

Evaluation of Acquired Inhibitors of Coagulation Proteins

The most commonly detected acquired inhibitors are the antiphospholipid antibodies (APLAs) (see Chapter 141). APLAs represent antibodies directed to epitopes of proteins that bind phospholipids. They include the lupus anticoagulant (LAC), anticardiolipin antibodies (aCL) and anti-β_2 glycoprotein I antibodies (aβ_2GPI). LAC variably interfere with the APTT and PT, depending on the nature of the commercial APTT or PT reagent. Despite their ability to inhibit coagulation factors, LAC (like other APLAs) do not increase bleeding risk. APLAs may have no clinical significance at all, or they may predispose to thrombosis. Laboratory assays of APLAs fall into

three categories: (1) clot-based assays that detect the LAC; (2) immunoassays that detect aCL; and (3) immunoassays that detect aβ_2GPI. There is currently a lack of standardization of these assays, and their findings do not always correlate with clinical symptoms. However, laboratory identification of APLAs is a key component of diagnosing antiphospholipid syndrome, an autoimmune syndrome that increases the risk of thrombotic and pregnancy complications.[12] Current laboratory principles of detecting APLAs are well described in Chapters 140 and 141. Highlights are outlined here.

LAC screening comprises two tests based on different principles: the dilute Russell viper venom time, and a sensitive APTT, using an APTT reagent containing silica as the activator.[12] Both tests are phospholipid-dependent. If at least one of the two tests suggests the presence of a LAC, a 1:1 mixing test using pooled normal plasma should be performed. Confirmatory testing must also be done with an assay that is less sensitive but more specific to LAC, by increasing the phospholipid content. aCL and aβ_2GPI antibodies are detected using immunoassays. Traditionally, the enzyme-linked immunosorbent assay (ELISA) technique was used. However, newer automated assays have been introduced; these are expected to improve test reproducibility, specificity, and accuracy of detection. At this time, aCL and aβ_2GPI testing is not well standardized, and there is a lack of uniformity in reference material used for calibration. Reporting is also not standardized. aCL assays are expressed in GPL (units of aCL immunoglobulin [Ig] G antibodies, calculated against the original Harris standards) or MPL (units of aCL IgM antibodies, calculated against the original Harris standards). aβ_2GPI can be expressed in U/mL, ng/mL, and µg/mL among others.

PRACTICAL APPROACH TO LABORATORY TESTING OF COAGULATION PROTEINS

The first step in interpreting laboratory tests of coagulation proteins is synthesizing the results of the PT, APTT, and TCT. When all three assays are performed simultaneously, they can give the clinician a high level snapshot of the patient's coagulation factors, and inform a practical differential diagnosis (Table 129.1.) An abnormality in one test suggests an abnormality in one branch of the Ratnoff-Davie-Macfarlane coagulation cascade, whereas abnormalities in more than one test suggest a problem in the common pathway of coagulation.

Isolated prolongation of the APTT is caused by abnormalities in the intrinsic pathway, only some of which are associated with an increased bleeding risk. It is essential to consider the APTT in the context of a thorough clinical bleeding assessment. If the prolonged APTT is associated with bleeding, then the differential diagnosis in decreasing likelihood of frequency is: factor VIII deficiency; factor IX deficiency; or factor XI deficiency. Factor VIII and IX deficiencies are X-linked, and affect 1:5000–10,000 males and 1:25,000–30,000 males respectively.[13] Factor XI deficiency is an autosomal disorder that affects both males and females, and has a variable prevalence.[13] It causes a clinically significant bleeding disorder in 1:1 million in the general population, but has a rate of heterozygosity as high as 8% to 9% in Ashkenazi Jews (see Chapters 135 and 137 for a full discussion of these factor deficiencies). If the isolated prolonged APTT is not associated with bleeding symptoms, the most common cause is an APLA, often found in otherwise healthy individuals. Coagulation protein deficiencies that prolong the APTT but do not cause bleeding include factor XII, prekallikrein, and high-molecular-weight kininogen deficiency (see Table 129.1). It is important to consider these three proteins in the evaluation of an isolated prolonged APTT, to preclude misguided attempts to "correct" the prolonged APTT by giving patients unnecessary blood products or factor concentrates.

An isolated PT prolongation associated with bleeding usually indicates factor VII deficiency (see Chapter 137); these deficiencies are partial, as complete factor VII deficiency appears to be incompatible with life.[13] Sometimes, mild defects in common pathway proteins (e.g., factors II, V, and X) may initially appear as an isolated PT prolongation, though as they progress they eventually prolong the

TABLE 129.1	Synthesizing Results of PT, APTT, and TCT			
Test				
PT	**APTT**	**TCT**	**Possible Diagnoses**	
Normal	Normal	Normal	Normal hemostasis, disorder of platelet function, factor XIII deficiency, disorder of vascular hemostasis, mild coagulation protein deficiency, mild vWD, disorder of fibrinolysis (α_2-antiplasmin deficiency/defect, plasminogen activator inhibitor-1 deficiency/defect)	
Prolonged	Normal	Normal	Factor VII deficiency, early oral anticoagulation, lupus anticoagulant, mild factor II, V or X deficiency, specific factor inhibitor	
Normal	Prolonged	Normal	Factor VIII, IX, XI, XI, prekallikrein or HMWK deficiency, lupus anticoagulant, amyloid-adsorbed factor IX, specific factor inhibitor	
Prolonged	Prolonged	Normal	Multiple factor deficiency (e.g., liver failure, vitamin K deficiency, oral anticoagulants), factor V, X or II deficiency, amyloid-adsorbed factor X, specific factor inhibitor	
Prolonged	Prolonged	Prolonged	Anticoagulants, DIC, dilutional coagulopathy, liver disease, fibrinogen deficiency/disorder, inhibition of fibrin polymerization, hyperfibrinolysis	

APTT, Activated partial thromboplastin time; DIC, disseminated intravascular coagulation; HMWK, high-molecular-weight kininogen; PT, prothrombin time; TCT, thrombin clotting time; vWD, von Willebrand disease.

APTT as well. This asynchronous prolongation occurs because PT reagents with an ISI approaching 1 are more sensitive to factor deficiencies than the APTT. Conversely, the PT and APTT are relatively insensitive to mild defects in fibrinogen. With some reagents, APLAs may also prolong the PT.

When confronted with prolongation in both the PT and APTT, the hematologist should first consider clinical situations that broadly affect these tests: anticoagulant therapy, vitamin K deficiency, liver disease, or disseminated intravascular coagulation (DIC). These conditions are far more common than isolated factor deficiencies of the factors in the common pathway (factor II, V and X). Anticoagulants act by inhibiting one or many coagulation proteins in the common pathway, while vitamin K deficiency decreases functional factor II, VII, IX and X. Vitamin K deficiency is found in individuals receiving warfarin therapy, who are profoundly nutritionally deplete (caused by a poor diet, or the receipt of incomplete parenteral nutrition), who have altered gut microbiota as a result of intestinal surgery or antibiotic therapy, or, very rarely, who have defects in transport proteins or enzymes for vitamin K metabolism. The liver synthesizes all coagulation proteins, so liver disease can have a profound effect on laboratory tests of hemostasis by causing multiple factor deficiency. Prekallikrein, factor XI, factor VII, and factor V production drop in hepatic failure, and fibrinogen synthesis becomes abnormal. DIC, an important cause of APTT and PT prolongation, is discussed in detail toward the end of this chapter.

TCT prolongation can be caused by reduced fibrinogen levels (e.g., because of liver disease), abnormal fibrinogen function, or large amounts of thrombin inhibitors like heparin. The TCT also detects defects in fibrinopeptide A and B release, as well as polymerization defects. The reptilase time uses Batroxobin (Reptilase), a purified enzyme from the snake *Bothrops atrox*, to "clot" fibrinogen by liberating only fibrinopeptide A. An abnormal TCT with a normal reptilase time indicates a fibrinopeptide B–release defect, an abnormality that gives very long APTT and PT values but is not associated with bleeding. The reptilase time also will not be altered by the presence of heparin, and can thus be used to determine if a prolonged TCT is the result of heparin. Another practical way to determine if a prolonged TCT is a result of heparin is to use the protamine neutralization test. This test is based on the TCT, but varying amounts of protamine sulfate are added to patient plasma before the addition of thrombin. Protamine sulfate can neutralize heparin, and thus normalize the TCT. The concentration of heparin in the plasma can be calculated from the amount of protamine sulfate required to produce this effect.

When presented with a prolonged clot-based assay, the hematologist must also be able to differentiate between a coagulation protein deficiency and an inhibitor to a specific coagulation protein. Two approaches can be used to obtain a specific diagnosis. The first approach uses the 1:1 mix, a test in which patient and normal plasma are mixed in equal proportions. Mixing studies based on the PT or APTT are interpreted based on the fact that 50% levels of any coagulation factor will yield normal PT and APTT values. Only when the level drops below 50% will clot formation become prolonged, though the sensitivity of the assay then depends on the factor and the test reagent. Practically, this means that if a patient has less than 1% of a factor, and their plasma is mixed 1:1 with normal plasma, the PT or APTT will be normal. However, if a patient has something in their plasma that interferes with protein function in normal plasma (e.g., an inhibitor, an anticoagulant), the PT or APTT will be prolonged. The 1:1 mix can thus be used to screen for the presence of factor deficiency and inhibitors. This approach is far from perfect. No studies provide standardized evidence-based laboratory procedures for these screening assays, so the ratio of patient plasma to normal plasma used, the time of incubation from mixing to assay, and the sensitivity and specificity for assessing factor deficiencies and circulating anticoagulants is variable. This makes it difficult to translate the results of mixing studies into meaningful diagnostic data. If a factor deficiency or inhibitor is suspected, it is essential to perform the appropriate specific testing, as outlined previously.

Other comorbid illnesses may also result in a bleeding diathesis. For example, systemic amyloidosis is associated with decreases in plasma factor X or IX as a result of adsorption of the coagulation proteins onto the amyloid protein. In the case of factor X adsorption, the PT and APTT may be affected, while in the case of factor IX adsorption, only the APTT is affected. Hypergammaglobulinemic states seen with multiple myeloma or Waldenström macroglobulinemia (IgM) can be associated with inhibitors to coagulation protein function. Dysfibrinogenemias are common in these patients because fibrinogen readily binds the immunoglobulin.

LABORATORY EVALUATION OF PLATELETS AND VON WILLEBRAND FACTOR

Screening for Disorders of Primary Hemostasis

Disorders of platelets and von Willebrand factor (vWF), the key components of primary hemostasis, are characterized by disproportionate bleeding after injury or surgery, petechiae, purpura, ecchymoses, mucosal bleeding (including epistaxis and gum bleeding), and heavy menstrual bleeding. Most patients have a family history of similar mucocutaneous bleeding. In the past, the Ivy bleeding time—a test in which the forearm is cut, and the time until bleeding stops is measured—was used to screen for disorders of primary hemostasis, including platelet function disorders (PFDs) and vWD.[14] This test is no longer considered to be useful in the investigation of bleeding disorders. It is invasive, operator dependent, can be affected by nonhematologic factors (e.g., Ehlers-Danlos syndrome, osteogenesis imperfecta, scurvy, skin quality, skin temperature, vascular function), and has low predictive value for surgical bleeding.[15] It is also not useful in detecting platelet dysfunction in the setting of thrombocytopenia. Importantly, the bleeding time is neither sensitive nor specific enough to preclude further testing for vWF or platelet abnormalities.[16] A normal bleeding time should not reassure the clinician that an important bleeding disorder is not present.

Several automated analyzers have been proposed as replacements for the bleeding time, and potentially useful screening tools for disorders of primary hemostasis. The platelet function analyzer PFA-100 (Siemens, Deerfield, IL), has been best evaluated. The PFA-100 attempts to recreate the high shear conditions under which primary hemostasis occurs in vivo. Using citrated whole blood, it measures the closure time required for platelets to adhere to agonist-coated membranes and aggregate under high shear stress (5000–6000/s). Two cartridges are available: one with collagen–adenosine diphosphate (ADP) membranes, and the other and collagen–epinephrine coated membranes. Platelet function is measured as a function of the time needed to occlude the aperture, termed *closure time*. Abnormalities can lead to lengthening of the closure time. The PFA-100 is more sensitive than the bleeding time in patients with previously diagnosed vWD, but less sensitive in those with mild platelet secretion disorders (which are the most frequent PFDs) and platelet storage pool deficiency. In a prospective study by Quiroga et al, the overall sensitivity of closure time in vWD and PFDs was 50% and 18%, respectively.[16] This suggests that the PFA-100 is only marginally more useful than the bleeding time. It is still not sensitive or specific enough to preclude further testing for vWF or platelet abnormalities, and cannot definitively rule out important bleeding disorders.

At this time, laboratory screening tests for disorders of primary hemostasis have limited usefulness. Diagnosis of these disorders must be grounded in a thorough clinical history and physical exam, and ultimately relies on the performance of the specific and sensitive tests outlined in the following.

Evaluation of Platelets

The first step in the investigation of platelet disorders is determining the platelet count, as thrombocytopenia alone may increase bleeding risk (thrombocytopenia is discussed in detail in Chapters 131 and 132). Obtaining a detailed list of medications the patient is taking, allopathic and naturopathic, prescription and over-the-counter, is also essential, as many drugs impact platelet number and function. Platelet function can also be altered in the setting of systemic disorders, such as renal disease, liver disease, myeloproliferative and myelodysplastic disorders, and malignancy. Inherited platelet disorders are often syndromic, and are associated with manifestations like albinism, bone changes, sensorineural hearing loss, renal disease, and immunodeficiency.

Platelet function can be evaluated with platelet aggregation studies. These tests measure the ability of agonists to cause in vitro platelet activation and aggregation. Two forms of platelet aggregation studies are available: light transmission aggregometry (LTA) in platelet-rich plasma and impedance aggregometry in platelet-rich plasma or whole blood. LTA in platelet-rich plasma is considered the gold standard of platelet function testing, whereas impedance aggregometry is less well characterized. A number of recent guidelines have laid out standards on how to perform and interpret LTA.[17] Briefly, when a platelet agonist is added to platelet-rich plasma, aggregation occurs and light transmission increases. When factors like temperature, platelet count, and mixing speed are controlled, the amount and rate of this increase depends on how reactive platelets

are to the added agonist. The increase in light transmission can be measured spectrophotometrically. Recommended agonists include ADP, epinephrine, arachidonic acid, collagen, and thromboxane analogue U46619 at predetermined concentrations.[17] Ristocetin, an antibiotic that facilitates vWF binding to the glycoprotein Ib/IX/V complex, is also used in LTA to cause platelet agglutination. ADP and epinephrine result in a biphasic aggregation pattern; primary aggregation occurs in response to activation of the platelet glycoprotein IIb/IIIa receptor, then platelets degranulate and cause secondary aggregation. Conversely, arachidonic acid, thromboxane analogue, and collagen result in a monophasic aggregation pattern. Several defects of platelet function have well-characterized LTA patterns.[18] Bernard-Soulier syndrome, a defect in glycoprotein Ib, results in normal aggregation to ADP and collagen, but absent agglutination to ristocetin (this pattern can also be seen in vWD.) Glanzmann thrombasthenia, a defect in glycoprotein IIb/IIIa, results in an absent primary response to ADP and collagen. Impaired aggregation to arachidonic acid suggests an aspirin effect, or cyclooxygenase deficiency. Platelet storage pool disorders can be diagnosed with LTA and studies that measure proteins within or released from platelet α-granules or dense granules. Tests of ATP secretion from platelets can also be valuable in assessing PFDs, as they complement and expand on LTA results.[19] ATP secreted by dense granules is measured by a sensitive luminescent (firefly luciferin-luciferase) assay for extracellular ATP. Platelet electron microscopy is increasingly used to evaluate the ultrastructure of platelets, including the dense granules. Finally, with appropriate monoclonal antibodies, flow cytometry can examine the surface of the platelet. Flow cytometry has a variety of uses, including detection of platelet activation by using antibodies to proteins expressed on the platelet surface (e.g., P-selectin, thrombospondin), diagnosis of platelet surface glycoprotein deficiencies, and measurement of dense granules.

Evaluation of Von Willebrand Factor

vWD is discussed in detail in Chapter 138. It is diagnosed when patients have a history of mucocutaneous bleeding (usually with a positive family history), and quantitative or qualitative abnormalities of vWF. Laboratory testing of vWD includes the factor VIII assay, vWF antigen (vWF:Ag), and vWF activity (most commonly measured with the ristocetin cofactor assay, vWF:Rco).[20] Many laboratories also test vWF further with the collagen binding assay (vWF:CB, abnormal when there is a loss of high-molecular-weight vWF multimers or impaired binding of vWF to vascular endothelium), the low-dose ristocetin-induced platelet aggregation assay (abnormal in loss-of-function and gain-of-function defects that characterize type 2B vWD and platelet-type pseudo-vWD), and vWF multimer analysis (which is useful in type 2A and 2M vWD).[20] Assays that measure factor VIII binding to vWF can identify patients with defects in factor VIII binding, such as type 2N vWD.[20] Highly specialized coagulation laboratories may also perform vWF gene sequence analysis and vWF propeptide analysis; the latter shows promise in detecting defects associated with accelerated vWF clearance.[20]

The diagnosis of vWD—particularly type 1 vWD, which is defined as a partial, quantitative deficiency of vWF—can be challenging.[14] Studies have shown a high prevalence of bleeding symptoms in normal, healthy individuals. By definition, 2.5% of the population will also have a level of vWF:Ag that falls below the lower limit of laboratories' normal reference range. Thus, there is a danger of coincidentally associating low vWF with bleeding symptoms, and overdiagnosing type 1 vWD in the general population.[21] To further complicate the situation, the normal range of plasma vWF is quite broad. vWF is an acute phase reactant, and can go up in patients who are inflamed, infected, pregnant, under stress, or suffering from comorbid diseases like cancer. vWF goes up with age, and is lower in individuals with blood type O. It is recommended that the label of type 1 vWD be applied only when the clinical presentation is consistent, and when vWF levels are persistently low and <30 IU/dL.[14]

LABORATORY EVALUATION OF FIBRINOLYSIS

Disorders of fibrin cross-linking and fibrinolysis are not recognized by routine coagulation protein and platelet testing (see Table 129.1). Congenital factor XIII deficiency, a rare disease with a prevalence of 1 : 2 or 3 million people worldwide, is one example.[22] Screening tests for factor XIII deficiency aim to dissolve fibrin clots in acetic acid, monochloracetic acid, or urea.[22] In the urea clot solubility test, patient plasma and a normal plasma control are induced to clot with or without added thrombin. Both samples are exposed to a 5 M urea solution and observed over time. The control clot should remain undissolved at 24 hours, as fibrin clots cross-linked in the presence of thrombin and factor XIII are stable. If the patient is factor XIII–deficient, the clot will dissolve rapidly. The urea clot solubility test, and related assays, are not standardized and have poor sensitivity; their detection limit is generally less than 5% of factor XIII activity. Suspected factor XIII deficiency must be confirmed by functional assays (which measure the release of ammonia during the transglutaminase reaction, or incorporation of radioactive amines into proteins), or immunologic factor XIII antigen assays.[22]

Tests that give a global picture of fibrinolysis can also be performed; they measure the combined effect of plasminogen activators (e.g., urokinase, tissue plasminogen activator) and inhibitors (e.g., α_2-antiplasmin defects, plasminogen activator inhibitor 1). Defects in the latter group of proteins can produce hyperfibrinolytic states and increased bleeding potential. In the euglobulin clot lysis assay, plasma is diluted and acidified. This causes precipitation of the acid insoluble or euglobulin fraction of plasma, which includes fibrinogen, plasminogen, plasminogen activators, and plasminogen activator inhibitor-1. The precipitate is redissolved, and the fibrinogen is clotted by adding calcium. The time to spontaneous lysis of the fibrin clot is then monitored. Shortened lysis times are observed in hyperfibrinolytic states such as DIC, or when there is a deficiency of plasminogen activator inhibitor-1; however, like the urea clot solubility test, the euglobulin clot lysis time is hampered by a lack of standardization and susceptibility to interference by other factors. Specialized coagulation laboratories may offer specific assays for plasminogen inhibitors as well.

OTHER ACTIVITIES FOR HEMOSTASIS LABORATORIES

Global Hemostasis Assays

Standard coagulation tests are capable of measuring the individual components of hemostasis. There is tremendous interest in evaluating hemostasis more globally, to accurately evaluate in vivo hemostatic function, sensitively and specifically diagnose hemostatic disorders, monitor treatment, and better predict clinical manifestations of disordered hemostasis. Global hemostasis assays aim not only to measure components of hemostasis, but also determine how they interact with each other. They do so by assessing the rate of thrombin generation, the quantity of thrombin generation, the formation of clots in whole blood, and/or the polymerization of fibrin.

Measurement of thrombin generation was first described in the early 1950s by MacFarlane and Biggs (who used whole blood), and Pitney and Dacie (who used plasma). Over the years, methods were refined; ultimately, continuous measurement of thrombin generation was accomplished by using a thrombin-chromogenic substrate in defibrinated plasma, or a fluorogenic substrate in whole plasma. In general, modern thrombin generation assays (TGAs) use recalcified platelet-rich or platelet-poor plasma, and then trigger clotting using tissue factor. TGAs can capture not only the rate and amount of thrombin generated, but also the role of platelets (which act as an amplifying surface for thrombin activity). TGAs have been widely used in research. Clinically, they may play a role in thrombophilic states (e.g., ATII deficiency, protein C or S deficiency, activated protein C resistance, cancer-associated thrombosis) and in hemorrhagic tendencies (hemophilia, other factor deficiencies, cardiac surgery). In hemophilia, TGAs might more accurately predict

bleeding risk and efficacy of inhibitor bypassing than traditional tests.[23] TGAs are not yet used broadly in the clinical context; test procedures are not yet well standardized, and validated reference ranges for specific conditions have not been developed.

Viscoelastic assays like thromboelastography and thromboelastometry are increasingly used in the clinical context. Viscoelastic tests are based on the premise that the end result of normal hemostasis is to rapidly create a strong, stable clot; changes in the speed of clot creation, or its strength or stability, may indicate abnormal hemostatic function. Thromboelastography was first described in 1948 by Hartert, who presented a method in which clotting was triggered in fresh whole blood with the addition of celite (an activator of the intrinsic pathway). The blood was then put into a continuously rotating cup, and a torsion wire was introduced into the system. As the clot gradually became stronger, the movement of the torsion wire dampened and ultimately stopped. A tracing of the torsion wire's movement over time reflected the velocity of clot formation, its maximal stability, and its gradual dissolution. This tracing was recorded onto light-sensitive photographic paper by a mirror-galvanometer; the image developed over hours to days.

Currently, two semi-automated commercial viscoelastic devices on the market allow results to be obtained in 10–15 minutes: the ROTEM-analyzer (TEM International, Munich, Germany), which uses a fixed cup with a rotating pin and optical detector, and the TEG-analyzer (Haemonetics Corp., Braintree, MA, USA), which uses a torsion wire and a rotating cup. Both are kinetic tests, and their tracings measure clot formation over time. They also measure maximal clot strength, clot elasticity, and clot lysis. Both use citrated whole blood that is recalcified and added to a cuvette. An activator (e.g., tissue factor) is commonly used to standardize the test, and speed up the assay. These analyzers can perform additional tests (using different activators or additives) to provide information similar to that of the APTT or PT, to neutralize heparin, to inhibit fibrinolysis, and to qualitatively analyze the functional fibrinogen component.

Viscoelastic methods are increasingly used at the bedside. They have shown some promise in detecting coagulopathies and guiding the use of blood products and other prohemostatic therapy intraoperatively, in obstetric hemorrhage, in the trauma setting, and in the intensive care unit.[24,25] They may also be helpful in screening for hypercoagulable states, as some individuals with a history of thromboembolism demonstrate accelerated clot propagation. Viscoelastic methods do have some drawbacks. They are insensitive to platelet and vWF dysfunction, as well as factor XIII problems. Assay standardization and variability of results continue to be a challenge.[26,27]

Evaluation of Prothrombotic States

In addition to the diagnosis of bleeding disorders, the hemostasis laboratory can help evaluate acquired and inherited prothrombotic states (see Chapter 140). It is known that certain prothrombotic states (e.g., antithrombin, protein C, and protein S deficiencies; antiphospholipid antibody syndrome) may confer a higher risk for recurrent thrombosis. Patients with these abnormalities may benefit from long-term anticoagulation after their first episode of thrombosis. Less severe prothrombotic states (e.g., heterozygous factor V Leiden and prothrombin 20210 polymorphisms, functional defects in fibrinogen and plasminogen) do not appear to impact the risk of recurrence. Clinicians often consider testing for prothrombotic states in patients who develop thrombosis at a young age, who have a strong family history of thrombosis, who have thrombosis at an unusual site, or who experience recurrent or unexplained thrombosis. However the utility of this testing is limited, as the results usually do not affect patient management or result in improved patient outcomes.[28] Testing can also result in potential harm, including inappropriate use of anticoagulation and undue patient anxiety. For these reasons, testing for prothrombotic states is not routinely recommended in unselected patients with thrombosis. Testing should only be undertaken with patients whose clinical presentation strongly suggests an underlying prothrombotic condition. Before testing is done, clinicians should consider how it will affect management, and if it is aligned with the patient's values and preferences.

Monitoring Anticoagulant Therapy

The coagulation laboratory plays an important role in the monitoring of patients on anticoagulant therapy. Historically, monitoring was limited to unfractionated heparin and warfarin, which are monitored using the clot-based APTT and INR assays, respectively. However, coagulation laboratories are increasingly developing assays to monitor low-molecular-weight heparin (LMWH), fondaparinux, parenteral direct thrombin inhibitors, and the target-specific oral anticoagulants (TSOACs), which include dabigatran, rivaroxaban, and apixaban. Therapeutic ranges for these agents are not clinically validated, and vary by laboratory and by indication. However, clinicians may consider measurement of on-therapy drug levels in patients who are obese, have renal or hepatic insufficiency, experience thrombosis or bleeding while on therapy, or require urgent surgery.

The ability to neutralize the enzymatic activity of factor Xa or thrombin is the most reliable way to assay for the plasma level of anticoagulants. Antifactor Xa chromogenic assays can be used to measure Xa inhibitors like LMWH, fondaparinux, rivaroxaban, and apixaban, while antithrombin chromogenic and clot-based assays can measure direct thrombin inhibitors like argatroban, bivalirudin, hirudin, and dabigatran. Standard curves for anticoagulants are constructed by combining known amounts of the anticoagulant and the factor it inhibits. Residual factor activity is inversely proportional to the concentration of drug in the sample. Antifactor Xa assays to monitor LMWHs can be developed against WHO's International Standard for LMWH, which serves as a calibrator of drug levels. Other anticoagulants require unique calibrated assays, established by the individual laboratory.

The TSOACs also affect more commonly used clot-based assays. The TCT and APTT are more sensitive to dabigatran than the PT, and the TCT can be used to exclude the presence of dabigatran and its anticoagulant effect.[29] The PT is sensitive to rivaroxaban (though sensitivity varies by laboratory reagent), while it is less sensitive to apixaban.[30] The PT should not be used to exclude clinically significant drug concentrations of either rivaroxaban or apixaban; appropriately calibrated antifactor Xa assays are more appropriate.

Evaluating Activated Coagulation States

Specialized coagulation laboratories can monitor activated coagulation states that result in acute hemostasis and thrombosis, such as antiphospholipid antibody syndrome (see Chapter 141), heparin-induced thrombocytopenia (see Chapter 132), and warfarin–skin necrosis. The classic activated coagulation state is DIC (see Chapter 139). DIC is a clinicopathologic state characterized by excessive and dysregulated activation of coagulation and fibrinolysis, with consequent consumption of prothrombotic and antithrombotic factors. DIC is triggered by an underlying cause, such as sepsis, malignancy, trauma, obstetric complications or intravascular hemolysis. There are two forms of DIC: an *acute* and a *chronic* form. The acute form is characterized by overwhelming defibrination and a tendency to hemorrhage. The APTT and PT are elevated, and the fibrinogen and platelet count are low. The more indolent chronic form is characterized by partially compensated coagulation and a tendency to thrombosis. The APTT, PT, and platelet count may be normal or slightly low, and the fibrinogen can be normal or even elevated.

The laboratory diagnosis of DIC requires evidence of simultaneous coagulation and fibrinolysis. Evaluation begins with a complete blood count, PT, APTT and fibrinogen. The D-dimer assay is a useful adjunct to confirm fibrinolysis. D-dimers are insoluble degradation products that arise when fibrin is cross-linked by thrombin-activated factor XIII, then cleaved with plasmin. Though D-dimer elevation is a sensitive test for DIC, it is not specific for this condition; D-dimer elevation occurs in pregnancy, large vessel thrombosis, hepatic failure, and many other conditions. Isolated D-dimer elevation in the absence of another etiology can also suggest chronic DIC. Laboratory testing can be repeated serially to monitor the severity of DIC, and its response to treatment.

ACKNOWLEDGMENTS

The author wishes to recognize the invaluable assistance and expertise of Karen A. Moffat, who provided many thoughtful comments on versions of this chapter.

REFERENCES

1. Macfarlane RG: An enzyme cascade in the blood clotting mechanism, and its function as a biochemical amplifier. *Nature* 202:498–499, 1964.
2. Davie EW, Ratnoff OD: Waterfall sequence for intrinsic blood clotting. *Science* 145:1310–1312, 1964.
3. Osterud B, Rapaport SI: Activation of factor IX by the reaction product of tissue factor and factor VII: additional pathway for initiating blood coagulation. *Proc Natl Acad Sci USA* 74:5260–5264, 1977.
4. Gailani D, Broze GJ, Jr: Factor XI activation in a revised model of blood coagulation. *Science* 253:909–912, 1991.
5. Schmaier AH: Physiologic activities of the contact activation system. *Thromb Res* 133(Suppl 1):S41–S44, 2014.
6. Poller L, Ibrahim S, Keown M, et al: Simplified method for international normalized ratio (INR) derivation based on the prothrombin time/INR line: an international study. *Clin Chem* 56:1608–1617, 2010.
7. Poller L, Van Den Besselaar AM, Jespersen J, et al: The effect of sample size on fresh plasma thromboplastin ISI determination. *Br J Haematol* 105:655–663, 1999.
8. Verhovsek M, Moffat KA, Hayward CP: Laboratory testing for fibrinogen abnormalities. *Am J Hematol* 83:928–931, 2008.
9. Hayward CP, Moffat KA: Laboratory testing for bleeding disorders: strategic uses of high and low-yield tests. *Int J Lab Hematol* 35:322–333, 2013.
10. Green D: Factor VIII inhibitors: a 50-year perspective. *Haemophilia* 17:831–838, 2011.
11. Verbruggen B, Novakova I, Wessels H, et al: The Nijmegen modification of the Bethesda assay for factor VIII:C inhibitors: improved specificity and reliability. *Thromb Haemost* 73:247–251, 1995.
12. Pengo V, Tripodi A, Reber G, et al: Update of the guidelines for lupus anticoagulant detection. Subcommittee on Lupus Anticoagulant/Antiphospholipid Antibody of the Scientific and Standardisation Committee of the International Society on Thrombosis and Haemostasis. *J Thromb Haemost* 7:1737–1740, 2009.
13. Palla R, Peyvandi F, Shapiro AD: Rare bleeding disorders: diagnosis and treatment. *Blood* 125:2052–2061, 2015.
14. Nichols WL, Hultin MB, James AH, et al: von Willebrand disease (VWD): evidence-based diagnosis and management guidelines, the National Heart, Lung, and Blood Institute (NHLBI) Expert Panel report (USA). *Haemophilia* 14:171–232, 2008.
15. Peterson P, Hayes TE, Arkin CF, et al: The preoperative bleeding time test lacks clinical benefit: College of American Pathologists' and American Society of Clinical Pathologists' position article. *Arch Surg* 133:134–139, 1998.
16. Quiroga T, Goycoolea M, Munoz B, et al: Template bleeding time and PFA-100 have low sensitivity to screen patients with hereditary mucocutaneous hemorrhages: comparative study in 148 patients. *J Thromb Haemost* 2:892–898, 2004.
17. Hayward CP, Moffat KA, Raby A, et al: Development of North American consensus guidelines for medical laboratories that perform and interpret platelet function testing using light transmission aggregometry. *Am J Clin Pathol* 134:955–963, 2010.
18. Hayward CP, Pai M, Liu Y, et al: Diagnostic utility of light transmission platelet aggregometry: results from a prospective study of individuals referred for bleeding disorder assessments. *J Thromb Haemost* 7:676–684, 2009.

19. Pai M, Wang G, Moffat KA, et al: Diagnostic usefulness of a lumi-aggregometer adenosine triphosphate release assay for the assessment of platelet function disorders. *Am J Clin Pathol* 136:350–358, 2011.

20. Ng C, Motto DG, Di Paola J: Diagnostic approach to von Willebrand disease. *Blood* 125:2029–2037, 2015.

21. Sadler JE: Von Willebrand disease type 1: a diagnosis in search of a disease. *Blood* 101:2089–2093, 2003.

22. Muszbek L, Bagoly Z, Cairo A, et al: Novel aspects of factor XIII deficiency. *Curr Opin Hematol* 18:366–372, 2011.

23. Young G, Sorensen B, Dargaud Y, et al: Thrombin generation and whole blood viscoelastic assays in the management of hemophilia: current state of art and future perspectives. *Blood* 121:1944–1950, 2013.

24. Afshari A, Wikkelso A, Brok J, et al: Thrombelastography (TEG) or thromboelastometry (ROTEM) to monitor haemotherapy versus usual care in patients with massive transfusion. *Cochrane Database Syst Rev* CD007871, 2011.

25. Perry DJ, Fitzmaurice DA, Kitchen S, et al: Point-of-care testing in haemostasis. *Br J Haematol* 150:501–514, 2010.

26. Mauch J, Spielmann N, Hartnack S, et al: Intrarater and interrater variability of point of care coagulation testing using the ROTEM delta. *Blood Coagul Fibrinolysis* 22:662–666, 2011.

27. Kitchen DP, Jennings I, Kitchen S, et al: Bridging the gap between point-of-care testing and laboratory testing in hemostasis. *Semin Thromb Hemost* 2015.

28. Middeldorp S, van Hylckama Vlieg A: Does thrombophilia testing help in the clinical management of patients? *Br J Haematol* 143:321–335, 2008.

29. Cuker A, Siegal DM, Crowther MA, et al: Laboratory measurement of the anticoagulant activity of the non-vitamin K oral anticoagulants. *J Am Coll Cardiol* 64:1128–1139, 2014.

30. Samama MM, Martinoli JL, LeFlem L, et al: Assessment of laboratory assays to measure rivaroxaban–an oral, direct factor Xa inhibitor. *Thromb Haemost* 103:815–825, 2010.

CHAPTER 130

ACQUIRED DISORDERS OF PLATELET FUNCTION

Reyhan Diz-Küçükkaya and José A. López

Acquired disorders of platelet function are among the most common hematologic abnormalities, a reflection of the sensitivity of platelets to external and internal perturbations. The clinical challenge in evaluating acquired disorders of platelet function is to determine whether observed derangements in platelet function pose a threat to the patient. Although platelet function can be altered to predispose to either hemostatic or thrombotic disorders, this chapter deals primarily, but not exclusively, with platelet disorders that may compromise hemostasis. We attempt also to guide clinicians in trying to determine the clinical importance of these disorders, but the marked variation in bleeding risks associated with any particular disorder of platelet function make this a difficult task. Bleeding in patients with acquired platelet dysfunction is likely to occur less frequently and predictably than in those affected by severe inherited platelet disorders such as Bernard-Soulier syndrome or Glanzmann thrombasthenia, and may manifest only in the setting of trauma or surgery or in the presence of additional hemostatic defects. However, even some patients with inherited platelet disorders only bleed when stressed by surgery or trauma, making the distinction between inherited and acquired disorders less clear cut.

The laboratory evaluation of these patients may illuminate these disorders (see Chapter 129) but may offer little concrete guidance in management. Acquired platelet defects (Table 130.1) may produce abnormal laboratory test results, such as a prolonged closure time on a platelet function analyzer (PFA) or abnormal aggregation in response to added agonists. Historically, the bleeding time was used to evaluate bleeding risk in patients with jaundice or uremia, but it measures hemostasis only in one vascular bed (the skin) and bears inherent interoperator variability. These platelet assays are useful research tools; however, defects quantified by laboratory tests, including the bleeding time, are not predictive of bleeding in these patients. Additionally, some acquired platelet disorders increase the risk of thrombosis rather than bleeding, a risk for which there is currently no effective screening test. Lastly, tests that depend on assessing the functions of platelets ex vivo do not assess the contributions of labile substances from the endothelium (see Chapter 123) and occasionally (as in platelet aggregometry) do not account for flow, a key component of in vivo platelet function.

DRUGS, FOODS, AND ADDITIVES THAT AFFECT PLATELET FUNCTION

The most common causes of acquired platelet dysfunction are drugs. In a large prospective study, 5649 unselected adult patients were screened preoperatively for hemostatic defects with activated partial thromboplastin time (aPTT), prothrombin time (PT), platelet counts, platelet function analyzer (PFA)-100 testing, and a questionnaire regarding bleeding history.[1] Bleeding history was positive in 628 patients (11.1%), and impaired hemostasis was verified in 256 (40.8%) of these patients. Of these 256 patients, 162 (63.28%) were found to have acquired platelet dysfunction. Antiplatelet drugs or nonsteroidal antiinflammatory drugs (NSAIDs) were responsible for the acquired platelet dysfunction in 147 patients and antibiotics in 10 patients.

Numerous drugs affect platelet function (Table 130.2). For several, inhibition of platelet function is their intended effect (Fig. 130.1); for most, platelet dysfunction is an unintended and undesired side effect. Drug-induced platelet function abnormalities do not usually cause a clinically significant problem in healthy individuals. However, these drugs may increase the bleeding risk with interventions (e.g., surgery, biopsy), trauma, or in the presence of other hemostatic defects, such as those associated with cirrhosis or uremia. Antiplatelet agents are discussed more fully in Chapter 149. For all of these drugs, their effects on platelet function are defined by an abnormality of platelet aggregation, but their contribution to a risk of excessive bleeding is definitively established only for aspirin, clopidogrel, ticlopidine, and inhibitors of $\alpha IIb\beta3$ function.

ANTIPLATELET DRUGS

Aspirin

Aspirin has been in routine use worldwide for more than 100 years and is still by far the most common agent associated with platelet dysfunction.[2] The antipyretic and analgesic effect of willow bark was first recorded by Galen. In 1826 and 1828 Leroux and Buchner isolated a compound from willow bark that they called *salicin* (which means *willow* in Latin).[3] In 1897 a German chemist, Felix Hoffman from the Bayer Company, inspired by his father's severe arthritis and the untoward side effects of salicylic acid, discovered a method to convert salicylic acid, the active compound in willow bark, to a compound with less gastrointestinal (GI) toxicity, acetyl salicylic acid (aspirin).[4] However, with Hoffmann's subsequent synthesis of heroin from morphine, commercial development of aspirin was relegated to the back burner for a number of decades.[5] Aspirin was widely used for rheumatic fever in the 1940s. In the 1950s, case reports and uncontrolled studies were published suggesting that aspirin could prevent myocardial infarction and stroke.[5,6] The clinical importance of the antithrombotic effect of aspirin was clearly demonstrated in a study of 22,071 physicians who received either 325 mg of aspirin or placebo every other day over the course of 5 years.[7] Those receiving aspirin had a 44% decreased incidence of myocardial infarction. In a large metaanalysis, it was shown that aspirin reduced death from vascular events by 15% and nonfatal vascular events by 30%.[7] The primary mechanism by which aspirin impairs hemostasis is through irreversible acetylation of the enzyme cyclooxygenase-1 (COX-1), an early enzyme in the synthetic pathway that produces the potent platelet agonist, thromboxane A_2 (TXA_2). Because platelets have no nuclei and therefore retain only a limited capacity to synthesize new proteins, a single low dose of aspirin (30–100 mg)[8] or as little as 10 mg taken daily for 1 week can completely inhibit TXA_2 production and therefore impair the function of a cohort of platelets for their circulating life span.[9] Aspirin also acetylates the isoform of COX mostly present in endothelial cells, COX-2; COX-2 acetylation blocks synthesis of prostacyclin, a strong inhibitor of platelet function.[10] However, COX-2 is markedly less sensitive than COX-1 to inhibition by aspirin,[2] and endothelial cells, unlike platelets, are able to synthesize new enzymes quite rapidly.[11]

Platelets exposed to aspirin either in vivo or in vitro predictably demonstrate impaired aggregation in response to epinephrine, ADP, arachidonic acid, and low concentrations of collagen and thrombin,[12] a result of defective TXA_2 production. These agonists have therefore been defined as *weak* agonists, requiring that TXA_2 diffuse out of the

TABLE 130.1 Acquired Disorders of Platelet Function

Drugs, Foods, and Additives

Drugs: see Table 130.2

Food and additives: omega-3 fatty acids, ethanol, ginger, onion, garlic, black tree fungus, *Gingko biloba*, cumin, turmeric, tonic water, caffeine, pineapple, others

Clonal Disorders

Clonal hematologic diseases

Myeloproliferative neoplasms

Paroxysmal nocturnal hemoglobinuria

Paraproteinemias

Leukemias and myelodysplastic syndromes

Solid tumors

Systemic Metabolic Disorders

End-stage renal disease

Liver diseases

Diabetes and hyperlipidemias

Platelet Dysfunction Related With Extracorporeal Circuits

Miscellaneous

Hypothermia

Scurvy

Acquired platelet dysfunction with eosinophilia

TABLE 130.2 Drug-Induced Platelet Dysfunction

Anti-Platelet Drugs

COX inhibitors: aspirin

ADP receptor antagonists

Thienopyridines: clopidogrel, ticlopidine, prasugrel

Nonthienopyridines: ticagrelor, cangrelor

$\alpha_{IIb}\beta_3$ inhibitors: abciximab, eptifibatide, tirofiban

PDE inhibitors

Nonselective PDE inhibitors: pentoxifylline, caffeine, theophylline

PDE3 inhibitors: cilostazol, milrinone, anagrelide

PDE5 inhibitors: dipyridamole, sildenafil

Adenyl cyclase stimulators: epoprostenol, iloprost, beraprost

Drugs that adversely affect platelet function

NSAIDs: ibuprofen, naproxen, indomethacin,

Cardiovascular agents

Calcium channel blockers: nifedipine, diltiazem, verapamil

β-Blockers: propranolol

Vasodilators: nitrates, nitroprusside

Diuretics: furosemide

Angiotensin II receptor antagonist: losartan, valsartan, and olmesartan

Antibiotics: β-lactams, amphotericin, hydroxychloroquine, nitrofurantoin

Antifungal drugs: Miconazole, amphotericin B

Psychiatric drugs: TCAs, fluoxetine, chlorpromazine, promethazine, trifluoperazine

Oncologic drugs: mithramycin, daunorubicin, BCNU, asparaginase, vincristine, dasatinib, ibritunib

Anesthetics: dibucaine, procaine, halothane, sevoflurane, propofol

Plasma expanders: dextran, hydroxyl ethyl starch

Heparins and thrombolytic agents

Miscellaneous: clofibrate, statins, cocaine, ketanserin, radiographic contrast agents, antihistamines, immunosuppressive drugs

ADP, Adenosine diphosphate; BCNU, carmustine; COX, cyclooxygenase; NSAID, nonsteroidal antiinflammatory drug; PDE, phosphodiesterase; TCA, tricyclic antidepressant.

platelet, bind to its receptor on the platelet membrane, and reinforce aggregation by promoting secretion from α and dense granules. Aspirin-treated platelets stimulated with these agonists demonstrate only a primary, reversible wave of aggregation without granule secretion. Stronger agonists (high concentrations of thrombin and collagen) do not require TXA_2 synthesis to cause platelet secretion and irreversible aggregation, and thus some hemostatic function is maintained in aspirin-treated patients.

Aspirin may also have COX-independent actions that may affect coagulation. At the site of microvascular injury, platelets bind to exposed collagen, and coagulation is initiated by tissue factor concurrently. It was reported that low-dose aspirin (30 mg/day for 7 days) decreased thrombin formation in healthy volunteers.[13] Undas et al[14] used the same microvascular injury model and showed that aspirin at 75 mg/day for 7 days decreased the velocity of prothrombin consumption by 29%, thrombin generation by 29%, and delayed both activation and maximum cleavage of factor XIII by thrombin. Interestingly, high cholesterol levels (>240 mg/dL) impaired the antithrombotic effect of low-dose aspirin in a microvascular injury model.[15]

In contrast to the antiplatelet effect of aspirin, which appears unrelated to the dose above small threshold doses, GI mucosal toxicity is dose related.[16] The mechanism of mucosal injury appears to be distinct from the effect on hemostasis, involving ionic trapping of aspirin within gut mucosal cells[17] and diminished synthesis of protective gut prostaglandins.[18,19] The inhibitory effect of even a single dose of aspirin on gastric prostaglandin synthesis is prolonged, with one study showing that gastric COX activity was still 57% suppressed 72 hours after a single 325-mg dose of aspirin.[20] Bleeding may originate from discrete ulcers or diffuse mucosal damage and is more common to arise from the upper GI tract. The risk of bleeding is increased even with doses of aspirin as low as 10–30 mg/day;[21] the protective effect of resistant coatings is unproven.[22] The GI risk of aspirin is increased in elderly adults (older than 65 years of age) and in those with concomitant medical conditions, such as cardiovascular disease, as well as in those taking certain other medications, such as other NSAIDs.[22] Aspirin appears to delay the healing of gastric ulcers, possibly because it interferes with the release of growth factors from platelets, such as endostatin and vascular endothelial growth factor.[23]

Regular use of aspirin (≥75 mg) impairs primary hemostasis dose-dependently.[8] Aspirin treatment was associated with a small but significant increase in mucocutaneous bleeding as evidenced by easy bruising, hematemesis, melena, epistaxis, and an increased frequency of blood transfusion surrounding surgeries. Because low doses have been shown to be effective in preventing thrombosis, it is likely that the risk of bleeding can be reduced while maintaining an antiplatelet effect.

Aspirin may unmask mild hereditary disorders of platelet function.[24] For example, patients with mild von Willebrand disease often have a normal bleeding time that becomes markedly increased with aspirin therapy.[24] The bleeding risk associated with aspirin is increased in the presence of other hemostatic defects, or if aspirin is given simultaneously with anticoagulant drugs.

Aspirin Resistance

The response to aspirin therapy varies among individuals. Every day, the human body can produce approximately 10×10^{11} platelets, and this production can increase 10-fold if needed. The life span of platelets is 8–10 days, and every day nearly 10%–12% of the platelets are replaced by new platelets. The capacity of the bone marrow to produce new platelets, the aspirin dosage, the aspirin exposure time (spot doses or regular use), and individual parameters will determine the antihemostatic effect of aspirin in any particular individual.

The issue of aspirin resistance is hotly debated, with reported incidence rates varying from 0% to 57%.[25–28] The presence of aspirin resistance is associated with high rates of cardiovascular events.[27,28]

The most important issue in determining whether laboratory aspirin resistance is real is compliance. Schwartz et al[29] evaluated 190

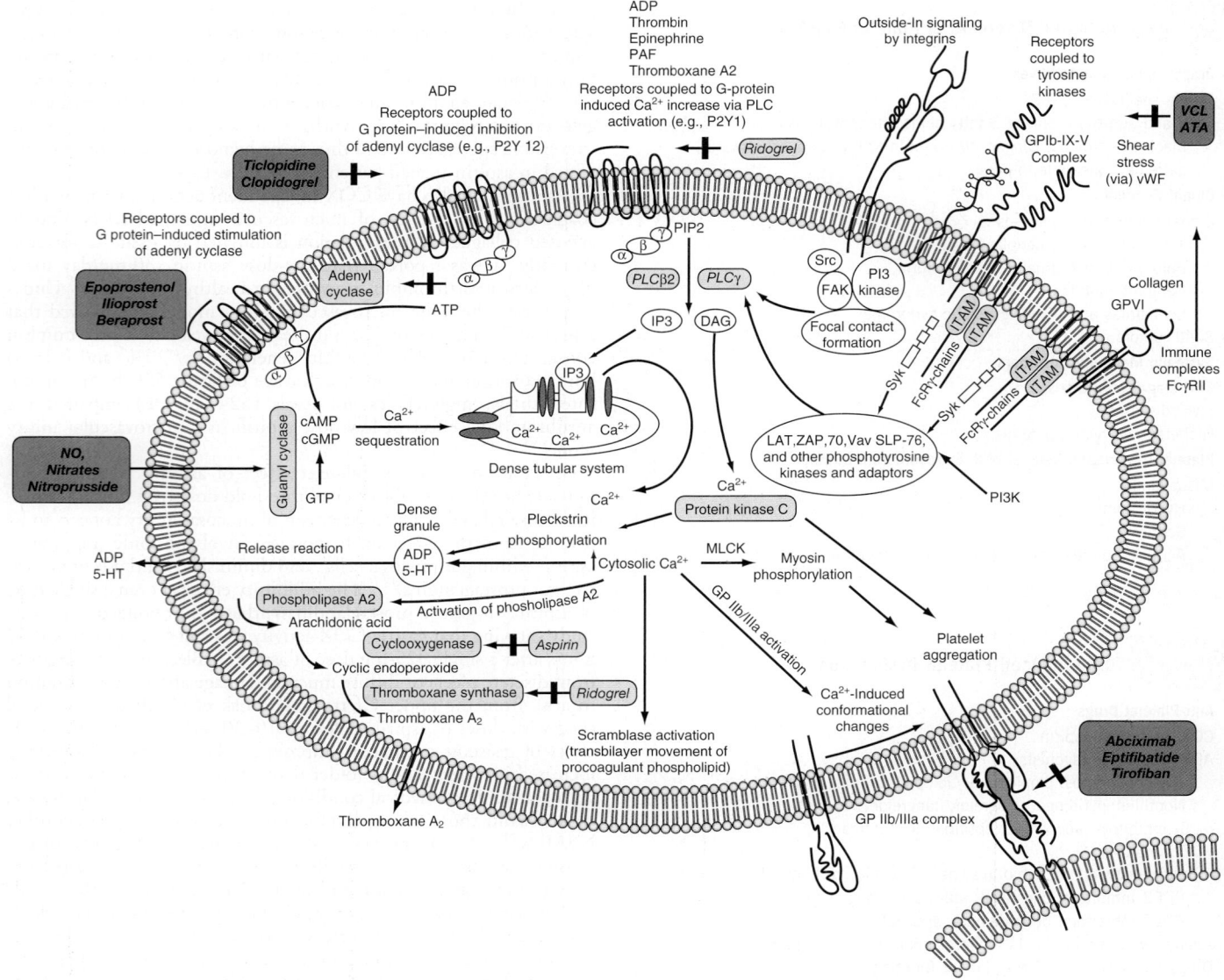

Fig. 130.1 MECHANISM OF INHIBITION OF PLATELET FUNCTION BY VARIOUS DRUGS. Some of the drugs shown, such as Ridogrel, VCL (rA1 domain of von Willebrand factor), and ATA (aurin tricarboxylic acid), are not now used clinically. *5-HT*, serotonin (5-hydroxytryptamine); *ADP*, adenosine diphosphate; *ATP*, adenosine triphosphate; *cAMP*, cyclic adenosine monophosphate; *cGMP*, cyclic guanyl monophosphate; *DAG*, diacylglycerol; *GP*, glycoprotein; *GTP*, guanyl triphosphate; *IP3*, inositol triphosphate; *ITAM*, immunoreceptor tyrosine-based activation motif; *MLCK*, myosin light chain kinase; *NO*, nitric oxide; *PAF*, platelet activating factor; *PI3K*, phosphatidylinositol 3-kinase; *PLA2*, phospholipase A2; *PLC*, phospholipase C; *TXA₂*, thromboxane A₂; *vWF*, von Willebrand factor.

patients with a history of coronary disease and receiving aspirin therapy. They investigated these patients on regular aspirin therapy, after withdrawal of aspirin for 7 days, and after an observed ingestion of 325 mg of aspirin. They found that 17 patients (9%) receiving regular aspirin therapy had aspirin resistance as defined by defective inhibition of arachidonic acid–stimulated platelet aggregation. After being observed to take the 325 mg aspirin, however, all patients but one displayed inhibition of aggregation. Similar results were observed in other studies.[30] These investigators concluded that noncompliance was the predominant cause of aspirin resistance, and higher doses of aspirin may eliminate the resistance. Although it has been shown that aspirin inhibits platelet functions in a dose-dependent manner,[31] higher aspirin doses failed to reduce the risk of thrombosis in large trials.[32]

Higher aspirin resistance rates are reported in elderly patients, probably owing to the fact that increased gastric pH affects aspirin absorption in patients taking enteric-coated forms of aspirin.[8,33] Other causes of aspirin resistance may include increased platelet

turnover and increased COX-1 expression in new platelets[34] and overexpression of COX-2 in macrophages and endothelial cells.[35] It has also been reported that concomitant use of some NSAIDs such as ibuprofen and naproxen may prevent COX-1 inactivation in patients receiving low-dose aspirin.[36,37] Interindividual variation of aspirin response can also be explained by genetic variations involved in the genes for COX-1 and COX-2, platelet integrin α2 or β3, the ADP receptors P2Y1 and P2Y12, the TXA₂ receptor and some coagulation proteins.[26,38–41] However, these studies showed conflicting results and have failed to confirm that aspirin therapy tailored to account for genetic variation improves clinical outcomes.

In patients treated with aspirin who experience recurrent arterial thrombosis, it is important to keep in mind that arterial thrombosis is a multifactorial process and that the inhibition of one pathway of platelet activation may be insufficient to prevent recurrent events.

Assessment of aspirin's inhibitory effects on platelets is important in two clinical situations: (1) in patients with arterial thrombosis, or at high risk for arterial thrombosis, to insure that sufficient platelet inhibition is achieved by a given aspirin dose; (2) for estimating the bleeding risks in patients who need surgery or who have experienced trauma.

The antiplatelet effect of aspirin can be screened by different techniques, including light-transmission aggregometry, whole-blood aggregometry, platelet function analyzer (PFA)-100, VerifyNow Aspirin, measurement of serum/plasma or urinary TXB_2 metabolites, thromboelastography, flow cytometry, or other tests (see Chapters 128 and 129).

Adenosine Diphosphate Receptor Antagonists

The thienopyridines selectively and irreversibly inhibit ADP-mediated platelet activation and aggregation.[42] ADP activates platelets by raising the concentration of cytoplasmic Ca^{2+} through influx from the extracellular fluid and mobilization from internal stores, and by decreasing the concentration of intracellular cyclic adenosine monophosphate (cAMP) coupled to inhibition of adenylyl cyclase. ADP receptors can be divided into two groups: the G protein–coupled receptors, termed *P2Y*, and the ionotropic receptors, *P2X*. Platelets contain two P2Y receptors, $P2Y_1$ and $P2Y_{12}$, complexed to the heterotrimeric G proteins G_q and G_{i2}, respectively. ADP binding to $P2Y_1$ is necessary for platelet aggregation but is not sufficient. Rather, $P2Y_1$ is responsible for ADP-induced platelet shape change, and its engagement by ADP triggers a transient aggregatory response. $P2Y_{12}$, coupled to inhibition of adenylyl cyclase, mediates the amplification of the aggregation response.[43] The thienopyridine derivatives have no effects on arachidonic acid metabolism and hence act synergistically with aspirin to inhibit platelet function.

The thienopyridines are all prodrugs of similar structure that produce active metabolites that bind irreversibly to $P2Y_{12}$, inhibiting ADP-mediated aggregation for up to 10 days after withdrawal of the drug, paralleling the platelet life span.[44] Because most platelet agonists require ADP for their full activity, the thienopyridines inhibit platelet activation by all agonists except strong agonists at high concentrations.[45] They have a further hypothetical advantage over aspirin in that they inhibit shear-induced platelet aggregation.[46]

There are three generations of thienopyridine drugs, represented by ticlopidine, clopidogrel, and prasugrel. The use of ticlopidine has been greatly curtailed because of serious side effects such as agranulocytosis, thrombocytopenia, and thrombotic thrombocytopenic purpura.[47]

Platelet $\alpha_{IIb}\beta_3$ (Glycoprotein IIb/IIIa) Inhibitors

A myriad of pathways lead to platelet aggregation, the final common step being activation of the major platelet integrin $\alpha_{IIb}\beta_3$ to a ligand-competent form, which can bind multivalent ligands such as fibrinogen or von Willebrand factor (vWF) to cross-link the platelets into an aggregate. Conventional antiplatelet agents such as aspirin and clopidogrel each inhibit only one pathway leading to platelet aggregation, aspirin preventing thromboxane production, and clopidogrel blocking ADP receptors. Dual therapy with aspirin and clopidogrel improves the clinical benefit of antiplatelet therapy, but aggregation is still able to proceed through the action of other agonists such as thrombin. Because $\alpha_{IIb}\beta_3$ engagement is required for aggregation through all pathways, blocking this receptor inhibits platelet aggregation more effectively.

Inhibitors of $\alpha_{IIb}\beta_3$ work selectively and competitively to inhibit platelet aggregation.[48,49] These agents are intended to produce a transient effect akin to the defect in Glanzmann thrombasthenia, but there are important differences between the drug effect and the disease.

Although these agents share many similarities in their antithrombotic properties, they also have a number of clinically important pharmacokinetic and off-target effect differences. Three drugs are available: eptifibatide, tirofiban, and abciximab.

Abciximab

The first $\alpha_{IIb}\beta_3$ inhibitor approved for clinical use, abciximab (ReoPro), is a human-murine chimeric Fab fragment of a monoclonal antibody that targets the β_3 subunit of $\alpha_{IIb}\beta_3$ and therefore also reacts with another integrin that shares the β_3 subunit, $\alpha_V\beta_3$. Although $\alpha_{IIb}\beta_3$ expression is restricted to megakaryocytes and platelets, $\alpha_V\beta_3$ is expressed on platelets; at low levels; and in cells of the vascular wall, including endothelial cells and fibroblasts.[50] In addition to its antithrombotic properties, abciximab may also reduce infarct size, prevent stent thrombosis, and modulate inflammatory responses by virtue of β_3 subunit inhibition in other tissues.[48]

Abciximab administered intravenously as a standard 0.25 mg/kg bolus blocks approximately 80% of surface $\alpha_{IIb}\beta_3$ and inhibits platelet aggregation to a similar extent, although the extent of inhibition is variable.[51] This level of blockade increases the bleeding time only mildly. The bleeding time only becomes markedly prolonged when receptor blockade exceeds 90%. After the bolus dose, abciximab is infused at 0.125 µg/kg/min for 12 hours. Several trials have established this as a clinically effective regimen.[52] Plasma levels of free abciximab drop rapidly after its administration, with an initial half-life of approximately 30 min. Most of the drug is bound to platelets. This explains why patients with thrombocytosis may require larger weight-adjusted doses of abciximab to attain a therapeutic antiplatelet effect[53] and why patients with lower platelet counts treated with the usual dose of abciximab display more profound platelet inhibition. Abciximab is not excreted in the urine and is probably metabolized by the reticuloendothelial system at the time platelets (with bound abciximab) are cleared from the circulation. The dose of abciximab does not have to be adjusted in patients with renal impairment. Although a daily platelet turnover rate of 10% would predict that no abciximab would be detected in blood after 10 days of its administration, platelet-bound abciximab has been observed up to 3 weeks after its initial administration, suggesting platelet-to-platelet redistribution of the drug or release of new platelets from megakaryocytes that had previously bound the drug. Several in vitro and in vivo studies confirm abciximab's ability to exchange between platelets.[51] Because of the low plasma levels of unbound abciximab, the drug's inhibitory effect can be rapidly reversed by platelet transfusion, and hemostasis should be normal when the concentration of infused platelets exceeds 50,000/µL, as it is in normal individuals. However, because of abciximab's ability to redistribute to the newly transfused platelets, the platelet-bound abciximab may produce a gradual inhibitory effect on the infused platelets;[51] in severe or refractory bleeding, it may be necessary to infuse a very large dose of platelets, sufficient to leave 50% of $\alpha_{IIb}\beta_3$ receptors free, a number shown to be sufficient for normal hemostasis in studies of Glanzmann thrombasthenia heterozygotes. Without platelet transfusions, platelet aggregation generally returns to baseline levels within 12–24 hours after discontinuing abciximab.

Eptifibatide

Eptifibatide (Integrilin) is a cyclic heptapeptide based on the Lys-Gly-Asp (KGD) sequence found in barbourin, a platelet-inhibitory disintegrin from the venom of the Southeastern Pigmy rattlesnake, *Sistrurus miliarius barbouri*.[54] Barbourin differs from other integrin-binding proteins with the Arg-Gly-Asp (RGD) canonical sequence in that the arginine is conservatively substituted by lysine, a change that renders the protein a specific inhibitor of $\alpha_{IIb}\beta_3$. Eptifibatide incorporates the KGD sequence within a cyclic seven-member peptide of high potency. Eptifibatide differs pharmacokinetically from abciximab in several important ways.[55] For example, unlike abciximab, intravenous eptifibatide infusion produces high levels of unbound drug because of its lower affinity for the receptor. Platelet transfusions therefore are not a good method for acutely reversing eptifibatide's antiplatelet effect because the newly transfused platelets are rapidly inhibited. However, its short plasma half-life ($\approx$2.5 hours) allows for rapid clearance of eptifibatide and the reversal of its antiplatelet effect when administration is discontinued. Platelet aggregation returns to normal in approximately 4 hours, with the bleeding time normalizing within 1 hour.[55]

Tirofiban

Tirofiban (Aggrastat) is a peptidomimetic agent based on the RGD sequence, with a pharmacokinetic profile similar to that of eptifibatide.[56] Tirofiban antagonizes $\alpha_{IIb}\beta_3$ and does not cross-react with $\alpha_V\beta_3$.[56] As with eptifibatide, the maximum antiplatelet effect is seen at concentrations that leave a high concentration of unbound drug in the plasma. Therefore platelet transfusions are not often effective in reversing tirofiban's antiplatelet effect. However, its half-life is even shorter than that of eptifibatide (≈ 2 hours), and its antiplatelet effect diminishes rapidly after discontinuation of infusion.

The major adverse effects of $\alpha_{IIb}\beta_3$ inhibitors are thrombocytopenia and bleeding complications. Up to 5% of patients receiving abciximab may experience mild thrombocytopenia (<100,000/μL), and 1% may develop profound thrombocytopenia (platelet count <20,000/μL).[57,58] The incidence of severe thrombocytopenia is lower with tirofiban and eptifibatide, being approximately 0.2%.[58,59] A decrease in the platelet count is appreciable within the first hours after administration. It is therefore essential that a platelet count be obtained 2–4 hours after initiating treatment. Most patients with severe thrombocytopenia respond well to platelet transfusions and their platelet counts usually recover within 5 days, although they may take more than 1 week to do so.

Bleeding complications with $\alpha_{IIb}\beta_3$ inhibitors are quite common, especially in the inguinal area when the femoral artery has been breached during procedures. Rates of major bleeding vary between 0.7% and 5.2% in different randomized controlled studies.[59,60] Intracranial bleeding is very rare (0.09%).[59] Bleeding risk increases in patients older than 65 years of age; in patients weighing less than 50 kg; in patients taking anticoagulant, antiplatelet, or thrombolytic therapies; and in patients with inherited or acquired bleeding disorders such as hemophilia and uremia, respectively.[59,60]

Phosphodiesterase Inhibitors

Elevation of cAMP or cyclic guanosine monophosphate (cGMP) inhibits many pathways involving platelet activation, including shape change, $\alpha_{IIb}\beta_3$ activation, and degranulation. Phosphodiesterases (PDEs) catalyze degradation of cAMP and cGMP, thus preventing platelet inhibition. Eleven PDE isoforms have been described, and three are expressed in platelets: PDE2, PDE3, and PDE5.[61] Many PDE inhibitors have antiplatelet effects.

Nonselective Phosphodiesterase Inhibitors

These include the methylxanthines caffeine (1,3,7-trimethylxanthine), theophylline (1,3-dimethylxanthine), and pentoxifylline (3,7-dimethyl-1-(5-oxohexyl)xanthine). Caffeine, at a dosage of 250 mg orally three times a day for 1 week, was demonstrated to reduce platelet aggregation in healthy subjects.[62]

PDE3 inhibitors are anagrelide, cilostazol, and milrinone. Although anagrelide inhibits platelet aggregation in vitro, it surprisingly also inhibits megakaryocyte maturation and proliferation, and causes thrombocytopenia in humans by a mechanism that is poorly understood.[63] Anagrelide is used to treat essential thrombocythemia.[64]

Cilostazol is a cyclic nucleotide PDE inhibitor with both platelet inhibitory and vasodilatory effects; its current clinical use for peripheral artery disease in the United States was preceded by its use in Japan and other Asian countries. In addition to selectively inhibiting PDE, cilostazol also inhibits adenine nucleotide uptake, a property not shared with other PDE inhibitors that further enhances its antiplatelet activity.[65]

Milrinone inhibits platelet aggregation and shape change. The drug is used for congestive heart failure.

PDE5 Inhibitors

Dipyridamole has several biologic effects, including PDE inhibition, targeting the PDE5 isoform that degrades cGMP.[66] It also enhances the release and prevents the breakdown of prostaglandin I$_2$ (prostacyclin).[61,67] Primarily used for prevention of stroke, its usefulness was demonstrated by a metaanalysis of randomized trials showing that the combination of dipyridamole (particularly the modified release form) and low-dose aspirin was more effective than aspirin alone in secondary prevention of vascular events after transient ischemic attack or stroke.[68] Dipyridamole has been associated with a significantly increased risk of GI bleeding when used either as a single agent or in combination with aspirin.[69]

Recently, inhibitors of PDE5 have become popular in the treatment of erectile dysfunction.[70] PDE5 is expressed in platelets, and its inhibition results in increases in the level of platelet cGMP, an effect similar to the effect of the well-known inhibitor of platelet function, nitric oxide. One study examined the activation response of platelets drawn from patients taking sildenafil (Viagra) when stimulated with either ADP or low-dose thrombin. The results showed significantly reduced activation in response to ADP in sildenafil-treated platelets, suggesting that the drug impairs selected pathways of platelet function in vivo. Several reports of sildenafil-associated bleeding have appeared, including epistaxis,[71,72] hemorrhoidal bleeding,[73] spontaneous intracranial hemorrhage,[74] and acute variceal bleeding.[75]

Adenyl Cyclase Stimulators or Prostacyclin Analogues

Epoprostenol (the synthetic salt of prostacyclin), prostacyclin (iloprost), and an orally active stable analogue (beraprost) are prostacyclin-like agents in clinical use. Despite the potent inhibition of platelet aggregation by prostacyclin in vitro, the effects on the bleeding time are minimal and inconsistent. These drugs are used for pulmonary arterial hypertension and peripheral artery disease.[76]

Other Drugs That Adversely Affect Platelet Function

Nonsteroidal Antiinflammatory Drugs

In addition to aspirin, many other drugs used for their antiinflammatory and analgesic properties can impair platelet function.[77] As with aspirin, their mechanism of action appears to be the inhibition of COX-1; but in contrast to aspirin, these agents only temporarily affect COX-1 function, inhibiting the enzyme only as long as the active drug circulates. Among these agents, therefore, only drugs such as piroxicam, which has a plasma half-life of more than 2 days,[78] affect platelets for more than a few hours. Like with aspirin, the most sensitive indicator of impaired platelet function is the inhibition of in vitro platelet aggregation and secretion. These agents induce little or no prolongation of the bleeding time, consistent with the bleeding time being a less sensitive measure of the aspirin-induced defect.[77] PFA-100 may detect the defect, manifested as a prolonged closure time with the collagen/epinephrine cartridge.[79]

Reports of bleeding correlate with the effects of these agents on platelet function, suggesting that they increase the risk for excessive bleeding less than aspirin. As with aspirin, they may increase the bleeding times in patients with severe hemophilia, but in two studies, therapeutic doses of ibuprofen had no effect on the bleeding time in 19 of 20 patients with hemophilia.[80] Therefore, the clinical approach to patients taking any drug that can inhibit COX-1 should be similar, but the reversibility of the effect of NSAIDs provides an added margin of safety when these agents are used. Because of the increased bleeding risk, these drugs should be stopped before surgery. The timing for cessation of NSAIDs is based on the half-lives of the individual drug. Indomethacin, ibuprofen, ketoprofen, and diclofenac all have short half-lives (2–6 hours), and discontinuing these drugs 1 day before surgery is sufficient. Naproxen, sulindac, diflunisal, and celecoxib have intermediate half-lives (7–15 hours) and should be stopped 2 or 3 days before surgery. Nabumetone, meloxicam, and piroxicam have very long half-lives (>20 hours). The ACCP guidelines recommend discontinuing these drugs 10 days before surgery.[52] Analgesics such as acetaminophen and sodium or choline salicylate do not inhibit platelet function and have no adverse effects on hemostasis.[80]

Cardiovascular Drugs

Many cardiovascular drugs affect platelet functions through a variety of mechanisms.[81] Administration of nitroglycerin, isosorbide dinitrate, or nitroprusside can decrease platelet aggregation and secretion in vitro, but their effects in vivo are minimal and inconsistently observed.[77] The mechanism of platelet inhibition appears to involve the production of nitric oxide from the drug, with concomitant increases in platelet cAMP and, more markedly, cGMP.[82] β-Adrenergic receptor blockers such as propranolol, metoprolol, atenolol, and pindolol have also been shown to inhibit platelet aggregation, apparently through mechanisms independent of β-adrenergic receptor blockade.[83,84] Several of these agents have been shown to blunt platelet aggregation to ADP and collagen,[85] and to decrease platelet TXA_2 production in response to agonists.[83] Blunting of serotonin uptake by platelets and inhibition of the response to serotonin have also been demonstrated. There are numerous reports of antiplatelet effects of calcium channel blockers, such as nifedipine, verapamil, and diltiazem. Most of these studies demonstrated inhibition of platelet aggregation in washed platelets at high concentrations (micromolar) of the drug. This effect is mainly with epinephrine as the agonist, and it does not appear to be related to inhibition of calcium ion influx. Proposed mechanisms include inhibition of epinephrine binding to α_2-adrenergic receptors, inhibition of the platelet response to TXA_2, and inhibition of serotonin-induced aggregation. In therapeutic doses, the calcium channel blockers do not prolong the bleeding time. At high concentrations, quinidine can act as an antagonist of platelet α_2-adrenergic receptors. In one report, a patient taking 800 mg of quinidine and 650 mg of aspirin daily developed melena and generalized petechiae with a normal platelet count and a bleeding time over 35 minutes.[86] In a subsequent study in two healthy volunteers, quinidine caused a mild prolongation of the bleeding time that was apparently potentiated by aspirin. Quinidine and its stereoisomer, quinine, can also impair hemostasis by inducing drug-dependent antibodies that cause thrombocytopenia.

The commonly used angiotensin receptor antagonists losartan, valsartan, and olmesartan interact with the TXA_2 receptor and inhibit thromboxane-dependent platelet adhesion and aggregation.[87] Valsartan also inhibits the expression of major platelet receptors including $\alpha_{IIb}\beta_3$ and glycoprotein (GP)Ib.[88]

Antibiotics

Antibiotics can also affect platelet function. Those implicated most often are the penicillins and cephalosporins, which share a β-lactam ring structure. Some of these drugs produce predictable dose- and duration-related effects on the bleeding time.[89–91] Because the effect on bleeding time is seen only in patients who are receiving large parenteral doses of antibiotics, this is a potential problem only for hospitalized patients. In a study of 74 hospitalized patients with a consistently prolonged bleeding time, the likely cause was penicillin in 39 patients (30 patients were receiving >15,000,000 U/day of penicillin G, and 9 were receiving 6–8 g/day of ampicillin) and aspirin or related drugs in 7 patients.[91] Floxacillin (an isoxazolyl penicillin) has been shown to significantly impair platelet function and cause severe bleeding when used in high dose in a patient with infective endocarditis.[92]

The structural properties that cause some, but not all, penicillins and cephalosporins to affect platelet function are unknown. The side chain structure alters the antibacterial and pharmacologic properties of the penicillins and cephalosporins, and may also determine their effects on platelet function. It is postulated that the antibiotic associates with the platelet plasma membrane via a lipophilic mechanism where it perturbs receptor–agonist interactions or signal transduction.[93] The characteristic laboratory findings are a prolonged bleeding time and abnormal platelet aggregation studies that occur after several days of high-dose parenteral therapy.[90,91,94] These abnormalities do not usually subside until several days after the antibiotic is discontinued.

The frequency of clinically important bleeding in patients taking β-lactam antibiotics is low and is not predicted by a prolonged bleeding time; consequently, the causal relation to antibiotic treatment is unproved.[95] For each report implicating an antibiotic as a cause of hemorrhage, many more patients receive the same antibiotics in large doses without bleeding complications.[95]

Although antibiotic-induced platelet dysfunction usually is of little clinical importance, there are some exceptions to this rule. The frequency of clinically important hemorrhagic complications with moxalactam appears to be higher than with other antibiotics.[96] This drug has been demonstrated to inhibit ADP- and collagen-induced platelet aggregation in a dose-dependent fashion and to decrease TXA_2 generation,[97] which suggests that, like aspirin, it acts on the thromboxane synthesis pathway. Furthermore, in contrast to most other β-lactam antibiotics, moxalactam contains a methylthiotetrazole-leaving group that has been implicated in the inhibition of synthesis of the vitamin K–dependent coagulation factors.[98] Therefore, moxalactam-induced bleeding may be caused by the combination of deficiencies in vitamin K–dependent coagulation factors and impaired platelet function.

Nitrofurantoin, an antibiotic structurally unrelated to the β-lactam antibiotics, may mildly prolong the bleeding time and impair platelet aggregation at plasma concentrations in excess of 20 μM.[99]

Antifungal Drugs

Miconazole has been shown to inhibit platelet aggregation in rabbits;[100] but there is no evidence that the drug causes platelet dysfunction in humans. Concomitant use of miconazole and vitamin K antagonists may cause significant bleeding because miconazole is a strong inhibitor of CYP2C9.[101]

Amphotericin B inhibits thrombin-induced platelet aggregation, serotonin uptake, and thrombin-induced serotonin release in in vitro studies.[102] Studies have shown that platelet transfusion immediately after amphotericin B infusion caused poor platelet recovery and survival. An interval of at least 2 hours should separate platelet transfusion from amphotericin B therapy.[103]

Psychiatric Drugs

Platelets from patients taking tricyclic antidepressant drugs (imipramine, amitriptyline, nortriptyline) or phenothiazines (chlorpromazine, promethazine, trifluoperazine) can exhibit impaired in vitro aggregation and secretion responses to ADP, epinephrine, and collagen, but this effect is not associated with an increased risk for bleeding.[77] However, there are numerous reports of antiplatelet effects of the widely used selective serotonin reuptake inhibitors (SSRIs; paroxetine, sertraline, fluoxetine, citalopram), which block the only means of platelet serotonin uptake for storage;[104–108] the effect of these drugs in decreasing platelet serotonin levels has been documented.[109,110] Prolonged bleeding times,[111] excessive bruising,[112] and defective platelet aggregation have all been noted in patients taking fluoxetine.[113] SSRI use increases perioperative and postoperative bleeding,[114] increases red cell transfusion rates during and after surgery,[115] and increases the risk of postpartum hemorrhage in pregnant women.[116] On the other hand, the cessation of the SSRI antidepressant drug may cause discontinuation syndrome or depression relapse. Thus the risk–benefit profile should be considered before cessation of an SSRI drug prior to elective surgery.

Additionally, the risk of GI bleeding is increased in patients taking SSRIs, particularly when they are combined with NSAIDs.[117] A recent prospective population study showed that the use of antidepressants, especially SSRIs was associated with a low risk for myocardial infarction.[118]

Oncologic Drugs

Administration of mithramycin has been associated with decreased platelet aggregation, a prolonged bleeding time, and mucocutaneous bleeding.[119] Daunorubicin and bis-chloroethyl-nitrosourea can both inhibit platelet aggregation and secretion when added to platelet-rich plasma, but these effects do not appear to be clinically important.[77] Vincristine inhibits platelet aggregation by interfering with the microtubule network.[120]

Tyrosine kinase inhibitors, which are used for the treatment of chronic myeloid leukemia, can cause thrombocytopenia and/or platelet dysfunction. Dasatinib and imatinib both have been demonstrated to impair platelet aggregation.[121] Dasatinib may cause clinically relevant bleeding because of platelet dysfunction.[122]

Ibritunib is an orally administered Bruton kinase inhibitor used for the treatment of B-cell malignancies. It also inhibits signaling downstream of platelet GPVI and affects platelet adhesion to vWF under arterial flow, increasing the risk for bleeding.[123]

Anesthetics

Although some local and general anesthetic agents have been shown to inhibit platelet function in vitro, this effect is generally produced at high drug concentrations.[124,125] Sevoflurane suppresses formation of TXA_2; propofol and nitrous oxide inhibit calcium mobilization.[124] Procaine inhibits calcium and P-selectin release from platelet storage pools.[126] Dibucaine is a calpain activator, induces platelet apoptosis, and inhibits platelet functions.[127] At usual doses, halothane reversibly inhibits platelet aggregation.[128]

Plasma Expanders

Dextrans are partially hydrolyzed branched polymers of glucose. Of the two preparations in clinical use, dextran 70 has an average molecular mass of 70–75 kDa and dextran 40 has an average molecular mass of 40 kDa. Both preparations are effective plasma expanders and can affect platelet function, but the high-molecular-weight molecules have a greater effect on hemostasis.[129] Dextran infusion also impairs platelet aggregation and platelet procoagulant activity, and can cause a modest reduction in plasma vWF concentration. However, dextran has no effect on platelet function when added directly to platelet-rich plasma in vitro.[130] Because of its effects on platelet function, dextran was explored as an antithrombotic agent, but it is no longer used for this purpose.

Hydroxyethyl starch, known as *hetastarch*, is a synthetic glucose polymer with an average molecular weight of 450,000 (range: 10,000–1,000,000) that is also used for plasma expansion. Hetastarch use has been associated with abnormal platelet function (albeit inconsistently), a problem more evident with the higher-molecular-weight forms.[131] Like dextran, it can prolong the bleeding time, particularly if administered at doses higher than 20 mL/kg in a 6% solution, and predisposes to bleeding if administered simultaneously with heparin or in the presence of a preexisting hemostatic defect.[132]

Heparins and Thrombolytic Agents

Although heparin is best known for its anticoagulant effect and its association with HIT and thrombosis (see Chapters 133 and 149), it also has the potential to affect platelet function. Heparin can bind to the platelet surface,[133] induce platelet aggregation and secretion,[134] and impair vWF-dependent platelet function.[135] Heparin can also increase the bleeding time.[136] Whether these phenomena contribute to heparin-induced bleeding is unknown. The prolonged bleeding time is probably the result of inhibition of thrombin generation, analogous to the slight but significant increase in bleeding times seen in patients with hemophilia.[134]

Paradoxically, heparin is also capable of inducing the association of vWF with the GPIb complex.[137] Whether this is restricted to certain individuals or occurs only at certain heparin concentrations is unclear, but it raises the possibility that this mechanism may contribute to heparin-induced thrombosis.

Bleeding during therapy with plasminogen activators is predominantly caused by fibrin degradation, hypofibrinogenemia, and increased levels of fibrin(ogen) degradation products, usually in the setting of structural lesions. At pharmacologic concentrations, streptokinase, urokinase, and tissue plasminogen activator (t-PA) may also impair platelet function through several potential mechanisms, all related to excessive production of plasmin.[138] First, high levels of fibrin(ogen) degradation products and low levels of fibrinogen can impair platelet aggregation. Second, the binding of plasminogen to the platelet surface may facilitate its conversion to plasmin.[139] Plasmin can degrade GPIbα (thereby impairing the interaction of the platelet with vWF[140]) and fibrinogen (thereby dispersing platelet aggregates).[141] Third, plasmin can inhibit platelet aggregation by blocking the release of arachidonic acid from platelet membranes, thereby limiting TXA_2 production.[142] The clinical importance of these observations is unknown.

In addition to decreasing platelet function, plasmin has been shown to directly activate platelets,[143,144,145,146] an effect that may contribute to vessel reocclusion after t-PA treatment for myocardial infarction.[147] Platelet activation is the result of plasmin-mediated cleavage of protease-activated receptors (PAR), particularly PAR4.[148]

Miscellaneous Drugs

The statins, which inhibit 3-hydroxy-3-methylglutaryl coenzyme A reductase, are widely used in patients with dyslipidemia.[149] These agents reduce the risk of cardiovascular events through a variety of mechanisms, including reducing the risk of atherothrombosis. Among its antithrombotic effects are decreases in platelet reactivity, brought about by its beneficial effects on endothelial cells, with increased production of nitric oxide and prostacyclin, and by direct effects on platelets.[150] Membrane cholesterol content, which is lowered by the statins, has been correlated with platelet reactivity,[151,152] with studies demonstrating that the content of cholesterol in platelet membranes correlates with localization of important adhesive and agonist receptors within membrane microdomains known as *lipid rafts*.[153,154] Statins, in addition to lowering plasma and membrane cholesterol levels, also reduce the activity of stimulatory signaling pathways involving the small guanyl triphosphate (GTP)–binding proteins Ras, Rho, and Rac, which require posttranslational prenylation to be targeted to cell membranes. Statins inhibit protein prenylation.[155] No bleeding complications have been associated with statin use, but a substudy of the Platelet Receptor in Ischemic Syndrome Management (PRISM) trial showed that their sudden withdrawal in the setting of acute coronary syndrome was associated with an increased cardiac risk compared with the risk in patients who continued to receive statins (relative risk: 2.93) or never received statins.[156] This increase in cardiac events was partially attributed to increased platelet reactivity. A recent meta-analysis found no correlation between statin therapy and increased intracranial hemorrhage.[157]

Clofibrate, another lipid-lowering drug, diminishes platelet responsiveness to ADP, collagen, and epinephrine when given to patients with type II hyperbetalipoproteinemia, and can diminish the responsiveness of normal platelets to ADP and epinephrine in vitro.[77]

Cocaine accounts for more drug-related visits to emergency departments in the United States than any other drug except alcohol. Its use is associated with a large increase in the incidence of myocardial infarction in individuals who are otherwise at low risk, and it has been hypothesized that cocaine-induced platelet aggregation is a major contributor to this risk.[158] In vitro, however, cocaine inhibits platelet aggregation in response to several agonists and dissociates preformed aggregates.[159] Another important prothrombotic mechanism associated with cocaine use is the ability of cocaine and its long-acting metabolites to induce release of vWF from endothelial cells.[160]

Ketanserin, which has been studied for its potential to prevent atherosclerotic complications, decreases platelet aggregation in response to serotonin. Antihistamines, some radiographic contrast agents, and immunosuppressive drugs can also impair platelet aggregation. The mechanisms responsible for these effects are unknown.

Foods and Food Additives

Certain foods and food additives can have important effects on platelet function, particularly when consumed in large quantities. In a classic study published in 1979, Dyerberg and Bang[161] reported that Greenland Eskimos on traditional diets had markedly prolonged bleeding times compared with gender- and age-matched Danish control subjects (mean: 8.1 min vs. 4.8 min, respectively), and they correlated this finding with an impaired secondary wave of platelet aggregation to ADP and collagen, and high plasma levels of ω-3 fatty acids. The proposed mechanisms by which ω-3 fatty acids (eicosapentaenoic acid, $C20:5\omega$-3; and docosahexaenoic acid, $C22:6\omega$-3) interfere with platelet function is through competition with arachidonic acid for the 2-acyl position of membrane phospholipids or access to COX-1.[162,163] ω-3 Fatty acids not only reduce TXA_2 synthesis in response to platelet agonist stimulation by competing with the substrate arachidonic acid, but also by producing inhibitory eicosanoids. The latter mechanism was substantiated in the original study of Eskimos by the demonstration that administration of aspirin decreased the bleeding time in all subjects tested but not to normal levels.[161] Additionally, ω-3 fatty acids may increase the production of antiaggregatory prostaglandins by cells in the vessel wall.[161]

Ethanol, one of the most commonly and excessively ingested substances in the world, acts synergistically with aspirin to prolong the bleeding time.[164] In addition, ethanol acts cooperatively with agents that block binding of fibrinogen to $\alpha_{IIb}\beta_3$ to further reduce platelet aggregation in response to several agonists, an effect not solely the result of reduced TXA_2 generation.[165] Ethanol can also impair collagen-induced platelet aggregation, secretion, arachidonate mobilization, and TXA_2 formation, but it did not inhibit platelet adhesion to deendothelialized rabbit aortae.[166]

Other food components or additives can also affect platelet function and increase the risk of minor bleeding. Easy bruising after eating Chinese food has been attributed to a platelet inhibitory effect of black tree fungus.[167] A component of onion extract can inhibit platelet arachidonic acid metabolism.[168] Ajoene, a component of garlic, is an inhibitor of fibrinogen binding to platelets and platelet aggregation.[169] Extracts from frequently consumed spices—cumin, turmeric, and clove—can decrease platelet thromboxane production and inhibit platelet aggregation.[170] Bromelain, an extract from pineapple, can inhibit ADP-induced platelet aggregation, and prolong both the PT and aPTT.[171] Parsley (*Petroselinum crispum*) may inhibit ADP-induced platelet aggregation.[172]

It can be concluded that platelets are sensitive to a variety of therapeutic and dietary compounds, the extent of inhibition primarily depending on the dose of the inhibitory agent.[173] However, an increased risk for clinically important bleeding has been demonstrated only for aspirin and agents specifically designed to inhibit platelet function. Reports of increased bleeding with all other agents must be viewed with caution. Despite this qualification, it is prudent for clinicians to have a thorough understanding of the antiplatelet effects of prescribed drugs and to always consider the potential impacts of drug- or diet-induced platelet dysfunction, particularly in patients with coexisting hemostatic defects.

CLONAL DISORDERS

Hematological Clonal Disorders

Myeloproliferative Neoplasms

Myeloproliferative neoplasms (MPNs; see Chapters 67–72) are clonal disorders arising from hematopoietic stem cells affected by somatic mutations that cause abnormal production of mature myeloid cells. Philadelphia chromosome–negative MPNs, which include polycythemia vera (PV), essential thrombocythemia (ET), and primary myelofibrosis, are the most common MPNs. These disorders are characterized by varying degrees of leukocytosis or thrombocytosis; patients with PV usually have a markedly elevated hematocrit. Particularly in PV and ET, thrombosis or bleeding account for a high percentage of the associated morbidity of the disorders, with thrombosis being the most common.

Bleeding in patients with MPN is primarily mucocutaneous. The bleeding time is prolonged in a small percentage of patients with MPNs, but bleeding complications can occur even in patients with normal bleeding times. Routine plasma coagulation tests, such as the PT and aPTT, may be falsely prolonged if the red blood cell mass is increased. Because the plasma volume in these patients is reduced, it is important to adjust the citrate concentration in the tubes used to collect the blood for coagulation testing.

The mechanisms of bleeding are multifactorial in patients with MPN. Some bleeding episodes can in part be attributed to thrombosis, such as variceal bleeding resulting from thrombosis-induced portal hypertension.[174] Acquired platelet abnormalities, acquired coagulation factor (especially factor V) and vWF deficiencies,[175] antiplatelet drug usage, and drugs used for the clonal disease (such as anagrelide) may cause bleeding problems.

The platelets of patients with MPNs can show various morphologic abnormalities, including variations in size and shape, as well as reduced numbers of secretory granules. Platelet survival can be decreased in ET. The most common platelet abnormality is decreased aggregation and secretion in response to agonists, particularly epinephrine, ADP, and collagen.[176] These abnormalities are not simply the result of the high platelet count because patients with reactive thrombocytosis have functionally normal platelets.[177] In what may appear to be a paradox, some patients demonstrate spontaneous in vitro platelet aggregation in platelet-rich plasma. Decreased platelet aggregation or secretion and decreased procoagulant activity may be caused by decreased (1) agonist-induced release of arachidonic acid from membrane phospholipids; (2) conversion of arachidonic acid to prostaglandin endoperoxides or lipoxygenase products; (3) platelet responsiveness to TXA_2; (4) dense-granule or α-granule contents; or (5) α_2-adrenergic receptors. Some of the described abnormalities may also be a consequence of platelet activation in vivo or ex vivo during platelet preparation.

Specific platelet membrane abnormalities have also been reported, including deficiencies of GPIb and GPIX, causing an acquired form of the Bernard-Soulier syndrome;[178] deficiencies of receptors for prostaglandin D_2;[179] c-*MPL* receptors;[180] and an increased number of Fc receptors.[181] Because MPNs are clonal in origin, the abnormal platelets can arise from a clone of abnormal megakaryocytes.[182] Alternatively, the findings may be the result of platelet hyperreactivity and previous activation.[183,184] It is important to emphasize several features about the platelet function defects reported in MPNs. First, no defect has consistently predicted the risk for bleeding or thrombosis. Second, no defect is unique to, and therefore predictive of, a particular MPN. Third, the relative frequency of the different defects varies widely. Therefore the clinical importance of the abnormalities of platelet function in MPNs is unknown.

Acquired von Willebrand syndrome (Chapter 138) can cause mucocutaneous bleeding or complicate surgical interventions in nonbleeding patients. In acquired von Willebrand syndrome, the largest multimers of vWF are absent, possibly as a consequence of their adsorption to binding sites on the elevated numbers of platelets,[185–189] or because of enhanced a disintegrin and metalloproteinase with a thrombospondin type 1 motif, member 13 (ADAMTS13) proteolysis of the large multimers.[190] In a prospective study of MPN patients, the incidence of acquired von Willebrand syndrome was 11%.[191] Although increased adsorption of plasma vWF multimers by platelets is the cause of the syndrome and decreased vWF:RCo/Ag or vWF:collagen binding/Ag ratio was found in patients with extreme thrombocytosis,[189] acquired von Willebrand syndrome has also been described in patients with platelet counts between 120 and $135 \times 10^9/\mu L$.[191]

Several intrinsic platelet function defects result, at least in part, from an increased sensitivity of the platelets to activation, a potential consequence of the *JAK2* gain-of-function mutation. For example, a study demonstrated an increased risk of thrombosis in patients with chronic MPN when the mutant kinase was detected in platelets or in platelets and granulocytes.[182] Likewise, the *JAK2* mutation in platelets correlated with increased platelet expression of tissue factor and P-selectin, decreased expression of CD41 and CD42b, and increased quantities of platelet–neutrophil aggregates, all indicators of a hyperreactive platelet phenotype.[183] Panova-Noeva et al[184] evaluated the platelets from 140 patients with MPN (80 ET, 60 PV) for global procoagulant potential by measuring thrombin generation and expression of tissue factor and P-selectin on the platelet surface. They found that patients with the *JAK2* V617F mutation had the highest values for thrombin generation and platelet tissue factor and P-selectin expression. These findings correlated with *JAK2* V617F allele burden.[184]

Paroxysmal Nocturnal Hemoglobinuria

Paroxysmal nocturnal hemoglobinuria (PNH; see Chapter 31) is another clonal disorder that involves all blood cells. The hematopoietic stems cells and their progeny are defective in the synthesis of the glycosylphosphatidylinositol attachments required for the plasma membrane expression of some membrane proteins, leading to a defect in all glycosylphosphatidylinositol-linked proteins on blood cells,[192] including platelets.[193]

Thrombosis is a leading cause of mortality in PNH, affecting at least half of these patients. The platelet function abnormalities described in PNH range from hypersensitivity to agonists to dysfunction.[194] One study showed platelets to be hypersensitive to epinephrine, ADP, and collagen, as judged by their abilities to aggregate and to release ^{14}C serotonin.[195] The total release of nucleotides was also markedly increased over normal with all aggregating agents. By contrast, another study examining platelets from PNH patients showed them to be profoundly hyporeactive, as measured by defective clot formation, adhesion, and aggregation.[196] This finding was interpreted as being a consequence of chronic overstimulation of the platelets while they circulate.

Platelet activation and increased platelet microparticle formation have also been demonstrated in PNH patients.[194,195,197]

Paraproteinemias

Although thrombotic complications can occur in patients with paraproteinemias because of hyperviscosity, bleeding complications also are seen. Platelet dysfunction is observed in approximately one-third of patients with immunoglobulin (Ig)A myeloma or Waldenström macroglobulinemia, in 15% of patients with IgG myeloma, and occasionally in patients with benign monoclonal gammopathy.[198,199] Additional hemostatic problems in these patients can be caused by the hyperviscosity syndrome,[200,201] a heparin-like coagulation inhibitor,[202] acquired von Willebrand syndrome,[189] or complications of amyloidosis (e.g., acquired factor X deficiency[203] or enhanced fibrinolysis).[204] Patients may have markedly abnormal results on laboratory tests (e.g., a prolonged thrombin time) with no evidence of clinical bleeding.[198]

Abnormalities of platelet function correlate with the concentration of the plasma paraprotein. Myeloma proteins can inhibit all

platelet functions (aggregation, secretion, procoagulant activity, and clot retraction), and normal platelets can acquire these defects when incubated with the purified monoclonal immunoglobulin.[205,206] In some cases, specific interactions of the monoclonal protein have been described. One IgA myeloma protein inhibited the ability of a suspension of aortic connective tissue to aggregate normal platelets.[207] The bleeding time and bleeding symptoms of the patient from whom this paraprotein was isolated were corrected when the IgA myeloma protein was removed by plasmapheresis. One patient had a fatal hemorrhage from an IgG1κ paraprotein that bound GPIIIa (β₃ integrin) and inhibited platelet aggregation.[208] A number of reports have described acquired von Willebrand disease in patients with myeloma, benign monoclonal gammopathy, or chronic lymphocytic leukemia.[209] In some patients, the plasma concentration of vWF was decreased; in others, the larger multimers were deficient. The myeloma protein can either accelerate vWF clearance from plasma or interfere with its binding to platelet GPIb.

Easy bruising, epistaxis, periorbital purpura (in patients with amyloidosis), and GI hemorrhage are the most common bleeding symptoms associated with the paraproteinemias. Because bleeding appears to be related to high plasma paraprotein concentrations,[210] chemotherapy for the underlying plasma cell neoplasm should be given to effect a longer lasting reduction of the paraprotein. In emergency situations, plasmapheresis should be performed expeditiously; the effectiveness of this therapy can be evaluated by improvement of bleeding. Intravenous immunoglobulin (IVIG) infusions are effective in controlling bleeding in patients with plasma cell dyscrasias and acquired von Willebrand disease. IVIG can produce a clinical and laboratory response in 12–72 hours, and the effect usually persists for 1–3 weeks. In patients with severe bleeding, IVIG can be combined with plasmapheresis, DDVAP, and infusions of vWF concentrates or factor VIIa.[189,191,199,209]

LEUKEMIAS AND MYELODYSPLASTIC SYNDROMES

Bleeding in patients with the leukemias and myelodysplastic syndromes (MDS) is almost always caused by thrombocytopenia, but abnormalities of platelet function have also been described. In acute myeloid leukemia and its variants, platelets may be larger than normal, abnormally shaped, and vary in their granule numbers. Abnormal platelet structure and function have been described, especially in association with acute megakaryoblastic leukemia (FAB M7),[211–213] with one study describing three patients with decreased aggregation to collagen, ADP, epinephrine, and the thromboxane analogue U46619, along with a decreased platelet serotonin content.[211] Platelet abnormalities can also be found in the MDS, with defective aggregation and glass bead retention most often associated with hypolobulated megakaryocytes and the 5q⁻ syndrome.[213,214] Abnormal platelet function has also been described in association with B-cell malignancies, such as hairy cell leukemia, which can persist after splenectomy,[215] and with chronic lymphocytic leukemia,[216] in which the platelets exhibit reduced responses to GPVI agonists such as collagen and convulxin.

Also, acquired platelet GP defects have been reported in hematological malignancies, including acquired Glanzmann thrombasthenia in a patient with Hodgkin lymphoma[217] and acquired Bernard-Soulier syndrome in a child with MDS.[218]

SOLID TUMORS

Bleeding complications in patients with cancer are related to decreased platelet production caused by bone marrow infiltration, the myelosuppressive effects of chemotherapy and radiotherapy, sepsis, disseminated intravascular coagulation, microangiopathic hemolytic anemia, drug-induced thrombocytopenia, immune thrombocytopenia, or hypersplenism. Although several defects of platelet functions have been described in cancer patients, none are specific.[219]

SYSTEMIC METABOLIC DISORDERS

End-Stage Renal Disease

The pathogenesis of the hemorrhagic diathesis in patients with end-stage renal disease (ESRD) is complex (Chapter 154). Factors such as platelet function abnormalities caused by uremic toxins, anemia, hemodialysis procedures (both the artificial circulation and the use of anticoagulation), and decreased drug clearance may impair hemostasis.

In ESRD patients both platelet hypofunction and platelet hyperreactivity can occur.[220]

Deficiencies in the number of GPIb complexes in uremic platelets have been reported, the number inversely correlating with the creatinine level.[221] Consistent with this finding, another study demonstrated that defective ristocetin-induced platelet aggregation of uremic platelet-rich plasma was not corrected by resuspending the platelets in normal platelet-poor plasma. Likewise, uremic platelets suspended in normal plasma were defective in their adhesion to deendothelialized rabbit vessels at high shear, a test of the competency of the interaction between GPIb and vWF.[222] Conversely, the same study demonstrated that plasma factors also influence platelet function by showing that normal platelets suspended in uremic plasma acquired an adhesion defect possibly related to an abnormal interaction of vWF with the subendothelium. This led to the suggestion that vWF may be abnormal in uremia. Two studies have demonstrated normal-to-elevated vWF antigen and activity (measured as ristocetin cofactor activity) in uremic patients but decreased levels of the largest, most hemostatically active multimers,[223,224] reflected in one study as a decreased ratio of activity to antigen level compared with the vWF from normal subjects.[223] Taken together, the various studies consistently indicate that the first step of platelet adhesion at sites of vessel wall injury is abnormal, a defect that could be clinically significant if coupled with other defects of platelet function.[220]

The platelets of uremic patients frequently exhibit reduced fibrinogen binding, aggregation, and secretion in response to a wide variety of agonists. This abnormality may persist when the platelets are removed from uremic plasma, and in some studies, uremic plasma has induced these defects in normal platelets. One potential mechanism is provided by the demonstration that fibrinogen fragment levels are elevated in patients with ESRD and bind to platelet $\alpha_{IIb}\beta_3$, inhibiting platelet aggregation.[225]

Uremic platelets can also exhibit a reduction in several of the biochemical responses necessary for aggregation and secretion, including the rise in cytoplasmic calcium ion concentration, release of arachidonic acid from membrane phospholipids, conversion of arachidonic acid to TXA_2, and dense-granule and α-granule secretion. Abnormal cytoskeletal assembly and deficient tyrosine phosphorylation have also been noted in uremic platelets, abnormalities only partially corrected by dialysis.[220,226]

The accumulation of dialyzable platelet-inhibitory substances in the plasma of uremic patients has long been recognized. The ability of uremic plasma to inhibit platelet function was demonstrated in the late 1960s by Horowitz and colleagues,[227] who showed reduced ADP-induced platelet aggregation and a prolonged Stypven clotting time, a measure of platelet procoagulant activity. This activity, previously called *platelet factor 3*, is vital for the support of coagulation factor complex assembly on the platelet surface and requires externalization of the anionic phospholipid phosphatidylserine. One uremic substance with platelet inhibitory properties described by Horowitz and coworkers[228] was guanidinosuccinic acid, which accumulates in uremic plasma as an alternative byproduct of L-arginine metabolism,[229] a consequence of the inhibitory effect of high urea levels on enzymes of the urea cycle. Similar to L-arginine, guanidinosuccinic acid is a precursor of nitric oxide, which is produced in increased quantities in the endothelial cells and platelets of uremic patients and experimental animals.[229] Consistent with an important role for nitric oxide in uremia, infusion of the nitric oxide synthesis inhibitor monomethyl L-arginine reduced the bleeding time in uremic rats.[230] Furthermore, suppression of nitric oxide production

appears to correlate with the benefit of conjugated estrogens in improving the bleeding time in uremia.[231] Increased expression of vascular prostacyclin has also been described in uremic rats, a factor that would further depress in vivo platelet function.[232]

Dialysis itself may be associated with alterations in platelet function. For example, hemodialysis can reduce the responsiveness of platelets to agonists in vitro,[233] and chronic hemodialysis and peritoneal dialysis are associated with an increase in reticulated platelets, suggesting accelerated platelet turnover.[234] Of the two forms of dialysis, hemodialysis appears to have the greatest effect on platelet function, with one study noting abnormal cytoskeletal assembly and defective tyrosine phosphorylation to thrombin stimulation in the platelets of patients on hemodialysis, parameters that returned almost to normal with the institution of ambulatory peritoneal dialysis.[226] The cause of the defect associated with hemodialysis is likely to be the chronic low-level platelet activation associated with the procedure. In particular, polymerization and depolymerization of actin, release of granule proteins and their binding to the platelet surface, and shedding of membrane proteins may render the platelets relatively refractory to activation.

Uremia and artificial surfaces during hemodialysis also affect platelet mRNA and microRNA profiles, and alter protein expression.[235]

As would be expected, platelets from uremic patients may be unusually sensitive to medicines that decrease platelet function. Aspirin has been reported to produce a greater prolongation of the bleeding time in uremic patients than in controls, an effect that may be attributable to more than the irreversible inhibition of COX-1.[236] Similarly, β-lactam antibiotics that prolong the bleeding time can also have a greater effect in uremic patients and may increase the risk of bleeding, particularly those antibiotics cleared by the kidney.[173,237]

Anemia, which does correlate with the severity of renal failure, is an independent cause of a prolonged bleeding time,[237–240] and the defect correlates with the severity of the anemia. The relationship of the bleeding time to hematocrit in uremic patients has been confirmed by its correction with the transfusion of red blood cells and by treatment with erythropoietin.[220,240,241]

In contrast to the studies of platelet function performed to understand the possible increased risk for bleeding in patients with chronic renal failure, the coagulation and fibrinolytic systems have been interrogated to understand the increased risk for thrombotic complications, a major cause of mortality.[242]

Uremia-related contributions to a thrombotic tendency include endothelial dysfunction, increased TF expression, increased microparticle generation, increased coagulation factors (fibrinogen, FXIIa, FVIIa) and proinflammatory markers, decreased natural anticoagulant levels, and changes related to renal replacement therapy as extracorporeal thrombin generation, decreased fibrinolysis, and membrane-induced platelet activation.[220,243]

Liver Disease

The bleeding diathesis observed with fulminant or end-stage liver disease (Chapter 153) is multifactorial, with contributing causes including thrombocytopenia, anemia, deficiencies in liver-synthesized coagulation factors, and excessive fibrinolysis.[244,245] Patients with chronic liver disease and hepatic cirrhosis of various causes have been reported to have prolonged bleeding times, and these disorders are associated with other platelet function abnormalities possibly related to a decrease in GPIb.[246] Although an association between prolonged bleeding time and GI hemorrhage has been demonstrated in some studies of cirrhotic patients,[247] other studies showed that the bleeding time and platelet aggregation abnormalities correlated best with the degree of thrombocytopenia,[248] suggesting that no specific platelet function defect exists in liver disease. An aspirin-like defect has been reported in patients with severe liver disease, with defective aggregation and TXA_2 production.[249] Interestingly, one study showed that platelets obtained from the portal circulation of patients with hepatocellular cancer on a background of cirrhosis showed decreased and delayed aggregation in response to collagen compared with circulating platelets.[250] In addition to portal hypertension and esophageal varices, this finding raises the possibility that localized vascular bed factors (including increased prostacyclin) may contribute to variceal bleeding.

Because patients with cirrhosis often have a complicated hemostatic picture that includes thrombocytopenia, decreased fibrinogen levels, and prolonged prothrombin and aPTTs, one might expect this to uniformly produce a severe bleeding diathesis. However, recent studies have shown that the hemostatic defects in these patients are at least partially compensated through several mechanisms. The potential to bleed because of thrombocytopenia is reduced because vWF levels are often elevated and ADAMTS13 activity is decreased,[251–253] perhaps as a consequence of decreased synthesis by hepatic stellate cells. The decreased concentrations of procoagulant factors are balanced by the decreased concentrations of anticoagulant proteins.[254] Dysfibrinogenemia produces a less severe hemostatic defect because of decreased plasminogen levels.[255,256] This balance may easily be tipped in either direction, favoring either bleeding or thrombosis.

Although patients with cirrhosis may have platelet dysfunction, it is usually not associated with serious bleeding. Bleeding in these patients cannot be predicted with routine diagnostic tests, such as the platelet count and bleeding time.[257,258]

PLATELET DYSFUNCTION RELATED WITH EXTRACORPOREAL CIRCUITS

Extracorporeal circuits such as cardiopulmonary bypass (CPB), extracorporeal membrane oxygenation (ECMO), continuous flow left ventricular assist devices (LVADs), and total artificial heart generate high shear stress and affect blood cells, endothelial cells, and plasma proteins.

Bleeding complications can be seen in 10%–20% of the patients undergoing CPB, and hemostatic disturbances are responsible from bleeding in nearly half of those patients.[259,260] CPB activates both coagulation and fibrinolytic systems, and causes consumption coagulopathy. Besides the surgery itself, high shear stress and exposure of the blood to artificial surfaces activates FXII and FXI directly, and induces blood cells to express TF.[259,261]

Typical findings after bypass surgery include a prolonged bleeding time (longer than expected for the degree of thrombocytopenia), decreased platelet aggregation, decreased platelet agglutination in response to ristocetin, and depletion of platelet α-granule and dense granule contents.[262]

As with hemodialysis, the platelet defect caused by CPB is most likely a consequence of platelet activation and fragmentation within the extracorporeal circuit. The severity of the platelet abnormalities correlates with the duration of the bypass procedure.[260] With uncomplicated surgery, platelet function returns to normal within 24 hours; however, a much longer time may be required in some patients, and the platelet count typically does not return to normal for several days.[263]

Thrombocytopenia is caused by hemodilution and deposition of platelets on the bypass circuit and, to a lesser extent, sequestration of damaged platelets in the liver. Platelet dysfunction during bypass may be caused by reversible adhesion and aggregation of platelets on fibrinogen adsorbed from plasma onto the bypass circuit material, mechanical trauma and shear stress, cardiotomy suction, trace concentrations of circulating thrombin and ADP, complement activation, hypothermia, blood conservation devices; bypass priming solutions; and, with bubble oxygenators, exposure of platelets to the blood–air interface.[173,259] CPB consistently induces the formation of platelet fragments, or membrane "microparticles," evidence that the platelet surface membrane is subjected to severe mechanical stress and activation during the procedure.[264] Thus considerable platelet activation and aggregation occur during CPB, which leads to deleterious effects from substances released from the platelets and the new adhesive molecules exposed on their surfaces, and renders the platelets relatively refractory to activation by agonists.

Another surgical cause of platelet dysfunction relates to the use of deep hypothermic circulatory arrest in some surgeries. This procedure involves cooling the vital organs to temperatures between 15°C and 22°C (59°F and 71.6°F) for reducing oxygen requirements of major organs such as the heart, brain, and kidney.[265]

In patients with mechanical circulatory support such as LVADs or ECMO, continuous exposure of blood to nonbiological surfaces creates additional hemostatic problems.[266,267] Continuously elevated shear stress both elongates and breaks down vWF multimers mechanically and facilitates the cleavage of high-molecular-weight vWF multimers by ADAMTS13, causing acquired von Willebrand disease.[267] Increased shear stress created by these devices also causes platelet receptor shedding. In a study evaluating patients with ECMO and continuous flow LVADs, platelet surface receptor shedding was demonstrated by elevated soluble GPVI levels in plasma, and significantly reduced expression of GPVI and GP Ibα on the platelet surface.[268]

MISCELLANEOUS

Hypothermia

Hypothermia is defined as core body temperature below 35°C or 95°F and is classified as mild (32–35°C or 90–95°F), moderate (28–32°C or 82–90°F), severe (20–28°C or 68–82°F), and profound (below 20°C or 68°F). Major causes of hypothermia are exposure to cold weather or immersion in cold water, but hypothermia can also be caused by dehydration, severe trauma, massive transfusion, head injury, burns, sepsis, and drugs (e.g., alcohol, sedatives, and hypnotics). Age is an important risk factor because elderly adults and newborns are particularly prone to hypothermia. Hypothermia is also intentionally induced in some cardiac operations.[265]

Mild hypothermia is usually well tolerated, but mortality increases when the core body temperature falls below 20°C. In animals, hypothermia causes thrombocytopenia because of platelet sequestration in the spleen and liver. Hypothermia inhibits platelet aggregation in response to thrombin and thromboxane, increases platelet expression of P-selectin, and decreases expression of the GPIb-IX-V complex.[269] Both the thrombocytopenia and the functional defects are reversible, returning to normal when the body temperature normalizes.[265]

ANTIPLATELET ANTIBODIES

Immunoglobulins can bind to platelets in a specific or nonspecific fashion and can disrupt platelet function. In conditions such as immune thrombocytopenic purpura (ITP), systemic lupus erythematosus (SLE), and platelet alloimmunization, the antibodies can trigger accelerated platelet destruction and subsequent thrombocytopenia. Surviving platelets, known as *stress platelets*, display enhanced function.[270] Indeed, bleeding times in ITP may be shorter than expected for the degree of thrombocytopenia. Sometimes, however, the hemorrhagic tendency is out of proportion to the degree of thrombocytopenia or persists after the platelet count returns to normal, suggesting that the bound antibody is perturbing platelet function.[271]

In some patients with ITP or SLE, platelet dysfunction may be suspected because mucocutaneous bleeding symptoms occur despite platelet counts that are usually sufficient for normal hemostasis (>50,000/μL), and the bleeding time may be longer than expected for the degree of thrombocytopenia. Patients with antiplatelet antibodies can exhibit defective platelet function in vitro even if they do not have prolonged bleeding times or clinical symptoms of excessive bleeding, a situation similar to what occurs with aspirin ingestion or renal disease. For example, in two studies, 13 of 19 patients with ITP demonstrated impaired platelet aggregation to ADP, epinephrine, or collagen.[272,273] In two other studies, 22 of 35 patients with SLE were found to have decreased platelet aggregation in response to these agonists.[274,275] The platelet function abnormalities appear to be antibody mediated because IgG purified from the plasma or eluted from the platelets of these patients inhibited the aggregation of normal platelets.

Platelet antibodies may affect several aspects of platelet function. The most frequently observed abnormality is absence of platelet aggregation in response to low concentrations of collagen and absence of the second wave of aggregation in response to ADP or epinephrine. This pattern is identical to the abnormalities caused by aspirin, described earlier. In ITP and SLE, the abnormal aggregation may be related to a reduction in the contents of dense and α-granules, or to an activation defect manifested by diminished synthesis of TXA_2.

Autoantibodies or alloantibodies usually impair the function of the antigen against which they are targeted. For example, alloantibodies (e.g., anti-Pl[A1]) and autoantibodies that bind to $\alpha_{IIb}\beta_3$ produce a syndrome similar to Glanzmann thrombasthenia.[276–280] These antibody-associated thrombopathies can be severe.[281]

It is not surprising that many of the antiplatelet antibodies target $\alpha_{IIb}\beta_3$ because this is the most abundant receptor on the platelet surface and required for all aggregation responses.[282] Antibodies that target GPIb have also been described, in one case producing a syndrome of severe refractory thrombocytopenia and a functional defect resembling that observed in Bernard-Soulier syndrome.[283] An interesting aspect of antibodies against GPIb is their association with more severe thrombocytopenia than that observed with antibodies directed against other antigens.[284] This finding is consistent with the observations that anti-GPIb antibodies inhibit megakaryopoiesis[285] and proplatelet formation in vitro.[286] Autoantibodies have been described that target GPIa (integrin α_2),[287,288] GPIV,[288] and GPVI.[289–291]

Platelet-activating antibodies have been described. Of particular interest is the report of a patient who presented with immune thrombocytopenia and an antibody against CD9 (a member of the tetraspanin protein family) that was capable of activating normal platelets.[292] After recovery of the platelet count, the patient relapsed, this time with an antibody described against the platelet Fc receptor, $Fc\gamma RIIA$. The latter antibody blocked the capacity of the first antibody to activate platelets, confirming that activation involved stimulation of the Fc receptor.

Platelets that have been activated and induced to secrete but have not been incorporated into aggregates are likely to be refractory to platelet agonists and deficient in secretory granule contents, essentially leading to an acquired storage pool deficiency, which has also been described in association with autoantibodies.[293]

SCURVY

Vitamin C deficiency results in defective collagen synthesis and abnormal bleeding from fragile capillaries. However, significant platelet aggregation defects can be seen in patients with scurvy, which normalize after vitamin C supplementation.[294]

ACQUIRED PLATELET DYSFUNCTION WITH EOSINOPHILIA

Acquired platelet dysfunction with eosinophilia is a self-limited disorder characterized by mucocutaneous bleeding and hypereosinophilia.[295,296] The platelet count is usually normal; however, the platelets are pale by light microscopy (as in gray platelet syndrome), and aggregation studies show an acquired storage pool defect. All reported cases have been from South-East Asia. In some cases

eosinophilia and platelet dysfunction returned to normal after anti-helmintic therapy, which suggests a parasitic infection.

SUGGESTED READINGS

Ashrani AA, Tefferi A, Pruthi RK, et al: Acquired factor V deficiency in myeloproliferative neoplasms: a Mayo Clinic series of 33 patients. *Br J Haematol* 171:875, 2015.

Bartoli CR, Restle DJ, Zhang DM, et al: Pathologic von Willebrand factor degradation with a left ventricular assist device occurs via two distinct mechanisms: mechanical demolition and enzymatic cleavage. *J Thorac Cardiovasc Surg* 149:281, 2015.

Baumann KL, Massicotte MP: Mechanical circulatory support: balancing bleeding and clotting in high-risk patients. *Hematology Am Soc Hematol Educ Program* 2015:61, 2015.

Fu R, Meng Y, Wang Y, et al: The dysfunction of platelets in paroxysmal nocturnal hemoglobinuria. *Thromb Res* 148:50, 2016.

Hanley GE, Smolina K, Mintzes B, et al: Postpartum Hemorrhage and Use of Serotonin Reuptake Inhibitor Antidepressants in Pregnancy. *Obstet Gynecol* 127:553, 2016.

Kaur H, Corscadden K, Lott C, et al: Bromelain has paradoxical effects on blood coagulability: a study using thromboelastography. *Blood Coagul Fibrinolysis* 27:745, 2016.

King S, Short M, Harmon C: Glycoprotein IIb/IIIa inhibitors: the resurgence of tirofiban. *Vascul Pharmacol* 78:10, 2016.

Kostos L, Burbury K, Srivastava G, et al: Gastrointestinal bleeding in a chronic myeloid leukaemia patient precipitated by dasatinib-induced platelet dysfunction: case report. *Platelets* 26:809, 2015.

Lukito P, Wong A, Jing J, et al: Mechanical circulatory support is associated with loss of platelet receptors glycoprotein Ibalpha and glycoprotein VI. *J Thromb Haemost* 2016. epub ahead of print.

Noordam R, Aarts N, Leening MJ, et al: Use of antidepressants and the risk of myocardial infarction in middle-aged and older adults: a matched case-control study. *Eur J Clin Pharmacol* 72:211, 2016.

Oudemans-van Straaten HM: Hemostasis and thrombosis in continuous renal replacement treatment. *Semin Thromb Hemost* 41:91, 2015.

Reuken PA, Kussmann A, Kiehntopf M, et al: Imbalance of von Willebrand factor and its cleaving protease ADAMTS13 during systemic inflammation superimposed on advanced cirrhosis. *Liver Int* 35:37, 2015.

Roose SP, Rutherford BR: Selective serotonin reuptake inhibitors and operative bleeding risk: a review of the literature. *J Clin Psychopharmacol* 36:704, 2016.

Sajan F, Conte JV, Tamargo RJ, et al: Association of Selective Serotonin Reuptake Inhibitors with Transfusion in Surgical Patients. *Anesth Analg* 123:21, 2016.

Tripodi A: Hemostasis abnormalities in cirrhosis. *Curr Opin Hematol* 22:406, 2015.

Tuffigo M, Lazaro E, James C, et al: Successful use of recombinant factor VIIa in a patient with acquired Glanzmann thrombasthenia. *Haemophilia* 21:e116–e118, 2015.

Van Poucke S, Stevens K, Wetzels R, et al: Early platelet recovery following cardiac surgery with cardiopulmonary bypass. *Platelets* 1:2016.

Yadav DD, Nayar PS, Manchanda RV: Acquired Platelet Dysfunction with Eosinophilia (APDE) syndrome: a case report. *Indian J Hematol Blood Transfus* 32:235, 2016.

REFERENCES

For the complete list of references, log on to www.expertconsult.com.

DISEASES OF PLATELET NUMBER: IMMUNE THROMBOCYTOPENIA, NEONATAL ALLOIMMUNE THROMBOCYTOPENIA, AND POSTTRANSFUSION PURPURA

Donald M. Arnold, Michelle P. Zeller, James W. Smith, and Ishac Nazy

Platelets are anucleate cells that are required for primary hemostasis. Platelets have a life span of 7–10 days in the circulation, after which time they are cleared by the cells of the reticuloendothelial system (RES), including the spleen. Platelet production is stimulated by thrombopoietin (TPO), a hormone that is constitutively secreted by the liver. TPO binds to c-Mpl, its receptor on platelets, hematopoietic progenitor cells, and bone marrow (BM) megakaryocytes. When bound to c-Mpl, TPO is internalized, degraded, and removed from the circulation; thus when the platelet count is low, free TPO levels are high, and more platelets are produced. In contrast, when platelet counts are high, circulating TPO levels are low, and platelet production declines. This primitive feedback system is very effective at maintaining the platelet count at a stable level. Recent evidence in mice has shown that the Ashwell-Morell receptor on murine hepatocytes binds platelets that have lost sialic acid residues on their surface. Binding activates a JAK-STAT signaling pathway, resulting in increased hepatic TPO mRNA expression and TPO production. The role of this pathway in normal human thrombopoiesis is not yet known.

Immune-mediated platelet disorders disrupt normal regulation of platelet number because of antibody-mediated or cell-mediated platelet destruction or platelet underproduction. Antibodies that target self (autoimmune) or nonself (alloimmune) antigens on platelets can cause severe thrombocytopenia. Immune thrombocytopenia (ITP) is an autoimmune disorder characterized by antibodies directed against platelet glycoproteins (GPs). Neonatal alloimmune thrombocytopenia (NAIT) is a thrombocytopenic syndrome caused by platelet alloantibodies. Posttransfusion purpura (PTP) has features of both alloantibody- and autoantibody-mediated processes. These platelet disorders have related immunologic features with distinct clinical characteristics (Table 131.1). The pathophysiology, clinical manifestations, and management of these disorders are discussed in this chapter.

IMMUNE THROMBOCYTOPENIA

ITP is a common autoimmune disease characterized by a low platelet count that can be associated with an increased risk of bleeding. Increased platelet destruction resulting from platelet autoantibodies is a hallmark of ITP. Recently, however, it has become evident that relative platelet underproduction is also an important mechanism for the thrombocytopenia in ITP. Conventional treatments, including corticosteroids, intravenous immunoglobulin (IVIg), immunosuppressant drugs, and splenectomy are aimed at preventing platelet destruction. TPO receptor agonists are medications that work by increasing platelet production. They represent the most significant advance in ITP management since the first description of IVIg as a treatment for ITP in the early 1980s. TPO receptor agonists have been shown to be effective in clinical trials[1,2] and were the catalyst for several key initiatives in ITP including the standardization of terminology (2009)[3] and the development of the American Society of Hematology (ASH) Guidelines on diagnosis and management of ITP (2011).[4]

Epidemiology

The natural history of ITP is different in children and adults. For the majority of children, ITP presents acutely and resolves within several weeks, often in the absence of intervention. Seasonal variability suggests that viral infections may trigger the disease in many children. Conversely, adult-onset ITP tends to be insidious in onset and is characterized by a chronic or remitting and relapsing course.

Incidence and Prevalence of Immune Thrombocytopenia in Children

The incidence of acute ITP in children is estimated at 1.9–6.4 per 100,000 per year. Nearly 70% of childhood ITP occurs between the ages of 1 and 10 years with the peak prevalence between 4 and 6 years. Most studies in children report an overall male predominance in early childhood and equalization or reversal to female predominance in older children. Reported prevalence estimates are 12.6 per 100,000 for girls and 9.3 per 100,000 for boys in the older age groups.

Incidence and Prevalence of Immune Thrombocytopenia in Adults

Incidence estimates for adult-onset ITP are reported to be between 1.6 and 3.9 per 100,000 per year. A retrospective analysis from the United Kingdom described a bimodal distribution for men, with peak incidences before the age of 18 years and between 75 and 84 years of age. Relatively stable incidence rates were found in women up to the age of 60 years with a steady increase thereafter. The incidence of ITP has been reported to double in patients over 60 years of age.

The overall prevalence of ITP in adults has been estimated at 9.5 per 100,000, and ranges from 4.1 per 100,000 in younger ages (19–24 years) to 16 per 100,000 in older age groups (55–64 years). Male and female prevalence rates are 16.6 and 27.2 per 100,000 adults, respectively, for those 18–64 years of age, with prevalence rates increasing significantly after the age of 65 years. The female predominance is attenuated in older age groups and may revert to a male predominance after the age of 65 years. Indeed, the prevalence of ITP in older men is reported to be as high as 38.3 per 100,000. Increasing incidence and prevalence rates may reflect a true rise in disease frequency with age or ascertainment bias because of the higher likelihood of discovering incidental thrombocytopenia with more frequent medical visits in older individuals.

Pathophysiology

ITP is caused by increased platelet destruction and impaired platelet production. Until recently, the pathogenesis of immune-mediated thrombocytopenia was mainly attributed to platelet-reactive autoantibodies; however, it is now evident that the pathophysiology of ITP

TABLE 131.1	Antibody-Mediated Thrombocytopenic Disorders Caused by Autoantibodies (Immune Thrombocytopenia), Alloantibodies (Neonatal Alloimmune Thrombocytopenia) or Potentially Both (Posttransfusion Purpura)		
	Immune Thrombocytopenia	**Neonatal Alloimmune Thrombocytopenia**	**Posttransfusion Purpura**
Immune reaction	Autoimmune	Alloimmune	Features of both allo- and autoimmunity
Incidence	5 per 100,000 population	40 per 100,000 births (or 1 per 2500)	1 per 100,000 blood transfusions
Principal antigenic target	GPIIb/IIIa	HPA-1a	HPA-1a plus autoantigens
Nature of the antibody	Intermittent	Persistent (past 1 year)	Persistent often at high titers
Mode of sensitization	Autoantibody	Alloantibody	Features of allo- and autoantibodies
Sensitizing event	Mostly unknown; some viral illnesses, chronic infection	Exposure to fetal platelet antigens early in first pregnancy	Blood transfusion (RBCs or platelets) 5–10 days earlier
Bleeding frequency	Uncommon	Common	Very common
Epidemiology	Higher incidence in children and elderly adults; female predominance in early adulthood	Majority affects fetus or newborn carrying the HPA-1a antigen	Almost all are HPA-1bb women sensitized by previous transfusion or pregnancy

GP, Glycoprotein; HPA, human platelet antigen; RBC, red blood cell.

is more complex and involves alterations in cellular immunity and immune-mediated megakaryocyte injury.

The antibody hypothesis began with the observation that blood from patients with ITP was able to cause a reduction in platelet count levels in other individuals. In one of the first experiments, William Harrington infused blood from ITP patients into normal volunteers and observed a decrease in the platelet counts in most recipients.[5] The circulating factor in blood responsible for this effect was later identified as an immunoglobulin (Ig) that bound to the surface of platelets. In further studies, investigators were able to quantify platelet-associated IgG (PAIgG) on or inside platelets. PAIgG was not able to discriminate between immune and non-ITP and eventually assays were developed to detect antibodies directed against specific platelet GPs, specifically GPIIb/IIIa or GPIb/IX. GP-specific assays exhibited improved specificity but had limited sensitivity (50%–66%) since many patients with ITP had no detectable antibody. Autoantibodies against platelet GPs target those cells for rapid opsonization and clearance in the RES, particularly the spleen. Peptides from phagocytosed platelets may be processed and presented to specific T cells, which in turn stimulate B cells to produce additional platelet autoantibodies. This process, known as *epitope spreading*, may explain why patients have circulating autoantibodies targeting a variety of platelet antigens. Other proposed mechanisms of antibody-induced platelet destruction are complement activation and platelet apoptosis.

In ITP, platelet production does not compensate for the increased platelet destruction, suggesting that BM megakaryocyte growth and/or ability to produce platelets are impaired. Evidence supporting reduced platelet production in ITP derives from radiolabeled autologous platelet studies demonstrating normal or reduced platelet turnover; and from clinical studies that have consistently demonstrated the capacity of TPO receptor agonists to increase platelet counts in patients with severe thrombocytopenia. Megakaryocytes also express GP receptors, which may render them targets of ITP autoantibodies. Indeed, in vitro studies demonstrated suppression of megakaryocyte growth and maturation when the cells were incubated with IgG from ITP patients.

In addition to the effect of autoantibodies, cytotoxic T cells from ITP patients may have direct cytolytic effects on platelets. Some patients with active ITP but without detectable platelet autoantibodies had CD8[+] T cells that induced platelet lysis in vitro. In contrast, CD8[+] T cells from patients in remission did not show significant platelet reactivity. Furthermore, compared with cells from controls, CD3[+] cells from ITP patients exhibited increased expression of genes involved in cell-mediated cytotoxicity including tumor necrosis factor-α (TNF-α), perforin, and granzyme A and B, and CD8[+] T cells exhibited increased expression of FasL (Fas–Fas ligand) and TNF-α.

In the broadest sense, autoimmunity develops because of a breakdown in regulatory checkpoints that occurs during development or maturation of the immune system. Although the precise events that trigger the loss of self-tolerance to platelet GPs are largely unknown, patients with ITP have been shown to exhibit several immune alterations to platelet antigens including dysfunctional cellular immunity because of T-helper (Th)0/Th1 polarization, decreased regulatory T-cell function, and autoreactive platelet-specific cytotoxic T cells. In addition, ITP patients may have increased circulating levels of cytokines and soluble factors that promote the survival of self-reactive T and B cells, including B-cell activating factor, a proliferation-inducing ligand, and B-cell lymphoma-2 interacting mediator of cell death. Reduced levels of proapoptotic cytokines that regulate self-reactive T-cells, including Fas, interferon-γ, interleukin-2 receptor β (IL2RB), Bax, and caspases 8 and A20, have also been demonstrated.

Primary and Secondary Immune Thrombocytopenia

Primary ITP, which was previously known as *idiopathic* but is now referred to as *immune thrombocytopenia* (Table 131.2) occurs for unknown reasons. Secondary ITP is important to recognize because treatment of the underlying cause is often necessary to increase the platelet count. Examples are ITP occurring in the setting of infection, pregnancy, drugs, or lymphoproliferative disease.

Infection may stimulate the formation of platelet reactive autoantibodies. Cross-reactive antibodies (molecular mimicry) have been described in *Helicobacter pylori*, human immunodeficiency virus (HIV), and hepatitis C virus (HCV) infections. Molecular mimicry between the highly antigenic *H. pylori* CagA protein and platelet antigens is the suspected mechanism of *H. pylori*–associated ITP. In most patients, *H. pylori* can be successfully eradicated with a 1–2 week course of clarithromycin (500 mg twice daily), amoxicillin (1000 mg twice daily), and a proton pump inhibitor (e.g., pantoprazole 40 mg twice daily); however, the effect of *H. pylori* eradication on the platelet count is variable. In a metaanalysis that included 788 patients, *H. pylori* eradication resulted in platelet counts that were 34 × 10⁹/L higher than those in untreated control participants and 52 × 10⁹/L higher than those in treated patients whose *H. pylori* was not eradicated. Another systematic review evaluating 696 patients reported that 42.7% of treated patients achieved platelet counts above 100 × 10⁹/L; however, the effect was highly dependent on geographic location with the beneficial effect mainly observed in patients from Japan. Evidence-based guidelines for the investigation and management of ITP recommend against routine screening for *H. pylori* in patients presenting with ITP because of the low yield of testing and the low likelihood of a platelet count increase with *H. pylori*

TABLE 131.2	Standardized Terminology and Definitions for Immune Thrombocytopenia Proposed by the International Working Group (Vicenza Consensus Conference) in 2009

Terminology	Definition
ITP	Immune thrombocytopenia (rather than idiopathic or immune thrombocytopenic purpura)
Platelet threshold for ITP diagnosis	$<100 \times 10^9$/L
Primary ITP	ITP with no associated cause (diagnosis of exclusion)
Secondary ITP	ITP in the setting of an underlying cause such as drugs, HIV, or SLE
Newly diagnosed ITP	Designation for patients at diagnosis (rather than "acute" ITP).
Persistent ITP	Sustained or recurrent thrombocytopenia lasting 3–12 months
Chronic ITP	Thrombocytopenia lasting >12 months
Complete response	Achievement of a platelet count of $\geq 100 \times 10^9$/L in the absence of bleeding
Response	Achievement of a platelet count of $\geq 30 \times 10^9$/L and at least a twofold increase from baseline in the absence of bleeding
Refractory ITP	Failure to achieve a response or relapse after splenectomy[a] and requirement for treatment(s) to minimize the risk of clinically significant bleeding

[a]Splenectomy failure may not be applicable in children.
HIV, Human immunodeficiency virus; ITP, immune thrombocytopenia; SLE, systemic lupus erythematosus.

eradication. Testing may be warranted in countries where *H. pylori* infection is endemic, particularly those where the response rates to eradiation therapy are high.

ITP also may present for the first time or relapse in pregnancy. Although mild ITP may be difficult to differentiate from incidental thrombocytopenia of pregnancy, pregnancy-related vascular disorders must be excluded.[6] Incidental thrombocytopenia of pregnancy (also called *gestational thrombocytopenia*) represents a physiologic change in platelet count. Pregnancy-related vascular disorders include pre-eclampsia, microangiopathy caused by HELLP syndrome (characterized by hemolysis, elevated liver enzymes, and a low platelet count), and acute fatty liver. Platelet counts tend to be mildly reduced and hypertension is common.

Pregnancy-associated ITP may present early in pregnancy and thrombocytopenia can be severe. Typically, platelet counts increase after ITP-specific therapies such as IVIg or corticosteroids. In contrast, incidental thrombocytopenia of pregnancy, which occurs late in pregnancy, is associated with a mild reduction in platelet count and does not respond to immune-modulating therapy. Platelet count thresholds for instituting treatment are the same as those for women with ITP who are not pregnant. In the absence of bleeding, treatment should be considered when the platelet count decreases to less than 20×10^9/L. Vaginal deliveries are thought to be safe for mothers with ITP, even if the platelet count is very low, and most clinicians try to maintain the count above $20–30 \times 10^9$/L. Epidural anesthesia is not recommended with platelet counts below $70–80 \times 10^9$/L; however, this practice is operator driven and based on little evidence. IVIg and corticosteroids are generally safe in pregnancy, but corticosteroids can be associated with hypertension, gestational diabetes, intrauterine growth restriction, and other pregnancy-associated morbidities. Splenectomy is rarely performed during pregnancy because most

women can successfully be managed with less aggressive treatments. Immunosuppressant medications, such as azathioprine, have been used in pregnancy but should be reserved for refractory pregnancy-associated ITP with bleeding. There is a risk of severe thrombocytopenia in the newborn because of passive transfer of maternal antiplatelet autoantibodies. This can occur in 10% of newborns.

Clinical and Laboratory Features

Thrombocytopenia

Thrombocytopenia is the defining feature of ITP. The international working group on standardization of terminology in ITP established a platelet count below 100×10^9/L as the cutoff for the diagnosis (see Table 131.2).[3] The rationale behind this threshold was that patients with mild thrombocytopenia ($100–150 \times 10^9$/L) have a low risk (approximately 7%) of developing persistent thrombocytopenia (platelets less than 100×10^9/L); platelet counts slightly below 150 $\times 10^9$/L may be normal for certain ethnic groups; and mild thrombocytopenia may be caused by physiologic processes, such as pregnancy. Nonetheless, primary ITP remains a diagnosis of exclusion, and as such, investigations are directed towards ruling out nonimmune causes, including pseudothrombocytopenia, myelodysplastic syndromes, thrombotic microangiopathies, splenomegaly, or hereditary thrombocytopenia; and secondary immune causes such as infection, concomitant autoimmune disease, or lymphoproliferative disorders.

Clinical Outcomes: Mortality, Bleeding and Quality of Life

Patients with ITP most commonly present with asymptomatic thrombocytopenia. Although some patients bleed with platelet counts less than 30×10^9/L, many do not. Bleeding symptoms characteristic of ITP ("platelet-type bleeding") include skin bleeding (i.e., bruises, nonpalpable purpura, or petechiae), oral hemorrhagic blood blisters or oral petechiae, epistaxis, menorrhagia, or gastrointestinal bleeding. The most severe complication is intracerebral hemorrhage (ICH).

In a systematic review of prospective studies, the incidence of ICH was 1.4% for adults (95% confidence interval [CI], 0.9–2.1) and 0.4% for children (95% CI, 0.2–0.7).[7] The proportion of patients with severe (non-ICH) bleeding was 9.6% for adults (95% CI, 4.1–17.1) and 20.2% for children (95% CI, 10.0–32.9). Risk factors for severe bleeding include severe thrombocytopenia, previous bleeding, and older age.

Chronic ITP has been associated with a risk of death that is up to four times higher than that in the general population. ITP patients are more likely to die of bleeding, infection, and hematologic malignancies. Some deaths are attributable to adverse effects of treatment rather than the disease. Quality of life is affected, at least in part, because of the prevalence of fatigue that appears to be independent of platelet count levels.

Investigations of Patients With Suspected Immune Thrombocytopenia

Patients presenting with newly identified thrombocytopenia require a careful history and physical examination to uncover the underlying cause of the thrombocytopenia and to assess the risk of bleeding. A complete blood count and review of the blood film is required (Fig. 131.1). HIV and HCV testing should be performed in any patient suspected of having ITP. There are insufficient data to support routine screening for antinuclear antibodies or antiphospholipid antibodies unless other signs and symptoms of systemic lupus erythematosus or antiphospholipid syndrome are present. BM aspiration and biopsy should be reserved for patients with abnormalities affecting other cell

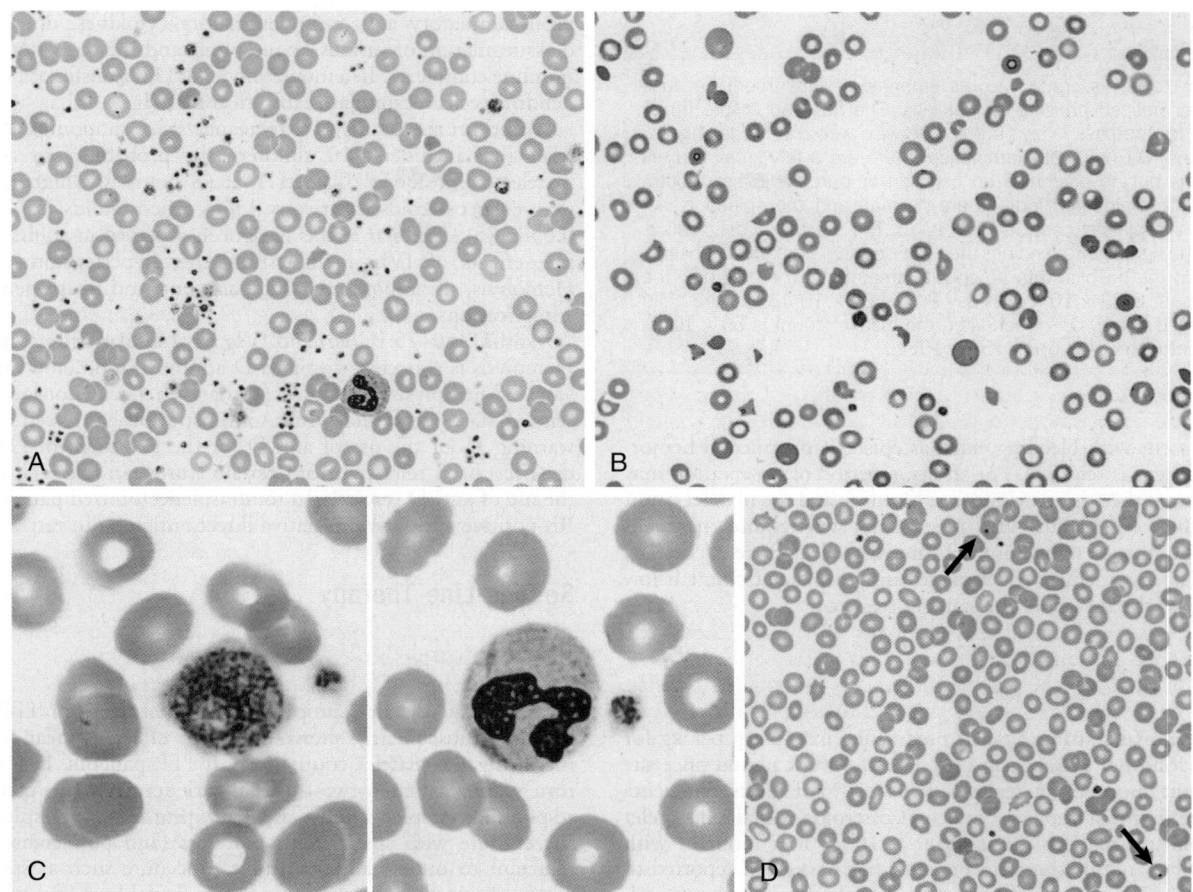

Fig. 131.1 BLOOD FILM EXAMINATIONS FROM PATIENTS WITH THROMBOCYTOPENIA. (A) Pseudothrombocytopenia showing marked platelet clumping. (B) Schistocytes (fragmented red blood cells) and reticulocytosis in a patient with thrombotic thrombocytopenic purpura. (C) Macrothrombocyte *(left panel)* and neutrophil-containing cytoplasmic inclusions (Döhle bodies, *right panel*) in a patient with May-Hegglin anomaly. (D) A patient with immune thrombocytopenia with low platelets and postsplenectomy Howell-Jolly bodies *(arrows)*.

lines such as anemia, leukopenia, or macrocytosis. Most patients with typical ITP do not require BM examination. Quantitative Ig levels may be useful in children to exclude common variable immune deficiency and thyroid testing can uncover subclinical hypothyroidism if surgery is planned.

First-Line Therapy

Corticosteroids with or without IVIg are first-line treatments for patients with newly diagnosed ITP. Second-line therapies include rituximab, splenectomy, TPO receptor agonists, or immunosuppressant medications. ASH guidelines for the management of ITP were developed using GRADE methodology to assess the level of evidence associated with each recommendation.[4] Aligned with these guidelines, the authors recommend a treatment approach starting with those that are least toxic (Fig. 131.2).

Observation

One of the ASH 2014 Choosing Wisely recommendations is that patients with ITP should not be treated unless they are bleeding or have very low platelet counts.[8] Most patients with platelet counts above 30 x 10⁹/L and no bleeding can be managed safely with observation alone. This is especially true for children with ITP who are at low risk of serious bleeding. Furthermore, in up to 80% of cases, childhood ITP resolves within 6 months with no treatment. If

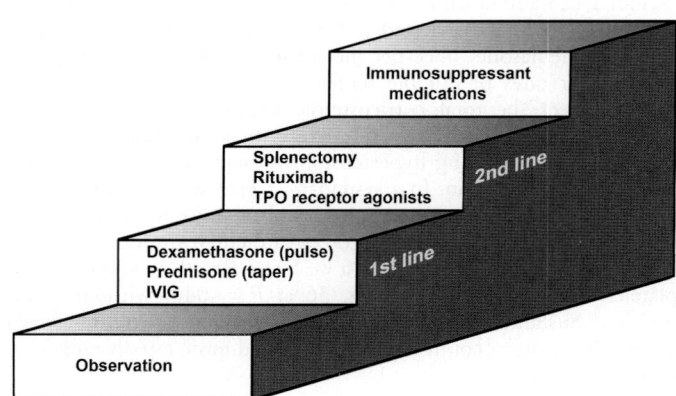

Fig. 131.2 STAIRCASE MODEL OF IMMUNE THROMBOCYTOPENIA TREATMENT. Therapies build on each other, often cumulatively, in a stepwise fashion starting from the least toxic. After a period of observation, corticosteroid-based treatment is the accepted first-line therapy. Splenectomy, rituximab, and thrombopoietin receptor agonists may be reasonable second-line therapies. Rituximab is not currently licensed for immune thrombocytopenia. Thrombopoietin (TPO) receptor agonists are indicated for immune thrombocytopenia (IVIg) patients who have failed to respond to other therapies, including splenectomy. *(Modified with permission from Arnold DM, Kelton JG: Current options for the treatment of idiopathic thrombocytopenic purpura. Semin Hematol 44:S12, 2007.)*

patients present with bleeding, such as epistaxis or mucosal hemorrhage, treatment is required. For adults, a period of observation may be reasonable if there is no evidence of bleeding and the platelet count is above 20×10^9/L; however, most adults will require treatment because spontaneous remissions are rare. To reflect current practice, the ASH 2011 guidelines recommend using a platelet count below 30×10^9/L as the threshold for starting treatment.

Corticosteroids

The conventional starting dose of prednisone is 1–2 mg per kg for 2–4 weeks followed by tapering over a several week period once the platelet count improves. In general, 60% to 70% of adults with acute ITP achieve an initial response with corticosteroids. Sustained platelet count responses (platelet count >100×10^9/L at 6 months) with corticosteroids are infrequent in practice, but have been reported to be as high as 47% in some studies. The risk of relapse increases with longer duration of follow up. Low-dose prednisone (0.5 mg/kg per day followed by a taper) may be as effective as the conventional dose for initial ITP treatment, but long-term remissions are rare. The optimal duration of prednisone treatment and the optimal tapering schedule have yet to be established.

High-dose dexamethasone, typically administered at a dose of 40 mg/day for 4 consecutive days, is also effective. In one study that included 125 adults with ITP, approximately 40% of patients had a sustained response that lasted 2–5 years.[9] Repeated cycles of high-dose dexamethasone (once per month for 6 months) may result in even higher rates of durable remissions, although this effect may simply reflect the total corticosteroid exposure. High-dose dexamethasone is associated with side effects that may limit the use of this treatment including hypertension, muscle weakness, insomnia, and impaired cognition. In a systematic review of randomized trials comparing high dose dexamethasone and prednisone in adults with previously untreated ITP ($n = 533$), treatment with dexamethasone resulted in improved overall (79% vs. 59%; $P = .048$) and complete platelet count response (64% vs. 36%; $P = .040$) without excess toxicity.[9a] Sustained responses at 6 months were not different between groups, but platelet count responses occurred more rapidly with high dose dexamethasone.

Intravenous Immunoglobulin and Anti-D

The predominant mechanism of action of high-dose IVIg and anti-D is thought to be via RES blockade. Individuals with low plasma IgG levels exhibit more rapid clearance of sensitized red blood cells (RBCs) (indicating enhanced RES capacity) than those with high levels of plasma IgG, such as those achieved with high-dose IVIg. A competitive model of RES clearance would also explain why anti-D administration to Rhesus (Rh)-positive individuals is effective in improving platelet counts in patients with ITP. Thus IgG-sensitized RBCs compete for Fc receptor occupancy. Other potential mechanisms of action of IVIg or anti-D include antiidiotypic antibodies, stimulation of

proinflammatory and antiinflammatory cytokines, upregulation or downregulation of various Fc receptors, and the induction of soluble immune complexes. In a mouse model of ITP, transfer of IVIg-primed dendritic cells recapitulated the effect of IVIg.

Based on the results of a metaanalysis of randomized controlled trials that included 410 children, the probability of achieving a platelet count above 20×10^9/L at 48 hours was higher with IVIg than corticosteroids (relative risk for corticosteroids, 0.74; 95% CI, 0.65–0.85).[10] Similar results have been observed in adults. Common side effects of IVIg include headache, hypertension, and chills. Hemolysis, thrombosis, renal impairment, and neutropenia are rare complications.

Anti-D (50–75 IU/kg) and IVIg have similar efficacy in children. Hemolysis is expected with anti-D administration, and rarely, intravascular hemolysis can be severe or even fatal. Consequently, the United States Food and Drug Administration has issued a black box warning about the use of anti-D for the treatment of ITP, and the drug has been removed from certain European markets. In general, the use of anti-D is restricted to nonsplenectomized patients who are Rh-positive and have a negative direct antiglobulin test.

Second-Line Therapy

Splenectomy

Splenectomy was first proposed as a treatment for ITP in 1913 and was subsequently shown to be an effective means of rapidly increasing the platelet count in most ITP patients. In a systematic review, approximately two-thirds of patients achieved a platelet count response after splenectomy, usually within days.[11] Despite the high success rate with splenectomy, patients (and physicians) are often reluctant to undertake an invasive procedure such as splenectomy, when pharmacologic alternatives are available. Only younger age has been identified as a predictor of splenectomy success, although some investigators have found a correlation between prior response to IVIg and a splenic pattern on radiolabeled platelet sequestration studies.

With currently available minimally invasive surgical techniques, complications after splenectomy are uncommon. The overall mortality rate is approximately 1% with open surgery and about 0.2% after laparoscopic splenectomy. The most frequent perioperative complications include pneumonia, subphrenic abscess or pleural effusion (4%), major bleeding (1.5%), and thromboembolism (1%). With laparoscopic techniques, patients have less postoperative pain, shorter hospital stays, and fewer wound complications.

Because the spleen is involved in clearance of encapsulated bacteria, asplenic individuals are at risk for infection with *Streptococcus pneumoniae, Neisseria meningitides,* and *Haemophilus influenzae* type b. Therefore all patients undergoing splenectomy should receive vaccinations against these bacteria at least 2 weeks before surgery. Poor compliance and vaccine failures contribute to the ongoing risk of serious postsplenectomy infections. The lifetime risk of overwhelming postsplenectomy infection is estimated to be 1% to 3% with the risk being higher in children younger than 15 years of age and in patients with hematologic malignancies. Although the risk of an infection requiring hospitalization was highest in the first 90 days after splenectomy in a cohort of 3812 splenectomized patients in Denmark, this risk remained 2.5 times higher than that in the general population even after 90 days.

The ITP International Working Group and the revised ASH guidelines consider splenectomy an acceptable second-line therapy for ITP. However, the former group considers splenectomy equal to other medical options, whereas the ASH guidelines favor splenectomy (grade 1B evidence) over rituximab or TPO receptor agonists (grade 2C evidence). Splenectomy leads to a high rate of durable remission. In a systematic review, 1731 (66%) of 2623 adults with ITP achieved a complete response following splenectomy at a median follow up of 28 months (range 1–153 months) and this response rate was maintained for 10 years or more after splenectomy.

Disadvantages of splenectomy include a lack of validated predictors of response, surgical risk with 30-day mortality, and complication rates of 0.2% and 9.6% for laparoscopic splenectomy, respectively, and 1.0% and 12.9% for open splenectomy, respectively, and an increased risk of postsplenectomy infection, and vascular thrombosis.

Rituximab

Rituximab has been widely used in patients with various autoimmune diseases, including ITP. Rituximab is an anti-CD20 monoclonal antibody that targets and destroys CD20$^+$ B lymphocytes, some of which are likely involved in autoantibody production. Data correlating cellular profiles with clinical outcomes suggest that the efficacy of rituximab reflects improvement in T-cell function and reversion of T-cell abnormalities; processes downstream to its direct effect on B-cell depletion. The effects of rituximab on platelets and autoantibodies require further investigations.

In a systematic review of 19 observational studies that enrolled 313 ITP patients of whom 46.2% were not splenectomized, rates of complete response (platelet count >150 × 10^9/L) and overall response (platelet count >50 × 10^9/L) with rituximab after a median follow up of 9.5 months were 43.6% (95% CI, 29.5–57.7) and 62.5% (95% CI, 52.6–72.5), respectively.[12] The typical rituximab regimen was 375 mg/m^2 administered by intravenous infusion once weekly for 4 consecutive weeks. The median time to response was 5.5 weeks, and responses lasted a median of 10.5 months. Other observational studies have reported lower rates of durable remission, ranging from 24% at 12 months to 35% at 57 months. A metaanalysis of five randomized trials demonstrated that complete platelet count response was more frequent with rituximab plus standard of care than with standard of care alone (relative risk 1.4, 95% CI, 1.1–1.8); however, there was limited evidence for sustained platelet count responses beyond 6–12 months.[13]

In a prospective observational study that included 60 nonsplenectomized adult patients with ITP who had a median of two prior therapies, 24 (40%) achieved a platelet count above 50 × 10^9/L and at least twice their baseline value at 1 year, and 20 (33%) maintained their platelet count response at 2 years with rituximab treatment. In a follow-up study of 72 adults and 66 children with chronic ITP who achieved an initial response to rituximab, 21% to 26% maintained a treatment-free response for at least 5 years.[14] Low-dose rituximab (100 mg per week for 4 weeks) has been shown to be effective in ITP, but the frequency of durable responses is uncertain.

Minor infusion-related side effects of rituximab occur in approximately 30% of patients with ITP and include hypotension, rash, sore throat, fever, and rigors. Severe or fatal infusion reactions are rare in patients treated for autoimmune diseases. Serum sickness, which is characterized by arthropathy, fever, and low serum complement levels, may be more common in children than in adults and often necessitates treatment interruption. Progressive multifocal leukoencephalopathy (PML) is a rapidly fatal neurologic syndrome caused by reactivation of latent JC virus in the brain. Rare reports have linked PML with rituximab treatment.

Rituximab also interferes with the response to polysaccharide vaccines. This is of potential concern in patients who may subsequently undergo splenectomy and supports the practice of administering immunizations before initiating rituximab therapy.

The 2011 ASH treatment guidelines gave rituximab a weak (grade 2C) recommendation for patients who have failed corticosteroids, IVIg, or splenectomy.

Thrombopoietin Receptor Agonists

Drugs aimed at increasing platelet production by stimulating the c-Mpl receptor have been investigated for the treatment of thrombocytopenia. Initial studies with pegylated recombinant human megakaryocyte growth and development factor were halted because of the development of cross-reactive antibodies against endogenous TPO, which led to severe and sustained thrombocytopenia in some healthy volunteers. These findings prompted the development of second-generation TPO receptor agonists that have no homology to endogenous TPO. Two such drugs are now approved for the treatment of patients with chronic ITP, romiplostim (Nplate, Amgen) and eltrombopag (Promacta/Revolade, GlaxoSmithKline). These agents increase the platelet count in most ITP patients including those with refractory disease. The effect on platelet count is generally sustained as long as the TPO receptor agonists are administered; when they are stopped, platelet counts tend to fall rapidly to baseline levels.

Romiplostim (administered as a once-weekly subcutaneous injection) is a synthetic peptibody consisting of four peptides linked to an IgG Fc fragment. The molecule binds the c-Mpl receptor at the same location as endogenous TPO and stimulates megakaryocyte proliferation and platelet production through intracellular JAK/STAT and mitogen-activated protein kinase signaling. In a phase III trial, a durable platelet count response (defined as the achievement of a platelet count of 50 × 10^9/L or higher for 6 or more of the last 8 weeks of treatment) was achieved in 41 of 83 patients (49.4%) receiving romiplostim compared with 1 of 42 (2.4%) patients receiving a placebo.[15] In a subsequent randomized trial that compared romiplostim plus standard of care with standard of care alone, romiplostim was associated with more platelet count responses, fewer treatment failures, fewer splenectomies, less bleeding, and better quality of life.[2] Weekly doses of romiplostim ranged between 1 and 10 µg/kg; however, most patients achieved a suitable response with a dose of 3 µg/kg. Weekly doses were titrated up or down to maintain the platelet count in the appropriate range (30–100 × 10^9/L).

Eltrombopag (administered as an oral daily tablet, 50–75 mg daily) is a small molecule, nonpeptide TPO receptor agonist. Eltrombopag also activates the c-Mpl receptor, but unlike romiplostim, eltrombopag binds to the transmembrane domain of the receptor and does not compete with circulating TPO for binding. In a phase III trial, eltrombopag was associated with an eightfold increase in platelet count response compared with placebo throughout the 6-month treatment period.[16] The time to response was 1–2 weeks (similar to romiplostim) and there was minimal need for dose titration. Durable responses were achieved in 57 of 95 patients (60%) receiving maintenance eltrombopag and in only 4 of 39 patients (10%) receiving placebo.

In a recent systematic review that summarized the data from randomized trials comparing TPO receptor agonists with standard of care in ITP patients, the authors concluded that although romiplostim and eltrombopag increased the platelet count response, neither agent significantly lowered the rate of severe, life-threatening, or fatal bleeding. These findings highlight the need for studies that evaluate patient focused outcomes.

TPO receptor agonists are generally well tolerated but have been associated with headache, fatigue, and insomnia. The development of BM reticulin in patients with ITP was an early concern; however, this problem was rarely encountered in prospective studies and the changes improved with discontinuation of the medication. TPO receptor agonists have also been associated with thromboembolic events (independent of platelet count), although the strength of this association remains uncertain. One study of eltrombopag in patients with advanced liver disease was ended early because of an increase in portal vein thrombosis. Eltrombopag has been associated with serum liver function test abnormalities in approximately 10% of patients. Treatment-related serious adverse events were infrequent even after prolonged exposure to romiplostim (n = 292) or eltrombopag (n = 299). Thromboembolic events occurred in 6.5% of patients on romiplostim and 4% of patients on eltrombopag.

Long-Term Follow-Up

The best treatment for patients with ITP who fail to respond to first-line therapy remains controversial and depends on the severity of symptoms, side effect profile, and patient preference. Splenectomy has been used for many years and is the treatment option most likely to be associated with durable remissions. Rituximab may achieve a platelet count response in up to 60% of patients, but responses are rarely sustained past 6–12 months. TPO receptor agonists (romiplostim or eltrombopag) are associated with a platelet count response in up to 60% of patients as long as treatment is maintained. These drugs are generally well tolerated; however, long-term safety data beyond 5 years are not yet available and long-term maintenance therapy is expensive since either agent costs approximately $3,000 per month.

Treatment of Refractory Immune Thrombocytopenia

As suggested by the International Working Group on standardization of terminology in ITP, the term *refractory ITP* is used to define patients who have failed splenectomy or relapsed thereafter and either exhibit severe thrombocytopenia or have a risk of bleeding that necessitates therapy (see Table 131.2).[3]

Evidence to help guide management of patients with chronic refractory ITP after splenectomy is limited, and treatment has been mainly unsatisfactory. However, TPO receptor agonists provide a new and effective option for this challenging group of patients. The overarching principle of therapy for this population is to prevent bleeding with the achievement of a stable, although not necessarily normal, platelet count, and that combination therapy may be more effective than single agent treatment for achievement of this goal.

In randomized trials, nonsplenectomized patients with ITP tended to show better platelet count responses to TPO receptor agonists than splenectomized patients; however, the difference was small, and response rates in splenectomized patients approached 50%. Although some patients included in the trials had failed up to five prior therapies, the results may not be applicable to all patients with refractory ITP seen in clinical practice.

Before the availability of TPO receptor agonists, a systematic review identified rituximab, azathioprine, and cyclophosphamide as the agents most often associated with complete responses in patients with refractory ITP. Good response rates have also been reported with a combination of cyclosporine, azathioprine, and mycophenolate (CellCept). Similarly, a combination of IVIg, intravenous methylprednisolone, vincristine, or intravenous anti-D followed by maintenance therapy with danazol and azathioprine have shown good response rates. Other treatment options include low-dose or alternate-day corticosteroids, repeated doses of IVIg, high-dose chemotherapy, or dapsone. High-dose chemotherapy followed by stem cell transplantation has also been used successfully in this population, but with the advent of TPO receptor agonists, transplantation is no longer used.

NEONATAL ALLOIMMUNE THROMBOCYTOPENIA

NAIT is an uncommon but serious thrombocytopenic disorder that can cause fetal or neonatal bleeding resulting in death or disability. It is important to recognize this disorder because treatment may prevent recurrence in subsequent pregnancies. With NAIT, intracranial bleeding can occur during the neonatal period or in utero, in which case the diagnosis is first suspected after abnormal fetal ultrasonography. The incidence of NAIT has been estimated to range from 1:1000–1:5000 births; however, it is often underdiagnosed.

Clinical Presentation

Thrombocytopenia may be severe in infants affected by NAIT and often the platelet count is less than $10–20 \times 10^9/L$ shortly after birth. The differential diagnosis is broad and includes septicemia, hypoxia, and birth trauma, among other factors (Table 131.3). Typically, NAIT presents as severe thrombocytopenia, possibly with associated bleeding, in an otherwise healthy neonate with no other explanation for the low platelet count. The thrombocytopenia often worsens hours or days after delivery, likely reflecting increased RES function in the newborn, particularly within the lungs. Without treatment,

TABLE 131.3	Differential Diagnosis of Thrombocytopenia in Newborns
Perinatal Hypoxemia	
Placental Insufficiency	
Congenital Infection	
Sepsis	
Toxoplasmosis	
Rubella	
Cytomegalovirus	
Autoimmune	
Maternal immune thrombocytopenia	
Maternal systemic lupus erythematosus	
Disseminated Intravascular Coagulation	
Maternal Drug Exposure	
Congenital Heart Disease	
Hereditary Thrombocytopenia	
MYH9 macrothrombocytopenia (including May-Hegglin anomaly)	
Thrombocytopenia absent radii syndrome	
Amegakaryocytic thrombocytopenia	
Wiskott-Aldrich syndrome	
Fanconi anemia	
Hemangioma with Thrombocytopenia	
Kasabach-Merritt syndrome	
Bone marrow Infiltration	
Congenital leukemia	

thrombocytopenia may last for days, but occasionally, it can be severe and can persist for many weeks. Bleeding symptoms range from petechiae and bruising to gastrointestinal or intracranial hemorrhage. Bleeding occurs in up to 20% of neonates with NAIT and can occur early in pregnancy. For infants with severe thrombocytopenia, mortality estimates of 10% have been reported and infants with intracranial bleeding may be left with developmental delays and permanent neurologic deficits.

Pathophysiology

Fetal and neonatal thrombocytopenia in NAIT reflects the clearance of IgG-sensitized fetal platelets by maternal alloantibodies directed against fetal/paternal platelet-specific antigens. The syndrome can be considered analogous to the destruction of fetal RBCs in hemolytic disease of the newborn (HDN) but with several differences. Perhaps most importantly, NAIT often presents in a first pregnancy, possibly because of early maternal sensitization to paternally derived antigens expressed on fetal platelets. In contrast, it is uncommon for HDN to occur in a first pregnancy without previous sensitization to the Rh antigen. This difference suggests that unlike RBCs, transplacental passage of fetal platelets or platelet antigens into the maternal circulation occurs early in pregnancy. Another difference is that pregnant women at risk for HDN (e.g., those who are Rh negative) can be identified early by screening and treatment with anti-Rh immune globulin reduces the risk of sensitization. To date, screening programs for NAIT have not been widely implemented because women at risk are not readily identifiable before sensitization has occurred, and therapies to prevent maternal alloimmunization are not currently available. Screening programs for NAIT continue to be an active area of research (see box on Neonatal Alloimmune Thrombocytopenia Versus Hemolytic Disease of the Newborn).

Laboratory Investigation of Suspected Neonatal Alloimmune Thrombocytopenia

The diagnosis of NAIT is established by documenting the presence of platelet-specific antigen incompatibility between mother and infant (or mother and father) and the presence of maternal antiplatelet alloantibodies directed against the incompatible antigen (Fig. 131.3).[17]

Diagnosis of Neonatal Alloimmune Thrombocytopenia (NAIT)
Testing for Human Platelet Antigens (HPA) and Antibodies

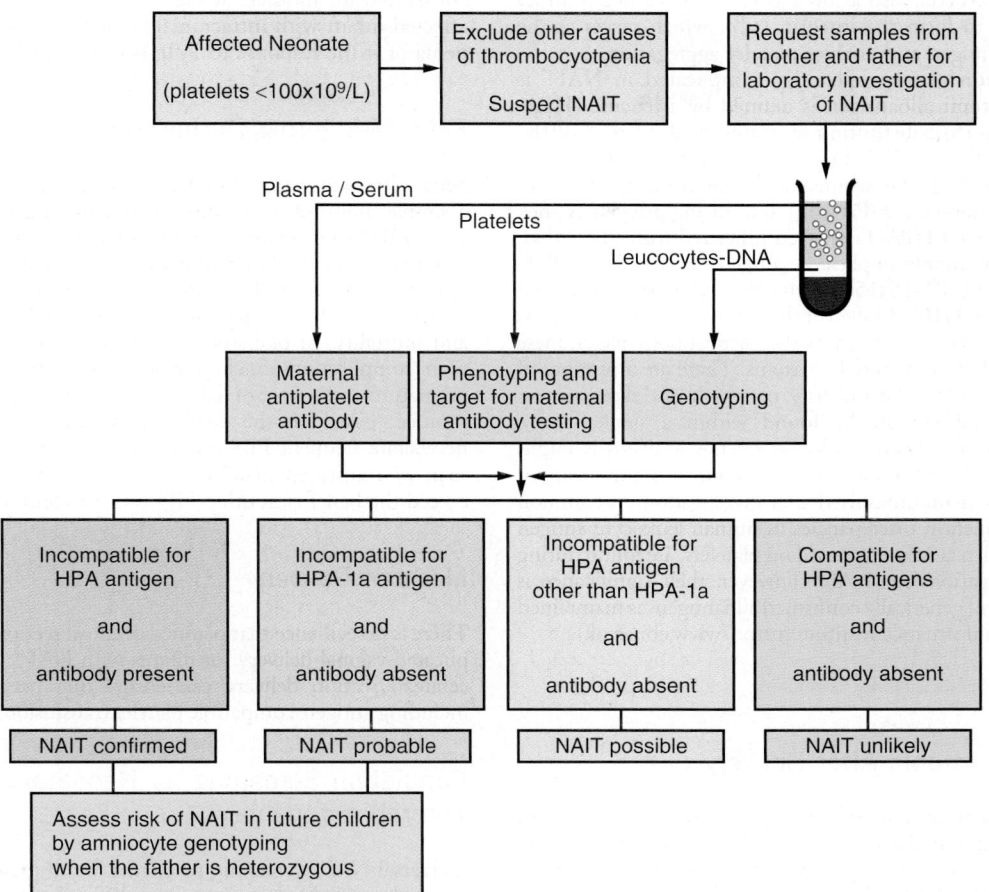

As currently practised at the McMaster University Platelet Immunology Reference Laboratory 2017

Fig. 131.3 DIAGNOSTIC TESTING ALGORITHM FOR INVESTIGATION OF NEONATAL ALLO-IMMUNE THROMBOCYTOPENIA AND MANAGEMENT RECOMMENDATIONS BASED ON RESULTS OF TESTING. This algorithm is currently used by the McMaster University Platelet Immunology Reference Laboratory, 2017. Maternal blood samples are tested for platelet antigens (phenotyping and polymerase chain reaction genotyping) and platelet alloantibodies. Amniocentesis and fetal genotyping are recommended when the father is known to be heterozygous for the incompatible antigen. *HPA*, Human platelet antigen; *NAIT*, neonatal alloimmune thrombocytopenia. *(Modified from Arnold DM, Smith JW, Kelton JG: Diagnosis and management of neonatal alloimmune thrombocytopenia. Transfus Med Rev 22:255, 2008, with permission.)*

Neonatal Alloimmune Thrombocytopenia Versus Hemolytic Disease of the Newborn

NAIT can be viewed as the platelet equivalent of HDN with some important differences: (1) maternal sensitization by fetal platelet antigens can occur early in the first trimester, (2) NAIT can affect first pregnancies, (3) women at risk for NAIT are not easily identifiable before sensitization and thus are not amenable to universal screening programs, and (4) a specific therapy that targets prevention of platelet antigen sensitization is lacking (e.g., Rh-immune globulin that target RBC antigen exposure).

Consequently, diagnosis requires allele-specific genotyping using polymerase chain reaction technology to identify a maternal–fetal (or maternal–paternal) antigenic mismatch. Serologic confirmation for the complete array of maternal alloantibodies is more difficult for two reasons. First, the technology is complex and relatively few laboratories perform these tests. In general, most commercial assays detect platelet alloantibodies directed against only a limited number of antigens. This limitation necessitates the use of more specific assays, such as monoclonal antibody immobilization of platelet antigen assays or antigen capture assays.[18] Even these tests are limited by the lack of monoclonal antibodies required to capture the different target proteins that express the alloantigens (e.g., human platelet antigen (HPA)-15 on CD109). An alternative method uses radioimmunoprecipitation, which can detect all of the known alloantibodies described to date. Second, for unknown reasons, up to 25% of HPA-1a–negative women with NAIT have no detectable antibodies using currently available laboratory methods. Recent studies have used surface plasmon resonance to identify alloantibodies in women suspected of having NAIT, but who tested negative in conventional immunoassays. Low affinity anti–HPA-1a antibodies were detected in some, suggesting that standard immunoassays may be limited in their capacity to detect such antibodies.[19] Low-incidence platelet-specific alloantigens expressed on platelets only from the paternal lineage may account for fetomaternal incompatibility. Detection of alloantibodies in these cases requires that maternal serum be tested against paternal platelets whenever possible.

Alloantibodies recognize epitopes on platelet GPs that are defined by genetic polymorphisms. To date, all of these antigens are the result of single nucleotide polymorphisms or in-frame deletions of the codon. Consequently, platelet typing using genetic analysis is relatively straightforward. The majority of platelet alloantigens occur on GPIIIa, which is the most abundant platelet GP (50,000–75,000 copies per platelet). GPIIIa, also known as β3, forms a heterodimer with platelet GPIIb to form the integrin $\alpha_2\beta_3$, which serves as the binding site for fibrinogen and enables platelet aggregation.

The most common platelet alloantigen implicated in NAIT is HPA-1a. This important alloantigen is defined by a leucine (HPA-1a) to proline (HPA-1b) substitution at amino acid 33 on GPIIIa. Maternal incompatibility to HPA-1a is implicated in more than 80% of women with NAIT. These women lack the common HPA-1a antigen (i.e., their genotype is HPA-1bb) and during pregnancy they are immunized with fetal HPA-1a antigen inherited from the father.

The next most commonly implicated antigens in NAIT are HPA-5a5b on GPIa/IIa and HPA-15a15b on the glycosylphosphatidylinositol–anchored protein, CD109. Only 6 of the 28 platelet antigen systems have been defined by maternal alloantibodies against both alleles; these include the HPA 1, 2, 3, 4, 5, and 15 systems. There are a number of other low-frequency alleles, the majority of which are expressed on platelet GPIIb/IIIa and are usually found within a single family. Although maternal immunization to low-frequency antigens is implicated in some cases of NAIT, these antigens account for a minority of the NAIT cases that remain unresolved after investigation for common HPA antigens.[20] Frequently, discrepancies in human leukocyte antigen (HLA) and ABO, which are also expressed on platelets, are found during the course of investigations for NAIT; however, their significance is uncertain. A database of genetically confirmed alloantigens is maintained by the European Bioinformatics Institute (http://www.ebi.ac.uk).

Management

Management of Infants After Delivery

When NAIT is suspected and depending on the platelet count, treatment should be initiated even before confirmatory test results are available. It is important to appreciate that moderate or severe thrombocytopenia at birth ($20–50 \times 10^9$/L) can worsen over the next few days. Treatment should be initiated immediately if thrombocytopenia is severe (platelets $<50 \times 10^9$/L); if there are petechiae or purpura; or if there is evidence of serious bleeding, such as intracranial bleeding on cranial ultrasonography. The initial treatment is platelet transfusion along with high-dose IVIg (1–2 g/kg).[21] Ideally, platelet products for transfusions should be alloantigen compatible; however, if these are unavailable, random donor platelets can be used because they often produce adequate increases in the platelet count.[22]

Antenatal Management of the Mother

Women with a previously affected infant with NAIT are at high risk of having another affected infant. Consequently, careful management in subsequent pregnancies is required. Similar to HDN, the disorder is often more severe in subsequent pregnancies than it is in the first. The exception is if the father is heterozygous for the implicated platelet antigen, in which case antigenic testing can be performed by amniocentesis to determine if the fetus is at risk and whether treatment is required.

Antenatal treatment options for at-risk mothers during subsequent pregnancies range from careful observation, to IVIg with or without corticosteroids, to fetal blood sampling (FBS) and intrauterine platelet transfusion. Invasive strategies that include FBS are associated with a high rate of complications, including fetal death and premature labor; thus a noninvasive approach is often recommended.

The mainstay of antenatal therapy for women with a previously affected infant is high-dose IVIg (1–2 g/kg) administered weekly throughout pregnancy starting at 18–22 weeks of gestation. A systematic review summarizing the results of four randomized trials that included 206 women compared weekly IVIg with a variety of other therapies, including alternate dosing of IVIg or IVIg plus corticosteroids.[23] Although no definitive conclusions could be drawn, most

clinicians use IVIg for antenatal treatment. Corticosteroids (prednisone or dexamethasone) given in combination with IVIg should be considered for mothers at high risk, such as those with a previously affected infant with intracranial hemorrhage or severe thrombocytopenia or if the response to IVIg is suboptimal.

Fetal Monitoring During Pregnancy

Serial ultrasonography is indicated for fetal surveillance. This provides a simple, noninvasive method for identifying fetal bleeds at an early stage. FBS by percutaneous cannulation of the umbilical or intrahepatic vein may be a way of capturing high-risk fetuses, identifying those who require treatment, and monitoring response to therapy. However, FBS is technically challenging and is associated with significant morbidity and mortality. In one study, 6% of FBS procedures were associated with complications, including fetal death from exsanguination and premature induction of labor.[24] Furthermore, a platelet transfusion protocol based on the detection of fetal thrombocytopenia would necessitate frequent FBS procedures because of the short (7-day) life span of transfused platelets. Because the risks associated with FBS exceed the benefits, routine FBS is not recommended.

Mode of Delivery

There is no evidence that planned cesarean section is safer than uncomplicated vaginal delivery for infants with NAIT. Nonetheless, planned cesarean section delivery can ensure that personnel and resources, including antigen-compatible platelet transfusions, are readily available.

Population Screening for Neonatal Alloimmune Thrombocytopenia

Universal NAIT screening programs for all pregnant women are not currently available because of the difficulty in early identification of at-risk women and the lack of specific and proven treatments. Screening algorithms also have to account for the large difference in numbers of women lacking an antigen and those who will later develop NAIT. About 2% of women will be identified as HPA-1bb, whereas only 1 in 20 of these will have an affected child because of HPA-1a immunization. One study screened 100,448 pregnant women and offered those with HPA-1a antibodies early cesarean section together with compatible platelet transfusions.[25] This approach identified 161 affected infants, of whom three (6%) died or had an intracranial bleed, compared with 10 of 51 infants (20%) born to mothers who were not screened. These results are encouraging, and additional studies of NAIT screening programs are ongoing.

POSTTRANSFUSION PURPURA

PTP is a rare thrombocytopenic syndrome that is provoked by an immune-mediated reaction against HPAs, most frequently HPA-1a. PTP presents 5–10 days following exposure to platelets or platelet antigenic material in blood transfusions with profound thrombocytopenia and clinically significant bleeding.

Epidemiology

PTP is rare with an estimated incidence of 1–2 per 100,000 transfusions. Data from the Serious Hazards of Transfusion surveillance program from the United Kingdom have shown that the incidence of PTP has decreased in the last decade (Fig. 131.4).[26] Reasons for this trend may be related to universal leukoreduction, which was implemented in the United Kingdom in 1999. The average annual incidences of PTP in the years preceding 1996–99 and following the implementation of universal leukoreduction between 2000 and 2005

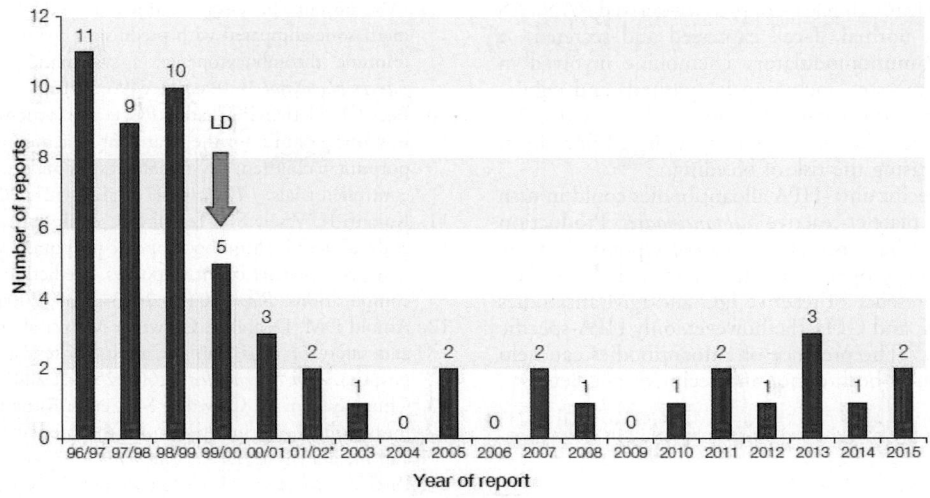

Fig. 131.4 CONFIRMED CASES OF POSTTRANSFUSION PURPURA REPORTED BY THE UK SERIOUS HAZARDS OF TRANSFUSION (SHOT) SURVEILLANCE PROGRAM. Universal leukoreduction began in the United Kingdom in late 1999 and coincided with a decrease in new cases of posttransfusion purpura. *(From www.shotuk.org.)*

Clinical Presentation of Posttransfusion Purpura

On postoperative day 8 after spinal surgery, a 43-year-old woman has a platelet count of 3 × 10⁹/L. During the operation, she received 3 units of non–leuko-reduced packed RBCs because of intraoperative bleeding. She is receiving intravenous ampicillin and prophylactic doses of the low-molecular-weight heparin dalteparin. On physical examination, she has extensive oral mucosal purpura and petechiae on both lower extremities. HIT testing results (anti-PF4/heparin enzyme-linked immunosorbent assay and serotonin release assay) are negative. The ampicillin is stopped, and she is treated with IVIG (2 g/kg) and platelet transfusions. Three days later, the platelet count is 4 × 10⁹/L, and the patient develops melena. The presumed diagnosis is posttransfusion purpura; therefore, HPA-1a–negative platelets and high-dose parenteral corticosteroids are administered, and daily plasma exchange is initiated. One week later, the thrombocytopenia and bleeding symptoms resolve. Platelet antibody testing reveals the presence of anti–HPA-1a antibodies.

---

were 10.3 and 2.3 cases per year, respectively. Since the implementation of universal leukoreduction, there has also been a shift from red cell concentrates to platelet concentrates as the inciting transfusion event, which may be attributable to the reduction in platelet contamination of red cell products with leukoreduction methods. A recent study estimated that the frequency of PTP corresponds to 1.8 per 100,000 transfusions.[27] In this study, platelet containing transfusions posed a significantly higher risk than RBC transfusions.

Approximately 85% of PTP episodes occur in women, the majority of whom had a history of pregnancy. In a report of 61 patients, the sensitizing event among women was pregnancy alone in 58%, pregnancy and/or transfusion in 34%, and transfusion alone in 7.5%. Males had associated transfusion histories in 55%, with some having no known exposure. PTP has not been reported in children.

Clinical Presentation

PTP presents with severe thrombocytopenia (platelets <10 x 10⁹/L) and bleeding, which may include petechiae, purpura, mucosal hemorrhage, hematuria, and rarely ICH. The thrombocytopenia is often refractory to platelet transfusions even with antigen-negative platelets. Mortality because of severe thrombocytopenia and bleeding has been estimated to be 5% to 20%. The thrombocytopenia occurs 5–10 days after blood transfusion and typically resolves within weeks, but occasionally can be prolonged and severe and can persist for months. Other causes of

thrombocytopenia with similar clinical presentation include primary ITP, drug-induced ITP, sepsis, disseminated intravascular coagulation, and thrombotic thrombocytopenic purpura; however, association with transfusion and bleeding severity suggest a diagnosis of PTP. Patients with PTP may present with features that overlap with heparin-induced thrombocytopenia (HIT), and positive HIT testing in the context of anti–HPA antibodies has been reported; however, thrombocytopenia is typically less severe with HIT and bleeding is rare.

Diagnosis

Most patients with PTP lack the common HPA-1a platelet antigen and are homozygous for HPA-1b. These patients develop anti-HPA 1a antibodies from sensitizing events such as previous pregnancies or transfusions. Anti–HPA 1a antibodies may persist for many years in these patients. In addition, platelet antibodies with specificities other than HPA-1a may also be found.[28]

Pathophysiology

Platelets contain abundant amounts of GPIIb/IIIa; thus even small numbers of platelets or platelet microparticles contained within RBC concentrates can be immunogenic and can lead to the development of PTP. Genotypic analyses have shown that HLA-II alleles DRβ3*0101 and DQβ1*0201 are commonly associated with this disorder. This is similar to NAIT: the frequency of immunization depends on platelet alloantigen discrepancy plus the presence of certain immune response genes.

The most intriguing feature of PTP is that the patient's own antigen-compatible platelets are destroyed. Furthermore, platelet reactive antibodies can be eluted from both antigen-positive and antigen-negative platelets. Although the mechanism is still poorly understood, theories to explain this "innocent bystander" phenomenon include immune complex formation, passive antigen adsorption, and autoantibody formation. As discussed later, some of these mechanisms may be overlapping.

Immune complexes can form if the anti–HPA-1a antibodies bind soluble antigen. Alternatively, platelet alloantigens contained within the transfused blood product may be passively adsorbed onto autologous platelets, converting them from antigen negative to antigen positive and rendering them targets for immune destruction. Immune complexes may then bind to platelets through Fc-receptors causing platelet destruction. Anti–HPA-1a antibodies have been shown to induce platelet activation through release of platelet-derived RANTES (regulated on activation, normal, T-cell expressed and secreted), a proinflammatory and immunomodulatory chemokine involved in multiple immunologic processes, including Ig synthesis and regulation of Th1/Th2 cytokine homeostasis. In some patients with PTP, the alloantibodies have been shown to interfere with cell-fibrinogen interaction, thereby increasing the risk of bleeding.

The stimulation of specific anti–HPA alloantibodies could in turn initiate the formation of platelet-reactive *autoantibodies*. Production of pan-reactive antibodies has been shown to correspond with the period of greatest thrombocytopenia and serologic analyses of PTP cases demonstrated the presence of reactive IgG and IgM antibodies against GPIIb/IIIa, GPIX, and GPIa/IIa; however, only HPA-specific IgG antibodies persisted.[29] The presence of autoantibodies can help to explain the destruction of both donor and recipient platelets.

Management

Treatment of PTP should be initiated even before serologic test results for anti–HPA-antigens are available. The primary goal of treatment is to abbreviate the period of severe thrombocytopenia and minimize the risk of bleeding. Multiple treatments are often administered simultaneously or in rapid succession because of the desperate nature of the disorder when it is severe.

Patients with PTP require admission to hospital for close observation, supportive treatments, and rapid management of bleeding symptoms should they occur. Nonessential transfusions should be discontinued. The mainstay of therapy is high dose IVIg, which is followed by a platelet count increase after 3–4 days.[30] High-dose corticosteroids have also been tried as a means of inhibiting RES phagocytosis and reducing IgG synthesis. Patients with bleeding should be transfused with HPA-compatible platelets. While awaiting the results of antigen typing, HPA-1a–negative platelet transfusions can be administered to reduce further antibody production. Patients with PTP may be at increased risk of transfusion reactions such as fever, dyspnea, and allergic reactions. Plasma exchange should be considered in patients who do not respond to IVIg and corticosteroids.

REFERENCES

1. Bussel JB, Provan D, Shamsi T, et al: Effect of eltrombopag on platelet counts and bleeding during treatment of chronic idiopathic thrombocytopenic purpura: a randomised, double-blind, placebo-controlled trial. *Lancet* 373:641, 2009.
2. Kuter DJ, Rummel M, Boccia R, et al: Romiplostim or standard of care in patients with immune thrombocytopenia. *N Engl J Med* 363(20):1889–1899, 2010.
3. Rodeghiero F, Stasi R, Gernsheimer T, et al: Standardization of terminology, definitions and outcome criteria in immune thrombocytopenic purpura of adults and children: report from an international working group. *Blood* 113(11):2386–2393, 2009.
4. Neunert C, Lim W, Crowther M, et al: The American Society of Hematology 2011 evidence-based practice guideline for immune thrombocytopenia. *Blood* 117(16):4190–4207, 2011.
5. Harrington WJ, Minnich V, Hollingsworth JW, et al: Demonstration of a thrombocytopenic factor in the blood of patients with thrombocytopenic purpura. *J Lab Clin Med* 38(1):1–10, 1951.
6. Burrows RF, Kelton JG: Fetal thrombocytopenia and its relation to maternal thrombocytopenia. *N Engl J Med* 329(20):1463–1466, 1993.
7. Neunert C, Noroozi N, Norman G, et al: Severe bleeding events in adults and children with primary immune thrombocytopenia: a systematic review. *J Thromb Haemost* 13(3):457–464, 2015.
8. Hicks LK, Bering H, Carson KR, et al: Five hematologic tests and treatments to question. *Hematology Am Soc Hematol Educ Program* 2014(1):599–603, 2014.
9. Cheng Y, Wong RS, Soo YO, et al: Initial treatment of immune thrombocytopenic purpura with high-dose dexamethasone. *N Engl J Med* 349(9):831–836, 2003.
9a. Mithoowani S, Gregory-Miller K, Goy J, et al: High-dose dexamethasone compared with prednisone for previously untreated primary immune thrombocytopenia: a systematic review and meta-analysis. *Lancet Haematol* 3(10):e489–e496, 2016.
10. Beck CE, Nathan PC, Parkin PC, et al: Corticosteroids versus intravenous immune globulin for the treatment of acute immune thrombocytopenic purpura in children: a systematic review and meta-analysis of randomized controlled trials. *J Pediatr* 147(4):521–527, 2005.
11. Kojouri K, Vesely SK, Terrell DR, et al: Splenectomy for adult patients with idiopathic thrombocytopenic purpura: a systematic review to assess long-term platelet count responses, prediction of response, and surgical complications. *Blood* 104(9):2623–2634, 2004.
12. Arnold DM, Dentali F, Crowther MA, et al: Systematic review: efficacy and safety of rituximab for adults with idiopathic thrombocytopenic purpura. *Ann Intern Med* 146(1):25–33, 2007.
13. Chugh S, Lim W, Crowther MA, et al: Rituximab plus standard of care for treatment of primary immune thrombocytopenia: a systematic review and meta-analysis. *Lancet Haematol* 2:e75–e81, 2015.
14. Patel VL, Mahevas M, Lee SY, et al: Outcomes 5 years after response to rituximab therapy in children and adults with immune thrombocytopenia. *Blood* 119(25):5989–5995, 2012.
15. Kuter DJ, Bussel JB, Lyons RM, et al: Efficacy of romiplostim in patients with chronic immune thrombocytopenic purpura: a double-blind randomised controlled trial. *Lancet* 371(9610):395–403, 2008.
16. Cheng G, Saleh MN, Marcher C, et al: Eltrombopag for management of chronic immune thrombocytopenia (RAISE): a 6-month, randomised, phase 3 study. *Lancet* 377(9763):393–402, 2011.
17. Arnold DM, Smith JW, Kelton JG: Diagnosis and management of neonatal alloimmune thrombocytopenia. *Transfus Med Rev* 22(4):255–267, 2008.
18. Warner MN, Moore JC, Warkentin TE, et al: A prospective study of protein-specific assays used to investigate idiopathic thrombocytopenic purpura. *Br J Haematol* 104(3):442–447, 1999.
19. Bakchoul T, Bertrand G, Krautwurst A, et al: The implementation of surface plasmon resonance technique in monitoring pregnancies with expected fetal and neonatal alloimmune thrombocytopenia. *Transfusion* 53(9):2078–2085, 2013.
20. Ghevaert C, Rankin A, Huiskes E, et al: Alloantibodies against low-frequency human platelet antigens do not account for a significant proportion of cases of fetomaternal alloimmune thrombocytopenia: evidence from 1054 cases. *Transfusion* 49(10):2084–2089, 2009.
21. Mueller-Eckhardt C, Kiefel V, Grubert A, et al: 348 cases of suspected neonatal alloimmune thrombocytopenia. *Lancet* 1(8634):363–366, 1989.
22. Kiefel V, Bassler D, Kroll H, et al: Antigen-positive platelet transfusion in neonatal alloimmune thrombocytopenia (NAIT). *Blood* 107(9):3761–3763, 2006.
23. Rayment R, Brunskill SJ, Soothill PW, et al: Antenatal interventions for fetomaternal alloimmune thrombocytopenia. *Cochrane Database Syst Rev* (5):CD004226, 2011.
24. Berkowitz RL, Kolb EA, McFarland JG, et al: Parallel randomized trials of risk-based therapy for fetal alloimmune thrombocytopenia. *Obstet Gynecol* 107(1):91–96, 2006.
25. Kjeldsen-Kragh J, Killie MK, Tomter G, et al: A screening and intervention program aimed to reduce mortality and serious morbidity associated with severe neonatal alloimmune thrombocytopenia. *Blood* 110(3):833–839, 2007.
26. Williamson LM, Stainsby D, Jones H, et al: The impact of universal leukodepletion of the blood supply on hemovigilance reports of post-transfusion purpura and transfusion-associated graft-versus-host disease. *Transfusion* 47(8):1455–1467, 2007.
27. Menis M, Forshee RA, Anderson SA, et al: Posttransfusion purpura occurrence and potential risk factors among the inpatient US elderly, as recorded in large Medicare databases during 2011 through 2012. *Transfusion* 55(2):284–295, 2015.
28. Woelke C, Eichler P, Washington G, et al: Post-transfusion purpura in a patient with HPA-1a and GPIa/IIa antibodies. *Transfus Med* 16(1):69–72, 2006.
29. Taaning E, Tonnesen F: Pan-reactive platelet antibodies in post-transfusion purpura. *Vox Sang* 76(2):120–123, 1999.
30. Mueller-Eckhardt C, Kiefel V: High-dose IgG for post-transfusion purpura-revisited. *Blut* 57(4):163–167, 1988.

THROMBOCYTOPENIA CAUSED BY PLATELET DESTRUCTION, HYPERSPLENISM, OR HEMODILUTION

Theodore E. Warkentin

Thrombocytopenia is defined as a platelet count below the lower limit of the normal range ($\approx 150 \times 10^9$/L). Sometimes an expanded definition of thrombocytopenia is appropriate. For example, an abrupt drop in the platelet count can signify the onset of a platelet-destructive process such as heparin-induced thrombocytopenia (HIT) or bacteremia even if the platelet count remains above 150×10^9/L. This is especially relevant in the second or third week after surgery because patients usually have platelet counts that peak at levels 2–3 times greater than their usual preoperative value (postoperative thrombocytosis).

In the clinical evaluation of a patient with thrombocytopenia, three questions must be asked. First, could the patient have pseudothrombocytopenia? Second, what is the most likely explanation for the thrombocytopenia? And third, what are the risks posed by the causative disorder and the severity of the thrombocytopenia? For example, severe thrombocytopenia caused by drug-dependent antibodies or platelet-reactive autoantibodies is often associated with bleeding. By contrast, thrombocytopenia caused by HIT antibodies or attributable to disseminated intravascular coagulation (DIC) secondary to adenocarcinoma is associated with thrombosis. Often, the underlying cause of the thrombocytopenia (e.g., bacteremia, cancer, cirrhosis), rather than the thrombocytopenia itself, poses the greater risk.

Thrombocytopenia can be caused by any of four general mechanisms: (1) platelet underproduction, (2) increased platelet destruction or consumption, (3) platelet sequestration, and (4) hemodilution. Platelet underproduction usually occurs in association with underproduction of other blood cell lines, which results in bicytopenia or pancytopenia. Thrombocytopenia caused by increased platelet destruction develops when the rate of platelet loss surpasses the ability of the bone marrow (BM) to produce platelets and may be caused by immune or nonimmune mechanisms (Table 132.1). Thrombocytopenia from platelet sequestration is caused by redistribution of platelets from the circulation into an enlarged splenic vascular bed. Hemodilution is characterized by a decrease in the number of platelets, as well as red blood cells (RBCs) and white blood cells (WBCs) as a result of the administration of colloid, crystalloid, or platelet-poor blood products.

In the postoperative period, platelet count changes reflect several processes, including initial hemodilution (immediate platelet count decrease) and increased platelet consumption (first 2–4 days), at which point the platelet count begins to rise because of increased platelet production; when the platelet count reaches its postoperative peak—usually about 14 days after surgery—platelet production decreases somewhat, and the platelet count returns to baseline (Fig. 132.1).[1] In addition to usual mechanisms, the differential diagnosis of thrombocytopenia in pregnancy includes some unique causes (Table 132.2).

APPROACH TO PATIENTS WITH THROMBOCYTOPENIA

History and Physical Examination

Certain information should be ascertained, including (1) the location and severity of bleeding (if any); (2) the temporal profile of the hemostatic defect (acute, chronic, or relapsing), particularly the temporal relationship with potential proximate triggers (e.g., new drug, recent infection); (3) the presence of symptoms of a secondary illness, such as a neoplasm, infection, or an autoimmune disorder such as systemic lupus erythematosus (SLE); (4) history of recent medication use, alcohol ingestion, or transfusion; (5) presence of risk factors for certain infections, particularly human immunodeficiency virus (HIV) infection or viral hepatitis; and (6) family history of thrombocytopenia.

As part of the physical examination, evidence of hemostatic impairment should be sought, as well as secondary causes of thrombocytopenia. The signs of platelet-related bleeding include petechiae and purpura. Petechiae typically occur in the dependent regions of the body or on traumatized areas. Spontaneous mucous membrane bleeding (wet purpura), epistaxis, and gastrointestinal bleeding indicate a more serious hemostatic defect. Although petechiae are common in patients whose platelet counts are less than $10–20 \times 10^9$/L, most patients with platelet counts over 50×10^9/L have no signs of hemostatic impairment. The physical examination may provide an explanation for the thrombocytopenia. For example, enlarged lymph nodes may indicate a viral infection, such as infectious mononucleosis or HIV infection, or a neoplastic process. An enlarged spleen raises the possibility of hypersplenism.

Timing of Onset and Severity of Thrombocytopenia

Many thrombocytopenic disorders, particularly those involving an immune pathogenesis, exhibit characteristic temporal features that can aid in the diagnosis. For example, if the platelet count begins to fall 5–10 days (median, 6–7 days) after starting a new drug or after a blood transfusion and reaches a nadir of less than 20×10^9/L a few days later, the diagnosis of drug-induced immune thrombocytopenia (D-ITP) or posttransfusion purpura (PTP), respectively, should be considered (Fig. 132.2).[2] Patients with these disorders typically have mucocutaneous bleeding and are at risk for fatal intracranial hemorrhage.

A similar temporal profile is also characteristic of typical-onset HIT, although there the platelet count only falls below 20×10^9/L in only 10% of affected patients (see Fig. 132.2); in approximately 80% of patients, the platelet count nadir ranges from $20–150 \times 10^9$/L, and in the remainder, the platelet count nadir never falls below 150×10^9/L despite a large reduction in the platelet count. When the platelet count falls abruptly after drug administration, the possibility of rapid-onset thrombocytopenia caused by preexisting drug-dependent antibodies should be considered, as is well described with HIT. Indeed, so-called rapid-onset HIT is the presenting feature of this adverse drug reaction in 25% to 30% of cases.[3] Rapid-onset thrombocytopenia is also a feature of glycoprotein (GP) IIb/IIIa antagonist-induced ITP.

Occasionally, thrombocytopenia worsens in the first few days after surgery; this can occur with multiorgan system failure (e.g., cardiogenic or septic shock) (see Fig. 132.2). If the patient develops concomitant DIC and hypotension, there is high risk for ischemic limb injury secondary to microvascular thrombosis ("symmetric peripheral gangrene"), especially if the patient has "shock liver" (ischemic hepatitis), which is a risk factor for severe depletion of protein C, an important endogenous anticoagulant.[4,5] If the platelet count falls to very low levels and is accompanied by microangiopathic hemolysis,

TABLE 132.1	Mechanisms of Platelet Destruction or Consumption	
Type of Thrombocytopenia		**Specific Example(s)**
Immune Mediated		
Autoantibody-mediated platelet destruction by RES		Primary and secondary idiopathic (immune) ITP[a]
Alloantibody-mediated platelet destruction by RES		NAIT,[a] PTP,[a] PAT; alloimmune platelet transfusion refractoriness[a]
Drug-dependent, antibody-mediated platelet destruction by RES		Drug-induced immune ITP (e.g., vancomycin) (see Fig. 132.5)
Platelet activation by binding of IgG Fc of drug-dependent IgG to platelet FcγIIa receptors		HIT
Non–Immune Mediated		
Platelet activation by thrombin or proinflammatory cytokines		DIC[a]; septicemia or systemic inflammatory response syndromes
Platelet destruction via ingestion by macrophages (hemophagocytosis)		Infections, certain malignant lymphoproliferative disorders
Platelet destruction through platelet interactions with altered vWF[b]		TTP,[a] HUS[a]
Platelet losses on artificial surfaces		CPB,[a] use of intravascular catheters
Decreased platelet survival associated with cardiovascular diseases		Congenital and acquired heart disease, cardiomyopathy, PE

[a]See Chapter 131 for a discussion of thrombocytopenia in these disorders.
[b]Although platelet destruction is not directly caused by antibodies, immune mechanisms can explain altered vWF (e.g., autoimmune clearance of vWF-cleaving metalloprotease).
CPB, Cardiopulmonary bypass surgery; DIC, disseminated intravascular coagulation; HIT, heparin-induced thrombocytopenia; HUS, hemolytic uremic syndrome; IgG, immunoglobulin G; ITP, idiopathic (immune) thrombocytopenic purpura; NAIT, neonatal alloimmune thrombocytopenia; PAT, passive alloimmune thrombocytopenia; PE, pulmonary embolism; PTP, posttransfusion purpura; RES, reticuloendothelial system; TTP, thrombotic thrombocytopenic purpura; vWF, von Willebrand factor.

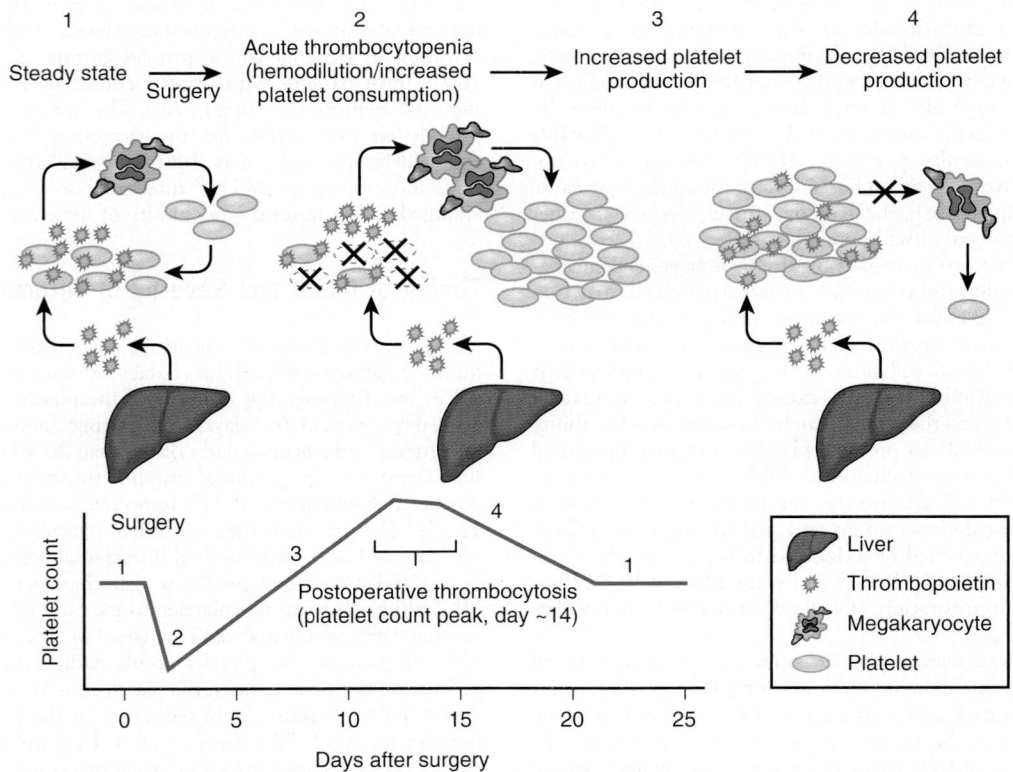

Fig. 132.1 POSTSURGERY PLATELET COUNT CHANGES. Initial platelet count declines result from hemodilution and increased platelet consumption, with the platelet count nadir occurring between days 1 to 4 (median, day 2). There is constitutive production of thrombopoietin (TPO) by the liver. TPO binds to platelets and megakaryocytes via a specific receptor (c-Mpl, not shown), and receptor-bound TPO is removed from circulation and degraded. The level of circulating TPO is thus inversely related to the mass of platelets and megakaryocytes. In early postsurgery thrombocytopenia, fewer TPO binding sites are available, resulting in high free TPO levels, which stimulates megakaryocyte proliferation and differentiation and leads to increased platelet production. With subsequent thrombocytosis, the high platelet mass acts as a "sink" for removing TPO, with decreased stimulus for platelet production. Thus after acute postsurgery thrombocytopenia, TPO levels rise about twofold, leading to increased platelet production that begins on days 2–4, with resulting thrombocytosis that generally peaks at approximately day 14 (postoperative thrombocytosis) and returns to baseline by about day 21. *(Reprinted, with modifications, with permission, from Arnold DM, Warkentin TE: Thrombocytopenia and thrombocytosis. In Wilson WC, Grande CM, Hoyt DB, editors: Trauma: Critical care, vol 2, New York, 2007, Informa Healthcare, p 983).*

the possibility of postoperative thrombotic thrombocytopenic purpura (TTP) should be considered.[6]

Mild to moderate platelet count decreases that occur soon after transfusion of blood products are common and can be explained by hemodilution; however, a marked platelet count fall after transfusion may be the result of passive alloimmune thrombocytopenia (PAT) or sepsis because of contaminated blood products (see Fig. 132.2).

Other characteristic temporal features of thrombocytopenia include postenterohemorrhagic *Escherichia coli*–associated hemolytic

uremic syndrome (HUS); thrombocytopenia and microangiopathic hemolysis that begin approximately 1 week after a prodromal diarrheal illness; and fungemia-associated thrombocytopenia (onset, 1–3 weeks after complex illness involving indwelling catheters and broad-spectrum antibiotic usage). In contrast, thrombocytopenia of insidious onset that progresses over several years suggests chronic liver disease, with evolution to portal hypertension and associated splenomegaly (e.g., cirrhosis secondary to alcohol or hepatitis C) or a slowly progressive BM disorder (e.g., myelodysplasia).

TABLE 132.2	Differential Diagnosis of Thrombocytopenia in Pregnancy

Incidental thrombocytopenia of pregnancy (gestational thrombocytopenia)
Preeclampsia or eclampsia[a]
DIC secondary to:
    Abruptio placentae
    Endometritis
    Amniotic fluid embolism
    Retained fetus
    Preeclampsia or eclampsia[a]
Peripartum or postpartum thrombotic microangiopathy
    TTP
    HUS

[a]Preeclampsia or eclampsia usually is not associated with overt DIC.
DIC, Disseminated intravascular coagulation; HUS, hemolytic uremic syndrome; TTP, thrombotic thrombocytopenic purpura.

Laboratory Evaluation

Laboratory evaluation of patients with thrombocytopenia is summarized in Table 132.3 (also see Chapter 129). The blood film is examined to exclude pseudothrombocytopenia, which is characterized by in vitro platelet clumping. This phenomenon, which is evident in approximately one in 1000 blood samples, is most often caused by naturally occurring GPIIb/IIIa ($\alpha_{IIb}\beta_3$)-reactive autoantibodies that induce aggregation of platelets in the presence of the calcium-chelating anticoagulant ethylenediamine tetraacetic acid (EDTA). Because the platelet aggregates are not counted by the electronic particle counter, the automated platelet count appears falsely low. The correct platelet count usually can be determined by collecting the blood into sodium citrate or heparin or by performing the count on nonanticoagulated finger prick samples; maintaining the blood sample at 37°C often attenuates platelet clumping. EDTA-dependent pseudothrombocytopenia has no pathologic significance other than potentially placing a patient in jeopardy for inappropriate

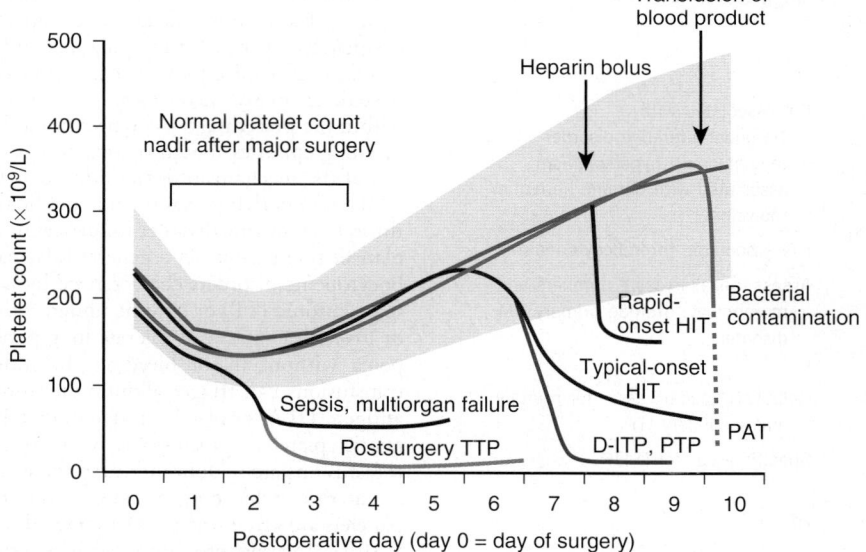

Fig. 132.2 TIMING OF ONSET AND SEVERITY OF THROMBOCYTOPENIA: IMPLICATIONS FOR DIFFERENTIAL DIAGNOSIS. The usual postoperative platelet count nadir is seen between postoperative days 1 to 3 (inclusive). Early and progressive platelet count declines often reflect severe postoperative complications such as sepsis and multiorgan failure; severe thrombocytopenia can (rarely) indicate postsurgery thrombotic thrombocytopenic purpura. Thrombocytopenic disorders that begin approximately 1 week after surgery are often immune mediated: moderate thrombocytopenia can indicate heparin-induced thrombocytopenia (HIT), both "typical onset" or (if heparin is not being given) "delayed onset"; very severe thrombocytopenia can indicate drug-induced immune thrombocytopenia (D-ITP) or (rarely) posttransfusion purpura. An abrupt decline in platelet count after receiving a heparin bolus in a patient who has received heparin within the past 7–100 days can indicate "rapid-onset" HIT; thrombocytopenia that begins abruptly after transfusion of a blood product can indicate sepsis from bacterial contamination or (rarely) passive alloimmune thrombocytopenia caused by transfusion of platelet-reactive alloantibodies. *D-ITP,* Drug-induced immune thrombocytopenia; *HIT,* heparin-induced thrombocytopenia; *PAT,* passive alloimmune thrombocytopenia; *PTP,* posttransfusion purpura; *TTP,* thrombotic thrombocytopenic purpura. *(Reprinted, with permission, from Greinacher A, Warkentin TE: Acquired non-immune thrombocytopenia. In: Marder VJ, Aird WC, Bennett JS, et al, editors: Hemostasis and thrombosis: Basic principles and clinical practice, ed 6, Philadelphia, 2013, Lippincott Williams & Wilkins, p 796.)*

TABLE 132.3 Laboratory Tests Used to Investigate a Patient With Thrombocytopenia

Test	Rationale
Common Tests	
CBC	Isolated thrombocytopenia usually is caused by platelet destruction, but involvement of all cell lines suggests underproduction or sequestration
Examination of the blood film	Pseudothrombocytopenia (platelet clumps)
	Toxic changes and granulocyte "left shift" suggest septicemia
	Atypical lymphocytes suggest viral infection
	RBC fragments suggest TTP or HUS
	Parasites (e.g., in malaria)
	White cell inclusions suggest hereditary macrothrombocytopenia
Blood cultures	Bacteremia, fungemia
ANA test	Systemic lupus erythematosus
Direct antiglobulin test	Exclude immune hemolysis accompanying ITP (Evans syndrome)
Coagulation Assays	
aPTT, PT (INR), thrombin time, fibrinogen, D-dimer assay	DIC
LA assay (nonspecific inhibitor), anticardiolipin and anti-β2-glycoprotein I assays	aPL antibody syndrome
Serum protein electrophoresis; IgG, IgM, IgA levels	ITP associated with lymphoproliferative disorder (monoclonal); hypersplenism associated with chronic hepatitis (polyclonal)
HIV serologic studies	HIV-associated thrombocytopenia
BM aspiration, biopsy	Assess megakaryocyte numbers and morphology; exclude primary BM disorder
Specialized Tests	
GP-specific platelet antibody assays (e.g., MAIPA)	Relatively specific assay for primary and secondary ITP
Drug-dependent increase in platelet-associated IgG	Specific assay for D-ITP
Drug-dependent platelet activation test (e.g., platelet serotonin release assay) or PF4–heparin (or PF4-polyanion) ELISA	HIT
Radionuclide platelet life span study with imaging (e.g., ^{111}In platelet survival study)	Define the mechanism of thrombocytopenia; identify an "accessory" spleen postsplenectomy

ANA, Antinuclear antibody; aPL, antiphospholipid; aPTT, activated partial thromboplastin time; BM, bone marrow; CBC, complete blood count; DIC, disseminated intravascular coagulation; D-ITP, drug-induced immune thrombocytopenia; ELISA, enzyme-linked immunosorbent assay; GP, glycoprotein; HIT, heparin-induced thrombocytopenia; HIV, human immunodeficiency virus; HUS, hemolytic uremic syndrome; IgG, immunoglobulin G; INR, international normalized ratio; ITP, idiopathic (immune) thrombocytopenic purpura; LA, lupus anticoagulant; MAIPA, monoclonal antibody immobilization of platelet antigens; PF4, platelet factor 4; PT, prothrombin time; RBC, red blood cell; TTP, thrombotic thrombocytopenic purpura.

treatment for thrombocytopenia that does not exist. A much less common (one in 10,000 blood samples) antibody-mediated pseudo-thrombocytopenic disorder is platelet satellitism, in which rosette-like clusters of platelets surround neutrophils. This entity is produced by immunoglobulin G (IgG) antibodies that recognize EDTA-induced cryptic epitopes on both platelet GPIIb/IIIa and neutrophil FcγIII receptors.

BM examination can be helpful for assessment of platelet production, particularly if megakaryocytes are reduced in number or abnormal in appearance. Examination of the BM can be diagnostic in some disorders (e.g., leukemia, metastatic tumor, Gaucher disease, megaloblastic anemia).

Elevated platelet-associated IgG (PAIgG) can be detected in patients with either immune or non-ITP; therefore, this assay is not useful diagnostically. In contrast, GP-specific platelet antibody assays, such as the monoclonal antibody immobilization of platelet antigens (MAIPA) assay or antigen capture enzyme immunoassay, are relatively specific for detection of autoimmune thrombocytopenic disorders. These assays can also be adapted for detection of drug-dependent GP-reactive antibodies.

When the mechanism of chronic thrombocytopenia is unclear, an autologous platelet survival study using ^{111}In-labeled platelets may be informative. Three patterns can be seen: (1) normal platelet survival and recovery (underproduction), (2) marked reduction in the platelet life span (increased destruction), and (3) reduced recovery but a normal or near-normal life span (sequestration). However, platelet survival studies are rarely performed.

Therapy

The risk of bleeding in patients with thrombocytopenia can be reduced by avoiding drugs that impair hemostasis (e.g., alcohol, antiplatelet agents, anticoagulants) and invasive procedures (e.g., intramuscular injections). If drug-induced thrombocytopenia is suspected, as many medications as possible, especially those started within the preceding 5–14 days, should be stopped. Life-threatening bleeding episodes should be treated with platelet transfusion regardless of the mechanism of the thrombocytopenia.

The underlying cause and anticipated natural history of the thrombocytopenic disorder influence the decision about prophylactic platelet transfusion. As a general rule, patients with chronic thrombocytopenic disorders characterized by increased platelet destruction (e.g., chronic ITP) or chronic underproduction (e.g., aplastic anemia or myelodysplasia) can tolerate long periods of severe thrombocytopenia without major bleeding. In addition, prophylactic platelet transfusions can trigger alloimmunization against human leukocyte antigen (HLA) or platelet antigens, thereby jeopardizing future therapeutic platelet transfusions. Consequently, prophylactic platelet transfusions are seldom indicated for such patients except when they are at risk of bleeding because of trauma or major surgery. When platelets are given, the platelet count should be maintained above 50 × 10^9/L. Invasive procedures such as thoracentesis, paracentesis, and liver biopsy are not usually associated with excess bleeding if the platelet count is greater than 50 × 10^9/L.

Prophylactic platelet transfusions should not be given to patients with strongly suspected or confirmed HIT, TTP, or HUS because they may exacerbate platelet-mediated thrombotic complications, and, particularly with HIT, mucocutaneous bleeding is uncommon. However, bleeding in the setting of severe thrombocytopenia may justify platelet transfusion even in these disorders.

ANATOMY AND PHYSIOLOGY

The Spleen: Anatomy and Function

The spleen is a small, well-perfused organ that receives about 5% of the total cardiac output. In adults, the spleen weighs between 150 and 200 g and measures approximately 11 cm in length.

The anatomy of the spleen is uniquely suited for its function; progressive branching of the splenic artery into trabecular and central arteries helps separate the plasma from the cellular elements (see Chapter 160). The central arteries arise perpendicularly from the trabecular arteries and skim the plasma layer from the cells. Soluble antigens in the plasma are delivered to the white pulp, where phagocytic cells process them and antibody production is initiated.

A cell-rich, hemoconcentrated fraction of the blood is delivered to the red pulp. Some of this blood flows directly to the splenic veins (the closed system), but most moves into the splenic cords (the open system). Here, the cellular elements percolate through a meshwork of reticulum fibers, reticuloendothelial cells, and supporting cells to reach the splenic sinuses. The cells enter the sinuses by passing through narrow fenestrations in the basement membrane of the endothelial cells lining the sinuses. The blood exits through the splenic vein into the portal system. Because the veins in the portal system lack valves, any increase in portal pressure is transmitted to the splenic microcirculation.

The spleen plays a number of important roles. It is the largest lymphoid organ in the body and contributes to host defense by clearing microorganisms and antibody-coated cells. The spleen is also important for antibody synthesis, especially antibodies directed against soluble antigens. The filtering function of the spleen includes (1) culling (removal of damaged or senescent cells and bacteria), (2) pitting (removal of RBC inclusion bodies or parasites), and (3) remodeling (reticulocyte sequestration and maturation). The spleen also serves as a reservoir of platelets (accommodating about one-third of the platelet mass in normal individuals). By contrast, the human spleen contains less than 2% of the total RBC mass, although in some animals (dogs and cats), the spleen is a much more important RBC reservoir.

Physiologic Platelet Sequestration

Radiolabeled platelet studies have shown that approximately 30% of the total platelet mass exists as a freely exchangeable pool in the spleen. Because the normal platelet life span is 9–10 days, platelets spend approximately one-third of their lives, or 3 days, within the spleen. In patients with hypersplenism, up to 90% of the platelets can be found in the spleen.

After labeled platelets are injected, there is accumulation in both the liver and the spleen. An initial, irreversible phase of hepatic uptake occurs. This equilibrates during the first 5 minutes and may reflect hepatic clearance of platelets damaged during the labeling procedure. Simultaneously, there is a slow increase in activity over the spleen that peaks in about 20 minutes. Splenic platelet uptake is thus dependent on input (spleen blood flow) and output (clearance).

The splenic platelet pool size can be decreased and the platelet count increased with intravenous infusions of epinephrine in normal persons and in patients with splenomegaly. By contrast, isoprenaline increases the splenic pool size. Splenic blood flow increases with increasing spleen size, although perfusion (flow per unit of tissue volume) falls. Blood flow can be increased in some inflammatory disorders (e.g., SLE) without an increase in spleen size. A marked increase or decrease in splenic perfusion alters the proportion of platelets within the spleen.

Fig. 132.3 shows why approximately 30% of the platelets are normally present in the spleen.[1] Because about 5% of cardiac output goes to the spleen and because the average splenic transit time (i.e., the time for the platelet to pass through the spleen) is approximately 10 minutes—compared with the usual average time of 1 minute for a platelet to make a complete circulatory pass—approximately one-third of the platelets are within the spleen

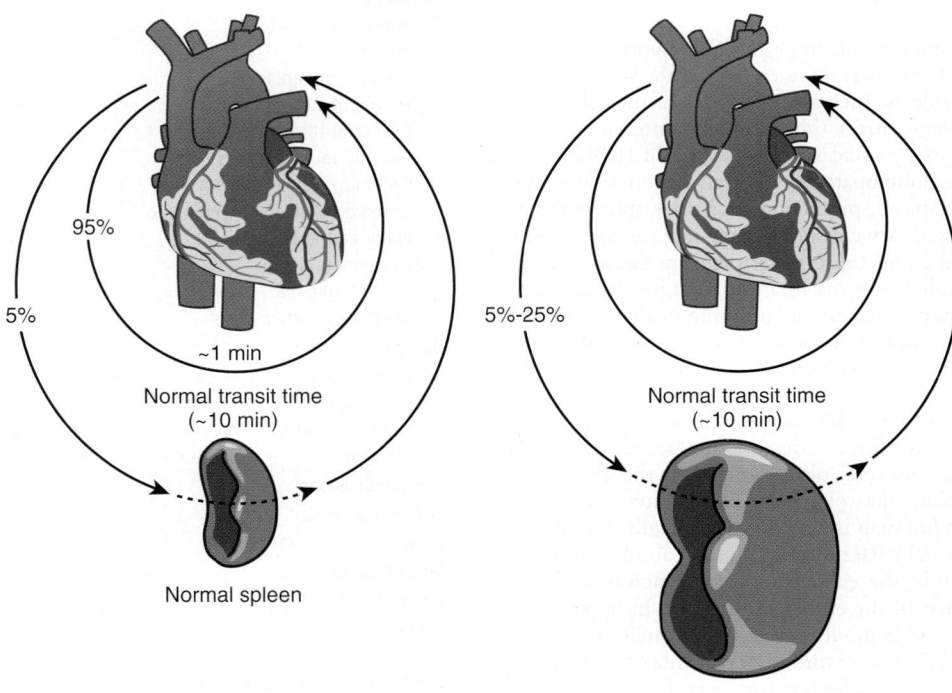

Fig. 132.3 PHYSIOLOGIC AND PATHOLOGIC PLATELET SPLENIC SEQUESTRATION. Normally, about 5% of cardiac output is to the spleen; however, a platelet that enters the spleen spends about 10 minutes there (splenic transit time = 10 min). In contrast, it usually takes only about 1 minute for a platelet to make a circulatory pass elsewhere. Thus about one-third of the platelets at any one time are located within the spleen: (5% × 10 min):(95% × 1 min), or an approximate 1:2 ratio. In hypersplenism, the splenic blood flow can increase by a factor of 5, that is, from 5% to 25% of total blood flow per minute. Thus, even without increase in splenic transit time, up to 70% or more of the platelets can be exchangeably sequestered within the spleen. *(From Arnold DM, Warkentin TE: Thrombocytopenia and thrombocytosis. In: Wilson WC, Grande CM, Hoyt DB, editors: Trauma: Critical care, vol. 2, New York, 2007, Informa Healthcare USA, p 983.)*

(i.e., 5% × 10 min/95% × 1 min, or a ratio of 50 : 95, or ≈1 : 2). With hypersplenism, the splenic blood flow can increase up to fivefold (i.e., from 5% to 25% of total blood flow). Thus even without an increase in splenic transit time, 70% or more of the platelets can be exchangeably sequestered within the spleen.

The most important determinant of the splenic platelet pool is the spleen size. The measurement of spleen size can thus be helpful in predicting the degree of thrombocytopenia expected from excess platelet pooling in the spleen. For example, if 90% of the platelet pool is in the spleen (i.e., 10% outside the spleen), the platelet count will be reduced by sevenfold because normally, 70% of platelets lie outside the spleen. Consequently and as a general rule, even if the spleen is massively enlarged, severe thrombocytopenia ($<20 \times 10^9$/L) is rare. On the other hand, mild thrombocytopenia may be explained by mild splenomegaly that may not be detectable on physical examination but can be seen with imaging studies.

PATHOLOGIC PLATELET SEQUESTRATION: HYPERSPLENISM

Definition

Hypersplenism is a syndrome characterized by splenomegaly and any or all of the following cytopenias: anemia, leukopenia, or thrombocytopenia. Implicit in the definition is that the cytopenias will correct after splenectomy. Although splenomegaly is almost always present in hypersplenism, many patients with splenomegaly do not have hypersplenism. Hypersplenism usually is the result of an identifiable pathologic process, but rarely, the cause of the splenomegaly remains elusive, and the hypersplenism is termed *primary*.

Pathogenesis

A list of disorders producing splenomegaly and hypersplenism is presented in Table 132.4. An increase in the size of the spleen can be caused by several mechanisms. Increased workload of the spleen can be caused by immunologic stress (infection, inflammation, or an autoimmune disorder) or by increased RBC removal (RBC membrane disorders, hemoglobinopathies). Portal hypertension also increases the size of the spleen, producing congestive splenomegaly. Benign and malignant infiltrative disorders may increase splenic size (infiltrative splenomegaly) and cause hypersplenism. Some of these disorders produce thrombocytopenia by more than just hypersplenism (e.g., BM infiltration with tumor, immune-mediated platelet clearance). Thus the demonstration of an enlarged spleen does not necessarily mean that the cytopenias are caused solely by hypersplenism.

Thrombocytopenia of hypersplenism is caused primarily by increased splenic platelet pooling. A massively enlarged spleen can hold more than 90% of the total platelet mass. In the absence of altered platelet production, the total body platelet mass usually is normal, and the platelet life span is near normal. Usually, the splenic transit time remains normal (≈10 minutes), but the absolute number of platelets retained within the enlarged spleen is increased. All of these platelets remain part of the exchangeable pool. In hypersplenism, the thrombocytopenia is moderately severe (platelet counts of 50×10^9/L to 150×10^9/L). Severe thrombocytopenia ($<20 \times 10^9$/L) suggests another diagnosis. Therefore it is unusual for patients with hypersplenism to have evidence of hemostatic impairment attributable to thrombocytopenia or to need specific interventions to raise the platelet count. Plasma volume expansion occurs in hypersplenism, but hemodilution plays a relatively minor role in the thrombocytopenia. In some patients with advanced liver disease, impaired hepatic production of thrombopoietin may contribute to thrombocytopenia in addition to hypersplenism.

The neutropenia of hypersplenism is caused by an increase in the marginated granulocyte pool, a portion of which is located in the spleen. The neutropenia of hypersplenism is usually asymptomatic.

TABLE 132.4   Differential Diagnosis of Splenomegaly and Hypersplenism

Infections
Acute

Viral (viral hepatitis, infectious mononucleosis, CMV infection)
Bacterial (septicemia, salmonellosis, brucellosis, splenic abscess)
Parasite (toxoplasmosis)

Subacute and Chronic

Subacute bacterial endocarditis
Tuberculosis
Malaria
Kala-azar
Fungal disease

Inflammation

Felty syndrome
SLE
Serum sickness
Rheumatic fever
Sarcoidosis
ALPS

Congestive Splenomegaly
Intrahepatic

Cirrhosis

Extrahepatic

Portal vein obstruction
Splenic vein obstruction
Hepatic vein occlusion (Budd-Chiari syndrome)

Chronic Passive Congestion

Heart failure

Hematologic Disorders

RBC disorders: hemolytic anemias, thalassemia, sickle cell disorders

Neoplasia
Malignant

MPDs
Myeloid metaplasia
Polycythemia rubra vera
Essential thrombocythemia
Chronic leukemia
Chronic myeloid leukemia
Chronic lymphocytic leukemia
Hairy cell leukemia
Lymphoma
Acute leukemia
Malignant histiocytosis

Benign

Hamartoma
Hemangioma
Lymphangioma
Fibroma

Storage Diseases

Gaucher disease
Niemann-Pick disease

Miscellaneous

Amyloidosis
Cysts

ALPS, Autoimmune lymphoproliferative syndrome; CMV, cytomegalovirus; MPD, myeloproliferative disorder; RBC, red blood cell; SLE, systemic lupus erythematosus.

Diagnosis

Thrombocytopenia is likely to be caused by hypersplenism when (1) splenomegaly is present, (2) the thrombocytopenia is mild to moderate in severity, (3) a moderately reduced neutrophil count and low-normal hemoglobin levels are found, and (4) there is no or minimal evidence of impaired hematopoiesis on BM examination.

Ultrasonography, computed tomography, and radionuclide imaging are of comparable sensitivity for documenting splenomegaly, and an imaging study should be performed if splenomegaly is not evident on physical examination. The mean platelet volume is often slightly decreased in hypersplenism, but this finding is not sufficiently specific to be diagnostically useful. An ^{111}In-labeled platelet survival study can be diagnostic of hypersplenism, demonstrating reduced platelet recovery and a normal platelet life span. Determining the cause of the splenomegaly is usually the most important issue.

Therapy

Several maneuvers can improve or correct the cytopenias attributable to hypersplenism, including total or partial splenectomy; partial splenic embolization; and in patients with congestive splenomegaly, surgical or transjugular intrahepatic portosystemic shunting. However, cytopenias secondary to hypersplenism and thrombocytopenia in particular, are almost never of sufficient severity to justify such treatment. Consequently the decision to perform one of these interventions usually depends on other considerations. For example, splenectomy should be considered for relief of pain or early satiety associated with massive splenomegaly (e.g., in myelo- or lymphoproliferative disorders) or for splenomegaly of unknown origin (for investigation of possible splenic lymphoma).

Short-term complications from splenectomy include infections, bleeding, and thromboembolism. The major long-term risk associated with splenectomy is overwhelming septicemia; this risk can be reduced by vaccination. All patients should be vaccinated against pneumococci, meningococci, and *Haemophilus* species at least 2 weeks before elective splenectomy. Moreover, "booster" doses of pneumococcus and meningococcus vaccines are recommended after 5 years.[7] Splenectomy for congestive hypersplenism in the setting of portal hypertension is associated with high morbidity and mortality rates. Splenectomy is also associated with high morbidity (50%) and mortality (10%–15%) rates in myeloid metaplasia and does not alter the natural history of this disorder. Thus splenectomy is usually performed for palliation of intractable symptoms.

Splenectomy in Gaucher disease usually corrects the cytopenias, relieves abdominal discomfort, and improves growth in children. Partial, rather than total, splenectomy has been used in an attempt to avoid shifting the deposition of glucocerebroside from the spleen to the bones. Often, however, splenomegaly and hypersplenism recur after partial splenectomy. Enzyme replacement therapy can reduce the morbidity from hypersplenism (see Chapter 53).

DRUG-INDUCED THROMBOCYTOPENIC SYNDROMES

Many drugs can cause thrombocytopenia. Some drugs (e.g., anticancer chemotherapeutic agents, valproic acid) cause dose-dependent thrombocytopenia, generally through myelosuppressive mechanisms. An important disorder encountered by hematologists is unexpected thrombocytopenia caused by immunologic (idiosyncratic) mechanisms.[8–10] The frequency of these reactions varies considerably among drugs and ranges from very rare (<1:10,000) for commonly used drugs such as acetaminophen, indomethacin, naproxen, quinine or quinidine, and trimethoprim-sulfamethoxazole (TMP-SMX) to common (1%–5%) for other drugs such as gold and unfractionated heparin (UFH).

Immunologic drug-induced thrombocytopenia can occur through different mechanisms (Fig. 132.4). For example, thrombocytopenia can occur when the Fab terminus of the pathogenic IgG binds to a complex composed of drug (or drug metabolite) and a platelet membrane component (typically, platelet GPIIb/IIIa or GPIb/IX/V). The Fc portions of the pathogenic IgG molecules do not bind to platelets but interact with Fc receptors on phagocytic cells of the reticuloendothelial system, which ingest the platelets, leading to accelerated platelet clearance. Severe thrombocytopenia (platelet counts <20 × 10^9/L) is typically observed. This mechanism is exemplified by quinine- and quinidine-induced thrombocytopenia. A complicating issue (discussed later in this chapter) is that quinine can also rarely cause thrombocytopenia with a clinical picture of microangiopathic hemolysis[11] and/or DIC.

Sometimes the Fab terminus binds to a neoepitope on platelet GPIIb/IIIa induced by the drug, and the drug itself is not part of the neoepitope. This mechanism is exemplified by the GPIIb/IIIa receptor antagonists, eptifibatide and tirofiban, which bind to the Arg-Gly-Asp recognition site on GPIIb/IIIa, forming a neoepitope to which the "fiban-dependent" antibodies bind.

Another distinct form of drug-induced thrombocytopenia is exemplified by HIT (see Chapter 133). In this disorder, the Fab portion of the pathogenic IgG binds to platelet factor 4 (PF4), an α-granule protein that is immunogenic when complexed to heparin or certain other polyanions. The Fc portions of the IgG molecules bind to platelet FcγIIa receptors, initiating intense platelet activation (see Fig. 132.4). Perhaps because HIT is a platelet activation syndrome or because of the relatively low number of HIT antibodies that bind to platelet surfaces, the thrombocytopenia is typically mild to moderate rather than severe (see Fig. 133.3 in Chapter 133).

DRUG-INDUCED IMMUNE THROMBOCYTOPENIA

A large number of drugs can cause a syndrome that mimics acute ITP (D-ITP); however, there are relatively few drugs for which causation is well established on both clinical and serologic grounds (Table 132.5).[10,12–14] Typically, severe thrombocytopenia (platelet count usually <20 × 10^9/L), together with petechiae and purpura, develop within approximately 1 week (although occasionally much longer) after initiation of therapy with the responsible drug. D-ITP is much less common than HIT. For example, a relatively "common" cause of this syndrome is TMP-SMX (co-trimoxazole), even though it occurs in only approximately one in 25,000 patients who receive this drug combination.

Important exceptions to these generalizations occur with D-ITP that results from GPIIb/IIIa receptor antagonists; these reactions are relatively common (affecting about 0.5%–1% of patients) and usually occur within hours of first use as a result of preexisting, naturally occurring antibodies. Another exception is carbimazole-induced thrombocytopenia, in which mild thrombocytopenia is explained by the presence of relatively small quantities of the platelet GP target (platelet endothelial cell adhesion molecule-1 [PECAM-1]) on the platelet surface. Besides the atypical immune-mediated syndromes of HIT and GPIIb/IIIa antagonist thrombocytopenia, the most common drugs (in absolute terms) implicated in the causation of classic D-ITP syndrome are quinine (outpatients) and vancomycin (inpatients).[15]

Pathogenesis

Drug-dependent binding of the Fab component of IgG to platelet GP leads to platelet destruction. This occurs because the IgG-sensitized platelets are recognized by Fc receptors of phagocytic cells. For quinine- and quinidine-induced ITP, both the GPIIb/IIIa and GPIb/IX/V complexes have been implicated as targets for the drug-dependent IgG (see Fig. 132.4). By contrast, for sulfa antibiotic- and naproxen-induced ITP, the GPIIb/IIIa complex is predominantly involved. Sometimes, drug metabolites form the antigen rather than the parent drug. A trimolecular complex is formed among IgG Fab, the drug (or metabolite), and the platelet GP. In contrast to HIT, platelet Fc receptors are not involved in D-ITP pathogenesis. Drug-dependent IgG binding is remarkably heterogeneous with respect to binding affinity, number of binding sites per platelet, and the range of drug concentrations required. A study of quinine-induced ITP identified two different types of antibodies: quinine-dependent antibodies that bound to platelets in the presence of drug and quinine-specific antibodies that reacted with quinine-conjugated albumin.[16] The pathophysiologic implications of this latter group of antibodies remain unclear.

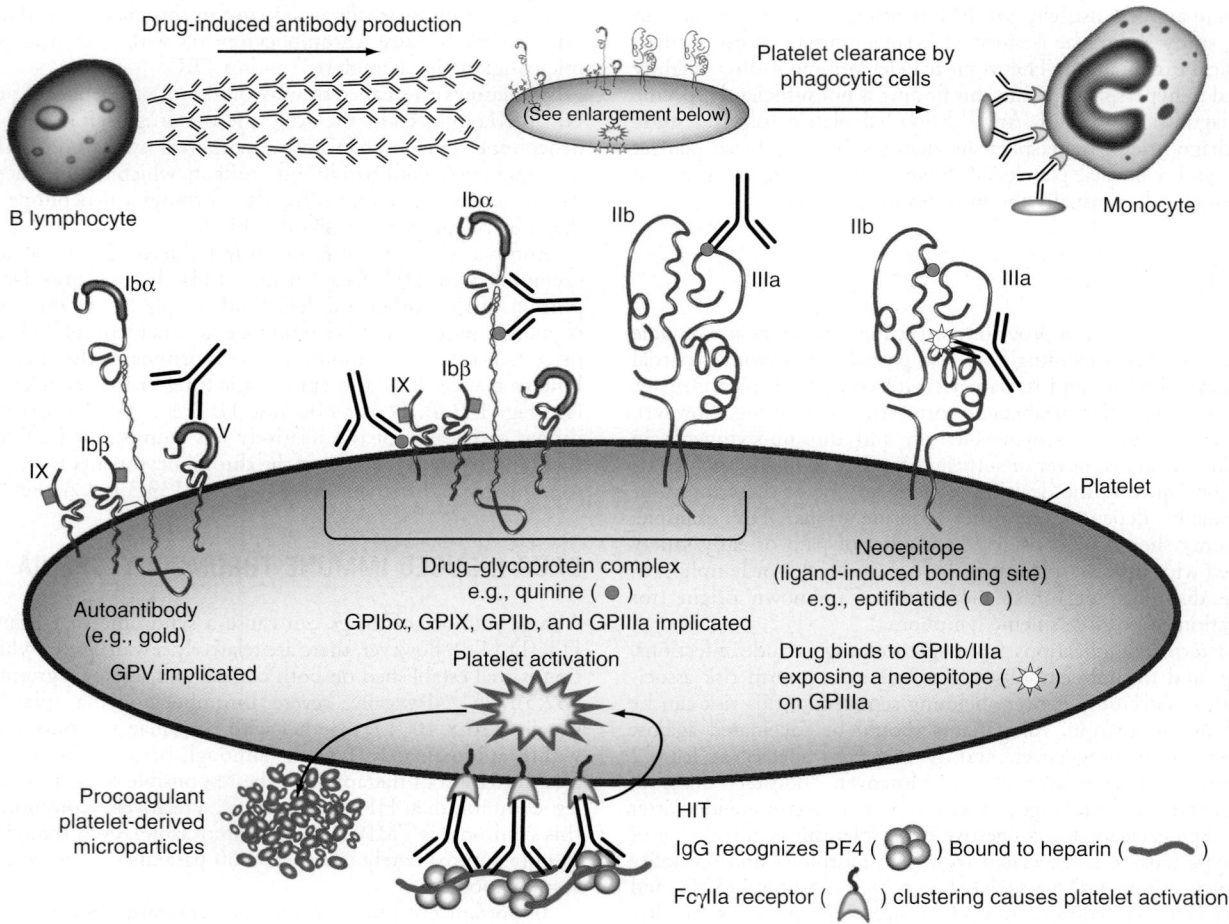

Fig. 132.4 MECHANISMS OF DRUG-INDUCED IMMUNE THROMBOCYTOPENIA. Four immune thrombocytopenic syndromes are illustrated. On the *bottom* of the schematic platelet, heparin-induced thrombocytopenia (HIT) is illustrated, indicating that immunoglobulin G (IgG) antibodies bind to complexes of platelet factor 4 (PF4) and heparin, with the Fc regions of the antibodies binding to the platelet FcγIIa receptors, resulting in platelet activation (including generation of procoagulant, platelet-derived microparticles). On the *top* of the schematic platelet, three mechanisms are illustrated that lead to increased platelet clearance by phagocytic cells. From left to right, these are (1) autoantibody-induced immune thrombocytopenia (e.g., gold-induced antiglycoprotein V [GPV] antibodies). (2) Drug-dependent antibodies reactive against drug (or drug metabolite)–platelet glycoprotein complex(es) (e.g., quinine-induced thrombocytopenia in which drug-dependent antibodies against GPIbα, GPIX, GPIIb, and GPIIIa have been implicated, resulting in an antibody/drug/glycoprotein ternary complex), and (3) antibodies against neoepitope(s) formed in the presence of a drug (e.g., eptifibatide-induced immune thrombocytopenia caused by formation of ligand-induced binding site elsewhere on the GPIIb/IIIa complex after eptifibatide binding). Note that preexisting (naturally occurring) antibodies can explain abrupt-onset thrombocytopenia in a patient receiving eptifibatide for the first time.

The fundamental mechanism that accounts for antibody formation in a small proportion of patients is unknown. One group has proposed that drug-dependent platelet-reactive antibodies are derived from a pool of naturally occurring autoantibodies with inherently weak (nonpathologic) affinity for certain platelet membrane GPs.[8,16] However, if a certain drug is able to enhance antibody–antigen interaction, and if B cells expressing such antibodies are induced to proliferate and undergo affinity maturation in such a patient, the resulting antibody can destroy the platelets in the presence of the drug.

Clinical Features

Patients with D-ITP typically present with petechiae, purpura, and severe thrombocytopenia (platelet count often $<20 \times 10^9/L$). Systemic symptoms, such as fever and chills, may occur in patients with abrupt-onset thrombocytopenia. Usually, the thrombocytopenia becomes clinically apparent 1–2 weeks after initiation of the drug, but the thrombocytopenia can start after a patient has been taking a drug for several years. Typically, the platelet count begins to rise in a few days after discontinuation of the implicated drug, but occasionally several weeks are required for recovery, possibly because of the generation of drug-independent IgG (platelet autoantibodies).

Sometimes drug exposure is relatively obscure. Among outpatients, the physician needs to inquire about potential exposure to quinine. Quinine is widely available: for example, as an ingredient in tonic water, as an additive to street drugs, and in some countries as therapy for leg cramps. Vancomycin is a relatively common cause of D-ITP in hospitalized inpatients; most often this occurs after the usual intravenous administration, but some reports have implicated exposure via orthopedic cement or with peritoneal administration of vancomycin.

Rarely, distinct drug-dependent IgG molecules destroy RBCs or WBCs in addition to platelets. For example, both platelet- and leukocyte-reactive quinidine-dependent IgG molecules have been detected in a patient with quinidine-induced bicytopenia. Sometimes the immune process is directed against a pluripotent hematopoietic stem cell, resulting in pancytopenia accompanied by BM aplasia or hypoplasia (e.g., gold-, carbamazepine-, or quinidine-induced pancytopenia). A BM aspirate should be performed in patients with suspected drug-induced bicytopenia or pancytopenia because a hypoplastic BM may be indicative of drug-induced aplastic anemia.

Diagnosis

A high index of clinical suspicion is required to make the diagnosis. Moreover, clinicians need to evaluate which drug (often among several that the patient is receiving) is most likely to explain a diagnosis of D-ITP.[10,12–14] The clinician should focus on drugs that have been started 5–10 days before the onset of the platelet count decrease (Fig. 132.5A). Also, with drugs such as quinine, in which there may be intermittent exposure (e.g., consumption of gin and tonic), a very recent exposure (previous 1 or 2 days) usually explains the abrupt onset of symptomatic thrombocytopenia.

After the physician has identified one or more potential agents, the next step is to determine whether these drugs have previously been implicated as causes of D-ITP. The box Search Strategies When Investigating Patient With Possible Drug-Induced Immune Thrombocytopenic Purpura includes some strategies for identifying drugs implicated in D-ITP.

Demonstration of drug-dependent binding of IgG to platelets in vitro can be important for diagnosis (see Fig. 132.5B). Labeled Ig-specific probes (e.g., phase II assays) or GP capture techniques (phase III assays) can be used (see Table 132.3). In other cases, D-ITP test results are negative, but the diagnosis still seems likely based on clinical features and supporting literature (see Fig. 132.6).

There are certain caveats in diagnostic testing. First, metabolites must sometimes be used instead of the parent drug to detect the IgG. Second, the target drug (or metabolite) must be included in the wash buffer used in these assays. Third, despite these maneuvers, the sensitivity of in vitro assays is relatively low, and the diagnosis of D-ITP must often be made on clinical grounds. Sometimes the diagnosis is confirmed by inadvertent or deliberate reexposure to the suspected drug. However, deliberate drug challenge is not often performed because of its potential risk.

A novel approach to identify drug-dependent platelet-reactive antibodies was reported by investigators at the Milwaukee Blood Center.[20] They used nonobese diabetic/severe combined immunodeficient (NOD/SCID) mice (which lack xenoantibodies, thereby allowing infused human platelets to circulate) to identify drug-dependent antibodies in patient sera, including antibodies that only recognize drug metabolites (presumably, mice produce the same or similar drug metabolites as humans, which are recognized by the drug-dependent antibodies).

TABLE 132.5	List of Drugs Implicated in Drug-Induced Immune Thrombocytopenia

Drugs Common to All Three Lists[12–14]

Quinine, quinidine, rifampin, trimethoprim-sulfamethoxazole, vancomycin

George[12]	Reese[13]	Arnold[14]
Acetaminophen	Abciximab[a]	Abciximab[a]
Alprenolol	Acetaminophen	Carbamazepine
Aminoglutethimide	Amiodarone	Ceftriaxone
Aminosalicylic acid	Ampicillin	Eptifibatide[b]
Amiodarone	Carbamazepine	Ibuprofen
Amphotericin B	Eptifibatide[b]	Mirtazapine
Amrinone	Ethambutol	Oxaliplatin
Chlorothiazide	Haloperidol	Penicillin
Chlorpromazine	Ibuprofen	Suramin
Cimetidine	Irinotecan	Tirofiban[b]
Danazol	Naproxen	Heparin[c]
Diatrizoate meglumine	Oxaliplatin	
Diazepam	Phenytoin	
Diazoxide	Piperacillin	
Diclofenac	Ranitidine	
Digoxin	Simvastatin	
Ethambutol	Sulfisoxazole	
Haloperidol	Tirofiban[b]	
Interferon-α	Valproic acid	
Iopanoic acid		
Levamisole		
Lithium		
Meclofenamate		
Methyldopa		
Minoxidil		
Nalidixic acid		
Naphazoline		
Nitroglycerin		
Oxprenolol		
Sulfasalazine		
Sulfisoxazole		
Tamoxifen		
Thiothixene		
Tolmetin		

[a]Subtype of D-ITP where patient's antibodies (either naturally occurring or that are formed after treatment with abciximab) bind to platelet GPIIb/IIIa subsequent to binding of abciximab (chimeric human-murine Fab that recognizes GPIIb/IIIa) to platelets.
[b]Subtype of D-ITP caused by fiban-dependent antibodies (either naturally-occurring or that are formed after treatment with eptifibatide or tirofiban) that recognize neoepitopes on platelet GPIIb/IIIa that form subsequent to binding of fiban drug to GPIIb/IIIa.
[c]HIT is considered a distinct subtype of D-ITP disorder, given its unusual pathogenesis centered on IgG-induced platelet activation.
D-ITP, Drug-induced immune thrombocytopenia; HIT, heparin-induced thrombocytopenia.

Search Strategies When Investigating a Patient With Possible Drug-Induced Immune Thrombocytopenic Purpura

Four sources of information as to whether a drug has been implicated as a cause of D-ITP:

- **PubMed search** (http://www.ncbi.nlm.nih.gov/pubmed): [name of drug] and [thrombocytopenia]. By way of example, the author encountered a patient who developed severe thrombocytopenia 5 days after starting treatment with mirtazapine (Fig. 132.6). Searching [mirtazapine] and [thrombocytopenia] in December 2014 identified two reports[17,18] of mirtazapine-induced D-ITP syndrome.
- **Drug-induced thrombocytopenia website** (http://www.ouhsc.edu/platelets/ditp.html): Investigators at the University of Oklahoma published a comprehensive survey of drugs implicated in D-ITP using clinical criteria[12]; a website maintained by these investigators is updated every 2 years.
- **Database from drug-dependent platelet-reactive antibody testing** at the BloodCenter of Wisconsin, 1995–2010 (http://www.ouhsc.edu/platelets/InternetPostingLab2_18_11Frames.htm): the BloodCenter of Wisconsin maintains a website reporting its experience in detecting drug-dependent platelet-reactive antibodies.[19]
- **Combined approach that uses clinical criteria,[12] laboratory criteria,[19] and Adverse Event Reporting System.[13]** Table 132.5 (middle column) lists two dozen drugs (including those drugs identified by two other comprehensive reviews[12,14]) for which convincing clinical and laboratory evidence exists.[13] To review the comprehensive list of all drugs investigated in this study,[13] interested readers can consult the online supplemental table (http://bloodjournal.hematologylibrary.org/content/suppl/2010/06/08/blood-2010-03-276691.DC1/TableS1.pdf).

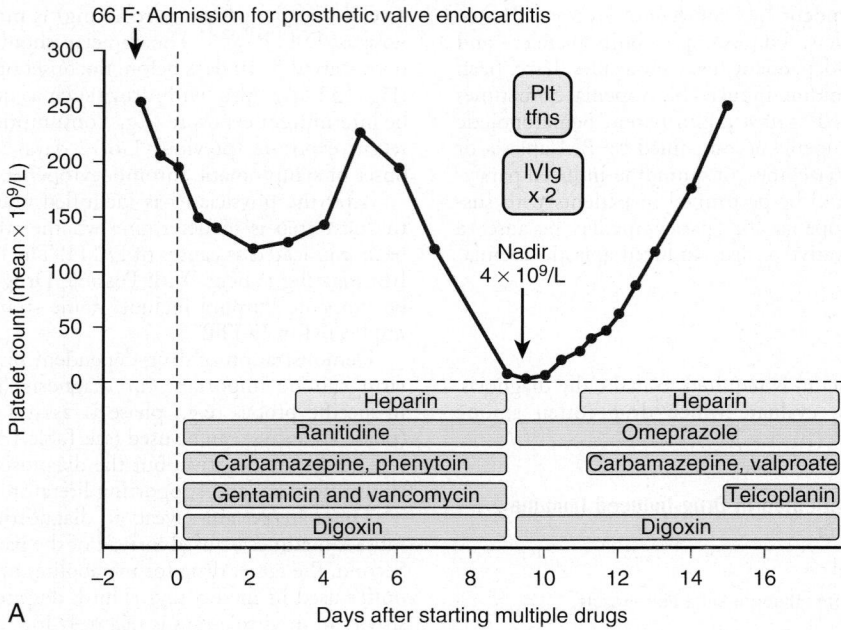

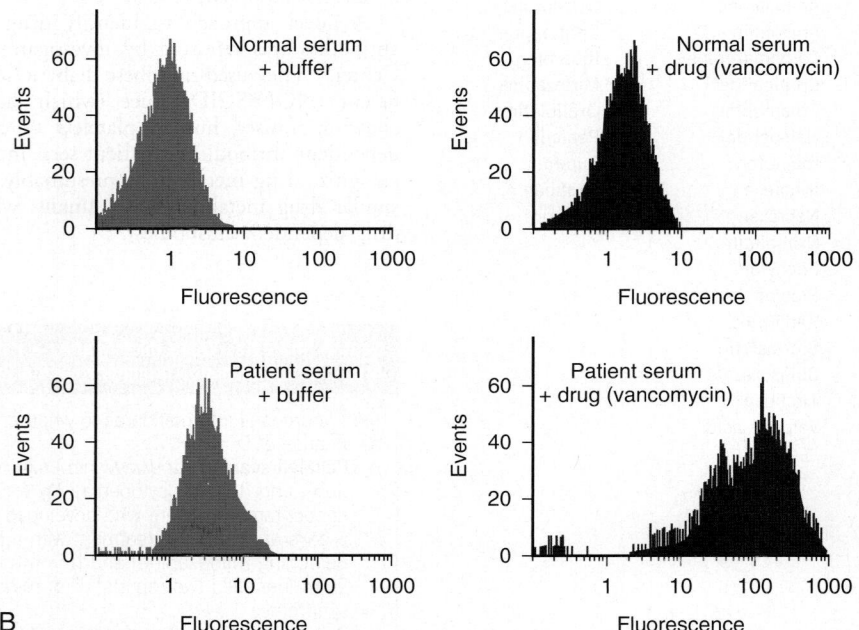

Fig. 132.5 DRUG-INDUCED IMMUNE THROMBOCYTOPENIA (D-ITP) SECONDARY TO VAN-COMYCIN. **A,** Timeline of D-ITP. A 66-year-old woman was admitted for prosthetic valve endocarditis 5 months after undergoing mitral valve replacement. The initiation of multiple new drugs and the onset 6 days later of progressively severe thrombocytopenia (platelet count nadir, 4×10^9/L on day 9) suggested D-ITP syndrome. However, the timing fit several drugs (ranitidine, carbamazepine, phenytoin, gentamicin, vancomycin, and digoxin). **B,** Drug-dependent binding of antibodies was demonstrated using patient serum and vancomycin. Also, test results for heparin-induced thrombocytopenia antibodies was negative. Thus the diagnosis of vancomycin-induced D-ITP syndrome was made based on clinical and serological grounds. The patient received treatment with high-dose intravenous immunoglobulin (IVIG) and platelet transfusions. *Plt tfns,* Platelet transfusions.

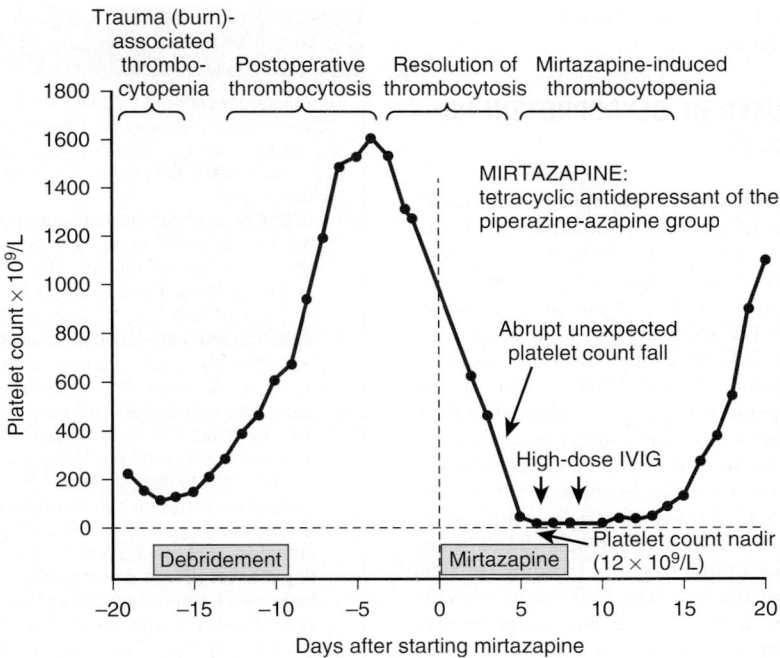

Fig. 132.6 DRUG-INDUCED IMMUNE THROMBOCYTOPENIA (D-ITP) SECONDARY TO MIRTAZAPINE. The onset of severe thrombocytopenia (platelet count nadir, $12 \times 10^9/L$) on day 6 of mirtazapine therapy implicated this tetracyclic antidepressant of the piperazine-azapine group as a cause of drug-induced immune thrombocytopenia (D-ITP) syndrome. The very rapid platelet count fall (which was already manifest on day 5 of mirtazapine therapy) is explained by reduced platelet production (because the patient's platelet count was declining from postoperative thrombocytosis). Although in vitro testing for mirtazapine-dependent antibodies was negative, the low sensitivity of these assays does not rule out mirtazapine as the cause of D-ITP syndrome, particularly in a high pretest probability scenario such as this. *IVIg,* Intravenous immunoglobulin.

Management

As many drugs as possible should be discontinued in patients with suspected D-ITP. If further drug treatment is necessary, an alternate, immunologically non–cross-reactive substitute should be used. Spontaneous improvement in the platelet count usually begins within a few days of discontinuing the offending drug, although in some cases, complete recovery may take 2 weeks or longer. Platelet transfusions should be given to patients with life-threatening bleeding. High-dose intravenous immunoglobulin (IVIg), 1 g/kg given over 6–8 hours, with a second dose 1 or 2 days later if required, may be helpful in some situations. Corticosteroids appear to be relatively ineffective for treatment of D-ITP.

GOLD-INDUCED THROMBOCYTOPENIA

Gold-induced ITP occurs in as many as 1% to 3% of treated patients. A genetic predisposition is suggested by the association with HLA-DR3, which is found in approximately 85% of affected patients. The thrombocytopenia typically occurs during the first 20 weeks of therapy before a total of 1000 mg of gold has been given. Rarely, the thrombocytopenia begins much later, sometimes several months after discontinuation of the gold. Although the onset of thrombocytopenia is typically abrupt, regular platelet count monitoring is important because an early diagnosis can be made in some patients. The thrombocytopenia often persists for several months after discontinuation of the gold, probably because of gold-induced autoimmune thrombocytopenia (drug-independent gold-induced autoantibodies against gold-induced antiglycoprotein V [GPV] have been implicated) (see Fig. 132.4). Although most patients will eventually respond to corticosteroids, immediate, albeit often transient, correction of severe thrombocytopenia can usually be achieved with high-dose IVIg. Some patients with persisting thrombocytopenia benefit from splenectomy or use of gold-chelating agents (dimercaprol, *N*-acetylcysteine). The disorder is rarely encountered because the use of gold to treat rheumatic disorders has declined.

DRUG-INDUCED AUTOIMMUNE THROMBOCYTOPENIA

Certain drugs other than gold have been reported to initiate autoimmune thrombocytopenia (e.g., levodopa, procainamide). Because the pathogenic antibodies are by definition drug independent, however, it is difficult to establish causation. The mumps–measles–rubella (MMR) vaccine can rarely ($\approx 1:40,000$) cause a severe but generally self-limited thrombocytopenia that is clinically and serologically indistinguishable from childhood acute ITP; MMR vaccination of unimmunized children with ITP and revaccination of children with prior ITP does not lead to recurrent thrombocytopenia.

DRUG-INDUCED IMMUNE THROMBOCYTOPENIA OF RAPID ONSET

A rapid onset of thrombocytopenia (within hours) can occur if a patient with preexisting drug-dependent antibodies is (re)exposed to the drug. This situation is relatively common in HIT ($\approx 25\%$ of patients identified)[3] because repeated treatment with heparin is common and heparin use itself can result in the complication (HIT-associated thrombosis) that might lead to further use of heparin. Because HIT antibodies are transient, however, rapid-onset HIT occurs in patients with recent heparin exposures, usually within the past 100 days.[3] By contrast, repeated episodes of quinine-induced thrombocytopenia of abrupt onset can occur many months or even years apart because these antibodies persist for much longer.

Thrombocytopenia of rapid onset is commonly seen with GPIIb/IIIa receptor antagonists (see next section).

THROMBOCYTOPENIA CAUSED BY GLYCOPROTEIN IIB/IIIA RECEPTOR ANTAGONISTS

Several thrombocytopenic syndromes have been reported with use of GPIIb/IIIa receptor antagonists (abciximab, eptifibatide, tirofiban) administered during percutaneous coronary intervention (e.g., angioplasty, stenting): (1) rapid-onset, severe thrombocytopenia within 12 hours of drug administration (in 0.4%–2% of patients), (2) rapid-onset pseudothrombocytopenia (in approximately 1% of patients exposed to abciximab [ReoPro]), (3) rapid-onset thrombocytopenia within 12 hours of a second exposure to a GPIIb/IIIa antagonist, and (4) delayed-onset thrombocytopenia beginning 5–7 days after drug administration (rare).[21] The frequency of rapid-onset thrombocytopenia is higher among patients who receive a second course of therapy, especially if it follows the initial exposure by only a few weeks. Thrombocytopenia is typically severe (median platelet count nadir, about $5 \times 10^9/L$ to $10 \times 10^9/L$), but clinical effects vary dramatically, ranging from absence of petechiae or other signs of bleeding (in 50% of patients) to fatal hemorrhage (in less than 5%). Some patients develop anaphylactoid reactions accompanying the abrupt platelet count declines. The antibodies may cause thrombosis in some patients, likely because the pathogenic antibodies also activate platelets.[21]

These syndromes are caused by at least three mechanisms. First, antibodies of IgG (and possibly IgM) class can bind to neoepitopes on the GPIIb/IIIa complex generated by these drugs (or their metabolites), that is, ligand-induced binding sites (see Fig. 132.4). Up to 5% of humans and nonhuman primates have naturally occurring IgG antibodies that will bind to GPIIb/IIIa receptors in the presence of drug, which could explain why rapid-onset thrombocytopenia occurs so frequently with these agents. A second mechanism is applicable to abciximab, a chimeric Fab fragment comprised of murine GPIIb/IIIa-reactive sequences and human framework sequences. Interestingly, although a high frequency of normal persons (74%) have antibodies that recognize platelets coated with abciximab, these "normal" antibodies were shown to differ from those detected in patients in whom thrombocytopenia developed after a second exposure to abciximab: whereas the pathogenic antibodies recognized murine sequences within abciximab, the "normal" (nonpathogenic) antibodies were specific for the carboxyl terminus (papain cleavage site) of Fab fragments prepared from normal human IgG. Drug-dependent antibodies can also be generated about 1 week after exposure. The antibodies differ among patients with respect to the precise neoepitopes recognized and display variable degrees of cross-reactivity among the different GPIIb/IIIa receptor antagonists ("fibans"); this explains why a repeat treatment course with another GPIIb/IIIa receptor antagonist may not necessarily cause thrombocytopenia. A third mechanism involves eptifibatide-dependent antibodies that activate platelets via their FcγIIa receptors.[21]

Some naturally occurring antibodies only bind to GPIIb/IIIa when the calcium concentration is low, thus explaining pseudothrombocytopenia—falsely low platelet count estimates caused by ex vivo aggregation of platelets in blood samples collected into calcium-chelating anticoagulants, especially EDTA. The rare syndrome of delayed-onset thrombocytopenia after brief exposure might result from high-titer GPIIb/IIIa-reactive antibodies that bind even in the absence of the drug.

Platelet transfusions are indicated in patients who are bleeding, although their efficacy has not been established. Platelet transfusions are most likely to be effective for the treatment of abciximab-induced thrombocytopenia because the drug binds so tightly to GPIIb/IIIa that little abciximab is free to bind to the transfused platelets. Platelet transfusions are not indicated in pseudothrombocytopenia, which underscores the importance of reviewing the blood film when a low platelet count is reported after treatment with one of these agents.

Approach to Patients With Thrombocytopenia Following Percutaneous Coronary Intervention

Four diagnoses should be considered in patients who develop thrombocytopenia within minutes or a few hours after a PCI and have received one or more of the following agents: (1) platelet GPIIb/IIIa inhibitor (e.g., abciximab, eptifibatide, tirofiban), (2) heparin, or (3) iodinated contrast agent.

- **GPIIb/IIIa inhibitor–induced pseudothrombocytopenia.** The patient has no symptoms or signs of bleeding, and platelet aggregates are seen in the blood film. The platelet count is falsely reported as low by the automated particle counter, which fails to count aggregated platelets. No treatment is required.

- **GPIIb/IIIa inhibitor–induced thrombocytopenia.** The platelet count falls abruptly, often to profoundly reduced levels (typical nadir, $<20 \times 10^9/L$). Hemostatic impairment is variable, ranging from petechiae to fatal hemorrhages; occasionally, patients develop anaphylactoid reactions or even associated thrombosis. Treatment involves stopping all platelet antagonists and anticoagulants and giving platelets if the patient has signs of bleeding. Prophylactic platelet transfusions can also be considered if the platelet count is very low (e.g., $<10 \times 10^9/L$). Testing for drug-dependent antibodies can be accomplished using flow cytometry or ELISA.

- **Rapid-onset HIT.** In patients who have preexisting HIT antibodies because of recent heparin exposure (generally within the past 100 days), rapid-onset HIT can occur when heparin is given during PCI. This is much less common than GPIIb/IIIa inhibitor–induced thrombocytopenia or pseudothrombocytopenia, so presumptive treatment of HIT with a nonheparin anticoagulant is rarely indicated in this situation. The platelet count nadir is usually much higher than with GPIIb/IIIa inhibitor–induced thrombocytopenia.

- **Radiocontrast-induced ITP.** Very rarely, patients who have previously received iodinated contrast can develop abrupt-onset, severe thrombocytopenia after exposure to contrast during PCI. Platelet transfusions (with or without high-dose IVIg) are appropriate for a bleeding patient.

ELISA, Enzyme-linked immunosorbent assay; HIT, heparin-induced thrombocytopenia; ITP, induced thrombocytopenia; IVIg, intravenous immunoglobulin; PCI, percutaneous coronary intervention.

Various in vitro assays using flow cytometry or enzyme-linked immunosorbent assay (ELISA) have been developed to detect these antibodies. Because some pathogenic antibodies are naturally occurring, it is theoretically possible to identify patients at high risk for rapid-onset thrombocytopenia in elective situations (see box on Approach to Patients With Thrombocytopenia Following Percutaneous Coronary Interventions).

MISCELLANEOUS DRUG-INDUCED THROMBOCYTOPENIC SYNDROMES

Drug-Induced Thrombotic Microangiopathy

Several drugs can trigger a syndrome of thrombocytopenia, fragmentation hemolysis, and renal failure known as *drug-induced thrombotic microangiopathy (TMA)*. This syndrome has been established for quinine,[11] in which multiple quinine-dependent antibodies reactive against platelets, RBCs, leukocytes, and endothelial cells have been reported. Although TMA has been reported with ticlopidine and clopidogrel, a recent systematic review[22] failed to confirm this association.

Although a similar syndrome may be caused by mitomycin, gemcitabine, cyclosporine, and tacrolimus, it should be noted that many patients who receive these drugs have an underlying illness (e.g., gastric adenocarcinoma, BM transplantation, collagen vascular disease) that itself can be complicated by TMA; moreover, high cumulative doses of the implicated drug have usually been received, suggesting a nonimmune (e.g., toxic) pathogenesis.[11] Furthermore, these patients tend to be less responsive to plasma exchange than those with idiopathic TTP.

Drug-Induced Disseminated Intravascular Coagulation

On rare occasions, quinine causes severe thrombocytopenia accompanied by marked coagulation abnormalities indicative of DIC. This syndrome overlaps that of quinine-induced thrombotic microangiopathy, and the explanation for the prominent coagulopathy is unknown. Although all patients with HIT have biochemical evidence of increased thrombin generation, only about 10% to 20% have overt DIC; however, these patients often present with large and small vessel thrombosis.

Nonidiosyncratic Drug-Induced Thrombocytopenia

Most antineoplastic drugs produce dose-dependent pancytopenia because of their effect on hematopoietic cells, including megakaryocytes and their progenitor cells. Typically, the platelet count nadir occurs at a predictable time after treatment, and the count then quickly recovers. Unexpectedly severe or prolonged thrombocytopenia in patients receiving chemotherapy should suggest alternate explanations (e.g., idiosyncratic thrombocytopenia caused by another drug).

Mild to moderate thrombocytopenia develops in approximately 20% of patients who take valproic acid (an antiepileptic agent); bleeding symptoms are uncommon. The mechanism of thrombocytopenia in this setting is unknown, but the condition appears to be nonidiosyncratic because the risk of thrombocytopenia correlates strongly with serum concentrations of valproic acid metabolite. Amrinone is another agent that can cause mild, dose-dependent thrombocytopenia.

Rapid Nonimmune Drug-Induced Thrombocytopenia

Some drugs produce rapid but generally mild and transient drops in the platelet count. These drugs include heparin, protamine, bleomycin, hematin, desmopressin (particularly in patients with type 2B von Willebrand disease), and porcine factor VIII. The mechanisms for thrombocytopenia in these syndromes are obscure.

Drug Hypersensitivity Reactions

Mild to moderate thrombocytopenia is sometimes observed in patients with systemic drug hypersensitivity reactions. Co-morbid clinical features can include generalized rash, fever, cholestasis, and leukopenia. Allopurinol, isoniazid, sulfasalazine, and phenothiazine drugs, among others, have been implicated in these reactions.

Thrombocytopenia Secondary to Biologic Response Modifiers

Use of purified or recombinant biologic response modifiers such as interferon, interleukin-2, and certain colony-stimulating factors has resulted in severe, reversible thrombocytopenia in some patients. Antilymphocyte globulins can also produce severe thrombocytopenia.

OTHER CAUSES OF DESTRUCTIVE THROMBOCYTOPENIA

Incidental Thrombocytopenia of Pregnancy

Maternal thrombocytopenia occurs in 4% to 8% of pregnancies.[23] Most affected women are healthy and have no history of thrombocytopenia, and their thrombocytopenia is incidentally detected by routine blood testing. The cause of the mild reduction in platelet count (approximately $75 \times 10^9/L$ to $150 \times 10^9/L$) is believed to represent a leftward shift in the normal platelet count range during pregnancy related to one or more of hemodilution, reduced platelet production, or increased platelet turnover.[23] This condition is benign and is not associated with an increased risk for maternal bleeding or neonatal thrombocytopenia. Accordingly, no special maneuvers are indicated in these women, and the route of delivery should be determined by obstetric indications. Epidural anesthesia is believed to be safe if the platelet count is at least $75 \times 10^9/L$.

Preeclampsia and Eclampsia

Preeclampsia is characterized by the onset of hypertension and proteinuria during pregnancy, especially in a primigravida near term. Preeclampsia complicates approximately 5% of pregnancies, and the frequency is higher in black women. Thrombocytopenia occurs in up to 50% of preeclamptic patients, and its severity generally parallels that of the underlying preeclampsia.[23] A subset of patients with preeclampsia has microangiopathic hemolysis, elevated liver enzymes, and low platelets, widely known as the HELLP syndrome. This condition usually indicates severe preeclampsia and is associated with a higher risk of fetal and maternal complications, including maternal hepatic rupture. Repeated clinical and laboratory assessment of these patients is important because this syndrome can mimic other life-threatening complications of pregnancy, such as overt DIC, TTP, septicemia, and acute fatty liver of pregnancy.

Increased platelet destruction is the mechanism for the thrombocytopenia in preeclampsia. However, activation of the coagulation system is relatively modest, suggesting that thrombin generation may not be a major driver of the thrombocytopenia. Endothelial dysfunction (e.g., impaired nitric oxide synthesis) is a potential explanation for increased platelet turnover in preeclampsia.

Pharmacologic control of hypertension and rapid delivery are the treatments for preeclampsia and usually result in resolution of the thrombocytopenia within a few days. If delivery is not an option, treatment with bed rest and aggressive antihypertensive therapy has been reported to result in an improved platelet count. However, the clinical course is markedly variable, and some patients develop life-threatening organ failure. Plasmapheresis has been used in some patients, especially if there is evidence of thrombotic microangiopathy and organ dysfunction. Plasma exchange is appropriate for patients whose clinical picture has features suggesting TTP.

Infection

Infection is a common cause of thrombocytopenia, occurring in approximately 50% to 75% of patients with bacteremia or fungemia and in almost all patients with septic shock or DIC. Even when caused by bacteremia, the thrombocytopenia is generally mild to moderate in severity and is usually not accompanied by significant coagulation abnormalities or bleeding. The likelihood of laboratory evidence for DIC increases as the platelet count falls below $50 \times 10^9/L$. The mechanisms for thrombocytopenia in septicemia in the absence of DIC are uncertain but could include chemokine-induced macrophage ingestion of platelets (hemophagocytosis) and direct activation of platelets by endogenous mediators of inflammation (e.g., platelet-activating factor) or certain microbial products. In rare situations, platelet-reactive autoantibodies are implicated. Various explanations for thrombocytopenia in different types of infection are listed in Table 132.6.

Unexplained thrombocytopenia in a hospitalized patient warrants studies to exclude infection, such as blood cultures. Prompt recognition and treatment of the infection constitute the most important therapy because platelet count recovery tends to parallel the resolution of the infection. Prophylactic platelet transfusions are generally not required unless the platelet count falls below $10 \times 10^9/L$ or comorbid clinical features increase the likelihood of serious bleeding

TABLE
132.6

Mechanisms for Thrombocytopenia Complicating Infections

Mechanism for Thrombocytopenia	Selected Example(s)[a]
Increased Platelet Destruction	
DIC	Meningococcemia
Hemophagocytosis	Septicemia, EBV infection
Platelet-reactive autoantibodies (acute)	Varicella, subacute bacterial endocarditis (rare)
Platelet-reactive autoantibodies (chronic)	HIV infection
HUS	Verocytotoxin-producing *Escherichia coli, Shigella* spp., HIV infection
Antibodies against platelet-adsorbed microbial antigens	Malaria
Hypersplenism	
Acute	Disseminated *Mycobacterium avium* infection in HIV infection
Chronic	Viral chronic active hepatitis, malaria
Decreased Platelet Production	
Replacement of BM by granulomas	Ehrlichiosis, tuberculosis
Infection of megakaryocytes	HIV infection
Transient virus-induced aplasia	Parvovirus B19 infection (erythroblastopenia predominates)
Multiple Mechanisms	
Platelet destruction plus hypersplenism	Recurrent malaria
Increased platelet destruction, decreased platelet production, hypersplenism	Chronic HIV infection

[a]References can be found in Hoffman R, Benz EJ Jr, Shattil SJ, et al, eds: *Hematology: Basic Principles and Practice*, ed 3. New York, 2000, Churchill Livingstone. BM, Bone marrow; DIC, disseminated intravascular coagulation; EBV, Epstein-Barr virus; HIV, human immunodeficiency virus; HUS, hemolytic uremic syndrome.

(e.g., concomitant coagulopathy, an invasive procedure, uremic platelet dysfunction). The use of heparin for patients with septic shock and DIC is controversial. However, heparin may be of benefit in patients with clinical evidence of DIC and microvascular thrombosis (e.g., acral tissue ischemia or necrosis). The possibility of acquired protein C deficiency complicating acute DIC should also be considered in septic patients with purpura fulminans, such as that secondary to meningococcemia, or preceding "shock liver,"[4,5] in whom treatment with heparin[24] and plasma could be beneficial. Vitamin K administration is reasonable, although it will not help in the absence of vitamin K deficiency.

Thrombocytopenia in patients infected with HIV poses a special diagnostic problem because there are many potential explanations for the thrombocytopenia. These include immune platelet destruction, impaired platelet production secondary to HIV infection of megakaryocytes, drug-induced myelosuppression (commonly implicated drugs include zidovudine, ganciclovir, and TMP-SMX), HIV-associated thrombotic microangiopathy, hypersplenism, and BM infiltration by tumor or opportunistic infections. Platelet kinetic studies have shown a complex interaction of decreased platelet production, increased platelet destruction, and splenic platelet sequestration. Immune mechanisms for platelet destruction include antibodies that cross-react with GPIIb/IIIa complexes ("molecular mimicry") and

immune complexes containing IgM antiidiotype antibodies (which could explain the paradox of high levels of platelet-associated IgG and IgM with low serum levels of platelet-reactive antibodies). Anti-HIV therapy (e.g., zidovudine, HAART) often raises the platelet count in patients with HIV-associated thrombocytopenia. Most patients with HIV-associated thrombocytopenia respond to conventional treatments for ITP, including corticosteroids, splenectomy, IVIg, and, particularly, anti-D.

Systemic Lupus Erythematosus

Immune-mediated thrombocytopenia, which occurs in as many as 25% of patients with SLE, is associated with a twofold increased risk of organ damage events. Many different types of platelet–IgG interactions are described (e.g., antiglycoprotein, antiglycolipid, β_2-glycoprotein I [β_2GPI]–containing immune complexes). In addition, antithrombopoietin, anti–c-Mpl (thrombopoietin receptor), and anti-CD40 ligand autoantibodies have been reported. Multiple causes for thrombocytopenia—increased platelet destruction, hypersplenism, and even impaired platelet production related to antibody-induced megakaryocytic hypoplasia—have been reported. The predominant explanation for thrombocytopenia in SLE remains unknown.

Several thrombocytopenic syndromes are seen in patients with SLE. For many patients, the thrombocytopenia is chronic, resembling ITP, and is the predominant clinical manifestation of the lupus. Often, these patients have a prolonged bleeding time despite mild thrombocytopenia. Some thrombocytopenic patients with SLE have antiphospholipid (aPL) antibodies and are at increased risk for thrombotic rather than bleeding complications (see Chapter 141). Acute, severe thrombocytopenia can be a prominent feature in patients with a severe multisystem exacerbation of lupus. Rarely, patients with SLE develop an illness that closely resembles TTP or HUS; these patients should be treated with plasma exchange. Thrombocytopenia as a feature of SLE-associated, viral-induced macrophage activation syndrome has been reported.

Treatment of the thrombocytopenia of SLE is similar to that of ITP (see Chapter 131). Corticosteroids constitute the first line of therapy, but many patients do not respond or require high doses. High-dose IVIg may be useful in patients who are bleeding to transiently increase the platelet count. Before resorting to splenectomy, one could try danazol (an attenuated androgen) in doses of 200–800 mg/day. Higher doses can cause hepatitis. Typically, several weeks of treatment are required before a benefit is seen. Splenectomy is probably as effective in achieving platelet count remission in SLE as in ITP. Patients with refractory thrombocytopenia sometimes benefit from more aggressive therapies, such as azathioprine, intermittent-pulse cyclophosphamide, plasmapheresis synchronized with pulse cyclophosphamide, cyclosporine, thrombopoietin mimetics, or rituximab.

Antiphospholipid Syndrome

Antiphospholipid syndrome (APS; see Chapter 141) is characterized by occurrence of one or more clinical events (e.g., venous, arterial or small vessel thrombosis, pregnancy loss, preterm delivery for patients with severe preeclampsia or placental insufficiency) associated with IgG, IgM, or IgA antibodies that recognize a complex of one or more protein cofactors (e.g., β_2GPI, annexin V, prothrombin, protein C, protein S) bound to negatively charged phospholipid. Many patients (30%–50%) with this syndrome have thrombocytopenia, which is typically mild and intermittent; approximately 15% have autoimmune hemolysis. The APS should be considered in patients who develop idiopathic lower limb or abdominal vein (mesenteric, renal, adrenal) thrombosis, cerebral venous (dural sinus) thrombosis, cardiac valvulitis, nonatheromatous arterial thrombosis (especially thrombotic stroke in a patient younger than 50 years of age), dermal microvascular thrombosis (acrocyanosis, digital ulceration or gangrene, livedo reticularis), or acute multiorgan failure associated with DIC or widespread thrombosis of the microvasculature (catastrophic APS).

The mechanism of the prothrombotic tendency in patients with APS remains elusive, but interference with endothelial cell function, impaired fibrinolysis, antibody-mediated platelet activation, formation of endothelial microparticles, interference with thrombin and factor Xa degradation by antithrombin, disturbance in the protein C anticoagulant pathway or anticoagulant activity of β_2GPI have all been described. Disruption of the antithrombotic annexin V antithrombotic "shield" by aPL antibodies has been proposed to explain pregnancy losses through placental vascular thrombosis. Evidence indicates that thrombocytopenia in patients with APS is associated with platelet GP-reactive autoantibodies.

aPL antibodies are detected by either of two methods: (1) solid-phase ELISA with purified phospholipids (usually cardiolipin) as target antigens or (2) a "functional" assay for so-called lupus anticoagulant (LA) activity, shown by demonstrating inhibition of certain phospholipid-dependent coagulation assays, such as the activated partial thromboplastin time or the Russell viper venom time. Although aPL antibodies are frequently detected in patients with SLE, they can also be found in patients with other autoimmune disorders, malignancy, or infections or as a complication of certain drugs (e.g., procainamide). Often no associated condition is identified ("primary" APS). aPL antibodies of low titer are sometimes found in normal persons, particularly elderly individuals, or during normal pregnancy. Autoantibody "cluster" studies show that anticardiolipin, LA, and anti–double-stranded DNA antibodies occur together more often than with other SLE-associated autoantibodies (e.g., anti-Sm, anti-Ro, anti-RNP).

There are intriguing parallels between the APS and HIT: in both disorders, the antibodies are directed at a protein target (β_2GPI and PF4, respectively) bound to a negatively charged species (anionic phospholipid and heparin, respectively). For both, high-titer IgG antibodies that result in a positive "functional" test result (LA activity and HIT-IgG–induced platelet activation, respectively) are most likely to be associated with clinical disease. Both disorders are characterized by the paradox of thrombocytopenia associated with increased risk for venous and arterial thrombosis.

To help physicians diagnose the APS, clinical and laboratory criteria have been developed. The laboratory criteria include the presence of anticardiolipin, anti-β_2GPI, or LA antibodies (moderate- to high-titer IgG or IgM) on two or more occasions at least 12 weeks apart. The major clinical criteria are thrombosis and complications of pregnancy. Thrombosis can involve large arteries or veins or small vessels within any organ. The complications of pregnancy include one or more unexplained deaths of normal fetus(es) after week 10 of gestation or premature births (before 34 weeks) or more than three spontaneous abortions before week 10 of gestation. Some experts advocate for thrombocytopenia to be included within the criteria for APS.[25]

Specific treatment for the thrombocytopenia is not usually required. For many patients, long-term anticoagulant or antiplatelet therapy, or both, are needed to prevent recurrent thrombosis. For patients with recurring pregnancy losses and aPL antibodies, randomized trials have documented the benefit of low-dose aspirin combined with either low-dose UFH or low-molecular-weight heparin (LMWH).

Malignancy

Thrombocytopenia complicating malignant disorders most frequently results from antineoplastic treatment or BM replacement by tumor. However, certain thrombocytopenic syndromes have been associated with malignancy, including autoimmune thrombocytopenia, DIC, and thrombotic microangiopathy.

ITP attributable to platelet GP-reactive autoantibodies can complicate neoplastic lymphoproliferative diseases such as Hodgkin disease, non-Hodgkin lymphoma, chronic lymphocytic leukemia,

and multiple myeloma. Sometimes the thrombocytopenia responds to treatment of the neoplasm, although in some patients (particularly those with Hodgkin disease), the thrombocytopenia is indistinguishable from ITP and is not related to the activity of the lymphoma.

DIC occurs with certain malignancies, particularly adenocarcinoma of the pancreas, stomach, lung, colon, breast, and prostate. Some patients present with venous or, less commonly, arterial thrombosis as the first clinical manifestation of their malignancy. In these patients, the presence of thrombocytopenia is an important clue that should prompt investigations for DIC, such as measurement of fibrinogen or D-dimer levels. In the author's experience, the platelet count typically rises to normal or even elevated levels with heparin therapy because heparin ameliorates the DIC process; however, recurrent thrombocytopenia and thrombosis can occur within hours of discontinuing the heparin therapy.[26] Cancer patients with DIC and venous thrombosis are also at increased risk for warfarin-associated venous limb gangrene.[26] The role of various tumor-associated procoagulant substances—such as "cancer procoagulant" (a 68-kDa cysteine proteinase that activates factor X independently of tissue factor/factor VIIa) and cancer-associated tissue factor (which is expressed on tumor cells, as well as circulating microparticles)—suggest pathophysiologic parallels with microthrombosis in HIT because both cancer-associated DIC and acute HIT are risk factors for phlegmasia cerulea dolens and venous limb gangrene during anticoagulation with warfarin. Thus cancer patients with DIC should receive heparin (especially LMWH) rather than warfarin anticoagulation (see box on Diagnostic Considerations in the Patient With Limb Ischemia and Thrombocytopenia in Chapter 133). DIC with hemorrhagic manifestations is characteristically seen in some patients with prostate cancer and in many patients with acute promyelocytic leukemia. It is crucial to recognize promyelocytic leukemia because treatment with all-*trans*-retinoic acid produces differentiation of the malignant cells, thereby rapidly reducing the life-threatening bleeding risks attributable to hyperfibrinolysis.

A destructive thrombocytopenic disorder that resembles HUS or TTP has been described in patients with advanced cancer. In some patients, mitomycin, gemcitabine, or other drugs may have contributed to the microangiopathy. DIC is not usually present. Some patients respond transiently to plasmapheresis, but for many, response to any therapy is poor.

Macrophage Activation (Hemophagocytic) Syndrome

The macrophage activation (or hemophagocytic) syndrome comprises a heterogeneous group of disorders characterized by variable cytopenias and morphologic evidence of macrophage phagocytosis of RBCs, granulocytes, and platelets; hyperferritinemia, hypercytokinemia, and sepsis-like features are characteristic, with potential for evolution to fatal multiple organ failure.[27] Some adult patients have an aggressive disease characterized by high fever, weight loss, prominent hepatosplenomegaly, severe pancytopenia, elevated liver enzymes, and often a terminal infection. Both T- and B-cell lymphomas can explain such a dramatic syndrome. However, similar patients with fulminant illness have been described after otherwise unremarkable bacterial or viral infections (particularly those caused by Epstein-Barr virus). In children, the high mortality rate associated with hemophagocytic lymphohistiocytosis warrants aggressive treatment, including antineoplastic chemotherapy and BM transplantation. Nonneoplastic but nonetheless severe hemophagocytosis can be seen in patients with certain infections (e.g., babesiosis, ehrlichiosis, HIV infection), as well as in patients with rheumatologic disorders (SLE, Still disease, ankylosing spondylitis). Laboratory indicators of macrophage activation syndrome include markedly elevated ferritin,[28] high levels of soluble CD163 and CD25, and morphologic evidence of hemophagocytosis. Treatment should be directed at the underlying illness. Early administration of corticosteroids and high-dose IVIg appears to benefit some patients with nonneoplastic macrophage activation syndrome.

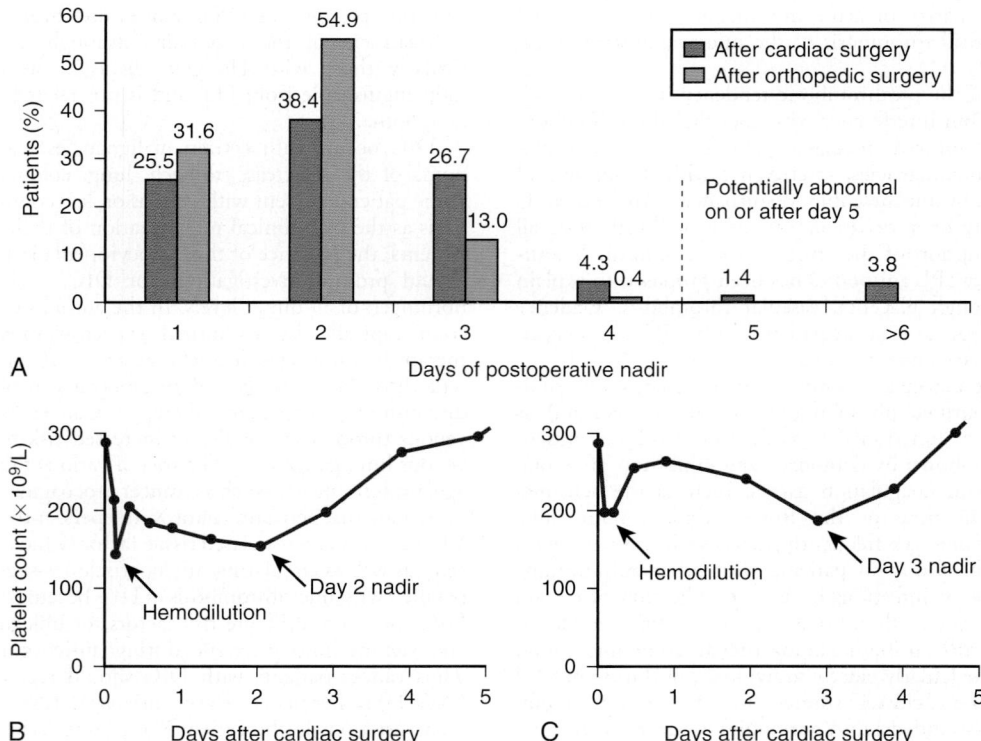

Fig. 132.7 EARLY POSTOPERATIVE PLATELET COUNT DECLINES. (A) Distribution of early postoperative count nadirs. For both orthopedic and cardiac surgery patients, day 2 represents the most common day for the postoperative platelet count nadir to occur (data exclude day 0); beyond postoperative day 4, it is likely that a superimposed thrombocytopenic disorder is occurring. (B and C) Representative postcardiac surgery platelet count declines. Both patients illustrate early hemodilution effects (day 0) and subsequent additional early platelet count declines with nadirs of day 2 (B) and day 3 (C). Neither patient received platelet transfusions. *(From Greinacher A, Warkentin TE: Acquired non-immune thrombocytopenia. In: Marder VJ, Aird WC, Bennett JS, et al, editors:* Hemostasis and thrombosis: Basic principles and clinical practice, *ed 6. Philadelphia, 2013, Lippincott Williams & Wilkins, p 796.)*

Solid Organ and Bone Marrow Transplantation

Thrombocytopenia commonly occurs during episodes of solid organ allograft rejection. It is possible that platelet activation and deposition in the transplanted organ vasculature contribute to the rejection process. Antirejection therapies can also cause thrombocytopenia through increased platelet destruction (antilymphocyte globulin) or BM suppression (azathioprine). Posttransplantation HUS develops in approximately 5% of renal transplant recipients and in even fewer recipients of liver or heart transplants. Although cyclosporine is sometimes implicated in HUS, it can usually be safely resumed after recovery.

Early, severe thrombocytopenia caused by BM-ablative therapy invariably accompanies BM transplantation (BMT). Platelet count recovery to greater than $50 \times 10^9/L$ is more rapid (16 vs. 35 days) in patients receiving autologous mobilized peripheral blood progenitor cells than in those undergoing autologous BMT. Severe persistent thrombocytopenia despite recovery of RBCs and WBCs is relatively common after BMT or peripheral blood transplantation; autoimmune thrombocytopenia has been implicated in some patients. Late-onset thrombocytopenia after BMT that responds to corticosteroids, IVIg, and splenectomy also has been attributed to autoimmune thrombocytopenia. Rarely, transplantation-associated alloimmune thrombocytopenia can be caused by donor–recipient incompatibility involving platelet-specific alloantigens such as Pl[A1] (HPA-1a) or Br[a] (HPA-5b).

A syndrome of thrombocytopenia, RBC fragmentation, and renal impairment can occur in as many as 10% of patients undergoing BMT, usually beginning 3–12 months after transplantation (BMT-associated thrombotic microangiopathy). The pathogenesis remains obscure; reduced ADAMTS13 (a disintegrin and metalloproteinase with thrombospondin 13) levels have not been implicated. The hematologic abnormalities can be mild and remit spontaneously, although patients often have residual azotemia and hypertension. More severely affected patients do not usually benefit from plasmapheresis. The syndrome has a poor overall prognosis, and many patients die irrespective of any intervention.

Cardiopulmonary Bypass Surgery

Excess bleeding is a common problem in patients who undergo heart surgery using cardiopulmonary bypass. Many of these patients receive blood transfusions, and approximately 5% require reoperation for postoperative bleeding.

Thrombocytopenia and transient platelet dysfunction (see Chapter 159) are observed in virtually every patient. Typically, the platelet count falls by 30% to 70%, primarily as a result of hemodilution but also because of bleeding and losses within the extracorporeal perfusion device. Because patients invariably receive heparin during cardiac surgery and have often received heparin in the remote or recent past, immune HIT is frequently considered in the differential diagnosis of early-onset and persisting postcardiac surgery thrombocytopenia; however, HIT is an unlikely explanation for thrombocytopenia even when anti-PF4/heparin antibodies are positive.[29]

The bleeding time increases markedly during heart surgery (to greater than 30 minutes) but usually improves to less than 15 minutes shortly after surgery and to normal several hours later. By contrast, the thrombocytopenia persists for 3–4 days followed by recovery of the platelet count to values exceeding the preoperative baseline.

The pathogenesis and clinical significance of the hemostatic defect in these patients remain uncertain, but the explanation is probably multifactorial. Studies have described transient, *intrinsic* defects in platelet function. These defects include decreased in vitro platelet aggregation, decreased platelet surface membrane proteins, selective depletion of platelet α-granules, and evidence of in vivo platelet activation and platelet vesiculation. The platelet dysfunction in heart surgery is also attributable to an *extrinsic* platelet defect resulting from thrombin inhibition by the high doses of heparin. Furthermore, an important role for hyperfibrinolysis in the pathogenesis of bleeding is shown by elevated D-dimer levels in bleeding patients, as well as the efficacy of antifibrinolytic agents in the prevention and treatment of heart surgery–associated bleeding. Other factors in some patients include residual heparin effect after bypass (including heparin rebound) and preoperative use of aspirin and/or clopidogrel. Treatment of platelet dysfunction after cardiopulmonary bypass is discussed in Chapter 159.

THROMBOCYTOPENIA ASSOCIATED WITH CARDIOVASCULAR DISEASE

Congenital Cyanotic Heart Disease

Thrombocytopenia caused by a decrease in platelet life span occurs in some patients with severe cyanotic congenital heart disease and is approximately related to the severity of the polycythemia. Bleeding occurs in a few patients and can be related to platelet function defects, coagulopathy, or hyperfibrinolysis. Reducing the hematocrit by phlebotomy sometimes helps to correct the hemostatic defects.

Valvular Heart Disease

Increased platelet turnover is common in valvular heart disease, and some patients have mild thrombocytopenia. The pathogenesis of the platelet consumption is not well understood, but the defect could be related to increased platelet–von Willebrand factor (vWF) interactions at high shear. Indeed, high-molecular-weight multimers of vWF are reduced in some of these patients, which explains why bleeding from gastrointestinal angiodysplasia in patients with aortic stenosis (Heyde syndrome) typically resolves after aortic valve replacement.[30] Thrombocytopenia secondary to consumptive coagulopathy can be seen in intracardiac thrombosis associated with valvular heart disease.

Pulmonary Vascular Disorders

Disorders characterized by pulmonary hypertension can be accompanied by thrombocytopenia, the pathogenesis of which is poorly defined. Thrombocytopenia can occur in association with pulmonary embolism, possibly as a result of DIC. When evaluating such patients, the clinician should inquire about current or recent heparin exposure because HIT and pulmonary embolism are strongly associated.

HEMODILUTION AND PLATELET CONSUMPTION AFTER SURGERY

Platelet count declines of 30% to 70% occur universally after major surgery and reflect the combined effects of hemodilution and increased platelet consumption. Such hemodilution-associated thrombocytopenia is especially prominent after cardiac surgery and is proportional to the amount of fluids (crystalloid, colloid, blood products) administered. The platelet count fall is abrupt and is evident a few hours after surgery. Dilutional coagulopathy also occurs, which is responsible for the minor to moderate increases in coagulation test results that occur transiently after surgery.

Perioperative hemodilution is also usually accompanied by increased platelet consumption related to the effects of surgery. This helps to explain why the postsurgery platelet count usually continues to decline over the next 1–3 days, with the postoperative nadir (lowest platelet count value) usually occurring at a median of postoperative day 2, with a range between postoperative days 1–4 (Fig. 132.7).[2] Subsequently, there is a rise in the platelet count that peaks at approximately day 14 at levels often 2–3 times the patient's preoperative baseline before it returns to baseline over the next 2 weeks (≈day 28). As described earlier in this chapter (see Fig. 132.1), these platelet count changes reflect thrombopoietin physiology.

REFERENCES

1. Arnold DM, Warkentin TE: Thrombocytopenia and thrombocytosis. In Wilson WC, Grande CM, Hoyt DB, editors: *Trauma: Critical care*, (vol 2). New York, 2007, Informa Healthcare USA, p 983.
2. Greinacher A, Warkentin TE: Acquired non-immune thrombocytopenia. In Marder VJ, Aird WC, Bennett JS, editors: *Hemostasis and thrombosis: Basic principles and clinical practice*, ed 6, Philadelphia, 2013, Lippincott Williams & Wilkins, p 796.
3. Warkentin TE, Kelton JG: Temporal aspects of heparin-induced thrombocytopenia. *N Engl J Med* 344:1286, 2001.
4. Siegel DM, Cook RJ, Warkentin TE: Acute hepatic necrosis and ischemic limb necrosis. *N Engl J Med* 367:879, 2012.
5. Warkentin TE: Ischemic limb gangrene with pulses. *N Engl J Med* 373:642, 2015.
6. Eskazan AE, Buyuktas D, Soysal T: Postoperative thrombotic thrombocytopenic purpura. *Surg Today* 45:8, 2015.
7. Harji DP, Jaunoo SS, Mistry P, et al: Immunoprophylaxis in asplenic patients. *Int J Surg* 7:421, 2009.
8. Aster RH, Bougie DW: Drug-induced immune thrombocytopenia. *N Engl J Med* 357:580, 2007.
9. Warkentin TE: Drug-induced immune-mediated thrombocytopenia—from purpura to thrombosis. *N Engl J Med* 356:891, 2007.
10. Arnold DM, Nazi I, Warkentin TE, et al: Approach to the diagnosis and management of drug-induced immune thrombocytopenia. *Transfus Med Rev* 27:137, 2013.
11. George JN, Nester CM: Syndromes of thrombotic microangiopathy. *N Engl J Med* 371:654, 2014.
12. George JN, Raskob GE, Shah SR, et al: Drug-induced thrombocytopenia: a systematic review of published case reports. *Ann Intern Med* 129:886, 1988.
13. Reese JA, Li X, Hauben M, et al: Identifying drugs that cause acute thrombocytopenia: an analysis using 3 distinct methods. *Blood* 116:2127, 2010.
14. Arnold DM, Kukaswadia S, Nazi I, et al: A systematic evaluation of laboratory testing for drug-induced thrombocytopenia. *J Thromb Haemost* 11:169, 2013.
15. Von Drygalski A, Curtis BR, Bougie DW, et al: Vancomycin induced immune thrombocytopenia. *N Engl J Med* 356:904, 2007.
16. Bougie DW, Wilker PR, Aster RH: Patients with quinine-induced immune thrombocytopenia have both "drug-dependent" and "drug-specific" antibodies. *Blood* 108:922, 2006.
17. Liu X, Sahud MA: Glycoprotein IIb/IIIa complex is the target in mirtazapine-induced immune thrombocytopenia. *Blood Cell Mol Dis* 30:241, 2003.
18. Stuhec M, Alisky J, Malesic I: Mirtazapine associated with drug-related thrombocytopenia: a case report. *J Clin Psychopharmacol* 34:662, 2014.
19. Aster RH, Curtis BR, McFarland JG, et al: Drug-induced immune thrombocytopenia: pathogenesis, diagnosis, and management. *J Thromb Haemost* 7:911, 2009.
20. Bougie DW, Nayak D, Boylan B, et al: Drug-dependent clearance of human platelets in the NOD/scid mouse by antibodies from patients with drug-induced immune thrombocytopenia. *Blood* 116:3033, 2010.
21. Aster RH, Curtis BR, Bougie DW, et al: Thrombocytopenia associated with the use of GPIIb/IIIa inhibitors: Position paper of the ISTH working group on thrombocytopenia and GPIIb/IIIa inhibitors. *J Thromb Haemost* 4:678, 2006.

22. Al-Nouri ZL, Reese JA, Terrell DR, et al: Drug-induced thrombotic microangiopathy: a systematic review of published reports. *Blood* 125:605, 2015.

23. McCrae KR: Thrombocytopenia in pregnancy. *Hematology Am Soc Hematol Educ Program* 397:2010, 2010.

24. Zarychanski R, Abou-Setta AM, Kanji S, et al: The efficacy and safety of heparin in patients with sepsis: a systematic review and metaanalysis. *Crit Care Med* 19:123, 2015.

25. Cervera R, Tektonidou MG, Espinosa G, et al: Task force on catastrophic antiphospholipid syndrome (APS) and non-criteria APS manifestations (II): thrombocytopenia and skin manifestations. *Lupus* 20:174, 2011.

26. Warkentin TE: Venous limb gangrene during warfarin treatment of cancer-associated deep venous thrombosis. *Ann Intern Med* 135(8 Pt 1):589, 2001.

27. Usmani GM, Woda BA, Newburger PE: Advances in understanding the pathogenesis of HLH. *Br J Haematol* 161:609, 2013.

28. Lehmberg K, McClain KL, Janka GE, et al: Determination of an appropriate cut-off value for ferritin in the diagnosis of hemophagocytic lymphohistiocytosis. *Pediatr Blood Cancer* 61:2101, 2014.

29. Selleng S, Malowsky B, Strobel U, et al: Early-onset and persisting thrombocytopenia in post-cardiac surgery patients is rarely due to heparin-induced thrombocytopenia, even when antibody tests are positive. *J Thromb Haemost* 8:30, 2010.

30. Warkentin TE, Moore JC, Anand SS, et al: Gastrointestinal bleeding, angiodysplasia, cardiovascular disease, and acquired von Willebrand syndrome. *Transfus Med Rev* 17:272, 2003.

CHAPTER 133

HEPARIN-INDUCED THROMBOCYTOPENIA

Theodore E. Warkentin

Heparin-induced thrombocytopenia (HIT) is the most important drug-induced immune-mediated cytopenia for several reasons. First, heparin is a widely used anticoagulant (see Chapter 149). Second, HIT is relatively common, occurring in approximately 1% to 3% of postoperative patients, and 0.2% to 0.5% of medical patients, who receive unfractionated heparin (UFH) derived from porcine intestine for 7–14 days.[1] Third, HIT frequently causes life- and limb-threatening venous or arterial thrombosis. Finally, there are several pitfalls of HIT management, including the potential for thrombocytopenia and/or thrombosis to worsen despite stopping heparin, the high risk for warfarin-associated microthrombosis (most often manifesting as venous limb gangrene), and the potential for failure of approved direct thrombin inhibitor (DTI) therapy because of the confounding of activated partial thromboplastin time (aPTT)-monitored dosing that results from HIT-associated coagulopathies.

HIT is caused by platelet-activating immunoglobulin G (IgG) antibodies that bind to multimolecular complexes of platelet factor 4 (PF4) bound to heparin.[2,3] Although anti-PF4/heparin antibodies are frequently triggered by heparin therapy, relatively few patients develop clinically evident HIT. Indeed, a major current problem with HIT is its "overdiagnosis"[4]: only 5% to 10% of patients who are referred for antibody testing have a serologic profile that supports a diagnosis of HIT.[5] The challenge for the clinician is to discern which of the (many) patients who develop thrombocytopenia in association with heparin therapy really have HIT, a conundrum magnified by the observation that at most 50% of anti-PF4/heparin antibody–positive patients have "true" HIT, as indicated by the presence of platelet-activating IgG antibodies.[1,5]

EPIDEMIOLOGY

Table 133.1 lists risk factors for HIT. The highest risk for HIT is seen in patients with multiple interacting risk factors (e.g., females given postoperative thromboprophylaxis with UFH for 2 weeks [frequency approximately 5%]).[6] Even higher frequencies (approximately 10%) are reported in patients with ventricular assist devices who are receiving therapeutic doses of UFH. Ironically, even though the risk for HIT appears to be somewhat higher in women (odds ratio, 1.5–2.0),[6] HIT is rare in pregnancy, particularly with the use of low-molecular-weight heparin (LMWH). The synthetic antithrombin-binding sulfated pentasaccharide, fondaparinux, although similarly immunizing as LMWH, is much less likely than LMWH to cause HIT, likely because fondaparinux does not usually increase the platelet-activating potential of HIT antibodies.[7] Indeed, fondaparinux appears to be an effective treatment for HIT (discussed later).

Only a minority of patients who form anti-PF4/heparin antibodies following heparin treatment develop clinically evident HIT.[2,3] The proportion of antibody-positive patients who develop HIT ranges from as high as one-third (e.g., postorthopedic surgery thromboprophylaxis with UFH) to as few as 1 in 50 (postcardiac surgery patients).[1,2] Notably, the risk for HIT in postcardiac surgery patients who receive UFH thromboprophylaxis is only approximately 1% even though as many as 50% to 80% of patients develop detectable anti-PF4/heparin antibodies within 2 weeks of surgery.[1] In general, those at highest risk for HIT are the subgroup of patients whose anti-PF4/heparin antibodies evince strong platelet-activating properties

in vitro.[2,3] However, patient-dependent susceptibility factors are also important, because at most only half of all patients who form platelet-activating antibodies develop HIT.

PATHOBIOLOGY

Fig. 133.1 illustrates several features of HIT pathogenesis. Heparin binds reversibly and saturably to platelets and can weakly activate platelets in vitro through potentiation of $\alpha_{IIb}\beta_3$-mediated outside-in signaling.[8] In general, the direct platelet-activating effects of heparin, as well as its immunogenicity, are proportional to its molecular mass and degree of sulfation; consequently, LMWH is less likely to cause HIT than UFH.[1,2,6]

Platelet activation by HIT antibodies occurs because platelet-activating HIT-IgG cross-link platelet FcγIIa receptors.[1–3] The HIT antigens reside on large multimolecular complexes formed between cationic PF4—a member of the CXC subfamily of chemokines—and anionic heparin. A unique laboratory characteristic of HIT is that high heparin concentrations (10–100 units/mL) inhibit platelet activation by the pathogenic IgG[9]; this laboratory feature is exploited in diagnostic testing for HIT (see Diagnosis).

There is a characteristic timeline that underlies the HIT immune response (Fig. 133.2).[3] Formation of pathogenic IgG antibodies is surprisingly fast, even in patients who have never previously been exposed to heparin. Bacterial cell walls, which are negatively charged, bind PF4, and there is evidence that bacterial infection could be responsible for preimmunization against PF4-dependent antigens.[10] This could explain both the high frequency of anti-PF4/heparin immunization and of clinical HIT (i.e., HIT could represent a misdirected antibacterial immune response).[10] Although heparin-treated patients can form heparin-dependent antibodies of the IgM or IgA subclass, these are unlikely to cause HIT.[1–3]

Excess thrombin generation contributes to the pathogenesis of some of the unusual sequelae of HIT, which can include venous thromboembolism,[11] warfarin-associated venous limb gangrene,[12] and overt (decompensated) disseminated intravascular coagulation (DIC). Increased thrombin generation in HIT is triggered by the shedding of procoagulant microparticles from platelets activated by HIT antibodies, as well as by the expression of tissue factor by endothelial cells or monocytes activated by HIT antibodies (see Fig. 133.1).[13]

As noted, thrombocytopenia develops in only a minority of patients who form HIT antibodies.[1] The variable risk for HIT in different patient populations may reflect variations in the susceptibility of platelets to activation by HIT-IgG and/or differences in the levels and immunoglobulin class composition of HIT antibodies.[2,3] Poorly defined clinical factors also influence the risk for HIT, which occurs more often in surgical patients than in medical or obstetric patients.[6] Major trauma was more likely than minor trauma to be associated with HIT antibody formation and clinical HIT in one study.[14] There is indirect evidence that formation of stoichiometrically optimal complexes of PF4/heparin influences the risk for immunization.[15] The clinical situation influences the type of HIT-associated thrombosis: venous thromboembolism typically develops in orthopedic patients with HIT, whereas thrombosis develops equally often in arteries and in veins in cardiovascular patients with HIT.[1]

TABLE 133.1	Risk Factors for Heparin-Induced Thrombocytopenia
Heparin type	Unfractionated > low-molecular-weight heparin > fondaparinux
Patient type	Postoperative (major > minor surgery) > medical > obstetric/pediatric
Dose[a]	Prophylactic dose > therapeutic dose > flushes
Duration	11–14 days[b] > 5–10 days > 4 days or fewer
Sex	Female > male

[a]Importance of heparin dose is uncertain because of confounding effect of patient type (e.g., postoperative patients tend to receive prophylactic-dose heparin whereas medical patients [e.g., with venous thromboembolism] are more likely to receive therapeutic-dose heparin); nevertheless, reported frequencies of heparin-induced thrombocytopenia (HIT) are relatively high in patients given postoperative prophylactic-dose heparin.
[b]Heparin exposure beyond 14 days does not usually increase the risk of HIT beyond that of an 11- to 14-day exposure.

CLINICAL AND LABORATORY MANIFESTATIONS

Most patients with HIT have moderate thrombocytopenia; The median platelet count nadir is approximately 60×10^9/L; for 90% of patients, the platelet count nadir is greater than 20×10^9/L (Fig. 133.3).[16] In the rare patient whose platelet count falls to less than 10×10^9/L, there is often evidence of overt DIC, and red cell fragments and circulating normoblasts may be evident on examination of the blood smear. Thrombosis can occur in HIT patients even if there is a minimal decrease in the platelet count, and even if the platelet count nadir never falls below 150×10^9/L.[1]

The platelet count fall usually begins 5–10 days after the initiation of an immunizing heparin exposure and while the patient continues to receive heparin (typical-onset HIT).[17] Usually the immunizing trigger is heparin given during surgery (e.g., cardiac or vascular surgery) or that is started soon after surgery (e.g., thromboprophylaxis). Interestingly, starting LMWH thromboprophylaxis before elective surgery (as is more frequently done in Europe) is less likely to be associated with antibody formation compared with postoperative first-dose administration.[15]

HIT is recognized in approximately one-quarter of patients when the platelet count fall occurs abruptly after restarting UFH or LMWH (rapid-onset HIT). Invariably, such patients have been exposed to heparin within the previous 5–100 days,[17] because HIT antibodies are transient and are only detectable for several weeks after an immunizing heparin exposure. Consequently, rapid-onset HIT, which is caused by administration of heparin to a patient with preformed HIT antibodies, is strongly associated with recent heparin exposure.

Sometimes, thrombocytopenia occurs several days after a brief exposure to heparin or worsens despite stopping heparin (delayed-onset HIT).[4,18] On exceptionally rare occasions, a transient prothrombotic disorder that resembles HIT clinically and serologically occurs without an apparent preceding heparin exposure; triggers of so-called "spontaneous HIT syndrome" include knee replacement surgery (perhaps because of release of heparin-like glycosaminoglycans from knee cartilage) and infection.[19,20]

HIT is a highly prothrombotic condition: At least 50% of HIT patients develop thrombosis.[1,11,16] Both venous (deep vein thrombosis and/or pulmonary embolism) and arterial (especially aortic and iliofemoral arterial thrombosis, stroke, or myocardial infarction) thrombosis can occur.[11] Other complications include necrotizing skin lesions at the sites of subcutaneous heparin injection and acute inflammatory/cardiorespiratory (anaphylactoid) or transient memory disturbances after intravenous heparin bolus administration to sensitized persons. Unexplained hypotension or abdominal pain in a patient with HIT suggests bilateral adrenal hemorrhagic infarction, which can lead to acute adrenal failure; the hemorrhagic adrenal necrosis is the result of adrenal vein thrombosis.[20]

Diagnostic Considerations in the Patient With Limb Ischemia and Thrombocytopenia

Concurrence of limb ischemia/necrosis and thrombocytopenia suggests one of several hematologic emergencies:

- **Heparin-induced thrombocytopenia.** Occlusion of large lower-limb arteries by platelet-rich "white clots" is characteristic of heparin-induced thrombocytopenia (HIT). The major clue is an otherwise unexplained platelet count fall that begins 5 or more days after initiation of heparin. Urgent thromboembolectomy may be limb sparing. Sensitive assays for HIT antibodies give strongly positive results. See subsequent entry for warfarin.
- **Adenocarcinoma-associated disseminated intravascular coagulation.** Severe venous or arterial thrombosis can develop in patients with metastatic adenocarcinoma who have disseminated intravascular coagulation (DIC).[21] This often occurs within hours after stopping heparin. A clinical clue is an otherwise unexplained rise in platelet count that occurs with initial or repeated heparin therapy. See next entry for warfarin.
- **Warfarin-induced phlegmasia cerulea dolens/venous limb gangrene.** Coumarin anticoagulants, such as warfarin, can lead to venous ischemia (phlegmasia cerulea dolens) or venous limb gangrene in patients with DIC caused by HIT[12] or adenocarcinoma.[21] Limb loss can occur even though the limb pulses are palpable.
- **Sepsis-associated microvascular thrombosis.** Acquired natural anticoagulant depletion (e.g., markedly reduced antithrombin or protein C levels) can complicate DIC associated with sepsis, leading to bilateral acral limb ischemia or necrosis involving feet and (sometimes) fingers/hands ("symmetric peripheral gangrene").
- **Septic embolism.** Rarely, infective endocarditis or aneurysmal thrombosis leads to the constellation of thrombocytopenia and acute limb ischemia.
- **Antiphospholipid syndrome.** Autoimmune thrombocytopenia and hypercoagulability can interact to produce acute limb ischemia and thrombocytopenia in patients with antiphospholipid syndrome.

Patients with HIT have an unusual predisposition to develop ischemic limb necrosis. Indeed, approximately 5% of such patients develop some degree of limb necrosis necessitating amputation. Occasionally multiple limbs are involved (see the box on Diagnostic Considerations in the Patient With Limb Ischemia and Thrombocytopenia).

DIFFERENTIAL DIAGNOSIS

Only approximately 10% of patients who undergo laboratory investigations for clinically suspected HIT have a serologic profile that supports the diagnosis (i.e., detectable heparin-dependent, platelet-activating IgG antibodies that recognize PF4/heparin complexes).[5] The differential diagnosis includes postoperative thrombocytopenia (hemodilution/platelet consumption), thrombocytopenia of critical illness, and septicemia. Some non-HIT disorders mimic HIT so closely that they warrant the term *pseudo-HIT*. One example of pseudo-HIT is adenocarcinoma-associated DIC, in which the combination of progressive thrombocytopenia and severe venous limb ischemia that occurs during the transitioning of patients from heparin (either UFH or LMWH) to warfarin may suggest a diagnosis of HIT.[21] Another disorder that can mimic HIT is the antiphospholipid syndrome: here, thrombocytopenia, thrombosis, and a false-positive PF4-dependent enzyme immunoassay (EIA) caused by anti-PF4 (not anti-PF4/heparin) antibodies can be present.[22]

CLINICAL SCORING SYSTEMS

The pretest probability of HIT can be estimated using validated scoring systems. The 4Ts system represents a mnemonic that is based

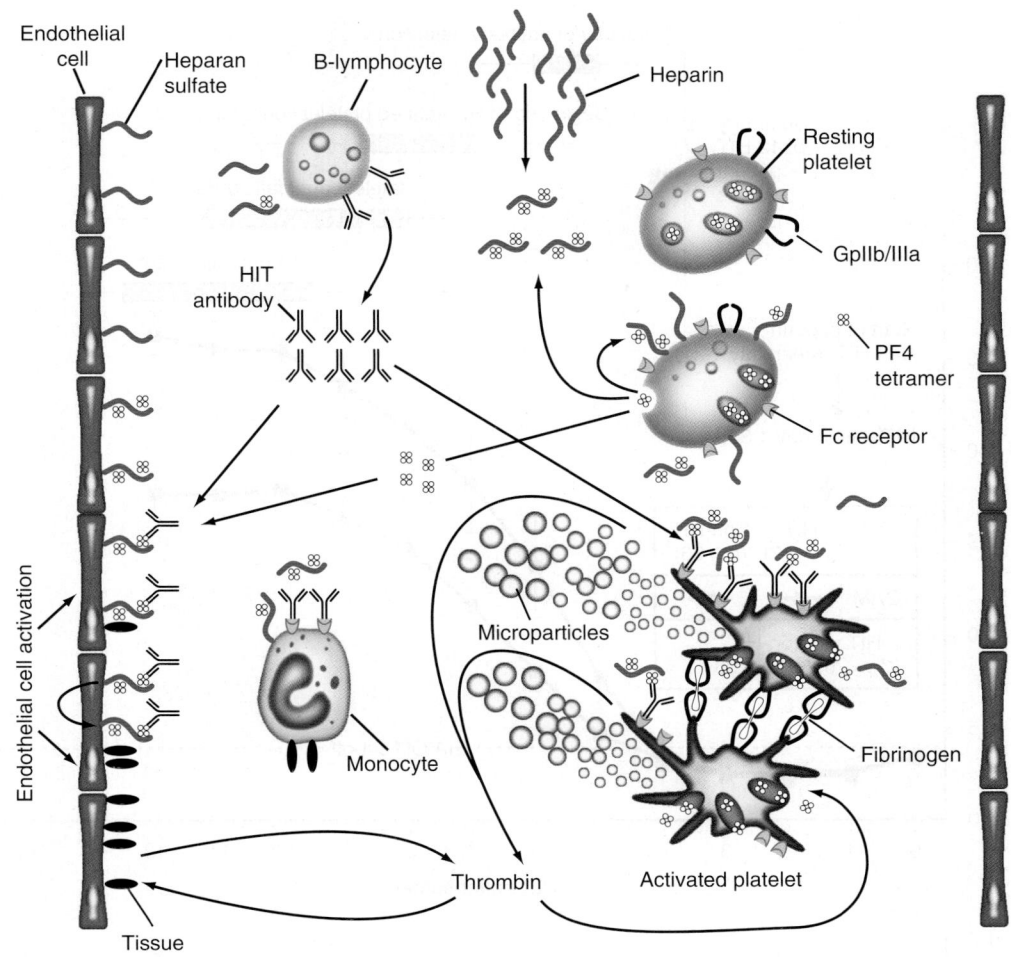

Fig. 133.1 PATHOGENESIS OF HEPARIN-INDUCED THROMBOCYTOPENIA. Heparin produces mild platelet activation, resulting in release of platelet factor 4 (PF4) from platelet α-granules and the formation of immunogenic PF4/heparin complexes. B lymphocytes generate immunoglobulins G (IgGs) that recognize the PF4/heparin complexes; the Fc "tails" of the IgG bind to platelet FcγIIa receptors, resulting in Fc receptor clustering and consequent "strong" platelet activation. Platelet-derived microparticles are generated that accelerate thrombin generation. The heparin-induced thrombocytopenia (HIT) antibodies also recognize PF4 bound to endothelial heparan sulfate, leading to immunoinjury that causes endothelial activation. Recent evidence suggests that HIT antibodies also activate monocytes. The greatly increased thrombin generation observed in HIT helps to explain its association with venous and arterial thrombosis, as well as some of its unusual clinical features (e.g., warfarin-induced venous limb gangrene, decompensated disseminated intravascular coagulation), and also provides a rationale for treatments that control thrombin generation (e.g., with indirect [antithrombin-dependent] or with direct thrombin inhibitors). *(Reprinted with permission from Greinacher A, Warkentin TE: Treatment of heparin-induced thrombocytopenia: An overview. In Warkentin TE, Greinacher A, editors: Heparin-induced thrombocytopenia, ed 4, New York, 2007, Informa Healthcare USA, p 287.)*

on *T*hrombocytopenia, *T*iming (of onset of thrombocytopenia or thrombosis), *T*hrombosis (or other clinical sequelae of HIT), and no o*T*her explanation for thrombocytopenia, with each of the 4Ts scoring as an integer of 0, 1, or 2 points, based upon the likelihood of HIT (thus the maximum score is 8 points) (Table 133.2).[23] The presence of platelet-activating HIT antibodies is unlikely (<3%) with a low score (≤3 points), but relatively probable (approximately 65%) with a high score (≥6). An intermediate score (4 or 5) indicates a clinical profile compatible with HIT, but also with other disorders, such as sepsis; here the frequency of platelet-activating HIT antibodies is still only approximately 10% to 20%.

A newer scoring system is called the HIT Expert Probability (HEP) score (Table 133.3).[24] In the initial evaluation, a HEP score of 4 points or higher indicated an approximately 50% probability of HIT, whereas a score of 3 points or lower was associated with only a 3% probability of HIT.

It is uncertain whether one scoring system offers advantages over the other. In general, low scores in either system indicate a low probability of HIT, whereas high scores indicate approximately a 50:50 chance of HIT. Thus laboratory testing is crucial to establish a diagnosis of HIT.

LABORATORY DIAGNOSIS

Assays for HIT antibodies can be classified as platelet "activation" (or "functional") and PF4-polyanion "antigen" assays (or immunoassays). Activation assays that measure serotonin release from ^{14}C-labeled, washed platelets (i.e., the serotonin-release assay [SRA]) are quite sensitive and specific for detecting clinically significant HIT antibodies.[25] Important quality control maneuvers include the selection of platelet donors whose platelets respond well to Fc receptor

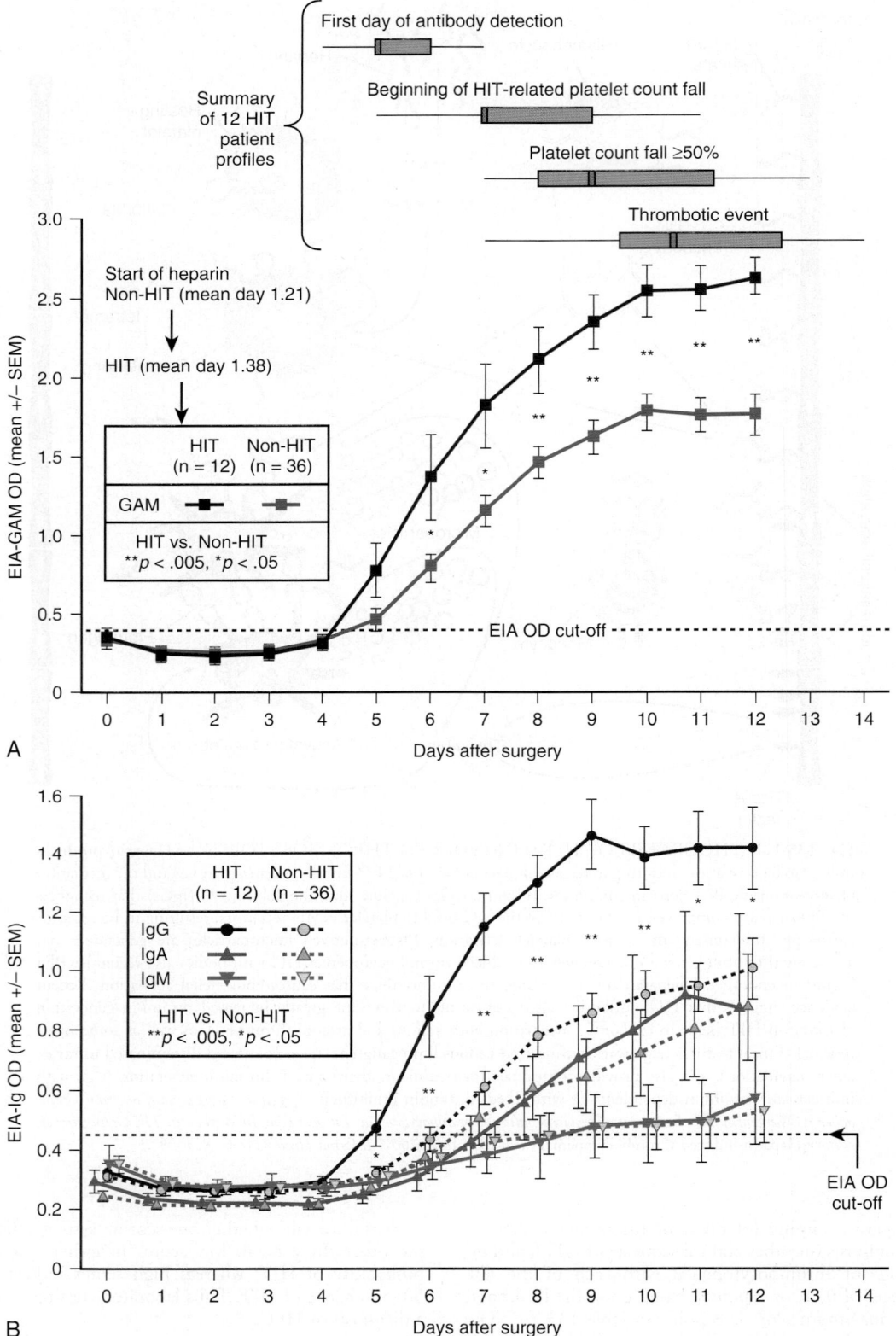

Fig. 133.2 CHARACTERISTIC TIMELINE OF HEPARIN-INDUCED THROMBOCYTOPENIA. Antiplatelet 4 (PF4)/heparin antibodies (by enzyme immunoassay [EIA]) per postoperative day in 12 patients with heparin-induced thrombocytopenia (HIT) and 36 seropositive non-HIT control patients. (A) Mean (± standard error of the mean [SEM]) optical density (OD) of anti-PF4/heparin antibodies detected using commercial immunoassay (EIA-GAM) that detects antibodies of all three immunoglobulin classes (IgG, IgA, IgM). HIT patients are indicated by *blue squares*, and seropositive non-HIT controls by *green squares*. On each day beginning on postoperative day 6, there is a significant difference in the mean of the OD levels between the patients with HIT and the seropositive non-HIT controls ($p < .05$ by nonpaired *t*-test). At the *top* of the figure, summary data for 12 HIT patient profiles are shown for four key events (first day of antibody detection, beginning of HIT-related platelet count fall, platelet count fall ≥50%, and thrombotic event), summarized as median *(small purple squares within rectangles)*, interquartile range *(rectangles)*, and range *(ends of thin black lines)*. (B) Mean (±SEM) OD values of anti-PF4/heparin antibodies detected using an in-house immunoassay (EIA-Ig) that detects antibodies of the individual immunoglobulin classes, IgG *(red circles)*, IgA *(green triangles)*, and IgM *(blue inverted triangles)* for HIT *(solid symbols)* and non-HIT *(open symbols)*. On each postoperative day beginning on day 5, there is a significant difference in the mean of the OD units for the IgG immunoassay between the patients with HIT and the seropositive non-HIT controls (**$p < .005$ for days 6–10; *$p < .05$ for days 5, 11, and 12). *(From Warkentin TE, Sheppard JI, Moore JC, et al: Studies of the immune response in heparin-induced thrombocytopenia.* Blood *113:4693, 2009.)*

stimulation, as well as the inclusion of negative and positive HIT sera of variable reactivity to ensure that the test platelets identify weaker HIT sera. The characteristic activation profile produced by HIT serum includes increased platelet activation at low heparin concentrations (0.05–0.3 units/mL), but background platelet activation at high heparin concentrations (10–100 units/mL).[9] Strong platelet activation induced by HIT sera even in the absence of pharmacologic heparin is a feature of delayed-onset HIT and may generally indicate more severe HIT.[18]

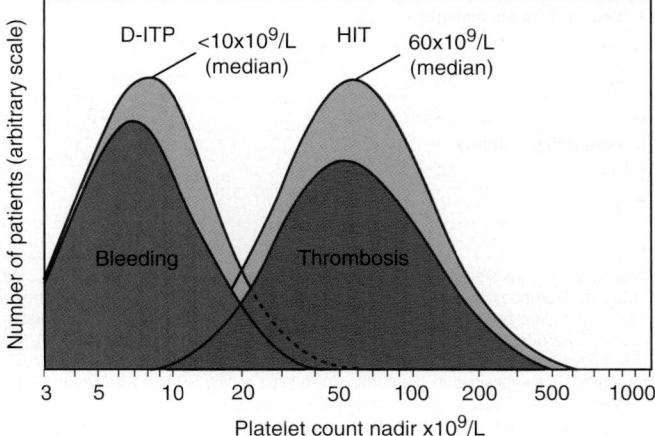

Fig. 133.3 SEVERITY OF THROMBOCYTOPENIA IN DRUG-INDUCED IMMUNE THROMBOCYTOPENIA: A COMPARISON OF HEPARIN-INDUCED THROMBOCYTOPENIA VERSUS OTHER DRUG-INDUCED IMMUNE THROMBOCYTOPENIA DISORDERS. Whereas drug-induced immune thrombocytopenia (D-ITP) is strongly associated with petechiae and purpura, heparin-induced thrombocytopenia (HIT) is strongly associated with thrombosis. Note: The heights of the D-ITP and HIT curves are not drawn to scale, because HIT is more common than all DITP disorders combined. *(From Warkentin TE: Drug-induced immune-mediated thrombocytopenia—from purpura to thrombosis. N Engl J Med 356:891, 2007.)*

Three enzyme(-linked) immuno(sorbent) assays (EIAs or ELISAs) are commercially available for detecting antibodies that recognize PF4 bound to heparin, to the polyanion, polyvinyl sulfonate, or to PF4 (from platelet lysate) bound to protamine. These assays are very sensitive for detecting HIT antibodies but are much more likely than washed platelet activation assays to detect clinically insignificant anti-PF4/heparin antibodies.[2,3,5] Thus results of laboratory tests must be interpreted in the clinical context—that is, HIT is a "clinicopathologic" syndrome.[4] Activation and antigen assays are not 100% concordant, and there are advantages if reference laboratories are able to perform both types of assay. In general, serum or plasma from patients with clinical HIT have strongly positive assay results, whereas clinically insignificant antibodies give weaker results.[2,5] Indeed, if the EIA yields only a weakly positive result (e.g., 0.40 to 1.0 absorbance units), the corresponding probability of "true" HIT is 5% to 10% at most. In contrast, if the EIA yields a strongly positive result (>2.0 units), the probability of HIT exceeds 90%.[5] Table 133.4[25] provides evidence from three studies supporting the greater diagnostic specificity of the SRA compared with the EIA: importantly, EIA+/SRA– status does *not* support a diagnosis of HIT.

PROGNOSIS

Approximately half of all patients with SRA+ HIT have clinically evident thrombosis at the time of initial diagnosis of HIT.[11] Among patients without thrombosis at diagnosis, there appears to be a high risk (approximately 25%–50%) for subsequent thrombosis if heparin is simply discontinued.[11] It is increasingly accepted that further anticoagulation is indicated in most patients strongly suspected as having "isolated" HIT[26,27]—that is, HIT recognized because of thrombocytopenia rather than because of HIT-associated thrombosis.

THERAPY

Although it is standard practice to discontinue heparin in patients strongly suspected of having HIT, including stopping heparin "flushes" of intravascular catheters (with substitution of saline flushes), heparin cessation is not necessarily beneficial, for two reasons:

TABLE 133.2	4Ts Scoring System: Estimating the Pretest Probability of Heparin-Induced Thrombocytopenia		
	Points (0, 1, or 2 for Each of Four Categories: Maximum Possible Score = 8)		
	2	**1**	**0**
Thrombocytopenia (acute)	Platelet fall >50% (nadir ≥20 × 10⁹/L) and no surgery within preceding 3 days	Nadir, 10–19 × 10⁹/L; or any 30%–50% fall; or, >50% fall within 3 days of surgery	Nadir, <10 × 10⁹/L; or any <30% fall
Timing[a] of platelet count fall, thrombosis, or other sequelae	Clear onset between days 5–10; or ≤1 day (if prior heparin exposure in the past 5–30 days)	Consistent with day 5–10 fall, but not clear (e.g., missing platelet counts); or ≤1 day (heparin exposure within past 31–100 days); or platelet fall after day 10	Platelet count fall begins in ≤4 days without recent heparin exposure
Thrombosis or other clinical sequelae	New proven thrombosis; skin necrosis[b]; anaphylactoid reaction after IV heparin bolus; adrenal hemorrhage	Progressive or recurrent thrombosis; erythematous skin lesions[b]; suspected thrombosis (awaiting confirmation with imaging)	None
O**T**her cause for thrombocytopenia not evident	No other explanation for platelet count fall is evident	Possible other cause is evident	Definite other cause is present

Pretest probability score: 6–8 = HIGH; 4–5 = INTERMEDIATE; 0–3 = LOW

The scoring system shown here has undergone minor modifications from previously published scoring systems.
[a]First day of immunizing heparin exposure considered day 0; immunizing heparin is usually that given during or soon after surgery (e.g., unfractionated heparin [UFH] during cardiac surgery is more immunogenic than UFH given during preceding acute coronary syndrome or with heart catheterization); the day the platelet count *begins* to fall is considered the day of onset of thrombocytopenia.
[b]Skin lesions occurring at heparin injection sites.
Reprinted, with permission, from Warkentin TE: Clinical picture of heparin-induced thrombocytopenia. In Warkentin TE, Greinacher A, editors: *Heparin-induced thrombocytopenia*, ed 4, New York, 2007, Informa Healthcare USA, pp 21–66.

TABLE 133.3	HIT Expert Probability (HEP) Scoring System	
Clinical Feature		**Score**
1. Magnitude of fall in platelet count (measured from peak platelet count to nadir platelet count since heparin exposure)		
a. <30%		−1
b. 30%–50%		1
c. >50%		3
2. Timing of fall in platelet count		
For patients in whom typical-onset HIT is suspected		
a. Fall begins <4 days after heparin exposure		−2
b. Fall begins 4 days after heparin exposure		2
c. Fall begins 5–10 days after heparin exposure		3
d. Fall begins 11–14 days after heparin exposure		2
e. Fall begins >14 days after heparin exposure		−1
For patients with previous heparin exposure in last 100 days in whom rapid-onset HIT is suspected		
f. Fall begins <48 h after heparin reexposure		2
g. Fall begins >48 h after heparin reexposure		−1
3. Nadir platelet count		
a. ≤20 × 10^9/L		−2
b. >0 × 10^9/L		2
4. Thrombosis (Select no more than one)		
For patients in whom typical-onset HIT is suspected		
a. New VTE or ATE ≥4 days after heparin exposure		3
b. Progression of preexisting VTE or ATE while receiving heparin		2
For patients in whom rapid-onset HIT is suspected		
c. New VTE or ATE after heparin exposure		3
d. Progression of preexisting VTE or ATE while receiving heparin		2
5. Skin necrosis		
a. Skin necrosis at subcutaneous heparin injection sites		3
6. Acute systemic reaction		
a. Acute systemic reaction after intravenous heparin bolus		2
7. Bleeding		
a. Presence of bleeding, petechiae, or extensive bruising		−1
8. Other causes of thrombocytopenia (Select all that apply)		
a. Presence of a chronic thrombocytopenic disorder		−1
b. Newly initiated nonheparin medication known to cause thrombocytopenia		−2
c. Severe infection		−2
d. Severe DIC (defined as fibrinogen <100 mg/dL and D-dimer >5.0 μg/mL		−2
e. Indwelling intraarterial device (e.g., IABP, VAD, ECMO)		−2
f. Cardiopulmonary bypass within previous 96 h		−1
g. No other apparent cause		3

ATE, Arterial thromboembolism; DIC, disseminated intravascular coagulation; ECMO, extracorporeal membrane oxygenation; HIT, heparin-induced thrombocytopenia; IABP, intraaortic balloon pump; VAD, ventricular assist device; VTE, venous thromboembolism. In its initial evaluation, a HEP score of ≥4 points indicated an approximately 50% probability of HIT, whereas a score of ≤3 points was associated with only a 3% probability of HIT.
Reprinted, with permission, from Cuker A, Arepally G, Crowther MA, et al: The HIT Expert Probability (HEP) Score: A novel pre-test probability model for heparin-induced thrombocytopenia based on broad expert opinion, *J Thromb Haemost* 8:2642, 2010.

TABLE 133.4	Frequency of Thrombocytopenia (>50% Platelet Count Fall) Among EIA+ Patients (Polyspecific or IgG-Specific Assay) Who Received Heparin (UFH or LMWH): A Comparison of SRA+ versus SRA–Status	
SRA Status	**Positive in Polyspecific EIA (IgG/A/M)**	**Positive in IgG-Specific EIA**
A. Postorthopedic Surgery		
SRA+	12/24	12/24
SRA–	0/58	0/16
p	< .0001	.0009
B. Venous Thromboembolism		
SRA+	4/4	4/4
SRA–	0/15	0/6
p	.0003	.0048
C. Postcardiac Surgery		
SRA+	4/11	NA
SRA–	0/152	NA
p	< .0001	NA

The data are consistent with the SRA having a high sensitivity for heparin-induced thrombocytopenia (>95%); the specificity of the SRA depends on the clinical situation but in most circumstances is at least 90%. Patients in studies A and B were tested in both the polyspecific and IgG-specific assays.
EIA, Enzyme immunoassay; LMWH, low-molecular-weight heparin; NA, not available; SRA+, positive in the serotonin-release assay; SRA–, negative in the serotonin-release assay; UFH, unfractionated heparin.
Reprinted, with modifications, with permission, from Warkentin TE: How I diagnose and manage HIT, *Hematology Am Soc Hematol Educ Program* 2011:143, 2011.

Currently there are two types of anticoagulant therapeutic approaches that are commonly used to treat HIT: (1) long-acting indirect (i.e., antithrombin-dependent) factor Xa inhibitors (danaparoid, fondaparinux), and (2) DTIs (argatroban, bivalirudin). In the author's opinion, indirect factor Xa inhibitors—although not approved in the United States for treatment of HIT—are the preferred treatment option for HIT, because they have numerous advantages over DTIs (Table 133.5). In addition, because approximately 90% of patients suspected of HIT do not have HIT,[5] another advantage for indirect factor Xa inhibitors is that these agents, unlike DTIs, are safe and effective for prevention and treatment of thrombosis in numerous non-HIT settings.

Indirect Factor Xa Inhibitors: Danaparoid and Fondaparinux

Danaparoid is an anticoagulant heparinoid (mixture of glycosaminoglycans) with predominant inhibitory activity against factor Xa that is effective for treating HIT; however, danaparoid was never approved for HIT treatment in the United States (although it was approved in many other countries, including Canada and in the European Union) and was discontinued in the United States in April 2002. Danaparoid was shown to be safe and effective for treatment of HIT in an open-label randomized controlled trial (versus dextran 70) and in a retrospective comparison against ancrod (defibrinogenating snake venom) and/or vitamin K antagonist therapy.

In recent years, however, physicians have increasingly been using fondaparinux as off-label therapy for HIT. The advantages of fondaparinux include its long half-life, the fact that it does not require coagulation monitoring nor does it influence the aPTT or international normalized ratio (INR), its low potential to cross-react with HIT antibodies, and low cost. In addition, because relatively few patients with suspected HIT actually have this diagnosis, the wide experience with fondaparinux and its approval for the prevention and treatment of thrombosis in non-HIT settings constitute other advantages. To date, the experience with fondaparinux to treat HIT has

(1) heparin likely has an anticoagulant effect even in patients with HIT, and (2) HIT antibodies often cause ongoing platelet activation and hypercoagulability in the absence of pharmacologic heparin. In addition, HIT antibody levels can decline even with continued heparin. The recognition that patients with HIT have increased thrombin generation[12] provides a rationale for use of nonheparin anticoagulant agents that rapidly inhibit thrombin or its generation.

TABLE 133.5	Comparison of the Two Classes of Anticoagulants Used to Treat Heparin-Induced Thrombocytopenia	
	Indirect (AT-Dependent) Factor Xa Inhibitors: Danaparoid, Fondaparinux	**Direct Thrombin Inhibitors: r-Hirudin (Lepirudin, Desirudin), Argatroban, Bivalirudin**
Half-life	✓ Long (danaparoid, 25 h[a]; fondaparinux, 17 h): reduces risk of rebound hypercoagulability	Short (<2 h): potential for rebound hypercoagulability
Dosing	✓ Both prophylactic- and therapeutic-dose regimens[b]	Prophylactic-dose regimens are not established (exception: subcutaneous desirudin)
Monitoring	✓ Direct (anti-Xa levels): accurate drug levels obtained	Indirect (aPTT): risk for DTI underdosing resulting from aPTT elevation caused by non-DTI factors, including HIT-associated DIC
Effect on INR	✓ No significant effect: thus simplifies overlap with warfarin	Increases INR: argatroban > bivalirudin > r-hirudin; complicates warfarin overlap
Protein C pathway	✓ Adverse effect unlikely (with reduced thrombin generation, there will be less thrombin to activate protein C)	Thrombin inhibition could impair thrombin-mediated activation of protein C pathway
Reversibility of action	✓ Irreversible inhibition: AT forms covalent bond with factor Xa	Irreversible inhibition only with r-hirudin
Efficacy and safety in non-HIT settings	✓ Treatment and prophylaxis of VTE (danaparoid, fondaparinux) and ACS (fondaparinux)	Not established for most non-HIT settings (exception: bivalirudin established for PCI)
Platelet activation	✓ Danaparoid inhibits platelet activation by HIT antibodies	No effect
Inhibition of clot-bound thrombin	No effect	✓ Inhibition of both free and clot-bound thrombin
Drug clearance	Predominantly renal	Variable (predominantly hepatobiliary: argatroban; predominantly renal: r-hirudin)
Cost	✓ Relatively low[c]	Relatively high[c]

Check mark (✓) indicates favorable feature in comparison of drug classes (author's opinion).
[a]For danaparoid, half-lives of its anti-thrombin (anti-IIa) and its thrombin generation inhibition activities (2–4 h and 3–7 h, respectively) are shorter than for its anti-Xa activity (approximately 25 h).
[b]Although therapeutic dosing is recommended for HIT, availability of prophylactic-dose regimens increases flexibility when managing potential non-HIT situations.
[c]Another cost consideration is that a patient can be discharged to home on subcutaneous danaparoid or fondaparinux, whereas an additional 5–7 in-hospital days may be required for DTI-warfarin overlap before discharge from hospital.
ACS, Acute coronary syndrome; aPTT, activated partial thromboplastin time; AT, antithrombin; DIC, disseminated intravascular coagulation; DTI, direct thrombin inhibitor; HIT, heparin-induced thrombocytopenia; INR, international normalized ratio; PCI, percutaneous coronary intervention; VTE, venous thromboembolism.
Reprinted, with modifications, with permission, from Warkentin TE: Agents for the treatment of heparin-induced thrombocytopenia, *Hematol Oncol Clin North Am* 24:755, 2010.

been favorable;[28–31] a recent retrospective propensity score-matched study of 133 fondaparinux-treated HIT patients (with 60 controls) concluded that fondaparinux has similar efficacy and safety as argatroban and danaparoid.[32] Also, fondaparinux is much less likely than UFH or LMWH to precipitate rapid-onset HIT in patients who have unrecognized HIT antibodies.[33] Although fondaparinux thromboprophylaxis has been associated with rare cases of de novo HIT,[28] this should not deter from its use as a treatment of HIT because the potential to trigger immunization is "dissociated" from whether an anticoagulant potentiates antibody-induced platelet activation,[7] and fondaparinux has low potential to exacerbate HIT.[33] Dosing information for danaparoid and fondaparinux is shown in Table 133.6.

In theory, oral direct factor Xa inhibitors, such as rivaroxaban (approved in the United States for thromboprophylaxis after knee or hip replacement surgery), should be effective for treatment of HIT. Anecdotal experience with rivaroxaban[20] for this indication is beginning to be reported.

Direct Thrombin Inhibitors: Recombinant Hirudin (Lepirudin, Desirudin), Bivalirudin, Argatroban

The recombinant hirudin-derivative lepirudin (Refludan) is a 65-amino-acid polypeptide that inactivates thrombin by forming a tight, noncovalent 1:1 complex with it. Although this agent is approved for the treatment of HIT-associated thrombosis in the European Union, the United States, and elsewhere[26] it was discontinued by the manufacturer in 2012.

Bivalirudin (Angiomax) is a 20-amino-acid thrombin inhibitor modeled after hirudin that is composed of two peptide fragments that recognize the active site of thrombin and its fibrinogen-binding site, linked by a tetraglycine spacer. The half-life of bivalirudin is about one-third that of lepirudin (25 versus 80 minutes), and only minor dose adjustments are needed in patients with renal insufficiency because bivalirudin is only partially cleared by the kidneys. It is approved as an alternative to heparin in patients undergoing percutaneous coronary intervention (PCI), including those with HIT. Its short half-life and predominantly extrarenal elimination are reasons why it is an option for intraoperative anticoagulation in patients undergoing cardiac surgery, when heparin is contraindicated because of acute or recent HIT. Experience using bivalirudin off-label to treat HIT outside the PCI setting is limited. Anaphylaxis has not been reported.

Argatroban (marketed as argatroban in the United States and as Novastan elsewhere) is a small-molecule (527-Da) DTI that undergoes predominantly hepatobiliary excretion and is therefore suitable for use without dose adjustment in patients with renal failure (the dose is reduced by three-quarters in patients with hepatic insufficiency). Argatroban is approved in the United States for both treatment and prevention of thrombosis in HIT. It is given in the same dosage for both indications (usual starting infusion rate of 2 µg/kg/min without an initial bolus). However, lower starting doses are usually given (e.g., 0.5–1.2 µg/kg/min), especially in critically ill patients. Argatroban (in substantially higher doses) is also approved for anticoagulation during PCI in patients with acute HIT or a history of HIT. Its half-life is 40–50 minutes. Argatroban prolongs the INR

TABLE 133.6   Treatment Schedules for Danaparoid and Fondaparinux

Anticoagulant	Therapeutic Dosing Protocol for HIT-Associated Thrombosis[a]	Anticoagulant Monitoring	Clearance	Half-Life (h)	Comment
Danaparoid	Initial bolus, 2250 units[b] IV; accelerated infusion (400 units/h × 4 h, 300 units/h 4 h; then 200 units/h IV, subsequently adjusted by antifactor Xa levels)	Antifactor Xa levels (target, 0.5–0.8 units/mL)	Renal (minor)	25	Widely approved for HIT treatment (although not in the United States); not available in the United States; low risk for in vivo cross-reactivity; prophylactic-dose therapy[c] may be appropriate when clinical suspicion for HIT is low
Fondaparinux	7.5 mg[d] subcutaneous once daily	Anti-Xa factor levels (target levels not well established)	Renal (major)	17	Not approved for HIT treatment (although increasingly used as off-label therapy). Prophylactic-dose therapy[e] may be appropriate when clinical suspicion for HIT is low, or if there is renal insufficiency

[a]Therapeutic dosing is usually appropriate for strongly suspected or confirmed HIT (including "isolated" HIT, i.e., HIT without apparent thrombosis), or when thrombosis is documented.
[b]Adjust IV danaparoid bolus for body weight: <60 kg, 1500 units; 60–75 kg, 2250 units; 75–90 kg, 3000 units; >90 kg, 3750 units.
[c]Prophylactic-dose regimen, 750 units subcutaneous every 8 h (for renal failure, reduce to 750 units every 12 h).
[d]Five milligrams for body weight <50 kg and 10 mg for body weight >100 kg; the author sometimes gives 10 mg as the first and/or second dose (rather than 7.5 mg) for severe HIT. Because HIT treatment is usually started in the afternoon, the author usually gives the second dose (and subsequent doses) at 8 AM (i.e., the interval between first and second doses is often only 14–20 h rather than 24 h), which helps to achieve steady-state therapy more quickly. Dose reduction and antifactor Xa monitoring (if available) is appropriate if being used in a patient with renal insufficiency.
[e]Prophylactic-dose regimen, 2.5 mg subcutaneous every day (assumes normal renal function).
HIT, Heparin-induced thrombocytopenia; IV, intravenous.

TABLE 133.7   Treatment Schedules for Lepirudin, Desirudin, Bivalirudin, and Argatroban

Anticoagulant	Dosing Protocol for HIT-Associated Thrombosis	Anticoagulant Monitoring[a]	Clearance	Half-Life (min)	Comment
Lepirudin	No bolus; initial infusion rate: 0.05–0.10 mg/kg/h[b,c]	1.5–2.5 × baseline aPTT	Renal[c]	80	Approved dosing regimen (not shown) is too high; no longer available (withdrawn by manufacturer
Desirudin	Not established	aPTT	Renal	120	Half-life shown is for subcutaneous administration; minimal experience for treating HIT
Bivalirudin	No bolus; initial infusion rate: 0.15–0.20 mg/kg/h	1.5–2.5 × baseline aPTT	Enzymic (80%); renal (20%)	25	Off-label treatment for HIT (although approved for PCI in patient with HIT); minor prolongation of INR (compared with argatroban)
Argatroban	No bolus; initial infusion rate: 2 µg/kg/min	1.5–3.0 × baseline aPTT	Hepatobiliary	40–50	Initial dose 0.5 µg/kg/min in hepatic insufficiency[d]; moderate or marked prolongation of INR, which complicates overlap with warfarin anticoagulation

Dosing protocols shown are appropriate for most patients with strongly suspected or confirmed HIT whether or not complicated by thrombosis. (Dosing for bivalirudin and argatroban is substantially different when given for PCI.)
[a]In general, the patient's baseline aPTT should be used for calculating target range, when appropriate; otherwise the mean laboratory normal range can be used.
[b]This dosing protocol differs from the package insert (which advises initial bolus of 0.4 mg/kg and initial infusion rate [assuming normal renal function] of 0.15 mg/kg/h); however, this dosing regimen is now considered too high.[26]
[c]Major dose reduction in renal insufficiency is required.[26]
[d]Reduced initial dosing (e.g., 0.5–1.2 µg/kg/min) is also appropriate in patients in intensive care units, with cardiac failure, or postcardiac surgery).
aPTT, Activated partial thromboplastin time; HIT, heparin-induced thrombocytopenia; INR, international normalized ratio; PCI, percutaneous coronary intervention.

more than lepirudin or bivalirudin, and a higher-than-usual target INR during warfarin co-therapy (which depends on the thromboplastin reagent used to measure the INR) can be expected (see Caveats in Treatment of Heparin-Induced Thrombocytopenia). Argatroban reduced the frequency of a composite end point (new thrombosis, limb amputation, and all-cause mortality) from 56.5% (in historical controls) to 43.8% and 41.5% in two studies of patients with HIT complicated by thrombosis; new thrombosis event rates were reduced from 34.8% to 19.4% and 13.1%, respectively.[26] In patients with isolated HIT, argatroban reduced the rate of new thrombosis from 22.4% to 6.9%, and the combined event rate of new thrombosis, limb amputation, and all-cause mortality from 38.8% to 26.9%.[26] Dosing information for the parenteral DTIs is shown in Table 133.7.

In theory, dabigatran, an oral thrombin inhibitor, should also be effective for treatment of HIT. To date, experience for treating HIT has been minimal.

Caveats in Treatment of Heparin-Induced Thrombocytopenia

Warfarin and other vitamin K antagonists (coumarins) should not be used during the acute thrombocytopenic phase of HIT.[12] A particularly high-risk situation is HIT associated with deep vein thrombosis, especially if there is overt (decompensated) DIC. If such patients are treated with warfarin, there is a risk for progression to venous limb gangrene.[12,26,27] The laboratory marker for this unusual syndrome is a high INR (generally, greater than 4.0), which corresponds to the combination of a marked reduction in the level of protein C together with increased thrombin generation (as evidenced by elevated levels of thrombin-antithrombin complexes) during warfarin therapy.[12] Although warfarin (in theory) should be safe in a patient whose thrombin generation is controlled (e.g., using a DTI), it is important to delay the initiation of warfarin until there is substantial resolution of the thrombocytopenia (to more than 150×10^9/L).[26,27] Warfarin treatment should be delayed because its prolongation of the aPTT may result in *underdosing* of the DTI, and because stopping the DTI before resolution of the HIT during warfarin overlap can lead to limb loss caused by fulminant venous limb gangrene.[4]

Several case observations suggest that aPTT confounding of DTI therapy can be a factor explaining progression of thrombosis in patients with severe HIT.[4,34] For example, patients can develop progressive thrombocytopenia and HIT-associated consumptive coagulopathy despite stopping heparin (Fig. 133.4). In such patients, aPTT monitoring of DTI therapy can fail because a brief course of DTI can abruptly lead to supratherapeutic aPTT levels—not because of anticoagulant overdosing but because of the combination of DTI and consumptive coagulopathy—and interruption/cessation of DTI therapy can be associated with rapid progression of microvascular thrombosis. In this setting, factor Xa inhibitors (danaparoid, fondaparinux) may be more effective because they do not require aPTT monitoring. Alternatively, DTI levels can be measured directly, but these assays are rarely performed in North American laboratories.

Using sensitive assays for HIT antibodies, LMWH reacts similarly to UFH in vitro. Furthermore, because LMWH can lead to worsening of clinical HIT, these agents should not be used to treat HIT.[26,27]

Although primary treatment for HIT should include an anticoagulant that inhibits thrombin or reduces its generation, certain treatment adjuncts can be used in special situations. These include surgical thromboembolectomy, high-dose intravenous immunoglobulin, antiplatelet drugs such as aspirin, and therapeutic plasma exchange.

These caveats, along with recommendations for management of patients with suspected HIT, are summarized in the box on Diagnosis and Treatment of Heparin-Induced Thrombocytopenia.

PLATELET COUNT MONITORING FOR HEPARIN-INDUCED THROMBOCYTOPENIA

The frequency of platelet count monitoring in patients receiving heparin should reflect the overall risk of HIT (i.e., the preparation, the dose, and the clinical situation).[26] At least alternate-day platelet count monitoring should be considered in patients at relatively high risk for developing HIT (e.g., after orthopedic or cardiac surgery). Monitoring at least two or three times a week should be considered for patients at moderate risk for developing HIT (e.g., medical patients receiving UFH, postoperative patients receiving UFH flushes or LMWH). The frequency of HIT is low with LMWH,[1,6] particularly in medical patients or during pregnancy, and routine platelet count monitoring may not be required in such settings.[26] In addition, HIT rarely begins 14 or more days after initiation of a course of heparin,[17] so routine monitoring beyond this period is not required. A more recent consensus conference[27] recommended somewhat less intensive platelet count monitoring than advised in this paragraph.

Diagnosis and Treatment of Heparin-Induced Thrombocytopenia

Heparin-induced thrombocytopenia (HIT) should be clinically suspected when thrombocytopenia occurs during (or soon after) heparin therapy and the temporal profile of the decrease in platelet count is consistent with immune sensitization to heparin. Four relevant questions, the 4Ts, should be asked:

Thrombocytopenia: Does the patient have thrombocytopenia? A greater than 50% fall in the platelet count can indicate HIT even if the platelet count has not fallen to below 150×10^9/L. (Note: Severe thrombocytopenia, such as a platelet count below 10×10^9/L, is only rarely caused by HIT.)

Timing: Is the timing of the platelet count fall consistent with immune sensitization? In HIT the platelet count usually begins to fall 5–10 days after starting heparin (first day of heparin is day 0); a more rapid fall in the platelet count can occur if the patient is already sensitized from heparin exposure within the past 100 days.

Thrombosis: Does the patient have thrombosis or other sequelae of HIT? (Note: In addition to venous and arterial thrombosis, patients with HIT can develop necrotizing skin lesions at heparin injection sites or systemic inflammatory or cardiorespiratory reactions that begin 5–30 minutes after an IV heparin bolus.)

OTher: Are there other explanations for the thrombocytopenia? HIT is less likely when there is compelling clinical evidence for another cause of the thrombocytopenia, such as positive blood cultures.

Steps in Management of Clinically Suspected Heparin-Induced Thrombocytopenia

1. Confirm that thrombocytopenia is present (repeat complete blood count), test for DIC, and test for HIT antibodies, preferably using a platelet activation test such as the serotonin-release assay.
2. Assess clinically and radiologically for thrombosis (e.g., compression ultrasound for lower-limb deep venous thrombosis).
3. Stop all heparin, including heparin flushes and possibly use of heparin-coated intravascular catheters (catheters left in situ for several days may not have much residual heparin).
4. Initiate treatment with an alternative anticoagulant, generally in therapeutic doses if HIT is strongly suspected (options: danaparoid,[a,b] fondaparinux,[a,c] lepirudin,[d] argatroban, bivalirudin[a]).
5. Although initial treatment decisions are made on clinical grounds, results of testing for HIT antibodies can influence subsequent treatment, including the decision to resume heparin if HIT has been ruled out.

Caveats

- Do not use low-molecular-weight heparin to treat HIT.
- Do not start (or continue) warfarin or other coumarins until the platelet count has returned to normal (greater than 150×10^9/L), and give only in low initial doses (warfarin, 5 mg or less) and overlap with a parenteral anticoagulant for at least 5 days.
- Do give vitamin K (e.g., 5–10 mg IV over 30–60 minutes) if HIT is diagnosed after warfarin has already been given, so as to reduce risk for coumarin necrosis and to avoid underdosing of DTI because of activated partial thromboplastin time (aPTT) prolongation by warfarin.
- Beware of confounding[34] of aPTT-monitored DTI therapy in patients with severe HIT complicated by HIT-associated consumptive coagulopathy (DIC) or who have other explanations for an elevated aPTT, such as warfarin therapy, liver disease, or antiphospholipid syndrome.
- Do not give prophylactic platelet transfusions (platelet transfusions are appropriate if the patient is bleeding or if there is diagnostic uncertainty).

[a]Not approved for treatment of HIT in the United States (except, in the case of bivalirudin, for anticoagulation during percutaneous coronary intervention).
[b]Withdrawn from the US market but available in many other countries.
[c]Fondaparinux is not approved for treatment of HIT, but case series suggest that it is at least as effective as DTI therapy; moreover, the risk for bleeding with fondaparinux is likely to be lower than that with DTI therapy, and fondaparinux costs less than the other agents. Also, there is greater experience with fondaparinux than DTIs for prevention and treatment of thrombosis in non-HIT situations, and only approximately 10% of patients with suspected HIT actually have the disorder. Fondaparinux also avoids the risk for confounding of aPTT-monitored DTI therapy. The author is a proponent of the use of fondaparinux to treat HIT.
[d]Lepirudin was discontinued by the manufacturer, April 2012.

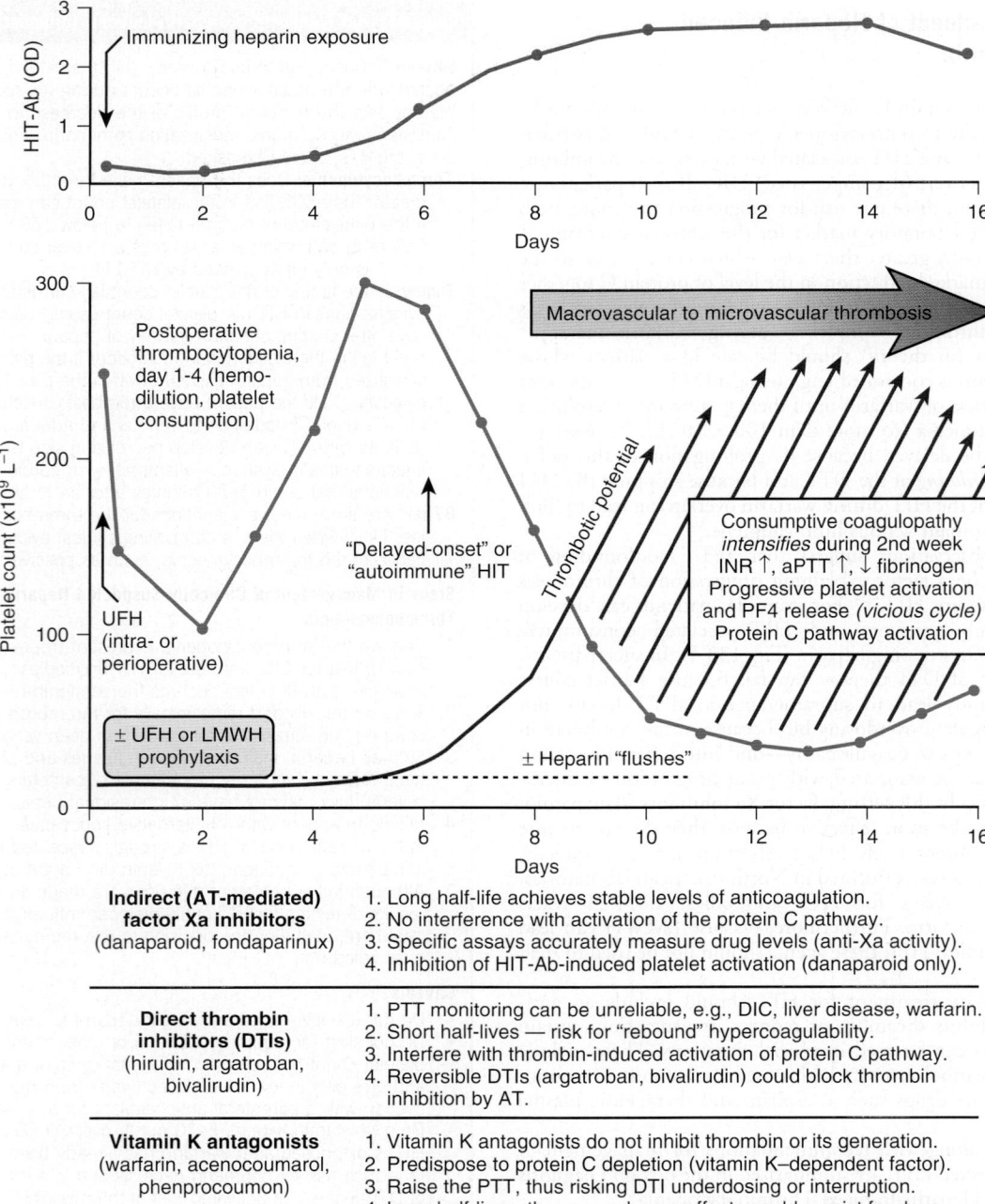

Indirect (AT-mediated) factor Xa inhibitors (danaparoid, fondaparinux)	1. Long half-life achieves stable levels of anticoagulation. 2. No interference with activation of the protein C pathway. 3. Specific assays accurately measure drug levels (anti-Xa activity). 4. Inhibition of HIT-Ab-induced platelet activation (danaparoid only).
Direct thrombin inhibitors (DTIs) (hirudin, argatroban, bivalirudin)	1. PTT monitoring can be unreliable, e.g., DIC, liver disease, warfarin. 2. Short half-lives — risk for "rebound" hypercoagulability. 3. Interfere with thrombin-induced activation of protein C pathway. 4. Reversible DTIs (argatroban, bivalirudin) could block thrombin inhibition by AT.
Vitamin K antagonists (warfarin, acenocoumarol, phenprocoumon)	1. Vitamin K antagonists do not inhibit thrombin or its generation. 2. Predispose to protein C depletion (vitamin K–dependent factor). 3. Raise the PTT, thus risking DTI underdosing or interruption. 4. Long half-lives, thus any adverse effects could persist for days.

Fig. 133.4 CONCEPTUAL FRAMEWORK OF HEPARIN-INDUCED THROMBOCYTOPENIA: FOCUS ON HEPARIN-*IN*DEPENDENT PLATELET ACTIVATION AND DELAYED-ONSET ("AUTOIMMUNE") HEPARIN-INDUCED THROMBOCYTOPENIA. The *upper panel* shows the timeline of heparin-induced thrombocytopenia (HIT) antibody (HIT-Ab) formation, as judged by optical density units in an antiplatelet factor 4/polyanion enzyme immunoassay. The *middle panel* illustrates a platelet count decline in the absence of heparin (or with small amounts of heparin, e.g., heparin flushes) indicating delayed-onset HIT, with intensification of HIT-associated hypercoagulability from day 7–14, especially after stopping heparin. Patients with this clinical profile often have HIT-associated consumptive coagulopathy (overt disseminated intravascular coagulopathy [DIC]), and are at risk for confounding of activated partial thromboplastin time (aPTT)-monitored direct thrombin inhibitor treatment. The *lower panel* compares different classes of anticoagulant for expected effects on HIT-associated hypercoagulability, including the risk for aPTT confounding in the setting of HIT-associated DIC. *AT,* Antithrombin; *DTI,* direct thrombin inhibitor; *INR,* international normalized ratio; *LMWH,* low-molecular-weight heparin; *PF4,* platelet factor 4; *PTT,* partial thromboplastin time; *UHF,* unfractionated heparin. (From Warkentin TE: *Agents for the treatment of heparin-induced thrombocytopenia.* Hematol Oncol Clin North Am *24:755, 2010.*)

ANTICOAGULATION AND PREVIOUS HEPARIN-INDUCED THROMBOCYTOPENIA

HIT antibodies are transient and usually are undetectable several weeks or a few months after an episode of HIT.[17] If HIT antibodies are no longer detected, it is appropriate to use heparin for a brief indication in situations where other anticoagulants have drawbacks, for example, cardiac surgery.[17,26,27,35] Heparin should be avoided preoperatively (e.g., argatroban or bivalirudin can be used for heart catheterization). The risk of recurrent HIT appears to be low (approximately 2%), but is possible beginning approximately one week post-reexposure for cardiac or vascular surgery even if postoperative heparin is not given, because of the possibility of regenerating strong HIT antibodies that can activate platelets in the absence of pharmacologic heparin.[35] Alternatively, if a patient with recent HIT remains SRA+ and heparin reexposure is desired (e.g., for urgent cardiac surgery), therapeutic plasma exchange can be used to remove HIT antibodies preoperatively; in this situation, achieving a negative SRA is the appropriate serologic endpoint (as the EIA can remain positive even when platelet-activating antibodies are no longer detectable by SRA).[36]

Patients with acute or recent HIT who require urgent heart surgery and still have detectable antibodies have been successfully treated with alternate anticoagulant approaches (e.g., bivalirudin, or heparin plus an antiplatelet agent such as epoprostenol or tirofiban), but each of these approaches has disadvantages. For example, epoprostenol causes hypotension, and there is limited experience with its use in cardiac surgery. Bivalirudin is the most promising agent for use in cardiac surgery, but special surgical and anesthesiologic maneuvers are required (because bivalirudin undergoes proteolysis, thus posing a risk for clotting of stagnant blood in the extracorporeal circuit).

A diagnostic and therapeutic approach to HIT is shown in the box on Diagnosis and Treatment of Heparin-Induced Thrombocytopenia.

REFERENCES

1. Linkins LA, Lee DH: Frequency of heparin-induced thrombocytopenia. In Warkentin TE, Greinacher A, editors: *Heparin-induced thrombocytopenia*, ed 5, Boca Raton, FL, 2013, CRC Press, p 110.
2. Warkentin TE, Sheppard JI, Moore JC, et al: Laboratory testing for the antibodies that cause heparin-induced thrombocytopenia: how much class do we need? *J Lab Clin Med* 146:341, 2005.
3. Warkentin TE, Sheppard JI, Moore JC, et al: Studies of the immune response in heparin-induced thrombocytopenia. *Blood* 113:4963, 2009.
4. Warkentin TE: HIT paradigms and paradoxes. *J Thromb Haemost* 9:105, 2011.
5. Warkentin TE, Sheppard JI, Moore JC, et al: Quantitative interpretation of optical density measurements using PF4-dependent immunoassays. *J Thromb Haemost* 6:1304, 2008.
6. Warkentin TE, Sheppard JI, Sigouin CS, et al: Gender imbalance and risk factor interactions in heparin-induced thrombocytopenia. *Blood* 108:2937, 2006.
7. Warkentin TE, Cook RJ, Marder VJ, et al: Anti-platelet factor 4/heparin antibodies in orthopedic surgery patients receiving antithrombotic prophylaxis with fondaparinux or enoxaparin. *Blood* 106:3791, 2005.
8. Gao C, Boylan B, Fang J, et al: Heparin promotes platelet responsiveness by potentiating αIIbβ3-mediated outside-in signaling. *Blood* 117:4946, 2011.
9. Sheridan D, Carter J, Kelton JG: A diagnostic test for heparin-induced thrombocytopenia. *Blood* 67:27, 1986.
10. Krauel K, Weber C, Brandt S, et al: Platelet factor 4 binding to lipid A of Gram-negative bacteria exposes PF4/heparin-like epitopes. *Blood* 120:3345, 2012.
11. Warkentin TE, Kelton JG: A 14-year study of heparin-induced thrombocytopenia. *Am J Med* 101:502, 1996.
12. Warkentin TE, Elavathil LJ, Hayward CPM, et al: The pathogenesis of venous limb gangrene associated with heparin-induced thrombocytopenia. *Ann Intern Med* 127:804, 1997.
13. Rauova L, Hirsch JD, Greene TK, et al: Monocyte-bound PF4 in the pathogenesis of heparin-induced thrombocytopenia. *Blood* 116:5021, 2010.
14. Lubenow N, Hinz P, Thomaschewski S, et al: The severity of trauma determines the immune response to PF4/heparin and the frequency of heparin-induced thrombocytopenia. *Blood* 115:1797, 2010.
15. Warkentin TE, Cook RJ, Marder VJ, et al: Anti-PF4/heparin antibody formation post-orthopedic surgery thromboprophylaxis: the role of non-drug risk factors and evidence for a stoichiometry-based model of immunization. *J Thromb Haemost* 8:504, 2010.
16. Warkentin TE: Drug-induced immune-mediated thrombocytopenia—from purpura to thrombosis. *N Engl J Med* 356:891, 2007.
17. Warkentin TE, Kelton JG: Temporal aspects of heparin-induced thrombocytopenia. *N Engl J Med* 344:1286, 2001.
18. Warkentin TE, Kelton JG: Delayed-onset heparin-induced thrombocytopenia and thrombosis. *Ann Intern Med* 135:502, 2001.
19. Warkentin TE, Basciano PA, Knopman J, et al: Spontaneous heparin-induced thrombocytopenia syndrome. *Blood* 123:3651, 2014.
20. Warkentin TE, Safyan EL, Linkins LA: Heparin-induced thrombocytopenia presenting as bilateral adrenal hemorrhages. *N Engl J Med* 372:492, 2015.
21. Warkentin TE, Cook RJ, Sarode R, et al: Warfarin-induced venous limb ischemia/gangrene complicating cancer: a novel and clinically distinct syndrome. *Blood* 126:486, 2015.
22. Pauzner R, Greinacher A, Selleng K, et al: False-positive tests for heparin induced thrombocytopenia in patients with antiphospholipid syndrome and systemic lupus erythematosus. *J Thromb Haemost* 7:1070, 2009.
23. Lo GK, Juhl D, Warkentin TE, et al: Evaluation of pretest clinical score (4 T's) for the diagnosis of heparin-induced thrombocytopenia in two clinical settings. *J Thromb Haemost* 4:759, 2006.
24. Cuker A, Arepally G, Crowther MA, et al: The HIT Expert Probability (HEP) Score: a novel pre-test probability model for heparin-induced thrombocytopenia based on broad expert opinion. *J Thromb Haemost* 8:2642, 2010.
25. Warkentin TE: How I diagnose and manage HIT. *Hematology Am Soc Hematol Educ Program* 2011:143, 2011.
26. Warkentin TE, Greinacher A, Koster A, et al: Treatment and prevention of heparin-induced thrombocytopenia: American College of Chest Physicians Evidence-Based Clinical Practice Guidelines (8th edition). *Chest* 133:340S, 2008.
27. Linkins LA, Dans AL, Moores LK, et al: Treatment and prevention of heparin-induced thrombocytopenia. Antithrombotic Therapy and Prevention of Thrombosis, 9th ed: American College of Chest Physicians Evidence-Based Clinical Practice Guidelines. *Chest* 141:e495S, 2012.
28. Warkentin TE: Fondaparinux: does it cause HIT? Can it treat HIT? *Expert Rev Hematol* 3:567, 2010.
29. Lobo B, Finch C, Howard A, et al: Fondaparinux for the treatment of patients with acute heparin-induced thrombocytopenia. *Thromb Haemost* 99:208, 2008.
30. Warkentin TE, Pai M, Sheppard JI, et al: Fondaparinux treatment of acute heparin-induced thrombocytopenia confirmed by the serotonin-release assay: a 30-month, 16-patient case series. *J Thromb Haemost* 9:2389, 2011.
31. Goldfarb MJ, Blostein MD: Fondaparinux in acute heparin-induced thrombocytopenia: a case series. *J Thromb Haemost* 9:2501, 2011.
32. Kang M, Alahmadi M, Sawh S, et al: Fondaparinux for the treatment of suspected heparin-induced thrombocytopenia: a propensity score-matched study. *Blood* 125:924, 2015.
33. Warkentin TE, Davidson BL, Büller HR, et al: Prevalence and risk of preexisting heparin-induced thrombocytopenia antibodies in patients with acute VTE. *Chest* 140:366–373, 2011.
34. Warkentin TE: Anticoagulant failure in coagulopathic patients: PTT confounding and other pitfalls. *Expert Opin Drug Saf* 13:25, 2014.
35. Warkentin TE, Sheppard JI: Serological investigation of patients with a previous history of heparin-induced thrombocytopenia who are reexposed to heparin. *Blood* 123:2485, 2014.
36. Warkentin TE, Sheppard JI, Chu FV, et al: Plasma exchange to remove HIT antibodies: dissociation between enzyme-immunoassay and platelet activation test reactivities. *Blood* 125:195, 2015.

CHAPTER 134

THROMBOTIC THROMBOCYTOPENIC PURPURA AND THE HEMOLYTIC UREMIC SYNDROMES

Robert Schneidewend, Narendranath Epperla, and Kenneth D. Friedman

In 1924 Moschowitz reported a case of a 16-year-old girl who died of a previously undescribed illness characterized by microangiopathic hemolytic anemia (MAHA), petechiae, hemiparesis, and fever. Postmortem examination revealed numerous hyaline thrombi, most prevalent in the terminal arterioles and capillaries of the heart and kidneys. In 1936 four similar cases were reported by Baehr and colleagues, who proposed that the hyaline thrombi were secondary to agglutinated platelets. In 1947 Singer suggested that the term *thrombotic thrombocytopenic purpura (TTP)* be used to describe this disorder. In 1955 Gasser used the term *hemolytic uremic syndrome (HUS)* to describe a related syndrome consisting of Coombs-negative hemolytic anemia, thrombocytopenia, and renal failure. The clinical features of Shiga toxin–associated HUS (ST-HUS) were described in six young children who presented with renal failure following a diarrheal illness in 1962. An association to Shigella was recognized in 1975 and the linkage to Shiga toxin–producing *E. coli* (STEC) was made in 1983. These disorders are now referred to as *thrombotic microangiopathies (TMAs),* based on their shared features of MAHA, thrombocytopenia, and microvascular thrombotic lesions with resultant organ dysfunction.

By definition, MAHA and thrombocytopenia are cardinal signs/features of all TMA syndromes, leading to overlapping clinical and pathologic features. However, a multitude of different pathogenic pathways lead to vascular endothelial injury in these conditions. The vast majority of cases of TTP appear to be caused by deficiency of ADAMTS13 (a disintegrin-like and metalloprotease with thrombospondin type1 motif, family member 13), resulting in failure to control the interaction of von Willebrand factor (vWF) with platelets and subsequent organ dysfunction as a consequence of platelet-rich thrombi formation in the microcirculation (and occasionally in large vessels). Recent studies indicate that "atypical" hemolytic uremic syndrome (aHUS) is mainly attributable to a defect in the regulation of the complement mechanism and unregulated deposition of complement factor C3b on cellular surfaces. A rare autosomal recessively inherited form of aHUS occurs in patients with defects in the gene encoding for diacylglycerol kinase epsilon (DGKE), which results in a shift of endothelial cells to a prothrombotic phenotype. Finally, in STEC-HUS, endothelial injury is caused by Shiga toxin and inflammatory cytokines, perhaps inciting disease with increased frequency in individuals with specific genetic predispositions. With improved understanding of the pathogenesis of TMAs and the availability of specific therapy that targets that pathogenesis, distinction of the various TMA syndromes is clinically important. Several pathogenesis-based classification schemes for TMAs have been developed; one example is illustrated in Fig. 134.1.

DIFFERENTIAL DIAGNOSIS

The differential diagnosis of MAHA and thrombocytopenia is extensive. An example of a decision tree is shown in Fig. 134.2. Vascular damage secondary to severe sepsis, autoimmune disorders (i.e., systemic lupus erythematosus, scleroderma, antiphospholipid antibody syndrome, see Chapter 141), septic or tumor emboli, immune complex-mediated vasculitis (e.g., infective endocarditis), malignant hypertension, complications of pregnancy (severe preeclampsia, eclampsia, HELLP syndrome [an acronym for *h*emolysis, *e*levated *l*iver function tests, and *low p*latelet counts]), cryoglobulinemia, or infection with rickettsial or, more rarely, hemorrhage-inducing viral organisms, may all mimic TMAs. Occasionally, patients with disseminated intravascular coagulation secondary to malignancy or sepsis present with microangiopathy of sufficient severity to be confused with primary TMAs (see Chapter 139). In the setting of renal transplantation, a biopsy may be required to distinguish TMAs from allograft rejection or recurrence of a preexisting renal vascular disorder. Occasional patients present with acute pancreatitis, acute respiratory distress syndrome, memory and personality changes, or other poorly defined neurologic symptoms, which have a broad differential diagnosis.

Clues suggesting STEC-HUS include age at the time of presentation, ingestion of undercooked ground beef or other food that might have become contaminated by cattle, contact with farm animals, or concurrent HUS in another family member. History of asynchronous presentation in a sibling would suggest inherited TTP or aHUS. Historical approaches to the distinction of TTP from aHUS have relied heavily upon the age of presentation and distribution of symptoms. However, as demonstrated by the recent trials showing the utility of eculizumab, aHUS is not uncommonly diagnosed in adults. Similarly, there is significant end-organ dysfunction overlap between these two disorders. While the kidney remains a major target organ in aHUS, renal injury of sufficient severity to require dialysis may occur in up to 10% of patients with TTP. Neurologic symptoms are reported in 25% to 79% of patients diagnosed with TTP but may also be seen in 10% to 30% of patients with aHUS.

Choosing the appropriate therapy depends on an accurate diagnosis. While symptoms may not support distinctions, several groups have reported that platelet counts and creatinine levels are significantly lower in patients with severe ADAMTS13 deficient TTP; it has been suggested that a platelet count under $30,000/\mu L$ or a creatinine under 2.3 mg/dL favors a diagnosis of TTP. An ADAMTS13 level below 10% in the appropriate clinical context provides strong evidence for a diagnosis of TTP, although TTP should not be excluded in patients with characteristic/prototypic presentation whose levels of ADAMTS13 are not severely reduced. STEC infection should be ruled out as soon as possible when infectious HUS is possible utilizing appropriate microbiologic studies (stool culture, immunoassay for Shiga toxin or fecal polymerase chain reaction). Children may also merit testing for a cobalamin C defect, as defects of cobalamin metabolism may present with a similar hematologic picture (including thrombocytopenia, presence of bizarre microcytic red cells on the peripheral blood film, and elevations of lactate dehydrogenase [LDH] and bilirubin)

THROMBOTIC THROMBOCYTOPENIC PURPURA

Clinical Manifestation

The classic pentad of signs and symptoms that compose the TTP syndrome include MAHA, thrombocytopenia, neurologic impairment, fever, and renal dysfunction. More recent data have shown that the majority of TTP cases, which are caused by an acquired

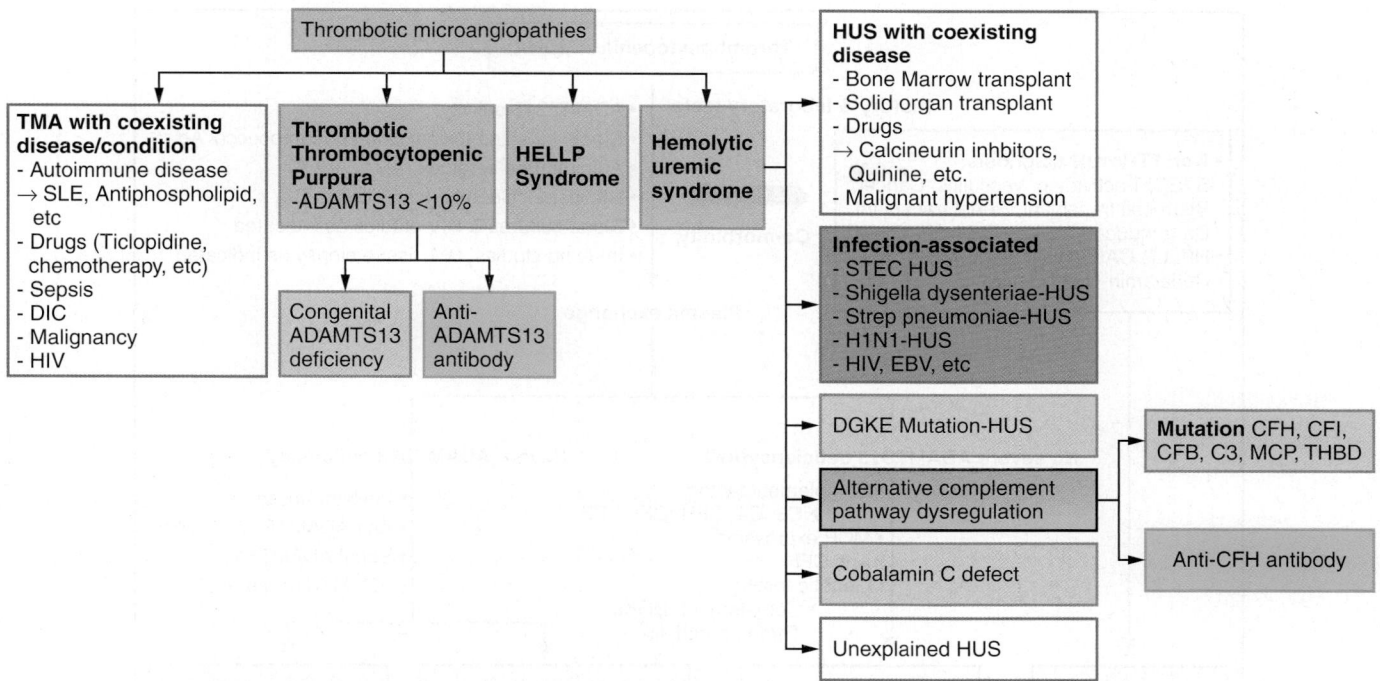

Fig. 134.1 AN ETIOLOGY-BASED CLASSIFICATION OF THE VARIOUS FORMS OF THROMBOTIC MICROANGIOPATHIES *Blue* indicates postinfectious. *Pink* indicates hereditary. *Green* indicates autoimmune. *ADAMTS13*, A disintegrin and metalloproteinase with Thrombospondin type 1 motifs, member 13; *CFB*, complement factor B; *CFH*, complement factor H; *CFI*, complement factor I; *DGKE*, diacyl glycerol kinase ε; *DIC*, disseminated intravascular coagulation; *EBV*, Epstein-Barr virus; *HIV*, human immunodeficiency virus; *HUS*, hemolytic uremic syndrome; *MCP*, membrane cofactor protein; *SLE*, systemic lupus erythematosus; *STEC*, Shiga toxin-producing *E. coli*; *THBD*, thrombomodulin; *TMA*, thrombotic microangiopathy. *(Figure modified from Loriat C, Fakhouri F, Ariceta G, et al: An international consensus approach to the management of atypical hemolytic uremic syndrome in children.* Pediatr Nephrol *31:15, 2016.)*

ADAMTS13 deficiency, present with neurologic symptoms (73.9%) and fever (72.3%). Earlier recognition of this syndrome and the established efficacy of plasma exchange, however, have led to the appreciation that MAHA and thrombocytopenia, in the absence of an obvious precipitating condition, are sufficient to make a presumptive diagnosis of TTP. The evolution of this diagnostic approach has led to a significant increase in the use of plasma exchange, and it is likely that TTP is now as frequently overdiagnosed as underdiagnosed.

Approximately 10% to 40% of patients with TTP recall an upper respiratory tract infection or flu-like syndrome in the weeks preceding the diagnosis. Patients may present with malaise, fatigue, fever, or other nonspecific symptoms days to weeks in duration and are unresponsive to antibiotics or symptomatic management. The diagnosis of TTP may be overlooked until these prodromal symptoms become unrelenting or neurologic dysfunction develops. Neurologic symptoms ranging from headache and confusion to somnolence, seizures, aphasia, or coma often dominate the clinical picture in TTP and may fluctuate in severity. This is attributed to the repetitive formation and dissolution of thrombi in the cerebral microvasculature. Other less common symptoms are abdominal pain and respiratory distress. Thrombocytopenia may be severe, with median platelet counts between 10,000 and 30,000/μL at presentation and mucocutaneous bleeding is common.

Epidemiology

Acquired TTP (caused by autoantibody inhibition of ADAMTS13 activity) accounts for 70% to 80% of all TTP cases and occurs with an estimated annual incidence of 4–10 cases per million, but the incidence appears to be increasing, perhaps as a result of increased awareness. Interestingly, a much lower incidence was reported by the Nara Medical University Registry in Japan, with 0.4 cases per million.

Acquired TTP has a higher incidence in adults compared with children and has a female/male ratio of 3:2 and a peak incidence in the fourth decade. Additional risk factors include blood group O, obesity, and African ancestry, which is also associated with an increased risk of relapse. Nonidiopathic acquired TTP (defined as TTP associated with a known precipitant), which appears to be more common and includes drug-mediated disease, should be differentiated from TMAs based on other pathologic processes (see discussion section later in chapter).

Pregnancy is another common precipitating factor for both acquired TTP (12%–31% of individuals) and hereditary TTP. TTP most frequently develops in the second or third trimester, with the decrease in ADAMTS13 levels and increase in vWF and factor VIII that occur in normal pregnancy perhaps acting as precipitants. TTP has also been reported in approximately 0.3% of human immunodeficiency virus (HIV)-infected patients, usually in those with advanced disease.

Congenital TTP, also known as *Upshaw-Schülman syndrome*, is considerably less common than idiopathic TTP. It is estimated that there are fewer than 100 cases worldwide. A 2011 study describing the natural history of congenital TTP in Japan identified 43 cases in patients ranging in age from childhood to 79 years. Of these cases, 42% were diagnosed during childhood, 36% between the ages of 15 and 45 (all female, most commonly presenting during pregnancy), and 12% beyond 45 years of age.

Pathobiology

Most patients with TTP exhibit inherited or acquired deficiency of ADAMTS13, leading to increased levels of "unusually large" vWF multimers that induce platelet aggregation in the microvasculature. Endothelial cells secrete unusually large vWF multimers that may adhere to cell surfaces and promote platelet attachment or enter

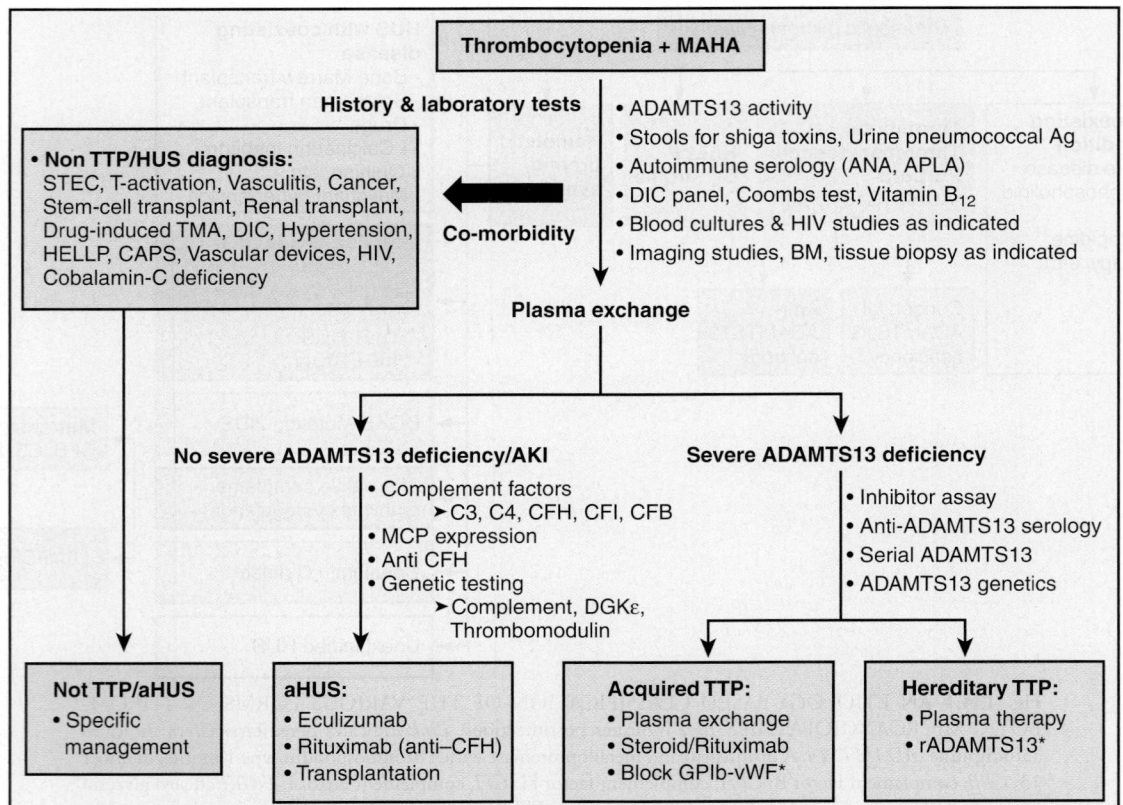

Fig. 134.2 AN APPROACH TO DIAGNOSIS AND MANAGEMENT OF THROMBOTIC MICROAN-GIOPATHIES. *ADAMTS13*, A disintegrin and metalloproteinase with Thrombospondin type 1 motifs, member 13; *Ag*, antigen; *ANA*, antinuclear antibody; *APLA*, antiphospholipid antibodies; *BM*, bone marrow; *CAPS*, catastrophic antiphospholipid syndrome; *CFB*, complement factor B; *CFH*, complement factor H; *CFI*, complement factor I; *DGKE*, diacyl glycerol kinase ε; *DIC*, disseminated intravascular coagulation; *GP*, glycoprotein; *HIV*, human immunodeficiency virus; *HUS*, hemolytic uremic syndrome; *MAHA*, mac-roangiopathic hemolytic anemia; *MCP*, membrane cofactor protein; *STEC*, Shiga toxin-producing *E. coli*; *TMA*, thrombotic microangiopathy; *TTP*, thrombotic thrombocytopenic purpura; *vWF*, von Willebrand factor. *Bullet points* are diagnoses or therapies. * indicates therapies under investigation.

the circulation and promote intravascular platelet aggregation. Under high shear, vWF multimers elongate along the endothelium and promote platelet adhesion through interactions with platelet glycoprotein (GP) Ib; shear stress–induced conformational changes also enhance the susceptibility of vWF to enzymatic cleavage. ADAMTS13 regulates the activity of vWF by cleaving the most hemostatically active high-molecular-weight multimers; failure of this feedback mechanism may lead to the microvascular thrombosis, tissue ischemia, and infarction characteristic of TTP. However, the factors that trigger sporadic episodes of TTP by causing endothelial damage or activation remain undefined. Moreover, some patients develop TTP despite normal levels of circulating ADAMTS13, while patients with congenital deficiencies of ADAMTS13 may not develop TTP until adulthood, or not at all. The latter observations suggest that ADAMTS13 deficiency should be considered an important predisposing factor, but not the sole cause of this syndrome. This concept is supported by studies of ADAMTS13-deficient mice, in which a TTP-like syndrome develops spontaneously in some genetic backgrounds (high vWF levels) but requires a triggering factor, such as Shiga toxin, in other strains.

Inherited ADAMTS13 Deficiency

Upshaw-Schülman syndrome is an autosomal recessive form of TTP first linked to vWF by Moake, who found unusually large vWF

multimers between disease flairs in the plasma of patients with chronic relapsing TTP. He proposed that the patients lacked a plasma enzyme that cleaves these unusually large multimers and that the abnormal multimers then caused uncontrolled intravascular platelet aggregation, thrombosis, and tissue infarction. Subsequently, a plasma metalloprotease was discovered that degrades vWF multimers by cleaving the Tyr^{1605}-Met^{1606} bond in the vWF A2 domain. This metal-loprotease is lacking in patients with Upshaw-Schülman syndrome.

When the vWF-degrading protease was isolated from plasma and cloned, it was found to be a member of the ADAMTS family of metalloproteases (Fig. 134.3). Genome-wide linkage analysis showed that Upshaw-Schülman syndrome is caused by mutations in the ADAMTS13 gene on chromosome 9q34.

ADAMTS13 is mainly synthesized by hepatic stellate cells but also in vascular endothelial cells and renal glomerular podocytes. Small amounts of functional ADAMTS13 are present in platelets. More than 150 mutations that can cause Upshaw-Schülman syndrome have been reported, and they have been found in almost all structural domains of ADAMTS13 (see Fig. 134.3). The majority of these mutations, approximately 60%, are single amino acid missense sub-stitutions. Mutations affecting the highly conserved N-terminal domains of ADAMTS13 are associated with lower residual enzyme activity, more severe clinical phenotype, and probably presentation of disease earlier in life. Expression studies have shown that missense mutations usually prevent the secretion of ADAMTS13, although some also impair catalytic activity.

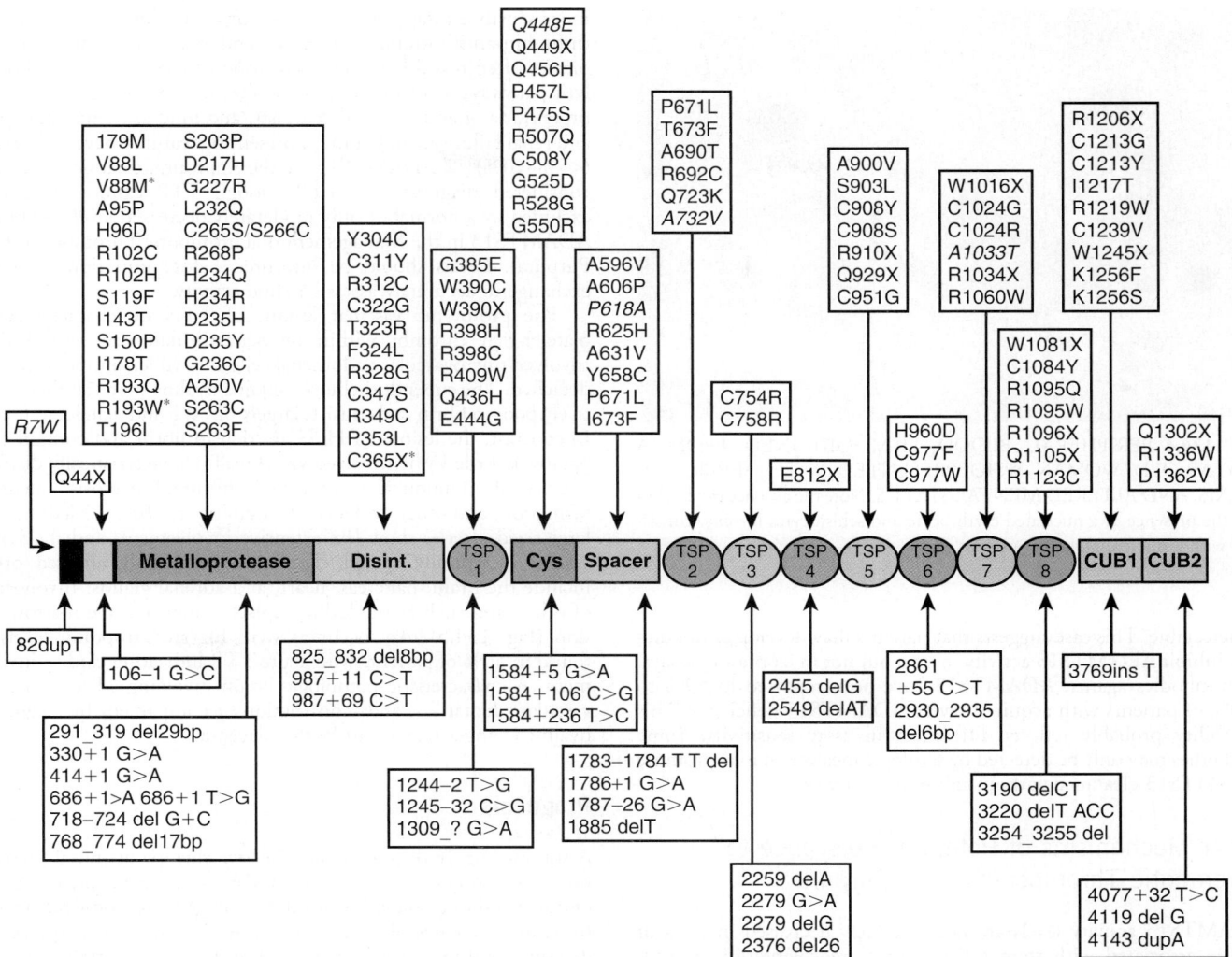

Fig. 134.3 ADAMTS13 STRUCTURE AND LOCATION OF THE MUTATIONS FOUND IN PATIENTS WITH CONGENITAL THROMBOTIC THROMBOCYTOPENIC PURPURA. ADAMTS13 is a multiple domain protein consisting of a metalloprotease domain followed by a disintegrin-like motif, a first thrombospondin-1 (TSP-1) repeat, Cys-rich and spacer domains, seven additional TSP-2 repeats, and two complement components C1r/C1s, urinary epidermal growth factor, and bone morphogenic protein-a domains. About 150 candidate mutations in ADAMTS13 spread throughout the gene have been reported in the inherited form of thrombotic thrombocytopenic purpura (Upshaw-Schülman syndrome). Most mutations are located within the N-terminal region of the protease comprising the metalloprotease domain to the Cys-rich-spacer domain of the protease. The N-terminal part of ADAMTS13 is the active part of the protein in vitro; the C-terminal part is not crucial for ADAMTS13 activity in vitro, but is essential for the normal function of ADAMTS13 in vivo. Mutations leading to amino acid substitutions (missense mutations) are found in about two-thirds of cases and truncating mutations (nonsense mutations inducing stop codon or splice/frameshift mutations) are also described. Missense and nonsense mutations are represented at the top of the figure, whereas splice/frameshift mutations are represented at the bottom of the figure. *(Reproduced from Loriat C, Coppo P, Veyradier A: TTP in children.* Curr Opin Pediatr *25:216, 2013.)*

Acquired ADAMTS13 Deficiency

Almost all patients with nonfamilial, idiopathic TTP have an acquired severe reduction or absence of ADAMTS13 activity (<5%–10%), usually associated with autoantibody immunoglobulin (Ig) G inhibitors. Some of the reported variation in ADAMTS13 activity levels may reflect inclusion or exclusion of patients with acute renal failure or other preexisting conditions. For example, severe ADAMTS13 deficiency was found in 18 of 48 adults with idiopathic TMAs unselected for renal function, but it was seen in 22 of 22 patients without acute anuric renal failure. Acquired severe ADAMTS13 deficiency (<5%–10%) is rare in other settings, with the possible exception of severe hepatic insufficiency or sepsis. For example,

ADAMTS13 levels below 5% were found in 17 of 109 patients with sepsis-induced disseminated intravascular coagulation (DIC). More modest decreases (typically >40%) occur in newborns and among adults with cirrhosis, chronic renal insufficiency, pregnancy, connective tissue diseases, and various inflammatory conditions; none had levels below 6%. Therefore severe ADAMTS13 deficiency appears to be specific for TTP in the appropriate clinical setting.

ADAMTS13 levels appear normal in some cases of idiopathic TTP. This was highlighted by the unusual case reported by Froelich-Zahnd and colleagues of a patient with multiple relapses of HIV-associated TTP. With the earlier relapses, the patient had detectable ADAMTS13 activity by multiple assays and responded to plasma exchange. In contrast, with later relapses ADAMTS13 levels were

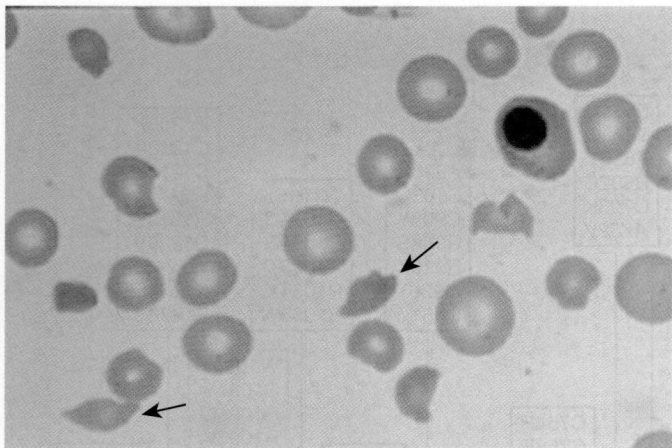

Fig. 134.4 PERIPHERAL BLOOD FILM OBTAINED FROM A 28-YEAR-OLD WOMAN WHO PRESENTED WITH FEVER, EPISTAXIS, AND ALTERED MENTAL STATUS. Note the absence of platelets and the presence of a nucleated erythrocyte and schistocytes *(arrows)* consistent with a microangiopathic process.

undetectable. This case suggests that patients may develop antibodies that inhibit ADAMTS13 activity in vivo but not in laboratory assays.

Antibodies against ADAMTS13 have been reported in 59% to 100% of patients with acquired severe ADAMTS13 deficiency. This variability probably reflects differences in assay sensitivity. Some antibodies may only be detected by serologic means and may promote ADAMTS13 clearance without inhibiting activity.

Other Mechanisms of Potential Relevance to Thrombotic Thrombocytopenic Purpura

ADAMTS13 activity levels are rarely severely decreased in cases of TMAs associated with stem cell or organ transplantation, cancer, infections, severe hypertension, and certain drugs. Therefore mechanisms other than ADAMTS13 deficiency can cause TMA, and various studies have implicated direct endothelial injury, platelet activation, and alterations in blood clotting as contributory factors. Evidence in support of these mechanisms include the demonstration of (1) increased levels of circulating endothelial proteins (thrombomodulin, PAI-1, vWF) and endothelial cell microparticles in TTP plasma; (2) circulating antiplatelet and antiendothelial cell antibodies, some of which may bind CD36 and impair ADAMTS13 binding to endothelial cells; (3) increased levels of circulating platelet-derived microparticles; (4) induction of microvascular endothelial cell apoptosis by plasma from patients with idiopathic, HIV-associated, or ticlopidine-associated TTP; (5) increased plasma procoagulant activity; (6) increased endothelin and decreased nitric oxide, leading to vasoconstriction; and (7) diminished plasma fibrinolytic activity because of elevated levels of PAI-1.

Laboratory Manifestations

The presence of schistocytes on the peripheral blood smear is a characteristic laboratory finding of TTP (Fig. 134.4). Schistocytes may not be apparent in rare patients at disease onset. The markedly elevated levels of plasma LDH typically seen in patients with TTP reflect both hemolysis and tissue ischemia. Nucleated red blood cells are present in many patients, and their number may be disproportionately increased in comparison with the degree of reticulocytosis. With rare exceptions, the direct antiglobulin test is negative. The prothrombin time, partial thromboplastin time, and fibrinogen levels are usually normal or only mildly perturbed; mild elevations in fibrinogen degradation products occur in 50% of patients although

more sensitive assays, such as those for prothrombin fragment 1+2, thrombin-antithrombin complexes and plasmin-antiplasmin complexes, often reveal low-grade activation of coagulation and fibrinolytic pathways. Evidence of renal involvement may include hematuria, proteinuria, granular or red cell casts, and mild azotemia, but anuria and renal failure are uncommon presenting features. Severe deficiency (<5%–10%) of ADAMTS13 in the appropriate clinical setting is considered diagnostic of TTP, though TTP cannot be entirely excluded by a normal or only moderately decreased level (see box on ADAMTS13 in the Management of Thrombotic Thrombocytopenic Purpura). Levels should be measured before initiation of plasma exchange to accurately assess baseline activity.

The prototypic vascular lesions of TTP are characterized by platelet-rich thrombi within or beneath damaged endothelium. Involved microvascular endothelial cells are swollen and in some cases detached. The subendothelium contains hyaline material that is relatively poor in fibrin and consists largely of vWF and platelet remnants. In contrast, the lesions of HUS are rich in fibrin and contain comparatively little vWF. Involved vessel walls characteristically display a paucity of mononuclear leukocytes; fibrinoid necrosis, aneurysm formation, and other evidence of vasculitis are absent. Medium- and large-sized arteries show less extensive involvement, and the venous system is typically spared. The most commonly affected organs include the brain, pancreas, heart, and adrenal glands. Involvement of other sites such as the kidney, spleen, gingiva, bone marrow, and skin (Fig. 134.5) may occur as well. Elevated troponin levels are found in 50% of patients with acute TTP, indicating cardiac involvement. A characteristic pathologic lesion involving adjacent areas of vascular dilatation and constriction accompanied by segmental hyaline changes may occur in the placenta.

Prognosis

Assuming timely diagnosis and effective therapy at initial presentation, the prognosis of primary TMA is relatively favorable. For example, although older historical data suggest a response rate in TTP to plasma exchange of approximately 80%, more recent studies have demonstrated response rates upward of 95% and mortality rates less than 5%. This apparent improvement in outcome may be generalized and reflects advances in supportive care as well as active therapies. Patients with acquired TTP continue to experience a significant relapse rate of 30% to 50%, though these numbers may be further reduced if rituximab is used for the initial treatment of patients with autoimmune disease.

Patients with congenital deficiency of ADAMTS13 may follow a chronic, relapsing course, but relapses may be prevented by periodic plasma infusions. Case reports suggest that some intermediate-purity factor VIII concentrates may also supply sufficient ADAMTS13 to prevent symptomatic relapses. Insufficient numbers of patients have been followed to determine whether overall survival is reduced in patients with congenital ADAMTS13 deficiency, and case reports suggest that these individuals may be at increased risk for stroke.

Therapy

Without therapy, the mortality rate of TTP exceeds 90%. Through the mid-1970s, splenectomy remained the only modality with more than an anecdotal response rate. Prognosis has been dramatically improved since the advent of plasma-based therapy, such that long-term survival may now exceed 90%.

Plasma Therapy in Thrombotic Thrombocytopenic Purpura

The beneficial effect of plasma therapy in TTP was first noted more than 25 years ago when the results of a prospective trial resolved the long-debated issue of the relative efficacy of plasma exchange versus

Management of Thrombotic Thrombocytopenic Purpura and Management of Atypical Hemolytic Uremic Syndrome)

Management of TTP

- A high index of suspicion is necessary to make a diagnosis of TTP.
  - ADAMTS13 activity should be determined before initiation of plasma therapy.
- Prompt initiation of therapy is required to prevent organ dysfunction or death.
- Prophylaxis is recommended during pregnancy.
- For suspected or confirmed acquired (autoimmune) TTP:
  - Plasma exchange is recommended (exchange 1–1.5 plasma volumes [40–60 mL/kg]) daily Plasma infusion may be used until exchange is initiated.
  - Continue plasma exchange until the neurologic symptoms have resolved and the serum LDH and platelet count is normal; many experts recommend continuing plasma exchange for an additional 2–3 days thereafter.
  - Corticosteroids are often used as part of initial therapy
  - Administration of rituximab together with plasma exchange early in the course of disease appears to induce a more rapid response and may delay relapse.
  - Use of rituximab is controversial for treatment of asymptomatic patients (in clinical remission) with ADAMTS 13 deficiency.
  - Splenectomy is generally reserved for patients who are refractory to plasma exchange and rituximab.
  - Immunosuppressive agents are only recommended for patients with critical illness that is unresponsive to plasma exchange, corticosteroids, and rituximab.
  - Platelet transfusion should be reserved for life-threatening bleeds. Packed red blood cells can safely be transfused in TTP.
- For hereditary TTP (Upshaw-Schulman syndrome)
  - Plasma infusion is often sufficient to treat acute symptoms.
  - Prophylactic plasma infusion may prevent symptomatic recurrence.

Management of aHUS

- A high index of suspicion is necessary for diagnosis of aHUS.
  - aHUS is a systemic disorder
    - Advanced renal failure, hypertension and increased vascular permeability suggest a diagnosis of aHUS rather than TTP
    - Neurologic and gastrointestinal symptoms are common.
- aHUS is a diagnosis of exclusion
  - TTP should be excluded with ADAMTS13 assay
  - STEC-HUS should be excluded with stool culture and/or tests for Shiga toxin
  - Other causes of microangiopathic hemolytic anemia should be excluded with history, coagulation studies, infectious disease studies, serologies, etc.
  - Plasma studies of C3, C4, and complement control proteins (CFH, CFI, CFB) and autoantibody to CFH may be normal, as may be genetic studies (CFH, CFI, CFB, C3, MCP, THBD, DGKE). Initiation of therapy should not be delayed while awaiting test results.
- Treatment of suspected or confirmed aHUS:
  - Plasma exchange is recommended until a diagnosis of TTP is excluded.
  - Eculizumab is currently the therapy of choice for aHUS
    - Vaccination to prevent meningococcal infection is required; antibiotic prophylaxis should also be considered.
    - Early treatment reduces the risk of long-term renal impairment.
    - Thrombocytopenia and hemolysis tend to respond early, but renal recovery may take months.
    - Long-term therapy is currently recommended. If eculizumab is discontinued, close follow up to detect early relapse is suggested.

ADAMTS13, A disintegrin and metalloproteinase with Thrombospondin type 1 motifs, member 13; aHUS, atypical hemolytic uremic syndrome; CFB, complement factor B; CFH, complement factor H; CFI, complement factor I; DGKE, diacyl glycerol kinase ε; LDH, lactate dehydrogenase; MCP, membrane cofactor protein; STEC, Shiga toxin-producing E. coli; THBD, thrombomodulin; TTP, thrombotic thrombocytopenic purpura.

only infusion of plasma. At 6 months, complete remissions were seen in 78% of patients treated with exchange versus 31% of those treated with plasma infusion. This study did not resolve the question as to whether removal of a disease-inciting agent or replacement of a missing factor accounted for the superior response, particularly because patients in the exchange arm received a threefold larger volume of plasma. Indeed, a retrospective study demonstrated no significant difference in outcome in patients with acquired TTP who received equal volumes of plasma by exchange or infusion. However, the current model for the pathogenesis of acquired idiopathic TTP suggests that plasma exchange is superior because it both removes an IgG inhibitor of ADAMTS13 and replaces the deficient protein. In contrast, plasma infusion (or potentially infusion of a factor concentrate containing ADAMTS13) suffices for patients with genetic ADAMTS13 deficiency. Large volumes of plasma are more easily administered by exchange, and unless a genetic deficiency of ADAMTS13 has been documented, plasma infusion should be reserved for situations in which exchange is not immediately available. The recovery of ADAMTS13 levels may lag behind other indicators of clinical response, and the utility of monitoring ADAMTS13 levels during treatment has not been established.

Plasma (either fresh frozen plasma [FFP] or thawed plasma) remains the most commonly used replacement product for plasma exchange. There is no clear advantage to the use of cryo-poor plasma (CPP), which is depleted of vWF. These findings are consistent with a recent study showing similar concentrations and stability of ADAMTS13 during storage at 1–5°C in CPP and FFP. Pilot studies suggest that solvent-detergent treated plasma (which contains ADAMTS13 at concentrations approximately 20% lower than those in FFP) is as efficacious as FFP and is associated with fewer allergic/urticarial reactions.

Treatment is generally initiated with the goal of exchanging 1–1.5 plasma volumes (40–60 mL/kg) daily, although the optimal regimen has not been determined. The volume of exchange can be increased to 1.5–2 plasma volumes daily if the initial response is poor. Neurologic improvement occurs most rapidly, often within hours to days. The serum LDH level typically falls by 50% within 3 days in responders, and the platelet count begins to rise at a mean of 5 days, though normalization may take up to several weeks. Impaired renal function and disappearance of schistocytes are generally the last to improve.

Daily plasma exchange should be continued until neurologic symptoms have resolved and both a normal serum LDH and platelet count have been achieved; many experts recommend an additional 2–3 days of plasma exchange thereafter. Approximately 85% to 90% of patients show a clinical and laboratory response to plasma exchange within 3 weeks, most often within 10 days (mean 15.8; range 3–36 days). However, 20% to 40% of patients will experience an exacerbation of disease within 30 days after stopping plasma exchange, whereas approximately 30% will relapse at later dates, usually within the first year. The decision to switch to CPP or to introduce another form of therapy is empiric but is generally not considered until the patient has received a minimum of 10–14 days of daily exchange with FFP. One prospective nonrandomized study suggested that administration of rituximab early in the course of disease in conjunction with plasma exchange induced more rapid responses and reduced relapses. Little or no data are available to support either abrupt discontinuation or "tapering" of plasma exchange after remission.

Complication rates associated with plasma exchange therapy have been reported to be as high as 30%, but recent reports suggest a lower rate. The majority of adverse events are related to central venous catheter insertion, infection, allergic reactions to plasma and occasionally thrombosis.

Plasma exchange is effective for patients with or without inhibitors, and clinical responses frequently occur despite persistence of both the inhibitor and severe ADAMTS13 deficiency, although

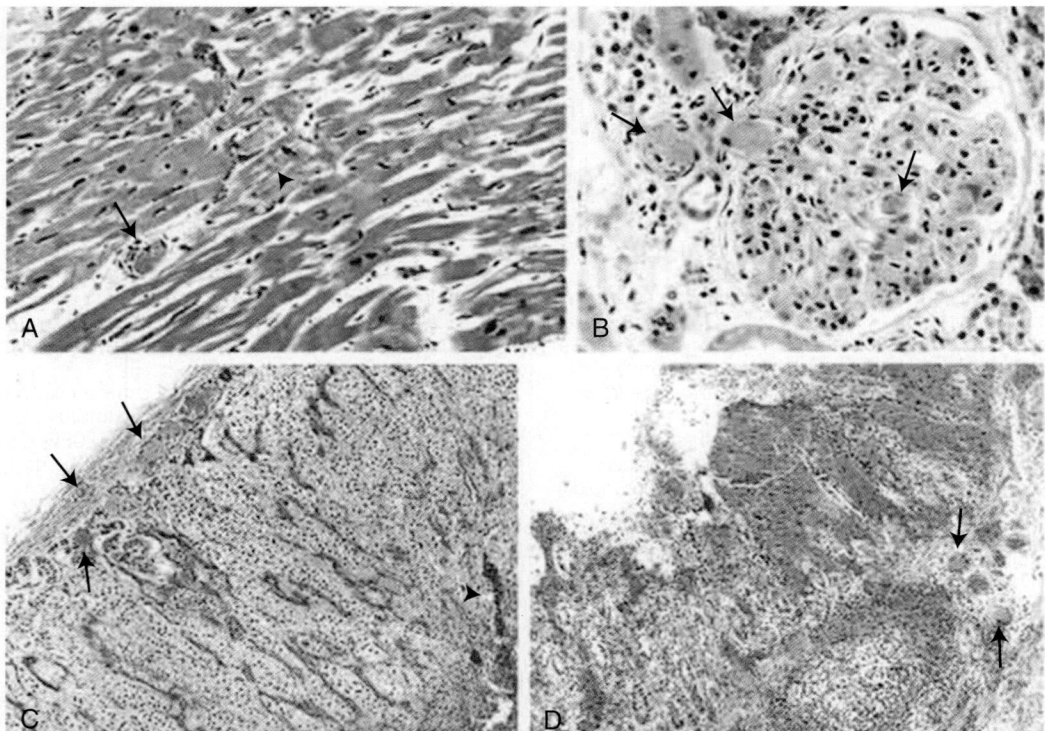

Fig. 134.5 TISSUE SPECIMENS OBTAINED AT AUTOPSY FROM A PATIENT WITH ABNORMALITIES CHARACTERISTIC OF THROMBOTIC THROMBOCYTOPENIC PURPURA. A specimen from the heart (A) shows multiple intramyocardial microthrombi (*arrow*), hemorrhage, and early ischemic changes, with scattered foci of contraction-band necrosis (*arrowhead*). A specimen from the kidney (B) shows characteristic microthrombi in an afferent arteriole, the glomerular hilum, and glomerular capillaries (*arrows*) together with vascular congestion and parenchymal hemorrhage in the surrounding interstitium. A tissue specimen from the adrenal gland (C) shows characteristic subcapsular microthrombi (*arrows*) with congestion of the cortical arterioles and medullary parenchymal hemorrhage (*arrowhead*). A specimen from the cecum (D) shows submucosal microthrombi (*arrows*) and hemorrhagic mucosal ulceration and necrosis. Microthrombi were also present in the pancreas, thyroid gland, and other organs. (*Reproduced from George, JN: Thrombotic thrombocytopenic purpura. N Engl J Med 354:1927, 2006, with permission. Photographs and interpretation by Patrick Stangeby.*)

patients with high titer inhibitors may respond more slowly and relapse more often. Both congenital and acquired ADAMTS13 deficiency are characterized by unpredictable periods of stability between relapses, probably reflecting exacerbation of the disease by co-morbid conditions that activate or damage the endothelium, thereby increasing the release of unusually large vWF multimers, and triggering microvascular thrombosis.

Rituximab

Several reports support the efficacy of rituximab, an anti-CD20 antibody, for decreasing the level of autoantibodies and restoring normal ADAMTS13 activity in TTP. In one study, remission was noted in more than 90% of patients treated with rituximab (with plasma exchange and corticosteroids) in an acute episode of TTP within 14–21 days. In addition, patients who received rituximab with plasma exchange experienced a fivefold lower relapse rate at a median of 18 months compared with historical controls. In cases of refractory TTP, increases in platelet count were noted in more than 80% of patients with the addition of rituximab to plasma exchange and corticosteroids; the time required to achieve a platelet count response was also decreased. Though there were fewer relapses in rituximab treated patients in the short term, this may represent a delay in immune reconstitution and the number of relapses may not differ from that in controls with longer term follow up.

Prophylactic treatment with rituximab may also result in fewer TTP relapses, although again, longer-term follow-up studies are needed. After initial prophylactic rituximab, 30% of patients had asymptomatic decreases in ADAMTS13 activity and required additional rituximab or other treatments, some of which have greater risks than rituximab. In some asymptomatic patients, sustained recovery of ADAMTS13 activity failed to occur, even with multiple courses of rituximab treatment. Therefore, the value of rituximab treatment during remission remains controversial.

Corticosteroids

Corticosteroids are often used as part of initial treatment or for patients who fail to show a brisk response to plasma-based therapy. These drugs are of little benefit when used alone, and retrospective studies do not provide compelling evidence that they improve the response to plasma exchange. However, the antiinflammatory and immunosuppressive effects of corticosteroids make them a logical adjunct for treatment of autoimmune TTP, and most experts continue to use them in patients receiving plasma exchange.

Splenectomy

Before the introduction of plasma therapy, splenectomy was the first-line treatment for TTP and induced remission in up to 50% of patients. Currently, open or laparoscopic splenectomy is reserved for patients who are refractory to plasma exchange and rituximab. Splenectomy may reduce the frequency of relapses in patients with chronic relapsing TTP. Plasma exchange should be continued after splenectomy until the TMA resolves.

Other Modalities

Antiplatelet Agents

The response rate to aspirin, dipyridamole, sulfinpyrazone, or ticlopidine as single antiplatelet agents approximates 10%, essentially indistinguishable from the natural history. Antiplatelet agents have not been convincingly shown to increase the response to plasma exchange and may promote bleeding in the setting of severe thrombocytopenia and invasive procedures.

Immunosuppressive Agents

Cyclosporine has been used as an alternative to rituximab for decreasing the risk of relapse and the time to achieve a durable remission. There is evidence that cyclosporin reduces the incidence of TTP relapse, decreases ADAMTS13 antibody levels and produces a parallel increase in ADAMTS13 activity. Cyclophosphamide and vincristine were used before the advent of rituximab. However in current practice, they are used only in patients with critical illness that is unresponsive to treatment with plasma exchange, corticosteroids, and rituximab. Reports of responses to other immunosuppressive agents including azathioprine, mycophenolate mofetil, staphylococcal protein A immunoadsorption and bortezomib also exist.

Intravenous Immunoglobulin

The efficacy of intravenous immunoglobulin remains unclear.

Supportive Care

Starting low-dose aspirin (81 mg daily) once the platelet count exceeds 50,000/µL has been recommended in the 2003 guidelines of the British Committee for Standards in Haematology. Folate supplementation and administration of the hepatitis B vaccine should be considered routine components of supportive care. Platelet transfusion in patients with TTP should be restricted to patients with life-threatening bleeds (see discussion later).

Blood Product Transfusion in Thrombotic Microangiopathy

Red Blood Cells

Patients with TTP often develop symptomatic anemia because of bleeding and partially compensated hemolytic anemia. Packed red blood cells can be transfused safely in this setting. In older adults and in those with impaired cardiac function, it may be prudent to provide an additional margin of safety when choosing a threshold for transfusion.

Platelet Transfusion

Historically, platelet transfusions have not been recommended for patients with TTP because they have been hypothesized to provoke fatal thrombotic events. This is based on two observations. First, there are anecdotal reports of a close temporal relationship between platelet transfusion and adverse outcomes. In these cases, there was clinical deterioration within 1–24 hours of allogeneic platelet transfusion. Second, postmortem examination in such patients revealed widespread microthrombi involving the brain, heart, lung, kidney, and multiple other organs. Furthermore, clinical deterioration after platelet transfusion has also been reported in patients with other TMAs (HUS, STEC-HUS and drug-induced TMAs). Rarely, sudden death has occurred in patients who responded to plasma therapy with a rapid rise in the platelet count.

Data from the Oklahoma TTP-HUS registry challenge this dogma. Thus none of 33 platelet transfusions administered to a cohort of 54 consecutive TTP patients (of whom 47 had ADAMTS13 activity <10%) was associated with an increase in the incidence of death or severe neurologic events. The authors of the study concluded that there was "uncertain evidence of harm" with platelet transfusion in TTP. More recently however, this question has been revisited in a study conducted over a 5-year period (2007–2011) using a large US inpatient database (Nationwide Inpatient Sample that includes both adults and children). Based on retrospective analysis of these data, platelet transfusion was associated with a sixfold higher risk of arterial (but not venous) thrombosis and a twofold higher risk of acute myocardial infarction, after adjusting for age and gender in a population with no reported prior history of thrombosis. In experienced hands, vascular access catheters for apheresis can safely be inserted even in the face of thrombocytopenia. Therefore based on accumulating evidence, platelet transfusion in TTP patients should be reserved for those with life-threatening bleeding.

SHIGA TOXIN HEMOLYTIC UREMIC SYNDROME

Clinical Manifestations

STEC-HUS is one of the main causes of acute renal failure in children. Patients generally present with the triad of hemolytic anemia, thrombocytopenia and acute renal injury. STEC-HUS occurs most commonly after E. coli O157:H7–induced gastroenteritis, with rare cases reported after infection of the urinary tract or skin, or after infection with organisms other than E. coli. The clinical presentation begins with the sudden onset of abdominal pain and watery diarrhea, on average 4 days (range, 2–12 days) after toxin exposure. Abdominal pain may be severe and precede the onset of diarrhea. In the absence of fever, STEC-HUS may be difficult to differentiate from inflammatory bowel disease, appendicitis, ischemic colitis, or intussusception. Bloody diarrhea generally ensues on the second day, accompanied in some cases by nausea and vomiting; though up to one-third of patients do not report blood in the stool. Fever is typically absent or mild. Colonoscopy reveals edematous colonic mucosa with occasional ulceration and pseudomembrane formation.

E. coli–associated hemorrhagic gastroenteritis is complicated by HUS in 8% to 18% of sporadic cases, and in over 20% in certain epidemic outbreaks. Therefore, the disease should be suspected in a patient who presents with characteristic clinical manifestations after an episode of bloody diarrhea, although the prototypic history of a preceding hemorrhagic gastroenteritis may be absent in up to 30% of cases. Young children and older adults are at greatest risk. HUS typically develops 7 days (range, 5–13 days) after the onset of diarrhea. Patients often present with oliguria or other evidence of renal impairment; 50% of patients require dialysis, at least temporarily. The severity of MAHA varies considerably, but many affected individuals require red cell transfusion. Thrombocytopenia is common, with a median platelet count of 30,000/µL in one study, but may be mild or absent in up to 30% of cases at presentation. Up to 25% of patients develop neurologic manifestations, which may include irritability and somnolence and less commonly, confusion, paresis, and seizures. The mortality rate is estimated at 3% to 5%.

Epidemiology

STEC-HUS accounts for at least 90% of cases of infection associated HUS. In one study conducted in the United States, the median age of patients with STEC-HUS was 4 years; 55% of patients were younger than 5 years of age, 33% between 5 and 17 years, 6% between 18 and 44 years, and 6% older than 45 years of age. The annual incidence of STEC-HUS is estimated to be 2–3 per 10^5 in children under age 5. STEC accounts for 80% to 86% of cases in the United States and Europe. The most common serotype of E. coli associated with HUS is O157:H7, although other serotypes including O26:H11, O103:H2, O111:NM, O21:H19, O145:NM and O104:H4 have been reported. The major reservoir of STEC is domestic cattle; approximately 2% to 3% harbor STEC in their gastrointestinal tract at the time of slaughter, and meat can become contaminated during processing. The organism has also been isolated from deer, sheep, goats, horses, dogs, birds, and flies. Large outbreaks have been reported in association with ingestion of contaminated ground beef, although contamination of poultry, cheese, fruits, and vegetables has also been reported. Other cases have been attributed to ingestion of contaminated water or unpasteurized apple cider or milk. The incidence of STEC-HUS may be increasing as a result of developments in food production methods. Industrial farming generates large quantities of potentially contaminated manure that periodically enters streams, where it can contaminate feed and uncooked vegetables. A 2011 outbreak of HUS in Northern Germany that affected more than 3000 individuals was caused by enteroaggressive *E. coli* O104:H4; the infection vector was traced to bean sprouts with evidence of intrahousehold transmission. Carriage of STEC may be asymptomatic, and fecal-oral transmission may contribute to epidemic spread in day care centers, nursing homes, and petting zoos. Aerosolization in barns has been implicated in outbreaks at fairs.

STEC strains are also associated with sporadic, nonepidemic cases of HUS. The disease occurs more frequently during the summer and autumn in temperate climates. Infection by Shiga toxin–producing *Shigella dysenteriae* serotype 1 is associated with HUS in developing countries and carries a higher mortality.

Pathobiology

STEC-HUS is caused by endothelial cell damage initiated by Shiga toxin and the inflammatory cytokines they induce. The type of Shiga toxin, as well as other virulence factors, contributes to risk.

After ingestion, the noninvasive enteropathic *E. coli* bacteria colonize the terminal ileum and follicle-associated epithelium of Peyer patches, after which they colonize the colon. Once colonization occurs, STEC bacteria express numerous virulence factors by horizontally transmitted gene cassettes termed *pathogenicity islands*. One pathogenicity island contains the locus of enterocyte effacement, which contains genes for the adhesin intimin, as well as a type III (three) secretion system that mediates transfer of bacterial proteins directly into enterocytes. Their capacity to cause HUS is mediated by two 70-kDa bacterial exotoxins. The toxins are transported across the intestinal epithelium through specific para- and intercellular mechanisms and then circulate, most likely by low affinity binding to the surface of neutrophils and platelets, before being transferred to higher affinity receptors expressed on glomerular endothelial cells that are upregulated by proinflammatory cytokines.

The toxin produced by these strains of *E. coli* is identical to Shigella toxin and is therefore generally referred to as *Shiga-like toxin 1 (Stx1)*. Most strains of pathogenic *E. coli* produce a second homologous toxin, Stx2, which is associated with a higher risk for HUS. The toxins are carried on a lysogenic bacteriophage capable of infecting other strains of *E. coli*. Intact, 70-kDa Stx holotoxins consist of a 32-kDa A subunit and five 7.7-kDa B receptor-binding subunits. The toxin binds to terminal Gala1-4Galb (galabiose) residues on globosyltriaosylceramide (Gb$_3$; also known as *CD77* and the human blood group *P^k antigen*). Increased expression of Gb$_3$ on glomerular microvascular and cerebral endothelium compared with other vascular beds contributes to their heightened sensitivity to apoptosis, cytotoxicity, upregulation of integrins, and procoagulant activity. The higher levels of Gb$_3$ expression in children compared with adults may explain why children are particularly prone to develop HUS.

Following binding to Gb$_3$, Stx1 and Stx2 are internalized and transported in a retrograde manner to the endoplasmic reticulum and translocated into the cytosol. The A subunit is proteolyzed to a 27-kDa A1 subunit that binds the 60S ribosomal subunit and cleaves adenine 4323 from the 28S ribosomal RNA. This prevents elongation factor 1-dependent binding of aminoacyl tRNA, which inhibits protein synthesis and leads to ribotoxic stress response, changes in cellular function, and apoptosis. Stx alters the usual balance between intestinal absorption and secretion to a net excretory phenotype. *E. coli* lipopolysaccharide and Stx also stimulate leukocyte and intrarenal expression of proinflammatory cytokines (including interleukin

[IL]-1, IL-1β, IL-6, and IL-8; MCP-1; and interferon-γ), which exacerbate toxin- and leukocyte-induced endothelial dysfunction. Changes in endothelial function include upregulation of expression of Stx receptors, which further sensitizes cells to Stx-induced injury, increased expression of P-selectin and tissue factor, increased release of vWF, and downregulation of thrombomodulin expression. Early in the course of the disease, Stx also acts in concert with lipopolysaccharide to trigger a procoagulant state that involves platelet activation.

It remains unclear why a minority of patients infected with STEC bacteria develops STEC-HUS. Activation of complement may contribute to the pathogenesis of Stx-HUS. Stx2 directly activates the alternative pathway (AP) of complement and binds to short consensus repeat (SCR) 6-8 and 19-20 of factor H, which mediate surface recognition, blocking its ability to inhibit complement activation on cell surfaces. It has been hypothesized that subtle allotypic variation in factor H (CFH) may modulate the sensitivity of CFH to Stx2-induced dysregulation in susceptible patients.

Laboratory Manifestations

Like TTP, STEC-HUS is characterized by MAHA and thrombocytopenia. Thrombocytopenia tends to be less severe than that observed in TTP, and renal disease is the major clinical manifestation.

Renal biopsy, although rarely required for diagnosis in endemic areas, illustrates the importance of endothelial damage. Involved glomeruli show widening of the subendothelial space, which is filled with cellular debris and fibrin. Glomerular capillary endothelial cells are swollen and occasionally detached, leading to obliteration of the capillary lumens.

Though clinical features are often sufficient for the diagnosis of STEC-HUS, bacteriologic confirmation should be sought through stool culture, testing for Stx (e.g., by enzyme-linked immunosorbent assay), stool analysis for Stx structural genes, or acute and convalescent serologies. Stool should be tested as soon as possible after the onset of diarrhea. The recovery rate for STEC appears to be at least 90% during the first 6 days but less than 33% thereafter. *E. coli* O157:H7 ferments sorbitol slowly, appearing as colorless overnight colonies on sorbitol-MacConkey agar; sorbitol-negative cultures may be further characterized using commercially available O157:H7-specific antisera. Methods to detect Stx or their structural genes improve diagnostic sensitivity.

Antibody titers against *E. coli* O157:H7 antigens and Stx rise after infection, persist for 8–12 weeks, and may be useful to confirm STEC infection in selected cases; however, they are not widely available. In some cases, further evaluation may be desired to differentiate STEC-HUS from the other TMAs, such as autoimmune disease, aHUS and TTP.

Prognosis

The outcome of patients with STEC-HUS is generally favorable, although STEC-HUS remains the most common cause of acute renal failure in children and up to 60% of children require dialysis during the acute phase. However, STEC-HUS is usually self-limited and as a result of advances in supportive care, mortality has been reduced to 3% to 5%, with death usually caused by severe involvement of the central nervous system, intestine, or myocardium. Renal insufficiency generally resolves within 2–3 weeks, although some patients have prolonged anuria, requiring several months before recovery. Despite a favorable short-term outcome, many children with STEC-HUS develop chronic renal insufficiency over time. In one report of 29 patients with "typical" childhood HUS followed for 15–28 years, 7 developed chronic renal failure and 12 developed hypertension, proteinuria, or reduced glomerular filtration rate, whereas only 10 showed no residual abnormalities. Therefore 50% to 60% of patients have complete recovery with long-term preservation of renal function. Long-term outcomes are worse in older patients. Proteinuria persisting for more than 1 year after the initial episode of TMA is likewise associated with progressive renal disease.

Therapy

Treatment of STEC-HUS is supportive. Volume expansion within the first 4 days of the onset of diarrhea significantly reduces the incidence of progression to oliguric HUS. However, no therapy has been shown to prevent HUS or to reduce the severity of kidney injury once established. In randomized trials, neither plasma infusion nor exchange was of benefit in children or adults with STEC-HUS. Corticosteroids, heparin, urokinase, aspirin, dipyridamole, antifibrinolytic drugs and intravenous immunoglobulin are ineffective. Antimotility agents and narcotics delay clearance of *E. coli* and toxin from the gastrointestinal tract and may increase the risk for progression to TMA; therefore these agents should be avoided. Nonsteroidal antiinflammatory agents may reduce renal blood flow and should also be avoided. Most experts believe that antibiotics increase the risk for progression to HUS, probably by lysing bacteria, releasing Stx and inducing bacteriophages on which Stx genes are expressed. Therefore, routine use of antibiotic is discouraged.

Activation of complement may contribute to the pathogenesis of STEC-HUS. In support of this concept, eculizumab, an antibody to complement factor 5, was reported to reverse neurologic abnormalities, low platelet counts, and elevated LDH levels in three patients with STEC-HUS. However, insufficient data are available to validate this hypothesis. During the 2011 German O105H4 STEC-HUS epidemic, eculizumab was administered most commonly to patients with the most severe organ compromise and often late in the course of disease. The outcome in these patients was similar to that in untreated patients, suggesting a potential role. Similarly immunoadsorption appeared to potentially benefit a small cohort of patients with severe neurologic compromise; however, most of these patients also received other therapeutic interventions. Additional data on the utility of eculizumab and immunoadsorption are needed before their routine use can be recommended.

Isolation of patients with STEC-HUS should be considered because shedding of the pathogenic bacteria may continue long after cessation of diarrhea.

ATYPICAL HEMOLYTIC UREMIC SYNDROME

Clinical Manifestations

Like TTP, aHUS may present with a prodrome suggestive of an upper respiratory tract infection or with nonspecific symptoms of malaise and fatigue. Though aHUS is generally not associated with a prodrome of bloody diarrhea, a history of recent gastroenteritis may be obtained from up to 30% of patients making distinction from STEC-HUS difficult. Extrarenal manifestations may occur in up to half of the patients; neurologic manifestations are typically less common and severe than in TTP and are less likely to dominate the course. Evidence of microangiopathy on the peripheral blood film is a universal finding, and the reticulocyte count and LDH concentration are elevated, but severe thrombocytopenia is less common than in TTP. Renal involvement is more severe than in TTP, with up to 60% of patients requiring dialysis. It has been suggested that in the absence of another cause for a renal TMA (such as STEC-HUS, systemic lupus erythematosus, scleroderma, medication effect, complications of transplantation, etc.), the presence of a creatinine over 2.3 mg/dL and a platelet count over 30,000/μL argues against a diagnosis of TTP and favors aHUS. However, cohort studies in patients with TTP indicated that some patients did require dialysis; suggesting that these disorders may be indistinguishable on clinical grounds alone, thereby highlighting the importance of ADAMTS13 assessment.

Typically, aHUS follows a chronic relapsing course, often complicated by hypertension and renal insufficiency. Moreover, exacerbations are often preceded by infection, pregnancy, or other seemingly incidental events. Affected patients have a high risk for recurrence after renal allografting, and HUS occasionally presents in related donors after surgery. The disorder may resemble TMA associated with pregnancy, cancer, and chemotherapy, which have similar clinical presentations, but different natural histories.

Epidemiology

aHUS is a systemic TMA in which renal failure develops in the absence of a coexisting disease. While historically considered a pediatric disease, approximately 40% of cases present in adulthood, with the remaining 60% occurring in pediatric patients. However, aHUS only accounts for 5% to 10% of all childhood HUS. Seventy percent of children have their first episode before 2 years of age, 25% of these developing before 6 months, an age at which STEC-HUS is very uncommon. Childhood aHUS is equally prevalent in males and females, with a slight female preponderance in adults. Abnormalities in complement regulation, most commonly arising from mutations in complement regulatory proteins, have been implicated in up to 70% of cases. Inheritance is autosomal dominant with approximately 50% penetrance, and aHUS may occur in siblings with or without identical genetic abnormalities. Clinical conditions that increase complement activation (including pregnancy) may unmask the genetic propensity to develop aHUS. An autosomal recessive form of aHUS attributable to defects in the gene encoding for DGKE (an enzyme involved in intracellular signaling) has recently been described. Defects in DGKE may account for up to 30% of cases of aHUS presenting before the first year of life.

The incidence of aHUS in the United States has been estimated at 2 per million. More than 1000 patients with aHUS investigated for complement abnormalities have been identified through registries in Europe and the United States.

Pathobiology

The complement system is an ancient defense mechanism that stimulates the inflammatory response and destroys pathogens by opsonization or lysis. Most commonly, aHUS is a consequence of aberrant activation of the complement AP, which leads to endothelial damage, and is the result of mutations that lead to loss or functional impairment of complement regulatory proteins, or less commonly, activating mutations in alternative complement proteins.

Complement may be activated via the classical pathway, AP or lectin pathways. The AP plays an important role in protecting the intravascular space against bacterial infection and depends on potent amplification loops (Fig. 134.6). The AP is in a constant low-level activation state because of spontaneous hydrolysis of the thioester bond in C3, and regulation by complement inhibitory proteins is required to prevent pathologic activation and complement-mediated injury to host tissues. C3b is deposited on cell membranes of both pathogens and host cells. An amplification loop consisting of complement factor B, factor D, and properdin leads to the deposition of additional C3b on the cell surface and the generation of C3b convertase (C3bBbP), which further amplifies C3b generation. In the presence of additional C3b, this convertase can cleave C5 to C5a and C5b, leading to formation of the lytic C5b-C9 complex. To protect host cells from collateral damage as a consequence of complement activation, multiple soluble and membrane-associated regulatory proteins inactivate C3b on the cell surface. These include plasma protein factor H and membrane-associated cofactor protein (MCP; CD46), both of which bind to membrane bound C3b. Then another plasma protein, factor I (CFI), cleaves and inactivates C3b. Similarly, cell-surface thrombomodulin enhances CFI-mediated inactivation of C3b. Another membrane-associated protein, decay-accelerating factor (DAF; CD55) accelerates the inactivation of C3 convertase, although mutations of DAF have not been shown to play a role in aHUS.

Mutations in several complement regulatory proteins predispose to aHUS. Mutations in CFH account for 25% of cases. Loss of

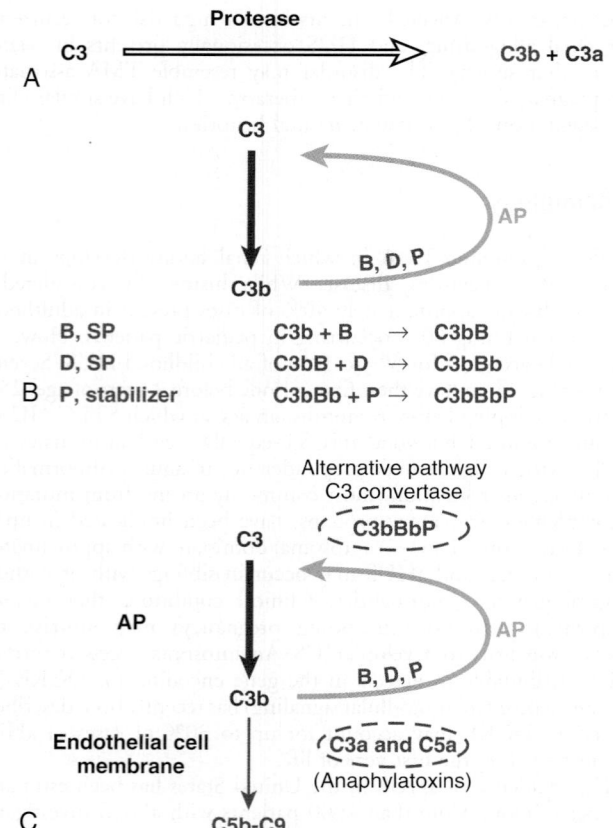

Fig. 134.6 THE ALTERNATIVE PATHWAY OF COMPLEMENT ACTIVATION. (A) The alternative pathway (AP) of the complement system originally consisted of a serine protease that cleaved C3 to the opsonin C3b and the proinflammatory anaphylatoxin C3a. (B) An amplification loop was evolved to more efficiently deposit C3b on a target and liberate C3a into the surrounding milieu. *B* indicates factor B; *D* indicates factor D, a serine protease; *P* indicates properdin, a stabilizer of the enzyme. (C) Development of a C5 convertase. The same enzyme that cleaves C3 (AP C3 convertase) can cleave C5 to C5a and C5b with the addition of a second C3b to the enzyme complex (AP C5 convertase).

function mutations have been identified throughout the protein, most commonly in the C-terminal SCRs 19 and 20, which mediate cell binding (Fig. 134.7). These mutations do not result in decreased CFH plasma concentrations, but reduce its capacity to regulate complement activation on platelet and endothelial cell surfaces and on subendothelial basement membranes. SCRs 1–4 compete with factor B for binding to C3b and serve as cofactors for CFI-mediated proteolysis of C3b. The CFH gene (*CFH*) resides in the regulators of complement activation (RCA) cluster at 1q32 close to five factor H–related proteins (CFHR 1–5). The latter contain multiple duplicated segments with homology to *CFH*. Therefore the RCA is susceptible to nonallelic homologous recombination; the mechanism likely responsible for the formation of a hybrid gene consisting of the first 21 exons of factor H (encoding the first 18 SCRs) and the last two exons of CFHR1 (encoding SCR 19 and 20), which has been associated with aHUS. In addition to genetic abnormalities in factor H, acquired deficiencies account for 5% to 10% of aHUS, which occur in a subset of individuals with homozygous deletions of *CFHR1* (either as recombination events including CFHR3 and CFHR1 [ΔCFHR1/3] or CFHR3 and CFHR4 [ΔCFHR1/4]). The autoantibodies may cross react with factor H SCR 19 and 20 and CFHR1 SCR 4 and 5, which share extensive homology.

Mutations in MCP are found in approximately 15% of patients with aHUS. MCP is present on the surface of all nucleated cells except erythrocytes. Mutations are found throughout the extracellular domain of the protein (see Fig. 134.7) and most commonly lead to diminished cell surface expression, although some impair protein activity.

MCP and factor H bind C3b and facilitate its cleavage on the cell membrane by factor I. Factor I mutations are observed in approximately 12% of aHUS patients and most commonly result in decreased protein expression; although some mutations cause decreased catalytic activity, which is mediated through the factor I light chain. Thrombomodulin also enhances CFI-mediated degradation of C3b, and mutations of thrombomodulin have been observed in 5% of patients with aHUS in one series.

Mutations in factor B and C3 are observed in approximately 3% and 10% of aHUS patients, respectively. Mutations in factor B lead to enhanced formation or greater stability of C3 convertase on cell surfaces. Mutations in C3 may result in resistance to regulation, principally mediated by diminished ability of regulatory proteins (CHF, MCP or CFI) to interact with mutant C3b.

Recently, mutations in the gene encoding for DGKE, a lipid kinase expressed in endothelium, platelets, and renal podocytes, has been identified as the cause of an autosomal recessive form of aHUS with high penetrance. The mechanism of disease is attributed to deregulation of intracellular signaling, leading to activation of protein kinase C with a subsequent shift of the balance of endothelial cells and platelets toward a more activated and prothrombotic phenotype. Altered podocyte homeostasis has been hypothesized to occur as a consequence of abnormal protein kinase C-dependent vascular endothelial growth factor (VEGF) receptor expression, disrupting this important cell nurturing pathway. In general, patients with *DGKE*-related aHUS have no evidence of complement dysregulation. Furthermore, unlike patients with defects of the complement mechanism, patients with DGKE-associated aHUS have persistent microhematuria and proteinuria between flares of disease.

Mutations have been detected in up to 70% of patients with aHUS and are transmitted in an autosomal manner, accounting for the commonly observed familial inheritance pattern, although disease penetrance is only 50%. The basis for incomplete penetrance of aHUS is poorly understood. Identified precipitating factors include infection, pregnancy, and additional single nucleotide genetic polymorphisms and haplotypes in complement regulatory genes. Up to 20% of patients harbor more than one mutation in complement regulatory genes. The cause of aHUS in the 30% of patients with no identifiable complement protein mutations remains uncertain.

Laboratory Manifestations

aHUS is characterized by MAHA and thrombocytopenia. Compared with TTP, thrombocytopenia and anemia may be less severe and renal insufficiency more prominent. Reports suggest that between 6% and 15% of children do not have the full triad of thrombocytopenia, anemia, and renal dysfunction at presentation. Recent guidelines have emphasized the importance of using both clinical and laboratory studies to diagnose aHUS and to distinguish it from other TMAs.

Diagnosis of aHUS requires several criteria, including: (1) the absence of other diseases associated with TMA, (2) the absence of criteria for pathogen-associated postinfectious HUS (i.e., negative stool culture and/or Stx assays), and (3) the absence of criteria for TTP (i.e., ADAMTS13 >10%). In addition, the complement system should be evaluated. A recent consensus statement suggests obtaining levels of C3, C4, CFH, and CFI, as well as flow cytometry studies for MCP (CD46) before initiating plasma exchange therapy. However, it is important to note that decreased C3 is only found in 30% to 40% of patients and that decreased CFH or CFI is only seen in 50% or 30% of patients with mutations in these genes respectively and between 30% and 60% of patients with autoantibodies to CFH. Also, decreased levels of C3 and decreased MCP expression may be observed in the acute phase of STEC-HUS. Serologic autoantibody

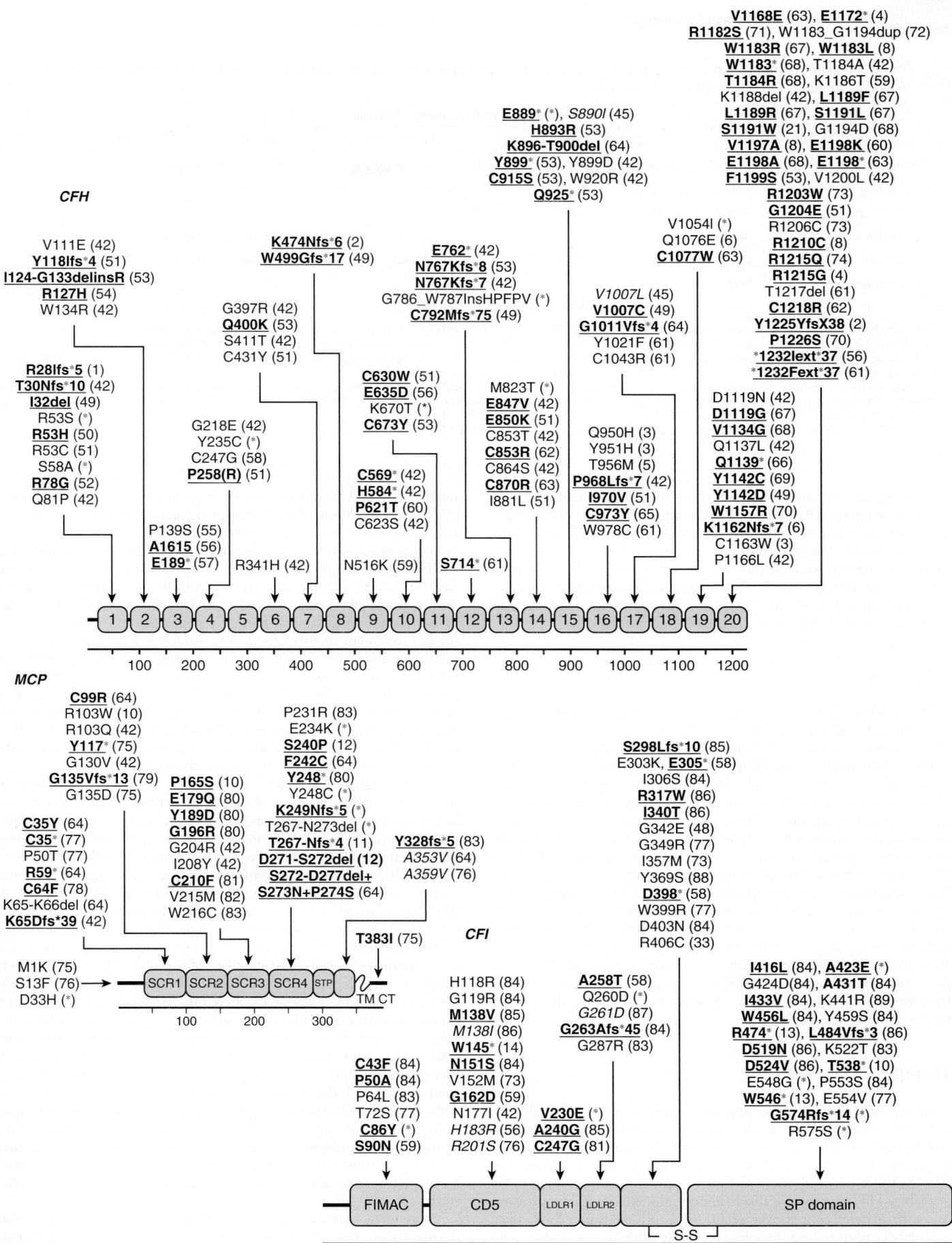

Fig. 134.7 *CFH, MCP* AND *CFI* MUTATIONS ASSOCIATED WITH aHUS. This figure provides a schematic representation of the location of the mutations in the protein domains of factor H, MCP and factor I. Mutations demonstrated to impair function or decrease expression levels are depicted in bold and underlined. Polymorphisms are shown in italics. References are in parenthesis, (*) indicates unpublished data by Rodriguez de Cordoba et al. *aHUS*, Atypical hemolytic uremic syndrome; *CFH*, complement regulatory protein factor H; *CFI*, complement factor I; *MCP*, membrane cofactor protein. (*Reproduced from Rodrigues de Cordoba S, Hidalgo MS, Pinot S, Torajada A: Genetics of atypical hemolytic uremic syndrome (aHUS). Semin Thromb Hemost 40:422, 2014, with permission.*)

TABLE 134.1	Plasma Concentration of C3, C4, CFH, CFI, and CFB and Expression of Membrane Cofactor Protein in the Various Subgroups of Atypical Hemolytic Uremic Syndrome

	Protein Level or Expression					
	C4	C3	CFH	CFI	CFB	MCP
CFH mutation	N	Normal (decreased)	Normal (decreased)	Normal	Normal (decreased)	Normal
CFI mutation	N	Normal (decreased)	Normal	Normal (decreased)	Normal (decreased)	Normal
MCP mutation	N	Normal (decreased)	Normal	Normal	Normal	Decreased (normal)
CFB mutation	N	Decreased	Normal	Normal	Normal (decreased)	Normal
C3 mutation	N	Decreased	Normal	Normal	Normal (decreased)	Normal
THBD mutation	N	Normal or decreased	ND	ND	ND	Normal
Anti-CFH Ab	N	Decreased (normal)	Normal (decreased)	Normal	Normal (decreased)	Normal

Note: Very low C3 levels are observed in patients with homozygous CFH mutation (complete CFH deficiency) or compound heterozygous CFH mutation, and in patients with CFB or C3 gain-of-function mutations. In most of the other patients, C3 concentration is mildly decreased or normal. CFH is undetectable only in patients with homozygous CFH mutation. Decreased CFH concentration can be observed in patients with heterozygous type 1 *CFH* mutation, and during flares of anti-CFH antibodies-HUS. Decreased C4 plasma levels have been reported in a few patients in each of the various subgroups.
"Normal" and "Decreased" without parentheses mean most frequently, normal or decreased. "Normal" and "Decreased" within parentheses mean possible, but not frequent. "Normal or decreased" without parentheses means that normal or decreased is equally frequent.
Ab, antibodies; *CFB*, factor B; *CFH*, Factor H; *CFI*, factor I; *ND*, not documented; *THBD*, thrombomodulin.
Data from Loirat C, Frémeaux-Bacchi V: Atypical hemolytic uremic syndrome. *Orphanet J Rare Diseases* 6:60, 2011.

to CFH should be sent. Abnormalities of complement regulation are involved in up to 70% of cases. Finally, genetic analyses of the genes that have been implicated in the pathogenesis of aHUS are recommended, despite the fact that no defects are found in 30% to 50% of cases. Because of variable penetrance, only 20% to 30% of patients will have a family history of aHUS. Plasma concentrations of complement and complement inhibitory proteins in various subgroups of aHUS classified by mutation are shown in Table 134.1.

Prognosis

aHUS has been historically associated with a poor prognosis, especially in older adults and those with severe renal dysfunction. The mortality rate approaches 25% and 50% of surviving patients develop chronic renal insufficiency. However, identification of the central role of control of complement and DGKE in the pathogenesis of aHUS allows prognostication based on genotype. Before the advent of specific anticomplement therapy, the prognosis of patients with genetic defects of factor H or factor I deficiency was poor, with a rate of recurrence and progression to end-stage renal disease or death of 70%, whereas MCP deficiency appeared to carry a better prognosis. Aggressive plasma-based treatment slows but does not prevent progression to renal failure. Eculizumab treatment has been shown to halt disease activity and improve renal function. In fact, some participants in the single armed trials were able to discontinue dialysis therapy. Initial experience suggests that eculizumab is ineffective in patients with disease caused by DGKE mutations, but no recurrences have been observed in the few reported DGKE cases where renal transplantation was performed.

Therapy

Until recently, patients presenting with TMAs (either TTP or aHUS) were offered a trial of plasma exchange therapy. Plasma exchange may still be indicated in patients where there is uncertainty about the diagnosis of TTP or aHUS pending the results of assays for ADAMTS13 or until more definitive anticomplement therapy is available. This approach is also being questioned in patients presenting with platelet counts over 30,000/μL and creatinine levels over 2.3 mg/dL, findings that are observed more often in association with aHUS than with TTP. Although plasma therapy replaces missing soluble regulators of the alternative mechanism of activation of complement and may ameliorate thrombocytopenia, it does not appear to halt renal disease progression, as evidenced by a high incidence of end-stage renal disease in pediatric patients treated with this approach. Plasma-based therapy is at best temporizing and is associated with a high rate of complications.

Therapy for aHUS is rapidly evolving with the recent approval of eculizumab, a recombinant humanized monoclonal immunoglobulin that binds C5 with high affinity and inhibits its cleavage to C5a (a proinflammatory mediator) and C5b (the first component of the C5b-9 membrane attack complex). This medication was introduced for the treatment of paroxysmal nocturnal hemoglobinurea (PNH). Its approval for HUS was based on two single-arm studies involving 37 adults and adolescents and a retrospective review of 19 pediatric patients and 11 adults. Eculizumab demonstrated activity in the majority of treated patients, whether or not they were refractory to plasma therapy and independent of whether or not a mutation of a complement control protein was demonstrated. Several patients with severe renal insufficiency were able to discontinue dialysis.

These results suggest that eculizumab is the treatment of choice for patients with established aHUS or with a high clinical likelihood in an appropriate setting (e.g., postpartum status, positive family history, younger than 2 years of age). Markers of active TMA (thrombocytopenia, LDH, and haptoglobin) respond rapidly to therapy. The results of trials and accumulating registry data suggest that the sooner treatment is initiated, the better the chance of recovery of renal function. Current data also suggest that remissions are sustained. Checking for full complement blockade should be considered in individuals where there is apparent disease reactivation. Assay of eculizumab levels or CH50 may be informative. There is a risk of relapse of aHUS with potential for irreversible renal failure upon discontinuation of eculizumab, therefore, life-long treatment is currently recommended. However, with further experience, it may be possible to identify subgroups of patients who can safely discontinue treatment. Finally, it is important to note that immunity to *Neisseria* meningitis depends upon the lytic terminal complement C5b-9 mechanism, and the reported incidence of *Neisseria* infection in patients taking this medication for treatment of PNH was 0.42 per 100 patient-years. Therefore, all patients should be vaccinated. Prophylaxis with antibiotics is suggested if therapy is initiated before antibody response develops, but because vaccination may only confer incomplete immunity, some recommend chronic antibiotic treatment.

In general, patients with aHUS who progress to end-stage renal disease are considered candidates for transplantation. Living related donor transplants are not recommended, except possibly in the case of DGKE-associated disease, because of the risk for aHUS in the donor's remaining kidney. Thus there are reports of aHUS developing in family-related renal donors within months of donation.

Since CFH, CFI, factor B and C3 are all soluble plasma proteins, deficiency or dysfunction is not corrected by renal allografting. The outcome of renal transplantation in aHUS has been poor, with a high rate of failure because of recurrent disease. In fact, the failure rate can approach 60% to 70% and failure often occurs within the first month after transplantation. The underlying genetic defect is predictive of relapse risk, being as high as 80% with mutations in CFH, C3 and factor B, but as low as 20% in patients with defects in MCP or in those without genetic abnormalities. Before the introduction of eculizumab, combined liver and kidney transplantation was recommended; however, the 1-year survival for this complicated procedure was disappointing. Anecdotal reports suggest that eculizumab prophylaxis may prevent posttransplantation recurrence.

OTHER THROMBOTIC MICROANGIOPATHIC DISORDERS

Posttransplantation Thrombotic Microangiopathy

TMA can occur in three transplant-related settings: (1) recurrent disease after transplantation for a TMA-related disorder, (2) in association with the use of immunosuppressive medications (calcineurin inhibitors [cyclosporine A and tacrolimus] and inhibitors of the mammalian target of rapamycin [mTOR inhibitors sirolimus and everolimus]) and (3) after hematopoietic stem cell transplantation.

Recurrent Disease and "De Novo Thrombotic Microangiopathy" After Renal Transplantation

As indicated previously, there is a high risk of developing recurrent aHUS after renal transplantation in patients with disorders of complement regulation. However, it is important to note that the diagnosis of recurrent TMA depends on the correct diagnosis of the index disorder. Patients with suspected de novo TMA that is subsequently attributed to aHUS may have initially presented with hypertension, renal failure and nephrosclerosis. In a French series of renal transplant recipients whose initial diagnosis was not aHUS, 7 of 24 of those diagnosed with de novo aHUS after renal transplantation were shown to have mutations of CFH or CFI. In the majority of these individuals, renal failure was attributed to hypertension or chronic glomerulonephritis. No mutations were identified in a control group of renal transplant recipients who did not develop TMA, suggesting that underlying defects of complement should be considered when TMA develops in the postrenal transplant setting. However, the most cases of posttransplant de novo TMA are attributable to drug toxicity, rejection, viral infection (such as parvovirus, cytomegalovirus and hepatitis C), or a combination of these processes. Antibody-mediated rejection may be confirmed by demonstrating the presence of major histocompatibility complex antibody, or by renal biopsy evidence of peritubular capillary C4d staining. Antibody-mediated rejection associated with TMA has a poorer prognosis than antibody-mediated rejection alone. Plasma exchange therapy appears beneficial in this setting.

Immunosuppressive Medications

Cyclosporine A and tacrolimus are common causes of drug-induced TMAs. The pathogenesis of calcineurin-induced TMA is uncertain. Cyclosporine A causes arteriolar vasoconstriction, probably through upregulation of endothelin and thromboxane, and downregulation of vasodilators (nitric oxide and prostacyclin). In vitro studies showed that cyclosporin A induces endothelial release of complement activating microparticles, suggesting both a toxic effect on the cells and a role for complement in the pathogenesis of renal dysfunction. Cyclosporin A also enhances platelet aggregation and thromboxane release.

TMA occurs in 1% to 5% of renal transplant recipients, as well as in occasional solid organ recipients treated with cyclosporin A or tacrolimus. Calcineurin-induced TMA typically develops insidiously

with progressive, otherwise unexplained renal insufficiency. MAHA or thrombocytopenia is found in only half these patients and are usually mild. The glomerular capillary and arteriolar thrombotic lesions are similar in appearance to those in primary cases of TMA. The distinction between calcineurin-induced TMA and acute tubular necrosis or rejection can often be made by biopsy, but not in all cases. Broad alloantibody reactivity and coinfection with cytomegalovirus may predispose to cyclosporin-associated TMA.

The extent to which calcineurin-induced TMA responds to a reduction of the dose or temporary discontinuation of medication is uncertain. The prognosis is generally good, although some patients develop permanent renal failure. In many patients, cyclosporin A can be reintroduced at a lower dose; in others, tacrolimus has been substituted successfully, although the latter may also precipitate TMA. Other strategies include substitution of an alternative immunomodulatory medication. The utility of plasma exchange is uncertain.

Recent evidence suggests that mTOR (mammalian target of rapamycin) inhibitors, such as sirolimus and everolimus, can also be associated with posttransplant TMA. It is likely that mTOR inhibitors impair endothelial function, but the mechanism remains to be elucidated.

Hematopoietic Stem Cell Transplantation

TMA occurs in approximately 6% of patients who undergo allogeneic marrow transplantation; the incidence is estimated to be 0.1% to 1% after autologous marrow or stem cell transplantation. Though guidelines have been developed, diagnosis is difficult because schistocytes and thrombocytopenia are common after bone marrow transplantation, and because the differential diagnosis of fever, renal failure, and neurologic complications is extensive. The clinical manifestations typically begin months after transplantation and the kidneys appear to be a major target organ. The pathophysiology is assumed to reflect systemic endothelial cell injury from a variety of causes. ADAMTS13 activity may fall after transplantation, but severe deficiency such as occurs in TTP is uncommon. Risk factors include the use of an unrelated or mismatched donor, total body irradiation as part of the pretransplant conditioning regimen, calcineurin inhibitor treatment, systemic cytomegalovirus or other infection, older age, female gender, and graft-versus-host disease (GVHD). Systemic microangiopathy is rare, but an intestinal biopsy may be needed to distinguish TMA from GVHD in patients with refractory diarrhea. Evidence of terminal complement deposition in the skin may suggest an aHUS-like mechanism.

Withdrawal or substitution of another immunosuppressive agent for cyclosporin A, if possible, should be considered, although at the risk for worsening of the underlying GVHD. Alternative causes should be sought, and aggressive treatment of infection and GVHD should be used in all but the most overt cases. It is difficult to determine the prognosis because of variable inclusion criteria. Although patients may appear to show an initial response to plasma therapy, the long-term effectiveness of plasma exchange has not been established and mortality exceeds 50%, often caused by complications of GVHD or opportunistic infection. Defibrotide has been used with reported success in a few cases, and there have been anecdotal successes with rituximab, anti-CD25 antibodies and eculizumab.

Cancer and Chemotherapy-Associated Thrombotic Microangiopathy

TMA may occur late in the course of some patients with disseminated malignant neoplasms and large tumor burdens, most commonly adenocarcinoma of the gastrointestinal tract, breast, or lung. Patients generally present with an abrupt onset of moderate to severe MAHA and thrombocytopenia. Renal insufficiency and neurologic dysfunction occur less commonly than in idiopathic or chemotherapy-induced TMA and may result from concurrent metabolic disturbances, central nervous system metastases, stroke, or hemorrhage.

The pathogenesis of cancer-associated TMAs is poorly understood. Laboratory evidence of DIC is found in 25% to 80% of patients based on findings of elevated fibrin degradation products or more sensitive measures of increased fibrinogen turnover. However, the observation that TMA occurs in only 5% of patients with disseminated malignancy and DIC suggests the involvement of additional factors, such as microvascular occlusion, intimal proliferation induced by tumor emboli within the pulmonary vasculature, or formation of an incompletely endothelialized tumor vasculature that predisposes to platelet adhesion, activation and aggregation. Severe deficiency of ADAMTS13 is not typical. Outcomes of patients who develop TMA in the setting of chemotherapy or advanced cancer are poor because the TMA tends to be unrelenting and the co-morbidity of the malignancy is significant. Survival is generally measured in weeks. The only effective therapy is reduction of the tumor burden, a goal often not attainable. A role for plasma exchange has not been established.

Specific cancer chemotherapeutic agents have also been implicated in the development of TMA. Patients are often receiving therapy for adenocarcinoma at the time TMA develops, making attribution to the neoplasm versus its therapy difficult to determine. However, unlike cancer-associated TMA, most patients with chemotherapy-associated TMA do not have a large tumor burden, and some may be in remission. Implicated agents include mitomycin-C, gemcitabine, cis-platinum, bleomycin, docetaxel, 5-fluourouracil, deoxycoformycin, carboplatin, oxaliplatin, interferon-α and bevacizumab, either alone or in combination.

Patients with chemotherapy-associated TMA generally present with moderate to severe MAHA, thrombocytopenia, and renal insufficiency (median creatinine value of 4.2 mg/dL). Approximately 15% to 20% of such patients develop neurologic dysfunction. A unique feature is noncardiogenic pulmonary edema, which is observed in over 50% of patients in some series. Pulmonary function may deteriorate rapidly after red blood cell or platelet transfusion, and patients should be transfused with caution.

Chemotherapy-associated TMA is presumed to result from direct toxicity to the endothelium. Mitomycin inhibits the production of prostacyclin by umbilical vein endothelium, and infusion of mitomycin-C into the rat kidney induces histologic changes similar to those found in chemotherapy-induced TMA. Alternatively, anti-VEGF antibodies and other VEGF inhibitors have revealed a critical dependence of podocytes and glomerular endothelial cells on VEGF. Toxicity of these agents includes a TMA localized primarily to the kidney and manifested mainly by hypertension and proteinuria.

ADAMTS13 levels are not severely reduced in chemotherapy-associated TMA. Fewer than 20% of affected patients appear to respond to plasma exchange and/or corticosteroids, and more than 50% die within 2 months.

Streptococcus pneumoniae

Infection with *S. pneumoniae* may lead to desialylation of the glycocalyx of cells that express the Thomsen-Freidenreich (T-F) antigen. The activity of neuraminidase related to influenza virus may present with the same complication. A naturally occurring, cold reactive IgM may recognize the exposed T-F antigen, leading to red cell agglutination in vitro and rarely hemolysis in vivo. Affected individuals have a positive antiglobulin test. Postpneumococcal HUS is the second most common cause of postinfectious HUS in children, accounting for between 5% and 15% of cases, and occurring after approximately 0.5% of infections with this organism. It generally occurs in children less than 2 years of age and is associated with significant morbidity and mortality. In two series, 75% of patients required dialysis. Extrarenal manifestations are common. The pathogenesis is not well defined but may involve interactions among the IgM, red cells, platelets, and endothelium. Alternatively, desialylation by neuraminidase may disrupt factor H binding sites, resulting in unregulated complement activation and cell injury because factor B can no longer regulate C3 convertase. Management is generally supportive, but many experts suggest avoidance of plasma infusion because of the concern that there may be unintended infusion of IgM anti–T-F.

Disordered Cobalamin Metabolism

An autosomal recessive TMA associated with disordered cobalamin-C metabolism can occur in individuals during the first weeks to months of life. Deficiency of cobalamin-C may result in markedly elevated levels of homocysteine and methylmalonic acid, which may be responsible for vascular injury. Approximately one quarter of such patients present with HUS. Although the majority of patients have a fulminant course leading to death, some present with a more chronic form of the disease later in childhood. One adult case was reported. Therapy consists of treatment with hydroxycobalamin. Neurologic sequelae are common, as is chronic hypertension.

Miscellaneous Drug-Associated Thrombotic Microangiopathy

Although TMA has been associated with more than 75 drugs, the 9 drugs that account for 75% of the cases include clopidogrel, estrogen/progesterone, gemcitabine, interferon, mitomycin, quinine, tacrolimus and ticlopidine. The mechanisms by which these agents induce TMA may differ, as may the natural history and response to therapy. Whereas mitomycin C, gemcitabine, and cyclosporin appear to induce TMA in a cumulative dose-dependent manner, quinidine and thienopyridines (ticlopidine and clopidogrel) induce TMA through either idiosyncratic, immune-mediated mechanisms or by acute endothelial toxicity (see Chapter 131).

The first report of quinine-associated TMA described the course of three patients with a syndrome resembling idiopathic HUS. Patients generally present with severe MAHA, platelet counts below 50,000/μL, and renal insufficiency, usually requiring dialysis. Neurologic dysfunction occurs in a minority of patients, but it can be severe; granulocytopenia and lymphopenia have been reported. In earlier reports, the prognosis was favorable once quinine was withdrawn and plasma exchange instituted. However, in another series, 17 of 225 patients with HUS had quinine-associated TMA, 4 of whom died, and 7 survivors were left with chronic renal failure. Although this disorder occurs most commonly after the ingestion of quinine tablets, cases have been reported after exposure to quinine in beverages such as tonic water or herbal health supplements (cinchona). A careful history is sometimes necessary to establish the link between quinine ingestion and the patient's clinical disease. The pathogenesis may involve idiosyncratic, quinine-dependent antibodies reactive with platelet GPs IIb/IIIa and Ib/IX and related antigens on endothelial cells and neutrophils that promote neutrophil aggregation and binding to endothelial cells in a drug-dependent manner. Patients with quinine-induced TMA have significant early mortality, though with appropriate supportive care and treatment of the acute episode, the disorder does not recur without reexposure to quinine.

The thienopyridines are another common cause of drug-induced TTP. TTP occurs in a higher percentage of patients exposed to ticlopidine, with an incidence ranging from 1:600 to 1:4814 patient exposures in contrast to an estimated incidence of 4 per 1,000,000 to 1 per 8500–26,000 exposures to clopidogrel. No cases of clopidogrel-associated TTP were encountered in the CAPRIE and CURE studies, each of which enrolled more than 6200 patients. Despite the low incidence, the frequency with which clopidogrel is prescribed renders it the most commonly reported drug associated with TTP in the Food and Drugs Administration MedWatch database, accounting for more than 30% of all cases. The pathogenesis and natural history of TTP associated with ticlopidine and clopidogrel differ. Reductions in ADAMTS13 activity below 15% occur in 85% of patients with ticlopidine-associated TTP but in only 15% of patients with clopidogrel-associated TTP. Reduced ADAMTS13 reflects the development of anti-ADAMTS13 antibodies. TTP generally develops within 2–12 weeks of starting ticlopidine and responds relatively quickly to plasma exchange. Spontaneous relapses may occur. In contrast, 90% of patients exposed to clopidogrel but only 10% of patients exposed to ticlopidine develop a syndrome characterized primarily by MAHA and renal insufficiency, without severe thrombocytopenia; these individuals have normal levels of ADAMTS13, usually develop disease within the first 2 weeks of exposure, and may require several weeks of plasma exchange to achieve remission. Whether plasma exchange actually improves the clinical outcome is uncertain. Spontaneous relapses are uncommon.

HIV-Associated Thrombotic Microangiopathy

An association between HIV infection and TMA has been recognized since 1984. TMA occurred in up to 7% of patients hospitalized with HIV infection. Conversely, the incidence of HIV infection in patients with TMA varied from 15% to 50% in endemic areas. In contrast, TMA is rare in HIV patients who are treated with highly active antiretroviral therapy. The mechanism of disease remains unclear, but endothelial injury is hypothesized. Coexisting opportunistic infections may be a contributing cofactor. TMA that occurs in patients with advanced or untreated HIV often responds quickly to the initiation of antiretroviral therapy and can relapse if therapy is discontinued.

In some patients with HIV infection, the associated immune dysfunction may predispose to the formation of autoantibodies against ADAMTS13. This can lead to severe ADAMTS13 deficiency and TTP, despite adequate treatment for HIV. These patients may respond to plasma exchange.

Pregnancy-Associated Thrombotic Microangiopathy

The differential diagnosis of MAHA associated with gestation is complex. TMA may be difficult if not impossible to distinguish from other causes of MAHA unique to pregnancy, such as preeclampsia, acute fatty liver associated with DIC, and HELLP syndrome. The severity of the renal and neurologic abnormalities and the time during gestation at which the signs and symptoms of TMA first appear may provide the clues needed to prevent critical delays in therapy.

Approximately 10% of cases of idiopathic TTP occur in association with pregnancy. In one series, 40 of 45 cases of TTP in pregnancy were diagnosed antepartum at a mean gestational age of 23.5 weeks. Additional studies have confirmed that TTP frequently develops in the second trimester, although some studies report more common occurrence in the third trimester or immediately postpartum. ADAMST13 levels fall progressively during pregnancy, but severe deficiency (<10%) is seen only in women with TTP. In the absence of appropriate therapy, maternal and fetal mortality approach 90%, and TTP during pregnancy is associated with a high risk of fetal loss. Pregnancies in women with congenital ADAMTS13 deficiency have been carried to term with prophylactic plasma infusion, sometimes combined with aspirin and low-molecular-weight heparin. The prognosis of pregnancy-associated autoimmune TTP has improved dramatically since the advent of plasma exchange, and continuing pregnancy does not impair response. There is no evidence that uterine evacuation leads to resolution. Many patients carry to term successfully, although the overall risk for fetal loss remains significant. Up to 20% of patients with chronic, relapsing TTP have recurrences during subsequent pregnancies, whereas recurrence occurs in almost all women with inherited ADAMTS13 deficiency.

aHUS also occurs with increased frequency in association with pregnancy. The disorder primarily affects primiparas who present with MAHA, thrombocytopenia, renal insufficiency and hypertension beginning at a mean of approximately 26 days after delivery in one series—this later onset may help to distinguish HUS from other causes of pregnancy-associated MAHA and thrombocytopenia, such as preeclampsia and HELLP, which occur late in gestation or soon after parturition. The outcome of aHUS associated with pregnancy is poor with mortality rates up to 50% and an additional 15% are left with chronic renal insufficiency. Recent studies suggest that as in the nonpregnant setting, pregnancy-associated aHUS is closely tied to complement AP activation, particularly factor H, and thus may respond to complement inhibitors, such as eculizumab.

HELLP syndrome complicates approximately 0.5% to 0.9% of pregnancies and approximately 10% to 20% of cases of preeclampsia. The pathogenesis is attributed to aberrant placental development, but the details remain unclear. Patients often present with abdominal pain and/or gastrointestinal symptoms, and concomitant hypertension and proteinuria. Seventy percent of cases occur before delivery and the majority of the postpartum cases occur within 48 hours of parturition. Diagnosis is based on evidence microangiopathic changes on the blood smear, thrombocytopenia and abnormal liver function studies. The differential diagnosis is broad, and includes acute fatty liver of pregnancy, TTP, aHUS, vasculitis, DIC, and infection. The timing of development of symptoms may assist in the diagnosis because TTP tends to occur earlier in pregnancy, whereas aHUS often occurs postpartum. Initial management is to stabilize the patient, treat hypertension and prepare for delivery—delivery is considered curative for HELLP syndrome.

FUTURE DIRECTIONS

Thrombotic microangiopathic syndromes are uncommon, but their associated morbidity and mortality are significant. Over the last 10 years, dramatic progress has been made in our understanding of the pathogenesis of these syndromes, and these discoveries are being translated into effective therapeutic interventions. A phase I trial of recombinant ADAMTS13 for treatment of congenital TTP has been initiated. Targeted disruption of the vWF-GP1b interaction may prevent microvascular occlusion in TTP, and a phase II trial of a targeted therapy with caplacizumab has been completed. Expanded use of anti-CD20 and other immunomodulatory approaches may reduce relapses and induce durable remissions. Drugs that block the action of Stx may be the most promising approach to ameliorating STEC-HUS. A tetravalent peptide has been shown to be effective in animal models. Alternatively, generation of highly neutralizing anti–Stx-2 antibody may provide passive immunity and a mechanism to interrupt outbreaks of STEC-HUS.

Complement factor H concentrates have received orphan drug designation in Europe. Eculizumab and other complement inhibitors may convert aHUS from a progressive disorder that often culminates in chronic renal failure or death to a manageable chronic disease. Better biomarkers are needed to aid in the diagnosis of aHUS and to monitor patients on eculizumab. Such biomarkers indicate early response before organ functional changes can be identified, allow better understanding of the optimal duration of therapy, and define who might not require life-long anticomplement therapy to prevent aHUS relapse.

The factors that trigger onset and relapse of TMAs remain to be elucidated. It is unclear why some patients with acquired TTP have multiple relapses while others do not. Although Stx triggers acute episodes of STEC-HUS, other factors must account for the fact that some individuals with congenital deficiency of ADAMTS13 present in early childhood, while others develop the disease in the fifth or sixth decades of life, if at all. Why is the penetrance of aHUS only 50% in the presence of a complement inhibitor gene mutation known to predispose to disease? Clearly, a better understanding of genetic susceptibility factors is essential, but equally important is identification of the environmental agents that incite disease, about which we currently have little information.

SUGGESTED READINGS

Ardissino G, Tesla S, Possenti I, et al: Discontinuation of eculizumab maintenance treatment for atypical hemolytic uremic syndrome: a report of 10 cases. *Am J Kidney Dis* 64:633–637, 2014.

Bitzan M, Schaefer F, Reymond D: Treatment of typical (enteropathic) hemolytic uremic syndrome. *Semin Thromb Hemost* 36:594, 2010.

Cataland SP, Wu HM: Diagnosis and management of complement mediated thrombotic microangiopathies. *Blood Rev* 28:67–74, 2014.

Chapin J, Shore T, Forsberg P, et al: Hematopoietic transplant-associated thrombotic microangiopathy: case report and review of diagnosis and treatments. *Clin Adv Hematol Oncol* 12:565–573, 2014.

Fakhouri F, Roumenina L, Provot F, et al: Pregnancy-associated hemolytic uremic syndrome revisited in the era of complement gene mutations. *J Am Soc Nephrol* 21:859, 2010.

Froissart A, Buffet M, Veyradier A, et al: Efficacy and safety of first-line rituximab in severe, acquired thrombotic thrombocytopenic purpura with a suboptimal response to plasma exchange. Experience of the French Thrombotic Microangiopathies Reference Center. *Crit Care Med* 40:104, 2012.

Furlan M, Robles R, Solenthaler M, et al: Deficient activity of von Willebrand factor-cleaving protease in chronic relapsing thrombotic thrombocytopenic purpura. *Blood* 89:3097, 1997.

Gasser C, Gautier E, Steck A, et al: Hämolytisch-urämische Syndrome: bilaterale Nierenrindennekrosen bei akuten erworbenen hämolytischen Anämien. *Schweiz Med Wochenschr* 85:905–909, 1955.

George JN, Nester CM: Syndromes of thrombotic microangiopathy. *N Engl J Med* 371:654, 2014.

Goel R, Ness PM, Takemoto CM, et al: Platelet transfusions in platelet consumptive disorders are associated with arterial thrombosis and in-hospital mortality. *Blood* 1251470–1251476, 2015.

Hovinga JA, Vesely SK, Terrell DR, et al: Survival and relapse in patients with thrombotic thrombocytopenic purpura. *Blood* 115:1500, 2010.

Ibarra C, Amaral MM, Palermo MS: Advances in the pathogenesis and therapy of hemolytic uremic syndrome caused by Shiga Toxin-2. *IUBMB Life* 65:827, 2013.

Karpman D, Sartz L, Johnson S: Pathophysiology of typical hemolytic uremic syndrome. *Semin Thromb Hemost* 36:575, 2010.

Kavanagh D, Goodship H, Richards A: Atypical hemolytic uremic syndrome. *Semin Nephrol* 33:508, 2013.

Kerr H, Richards A: Complement-mediated injury and protection of endothelium: lessons from atypical haemolytic uraemic syndrome. *Immunobiology* 217:195, 2012.

Lim W, Vesely SK, George JN: The role of rituximab in the management of patients with acquired thrombotic thrombocytopenic purpura. *Blood* 125:1526–1531, 2015.

Loirat C, Fakhouri F, Gema A, et al: An international consensus approach to the management of atypical hemolytic uremic syndrome in children. *Ped Nephrol* 31:15–39, 2016.

Lotta L, Wu H, Mackie I, et al: Residual plasmatic activity of ADAMTS13 is correlated with phenotype severity in congenital thrombotic thrombocytopenic purpura. *Blood* 120:440–448, 2012.

McCrae KR: Thrombocytopenia in pregnancy. *Hematology Am Soc Hematol Educ Program* 2010:397–402, 2010.

Moschcowitz E: Hyaline thrombosis of the terminal arterioles and capillaries: a hitherto undescribed disease. *Proc N Y Pathol Soc* 24:21–24, 1924.

Nadasdy T: Thrombotic microangiopathy in renal allografts: the diagnostic challenge. *Curr Opin Organ Transplant* 19:283–292, 2014.

Obrig TG, Karpman D: Shiga toxin pathogenesis: kidney complications and renal failure. *Curr Top Microbiol Immunol* 357:105, 2012.

Orth D, Wurzner R: Complement in typical hemolytic uremic syndrome. *Semin Thromb Hemost* 36:620, 2010.

Rock GA, Shumak KH, Buskard NA, et al: Comparison of plasma exchange with plasma infusion in the treatment of thrombotic thrombocytopenic purpura. *N Engl J Med* 325:393, 1991.

Scully M, Goodship T: How I treat thrombotic thrombocytopenia purpura and atypical haemolytic uremic syndrome. *Br J Haematol* 164:759, 2014.

Scully M, McDonald V, Cavenagh J, et al: A phase 2 study of the safety and efficacy of rituximab with plasma exchange in acute acquired thrombotic thrombocytopenic purpura. *Blood* 118:1746, 2011.

Tarr PI: Shiga toxin-associated hemolytic uremic syndrome and thrombotic thrombocytopenic purpura: distinct mechanisms of pathogenesis. *Kidney Int Suppl* 112:S29, 2009.

Tsai H-M, Lian ECY: Antibodies to von Willebrand factor-cleaving protease in acute thrombotic thrombocytopenic purpura. *N Engl J Med* 339:1585, 1998.

Wada H, Matsumoto T, Yamashita Y: Natural history of thrombotic thrombocytopenic purpura and hemolytic uremic syndrome. *Semin Thromb Hemost* 40:866–873, 2014.

Wong CS, Jelacic S, Habeeb RL, et al: The risk of the hemolytic uremic syndrome after antibiotic treatment of Escherichia coli 0157:H7 infections. *N Engl J Med* 342:930, 2000.

CHAPTER 135

HEMOPHILIA A AND B

Manuel Carcao, Paul Moorehead, and David Lillicrap

EPIDEMIOLOGY

Hemophilia is the most common severe inherited bleeding disorder recognized in humans. The hereditary and sex-linked nature of the disease has been appreciated since prebiblical times, and the previous occurrence of the disease in the European Royal family has added further interest in this condition.

The prevalence of hemophilia is worldwide, with no major geographic variances aside from rare clusters of disease in areas where founder mutations have been propagated (e.g., Twillingate, Newfoundland). In many parts of the developing world the true prevalence of the condition is unknown because of inadequate diagnostic facilities, but from experiences in the developed world, we can probably assume that the prevalence of hemophilia A is approximately one in 5000 males and for hemophilia B, one in 30,000 males These prevalence figures do show some variances among countries but except where local founder effects are important, these differences likely represent variable disease ascertainment and diagnosis. Because of the X-linked recessive inheritance of the disease, most affected subjects are male. However, for every male with hemophilia we estimate that there are on average at least two carrier females (in most cases the mother of the affected male as well as potentially some sisters of the male, his daughters and potentially his aunts). Hence the hemophilia carrier state is almost certainly much more common although there are no good data for this. Many carriers may not be diagnosed mainly because they never have affected sons. Although most hemophilia carrier women do not experience significant bleeding, some will have clotting factor levels low enough to cause symptoms.

International studies in the past decade indicate that the numbers of persons with hemophilia in the population are increasing by approximately 2% each year. There are likely several reasons for this trend, including the overall increase in population numbers, increasing longevity of persons with hemophilia, particularly because human immunodeficiency virus (HIV) and hepatitis C are having less impact on mortality than they did in the past, and increasing worldwide awareness and diagnosis of patients with milder forms of hemophilia.

The clinical signs and symptoms and inheritance patterns for hemophilia A and B are essentially identical, and it was not until the early 1950s that the two forms of hemophilia were differentiated. Subsequently, in the early 1980s, the two genes encoding factor VIII (FVIII) and factor IX (FIX) were cloned, and the specific mutations responsible for hemophilia began to be determined.

FACTOR VIII BIOLOGY: GENETICS, STRUCTURE, FUNCTION, AND PATHOPHYSIOLOGY

The Factor VIII Gene

The FVIII gene *(F8)* encoding the FVIII protein is located at Xq28, the most distal band of the long arm of the X chromosome (Fig. 135.1). It is a large and complex structure, 186 kb in length, consisting of 9 kb of exonic DNA arranged into 26 exons and 177 kb of intronic DNA in 25 introns. Most of the exons are small, ranging in size from 69 base pairs (bp) (exon 5; the smallest exon) to 3106 bp (exon 14; the largest exon—encoding the central B domain). The correspondence of these exons with the domains of the FVIII protein

is described later. The size of *F8* introns varies from 207 base pairs (intron 17) to 32.4 kb (intron 22).

In addition to the 9-kb FVIII transcript, this locus also encodes two additional messenger RNAs (mRNAs) that, unlike FVIII, are expressed ubiquitously. Within intron 22 of the *F8* gene there are two additional coding elements, *F8A* and *F8B*. The *F8A* transcript is made up entirely of intronic sequence from intron 22, and the *F8A* mRNA is transcribed in the opposite direction to *F8*. Although the function of the F8A transcript/protein is unknown, there is the potential that this mRNA could act as an antisense regulator of FVIII expression. In addition, two (or more) other copies of the *F8A* sequence are located further telomeric to *F8* and are involved in a frequent intrachromosomal recombination event in approximately 45% of patients with severe hemophilia A. The *F8B* transcript is expressed in the same orientation as the native *F8* mRNA, and this transcript comprises an initial intron 22 sequence that is spliced onto exons 23 to 26 of *F8*. As with F8A, the F8B transcript is also ubiquitously expressed. Although the function of the protein is unknown, because it contains the phospholipid binding region of FVIII it may play a role in membrane binding.

Factor VIII Expression

Transcription of the *F8* gene is regulated by a promoter that contains binding sites for both tissue-specific and ubiquitous transcription factors. The mRNA transcribed from *F8* is 9 kb in length and contains 7053 nucleotides of coding (i.e., translated) sequence and short 5′ and long 3′ untranslated sequences. The cellular site of FVIII expression has long been a matter of controversy. The situation is complicated by the very low abundance and instability of the FVIII transcript and protein. Nevertheless, F8 mRNA has been found to be expressed in a variety of human tissues, including liver, spleen, kidney cells, and muscle. It has long been known that hemophilia can be cured by liver transplantation. The cell types within the liver responsible for FVIII synthesis have previously been unclear, but there is now strong evidence that the liver sinusoidal endothelium is the source of FVIII production.[1] Nonetheless, FVIII levels are maintained during episodes of severe liver failure, suggesting the existence of extrahepatic sites of FVIII expression. Recently, two reports using different conditional knock-out approaches in mice have shown that the vascular endothelium is the predominant site of FVIII expression in this animal model.[2,3]

FVIII is an acute phase reactant, and studies have shown that FVIII expression can be induced through a nuclear factor kappa-B (NFκB). FVIII is an acute phase protein whose levels increase with hormone induction (estrogen use), but the mechanistic basis for this increase is not known.

The Biosynthesis of Factor VIII

FVIII biosynthesis has been extensively investigated in vitro using cell types that do not normally express this protein, such as baby hamster kidney (BHK) or Chinese hamster ovary (CHO). Therefore conclusions about the details of this process in a physiologic context should be made with caution. After production of the primary polypeptide chain and cleavage of the 19-amino-acid signal peptide, the protein undergoes a series of posttranslational modifications, including N- and O-linked glycosylation mainly in the B domain (Fig. 135.2) and sulfation of tyrosine residues. Furthermore, when the nascent protein transits the endoplasmic reticulum (ER), it interacts with ER chaperones, including calreticulin and immunoglobulin binding protein (BiP). Although these interactions limit the transport of malfolded

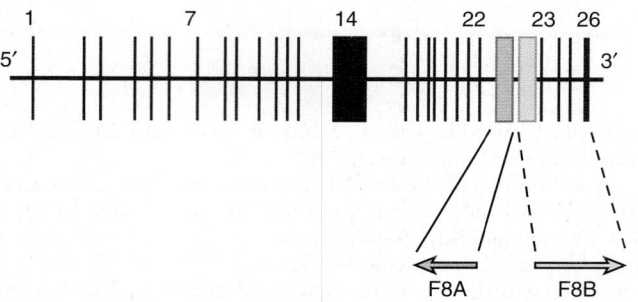

Fig. 135.1 FACTOR VIII GENE. The factor VIII (FVIII) gene *(F8)* is located on the X chromosome at cytogenic band Xq28-qter. The 26 exons span 184 kb of genomic DNA, and there are three open reading frames expressed from the locus: the 9 kb FVIII mRNA transcript incorporating all 26 exons of the gene; the F8A transcript that is transcribed in the opposite direction to FVIII and comprises sequences from intron 22; and finally, F8B comprising an initial 5′ exon derived from intron 22 sequence that is spliced to exons 23 to 26 of the *F8* gene.

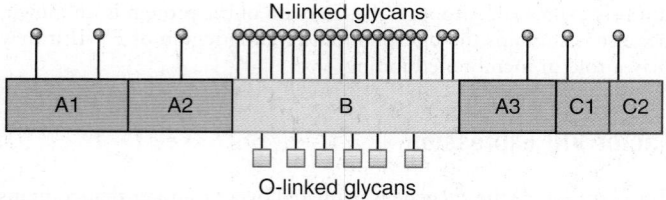

Fig. 135.2 FACTOR VIII GLYCAN MODIFICATION (molecular weight, 260 kDa; plasma concentration, 100–200 ng/mL; 1 nM). The factor VIII (FVIII) protein is modified by the addition of multiple N- and O-linked glycan chains. The majority of these glycan additions are located in the B domain and appear to play a role in facilitating intracellular trafficking and secretion of the protein.

or aggregated forms of the protein in heterologous cells with high levels of FVIII expression, their relevance in native FVIII-producing cells (i.e., vascular endothelium and liver sinusoidal endothelial cells) is unknown. Indeed, under conditions of high-level FVIII expression, cells can activate a classic unfolded protein response and can succumb to apoptotic cell death.

The other detail of FVIII trafficking that has attracted attention is its transit between the ER and Golgi en route to secretion. Efficient transit through the ER–Golgi boundary appears to require an interaction with glycans within the B domain of the protein. Absence of these glycans or lack of specific transport proteins responsible for this trafficking event can significantly reduce the levels of secreted FVIII.

The Factor VIII Protein Structure

The DNA sequence of the *F8* gene predicts a translated single-chain polypeptide with a molecular weight of 260 kDa consisting of 2351 amino acid residues, including a 19-residue signal peptide. Upon translocation to the ER, the signal peptide is cleaved. The remaining polypeptide is 2332 residues long.

The FVIII protein consists of three types of domains: the three A domains, which have a 35% to 40% amino acid sequence homology to ceruloplasmin and to factor V (FV); a central B domain with no known homologues; and two C-terminal discoidin-like (discoidin being a cell adhesion protein found in slime molds) C domains that are also 35% to 40% homologous to FV and to ceruloplasmin (Fig. 135.3). There are also three small "a" domains (each between 20 and 40 amino acids) consisting of predominantly acidic residues. The sequence of these domains within the protein is NH2-A1-a1-A2-a2-B-a3-A3-C1-C2-COOH. Tyrosine residues in the a2 and a3 domains, when sulfated, contribute to the cofactor function of FVIII and enable its interaction with von Willebrand factor (VWF). As indicated, the A and C domains of FVIII have structural similarities to similar A and C domains in coagulation FV. However, FV does not contain a domain homologous to the B domain. Given these structural similarities, it is not surprising that both FVIII and FV function as cofactors for serine protease enzymes in the coagulation cascade, FVIII in the intrinsic tenase complex and FV in the prothrombinase complex.

Subsequent proteolysis of the FVIII polypeptide chain in the Golgi generates a light chain consisting of the A3-C1-C2 domains with a mass of 80 kDa and a heavy chain consisting of the A1 and A2 domains. (see Fig. 135.3).

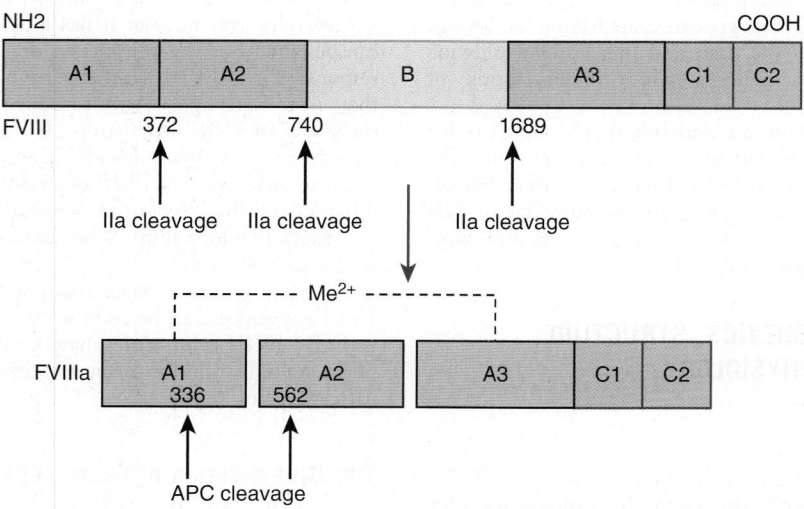

Fig. 135.3 FACTOR VIII PROTEIN ACTIVATION AND INACTIVATION. The factor VIII (FVIII) protein comprises a series of A and C domains that are homologous to factor V (FV) and ceruloplasmin and a central B domain that does not show sequence homology. The inactive precursor protein is activated by thrombin through proteolytic cleavages at three locations. Inactivation of FVIIIa occurs through two mechanisms: spontaneous dissociation of the noncovalently bound A2 domain and proteolysis mediated by activated protein C (APC).

Circulating FVIII exists as a heterodimer of the NH_2-terminus heavy chain and the COOH-terminus light chain. The two FVIII chains are bound to one another at the A1 and A3 domains by noncovalent bonds that are divalent metal ion dependent. The involved ion is likely copper, which has been found in association with FVIII.

Storage, Secretion, and Circulation of Factor VIII

After synthesis, FVIII is secreted into the circulation, where it forms a tight noncovalent complex with its multimeric partner VWF (kDa ≈0.2–0.5 nM). Whereas the plasma concentration of FVIII is 100–200 ng/mL (≈1 nM), the concentration of VWF is approximately 10 μg/mL (50 nM); thus the molar ratio of FVIII to VWF in the FVIII-VWF complex is about 1:50. The majority of VWF in plasma is synthesized and secreted by vascular endothelial cells. VWF binds to the a3 and C2 regions of FVIII through sequences in the D′/D3 region of the mature VWF monomer. Just as the cellular source of FVIII had long been argued, so necessarily has the site at which FVIII and VWF first interact. However, the recent finding that FVIII is expressed by endothelial cells suggests that at least some of the circulating FVIII may interact with VWF before secretion and may be co-stored with VWF in Weibel-Palade bodies. In the plasma, VWF protects FVIII from proteolysis by lipid-binding proteases including factor Xa (FXa). Without this interaction—for example, in cases of type 3 von Willebrand disease (VWD; in which VWF is absent) or type 2N VWD (in which mutations occur in the FVIII binding region of VWF)—the plasma half-life of FVIII is reduced and consequently, the plasma levels of FVIII are low.

Activation and Coagulant Function of Factor VIII

FVIII plays a critical role in the propagation (amplification) phase of coagulation. The physiologic activator of FVIII is thrombin, which proteolytically cleaves FVIII at three sites: Arg372 at the NH_2-terminus of the A2 domain, Arg740 at the NH_2-terminus of the B domain, and Arg1689 at the NH_2-terminus of the A3 domain (see Fig. 135.3). These cleavages release FVIII from VWF and result in the formation of a noncovalently associated A1-A2-A3/C1/C2 heterotrimeric activated FVIII (FVIIIa) molecule. FVIII can also be activated by FXa and FIXa, although the physiologic contribution of activation by these proteases is less clear.

In its activated form, FVIII provides essential cofactor activity in the intrinsic tenase complex where FIXa is the serine protease and FX is the substrate (Fig. 135.4). This reaction takes place on a procoagulant phospholipid surface, which in normal hemostasis is likely the activated platelet. Participation of FVIIIa in the complex enhances the catalytic efficiency of this reaction about 200,000-fold, and thus severe FVIII deficiency profoundly reduces the rate of FXa generation and renders this reaction biologically futile. The exact details of the cofactor role of FVIIIa remain to be elucidated, but it is assumed that it acts as a "scaffold" protein that optimally aligns the enzymatic and substrate components of the complex on the phospholipid surface. Indeed, the FIXa and FX interactive regions of FVIII have been defined, and the cofactor binds to the phospholipid surface through hydrophobic residues in the C2 domain. Of note, the FVIII B domain is not required for cofactor function, and to date, it appears that the principal role of this region of the protein is to facilitate trafficking and secretion of the nascent polypeptide.

FVIIIa is inactivated through two processes. The predominant mechanism is through spontaneous dissociation of the A2 domain. The secondary inactivation event is via activated protein C–mediated proteolysis at Arg336 and Arg562 in the FVIIIa heavy chain (see Fig. 135.3).

Our understanding of the clearance of FVIII/FVIIIa is limited. The low-density lipoprotein (LDL) receptor–related protein and other members of the LDL receptor family contribute, but this is unlikely to be the complete story. Indeed, evolving evidence indicates

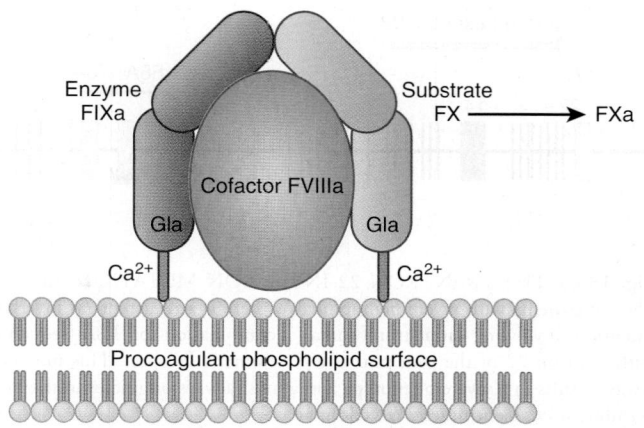

Fig. 135.4 THE INTRINSIC TENASE COMPLEX. This membrane-bound complex plays an essential role in the amplification phase of hemostasis. Participation of all components of the complex enhances the catalytic efficiency of the FXa-generating process by more than 200,000-fold. Deficiency or dysfunction of either the enzyme or cofactor involved in the complex results in a marked reduction in catalytic efficiency and the clinical manifestations of hemophilia. *FIXa,* Factor IXa; *FVIIIa,* factor VIIIa.

TABLE 135.1	Genetic Mechanisms Causing Hemophilia in Females

- *F8* or *F9* mutation homozygosity
- *F8* or *F9* mutation compound heterozygosity
- Extreme skewing of X inactivation process
- X/O karyotype: Turner syndrome
- X/autosome translocation

that FVIII clearance may be mainly influenced by its multimeric partner, VWF, and that a group of lectin and scavenger receptors on macrophages, and other cells, such as the sinusoidal endothelium in the liver and spleen, may remove FVIII in complex with VWF.

PATHOPHYSIOLOGY OF HEMOPHILIA A

Hemophilia A is a disorder characterized by congenital deficiency of FVIII. Almost all patients with hemophilia A have *F8* gene mutations. Because *F8* is located on the X chromosome, hemophilia A follows an X-linked inheritance pattern. As a result, most affected individuals are male. Severe and moderately severe cases of hemophilia A are unusual in females but can result from a number of genetic mechanisms; these are listed in Table 135.1. Approximately 30% to 50% of hemophilia A cases are caused by a sporadic mutation and occur without a family history of the disorder. The sporadic mutation is most commonly first evident in a female making her a carrier. However, as most carriers do not have excessive bleeding symptoms the new carrier is unlikely to be diagnosed until later when she has affected sons of her own or potentially affected grandsons. New female carriers often arise in the context of older paternal age (i.e., older paternal sperm cells). A good example of this was Queen Victoria's father who was 51 years old at the time that Queen Victoria was conceived.

The molecular genetic basis of hemophilia A has been extensively characterized over the past 25 years. A comprehensive Internet database of hemophilia A mutations is maintained and updated at http://www.factorviii-db.org.

A significant proportion of hemophilia A cases are the result of a recurrent mutation, an inversion mutation involving sequences in intron 22 of the gene (Fig. 135.5). The mechanism involved in generating this mutation involves an intrachromosomal recombination event in which there is an exchange between the *F8A* gene in

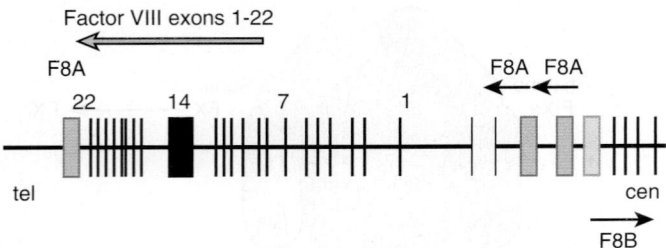

Fig. 135.5 THE *F8* INTRON 22 INVERSION MUTATION. In about 45% of patients with severe hemophilia A, there is a recurrent *F8* inversion mutation involving intrachromosomal recombination of F8A sequences within intron 22 of the gene and at a 5′ telomeric location. This mutation always results in a severe phenotype and almost always originates in the male germline. *Cen*, Centromere; *tel*, telomere.

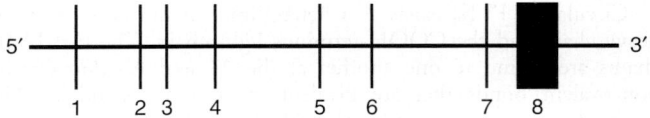

Molecular pathology of hemophilia B
• No predominant recurring mutation
• Majority of mutations are missense variants
• Some mild phenotypes are due to founder mutations

Fig. 135.6 THE FACTOR IX GENE *(F9)*. The *F9* gene is located on the long arm of the X chromosome at cytogenetic band Xq27 centromeric to the *F8* gene and the common X chromosome fragile site. The gene comprises 34 kb of genomic DNA arranged in eight exons.

TABLE 135.2	Factor VIII Mutant Genotype and Inhibitor Risk in Previously Untreated Hemophilia A Patients
Multidomain deletions	≈75%
Light chain nonsense mutations	30%–40%
Intron 22 inversion	20%–25%
Single domain deletions	15%–25%
Small non-A run insertions/deletions	15%–20%
Heavy chain nonsense mutations	10%–20%
Factor VIII missense mutations	<10%
Small A run insertions/deletions	<5%
Splicing mutations	<5%

intron 22 and one of two extragenic copies of this sequence that are located 5′ and telomeric to *F8*. The origin of this recurrent mutation is almost exclusively in the male germline (in sperm cells), where the single X chromosome has no partner to pair with, thereby potentially facilitating the F8A-mediated intrachromosomal recombination. The result of this event is the inversion of the *F8* gene between exons 1 and 22 and thus, although two distinct *F8* transcripts are expressed from separate promoters (exons 1–22 and exons 23–26), a contiguous FVIII protein sequence is not synthesized. The intron 22 inversion mutation is always associated with a severe phenotype and is responsible for approximately 45% of the cases of severe hemophilia A.

A second recurrent inversion mutation involving intron 1 of the *F8* gene is responsible for approximately 2% of severe hemophilia A cases. The remainder of the mutations responsible for hemophilia A involves more than 2000 different alterations with a wide array of missense, nonsense, frameshift, insertion or deletion, and splicing mutations. In addition, two transcriptional mutations have been identified in the *F8* promoter region. All regions of the gene are potential mutation targets, but, as elsewhere in the genome, certain sequences such as the CpG dinucleotide in arginine codons are more prone to mutation because of spontaneous methylation of the 5′ cytosine and spontaneous deamination to thymine. To date approximately 98% of cases of hemophilia A have been associated with mutations of the *F8* locus. The location of the missing mutations is not yet resolved, but the likelihood of locus heterogeneity for hemophilia A seems small. Indeed, the recent identification of mutations deep within introns of the gene suggests that all hemophilia A mutations are likely to be found within or adjacent to *F8*.

There have been extensive genotype and phenotype studies of hemophilia A with, in general, a good correlation between null mutations and severe disease and between nonnull missense mutations and a moderate or mild phenotype. The phenotype remains generally consistent with a specific mutation both within and among families.

In addition to its utility for family counseling issues, the *F8* genotype has also been found to be a predictive factor for the development of anti-FVIII antibodies (Table 135.2). Multidomain deletions are associated with the highest risk (approximately 75% risk) of inhibitor development, while the lowest risk (less than 10%) is associated with most missense and splicing mutations. The largest group is those with an average risk of 20% to 30%; this includes patients with intron 22 and intron 1 inversions, nonsense and insertion or deletion mutations. Even within these categories there is significant variability in risk of inhibitor development; for example, certain missense mutations in the C2 and C3 domains are associated with much higher risk of inhibitor development.[4]

FACTOR IX BIOLOGY: GENETICS, STRUCTURE, FUNCTION, AND PATHOPHYSIOLOGY

Factor IX Gene and Factor IX Expression

The gene that encodes FIX was cloned and characterized by two groups in the early 1980s. The gene is located on the X chromosome at cytogenetic band Xq27 and spans 34 kb of genomic sequence (Fig. 135.6). The eight exons of the *F9* gene encode an mRNA transcript of 1.4 kb that is expressed exclusively in hepatocytes. The transcriptional regulatory elements of the *F9* gene have been well characterized, and indeed there is a variant form of hemophilia B, hemophilia B Leyden, in which a postpubertal rescue of inherited FIX deficiency is the result of an activated androgen response element in the *F9* proximal promoter.[5] Aside from this hormone-responsive element, the *F9* promoter contains a typical combination of predominantly liver-specific transcription factor binding sites.

Factor IX Protein

FIX is synthesized exclusively in hepatocytes and circulates in plasma at a concentration of approximately 5 μg/mL (90 nM). The mature circulating protein consists of 416 amino acids and has a molecular weight of 57 kDa (Fig. 135.7). The protein is initially synthesized as a prepropolypeptide with a short signal sequence, which facilitates entry into the ER, and a propolypeptide sequence, which interacts with the γ-glutamylcarboxylase in the ER. The interaction with this microsomal enzyme catalyzes the posttranslational conversion of the amino-terminal 12 glutamic acid residues of mature FIX into γ-carboxyglutamyl residues (the GLA domain). This posttranslational modification enables FIX to form calcium-dependent interactions with procoagulant phospholipid membranes. A second posttranslational modification at residue 64 in the first epidermal growth factor (EGF)–like domain of the mature polypeptide involves β-hydroxylation of asparagine. This modification also plays a role in facilitating interactions with calcium and phospholipid membranes.

The structure of FIX is homologous to that of other vitamin K–dependent coagulation proteins. The domain structure includes an amino-terminal GLA sequence followed by two EGF-like domains, an activation peptide and the carboxyl-terminus catalytic domain, which is similar to the organization of procoagulant factor VII (FVII) and FX and to the anticoagulant protein C.

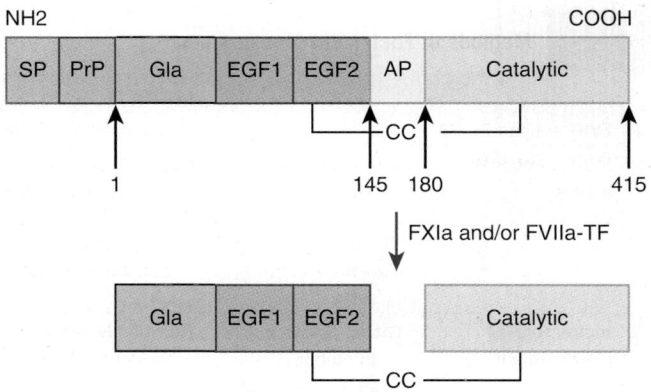

Fig. 135.7 THE FACTOR IX PROTEIN (415 amino acids; 57 kDa; plasma concentration, 5 μg/mL; 90 nM). Factor IX (FIX) is synthesized exclusively in hepatocytes. The protein is produced initially as a prepropolypeptide. The signal peptide is cleaved upon entry into the endoplasmic reticulum (ER), and the propeptide is also removed in the ER after γ-carboxylation of 12 glutamic acid residues in the N-terminal Gla domain. FIX is activated by proteolytic removal of the activation peptide and FIXa is inactivated through complex formation with antithrombin. *AP*, Activation peptide; *CC*, disulfide linkage; *EGF*, epidermal growth factor-like domain; *PrP*, propeptide; *SP*, signal peptide.

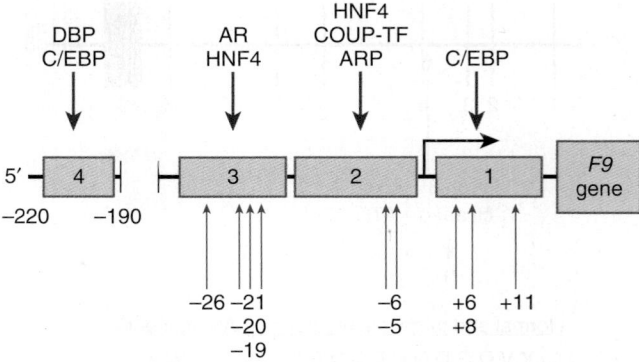

Fig. 135.8 MUTATIONAL BASIS OF HEMOPHILIA B LEYDEN. In this variant form of hemophilia B, patients experience a spontaneous recovery of FIX levels after puberty. The disease results from mutations in the *F9* promoter that disrupt transcription factor binding. Postpubertal recovery is at least partly attributable to the expression of testosterone, with the subsequent activation and binding of the androgen receptor to its cognate sequence in the *F9* promoter. Sites 1 to 4 are transcription factor binding regions. *AR*, androgen receptor; *C/EBP*, CCAAT enhancer binding protein; *COUP-TF*, chicken ovalbumin upstream transcription factor; *DBP*, D site binding protein; *HNF-4*, hepatocyte nuclear factor 4.

The FIX zymogen is activated by two processes, proteolytic cleavage mediated by factor XIa (FXIa) and by a similar process involving the FVIIa–tissue factor complex. The activation of FIX involves sequential proteolysis of two peptide bonds at arginine residues 145/146 and 180/181 (see Fig. 135.7). These cleavages release the FIX activation peptide and result in the formation of the disulfide-linked FIXa enzyme with an NH_2-terminus light chain and COOH-terminus heavy chain. Whereas the light chain binds to procoagulant phospholipid surfaces through a calcium-mediated process involving the GLA domain, the C-terminus catalytic domain cleaves and activates the substrate FX. This reaction involves the so-called intrinsic tenase complex in which activated FVIII participates as an essential cofactor. Absence of FVIIIa in the tenase complex reduces the catalytic efficiency of the reaction by approximately 200,000-fold.

FIXa is inhibited through an interaction with the natural anticoagulant protein antithrombin (AT). The fate of FIXa–AT complexes is not well characterized, but specific AT-protease receptors on the surface of hepatocytes participate in this process.

Hemophilia B Molecular Pathology

To date, all of the mutations responsible for hemophilia B have involved the FIX gene. Although there is a combined vitamin K–dependent protein deficiency state that involves mutations of the γ-glutamylcarboxylase gene, this condition is characterized by low levels of FVII, FX, and prothrombin as well as FIX. Mutational analyses of large numbers of patients with hemophilia B have detected mutations in the *FIX* gene in more than 98% of cases, and it may well be that the remaining mutations are located within intronic sequences that have not yet been analyzed.

In marked contrast to hemophilia A, in which approximately 50% of mutations resulting in severe disease are caused by two recurrent gene inversion events, approximately 75% of mutations in hemophilia B are missense substitutions. There are no common recurrent FIX mutations, although mild forms of hemophilia B may show a founder effect of missense variants in some populations.

Aside from the predominance of missense mutations, multiple other mutations can produce hemophilia B ranging from large gene deletions to a mix of nonsense, insertion or deletion, and splicing changes. The full array of FIX mutations responsible for hemophilia

B can be reviewed in the database available at http://www.factorix.org. The following text highlights several distinct and clinically important hemophilia B mutations.

The most biologically remarkable hemophilia B mutations are those that produce hemophilia B Leyden, a disorder wherein FIX levels gradually increase from less than 5% at birth to more than 30% by early adulthood. Because of the low FIX levels early in life, boys with this disorder often have bleeding episodes consistent with having moderate hemophilia B. After puberty, these problems improve or even resolve to the extent that the label of hemophilia is often removed from these patients. All of the hemophilia B Leyden point mutations are located in a 40-bp region of the FIX promoter around the transcriptional start site (Fig. 135.8). Each of these mutations interferes with the binding of a liver-specific transcription factor and thus up to the time of puberty, levels of FIX expression are markedly reduced. After puberty, there is synthesis of testosterone and androgen receptor activation. Binding of testosterone to an androgen response element in the FIX promoter provides a rescue mechanism for the disrupted FIX transcriptional status. Thus any family in which a previously diagnosed hemophilia B subject now appears normal should be investigated for a FIX promoter mutation.

Since the cloning of the *FIX* gene in the 1980s, the association of *F9* gene deletions with FIX antibody formation has been well recognized. Thus with partial and complete *F9* deletion mutations, there is a 30% to 50% risk of developing a FIX antibody response. In addition to neutralizing FIX enzymatic function, these antibodies can also be associated with anaphylactic or anaphylactoid reactions to FIX infusions.[6] The antibodies usually develop in young children (1–2 years old) after 10 to 20 exposures to FIX concentrate. In such patients FIX concentrate use is generally no longer of benefit, and attempts at inducing immunologic tolerance to FIX may be complicated by the development of nephrotic syndrome. The mechanism underlying this complication is currently unresolved.

Hemophilia B is the bleeding disorder associated with past members of the Royal families of Europe. Although the clinical picture in these individuals was consistent with severe hemophilia, the precise diagnosis was not reported until 2009. In fact, a diagnosis of hemophilia was confirmed, but not hemophilia A as had been thought and would have been expected on the basis of disease incidence, but hemophilia B (Fig. 135.9).[7] The "Royal" *F9* mutation is a splicing variant occurring at the 3′ end of intron

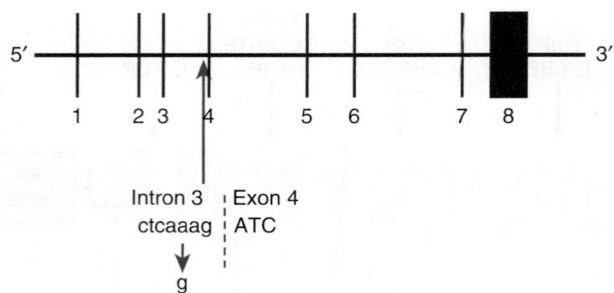

Intron 3 ¦ Exon 4
ctcaaag   ¦ ATC

↓
g

Normal and mutant exon 3/exon 4 AA sequences

.....Y V D G D Q C E S N P C L.....   Normal

.....Y V E M E I S V S P I H V Stop   Mutant

Fig. 135.9 THE "ROYAL" HEMOPHILIA MUTATION. There is now definitive evidence that the hemophilia previously present in the European royal families was hemophilia B. The point mutation found in an affected male from the Russian royal family introduces a new acceptor splice site at the 3′ end of intron 3 of the *F9* gene. The consequence of this change is the translation of 11 novel amino acids from the exon 3/4 boundary followed by a premature stop codon. A severe phenotype would be expected either because of accelerated mRNA decay or the synthesis of a nonfunctional truncated factor IX protein. *(Data from Rogaev EI, Grigorenko AP, Faskhutdinova G, et al: Genotype analysis identifies the cause of the "royal disease." Science 326:817, 2009.)*

3 that creates a new splice acceptor sequence that results in a novel out-of-frame transcript with 11 new amino acids followed by a premature stop codon. This mutation likely leads to either nonsense-mediated accelerated decay of the mutant FIX mRNA or to the translation of a significantly truncated nonfunctional FIX protein. In both instances, the clinical phenotype would likely have been severe.

Missense mutations elsewhere in the *FIX* gene have been informative with regards to our detailed understanding of protein structure and function. Mutations at both activation peptide cleavage sites have been described, and as with many genes, recurrent "hotspot" mutations have been documented at arginine codons with CpG dinucleotide sequences. Finally, some mild and frequently encountered FIX variants appear to be caused by founder mutations, as evidenced by a common adjacent polymorphic haplotype.

Hemophilia Diagnosis

The initial diagnosis of hemophilia depends to some extent on the family context. In families in which hemophilia has previously been identified, family counseling determines the risk of hemophilia transmission and usually results in a diagnosis being made in utero or early in neonatal life. In contrast, when there is no family history of the disease, the diagnosis will often not be made until there are signs of bleeding, and the timing of this depends on the extent of factor deficiency. In severe deficiency states, the diagnosis is usually made in the first 1–2 years of life, but with moderate and mild disease, the diagnosis may be made much later; with mild hemophilia, the diagnosis may be delayed until late adult life when bleeding occurs after a surgical intervention.

Phenotypic Diagnosis of Hemophilia

Two diagnostic strategies can be used for hemophilia. In the vast majority of cases, this involves measurement of FVIII or FIX coagulant levels in platelet poor plasma using a functional clotting assay (usually a one-stage partial thromboplastin time [PTT], i.e., clot-based assay). Although most clinical hemostasis laboratories use a one-stage PTT-based test to quantify FVIII, some laboratories use either a two-stage assay or a chromogenic assay that measures the

TABLE 135.3	Methods of Factor VIII Measurement		
			Comments
1. FVIII antigen ELISA			Rarely used clinically
2. FVIII functional assays	One-stage clotting assay		>98% of clinical laboratories. Assay CV <10%.
	Chromogenic assay Two-stage clotting assay		May detect FVIII instability mutants
3. Indirect measurement	Global assays e.g., thrombin generation assay		Not readily available or standardized

CV, Coefficient of variation; ELISA, enzyme-linked immunosorbent assay; FVIII, factor VIII.

generation of FXa in a purified system (Table 135.3). In these latter assays, the incubation time is often longer, which may influence test results. For example, some missense mutations causing mild hemophilia A result in the synthesis of an unstable FVIII with enhanced dissociation of the A2 domain from the remainder of the protein. These unstable mutants can sometimes be missed when a one-stage FVIII assay is used but are readily apparent with two-stage or chromogenic assays that use a prolonged incubation time.

The severity of hemophilia is based on the extent of clotting factor deficiency (severe, <1% [<0.01 IU/mL]; moderate, 1%–5% [0.01–0.05 IU/mL]; and mild, 5%–40% [0.05–0.40 IU/mL]). When making a diagnosis of hemophilia B, caution must be taken in neonates because levels of FIX can be low in normal newborns as a result of an immature carboxylase system. FIX levels double in the first few years of life. Consequently, a child may be initially labeled as having moderate hemophilia and after a few years may have FIX levels in the range of mild hemophilia. Likewise, a child may be initially misdiagnosed as having mild hemophilia B and after several years the FIX levels may normalize.

Genetic Diagnosis of Hemophilia

The other diagnostic strategy that can be used in hemophilia involves DNA analysis. Since the cloning of the FVIII and FIX genes in the early 1980s, molecular genetic approaches to hemophilia diagnosis have advanced dramatically. There are now more than 2000 different *F8* mutations associated with hemophilia A and more than 1000 *F9* mutations documented in hemophilia B.

Currently, mutations responsible for hemophilia A and B can be identified in the *F8* and *F9* genes in approximately 98% of cases. In cases in which mutations have not been found, it is likely that sequence changes are deep within introns or within distant regulatory elements, regions of the genes that are not routinely examined in diagnostic laboratories.

The strategy for genetic analysis depends on the type of hemophilia and the severity of the phenotype. For example, all patients with severe hemophilia A should be screened initially for the recurrent *F8* intron 22 and intron 1 inversion mutations. In contrast, most patients with hemophilia B require full-sequence analysis of the entire *FIX* promoter, coding region, and splice sites.

When a familial mutation has already been identified in the FVIII or FIX gene, a prenatal diagnosis can be made by either chorionic villus sampling or amniocentesis. Outside of the prenatal context, mutation testing in hemophilia can be used for carrier detection for family planning purposes and as one component of the risk analysis for inhibitor development. Determination of the hemophilic genotype is now regarded as the standard of care in comprehensive hemophilia treatment centers (see box on Hemophilia Carrier Detection and Prenatal Diagnosis).

Hemophilia Carrier Detection and Prenatal Diagnosis

The X-linked recessive nature of hemophilia naturally results in the majority of affected subjects being males. Females, however, carry and transmit the hemophilic trait and can sometimes also express clinical manifestations of the disease. Although there are rare genetic circumstances that can result in moderately severe or severe hemophilia in women (see Table 135.1), the majority of females with low FVIII or FIX levels have low factor levels because of variable skewing of the random X inactivation process that takes place early during embryonic development.

There are four ways in which hemophilia carriers can be identified. First, in light of the X-linked transmission of the disease, pedigree analysis will determine the carrier status of some women. Thus all daughters of hemophilic fathers are obligate carriers, and 50% of the daughters of a hemophilia carrier mother will also carry the mutant allele.

The second mode of identification can be through the manifestation of abnormal bleeding caused by a low FVIII or FIX level. Estimates of the percentage of hemophilia carriers who experience excessive bleeding (most often demonstrated through menorrhagia) vary but likely approximate 20% to 30%.

The third mode of carrier detection involves use of the laboratory phenotype, in which tests of the intrinsic pathway (PTT) may be abnormal and the plasma levels of FVIII or FIX may be reduced below the normal range. The etiology for low factor levels in carrier females is multifactorial and includes a woman's blood type and VWF levels in the case of carriers of FVIII deficiency as well as the ratio of inactivation of the hemophilic and normal X chromosomes, a random process that occurs early during embryonic development. If there is markedly skewed inactivation of the normal X chromosome, the plasma level of FVIII or FIX may be correspondingly reduced, and the carrier female may have a bleeding disorder. It is important to determine the FVIII or FIX levels in all carrier females to provide advice regarding potential bleeding symptoms and the risk of bleeding with surgical procedures. However, it should be noted that whereas a low plasma level of FVIII or FIX is predictive of a carrier state, the lack of a low factor level does not rule out a carrier state. In the case of carriers of FVIII deficiency, a low FVIII to VWF ratio has greater predictive power than a low FVIII level on its own, which is only found in about 20% of carrier females.

The fourth and most definitive approach to carrier diagnosis is to use molecular genetics to identify the causative FVIII or FIX mutation. Although carrier detection studies originally used analysis of linked polymorphisms to track mutant alleles, advances in sequencing technology now enable relatively easy access to direct mutation detection. This advance has significantly enhanced family counseling for hemophilic kindred and has also enabled women and their caregivers to prepare optimally for the delivery of newborns.

With current molecular genetic testing strategies, the results of mutation analyses are available within a few days in urgent circumstances. However, most often results are returned within a few weeks.

If a woman is a carrier, the causative mutation in the FVIII or FIX gene will be found in 98% of cases. If a mutation is not found, it is possible that the mutation is deep within an intron or involves a distant transcriptional element.

Ideally, carrier detection should be performed after puberty but before the woman is contemplating starting a family. In many countries, testing for the carrier status of genetic disease is prohibited before adolescence so that the girl can participate in discussions of testing options.

Prenatal diagnosis of hemophilia should begin with an evaluation of the fetal sex, which can usually be determined through a routine ultrasound examination. Recent studies suggest that free fetal DNA can be isolated from the mother's blood, with levels increasing toward term. Examination of this material for the presence of Y chromosome sequences allows for definitive sex determination. If the fetus is female, no additional studies should be performed. If the fetus is male, molecular genetic analysis can be used to identify the hemophilic mutation. Fetal DNA can be isolated from chorionic villus samples obtained after 10 weeks of gestation or from amniocytes obtained by amniocentesis from 12 to 34 weeks. The risk of miscarriage with both of these procedures is approximately 1%. If the studies are being used for making decisions about therapeutic abortion, they should be performed as early as possible. Determination of the hemophilic status of the fetus will also help plan for delivery, although consensus about the optimal obstetric management of an affected baby is lacking.

Differential Diagnosis of Hemophilia

The initial clinical suspicion of hemophilia will usually come from signs and symptoms of excessive bleeding, a family history of a bleeding problem, or abnormal coagulation test results.

There are many causes of mild bleeding manifestations, such as increased bruising and prolonged bleeding after dental and surgical procedures. These include isolated or combined deficiencies of other clotting factors (i.e., FXI, FVII, FX, FII, FV deficiency; see Chapter 137), VWD (see Chapter 138), or various quantitative or qualitative platelet pathologies (see Chapters 130 to 132). Acquired bleeding symptoms can be caused by antithrombotic drugs (e.g., antiplatelet agents and anticoagulants) or can result from autoantibodies against clotting factors (e.g., acquired hemophilia A or acquired VWD).

It should be pointed out that a low plasma FVIII level is not synonymous with a diagnosis of hemophilia A. There are a number of potential diagnoses that can result in low FVIII levels (Table 135.4). Levels of FVIII below 10% are most often the result of inherited or acquired hemophilia A or a severe form of inherited or acquired VWD (severe type 1 or type 3 VWD). Determination of VWF antigen and VWF ristocetin cofactor levels is essential for diagnosis. Occasionally, levels of FVIII below 10% can be attained with type 2N VWD. This diagnosis can be confirmed using FVIII binding studies or by genotypic analysis of the FVIII binding codons of VWF (exons 17 to 25, which encode the D'/D3 regions of the VWF protein).[8] Levels of FVIII between 10% and 50% are also likely the result of either hemophilia A or VWD (types 1 or one of the type 2 variants, 2A, 2B, 2M, or 2N). Assessment of VWF levels must be undertaken in these cases; if the VWF:RCo/VWF:Ag ratio is below 0.6, further evaluation of a possible type 2 variant must be pursued. Rarely, mild or moderate FVIII deficiency can be co-inherited with FV deficiency (see Chapter 137). Combined inherited deficiency of

TABLE 135.4	Differential Diagnosis of a Low Factor VIII Level

1. FVIII <10%
   - Severe or moderately severe hemophilia A
   - Severe type 1 VWD
   - Type 3 VWD
   - Type 2N VWD
   - Acquired hemophilia A
   - Acquired VWD
2. FVIII: 10% to 50%
   - Mild hemophilia A
   - Type 1 VWD
   - Type 2N VWD
   - Combined FVIII and FV deficiency

FV, Factor V; FVIII, factor VIII; VWD, von Willebrand disease.

FVIII and FV (levels are usually between 5% and 20%) has a prevalence of approximately 1 per million. This rare inherited trait is caused by recessive mutations in one of two genes involved in the facilitation of protein transport across the ER-Golgi interface: lectin mannose binding protein type 1 or multiple coagulation factor deficiency 2.

Isolated low plasma levels of FIX are almost always caused by congenital hemophilia B. Interestingly, in contrast to acquired hemophilia A, autoantibody development against FIX is rarely encountered. Other situations in which FIX deficiency is found usually involve concomitant reductions in the other vitamin K–dependent clotting factors, such as occurs with vitamin K antagonists, vitamin K deficiency, or significant liver disease. A much less common cause of a mild deficiency state of all of the vitamin K–dependent proteins is an inherited defect in the γ-carboxylase enzyme required for the posttranslational modification of these proteins.

CLINICAL FEATURES OF HEMOPHILIA

The clinical symptoms and signs of hemophilia A and B are essentially identical and relate to the propensity for prolonged and excessive bleeding. The bleeding tendency in hemophilia is determined in large part by the baseline activity level of the deficient or defective clotting factor. Thus in severe hemophilia (A and B), in which the baseline activity level of clotting factor is below 1% (0.01 IU/mL), spontaneous bleeding usually occurs multiple times each year. With a moderate factor deficiency state of 1% to 5% (0.01–0.05 IU/mL), spontaneous bleeding is typically infrequent, but excessive and prolonged bleeding can occur with trauma and invasive surgical or dental procedures. Finally, in mild disease, with factor levels of 5% to 40% (0.05–0.40 IU/ml), excessive bleeding is usually only documented with trauma or invasive procedures.

Pathologic bleeding can occur in the neonatal period, when intracranial bleeding can develop after traumatic delivery, especially in infants with severe hemophilia. However, most frequently, severe disease manifests with easy bruising or soft tissue or joint bleeding between 6 and 18 months of age when the young child becomes more mobile. In mild hemophilia, the disease may remain silent for many years, and occasionally a new diagnosis of hemophilia may be made in those older than 60 years of age when challenged with a surgical procedure.

The bleeding pattern in severe hemophilia is distinct and is not often seen in other bleeding disorders. In severe hemophilia, the development of hemarthroses is a classic clinical sign. Bleeding into the ankles, knees, and elbows is seen most frequently, although a hemarthrosis can occur in virtually any joint. The development of a hemarthrosis is accompanied by pain, swelling, and reduced mobility, but after repeated episodes of joint bleeding, most patients with hemophilia are able to discern intraarticular bleeding at a very early stage before any of the classic clinical signs are apparent. Repeated bleeding into a single joint results in the development of a "target joint," one in which further bleeding episodes are facilitated by previous events, leading to a vicious cycle of joint damage. With repeated episodes of bleeding, the joints become painful and less mobile. Eventually, this can result in immobility and muscle wasting of the affected limb (Fig. 135.10).

In addition to joint bleeding, patients with hemophilia are prone to excessive and prolonged soft tissue and mucocutaneous bleeding. Bleeding into unusual sites, such as the iliopsoas muscle, can result in prolonged disability and rarely, intracranial bleeding can develop, most often after trauma.

Although bleeding is the hallmark of hemophilia, the types of bleeds and issues vary somewhat according to the age of the patient. This is particularly true in newborns in whom issues related to the birthing process can occur, which are not encountered later in life. Also, the issues encountered in infancy (the highest risk period for developing inhibitors and the time for establishing home care and prophylaxis protocols) are different from those encountered in later childhood, adolescence, and the early and late adult years.

Hemophilia in Newborns

The neonatal period is a particularly hazardous period for newborn children with severe hemophilia. Newborn babies with hemophilia can be born to mothers who are known or suspected of being carriers or can be born to mothers who are not known to be carriers. The latter has become more frequent, likely as a result of demographic changes in populations including decreasing birth rates; this scenario is now encountered in about 30% to 50% of newborns with hemophilia. It is principally in the group of children born to families with no history of hemophilia that the risk of severe bleeding is greater

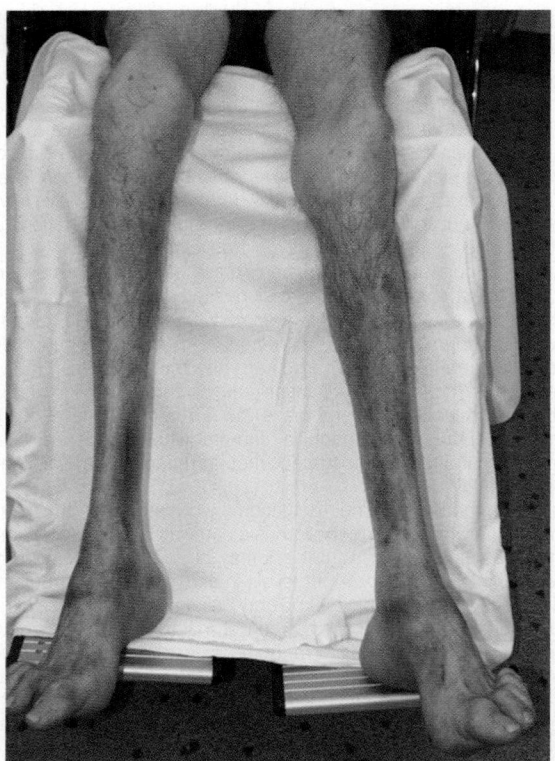

Fig. 135.10 CLINICAL OUTCOME OF CHRONIC SEVERE HEMOPHILIC ARTHROPATHY. This picture shows the legs of a 55-year-old patient with severe hemophilia A who is a wheelchair user. After a lifelong experience of multiple hemarthroses, the patient has very limited mobility. His ankles and knees show deformities, and his leg muscles are markedly atrophic because of a lack of use.

because no precautions are taken to avoid bleeding. How best to deliver children known or suspected of having severe hemophilia is still a matter of debate. For the most part, physicians still recommend atraumatic vaginal delivery because this can usually be performed safely and because it avoids the increased maternal morbidity associated with cesarean section. Furthermore, delivery of a child by cesarean section does not completely eliminate the risk of intracranial hemorrhage (ICH) (Fig. 135.11). The use of vacuum extraction or forceps should be avoided because these procedures increase the risk of both extracranial (e.g., subgaleal hemorrhage and cephalohematoma) and ICH. Fetal blood sampling has not been shown to be a significant risk factor for ICH.

Intracranial Hemorrhage in Newborns

The incidence of ICH in newborn children with severe hemophilia varies from 3.5% to 4%.[9] It is surprising that it is this low given the trauma of childbirth. Nevertheless, this is still 40- to 80-fold higher than that in the normal nonhemophilic population. If a child with known hemophilia shows any sign of ICH (e.g., unequal pupils, seizures, vomiting, and lethargy), prompt infusion of the appropriate factor concentrate should be undertaken.

In newborn boys without a family history of hemophilia, signs of ICH should prompt an urgent PTT determination along with central nervous system imaging. If the PTT is prolonged and imaging studies reveal an ICH, levels of FVIII, FIX, and VWF should be determined urgently. While waiting for the results of these levels, fresh plasma can be given at a dose of 10 mL/kg. Because FVIII deficiency is much more common than FIX deficiency, an alternative is to administer FVIII concentrate and determine the PTT 10 to 15 minutes later. If the patient has hemophilia A or type 3 VWD, the PTT should correct; in the case of type 3 VWD this correction might be

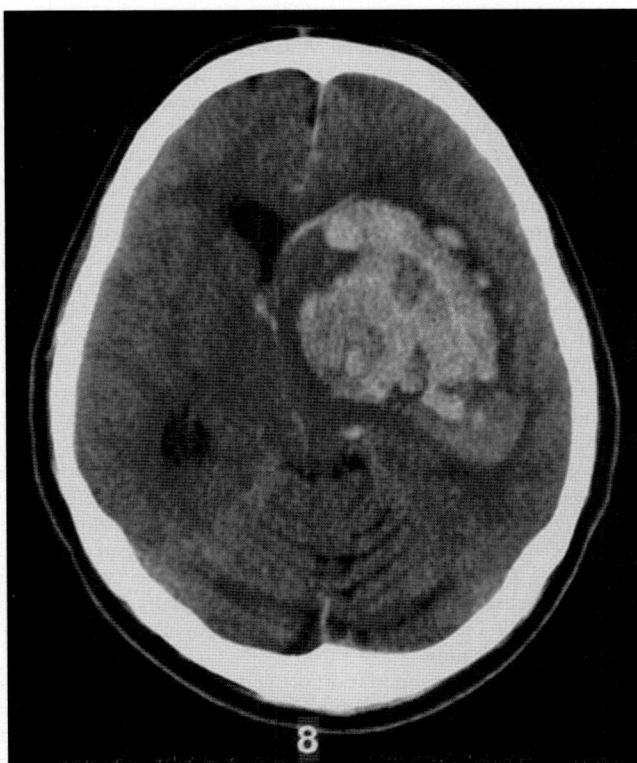

Fig. 135.11 INTRACRANIAL BLEEDING IN HEMOPHILIA. A computed tomography scan shows an intracranial bleed in a person with hemophilia. This complication most often occurs after trauma with an incidence of five per 1000 per year in patients younger than age 5 years and 1% to 2% per year in persons with hemophilia older than age 55 years.

temporary caused by the reduced half-life of FVIII in the setting of type 3 VWD. If the PTT does not correct, then it can be assumed that the child has FIX deficiency, and an appropriate FIX concentrate can be given. If FVIII concentrate is used, fresh plasma can be given while waiting for the PTT results to cover the possibility that the child has hemophilia B.

Circumcision in Newborns

Surprisingly, bleeding after circumcision only occurs in about half of patients with severe hemophilia. Consequently, the lack of bleeding after circumcision does not exclude hemophilia. In children who are suspected of having hemophilia, the hemophilic status should be confirmed before circumcision. If hemophilia is proven and the family still wishes to undertake circumcision, the appropriate factor concentrate should be administered to the child before the procedure. In general, a single dose is sufficient although some clinicians may elect to give some postoperative doses.

Other Bleeding Manifestations in Hemophilia

Although virtually all types of bleeds can occur in hemophilia, musculoskeletal bleeds (hemarthrosis, muscle bleeds, and hematomas) are most common and cause the most long-term complications. Other reasonably common bleeds include oral, dental, gastrointestinal (GI), genitourinary, and neurologic bleeding. In addition, insufficiently treated muscle and soft tissue bleeds may develop into pseudotumors (see box on Hemophilic Pseudotumors) or lead to compartment syndrome (see box on Compartment Syndrome). Finally, bleeds can occur in the context of surgery and dental procedures.

TABLE 135.5	Reasons for Differences in Bleeding Phenotype

1. Differences in factor levels
2. Differences in mutations causing hemophilia: null versus non-null mutations
3. Coinheritance of other bleeding disorders
   - VWD
   - mild functional platelet disorders
4. Coinheritance of prothrombotic disorders
   - factor V Leiden
   - prothrombin G20210A mutation
   - low levels of protein C, protein S, or antithrombin
5. Differences in the pharmacokinetic handling of factor that might be associated with patients' ABO blood group and endogenous levels of VWF in the case of hemophilia A
6. Differences in levels of physical activity
7. Differences in the structural integrity of joints, making patients more or less susceptible to joint bleeds and joint damage.

VWD, von Willebrand disease; VWF, von Willebrand factor.

Bleeding in hemophilia is broadly correlated with the endogenous level of clotting factor. Patients with severe forms of hemophilia defined as having an endogenous FVIII or FIX level of less than 1% (<0.01 IU/mL) will develop spontaneous bleeds throughout their lives beginning at about 6 to 12 months of age when beginning to crawl. Without prophylaxis, the annual incidence of bleeding increases in the first 5–6 years of life and plateaus at an average of 20–30 bleeds per patient per year. For the most part, patients with moderate hemophilia (FVIII or FIX level of between 1% and 5% [0.01 and 0.05 IU/mL]) and mild hemophilia (factor levels of >5% [>0.05 IU/mL]) only experience bleeding with trauma or surgery.

Hemophilia A and B are characterized by similar types of bleeds. However, the severity and frequency of bleeding may vary considerably among individuals with the same factor activity level. Although not conclusively proven, a number of studies suggest that the bleeding phenotype in hemophilia B seems to be less severe than that in hemophilia A patients with comparable factor levels. This is reflected in a lower median age at first joint bleed, a lower median age at start of prophylaxis, increased use of prophylaxis, and increased joint arthroplasty in patients with severe hemophilia A compared with those with severe hemophilia B. Similarly, a higher proportion of children with moderate hemophilia A than hemophilia B tend to be on prophylaxis, again suggesting differences in the severity of hemophilia A and B. The reason for this difference in clinical bleeding severity has not been well studied. For patients with severe hemophilia, one possible explanation is related to the genetics of hemophilia. Patients with severe hemophilia B generally have nonnull mutations (e.g., missense mutations) and as such are likely to have some, albeit minimal, endogenous FIX activity. In contrast, most patients with severe hemophilia A have null mutations and produce no functional FVIII. Another theoretical reason to explain the difference in the severity of bleeding is that FVIII levels tend to rise when patients with hemophilia B have a bleed because FVIII is an acute phase reactant. Because FVIII serves as a cofactor for FIX, the increase in FVIII may augment the activity of the very low levels of FIX found in patients with mild, moderate, or nonnull mutation severe FIX deficiency, thereby improving hemostatic potential and limiting bleeding.

Even in patients with the same mutation and thus with approximately the same endogenous level of clotting factor, there may be differences in bleeding predisposition. Reasons to account for this are described in Table 135.5. All of these reasons for phenotypic variability may explain why some patients bleed much less than would be expected on the basis of their factor levels while others might bleed much more; these differences may also explain why some patients can experience one significant joint bleed and end up developing signs and symptoms of chronic hemophilic arthropathy while other patients may not develop joint damage despite repeated joint bleeds.

Soft Tissue Hemorrhages and Muscle Bleeds

Bleeding into soft tissues includes spontaneous and trauma-related bleeding into subcutaneous tissues and muscles. Superficial hematomas (bruises) may resolve spontaneously without the need for treatment, and as such, bruising is not an indication for clotting factor replacement. However, in moderate and severe hemophilia, soft tissue hematomas often undergo progressive enlargement and may need to be treated. Furthermore, some soft tissue bleeds (e.g., retroperitoneal bleeds or hematomas of the neck) can cause extensive blood loss and be life or organ threatening because of their propensity to expand, thus causing compression of adjacent organs, blood vessels, and nerves and the airway in the case of a neck hematoma.

Muscle bleeds are quite common in hemophilia. The muscles most often involved are, in descending order of frequency, the calf, thigh, buttocks, and forearm. Bleeds into these locations can lead to compartment syndrome, which is an emergency situation (see box on Compartment Syndrome). A particularly problematic muscle bleed is a bleed into the iliopsoas muscle, a large muscle in the hip region. Such bleeds can rapidly expand because there is no surrounding connective tissue to restrict their growth. Consequently, significant bleeding can occur into this muscle, potentially leading to the need for blood transfusion. Patients with iliopsoas muscle bleeds have pain and restriction of movement around the hip joint; they tend to maintain the leg in a flexed position. Because of increased pressure on the femoral nerve, they may complain of paresthesia, hyperesthesia, or weakness of the quadriceps muscle. An iliopsoas bleed can be confused with a hemarthrosis of the hip (see box on Hip Joint Bleeds). Urgent ultrasonography or magnetic resonance imaging (MRI) examination is required to differentiate between the two conditions. Iliopsoas muscle bleeds need prolonged treatment with factor concentrates, as well as immobilization and physical therapy, and consequently they usually necessitate hospitalization (see box on Hemophilic Pseudotumors).[10]

Hemarthrosis

Bleeding into joints accounts for about 75% of all bleeding events in hemophilia and is the hallmark of hemophilia. Although any joints may be involved, the most commonly involved are the ankles, knees, and elbows. These three joints are therefore referred to as *index joints*. Less commonly involved joints are the shoulders, hips, and wrists. The least involved are the joints in the hands and feet.

There is significant variability in the time when children with severe hemophilia experience their first joint bleed. Although the median age to experience the first joint bleed is around 1.8 years, some children experience this within the first year of life (as they begin to ambulate) and others not until their fourth, fifth, or sixth years of life.[11] Hemarthroses become more common as children age if they are not placed on prophylactic therapy. Hemarthrosis can be either spontaneous or trauma related; however, the trauma may be

imperceptible, particularly in very young children who may not vocalize the occurrence of trauma. Mild trauma may even occur while the child is asleep, causing the child to wake up with joint pain and swelling. The onset of a hemarthrosis is often signaled by a feeling of warmth and tingling in the joint. This may last for several hours before increasing pain and limitation of joint movement set in. In patients with severe hemophilia, bleeding into the joint will continue until the patient receives hemostatic therapy or the pressure within the joint increases to the point of causing occlusion of bleeding vessels and bleeding cessation. In the later scenario, the pain in the joint may be excruciating. In patients with moderate or mild hemophilia, the bleeding may stop without the administration of hemostatic replacement but only after substantial bleeding has occurred. Consequently, joint bleeds should be treated as soon as possible to minimize the extent of bleeding and reduce the risk of long-term disabling sequelae.

Blood in a joint leads to joint damage through at least three mechanisms: iron toxicity, inflammation, and mechanical distension of the joint. Repeated joint bleeds may result in inflammation and hyperplasia of the synovial tissue within the joint (a situation referred to as *synovitis*).[12] Synovitis is the first step toward the development of hemophilic arthropathy. Any joint that undergoes repeated bleeds is referred to as a *target joint*. The strict definition of a target joint is still under discussion, but in general, most clinicians tend to accept that a joint that bleeds three or four times in a 6-month period qualifies as a target joint.[13]

A target joint is a manifestation of synovitis, and if not managed with long-term prophylaxis, such a joint will continue to bleed and will ultimately become a chronically damaged, arthropathic joint. Early stage hemophilic arthropathy is characterized by synovial hyperplasia, extensive destruction of articular cartilage, progressive loss of joint space, cystic changes within the subchondral bone, osteoporosis, and atrophy of surrounding muscles. The final stage of hemophilic arthropathy is a deformed and dysfunctional joint. At this stage, joint bleeds become less frequent as synovial hypertrophy becomes less prominent.

Determining the status of joints of patients with hemophilia at a given time or longitudinally over time necessitates both clinical and radiographic examinations. Over the past 10 to 20 years clinical and radiographic scoring systems have been developed to objectively evaluate these findings (Table 135.6). Clinical scores are the most readily available, do not require expensive radiologic equipment, and

---

Compartment Syndrome

A compartment syndrome arises when a bleed (usually trauma induced) occurs into a closed (encapsulated) space, such as the forearm or calf. The capsule restricts exit of blood, thereby raising the pressure within the compartment. This ultimately results in compression of blood vessels and obstruction of blood flow, leading to tissue ischemia and the potential for nerve and muscle damage. Compartment syndrome is characterized by severe pain and swelling, limb pallor, paresthesia, and reduced limb movement. Without treatment, a compartment syndrome may lead to permanent neuropathy, tissue necrosis, and even loss of the limb. This emergency condition requires urgent factor replacement and potentially surgical decompression (fasciotomy).

TABLE 135.6	Clinical and Radiological Joint Scores in Hemophilia A and B		
	Scores		**Reference**
Clinical	WFH joint score (Gilbert score)		Gilbert, *Semin Hematol*, 1993
	Modified WFH joint score Colorado PE-1 and PE-0.5		Manco-Johnson et al, *Haemophilia*, 2000
	HJHS		Feldman et al, *Arthritis Care Res*, 2011
Plain radiography	Arnold-Hilgartner		Arnold and Hilgartner, *J Bone Joint Surg Am*, 1977
	Pettersson		Petterson et al, *Acta Paediatrica*, 1981
MRI	Progressive Denver scoring system		Nuss et al, *Haemophilia*, 2000
	Additive European scoring system		Lundin et al, *Haemophilia*, 2004
	Single compatible IPSG MRI scoring system		Doria et al, *Haemophilia*, 2008

HJS, Hemophilia joint health score; IPSG, International Prophylaxis Study Group; MRI, magnetic resonance imaging; WFH, World Federation of Hemophilia.

Hip Joint Bleeds

Hemorrhage into the hip joint is uncommon compared with other joints. However, because the clinical features of hip bleeds are less distinctive than those of more exposed joints, it is possible that the incidence of hip bleeding is underestimated. Patients with a hip bleed maintain the joint in a partially flexed position, the position of lowest pressure. This position is similar to that seen in patients with an iliopsoas muscle bleed, causing these entities to be confused.

The management of acute hemarthrosis of the hip joint is somewhat different from that of other joints because of the vascular anatomy of the hip joint, which renders the head of the femur vulnerable to ischemia in the context of a bleed, causing raised intraarticular pressure.

Pain in the hip joint region may be caused by a range of conditions (hip joint bleed, iliopsoas muscle bleed, bleeds into surrounding muscles, retroperitoneal bleed, and appendicitis). Consequently, without appropriate imaging, a hip joint bleed may be easily misdiagnosed. Ultrasonography remains the preferred modality for investigation of hip pain because plain radiographs lack sufficient sensitivity to detect a joint bleed. Persistent pain despite appropriate factor replacement may indicate impending avascular necrosis, and urgent joint aspiration by an experienced interventionalist (using ultrasound guidance) or surgeon should be considered. Graded physiotherapy should be instituted when there is symptomatic improvement. Follow-up imaging studies (MRI, bone scan, or both) should be considered for assessment of avascular necrosis.

Hemophilic Pseudotumors

Pseudotumors are a rare but very problematic complication in hemophilia. The most common type of pseudotumor arises as a result of repeated hemorrhages into a muscle with insufficient resorption of blood between hemorrhages. Pseudotumors become walled-off cystic structures surrounded by a fibrous membrane. They may become multivacuolated over time, and parts may become calcified. These cystic lesions frequently expand into adjacent structures, leading to their destruction. Skeletal fractures and bony deformities may arise from such lesions. Another and rarer type of pseudotumor, generally only seen in adult patients, arises from within the bone itself and is often secondary to subperiosteal bleeding. This type of pseudotumor is typically observed in the long bones of the lower extremities and in the pelvis. Pseudotumors arising distally are more common in young children and most often occur in the hand. Pseudotumors may be associated with pain from rapid growth or nerve compression.

Pseudotumors are usually diagnosed by radiologic means (ultrasonography or MRI). A pseudotumor may be misdiagnosed as a neoplasm (e.g., Ewing sarcoma or osteosarcoma) or as an infection (e.g., osteomyelitis or tuberculous abscess). Biopsy of such lesions is contraindicated because of the potential for significant bleeding or infection. Small pseudotumors, particularly distal ones or pseudotumors in patients with inhibitors, are often treated conservatively with aggressive clotting factor replacement along with immobilization of the affected limb.

Unfortunately, in some instances, factor replacement alone is insufficient, and complete surgical excision is needed. This carries potential morbidity and even mortality and should only be undertaken by skilled surgeons in conjunction with appropriate hemophilia specialists. Attempts have been made at embolization of such pseudotumors, and radiation therapy has been successfully used for treatment of small pseudotumors of the hand.

may be the most reflective of a patient's joint disability status. Plain radiographs are relatively inexpensive and widely available but are insensitive to the soft tissue changes seen in the early stages of joint disease and furthermore involve radiation exposure. Magnetic resonance imaging (MRI) is most sensitive to early joint (soft tissue) changes and does not expose patients to radiation but is limited by high cost, more limited availability, and the need for general anesthesia in very young children. Work is ongoing on the use of point-of-care ultrasonography to evaluate acute and chronic changes in joints. Ultrasonography does not require sedation in young children; is much less expensive than MRI; and differentiates between synovium and hemosiderin, which is not always possible with MRI. However, ultrasonography also has limitations: (1) it is very operator dependent, and the interpretation of ultrasound findings can be subjective, and (2) some structures within a joint (e.g., cartilage) are not readily visualized. Automated ultrasonography is also being developed to address some of the former limitations of this imaging modality.

Mucous Membrane Bleeding

Epistaxis is not a prominent feature of hemophilia, but it certainly can occur. Oral bleeding is, however, quite common in patients with hemophilia. Often one of the first presentations of hemophilia is bleeding from the frenulum after trauma. Tongue bleeding, caused by a child biting the tongue, is also reasonably common. This can become an emergency, either because of significant blood loss or from tongue swelling to the point of airway obstruction. Excessive bleeding with loss of deciduous teeth and eruption of secondary dentition can occur but is again not common in hemophilia. Fortunately, most bleeding from the mouth can be controlled with antifibrinolytic agents, such as tranexamic acid (Cyklokapron) or epsilon aminocaproic acid (Amicar). Factor replacement may be required for more serious cases. For dental surgery, particularly if it requires a nerve block, factor replacement or DDAVP (1-deamino-8 D-arginine vasopressin, desmopressin) needs to be given to raise the factor level to at least 30% of normal.

Hematuria

In the past, hematuria was a reasonably common occurrence in patients with hemophilia. Hematuria may be associated with trauma but most often is spontaneous, episodic, and usually painless.

Hematuria can rarely be caused by renal calculi because these are thought to be more common in males with hemophilia compared with the normal nonhemophilic male population. There is no consensus on how best to manage hematuria in patients with hemophilia, but in general, increased oral fluids along with bed rest are recommended. If despite these measures, bleeding continues or is particularly severe, factor replacement should be given; the use of steroids to manage hematuria in patients with hemophilia has been reported, but there is no conclusive evidence that steroids provide any additional benefit. Fortunately, hematuria in patients with hemophilia is not associated with progressive loss of renal function, and as such, its natural history is probably benign.

The use of antifibrinolytic agents (tranexamic acid or epsilon aminocaproic acid) is contraindicated in hematuria because of the risk of ureteral obstruction by clots.

Gastrointestinal Bleeding

GI bleeding can occur in patients with hemophilia, particularly in adults, in whom it is often associated with the chronic use of nonsteroidal antiinflammatory drugs (NSAIDs) for hemophilic arthropathy. Another potential explanation for GI tract bleeding is esophageal varices in patients with portal hypertension secondary to longstanding hepatitis C. Such patients may present with massive life-threatening melena or hematemesis.

Neurologic Bleeding

ICH is the most dangerous hemorrhagic event in hemophilic patients. It is at present, along with HIV and hepatitis C, one of the three leading causes of death in persons with hemophilia. In both neonates and children with hemophilia, ICH is the leading cause of death. ICH is also one of the leading causes of morbidity (mental retardation, seizure disorders, and motor dysfunction) in children with hemophilia.[14] The incidence of ICH is highest in neonates and is associated with the birthing process, particularly with a traumatic vaginal delivery. ICH is also seen in young children with severe hemophilia, particularly in those who are not on prophylaxis or have an inhibitor. In older adults, ICH again becomes more common, particularly in patients with coexisting HIV or hepatitis C. In such patients, mild to moderate thrombocytopenia is frequently seen either as a result of portal hypertension–induced splenomegaly or from HIV-associated immune thrombocytopenia. The combination of thrombocytopenia together with hemophilia increases the risk of central nervous system bleeding. ICH is rare in patients with mild or moderate hemophilia.

ICH may be subdural, epidural, subarachnoid, or intracerebral. Intraspinal (usually epidural) bleeding is rare, but when it occurs, can cause spinal cord compression. Most cases of ICH occur after trauma, but the trauma may be quite trivial, such that the ICH appears to occur spontaneously. Patients with ICH usually present with neurologic symptoms soon after trauma. Typical neurologic symptoms include drowsiness, loss of consciousness, seizures, headache, and vomiting. Any of these symptoms should raise the suspicion of ICH. Thus, any person with hemophilia who has neurologic symptoms or signs should immediately be given a bolus of an appropriate factor concentrate to raise the factor level to about 100%. Replacement should always be given before any diagnostic procedure (e.g., computed tomography or MRI) is performed to confirm the diagnosis of ICH. If an ICH is present, in addition to appropriate factor replacement, patients should be hospitalized for 10 to 14 days during which time they should be maintained on factor concentrate (by continuous infusion or frequent bolus infusions) to maintain a factor level over 100% at all times.

Lumbar punctures and neurosurgical interventions can safely be performed in persons with hemophilia provided that 100% factor correction is achieved.

Surgery and Bleeding

With the exception of circumcision in neonates, excessive bleeding is almost inevitable in patients with severe or moderate hemophilia who undergo surgery without adequate replacement therapy with appropriate hemostatic agents. The bleeding can be acute or can be delayed for several hours or days. In addition to bleeding, surgery in such patients is characterized by poor wound healing as a result of poor clot formation along with prolonged bleeding and subsequent infection at the wound site. For surgical management of hemophilia see later section in this chapter.

CLINICAL MANAGEMENT OF HEMOPHILIA

As a lifelong, expensive, and disabling illness, the management of patients with hemophilia is complex and ideally best undertaken through comprehensive care in hemophilia treatment centers with multidisciplinary teams of health professionals. These teams should include a physician (usually a hematologist) with specialist training in hemophilia, a dedicated nurse, a physical therapist, and a social worker. Additional members that should be available for consultation include an orthopedic surgeon, a dentist, a genetic counselor, an obstetrician/gynecologist, a psychologist, a rheumatologist, a urologist, and (increasingly, for the management of elderly persons with hemophilia) a cardiologist. Fortunately, the role of the orthopedic surgeon in the management of hemophilia has been reduced in countries where prophylactic therapy can be provided.

Over the course of a lifetime, a patient and his family will experience numerous issues related to hemophilia. Significant psychologic sequelae ensue for both affected children and their families. These children may be overprotected, and this may result in their experiencing difficulties in adjusting to the school environment and to society in general as they age. Hemophilia impacts children's school experience and what sports and recreational activities they are allowed to undertake. Some studies have shown lower academic performance and behavioral and emotional problems in school-aged children.[15] There may be multifactorial causes for this, including potentially silent ICH. These children may grow up with resentment toward their peers and nonhemophilic siblings and they may harbor suppressed anger about having the condition. Hemophilia can also impact vocational choices and opportunities for adults with hemophilia with established arthropathy. In addition to all of the psychologic sequelae of hemophilia, unfortunate men with hemophilia who acquired HIV and hepatitis C also have to deal with the myriad emotional and social ramifications of these devastating infectious illnesses.

The child's mother may experience guilt knowing that as a carrier she passed the hemophilic mutation to her son. This can contribute to marriage breakdown, although it has not been ascertained whether separation occurs more frequently in marriages of parents of children with hemophilia than in parents of children without the condition. Clearly, persons with hemophilia and their families require significant education, counseling, and support throughout the individual's lifetime.

For society in general, hemophilia with or without HIV or hepatitis C has a substantial impact, mainly because of the high cost of care.

The key aspects of hemophilia management are preventive therapy, treatment of bleeds, and care of the complications of hemophilic bleeding.

Preventive Therapy

Preventing trauma does much to reduce bleeding frequency in persons with hemophilia. One of the strategies involved in bleed prevention is restricting the child from high-risk sports (e.g., ice hockey, American-style football, rugby, and martial arts). A number of other sports (e.g., soccer, basketball, baseball, and tennis) also entail a certain amount of risk but for the child's psychologic well-being are usually permitted. Other sports considered to be relatively safe include road cycling (with a protective helmet), running, and swimming. Ideally, persons with hemophilia should be encouraged to keep active throughout their lives because osteoporosis and obesity are growing problems in this population as a result of inactivity. All patients with severe and moderately severe hemophilia should be told to wear helmets for bicycle riding, rollerblading, skateboarding, and downhill skiing. There is controversy regarding the use of helmets (outside of sports) in very young children as they are learning to walk and are unsteady on their feet and prone to falling. Some clinics advocate that patients between the ages of 1 and 2.5 years with severe forms of hemophilia wear a helmet at all times, with the exception of when they are sleeping. Whether this policy reduces the incidence of ICH is not known. Advising families on the importance of good dental hygiene is important because good oral hygiene may prevent or reduce the need for dental procedures (extractions, root canals), which entail a risk of bleeding. Unfortunately, dental care, including regular cleaning by a dentist, is often not subsidized by society and as such may be an expensive undertaking for families.

Vaccinations

Children with hemophilia have normal immune systems and should receive all routine vaccines. In addition, they should receive hepatitis B vaccinations at a young age. Recombinant factor concentrates and currently available plasma-derived factor concentrates do not transmit hepatitis B. However, patients with hemophilia are at a higher risk of requiring blood transfusions because of trauma-associated blood loss, and there is still a small risk of acquiring hepatitis B from blood transfusions. It is not clear whether patients with hemophilia should receive the hepatitis A vaccination. However, the US National Hemophilia Foundation's Medical and Scientific Advisory Council has recommended that all persons with hemophilia who are seronegative for hepatitis A should be immunized against hepatitis A.

For persons with hemophilia, all vaccines should be given with care using the smallest gauge needle possible (#25 or #27) and applying pressure to the injection site for about 5 minutes. Vaccinations should be given subcutaneously rather than intramuscularly. This is a matter of some debate, however, because the majority of carefully administered intramuscular injections can be given safely. Nevertheless, there is an increased risk of hematoma formation after intramuscular injections. Subcutaneously administered vaccinations appear to produce the same immune response as those given intramuscularly.[16] The enhanced safety of subcutaneous injections renders this the preferred route.

Avoidance of Aspirin and Other Medications

Persons with hemophilia already have a severe bleeding disorder, and this can be exacerbated by aspirin. NSAIDs may also interfere with platelet function and should be avoided if possible. Cyclooxygenase-2 inhibitors have less of an effect on platelet function than traditional NSAIDs. For older persons with hemophilia with coexistent cardiovascular disease, aspirin, other antiplatelet agents, or anticoagulants may be indicated, but such patients require coordinated care by an experienced cardiologist and a hemophilia specialist.

Treatment of Bleeds

When a bleed occurs in a patient with hemophilia, immediate treatment is required to halt further bleeding. Rapid treatment prevents expansion of the bleed, accelerates healing, and reduces the risk of permanent disability. The longer the delay in providing treatment, the more bleeding that will ensue, and consequently the longer it will take to completely resorb the blood. Rapid treatment of joint bleeds will minimize damage to the joint and prompt treatment of muscle bleeds will limit expansion and reduce the risk of pseudotumor formation or compartment syndrome. Rapid treatment of ICH may be life saving and will minimize morbidity. The capacity to administer rapid treatment is enhanced if the patient/family is able to administer factor at home (see box on Home Care).

Coagulation Factor Concentrates

One of the main components of treating bleeds in hemophilia is replacement of the missing coagulation factor to achieve hemostasis.

Home Care

Hemophilic treatment is best administered in the patient's home. Having a patient or other caregiver able to administer factor allows for prompt treatment of bleeds and facilitates prophylaxis. Teaching patients and families how to administer clotting factor concentrates is labor intensive and usually falls to a dedicated hemophilia clinic nurse. It often takes a long time before families become skilled at factor infusions. Most boys with hemophilia older than the age of 3 years can be treated at home after the parents are taught how to administer factor. In some children, poor venous access precludes routine factor delivery; these children often require implantation of a central venous access device (CVAD) such as a port-a-cath or creation of an arterial-venous fistula (AVF). The teaching of home care is complex. Good sterile technique is critical to avoid CVAD or AVF infections. Later in life, children can be taught to self-administer factor through peripheral veins. This is generally done in children between the ages of 8 and 12 years of age.

Treatment of bleeds generally consists of more than just hemostatic support (factor concentrates or DDAVP). For example, epistaxis and oral bleeding benefit from the use of antifibrinolytic therapy, and rest and physiotherapy are important components of the treatment of joint bleeds (see section on hemarthroses). The use of ice, which is routine in hemostatically normal people with musculoskeletal injuries, is controversial in hemophilia because cooling may impair hemostasis.

Until the 1970s, this entailed the use of plasma or cryoprecipitate. Plasma contains small amounts of FVIII and FIX. Consequently, when plasma is used as the source of clotting factor replacement, large volumes are needed. Cryoprecipitate contains a higher concentration of FVIII, and in the past was commonly used for hemophilia A treatment. However, neither plasma nor cryoprecipitate is virally inactivated. Consequently, both of these blood products carry a risk of viral transmission. This limitation, together with issues of volume and convenience, has rendered these products obsolete for management of bleeding in persons with hemophilia.

Plasma-derived clotting factor concentrates became available in the 1970s. In the early 1980s, it became evident that these concentrates were contaminated with HIV and hepatitis C.[17,18] Consequently, thousands of hemophilia patients worldwide were exposed to these devastating viral illnesses, and many died of AIDS or of complications of hepatitis C.[19] Out of this tragedy came the development of safer factor concentrates—plasma-derived concentrates that were subjected to effective viral inactivation methods, including solvent detergent, pasteurization, vapor treatment, nanofiltration, and dry heating—as well as recombinant clotting factors. Currently administered plasma-derived clotting factor concentrates are not associated with HIV, hepatitis B, or hepatitis C seroconversion. In theory, there still is a small risk of transmission of viruses and prions from plasma-derived concentrates. Plasma-derived concentrates are generally classified as high purity (containing only the desired factor and very little else) or intermediate purity (containing the desired factor but with other factors present). In the case of FVIII, intermediate-purity products generally contain VWF (e.g., Alphanate [Grifols], Humate [CSL-Behring], and Wilate [Octapharma]), and intermediate-purity FIX products are prothrombin complex concentrates (PCCs, e.g., Beriplex [CSL Behring], Octaplex [Octapharma], and Proplex [Shire]), which in addition to FIX, contain factors II, VII, and X, as well as protein C and S. In general, PCCs are no longer used for the management of bleeding in patients with hemophilia B because of the risk of thrombosis. In the late 1980s, recombinant factor concentrates were developed. First-generation recombinant products were stabilized by the inclusion of albumin in the final product. Second-generation products no longer contained albumin in the reconstituted preparation but were still exposed to human plasma-derived albumin during the manufacturing process. Third-generation products have no exposure to human or animal proteins and are stabilized with sucrose. Until now, most recombinant FVIII concentrates have been derived from a full-length (as opposed to B domain–deleted) complementary DNA (cDNA) constructs. However, many of the extended half-life FVIII concentrates (including the recently licensed Fc Fusion FVIII Eloctate [Biogen]) currently being developed are B domain deleted. Recombinant factor concentrates have traditionally been more expensive than their plasma-derived counterparts, but they have generally supplanted plasma-derived concentrates for hemophilia treatment because of increased safety and small volume of infusion. Until recently, there was only one licensed recombinant FIX (Benefix [Pfizer]). A second recombinant (regular acting) FIX (Rixubis [Shire]) and two extended half-life FIX (Alprolix [Biogen] and Idelvion [CSL-Behring]) were recently licensed and several more extended half-life products are close to approval.

All brands of traditional recombinant FVIII concentrates have exhibited similar efficacy and have generally been thought to have similar rates of inhibitor development.

The efficacy of a factor concentrate primarily relates to its pharmacokinetic properties (recovery and half-life), and in this respect until recently all available plasma-derived and recombinant concentrates have had similar pharmacokinetic properties.

The recovery of factor concentrate refers to the increase in factor level achieved immediately after infusion of a given amount of factor. With all FVIII concentrates, administration of 1 IU/kg of FVIII increases the FVIII level by approximately 2%. Therefore to achieve a FVIII level of 100% in an individual with severe hemophilia, a dose of 50 IU/kg is needed. FIX has a volume of distribution twice that of FVIII, and 1 IU/kg has traditionally been thought to increase the FIX level by 1%. However, the recovery of recombinant FIX is generally lower, with 1 IU/kg increasing the FIX level by 0.8%. With the newer modified extended half-life FIX concentrates, recoveries appear to be variable, perhaps because of differences in their extravascular distribution. Children exhibit lower recoveries of clotting factor. FVIII concentrates have much shorter half-lives (approximately 8–12 hours) than FIX concentrates (approximately 18–24 hours). There are large interindividual variations in clotting factor half-life because the half-life is affected by a number of variables. In the case of FVIII, it appears to be affected by the patient's endogenous VWF level, which in turn is related to the patient's ABO blood group. Both FVIII and FIX half-lives are also affected by patient age; half-lives generally increase with age.

Recent cohort studies and a randomized open label study have challenged the assumption that the rate of inhibitor development is similar with all plasma derived and recombinant FVIII concentrates.[20–22] The Sippet (Study on Inhibitors in Plasma-Product Exposed Toddlers) study showed a 1.87-fold higher rate of inhibitor development with recombinant FVIII versus plasma derived FVIII while the Rodin study showed a 1.6-fold higher rate of inhibitor development with a second generation recombinant FVIII as compared to a third generation recombinant FVIII. The findings of both studies have been challenged because of methodologic study design issues and also on the basis of previous studies showing contrasting results. Over the next few years these studies may impact on the choice of FVIII chosen for newborn previously untreated patients (PUP) with severe hemophilia A.

Up until the present, the choice of recombinant FVIII concentrate to use has been primarily influenced by cost. In the future, with newer extended half-life FVIII concentrates (see later section) the efficacy and inhibitor incidence between newer products may be more variable and thus may impact increasingly on choice of product.

The dose and duration of substitution therapy depend on the severity of the bleed or the extent of the surgery. Table 135.7 shows the desired factor levels for various types of bleeding events and surgeries. After the initial bolus of factor, repeat doses have traditionally been needed. For major bleeds, such as an ICH, or for major surgeries, such as joint replacement, 10 to 14 days of full factor replacement may be required, but for less severe bleeds, such as an uncomplicated hemarthrosis, two or three treatments are usually sufficient. For minor bleeds or minor surgeries (e.g., dental extraction) only 1 to 3 days of factor is required. For patients who require factor for a number of days, in addition to the initial dose of factor, bolus infusions are generally required every 6 to 24 hours depending on the severity of the bleed or the surgery. Because of variable pharmacokinetics, factor levels should be monitored. This avoids high factor levels, which might be prothrombotic and represent an unnecessary expense, as well as low factor levels, which increase the risk of bleeding. In addition, monitoring helps detect development of

inhibitors. Determining the factor level at trough every several days ensures that the patient is achieving a hemostatic level of replacement.

An alternative method for maintaining hemostasis is by continuous clotting factor infusion. A lower dose of factor is required with this form of treatment, and the peaks and troughs of repeated bolus administration are avoided. In general, a FVIII infusion rate of 2 to 3 U/kg/h is sufficient once the FVIII level is increased to 100% with a bolus infusion of 50 U/kg. There has been concern about inhibitor development with continuous infusion therapy, particularly in patients with mild/moderate hemophilia A but there is no conclusive evidence that continuous infusion poses a risk for inhibitor development.

The above recommendations are based on the use of conventional half-life FVIII and FIX concentrates; different recommendations are needed for extended half-life FVIII and FIX and continuous infusion of these products is unlikely to be necessary to maintain hemostasis in patients undergoing surgery.

Extended Half-life FVIII and FIX Concentrates

A number of extended half-life or longer acting FVIII and FIX concentrates have been developed or (at the time of writing this chapter) are undergoing prospective clinical studies (Table 135.8). Consequently, many such products are likely to be available in the next few years. These agents will alter the management of hemophilia, particularly hemophilia B. Although all of the extended half-life or longer acting agents are recombinant proteins, the technology

TABLE 135.7	Recommendations for Clotting Factor Replacement		
Site of Bleed	Level Desired (%)	Hemophilia A (rFVIII) (U/kg)	Hemophilia B (rFIX) (U/kg)
Oral mucosa	>30	20	40
Epistaxis	>30	20	40
Joint or muscle	>50	30	50
GI	>50	30	50
GU	>50	50	75
CNS	>100	75	125
Trauma or surgery	>100	75	125

CNS, Central nervous system; GI, gastrointestinal; GU, genitourinary; rFIX, recombinant factor IX; rFVIII, recombinant factor VIII.

TABLE 135.8	Extended Half-Life FVIII and FIX Concentrates in Development			
Product	Technology	Manufacturer	$T_{1/2}$ (h)	$T_{1/2}$ vs. Native FVIII/FIX
Extended Half-Life FIX				
rFIXFc	Fusion protein with Fc fragment of IgG1	Biogen Idec/Sobi	57–83	3-fold
rIX-FP	Fusion protein with albumin	CSL-Behring	89–96	>5-fold
N9-GP	Site-specific glycopegylation with a 40-kDa PEG molecule	Novo-Nordisk	96–110	>5-fold
Extended Half-Life FVIII				
rFVIII-Fc	B domain deleted FVIII fused to a monomeric Fc fragment of IgG	Biogen Idec/Sobi	18.8–19	1.5–1.7-fold
BAY-94-9027	Site specific pegylation (60 kDa PEG) of a B domain–deleted FVIII	Bayer	19	1.4-fold
BAX 855	Controlled pegylation (2–20 kDa branched chain PEG) of a full-length FVIII	Baxter (now Shire)	NA	1.5-fold
N8-GP	Single site specific glycopegylation (40 kDa PEG) of a B domain–truncated (21 AA) FVIII	Novo Nordisk	19	1.6-fold

AA, Amino acids; FIX, Factor IX; FVII, factor VIII; IgG, immunoglobulin G; NA, not available; PEG, polyethylene glycol; $T_{1/2}$, half-life.
Adapted from: Carcao M. Changing paradigm of prophylaxis with longer acting factor concentrates. *Haemophilia* 20 (Suppl. 4):99, 2014.

used to extend the half-life differs among products. The two main methods involve fusion technology and pegylation. Both technologies work by interfering with the natural clearance of factor concentrates by cells of the mononuclear phagocyte system and by sinusoidal endothelial cells.

Fusion technology involves linking the cDNA sequences of clotting factors to the cDNAs of proteins (the Fc portion of immunoglobulin or albumin) that have long half-lives primarily because they bind to the neonatal Fc receptor in endothelial endosomes. This protects them and whatever is attached to them from degradation within endothelial cells, and then recycles the proteins back into the plasma. There are currently two extended half-life fusion FIX concentrates: in one, recombinant FIX is bound to recombinant Fc and in the other, recombinant FIX is bound to recombinant albumin. There is also one Fc fusion FVIII. For pegylation, polyethylene glycol molecules of different sizes are bound to either recombinant FVIII or FIX. There is one pegylated FIX and at least three pegylated or glycopegylated FVIII concentrates in development.

These newer concentrates have significantly prolonged half-lives. The half-life of FIX is extended three- to fivefold, while that of FVIII is extended by about 1.5-fold likely reflecting the dominant role of VWF in FVIII clearance.

These products, particularly the newer FIX concentrates, offer the possibility for fewer infusions and the achievement of higher trough levels. The extent to which these products will transform hemophilia management including such things as prophylaxis regimens, proportion of patients on prophylaxis, adherence to prophylaxis, long-term joint outcomes, and patient quality of life remains to be determined.

Adjunctive Treatments

Desmopressin

In the mid-1970s, Mannucci and colleagues showed that DDAVP (1-deamino-8 D-arginine vasopressin, desmopressin, Ferring Pharmaceuticals, Langley, UK), a synthetic analogue of the natural antidiuretic hormone vasopressin, raises circulating levels of VWF and FVIII:C.[23] DDAVP causes the release of endogenous VWF and endogenous FVIII from the Weibel-Palade bodies in endothelial cells into the blood. DDAVP also increases platelet adhesiveness and shortens the bleeding time independent of its effect on raising FVIII:C and VWF levels. Because DDAVP is not a blood-derived product or a factor concentrate, it is free of both infectious complications and potential inhibitor development. Furthermore, it is much less costly than factor concentrates and has few, generally mild and transient adverse events (flushing, headache, mild tachycardia, and hypotension). DDAVP has antidiuretic activity and thus carries a risk of hyponatremia and seizures, particularly if given to very young children or to those with excessive fluid intake. Because of concern about hyponatremia, many clinicians do not give DDAVP to children younger than 3 years of age, and administer DDAVP only once daily unless patients are hospitalized and serum sodium levels and fluid intake are monitored. The effectiveness of DDAVP decreases with repeated administration (tachyphylaxis) because of exhaustion of VWF/FVIII stores. Therefore, DDAVP should not be given for more than 3 consecutive days.

Most patients with mild hemophilia respond to DDAVP with a doubling or tripling of their FVIII:C levels to 30% or greater. In patients with moderate hemophilia, DDAVP rarely increases FVIII:C levels into a hemostatically effective range. All individuals with mild hemophilia A should be assessed for DDAVP responsiveness to determine whether they will benefit from this synthetic product. This involves determining FVIII and VWF levels before and 30 minutes to 1 hour after DDAVP administration.

DDAVP can be administered intravenously, subcutaneously, or intranasally. The usual dose for intravenous administration is 0.3 µg/kg given in 50 mL of normal saline over 30 minutes. For intranasal administration, the usual dose is 150 µg (1 nasal puff) for patients weighing less than 50 kg and 300 µg (1 nasal puff into each nostril) for patients weighing 50 kg or more. The maximum effect of DDAVP is achieved within 30 minutes when given intravenously and within 60 minutes when given intranasally. In general the safest approach to avoid hyponatremia is to restrict fluids in patients receiving DDAVP and to administer only isotonic solutions such as normal saline.

Because DDAVP stimulates VWF release from endothelial cells, it may increase platelet adhesiveness. In patients with hemophilia with risk factors for coronary or cerebral artery thrombosis, this may result in angina, myocardial infarction, or stroke. Consequently, DDAVP should be used with caution in elderly men with hemophilia. Because DDAVP also stimulates the release of tissue plasminogen activator, it may exacerbate bleeding. Consequently, DDAVP is often administered in conjunction with antifibrinolytic agents.

Antifibrinolytic Agents

Antifibrinolytic agents are useful in the management of bleeding from mucosal sites where there is high fibrinolytic potential (e.g., the oropharynx, nose, GI tract, and uterine-vaginal lining). In hemophilia, antifibrinolytic agents (e.g., tranexamic acid or epsilon aminocaproic acid) are generally used in the context of oral bleeding or dental surgery. Oral tranexamic acid (25 mg/kg every 6 to 8 hours) should be started 24 hours before the scheduled procedure whereas intravenous tranexamic acid (10 mg/kg every 8 hours) can be given immediately before the procedure. Tranexamic acid is available in 500-mg tablets, which can be crushed and dissolved in liquids for administration to young children. The usual dosage of epsilon aminocaproic acid is 75 mg/kg every 6 hours. In general, antifibrinolytic agents should be administered for 3 to 10 days after a bleeding episode or an invasive procedure. Longer durations of therapy are required for tonsillectomy–adenoidectomy because bleeding often occurs about 7 days after the procedure when the eschar detaches. The major contraindication to the use of antifibrinolytic agents is hematuria.

Fibrin Sealants

Experience with fibrin sealants in patients with hemophilia is increasing. Fibrin sealants function both as local hemostatic agents and as promoters of wound healing. They are particularly useful for dental procedures. Fibrin sealants have been used successfully to reduce bleeding with dental procedures, circumcision, and after excision of hemophilic pseudotumors.

Adjunctive and Alternative Management Strategies for Joint Bleeds

In the management of joint bleeds, appropriate hemostatic support is critical, but other important measures include appropriate joint rest, analgesia, and graduated physiotherapy. The application of rest, ice (for 20 minutes every 3–4 hours), compression, and elevation (RICE protocol) during the first 24 hours after a joint bleed can provide substantial benefits. The role of joint aspiration in the management of joint bleeds remains controversial, but the procedure is advocated by some groups for management of persistent pain in large-volume hemarthrosis or for exclusion of septic arthritis. Orthotics and physical therapy are of vital importance in the management of acute joint bleeds and in dealing with long-term joint damage in patients with hemophilia. Ankle guards and arch supports are useful for patients with ankle arthropathy to improve gait and weight-bearing capacity. Shoe lifts can equalize the length of the lower extremities when there is a leg length discrepancy. Muscle strength training enhances the mechanics of joint movement and provides protection and stabilization of the joint.

Surgical Management in Hemophilia

With appropriate management (factor replacement with or without other adjunctive hemostatic agents), intra- and postoperative hemorrhages can be prevented in patients with hemophilia thus allowing for surgery to be performed safely in patients with hemophilia. Ideally a multidisciplinary team is required to undertake surgery in a safe manner; physicians with expertise in the management of hemophilia patients should always be involved. Some surgeries might need to be adapted for patients with hemophilia (e.g., bioprosthetic heart valves are preferable to mechanical valves to avoid the need for anticoagulant therapy).

The most common surgical procedures in hemophilia are those undertaken to manage the complications of joint bleeds. These include surgical or arthroscopic synovectomy, nonsurgical (chemical or radionucleotide) synovectomy, various arthrodesis procedures, and joint replacement.

An open surgical or arthroscopic synovectomy endeavors to remove the inflamed and thickened synovial tissue that is the source of bleeding within the joint. Although it may reduce the frequency of bleeding, it does not improve joint mobility and may even worsen it.

Radionucleotide synovectomy has largely replaced chemical synovectomy. This involves injection of a radioisotope (e.g., yttrium[90], chromic phosphate P[32]) into the joint space to obliterate synovial tissue. Compared with surgical synovectomy, radionucleotide synovectomy is less invasive, associated with a shorter hospital stay, and reduced clotting factor coverage. Consequently, the procedure is less costly than surgical synovectomy. Radionucleotide synovectomy is particularly useful for patients with inhibitors because there is a lower risk of bleeding. However, long-term safety data are lacking in hemophilia.

Arthrodesis (surgical joint fixation) is particularly useful for painful joints with greatly compromised mobility in which joint replacement is not easily undertaken (e.g., ankles).

Joint replacements (particularly of the knee and hip) are still commonly performed procedures in adults with hemophilia. The elbow, which is not amenable to arthrodesis or for the most part to joint replacement, is often the most difficult joint to manage in patients with hemophilia. It is likely that there will be less need for surgical procedures with the initiation of prophylaxis regimens in early childhood.

Prophylactic Clotting Factor Replacement

Experience has shown that if treated solely on demand, patients with hemophilia will experience frequent bleeds and will, over time, develop disabling joint disease. Prophylaxis regimens reduce bleeding and prevent or limit joint damage in patients with hemophilia. The longest experience with the use of prophylaxis comes from European centers in Sweden, the Netherlands, and Germany.[24] Based on numerous cohort studies, there is good evidence that patients who receive prophylaxis experience fewer bleeds and maintain better joint function than those treated on demand. There are several different prophylaxis regimens distinguished by dose and frequency of factor administration. The full-dose prophylactic regimen, often referred to as the Malmö regimen, involves administration of 25 to 40 IU/kg of conventional FVIII every other day (minimum, 3 days/week) for patients with hemophilia A and the same amount of FIX 2 days a week for those with hemophilia B. Less intense "intermediate-dose" prophylaxis regimens involve the administration of 15 to 25 U/kg 2 to 3 times a week, and low-dose prophylaxis regimens call for the administration of dosages of 10 to 15 IU/kg given once or twice a week.

Of course, new protocols will be needed for the extended-half-life concentrates and full-dose, intermediate-dose and low-dose prophylaxis regimens with these products remain to be defined. In addition, these concentrates enable achievement of higher prophylactic trough levels, which could further reduce the risk of bleeding and allow patients more flexibility in pursuing activities.

Ample evidence shows that prophylaxis must be commenced early in life to prevent joint disease. This is referred to as primary prophylaxis; prophylaxis started at a very young age (usually 2 years of age or earlier) before joint disease has developed (generally, before or immediately after the first joint bleed). In contrast, secondary prophylaxis refers to continuous long-term prophylaxis started at a later age (after 2 years of age) or after more than one joint bleed has occurred. The term tertiary prophylaxis has recently been coined to refer to prophylaxis starting after there is established joint disease. The term *prophylaxis* also encompasses short-term prophylaxis regimens given after surgery or ICH.

Comparisons of different starting prophylactic regimens have shown that patients can be started on less intensive prophylaxis regimens and gradually escalated to full-dose regimens. Although full-dose regimens prevent bleeds more effectively than intermediate- and low-dose schedules, they cost more and may not be feasible in less affluent countries. In these countries, intermediate- or low-dose prophylaxis regimens may be more affordable, and may still confer significant benefit.

Although prophylaxis has been used for decades it was only in the last 10 years that a randomized study comparing primary full-dose prophylaxis with on-demand therapy in young children with severe hemophilia was undertaken. This study demonstrated 90% fewer bleeds in patients given primary prophylaxis and after only a few years, these patients already had less joint damage than those treated on demand.[25] The benefits of prophylaxis include reduced hospitalization, less time lost from school or work, improved school performance, and a reduced need for orthopedic surgery. Because of these benefits, the World Health Organization, World Federation of Hemophilia, and many other national hemophilia organizations have endorsed primary prophylaxis as the standard of care for children with severe hemophilia. One other potential benefit of prophylaxis is that early initiation of prophylaxis may reduce the risk of inhibitor development, at least in the subgroup of patients with severe hemophilia with "good risk" *F8* mutations.[20,26]

The approach to prophylaxis varies by center and country. In some centers and countries, all patients are given full-dose prophylaxis, while in others, prophylaxis is individualized based on the severity and frequency of bleeding episodes.[27]

Burdens of prophylaxis include the need for venous access and cost. Patients receiving full-dose prophylaxis often require a CVAD or AVF for repeated factor administration. Furthermore, in the short term, full-dose prophylaxis regimens in young children are threefold more expensive than on-demand therapy. However, the cost of on-demand therapy increases over time because once joint bleeds occur, the subsequent joint damage triggers more bleeding. The social costs of joint damage are high in terms of lost time from school or work and limitations in vocational opportunities for adults with arthropathy. Whereas the costs of treating patients on demand rise over time, the cost of prophylaxis may stabilize or decrease when adults become less active.

Although most children in Europe and North America are on prophylactic regimens, prophylaxis is less routinely used in developing countries. However, this trend appears to be changing with increasing use of intermediate- and low-dose prophylaxis regimens in developing countries.

Considerations for Treatment of Hemophilic Bleeding in Adults

There is little doubt that regular prophylactic infusion of clotting factor concentrate is the treatment of choice for children and adolescents. However, the role of prophylaxis in adults is less clear. Although it may seem intuitive to maintain prophylaxis throughout life, this strategy is expensive, and its benefits have not been formally evaluated. Furthermore, there is some evidence that not all children who received prophylaxis require continued prophylactic therapy as adults.

When prophylactic therapy is undertaken in adults, it should be administered in a manner best suited to the individual needs of the patient. Thus some patients prefer to treat themselves with a small amount of clotting factor every day (e.g., 500 IU of FVIII/daily), while others prefer a once- or twice-weekly regimen with additional infusions before high-risk activities, such as sports. Prophylaxis should be used in patients with a target joint into which repeated bleeding is documented. In this instance, prophylactic concentrate infusions at regular intervals (three times a week for FVIII and twice a week for FIX) should be initiated and continued for several months or longer.

If an on-demand regimen is used, patients must be carefully counseled. Treatment should be started as soon as possible after the first signs of bleeding and, if appropriate, adjunctive measures such as rest, ice, compression, or limb elevation should be used to hasten symptom control.

Complications of Treatment

Until the mid-1970s, the biggest impediment to the management of patients with hemophilia was the lack of readily administered treatment, which virtually guaranteed that patients with severe hemophilia would develop hemophilic arthropathy, and many would die from bleeding, including ICH. By the 1980s, treatments were available, and prophylaxis programs were initiated in many countries. Unfortunately, the 1980s was the era of HIV and hepatitis C, and most patients with hemophilia treated before 1985 became infected with both, with smaller numbers also becoming infected with hepatitis A and B. Many of these patients have died. This tragedy prompted widespread implementation of blood donor screening programs and viral inactivation processes and accelerated the development of recombinant clotting factor concentrates.

The management of HIV since the 1980s has undergone tremendous advances. Currently, patients with HIV who are treated with highly active antiretroviral therapy live almost normal life spans. Infection with hepatitis C has been more problematic because it results in chronic disease in approximately 60% of those infected. A combination of interferon and ribavirin has been used with good results in patients with certain hepatitis C genotypes 2 and 3 and less satisfactory results in those with genotype 1. Several new-generation anti–hepatitis C virus therapies are now available, and these may facilitate the cure of increasing numbers of infected patients with hemophilia.[28] Nonetheless, many patients still develop long-term complications of chronic hepatic infection, including hepatocellular carcinoma. Co-infection with HIV and hepatitis C together with alcohol use increases the risk of liver complications. All noninfected persons with hemophilia should routinely receive hepatitis A and B vaccination to reduce the risk of infection.

Other Comorbidity in Patients With Hemophilia

With progressive improvements in hemophilia care, persons with hemophilia are living longer, and morbidities associated with aging are now complicating the clinical management of hemophilia. Although patients with hemophilia are somewhat protected from atherothrombotic events, there are increasing numbers of older patients with coronary artery disease. This problem is necessitating the development of guidelines to safely introduce antiplatelet regimens for secondary prevention in patients with coronary artery disease.

There is also an increased prevalence of hypertension in hemophilia, the pathogenic mechanism of which is currently unresolved.

Limitations to Treatment for Hemophilia

Currently, the major impediments in the management of patients with hemophilia are cost, inhibitor development, and the need for CVADs.

1. Cost: Worldwide, cost is the major issue. Currently available factor concentrates, particularly recombinant factor concentrates, are very expensive, and prophylaxis regimens can cost as much as $300,000 per patient per year. However, the cost has decreased in countries with tendering systems. In the next few years, widespread introduction of extended half-life factor concentrates will likely have a major impact on the price of factor concentrates—both the newer products and the current products.

2. Inhibitor development: Management of patients with inhibitors remains a challenge. Although inhibitor development is more common in patients with hemophilia A (particularly severe forms), patients with hemophilia B are difficult to manage because they often develop anaphylaxis and nephrotic syndrome. Although the genetic and environmental risk factors for inhibitor development are increasingly well understood, our capacity to prevent inhibitor development remains limited.

3. CVADs: These are useful for the management of young children with severe hemophilia. They are of particular benefit in children who develop inhibitors and require immune tolerance therapy (ITT). Most ITT regimens call for daily administration of factor, which can rarely be given by repeated peripheral venipuncture in young children. CVAD complications include infections and thrombosis. Catheter infections caused by skin organisms can produce considerable morbidity, and the CVAD often needs to be removed. In a meta-analysis of studies evaluating CVAD complications, Valentino and colleagues reported a 40% CVAD infection rate with a mean of one CVAD infection for every four patients with a CVAD in place for 1 year. Thrombosis associated with CVADs varies in significance from small fibrin sheaths to thrombi that occlude large vessels and can lead to pulmonary embolism or death. Several studies have shown that radiographically proven CVAD-associated thrombosis develops in up to 50% of patients with hemophilia with these devices. Such thrombi may impair CVAD function, thereby necessitating their removal. Because of the complications associated with CVAD implantation, some institutions recommend AVFs as an alternative. However, experience with AVFs is still limited.

Immune Responses to Exogenous Factor VIII and Factor IX

Adverse immunologic responses to replacement products are a major complication for patients with hemophilia who have access to replacement factor concentrates. These responses occur because the infused factors contain foreign epitopes. However, not all patients develop an immune response to replacement; the reasons for this are unknown.

Immune responses include anaphylactic reactions and nonanaphylactic antibody-producing responses. The latter are classified according to their effects in vitro: whereas immunoglobulin (Ig) G antibodies that "inhibit" the coagulant function of the replacement factor are referred to as *inhibitors,* those that do not interfere with coagulant activity are called *nonneutralizing antibodies. Catalytic antibodies* directly hydrolyze the target protein.

Anaphylactic Reactions

Type I hypersensitivity reactions are rare in patients with hemophilia A but have been reported with infusion of either plasma-derived or recombinant FVIII concentrates. Rarely, there is evidence of IgE mediation, suggesting that in some cases, these reactions may reflect complement activation, immune complex formation, or other mechanisms.

Approximately 3% of patients with hemophilia B experience anaphylactic reactions to FIX products; these occur with equal frequency with plasma-derived and recombinant products. The median number of FIX exposure days at the time of anaphylactic reactions is 11.[29] These reactions often occur in patients who have FIX inhibitors and show evidence of IgE mediation. In some cases, transient IgG1 antibodies to FIX have been detected near the time of the allergic reaction. Because

IgG1 antibodies can bind complement, this may point to an alternative mechanism for anaphylactic-type reactions without evidence of IgE mediation. Factors that may confer an increased risk for anaphylactic reactions to FIX include Hispanic race, personal or family history of other allergies, and severe hemophilia B (FIX: C <1%) caused by large deletions and nonsense mutations of the *F9* gene.[30] It is unclear why anaphylactic reactions are more common with FIX deficiency than in FVIII deficiency. It is possible that the extravascular distribution of FIX is more likely to provoke such a reaction. In addition, therapeutic doses of FIX contain much more protein than therapeutic doses of FVIII, which may trigger anaphylaxis. Total deletions of the *F9* gene may also include deletions of adjacent genes whose absence may predispose patients to anaphylaxis.

The acute management of anaphylaxis involves supportive care and the use of non–FVIII or non–FIX-containing bypassing agents to treat bleeding. Desensitization by repeated administration of concentrate may be successful, particularly in patients with hemophilia B. Because of the timing of anaphylactic reactions in hemophilia B, it is recommended that the first 10 (in those with missense mutations) to 20 (in those with deletion and nonsense mutations) FIX treatments be given in a controlled setting.

Inhibitory Antibody Development

This important treatment-related complication is dealt with in detail in Chapter 136. The current chapter deals with selected issues concerning pathophysiologic mechanisms and inhibitor detection only.

Factor VIII Inhibitors: Pathophysiology

FVIII inhibitors in patients with hemophilia A are antibodies of the IgG isotype and are typically of the IgG1 and IgG4 subclasses, although inhibitory antibodies of other subclasses are observed as well. Some evidence indicates that IgG4 antibodies are predominant in patients with high-titer inhibitors, while IgG1 antibodies are more abundant in patients with low-titer inhibitors. The predominance of IgG4 antibodies may be a consequence of prolonged exposure to exogenous FVIII because this phenomenon has been observed with repeated administration of other antigens. Inhibitory antibodies may have higher binding affinity than noninhibitory antibodies.

Inhibitors may be classified by the kinetics of their binding to FVIII. *Type I* inhibitory kinetics is characterized by a linear relationship between the antibody concentration and the logarithm of the residual FVIII activity; at high antibody concentrations, the inhibition of FVIII is near total. FVIII inhibitors in patients with congenital hemophilia A usually have type I kinetics. Inhibitors with *type II* kinetics do not display a linear relationship, and even high antibody concentrations do not result in complete inhibition of FVIII activity. Type II kinetics are commonly seen in acquired hemophilia A.

Inhibitors are produced when a FVIII-specific memory B cell is stimulated to differentiate into an anti-FVIII antibody–secreting cell (plasma cell). This differentiation is dependent on binding of FVIII to the B-cell receptor, and subsequent interaction with a CD4 positive helper T cell. The important role of helper T cells in the genesis of inhibitors is supported by diverse data: T-cell proliferation in response to FVIII is increased in hemophilia A patients who have inhibitors compared with those without. Blockade of CD3, a component of the T-cell receptor complex, has been shown to decrease inhibitor formation in vitro, as has stimulation of cytotoxic T-lymphocyte antigen 4 (CTLA-4), an inhibitory receptor involved in the downregulation of T-cell stimulation. Decrease of inhibitor titers, and even loss of inhibitors altogether, has been observed in hemophilia A patients with inhibitors who have HIV infection, particularly those with very low numbers of CD4-positive T cells. T-cell activation that effectively produces inhibitors requires co-stimulation from antigen-presenting cells (e.g., via the CD40/CD40 ligand pathway or the CD28/B7 pathway).

Regulatory T cells (Tregs), which can suppress the activity of helper T cells, may have a role in determining whether an individual patient will be immunologically reactive or tolerant to FVIII. T-cell proliferation in response to FVIII stimulation has been observed in Treg-depleted peripheral blood from normal (nonhemophilic) human subjects. In contrast, high levels of Tregs have been shown to suppress inhibitor development in mice models; hemophilia A mice treated with rapamycin (a small molecule inhibitor of the serine kinase mammalian target of rapamycin [mTOR]) failed to develop inhibitors on exposure to FVIII and had increased number of Tregs compared with control mice. Hemophilia A mice had lower inhibitor titers in response to FVIII with infusion of Tregs taken from wild-type mice than without, and Tregs created with chimeric antigen receptor technology have been shown to suppress anti-FVIII immune responses in vitro.

Immunologic tolerance to FVIII in people without hemophilia A is not complete. Rarely, usually as a result of autoimmune disease, immunologic tolerance to FVIII fails and autoantibodies to FVIII develop; this is known as *acquired hemophilia A*. Furthermore, antibodies to FVIII, detectable by enzyme-linked immunosorbent assay (ELISA) and Bethesda assay as well as other methods, can be found in the plasma of some individuals who do not have hemophilia A. T cells that are reactive to FVIII can also be found in normal individuals, although this reactivity is transient and less intense than in hemophilia A patients. The relevance of these observations for hemophilia A patients who have inhibitors is not known. Further understanding of the mechanisms that might prevent normal individuals from developing clinically important autoantibodies to FVIII, such as T-cell suppression by Tregs or neutralization of inhibitory antibodies by antiidiotypic antibodies (antibodies to the antigen-binding region of the inhibitory antibody), might provide insight into inhibitor suppression in hemophilia A patients.

Fortunately, the majority of patients with hemophilia A who are exposed to replacement FVIII products do not develop inhibitors. The reasons for tolerance to FVIII in some patients are not clear. Genetic factors play a role in inhibitor risk (see Chapter 136). It has been hypothesized that some patients are exposed in utero, via maternal–fetal hemorrhage, to small quantities of maternal FVIII that induce immunologic tolerance in the fetus. However, there has been no observed association between inhibitor risk and intrauterine procedures such as amniocentesis, or with breastfeeding.

Another theory to explain the development of FVIII inhibitors in some patients is that of immunologic "danger signals": if a patient has exposure to FVIII at the same time as exposure to pathogen-associated molecular patterns, such as infectious agents or vaccines, or to damage-associated molecular patterns, such as might occur in the setting of surgery or in the setting of a major bleed, this may induce an immunogenic, rather than a tolerogenic, immune response to FVIII. Although specific danger signals, for example molecular patterns that are agonists for toll-like receptors or other receptors in the innate immune system have not yet been definitively identified in association with FVIII inhibitor development; some clinical data are consistent with the danger signal hypothesis.

Transient Inhibitors

Some FVIII inhibitors may disappear spontaneously without specific management. Inhibitors may ultimately prove to be transient despite continued on-demand FVIII exposure. This typically occurs with low titer inhibitors (<5 Bethesda units [BU]) but can occur with some higher titer inhibitors as well (≤10 BU). Transient inhibitors are also possible in patients with hemophilia B, but this phenomenon is not well characterized.

Factor IX Inhibitors: Pathophysiology

As severe hemophilia B is much less common than severe hemophilia A and as a much lower percentage of hemophilia B patients develop inhibitors, much less is known about the basic science of FIX inhibitors than about FVIII inhibitors. There is, as previously described, a relationship between FIX inhibitors and anaphylaxis to FIX that generally does not occur with FVIII inhibitors.

FIX inhibitors are primarily IgG4 subclass antibodies although some are IgG2 subclass.

Epitopes for FIX inhibitors have been identified in the γ-carboxyglutamic acid domain, which is involved in binding to phospholipid surfaces, the serine protease domain, and possibly in the activation peptide region, at which FIX is activated by activated FXI. As is the case with inhibitory FVIII antibodies, the specificity of these antibodies for epitopes in functionally important regions of the FIX molecule explains their ability to inhibit FIX's coagulant activity.

Because FIX inhibitors are antibodies of the IgG isotype, they are products of interaction between FIX-specific B cells and helper T cells, but this process is less well described than is the case for FVIII inhibitors. The roles of co-stimulatory molecules, immunoregulatory genes, and Tregs in FIX inhibitors have not been demonstrated.

Detection of Inhibitors and Antibodies

Inhibitors are detected using the Bethesda assay (see Chapter 136). The Bethesda assay will not, by definition, detect nonneutralizing antibodies (i.e., those antibodies to FVIII or FIX that do not inhibit the coagulant function of these proteins). New modifications of the Bethesda assay, including an "ultrasensitive" Bethesda assay that uses concentrated patient plasma, are being developed and may improve the reliable identification of low-titer inhibitors (Fig. 135.12).

Both neutralizing and nonneutralizing antibodies to FVIII or FIX may also be detected by ELISA. This assay can only detect and quantify the antibodies present and cannot determine their inhibitory activity, but assays that identify the epitopes to which antibodies bind can discriminate between antibodies that interfere with important functional domains of the FVIII or FIX protein and those that do not. Techniques for measuring binding affinity of antibodies may also be of clinical use in the future.

Immunogenicity of New Factor Concentrates

Many new FVIII and FIX concentrates are in different stages of development for clinical use. In view of recent research that suggests the possibility of different rates of immunogenicity between different FVIII products that are currently in use, the immunogenicity of any new products will be of interest and importance.

Every factor concentrate's immunogenicity is initially evaluated in previously treated patients (PTPs, i.e., those with a minimum of 100 to 150 prior exposure days to a FVIII or FIX concentrate). In studies of PTPs exposed to new factor concentrates, very few inhibitors have so far occurred. This suggests that in widespread clinical use, inhibitors will occur only rarely, if at all, in PTPs who switch to new concentrates.

There is less experience using new concentrates in hemophilia patients that have not yet been exposed to a factor concentrate (PUPs). Since the risk of both FVIII and FIX inhibitors is greatest early in a patient's treatment course, the immunogenicity of new concentrates in PUPs may differ from what occurs in PTPs.

There are some reasons to suspect that immunogenicity of new concentrates may not be worse than that of existing concentrates, despite the presence of additional modifications such as Pegylation or fusion to Fc or albumin. For example, pegylated versions of other protein therapeutics (e.g., asparaginase, granulocyte-colony stimulating factor) have not proven to be more immunogenic than their nonpegylated counterparts, and there is some animal evidence to suggest that FVIII and FIX concentrates that have been fused to the Fc region of IgG may be less immunogenic than standard FVIII or FIX, perhaps because of interactions with Fc receptors present on cells involved in immune responses. In addition to developing EHL factor concentrates some manufacturers are developing FVIII concentrates that are produced in human cell lines, rather than in cells obtained from other mammalian species, with the hope that factor produced in human cell lines will show reduced immunogenicity because of more "native" posttranslational modifications of the factor protein.

Of course all of this remains speculative and the results of studies of the immunogenicity of new factor concentrates in PUPs are eagerly awaited.

Nonclotting Factor Concentrate Treatments for Hemophilia

Since about 2010, there has been significant interest in developing novel strategies for treating hemophilia that do not rely upon clotting factor replacement. In 2017 some of these therapies are just beginning to enter the clinic.

There are two principal approaches that are being used to enhance hemostasis through these alternative strategies: (1) through "rebalancing hemostasis" by inhibiting natural anticoagulant pathways (e.g., through tissue factor pathway inhibitor [TFPI] or AT inhibition) and (2) through the delivery of a bispecific antibody that mimics FVIII cofactor activity (Table 135.9).

The studies involving anticoagulant pathway inhibition have, to date, focused on TFPI and AT, and have used contrasting methods to reduce production or inhibit the function of these proteins. The anti-AT approach has used the subcutaneous delivery of small interfering RNA (siRNA) to reduce synthesis of the protein.[31] The magnitude of AT knock down is dose dependent, and the effect persists

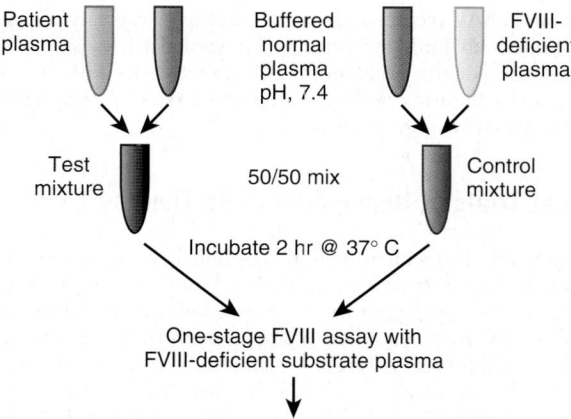

Fig. 135.12 THE NIJMEGEN-MODIFIED BETHESDA ASSAY. This is the currently recommended methodology for quantifying anti–factor VIII (anti–FVIII) inhibitory antibodies.

TABLE 135.9	Alternative, Nonclotting Factor Concentrate Therapies for Treating Hemophilia

1. Rebalancing hemostasis strategies:
   a. TFPI Inhibition approaches: anti-TFPI aptamer, antibody and peptide.
   b. Antithrombin siRNA biosynthesis inhibition.
   Both approaches can be delivered by infrequent (weekly or less often) subcutaneous injections.
2. Factor VIII mimetic molecule: bispecific antibody to FIXa and FX.
   Can be administered by subcutaneous injection and has shown activity in FVIII inhibitor patients.

FX, Factor X; FIXa, Factor IXa; FVIII, factor VIII; siRNA, small interfering ribonucleic acid; TFPI, tissue factor pathway inhibitor.

for up to 4 weeks. In contrast, the approaches used to inhibit TFPI have focused on functional neutralization using anti-TFPI aptamers, antibodies and peptides.[32] These approaches offer much promise but are not without risks; a phase III study on an anti-TFPI aptamer was halted because of unexpectedly increased bleeding with the product. It remains unclear whether any of these rebalancing approaches to hemostasis will provide sufficient procoagulant activity to eliminate bleeds in the absence of FVIII or FIX, or whether they would need to be administered as adjunctive therapies with small doses of clotting factor concentrate. Finally, the risk of generating a pathologic procoagulant response with these approaches remains a possibility that will require careful monitoring.

The other innovative approach is the use of a bispecific antibody that substitutes for the cofactor activity of FVIIIa.[33] This antibody binds to FIXa and FX and at least partially mimics the scaffold function of FVIIIa in the intrinsic tenase complex. The antibody can be administered by weekly subcutaneous injection and phase II clinical studies have shown no adverse effects and a reduction in bleeding events in hemophilia A patients both with and without FVIII inhibitors. Therefore the bispecific antibody could serve as an alternative to FVIII replacement in hemophilia A patients with or without inhibitors.

Gene Therapy for Hemophilia

Since the cloning of the FVIII and FIX genes in the early 1980s, hemophilia has been a leading candidate for the application of somatic cell gene transfer. The rationale for gene therapy in hemophilia includes the following: small increments in FVIII or FIX levels have a significant clinical benefit; regulation of FVIII or FIX levels is not critical as long as they do not reach supraphysiologic levels for extended periods of time; the site of coagulation transgene expression need not be restricted as long as sufficient amounts of the protein reach the circulation; and small (genetically modified hemophilic mice) and large (spontaneously generated hemophilic dogs) animal models of hemophilia are available for preclinical evaluation of gene transfer approaches.

Modes of Transgene Delivery

A key component to any gene transfer strategy is the development of a delivery system that enables efficient transfer of the therapeutic transgene to the recipient cell type of choice. After 30 years of investigation, viral vectors remain the most effective means of achieving high-level gene transfer. Although efforts have been made to enhance the efficiency of nonviral delivery methods such as liposome encapsulation, various physicochemical conjugates, and hydrodynamic injection, all of these approaches have limitations that preclude their advancement into the clinic at this time.

Hemophilia gene transfer studies have used three main types of viral vector: adenovirus, several forms of retrovirus and adeno-associated virus (AAV). Trials of adenoviral gene transfer have been successful in animal models of hemophilia, but the single hemophilia A patient treated with an adenoviral vector experienced significant hematologic toxicity, and no further clinical studies have been undertaken with this vector type. Thus although adenoviral gene transfer is highly efficient, these vectors elicit a major innate immune response upon cell entry, and the proinflammatory consequences of this response remain a significant safety concern. Therefore until the innate immune reactivity of adenoviral gene delivery has been mitigated, this vector system will not be used for the treatment of hemophilia.

The second viral vector approach that has shown promise in hemophilia is the retroviral system. Initial studies were performed with replication-defective γ-retroviral vectors, and one human clinical study in hemophilia A also used this vector system. The major problem with these vectors is the requirement for recipient cell replication to facilitate nuclear entry of the vector. Consequently, gene

TABLE 135.10	Features of Adeno-Associated Virus–Mediated Gene Therapy

- AAV is a nonpathogenic virus.
- AAV rarely integrates into the host genome.
- There are no immediate adverse effects after AAV delivery.
- Innate immune reactivity to AAV is minimal.
- Vector readministration can be achieved with different vector serotypes (different capsids).
- Cytotoxic T-cell responses to capsid protein presentation can limit the duration of expression.
- Transgene size is limited to ~5 kb.

AAV, Adeno-associated virus.

transfer with these vectors is limited to tissues in which a significant proportion of cells are cycling. In contrast, lentiviral vectors are equally capable of transducing both postmitotic and replicating cells. For this reason, most of the more recent studies of retroviral hemophilia gene transfer have used lentiviral vector protocols in which the vector construct is usually derived from elements of the human immunodeficiency virus. The other major difference between lentiviral gene delivery and gene transfer with other viral vectors is that lentiviruses integrate their genome into the recipient cell genome as a natural part of their life cycle. Although viral vectors do not possess the structural components that enable further rounds of viral replication, there is a risk of insertional mutagenesis, which can trigger activation of adjacent oncogenes or inactivation of tumor suppressor loci. Studies performed in the past 5 years indicate that lentiviral integrations are not random but tend to cluster in transcribed regions of the genome and more often occur within introns and coding regions of genes rather than in the upstream regulatory regions where γ-retroviruses insert.

Currently, the lead candidate for hemophilia gene transfer is AAV (Table 135.10). This is a small nonpathogenic human parvovirus with a small, single-stranded DNA genome of approximately 4.8 kb. Infection in humans, which for some serotypes of the virus is frequent, is not associated with any clinical disease. The various serotypes of AAV have distinct tissue tropisms, and thus by using the capsid sequence for a particular serotype, gene therapists can target specific tissues for transgene expression. As one example, AAV-8 has excellent hepatotropic properties and has been successfully used for liver transgene delivery and expression. Upon entry into recipient cells, AAV is maintained within the nucleus in the form of stable extrachromosomal concatemers, and only a small proportion of the virus integrates into the recipient genome at sites of natural chromosomal breaks. Wild-type AAV preferentially integrates into a site on chromosome 19, but the replication-defective AAV vectors appear to insert into sites of natural chromosomal breakages. One significant limitation to AAV vectors is their small packaging capacity. Transgenes larger than 5 kb limit the capacity for viral particle assembly, and although this is not a problem for FIX (cDNA ≈1.4 kb), even the B domain deleted forms of FVIII (cDNA of ≈4.7 kb) are not easily accommodated by this vector type.

Clinical Trials of Hemophilia Gene Therapy

Approximately 100 patients with hemophilia have undergone clinical evaluation of gene transfer strategies.[34] An initial trial of ex vivo gene transfer for FIX was performed on two subjects in China in the 1990s. A FIX γ-retroviral vector was used to transduce autologous skin-derived fibroblasts before reimplantation. No significant increases in FIX levels were observed. Since then, one patient has been treated with an intravenous FVIII adenoviral vector; a plasmid vector was used as a second ex vivo approach in which autologous fibroblasts were implanted into the omentum, and a small cohort of patients with hemophilia was treated with intravenous FVIII γ-retrovirus. Aside from the transient thrombocytopenia associated with adenoviral

TABLE 135.11	Challenges to Successful Hemophilia Gene Therapy

1. Efficient transgene delivery
2. Persistent therapeutic transgene expression
3. Host immunologic responses
   a. To the transgene product: inhibitors
   b. To the vector
      - Antivector antibodies
      - Antivector cytotoxic T-cell response

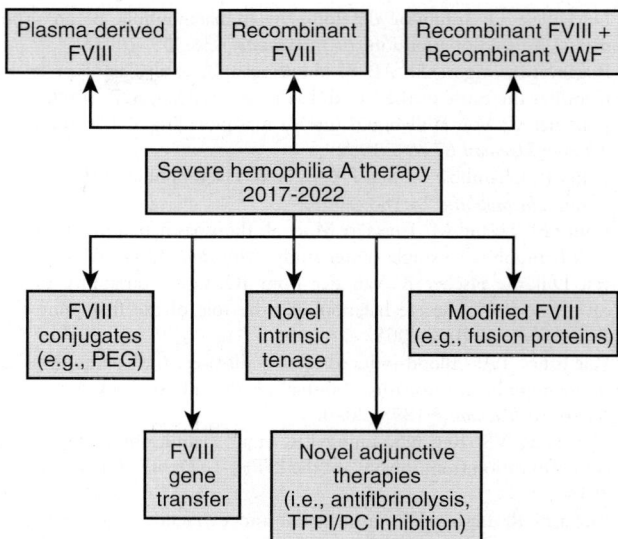

Fig. 135.13 THE FUTURE OF HEMOPHILIA A TREATMENT. This figure speculates on the therapeutic options that may well face clinicians treating patients with hemophilia A within the next 5 to 10 years. *FVIII,* Factor VIII; *PC,* Protein C; *PEG,* polyethylene glycol; *TFPI,* tissue factor pathway inhibitor; *VWF,* von Willebrand factor.

vector infusion, there were no adverse events, but none of those approaches increased FVIII or FIX levels beyond a few days, and even then, levels were in the 1% to 4% range.

In contrast, the AAV trials of gene transfer have shown evidence of therapeutic efficacy. There have now been three completed AAV FIX trials, the first into skeletal muscle and the latter two into liver. Both of the liver-directed trials, the first using hepatic artery delivery of AAV-2 and the second systemic intravenous delivery of AAV-8, have resulted in longer term expression of FIX at therapeutically relevant levels (between 2% and 10%) in some patients. Indeed, in the most recent AAV-8 liver trial, therapeutic FIX levels have now persisted beyond 3 years.[35] There are currently six ongoing FIX gene therapy trials, all using AAV vectors and in two instances using a gain-of-function FIX transgene encoding the FIX Padua variant that has approximately sevenfold higher specific activity compared to wild-type FIX. A recent AAV FVIII gene therapy trial has documented persistent FVIII levels of 20% to 200% in six patients.

Despite these advances, challenges persist (Table 135.11). Most significant has been the recipient immune response against the vector capsid. In some instances, potential gene therapy recipients are excluded from participation because of evidence of prior AAV exposure (neutralizing anti-AAV antibodies), but even in those without documented prior AAV immunity, several patients have developed a delayed cytotoxic T cell–mediated response with transient hepatotoxicity and subsequent reduction of transgene expression. This immune response may be mitigated by transient immunosuppression, and recent evidence from the AAV-8 trial suggests that a brief course of prednisone may be sufficient to minimize the hepatotoxicity in most patients. Of note, none of these patients has had an anti-FIX immune response.

The future for hemophilia gene therapy is promising. After two decades of excellent progress in preclinical studies, there is now realistic hope that clinical success is achievable, at least for FIX gene therapy. Although AAV vector production will need to be scaled up and methods to limit the antivector immune response remain to be optimized, larger cohort studies are now possible. All of the current clinical studies of gene therapy for hemophilia involve FIX gene transfer, and there has been no successful FVIII gene transfer in humans to date. A number of substantive challenges remain to be overcome before FVIII gene transfer is successful. These include the AAV packaging limitation for a FVIII expression cassette that will be minimally 5 kb in size, and the inherent increased immunogenicity of FVIII (see Table 135.9).

FUTURE DIRECTIONS

Already in 2017, hemophilia represents a superb example of the application of molecular science to clinical benefit. Mutation-specific diagnosis is now being incorporated into the initial workup of many patients, and family counseling for kindreds with hemophilia has been dramatically enhanced by advances in the application of molecular genetic technology. In addition, use of the hemophilic mutation as a significant risk factor for inhibitor development is prompting clinicians to evaluate novel strategies to mitigate the likelihood of this treatment complication. As our ability to analyze the genome in far greater detail at greater speed and with reduced costs

increases, we can look forward to an even greater potential for inhibitor risk definition.

The increasing use of recombinant factor concentrates worldwide is a strong indicator of our growing reliance on novel technologies to provide safe and effective therapies for hemophilia. In the next 5 to 10 years, we can look forward to a large number of additional innovations in the area of hemophilia treatment (Fig. 135.13). The first wave of novel products is aimed at extending the circulating half-life of the concentrates with the objective of reducing the frequency of replacement therapy.

A second, more challenging approach to improving hemophilia therapy is to develop components of an improved intrinsic tenase complex. This area of innovation is currently focused on the development of a FVIII mimetic that incorporates the various roles that FVIII plays as a "scaffold" protein in this membrane-bound complex.

Finally, various adjunctive strategies for hemophilia treatment are being pursued. These include inhibition of coagulation inhibitory proteins (tissue factor pathway inhibitor and antithrombin) with antibodies, aptamers, peptides, and inhibitory nucleic acid strategies (siRNA) and the development of novel approaches to inhibit fibrinolysis.

Overall, the future for a more diverse array of hemophilia therapeutics is highly promising. How each of these products will be used in individual patients will provide future hemophilia treaters with some interesting and ultimately gratifying challenges.

REFERENCES

1. Fahs SA, Hille MT, Shi Q, et al: A conditional knockout mouse model reveals endothelial cells as the principal and possibly exclusive source of plasma factor VIII. *Blood* 123:3706, 2014.
2. Everett LA, Cleuren AC, Khoriaty RN, et al: Murine coagulation factor VIII is synthesized in endothelial cells. *Blood* 123:3697, 2014.
3. Do H, Healey JF, Waller EK, et al: Expression of factor VIII by murine liver sinusoidal endothelial cells. *J Biol Chem* 274:19587, 1999.
4. Eckhardt CL, van Velzen AS, Peters M, et al: Factor VIII gene (F8) mutation and risk of inhibitor development in nonsevere hemophilia A. *Blood* 122:1954, 2013.
5. Picketts DJ, Mueller CR, Lillicrap D: Transcriptional control of the factor IX gene: analysis of five cis-acting elements and the deleterious effects of naturally occurring hemophilia B Leyden mutations. *Blood* 84:2992, 1994.

6. DiMichele D: Inhibitor development in haemophilia B: an orphan disease in need of attention. *Br J Haematol* 138:305, 2007.

7. Rogaev EI, Grigorenko AP, Faskhutdinova G, et al: Genotype analysis identifies the cause of the "royal disease. *Science* 326:817, 2009.

8. Mazurier C: Von Willebrand disease masquerading as haemophilia A. *Thromb Haemost* 67:391, 1992.

9. Ljung R, Chambost H, Stain A-M, et al: Haemophilia in the first years of life. *Haemophilia* 14:188, 2008.

10. Dauty M, Sigaud M, Trossaërt M, et al: Iliopsoas hematoma in patients with hemophilia: a single-center study. *Joint Bone Spine* 74:179, 2007.

11. van Dijk K, Fischer K, van der Bom JG, et al: Variability in clinical phenotype of severe haemophilia: the role of the first joint bleed. *Haemophilia* 11:438, 2005.

12. Valentino LA: Blood-induced joint disease: the pathophysiology of hemophilic arthropathy. Journal of thrombosis and haemostasis. *J Thromb Haemost* 8:1895, 2010.

13. Blanchette VS, Key NS, Ljung LR, et al: Definitions in hemophilia: communication from the SSC of the ISTH. *J Thromb Haemost* 12:1935, 2014.

14. Kulkarni R, Lusher JM: Intracranial and extracranial hemorrhages in newborns with hemophilia: a review of the literature. *J Pediatr Hematol Oncol* 21:289, 1999.

15. Shapiro AD, Donfield SM, Lynn HS, et al: Defining the impact of hemophilia: the academic achievement in children with hemophilia study. *Pediatrics* 108:E105, 2001.

16. Ragni MV, Lusher JM, Koerper MA, et al: Safety and immunogenicity of subcutaneous hepatitis A vaccine in children with haemophilia. *Haemophilia* 6:98, 2000.

17. Johnson RE, Lawrence DN, Evatt BL, et al: Acquired immunodeficiency syndrome among patients attending hemophilia treatment centers and mortality experience of hemophiliacs in the United States. *Am J Epidemiol* 121:797, 1985.

18. Brettler DB, Alter HJ, Dienstag JL, et al: Prevalence of hepatitis C virus antibody in a cohort of hemophilia patients. *Blood* 76:254, 1990.

19. Gouw SC, van der Bom JG, Ljung R, et al: Factor VIII products and inhibitor development in severe hemophilia A. *N Engl J Med* 368:231, 2013.

20. Collins PW, Palmer BP, Chalmers EA, et al: Factor VIII brand and the incidence of factor VIII inhibitors in previously untreated UK children with severe hemophilia A, 2000-2011. *Blood* 124:3389, 2014.

21. Calvez T, Chambost H, Claeyssens-Donadel S, et al: Recombinant factor VIII products and inhibitor development in previously untreated boys with severe hemophilia A. *Blood* 124:3398, 2014.

22. Plug I, van der Bom JG, Peters M, et al: Mortality and causes of death in patients with hemophilia, 1992-2001: a prospective cohort study. *J Thromb Haemost* 4:510, 2006.

23. Mannucci PM, Aberg M, Nilsson IM, et al: Mechanism of plasminogen activator and factor FVIII increase after vasoactive drugs. *Br J Haematol* 30:81, 1975.

24. Van Creveld S: Prophylaxis of joint hemorrhages in hemophilia. *Acta Haematol* 45:120, 1971.

25. Manco-Johnson MJ, Abshire TC, Shapiro AD, et al: Prophylaxis versus episodic treatment to prevent joint disease in boys with severe hemophilia. *N Engl J Med* 357:535, 2007.

26. Gouw SC, van der Bom JG, Auerswald G, et al: Recombinant versus plasma-derived factor VIII products and the development of inhibitors in previously untreated patients with severe hemophilia A: the CANAL cohort study. *Blood* 109:4693, 2007.

27. Feldman BM, Pai M, Rivard GE, et al: Tailored prophylaxis in severe hemophilia A: interim results from the first 5 years of the Canadian hemophilia primary prophylaxis study. *J Thromb Haemost* 4:1228, 2006.

28. Liang TJ, Ghany MG: Therapy of hepatitis C — back to the future. *N Engl J Med* 370:2043, 2014.

29. Warrier I, Ewenstein BM, Koerper MA, et al: Factor IX inhibitors and anaphylaxis in hemophilia B. *Haemophilia* 3:131, 1997.

30. Recht M, Pollmann H, Tagliaferri A, et al: A retrospective study to describe the incidence of moderate to severe allergic reactions to factor IX in subjects with haemophilia B. *Haemophilia* 17:494, 2011.

31. Sehgal A, Barros S, Ivanciu L, et al: An RNAi therapeutic targeting antithrombin to rebalance the coagulation system and promote hemostasis in hemophilia. *Nat Med* 21:492, 2015.

32. Chowdary P, Lethagen S, Friedrich U, et al: Safety and pharmacokinetics of anti-TFPI antibody (concizumab) in healthy volunteers and patients with hemophilia: a randomized first human dose trial. *J Thromb Haemost* 13:743, 2015.

33. Muto A, Yoshihashi K, Takeda M, et al: Anti-factor IXa/X bispecific antibody (ACE910): hemostatic potency against ongoing bleeds in a hemophilia A model and the possibility of routine supplementation. *J Thromb Haemost* 12:206, 2014.

34. Hough C, Lillicrap D: Gene therapy for hemophilia: an imperative to succeed. *J Thromb Haemost* 3:1195, 2005.

35. Nathwani AC, Reiss UM, Tuddenham EG, et al: Long-term safety and efficacy of factor IX gene therapy in hemophilia B. *N Engl J Med* 371:1994, 2014.

CHAPTER 136

INHIBITORS IN HEMOPHILIAS

Guglielmo Mariani, Barbara A. Konkle, and Craig M. Kessler

With the availability of plasma-derived and recombinant replacement products safe from transmission of known infectious agents, the development of antibodies neutralizing factor VIII (FVIII) or factor IX (FIX) has become the major complication of hemophilia treatment.

Antibodies to FVIII can be detected (1) in healthy individuals, (2) as expression of an autoimmune disorder, and (3) in patients with FVIII or FIX deficiency (hemophilia A and B). Clinically speaking, only those antibodies that affect the clotting activity, which are therefore termed *inhibitors,* are considered relevant because they render patients refractory to treatment. In hemophilias, inhibitors occur after factor replacement therapy with FVIII or FIX concentrates. Patients with a severe deficiency (FVIII or FIX less than 1% of normal) are particularly at risk.

Inhibitor formation in hemophilia was first reported in 1941.[1] A 44-year-old man with classic hemophilia had been treated numerous times with blood products, and his hemostasis subsequently became refractory to transfusions. The authors realized that transfusion may have caused this heretofore-unknown complication and suggested that coagulation times should be checked after administration of blood products to monitor for the phenomenon. This report was soon followed by numerous cases[2–5] reporting the development of a substance that counteracted infused blood product components. The nature of the inhibitor was shown to be an immunoglobulin (Ig) G antibody mainly of the IgG4 subclass.[6]

Alloantibody inhibitors arise much more frequently in patients with severe hemophilia A (15%–20% with a range of 8%–52%)[7] than in those with severe hemophilia B (≈3%–7%). Their occurrence is associated with higher morbidity and mortality if modern therapies are not available, increased cost of care, and more complicated treatment regimens.

HEMOPHILIA A

Epidemiology

It is curious that hemophilia A and B, which share an almost identical clinical phenotype, would have such a disparate incidence of alloantibody inhibitor development. The explanation may reside in the type of genetic mutation responsible for each disease. In hemophilia A, the severe phenotype is most often caused by a null mutation, which is less common in hemophilia B. Null mutations result in complete absence of a translated protein product and are more likely to predispose to inhibitor formation. Also, FIX shares significant homology with the other vitamin K–dependent clotting factors, possibly protecting against inhibitor development.[8] Finally, it is hypothesized that because FIX is smaller and more abundant than FVIII, some FIX may cross the placenta, thereby inducing tolerance in the developing fetus.[8]

Among patients with severe hemophilia A, approximately 30% will develop an alloantibody inhibitor (compared with 3% of those with moderate hemophilia and 0.3% with mild hemophilia).[9] Inhibitor formation occurs early after initiation of replacement therapy. Data from prospective clinical trials of recombinant FVIII reveal that inhibitor development typically arises within a median of 8 to 10 "exposure-days" (treatment-days), but a wide range is not uncommon.[10] The risk for inhibitor development decreases inversely with increasing number of exposure days and is uncommon (≈2/1000 patient-years) after 150 exposure-days.

There appears to be a bimodal distribution of inhibitor occurrence in severe hemophilia. The incidence peaks in early childhood in those younger than 5 years of age (64.3/1000 treatment-years), falls substantially between the ages of 10 and 49 years of age (5.3/1000 treatment-years), and rises again in older age (10.5/1000 treatment-years).[11] The latter finding raises the possibility that there is a breakdown of tolerance with aging.[11] Another epidemiologic study conducted by the same organization and covering a period of 22 years, showed that the rate of inhibitor development may vary over time, although the reasons appear unclear.[12] At any rate, there is no doubt that inhibitor formation has a negative impact on overall mortality in severe hemophilia A patients, essentially cancelling out the improved life expectancy realized in patients with severe hemophilia A population over the last 30 years.[13]

Genetic Factors

One of the most significant risk factors associated with the development of inhibitory alloantibodies in hemophilia A is the presence of a positive family history. The increased concordance rate of inhibitor occurrence in brother and twin pairs[14,15] provided the initial indication that genetic factors play a role in inhibitor development. Having a first-degree relative with an inhibitor raises the risk for inhibitor development threefold, resulting in an approximately 50% chance of inhibitor development compared with a control cohort in which there is a 15% risk.[14,15]

Patient ethnicity first emerged as a possible risk factor for inhibitor development in retrospective analyses of the prevalence of inhibitors in various racial cohorts included within large pooled populations of hemophiliacs.[15–18] African Americans (AA) and Latinos were observed to have a twofold higher rate of inhibitor formation compared with whites. For instance, in the Malmö International Brother Study (MIBS), inhibitors were noted in 27.4% of whites and in 55.6% of AA.[15] This same trend was subsequently appreciated in prospective analyses of inhibitor development in the initial recombinant FVIII concentrate safety and efficacy trials.[19]

One potential and provocative explanation for the increased propensity of AA with hemophilia to produce FVIII relative to immunoreactivity is a mismatch between the host endogenous wild-type FVIII haplotype polymorphisms found only in AA (H3, H4, and H5) and their exposure to the exogenous FVIII polymorphisms found in the commercially available brands of recombinant FVIII concentrates (either H1 or H2) used for replacement therapy. The risk for alloantibody inhibitor development is significantly higher among AA with haplotypes H3 or H4 than it is in those with the H1 or H2 haplotype (odds ratio [OR] of 3.4). These observations await confirmation in larger studies.[20]

Emerging data consistently indicate that certain FVIII mutations producing phenotypically severe hemophilia A[7,8] are strong predictors of inhibitor development.[21–23] Three general categories of mutations in FVIII have been considered for patients at "high risk" for inhibitor formation: (a) inversions of intron 22 (intrachromosomal recombinations), (b) large deletions affecting more than one domain, and (c) nonsense mutations involving the light chain (the risk for inhibitor formation is twofold higher with light chain mutations than with heavy chain mutations).[7,21] All of these mutations either eliminate FVIII protein altogether or alter the molecular conformation of the FVIII protein in such a way that innate immune tolerance cannot be achieved during fetal development. Consequently, the immune system recognizes exogenously administered native FVIII protein as "foreign."[22] The "low-risk" FVIII mutations consist of small gene deletions/insertions, missense mutations, and splice site mutations. It is postulated that some "nonfunctional" FVIII protein is produced with these FVIII gene mutations, which may be sufficient to induce partial central immune tolerance.[21]

Even with genetic information, it is not possible to predict which patients are at highest risk for development of alloantibody inhibitors. Inhibitors in the high-risk category occur 7- to 10-fold more frequently for large deletions and nonsense mutations (pooled OR, 3.6; 95% confidence interval [CI], 2.3–5.7 and 1.4 CI, 1.1–1.8, respectively)[21] ($\approx$35%)[22] compared with those with intron 22 inversions. Furthermore, inhibitors occur less frequency with small FVIII gene deletions/insertions ($\approx$7%)[22] or missense mutations ($\approx$4%) (pooled OR, 0.5 [95% CI, 0.4–0.6] and 0.3; 95% CI, 0.2–0.4, respectively).[21,22] Intron 22 inversions are associated with a lower inhibitor frequency than would be anticipated for a genotype that produces no circulating FVIII protein. However, recent data suggest that some of these hemophiliacs may possess intrahepatocyte-endogenous FVIII protein fragments, which can induce partial immune tolerance[21]; most recently, experimental data confirmed the low-risk categorization of intron 22 inversion by demonstrating that patients bearing this change produce intracellular peptides that may act as tolerogens.[24,25] There does not appear to be any relationship between the type of FVIII gene mutation and the relative risks for developing high-titer versus low-titer alloantibody FVIII inhibitors.[21]

Environmental Factors

Despite the strong FVIII-related genetic influences that underlie inhibitor formation, clinical observations indicate that various environmental or epigenetic pressures contribute to the development of alloantibody inhibitors. For example, within the MIBS cohort, there are discordant monozygotic twins (i.e., identical twin brothers with the same mutations) in which only one brother developed an inhibitor.[14] In addition, among families with high-risk gene mutations, only about 30% of siblings with severe hemophilia A because of the intron 22 inversion develop inhibitors. Even with multidomain deletions, the highest estimated inhibitor risk only approaches 75%,[15] implying that other patients with the same mutation are somehow protected against inhibitor formation.

A concerted effort has been made to explore the importance of other genetic determinants in hemophilia A patients that may contribute to alloantibody inhibitor development. Of the immune response genes, the presence of a microsatellite polymorphism in the promoter region (134 base pair variant) of the interleukin (IL)-10 gene, which may lead to upregulated B-lymphocyte activity, has been associated with a 73% incidence of inhibitor formation (OR, 4.4). A G308A polymorphism in the promoter region of the tumor necrosis factor α gene (A/A genotype) has been associated with 72.7% inhibitors and an OR of 4.0. On the other hand, there is no robust evidence that polymorphisms of major histocompatibility complex (MHC) class II alleles or of other inflammatory cytokine genes contribute to alloantibody inhibitor development.[22–26] All in all, the associations of distinct human leucocyte antigen haplotypes and of polymorphisms of immunoregulatory genes with the risk of patients developing FVIII inhibitors seems to be modest.

Among possible environmental risk factors, age at first treatment has been implicated as a major independent contributor for inhibitor development: initial observations suggested that the earlier the first exposure to FVIII-containing products occurred, the greater the risk was for alloantibody inhibitor formation.[26–29] Children treated before 6 months of age have a cumulative inhibitor incidence of 41% compared with a 12% incidence if initial exogenous FVIII exposure is delayed until after the first year of life. Results of a subsequent

case-control study suggested that early age of first exposure to FVIII treatment reflected the severity of the hemophilia conveyed by the particular FVIII gene mutation. Thus more intense FVIII replacement and high-risk FVIII gene polymorphisms were more strongly associated with inhibitor formation than was age. In fact, there appeared to be a protective effect against the formation of inhibitors when children were started on primary FVIII prophylaxis regimens early in life.[30] The United Kingdom Haemophilia Centre Doctors' Organisation (UKHCDO) study reported that peak inhibitor formation occurs in children younger than 5 years of age.[11]

The method of FVIII infusion (continuous infusion versus bolus administration) and the clinical scenarios for FVIII replacement have also been examined for their contribution to inhibitor formation. Although administration of FVIII by continuous infusion has the advantage of requiring less factor replacement over time and avoids the peaks and troughs seen with bolus administration,[31] intense replacement of FVIII by continuous infusion was more likely to induce inhibitor development than bolus injections (57% versus 14%) in patients who were otherwise considered to be at low risk (i.e., mild hemophiliacs).[32,33] These results were gleaned from the retrospective examination of the medical records of 54 mild hemophiliacs, of whom only seven had received FVIII by CI; a prospective study in a larger population remains to be conducted to confirm this finding. On the other hand, intensive FVIII replacement in the context of injury, surgery, or inflammation appears conducive to inhibitor formation. In the retrospective CANAL study (concerted action on neutralizing antibodies in severe hemophilia A) of previously untreated patients (PUPs), 65% of those whose first exposure to FVIII therapy was associated with surgery developed an allogeneic FVIII antibody inhibitor (relative risk, 3.7), compared with a 23% inhibitor incidence when first exposure was not related to a "danger signal" indication.[33]

As concerns surgery, a very common procedure of minor surgery, circumcision, was analyzed with respect to the occurrence of inhibitors: 3 of 25 patients among those circumcised developed an inhibitor versus 4 of 36 of age-, therapy- and intron 22 inversion-matched patients not circumcised; all inhibitors were high-titer and median ED was 16 days for both groups.[34] This observational study would suggest that minor surgery does not increase the risk associated with replacement therapy or intron 22 inversion.

Perhaps the most controversial "environmental" risk factor for alloantibody inhibitor development involves the type of FVIII concentrate replacement used by the patient (low- to intermediate-purity plasma-derived FVIII versus high-purity plasma-derived FVIII versus recombinant FVIII concentrates). After more than 20 years the question of whether the use of recombinant FVIII concentrates (highest purity) leads to a higher inhibitor incidence than the lower purity concentrates remains largely unresolved.[35,36] This debate originated with the prospective trials of first-generation recombinant FVIII concentrates in PUPs, which mandated frequent monitoring for inhibitor formation (at least every 3 months).[37,38] In the Kogenate trial, the total incidence of any inhibitor formation in patients with severe hemophilia A was 29.2% within a median of 9 exposure days.[39] A similar inhibitor incidence rate of 31.5% was found in a prospective trial of Recombinate.[40] Thus when compared with the inhibitor incidence rate of approximately 10% reported in older retrospective studies, which used low-purity plasma-derived FVIII concentrates and screened less frequently for inhibitors,[41] recombinant FVIII seemed to be significantly more immunogenic. Prospective monitoring of patients receiving high-purity plasma-derived FVIII concentrates revealed a similar inhibitor rate as seen in those given recombinant concentrates.[42]

A number of variables may have contributed to these observations, thus reducing their clinical relevance. The recombinant FVIII trials in PUPs were the first large prospective clinical trials of hemophilia treatment, so their comparison with results of anecdotal or retrospective case reports and case series is inappropriate.[33–39] These trials were also the first to use routine and frequent prospective monitoring for inhibitor development. In prior studies, testing for inhibitors was done only when deemed clinically important. Continued analysis of the results of the recombinant FVIII trials showed that almost half (11/23) of the inhibitors in the Kogenate trial were transient in nature, decreasing the prevalence of inhibitors upon extended observation.[39] A similar pattern was observed in the Recombinate trial; alloantibodies disappeared in 14 of 22 study subjects who developed an inhibitor despite continued treatment, eventually reducing the prevalence rate to 11.1%.[40] The older studies likely missed these ephemeral inhibitors. A Dutch study suggested that although transient inhibitors may develop earlier during treatment with ultrapure plasma-derived and recombinant FVIII concentrates compared with lower-purity plasma products, the overall risk for inhibitor development is similar.[43] The debate continues with conflicting results in both PUPs and previously treated patients (PTPs).[44-46] A recent UKHCDO case-control study examined inhibitor occurrence over 25 years of observation and identified "high-intensity treatments" rather than the type of FVIII product as the main risk factor for inhibitor development.[47] Similarly an analysis of pooled data from over 2900 hemophiliacs indicated that the duration of study observation and follow-up and testing frequency for inhibitor presence, but not the source or purity of concentrate, explained most of the differences in inhibitor development seen in earlier studies.[42]

Proposed causes of variable immunogenicity among FVIII products have included neoantigen formation during their manufacture and their content of von Willebrand factor (vWF) protein, which is present in low- and intermediate-purity plasma-derived products but absent in recombinant FVIII concentrates.[28] It has been suggested that vWF may interfere with FVIII-dendritic cell interactions, alter FVIII molecular conformation, or mask T- or B-lymphocyte epitopes. The former scenario has been illustrated by the fact that some, previously low immunogenic plasma-derived FVIII concentrates were rendered more immunogenic after extra viral-attenuation steps were added to their manufacturing processes.[48-50] However, when recombinant FVIII products were administered to patients previously and extensively treated with lower-purity FVIII products, the rate of inhibitor formation was low, consistent with a low immunogenicity in this setting (relative overall risk for inhibitors, 0.8; for high-titer inhibitors 0.9; for plasma-derived products versus recombinant FVIII products 1.0; for switching FVIII products, 1.1).[45,51] A large prospective, randomized study comparing the immunogenicity of vWF-containing products with recombinant FVIII concentrates in PUPs and minimally treated patients is ongoing. Nonetheless, most experts believe that the risk for inhibitor formation with the various FVIII concentrates is similar.

Recently, clinical prediction models for inhibitor development in the pediatric and adolescence ages[52] evidenced the fact that treaters consider family history of inhibitors (and related major FVIII defects) and early intensive treatment as elements associated with a high risk, whereas early onset of prophylaxis and avoidance of elective surgery were considered as factors that are associated with a low risk of inhibitor development. Interestingly, the type of concentrate was not included in the prediction model. Though the results stemmed from the surveys are interesting, their probabilistic nature and the fact that a number of minor risk factors were not considered suggests that interventional studies including very large numbers of patients are needed to validate these exercises, because combinations of risk factors are many.

A recent prospective study on the influence of treatment-related determinants demonstrated that intensive on-demand treatment for hemorrhage or surgery increased the risk, whereas prophylaxis decreased the risk especially in patients with low-risk mutations.[53] A similarly focused prospective study on inhibitor development[54] showed that risky gene mutations, first treatment before the age of 3 months, and the dose of FVIII had a significant impact whereas the type of concentrate did not.

Recently, a prospective study focused to the type or brand of concentrate, either in PUPs or PTPs, demonstrated that different concentrates failed to elicit inhibitors with different cumulative incidence or incidence rates.[55] In contrast with this study, Peyvandi et al, in PUPs, elegantly demonstrated that exclusive use of recombinant FVIII during the period of maximum risk of inhibitor development increases the incidence of inhibitors in comparison with plasma-derived preparations (37.2% vs. 23.2%; hazard ratio [HR], 1.87). The same effect was noted when the analysis was restricted to the high-titer alloantibodies.[56] If the contrasting outcomes of the previous trials on the topic are considered, it appears difficult to foresee the influence of this study on the clinical practice.

A longstanding issue has been that concerning the switch from one concentrate brand to another. This issue has been clarified by a study focused on the full-length and the B-domain recombinant preparations that showed that switching was not associated with an increased inhibitor development.[57]

Mild Hemophilia

In patients with mild or moderate hemophilia A, inhibitors appear to develop at a cumulative incidence of 3% to 13%, commonly after periods of intense FVIII replacement associated with surgery or inflammatory states.[58] A recent, large international cohort study on 1112 patients (median age 38, interquartile range [IQR] 18–56 years) evidenced a cumulative incidence of 5.3% after a median exposure of 28 days, that increased to 6.7% at 50 and to 13.3% at 100 days. Most of the tested mutations (15/19) were located in the light chain, evenly distributed among the A3, C1 and C2 domains.[59] A particularly risky mutation (T295A) was described in 3 of 16 patients (17%).[60] This study suggests that the capacity for immune tolerance in these infrequently treated individuals may be compromised with aging and that immune challenge with FVIII replacement should be avoided whenever possible by using desmopressin (DDAVP) to enhance endogenous FVIII activity levels. Continuous lifelong vigilance for the inhibitor occurrence is warranted, particularly after occasional, intensive FVIII exposure.

Venous Access

A disturbingly high incidence of infections may occur in FVIII inhibitor patients with central venous access catheter devices (CVADs), particularly those with external devices set for immune tolerance induction (ITI) (124 episodes in 41 patients).[61] This fact may be related to frequent, unprofessional catheter accessing related to the administration of replacement therapy. CVAD-associated infection did not seem to affect the ability to achieve tolerance.[61] The presence of CVADs per se does not appear to be associated with increased inhibitor formation.[47]

Other Factors

Other miscellaneous proposed environmental influences on inhibitor development, such as breastfeeding and receiving replacement therapy during a vaccination course, remain to be confirmed as significant risk factors.

Pathobiology of Factor VIII Alloantibody Inhibitor Formation

Circulating antigens provided by the exogenous FVIII undergo initial endocytosis and subsequent proteolysis by antigen-presenting cells, and digested peptides bind to MHC II molecules for presentation to T-cell receptor on $CD4^+$ T lymphocytes.[62] Co-stimulation signals subsequently mediate differentiation of T-lymphocytes into either T_H1 or T_H2 subsets. T_H2 cells secrete IL-4, IL-5, and IL-10 cytokines, which promote the synthesis of noncomplement-binding immunoglobulins, predominantly IgG4, by B lymphocytes.[62] IgG4-mediated humoral responses display the following features: (1) are unable to form large immune-complexes, (2) have low potential of inducing immune inflammation, (3) are expressed in conditions of chronic antigen exposure and (4) maintain a "normal" half-life. These features accord with the clinical observations of uncomplicated anamneses in hemophiliacs and account for an inhibitor half-life in the range of 25–30 days.[63] Interestingly, IgG4 subclass antibodies (either inhibiting or noninhibiting) are absent in hemophiliacs without inhibitors and in healthy subjects.[64] Most recently it has been shown that the presence of anti-FVIII IgG1 subclass may herald the appearance of

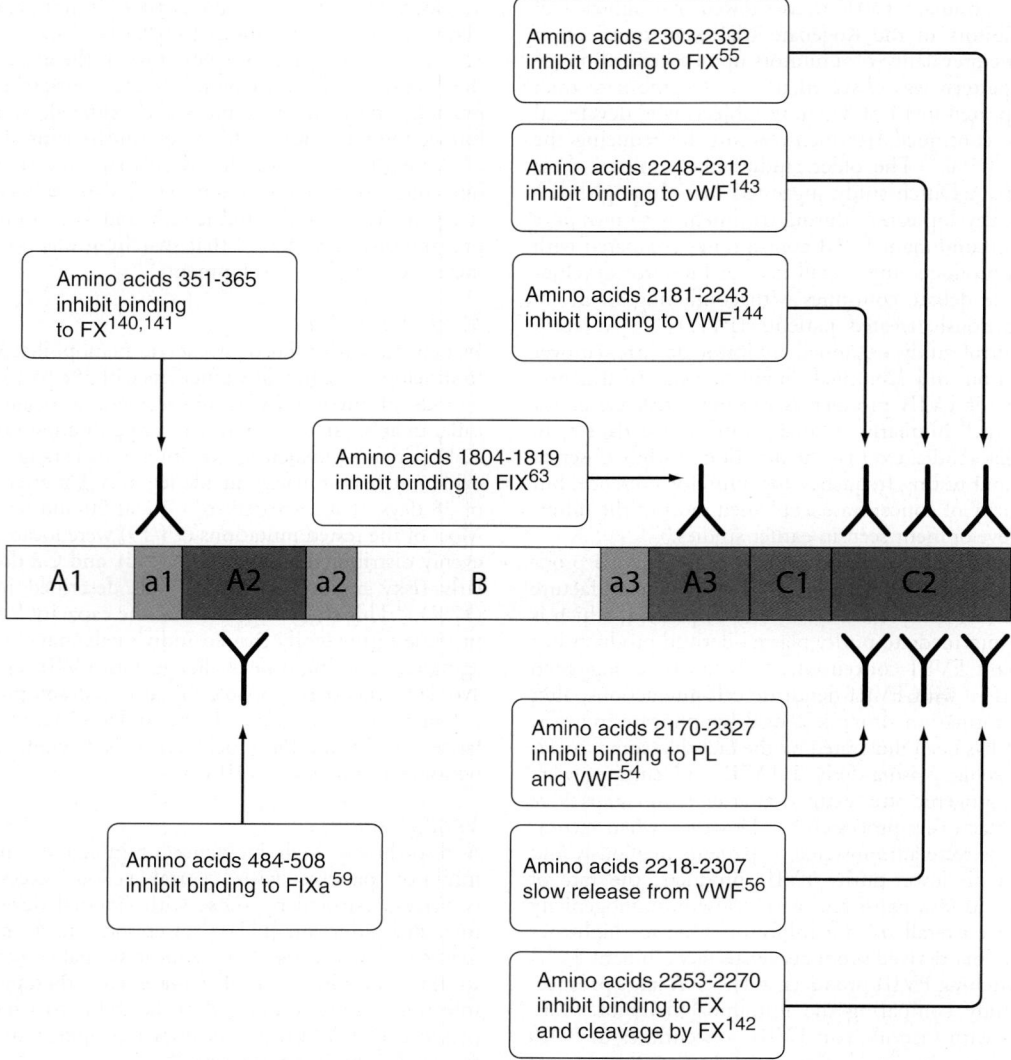

Fig. 136.1 FACTOR VIII DOMAINS AND BINDING SITE BY AMINO ACID LOCATION AND EFFECT ON FACTOR VIII. Intensity of color reflects the frequency of inhibitors to the epitope.[170–174] *FIX*, Factor IX; *FIXa*, activated factor IX; *FX*, factor X; *PL*, phospholipid; *vWF*, von Willebrand factor.

an inhibitor.[65] This polyclonal antibody response can result in the inhibition of FVIII function via diverse clotting impairing mechanisms because the epitopes may be different.[66] It is important to note that inhibiting antibodies to FVIII have an up to 100-fold higher affinity for FVIII than those in patients without inhibitors or healthy individuals.[67]

The weak association between MHC II phenotypes and FVIII inhibitor formation is dependent on the availability of "risk" MHC class I/II alleles.[68,69] T-lymphocyte involvement in inhibitor formation is manifested by the isotype switching and the somatic hypermutation of the B cells.[70] There are several FVIII epitopes against which CD4+ T cells react strongly.[70] In addition, non–FVIII-associated gene polymorphisms can exert a protective influence on inhibitor development—for example, the C→T single-nucleotide polymorphism (SNP) at position −318 in the promoter region of the gene encoding for cytotoxic T-lymphocyte–associated protein-4 (CTLA4).[71] This polymorphism "downregulates" the effects of the co-stimulatory signal of the B7-CD28 complex, which mediates T-cell immune responsiveness to infused FVIII. The MIBS study group reported an OR of 0.3 for inhibitor formation among a cohort of severe hemophiliacs with the T allele SNP despite their risk for inhibitors related to a FVIII intron 22 gene inversions.[71] MIBS also identified polymorphisms in the IL-10 cytokine gene that are associated with inhibitor formation in severe hemophiliacs.[72] The same group

investigated SNPs in more than 1000 genes in a cohort of 833 HA patients for the association with inhibitor occurrence, and identified 53 polymorphisms significantly associated with the risk of developing inhibitors.[73] This study highlighted the complexity of the mechanisms that are involved in the antibody formation against FVIII and FIX. In support of the polygenic nature of inhibitor formation, evidence is emerging that the regulatory T cell (Treg) lymphocyte system downmodulates the immune reaction to FVIII and plays a role in ITI induction.[74]

FVIII exists as a heterodimer, with a heavy chain containing the A1, A2, and B domains connected to a light chain containing the A3, C1, and C2 domains (Fig. 136.1). Short intervening acidic regions (a1, a2, and a3) aid in FVIII binding to factor X and serve as important sites for FVIII proteolysis by thrombin and factor Xa (FXa).[75] By serving as a cofactor for FIX in the intrinsic tenase complex, FVIIIa promotes the conversion of FX to FXa, which together with factor Va forms the prothrombinase complex on the activated platelet surface. This complex then converts prothrombin to thrombin, which in turn amplifies the coagulation system (see Chapter 122).[76,77]

Normally, when FVIII is secreted, it is noncovalently bound to vWF via the light chain, particularly through interactions with the A3 and C2 domain.[77] Upon thrombin activation, FVIIIa dissociates from vWF and via the C2 domain, which is no longer linked to vWF, binds to platelet membrane-associated phosphatidylserine.[78] Neutralizing alloantibody inhibitors can interrupt this complex process (see Fig. 136.1) by (a) preventing FVIII interaction with vWF, thereby significantly decreasing its circulating half-life, (b) hampering the release of FVIIIa from vWF following thrombin activation, (c) increasing the time available for FVIII inactivation, and/or (d) preventing C2 domains from binding to the phospholipid layer.[79–83]

Other FVIII alloantibody inhibitors interact with the A2 domain, predominantly at the Arg4844–Ile5085 epitope and interrupt FVIIIa–FIXa interactions, thereby impairing intrinsic tenase activity.[84] Regions outside the A2 and C2 domains are minor epitopes for FVIII inhibitors; however, those binding to the A3 domain also blocks the FVIIIa–FIXa interaction.[84] In most hemophilia A patients, alloantibodies recognize multiple epitopes in both the A2 and C2 domains, in contrast to autoantibodies to FVIII, which target either the C2 or A2 domain but not both.[84] Although antibodies that target B domain epitopes have been reported, these do not exert any neutralizing activity.

Another mechanism of FVIII inhibition involves alloantibodies that catalyze the proteolysis of FVIII.[85,86] FVIII-hydrolyzing IgGs are detected in more than 50% of alloantibody inhibitor patients and functionally resemble serine proteases. In contrast to the A2, A3, and C2 epitope specificity of the classic alloantibody inhibitors in severe hemophilia A, IgG-mediated hydrolysis occurs evenly throughout the FVIII molecule with final loss of FVIII activity.[87]

Clinical Manifestations

The frequency and severity of bleeding complications do not necessarily increase when an alloantibody to FVIII develops in a patient with severe hemophilia A. Similarly, no predictive relationship exists between the Bethesda unit (BU) titer and the severity of bleeding. Any person with hemophilia, regardless of severity, who is undergoing treatment and fails to respond to the FVIII dose that had previously been effective should be promptly evaluated for the development of an inhibitor.[88] Routine laboratory testing for the presence of an inhibitor is recommended before any major surgical procedure. A truncated pharmacokinetic study may be useful for inhibitor screening because even low-titer (<5 BU) inhibitors may be detected when less than 66% of the calculated incremental rise in FVIII activity is achieved within 30 minutes of administration of exogenous FVIII (i.e., decreased recovery). In general, patients with hemophilia A who have FVIII inhibitors will experience more frequent hemarthroses, more severe and progressive arthropathy, and an overall reduced quality of life compared with noninhibitor patients.[89,90] Those with inhibitors will also have more hospital visits and absences from school or work, and will more likely require assistive devices, such as wheelchairs or crutches.[90] In the past, development of an inhibitor increased the mortality risk, but with current therapies the mortality rate is falling. However, the mortality rate for patients with inhibitors still exceeds that for those without.[91]

If patients with mild to moderately severe hemophilia A develop an alloantibody FVIII inhibitor, it usually occurs after a period of intense factor replacement. Genetic factors likely play a role as well. The clinical manifestations become the same as in severe hemophiliacs, including reduced recovery of FVIII activity after FVIII infusion. Thus a patient with a mild disease usually converts to a severe phenotype following the inhibitor development and may present with spontaneous bleeding.

Laboratory Diagnosis

In 1975, the Bethesda assay (BA) was devised as a simple and reproducible method for determining antibody titer and quantifying the extent of its inhibitory/neutralizing capacity. The assay is based on the ability of patient plasma to inactivate FVIII in normal plasma. The result is expressed in BUs.[92] Patient plasma is serially diluted with normal plasma, incubated for 2 hours at 37°C and residual FVIII

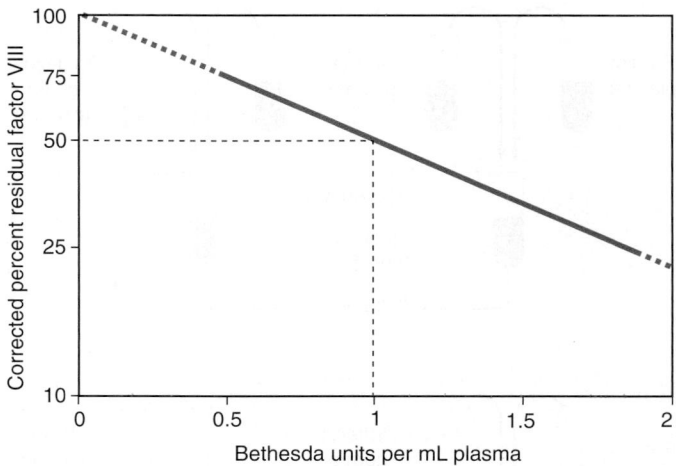

Fig. 136.2 BETHESDA ASSAY FOR FACTOR VIII INHIBITOR QUANTITATION. Relationship between corrected residual factor VIII activity and Bethesda titer is shown. If the result is less than 25%, serial dilutions of the patient's plasma are tested until the result is between 25% and 75%. The result is multiplied by the dilution to assign the Bethesda titer. One Bethesda unit (BU) is defined by a corrected residual factor VIII of 50% in the assay *(dotted line)*. *(From Konkle BA: Clinical approach to the bleeding patient. In Colman RW, Marder VJ, Clowes AW, et al, editors: Hemostasis and thrombosis, Philadelphia, 2006, Lippincott, Williams & Wilkins, p 1147.)*

activity is measured using a one-stage assay. One BU correlates with patient FVIII activity reduced by 50%. A standard curve is drawn, and the patient's plasma is diluted until FVIII activity is between 25% and 75%, that is, the linear portion of the standard curve. The inhibitor units are read from the graph and multiplied by the reciprocal of the dilution factor to determine the BU in undiluted plasma (Fig. 136.2).

To improve the specificity and reliability of the BA, two groups developed the Nijmegen modification of the BA.[93] The BA, because of a decreased FVIII activity caused by a pH increase and/or protein concentration decrease, may yield false-positive results, labelled as low-titer inhibitors. The Nijmegen modification made two important changes to the BA: plasma mixtures were buffered with imidazole to a pH of 7.4, and plasma depleted of FVIII was used to yield similar protein concentrations (Fig. 136.3). These modifications are now recommended for diagnosis of inhibitors.[94] A new standardized assay was recently proposed to reduce the cost that is mostly related to the use of FVIII-deficient plasma; instead of the latter, a 4% albumin solution was proposed. Comparison of results on 59 inhibitor samples evidenced a good agreement with the Nijmegen method together with a good reproducibility.[95]

Care is needed to ensure that isolated prolongations of the activated partial thromboplastin time (aPTT) are not misdiagnosed as lupus anticoagulants or vice versa. The key maneuver to distinguish between the two possibilities is based on the incubation time: whereas the aPTT results performed immediately and after 2 hours of incubation are similar in the presence of a lupus anticoagulant, inhibitors exert their effect only after incubation. This is a critical issue because patients with lupus anticoagulants do not usually bleed, whereas the bleeding related to a FVIII inhibitor may be severe.

Based on the results of the inhibitor assay, a value less than 5 BU is considered a low-titer inhibitor. If the inhibitor titer fails to rise despite repeated challenges with clotting factor protein, the patient is termed a *low responder*. In contrast, a patient with an inhibitor titer greater than 5 BU is considered a *high responder*.[94]

Overall, 75% to 80% of the immune responses are causative of the classic features of refractory hemophilia, that is, a bleeding phenotype that can hardly be treated with FVIII/FIX concentrates: this corresponds to a titer of about 5–10 BU of inhibitor or greater. Of the remaining, some may be transient, resolving within 6 months.

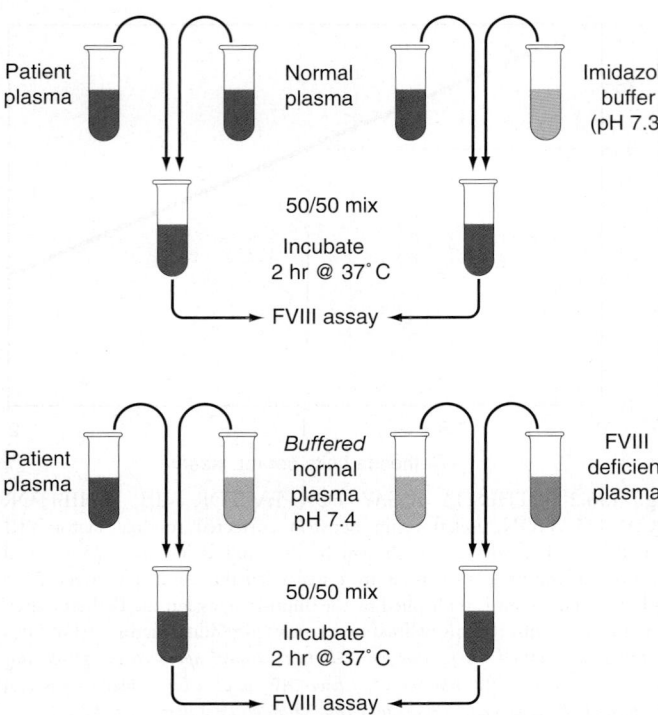

Fig. 136.3 METHODOLOGIC DIFFERENCES BETWEEN THE CLASSIC BETHESDA ASSAY[94] AND THE MODIFIED NIJMEGEN ASSAY.[96] *(From Giles AR, Verbruggen B, Rivard GE, et al: A detailed comparison of the performance of the standard versus the Nijmegen modification of the Bethesda assay in detecting factor VIII:C inhibitors in the haemophilia A population of Canada. Association of Hemophilia Centre Directors of Canada. Factor VIII/IX Subcommittee of Scientific and Standardization Committee of International Society on Thrombosis and Haemostasis,* Thromb Haemost *9:872, 1998.)*

External quality control assessments examining the reliability of clotting-based inhibitor testing (Bethesda and Nijmegen) have noted considerable interlaboratory variability that could influence patient management and may contribute to differences in the incidence of FVIII inhibitors reported in various clinical settings.[96]

Enzyme-linked immunofluorescence assay (ELISA)[97] or fluorescence immunoassay-based[98] methods may complement the clotting assays because these techniques also detect nonneutralizing antibodies against FVIII, but there may be discordance between the results of ELISA-based inhibitor assays, and the functional clot-based assays. Pharmacokinetic studies may be useful in patients with antibodies that are not overtly neutralizing in the BA because these antibodies may influence the circulating half-life of infused FVIII.[99]

Monitoring for inhibitor development in PUPs is of paramount importance, especially when starting treatment or prophylaxis regimens because inhibitor development occurs early in the course of treatment. Guidelines recommend screening PUPs every 5th exposure day up to the 20th exposure day, and then every 3 months until the 150th exposure day.[100] Repeat testing should be performed before any invasive procedure or elective operation.[100] Considering the fact that inhibitors are antibody mixtures mainly made up of IgG4 subclass antibodies, an unstimulated inhibitor titer will decrease by 50% every 25–30 days.

Treatment

Patients with hemophilia should receive comprehensive and routine therapy at a hemophilia treatment center (HTC) of excellence, where expertise in the treatment of individuals with severe bleeding disorders and inhibitors is available. If emergency treatment or surgery is needed, patients should be transferred to the HTC as soon as possible and in a stabilized condition (see box on Treatment of Bleeding in a

Patient With Factor VIII Deficiency and an Inhibitor). Typically, the HTC and its physicians serve as a community resource to help guide the care of complex inhibitor patients at other institutions when timely transport is not feasible because of active bleeding and hemodynamic instability.

In general, there are two main aspects that should be considered: first that bleeds may be more frequent and are more difficult to treat and, second, that any available treatment is not as efficacious as FVIII in hemophilia with no inhibitors.

Minor Bleeding Episodes

In established low-titer alloantibody FVIII inhibitor patients (consistently *less than* 5 BU after repeated challenges) or in patients with low-titer transient inhibitors, larger doses of FVIII concentrate replacement can be given to overcome the neutralizing properties of the inhibitor. Such treatment may provide therapeutic levels of FVIII activity. The following equation approximates the dose necessary to overcome the neutralization effects of a low-titer FVIII inhibitor:

$$FVIII\ Replacement\ Loading\ Dose$$
$$= 2\,(Body\ Weight\ in\ kg\,[(80)(100 - Hematocrit)/100])/BU$$

FVIII activity levels should be determined after the infusion to ensure that adequate therapeutic levels are achieved and sustained. For invasive procedures, maintenance of FVIII level sufficient to maintain hemostasis adequately may require continuous infusion of replacement product. If a bolus dosing protocol is chosen, the treatment interval will need to be short, every 4 hours, to start with, followed by a schedule tailored to the aPTT or the FVIII level. Once the optimal bolus dose of FVIII replacement is established, home therapy may be possible.

High-titer FVIII inhibitors are characterized by titers above 5 BU and by anamnestic responsiveness after repeated exposures to exogenous FVIII. Often, high-titer inhibitors may spontaneously fall below 5 BU, especially after prolonged lapses in FVIII reexposure. In this scenario, FVIII replacement should be avoided, if possible, so that anamnesis can be abated and the chances for successful ITI and eradication of the inhibitor can be enhanced.[101] On the other hand, in urgent situations when "bypass" products are not available, low-titer inhibitor expression (<5 BU) may allow for effective use of FVIII concentrate replacement therapy, particularly in bleeds that are threatening to life or limb, because the anamnestic response will be delayed for several days. In these situations, administration of sufficient amounts of exogenous FVIII to overcome the immediate neutralization by the low-titer inhibitor will allow hemostasis to be achieved. Anamnestic rises in FVIII inhibitor titers have been observed after infusion of activated prothrombin complex concentrates (APCCs) to high-titer antibody patients, which are administered to bypass the inhibitor and to treat or prevent bleeding. These products contain a small amount of FVIII.[101–104]

Low-titer FVIII alloantibody inhibitors never rise above 5 BU and do not exhibit anamnestic increases after reexposure to exogenous FVIII. DDAVP administration may also be effective in selected patients with mild to moderately severe hemophilia complicated by an inhibitor (high or low titer). A DDAVP challenge should be undertaken before any intervention before assessing the adequacy of incremental rises in FVIII activity in such patients.

Severe Bleeding Episodes

For patients who have an inhibitor titer less than 5 BU, administration of exogenous FVIII should be considered if FVIII levels can be monitored closely. This approach provides the most specific and effective therapy; however, anamnesis can occur within a week in patients with a history of a high-titer inhibitor, and switching to a bypassing agent is indicated. Anamnesis may render subsequent use

Treatment Options for Bleeding in a Patient With Factor VIII Deficiency and an Inhibitor

Low Titer, Low Responder

Mild Bleeding

- Local and conservative measures, such as rest, ice, compression, and elevation
- If the patient is known to respond to DDAVP (i.e., mild hemophilia A), 0.3 µg/kg IV or 300 µg intranasal (150 µg per nostril; 150 µg for patients <50 kg) for minor bleeding or treatment before minor surgery
- Oral antifibrinolytic therapy (ε-aminocaproic acid or tranexamic acid) for mucosal bleeding
- FVIII dosing to raise the level to 50%
- Recombinant FVIIa (90 to 120 µg/kg, followed by 90 µg/kg every 2 to 3 hours)
- Activated prothrombin complex concentrates (50 to 100 units/kg, with maximum daily dose of 200 units/kg)
- Concurrent treatment with antifibrinolytics should be administered with caution

Life- or Limb-Threatening Bleeding

- FVIII dosing to maintain FVIII activity levels at 100%
- Recombinant FVIIa (270 µg/kg for one dose may be considered with caution versus 90 µg/kg every 2 to 3 hours)
- Activated prothrombin complex concentrates (100 units/kg, with maximum daily dose of 200 units/kg)
- Concurrent treatment with antifibrinolytics should be administered with caution

Low Titer, High Responder

Mild Bleeding

- Local and conservative measures, such as rest, ice, compression, and elevation
- If the patient is known to respond to DDAVP (i.e., mild hemophilia A), 0.3 µg/kg IV or 300 µg intranasal (150 µg for patients <50 kg) for minor bleeding or treatment before minor surgery
- Oral antifibrinolytic therapy (ε-aminocaproic acid or tranexamic acid) for mucosal bleeding
- Recombinant factor VIIa (270 µg/kg, bolus may be considered with caution versus 90 µg/kg every 2 to 3 hours)
- Activated prothrombin complex concentrates (100 units/kg, with a maximum daily dose of 200 units/kg, may induce anamnesis)

Life- or Limb-Threatening Bleeding

- FVIII in high doses to maintain levels of 100%
- Frequent monitoring for an anamnestic response, usually within 5 to 7 days
- After the anamnestic response develops:
  - Recombinant FVIIa (270 µg/kg, may be considered with caution versus 90 µg/kg every 2 to 3 hours)
  - Activated prothrombin complex concentrates (50 to 100 units/kg, with a maximum daily dose of 200 units/kg)

High Titer, High Responder

Mild Bleeding

- Local and conservative measures, such as rest, ice, compression, and elevation
- Oral antifibrinolytic therapy (ε-aminocaproic acid or tranexamic acid) for mucosal bleeding
- Recombinant FVIIa (270 µg/kg, should be considered with caution versus 90 µg/kg every 2 to 3 hours)
- Activated prothrombin complex concentrates (100 units/kg, with a maximum daily dose of 200 units/kg)
- Concurrent treatment with antifibrinolytics should be administered with caution

Life- or Limb-Threatening Bleeding

- Recombinant FVIIa (270 µg/kg, should be considered with caution versus 90 µg/kg IV every 2 to 3 hours)
- Activated prothrombin complex concentrates (100 units/kg, with a maximum daily dose of 200 units/kg)
- If available, immunoadsorption can be attempted to rapidly lower the inhibitor titer so as to allow use of FVIII

Main Features of the Agents Effective for Inhibitor Treatment/Prophylaxis

- **Content** APCC: activated vitamin k-dependent clotting factors; rFVIIa: recombinant FVIIa alone
- **Mechanism of action** APCC: activate plasma FX and FII; rFVIIa: activates FX on platelets
- **Half-Life** APCC: putatively 8-12 hours; rFVIIa: 2-3 hours
- **Efficacy** APCC: about 80%; rFVIIa: about 80%

---

of exogenous FVIII therapy ineffective, so that even when exogenous FVIII replacement is anticipated to be effective in the short term, treatment should start with factor VIIa (FVIIa) or an APCC if prolonged periods of replacement therapy are necessary.

In the case of a severe bleed or a life-threatening emergency, the inhibitor titer should be determined as rapidly as possible, but treatment should not be delayed until the results are available. For patients with a known persistent high-titer antibody, prompt replacement treatment should consist of a bypass agent, either an APCC or recombinant FVIIa (rFVIIa).

Surgery

Surgery in patients with hemophilia, especially those who have an inhibitor, requires the involvement of an entire facility experienced in the preoperative and postoperative care of such patients. Replacement therapy recommendations for surgical procedures are similar to those for hemorrhage. For known low responders, adequate hemostasis can be achieved with higher doses of FVIII. For the high-responding patient, APCC or rFVIIa are the most effective in the postoperative setting.[8-10]

Prothrombin Complex Concentrates

Prothrombin complex concentrates (PCCs) were designed for treatment of bleeding events associated with hemophilia B, congenital deficiencies of the other vitamin K–dependent clotting disorders, or with severe liver disease. PCCs were hypothesized to be useful to treat FVIII inhibitor-related bleeding because of their thrombogenic properties. Prepared from large pools of normal donor plasma, the PCCs contain the vitamin K–dependent clotting factors prothrombin, FVII, FIX, and FX, as well as anticoagulant proteins C and S. Heparin or antithrombin is added to some preparations to limit activation of the coagulation factors during the manufacturing process and with administration. All PCCs undergo a viral inactivation process. In comparison with placebo, PCCs were shown to be partially effective in controlling approximately 50% of bleeding episodes in patients with FVIII alloantibody inhibitors, compared with 25% for product containing albumin alone.[105] A major caveat is that administration of PCCs to treat hemorrhage in hemophiliacs with inhibitors is *not* the treatment of choice and is justified *only* in the absence of more effective therapies.[105]

Activated Prothrombin Complex Concentrates and Factor VIIa

APCCs are PCCs that are supercharged by virtue of their partial activation during the manufacturing process with activated FVII credited for the maximum clotting potential. In a randomized, double-blind trial, an APCC showed significantly better control of bleeding events in severe hemophiliacs with inhibitors than did PCCs ($p = .0085$); however, APCC was judged effective in only 64% of the episodes versus 52% effectiveness for PCC.[106] Uncontrolled clinical studies have shown that APCCs are effective in treating 81% to 93% of joint bleeds.[107,108] One should bear in mind, however, that APCCs are never as effective in inhibitor patients as is FVIII replacement in noninhibitor patients. Use of APCCs facilitates surgery in inhibitor patients and has been reported to be effective[108,109] and safe in large populations.[109]

APCC administration in a secondary prophylaxis regimen has also been deemed feasible, successful, and safe in reducing the frequency of bleeding events in severe hemophilia A patients with high-titer FVIII inhibitors. In the randomized, prospective, crossover Pro-FEIBA study, a statistically significant 62% reduction in all bleeding events was observed during the prophylaxis phase of the study (85 units/kg on 3 nonconsecutive days/week) compared with the on-demand period (85 units/kg every 6 to 12 hours).[110]

Use of PCCs and APCCs is hampered by the lack of laboratory tests to measure efficacy or to predict the potential for anamnesis (because of the presence of small amounts of FVIII) and the risk for precipitating thrombotic complications. The incidence of thrombosis is increased with regimens that exceed the recommended dosage and in patients at risk for thrombotic events, such as older individuals with coronary artery disease.

For acute bleeds, APCCs are administered at doses of 50 to 100 units/kg every 6 to 12 hours based on the clinical severity, with the maximum daily dose capped at 200 units/kg. This broader time frame allows for use at home for treatment of acute bleeds and for prophylaxis.

rFVIIa was purified from plasma and first used to treat a patient with hemophilia A with an inhibitor in 1983.[111] Later, FVIIa produced by recombinant technology was found to be effective for preventing and treating acute bleeding. A randomized dose-finding trial determined that FVIIa effectively reversed 71% of joint and muscle bleeds within two to three doses, given every 2 to 3 hours.[112] Another prospective study established that 90 µg/kg rFVIIa promoted adequate hemostasis during major surgical procedures, with an efficacy rate of 83% to 100%.[113]

Randomized prospective studies have directly compared the efficacy and safety of one dose of an APCC (factor eight inhibitor bypassing activity [FEIBA, Baxter], 85 to 90 IU/kg) with 1 to 2 doses of FVIIa (NovoSeven [Novo Nordisk Health Care AG] 90 to 105 µg/kg/dose) to treat acute joint bleeds. Although both products showed around 80% efficacy after 12 hours, equivalence was not shown at the 6-hour primary outcome point, but this was probably because of study design and underpowered cohorts.[114] When the primary outcome was the percentage of patients who required additional hemostatic replacement therapy 9 hours after initiation of treatment, significantly lower percentages of the 270 µg/kg (8.3%) and 3 × 90 µg/kg (9.1%) FVIIa treatment dose cohorts required rescue therapies compared with the APCC treatment group (36.4%).[115]

Use of FVIIa is associated with some drawbacks, such as the lack of effective laboratory monitoring, very short half-life (≈2 to 3 hours, which necessitates frequent administration), potential for thrombotic events (more frequently observed in noninhibitor patients), and expense.

For acute bleeding events in inhibitor patients, debate exists as to whether the more convenient dosing regimen of a single large bolus dose of FVIIa (270 µg/kg) is as safe and efficacious as the multiple-dose regimen (90 µg/kg every 2 to 3 hours as recommended in the package insert). The initial concern was related to the thrombogenic potential of larger single doses, particularly in older individuals, since the large single-dose regimen was studied predominantly in children. In reality, a recent analysis of the FVIIa dosages used in FVIII inhibitor patients in the United States[116] (n = 20,469 doses, recommended dosages were the large ones, up to >270 µg/kg) revealed a very low incidence of thromboembolic complications (0.2%).[116] Thus for serious life- and limb-threatening hemorrhages, a single 270 µg/kg bolus dose is recommended, at least to start with. Treatment of acute bleeds with FVIIa concentrate should be initiated as soon as possible because efficacy is inversely related to time to treatment.

Recently, a comparative study was conducted between Novoseven and an iranian biosimilar of rFVIIa[117] in the range of 90–120 µg/kg/body weight: no differences were noted in terms of efficacy score, pain reduction, increased range of motion and side-effects. For

surgery, some experts advise an initial dose of rFVIIa of 120 µg/kg, followed by repeated 90 µg/kg doses every 2 to 3 hours.[117]

Parallel-Sequential Use of Activated Prothrombin Complex Concentrates and Factor VIIa Concentrates

For active inhibitor-associated bleeding episodes that appear to be unresponsive to treatment with either the APCC or rFVIIa alone, the administration of both products simultaneously or in an alternating regimen (within 12 hours) was reported to be successful.[119–121] This combination is not recommended by the product manufacturers, and its clinical usefulness has not been set in a scientifically valid manner. In vitro sequential spiking experiments[122] or ex vivo systematic infusion studies using plasma specimens from inhibitor patients who have received these two types of bypassing agents alone, simultaneously, or in tandem[123] have demonstrated enhanced hemostasis for the combined approach. One study suggests that individualized bypass replacement therapy regimens can be designed for inhibitor patients based on the ex vivo responses observed in thromboelastogram tracings.[123] Even though the efficacy of parallel treatment with bypassing agents may be good in inhibitor-related refractory bleeds, these regimens may increase the risk for thrombotic complications. A recent critical review of 49 inhibitor patients (9 acquired and 40 congenital), who received both bypassing agents in combined or alternating dosing regimens, reported 10 thromboembolic events, of which 1 was fatal.[124]

Prophylaxis With Activated Prothrombin Complex Concentrate and Factor VIIa

Prophylaxis regimens using either APCC or rFVIIa to prevent acute and chronic arthropathy in inhibitor patients can be classified as primary (children awaiting ITI) or secondary (patients in whom ITI failed). Though not formally compared, prophylaxis with bypassing agents in inhibitor patients is not as efficacious as FVIII replacement in patients without an inhibitor. However, an accumulation of case reports and small clinical studies has suggested that prophylaxis with bypassing agents is safe and feasible in the subset of inhibitor patients with frequent bleeds, such as in target joints. The first prospective controlled study of prophylaxis in inhibitor patients[125] showed that a daily bolus dose of 270 µg/kg of FVIIa is superior to a 90 µg/kg dose (59% versus 45%) in reducing the bleeding frequency in comparison to the preprophylaxis period. An uncontrolled study[126] described equivalent efficacy and safety for FVIIa and APCC for prophylaxis in patients with hemophilia A with inhibitors. Patients were placed on prophylaxis while awaiting initiation of ITI. In this context, the investigators favored the use of FVIIa to avoid potential anamnestic responses with APCC.[126] A recent prospective controlled trial demonstrated that a prophylaxis APCC regimen at the dose of 85 IU/kg three times/week reduced bleeding events by 62% in inhibitor patients, compared to the on-demand treatment regimen.[102]

Fibrinolytic Inhibitors

ε-Aminocaproic and tranexamic acid have long safety records and are commonly used in patients with hemophilia, including those with inhibitors, as a sole treatment modality or as adjuncts to factor replacement for mucosal bleeding, dental procedures, and some orthopedic surgeries.[127]

For children, ε-aminocaproic acid can be administered orally at doses of 50 to 100 mg/kg every 6 hours. If used before a surgical intervention, the first dose should be given 4 hours before the start of the procedure. In adults, a loading dose of 4 to 5 g can be given initially, followed by similar or lower doses every 6 to 12 hours until bleeding is controlled (total suggested dose is 100 mg/kg/day). Fibrinolytic inhibitors are useful adjuncts for the treatment or prevention of bleeds treated with DDAVP in patients with low-titer inhibitors but, considering their prothrombotic potential, should be administered cautiously when APCCs are used in large doses. Antifibrinolytic inhibitors are considered to be safe for use in conjunction with FVIIa.[103]

Newly Proposed Tools

Among the alternative treatments recently developed there is a recombinant porcine FVIII preparation (rpFVIII); a preliminary study demonstrated its efficacy in acquired hemophilia with severe bleeds.[128] The clinical rationale for this preparation is based on the fact that porcine FVIII has a limited cross-reactivity with inhibitors to human FVIII. A similar concentrate from plasma had been used for years in the UK and proved efficacious and safe[129] but in the long run anamneses to porcine FVIII were shown to occur. Whether a similar situation will occur with rpFVIII is difficult to say, as there are no data available on the molecular structure of the preparation and the clinical experience is too short. The very short half-life of rFVIIa prompted the industry to develop new products with a prolonged activity, but their development was halted because of the occurrence of antibodies to FVIIa.[130] Further, a phase I trial of a new formulation of rFVII for subcutaneous injection was performed that showed a prolonged half-life (5.6 vs. 2.7 hours for the intravenous administration and a good safety profile).[131]

A novel therapeutic approach has recently been reported based on the use of a conformational replica of FVIII, Emicizumab. This humanized, bispecific antibody binds both FIX and FX forming a thrombin-generation complex. This complex, in vitro and in vivo, elicits thrombin formation independent of the FVIII levels and, most importantly, the presence of an inhibitor to FVIII. A recent clinical trial showed a strong reduction of spontaneous bleeding in patients with hemophilia A with or without inhibitors.[132] Other advantages of this drug are its bioavailability by the subcutaneous route and the long-lasting efficacy; further, aPTT remained short during the study period. This approach could represent a novel, alternative therapy for inhibitor patients.

Immune Tolerance Therapy

ITI means the frequent, regular, long-term administration of a concentrate with the goal of inducing tolerance to FVIII or FIX . Today, ITI is considered the ultimate therapy for a patient with hemophilia complicated by an inhibitor. Immunologic mechanisms that underlie ITI-induced tolerance include peripheral T-cell anergy, inhibition of B-cell memory, the formation of antiidiotypic antibodies or activity of suppressor T-cells.

The goal of the procedure is to eradicate the alloantibodies. Successful ITI enables reinitiating on-demand or prophylactic replacement therapies for bleeding.

Taking into account that about 25% of inhibitors are persistently low titer and/or transient, ITI should be exclusively proposed to those patients who are high responders (anamneses >10 BU), and clearly symptomatic.

The first successful implementation of ITI was accomplished in 1974 when a child with a high-titer inhibitor (>500 BU) required emergency reversal of a life-threatening bleed.[133,134] Very large doses of FVIII concentrate and APCC were administered and the hemorrhage was eventually controlled. A serendipitous finding was that the inhibitor titer decreased to almost 40 BU. This was the first documentation that high-dose FVIII administration could decrease inhibitor titers and provided proof of principle for the Bonn protocol, which originally used high doses of FVIII (100 IU/kg) twice daily.[133,134] Bypass agents are administered as needed, to treat acute bleeds that occur during ITI. This regimen is continued until the inhibitor disappears, which can take up to a maximum of 3 years.[134,135]

The Malmö ITI protocol was developed to induce a more rapid elimination of an inhibitor in a patient with severe hemophilia B who required urgent orthopedic surgery.[136] Unique among the ITI regimens, the Malmö protocol, to lower the inhibitor level, uses immune-modulatory therapies in conjunction with large doses of clotting factor concentrate.[137,138]

As experience with ITI regimens increased, it became evident that low-dose FVIII protocols could also induce tolerance. Such regimens start with a dose of 25 IU/kg every other day, a 16- to 24-fold lower dose than those used in high-dose ITI protocols.[139,140]

Because of different ITI treatment protocols and outcomes, a retrospective International Immune Tolerance Registry was established in 1989. The registry eventually collected 314 inhibitor patients (>90% high titer) who underwent mostly high-dose ITI treatment regimens.[141] The success rate was shown to range from 50% to 60% over time. Predictors of successful ITI included a low maximum inhibitor titer (85% success with ≤20 BU titer); low immediate pre-ITI BU (59% failure rate for >20 BU); higher FVIII dosages (86% success with ≥200 IU/kg/day); age of patient at initiation of ITI (60% failure for age >20 years); and shorter time interval between inhibitor detection and ITI initiation (>70% success for <5-year interval).[142,143] Although other registries yielded similar findings,[144–146] uncertainty remained as to the optimal daily dose of FVIII, the use of concomitant immunosuppressive/immune-modulating agents, and the type of clotting factor replacement therapy (plasma-derived versus recombinant concentrates). Another major issue was the definition of success: stringent criteria (disappearance of the inhibitor, normal FVIII recovery and half-life) were not always accepted and therefore had an impact on the retrospective outcome evaluations. Although never formally proven, some believe that low- and/or intermediate-purity factor concentrates containing vWF may be more efficacious than recombinant FVIII for successful ITI.[147–150]

A number of treatment-related elements that may influence ITI outcomes cannot be addressed by registries. These include the number of acute bleeds during ITI, use of CVADs, onset of infections during ITI, and the use of plasma-derived PCCs or FVIIa to treat bleeds. Most of these questions were addressed in a randomized prospective multinational ITI trial that compared high- to low-dose ITI regimens, with the decision to use recombinant or a vWF-containing FVIII replacement product left to the discretion of the treating physician.[151,152] The results published to date have confirmed that ITI can eradicate inhibitors in almost 70% of cases, even when very stringent outcome definitions are applied. Recombinant FVIII preparations were used in 90% of the enrolled individuals, making it very unlikely that plasma-derived vWF-containing concentrates could yield results superior to the recombinant preparations. The success rates gained with high-dose (200 IU/kg daily) or low-dose (50 IU/kg three times a week) ITI regimens were similar; however, successful ITI was achieved 50% earlier with the high-dose regimen. The low-dose regimen was associated with an increased frequency of breakthrough bleeding events during ITI. This safety signal led to premature discontinuation of the study.

A high proportion of patients with a CVAD (41/99, 41%) developed access device infection, but this complication did not affect the likelihood of success[152] and therefore should not reduce the ITI use as an indication; however, this untoward side effect pinpoints the need for trained and professional device nursing when long-term treatments are needed. Further prospective studies are warranted to determine the optimal and most cost-effective dosing regimens for ITI. At any rate, a recent large retrospective study[153] reporting on ITI in patients with freshly diagnosed inhibitors, stressed the importance of starting the procedure as soon as possible, no matter the inhibitor titer or other risk factors.

In mild and moderate hemophilia A, inhibitors are less common than in severely affected patients but the change in the bleeding phenotype may pose significant challenges. ITI role in this clinical context is less clear as shown by a UKHCDO study from 1998[154] and a more recent one published in 2012.[155]

A number of high-risk and/or ITI-relapsed patients have been treated with Rituximab, an anti-CD20 monoclonal antibody, with or without FVIII concentrate. Success rates have ranged from 33% to 57%,[156] although only a few patients exhibited long-lasting remissions. Recently, Rituximab was used at the time of the first anamnesis occurred during ITI but a major response (titer <5 BU) was seen in only 3 out of 16 (18%) patients.[157]

Data on the risk of inhibitor recurrence during follow up are scanty. Essentially, once the inhibitor has been eradicated, the risk of a recurrence is very low, in the range of 1% to 5%, and may occur many years afterwards, as shown by some studies that tackled the matter.[141,142,144,152,158]

The new FVIII products (glycol-pegylated, fused to an Fc protein or to albumin) have not yet been used in ITI. The question is whether these concentrates display a reduced immunogenicity in vivo, as suggested by preliminary studies in animals or in vitro.[159,160]

HEMOPHILIA B

The development of inhibitors to FIX in severe hemophilia B follows the same general principles as in hemophilia A. Inhibitory alloantibodies may arise after administration of FIX-containing replacement products, and this phenomenon was appreciated very soon after hemophilia B was documented to be a separate entity from hemophilia A.[161] However, several distinct features in the epidemiology and treatment of FIX inhibitors in severe hemophilia B deserve a specific mention. These include (1) the lower incidence and prevalence of FIX inhibitors; (2) the increased risk for developing anaphylaxis after administration of FIX-containing concentrates to FIX inhibitor patients; (3) the risk for developing nephrotic syndrome after exposure to FIX-containing replacement products; and (4) the lower success rate of ITI for the eradication of FIX alloantibodies.[162,163]

Epidemiology

Patients with severe hemophilia B have a 10-fold lower risk for developing inhibitors compared with those with severe hemophilia A (3% vs. 30%).[164] FIX gene mutations associated with a very low risk for inhibitor formation are single amino acid substitutions, whereas the risk for inhibitor development approaches 20% with more significant mutations, such as frameshift mutations, premature stop codons, large deletions, and splice site mutations.[164] Patients with hemophilia B who are at highest risk for inhibitor development have a severe phenotype as a result of large gene deletions or other aberrations of the gene product, such as nonsense mutations. Although the latter mutations are found only in a small fraction of the hemophilia B population, they account for approximately 50% of the inhibitor population.[164]

Diagnosis

As in hemophilia A, an inhibitor should be suspected in hemophilia B when a patient ceases to respond to conventional replacement treatment. Given the possibility of anaphylaxis that may occur with initial treatment of bleeding episodes, patients with high-risk FIX gene mutations should be regularly screened for alloantibody inhibitors. The laboratory diagnosis for inhibitors in hemophilia B involves a modification of the BA used for the titration of FVIII inhibitors. In this case, FIX-deficient plasma is used instead of FVIII-deficient plasma.[165] In contrast to the FVIII inhibitor scenario, FIX inhibitors rapidly neutralize FIX in the normal plasma/patient plasma mixing studies: there is no time-dependent increase in the inhibitory increase of FIX alloantibodies over incubation at 37°C with either high- or low-titer FIX inhibitors.

Treatment

Treatment of hemophilia B in patients with FIX inhibitors mirrors that of hemophilia A complicated by FVIII inhibitors. Both APCC and rFVIIa are the key therapeutic modalities to reverse, control, and

prevent bleeding regardless of whether it is spontaneous in nature or induced by trauma or surgery.[165] However, because APCC contains significant amounts of FIX, which may induce anamnesis, some experts prefer rFVIIa.

Few treatment options exist for patients with FIX inhibitors who have experienced allergic reactions to the FIX antigenic material found in plasma, as in PCC, APCC, high-purity plasma-derived FIX concentrate, or even in recombinant FIX concentrates. Anaphylaxis is in fact, a major complication that can occur soon after the infusion of FIX-containing replacement therapies, manifesting as either a type II (dyspnea and hypoxia, and generalized hypersensitivity) or a type III (anaphylaxis and hypotension) allergic reaction. The rarity of anaphylactic complications in patients with hemophilia B with FIX inhibitors (only an estimated 35 cases have been reported) does not negate the seriousness of this complication.[162,166,167] In addition, this is likely an underreported and perhaps underrecognized event. The major risk factor for developing an anaphylactic reaction is the presence of a FIX gene null mutation, leading to an absence of circulating FIX antigenic material.[168]

Because these severe reactions occur only after initiation of treatment, they have been observed only in children (median age 12 months), occurring early, following a median of 11 exposure days. The development of anaphylaxis occurs at the same time as the appearance of an inhibitor. A recent survey on the topic has shown that allergic reactions can be elicited with either recombinant or plasma-derived FIX concentrates at similar rates (3.9%).[169]

Because experience with anaphylaxis is limited by its low incidence, some general practice guidelines have been developed:

1. For newly diagnosed hemophilia B patients, especially those with high-risk FIX gene mutations, the initial FIX replacement treatments should be conducted in a medical facility where hemophilia expertise and resuscitation equipment are available.[162]
2. Once a FIX inhibitor has been documented, FVIIa is the treatment of choice for active bleeding and for prophylaxis against bleeding.
3. ITI is generally ineffective in these patients, although tolerance to FIX has been reported with progressively increasing doses of FIX (desensitization procedure) administered with hydrocortisone.[162,167]
4. FIX alloantibody formation may be complicated by a nephrotic syndrome, especially in patients who previously experienced an allergic reaction to FIX replacement. The limited data available suggest that this syndrome is not the result of immune complex deposition, and it does not respond to corticosteroid treatment.[170,171] If nephrosis occurs, FIX doses should be reduced or treatment should be discontinued and rFVIIa therapy should be used instead.[171]
5. In a few refractory cases with or without nephrosis, immune modulation (anti-CD20,[172,173] cyclosporine A[174] or mycophenolate mofetil[175]) resulted in temporary tolerance to FIX.
6. Prophylaxis regimens with FVIIa (or APCC, if anaphylaxis and/or anamnesis is not an issue) may be useful in the context of high-titer FIX inhibitors; however, controlled trials are necessary before this approach becomes the standard of care.

As information available on inhibitors to FIX is scant, the literature on ITI procedures does not support clinically useful decisions. However, ITI should be used only in those patients who never displayed allergic symptoms related to FIX concentrates. All in all, ITI is less effective than in hemophilia A as shown by the North American Immune Tolerance Registry (NAITR) where an overall success rate of 31% was reported.[144,145]

FACTOR VII DEFICIENCY

Congenital Factor VII deficiency is the third most frequent among the congenital clotting disorders. Recent epidemiologic studies provided a higher than expected prevalence in the general population, of about 1–2 cases/10^5, with severe phenotypes accounting for about

20% to 25%.[176] The latter cases may have a bleeding tendency that is more severe than hemophilia, characterized by central nervous system or gastrointestinal bleeding soon after birth, or precocious joint bleeds.[177] With the availability of specific concentrates, especially rFVIIa, treatment has become widespread and the occurrence of complications fairly well known. As FVII shares considerable homology with FIX, both at the gene and protein levels,[178] and displays a comparable distribution of disease-causing mutations, with a large predominance of missense changes,[177] the occurrence of inhibitors to FVII was an expected finding. The lack of severe gene lesions, as large deletions, may account for the apparently lower prevalence of inhibitors in comparison with hemophilia B. Only a recent prospective study with a centralized inhibitor screening,[178] provided clear cut data on the inhibitor prevalence and features; in fact, inhibitors to FVII were detected in 3 of 115 (2.6%) patients (one de novo inhibitor and two preexisting inhibitors), all high titer, and their anamneses were kinetically similar to those described in hemophilias. Importantly, FVII inhibitors were in no case associated with allergic reactions. In the presence of a high-titer inhibitor to FVII, treatment becomes a problem as there are no bypassing agents capable of triggering blood coagulation.

SUGGESTED READINGS

Alexander S, Hopewell S, Hunter S, et al: Rituximab and desensitization for a patient with severe factor IX deficiency, inhibitors and history of anaphylaxis. *J Pediatr Hematol Oncol* 30:93, 2008.

Astermark J, Donfield SM, Gomperts ED, et al: The polygenic nature of inhibitors in hemophilia A: results from the Hemophilia Inhibitor Genetics Study (HIGHS) Combined Cohort. *Blood* 121:1445–1454, 2013.

Darby SC, Kan SW, Spooner RJ, et al: Mortality rates, life expectancy and causes of death in people with haemophilia A or B in the United Kingdom who were not infected with HIV. *Blood* 110:815, 2007.

Di Michele D: Hemophlia therapy – Navigating Speed Bumps on the Innovation Highway. *N Engl J Med* 374:2087–2089, 2016.

Faranoush M, Abolghasemi H, Mahboudi F, et al: A comparison of efficacy between recombinant activated factor VII (Aryoseven) and Novoseven in patients with hereditary FVIII deficiency with inhibitor. *Clin App Thromb Hemost* 22:184, 2016.

Gouw SC, van den Berg HM, Fischer K, et al for the RODIN Study Group: Intensity of factor VIII treatment and inhibitor development in children with severe hemophilia A: the RODIN study. *Blood* 121:4046–4056, 2013.

Hay CR, Brown S, Collins PW, et al: The diagnosis and management of factor VIII and IX inhibitors: A guideline from the United Kingdom Haemophilia Centre Doctors Organisation. *Br J Haematol* 133:591, 2006.

Hay CR, DiMichele DM: The principal results of the International Immune Tolerance Study: a randomized dose comparison. *Blood* 119:1335, 2011.

Hay CRM, Palmer B, Chalmers E, et al on behalf of the United Kingdom Hemophilia Centre Doctor's Organisation (UKHCDO): Incidence of FVIII inhibitors throughout life in severe haemophilia A in the United Kingdom. *Blood* 117:6367, 2011.

Ingerslev J: Hemophilia. Strategies for the treatment of inhibitor patients. *Haematologica* 85:15, 2000.

Kempton CL, Meeks SL: Towards optimal therapy for inhibitors in Hemophilia. *Hematology Am Soc Hematol Educ Program* 2014:364, 2014.

Konkle B, Ebbesen LS, Erhardtsen E, et al: Randomized, prospective clinical trial of recombinant factor VIIa for secondary prophylaxis in haemophilia patients with inhibitors. *J Thromb Haemost* 5:1904, 2008.

Lacroix-Desmazes S, Bayry J, Misra N, et al: The prevalence of proteolytic antibodies against factor VIII in hemophilia A. *N Engl J Med* 346:662, 2002.

Mariani G, Ghirardini A, Bellocco R: Immune tolerance in hemophilia-principal results from the International Registry. Report of the factor VIII and IX Subcommittee. *Thromb Haemost* 72:155, 1994.

Mariani G, Siragusa S, Kroner B: Immune tolerance induction in hemophilia A: a review. *Semin Thromb Hemost* 29:69, 2003.

Miao CH: Immunomodulation for inhibitors in haemophilia A: the important role of Treg cells. *Expert Rev Hematol* 3:469, 2010.

Oldenburg J, Schroeder J, Brackmann HH, et al: Environmental and genetic factors influencing inhibitor development. *Semin Hematol* 41:82, 2004.

Oldenburg J, Schwaab R, Brackmann HH: Induction of immune tolerance in haemophilia A inhibitor patients by the "Bonn Protocol": Predictive parameter for therapy duration and outcome. *Vox Sang* 77:49, 1999.

Roberts HR, Monroe DM, White GC: The use of recombinant factor VIIa in the treatment of bleeding disorders. *Blood* 104:3858, 2004.

Thompson AR, Murphy ME, Liu M, et al: Loss of tolerance to exogenous and endogenous factor VIII in a mild hemophilia A patient with an Arg593 to Cys mutation. *Blood* 90:1902, 1997.

Warrier I, Ewenstein BM, Koerper MA, et al: Factor IX inhibitors and anaphylaxis in hemophilia B. *J Pediatr Hematol Oncol* 19:23, 1997.

REFERENCES

For the complete list of references, log on to www.expertconsult.com.

CHAPTER 137

RARE COAGULATION FACTOR DEFICIENCIES

David Gailani, Allison P. Wheeler, and Anne T. Neff

INTRODUCTION

In this chapter the term *rare coagulation factor deficiency* is applied to disorders caused by mutations in single genes, other than those for von Willebrand factor, factor VIII, or factor IX, that cause reduced plasma activity of one or more coagulation proteins, ultimately leading to a defect in thrombin and/or fibrin formation.[1-3] The most common inherited deficiencies affecting plasma coagulation are those for factors VIII (hemophilia A) and IX (hemophilia B), with frequencies of 1 in 10,000 and 1 in 30,000 male births, respectively (Chapter 135). In comparison, severe deficiency of fibrinogen; one of the protease zymogens prothrombin, prekallikrein or factors VII, X, XI, or XII; one of the cofactors (factor V or high-molecular-weight kininogen); or the transaminase factor XIII occurs in one in 500,000 to 2 million individuals (Table 137.1). These conditions are primarily inherited as autosomal recessive conditions, implying carrier frequencies of approximately 1 in 1000 persons; 10-fold higher than the carrier frequency for the alleles causing X-linked hemophilia A or B. The rarity of these disorders, therefore, is due to their recessive nature, and not low allele frequency. This is important to keep in mind, as partial (heterozygous) deficiencies of these proteins are relatively common and may contribute to bleeding symptoms. As with any recessive trait, incidences are up to 10-fold higher in areas where consanguinity is common.[1,3]

Fig. 137.1A shows a scheme reflecting our current understanding of the major enzymatic reactions involved in thrombin generation and fibrin formation. During hemostasis, factor VIIa binds to tissue factor in the wall of a damaged blood vessel. The factor VIIa/tissue factor complex converts factor X to Xa, which in turn converts prothrombin to thrombin in the presence of factor Va. Mice lacking prothrombin, or factor VII, X, or V die in utero or soon after birth, demonstrating the importance of these proteins. Thrombin, among its many functions, converts fibrinogen to fibrin. Factor IX is also activated by factor VIIa/tissue factor and, with factor VIIIa, sustains thrombin generation by activating factor X. In some situations factor IX activation by factor XIa is required. The older model shown in Fig. 137.1B highlights the order of reactions during coagulation in a prothrombin time (PT) or activated partial thromboplastin time (aPTT) assay. Here factor XI activation requires the contact factors, factor XII, prekallikrein, and high-molecular-weight kininogen. Deficiency of a contact factor does not result in abnormal bleeding indicating that other mechanisms exist for factor XI activation. For example, thrombin activates factor XI (Fig. 137.1A). Finally, factor XIII is activated by thrombin and cross-links fibrin monomers within a fibrin polymer, increasing the strength of the fibrin strands (Fig. 137.1A).

The disorders discussed in this chapter represent 3% to 5% of coagulation factor deficiencies. Their rarity, clinical heterogeneity, and the limited availability of standardized testing present challenges for establishing evidence-based treatment guidelines.[1-3] Common symptoms include hemorrhage with invasive procedures and childbirth, and bleeding from mucosal surfaces. Bleeding involving the central nervous system (CNS) often accompanies severe deficiencies of fibrinogen and factors XIII, X, or VII. Gastrointestinal (GI) bleeding is a particular problem in factor X deficiency, and umbilical cord bleeding is most common with fibrinogen, factor XIII, or factor X deficiency. Hemarthroses can occur with afibrinogenemia and severe deficiency of factors II or X. The World Federation of Hemophilia

(WHF, www.wfh.org) and the International Rare Bleeding Disorder Database (RBDD, www.rbdd.org) have collected information on the worldwide prevalence of rare coagulation factor deficiencies (Fig. 137.2).[1,3,4] The European Network of Rare Bleeding Disorders (EN-RBD) recently reclassified these disorders based on clinical severity to facilitate development of evidenced-based diagnostic and treatment strategies (Table 137.2).[4] They noted the strongest associations between bleeding severity and coagulation factor activity with fibrinogen, factor X, and factor XIII deficiencies, and weaker associations with deficiencies of factor V and factor VII. The association between factor XI levels and propensity to bleed is very weak. This chapter contains sections describing deficiency states for each coagulation factor. The number from the Online Mendelian Inheritance in Man (OMIM) database for the deficiency is given in the section title. Updated lists of mutations associated with the factor deficiencies can be found at several websites such as http://www.hgmd.org and http://www.clotbase.bicnirrh.res.in. Table 137.1 lists properties of coagulation factors and features of their deficiency states; while Table 137.3 contains treatment recommendations.

FIBRINOGEN DEFICIENCY (OMIM 202400)

Fibrinogen was first purified from plasma in the late 19th century. Fibrinogen and fibrin are designated factor I and Ia, respectively, by the International Committee for the Nomenclature of Blood Clotting. Congenital absence of fibrinogen (afibrinogenemia) was first described in 1920 and has an estimated incidence of 1 in 1 million people (Table 137.1).[5,6] Partial deficiency is called *hypofibrinogenemia*. Fibrinogen is synthesized in hepatocytes as a 340,000-Da protein composed of two trimers, each containing an Aα, Bβ, and γ chain (Fig. 137.3), which are encoded by separate genes (*FGA, FGB, FGG*) within a 50-kb region of chromosome 4. Thrombin converts fibrinogen to fibrin by cleaving fibrinopeptides A and B from the Aα and Bβ chains, respectively. Fibrinogen also binds glycoprotein IIb/IIIa, facilitating platelet aggregation. Fibrinogen in platelet α-granules is taken up from plasma via a glycoprotein IIb/IIIa-dependent mechanism. Between 8% and 15% of plasma fibrinogen contains at least one γ chain that is a product of an alternatively spliced mRNA called γ'-fibrinogen. γ'-fibrinogen modulates thrombin and factor XIII activity and influences clot architecture.

The normal plasma fibrinogen concentration is 1.5 to 4.0 g/L (150–400 mg/dL). Afibrinogenemic patients have levels <0.1 g/L as determined by both clotting and immunoreactive assays, due to homozygosity or compound heterozygosity for fibrinogen gene mutations.[5,6] Hypofibrinogenemia is a milder condition due to heterozygosity for a mutation. The first causative mutation for fibrinogen deficiency was reported in 1999, and over 200 fibrinogen gene deletions, frameshifts, nonsense, missense, and frameshift mutations have subsequently been identified in afibrinogenemic and hypofibrinogenemic patients (www.geht.org/databaseang/fibrinogen).[6] The *FGA* gene is most commonly affected. Missense mutations are more prevalent in the *FGB* and *FGG* genes and cluster in the polypeptide C-termini affecting D-domain formation (Fig. 137.3) and interfering with secretion.[6] In afibrinogenemia, fibrinogen is not secreted due to lack of synthesis of one of the fibrinogen chains or the presence of a mutant chain that alters fibrinogen structure. Nonsecretable fibrinogen polypeptides are usually degraded in the hepatocyte. Some *FGG*

TABLE 137.1 Properties of Plasma Coagulation Factors and Characteristics of Deficiency States.

Protein	Factor Plasma Half-Life (hours)	Vitamin K–Dependent Modification	Factor Level in Pregnancy	Incidence of Severe Congenital Deficiency	Autosomal Inheritance Pattern of Deficiency	Other Names for Deficiency State	Bleeding Diathesis in Severe Deficiency	Screening Tests in Deficiency	
								PT	aPTT
Fibrinogen	72–120	No	↑	~1:1 × 10^6	Recessive or dominant	Afibrinogenemia	Severe	↑	↑
Prothrombin	60–100	Yes	↔	~1:2 × 10^6	Recessive	Hypoprothrombinemia	Severe	↑	↑
Factor V	12–14	No	↔	~1:1 × 10^6	Recessive	Parahemophilia	Moderate to severe	↑	↑
Factor VII	3–4	Yes	↑	~1:5 × 10^5	Recessive	Serum prothrombin conversion accelerator deficiency	Moderate to severe	↑	↔
Factor X	20–40	Yes	↑	~1:1 × 10^6	Recessive	Stuart-Prower factor deficiency	Severe	↑ ↔	↑ ↔
Factor XI	45–52	No	Inconsistent	~1:1 × 10^6	Recessive or dominant	Hemophilia C, Plasma thromboplastin antecedent deficiency	Asymptomatic to moderate	↔	↑
Factor XII	60	No	↑	Unknown	Recessive	Hageman trait	Asymptomatic	↔	↑
Prekallikrein	Not known	No	↔	Unknown	Recessive	Fletcher trait	Asymptomatic	↔	↑
High-molecular-weight kininogen	170	No	↔	Unknown	Recessive	Flaujeac trait Williams trait Fitzgerald trait	Asymptomatic	↔	↑
Factor XIII	150	No	↓	1:2 × 10^6	Recessive	Fibrin stabilizing factor deficiency	Severe	↔	↔

aPTT, Activated partial thromboplastin time; PT, prothrombin time.

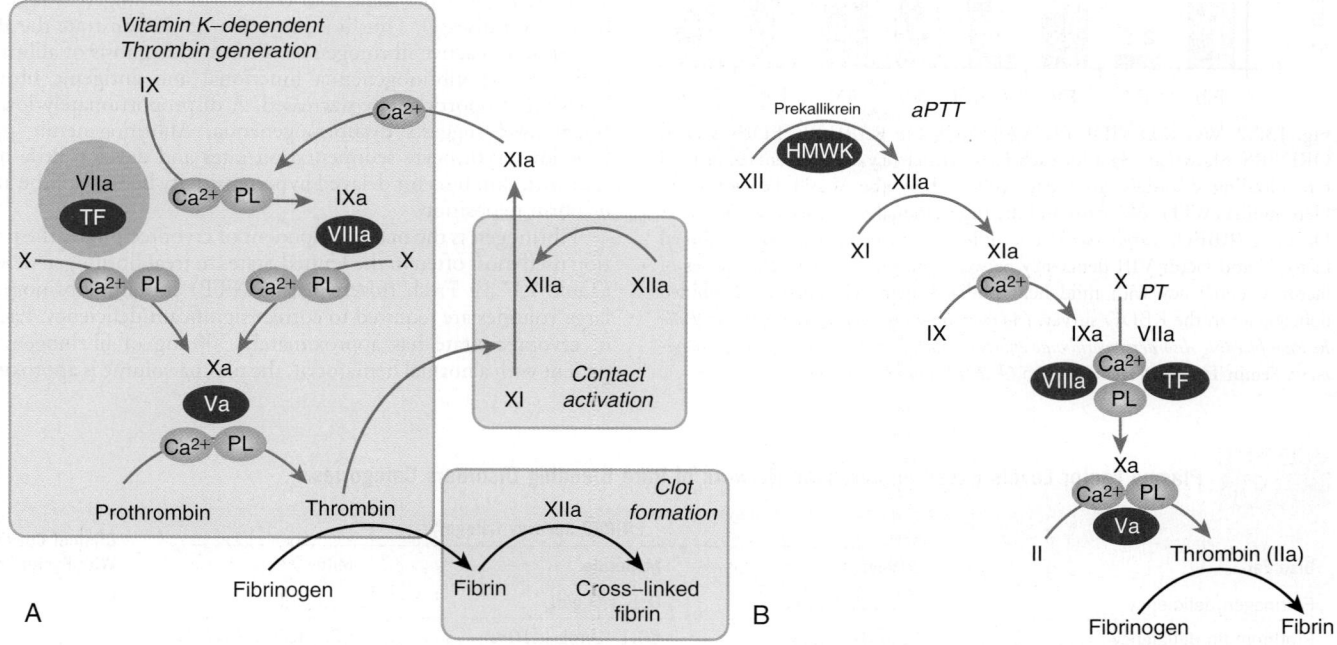

Fig. 137.1 MODELS OF PLASMA COAGULATION. Unactivated plasma factors are indicated by *Roman numerals* and activated factors by *Roman numerals* followed by a lowercase *a*. Enzymes are indicated by *black lettering* and cofactors by *white lettering* in *red ovals*. *Orange arrows* indicate reactions involving enzyme activation. Some reactions require calcium ions (Ca^{2+}) or phospholipid (PL) to proceed optimally. The *green arrow* indicates feedback activation of factor XI by thrombin. *Black arrows* indicate fibrin formation. (A) A model of tissue factor (TF) initiated hemostasis. Please read the introduction to this chapter for a description of the events leading to formation and stabilization of a fibrin clot depicted in this figure. (B) The cascade/waterfall model of hemostasis. This model serves as the basis for the prothrombin time (PT) and activated partial thromboplastin time (aPTT) assays. In the PT assay a reagent containing TF is added to plasma, and the factor VIIa/TF complex induces clot formation through activation of factor X. In the aPTT assay a reagent containing a negatively charged substance initiates clot formation through activation of factor XII (contact activation; see Fig. 137.5 for details). *HK,* High-molecular-weight kininogen; *PK,* prekallikrein; *TF,* tissue factor.

gene mutations such as Gly284Arg (fibrinogen Brescia), Arg375Trp (fibrinogen Aguadilla), or Thr314Pro (fibrinogen Al DuPont) are associated with accumulation of the mutant γ-polypeptide in hepatocytes, leading to hepatic dysfunction and cirrhosis similar to the process associated with α1-antitrypsin deficiency (endoplasmic reticulum [ER] storage disease).

Acquired hypofibrinogenemia occurs in disseminated intravascular coagulation (DIC) and primary fibrinolysis (see Chapter 139). Fibrinogen levels are usually normal or increased in liver disease, but levels less than 1 g/L may be seen in cirrhosis with hepatic failure or fulminant hepatic necrosis, and indicate a poor prognosis. Patients receiving L-asparaginase for hematologic malignancies may develop severe hypofibrinogenemia (<0.2 g/L), while other coagulation factors are normal or only slightly reduced.

Hemorrhagic symptoms in fibrinogen deficiency are most significant when the plasma level is less than 0.5 g/L.[5,6] Data from the EN-RBD database indicate spontaneous bleeds rarely occur when levels are over 0.7 g/L, while bleeding even with surgery is unusual with levels over 1.0 g/L. Most (85%) afibrinogenemic patients bleed from their umbilical cord and mucosal surfaces.[6] Menorrhagia and bleeding from the skin, GI tract and genitourinary tract are common.[6] Hemarthroses and muscle hematomas were common in one series (54% and 72%, respectively), but were less frequent (25%) in another study.[6] Hemarthrosis-related arthropathy appears to be less pronounced than in hemophilia A or B. Intracranial bleeding occurs in up to 10% of patients, and is a major cause of death, providing a justification for prophylaxis.[6] Afibrinogenemic patients are prone to spontaneous rupture of the spleen. Hypofibrinogenemic patients are usually asymptomatic, but may have excessive bleeding with trauma or surgery, particularly if the fibrinogen level is below 0.5 g/L. In the absence of factor replacement, pregnancy loss is common in afibrinogenemic women, usually occurring in the first trimester.[2,7] Fibrinogen-deficient mice also have difficulty sustaining pregnancy, confirming the importance of maternal fibrinogen to fetal viability. Pre- and postpartum bleeding is common,[7] and intraabdominal bleeding from ruptured corpus luteal cysts has been reported.

Curiously, arterial and venous thromboses occur in afibrinogenemic patients, and there may actually be an increased risk of myocardial infarction. While some events are likely precipitated by known risk factors or by factor replacement, no identifiable cause is evident in most instances. Fibrinogen and fibrin downregulate thrombin activity, providing a possible explanation for these events.

Assays such as the PT, aPTT, and thrombin time will be infinitely prolonged in afibrinogenemia. In hypofibrinogenemia, the thrombin time is often prolonged, but the PT and aPTT are insensitive to low fibrinogen and may be normal. Results for the template bleeding time and standard platelet aggregometry are usually abnormal. However, the aperture closure times in the PFA-100 platelet function screen are usually normal, as this test depends on von Willebrand factor and not fibrinogen to support platelet function. The von Clauss method is most commonly used for measuring fibrinogen, based on determining the time to clot formation after addition of thrombin to plasma. The assay is not reliable at low fibrinogen levels (<10 mg/dL) and may give falsely low readings with fibrinogen variants that polymerize slowly (dysfibrinogenemia), if high levels of substances that interfere with fibrin polymerization (paraproteins, fibrin degradation products) are present, or if the sialic acid content of fibrinogen is high (newborns, liver disease). Thus it is important to demonstrate the absence of immune-reactive fibrinogen to confirm a diagnosis of afibrinogenemia. In hypofibrinogenemia functional and antigenic fibrinogen levels are proportionately decreased. A disproportionately low functional level suggests dysfibrinogenemia. Afibrinogenemic patients have low erythrocyte sedimentation rates and develop little induration with skin tests for delayed hypersensitivity because of the absence of fibrin deposition.

Fibrinogen is the main component of cryoprecipitate, the preparation used most often in the United States to treat fibrinogen deficiency (Table 137.3). Fresh frozen plasma (FFP) contains fibrinogen, but large volumes are required to correct significant deficiency. Each unit of cryoprecipitate has approximately 300 mg of fibrinogen. For a patient with a normal hematocrit, the plasma volume is approximately

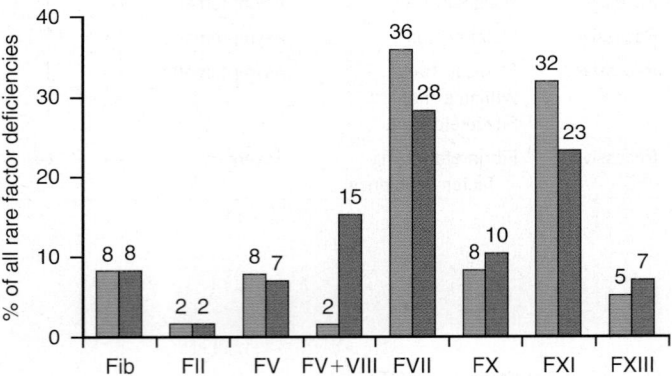

Fig. 137.2 WORLDWIDE PREVALENCE OF RARE BLEEDING DISORDERS. Shown are data for each factor deficiency as a percentage of total rare bleeding disorders from data collected by the World Federation of Hemophilia (WFH, *blue bars*) and the International Rare Bleeding Disorders Database (RBBD, *purple bars*). The difference in percentage for combined factor V and factor VIII deficiency between the surveys may reflect cases of factor V deficiency with mild hemophilia A being classified as combined deficiencies in the RBDD survey. (*Adapted from Peyvandi F, Menegatti M, Palla R: Rare bleeding disorders: worldwide efforts for classification, diagnosis and management. Semin Thromb Haemost. 39:579, 2013, with permission.*)

TABLE 137.2	Plasma Factor Levels Based on European Network of Rare Bleeding Disorders Categories.			
	EN-RBD Severity Category			**Clinical Correlation With Factor Level**
Disorder	**Severe**	**Moderate**	**Mild**	
Fibrinogen deficiency	Undetectable	0.1–1.0 g/dL	>10 g/dL	Strong
Prothrombin deficiency	Undetectable	≤0.1 IU/mL (≤10%)	>0.1 IU/mL (>10%)	Strong
Factor V deficiency	Undetectable	<0.1 IU/mL (<10%)	≥0.1 IU/mL (≥10%)	Weak
Factor VII deficiency	<0.1 IU/mL (<10%)	0.1–0.2 IU/mL (10%–20%)	>0.2 IU/mL (>20%)	Weak
Factor X deficiency	<0.1 IU/mL (<10%)	0.1–0.4 IU/mL (10%–40%)	>0.4 IU/mL (>40%)	Strong
Factor XI deficiency	–	–	–	Very weak
Factor XIII deficiency	Undetectable	<0.3 IU/mL (≤30%)	≥0.3 IU/mL (>30%)	Strong
Combined factor V and VIII deficiency	<0.2 IU/mL (<20%)	0.2–0.4 IU/mL (20%–40%)	>0.4 IU/mL (>40%)	Weak
Vitamin K–dependent factor deficiencies	–	–	–	Weak

EN-RBD, European Network of Rare Bleeding Disorders.

TABLE 137.3   Treatment Considerations for Rare Coagulation Factor Deficiencies.

Protein	Blood Product Sources	Concentrate (Manufacturer)	Minimum Plasma Level Required for Hemostasis	Minimum Plasma Level Required for Surgery	Dose of Preferred Treatment for Surgery or Bleeding	Dosing Frequency for Surgery or Bleeding	Prophylaxis for Severe Deficiency	Pregnancy: Suggested Plasma Levels for Invasive Procedures and Delivery
Fibrinogen	CRYO FFP	RiaSTAP (CSL Behring)[a]	>50 mg/dL	100 mg/dL until healing complete	20–30 mg/kg[b] FFP 15–20 mL/kg Cryo 1 bag/10 kg	Q 24–72 h depending on consumption	Keep level 50 mg/dL for recurrent bleeders	Maintain at 100 mg/dL throughout pregnancy
Prothrombin	FFP	PCC[a]	~5%	30%	20–30 factor IX units/kg	Q 48–72 h	40 factor IX units/kg Q 5–6 days	20%–30%
Factor V	FFP[a] platelets	None	~10%	25%	20 mL FFP/kg then 5–10 mL/kg q12 h	Q 12–24 h	Not usually required	15%–25%
Factor VII	FFP	NovoSeven, recombinant Factor VIIa (Novo Nordisk)[a]; PCC	5%–10%	15%–25%	15–30 µg factor VIIa/kg	Q 2–12 h	20–30 µg/kg 2–3 times per wk	10%–20%
Factor X	FFP	PCC[a]; Coagadex, Factor X concentrate (BioProducts Laboratory)	~10%	25%–40%	PCC: 15–20 factor IX units/kg Fx: 25 factor X units/kg	Q 24 h	15–20 factor X units/kg weekly. 40–50 Factor X units twice weekly	10%–20%
Factor XI	FFP[a]	Hemoleven (LFB Biomedicaments); Factor XI concentrate (Bio Products Laboratory)	15%	30%–40%	15–20 factor XI units/kg	Q 1–2 days	Not required	May withhold treatment unless bleeding. 20%–40% if bleeding occurs
Factor XIII	CRYO FFP	Corifact[a] (Formerly Fibrogammin P, CSL Behring); Recombinant Factor XIII (Tretten, Novo Nordisk)	1%–2%	20%–50%	20–30 factor XIII units/kg	Single dose may be sufficient	40 factor XIII units/kg q 28 days	250 units/wk through wk 22, then 500 units/wk with a 1000 unit bolus during labor

[a]Preferred treatment for congenital deficiency
[b]Assuming baseline fibrinogen is not known.
CRYO, Cryoprecipitate; FFP, fresh frozen plasma; PCC, prothrombin complex concentrate.

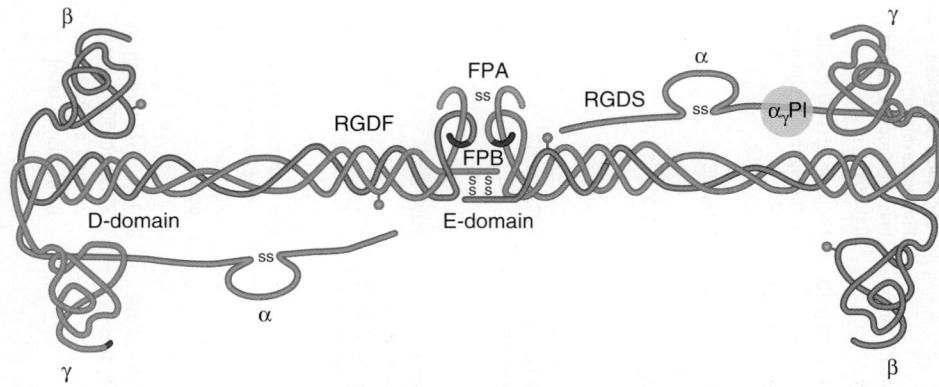

Fig. 137.3 MODEL OF HUMAN FIBRINOGEN. A fibrinogen molecule consists of two trimers, each containing an Aα-chain *(blue)*, Bβ-chain *(pink)*, and γ-chain *(yellow)*. The amino-termini of the six chains that compose the whole molecule are linked by disulfide bonds in the central E domain, and the C-termini of the polypeptides form two nodular D domains at opposite ends of the molecule. Fibrinopeptides A (FPA; *green)* and B (FPB; *purple)* reside in the E domain and are removed by the proteolytic activity of thrombin during conversion of fibrinogen to fibrin monomer. *(Adapted from Mosesson MW: The roles of fibrinogen and fibrin in hemostasis and thrombosis. Semin Hematol. 29:177, 1992, with permission.)*

0.04 L/kg body mass (40 mL/kg). Administering cryoprecipitate at 1 unit/5 kg of body mass will increase plasma fibrinogen in an afibrinogenemic patient to approximately 1 g/L. The fibrinogen concentrate RiaSTAP (Haemocomplettan) was approved by the Food and Drug Administration (FDA) in 2009 for treating bleeding and for prophylaxis in severe fibrinogen deficiency. This preparation has gone through viral inactivation steps. In a study of 15 patients given RiaSTAP (70 mg/kg), the median plasma fibrinogen concentration 1 hour postinfusion was 1.3 g/L with a half-life of 77.1 hours. In one study, the concentrate was effective in congenital fibrinogen deficiency in 26 of 26 bleeding episodes, 10 of 11 surgical procedures, and all 90 prophylactic administrations. Subsequent studies involving trauma, cardiothoracic surgery, and obstetrical hemorrhage confirmed its ability to improve coagulation and reduce blood loss.[5,6] Low-molecular-weight heparin may be administered with fibrinogen concentrate if there is concern that therapy may precipitate a thrombotic event. The required dose of concentrate can be determined using the following formula:

$$\text{Dose (mg/kg)} = \frac{(\text{Target level [mg/dL]} - \text{Measured level [mg/dL]})}{1.7\ (\text{kg body weight/dL})}$$

For treating bleeding, the United Kingdom Haemophilia Centre Doctors Organization guidelines recommend that plasma fibrinogen be maintained at 1.0 g/L until hemostasis is achieved and greater than 0.5 g/L until wound healing is complete.[2] A similar strategy makes sense for managing surgery. A review of replacement therapy and outcomes for 50 patients with congenital fibrinogen deficiency generally agrees with these recommendations. A fibrinogen concentration of 0.5 to 1.0 g/L was sufficient for prevention or treatment of bleeding in nonsurgical or obstetrical settings, while 1.0 to 2.0 g/L was effective for preventing bleeding during surgery. One review reported that thrombotic episodes (related or unrelated to replacement) occurred in 30% of patients. As the half-life of transfused fibrinogen is approximately 3 days, dosing every 2 to 4 days is usually adequate to maintain levels in the absence of consumption. Increased dosing frequency may be necessary in cases of massive hemorrhage, major surgery or advanced pregnancy, and monitoring of the fibrinogen level is recommended to facilitate dosing. The utility of thromboelastography to provide guidance for patients receiving fibrinogen concentrate for bleeding is being investigated.

Prophylactic fibrinogen administration is recommended to maintain pregnancies in afibrinogenemic women and to reduce postpartum hemorrhage.[2,5,7] Therapy should be initiated early as fetal loss in the first trimester is common. One study suggested that initiating therapy before conception is beneficial. Although some authors recommend keeping fibrinogen levels above 0.5 g/L during pregnancy and peripartum, others suggest a higher level (1.0 g/L) based on reports of fetal loss in patients with levels near 0.5 g/L. Long-term prophylaxis may be useful in preventing initial bleeding in young patients or to prevent recurrence, particularly after CNS hemorrhage. Administration of 20–30 mg/kg of concentrate every 7 to 14 days to maintain plasma levels of approximately 0.5 g/L is recommended.[5,6]

Increased use of fibrinogen concentrate has raised concerns regarding adverse events. An analysis of 27 years of pharmacovigilance data identified 21 cases of suspected viral transmission (1 per 124,300), 28 cases of thromboembolism (1 per 93,300), and 20 cases of hypersensitivity (1 per 130,600 doses) suggesting a promising safety profile.[8] Acquired antibody inhibitors have been reported in only two patients with afibrinogenemia after replacement therapy.

Antifibrinolytic therapy with ε-amino caproic acid may be an effective replacement for blood products for some mucosal bleeds and for dental extractions. However, this therapy may increase the risk for thrombosis and must be used cautiously in patients with a history of thrombosis, or during pregnancy, surgery, or immobilization. Fibrin glue may be useful for tooth extraction, and estrogen/progesterone therapy may be helpful for controlling menorrhagia.[5]

DYSFIBRINOGENEMIA (OMIM 134820 Aα-CHAIN, 134830 Bβ-CHAIN, AND 134850 γ-CHAIN)

In dysfibrinogenemia structural variants of fibrinogen circulate in plasma.[9,10] Cases in which the dysfunctional protein is present at low levels may be referred to as *hypodysfibrinogenemia*. The first family with dysfibrinogenemia (15 amino acid insertion after Gln350 in the γ-chain [fibrinogen Paris I]) was described in 1964. The actual incidence of congenital dysfibrinogenemia is not known because the majority of affected individuals are probably asymptomatic.

Congenital dysfibrinogenemias are almost all autosomal dominant traits due to missense mutations in a fibrinogen gene (www.geht.or/databaseand/fibrinogen).[6,9,10] Amino acid substitutions that alter fibrinopeptide release, cross-linking, polymerization, or degradation have been described. The diagnosis is established by identifying low fibrinogen in a rate-based clotting assay relative to immunoreactive fibrinogen. The functional defects most often reported are clearly influenced by the assays available in clinical laboratories and are unlikely to represent the full spectrum of mutations causing

The antifibrinolytic agents ε-amino caproic acid and tranexamic acid can be effective adjuncts to factor replacement when treating congenital or acquired bleeding disorders, and are useful alternatives to replacement therapy for mild bleeding or minor procedures. These drugs inhibit clot dissolution by interfering with plasminogen activation and plasmin activity, and are particularly effective when bleeding involves tissues with high fibrinolytic activity such as the oral and nasal cavity. They are also useful for treating menorrhagia, imiting blood loss with surgery, controlling epistaxis and reducing some types of GI bleeding. A typical loading dose of ε-amino caproic acid is 50 to 100 mg/kg followed by 50 mg/kg every 6 hours (for adults dose 2 to 4 g every 6 hours). If bleeding subsequently occurs, the dose can be increased, but should not exceed 24 grams in 24 hours. ε-Amino caproic acid is available in oral and intravenous formulations. Identical dosing for either preparation may be used due to excellent bioavailability. For dental extraction in factor VIII or IX deficiency, many centers utilize a single 50% to 100% dose of factor concentrate followed by seven days of ε-amino caproic acid, and it is reasonable to use this approach for patients with some rare bleeding disorders. Patients with factor XI deficiency do well with antifibrinolytic agents alone for tooth extraction (see Treating Factor XI Deficient Patients). Prolonged therapy with antifibrinolytics must be undertaken with caution in patients who are not mobile, who have a history of thrombosis, or who have significant urogenital bleeding. These drugs interfere with urokinase-mediated fibrinolysis in the genitourinary tract that can lead to thrombotic occlusion of the ureter. Concomitant use of antifibrinolytic agents with activated prothrombin complex concentrates or recombinant factor VIIa may result in a particularly high risk of thrombus formation. Patients may develop nausea or vertigo with high doses of ε-amino caproic doses, and rarely, rhabdomyolysis.

Recombinant factor VIIa may stop or prevent hemorrhage in rare bleeding disorders. The mechanism by which this agent works is not completely understood, particularly for deficiencies of common pathway factors (prothrombin and factors V and X). For patients with rare bleeding disorders and an antibody inhibitor directed against the missing factor, factor VIIa may be the treatment of choice. Doses range from 15 to 120 μg/kg every 2 to 6 hours depending upon the severity of bleeding. Because of the risk of thromboembolism with factor VIIa, we recommend frequent reevaluation and reduction to the lowest effective dose. Doses of 90 μg/kg every 2 to 3 hours have been used in patients with congenital factor V deficiency or combined deficiencies of factors V and VIII; with acquired factor X deficiency associated with amyloidosis, and with antibody-mediated acquired prothrombin deficiency associated with lupus anticoagulants. With factor VIIa, as compared to FFP, the volume of infused material is smaller, and the risk is lower for complications such as of fever, urticaria, transfusion-related acute lung injury (TRALI) and anaphylaxis. Caution must be exercised when using factor VIIa in older patients with cardiovascular disease, as arterial thrombosis can result, particularly when therapy is combined with antifibrinolytic therapy or prothrombin complex concentrate.

fibrinogen dysfunction. Variants easily detected in clinical laboratories typically have defects in fibrinopeptide release (e.g., FGA-Arg16His and FGA-Arg16Cys [fibrinogens Bicêtre and Metz]), or polymerize slowly (e.g., FGG-Ser434Asn [fibrinogen Caracas II], FGG-Arg275Cys and FGG-Arg275His). Indeed, approximately 45% of the mutations in the dysfibrinogenemia database involve substitutions at FGA-Arg16 or FGG-Arg275, at least partly reflecting the ease with which these variants are detected by common functional assays.

Most individuals with dysfibrinogenemia are asymptomatic.[9,10] In a recent multicenter study of congenital dysfibrinogenemia 58% were identified incidentally by an abnormal coagulation test. Over a mean follow-up of 8.8 years, the incidences of major bleeding and thrombosis were 2.5 and 18.7 per 1000 patient years, respectively,[10] with estimated cumulative incidences of 19.2% and 30.1% at age 50 years. There were no clear associations between symptoms and fibrinogen level, functional abnormalities, or gene mutations, consistent with older observations that common substitutions such as FGA-Arg16His

and FGA-Arg16Cys occur in asymptomatic individuals as well as patients with bleeding or thrombosis.

Bleeding symptoms tend to be relatively mild, with epistaxis, easy bruising, and menorrhagia being common.[9,10] More serious bleeding events including soft tissue hematomas, hemarthroses, postoperative hemorrhage, and bleeding during and after pregnancy do occur, but are rarer. Major bleeding seems to occur primarily between the ages of 20 and 40 years, partly due to hemostatic challenges related to childbirth. Abnormal wound healing and spontaneous abortions have been reported.

Thrombotic events primarily involve the venous circulation, although arterial events occur.[9,10] The mean age for venous and arterial events in one study (34 and 49 years) was significantly lower than for the general population.[10] There was a high prevalence of venous thromboembolism (VTE) at the time of diagnosis, with an incidence during follow-up similar to that for carriers of the factor V Leiden (G1691A) polymorphism. A strong relationship exists between certain fibrinogen variants and venous thrombosis. Thrombosis-associated mutations tend to cluster at the C-terminus of the Aα-chain and near the thrombin cleavage site on the Bβ chain. Abnormalities in fibrin polymerization and cross-linking, clot structure, and susceptibility to fibrinolysis have been described. The "Dusart Syndrome" caused by FGA-Arg554Cys (fibrinogen Paris V) was associated with venous thrombosis and sudden death in adolescents and young adults in several families. Dysfibrinogenemia was reported in 5 of 33 patients with chronic thromboembolic pulmonary hypertension, with the FGB-Pro235Leu substitution identified in three unrelated patients. Altered fibrin structure and susceptibility to fibrinolysis may result in poor clot dissolution in these patients. Despite these associations, a review of 2376 patients with venous thrombosis found dysfibrinogenemia in less than 1%, so testing for abnormal fibrinogen in patients with venous thrombosis is not widely recommended.

As discussed in the section on Fibrinogen Deficiency, maternal fibrinogen is required to maintain pregnancies. Pregnancy loss, as well as peripartum bleeding and thrombosis, have been reported in dysfibrinogenemic women. In contrast to older reports, the survey cited above did not identify an increased risk of spontaneous abortion, but there was a significant risk of postpartum bleeding, particularly in patients with histories of prior bleeding.

A group of mutations in the C-terminus of the fibrinogen Aα-chain is associated with autosomal dominant hereditary amyloidosis. The amyloid deposits contain fragments of the variant fibrinogen. The kidneys are initially affected, but wider visceral and nerve involvement may occur. Renal grafts subsequently become involved with amyloid, and liver transplantation may be a better treatment option. The allele for one responsible mutation, FGA-Glu526Val, is relatively common and may account for 5% of patients with apparent sporadic amyloid. Acquired dysfibrinogenemia is most frequently diagnosed in liver disease, with 80% to 90% of patients with cirrhosis or liver failure showing fibrinogen dysfunction. Increased sialic acid content similar to fetal fibrinogen seems to impair fibrin polymerization in vitro, but the process probably does not contribute substantially to abnormal hemostasis. The monoclonal paraprotein in patients with multiple myeloma can interfere nonspecifically with fibrin polymerization but usually does not cause abnormal hemostasis. Acquired dysfibrinogenemia has been associated with other malignancies and bone marrow transplantation.

Dysfibrinogenemia often presents as an abnormality on routine coagulation testing (PT or aPTT). The thrombin time is frequently used as a screening test for dysfibrinogenemia, although its sensitivity is not established. The test involves measuring time to clot formation in plasma after addition of a standard amount of thrombin. The specificity for dysfibrinogenemia is low, as heparin, direct thrombin inhibitors (argatroban, dabigatran, hirudin), elevated fibrin degradation products, paraproteins, and low levels of fibrinogen all prolong the thrombin time. The reptilase time has been used as an alternative screen and is useful in combination with the thrombin time. The assay involves inducing clot formation with an enzyme from a snake venom (*Bothrops jararaca* or *Bothrops atrox*) that releases fibrinopeptide A (but not fibrinopeptide B) from fibrinogen, and is not sensitive to heparin or direct thrombin inhibitors. The apparent plasma concentration of fibrinogen as determined by the von Clauss method (see section on Fibrinogen Deficiency) may be low in some types of dysfibrinogenemia. Levels of immunoreactive fibrinogen are usually normal, but are decreased in cases of hypodysfibrinogenemia. With some variants, serum fibrin degradation products may appear to be elevated because the variant fibrinogen is incompletely incorporated into the clot. This can lead to the false impression that DIC is present.

Most dysfibrinogenemic patients are asymptomatic, and symptoms correlate poorly with coagulation assay abnormalities, making it difficult to make general therapeutic recommendations. The patient's personal and family histories are useful for guiding therapy. Active bleeding can be treated with replacement therapy as in afibrinogenemia, and such treatment may be indicated in some patients before invasive procedures. In general, patients with thrombosis and dysfibrinogenemia should be treated in the same manner as other patients with thrombosis. There are no data on which to formulate recommendations as to duration of therapy; thus past history, family history, coexisting conditions, and the nature (idiopathic, pregnancy-related or surgery-related) and seriousness of the thrombotic event are taken into consideration. As with any thrombotic event, the risk for bleeding associated with prolonged therapy must be considered. Recurrent spontaneous abortions have been associated with dysfibrinogenemia in several families, and pregnancies have been carried to term using replacement therapy. While some investigators recommend replacing fibrinogen starting early in pregnancy, as in afibrinogenemic patients, the prothrombotic nature of the peripartum period may dictate against this approach in certain patients.

PROTHROMBIN DEFICIENCY (OMIM 176930)

More than a century ago Morawitz proposed that insoluble fibrin is formed from fibrinogen through the activity of fibrin ferment or thrombin. Thrombin was generated from a precursor, prothrombin, by thrombokinase (probably factor Xa). Prothrombin and thrombin are designated factors II and IIa. Total prothrombin deficiency is probably not compatible with life. Complete absence of the protein has not been observed in a human, and prothrombin-deficient mice succumb to bleeding in utero or shortly after birth. Severe deficiency associated with reduced plasma prothrombin antigen (hypoprothrombinemia) or circulating dysfunctional prothrombin (dysprothrombinemia) affects about 1 in 2 million people (Table 137.1).[11] Prothrombin deficiency is the third most common coagulation factor disorder in Puerto Rico (carrier frequency about 1 in 700), accounting for 6% of congenital bleeding disorders other than von Willebrand disease at the University of Puerto Rico Hemophilia Center. In the North American Rare Bleeding Disorder Registry, 62% of patients with prothrombin deficiency were Latino, possibly reflecting the prevalence of the pArg457Gln variant prothrombin Puerto Rico I. Globally almost 70% of patients with prothrombin deficiency are of Latin or Hispanic origin.[11] Prothrombin is a 72,000-Da protein that is converted to thrombin by factor Xa in complex with factor Va on phospholipid surfaces (Fig. 137.1A). Thrombin is the pivotal protease in hemostasis, with multiple procoagulant activities including cleavage of fibrinopeptides A and B from fibrinogen to form fibrin (Fig. 137.3), activation of factors V, VIII, XI, and XIII, and cleavage of protease activated receptors on a variety of cells including platelets.[11] Thrombin forms a complex with thrombomodulin on endothelial cells that downregulates fibrinolysis by activating thrombin-activatable fibrinolysis inhibitor (TAFI) and downregulates coagulation by activating protein C.

Prothrombin deficiency is an autosomal recessive disorder manifested as hypoprothrombinemia (reduced activity and antigen; cross-reactive material [CRM]–negative [CRM–] deficiency), dysprothrombinemia (activity reduced relative to antigen; CRM+ deficiency) or a combination of both.[11] Plasma prothrombin activity is typically 1% to 10% of normal in hypoprothrombinemia and 1% to 20% in dysprothrombinemia. Heterozygotes for either condition have 40%

to 60% normal activity. Approximately 50 prothrombin gene mutations have been described in patients with prothrombin deficiency, three-quarters of which are missense mutations.[11] In dysprothrombinemia, missense mutations typically cause defects in prothrombin conversion to thrombin (e.g., prothrombin pArg457Gln [Puerto Rico I] and pArg271Cys [Madrid]), or result in functionally defective thrombin (e.g., prothrombin pArg418Trp [Tokushima]).[11] Prothrombin deficiency can be inherited in combination with deficiencies of other vitamin K–dependent proteins (see Combined Deficiency of Vitamin K–Dependent Proteins).

Acquired prothrombin deficiency occurs with warfarin therapy, poisoning with rodenticides such as brodifacoum, vitamin K deficiency, liver disease, and DIC. Cephalosporins, particularly those with N-methyl-thiotetrazole side chains, can decrease prothrombin levels. Antiprothrombin antibodies are common phospholipid-dependent antibodies in patients with lupus anticoagulants or the antiphospholipid syndrome. More rarely, patients with a lupus anticoagulant or systemic lupus erythematosus have antibodies that enhance prothrombin clearance causing true deficiency. This acquired hypoprothrombinemia occurs primarily in children under 10 years of age, usually in association with lupus anticoagulants after a viral illness. These episodes typically resolve spontaneously but excessive bleeding can occur. There are no reports of neutralizing antibodies forming after replacement therapy in congenital prothrombin deficiency, consistent with patients having at least a trace of circulating prothrombin.

Severe hypoprothrombinemia is inevitably associated with bleeding that may be life threatening. In the EN-RBD survey prothrombin deficiency is classified as severe (<1% or normal), moderate (1% to 10%) or mild (> 10%) (Table 137.2).[12] CNS hemorrhage was reported in 8% to 12% of patients, and in 20% with prothrombin levels less than 1% of normal activity.[11,12] Soft tissue hematomas, bruising (60%), and hemarthroses (42%) are common.[11] The bleeding diathesis can present at circumcision in neonates, with trauma or surgery, or as easy bruising, epistaxis, menorrhagia, or GI hemorrhage. Heterozygotes occasionally have excessive bleeding with surgery or tooth extraction, but most are asymptomatic.[11] Bleeding tends to be less severe in dysprothrombinemia, and some variants are particularly mild. For example, homozygosity for pArg67His causes severe reduction in plasma prothrombin activity (<20% of normal) but causes relatively few symptoms.

In the PT and aPTT assays, prothrombin is converted to thrombin by factor Xa in complex with factor Va on phospholipid surfaces (Fig. 137.1B), and severe prothrombin deficiency will prolong the clotting time in both tests. Some PT and aPTT reagents are relatively insensitive to reductions in prothrombin, and mild deficiencies may be missed. The diagnosis is usually confirmed, and the degree of deficiency established, by a modified PT assay using prothrombin-deficient plasma. A prothrombin antigen level is needed to distinguish between hypoprothrombinemia (activity and antigen are equivalent) and dysprothrombinemia (activity is less than antigen). Prothrombin deficiency must be distinguished from deficiencies of fibrinogen, factor V, or factor X, which also prolong the PT and aPTT.

Prothrombin complex concentrate (PCC) approved for use in factor IX deficiency typically contains an amount of prothrombin comparable to, or higher than, the factor IX activity. It is the preferred product for treating prothrombin deficiency (Table 137.3). PCC is derived from human plasma and undergoes viral inactivation. Hemostatic levels of prothrombin are estimated to be 20% to 40% of normal for major surgery or trauma, but 10% to 15% may be adequate for milder hemostatic challenges.[11] A PCC dose of 20 to 30 factor IX units/kg usually produces plasma prothrombin levels of 20% to 30% of normal in a severely deficient patient. The half-life of prothrombin is about 3 days, and dosing every 2 to 3 days can maintain adequate levels until healing is complete. Alternatively, one-fourth of the loading dose each day should keep the level therapeutic. Prophylactic infusion of PCC every 5 to 6 days prevented spontaneous bleeding in one severely deficient patient. PCC administration has been associated with thrombosis, although a meta-analysis of studies using PCC to reverse the effect of warfarin suggests the risk is relatively low (<2%). It is reasonable to maintain the factor VII, IX, and X levels at less than 150% of normal to reduce risk. Dental procedures or minor hemorrhage may respond to antifibrinolytic therapy with ε-amino caproic acid.[1] Prothrombin deficiency may also be treated with FFP for bleeding episodes or surgical intervention (15 to 20 mL/kg loading dose followed by 3 mL/kg/day). Because of the long half-life, additional doses may not be required in all situations. Cryoprecipitate is not a source of prothrombin, and plasma prothrombin levels do not increase after infusion or inhalation of desmopressin (1-desamino-8-D-arginine vasopressin [DDAVP]).

The postviral hypoprothrombinemia seen in young children often spontaneously resolves. Intravenous immunoglobulin has been effective is this population. Treatment of acquired prothrombin deficiency associated with lupus anticoagulants in patients with autoimmune diseases often requires immune suppression. Steroids are effective in most patients, although many relapse during weaning or after stopping treatment. Subsequent treatment with azathioprine or cyclophosphamide has successfully eradicated the antibody. Rituximab has also been reported to be effective. In a rare case of quinidine-induced lupus anticoagulant with concomitant antiprothrombin antibody, cessation of the drug led to spontaneous resolution of acquired prothrombin deficiency, but not the lupus anticoagulant. The low prothrombin activity in these patients may protect them from thrombosis, as suggested by reports of thrombosis after successful eradication of the antiprothrombin antibody.

FACTOR V DEFICIENCY (OMIM 227400)

In 1943 Quick reported that aged plasma clotted more slowly than fresh plasma in a PT assay, and proposed that a labile factor distinct from prothrombin was required for coagulation. At the same time, Owren noted that a patient with a lifelong bleeding problem lacked a plasma factor that, unlike prothrombin, did not adsorb onto aluminum hydroxide. Owren's patient was deficient in the labile factor described by Quick, which is now called *factor V*. Moderate to severe congenital factor V deficiency (1%–10% of normal level) occurs in 1 in 1 million persons (Table 137.1).[13,14] Full length factor V, a homolog of factor VIII, is the 330,000-Da precursor of the cofactor factor Va, which facilitates prothrombin activation by factor Xa on phospholipid surfaces (Fig. 137.1).[13,14] During coagulation, the B-domain of factor V is removed by thrombin or factor Xa to produce factor Va (Fig. 137.4). An approximately 250,000-Da form of factor V lacking 703 amino acids from the B-domain is a minor constituent in normal plasma (Fig. 137.4). Referred to as factor V-short (or factor V East Texas), it is a product of an alternatively spliced mRNA. Most (80%) factor V in blood is in plasma, with the remainder stored in platelet α-granules.[13] In humans, platelet factor V is primarily of plasma origin. It is taken up by megakaryocytes in a process requiring low-density lipoprotein receptor-related protein-1 (LRP-1), then converted to a partially activated form.[13]

Severe factor V deficiency is an autosomal recessive trait with undetectable (<1% of normal) plasma factor V. In moderate deficiency the level is between 1% and 10% of normal (Table 137.2).[13,14] More than 100 factor V gene mutations have been described in factor V–deficient patients.[13] Nonsense and frameshift mutations and splice variants are common and are distributed throughout the gene. Missense mutations cluster in the A2 and C2 domains,[13,14] and usually result in abnormal polypeptides that are degraded within the cell, resulting in low plasma factor V antigen (CRM – deficiency). While it is estimated that approximately 25% of cases of factor V deficiency are CRM+ mutations (plasma antigen exceeds activity), only two have been characterized. The Ala221Val (factor V New Brunswick) and His147Arg substitutions appear to reduce factor Va activity by affecting protein stability.

Combined deficiency of factor V and factor VIII is caused by mutations in proteins required for secretion of both (see Combined Factor V and Factor VIII Deficiency).[13,14] A few patients have been described with abnormalities specific to platelet factor V.[13] The Quebec platelet disorder is an autosomal dominant condition with

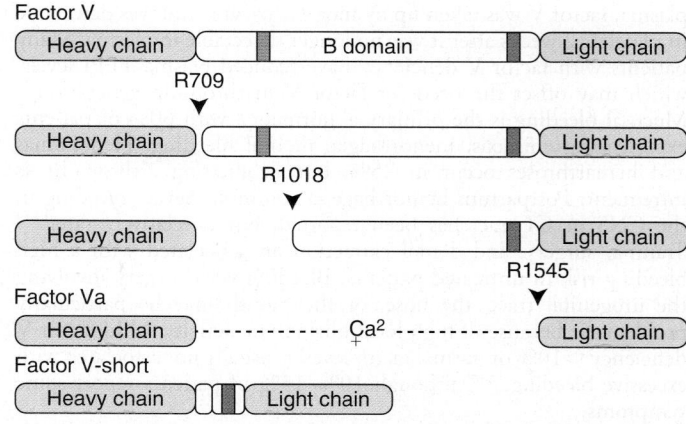

Fig. 137.4 SCHEMATIC DIAGRAMS OF HUMAN FACTOR V AND FACTOR Va. In factor V the heavy and light chains (*yellow*) are separated by a central B domain (*white*, amino acids 710 to 1545) that contains a basic region (blue, amino acids 963 to 1008) and acidic region (*red*, amino acids 1493 to 1537) Removal of the B domain by thrombin to generate factor Va involves sequential cleavages after Arginine 709, 1018 and 1545. Factor V-short is the product of an alternatively spliced factor V mRNA that lacks residues 756 through 1458, which comprise most of the B domain including the basic region. In factor V-short, the loss of the B domain basic region leaves the acidic region free to bind to TFPI.

low platelet factor V and normal plasma factor V levels. In this syndrome, excessive proteolysis of α-granule proteins is caused by overexpression of urokinase. Platelet factor V activity is also reduced in factor V New York, but the underlying mechanism is not known.

The autosomal dominant condition East Texas bleeding disorder is caused by an A2440G nucleotide substitution in exon 13 of the factor V gene. The substitution increases levels of the alternatively spliced mRNA encoding Factor V-short (Fig. 137.4), leading to increased plasma levels of this protein. In East Texas bleeding disorder plasma levels of a key regulator of coagulation, tissue factor pathway inhibitor (TFPI), are 10-fold higher than normal. TFPI-mediated inhibition of factor Xa and the factor VIIa-tissue factor complex likely contributes to the bleeding. In factor V, the B-domain contains basic and acid regions that are thought to bind to each other (Fig. 137.4).[13] In factor V-short, the basic region is missing, leaving the acidic region free to bind to TFPI, stabilizing it in plasma. A similar bleeding disorder was observed in a Dutch family with a C2588G substitution in exon 13 of the factor V gene, leading to alternative mRNA splicing and loss of 632 amino acids from the B domain (factor V Amsterdam). These patients also have markedly elevated plasma TFPI levels.

Acquired factor V deficiency may occur with liver disease, DIC, myeloproliferative disorders or systemic amyloidosis. Patients with acquired antibodies to factor V may have bleeding that can be severe, or may be asymptomatic. Alloantibodies to factor V were often associated with exposure to topical bovine thrombin during surgery, a problem that rarely occurs now because recombinant human thrombin preparations are used. Alloantibodies to factor V also occur in some factor V–deficient patients exposed to human plasma. Factor V autoantibodies may form after surgery or blood transfusions or with cancer, autoimmune disorders, or therapy with β-lactam or aminoglycoside antibiotics.

There is striking variability in bleeding symptoms among patients with severe factor V deficiency.[13,14] Significant bleeding does occur, but the frequency tends to be less than in patients lacking factor VIII or factor IX. Several factors may contribute to the variability. Some patients with mild bleeding symptoms despite low plasma factor V levels have sufficient platelet factor V to support thrombin generation. This implies that their factor V is unstable in plasma, but can be taken up by platelets. Patients with severe bleeding may lack plasma and platelet factor V. In one such individual treated with plasma, factor V was taken up by megakaryocytes and was detectable in platelets 2 weeks after it was no longer detectable in plasma. Many patients with factor V deficiency have reduced plasma TFPI levels, which may offset the need for factor V in thrombin generation.[13] Mucosal bleeding is the primary abnormality, with 60% of patients experiencing epistaxis, menorrhagia, or oral bleeding. Hematomas and hemarthroses occur in 25%, but debilitating arthropathy is infrequent. Postpartum hemorrhage is common. Severe bleeding in the CNS or GI tract has been reported, but is relatively rare.[13,14] Trauma, surgery, and dental extraction are associated with a high bleeding risk in untreated patients. Bleeding with surgery involving the urogenital tract, the nose, or the mouth may be particularly problematic because of high local fibrinolytic activity. Mild factor V deficiency (>10% of normal factor level) is usually not associated with excessive bleeding,[13,14] although 10%–15% of patients report some symptoms.

Thrombosis has been reported in factor V–deficient patients.[13,14] In some cases, the deficiency may not have prevented thrombosis. Indeed, with the exception of prothrombin or factor X deficiency, thrombotic events have been reported in all severe coagulation factor deficiency states. However, the situation with factor V is more complex. Deficiency can occur in patients with the common procoagulant polymorphism factor V Arg506Gln (factor V Leiden). If Arg506Gln and a mutation causing deficiency occur on opposite alleles (in-*trans*), most plasma factor V will have the Gln506 substitution, increasing the thrombotic risk (pseudohomozygous activated protein C resistance). Such patients usually do not bleed excessively, despite reduced plasma factor V antigen.

Factor V is required for normal prothrombin activation (Fig. 137.1B), and factor V deficiency causes prolongation of the PT and aPTT. The diagnosis and severity are established with a modified PT assay with factor V–deficient plasma. With severe deficiency the template bleeding time may be prolonged. Patients with factor V deficiency should be tested for factor VIII deficiency so that combined deficiency is not missed. Factor V inhibitors cause prolongations of the PT and aPTT that do not correct on mixing with normal plasma. As for factor VIII inhibitors, factor V inhibitor titers are established using the Bethesda method.[16] However, unlike inhibitors to factor VIII, which typically take 1 to 2 hours to fully inactivate their target, factor V inhibitors inhibit factor V almost immediately. The thrombin time should be normal, except in cases of inhibition induced by bovine topical thrombin, where antithrombin antibodies are also present. In patients with the East Texas bleeding disorder or factor V Amsterdam the prolonged PT and aPTT are due to the inhibitory effects of TFPI. In these patients the PT and aPTT will not completely correct on mixing with normal plasma, and the factor V activity level will be normal.

No factor V concentrate is commercially available (Table 137.3). Administration of FFP is recommended for serious bleeding or prior to surgery. The minimum factor V level for hemostasis is 10%–15% of normal.[1,2] In a patient with less than 1% plasma factor V, this can be achieved by administering 15 to 20 mL/kg FFP, followed by 5 mL/kg every 12 hours. A plasma level of at least 25% is recommended for major surgery. Estimates of the factor V plasma half-life vary widely, but 12 to 14 hours should be assumed for replacement purposes. Infusion of 20 mL/kg FFP (over 3 to 4 hours) before surgery, followed by 5 to 10 mL/kg every 12 hours is usually adequate. Infusions should be continued for 7 to 10 days to permit wound healing. Care must be taken to avoid fluid overload from large volumes of FFP. Plasma exchange has been successful in a few factor V–deficient patients requiring surgery. Mucosal bleeding from the nose and mouth may respond to ε-amino caproic acid, and superficial lacerations usually respond to local pressure. Although the defect caused by factor V deficiency would hypothetically render therapy with recombinant factor VIIa ineffective, this agent has been used successfully in a patient with severe factor V deficiency requiring surgery.

Menorrhagia is common in factor V–deficient women. Symptoms may be managed with antifibrinolytic therapy (ε-amino caproic acid 50 to 60 mg/kg every 4 to 6 hours or tranexamic acid 15 mg/kg every

6 to 8 hours), oral contraceptives, levonorgestrel-releasing intrauterine devices, replacement therapy, or surgical intervention (endometrial ablation or hysterectomy).[7] Replacement should be adjusted to maintain a factor V level of 10%–15% of normal. Factor V–deficient women may have significant bleeding with childbirth and should be treated in a similar manner.

Platelets are a source of factor V and may be particularly useful in patients with severe bleeding or factor V inhibitors. Platelet factor V may either be protected from inhibition or may be sufficiently different in structure from its plasma counterpart to not cross-react with antibodies directed against factor V. However, platelet transfusions are not recommended as routine first-line treatment for factor V deficiency because of the possibility of developing antiplatelet alloantibodies. Cryoprecipitate is not a source of factor V, and plasma levels do not respond to administration of DDAVP.

FACTOR VII DEFICIENCY (OMIM 227500)

Factor VII deficiency was first reported by Alexander and colleagues in 1951. Severe factor VII deficiency is the most common of the nonhemophilic coagulation factor deficiencies (Table 137.1), with an estimated prevalence of 1 in 500,000 persons.

Factor VII is the 50,000-Da precursor of the protease factor VIIa. Factors VII and VIIa bind to tissue factor, and initiate coagulation through activation of factors X and IX (Fig. 137.1A). Factor VII levels correlate weakly with clinical presentation (Table 137.2). Mice lacking factor VII develop normally in utero but succumb to bleeding at birth. An infant born lacking factor VII died from intracranial hemorrhage 12 days after birth, while another survived with replacement therapy. Thus low levels of factor VII appear to be necessary to sustain life. Activity levels of <10%, 10%–20%, and >20% have been proposed as criteria to classify deficiency as severe, moderate, or mild, respectively.[12] However, many patients with levels <10% will not have significant bleeding, even with invasive procedures. A classification system based on clinical presentation has also been suggested. Although factor VII deficiency is considered an autosomal recessive trait, the observation that bleeding symptoms are reported in up to one-third of patients with heterozygous deficiency raises questions about this concept.

More than 200 factor VII gene mutations associated with factor VII deficiency have been described, well over half of which are missense mutations. Most have been identified in single families, but some are widespread. In surveys of patients from Europe and Latin America, pAla244Val accounted for 84% of abnormal factor VII alleles in 88 unrelated Jewish patients, and in 14% and 7% of abnormal factor VII alleles in Germany and France, respectively. CRM+ variants are common. Some factor VII variants demonstrate variable activity in PT assays, depending on the species of origin of the tissue factor used. The name "factor VII Padua" has been applied to these variants, many of which have an Arg304Gln substitution that causes a defect in the interaction with tissue factor from rabbits, but not humans or oxen.

Factor VII deficiency may occur in combination with deficiencies of other vitamin K–dependent proteins (see Combined Deficiency of Vitamin K–Dependent Proteins) and in combination with factor X deficiency as a result of loss of both genes due to a chromosome 13 q34 deletion. Factor VII deficiency has also been reported in cases of trisomy 8 and in conjunction with abnormalities of bilirubin metabolism, mental retardation, microcephaly, epicanthus, cleft palate, and patent ductus arteriosus.

Reduced levels of factor VII occur with warfarin therapy, poisoning with rodenticides such as brodifacoum, liver disease, DIC, biliary tract disease, vitamin K deficiency, and cephalosporin therapy. In these situations other vitamin K–dependent factors are usually decreased, although the effect on factor VII is often greater because of its short half-life. Alloantibody inhibitors to factor VII have been reported in deficient patients after replacement therapy. Acquired factor VII deficiency has been reported as a paraneoplastic syndrome with atrial myxoma and Wilms tumor. Other scenarios rarely associated with low factor VII include hematopoietic stem cell transplantation, aplastic anemia, and sepsis.

The clinical spectrum of bleeding in factor VII deficiency is broad.[15] Not surprisingly, significant bleeds tend to be most frequent with severe deficiency and patients with levels less than 1% of normal may have a syndrome similar to severe hemophilia, with joint and soft tissue bleeding and hemarthrosis-related arthropathy. The best predictor of future bleeding risk seems to be the nature of bleeding (or its absence) at the time of diagnosis.[15] CNS hemorrhage is relatively common (4% to 17%). Patients with factor VII activity of ≥5% of normal tend to have milder symptoms (epistaxis, menorrhagia, and bruising). Although little bleeding occurs in most patients with factor VII levels ≥10% of normal, some have significant bleeding spontaneously or in response to hemostatic challenges. In one study, 36% of heterozygotes (factor VII activity 21% to 69%) reported bleeding problems, mostly involving skin and mucous membranes, whereas another study reported a greater risk for subcutaneous bleeding in heterozygotes. Bleeding often complicates tooth extraction and surgery on the oropharynx or urogenital tract in untreated patients. Abdominal surgery and hysterectomy are associated with fewer problems. Postpartum bleeding is not common in factor VII–deficient women because factor VII levels rise in late pregnancy in all but the most severely deficient patients. Risk of postpartum hemorrhage correlates poorly with FVII level, leading some to suggest that recombinant factor VIIa be available for excessive bleeding if it occurs.

Thrombosis associated with factor VII deficiency is well documented. A study of 33 reported cases (6 arterial, 27 venous) revealed 15 with molecular studies. Nearly all patients had other thrombotic risk factors, usually acquired, and four had congenital thrombophilia. Of the 15 patients, 11 had either pArg304Gln (factor VII Padua) or pAla294Val. Those with factor VII Padua had no bleeding history, while mild bleeding was reported with pAla294Val. Treatment with vitamin K antagonists is problematic because the baseline PT is abnormal as a result of the mutation. Therapy with low-molecular-weight heparin or one of the newer direct oral anticoagulants may be a better option.

In factor VII deficiency, the PT is prolonged and the aPTT is normal. The diagnosis is confirmed, and the severity determined, by a modified PT assay using factor VII–deficient plasma. With very sensitive thromboplastin reagents, the PT may be prolonged with factor VII levels at the lower end of the normal range. When assessing patients for factor VII deficiency, the source of the tissue factor must be considered. Factor VII Padua–type variants interact poorly with the rabbit tissue factor–based reagents widely used in North America; they function better with human tissue factor and best with ox tissue factor. We routinely retest patients with apparent factor VII deficiency in rabbit tissue factor-based assays with a human tissue factor thromboplastin reagent to detect Padua-type variants.

Major considerations when treating factor VII–deficient patients include the short plasma half-life of the protein (3 to 4 hours), relatively low recovery of infused material (possibly due to a large volume of distribution), and rapid clearance in children.[16] A plasma factor VII level of 15% of normal is probably the minimum required for surgery, with 15% to 25% being adequate in most cases. Of 157 surgeries performed on 83 factor VII–deficient patients with a mean baseline activity of 5% who did not receive prophylaxis, 15.3% had bleeding complications, suggesting that supplementing patients with baseline levels below 10% should prevent bleeding. Factor replacement can be accomplished with several products (Table 137.3). FFP is widely used, but its effectiveness is limited because of the large volumes required. PCC contains variable amounts of factor VII; however, these products contain other vitamin K–dependent factors in higher concentrations than factor VII, which could increase the risk for thrombosis. Recombinant factor VIIa (rfVIIa) is the preferred therapy for treating or preventing bleeding in factor VII deficiency. A prospective registry of FVII deficient patients recorded the replacement therapy given for various bleeding events (hemarthrosis, soft-tissue hematomas, epistaxis, gum bleeding, menorrhagia and others) and found that the majority responded adequately to a single relatively large dose of rfVIIa (60 μg/kg).[16] The exception was treating

menorrhagia, which often required subsequent doses.[16] Prophylaxis for invasive procedures may require treatment every 2 to 3 hours. In a study of 41 surgeries in 34 factor VII–deficient subjects receiving rfVIIa, bleeding occurred in only three instances, and in those, the rfVIIa dose was considered low. The minimum treatment that adequately prevented bleeding was 13 μg/kg/dose, and no less than three doses given on the day of surgery. However, patients may do quite well with much less. In one report, two doses on the day of surgery followed by daily dosing successfully controlled bleeding. Continuous infusion rfVIIa has been used to cover surgical procedures and may reduce the total amount of drug administered by 70% to 90% compared with bolus infusions.

Patients with severe factor VII deficiency who have experienced life-threatening bleeding may benefit from secondary prophylaxis, particularly if bleeding involved the CNS (50% to 70% mortality). FFP and plasma-derived factor VII concentrate have been used, but rfVIIa is the preferred agent. Interestingly, despite its short half-life, rfVIIa is effective at doses of 20 to 30 μg/kg given 2 to 3 times per week.[17] The large volume of distribution for both rfVIIa and plasma-derived FVII may explain this effect. In one registry, inhibitors were reported in 4 of 225 patients with activity levels less than 4% who received replacement. All were high titer responders (three developed in infancy). Not all bleeding episodes in factor VII–deficient patients require factor replacement. Minor injuries may be controlled with local measures. Fibrinolytic inhibitors, such as ε-amino caproic acid, may be effective for minor bleeding, dental surgery, or other procedures involving mucous membranes. Fibrin glue may also be effective.[2] Cryoprecipitate is not a source of factor VII. Plasma levels do not respond to administration of DDAVP. An infant with severe deficiency was cured with liver transplantation. AAV-vector gene therapy has shown promising results in mice and macaques, raising FVII levels to therapeutic ranges.

FACTOR X DEFICIENCY (OMIM 227600)

Factor X deficiency was first described in two patients more than 50 years ago. The missing plasma factor was called *Stuart-Prower factor* after the two index cases, and subsequently designated factor X. Patient Stuart was thought to have factor VII deficiency, but mixing his plasma with factor VII–deficient plasma corrected the clotting defect. Patient Prower had multiple coagulation assay abnormalities. The prevalence of severe factor X deficiency is estimated at approximately 1 in 1 million persons (Table 137.1).[18] Factor X is a 58,000-Da protein that is the precursor of the protease factor Xa. Factor X is activated by the factor VIIa/tissue factor complex and by the factor IXa/factor VIIIa complex (Fig. 137.1A). Factor Xa catalyzes conversion of prothrombin to thrombin, and the conversion of factor V to factor Va.

Congenital factor X deficiency is an autosomal recessive trait. Factor X–deficient mice die in utero or shortly after birth from bleeding, indicating the protein is necessary for life. Humans with the severest form of factor X deficiency (activity <1% of normal) probably have a trace of factor X in their plasmas. More than 100 factor X gene mutations have been identified in factor X–deficient patients. Most are missense mutations and many are CRM+ variants.[18] A three part classification system has been proposed. Type I deficiencies involve CRM–mutations, and include patient Stuart (homozygous for Val298Met). Type II deficiencies are CRM+ variants lacking activity, and include patient Prower (compound heterozygote for Arg287Trp and Asp282Asn). Type III deficiency includes variants that are activated normally by Russell viper venom but not by factor VIIa/tissue factor or factor IXa/VIIIa, variants defective only in activation by factor VIIa/tissue factor, variants defective only in activation by factor IXa/VIIIa, and variants with higher activity in chromogenic assays than clotting assays. Factor X deficiency can be inherited with deficiencies of other vitamin K–dependent proteins (see Combined Deficiency of Vitamin K–dependent Proteins) and in combination with factor VII deficiency when both genes are lost due to a chromosome 13 q34 deletion.

Acquired factor X deficiency occurs with warfarin therapy, poisoning with rodenticides such as brodifacoum, vitamin K deficiency, liver disease, and DIC, all of which reduce levels of other coagulation factors. Factor X deficiency has been reported with malignancies, infections, burn injury,[204] proteinuria, and medications. There are rare reports of acquired factor X inhibitors, most of which resolve after treatment of underlying conditions.[19] Acquired factor X deficiency may accompany systemic amyloidosis, occurring in 8.7% to 14% of patients with AL amyloidosis, but rarely in secondary (AA) amyloidosis.[20] Factor X binds to amyloid fibrils, which reduces the plasma half-life of the protein. Distinguishing this disorder from inherited factor X deficiency is based on the clinical setting and evidence of poor clinical response to infusion of factor X–containing products in amyloidosis patients.

A clinical classification system for factor X deficiency has been proposed based on factor X activity (severe, <10%; moderate, 10%–40%; mild, >40% of normal activity) (Table. 137.2). Bleeding in factor X deficiency is severe and occurs earlier in life in patients with the lowest plasma levels.[18] There is an impression that factor X–deficient patients bleed more severely than patients with other congenital coagulopathies. In a series of 102 factor X–deficient patients, the most frequent symptom was easy bruising (55%) followed by hematomas (43%). Epistaxis and hemarthrosis were common. Intracranial hemorrhage was seen in patients homozygous for the pGly380Arg mutation. Among homozygotes, hemarthrosis was very common, and all women suffered from menorrhagia. Umbilical stump bleeding occurred in 28% of newborns. Moderate to mildly affected persons (activity >10%) may have increased bruising or bleeding with trauma. While heterozygotes tend to be asymptomatic, up to one-third may have excessive bleeding from mucous membranes with invasive procedures, or with childbirth.

Because factor X is a component of the common pathway of coagulation (Fig. 137.1B), its absence prolongs the PT and aPTT, and factor X deficiency must be distinguished from deficiencies of fibrinogen, prothrombin, or factor V. Definitive diagnosis and determination of severity are established using a modified PT or aPTT assay with factor X–deficient plasma. Some factor X variants preferentially prolong either the PT or the aPTT. Congenital factor X deficiency cannot be distinguished from acquired deficiency due to amyloidosis in the laboratory, because factor X-dependent assays correct after mixing with normal plasma in both conditions. The absence of a lifelong bleeding disorder, findings of a serum M-protein, signs of amyloidosis, and histologic confirmation of amyloid in tissues point toward AL amyloidosis. A poor response to factor X infusion in the absence of an inhibitor also distinguishes the two conditions.

Factor X–deficient patients are treated with FFP or PCC for bleeding episodes (Table 137.2).[18] A trough level of 10% to 20% is usually sufficient for hemarthroses and soft tissue bleeding. The half-life of factor X is 20 to 40 hours. FFP administered as a loading dose of 10 to 20 mL/kg followed by 3 to 6 mL/kg every 12 to 24 hours usually keeps trough levels above 10 to 20%.[2,18] Higher factor X levels may be required for severe bleeding or surgery, and accumulation of factor X in plasma can be achieved by increasing the transfusion frequency to every 12 hours. PCCs with a factor X to factor IX ratio of approximately 1 : 1 will increase plasma factor X levels by 1.5% for each factor IX unit/kg body weight. A dose of 15 to 20 factor IX units/kg every 1 to 2 days has been suggested for major surgery.[2,18] While no patient with congenital factor X deficiency has been reported to have thrombosis, there is a risk of thrombosis or DIC with PCC, and it is recommended that the plasma factor X level not exceed 50% of normal when using these products, unless absolutely necessary. Factor X levels will rise slightly in pregnancy, but severely deficient patients will require prophylaxis with invasive procedures and at delivery to prevent hemorrhage. A factor X level of 20%–40% is recommended. For patients with severe deficiency and recurrent hemorrhage, prophylactic PCC or factor X concentrate infusion is effective.[18] Minor bleeding can be treated with local measures and/or ε-amino caproic acid. Cryoprecipitate lacks factor X, and DDAVP infusion does not affect factor X levels. A factor X concentrate is now

approved for clinical use in the United States and Europe and is considered the treatment of choice. As with prothrombin deficiency, there are no reports of acquired alloantibody inhibitors to factor X after replacement therapy in congenitally deficient patients, consistent with the concept that these patients have trace amount of plasma factor X at baseline. Severe factor X deficiency was cured by liver transplantation in a child.

Patients with acquired factor X deficiency and amyloidosis have variable responses to infusion of products containing factor X, making individual pharmacokinetic studies of factor X replacement therapy important. Treatment may involve chemotherapy, splenectomy, plasma exchange, PCCs,[21] activated factor VIIa and factor X concentrate. The optimal hemostatic management for invasive procedures has not been determined. In one series, complications occurred in only 13% of procedures, and there was a poor correlation between the risk for bleeding and factor X levels.

FACTOR XI DEFICIENCY (OMIM 264900)

In 1953 Rosenthal and colleagues described three members of a family with abnormal hemostasis, prolonged time to clot formation in a glass tube, and a normal PT. In mixing studies, patient plasma shortened the clotting times of hemophilia A and B plasmas, indicating the missing factor was distinct from factors VIII and IX. Unlike the X-linked hemophilias, the new disorder (sometimes called hemophilia C) was transmitted as an autosomal trait. The missing factor was called *plasma thromboplastin antecedent* and subsequently *factor XI*. It is estimated that severe factor XI deficiency (<15% of normal plasma level) occurs in 1 per million persons (Table 137.1), although perhaps this number should be higher, as patients with milder deficiencies are often symptomatic. Severe factor XI deficiency is common in persons of Ashkenazi Jewish ancestry (incidence of 1 in 450).[22] Factor XI is the precursor of the 160,000-Da protease factor XIa, which contributes to clotting by activating factor IX (Fig. 137.1A). The protein is a homodimer, a feature that has implications for inheritance of factor XI deficiency. Factor XI is activated by factor XIIa in the aPTT assay (Fig. 137.1B); however, it is probably activated by other proteases in vivo because factor XII deficiency does not cause abnormal bleeding. For example, factor XI is also activated by thrombin (Fig. 137.1A).

Factor XI deficiency in the Jewish population and in many other patients is an autosomal recessive condition.[22] Two point mutations account for over 90% of mutant factor XI alleles in Ashkenazi Jews. Glu117Stop encodes a truncated protein, and homozygotes lack plasma factor XI.[237] Glu117Stop is at least 2500 years old and is found in Jews from different ethnic backgrounds, and non-Jewish patients. Phe283Leu, occurs primarily in Jews of European ancestry and is likely of recent origin. It causes a defect in dimer formation resulting in poor secretion; with homozygotes having about 10% of normal plasma factor XI activity. Compound heterozygotes for Glu117Stop and Phe283Leu have about 3% normal activity, while heterozygotes for either mutation have activities of 50% to 60%. The allele frequencies of Glu117Stop and Phe283Leu in Ashkenazi Jews (2.2% and 2.5%, respectively) indicate a carrier frequency for an abnormal factor XI allele of approximately 5%.

More than 200 human factor XI gene mutations have been identified, and several are relatively widespread with evidence of founder effects.[22] Cys38Arg has an allele frequency of 0.5% in French Basques, Cys128Stop accounts for 10% of abnormal alleles in Great Britain, and Gln88Stop is present in several families from France. In most deficient patients, factor XI activity and antigen are comparably reduced (CRM − deficiency). CRM+ factor XI mutations are rare. A three-category scheme has been proposed for classifying CRM − factor XI deficiency. Category one contains mutations that prevent protein synthesis (e.g., Glu117Stop), while mutations in category two interfere with dimer formation (e.g., Phe283Leu). Inheritance in both categories follows a recessive pattern, because mutant polypeptides do not interfere with the product of the normal allele in heterozygotes. Category three includes mutations that impair secretion but do not prevent dimer formation (e.g., Gly400Val). In heterozygotes, mutant and wild-type polypeptides form nonsecretable dimers, trapping normal protein in the cell. This phenomenon likely accounts for families in which severe to moderate factor XI deficiency appears to be a dominant trait.

Factor XI levels decrease in liver disease and DIC but are not affected by vitamin K deficiency or warfarin therapy. Mild to moderate factor XI deficiency occurs in approximately 25% of patients with Noonan syndrome and is common in carbohydrate-deficient glycoprotein syndrome, a group of inherited disorders involving defects in glycosylation of secretory glycoproteins. Antibody inhibitors to factor XI are common after replacement therapy, particularly in patients with no circulating factor XI. For example, one-third of individuals homozygous for Glu117Stop develop inhibitors, often after a single exposure to plasma.

Bleeding in severe factor XI deficiency is usually injury-related and is most frequent in tissues with robust fibrinolytic activity, such as the oral and nasal cavities, and the urinary tract.[22] Injury to these areas causes excessive bleeding in two-thirds of patients, regardless of genotype. Bleeding with injury at other locations is less frequent and tends to occur in those with the lowest factor XI levels. Bleeding may start at the time of injury or be delayed by hours, and oozing from tooth extraction may persist for days. Excessive bleeding with skin laceration, circumcision, appendectomy, and orthopedic surgery is infrequent; spontaneous bleeding (except for menorrhagia) is uncommon. In a clinical trial testing reduction of plasma factor XI as prophylaxis for venous thrombosis in knee replacement surgery, bleeding was rare despite the fact that factor XI levels were less than 5% at the time of surgery in some patients.

Bleeding correlates poorly with plasma factor XI activity (Table 137.2).[22,23] Patients with severe deficiency may not bleed excessively, even during surgery, and a patient may exhibit different bleeding tendencies over time. Opinions differ regarding the propensity to bleed with mild deficiency (plasma level 20%–50%). Some studies describe minimal bleeding with tooth extraction, tonsillectomy, nasal surgery, and urologic surgery, while others report difficulty distinguishing severe and mild deficiency on clinical grounds.[22,23] In a study of 45 families, the odds ratios for excessive bleeding were 13.0 and 2.6 for homozygotes and heterozygotes, respectively. Thus mild deficiency may confer a slightly increased risk for bleeding, but not as much as severe deficiency. A recent analysis indicated that ristocetin cofactor activity is significantly lower in symptomatic patients with heterozygous factor XI deficiency, compared with nonbleeders, raising the possibility that von Willebrand factor levels influence bleeding propensity. Recent work suggests that thrombin generation tests and analyses of fibrin clot structure can predict the propensity to bleed, but these findings require confirmation in prospective studies.

In the aPTT assay, factor XI is bound to the contact surface through high-molecular-weight kininogen (HK) and is activated by factor XIIa (Figs. 137.1B and 137.5). Factor XIa, in turn, activates factor IX. Therefore, factor XI deficiency prolongs the aPTT, but not the PT. Diagnosis and severity are established by a modified aPTT assay using factor XI–deficient plasma. The aPTT is often normal in heterozygotes.

Perioperative therapy should be individualized for factor XI–deficient patients (see box on Treating Factor XI–Deficient Patients). For those requiring replacement, FFP or factor XI concentrate (Hemoleven or FXI concentrate) (Table 137.2), effectively prevent bleeding.[24] The half-life of factor XI is 45 to 52 hours, facilitating daily or every-other-day dosing. Hemoleven has orphan drug status in the United States. A 3-year postmarketing analysis of this concentrate indicated that it was effective as prophylaxis for surgery, invasive procedures, and pregnancy, and for treating bleeding.[24] However, it is recommended that concentrates be used sparingly due to potential prothrombotic effects. In the past, factor XI concentrates were associated with thrombosis and DIC, mostly in older patients with cardiovascular disease receiving doses over 30 units/kg.[22] However, more recent analyses indicate that patients receiving 20 to 30 units/kg also have thrombotic events. Based on this, it has been suggested that the

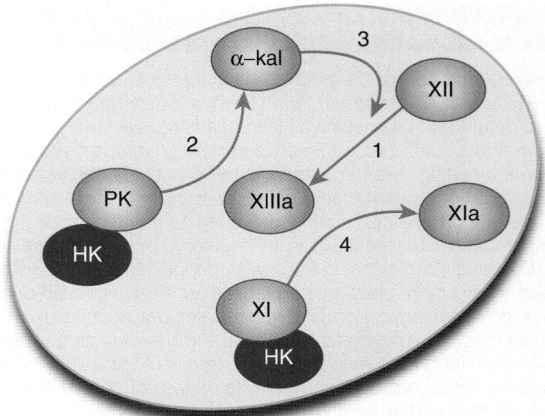

Fig. 137.5 CONTACT ACTIVATION. In the activated partial thromboplastin time assay, contact activation is initiated by conversion of factor XII (XII) to α-factor XIIa (XIIa) (reaction 1) when plasma is exposed to a negatively charged surface *(light green disk)*. Factor XIIa converts prekallikrein (PK) to the active protease α-kallikrein (reaction 2), and α-kallikrein reciprocally activates additional factor XII (reaction 3). Factor XIIa initiates coagulation through conversion of factor XI (XI) to factor XIa (XIa) (reaction 4). PK and factor XI require high-molecular-weight kininogen (HK) to bind properly to the surface. Factor XIa ultimately promotes thrombin generation and fibrin clot formation through activation of factor IX (see Fig. 137.1).

initial dose should not exceed 10 to 15 units/kg, and concentrates should be used with caution (or avoided) in patients with a history of thrombosis, or risk factors for thrombosis.[2] Antifibrinolytic therapy should probably not be used concomitantly with concentrate. Cryoprecipitate does not contain factor XI.

Circumcision, orthopedic surgery, and appendectomy carry a low bleeding risk, and replacement can often be withheld unless bleeding occurs.[22] A similar "wait and see" approach has been proposed for factor XI–deficient women during labor and delivery, which is associated with a relatively low (~20%) rate of excessive bleeding.[22] However, others advocate replacement for childbirth.[2] Dental procedures such as tooth extraction can be covered with antifibrinolytic therapy.[22] The effectiveness of DDAVP in mild factor XI deficiency is not established, but there are reports that levels increase in response to this drug. Factor XI–deficient patients with inhibitors do not usually have increased spontaneous bleeding. Recombinant factor VIIa has been used successfully for surgery in factor XI–deficient patients with and without inhibitors, and to cover epidural block in deficient women during labor and delivery.

DEFICIENCIES OF FACTOR XII, PREKALLIKREIN OR HIGH-MOLECULAR-WEIGHT KININOGEN

Factor XII, prekallikrein, and HK are required for normal factor XI activation in the "contact phase" that initiates coagulation in the aPTT assay (Figs. 137.1B and 137.5). Patients lacking one of these proteins have prolonged aPTTs, but do not have abnormal hemostasis, even with surgery or injury. Therefore, these proteins either do not participate in hemostasis, or redundant mechanisms compensate for their absence. No specific therapy is required to prepare deficient patients for invasive procedures. Factor XII, prekallikrein or HK deficiency must be distinguished from deficiencies of factors VIII, IX, or XI, which prolong the aPTT, but cause abnormal hemostasis.

Factor XII Deficiency (OMIM 234000)

In 1955 Ratnoff and Colopy described asymptomatic individuals with a novel abnormality of surface-induced coagulation. The missing plasma component was called *Hageman factor*, after the index case,

Treating Factor XI–Deficient Patients

When preparing patients with severe factor XI deficiency (plasma factor XI level <15%–20% of normal) for an invasive procedure it is important to keep in mind that (1) a negative bleeding history does not indicate a low risk with subsequent procedures, (2) certain procedures are associated with lower bleeding risks than others, and (3) patients with very low factor XI levels (<1%) frequently develop neutralizing inhibitors after replacement therapy. These observations have led to refinements in treatment recommendations that limit exposure to factor XI by targeting replacement to certain clinical situations. In the Jewish population, patients with severe deficiency have more bleeding problems than those with mild deficiency, but this does not appear to hold for the general population. The poor correlation between plasma factor XI level and bleeding propensity means that some patients with mild deficiency (levels of 20%–40% of normal) may require factor replacement for certain types of procedures, such as surgery on the prostate or on the oral and nasal cavity.

Antiplatelet drugs should be stopped one week before surgery. The prothrombin time and platelet count should be normal, and the possibility of co-existing hemostatic abnormalities thoroughly investigated. Patients with factor XI levels greater than 40% to 50% of normal generally do not experience abnormal bleeding, and a history of excessive bleeding in such an individual suggests other hemostatic abnormalities are present. If the patient has been exposed to factor XI in the recent past, the possibility that a neutralizing inhibitor is present should be considered.

Factor replacement is required for most major surgery in factor XI deficient patients, and should be initiated prior to the procedure. Surgery on the oropharynx, nasopharynx or urinary tract should be treated with fresh frozen plasma (FFP) or factor XI concentrate to keep the plasma trough factor XI level above 40% of normal for at least seven days. Administering FFP at 15 mL/kg every 1 to 2 days is the most common way to achieve this. A similar strategy is appropriate for neurosurgery, head and neck surgery, cardiothoracic procedures, and major abdominal or pelvic surgery. For nasal surgery and oral procedures such as tonsillectomy, supplementing FFP therapy with antifibrinolytic therapy should be considered. Antifibrinolytics must be used with caution in patients receiving factor XI concentrate because of the potential for thrombotic events. For prostatectomy and other surgery on the lower urinary tract, flushing the bladder with saline containing an antifibrinolytic agent may be beneficial. In some types of minor surgery patients may receive replacement to maintain levels of 30% for 5 days. However, a "wait and see" strategy in which replacement is withheld unless bleeding occurs appears to be appropriate for procedures such as circumcision, appendectomy and some orthopedic surgery, and with normal vaginal deliveries. In a recent phase 2 trial in which antisense oligonucleotide therapy was used to reduce plasma factor XI as prophylaxis to prevent venous thrombosis in total knee arthroplasty, patients underwent surgery with factor XI levels as low as a few percent of normal, without excessive bleeding. This demonstrates that factor XI probably plays a minor role, at most, in hemostasis during certain types of procedures. In pregnancy, there is little data to evaluate the safety of epidural anesthesia in the absence of factor coverage, and replacement therapy is generally advised.

Low doses of recombinant factor VIIa (15–30 µg/kg) every 2 to 4 hours in conjunction with antifibrinolytic therapy has been used successfully in lieu of replacement therapy in patients without factor XI inhibitors undergoing surgery. This strategy may be preferable to factor replacement in some patients with very low plasma factor XI levels (<1% of normal) because of their propensity to develop neutralizing antifactor XI antibodies. In patients with known factor XI inhibitors, a strategy based on a single dose of recombinant factor VIIa (15–30 µg/kg) followed by antifibrinolytic therapy maintained hemostasis in several patients undergoing major surgery, including a patient who required repair of an aortic dissection. The higher doses of factor VIIa typically used to treat patients with factor VIII inhibitors are not required in factor XI deficient patients with or without inhibitors, and should not be used as they may increase the risk of thrombotic complications.

Alternatives to factor replacement are recommended in several situations. Tooth extraction or skin biopsies can be managed with antifibrinolytic drugs alone (ε-amino caproic acid 5 to 6 g q6 hours or tranexamic acid 1 to 1.3 g q6 hours), starting 12 hours before the procedure and continuing for seven days. Dental procedures such as scaling or root canal can be performed safely using ε-amino caproic acid or tranexamic acid mouthwash prepared from the intravenous formulation three to four times daily with or without systemic antifibrinolytic therapy. Fibrin glues can be used in place of fibrinolytic therapy for skin biopsy or resection of skin lesions.

Patients with factor XI deficiency can experience thromboembolic episodes. Aspirin or clopidogrel can be used in factor XI-deficient patients with myocardial infarction or other manifestations of atherosclerosis, while atrial fibrillation or venous thromboembolism should be treated with warfarin, with the goal of not allowing the international normalized ratio (INR) to exceed 2.5.

---

and later designated *factor XII*. The incidence of severe factor XII deficiency is not known as many deficient persons likely go undiagnosed. Factor XII deficiency was reported in 1.5% to 3.0% of healthy blood donors. This high number may be partly explained by antifactor XII or antiphospholipid antibodies that interfere with factor XII activity assays. α-Factor XIIa, the activated form of factor XII, is an 80,000-Da protease that activates factor XI and prekallikrein in the contact phase of the PTT assay (Fig. 137.5). A C/T polymorphism in the 5'-untranslated region of the factor XII gene (referred to as 46C/T [or −4C/T]) strongly influences plasma factor XII levels. The frequency of 46T is high (73%) in Japanese and Han Chinese individuals who have lower factor XII levels than members of other ethnic groups, compared to 20% in whites. Factor XII activity and antigen are usually reduced in parallel, and circulating dysfunctional variants are rare.

About thirty factor XII gene mutations have been identified. Factor XII deficiency is not associated with spontaneous or excessive posttraumatic bleeding, and most cases are identified by the incidental finding of a prolonged aPTT. There is conflicting literature regarding an association between factor XII deficiency and thrombosis. Two studies reported an inverse relationship between plasma factor XII levels within the broad normal range and the risk of cardiovascular events; however, most work indicates that severe deficiency does not prevent thrombosis or increase its risk. A meta-analysis of studies examining the 46C/T factor XII gene polymorphism suggests that the correlation between the polymorphism and venous thrombosis or myocardial infarction, if present, is weak. There are reports linking low factor XII levels to pregnancy loss or failure of in vitro fertilization. Interestingly, factor XII deficient mice do not display an abnormality in reproduction. It is possible that antibodies that interfere with factor XII function, rather than true deficiency, are responsible for pregnancy-related complications in humans.

Factor XII undergoes autoactivation when exposed to the contact surface used to initiate clotting in the aPTT assay. Factor XIIa activates prekallikrein to α-kallikrein, which reciprocally activates additional factor XII (Fig. 137.3). Factor XIIa also activates factor XI to XIa. In severe factor XII deficiency the aPTT is very long. Definitive diagnosis is established using a modified aPTT with factor XII–deficient plasma. Antiphospholipid antibodies may disproportionately affect factor XII measurements in aPTT-based assays. Factor XII antibodies are present in up to half of plasmas with antiphospholipid antibodies, and may account for many cases of presumed mild factor XII deficiency.

Prekallikrein Deficiency (OMIM 229000)

In 1965 Hathaway and coworkers described members of a family with long plasma clotting times that corrected on prolonged incubation with glass. They did not have histories of abnormal hemostasis. The missing plasma component, initially called *Fletcher factor* after the index cases, was subsequently shown to be prekallikrein. Severe prekallikrein deficiency appears to be rare. Mild cases may be missed because a low level of prekallikrein activity is often sufficient to bring many PTT assays into the normal range. Prekallikrein is the 95,000-Da precursor of the protease α-kallikrein. Prekallikrein deficiency is an autosomal trait, presenting in the homozygous or compound heterozygous forms with plasma levels usually less than 1% of normal. CRM+ variants account for about half of cases, and are common in white and Japanese patients, while most black patients are CRM −. Partial deficiency (10%–50 %) may be seen in patients with severe HK deficiency, likely due to increased clearance because prekallikrein circulates in complex with HK. Severe prekallikrein deficiency presents as a prolongation of the aPTT in a person without a history of excessive bleeding. While thrombotic events have been described in deficient patients, it is not clear that the deficiency contributed to thrombosis. Indeed, studies in mice indicate that reducing prekallikrein levels actually attenuates thrombus formation. A recent analysis raised the possibility that the incidence of hypertension may be higher in prekallikrein deficient individuals than the general population, possibly related to reduced bradykinin formation.

In the aPTT assay, prekallikrein is converted to α-kallikrein by factor XIIa, which then activates factor XII (Fig. 137.5). Severe prekallikrein deficiency causes a prolonged aPTT, and the diagnosis is confirmed using a modified aPTT with prekallikrein deficient plasma. The prolonged aPTT in prekallikrein deficiency may be shortened by increased incubation time with the contact reagent, which facilitates factor XII activation independently of prekallikrein. This distinguishes prekallikrein deficiency from deficiencies of factors VIII, IX, XI XII, and HK, in which the prolonged aPTT does not correct with prolonged incubation. Those aPTT reagents that use ellagic acid as the contact activator are relatively insensitive to prekallikrein, and may fail to detect some deficient patients.

High-Molecular-Weight Kininogen Deficiency (OMIM 228960)

In 1974 Schiffman and Lee reported that a plasma factor distinct from prekallikrein was required for factor XI activation by factor XIIa. In 1975 asymptomatic individuals from three distinct families were described with in vitro abnormalities of coagulation, fibrinolysis, and kinin generation who appeared to lack the unknown factor. The condition, originally named for the affected families (Fitzgerald trait, Williams trait, and Flaujeac trait), was subsequently determined to be due to HK deficiency. The disorder appears to be very rare. HK is a 110,000-Da protein containing the vasoactive peptide bradykinin. Prekallikrein and factor XI circulate in complex with HK. Low-molecular-weight kininogen and HK are products of a single kininogen gene; however, low-molecular-weight kininogen does not play a role in coagulation in vitro. HK deficiency is an autosomal recessive trait. Depending on the genetic abnormality, patients may have isolated HK deficiency or combined HK and low-molecular-weight kininogen deficiency. HK deficient patients are usually identified by the incidental finding of a prolonged aPTT, and they do not bleed excessively.

In the aPTT assay, HK facilitates binding of prekallikrein and factor XI to the contact surface, enhancing their activation by factor XIIa (Fig. 137.5). Severe deficiency is characterized by a very prolonged aPTT, and definitive diagnosis is established using a modified aPTT with HK deficient plasma. Partial prekallikrein deficiency is common in severe HK deficiency, likely due to increased catabolism of prekallikrein when it is not in complex with HK.

FACTOR XIII DEFICIENCY (OMIM 134570 [A SUBUNIT] AND 134580 [B SUBUNIT])

In 1944 Robbins demonstrated that fibrin formed from purified fibrinogen was soluble in weak acid, while fibrin formed in the presence of serum or plasma was not. He proposed that a fibrin-stabilizing factor was present in plasma. In 1960 Duckert and colleagues described the first patient with deficiency of fibrin-stabilizing factor, which was subsequently designated factor XIII. The incidence

of severe factor XIII deficiency is estimated at 1 in 2 million (Table 137.1).[25,26] Factor XIII in blood is distributed between plasma and platelets, with a small amount in monocytes. The plasma protein is a 330,000-Da tetramer composed of two catalytic A subunits and two carrier B subunits.[25,26] Factor XIII in platelets, monocytes, and placenta has only A subunits. The A subunit of the protein in plasma appears to be synthesized primarily in hematopoietic cells, while the B subunit comes from the liver. Factor XIII is converted to the transglutaminase factor XIIIa by thrombin, and catalyzes formation of γ-glutamyl-ε-lysyl bonds between fibrin monomers (Fig. 137.1A), resulting in a fibrin mesh resistant to dissolution in mild acid or urea. Factor XIIIa also cross-links fibrin to plasma, extracellular matrix, and cytoskeletal proteins, enhancing clot adherence to an injury site. Congenital factor XIII deficiency is an autosomal recessive condition. The current classification scheme recognizes factor XIII-A and factor XIII-B defects. Factor XIII-A deficiency is divided into type I (quantitative) and type II (qualitative) deficiencies. In patients with apparent combined FXIII-A and -B deficiency, low levels of the A subunit are likely the result of rapid clearance because of the absence of the stabilizing B subunit.

Most cases of congenital factor XIII deficiency are due to mutations in the A subunit gene, with less than 5% in the B subunit gene. More than 75 different mutations have been reported in the factor XIII-A gene, and more than 20 in the factor XIII-B gene (www.f13-database.de). The incidence of factor XIII mutations affecting plasma activity is probably higher than suspected, considering that screening test abnormalities occur mostly in those with severely decreased plasma activity (<5% of normal). A few mutations show evidence of a founder effect, with the IVS5–1 G>A splice-site defect and Arg-661Stop nonsense mutation each identified in 10 apparently unrelated individuals.

Plasma factor XIII levels decrease in DIC and liver disease. Significant deficiency is rare in liver disease and may indicate a poor prognosis. Acquired deficiency has been reported in leukemia, Crohn disease, ulcerative colitis, and Henoch-Schönlein purpura, but levels are usually greater than 30% of normal and replacement is not required. Alloantibodies to factor XIII induced by replacement therapy are relatively uncommon in factor XIII–deficient patients. Neutralizing autoantibodies that block the activation, activity, or fibrin binding capacity of the factor XIII-A subunit, or that enhance factor XIII clearance from plasma, have been reported in older adults, in patients with systemic lupus erythematosus and lymphoproliferative disorders, and with medications such as isoniazid, penicillin, procainamide, phenytoin, and practolol. An autoantibody to the B subunit that developed in a patient with systemic lupus erythematosus enhanced clearance of the protein from plasma and was associated with life-threatening bleeding.

In patients with factor XIII levels ≤5% of normal, delayed bleeding from the umbilical stump occurs in 80% to 90% of newborns with severe factor XIII deficiency and is considered a diagnostic feature of the disorder.[25,26] Ecchymoses, soft tissue hematomas, and prolonged bleeding with trauma are common, and recurrent soft tissue bleeding may lead to formation of hemorrhagic cysts (pseudotumors).[25,26] Hemarthroses is less frequent than in factor VIII or IX deficiency. Bleeding that is delayed 12 to 36 hours postinjury is characteristic of factor XIII deficiency, although hemorrhage is immediate in some cases. Bleeding at the time of invasive procedures may be minimal, but delayed hemorrhage often occurs. Intracranial bleeding is more frequent in factor XIII deficiency than in other inherited coagulation disorder, with an incidence as high as 30%,[25,26] justifying prophylactic replacement. Delayed wound healing has been observed, possibly related to a defect in angiogenesis. Spontaneous abortions occur with most pregnancies in untreated factor XIII–deficient women,[25,26] possibly due to abnormal formation of the cytotrophoblastic shell and poor attachment of the placenta to the uterus. The issue of excessive bleeding in patients with milder (>5% of normal) factor XIII deficiency is more controversial. In at least two studies, patients heterozygous for factor XIII deficiency reported excessive bleeding, but these studies lacked control groups. Experience with pregnant women with severe factor XIII deficiency shows that the factor XIII level needs to be higher than 10% to reliably prevent pregnancy loss, indicating that clinically significant problems can occur in patients with levels higher than 5% of normal.

The PT and aPTT measure time to fibrin clot formation, but do not assess clot stability. Thus results for these assays are normal in factor XIII–deficient patients. Clots formed in plasma lacking factor XIII are soluble in 5 M urea or 1% monochloroacetic acid, while clots from normal plasma are stable. Solubility in 5 M urea (urea clot stability assay) is often used to screen for factor XIII deficiency or inhibitors. Plasma clots lacking α_2-antiplasmin are also soluble in the urea clot stability assay, and can be identified with specific assays. Solubility tests have low sensitivity for factor XIII deficiency, even failing to detect some samples with <2% of normal activity and probably almost all samples with levels ≥5% of normal.[27] Chromogenic assays that quantitatively measure factor XIIIa activity are available and are replacing the urea clot stability assays in many institutions.[27] These assays can also be used to detect and quantify neutralizing factor XIII inhibitors, using a mixing method with normal plasma.

The plasma half-life of factor XIII is 10 to 14 days,[25,26] facilitating prophylactic replacement therapy. Although some consider a level of 5% adequate for hemostasis, others suggest levels greater than 10% are required to reduce bleeding risk. FFP and cryoprecipitate contain factor XIII; however, the factor XIII concentrate Fibrogammin P (marketed as Corifact in the United States; Table 137.2) is preferred for replacement.[25,26] Fibrogammin P contains factor XIII purified from human plasma and is pasteurized. Recombinant factor XIII-A subunit (Tretten) received FDA approval in December 2013 to prevent bleeding in patients with congenital factor XIII A-subunit deficiency. Tretten is produced in yeast and contains no human blood component. In a prospective study, prophylactic replacement with recombinant factor XIII to maintain activity at >0.05–0.2 IU/mL prevented spontaneous bleeding without adverse effects.[28]

Dosing regimens are the same for plasma derived and recombinant factor XIII. A regimen of 40 units/kg every 4 weeks is recommended for prophylaxis. Although concentrated recombinant or plasma-derived factor XIII are preferred for prophylaxis (or treatment of acute bleeding), if it is not available, FFP (10–20 mL/kg every 4 to 6 weeks) or cryoprecipitate (1 unit for every 10 to 20 kg body weight every 3 to 4 weeks) can be used. A dose of 20 to 30 units/kg/day should be used with major surgery to keep the plasma activity 20% to 50% of normal. For minor surgery, 10 to 20 units/kg/day for 2 to 3 days is sufficient. Bleeding can be treated with 10 to 30 units/kg/day depending on severity. In pregnancy, replacement should be started early, preferably before gestational week 5, because decidual bleeding from implantation will occur without replacement. The optimal plasma factor XIII concentration in pregnancy is not established, but >10% of normal is recommended. This can be achieved by infusing 250 units of concentrate every 7 days through week 22 of gestation, then 500 units per week until delivery, with a 1000 unit bolus during labor.

CONGENITAL DEFICIENCIES INVOLVING MULTIPLE COAGULATION FACTORS

Numerous cases of congenital deficiencies of more than one coagulation factor have been described. While most represent chance coinheritance of distinct deficiencies, several represent familial syndromes (Table 137.4). Such syndromes are likely caused by abnormalities in intracellular protein processing or alterations in posttranslational modification. Common nonspecific inhibitors such as lupus anticoagulants interfere with coagulation assays and can lead to erroneous interpretations when they suggest multiple factor deficiencies. Similarly, potent inhibitors directed at a single coagulation factor (e.g., factor VIII) occasionally interfere with assays for other factors. Two familial states, combined factor V and VIII deficiency (type 1) and deficiency of vitamin K dependent factors (type 3), are well characterized.

TABLE 137.4 Combined Familial Deficiency States.

Type	Deficient Factors	OMIM Designation	Underlying Cause
1	V and VIII	227300	Mutations in LMAN1 or MCFD2 genes
2	VIII and IX	134510	Unknown
3	II, VII, IX, X, Protein C, and Protein S	277450 (gamma-glutamyl carboxylase) 607473 (vitamin K oxidoreductase)	Mutations in γ-glutamyl carboxylase (GGCX) or vitamin K oxidoreductase (VKORC1) genes
4	VII and VIII	134430	Unknown
5	VIII, IX and XI	134520	Unknown
6	IX and XI	134540	Unknown
	VII and X		Gene deletion 13q34

OMIM, Online Mendelian Inheritance in Man.

Combined Factor V and Factor VIII Deficiency (OMIM 227300)

Combined factor V and factor VIII deficiency was first reported in 1954. The familial form is an autosomal recessive trait caused by mutations in either the LMAN1 (mannose-binding lectin) or MCFD2 (multiple combined factor deficiency protein) gene.[29] These proteins form a cargo receptor that transports factors V and VIII from the ER to the ER-Golgi intermediate compartment. Although the incidence of this disorder is thought to be 1 in 1 million persons, the allele frequency is particularly high (~1%) in Tunisian Jews originating from a community on the island of Djerba.

Deficiency of LMAN1 or MCFD2 activity causes a defect in factor V and factor VIII secretion, lowering plasma levels to 5%–30% of normal. In Tunisian Jews, a T-to-C substitution at a donor splice site in intron 9 causes LMAN1 deficiency. A history of consanguinity, co-segregation of factor deficiencies, and similar reductions in factor V and VIII favor the familial disorder. Affected individuals bleed primarily after trauma, and epistaxis, gingival bleeding, easy bruising, and menorrhagia are common. Hemarthrosis unrelated to trauma may occur in 20% of patients, but bleeding from the GI tract or intracranial hemorrhage is less common.[29] Postpartum hemorrhage occurs in most affected women, and invasive procedures, including tooth extraction, are usually accompanied by bleeding in the absence of factor replacement. The PT and aPTT are prolonged. As isolated factor V deficiency also prolongs these tests, patients with factor V deficiency should have factor VIII levels measured to avoid missing combined deficiency. Patients with mucosal bleeding and menorrhagia may respond to antifibrinolytic therapy. For more significant bleeds, or in preparation for surgery or tooth extraction, a combination of FFP and factor VIII concentrate should be used. DDAVP may raise factor VIII, but not factor V levels. Trough levels of approximately 50% for factor VIII and 25% for factor V have been recommended for surgery. Plasma exchange may be used to increase factor V in situations in which volume overload from large volumes of FFP is a concern. Recombinant factor VIIa was used successfully to stop bleeding in one surgery patient.

Combined Deficiency of Vitamin K–Dependent Proteins (OMIM 277450 and 607473)

In 1966 McMillan and Roberts described a newborn girl with prolonged PT and aPTT; low levels of prothrombin and factors VII, IX, and X; and no evidence of liver disease or malabsorption.

Laboratory Testing in Rare Coagulation Factor Deficiencies

When deficiency of a coagulation factor is under consideration, it is important to keep in mind that (1) acquired conditions causing multiple factor deficiencies are more common than congenital deficiency of a single factor, and (2) common inhibitors of coagulation, such as lupus anticoagulants, heparins, and the direct oral anticoagulants (DOACs) interfere with coagulation factor assays. Unexplained prolongation of the PT or aPTT should be evaluated in a qualified laboratory. If at all possible, the plasma should be prepared from blood collected by venipuncture. In our experience, the common practice of collecting blood from central venous catheters/ports or peripheral intravenous catheters frequently introduces fluids or drugs that adversely affect clotting assays and contribute to misdiagnosis. We frequently use the thrombin time assay and factor Xa-based assays to screen samples for the presence of heparins or DOACs.

The initial evaluation of a plasma sample with a prolonged PT or aPTT should start by repeating the abnormal test on a mixture of patient and normal plasma to determine if the prolonged clotting time is related to a clotting factor deficiency (clotting time becomes normal after mixing) or an inhibitor that neutralizes clotting factor activity (clotting time remains prolonged after mixing). The mixing study should be performed with and without incubation (2 hours), as some antibody inhibitors demonstrate a time-dependent pattern of inhibition. Slight (a few second) prolongations of the PT or aPTT can be difficult to evaluate with a mixing study. We evaluate such samples with assays for lupus anticoagulants prior to measuring specific levels of coagulation factors.

The antibodies to clotting factors that most physicians are familiar with neutralize factor activity, and generate abnormal results on a mixing study (i.e., mixing with normal plasma fails to correct the abnormal clotting time). However, nonneutralizing antibodies can cause severe factor deficiency. These antibodies typically enhance clearance of the clotting factor from the plasma in vivo, and are not detected in a mixing study. A failure to respond to replacement therapy in the absence of a measurable inhibitor suggests a nonneutralizing antibody is present. In our practice, we have observed severe acquired deficiencies of prothrombin, factor V, factor X, factor XI, and factor XIII caused by (or presumed to be caused by) nonneutralizing antibodies.

If the level of a vitamin K–dependent protein (prothrombin or factors VII, IX or X) is low, levels of factor V and at least one other vitamin K-dependent factor should be measured. If multiple vitamin K–dependent factors are low and factor V is normal, a process affecting vitamin K is likely. If factor V is also low, liver disease or DIC should be considered. Tests for hepatic function (albumin) or injury (transaminases) can facilitate interpretation of the coagulation factor studies. Distinguishing DIC from liver disease can be difficult, because results of standard tests such as the PT, aPTT, platelet count, fibrinogen and D-dimer may be abnormal in both conditions. Measuring factor V and factor VIII may be useful in this situation, because both are often low in DIC, while factor VIII is normal or elevated in liver disease.

It is likely that the apparent rarity of congenital factor XIII deficiency is partly due to the insensitivity of clot solubility assays still used in many places to screen for this disorder. Quantitative measurements of factor XIII activity are preferable, and are replacing solubility assays at many institutions.

Patients with factor XI, factor XII, prekallikrein or high-molecular-weight kininogen deficiency may require anticoagulation for treatment or prophylaxis for thromboembolism. Assays based on contact activation such as the aPTT or the activated clotting time (ACT) cannot be used for monitoring therapy with heparin or the direct thrombin inhibitor argatroban in these patients, because the baseline PTT and ACT are prolonged. Chromogenic heparin assays based on factor Xa inhibition are now widely available for monitoring heparin, and should be used in place of the aPTT in patients with these deficiencies. Alternatively, low-molecular-weight heparin, fondaparinux or a DOAC, which do not generally require monitoring, can be used instead of unfractionated heparin or argatroban.

She responded partially to large doses of vitamin K. Subsequently, low protein C and protein S levels were reported in association with mutations in the γ-*glutamyl carboxylase* (GGCX) gene. Although the condition is considered autosomal recessive, severe bleeding was reported in a neonate heterozygous for a GGCX mutation. Prothrombin; factors VII, IX, and X; proteins C and S; and the bone proteins osteocalcin and matrix Gla protein require γ-carboxylation of glutamic acid residues in their N-terminal Gla-domains. This process is mediated by GGCX, which uses reduced vitamin K as a cofactor. The reactions result in formation of vitamin K 2,3-epoxide, which must be reduced by *vitamin K epoxide reductase complex subunit 1* (VKORC1) to replenish the vitamin K pool. Mutations in the GGCX or VKORC1 genes can impair γ-carboxylation, resulting in reduced levels (10% to 50% of normal) of all vitamin K–dependent proteins, and a bleeding tendency that may be severe. Some patients have skeletal abnormalities resembling warfarin embryopathy, probably due to abnormalities of osteocalcin and matrix Gla protein. Vitamin K–dependent proteins are reduced in patients taking warfarin, poisoning with rodenticides such as brodifacoum, and with vitamin K deficiency. Recently, a cluster of cases of severe vitamin K deficiency causing hemorrhagic disease of the newborn were linked to a failure to administer prophylactic vitamin K after birth.[30] The levels of these proteins are also low in liver failure, in conjunction with other proteins synthesized in the liver (such as factor V), and in malabsorption syndromes. An acquired antibody that resulted in fatal bleeding in a patient with a lymphoproliferative disorder bound to an epitope on the Gla domain of prothrombin and factors IX and X.

Combined deficiencies of prothrombin and factors VII, IX, and X cause prolongation of the PT and aPTT. Protein C and protein S are also reduced. The abnormalities correct on mixing with normal plasma. Failure to do so suggests that a nonspecific inhibitor such as a lupus anticoagulant is present. Patients with deficiencies of vitamin K–dependent proteins should be evaluated for liver disease, malabsorption, and exposure to vitamin-K antagonists such as warfarin or brodifacoum. Toxicology screens can identify these agents in blood long after ingestion because of their long half-lives. Some patients have adequate clinical response to vitamin K_1 (10 mg weekly), but others require unusually high doses. Nonresponders, or responders with significant bleeding episodes, can be treated with FFP or PCC.

REFERENCES

1. Peyvandi F, Menegatti M, Palla R: Rare bleeding disorders: worldwide efforts for classification, diagnosis and management. *Semin Thromb Haemost* 39:579, 2013.
2. Mumford AD, Ackroyd S, Alikhan R, et al: Guideline for the diagnosis and management of the rare coagulation disorders: a United Kingdom Haemophilia Centre Doctors' Organization guideline on behalf of the British Committee for Standards in Haematology. *Br J Haematol* 167(3):304–326, 2014.
3. Palla R, Peyfandi F, Shapiro AD: Rare bleeding disorders: diagnosis and treatment. *Blood* 125(13):2052–2061, 2015.
4. Peyvandi F, Palla R, Menegatti M, et al: Coagulation factor activity and clinical bleeding severity in rare bleeding disorders: results from the European Network of Rare Bleeding Disorders. *J Thromb Haemost* 10(4):615–621, 2012.
5. Peyvandi F: Epidemiology and treatment of congenital fibrinogen deficiency. *Thromb Res* 130(Suppl 2):S7–S11, 2012.
6. De Moerloose P, Casini A, Neerman-Arbez M: Congenital fibrinogen disorders: an update. *Semin Thromb Haemost* 39(6):585–595, 2013.
7. Kadir RA, Davies J, Winikoff R, et al: Pregnancy complications and obstetric care in women with inherited bleeding disorders. *Haemophilia* 19(Suppl 4):1–10, 2013.
8. Solomon C, Groner A, Ye J, et al: Safety of fibrinogen concentrate: analysis of more than 27 years of pharmacovigilance data. *Thromb Haemost* 113(4):759–771, 2015.
9. Casini A, Neerman-Arbez M, Ariens RA, et al: Dysfibrinogenemia: from molecular anomalies to clinical manifestations and management. *J Thromb Haemost* 13(6):909–919, 2015.

10. Casini A, Blondon M, Lebreton A: Natural history of patients with congenital dysfibrinogenemia. *Blood* 125(3):553–561, 2015.

11. Lancellotti S, Basso M, de Crisofaro R: Congenital Prothrombin Deficiency: an update. *Semin Thromb Hemost* 39(6):596–606, 2013.

12. Peyvandi F, DiMichele D, Bolton-Maggs PHB, et al: Classification of rare bleeding disorders (RBDs) based on the association between coagulant factor activity and clinical bleeding severity. *J Thromb Haemost* 10(9):1938–1943, 2012.

13. Thalji N, Camire RM: Parahemophilia: new insights into factor V deficiency. *Semin Thromb Hemost* 39(6):607–612, 2013.

14. Lippi G, Favaloro EJ, Montagnana M, et al: Inherited and acquired factor V deficiency. *Blood Coagul Fibrinolysis* 22(3):160–166, 2011.

15. DiMinno MN, Dolce A, Mariani G, et al: Bleeding symptoms at disease presentation and prediction of ensuing bleeding in inherited factor VII deficiency. *Thromb Haemost* 109(6):1051–1059, 2013.

16. Mariani G, Napolitano M, Dolce A, et al: Replacement therapy for bleeding episodes in factor VII deficiency. A prospective evaluation. *Thromb Haemost* 109(2):238–247, 2013.

17. Siboni SM, Biguzzi E, Mistretta C, et al: Long-term prophylaxis in severe factor VII deficiency. *Haemophilia* 21(6):812–819, 2015.

18. Menegatti M, Peyvandi F: Factor X deficiency. *Semin Thromb Hemost* 35(4):407–415, 2009.

19. Lee G, Duan-Porter W, Metjian A: Acquired, non-amyloid related factor X deficiency: Review of the literature. *Haemophilia* 18(5):655–663, 2012.

20. Thompson CA, Kyle R, Gertz M, et al: Systemic AL amyloidosis with acquired factor X deficiency: A study of perioperative bleeding risk and treatment outcomes in 60 patients. *Am J Hematol* 85(3):171–173, 2010.

21. Litvak A, Kumar A, Wong RJ, et al: Successful perioperative use of prothrombin complex concentrate in the treatment of acquired factor X deficiency in the setting of systemic light-chain (AL)amyloidosis. *Am J Hematol* 89(12):1153–1154, 2014.

22. Duga S, Salomon O: Congenital factor XI deficiency: an update. *Semin Thromb Hemost* 39(6):621–631, 2013.

23. Santoro C, Di Mauro R, Baldacci E, et al: Bleeding phenotype and correlation with factor XI (FXI) activity in congenital FXI deficiency: results of a retrospective study from a single centre. *Haemophilia* 21(4):496–501, 2015.

24. Bauduer F, de Raucourt E, Boyer-Neumann C, et al: Factor XI replacement for inherited factor XI deficiency in routine clinical practice: results of the HEMOLEVEN prospective 3-year postmarketing study. *Haemophilia* 21(4):481–489, 2015.

25. De Jager T, Pericleous L, Kokot-Kierepa M, et al: The burden and management of factor XIII deficiency. *Haemophilia* 20(6):733–740, 2014.

26. Schroeder V, Kohler HP: New developments in the area of factor XIII. *J Thromb Haemost* 11(2):234–244, 2013.

27. Hsu P, Zantek ND, Meijer P, et al: Factor XIII Assays and associated problems for laboratory diagnosis of factor XIII deficiency: an analysis of International Proficiency testing results. *Semin Thromb Hemost* 40(2):232–238, 2014.

28. Inbal A, Oldenburg J, Carcao M: Recombinant factor XIII: a safe and novel treatment for congenital factor XIII deficiency. *Blood* 119(22):5111–5117, 2012.

29. Zheng C, Zhang B: Combined deficiency of coagulation factors V and VIII: an update. *Semin Thromb Hemost* 39(6):613–620, 2013.

30. Schulte R, Jordan LC, Morad A, et al: Rise in late onset vitamin K deficiency bleeding in young infants because of omission or refusal of prophylaxis at birth. *Pediatr Neurol* 50(6):564–568, 2014.

STRUCTURE, BIOLOGY, AND GENETICS OF VON WILLEBRAND FACTOR

Paula James and Natalia Rydz

Von Willebrand factor (VWF) is an adhesive multimeric plasma glycoprotein that mediates platelet adhesion to injured subendothelium via glycoprotein (GP) 1bα, and binds and stabilizes factor VIII (FVIII) in the circulation, protecting it from proteolytic degradation. This important multifunctional protein was named after the Finnish physician, Dr. Erik von Willebrand, who first described von Willebrand disease (VWD) in 1926. In the original publication he described a severe mucocutaneous bleeding problem in a family living on the Åland archipelago in the Baltic Sea. The index case, a young woman named Hjördis, bled to death during her fourth menstrual period at the age of 13. Dr. von Willebrand referred to the condition as *pseudohemophilia*, but noted that in contrast to hemophilia, this condition affected both genders, with females typically being more severely affected.

In the mid-1950s it was recognized that VWD was usually accompanied by a reduced level of FVIII activity and that the bleeding phenotype could be corrected by the infusion of normal plasma. In the early 1970s the critical immunologic distinction between FVIII and VWF was made, and since that time significant progress has been made in our understanding of the molecular pathophysiology of this disorder. Cloning and characterization of the *VWF* gene in the 1980s has facilitated further investigation into the function of VWF and the genetic basis of VWD.

FUNCTIONS OF VON WILLEBRAND FACTOR

VWF is a multifunctional adhesive protein that plays an important role in both primary hemostasis and blood coagulation. In primary hemostasis, VWF initiates platelet adhesion at the site of endothelial injury, whereas in coagulation, VWF stabilizes FVIII in the circulation (Fig. 138.1).

Platelet Adhesion

At the site of endothelial injury, VWF adheres to exposed collagen. The hemostatically important forms of collagen include types I, III, and VI, but VWF preferentially binds to type III collagen. The interactions of VWF with collagen are predominately mediated by the VWF A3 domain (Fig. 138.2). Once immobilized, VWF is subjected to the high shear rates of the arterial circulation and undergoes a conformational change that exposes the platelet GPIbα binding site within the VWF A1 domain. High affinity, rapid and reversible interaction between VWF and GPIbα tethers platelets to the endothelium where they roll until they are immobilized and activated by direct platelet-collagen binding which is mediated by two collagen receptors on platelets, GPVI and the integrin α2β1 (or GPIa/IIa). The Arg-Gly-Asp (RGD) sequence within the VWF C1 domain also contributes to platelet adhesion by interacting with GPIIb-IIIa of activated platelets.

Factor VIII Stabilization

VWF binds FVIII through the VWF D′D3 domains and protects it from proteolytic degradation, thereby prolonging its half-life. In the absence of VWF, FVIII has a half-life of approximately 2 hours in contrast to a normal half-life of 12–20 hours when bound to VWF.

BASAL VON WILLEBRAND FACTOR LEVELS

The normal level for VWF is highly variable and ranges from 50 to 150 IU/dL. Factors that contribute to the variable VWF levels include ABO genotype (see section on ABO blood groups later), Secretor genotype, race, and age. Plasma VWF concentrations have been reported to be approximately 20% higher in subjects homozygous for the Secretor (Se) allele as compared with those who are heterozygous. VWF levels in blacks are 15% higher than those in whites. Increased age has also been associated with higher VWF levels, with studies suggesting that the levels may increase by as much as 15–17 U/mL per decade.

Within subjects, VWF levels often vary over time as a result of β-adrenergic stimuli, drugs, or more sustained physiologic factors, such as pregnancy, hypothyroidism, chronic illness, or long-term use of certain medications. The vasopressin analogue, 1-deamino-(8-D-arginine)-vasopressin (DDAVP, desmopressin) transiently and reliably increases VWF and FVIII levels—a fact that, in addition to an acceptable side effect profile, has led to the use of DDAVP as a first-line treatment in certain types of VWD and mild hemophilia A. Several physiologic stressors involving β-adrenergic stimulation, such as exercise, surgery, and psychological distress, can produce an acute increase in VWF levels. VWF levels remain elevated for up to 6 days after surgery, suggesting that after the acute secretory response, there is upregulation of VWF production. A sustained elevation of VWF levels can occur with chronic diseases, such as hyperthyroidism, renal failure, diabetes, liver disease, atherosclerosis, chronic inflammatory states, and cancer. Conversely, acquired VWD, characterized by qualitative or quantitative VWF defects, can occur with certain medications, such as valproic acid, and with some chronic medical conditions (see section later on acquired VWD).

VWF levels are increased by estrogen. In premenopausal women, VWF levels vary in a cyclical fashion, with the lowest levels occurring in the early follicular phase of the menstrual cycle (days 1–7) and peak values occurring during the luteal phase. Oral contraceptives increase VWF levels and dampen the cyclical variation. This dose-dependent effect is mediated by the estrogen component and is evident with ethynylestradiol doses of 0.5 μg or higher. Lower estrogen doses have little or no effect on VWF levels. VWF levels increase in pregnancy starting in the second trimester and achieve levels threefold higher than baseline values by the end of the third trimester. VWF levels return to baseline 1–3 weeks after delivery.

VON WILLEBRAND FACTOR GENE

Located on the short arm of chromosome 12 at p13.3, the *VWF* gene spans 178 kb and is composed of 52 exons that range in size from 1.3 kb (exon 28) to 40 bp (exon 50) (Fig. 138.2A). There is a partial, unprocessed pseudogene, *vWFP*, located on the long arm chromosome 22 at q 11.2, measuring 21–29 kb, which duplicates the *VWF*

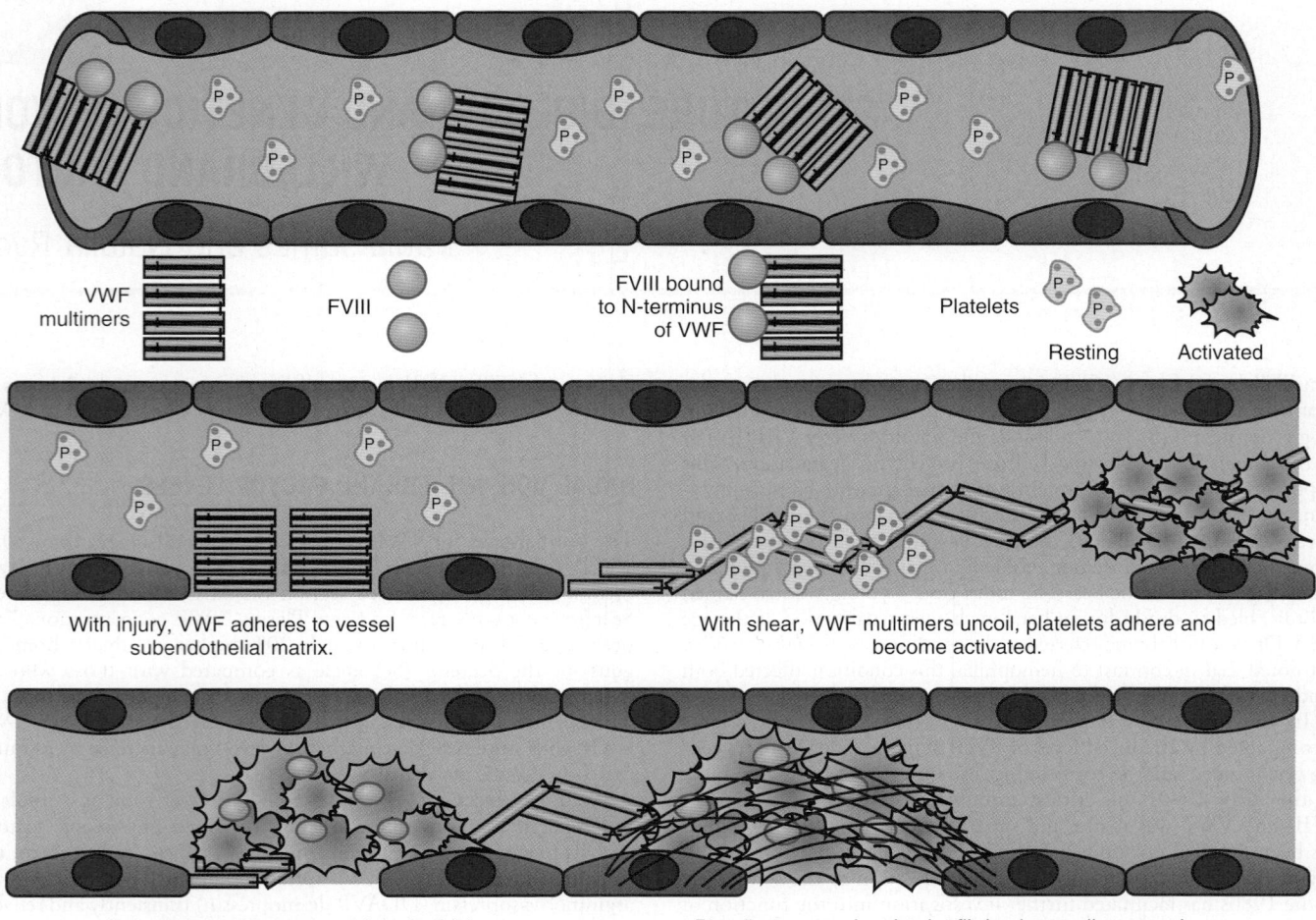

VWF multimers

FVIII

FVIII bound to N-terminus of VWF

Platelets

Resting

Activated

With injury, VWF adheres to vessel subendothelial matrix.

With shear, VWF multimers uncoil, platelets adhere and become activated.

Activated platelets expose phosphatidyl serine and bind FVIII to facilitate clotting.

Bleeding ceases by platelet-fibrin plug sealing vascular injury and is followed by thrombolysis and tissue repair.

Fig. 138.1 FUNCTION OF VON WILLEBRAND FACTOR. Role of VWF in mediating the initial events in the hemostatic process. VWF is the carrier protein for FVIII *(top)*. After endothelial injury, VWF adheres to the exposed subendothelium, where it is uncoiled by the shear forces, thereby exposing GP1bα binding sites that interact with platelets *(middle)*. The bound platelets are activated and the GPIIb-IIIa complex is exposed on the platelet surface. Interaction of fibrinogen and VWF with GPIIb-IIIa then consolidates the platelet adhesive event and initiates platelet aggregation *(bottom)*. *FVIII,* Factor VIII; *GP,* glycoprotein; *VWF,* von Willebrand factor. *(Used with the permission of Robert Montgomery).*

gene sequence for exons 23–34 with 97% sequence homology. The pseudogene contributes to the mutation spectrum of VWD through gene conversion. The *VWF* gene is highly polymorphic with more than 160 polymorphisms in the exons and closely flanking intronic sequences; these normal variants include promoter polymorphisms, a highly variable tetranucleotide repeat in intron 40, two insertion/deletion polymorphisms and 132 distinct single-nucleotide polymorphisms involving exon and intron sequences. An International Society on Thrombosis and Haemostasis Scientific and Standardization Committee (ISTH-SSC) database of both polymorphisms and mutations is maintained at the University of Sheffield (http://www.vwf.group.shef.ac.uk/). The high degree of polymorphism, the large size, and the presence of the pseudogene render full *VWF* gene sequencing and data interpretation challenging.

VWF expression is tightly restricted to endothelial cells, platelets, and megakaryocytes. Cell-specific transcriptional regulation is complex and poorly understood. A 734–base pair region, spanning approximately 500 bases of the 5′-flanking region and 247 bases into the first exon, functions as a promoter and includes a minimal core promoter, as well as negative and positive regulatory regions. The positive regulatory region confers cell-specificity by relieving inhibition in specific cells, thereby allowing transcription of the *VWF* gene.

DOMAIN STRUCTURE

Encoded VWF messenger ribonucleic acid is 8.8 kb in length and the translated prepro-VWF molecule contains 2813 amino acids (AA), comprising a 22 AA signal peptide, a 741 AA propeptide, and a 2050 AA secreted mature subunit that possesses all of the adhesive sites required for the hemostatic function of VWF. The AA sequence is rich in cysteine residues, which make up 8.3% of the prepro-VWF and are abundant in all of the domains except the A domains, where only six cysteine residues are found. The cysteine residues are involved not only in interchain disulfide bonds, but also in intrachain disulfide bonds.

The VWF amino acid sequence contains four homologous repeated segments, named A through D, which make up approximately 90% of the precursor. These homologues also occur in a number of unrelated proteins. For example, VWF A domains appear in up to 22 human genes, such as leukocyte adhesion receptors, collagen receptors, and cartilage matrix protein. Likewise, homologues of VWF domains B, C, D, and CK exist throughout the genome, and are found in proteins with various functions. This suggests that the *VWF* gene is the product of a complex series of partial gene duplications.

Based on four homologous repeated segments, A through D, the domain structure of VWF has been annotated in the following sequence: S-D1-D2-D′-D3-A1-A2-A3-D4-B1-B2-B3-C1-C2-CK.

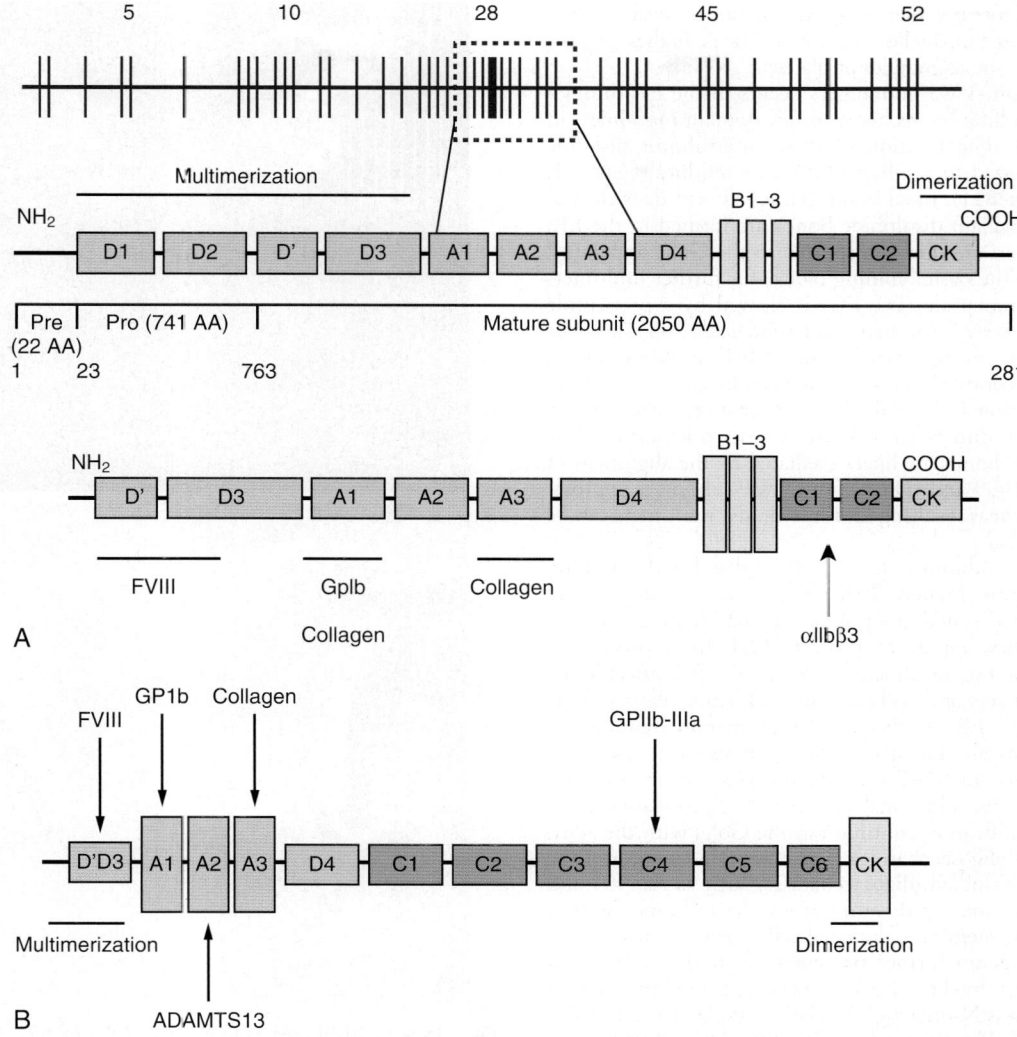

Fig. 138.2 VON WILLEBRAND FACTOR GENE, mRNA AND PROTEIN. (A) The *VWF* gene is located on chromosome 12 at p13.3 and spans 178 kb and includes 52 exons. The mRNA is 8.8 kb in length. Prepro-VWF contains 2813 amino acids (AA) with a 22-AA signal peptide, a 741-AA propeptide, and a 2050-AA mature subunit. The mature subunit consists of repeated domains (A–D), several of which have distinct functions and binding sites. (B) Diagram showing the revised annotation of the VWF subunit that was derived from electron microscopy. *ADAMTS13*, a Disintegrin and metalloproteinase with a thrombospondin member 13; *FVIII*, factor VIII; *GP*, glycoprotein, *mRNA*, messenger RNA.

Recently, the annotation of VWF's protein structure has been revised based on structures seen using electron microscopy. The A domains are seen as globular structures and represent the major functional binding sites with VWF, to platelets and collagen. The domains previously known as B and C are reannotated as six-tandem von Willebrand C (vWC) and vWC-like domains. These domains elongate and provide flexibility to the VWF protein, an important characteristic to the functioning of VWF under different shear stresses within the circulation (Fig. 138.2B).

Functional domains important for multimerization, cleavage, and binding have been identified. The signal peptide (S) targets prepro-VWF to the endoplasmic reticulum (ER), where it is promptly cleaved. The cysteine knot (CK) domains of adjacent VWF monomers form disulfide bonds, resulting in tail-to-tail dimers. The VWF propeptide (domains D1–D2) plays an important role in VWF multimer assembly by promoting the formation of head-to-head oligomers through disulfide bonds involving D3. The A2 domain contains the Tyr1605-Met1606 cleavage site for ADAMTS13 (a disintegrin and metalloproteinase with a thrombospondin type 1 motif, member 13).

The VWF subunit possesses several binding sites, almost entirely encoded by exon 28 and including domains D'-D3-A1-A2-A3. In addition, the C1 domain, encoded by exons 42–44, contains a binding site. The D' and D3 domains contain the FVIII-binding site, which interacts with the N-terminus portion of the FVIII light chain. VWF interacts with platelets via two platelet receptors; GPIbα and GPIIb/IIIa, which mediate platelet adhesion to injured subendothelium and the aggregation of activated platelets, respectively. The binding site for GPIbα is localized within the large disulfide loop of A1, whereas the binding site for GPIIb/IIIa is found within the RGD sequence of C1. VWF binds to collagen I and III via the VWF A1 and A3 domains and collagen VI via the A1 domain. Although the major binding site for collagen is thought to be within the A3 domain, the two sites likely have complementary roles and blood flow-mediated shear stress is important for the conformation and function of both.

BIOSYNTHESIS

VWF is synthesized in endothelial cells and megakaryocytes and undergoes a complex series of posttranslational modifications, including dimerization, glycosylation, sulfation, and ultimately, multimerization.

The fully processed protein is then either released into the circulation or is stored in specialized organelles: the Weibel-Palade bodies (WPBs) of endothelial cells or the α-granules of platelets.

Dimerization of pro-VWF monomers occurs in the ER through the formation of disulfide bonds between CK domain monomers in a tail-to-tail fashion. The location of these intersubunit disulfide bonds has been localized to a subset of cysteine residues (Cys2771, Cys2773, and/or Cys2811). In addition, the signal peptide is cleaved and most of the intrachain disulphide bonds are formed in the ER. Only pro-VWF dimers are then transported to the Golgi apparatus, where they make up the basic building blocks for further multimerization. Here, the propeptide (D1–D2) is cleaved by a propeptide processing protease, likely furin, between amino acids 763–764. The propeptide continues to be essential for VWF multimerization because under acidic conditions, it serves as an endogenous chaperone that promotes additional disulfide bond formation between D3 domains of adjacent dimers in a head-to-head orientation. The intersubunit disulfide bonds are likely mediated by the alignment of the cysteine pairs C1099 and C1142. The VWF subunit is approximately 250 kDa, whereas resulting disulfide-linked multimers can be more than 20,000 kDa.

The mature VWF subunit is heavily glycosylated with carbohydrate making up approximately 20% of the mass of the mature subunit. Although the function of these oligosaccharide chains is largely unknown, they appear to protect VWF from proteolytic degradation, maintain the multimeric structure of VWF, affect VWF interaction with platelets and collagen, and influence plasma clearance of VWF. In the ER, 12 N-linked high-mannose-containing oligosaccharide chains are added to each VWF subunit, and these appear to be necessary for VWF subunit dimerization. In addition, the propeptide has three additional potential N-glycosylation sites. Posttranslational modification continues in the Golgi with the addition of 10 O-linked oligosaccharides to the peptide chain, and the sulfation of certain N-linked oligosaccharides, such as Asn384 and Asn468. Glycan expression is determined by the cell-type. Within the postGolgi compartment of endothelial cells, the previously added N-linked glycans undergo further processing with the addition of ABO groups, as determined by the ABO genotype. Preliminary data suggest that there is less N-linked glycosylation in platelets and ABO groups are not added. The net result of this differential glycosylation is that platelet VWF is more resistant to ADAMTS13 proteolysis than plasma VWF. The cleaved propeptide remains noncovalently associated with VWF multimers and is stored and secreted with the mature VWF in a 1:1 molar ratio.

STORAGE AND SECRETION

Most of the VWF in endothelial cells consists of small multimers that are constitutively secreted. The more biologically active high-molecular-weight (HMW) VWF multimers are preferentially targeted for storage in endothelium-specific cytoplasmic granules, the WPBs. In addition to VWF and the VWF propeptide, WBPs also store P-selectin, CD63, interleukin-8, tissue plasminogen activator, and angiopoietin-2. Thus WPBs store proteins that are involved not only in hemostasis, but also in inflammation, hemodynamics, and angiogenesis. WPBs have a characteristic cigar-like shape, measuring 0.2 μm in width and 5 μm in length (Fig. 138.3), and are composed of tightly packed tubules, measuring 150–200 Å in cross-section. Platelet VWF is stored within similar tubules that are found in the periphery of α-granules and constitutes approximately 15% to 20% of total blood VWF. Tubular packing condenses the length of VWF multimers by 50-fold and is dependent on the acidic pH within the trans-Golgi, as well as the propeptide (D1D2) and the NH₂-terminal region (D′D3A1). Long VWF multimers, which can be up to 100 μm in length, are reversibly packaged into coils. With WPB exocytosis, the filamentous strings of VWF are secreted into the circulation, where they rapidly unfurl and are capable of binding to platelets. If the tubular structure is perturbed, WPBs release short, tangled VWF that does not support platelet binding to the endothelium.

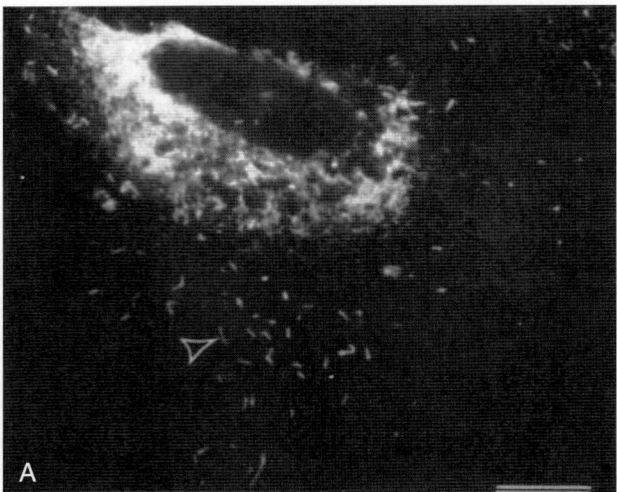

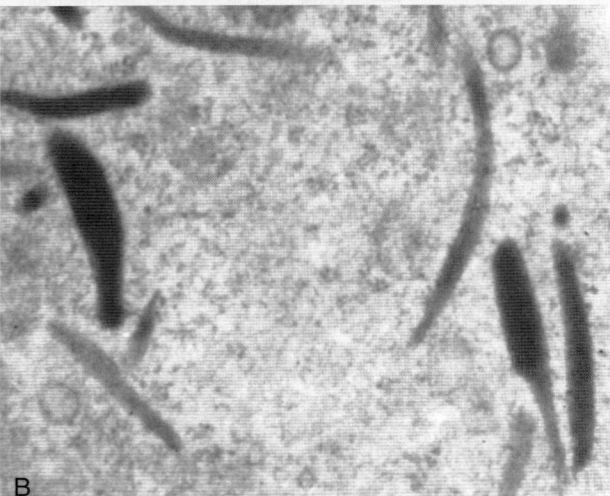

Fig. 138.3 WEIBEL-PALADE BODIES OF ENDOTHELIAL CELLS. (A) Immunofluorescence staining of a human umbilical vein endothelial cell with anti-VWF antiserum. VWF is present in the perinuclear region, where it is synthesized, and in the Weibel-Palade bodies *(arrowhead)* throughout the cytoplasm. Bar = 10 μm. (B) Electron micrograph of Weibel-Palade bodies of the same origin. Bar = 0.5 μm.

A variety of agonists can induce the secretion of VWF from endothelial cells. These agonists include histamine, thrombin, fibrin, the terminal complement proteins C5b-9, and β-adrenergic agonists. With endothelial cell stimulation, WPBs fuse with the plasma membrane to form a secretion pore. This leads to a rapid rise in pH and release of intracellular calcium stores. The freshly secreted unusually large (or ultra-large) VWF multimers (ULvWF) are highly active and can spontaneously bind platelets. Some of the released protein remains associated with the endothelial membrane, and some self-associate.

ADAMTS13

ADAMTS13 is a plasma protease that cleaves circulating VWF between Tyr 1605 and Met 1606 in the A2 domain. Its main target is the ULvWF multimers, which spontaneously bind GPIbα on platelets. ADAMTS13 cleaves ULvWF multimers when there is sufficient shear to unfold the A2 domain and to expose the cleavage site. ULvWF multimers that appear in plasma after WPB secretion are cleaved within 2 hours by ADAMTS13 to form shorter, less hemostatically active multimers. Proteolysis of VWF multimers is responsible for the characteristic "triplet" pattern of satellite bands

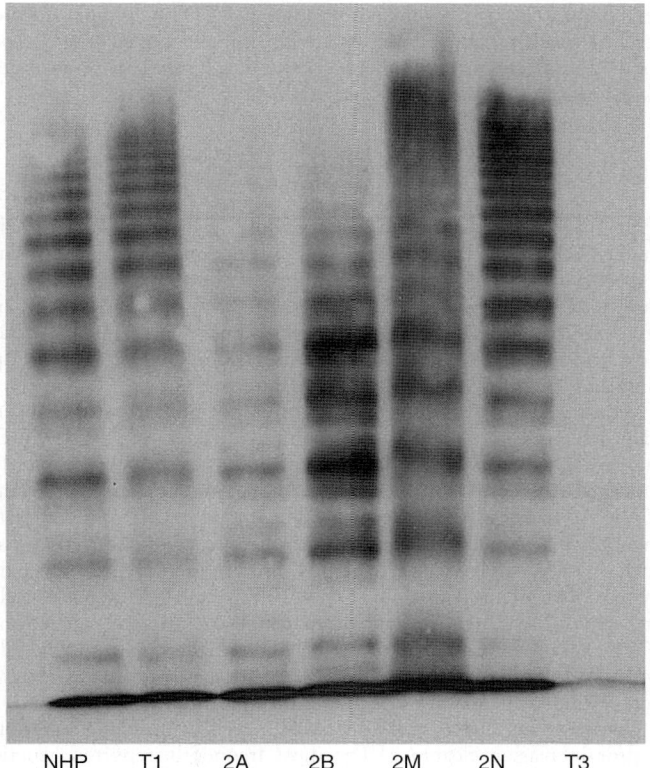

Fig. 138.4 EXAMPLE OF A MULTIMER ANALYSIS (2.25% AGAROSE GEL). Lane 1 normal human plasma (NHP) represents normal plasma multimer patterns with a characteristic "triplet" pattern of satellite bands flanking each main multimer. Lanes 2–7 show the plasma VWF multimer analysis for patients with the different subtypes of VWD (T1, type 1; 2A, type 2A; 2B, type 2B; 2M, type 2M; 2N, type 2N; T3, type 3). Type 2A and type 2B VWD both show variable loss of high-molecular-weight multimers. Types 1, 2M, and 2N demonstrate the presence of high molecular weight multimers. Finally, with type 3 VWD, there is an absence of any VWF.

flanking each main multimer band that is observed on multimer analysis gels. (Fig. 138.4).

VWF proteolysis is influenced by glycosylation and specific polymorphisms. For example, nonglycosylated recombinant VWF is cleaved more rapidly than its plasma-derived glycosylated counterparts. Likewise, addition of A or B blood group antigens to N-linked oligosaccharide chains of VWF attenuates ADAMTS13 proteolysis compared with VWF bearing the O blood group antigen. Finally, the differential glycosylation of platelet VWF renders it resistant to ADAMTS13 proteolysis. Single-nucleotide polymorphisms, such as the A/G polymorphism at position 24/1282 resulting in Tyr/Cys at 1584, have also been shown to affect the susceptibility of VWF to proteolysis.

Alterations in the balance between ADAMTS13 activity and VWF proteolysis can lead to a number of disease states. Congenital or acquired deficiency of ADAMTS13 can result in thrombotic thrombocytopenic purpura (see Chapter 134). On the other hand, enhanced proteolysis can give rise to a bleeding phenotype. For example, mutant VWF in a subtype of type 2A VWD exhibits enhanced susceptibility to ADAMTS13 cleavage, which results in loss of large VWF multimers.

CLEARANCE

VWF clearance is complex and involves multiple receptors and cell-types. Data suggest that macrophages and hepatocytes internalize and clear VWF in a process that is independent of multimer size and mediated by lipoprotein receptor-related protein and asialoglycoprotein receptor in both cell types and sialic-acid-binding-immunoglobulin-like-lectin 5 in macrophages. C-type lactic domain family 4 member M on endothelial cells has also been shown to mediate VWF clearance in a glycan-dependent manner. Further studies are needed to decipher the relative contribution of each of these mechanisms as determinants of VWF levels.

The VWF propeptide remains associated with VWF multimers stored in WPBs and is secreted in a 1:1 molar ratio with the mature VWF subunit. After secretion, the propeptide (VWFpp) dissociates from VWF and circulates at a concentration of approximately 1 μg/mL and with a half-life of 2–3 hours. In contrast, VWF circulates at a plasma concentration of approximately 10 μg/mL and has a half-life of approximately 12–20 hours. The ratio between VWFpp and mature VWF (vWFpp/VWF:Ag) can be used to estimate the relative half-life of mature VWF; elevated ratios indicate enhanced clearance.

Changes in VWF glycosylation or point mutations can be associated with increased clearance. Blood group O subjects (see the following section on ABO Blood Groups) exhibit increased VWF clearance compared with the other blood types and have consistently elevated vWFpp/VWF:Ag ratios and shorter VWF survival after DDAVP administration. Several point mutations may lead to accelerated VWF clearance and are associated with either a type 1 or type 2A VWD phenotype. The vast majority of these are localized to the D3 domain (e.g., R1205H and C1130F), but point mutations in the A1 (I1416N), CK (C2617), and D4 domains (S2179F) have also been implicated.

VWF mutations associated with accelerated clearance are not necessarily associated with increased susceptibility to proteolysis by ADAMTS13 and vice versa. For example, the VWD Vicenza mutation, R1205, is the prototypical clearance mutation. Patients with this mutation have severely reduced plasma FVIII and VWF levels, an increased vWFpp/VWF:Ag, and a VWF half-life of 1–2 hours. However, there is no association between increased clearance of this mutant VWF and altered susceptibility to ADAMTS13 proteolysis.

ABO BLOOD GROUPS

Blood group O subjects have VWF levels that are on average 25% lower than those with non-O blood types: the mean VWF level in blood group O subjects is 74.8 IU/dL as compared with 105.9 IU/dL, 116.9 IU/dL, and 123.3 IU/dL in blood group A, B, and AB subjects, respectively. ABO antigens are added to N-linked oligosaccharide chains on the VWF subunit. Thus patients with the type O blood group genotype lack the functional glycosyltransferase that adds N-acetylgalactosamine and D-galactose to the H antigen on VWF in blood group A and B subjects, respectively. Altered glycosylation of VWF in subjects with blood type O leads to lower plasma VWF levels as a result of increased proteolysis and/or more rapid clearance. Blood group O VWF is more susceptible to ADAMTS13 proteolysis, and blood group O subjects have elevated VWFpp:vWFAg ratios and shorter VWF survival after DDAVP. The mean half-life of VWF in type O subjects is approximately 10 hours compared with a half-life of approximately 25.5 hours in those with other ABO blood types. Clinically, the difference in VWF levels results in an overrepresentation of blood group O patients with type 1 VWD, which is defined by a reduction in VWF levels.

AREAS OF ONGOING INVESTIGATION

There is emerging evidence that VWF may have a role in the regulation of vascular endothelial growth factor-dependent angiogenesis directly through its interaction with integrins on endothelial cells and indirectly via regulation of WPB formation and secretion of constituents such as angiopoietin-2. In addition, VWF may protect against tumor metastasis. Patients with increased VWF levels are at risk for cardiovascular events; it is unclear whether VWF contributes to atherosclerosis or whether it is a marker of endothelial dysfunction. Nonetheless, VWF plays an important role in atherothrombosis, and drugs targeting VWF attenuate arterial thrombosis in animal models. Their utility in humans is unknown.

VON WILLEBRAND DISEASE

VWD is caused by deficient or defective plasma VWF and represents the most common inherited bleeding disorder. Bleeding symptoms reflect the defect in primary hemostasis: mucocutaneous bleeding, especially epistaxis and menorrhagia. When FVIII levels are sufficiently low, the bleeding phenotype overlaps with that of mild to moderate hemophilia; patients may experience joint or muscle bleeds. The current VWD classification recognizes three subtypes. Type 1 VWD is characterized by quantitative deficiency of VWF, type 2 VWD is characterized by qualitative defects, and type 3 VWD is characterized by an almost complete absence of VWF.

Epidemiology

VWD is the most common inherited bleeding disorder. However, because VWF levels are variable in the population and symptom severity ranges from infrequent, mild bleeding to frequent or severe bleeds, the reported prevalence depends on the diagnostic criteria and the study population. In two large epidemiologic studies, the prevalence of VWD was approximately 1% in healthy school-age children based on low VWF activity, and a personal and family history of bleeding symptoms. The prevalence of VWD in individuals who present to a primary care physician with bleeding symptoms is approximately 0.1%, whereas in patients whose bleeding symptoms are sufficiently severe to warrant referral to specialized centers, the prevalence is 20–113 per million.

Classification and Pathophysiology

The 2006 ISTH VWD classification relies on the VWF protein phenotype, which in turn often reflects the underlying pathophysiology and has implications for treatment. Type 1 VWD is a partial quantitative deficiency; type 2 (with four subtypes: 2A, 2B, 2M, and 2N) is a qualitative defect; and type 3 is a virtual deficiency of VWF (Table 138.1). The diagnosis and categorization of VWD into a type can be achieved with widely available laboratory testing. However, the differentiation among type 2 subtypes may require referral to a specialized laboratory. The current classification does not incorporate genotypic data: the diagnosis of VWD is not limited to individuals with mutations within the *VWF* gene. VWF mutations may not be identified in VWD patients because of the complexity of the *VWF* gene or because of mutations in other genes, such as those affecting

TABLE 138.1	Classification of von Willebrand Disease
Type	**Description**
1	Partial quantitative deficiency of VWF. Mild abnormalities in multimer structure or distribution may occur.
2	Qualitative VWF defects.
2A	Decreased VWF-dependent platelet adhesion and deficiency of HMW VWF multimers.
2B	Increased affinity for platelet GPIbα.
2M	Decreased VWF-dependent platelet adhesion with a normal multimer distribution.
2N	Decreased affinity for FVIII.
3	Almost complete deficiency of VWF.

FVIII, Factor FVIII; *GPIbα*, glycoprotein 1bα; HMW, high molecular weight; VWF, von Willebrand factor.

secretion or clearance, which also lead to a VWD phenotype. A third level of classification denoted by roman numerals (e.g., VWD type 2A IIA) indicates specific phenotypes and is a remnant of an older classification system that is mainly used in the research setting.

von Willebrand Disease Type 1

Type 1 VWD, a quantitative deficiency of VWF, represents approximately 70% of VWD cases. The VWF is functionally normal without a specific abnormality in ligand binding sites or a significant decrease in HMW multimers. Functional assays of VWF, such as VWF:RCo, are decreased in proportion to the decrease in VWF:Ag concentration, and the ratio of functional activity as compared with VWF:Ag is normal (i.e., VWF:RCo/VWF:Ag ratio is >0.6).

Point mutations, most frequently missense mutations, have been identified in approximately 65% of individuals with type 1 VWD and occur throughout the *VWF* gene. Fully penetrant, dominantly inherited missense mutations are more often identified when VWF:Ag and VWF:RCo levels are less than 25 IU/dL. In contrast, incompletely penetrant, dominantly inherited missense mutations, such as p.Tyr1584Cys and p.Arg924Gln, are identified in approximately 50% of individuals whose VWF:Ag and VWF:RCo levels are above 25 IU/dL. The extent to which incompletely penetrant VWF mutations contribute to the bleeding phenotype in individuals with VWF levels of approximately 50 IU/dL is not clear, and genetic analyses in such cases are difficult to interpret.

Missense mutations may affect VWF levels by reducing secretion and/or increasing clearance. The most frequently reported genetic mutation is a missense mutation that results in the substitution of tyrosine with cysteine at codon 1584 (Y1584C), which is found in 10% to 20% of type 1 VWD patients. Intracellular retention is a common mechanism for type 1 VWD pathogenicity and can result from missense mutations in various VWF domains. Haploinsufficiency from a heterozygous null allele results in reduced VWF expression in a small proportion of cases. A common heterozygous in-frame large deletion of exons 4–5 was reported in a cohort of type 1 VWD patients in the United Kingdom, and this and similar partial gene deletions may contribute to the spectrum of mutations in a minority of cases. A well-described pathophysiologic mechanism for VWD type 1 is increased VWF clearance, referred to as type 1C (C for increased clearance), although this designation is not included in the ISTH classification. Patients typically have very low VWF levels, an increased vWFpp/VWF:Ag ratio, and a marked but short-lived response to DDAVP. Of note, the half-life of VWF/FVIII concentrates is normal in these individuals. Missense mutations mainly occur in the D3 domain and reduce the half-life of VWF up to 15-fold. R1205H, which is known as the "Vicenza" variant, is the most common, most severe, and best characterized of these mutations. Because of the transient response to DDAVP, the utility of this medication for treatment of major bleeds is questioned in this subgroup of patients.

VWF levels increase with age in normal individuals and the same phenomena is seen in patients with type 1 VWD (but not type 2 or 3). The increase has been reported as 3.5 U/dL VWF:Ag and 7.1 U/dL FVIII:C per decade. The effect of this increase on bleeding phenotype needs further investigation.

von Willebrand Disease Type 2

Type 2 VWD is characterized by a qualitative defect of VWF activity and is further classified into variants that affect VWF-platelet interactions (2A, 2B, and 2M) and that affect VWF binding to FVIII (2N) (Fig. 138.5).

Type 2A
VWD type 2A is the most common type 2 variant, accounting for approximately 10% of all VWD cases. VWD type 2A usually is inherited as a dominant trait and is characterized by a lack of HMW

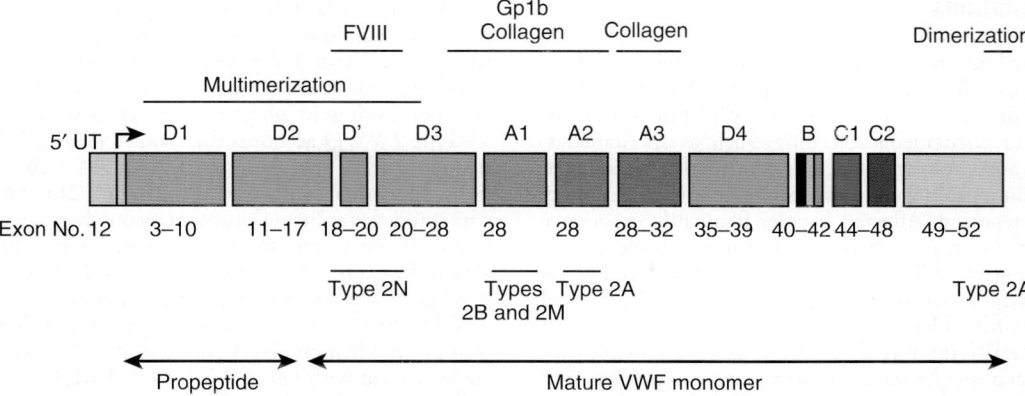

Fig. 138.5 FUNCTIONAL DOMAINS OF VON WILLEBRAND FACTOR AND LOCATION OF TYPE 2 VON WILLEBRAND DISEASE MUTATIONS. VWF protein comprises a large N-terminal propeptide and mature subunit. Repeated protein domains are designated A through D. Highlighted are binding sites for factor VIII, platelet Gp1b, collagen, and the areas critical for dimerization and multimerization. Sites of the common mutations that result in type 2 VWD are shown. *Arrow* indicates translational start site. *FVIII,* Factor VIII; *GP,* glycoprotein; *VWF,* von Willebrand factor.

and/or intermediate-molecular-weight (IMW) multimers, which are the most hemostatically active. This results in a disproportionately low functional activity compared with antigen level (i.e., VWF:RCo to VWF:Ag ratio of <0.6). The FVIII level may be low or normal. The multimer profile shows a loss of HMW and sometimes IMW multimers. This subtype may encompass missense mutations that impair dimer (CK domain) or multimer assembly (recessive mutations in the D1 and D2 domains), disrupt intersubunit disulphide bonds (D3 and D2 domains) enhance susceptibility to ADAMTS13-mediated proteolysis (A2 and A1 domains), and/or result in intracellular retention of VWF, particularly the HMW multimers (D3, A1, and A2 domains).

Type 2B

Type 2B VWD is the result of gain-of-function mutations within the GpIbα binding site on VWF. Missense mutations are located in exon 28, in or close to the A1 domain. This results in spontaneous binding of VWF to platelets without the need for a VWF-collagen interaction. The VWF-platelet interactions selectively deplete the HMW multimers by increasing ADAMTS13 proteolysis. The increased binding of mutant VWF to platelets also triggers the formation of platelet aggregates, which are removed from the circulation resulting in thrombocytopenia. Altered megakaryocytopoiesis characterized by giant platelets with abnormal ultrastructure contributes to the thrombocytopenia.

The laboratory profile reveals a decreased VWF:RCo to VWF:Ag ratio and absence of HMW multimers, but in contrast to 2A, ristocetin-induced platelet aggregation (RIPA) reveals increased sensitivity to low doses of ristocetin. Although these features may be present to varying degrees in the majority of patients, not all cases demonstrate these classic features. For example, mutations affecting p.Pro1266Leu may enhance GpIbα binding (RIPA) without inducing thrombocytopenia or HMW multimer loss.

Type 2M

Type 2M VWD (the M refers to multimer) is characterized by a loss of function mutation within the VWF GpIbα binding site. The laboratory workup shows a reduced ratio of VWF:RCo to VWF:Ag but a normal multimer pattern. A number of missense mutations are reported in exon 28, and there are case reports of mutations in exons 27, 30–31, and 52. VWF exhibits reduced affinity for GpIbα because of mutations in the A1 domain that alter protein conformation, but HMW multimers are normal. Rare mutations in the A3 domain that impair the VWF/collagen interaction are also classified as 2M VWD. In these cases, VWF:RCo may be normal, and the diagnosis requires VWF/collagen binding assays (VWF:CB).

Type 2N

Type 2N VWD (with the N referring to Normandy, where the first cases were reported) has been described as an autosomal form of hemophilia A and is an important consideration in the differential diagnosis of individuals of either sex who present with low FVIII levels. The affinity of VWF for FVIII is reduced because of mutations in the FVIII binding site or conformational changes that impair the VWF-FVIII interaction. The characteristic laboratory feature is a disproportionate decrease in the FVIII level relative to the VWF level (which may be low or normal) with a resultant reduction in the FVIII/VWF:Ag ratio. The majority of patients with VWD type 2N have a normal multimer profile, but occasional cases will demonstrate loss of HMW multimers. The majority (≈ 80%) of missense mutations are located in exons 18–20 (D′ and D3) with a much lower proportion of mutations in exons 17 and 24–27. Type 2N exhibits autosomal recessive inheritance, and affected individuals are either homozygous or compound heterozygous for missense mutations, or compound heterozygous for a missense mutation and a mutation resulting in a null allele. Definitive diagnosis requires evidence of reduced FVIII binding to VWF (VWF:FVIIIB) or identification of causative mutations in the FVIII binding region of the *VWF* gene.

von Willebrand Disease Type 3

Type 3 VWD is defined by a virtual absence of VWF. The inheritance of type 3 VWD is autosomal recessive in about half of type 3 patients and autosomal codominant in the remainder: approximately 50% of carriers will be symptomatic and meet the criteria for type 1 VWD. This condition is characterized by prolongation of the aPTT, undetectable levels of VWF:Ag and VWF:RCo, and FVIII levels less than 10 IU/dL (i.e., less than 10% of normal). Mutations associated with type 3 VWD are found throughout the coding region of VWF, including the propeptide. Up to 80% of type 3 VWD patients have two null alleles and produce little or no VWF. Null alleles can result from a variety of mutations, with nonsense mutations accounting for about one-third. Approximately 20% of alleles carry missense mutations predominantly located in the D1–D2 (exons 3–11) and D4–CK (exons 37–52) domains. These mutations may impair dimer or multimer formation, resulting in intracellular VWF retention and decreased secretion into plasma. Large deletions, predominantly resulting in frameshift mutations affecting one or more exons, contribute to approximately 12% of the type 3 VWD mutation spectrum. Because there is little or no circulating VWF, patients with these mutations may develop alloantibodies against infused VWF.

Clinical Manifestations

The bleeding history depends on disease severity; type 3 VWD is often diagnosed early in life, whereas mild type 1 VWD may not be diagnosed until adulthood. Individuals with VWD primarily complain of excessive mucocutaneous bleeding, such as spontaneous, recurrent epistaxis, and prolonged bleeding after dental cleaning or extraction. In addition, prolonged or excessive bleeding after surgery or trauma is often reported. Affected females frequently experience menorrhagia from the time of menarche, and can have prolonged or excessive bleeding after childbirth. Musculoskeletal bleeding is unusual, except in type 2N or type 3 VWD when the FVIII:C level may be below 10 IU/dL. Bleeding assessment tools (BATs) help to standardize and quantify the bleeding history. BATs are helpful for making a VWD diagnosis. In addition, high scores are predictive of the risk of future bleeding. (see Chapter 128)

Example of the Presentation and Impact of Type 1 von Willebrand Disease

J.C., a 26-year-old female, presents with delayed postpartum hemorrhage (PPH) after the delivery of her first child. The pregnancy and delivery were unremarkable. One week postpartum, the patient experienced heavy bleeding, and required a dilation and curettage. At the same time, she was started on tranexamic acid, which was continued for 2 weeks. By approximately 3 weeks postpartum, there was complete cessation of bleeding. A bleeding history was significant for the following: excessive postsurgical bleeding following tonsillectomy and adenoidectomy, which required red blood cell transfusion; excessive bleeding postdental extractions, requiring consultation with the dentist and repacking; and menorrhagia from the time of menarche, which had been well controlled with the combined oral contraceptive pill. There was no family history of VWD. Investigations revealed VWF:Ag 0.40 IU/dL, VWF:RCo 0:39 IU/dL, and FVIII:C 0.60 IU/dL. Multimer gel was unremarkable. A DDAVP challenge demonstrated that the patient was a responder. She became pregnant again 4 years later. At the time of delivery she was treated with tranexamic acid and a dose of DDAVP after the cord was clamped. Her postpartum course was uncomplicated.

This case illustrates several important points. First, type 1 VWD is a mild to moderate bleeding disorder. Patients often do not have significant symptoms on a regular basis, or symptoms may be masked or ameliorated by concomitant combined oral contraceptive use, which is common in this patient demographic. A careful bleeding history focusing on past hemostatic challenges and subsequent complications is vital in making the diagnosis. A high index of suspicion is required for unusual bleeding complications, such as delayed PPH. The importance of making the diagnosis is highlighted here. With little burden of prophylactic treatment, bleeding complications can be avoided.

Type 1 VWD accounts for up to 70% of VWD. It typically manifests as mild mucocutaneous bleeding; however, symptoms may be more severe if VWF levels are below 15 IU/dL. Epistaxis and bruising are common symptoms in children. Menorrhagia is the most common finding in women of reproductive age.

Type 2 VWD accounts for about 25% of all VWD. The relative frequency of the subtypes is 2A > 2N > 2M > 2B in European populations. Individuals with type 2A, 2B, and 2M VWD usually present with mild to moderate mucocutaneous bleeding, but bleeding episodes can be severe, particularly when VWF:RCo is very low or absent. In many patients with type 2B VWD, thrombocytopenia can develop or worsen with infection, surgery, pregnancy, or treatment with DDAVP. The symptoms of type 2N VWD are similar to those seen in mild hemophilia A (see Chapter 135) because both disorders are associated with reduced levels of FVIII:C.

Type 3 VWD is the rarest subtype and accounts for less than 5% of VWD. Prevalence estimates range from 0.55 to 6 per million, with higher rates seen with consanguineous marriage. Type 3 VWD manifests with severe bleeding, including excessive mucocutaneous bleeding and musculoskeletal bleeding.

Penetrance

In autosomal dominant type 1 VWD, mutations resulting in plasma VWF level less than 25 IU/dL are often fully penetrant, whereas those resulting in higher VWF levels are often incompletely penetrant. Mutations responsible for autosomal dominant types of VWD (2A, 2B, and 2M) are often fully penetrant. Thus in contrast to the variably positive family histories in patients with type 1 VWD, those with type 2 VWD usually have a positive family history.

Laboratory Investigations

The laboratory evaluation for VWD involves a battery of qualitative and quantitative measurements of VWF and FVIII that should be interpreted by a physician with experience in this area given the heterogeneity of possible results (Table 138.2).

Screening Tests

The complete blood cell count may show microcytic anemia as a result of iron deficiency or thrombocytopenia in type 2B VWD. The aPTT is often normal, but may be prolonged if the FVIII level is reduced below 30–40 IU/dL, as can be seen with severe type 1, type 2N, or type 3 VWD. The prothrombin time is normal in VWD.

TABLE 138.2   Table of Investigations

VWD Type	vWF:RCo IU/dL[a]	vWF:Ag IU/dL[a]	RCo/Ag IU/dL[a]	FVIII:C IU/dL[a]	Multimer Pattern[b]	Other
1	Low	Low	Equivalent	~1.5× VWF:Ag	Normal	
2A	Low	Low	VWF:RCo < VWF:Ag	Low or normal	Abnormal ↓ HMWM	
2B	Low	Low	VWF:RCo < VWF:Ag	Low or normal	Abnormal ↓ HMWM	↑ RIPA[c] (↓ platelet count)
2M	Low	Low	VWF:RCo < VWF:Ag	Low or normal	Normal	
2N	Normal/low	Normal/low	Equivalent	<30	Normal	↓ VWF:FVIIIB[d]
3	Absent	Absent	NA	<10	Absent	

[a]Relative to the reference range (approximate values); VWF:RCo (50–200 IU/dL); VWF:Ag (50–200 IU/dL); FVIII:C (50–150 IU/dL).
[b]HMWM, High-molecular-weight multimers.
[c]Increased agglutination at low concentrations of ristocetin.
[d]The ability of VWF to bind and protect FVIII is reduced. VWF and FVIII levels can look exactly like those in males with mild haemophilia A or in symptomatic hemophilia A carrier females.

Ag, Antigen; FVIII:C, FVIII level; NA, not applicable; RCo, ristocetin cofactor; RIPA, ristocetin-induced platelet aggregation; VWD, von Willebrand disease; VWF:FVIIIB, FVIII-binding assay.

Although some laboratories may also include a skin bleeding time and platelet function analysis (PFA closure time) in their evaluation of an individual with suspected VWD, these tests lack sensitivity in persons with mild bleeding or specificity for VWD.

Confirming a Diagnosis of von Willebrand Disease

The following specific factor assays should be performed even if the screening tests are normal.

von Willebrand Factor: Antigen

This assay determines the quantity of VWF protein antigen in the plasma, and is performed using an enzyme-linked immunosorbent assay (ELISA) or latex immunoassay (LIA). The normal range (which should be determined independently by each laboratory) is approximately 50–200 IU/dL.

von Willebrand Factor: Ristocetin Cofactor

The VWF:RCo activity assay measures the capacity of VWF to agglutinate platelets in response to ristocetin. The normal range is approximately 50–200 IU/dL.

Factor VIII: C Level

The functional FVIII assay determines the activity of FVIII in clot-based assays. The normal range is approximately 50–150 IU/dL.

Several analytic variables can complicate the diagnosis of VWD. Based on established reference ranges, approximately 2.5% of the normal population will have low VWF levels. In addition, assay variability, particularly for VWF:RCo, renders differentiation of type 1 VWD from type 2 VWD difficult. VWF:RCo and VWF:Ag determined by LIA have limited sensitivity, which may result in the misdiagnosis of type 3 VWD as type 1 or type 2 VWD. Finally, inappropriate sample handling can lead to decreases in VWF:Ag, VWF:RCo, and FVIII, with VWF:RCo predominantly affected. All of these factors must be considered when interpreting VWF laboratory results and at least two sets of tests using fresh samples are needed to confirm the diagnosis of VWD. Diagnostic testing should be avoided in stressed, ill, or pregnant patients (see box on Factors to Consider When Interpreting von Willebrand Disease Results).

Discriminating Tests to Identify von Willebrand Disease Subtype

von Willebrand Factor Multimer Analysis

Sodium dodecyl sulfate-agarose electrophoresis is used to assess VWF oligomers in plasma (see Fig. 138.4). Normal plasma contains multimers composed of over 40 VWF dimers. Multimers are classified as HMW, IMW, and low molecular weight (LMW) by counting bands 1–5 as LMW, 6–10 as IMW, and those above 10 as HMW. HMW and/or IMW multimers are decreased or missing in types 2A and 2B VWD.

Low Dose Ristocetin-Induced Platelet Aggregation

The RIPA assay tests the capacity of VWF to agglutinate platelets with varying concentrations of ristocetin. In contrast to the VWF:RCo (which evaluates the interaction between the patient's VWF and formalin-fixed platelets), the low dose RIPA assay evaluates the sensitivity of the patient's platelets to low-dose ristocetin. In cases of type 2B or platelet-type VWD, the platelet membrane is "overloaded" with high-affinity mutant VWF, resulting in abnormal

Factors to Consider When Interpreting von Willebrand Disease Results

	Considerations	Results
Preanalytical	When was the sample collected and processed? Was there a significant delay before samples were run? Were they frozen in a timely fashion?	VWF:RCo may be decreased resulting in a false-positive diagnosis of type 2 VWD
Analytical	Convention of established references	False-positive diagnosis of VWD in 2.5% of population
	High degree of assay variability, particularly for VWF:RCo	False-positive diagnosis of type 2 in a type 1 patient may result in the misdiagnosis of type 3 for type 1 or type 2 VWD
	A high lower limit of detection for certain VWF:Ag and VWF:RCo assays, in particular LIA-based assays	
Patient factors	Drugs (OCP, HRT, or valproic acid)	False negative or positive
	ABO type	False negative
	Pregnancy	Reversible acquired von Willebrand syndrome
	Hypothyroidism	
	Comorbid illness (e.g., valvular heart disease, lymphoma)	

Ag, Antigen; LIA, latex immunoassay; OCP, oral contraceptive pill; HRT, hormone replacement therapy; RCo, ristocetin cofactor; VWD, von Willebrand disease; VWF, von Willebrand factor.

platelet agglutination with low ristocetin concentrations. In some cases of type 2B VWD, all variables except low dose RIPA may be normal. RIPA at normal ristocetin concentrations should be normal in type 1 VWD unless VWF levels are below 10–20 IU/dL.

Binding of Factor VIII by von Willebrand Factor

The VWF:FVIIIB ELISA test determines the ability of VWF to bind FVIII and is useful for the diagnosis of type 2N VWD. There are no standard units for the output of this test.

Collagen Binding Assay

The VWF:CB ELISA test determines the ability of VWF to bind to collagen and is dependent on HMW VWF multimers. Consequently, the test helps to identify functional VWF discordance (i.e., to distinguish between types 1 and 2 VWD). Reduced collagen binding reflects the loss of HMW multimers or can reflect a specific collagen-binding deficiency (type 2M VWD). The normal range is approximately 50–200 IU/dL.

von Willebrand Factor Propeptide/Antigen Ratio

An increased ratio of steady-state plasma VWFpp to VWF:Ag identifies patients with mutations that increase VWF clearance. The mean ratio in normal individuals is 1.3, with a normal range of 0.54–1.98.

Desmopressin Responsiveness

DDAVP administration releases VWF stores from endothelial cells. The pattern of DDAVP response in VWD subtypes (Table 138.3)

TABLE 138.3	Desmopressin Responsiveness in the Various Subtypes of von Willebrand Disease					
VWD Type	**vWF:RCo**	**vWF:Ag**	**RCo/Ag**	**FVIII:C IU/dL**	**vWF:CB**	**vWF:CB/vWF:Ag**
1	Increase	Increase	Remains >0.7	Increase	Increase	Remains >0.7
2A	No/little change	Increase	Remains <0.7	Increase	No/little change	Remains <0.7
2M (GP1B binding dysfunction)	No/little change	Increase	Remains <0.7	Increase	Increase	Remains >0.7
3	No/little change	No/little change		Increase	No/little change	No/little change

Ag, Antigen; *VWF:CB*, collagen binding assays; *FVIII:C*, factor VIII level; *GP1B*, glycoprotein 1B; *RCo*, ristocetin cofactor; *VWD*, von Willebrand disease; *VWF*, von Willebrand factor.
Modified from Favaloro EJ: Rethinking the diagnosis of von Willebrand disease. *Thromb Res* 127;Suppl 2:17, 2011.

may help to assign VWD subtype. In addition, a decrease in the duration of the DDAVP response may indicate an increased clearance mutation.

Genotyping

The identification of a mutation is not necessary for the diagnosis of VWD. However, genotyping should be considered when specialized testing with the VWF:FVIIIB assay is unavailable and type 2N VWD is suspected. Genotyping is also useful to discriminate between type 2B VWD and platelet-type VWD, and for prenatal assessment and alloantibody risk assessment in type 3 VWD. In mild-type 1 VWD, the likelihood of finding a mutation is low because mutations are not localized to a particular domain or exon and the results are of little clinical utility.

Differential Diagnosis

Hemophilia A

Both type 2N VWD and mild hemophilia A (caused by mutations in F8) result in reduced levels of FVIII:C (approximately 5–40 IU/dL) with normal or borderline low levels of VWF. Although the VWF:FVIIIB test distinguishes between the two disorders, the test is not widely available and the results may be equivocal.

In families with reduced FVIII:C, an X-linked pattern of inheritance helps identify those with mild hemophilia A. When family history is uninformative and VWF levels and function are normal, it may be preferable to perform sequence analysis of the *F8* gene before the *VWF* gene, even in symptomatic females who are simplex cases (i.e., a single occurrence in a family), because *F8* mutation and skewed X-chromosome inactivation (lyonization) are often responsible for symptoms. *F8* mutations may be detected in more than 50% of cases referred for "possible 2N VWD or hemophilia A." When *F8* mutations are absent, or if the VWF level and function are also abnormal, *VWF* can be analyzed.

Platelet-Type von Willebrand Disease

Platelet-type VWD (PT-VWD, also called *pseudo VWD*) mimics type 2B VWD but is caused by mutations in the platelet *GPIBA*. The disorders can be distinguished by mixing patient platelets or plasma with control plasma or platelets and using aggregometry or flow cytometry to identify the defective component. However, these assays are technically challenging. In the absence of mutations in exon 28 of VWF, mutations in exon 2 of *GPIBA* are identified in approximately 10% of persons misdiagnosed with type 2B VWD. To date, missense mutations reported to affect GpIbα include p.Gly249 and p.Met255 plus a 27 bp in-frame deletion p.Pro449_Ser457del (c.1345_1371del27). Misdiagnosis of PT-VWD may result in ineffective treatment of patients. VWF concentrate is needed to correct

the reduced VWF level, but platelet transfusion may also be required if there is significant thrombocytopenia. The half-life of replaced VWF is reduced in PT-VWD because of binding to abnormal GpIbα. Consequently, VWF concentrate must be administered more frequently.

Acquired von Willebrand Syndrome

This mild to moderate bleeding disorder is a result of an acquired deficiency or dysfunction of VWF. Exclusion of a lifelong personal and family history of bleeding is an important aspect of the diagnosis. Although acquired von Willebrand syndrome (AvWS) was thought to be uncommon, cohort studies suggest that the prevalence may be significantly underestimated. When selected patient populations were screened, approximately 10% of patients with hematologic disorders, approximately 79% with aortic stenosis, and up to 100% with left ventricular assist devices were diagnosed with AvWS. The median age of diagnosis is 62 years, but the disorder may occur in any age group (range 2–96 years). AvWS has diverse pathology and may result from autoantibodies that impair VWF function or increase its clearance, adsorption of HMW VWF multimers to malignant cells or platelets, proteolytic cleavage of VWF after shear stress-induced unfolding, or decreased VWF synthesis. Diseases that have been implicated include (1) lymphoproliferative disorders and plasma cell dyscrasias, including monoclonal gammopathy of unknown significance, multiple myeloma, and Waldenström macroglobulinemia; (2) autoimmune disorders, including systemic lupus erythematosus, scleroderma, and antiphospholipid antibody syndrome; (3) aortic stenosis and ventricular septal defects, which can trigger shear-induced conformational changes that increase VWF proteolysis; (4) thrombocytosis, including myeloproliferative neoplasms that lead to a type 2 phenotype; (5) Wilms tumor or lymphoproliferative disorders that can be associated with increased VWF clearance by aberrant binding to tumor cells; (6) decreased VWF synthesis, for instance, with hypothyroidism, and drugs including valproic acid, ciprofloxacin, griseofulvin, and hydroxyethyl starch. The treatment goals can be divided into two categories: treatment or prevention of bleeding and induction of long-term remission. The agents used for prevention and treatment of bleeding in AvWS overlap with those used in VWD and include DDAVP or VWF-containing concentrates, which can transiently increase VWF levels. Other options include recombinant factor VIIa, antifibrinolytic agents, intravenous immunoglobulin, or plasmapheresis for AvWS associated with monoclonal gammopathies. Often a combination of agents is required to affect hemostasis. Maneuvers to induce long-term remission will depend on the underlying pathogenic etiology of AvWS. Whenever possible, treatment of the underlying disorder should be considered and may result in remission of the AvWS.

Management of von Willebrand Disease

The approach to the management of VWD is summarized in Fig. 138.6.

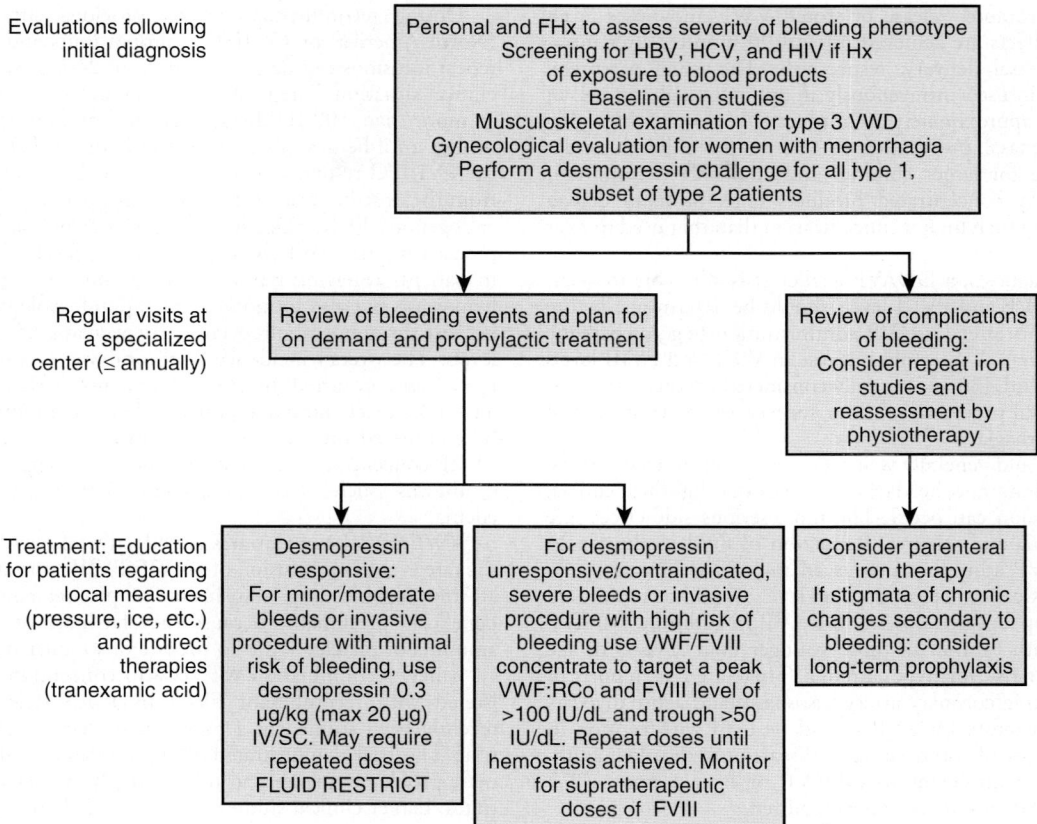

Evaluations following initial diagnosis

Personal and FHx to assess severity of bleeding phenotype
Screening for HBV, HCV, and HIV if Hx
of exposure to blood products
Baseline iron studies
Musculoskeletal examination for type 3 VWD
Gynecological evaluation for women with menorrhagia
Perform a desmopressin challenge for all type 1,
subset of type 2 patients

Regular visits at a specialized center (≤ annually)

Review of bleeding events and plan for on demand and prophylactic treatment

Review of complications of bleeding: Consider repeat iron studies and reassessment by physiotherapy

Treatment: Education for patients regarding local measures (pressure, ice, etc.) and indirect therapies (tranexamic acid)

Desmopressin responsive: For minor/moderate bleeds or invasive procedure with minimal risk of bleeding, use desmopressin 0.3 μg/kg (max 20 μg) IV/SC. May require repeated doses FLUID RESTRICT

For desmopressin unresponsive/contraindicated, severe bleeds or invasive procedure with high risk of bleeding use VWF/FVIII concentrate to target a peak VWF:RCo and FVIII level of >100 IU/dL and trough >50 IU/dL. Repeat doses until hemostasis achieved. Monitor for supratherapeutic doses of FVIII

Consider parenteral iron therapy If stigmata of chronic changes secondary to bleeding: consider long-term prophylaxis

Fig. 138.6 APPROACH TO THE MANAGEMENT OF VON WILLEBRAND DISEASE. *FHx,* Family history; *FVIII,* factor VIII; *HBV,* hepatitis B virus; *HCV,* hepatitis C virus; *HIV,* human immunodeficiency virus; *Hx,* history; *IV,* intravenous; *RCo,* ristocetin cofactor; *SC,* subcutaneous; *VWD,* von Willebrand disease; *VWF,* von Willebrand factor.

Evaluations Following Initial Diagnosis

To establish the extent of disease in an individual diagnosed with VWD, the following evaluations are recommended: (1) a personal and family history of bleeding to help predict severity and tailor treatment (use of a standardized bleeding assessment tool can be helpful); (2) a joint and muscle evaluation for those with type 3 VWD (musculoskeletal bleeding is rare in types 1 and 2 VWD); (3) screening for hepatitis B and C, as well as HIV if the diagnosis is type 3 VWD or if the individual received blood products or plasma-derived clotting factor concentrates before 1985 (this screening should be followed by vaccinations for hepatitis A and B); (4) determination of serum iron and ferritin (to assess iron stores), because many individuals with VWD are iron deficient, particularly women with menorrhagia; and (5) gynecologic evaluation for women with menorrhagia. Individuals with VWD benefit from referral to a comprehensive bleeding disorders program for education, treatment, and genetic counseling.

Treatment of von Willebrand Disease

The management of VWD can be divided into three main categories: (1) localized measures to stop or minimize bleeding; (2) pharmacologic agents that provide indirect hemostatic benefit; and (3) treatments that directly increase plasma VWF and FVIII levels.

Localized Measures

The importance of localized measures to control bleeding in VWD, such as the application of direct pressure to a site of bleeding or injury, should not be understated. Biting down on a piece of gauze may halt

bleeding from a tooth socket, and application of a compression bandage and cold pack to an injured limb may reduce subsequent hematoma formation. With epistaxis, patients may benefit from a step-wise action plan that escalates from pressure to packing after a certain time period. In selected cases, nasal cautery may be required for prolonged or excessive epistaxis.

A number of topical hemostatic agents that are predominately used to achieve surgical hemostasis may have a limited role in the treatment of VWD and bleeding; these include gelatin foam/matrix, topical thrombin, and fibrin sealants.

Indirect Therapies

Fibrinolytic inhibitors (e.g., tranexamic acid), which inhibit the conversion of plasminogen to plasmin, can be used either as sole therapy or as adjuncts to DDAVP or VWF/FVIII concentrates and may be particularly useful to control mucosal bleeding in the oral cavity or gastrointestinal (GI) or genitourinary tracts. The most common adverse events to tranexamic acid are GI side-effects and headache. Tranexamic acid is contraindicated in disseminated intravascular coagulation and bleeding from the upper urinary tract, where it can lead to obstruction by clots. Hormonal treatments (i.e., the combined oral contraceptive pill) are effective for the treatment of menorrhagia. Nonmedical treatments, such as levonorgestrel-releasing intrauterine systems or endometrial ablation, may be useful in selected patients with VWD.

Desmopressin

Most individuals with type 1 VWD and some with type 2 VWD respond to intranasal, intravenous or subcutaneous treatment with

DDAVP, which promotes release of stored VWF and raises levels 3–10-fold. Peak effects are achieved 30 and 90 minutes after intravenous and intranasal delivery, respectively. The usual parenteral dose is 0.3 μg/kg infused intravenously in approximately 50 mL of normal saline over approximately 30 minutes. The dose of the highly concentrated intranasal preparation is 150 μg for children under 50 kg and 300 μg for larger children and adults. It is important to note that highly concentrated products (e.g., Stimate) deliver 150 μg per spray, a much higher concentration than that used to treat enuresis.

After VWD diagnosis, a DDAVP challenge is advisable to assess VWF response. VWF and FVIII levels should be determined before and at several points after DDAVP administration (e.g., at baseline and at 1 and 4 hours). A threefold increase in VWF and FVIII levels to at least 0.30 IU/mL (30%) is usually considered adequate for situations such as dental procedures, minor surgery, or the treatment of epistaxis or menorrhagia.

DDAVP is safe and generally well tolerated. Common side effects include facial flushing and headache. Tachycardia, lightheadedness, and mild hypotension can occur. The most serious side effects are severe hyponatremia and seizures. Reduction of fluid intake for 24 hours after DDAVP administration is an important precaution to prevent water intoxication. Serum sodium levels should be monitored in patients receiving repeated doses of DDAVP. In addition, DDAVP should be used with caution in those younger than 2 years of age because of a higher risk for hyponatremia. There are case reports of DDAVP precipitating coronary artery vasospasm and acute myocardial infarction. Therefore DDAVP should be used with caution in patients with a history of coronary artery disease or in the older adult. In persons who are intolerant to DDAVP or have a poor VWF response, clotting factor concentrate is required.

An important limitation in the use of DDAVP is the development of tachyphylaxis with repeated administration. When given repeatedly at intervals of less than 24 hours, the magnitude of the VWF and FVIII increments can fall to approximately 70% of those obtained with the initial dose. For practical purposes, a single dose of DDAVP before dental extractions or minor procedures is usually sufficient. Although repeated doses can be given at 12 or 24 hours, the potential for tachyphylaxis must be considered. Additionally, in situations where repeat dosing is considered, more prolonged fluid restriction is required.

Although most type 1 VWD patients respond adequately to DDAVP, type 3 VWD patients typically do not respond to this drug, and the response in type 2 VWD patients is variable. Type 2A patients often exhibit an adequate response and may benefit from a DDAVP trial. Type 2M patients typically do not respond well to DDAVP. DDAVP is generally contraindicated in type 2B VWD because of the transient thrombocytopenia that accompanies the release of mutant VWF. In type 2N VWD, DDAVP produces a two-fold to ninefold increase in FVIII, but the increase persists for approximately 3 hours. Therefore DDAVP should be reserved for situations in which a transient rise in FVIII is sufficient.

von Willebrand Factor/Factor VIII Concentrates

VWF/FVIII concentrates are required for patients who do not have an adequate response, experience side effects, or have contraindications to DDAVP. Because of tachyphylaxis and the risk of hyponatremia with DDAVP, patients with severe bleeding or those requiring major or repeated surgery often need VWF replacement therapy. Purified, viral-inactivated, plasma-derived VWF/FVIII is the product most frequently used (e.g., Humate-P, Wilate). The quantity of ristocetin cofactor activity (VWF:RCo) relative to FVIII:C varies by product; Humate-P contains 2.4 VWF:RCo units for each 1 FVIII:C unit, whereas Wilate contains a 1:1 ratio. Both products contain a full spectrum of VWF multimers, including HMW multimers, and closely resemble normal plasma. Highly purified FVIII concentrates (monoclonal antibody purified and recombinant) should not be used to treat VWD because they lack VWF.

Dosing recommendations are provided either in VWF:RCo (North America) or FVIII:C (Europe) units and are weight-based; repeat infusions can be given every 8 to 24 hours, depending on the clinical situation. The goal is to maintain VWF:RCo and FVIII:C at more than 100 IU/dL at peak and at more than 50 IU/dL at trough until hemostasis is achieved. With VWF/FVIII concentrates, the FVIII:C response is higher and more sustained than predicted from the dose because of the stabilizing effect of exogenous VWF on endogenous FVIII. Details regarding dosing can be found in the product inserts. VWF:RCo and FVIII:C levels should be measured in patients receiving repeat infusions, not only to ensure adequate hemostasis but also to monitor for supraphysiological levels of FVIII because thromboembolic events have been associated with high FVIII levels. The overall incidence of thrombotic events is very low, and most cases occurred in surgical patients with other risk factors. Therefore mechanical and anticoagulant thromboprophylaxis should be considered on a case-by-case basis. Adverse reactions to VWF/FVIII concentrates are rare but include allergic and anaphylactic symptoms, such as urticaria, chest tightness, rash, pruritus, and edema.

VWF:FVIII concentrates are effective in over 97% of events. In the rare event that infusion of a VWF/FVIII concentrate is ineffective at stopping bleeding, transfusion of platelet concentrates may be beneficial, presumably because they facilitate the delivery of small amounts of platelet VWF to the site of vascular injury.

A new recombinant VWF (rvWF) concentrate, which is administered with recombinant FVIII in a 1.3 RCo:FVIII ratio, has recently been studied in a prospective phase 1 randomized clinical trial. The trial demonstrated safety, tolerability, and a pharmacokinetic profile comparable to that with plasma-derived VWF concentrates. Larger clinical studies are needed and are ongoing, but rvWF represents an important advance in the treatment options for VWD.

Prophylaxis

Short-term prophylaxis with a combination of an antifibrinolytic, DDAVP, and/or VWF/FVIII concentrates, in anticipation of a defined bleeding challenge, such as surgery, is the standard of care in the treatment of VWD. The role of long-term continuous prophylaxis, defined as primary if initiated before long-term sequelae have developed (e.g., joint damage) or secondary if initiated after the development of chronic changes, is less established in VWD than it is in severe hemophilia. Individuals with severe cases of VWD, in particular type 3 VWD and certain patients with severe type 1 or type 2 VWD, may experience recurrent joint bleeds, as well as severe and frequently recurrent nasal/oral, GI, or menstrual bleeding. The resultant anemia, hospitalizations, and absences from school or work may have a significant impact on quality of life. Although there is limited evidence, several cohort and case studies suggest that both primary and secondary long-term prophylaxis improve quality of life, alleviate anemia, reduce hospitalizations, and prevent chronic joint disease. Complications are unusual aside from rare cases of VWF inhibitor formation (approximately 3%). Controversy exists about the specific indications, schedules, and dosing of prophylactic regimens. This is the subject of an ongoing international trial, known as the VWD International Prophylaxis trial, which began recruitment of patients in 2007.

Pediatric Issues

Prenatal diagnosis for pregnancies at increased risk (generally only for type 3 VWD) is possible by analysis of DNA extracted from fetal cells obtained by chorionic villus sampling at 11–13 weeks of gestation or amniocentesis at 15–18 weeks of gestation. The disease-causing allele(s) of an affected family member must be identified before prenatal testing. Preimplantation genetic diagnosis may be available for families in which the disease-causing mutation(s) have been identified.

The diagnosis and care of infants and children with VWD require special consideration. An accurate assessment of hemorrhagic symptoms is a key component in the diagnosis of VWD, but it often presents a significant challenge in the pediatric population. Because young children may have been exposed to few hemostatic challenges and may be prepubertal, the bleeding history may be unimpressive. The effect this negative history may have on perceived risk for bleeding is highlighted in two of the previously published bleeding scores, which assign a negative value to lack of bleeding symptoms and are based on the accumulation of bleeding symptoms or complications. Finally, the initial diagnostic assessment of an infant is complicated by the fact that VWF levels are higher in the neonatal period. Consequently, phenotypic testing of VWD should be delayed until later in childhood (see Fig. 138.6).

DDAVP should be avoided in children younger than the age of 2 because of the potential difficulty in restricting fluids. Infant males should be circumcised only after consultation with a pediatric hemostasis specialist. Typically, only patients with type 3 VWD experience spontaneous musculoskeletal bleeding, such as that seen in patients with severe hemophilia, and should be considered for long-term prophylaxis with VWF/FVIII concentrates, as discussed in the preceding section (see box on Assessment of a Neonate).

SUGGESTED READINGS

Abshire TC, Federici AB, Alvarez MT, et al: Prophylaxis in severe forms of von Willebrand's disease: results from the von Willebrand Disease Prophylaxis Network (PN). *Haemophilia* 19:76, 2013.

Berntorp E: Haemate P/Humate-P: a systematic review. *Thromb Res* 124:S11, 2009.

Bowen D: An influence of ABO blood group on the rate of proteolysis of von Willebrand factor ADAMTS13. *J Thromb Haemost* 1:33, 2003.

Bowman M, Mundell G, Grabell J, et al: Generation and validation of the condensed MCMDM-1VWD bleeding questionnaire for von Willebrand disease. *J Thromb Haemost* 6:2062, 2008.

Bowman M, Tuttle A, Notley C, et al: The genetics of Canadian type von Willebrand disease: further evidence for co-dominant inheritance of mutant alleles. *J Thromb Haemost* 11:512, 2013.

Casari C, Lenting PJ, Wohner N, et al: Clearance of von Willebrand factor. *J Thromb Haemost* 11(Suppl 1):202, 2013.

Castaman G, Lethagen S, Federici AB, et al: Response to desmopressin is influenced by the genotype and phenotype in type 1 von Willebrand disease (VWD): results from the European study MCMDM-1VWD. *Blood* 111:3531, 2008.

Castaman G, Tosetto A, Rodeghiero F: Pregnancy and delivery in women with von Willebrand's disease and different von Willebrand factor mutations. *Haematologica* 95:963, 2010.

Cumming A, Grundy P, Keeney S, et al: An investigation of the von Willebrand factor genotype in UK patients diagnosed to have type I von Willebrand disease. *Thromb Haemost* 96:630, 2006.

Eikenboom J, Van Marion V, Putter H, et al: Linkage analysis in families diagnosed with type 1 von Willebrand disease in the European study, molecular and clinical markers for the diagnosis and management of type 1 VWD. *J Thromb Haemost* 4:774, 2006.

Federici AB: The use of desmopressin in von Willebrand disease: the experience of the first 30 years (1977-2007). *Haemophilia* 14(5):2008.

Federici AB, Bucciarelli P, Castaman G, et al: The bleeding score predicts clinical outcomes and replacement therapy in adults with von Willebrand disease. *Blood* 123:4037, 2014.

Federici AB, Rand JH, Bucciarelli P, et al: Acquired von Willebrand syndrome: data from an international registry. *Thromb Haemost* 84:345, 2000.

Giannini S, Cecchetti L, Mezzasoma AM, et al: Diagnosis of platelet-type von Willebrand disease by flow cytometry. *Haematologica* 95:1021, 2010.

Goodeve AC: The genetic basis of von Willebrand disease. *Blood Rev* 24:123, 2010.

Haberichter SL, Castaman G, Budde U, et al: Identification of type 1 von Willebrand disease patients with reduced von Willebrand factor survival by assay of the VWF propeptide in the European study: molecular and clinical markers for the diagnosis and management of type 1 VWD (MCMDM-1VWD). *Blood* 111:4979, 2008.

Halimeh S, Krümpel A, Rott H, et al: Long-term secondary prophylaxis in children, adolescents and young adults with von Willebrand disease. Results of a cohort study. *Thromb Haemost* 105:597, 2011.

James AH, Jamison MG: Bleeding events and other complications during pregnancy and childbirth in women with von Willebrand disease. *J Thromb Haemost* 5:1165, 2007.

James AH, Kouides PA, Abdul-Kadir R, et al: von Willebrand disease and other bleeding disorders in women: consensus on diagnosis and management from an international expert panel. *Am J Obstet Gynecol* 201:12. e1, 2009.

James PD, Notley C, Hegadorn C, et al: The mutational spectrum of type 1 von Willebrand disease: results from a Canadian cohort study. *Blood* 109:145, 2007.

Keeney S, Bowen D, Cumming A, et al: The molecular analysis of von Willebrand disease: a guideline from the UK haemophilia centre doctors' organisation haemophilia genetics laboratory network. *Haemophilia* 14:1099, 2008.

Mannucci PM, Kempton C, Millar C, et al: Pharmacokinetics and safety of a novel recombinant human von Willebrand factor manufactured with a plasma-free method: a prospective clinical trial. *Blood* 122:648, 2013.

McGrath RT, van den Biggelaar M, Byrne B, et al: Altered glycosyaltion of platelet-derived von Willebrand factor confers resistance to ADAMTS13 proteolysis. *Blood* 122:4107, 2013.

Millar CM, Brown SA: Oligosaccharide structures of von Willebrand factor and their potential role in von Willebrand disease. *Blood Rev* 20:83, 2006.

Nichols WL, Hultin MB, James AH, et al: von Willebrand disease (VWD): evidence-based diagnosis and management guidelines, the national heart, lung, and blood institute (NHLBI) expert panel report (USA). *Haemophilia* 14:171, 2008.

Sadler JE, Budde U, Eikenboom JCJ, et al: Update on the pathophysiology and classification of von Willebrand disease: a report of the subcommittee on von Willebrand factor. *J Thromb Haemost* 4:2103, 2006.

Sanders Y, Giezenaar M, Laros-van Gorkom B, et al: von Willebrand disease and aging: an evolving phenotype. *J Thromb Haemost* 12:1066, 2014.

Springer TA: Biology and physics of von Willebrand factor concatamers. *J Thromb Haemost* 9:130, 2011.

Tiede A, Rand JH, Budde U, et al: How I treat the acquired von Willebrand syndrome. *Blood* 117:6777, 2011.

Zhou YF, Eng TE, Zhe J, et al: Sequence and structure relationships within von Willebrand factor. *Blood* 120:449, 2012.

CHAPTER 139

DISSEMINATED INTRAVASCULAR COAGULATION

Marcel Levi

A variety of disorders, including infectious or inflammatory conditions and malignant disease, will lead to activation of coagulation. In many cases, this activation of coagulation will not lead to clinical complications and will not even be detected by routine laboratory tests, but can only be measured with sensitive molecular markers for activation of coagulation factors and pathways.[1,2] However, if the stimulus for activation of coagulation is sufficiently strong, the platelet count may decrease and global clotting times may become prolonged. In its most extreme form, systemic activation of coagulation is known as disseminated intravascular coagulation (DIC). DIC is characterized by the simultaneous occurrence of widespread (micro) vascular thrombosis, thereby compromising blood supply to various organs, which may contribute to organ failure.[3,4] Because of ongoing activation of the coagulation system and other factors, such as impaired synthesis and increased degradation of coagulation proteins and protease inhibitors, consumption of clotting factors and platelets may occur, resulting in bleeding from various sites.

In view of the multiple, often contrasting mechanisms that occur in patients with DIC, a consensual definition of DIC had been a matter of debate. In 2001 the subcommittee on DIC of the International Society on Thrombosis and Hemostasis proposed a definition that reflects the central role of the microvascular milieu, i.e., endothelial cells, blood cells, and the plasma protease system, in the pathogenesis of DIC. This definition of DIC reads as follows: "DIC is an acquired syndrome characterized by the intravascular activation of coagulation without a specific localization and arising from different causes. It can originate from and cause damage to the microvasculature, which if sufficiently severe, can produce organ dysfunction."[5]

The diagnosis of DIC may be hampered by the nonspecific nature of many indicators of coagulation activation, although newly developed scoring algorithms based on readily available routine laboratory parameters show promising diagnostic accuracy.[5] Owing to the complexity of the clinical presentation, the variable and unpredictable course, and the multitude of therapies given to patients with DIC, properly conducted clinical trials are difficult to perform and even to devise. Management relies on limited evidence from clinical trials in combination with small studies employing surrogate outcome endpoints and experience from case series, as well as from an understanding of the underlying pathophysiologic mechanisms.[6]

EPIDEMIOLOGY

Activation of coagulation in concert with inflammatory activation can result in microvascular thrombosis, which contributes to multiple organ failure in patients with severe sepsis.[7] In support of this concept, postmortem findings in patients with coagulation abnormalities and DIC on the background of severe sepsis include diffuse bleeding, hemorrhagic necrosis of tissues, microthrombi in small blood vessels, and thrombi in midsize and larger arteries and veins. Ischemia and necrosis were invariably the result of fibrin deposition in small and midsize vessels. Importantly, intravascular thrombi appear to be the driver of the organ dysfunction. Fibrin deposition in various organs also is a characteristic finding in animal models of DIC. Thus experimental bacteremia or endotoxemia causes intra- and extravascular fibrin deposition in the kidneys, lungs, liver, brain, and other organs. Amelioration of the hemostatic defect with various interventions reduces fibrin deposition, improves organ function in these models,

and, in some cases, reduces mortality. Finally, results of clinical studies also support the concept that activation of coagulation is an important determinant of clinical outcome. DIC has been shown to be an independent predictor of organ failure and mortality.[8] In a consecutive series of patients with severe sepsis, 43% of the patients with DIC were compared with the 27% without DIC. In that study, the severity of the coagulopathy was directly related to mortality.[9]

In addition to microvascular thrombosis and organ dysfunction, coagulation abnormalities may have other harmful consequences. Thrombocytopenia in patients with sepsis places them at risk of bleeding. For example, critically ill patients with a platelet count of $<50 \times 10^9$/L have a four- to fivefold higher risk for bleeding than those with higher platelet counts.[10] Although the overall risk of intracerebral bleeding in intensive care unit (ICU) patients is less than 0.5%, up to 88% of patients with this complication have platelet counts below 100×10^9/L. The use of anticoagulants in patients with thrombocytopenia further increases the risk of bleeding. Regardless of the cause, multivariate analyses indicate that thrombocytopenia is an independent predictor of ICU mortality and increases the risk of death by 1.9- to 4.2-fold. In particular, thrombocytopenia that persists for more than 4 days after ICU admission, or a 50% or greater decrease in platelet count during the ICU stay, is associated with a four- to sixfold increase in mortality. In fact the platelet count appears to be a stronger predictor of ICU mortality than composite scoring systems, such as the Acute Physiology and Chronic Evaluation (APACHE) II or Multiple Organ Dysfunction Score (MODS). Decreased levels of coagulation factors, as reflected by prolonged global coagulation times, also increase the risk of bleeding. Prolongation of the prothrombin time (PT) or activated partial thromboplastin time (aPTT) to over 1.5 times the control is associated with an increased risk of bleeding and mortality in critically ill patients.

PATHOBIOLOGY

Traditionally, DIC was thought to be the result of activation of both the extrinsic and intrinsic pathways of coagulation. The classical concept was that the extrinsic pathway was initiated by a tissue-derived component, which activated factor VII leading to the direct conversion of prothrombin to thrombin. This process would proceed as long as there was tissue damage from systemic infection, trauma, circulating placental components, or malignancy. In contrast, the intrinsic or contact pathway of coagulation was initiated by contact activation of factor XII which, together with its cofactors, kallikrein and high molecular weight kininogen, then activated factor XI leading to subsequent activation of factor IX. Until recently, the initiators of contact activation were thought to include collagen and artificial surfaces. In recent years the molecular mechanisms of coagulation pathway activation have been better defined (Fig. 139.1), thereby providing new insight into the pathogenesis of DIC. In general, current thinking is that thrombin and fibrin generation in patients with DIC is largely driven via the extrinsic pathway; the role of the contact system is uncertain.

Tissue Factor-Factor VII(a) Pathway

The extrinsic pathway is initiated by the tissue factor (TF)–factor VIIa complex. TF is a membrane-bound 4.5-kDa protein that is

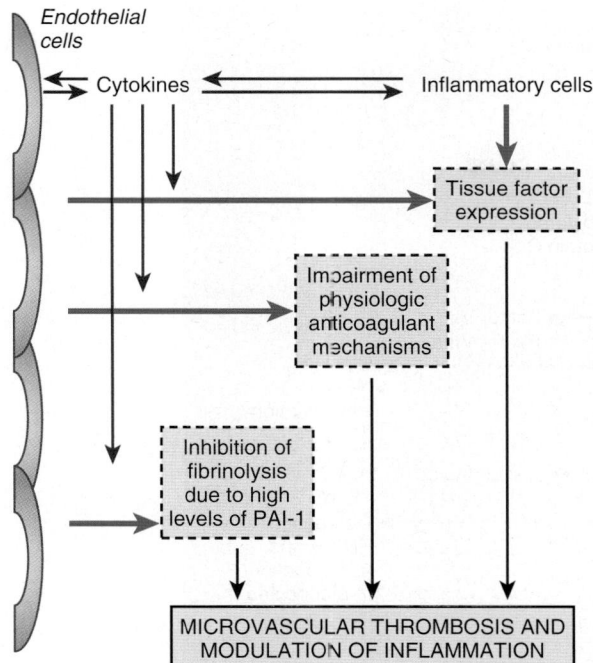

Fig. 139.1 PATHOGENESIS OF DISSEMINATED INTRAVASCULAR COAGULATION (DIC). Pathways involved in the activation of coagulation in DIC. Both perturbed endothelial cells and activated mononuclear cells may produce proinflammatory cytokines that induce tissue factor expression, thereby initiating coagulation. In addition, downregulation of physiologic anticoagulant mechanisms and inhibition of fibrinolysis promotes intravascular fibrin deposition. *PAI-1*, plasminogen activator inhibitor, type 1.

constitutively expressed on cells that are mostly in tissues and not in direct contact with blood, such as the adventitial layer of larger blood vessels.[12] Subcutaneous tissue also contains substantial amounts of TF. When expressed on the cell surface, TF interacts with factor VII, either in its zymogen or activated form. The TF–factor VIIa complex catalyzes the activation of both factor IX and factor X. Factors IXa and Xa enhance the activation of factors X and prothrombin, respectively. In cells in contact with the blood, TF is induced by the action of mediators such as cytokines, C-reactive protein and advanced glycosylation end products. Inducible TF is predominantly expressed by monocytes and macrophages. Monocyte TF expression is enhanced in the presence of platelets and granulocytes in a P-selectin dependent fashion. This may reflect nuclear factor kappa-B (NFκB) activation that occurs when activated platelets bind to neutrophils or mononuclear cells. These cell-cell interactions also stimulate the production of interleukin (IL)-1b, IL-8, MCP-1, and tumor necrosis factor (TNF)-α. Under cell culture conditions, cytokines such as TNF-α, and IL-1 can induce TF expression by vascular endothelial cells, but the in vivo relevance of this finding is uncertain. Studies in vivo suggest that IL-6 is the dominant mediator of TF expression by mononuclear cells.

Increased monocyte TF expression and procoagulant activity has been demonstrated in DIC associated with sepsis, cancer, or coronary disease. Tissue expression of TF appears to be localized to certain organs and vascular beds, but it is uncertain whether its expression is under genetic control in an organ-specific fashion. With trauma, such as extensive surgery, brain injury, or burns, it is likely that constitutively expressed TF at the site of injury is the primary source of procoagulant material, but direct support for this concept is lacking.

The Intrinsic Pathway

The role of the intrinsic pathway in the pathogenesis of DIC is uncertain. Negatively charged substances, such as phospholipids,

polyphosphates, and glycosaminoglycans, are potential activators of the contact pathway. Studies in patients with suspected DIC have identified elevated levels of markers of activation of the contact system. In patients with meningococcal septicemia, there was a negative correlation between plasma factor XII levels and factor XIIa–C1 inhibitor complexes. Although this finding implies consumption of factor XII, and subsequent downstream activation of factor XI, an alternative explanation is that there is a negative acute phase effect with reduced synthesis of factor XII, in conjunction with thrombin-mediated activation of factor XI.

However, blockade of the contact system with a factor XIIa–directed antibody failed to prevent DIC in a balloon model of *Escherichia coli* sepsis, but diminished development of lethal hypotension. These findings provide reasonable support for the current view that the contact pathway does not contribute to DIC, but may play important roles in proinflammatory mechanisms related to vascular permeability, vascular proliferation (kininogen induces smooth muscle cell proliferation), and enhancement of fibrinolysis.[11]

Cytokines and Other Amplification Pathways

Activation of blood coagulation requires several cofactors. For development of DIC, the surfaces of cell remnants or intact cells, inflammatory mediators, and coagulation proteins are required. The stimulus for activation depends on the underlying disease and may encompass bacterial cell compounds, such as endotoxin, TF on host or cancer cells, other cancer cell procoagulants, fat, or amniotic fluid emboli by unknown pathways. Each of these triggers interacts with other mediators: TF assembles on anionic phospholipid surfaces, which can be provided by activated platelets, leukocytes, or cancer cells; cytokines interact with receptors and induce signaling pathways that induce TF expression and other proinflammatory components via the NFκB complex.

Endotoxin is a lipopolysaccharide compound of gram-negative bacteria that induces the sepsis syndrome and DIC. Gram-negative bacteria liberate endotoxins from their membrane, which interact with cell surfaces via various pathways. In blood, endotoxin directly binds to CD14 on monocytes, and binds to endothelial cells after complexing with lipopolysaccharide binding protein (LBP) and the Toll-like receptor 4 (TLR 4) complex. Through these interactions, endotoxin induces signaling pathways that culminate in NFκB activation, and initiates the expression of proinflammatory cytokines and TF. Likewise, exotoxins, such as lipoteichoic acid (LTA) from gram-positive bacteria can also induce proinflammatory cytokine expression.

The molecular mechanisms underlying endotoxin-induced activation of coagulation have been studied in nonhuman primates. In endotoxin or *E. coli* models of sepsis, inhibition of the TF pathway abolishes the activation of coagulation, highlighting the importance of TF. IL-6 is an important mediator of procoagulant effects, whereas TNF-α is involved in the fibrinolytic response to endotoxin. Inhibition of TF with tissue factor pathway inhibitor (TFPI) reduces IL-6 levels in the baboon model, suggesting that there is extensive crosstalk between coagulation and inflammatory mediators (see later). Monocytes that express TF bind factor VII(a), shed TF, or bind to the damaged vessel wall. After interacting with platelets, circulating monocytes can trigger DIC. Microvesicles may accelerate this process, and the complex interaction between cells, membrane fragments, soluble mediators, and proteins may trigger the DIC syndrome. The severity and duration of the consumptive process are mainly determined by the potency of the triggers and the capacity of inhibitory mechanisms.

Cross Talk Among Coagulation Proteases Results in Proinflammatory Effects

In addition to activating coagulation protein zymogens, coagulation proteases also interact with specific cell receptors and trigger signaling

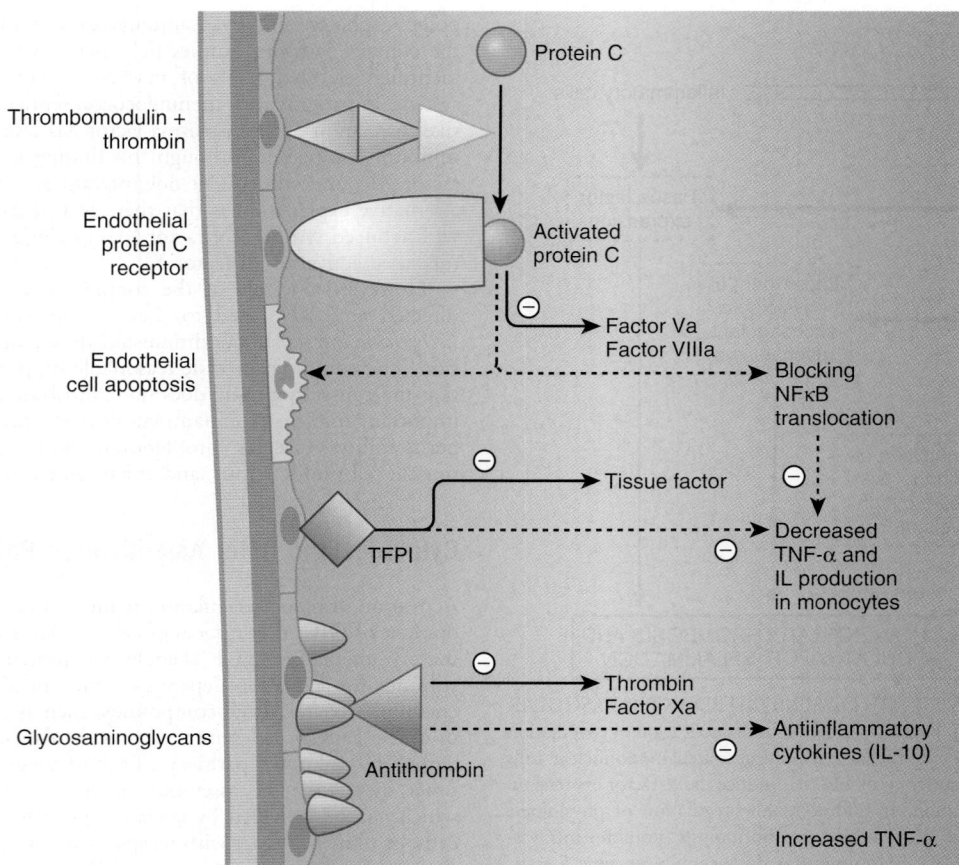

Fig. 139.2 PHYSIOLOGIC ANTICOAGULANT MECHANISMS IN DISSEMINATED INTRAVASCU-LAR COAGULATION. Physiologic anticoagulant mechanisms (activated protein C system, tissue factor pathway inhibitor (TFPI), and antithrombin) are not only involved in blocking thrombin generation and thrombin activity but also affect inflammatory pathways.

pathways that elicit proinflammatory mediators.[7] Factor Xa, thrombin, and the factor VIIa–TF complex have such effects. Factor Xa injection into rats induces localized inflammation, probably as a result of its interaction with EPR-1 and not because of thrombin generation. Exposure of cultured endothelial cells to factor Xa stimulates the production of monocyte chemotactic protein 1 (MCP-1), IL-6 and IL-8, and upregulates the expression of adhesion proteins that tether neutrophils to the cell surface. Further evidence for the crosstalk between inflammation and coagulation comes from the observations that IL-6 and IL-8 elicit TF-dependent procoagulant activity in monocytes and the fact that IL-6 has been identified as the critical mediator of procoagulant activity either on its own or after endotoxin challenge in vivo. Therefore cytokine production induced by factor Xa may be an important driver of coagulation in DIC.

In addition to its procoagulant functions, thrombin has a variety of noncoagulant effects. Thrombin induces the release of MCP-1 and IL-6 from fibroblasts, epithelial cells, and mononuclear cells in vitro. Thrombin also induces IL-6 and IL-8 production in endothelial cells. When generated in whole blood, IL-8 production has a procoagulant effect that is TF dependent. Cell activation by thrombin is likely mediated by protease activated receptors (PARs). The factor VIIa–TF complex also activates cells by binding and activating PAR 2.

Direct evidence of the in vivo relevance of these phenomena comes from a study showing that recombinant factor VIIa infusion in volunteers induces an increase in plasma levels of IL-6 and IL-8. Although the concentrations of factor VIIa infused far exceed those found in patients with sepsis, it is possible that factor VIIa-induced cytokine production is of physiologic importance. Therefore this information adds to the concept that several coagulation proteases induce proinflammatory mediators that augment procoagulant

activity and amplify the consumptive process. Endogenous anticoagulant pathways are essential to regulate these proteases and to prevent uncontrolled DIC.

Endogenous Anticoagulant Pathways in Disseminated Intravascular Coagulation

The development of DIC is counteracted by several mechanisms. First, coagulation inhibitors regulate the coagulation mechanism. Those inhibitors include antithrombin (AT), the protein C system, and TFPI (Fig. 139.2).[7] AT, which complexes and inhibits thrombin and factor Xa, is one of the most important inhibitors and reduced AT levels are a characteristic of DIC. Reduction in AT levels reflects a combination of reduced protein synthesis as well as increased clearance through the formation of protease–AT complexes, and by degradation by neutrophil elastase. In addition, cytokines may impair proteoglycan synthesis in the vessel wall thereby reducing the availability of heparan sulfate for potentiation of AT activity.

In animal models of experimental bacteremia, AT concentrate infusion increases survival, reduces the severity of DIC, and lowers the levels of IL-6 and IL-8. Therefore in addition to its anticoagulant function, AT may also have an antiinflammatory effect.

Activated protein C and its cofactor protein S provide a second line of defense. Thrombin binds to thrombomodulin on the endothelial cell membrane and the thrombin–thrombomodulin complex converts protein C to its active form, activated protein C (APC).[12] In addition the thrombin–thrombomodulin complex converts the latent carboxypeptidase B–like enzyme thrombin activatable fibrinolytic inhibitor (TAFI) to its activated form. APC inactivates factors

Va and VIIIa by proteolytic cleavage, thereby downregulating the coagulation cascade. Endothelial cells, primarily of large blood vessels, express endothelial protein C receptor (EPCR) on their surface. EPCR augments protein C activation by binding protein C and presenting it to the thrombin–thrombomodulin complex on the cell surface. APC has antiinflammatory effects on mononuclear cells and granulocytes, which may be distinct from its anticoagulant activity. Administration of APC prevented thrombin-induced thromboembolism in mice, mainly through its antithrombotic effect.

Defects in the protein C mechanism enhance the vulnerability to inflammatory reactions and DIC. In patients, reduced levels of protein C and protein S are associated with increased mortality. Mice with a one-allele targeted disruption of the protein C gene, causing heterozygous protein C deficiency, developed a more severe form of DIC and associated inflammatory response compared with their wild-type counterparts. Blockade of protein C activity by infusion of C4 binding protein converted a sublethal model of E. coli in baboons into a lethal model. In addition, blockade of EPCR with a neutralizing monoclonal antibody also increased mortality in the E. coli baboon model, whereas infusion of PC protected against DIC and lethality. Therefore the protein C pathway is important in the host defense against sepsis and DIC. In situations associated with DIC and systemic inflammation, cell culture experiments suggest that TNF-α and IL-1 may downregulate thrombomodulin expression. However, in vivo studies suggest that EPCR is upregulated in sepsis; an effect mediated by thrombin. The generation of thrombin may also trigger EPCR shedding due to the activation of metalloproteinases by thrombin. It is presently unknown whether thrombomodulin is also cleaved by similar mechanisms.

TFPI provides a third inhibitory mechanism. TFPI exists in several pools including endothelial cell associated and lipoprotein bound in plasma. It inhibits the TF–factor VIIa complex by forming a quaternary complex in which factor Xa is the fourth component. Clinical studies in patients with sepsis have not provided clues as to its importance because in the majority of patients the TFPI levels are normal. This may be explained by the lack of downregulatory effects of inflammatory mediators on cultured endothelial cells. The relevance of TFPI in DIC is illustrated by two lines of experimentation. First, depletion of TFPI sensitizes rabbits to DIC induced with tissue factor infusion. Second, TFPI infusion protects against the harmful effects of E. coli in primates. TFPI not only blocks DIC in baboons given lethal doses of E. coli, but improves vital functions and survival. A study in human volunteers confirmed the potential of TFPI to block the procoagulant effects of endotoxin.

In general, normal levels and function of inhibitors is important in the defense against DIC. It should be noted, however, that there are no strong indications that patients with congenital deficiencies of inhibitors are at increased risk of DIC, but this issue requires greater exploration. In addition, the capacity of inhibitors to modify the interaction between coagulation and inflammation deserves further attention.

Fibrinolysis

In experimental models of DIC, fibrinolysis is activated, demonstrated by an initial activation of plasminogen, followed by impairment caused by the release of type 1 plasminogen activator inhibitor (PAI-1). This results in a net procoagulant state. The molecular basis for this procoagulant state is cytokine-mediated activation of vascular endothelial cells, thus TNF-α and IL-1 decrease tPA production and increase PAI-1 production. Although TNF-α increases urokinase type plasminogen activator (uPA) production by endothelial cells, endotoxin and TNF-α stimulate PAI-1 production in the liver, kidney, lung, and adrenals of mice.

The net procoagulant state is manifested by a late rise in fibrin breakdown fragments after E. coli challenge in baboons. Experimental data also suggest that the fibrinolytic mechanism is active in clearing fibrin from organs and the circulation. Endotoxin-induced fibrin formation in the kidneys and adrenals is most dependent on decreased levels of uPA. In contrast to wild-type mice challenged with endotoxin, PAI-1 knockout mice do not develop thrombi in the kidney. Endotoxin administration to mice with a functionally inactive thrombomodulin gene (TMProArg mutation) and defective protein C activator cofactor function caused fibrin plugs in the pulmonary circulation, whereas wild-type mice did not develop macroscopic fibrin. This phenomenon in thrombomodulin deficient mice proved to be temporary; thrombi developed 4 hours after endotoxin administration and disappeared at 24 hours in animals killed at that time point. These experiments demonstrate that the fibrinolytic system is essential for clearance of intravascular fibrin.

Fibrinolytic activity is regulated by PAI-1, the principal inhibitor of this system. Previous studies have shown that a functional mutation in the PAI-1 gene, the 4G/5G polymorphism, not only influences plasma levels of PAI-1, but also affects the clinical outcome of meningococcal septicemia. Patients with the 4G/4G genotype had significantly higher PAI-1 concentrations in plasma and an increased risk of death. Further investigations demonstrated that the PAI-1 polymorphism did not influence the risk of contracting meningitis, but probably increased the likelihood of developing septic shock from meningococcal infection. These studies provide the first evidence that genetically determined differences in the level of fibrinolysis influence the risk of developing complications of gram-negative infection. In other clinical studies in cohorts of patients with DIC, high plasma levels of PAI-1 were one of the best predictors of mortality. These data suggest that DIC contributes to mortality in this situation, but as indicated earlier, because PAI-1 is an acute-phase protein, higher plasma levels may also be a marker of disease rather than a causal factor.

CLINICAL MANIFESTATIONS

The clinical manifestations of DIC vary depending on the underlying disorder. At the extreme end of the spectrum is acute, severe DIC, which often occurs in the setting of sepsis, major trauma, obstetric calamities, and severe immunologic responses. Diffuse multiorgan bleeding, hemorrhagic necrosis, microthrombi in small blood vessels, and thrombi in medium and large blood vessels are common findings at autopsy, although patients with unequivocal clinical and laboratory signs of DIC may not have confirmatory postmortem findings. Conversely, some patients in whom clinical and laboratory signs were not consistent with DIC have typical autopsy findings. Although this occasional lack of correlation among clinical, laboratory, and pathologic findings can partly be explained by excessive fibrinolysis post mortem, this does not account for all cases. The organs most frequently involved by diffuse microthrombi are the lungs and kidneys, followed by the brain, heart, liver, spleen, adrenal glands, pancreas, and gut. Specific immunohistological techniques and ultrastructural analysis have revealed that most thrombi consist of fibrin monomers or polymers in combination with platelets. In addition, involvement of activated mononuclear cells and other signs of inflammation are frequently present. In cases of long-lasting DIC, organization and endothelialization of the microthrombi are often observed. Acute tubular necrosis is more frequent than renal cortical necrosis. Clinically, thrombotic occlusive events occur first as a consequence of microvascular obstruction by microthrombi consisting of fibrin or platelets. These thrombi result from clots that form either in the circulation or in situ in arterioles, capillaries, or venules. Circulatory obstruction reduces organ perfusion and may lead to ischemia, infarction, and necrosis. The process is disseminated throughout the microcirculation, therefore all organs are potentially vulnerable.

In contrast to acutely ill patients with severe DIC, others may have mild or protracted clinical manifestations of consumption or even subclinical disease manifested only by laboratory abnormalities.[1] The clinical picture of subacute to chronic DIC generally occurs in patients with malignancy, in particular those with mucin-producing adenocarcinomas or acute promyelocytic leukemia (APL). The latter usually is dominated by a hemorrhagic presentation, whereas venous thrombotic manifestations are more common in the former. In addition, patients with solid tumors may develop nonbacterial thrombotic endocarditis with systemic arterial embolization and infarction. Another cause of subacute to chronic DIC is the retained dead fetus syndrome. These patients have an extremely variable presentation ranging from asymptomatic to mild or moderate skin and mucous membrane bleeding.

It is important to stress that DIC is not a disease in itself but is always secondary to an underlying disorder, which causes the activation of coagulation. The underlying disorders most commonly known to be associated with DIC are listed in Box 139.1 and are described in detail below.

Disseminated Intravascular Coagulation in Infectious Disease

Systemic infections are among the most common causes of DIC. Immunocompromised patients, asplenic patients whose ability to clear bacteria (particularly pneumococci) is impaired, and newborns whose anticoagulant systems are immature are particularly prone to infection-induced DIC. Infections may be superimposed on trauma or malignancies, which themselves are potential triggers of DIC. In addition, infections can aggravate bleeding and thrombosis by directly inducing thrombocytopenia, hepatic dysfunction, and shock, which can lead to diminished blood flow in the microcirculation.

Clinically overt DIC occurs in 30%–50% of patients with gram-negative or gram-positive sepsis. Extreme examples of sepsis-related DIC are streptococcus A toxic shock syndrome, which is characterized by deep tissue infection, vascular collapse, vascular leakage, and multiple organ dysfunction. M protein released from streptococci forms complexes with fibrinogen that bind to β_2 integrins on neutrophils leading to their activation, and meningococcemia, a fulminant gram-negative infection characterized by extensive hemorrhagic necrosis, DIC, and shock. More frequent gram-negative infections associated with DIC are caused by *Pseudomonas aeruginosa, E. coli,* and *Proteus vulgaris.* Patients with these infections may only have laboratory evidence of activated coagulation or they may present with severe DIC.

Activation of the coagulation system has also been documented with nonbacterial pathogens, such as viruses, protozoa (malaria), and fungi.[13] Common viral infections, such as influenza, varicella, rubella, and rubeola, are rarely associated with DIC. Some viral infections can cause hemorrhagic fever characterized by fever, hypotension, bleeding, and renal failure. Laboratory evidence of DIC can accompany Korean, rift valley, and dengue-related hemorrhagic fevers. Protozoan infections, such as cerebral malaria, may be associated with overt DIC. In these cases, secondary deficiency of a disintegrin-like metalloprotease with thrombospondin type 1 repeats (ADAMTS13), the von Willebrand cleaving protease, may occur. Such deficiency

may also complicate other types of sepsis-induced DIC and may enhance platelet–vessel wall interactions, thereby contributing to microvascular thrombosis.[14]

Purpura fulminans is an extreme form of DIC, which is often lethal. This disorder is characterized by extensive hemorrhagic necrosis of the skin over the extremities and buttocks. The disease predominantly affects infants and children and is rare in adults. Diffuse microthrombi in small blood vessels leads to necrosis and vasculitis may also be found in biopsies of skin lesions. The disorder can occur 2 to 4 weeks after mild infection, such as scarlet fever, varicella, or rubella, or can occur during an acute viral or bacterial infection in patients with acquired or hereditary deficiencies of protein C or protein S. The syndrome mimics neonatal homozygous protein C or protein S deficiency where purpura fulminans, with or without extensive thrombosis, develops soon after birth.

Disseminated Intravascular Coagulation in Trauma, Brain Injury, Burns, and Heat Stroke

The time interval between trauma and medical intervention correlates with the development and magnitude of DIC. Experience during wars proved that fast evacuation and prompt medical care reduce the risk of DIC. Extensive exposure of TF to the blood and hemorrhagic shock are the most immediate triggers of DIC in such instances, although direct proof of this mechanism is lacking. An alternative hypothesis is that cytokines play a pivotal role in the occurrence of DIC in trauma patients. In fact, the changes in cytokine levels in trauma patients are virtually identical to those in patients with sepsis.[15] The levels of TNF-α, IL-1β, PAI-1, circulating TF, neutrophil elastase, and soluble thrombomodulin can be elevated in patients with signs of DIC, predicting multiorgan dysfunction (adult respiratory distress syndrome [ARDS] included) and death. Careful monitoring for laboratory signs of DIC, reduced fibrinolytic activity, and perhaps low AT levels may be useful to predict the outcome of such patients.

In adults and children with head injuries, mortality is high when DIC occurs. A laboratory DIC score has predictive value for prognosis in patients with head injuries, thereby supplementing the Glasgow coma score. Brain injury can be associated with DIC, most likely because the injury exposes the abundant TF of the brain to blood. Specimens of contused brain, obtained during surgery in patients with head injury, and of liver, lungs, kidneys, and pancreas obtained during autopsy, reveal microthrombi in arterioles and venules.

Bleeding, laboratory tests indicative of DIC, and vascular microthrombi in biopsies of undamaged skin have been described in patients with extensive burns. Kinetic studies with labeled fibrinogen and platelets suggest that in addition to systemic consumption of hemostatic factors, there is significant local consumption in burned areas. TF exposed at sites of burned tissue, the systemic inflammatory response syndrome induced by the burn, and the presence of superimposed infections can trigger DIC. Local activation of coagulation in the bronchoalveolar compartment may contribute to acute lung injury in these patients.

A severe hemorrhagic diathesis and multiple organ failure indicative of DIC can complicate heat stroke.[16] Diffuse fibrin deposition and hemorrhagic infarctions are found in fatal cases. DIC associated with profound fibrin(ogen) degradation is evident in such patients. Potential triggers of DIC in patients with heat stroke include endothelial cell damage and TF released from heat-damaged tissues. In 18 critically ill patients with heat stroke during the 2003 heat wave in Western Europe that caused numerous deaths in France,[16] there were high levels of IL-6 and IL-8. In addition, there was marked activation of white blood cells, as evidenced by β2-integrin upregulation and increased production of reactive oxygen species. All patients had evidence of systemic activation of coagulation and DIC was present in about 35%. There was good correlation between the extent of activation of inflammation and coagulation and the clinical severity of the heat stroke.

Disseminated Intravascular Coagulation in Obstetric Complications

Placental abruption is a leading cause of perinatal death.[17] Older multiparous women or patients with one of the hypertensive disorders of pregnancy are thought to be at highest risk. The severe hemostatic failure accompanying abruptio placentae is the result of acute DIC emanating from the introduction of large amounts of TF into the circulation from the damaged placenta and uterus. Amniotic fluid has been shown to activate coagulation in vitro, and the degree of placental separation correlates with the extent of DIC, suggesting that leakage of thromboplastin-like material from the placental system is responsible for the DIC. Abruptio placentae occurs in 0.2% to 0.4% of pregnancies, but only 10% of these cases are associated with DIC. Different grades of severity are found among those who develop DIC, with only the more severe forms resulting in shock and fetal death.

Amniotic fluid embolism is a rare but serious complication of pregnancy and delivery. A maternal mortality rate of 86% was reported in a 1979 review of 272 cases, but in a more recent population-based study, the maternal mortality was 26%. Patients predisposed to amniotic fluid embolism are multiparous women whose pregnancies are postmature with large fetuses and women undergoing a tumultuous labor after pharmacologic or surgical induction. Amniotic fluid is introduced into the maternal circulation through tears in the chorioamniotic membranes, rupture of the uterus, and injury of uterine veins. TF in amniotic fluid is the likely trigger for DIC. Mechanical obstruction of pulmonary blood vessels by fetal debris, meconium, and other particulate matter in the amniotic fluid enhances local fibrin–platelet thrombus formation and fibrinolysis. The extensive occlusion of the pulmonary arteries and an acute anaphylactoid response reminiscent of severe systemic inflammatory response syndrome provoke sudden dyspnea, cyanosis, acute cor pulmonale, left ventricular dysfunction, shock, and convulsions. These symptoms are followed within minutes to several hours by severe bleeding in 37% of patients. Hemorrhage is particularly severe from the atonic uterus, puncture sites, gastrointestinal tract, and other organs.

Some studies provide evidence of activation of coagulation, in its most extreme form DIC, in preeclampsia and eclampsia. In a large series of patients, a good correlation was noted between the clinical severity and abnormalities in platelet counts and fibrin(ogen) degradation products. Also consistent with DIC were results of assays of sensitive parameters of thrombin generation and activation of fibrinolysis, such as TAT complexes, D-dimer, and fibrinopeptide Bβ1–42. Despite these observations, administration of heparin to patients with preeclampsia and eclampsia has not resulted in convincing benefits. The HELLP syndrome, which is comprised of hemolysis, elevated liver enzymes, low platelet count, and severe epigastric pain, is another complication of pregnancy-induced hypertension. Liver biopsy findings of fibrin deposition in hepatic blood vessels and laboratory tests consistent with DIC are found in a significant proportion of patients suggesting that DIC plays a role in the pathogenesis of the syndrome. However, according to current insights, thrombotic microangiopathy rather than DIC causes the coagulation abnormalities in patients with hypertensive disorders of pregnancy.

Disseminated Intravascular Coagulation in Malignancy

Patients with solid tumors are vulnerable to risk factors and additional triggers for DIC that can aggravate thromboembolism and bleeding.[18] Risk factors include advanced age, stage of the disease, and use of chemotherapy or antiestrogen therapy. Triggers include septicemia, immobilization, and hepatic metastases, which can compromise the capacity of the liver to control DIC. Microangiopathic hemolytic anemia frequently is induced by DIC in patients with malignancies and is particularly severe in patients with widespread intravascular metastases of mucin-secreting adenocarcinomas. Solid tumor cells can express different procoagulant molecules including tissue factor,

which forms a complex with factor VII(a) to activate factors IX and X, and a cancer procoagulant (CP), a cysteine protease with factor X–activating properties. In breast cancer, TF is expressed by vascular endothelial cells as well as by the tumor cells. TF also appears to be involved in tumor metastasis and angiogenesis. CP is an endopeptidase that can not only be found in extracts of neoplastic cells but also in the plasma of patients with solid tumors. The exact role of CP in the pathogenesis of cancer-related DIC is unclear. Interactions of P- and L-selectins with mucin from mucinous adenocarcinoma can induce the formation of platelet microthrombi, which probably constitute a third mechanism of cancer-related thrombosis. Depending on the rate and quantity of exposure or influx of shed vesicles from tumors containing TF, a covert or overt DIC develops.

There are numerous reports of DIC and excessive fibrinolysis complicating the course of acute leukemia. In 161 consecutive patients presenting with acute myeloid leukemia, DIC was diagnosed in 52 (32%). In acute lymphoblastic leukemia, DIC was diagnosed in 15% to 20%.[19] Some reports suggest that the incidence of DIC in acute leukemia patients may increase even more during remission induction with chemotherapy. In patients with APL, DIC is present in more than 90% of patients at the time of diagnosis or after initiation of remission induction. The pathogenesis of hemostatic disturbance in APL is related to properties of the malignant cells and their interaction with host endothelial cells. APL cells express TF and CP, which can initiate coagulation, and they release IL-1β and TNF-α, which downregulate endothelial thrombomodulin, thereby compromising the protein C anticoagulant pathway. APL cells also express increased amounts of annexin II, which binds plasminogen and tPA and promotes plasmin generation. The net result of these processes is DIC and hyperfibrinolysis, which can lead to bleeding that can be fatal. All-*trans*-retinoic acid, which is used for induction and maintenance therapy of APL, inhibits the deleterious effect of APL cells in vitro and in vivo and has reduced the frequency of early hemorrhagic death.

Disseminated Intravascular Coagulation With Vascular Disorders

Rarely, vascular anomalies can trigger DIC. With some large aortic aneurysms, localized consumption of platelets and fibrinogen can produce coagulation abnormalities and bleeding.[20] In a series of patients with aortic aneurysms, 40% had elevated levels of fibrin(ogen) degradation products, but only 4% had laboratory evidence of DIC or bleeding.[20] Factors that predispose such patients to the development of DIC include large aneurysms, dissection, and expansion. Coagulation in these cases likely is triggered by the abundant TF in atherosclerotic plaques.

Kasabach and Merritt were the first to describe bleeding in association with giant cavernous hemangiomas, benign tumors found in newborns or children that can evolve into convoluted masses of abnormal vascular channels that sequester and consume platelets and fibrinogen. Localized pain may occur, likely from thrombosis of these vascular channels and there may be bleeding after trauma or surgery because of the consumptive process. Increased fibrinogen consumption reflects hyperfibrinolysis, which may be driven by tPA released from the abnormal endothelium lining the tumor walls. Patients with this syndrome exhibit accelerated platelet turnover, and accumulation of labeled platelets and fibrinogen in the hemangiomas.

Hemangiomas may regress spontaneously; some respond to radiation or laser therapy.

Disseminated Intravascular Coagulation With Liver Disease

The levels of most coagulation factors, endogenous anticoagulants, and major components of the fibrinolytic system are reduced in patients with severe liver disease reflecting reduced synthesis. In addition, the capacity of the liver to clear factors IXa, Xa, XIa, and tPA is decreased. Thrombocytopenia is common because of hypersplenism and decreased hepatic production of thrombopoietin. The similarities between the hemostatic defects of liver disease and those of DIC have evoked controversy as to the contribution of DIC to the coagulopathy of liver disease. Several laboratory and clinical observations support the concept that DIC accompanies hepatic disorders. These include a reduced half-life of radiolabeled fibrinogen that is reversed with heparin administration; failure of replacement therapy to significantly increase the levels of hemostatic factors (suggesting ongoing consumption); and increased levels of markers of activation of coagulation. All of these findings are consistent with increased thrombin generation. Against the DIC hypothesis are the observations that microthrombi are found in only 2% of the tissues from patients who die of liver disease, and the fact that the increased fibrinogen turnover can be explained by extravascular accumulation. Current thinking is that DIC is rare in patients with liver disease, but such patients are sensitive to the triggers of DIC because of the decreased synthetic capacity of the diseased liver and its inability to clear activated clotting factors. In patients who undergo peritoneovenous shunting for ascites, those with underlying liver disease are more likely to develop DIC than those with normal liver function.

Disseminated Intravascular Coagulation With Toxic Reactions or Snake Bites

The venom of certain snakes, particularly vipers and rattlesnakes, can produce a coagulopathy similar to DIC.[21] Prominent among these species are the *Vipera, Echis (E. carinatus* or *E. coloratus), Aspis, Crotalus, Bothrops,* and *Agkistrodon.* Venoms of these snakes contain enzymes or peptides that (1) release fibrinopeptide A *(Agkistrodon rhodostoma)*; (2) activate prothrombin even in the absence of calcium *(E. carinatus)*; (3) activate factors X and V (Russell viper venom); (4) degrade fibrinogen *(Agkistrodon acutus)*; (5) induce platelet aggregation; (6) inhibit platelet aggregation because of the presence of arginine-glycine-aspartic acid–containing peptides; (7) activate protein C; and (8) damage endothelial cells which leads to bleeding, tissue ischemia, and edema. Interestingly, victims of snake bites rarely have excessive bleeding or thromboembolism despite the abnormal coagulation tests and DIC-like picture.

LABORATORY MANIFESTATIONS

Thrombocytopenia or a rapidly declining platelet count is an important diagnostic hallmark of DIC. However, only 35% to 44% of critically ill patients develop thrombocytopenia (platelet count <150 $\times$ 10^9/L). Consequently, the specificity of thrombocytopenia for the diagnosis of DIC is limited.[16] A platelet count of <100 $\times$ 10^9/L is seen in 50% to 60% of patients with DIC, whereas 10% to 15% of patients have a platelet count <50 $\times$ 10^9/L. In surgical or trauma patients with DIC, over 80% have platelet counts less than 100 $\times$ 10^9/L.

Consumption of coagulation factors leads to low levels of coagulation factors in patients with DIC. In addition, impaired hepatic synthesis, for example due to impaired liver function or vitamin K deficiency, and loss of coagulation proteins, due to massive bleeding, may also play a role in DIC. Although the accuracy of the measurement of one-stage clotting assays in DIC has been contested (because of the presence of activated coagulation factors in plasma), the levels of coagulation factors appear to correlate with the severity of the DIC. The low levels of coagulation factors are reflected by prolonged global tests of coagulation, such as the PT and the aPTT. A prolonged PT or aPTT is found in 14% to 28% of intensive care patients but is present in more than 95% of patients with DIC.

Plasma levels of factor VIII are paradoxically increased in most patients with DIC, probably due to massive release of von Willebrand factor from the endothelium in combination with the acute phase **behavior** of factor VIII. Recent studies have pointed to a relative deficiency of ADAMTS-13, the von Willebrand cleaving protease, which results in high concentrations of ultralarge von Willebrand multimers in plasma. These large multimers promote platelet-vessel wall interaction, which can lead to thrombotic microangiopathy and organ dysfunction.[14]

Although determination of the fibrinogen concentration has been advocated as a useful tool for the diagnosis of DIC, this test is rarely helpful.[22] Fibrinogen is as an acute-phase protein whose levels increase with inflammation. Therefore the fibrinogen level may remain within the normal range for a long period of time despite ongoing consumption. In a consecutive series of patients, the sensitivity of a low fibrinogen level for the diagnosis of DIC was 28%, and hypofibrinogenemia was only found in very severe cases of DIC.

Markers of Fibrin Generation and Degradation

Plasma levels of fibrin split products are frequently used for the diagnosis of DIC.[23] Fibrin split products were detectable in 42% of consecutive patients in the intensive care unit, in 80% of trauma patients, and in 99% of patients with sepsis and DIC. The levels of fibrin degradation products (FDP) can be quantified by immunoassay. Latex agglutination assays can be used for rapid point-of-care determination in emergency cases. None of the available FDP assays discriminate between degradation products derived from cross-linked fibrin or from fibrinogen, which may cause spuriously high levels. Therefore the FDP assay lacks specificity because in addition to DIC, high levels can be found with trauma, recent surgery, inflammation, venous thromboembolism, and many other conditions. Because FDP are metabolized in the liver and cleared by the kidneys, FDP levels are influenced by liver and kidney function.

D-dimer is a degradation product of cross-linked fibrin. Therefore this test is not influenced by fibrinogen degradation products. D-dimer levels are high in patients with DIC, but high levels can also be found in patients with venous thromboembolism, recent surgery, or inflammatory conditions. Theoretically, soluble fibrin or fibrin monomers would be useful markers of intravascular fibrin formation in DIC. Indeed, initial clinical studies suggest that if the soluble fibrin concentration exceeds a threshold level, a diagnosis of DIC can be made. Unfortunately there are no reliable tests to quantify plasma levels of soluble fibrin. Since plasma levels of soluble fibrin reflect intravascular fibrin formation, the test is not influenced by extravascular fibrin formation, which can occur with local inflammation or trauma.

Endogenous Coagulation Inhibitors

Plasma levels of physiologic coagulation inhibitors, such as protein C or antithrombin, may be useful indicators of ongoing activation of coagulation.[23] Reduced levels of these inhibitors are found in 40% to 60% of critically ill patients and in 90% of DIC patients.

Levels of protein C may correlate with the severity of the DIC. In patients with meningococcal septicemia, plasma levels of protein C are markedly reduced, which likely contributes to the purpura fulminans that occurs in these patients. Downregulation of thrombomodulin and reduced levels of protein S further compromise the capacity to generate APC. Therefore it is not surprising the low levels of protein C are a strong predictor of poor outcome in DIC patients.

Plasma levels of antithrombin also are reduced in patients with DIC. The low levels reflect consumption due to ongoing thrombin generation, decreased synthesis, and degradation by neutrophil elastase. Like protein C, low levels of antithrombin also a strong predictor of mortality in patients with sepsis and DIC.

Fibrinolytic Markers

Increased fibrinolytic activity in DIC can be monitored by measuring plasma levels of plasminogen and α_2-antiplasmin. Low levels may indicate consumption of these proteins. The concentration of

α_2-antiplasmin is a helpful test for assessing the dynamics of fibrinolysis. Markers of plasmin generation include plasmin–α_2-antiplasmin (PAP) complexes, which are moderately elevated in patients with DIC. However, because the normal plasma concentration of α_2-antiplasmin is about half that of plasminogen, α_2-antiplasmin is susceptible to consumption when there is excessive plasmin generation. Therefore PAP levels may underestimate total fibrinolytic activity. With α_2-antiplasmin consumption, other protease inhibitors, such as antithrombin, α_2-macroglobulin, α_1-antitrypsin, and C1-inhibitor may act as plasmin inhibitors as well. Fibrinolytic activity may be insufficient to degrade intravascular fibrin in patients with DIC. Fibrinolysis is suppressed by high levels of PAI-1, the major inhibitor of tPA and uPA, PAI-1 levels are often elevated in patients with DIC, and correlate with an unfavorable outcome. A functional mutation in the PAI-1 gene, the 4G/5G polymorphism, is associated with high levels of PAI-1, DIC and an increased risk of death in patients with meningococcal septicemia.

Point of Care Tests

Although thrombelastography (TEG) was developed decades ago, modern techniques, such as rotational thrombelastography (ROTEM), enable bedside assessment of coagulation and fibrinolysis, which can be helpful in acute care settings.[24] A theoretical advantage of TEG over conventional coagulation assays is that because TEG uses whole blood, it provides a global assessment of platelet function, coagulation, and fibrinolysis. Increased and decreased coagulation as demonstrated with TEG was shown to correlate with clinically relevant morbidity and mortality in several studies, although the superiority of TEG over conventional tests has not been unequivocally proven. TEG may be overly sensitive to some interventions, such as fibrinogen administration, which is of questionable therapeutic value. Although there are no systematic studies on the diagnostic accuracy of TEG for the diagnosis of DIC, the test may be useful for assessing the global status of the coagulation and fibrinolytic systems in critically ill patients.

The aPTT biphasic waveform analysis is a sensitive and specific test for hypercoagulability in critically ill patients. This test, which requires specific instrumentation, detects the presence of precipitates of complexes of very low density lipoprotein and C-reactive protein that form early in DIC. The appearance of such complexes in the plasma of individuals with diseases known to predispose to hypercoagulability confer a greater than 90% sensitivity and specificity for subsequent development of DIC and fatal outcome.

Diagnostic Algorithm for Disseminated Intravascular Coagulation

A simple scoring system for the diagnosis of overt DIC was developed by the subcommittee on DIC of ISTH (Box 139.2).[5] The score can be calculated using routinely available laboratory tests including the platelet count, the PT, a fibrin-related marker (usually D-dimer), and the fibrinogen concentration. Tentatively, a score of 5 or higher is compatible with DIC, whereas a score below 5 may be indicative but is not affirmative for nonovert DIC. More refined scoring systems have been developed for the diagnosis of nonovert DIC. A recent study showed that the international normalized ratio (INR) can be used in place of the PT, further facilitating international exchange and standardization. Using receiver-operating characteristic curves, an optimal D-dimer cut-off was identified, thereby optimizing the sensitivity and the negative predictive value of the test. Prospective studies show that the sensitivity and specificity of the DIC score are 93% and 98%, respectively. Studies in series of patients with specific underlying disorders causing DIC (e.g., cancer or obstetrical complications) show similar results. The severity of DIC according to this scoring system is related to the mortality in patients with sepsis.[9] Linking prognostic determinants from critical care measurement scores such as APACHE-II to DIC scores is an important means to

---

BOX 139.2   Diagnostic Algorithm for the Diagnosis of Overt Disseminated Intravascular Coagulation[a]

1. Presence of an underlying disorder known to be associated with disseminated intravascular coagulation (DIC) (Table 139.2) (no = 0, yes = 2)
2. Score global coagulation test results
   - Platelet count (>100 = 0; <100 = 1; <50 = 2)
   - Level of fibrin markers (e.g., D-dimer, fibrin degradation products)
   (no increase: 0; moderate increase: 2; strong increase: 3)[b]
   - Prolonged prothrombin time
   (<3 s = 0; >3 s but <6 s = 1; >6 s = 2)
   - Fibrinogen level
   (>1.0 g/L = 0; <1.0 g/L = 1)
3. Calculate score
4. If ≥5: compatible with overt DIC; repeat scoring daily
   If < 5: suggestive (not affirmative) for nonovert DIC; repeat next 1–2 days

[a]According to the Scientific Standardization Committee of the International Society of Thrombosis and Haemostasis.[5]
[b]Strong increase, greater than 5x upper limit of normal; moderate increase, greater than upper limit of normal but less than 5x upper limit of normal.

---

assess prognosis in critically ill patients. Similar scoring systems have been developed and extensively evaluated in Japan. The major difference between the international and Japanese scoring systems is a slightly higher sensitivity of the Japanese algorithm, which may reflect differences in the patient populations because the Japanese series include relatively large numbers of patients with hematologic malignancies.

DIFFERENTIAL DIAGNOSIS

There are several other causes of coagulation abnormalities in patients with underlying disorders known to be associated with DIC. A complicating factor is that patients may have multiple explanations for their coagulopathy. For example, a patient with sepsis with DIC may also have liver failure and vitamin K deficiency.

The differential diagnosis of thrombocytopenia in patients with suspected DIC is shown in Table 139.1. Sepsis itself is a risk factor for thrombocytopenia in critically ill patients and the severity of sepsis correlates with the extent of thrombocytopenia. The principal factors that contribute to thrombocytopenia in patients with sepsis are decreased platelet production, increased consumption or destruction, or sequestration platelets in the spleen or on the endothelial surface. The decreased production of platelets in the bone marrow in patients with sepsis occurs despite high levels of proinflammatory cytokines, such as TNF-α and IL-6, and increased levels of thrombopoietin. Platelet production is impaired because of hemophagocytosis, a pathologic process characterized by phagocytosis of megakaryocytes and other hematopoietic cells by monocytes and macrophages. Hemophagocytosis may be driven by the high levels of macrophage colony-stimulating factor (M-CSF) in patients with sepsis.

Heparin-induced thrombocytopenia (HIT) is caused by a heparin-induced antibody that binds to the heparin-platelet factor 4 (PF4) complex on the platelet surface (see Chapter 133). This may result in platelet activation and consumption and arterial and venous thrombosis. A consecutive series of critically ill patients who received heparin revealed an incidence of HIT of 1%. The risk of HIT is higher with unfractionated heparin than with low-molecular-weight heparin (LMWH). Thrombosis may occur in 25% to 50% of patients with HIT (with fatal thrombosis in 4%–5%). The diagnosis of HIT is based on detection of HIT antibodies in combination with the occurrence of thrombocytopenia in a patient receiving heparin, with or without concomitant arterial or venous thrombosis. The immunoassay for heparin-PF4 antibodies has a high negative predictive

TABLE 139.1
Differential Diagnosis of Thrombocytopenia in Suspected Disseminated Intravascular Coagulation

Differential Diagnosis	Additional Diagnostic Clues
DIC	Prolonged aPTT and PT, increased FDP, low levels of antithrombin or protein C
Sepsis without DIC	Positive (blood) cultures, positive sepsis criteria, hematophagocytosis in bone marrow
Massive blood loss	Major bleeding, low hemoglobin, prolonged aPTT and PT
Thrombotic microangiopathy	Schistocytes evident on blood smear, Coombs-negative hemolysis, fever, neurologic symptoms, renal insufficiency, coagulation tests usually normal, ADAMTS13 levels decreased
Heparin-induced thrombocytopenia	Use of heparin, venous or arterial thrombosis, positive HIT test (usually immunoassay for heparin-platelet factor 4 antibodies), increase in platelet count after cessation of heparin; coagulation tests usually normal
Immune thrombocytopenia	Antiplatelet antibodies, normal or increased number of megakaryocytes in bone marrow aspirate, normal levels of TPO (TPO levels are usually normal or slightly increased in ITP); coagulation tests usually normal
Drug-induced thrombocytopenia	Decreased number of megakaryocytes in bone marrow aspirate or detection of drug-induced antiplatelet antibodies, increase in platelet count after cessation of drug; coagulation tests usually normal

ADAMTS13, A disintegrin and metalloproteinase with thrombospondin 13; aPTT, activated partial thromboplastin time; DIC, disseminated intravascular coagulation; FDP, fibrin degradation products; HIT, heparin-induced thrombocytopenia; PT, prothrombin time; ITP, immune thrombocytopenia; TPO, thrombopoietin.

TABLE 139.2
Differential Diagnosis of Prolonged aPTT and/or PT in Suspected Disseminated Intravascular Coagulation

Test Result	Cause
PT prolonged, aPTT normal	Factor VII deficiency
	Mild vitamin K deficiency
	Mild liver insufficiency
	Low doses of vitamin K antagonists
PT normal, aPTT prolonged	Factor VIII, IX, or XI deficiency
	Unfractionated heparin
	Inhibitory antibody and/or antiphospholipid antibody
	Factor XII or prekallikrein deficiency
Both PT and aPTT prolonged	Factor X, V, II, or fibrinogen deficiency
	Severe vitamin K deficiency
	Vitamin K antagonists
	Global clotting factor deficiency
	• Decreased synthesis: liver failure
	• Increased loss: massive bleeding, DIC

aPTT, Activated partial thromboplastin time; PT, prothrombin time.

value (100%) but a low positive predictive value (10%). Although the gold standard for the diagnosis of HIT is a sensitive platelet activation assay, this test is not routinely available in most hospitals. Normalization of the platelet count 1–3 days after discontinuation of heparin may further support the diagnosis of HIT.

The group of thrombotic microangiopathies includes thrombotic thrombocytopenic purpura (see Chapter 134), hemolytic–uremic syndrome (see Chapter 134), malignant hypertension, chemotherapy-induced microangiopathic hemolytic anemia, and the HELLP syndrome. A common pathogenic feature of these disorders is endothelial damage, which triggers platelet adhesion and aggregation, thrombin generation, and an impaired fibrinolysis. The clinical consequences of extensive endothelial dysfunction include thrombocytopenia, mechanical fragmentation of red cells with hemolytic anemia, and microvasular occlusion, which leads to multiorgan dysfunction, including renal insufficiency and neurologic symptoms. Despite this common final pathway, the various thrombotic microangiopathies have different underlying etiologies (see Chapter 134).

Drug-induced thrombocytopenia is another frequent cause of thrombocytopenia in critically ill patients (see Chapter 131). Thrombocytopenia may be caused by drug-induced myelosuppression, (e.g.,

by cytostatic agents), or by immune-mediated mechanisms. Drug-induced thrombocytopenia is a difficult diagnosis in patients suspected of DIC because these patients are often receiving multiple drugs and have several other potential reasons for the thrombocytopenia. Drug-induced thrombocytopenia is often diagnosed based upon the timing of initiation of a new agent in relationship to the development of thrombocytopenia, after exclusion of other causes of thrombocytopenia. The observation of rapid restoration of the platelet count after discontinuation of the suspected agent is highly suggestive of drug-induced thrombocytopenia.

A prolongation of global coagulation tests may be due to a deficiency of one or more coagulation factors (Table 139.2). In addition, but more rarely, the prolonged tests may be due to an inhibitory antibody. Some of these antibodies may be clinically important, such as antibodies to factor VIII that lead to acquired hemophilia (see Chapter 136), whereas others may be less important, such as antiphospholipid antibodies (see Chapter 141). However, patients with antiphospholipid antibodies may have thrombocytopenia and may be at increased risk of thrombosis particularly if they also have a lupus anticoagulant. Inhibitory antibodies and lupus anticoagulants can be identified and distinguished with mixing studies (see Chapters 136 and 141).

In general, acquired deficiencies of coagulation factors can be due to impaired synthesis, massive loss, or increased turnover (consumption). Impaired synthesis is often due to hepatic insufficiency or vitamin K deficiency. Vitamin K deficiency may be caused by poor nutrition in combination with the use of antibiotics that impair bacterial vitamin K production in the intestine. The PT is sensitive to both conditions because this test is highly dependent on the plasma levels of factor VII, the vitamin K–dependent coagulation factor with the shortest half-life. Liver failure may be differentiated from vitamin K deficiency by measuring the levels of factor V, which is not vitamin K dependent. In fact, the factor V level is included in several scoring systems for acute liver failure. Uncompensated loss of coagulation factors may occur after massive bleeding, which can occur in trauma patients or those undergoing major surgical procedures. This is common in patients with major bleeding who receive intravascular volume replacement with crystalloids, colloids, and red cells without simultaneous administration of coagulation factors. This results in a dilutional coagulopathy, which can exacerbate the bleeding. In addition, transfusion in these patients may lead to systemic activation of inflammatory processes and may contribute to further coagulation derangements. In hypothermic patients (e.g., trauma patients) measurement of the global coagulation tests may underestimate the extent of the coagulopathy because these assays are performed at 37°C to mimic normal body temperature.

BOX 139.3	Mainstays of Supportive Treatment of Disseminated Intravascular Coagulation	
Modality	**Details**	**Expectations/Rationale**
Treating the underlying disorder	Depencent on the primary diagnosis	Inhibit or block the complicating pathologic mechanism of disseminated intravascular coagulation (DIC) in parallel with the response (if any) of the disorder
Antithrombotic agents	Prophylactic heparin to prevent venous thromboembolic complications (Low dose) therapeutic heparin in case of confirmed thromboembolism or if clinical picture is dominated by (micro) vascular thrombosis and associated organ failure	Risk of thromboembolism is increased in critically ill patients, trauma patients, or patients with cancer Prevent fibrin formation; tip the balance within the microcirculation toward anticoagulant mechanisms and physiologic fibrinolysis; allow reperfusion of the skin, kidneys, and brain
Transfusion	Infuse platelets, plasma and fibrinogen (cryoprecipitate) if there is overt bleeding or a high risk of bleeding	Bleeding should diminish and stop over the course of hours Platelet count, coagulation tests and fibrinogen should return toward normal
Anticoagulant factor concentrates	Recombinant human activated protein C may be effective in sepsis and DIC (24 µg/kg/h for 4 days); Currently withdrawn from the market	Restore anticoagulation in microvascular environment and may have antiinflammatory activity Latest trials were negative.
Fibrinolytic inhibitors	Tranexamic acid (e.g., 500–1000 mg q8–12 h or ε-aminocaproic acid 1000–2000 mg q8–12 h)	May be useful if there is (hyper) fibrinolysis Bleeding ceases, but there is a risk of microvascular thrombosis and renal failure

THERAPY

Management of patients with DIC depends on vigorous treatment of the underlying disorder to alleviate or remove the inciting injurious cause. For sepsis-induced DIC, treatment includes aggressive use of intravenous organism-directed antibiotics and source control (e.g., by surgery or drainage). Other examples of vigorous treatment of the underlying condition include cancer surgery or chemotherapy, uterus evacuation in patients with abruptio placentae, resection of aortic aneurysm, and debridement of crushed tissue in the case of trauma. In addition to intensive support of vital functions, supportive treatment aimed at the coagulopathy may be helpful (Box 139.3),[6] as outlined later.

Platelet and Plasma Transfusion

Low levels of platelets and coagulation factors may increase the risk of bleeding. However, plasma or platelet transfusion should not be instituted on the basis of laboratory results alone; it is only indicated in patients with active bleeding and in those requiring an invasive procedure or at risk for bleeding complications.[6] The presumed efficacy of treatment with plasma, fibrinogen concentrate, cryoprecipitate, or platelets is not based on the results of randomized controlled trials. Nonetheless, transfusion of these products is rational in bleeding patients or in patients at risk of bleeding who have significant depletion of these hemostatic factors. The suggestion that administration of blood components might "add fuel to the fire" has never been proven in clinical or experimental studies.

Replacement therapy for thrombocytopenia consists of 5 to 10 U platelet concentrate to raise the platelet count to $20–30 \times 10^9/L$ and to $50 \times 10^9/L$ in patients requiring an invasive procedure.

One of the major challenges of infusion of fresh-frozen plasma in patients with DIC who are bleeding is the propensity of the added volume, which is necessary to correct the coagulation defect, to exacerbate the capillary leak syndrome. This increases the risk of causing or worsening pulmonary edema and, by extension, predisposes to ARDS and induces ascites. Coagulation factor concentrates, such as prothrombin complex concentrate, may partially overcome this obstacle, but these concentrates do not contain essential factors, such as factor V. Moreover, caution is advocated with the use of prothrombin complex concentrates in DIC because they can contain trace amounts of activated coagulation factors, which may worsen the coagulopathy. Specific deficiencies of coagulation factors, such as fibrinogen, may be corrected by administration of purified coagulation factor concentrates.

Cryoprecipitate (if available) can be used to rapidly raise the levels of fibrinogen, von Willebrand factor, and factor VIII levels in patients with DIC, particularly when there is bleeding and the fibrinogen level is less than 1 g/L. Cryoprecipitate has at least four- to fivefold more fibrinogen in each milliliter than fresh-frozen plasma. Nonetheless, fresh-frozen plasma contains sufficient amounts of fibrinogen to treat mild to moderate hypofibrinogenemia.

Anticoagulant Treatment

Heparin therapy in patients with DIC remains controversial. Experimental studies have shown that heparin can at least partly inhibit activation of coagulation in DIC. However, clinical trials have failed to demonstrate a beneficial effect of heparin on clinically important outcome events in patients with DIC and the safety of heparin is debatable in those at risk for bleeding. A large trial in patients with severe sepsis showed a small but nonsignificant benefit of low dose heparin on 28-day mortality in patients and no major safety concerns.[25]

There is general consensus that administration of heparin is beneficial in some categories of DIC, such as metastatic cancer, purpura fulminans, and aortic aneurysm (prior to resection). Heparin also is indicated for treating thromboembolic complications in large vessels and before surgery in patients with chronic DIC. Heparin administration may be helpful in patients with acute DIC when intensive blood component replacement fails to improve excessive bleeding or when thrombosis threatens to cause irreversible tissue injury (e.g., acute cortical necrosis of the kidney or digital gangrene).

Heparin should be used cautiously in these conditions. In patients with chronic DIC because of metastatic cancer or aortic aneurysm, continuous infusion of unfractionated heparin (500 to 750 U/hour without a bolus) has been advocated. If no response is obtained within 24 hours, higher dosages can be used. In hyperacute DIC cases, such as amniotic fluid embolism, septic abortion, and purpura fulminans, intravenous bolus injection of 5000 to 10,000 U heparin may be given simultaneously with replacement therapy with blood products. Some experts, however, recommend against administration of a bolus dose of heparin under these circumstances. A heparin infusion of 500 to 1000 U/hour may be necessary to maintain the benefit until the underlying disease responds to treatment. Aside from these considerations, current guidelines recommend universal thromboprophylaxis with low doses of heparin or LMWH in critically ill patients.[6]

Theoretically, the most logical anticoagulants to use in DIC would be those directed against TF. Potential agents include recombinant TFPI, inactivated factor VIIa, and recombinant NAPc2, a potent and specific inhibitor of the ternary complex of TF/factor VIIa and factor Xa. Phase II trials of recombinant TFPI in patients with sepsis showed promising results but phase III trials in patients with severe sepsis or severe pneumonia and organ failure failed to show a survival advantage with TFPI adminsitration.[26]

Recombinant human soluble thrombomodulin binds thrombin to form a complex that blocks the coagulant activity of thrombin and promotes its capacity to activate protein C. In a phase III randomized double-blind clinical trial in patients with DIC, soluble thrombomodulin was superior to heparin at reducing bleeding and improving the coagulation parameters. A systematic review and meta-analysis of mostly retrospective studies on the effect of recombinant human soluble thrombomodulin in severe sepsis demonstrated a pooled relative risk of 0.81 (95% confidence interval (CI) 0.62–1.06) in three randomized trials encompassing 838 patients, and a relative risk of 0.59 (95% CI 0.45–0.77) in nine observational studies including 571 patients.[27] Interestingly, meta-regression of the combined results revealed a strong relationship between the effect size of recombinant soluble thrombomodulin treatment and baseline mortality risk, which is reminiscent of a similar relationship in patients who were treated with activated protein C.[9,28] Importantly, there was no evidence of an increased risk of major bleeding or other safety concerns with soluble thrombomodulin. Ongoing randomized trials with soluble thrombomodulin are focusing on its effects on DIC, organ failure, and mortality.

Physiologic Anticoagulant Factor Concentrates

Restoration of the levels of physiologic anticoagulants in DIC may be a rational approach.[29,30] Based on successful preclinical studies, AT concentrates without or with concomitant heparin have been evaluated in patients with DIC. All trials have shown some beneficial effect in terms of improvement of laboratory parameters, shortening of the duration of DIC, or even improvement in organ function. In several small clinical trials, use of very high doses of AT concentrate produced a modest but not statistically significant reduction in mortality. A large, multicenter, randomized controlled trial also showed no significant reduction in mortality with AT concentrate in patients with sepsis.[31] Interestingly, post hoc subgroup analysis suggested that AT was of benefit in patients who did not receive concomitant heparin, but this observation needs validation. In a small randomized trial in patients with burns and DIC, AT administration decreased mortality, reduced multiple organ failure, and improved coagulation parameters compared with placebo.

Because decreased function of the protein C system contributes to the pathogenesis of DIC, recombinant APC was predicted to be beneficial.[32] Indeed, in a dose-ranging study, a continuous infusion of recombinant human APC at a dose of 24 μg/kg per hour was considered optimal based on reductions in D-dimer levels. A subsequent placebo-controlled phase III trial of APC concentrate in patients with severe sepsis was stopped early because of a 19% reduction in 28-day all cause mortality from 30.8% to 24.7% with APC. Interestingly, patients who manifested with "overt DIC" (see Diagnosis section, earlier) benefited more from APC than those without overt DIC.[9] However, meta-analyses of the APC trials concluded that APC had little or no effect. A series of negative trials in patients with severe sepsis has added to the skepticism regarding the use of APC. In addition to questionable efficacy, APC increases the risk of bleeding in patients with severe sepsis. A placebo-controlled trial in patients with severe sepsis and septic shock was stopped early because there was no benefit with APC. Subsequently, the manufacturer elected to withdraw APC from the market, which has resulted in a revision of current guidelines for treatment of DIC.

Fibrinolytic Inhibitors

Most guidelines recommend against the use of antifibrinolytic agents, such as ε-aminocaproic acid or tranexamic acid, in patients with DIC. This is because these drugs block already suppress endogenous fibrinolysis, and may further compromise tissue perfusion. In support of this concept there are reports of severe thrombosis in DIC patients treated with these agents. However, in patients with DIC accompanied by primary fibrino(geno)lysis, which occurs in some cases of acute promyelocytic leukemia, giant cavernous hemangioma, heat stroke, and metastatic carcinoma of the prostate, the use of fibrinolytic inhibitors can be considered if the patient has profuse bleeding that does not respond to replacement therapy and there is evidence of excessive fibrino(geno)lysis. In these situations, it is important to replace depleted blood components before initiating treatment with fibrinolytic inhibitors.

REFERENCES

1. Seligsohn U: Disseminated intravascular coagulation. In Handin RI, Lux SE, Stossel TP, editors: *Blood: Principles and practice of hematology*, Philadelphia, 2000, J.B. Lippincott.
2. Levi M, Seligsohn U: Disseminated intravascular coagulation. In Kaushansky K, Lichtman M, Beutler E, et al, editors: *Williams hematology*, Philadelphia, 2010, McGraw Hill.
3. Levi M, ten Cate H: Disseminated intravascular coagulation. *N Engl J Med* 341(8):586–592, 1999.
4. Levi M: Disseminated intravascular coagulation. *Crit Care Med* 35:2191–2195, 2007.
5. Taylor FBJ, Toh CH, Hoots WK, et al: Towards definition, clinical and laboratory criteria, and a scoring system for disseminated intravascular coagulation. *Thromb Haemost* 86(5):1327–1330, 2001.
6. Levi M, Toh CH, Thachil J, et al: Guidelines for the diagnosis and management of disseminated intravascular coagulation. *Br J Haematol* 145(1):24–33, 2009.
7. Levi M, van der Poll T: Inflammation and coagulation. *Crit Care Med* 38(2 Suppl):S26–S34, 2010.
8. Fourrier F, Chopin C, Goudemand J, et al: Septic shock, multiple organ failure, and disseminated intravascular coagulation. Compared patterns of antithrombin III, protein C, and protein S deficiencies. *Chest* 101(3):816–823, 1992.
9. Dhainaut JF, Yan SB, Joyce DE, et al: Treatment effects of drotrecogin alfa (activated) in patients with severe sepsis with or without overt disseminated intravascular coagulation. *J Thromb Haemost* 2:1924–1933, 2004.
10. Levi M, Opal SM: Coagulation abnormalities in critically ill patients. *Crit Care* 10(4):222, 2006.
11. Colman RW, Schmaier AH: Contact system: a vascular biology modulator with anticoagulant, profibrinolytic, antiadhesive, and proinflammatory attributes. *Blood* 90(10):3819–3843, 1997.
12. Esmon CT: The regulation of natural anticoagulant pathways. *Science* 235(4794):1348–1352, 1987.
13. Keller TT, Mairuhu AT, de Kruif MD, et al: Infections and endothelial cells. *Cardiovasc Res* 60(1):40–48, 2003.
14. Lowenberg EC, Meijers JC, Levi M: Platelet-vessel wall interaction in health and disease. *Neth J Med* 68(6):242–251, 2010.
15. Gando S, Nakanishi Y, Tedo I: Cytokines and plasminogen activator inhibitor-1 in posttrauma disseminated intravascular coagulation: relationship to multiple organ dysfunction syndrome. *Crit Care Med* 23(11):1835–1842, 1995.
16. Huisse MG, Pease S, Hurtado-Nedelec M, et al: Leucocyte activation: the link between inflammation and coagulation during heatstroke. A study of patients during the 2003 heat wave in Paris. *Crit Care Med* 36:2288–2295, 2008.
17. Levi M: Disseminated intravascular coagulation (DIC) in pregnancy and the peri-partum period. *Thromb Res* 123(Suppl 2):S63–S64, 2009.
18. Colman RW, Rubin RN: Disseminated intravascular coagulation due to malignancy. *Semin Oncol* 17(2):172–186, 1990.
19. Barbui T, Falanga A: Disseminated intravascular coagulation in acute leukemia. *Semin Thromb Hemost* 27(6):593–604, 2001.
20. Fisher DF, Jr, Yawn DH, Crawford ES: Preoperative disseminated intravascular coagulation associated with aortic aneurysms. A prospective study of 76 cases. *Arch Surg* 118(11):1252–1255, 1983.

21. Isbister GK: Snake bite doesn't cause disseminated intravascular coagulation: Coagulopathy and thrombotic microangiopathy in snake envenoming. *Semin Thromb Hemost* 36:444–451, 2010.

22. Levi M, de Jonge E, Meijers J: The diagnosis of disseminated intravascular coagulation. *Blood Rev* 16(4):217–223, 2002.

23. Levi M, Meijers JC: DIC: Which laboratory tests are most useful. *Blood Rev* 2010.

24. Dempfle CE, Borggrefe M: Point of care coagulation tests in critically ill patients. *Semin Thromb Hemost* 34(5):445–450, 2008.

25. Levi M, Levy M, Williams MD, et al: Prophylactic heparin in patients with severe sepsis treated with drotrecogin alfa (activated). *Am J Respir Crit Care Med* 176(5):483–490, 2007.

26. Abraham E, Reinhart K, Opal S, et al: Efficacy and safety of tifacogin (recombinant tissue factor pathway inhibitor) in severe sepsis: a randomized controlled trial. *JAMA* 290(2):238–247, 2003.

27. Yamakawa K, Aihara M, Ogura H, et al: Recombinant human soluble thrombomodulin in severe sepsis: a systematic review and meta-analysis. *J Thromband Haemost* 13(4):508–519, 2015.

28. Bernard GR, Vincent JL, Laterre PF, et al: Efficacy and safety of recombinant human activated protein C for severe sepsis. *N Engl J Med* 344:699–709, 2001.

29. Levi M, de Jonge E, van der Poll T: Rationale for restoration of physiological anticoagulant pathways in patients with sepsis and disseminated intravascular coagulation. *Crit Care Med* 29:S90–S94, 2001.

30. de Jonge E, van der Poll T, Kesecioglu J, et al: Anticoagulant factor concentrates in disseminated intravascular coagulation: rationale for use and clinical experience. *Semin Thromb Hemost* 27:667–674, 2001.

31. Warren BL, Eid A, Singer P, et al: Caring for the critically ill patient. High-dose antithrombin III in severe sepsis: a randomized controlled trial. *JAMA* 286(15):1869–1878, 2001.

32. Levi M: Activated protein C in sepsis: a critical review. *Curr Opin Hematol* 15(5):481–486, 2008.

CHAPTER 140

HYPERCOAGULABLE STATES

Julia A. Anderson, Kerstin E. Hogg, and Jeffrey I. Weitz

Arterial and venous thromboses are common problems for all clinicians. Some patients with thrombosis have an underlying hypercoagulable state. These hypercoagulable states can be divided into three categories: inherited disorders, acquired disorders, and those that are mixed in origin.

Inherited hypercoagulable states, also known as thrombophilic disorders, can be due to loss of function of natural anticoagulant pathways or gain of function in procoagulant pathways (Table 140.1). Acquired hypercoagulable states represent a heterogeneous group of disorders in which the risk for thrombosis appears to be higher than that in the general population. These include such diverse risk factors as a prior history of thrombosis, obesity, pregnancy, cancer and its treatment, antiphospholipid antibody syndrome, drug-induced thrombosis such as heparin-induced thrombocytopenia or thrombosis associated with chemotherapeutic agents, or myeloproliferative disorders. The pathogenesis of thrombosis in these situations is largely unknown and, in many cases, is likely multifactorial in origin. Mixed disorders are those with both an inherited and an acquired component; one example is hyperhomocysteinemia. Although severe hyperhomocysteinemia and associated homocysteinuria are rare genetic disorders, most cases of mild to moderate hyperhomocysteinemia result from acquired folate and/or vitamin B_{12} deficiency superimposed on common genetic mutations in biochemical pathways involved in methionine metabolism.

Genetic hypercoagulable states and acquired risk factors combine to establish an intrinsic risk for thrombosis for each individual. This risk can be modified by extrinsic or environmental factors, such as surgery, immobilization, or hormonal therapy, which also increase the risk for thrombosis. When the intrinsic and extrinsic forces exceed a critical threshold, thrombosis occurs (Fig. 140.1). Appropriate thromboprophylaxis can prevent the thrombotic risk from exceeding this critical threshold, but breakthrough thrombosis can still occur if procoagulant stimuli overwhelm protective mechanisms.

This chapter describes the inherited, acquired, and mixed hypercoagulable states, details their laboratory evaluation, and provides practical advice for the management of these conditions.

INHERITED HYPERCOAGULABLE STATES

Inherited disorders are found in up to half of patients who present with venous thromboembolism before the age of 40, particularly those whose event occurred either in the absence of well-recognized risk factors, such as surgery or immobilization, or with minimal provoking factors, such as minor trauma, long-distance flight, or estrogens. Patients with inherited thrombophilic disorders often have a family history of thrombosis. Of greatest significance is a family history of sudden death due to pulmonary embolism or a history of multiple family members requiring long-term anticoagulation therapy because of recurrent thrombosis. Patients who present with venous thrombosis in unusual sites, such as the cerebral or mesenteric veins, those with recurrent thrombosis, and patients who develop skin necrosis upon initiation of warfarin therapy should also be suspected of having an inherited hypercoagulable state.

From a pathophysiologic perspective, inherited hypercoagulable states fall into two categories. First are those associated with loss of function of endogenous anticoagulant proteins. These include deficiencies of antithrombin, protein C, and protein S. The second

category involves gain of function in procoagulant pathways. These disorders include factor V_{Leiden} and the FIIG20210A mutation, as well as increased levels of procoagulant proteins, such as factors VIII, IX, and XI. Each of these conditions will be briefly described.

Loss of Function of Endogenous Anticoagulants

Antithrombin Deficiency

Antithrombin, a single-chain glycoprotein with a molecular weight of 52,000 Da, is a member of the serine proteinase inhibitor (serpin) superfamily that was first described by Brinkhous in 1939. Antithrombin is synthesized in the liver and endothelial cells, and its gene (*SERPINC1*, previously known as *AT3*) is localized on the long arm of chromosome 1 (1q23–1q25). *SERPINC1* is composed of 7 exons and 7 introns and spans 16 kb.

Antithrombin plays a critical role in regulating coagulation by forming a 1:1 covalent complex with thrombin, factor Xa, and other activated clotting factors. Once covalent complexes are generated, they are cleared from the circulation via the liver. The rate of antithrombin interaction with its target proteases is accelerated by heparin by 1000-fold. Heparan sulfate proteoglycan, which coats the vasculature, is the physiologic counterpart of medicinal heparin.

Newborn infants have approximately 50% of normal adult antithrombin levels, and much lower levels are found in preterm infants because of liver immaturity; adult levels are attained at 6 months.

Antithrombin deficiency can be inherited or acquired, and congenital deficiency of antithrombin was the first reported inherited risk factor for venous thromboembolism. Congenital antithrombin deficiency is relatively rare, occurring in about 1 in 2000, and can be one of two types (Table 140.2), both of which are inherited in an autosomal dominant fashion and affect both sexes equally. Type I deficiency, which represents the classic deficiency state, is the result of reduced synthesis of biologically normal antithrombin. Heterozygotes with this condition have parallel reductions in antithrombin antigen and activity with levels reduced to about 50% of normal. A heterogeneous group of nonsense mutations, small deletions, insertions, or single-base substitutions are the molecular cause of most cases, although gene deletions can also be responsible. In total, more than 113 mutations have been identified as causes of type I antithrombin deficiency. An antithrombin mutation database compiled by members of the Plasma Coagulation Inhibitors Subcommittee of the Scientific and Standardization Committee of the International Society on Thrombosis and Hemostasis summarizes the mutations and can be accessed on the Imperial College London website (www.imperial.ac.uk/departmentofmedicine/research/experimental-medicine/haematology/haemostasis-and-thrombosis/database/) or in the human gene mutation database (www.hgmd.cf.ac.uk).

Type II antithrombin deficiencies are characterized by normal levels of antithrombin with impaired functional activity due to the presence of a variant protein. This condition is mainly caused by missense mutations that result in single amino acid substitutions. The clinical consequences of type II antithrombin deficiency depend on the location of the mutation, which may involve the reactive center loop or the heparin-binding domain. For example, some mutations in the reactive center loop of antithrombin slow its interaction with target proteases and are characterized by reduced antithrombin

TABLE 140.1 Classification of Hypercoagulable States

Hereditary	Mixed	Acquired
Loss of Function		
Antithrombin deficiency	Hyperhomocysteinemia	Previous venous thromboembolism
Protein C deficiency	Obesity	Pregnancy, puerperium
Protein S deficiency	Cancer	
		Drug-induced:
		Heparin-induced thrombocytopenia
		Prothrombin complex concentrates
		L-asparaginase
		Hormonal therapy
Gain of Function		
Factor V Leiden	Postoperative	
Prothrombin FII G20210A	Myeloproliferative disorders	
Elevated factor VIII, IX, or XI		

TABLE 140.2 Types of Inherited Antithrombin Deficiency

Type	Antigen	Activity (No Heparin)	Activity (With Heparin)
I	Low	Low	Low
II (active site defect)	Normal	Low	Low
II (heparin-binding site defect)	Normal	Normal	Low

TABLE 140.3 Causes of Acquired Antithrombin Deficiency

Decreased Synthesis	Increased Consumption	Enhanced Clearance
Hepatic cirrhosis	Major surgery	Heparin
Severe liver disease	Acute thrombosis	Nephrotic syndrome
L-asparaginase	Disseminated intravascular coagulation	
	Severe sepsis	
	Multiple trauma	
	Malignancy	
	Prolonged extracorporeal circulation	

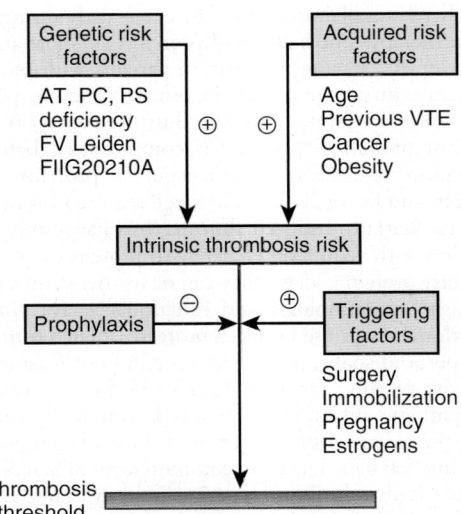

Fig. 140.1 THROMBOSIS THRESHOLD. Genetic and acquired risk factors continue to determine an intrinsic risk for thrombosis for each individual. This risk is increased by extrinsic or environmental factors and decreased by thromboprophylaxis. If the intrinsic and extrinsic forces exceed a critical threshold at which thrombin generation overwhelms the protective mechanisms, thrombosis will result. *AT,* Antithrombin; *PC,* protein C; *PS,* protein S; *VTE,* venous thromboembolism. *(From Anderson JA, Weitz JI: Hypercoagulability and uncommon vascular diseases. In Jaff MR, White CJ, editors: Vascular disease: Diagnostic and therapeutic approaches, Minneapolis, MN, 2011, Cardiotext Publishing.)*

activity in the absence or presence of heparin. In contrast, mutations in the heparin-binding domain are associated with reduced antithrombin activity in the presence of heparin but normal activity in its absence. Unlike other inherited forms of antithrombin deficiency, which are embryonic lethal in the homozygous state, mutations in the heparin-binding domain only have clinical consequences in individuals homozygous for these mutations and do not increase the risk for thrombosis in the heterozygous state.

Because of the wide variety of heritable forms of antithrombin deficiency, functional antithrombin assays are the preferred method for screening. Most functional assays use synthetic substrates to monitor the rates at which added thrombin or factor Xa are inhibited in patient plasma. However, the assays differ in terms of whether bovine or human thrombin is used and whether or not heparin is added. Defects in the heparin-binding domain of antithrombin will be detected only in the presence of heparin. When antithrombin deficiency is identified with functional assays, immunologic assays are performed to distinguish between type I and type II deficiency.

Congenital antithrombin deficiency can cause spontaneous venous thromboembolism, but thrombosis often occurs in the setting of pregnancy and the puerperium; with the use of estrogen-containing oral contraceptives; or after major trauma or surgery. Thrombotic events are rare in children, with events typically occurring from mid- to late teenage years and into the early twenties. The European Prospective Cohort on Thrombophilia (EPCOT) study compared the risks of a first episode of venous thromboembolism in asymptomatic individuals with antithrombin, protein C, or protein S deficiency with that in subjects with factor V_{Leiden} over a 6-year period. The annual incidence of venous thromboembolism was highest in those with antithrombin deficiency.[1] Likewise, in a cohort of Italian patients, the risk of venous thrombosis was higher with antithrombin deficiency than with other thrombophilic defects.[2] The most common sites for venous thrombosis in patients with antithrombin deficiency are the deep veins of the leg, but thrombosis can occur in mesenteric veins, as well as the renal and retinal veins. The risk for recurrence is high,[3] particularly in those with lower antithrombin levels,[4] and the risk varies depending on the subtype of antithrombin deficiency.

Acquired antithrombin deficiency can reflect decreased antithrombin synthesis, increased consumption, or enhanced clearance (Table 140.3). Decreased synthesis can occur in patients with severe hepatic disease, particularly cirrhosis, or in those given L-asparaginase, the latter as a result of drug-induced retention of antithrombin within the endoplasmic reticulum. Increased thrombin generation can result in antithrombin consumption. Disorders associated with excessive thrombin generation include acute thrombosis, disseminated intravascular coagulation (DIC), severe sepsis, multiple trauma, disseminated malignancy, extensive burns, or prolonged extracorporeal circulation. Heparin treatment can reduce antithrombin levels up to 20% by enhancing its clearance. Severe antithrombin deficiency can also occur in some patients with nephrotic syndrome because of the loss of protein in the urine.

Protein C Pathway

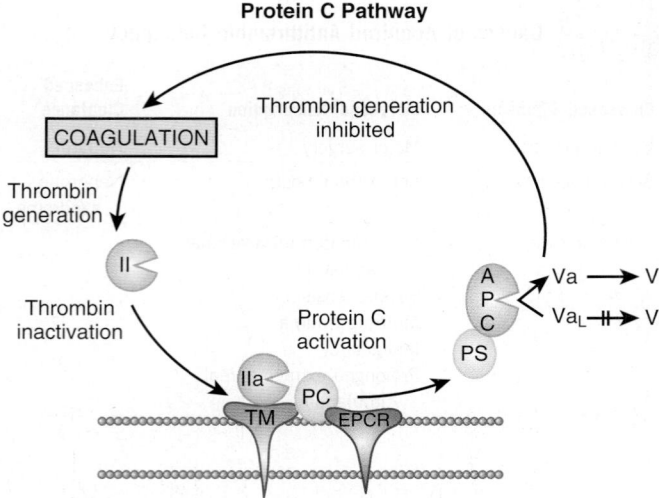

Fig. 140.2 PROTEIN C PATHWAY. Activation of coagulation triggers thrombin (IIa) generation. Excess thrombin binds to thrombomodulin (TM) on the endothelial cell surface. Once bound, the substrate specificity of thrombin is altered so that it no longer acts as a procoagulant but becomes a potent activator of protein C (PC). Endothelial protein C receptor (EPCR) binds PC and presents it to thrombomodulin-bound thrombin, where it is activated. Activated protein C (APC), together with its cofactor, protein S (PS), binds to the activated platelet-surface and proteolytically degrades factor Va (Va) into inactive fragments (Vi). Because factor Va is a critical component of the prothrombinase complex, factor Va inactivation by APC attenuates thrombin generation. Because factor Va_{Leiden} (FVa_L) is resistant to inactivation by APC, patients with the factor V_{Leiden} mutation have reduced capacity to regulate thrombin generation. *(From Anderson JA, Weitz JI: Hypercoagulability and uncommon vascular diseases. In Jaff MR, White CJ, editors:* Vascular disease: Diagnostic and therapeutic approaches, *Minneapolis, MN, 2011, Cardiotext Publishing.)*

Users of oral contraceptive pills or hormone replacement therapy may have moderate reductions in antithrombin levels; during pregnancy, the antithrombin levels do not fall significantly but decreases are found in preeclampsia and pregnancy-induced hypertensive illnesses.

Protein C Deficiency

The protein C pathway is an important natural anticoagulant pathway. This on-demand pathway is activated when thrombin is generated (Fig. 140.2). Thrombin binds to thrombomodulin, a transmembrane thrombin receptor found on the surface of endothelial cells. Once bound to thrombomodulin, the substrate specificity of thrombin is altered so that it no longer serves as a procoagulant enzyme, but becomes a potent activator of protein C, a vitamin K–dependent glycoprotein. Thus thrombin bound to thrombomodulin activates protein C 1000-fold more efficiently than free thrombin. The endothelial cell protein C receptor (EPCR), another transmembrane receptor on the endothelial cell surface, binds protein C and presents it to the thrombin–thrombomodulin complex for activation, thereby producing an additional 20-fold increase in the rate of protein C activation. The physiologic importance of thrombomodulin and EPCR is highlighted by the fact that deficiency of either receptor results in embryonic lethality in mice.

Activated protein C (APC) dissociates from this activation complex and acts as an anticoagulant by proteolytically degrading and inactivating factors Va and VIIIa, thereby attenuating thrombin generation. For efficient inactivation of factors Va and VIIIa, APC must bind to protein S, its cofactor. This interaction facilitates APC binding to activated cell surfaces, particularly the platelet surface, where factors Va and VIIIa are localized.

TABLE 140.4   Types of Inherited Protein C Deficiency

Type	Antigen	Activity
I	Low	Low
II	Normal	Low

APC has a half-life in the circulation of about 15 minutes, whereas thrombin has a half-life of about 10 seconds. APC is inhibited by protein C inhibitor and α_1-proteinase inhibitor (α_1-antitrypsin), both of which are relatively slow inhibitors. Only the activity of protein C inhibitor is enhanced by heparin, but both inhibitors appear to contribute to APC inhibition in vivo.

Protein C deficiency can be inherited or acquired. Like antithrombin deficiency, protein C deficiency is inherited in an autosomal-dominant fashion and has a proven association with venous thrombosis.[5] Based on studies in healthy blood donors, heterozygous protein C deficiency can be found in 1 in 200 to 500 of the adult population, but many of these individuals do not have a history of thrombosis. Thus the phenotypic expression of hereditary protein C deficiency is highly variable and may depend on other, as yet unrecognized, modifying factors. In contrast to antithrombin deficiency in which the homozygous state is embryonic lethal, homozygous or doubly heterozygous protein C deficiency can occur. The prevalence of homozygous protein C deficiency is estimated to be 1 in 160,000 to 360,000 births. Newborns with these disorders may present with purpura fulminans characterized by widespread thrombosis.

Individuals with heterozygous protein C deficiency can develop skin necrosis upon initiation of treatment with vitamin K antagonists, such as warfarin. Typically, skin lesions are found on the extremities, breasts, or trunk. Starting as erythematous macules, the central regions of the cutaneous lesions become purpuric and then necrotic over a period of hours unless protein C is administered. Biopsies reveal fibrin thrombi within the vessels of the skin associated with interstitial hemorrhage. The skin lesions are clinically and histologically similar to those seen in infants with purpura fulminans and are attributable to the transient hypercoagulable state that is induced by warfarin, thereby explaining why they occur early during the course of warfarin therapy. The half-life of protein C is short and similar to that of factor VII. Starting warfarin in patients with protein C deficiency causes a further reduction in protein C levels, particularly if loading doses of warfarin are given. Thus the activity of the natural anticoagulant protein C pathway is compromised before warfarin lowers vitamin K–dependent procoagulant proteins, particularly prothrombin and factor X, into the range required for its antithrombotic effects. Warfarin-induced skin necrosis has also been reported in association with acquired deficiency of protein C.

Hereditary protein C deficiency can be further delineated into two subtypes using immunologic and functional assays (Table 140.4). Most functional assays use Protac, a protease isolated from the venom of the copperhead snake, to activate protein C in plasma. The enzymatic activity of APC can then be assayed directly using an APC-directed synthetic substrate, or it can be indirectly quantified by measuring the extent of prolongation of the activated partial thromboplastin time (aPTT). The most common form of hereditary protein C deficiency is the classic or type I deficiency state. This disorder reflects reduced synthesis of a normal protein and is characterized by a parallel reduction in protein C antigen and activity, resulting in a quantitative deficiency due to reduced synthesis or stability of protein C. A variety of genetic defects can produce type I protein C deficiency, including promoter mutations, splice-site abnormalities, in-frame deletions, frameshift deletions, in-frame insertions, and frameshift insertions in the protein C gene (*PROC*), but missense or nonsense mutations are the most common.

Type II protein C deficiency reflects synthesis of a dysfunctional protein and is characterized by normal protein C antigen with reduced functional activity, a qualitative deficiency. Most type II protein C deficiency states are caused by point mutations. Mutations in the active site of APC reduce its activity against synthetic substrates and decrease its capacity to prolong the aPTT. In contrast, mutations that affect other protein C domains essential for its activity may reduce its anticoagulant activity but may not affect its capacity to cleave synthetic substrates activity. Therefore coagulation-based functional assays are preferred when screening patients for protein C deficiency.

Diagnosis of protein C deficiency is complicated. Protein C circulates in human plasma at an average concentration of 4 µg/mL. Plasma protein C antigen levels are widely distributed in healthy adults such that 95% of the values range from 70% to 140%. Furthermore, protein C levels increase with age particularly in postmenopausal women.[6] The wide range of values makes it difficult to establish a normal range. Levels less than 55%, however, are likely to reflect deficiency, whereas those between 55% and 70% are considered borderline and may be consistent with a deficiency state or the lower end of the normal distribution. Acquired causes of protein C deficiency must be excluded, and to document the presence of protein C deficiency, it is necessary to repeat the testing. Family studies may also be helpful to highlight the autosomal dominant pattern of inheritance.

Acquired protein C deficiency can be due to decreased synthesis or increased consumption. Decreased synthesis can occur in patients with liver disease or in those given warfarin. Warfarin decreases functional activity more than immunologic activity; newborns have protein C levels 20% to 40% lower than those of adults, and premature infants have even lower levels. Protein C consumption can occur with severe sepsis, with DIC, and after surgery. Reduced protein C levels have also been reported in cancer patients receiving cyclophosphamide, methotrexate, 5-fluorouracil, or L-asparaginase. A particularly severe form of acquired protein C deficiency has been described in association with meningococcal septicemia. In contrast to antithrombin, which is excreted in the urine of patients with nephrotic syndrome, the levels of protein C are normal or elevated in patients with nephrotic syndrome.

Protein S Deficiency

Protein S serves as a cofactor for APC and enhances its capacity to inactivate factors Va and VIIIa. In addition, protein S may have direct anticoagulant activity by inhibiting prothrombin activation through its capacity to bind anionic phospholipid, factor Va, or factor Xa, components of the prothrombinase complex. The importance of the direct anticoagulant activity of protein S is uncertain.

In the circulation, about 60% of total protein S is bound to C4b-binding protein, an acute phase complement component. Because only 40% of the protein S that is free is functionally active, only patients with low free protein S levels are prone to venous thrombosis. Therefore the diagnosis of protein S deficiency requires measurement of both free and bound forms of protein S. Total protein S levels can be measured immunologically under conditions that dissociate protein S from C4b-binding protein. The free fraction can then be quantified with a monoclonal antibody that only recognizes free protein S while the functional activity of protein S can be measured using an APC cofactor assay. This assay depends on prolongation of the aPTT when diluted patient plasma is added to protein S–depleted plasma containing APC and factor Va.

Protein S deficiency can be inherited or acquired. Heterozygous protein S deficiency is inherited in an autosomal dominant manner; the prevalence varies between 1% and 7% among patients with thrombotic events. There is an association with unprovoked venous thromboembolism.[7] Based on measurements of total and free protein S antigen and protein S activity, three subtypes of inherited protein S deficiency have been identified (Table 140.5). Type I or classical deficiency results from decreased synthesis of a normal protein and is characterized by reduced levels of total and free protein S antigen together with reduced protein S functional activity. Molecular analysis

TABLE 140.5	Types of Inherited Protein S Deficiency		
Type	Total Protein S	Free Protein S	Protein S Activity
I	Low	Low	Low
II	Normal	Normal	Low
III	Normal	Low	Low

of protein S deficiency is complicated because there are two homologous protein S genes, one of which is likely a pseudogene. Nonetheless, most cases of type I protein S deficiency are caused by partial gene deletions, missense mutations, base pair insertions or deletions, premature stop codons, or mutations affecting a splice site in the gene encoding protein S (PROS1). Type II protein S deficiency is characterized by normal levels of total and free protein S, associated with reduced protein S activity. This type of deficiency is uncommon, and most of the causative mutations encode protein S domains involved in its interaction with APC.

Type III protein S deficiency is characterized by normal levels of total protein S, but low levels of free protein S associated with reduced protein S activity. The molecular basis of this type of deficiency appears to be similar to that of the type I deficiency states. In fact, type I and type III protein S deficiency are likely to be manifestations of the same disease because they often coexist in families. Thus younger family members present with type I deficiency, whereas older family members have type III deficiency because protein S levels increase with age.

Acquired protein S deficiency can be due to decreased synthesis, increased consumption, loss, or shift of free protein S to the bound form. Decreased synthesis can occur in patients with severe liver disease, in those given L-asparaginase, and in patients given vitamin K antagonists. Increased consumption of protein S occurs in patients with acute thrombosis or in those with DIC. Patients with nephrotic syndrome can lose free protein S in their urine, causing decreased protein S activity. Total protein S levels in these patients are often normal because the levels of C4b-binding protein increase, shifting more protein S to the bound form. C4b-binding protein levels also increase in pregnancy and with the use of oral contraceptives. This shifts more protein S to the bound form and lowers the levels of free protein S and protein S activity. The pathophysiologic consequences of this phenomenon are uncertain. An association between antiphospholipid antibodies and acquired protein S deficiency has been reported in patients with severe forms of varicella zoster virus infection complicated by purpura fulminans. In healthy neonates the total protein S antigen levels are 15% to 30% of normal, and the C4b-binding protein is significantly reduced to less than 20%, such that the free form of protein S predominates and the functional levels are only slightly reduced compared with normal adult levels.

Gain of Function Mutations

Gain of function mutations includes factor V_{Leiden}, FIIG20210A, elevated levels of procoagulant proteins, and other less well-characterized genetic disorders. The gain of function mutations are more prevalent in the general population than those associated with loss of function.

Factor V_{Leiden}

In 1993 Dahlback and colleagues described three families with a history of venous thromboembolism. Affected family members exhibited limited prolongation of the aPTT when APC was added to their plasma. Accordingly, this phenotype was designated APC resistance (APCR). Bertina and colleagues demonstrated that APCR co-segregated with the factor V gene and was due to a single base substitution, guanine to adenine at position 1691, that produced an

Arg 506 Gln mutation at one of the APC cleavage sites on factor Va. This mutation, which is designated factor V$_{Leiden}$, endows activated factor V$_{Leiden}$ with a 10-fold longer half-life in the presence of APC than its wild-type counterpart.

The factor V$_{Leiden}$ mutation is responsible for most cases of APCR. Other causes are mutations at Arg 306, another APC cleavage site. Arg 306 is replaced by a Gly residue in factor V$_{Hong Kong}$ and by a Thr residue in factor V$_{Cambridge}$. Neither of these mutations is strongly associated with thrombosis.

The factor V$_{Leiden}$ mutation is inherited in an autosomal-dominant fashion. The prevalence of the mutation ranges from 2% to 5% in whites, but it is rare in Asians and Africans. This racial difference likely reflects a founder effect with the mutation arising 20,000 to 30,000 years ago, after the divergence of non-Africans from Africans and Caucasoids from Mongoloid subpopulations. The prevalence of factor V$_{Leiden}$ homozygosity is about 1 in 2500. The risk for thrombotic complications is lower with factor V$_{Leiden}$ than it is with deficiencies of antithrombin, protein C, or protein S,[8] and in the heterozygous state, does not appear to be a strong risk factor for recurrent venous thrombosis.[9] The risk for thrombosis is higher in homozygotes than in heterozygotes. Acquired APC resistance may be caused by hormonal changes during pregnancy or by the administration of estrogens, such as oral contraceptive pills or hormone replacement therapy.

A diagnosis of APCR is established using a functional assay based on the ratio of the aPTT after APC addition divided by that determined before APC addition. Second-generation tests, which add dilute patient plasma to factor V–deficient plasma, are more specific for factor V$_{Leiden}$. A normal functional test excludes factor V$_{Leiden}$; a positive functional test for APCR should be confirmed with a genetic test for the factor V$_{Leiden}$ mutation. Some laboratories only use the genetic test for diagnosis of factor V$_{Leiden}$.

FII G20210A Mutation

After extensive screening of 28 families with unexplained venous thromboembolism, Poort and colleagues identified a heterozygous G to A nucleotide transition at position 20210 in the 3′-untranslated region of the prothrombin gene in five of the probands. This mutation, FII G20210A, results in elevated levels of prothrombin. Elevated levels of prothrombin, in turn, may increase the risk for thrombosis by enhancing thrombin generation or by inhibiting factor Va inactivation by APC.

The mechanism by which the FII G20210A mutation causes increased prothrombin levels appears to vary. Enhanced protein synthesis may result from more efficient 3′-end formation, increased messenger RNA stability, increased translation efficiency, or some combination of these mechanisms. An intronic FII gene polymorphism, A19911G, which influences splicing efficiency, may modulate the effect of the FII G20210A mutation such that heterozygous carriers of both mutations have a greater risk for thrombosis than those with only the FII G20210A mutation.

Like the factor V$_{Leiden}$ mutation, the prevalence of the FII G20210A mutation is higher in whites and low in Asians, American Indians, and African Americans. A founder effect likely explains the higher prevalence in whites. The mutation may have provided a survival advantage based on a protective effect with childbirth or severe sepsis.

FII G20210A is found in 1% to 6% of whites. The mutation is more common in southern Europe than in northern Europe, a gradient opposite to that of factor V$_{Leiden}$. Rare individuals homozygous for the FII G20210A mutation have been identified. In the Leiden Thrombophilia Study, 6.2% of venous thrombosis patients and 2.3% of healthy matched controls had the FII G20210A mutation.[10] The mutation independently confers a 2.8-fold increased risk for venous thrombosis, with no gender bias; a risk lower than that with antithrombin, protein C, or protein S deficiency. The abnormality confers a weaker increased risk of venous thrombosis than protein C, protein S or antithrombin deficiencies.

Laboratory diagnosis of FIIG 20210A depends on genetic screening after PCR amplification of the 3′-untranslated region of the FII gene. Although FII G20210A heterozygotes have 30% higher levels of prothrombin than non-carriers, the wide range of prothrombin

levels in healthy individuals precludes the use of this phenotype to identify carriers.

Elevated Levels of Procoagulant Proteins

Elevated levels of factor VIII and other coagulation factors, including factors XI, IX, and VII, have been implicated as independent risk factors for thrombosis. Although the molecular bases for the high levels of these coagulation factors have yet to be identified, genetic mechanisms are likely responsible because the hereditability of these quantitative abnormalities is high.

Other Hereditary Disorders

The dysfibrinogenemias represent a heterogeneous group of disorders characterized by abnormal fibrinogen structure and are diagnosed by low functional and/or immunologic levels of fibrinogen, in association with prolonged thrombin and reptilase times. Acquired causes of dysfibrinogenemia, such as liver disease, must be excluded in the diagnostic work-up. Most congenital dysfibrinogenemias are asymptomatic, and are often identified as an incidental finding when coagulation testing is performed for other reasons. Up to 40% of the known dysfibrinogenemias are associated with a bleeding diathesis. Approximately 15 variant fibrinogens, which represent less than 10% of known dysfibrinogenemias, have been reported to be associated with thrombotic complications, including fibrinogen Marburg, Caracas V, Chapel Hill III, Hannover II, Nijmegen, New York I, Christchurch II and III, and Milano III. The exact mechanism by which these dysfibrinogenemias increase the risk for thrombosis depends on the nature of the fibrinogen defect. Most affect the C-terminal domain of the Aα chains or the thrombin cleavage site on the Bβ chains. Some biochemical defects have been further characterized, such as defects in the release of fibrinopeptides A or B by thrombin, impaired binding of thrombin or tissue plasminogen activator to fibrin, or resistance to lysis by plasmin. It is likely that acquired and/or other hereditary factors contribute to thrombosis that occurs in patients with dysfibrinogenemia.

Polymorphisms in the gene encoding EPCR have been associated with thrombosis. An EPCR polymorphism associated with high levels of soluble EPCR has been identified. By binding circulating protein C and APC, soluble EPCR competes with cell surface EPCR for protein C and prevents circulating APC from functioning as an anticoagulant.

ACQUIRED HYPERCOAGULABLE STATES

Acquired hypercoagulable states include antiphospholipid antibody syndrome and cancer, as well as pregnancy and estrogen therapy (oral contraception or hormone replacement therapy). These disorders can occur in isolation or can be superimposed on hereditary hypercoagulable states. Heparin-induced thrombocytopenia is an immune-mediated adverse drug reaction, and is a strong, independent risk factor for arterial and venous thrombosis.

Lupus Anticoagulants and the Antiphospholipid Syndrome

First described in a study by Wasserman and colleagues in 1906 among patients with positive serologic tests for syphilis, antiphospholipid antibodies are a heterogeneous group of autoantibodies directed against proteins that bind phospholipid. Antibodies can be categorized into those that prolong phospholipid-dependent coagulation assays, known as the lupus anticoagulant (LA), or anticardiolipin antibodies (ACLs), which target cardiolipin. A subset of ACL recognizes other phospholipid-bound proteins, particularly β$_2$-glycoprotein I.

Patients who have thrombosis in association with an LA and/or ACL (antibodies of the immunoglobulin [Ig]G or IgM subclass directed against cardiolipin or β$_2$-glycoprotein 1) are diagnosed with antiphospholipid syndrome (APS). The criteria for diagnosis of APS were updated in 2006.[11] APS is considered primary when it occurs in isolation and secondary when it is associated with autoimmune disorders, such as systemic lupus erythematosus or other connective tissue diseases. Clinical manifestations of APS include one or more episode of thrombosis, one or more unexplained fetal deaths at 10 or more weeks of gestation, or three or more first-trimester miscarriages (less than 10 weeks of gestation). Placental thrombosis is hypothesized to be the root cause of the pregnancy-related complications that characterize APS. Intrauterine growth retardation, preeclampsia, and eclampsia have also been associated with APS. APS can also occur with cancer, with some infections, and with drugs, such as phenothiazines, phenytoin, hydralazine, or amoxicillin. Thrombosis in APS patients can be arterial, venous, or placental.

To make the diagnosis of APS, at least one clinical criterion and one laboratory criterion must be met. Laboratory diagnosis of APS requires the presence of LA or ACL on tests taken at least 6 to 12 weeks apart. Tests for LA are well standardized, and a LA is associated with a higher risk of thrombosis than ACL. In contrast, there is considerable variability among laboratory results of ACL tests reflecting, at least in part, different methods and lack of consensus on what constitutes a negative or positive test.[12]

The LA is detected using phospholipid-dependent clotting tests. Most screening assays are based on the aPTT. aPTT reagents differ in their sensitivity for detection of LA, and many laboratories have adopted less-sensitive aPTT reagents for routine aPTT testing. LA is suspected when the aPTT is prolonged. To explore the cause of the prolonged aPTT, patient plasma is mixed with normal plasma and the aPTT is again determined (see Chapter 129). If the aPTT remains prolonged, an LA is suspected. The diagnosis is confirmed by demonstrating that addition of excess hexagonal-phase phospholipid normalizes the aPTT, thereby documenting the phospholipid dependence of the abnormal test result.[13] In addition to the aPTT, a battery of phospholipid-dependent clotting tests is often used for diagnosis of LA. These include the dilute Russell viper venom time and kaolin clotting time.

ACL antibodies are detected using immunoassays. Only ACL of medium to high titer and of the IgG or IgM subclass are associated with thrombosis, and the risk is higher with antibodies against β_2 glycoprotein-1 than against cardiolipin. For ACL, the amount of IgG or IgM antibody binding to cardiolipin-coated platelets is expressed in standardized GPL or MPL units, with 1 unit representing the cardiolipin-binding capacity of 1 µg/mL affinity-purified antiphospholipid antibody from reference sera. The extent of antibody binding is influenced by both the titer of the antibody and its affinity for cardiolipin.[14] Lack of standardization of ACL assays makes it difficult to compare results between laboratories.

ACL antibodies are found in 3% to 10% of healthy individuals. They also are common with certain infections (such as mycobacterial pneumonia, malaria, or parasitic disorders) and after exposure to some medications. Often, these antibodies are of low titer and are transient. ACL antibodies are detected in about 30% to 50% of patients with systemic lupus erythematosus. Of these, 10% to 20% also have an LA.

The mechanism by which antiphospholipid antibodies trigger thrombin generation is unclear. In cell cultures, these antibodies can directly activate endothelial cells and induce the expression of adhesion molecules that can tether tissue factor–bearing leukocytes or microparticles onto their surface. Tissue factor can then induce clotting in vitro.

Antiphospholipid antibodies also have been shown to (a) activate platelets, (b) interfere with the protein C pathway, (c) inhibit antithrombin catalysis by vessel wall heparan sulfate, (d) impair fibrinolysis, and (e) enhance transmigration of oxidized LDL into the vessel wall, thereby promoting atherothrombosis. Whether these mechanisms are operative in vivo has yet to be established.

In contrast to most hypercoagulable states, APS can be associated with spontaneous arterial thrombosis, as well as with venous thromboembolism. Arterial thrombosis can manifest as a stroke or transient ischemic attack. Thrombosis of the sagittal sinus or other cerebral veins, a form of venous thrombosis, can cause stroke in these patients.

Heparin-Induced Thrombocytopenia

A clinicopathologic syndrome, heparin-induced thrombocytopenia (HIT) is diagnosed on the basis of clinical features and laboratory detection of HIT antibodies[15] (see Chapter 133). The risk for HIT is higher with unfractionated heparin than with low-molecular-weight heparin (LMWH) and almost never occurs with fondaparinux. HIT is more common in surgical patients than in medical patients and occurs more frequently in women.

Typical clinical features of HIT include thrombocytopenia and thrombosis (arterial or venous). Less common features include necrotic skin lesions at the site of subcutaneous heparin injection, acute systemic reactions to heparin, and rarely, DIC.[16,17] Thrombocytopenia is the most common finding, occurring in 90% of patients. Typically, the platelet count falls 5 to 10 days after heparin is started.[18] However, thrombocytopenia can occur earlier if the patient has been exposed to heparin in the past 3 months. Rarely, the onset of HIT can be delayed and occurs several days after stopping heparin.

HIT is an autoimmune-like disorder and is caused by heparin-dependent, platelet-activating antibodies of the IgG subclass. These antibodies are directed against neoantigens that are exposed on platelet factor 4 (PF4) when it forms a complex with heparin. By binding to FcγII receptors on platelets, these antibodies trigger platelet activation. Activated platelets and platelet-derived microparticles provide an anionic phospholipid surface on which coagulation factors assemble and promote thrombin generation. This produces a hypercoagulable state and explains why 30% to 70% of HIT patients develop thrombosis.

The diagnosis of HIT is supported by assays that capitalize on the platelet-activating properties of HIT antibodies. Functional assays, such as the platelet serotonin release assay or heparin-induced platelet activation assay, detect antibody-induced platelet activation in the presence of heparin and are the gold standard for diagnosis of HIT. In contrast, although enzyme immunoassays for detection of antibodies against PF4/heparin complexes are more sensitive than functional assays, they are less specific because only a small subset of these antibodies has the capacity to produce HIT. Consequently a negative immunoassay is useful to exclude the diagnosis of HIT, but a positive test should be confirmed with a functional assay.

When the diagnosis of HIT is established, heparin must be stopped and an alternative anticoagulant should be given. Options include direct thrombin inhibitors (such as argatroban or bivalirudin) or factor Xa inhibitors (such as fondaparinux or danaparoid). Treatment with these agents should be continued until the platelet count returns to baseline levels at which point, low-dose warfarin can be initiated.

Cancer and Its Treatment

About 25% of patients who present with venous thromboembolism have cancer. Cancer patients who develop venous thromboembolism have reduced survival compared with those without this complication. Patients with brain tumors, pancreatic cancer, and advanced ovarian, lung, gastrointestinal tract, or prostate cancer have particularly high rates of venous thromboembolism.[19] Treatment with chemotherapy, hormonal therapy, and biologic agents, such as erythroid stimulating agents and antiangiogenic drugs, and surgery further increases the risk for venous thromboembolism. Additional risk factors include indwelling central venous catheters and major abdominal, pelvic, or orthopedic surgery.

The pathogenesis of thrombosis in cancer patients is multifactorial in origin and represents a complex interplay among the tumor, patient characteristics, and the host hemostatic system. Tumors can initiate coagulation by expressing tissue factor or cysteine proteases on their surface or by shedding tissue factor–bearing microparticles. In addition to its role in coagulation, tissue factor also acts as a cell-signaling molecule that promotes tumor proliferation and spread.

Patient factors that contribute to venous thromboembolism include immobility and venous stasis secondary to extrinsic compression of major veins by tumor. Surgical procedures, indwelling central venous catheters, and chemotherapy can produce vessel wall injury. In addition, tamoxifen, selective estrogen receptor modulators (SERM), L-asparaginase, and other drugs may induce an acquired hypercoagulable state by reducing the levels of natural anticoagulant proteins.

L-Asparaginase and combination chemotherapeutic regimens, such as breast cancer regimens of cyclophosphamide, methotrexate, and 5-fluorouracil increase the risk for thrombosis. The incidence of thromboembolic events in children receiving L-asparaginase for treatment of acute lymphocytic leukemia ranges from 1.1% to 36.7%, depending on whether or not catheter-related events are included. The mechanism likely involves decreased synthesis of antithrombin, protein C, and protein S, in addition to the retention of antithrombin within the endoplasmic reticulum. Concomitant administration of steroids increases the risk for thrombosis, and age seems to be an important risk factor; older children demonstrate a more marked decrease in anticoagulant and fibrinolytic proteins than younger children, as well as a slower recovery to normal.

Patients with multiple myeloma and other plasma cell dyscrasias are at increased risk for arterial and venous thrombosis. The reason for this is unclear, but may include acquired activated protein C resistance, elevated levels of factor VIII and/or von Willebrand factor, and the influence of the paraprotein on blood viscosity and fibrinolysis. Patients treated with thalidomide or lenalidomide are at high risk for venous thromboembolism, particularly when these drugs are given in combination with dexamethasone. Current guidelines recommend low-dose aspirin or LMWH thromboprophylaxis for patients receiving these agents.[20,21]

A proportion of patients who present with unprovoked venous thromboembolism have occult cancer. This observation has prompted some experts to recommend extensive screening for cancer in such patients. Benefits of this approach, however, are likely to be offset by potential harms. These include procedure-related morbidity, the psychological impact of false-positive tests and the cost of screening. Furthermore, early detection of cancer is only of benefit if there is potentially curative therapy. To date, only screening for breast, cervical, and possibly colon cancer has been shown to reduce mortality.

A careful history should be taken to identify any symptoms suggestive of underlying cancer. If such symptoms are present, further investigation is warranted. If there are no symptoms suggestive of underlying cancer, patients should be encouraged to undergo age-appropriate screening tests for breast, cervical, colon, or prostate cancer.

Myeloproliferative Disorders

The most common Philadelphia chromosome-negative (Ph-neg) myeloproliferative disorders, essential thrombocythemia (ET) and polycythemia vera (PV), are associated with an increased risk for thrombosis, especially arterial thrombosis, and venous thrombosis affecting the splanchnic vessels, including the hepatic and portal veins, which can lead to the Budd-Chiari syndrome, or the mesenteric veins.[20] Thrombosis involving the microcirculation is common in patients with ET, and patients may complain of erythromelalgia, characterized by burning pain, redness and swelling of the fingers and toes, transient visual defects, or recurrent headache. Although ET and PV may evolve to myelofibrosis or transform into acute myeloid leukemia, fatal cardiovascular events are a leading cause of mortality. The reported cumulative risk for thrombosis ranges from 2.5% to 5.0% per patient-year in PV and from 1.9% to 3% per patient-year in ET, depending on the patient risk category.[21] Age over 60 years and a previous history of thrombosis are risk factors for serious thrombosis, whereas usual cardiovascular risk factors, such as hypertension, diabetes, dyslipidemia and smoking, may place patients at intermediate risk.

The pathogenesis of thrombosis in patients with myeloproliferative disorders is multifactorial in origin and includes leukocytosis, leukocyte activation, rheologic abnormalities due to raised red cell mass in PV, enhanced platelet activation, and a prothrombotic endothelial phenotype.

An acquired point mutation in the Janus kinase 2 gene (JAK2 V617F) is found in up to 95% of patients with Ph-neg PV and in 50% to 60% of those with ET. The JAK2 gene encodes a cytoplasmic tyrosine kinase that is critical for signaling between type 1 cytokine receptors and intracellular proliferation mechanisms. Clinical observations, supported by laboratory studies, suggest an association between the JAK2 mutation and increased leukocyte and platelet activation, particularly in reticulated platelets, and there is a correlation between the burden of the mutant allele and thrombin generation. Acquired activated protein C resistance secondary to a reduction in free protein S levels has also been demonstrated in patients with ET and PV. Overall, there is little to support routine JAK2 screening unless splenomegaly or an elevated hemoglobin, white blood cell, and/or platelet count raises the possibility of an underlying myeloproliferative disorder. However, it may be justifiable to check for the JAK2 mutation in patients with unexplained splanchnic or mesenteric vein thrombosis, even in the absence of evidence of these findings.

Current management of PV and ET is aimed at prevention of major cardiovascular events and is based on the patient's risk category. Low-risk patients with PV are managed with phlebotomy, whereas high-risk patients are given cytoreductive therapy. Low-dose aspirin (70–100 mg daily) is recommended for all PV patients regardless of risk category, and such therapy is highly effective for treatment of the microcirculatory disturbances in patients with ET.

Paroxysmal Nocturnal Hemoglobinuria

A rare but serious disorder, paroxysmal nocturnal hemoglobinuria (PNH) is associated with intravascular hemolysis and cytopenia.[22] PNH is caused by the clonal expansion of a hematopoietic stem cell that has a somatic mutation in the X-linked PIG-A gene, which encodes cell surface proteins that serve as phosphatidylinositol anchors (see Chapter 31). Patients with PNH may have life-threatening thrombosis that can be difficult to recognize when it affects the splanchnic or cerebral veins. Severe persistent abdominal pain or headache in patients with PNH should prompt appropriate radiologic investigations to exclude thrombosis. Although patients with PNH who have documented thrombosis should be treated with anticoagulants, phlebotomy, cytoreductive therapy, and eculizumab are important adjunctive measures to reduce the risk for recurrence.

Pregnancy

Pregnancy is an independent risk factor for venous thromboembolism: the risk for venous thromboembolism in pregnant women is up to sixfold higher than that in age-matched nonpregnant women. About 1 in 1000 pregnancies are complicated by venous thromboembolism,[23] and the risk is highest in the postpartum period. Thus venous thromboembolic disease is the leading cause of maternal morbidity and mortality and is estimated to account for 12% of fatalities in pregnancy.

The individual risk for venous thromboembolism in pregnancy and the puerperium, defined as the 6-week period after delivery, is influenced by patient-related factors. These factors include age over 35 years, body mass index over 29, cesarean delivery, prolonged immobilization, obesity, and thrombophilia or family history of venous thromboembolism. Multiparity, ovarian hyperstimulation, and a past history or family history of venous thromboembolism are other risk factors.

Over 90% of deep vein thrombosis in pregnancy occurs in the left leg because the enlarged uterus further compresses the left iliac vein by placing pressure on the overlying right iliac and ovarian arteries. A similar mechanism likely explains the isolated left iliofemoral thrombosis that can occur in pregnancy.

Hypercoagulability of the blood occurs in pregnancy and reflects a combination of venous stasis and changes in the hemostatic system. The enlarging uterus reduces venous blood flow from the lower extremities. This is not the only mechanism responsible for venous stasis because blood flow from the lower extremities begins to decrease by the end of the first trimester, likely reflecting hormonally induced venous dilatation. Systemic factors also contribute to hypercoagulability. Thus the levels of circulating procoagulant proteins increase in the third trimester of pregnancy. These include factor VIII, fibrinogen, and von Willebrand factor, among others. Coincidentally, suppression of natural anticoagulant pathways and decreased fibrinolytic activity occur. Thus there is an acquired resistance to activated protein C that is related, at least in part, to reduced levels of free protein S. The net effect of these changes is enhanced thrombin generation, in addition to release of tissue factor from the uteroplacental circulation, as evidenced by elevated levels of prothrombin fragments and thrombin/antithrombin complexes. Platelet activation and increased platelet turnover occur, and mild thrombocytopenia, likely secondary to consumption, occurs in 8.3% of women at term. The altered levels of hemostatic proteins normalize 4 to 6 weeks after delivery.

About half of the episodes of venous thromboembolism in pregnancy occur in women with thrombophilia. The risk for venous thromboembolism in women with thrombophilic defects depends on the type of abnormality and the presence of other risk factors. The risk appears to be highest in women with a positive family history of venous thromboembolism who are homozygous for the factor V_{Leiden} or FIIG 20210A mutation. There is also an increased risk in women with antithrombin, protein C, or protein S deficiency and a positive family history and a lower risk in those who are heterozygous for the factor V_{Leiden} or FIIG 20210A mutation. The risk of venous thromboembolism during pregnancy is similar in all three trimesters and begins in early pregnancy. In general, the daily risk is higher in the postpartum period than it is during pregnancy. Therefore, if thromboprophylaxis is given during pregnancy, it must be administered throughout the pregnancy and continued for at least 6 weeks postpartum.

Assisted Conception and Ovarian Hyperstimulation Syndrome

The overall risk for venous thrombosis in women undergoing ovarian hyperstimulation is small (estimated as 0.1% per treatment cycle). Often, thrombosis affects veins of the upper extremities or the jugular veins; the explanation for this phenomenon remains unclear. Thrombophilia testing is not routinely recommended in women undergoing ovarian stimulation as its predictive value is low.

Hormonal Therapy

Oral contraceptives, estrogen replacement therapy, and SERM are all associated with an increased risk for thrombosis. The relatively high risk for venous thromboembolism associated with early oral contraceptives prompted development of low-dose formulations containing reduced doses of estrogen and progestin. Currently available low-estrogen combination oral contraceptives contain 20 to 50 µg of ethinylestradiol and one of several different progestogens. Even these low-dose combination contraceptives are associated with a three- to four-fold increased risk for venous thromboembolism compared with the risk in non-users. In absolute terms, this translates to an incidence of 3 to 4 per 10,000. In contrast, progesterone only methods of contraception, including pills, cutaneous implants and progesterone-releasing intrauterine devices, are associated with little or no risk of thrombosis.[24]

Although smoking increases the risk for myocardial infarction and stroke in women taking oral contraceptives, it is unclear whether smoking affects the risk for venous thromboembolism. In contrast, obesity increases the risk for both arterial and venous thrombosis and

the risk of venous thrombosis increases steeply in those over the age of 40 years. The risk for venous thromboembolism is highest during the first 3 months of oral contraceptive use and persists only for the duration of use.

Case-control studies suggest that the risk for venous thromboembolism is 20- to 30-fold higher in women with inherited thrombophilia who use oral contraceptives than the risk for non-users with thrombophilia or users without these defects. Despite the increased risk, however, routine screening for thrombophilia is not indicated in women considering the use of oral contraceptives. Based on the estimated incidence and case fatality rate of thrombotic events, it is estimated that 400,000 women would need to be screened to detect 20,000 carriers of factor V_{Leiden}. Oral contraceptives would need to be withheld in all of these women to prevent a single death. For less prevalent thrombophilic defects, even larger numbers of women would need to be screened. Based on these considerations, routine screening cannot be recommended.

Oral contraceptive pills may cause prothrombotic side effects by inducing modest increases in levels of procoagulant factors (such as factors VII, VIII, X, prothrombin, and fibrinogen) and decreases in the levels of anticoagulant proteins (such as antithrombin and protein S). Acquired APC resistance is an almost universal finding in women taking oral contraceptives; the clinical significance of this phenomenon is uncertain.

There is good evidence that oral hormonal replacement therapy with conjugated equine estrogen (with or without a progestogen) increases the risk for myocardial infarction, ischemic stroke, and venous thrombosis. Carriers of the factor V_{Leiden} mutation receiving hormone replacement therapy have a significantly increased risk for venous thromboembolism. Data from the Heart and Estrogen Replacement Study (HERS) and the Estrogen Replacement and Atherosclerosis Trial indicate that heterozygous carriers of the factor V_{Leiden} mutation who were taking hormone replacement therapy had a 14-fold higher risk for venous thromboembolism compared with non-carriers receiving placebo. Based on this information, the use of oral hormone replacement preparations has markedly decreased. Use of transdermal hormone replacement therapy does not appear to increase the risk of venous thrombosis.[25]

Selective estrogen receptor modulators (SERMs) are estrogen-like compounds. The prototypical SERM is tamoxifen, which serves as an estrogen antagonist in the breast, but has an estrogen agonist effect in other tissues, such as bone and uterus. Like estrogens, tamoxifen increases the risk for venous thromboembolism three- to four-fold. The risk is higher in postmenopausal women, particularly when they are receiving systemic combination chemotherapy.

Aromatase inhibitors are replacing tamoxifen for treatment of estrogen receptor–positive breast cancer. These agents are associated with a lower risk for venous thromboembolism than is tamoxifen. Raloxifene, a SERM used to prevent osteoporosis, increases the risk for venous thromboembolism threefold compared with placebo. Therefore this agent is contraindicated for prevention of osteoporosis in women with a prior history of venous thromboembolism.

Prior History of Venous Thromboembolism

A history of previous venous thromboembolism places patients at risk for recurrence. Those with unprovoked venous thromboembolism have a particularly high risk for recurrence when anticoagulant treatment is stopped.[26–28] Their risk for recurrence is about 10% at 1 year and 30% at 5 years. This risk occurs regardless of whether or not there is an underlying thrombophilic defect, such as factor V_{Leiden} or the FIIG 20210A mutation.

The risk for recurrent venous thromboembolism is lower in patients whose incident event occurred in association with a well-recognized and transient risk factor, such as major surgery or prolonged immobilization. These patients have a risk for recurrence of about 4% at 1 year and 10% at 5 years. Patients at highest risk for recurrence are those homozygous for factor V_{Leiden} or the FII G20210A mutation and those with antiphospholipid syndrome, advanced

Routine Investigations to Evaluate a Patient With Thrombosis		
Test	**Abnormality**	**Diagnostic Information**
Complete blood count	Elevated hematocrit Increased white count Increased platelet count Leukopenia Thrombocytopenia	Myeloproliferative disorder (e.g., essential thrombocythemia, polycythemia vera); may be found in paroxysmal nocturnal hemoglobinuria; if associated with heparin administration, consider heparin-induced thrombocytopenia
Blood film	Leukoerythroblastic changes	Underlying neoplasm invading bone marrow
Liver function tests	Abnormal tests	May point to malignancy
Renal function	Impaired renal function	Assess prior to anticoagulation with heparin or low-molecular-weight heparin or new oral anticoagulants
Urinalysis	Proteinuria	Nephrotic syndrome; may be associated with venous thromboembolism or renal vein thrombosis
PT and aPTT	Prolonged PT and aPTT	To enable safe anticoagulation to proceed if required Need to exclude lupus anticoagulant

aPTT, Activated partial thromboplastin time; PT, prothrombin time.

malignancy, or inherited deficiencies of antithrombin, protein C, or protein S. These patients' risk for recurrence is likely to be 15% at 1 year and up to 50% at 5 years.

COMBINED INHERITED AND ACQUIRED HYPERCOAGULABLE STATES

Hyperhomocysteinemia is the prototypical hypercoagulable state that occurs due to a combination of inherited and acquired factors. Homocysteine is an intermediate sulfur-containing amino acid that acts as a methyl group donor during the metabolism of methionine, an essential amino acid derived from the diet. The interconversion of methionine and homocysteine depends on the availability of 5-methyltetrahydrofolate, a methyl group donor, vitamin B_{12} and folate, cofactors in the interconversion, and the enzyme methionine synthase. Increased levels of homocysteine can be the result of increased production or reduced metabolism. Severe hyperhomocysteinemia and cysteinuria are rare and are usually caused by deficiency in the enzyme, cystathione β-synthetase. More common is mild to moderate hyperhomocysteinemia. This can be caused by genetic mutations in methyltetrahydrofolate reductase (MTHFR) when they are accompanied by nutritional deficiency of folate, vitamin B_{12}, or vitamin B_6. Common polymorphisms in MTHFR, C677T and A1298C, are associated with reduced enzymatic activity and increased thermolability. The cofactor requirements are therefore increased with these mutations. Hyperhomocysteinemia also can be associated with certain drugs, such as methotrexate, theophylline, cyclosporine, and most anticonvulsants, as well as some chronic diseases, such as end-stage renal disease, severe hepatic dysfunction, and hypothyroidism.

A fasting serum homocysteine level over 15 mmol/L is considered elevated. Although elevated levels were a common finding, routine fortification of flour with folic acid has resulted in lower homocysteine levels in the general population. Elevated serum levels of homocysteine have been associated with an increased risk for arterial thrombosis (myocardial infarction, stroke, and peripheral arterial disease) and venous thromboembolism.

Elevated levels of homocysteine can be reduced by administration of folate with vitamin B_{12} and vitamin B_6. Randomized trials, however, have shown that reduction of homocysteine levels with vitamin therapy does not reduce the risk for recurrent cardiovascular events in patients with coronary artery disease or stroke, nor does it lower the risk for recurrent venous thromboembolism; whether reduction of homocysteine levels is of benefit in peripheral artery disease with bypass grafts is less certain. Nonetheless, based on these negative trials and the declining incidence of hyperhomocysteinemia, the enthusiasm for screening for hyperhomocysteinemia has waned.

CLINICAL EVALUATION OF PATIENTS WITH HYPERCOAGULABLE STATES

A carefully taken history is essential to evaluate a patient with a history of thrombosis. The patient's age at the time of thrombosis, the location of the thrombosis, and results of objective diagnostic tests should be recorded. A historical record of previous thromboses and sites, and potential risk factors, such as recent surgery, trauma, prolonged immobility, pregnancy, or estrogen use should be noted. A family history of thrombosis, especially in first-degree relatives may point to a heritable thrombophilic defect; systemic symptoms, such as anorexia, weight loss, change in bowel habits, or gastrointestinal bleeding may suggest an underlying malignant condition.

A full physical examination should be conducted with attention to abdominal or pelvic masses, lymphadenopathy, and skin changes such as skin necrosis and livedo reticularis. Basic investigations are necessary to exclude acquired causes of thrombosis and to assess the patient's general health and tolerance to anticoagulation (see box on Routine Investigations to Evaluate a Patient With Thrombosis).

THROMBOPHILIA SCREENING

In the past, the indications for thrombophilia screening were somewhat controversial, and the implications of such tests were often misinterpreted. It is now apparent that testing for heritable thrombophilia does not predict the likelihood of recurrence in unselected patients with symptomatic venous thrombosis. For patients with a first episode of venous thromboembolism, thrombophilia screening is indicated only if the results influence the duration of treatment or have an impact on family counselling regarding use of estrogen-containing compounds. It is reasonable to screen patients whose first episode of thrombosis occurred before the age of 40 years, patients with thrombosis in an unusual site, such as cerebral or mesenteric veins, and those with two or more first-degree relatives with unprovoked thrombosis; retinal vein thrombosis is not an indication for such screening. Screening should not be done when patients are taking an anticoagulant. If indefinite anticoagulation therapy is planned, screening is generally not required. Neonates and children with purpura fulminans should be urgently tested for protein C or S deficiency, as should adults who develop skin necrosis in association with vitamin K antagonists (see box on When to Perform a Thrombophilia Screen).

LABORATORY EVALUATION OF THROMBOPHILIA

Screening should include functional assays for antithrombin and protein C, an immunoassay for free protein S, testing for activated protein C resistance using the modified APC sensitivity ratio with DNA testing for the factor V_{Leiden} mutation if the screening test is positive, DNA testing for the FIIG 20210A gene mutation, phospholipid-based clotting tests to detect a lupus anticoagulant and enzyme immunoassay for ACL (see box on Essential Tests for Thrombophilia Screening). The benefits and potential harms of thrombophilia testing should always be discussed in advance with the patient because the psychological impact of knowing that they are a carrier of a genetic defect is one of the disadvantages of testing, and because test results may also impact on the cost of life insurance.

The timing of thrombophilia screening is critical. Levels of natural anticoagulants may be lower at the time of an acute thrombotic event; additionally, heparin can reduce the level of antithrombin, while vitamin K antagonists, such as warfarin, reduce the levels of protein C and protein S. Therefore testing is best performed after the acute event and when anticoagulant treatment has stopped. During pregnancy, protein S levels fall, which complicates the diagnosis of protein S deficiency.

MANAGEMENT OF THROMBOSIS IN PATIENTS WITH HYPERCOAGULABLE STATES

Thrombosis treatment is usually divided into two overlapping stages, initial treatment and extended therapy. The impact of hypercoagulable states on these two stages is discussed separately as is their impact on duration of anticoagulant therapy and recommendations for prevention of recurrence.

Initial Treatment

With few exceptions, management of initial thrombotic events in patients with hypercoagulable states is no different from the management of these events in patients without underlying hypercoagulable disorders. The exceptions are purpura fulminans in newborns with homozygous protein C or protein S deficiency, warfarin-induced skin necrosis, heparin-induced thrombocytopenia and thrombosis in patients with severe antithrombin deficiency. Newborns with purpura fulminans require protein C or protein S concentrates or sufficient amounts of plasma to increase the levels of protein C or protein S.

Patients with severe antithrombin deficiency can usually be managed with LMWH or unfractionated heparin, although some patients may require considerably higher doses to achieve therapeutic anticoagulation. Some individuals may require antithrombin concentrates to increase plasma levels of antithrombin to a point where heparin or LMWH can be used for treatment. Antithrombin concentrates are commercially available in plasma-derived and recombinant forms. The aim of treatment with antithrombin concentrate is to initially increase antithrombin activity to greater than 120% of the normal level (based on an expected 1.4% increase above baseline activity level per IU/kg of antithrombin administered) and to then maintain antithrombin activity at over 80% of the normal level. Plasma antithrombin levels need to be monitored to ensure that levels over 80% are maintained; antithrombin has a half-life of 2 to 4 days. The role of the non–vitamin K antagonist oral anticoagulants, such as dabigatran, rivaroxaban, apixaban, or edoxaban, in patients with antithrombin deficiency and thrombosis is uncertain.

Treatment of heparin-induced thrombocytopenia involves discontinuation of heparin (including heparin flushes of indwelling central venous catheters) and the initiation of an alternative anticoagulant, such as argatroban or fondaparinux.

The management of acute venous thromboembolism in patients with APS is similar to that in other patients. However, monitoring treatment with heparin or vitamin K antagonists can be problematic because the aPTT or INR may be prolonged at baseline. Under these circumstances, heparin can be monitored using an antifactor Xa assay and warfarin can be monitored using a factor X assay. Alternatively, LMWH or fondaparinux can be used in place of heparin because these agents do not require coagulation monitoring. Although the non–vitamin K antagonist oral anticoagulants may be reasonable alternatives to warfarin, clinical data on their effectiveness in APS patients are lacking. In asymptomatic subjects with laboratory evidence of ACL or LA, but no history of venous or arterial thrombosis, appropriate thromboprophylaxis should be given at time of thrombotic challenge, such as major surgical procedures, prolonged immobilization, or pregnancy and the puerperium. There is no indication for primary preventive treatment with anticoagulants or antiplatelet agents in such individuals.

Extended Therapy

Extended treatment of thrombosis in patients with hypercoagulable states is similar to that of patients without these underlying disorders. Caution is needed when starting patients with protein C or protein S deficiency on warfarin or other vitamin K antagonists to prevent skin necrosis. Warfarin should not be started in these patients until therapeutic anticoagulation has been fully achieved with heparin or LMWH. Once started, low doses of warfarin should be given to prevent precipitous decreases in the levels of protein C or protein S; the heparin or LMWH should only be stopped when the INR has been therapeutic for at least two consecutive days.

Randomized trials have shown that usual-intensity warfarin (target INR of 2.0 to 3.0) is as effective as higher-intensity warfarin in patients with antiphospholipid syndrome. The risk for major bleeding is lower with usual-intensity warfarin than it is with higher-intensity regimens. A target INR of 2.5 with an INR range from 2.0 to 3.0 is appropriate for patients with other hypercoagulable states.

Patients with thrombosis who have a history of metastatic cancer may do better with extended treatment with LMWH. Randomized clinical trials have shown that, compared with warfarin, LMWH reduces the risk for recurrent venous thromboembolism without increasing bleeding.[29] Furthermore, LMWH simplifies treatment because it can be given subcutaneously once-daily without coagulation monitoring. The drug can be held before invasive procedures, and the dose may be reduced if thrombocytopenia is present. The major drawbacks of LMWH are cost and its requirement for

TABLE 140.6	Management of Women With a History of Venous Thrombosis During Pregnancy and the Puerperium			
Clinical History	**Thrombophilia**		**Antepartum**	**Postpartum**[a]
Prior VTE due to a transient risk factor	No		Surveillance	Yes
Prior VTE due to pregnancy or estrogens	Yes or no		Prophylactic LMWH	Yes
Prior idiopathic VTE	Yes or no		Prophylactic LMWH	Yes
Recurrent VTE	Yes or no		Treatment dose LMWH	Resume long-term anticoagulation
No prior VTE Positive family history	Antithrombin deficiency; homozygous FII G20210A; or Factor V_{Leiden}; or dual heterozygosity for both mutations		Prophylactic or intermediate dose LMWH	Yes

[a]Postpartum prophylaxis involves a 6-week course of prophylactic doses of LMWH or dose-adjusted warfarin (target INR: 2.0 to 3.0).
LMWH, low-molecular-weight heparin; VTE, venous thromboembolism.

parenteral administration, although the drug has been shown to be cost-effective in patients at high risk for recurrent venous thromboembolism.

Duration of Treatment

The presence of a hypercoagulable state has no influence on the duration of anticoagulant treatment in patients whose venous thromboembolic event occurred in the setting of a well-recognized and transient risk factor, such as major surgery or prolonged immobilization due to medical illness. These patients are treated with anticoagulants for at least 3 months. For those with unprovoked venous thromboembolism, a minimum of 3 months of anticoagulation treatment is recommended at which point individualized assessment of the risk of recurrence without anticoagulation and the risk of bleeding with anticoagulation should be undertaken. Unless the risk of bleeding is high, most patients should receive extended anticoagulation therapy. Heterozygosity for factor V_{Leiden} or the FIIG20210A mutation does not influence the risk for recurrence. In contrast, patients with deficiency of antithrombin, protein C, or protein S or those homozygous for factor V_{Leiden} or the FII G20210A mutation appear to be at higher risk for recurrence and likely should receive longer-term anticoagulation treatment. Likewise, patients with APS with a persistent ACL or LA are also at high risk for recurrence and require long-term treatment.

The decision to continue anticoagulation indefinitely requires consideration of the site and severity of the first episode of venous thromboembolism, information on whether or not the event was provoked, assessment of the risk for anticoagulant-related bleeding and other risk factors such as an elevated D-dimer level after stopping anticoagulant therapy.[25] The decision should also take into account patient adherence and patient preferences.

Treatment and Prevention of Thrombosis During Pregnancy

Thrombophilic disorders have no influence on the treatment of venous thrombosis during pregnancy. Due to its better bioavailability and longer half-life, LMWH is preferred over subcutaneous heparin; fondaparinux is reserved for women with an allergy to heparin. LMWH can be given once or twice daily in a weight-adjusted fashion. The need for dose adjustments and monitoring during the course of pregnancy remains controversial. The non–vitamin K antagonist oral anticoagulants should not be used in pregnancy or in nursing mothers because these drugs have the potential to cross the placenta and it is unknown whether they pass into breast milk.

After delivery, LMWH or warfarin should be given for at least 6 weeks. No studies have addressed the optimal duration of

anticoagulation for pregnancy-related venous thrombosis. In total, treatment should be given for 3 to 6 months from the time of diagnosis. Warfarin and LMWH can be safely administered in nursing mothers, with no detectable anticoagulant effect in breast milk.

Women with a past history of unprovoked or recurrent venous thromboembolism, those homozygous for factor V_{Leiden} or the FII G20210A mutation, and those with deficiencies of antithrombin, protein C, or protein S and a family history of venous thrombosis, should receive antepartum prophylaxis with LMWH. Postpartum, LMWH or warfarin should be given for 6 weeks. Postpartum treatment with LMWH or warfarin for 6 weeks is likely adequate for women with a history of venous thrombosis secondary to a well-defined risk factor. Prophylaxis during pregnancy, as well as postpartum, should be considered for women who developed venous thromboembolism after taking oral contraceptives particularly if they have underlying thrombophilia. Women with thrombophilic defects, but no prior history of venous thromboembolism, or family history of the same likely do not require antepartum prophylaxis or postpartum treatment, but definitive data are lacking. A summary of these recommendations is provided in Table 140.6.[30]

Thrombophilia and Fetal Loss

About 30% of women have at least one fetal loss, and approximately 5% of women of reproductive age experience recurrent fetal loss. Women with hereditary or acquired thrombophilia have a two- to five-fold increased risk for fetal loss. Screening for APS is recommended if there is a history of three or more miscarriages before 10 weeks' gestation. Although once-daily LMWH in prophylactic doses, with or without aspirin, is often prescribed for women with recurrent fetal loss on the background of an underlying thrombophilic defect, such therapy is of no benefit and it is costly and potentially harmful.

CONCLUSIONS AND FUTURE DIRECTIONS

Inherited or acquired hypercoagulable states can now be identified in up to 50% of patients with venous thromboembolism thanks to an increased understanding of the regulation of coagulation. The role of these disorders in the pathogenesis of arterial thrombosis is less clear, and further research is necessary to identify those individuals vulnerable to arterial thrombosis after plaque rupture. Despite an improved ability to diagnose hypercoagulable states, the impact of this information on clinical decisions remains limited. Common congenital hypercoagulable states increase the risk for a first thrombotic episode but appear to have little impact on the risk for recurrence. Identification of biomarkers for patients at risk for recurrent thrombosis and elucidating new hypercoagulable states are goals for the future.

REFERENCES

1. Vossen CY, Conard J, Fontcuberta J, et al: Risk of a first venous thrombotic event in carriers of a familial thrombophilic defect. The European Prospective Cohort on Thrombophilia (EPCOT). *J Thromb Haemost* 3:459, 2005.

2. Rossi E, Ciminello A, Za T, et al: In families with inherited thrombophilia the risk of venous thromboembolism is dependent on the clinical phenotype of the proband. *Thromb Haemost* 106(4):646–654, 2011.

3. Vossen CY, Walker ID, Svensson P, et al: Recurrence rate after a first venous thrombosis in patients with familial thrombophilia. *Arterioscler Thromb Vasc Biol* 25(9):1992–1997, 2005.

4. Di Minno MN, Dentali F, Lupoli R, et al: Mild antithrombin deficiency and risk of recurrent venous thromboembolism: a prospective cohort study. *Circulation* 129(4):497–503, 2014.

5. Lijfering WM, Brouwer JL, Veeger NJ, et al: Selective testing for thrombophilia in patients with first venous thrombosis: results from a retrospective family cohort study on absolute thrombotic risk for currently known thrombophilic defects in 2479 relatives. *Blood* 113(21):5314–5322, 2009.

6. Franchi F, Biguzzi E, Martinelli I, et al: Normal reference ranges of antithrombin, protein C and protein S: effect of sex, age and hormonal status. *Thromb Res* 132(2):e152–e157, 2013.

7. Pintao MC, Ribeiro DD, Bezemer ID, et al: Protein S levels and the risk of venous thrombosis: results from the MEGA case-control study. *Blood* 122(18):3210–3219, 2013.

8. Vossen CY, Conard J, Fontcuberta J, et al: Familial thrombophilia and lifetime risk of venous thrombosis. *J Thromb Haemost* 2(9):1526–1532, 2004.

9. Lijfering WM, Middeldorp S, Veeger NJ, et al: Risk of recurrent venous thrombosis in homozygous carriers and double heterozygous carriers of factor V Leiden and prothrombin G20210A. *Circulation* 121(15):1706–1712, 2010.

10. van der Meer FJ, Koster T, Vandebroucke JP, et al: The Leiden Thrombophilia Study (LETS). *Thromb Haemost* 78:631, 1997.

11. Miyakis S, Lockshin MD, Atsumi T, et al: International consensus statement on an update of the classification criteria for definite antiphospholipid syndrome (APS). *J Thromb Haemost* 4:295, 2006.

12. Favaloro EJ, Wong RCW: Antiphospholipid antibody testing for the antiphospholipid syndrome: a comprehensive practical review including a synopsis of challenges and recent guidelines. *Pathology* 46(6):481–495, 2014.

13. Pengo V, Tripodi A, Reber G, et al: Update of the guidelines for lupus anticoagulant detection. Subcommittee on Lupus Anticoagulant/Antiphospholipid Antibody of the Scientific and Standardisation Committee of the International Society on Thrombosis and Haemostasis. *J Thromb Haemost* 7(10):1737–1740, 2009.

14. Devreese KM, Pierangeli SS, de Laat B, et al: Testing for antiphospholipid antibodies with solid phase assays: guidance from the SSC of the ISTH. *J Thromb Haemost* 12(5):792–795, 2014.

15. Lo GK, Juhl D, Warkentin TE, et al: Evaluation of pretest clinical score (4 T's) for the diagnosis of heparin-induced thrombocytopenia in two clinical settings. *J Thromb Haemost* 4(4):759–765, 2006.

16. Warkentin TE: Heparin-induced thrombocytopenia. In Marder VJ, Aird WC, Bennett SC, et al, editors: *Hemostasis and thrombosis: basic principles and practice*, ed 6, Chapter 108. Philadelphia, 2012, Lippincott Williams, and Wilkins.

17. Warkentin TE: Heparin-induced thrombocytopenia: pathogenesis and management. *Br J Haematol* 121:535, 2003.

18. Cuker A: Clinical and laboratory diagnosis of heparin-induced thrombocytopenia: an integrated approach. *Semin Thromb Hemost* 40(1):106–114, 2014.

19. Lee AYY: Management of thrombosis in cancer: primary prevention and secondary prophylaxis. *Br J Haematol* 128:291, 2006.

20. Zamagni E, Brioli A, Tacchetti P, et al: Multiple myeloma, venous thromboembolism, and treatment-related risk of thrombosis. *Semin Thromb Hemost* 37:209, 2011.

21. Carrier M, Le Gal G, Lee AYY: Rates of venous thromboembolism in multiple myeloma patients undergoing immunomodulatory therapy with thalidomide or lenalidomide; a systematic review and meta-analysis. *J Thromb Haemost* 9:653, 2011.

22. Luzzatto L, Gianfaldoni G, Notaro R: Management of paroxysmal nocturnal haemoglobinuria: a personal view. *Br J Haematol* 153:709, 2011.

23. James AH, Jamison MG, Brancazio LR, et al: Venous thromboembolism during pregnancy and the postpartum period: incidence, risk factors, and mortality. *Am J Obstet Gynecol* 194:1311, 2006.

24. Middeldorp S: Thrombosis in women: what are the knowledge gaps in 2013? *J Thromb Haemost* (11 Suppl 1):180–191, 2013.

25. Canonico M, Plu-Bureau G, Lowe GDO, et al: Hormone replacement therapy and risk of venous thromboembolism in postmenopausal women: systematic review and meta-analysis. *BMJ* 336(7655):1227–1231, 2008.

26. Kearon C, Spencer FA, O'Keeffe D, et al: D-dimer testing to select patients with a first unprovoked venous thromboembolism who can stop anticoagulant therapy: a cohort study. *Ann Intern Med* 162(1):27–34, 2015.

27. van der Hulle T, Tan M, den Exter PL, et al: Recurrence risk after anticoagulant treatment of limited duration for late, second venous thromboembolism. *Haematologica* 100(2):188–193, 2015.

28. Rodger MA, Kahn SR, Wells PS, et al: Identifying unprovoked thromboembolism patients at low risk for recurrence who can discontinue anticoagulant therapy. *CMAJ* 179(5):417–426, 2008.

29. Lee AYY, Levine MN, Baker RI, et al: Low-molecular-weight heparin versus a coumarin for the prevention of recurrent venous thromboembolism in patients with cancer. *N Engl J Med* 349:146, 2003.

30. Bates SM, Greer IA, Middeldorp S, et al: VTE, thrombophilia, antithrombotic therapy, and pregnancy: antithrombotic therapy and prevention of thrombosis, 9th ed: American college of chest physicians evidence-based clinical practice guidelines. *Chest* 141(2 Suppl):e691S–e736S, 2012.

CHAPTER 141

THE ANTIPHOSPHOLIPID SYNDROME

Jacob H. Rand and Lucia R. Wolgast

The antiphospholipid (aPL) syndrome (APS) is an autoimmune thrombophilic condition that is defined by a combination of clinical and laboratory criteria. This chapter reviews the current understanding of aPL-mediated pathogenic mechanisms, diagnostic tests for the condition, its clinical manifestations, and current treatment approaches.

DEFINITION OF ANTIPHOSPHOLIPID SYNDROME

APS is an autoimmune thrombophilic condition in which patients have circulating antibodies against plasma proteins that bind to phospholipids. The precise mechanism(s) by which these autoantibodies cause disease has (have) not yet been precisely established. Investigational diagnostic criteria (referred to as the Sydney Criteria), detailed in Table 141.1, have been formulated to provide consistency for clinical trials. These require that patients have documented evidence of vascular thrombosis and/or obstetric complications attributable to placental vascular insufficiency; the latter include otherwise unexplained recurrent miscarriages, intrauterine growth restriction, intrauterine fetal demise, preeclampsia/toxemia, placental abruption, and preterm labor. The laboratory criteria require persistent abnormality (defined as at least two abnormal measurements at least 12 weeks apart) of one or more of the aPL assays, which include elevated anticardiolipin (aCL) immunoglobulin (Ig) G or IgM, antibodies, anti–β_2-glycoprotein I (anti-β_2GPI) IgG or IgM antibodies or an abnormal lupus anticoagulant (LA).

Because these criteria were intended to provide a uniformly rigorous definition of APS for standardizing clinical research and not for the diagnosis of APS in "real world" clinical practice settings, some patients may be diagnosed clinically with presumptive APS without meeting the strict investigational criteria. For example, some patients with APS have positive results on "noncriteria" clinical laboratory tests (described later) that have not been included by consensus panels as diagnostic criteria for the disorder. Also, some patients present with manifestations that have been associated with aPL antibodies that were not included in the investigational criteria. These "noncriteria manifestations" include thrombocytopenia, livedo reticularis, skin ulcers, nephropathy, migraine, cognitive defects, diffuse alveolar hemorrhage, and valvular heart disease (Libman-Sachs endocarditis).

At the present time, APS may be divided into the following subcategories: (1) Primary APS is the "stand alone" disorder, in the absence of systemic lupus erythematosus (SLE), (2) secondary APS occurs in the presence of SLE, (3) catastrophic APS (CAPS), manifests as disseminated thrombosis in large and small vessels with resulting multiorgan failure (Table 141.2), and (4) SNAPS includes patients whose diagnostic tests are entirely negative but who, on clinical grounds, are still suspected to have the disorder.

ANTIGENIC SPECIFICITIES OF ANTIPHOSPHOLIPID ANTIBODIES

β_2-Glycoprotein I

β_2-Glycoprotein I (β_2GPI), a 50-kDa glycoprotein member of the complement control protein (CCP) superfamily, is a major antigenic target for aPL antibodies. The protein consists of five homologous CCP domains, each consisting of about 60 amino acids, with a fifth domain that includes a phospholipid binding site near the carboxy-terminus of the protein. Binding of β_2GPI to membranes that express anionic phospholipids occurs via the affinity of cationic residues near the carboxy-terminus for anionic polar heads of phospholipids that adjoin a hydrophobic loop that inserts into the lipid bilayer. Although patients with APS have been described to have antibodies that recognize all of the five domains of β_2GPI, IgG antibodies against an epitope on domain I comprising Gly40-Arg43 has been particularly correlated with an increased risk for thrombosis; this domain I epitope is cryptic in the circulating protein and becomes exposed after β_2GPI binds to phospholipid bilayers. The specific conformation of the unbound form of β_2GPI is not entirely clear; transmission electron microscopy of negatively stained β_2GPI molecules indicates that the unbound protein has a circular conformation that was attributed to the affinity of its carboxy-terminus domain (domain V) for the protein's amino-terminus domain, whereas β_2GPI bound to phospholipid has a "J-shaped" conformation with the binding site for phospholipid near the carboxy-terminus of the J. On the other hand, small angle x-ray scattering studies indicate an "S" shape configuration for the free form (Fig. 141.1).

Other Antigenic Targets of Antiphospholipid Antibodies

Besides β_2GPI, prothrombin (factor II), factor V, protein C, protein S, annexin A2, annexin A5, high- and low-molecular-weight kininogen, heparin, factor VII/VIIa, plasmin, vimentin, and other proteins have been identified as targets for autoantibodies in APS patients. Antibodies have also been found to bind to sulfatides, acidic glycosphingolipids that can interact with sulfatide-binding proteins such as von Willebrand factor, thrombospondin, and P-selectin.

PATHOGENIC EFFECTS OF ANTIPHOSPHOLIPID ANTIBODIES

As described later, numerous mechanisms have been proposed to explain the thrombotic manifestations of APS (Table 141.3). Although all of these are based on in vitro findings or on animal models, their in vivo significance in the human disease process remain to be established.

Antiphospholipid-Mediated Promotion of Tissue Factor Expression

aPL antibodies can bind to, injure, and/or activate cultured vascular endothelial cells. Antibody binding to β_2GPI on the endothelial surface may trigger signaling cascades that promote the expression of tissue factor and adhesion molecules. There is evidence that annexin A2, which forms tetramers with S100 and is an endothelial surface receptor for tissue plasminogen activator and plasminogen, serves as a receptor for β_2GPI on vascular endothelium. Annexin A2 and the signaling coreceptors, Toll-like receptor-4 (TLR4) and Toll-like receptor-2 (TLR2) have been implicated as triggers of the signaling cascade. Downstream signaling appears to involves TRAF6 (tumor necrosis factor receptor–associated factor 6) and MyD88 (myeloid differentiation factor 88). Tissue factor expression is mediated by p38

TABLE 141.1	Sydney Investigational Criteria for the Diagnosis of the Antiphospholipid Syndrome[a]

Clinical

- Vascular thrombosis (one or more episodes of arterial, venous, or small-vessel thrombosis). For histopathologic diagnosis, there should be no evidence of inflammation in the vessel wall.
- Pregnancy morbidities attributable to placental insufficiency, including: (a) three or more otherwise unexplained recurrent spontaneous miscarriages, before 10 weeks of gestation, (b) one or more fetal losses after the 10th week of gestation, (c) stillbirth, and (d) episode of preeclampsia, preterm labor, placental abruption, intrauterine growth restriction, or oligohydramnios that are otherwise unexplained.

Laboratory

- Medium- or high-titer aCL or anti-β_2GPI IgG and/or IgM antibody present on two or more occasions, at least 12 weeks apart, measured by standard ELISA.
- Lupus anticoagulant in plasma, on two or more occasions, at least 12 weeks apart, detected according to the guidelines of the ISTH SSC Subcommittee on Lupus Anticoagulants and Phospholipid-Dependent Antibodies.

"Definite APS" is considered to be present if at least one of the clinical criteria and one of the laboratory criteria are met.

aCL, Anticardiolipin; aPL, antiphospholipid; β_2GPI, β_2-glycoprotein I; ELISA, enzyme-linked immunosorbent assay; Ig, immunoglobulin.
[a]Modified from Miyakis et al: International consensus statement on an update of the classification criteria for definite antiphospholipid syndrome (APS). *Thromb Haemost* 4:295, 2006.

TABLE 141.2	Proposed Criteria for the Classification of Catastrophic Antiphospholipid Syndrome*

1. Evidence of involvement of three or more organs, systems and/or tissues[a]
2. Development of manifestations simultaneously or in less than a week
3. Confirmation by histopathology of small vessel occlusion in at least one organ or tissue[b]
4. Laboratory confirmation of the presence of antiphospholipid antibodies (lupus anticoagulant and/or anticardiolipin antibodies)[c]

Definite catastrophic APS

- All four criteria

Probable catastrophic APS

- All four criteria, except for only two organs, systems and/or tissues involvement
- All four criteria, except for the absence of laboratory confirmation at least 6 weeks apart because of the early death of a patient never previously tested for aPL prior to the catastrophic APS event
- Criteria 1, 2, and 4
- Criteria 1, 3, and 4 and the development of a third event in more than a week but less than a month, despite anticoagulation

[a]Usually, clinical evidence of vessel occlusions, confirmed by imaging techniques when appropriate. Renal involvement is defined by a 50% rise in serum creatinine, severe systemic hypertension ($\geq$180/100 mmHg) and/or proteinuria ($\geq$500 mg/24 h).
[b]For histopathologic confirmation, significant evidence of thrombosis must be present, although, in contrast with Sydney criteria, vasculitis may coexist occasionally.
[c]If the patient had not been previously diagnosed as having an APS, the laboratory confirmation requires that the presence of antiphospholipid antibodies must be detected on two or more occasions at least 6 weeks apart (not necessarily at the time of the event), according to the proposed preliminary criteria for the classification of definite APS.
aPL, Antiphospholipid; APS, antiphospholipid syndrome.
*Modified from Asherson RA, Cevera R, de Groot PG et al. Catastrophic antiphospholipid syndrome: international consensus statement on classification criteria and treatment guidelines. *Lupus* 12:530, 2003.

mitogen-activated protein kinase (MAPK). This mechanism is supported by the finding that a mutation in murine TLR-4 that disrupts LPS binding, attenuated the prothrombotic state in mice injected with aPL antibodies.

Apolipoprotein E receptor 2' (apoER2'), a member of the low-density lipoprotein (LDL)–receptor family and a multiligand receptor with a wide tissue distribution may also be a target for anti-β_2GPI/β_2GPI complexes to trigger tissue factor and cell adhesion molecule expression on the endothelial surface. ApoER2' is expressed on endothelial cells, platelets, and monocytes where it has been proposed to mediate the pathogenic effects of the antibodies. Evidence from apoER2'$^{-/-}$ knockout mice supports such a role and identifies this interaction as a potential target for novel nonanticoagulant therapy.

There is evidence from a mouse model that aPL-mediated promotion of tissue factor expression can induce trophoblast injury and fetal death. In addition, tissue factor contributed to C5a-induced oxidative burst in neutrophils leading to trophoblast and fetal injury in APS. A monoclonal antibody against factor B, that disrupted the alternative pathway of complement activation, protected against aPL antibody-induced fetal loss in mice.

Activation of Platelets and Monocytes by Antiphospholipid Antibodies

Recent evidence from a mouse model indicated that aPL-induced thrombosis is a consequence of platelet activation that then promotes endothelial activation and fibrin formation. aPL antibodies can also induce platelet aggregation, an effect that might be promoted via signaling through apoER2; the β_2GPI binding site for apoER2 on platelets was localized to its domain V. β_2GPI also has a dampening effect on platelet adhesion by interfering with the platelet–von Willebrand factor interaction, and consequently aPL antibodies, by interfering with this dampening, can increase platelet adhesion in flow systems.

aPL antibodies increased the expression of tissue factor and other cytokines in monocytes, a process that occurred through activation of the p38MAPK and MEK-1/ERK pathways. Enhanced monocyte expression of tissue factor resulted in increased expression of vascular endothelial growth factor (VEGF) and Flt-1 tyrosine kinase receptor. aPL antibodies may also promote mitochondrial dysfunction and oxidative stress in monocytes resulting in a proinflammatory state.

Inhibition of Endogenous Anticoagulant and Fibrinolytic Mechanisms

aPL antibodies can accelerate coagulation reactions on endothelial cells and trophoblasts by disrupting an antithrombotic shield composed of annexin A5, a potent anticoagulant protein with high affinity for phospholipid membranes. The protein forms two-dimensional crystalline arrays over the phospholipid bilayers (Fig. 141.2) that shield the anionic phospholipids on cell membranes from availability for phospholipid-dependent coagulation enzyme reactions. Annexin A5 is highly expressed by endothelial cells and on the apical membranes of placental syncytiotrophoblasts, the location where maternal blood interfaces with fetal cells. Pregnant mice treated with anti-annexin A5 antibodies develop placental necrosis, fibrosis, and pregnancy loss and pregnant annexin A5-null mice develop placental infarctions and have reduced litter sizes.

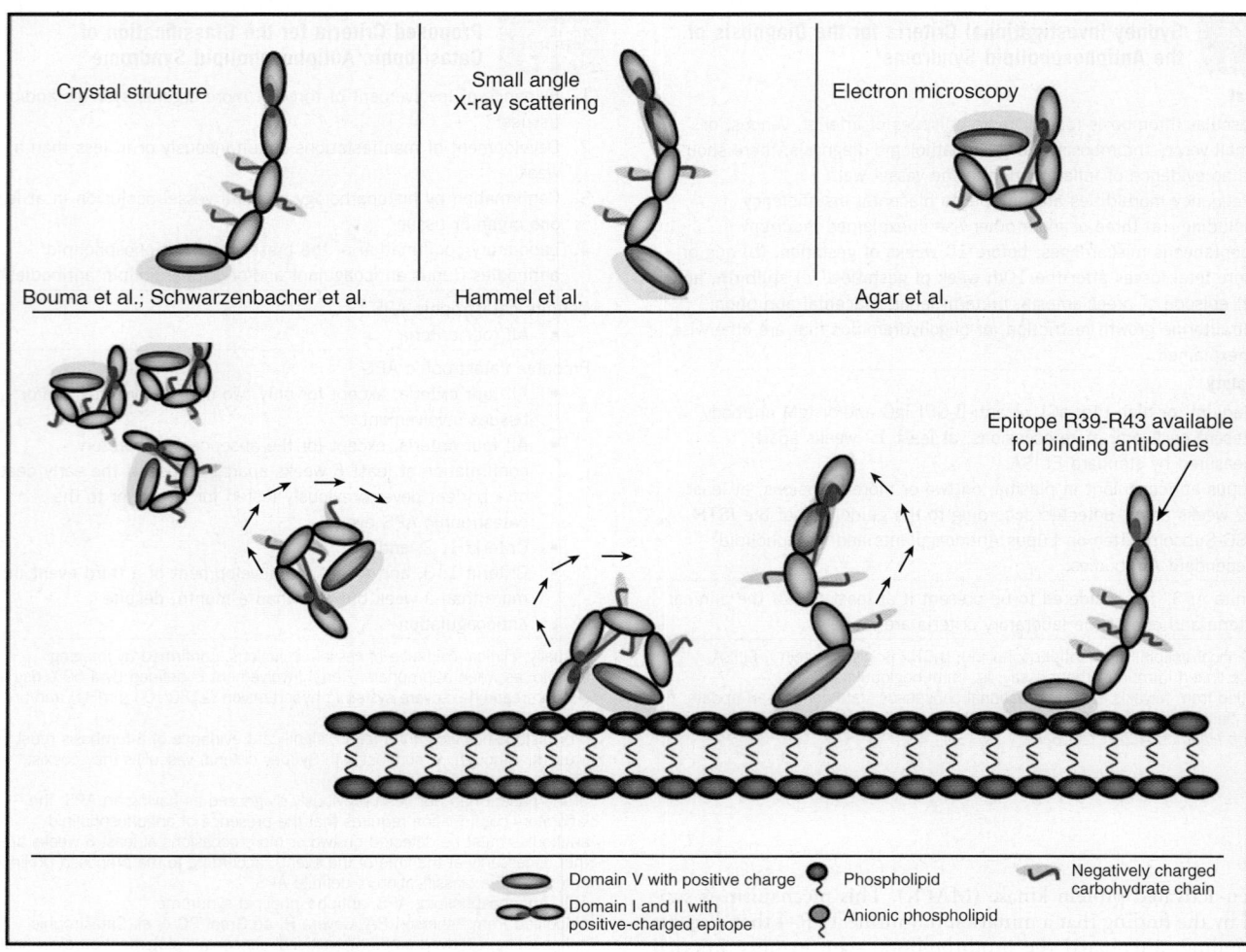

Fig. 141.1 MODELS FOR PROPOSED β_2-GLYCOPROTEIN I STRUCTURES. By x-ray crystallography, the structure of β_2GPI showed a J shape. However, small angle x-ray scattering (SAXS) of β_2GPI in solution revealed an S-shape conformation, with a carbohydrate chain on top of the interface between domains I and II. In contrast to the SAXS structure, transmission electron microscopy (TEM) of negatively stained unbound β_2GPI mounted on grids showed a circular conformation, but a J shape for β_2GPI bound to phospholipid. The arginine 39-arginine 43 epitope on domain I that is recognized by thrombogenic antiphospholipid antibodies is cryptic in the free-β_2GPI proposed conformations. This epitope then becomes exposed and available for antibody recognition after the protein is bound to phospholipid. *(Reprinted from de Laat, B, de Groot, PG: Curr Rheumatol Rep 2011 13:70, 2011.)*

The reduction in annexin A5 on cell membranes is a consequence of its competitive displacement by aPL IgG–β_2GPI immune complexes (see Fig. 141.2). As described later, a mechanistic assay has been developed that measures the interference with annexin A5 anticoagulant activity.

aPL antibodies can affect fibrinolytic mechanisms in several ways. APS patients have increased levels of antibodies against annexin A2, an endothelial surface receptor for tissue plasminogen activator and plasminogen; in distinction to the effect on cell signaling described earlier, aPL antibodies may also interfere with binding of plasminogen and t-PA and thereby reduce plasmin formation and fibrinolysis. Fibrinolysis may also be impaired by autoantibodies directed against the catalytic site of plasmin or t-PA, by increased levels of plasminogen activator inhibitor-1, and by inhibition of autoactivation of factor XII. Also, because β_2GPI is a cofactor for t-PA-mediated activation of plasminogen, aPL antibodies against β_2GPI can interfere with t-PA activity and downregulate plasmin formation.

aPL antibodies have also been reported to inhibit several steps in the protein C pathway. These include: (a) reducing the activation of protein C by the thrombomodulin-thrombin complex; (b) inhibiting the assembly of the protein C complex; (c) inhibiting the activity of protein C directly or via its cofactor protein S, (d) binding to factors Va and VIIIa in a manner that protects them from proteolysis by APC, and (e) reducing levels of both protein C and protein S. Some aPL antibodies can directly recognize protein C or S. APC resistance has been described in APS plasmas and has been correlated with anti-β_2GPI domain I antibodies.

Antiphospholipid-Mediated Activation of Complement

Complement activation has also been proposed to play a significant role in the APS disease process. Evidence from a mouse model has indicated that blockade of complement activation using a C3 convertase inhibitor or genetic deletion of C3 protected against pregnancy complications induced by aPL antibodies. Complement activation in APS appears to involve aPL antibody-stimulated direct injury to endothelial cells and monocytes, promotion of cell lysis and inflammation, modulation of downstream signaling via protease activated receptor-2 (PAR-2), and enhanced expression of tissue factor by

**TABLE
141.3**   **Proposed Pathogenic Mechanisms of Antiphospholipid Syndrome**

I. aPL-mediated promotion of tissue factor expression
  A. Direct injury and subsequent anti-β₂GPI binding on endothelial cells
  B. Signaling via annexin A2/TLR4/apoER2 inducing proadhesive prothrombotic phenotype
  C. Induction of adhesion molecules and tissue factor on endothelial cells and cytokine release

II. Activation of platelets and monocytes by aPL antibodies
  A. Activation of platelets: via apoER2′, GPIbα, and/or β₂GPI-platelet factor 4 interaction
  B. Interference of β₂GPI in regulating vWF-mediated platelet adhesion
  C. Activation of monocytes: results in increased tissue factor, VEGF, cytokine expression
  D. Activation of monocytes causes mitochondrial dysfunction and oxidative stress

III. Inhibition of endogenous anticoagulant and fibrinolytic mechanisms
  A. Disruption of the annexin A5 anticoagulant shield
  B. Interference with fibrinolysis via annexin A2, β₂GPI cofactor activity, autoactivation of XIIa, direct inhibition of plasmin and increase of PAI-1
  C. Inhibition of the protein C pathway: decreased activation of protein C, barrier of APC proteolysis of factor Va and VIIIa, prevention of protein C and EPCR binding
  D. Interference with tissue factor pathway inhibitor

IV. aPL-mediated activation of complement
  A. Antibodies against β₂GPI–HLA-DR7 complexes on cell surfaces trigger complement-mediated cytotoxicity

V. Direct activation of trophoblasts and endometrial cells by aPL antibodies
  A. Abnormal trophoblast proliferation, migration and invasiveness, increased trophoblast apoptosis, and reduced secretion of HCG and adhesion molecules
  B. Disruption in the differentiation of decidual endometrial cells
  C. Disruption of maternal spiral artery transformation and maturation

VI. Other mechanisms
  A. mTORC pathway–mediated vasculopathy
  B. Release in procoagulant microparticles by endothelial cells and platelets

APC, activated protein C; aPL, antiphospholipid; apoER2, apolipoprotein E receptor 2; EPCR, endothelial cell protein C receptor; β₂GPI, β₂-glycoprotein I; HCG, human chorionic gonadotropin; HLA, human leukocyte antigen; mTORC, mammalian target of rapamycin complex; PAI-1, plasminogen activator inhibitor 1; TLR, Toll-like receptor; VEGF, vascular endothelial growth factor; vWF, von Willebrand factor.

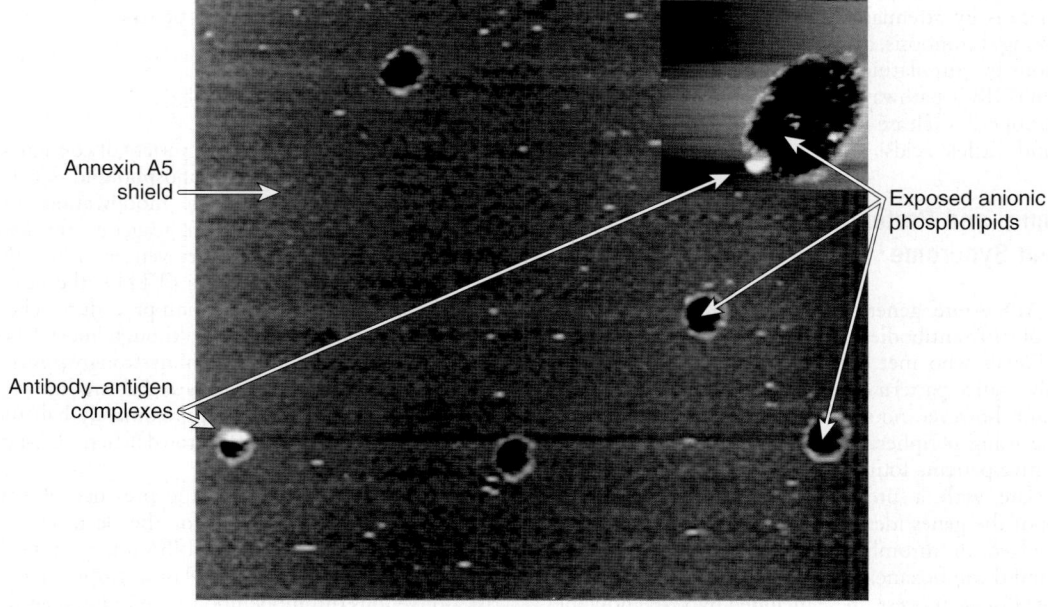

500 nm

Fig. 141.2 DISTRUPTION OF ANNEXIN A5 SHIELD BY MONOCLONAL ANTIPHOSPHOLIPID ANTIBODIES AND β₂-GLYCOPROTEIN I (β₂-GPI). Atomic force microscopy picture showing the effect of antiphospholipid monoclonal antibody IS3 on a preformed annexin A5 crystal. The figure demonstrates the smooth lipid bilayer covered by the annexin A5 crystals, disrupted by antibody–β₂GPI complexes *(white rims)* and exposing anionic phospholipids *(black holes)* to coagulation factors and accelerated coagulation. *(Adapted from Rand JH, Wu XX, Quinn AS, et al: Human monoclonal antiphospholipid antibodies disrupt the annexin A5 anticoagulant crystal shield on phospholipid bilayers: evidence from atomic force microscopy and functional assay.* Am J Pathol *163:1193, 2003.)*

myeloid cells. In addition, anti-β_2GPI antibodies may interfere with the role of β_2GPI as a regulator of the complement cascade.

Complexes of β_2GPI and human leukocyte antigen (HLA)-DR7 have been found in uterine decidual tissues from placentas of patients with APS, but not on normal placentas. aPL antibodies that recognize these β_2GPI–HLA-DR7 complexes on cell surfaces can trigger complement-mediated cytotoxicity. This mechanism may play a role in the pregnancy complications of APS.

Direct Activation of Trophoblasts and Endometrial Cells by Antiphospholipid Antibodies

In addition to the prothrombotic effects of aPL antibodies, aPL antibodies may have direct effects on trophoblasts that induce abnormal trophoblast proliferation, migration and invasiveness, increased trophoblast apoptosis, and reduced secretion of HCG and adhesion molecules. Activation of MYD88 by TLR4 has been linked to increased levels of proinflammatory molecules (IL-8, IL-1β, monocyte chemoattractant proteins) that influence trophoblast survival. Downregulation of STAT3 phosphorylation decreases IL-6 expression and reduced trophoblast migration. aPL antibodies have been implicated in the disruption of maternal spiral artery transformation and maturation and differentiation of decidual endometrial cells through activation of signaling pathways such as nuclear factor kappa-B (NFκB). Defective placentation may result in impaired blastocyte implantation.

Other Mechanisms

Autoantibodies against tissue factor pathway inhibitor have also been reported in APS patients; these antibodies may prevent the regulation of tissue factor-mediated activation of factor IX and factor X. Some aPL antibodies cross-react with heparin and heparinoid molecules, which are highly polyanionic, and inhibit their capacity to catalyze antithrombin. aPL antibodies show cross-reactivity with oxidized LDL and antibodies against the β_2GPI-oxidized LDL complex may promote atherosclerosis by attenuating oxidized LDL clearance. In addition to promoting thrombosis, aPL antibodies may contribute to other vascular lesions by stimulating the mammalian target of rapamycin complex (mTORC) pathway. Endothelial cells and platelets activated by aPL antibodies release microparticles containing procoagulant proteins and nucleic acids.

Genetic, Genomic, and Proteomic Studies in Antiphospholipid Syndrome

Although familial APS is rare, genetic factors appear to play a role in the development of aPL antibodies. One study of 7 families that included 30 individuals who met consensus criteria for APS concluded that the inheritance pattern of aPL antibodies appeared to be autosomal dominant; however, no specific linkages could be identified. A study done using peripheral blood mononuclear cells from aPL antibody–positive patients found a gene-expression pattern that appeared to correlate with a predisposition towards developing thrombosis. Some of the genes identified encoded proteins that are known to be involved in thrombosis, such as apolipoprotein E (apoE), factor X, and thromboxane. Other genes did not have a clear connection with the disease process; these included hypoxia inducible factor-1alpha (HIF-1α), zinc finger proteins, matrix metalloproteinase 19 (MMP19), interleukin-22 (IL-22) receptor, and hematopoietic progenitor cell antigen (CD34) precursor.

Proteomic studies may also provide insights on the proteins that might predict thrombotic risk in APS patients. Proteins reported to be differentially expressed in monocytes of APS patients with a history of thrombosis included annexin A1, annexin A2, ubiquitin Nedd8, Rho A protein, protein disulfide isomerase, and Hsp60.

ANTIPHOSPHOLIPID ASSAYS

History

The development of the current consensus-based clinical tests for APS stemmed from anomalous observations involving syphilis testing and coagulation assays. The immunoassays were developed in the early 1980s in efforts to quantify testing for syphilis by measuring the binding of antibodies in the test serum to cardiolipin (diphosphatidyl glycerol), the key antigen in the serologic test for syphilis. This assay turned out to be ineffective for detecting syphilis, but did quantify the biologic false-positive serologic test for syphilis (BFP-STS), a laboratory phenomenon that was associated with autoimmunity. Subsequent clinical studies revealed that increased levels of aCL antibodies detected with these assays were associated with thrombosis, spontaneous abortion, and neurologic disease. This constellation of clinical and laboratory abnormalities was recognized as a new disorder, named the "antiphospholipid syndrome." It was later discovered that, in contrast to patients who were infected with syphilis, antibodies from patients with this syndrome did not recognize cardiolipin directly, but rather a "cofactor" serum protein, β_2GPI, that binds cardiolipin in the assay. It was subsequently determined that, although β_2GPI is the primary target antigen, aPL antibodies also may recognize several other phospholipid-binding proteins.

In the early 1950s the LA assays were derived from Conley's and Hartmann's report of two patients with SLE with prolonged activated partial thromboplastin time (aPTT) values. That led to the recognition that these were a result of anticoagulants that were associated with a BFP-STS and recurrent pregnancy loss and also with thrombosis, and ultimately to the recognition that the anticoagulant was a result of antibody-mediated inhibition of phospholipid-dependent coagulation reactions and was part of the APS. The term *lupus anticoagulant* was erroneously coined to describe these antibodies because initial studies were done with patients who had SLE; the terminology has nevertheless persisted. The current aPL tests are inherently limited because they do not measure a known disease mechanism. However, as detailed later, these assays are useful as surrogate reporters for thrombotic risk.

Lupus Anticoagulant Tests

The LA tests are performed in a variety of configurations, all of which aim to detect the inhibition of phospholipid-dependent blood coagulation reactions, These include modifications of the aPTT with LA-sensitive and LA-insensitive reagents, the kaolin clotting time (KCT), the dilute Russell viper venom time (dRVVT), the tissue thromboplastin inhibition time (TTIT), the hexagonal phase array test, and the platelet neutralization procedure. The results of LA tests can vary among laboratories; although most laboratories agree on identification of plasmas containing strongly positive LA activity, they frequently disagree about samples that are known to have weak LA activity (these are missed in approximately half the cases) and laboratories often misdiagnose factor-deficient LA-negative plasmas as being LA positive.

Despite these limitations, the presence of LA activity is more predictive and more specific for the occurrence of thrombosis or pregnancy loss than the aCL ELISA assays, in both patients with or without lupus erythematosus. For example, a meta-analysis of the risks for venous thromboembolism in individuals with aPL antibodies without underlying autoimmune disease or previous thrombosis for a 15 year period reported mean ORs of 11 for LA, 3.2 for high-titer aCL antibodies and 1.6 for elevated aCL antibodies. In a systematic literature review, 12 of 12 studies showed significant associations between LA and thrombosis, with ORs ranging from 5.7 to 9.4. LA increased the risks of arterial and venous events to the same extent. In contrast, only 15 of 28 studies showed significant associations between aCL antibodies and thrombosis. In the Antiphospholipid Antibodies Stroke Study (APASS), positivity for both LA and aCL antibodies, but not for aCL antibodies alone, predicted a higher risk of recurrent thrombooclusive events in patients with first ischemic stroke. In the Risk of Arterial Thrombosis In relation to Oral contraceptives (RATIO) study, the presence of LA was found to be a major risk factor for arterial thrombotic events in young women with an OR of 5.3 for myocardial infarction and 43.1 for ischemic stroke. In LA-positive women on oral contraceptives, the OR for myocardial infarction increased to 21.6 and the OR for ischemic stroke increased to 201.0. For LA-positive women who were also cigarette smokers, the ORs for myocardial infarction and ischemic stroke increased to 33.7 and 87.0, respectively. Finally, the PROMISSE study demonstrated that of the available aPL markers, a positive LA was the single strongest predictor of adverse pregnancy outcomes in patients with APS.

Patient Selection

LA testing should not be routinely performed in patients without a history of thrombosis and/or pregnancy complications that may be attributable to APS or a history of SLE. The Antiphospholipid Antibodies Subcommittee of the International Society of Thrombosis and Hemostasis (ISTH) has prioritized the appropriateness of testing for LA into low, moderate, and high groups. Patients in the low-appropriateness group include elderly patients with venous or arterial thromboembolism. The moderate group includes asymptomatic patients who are incidentally found to have a prolonged aPTT (often during routine testing) and young patients with recurrent spontaneous early pregnancy loss or provoked VTE. Patients in the high-appropriateness group include those with unprovoked VTE, arterial thrombosis in young patients (<50 years of age), thrombosis in unusual sites, late pregnancy loss, and thrombosis or pregnancy morbidity in patients with autoimmune diseases (SLE, rheumatoid arthritis, autoimmune thrombocytopenia, autoimmune hemolytic anemia). In our opinion these same guidelines should also be applied to aPL testing.

Choosing the Appropriate Lupus Anticoagulant Assays

The Subcommittee on Antiphospholipid Antibodies of ISTH has proposed specific criteria for standardizing the diagnosis of LA. They recommend performing two different LA tests that are based on different assay principles. The dRVVT is widely used in clinical laboratories and is believed to be specific for detecting LA in patients at high risk for thrombosis. aPTT tests performed with silica as an activator and low phospholipid content were recommended as the second test of choice because of their sensitivity for LA.

Activated Partial Thromboplastin Time

A prolonged aPTT in an otherwise healthy individual without a history of bleeding is most frequently caused by an LA. Commercial aPTT reagents vary in their sensitivities to LA, so it is important to know the characteristics of the particular reagent that is being utilized. The LA needs to be differentiated from inhibitors of specific coagulation factors and from anticoagulant medications such as heparin. In addition to specific assays to evaluate these possibilities, the clinician can check whether the aPTT normalizes when an LA-insensitive aPTT reagent is used or when the assay is performed using frozen washed platelets as the source of phospholipid, a procedure referred to as the *platelet neutralization procedure*. Mixing and incubating the test plasma with normal plasma may be helpful in differentiating LAs from coagulation factor inhibitors. aPTTs performed on mixtures of normal plasma and plasma containing a factor VIII inhibitor usually require incubation for 1 to 2 hours at 37°C to show prolongation, whereas LA-containing plasmas typically prolong the aPTT immediately without requiring incubation. The clinician should be aware that in rare patients both types of anticoagulants, i.e., LA and specific

coagulation factor inhibitors, may coexist and yield a confusing laboratory picture. LAs may also cause artifactual decreases in contact activation pathway coagulation factor levels because those assays are based on the aPTT; these patients are sometimes misdiagnosed as having multiple coagulation factor deficiencies. This problem can be handled by repeating the coagulation factor assays after dilution of the plasma or by using an aPTT reagent that is insensitive to LA for the coagulation factor assays.

Dilute Russell Viper Venom Time

The dRVVT is considered to be one of the most sensitive LA tests. The assay uses Russell viper venom (RVV) in a system containing limiting quantities of diluted rabbit brain phospholipid. RVV directly activates factor X, leading to clotting. aPL antibodies can prolong the dRVVT by interfering with assembly of the prothrombinase complex; this prolongation is reversed by adding excess phospholipid to the reaction (sometimes referred to as a "confirmatory test"). To ensure that prolongation of the clotting time is not a result of a factor deficiency, the procedure includes mixing of patient plasma with control plasma. Anticoagulant therapy with heparin, warfarin, or direct thrombin inhibitors can yield falsely abnormal test results.

Antiphospholipid Immunoassays

Antiphospholipid Antibody and Cofactor Assays

The quantities of aCL IgG and aCL IgM bound are expressed in GPL and MPL units, respectively; one unit representing the cardiolipin binding activity of 1 µg/mL of affinity-purified aPL antibodies from reference sera. Binding reflects both the titer and affinity/avidity of the antibody. The levels of aCL antibodies detected in reference sera can vary among laboratories, particularly when the tests are done with different commercial ELISA kits.

It is important for the clinician to recognize that the majority of patients with elevated aCL antibodies detected on routine screening do not have APS. The prevalence of positive immunoassays in the asymptomatic "normal" population ranges from 3% to nearly 20%. In a prospective study of 2132 consecutive Spanish patients with VTE, 4.1% had elevated levels of aCL antibodies (i.e., about the same prevalence as in the asymptomatic healthy population). In one group of healthy young women, 18.2% had elevated levels of aCL antibodies and 12.8% were LA positive. Many individuals have elevated antibody levels in response to infections; these antibodies are not associated with thrombotic complications. Patients with syphilis, Lyme disease, and other infections may be misdiagnosed with APS based on elevated aCL antibody levels when concurrent stroke or arterial thrombosis is present.

High levels of aCL antibodies are associated with an increased risk of thrombosis. During a 10-year follow-up of patients with elevated levels of aCL antibodies, approximately 50% of those without clinical manifestations of APS at baseline went on to develop APS. The presence of elevated titers of aCL antibodies 6 months after an episode of VTE is a predictor of an increased risk of recurrence and of death. In a systematic review, 15 of 28 studies showed significant associations between aCL antibodies and thrombosis. In all cases, higher antibody titers were associated with an increased risk of thrombosis. Elevated levels of aCL antibodies, whether of high or low titer, were significantly associated with both myocardial infarction and ischemic stroke. Only high-titer aCL antibodies significantly increased the risk of deep vein thrombosis (DVT). With respect to pregnancy losses, a meta-analysis that reviewed 25 studies evaluating the impact of aPL antibodies on recurrent fetal loss showed a significant correlation with increased levels of aCL IgG, but the highest correlation was with LA.

Elevated levels of aCL antibodies of the IgG or IgM isotype are reported to be a significant risk factor for stroke. aPL antibodies are also reported to be an independent risk factor for stroke in young women. In the APASS, 41% of patients who experienced an ischemic stroke within 30 days were aCL antibody-positive.

Anti–β₂-Glycoprotein I Antibody Assay

β₂GPI is the major protein cofactor recognized by aPL antibodies. ELISAs for anti-β₂GPI antibodies are considered to be less sensitive but more specific for APS than aCL antibody assays. Although antibodies against β₂GPI are usually found in conjunction with aCL and antiphosphatidylserine antibodies, some patients with APS only have antibodies against β₂GPI. Despite the higher specificity (98%), β₂GPI antibodies cannot be relied upon as a stand-alone test for APS because of its low sensitivity (40%–50%) and concurrent testing for both antibodies, along with LA is advised.

In a systematic literature review, 34 of 60 studies, of which none was prospective, showed significant associations between anti-β₂GPI antibodies and thrombosis. Of 10 studies that included multivariate analysis, only 2 confirmed that IgG anti-β₂GPI antibodies were independent risk factors for venous thrombosis. Anti-β₂GPI antibodies were more often associated with venous than arterial events.

Multipositivity for Antiphospholipid Tests and Clinical Risk

Strong positivity for more than one of the aPL antibody criteria assays has been correlated with increased risk for developing clinical events in several retrospective studies and in one prospective study. One study showed that multipositivity for aPL antibodies, but not single positivity, was associated with antenatal and postnatal DVT. Another study of pregnant women with APS reported that patients with triple aPL antibody positivity and/or previous thromboembolism appeared to have a higher probability of poor neonatal outcome than patients with double or single aPL antibody positivity and no thrombosis history. A retrospective analysis of 162 APS patients who were triple-positive for LA, aCL, and anti-β₂GPI antibodies reported a higher risk of recurrent thromboembolic events with a cumulative incidence of events of 44.2% after 10 years. This finding was confirmed in a recent prospective analysis of 104 triple positive patients without a prior history of thrombosis or pregnancy complications. When followed for a mean duration of 4.5 years, the cumulative incidence of a first thrombotic event was 37.1% (95% confidence interval (CI), 19.9%–54.3%). Male sex and the presence of other risk factors for venous thrombosis were associated with an increased risk of thrombosis in this cohort.

A risk scale has been proposed to aid in the diagnosis and management of patients with APS (Table 141.4). Both symptomatic and asymptomatic patients with triple-positive laboratory results (LA positive, aCL [IgG or IgM >40 GPL] and anti-β₂GPI [IgG or IgM >99th percentile]) should be considered high-risk for future manifestations of APS, whereas patients who are double positive for LA, aCL (IgG or IgM >40 GPL) and/or anti-β₂GPI (IgG or IgM >99th percentile) or single positive for LA should be considered at medium risk for APS. Finally, single positivity for aCL (IgG or IgM >40 GPL) or anti-β₂GPI (IgG or IgM >99th percentile) should be considered low risk for APS, but treatment may be warranted if such patients develop thrombosis or pregnancy complications or have other high risk factors.

"Noncriteria" Antiphospholipid Assays

Occasionally clinicians may consider testing selected patients with one of the assays that are not included within the formal diagnostic criteria. An example of such a situation would be a patient with SLE or another autoimmune disorder who has clinical manifestations that suggest APS but who has negative assays for aCL and β₂GPI IgG and IgM along with negative LA tests.

Immunoglobulin A Antibodies Against Cardiolipin and β₂-Glycoprotein I

The clinical utility of testing aPL antibodies of IgA isotype remains controversial. The prevalence of true positivity to aCL IgA antibodies is very low; for example one study of 795 patients reported positive aCL IgA in only 2 patients, both of whom were also positive for IgG aCL. However, anti-β2GPI IgA antibodies were reported to be significantly associated with thrombosis. A recent retrospective case-control study of 56 patients with isolated anti-β₂GPI IgA found that patients with this marker had significantly more thromboembolic events and higher polyclonal IgA levels than controls. Anti-β₂GPI IgA was associated with an increased risk of thromboembolic events in patients with SLE.

aPL antibodies of IgA isotype (either aCL or anti-β2GPI) were not included in the international consensus statement on the criteria for APS classification. However, testing for the IgA isotype (particularly IgA anti-β2GPI) was recommended in cases where APS is suspected but the IgG and IgM tests are negative.

Annexin A5 Resistance Assay

The annexin A5 resistance (A5R) assay was designed to test for a specific pathogenic mechanism: the aPL antibody-mediated disruption of annexin A5 crystallization on phospholipid surfaces. As discussed earlier (section on Pathophysiologic Mechanisms), annexin A5 forms a crystal shield on endothelial surfaces which is disrupted by anti-β₂GPI/β₂GPI complexes, thereby exposing more anionic phospholipids and accelerating coagulation reactions (see Fig. 141.2). The failure of annexin A5 to sufficiently prolong coagulation times because of interference by aPL antibodies can be detected through reduction of the annexin A5 anticoagulant ratio (A5R). A study of 96 patients demonstrated significantly lower A5R values in APS patients with a history of thrombosis than in aPL antibody-positive patients without a history of thrombosis, aPL antibody-negative patients with a thrombosis history and healthy controls. A recent study of 166 patients demonstrated a significantly lower A5R ratio in obstetric primary APS patients and thrombotic primary APS patients than in healthy controls (Fig. 141.3). Clinicians should be aware that this assay falls into the category of laboratory developed tests (LDTs) and is not commercially available in kit forms.

Anti–Domain I of β₂-Glycoprotein I Assay

This immunoassay identifies IgG antibodies against a specific amino acid sequence, G40-R30, within domain I of β₂GPI. A recent analysis of 198 samples from patients with a variety of autoimmune conditions revealed that the 52 patients with anti-β₂GPI IgG antibodies could be divided into two groups: one whose antibodies recognized domain I alone and another whose antibodies reacted with all domains; only the former had positivity for LA and an increased OR for thrombosis. A recent multicenter study of 442 patients who tested positive for anti-β₂GPI antibodies reported that specific anti-domain I IgG antibodies were more strongly associated with thrombosis and obstetric complications than anti-β₂GPI antibodies detected using the standard anti-β₂GPI antibody assays. Anti–domain I IgG antibodies were present in the plasma of 55% of patients, of which 83% had a history of thrombosis (OR, 3.5) and 57% had pregnancy complications (OR, 2.4).

Antiprothrombin Antibody Assay

Prothrombin is considered the second major cofactor for aPL antibodies after β₂GPI. In a systematic literature review, 17 of 46 studies showed significant associations between antiprothrombin antibodies and thrombosis. Of the eight studies that included multivariate analyses, 2 confirmed that antiprothrombin antibodies were

TABLE 141.4	Laboratory Interpretation in Antiphospholipid Syndrome Diagnosis and Treatment*		
Risk	Laboratory Result[a]	Clinical Manifestation	Treatment
High risk OR>9	Triple positive for LA, aCL (IgG or IgM >40 GPL) and anti-β_2GPI (IgG or IgM >99th percentile)	Venous thromboembolism	Long-term vitamin K antagonist, INR 2.0–3.0
		Arterial thromboembolism	Stroke: Long-term vitamin K antagonist, INR 2.0–3.0 plus aspirin 100 mg per day
			Myocardial infarction: Long-term vitamin K antagonist, INR 2.0–3.0 plus aspirin 100 mg per day
			or
			Long-term vitamin K antagonist, INR 3.0–4.0
			Myocardial infarction with percutaneous coronary interventions and stent placement: Long-term vitamin K antagonist, INR 2.0–3.0, aspirin 100 mg per day, and clopidogrel 75 mg per day
		Pregnant women with history of pregnancy complications or thrombotic events	Unfractionated heparin plus low-dose aspirin
		Asymptomatic	Consider anticoagulant prophylaxis for high risk situations, e.g., immobilization, surgery, air travel
			Consider long-term vitamin K antagonist recommended to prevent thromboembolic events
			Consider low-dose aspirin and possible unfractionated heparin for pregnant patients
Medium risk OR 5–9	Double positive for LA, aCL (IgG or IgM >40 GPL) or anti-β_2GPI (IgG or IgM >99th percentile) or Single positive for LA	Venous thromboembolism	Long-term vitamin K antagonist, INR 2.0–3.0
		Arterial thromboembolism	Long-term vitamin K antagonist, INR 2.0–3.0 plus aspirin 100 mg per day
		Pregnant women with history of pregnancy complications	Unfractionated heparin plus low-dose aspirin
		Asymptomatic	No treatment, consider prophylaxis treatment in situations with increased risk: surgery or prolonged immobilization
Low risk OR 1–5	Single positive for aCL (IgG or IgM >40 GPL) or anti-β_2GPI (IgG or IgM >99th percentile)[b]	Venous thromboembolism	Long-term vitamin K antagonist, INR 2.0–3.0
		Arterial thromboembolism	Long-term vitamin K antagonist, INR 2.0–3.0
		Pregnant women with history of pregnancy complications	Early miscarriage (does not meet clinical criteria for obstetric APS): consider low-dose aspirin
			Late miscarriage: unfractionated heparin plus low-dose aspirin
		Asymptomatic	No treatment; however, consider prophylaxis treatment in situations with increased risk: surgery or prolonged immobilization

[a]Laboratory tests should be deferred until at least 12 weeks after the clinical event to avoid interferences of the acute phase of the disease. Earlier testing may yield false positive results.
[b]More information from clinical studies on homogeneous cohort of patients with single positivity is needed.
aCL, Anticardiolipin; β_2GPI, β_2-glycoprotein ; Ig, immunoglobulin; INR, international normalized ratio; LA, lupus anticoagulant; OR, odds ratio.
*Adapted from Sciascia S, Cosseddu D, Montaruli B et al: Risk scale for the diagnosis of antiphospholipid syndrome. *Ann Rheum Dis* 70:1517–1518, 2011; Pengo V, Banzato A, Bison E, et al: Antiphospholipid syndrome: critical analysis of the diagnostic path. *Lupus* 19:428, 2010; Pengo V, Ruffatti A, Legnani C et al: Incidence of a first throboembolic event in asymptomatic carriers of high risk antiphospholipid antibody profile: a mulitcenter prospective study. *Blood* 118:4714, 2011; Tripodi A, de Groot PG, Pengo V: Antiphospholipid syndrome: laboratory detection, mechanisms of action and treatment. *J Intern Med* 270:110, 2011.

independent risk factors for thrombosis, and 3 other studies showed that antiprothrombin antibodies added to the risk borne by LA or aCL antibodies. However, 29 of the aforementioned studies did not demonstrate an association between antiprothrombin antibodies and risk of thrombosis.

Antiphosphatidylserine Antibody Assay

Cardiolipin is normally present in mitochondrial membranes and probably does not become exposed to plasma coagulation proteins in vivo. It was hypothesized that immunoassays for antibodies against phosphatidylserine may be more relevant because this anionic phospholipid is expressed on apoptotic cells, activated platelets, and syncytial cells. Although some studies have shown a relationship between antiphosphatidylserine antibodies and pregnancy complications, mainly recurrent miscarriages and reproductive failure, others have not. However, in arterial thrombosis, antiphosphatidylserine antibodies have been shown to correlate with APS better than aCL antibodies. Additionally, it was reported that antibodies against the phosphatidylserine–prothrombin complex (aPS/PT) were associated

with APS and LA. Additional studies are needed to confirm these findings.

CLINICAL MANIFESTATIONS OF THE ANTIPHOSPHOLIPID SYNDROME

The clinical manifestations of APS can be categorized into criteria manifestations and noncriteria manifestations. The criteria manifestations include thrombotic events, obstetric APS, and CAPS, and the noncriteria manifestations include other pathologic conditions that have been associated with aPL antibodies but have not been included in the definition of "definite APS" by the expert consensus groups.

Criteria Manifestations of Antiphospholipid Syndrome

Systemic Vascular Thrombosis

Thrombosis in APS may occur spontaneously or in the presence of predisposing factors such as estrogen therapy, oral contraceptives,

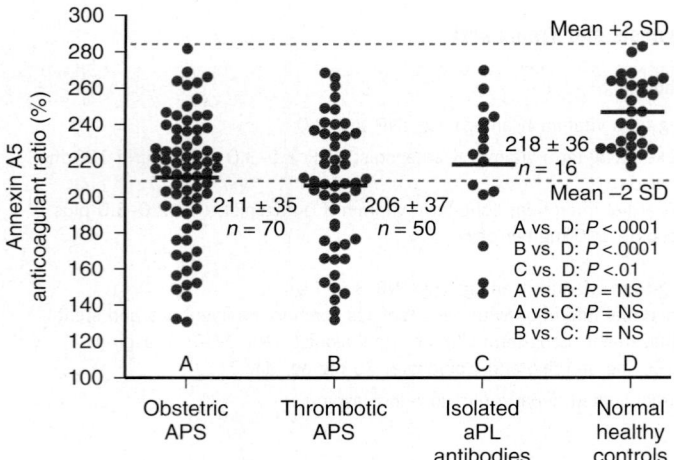

Fig. 141.3 REDUCTION OF ANNEXIN A5 ANTICOAGULANT RATIO ("ANNEXIN A5 RESISTANCE") IN PLASMAS FROM PATIENTS WITH ANTIPHOSPHOLIPID SYNDROME. The mean AnxA5 anticoagulant ratio for obstetric patients with primary antiphospholipid syndrome (APS) (group A) and thrombotic primary APS (group B) was significantly decreased compared with normal healthy controls (both *p* < .0001). The patients with isolated antiphospholipid (aPL) antibodies (group C) also showed significant reduction of AnxA5 anticoagulant ratios compared with the normal controls (*p* = .007). There were no significant differences in AnxA5 anticoagulant ratio between the groups A and B and between the groups A and C and between the groups B and C. The *horizontal lines* show the mean of each group; the *dashed lines* show the mean ± 2 SD of the 30 normal healthy controls. *(From Hunt BJ, Wu, XX, de Laat B et al: Resistance to annexin A5 anticoagulant activity in women with histories for obstetric antiphospholipid syndrome. Am J Obstet Gynecol 205:485, 2011.)*

pregnancy, the postpartum state, surgery, or trauma. Not surprisingly, occasional patients with APS-associated venous thrombosis, but generally not with arterial thrombosis, have concurrent hereditary thrombophilic conditions such as heterozygosity for the factor V Leiden mutation. Patients may present with venous and/or arterial thromboembolism in any vascular bed but the most common presentation is DVT of the lower extremities, which occurs in about half of the patients and can lead to pulmonary embolism; other sites of venous thrombosis include the thoracic veins (superior vena cava, subclavian or jugular veins), and abdominal or pelvic veins. In one study of patients with aPL antibodies and radiologic evidence of thrombosis, 59% had thrombi limited to the venous circulation, 28% had solely arterial thrombi, and 13% had both types of events.

The most significant risk factor for recurrent thromboembolism in APS is a history of a prior thromboembolic event. The risk of recurrence after a first episode of VTE in patients with aCL antibodies is about 30% at 4 years and is likely to be higher in those with a LA or with anti-β2GPI domain I antibodies.

Reproductive Manifestations

Routine aPL antibody screening of asymptomatic obstetrical patients is not warranted because of the high frequency of false positives with the current tests and the absence of any specified treatment for asymptomatic positives. Most studies have estimated the prevalence of aPL antibodies among general obstetric populations to be approximately 5% or less and most of these aPL antibody–positive patients are asymptomatic. Reports from cohorts of obstetric patients with recurrent fetal losses indicate that approximately 16%–38% have elevated aPL antibodies. Pregnant women then with elevated aPL antibodies had significantly more obstetric complications, including preeclampsia, placental abruption, miscarriage, prematurity, intrauterine

fetal demise, intrauterine growth restriction, and oligohydramnios than aPL antibody–negative pregnant women.

Women with obstetric APS generally present with a history of recurrent (i.e., three or more) miscarriages. In approximately half of the patients, the pregnancy losses occur in the first trimester; other patients present with later losses, most in the second trimester, but some even later, including stillbirth. The specific pregnancy complications that define obstetric APS include: the absence of another explanation for the complications, three or more recurrent spontaneous first trimester miscarriages, or one midtrimester loss, stillbirth, episode of preeclampsia, preterm labor, placental abruption, intrauterine growth restriction, or oligohydramnios. Pregnant women with APS are also more prone to develop DVT during pregnancy or the puerperium. Rarely, pregnant patients can develop CAPS.

As with the thrombotic manifestations, a prior clinical history of previous pregnancy loss, complications, or thrombosis is a better predictor for future pregnancy loss than the degree of laboratory abnormality. Furthermore, recent studies have shown that positivity on more than one assay (so-called multipositivity) correlates with increased pregnancy complications. For example, one study showed that multipositivity, but not single positivity for aPL antibodies, was associated with antenatal and postnatal DVT. Another retrospective study of 128 pregnant women with APS found that patients with triple antiphospholipid positivity and/or previous thromboembolism appeared to have a higher likelihood of poor neonatal outcome than those with double or single antiphospholipid positivity and no thrombosis history.

The current consensus is that aPL antibodies do not contribute to early reproductive failure (i.e., infertility). Recently, the 14th International Congress on Antiphospholipid Antibodies Task Force also concluded that "there are no data to support the inclusion of infertility as a criterion for APS and investigation of APS in patients with infertility should not be done in routine clinical practice, being reserved only for research purposes." Although one group reported data suggesting that women with recurrent implantation failure were more likely to have positive assays for aPL antibodies compared with fertile controls, a review of 29 studies showed mixed results. Many of the studies had limitations, including problems with study design and statistical power.

Studies suggest a possible nonthrombogenic mechanism of impaired trophoblastic differentiation, proliferation, and migration that may lead to the recurrent implantation failure seen in infertile women.

Neurologic Manifestations

Ischemic stroke is frequent in APS. In a large European cohort, stroke or transient ischemic attack (TIA) was the initial manifestation of APS in 29.9% of adults with APS; in the same study, stroke or TIA was the most frequent recurrent event and contributed to a large proportion of deaths. A Latin American study of adults with APS reported that 18% presented with stroke or TIA. A multinational lupus cohort showed that aPL antibody–associated stroke accounted for 11.8% of deaths. In the European CAPS registry, cerebral manifestations occurred in 62% of patients and caused 13% of deaths.

Prospective analysis for the presence of aPL antibodies in stroke patients in the APASS demonstrated that elevated levels of anticardiolipin antibodies are associated with an increased risk for stroke but not with subsequent thromboembolic events. There was a trend for more recurrent thrombotic events in patients who tested positive for both aCL and LA than in those who tested negative for both (31.7% vs. 24.0%, *p* = .07). A subsequent study from the same group reported that elevated antibodies against β2GPI and LA, and not aCL or antiphosphatidylserine, were the most significant risk factors for stroke. It is important for clinicians to be aware that the presence of conventional risk factors for vascular disease adds to the baseline risk associated with the antibodies. In the RATIO study, women with LA positivity and other modifiable risk factors such as smoking or use of oral contraceptives had an increased risk of ischemic stroke. Lupus and APS patients with valvular heart lesions were also shown to be at increased risk of cerebrovascular disease, and echocardiography should be considered for patients with APS and stroke because a high proportion of APS patients have cardiac valvular abnormalities (see later).

The diagnosis of APS is should be considered when young patients present with a TIA or a stroke, particularly those without other risk factors. Rates of stroke were higher in younger patients with APS, with a rate of up to 32% in a multinational childhood registry versus 16%–21% in adult APS patients. Case-control and prospective studies have shown strong associations between aPL antibody or LA positivity and ischemic stroke in young adults with an OR of 43.1 for positive LA tests and ischemic strokes. Younger patients presenting with stroke tended to have venous, rather than arterial, occlusion with 7% of children presenting with cerebral vein thrombosis in the multinational childhood registry. In addition to the immediate impact, recurrent strokes may lead to multi-infarct dementia that can mimic other causes of dementia.

Cardiovascular Manifestations

APS should be considered in patients without the more typical risk factors for coronary artery disease and in patients with evidence of thrombotic or embolic coronary occlusion who lack angiographic evidence of atherosclerotic disease. In the RATIO population-based case-control study, the presence of a LA was a significant risk factor for arterial occlusion. LA correlated with an increased risk of myocardial infarction with an OR of 5.3, which increased to 21.6 in women who used oral contraceptives and to 33.7 in women who smoked. Elevated anti-β_2GPI correlated with a mild increase in stroke but not with myocardial infarction. Antiprothrombin and anticardiolipin antibodies did not correlate with an increased risk of arterial thrombosis. However, antiprothrombin antibodies were reported to be a predictor of myocardial infarction in middle-aged men, and one study found that the interaction in risk between antiprothrombin antibodies and other risk factors was multiplicative.

Hepatic and Gastrointestinal Manifestations

The liver is the most commonly affected abdominal organ in APS. Occlusion of hepatic vessels supplying the biliary tree may present as acute acalculous cholecystitis with gallbladder necrosis. Gastrointestinal manifestations of APS also include esophageal necrosis with perforation, intestinal ischemia and infarction, pancreatitis, colonic ulceration, and giant gastric ulcerations. APS has been reported in patients with mesenteric inflammatory venoocclusive disease and with mesenteric and portal vein obstruction.

Renal Abnormalities

Patients with APS may present with vasoocclusive manifestations such as renal artery stenosis and/or thrombosis, renal infarction and renal vein thrombosis, and with nonthrombotic manifestations, described in the section on noncriteria manifestations. An entity named *APS nephropathy* consists of vasoocclusive disease of small intrarenal vessels characterized by fibrous intimal hyperplasia, focal cortical atrophy, and thrombotic microangiopathy. The acute form of this vascular nephropathy resembles other thrombotic microangiopathies, such as hemolytic uremic syndrome or thrombotic thrombocytopenic purpura. A chronic form that is frequently clinically silent until late stages manifests as a vasoocclusive process that develops at all levels of the renal vasculature, from the main renal artery to glomerular capillaries and renal veins.

Retinal Abnormalities

The diagnosis of APS retinopathy should be suspected in patients with diffuse retinal vasoocclusion, particularly when characterized by involvement of arteries and veins, neovascularization at presentation, and symptoms of systemic rheumatologic disease. Elevated aPL antibody levels were present in 5% to 33% of patients with retinal vein occlusion. Cilioretinal artery occlusion, optic neuropathy, and severe vasoocclusive retinopathy have been described with APS.

Other Organ Manifestations

aPL antibodies have been described in patients with pulmonary hypertension. A multi-institutional study of 687 patients with chronic thromboembolic pulmonary hypertension reported that aPL antibodies were a significant risk factor. In one prospective trial of 38 consecutive patients with precapillary pulmonary hypertension, approximately 30% had aPL antibodies with various phospholipid specificities.

Acute adrenal failure secondary to bilateral infarction of the adrenal glands has been reported as the first manifestation of primary APS. Adrenal hemorrhage has also been reported. aPL antibodies have also been associated with osteonecrosis. Skin manifestations may be a first sign of APS. Skin ulcerations associated with skin necrosis are a presenting feature in 3.5% of cases.

Catastrophic Antiphospholipid Syndrome

Rare patients present with a catastrophic form of APS, which is characterized by severe widespread vascular occlusion and a high mortality. The formal diagnostic criteria include evidence of involvement of at least three organs, systems and/or tissues, development of manifestations simultaneously or within 1 week, histopathological confirmation of small vessel occlusion, and laboratory confirmation of the presence of aPL antibodies (Table 141.2).

In contrast to the diagnostic criteria for APS, the diagnostic criteria for CAPS permit the presence of histologic evidence of vasculitis together with thrombosis. These patients present with evidence of severe multiorgan ischemia/infarction, usually with concurrent microvascular thrombosis. Patients with CAPS can present with massive venous thromboembolism, along with respiratory failure, stroke, abnormal liver enzymes, renal impairment, adrenal insufficiency, and areas of cutaneous infarction. The respiratory failure is usually caused by acute respiratory distress syndrome (ARDS) and diffuse alveolar hemorrhage. Laboratory evidence for disseminated intravascular coagulation is frequently present.

According to the CAPS Registry, a web based database of 433 patients with CAPS (https://ontocrf.costaisa.com/en/web/caps/), the majority of CAPS patients are female (69%), in their late thirties (mean age of 38.5 years), but patients can present at any age (range 0 to 85 years). In half of the CAPS cases, the catastrophic event was their first manifestation of APS. Precipitating factors for CAPS include infection, drugs (sulfur-containing diuretics, captopril, and oral contraceptives), surgical procedures, and cessation of anticoagulant therapy. In 26.9% of cases, the patients also had SLE. The most frequently affected organ was the kidney (73% of episodes), followed by the lungs (58.9%), brain (55.9%), heart (49.7%), and skin (45.4%). Other organs were also affected including the peripheral vessels, intestines, spleen, adrenal glands, pancreas, retina, and bone marrow. An LA is present in 81.7% of patients, and aCL IgG is the most common positive aPL antibody. Improved treatment has reduced mortality from approximately 50% to 20%. Fortunately, relapse is rare in survivors. The only identified predictive factor for adverse outcome is underlying SLE.

Pediatric Antiphospholipid Syndrome

APS is a significant cause of thrombosis in the pediatric population. In a European registry, children with primary APS tended to be younger and had a higher frequency of arterial thrombotic events, whereas those with secondary APS were older and were more likely to have venous thrombotic events associated with hematologic and skin manifestations. Children with rheumatic diseases with persistently positive criteria aPL assays were reported to have resistance to annexin A5 anticoagulant activity compared with patients with transiently positive antibodies. The catastrophic form of the syndrome has been reported in children, but occurs less frequently than it does in adults. Thrombosis is rare in newborns delivered by mothers with APS, although aPL antibodies have been found in up to 30% of such offspring.

"Noncriteria" Clinical Manifestations Associated With Antiphospholipid Antibodies and Antiphospholipid Syndrome

Cardiovascular Manifestations

In the absence of thrombotic occlusion, coronary artery disease is not a criterion for APS. However, aPL antibodies have been associated with increased susceptibility to atherosclerosis. aPL antibodies also appear to be a risk factor for adverse outcomes after all coronary revascularization procedures, interventional and surgical.

A remarkably large proportion of patients with the primary APS, approximately 35%, have cardiac valvular abnormalities detectable by echocardiography. When patients with cardiac valvular diseases that were not suspected to be associated with APS were evaluated for aPL antibodies, about 20% had evidence of aPL antibodies compared with about 10% of matched controls. Valvular abnormalities were reported in about half of patients with the combination of SLE and aPL antibodies; these abnormalities included leaflet thickening, vegetations, regurgitation, and stenosis. The mitral valve is most commonly affected, followed by the aortic valve. In a prospective follow-up of 89 patients with severe, nonspecific valvular heart disease, thromboembolic events were significantly more frequent in the aPL antibody–positive group than in the aPL antibody-negative group; however, the presence of aPL antibodies was not an independent risk factor for thromboembolic events. There was one dissenting study that failed to find a relationship between increased aCL antibodies and valvular abnormalities in patients with SLE, progressive systemic sclerosis, rheumatoid arthritis, and primary APS.

Neurologic Manifestations

aPL antibody-associated neurologic abnormalities, other than stroke, include migraine headache, seizures, chorea, Guillain-Barré Syndrome, transient global amnesia, dementia, diabetic peripheral neuropathy, and orthostatic hypotension. In the pediatric APS registry, migraine headache (7%), chorea (4%), and epilepsy (3%) were the most common nonthrombotic neurologic manifestations.

Elevated aCL antibodies are often seen in patients with multiple sclerosis but these are not associated with an increased risk for thrombosis or stroke. In one series of patients with multiple sclerosis, 9% had IgG antibodies and 44% had IgM antibodies, but there was no clinical distinction between those with or without these antibodies. Patients with psychotic disorders have also been reported to have an increased prevalence of LA and aCL antibodies. In one study, 32% (11/34) of the unmedicated psychotic patients had elevated aPL antibodies, but these patients did not appear to have an increased risk of thrombosis.

Hepatic Manifestations

aPL antibody levels are frequently elevated in patients with chronic liver diseases. In one prospective study of patients with liver disease, approximately half of patients with alcoholic liver disease and one-third of patients with chronic hepatitis C virus had elevated aPL

antibody levels. The frequency was even higher in patients with more severe cirrhosis. One review reported that about 20% of patients with chronic hepatitis B and hepatitis C had elevated aPL antibodies, most of which were cofactor independent, i.e., similar to antibodies in infections that recognize phospholipid directly rather than antibodies that recognize phospholipid-binding proteins such as β_2GPI. Hepatitis C may be an exception because patients can present with "true" autoimmune aPL antibodies; the most common features reported were intraabdominal thrombosis and myocardial infarction. Primary biliary cirrhosis has also been associated with aPL antibodies.

Renal Manifestations

Several nonthrombotic types of renal lesions have also been identified in APS patients. Patients with aPL antibodies may present with glomerulonephritis without vasoocclusive disease. A review of 29 consecutive renal biopsies from patients with primary APS, performed at 2 institutions over 22 years, described 20 cases of APS nephropathy and identified 9 cases with distinct pathologic features including membranous nephropathy, minimal change disease/focal segmental glomerulonephritis, mesangial C3 nephropathy, and pauci-immune crescentic glomerulonephritis.

Dermatologic Manifestations

Livedo reticularis is relatively common, occurring in 24% of a series of 1000 aPL patients (Fig. 141.4). Livedo reticularis is usually widespread and can localize on nonadjacent areas on the limbs, trunk, and buttocks. Its prevalence was found to be higher in APS that was associated with SLE compared with primary APS, in women compared with men, and in patients with high levels of aCL antibodies. Livedo reticularis may be associated with other manifestations of APS such as cerebral or ocular ischemic arterial events (OR, 10.8; 95% CI, 5.2–22.5), seizures (OR, 6.5; 95% CI, 2.6–16), arterial events (OR, 6; 95% CI, 2.9–12.6), heart valve abnormalities detected on echocardiography (OR, 7.3; 95% CI, 3.6–14.7), and arterial systemic hypertension (BP >160/90 mmHg) (OR, 2.9; 95% CI, 1.5–5.7). Necrotizing vasculitis, livedoid vasculitis, thrombophlebitis, cutaneous ulceration and necrosis, erythematous macules, purpura, ecchymoses, painful skin nodules, subungual splinter hemorrhages, anetoderma (macular atrophy), discoid lupus erythematosus, and cutaneous T cell lymphoma have all been reported.

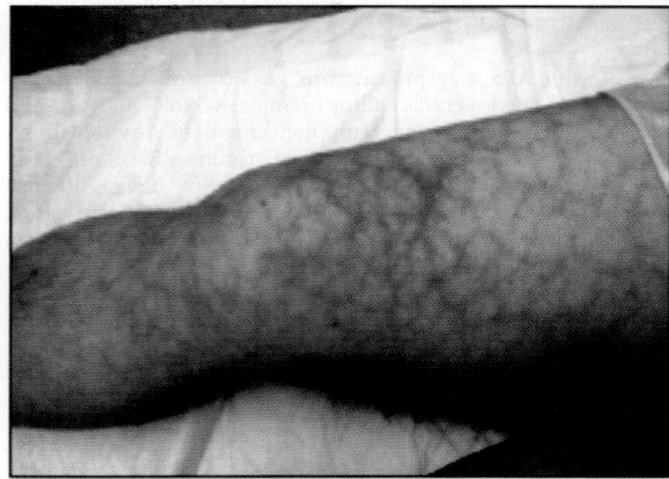

Fig. 141.4 LIVEDO RETICULARIS IN A WOMAN WITH ANTIPHOSPHOLIPID SYNDROME. *(From Ruiz-Irastorza G, Crowther M, Branch W, Khamashta MA: Antiphospholipid syndrome.* Lancet *376:1498, 2010.)*

Hematologic Abnormalities

Thrombocytopenia occurs in a large fraction of patients with APS, but is rarely significant enough to cause bleeding complications or to affect anticoagulant therapy. Most cases appear to be immune mediated and are likely to reflect mild chronic immune thrombocytopenia (ITP). In a prospective cohort study, the 5-year thrombosis-free survival of aPL antibody–positive and aPL antibody–negative ITP patients was 39% and 98%, respectively, indicating that thrombocytopenia itself is not protective against thrombosis in these patients. This has been further substantiated by a recent systematic review and meta-analysis that reported that an increased risk of thrombosis in patients with primary immune thrombocytopenia who also tested positive for antiphospholipid antibodies, particularly for LA for which the pooled OR for the risk of thrombosis was 6.11 (95% CI, 3.40–10.99).

LA by themselves are not associated with abnormal hemostasis. Therefore when patients with APS exhibit a bleeding tendency a concurrent coagulopathy must be considered. In patients with normal platelet counts, the differential diagnosis should include hypoprothrombinemia, acquired thrombocytopathy, acquired factor VIII inhibitor, and acquired von Willebrand syndrome.

TREATMENT OF PATIENTS WITH ANTIPHOSPHOLIPID SYNDROME

There is general agreement that patients with recurrent or spontaneous thrombosis require long-term anticoagulant therapy and that patients with recurrent spontaneous pregnancy losses require antithrombotic therapy for most of the gestational period and for the puerperium. There are unsettled differences of opinion regarding the approach to treatment of patients with single thrombotic events, or a history of previous thrombotic events in the remote past (i.e., >5 years), or patients with provoked thrombotic events after risk factors such as surgery, pregnancy, or estrogens. The recent categorization of patients into high, medium, and low risk groups based on multipositivity on laboratory results may help guide management (see Table 141.4).

Thrombosis

The accumulated evidence from randomized controlled trials indicates that regardless of single or multiple positivity for aPL antibodies, patients with APS and thrombosis should be treated with long-term warfarin with the dose adjusted to achieve an INR of 2.0–3.0. Although patients with unprovoked venous thromboembolism should probably be treated for the long term, duration of therapy for provoked events is debatable.

Although there is a general consensus on this therapeutic range for venous thrombosis, there is controversy as to whether patients with arterial thrombosis may warrant a higher intensity of anticoagulation because a retrospective study of a variety of patients with APS showed that an INR >3.0 was required to prevent recurrence in this group of patients. Although two major prospective, randomized, controlled trials reported no benefit, and even some downside for high-intensity warfarin, there has been debate on whether these two studies had sufficient numbers of patients with arterial thrombotic events to allow those findings to be generalized beyond venous thromboembolism. Some investigators have recommended that patients with myocardial infarction and triple positivity be treated with higher-intensity warfarin of INR 3.0–4.0 or lower-intensity warfarin of INR 2.0–3.0 plus low-dose aspirin. In addition, the triple-positive myocardial infarction patients who undergo percutaneous coronary interventions and stent implantations should be treated with triple antithrombotic regimens that include warfarin (INR 2.0–3.0), low-dose aspirin, and clopidogrel.

Clinicians should be aware that the LA may impact monitoring of anticoagulation with both warfarin and unfractionated heparin (UFH) but has no impact on treatment with low-molecular-weight heparin (LMWH). The prothrombin time and INR results can be artifactually elevated in some patients with APS and LA. A multicenter study reported that all but one of the commercial thromboplastins in use in nine centers provided acceptable INR values for APS patients with LA. Chromogenic factor X (CFX) assays can be used as an alternative to the INR to monitor warfarin in APS patients with a prolonged baseline PT, those who are persistently positive for LA and those patients with recurrent VTE. Therapeutic CFX values range from 20% to 40%; thus a CFX of 40% would approximate an INR of 2.0, and a CFX of 20% would approximate an INR of 3.0.

LMWH is generally recommended for treatment in the acute setting. For those patients who require treatment with intravenous UFH (e.g., high risk patients for whom the short half-life of UFH may be advantageous for bridging purposes), the physician must first determine that the baseline aPTT used for monitoring and adjusting heparin dosage is not prolonged by a LA. If this is a problem, the heparin concentration may be estimated with one of the LA-insensitive aPTT reagents or measured directly with a specific heparin assay.

Fibrinolytic therapy has been used in patients with primary APS who present with extensive thrombosis of the common femoral and iliac veins extending to the lower vena cava, acute ischemic stroke, and acute myocardial infarction.

Although the direct-acting oral anticoagulants (DOACs) are as effective as warfarin for VTE treatment, they have not been extensively evaluated in APS patients. In two recent case studies, DOACs failed to prevent thrombosis in APS patients. Of 6 APS patients studied, 5 suffered recurrent venous thromboembolism and 1 suffered a recurrent TIA after transitioning to DOACs. At least two prospective randomized trials comparing warfarin with rivaroxaban are currently in progress (ClinicalTrials.gov Identifier: NCT02116036 NCT02157272), but until the results are available, DOACs should be used with caution in APS patients.

Stroke

There is controversy about the appropriate antithrombotic treatment of aPL antibody–associated stroke. Currently most hematologists and rheumatologists view APS stroke as no different from other arterial thrombotic manifestations of APS and treat with warfarin, with some debate as to whether to use an INR target of 2.0–3.0 or a higher intensity. Conversely many neurologists view APS stroke as no different from other arterial strokes and accept the APASS study conclusion that treating with aspirin alone is as effective as warfarin but associated with a lower risk of bleeding (the daily dose in that study was 325 mg; however, most guidelines recommend 81 mg/day). Guidelines issued in 2006 from the American Heart Association/American Stroke Association stated that for patients with cryptogenic ischemic stroke or TIA associated with aPL antibodies, antiplatelet therapy is reasonable and for patients who meet the criteria for APS with venous and arterial occlusive disease in multiple organs, miscarriages, and livedo reticularis, warfarin with a target INR of 2.0–3.0 is reasonable.

Pregnancy Complications

The current approach to treating pregnant women with APS and recurrent pregnancy losses or the other aPL antibody–associated complications of pregnancy includes daily low-dose aspirin (75–81 mg/day) and either UFH or LMWH. Although clinical studies have shown efficacy with UFH, most clinicians treat with LMWH because it has a better pharmacokinetic profile (it can be given once daily subcutaneously rather than twice daily) and lower risk of heparin-induced thrombocytopenia and osteopenia. Heparin is then withheld when labor begins or 24 hours prior to a cesarean section. Anticoagulation with either LMWH or warfarin (although most patients and physicians prefer LMWH for convenience, despite the need for injection) is then resumed for 6 weeks because of the increased risk of VTE in this time period. This latter recommendation may be modified if DOACs are proven to be useful in this setting. Interestingly, the current standard of care for pregnant patients with APS is based on only two randomized controlled trials conducted prior to 2000 and included only 150 patients. More recent trials have shown conflicting results with some showing no difference in prevention of pregnancy loss in APS patients receiving aspirin alone versus aspirin and LMWH and others showing a small benefit. However, the likelihood of a good pregnancy outcome in treated women with APS has been estimated to be about 75%–80%.

The presence of elevated aPL antibodies in pregnant women without any history of spontaneous pregnancy losses, other attributable pregnancy complications, thrombosis or embolism is currently not sufficient justification for treatment. A recent systematic review found no benefit of prophylactic treatment with aspirin to prevent pregnancy complications in aPL antibody carriers in the absence of other risk factors. Because 2%–3% of the general obstetric population has low titers of aPL antibodies, with a live birth rate of 60% among these patients, it is not recommended that physicians screen for aPL antibodies or LA in their routine prenatal screening panel.

Catastrophic Antiphospholipid Syndrome

Patients with CAPS require aggressive treatment because of the high mortality. Treatment for CAPS is directed toward the thrombotic events and suppression of the cytokine cascade. Conventional anticoagulant therapy is usually insufficient and treatment modalities may include anticoagulation with heparin, immunosuppressive therapy in the form of high-dose steroids, IVIG, cyclophosphamide, azathioprine, or rituximab. Plasmapheresis may be a helpful adjunct in some patients. A triple therapy strategy of anticoagulation, steroids, and either intravenous immunoglobulin or plasma exchange or both has improved outcomes. The higher rate of this triple therapy strategy has resulted in a significant reduction in mortality rate to 30% in CAPS. Cyclophosphamide is recommended for CAPS patients with inflammatory features of SLE or high-titer aPL antibodies. Rituximab may be useful for refractory or relapsing cases of CAPS.

Asymptomatic Antiphospholipid Antibody–Positive Patients

A recent task force at the 13th International Congress on Antiphospholipid Antibodies has recommended that asymptomatic patients with no previous thrombosis but a high risk aPL antibody profile (LA positive, triple positive (LA+, aCL antibody+, anti-β₂GPI antibody+), or persistently positive medium-high titers of aCL antibodies be given long-term prophylaxis with low-dose aspirin, especially if there are other thrombotic risk factors. Furthermore, aPL-antibody carriers should receive thromboprophylaxis with usual doses of LMWH in high-risk situations, such as surgery, prolonged immobilization and the puerperium. In addition to low-dose aspirin, aPL-antibody carriers with SLE should receive hydroxychloroquine (HCQ) as primary prophylaxis. A recent meta-analysis of five international studies that included 495 patients confirmed the benefit of low-dose aspirin in asymptomatic aPL antibody carriers with and without SLE. The risk of a first thrombotic event is significantly decreased in SLE patients and asymptomatic aPL antibody carriers treated with low-dose aspirin. Specifically, low-dose aspirin showed a protective effect against arterial but not venous thrombosis. The meta-analysis failed to show an independent protective effect of HCQ.

NONANTICOAGULANT TREATMENTS UNDER STUDY FOR ANTIPHOSPHOLIPID SYNDROME

Hydroxychloroquine

HCQ, a synthetic antimalarial drug with many antiinflammatory and antithrombotic effects has been associated with a reduced risk of thrombosis in patients with APS and SLE. The potential effectiveness of this treatment has been supported by an animal model for aPL antibody thrombosis and by a recent reports that HCQ directly disrupts aPL IgG–β₂GPI complexes, and also reverses the aPL antibody–mediated disruption of annexin A5 binding on phospholipid bilayers and on human placental syncitiotrophoblasts. In a longitudinal cohort study that included 272 patients with APS and 152 taking HCQ (17 of 272 patients on warfarin, 203 were on prednisolone, 112 on azathioprine, 38 on aspirin) there were fewer thrombotic complications in those taking HCQ (OR, 0.17; 95% CI, 0.07–0.44; $p < .0001$). In asymptomatic aPL antibody-positive patients with SLE, primary prophylaxis with aspirin and HCQ appeared to reduce the frequency of thrombotic events. A recently published prospective, nonrandomized study compared oral anticoagulant plus HCQ versus oral anticoagulant alone. In this study, 30% (6/20) of patients had a thrombotic event if they were on oral anticoagulant alone, despite therapeutic range INR, versus no thrombotic events in the oral anticoagulant plus HCQ group (0/20). However this study was limited by the small sample size and short follow-up. A prospective randomized controlled trial comparing HCQ to placebo in aPL-positive patients without a prior history for thrombosis (clinicaltrials.gov NCT01784523) was recently terminated because of insufficient recruitment.

Rituximab

Rituximab is an anti-CD20 chimeric monoclonal antibody effective against non-Hodgkin lymphomas and approved for the treatment of rheumatoid arthritis. Limited case reports have shown rituximab as effective in treating thrombocytopenia and hemolytic anemia in aPL antibody–positive patients; however, it is unknown if rituximab is effective against aPL antibody–mediated thrombosis. An open-label, phase II pilot study demonstrated safety and effectiveness of rituximab in aPL antibody–positive patients with anticoagulant resistant manifestations but did not show any effect on aPL laboratory parameters.

Main Points and Clinical Pearls

- The antiphospholipid (aPL) syndrome (APS) is an acquired thrombophilic disorder in which patients have vascular thrombosis and/or pregnancy complications attributable to placental insufficiency, accompanied by laboratory evidence for the presence of antiphospholipid antibodies in blood.
- Rare patients have a catastrophic form of APS (CAPS) in which there is disseminated thrombosis in large- and small-vessel thrombi, often after a triggering event such as infection or surgery, and often with multiorgan ischemia and infarction.
- Laboratory testing for aPL antibodies should generally be limited to patients who present with the thrombotic and/or the pregnancy manifestations of the disorder or asymptomatic patients with autoimmune disease such as systemic lupus erythematosus because they are at increased risk for having aPL antibodies and for experiencing thrombosis.
- The syndrome is identified by persistent positivity of criteria laboratory tests including high titers for aCL and anti-β₂GPI IgG or IgM antibodies detected by immunoassays and by positive LA using two different coagulation tests.
- Weak positive test results for aPL immunoassays are unlikely to have any clinical significance. Transient aPL antibodies can develop as a result of infection, HIV, liver disease, cancer, and certain medications such as phenothiazines, quinine, procainamide, oral contraceptives, and anti-TNF agents.
- In clinical practice selected patients may be suspected to have APS without necessarily meeting the strict investigational criteria.
- When a patient has the clinical appearance of APS but negative standard aPL assay results, think about the possibility of seronegative APS. Noncriteria tests such as anticardiolipin (aCL) and anti–β₂-glycoprotein I (anti-β₂GPI) immunoglobulin A

SUGGESTED READINGS

Agar C, de Groot PG, Morgelin M, et al: Beta2-glycoprotein I: a novel component of innate immunity. *Blood* 2011.

Agnelli G, Becattini C, Franco L: New oral anticoagulants for the treatment of venous thromboembolism. *Best Pract Res Clin Haematol* 26:151–161, 2013.

Amengual O, Fujita D, Ota E, et al: Primary prophylaxis to prevent obstetric complications in asymptomatic women with antiphospholipid antibodies: a systematic review. *Lupus* 24(11):1135–1142, 2015.

Arnaud L, Mathian A, Devilliers H, et al: Patient-level analysis of five international cohorts further confirms the efficacy of aspirin for the primary prevention of thrombosis in patients with antiphospholipid antibodies. *Autoimmun Rev* 14:192–200, 2015.

Andreoli L, Piantoni S, Dall'Ara F, et al: Vitamin D and antiphospholipid syndrome. *Lupus* 21:736–740, 2012.

Brandt KJ, Fickentscher C, Boehlen F, et al: NF-kappaB is activated from endosomal compartments in antiphospholipid antibodies-treated human monocytes. *J Thromb Haemost* 12:779–791, 2014.

Breen KA, Sanchez K, Kirkman N, et al: Endothelial and platelet microparticles in patients with antiphospholipid antibodies. *Thromb Res* 135:368–374, 2015.

Bezati E, Wu XX, Quinn AS, et al: A new trick for an ancient drug: quinine dissociates antiphospholipid immune complexes. *Lupus* 24:32–41, 2015.

Canaud G, Bienaime F, Tabarin F, et al: Inhibition of the mTORC pathway in the antiphospholipid syndrome. *N Engl J Med* 371:303–312, 2014.

Cervera R, Rodriguez-Pinto I, Colafrancesco S, et al: 14th International Congress on Antiphospholipid Antibodies Task Force Report on Catastrophic Antiphospholipid Syndrome. *Autoimmun Rev* 13:699–707, 2014.

Crowl A, Schullo-Feulner A, Moon JY: A Review of Warfarin Monitoring in Antiphospholipid Syndrome and Lupus Anticoagulant. *Ann Pharmacother* 2014.

de Jesus GR, Rodrigues G, de Jesus NR, et al: Pregnancy morbidity in antiphospholipid syndrome: what is the impact of treatment? *Curr Rheumatol Rep* 16:403, 2014.

de Laat B, de Groot PG: Autoantibodies directed against domain I of beta2-glycoprotein I. *Curr Rheumatol Rep* 13:70–76, 2011.

Di Simone N, Marana R, Castellani R, et al: Decreased expression of heparin-binding epidermal growth factor-like growth factor as a newly

identified pathogenic mechanism of antiphospholipid-mediated defective placentation. *Arthritis Rheum* 62:1504–1512, 2010.

Erkan D, Aguiar CL, Andrade D, et al: 14th International Congress on Antiphospholipid Antibodies: task force report on antiphospholipid syndrome treatment trends. *Autoimmun Rev* 13:685–696, 2014.

Gropp K, Weber N, Reuter M, et al: beta(2)-glycoprotein I, the major target in antiphospholipid syndrome, is a special human complement regulator. *Blood* 118:2774–2783, 2011.

Mekinian A, Lachassinne E, Nicaise-Roland P, et al: European registry of babies born to mothers with antiphospholipid syndrome. *Ann Rheum Dis* 72:217–222, 2013.

Mekinian A, Lazzaroni MG, Kuzenko A, et al: The efficacy of hydroxychloroquine for obstetrical outcome in anti-phospholipid syndrome: Data from a European multicenter retrospective study. *Autoimmun Rev* 14:498–502, 2015.

Moulis G, Audemard-Verger A, Arnaud L, et al: Risk of thrombosis in patients with primary immune thrombocytopenia and antiphospholipid antibodies: A systemic review and meta-analysis. *Autoimmun Rev* 15:203–209, 2016.

Proulle V, Furie RA, Merrill-Skoloff G, et al: Platelets are required for enhanced activation of the endothelium and fibrinogen in a mouse thrombosis model of APS. *Blood* 124:611–622, 2014.

Pengo V, Ruffatti A, Legnani C, et al: Incidence of a first thromboembolic event in asymptomatic carriers of high-risk antiphospholipid antibody profile: a multicenter prospective study. *Blood* 118:4714–4718, 2011.

Pengo V, Banzato A, Bison E, et al: Antiphospholipid syndrome: critical analysis of the diagnostic path. *Lupus* 19:428–431, 2010.

Perez-Sanchez C, Ruiz-Limon P, Aguirre MA, et al: Mitochondrial dysfunction in antiphospholipid syndrome: implications in the pathogenesis of the disease and effects of coenzyme Q(10) treatment. *Blood* 119:5859–5870, 2012.

Rand JH, Wu XX, Quinn AS, et al: Human monoclonal antiphospholipid antibodies disrupt the annexin A5 anticoagulant crystal shield on phospholipid bilayers: evidence from atomic force microscopy and functional assay. *Am J Pathol* 163:1193–1200, 2003.

Ruiz-Irastorza G, Cuadrado MJ, Ruiz-Arruza I, et al: Evidence-based recommendations for the prevention and long-term management of thrombosis in antiphospholipid antibody-positive patients: report of a task force at the 13th International Congress on antiphospholipid antibodies. *Lupus* 20(2):206–218, 2011.

Schmidt-Tanguy A, Voswinkel J, Henrion D, et al: Antithrombotic effects of hydroxychloroquine in primary antiphospholipid syndrome patients. *J Thromb Haemost* 11:1927–1929, 2013.

Sciascia S, Cosseddu D, Montaruli B, et al: Risk Scale for the diagnosis of antiphospholipid syndrome. *Ann Rheum Dis* 70:1517–1518, 2011.

Tanimura K, Jin H, Suenaga T, et al: beta2-glycoprotein I / HLA class II complexes are novel autoantigens in antiphospholipid syndrome. *Blood* 125:2835–2844, 2015.

Ueki H, Mizushina T, Laoharatchatathanin T, et al: Loss of maternal annexin A5 increases the likelihood of placental platelet thrombosis and foetal loss. *Sci Rep* 2:827, 2012.

Wolgast LR, Arslan AA, Wu XX, et al: Reduction of annexin A5 anticoagulant ratio identifies antiphospholipid antibody-positive patients with adverse clinical outcomes. *J Thromb Haemost* 2017, In Press.

Xie H, Sheng L, Zhou H, et al: The role of TLR4 in pathophysiology of antiphospholipid syndrome-associated thrombosis and pregnancy morbidity. *Br J Haematol* 164:165–176, 2014.

CHAPTER 142

VENOUS THROMBOEMBOLISM

Deborah Siegal and Wendy Lim

Venous thromboembolism (VTE), encompassing both deep venous thrombosis (DVT) and pulmonary embolism (PE), remains a common medical condition that is associated with significant morbidity and mortality.

Although DVT can occur in any vein, it most commonly occurs in the leg veins. Superficial venous thrombosis occurs most frequently in varicosities and usually is self-limiting and benign. In contrast, DVT is a more serious condition. Thrombi localized to the deep calf veins often are small and therefore less commonly associated with clinically important PE or postthrombotic syndrome, but PE occurs in about 60% of patients with proximal DVT involving the popliteal, femoral, or iliac venous system.

Increased clinical suspicion and availability of reliable, noninvasive diagnostic tests have increased the frequency of diagnosis of acute VTE. In hospitalized patients this condition is largely preventable through the use of anticoagulant prophylaxis. In patients with established VTE advances in anticoagulant therapy have facilitated outpatient-based therapy.

PATHOGENESIS OF VENOUS THROMBOEMBOLISM AND CLINICAL RISK FACTORS

Venous thrombi are composed predominantly of fibrin and red cells, and usually arise in the large venous sinuses in the calf, in valve cusp pockets in the deep veins of the calf, or at sites of vessel damage. Venous thrombosis occurs when activation of blood coagulation exceeds the ability of the natural anticoagulant mechanisms and the fibrinolytic system to prevent clot formation. The current understanding of VTE pathogenesis was first described by Virchow more than 150 years ago. He proposed that thrombotic disorders were associated with the triad of stasis, vascular injury, and hypercoagulability. Stasis and vascular injury are the most frequent precipitants of VTE. In addition to activating coagulation, tissue damage and/or vascular damage can also impair fibrinolysis by reducing synthesis of tissue plasminogen activator (t-Pa) and by increasing endothelial cell production of plasminogen activator inhibitor type 1 (PAI-1), the major inhibitor of the fibrinolytic pathway.

Under normal circumstances, activated coagulation factors are diluted in the flowing blood and are neutralized by inhibitors on the surface of endothelial cells or by circulating proteinase inhibitors. Activated coagulation factors that escape regulation because of reduced levels of inhibitors or because they are generated in overwhelming amounts trigger the coagulation system and fibrin formation. Homeostatic mechanisms, including activation of the fibrinolytic system with release of t-PA and urokinase, are immediately invoked to reduce the likelihood of pathologic thrombus formation.

THROMBOGENIC FACTORS

Activation of Blood Coagulation

With the exception of small amounts of active factor VII, the coagulation factors circulate as inactive protein precursors, or zymogens. Each zymogen is converted into an active enzyme that then activates the next zymogen in the coagulation pathway (see Chapter 122). Traditionally the coagulation system has been divided into the intrinsic, extrinsic, and common pathways. Although these pathways reflect the way coagulation is measured in the laboratory, they do not reflect how coagulation occurs in vivo. In vivo, coagulation is primarily initiated via the tissue factor pathway. In this pathway, circulating activated factor VII (factor VIIa) binds to tissue factor at sites of vascular injury. The tissue factor–factor VIIa complex then activates factor IX and factor X. Levels of factor VIIa can be increased by factor Xa; however, this reaction is rapidly downregulated by tissue factor pathway inhibitor (TFPI). TFPI binds and inactivates factor Xa; the TFPI–factor Xa complex then binds the factor VIIa–tissue factor complex and prevents further activation of factor X.

In the presence of calcium, factor Xa binds to factor Va on the surface of activated platelets to form the prothrombinase complex, which converts prothrombin to thrombin. Thrombin then converts fibrinogen to fibrin, and activates platelets and factor XIII. Factor XIIIa, in the presence of calcium, cross-links fibrin, thereby stabilizing the clot. To ensure continuous generation of thrombin, thrombin and, to a lesser extent, factor Xa activate factor VIII and factor V, markedly accelerating the coagulation reactions involving these two cofactors. Thrombin also activates factor XI, which in turn activates additional factor IX, establishing a positive feedback loop.

Coagulation may be activated by contact of factor XII with collagen on exposed subendothelium of damaged vessels, by contact with prosthetic surfaces, by polyphosphates released from activated platelets, or by DNA or RNA released from damaged cells. There is mounting evidence that this pathway contributes to thrombosis. Thus mice deficient in factor XII or factor XI exhibit attenuated thrombus formation at sites of injury and factor XI knockdown with an antisense oligonucleotide attenuated VTE after elective knee arthroplasty. Therefore the contact pathway appears to be important for thrombus growth and stabilization.

Under most situations coagulation is initiated by exposure of blood to tissue factor made available locally as a result of vascular wall damage, by activation of endothelial cells, or by activated monocytes that migrate to areas of vascular injury. Factor X can be activated directly by extracts of malignant cells that contain a cysteine protease, which may be one of the mechanisms by which thrombosis is induced in patients with cancer. A factor elaborated by hypoxic endothelial cells also can directly activate factor X, potentially leading to thrombosis in patients with severe venous stasis where hypoxia occurs in the valve cusps.

Venous Stasis

Venous stasis is produced by immobility, venous obstruction, increased venous pressure, venous dilation, and increased blood viscosity. Venous return from the lower extremities is enhanced by venous valves, which prevent blood from pooling in the lower legs, and by contraction of the calf muscles, which propels blood upward from the extremities. Venous stasis may contribute to thrombogenesis by allowing stagnation of the blood with associated local hypoxia.

Immobility

Venous thrombosis can occur in immobilized persons because blood pools in the intramuscular sinuses of the calf, which are dilated during recumbency. Many clinical examples highlight the role of stasis in the pathogenesis of VTE. For example, the prevalence of VTE at autopsy is markedly increased in persons who were confined to bed for more than 1 week before death. Preoperative immobility is associated with a higher frequency of perioperative VTE, and postoperative immobility contributes to the high incidence of postoperative VTE in patients who have undergone hysterectomy, transabdominal prostatectomy, hip or knee arthroplasty, or surgery for fractures of the lower limb. The effect of immobility on thrombus formation is well illustrated by comparing the location of thrombosis in patients with paraplegia with that in patients who have had a stroke. Whereas thrombosis occurs with equal frequency in both legs in patients with paraplegia, it occurs more frequently in the paralyzed limb in patients with a stroke.

Venous Obstruction and Increased Venous Pressure

Venous obstruction contributes to the risk of VTE in patients with pelvic tumors and to recurrent venous thrombosis in patients with persistent obstruction because of residual proximal vein thrombosis. Raised central venous pressure produces venous stasis in the extremities, which may explain the high prevalence of venous thrombosis in patients with congestive heart failure. A similar mechanism may underlie the propensity for thrombosis in the left leg during pregnancy, presumably from obstruction of the left common iliac vein by the right common iliac artery, which is accentuated by the gravid uterus.

Increased Blood Viscosity and Venous Dilation

Venous stasis can be caused by increased blood viscosity or venous dilation. The blood viscosity can be increased by polycythemia, hypergammaglobulinemia, dysproteinemias, or increased fibrinogen levels. Stasis because of venous dilation may contribute to the increased risk of thromboembolism in patients with varicose veins and in elderly patients, particularly if they are bedridden. The capacity of estrogens to cause venous dilation may contribute to the increased prevalence of thrombosis during pregnancy, in women taking estrogen-containing oral contraceptive pills or estrogen replacement therapy.

Vessel Wall Damage

Damage or injury to the vascular endothelium exposes tissue factor, which triggers coagulation. Furthermore, the exposure of blood to the subendothelium leads to platelet adhesion, activation, and aggregation.

The vascular endothelium can be damaged by direct trauma, or it can be perturbed by exposure to endotoxin, inflammatory cytokines such as interleukin-1 and tumor necrosis factor, thrombin, or low oxygen tension. Perturbed endothelial cells synthesize tissue factor and PAI-1 and internalize thrombomodulin, promoting thrombogenesis. Furthermore, damaged endothelial cells may produce less t-PA, the principal activator of intravascular fibrinolysis.

Direct venous damage may lead to venous thrombosis in patients undergoing hip surgery, knee surgery, or varicose vein stripping, and in patients with severe burns, lower limb trauma, or central venous catheters.

PROTECTIVE MECHANISMS

Endothelial Protective Mechanisms

Normal vascular endothelium is not thrombogenic to flowing blood. Endothelial cell surface glycosaminoglycans, thrombomodulin, and endothelial protein C receptor (EPCR) are potent inhibitors of coagulation, and vessel wall generation of prostacyclin and nitric oxide and synthesis of plasminogen activators limit platelet aggregation and fibrin deposition.

Heparan sulfate, thrombomodulin, and EPCR present on the luminal surface of endothelial cells are important modulators of thrombin activity. Heparan sulfate, a glycosaminoglycan similar to heparin, catalyzes the inhibition of thrombin and factor Xa by antithrombin. Thrombomodulin serves as a surface-bound receptor for thrombin. Once bound to thrombomodulin, thrombin undergoes a change in substrate specificity that renders it incapable of activating platelets, of converting fibrinogen to fibrin, or of activating factors V, VIII, and XIII. Instead, once bound to thrombomodulin, thrombin becomes a potent activator of protein C. Activated protein C, together with protein S, its cofactor, downregulates coagulation by, proteolytically inactivating factors Va and VIIIa. EPCR enhances protein C activation by binding protein C and presenting it to the thrombin–thrombomodulin complex for activation.

Generation of plasminogen activators by vascular endothelium limits fibrin deposition, and platelet aggregation is inhibited by the release of prostacyclin (prostaglandin I_2) and endothelium-derived nitric oxide. Plasminogen binds to the cell surface, where it can be activated to plasmin by t-PA, thereby promoting local fibrinolytic activity.

Inhibitors of Blood Coagulation

Activated coagulation factors are serine proteases and their activity is modulated by several naturally occurring plasma inhibitors. The most important inhibitors of the blood coagulation system are antithrombin, protein C, and protein S. Congenital deficiency in one of these three proteins was found in 11% of patients enrolled in a prospective study of 2132 consecutive patients presenting with VTE. Abnormalities in the fibrinolytic system including congenital dysfibrinogenemias and deficiency of plasminogen can also predispose the affected person to thromboembolism.

HYPERCOAGULABLE STATES

In addition to deficiencies of antithrombin and proteins C and S, other hypercoagulable states associated with VTE include factor V Leiden (activated protein C resistance) and prothrombin G20210A mutations, hyperhomocysteinemia, antiphospholipid syndrome, pregnancy, and malignancy. Hypercoagulable states are the subject of Chapter 140.

NATURAL HISTORY OF VENOUS THROMBOEMBOLISM

Most DVTs are asymptomatic and confined to the intramuscular veins of the calf. These distal thrombi often undergo spontaneous lysis and rarely produce long-term sequelae. In contrast, complete lysis of proximal vein thrombosis is uncommon even when anticoagulant treatment is given.

The symptoms and signs of VTE are caused by obstruction to venous outflow, inflammation of the vessel wall or perivascular tissues, and embolization of thrombus into the pulmonary circulation. Asymptomatic PE is detected by perfusion lung scanning in approximately 50% of patients with documented proximal vein thrombosis. Most clinically significant and fatal PEs arise from DVT in the proximal veins of the legs. PE occurs less commonly and tends to be less extensive in patients with calf DVT than in those with proximal DVT. Asymptomatic DVT is found in 70% of patients who present with confirmed PE. The DVT in such patients tends to be extensive and involves the proximal veins.

Extensive DVT can lead to venous valvular damage, which is a hallmark of postthrombotic syndrome. Patients with a previous history of DVT are at increased risk of recurrence, particularly when patients are exposed to high-risk situations.

PROGNOSIS OF VENOUS THROMBOEMBOLISM

Untreated or inadequately treated VTE is associated with a high complication rate, which can be decreased markedly by adequate anticoagulant therapy. Approximately 20% of untreated asymptomatic calf vein thrombi and 20%–30% of untreated symptomatic calf vein thrombi extend into the popliteal vein; in the majority of cases this occurs within 1 week. When extension occurs and is untreated, it is associated with a 40%–50% risk of clinically detectable PE. Patients with proximal DVT who receive inadequate treatment have a 47% risk of recurrent VTE over 3 months. Approximately 10% of symptomatic PE cases are estimated to be fatal within 1 hour of symptom onset. Anticoagulant therapy reduces the mortality associated with PE; without therapy, mortality rates are as high as 30%. Clinically detectable recurrence occurs in fewer than 3% of patients with proximal DVT during anticoagulant therapy. The most important determinant of VTE recurrence following discontinuation of anticoagulant therapy is the presence or absence of identifiable risk factors at diagnosis. VTE associated with transient surgical or nonsurgical risk factors are associated with lower rates of VTE recurrence compared with those that are unprovoked (idiopathic). After 3 months of treatment for VTE associated with a transient surgical or nonsurgical (e.g., exogenous hormone use, immobility) risk factor, 12-month VTE recurrence rates are 1% and 5%, respectively. Subsequent recurrence rates are 0.5% and 2.5% per year. In contrast, the recurrence rate after at least 3 months of anticoagulant therapy for a first episode of unprovoked VTE is approximately 10% within the first 12 months and 5% per year thereafter. Patients with malignancy and those with a second episode of unprovoked VTE have high recurrence rates, up to 15% within 12 months and 7.5% per year thereafter following anticoagulant discontinuation.

LONG-TERM COMPLICATIONS OF VENOUS THROMBOEMBOLISM

Postthrombotic Syndrome

The postthrombotic syndrome is caused by venous hypertension, usually resulting from valve damage. Valve damage results in malfunction of the muscular pump mechanism, which leads to increased pressure in the deep calf veins during ambulation. The high pressure ultimately renders the perforating veins of the calf incompetent, so that blood flow is directed from the deep veins into the superficial venous system during muscular contraction. This leads to edema and impaired viability of subcutaneous tissues and, in its most severe form, to venous ulceration. Outflow obstruction initially may be bypassed by the development of collateral veins, but with time, the veins distal to the obstruction become dilated, and their valves become incompetent.

In patients whose thrombosis extends into the iliofemoral veins, the leg swelling at initial presentation may not resolve entirely. This is in contrast to patients with less extensive proximal vein thrombosis, in whom the swelling may subside after initial treatment but recur months or years later. Other symptoms and signs of the postthrombotic syndrome may be delayed for 5–10 years after the initial thrombotic event. These symptoms include pain in the calf that is relieved with rest and leg elevation, skin pigmentation and induration around the ankle and lower third of the calf, and ulceration in the region of the medial malleolus.

Patients with extensive thrombosis involving the iliofemoral vein frequently have greater disability and may have venous claudication, characterized by incapacitating, bursting pain with exercise. This complication rarely occurs in patients with thrombosis involving the more distal veins.

The clinical spectrum of the postthrombotic syndrome varies from a course that may mimic acute DVT to one of persistent leg pain that is worse at the end of the day and is associated with dependent edema, stasis pigmentation, and, in its most severe form, skin ulceration. Rarely, patients may complain of venous claudication

on walking. When symptoms are acute or subacute in onset, a diagnosis of postthrombotic syndrome should be considered only after recurrent DVT has been excluded by objective testing. There is no single definitive diagnostic test for the postthrombotic syndrome, but a history of objectively documented DVT, appropriate clinical findings, and evidence of venous reflux or outflow obstruction on venous ultrasonography constitute sufficient evidence to make this diagnosis.

The frequency with which postthrombotic syndrome occurs after VTE is controversial, with contemporary studies reporting incidence rates of 20%–80%. Severe postthrombotic syndrome occurs in approximately 5%–10% of patients. Risk factors for postthrombotic syndrome include proximal location of thrombosis (especially femoral or iliac veins), ipsilateral recurrent thrombosis, older age, obesity, and inadequate anticoagulant treatment.

Postthrombotic syndrome can cause significant disability and impairs quality of life. The clinical severity of postthrombotic syndrome can be assessed using the Villalta scale, a validated scoring system. Treatment for acute DVT may reduce the long-term risk of postthrombotic syndrome. In addition, there is conflicting evidence regarding the effectiveness of below-knee graduated compression stockings for reducing the risk of postthrombotic syndrome in patients with DVT. Other conservative measures may include exercise, limb elevation, compression bandages, pharmacologic management of edema, and careful attention to skin care.

Chronic Thromboembolic Pulmonary Hypertension

Chronic thromboembolic pulmonary hypertension (CTEPH) is a rare complication typically occurring within 2 years of acute PE. Patients with CTEPH present with exertional dyspnea that may progress to dyspnea at rest. With worsening pulmonary hypertension, patients may report signs or symptoms of right ventricular dysfunction such as lower extremity edema. CTEPH should be considered in patients presenting with signs and symptoms consistent with pulmonary hypertension, especially if they have a history of VTE or risk factors for VTE.

Echocardiography is a useful, noninvasive method of evaluating estimated systolic pulmonary artery pressure, right atrial enlargement, right ventricular systolic dysfunction, and septal displacement suggesting pulmonary hypertension. Ventilation/perfusion (V/Q) lung scanning has higher sensitivity for CTEPH than computed tomography (CT) pulmonary angiogram and is the preferred initial diagnostic test in this setting. Subsequent CT pulmonary angiogram is then used to exclude competing diagnoses that can cause perfusion defects on V/Q scanning.

Medical therapy for CTEPH includes anticoagulation, and pulmonary vasodilatory and remodeling therapies that are not curative and modestly improve symptoms. Medical therapy is administered at specialized centers and is reserved for patients who are not surgical candidates or as a bridge to surgical intervention. Surgical management with pulmonary thromboendarterectomy is the only potentially curative treatment option and is conducted at specialized centers.

DIAGNOSIS OF VENOUS THROMBOEMBOLISM

The diagnosis of VTE is based on objective testing as opposed to clinical assessment, which may be subjective.

Deep Venous Thrombosis

Clinical Manifestations

DVT classically causes swelling, pain, and erythema of the affected extremity. Proximal vein lower extremity DVT is more likely to be symptomatic than calf vein thrombosis. Patients with massive thrombosis involving the iliac and femoral veins may present with phlegmasia cerulea dolens, which is severe leg pain with swelling, cyanosis, venous gangrene, compartment syndrome, and arterial compromise. Patients with phlegmasia cerulea dolens may experience circulatory collapse and shock, which may result in death or loss of the affected limb.

Differential Diagnosis

The differential diagnosis of patients with suspected DVT includes musculoskeletal disorders (muscle or tendon strains or tears), lymphatic obstruction, venous insufficiency, a ruptured popliteal (Baker) cyst, cellulitis, sciatica, muscle hematoma, and postthrombotic syndrome.

OBJECTIVE DIAGNOSTIC TESTS FOR DEEP VENOUS THROMBOSIS

Both invasive and noninvasive tests are useful for the diagnosis of DVT. Venography is the only invasive test of proven value, and venous compression ultrasonography is the most widely studied and used noninvasive test. Although other imaging modalities have been studied (e.g., magnetic resonance direct thrombus imaging), these are not commonly performed.

Venography

Venography remains the reference standard for the diagnosis of DVT, although it is rarely performed because of the availability of reliable noninvasive tests. Venography is technically difficult, and its proper execution and interpretation require considerable experience. Venography may produce superficial phlebitis and can cause DVT, but with good technique ascending venography outlines the entire deep venous system of the lower extremities, including the calf and iliac veins. It is currently used only when noninvasive testing is not feasible or the results of such testing are inconclusive.

Venous Compression Ultrasonography

Venous ultrasonography is performed using a high-resolution real-time scanner equipped with a 5-MHz electronically focused linear array transducer. The common femoral vein and femoral artery are first located in the groin, with the patient in a supine position. The femoral vein (a deep vein) is then examined along its course. Next, the popliteal vein is located and examined down to the level of its trifurcation into the peroneal and tibial veins. At each of these locations, the vein being examined is compressed gently but firmly with the transducer probe, and the results are observed on the monitor. Hard copies from freeze-frame images of both stages of the procedure are obtained and serve as a permanent record.

In symptomatic patients, venous compression ultrasonography has a sensitivity and specificity for detection of proximal DVT (femoral or popliteal vein) of more than 95%. However, ultrasonography is less sensitive for detection of calf vein thrombosis. Ultrasound examination can be repeated 7 days after the initial study to increase its sensitivity for detection of clinically important calf vein thrombosis and to improve the safety of diagnostic strategies that do not include venography in patients with suspected calf vein thrombosis. This strategy will detect the 10%–30% of calf vein thrombi that extend proximally. If the ultrasound examination result remains negative after 7 days, the risk of clinically important proximal extension is negligible, and it is safe to withhold antithrombotic treatment.

If the field of examination is extended to the distal popliteal vein and the proximal deep calf veins, venous ultrasonography detects approximately 50% of calf vein thrombi in symptomatic patients. Although there are reports that ultrasound examination of the calf

can reliably detect thrombi, most such reports have not used venography as their reference standard. Furthermore, whether the value of this test is maintained when it moves from highly specialized vascular laboratories into community ultrasonography laboratories is unknown. A potential limitation of venous ultrasonography is its inability to visualize the iliac veins and the segment of the superficial femoral vein within the femoral canal. This is not a serious limitation because isolated thrombi within the femoral canal or the iliac vein are rare. Furthermore, the obstruction produced by iliac vein thrombi often limits the compressibility of the common femoral vein segment and hence will be detected indirectly. Doppler color flow can also be used to assess for blood flow and occlusion within a vein. The combination of compression ultrasonography and Doppler is often referred to as duplex ultrasonography.

D-Dimer Assays

D-dimer assays use mono- or polyspecific antibodies against D-dimer to provide quantitative or qualitative data on the concentration of D-dimer in whole blood or plasma. D-dimer is the product of lysis of cross-linked fibrin and the levels of D-dimer are increased in patients with acute VTE. However, the test is nonspecific because the level of D-dimer can be increased in a variety of other conditions, including malignancy, inflammatory conditions, and infections. Therefore the D-dimer assay is most useful as a tool to rule out suspected DVT.

D-dimer assays have two principal limitations: (1) a positive test result is nonspecific and should not be used as the sole criterion for diagnosis of VTE, and (2) numerous test kits are available that have different sensitivities for VTE. Thus D-dimer results are not interchangeable between kits. D-dimer assays employ different standards with some using fibrinogen and others using D-dimer. This results in differences in reporting because laboratory cut-offs depend on which standard is used. This has led to confusion among clinicians regarding the use of D-dimer assays. Further, the use of an insensitive D-dimer assay to rule out VTE could result in omission of required diagnostic testing, thereby placing patients at risk for PE and death.

The optimal setting for use of a D-dimer assay is in the assessment of patients with a low clinical pretest probability of VTE. The combination of a low pretest probability (determined using a validated scoring system) and a negative result with a validated D-dimer assay rules out the diagnosis of acute VTE, obviating the need for additional testing. Evaluation of the levels of D-dimer may be of value in patients with suspected recurrent VTE, and it may assist in decision-making about optimal duration of anticoagulation.

DIAGNOSTIC STRATEGIES FOR ACUTE DEEP VENOUS THROMBOSIS

Diagnostic algorithms for the noninvasive diagnosis of clinically suspected VTE are presented in Fig. 142.1. If compression ultrasonography is not immediately available, patients can be empirically anticoagulated pending diagnostic testing on the subsequent day. In assessing patients with suspected acute DVT, clinical prediction rules assign a clinical pretest probability (high, intermediate, or low probability) based on the clinical manifestations and the presence or absence of risk factors. The Wells clinical prediction rule for DVT assigns a risk category based on the following factors: active cancer (or cancer treated within the previous 6 months), calf swelling ≥3 cm compared to the asymptomatic leg, swelling of superficial veins (nonvaricose), unilateral pitting edema, tenderness along the deep venous system, such as recent immobilization (≥3 days) or major surgery (within 12 weeks), and absence of alternative diagnosis. Acute DVT can be excluded in patients with a low clinical probability (based on a validated clinical prediction rule such as the Wells score) and negative D-dimer. Patients with moderate or high clinical probability should proceed to objective testing. Patients

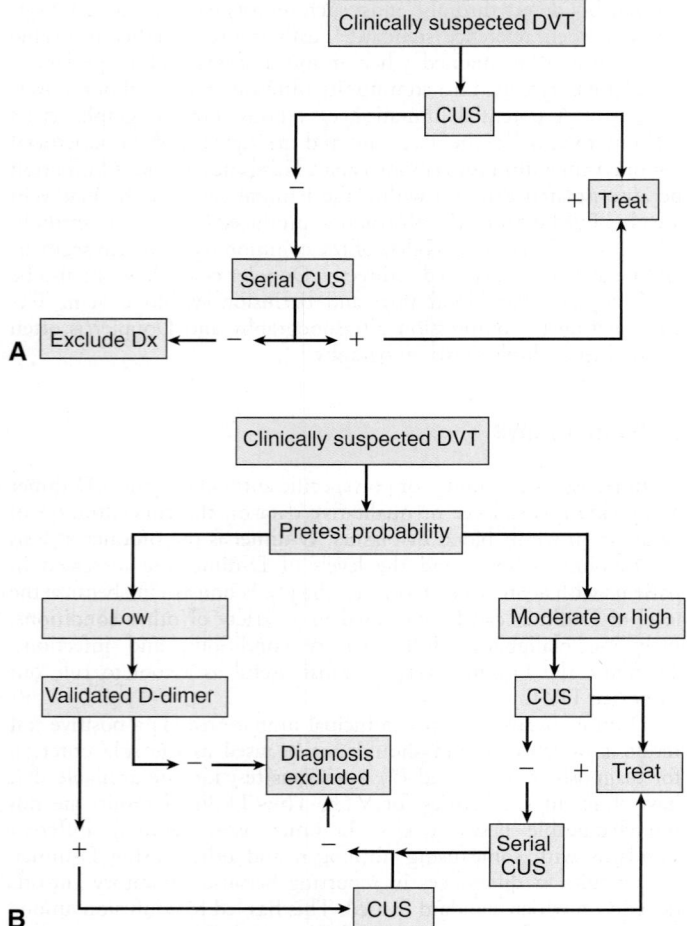

Fig. 142.1 DIAGNOSTIC ALGORITHMS FOR THE MANAGEMENT OF PATIENTS WITH SUSPECTED DEEP VENOUS THROMBOSIS. (A) Ultrasound examination–based strategy. (B) Clinical probability–based strategy. *CUS,* Compression ultrasound; *DVT,* deep venous thrombosis.

with a high clinical pretest probability and a negative noninvasive test result should prompt further investigation with or serial ultrasonography.

In approximately 70% of patients referred for clinically suspected DVT, the diagnosis will be excluded by objective tests. Of the 30% who have DVT, approximately 85% will have proximal vein thrombosis, and the remainder will have thrombosis confined to the calf.

PULMONARY EMBOLISM

Clinical Manifestations

The most frequently reported symptom of PE is dyspnea. Chest pain is common and typically pleuritic in nature but may be substernal and compressing. Hemoptysis is a less frequent feature.

The physical signs of PE are nonspecific. Syncope usually is associated with massive PE and is caused by a reduction in cardiac output. This in turn results in hypotension and transient impairment of cerebral blood flow. Approximately 5%–10% of patients present with shock.

Although 70% of patients with PE have venographic evidence of DVT at presentation, fewer than 20% of these patients have leg symptoms. Massive PE causes tachypnea, tachycardia, cyanosis, and hypotension. In these patients, cardiac examination may reveal a right ventricular heave, a loud pulmonary second sound, and a gallop rhythm. Physical examination of the chest may be normal, or

nonspecific abnormalities may be detected. Patients with pulmonary infarction or atelectasis may have reduced movement of the affected portion of the chest.

Differential Diagnosis

The differential diagnosis of dyspnea and pleuritic chest pain, in addition to PE, includes pneumonia, pleurisy, chest wall pain, pericarditis, atelectasis, pneumothorax, acute bronchitis, acute bronchiolitis, and acute bronchial obstruction as a result of mucous plugging or bronchoconstriction.

Diagnosis

The clinical diagnosis of PE requires objective testing. The chest radiograph is not specific for PE and usually does not show any diagnostic abnormality. Nevertheless, it is useful in excluding other causes for the presenting symptoms (e.g., pneumothorax) and is essential for interpreting V/Q lung scan findings. The electrocardiogram (ECG) is frequently normal or may show nonspecific abnormalities (e.g., sinus tachycardia). However, in the appropriate clinical setting, ECG evidence of right ventricular strain is strongly suggestive of PE. Elevated levels of cardiac troponin, brain natriuretic peptide (BNP) or N-terminal pro-BNP (NT-proBNP) can result from right ventricular strain and associated cardiomyocyte stretch.

OBJECTIVE DIAGNOSTIC TESTS FOR PULMONARY EMBOLISM

Pulmonary Angiography

Although pulmonary angiography is the reference standard for establishing the presence or absence of PE, it is no longer routinely used in clinical practice because of the availability of noninvasive imaging modalities such as CT and V/Q lung scanning.

Helical Computed Tomography Scanning

Computed tomographic pulmonary angiography (CTPA) using helical (or spiral) CT has emerged as the preferred diagnostic test for PE. When performed in experienced clinical centers with use of validated scanning protocols, helical CTPA is a useful tool to rule out PE in patients with compatible clinical symptoms with a sensitivity of 83% and specificity of 96%. The use of multiple detectors allows direct detailed visualization of the pulmonary arteries. Although less than 2% of patients with negative CTPA develop symptomatic VTE during follow-up, patients with a negative CTPA and high clinical probability should undergo bilateral leg compression ultrasonography to exclude DVT.

Ventilation/Perfusion Lung Scan

The V/Q lung scan consists of a perfusion and a ventilation component. For the perfusion component, particles of isotopically labeled microaggregates of human albumin are injected intravenously and become trapped in the pulmonary capillary bed. Their distribution reflects lung blood flow and is recorded with an external photoscanner. A normal perfusion scan excludes PE, but an abnormal perfusion scan is nonspecific.

Ventilation lung scanning is performed using either radioactive gases or aerosols that are inhaled and exhaled by the patient while a gamma camera records the distribution of radioactivity within the alveolar gas exchange units. The purpose of ventilation imaging is to improve the specificity of perfusion scanning for the diagnosis of PE. A high-probability V/Q scan (in which a segmental or greater area is ventilated but not perfused) has a positive predictive value for PE of more than 90%, obviating the need for additional testing.

The relative ease and accessibility of CT scanning has reduced the use of V/Q scanning for the diagnosis of PE. However, V/Q scanning is frequently preferred in two patient populations: young patients and those with impaired renal function. CT scanning exposes patients to a higher dose of radiation than V/Q scanning, raising concern regarding the risk of subsequent cancer. Although this risk varies depending on a number of factors, concern about increasing the risk of breast cancer in young women has prompted use of V/Q scanning preferentially in this population. In patients with impaired renal function, contrast dye administration for the CT scan can induce contrast nephropathy, increasing mortality up to 30% after such a procedure. V/Q lung scanning should ideally be reserved for patients with normal chest radiographs because preexisting lung disease may result in indeterminate scans.

Patients with large perfusion defects (involving one or more segments or more extensive defects) and a V/Q mismatch have a 90% probability of PE. Patients with a normal perfusion scan have less than a 2% probability of having PE, excluding the diagnosis. However, most patients who have V/Q scanning performed will have neither of these findings; rather, they will have either matched defects or small perfusion defects (indeterminate scan). Patients with these findings require further investigation with either pulmonary angiography or objective tests for DVT of the lower extremities. A patient with suspected PE, an indeterminate V/Q scan result, and positive findings on compression ultrasound examination of the lower extremities can be assumed to have PE. A patient with suspected PE, an indeterminate scan, and a negative result on leg compression ultrasound examination requires additional testing (e.g., serial compression ultrasound examination after 7 days) because the thrombus may have completely embolized to the lungs.

Diagnostic Strategy for Pulmonary Embolism

A diagnostic algorithm for the management of clinically suspected PE is shown in Fig. 142.2. After a history and physical examination, ECG, and chest radiography, the clinical probability of PE should be assessed using a validated clinical prediction rule. The Wells clinical prediction rule assigns a pretest clinical probability based on the presence of the following: clinical signs of DVT, recent immobilization or surgery, heart rate above 100 beats/min, previous history of VTE, hemoptysis, active malignancy, absence of alternative diagnosis.

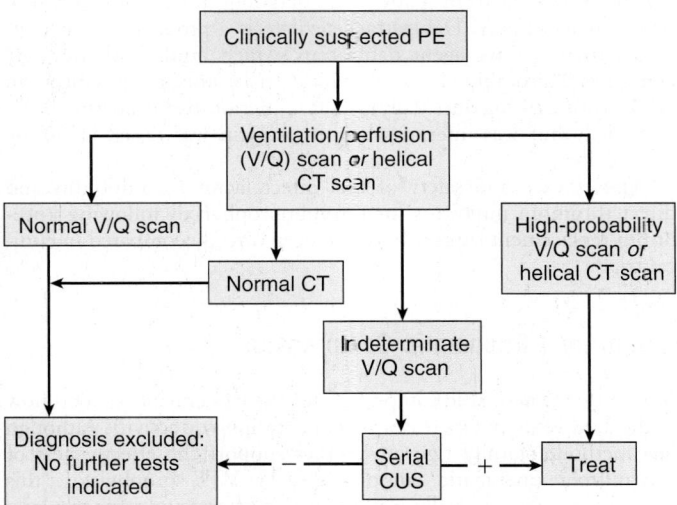

Fig. 142.2 DIAGNOSTIC ALGORITHM FOR THE MANAGEMENT OF PATIENTS WITH SUSPECTED PULMONARY EMBOLISM. *CT*, Computed tomography; *CUS*, compression ultrasound; *PE*, pulmonary embolism *V/Q*, ventilation/perfusion.

A low clinical pretest probability combined with a normal D-dimer excludes PE. Patients with intermediate or high pretest probability should undergo further testing. A negative helical CTPA or a normal perfusion lung scan result rules out clinically significant PE, and anticoagulant therapy can be withheld. If an intraluminal filling defect is seen on helical CTPA or the perfusion scan demonstrates one or more segmental (or larger) defects and ventilation to these regions is normal, a diagnosis of PE is made. Although a V/Q mismatch supports a diagnosis of PE, a V/Q "match" does not exclude PE, and further objective testing is required in these patients. Similarly, the diagnosis of PE cannot be excluded in patients with small perfusion defects (one or more subsegmental defects) or those with indeterminate lung scan findings (in which the perfusion defects correspond with abnormalities on the chest radiograph). In these patients, venous ultrasonography should be performed. If DVT is documented, a diagnosis of PE can be assumed, and anticoagulant therapy should be started. However, if results on these tests are negative, additional objective investigations (e.g., pulmonary angiography) are required in patients with a high clinical pretest probability. For those with a lower pretest probability of PE, an alternative strategy is to withhold anticoagulants and to perform serial noninvasive tests to detect venous thrombosis.

DIAGNOSIS OF ACUTE RECURRENT VENOUS THROMBOEMBOLISM

The diagnosis of acute recurrent VTE is challenging because the clinical manifestations of recurrence are nonspecific. In addition, there are no clinical prediction rules specifically validated for patients with suspected recurrence, and diagnostic tests for acute VTE have limitations in this setting. Following treatment of acute DVT, incomplete resolution of thrombosis may be evident as chronic venous occlusion on compression ultrasound, making it difficult to identify new abnormalities. With respect to PE, the interpretation of repeat CTPA or V/Q scanning may be difficult because of thrombus migration and variable rates of clot resolution. Therefore comparison with prior imaging can facilitate diagnosis of acute recurrence. D-dimer testing has limited utility in this setting because of the high frequency of positive D-dimer results in patients with suspected recurrence.

When assessing patients for recurrence, the adequacy of anticoagulant therapy is an important consideration (e.g., nonadherence, subtherapeutic international normalized ratio [INR] measurements, temporary interruption for procedure or surgery). Recurrent thrombosis despite adequate therapeutic anticoagulation can be seen in patients with cancer or those with the antiphospholipid antibody syndrome.

Many patients with a history of VTE will have a heightened level of concern about the risk of recurrent thrombosis, prompting them to seek testing for recurrent thrombosis even with trivial symptoms. Such patients require careful clinical and radiologic evaluation. If there is no evidence of acute recurrence, they may require counseling and education about their condition.

Patients with suspected recurrence should be treated empirically with anticoagulant therapy pending investigations.

Acute Recurrent Deep Venous Thrombosis

The optimal diagnostic strategy for suspected recurrent DVT is uncertain. The clinical history may be helpful in determining the likelihood of recurrent thrombosis. Leg pain with ambulation and leg swelling that is relieved with overnight rest is typical of the postthrombotic syndrome. New clinically significant and persistent leg swelling, particularly if the symptoms do not abate overnight, is consistent with recurrent thrombosis and should prompt diagnostic evaluation.

To establish a diagnosis of recurrent DVT, one must demonstrate a new thrombus in a previously unaffected venous segment. A normal result on ultrasound study does not rule out recurrent calf vein thrombosis and requires that additional testing with serial ultrasonography be performed if this is suspected. If the lack of compressibility of the veins or an intraluminal filling defect with flow seen on Doppler ultrasound studies is visualized in the venous segment previously affected, these tests are not sufficiently reliable to either confirm or rule out acute thrombosis. In these cases, serial testing to detect extension may be useful. Alternately, if the patient had a follow-up ultrasound examination, comparison with previous imaging may be useful.

Acute Recurrent Pulmonary Embolism

Patients presenting with clinical symptomatology consistent with an acute recurrent PE should be assessed urgently. Empiric anticoagulant therapy should be provided if diagnostic testing is delayed. A significant proportion of patients have persistent residual defects on CTPA or V/Q scanning even up to 11 months after the acute PE. Therefore baseline imaging (e.g., at the completion of anticoagulant treatment) can facilitate diagnosis of recurrence by evaluating differences between tests. It is important to use the same imaging modality as baseline if possible because of poor agreement between CTPA and V/Q scanning for detecting residual defects. However, cost, availability, and clinical considerations (e.g., renal failure, radiation exposure, young age, pregnancy, underlying lung disease) also influence the choice of test.

Similar to the diagnosis of initial PE, recurrent PE can be diagnosed on CTPA in the presence of a new central filling defect or occlusion of segmental or more proximal branches of the pulmonary arteries.

PROPHYLAXIS OF VENOUS THROMBOEMBOLISM

PE is a common preventable cause of death in hospitalized patients. Hospitalized patients can be classified as having a low, moderate, or high risk for developing VTE. Effective prophylaxis is cost effective and is available for high-risk groups.

Low-Molecular-Weight Heparins and Fondaparinux

Low-molecular-weight heparins (LMWHs) exert their anticoagulant effect by preferentially catalyzing the inactivation of factor Xa by antithrombin. When used in prophylactic doses once or twice daily, LMWH is an effective and safe agent for VTE prophylaxis in medical and surgical patients. Anticoagulant monitoring is not required when used in prophylactic doses. It is at least as effective as standard low-dose UFH and warfarin in most patient populations.

The anticoagulant effect of LMWH is mediated by a unique pentasaccharide sequence in the heparin molecule that binds antithrombin. The pentasaccharide moiety has been synthesized chemically as fondaparinux. Extended use of fondaparinux following hip fracture surgery significantly reduces the risk of symptomatic VTE. In patients with acute coronary syndromes, fondaparinux given at prophylactic doses was associated with decreased bleeding complications compared with therapeutic doses of enoxaparin.

Low-Dose Unfractionated Heparin

Low doses of UFH prevent thrombosis by antithrombin-mediated inhibition of thrombin, factor Xa, and other serine proteases. For prophylaxis, UFH is usually given subcutaneously at a dose of 5000 units every 8–12 hours. Low-dose UFH prophylaxis does not require laboratory monitoring and is simple and convenient to administer. It is an acceptable option for moderate-risk general surgical and medical patients, and it reduces the risk of VTE by 50%–70%. When used in these doses, UFH is both highly effective and associated with only a small increase in the risk of bleeding. Although low-dose UFH is

effective in patients undergoing elective hip surgery and reduces the incidence of venous thrombosis by approximately 40%, it is less effective than other current prophylactic strategies and thus should be reserved for patients with renal failure in whom LMWH and fondaparinux are contraindicated. Low-dose UFH has not been shown to be effective in patients undergoing surgery for hip fracture or hip or knee arthroplasty. In addition, use of subcutaneous heparin may be associated with heparin-induced thrombocytopenia, particularly in the postoperative period.

Vitamin K Antagonists (Warfarin)

When administered in doses that increase the INR to 2.0–3.0, vitamin K antagonists (VKAs) effectively prevent postoperative VTE in patients in all risk categories. VKAs can be given preoperatively, at the time of surgery, or in the early postoperative period. The antithrombotic effect of VKAs is not achieved until the fourth or fifth day of administration. Nevertheless, when used in this fashion, VKAs are effective in very high-risk patient groups. Prophylaxis with VKAs is relatively inconvenient, however, because frequent INR monitoring and dose adjustments are necessary.

Direct Oral Anticoagulants for Orthopedic Thromboprophylaxis

Rivaroxaban and apixaban are oral direct factor Xa inhibitors with excellent bioavailability that have been studied in patients undergoing total knee- or hip-replacement surgery. In a pooled analysis of randomized trials, 10 mg/day of rivaroxaban was superior to enoxaparin (40 mg once daily or 30 mg every 12 hours) for prevention of symptomatic VTE and all-cause mortality with similar major bleeding rates. Apixaban is also associated with a similar risk of symptomatic VTE and major bleeding, and reduced risk of clinically relevant bleeding compared with enoxaparin. Overall, the net clinical benefit with rivaroxaban and apixaban is similar to that with enoxaparin. However, rivaroxaban and apixaban simplify extended out-of-hospital thromboprophylaxis compared with enoxaparin because they obviate the need for daily subcutaneous injections.

Although rivaroxaban and apixaban have also been evaluated for extended thromboprophylaxis in medically ill patients, the benefit-risk profile in this setting is less certain because of an increased risk of bleeding compared with shorter courses of prophylactic dose enoxaparin.

Dabigatran etexilate is an oral direct thrombin inhibitor that also has been evaluated in patients undergoing total knee- or hip-replacement surgery. Dabigatran etexilate is a prodrug that is converted to the active agent dabigatran, which binds both free and clot-bound thrombin. In large clinical trials, once-daily dabigatran (150 mg or 220 mg once daily) was noninferior to enoxaparin 40 mg once daily but was inferior when enoxaparin was dosed at 30 mg twice daily.

The efficacy and safety of oral direct factor Xa inhibitors and direct thrombin inhibitors for thromboprophylaxis following knee- or hip-replacement surgery have not been directly compared in clinical trials.

Intermittent Pneumatic Compression

Intermittent pneumatic compression of the legs enhances blood flow in the deep veins and increases systemic fibrinolytic activity. Although few methodologically rigorous studies support the effectiveness of intermittent pneumatic compression for VTE prophylaxis, this modality has few clinically important side effects and is particularly useful in patients who have a high risk of bleeding. It also is frequently used, albeit with little supporting evidence, during the operative procedure in patients undergoing extended-duration surgery and in patients after trauma. Intermittent compression is the prophylactic measure of choice in selected patients undergoing neurosurgical procedures; however, most of these patients should eventually receive pharmacologic thromboprophylaxis as well.

Graduated Compression Stockings

Graduated compression stockings also reduce venous stasis in the legs and are effective for preventing postoperative VTE in low- and moderate-risk general surgical patients and in medical or surgical patients with neurologic disorders, including paralysis of the lower limbs. However, graduated compression stockings may increase the risk of skin ulcers when used in hospitalized patients with stroke. In surgical patients, the combination of graduated compression stockings and low-dose UFH is significantly more effective than low-dose UFH alone. Use of graduated compression stockings alone, however, constitutes inadequate prophylaxis in patients undergoing surgery associated with a very high risk of thromboembolism. Graduated compression stockings are inexpensive and should be considered for use in all high-risk surgical patients even if other forms of prophylaxis are used.

TREATMENT OF VENOUS THROMBOEMBOLISM

The goals of treatment for VTE are to prevent death from PE, reduce morbidity from the acute event, decrease the risk of postthrombotic symptoms, and prevent CTEPH. All of these goals can be achieved with adequate anticoagulant therapy. Use of thrombolytic therapy or surgical thrombectomy is reserved for patients with severe disease or severe complications.

Anticoagulant Therapy for Treatment of Acute Venous Thromboembolism

The treatment of acute VTE currently involves administration of effective doses of anticoagulants as soon as the diagnosis is confirmed (or if testing is delayed and the clinical likelihood of disease is moderate or high, before confirmation of the diagnosis). Traditionally patients with acute VTE were admitted to hospital and given intravenous UFH, to achieve a therapeutic activated partial thromboplastin time (aPTT). A VKA, typically warfarin, was then started and the heparin continued until the INR was more than 2.0 on two consecutive measurements. Although this treatment strategy remains a practice standard, the vast majority of patients with acute DVT and/or PE can be managed in the outpatient setting because of the availability of safe and effective treatment options such as direct oral anticoagulants (DOACs; dabigatran, rivaroxaban, apixaban, edoxaban), LMWH, and fondaparinux. Patients who are hemodynamically stable, lack contraindications to treatment (e.g., severe thrombocytopenia, recent bleeding, severe renal or liver disease), have manageable symptoms, and are likely to be compliant with treatment are good candidates for outpatient therapy.

Low-Molecular-Weight Heparin and Fondaparinux

Treatment with LMWH or fondaparinux involves administration of weight-adjusted, once- or twice-daily subcutaneous injections that do not require routine monitoring of anticoagulant effect. However, the anticoagulant effect can be measured using anti–factor Xa activity assays calibrated for the specific drug for selected patients with anticoagulant-related complications such as bleeding or need for urgent surgery/procedure, those at the extremes of weight (<40 kg or >100 kg), or renal insufficiency. LMWH and fondaparinux should generally be avoided in patients with significant renal impairment (creatinine clearance <30 mL/min). For LMWH, typically one would target a peak anti-Xa level of 0.5–1.0 unit/mL measured 4 hours after a subcutaneous injection of LMWH using a twice-daily

dosing schedule. LMWH and fondaparinux do not have predictable effects on the aPTT and therefore cannot be monitored using this test.

Low-Molecular-Weight Heparin is the Treatment of Choice for Venous Thromboembolism Associated With Pregnancy and Cancer

VKAs, DOACs, and fondaparinux are contraindicated in pregnancy. In patients with cancer, use of LMWH is associated with a reduced risk of VTE recurrence and bleeding compared with VKA. Further, the anticoagulant effect of VKAs can be affected by reduced oral intake and concomitant medications which can lead to suboptimal anticoagulant therapy in cancer patients receiving chemotherapy.

Unfractionated Heparin

Although increasingly less common, selected patients may be admitted to the hospital for intravenous UFH therapy. There is no evidence that UFH therapy is superior to LMWH in any clinical setting. Practical considerations include the need for reliable intravenous access, frequent blood work, and infusion adjustment. Hence, intravenous UFH is typically reserved for patients at high risk of bleeding in whom rapid anticoagulant reversal may be necessary. Patients with significant renal impairment are also treated with UFH because LMWH is eliminated by the kidneys, leading to a risk of anticoagulant accumulation. UFH therapy can be monitored using the activated clotting time, the aPTT, or by heparin assays that measure the ability of heparin to accelerate the inactivation of factor Xa. It is important to give adequate doses of UFH at initial presentation because the risk of recurrent VTE is increased if there is failure to achieve a therapeutic level of anticoagulation. Accordingly, the aPTT ratio of 1.5 to 2.5 times the control should be maintained above a level equivalent to a heparin level of 0.3 to 0.7 units/mL, as determined by measuring anti-Xa activity. For most currently used aPTT reagents, this is equivalent to an aPTT ratio of 1.8–2.5 times the control value. To monitor UFH given by continuous intravenous infusion, the aPTT should be measured 6 hours after the bolus dose so that it reflects the anticoagulant effects of the infusion. If twice-daily subcutaneous UFH is given, a mid-interval aPTT is typically measured 6 hours after the injection. UFH can also be given in fixed doses without laboratory monitoring; in a study of more than 700 VTE patients, UFH was administered using a fixed, weight-adjusted dose without aPTT monitoring. The risks of bleeding and recurrent thrombosis were similar to those in patients treated with twice-daily LMWH.

Vitamin K Antagonists (Warfarin)

Because rapid anticoagulant effect is desired in the setting of acute VTE, initiation of warfarin therapy requires concomitant administration with a parenteral agent (UFH, LMWH), which should be continued for at least 5 days and until the INR has been between 2.0 and 3.0 on 2 consecutive days. An initial dose of 5–10 mg daily for 2 days can be given to most individuals, with doses less than 5 mg reserved for elderly patients. Subsequent dosing should be based on results of INR testing. The required maintenance dose of warfarin may be influenced by age, gender, race, nutritional status, organ function, and concomitant medications, and should be determined based on the results of routine INR monitoring. Women generally require lower warfarin doses than men. The warfarin dose variability is also affected by variation in the genotypes of the cytochrome P450 CYP2C9 and the vitamin K epoxide reductase complex, VKORC1. These enzymes influence the rate of warfarin metabolism and sensitivity, respectively. Studies using warfarin genotyping to optimize warfarin dosing have yielded conflicting results, and further study along with economic evaluation is ongoing.

Warfarin has numerous drug interactions including many commonly administered medications. Noninteracting medications should be prescribed preferentially in patients receiving warfarin to avoid adverse events. When noninteracting medications are unavailable, increased frequency of INR monitoring and dose adjustments enhance safety. Warfarin is contraindicated during pregnancy, but may be used during breastfeeding.

Direct Oral Anticoagulants

DOACs that target thrombin (dabigatran) and factor Xa (rivaroxaban, apixaban, edoxaban) are available for the treatment of acute VTE. These agents do not require routine anticoagulation monitoring and have fewer interactions with food and drugs compared with warfarin. Large phase III clinical trials have demonstrated that dabigatran, rivaroxaban, apixaban, and edoxaban are noninferior to the combination of LMWH/warfarin for the treatment of acute VTE. Treatment with LMWH is given for at least 5 days before dabigatran or edoxaban. DOACs should be avoided in patients with severe renal impairment (creatinine clearance <30 mL/min) and used with caution in those with weight above 120 kg, body mass index >40 kg/m^2, or active malignancy because of a lack of clinical efficacy and safety data in these populations.

Duration of Treatment

The optimal duration of oral anticoagulant therapy for treatment of VTE is unknown. Patients with VTE provoked by a clear transient risk factor are generally treated for 3 months. Patients with unprovoked (idiopathic) VTE should be treated for a minimum of 3 months, with consideration of extended therapy especially for patients at low bleeding risk in whom the clinical benefit of preventing VTE recurrence outweighs the risk of bleeding. Patients with a persistent, major risk factor for recurrence (e.g., malignancy, immobility) and patients who prefer to decrease their thrombotic risk should receive anticoagulation for longer periods or indefinitely with regular reassessments of the benefits and risks of ongoing therapy. At this time, there are no absolute predictors of recurrence, but recurrence appears to be more common in male patients and those with an elevated D-dimer assay at or around the time of anticoagulant discontinuation. The relationship between residual venous obstruction on ultrasound at the completion of initial treatment and recurrence risk requires further study.

Decisions regarding extended anticoagulant therapy should incorporate counselling regarding the expected risks and benefits, and patient values and preferences. Extended treatment reduces the risk of recurrent VTE by at least 80% with a small increased risk of bleeding. When prescribing apixaban, a reduced dose (2.5 mg twice daily) is used for secondary VTE prevention after initial 6 months of anticoagulant therapy. Low-dose aspirin reduces the risk of recurrence by approximately 30%. However, it is not considered an equivalent alternative to anticoagulant therapy given the reduced efficacy and should be reserved for patients wishing to discontinue anticoagulants who have no contraindication to aspirin therapy and/or have another indication for aspirin.

Inferior Vena Cava Filter

Anticoagulants are effective in reducing mortality from PE. However, some patients have relative or absolute contraindications to anticoagulant therapy. In these cases, there may be a role for inferior vena cava (IVC) filters (see Chapter 143). IVC filters do not treat VTE but are used to prevent PE in patients with DVT who cannot receive adequate anticoagulant therapy. In patients with active bleeding or a transient risk factor for bleeding (e.g., surgery), insertion of a temporary IVC filter followed by its removal and subsequent therapeutic anticoagulation when the bleeding risk is diminished should be considered. Although not formally evaluated in randomized trials, this strategy likely reduces the initial risk of bleeding while eliminating the long-term increased risk of DVT associated with permanent caval interruption. In contrast, patients who have a persistent major risk factor for bleeding may be considered for insertion of a permanent IVC filter because the mortality rate associated with major bleeding during therapeutic anticoagulation is approximately 20%. This procedure is associated with a significant risk of immediate worsening of leg symptoms because of blockage of the IVC by thrombus and a long-term increase in the risk of recurrent DVT.

Thrombolytic Therapy for Massive Pulmonary Embolism

Thrombolytic therapy with streptokinase, urokinase, or t-Pa is more effective than UFH alone in correcting the angiographic defects produced by PE, and may be better than UFH in preventing death in patients with massive PE associated with shock. Based on these findings, thrombolytic therapy is the treatment of choice for patients with massive PE associated with cardiovascular collapse.

Bleeding occurs more frequently with thrombolytic therapy than with UFH. The risk of hemorrhage increases with the duration of thrombolytic infusion and usually occurs at a site of previous surgery or trauma. Intracranial hemorrhage occurs in approximately 1% of patients at risk, approximately twice as frequently as with UFH treatment.

Catheter-Directed Thrombolysis for Deep Vein Thrombosis

Catheter-directed thrombolysis (CDT) involves direct injection of a thrombolytic agent through a catheter into the vein affected by DVT, which can also be combined with mechanical thrombus removal. In a small nonblinded randomized study, CDT reduced the risk of postthrombotic syndrome but not health-related quality of life after 24 months of follow-up compared with standard therapy. It has not been shown to reduce the risk of PE or mortality, and increases the risk of bleeding. At present there is insufficient high-quality evidence supporting a net clinical benefit of CDT given the bleeding risk. CDT may be considered at centers with technical expertise in CDT in consultation with a thrombosis expert for select patients presenting with recent (less than 14 days) iliofemoral DVT with severe symptoms and low bleeding risk.

Thromboendarterectomy for Pulmonary Embolism

Thromboendarterectomy is effective in selected cases of CTEPH with proximal pulmonary arterial obstruction. Urgent pulmonary embolectomy is usually reserved for patients with a saddle embolism lodged in the main pulmonary artery or for those with massive embolism whose blood pressure cannot be maintained despite thrombolytic therapy and vasopressor agents. Although this procedure can be successfully performed by experienced surgical teams, in inexperienced hands it is associated with high complication and mortality rates. Patients with repeated episodes of PE and significant chronic pulmonary hypertension with right ventricular compromise should be anticoagulated and monitored. If pulmonary pressures do not decrease, patients should be evaluated for surgical fitness. If deemed necessary, thromboendarterectomy should be carried out in centers with expertise with optimal perioperative management, within which the likelihood of success of the procedure is high.

VENOUS THROMBOSIS IN PREGNANCY

The risk of VTE is increased during pregnancy and the postpartum period. DVT is more common than PE and affects the left leg in greater than 80% of cases. Clinical prediction rules such as the Wells score and the use of D-dimer testing have not been validated in this setting. A high index of suspicion should be maintained in pregnant women presenting with signs or symptoms of VTE.

Pregnant women with suspected DVT should undergo proximal compression ultrasonography. However, standard compression ultrasound techniques are less sensitive for pelvic and iliac vein thromboses, which are more common in pregnancy. Pregnant women with suspected DVT and negative proximal compression ultrasound should undergo serial compression ultrasounds at 3 and 7 days. Anticoagulants can be safely withheld in patients with negative serial compression ultrasounds.

Pregnant women with suspected PE should undergo chest radiography with shielding of the abdomen to exclude alternative causes of presenting symptoms. Bilateral proximal compression ultrasounds should be done to assess for concurrent DVT in women with clinical suspicion of DVT which, if positive, would obviate the need for CTPA or V/Q scanning. Because of the low prevalence of coexistent DVT in pregnant women with suspected PE, routine compression ultrasonography in the absence of DVT symptoms may lead to delays in definitive diagnosis and treatment of PE. V/Q scanning is preferred over CTPA for diagnosis of PE in pregnancy because of reduced maternal exposure and similar fetal exposure to radiation.

Weight-adjusted LMWH is the treatment of choice for pregnancy-associated VTE. Although warfarin use during the first trimester is associated with teratogenicity, it is safe during breastfeeding. DOACs and fondaparinux, however, should be avoided during both pregnancy and breastfeeding. The duration of anticoagulant treatment for pregnancy-associated VTE is a minimum of 3 months, including the 6-week postpartum period.

CANCER-ASSOCIATED VENOUS THROMBOSIS

VTE occurs in up to 20% of patients with cancer and confers an increased risk of death, VTE recurrence, and bleeding. LMWH is the recommended treatment for acute cancer-associated VTE based on clinical data showing reduced risk of VTE recurrence with no increased risk of bleeding compared with VKA therapy. Anticoagulant treatment should be given for at least 3 months, with consideration of prolonged therapy for patients receiving ongoing cancer treatment or those with metastatic disease and who are not at high risk of bleeding.

Postoperative VTE prophylaxis with LMWH or low-dose UFH should be provided for cancer patients undergoing surgery. Extended-duration prophylaxis (4 weeks) can be considered for cancer patients at high risk for VTE and low risk for bleeding who are undergoing abdominal or pelvic surgery for cancer. Hospitalized cancer patients with reduced mobility should receive VTE prophylaxis with LMWH or low-dose UFH. In the outpatient setting, pharmacologic VTE prophylaxis is generally reserved for cancer patients with additional risk factors for VTE such as previous VTE, immobilization, or hormonal therapy treatment with angiogenesis inhibitors (thalidomide and lenalidomide).

SUGGESTED READINGS

Bell WR, Simon TL, DeMets DL: The clinical features of submassive and massive pulmonary emboli. *Am J Med* 62:355, 1977.

Castellucci LA, Cameron C, Le Gal G, et al: Clinical and safety outcomes associated with treatment of acute venous thromboembolism: a systematic review and meta-analysis. *JAMA* 312(11):1122–1135, 2014.

Collins R, Scrimgeour A, Yusuf S, et al: Reduction in fatal pulmonary embolism and venous thrombosis by perioperative administration of subcutaneous heparin. Overview of results of randomized trials in general, orthopedic, and urologic surgery. *N Engl J Med* 318:1162, 1988.

Colman RW, Marder VJ, Salzman EW, et al: Overview of hemostasis. In Colman RW, Hirsh J, Marder VJ, et al, editors: *Hemostasis and thrombosis:* *basic principles and clinical practice*, ed 3, Philadelphia, 1994, JB Lippincott, p 3.

Daly E, Vessey MP, Hawkins MM, et al: Risk of venous thromboembolism in users of hormone replacement therapy. *Lancet* 348:977, 1996.

Eriksson BI, Dahl OE, Rosencher N, et al: Dabigatran etexilate versus enoxaparin for prevention of venous thromboembolism after total hip replacement: a randomised, double-blind, non-inferiority trial. *Lancet* 370:949, 2007.

Eriksson BI, Dahl OE, Rosencher N, et al: Oral dabigatran etexilate vs. subcutaneous enoxaparin for the prevention of venous thromboembolism after total knee replacement: the RE-MODEL randomized trial. *J Thromb Haemost* 5:2178, 2007.

Freiman D: The structure of thrombi. In Colman RW, Hirsh J, Marder VJ, et al, editors: *Hemostasis and thrombosis: basic principles and clinical practice*, ed 2, Philadelphia, 1987, JB Lippincott.

Ginsberg JS, Brill-Edwards P, Burrows RF, et al: Venous thrombosis during pregnancy: leg and trimester of presentation. *Thromb Haemost* 67:519, 1992.

Ginsberg JS, Wells PS, Brill-Edwards P, et al: Application of a novel and rapid whole blood assay for D-dimer in patients with clinically suspected pulmonary embolism. *Thromb Haemost* 73:35, 1995.

Gómez-Outes A, Terleira-Fernández AI, Suárez-Gea ML, et al: Dabigatran, rivaroxaban, or apixaban versus enoxaparin for thromboprophylaxis after total hip or knee replacement: systematic review, meta-analysis, and indirect treatment comparisons. *BMJ* 344:e3675, 2012.

Grodstein F, Stampfer MJ, Goldhaber SZ, et al: Prospective study of exogenous hormones and risk of pulmonary embolism in women. *Lancet* 348:983, 1996.

Hull RD, Hirsh J, Carter CJ, et al: Diagnostic value of ventilation-perfusion lung scanning in patients with suspected pulmonary embolism. *Chest* 88:819, 1985.

Hull RD, Hirsh J, Jay RM: Different intensities of anticoagulation in the long-term treatment of proximal vein thrombosis. *N Engl J Med* 307:1676, 1982.

Kearon C, Ginsberg JS, Anderson DR, et al; SOFAST Investigators: Comparison of 1 month with 3 months of anticoagulation for a first episode of venous thromboembolism associated with a transient risk factor. *J Thromb Haemost* 2:743, 2004.

Kearon C, Ginsberg JS, Julian JA, et al: Comparison of fixed-dose weight-adjusted unfractionated heparin and low-molecular-weight heparin for acute treatment of venous thromboembolism. *JAMA* 296:935, 2006.

Lee AY, Levine MN, Baker AI, et al: Low-molecular-weight heparin versus a coumarin for the prevention of recurrent venous thromboembolism in patients with cancer. *N Engl J Med* 349:146, 2003.

Lensing AW, Prandoni P, Brandjes D, et al: Detection of deep-vein thrombosis by real-time B-mode ultrasonography. *N Engl J Med* 320:342, 1989.

Miller GA, Sutton GC, Kerr IH, et al: Comparison of streptokinase and heparin in treatment of isolated acute massive pulmonary embolism. *BMJ* 33:616, 1971.

Prandoni P, Lensing AW, Cogo A, et al: The long-term clinical course of acute deep venous thrombosis. *Ann Intern Med* 125:1, 1996.

Quiroz R, Kucher N, Zou KH, et al: Clinical validity of a negative computed tomography scan in patients with suspected pulmonary embolism: a systematic review. *JAMA* 293:2012, 2005.

Simonneau G, Sors H, Charbonnier B, et al: A comparison of low-molecular weight heparin with unfractionated heparin for acute pulmonary embolism. *N Engl J Med* 337:663, 1997.

The PIOPED Investigators: Value of the ventilation/perfusion scan in acute pulmonary embolism. Results of the Prospective Investigation of Pulmonary Embolism Diagnosis (PIOPED). *JAMA* 263:2753, 1990.

Tibbutt DA, Davies JA, Anderson JA, et al: Comparison by controlled clinical trial of streptokinase and heparin in treatment of life-threatening pulmonary embolism. *BMJ* 1:343, 1974.

Turkstra F, van Beek EJ, ten Cate JW, et al: Reliable rapid blood test for the exclusion of venous thromboembolism in symptomatic outpatients. *Thromb Haemost* 76:9, 1996.

Turpie AG, Bauer KA, Eriksson BI, et al: Fondaparinux vs enoxaparin for the prevention of venous thromboembolism in major orthopedic surgery: a meta-analysis of 4 randomized double-blind studies. *Arch Intern Med* 162:1833, 2002.

Turpie AG, Lassen MR, Eriksson BI, et al: Rivaroxaban for the prevention of venous thromboembolism after hip or knee arthroplasty. Pooled analysis of four studies. *Thromb Haemost* 105:444, 2011.

Virchow R: *Gesammalte abhandlungen zur wissenschaftlichen medtzin.* Frankfurt, 1856, Medinger Sohn & Company.

Wells PS, Brill-Edwards P, Stevens P, et al: A novel and rapid whole-blood assay for D-dimer in patients with clinically suspected deep vein thrombosis. *Circulation* 91(8):2184–2187, 1995.

Wells PS, Hirsh J, Anderson DR, et al: Accuracy of clinical assessment of deep-vein thrombosis. *Lancet* 345:1326, 1995.

CHAPTER 143

MECHANICAL INTERVENTIONS IN ARTERIAL AND VENOUS THROMBOSIS

Steven Sauk and Suresh Vedantham

Arterial and venous thromboses are common medical conditions that are associated with significant morbidity. Patients who suffer from acute occlusions of the peripheral arteries may present with ischemic extremities, culminating in limb loss or death if left untreated. Those who suffer from venous thrombosis are not only at significant risk for recurrent thrombotic episodes and pulmonary embolism (PE), but are also at risk for the postthrombotic syndrome (PTS), which can cause significant impairment of their long-term quality of life (QOL).

For many patients with symptomatic arterial or venous occlusions, surgical therapies are required in addition to standard medical treatments to provide optimal patient outcomes. Spurred by advances in vascular imaging and catheter/device technology, and driven by the clinical needs of the large number of vascular patients with concomitant comorbidities, many patients are now referred for nonsurgical, imaging-guided endovascular interventions to eliminate thrombi and to treat associated vascular lesions. In this chapter, we discuss the use of catheter-based interventions in the management of arterial and venous thromboses.

OVERVIEW OF CATHETER-BASED THROMBOLYTIC INTERVENTIONS

Systemic thrombolysis, which refers to the dissolution of thrombus via the administration of a fibrinolytic drug into an intravenous line distant from the affected site, can be a valuable treatment option for acute myocardial infarction (MI), massive PE, and acute ischemic stroke. A primary advantage of the systemic administration route is the ability to rapidly initiate therapy in almost any clinical setting, without the need for specialized technical expertise or hospital resources. However, only a fraction of systemically administered drug reaches the target vessel. This problem is compounded when there is complete occlusion of blood flow in the target vessel such that access of the fibrinolytic drug to the interior of the thrombus is precluded. For acute MI and stroke, this limitation is overcome by the use of relatively high concentrations of fibrinolytic drugs (e.g., 50–100 mg of recombinant tissue plasminogen activator [rt-PA]) and the ability of arterial pulsations to force sufficient amounts of the drug into the fresh thrombus that occludes a small (2–4 mm) coronary or cerebral artery to effect fibrinolysis. However, with these high doses of fibrinolytic drugs, there is a small but significantly increased risk of major bleeding, a price that physicians are willing to pay given the potentially fatal consequences of ongoing vascular occlusion in these critical sites.

For occlusions in the peripheral arteries and veins, however, systemic fibrinolysis is not sufficiently effective to justify the attendant risks, presumably because of the larger vessel size, greater thrombus burden, and the presence of mature thrombus that is less susceptible to dissolution. For these reasons, catheter-directed fibrinolysis and mechanical methods for thrombus extraction and dissolution have been developed.

Catheter-Directed Intrathrombus Thrombolysis

Catheter-directed intrathrombus thrombolysis (CDT) refers to the infusion of a fibrinolytic drug directly into the thrombosed vessel via a catheter that has been inserted into that vessel using imaging guidance. The rationale for CDT is to improve the efficacy of thrombus dissolution by achieving a higher intrathrombus concentration of fibrinolytic drug, and to reduce the risk of hemorrhage by enabling the use of lower total fibrinolytic drug doses than those required for systemic fibrinolysis. Although several catheters and devices have been approved by the US Food and Drug Administration (FDA) for this purpose, none of the currently available fibrinolytic drugs is FDA approved for the specific indication of peripheral arterial or venous thrombosis.

Although the procedural details are beyond the scope of this chapter, the principles of CDT are reviewed here[1] (Fig. 143.1). First, a vascular access site is selected based upon the thrombus location and extent, and needle access into the vessel is obtained. With ultrasound-guided venipuncture, access site bleeding is rare. Under fluoroscopic guidance, the needle is exchanged over a guidewire for an angiographic catheter and iodinated contrast is injected to delineate the location, extent, and morphology of the thrombus and the status of other relevant vessels in the limb. The angiographic catheter is then exchanged for a specially designed infusion catheter with multiple side holes (akin to a soaking garden hose) that is positioned such that the side holes are embedded within the thrombus-containing vascular segment. Fibrinolytic drug is then infused. The drugs and doses commonly used for this purpose include rt-PA (0.01 mg/kg/hour up to 1.0 mg/hour), and rt-PA variants such as reteplase (0.25–0.75 units/hour), and tenecteplase (0.25–0.50 mg/hour).[1,2] The procedure is done under conscious sedation and with local anesthesia, and the heart rate, blood pressure, and oxygen saturation are continuously monitored.

Patients are then transferred to an observation unit, usually an intensive care or step-down unit, for monitoring during the fibrinolytic drug infusion. Typically a concomitant infusion of unfractionated heparin at subtherapeutic doses is administered and the hemoglobin, activated partial thromboplastin time (aPTT), and in some centers, the fibrinogen level are measured every 6–8 hours while the fibrinolytic drug is given. Patients are monitored closely for evidence of bleeding and for changes in limb status, and the drug infusion rate is adjusted (or stopped entirely) as necessary. After 6–18 hours, patients return to the procedure room for a follow-up venogram or angiogram to assess the extent of thrombus dissolution. The infusion catheter may be repositioned and the infusion continued if there is residual thrombus. Once thrombolysis is nearly complete, the fibrinolytic drug infusion is stopped and, based on the results of the venogram or angiogram, a decision is made as to whether adjunctive treatment with balloon angioplasty or stent placement is needed—if so, this is performed, usually through the same vascular access site during the same procedure session. The catheter and sheath are then removed and systemic anticoagulation at fully therapeutic levels is reinstituted. The treated limb is closely monitored for improvement in pain, perfusion abnormalities (arterial), and/or swelling (venous).

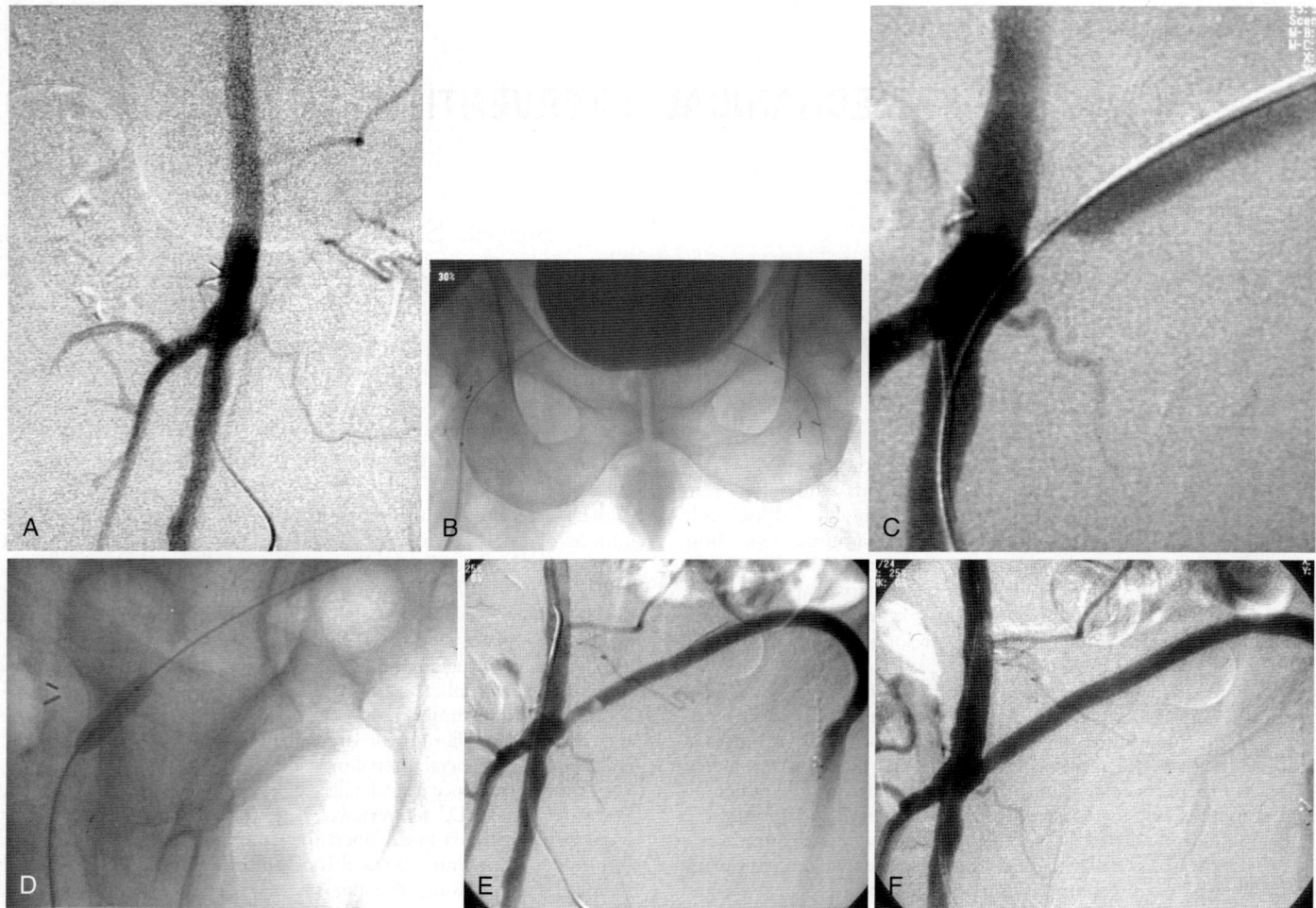

Fig. 143.1 A 67-YEAR-OLD MAN WITH A CHRONIC LEFT ILIAC ARTERY OCCLUSION AND A RIGHT-TO-LEFT FEMORAL-FEMORAL ARTERIAL BYPASS PRESENTS WITH LEFT FOOT PAIN AND PULSELESSNESS. (A) Digital subtraction arteriography reveals patency of the right iliac artery but only a "stump" of the bypass graft is seen, consistent with graft thrombosis. (B) The lowermost aspect of the right common femoral artery was accessed and a multi–side-hole infusion catheter was positioned across the occluded graft. The radiopaque markers show the infusion zone. An infusion of recombinant tissue plasminogen activator was given at 0.5 mg/hour through this catheter. The patient received heparin (500 units/hour) through a peripheral intravenous catheter. (C) After 16 hours of thrombolysis, a repeat arteriogram reveals successful thrombus removal with residual tight focal stenosis at the proximal graft anastomosis. (D) The stenosis was subjected to angioplasty using a 6-mm balloon. (E) Repeat arteriogram shows improvement in the stenosis, but small thrombi are evident within the graft. (F) After use of the AngioJet Rheolytic Thrombectomy System to aspirate residual thrombus, the graft is widely patent. Subsequent physical examination revealed good pedal pulses and capillary refill, consistent with successful reperfusion of the limb.

Although there have been few changes to the basic CDT technique over the past 25 years, there has been a switch from biologically derived fibrinolytic drugs (streptokinase and urokinase) to recombinant drugs that are less allergenic and have greater affinity for fibrin. In addition to the standard multi–side-hole infusion catheter, a specialized multi–side-hole infusion catheter (the Ekosonic Mach 4e catheter, EKOS Corporation, WA, USA) that emits low-power ultrasound energy to ostensibly loosen fibrin strands and permit more rapid intrathrombus drug dispersion is available. Although this catheter also permits successful thrombolysis to be obtained, conclusive evidence that the addition of ultrasound energy improves patient outcomes is lacking.[3,4]

Variation on a Theme: Percutaneous Mechanical Thrombectomy

Hemorrhagic complications are the Achilles' heel of currently available thrombolytic agents. To reduce exposure to these drugs,

specialized catheters, known as *percutaneous mechanical thrombectomy (PMT) devices*, have been developed. PMT is defined as the use of a percutaneous catheter-based device that contributes to thrombus removal via thrombus fragmentation, maceration, and/or aspiration. Although originally developed to supplant thrombolytic drugs, until recently, none of the available PMT devices has enabled safe, successful clot removal when used as a stand-alone treatment.[1] Consequently, fibrinolytic drugs are used in conjunction with PMT, except in situations where there are absolute contraindications to the use of fibrinolytic drugs and no other treatment options are available.

Recently a new thrombectomy device (AngioVac, Angiodynamics) was introduced into some clinical practices.[5] This device, which relies upon creation of a bypass circuit to enable more robust suction thrombectomy, may provide greater thromboaspiration capability than previous devices. However, the device is somewhat inflexible and requires placement of two large access sheaths into the venous system. Given the lack of prospective data on its use, at present this device may be best targeted to urgent clinical problems for which there is no other solution (e.g., large thrombus in the suprarenal inferior vena

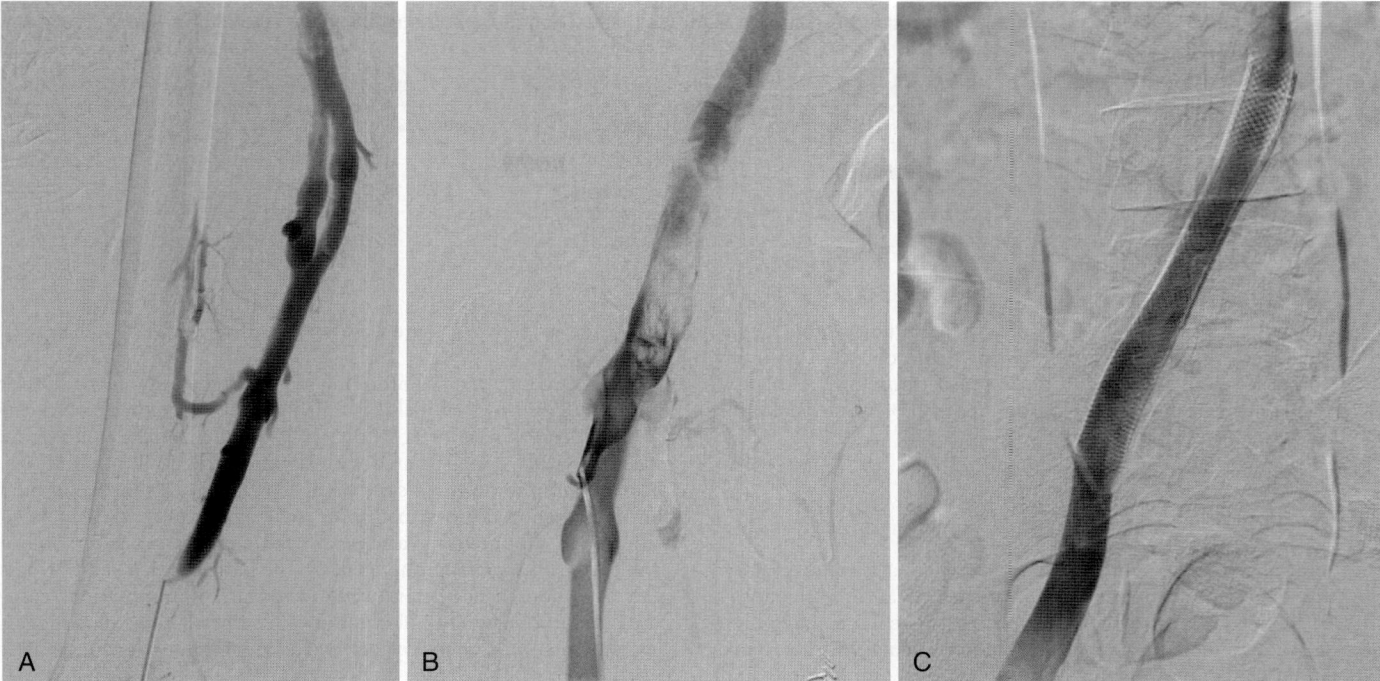

Fig. 143.2 A 35-YEAR-OLD MAN PRESENTS WITH A 3-DAY HISTORY OF SEVERE LEFT LOWER EXTREMITY PAIN AND SWELLING. (A) Digital subtraction venogram from a left popliteal vein approach shows patency of the lower part of the femoral vein with a short segment of duplication; a normal variant. (B) The left common femoral and iliac veins have large globular filling defects, consistent with acute iliofemoral deep vein thrombosis. (C) The Trellis device was used to deliver and disperse 10 mg of recombinant tissue plasminogen activator into the thrombus. After balloon maceration of the thrombus and subsequent placement of two 12-mm stents to treat stenosis of the left common iliac vein, the left common femoral vein and iliac vein are seen to be widely patent. The pain and swelling resolved within a few days.

cava [IVC] or right atrium in patients with contraindications to use of fibrinolytic drugs).

Variations on a Theme: Pharmacomechanical Catheter-Directed Thrombolysis

Pharmacomechanical catheter-directed thrombolysis (PCDT) refers to thrombus dissolution via the combined use of CDT and PMT devices. The rationale for utilizing both modalities is twofold: (1) fibrinolytic drugs given via CDT soften the thrombus, rendering it more susceptible to mechanical fragmentation and removal with PMT, while also dissolving thrombus fragments that may otherwise embolize; and (2) PMT devices macerate the thrombus, enhance dispersion of the fibrinolytic drug, and accelerate pharmacologic thrombolysis. Although a broad range of PCDT techniques have been used, they largely fall into two general categories. First, "first-generation" PCDT techniques incorporate PMT devices to assist traditional CDT; either a PMT device is initially used to de-bulk thrombus before starting the CDT infusion, or a PMT device is used after CDT to aspirate and/or macerate residual thrombus. Second, "single-session" PCDT techniques utilize PMT devices that can rapidly disperse the thrombolytic drug within the thrombus to enable the entire clot-removal treatment to be completed in a single on-table procedure session, thereby obviating the need for an overnight thrombolytic infusion with the required monitoring in an intensive-care unit.

Single-session PCDT techniques have attracted considerable interest. Two devices can be used for single-session PCDT. The AngioJet Rheolytic Thrombectomy System (Possis Medical, MN, USA) uses high-velocity saline jets to fracture the thrombus through a combination of rapid fluid streaming and hydrodynamic forces. Based on the Bernoulli principle of low pressure, these jets create a localized negative-pressure zone at the catheter tip, enabling clot aspiration. With the Powerpulse PCDT technique, the AngioJet is first used to deliver a thrombolytic drug into the thrombus via a powerful pulse-spray injection.[6] After a 20–30-minute dwell time, the AngioJet is then used to aspirate and remove the softened thrombus. The Isolated Thrombolysis technique refers to the use of the Trellis Peripheral Infusion System (Bacchus Vascular, CA, USA) to provide single-session PCDT[7] (Fig. 143.2). The Trellis device is composed of a multilumen catheter with two balloons that, when inflated, effectively isolate a thrombus-containing treatment zone from the remainder of the venous circulation. After the device is advanced across the venous thrombus, the occluding balloons are inflated and a thrombolytic drug is injected into the thrombus via side holes in the catheter. A sinusoidal wire within the catheter oscillates to disperse the drug within the thrombus, after which liquefied thrombotic debris can be aspirated through a port in the catheter. Both single-session PCDT techniques feature rapid intrathrombus drug dispersion that promotes faster thrombolysis, thereby reduced patient exposure to the fibrinolytic drug. Because the mechanical manipulation can induce thrombus fragmentation and embolization, these methods are best suited for venous applications.

Mechanical Interventions in Peripheral Arterial Occlusion

Acute peripheral arterial occlusion (PAO) is associated with high rates of morbidity and mortality. It is usually caused by atherosclerotic disease but can also arise from other etiologies (i.e., dissection, intimal hyperplasia, in situ thrombosis secondary to a hypercoagulable state, trauma, vasculitis, or aneurysm thrombosis). Up to 15%–20% of patients with chronic peripheral artery disease will develop acute exacerbation of symptoms (acute limb ischemia), usually due to thrombosis of the involved artery, and are at high risk of limb loss. Even with treatment, the 30-day mortality rate of acute arterial

TABLE 143.1	Clinical Outcomes in Patients With Acute or Chronic Limb Ischemia Treated by Catheter-Directed Thrombolysis or Surgery in the STILE Trial					
	Acute Ischemia ($\leq$14 days), $n = 112$			Chronic Ischemia (>14 days), $n = 266$		
	Surgery (%)	Lysis (%)	*p*-Value	Surgery (%)	Lysis (%)	*p*-Value
Death	10.0	5.6	0.45	7.9	6.9	0.81
Amputation	30.0	11.1	0.02	3.0	12.1	0.01
Death + amputation	37.5	15.3	0.01	9.9	17.8	0.08

thrombosis is approximately 15% and the amputation rate ranges from 10% to 30%.[8] In one study, the time from diagnosis to treatment correlated with amputation rates: 6% if thrombolytic therapy was started within 12 hours of symptom onset, 12% if started within 13–24 hours, and 20% if started after 24 hours.[9]

Rationale, Benefits, and Risks of CDT for PAO

The traditional treatment for acute limb ischemia is open surgery. However, the emergent nature of these procedures and the characteristics of the affected patient population, which tends to have high rates of concomitant coronary and cerebrovascular disease, have contributed to significant rates of perioperative complications and death. By dissolving platelet–fibrin aggregates in the microcirculation and thrombi in collateral vessels, CDT allows rapid but gradual reperfusion of the distal limb, thereby minimizing the risk of reperfusion complications and compartment syndrome.[2] CDT enables both rapid restoration of arterial blood flow to the ischemic limb and unmasking of arterial stenotic or occlusive lesions that require treatment. Because many such lesions can be treated with endovascular techniques, such as balloon angioplasty or stent placement, CDT allows many patients to avoid the risks and inconveniences of open surgery. When surgery is required, a more limited procedure can often be performed on an elective basis in a well-prepared patient, with reduced rates of complications and death.

The major complication of CDT is bleeding.[10] In the setting of PAO, the incidence of CDT-related hemorrhagic stroke is approximately 1%. The rate of major hemorrhage, defined by hypotension, need for surgical therapy, or need for blood transfusion, is approximately 5%, with minor hemorrhage (e.g., local hematoma) occurring in 15% of patients. In modern practice, the use of subtherapeutic doses of heparin during thrombolysis may help to minimize bleeding complications.[11] Distal embolization of thrombus fragments occurs in about 5% of cases; most of these resolve with continued lytic therapy. However, worsening ischemia can occur and generally requires percutaneous thrombus aspiration or operative intervention if the condition does not improve with thrombolysis within a few hours. Compartment syndrome, a complication that results from rapid reperfusion of the ischemic limb, occurs in 2% of patients. Death occurs in less than 1% of patients, usually in the setting of intracranial or abdominal hemorrhage, or reperfusion syndrome. Complications of CDT, which usually are minor, can also be related to intraarterial catheter insertion. Catheter-related trauma, resulting in mural dissection, puncture site pseudoaneurysm, and/or major hematoma occurs in 1%–2% of patients.

Randomized Trials: CDT Versus Surgery for Arterial Thrombosis

Three randomized controlled trials compared clinical outcomes in patients with acute PAO who were randomized to receive either CDT or surgical intervention.

The Rochester trial randomized 114 patients presenting with acute limb ischemia to catheter-directed urokinase infusion or surgery.[12] While there was no difference in limb salvage rates at 1 year, mortality at 1 year was significantly lower with urokinase than

with surgery. However, there was more bleeding with CDT than with surgery.

The Surgery versus Thrombolysis for Ischemia of the Lower Extremity (STILE) trial included 393 patients who either underwent CDT with urokinase or rt-PA, or surgery.[13] In patients with acute ischemia, CDT was associated with significantly fewer amputations, increased amputation-free survival at 1 year, and a shorter hospital stay. However, in those with chronic ischemia, surgery was associated with fewer amputations and improved amputation-free survival (Table 143.1). In a subgroup analysis, the patients with acute bypass graft occlusions had a significantly lower rate of amputations compared with those patients who underwent surgery. These data suggest that patients with acute bypass occlusion may derive the greatest benefit from CDT.

The Thrombolysis or Peripheral Arterial Surgery (TOPAS) trial randomized 544 patients with acute limb ischemia to CDT with recombinant urokinase or to surgery.[11] There was no difference in amputation-free survival at 1 year. However, CDT was associated with more bleeding complications, including a 1.6% rate of intracranial hemorrhage.

In summary, the results of these three trials suggest that CDT reduces the need for amputation and surgical intervention in patients with acute limb ischemia, particularly those with acute bypass graft occlusion. However, the risk of bleeding is higher with CDT than with surgery. Although outcomes in patients with acute limb ischemia are better with CDT, surgery is recommended for those with chronic ischemia. Because revascularization of nonviable limbs can precipitate a reperfusion syndrome associated with release of potassium, myoglobin, and other toxic elements from the nonviable limb, which can lead to multiorgan damage and death, patients with nonviable limbs (Rutherford class III) generally require primary amputation.

PMT, PCDT, and Ultrasound-Assisted CDT for Arterial Thrombosis

There is a paucity of data concerning the relative effectiveness and safety of newer thrombolytic techniques for PAO. The AngioJet device is FDA approved for peripheral arterial thrombus removal and is routinely utilized as an adjunct to CDT. There are limited data related to the safety and efficacy of the AngioJet, Trellis, and Ekosonic devices for the treatment of PAO. Aside from bleeding, the major complications associated with PMT and PCDT are distal embolization and local vascular injury (i.e., dissection or rupture). Although there are no randomized PAO trials comparing ultrasound-accelerated CDT with standard CDT, preliminary data from several studies suggest that ultrasound-accelerated CDT significantly reduces treatment time without increasing the rate of serious adverse events when compared with CDT alone.[3,14]

A multicenter registry of 99 patients treated with AngioJet reported substantial or complete revascularization (defined as <50% residual defect) in 70% of patients and in-hospital and 30-day mortality rates of less than 5%.[15] Another study documents higher amputation-free success rates associated with initial endovascular PCDT procedures, with low repeat intervention rates.[16] However, these studies are limited by methodological deficiencies including lack of randomization. Studies using the Trellis device are limited and only case reports have described its use for acute limb ischemia; given

TABLE 143.2	Rutherford Classification of Acute Limb Ischemia					
		Clinical Examination			**Doppler Signal**	
Category	Description/Prognosis	Sensory Loss	Muscle Weakness	Arterial	Venous
I. Viable	Not immediately threatened	None	None	Audible	Audible
II. Threatened					
IIa. Marginally	Salvageable if promptly treated	Minimal (toes) or none	None	(Often) audible	Audible
IIb. Immediately	Salvageable with immediate revascularization	More than toes, associated with rest pain	Mild, Moderate	(Usually) audible	Audible
III. Irreversible	Major tissue loss or permanent nerve damage inevitable	Profound, anesthetic	Profound, paralysis (rigor)	Inaudible	Inaudible

TABLE 143.3	Contraindications to Thrombolytic Therapy

Absolute Contraindications

Active bleeding
History of stroke within the previous 3 months
Neurosurgery (intracranial, spinal) within the previous 3 months
Intracranial trauma within the previous 3 months

Relative Contraindications

Recent (<7–10 days) major surgery, trauma, CPR, obstetrical delivery, or cataract surgery
Recent (<7–10 days) major invasive procedure or puncture of uncompressible vessel
Recent (<3 months) internal eye surgery or hemorrhagic retinopathy
Acute gastroduodenal ulcer or recent (<7–10 days) gastrointestinal bleeding
Intracranial neoplasm, arteriovenous malformation, aneurysm, or other lesion
Uncontrolled hypertension (systolic >180 mmHg or diastolic >110 mmHg)
Hepatic failure, particularly in cases with coagulopathy
Bacterial endocarditis or septic thrombophlebitis
Pregnancy
Severe anemia or thrombocytopenia

the potential for thrombus fragmentation and embolization, this technique does not appear to be well suited for management of arterial occlusions.[17]

Summary: Indications and Contraindications for Thrombolytic Therapy in PAO

The use of arterial CDT should be individualized. Reasonable candidates include those with (1) acute (<14 days) thrombosis of a previously patent bypass graft or native artery; (2) acute embolus in a vessel not readily accessible to surgical embolectomy; (3) acute thrombosis of a popliteal artery aneurysm resulting in severe ischemia when all distal run-off vessels are also thrombosed; and (4) acute arterial thromboembolic occlusions in patients who are poor surgical candidates. The clinical status of PAO patients should be classified using the Rutherford scheme (Table 143.2). Patients with Rutherford class I, class IIa, and in specific cases class IIb disease are potential candidates for CDT. Patients with category III ischemia should not be treated percutaneously because catheter-based thrombolysis often takes many hours and ischemic changes may become irreversible over the course of treatment. In patients with irreversible limb ischemia, mild-to-moderate ischemia with claudication, early postoperative bypass graft thrombosis, or large-vessel thrombi that are easily accessible by surgery, open surgery is preferred over CDT. Absolute and relative contraindications to CDT are outlined in Table 143.3.

Mechanical Interventions in Deep Vein Thrombosis

Venous thromboembolism (VTE) occurs in 350,000–600,000 persons per year in the United States alone, of which more than 250,000 cases represent a first-episode of deep vein thrombosis (DVT). The management of DVT has traditionally been anchored in a longstanding view of the disease as an "acute" condition involving an initial period of high risk of PE (which is estimated to kill over 100,000 persons in the United States each year), followed by a steadily diminishing risk over time that ultimately permits discontinuation of anticoagulant therapy in most patients. In recent years, there is better appreciation of the long-term impact of DVT in terms of the risk of recurrence, particularly in those with unprovoked VTE, and the high incidence of PTS in patients with extensive DVT.

Anticoagulation is the mainstay of initial DVT therapy. During the last few years, the number of anticoagulant options for DVT therapy has increased substantially. Historically, initial anticoagulation has consisted of administration of a parenteral anticoagulant drug (unfractionated heparin, low-molecular-weight heparin [LMWH], or fondaparinux) with subsequent transition to long-term oral vitamin K antagonist therapy for at least 3 months, with the duration of therapy dependent on the presence or absence of ongoing risk factors for recurrence.[18] The preferred initial approach for most patients with cancer-related DVT has been LMWH monotherapy for at least 3–6 months. These longstanding treatment options are now supplemented by the availability of an oral direct thrombin inhibitor (dabigatran) and three oral direct factor Xa inhibitors (rivaroxaban, apixaban, and edoxaban).[19]

The therapeutic goals of anticoagulant therapy are to prevent symptomatic and fatal PE, thrombus progression, and late recurrent DVT. All of the currently available anticoagulants are effective in achieving these goals in most patients. In general, during the first year after discontinuation of anticoagulant therapy, recurrent VTE events occur in 3%–5% of patients whose DVT episode was provoked by a major reversible risk factor and in 10%–15% of patients with unprovoked/idiopathic DVT or cancer-related DVT.

Rationale, Benefits, and Risks of CDT for DVT:

PTS develops in 20%–50% of patients after a first episode of lower extremity DVT.[20] The symptoms and signs of PTS include chronic aching, swelling, fatigue, heaviness, edema, hyperpigmentation, and/or subcutaneous fibrosis in the affected limb. In severe cases, patients may experience short-distance venous claudication and venous leg ulcers, both of which limit ambulation and the ability to work and perform the activities of daily living. Consequently PTS reduces health-related QOL. In fact, in a recent large prospective cohort study, the presence and severity of PTS were the leading determinants of QOL 2 years after an initial lower extremity DVT.[21] PTS also occurs with moderate frequency in patients with upper-extremity DVT, particularly those who present with axillosubclavian vein involvement in the dominant arm. The management of PTS results in major economic costs to patients and society because of the direct medical costs of caring for its clinical sequelae (e.g., venous ulcers) and the indirect costs of work disability.

The pathogenesis of PTS is complex and incompletely understood. Inflammatory mediators, growth factors, extracellular matrix components, blood-borne elements, and endothelial cell factors contribute to the inflammatory response to DVT, which influences thrombus resolution, organization, and subsequent venous wall injury. Even with anticoagulant therapy, incomplete clearance of thrombus is common, and residual thrombus often blocks venous blood flow. In addition, venous valves may be damaged, resulting in valvular reflux. The combination of valvular reflux and obstruction causes ambulatory venous hypertension, which leads to edema, tissue hypoxia and injury, progressive calf pump dysfunction, subcutaneous fibrosis, and skin ulceration. Therefore, it is logical to postulate that rapid thrombus elimination and restoration of deep venous flow may prevent these untoward physiologic effects and preserve long-term venous function.

In support of this "open vein hypothesis" are studies that have observed a strong correlation between the amount of residual thrombus after a course of anticoagulant therapy and the subsequent incidence of recurrent venous thromboembolism. Moreover, data from a number of small randomized trials suggest that systemic thrombolysis and contemporary surgical venous thrombectomy are associated with improved long-term venous patency, preservation of venous valvular function, and reduced PTS compared with anticoagulation alone. However, these studies are small and all have methodologic limitations. For patients with DVT, CDT is performed using the same procedures as those used for arterial thrombosis. Ultrasound-guided access to an extremity vein, usually the popliteal vein for the lower extremity, is obtained.[1] A venogram is performed and the CDT or PCDT methods described previously are used to remove the thrombus. After clot lysis, venography is performed to evaluate the underlying vein. Any residual stenosis is then treated with angioplasty or stenting. In general, the use of stents after DVT thrombolysis is optimally limited to the iliac vein, although it is sometimes necessary to extend contiguous stents into the common femoral vein. Patients with femoral vein stenosis, or isolated common femoral vein lesions that do not extend into the iliac vein, are best treated with angioplasty. Axillosubclavian vein thrombosis of known cause (e.g., previous central venous catheter) is amenable to balloon angioplasty if there is underlying stenosis. In patients with primary axillosubclavian vein thrombosis ("effort thrombosis"), stenosis of the subclavian vein is typically identified and is best treated with surgical thoracic outlet decompression rather than aggressive balloon angioplasty or stenting. With rare exceptions, stent placement in the subclavian vein is contraindicated because of the high frequency of stent fractures.

In a historic 473-patient multicenter registry, the use of CDT resulted in successful clot lysis in more than 80% of patients with acute proximal DVT.[22] However, major bleeding was observed in 11.4% of patients, mostly access site bleeding. Intracranial bleeding was observed in 0.4% of patients and fatal PE occurred in 0.2% of patients.

In 2012, the first rigorously designed multicenter randomized controlled trial was published describing long-term outcomes with adjunctive CDT.[23] In this Norwegian study, 209 patients with acute iliac or femoral DVT were randomized to receive standard anticoagulant therapy with or without the addition of infusion-only CDT. This study demonstrated a 26% relative risk reduction (55.6% vs. 41.1%, $p = 0.04$) in the occurrence of PTS over 2 years of follow-up. Major bleeding occurred in 3% of patients, resulting in one blood transfusion and one surgical intervention. There were no intracranial bleeds. Adjunctive CDT was associated with a small QOL benefit and reduced job absenteeism over the first 6 months of follow-up; however, QOL was not different at 24 months follow-up. Overall, these findings suggest that endovascular thrombolysis may indeed improve long-term outcomes, but they are not entirely clear as to whether the degree of benefit is likely to be sufficient to justify the attendant risks and costs in large populations of DVT patients.

Limitations of this study are its modest sample size, geographical limitation to four treatment centers in Southern Norway, and possibly reduced relevance to clinical practice in the United States and other countries due to the lack of use of thrombectomy devices and limited use of stents.

Contemporary methods of PCDT have been integrated into pivotal multicenter randomized trials, including the ongoing National Institutes of Health–sponsored Acute Venous Thrombosis: Thrombus Removal with Adjunctive Catheter-Directed Thrombolysis (ATTRACT) trial, which completed patient enrollment in December 2014.[24] Patient follow-up is ongoing and the results should be available soon.

Acute Iliofemoral DVT as a High-Risk Condition

It is important for physicians to recognize the range of clinical presentations of proximal DVT. The extent of thrombosis is an important predictor of clinical course and long-term outcome with anticoagulant therapy. In particular, with femoral vein thrombosis, the primary collateral route by which blood leaves the limb (and by which the venous obstruction is decompressed) is via the deep (profunda) femoral vein, which empties into the common femoral vein in the groin. Consequently, thrombosis above the entry point of the deep femoral vein (i.e., in or above the common femoral vein) causes more severe outflow obstruction, which often results in more leg swelling and pain, and a higher incidence of late clinical sequelae.

Iliofemoral DVT is defined as DVT involving the iliac vein and/or common femoral vein, with or without involvement of other lower extremity veins.[1] Although physicians typically classify DVT as either distal or proximal because the risk of PE is higher with proximal DVT, patients with iliofemoral DVT have poorer clinical outcomes than patients with less extensive proximal DVT. Involvement of the common femoral vein and/or iliac vein portends a much higher risk of recurrent VTE and more severe PTS than those with less extensive DVT.[20] Hence, it is important to view iliofemoral DVT as a high-risk condition and to ensure the utilization of evidence-based PTS prevention measures, especially therapeutic anticoagulation of appropriate intensity and duration. These patients are readily identified because they usually present with swelling of the entire limb and most have compression ultrasound evidence of thrombus in the common femoral vein.

Patients with acute (symptom duration ≤14 days) iliofemoral DVT who are not at increased risk for bleeding are the best candidates for CDT and PCDT.[1,18,25] There are no well-designed prospective studies of CDT for treatment of upper-extremity DVT; generally, such treatment is restricted to symptomatic patients with axillosubclavian vein thrombosis of recent onset, often in the context of a combined interventional-surgical strategy (i.e., for Paget-Schroetter syndrome).

Summary: Indications and Contraindications for CDT in DVT

The lack of data to establish the utility and proper indications for CDT in DVT patients does not absolve physicians of their responsibility to ensure that the long-term risks of PTS are carefully considered when crafting an individualized treatment strategy for DVT patients. The strategy should incorporate a high degree of confidence in anticoagulation drugs; a familiarity with the available (albeit imperfect) data that suggest that CDT is reasonable for selected DVT patients; and an individualized assessment of the clinical DVT severity, extent of thrombosis, comorbidities, and personal preferences of the patient.

Patients who do not meet a clinical threshold justifying the use of CDT include those with asymptomatic DVT or DVT isolated to the calf (because the risk of PTS is relatively low in these groups), and patients with chronic femoropopliteal DVT (because studies have shown that organized thrombus is not susceptible to thrombolytic drugs).[22]

The most important safety factor to consider in a patient being evaluated for DVT thrombolysis is the risk of major bleeding. Factors associated with an increased risk of bleeding include ongoing or recent bleeding; recent major surgery, trauma, pregnancy, obstetrical delivery, or cardiopulmonary resuscitation; or the presence of lesions in critical areas such as the central nervous system, which may bleed. Because CDT involves the administration of iodinated contrast material for venography, renal function is also an important consideration as are life expectancy, baseline ambulatory capacity, and comorbidities.[1,25] Patients with limited long-term mobility or those with a life expectancy of less than 6 months are unlikely to benefit from aggressive therapy to prevent PTS. Comorbidities that increase procedure risks, such as respiratory compromise that limits the use of sedation, may also render CDT less attractive.

Urgent endovascular thrombolysis is indicated to prevent life-, limb-, or organ-threatening complications of acute DVT in situations such as phlegmasia cerulea dolens or extensive IVC thrombosis (especially with suprarenal extension, which may lead to fatal PE or acute renal failure). The use of endovascular thrombolysis in these situations is justifiable when other treatment options are lacking. In contrast, there is significant uncertainty regarding the appropriate indications for nonurgent CDT for the treatment of DVT. At present, guidelines of the American Heart Association (2011), Society of Interventional Radiology (2014), American Venous Forum and Society for Vascular Surgery (2012), and the United Kingdom's National Institute of Clinical Excellence (2012) suggest the use of CDT/PCDT as an adjunct to anticoagulant therapy for carefully selected patients with major symptomatic axillosubclavian DVT or extensive proximal lower extremity DVT, such as those with acute iliofemoral DVT, who have a low risk of bleeding and a long life-expectancy.[1,25-27] However, the 2016 guidelines update from the American College of Chest Physicians recommends against the routine use of CDT, with the caveat that patients who attach a high value to PTS prevention relative to bleeding risks and procedural inconvenience may choose CDT.[18]

Treatment of Established PTS

Patients with established PTS suffer major symptoms that significantly impair their ability to conduct their daily activities and to enjoy a normal QOL. Unfortunately once PTS has developed, there are no treatments that have consistently been shown to be effective. Despite limited evidence of benefit, elastic compression stockings are often utilized because of their low risk and ready availability. Low-dose diuretics may be useful to reduce edema. Patients with venous ulcers can be given pentoxifylline, dedicated wound care with topical antibiotics, exfoliants, and growth factors, and multilayer compression bandaging.[28] Despite these measures, PTS symptoms and venous ulcers often resist improvement and cause long-term hardships.

Because the severity of PTS symptoms often parallels the degree of ambulatory venous hypertension, endovascular interventions that eliminate venous obstruction and valvular reflux have been used for treatment of patients with severe PTS. Studies suggest that stent recanalization of chronically occluded iliac veins in patients with advanced PTS can be achieved in over 80% of patients and can reduce PTS symptoms, improve QOL, and enhance healing of venous ulcers[29] (Fig. 143.3). Accordingly, physicians who see patients

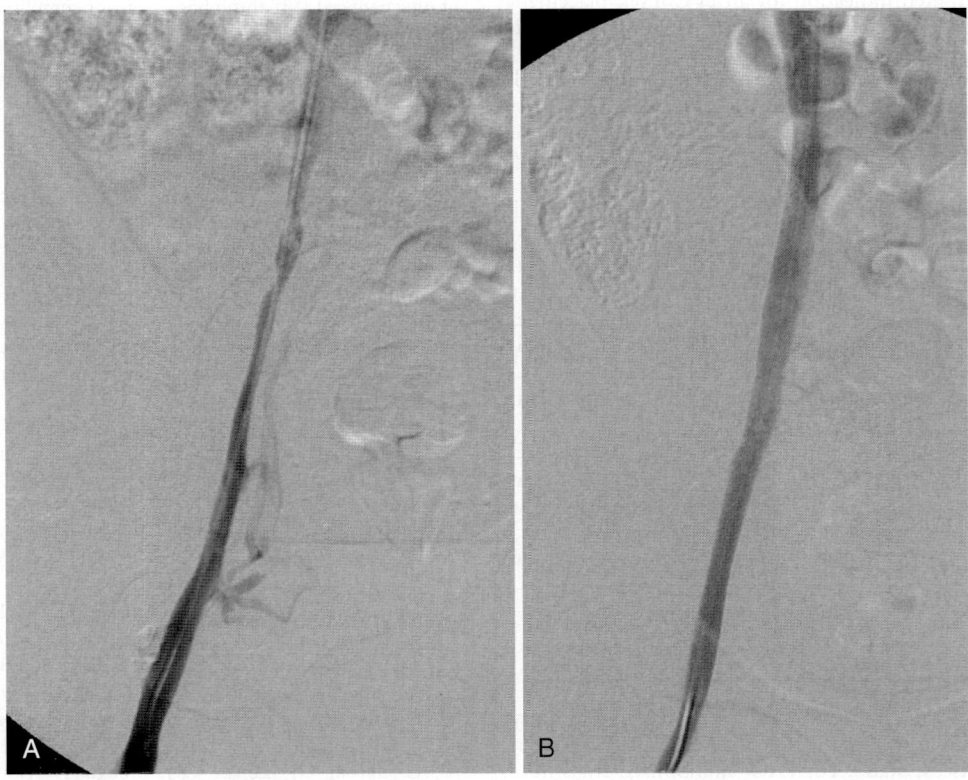

Fig. 143.3 A 46-YEAR-OLD WOMAN WITH A PAST HISTORY OF RIGHT ILIOFEMORAL DEEP VEIN THROMBOSIS (DVT) 2 YEARS AGO. She now presents to the clinic complaining of daily aching and swelling in the right lower extremity that preclude ambulation for even one block and render her unable to work. These symptoms have been present since her previous DVT. (A) A transjugular pelvic venogram demonstrates chronic narrowing of the right iliac vein with collateral formation. (B) After placement of four 12-mm stents, the right iliac vein is widely patent. The pain and swelling improved, and the patient was subsequently able to return to work.

with severe PTS, with or without ulcers, should consider consulting a venous endovascular specialist.

Inferior Vena Cava Filters

IVC filters are indicated for patients with proximal DVT or PE who have contraindications to or complications of anticoagulation, who develop symptomatic PE despite therapeutic-level anticoagulation, and/or who have severe cardiorespiratory compromise. In other circumstances, caution should be used when placing IVC filters because of ongoing uncertainty about their long-term risk–benefit ratio. Two randomized trials evaluating IVC filters are worthy of note. In the PREPIC Study, which was carried out in patients concomitantly receiving anticoagulant therapy and which was underpowered to detect an effect on fatal PE, filters appeared to provide additional protection against symptomatic PE but did not alter mortality.[30] Symptomatic recurrent DVT was increased in the filter group, but the overall rates of PTS and symptomatic recurrent VTE did not differ significantly. Because fatal PE rarely occurs in patients with DVT who are properly anticoagulated, IVC filters should not be routinely placed in patients with DVT. Patients who experience clinical failure of first-line anticoagulation can usually be switched to an effective alternative regimen, such as LMWH or another oral anticoagulant.

Retrievable IVC filters have the intended advantages of allowing PE prophylaxis during the period of highest risk, with subsequent removal thereafter. However, it should be noted that the stability and mechanical integrity of retrievable devices do not yet match those of older filters designed for permanent implantation, and many cases of retrievable filter migration have been reported. Therefore if there is a strong likelihood that permanent IVC filtration will be needed, it is best to select a permanent, nonretrievable IVC filter device. In DVT patients with a time-limited indication for an IVC filter, placement of a retrievable IVC filter is reasonable. However, it is important that the need for the IVC filter be reassessed every few weeks after placement so that the filter can be removed when it is no longer needed. Although many filters are placed with the intent to be retrieved, less than 50% are removed. Consequently physicians must monitor patients with these devices to ensure that they are removed when appropriate.

The recently completed PREPIC-2 study was a multicenter RCT that evaluated the use of retrievable IVC filters for the prevention of recurrent PE in hospitalized patients with acute PE and clinical features deemed to pose high risk for recurrence or death.[31] This study did not identify a clinical benefit from IVC filter placement, either in terms of mortality or recurrent symptomatic PE. Hence a compelling justification should be present to support placement of IVC filters in VTE patients who are eligible to receive anticoagulant therapy.

At a health care system level, better studies of the use of IVC filters in different clinical scenarios should be considered an urgent priority because the devices are being used more frequently. The balance between PE prophylaxis and the long-term risks of IVC filter placement is complex and deserves more rigorous evaluation (Fig. 143.4).

CONCLUSION

Imaging-guided endovascular interventions have evolved significantly over the last 25 years and now offer the potential for improved patient outcomes in several disease states. For PAO, randomized trials have defined the role for CDT for the treatment of acute limb ischemia. For DVT, a robust body of preliminary research and one randomized trial support the potential for catheter-based thromboreductive therapies to improve long-term patient outcomes, but larger randomized trials have not yet been completed. Therefore, an individualized approach is recommended to ensure that harms are minimized and appropriate patients are selected for intervention. Multidisciplinary

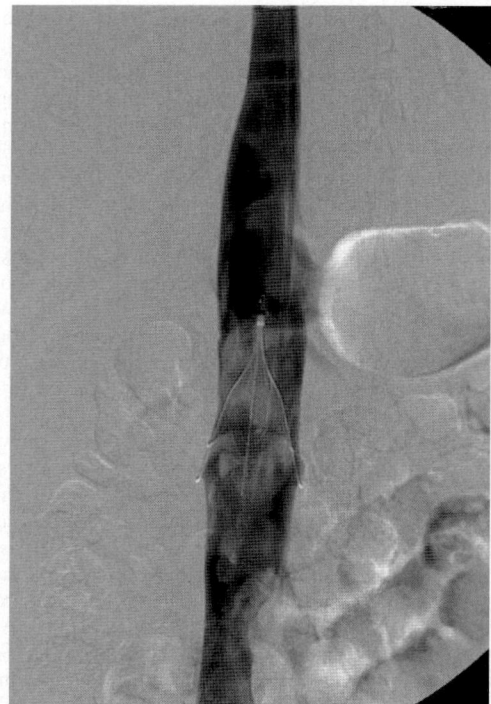

Fig. 143.4 ILLUSTRATING THE COMPLEXITIES OF DETERMINING WHETHER INFERIOR VENA CAVA (IVC) FILTERS ARE OF BENEFIT OR NOT. A digital subtraction venogram shows a large globular filling defect within an IVC filter that was placed 3 days ago. Filter proponents might argue that this represents a large, potentially fatal pulmonary embolism trapped within the filter, while filter opponents might argue that this is a case of filter-induced IVC thrombosis, a major complication. Who is right?

collaboration between internists and endovascular physicians is needed to ensure optimal patient care.

REFERENCES

1. Vedantham S, Thorpe PE, Cardella JF, et al: Quality improvement guidelines for the treatment of lower extremity deep vein thrombosis with use of endovascular thrombus removal. *J Vasc Interv Radiol* 17:435, 2006.
2. Rajan DK, Patel NH, Valji K, et al: Quality improvement guidelines for percutaneous management of acute limb ischemia. *J Vasc Interv Radiol* 20:S208–S218, 2009.
3. Engelberger RP, Spirk D, Willenberg T, et al: Ultrasound-assisted versus conventional catheter-directed thrombolysis for acute iliofemoral deep vein thrombosis. *Circ Cardiovasc Interv* 8:e002027, 2015.
4. Schrijver AM, van Leersum M, Fioole B, et al: Dutch randomized trial comparing standard catheter-directed thrombolysis versus ultrasound-accelerated thrombolysis for arterial thromboembolic infrainguinal disease. *J Endovasc Ther* 22(1):87–95, 2015.
5. Donaldson CW, Baker JN, Narayan RL, et al: Thrombectomy using suction filtration and veno-venous bypass: single-center experience with a novel device. *Catheter Cardiovasc Interv* 86:E81, 2015.
6. Cynamon J, Stein EG, Dym J, et al: A new method for aggressive management of deep vein thrombosis: retrospective study of the power pulse technique. *J Vasc Interv Radiol* 17:1043–1049, 2006.
7. O'Sullivan GJ, Lohan DG, Gough N, et al: Pharmacomechanical thrombectomy of acute deep vein thrombosis with the Trellis-8 isolated thrombolysis catheter. *J Vasc Interv Radiol* 18:715–724, 2007.
8. Dormandy J, Heeck L, Vig S: Acute limb ischemia. *Semin Vasc Surg* 12:148–153, 1999.
9. Ouriel K, Shortell CK, DeWeese JA, et al: A comparison of thrombolytic therapy with operative revascularization in the initial treatment of acute peripheral arterial ischemia. *J Vasc Surg* 19:1021–1030, 1994.

10. Working Party on Thrombolysis in the Management of Limb Ischemia: Thrombolysis in the management of lower limb peripheral arterial occlusion–a consensus document. *J Vasc Interv Radiol* 14:S337–S349, 2003.

11. Ouriel K, Veith FJ, Sasahara AA: A comparison of recombinant urokinase with vascular surgery as initial treatment for acute arterial occlusion of the legs. Thrombolysis or Peripheral Arterial Surgery (TOPAS) Investigators. *N Engl J Med* 338:1105–1111, 1998.

12. Ouriel K, Shortell CK, DeWeese JA, et al: A comparison of thrombolytic therapy with operative revascularization in the initial treatment of acute peripheral arterial ischemia. *J Vasc Surg* 19:1021–1030, 1994.

13. The STILE Investigators: Results of a prospective randomized trial evaluating surgery versus thrombolysis for ischemia of the lower extremity. The STILE trial. *Ann Surg* 220:251–266, discussion 266-268, 1994.

14. Schernthaner MB, Samuels S, Biegler P, et al: Ultrasound-accelerated versus standard catheter-directed thrombolysis in 102 patients with acute and subacute limb ischemia. *J Vasc Interv Radiol* 25:1149–1156, 2014.

15. Ansel GM, George BS, et al: Rheolytic thrombectomy in the management of limb ischemia: 30-day results from a multicenter registry. *J Endovasc Ther* 9(4):395–402, 2002.

16. Anset GM, Botti CF, Jr, Silver MJ: Treatment of acute limb ischemia with a percutaneous mechanical thrombectomy-based endovascular approach: 5-year limb salvage and survival results from a single center series. *Cathet Cardiovasc Interv* 72(3):325–330, 2008.

17. Daly B, Patel M, Prasad A: The use of the Trellis-6 thrombectomy device in the management acute limb ischemia due to native vessel occlusion: challenges, tips, and limitations. *Cathet Cardiovasc Interv* 81:42–47, 2013.

18. Kearon C, Akl EA, Ornelas J, et al: Antithrombotic therapy for VTE: CHEST guideline and expert panel report. *Chest* 149:315–352, 2016.

19. Mantha S, Ansell J: Indirect comparison of dabigatran, rivaroxaban, apixaban and edoxaban for treatment of acute venous thromboembolism. *J Thromb Thrombolysis* 39:155–165, 2015.

20. Kahn SR, Shrier I, Julian JA, et al: Determinants and time course of the postthrombotic syndrome after acute deep venous thrombosis. *Ann Intern Med* 149:698–707, 2008.

21. Kahn SR, Shbaklo H, Lamping DL, et al: Determinants of health-related quality of life during the 2 years following deep vein thrombosis. *J Thromb Haemost* 6:1105–1112, 2008.

22. Mewissen MW, Seabrook GR, Meissner MH, et al: Catheter-directed thrombolysis for lower extremity deep venous thrombosis: report of a national multicenter registry. *Radiology* 211:39–49, 1999.

23. Enden T, Haig Y, Klow N, et al: Long-term outcomes after additional catheter-directed thrombolysis versus standard treatment for acute iliofemoral deep vein thrombosis (the CaVenT study): a randomised controlled trial. *Lancet* 379:31–38, 2012.

24. Vedantham S, Goldhaber SZ, Kahn SR, et al: Rationale and design of the ATTRACT Study: a multicenter randomized trial to evaluate pharmacomechanical catheter-directed thrombolysis for the prevention of postthrombotic syndrome in patients with proximal deep vein thrombosis. *Am Heart J* 165(4):523–553, 2013.

25. Jaff MR, McMurtry MS, Archer SL, et al: Management of massive and submassive pulmonary embolism, iliofemoral deep vein thrombosis, and chronic thromboembolic pulmonary hypertension: a scientific statement from the American Heart Association. *Circulation* 123(16):1788–1830, 2011.

26. Meissner MH, Gloviczki P, Comerota AJ, et al: Early thrombus removal strategies for acute deep venous thrombosis: clinical practice guidelines of the Society for Vascular Surgery and the American Venous Forum. *J Vasc Surg* 55(5):1449–1462, 2012.

27. National Clinical Guideline Centre: *The Management of Venous Thromboembolic Diseases and the Role of Thrombophilia Testing. Clinical guideline - methods, evidence, and recommendations*, London, June 2012, Royal College of Physicians.

28. Kahn SR, Comerota AJ, Cushman M, et al: The post-thrombotic syndrome: evidence-based prevention, diagnosis, and treatment strategies: a scientific statement from the American Heart Association. *Circulation* 130(18):1636–1661, 2014.

29. Raju S, Neglen P: Percutaneous recanalization of total occlusions of the iliac vein. *J Vasc Surg* 50:360–368, 2009.

30. The PREPIC Study Group: Eight-year follow-up of patients with permanent vena cava filters in the prevention of pulmonary embolism. *Circulation* 112:416–422, 2005.

31. Mismetti P, Laporte S, Pellerin O, et al: Effect of a retrievable inferior vena cava filter plus anticoagulation vs anticoagulation alone on risk of recurrent pulmonary embolism: a randomized clinical trial. *JAMA* 313(16):1627–1635, 2015.

CHAPTER 144

ATHEROTHROMBOSIS

Roy L. Silverstein

Morbidity and mortality from atherosclerosis, the pathologic process underlying acute myocardial infarction, sudden death, stroke, and limb loss, represent an enormous burden on society and health care systems. Even though death rates from heart attack and stroke have dropped precipitously over the past 60 years (72% and 78%, respectively, from 1950 to 2008)[1], cardiovascular diseases are still the number one cause of death in the United States, accounting for more than 30% of all deaths—approximately 2200 per day (or one every 40 seconds). Unfortunately as the developing world adopts a more "Western" lifestyle (i.e., one marked by a high-fat, calorie-rich diet, and limited physical activity), these statistics are becoming the norm worldwide. The annual financial burden of cardiovascular disease in the United States in 2010 was estimated by the American Heart Association (AHA) to be $445 billion, including $172 billion due to lost productivity. These costs are predicted to triple over the ensuing 20 years; analyses of population survey data predict an increase in cardiovascular disease prevalence from 36.9% to 40.5%. It is interesting to note that as treatment of the acute complications of atherosclerosis improves, the burden of chronic complications, particularly heart failure, is expected to increase by as much as 25% over the next 20 years.[1]

Much of our knowledge of the epidemiology of cardiovascular disease comes from large-scale, long-term population studies, the most important being the Framingham Heart Study sponsored by the National Heart, Lung, and Blood Institute (NHLBI). This ongoing prospective study began in 1948 with a cohort of ≈5200 men and women between the ages of 30 and 62 years in Framingham (MA, USA), and has since added two subsequent generations and several other cohorts. Through this study and others elsewhere in the United States and Europe major risk factors for cardiovascular disease have been identified, including cigarette smoking, low-density lipoprotein (LDL) cholesterol, systolic blood pressure, male sex, menopause, physical inactivity, body mass index, high-sensitivity C-reactive protein (hsCRP), and coronary artery calcification scores determined by radiographic imaging. Additionally, high-density lipoprotein (HDL) was identified as a protective factor. Based on these data, risk scores have been developed to guide physicians and patients, and public health campaigns developed targeting hypertension, elevated cholesterol, and lifestyle modifications. These measures have clearly contributed to the reductions in cardiovascular mortality just noted, although they cannot account for the entire decrement. Racial and ethnic disparities are well described in cardiovascular risk, with blacks having higher rates than all other groups.

PATHOBIOLOGY

Atherosclerosis is caused by the progressive formation of arterial plaques, which are characterized by accumulation of lipids, in particular cholesterol and its derivatives, and inflammatory cells in the tunica intima of large- and medium-sized arteries (Fig. 144.1). Although occlusion of blood flow by plaque encroachment into the lumen can occur and cause ischemia of downstream tissues, most of the severe clinical events associated with atherosclerosis derive from acute or subacute thrombosis at a site of an unstable, inflamed, or ruptured plaque, or at a site of recent mechanical or pharmacologic intervention, a process termed *atherothrombosis*. The past 45 years have seen a remarkable increase in our understanding of the basic pathophysiologic mechanisms that govern plaque formation, plaque progression, and acute arterial thrombosis.[2] Translation of this knowledge into diagnostic, preventive, and therapeutic strategies has been impressive, but there is still a need for improvement. This chapter will summarize the current prevailing models of atherogenesis and atherothrombosis, highlighting some key knowledge gaps and potential new therapeutic targets.

LIPOPROTEIN HOMEOSTASIS AND THE "CHOLESTEROL HYPOTHESIS"

Human epidemiologic and clinical trial data and animal model studies show unequivocally that elevated levels of plasma lipids, especially LDL cholesterol, are essential for plaque development. Atherosclerotic lesions can be induced in "atheroresistant" animals, including mice and rabbits, by manipulating their diets and/or genomes to cause hypercholesterolemia. The development of mouse genetic models nearly 25 years ago[3] has provided great mechanistic insights into the underlying pathobiology of plaque formation. In humans, raising LDL cholesterol levels increases the risk for atherosclerosis proportionally and lowering levels either by lifestyle change or pharmacologic intervention reduces risk proportionally. In general, lowering LDL cholesterol levels by 10% reduces risk for cardiovascular events by 25% and cardiovascular death by 10%.

Normally cholesterol levels are tightly controlled in response to diet and cellular needs by a complex transcriptional pathway mediated by sterol response element-binding protein 2 (SREBP2). At low levels of cellular cholesterol, SREBP2 is activated and binds to specific DNA sequences in target genes known as *sterol response elements* to activate their transcription. Two key target genes are *HMGCR* and *LDLR*, which encode 3-hydroxy-3-methylglutaryl coenzyme A (HMGCoA) reductase (the rate-limiting enzyme in cholesterol biosynthesis) and the LDL receptor, respectively, thereby increasing both cholesterol production and cellular LDL uptake. At high levels of cellular cholesterol, SREBP2 is inactive, cholesterol biosynthesis is turned off, and LDL receptor expression is downregulated. As shown in Fig. 144.2, statins decrease cellular cholesterol biosynthesis by inhibiting HMGCoA reductase and thereby induce an increase in LDL receptor expression, driving down plasma LDL cholesterol levels.

Multiple randomized clinical trials have demonstrated efficacy of statin class drugs in reducing risk for cardiovascular events in high-risk individuals. Initial studies focused on secondary prevention in patients with a history of a previous atherosclerotic event, but later trials demonstrated efficacy as part of a primary prevention strategy in subjects with elevated LDL cholesterol or in subjects with normal LDL cholesterol in the setting of other risk factors, such as diabetes, hypertension, or elevated plasma levels of hsCRP. The latter studies, along with those showing benefit of lowering LDL cholesterol to levels well below "normal" (e.g., to 70 mg/dL in high-risk individuals),[4] are consistent with the concept that "normal" levels of LDL cholesterol, as defined by population means in the Western world, are not reflective of a true normal biology.

Genetic studies of rare individuals with extremely low LDL cholesterol levels identified a null mutation in a gene known as *PCSK9* that encodes a serine protease enzyme involved in downregulating LDL receptor expression. Individuals with this mutation seem to be otherwise normal, despite nearly absent LDL, suggesting that targeting this enzyme could represent an effective strategy for cholesterol-lowering therapeutics. Indeed, humanized monoclonal antibodies inhibiting PCSK9 function were quickly developed, moved through clinical trials (OSLER and ODYSSEY) and approved by the US Food and Drug Administration (FDA) in 2015 as second-line therapy for hypercholesterolemia.[5] In clinical trials these agents were well tolerated and lowered LDL cholesterol by approximately 60% and decreased cardiovascular events by half, but it must be noted that long-term toxicity data are not yet available.

Cells in the periphery have the capacity to eliminate excess cholesterol through a process known as *reverse cholesterol transport* (RCT). In this pathway, summarized in Fig. 144.3, postlysosomal trafficking of intracellular cholesterol to the plasma membrane, mediated in part by actions of acyl-CoA cholesterol acyltransferase (ACAT) and Niemann-Pick type C (NPC) protein, allows the cell surface adenosine triphosphate (ATP)-binding cassette (ABC) proteins ABCA1 and ABCG1 to transport excess cholesterol to apolipoprotein (apo) A-containing lipoproteins, either nascent HDL (in the case of ABCA1) or mature HDL (in the case of ABCG1). HDL then "delivers" the cholesterol back to the liver, where it is selectively taken up by hepatocytes through a protein known as *scavenger receptor B1* (SRB1) and ultimately secreted into the bile and excreted in feces. The role of HDL in RCT probably accounts for its association with lowered risk for cardiovascular disease, but HDL particles also contain antiinflammatory and antioxidant proteins that may also contribute to lowering atherosclerosis risk.

Pharmacologic and lifestyle approaches to enhance RCT have received significant attention as potential antiatherosclerosis strategies. HDL levels can be raised by physical exercise, as well as by moderate alcohol ingestion, and these are both associated with lower

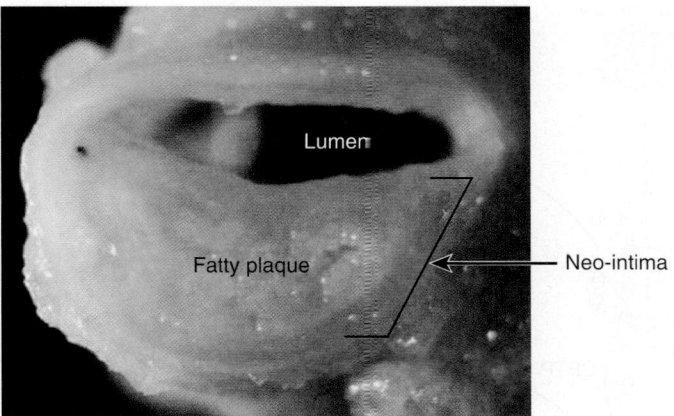

Fig. 144.1 ATHEROMATOUS PLAQUE. Cross-sectional view of a human artery taken from an autopsy, showing accumulation of yellow-colored fatty materials in the neointima.

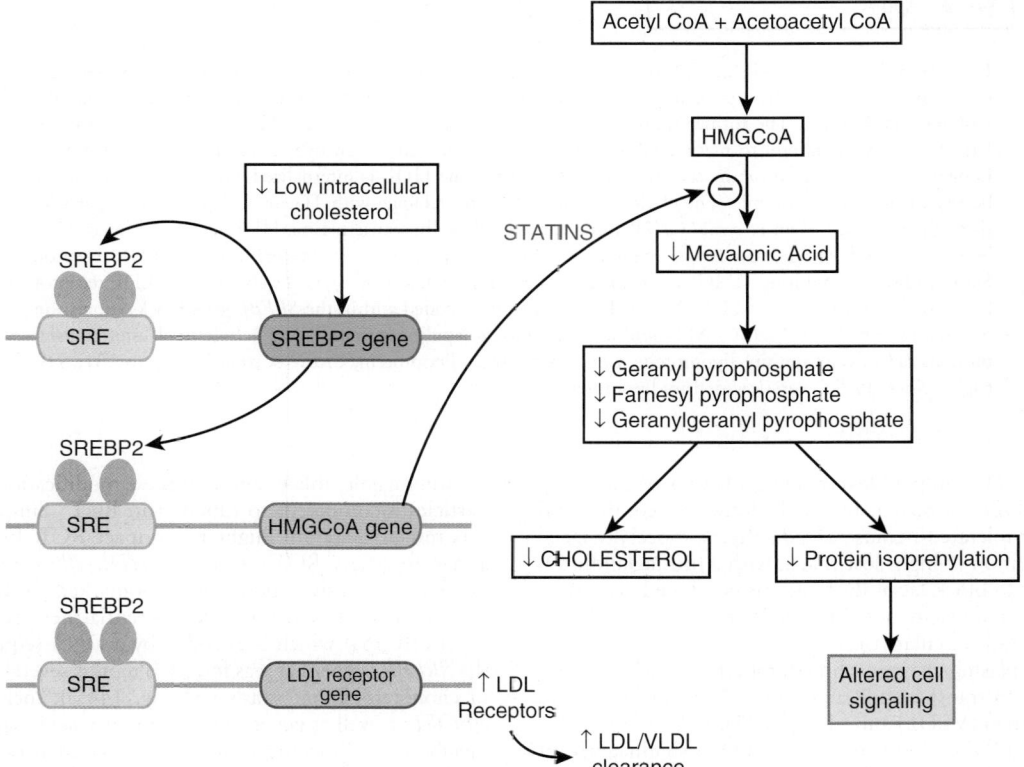

Fig. 144.2 STATINS TARGET CHOLESTEROL AND ISOPRENYLATION PATHWAYS. The statin class of drugs inhibits the intracellular enzyme HMGCoA reductase. This enzyme converts HMGCoA to mevalonic acid, which is a precursor in the biosynthesis of the isoprenoids geranyl and farnesyl pyrophosphates, which in turn are precursors of cholesterol, as well as intermediates in isoprenyl modification of proteins, including small-molecular-weight G proteins. Because HMGCoA reductase is the rate-limiting step in these pathways, its inhibition leads to decreases in cholesterol biosynthesis, hepatic VLDL production, and protein isoprenylation *(arrows).* Low levels of intracellular cholesterol activate the SREBP2 gene *(green),* which encodes a transcription factor that binds to SRE in multiple genes, including HMGCoA receptor and LDL receptor. The ensuing increased expression of LDL receptor results in increased clearance of apolipoprotein B–containing lipoproteins (LDL and VLDL) from plasma, further lowering plasma cholesterol levels. *CoA,* Coenzyme a; *HMGCoA,* 3-hydroxy-3-methylglutaryl coenzyme A; *LDL,* low-density lipoprotein; *SREBP2,* sterol response element binding protein 2; *SRE,* sterol response element; *VLDL,* very low-density lipoprotein.

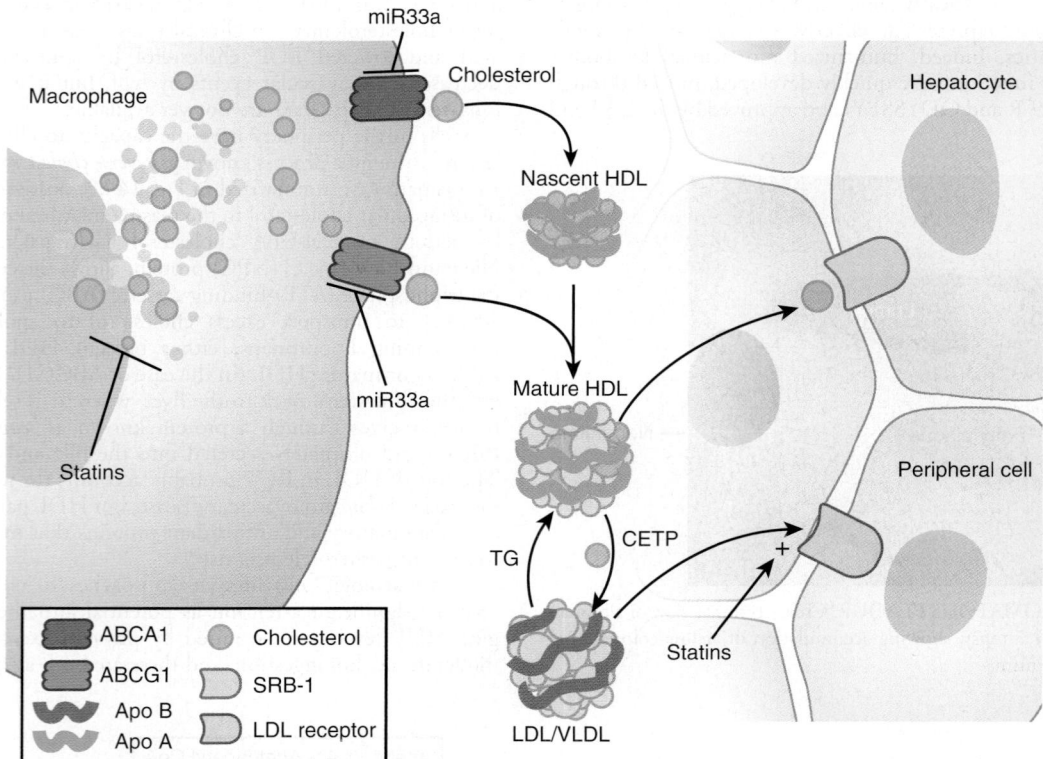

Fig. 144.3 REVERSE CHOLESTEROL TRANSPORT. Cells in the periphery, including macrophage foam cells, have the capacity to unload intracellular cholesterol via two members of the ABC transporter family: ABCA1 and ABCG1. The former transfers cholesterol to apoA and/or nascent HDL particles, whereas the latter transfers cholesterol to mature HDL. HDL interacts with SRB1 on liver cells, and through a process known as *selective cholesterol uptake*, the cholesterol within the HDL is internalized, where it can ultimately be reused or excreted via bile. The cholesterol in HDL can exchange with TG in LDL and VLDL particles through the action of an enzyme, CETP. Inhibitors of CETP thus raise plasma HDL levels and lower LDL levels. LDL and VLDL are normally cleared by cells in the periphery via internalization by LDL receptor. Statin drugs, by inhibiting HMGCoA reductase, lower intracellular cholesterol levels and raise LDL receptor levels, thus lowering plasma LDL. A microRNA, miR33a, encoded within the *SREBP* gene blocks expression of *ABCA1* and *ABCG1*. *ABC*, ATP-binding cassette; *apo*, apolipoprotein; *CETP*, cholesterol ester transfer protein; *HDL*, high-density lipoprotein; *LDL*, low-density lipoprotein; *SRB1*, scavenger receptor B1; *TG*, triglycerides; *VLDL*, very low-density lipoprotein.

cardiovascular risk. The only FDA-approved pharmacologic agent capable of raising HDL is niacin, but high doses are required and these are not easily tolerated because of side effects, especially facial flushing. A combination of high-dose niacin with a prostaglandin D_2 receptor antagonist to block facial flushing was developed, as was an extended release form of niacin, but although both raised HDL levels, neither decreased cardiovascular risk.

The circulating plasma enzyme, cholesterol ester transfer protein (CETP), functions to transfer cholesterol esters from HDL to very low-density lipoprotein (VLDL) and LDL (see Fig. 144.3). Inhibiting this enzyme raises HDL levels (and lowers LDL) significantly in humans, but a large phase III randomized clinical trial with the initially developed pharmacologic CETP inhibitor torcetrapib was halted in 2006 because of excessive all-cause mortality in the treatment group receiving a combination of atorvastatin and the study drug. This result may have been due to an off-target effect of the drug, but more recent studies with several different agents either failed to show efficacy despite raising HDL levels, or were halted in development. One agent remains in phase III trial with accrual scheduled to complete in 2017.

Failure of CTEP inhibitors and niacin in clinical trials raised doubts about the potential value of RCT or HDL as targets for antiatherosclerosis therapy. An emerging concept, however, is that HDL particles are sensitive to oxidative modification in the proatherogenic milieu, and that these modifications can render HDL particles incompetent to function in RCT.[6] Simply raising HDL in this milieu therefore might not impact RCT. In this regard, novel assays to assess RCT—so-called *HDL efflux capacity*—have been developed[7] and show potential as biomarkers for RCT in future drug development efforts. One such potential new target is microRNA-33a (miR-33a) which is encoded by a DNA sequence embedded in the *SREBP2* gene that was found to repress several key genes involved in cholesterol homeostasis (see Fig. 144.3), including *ABCA1* and *ABCG1*, as well as genes involved in fatty acid oxidation and glucose metabolism.[8] Blocking miR-33a in mice increased HDL levels and inhibited atherosclerosis, suggesting that this could be a good target for therapeutic development. Other strategies to enhance RCT that are under development include direct infusion of cholesterol acceptors from ABCA1 or ABCG1, such as recombinant apoA or small apoA mimetic amphipathic peptides.

Niemann-Pick C1-like1 protein is expressed on the surface of enterocytes and hepatocytes, and functions to promote cholesterol absorption. Ezetimibe, a well-tolerated FDA-approved drug inhibits this protein and lowers LDL cholesterol by approximately 20%. Early enthusiasm for this drug waned when studies failed to show improved cardiovascular outcomes, raising doubts in general about the relationship between biochemical endpoints and clinical efficacy. These results, and others, contributed to changes in clinical guidelines that

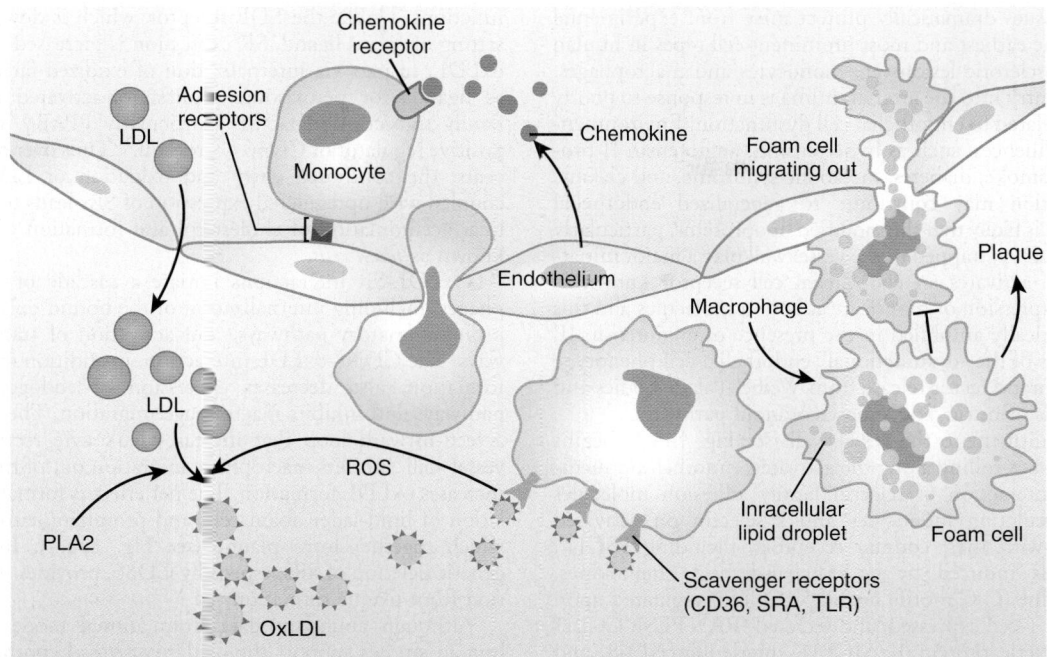

Fig. 144.4 FOAM CELL FORMATION IS AN EARLY EVENT IN ATHEROGENESIS. LDL particles, which are transudated through a dysfunctional endothelium at arterial branch points or areas of disrupted shear, enter the intima and become trapped within the extracellular matrix. In the presence of inflammation, the LDL particles become oxidized or otherwise modified and contribute to endothelial dysfunction by interacting with receptors on endothelial cells, such as LOX1. Monocytes, in response to chemokines secreted by activated endothelial cells and/or inflammatory leukocytes and platelets, adhere to the endothelium via selectin family adhesion receptors, as well as β2 integrins and their counterreceptors (intercellular adhesion molecule and vascular cell adhesion molecule). The monocytes then diapedese into the intima, where they differentiate into inflammatory macrophages that generate oxidant stress within the vessel wall and release proinflammatory mediators. Scavenger receptors, in particular CD36, expressed on macrophages recognize and internalize oxLDL, leading to a feed-forward loop of increased LDL oxidation and increased scavenger receptor expression, resulting ultimately in the formation of cholesterol-laden foam cells. These accumulate in the intima, in part because of signals induced by oxLDL that inhibit migration, forming plaque. *LDL*, Low-density lipoprotein; *oxLDL*, oxidized LDL; *PLA2*, phospholipase A2; *ROS*, reactive oxygen species; *SRA*, scavenger receptor A1; *TLR*, Toll-like receptor.

now no longer recommend specific LDL cholesterol targets and discourage use of nonstatin agents.[9] A more recent trial of ezetimibe in combination with a statin, however, showed a 10% reduction in cardiovascular events at 7 years associated with a mean decrease in LDL cholesterol of 16 mg/dL compared with statin alone.[10]

Multiple epidemiologic and genetic studies have shown positive associations of circulating triglyceride levels with coronary artery disease risk. Genetic variants in the gene encoding lipoprotein lipase, a key regulator of triglyceride metabolism, have also been associated with circulating triglyceride levels and with coronary artery disease risk, as have genetic variants in the APOC3 and APOA5 genes, which encode "minor" apolipoproteins in triglyceride-rich lipoproteins that critically regulate lipoprotein lipase in a reciprocal manner.[11] Therapeutic interventions targeting the lipoprotein lipase pathway, including an APOC3 antisense oligonucleotide, are under development.

FOAM CELL FORMATION AND THE FATTY STREAK

Atherosclerotic plaques develop in a geographically discontinuous manner very slowly and continuously evolve over many decades.[2] Autopsy studies of motor vehicle accident victims showed early "preatherosclerotic" lesions present in the aorta of otherwise healthy young children. These small superficial lesions consist predominantly of lipid-laden macrophages, so-called foam cells, and are termed *fatty streaks*. These are considered precursors of atherosclerotic plaque.

The initial event in formation of the fatty streak and atherosclerotic plaque is most likely transudation of apoB-containing lipoproteins across the endothelial cell monolayer into the arterial wall (Fig. 144.4). These lipoproteins are predominantly LDL, which is derived by remodeling of VLDL particles secreted into the plasma by hepatocytes. So-called remnant lipoproteins derived from chylomicrons produced by the intestinal epithelium may also play a role. The primary sites of lipoprotein entry are at arterial branch points or curvatures, explaining the discontinuous nature of atherosclerotic lesions. These locations are where normal laminar blood flow is disturbed. Normal laminar flow activates a specific genetic "protection" program in endothelial cells that enhances barrier function and promotes an antiinflammatory, antioxidant, antiatherogenic phenotype. Loss of these shear-dependent signals disrupts the normal endothelial architecture and increases permeability, allowing unregulated entry of lipoproteins into the tunica intima. Within the intima the lipoproteins become "trapped" by specific interactions with normal components of the vessel wall, such as glycosoaminoglycans, and undergo structural modifications, including aggregation, oxidation, and, in settings of hyperglycemia, glycation.

Just as data show an unequivocal role for LDL cholesterol in atherogenesis, equally compelling studies in humans and animal models show that mononuclear phagocytes are necessary for plaque formation and progression, and that atherosclerosis is associated with a chronic inflammatory state in the vessel wall and in the systemic circulation.[12] Targeted genetic mutations that block monocyte development from hematopoietic precursors or that prevent monocyte trafficking into tissues dramatically protect mice from experimental atherosclerosis. The earliest and most prominent cell types in human and mouse atherosclerotic lesions are monocytes and macrophages. Initial monocyte entry into the arterial intima is in response to poorly understood cues related to endothelial cell dysfunction. Environmental and genetic influences, such as hypertension, angiotensin II production, cigarette smoke, diabetes, metabolic syndrome, and chronic periodontal infection may contribute to generalized endothelial dysfunction, but it is likely that the modified lipoproteins, particularly oxidized LDL (oxLDL), trapped in the vessel wall play a major initiating role.[13] oxLDL activates an endothelial cell receptor known as *LOX1* to induce expression of monocyte adhesion molecules and this response is dramatically amplified in the presence of angiotensin II. Other components of the "dysfunctional" endothelial cell phenotype include von Willebrand factor release from Weibel-Palade bodies and altered homeostasis of nitric oxide and eicosanoid pathways.

Monocyte recruitment to the vessel wall (see Fig. 144.4) begins with their capture and rolling along the activated endothelium mediated by specific interaction of selectin family adhesion molecules (L-selectin on circulating monocytes and P-selectin on activated endothelial cells) with their counter receptors, including PSGL1. Subsequent signals induced by endothelial-derived chemokines, including chemokine (C-C motif) ligand 5 (CCL5)/ regulated upon activation, normal T-cell expressed, and secreted (RANTES), CCL2/ monocyte chemotactic protein 1 (MCP1), interleukin (IL)-8, and CXC-chemokine ligand 1 (CXCL1), lead to further recruitment of monocytes and facilitate firm adhesion of the rolling monocytes to the vessel wall. The latter is mediated by interaction of intercellular adhesion molecule 1 (ICAM1) and vascular cell adhesion molecule (VCAM) on the activated endothelial surface with specific integrin family counter receptors on monocytes; β2 integrins for ICAM1 and α4β1 for VCAM. By diapedesis, the adherent monocytes then traverse the disrupted endothelial junctions and enter the intima. Recent studies have suggested that a particular subset of circulating "inflammatory" monocytes, defined by high expression of the Ly6C antigen (in mice) or CD14 (in humans), are the predominant source of entering cells. The normal vasculature also contains a small number of resident macrophages, as well as "patrolling" monocytes. The latter are distinct from the Ly6C⁺/CD14ʰⁱ cells and exhibit a less inflammatory phenotype.

The ultimate fate of monocytes within the intima is probably determined in part by lineage-commitment programs carried by the entering monocytes and in part by local environmental cues. Most, however, seem to polarize toward the so-called *M1 inflammatory macrophage phenotype*. Investigators have, however, detected dendritic cell-like phenotypes (expressing CD11c), M2-like cells that express arginase and endothelial nitric oxide synthase (eNOS) and are highly phagocytic and antiinflammatory, and proangiogenic VEGF-expressing macrophage phenotypes within plaque.[14] In addition to monocytes, lymphocytes,[15] particularly T cells, also enter the intima, where they contribute to plaque formation by secreting cytokines and other mediators. Of these infiltrating lymphocytes, interferon-γ–producing T-helper (Th)1 cells and IL-17–producing Th17 cells have been shown to promote atherosclerosis, whereas the regulatory T cell subset is protective.

Reactive oxygen species (ROS) are generated by the inflammatory milieu within the atherogenic vessel wall and modify the trapped LDL by oxidizing both protein and lipid moieties (see Fig. 144.4), creating what are called collectively *oxLDL*.[13] Modified LDL lose their affinity for the LDL receptor but gain affinity for a genetically unrelated family of receptors known as *scavenger receptors* (SRs), including SRA1 and CD36, which are present at high levels on the macrophage surface. These receptors are part of the innate immune system, and their recognition of specific structures within oxLDL presumably relates to their mimicry of similar structures found on pathogenic organisms. CD36, for example,[16] also recognizes mycobacterial and *Staphylococcus* cell wall components, certain fungal structures, and falciparum malaria-infected erythrocytes. Toll-like receptor (TLR) family members, including TLR2, TLR4, and TLR6, can also recognize modified LDL and can partner with CD36 in these

functions. Unlike the LDL receptor, which is downregulated in the setting of excess ligand, SR expression is increased in the presence of oxLDL, in part via internalization of oxidized fatty acids that serve as ligands for peroxisome proliferator-activated receptor (PPAR) family transcription factors, particularly PPARγ, which is a major positive regulator of CD36 expression.[17] Thus over many months and years, the continued entry and oxidation of LDL in the intima coupled with upregulated expression of SRs leads to massive intracellular accumulation of cholesterol and formation of lipid-laden cells known as *foam cells*.

OxLDL-SR interactions initiate a cascade of events in macrophages, including internalization of the bound oxLDL, activation of proinflammatory pathways, and activation of transcriptional pathways. The CD36–oxLDL interaction, in addition to promoting ROS formation, also decreases expression of endogenous antioxidant pathways and inhibits macrophage migration. These events result in a feed-forward loop that increases leukocyte recruitment into the vessel wall, inhibits macrophage migration out of the vessel wall, and increases oxLDL formation. The net effect is formation and accumulation of lipid-laden foam cells and proinflammatory immune cells, which together form plaque (see Fig. 144.4). In mouse models, genetic deletion of SRs, especially CD36, provides substantial protection from plaque formation.

Although abundant data from animal models and correlative human studies support the oxidative stress hypothesis, considerable controversy remains because large- and medium-sized interventional trials of antioxidant therapy in humans have generally failed to prevent the complications of atherosclerosis.[18] These trials, however, are difficult to interpret because of lack of convincing evidence that the tested "antioxidant" therapies actually targeted the relevant vascular or circulating oxidant pathways. These oxidant systems include NADPH oxidase, xanthine oxidase, myeloperoxidase (MPO), and uncoupled nitric oxide synthase. MPO is of particular interest because it generates a highly specific oxidized phospholipid ligand for CD36 from LDL, and because circulating MPO levels associate with risk for atherosclerosis and with risk for acute cardiovascular events.

Another potential problem with the antioxidant clinical trials is that the choice of antioxidants may have been flawed. The most used vitamin E formulations contain mainly α-tocopherol. Recent studies showed that tocopherols, in addition to having activity as antioxidants, have important cell-signaling functions mediated by specific cellular receptors. Therapy with formulations containing primarily α-tocopherol may downregulate endogenous γ-tocopherol levels, leading to imbalance in natural tocopherol signaling pathways. Furthermore, tocopherols are lipid-based structures that are themselves subject to oxidation, producing lipid peroxides that can actually promote further oxidative stress. Nevertheless, it is possible that pathways of cholesterol uptake unrelated to LDL oxidation and SR expression, such as by micro- and macro-pinocytosis of "native" LDL or aggregated LDL, may play a significant role in foam cell formation.

Important unresolved issues in the pathogenesis of early atherosclerotic lesions include understanding why macrophages do not exit the vessel wall and travel to regional nodes after ingesting modified LDL, as they would after ingesting exogenous pathogens, and why cholesterol efflux cannot keep up with LDL uptake to maintain a homeostatic state. oxLDL inhibition of macrophage migration (see Fig. 144.4) may explain the former, suggesting that blocking oxLDL-mediated signaling pathways might have therapeutic potential by facilitating macrophage exit from developing plaque. Indeed, in experimental animals, transplantation of atherosclerotic aortae from hypercholesterolemic animals into normal recipients induces migration of lipid-laden macrophages out of the vessel wall and plaque regression.[19] The second issue might relate to differential gene regulation of SRs compared with cholesterol efflux transporters, and/or to intracellular cholesterol trafficking that might make it inaccessible to efflux transporters. In addition, as noted previously, HDL particles, similar to LDL, are sensitive to oxidative modification and such oxidation may produce dysfunctional HDL that does not function optimally in RCT and thus loses its atheroprotective activity.[6]

An intriguing recent development in understanding the cellular composition of plaque comes from so-called lineage marker studies that show that a surprisingly large percentage of foam cells expressing macrophage markers were actually derived from a smooth muscle cell lineage.[20] These studies suggest that local cues in plaque might interact with intimal or adventitial smooth muscle cells to redirect their genetic programs towards a macrophage-like phenotype. It is possible that such cells do not possess the full migratory capacity of macrophages and this could contribute to foam cell trapping in plaque.

LESION EVOLUTION: REMODELING AND THE VULNERABLE PLAQUE

In humans, plaque develops and evolves very slowly over many decades, explaining in part why animal models in which advanced lesions develop rapidly over weeks and months may not accurately reflect the human condition. Accumulation of foam cells is only one component of the atherogenic process. Early on, signals from macrophages (Fig. 144.5) and the injured endothelium, primarily platelet-derived growth factor (PDGF), stimulate adventitial smooth muscle cells to migrate into the intima and proliferate.[2] These cells contribute to the mass of the lesions, and secrete collagen and other factors that change the nature of the intimal extracellular matrix, and may even contribute to the burden of foam cells. Lymphocytes infiltrating from the circulation and mast cells from the adventitia also contribute to the inflammatory milieu and matrix remodeling. Platelet antigens are also readily detectable in plaque, suggesting that platelets enter the intima, where they may contribute to matrix remodeling and the inflammatory state by secreting PDGF, transforming growth factor-β, and other growth factors, along with platelet factor 4, which is a potent chemokine, also known as *CXCL4*,

for monocytes. Animal studies suggest that platelets may facilitate monocyte recruitment, acting as a bridge between the endothelium and circulating monocytes (see Fig. 144.5).[21] Sophisticated single-cell imaging studies in mice showed that monocytes continue to traffic through the "shoulders" of even advanced stage lesions.

Plaque generally grows in an eccentric pattern within the intima and in certain instances can create significant obstruction to blood flow (Fig. 144.6, *left*). In such cases, as oxygen demand increases, tissue ischemia results, leading to angina and/or lower extremity claudication. Recent in vivo studies using advanced imaging techniques, such as intravascular ultrasound, however, demonstrate that in most cases the vessel wall remodels as plaque grows (see Fig. 144.6, *right*) so that the arterial lumen is mostly preserved and the bulk of the atheromatous mass is ablumenal. These studies show that traditional two-dimensional angiographic techniques vastly underestimate plaque burden. Of note, such studies, along with careful histopathologic examinations, have led to the concept that the "quality" of the plaque may be more important than its quantity in predicting cardiovascular outcomes. Some plaques, particularly those with thick fibrous caps and cellular cores, seem to be stable (Fig. 144.7), whereas others, particularly those with thin fibrous caps, abundant leukocytes, and necrotic, lipid-rich cores, seem to be unstable and vulnerable to erosion and rupture (see Fig. 144.7). Rupture refers to the sudden loss of integrity of the fibrous cap with release of plaque material into the lumen, often followed by acute occlusive thrombosis. Erosion is a more subtle concept referring to loss of endothelial cells at the shoulder of the lesion or minimal leakage of plaque through a partially disrupted cap. Plaque erosion may lead to subocclusive thrombus formation and/or intraplaque hemorrhage and thrombosis. Repeated cycles of erosion and intraplaque hemorrhage/thrombosis may account for the apparent stepwise growth of some lesions.

Understanding factors that contribute to plaque vulnerability is an extremely important topic of research,[22] but one that is difficult

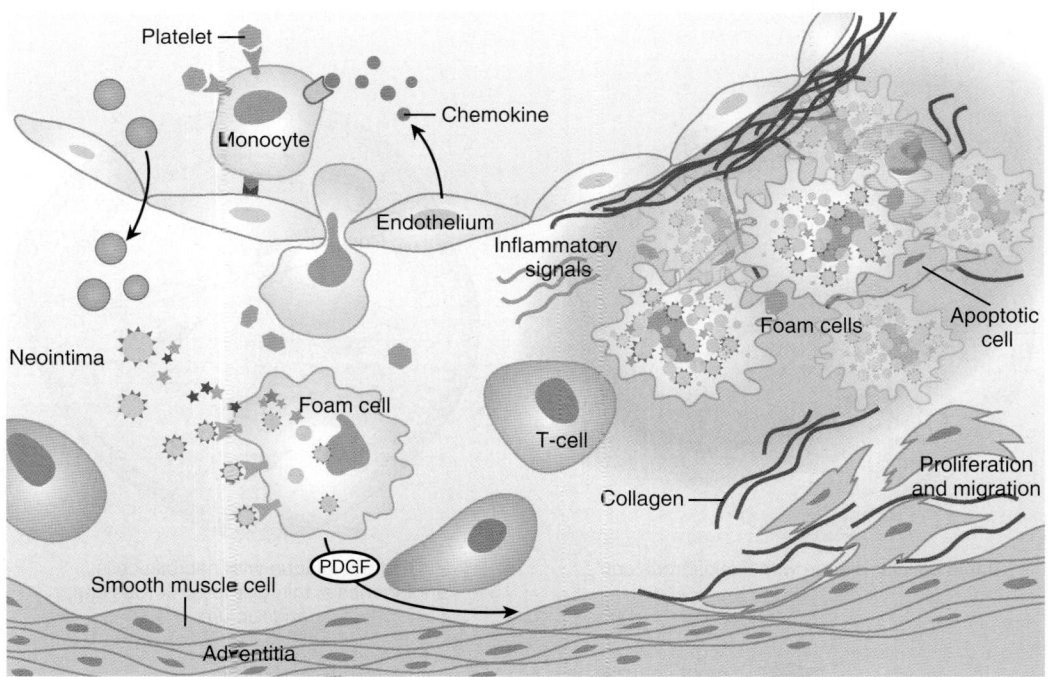

Fig. 144.5 LATER EVENTS IN ATHEROGENESIS. Fatty streaks formed in the vessel wall via accumulation of foam cells (see Fig. 144.4) evolve over many years into complex plaque. In response to chemokines, monocytes continue to enter plaque, perhaps accompanied by platelets. T cells, B cells, and other inflammatory cells also accumulate. Cholesterol loading of macrophages induces apoptosis and apoptotic cells accumulate because of dysfunction of normal efferocytotic clearance pathways. Smooth muscle cells respond to PDGF, transforming growth factor β, and other signals, and proliferate and migrate into the neointima. These cells produce collagen and other matrix components, contributing to plaque growth and formation of a fibrous cap. To support plaque growth, an angiogenic response is elicited from the vasa vasora within the adventitia. *PDGF*, Platelet-derived growth factor.

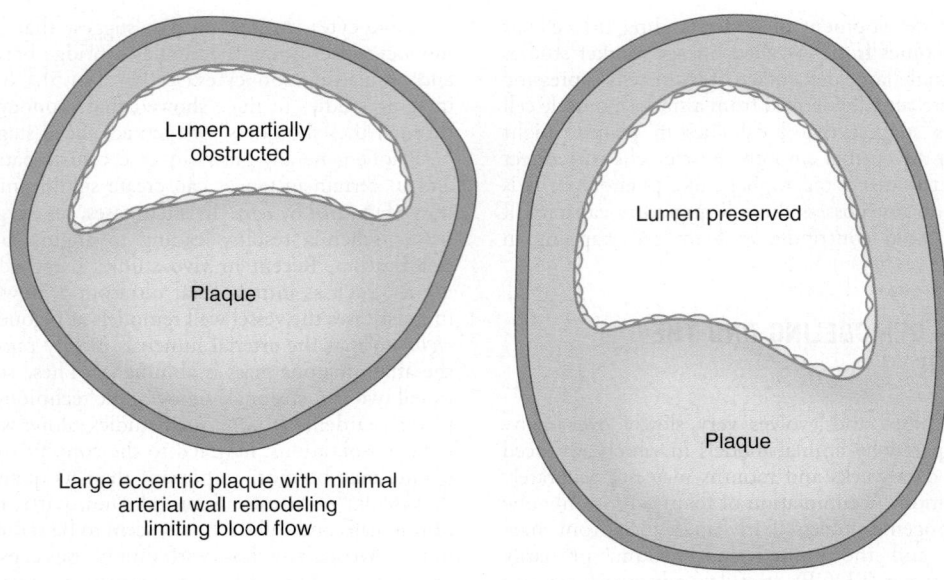

Lumen partially
obstructed

Plaque

Large eccentric plaque with minimal
arterial wall remodeling
limiting blood flow

Lumen preserved

Plaque

Large eccentric plaque with significant
arterial wall remodeling
preserving flow

Fig. 144.6 VESSEL WALL REMODELING CAN PRESERVE ARTERIAL LUMEN. On the *left* is a cross-section cartoon image of an artery containing a large eccentric plaque *(orange)*. The vessel has undergone minimal remodeling. The atheromatous lesion is extending into the arterial lumen and would be visible on an angiogram as an obstructing lesion. On the *right* is a lesion of similar mass, but its formation was accompanied by significant vessel wall remodeling so that the lesion extends mainly into the vessel wall, preserving the lumen. On an angiogram this would be nearly invisible.

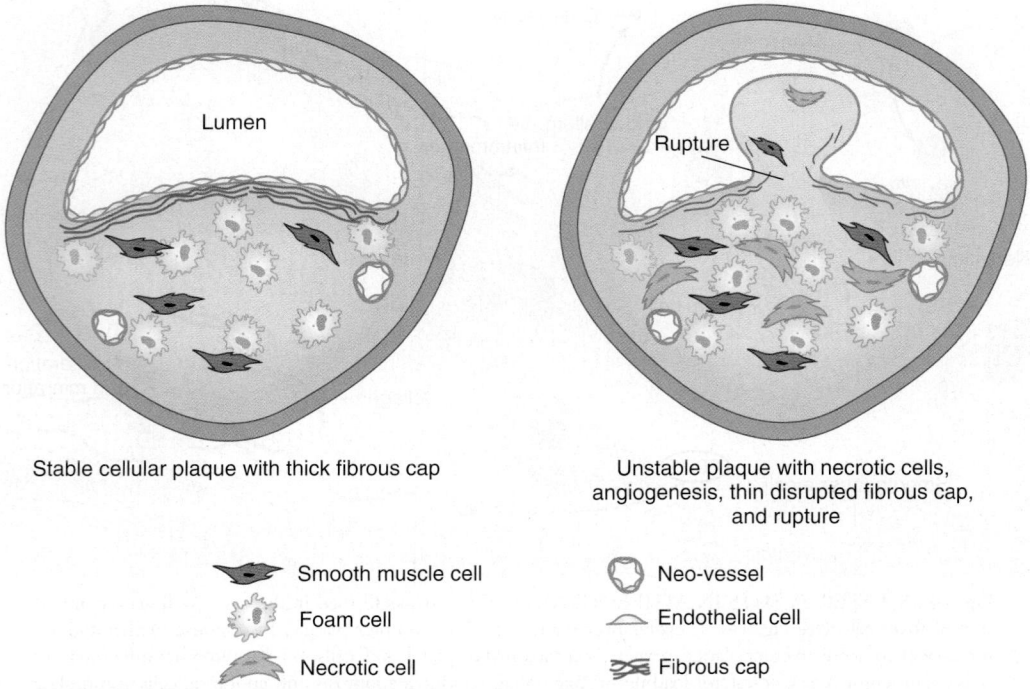

Lumen

Stable cellular plaque with thick fibrous cap

Rupture

Unstable plaque with necrotic cells,
angiogenesis, thin disrupted fibrous cap,
and rupture

Smooth muscle cell   Neo-vessel

Foam cell   Endothelial cell

Necrotic cell   Fibrous cap

Fig. 144.7 UNSTABLE PLAQUE IS PRONE TO RUPTURE. On the *left* is a cross-section cartoon image of an artery with a plaque containing abundant smooth muscle cells and foam cells and a thick fibrous cap. On the *right* is a similar-size plaque, but with a thin fibrous cap that has ruptured allowing plaque contents to extrude into the lumen. This plaque contains smooth muscle cells and foam cells, as in the stable plaque on the left, but there is abundant angiogenesis, along with apoptotic and necrotic cells.

to model in animals. Some key features that have emerged are the degree of angiogenesis within the plaque, balance of matrix-degrading enzymes and enzyme inhibitors, level of apoptosis of cells within the plaque, deposition of calcium within the plaque, and level of systemic and local inflammation.

Plaque angiogenesis is a recently appreciated process that can be visualized by certain imaging modalities, such as ultrafast computed tomography (CT) and magnetic resonance imaging (MRI), in real time.[23] Based on analogy to tumor growth, it is not surprising that the growing plaque requires a blood supply and also that the neovessels within the plaque may, similar to their counterparts in cancer, be leaky and unstable. This neovascular instability may contribute to plaque instability by facilitating entry of inflammatory cells, platelets, and plasma components, such as fibrinogen and cell-derived microparticles (MPs). In animal models, treatment with antiangiogenic agents significantly slows plaque growth. In some disease states, such as diabetes, accelerated atherosclerosis may reflect a "microvascular" disease of the vasa vasora.

Integrity of the fibrous cap is maintained by a balance between collagen synthesis by smooth muscle cells and fibroblasts, and collagenolysis by matrix-degrading enzymes. The latter is maintained by a balance between enzymes and their endogenous inhibitors. The predominant enzymes are members of the large family of zinc-dependent matrix metalloproteinases (MMPs), which are capable of degrading most matrix components, including collagen. These enzymes are tightly regulated by a network of activators and inhibitors, and in settings in which activation exceeds inhibition, excessive matrix degradation may occur. Metalloproteases of the ADAM (a disintegrin and metalloprotease domain) family and ADAMTS (a disintegrin and metalloprotease domain with thrombospondin structural homology domains) family may also contribute to plaque instability. Although several clinical trials have studied MMP inhibitors in atherosclerosis, none has shown clear benefit to date.

A prominent feature of advanced atherosclerotic lesions is the presence of apoptotic cells, mostly of macrophage and smooth muscle cell origin. The nature of the proapoptotic signals within plaque is incompletely understood, but excess intracellular cholesterol can initiate the endoplasmic reticulum stress response, leading to apoptosis.[24] oxLDL signaling through SRs and/or TLRs can also induce apoptosis.[25] In most inflammatory sites, apoptotic leukocytes are quickly removed by phagocytes in a process known as *efferocytosis*. The efferocytotic macrophages are generally thought to be of the M2 antiinflammatory type; thus their engagement by apoptotic cells not only removes the apoptotic cell from the microenvironment, but also directly contributes to downregulation of the inflammatory state by inducing secretion of antiinflammatory cytokines and effectors. In atherosclerotic plaque, this process seems to be inefficient so that apoptotic cells accumulate, contributing to the lipid load and releasing potentially toxic contents.

Although therapeutic interventions to stabilize vulnerable plaque or prevent plaques from becoming vulnerable have not yet materialized, several imaging approaches have been studied in attempt to develop useful biomarkers to identify vulnerable plaque and therefore to identify patients who might benefit from aggressive antithrombotic and lipid-lowering therapeutic interventions. Neovascular imaging using CT or MRI is a promising technology, as is plaque characterization by optical coherence tomography, high-resolution MRI, linear infrared imaging, and thermography.[23]

PLAQUE RUPTURE AND ACUTE ARTERIAL THROMBOSIS

The devastating complications of atherosclerosis, including acute coronary syndrome (ACS), stroke, gangrene, and sudden death, result primarily from acute and subacute thrombosis occurring at the site of plaque rupture (Fig. 144.8). As described in later chapters in this section, treatment and prevention strategies using aggressive antiplatelet, anticoagulant, fibrinolytic, and/or mechanical approaches have been remarkably effective at reducing major cardiovascular events, but tremendous unmet need still exists,

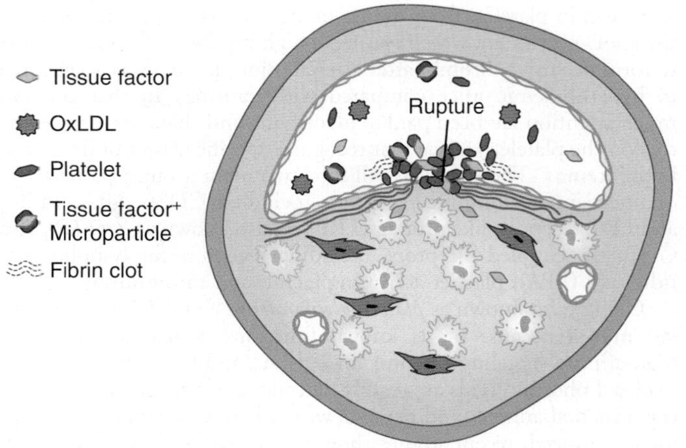

Fig. 144.8 ACUTE PLATELET-RICH THROMBUS AT SITE OF PLAQUE RUPTURE. An atherosclerotic artery with a ruptured plaque (as described in Fig. 144.7) serves as a nidus for formation of an acute thrombus. Tissue factor (TF) contained in plaque or expressed on circulating microparticles (MPs) leads to thrombin generation and formation of fibrin at the site of rupture. Platelets accumulate at the rupture site and are activated by plaque components, such as collagen, forming an aggregate that, if large enough, can obstruct blood flow. Blood in patients with advanced atherosclerosis is prothrombotic, in part because of oxidized low-density lipoprotein (LDL)–induced release of TF-positive MPs from monocytes. Oxidized LDL also interacts with platelets to make them more sensitive to activation and aggregation by plaque contents.

particularly in the areas of primary and secondary prevention of thrombosis.

Pathophysiologic mechanisms underlying acute arterial thrombosis center on two key concepts: (1) exposure of prothrombotic materials to the local circulation as a consequence of plaque rupture acts as a thrombotic trigger, and (2) advanced atherosclerosis is associated with a systemic prothrombotic state that accelerates or enhances pathologic thrombosis.[25] The former mechanism undoubtedly plays a major role. Immunohistochemical studies have convincingly shown that plaque contains abundant tissue factor (TF), and acute anticoagulation therapy directed toward blocking thrombin generation or inhibiting thrombin has proven to be effective in ACS. Plaque TF is derived mainly from smooth muscle cells, fibroblasts, and activated macrophages. Recent studies have also suggested that platelets can synthesize TF after stimulation by inflammatory mediators and thus may also contribute to the plaque procoagulant load. A significant proportion of plaque TF may be in the form of membrane-bound MPs derived from apoptotic and/or activated cells (see next section for more detailed explanation).[26] Exposure of flowing blood to TF exposed in or released from ruptured plaque leads to rapid activation of factor X, thrombin generation, and activation of platelets. In addition to TF, other components of plaque that become exposed to blood at sites of rupture include collagen and oxidized phospholipids, both of which can activate platelets directly. Thus aggressive antiplatelet therapy with aspirin, P2Y12 inhibitors, and glycoprotein αIIbβ3 inhibitors are mainstays of the pharmacologic approach to treatment of ACS; and aspirin and P2Y12 inhibitors are of proven efficacy for secondary prevention.

HYPERLIPIDEMIA, ATHEROSCLEROSIS, AND A SYSTEMIC PROTHROMBOTIC STATE

Platelet hyperreactivity has long been thought to play a role in acute atherothrombosis. Clinical studies support an association between in vitro platelet reactivity and prognosis in patients with coronary disease, and it was shown in the 1970s that platelets from patients with familial hypercholesterolemia were more sensitive to activation by epinephrine or adenosine diphosphate (ADP). Similar findings were seen in platelets from mouse models of hyperlipidemia, such as the apoE-null strain, which was fed a high-fat diet. Of note, the time to form occlusive thrombi after arterial injury in vivo was accelerated in hyperlipidemic mice compared with controls. In that context, much attention has been paid to identifying and characterizing receptors on the platelet surface that recognize specific classes of lipids and lipoproteins.[25] The receptors fall into two main groups: pattern recognition innate immune receptors, including CD36, SRA, TLR4, and LDL receptor–like protein (LRP)-8 (also known as *apoER2*), and G-protein–coupled receptors, including receptors for lysophosphatidic acid (LPA), platelet-activating factor, and thromboxane.

CD36 (also known as *platelet glycoprotein IV or IIIb*) is of particular interest because of its known function on macrophages as a high-affinity signaling receptor for oxLDL, and because oxLDL and oxidized phospholipids are readily detectable in circulating plasma of experimental animals and patients with atherosclerosis and hyperlipidemia. Indeed, recent studies showed that oxLDL bound to CD36 on the surface of platelets in a specific, concentration-, and time-dependent manner. At high concentrations, such as might occur during acute plaque rupture, oxLDL activates platelets, and at lower concentrations, such as those observed in the circulation of individuals with atherosclerosis, oxLDL augmented platelet-aggregation responses to low doses of "classic" platelet agonists, such as ADP and collagen. More recently platelet CD36 was shown to bind MP and advanced glycated proteins, suggesting that circulating endogenous "danger signals" generated by oxidant stress, hyperglycemia, and inflammation could induce a prothrombotic state through this pathway.[27]

Platelets also express SRB1, a CD36 family protein that functions in the liver as a cholesterol acceptor for HDL. The function of SRB1 on platelets is not well understood, but at least one study showed that oxHDL, but not native HDL, inhibited platelet reactivity to multiple agonists, including ADP, collagen, and thrombin via binding to SRB1. HDL is at least as susceptible to oxidation in vitro and in vivo as LDL, and it is possible that the balance between oxLDL and oxHDL and the relative expression levels of CD36, SRB1, and other receptors may determine platelet reactivity in patients with hyperlipidemia and oxidant stress.

Atherosclerotic plaque and so-called "minimally" oxLDL contain LPA, a family of biologically active lipids generated by the action of phospholipases on LDL and cell membrane lipids. Platelets express at least three different G-protein–coupled LPA receptors but the in vivo relevance of this system has not been demonstrated. Ex vivo studies, however, demonstrated that minimally oxLDL at high concentrations could induce platelet shape change and sensitize platelets to aggregate in response to other agonists. Epidemiologic studies have also associated levels of soluble phospholipase A2 with cardiovascular risk. In addition to participating in LPA biosynthesis, this family of enzymes generates free fatty acids from phospholipids that serve as substrates for cyclooxygenase and lipoxygenases, producing both pro- and antiatherogenic eicosanoids.

LRP-8 (particularly a splice variant known as apoER2) binds lipidated apoE3 (e.g., chylomicrons and remnant particles), resulting in enhanced nitric oxide production and inhibition of platelet activation by ADP and other agonists. On the other hand, LRP-8 has also been shown to bind apoB-containing lipoproteins, leading to enhanced thromboxane generation and sensitization of platelets to other agonists. Consistent with this, in mice genetic deletion of LRP-8 has an antithrombotic effect in models of arterial injury.

In addition to platelet hyperreactivity, it is also quite likely that systemic activation of the coagulation cascade contributes to the prothrombotic state associated with advanced atherosclerosis. This is consistent with studies showing that atherosclerosis is associated with increased risk for venous thromboembolic disorders, as well as arterial thrombosis. Elevated levels of circulating D-dimer and thrombin–antithrombin complexes have been reported in patients with ACS, and D-dimer levels tend to track with hsCRP. Large-scale population studies have identified elevated fibrinogen and factor VIII levels as risk factors for atherosclerosis. Recent studies suggest that a key initiator of thrombin generation in these settings is circulating TF

(see Fig. 144.8) in the form of TF-expressing MPs.[26] MPs are vesicular fragments that bud off from cells during either activation or apoptosis. They are 200–1000 nm in size and possess different antigenic properties depending on the cell from which they are derived. MPs can be generated from platelets, monocytes, erythrocytes, leukocytes, or endothelial cells during vascular injury and have been shown to become incorporated into developing thrombi in vivo. MPs, mostly of platelet origin, can be detected in the circulation of normal human subjects, but markedly increased numbers of circulating MPs have been reported in patients with a variety of inflammatory and prothrombotic disorders including ACS.

MPs contribute to thrombus formation through several mechanisms. A general feature of MP generation is loss of membrane asymmetry so that anionic phospholipids normally oriented in the inner membrane leaflet become exposed on the outer leaflet. Surface-exposed phosphatidylserine (PS) is a site for catalytic assembly of the prothrombinase complex and thrombin generation. Furthermore, PS on the surface of MP also has the capacity to bind to platelet CD36 and enhance platelet reactivity via the same mechanism as oxLDL.

It is important to note that MPs derived from some cells (e.g., monocytes, macrophages, smooth muscle cells, and tumor cells) are a source of circulating TF. A mechanistic link between atherogenesis and thrombosis may be oxLDL, which in vitro can induce TF-positive MP generation from blood-derived monocytes.[28] Of interest, a recent large clinical trial (JUPITER) testing the efficacy of statins in subjects with normal LDL, but elevated levels of hsCRP, showed that rates of venous thrombosis, as well as coronary events, were significantly decreased. In animal models, statins decrease circulating levels of oxLDL and also decrease circulating MP levels and levels of other prothrombotic and proinflammatory biomarkers, even in the absence of lowering cholesterol, suggesting that oxLDL-mediated prothrombotic activities may be important targets for thromboprevention in patients with atherosclerosis. These studies also support those showing that statins may have antiinflammatory and antithrombotic activities independent of lipid lowering. Because HMGCoA reductase is also the limiting step in biosynthesis of isoprenoids, it has been postulated that statins may dampen signaling pathways mediated by small-molecular-weight G proteins (e.g., Ras) in which membrane targeting by protein isoprenylation is required (see Fig. 144.2).

In mice, the contact activating system and intrinsic coagulation cascade have been shown to participate in arterial thrombosis after injury and to have proatherogenic properties.[14] Targeting these systems is attractive in that patients with known deficiencies in factor XII or contact system proteins have no obvious phenotype and do not have a bleeding diathesis, thus presumably an antithrombotic effect could be achieved without altering normal hemostasis.

CROSS-TALK BETWEEN COAGULATION AND INFLAMMATION SYSTEMS IMPACT ATHEROGENESIS

As noted previously, atherosclerosis can be thought of as a chronic, low-grade inflammatory disease of the artery wall. Clinical studies based on biomarkers, such as hsCRP, MPO, and IL-6, also suggest that advanced atherosclerosis is associated with a systemic state of chronic inflammation and that the degree of inflammation reflects the level of risk for major complications, possibly because the more inflamed the plaque, the more vulnerable the lesion. It is also now clear that mediators of inflammation, such as IL-1, LPA, oxLDL, and circulating MPs may interact with platelets and the coagulation cascade to promote a hypercoagulable, prothrombotic state. Furthermore, mediators of coagulation, such as thrombin, TF–factor VIIa complexes, and factor Xa, may contribute to the proinflammatory state by interacting with protease-activated receptors on endothelial cells and leukocytes. Activated platelets can contribute to inflammation by facilitating monocyte adhesion to endothelium and by secreting small molecules (ATP, pyrophosphates, and serotonin), cytokines, and growth factors that have proinflammatory activity. Thus bidirectional cross-talk between the inflammation and coagulation systems serves to enhance each other and to promote atherosclerosis.

Not surprisingly, patients with systemic autoimmune inflammatory disorders, including rheumatoid arthritis, Wegener's granulomatosis, and lupus erythematosus have been shown to have accelerated atherosclerosis, as assessed by biomarkers, such as ultrasound evidence of carotid artery intima-medial thickening, as well as major cardiovascular events. Obesity, a risk factor for atherosclerosis, is now also known to be a systemic inflammatory disorder, with evidence of inflammation readily detectable within obese central adipose tissue. Obese patients also have elevated, circulating levels of coagulation and inflammation biomarkers, including plasminogen activator inhibitor-1 (PAI-1).

Given these observations, there has been renewed interest in exploring the use of antiinflammatory agents and antithrombotic agents to slow the progress of atherosclerosis. The approach has been tempered by clinical studies showing small increases in atherosclerotic complications in patients taking cyclooxygenase (COX) inhibitors (especially those with preferential activity against COX2), but this may relate to the specific target and the complication of altered eicosanoid production, perhaps changing the balance away from antiatherothrombotic end products, such as prostacyclin and resolvins, towards proatherothrombotic products, such as thromboxane, HETE, and lipoxins. Also, although aspirin and ADP receptor antagonists definitively reduce risk for major cardiovascular events, no studies have shown an impact on burden of atheroma. Nevertheless, novel agents targeted to more specific atherothrombotic pathways, such as chemokines, LDL oxidation, SRs, lipoxygenases, phospholipase 2, leukotrienes, selectins, and IL-1 are being considered.[29]

PLAQUE REGRESSION

Finding pharmacologic approaches to decrease the amount of arterial plaque has proved to be an elusive goal. Intravenous ultrasound has shown that very aggressive lowering of LDL cholesterol with high-dose statins and extremely rigorous dietary alterations can halt plaque progression and, in some cases, cause some regression.[4] As noted previously, strategies to enhance RCT or to induce macrophage emigration from plaque are being developed, and strategies to stabilize plaque by targeting the neovasculature, cellular apoptosis, and efferocytosis are being considered. Specific antioxidant approaches based on fundamental understanding of the oxidation processes relevant to atherosclerosis remain viable as well, and much effort is being put into developing new animal models to study plaque regression.

ADDITIONAL FUTURE DIRECTIONS

Initial enthusiasm for large-scale genome-wide association studies (GWAS) as discovery platforms to identify novel genes and pathways that could be targeted with therapeutic or preventive effect has waned as multiple expensive studies have failed to produce impressive results. The most consistent data to come from GWAS identified a fairly large genomic region on chromosome 9p21 as a risk site, but identification of specific genes has not yet been accomplished with certainty. More recently, approaches moving beyond GWAS have coupled whole-genome or whole-exome sequencing of highly selective subjects (such as genetically isolated Icelanders[30] or subjects with high or low lipoprotein levels) followed by deep sequencing of specific candidate genes in larger cohorts. This approach has yielded new data identifying potential novel antiatherothrombosis targets; for example, loss of function variants of asialoglycoprotein receptor-1, NPC1L1, and APOC3 were found to be associated with decreased levels of non-HDL cholesterol and decreased risk of coronary artery disease.

An area of research that has generated significant intriguing data of potential relevance to atherosclerosis diagnostics and therapeutics is microRNA (MiR) biology. MiRs are small noncoding RNAs that regulate gene expression levels in a sequence-specific manner by posttranscriptional mechanisms. Dozens of specific MiRs have been identified that are expressed in highly regulated tissue-specific manners, and that regulate expression of genes involved in all aspects of atherosclerosis, including hepatic lipoprotein homeostasis; macrophage, endothelial cell, and smooth muscle cell functions; mechanosensory functions; and cytokine expression.[31] Therapeutic interventions based on specific MiRs are under development, including, as noted previously, an inhibitor of MiR-33 to raise HDL levels and promote RCT. Unbiased "omics" studies to identify expression levels of MiR–mRNA pairs that associate with cardiovascular risk or with circulating lipoprotein levels also show promise for both biomarker development and therapeutic target discovery.

Another very promising avenue of research in atherothrombosis is the gut microbiome. Elegant studies using mouse models and human subjects have identified a "metaorganismal" pathway that contributes both to the development of plaque[32] and to the prothrombotic state associated with atherosclerosis.[33] Diets rich in phosphatidyl choline, choline, and carnitine (which are present in meats, eggs, and cheese) can be metabolized in the gut by specific genera of microbes to generate trimethyl amine (TMA). TMA enters the circulation and is then converted to trimethyl amine oxide (TMAO) in the liver by flavin monooxidase enzymes. TMA and TMAO levels in blood associate strongly with both risk of cardiovascular disease and arterial thrombosis in human subjects, and TMAO was shown to promote platelet activation in vitro and thrombosis in vivo in animal models. Importantly, the constitution of the gut microbiome can be influenced by diet, and thus the ability to generate TMA and TMAO can also be influenced by diet. Human subjects on vegan diets have much less ability to generate TMA/TMAO than do carnivores and omnivores, and this could be restored simply by adding back meat, eggs, or carnitine to the diet. Interestingly, atherothrombotic risk in mice could be transmitted from susceptible to resistant strains by fecal microbiome transplant,[34] and resistant strains could be converted to susceptible by antibiotic or dietary manipulation of the microbiome. These studies suggest that microbial enzymes and/or ecosystems could be targeted for atherothrombosis treatment and prevention strategies.

Finally, although B cells are not prominent cellular constituents of plaque, B1 subclass cells responsible for innate antibody generation are present in plaque from humans and experimental animals. These cells produce innate IgM antibodies, including a prevalent species called E06 that reacts with oxLDL. E06 and other autoantibodies against plaque constituents may be protective, perhaps by facilitating clearance of oxLDL via pathways that do not lead to foam cell formation, and/or by interfering with oxLDL-mediated activation of circulating monocytes and platelets.[15] Based on these observations, passive immunization strategies against oxLDL are also being considered.

REFERENCES

1. Mozaffarian D, Benjamin EJ, Go AS, et al: Heart disease and stroke statistics – 2016 update: a report from the American Heart Association. *Circulation* 133:e38–e360, 2015.
2. Libby P, Ridker PM, Hansson GK: Progress and challenges in translating the biology of atherosclerosis. *Nature* 473:317–325, 2011.
3. Plump AS, Smith JD, Hayek T, et al: Severe hypercholesterolemia and atherosclerosis in apolipoprotein E-deficient mice created by homologous recombination in ES cells. *Cell* 71:343–353, 1992.
4. Nicholls SJ, Ballantyne CM, Barter PJ, et al: Effect of two intensive statin regimens on progression of coronary disease. *N Engl J Med* 365:2078–2087, 2011.
5. Sabatine MS, Giugliano RP, Wiviott SD, et al: Efficacy and safety of evolucumab in reducing lipids and cardiovascular events. *N Engl J Med* 372:1500–1508, 2015.
6. Undurti A, Huang Y, Lupica JA, et al: Modification of high density lipoprotein by myeloperoxidase generates a pro-inflammatory particle. *J Biol Chem* 284:30825–30835, 2009.

7. Rohatgi A, Khera A, Berry JD, et al: HDL cholesterol efflux capacity and incident cardiovascular events. *N Engl J Med* 371:2383–2393, 2014.

8. Fernández-Hernando C, Moore KJ: MicroRNA modulation of cholesterol homeostasis. *Arterioscler Thromb Vasc Biol* 31:2378–2382, 2011.

9. Goff DC, Jr, Lloyd-Jones DM, Bennett G, et al: ACC/AHA guideline on the assessment of cardiovascular risk: a report of the American College of Cardiology/ American Heart Association Task Force of Practice Guidelines. *Circulation* 129:S49–S73, 2014.

10. McPherson R, Hegele RA: Ezetimibe: rescued by Randomization (Clinical and Mendelian). *Arterioscler Thromb Vasc Biol* 35:e13–e15, 2015.

11. Khetarpal SA, Rader DJ: Triglyceride-rich lipoproteins and coronary artery disease risk: new insights from human genetics. *Arterioscler Thromb Vasc Biol* 35:e3–e9, 2015.

12. Moore KJ, Tabas I: Macrophages in the pathogenesis of atherosclerosis. *Cell* 145:341–355, 2011.

13. Steinberg D, Witztum JL: Oxidized low-density lipoprotein and atherosclerosis. *Arterioscler Thromb Vasc Biol* 30:2311, 2010.

14. Borissoff JI, Spronk HM, ten Cate H: The hemostatic system as a modulator of atherosclerosis. *N Engl J Med* 364:1746, 2011.

15. Hedrick CC: Lymphocytes in atherosclerosis. *Arterioscler Thromb Vasc Biol* 35:253–257, 2015.

16. Silverstein RL, Febbraio M: CD36, a scavenger receptor involved in immunity, metabolism, angiogenesis, and behavior. *Sci Signal* 2re3, 2009.

17. Nagy L, Tontonoz P, Alvarez JG, et al: Oxidized LDL regulates macrophage gene expression through ligand activation of PPARgamma. *Cell* 93:229–240, 1998.

18. Mitra S, Deshmukh A, Sachdeva R, et al: Oxidized low-density lipoprotein and atherosclerosis implications in antioxidant therapy. *Am J Med Sci* 342:135–142, 2011.

19. Llodrá J, Angeli V, Liu J, et al: Emigration of monocyte-derived cells from atherosclerotic lesions characterizes regressive, but not progressive, plaques. *Proc Natl Acad Sci USA* 101:11779–11784, 2004.

20. Bennett MR, Sinha S, Owens GK: Vascular smooth muscle cells in atherosclerosis. *Circ Res* 118:692–702, 2016.

21. Massberg S, Brand K, Grüner S, et al: A critical role of platelet adhesion in the initiation of atherosclerotic lesion formation. *J Exp Med* 196:887–896, 2002.

22. Finn AV, Nakano M, Narula J, et al: Concept of vulnerable/unstable plaque. *Arterioscler Thromb Vasc Biol* 30:1282–1292, 2010.

23. Dweck MR, Doris MK, Motwani M, et al: Imaging of coronary atherosclerosis – evolution towards new treatment strategies. *Nat Rev Cardiol* 13:533–548, 2016.

24. Scull CM, Tabas I: Mechanisms of ER stress-induced apoptosis in atherosclerosis. *Arterioscler Thromb Vasc Biol* 31:2792–2797, 2011.

25. Podrez EA, Byzova TV, Febbraio M, et al: Platelet CD36 links hyperlipidemia, oxidant stress and a prothrombotic phenotype. *Nat Med* 13:1086–1095, 2007.

26. Rautou PE, Vion AC, Amabile N, et al: Microparticles, vascular function, and atherothrombosis. *Circ Res* 109:593–606, 2011.

27. Silverstein RL: Type 2 scavenger receptor CD36 in platelet activation: the role of hyperlipidemia and oxidative stress. *Clin Lipidol* 4:767, 2009.

28. Owens AP, 3rd, Passam FH, Antoniak S, et al: Monocyte tissue factor-dependent activation of coagulation in hypercholesterolemic mice and monkeys is inhibited by simvastatin. *J Clin Invest* 122:558–568, 2012.

29. Charo IF, Taub R: Anti-inflammatory therapeutics for the treatment of atherosclerosis. *Nat Rev Drug Discov* 10:365–376, 2011.

30. Nioi P, Sigurdsson A, Thorleifsson G, et al: Variant *ASGR1* associated with a reduced risk of coronary artery disease. *N Engl J Med* 374:2131–22141, 2016.

31. Feinberg MW, Moore KJ: MicroRNA regulation of atherosclerosis. *Circ Res* 118:703–720, 2016.

32. Koeth RA, Wang Z, Levison BS, et al: Intestinal microbiota metabolism of L-carnitine, a nutrient in red meat, promotes atherosclerosis. *Nat Med* 19:576–585, 2013.

33. Zhu W, Gregory JC, Org E, et al: Gut microbial metabolite TMAO enhances platelet hyperreactivity and thrombosis risk. *Cell* 165:111–124, 2016.

34. Gregory JC, Buff JA, Org E, et al: Transmission of atherosclerosis susceptibility with gut microbial transplantation. *J Biol Chem* 290:5647–5660, 2015.

Stroke is the leading cause of acquired adult disability worldwide and the fourth most common cause of death in developed countries. Primary stroke subtypes include ischemic stroke, intracerebral hemorrhage (ICH), and subarachnoid hemorrhage (SAH). Each stroke subtype has differing etiologies, outcomes, and management strategies. The past 20 years has seen considerable advances in diagnosis (emergence of widely available neuroimaging) and treatment of acute stroke. In addition, there is an increased awareness of the importance of covert stroke (stroke on neuroimaging without a history of acute clinical stroke). In this chapter we provide an overview of stroke, with a primary focus on ischemic stroke, which is the most common cause of stroke worldwide.

DEFINITION

Stroke is defined by the World Health Organization (WHO) as "rapidly developing clinical signs of focal (at times global) disturbance of cerebral function, lasting more than 24 hours or leading to death with no apparent cause other than that of vascular origin." This definition is conventionally considered to include ischemic stroke, ICH, and SAH. However, because of advances in our knowledge about the nature, timing, and clinical presentation of stroke and its mimics, as well as significant advances in neuroimaging (particularly magnetic resonance imaging [MRI]), an updated definition of central nervous system (CNS) infarction has been proposed by the American Heart Association (AHA)/American Stroke Association (ASA). CNS infarction (including hemorrhagic infarction) is defined as "brain, spinal cord, or retinal cell death attributable to ischemia, based on: (1) pathologic, imaging, or other objective evidence of cerebral, spinal cord, or retinal focal ischemic injury in a defined vascular distribution; or (2) clinical evidence of cerebral, spinal cord, or retinal focal ischemic injury based on symptoms persisting ≥24 hours or until death, and other etiologies have been excluded." According to the AHA/ASA, a transient ischemic attack (TIA) is defined as a transient episode of neurologic dysfunction caused by focal brain, spinal cord, or retinal ischemia, without acute infarction.

EPIDEMIOLOGY

Frequency

The WHO estimates that 15 million people suffer a stroke each year, and of these, 5 million people are left with permanent disability. In the absence of further effective population-based interventions, a projected 6.5 million stroke deaths will occur in 2015 and 7.8 million deaths in 2030. A small decrease in age-specific stroke mortality rates has been projected from 2005 to 2030, which is largely because of a decline in mortality rates in high-income countries. However, because of an increasingly aging population worldwide, the crude stroke mortality rates are projected to increase across all ages, from 89 per 100,000 in 2005 to an estimated 98 per 100,000 in 2030. The increase in stroke mortality will be most marked in developing countries, where increases in stroke incidence are most prominent. Worldwide, stroke shows significant geographical variation in terms of incidence (and temporal trends), case fatality, and case mix (i.e., stroke subtypes). A systematic review of population-based studies reported that from 1970 to 2008 there was a 42% decrease in the incidence of stroke in high-income countries, compared with a more than 100% increase in the incidence of stroke in middle- and low-income countries.

Traditional Risk Factors for Stroke

Both ischemic stroke and ICH are associated with a number of potentially modifiable risk factors, including hypertension, diabetes mellitus, smoking, poor diet, and physical inactivity. The INTER-STROKE study, which included 26,919 participants from 32 countries, reported that 10 key risk factors are associated with 90% of the population-attributable risk (PAR) of ischemic stroke, namely hypertension, smoking, waist-to-hip ratio, diet, physical activity level, diabetes mellitus, alcohol intake, psychosocial stress/depression, cardiac causes such as atrial fibrillation, and ratio of apolipoprotein B to apolipoprotein A1 (Table 145.1). Of these risk factors, five were associated with about 80% of the PAR for all stroke (hypertension, smoking, abdominal obesity, physical inactivity, and diet), and each was an important risk factor for both ischemic and hemorrhagic stroke. Thus a large proportion of stroke is potentially preventable through population-based interventions aimed at modifying these risk factors. Hypertension is the strongest risk factor for both ischemic stroke and ICH and, arguably, the most modifiable though lifestyle intervention (e.g., reducing salt intake) and use of antihypertensive medications.

PATHOBIOLOGY

Stroke can be primarily classified into ischemic stroke (Fig. 145.1) and hemorrhagic stroke. Hemorrhagic stroke is further subtyped into ICH (Fig. 145.2) and SAH. In North America and Europe, approximately 87% of strokes are caused by ischemia, with the remaining 13% occurring caused by hemorrhage.

Etiological Classification of Ischemic Stroke

Unlike acute coronary syndrome, which is primarily caused by large-vessel atherosclerosis, the underlying mechanisms for ischemic stroke are more heterogeneous. The most commonly used etiological classification is the Trial of Org 10172 in Acute Stroke Treatment (TOAST) classification system, which focuses on the pathophysiologic mechanism of ischemic stroke, based on clinical features and the results of diagnostic investigations (brain imaging, cardiac investigations, and neurovascular imaging). The five etiological subcategories in the TOAST classification system are: large-artery, cardioembolism, small-artery occlusion (or lacunar ischemic stroke), stroke of other determined etiology, and stroke of undetermined etiology.

Large-Artery Stroke

Large-artery stroke is usually a consequence of atherosclerosis in the extracranial (carotid or vertebral) and/or intracranial arteries (e.g., middle cerebral or basilar artery), with plaque rupture and thrombus formation. Ischemic stroke may result from artery-to-artery thromboembolism with distal occlusion or, less commonly, by acute

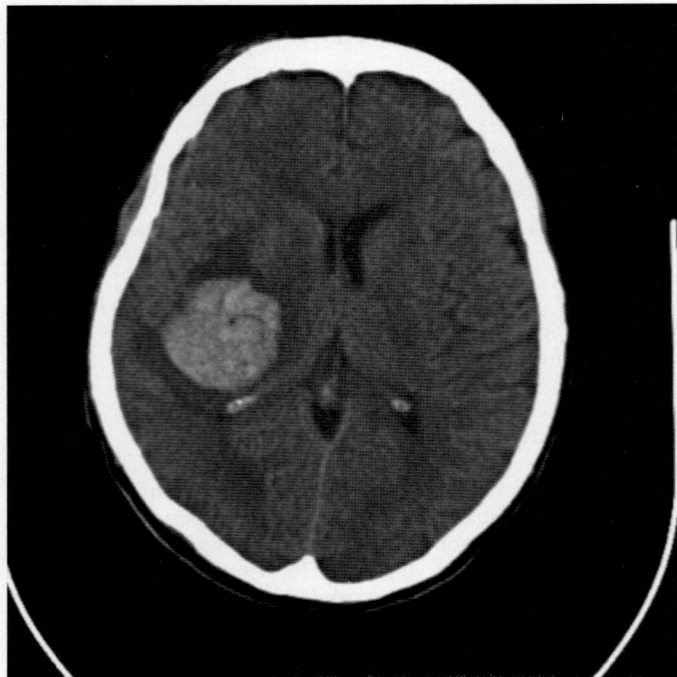

Fig. 145.1 COMPUTED TOMOGRAPHY OF BRAIN WITH RIGHT INTRACEREBRAL HEMORRHAGE.

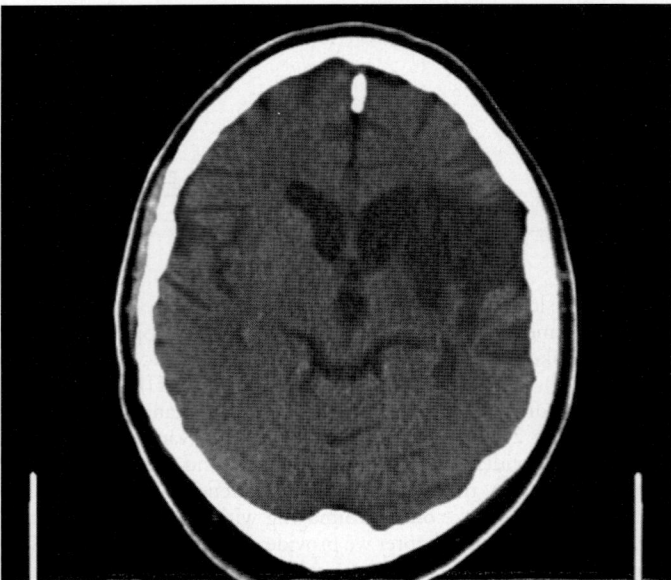

Fig. 145.2 COMPUTED TOMOGRAPHY OF BRAIN WITH LEFT HEMISPHERIC ISCHEMIC STROKE.

TABLE 145.1	Traditional Risk Factors for Ischemic Stroke
Risk Factor	**PAR (99% CI)**
Hypertension (self-reported history or blood pressure ≥140/90 mmHg)	47.9% (45.1–50.6)
Current smoking[a]	12.4% (10.2–14.9)
Diabetes mellitus	3.9% (1.9–7.6%)
Ratio of apoB to apoA1	26.8% (22.2–31.9)
Obesity (waist to hip ratio)	18.6% (13.3–25.3)
Physical inactivity	35.8% (27.7–44.7)
Diet risk score	23.2% (18.2–28.9)
Alcohol consumption (current)	5.8% (3.4–9.7)
Psychosocial factors	17.4% (13.1–22.6)
Cardiac etiologies	9.1% (8.0–10.2)

[a]Comparator for current smoker and alcohol intake is never or former.
Apo, Apolipoprotein; CI, confidence interval; PAR, population-attributable risk.
From O'Donnell MJ, Chin SL, Rangarajan S, et al: Global and regional effects of potentially modifiable risk factors associated with acute stroke in 32 countries (INTERSTROKE): a case-control study. *Lancet* 388:761, 2016.

occlusion with resultant hypoperfusion (e.g., watershed infarction). Large-vessel atherosclerosis accounts for about 20% of all ischemic strokes in high-income countries, and is predominantly extracranial in origin. Intracranial atherosclerosis has been reported to account for up to 33%–50% of ischemic strokes in parts of Asia (e.g., China and Thailand), but it is a much less common cause of acute stroke in North America and Europe. Arterial dissection, the third leading cause of ischemic stroke in young people, can lead to ischemic stroke either by local occlusion or distal thromboembolism. Predisposing factors for dissection include trauma and underlying arteriopathies, such as fibromuscular dysplasia. Less common large-vessel mechanisms of ischemic stroke include moyamoya disease, Fabry disease, and large-vessel arteritis (e.g., Takayasu arteritis and giant-cell arteritis).

Cardioembolism

Approximately 14%–30% of all ischemic strokes are caused by cardioembolism, with marked regional variation. A number of conditions predispose to cardioembolism, originating from the venous system (paradoxical embolism), intracardiac (e.g., atrial fibrillation), or postcardiac (aortic arch disease).

Precardiac

Paradoxical emboli occur when emboli that arise in the venous circulation (e.g., from deep vein thrombosis) cross into the arterial circulation through a patent foramen ovale (PFO), atrial septal defect (ASD), or a pulmonary arteriovenous malformation (AVM). PFO is found in up to 20% of the general population. A number of observational studies have reported an association between first ischemic stroke and PFO, particularly in younger patients, but PFO has not been shown to be a risk factor for recurrent ischemic stroke. Atrial septal aneurysm, a protrusion of part of the atrial septum through the fossa ovalis into the right or left atrium, is associated with an increased risk of ischemic stroke, particularly when it occurs in conjunction with a PFO.

Intracardiac

Left-sided cardiac sources of emboli include left atrial thrombus secondary to atrial fibrillation or flutter, left ventricle thrombus subsequent to a transmural myocardial infarction, akinetic segments of myocardium with a low ejection fraction in the setting of an old myocardial infarction, cardiac tumors such as left atrial myxoma, and abnormalities of the mitral valve (both native and artificial). Atrial fibrillation or flutter is a significant risk factor for stroke, associated with a fivefold increase in risk. In North America and Europe, about 25% of all ischemic strokes are attributed to atrial fibrillation, a proportion that increases with older age. After acute myocardial infarction, mural thrombi can arise in the presence of left ventricular aneurysms, akinetic segments of left ventricular myocardium, or new-onset atrial fibrillation or flutter. Congestive heart failure is also an independent risk factor for stroke and is associated with a two- to threefold increased relative risk of ischemic stroke. Valvular heart disease can involve both native (e.g., rheumatic heart disease) and prosthetic heart valves. Of native valvular disease, mitral stenosis has the strongest association with ischemic stroke; mitral annular calcification and mitral valve prolapse have weaker associations. Mitral stenosis is also commonly associated with atrial fibrillation, further increasing the risk of ischemic stroke. Emboli can also arise from valvular vegetations in nonbacterial thrombotic endocarditis or infective endocarditis. Mechanical mitral and aortic valves are associated with a sufficiently high risk for ischemic stroke that indefinite oral anticoagulant therapy is indicated. Rheumatic heart disease still accounts for half of all cases of endocarditis in some regions of the world (e.g., India and Africa). Several epidemiologic studies have shown a link between ischemic stroke and *Trypanosoma cruzi* infection (Chagas disease) in South America.

Postcardiac

Atherosclerotic plaques in the aortic arch, proximal to the left subclavian artery, can be postcardiac sources of emboli, either atheromatous debris or platelet emboli, which then enter the cerebral circulation resulting in an ischemic stroke. Severe aortic arch atheromas (>4 mm in diameter) are associated with a fourfold increase in the risk of ischemic stroke and peripheral embolism. Although anatomically a large vessel source, aortic arch disease is usually included in cardiac causes of ischemic stroke because it is often identified via transesophageal echocardiography.

Small-Vessel Disease

Approximately 20% of all ischemic strokes are caused by lacunar or small-vessel infarcts. Lacunar infarcts are the result of occlusion of small, deep-penetrating arteries, such as the lenticulostriate branches of the anterior cerebral and middle cerebral arteries. The terminal pathophysiological mechanism underlying small-artery occlusion is believed to be local thrombosis secondary to microatheroma (lipid-laden macrophages, cholesterol deposits, and subintimal fibroblast proliferation) and lipohyalinosis (the intermediate stage between fibrinoid necrosis and microatheroma, which has characteristics of both arterial atheromatous lipid deposits and arteriolar hyalinization disease). Growing evidence supports the concept that damage to the glycocalyx, by factors such as hyperglycemia, hypertension, and smoking, may contribute to vascular endothelial damage. Other causes of small-artery occlusion include microemboli from atherosclerotic plaques, polycythemia vera, antiphospholipid antibodies, amyloid angiopathy, cerebral autosomal dominant arteriopathy with subcortical infarcts and leukoencephalopathy (CADASIL), cerebral autosomal recessive arteriopathy with subcortical infarcts and leukoencephalopathy (CARASIL), Sneddon syndrome, and various types of small-vessel arteritis. The combination of mitochondrial myopathy, encephalopathy, lactic acidosis, and stroke-like episodes (MELAS) is an inherited progressive disorder characterized by mitochondrial dysfunction and early onset of stroke, typically before the age of 40 years. The mitochondrial angiopathy hypothesis suggests that the lesions are secondary to ischemia, which is caused by mitochondrial and vascular dysfunction of cerebral small arteries.

Ischemic Stroke of Other Determined Etiology

Cerebral Vein Thrombosis

Cerebral vein thrombosis accounts for less than 1% of ischemic strokes, and typically affects younger people. The superior sagittal, transverse, and cavernous sinuses are those most commonly affected by thrombosis. Venous thrombosis results in localized edema and venous infarction, which often becomes hemorrhagic, and may raise intracranial pressure (ICP). Reported risk factors for cerebral vein thrombosis include inherited thrombophilia; acquired prothrombotic states such as antiphospholipid syndrome, pregnancy, and the puerperium; infections such as otitis, sinusitis, and mastoiditis; chronic inflammatory conditions such as Wegener granulomatosis and sarcoidosis; trauma such as a head injury; dehydration, and injury to the jugular veins or sinuses during neurosurgical procedures.

Intracerebral Hemorrhage

ICH accounts for approximately 10%–15% of all strokes (a larger proportion is reported in middle- and low-income countries), and can be classified as either primary or secondary, depending on the underlying cause. Primary ICH accounts for about 80%–90% of cases and is the result of spontaneous rupture of small intracerebral blood vessels, usually damaged by chronic hypertension (and other vascular risk factors) or amyloid angiopathy. Antithrombotic therapy, particularly anticoagulant therapy, is an important risk factor for ICH. Secondary ICH occurs as a result of vascular abnormalities (ruptured saccular aneurysm, arteriovenous malformation, tumors (e.g., cavernous angioma, intracerebral neoplasm), impaired coagulation (e.g., because of use of oral anticoagulants or bleeding disorders such as hemophilia or von Willebrand disease), hemorrhagic transformation of ischemic stroke, septic emboli, vasculitis, moyamoya disease, and alcohol or illicit drug use (e.g., cocaine, amphetamines).

Subarachnoid Hemorrhage

SAH refers to bleeding within the subarachnoid space, which is the space between the arachnoid and pia mater. SAH accounts for about 3%–5% of all strokes and is most commonly caused by rupture of an intracranial aneurysm (approximately 80%–85% of cases). Idiopathic nonaneurysmal perimesencephalic hemorrhage accounts for about 10% of cases, and the remaining 5% are caused by rare causes such as inflammatory lesions of cerebral arteries (e.g., mycotic aneurysm, polyarteritis nodosa, primary angiitis), noninflammatory lesions of intracerebral vessels (e.g., arterial dissection, cerebral arteriovenous malformations, cerebral amyloid angiopathy, cerebral venous thrombosis, moyamoya disease), vascular lesions of the spinal cord (e.g., saccular aneurysm of the spinal artery, spinal arteriovenous malformation), coagulopathy (e.g., hemophilia, von Willebrand disease), sickle cell disease, tumors (e.g., malignant glioma), trauma, and drug use (cocaine, anticoagulants).

Covert Stroke

Clinically overt stroke is considered to represent only a fraction of all episodes of cerebral infarction. The advent of contemporary MRI sequences has identified a large burden of subclinical cerebrovascular disease, which includes covert infarction, white matter hyperintensities, cerebral atrophy, and microbleeds. Covert stroke is common; for example, a systematic review of eight population-based studies reported a prevalence of silent brain infarcts in an older population of 3%–28%. Moreover, covert stroke has been associated with an increased risk of cognitive decline, dementia, depression, and gait impairment (Box 145.1).

Hematologic Disorders and Ischemic Stroke

Inherited Thrombophilia

In general, studies have reported either no association or a modest association between inherited thrombophilia and ischemic stroke.

BOX 145.1 What Is Cryptogenic Ischemic Stroke?

In some cases, the cause of stroke cannot be definitively determined and the stroke is classified as "stroke of undetermined etiology." A stroke may be classified in this category when one of the following two conditions is met: (1) an extensive evaluation is negative, which includes large-vessel imaging, and complete cardiovascular assessment is negative; or (2) the diagnostic evaluation is incomplete. The most important determinant of the proportion of patients labeled as having cryptogenic stroke is the extent of the etiological diagnostic testing, including transesophageal echocardiography. In studies that have completed an extensive etiological workup, the proportion of patients designated as having cryptogenic stroke is small (5%–15%). In older patients with complete evaluation, paroxysmal atrial fibrillation is suspected to be a common underlying cause of ischemic stroke in older adults with "cryptogenic" ischemic stroke.

Meta-analyses of observational studies have failed to demonstrate a significant association between the factor V Leiden mutation and ischemic stroke in adults, although some small case-control studies have reported an increased risk of ischemic stroke in women with factor V Leiden using oral contraceptives. Two large prospective population studies, the Physicians' Health Study and the Cardiovascular Health Study, failed to demonstrate a significant association between the prothrombin *G20210A* mutation and ischemic stroke risk, although a large meta-analysis of 19 case-control studies reported a modest association. There is no evidence to support an association between protein C, protein S, or antithrombin deficiency and ischemic stroke risk in adults.

Antiphospholipid Syndrome

Antiphospholipid syndrome is reviewed in Chapter 141. Stroke is the main acute arterial thrombotic complication of antiphospholipid syndrome, and is reported to be the initial clinical manifestation in 13% of patients subsequently diagnosed with antiphospholipid syndrome. However, the overall association between antiphospholipid antibodies (without other features of the syndrome) and ischemic stroke is less certain. Anticardiolipin antibodies have been associated with ischemic stroke in some studies, especially in young women, but not in others. The lupus anticoagulant is a more potent risk factor for ischemic stroke. For example, in the Risk of Arterial Thrombosis in Relation to Oral Contraceptives (RATIO) study, the odds ratio (OR) for an association between the lupus anticoagulant and ischemic stroke was 43.1 (95% CI, 12.2–152.2) compared with an OR of 2.3 (95% CI, 1.4–3.7) for anti-β_2-glycoprotein I antibodies and no significant association reported for anticardiolipin antibodies. Current AHA guidelines recommend antiplatelet therapy for secondary prevention of ischemic stroke in patients with cryptogenic ischemic stroke who do not meet the criteria for antiphospholipid syndrome but have antiphospholipid antibodies. For patients with cryptogenic ischemic stroke who meet the diagnostic criteria for antiphospholipid syndrome and who have persistently moderate-to-high antiphospholipid antibody titers for more than 12 weeks, oral anticoagulant therapy for secondary prevention of ischemic stroke can be considered. The most recent American College of Chest Physicians (ACCP) guideline recommends oral anticoagulant therapy with a target international normalized ratio (INR) of 2–3 for the latter group

Sickle Cell Disease

Sickle cell disease is associated with an increased risk of stroke, particularly in those homozygous for the sickle cell gene. The risk of stroke is 11% at 20 years of age, 15% at 30 years, and 24% at 45 years. The most common mechanism underlying ischemic stroke in sickle cell disease is believed to be large-artery arteriopathy secondary to hyperplasia of the intima from repeated endothelial injury.

Myeloproliferative Disorders

Myeloproliferative disorders, such as polycythemia vera and essential thrombocytopenia, are uncommon conditions associated with an increased risk of stroke. In a randomized controlled trial of daily aspirin in 518 patients with polycythemia vera, the combined rate of ischemic and hemorrhagic stroke was 1.2% in the aspirin group compared with 3.8% in the control group over 3 years. Defective platelet function in these disorders also results in an increased risk of ICH.

Thrombotic Thrombocytopenic Purpura

Thrombotic thrombocytopenic purpura is an uncommon systemic disorder associated with an increased risk of ischemic stroke. It is characterized by a pentad of thrombocytopenia, microangiopathic hemolytic anemia, fever, renal failure, and neurologic abnormalities including ischemic stroke (see Chapter 134)

Paraproteinemias

The paraproteinemias, including Waldenström macroglobulinemia, multiple myeloma, and POEMS syndrome (characterized by a plasma-cell proliferative disorder, typically myeloma, polyneuropathy, with involvement of multiple other organ systems) are also associated with an increased risk of ischemic stroke and hemorrhagic stroke (because of thrombocytopenia).

Genetic Risk Factors

A substantial body of evidence from twin, family, and animal studies supports a genetic contribution to stroke risk. A recent meta-analysis of genome-wide association studies from more than 12,000 patients with ischemic stroke identified three loci with genome-wide significance for ischemic stroke—*PITX2* and *ZFHX3*, previously associated with an increased risk of atrial fibrillation, were associated with an increased risk of ischemic stroke, whereas *HDAC9* was associated with an increased risk of large-artery stroke. Another meta-analysis reported that APOEε2 carrier status was associated with an increased burden of white matter hyperintensities (a marker for prior cerebrovascular disease) and risk of ischemic stroke

The concordance rate for stroke is 65% higher in monozygotic twins compared with dizygotic twins, with a range of 12.8%–19.0% in monozygotic twins and 3.6%–13.0% in dizygotic twins. Family history of stroke increases the risk of ischemic stroke by about 75% and the presence of a first-degree relative with a history of hemorrhagic stroke is associated with a sixfold increase in risk of hemorrhagic stroke. A number of monogenic disorders have been associated with an increased risk of ischemic stroke, including Marfan syndrome, Fabry disease, familial moyamoya disease, homocysteinuria, sickle cell disease, and MELAS. Rare Mendelian forms of stroke have been described such as CADASIL and CARASIL, which manifest as small-vessel ischemic stroke. However, most monogenic disorders are infrequent and thus have limited impact on the wider population, despite their marked effect on individual risk in young populations.

CLINICAL MANIFESTATIONS

Clinical Presentation

Stroke is a clinical diagnosis, supported by the results of neuroimaging (computed tomography [CT] or MRI of the brain). CT of the brain may be normal in patients with acute ischemic stroke, and cases of MRI-negative stroke also occur. With advances in neuroimaging, an increasing proportion of patients (about one-quarter) presenting with transient neurologic deficits (previously diagnosed as TIA) have small infarcts identifiable on high-quality MRI. Clinically, stroke is characterized by the sudden onset of typically a focal neurologic deficit, lasting more than 24 hours or leading to death because of a presumed vascular cause. Common presenting features are lateralizing weakness of the upper extremities and/or lower extremities, facial weakness, speech abnormalities (aphasia, dysarthria), visual loss (monocular visual loss or homonymous hemianopia), reduced level of consciousness, ataxia, diplopia, vertigo, and headache. A number of clinical conditions can mimic stroke. Among patients admitted to a hospital with suspected stroke, only about two-thirds are subsequently diagnosed with stroke. Common stroke mimics include migraine, seizure, syncope, hypoglycemia, primary or secondary brain tumors, transient global amnesia, and toxic-metabolic disturbances with delirium.

Ischemic Stroke versus Intracerebral Hemorrhage

Ischemic stroke and ICH can have similar presentations. Although some clinical features are more typically associated with ICH (e.g., coma, neck stiffness, seizures, vomiting, and headache) than ischemic stroke, neuroimaging is required to discriminate between them. Therefore emergent CT or MRI of brain is mandatory in all patients presenting with suspected acute stroke.

Measuring Stroke Severity

Many scales are available for measuring stroke severity, including the Scandinavian Stroke Scale, the Canadian Stroke Scale, and the National Institutes of Health Stroke Scale (NIHSS). The NIHSS is the scale most widely used in clinical practice. Other scales (e.g., Hunt and Hess, Fisher) are used to measure stroke severity in patients with SAH.

Risk of Stroke After Transient Ischemic Attack

The ABCD2 score is a validated clinical prediction score for risk of stroke in patients with TIA. Points are score for each of the following risk factors: age >60 years (1); blood pressure ≥140/90 mmHg on first evaluation (1); clinical symptoms of focal weakness (2) or speech impairment without weakness (1); duration of 10–59 minutes (1) or ≥60 minutes (2); and diabetes mellitus (1). In combined validation cohorts, the 2-day risk of stroke was 0% for scores of 0 or 1, 1.3% for scores of 2 or 3, 4.1% for scores of 4 or 5, and 8.1% for scores of 6 or 7.

INVESTIGATIONS

Computed Tomography of the Brain

Neuroimaging is required to distinguish between ischemic and hemorrhagic stroke. On CT of the brain, early features of ischemia include loss of distinction between the gray and white matter border, sulcal effacement, loss of definition of the insula, and evolving areas of hypodensity. Scoring systems (e.g., ASPECT score) may be used to quantify the burden of ischemia, which predicts the risk of ICH in patients receiving thrombolysis. SAH is not reliably excluded by CT alone. If there is a high index of suspicion for SAH, a lumbar puncture is needed to reliably exclude this diagnosis.

Magnetic Resonance Imaging

MRI is superior to CT for detecting acute ischemia. In the acute setting, however, its use is limited by patient contraindications and availability. Diffusion-weighted imaging (DWI) may identify acute ischemia within 3–6 hours of symptom onset. For diagnosis of ICH, MRI with gradient-related echo or susceptibility-weighted imaging has been reported to provide results similar to those provided by CT of the brain (96% concordance).

Neurovascular Imaging

Extracranial and intracranial stenosis may be detected using ultrasound, CT angiography, magnetic resonance angiography, or conventional angiography. Ultrasound is a noninvasive, relatively inexpensive, and widely available imaging modality, but is dependent on ultrasonographer experience and skill. Transcranial Doppler may be used to detect intracranial large vessel stenosis, and has also been shown to risk-stratify patients with carotid stenosis with microembolic signals.

Cardiac Workup

An electrocardiogram can identify atrial fibrillation/flutter or evidence of previous myocardial infarction whereas in-hospital telemetry can identify a larger proportion of patients with paroxysmal atrial fibrillation. Based on the results of the recent CRYSTAL AF and EMBRACE trials, extended cardiac rhythm monitoring using loop recorders increases detection rates of paroxysmal atrial fibrillation in patients with cryptogenic ischemic stroke older than 55 years. Longer durations of cardiac monitoring result in higher diagnostic yield, but the optimal duration is uncertain. Transthoracic echocardiography has a low yield in patients with no previous cardiac history and a normal cardiac examination. The routine use of transesophageal echocardiography is controversial; however, this is an essential investigation in patients with suspected endocarditis. A PFO can be identified with a bubble study when performing transthoracic or transesophageal echocardiography. Although transesophageal echocardiography identifies potential etiologies of ischemic stroke in a relatively large proportion of patients, such as PFO, atrial septal aneurysm, or aortic arch disease, the treatment implications of these findings are less certain. All patients presenting with stroke should have vascular risk factor profiling, including measurement of blood pressure, fasting lipids, blood glucose, and glycated hemoglobin (HbA1c). All patients should have a complete blood count, troponin, and coagulation profile. Other useful tests, depending on clinical suspicion, may include erythrocyte sedimentation rate, antiphospholipid antibody panel, blood cultures, antineutrophilic cytoplasmic antibodies, antinuclear antibodies, homocysteine, and lipoprotein A.

THERAPY

A complete review of the management of stroke is beyond the scope of this chapter. Instead we provide an overview of the acute and chronic management of stroke.

Reperfusion Therapy for Acute Ischemic Stroke

Thrombolysis for Acute Ischemic Stroke

Intravenous tissue plasminogen activator (t-PA) is the most rigorously evaluated thrombolytic intervention in acute ischemic stroke. Current guidelines recommend administration of t-PA in patients with acute ischemic stroke presenting within 3 hours of symptom onset. Based on the results of the ECASS III trial, current guidelines recommend administration of t-PA to eligible patients up to 4.5 hours after symptom onset, provided none of the following additional exclusion criteria are met: age >80 years, NIHSS >25, history of both prior stroke and diabetes mellitus, use of oral anticoagulant therapy at the time of acute stroke, or imaging evidence of ischemic injury involving more than one-third of the middle cerebral artery territory. The main complication of t-PA is ICH. In the Third International Stroke Trial (IST-3), which enrolled patients up to 6 hours after symptom onset, there was an increased risk of spontaneous ICH and death at 7 days compared with the control group, although total mortality was similar between the two groups at 6 months. Currently t-PA is not approved by the European Medicines Agency (EMA) beyond 4.5 hours after symptom onset (Table 145.2).

Intraarterial Fibrinolysis

Current guidelines recommend intraarterial fibrinolysis in carefully selected patients with major ischemic strokes caused by middle cerebral artery occlusion if the duration of symptoms is less than 6 hours and they are ineligible for intravenous t-PA. Rescue intraarterial fibrinolysis is an option for recanalization in patients with large-artery occlusion who have not responded to intravenous t-PA. Use of intraarterial t-PA is currently not FDA approved. Limited access to

TABLE 145.2	Eligibility Criteria for Acute Thrombolysis in Acute Ischemic Stroke

Eligibility Criteria

Diagnosis of ischemic stroke causing measurable neurological deficit

The neurological signs should not be minor and isolated. Caution should be exercised in treating a patient with major deficits

Onset of symptoms <4.5 hours before beginning treatment

The neurologic signs should not be clearing spontaneously

The symptoms of stroke should not be suggestive of subarachnoid hemorrhage

The patient or family members should understand the potential risks and benefits from treatment

Contraindications for Thrombolysis

Evidence of intracranial hemorrhage on CT

Head trauma or prior stroke in previous 3 months

Myocardial infarction in the previous 3 months

Gastrointestinal or urinary tract hemorrhage in previous 21 days

Arterial puncture at a noncompressible site in the previous 7 days

Major surgery in the previous 14 days

History of previous intracranial hemorrhage

Elevated blood pressure (systolic >185 mmHg and diastolic >110 mmHg)

Evidence of active bleeding or acute trauma (fracture) on examination

Taking an oral anticoagulant or, if taking anticoagulant, INR ≥1.7 is a contraindication

If receiving heparin in previous 48 hours, aPTT must be in normal range.

Platelet count ≤100 000 mm³

Blood glucose concentration ≥50 mg/dL (2.7 mmol/L)

Seizure with postictal residual neurologic impairments

CT shows a multilobar infarction (hypodensity >1/3 cerebral hemisphere)

aPTT, Activated partial thromboplastin time; CT, computed tomography; INR, international normalized ratio.

interventional neuroradiology has been a major limitation to the use of this intervention and it has not yet been evaluated in large-scale clinical trials.

Mechanical Thrombectomy

The MR-CLEAN, ESCAPE, SWIFT PRIME, and EXTEND IA trials demonstrated the benefit of early intraarterial mechanical thrombectomy compared with intravenous thrombolysis alone in patients with acute ischemic stroke caused by large proximal artery occlusion meeting the following criteria: (1) small infarct size with no evidence of hemorrhage on baseline CT of brain; (2) evidence of proximal large-artery occlusion in the anterior circulation on vessel imaging (e.g., CT angiography); (3) symptom onset within the past 6–12 hours (three of the trials utilized a 6-hour cut-off and most of the patients in ESCAPE were enrolled within the 6-hour window); (4) rapid access to a stroke center with necessary expertise in use of second-generation stent retriever devices. Compared with intravenous thrombolysis alone, intraarterial treatment resulted in significantly higher rates of functional independence at 90 days in all four trials, with no significant difference in the risk of symptomatic ICH or death between treatment groups. The number needed to treat for one additional person to reach functional independence ranged from 3 to 7.5.

Acute Stroke Unit

Organized stroke unit (OSU) care in a dedicated, geographically identified ward with multidisciplinary teams that exclusively manage patients with stroke is associated with improved outcomes in patients with acute stroke. A meta-analysis of 26 trials (n = 5592) investigating OSU care reported a reduction in death (OR, 0.86; 95% CI,

0.76–0.98) and death or dependency at one year (OR, 0.82; 95% CI, 0.73–0.92) independent of age, sex, or stroke severity. Organized stroke care is associated with improved outcome for a number of reasons, including a reduced risk of medical complications such as deep vein thrombosis (caused by earlier mobilization), as well as a reduced risk of aspiration pneumonia, fever, urinary tract infection, falls, and delirium. Prompt evaluation of swallowing function and compliance with speech pathology safe swallowing guidelines help to reduce the risk of aspiration pneumonia in patients with stroke.

Blood Pressure in Acute Stroke

Although hypertension is the most important risk factor for both ischemic and hemorrhagic stroke, the optimal approach to managing blood pressure in the acute setting remains uncertain. A number of randomized controlled trials have evaluated acute blood pressure lowering in acute ischemic stroke, and meta-analyses of these trials reports no benefit of lowering blood pressure in acute phase of ischemic stroke, and current AHA guidelines recommend cautious introduction of antihypertensive therapy in those with an initial blood pressure >220/120 mmHg, unless there is an alternate indication for blood pressure lowering or the patient has received thrombolytic therapy (target <180/105 mmHg). The INTERACT-II phase III trial enrolled patients with spontaneous ICH within 6 hours of symptom onset and systolic blood pressure between 150 and 220 mmHg. There was no difference in the risk of death or major disability between patients randomized to intensive treatment (target systolic blood pressure <140 mmHg) compared with current guideline-recommended treatment (target systolic blood pressure <180 mmHg), although it was safe and an ordinal analysis of functional outcome (modified Rankin score) suggested improved functional outcomes with a blood pressure target of <140 mmHg. In the ATACH phase III trial of patients with ICH within 4.5 hours of symptom onset, an acute blood pressure-lowering target of 110–139 mmHg was not superior to a target of 140–179 mmHg for reduction in death and disability. The recent ENOS trial reported no difference in the risk of disability at 90 days between patients randomized to early (within 48 hours) blood pressure lowering after acute stroke versus no early intervention, or between patients randomized to continuation of home antihypertensives versus cessation of home medications in the acute period.

Antithrombotic Therapy in Acute Ischemic Stroke

Based on the results of two large randomized controlled trials, the International Stroke Trial (IST) and the Chinese Acute Stroke Trial (CAST), aspirin reduces the risk of recurrent stroke and death in patients with acute ischemic stroke. In general, therapeutic parenteral anticoagulant therapy is not indicated in acute ischemic stroke, with the exception of cerebral vein thrombosis. Therapeutic heparin is commonly used in patients with acute ischemic stroke and extracranial carotid or vertebral artery dissection, or symptomatic extracranial vertebral or carotid artery atherosclerotic stenosis with crescendo TIAs. However, there is limited evidence to guide clinical decision-making on optimal antithrombotic therapy in these patients. The recent CADISS trial, which included 250 patients with symptomatic carotid and vertebral artery dissection, reported no difference in the risk of recurrent stroke or death between patients randomized to antiplatelet and anticoagulant therapy. However, limitations of this study included the failure to confirm a diagnosis of dissection in 20% of participants along with very low rates of recurrent stroke.

Carotid Endarterectomy and Stenting

The European Carotid Surgery Trial (ECST) and the North American Symptomatic Carotid Endarterectomy Trial (NASCET) are the largest trials to evaluate carotid endarterectomy (CEA) in patients with recent ischemic stroke and TIA. Based on the results of these trials, current guidelines recommend CEA in patients with 70%–99% stenosis of the ipsilateral carotid artery, provided the perioperative morbidity and mortality are estimated to be less than 6%. Although patients with 50%–69% stenosis also derive benefit from CEA, it is only recommended for selected patients based on age, comorbidities, time from stroke/TIA, and operative risk. Time from symptom onset to CEA is the primary determinant of the absolute risk reduction obtained with this procedure, with maximal benefit realized when CEA is performed within the first 2 weeks of symptom onset. Although CEA is the gold standard for patients with symptomatic significant carotid stenosis, carotid stenting is an alternative option for patients with over 70% stenosis considered to be a high operative risk for CEA.

Intracranial Stenting

Two trials have failed to show a benefit of intracranial stenting in patients with symptomatic and significant (≥70%) intracranial stenosis. The SAMMPRIS trial reported no benefit of endovascular stenting (self-expanding stent) in addition to aggressive medical therapy, compared with aggressive medical therapy alone. The trial was stopped early because of a higher rate of stroke and death at 30 days in the endovascular group. The more recent VISSIT, which compared a balloon-expandable stent in addition to medical therapy with medical therapy alone, was terminated early because of higher rates of stroke or death at 30 days and 1 year in the endovascular group.

Prevention of Venous Thromboembolism

See Chapter 142.

Acute Management of Intracerebral Hemorrhage

Management of ICH includes both medical and surgical components. Initial strategies include monitoring in an intensive care setting in appropriate patients, intubation in those with reduced consciousness, discontinuation of antithrombotic therapy and immediate reversal of anticoagulant therapy (Chapter 149), administration of antipyretics for fever and insulin for hyperglycemia, and venous thromboembolism prophylaxis (e.g., compression stockings). Raised ICP can occur as a result of the hemorrhage itself or because of secondary edema. Management of increased ICP includes elevation of the head of the bed to 30 degrees, analgesia, and sedation. More aggressive therapies include osmotic diuretics with mannitol, drainage of cerebrospinal fluid using a ventricular catheter (ventriculostomy), hyperventilation, and neuromuscular blockade. Antiepileptic therapy should be used for seizure control, but prophylaxis is not recommended in current guidelines. The Surgical Trial in IntraCerebral Hemorrhage (STICH) showed no benefit of early surgery compared with medical management alone within 72–96 hours of onset of spontaneous ICH. However, uncertainty remains in some patient groups, and current guidelines suggest craniotomy for those with a lobar bleed of over 30 mL within 1 cm of the brain surface. Surgical evacuation is recommended in patients with cerebellar hemorrhage over 3 cm in diameter who have evidence of deterioration, brainstem compression, or hydrocephalus. Ventriculostomy with external drainage may be required for patients with intraventricular extension of ICH and a deteriorating level of consciousness. Based on a large phase III trial, current guidelines suggest that use of recombinant factor VIIa for acute ICH not associated with warfarin use is investigational and should not be used outside of a clinical trial.

Stroke Rehabilitation

Intensive rehabilitation should commence as early as possible after acute stroke. Animal models of neuroplasticity suggest that training results in upregulation of growth-promoting factors primarily in the first 4 weeks following acute stroke, but recovery can continue for months or years after the acute event. High levels of patient (and family) motivation and engagement are associated with better outcomes from stroke rehabilitation. Substantial evidence supports a well-coordinated multidisciplinary team care (nursing, physical therapy, occupational therapy, speech therapy, dietetics, and social work) approach for optimal delivery of stroke rehabilitation. This care can be provided in the stroke unit setting or by early supported discharge teams in the patient's own home. Both strategies have been shown to improve independence in stroke patients. For older patients with stroke, physical rehabilitation in a long-term care facility effective has been shown to improve independence.

Chronic Secondary Prevention of Ischemic Stroke

Case Study

A 72-year-old man presented with right-sided weakness and expressive aphasia 4 weeks ago. CT scan of brain revealed an ischemic stroke in the left hemisphere. He was admitted to a stroke unit, and after completing a rehabilitation program, he was discharged home. Etiological investigations included ultrasound of carotids (<20% stenosis of carotids), Holter monitor (no arrhythmia), and transthoracic echocardiography with bubble study, which revealed a small PFO. He is known to have hypertension; his serum glucose and HbA1c were normal. He was initiated on aspirin at the time of diagnosis. His blood pressure in clinic today is 152/92 mmHg, and he is currently receiving perindopril 8 mg daily. His fasting LDL level was 140 mg/dL.

Antithrombotic Therapy

Current guidelines recommend aspirin, clopidogrel, or combination aspirin-dipyridamole for secondary prevention of noncardioembolic ischemic stroke. The MATCH trial, which compared the combination of clopidogrel (75 mg per day) plus aspirin (75 mg per day) with aspirin alone in patients with recent ischemic stroke or TIA found no reduction in the risk of major vascular events but an increased risk of life-threatening and major bleeding in patients treated with combination therapy over 18 months of follow-up. Similar results were noted in the SPS3 trial, which included patients with recent symptomatic lacunar infarction. The subsequently published CHANCE trial reported a lower risk of recurrent stroke at 90 days in patients with TIA or minor ischemic stroke (NIHSS ≤3) treated with the combination of clopidogrel (initial dose 300 mg then 75 mg per day for 90 days) and aspirin (75 mg per day for first 21days) compared with aspirin alone. The POINT trial is currently enrolling patients with TIA and minor ischemic stroke to compare the effectiveness of combination clopidogrel (initial dose 600 mg then 75 mg per day for 90 days) plus aspirin (50–325 mg per day) versus aspirin alone for the prevention of ischemic vascular events (ischemic stroke, myocardial infarction, and ischemic vascular death), with results expected in 2017. In patients with atrial fibrillation or mechanical heart valves, oral anticoagulation is generally recommended for secondary prevention of ischemic stroke (Box 145.2). The direct thrombin inhibitor dabigatran and the oral factor Xa inhibitor apixaban have been shown to be superior to warfarin, whereas the oral factor Xa inhibitor rivaroxaban has been shown to be noninferior to warfarin for the prevention of stroke and systemic embolism in patients with atrial fibrillation. These agents are being increasingly used in clinical practice and offer a number of advantages over warfarin, including a more rapid onset of action, more predictable anticoagulant effect enabling fixed daily dosing without need for routine coagulation monitoring, and a lower risk of food and drug interactions. Randomized controlled trials of extended cardiac rhythm monitoring (event loop recording) have reported increased detection rates of paroxysmal atrial fibrillation in patients with formerly unexplained ischemic

| BOX 145.2 | When Should Warfarin Be Started After Acute Ischemic Stroke With Atrial Fibrillation? |

We initiate all patients on aspirin in the acute setting. In patients with acute transient ischemic attack or minor ischemic stroke and in the absence of a large area of acute infarction, we usually initiate warfarin immediately, where a decision is made to use warfarin. For those with severe stroke or moderate stroke with a large area of infarction, initiating aspirin is recommended without anticoagulant therapy in the acute phase. Warfarin can be cautiously introduced 5–7 days after stroke onset after hemorrhagic transformation of the infarct has been excluded on neuroimaging in those suspected to be at increased risk of intracerebral hemorrhage. For patients who have had large infarcts, evidence of hemorrhagic transformation, progression of stroke, or uncontrolled hypertension, further delays beyond 14 days poststroke may be required prior to initiation of therapy with warfarin. We stop aspirin once a therapeutic anticoagulant effect is achieved, unless there is a compelling indication for combination of aspirin and warfarin (e.g., coronary stent). We do not bridge the initial period with treatment doses of heparin, although it may be reasonable in patients with transient ischemic attack and atrial fibrillation, as they would be expected to be a lower risk of intracerebral hemorrhage (although unproven).

stroke. Oral anticoagulants are not superior to aspirin for the secondary prevention of stroke in patients with noncardioembolic stroke (WARSS and ESPRIT) or in patients with intracranial stenosis (WASID).

Lipid Modification

Current guidelines recommend statin therapy in patients with LDL ≥100 mg/dL. The SPARCL trial comparing atorvastatin 80 mg daily with placebo reported a reduced risk of recurrent stroke over 5 years of follow-up in the atorvastatin group.

Blood Pressure

PROGRESS, the largest trial of antihypertensive therapy for secondary stroke prevention, compared perindopril (with or without indapamide) with placebo. Combination therapy reduced blood pressure by 12/5 mmHg and stroke risk by 43%, and produced greater reduction in blood pressure and stroke risk compared with perindopril alone. Current guidelines recommend a target blood pressure of 140/90 mmHg or less.

Patent Foramen Ovale Closure

Despite the results of three randomized controlled trials, the role of PFO closure devices remains uncertain. The randomized controlled trial CLOSURE I ($n = 909$) reported that PFO closure with the STARFlex closure device (no longer clinically available) was not superior to medical therapy alone in reducing the risk of recurrent TIA/stroke at 24 months (5.5% vs. 6.8%; hazard ratio [HR], 0.78; 95% CI, 0.45–1.35), and was associated with an increased risk of major vascular complications (3.2% vs. 0.0%; $p < .001$) and new-onset atrial fibrillation (5.7% vs. 0.7%; $p < .001$). Furthermore, in the RESPECT trial ($n = 980$), PFO closure with the Amplatzer PFO occluder was not found to be superior to medical management in reducing the risk of recurrent stroke or death during follow-up (1.8% vs. 3.3%, HR, 0.49; 95% CI, 0.22–1.11). Interestingly, PFO closure was superior to medical management in preventing recurrent stroke in the subgroup of patients with a substantial shunt (0.8% vs. 4.3%; HR, 0.18; 95% CI, 0.04–0.81) and concomitant ASA (1.1% vs. 5.3%; HR, 0.19; 95% CI, 0.04–0.87), suggesting a benefit in high-risk patients. The PC trial also did not demonstrate a benefit with device closure of PFO. However, low event rates in these three trials have precluded a definitive conclusion.

Lifestyle Modification

Lifestyle modification remains a cornerstone of stroke prevention. Important components include smoking cessation, moderate physical activity, weight reduction in overweight or obese patients, adopting a healthy heart diet with increased fruit and vegetable intake, reduced salt intake in those consuming high-salt diets, and moderate alcohol consumption.

PROGNOSIS

Prognosis after stroke depends on patient age, underlying stroke etiology, severity of neurological deficit and level of dependence, and comorbidity burden. In a large cohort of over 10,000 US patients hospitalized with ischemic stroke, 1- and 4-year mortality rates were 24.5% and 41.3%, respectively, with rates of recurrent stroke of 8.0% and 18.1% at 1 and 4 years, respectively. Early death usually occurs because of neurological complications (e.g., cerebral edema, raised ICP) or medical complications of dependency and immobilization (e.g., aspiration pneumonia). Longer-term mortality is usually caused by cardiovascular disease. Two-thirds of stroke survivors are left with chronic residual disability. In addition, patients with stroke are at an increased risk of myocardial infarction, deep vein thrombosis, urinary tract infections, hip fracture, pneumonia, and subsequent rehospitalization. Common complications of stroke in the longer term include seizure disorders, cognitive impairment and dementia, depression, and chronic pain syndromes (e.g., central poststroke pain).

FUTURE DIRECTIONS

To date, our knowledge of the epidemiology of stroke has been derived from studies in North America and Europe, with comparatively fewer studies in middle- and low-income countries, although the vast majority of the global burden of stroke occurs in these regions. In addition, a number of large ongoing epidemiologic collaborative studies (International Stroke Genetics Consortium) will clarify the role of genetics in the pathogenesis of stroke. Population-based interventions to reduce the burden of stroke will be an important focus of future research, and will include evaluation of interventions to reduce salt intake and use of combination cardioprotective therapies (e.g., Polycap) in high-risk populations. In patients with TIA and minor ischemic stroke, a phase II trial (FASTER) suggested that combination aspirin and clopidogrel may be superior to aspirin alone and this question will be addressed in a phase III trial. For acute ischemic stroke, the IST-3 trial will provide important information on use of thrombolysis within 6 hours of symptom onset in a large generalizable population. Other ongoing trials will determine the role of acute interventions designed to reduce the severity of stroke (e.g., albumin in ALIAS and hypothermic interventions). For secondary prevention, ongoing trials will clarify optimal antithrombotic therapy and target blood pressure in patients with small-vessel disease (SPS-3), closure devices for PFO, and anticoagulant therapy for aortic arch disease (ARCH).

SUGGESTED READINGS

Amarenco P, Bogousslavsky J, Callahan A, III, et al: High-dose atorvastatin after stroke or transient ischemic attack. *N Engl J Med* 355:549, 2006.

Anderson CS, Chalmers J, Stapf C: Blood-pressure lowering in acute intracerebral hemorrhage. *N Engl J Med* 369(13):1274–1275, 2013.

Berge E, Cohen G, Roaldsen MB, et al: Effects of alteplase on survival after ischaemic stroke (IST-3): 3 year follow-up of a randomised, controlled, open-label trial. *Lancet Neurol* 15(10):1028–1034, 2016.

Broderick JP, Meyers PM: Acute stroke therapy at the crossroads. *JAMA* 306:2026, 2011.

Chimowitz MI, Lynn MJ, Derdeyn CP, et al: Stenting versus aggressive medical therapy for intracranial arterial stenosis. *N Engl J Med* 365:993, 2011.

Ederle J, Dobson J, Featherstone RL, et al: Carotid artery stenting compared with endarterectomy in patients with symptomatic carotid stenosis (International Carotid Stenting Study): an interim analysis of a randomised controlled trial. *Lancet* 375:985, 2010.

Gladstone DJ, Spring M, Dorian P, et al: Atrial fibrillation in patients with cryptogenic stroke. *N Engl J Med* 370(26):2467–2477, 2014.

Halkes PH, van Gijn J, Kappelle LJ, et al: Aspirin plus dipyridamole versus aspirin alone after cerebral ischaemia of arterial origin (ESPRIT): randomised controlled trial. *Lancet* 367:1665, 2006.

Hemphill JC, III, Greenberg SM, Anderson CS, et al: Guidelines for the Management of Spontaneous Intracerebral Hemorrhage: A Guideline for Healthcare Professionals From the American Heart Association/American Stroke Association. *Stroke* 46(7):2032–2060, 2015.

Jauch EC, Saver JL, Adams HP, Jr, et al: Guidelines for the early management of patients with acute ischemic stroke: a guideline for healthcare professionals from the American Heart Association/American Stroke Association. *Stroke* 44(3):870–947, 2013.

Kernan WN, Ovbiagele B, Black HR, et al: Guidelines for the prevention of stroke in patients with stroke and transient ischemic attack: a guideline for healthcare professionals from the American Heart Association/American Stroke Association. *Stroke* 45(7):2160–2236, 2014.

Koton S, Rothwell PM: Performance of the ABCD and ABCD2 scores in TIA patients with carotid stenosis and atrial fibrillation. *Cerebrovasc Dis* 24:231, 2007.

Langhorne P, Bernhardt J, Kwakkel G: Stroke rehabilitation. *Lancet* 377:1693, 2011.

Lansberg MG, O'Donnell MJ, Khatri P, et al: Antithrombotic and thrombolytic therapy for ischemic stroke: Antithrombotic Therapy and Prevention of Thrombosis, 9th ed: American College of Chest Physicians Evidence-Based Clinical Practice Guidelines. *Chest* 141(2 Suppl):e601S–e636S, 2012.

Lees KR, Emberson J, Blackwell L, et al: Effects of Alteplase for Acute Stroke on the Distribution of Functional Outcomes: A Pooled Analysis of 9 Trials. *Stroke* 47(9):2373–2379, 2016.

Lip GY, Tse HF, Lane DA: Atrial fibrillation. *Lancet* 379:648, 2012.

O'Donnell MJ, Chin SL, Rangarajan S, et al: Global and regional effects of potentially modifiable risk factors associated with acute stroke in 32 countries (INTERSTROKE): a case-control study. *Lancet* 388(10046):761–775, 2016.

Rothwell PM, Algra A, Amarenco P: Medical treatment in acute and long-term secondary prevention after transient ischaemic attack and ischaemic stroke. *Lancet* 377:1681, 2011.

Rothwell PM, Eliasziw M, Gutnikov SA, et al: Endarterectomy for symptomatic carotid stenosis in relation to clinical subgroups and timing of surgery. *Lancet* 363:915, 2004.

Sandercock PA, Counsell C, Tseng MC, et al: Oral antiplatelet therapy for acute ischaemic stroke. *Cochrane Database Syst Rev* (3):CD000029, 2014.

Sandercock PA, Gibson LM, Liu M: Anticoagulants for preventing recurrence following presumed non-cardioembolic ischaemic stroke or transient ischaemic attack. *Cochrane Database Syst Rev* (2):CD000248, 2009.

Tomaselli GF: Prevention of cardiovascular disease and stroke: meeting the challenge. *JAMA* 306:2147, 2011.

Yuan ZH, Jiang JK, Huang WD, et al: A meta-analysis of the efficacy and safety of recombinant activated factor VII for patients with acute intracerebral hemorrhage without hemophilia. *J Clin Neurosci* 17:685, 2010.

CHAPTER 146

ACUTE CORONARY SYNDROMES

John W. Eikelboom and Jeffrey I. Weitz

Acute coronary syndromes (ACS) lead to millions of hospital admissions worldwide each year and are a leading cause of death. Antithrombotic therapies are a cornerstone in the immediate and long-term management of ACS, reducing the risk of myocardial infarction (MI) and death in both medically and invasively managed patients. This chapter reviews fibrinolytic, antiplatelet, and anticoagulant therapies in the treatment of patients with ACS and provides a practical guide to several common hemostatic and thrombotic problems encountered in this patient population.

CLASSIFICATION

The clinical classification of ACS is based on the electrocardiogram (ECG) at the time of presentation and on blood levels of cardiac biomarkers (troponin, creatine kinase). Patients with ST-segment elevation on the ECG and elevated cardiac biomarkers are diagnosed with ST-segment elevation MI (STEMI). Patients with non–ST-segment elevation (NSTE) ACS are subdivided according to whether or not they have elevated blood levels of cardiac biomarkers; those with elevated cardiac biomarkers are diagnosed with non–ST-segment elevation MI (NSTEMI), and those without elevated cardiac biomarkers are diagnosed with unstable angina.[1-3]

PATHOPHYSIOLOGY

Atherothrombosis plays a central role in the pathogenesis of ACS.[4] Hypertension, abnormal blood glucose levels, dyslipidemia, and toxins contained in tobacco cause endothelial injury. Lipid accumulation promotes an inflammatory response characterized by the recruitment of macrophages, smooth muscle cells, and fibroblasts to the site of injury and the formation of increasingly complex and unstable plaques with a necrotic core and fibrous cap. Disruption of the fibrous cap by shear forces and its degradation by enzymatic and cellular processes expose the plaque contents to the blood. Platelets adhere to exposed subendothelial proteins and become activated and aggregate. Exposed tissue factor induces thrombin generation on cellular surfaces, further promoting the formation of a platelet-fibrin thrombus that can occlude coronary blood flow. These processes are described in more detail in Chapter 144.

The clinical manifestations of coronary atherothrombosis are influenced by the extent and duration of obstruction to blood flow and the presence or absence of a collateral circulation. Patients with small plaques that do not significantly impair blood flow generally remain asymptomatic. Patients with significant flow-limiting plaques may develop ischemic symptoms (e.g., chest pain, breathlessness) during exertion when myocardial oxygen demand exceeds supply. Patients with acute plaque disruption with superimposed thrombus formation that completely obstructs coronary blood flow typically present with STEMI unless there is an adequate collateral circulation. If obstruction to blood flow is transient or partial, patients typically present with NSTE ACS. If myocardial ischemia results in ventricular fibrillation, sudden cardiac death supervenes.

ANTITHROMBOTIC MANAGEMENT

The goal of antithrombotic therapies in patients with ACS is to prevent new thrombus formation at the site of plaque disruption and facilitate lysis of intracoronary thrombus. Antithrombotic drugs are also used to prevent thrombus formation on the guide wires, catheters, and stents used to open occluded arteries, and to prevent and treat left ventricular thrombus formation.

Although the pathophysiology is similar irrespective of whether patients present with STEMI or NSTE ACS, only STEMI patients benefit from immediate reperfusion therapy. This difference reflects the fact that most patients with NSTEMI do not have an occluded infarct-related coronary artery. Instead, they develop MI as a consequence of distal embolization of thrombus.

REPERFUSION THERAPY FOR ST-SEGMENT ELEVATION MYOCARDIAL INFARCTION

Effective approaches to coronary reperfusion include mechanical (primary percutaneous coronary intervention [PCI]) and pharmacologic (fibrinolytic therapy) methods.

Primary Percutaneous Coronary Intervention

Primary PCI is preferred over fibrinolytic therapy in patients with STEMI because it produces higher patency rates and does not cause intracranial bleeding. Unlike fibrinolysis, which only treats the thrombus, primary PCI also allows treatment of the underlying atherosclerotic plaque. However, many centers lack the facilities and expertise to perform urgent coronary interventions, and only a minority of STEMI patients worldwide is treated with primary PCI.[5,6] Patients undergoing primary PCI are routinely treated with anticoagulant and antiplatelet therapy (discussed in sections on antiplatelet therapy and anticoagulant therapy).

Fibrinolytic Therapy

Fibrinolytic drugs are plasminogen activators that initiate fibrinolysis by converting plasminogen to plasmin. Plasmin degrades fibrin resulting in clot lysis and recanalization of thrombotic occlusion. Restoration of coronary blood flow limits infarct size and improves myocardial function and survival.

The pharmacologic characteristics of the fibrinolytic drugs most commonly used in the management of ACS are summarized in Table 146.1. Streptokinase was the first agent to be evaluated in large-scale randomized controlled trials. A non–fibrin-specific agent, streptokinase, indirectly activates plasminogen, whereas the more fibrin-specific agents alteplase, reteplase, and tenecteplase directly convert plasminogen to plasmin. Reteplase and tenecteplase have longer half-lives than alteplase, enabling them to be given by double- or single-bolus injection, respectively, which simplifies administration. The direct-acting fibrinolytic agents are more fibrin specific than streptokinase because they bind to fibrin, where they convert fibrin-bound plasminogen to plasmin. Consequently, these agents produce a less marked systemic lytic state than streptokinase, which has no fibrin affinity. Avoidance of a systemic lytic state, which is characterized by a reduction in the circulating level of fibrinogen, is an important potential advantage of fibrin-specific drugs because this can be expected to be associated with a lower risk of bleeding complications.

TABLE 146.1	Pharmacologic Characteristics of Fibrinolytic Drugs Used in the Management of Patients With ST-Segment Elevation Myocardial Infarction			
Characteristic	Streptokinase	Alteplase	Reteplase	Tenecteplase
Fibrin specificity[a]	–	++	+	+++
Dose	1.5 million units	100 mg	20 U	30–50 mg
Administration	Infusion over 30–60 minutes	Bolus 15 mg; then infusion 0.75 mg/kg (maximum, 50 mg) over 30 minutes, 0.5 mg/kg (maximum, 35 mg) over the next 60 minutes	Double bolus, 10 U over 2 minutes; then repeat 10 U bolus after 30 minutes	Single weight-adjusted bolus, <60 kg = 30 mg, 60–69 kg = 35 mg, 70–79 kg = 40 mg, 80–89 kg = 45 mg, ≥90 kg = 50 mg
Half-life (min)	18–23	3–4	18	20
Adjunctive antiplatelet therapy[b]	Aspirin	Aspirin	Aspirin	Aspirin
Adjunctive anticoagulant therapy	Heparin in patients at high risk of thromboembolism[c]	Heparin 60 U/kg bolus (maximum, 4000 U); 12 U/kg/hour (maximum, 1000 U/hour)	Heparin 60 U/kg bolus (maximum, 4000 U); 12 U/kg/hour (maximum, 1000 U/hour)	Heparin 60 U/kg bolus (maximum, 4000 U); 12 U/kg/hour (maximum, 1000 U/hour)

[a]Less fibrin specificity is associated with more systemic fibrinogen depletion.
[b]Fibrinolytic drugs were evaluated on a background of aspirin, but the addition of clopidogrel to aspirin was subsequently shown to provide incremental benefit.
[c]High-risk patients include those with large or anterior myocardial infarction, atrial fibrillation, known left ventricular thrombus, or previous thromboembolism.

Initial trials with streptokinase established the efficacy of fibrinolytic therapy for reduction in the risk of MI and death; subsequent trials compared the efficacy and safety of newer fibrinolytic drugs with those of streptokinase or alteplase.

Streptokinase

Streptokinase is a single-chain polypeptide derived from β-hemolytic *Streptococcus* cultures. After intravenous (IV) administration, streptokinase binds to plasminogen, and the resulting streptokinase–plasminogen enzymatic complex converts plasminogen to plasmin. Because plasmin nonspecifically degrades circulating fibrinogen as well as fibrin, streptokinase produces a systemic lytic state. Streptokinase induces the formation of antistreptokinase antibodies and can cause allergic reactions, particularly with repeated administration. Severe reactions are rare, but rash, shivering, pyrexia, and mild hypotension occur in up to 10% of patients. It is uncertain whether neutralizing antibodies reduce the efficacy of streptokinase.

The GISSI-1 (Gruppo Italiano per lo Studio della Sopravvivenza nell'Infarto Miocardico 1) trial, which was conducted in 11,806 patients with STEMI, demonstrated that compared with no lytic therapy, streptokinase (1.5 million units over 1 hour) significantly reduced 21-day in-hospital mortality (10.7% vs. 13.0%; $p = .0002$). A similar reduction in mortality was seen when the same dose of streptokinase was compared with no lytic therapy in 17,187 patients with suspected MI in the ISIS-2 (International Studies of Infarct Survival 2) trial (9.2% vs. 12.0%; $p < .00001$).

Alteplase

Alteplase is a recombinant tissue-type plasminogen activator that directly converts plasminogen to plasmin. Although more fibrin-specific than streptokinase, alteplase still induces a systemic lytic state. It has a short circulating half-life of 3–4 minutes, which necessitates its administration by continuous IV infusion.

The ISIS-3 ($n = 41,299$) and GISSI-2 ($n = 20,891$) trials found no benefit of alteplase over streptokinase; findings possibly explained by the suboptimal use of heparin in conjunction with a short-acting fibrinolytic agent (heparin was given subcutaneously after a delay of 4–12 hours) and lack of front-loading of alteplase. The GUSTO-1 (Global Utilization of Streptokinase and Tissue Plasminogen Activator to Treat Occluded Arteries 1) trial ($n = 41,021$) demonstrated that front-loaded alteplase (15 mg bolus, followed by 0.75 mg/kg

[maximum, 50 mg] as an infusion over 30 minutes and then 0.50 mg/kg [maximum. 35 mg] over 60 minutes [maximum, 100 mg over 90 minutes]) plus IV heparin (5000 U IV bolus, followed by 1000 U/hour as an infusion, with the dose titrated to achieve an activated partial thromboplastin time [aPTT] of 60–85 seconds) compared with streptokinase (1.5 million units over 1 hour) with or without IV heparin, reduced 30-day mortality (6.3% vs. 7.3%; $p = .001$). The mortality benefits of alteplase were greatest in patients younger than the age of 75 years and in those with anterior MI. Despite its enhanced fibrin specificity, alteplase was not associated with less bleeding than streptokinase.

The greatest benefits of fibrinolytic therapy are seen in patients treated within 1 hour of symptom onset; there is a much smaller benefit or no benefit if treatment is commenced more than 6 hours after symptom onset.[7]

Reteplase

Reteplase is a second-generation nonglycosylated deletion mutant of alteplase. Reteplase is less fibrin specific than alteplase but has a longer half-life (18 minutes) that enables administration by double-bolus IV injection.

The INJECT trial ($n = 6010$) demonstrated that reteplase and streptokinase were associated with similar 35-day rates of mortality (9.0% vs. 9.5%), in-hospital stroke (1.2% vs. 1.0%), and major bleeding (0.7% vs. 1.0%), although reteplase was associated with a twofold higher rate of intracranial bleeding (0.8% vs. 0.4%). The GUSTO-III trial ($n = 15,059$) demonstrated that reteplase (two 10-mg IV bolus injections given 30 minutes apart) and front-loaded alteplase were associated with similar 30-day rates of mortality (7.5% vs. 7.2%) and stroke (1.6% vs. 1.7%).

Tenecteplase

Tenecteplase is a third-generation multiple point mutant of alteplase. Tenecteplase has a half-life of 20 minutes and is given by single bolus injection. Tenecteplase is the most fibrin-specific fibrinolytic drug approved for clinical use.

The ASSENT-2 (Assessment of the Safety and Efficacy of a New Thrombolytic) study, which enrolled 16,949 STEMI patients, showed that tenecteplase and alteplase were associated with similar 30-day rates of mortality (6.2% vs. 6.2%) and stroke (1.8% vs. 1.7%). Tenecteplase did not reduce the risk of intracerebral bleeding

TABLE 146.2	Management of Major Bleeding in Patients With ST-Segment Elevation Myocardial Infarction Treated With Fibrinolytic Therapy	
Steps	**Approach**	**Considerations**
Stop treatment	Stop fibrinolytic drug	Recovery of fibrinogen levels can take 24–48 hours after stopping streptokinase
	Stop antiplatelet drugs	Antiplatelet effects of aspirin and clopidogrel last for life span of platelets (5–10 days)
	Stop anticoagulant	Heparin has a half-life of about 40 minutes; LMWH has a half-life of 3–6 hours
Local measures	Local pressure	Sustained local pressure (e.g., for 30 minutes) may be required
	Endoscopy and local injection[a]	Can be used for upper or distal lower GI bleeding
	Embolization[a]	Used in rare situations such as life-threatening pulmonary or intraabdominal bleeding
Laboratory evaluation	Fibrinogen	Levels may be undetectable (<100 mg/dL)
	PT and aPTT	Results are uninterpretable if fibrinogen levels are low (<100 mg/dL)
	Anti-Xa level	PT (INR) and aPTT are elevated with warfarin; aPTT is prolonged with therapeutic doses of heparin but not with LMWH or fondaparinux
	Cross-match blood	Chromogenic antifactor Xa assay for LMWH and fondaparinux; this test is unaffected by low fibrinogen levels
		To restore blood volume and maintain hemoglobin
Reversal of fibrinolytic effect	Cryoprecipitate	Recommended initial dose is 10 U; monitor by repeating fibrinogen level
	FFP	The half-life of fibrinogen is about 4 days
		Requires large volumes (e.g., 2 L) to restore fibrinogen levels
Reversal of antiplatelet effect	Platelet transfusion	Increases the number of functional platelets but does not reverse the antiplatelet effects of aspirin and clopidogrel
		Also see text under heading "Antiplatelet Therapy"
Reversal of anticoagulant effect	Protamine	Protamine reverses heparin and partially reverses LMWH; it has no effect on fondaparinux (also see Table 146.6)

[a]Also requires restoration of adequate hemostasis.
aPTT, Activated partial thromboplastin time; FFP, fresh frozen plasma; GI, gastrointestinal; INR, international normalized ratio; LMWH, low-molecular-weight heparin; PT, prothrombin time.

compared with alteplase (1% vs. 1%), but reduced the rate of major noncerebral bleeding (4.7% vs. 5.9%; $p < .0002$), possibly reflecting its enhanced fibrin specificity.

Adjunctive Antithrombotic Therapy in Patients Receiving Fibrinolytic Drugs

A compelling rationale exists to administer adjunctive antithrombotic therapy to STEMI patients treated with fibrinolytic therapy. Platelet-rich thrombi that form after plaque rupture are relatively resistant to degradation, and the use of concomitant antiplatelet and anticoagulant therapy may help to promote clot lysis. Fibrinolytic drugs have an early activating effect on platelets, and the plaque rupture site remains prothrombotic after successful reperfusion therapy. Evidence in support of the efficacy of adjuvant antiplatelet and anticoagulant therapy in patients with STEMI is summarized in the sections on antiplatelet and anticoagulant therapy, respectively.

Intracranial Bleeding

The most important side effect of fibrinolytic therapy is intracranial bleeding, which affects up to 1% of patients and, in the majority of cases, is either fatal or permanently disabling.[8] Risk factors for intracranial bleeding include increasing age (particularly patients older than the age of 75 years), history of prior stroke, uncontrolled blood pressure, female sex, and low body weight. Bolus dose fibrinolytic therapy may be associated with a higher risk of intracranial bleeding than fibrinolytic therapy administered by continuous IV infusion (see Table 146.2 and box on Case 1: Bleeding After Fibrinolytic Therapy).[9]

ANTIPLATELET THERAPY

Aspirin, oral adenosine diphosphate (ADP) receptor antagonists, such as clopidogrel, prasugrel, and ticagrelor, and glycoprotein (GP) IIb/IIIa (GP IIb/IIIa) antagonists, such as abciximab, eptifibatide,

and tirofiban, are the foundation antiplatelet therapies for the management of ACS. Although the use of GP IIb/IIIa antagonists has decreased since the introduction of clopidogrel, they retain a role in high-risk ACS patients, particularly STEMI patients undergoing primary PCI.[5,6,10] In 2015, the US Food and Drug Administration approved cangrelor, a short-acting parenteral ADP receptor antagonist, for ACS patients undergoing PCI who have not received an oral ADP receptor antagonist and who are not given a GP IIb/IIIa inhibitor. The pharmacologic characteristics of antiplatelet drugs commonly used in the management of ACS are summarized in Tables 146.3 (oral drugs) and 147.4 (IV drugs).

Oral Antiplatelet Drugs

Aspirin

Aspirin inhibits platelets by irreversibly blocking the platelet enzyme cyclooxygenase-1, thereby preventing the formation of thromboxane A_2, a potent platelet agonist and vasoconstrictor. Despite having a half-life of only 20 minutes, the antiplatelet effect of aspirin lasts for the lifetime of the platelet (5–10 days) because platelets are anucleate and lack the machinery to synthesize new enzyme.[11]

Multiple randomized trials have demonstrated the efficacy of aspirin for the prevention of recurrent MI, stroke, or death in patients with ACS.[12] The ISIS-2 investigators evaluated the efficacy and safety of aspirin in 17,187 STEMI patients who were also randomized to receive or not to receive fibrinolytic therapy. Aspirin (162 mg/day), compared with no aspirin, significantly reduced 35-day mortality (9.4% vs. 11.8%; $p < .00001$) as well as nonfatal reinfarction (1.0% vs. 2.0%) and stroke (0.3% vs. 0.6%) without increasing bleeding. The Antithrombotic Trialists' Collaboration (ATTC) pooled the data from 15 randomized trials of antiplatelet therapy (predominantly with aspirin) involving 19,302 acute MI patients who were also treated with fibrinolytic therapy. Compared with placebo or no antiplatelet therapy, antiplatelet therapy given for a mean duration of 1 month significantly reduced the composite outcome of MI, stroke, or death (10.4% vs. 14.2%; $p < .0001$).

Case 1: Bleeding After Fibrinolytic Therapy

A 63-year-old man with a history of hypertension presents to a rural hospital with sudden onset of severe retrosternal chest pain. An electrocardiogram (ECG) performed in the emergency department demonstrates 4-mm ST segment elevation in the anterior leads. The nearest hospital with a cardiac catheterization laboratory is more than 6 hours away. After treatment with aspirin (300 mg loading dose), clopidogrel (300 mg loading dose), and an intravenous (IV) infusion of front-loaded alteplase, he has rapid resolution of his pain and the ECG reveals normalization of the ST-segment elevation. Toward the end of the alteplase infusion, he complains of abdominal pain, becomes hypotensive, and develops melena. Hemoglobin is 10.2 g/dL, the activated partial thromboplastin time (aPTT) is 89 seconds, the international normalized ratio (INR) is 1.7, and the fibrinogen level is 80 mg/dL.

Aspirin and clopidogrel are held; the patient receives 10 units of cryoprecipitate and is started on an IV infusion of a proton pump inhibitor. He undergoes urgent upper gastrointestinal tract endoscopy with injection of a bleeding ulcer. He does not receive platelets because of concerns about the risk of recurrent myocardial infarction (MI). No further bleeding occurs, and after 48 hours he resumes aspirin. Clopidogrel is restarted 1 week later after repeat endoscopy demonstrates healing of the ulcer.

Comment

Fibrinolytic trials in patients with acute MI report a 1%–6% incidence of major bleeding and a 10% incidence of moderate bleeding during the first 30 days. The most common sources of major bleeding are the gastrointestinal tract and procedure-related bleeding. The principles of management of major bleeding in STEMI patients treated with fibrinolytic therapy are summarized in Table 146.2. Steps include (1) stop antithrombotic therapies; (2) use local measures when possible to control bleeding; (3) draw blood to measure fibrinogen, prothrombin time (PT), aPTT, and possibly anti-Xa levels (to measure the anticoagulant effect of low-molecular-weight heparin [LMWH]) and for blood typing and crossmatch; and (4) administer therapies to mitigate or reverse the effects of fibrinolytic, antiplatelet, and anticoagulant drugs.

The extent and duration of the systemic lytic state induced by fibrinolytic drugs are determined by their fibrin specificity. Whereas streptokinase produces profound and sustained depletion of fibrinogen (<100 mg/dL) that lasts for up to 24–48 hours, alteplase and other more fibrin-specific agents exert less pronounced and more short-lived effects on fibrinogen levels. The aPTT and PT can be markedly prolonged in patients with hypofibrinogenemia. Normal coagulation can be restored by elevating the fibrinogen level to at least 100 mg/dL. This can readily be achieved by infusing cryoprecipitate (recommended dose: 10 units). Although fresh frozen plasma also contains fibrinogen, much larger volumes are needed to increase the fibrinogen concentration to the desired range.

Platelet dysfunction caused by aspirin, clopidogrel, and fibrinolytic therapy cannot be specifically reversed, but infusion of donor platelets can help to restore platelet function. Platelet transfusion is generally reserved for patients with life-threatening bleeding because of concerns about the risk of recurrent MI. A single unit of single donor platelets can be expected to increase the platelet count by $50-60 \times 10^9$/L. Even a small number (e.g., 10%–20%) of functional (nonaspirinated) platelets is sufficient to generate sufficient thromboxane to sustain normal platelet aggregation, but a much larger number of transfused platelets is needed to overcome the antiplatelet effects of clopidogrel. In this case, bleeding was controlled with cryoprecipitate and local measures, and platelet transfusion was not required.

TABLE 146.3	Pharmacologic Characteristics of Oral Antiplatelet Drugs Commonly Used in the Management of Acute Coronary Syndromes			
			ADP Receptor Antagonists	
Characteristic	**Aspirin**	**Clopidogrel**	**Prasugrel**	**Ticagrelor**
Class	COX inhibitor	Thienopyridine (second generation)	Thienopyridine (third generation)	Cyclopentyl triazolopyrimidine
Target	COX-1	P2Y12	P2Y12	P2Y12
Dose	162–325-mg loading dose; 75–325 mg/day maintenance dose	300–600-mg loading dose; 75 mg/day maintenance dose	60-mg loading dose; 10 mg/day maintenance dose	180-mg loading dose; 90 mg bid maintenance dose
Prodrug	No	Yes	Yes	No
Time to effect[a]	<1 hour	4–6 hours[b]	<1 hour	<1 hour
Drug half-life	20 min	Minutes	Minutes	12 hours
Reversible	No	No	No	Yes

[a]After loading dose.
[b]Increased antithrombotic benefit was seen after the first hour in patients enrolled in the COMMIT trial who did not receive a loading dose, but maximum effect is not seen until after 4–6 hours.
ADP, Adenosine diphosphate; bid, twice daily; COX, cyclooxygenase.

At least four randomized controlled trials have demonstrated the efficacy of aspirin in patients with NSTE ACS. Pooled data from four trials that included a combined total of 3096 patients indicate that aspirin compared with placebo or no aspirin significantly reduced the composite endpoint of MI, stroke, or vascular death (6.4% vs. 12.5%; $p = .0005$).

The efficacy and safety of aspirin in combination with dipyridamole have been evaluated in PCI patients in one randomized controlled trial involving 376 patients. Aspirin (300 mg) plus dipyridamole (75 mg given three-times daily except during a 24-hour period around the time of the procedure when dipyridamole was given intravenously) reduced the risk of MI by more than half compared with placebo (1.6% vs. 6.9%; $p = .01$). These results led to the adoption of aspirin as standard therapy for patients undergoing PCI.

The CURRENT OASIS-7 (Clopidogrel Optimal Loading Dose Usage to Reduce Recurrent EveNTs/Optimal Antiplatelet Strategy for InterventionS) trial explored the optimal dose of aspirin in 25,086 ACS patients with or without ST-segment elevation on the presenting ECG and included 17,263 patients undergoing early PCI.[13] After an initial aspirin loading dose, patients were randomized to receive aspirin at a dose of 300–325 mg/day or 75–100 mg/day for 30 days. The two doses were associated with similar rates of MI, stroke, or death at 30 days (4.2% vs. 4.4%), but the higher aspirin dose increased the rate of gastrointestinal bleeding (0.4% vs. 0.2%; $p = .04$). Based on these results, the optimal dose of aspirin for the management of patients with ACS (after an initial loading dose of 160–325 mg) appears to be 75–100 mg/day.

Clopidogrel

Clopidogrel undergoes metabolic activation in the liver to form the active moiety that irreversibly blocks P2Y12, the major ADP receptor on the platelet surface as evidenced by a decrease in ADP-induced platelet activation and aggregation. Like aspirin, the antiplatelet effect of clopidogrel lasts for the lifetime of the platelet. Clopidogrel is an effective antiplatelet drug for the prevention of MI and death when used in combination with aspirin, but has a slow onset of action and a variable antiplatelet effect that may limit its effectiveness.

The COMMIT trial, which involved 45,582 patients with STEMI, all of whom were treated with aspirin (162 mg/day), demonstrated that compared with placebo, 30 days of treatment with clopidogrel (75 mg/day) reduced the risk of MI, stroke, or death (9.2% vs. 10.1%; $p = .002$) with no increase in major bleeding (0.58% vs. 0.55%).[14] There was no age restriction in the COMMIT trial, and clopidogrel was given without a loading dose. In the CLARITY (Clopidogrel as Adjunctive Reperfusion Therapy) trial ($n = 3491$), which was conducted in parallel with COMMIT, clopidogrel was given as a loading dose of 300 mg followed by 75 mg/day for 2–8 days and was compared with placebo in patients receiving fibrinolysis. Clopidogrel reduced the risk of MI or death (15% vs. 21.7%; $p < .001$). Consistent benefits of clopidogrel were demonstrated in the 1863 patients who underwent PCI after mandated angiography.

The CURE (Clopidogrel in Unstable Angina to Prevent Recurrent Events) trial, which involved 12,562 patients with NSTE ACS, all of whom were treated with aspirin (recommended dose: 75–325 mg/day), demonstrated that compared with placebo, a median of 9 months of treatment with clopidogrel (300 mg loading dose followed by 75 mg/day) reduced the risk of MI, stroke, or death (9.3% vs. 11.4%; $p < .001$) at the cost of an increase in major bleeding (3.7% vs. 2.7%; $p = .001$).[15] Consistent benefits of clopidogrel were seen in the 2658 patients who underwent PCI irrespective of whether or not they underwent coronary stenting.

Prompted by concerns that some patients achieve suboptimal inhibition of platelet function with conventional doses of clopidogrel, the CURRENT-OASIS 7 trial compared the efficacy and safety of a higher loading and maintenance dose of clopidogrel (600-mg loading dose followed by 150 mg/day for 6 days and 75 mg/day for 23 days thereafter) with standard-dose clopidogrel (300-mg loading dose and 75 mg daily thereafter) in 25,086 patients with ACS referred for an invasive management strategy.[13] Both regimens were associated with similar rates of the primary outcome, MI, stroke, or vascular death (4.2% vs. 4.4%), but the higher dose regimen was associated with an increase in major bleeding (2.5% vs. 2.0%; $p = .01$). However, in the 17,263 patients who underwent PCI, the higher dose regimen reduced MI, stroke, or vascular death (3.9% vs. 4.5%; $p = .039$) and stent thrombosis (0.7% vs. 1.3%; $p = .0001$) compared with the lower dose regimen.

Prasugrel

Prasugrel is a third-generation thienopyridine that is more potent and has a more rapid onset of action than clopidogrel. Prasugrel is a prodrug, but unlike clopidogrel, it requires only single-step bioconversion to form the active metabolite that irreversibly blocks the platelet P2Y12 receptor.

The TRITON-TIMI 38 (Trial to Assess Improvement in Therapeutic Outcomes by Optimizing Platelet Inhibition With Prasugrel–Thrombolysis In Myocardial Infarction 38) trial evaluated the efficacy and safety of prasugrel in 13,608 ACS patients with or without ST-segment elevation who were undergoing PCI, all of whom were treated with aspirin (recommended dose: 75–162 mg/day).[16] Compared with clopidogrel (300 mg followed by 75 mg once daily thereafter), prasugrel (60 mg followed by 10 mg once daily thereafter) continued for a median of 14.5 months reduced the risk of MI, stroke, or cardiovascular death (9.9% vs. 12.1%; $p < .001$) and stent thrombosis (1.1% vs. 2.4%; $p < .001$) but did not reduce mortality and increased noncoronary artery bypass graft (CABG) major bleeding (2.4% vs. 1.8%; $p = .03$) as well as intracranial and fatal bleeding.

The TRILOGY ACS[17] (Targeted Platelet Inhibition to Clarify the Optimal Strategy to Medically Manage Acute Coronary Syndromes) trial evaluated the efficacy and safety of prasugrel in 9326 aspirin-treated patients with NSTE ACS who were managed noninvasively. At a median of 17 months of follow-up, prasugrel (30 mg followed by 10 mg once daily in patients less than 75 years or 5 mg once daily for those 75 years or older or who weighed less than 60 kg) and clopidogrel (300 mg followed by 75 mg once daily) were associated with similar rates of MI, stroke or cardiovascular death (13.9% vs. 16.0%; $p = .21$) and similar rates of major bleeding.

Ticagrelor

Ticagrelor is a nonthienopyridine platelet P2Y12 receptor antagonist. Like prasugrel, ticagrelor is more potent and has a more rapid onset of action than clopidogrel, but unlike both clopidogrel and prasugrel, ticagrelor binds reversibly to the platelet P2Y12 receptor.

The PLATO trial evaluated the efficacy and safety of ticagrelor in 18,624 ACS patients with or without ST-segment elevation.[18] Compared with clopidogrel (300 or 600 mg loading dose followed by 75 mg once daily), ticagrelor (180 mg loading dose followed by 90 mg twice daily) reduced the risk of MI, stroke, or vascular death by 16% (9.8% vs. 11.7%; $p < .001$) and produced a significant reduction in vascular death (4.0% vs. 5.1%; $p = .001$) and stent thrombosis (1.3% vs. 1.9%; $p = .009$). There was no increase in major bleeding (11.6% vs. 11.2%) or in intracranial or fatal bleeding, but ticagrelor increased non-CABG major bleeding (4.5% vs. 3.8%; $p = .03$).

Intravenous Antiplatelet Drugs

Glycoprotein IIb/IIIa Inhibitors

Three GP IIb/IIIa inhibitors are available for clinical use (see Table 146.4). Abciximab is a humanized version of a Fab fragment of a murine antibody directed against GP IIb/IIIa; tirofiban is a nonpeptide tyrosine derivative that selectively binds to GP IIb/IIIa; and eptifibatide is a synthetic disulfide-linked cyclic heptapeptide with high specificity for GP IIb/IIIa.

The efficacy and safety of GP IIb/IIIa inhibitors have been extensively evaluated in patients with ACS. A meta-analysis restricted to trials ($n = 6$) involving at least 1000 patients suggests a modest effect of these agents for the prevention of MI, urgent revascularization, or vascular death in patients with NSTE ACS (10.8% vs. 11.8%;

TABLE 146.4	Pharmacologic Characteristics of Intravenous Antiplatelet Drugs Used in the Management of Acute Coronary Syndrome				
	GP IIb/IIIa inhibitors			**ADP Receptor Antagonists**	
Characteristic	**Abciximab**	**Eptifibatide**	**Tirofiban**	**Cangrelor**	
Class	Fab fragment	Nonpeptide	Cyclic heptapeptide	Nonthienopyridine	
Onset	Rapid	Rapid	Rapid	Rapid	
Drug half-life	10–30 min	2 hours	2.5 hours	3–6 min	
Reversibility of platelet inhibition	Slow	Rapid	Rapid	Rapid	
Excretion	Unknown	40%–70% renal	50% renal	Dephosphorylation	

$p = .015$).[19] Pooled data from a meta-analysis of 16 randomized trials involving 10,085 STEMI patients undergoing primary PCI demonstrated that adjunctive GP IIb/IIIa blockade did not reduce 30-day mortality (2.8 vs. 2.9%; $p = .75$) or reinfarction (1.5 vs. 1.9%; $p = .22$) and increased major bleeding (4.1 vs. 2.7%; $p = .0004$). However, meta–regression analysis confirmed the impression from individual trials of a mortality benefit of IV GP IIb/IIIa inhibitors in those at highest risk (see boxes on Case 2: Stent Thrombosis and Case 3: Thrombocytopenia After Stenting).[20]

Cangrelor

Cangrelor is an IV P2Y12 receptor antagonist that has been compared with clopidogrel or placebo in three randomized trials that included patients with NSTE ACS. An individual patient metaanalysis of the three trials[21] demonstrated that compared with control, cangrelor reduced the risk of ischemia-driven revascularization, stent thrombosis, MI or death at 48 hours (3.8% vs. 4.7%, $p = .0007$) at the cost of an increase in GUSTO mild bleeding (16.8% vs. 13.0%, $p < .0001$) but no increase in more severe bleeding.

Case 2: Stent Thrombosis

A 49-year-old man with a history of type 2 diabetes presents with non–ST-segment elevation myocardial infarction and undergoes percutaneous coronary intervention (PCI) with placement of a drug-eluting stent in the left anterior descending coronary artery. He receives a 300-mg loading dose of aspirin and a 600-mg loading dose of clopidogrel and is discharged on aspirin 100 mg/day and clopidogrel 75 mg/day. He presents to the emergency department 3 weeks later with recurrent chest pain and anterior ST-segment elevation on the electrocardiogram. He denies missing any doses of clopidogrel. He is taken urgently to the cardiac catheterization laboratory where a diagnosis of stent thrombosis is confirmed, and he undergoes repeat PCI with thrombus aspiration.

Prompted by concern about the possibility of "clopidogrel resistance", genotyping studies are performed and demonstrate heterozygosity for the CYP2C19 *2 loss-of-function allele. Clopidogrel is stopped, and he is started on prasugrel (10 mg once daily) instead. He is discharged on indefinite dual antiplatelet therapy with aspirin and prasugrel.

Comment

Stent thrombosis is a potentially life-threatening complication of PCI, affecting 1%–2% of patients during the first year and presenting in almost all cases as death or myocardial infarction.[22] Risk factors for stent thrombosis can be categorized as patient related, technical (procedure, stent, or lesion), or drug related. The single most important predictor of stent thrombosis is premature discontinuation of clopidogrel. High on-treatment platelet reactivity during clopidogrel therapy has also emerged as a predictor of stent thrombosis and is affected by clinical (e.g., age, diabetes, renal insufficiency) and genetic factors. Carriers of reduced-function CYP2C19 alleles have low levels of the active metabolite of clopidogrel, diminished platelet inhibition, and an increased risk of stent thrombosis. Unlike clopidogrel, which undergoes two-step, cytochrome P450 (CYP)–dependent metabolic bioconversion in the liver, prasugrel and ticagrelor are not affected by CYP polymorphisms and consistently produce greater and more consistent inhibition of ADP-induced platelet aggregation than standard doses of clopidogrel. Higher doses of clopidogrel (e.g., 225 or 300 mg/day) in patients heterozygous for CYP2C19*2 alleles produce levels of platelet inhibition similar to those seen with standard (75 mg) doses but have not been evaluated in clinical outcome studies.

The role of genetic testing to detect poor clopidogrel responders remains controversial. Although observational studies have demonstrated an independent association between CYP2C19 loss-of-function alleles and the risk of stent thrombosis, analyses from multiple randomized controlled trials provide no evidence of an interaction between genotype and treatment for major cardiovascular events, including stent thrombosis.[23] It is reasonable to switch patients who have experienced stent thrombosis despite clopidogrel therapy to one of the newer P2Y12 receptor antagonists (i.e., prasugrel or ticagrelor) that have been demonstrated to reduce the risk of stent thrombosis compared with clopidogrel even without laboratory testing.

ANTICOAGULANT THERAPY

Anticoagulant therapy is effective for the initial and long-term management of patients with ACS with or without ST-segment elevation.[5,6,10] The pharmacologic characteristics of parenteral anticoagulants commonly used in the management of ACS are summarized in Table 146.5. Early trials suggested that heparin and aspirin were similarly effective for the prevention of MI, but aspirin was adopted as the foundation antithrombotic therapy because it caused less bleeding than heparin. Subsequent randomized controlled trials demonstrated that the combination of heparin plus aspirin provided additive benefit. More recent trials have established the efficacy and safety of newer parenteral anticoagulants, including low-molecular-weight heparin (LMWH), fondaparinux, and bivalirudin, on a background of single- or dual-agent antiplatelet therapy for the initial management of patients with ACS.

The pharmacologic characteristics of warfarin and new oral anticoagulants evaluated in the management of ACS are summarized in Table 146.6.[25] Warfarin is effective for the prevention of major cardiovascular events for the long-term management of patients with ACS who are also treated with aspirin, but no adequately powered randomized controlled trials have evaluated the efficacy and safety of warfarin in the context of dual antiplatelet therapy. Two new oral anticoagulants (rivaroxaban and apixaban) have been evaluated in phase III trials for long-term secondary prevention in ACS patients,[26,27] and rivaroxaban has been approved for this indication in Europe.

Heparin

Heparin is derived from porcine intestinal mucosa and is administered by IV or subcutaneous injection. It inhibits coagulation by binding

---

Case 3: Thrombocytopenia After Stenting

A 65-year-old woman presenting with ST-segment elevation myocardial infarction undergoes primary percutaneous coronary intervention with placement of a bare metal stent in her circumflex coronary artery. During the procedure, she receives an intravenous bolus of abciximab in addition to aspirin, clopidogrel, and heparin. A blood count performed after returning to the coronary care unit (within 6 hours of the procedure) reveals a platelet count of 6×10^9/L, which is confirmed on repeat testing using a sample collected in sodium citrate (to eliminate platelet clumping as a cause of spurious thrombocytopenia). She is diagnosed with abciximab-induced thrombocytopenia.

Heparin is stopped, and the patient receives 1 unit of single-donor platelets with a prompt increase in her platelet count. She is continued on aspirin and clopidogrel and is started on a proton pump inhibitor. The platelet count begins to rise spontaneously on day 4 and returns to baseline levels within 1 week.

Comment

Severe thrombocytopenia (platelet count $<50 \times 10^9$/L) occurs in about 0.5% and less severe thrombocytopenia in 2%–4% of patients treated with glycoprotein (GP) IIb/IIIa inhibitors.[24] Thrombocytopenia caused by GP IIb/IIIa inhibitors is readily distinguished from other causes by its rapid onset, typically within 24 hours of exposure and sometimes within the first hour, and severity (count often $<10 \times 10^9$/L). By contrast, heparin-induced thrombocytopenia is usually delayed until at least 4 days after starting heparin therapy (with the exception of patients with prior exposure to heparin in the past 3 months) and platelet counts rarely fall below 30×10^9/L. The rapid onset of thrombocytopenia is believed to be caused by preformed antibodies that react with GP IIb/IIIa inhibitor-coated platelets. Spontaneous recovery of the platelet count usually occurs within days but can take several weeks. Patients with GP IIb/IIIa inhibitor–induced thrombocytopenia respond normally to platelet transfusions, which should be considered when the count is below 10×10^9/L to reduce the risk of spontaneous bleeding. There is no evidence that steroids or IV gamma globulin alter the natural history of GP IIb/IIIa inhibitor-induced thrombocytopenia. Repeated exposure to GP IIb/IIIa inhibitors should be avoided because there is a risk of recurrent thrombocytopenia, which may be more severe than the initial episode.

TABLE 146.5	Pharmacologic Characteristics of Parenteral Anticoagulants Commonly Used in the Management of Patients With Acute Coronary Syndromes			
	Unfractionated Heparin	**Enoxaparin**	**Bivalirudin**	**Fondaparinux**
Route of administration	IV	SC (first dose IV[a])	IV	SC (first dose IV[a])
Frequency of dosing	Continuous IV infusion	Twice daily; once daily if CrCl <30 mL/min	Continuous IV infusion	Once-daily injection
Clearance	Primarily nonrenal	Renal	Renal, proteolytic cleavage	Renal
Use in ACS patients with moderate renal impairment	Yes	Yes (dose reduction)	Yes (dose reduction)	Yes[b]
Use in ACS patients undergoing dialysis	Yes	No experience	Yes (dose reduction)	No experience[c]
Routine laboratory monitoring	Yes	No	No[d]	No
Dose	Adjust dose according to the results of the aPTT	Fixed weight adjusted	Fixed weight adjusted	Fixed
Accumulation in renal failure	No	Yes	Yes	Yes
Nonanticoagulant side effects	Allergy, HIT	HIT (rare)	—	—
Nonbleeding contraindications	Allergy, immune HIT	Allergy, immune HIT	Allergy	Allergy
Antidote	Protamine sulfate	Protamine sulfate partially reverses	No	No

[a]The first dose of enoxaparin was given by the intravenous route in the TIMI-11B (Thrombolysis In Myocardial Infarction 11B) and EXTRACT-TIMI 25 (Enoxaparin and Thrombolysis Reperfusion for Acute Myocardial Infarction Treatment, Thrombolysis in Myocardial Infarction 25) studies. The first dose of fondaparinux was given by the intravenous route in the OASIS-6 (Optimal Antiplatelet Strategy for InterventionS 6) trial.
[b]Acute coronary syndrome patients with creatinine up to 265 μmol/L were eligible for inclusion in the OASIS-5 and -6 trials (equivalent to an estimated creatinine clearance of 15–20 mL/min in a 70-kg patient who is 70 years of age).
[c]Fondaparinux is contraindicated in patients with venous thromboembolism who have severe renal impairment.
[d]Monitoring and dose adjustment required in patients with creatinine clearance below 30 mL/min.
ACS, Acute coronary syndromes; aPTT, activated partial thromboplastin time; CrCl, creatinine clearance; HIT, heparin-induced thrombocytopenia; IV, intravenous; SC, subcutaneous.

TABLE 146.6	Pharmacological Characteristics of Warfarin and New Oral Anticoagulants Evaluated in Phase III Trials for the Long-Term Management of Acute Coronary Syndromes		
Characteristic	**Warfarin**	**Rivaroxaban**	**Apixaban**
Target	VKORC1	Factor Xa	Factor Xa
Prodrug	No	No	No
Bioavailability (%)	100	80	60
Dosing	Variable, once daily	Fixed, 2.5 or 5 mg twice daily[a]	Fixed, 5 mg twice daily (2.5 mg twice daily in selected patients)
Half-life	Mean: 40 hours (range: 20–60 hours)	7–11 hours	12 hours
Renal clearance (%)	Nil	66[b]	25
Routine coagulation monitoring	Yes (INR)	No	No
Drug interactions	Multiple	Potent inhibitors of CYP3A4 and P-gp[c]	Potent inhibitors of CYP3A4 and P-gp[c]
Antidote	Yes (vitamin K, PCC, FFP)	No[d]	No[d]
Approved for ACS management	Yes	Yes, in Europe	No

[a]A once-daily regimen was tested in atrial fibrillation.
[b]Half of renally cleared rivaroxaban is cleared as unchanged drug and half as inactive metabolites.
[c]Potent inhibitors of both CYP3A4 and P-glycoprotein include azole antifungals (e.g., ketoconazole, itraconazole, voriconazole, posaconazole) and protease inhibitors, such as ritonavir. Potent inhibitors of CYP3A4 include azole antifungals, macrolide antibiotics (e.g., clarithromycin), and protease inhibitors (e.g., atanazavir).
[d]Andexanet alfa is being developed as an antidote for rivaroxaban and apixaban.
ACS, Acute coronary syndromes; CYP-3A4, cytochrome P450 3A4; FFP, fresh frozen plasma; fXa, activated factor X; INR, international normalized ratio; PCC, prothrombin complex concentrates; P-gp, P-glycoprotein; VKORC1, C1 subunit of vitamin K epoxide reductase.

to antithrombin to induce a conformational change that converts antithrombin from a slow to a rapid inhibitor of thrombin and factor Xa.

Heparin has several limitations, including immune-mediated platelet activation, which leads to heparin-induced thrombocytopenia, and nonspecific protein binding, resulting in a variable anticoagulant response and the need for routine coagulation monitoring. Despite these limitations, heparin remains widely used because it has important advantages over more recently introduced anticoagulants. First,

the anticoagulant effect of heparin can be rapidly and completely reversed with protamine sulfate. Second, heparin is suitable for use in patients with renal failure because it is predominantly nonrenally cleared. Third, unlike LMWH and fondaparinux, heparin is also highly effective for prevention of contact activation of coagulation induced by catheters and stents.[28]

Meta-analysis of four randomized controlled trials involving 1239 STEMI patients treated with aspirin and fibrinolytic therapy demonstrated that short-term IV heparin (given for about 1 week) did not significantly reduce death or reinfarction compared with placebo or no heparin, but increased bleeding.[29] However, these trials were underpowered to demonstrate a benefit of heparin. Definitive data concerning the efficacy of heparin in STEMI patients treated with fibrinolysis come from a metaanalysis of 26 trials involving 73,000 patients, in which heparin, given either intravenously or subcutaneously, reduced mortality and reinfarction compared with placebo or no heparin.[30] Consistent benefits were evident in a subset of five trials in which patients also received aspirin; heparin compared with placebo or no heparin reduced both mortality (8.6% vs. 9.1%; $p = .03$) and reinfarction (3.0% vs. 3.3%; $p = .04$).

Short-term heparin therapy is also beneficial when added to aspirin in patients with NSTE ACS. A meta-analysis of six trials involving 1353 patients demonstrated that compared with placebo or no heparin, up to 7 days of IV heparin reduced death or MI (4.5% vs. 7.4%; $p = .045$) with a nonsignificant excess of major bleeding.[31] Heparin has not been rigorously evaluated in ACS patients undergoing PCI but is routinely used in this setting.

Low-Molecular-Weight Heparin

LMWH is derived from heparin by enzymatic or chemical methods, yielding shorter polysaccharide chains that produce a more predictable anticoagulant effect than heparin and a lower propensity for heparin-induced thrombocytopenia. LMWH is given in fixed weight-adjusted doses without routine coagulation monitoring. The anticoagulant effects of LMWH can be partially reversed with protamine sulfate.

The CREATE trial ($n = 15,570$) was the largest of four trials that evaluated the efficacy and safety of various LMWH preparations in patients with STEMI also treated with aspirin and fibrinolysis.[32] Approximately half of patients in the CREATE trial were treated with dual antiplatelet therapy. The pooled data ($n = 16,943$) demonstrated that compared with placebo, initial LMWH continued for up to 7 days reduced the risk of reinfarction (1.6% vs. 2.2%; $p < .05$) and death (7.8% vs. 8.7%; $p < .05$) at the cost of an increase in major bleeding (1.1% vs. 0.4%; $p < .05$).

Most of the trials comparing LMWH with heparin for the treatment of STEMI tested enoxaparin. Pooled data from eight trials involving 27,758 patients demonstrated that compared with heparin, initial LMWH reduced the risk of MI (2.1% vs. 3.9%; $p < .05$) with similar rates of death (5.3% vs. 5.8%) at the cost of an increase in major bleeding (2.2% vs. 1.6%).[33] Consistent results were evident at 30 days.

The FRISC-1 (Fragmin during Instability in Coronary Artery Disease 1) trial evaluated the efficacy and safety of dalteparin in patients with NSTE ACS. Pooled data from FRISC-1 ($n = 1539$) and a second much smaller phase II study demonstrated that compared with placebo or no LMWH, LMWH reduced the risk of MI or death (1.6% vs. 5.2%; $p < .0001$) with no significant increase in major bleeding.

Multiple trials have compared LMWH with heparin in patients with NSTE ACS. A pooled analysis of five trials involving 12,171 patients demonstrated that LMWH and heparin were associated with similar rates of MI or death (2.2% vs. 2.3%) and major bleeding.[31] A subsequent meta-analysis involving 21,946 patients with NSTE ACS demonstrated that compared with heparin, enoxaparin reduced the risk of death or MI (10.1% vs. 11.0%; $p < .05$) with no increase in major bleeding.[32] The latter meta-analysis included some trials that did not involve the use of GP IIb/IIIa inhibitors and other in which they were widely used. The proportion of patients who underwent an invasive management strategy also varied among the trials.

Fondaparinux

Fondaparinux is a synthetic pentasaccharide that contains the essential five-sugar chain that binds antithrombin with high affinity and enhances the rate at which it inhibits factor Xa. Fondaparinux has a half-life of 17 hours, which enables once-daily administration and produces an even more predictable anticoagulant effect than LMWH and does not appear to cause heparin-induced thrombocytopenia. Protamine sulfate has no effect on the anticoagulant activity of fondaparinux.

Fondaparinux has been evaluated in patients with ACS in three large phase III randomized controlled trials. The OASIS-6 trial evaluated fondaparinux in 12,092 STEMI patients treated with single or dual antiplatelet therapy and fibrinolytic therapy.[34] Compared with placebo or heparin, fondaparinux (2.5 mg/day) reduced the risk of reinfarction or death (9.7% vs. 11.2%; $p = .008$) with consistent effects in patients with or without an indication for heparin therapy and in patients who received aspirin alone or the combination of aspirin and clopidogrel. Fondaparinux did not increase major bleeding. However, fondaparinux was associated with no benefit and a trend for harm in patients undergoing primary PCI.

The OASIS-5 trial evaluated fondaparinux in 20,078 patients with NSTE ACS treated with aspirin with or without clopidogrel. Fondaparinux (2.5 mg once daily) and enoxaparin (1 mg/kg twice a day) given for a mean of 6 days were associated with similar rates of the primary outcome of refractory ischemic, MI, or death at 9 days (5.8% vs. 5.7%), but there was a lower rate of major bleeding with fondaparinux (2.2% vs. 4.1%; $p < .001$).[35] At 30 days, fondaparinux was associated with a reduced rate of death compared with enoxaparin (2.9% vs. 3.5%; $p = .02$), which appeared to be explained primarily by the lower rate of bleeding. In 6238 invasively managed patients, fondaparinux and enoxaparin were associated with similar rates of the primary outcome but fondaparinux was associated with a small excess of catheter-related thrombosis (0.9% vs. 0.4%) and a reduction in major bleeding (2.4% vs. 5.1%; $p < .00001$). The risk of catheter thrombosis was largely prevented by the administration of heparin at the time of intervention.

The FUTURA OASIS-8 (Fondaparinux Trial With Unfractionated Heparin During Revascularization in Acute Coronary Syndromes) study compared the effect of standard-dose heparin (85 units/kg bolus with additional boluses based on an activated clotting time dosing algorithm) with reduced-dose heparin (50 units/kg without activated clotting time adjustment) on the primary outcome, a composite of bleeding or major vascular site access complications, in 2026 patients with NSTE ACS who were treated with fondaparinux and scheduled to undergo PCI within 72 hours.[36] The incidences of the primary outcome and of catheter-related thrombosis were similar in the two heparin dose groups, but death, MI, or target vessel revascularization occurred more often in the low-dose group. These data support the use of standard-dose heparin in patients with NSTE ACS who are treated with fondaparinux and scheduled to undergo PCI.

Bivalirudin

Bivalirudin is an IV direct thrombin inhibitor that binds thrombin and prevents it from interacting and its substrates. Bivalirudin has a short half-life of only 25 minutes after IV injection, making the lack of an antidote less problematic than it is for longer-acting anticoagulants. It is about 20% renally cleared, and the half-life is prolonged in patients with renal impairment. Bivalirudin does not cause heparin-induced thrombocytopenia.

The efficacy and safety of direct thrombin inhibitors in ACS patients and those undergoing PCI was examined in the Direct Thrombin Inhibitor Trialists' Collaboration metaanalysis involving data from 11 trials and 35,970 patients.[37] The pooled data indicated a significant benefit of direct thrombin inhibitors (including bivalirudin) compared with heparin for the prevention of MI or death. Clopidogrel and GP IIb/IIIa inhibitors were not used in the trials included in this meta-analysis.

The HORIZONS AMI (Harmonizing Outcomes with Revascularization and Stents in Acute Myocardial Infarction) trial evaluated the use of bivalirudin in 3602 STEMI patients undergoing PCI who were treated with the combination of aspirin and clopidogrel.[38] Compared with heparin plus GP IIb/IIIa, bivalirudin plus provisional

GP IIb/IIIa inhibitor was associated with similar rates of the primary outcome, MI, target vessel revascularization, stroke, or death (5.4% vs. 5.5%) at 30 days, but bivalirudin significantly reduced major bleeding (4.9% vs. 8.3%; $p < .0001$).

The EUROMAX (European Ambulance Acute Coronary Syndrome Angiography) trial[39] evaluated the use of prehospital bivalirudin in 2218 participants treated with aspirin and a P2Y12 receptor antagonist (more than 50% received ticagrelor or prasugrel) being transported for primary PCI. Compared with heparin (unfractionated or low-molecular-weight) plus optional GP IIb/IIIa inhibitor, bivalirudin reduced the risk of death or non-CABG major bleeding (5.1% vs. 8.5%; $p = .001$), a difference that was primarily driven by a reduction in major bleeding (2.6% vs. 6.0%; $p < .001$). Bivalirudin was associated with an increase in stent thrombosis within 24 hours (1.1% vs. 0.2%; $p = .007$).

The single-center, open-label HEAT-PPCI (unfractionated heparin versus bivalirudin in primary percutaneous coronary intervention) trial[40] evaluated the use of bivalirudin in 1829 participants treated with aspirin and a P2Y12 receptor antagonist (almost 90% received ticagrelor or prasugrel) undergoing emergency angiography. Compared with heparin (13% also received a GP IIb/IIIa inhibitor), bivalirudin (15% also received a GP IIb/IIIa inhibitor) was associated with an increase in the composite of death, stroke, reinfarction, or unplanned target lesion revascularization (8.7% vs. 5.7%; $p = .01$). The rates of major bleeding were similar (3.5% vs. 3.1%; $p = .59$), but there was more stent thrombosis with bivalirudin (3.4% vs. 0.9%; $p = .001$)

The BRIGHT (Bivalirudin vs Heparin With or Without Tirofiban) trial[41] evaluated the use of bivalirudin continued for 30 minutes to 4 hours after PCI in 2194 participants with acute MI. Compared with heparin alone or heparin plus a GP IIb/IIIa inhibitor, bivalirudin reduced the risk of death, reinfarction, stroke, ischemia-driven target vessel revascularization or any bleeding (8.8% vs. 13.2%; $p = .008$, and 8.8% vs. 17%; $p < .001$), primarily driven by a reduction in bleeding (4.1% vs. 7.5% vs. 12.3%; $p < .001$) with similar rates of major adverse cardiac or cerebral events (5.0% vs. 5.8% vs. 4.9%; $p = .74$) and stent thrombosis (0.6% vs. 0.9% vs. 0.7%; $p < .77$). Prolonged bivalirudin therapy following PCI might explain the lack of excess stent thrombosis that was seen in most of the earlier bivalirudin trials.

The ACUITY (Acute Catheterization and Urgent Intervention Triage Strategy) trial evaluated the use of bivalirudin in 13,819 patients with NSTE ACS undergoing PCI who were treated with the combination of aspirin plus clopidogrel as well as a GP IIb/IIIa inhibitor.[42] Bivalirudin was noninferior to heparin or enoxaparin plus a GP IIb/IIIa inhibitor for the prevention of MI, unplanned revascularization, or death at 30 days (7.8% vs. 7.3%) but was associated with a lower rate of major bleeding (3.0% vs. 5.7%; $p < .001$).

A metaanalysis of 16 trials involving 33,958 participants[43] showed that compared with heparin-based treatment regimens, bivalirudin was associated with increased major adverse cardiac events and stent thrombosis and a reduction in major bleeding, with no different in death.

Oral Anticoagulation

Warfarin is an oral vitamin K antagonist that has been evaluated in the long-term management of patients with ACS who are treated with aspirin but has not been rigorously tested on a background of dual antiplatelet therapy. Furthermore, the efficacy and safety of the combination of aspirin plus warfarin have not been compared with those of dual antiplatelet therapy.

The results from a metaanalysis of 14 trials involving 25,307 patients demonstrated that compared with placebo or no warfarin, long-term warfarin (target INR, 2.0–3.0) reduced the risk of MI, ischemic stroke or death (9.4% vs. 12.3%; $p < .0001$) at the cost of a twofold increase in major bleeding (2.6% vs. 1.1%; $p < .00001$).[44]

Rivaroxaban and apixaban are orally active direct factor Xa inhibitors that have undergone evaluation in phase III trials for the long-term management of patients with ACS. The ATLAS TIMI-51 trial compared rivaroxaban (2.5 or 5 mg twice a day) with placebo in

TABLE 146.7	Strategies Aimed at Minimizing the Risk of Bleeding in Patients Treated With Triple Therapy (Dual Antiplatelet Therapy and an Oral Anticoagulant)
Proposed Approach	**Rationale**
Aspirin maintenance dose ≤100 mg/day	Higher aspirin maintenance doses increase bleeding, and there is no evidence that they improve efficacy
PPI with a preference for agents that interfere less with CYP 2C19 (e.g., pantoprazole)	Much of the excess bleeding is from the GI tract. The use of acid-suppressive agents that interfere less with CYP 2C19 minimizes the potential for a negative interaction with clopidogrel
Preference for a non–vitamin K antagonist oral anticoagulant	Dabigatran 110 mg twice daily and apixaban 2.5 or 5.0 mg twice daily are associated with lower rates of bleeding than warfarin
For warfarin, use a target INR of 2–2.5	Some evidence that a restricted target INR range reduces the risk of bleeding
Manage warfarin in a specialized anticoagulation clinic	Compared with usual care, specialist clinics achieve a higher TTR of the INR
Minimize duration of triple therapy	The risk of bleeding is highest during the first 30 days but remains elevated with long-term treatment
Avoid NSAIDs	NSAIDs are a common cause of upper GI bleeding
Avoid prasugrel and ticagrelor	Prasugrel and ticagrelor cannot be recommended because they are more potent than clopidogrel and cause more bleeding

CYP, Cytochrome P450; GI, gastrointestinal; INR, international normalized ratio; NSAID, nonsteroidal antiinflammatory drug; PPI, proton pump inhibitor; TTR, time in therapeutic range.

15,526 ACS patients, the majority of whom were also treated with the combination of aspirin and clopidogrel.[26] Treatment was started a median of 4.7 days after onset of symptoms and was continued for a mean of 13 months. Rivaroxaban significantly reduced the risk of MI, stroke, or cardiovascular death (8.9% vs. 10.7%; $p = .008$) at the cost of an increase in non-CABG major bleeding (2.1% vs. 0.6%; $p < .001$) and intracranial bleeding (0.6% vs. 0.2%; $p = .009$). Based on these results, rivaroxaban (2.5 mg twice daily) has been approved in Europe for post ACS patients.

The APPRAISE trial compared apixaban (5 mg twice a day; 2.5 mg twice a day in selected patients) with placebo in patients with ACS. The trial was stopped early because of an excess of bleeding with no significant reduction in ischemic events.[27]

The oral direct thrombin inhibitor dabigatran etexilate has been tested in a phase II trial but has not undergone evaluation in a phase III trial in ACS patients (see Table 146.7 and box on Case 4: Triple Therapy).

CONCLUSIONS AND FUTURE DIRECTIONS

Antiplatelet and anticoagulant drugs are effective for the prevention of MI and death across the spectrum of patients presenting with ACS, including STEMI patients treated with fibrinolytic therapy and those undergoing mechanical reperfusion. Aggressive antithrombotic treatment regimens involving multiple antiplatelet drugs given in combination with an anticoagulant during the acute phase have substantially reduced the risk of early and late recurrent ischemic events and stent thrombosis in ACS patients but at the cost of an increased risk of bleeding. Clinicians require detailed knowledge of the pharmacology

Davi G, Patrono C: Platelet activation and atherothrombosis. *N Engl J Med* 357:2482, 2007.

Case 4: Triple Therapy

A 55-year-old woman with a recent anterior myocardial infarction treated who underwent primary percutaneous coronary intervention with implantation of a drug-eluting stent in the left anterior descending coronary artery is found to have a left ventricular thrombus on transthoracic echocardiogram. She is taking aspirin and clopidogrel. She is started on intravenous heparin, which is overlapped with warfarin until an international normalized ratio of 2 is achieved. She is discharged home on triple antithrombotic therapy with aspirin, clopidogrel, and warfarin.

Comment

Anticoagulation is indicated for the management of left ventricular thrombosis, and the combination of aspirin and clopidogrel is indicated for the management of patients with drug-eluting stents. The combination of an anticoagulant with dual antiplatelet therapy is associated with a 2%–3% incidence of major bleeding during the first 30 days and a 4%–12% incidence during the first year.[45] Strategies that may help to minimize the risk of bleeding in patients receiving triple antithrombotic are summarized in Table 146.7. The new oral anticoagulants, dabigatran etexilate (110 or 150 mg twice a day), apixaban (2.5 or 5.0 mg twice a day), or rivaroxaban (15 or 20 mg once daily), may offer an advantage if they are used instead of warfarin in patients who require triple antithrombotic therapy because they cause less serious bleeding than warfarin in direct head-to-head comparisons.[46,47] However, all anticoagulants, including the new oral agents, increase the risk of bleeding when added to dual antiplatelet therapy.

and side-effects profile of antithrombotic therapies used in the management of patients with ACS to optimize clinical outcomes. Comparative effectiveness studies are urgently required to further define those combinations of antithrombotic drugs that will maximize the net clinical benefit for patients with ACS by minimizing the risk of both thrombotic and bleeding events.

SUGGESTED READINGS

Alexander JH, Lopes RD, James S, et al: Apixaban with antiplatelet therapy after acute coronary syndrome. *N Engl J Med* 365:699, 2011.

Anderson JL, Adams CD, Antman EM, et al: 2011 ACCF/AHA focused update incorporated into the ACC/AHA 2007 guidelines for the management of patients with unstable angina/non-ST-elevation myocardial infarction: a report of the American College of Cardiology Foundation/American Heart Association Task Force on Practice Guidelines. *Circulation* 12:e426, 2011.

Antithrombotic Trialists' Collaboration: Collaborative meta-analysis of randomised trials of antiplatelet therapy for prevention of death, myocardial infarction, and stroke in high risk patients. *BMJ* 324:71, 2002.

Antman EM, Anbe DT, Armstrong PW, et al: ACC/AHA guidelines for the management of patients with ST-elevation myocardial infarction: a report of the American College of Cardiology/American Heart Association Task Force on Practice Guidelines (Committee to Revise the 1999 Guidelines for the Management of Patients with Acute Myocardial Infarction). *Circulation* 110:e82, 2004.

Aster RH, Curtis BR, Bougie DW, et al: Thrombocytopenia associated with the use of GPIIb/IIIa inhibitors: position paper of the ISTH working group on thrombocytopenia and GPIIb/IIIa inhibitors. *J Thromb Haemost* 4:678, 2006.

Boersma E, Harrington RA, Moliterno DJ, et al: Platelet glycoprotein IIb/IIIa inhibitors in acute coronary syndromes: a meta-analysis of all major randomised clinical trials. *Lancet* 359:189, 2002.

Chen ZM, Jiang LX, Chen YP, et al: Addition of clopidogrel to aspirin in 45,852 patients with acute myocardial infarction: randomised placebo-controlled trial. *Lancet* 366:1607, 2005.

Collins R, MacMahon S, Flather M, et al: Clinical effects of anticoagulant therapy in suspected acute myocardial infarction: Systematic overview of randomised trials. *BMJ* 313:652, 1996.

De LG, Navarese E, Marino P: Risk profile and benefits from Gp IIb-IIIa inhibitors among patients with ST-segment elevation myocardial infarction treated with primary angioplasty: a meta-regression analysis of randomized trials. *Eur Heart J* 30:2705, 2009.

Eikelboom JW, Quinlan DJ, Mehta SR, et al: Unfractionated and low-molecular-weight heparin as adjuncts to thrombolysis in aspirin-treated patients with ST-elevation acute myocardial infarction: a meta-analysis of the randomized trials. *Circulation* 112:3855, 2005.

Eikelboom JW, Weitz JI: New anticoagulants. *Circulation* 121:2010, 1523.

Hirsh J, O'Donnell M, Eikelboom JW: Beyond unfractionated heparin and warfarin: current and future advances. *Circulation* 116:552, 2007.

Holmes MV, Perel P, Shah T, et al: CYP2C19 genotype, clopidogrel metabolism, platelet function, and cardiovascular events: a systematic review and meta-analysis. *JAMA* 306:2704, 2011.

Indications for fibrinolytic therapy in suspected acute myocardial infarction: collaborative overview of early mortality and major morbidity results from all randomised trials of more than 1000 patients. Fibrinolytic Therapy Trialists' (FTT) Collaborative Group. *Lancet* 343:311, 1994.

Kushner FG, Hand M, Smith SC, Jr, et al: 2009 focused updates: ACC/AHA guidelines for the management of patients with ST-elevation myocardial infarction (updating the 2004 Guideline and 2007 Focused update) and ACC/AHA/SCAI guidelines on percutaneous coronary intervention (updating the 2005 guideline and 2007 focused update): a report of the American College of Cardiology Foundation/American Heart Association Task Force on Practice Guidelines. *Circulation* 120:2271, 2009.

Marchini JF, Manica A, Croce K: Stent thrombosis: Understanding and managing a critical problem. *Curr Treat Options Cardiovasc Med* 14:91, 2012.

Mega JL, Braunwald E, Wiviott SD, et al: Rivaroxaban in patients with a recent acute coronary syndrome. *N Engl J Med* 366:9, 2011.

Mehta SR, Bassand JP, Chrolavicius S, et al: Dose comparisons of clopidogrel and aspirin in acute coronary syndromes. *N Engl J Med* 363:930, 2010.

Mehta SR, Eikelboom JW, Yusuf S: Risk of intracranial haemorrhage with bolus versus infusion thrombolytic therapy: a meta-analysis. *Lancet* 356:449, 2000.

Patel SC, Mody A: Cerebral hemorrhagic complications of thrombolytic therapy. *Prog Cardiovasc Dis* 42:217, 1999.

Patrono C, Garcia Rodriguez LA, Landolfi R, et al: Low-dose aspirin for the prevention of atherothrombosis. *N Engl J Med* 353:2373, 2005.

Roe MT, Armstrong PW, Fox KA, et al: Prasugrel versus clopidogrel for acute coronary syndromes without revascularization. *N Engl J Med* 367:1297, 2012.

Sami S, Willerson JT: Contemporary treatment of unstable angina and non-ST-segment-elevation myocardial infarction (part 1). *Tex Heart Inst J* 37:141, 2010.

Sami S, Willerson JT: Contemporary treatment of unstable angina and non-ST-segment-elevation myocardial infarction (part 2). *Tex Heart Inst J* 37:262, 2010.

Steg PG, Bhatt DL, Hamm CW, et al: Effect of cangrelor on periprocedural outcomes in percutaneous coronary interventions: a pooled analysis of patient-level data. *Lancet* 382:2013, 1981.

Wallentin L, Becker RC, Budaj A, et al: Ticagrelor versus clopidogrel in patients with acute coronary syndromes. *N Engl J Med* 361:1045, 2009.

White HD, Chew DP: Acute myocardial infarction. *Lancet* 372:570, 2008.

Wiviott SD, Braunwald E, McCabe CH, et al: Prasugrel versus clopidogrel in patients with acute coronary syndromes. *N Engl J Med* 357:2007, 2001.

Yusuf S, Zhao F, Mehta SR, et al: Effects of clopidogrel in addition to aspirin in patients with acute coronary syndromes without ST-segment elevation. *N Engl J Med* 345:494, 2001.

REFERENCES

For the complete list of references, log on to www.expertconsult.com.

CHAPTER 147

ATRIAL FIBRILLATION

Dipak Kotecha, Keitaro Senoo, and Gregory Y.H. Lip

Atrial fibrillation (AF) is the most common cardiac rhythm disturbance. Patients with AF have impaired prognosis, with increased risk of death, stroke, and hospital admission, in addition to poor quality of life.[1,2] The impact of AF on numerous specialties is set to increase further, as the number of patients with AF escalates to epidemic proportions and the populations that are susceptible to AF increase in prevalence. Most notably, this includes older adults and those with heart failure, both in themselves potent risk factors for stroke and systemic thromboembolism (SSE). Cardiologists and general physicians will often manage those patients with straightforward indications (and a lack of contraindications) for anticoagulation, leaving hematologists to face more difficult decisions regarding anticoagulation in patients with high bleeding risk and the consequences of therapy.

In this chapter, we provide a brief overview and background to the overall management of AF, with a focus on issues relating to SSE.

EPIDEMIOLOGY

There have been progressive increases in the incidence and prevalence of AF, and the burden of this condition is expected to increase further.[3] From 2010 to 2060, the number of older adults with AF in the European Union is expected to more than double.[4] Given that AF is a growing epidemic, the societal impact and cost of this condition will continue to increase.[5] AF is commonly accompanied by other comorbidities, including cardiovascular (CV) diseases such as coronary artery disease and valvular heart disease, in addition to non-CV conditions affecting the lungs, kidneys, and liver.[6]

PATHOBIOLOGY

AF can be classified based on etiology, depending on whether it occurs in patients without structural heart disease or whether it complicates other cardiac conditions. AF episodes are defined as paroxysmal if they terminate spontaneously (usually within 7 days) or persistent if they continue and require electrical or pharmacologic termination. Where cardioversion to sinus rhythm is not part of the management plan, AF is considered permanent.

The pathogenesis of AF is now thought to involve an interaction between initiating triggers, often in the form of rapidly firing ectopic foci located inside a pulmonary vein, and an abnormal atrial tissue substrate capable of maintaining the arrhythmia. Although there is considerable overlap, pulmonary vein triggers may play a dominant role in younger patients with relatively normal hearts and short paroxysms of AF, and an abnormal atrial tissue substrate may play a more important role in patients with structural heart disease and persistent/permanent AF.[7] After a period of continuous AF, electrical remodeling occurs, further facilitating the continuance of AF ("AF begets AF"). These changes are initially reversible if sinus rhythm is restored, but may become permanent and associated with structural changes if AF continues (left atrial dilatation, cardiac fibrosis, and impairment of systolic/diastolic function).

CLINICAL MANIFESTATIONS

Symptoms

Symptoms are a major reason that patients with AF seek medical advice. The most common symptoms include lethargy, dyspnea, and palpitations, associated with a reduction in exercise capacity. AF and its related symptoms therefore represent a major therapeutic challenge and burden to health care systems. However, the relationship between symptoms and the onset or recurrence of AF is not always obvious, and these symptoms may reflect other comorbidities. Given the lack of a standardized symptom classification, the European Heart Rhythm Association (EHRA) score has recently been modified for use as a clinical adjunct to classify symptoms of AF (Table 147.1). As yet, there are no outcome data supporting its use to determine management, although the modified EHRA score correlates well with more detailed quality of life assessments.[8]

Stroke and Thromboembolism

The Framingham Study has clearly shown that AF is associated with an increased risk of stroke (both ischemic and hemorrhagic). It is estimated that 20% of all strokes occur in the setting of AF; this rate increases to 25% in patients aged ≥80 years. Patients with AF have an age-adjusted risk of stroke that is fivefold higher than the normal population, regardless of the type of AF.[9] Strokes in AF patients are associated with greater neurologic disability, reduced functional outcomes, and higher mortality than strokes in patients with sinus rhythm.[10] Cognitive dysfunction, including vascular dementia, is present in 10%–15% of patients with AF, twice the rate in patients without AF. Cognitive disturbances can occur in the absence of an obvious stroke, as a consequence of multiple asymptomatic cerebral emboli.[11]

In patients with AF, thrombi have a predilection to form within the left atrial appendage (LAA) due to stagnant flow and reduced emptying of this blind-ended structure (See box on Concomitant Atrial Fibrillation and Risk of Stroke, and Fig. 147.1). The vast majority of atrial thrombi in nonvalvular AF (approximately 90%) are formed within the LAA. Thrombus formation in AF is consistent with the fulfillment of the Virchow triad of thrombogenesis, with intraatrial stasis, endothelial dysfunction, and a prothrombotic or hypercoagulable state due to elevated levels of D-dimer, P-selectin, and von Willebrand factor.

Heart Failure, Other Consequences, and Death

Beyond stroke, AF is associated with a range of CV and non-CV outcomes. Heart failure and AF are convergent disorders that are associated with substantial morbidity, and each of these conditions strongly predisposes to the other. AF directly leading to acute heart failure is termed tachycardiomyopathy, and is a direct result of the rapid heart rate that often responds to cardioversion to sinus rhythm. However, in the vast majority of patients, the link between AF and heart failure is less clear. The occurrence of new AF in

TABLE 147.1 Symptom Scoring in Atrial Fibrillation

mEHRA score	Symptoms	Description
1	None	
2a	Mild	Normal daily activity not affected
2b	Moderate	Normal daily activity not affected, but patient troubled by symptoms
3	Severe	Normal daily activity affected
4	Disabling	Normal daily activity discontinued

mEHRA, Modified European Heart Rhythm Association score.

Case 1: Concomitant Atrial Fibrillation and Risk of Stroke

A 77-year-old woman with syncope, progressive exertional breathlessness, and a systolic murmur was referred for urgent cardiology opinion by her family doctor. Past medical history included type 2 diabetes. On transthoracic echocardiography, the aortic valve was critically stenosed, with good biventricular function. She denied any history of palpitations and multiple electrocardiograms (ECGs) confirmed sinus rhythm. She was reviewed by a cardiac surgeon and urgently listed for a bioprosthetic aortic valve replacement. During all preoperative assessments, she remained in sinus rhythm. On the day of operation she was noted to be in atrial fibrillation (AF). Intraoperative transesophageal echocardiogram revealed a large thrombus arising from her left atrial appendage (LAA), measuring over 5 cm. The surgeon modified the approach and first opened the left atrium, physically removed the thrombus, surgically amputated the LAA, and overstitched the orifice, before proceeding to aortic valve replacement. The patient made a good recovery and was commenced on long-term warfarin due to a CHA$_2$DS$_2$-VASc score of 4.

Comment

In the context of other cardiovascular conditions, identifying symptoms of AF can be difficult. AF frequently complicates other conditions, particularly those that have a structural impact on the heart, such as heart failure and valve disease. This patient most likely had paroxysmal AF that was not detected despite numerous preoperative ECGs. The large thrombus in the LAA would have placed her at high risk of a fatal stroke. Surgical amputation of the LAA is a viable option during cardiac surgery; however, as more than 10% of clots arise from outside the LAA, patients still require long-term anticoagulation depending on predicted risk. In this patient, a CHA$_2$DS$_2$-VASc score of 4 is equivalent to an estimated stroke rate of 4%–5% per year.

patients with heart failure is associated with increased mortality,[12] irrespective of the type of heart failure (whether systolic or diastolic dysfunction).[13] Regardless of the development of heart failure, AF is linked with higher mortality in women (1.9-fold) and men (1.5-fold).[14]

DIAGNOSIS AND DIFFERENTIALS

Diagnosing Atrial Fibrillation

Advances in diagnostic technology are leading to more decisive therapeutic approaches. Among the various diagnostic tools, the simplest method of detecting AF is the electrocardiogram (ECG), which is often prompted by an irregular pulse. Diagnostic ECG criteria include absence of P waves, fibrillatory waves between QRS complexes, and irregular R-R intervals (Fig. 147.2). In paroxysmal AF, ambulatory ECG monitors are helpful, with longer-term monitoring now easily achieved with loop recorders implanted using a local anesthetic. In cases of embolic stroke with undetermined source (previously called cryptogenic stroke), implantable loop recorders are recommended to capture episodes of silent AF that would benefit from anticoagulation.

Key Investigations

Cardiac ultrasound (echocardiography) in AF contributes to risk stratification, diagnosis of complications, and management of associated conditions. Transthoracic echocardiography is a noninvasive method that provides a comprehensive assessment of cardiac structure and function. In patients where exclusion of the left atrial appendage thrombus is required, transesophageal echocardiography is the modality of choice; in addition to visualization of dense spontaneous echo contrast, LAA-emptying velocities of <20 cm/s are strongly associated with incident SSE.[15] Other imaging techniques, such as computed tomography and magnetic resonance imaging, are being used more frequently and have complementary roles in the management of patients with AF.

Blood tests are important in the initial assessment of AF, and should include tests for thyroid, renal, and hepatic function, in addition to serum electrolytes, full blood count, and global tests of coagulation, such as prothrombin time/international normalized ratio (INR) and activated partial thromboplastin time. Biomarkers (such as troponin, B-type natriuretic peptide, and D-dimer) have the potential for refining risk prediction for SSE, but their role in management requires further evaluation before routine measurement can be recommended.[16]

Differential Diagnoses

Other atrial rhythms may resemble AF on an ECG, but these can often be distinguished by the presence of discrete P waves (e.g., atrial tachycardias). Atrial flutter, in the typical form, is characterized by a sawtooth pattern of regular atrial activation, visible as flutter waves in leads II, III, aVF, and V1. Atrial flutter commonly occurs with 2:1 AV block, resulting in a ventricular rate of approximately 150 beats/min (unless rate control medications have been taken). It should be remembered that persistent atrial flutter is also associated with SSE, and hence requirements for anticoagulation are similar to those for AF. Supraventricular tachycardias can be readily distinguished from other narrow complex tachycardias (and often effectively treated) by the use of intravenous adenosine. Broad complex tachycardia should be treated urgently as ventricular tachycardia, unless there is good reason to suspect a bundle-branch block pattern (for example, hemodynamically stable irregular AF with preexisting left bundle branch block).

HEART RATE AND RHYTHM CONTROL

Aside from anticoagulation (see later), management of AF involves control of the rapid heart rate in the majority of patients and therapy to restore sinus rhythm in selected individuals. Compared with rate control therapy, rhythm control does not appear to reduce adverse outcomes; hence the strategy for managing patients with AF is dependent on the presence of ongoing symptoms.[17,18] Thus, modern management of AF is largely patient-centered and symptom-directed.

Rate Control

Rate control can be achieved with beta-blockers, non–dihydropyridine calcium channel blockers (CCB; diltiazem and verapamil), and cardiac glycosides (digoxin and digitoxin). Unfortunately there are few robust randomized trials in this field, leaving the choice of therapy up to individual clinicians based on patient factors such as the presence of heart failure or hypertension. Traditionally beta-blockers have been the preferred therapy due to a presumption of improved prognosis in patients with concomitant heart failure. Recent data, however, suggest that unlike their effect in patients with sinus rhythm, beta-blockers do not reduce mortality or cardiovascular hospitalization in heart failure patients with AF.[19] CCB are typically avoided in patients with reduced ejection fraction due to negative inotropic effects, but can be useful drugs in those with preserved

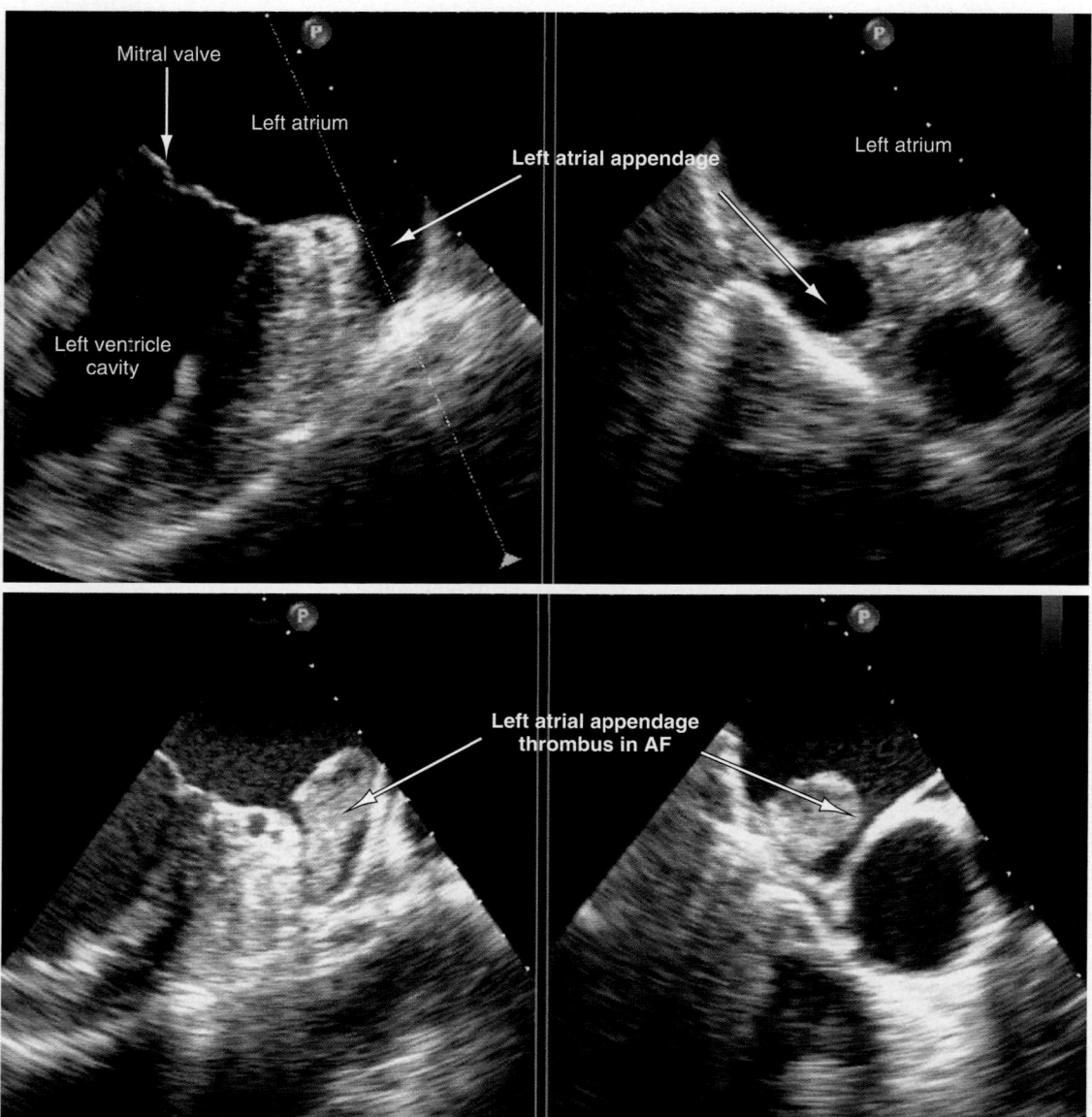

Fig. 147.1 LEFT ATRIAL APPENDAGE AND THROMBUS. The *top panel* shows the left atrial appendage (LAA) using two orthogonal planes from a mid-esophageal view using transesophageal echocardiography. The *bottom panel* shows the same view taken after the patient was found to be in atrial fibrillation (AF), with a large clot arising from the LAA and extending into the body of the left atrium.

cardiac function. Digoxin has not been tested in randomized trials in AF, but in heart failure with sinus rhythm, digoxin reduces symptoms and hospital admissions without affecting mortality. Digoxin is often useful as adjunctive therapy in patients with ongoing symptoms and uncontrolled heart rates. Conventional approaches to target to a strict heart rate (<80 beats/min) have not proved to be better than a more lenient approach, both for prognosis and symptom control.[20] Hence in most patients, the heart rate should be kept at <110 beats/min, with uptitration of therapy if symptoms persist.

Rhythm Control

The aim of rhythm control is to restore normal sinus rhythm and improve symptoms (or heart function). This can be achieved using antiarrhythmic drugs, electrical cardioversion, and catheter or surgical ablation. A full review of this expanding field is beyond the scope of this review, and readers are advised to refer to guideline documents, which are frequently updated (http://www.escardio.org/guidelines/clinical-practice-guidelines/atrial-fibrillation-management).

In brief, all antiarrhythmic drugs have the potential for side effects (e.g., thyroid dysfunction and pulmonary fibrosis with long-term amiodarone use, and the proarrhythmic effects of class I antiarrhythmics). However, in selected patients, they can be helpful to restore and maintain sinus rhythm.[21] Direct current electrical cardioversion is an effective method to achieve rhythm control, although patients will require heavy sedation/anesthetic, and recurrence of AF is common. Catheter ablation of AF involves radiofrequency ablation or cryoablation to the endocardium, typically involving isolation of the pulmonary veins (see box on Interventional Approach to Atrial Fibrillation). Although direct evidence of improvement in long-term outcomes is pending, there are studies that suggest that ablation improves symptoms and ejection fraction, even in patients with AF and heart failure.[22] Surgical ablation, either targeting the pulmonary veins or with the more extensive Cox-Maze approach, is typically performed in patients undergoing cardiac surgery for other reasons (e.g., valve replacement or coronary artery bypass grafting). Regardless of the method of rhythm control, there remains a risk of recurrent (often asymptomatic) AF, and clinicians should not stop long-term anticoagulation in patients with risk

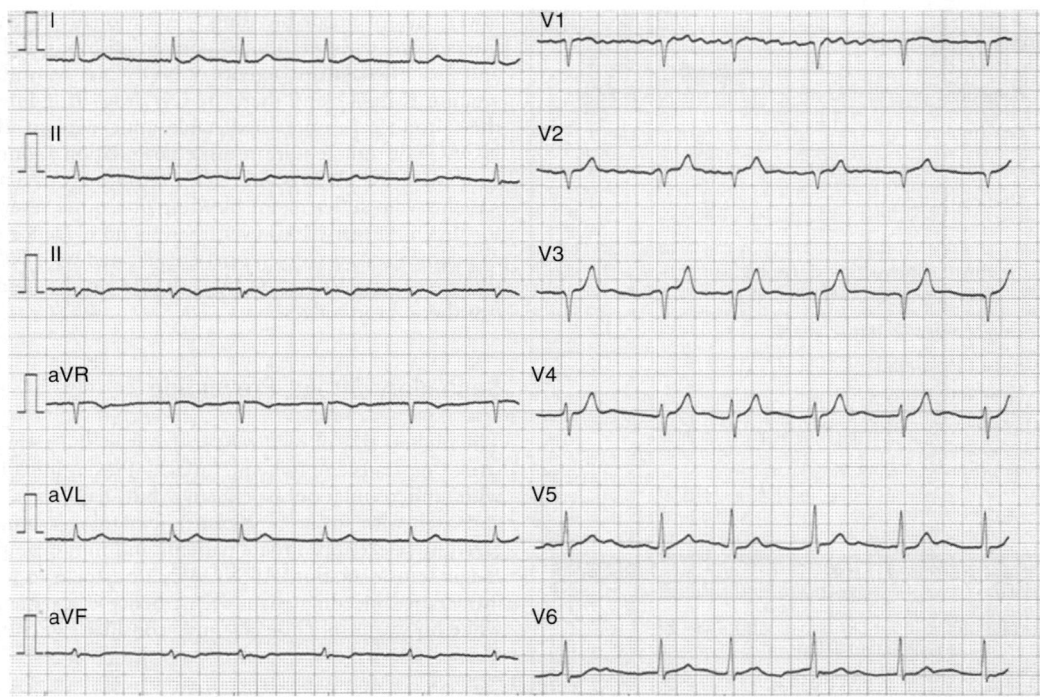

Fig. 147.2 ELECTROCARDIOGRAM OF ATRIAL FIBRILLATION.

factors for SSE, even if the patient appears to be in normal sinus rhythm.

PREVENTION OF STROKE AND THROMBOEMBOLISM

The risk of SSE in AF varies, depending on several clinical factors, including age, gender, previous embolic events and vascular disease, hypertension, diabetes mellitus, and heart failure. In most cases of AF related to valvular heart disease (such as mitral stenosis), there are rarely any reasons not to anticoagulate patients due to the high baseline risk of SSE, regardless of other patient characteristics. Risk stratification scores can be helpful in clinical practice in nonvalvular AF to initially identify those patients at lowest risk of SSE that do not require antithrombotic therapy (i.e., a CHA_2DS_2-VASc score 0 in men, 1 in women; Table 147.2). Subsequent to this step, effective stroke prevention (oral anticoagulation) can be offered to patients with one or more additional stroke risk factors (i.e., CHA_2DS_2-VASc score ≥1 in males, ≥2 in females). This approach is better than a categorical approach to stroke risk (i.e., low/moderate/high) and basing treatment decisions on these artificial risk categories, given that stroke risk is a continuum and because clinical risk scores have limited predictive value for identifying "high-risk" subjects.

Oral anticoagulation can be achieved using a well-controlled, adjusted-dose vitamin K antagonist (VKA, e.g., warfarin), with time in therapeutic range (TTR) >70%, or one of the non-VKA oral anticoagulants (NOACs) (see later). Deciding between a VKA and an NOAC can be assisted using the SAMe-TT_2R_2 score,[23] which is a simple clinical risk score to help identify those patients likely to do well on a VKA (patients with a high TTR [SAMe-TT_2R_2 score 0–2]), or those for whom an NOAC would be a better treatment option (less likely to achieve a good TTR (SAMe-TT_2R_2 score >2])[24,25] (Table 147.3). Although in some health care systems NOACs are routinely used as first-line therapy, the majority of patients with AF globally are still treated with VKAs.

Anticoagulants

The most commonly used anticoagulants in AF are VKAs such as warfarin, which reduce the risk of stroke by nearly two-thirds (i.e.,

TABLE 147.2   Risk Stratification for Incident Stroke and Systemic Thromboembolism and Bleeding

CHA_2DS_2-VASc Score for SSE Prediction		HAS-BLED Score for Bleeding Prediction	
Clinical Characteristic	Points	Clinical Characteristic	Points
CHF or LVEF ≤40%	1	Hypertension	1
Hypertension	1	Abnormal renal/liver function	1 or 2
Age ≥75	2	Stroke	1
Diabetes	1	Bleeding	1
Stroke/TIA/TE	2	Labile INRs	1
Vascular disease	1	Elderly (age >65 years)	1
Age 65–74	1	Drugs or alcohol	1 or 2
Sex category (female)	1		
Cumulative score	Range 0–9	Cumulative score	Range 0–9

For the CHA_2DS_2-VASc score, estimated stroke and thromboembolism event rates at 1 year follow-up are 0.78% (0 points), 2.01% (1 point), 3.71% (2 points), 5.92% (3 points), 9.27% (4 points), 15.26% (5 points), 19.74% (6 points), 21.50% (7 points), 22.38% (8 points), 23.64% (9 points); see Olesen JB, Lip GY, Hansen ML, et al: Validation of risk stratification schemes for predicting stroke and thromboembolism in patients with atrial fibrillation: nationwide cohort study. *BMJ.* 342:d124, 2011.

Hypertension = systolic blood pressure >160 mmHg; vascular disease = prior myocardial infarction, peripheral artery disease, and/or aortic plaque; abnormal renal function = dialysis, transplant, creatinine >2.6 mg/dL or >200 μmol/L; abnormal liver function = cirrhosis or bilirubin >2× normal with AST/ALT/AP >3× normal; labile INR = unstable/high INRs, time in therapeutic range <60%; drugs = antiplatelet agents, nonsteroidal antiinflammatories; alcohol = eight or more drinks/week.

AST, Aspartate aminotransferase; ALT, alanine aminotransferase; AP, alkaline phosphatase; CHF, congestive heart failure; INR, international normalized ratio; LVEF, left ventricular ejection fraction; SSE, stroke or systemic thromboembolism; TE, thromboembolism; TIA, transient ischemic attack.

TABLE 147.3	The SAMe-TT$_2$R$_2$ Score	
Acronym	Definitions	Points
S	Sex (female)	1
A	Age (less than 60 years)	1
M	Medical history[a]	1
e		
T	Treatment (interacting drugs e.g., amiodarone for rhythm control)	1
T	Tobacco use (within 2 years)	2
R	Race (non-white)	2
	Maximum points	8

[a]Two of the following: hypertension, diabetes mellitus, coronary artery disease/myocardial infarction, peripheral artery disease, congestive heart failure, previous stroke, pulmonary disease, hepatic or renal disease.

Case 2: Interventional Approach to Atrial Fibrillation

A 66-year-old man was referred to a cardiac electrophysiologist with a 6-month history of irregular palpitations that cause considerable distress. He had presented to his local emergency department twice and on both occasions was found to be in rapid atrial fibrillation (AF) that reverted spontaneously. Treatment with beta-blockers had not reduced the frequency of symptoms and the patient had developed profound lethargy with higher dosage. He was treated with two antihypertensive agents. The family doctor had already commenced warfarin, with a target international normalized ratio (INR) of 2.5. The patient elected to have catheter ablation after a discussion of alternative pharmacological options and the procedural risks. He underwent radiofrequency ablation, achieving isolation of the four pulmonary veins, accessed through the femoral vein with a transseptal puncture of the interatrial septum. Warfarin was continued without interruption, maintaining an INR of 2.0 to 3.0. The procedure was uncomplicated and the patient was discharged the following day. At 3 months he remained free of symptoms. The CHA$_2$DS$_2$-VASc score was 2 and the patient elected to switch to a non–vitamin K antagonist (VKA) oral anticoagulant (NOAC) to reduce the need for regular blood tests.

Comment

In some patients, AF can substantially reduce quality of life, and a strategy of rhythm control is the most appropriate choice. The number of catheter ablation procedures is rapidly increasing worldwide, and it can be offered as first-line therapy in place of antiarrhythmic drugs in selected patients. Complication rates are low in experienced centers, with 1 in 100 risk of cardiac tamponade and 1 in 500 risk of stroke. The procedure is frequently performed without interruption of VKAs and with only brief or no interruption of NOACs. There is mounting evidence that uninterrupted anticoagulant therapy periprocedurally is safer than stopping the anticoagulant and bridging with heparin. Long-term freedom from AF is 50% to 80% after catheter ablation, but this is variable and multiple ablation procedures may be necessary. Regardless of the apparent restoration of sinus rhythm, anticoagulation should continue in patients with two or more CHA$_2$DS$_2$-VASc risk factors. In this patient, a CHA$_2$DS$_2$-VASc score of 2 is equivalent to an estimated stroke rate of 3% to 4% per year.

reduce the overall risk of stroke from 4.5% to 1.4% per year).[26] A key consideration in the use of warfarin is the TTR (maintaining the INR between 2.0 and 3.0 in nonvalvular AF). To achieve optimal reduction in SSE, TTR should be maintained above 65%–70%. Antiplatelet agents such as aspirin are inferior to oral anticoagulation for stroke prevention and are associated with similar bleeding risks;[27] hence their use for primary prevention of SSE in AF is now discouraged. Recently, four NOACs have become available, including the oral direct thrombin inhibitor dabigatran and the oral factor Xa inhibitors apixaban, edoxaban, and rivaroxaban. All have shown equal or greater efficacy than warfarin in reducing SSE and generally have

lower risks of major bleeding.[28] Additionally, VKAs have numerous interactions with vitamin K–containing foods and other medicines, and the anticoagulant activity of NOACs is not influenced by dietary vitamin K intake and there are few drug–drug interactions. Because they produce a more predictable anticoagulant effect than VKAs, NOACs do not require routine coagulation monitoring. A specific issue with NOACs is the lack of routinely-available antidotes for patients who suffer major bleeding or require reversal in preparation for urgent surgery. However, there is no evidence that the outcome of major bleeds is worse in patients treated with NOACs than it is in those receiving VKAs. NOACs should not be used in patients with prosthetic heart valves.

Secondary Stroke Prevention

The highest risk of recurrent stroke is in the early phase after a first stroke or transient ischemic attack. Prevention of recurrent stroke with anticoagulation is effective but requires a multidisciplinary approach with stroke physicians, hematologists, and cardiologists to carefully select appropriate patients and minimize the risk of hemorrhagic transformation. All NOACs are associated with a lower risk of intracranial bleeding than VKAs; hence if a patient suffers a stroke while on warfarin, clinicians may consider switching to an NOAC.

Nonpharmacologic Strategy

Left atrial appendage occlusion can be used to reduce the risk of stroke for patients with AF that are unable to tolerate anticoagulation.[29] The US Food and Drug Administration (FDA) has recently approved the Watchman device for this indication, although it should be remembered that antiplatelet or anticoagulant therapy is often required in the initial stage of endothelialization. Surgical approaches to ligate or excise the LAA may be considered for patients with AF undergoing cardiac surgery or thoracoscopic maze surgery. However, in most cases it is advisable to continue oral anticoagulation (based on the CHA$_2$DS$_2$-VASc risk score), as not all SSE in AF arise from the LAA.

Periprocedural Anticoagulation

Interruption of anticoagulation temporarily increases thromboembolic risk, whereas continuing anticoagulation increases the risk of bleeding associated with surgical procedures. Individuals undergoing low bleeding risk procedures (e.g., dental and cutaneous procedures) can continue anticoagulation (warfarin within the target INR range and probably NOACs as well). Individuals at high or moderate thromboembolic risk should limit the period without anticoagulation to the shortest possible interval,[30] with or without bridging with low-molecular-weight heparin (LMWH). For individuals undergoing major surgery or those with a high bleeding risk procedure, full-dose LMWH bridging should be delayed for 2 to 3 days after hemostasis has been secured.[31]

Details on the pharmacologic properties of available anticoagulants are provided in Chapter 149.

ANTICOAGULANT-RELATED BLEEDING

Risk of Bleeding

Risk management of anticoagulation-related bleeding is complicated because many of the risk factors for bleeding are also risk factors for stroke. The HAS-BLED score (see Table 147.2) was derived and validated in the Euro Heart survey population,[32] with scores ≥3 indicating a high risk of bleeding and the requirement for attention to minimize bleeding complications. Of note, the HAS-BLED score should not be used to withhold anticoagulation, but rather to identify bleeding risk factors that can be modified to reduce bleeding risk.

Reversal of Anticoagulation

The management of bleeding is still a clinical challenge in the setting of anticoagulation. In patients taking VKAs, physicians have many years of experience with reversing the agent by using a number of therapies, such as intravenous vitamin K, fresh frozen plasma (FFP), and prothrombin complex concentrate (PCC). When rapid reversal is needed, PCC is preferred over FFP; recombinant factor VIIa is not recommended. In contrast, reversal agents for specific NOACs have only recently become available, and action is usually limited to supportive care (e.g., ceasing therapy, volume resuscitation, and hemodynamic support). Nonetheless, PCC is often administered in patients with life-threatening bleeds. Given their short elimination half-lives, time is the most important factor in bleeding associated with NOACs. This emphasizes the importance of asking patients about the exact time of last intake and ascertaining factors influencing plasma concentrations and hemostasis (e.g., age, comorbidities, and concomitant use of antiplatelet drugs).[33]

FUTURE DIRECTIONS

Current gaps in the evidence base for management of AF include comparison of different rate control therapies, defining the place of rhythm control with hybrid approaches to restoration of sinus rhythm, and determining how best to manage patients with AF and concomitant heart failure. We have seen an evolution in the antithrombotic management of AF in recent years due to widespread availability of NOACs. It is hoped that greater uptake of all forms of anticoagulation will result in reductions in the burden of stroke and thromboembolism due to AF. Though reduction in stroke will remain a major priority for these patients in the future, the risk of death remains unacceptably high, with etiology typically due to sudden cardiac death and progressive heart failure. Further attention on these areas is vital, considering the rapidly increasing incidence and prevalence of AF, and the burden this condition places on patients and health care systems.

REFERENCES

1. Kirchhof P, Benussi S, Kotecha D, et al: 2016 ESC Guidelines for the management of atrial fibrillation developed in collaboration with EACTS. *Eur Heart J* 37:2893–2962, 2016.
2. Fuster V, Ryden LE, Cannom DS, et al: 2011 ACCF/AHA/HRS focused updates incorporated into the ACC/AHA/ESC 2006 guidelines for the management of patients with atrial fibrillation: a report of the American College of Cardiology Foundation/American Heart Association Task Force on practice guidelines. *Circulation* 123:e269–e367, 2011.
3. Lane DA, Skøjth F, Larsen TB, et al: Temporal trends in atrial fibrillation incidence, comorbidity and mortality: comprehensive linked data from primary care. *J Am Heart Assoc* 2017, In Press. doi:10.1161/JAHA.116.005155.
4. Krijthe BP, Kunst A, Benjamin EJ, et al: Projections on the number of individuals with atrial fibrillation in the European Union, from 2000 to 2060. *Eur Heart J* 34:2746–2751, 2013.
5. Wodchis WP, Bhatia RS, Leblanc K, et al: A review of the cost of atrial fibrillation. *Value Health* 15:240–248, 2012.
6. Chiang CE, Naditch-Brule L, Murin J, et al: Distribution and risk profile of paroxysmal, persistent, and permanent atrial fibrillation in routine clinical practice: insight from the real-life global survey evaluating patients with atrial fibrillation international registry. *Circ Arrhyth Electrophysiol* 5:632–639, 2012.
7. Kotecha D, Piccini JP: Atrial fibrillation in heart failure: what should we do? *Eur Heart J* 36:3250–3257, 2015.
8. Wynn GJ, Todd DM, Webber M, et al: The European Heart Rhythm Association symptom classification for atrial fibrillation: validation and improvement through a simple modification. *Europace* 16:965–972, 2014.
9. Wolf PA, Abbott RD, Kannel WB: Atrial fibrillation as an independent risk factor for stroke: the framingham study. *Stroke* 22:983–988, 1991.
10. Jørgensen HS, Nakayama H, Reith J, et al: Acute stroke with atrial fibrillation: the copenhagen stroke study. *Stroke* 27:1765–1769, 1996.
11. Ott A, Breteler MM, de Bruyne MC, et al: Atrial fibrillation and dementia in a population-based study. The Rotterdam Study. *Stroke* 28:316–321, 1997.
12. Wang TJ, Larson MG, Levy D, et al: Temporal relations of atrial fibrillation and congestive heart failure and their joint influence on mortality: the framingham heart study. *Circulation* 107:2920–2925, 2003.
13. Mamas MA, Caldwell JC, Chacko S, et al: A meta-analysis of the prognostic significance of atrial fibrillation in chronic heart failure. *Eur J Heart Fail* 11:676–683, 2009.
14. Benjamin EJ, Wolf PA, D'Agostino RB, et al: Impact of atrial fibrillation on the risk of death: the Framingham Heart Study. *Circulation* 98:946–952, 1998.
15. Transesophageal echocardiographic correlates of thromboembolism in high-risk patients with nonvalvular atrial fibrillation. the stroke prevention in atrial fibrillation investigators committee on echocardiography. *Ann Intern Med* 128:639–647, 1998.
16. Hijazi Z, Oldgren J, Siegbahn A, et al: Biomarkers in atrial fibrillation: a clinical review. *Eur Heart J* 34:1475–1480, 2013.
17. Al-Khatib SM, Allen LaPointe NM, Chatterjee R, et al: Rate- and rhythm-control therapies in patients with atrial fibrillation: a systematic review. *Ann Intern Med* 160:760–773, 2014.
18. Kotecha D, Kirchhof P: Rate and rhythm control have comparable effects on mortality and stroke in atrial fibrillation but better data are needed. *Evid Based Med* 19:222–223, 2014.
19. Kotecha D, Holmes J, Krum H, et al: Efficacy of β blockers in patients with heart failure plus atrial fibrillation: an individual-patient data meta-analysis. *Lancet* 384:2235–2243, 2014.
20. Van Gelder IC, Groenveld HF, Crijns HJ, et al: Lenient versus strict rate control in patients with atrial fibrillation. *N Engl J Med* 362:1363–1373, 2010.
21. Zimetbaum P: Antiarrhythmic drug therapy for atrial fibrillation. *Circulation* 125:381–389, 2012.
22. Wazni O, Wilkoff B, Saliba W: Catheter ablation for atrial fibrillation. *N Engl J Med* 365:2296–2304, 2011.
23. Apostolakis S, Sullivan RM, Olshansky B, et al: Factors affecting quality of anticoagulation control among patients with atrial fibrillation on warfarin: the SAMe-TT(2)R(2) score. *Chest* 144:1555–1563, 2013.
24. Proietti M, Lip GY: Simple decision making between a Vitamin K Antagonist and Non-Vitamin K Antagonist Oral Anticoagulant (NOACs): Using the SAMe-TT2R2 Score. *Eur J Heart Cardiovasc Pharmacother* pvv012, 2015.
25. Fauchier L, Angoulvant D, Lip GY: The SAMe-TT2R2 score and quality of anticoagulation in atrial fibrillation: a simple aid to decision-making on who is suitable (or not) for vitamin K antagonists. *Europace* 17:671–673, 2015.
26. Hart RG, Pearce LA, Aguilar MI: Meta-analysis: antithrombotic therapy to prevent stroke in patients who have nonvalvular atrial fibrillation. *Ann Intern Med* 146:857–867, 2007.
27. Friberg L, Rosenqvist M, Lip GY: Evaluation of risk stratification schemes for ischaemic stroke and bleeding in 182 678 patients with atrial fibrillation: the Swedish Atrial Fibrillation cohort study. *Eur Heart J* 33:1500–1510, 2012.
28. Miller CS, Grandi SM, Shimony A, et al: Meta-analysis of efficacy and safety of new oral anticoagulants (dabigatran, rivaroxaban, apixaban) versus warfarin in patients with atrial fibrillation. *Am J Cardiol* 110:453–460, 2012.
29. Holmes DR, Jr, Lakkireddy DR, Whitlock RP, et al: Left atrial appendage occlusion: opportunities and challenges. *J Am Coll Cardiol* 63:291–298, 2014.

30. Spyropoulos AC, Douketis JD: How I treat anticoagulated patients undergoing an elective procedure or surgery. *Blood* 120:2954–2962, 2012.
31. Douketis JD, Spyropoulos AC, Spencer FA, et al: Perioperative management of antithrombotic therapy: antithrombotic therapy and prevention of thrombosis, 9th ed: American college of chest physicians evidence-based clinical practice guidelines. *Chest* 141:e326S–e350S, 2012.
32. Pisters R, Lane DA, Nieuwlaat R, et al: A novel user-friendly score (HAS-BLED) to assess 1-year risk of major bleeding in patients with atrial fibrillation: the Euro Heart Survey. *Chest* 138:1093–1100, 2010.
33. Heidbuchel H, Verhamme P, Alings M, et al: EHRA practical guide on the use of new oral anticoagulants in patients with non-valvular atrial fibrillation: executive summary. *Eur Heart J* 34:2094–2106, 2013.

CHAPTER 148

PERIPHERAL ARTERY DISEASE

Reena L. Pande and Mark A. Creager

Peripheral artery disease (PAD) is an important manifestation of systemic atherosclerosis with significant morbidity and mortality.[1-4] PAD affects the lower extremities and is defined as a stenosis or occlusion in the aorta or in the arteries supplying blood to the legs, including the iliac, femoral, popliteal, or infrapopliteal vessels (peroneal, posterior tibial, and anterior tibial arteries). Stenosis is typically caused by atherosclerosis. Nonatherosclerotic causes of vascular disease also can obstruct the peripheral arteries (see later discussion). There are two major clinical consequences of PAD. First, PAD can cause leg symptoms that include intermittent claudication, which impairs walking ability and diminishes quality of life, and rest pain, which occurs when there is critical limb ischemia (CLI). Second, as an atherosclerotic disorder, PAD is associated with as much as a four- to sixfold increased risk of cardiovascular death, myocardial infarction (MI), and stroke. This chapter reviews the epidemiology, pathophysiology, and management of PAD.

EPIDEMIOLOGY

Prevalence and Incidence

The prevalence of PAD has been determined from several epidemiologic studies. Early studies determined the prevalence of PAD from the presence of symptoms, such as intermittent claudication, or history of peripheral revascularization. Many patients with PAD are asymptomatic, and the use of noninvasive diagnostic testing, specifically measurement of the ankle–brachial index (ABI), has provided further clarification of the overall prevalence of disease. In most of these studies, an ABI of 0.90 or less was used to define PAD. Based on data from the National Health and Nutrition Examination Survey (NHANES), the prevalence of PAD in adults 40 years of age or older is estimated to be 5.9%, accounting for approximately 7.1 million adults in the United States alone.[5] In addition, PAD is estimated to affect as many as 202 million individuals worldwide, with increasing prevalence in both high and low-middle income countries.[6] There is a sharp increase in the prevalence of PAD with increasing age, approximating 16.8% of women and 19.8% of men older than age 65 years in the German Epidemiological Trial on ABI (GetABI study). In a US-based observational study that examined a selected population of adults older than 70 years or adults ages 50 to 69 years with a history of diabetes or smoking, the prevalence of PAD was 29%.[7] Recent studies have also shown higher PAD prevalence in populations of lower socioeconomic status, including lower education and lower income levels,[8] as well as a disproportionate burden among some race/ethnicity groups, particularly blacks, as compared with Hispanic or non-Hispanic white populations.

The incidence of PAD, which is largely based on the development of symptomatic disease, is less well established. Data from the Framingham Heart Study show an incidence rate of intermittent claudication of less than 0.4 per 1000 per year in younger men (35–45 years) and a rate as high as 6 per 1000 per year in older men (older than 65 years). The incidence of symptomatic PAD is lower in women at most age groups, although the estimates are more comparable in the oldest age group. Estimates of the incidence of PAD based on ABI are less commonly reported. One such study reports an incidence of 1.7 per 1000 person-years for ages 40 to 54 years, 1.5 per 1000 person-years for ages 55 to 64 years, and 17.8 per 1000 person-years for ages 65 years and older. When the diagnosis of PAD is based on

ABI alone, the differences in incidence between men and women are less evident. In the Cardiovascular Health Study, for example, there are no gender differences in the incidence of PAD based on ABI after adjusting for cardiovascular risk factors. At the other end of the spectrum, CLI represents only 1% to 2% of the patients with PAD. The incidence of CLI is estimated to be approximately 400 to 1000 per million individuals per year.[2]

Risk Factors

Atherosclerotic risk factors, including smoking, diabetes, hypertension, hyperlipidemia, renal insufficiency, and inflammation, contribute to the development of PAD.

In virtually all population-based studies, smoking has been one of the strongest risk factors for PAD. The risk is highest for current smokers compared with nonsmokers, with a two to four times increased odds of PAD, and the risk of PAD increases in a dose-dependent manner relative to the number of cigarettes smoked and the duration of tobacco use. In the Women's Health Study, smoking more than 15 cigarettes per day increased the risk of incident PAD approximately 17-fold, and the risk was lower in former smokers than in active smokers. In the Edinburgh Artery Study, smoking was two to three times more likely to cause lower extremity PAD compared with coronary artery disease (CAD).

Diabetes is also a potent risk factor for PAD and increases the risk of PAD by two- to fourfold. Data from the Rotterdam study and the San Luis Valley Diabetes study reveal that upwards of 12% to 20% of individuals with PAD have coexisting diabetes. Moreover, the risk of PAD increases depending on the duration and severity of diabetes. In the Strong Heart Study, individuals with PAD had a more than twofold higher prevalence of diabetes compared with those without PAD, and the diabetes tended to be of longer duration (11.7 vs. 8.4 years, $p < .001$) and associated with higher glycosylated hemoglobin levels. Patients with PAD who have concomitant diabetes are also more likely to develop intermittent claudication and ischemic ulceration and to require major amputation compared with those without diabetes.

Hypertension is a more modest risk factor for the development of PAD compared with its importance as a risk factor for coronary and cerebrovascular disease.[1] Although evidence suggests that hypertension increases the prevalence of PAD by 1.5- to 2.2-fold, the association of hypertension with incident or symptomatic PAD is less clear. Among American Indians in the Strong Heart Study, those with PAD had a higher mean systolic blood pressure, and the prevalence of PAD was significantly higher in those with established hypertension. In the Framingham Heart Study, hypertension increased the risk of developing intermittent claudication. However, in the Whitehall study of more than 18,000 men ages 40 to 64 years, there was no significant association between elevated blood pressure and claudication symptoms. Similarly, in the ARIC (Atherosclerosis Risk in Communities) study, there was no association of hypertension with incident PAD in subjects with diabetes. In the Women's Health Study, however, the risk of incident PAD increased by 43% with every 10-mmHg increase in systolic blood pressure.

Dyslipidemia, specifically elevated total cholesterol, low-density lipoprotein (LDL) cholesterol and triglycerides, and reduced high-density lipoprotein (HDL) cholesterol, is associated with PAD. Epidemiologic studies, such as the Cardiovascular Health Study and the Framingham Heart Study, have shown that a 10-mg/dL increase in total cholesterol increases the risk of PAD by 5% to 10%. In the Strong Heart study, individuals with PAD had significantly higher levels of total cholesterol, triglycerides, and LDL cholesterol than those without. The Whitehall study also demonstrated that an elevated total cholesterol level was associated with symptoms of intermittent claudication.

Chronic renal insufficiency has been recognized to be significantly associated with PAD in several studies. In the NHANES, renal insufficiency (defined as a glomerular filtration rate <60 mL/min) was associated with a 2.5-fold higher odds of PAD even after adjustment for other cardiovascular risk factors. In the Heart and Estrogen/Progesterone Replacement (HERS) study, renal insufficiency was also associated with an increased risk of incident peripheral vascular events, including revascularization and amputation. Moreover, renal insufficiency increases the mortality risk in patients with PAD irrespective of other risk factors, including diabetes.

Several other nontraditional factors have been associated with PAD. Markers of systemic inflammation, such as C-reactive protein (CRP), are elevated in patients with PAD. In the Physicians' Health Study, the risk of developing symptomatic PAD was approximately twofold higher in those in the highest CRP quartile compared with those in the lowest quartile. Other markers of inflammation, such as soluble intercellular adhesion molecule 1 (sICAM-1), a leukocyte adhesion molecule, are also associated with PAD in this population and in the Women's Health Study. Insulin resistance is associated with both prevalent PAD as shown in data from the NHANES study and with incident PAD as demonstrated in the Cardiovascular Health Study. The protective effect of bilirubin, an endogenous antioxidant, was explored in NHANES; there was evidence of an inverse association between total serum bilirubin levels and PAD. The impact of genetics on the development of PAD has not been well explored, but a family history of PAD has been associated with development of PAD.

PATHOBIOLOGY

Atherosclerosis is a progressive vascular disease characterized by lipid accumulation and formation of plaque in the arterial walls (see Chapter 144). The pathophysiology of atherosclerosis includes endothelial dysfunction, vascular inflammation, and cellular proliferation. Early in the atherogenic process, recruitment of inflammatory cells and accumulation of lipids promote development of a lipid-rich atheroma. Inflammation promotes the elaboration of proteases that weaken the vessel wall and allow positive remodeling with outward expansion of the arterial wall to accommodate the intimal expansion that occurs as a result of plaque formation. Although positive remodeling initially preserves the arterial lumen, continued plaque growth results in progressive narrowing of the lumen, which then limits blood flow and oxygen supply to target organs. This process may be enhanced by biomechanical factors, such as turbulent blood flow, particularly in areas of altered shear stress. This phenomenon is of particular significance at branch points along the arterial tree, which are predisposed to atherosclerotic plaque formation.

Increasingly, it has been recognized that atherosclerotic plaque formation is a dynamic biologic process that exhibits marked heterogeneity; some plaques remain "stable", but others have a more "unstable" pathophysiology. Stable atherosclerotic plaques may be asymptomatic or symptoms can occur with exertion if demand exceeds supply. On the other hand, "vulnerable" or unstable plaques are prone to acute rupture, and superimposed thrombi may cause sudden arterial insufficiency. Studies have shown that acute atherothrombosis is not restricted to plaques that produce stenosis; many lesions without flow-limiting disease are prone to rupture. Evidence suggests that disruption of the fibrous cap overlying the atheroma is promoted by proinflammatory cytokines. Plaque disruption exposes the highly prothrombotic lipid-rich core of the atheroma to the blood, a process that triggers platelet aggregation and fibrin formation.

Although PAD is mostly caused by atherosclerosis, other causes include thromboembolism, atheroembolism, vasculitides (e.g., thromboangiitis obliterans, giant cell arteritis, Takayasu arteritis), trauma, popliteal artery entrapment, cystic adventitial disease, fibromuscular dysplasia, and endofibrosis of the iliac artery (Table 148.1). Nonvascular causes of leg pain should also be considered in the differential diagnosis, including lumbosacral spine disease (causing pseudoclaudication), acute and chronic venous diseases, hip or knee osteoarthritis, myositis, and others (Table 148.2).

CLINICAL MANIFESTATIONS

The majority of patients with PAD are asymptomatic at presentation. Typical claudication symptoms are present in only 10% to 35% of patients and CLI in 1% to 2%.[1] The classic symptoms of PAD include intermittent claudication and rest pain, the latter occurring in patients with CLI. Intermittent claudication is defined as exertional discomfort in the muscles of the lower extremities that is variably described as pain, aching, burning, fatigue, or heaviness. Symptoms arise with leg exercise, typically walking, and are relieved after a predictable duration of rest (usually <10 minutes). Intermittent claudication occurs with effort and not at rest, and symptoms do not abate until activity ceases; a change in position is unnecessary. Although many patients with PAD report atypical symptoms, most have impaired walking ability exemplified by reduced walking speed or distance. CLI arises when there is inadequate perfusion to meet the resting metabolic demands of the tissues. Patients with CLI have pain at rest, typically affecting the toes, feet, or both; they may have accompanying tissue loss with nonhealing ulcers, tissue necrosis, or gangrene (Fig. 148.1).

DIAGNOSIS

The diagnosis of PAD is often evident from the history and physical examination. An important diagnostic feature is diminished or absent pulses in the legs. The examiner should palpate the femoral, popliteal, dorsalis pedis, and posterior tibial pulses. Absence of selected pulses provides insight into the location of critical stenoses. The groin should be auscultated for femoral artery bruits, which may be indicative of turbulent flow from atherosclerotic plaque. Other findings

TABLE 148.1	Nonatherosclerotic Causes of Peripheral Artery Disease

- Thromboembolism
- Atheroembolism
- Vasculitides
  - Large vessel vasculitides, such as giant cell arteritis and Takayasu arteritis
  - Small vessel vasculitides, such as thromboangiitis obliterans (Buerger's disease)
- Trauma
- Popliteal artery entrapment
- Cystic adventitial disease
- Fibromuscular dysplasia
- Iliac artery endofibrosis

TABLE 148.2	Nonarterial Causes of Leg Pain (Differential Diagnosis for Intermittent Claudication Symptoms)

- Lumbar radiculopathy
- Spinal stenosis
- Hip or knee osteoarthritis
- Myositis
- Venous claudication

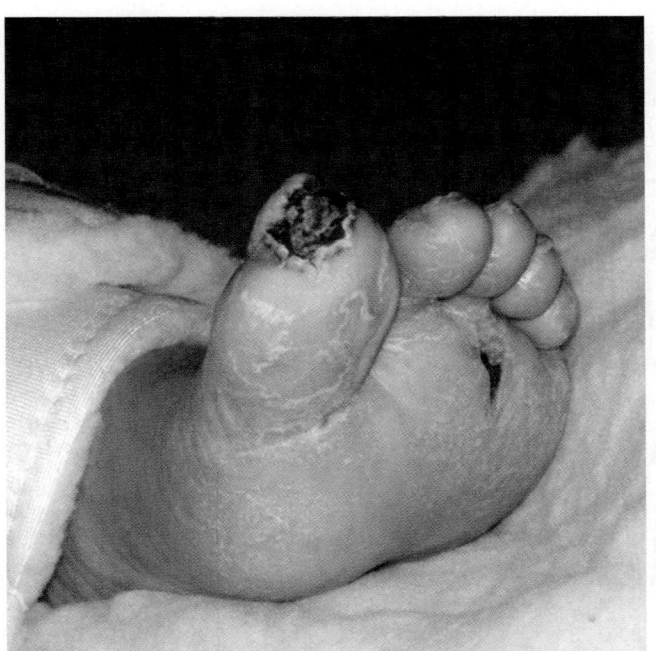

Fig. 148.1 Ulceration and gangrene of the foot representative of critical limb ischemia in a patient with peripheral artery disease.

suggestive of PAD include pallor of the soles of the feet upon leg elevation and the development of rubor when the feet are then placed in the dependent position. Signs of chronic limb ischemia include muscle atrophy; hair loss; thickened nails; and in severe stages, cyanosis, pallor, and coolness of the skin of the feet.

Ankle–Brachial Index

The ABI is a simple, noninvasive test for the diagnosis of PAD.[9] Normally, when measured in the supine position, the systolic blood pressure in the legs is the same as that in the arms. However, pulse wave amplification may yield a higher systolic pressure at the ankle. Therefore the ratio of the ankle to the brachial systolic pressure, designated as the ABI, should be 1.0 or slightly higher. A diminution of the ankle systolic blood pressure relative to the brachial artery pressure indicates a stenosis or occlusion in the aorta or in arteries of the lower extremities.

The ABI is determined by measuring the systolic blood pressure in both arms (brachial arteries) and in both ankle arteries (dorsalis pedis and posterior tibial arteries) after the patient has been in the supine position for at least 5 to 10 minutes.[1] To measure these pressures, sphygmomanometric cuffs are sequentially inflated at each location to suprasystolic pressures. The onset of systole with subsequent cuff deflation is determined with a Doppler device that is placed over the artery. The ABI for each leg is calculated by dividing the higher of the two ankle pressures by the higher of the two arm pressures. Taking into account the intrinsic variability in blood pressure over time, an ABI of 0.90 or less is indicative of PAD. At this threshold, the ABI has excellent sensitivity (90%) and specificity (>95%) compared with angiography. An ABI of 0.91 to 1.0 is considered borderline.[10] Vascular calcification, as often occurs in patients with diabetes or renal insufficiency, may preclude accurate determination of systolic blood pressure at the ankle. For this reason, an ABI that is markedly elevated (e.g., >1.4) is considered inaccurate and indicative of vascular calcification. In this circumstance, other simple noninvasive diagnostic tests, such as assessment of the toe–brachial index or pulse volume recordings, may be useful to detect PAD. In some cases of PAD, the ABI is normal at rest. This is particularly common in patients who have proximal disease, such as iliac artery stenosis, and an extensive collateral circulation. In such cases, measurement of the ABI after walking will detect a decrease in the ankle systolic pressure relative to brachial artery systolic pressure, thereby revealing the presence of PAD.

Noninvasive Testing and Imaging for Diagnosis of Peripheral Artery Disease

Several other noninvasive tests may help in the diagnosis of PAD and in the identification of sites of stenosis. These tests include segmental pressures with pulse volume recordings, duplex ultrasonography, computed tomography angiography (CTA), magnetic resonance angiography (MRA), and conventional contrast angiography. When measuring segmental leg pressures, systolic blood pressure measurements are obtained at multiple levels in the leg, typically in the upper thigh, lower thigh, upper calf, ankle, and across the metatarsal region of the foot. Systolic blood pressures in these sites are then compared with the higher of the arm systolic blood pressures. A significant drop in blood pressure (>20 mmHg) from one level to the next can localize arterial stenosis with a high degree of precision. An upper thigh pressure that is lower than the arm pressure indicates stenosis in the distal aorta or in the iliac or femoral arteries (or both). In patients with vascular calcification, measurement and interpretation of segmental pressures are unreliable. Pulse volume recordings can also be obtained at each level using a plethysmographic instrument that records the change in volume of that limb segment with each arterial pulsation. A normal waveform resembles an arterial waveform with a brisk upstroke and a prominent dicrotic notch in the downstroke (Fig. 148.2). Abnormal waveforms, which appear distal to a hemodynamically significant stenosis, have a parvus et tardus appearance with a blunted upstroke and decreased pulse amplitude.

Duplex ultrasonography is used both for diagnosis of PAD and for the surveillance of bypass grafts or stents after revascularization procedures. Color Doppler can identify abnormal flow with turbulence and Doppler aliasing suggesting an area of stenosis (Fig. 148.3). Pulse Doppler sampling can then confirm flow acceleration in a diseased segment. A peak systolic velocity (PSV) in a diseased segment that is more than twice the PSV in the proximal segment indicates a hemodynamically significant stenosis of at least 50%. Duplex ultrasonography has been shown to be accurate and reproducible with sensitivity and specificity of 88% and 96%, respectively, compared with angiography.[11] However, duplex ultrasonography is a time-consuming and operator-dependent procedure.

The most commonly used imaging modalities for diagnosis of PAD are MRA and CTA. The two tests have relatively comparable diagnostic accuracy for identification of arterial stenosis. MRA has been shown to have a sensitivity of 95% and specificity of 97% to detect stenosis greater than 50%, and CTA was shown to have a sensitivity of 91% and specificity of 91%.

MRA takes advantage of the inherent magnetic properties of human tissue. Pulsed magnetic sequences cause protons within cells to spin and align, generating a frequency of energy that can be detected by the scanner. Various tissues have different frequencies that allow delineation of the structures and tissues within the body. The addition of the paramagnetic contrast agent gadolinium allows selective imaging of moving blood (Fig. 148.4). This flow-related enhancement of the vasculature produces angiographic images. Although MRA has the advantage of using nonionizing radiation, it has several limitations. For example, MRA cannot be performed in patients with implanted cardiac devices or other metal objects. Although MRA can be used in patients with vascular stents, ferromagnetic metals in the stents may produce artifacts that limit assessment of the stented vessel. MRA is contraindicated with renal insufficiency because gadolinium administration in such patients can rarely be associated with nephrogenic systemic fibrosis. Claustrophobia may also preclude MRA.

Similar to MRA, CTA also has excellent specificity and sensitivity for detection of arterial stenosis. The advent of large-volume imaging with multidetector scanners enables rapid image acquisition and high

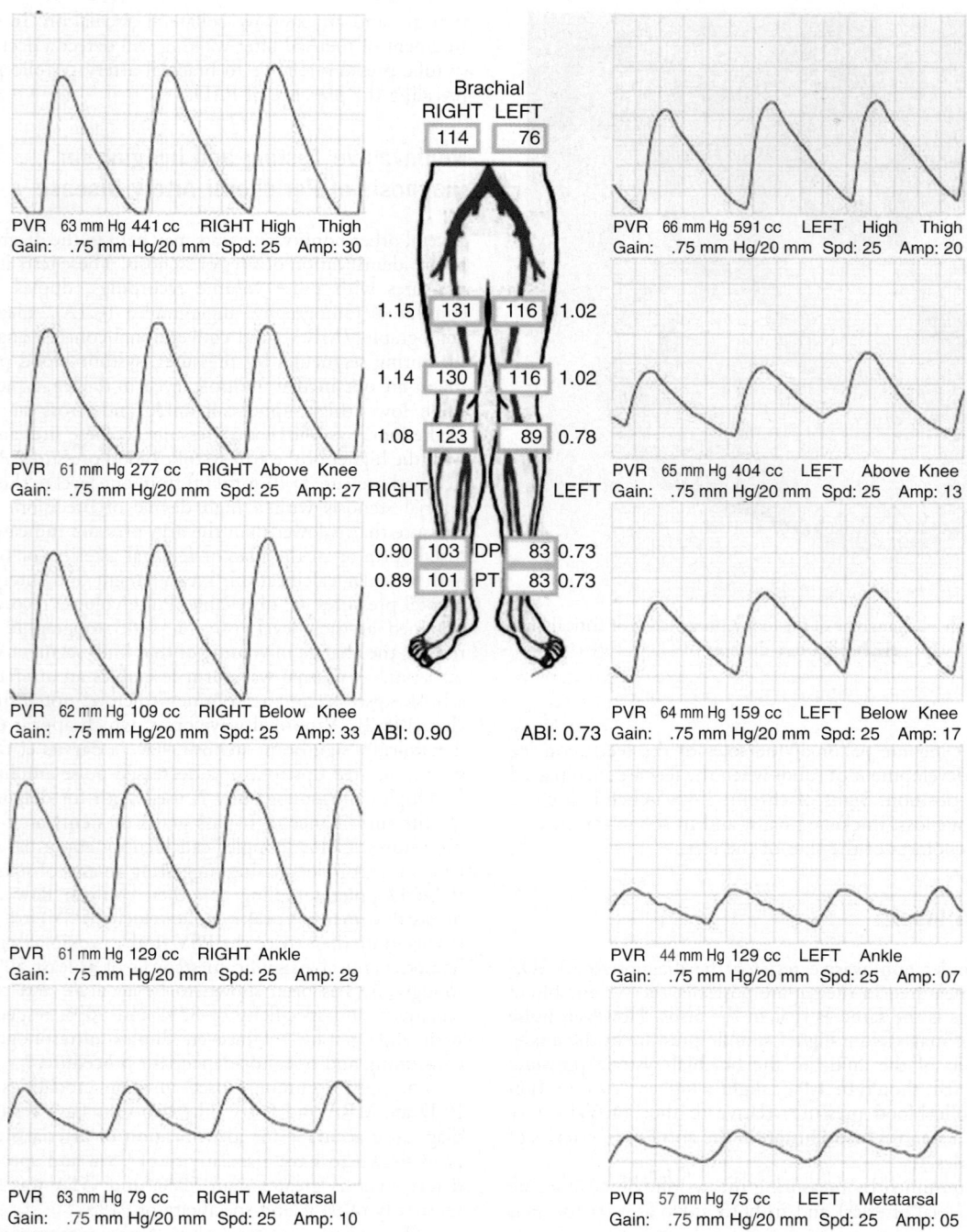

Fig. 148.2 SEGMENTAL LEG PRESSURE MEASUREMENTS AND PULSE VOLUME RECORD-INGS. The ankle–brachial index (ABI) is normal in the right leg. The greater than 20-mmHg drop in systolic blood pressure between the lower thigh and the calf in the left leg suggests stenosis involving the distal left femoral artery, popliteal artery, or both. There is also evidence of blunting of the pulse volume recording with a parvus et tardus waveform. The significant difference in brachial artery systolic blood pressure is suggestive of left subclavian artery stenosis. *Amp,* Amplitude; *DP,* dorsalis pedis; *PT,* posterior tibial; *PVR,* pulse volume recordings; *Spd,* speed.

resolution. Advantages of CTA include the capacity to rapidly visualize the entire arterial tree and to delineate vascular calcification and intraluminal thrombus. Limitations of the test include the exposure to ionizing radiation and the need for iodinated contrast agents, which is problematic in patients with renal impairment. In addition, extensive arterial calcification may prevent accurate determination of the degree of stenosis.

MRA and CTA have largely supplanted conventional catheter-based angiography for PAD diagnosis. Nonetheless, invasive contrast angiography remains the gold standard for the diagnosis of PAD.

Catheter-based angiography is most useful in situations in which concurrent endovascular interventions are planned or in preparation for surgical revascularization. Limitations to catheter-based angiography include the invasive nature of the procedure, the need to administer iodinated contrast, and the radiation exposure. Potential complications include arteriovenous fistula or pseudoaneurysm formation at the access site, atheroembolism, dissection, and contrast-induced renal insufficiency. Alternatives to iodine-based contrast agents, such as carbon dioxide and gadolinium, can be used when administration of iodinated contrast is contraindicated.

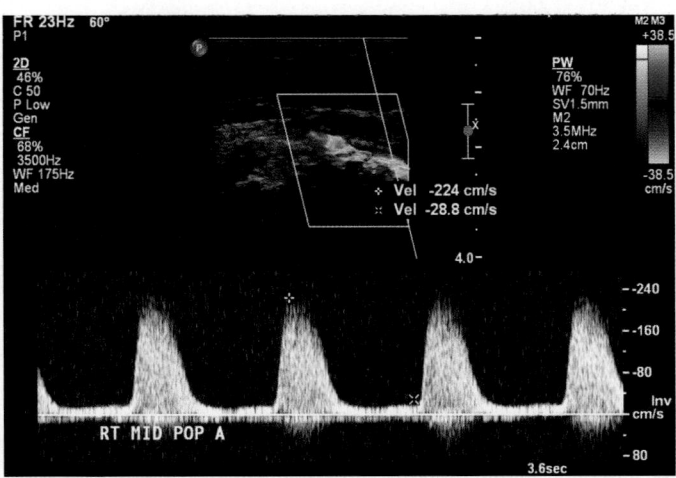

Fig. 148.3 DUPLEX ARTERIAL ULTRASOUND DEMONSTRATING DOPPLER INTERROGATION OF THE POPLITEAL ARTERY. Turbulence of color Doppler flow indicates possible stenosis, confirmed by elevated peak systolic velocity, monophasic waveform, and spectral broadening.

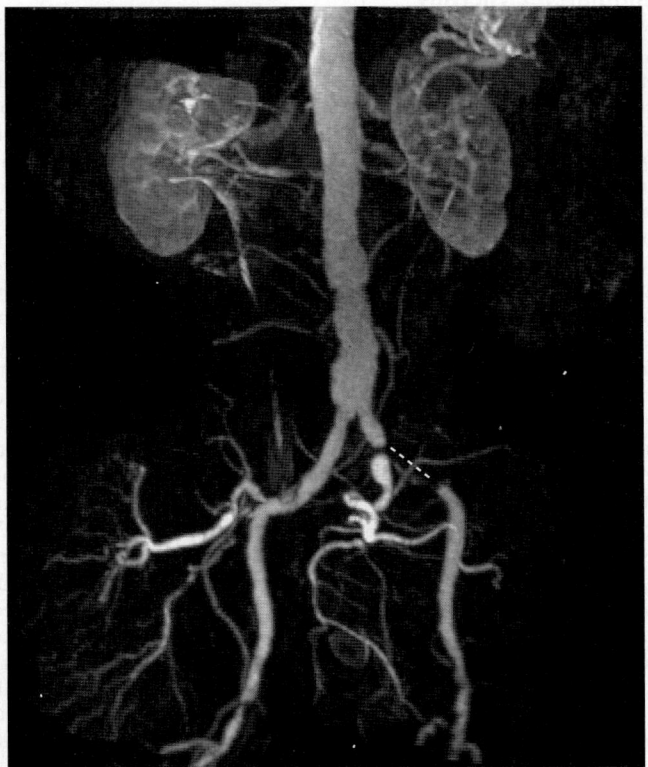

Fig. 148.4 Representative projection imaging from a gadolinium-enhanced magnetic resonance angiogram demonstrating segmental occlusion of the left common iliac artery (indicated by *dashed white line*), as well as nonobstructive atherosclerotic disease in the distal aorta and more distally in the external iliac arteries.

PROGNOSIS

Prognostic considerations are broadly divided into limb outcomes and overall cardiovascular outcomes. Limb prognosis is dependent on the severity of symptoms at initial presentation; concurrent risk factors, such as cigarette smoking and diabetes; and the likelihood of successful revascularization in those with threatened limb viability. Among patients with claudication symptoms, leg discomfort remains stable in the majority (≈70%–80%), worsens in about 10% to 20%, and progresses to CLI in a small percentage.[1] Data from the

Reduction of Atherothrombosis for Continued Health (REACH) registry, which enrolled patients with established PAD on the basis of clinical symptoms, abnormal ABI, and prior revascularization, demonstrated a 23.6% rate of new adverse limb events over 4 years including new revascularization procedures as well as ischemic amputations.[12] These data are consistent with findings from the TRA2°P-TIMI 50 trial, which evaluated the impact of the novel agent vorapaxar in patients with PAD, where the rate of peripheral artery revascularization in the placebo treated group was 22.2%[13] over a median period of three years. Prognosis is worst for those with CLI, where mean amputation-free survival at 1 year is only 50%. Outcomes are worse for patients with PAD who continue to smoke or have coexisting diabetes; such patients have even higher rates of ischemic ulceration and amputation.

Given the high risk of concomitant coronary and cerebral artery disease, individuals with PAD are also at increased risk of MI, stroke, and cardiovascular death. The mortality rate is increased two- to fourfold in patients with PAD compared with those without PAD, as confirmed in a meta-analysis of 16 cohort studies from the ABI collaboration.[14] Furthermore, a graded association has been noted with lower ABI associated with increased mortality.[14] In patients with PAD, the risk of MI is increased by 20% to 60%, and the risk of stroke is increased by 40%. The REACH registry found that the 1-year event rate for the composite of cardiovascular death, MI, and stroke was 6.2% in individuals with PAD. The highest event rates were in those with polyvascular disease compared with rates in patients with atherosclerosis involving only one vascular bed.[15]

THERAPY

The major goals in the management of patients with PAD are to (1) reduce the risk of cardiovascular morbidity and mortality and (2) improve lower extremity symptoms and preserve limb viability. Aggressive cardiovascular risk factor modification is indicated for all patients with PAD. This includes treatment of dyslipidemia, hypertension, and diabetes (including regular foot care) and the use of antiplatelet therapy. Encouragement of healthy lifestyle habits remains a cornerstone of the management of individuals with PAD; these include smoking cessation, a diet enriched in fruits and vegetables and limited in saturated fats, and regular physical activity.[1]

Dyslipidemia

Treatment of dyslipidemia with statins decreases major cardiovascular events in patients with all manifestations of atherosclerosis. The 4S study (Scandinavian Simvastatin Survival Study) was one of the first to demonstrate a clear benefit of lipid-lowering therapy for secondary prevention in patients with atherosclerosis and dyslipidemia. Subsequently, the Heart Protection Study demonstrated that statin therapy was associated with a 22% relative risk reduction in adverse cardiovascular events in patients with vascular disease, including PAD. Recent practice guidelines recommend the use of high-intensity statin therapy, such as atorvastatin 80 mg daily or rosuvastatin 20 mg daily, for individuals with established atherosclerotic vascular disease, including those with PAD to lower cholesterol and to reduce the risk of atherosclerotic events in this population.[16] Statin use is not only associated with lower cardiovascular event rates, but also with approximately 18% lower rates of adverse limb outcomes, including worsening symptoms, peripheral revascularization, and amputations.

The appropriate management of non-LDL cholesterol (HDL and triglycerides) is less clear. Although reduced HDL levels are a risk factor for atherosclerosis, studies with medications that increase HDL levels and lower triglyceride levels have yielded conflicting results. The VA-HIT study (Veterans Affairs High-Density Lipoprotein Intervention Trial) showed that gemfibrozil reduced the risk of fatal coronary disease or nonfatal MI by 22% over a median of 5.1 years in patients with known CAD. However, in a study of patients with

PAD, bezafibrate did not affect the rate of coronary events or stroke. In addition, in the FIELD (Fenofibrate Intervention and Event Lowering in Diabetes) study, fenofibrate did not reduce coronary events in diabetics, although its use was associated with fewer nonfatal MIs and revascularization procedures. Although niacin also reduces lipid levels, its efficacy for reducing cardiovascular events has been called into question based on recent studies showing no added benefit in patients with established atherosclerotic vascular disease.[17] Subgroup analyses showed no meaningful differences in the subset of patients with established PAD.

Hypertension

Treatment of hypertension is a critical component of the management of patients with atherosclerotic PAD. Such treatment reduces the risk of stroke, MI, and congestive heart failure. Management of hypertension should follow current guidelines. Although there is concern that lower systemic blood pressure may exacerbate symptoms of claudication or CLI, the majority of patients experience no change in their symptoms. Several studies have found that antihypertensive drugs reduce cardiovascular events in patients with PAD. The HOPE (Heart Outcomes Prevention) study demonstrated a 22% reduction in cardiovascular events with ramipril in patients with atherosclerotic disease, including those with PAD. ONTARGET (Ongoing Telmisartan Alone and in Combination with Ramipril Global Endpoint Trial) demonstrated that telmisartan and ramipril produced similar reductions in cardiovascular death, MI, stroke, or hospitalization for heart failure (16.7% and 16.5%, respectively; relative risk [RR], 1.01; 95% confidence interval, 0.94–1.09), albeit at the cost of greater risk of hypotension, syncope, and renal insufficiency when the combination of telmisartan and ramipril was used. In a substudy of the ABCD (Appropriate Blood Pressure Control in Diabetes) trial, intensive blood pressure lowering in patients with PAD was associated with a 65% relative reduction in the risk of MI, stroke, or cardiovascular death compared with modest blood pressure–lowering therapy. The INVEST study (International Verapamil-SR/Trandolapril Study) demonstrated that a calcium channel blocker–based antihypertensive strategy was comparable to a beta-blocker–based strategy in patients with concomitant PAD. A J-shaped relationship was noted between achieved systolic blood pressure and outcomes with the best outcomes noted in individuals achieving a systolic blood pressure between 135 and 145 mmHg.

Diabetes

In patients with PAD with concomitant diabetes, the goals of diabetes care include control of hyperglycemia and attention to diabetic foot care. Not only is diabetes associated with adverse limb outcomes (increased risk of ischemic ulceration and amputation in patients with PAD), but it also is associated with increased mortality. Aggressive glycemic control reduces both macrovascular events (MI, stroke, and death) and microvascular events (nephropathy, neuropathy, and retinopathy) in patients with type I diabetes. Although aggressive glycemic control reduces microvascular events in individuals with type II diabetes, reductions in macrovascular events have not been shown. Several recent studies, such as the ADVANCE (Action in Diabetes and Vascular Disease: Preterax and Diamicron Modified Release Controlled Evaluation), Action to Control Cardiovascular Risk in Diabetes and Veterans Affairs Diabetes trials, have failed to show a reduction in cardiovascular events with aggressive treatments aimed at lowering the hemoglobin A1c to 6%. Likewise in patients with type II diabetes who were at risk for cardiovascular events, the PROactive study (Prospective Pioglitazone Clinical Trial in Macrovascular Events) failed to show a reduction in the primary composite endpoint of cardiovascular or limb outcomes (lower rates of extremity revascularization or amputation) with pioglitazone. However, the study did show a significant 16% reduction in the secondary endpoint, a composite of total mortality, nonfatal MI, or stroke, with

pioglitazone. Several recent studies have evaluated the cardiovascular effects of newer classes of glucose-lowering agents including the glucagon-like peptide-1 (GLP-1) analogues, such as semaglutide and liraglutide, and sodium glucose co-transporter-2 (SGLT-2) agents, such as empagliflozin. These studies have demonstrated the safety and efficacy in reducing cardiovascular events in patients with diabetes with existing cardiovascular disease or at high cardiovascular risk.[9a-c] A recent meta-analysis also showed no significant differences among nine different classes of glucose-lowering drugs and risk of cardiovascular or all-cause mortality.[9d] Consequently, although the optimal glycemic control required to reduce macrovascular complications in patients with type II diabetes remains unclear, guidelines recommend treatments that maintain the level of hemoglobin A1c below 7%.

Foot care is a critical component of diabetes management, particularly in those with PAD. Diabetes increases the risk of foot injury because of the associated peripheral neuropathy and decreased sensation, thereby increasing the risk of ulcer formation. Resting limb ischemia and amputation are more frequent in patients with PAD with diabetes than in those without diabetes. Therefore careful attention to foot care is imperative to prevent skin breakdown, infections, ulceration, and amputation.

Antiplatelet Therapy

Antiplatelet therapy is recommended for patients with atherosclerosis, including patients with symptomatic PAD.[10] The Antiplatelet Trialists' Collaboration meta-analysis showed that antiplatelet therapy produces a 22% to 32% reduction in the relative risk of stroke, MI, or vascular death in patients with high-risk vascular disease, including prior stroke or transient ischemic attack or MI. In a subset of patients with evidence of PAD based on symptoms of claudication or prior lower extremity bypass or angioplasty, antiplatelet therapy also produced a 22% relative risk reduction. The meta-analysis included studies that evaluated a variety of antiplatelet agents, such as aspirin, dipyridamole, picotamide, and ticlopidine. The benefits of aspirin have been called into question with a recent meta-analysis showing no significant effect of aspirin on cardiovascular events in patients with PAD.[18] The largest of the studies included in this meta-analysis was the POPADAD (The Prevention Of Progression of Asymptomatic Diabetic Arterial Disease) study,[19] which randomized patients with ABI below 0.99 and no known cardiovascular disease to 100 mg of aspirin or placebo, and showed no significant difference between the groups (hazards ratio [HR], 0.98; 95% CI, 0.76–1.26). The AAA (Aspirin for Asymptomatic Atherosclerosis) trial explored whether aspirin (100 mg/day) was of benefit in asymptomatic individuals with PAD diagnosed solely on the basis of an abnormal ABI.[20] Compared with placebo, aspirin had no effect on the composite endpoint of fatal or nonfatal MI, stroke, or revascularization.

When clopidogrel was compared with aspirin in the CAPRIE trial, clopidogrel was associated with an 8% reduction in cardiovascular events. The CHARISMA study showed no benefit of dual antiplatelet therapy with aspirin plus clopidogrel in a population of patients with established CAD, cerebrovascular disease, or PAD or in those with risk factors for these disorders. In a post-hoc analysis that focused on patients with symptomatic or asymptomatic PAD, there also was no benefit of dual antiplatelet therapy for the primary endpoint. However, the risk of MI and repeat hospitalization for ischemic events was lower with dual antiplatelet therapy (HR, 0.63; 95% CI, 0.42–0.96 and HR, 0.81; 95% CI, 0.68–0.95, respectively).

Newer antiplatelet agents have also been evaluated in patients with PAD. The TRA2P-TIMI 50 study found that the addition of vorapaxar, a protease-activated receptor-1 antagonist, significantly reduced the composite endpoint of cardiovascular death, MI, or stroke by 13% in patients with established atherosclerosis manifesting as a prior MI, ischemic stroke, or established PAD. Among the subset of patients with PAD, vorapaxar did not significantly affect the composite endpoint, but did reduce the risk of hospitalization for acute limb ischemia by 42% ($p = .006$) and peripheral artery revascularization by 16% ($p = .017$), albeit with an increased risk of bleeding (HR

1.62, $p = .001$). More recently, the EUCLID study compared ticagrelor (90 mg twice daily) to clopidogrel in patients with symptomatic PAD. There was no statistically significant difference between the two therapies in reducing a composite endpoint including cardiovascular death, MI, or ischemic stroke (HR 1.02, $p = 0.65$), and no difference in rates of acute limb ischemia (HR 1.03, $p = 0.85$). Additionally there was no difference bleeding risk between clopidogrel and ticagrelor. The PEGASUS-TIMI 54 study also demonstrated the benefits of ticagrelor in reducing major cardiovascular events among patients with PAD.[20a,20b]

Treatment of Lower Extremity Symptoms

Treatments that target the symptoms and signs of PAD are implemented to improve function and mobility and preserve limb viability. Established treatments can be broadly categorized into supervised exercise therapy, pharmacotherapy, and revascularization. Therapeutic angiogenesis has also been explored as a potential therapeutic option.

Exercise Therapy

Supervised exercise therapy improves walking distance by as much as 100% to 150% in patients with PAD. Patients are recommended to walk on a treadmill or track three to five times per week for a duration of at least 45 minutes per session for 3 to 6 months. Exercise should continue until patients develop moderate to severe claudication; after a rest period, they should resume walking with the cycle repeated until the session is over. As patients improve, walking speed and treadmill grade can be increased. Recent studies have shown that home-based exercise therapy is also effective when home activities are monitored and quantified[21] or when paired with periodic and facilitated group behavioral training.[22] The CLEVER (The Claudication: Exercise Versus Endoluminal Revascularization) trial showed that a 6-month supervised exercise training program in patients with aortoiliac disease and claudication produced a greater improvement in walking time than optimal medical therapy alone or stenting.[23] In contrast, in the IRONIC (Invasive Revascularization or Not in Intermittent Claudication) study, improvement in disease-specific quality-of-life measures was greater for stenting than supervised exercise therapy in patients with life-limiting claudication. While prior studies had evaluated the benefits of supervised exercise therapy in comparison to revascularization, the ERASE study assessed the impact of exercise therapy in addition to endovascular revascularization. The study showed that combination treatment resulted in greater walking distance and quality of life at 1 year than supervised exercise therapy alone.[23a] It remains clear that physical activity should be recommended as a part of a multifaceted approach to improving symptoms in patients with PAD.

The mechanisms responsible for the benefits of exercise remain unclear. Potential mechanisms include collateral blood vessel development as a consequence of upregulation of angiogenic growth factors, endothelium-dependent vasodilation because of enhanced nitric oxide bioavailability, more efficient walking biomechanics, and improved skeletal muscle metabolism.

Pharmacologic Therapies

Although many medications have been evaluated, few have improved the symptoms of claudication in patients with PAD. Only two medications are approved by the Food and Drugs Administration; cilostazol and pentoxifylline. Cilostazol is a phosphodiesterase 3 (PDE3) inhibitor with both vasodilator and antiplatelet properties. The precise mechanism by which cilostazol confers benefit in patients with PAD is unknown. Several randomized trials have shown that compared with placebo, cilostazol produces an approximately 50% increase in walking time and improves perceived quality of life. Because other PDE3 inhibitors (e.g., milrinone) have been linked to increased mortality in patients with congestive heart failure, cilostazol should not be used in this subpopulation of patients with PAD. However, cilostazol has not been associated with an increase in mortality. Evidence for the efficacy of pentoxifylline, a hemorrheologic agent, is less robust than that for cilostazol, and pentoxifylline is less likely to be of clinical benefit.

Statins have also been explored for the treatment of claudication to exploit their pleiotropic effects, such as attenuation of inflammation. One study showed an improvement in pain-free walking time with atorvastatin but no significant increase in maximal walking time. Other studies revealed an increase in walking time with simvastatin. Another study, however, showed no benefit of niacin plus lovastatin on walking times compared with placebo.

Revascularization

Lower extremity revascularization is reserved for patients with CLI or lifestyle-limiting claudication symptoms despite maximal medical therapy. For those with CLI, prompt revascularization is necessary. Revascularization in such patients may alleviate resting limb pain, accelerate the healing of ulcers, and reduce infection. In patients with claudication, revascularization can lessen leg discomfort and improve quality of life. Options for revascularization include endovascular (percutaneous) intervention or open surgical revascularization.

Endovascular intervention, which includes percutaneous transluminal balloon angioplasty (PTA) and endovascular stenting, is increasingly being used as a less invasive option for revascularization in patients with PAD (Fig. 148.5). The advances in technology of balloon-expandable and self-expanding stents have widened the population of patients with suitable anatomic lesions that stand to benefit from these procedures. Eligible patients include those with severe or disabling symptoms of claudication and those with limb-threatening ischemia. Clinical outcomes for endovascular revascularization depend on the type and length of the lesions. Treatment of stenoses is more likely to be successful than treatment of total occlusions, and success is influenced by a variety of morphologic characteristics, as delineated in the TASC (TransAtlantic Inter-Society Consensus) Working Group classification for iliac and femoropopliteal lesions.[2] Durability and patency are greatest for iliac artery lesions; the likelihood of long-term patency with endovascular interventions is lower with disease in more distal arteries. Patency rates decrease with increasing lesion length, the presence of diffuse disease or multiple lesions, and poor run-off, as well as other adverse patient characteristics, such as diabetes, active smoking, and renal failure.[1]

For aortoiliac interventions, endovascular treatment affords excellent long-term patency, especially when combined with stenting. Five-year patency rates are approximately 94% and are comparable to rates achieved with surgical intervention. Results are less durable for femoropopliteal PTA with studies showing variable benefit of standard nitinol stents in the femoropopliteal arteries depending on lesion length and other factors.[23b] Compared with bare-metal stents, drug-eluting stents (DES) have shown promise for femoral artery revascularization; a recent study showed improved survival free of major vascular events (death, amputation, or revascularization) with DES.[25] Several trials have demonstrated the benefits of drug-eluting balloon over standard (uncoated) balloon angioplasty for femoropopliteal artery revascularization resulting in reduced rates of restenosis and target vessel revascularization with comparable safety.[23c]

Endovascular treatment of infrapopliteal artery stenosis is typically reserved for patients with limb ischemia. Recent studies have shown that DES use is safe for below-knee limb ischemia and may improve outcomes. For example, in the PARADISE (Preventing Amputations Using Drug Eluting Stents) study, a prospective, nonrandomized study of 106 patients, the 3-year amputation-free survival rate after DES implantation for treatment of limb ischemia involving the infrapopliteal vessels was 68%. In the IN.PACT DEEP study, infrapopliteal artery revascularization with a drug-eluting balloon was noninferior to standard balloon angioplasty with respect to the primary endpoints of target lesion revascularization and late lumen loss.

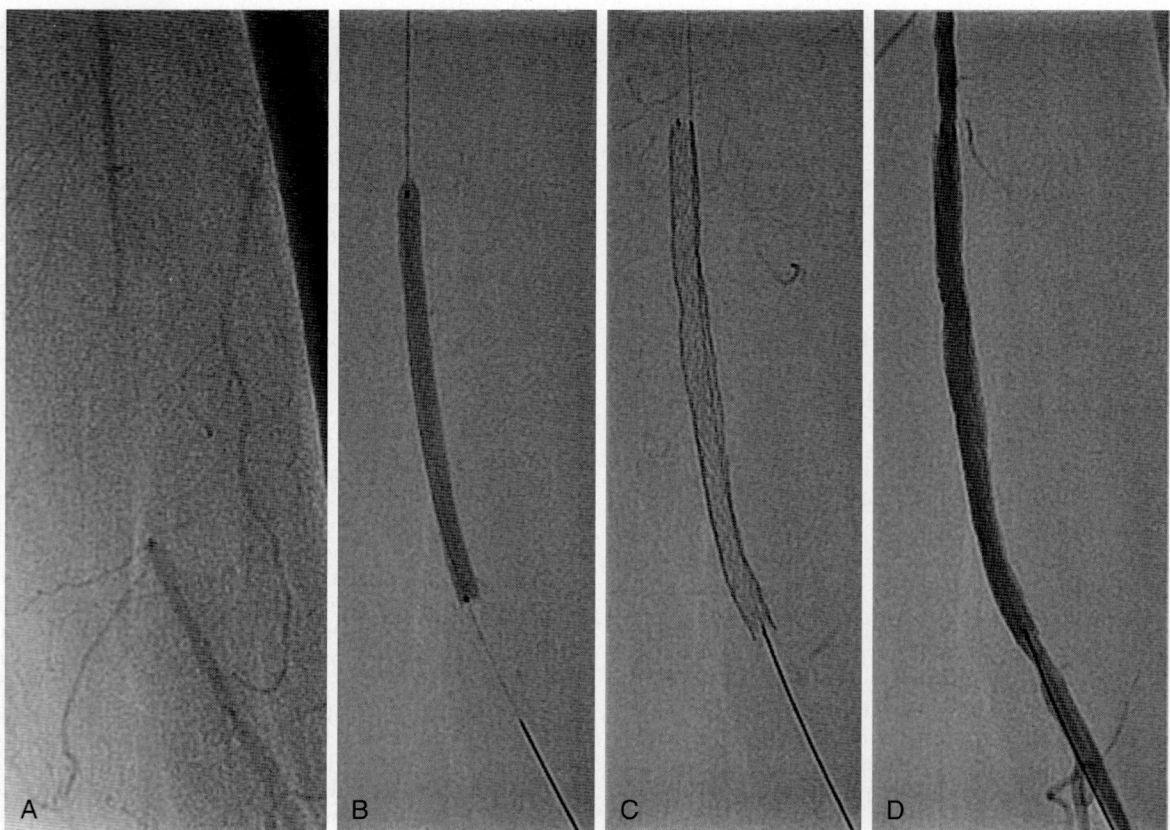

Fig. 148.5 CONVENTIONAL CONTRAST ANGIOGRAPHY ILLUSTRATING USE OF A SELF-EXPANDING NITINOL STENT TREATMENT OF AN OCCLUSION OF THE SUPERFICIAL FEMORAL ARTERY. (A) Occlusion in the mid-superficial femoral artery. (B) Balloon angioplasty. (C) Stent deployment in the lesion. (D) Angiogram after stent deployment *(Reproduced from Thukkani and Kinlay[24].)*

Surgical revascularization remains the gold standard for peripheral revascularization with the choice of operation depending on the location of the stenosis. Options include (1) aortoiliac or aortofemoral reconstruction for proximal disease involving the aorta or iliofemoral vessels, (2) femoral-popliteal bypass (either above- or below-knee popliteal) for superficial femoral artery or popliteal artery disease, and (3) femoral-distal (tibial or peroneal) bypass for distal arterial stenosis. Aortobiiliac or aortobifemoral bypass graft surgery for aortoiliac occlusive disease ("inflow") produces excellent long-term results with 5-year patency rates ranging from 85% to 90%. Surgical treatment of infrainguinal disease ("outflow") also produces durable results, although outcomes depend on the type of bypass conduit used. Vein grafts are the most durable; femoral-popliteal vein bypass grafts have an expected 5-year patency rate of approximately 66%. The 5-year patency rate for prosthetic grafts, such as polytetrafluoroethylene (PTFE), is lower, about 47%.[1] Limitations of surgical interventions include the need for general anesthesia and the attendant risk of cardiovascular events and death associated with major noncardiac surgery in patients with atherosclerosis. Given the potential for coexistent cardiovascular disease, preoperative assessment is important to identify and limit the risk of cardiovascular events in vascular surgery patients.[26]

Whereas revascularization is indicated for most patients with CLI to preserve limb viability, the comparative efficacy and safety of endovascular revascularization and surgical reconstruction for CLI is not known. A contemporary registry has sought to evaluate the comparative safety and effectiveness of surgical and endovascular interventions in patients with symptomatic PAD.[26a] The BEST-CLI Trial (Best Endovascular versus Best Surgical Therapy in Patients with Critical Limb Ischemia) is an ongoing trial that is comparing the relative benefits of surgical versus endovascular treatment in this population.[27]

Therapeutic Angiogenesis

Several clinical trials have explored the utility of angiogenic growth factors for improvement of walking time in patients with claudication or for promotion of healing and preservation of limb viability in patients with CLI. Angiogenic factors investigated have included vascular endothelial growth factor, fibroblast growth factor, hepatocyte growth factor, and hypoxia inducible factor-1α.[28] Despite encouraging results with these agents in animal models of hind-limb ischemia, none of the human studies has demonstrated a benefit of gene therapy. It is not known whether the lack of success is because of the choice of gene, mode of delivery, or other factors.

Early data on infusion of endothelial progenitor cells (EPCs) have been mixed. In experimental models, EPC infusion in hind-limb ischemia models promoted angiogenesis, as indicated by capillary density, and reduced the need for amputation. Preliminary studies in humans suggested that infusion of autologous CD34 cells may reduce amputation rates in patients with CLI. In a pilot study, intramuscular injection of CD34 cells in patients with CLI was also shown to be safe with a nonsignificant trend towards improved amputation-free survival. A meta-analysis of 12 trials showed that while there was an overall benefit of bone marrow–derived cell therapy, these benefits were considerably less and nonsignificant when only placebo-controlled randomized trials were assessed. In fact, more recent data from the placebo-controlled JUVENTAS study found that repetitive infusion of bone marrow mononuclear cells into the common femoral artery did not reduce amputation rates in patients with severe limb ischemia not amenable to revascularization. A recent meta-analysis reviewed the existing literature on cell-based therapies in the treatment of critical limb ischemia and demonstrated improved amputation-free survival and wound healing without significant impact on mortality.[29]

FUTURE DIRECTIONS

A better understanding of the factors that contribute to intermittent claudication and CLI is needed to craft innovative and durable therapeutic interventions for management of the limb complications of PAD. In addition, greater knowledge is needed about the unique contributors to atherogenesis and thrombosis in the lower extremities compared with other arterial beds. Further understanding of downstream effects of compromised blood flow, such as changes in skeletal muscle energetics and impaired neural function, will inform the design and development of novel pharmacotherapies for individuals with PAD. Finally, more comparative efficacy studies are needed to clarify ongoing debates with respect to the relative benefits of exercise training versus invasive therapies; endovascular versus surgical revascularization; and the impact of cell-based therapies in the treatment of PAD. Greater knowledge dissemination regarding PAD diagnosis and risks associated with PAD remain key to early detection and implementation of risk factor modification therapies to improve the care of this high-risk population.

SUGGESTED READINGS

COMPREHENSIVE GUIDELINES FOR THE MANAGEMENT OF PATIENTS WITH ATHEROSCLEROTIC VASCULAR DISEASE, INCLUDING EPIDEMIOLOGY, PATHOPHYSIOLOGY, AND MANAGEMENT OF PERIPHERAL ARTERY DISEASE

Gerhard-Herman MD, Gornik HL, Barrett C, et al: 2016 AHA/ACC guideline on the management of patients with lower extremity peripheral artery disease: executive summary. *J Am Coll Cardiol* 69:1465–1508, 2017.

Hirsch AT, Haskal ZJ, Hertzer NR, et al: ACC/AHA 2005 Practice guidelines for the management of patients with peripheral arterial disease (lower Extremity, renal, mesenteric, and abdominal aortic): a collaborative report from the American Association for Vascular Surgery/Society for Vascular Surgery, Society for Cardiovascular Angiography and Interventions, Society for Vascular Medicine and Biology, Society of Interventional Radiology, and the ACC/AHA Task Force on Practice Guidelines (Writing Committee to Develop Guidelines for the Management of Patients with Peripheral Arterial Disease): endorsed by the American Association of Cardiovascular and Pulmonary Rehabilitation; National Heart, Lung, and Blood Institute; Society for Vascular Nursing; Transatlantic Inter-Society Consensus; and Vascular Disease Foundation. *Circulation* 113:e463, 2006.

Kullo IJ, Rooke TW: Peripheral artery disease. *N Engl J Med* 374:861, 2016.

Norgren L, Hiatt WR, Dormandy JA, et al: Inter-society consensus for the management of peripheral arterial disease (TASC II). *J Vasc Surg* 45:S5, 2007.

Rooke TW, Hirsch AT, Misra S, et al: 2011 ACCF/AHA Focused update of the guideline for the management of patients with peripheral artery disease (updating the 2005 guideline): a report of the American College of Cardiology Foundation/American Heart Association Task Force on Practice Guidelines. *Circulation* 124:2020, 2011.

PREVALENCE, INCIDENCE, AND RISK FACTORS FOR PERIPHERAL ARTERY DISEASE

Criqui M, Aboyans V: Epidemiology of peripheral artery disease. *Circ Res* 116:1509, 2015.

Fowkes FG, Rudan D, Rudan I, et al: Comparison of global estimates of prevalence and risk factors for peripheral artery disease in 2000 and 2010: a systematic review and analysis. *Lancet* 382(9901):1329–1340, 2013.

Pande RL, Perlstein TS, Beckman JA, et al: Secondary prevention and mortality in peripheral artery disease: National Health and Nutrition Examination Study, 1999 to 2004. *Circulation* 124:17, 2011.

PROGNOSIS AND OUTCOMES IN PERIPHERAL ARTERY DISEASE

Cacoub PP, Abola MT, Baumgartner I, et al: Cardiovascular risk factor control and outcomes in peripheral artery disease patients in the Reduction of Atherothrombosis for Continued Health (REACH) registry. *Atherosclerosis* 204:e86, 2009.

Fowkes FG, Murray GD, Butcher I, et al: Ankle brachial index combined with Framingham risk score to predict cardiovascular events and mortality: a meta-analysis. *JAMA* 300:197, 2008.

Kumbhani DJ, Steg PG, Cannon CP, et al: Statin therapy and long-term adverse limb outcomes in patients with peripheral artery disease: insights from the REACH registry. *Eur Heart J* 35(41):2864–2872, 2014.

THERAPY FOR PATIENTS WITH PERIPHERAL ARTERY DISEASE

Belch J, Hiatt WR, Baumgartner I, et al: Effect of fibroblast growth factor Nv1FGF on amputation and death: a randomised placebo-controlled trial of gene therapy in critical limb ischaemia. *Lancet* 377:1929, 2011.

Berger JS, Krantz MJ, Kittelson JM, et al: Aspirin for the prevention of cardiovascular events in patients with peripheral artery disease: a meta-analysis of randomized trials. *JAMA* 301:1909, 2009.

Bhatt DL, Flather MD, Hacke W, et al: Patients with prior myocardial infarction, stroke, or symptomatic peripheral arterial disease in the Charisma trial. *J Am Coll Cardiol* 49:1982, 2007.

Bonaca MP, Bhatt DL, Storey RF, et al: Ticagrelor for prevention of ischemic events after myocardial infarction in patients with peripheral artery disease. *J Am Coll Cardiol* 67:2719, 2016.

Cooke JP, Losordo DW: Modulating the vascular response to limb ischemia. *Circ Res* 116:1561, 2015.

Fakhry F, Spronk S, van der Laan L, et al: Endovascular revascularization and supervised exercise for peripheral artery disease and intermittent claudication: a randomized clinical trial. *JAMA* 314:1936, 2015.

Fowkes FG, Price JF, Stewart MC, et al: Aspirin for prevention of cardiovascular events in a general population screened for a low ankle brachial index: a randomized controlled trial. *JAMA* 303:841, 2010.

Hiatt WR, Fowkes FGR, Heizer G, et al: Ticagrelor versus clopidogrel in symptomatic peripheral artery disease. *N Engl J Med* 376:32, 2017.

Murphy TP, Cutlip DE, Regensteiner JG, et al: Supervised exercise versus primary stenting for claudication resulting from aortoiliac peripheral artery disease: six-month outcomes from the claudication: Exercise Versus Endoluminal Revascularization (CLEVER) study. *Circulation* 125:130, 2011.

Pande RL, Hiatt WR, Zhang P, et al: A pooled analysis of the durability and predictors of treatment response of cilostazol in patients with intermittent claudication. *Vasc Med* 15:181, 2010.

Heart Study Collaboration Group: Randomized trial of the effects of cholesterol-lowering with simvastatin on peripheral vascular and other major vascular outcomes in 20,536 people with peripheral arterial disease and other high-risk conditions. *J Vasc Surg* 45:645, 2007.

Stewart KJ, Hiatt WR, Regensteiner JG, et al: Exercise training for claudication. *N Engl J Med* 347:1941, 2002.

Tepe G, Zeller T, Albrecht T, et al: Local delivery of paclitaxel to inhibit restenosis during angioplasty of the leg. *N Engl J Med* 358:689, 2008.

Yusuf S, Sleight P, Pogue J, et al: Effects of an angiotensin-converting-enzyme inhibitor, ramipril, on cardiovascular events in high-risk patients. The Heart Outcomes Prevention Evaluation study investigators. *N Engl J Med* 342:145, 2000.

Bonaca MP, Scirica BM, Creager MA, et al: Vorapaxar in patients with peripheral artery disease: results from TRA2P-TIMI 50. *Circulation* 127(14):1522–1529, 2013.

REFERENCES

For the complete list of references, log on to www.expertconsult.com.

CHAPTER 149

ANTITHROMBOTIC DRUGS

Iqbal H. Jaffer and Jeffrey I. Weitz

Arterial or venous thromboembolism is a major cause of morbidity and mortality. Arterial thrombosis is the most common cause of acute myocardial infarction, ischemic stroke, and limb gangrene, whereas deep vein thrombosis can lead to pulmonary embolism, which can be fatal, and to the postthrombotic syndrome. Most arterial thrombi are superimposed on disrupted atherosclerotic plaque because plaque rupture exposes thrombogenic material in the plaque core to the blood.[1] This material then triggers platelet aggregation and fibrin formation, which results in the generation of a platelet-rich thrombus that can temporarily or permanently occlude blood flow. In contrast to arterial thrombi, venous thrombi rarely form at sites of obvious vascular disruption.[1] Although they can develop after surgical trauma to veins or secondary to indwelling central venous catheters, venous thrombi usually originate in the valve cusps of the deep veins of the calf or in the muscular sinuses, where they are triggered by stasis. Sluggish blood flow in these veins reduces the oxygen supply to the avascular valve cusps. Endothelial cells lining the valve cusps become activated and express adhesion molecules on their surface. These adhesion molecules tether tissue factor–bearing leukocytes and microparticles to the surface of activated endothelial cells, where the tissue factor triggers coagulation. Local thrombus formation is exacerbated by reduced clearance of activated clotting factors as a result of impaired blood flow. If the calf vein thrombi extend into more proximal veins of the leg, thrombus fragments can dislodge, travel to the lungs, and produce a pulmonary embolism.

Arterial and venous thrombi are composed of platelets and fibrin, but the proportions differ. Arterial thrombi are rich in platelets because of the high shear in the injured arteries. In contrast, venous thrombi, which form under low-shear conditions, contain relatively few platelets and are composed predominantly of fibrin and trapped red cells. Because of the predominance of platelets, arterial thrombi appear white, whereas venous thrombi are red in color, reflecting the trapped red cells.

Antithrombotic drugs are used for prevention and treatment of thrombosis. Targeting the components of thrombi, these agents include (1) antiplatelet drugs, which inhibit platelets; (2) anticoagulants, which attenuate coagulation; and (3) fibrinolytic agents, which induce fibrin degradation (Fig. 149.1). With the predominance of platelets in arterial thrombi, strategies to inhibit or treat arterial thrombosis are focused mainly on antiplatelet agents, although in the acute setting they often include anticoagulants and fibrinolytic agents. Anticoagulants are the mainstay of prevention and treatment of venous thromboembolism because fibrin is the predominant component of venous thrombi. Antiplatelet drugs are less effective than anticoagulants in this setting because of the limited platelet content of venous thrombi. Fibrinolytic therapy is used in selected patients with venous thromboembolism. For example, patients with massive pulmonary embolism can benefit from systemic or catheter-directed fibrinolytic therapy. Catheter-directed fibrinolytic therapy also can be used as an adjunct to anticoagulants for treatment of certain patients with extensive deep vein thrombosis involving the iliac and femoral veins.

This chapter is focused on antithrombotic agents. In addition to describing antiplatelet, anticoagulant, and fibrinolytic drugs that are in current use, new agents in advanced stages of development also are discussed.

ANTIPLATELET DRUGS

Role of Platelets in Arterial Thrombosis

In healthy vasculature, circulating platelets are maintained in an inactive state by nitric oxide (NO) and prostacyclin released by endothelial cells lining the blood vessels. In addition, endothelial cells also express ADPase on their surface, which degrades ADP released from activated platelets. When the vessel wall is damaged, release of these substances is impaired and the subendothelial matrix is exposed. Platelets adhere to exposed collagen and to von Willebrand factor via glycoprotein (GP) VI and GPIb–IX, respectively; receptors are constitutively expressed on the platelet surface. Adherent platelets undergo a change in shape, secrete ADP from their dense granules, and synthesize and release thromboxane A_2. Released ADP and thromboxane A_2, which are platelet agonists, activate ambient platelets and recruit them to the site of vascular injury.

Disruption of the vessel wall also exposes tissue factor–expressing cells to the blood. Tissue factor initiates coagulation. Activated platelets potentiate coagulation by binding clotting factors and supporting the assembly of activation complexes that enhance thrombin generation. In addition to converting fibrinogen to fibrin, thrombin amplifies its own generation and serves as a potent platelet agonist, thereby recruiting additional platelets to the site of injury.

When platelets are activated, GPIIb/IIIa ($\alpha_{IIb}\beta_3$), the most abundant receptor on the platelet surface, undergoes a conformational change that enables it to ligate fibrinogen. Divalent fibrinogen molecules bridge adjacent platelets together to form platelet aggregates. Fibrin strands, generated through the action of thrombin, then weave these aggregates together to form a platelet–fibrin mesh.

Antiplatelet drugs target various steps in this process (Fig. 149.2). The commonly used drugs include aspirin, thienopyridines (clopidogrel and prasugrel), ticagrelor, cangrelor, dipyridamole, GPIIb/IIIa antagonists, and vorapaxar. Each is briefly described in the following.

Aspirin

The most widely used antiplatelet agent is aspirin. As a cheap and effective antiplatelet drug, aspirin serves as the foundation of most antiplatelet strategies.

Mechanism of Action

Aspirin produces its antithrombotic effect by irreversibly acetylating and inhibiting platelet cyclooxygenase-1 (COX-1), a critical enzyme in the biosynthesis of thromboxane A_2 (see Fig. 149.2). At high doses (about 1 g/day), aspirin also inhibits COX-2, an inducible COX isoform found in endothelial cells and inflammatory cells. In

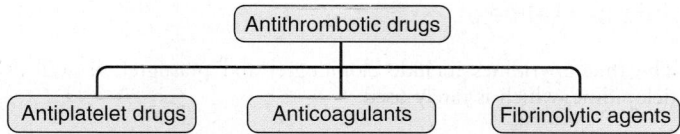

Fig. 149.1 CLASSIFICATION OF ANTITHROMBOTIC DRUGS.

endothelial cells, COX-2 initiates the synthesis of prostacyclin, a potent vasodilator and inhibitor of platelet aggregation.

Indications

Aspirin is widely used for secondary prevention of cardiovascular events in patients with coronary artery disease, cerebrovascular disease, or peripheral vascular disease. Compared with placebo, aspirin produces about a 25% reduction in the risk of cardiovascular

FIGURE 151-2

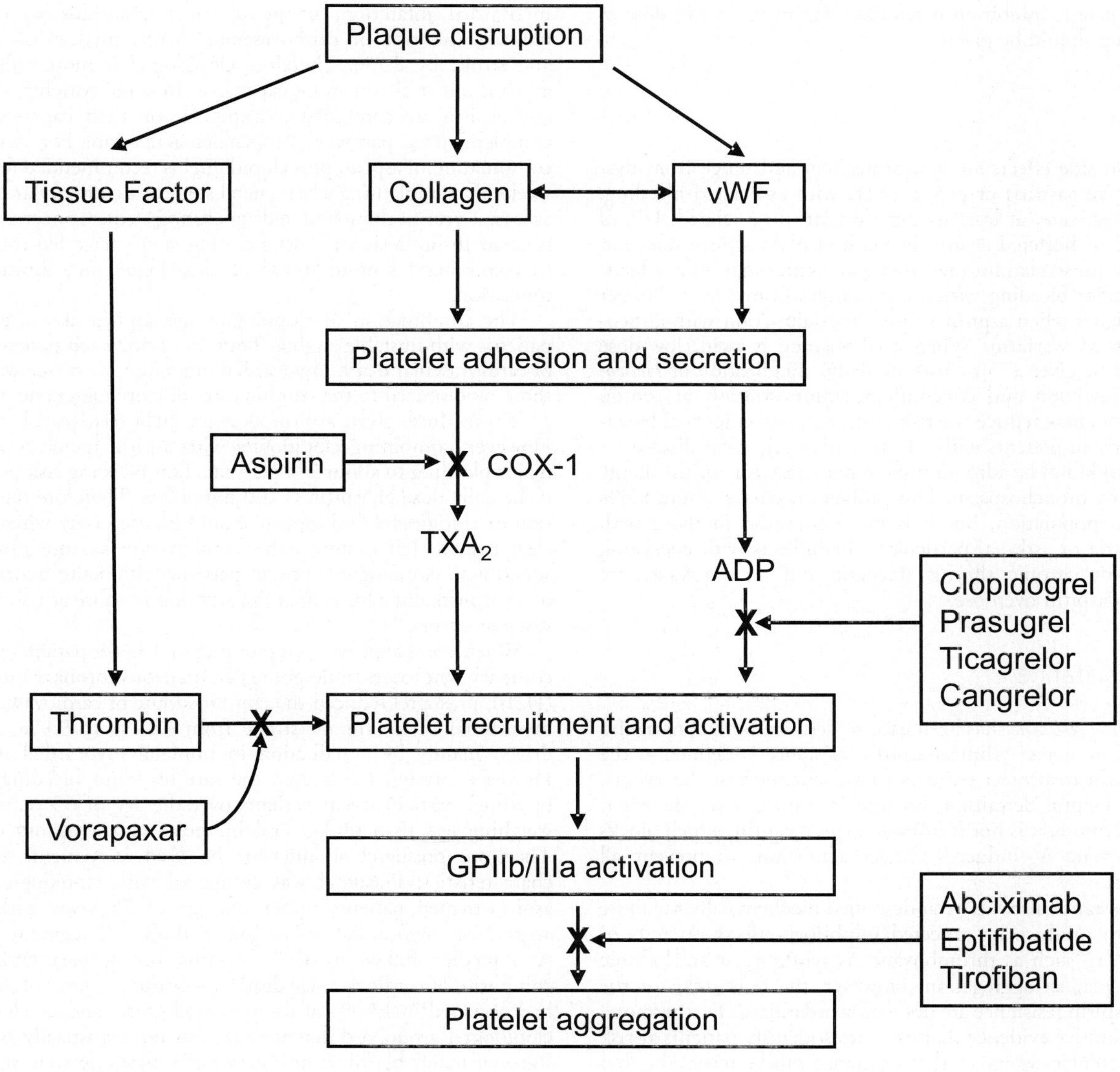

Fig. 149.2 SITE OF ACTION OF ANTIPLATELET DRUGS. Aspirin inhibits thromboxane A_2 (TXA$_2$) synthesis by irreversibly acetylating cyclooxygenase-1 (COX-1). Reduced TXA$_2$ release attenuates platelet activation and recruitment to the site of vascular injury. Clopidogrel, prasugrel, ticagrelor, and cangrelor block P2Y$_{12}$, a key adenosine diphosphate (ADP) receptor on the platelet surface. Therefore these agents also attenuate platelet recruitment. Vorapaxar inhibits type 1 protease-activated receptor (PAR-1), the major thrombin receptor on platelets. Abciximab, eptifibatide, and tirofiban inhibit the final common pathway of platelet aggregation by blocking fibrinogen binding to activated glycoprotein (GP) IIb/IIIa. *vWF,* von Willebrand factor.

death, myocardial infarction, or stroke in these patients. There is mounting evidence that aspirin is of limited benefit for primary prevention in subjects without clinical evidence of cardiovascular disease.[2] Although metaanalyses demonstrate a reduction in nonfatal myocardial infarction with daily aspirin use, this benefit is partially offset by an increase in gastrointestinal bleeding. Nonetheless, there also is evidence that aspirin reduces cancer mortality. If used for primary prevention, aspirin should be restricted to those at moderate to high risk of cardiovascular events.[2]

Dosages

Aspirin is usually administered at doses of 75 to 325 mg once daily. There is no evidence that higher-dose aspirin is more effective than lower aspirin doses, and some analyses suggest reduced efficacy with higher doses. Because the side effects of aspirin are dose-related, daily aspirin doses of 75 to 150 mg are recommended for most indications. When rapid platelet inhibition is required, an initial aspirin dose of at least 160 mg should be given.

Side Effects

Most common side effects are gastrointestinal and range from dyspepsia to erosive gastritis or peptic ulcers with associated bleeding. These side effects are, at least to some extent, dose related. Use of enteric-coated or buffered aspirin in place of plain aspirin does not eliminate the prostaglandin-mediated gastrointestinal side effects. The risk of major bleeding with aspirin ranges from 1% to 3% per year and is higher when aspirin is used in conjunction with anticoagulants, such as warfarin. When dual therapy is used, low-dose aspirin should be given (75 to 100 mg daily). Eradication of *Helicobacter pylori* infection and concomitant administration of proton pump inhibitors may reduce the risk of upper gastrointestinal bleeding, particularly in patients with a history of peptic ulcer disease.

Aspirin should not be administered to patients with aspirin allergy characterized by bronchospasm. This problem occurs in about 0.3% of the general population, but it is more common in those with chronic urticaria or asthma, particularly in subjects with coexisting nasal polyps or chronic rhinitis. Hepatic and renal toxicity are observed with aspirin overdose.

Aspirin Resistance

The term *aspirin resistance* has been used to describe both clinical and laboratory phenomena.[3] Clinical aspirin resistance is defined as the failure of aspirin to protect patients from ischemic vascular events. This is not a helpful definition, because it is made after the event occurs. Furthermore, it is not realistic to expect aspirin, which blocks only thromboxane A_2–induced platelet activation, to prevent all vascular events.

Aspirin resistance also has been described biochemically as failure of the drug to produce its expected inhibitory effects on tests of platelet function, such as thromboxane A_2 synthesis or arachidonic acid–induced platelet aggregation. However, the tests used for the diagnosis of aspirin resistance are not well standardized. Furthermore, there is no definitive evidence that these tests identify patients at risk of recurrent vascular events, or that resistance can be reversed either by giving higher doses of aspirin or by adding other antiplatelet drugs. Until such information is available, testing for aspirin resistance remains a research tool.

ADP Receptor Antagonists

$P2Y_{12}$ is the major ADP receptor on platelets. Agents that inhibit $P2Y_{12}$ include oral agents such as the thienopyridines as well as ticagrelor, and cangrelor, which is a parenteral inhibitor.

Thienopyridines

The thienopyridines include clopidogrel and prasugrel, as well as ticlopidine, which is rarely used.

Mechanism of Action

The thienopyridines are structurally related drugs that selectively inhibit ADP-induced platelet aggregation by irreversibly blocking $P2Y_{12}$ (see Fig. 149.2). Clopidogrel and prasugrel are prodrugs that must be metabolized by the hepatic cytochrome P450 (CYP) enzyme system to acquire activity. Consequently, their onset of action is delayed unless loading doses are given. The metabolic activation of prasugrel is more efficient than that of clopidogrel. Consequently, prasugrel produces more rapid, higher, and more uniform $P2Y_{12}$ blockade than clopidogrel.

Indications

When compared with aspirin in patients with recent ischemic stroke, myocardial infarction, or peripheral arterial disease, clopidogrel reduced the risk of cardiovascular death, myocardial infarction, and stroke by 8.7%. Therefore clopidogrel is more effective than aspirin, but it also is more expensive. In some patients, clopidogrel and aspirin are combined to capitalize on their capacity to block complementary pathways of platelet activation. For example, the combination of aspirin plus clopidogrel is recommended for at least 4 weeks after implanting a bare metal stent in a coronary artery and for at least 1 year in those with a drug-eluting stent. Concerns about late in-stent thrombosis with drug-eluting stents have led some experts to recommend long-term use of clopidogrel plus aspirin for this indication.

The combination of clopidogrel and aspirin also is effective in patients with unstable angina. Thus in 12,562 such patients, the risk of cardiovascular death, myocardial infarction, or stroke was 9.3% in those randomized to the combination of clopidogrel and aspirin and 11.4% in those given aspirin alone, a 20% relative risk reduction.[4] However, combining clopidogrel with aspirin increases the risk of major bleeding to about 2% per year. This bleeding risk persists even if the daily dose of aspirin is 100 mg or less. Therefore the combination of clopidogrel and aspirin should be used only when there is a clear benefit. For example, this combination has not proven to be superior to clopidogrel alone in patients with acute ischemic stroke or to aspirin alone for primary prevention in those at risk for cardiovascular events.

When compared with clopidogrel in 13,608 patients with acute coronary syndromes undergoing percutaneous coronary interventions (PCIs), prasugrel reduced the combined rate of cardiovascular death, myocardial infarction, or stroke from 12.1% to 9.9%, a decrease driven mainly by a reduction in nonfatal myocardial infarction.[5] However, prasugrel increased the rate of major bleeding and fatal bleeding, particularly in patients over the age of 65 years, in those weighing less than 60 kg, and in those with a history of stroke.[5] Therefore prasugrel should not be used in patients with these characteristics. Prasugrel was compared with clopidogrel in 7243 aspirin-treated patients under the age of 75 years with unstable angina or myocardial infarction without ST-segment elevation. At a median follow-up of 17 months, the primary endpoint, the composite of cardiovascular death, myocardial infarction, and stroke had occurred in 13.9% of the prasugrel group and in 16.0% of the clopidogrel group, a difference that was not statistically significant.[6] Rates of major bleeding and intracranial bleeding were similar with the two treatment regimens. Therefore prasugrel has no advantage over clopidogrel in medically managed patients with acute coronary syndrome.

Dosing

Clopidogrel is given once daily at a dose of 75 mg. Because its onset of action is delayed for several days, loading doses of clopidogrel are given when rapid ADP receptor blockade is desired. For example, patients undergoing coronary artery stenting are often given a loading dose of 600 mg, which produces inhibition of ADP-induced platelet aggregation within 6 hours. Prasugrel is given as a loading dose of 60 mg followed by 10 mg once daily. Partial inhibition of ADP-induced platelet aggregation is evident within 1 hour of prasugrel administration.

Side Effects

Gastrointestinal and hematologic side effects, other than bleeding, are rare with clopidogrel and prasugrel.

Clopidogrel Resistance

There is considerable between patient variability in the capacity of clopidogrel to inhibit ADP-induced platelet aggregation.[7] Nonresponsiveness to clopidogrel is termed *clopidogrel resistance*, and platelets from patients with this phenomenon exhibit high reactivity to ADP. Reduced responsiveness to clopidogrel reflects, at least in part, genetic polymorphisms in CYP2C19, which is critical for metabolic activation of clopidogrel in the liver. Thus loss-of-function *CYP2C19*2* and *CYP2C19*3* alleles are found in 2% of white individuals, 4% of black individuals, and 14% of Asian individuals, and the levels of the active metabolite of clopidogrel are reported to be up to 33% lower in carriers of either of these alleles than in those with healthy alleles. Patients with clopidogrel resistance are reported to have a higher risk of ischemic complications after PCI, including myocardial infarction and stent thrombosis. On the basis of these findings, some experts recommend pharmacogenetic testing and point-of-care assessment of platelet reactivity to predict or assess clopidogrel responsiveness. However, attempts to manage such patients with higher doses of clopidogrel or with additional antiplatelet drugs have not resulted in improved outcomes. Instead, patients with clopidogrel resistance may benefit from a switch to prasugrel, which produces more uniform inhibition of ADP-induced platelet aggregation, or to ticagrelor.

Ticagrelor

An orally active agent belonging to the cyclopentyl-triazolopyrimidine class, ticagrelor acts as a direct inhibitor of P2Y$_{12}$.

Mechanism of Action

Ticagrelor reversibly binds to P2Y$_{12}$ at a location distinct from the ADP binding site and blocks ADP-mediated receptor activation in a noncompetitive fashion, likely through an allosteric mechanism. Because it does not require metabolic activation, ticagrelor has a more rapid onset of action than clopidogrel or prasugrel.

Indications

When compared with clopidogrel in 18,624 patients with acute coronary syndromes, ticagrelor reduced the rate of cardiovascular death, myocardial infarction, or stroke from 11.7% to 9.8%.[8] All-cause mortality was also reduced with ticagrelor compared with clopidogrel (4.5% and 5.9%, respectively; $p < .001$), but ticagrelor produced more major bleeding not related to bypass surgery (2.8% and 2.2%, respectively).[8] An invasive strategy was planned for 72% of the patients entered in the trial. In this subset, the primary composite endpoint occurred in 9.0% of patients randomized to ticagrelor and in 10.7% of those given clopidogrel, a 16% relative risk reduction.[9] Rates of major bleeding were similar with ticagrelor and clopidogrel (11.6% and 16.5%, respectively; $p = .88$). Therefore ticagrelor also was superior to clopidogrel in patients undergoing coronary interventions.

If cost is not an issue and patients are compliant with twice-daily dosing, ticagrelor is a reasonable alternative to clopidogrel in patients with acute coronary syndrome, regardless of whether they are managed medically or undergo PCI with stent implantation. For these indications, ticagrelor should be given for at least 1 year. It also is reasonable to use ticagrelor in place of clopidogrel in patients with clopidogrel resistance or in those who develop in-stent thrombosis despite clopidogrel therapy.

Dosing

Ticagrelor is given as a 180-mg oral loading dose followed by 90 mg twice daily. Although the trial comparing ticagrelor with clopidogrel was not powered to compare outcomes in different geographical regions, patients enrolled in North America did not have the same benefit as those from other countries. On the basis of post hoc analysis, the only baseline covariate associated with this difference was the higher dose of aspirin used in the United States.[10] Consequently, it is recommended that when ticagrelor is combined with aspirin, the daily aspirin dose should be less than 100 mg.

Side Effects

Ticagrelor produces dyspnea, which is usually mild and dose related, asymptomatic bradycardia with ventricular pauses, and a modest increase in the levels of uric acid. The mechanisms responsible for these side effects are unclear. One possible explanation relates to the capacity of ticagrelor to inhibit adenosine reuptake by erythrocytes, thereby increasing circulating levels of adenosine. In addition to explaining the dyspnea and the bradycardia, the resultant adenosine-induced vasodilation and increased myocardial perfusion could also endow ticagrelor with beneficial effects that are independent of P2Y$_{12}$ blockade.

Cangrelor

Cangrelor is the only available parenteral inhibitor of P2Y$_{12}$.

Mechanism of Action

Cangrelor is a rapidly acting reversible inhibitor of P2Y$_{12}$. It has an immediate onset of action after intravenous administration, a half-life of 3 to 5 minutes, and an offset of action within 1 hour.

Indications

Cangrelor is licensed for use in patients undergoing PCI, in whom it produces rapid ADP receptor blockade in those who have not received pretreatment with clopidogrel, prasugrel, or ticagrelor and are not receiving a GPIIb/IIIa inhibitor.

Dosing

Cangrelor is administered as a 30 µg/kg intravenous bolus before PCI followed by an infusion of 4 µg/kg/min for at least 2 hours or for the duration of PCI, whichever is longer. When transitioning to oral P2Y$_{12}$ inhibitor therapy, ticagrelor can be given at a loading dose of 180 mg at any time during the cangrelor infusion or immediately after discontinuation. In contrast, loading doses of prasugrel or clopidogrel (60 and 600 mg, respectively) should be given only after cangrelor is stopped, because cangrelor blocks the interaction of their active metabolites with P2Y$_{12}$.

Side Effects

The major side effect of cangrelor is bleeding.

Dipyridamole

Dipyridamole is a relatively weak antiplatelet agent on its own. An extended-release formulation of dipyridamole combined with low-dose aspirin, a preparation known as Aggrenox, is used for prevention of stroke in patients with transient ischemic attacks.

Mechanism of Action

By inhibiting phosphodiesterase, dipyridamole blocks the breakdown of cyclic AMP (cAMP). Increased levels of cAMP reduce intracellular calcium and inhibit platelet activation. Dipyridamole also blocks the uptake of adenosine by platelets and other cells. This produces a further increase in local cAMP levels because the platelet adenosine A$_2$ receptor is coupled to adenylate cyclase (Fig. 149.3).

Indications

Dipyridamole plus aspirin was compared with aspirin or dipyridamole alone, or with placebo, in patients with an ischemic stroke or transient ischemic attack. The combination reduced the risk of stroke by 22.1% compared with aspirin alone and by 24.4% compared with dipyridamole alone. In a second trial, researchers compared dipyridamole plus aspirin with aspirin alone for secondary prevention in patients with ischemic stroke. Vascular death, stroke, or myocardial infarction occurred in 13% of patients given combination therapy and in 16% of those treated with aspirin alone. When Aggrenox was compared with clopidogrel, however, there was no difference in efficacy, and there was more intracranial bleeding with Aggrenox.[11] Although Aggrenox is used for stroke prevention, because of its vasodilatory effects and the paucity of data supporting the use of dipyridamole in patients with symptomatic coronary artery disease, Aggrenox should not be used for stroke prevention in such patients.

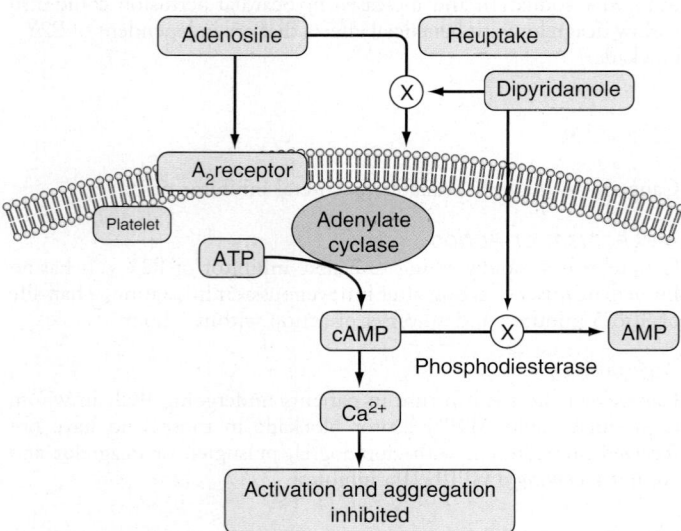

Fig. 149.3 MECHANISM OF ACTION OF DIPYRIDAMOLE. Dipyridamole increases levels of cyclic adenosine monophosphate (cAMP) in platelets by (A) blocking the reuptake of adenosine and (B) inhibiting phosphodiesterase-mediated cAMP degradation. By promoting calcium uptake, cAMP reduces intracellular levels of calcium. This, in turn, inhibits platelet activation and aggregation. *AMP,* Adenosine monophosphate; *ATP,* adenosine triphosphate.

Dosing

Aggrenox is given twice daily. Each capsule contains 200 mg of extended-release dipyridamole and 25 mg of aspirin.

Side Effects

Because dipyridamole has vasodilatory effects, it must be used with caution in patients with coronary artery disease. Gastrointestinal complaints, headache, facial flushing, dizziness, and hypotension also can occur. These symptoms often subside with continued use of the drug.

GPIIb/IIIa Receptor Antagonists

As a class, parenteral GPIIb/IIIa receptor antagonists have an established niche in patients with acute coronary syndromes. The three agents in this class are abciximab, eptifibatide, and tirofiban.

Mechanism of Action

A member of the integrin family of adhesion receptors, GPIIb/IIIa is found on the surface of platelets and megakaryocytes. With about 40,000 to 80,000 copies per platelet, GPIIb/IIIa is the most abundant receptor. Consisting of a noncovalently linked heterodimer, GPIIb/IIIa is inactive on resting platelets. When platelets are activated, inside–outside signal transduction pathways trigger a conformational activation of the receptor. Once activated, GPIIb/IIIa binds adhesive molecules, such as fibrinogen and, under high shear conditions, von Willebrand factor. Binding is mediated by Arg-Gly-Asp (RGD) sequences found on the fibrinogen and von Willebrand factor, as well as by the Lys-Gly-Asp (KGD) sequence located within a unique dodecapeptide domain on the γ-chains of fibrinogen. Once bound, fibrinogen and/or von Willebrand factor bridge adjacent platelets together to induce platelet aggregation.

Although abciximab, eptifibatide, and tirofiban all target the GPIIb/IIIa receptor, they are structurally and pharmacologically distinct (Table 149.1). Abciximab is a Fab fragment of a humanized murine monoclonal antibody directed against the activated form of GPIIb/IIIa. Abciximab binds to the activated receptor with high affinity and blocks the binding of adhesive molecules. In contrast to abciximab, eptifibatide and tirofiban are synthetic small molecules. Eptifibatide is a cyclic heptapeptide that binds GPIIb/IIIa because it incorporates the KGD motif, whereas tirofiban is

TABLE 149.1	**Features of GPIIb/IIIa Antagonists**		
Feature		**GPIIb/IIIa Antagonists**	
Generic name	Abciximab	Eptifibatide	Tirofiban
Trade name	ReoPro	Integrilin	Aggrastat
Description	Fab fragment of humanized mouse monoclonal antibody	Cyclical KGD-containing heptapeptide	Nonpeptidic RGD mimetic
Specific for GPIIb/IIIa	No	Yes	Yes
Plasma half-life	Short (min)	Long (2.5 h)	Long (2.0 h)
Platelet-bound half-life	Long (days)	Short	Short
Renal clearance	No	Yes	Yes
Dosing	0.25 mg/kg bolus followed by a 12-h infusion of 10 µg/min	Two 180 µg/kg boluses given 10 min apart	25 µg/kg boluses followed by an 18-h infusion of 0.15 µg/kg/min
Adjustment for renal impairment	No	Yes	Yes

KGD, Lys-Gly-Asp; RGD, Arg-Gly-Asp.

a nonpeptidic tyrosine derivative that acts as an RGD mimetic. Abciximab has a long half-life and can be detected on the surface of platelets for up to 2 weeks. Eptifibatide and tirofiban have shorter half-lives.

In addition to targeting the GPIIb/IIIa receptor, abciximab also inhibits the closely related $\alpha_v\beta_3$ receptor, which binds vitronectin, and $\alpha_M\beta_2$, a leukocyte integrin. In contrast, eptifibatide and tirofiban are specific for GPIIb/IIIa. Inhibition of $\alpha_v\beta_3$ and $\alpha_M\beta_2$ may endow abciximab with antiinflammatory and/or antiproliferative properties that extend beyond platelet inhibition.

Indications

These agents are used in high-risk patients undergoing PCIs, particularly those with ST-segment elevation acute myocardial infarction who have not been adequately pretreated with antiplatelet drugs or in those requiring rapid platelet inhibition. Tirofiban and eptifibatide are occasionally used upstream for intervention in high-risk patients with unstable angina.

Dosing

All of the GPIIb/IIIa antagonists are given as an intravenous bolus followed by an infusion. Because they are cleared by the kidneys, the doses of eptifibatide and tirofiban must be reduced in patients with renal impairment.

Side Effects

In addition to bleeding, thrombocytopenia is the most serious complication. Thrombocytopenia is immune mediated and is caused by antibodies directed against neoantigens on GPIIb/IIIa that are exposed upon antagonist binding. With abciximab, thrombocytopenia occurs in up to 5% of patients. Thrombocytopenia is severe in about 1% of these individuals. Thrombocytopenia is less common with the other two agents, occurring in about 1% of treated patients.

Vorapaxar

An orally active inhibitor of the type 1 protease-activated receptor (PAR-1), vorapaxar inhibits the major thrombin receptor on platelets.[12–14]

Mechanism of Action

Thrombin is a potent platelet activator that acts through the PARs.[14] PAR-1 is the highest-affinity thrombin receptor on platelets; PAR-1 also is expressed on endothelial cells and atherosclerotic plaques.[15] Vorapaxar is a synthetic analogue of himbacine, which is a natural product. Given orally, vorapaxar is rapidly absorbed form the gastrointestinal tract and inhibits platelet PAR-1 in a reversible fashion; however, because of its long half-life (8 to 12 days) and its high-affinity interaction with PAR-1, vorapaxar is effectively an irreversible inhibitor of PAR-1.

Indications

Vorapaxar is indicated for reduction of thrombotic cardiovascular events in patients with a history of myocardial infarction or peripheral artery disease. The drug is administered in conjunction with aspirin and/or clopidogrel. Vorapaxar is contraindicated in patients with a prior history of intracranial bleeding, stroke, or transient ischemic attack.

Dosing

Vorapaxar is given orally at a dose of 2.5 mg once daily.

Side Effects

The major side effect is bleeding, including intracranial and fatal bleeding.

ANTICOAGULANTS

There are both parenteral and oral anticoagulants. Currently available parenteral anticoagulants include heparin, low-molecular-weight heparin (LMWH), fondaparinux, and direct thrombin inhibitors (hirudin, bivalirudin, and argatroban). The oral anticoagulants include the vitamin K antagonists, of which warfarin is the agent most often used in North America, and the non–vitamin K antagonist oral anticoagulants (NOACs) that target either thrombin (dabigatran etexilate) or factor Xa (rivaroxaban, apixaban, and edoxaban).[14]

Parenteral Anticoagulants

Heparin

A sulfated polysaccharide, heparin is isolated from mammalian tissues rich in mast cells. Most commercial heparin is derived from porcine intestinal mucosa and is a polymer of alternating D-glucuronic acid and N-acetyl-D-glucosamine residues.

Mechanism of Action

Heparin acts as an anticoagulant by activating antithrombin (previously known as *antithrombin III*) and accelerating the rate at which antithrombin inhibits clotting enzymes, particularly thrombin and factor Xa. Antithrombin, the obligatory plasma cofactor for heparin, is a 58,000-Da single-chain polypeptide that is a member of the serine protease inhibitor (serpin) superfamily. Synthesized in the liver and circulating in plasma at a concentration of 2.6 ± 0.4 µM, antithrombin acts as a suicide substrate for its target enzymes.

To activate antithrombin, heparin binds to the serpin via a unique pentasaccharide sequence that is found on one-third of the chains of commercial heparin (Fig. 149.4); heparin chains lacking this pentasaccharide sequence have little or no anticoagulant activity. Once bound to antithrombin, heparin induces a conformational change in the reactive center loop of antithrombin that renders it more readily accessible to its target proteases. This conformational change enhances the rate at which antithrombin inhibits factor Xa by at least two orders of magnitude, but it has little effect on the rate of thrombin inhibition by antithrombin (Fig. 149.5). To catalyze thrombin inhibition, heparin serves as a template that binds antithrombin and thrombin simultaneously. Formation of this ternary complex brings the enzyme in close apposition to the inhibitor, thereby promoting the formation of a stable covalent thrombin–antithrombin complex.

Only pentasaccharide-containing heparin chains composed of at least 18 saccharide units (which correspond to a molecular weight of 5400) are of sufficient length to bridge thrombin and antithrombin together. With a mean molecular weight of 15,000 and a range of 5000 to 30,000, almost all of the chains of unfractionated heparin are long enough to affect this bridging function. Consequently, by definition, heparin has equal capacity to promote the inhibition of thrombin and factor Xa by antithrombin and is assigned an anti-factor Xa to anti-factor IIa (thrombin) ratio of 1:1.

In addition to activating antithrombin, heparin also can catalyze heparin cofactor II. This 66,000-Da serpin, which is found in plasma at a concentration of 1.2 ± 0.4 µM, is a specific inhibitor of thrombin. Two features account for the specificity of heparin cofactor II. First, the reactive site of heparin cofactor II contains the sequence Leu444–Ser445, a peptide bond that is not readily susceptible to

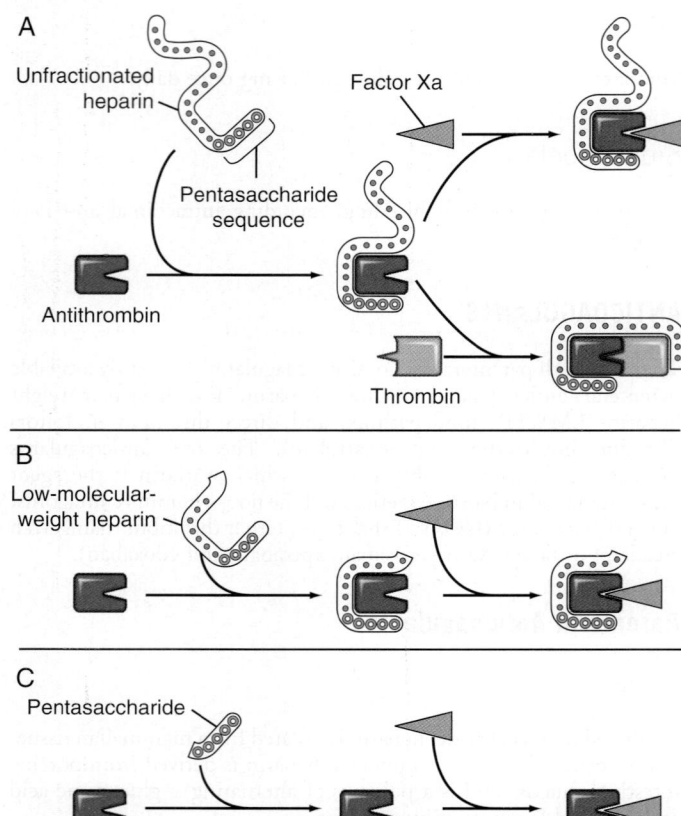

Fig. 149.4 MECHANISM OF ACTION OF HEPARIN, LOW-MOLECULAR-WEIGHT HEPARIN, AND FONDAPARINUX, A SYNTHETIC PENTASACCHARIDE. (A) Heparin binds to antithrombin via its pentasaccharide sequence. This induces a conformational change in the reactive center loop of antithrombin that accelerates its interaction with factor Xa. To potentiate thrombin inhibition, heparin must simultaneously bind to antithrombin and thrombin. Only heparin chains composed of at least 18 saccharide units, which correspond to a molecular weight of 5400, are of sufficient length to perform this bridging function. With a mean molecular weight of 15,000, all of the heparin chains are long enough to do this. (B) Low-molecular-weight heparin (LMWH) has greater capacity to potentiate factor Xa inhibition by antithrombin than thrombin does because, with a mean molecular weight of 4500 to 5000, at least half of the LMWH chains are too short to bridge antithrombin to thrombin. (C) The pentasaccharide accelerates only factor Xa inhibition by antithrombin because the pentasaccharide is too short to bridge antithrombin to thrombin.

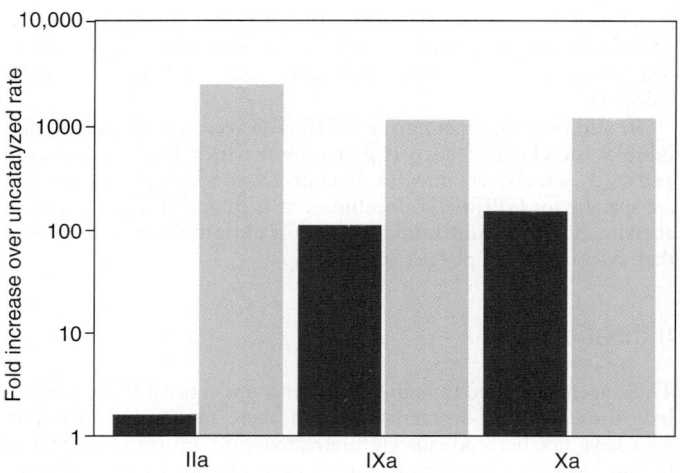

Fig. 149.5 COMPARISON OF THE STIMULATORY EFFECTS OF PENTASACCHARIDE AND UNFRACTIONATED HEPARIN ON CATALYSIS OF ANTITHROMBIN-MEDIATED INHIBITION OF THROMBIN (IIa), FACTOR IXa (IXa), AND FACTOR Xa (Xa). Second-order rate constants of inhibition of factor IIa, IXa, or Xa by antithrombin, measured in the presence of heparin *(green bars)* or fondaparinux *(pink bars)* were divided by those determined in the absence of glycosaminoglycan and are plotted as fold increases over the uncatalyzed rate of inhibition. *(Reprinted with permission from Wiebe et al: J Biol Chem 228:35767, 2003.)*

The interaction of heparin with heparin cofactor II is not mediated by the antithrombin-binding pentasaccharide sequence. Because heparin lacks a specific heparin cofactor II binding domain, heparin's affinity for heparin cofactor II is lower than that for antithrombin. Consequently, 10-fold higher heparin concentrations are needed to accelerate thrombin inhibition by heparin cofactor II in plasma than are necessary to enhance thrombin's inactivation by antithrombin. Therefore it is likely that heparin cofactor II contributes to the anticoagulant activity of heparin only when the drug is given in high doses.

Heparin causes the release of tissue factor pathway inhibitor (TFPI) from the endothelium. A factor Xa–dependent inhibitor of tissue factor–bound factor VIIa, TFPI may contribute to the antithrombotic activity of heparin. Longer heparin chains induce the release of more TFPI than shorter chains.

Pharmacology

Heparin must be given parenterally. It is usually administered subcutaneously or by continuous intravenous infusion. When used for therapeutic purposes, the intravenous route is most often employed. If heparin is given subcutaneously for treatment of thrombosis, the dose of heparin must be high enough to overcome the limited bioavailability associated with this method of delivery.

After entering the circulation, heparin binds to a variety of plasma proteins other than antithrombin, which decreases the anticoagulant activity of heparin. The levels of heparin-binding proteins vary between patients because some of these proteins are acute-phase reactants whose levels are elevated in ill patients, whereas others, such as high-molecular-weight multimers of von Willebrand factor, are released when platelets or endothelial cells are activated by thrombin. Activated platelets also release platelet factor 4 (PF4), a highly cationic protein that binds heparin with high affinity. The large amount of PF4 found in the vicinity of platelet-rich arterial thrombi has the potential to locally neutralize the anticoagulant activity of heparin.

Because the levels of heparin-binding proteins are so variable between patients, the anticoagulant response to fixed or weight-adjusted doses of heparin is unpredictable. Consequently, coagulation monitoring is essential to ensure that a therapeutic response is obtained when heparin is administered for treatment purposes.

cleavage by coagulation proteases other than thrombin. Second, heparin cofactor II possesses a unique anionic sequence at its N-terminal. In its unactivated state, this sequence forms an intramolecular bond with the positively charged glycosaminoglycan binding site located on the body of heparin cofactor II. When heparin or dermatan sulfate, a glycosaminoglycan that interacts only with heparin cofactor II, binds to heparin cofactor II, this N-terminal sequence is displaced, which enables its tethering to a positively charged domain on thrombin known as *exosite 1*. This tethering interaction occurs only with thrombin and facilitates thrombin inhibition by heparin cofactor II (Fig. 149.6).

Maximum catalysis of heparin cofactor II by heparin requires heparin chains composed of at least 26 saccharide units, which corresponds to a molecular weight of 7800. Longer heparin chains activate heparin cofactor II to a greater extent than shorter chains because the longer chains are of sufficient length not only to bind to heparin cofactor II but also to bind to thrombin to form a ternary complex. Formation of this complex brings thrombin and heparin cofactor II into close apposition.

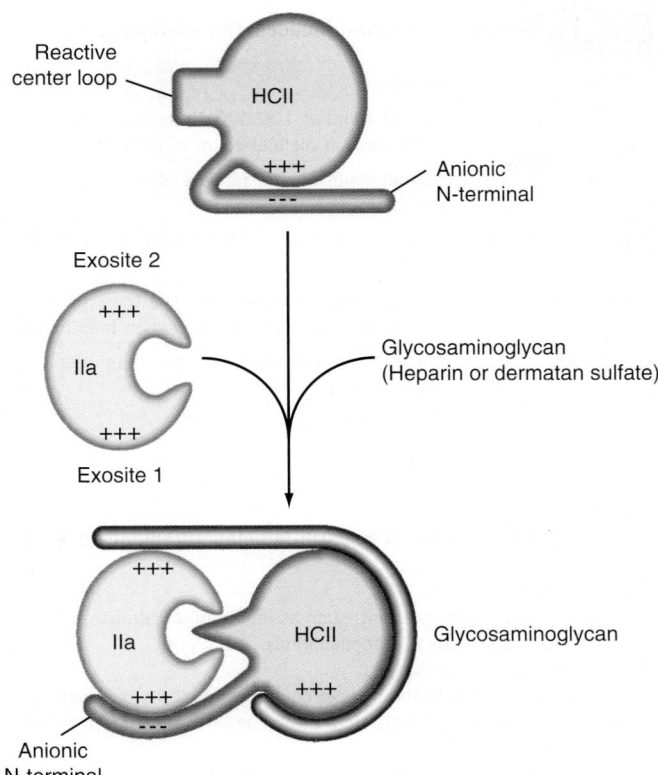

Fig. 149.6 CATALYSIS OF HEPARIN COFACTOR II (HCII) BY GLYCOSAMINOGLYCANS. In its unactivated form, the acidic N-terminal tail of HCII is tethered to the positively charged glycosaminoglycan-binding site on the body of the serpin. The binding of heparin or dermatan sulfate to this binding site displaces the N-terminal tail, thereby facilitating the interaction of this anionic domain with exosite 1 on thrombin. Glycosaminoglycan binding also evokes a conformational change in the reactive center loop of HCII that contributes to the formation of the HCII–thrombin complex. Longer heparin chains bind not only to HCII but also to the heparin-binding domain on thrombin, so-called exosite 2. Heparin-mediated bridging of HCII to thrombin enhances the rate of inhibition. Consequently, longer heparin chains that contain at least 26 saccharide units promote thrombin inhibition by HCII to a greater extent than shorter chains. Unlike heparin, dermatan sulfate does not need to bind to thrombin for maximal enhancement in the rate of thrombin inhibition, because shorter dermatan sulfate fragments are just as active as longer ones.

Heparin is cleared through a combination of a rapid, saturable and a much slower first-order mechanism. The saturable phase of heparin clearance is thought to be caused by binding to endothelial cell receptors and macrophages. Bound heparin is internalized and depolymerized. The slower, nonsaturable mechanism of clearance is largely renal. At therapeutic doses, a large proportion of heparin is cleared through the rapid, saturable, dose-dependent mechanism. The complex kinetics of clearance renders the anticoagulant response to heparin nonlinear at therapeutic doses, with both the intensity and duration of effect rising disproportionately with increasing dose. Thus the apparent biological half-life of heparin increases from approximately 30 minutes after an intravenous bolus of 25 U/kg, to 60 minutes with an intravenous bolus of 100 U/kg, to 150 minutes with a bolus of 400 U/kg.

Monitoring

Heparin therapy can be monitored using the activated partial thromboplastin time (aPTT), anti–factor Xa level, or the activated clotting time (ACT). Although the aPTT is the test most often employed for this purpose, there are problems with this assay. aPTT reagents vary in their sensitivity to heparin, and the type of coagulometer used for testing can influence the results. Consequently, laboratories must establish a therapeutic aPTT range with each reagent–coagulometer combination by measuring the aPTT and anti–factor Xa level in plasma samples collected from heparin-treated patients. For most of the aPTT reagents and coagulometers in current use, therapeutic heparin levels are achieved with a two- to threefold prolongation of the aPTT.

Anti–factor Xa levels also can be used to monitor heparin therapy. With this test, therapeutic heparin levels range from 0.3 to 0.7 U/mL. Although this test is gaining in popularity, anti–factor Xa assays have yet to be standardized, and results can vary widely between laboratories.

The ACT is used to monitor heparin when high doses are given (>100 U/kg) to patients undergoing PCI or cardiac surgery with cardiopulmonary bypass (CPB) and those requiring extracorporeal membrane oxygenation (ECMO). The ACT varies depending on which test kit is used. For PCI, the target ACT is 250 to 300 seconds in patients not receiving GPIIb/IIIa inhibitors and 200 to 250 seconds if a GPIIb/IIIa inhibitor is given. For CPB, a target ACT longer than 480 seconds is desirable, whereas for ECMO, the target ACT ranges from 140 to 240 seconds.

Up to 25% of heparin-treated patients with venous thromboembolism require more than 35,000 U/day to achieve a therapeutic aPTT. These patients are considered heparin resistant. It is useful to measure anti–factor Xa levels in these patients because many will have a therapeutic anti–factor Xa level despite a subtherapeutic aPTT. This dissociation in test results occurs because elevated plasma levels of fibrinogen and factor VIII, both of which are acute-phase proteins, shorten the aPTT but have no effect on anti–factor Xa levels. Heparin therapy in patients who exhibit this phenomenon is best monitored using anti–factor Xa levels instead of the aPTT. Patients with congenital or acquired antithrombin deficiency and those with unusually high levels of heparin-binding proteins often require very high doses of heparin to achieve a therapeutic aPTT or anti–factor Xa level. If there is good correlation between the aPTT and the anti–factor Xa levels, either test can be used to monitor heparin therapy.

Dosing

For prophylaxis, heparin is usually given in fixed doses of 5000 U subcutaneously two or three times daily. With these low doses, coagulation monitoring is unnecessary. In contrast, monitoring is essential when heparin is given in therapeutic doses because a subtherapeutic anticoagulant response has been associated with a higher risk of recurrent thrombosis. Fixed-dose or weight-based heparin nomograms are used to standardize heparin dosing and to shorten the time required to achieve a therapeutic anticoagulant response. At least two heparin nomograms have been validated in patients with venous thromboembolism and reduce the time required to achieve a therapeutic aPTT. Weight-adjusted heparin nomograms also have been evaluated in patients with acute coronary syndromes.

Unmonitored twice-daily subcutaneous heparin proved as effective and safe as once-daily LMWH for initial treatment of venous thromboembolism in one study.[15a] High doses of heparin were used; treatment was started with a dose of 333 U/kg followed by 250 U/kg twice daily thereafter. This regimen may be an option for patients with renal insufficiency where LMWH or fondaparinux is problematic.

Limitations

Heparin has pharmacokinetic and biophysical limitations (Table 149.2). The pharmacokinetic limitations reflect heparin's propensity to bind in a pentasaccharide-independent fashion to cells and plasma proteins. Heparin binding to cells explains its dose-dependent clearance, whereas binding to plasma proteins results in a variable anticoagulant response and can lead to heparin resistance.

The biophysical limitations of heparin reflect the inability of the heparin–antithrombin complex (1) to inhibit factor Xa when it is incorporated into the prothrombinase complex, the complex that converts prothrombin to thrombin, and (2) to inhibit thrombin bound to fibrin. Consequently, factor Xa bound to activated platelets

TABLE 149.2	Pharmacokinetic and Biophysical Limitations of Heparin	
	Limitations Mechanism	
Poor bioavailability at low doses	Limited absorption of long heparin chains	
Dose-dependent clearance	Binds to endothelial cells	
Variable anticoagulant response	Binds to plasma proteins whose levels vary from patient to patient	
Reduced activity in the vicinity of platelet-rich thrombi	Neutralized by platelet factor 4 released from activated platelets	
Limited activity against factor Xa incorporated in the prothrombinase complex and thrombin bound to fibrin	Reduced capacity of heparin–antithrombin complex to inhibit factor Xa bound to activated platelets and thrombin bound to fibrin	

TABLE 149.3	Features of Heparin-Induced Thrombocytopenia	
Features	**Details**	
Thrombocytopenia	Platelet count of 100,000/µL or less or a decrease in platelet count of 50% or more	
Timing	Platelet count falls 5–10 days after starting heparin	
Type of heparin	More common with unfractionated heparin than LMWH	
Type of patient	More common in surgical patients than medical patients; more common in women than in men	
Thrombosis	Venous thrombosis more common than arterial thrombosis	

LMWH, Low-molecular-weight heparin.

TABLE 149.4	Management of Heparin-Induced Thrombocytopenia

Stop all heparin
Give an alternative anticoagulant, such as lepirudin, argatroban, bivalirudin, danaparoid, or fondaparinux.
Do not give platelet transfusions.
Do not give warfarin until the platelet count returns to its baseline level. If warfarin is administered, give vitamin K to restore the INR to normal.
Evaluate for thrombosis, particularly deep vein thrombosis.

INR, International normalized ratio.

within platelet-rich thrombi has the potential to generate thrombin, even in the face of heparin. Once this thrombin binds to fibrin, it too is protected from inhibition by the heparin–antithrombin complex. Clot-associated thrombin can then trigger thrombus growth by locally activating platelets and amplifying its own generation through feedback activation of factors V, VIII, and XI. Further compounding the problem is the potential for heparin neutralization by the high concentrations of PF4 released from activated platelets within the platelet-rich thrombus.

Side Effects

The most common side effect of heparin is bleeding. Other complications include thrombocytopenia, osteoporosis, and elevated levels of transaminases.

Bleeding. The risk of heparin-induced bleeding increases with higher heparin doses. Concomitant administration of drugs that affect hemostasis, such as antiplatelet or fibrinolytic agents, increases the risk of bleeding, as does recent surgery or trauma. Heparin-treated patients with serious bleeding can be given protamine sulfate to neutralize the heparin. Protamine sulfate, a mixture of basic polypeptides originally isolated from salmon sperm, binds heparin with high affinity, and the resultant protamine-heparin complexes are then cleared. Typically, 1 mg of protamine sulfate neutralizes 100 U of heparin. Protamine sulfate is given intravenously. Anaphylactoid reactions to protamine sulfate can occur, and drug administration by slow intravenous infusion is recommended to reduce the risk of these problems.

Thrombocytopenia. Heparin can cause thrombocytopenia. Heparin-induced thrombocytopenia (HIT) is an antibody-mediated process that is triggered by antibodies directed against neoantigens on PF4 that are exposed when heparin binds to this protein (Table 149.3). These antibodies, which usually are of the immunoglobulin G subtype, bind simultaneously to the heparin–PF4 complex and to platelet Fc receptors. Such binding activates the platelets and generates platelet microparticles. Circulating microparticles are prothrombotic because they express anionic phospholipids on their surface and can bind clotting factors, thereby promoting thrombin generation.

HIT can be associated with thrombosis, either arterial or venous. Venous thrombosis, which manifests as deep vein thrombosis and/or pulmonary embolism, is more common than arterial thrombosis. Arterial thrombosis can manifest as ischemic stroke or acute myocardial infarction. Rarely, platelet-rich thrombi in the distal aorta or iliac arteries can cause critical limb ischemia.

The diagnosis of HIT is established using enzyme-linked assays to detect antibodies against heparin–PF4 complexes or with platelet activation assays. Enzyme-linked assays are sensitive, but they can be positive in the absence of any clinical evidence of HIT. The most specific diagnostic test is the serotonin release assay. This test is performed by quantifying serotonin release when washed platelets loaded with labeled serotonin are exposed to patient serum in the absence or presence of varying concentrations of heparin. If the patient serum contains the HIT antibody, heparin addition induces platelet activation and subsequent serotonin release.

Management of HIT is outlined in Table 149.4. Heparin should be stopped in patients with suspected or documented HIT, and an alternative anticoagulant should be administered to prevent or treat thrombosis.[16] The agents most often used for this indication are parenteral direct thrombin inhibitors, such as lepirudin, argatroban, or bivalirudin, or factor Xa inhibitors, such as fondaparinux or danaparoid. Oral factor Xa inhibitors, such as rivaroxaban, have been used successfully to manage HIT.

Patients with HIT, particularly those with associated thrombosis, often have evidence of increased thrombin generation that can lead to consumption of protein C. If these patients are given warfarin without a concomitant parenteral anticoagulant to suppress thrombin generation, the further decrease in protein C levels induced by warfarin can trigger skin necrosis. To avoid this problem, patients with HIT should be treated with a direct thrombin inhibitor or fondaparinux until the platelet count returns to normal levels. At this point, low-dose warfarin therapy can be introduced, and the thrombin inhibitor or fondaparinux can be discontinued when the anticoagulant response to warfarin has been therapeutic for at least 2 days. HIT also is covered extensively in Chapter 133.

Osteoporosis. Treatment with therapeutic doses of heparin for over 1 month can cause a reduction in bone density. This complication has been reported in up to 30% of patients given long-term heparin therapy, and symptomatic vertebral fractures occur in 2% to 3% of these individuals.

Studies in vitro and in laboratory animals have provided insights into the pathogenesis of heparin-induced osteoporosis. These investigations suggest that heparin causes bone resorption, both by decreasing bone formation and by enhancing bone resorption. Thus heparin affects the activity of both osteoblasts and osteoclasts.

Elevated Levels of Transaminases. Therapeutic doses of heparin frequently cause modest elevation in the serum levels of hepatic transaminases, without a concomitant increase in the level of bilirubin. The levels of transaminases rapidly return to normal when the drug is stopped. The mechanism responsible for this phenomenon is unknown.

Low-Molecular-Weight Heparin

Consisting of smaller fragments of heparin, LMWH is prepared from unfractionated heparin by controlled enzymatic or chemical depolymerization. The mean molecular weight of LMWH is about 5000, one-third the mean molecular weight of unfractionated heparin. LMWH has several advantages over heparin (Table 149.5) and is used instead of heparin for most indications.

Mechanism of Action

Like heparin, LMWH exerts its anticoagulant activity by activating antithrombin. With a mean molecular weight of 5000, which corresponds to about 17 saccharide units, at least half of the pentasaccharide-containing chains of LMWH are too short to bridge thrombin to antithrombin (see Fig. 149.4). However, these chains retain the capacity to accelerate factor Xa inhibition by antithrombin because this activity is largely the result of the conformational changes in antithrombin evoked by pentasaccharide binding. Consequently, LMWH catalyzes factor Xa inhibition by antithrombin more than thrombin inhibition. Depending on their unique molecular weight distributions, LMWH preparations have anti–factor Xa to anti–factor IIa ratios ranging from 2:1 to 4:1.

Pharmacology

Although usually given subcutaneously, LMWH also can be administered intravenously if a rapid anticoagulant response is needed. LMWH has pharmacokinetic advantages over heparin. These advantages reflect the fact that shorter heparin chains bind less avidly to endothelial cells, macrophages, and heparin-binding plasma proteins. Reduced binding to endothelial cells and macrophages eliminates the rapid, dose-dependent, and saturable mechanism of clearance that is a characteristic of unfractionated heparin. Instead, the clearance of LMWH is dose independent, and its plasma half-life is longer. Based on measurement of anti–factor Xa levels, LMWH has a plasma half-life of about 4 hours. LMWH is cleared almost exclusively by the kidneys, and the drug can accumulate in patients with renal insufficiency.

LMWH exhibits about 90% bioavailability after subcutaneous injection. Because LMWH binds less avidly than heparin to

heparin-binding proteins in plasma, LMWH produces a more predictable dose response, and resistance to LMWH is rare. With a longer half-life and more predictable anticoagulant response, LMWH can be given subcutaneously once or twice daily without coagulation monitoring, even when the drug is given in treatment doses. These properties render LMWH more convenient than unfractionated heparin. Capitalizing on this feature, studies in patients with venous thromboembolism have shown that home treatment with LMWH is as effective and safe as in-hospital treatment with continuous intravenous infusions of heparin. Outpatient treatment with LMWH streamlines care, reduces health care costs, and increases patient satisfaction.

Monitoring

In the majority of patients, LMWH does not require coagulation monitoring. If monitoring is necessary, anti–factor Xa levels must be measured because most LMWH preparations have little effect on the aPTT. Therapeutic anti–factor Xa levels with LMWH range from 0.5 to 1.2 U/mL when measured 3 to 4 hours after drug administration. When LMWH is given in prophylactic doses, peak anti–factor Xa levels of 0.2 to 0.5 U/mL are desirable.

Indications for LMWH monitoring include renal insufficiency and morbid obesity. LMWH monitoring in patients with a creatinine clearance of 50 mL/min or less is advisable to ensure that there is no drug accumulation. Although weight-adjusted LMWH dosing appears to produce therapeutic anti–factor Xa levels in patients who are overweight, this approach has not been evaluated extensively in those with morbid obesity. It may also be advisable to monitor the anticoagulant activity of LMWH during pregnancy because dose requirements can change, particularly in the third trimester. Monitoring also is important in high-risk settings, such as in patients with mechanical mitral valves who are given LMWH for prevention of valve thrombosis.

Dosing

The doses of LMWH recommended for prophylaxis or treatment vary depending on the LMWH preparation. For prophylaxis, once-daily subcutaneous doses of 4000 to 5000 U are often used, whereas doses of 2500 to 3000 U are given when the drug is administered twice daily. For treatment of venous thromboembolism, a dose of 150 to 200 U/kg is given if the drug is administered once daily. If a twice-daily regimen is employed, a dose of 100 U/kg is given. In patients with unstable angina, LMWH is given subcutaneously on a twice-daily basis at a dose of 100 to 120 U/kg.

Side Effects

The major complication of LMWH is bleeding. Recent metaanalyses suggest that the risk of major bleeding may be lower with LMWH than with unfractionated heparin. HIT and osteoporosis are less common with LMWH than with unfractionated heparin.

Bleeding

The risk of bleeding with LMWH is increased with concomitant use of antiplatelet or fibrinolytic drugs. Recent surgery, trauma, or underlying hemostatic defects also increase the risk of bleeding with LMWH.

Although protamine sulfate can be used as an antidote for LMWH, protamine sulfate incompletely neutralizes the anticoagulant activity of LMWH because it binds only the longer chains of LMWH. Because longer chains are responsible for catalysis of thrombin inhibition by antithrombin, protamine sulfate completely reverses the anti–factor IIa activity of LMWH. In contrast, protamine sulfate only partially reverses the anti–factor Xa activity of LMWH because the shorter pentasaccharide-containing chains of LMWH do not bind to

TABLE 149.5	Advantages of Low-Molecular-Weight Heparin Over Heparin	
	Advantage Consequence
Better bioavailability and longer half-life after subcutaneous injection	Can be given subcutaneously once or twice daily for both prophylaxis and treatment
Dose-independent clearance	Simplified dosing
Predictable anticoagulant response	Coagulation monitoring is unnecessary in most patients
Lower risk of heparin-induced thrombocytopenia	Safer than heparin for short- or long-term administration
Lower risk of osteoporosis	Safer than heparin for extended administration

protamine sulfate. Consequently, patients at high risk for bleeding may be more safely treated with continuous intravenous unfractionated heparin than with subcutaneous LMWH. In addition to the potential for complete reversal with protamine sulfate, the short half-life of intravenous heparin also is an advantage if major bleeding occurs.

Thrombocytopenia

The risk of HIT is about fivefold lower with LMWH than with heparin. LMWH binds less avidly to platelets and causes less PF4 release. Furthermore, with lower affinity for PF4 than heparin, LMWH is less likely to induce the conformational changes in PF4 that trigger the formation of HIT antibodies. LMWH should not be used to treat patients with HIT, because most HIT antibodies exhibit cross-reactivity with LMWH, and there are case reports of thrombosis when patients with HIT were treated with LMWH.

Osteoporosis

The risk of osteoporosis is lower with long-term LMWH than with heparin. For extended treatment, therefore, LMWH is a better choice than heparin because of the lower risk of both osteoporosis and HIT.

Fondaparinux

A synthetic analogue of the antithrombin-binding pentasaccharide sequence, fondaparinux differs from LMWH in several ways (Table 149.6). Fondaparinux is licensed for (1) thromboprophylaxis in medical, general surgical, and high-risk orthopedic patients and (2) as an alternative to heparin or LMWH for initial treatment of patients with established venous thromboembolism. In some countries, fondaparinux also is approved as an alternative to heparin or LMWH for treatment of patients with acute coronary syndromes.

Mechanism of Action

As a synthetic analogue of the antithrombin-binding pentasaccharide sequence found in heparin and LMWH, fondaparinux has a molecular weight of 1728. Fondaparinux binds only to antithrombin (see Fig. 149.4) and is too short to bridge thrombin to antithrombin. Consequently, fondaparinux catalyzes factor Xa inhibition by antithrombin and does not enhance the rate of thrombin inhibition.

Pharmacology

Fondaparinux exhibits complete bioavailability after subcutaneous injection. With no binding to endothelial cells or plasma proteins, the clearance of fondaparinux is dose independent, and its plasma

half-life is about 17 hours. The drug is given subcutaneously once daily. Because fondaparinux is cleared unchanged via the kidneys, it is contraindicated in patients with a creatinine clearance less than 30 mL/min, and it should be used with caution in those with a creatinine clearance less than 50 mL/min.

Fondaparinux produces a predictable anticoagulant response after administration in fixed doses because it does not bind to plasma proteins. The drug is given at a dose of 2.5 mg once daily for prevention of venous thromboembolism. For initial treatment of established venous thromboembolism, fondaparinux is given at a dose of 7.5 mg once daily. The dose can be reduced to 5 mg once daily for those weighing less than 50 kg and increased to 10 mg for those weighing more than 100 kg. When given in these doses, fondaparinux is as effective as heparin or LMWH for initial treatment of patients with deep vein thrombosis or pulmonary embolism and produces similar rates of bleeding.

Although not licensed for this indication in the United States, fondaparinux has been used in place of heparin or LMWH in patients with acute coronary syndrome. When the prophylactic dose of fondaparinux (2.5 mg daily) was compared with treatment doses of enoxaparin in patients with non–ST-segment elevation acute coronary syndrome, there was no difference in the rate of cardiovascular death, myocardial infarction, or stroke at 9 days.[17] However, the rate of major bleeding was 50% lower with fondaparinux than with enoxaparin, a difference that likely reflects the fact that the dose of fondaparinux was lower than that of enoxaparin. In patients with acute coronary syndrome who require PCI, there is a risk of catheter thrombosis with fondaparinux unless adjunctive heparin is given.

Side Effects

Fondaparinux does not cause HIT, and, in contrast to LMWH, there is no cross-reactivity of fondaparinux with HIT antibodies. Interestingly, fondaparinux induces the formation of HIT antibodies to the same extent as LMWH. In contrast to heparin or LMWH, however, fondaparinux is too short to cluster PF4 tetramers together, which is a prerequisite for HIT antibody binding. This phenomenon explains not only why HIT antibodies do not cross-react with fondaparinux but also why fondaparinux does not cause HIT despite the fact that it induces the formation of HIT antibodies. Although fondaparinux has been used successfully for HIT treatment, large clinical trials are lacking, and the drug is not licensed for this indication.

The major side effect of fondaparinux is bleeding. There is no antidote for fondaparinux. Protamine sulfate has no effect on the anticoagulant activity of fondaparinux, because it fails to bind to the drug. Recombinant activated factor VII reverses the anticoagulant effects of fondaparinux in volunteers, but it is unknown whether this agent will control fondaparinux-induced bleeding.

Parenteral Direct Thrombin Inhibitors

Heparin and LMWH are indirect inhibitors of thrombin because their activity is mediated by antithrombin. In contrast, direct thrombin inhibitors do not require a plasma cofactor; instead, these agents bind directly to thrombin and block its interaction with its substrates. Approved parenteral direct thrombin inhibitors include hirudin derivatives (lepirudin and desirudin), argatroban, and bivalirudin (Table 149.7). Lepirudin and argatroban are licensed for treatment of patients with HIT, whereas bivalirudin is approved as an alternative to heparin in patients undergoing cardiac surgery or PCI, including those with HIT. Desirudin is licensed for thromboprophylaxis after elective hip replacement surgery.

Lepirudin and Desirudin

Recombinant forms of hirudin, lepirudin, and desirudin are bivalent direct thrombin inhibitors, which interact with both the active site

TABLE 149.6	Comparison of Low-Molecular-Weight Heparin and Fondaparinux	
Features	**LMWH**	**Fondaparinux**
Molecular mass (Da)	4500 to 6000	1728
Catalysis of factor Xa inhibition	Yes	Yes
Catalysis of thrombin inhibition	Yes	No
Bioavailability after subcutaneous administration (%)	90	100
Plasma half-life (h)	4	17
Renal excretion	Yes	Yes
Induces release of tissue factor pathway inhibitor	Yes	No
Neutralized by protamine sulfate	Partially	No

LMWH, Low-molecular-weight heparin.

TABLE 149.7	Comparison of the Properties of Hirudin, Bivalirudin, and Argatroban		
	Hirudin	**Bivalirudin**	**Argatroban**
Molecular mass (Da)	7000	1980	527
Site(s) of interaction with thrombin	Active site and exosite 1	Active site and exosite 1	Active site
Renal clearance	Yes	No	No
Hepatic metabolism	No	No	Yes
Plasma half-life (min)	60	25	45

and exosite 1, the substrate-binding site on thrombin. Lepirudin is given by continuous intravenous infusion, whereas desirudin is administered subcutaneously twice daily. Lepirudin has a plasma half-life of 60 minutes after intravenous infusion, whereas the half-life of desirudin is about 2 hours. Both drugs are cleared by the kidneys and can accumulate in patients with renal insufficiency. A high proportion of lepirudin-treated patients develop antibodies against the drug. Although these antibodies rarely cause problems, in a small subset of patients they can delay lepirudin clearance and prolong its anticoagulant activity. Serious bleeding has been reported in some of these patients.

Desirudin is given subcutaneously in low doses and does not require monitoring. In contrast, lepirudin is usually monitored using the aPTT, and the dose is adjusted to maintain an aPTT that is 1.5 to 2.5 times the control. The aPTT is not an ideal test for monitoring lepirudin therapy, because the clotting time plateaus with higher drug concentrations. Although the ecarin clotting time provides a better index of lepirudin dose than does the aPTT, the ecarin clotting time has yet to be standardized.

Argatroban

A univalent inhibitor that targets the active site of thrombin, argatroban is metabolized in the liver. Consequently, this drug must be used with caution in patients with hepatic insufficiency. Argatroban is not cleared via the kidneys, so this drug is safer than lepirudin for patients with HIT who have renal insufficiency.

Argatroban is administered by continuous intravenous infusion and has a plasma half-life of about 45 minutes. The aPTT is used to monitor its anticoagulant effect, and the dose is adjusted to achieve an aPTT 1.5 to 3 times the baseline value, but not to exceed 100 seconds. Argatroban also prolongs the international normalized ratio (INR), a feature that can complicate the transitioning of patients from argatroban to warfarin. This problem can be circumvented by using the levels of factor X to monitor warfarin in place of the INR. Alternatively, the argatroban infusion can be stopped for 2 to 3 hours before INR determination.

Bivalirudin

A synthetic 20–amino acid analog of hirudin, bivalirudin is a divalent thrombin inhibitor. Thus the N-terminal portion of bivalirudin interacts with the active site of thrombin, whereas its C-terminal tail binds to exosite 1. Bivalirudin has a plasma half-life of 25 minutes, the shortest half-life of all the parenteral direct thrombin inhibitors. Bivalirudin is degraded by peptidases and is partially excreted via the kidneys. When given in high doses for PCI or cardiac surgery, the anticoagulant activity of bivalirudin is monitored using the ACT. With lower doses, its activity can be assessed using the aPTT.

Studies comparing bivalirudin with heparin plus GPIIb/IIIa antagonists suggest that bivalirudin produces less bleeding. This feature plus its short half-life makes bivalirudin an attractive alternative to heparin in patients undergoing PCI, and it is licensed for this indication. Bivalirudin also is approved for management of patients with HIT who require PCI or cardiac surgery.

ORAL ANTICOAGULANTS

Current oral anticoagulant practice dates back to the mid- to late-1930s when the vitamin K antagonists were discovered as a result of investigations into the cause of hemorrhagic disease in cattle. Characterized by a decrease in prothrombin levels, this disorder is caused by ingestion of hay containing spoiled sweet clover. Hydroxycoumarin, which was isolated from bacterial contaminants in the hay, interferes with vitamin K metabolism, thereby causing a syndrome similar to vitamin K deficiency. A variety of coumarin derivatives is available. The agent most widely used in North America is warfarin.

The repertoire of oral anticoagulants has expanded with the introduction of the non-vitamin k antagonist oral anticoagulants (NOACs), which are also known as *direct oral anticoagulants* (DOACs). These agents include dabigatran, which targets thrombin, and rivaroxaban, apixaban and edoxaban, which target factor Xa.[14] The NOACs are licensed for thromboprophylaxis after hip or knee replacement, stroke prevention in patients with atrial fibrillation, and for treatment and secondary prevention of venous thromboembolism.

Warfarin

A water-soluble vitamin K antagonist, warfarin was initially developed as a rodenticide. Like other vitamin K antagonists, warfarin interferes with the synthesis of the vitamin K–dependent clotting proteins, which include prothrombin (factor II) and factors VII, IX, and X. Warfarin also reduces the synthesis of the vitamin K–dependent anticoagulant proteins, proteins C, S, and Z.

Mechanism of Action

All of the vitamin K–dependent clotting factors possess glutamic acid residues at their N-termini. A posttranslational modification adds a carboxyl group to the γ-carbon of these residues to generate γ-carboxyglutamic acid. This modification is essential for expression of the activity of these clotting factors because it permits their calcium-dependent binding to negatively charged phospholipid surfaces. The γ-carboxylation process is catalyzed by a vitamin K–dependent carboxylase. Thus vitamin K from the diet is reduced to vitamin K hydroquinone by vitamin K reductase (Fig. 149.7). Vitamin K hydroquinone serves as a cofactor for the carboxylase enzyme, which in the presence of carbon dioxide replaces the hydrogen on the γ-carbon of glutamic acid residues with a carboxyl group. During this process, vitamin K hydroquinone is oxidized to vitamin K epoxide, which is then reduced to vitamin K by vitamin K epoxide reductase (VKOR).

Warfarin inhibits VKOR, thereby blocking the γ-carboxylation process. This results in the synthesis of vitamin K–dependent clotting proteins that are only partially γ-carboxylated. Warfarin acts as an anticoagulant because these partially γ-carboxylated proteins have reduced or absent biologic activity. The onset of action of warfarin is delayed until the newly synthesized clotting factors with reduced activity gradually replace their fully active counterparts.

The antithrombotic effect of warfarin depends on a reduction in the functional levels of factor X and prothrombin, clotting factors that have half-lives of 24 and 72 hours, respectively. Because of the delay in achieving an antithrombotic effect, initial treatment with warfarin is supported by concomitant administration of a rapidly acting parenteral anticoagulant, such as heparin, LMWH, or fondaparinux, in patients with established thrombosis or at high risk for thrombosis. This strategy also helps to prevent warfarin-induced skin necrosis (see later).

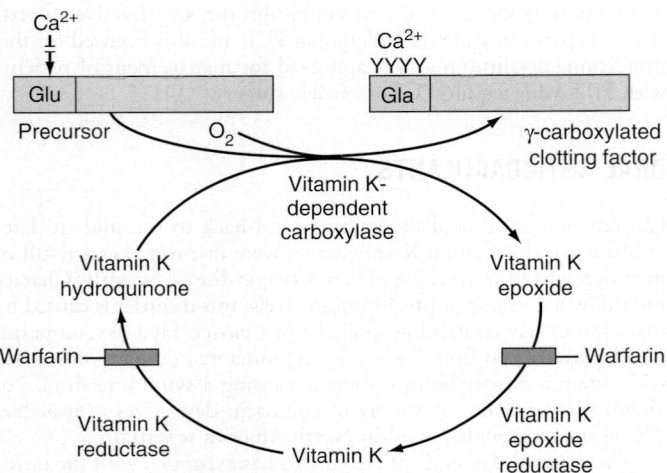

Fig. 149.7 THE VITAMIN K CYCLE AND ITS INHIBITION BY WARFARIN. Dietary vitamin K is reduced by vitamin K reductase to generate vitamin K hydroquinone. Vitamin K hydroquinone serves as a cofactor for the vitamin K–dependent carboxylase that converts glutamic acid residues at the N-termini of the vitamin K–dependent precursors to γ-carboxyglutamic acid residues, thereby creating the so-called Gla domain. By binding calcium, the Gla domain is critical for the interaction of the vitamin K–dependent clotting factors with negatively charged phospholipid membranes. During vitamin K–dependent carboxylation, vitamin K is oxidized to vitamin K epoxide. Vitamin K epoxide is then converted to vitamin K by vitamin K epoxide reductase. Vitamin K antagonists, such as warfarin, interfere with this cycle by inhibiting vitamin K epoxide reductase and vitamin K reductase. Of these two enzymes, vitamin K antagonists more readily block vitamin K epoxide reductase than vitamin K reductase. Consequently, supplemental vitamin K can overcome the inhibitory effects of vitamin K antagonists.

Pharmacology

Warfarin is a racemic mixture of R and S isomers; of these, the S isomer is more active. Warfarin is rapidly and almost completely absorbed from the gastrointestinal tract. Levels of warfarin in the blood peak about 90 minutes after drug administration. Racemic warfarin has a plasma half-life of 36 to 42 hours, and over 97% of circulating warfarin is bound to albumin. Only unbound warfarin is biologically active.

Warfarin accumulates in the liver, where the two isomers are metabolized via distinct pathways. Oxidative metabolism of the more active S isomer is effected by CYP2C9.[18] Two relatively common variants, *CYP2C9*2* and *CYP2C9*3*, have reduced activity. Patients with these variants require a lower maintenance dose of warfarin. The target of warfarin is VKOR. Polymorphisms in the C1 subunit of this enzyme (VKORC1) also can render patients less or more responsive to the anticoagulant effects of warfarin.[18] These findings have prompted a recommendation that patients starting on warfarin should be tested for these polymorphisms and that this information should be incorporated into their warfarin-dosing algorithms. Whether this approach will increase the efficacy and/or safety of warfarin therapy is uncertain.

In addition to genetic factors, diet, drugs, and various disease states influence the anticoagulant effect of warfarin. Fluctuations in dietary vitamin K intake affect the activity of warfarin. A wide variety of drugs can alter absorption, clearance, or metabolism of warfarin. Because of the variability in the anticoagulant response to warfarin, coagulation monitoring is essential to ensure that a therapeutic response is obtained.

Monitoring

Warfarin therapy is most often monitored using the prothrombin time, a test that is sensitive to reductions in the levels of prothrombin,

factor VII, and factor X.[19] The test is performed by adding thromboplastin, a reagent that contains tissue factor, phospholipid, and calcium, to citrated plasma and determining the time to clot formation. Thromboplastins vary in their sensitivity to reductions in the levels of the vitamin K–dependent clotting factors. Consequently, less sensitive thromboplastins will prompt the administration of higher doses of warfarin to achieve a target prothrombin time. This is problematic because higher doses of warfarin increase the risk of bleeding.

The INR was developed to circumvent many of the problems associated with the prothrombin time assay. To calculate the INR, the patient's prothrombin time is divided by the mean normal prothrombin time, and this ratio is then multiplied by the international sensitivity index (ISI), an index of the sensitivity of the thromboplastin used for prothrombin time determination to reductions in the levels of the vitamin K–dependent clotting factors. Highly sensitive thromboplastins have an ISI of 1.0. Most current thromboplastins have ISI values that range from 1.0 to 1.4.

Although the INR has helped to standardize anticoagulant practice, problems persist. The precision of INR determination varies depending on reagent–coagulometer combinations. This leads to variability in the INR results. Also complicating INR determination is unreliable reporting of the ISI by thromboplastin manufacturers. Furthermore, every laboratory must establish the mean normal prothrombin time with each new batch of thromboplastin reagent. To accomplish this, the prothrombin time must be measured in fresh plasma samples from at least 20 healthy volunteers using the same coagulometer that is used for patient samples.

For most indications, warfarin is administered in doses that produce a target INR of 2.0 to 3.0.[19] An exception is patients with mechanical heart valves in the mitral position, where a target INR of 2.5 to 3.5 is recommended.[20] Vitamin K antagonists have a narrow therapeutic window. Thus studies in atrial fibrillation demonstrate an increased risk of cardioembolic stroke when the INR falls below 1.7 and an increase in bleeding with INR values over 4.5. Likewise, a study with patients receiving long-term warfarin therapy for unprovoked venous thromboembolism demonstrated a higher rate of recurrent venous thromboembolism when the warfarin dose was adjusted to achieve a target INR of 1.5 to 1.9 than with a target INR of 2.0 to 3.0. Rates of major bleeding were similar.

Dosing

Warfarin is usually started at a dose of 5 to 10 mg. The dose is then titrated to achieve the desired target INR. Because of its delayed onset of action, patients with established thrombosis or those at high risk for thrombosis are given concomitant treatment with a rapidly acting parenteral anticoagulant, such as heparin, LMWH, or fondaparinux. Initial prolongation of the INR reflects reduction in the functional levels of factor VII. Consequently, concomitant treatment with the parenteral anticoagulant should be continued until the INR has been therapeutic for at least 2 consecutive days. A minimum 5-day course of parenteral anticoagulation is recommended to ensure that the levels of prothrombin have been reduced into the therapeutic range with warfarin.

Because warfarin has a narrow therapeutic window, frequent coagulation monitoring is essential to ensure that a therapeutic anticoagulant response is obtained. Even patients with stable warfarin dose requirements should have their INR determined every 2 to 4 weeks.[19] More frequent monitoring is necessary when new medications are introduced because many drugs enhance or reduce the anticoagulant effects of warfarin.

Side Effects

Like all anticoagulants, the major side effect of warfarin is bleeding. A rare complication is skin necrosis. Warfarin crosses the placenta and can cause fetal abnormalities. Consequently, warfarin should be avoided during pregnancy, particularly during the first trimester.

Bleeding

At least half of the bleeding complications with warfarin occur when the INR exceeds the therapeutic range. Bleeding complications may be mild, such as epistaxis or hematuria, or more severe, such as retroperitoneal or gastrointestinal bleeding. Life-threatening intracranial bleeding also can occur.

To minimize the risk of bleeding, the INR should be maintained in the therapeutic range. In asymptomatic patients whose INR is between 3.5 and 4.5, warfarin should be withheld until the INR returns to the therapeutic range. If the INR is over 4.5, a therapeutic INR can be achieved more rapidly by administration of low doses of sublingual vitamin K.

Patients with serious bleeding need treatment that is more aggressive. These patients should be given 5 to 10 mg of vitamin K by slow intravenous infusion. Additional vitamin K should be given until the INR is in the normal range. Treatment with vitamin K should be supplemented with prothrombin complex concentrate to replace the missing vitamin K–dependent clotting factors.[19]

Warfarin-treated patients who experience bleeding when their INR is in the therapeutic range require investigation into the cause of the bleeding. Those with gastrointestinal bleeding often have underlying peptic ulcer disease or a tumor. Similarly, investigation of hematuria or uterine bleeding in patients with a therapeutic INR may unmask a tumor of the genitourinary system.

Skin Necrosis

A rare complication of warfarin, skin necrosis usually is seen 2 to 5 days after initiation of therapy. Well-demarcated erythematous lesions form on the thighs, buttocks, breasts, or toes. Typically the center of the lesion becomes progressively necrotic. Examination of skin biopsies taken from the border of these lesions reveals thrombi in the microvasculature.

Warfarin-induced skin necrosis is seen in patients with congenital or acquired deficiencies of protein C or protein S. Initiation of warfarin therapy in these patients produces a precipitous fall in plasma levels of proteins C or S, thereby eliminating this important anticoagulant pathway before warfarin exerts an antithrombotic effect through lowering of the functional levels of factor X and prothrombin. The resultant procoagulant state triggers thrombosis. Why the thrombosis is localized to the microvasculature of fatty tissues is unclear.

Treatment involves discontinuation of warfarin and reversal with vitamin K, if needed. An alternative anticoagulant, such as heparin or LMWH, should be given in patients with thrombosis. Protein C concentrates or recombinant activated protein C can be given to patients with protein C deficiency to accelerate healing of the skin lesions; fresh frozen plasma may be of value for those with protein S deficiency. Occasionally, skin grafting is necessary when there is extensive skin loss.

Because of the potential for skin necrosis, patients with known protein C or protein S deficiency require overlapping treatment with a parenteral anticoagulant when initiating warfarin therapy. Warfarin should be started in low doses in these patients, and the parenteral anticoagulant should be continued until the INR is therapeutic for at least 2 to 3 consecutive days.

Pregnancy

Warfarin crosses the placenta and can cause fetal abnormalities or bleeding. The fetal abnormalities include a characteristic embryopathy, which consists of nasal hypoplasia and stippled epiphyses. The risk of embryopathy is highest if warfarin is given in the first trimester of pregnancy. Central nervous system abnormalities also can occur with exposure to coumarins at any time during pregnancy. Finally, maternal administration of warfarin produces an anticoagulant effect in the fetus that can cause bleeding. This is of particular concern at delivery, when trauma to the head during passage through the birth canal can lead to intracranial bleeding. Because of these potential problems, warfarin is rarely used in pregnancy, particularly in the first and third trimesters. Instead, heparin, LMWH, or fondaparinux can be given during pregnancy for prevention or treatment of thrombosis.

Warfarin does not pass into the breast milk. Consequently, warfarin can safely be administered to nursing mothers.

Special Problems

Patients with a lupus anticoagulant or those who need urgent or elective surgery present special challenges. Although observational studies suggested that patients with thrombosis complicating the antiphospholipid antibody syndrome required higher-intensity warfarin regimens to prevent recurrent thromboembolic events, two recent randomized trials demonstrated that targeting an INR of 2.0 to 3.0 is as effective as higher-intensity treatment and produces less bleeding. Monitoring warfarin therapy can be problematic in patients with antiphospholipid antibody syndrome if the lupus anticoagulant prolongs the baseline INR.

If patients receiving long-term warfarin treatment require an elective invasive procedure, warfarin can be stopped 5 days before the procedure to allow the INR to return to normal levels. Those at high risk for recurrent thrombosis can be bridged with once- or twice-daily subcutaneous injections of LMWH when the INR falls below 2.0. The last dose of LMWH should be given 12 to 24 hours before the procedure, depending on whether LMWH is administered twice or once daily, respectively. After the procedure, warfarin can be restarted.

Dabigatran

The active moiety of dabigatran etexilate, dabigatran targets the active site of thrombin and blocks its procoagulant activities. Dabigatran inhibits both free and fibrin-bound thrombin.

Mechanism of Action

Dabigatran etexilate is a prodrug with an oral bioavailability of 6% to 7%. Once absorbed, the drug is rapidly biotransformed by esterases to dabigatran, the levels of which peak 1 to 2 hours after oral administration. Dabigatran has a half-life of 12 to 14 hours. About 80% of the drug is excreted unchanged by the kidneys (Table 149.8). Potent permeability glycoprotein (P-GP) inhibitors, such as ketoconazole, are contraindicated.

Indications

Dabigatran is licensed for thromboprophylaxis after hip arthroplasty in the United States, and it is licensed for this indication and for thromboprophylaxis after knee arthroplasty in most other countries. Dabigatran also is licensed for stroke prevention in patients with nonvalvular atrial fibrillation and as an alternative to warfarin for treatment of venous thromboembolism.

When compared with warfarin in patients with atrial fibrillation, dabigatran at the 150-mg twice-daily dose was superior for reduction

TABLE 149.8	Comparison of Dabigatran, Rivaroxaban, Apixaban, and Edoxaban			
	Dabigatran	**Rivaroxaban**	**Apixaban**	**Edoxaban**
Target	Thrombin (IIa)	Factor Xa	Factor Xa	Factor Xa
Active drug	No	Yes	Yes	Yes
Onset Time (h)	0.5–2	2–4	3–4	1–3
Half-life (h)	12–17	5–13	~12	9–11
Renal excretion (%)	80	33	27	50

in both hemorrhagic and ischemic stroke.[21] Rates of major bleeding were similar with dabigatran and warfarin, whereas rates of intracranial and life-threatening bleeding were lower with dabigatran. At the 110-mg twice-daily dose, dabigatran was noninferior to warfarin for stroke prevention but was associated with significantly less intracranial and major bleeding.[21] In those over the age of 75 years, there was more gastrointestinal bleeding with dabigatran than with warfarin with the 150-mg dose but not with the 110-mg dose.[22]

For treatment of acute venous thromboembolism, dabigatran was compared with warfarin after a 5- to 7-day course of heparin or LMWH. Dabigatran was noninferior to warfarin for prevention of recurrent venous thromboembolism, but it produced less major plus clinically relevant nonmajor bleeding.[23]

When dabigatran was compared with warfarin in patients with mechanical heart valves, there was a trend for more ischemic strokes and more bleeding with dabigatran.[24] Consequently, dabigatran and the other NOACs are contraindicated in patients with mechanical heart valves; warfarin remains the anticoagulant of choice for such patients.

Dosing

For thromboprophylaxis after hip or knee arthroplasty, dabigatran is given once daily at a dose of 220 mg; a half-dose is given on the day of surgery. For stroke prevention in atrial fibrillation, dabigatran is given at a dose of 150 mg twice daily. A dose of 75 mg twice daily is used in the United States for patients with a creatinine clearance of 15 to 30 mL/min, whereas the 150-mg twice-daily dose is recommended for those with a creatinine clearance over 30 mL/min. In other countries, a dose of 110 mg twice daily is used for patients over the age of 80 years or in those 75 years of age or older who have risk factors for bleeding. For treatment of venous thromboembolism, dabigatran is given at a dose of 150 mg twice daily.

Monitoring

Routine coagulation monitoring is unnecessary. However, determination of the anticoagulant activity of dabigatran can be helpful to assess adherence, detect accumulation or overdose, determine its contribution to bleeding, and optimize the timing of surgery or intervention. The aPTT and thrombin time can be used for qualitative assessment of the anticoagulant activity of dabigatran, whereas the diluted thrombin time or ecarin clotting time can be used to quantify dabigatran levels if the tests are performed with dabigatran calibrators.

Drug Interactions

Dabigatran is a substrate of the efflux P-GP transporter. Consequently, coadministration with potent P-GP inhibitors such as quinidine, ketoconazole, amiodarone, and verapamil can increase plasma concentrations of dabigatran by decreasing its reabsorption into the gastrointestinal tract. In contrast, potent P-GP inducers such as rifampicin can reduce plasma dabigatran concentrations by increasing its reabsorption.

Side Effects

Dabigatran can be associated with dyspepsia. Taking the drug with food often helps to alleviate this problem. Bleeding is the major side effect of dabigatran. Dabigatran can rapidly be reversed with idarucizumab, a humanized monoclonal antibody fragment that binds dabigatran with high affinity.[25] Idarucizumab is given as an intravenous bolus of 5 g and is licensed for dabigatran reversal in patients with serious bleeding or in those requiring urgent surgery or intervention.

Dabigatran crosses the placenta and should not be used in pregnant women. The safety of dabigatran in women who are breastfeeding and in children has not been established.

Rivaroxaban

An oral factor Xa inhibitor, rivaroxaban is an active drug that targets the active site of factor Xa even when the enzyme is incorporated into the prothrombinase complex.

Mechanism of Action

Rivaroxaban has an oral bioavailability of 80%, and plasma levels peak 2 to 3 hours after drug administration. Absorption of rivaroxaban is enhanced by food; consequently, when given in doses of 15 or 20 mg once daily, rivaroxaban should be taken with a meal. The half-life of rivaroxaban is 5 to 9 hours in healthy young subjects and 11 to 13 hours in elderly subjects (Table 149.8). About one-third of the drug is cleared unchanged by the kidneys. The remainder is metabolized in the liver, and half of the inactive metabolites is cleared by the kidneys; the rest is excreted in the feces. The pharmacokinetic and pharmacodynamic profile is dose dependent and is not influenced by age, gender, or body weight.

Indications

Rivaroxaban is licensed for thromboprophylaxis after elective hip or knee arthroplasty, for treatment of venous thromboembolism, and for stroke prevention in patients with nonvalvular atrial fibrillation. When compared with enoxaparin for thromboprophylaxis after hip or knee arthroplasty, rivaroxaban significantly reduced the risk of venous thromboembolism with similar or slightly higher rates of major bleeding.[26] In patients with atrial fibrillation, rivaroxaban was noninferior to warfarin for prevention of stroke and systemic embolism, but it was associated with less intracranial bleeding and hemorrhagic stroke and a similar rate of major bleeding.[27] In patients with acute venous thromboembolism, an all-oral rivaroxaban regimen was as effective as conventional anticoagulant therapy consisting of heparin followed by a vitamin K antagonist, but it was associated with less major bleeding.[28,29] When compared with placebo as an adjunct to dual antiplatelet therapy in patients with acute coronary syndrome, rivaroxaban (at a dose of 2.5 mg twice daily) reduced the primary efficacy endpoint—the composite of cardiovascular death, myocardial infarction and stroke—from 10.7% to 9.1%.[30] Rivaroxaban increased the risk of bleeding, including intracranial bleeding, compared with placebo, but there was no increase in fatal bleeding.

Dosing

For thromboprophylaxis after hip or knee replacement surgery, rivaroxaban is given once daily at a dose of 10 mg.[26] When used for stroke prevention in patients with atrial fibrillation, the dose is 20 mg once daily. The dose is reduced to 15 mg once daily for those with a creatinine clearance of 15 to 49 mL/min. For treatment of venous thromboembolism, rivaroxaban is started at a dose of 15 mg twice daily for 3 weeks, followed by 20 mg once daily thereafter. When used as an adjunct to antiplatelet therapy in stabilized patients with acute coronary syndrome, rivaroxaban is given at a dose of 2.5 mg twice daily.

Monitoring

Rivaroxaban prolongs the prothrombin time more than the aPTT, but its effect on these tests is reagent dependent. Plasma concentrations of rivaroxaban can be quantified using a chromogenic anti–factor Xa assay with drug-specific calibrators.

Drug Interactions

Coadministration of rivaroxaban with dual inhibitors of CYP3A4 and P-GP, such as ketoconazole, itraconazole, ritonavir, and clarithromycin, increases drug exposure and the risk of bleeding, whereas coadministration with dual inducers of CYP3A4 and P-GP, such as rifampin, carbamazepine, phenytoin, and St. John's wort, decreases exposure and increases the risk of stroke and other thromboembolic events.

Side Effects

The major side effect is bleeding. Although prothrombin complex concentrate partly reverses the anticoagulant effects of rivaroxaban in volunteers, its utility for treatment of bleeding is uncertain. Nonetheless, prothrombin complex concentrate (30 to 50 U/kg) should be considered for patients with life-threatening bleeds. If the bleeding continues, activated prothrombin complex concentrate or recombinant factor VIIa can be used.

Specific reversal agents for rivaroxaban are in development. Most advanced is andexanet alfa. A recombinant variant of factor Xa that has its active site serine residue replaced with an alanine residue to eliminate catalytic activity and its membrane-binding domain removed to circumvent incorporation into the prothrombinase complex, andexanet competes with factor Xa for binding rivaroxaban and sequesters it until it can be cleared.[25,31] Andexanet also reverses heparin, LMWH, and fondaparinux by competing with factor Xa and thrombin for the antithrombin–heparin complex.

Ciraparantag is a second reversal agent that is at an earlier stage of development than andexanet. A synthetic, cationic small molecule, ciraparantag binds rivaroxaban and neutralizes its anticoagulant activity.[32] Ciraparantag also binds dabigatran, apixaban, edoxaban, heparin, LMWH, and fondaparinux.

Rivaroxaban crosses the placenta and should not be used in pregnant women. The safety of rivaroxaban in women who are breastfeeding and in children has not been established.

Apixaban

An oral factor Xa inhibitor, apixaban inhibits free factor Xa and factor Xa incorporated into the prothrombinase complex. It is licensed in many countries, for thromboprophylaxis after hip or knee replacement surgery, for treatment and secondary prevention of venous thromboembolism, and for stroke prevention in atrial fibrillation.

Mechanism of Action

Apixaban binds reversibly to the active site of free factor Xa or factor Xa incorporated into the prothrombinase complex. The drug has 50% oral bioavailability, and plasma levels peak 3 to 4 hours after drug administration. The half-life of apixaban is about 12 hours (Table 149.8). Apixaban is metabolized in the liver via CYP3A4/5-dependent and independent pathways. About 27% of the drug is cleared unchanged by the kidneys, and the remainder is excreted in the feces.

Indications

Apixaban is licensed for thromboprophylaxis after elective hip or knee arthroplasty, for stroke prevention in patients with nonvalvular atrial fibrillation, and for treatment of venous thromboembolism. When compared with enoxaparin for thromboprophylaxis after hip or knee arthroplasty, apixaban was at least as effective and safe.[33-35] For treatment of venous thromboembolism, an all-oral regimen of apixaban (10 mg twice daily for 7 days followed by 5 mg twice daily thereafter) was compared with conventional anticoagulant therapy consisting of enoxaparin followed by warfarin. Apixaban was noninferior to conventional therapy for prevention of recurrent venous

thromboembolism, but it was associated with less bleeding. Apixaban was superior to aspirin for stroke prevention in atrial fibrillation patients unwilling or unable to take warfarin and did not significantly increase the risk of bleeding.[36] When compared with warfarin in patients with atrial fibrillation, apixaban significantly reduced the risk of stroke and systemic embolism, and it was associated with less major bleeding and lower all-cause mortality.[37]

Dosing

For thromboprophylaxis, apixaban is given twice daily at a dose of 2.5 mg. For stroke prevention in patients with atrial fibrillation, the dose is 5 mg twice daily, and the dose is reduced to 2.5 mg twice daily in patients with at least two of the following criteria; age of 80 years or older, body weight of 60 kg or less, and serum creatinine of 1.5 mg/dL or higher. In patients with venous thromboembolism, apixaban is started at a dose of 10 mg twice daily for 7 days followed by 5 mg twice daily thereafter. After 6 months, the dose can be reduced to 2.5 mg twice daily.

Monitoring

Routine monitoring is unnecessary. Apixaban has little effect on the prothrombin time or aPTT. Plasma drug levels can be quantified using an anti–factor Xa assay with apixaban calibrators.

Drug Interactions

Coadministration of apixaban with dual inhibitors of CYP3A4 and P-GP, such as ketoconazole, itraconazole, ritonavir, and clarithromycin, increases drug exposure and may increase the risk of bleeding. In contrast, coadministration with dual inducers of CYP3A4 and P-GP, such as rifampin, carbamazepine, phenytoin, and St. John's wort, decreases exposure and may increase the risk of stroke and other thromboembolic events.

Side Effects

The major side effect is bleeding. Management of bleeding with apixaban is identical to that with rivaroxaban. Apixaban crosses the placenta and should not be used in pregnant women. The safety of apixaban in women who are breastfeeding and in children has not been established.

Edoxaban

Another oral factor Xa inhibitor, edoxaban inhibits free factor Xa and factor Xa incorporated into the prothrombinase complex.

Mechanism of Action

Edoxaban binds reversibly to the active site of free factor Xa or factor Xa incorporated into the prothrombinase complex. The oral bioavailability is 62%, and plasma levels of edoxaban peak 1 to 2 hours after drug administration. The half-life of edoxaban is 10 to 14 hours. Of the administered edoxaban dose, about 50% is excreted via the kidneys as unchanged drug, and the remainder is excreted in the feces (Table 149.8).

Indications

Edoxaban is licensed for stroke prevention in patients with nonvalvular atrial fibrillation and for treatment of venous thromboembolism.

When compared with warfarin in patients with atrial fibrillation, the higher-dose edoxaban regimen (60 mg once daily with dose reduction to 30 mg once daily for the indications listed earlier) was noninferior for prevention of stroke and systemic embolism, but it was associated with less intracranial bleeding and less major bleeding.[38] In patients with venous thromboembolism who had received at least 5 days of heparin, edoxaban was noninferior to warfarin for prevention of recurrent venous thromboembolism and was associated with less bleeding.[39]

Dosing

Edoxaban is given once daily at a dose of 60 mg, both for treatment of venous thromboembolism and for stroke prevention, in patients with atrial fibrillation. The dose is reduced to 30 mg once daily in patients who have a body weight of 60 kg or less, have a creatinine clearance of 15 to 50 mL/min, or are taking potent P-GP inhibitors such as verapamil, quinidine, or dronedarone. In the United States, there is a black box warning against the use of edoxaban in patients with atrial fibrillation who have a creatinine clearance over 95 mL/min.

Monitoring

Edoxaban prolongs the prothrombin time more than the aPTT, but its effects on the prothrombin time are reagent dependent. Plasma edoxaban concentrations can be quantified using an anti–factor Xa assay with edoxaban calibrators.

Drug Interactions

Edoxaban is a substrate of P-GP, and coadministration with potent P-GP inhibitors such as quinidine, verapamil, or dronedarone increases drug exposure and has the potential to increase the risk of bleeding.

Side Effects

The major side effect is bleeding. Management of bleeding with edoxaban is identical to that with rivaroxaban and apixaban. Edoxaban crosses the placenta and should not be used in pregnant women. The safety of edoxaban in women who are breastfeeding and in children has not been established.

FIBRINOLYTIC DRUGS

Role of Fibrinolytic Therapy

Used to degrade thrombi, fibrinolytic drugs can be administered systemically or they can be delivered via catheters directly into the substance of the thrombus. Systemic delivery is used for treatment of acute myocardial infarction, acute ischemic stroke, and most cases of massive pulmonary embolism. The goal of therapy is to produce rapid thrombus dissolution, thereby restoring antegrade blood flow. In the coronary circulation, restoration of blood flow reduces morbidity and mortality by limiting myocardial damage, whereas in the cerebral circulation, rapid thrombus dissolution decreases the neuronal death and brain infarction that produce irreversible brain injury. For patients with massive pulmonary embolism, the goal of fibrinolytic therapy is to restore pulmonary artery perfusion.

Peripheral arterial thrombi and thrombi in the proximal deep veins of the leg are most often treated using a catheter-directed approach. Catheters with multiple side holes can be used to deliver fibrinolytic drugs. In some cases, intravascular devices that fragment and extract the thrombus are used to hasten treatment.

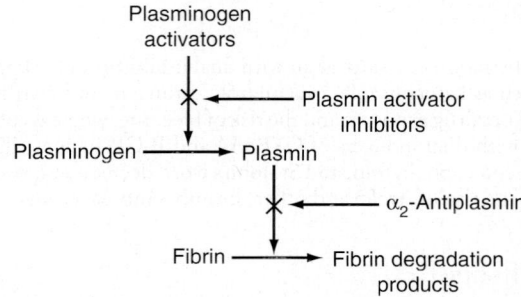

Fig. 149.8 FIBRINOLYTIC SYSTEM AND ITS REGULATION. Plasminogen activators convert plasminogen to plasmin. Plasmin then degrades fibrin into soluble fibrin degradation products. The system is regulated at two levels. Type 1 plasminogen activator inhibitor (PAI-1) regulates the plasminogen activators, whereas α_2-antiplasmin serves as the major inhibitor of plasmin.

Mechanism of Action

Commonly used fibrinolytic agents include streptokinase, recombinant tissue-type plasminogen activator (rt-PA), which is also known as alteplase or activase, and two recombinant derivatives of rt-PA, tenecteplase and reteplase. All of these agents act by converting the proenzyme, plasminogen, to plasmin, the active enzyme (Fig. 149.8). Plasmin then degrades the fibrin matrix of thrombi, thereby producing soluble fibrin degradation products.

Endogenous fibrinolysis is regulated at two levels. Plasminogen activator inhibitors, particularly the type 1 form, known as PAI-1, prevent excessive plasminogen activation by regulating the activity of tissue-type plasminogen activator (t-PA) and urokinase-type plasminogen activator (u-PA). Once plasmin is generated, plasmin inhibitors, particularly α_2-antiplasmin, regulate it. The plasma concentration of plasminogen is twofold higher than that of α_2-antiplasmin. Consequently, with pharmacologic doses of plasminogen activators, the concentration of plasmin that is generated can exceed that of α_2-antiplasmin. In addition to degrading fibrin, unregulated plasmin also can degrade fibrinogen and other clotting factors. This process, which is known as the systemic lytic state, reduces the hemostatic potential of the blood and increases the risk of bleeding.

The endogenous fibrinolytic system is geared to localize plasmin generation to the fibrin surface. Both plasminogen and t-PA bind to fibrin to form a ternary complex that promotes efficient plasminogen activation. In contrast to free plasmin, plasmin generated on the fibrin surface is relatively protected from inactivation by α_2-antiplasmin, a feature that promotes fibrin dissolution. Furthermore, C-terminal lysine residues exposed as plasmin degrades fibrin serve as binding sites for additional plasminogen and t-PA molecules. This creates a positive feedback that enhances plasmin generation. When used pharmacologically, the various plasminogen activators capitalize on these mechanisms to a lesser or greater extent.

There are two pools of plasminogen: circulating plasminogen and fibrin-bound plasminogen (Fig. 149.9). Plasminogen activators that preferentially activate fibrin-bound plasminogen are considered fibrin specific. In contrast, nonspecific plasminogen activators do not discriminate between fibrin-bound and circulating plasminogen. Activation of circulating plasminogen results in the generation of unopposed plasmin that can trigger the systemic lytic state. Alteplase and its derivatives are fibrin-specific plasminogen activators, whereas streptokinase is a nonspecific agent.

Streptokinase

Unlike other plasminogen activators, streptokinase is not an enzyme and does not directly convert plasminogen to plasmin. Instead, streptokinase forms a 1 : 1 stoichiometric complex with plasminogen.

Formation of this complex induces a conformational change in plasminogen that exposes its active site (Fig. 149.10). This conformationally altered plasminogen then converts additional plasminogen molecules to plasmin.

Streptokinase has no affinity for fibrin, and the streptokinase–plasminogen complex activates both free and fibrin-bound plasminogen. Activation of circulating plasminogen generates sufficient amounts of plasmin to overwhelm α_2-antiplasmin. Unopposed plasmin not only degrades fibrin in the occlusive thrombus but also induces a systemic lytic state.

When given systemically to patients with acute myocardial infarction, streptokinase reduces mortality. For this indication, the drug is usually given as an intravenous infusion of 1.5 million units over 30 to 60 minutes. Patients who receive streptokinase can develop antibodies against the drug, as can patients with prior streptococcal infection. These antibodies can reduce the effectiveness of streptokinase.

Allergic reactions occur in about 5% of patients treated with streptokinase. These may manifest as a rash, fever, chills, and rigors. Although anaphylactic reactions can occur, these are rare. Transient hypotension is common with streptokinase and has been attributed to plasmin-mediated release of bradykinin from kallikrein. The hypotension usually responds to leg elevation and administration of intravenous fluids and low-doses of vasopressors, such as dopamine or norepinephrine.

Alteplase

A recombinant form of single-chain t-PA, alteplase has a molecular weight of 68,000. Alteplase is rapidly converted into its two-chain form by plasmin. Although single- and two-chain forms of t-PA have equivalent activity in the presence of fibrin, in its absence, single-chain t-PA has 10-fold lower activity.

Alteplase consists of five discrete domains (Fig. 149.11). The N-terminal A-chain of two-chain alteplase contains four of these domains: residues 4 through 50 make up the finger domain, a region that resembles the finger domain of fibronectin; residues 50 through 87 are homologous with epidermal growth factor; and residues 92 through 173 and 180 through 261, which have homology to the kringle domains of plasminogen, are designated as the first and second kringle domains, respectively. The fifth alteplase domain is the protease domain; it is located on the C-terminal B-chain of two-chain alteplase.

The interaction of alteplase with fibrin is mediated by the finger domain and, to a lesser extent, by the second kringle domain. The affinity of alteplase for fibrin is considerably higher than that for fibrinogen. Consequently, the catalytic efficiency of plasminogen activation by alteplase is two to three orders of magnitude higher in the presence of fibrin than in the presence of fibrinogen. This phenomenon helps to localize plasmin generation to the fibrin surface.

Although alteplase preferentially activates plasminogen in the presence of fibrin, alteplase is not as fibrin-selective as was first predicted. Its fibrin specificity is limited because, like fibrin, (DD)E, the

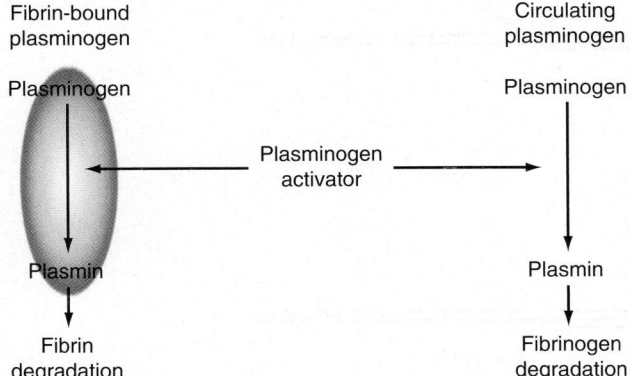

Fig. 149.9 CONSEQUENCES OF ACTIVATION OF FIBRIN-BOUND OR CIRCULATING PLASMINOGEN. The fibrin specificity of plasminogen activators reflects their capacity to distinguish between fibrin-bound and circulating plasminogen. This, in turn, reflects their affinity for fibrin. Plasminogen activators with high affinity for fibrin preferentially activate fibrin-bound plasminogen. This results in the generation of plasmin on the fibrin surface. Fibrin-bound plasmin, which is protected from inactivation by α_2-antiplasmin, degrades fibrin to yield soluble fibrin degradation products. In contrast, plasminogen activators with little or no affinity for fibrin do not distinguish between fibrin-bound and circulating plasminogen. Activation of circulating plasminogen results in systemic plasminemia and subsequent degradation of fibrinogen and other clotting factors.

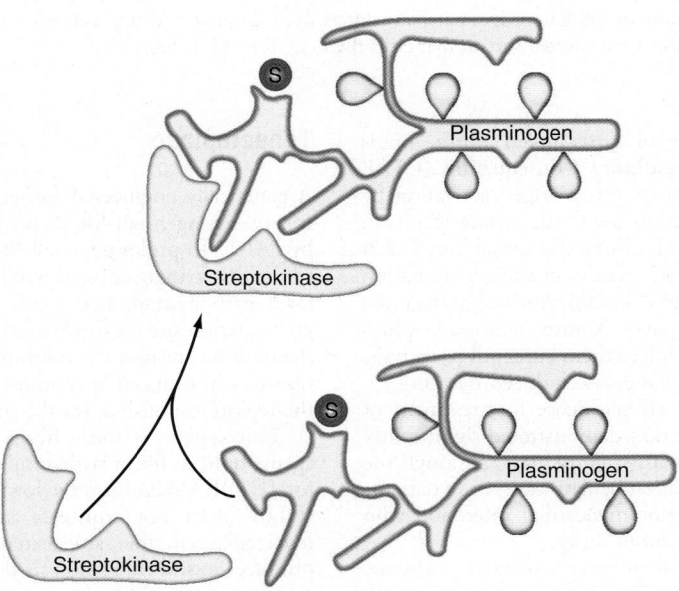

Fig. 149.10 MECHANISM OF ACTION OF STREPTOKINASE. Streptokinase binds to plasminogen and induces a conformational change in plasminogen that exposes its active site. The streptokinase–plasmin(ogen) complex then serves as the activator of additional plasminogen molecules.

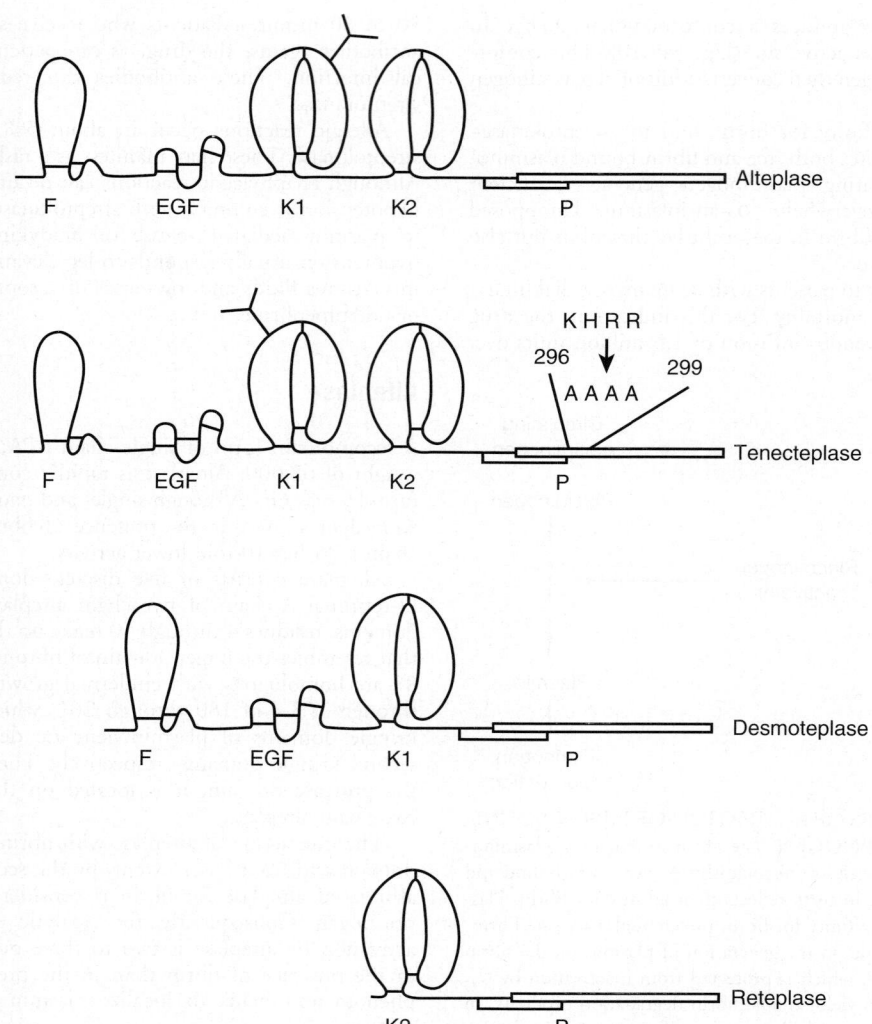

Fig. 149.11 DOMAIN STRUCTURES OF ALTEPLASE (TISSUE-TYPE PLASMINOGEN ACTIVATOR [t-PA]), TENECTEPLASE, DESMOTEPLASE, AND RETEPLASE. The finger (F), epidermal growth factor (EGF), first and second kringles (K1 and K2, respectively), and protease (P) domains are illustrated. The glycosylation site (Y) on K1 has been repositioned in tenecteplase to endow it with a longer half-life. In addition, a tetra-alanine substitution in the protease domain renders tenecteplase resistant to type 1 plasminogen activator inhibitor inhibition. Desmoteplase differs from alteplase and tenecteplase in that it lacks a K2 domain. Reteplase is a truncated variant that lacks the F, EGF, and K1 domains.

major soluble degradation product of cross-linked fibrin, binds alteplase and plasminogen with high affinity. Consequently, (DD)E is as potent as fibrin as a stimulator of plasminogen activation by alteplase. Whereas plasmin generated on the fibrin surface results in thrombolysis, plasmin generated on the surface of circulating (DD)E degrades fibrinogen. Fibrinogenolysis results in the accumulation of fragment X, a high-molecular-weight clottable fibrinogen degradation product. Incorporation of fragment X into hemostatic plugs formed at sites of vascular injury renders them susceptible to lysis. This phenomenon may contribute to alteplase-induced bleeding.

A trial comparing alteplase with streptokinase for treatment of patients with acute myocardial infarction demonstrated significantly lower mortality with alteplase than with streptokinase, although the absolute difference was small. The greatest benefit was seen in patients less than 75 years of age with anterior myocardial infarction who presented less than 6 hours after symptom onset.

For treatment of acute myocardial infarction or acute ischemic stroke, alteplase is given as an intravenous infusion over 60 to 90 minutes. The total dose of alteplase usually ranges from 90 to 100 mg. Allergic reactions and hypotension are rare, and alteplase is not immunogenic.

Tenecteplase

A genetically engineered variant of t-PA, tenecteplase was designed to have a longer half-life than t-PA and to be resistant to inactivation by PAI-1. To prolong its half-life, a new glycosylation site was added to the first kringle domain (see Fig. 149.11). Because addition of this extra carbohydrate side chain reduced fibrin affinity, the existing glycosylation site on the first kringle domain was removed. To render the molecule resistant to inhibition by PAI-1, a tetra-alanine substitution was introduced at residues 296 to 299 in the protease domain, the region responsible for the interaction of t-PA with PAI-1.

Tenecteplase is more fibrin specific than t-PA. Although both agents bind to fibrin with similar affinity, the affinity of tenecteplase for (DD)E is significantly lower than that of t-PA. Consequently, (DD)E does not stimulate systemic plasminogen activation by tenecteplase to the same extent as t-PA. As a result, tenecteplase produces less fibrinogenolysis than t-PA.

For coronary fibrinolysis, tenecteplase is given as a single intravenous bolus. In a large phase III trial in which almost 17,000 patients were enrolled, the 30-day mortality rate with single-bolus tenecteplase was similar to that with accelerated dose t-PA.[40,41] Although rates of intracranial hemorrhage also were similar with both treatments, patients given tenecteplase had fewer noncerebral bleeds and a reduced need for blood transfusions compared with those treated with t-PA. The improved safety profile of tenecteplase likely reflects its enhanced fibrin specificity. These properties have prompted studies comparing tenecteplase with alteplase in patients with acute ischemic stroke.[41]

Reteplase

A recombinant t-PA derivative, reteplase is a single-chain variant that lacks the finger, epidermal growth factor, and first kringle domains (see Fig. 149.11). This truncated derivative has a molecular weight of 39,000. Reteplase binds fibrin more weakly than t-PA because it lacks the finger domain. Because it is produced in *Escherichia coli*, reteplase is not glycosylated. This endows it with a plasma half-life longer than that of t-PA. Consequently, reteplase is given as two intravenous boluses, which are separated by 30 minutes. Clinical trials have demonstrated that reteplase is at least as effective as streptokinase for treatment of acute myocardial infarction, but the agent is not superior to t-PA.[42]

Desmoteplase

A recombinant form of the full-length plasminogen activator isolated from the saliva of the vampire bat, desmoteplase (see Fig. 149.11) is more fibrin specific than t-PA.[43] Although preliminary studies with desmoteplase for treatment of acute ischemic stroke were promising, further development has been halted.

CONCLUSIONS AND FUTURE DIRECTIONS

Arterial and venous thrombosis reflects a complex interplay among the vessel wall, platelets, the coagulation system, and the fibrinolytic pathways. Activation of coagulation also triggers inflammatory pathways that may contribute to thrombogenesis. A better understanding of the biochemistry of blood coagulation and advances in structure-based drug design have identified new targets and resulted in the development of novel antithrombotic drugs. Well-designed clinical trials have provided detailed information on which drugs to use and when to use them. Despite these advances, however, arterial and venous thromboembolic disorders remain a major cause of morbidity and mortality. Therefore the search for better targets and more potent or more convenient antiplatelet, anticoagulant, and fibrinolytic drugs continues.

REFERENCES

1. Mackman N: Triggers, targets and treatments for thrombosis. *Nature* 451:914–918, 2008.
2. Sutcliffe P, Connock M, Gurung T, et al: Aspirin for prophylactic use in the primary prevention of cardiovascular disease and cancer: a systematic review and overview of reviews. *Health Technol Assess* 17(43):2013.
3. Fitzgerald R, Pirmohamed M: Aspirin resistance: effect of clinical, biochemical and genetic factors. *Pharmacol Ther* 130:213–225, 2011.
4. Yusuf S, Zhao F, Mehta SR, et al: Effects of clopidogrel in addition to aspirin in patients with acute coronary syndromes without ST-segment elevation. *N Engl J Med* 345:494–502, 2001.
5. Wiviott SD, Braunwald E, McCabe CH, et al: Prasugrel versus clopidogrel in patients with acute coronary syndromes. *N Engl J Med* 357:2001–2015, 2007.
6. Roe MT, Armstrong PW, Fox KA, et al: Prasugrel versus clopidogrel for acute coronary syndromes without revascularization. *N Engl J Med* 367:1297–1309, 2012.
7. Gurbel PA, Tantry US: Clopidogrel response variability and the advent of personalised antiplatelet therapy: a bench to bedside journey. *Thromb Haemost* 106:265–271, 2011.
8. Wallentin L, Becker RC, Budaj A, et al: Ticagrelor versus clopidogrel in patients with acute coronary syndromes. *N Engl J Med* 361:1045–1057, 2009.
9. Cannon CP, Harrington RA, James S, et al: Comparison of ticagrelor with clopidogrel in patients with a planned invasive strategy for acute coronary syndromes (PLATO): a randomised double-blind study. *Lancet* 375:283–293, 2010.
10. Mahaffey KW, Wojdyla DM, Carroll K, et al: Ticagrelor compared with clopidogrel by geographic region in the Platelet Inhibition and Patient Outcomes (PLATO) trial. *Circulation* 124:544–554, 2011.
11. Sacco RL, Diener HC, Yusuf S, et al: Aspirin and extended-release dipyridamole versus clopidogrel for recurrent stroke. *N Engl J Med* 359:1238–1251, 2008.
12. Tricoci P, Huang Z, Held C, et al: Thrombin-receptor antagonist vorapaxar in acute coronary syndromes. *N Engl J Med* 366:20–33, 2012.
13. Morrow DA, Braunwald E, Bonaca MP, et al: Vorapaxar in the secondary prevention of atherothrombotic events. *N Engl J Med* 366:1404–1413, 2012.
14. Eikelboom JW, Weitz JI: New anticoagulants. *Circulation* 121:1523–1532, 2010.
15. Baker NC, Lipinski MJ, Lhermusier T, et al: Overview of the 2014 Food and Drug Administration Cardiovascular and Renal Drugs Advisory Committee meeting about vorapaxar. *Circulation* 130:1287–1294, 2014.
15a. Kearon C, Ginsberg JS, Julian JA, et al: Comparison of fixed-dose weight-adjusted unfractionated heparin and low-molecular-weight heparin for acute treatment of venous thromboembolism. *JAMA* 296(8):935–942, 2006.
16. Cuker A, Cines DB: How I treat heparin-induced thrombocytopenia. *Blood* 119:2209–2218, 2012.
17. Yusuf S, Mehta SR, Chrolavicius S, et al: Comparison of fondaparinux and enoxaparin in acute coronary syndromes. *N Engl J Med* 354:1464–1476, 2006.
18. Manolopoulos VG, Ragia G, Tavridou A: Pharmacogenetics of coumarinic oral anticoagulants. *Pharmacogenomics* 11:493–496, 2010.
19. Ageno W, Gallus AS, Wittkowsky A, et al: Oral anticoagulant therapy: antithrombotic therapy and prevention of thrombosis, 9th ed: American College of Chest Physicians Evidence-Based Clinical Practice Guidelines. *Chest* 141(2 Suppl):e44S–e88S, 2012.
20. Whitlock RP, Sun JC, Fremes SE, et al: Antithrombotic and thrombolytic therapy for valvular disease. *Chest* 141(2 Suppl):e576S–e600S, 2012.
21. Connolly SJ, Ezekowitz MD, Yusuf S, et al: Dabigatran versus warfarin in patients with atrial fibrillation. *N Engl J Med* 361:1139–1151, 2009.
22. Eikelboom JW, Wallentin L, Connolly SJ, et al: Risk of bleeding with 2 doses of dabigatran compared with warfarin in older and younger patients with atrial fibrillation: an analysis of the randomized evaluation of long-term anticoagulant therapy (RE-LY) trial. *Circulation* 123:2363–2372, 2011.
23. Schulman S, Kearon C, Kakkar AK, et al: Dabigatran versus warfarin in the treatment of acute venous thromboembolism. *N Engl J Med* 361:2342–2352, 2009.
24. Eikelboom JW, Connolly SJ, Brueckmann M, et al: Dabigatran versus warfarin in patients with mechanical heart valves. *N Engl J Med* 369:1206–1214, 2013.
25. Greinacher A, Thiele T, Selleng K: Reversal of anticoagulants: an overview of current developments. *Thromb Haemost* 113:931, 2015.
26. Duggan ST, Scott LJ, Plosker GL: Rivaroxaban: a review of its use for the prevention of venous thromboembolism after total hip or knee replacement surgery. *Drugs* 69:1829–1851, 2009.
27. Patel MR, Mahaffey KW, Garg J, et al: Rivaroxaban versus warfarin in nonvalvular atrial fibrillation. *N Engl J Med* 365:883–891, 2011.
28. Bauersachs R, Berkowitz SD, Brenner B, et al: Oral rivaroxaban for symptomatic venous thromboembolism. *N Engl J Med* 363:2499–2510, 2010.
29. Buller HR, Prins MH, Lensing AW, et al: Oral rivaroxaban for the treatment of symptomatic pulmonary embolism. *N Engl J Med* 366:1287–1297, 2012.
30. Mega JL, Braunwald E, Wiviott SD, et al: Rivaroxaban in patients with a recent acute coronary syndrome. *N Engl J Med* 366:9–19, 2012.

31. Siegal DM, Curnutte JT, Connolly SJ, et al: Andexanet alfa for the reversal of factor Xa inhibitor activity. *N Engl J Med* 373:2413–2424, 2015.

32. Enriquez A, Lip GY, Baranchuk A: Anticoagulation reversal in the era of the non-vitamin K oral anticoagulants. *Europace* 18:955, 2016.

33. Raskob GE, Gallus AS, Pineo GF, et al: Apixaban versus enoxaparin for thromboprophylaxis after hip or knee replacement: pooled analysis of major venous thromboembolism and bleeding in 8464 patients from the ADVANCE-2 and ADVANCE-3 trials. *J Bone Joint Surg Br* 94:257–264, 2012.

34. Agnelli G, Buller HR, Cohen A, et al: Oral apixaban for the treatment of acute venous thromboembolism. *N Engl J Med* 369:799–808, 2013.

35. Agnelli G, Buller HR, Cohen A, et al: Apixaban for extended treatment of venous thromboembolism. *N Engl J Med* 368:699–708, 2013.

36. Connolly SJ, Eikelboom J, Joyner C, et al: Apixaban in patients with atrial fibrillation. *N Engl J Med* 364:806–817, 2011.

37. Granger CB, Alexander JH, McMurray JJ, et al: Apixaban versus warfarin in patients with atrial fibrillation. *N Engl J Med* 365:981–992, 2011.

38. Giugliano RP, Ruff CT, Braunwald E, et al: Edoxaban versus warfarin in patients with atrial fibrillation. *N Engl J Med* 369:2093–2104, 2013.

39. Buller HR, Decousus H, Grosso M, et al: Edoxaban versus warfarin for the treatment of symptomatic venous thromboembolism. *N Engl J Med* 369:1406–1415, 2013.

40. Van De Werf F, Adgey J, Ardissino D, et al: Single-bolus tenecteplase compared with front-loaded alteplase in acute myocardial infarction: the ASSENT-2 double-blind randomised trial. *Lancet* 354:716–722, 1999.

41. Parsons M, Spratt N, Bivard A, et al: A randomized trial of tenecteplase versus alteplase for acute ischemic stroke. *N Engl J Med* 366:1099–1107, 2012.

42. Topol EJ, Ohman EM, Armstrong PW, et al: Survival outcomes 1 year after reperfusion therapy with either alteplase or reteplase for acute myocardial infarction: results from the Global Utilization of Streptokinase and t-PA for Occluded Coronary Arteries (GUSTO) III Trial. *Circulation* 102:1761–1765, 2000.

43. Medcalf RL: Desmoteplase: discovery, insights and opportunities for ischaemic stroke. *Br J Pharmacol* 165:75–89, 2012.

CHAPTER 150

DISORDERS OF COAGULATION IN THE NEONATE

Mihir D. Bhatt, Karin Ho, and Anthony K.C. Chan

The neonatal stage is a period of rapid physiologic changes, some of which affect the hemostatic system. The hemostatic system is a dynamic system that evolves gradually from birth into the mature adult form. Evaluation of disorders of coagulation in the neonate requires an understanding of the evolution of physiologic normal values for age, the congenital disorders that present in early life, and the clinical settings common in neonatology that affect hemostasis and thrombosis risks. The rapid evolution of the blood coagulation system after birth leads to a dynamic group of age-dependent reference ranges for the levels of the various components that should be considered physiologically normal. *Developmental hemostasis* is the term applied to the evolution of the hemostatic and fibrinolytic systems through infancy and childhood into adult age.

DEVELOPMENTAL HEMOSTASIS

The coagulation system in children provides innate protection from thrombosis without an increased risk for bleeding. The hemostatic system evolves throughout childhood and most rapidly during the neonatal period. Changes in the plasma concentrations of proteins involved in blood coagulation lead to a dynamic group of reference ranges for preterm and term infants. Although different from adult values, these reference ranges are neither abnormal nor pathologic. The relative rarity of hemorrhagic or thrombotic complications in this population suggests that the neonatal coagulation system is physiologically replete.

Laboratory Evaluation

The pioneering work of the late Dr. Maureen Andrew paved the way for research into developmental hemostasis. The concept of developmental hemostasis is now widely accepted, and her seminal papers describing the reference ranges for healthy premature and full-term neonates are still widely quoted.[1,2] Laboratory evaluation of thrombosis or bleeding in neonates must take into account the age-related reference ranges for healthy newborns, which differ significantly from adult levels. In addition, because coagulation assay results vary depending on the type of analyzer and reagents used, caution should be taken when prior publications of defined reference ranges for neonates are used.[3] Each laboratory that performs coagulation tests on neonatal samples must therefore develop their own age-related reference ranges specific to their analyzer and reagent combination in order to effectively diagnose and manage neonates with suspected hemostatic abnormalities. Neonatal samples should be drawn by experienced staff. Samples are processed in 1-mL tubes containing 0.1 mL of 3.2% buffered sodium citrate, aiming for a final ratio of one part citrate to nine parts blood.

Although recently researchers have started to look into age-specific differences in the quantitative levels of hemostatic proteins,[4] functional assays that are reagent and analyzer specific are still predominantly used in pediatric studies for hemostatic diagnosis. Changes in functional protein levels correspond to changes in global tests of coagulation. The prothrombin time (PT), expressed in seconds, in full-term and premature neonates is similar to that in adults, despite the fact that neonates have relative deficiencies of the vitamin K–dependent coagulation factors. However, samples from cord blood exhibit a prolonged PT compared with samples from adults.[1] The activated partial thromboplastin time (aPTT) is prolonged in newborns, which is attributed to relative deficiencies in the contact factors. Other tests, such as the thrombin time and thromboelastography, are less sensitive to age-related changes. The thrombin time in neonates is similar to that in adults when measured in the presence of calcium, which compensates for the unique fetal form of fibrinogen that has increased sialic acid content. Thromboelastography values vary very little with age. The template bleeding time is reported to be normal in neonates, but this is an unreliable test in neonates and is not recommended for evaluation of bleeding disorders. Investigations into neonatal hemostatic pathology are limited by the lack of normal reference values for the neonatal population and the difficulties associated with obtaining clean blood samples for testing.

Blood Coagulation Proteins

The synthesis of fetal and neonatal coagulation proteins begins at approximately 10 weeks of gestation, and plasma concentrations of these proteins increase with gestational age. Maternal coagulation proteins cannot cross the placenta. However, maternal drug intake can affect the synthesis of fetal vitamin K–dependent coagulation proteins, with warfarin, phenytoin, barbiturates, and antibiotics serving as examples.

In the healthy newborn, plasma levels of procoagulant factors such as thrombin, factor (F)VII, FIX, FX, and prothrombin (the vitamin K–dependent coagulation factors), as well as FXI, FXII, prekallikrein, and high-molecular-weight kininogen (the contact factors), are about 50% lower than adult values (Table 150.1).[1,2] The levels rise as the infant ages, and they reach about 80% of normal adult values by 6 months of age but remain decreased throughout childhood.[5] The levels of fibrinogen, FV, FVIII, and FXIII in neonates are similar to those in adults and remain so throughout childhood.[2,5] The level of von Willebrand factor (vWF) in newborns is about twofold higher than adult values and gradually decrease over the first 6 months of life,[2] whereas the levels of antithrombin (AT) are lower than adult levels in the first 3 months of life and are comparable to the levels seen in patients with heterozygous AT deficiency. The physiologic ranges for coagulation factors in healthy newborns who have received intramuscular vitamin K after delivery are shown in Table 150.2.

Regulation of Thrombin

Despite decreased and delayed thrombin generation, neonates have excellent hemostasis. Thrombin regulation in neonatal plasma is similar to that in plasma from adults who are receiving therapeutic doses of anticoagulants. The concentration of thrombin generated in neonatal plasma is proportional to the available prothrombin concentration, whereas the rate of thrombin generation depends on the level of other procoagulant proteins. Clots formed from neonatal plasma bind less thrombin than clots formed from adult plasma, in part because of reduced thrombin generation. The reduced capacity to generate thrombin and the reduction in fibrin-bound thrombin may protect neonates from thrombosis.

Thrombin is inhibited by AT, α_2-macroglobulin, and heparin cofactor II. In neonates, the α_2-macroglobulin concentration is

TABLE
150.1
Neonatal Versus Adult Hemostasis

Component		Neonatal Versus Adult Level
Primary hemostasis	↔	Platelet count
	↑	vWF
Coagulation factors	↓	FII, FVII, FIX, FX
	↓	FXI, FXII
	↓ to ↔	FV, FXIII
	↔	Fibrinogen
	↔	FVIII
Anticoagulant factors	↓	TFPI, AT, PC, PS
	↑	α₂M
Fibrinolysis	↓	Plasminogen
	↔ to ↑	PAI

α_2M, α_2-Macroglobulin; AT, antithrombin; F, factor; PAI, plasminogen activator inhibitor; PC, protein C; PS, protein S; TFPI, tissue factor pathway inhibitor; vWF, von Willebrand factor.
Modified from Guzzetta NA, Miller BE: Principles of hemostasis in children: Models and maturation. *Paediatr Anaesth* 21:3, 2011.

twofold higher than that in adults. The overall capacity of newborn plasma to inhibit thrombin is similar to that of adult plasma, owing in part to the increased binding of thrombin by α_2-macroglobulin. Thrombin inhibition by heparin cofactor II is catalyzed by a dermatan sulfate–like proteoglycan, which is produced by the placenta and is found in both maternal and fetal plasma.

Regulation of thrombin generation is accomplished by upstream inhibition of the clotting proteins in the prothrombinase and tenase complexes (see Chapter 126). Plasma concentrations of protein C are low at birth and gradually increase to adult levels by 6 months of age. Although the total concentration of protein S is low at birth, the functional activity of protein S is comparable to that in adults because low levels of C4b-binding protein result in more free protein S. The interaction of protein S with activated protein C in neonatal plasma may be limited by the elevated levels of α_2-macroglobulin. Free tissue factor pathway inhibitor levels are lower than in adults, although total levels of tissue factor pathway inhibitor in neonatal plasma are similar to those in adult plasma.

The Fibrinolytic System

Although the levels of some of the components of the fibrinolytic system in neonates are different from those in adults, the clinical relevance of this finding is probably minimal. The fibrinolytic system regulates fibrin deposition by generating plasmin, which solubilizes fibrin. At birth, the fibrinolytic system has all the key components, but there are important age-related differences in the quantity and quality of the fibrinolytic proteins and enzymes. Plasma concentrations of plasminogen, tissue plasminogen activator (t-PA), and α_2-antiplasmin (α_2AP) are decreased, whereas plasma concentrations of plasminogen activator inhibitor 1 (PAI-1) are increased. As well, plasmin generation and overall fibrinolytic activity are decreased.[6] The capacity to generate plasmin in newborn plasma is generally reduced compared with adult plasma, which likely reflects the decreased plasminogen concentration. Despite lower levels of fibrinolytic components, the newborn fibrinolytic system is still effective.

The whole-blood clotting time and euglobulin clot lysis time are global assays of fibrinolytic activity but reflect only part of the physiologic fibrinolytic potential. Maneuvers that induce the release of endogenous fibrinolytic components, such as venous occlusion, desmopressin infusion, or exercise, provide more sensitive measures of in vivo fibrinolytic activity.[6]

Plasminogen levels are lower in neonates than in adults, and fetal plasminogen binds to cellular receptors with lower affinity because of

its increased sialic acid and mannose content. Although healthy neonates have lower plasmin-generating potential than adults, baseline levels of t-PA can increase up to eightfold with illness. Neonates with severe plasminogen deficiency have only a minimally increased risk for thrombosis, and most of their clinical findings are the result of impaired extravascular fibrinolysis. The major plasmin inhibitors circulate at near-adult levels in the neonate.

The contribution of differences in the neonatal and adult fibrinolytic systems to the protection from thromboembolic complications in childhood remains to be elucidated. Imbalance in the fibrinolytic system, whether hereditary or acquired, can lead to thrombotic or bleeding complications. Hereditary disorders, although rare, include plasminogen deficiency, PAI-1 deficiency, and α_2AP deficiency. The efficacy and safety of fibrinolytic therapy may be influenced by age-dependent differences in the fibrinolytic system. Data are lacking on the optimal doses of fibrinolytic agents for the pediatric population, especially for neonates. t-PA is the agent of choice, with the most common dose and duration of treatment being 0.5 mg/kg per hour infused over 6 hours.[7]

Platelets

Platelet production starts around the end of the first trimester of gestation and reaches adult values in the middle of the third trimester. Therefore platelet counts in term and premature newborns are not different from those in adults. Similarly, mean platelet volume and platelet ultrastructure in neonates closely resemble those in adults. Yet, all the main platelet functions are deficient at birth. Neonatal platelets exhibit reduced phospholipid metabolism, calcium mobilization, granule secretion, and aggregation in response to agonists compared with adult platelets.[8] Although thrombocytopenia is common in neonates, thrombocytosis is rare and is associated with prematurity.

There are two proposed theories behind the reduced platelet function at birth. One hypothesis suggests that platelet activation and degranulation at the time of labor and delivery lead to exhausted circulating platelets; the other suggests that intrinsic platelet peculiarities account for neonatal platelet deficiency. Indeed, differences in intrinsic signal transduction in the neonatal platelets alter platelet aggregation and activation responses. Platelet aggregation studies showed that aggregation of neonatal platelets was reduced in response to a number of agonists, including ADP, epinephrine, collagen, and thrombin and thromboxane analogues. This is especially true in preterm infants. Flow cytometric studies using monoclonal antibodies directed against platelet activation markers also indicate that platelets from cord blood or from neonates on the first postnatal day are hyporeactive compared with adult platelets.[8] This hyporesponsiveness is transient, and the platelets regain normal reactivity 10 to 14 days after delivery. However, the exact duration of hyporeactivity remains to be elucidated because some studies suggest that functional defects persist beyond the neonatal period.[9]

Despite the reduced platelet reactivity at birth, platelet adhesion may be enhanced because of the presence of higher concentration of functionally more potent high-molecular-weight vWF multimers in the plasma. Consistent with this concept, the bleeding time and the platelet function analyzer (PFA-100) closure time are shorter in neonates than in adults.[8] In healthy neonates, enhanced platelet adhesion immediately after delivery may compensate for the reduced platelet activation in response to agonists. Nonetheless, sick neonates may be at increased risk for bleeding.[8]

If available, the PFA-100 closure time is preferred over the bleeding time as a means of assessing platelet-related hemostasis. Bleeding time is an in vivo screening test that reflects the interaction between platelets and the blood vessel wall, but it is as variable in neonates as it is in adults. Also, the devices used for measuring bleeding time are not suitable for use in small infants. Consequently, the bleeding time is rarely determined. Although the PFA-100 will not detect mild defects in platelet function, such defects rarely cause serious bleeding in neonates.

TABLE 150.2   Reference Values (Ranges) for Common Coagulation Tests and Blood Coagulation Protein Levels by Age, Comparing Two Comprehensive Prospective Studies With Different Methodologies

	Day 1		Day 3 (Ref. 3) vs. Day 5 (Ref. 2)		1 Month–1 Year		Adult (Measured)	
	Ref. 3	Ref. 2	Ref. 3	Ref. 2	Ref. 3	Ref. 2	Ref. 3	Ref. 2
Prothrombin time (s)	15.6 (14.4–16.4)	13 (11.6–14.4)	14.9 (13.5–16.4)	12.4 (10.5–13.9)	13.1 (11.5–15.3)	12.3 (10.7–13.9)	13 (11.5–14.5)	12 (11–14)
PTT (s)	38.7 (34.3–44.8)	42.9 (31.3–54.5)	36.3 (29.5–42.2)	42.6 (25.4–59.8)	39.3 (35.1–46.3)	35.5 (28.1–42.9)	33.2 (28.6–38.2)	33 (27–40)
Thrombin time (s)	N/A	23.5 (19–28.3)	N/A	23.1 (18–29.2)	17.1 (16.3–17.6)	24.3 (19.4–29.2)	16.6 (16.2–17.2)	N/A
Fibrinogen (mg/dL)	280 (192–374)	283 (225–341)	330 (283–401)	312 (237–387)	242 (82–383)	251 (150–387)	310 (190–430)	278 (156–400)
Prothrombin (%)	54 (41–69)	48 (37–59)	62 (50–73)	63 (48–78)	90 (62–103)	88 (60–116)	110 (78–138)	108 (70–146)
Factor V (%)	81 (64–103)	72 (54–90)	122 (92–154)	95 (70–120)	113 (94–14)	91 (55–127)	118 (78–152)	106 (62–150)
Factor VII (%)	70 (52–88)	66 (47–85)	86 (67–107)	89 (62–116)	128 (83–160)	87 (47–127)	129 (61–199)	105 (67–143)
Factor VIII (%)	182 (105–329)	100 (61–139)	159 (83–274)	88 (55–121)	94 (54–145)	73 (53–109)	160 (52–290)	99 (50–149)
Factor IX (%)	48 (35–56)	53 (34–72)	72 (44–97)	53 (34–72)	71 (43–121)	86 (36–139)	130 (59–254)	109 (55–163)
Factor X (%)	55 (46–67)	40 (26–54)	60 (46–75)	49 (34–64)	95 (77–122)	78 (38–118)	124 (96–171)	106 (70–152)
Factor XI (%)	30 (7–41)	38 (24–52)	57 (24–79)	55 (39–71)	89 (62–125)	86 (49–134)	112 (67–196)	97 (67–127)
Factor XII (%)	58 (43–80)	53 (33–73)	53 (14–80)	47 (29–65)	79 (20–135)	77 (39–115)	115 (35–207)	108 (52–164)
Antithrombin III (%)	76 (58–90)	63 (51–75)	74 (60–89)	67 (54–80)	109 (72–134)	104 (84–124)	96 (66–124)	100 (74–126)
Protein C activity (%)	36 (24–44)	35 (26–44)	44 (28–54)	42 (31–53)	71 (31–112)	59 (37–81)	104 (74–164)	96 (64–128)
Protein S activity (%)	36 (28–47)	36 (24–48)	49 (33–67)	50 (36–64)	102 (29–162)	87 (55–119)	75 (54–103)	81 (60–113)
D-dimer (μg/mL)	1.47 (0.41–2.47)	N/A	1.34 (0.58–2.74)	N/A	0.22 (0.11–0.42)	N/A	0.18 (0.05–0.42)	N/A

N/A, Not available; PTT, partial thromboplastin time.
Modified from Ref. 2: Andrew M, Paes B, Milner R, et al: Development of the human coagulation system in the full-term infant. *Blood* 70:165, 1987; Ref. 3: Monagle P, Barnes C, Ignjatovic V, et al: Developmental haemostasis: Impact for clinical haemostasis laboratories. *Thromb Haemost* 95:362, 2006 (range inferred from published statistical documentation).

The Vessel Wall

Studies in vitro and in neonatal animals suggest that the endothelium from neonates has greater antithrombotic potential than the endothelium from adult vessels. In both rabbit venous and aortic models, neonatal endothelium expresses more heparan sulfate proteoglycans than adult endothelium, which results in greater AT-mediated anticoagulant activity in rabbit kits than in adults. Circulating levels of endothelial cell adhesion markers vary with age, implying dynamic expression and/or secretion of these proteins as a function of age.

NEONATAL HEMORRHAGIC DISORDERS

Significant bleeding in neonates should prompt clinical evaluation. In sick infants, acquired factor deficiencies or thrombocytopenia are frequently to blame, but rare congenital factor deficiencies can also manifest with neonatal bleeding. Attention to maternal factors (e.g., infection, thrombocytopenia, drugs) is critical when evaluating neonates. Initial empirical therapy consists of platelet and/or factor supplementation, which is often administered while diagnostic studies are under way.

EVALUATION OF THE BLEEDING NEONATE

Neonatal, peripartum, maternal, and family history are each important in the evaluation of a newborn with hemorrhagic complications. Maternal history of prior pregnancies, medications, and illnesses can provide clues to the hemostatic disorder in the neonate. The family history, such as parental ethnicity and consanguineous marriage, may help to identify congenital bleeding disorders. Maternal infection, drug use, or immune thrombocytopenia can lead to neonatal thrombocytopenia. Maternal deficiency of vitamin K or consumption of drugs that impair vitamin K metabolism can reduce the levels of the vitamin K–dependent coagulation proteins at birth. Vitamin K administration in the delivery room should be confirmed.

On physical examination, the location and characteristics of bleeding (e.g., procedural, mucosal, cutaneous, intraventricular), whether diffuse or localized, in addition to the general appearance of the baby as sick or well, will help to identify the underlying etiology of the hemorrhage. In ill-appearing newborns, disseminated intravascular coagulation (DIC) or liver disease may result in acquired factor deficiencies. These disorders tend to present with diffuse bleeding. Well-appearing newborns are more likely to have localized bleeding or ecchymoses because of thrombocytopenia from a transplacental antibody, vitamin K deficiency, or a rare inherited factor deficiency.

Laboratory evaluation of the hemorrhage in newborns should include sepsis evaluation and determination of the platelet count, PT, aPTT, thrombin time, and fibrinogen concentration. If the test results are normal, bleeding neonates or infants should be assessed for FXIII and α_2AP activity. Deficiencies of FXIII, α_2AP, or PAI-1 are not detected with routine screening, and specific testing is needed if deficiencies are suspected. The approach to laboratory screening is summarized in Fig. 150.1, which has been modified from Blanchette and Rand.[10] Platelet function should be evaluated when primary hemostatic defects are suspected.[11] In male infants with a family history of hemophilia or when hemophilia is suspected, the levels of FVIII and FIX should be determined, regardless of the degree of aPTT prolongation.

Neonatal Thrombocytopenia

The following factors are important to consider when evaluating neonates with thrombocytopenia: congenital or acquired, sick or well,

maternal antibody or drug, and platelet size. A classification of neonatal thrombocytopenia is provided in Table 150.3. Thrombocytopenia is defined as a platelet count less than 150×10^9/L.[12] Platelet counts in the range of 100 to 150×10^9/L are common in healthy neonates; these mostly reflect transient thrombocytopenia and require no further investigation unless there is a further decrease in the count. More severe thrombocytopenia (platelet count $<50 \times 10^9$/L) in neonates rarely manifests with bleeding, particularly in the absence of maternal antiplatelet antibodies. The estimated prevalence of thrombocytopenia is in the range of 1% to 5% of all newborns. The prevalence of thrombocytopenia increases to 22% to 35% in neonates admitted to the neonatal intensive care unit (NICU), with the rates increasing with decreasing gestational age. With severe thrombocytopenia, platelet transfusion may be necessary to treat or decrease the risk of bleeding.

Causes of neonatal thrombocytopenia include decreased platelet production, increased platelet consumption, and/or hypersplenism (see Chapters 131 and 132). Other contributing factors include infection, placental insufficiency, genetic disorders, medications, DIC, or immune deficiency. In well-appearing newborns, thrombocytopenia is usually immune mediated and related to maternal transplacental immunoglobulin G antibodies or drugs (e.g., quinine, hydralazine, thiazides, tolbutamide). In sick newborns, platelet destruction is often related to infection, DIC, extracorporeal membrane oxygenation (ECMO), thrombosis, or mechanical ventilation for hyaline membrane disease. Large-vessel thrombosis can also lead to thrombocytopenia, as can specific syndromes, such as renal vein thrombosis (RVT), necrotizing enterocolitis, or vascular anomalies (Kasabach-Merritt syndrome). Platelet production can be impaired with hypoxic-ischemic

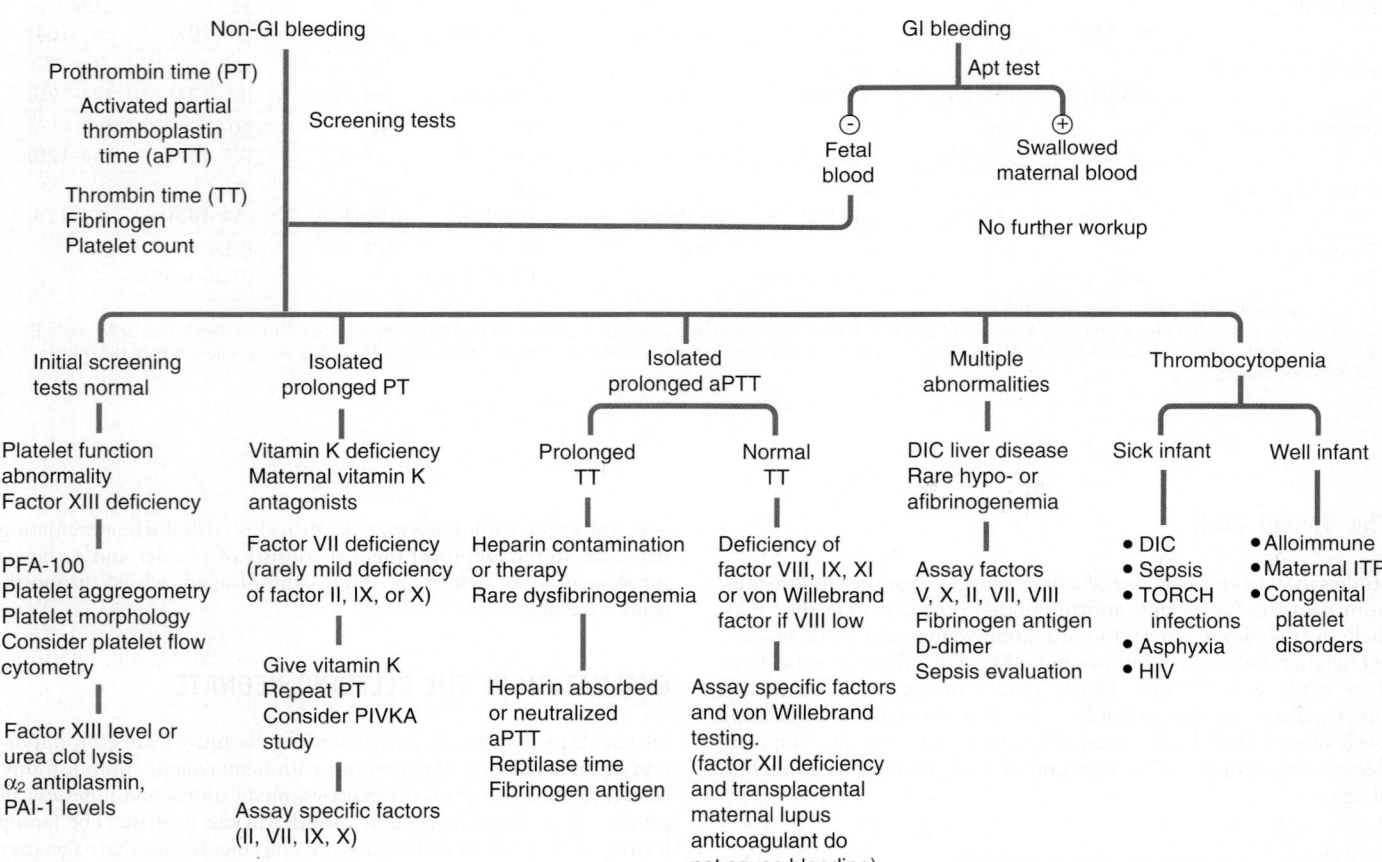

Fig. 150.1 DIAGNOSTIC APPROACH TO THE BLEEDING NEONATE. *DIC,* Disseminated intravascular coagulation; *GI,* gastrointestinal; *HIV,* human immunodeficiency virus; *ITP,* immune thrombocytopenia purpura; *PAI-1,* plasminogen activator inhibitor 1; *PIVKA,* proteins induced by vitamin k absence (antagonist); *TORCH,* toxoplasmosis, other agents, rubella, cytomegalovirus, herpes simplex. *(Modified from Blanchette VS, Rand ML: Platelet disorders in newborn infants: diagnosis and management.* Semin Perinatol *21:53, 1997.)*

TABLE 150.3	Classification of Fetal and Neonatal Thrombocytopenia		
	Fetal	**Early-Onset Neonatal(<72 h)**	**Late-Onset Neonatal(>72 h)**
Conditions	• **Alloimmune** • **Congenital infection** (e.g., CMV, toxoplasma, rubella, HIV) • **Aneuploidy** (e.g., trisomies 18, 13, 21) • Autoimmune (e.g., ITP, SLE) • Severe rhesus hemolytic disease • Inherited (e.g., Wiskott-Aldrich syndrome)	• **Chronic fetal hypoxia** (e.g., PIH, IUGR, diabetes) • Perinatal asphyxia • **Perinatal infection** (e.g., *Escherichia coli*, GBS, *Haemophilus influenzae*) • DIC • Alloimmune • Autoimmune (e.g., ITP, SLE) • Congenital infection (e.g., CMV, toxoplasma, rubella, HIV) • Thrombosis (e.g., aortic, renal vein) • Bone marrow replacement (e.g., congenital leukemia) • Kasabach-Merritt syndrome • Metabolic disease (e.g., propionic and methylmalonic acidemia) • Inherited (e.g., TAR, CAMT)	• **Late-onset sepsis** • **NEC** • Congenital infection (e.g., CMV, toxoplasma, rubella, HIV) • Autoimmune • Kasabach-Merritt syndrome • Metabolic disease (e.g., propionic and methylmalonic acidemia) • Inherited (e.g., TAR, CAMT)

CAMT, Congenital amegakaryocytic thrombocytopenia; CMV, cytomegalovirus; DIC, disseminated intravascular coagulation; GBS, group B Streptococcus; HIV, human immunodeficiency virus; ITP, idiopathic thrombocytopenic purpura; IUGR, intrauterine growth restriction; NEC, necrotizing enterocolitis; PIH, pregnancy-induced hypertension; SLE, systemic lupus erythematosus, TAR, thrombocytopenia with absent radii. The most frequently occurring conditions are in **bold**.
Modified from Roberts I, Stanworth S, Murray NA: Thrombocytopenia in the neonate. *Blood Rev* 22:173, 2008.

injury, perhaps because fetal megakaryocytes are particularly sensitive to hypoxia. Transient mild to moderate thrombocytopenia is common in newborns from pregnancies that were complicated by intrauterine growth restriction or pregnancy-induced hypertension. Other rare causes of decreased platelet production in neonates include primary congenital platelet or marrow disorders and infiltrative disorders. These are summarized in Table 150.4.

Neonatal Alloimmune Thrombocytopenia

Neonatal alloimmune thrombocytopenia is the platelet equivalent of hemolytic disease of the newborn. It affects approximately 1 in 2000 pregnancies. When fetal platelets express paternal human platelet antigens (HPAs) that the mother lacks, transplacental passage of maternal immunoglobulin G directed against fetal platelets can occur and usually results in severe neonatal thrombocytopenia (platelet count $<30 \times 10^9$/L). This may result in major bleeding, particularly intracranial hemorrhage (ICH), which can occur in 10% to 20% of untreated pregnancies.[12] Incompatibilities for HPA-1a account for the majority of cases of neonatal alloimmune thrombocytopenia in white populations. About half of the cases of neonatal alloimmune thrombocytopenia occur in the first pregnancy because fetal platelets pass into the maternal circulation early in the pregnancy. Treatment options include transfusion of antigen-negative platelets if available (HPA-1a ± 5b). Although large randomized studies are lacking, the threshold count for platelet transfusion in most studies is 30×10^9/L. High-dose intravenous immunoglobulin and/or a trial of random donor platelets can be given if compatible platelets are unavailable. The recommended total dose of intravenous immunoglobulin is 1 to 2 g/kg administered either at a dose of 0.4 g/kg daily for 3 to 5 days or at a dose of 1 g/kg daily for 1 or 2 days.[13]

Inherited Thrombocytopenia

Most cases of inherited thrombocytopenia are the result of decreased platelet production because of abnormal hematopoietic stem or progenitor cell development. Such disorders are often associated with congenital anomalies, which can inform the course of investigation and aid in the diagnosis.[12] Disorders that present with neonatal thrombocytopenia include Bernard-Soulier syndrome, type 2B von Willebrand disease (vWD), Wiskott-Aldrich syndrome, Fanconi anemia, thrombocytopenia with absent radii syndrome, amegakaryocytic thrombocytopenia with radioulnar synostosis, congenital

TABLE 150.4	Syndromic, Genetic Conditions and Acquired Marrow Disorders as Causes of Neonatal Thrombocytopenia
Inborn Errors of Metabolism	
Isovaleric acidemia	
Methylmalonic acidemia (with acute acidosis) and cobalamin metabolic defects	
Holocarboxylase deficiency	
Mitochondrial disorders	
Pearson syndrome	
Kearns-Sayre syndrome	
Genetic Marrow Failure Syndromes	
Amegakaryocytic thrombocytopenia	
Fanconi anemia	
Other Syndromic Thrombocytopenias	
Thrombocytopenia with absent radii syndrome	
Paris-Trousseau syndrome	
X-linked thrombocytopenias	
Wiskott-Aldrich syndrome	
GATA1 mutations	
Aneuploidy	
Trisomy 21, 13, or 18	
Genetic Macrothrombocytopenias	
May-Hegglin, Sebastian, and Fechtner syndromes	
Bernard-Soulier syndrome	
Acquired Marrow Disorders	
Oncologic	
Neonatal leukemia	
Neuroblastoma	
Histiocytic lymphohistiocytosis	

amegakaryocytic thrombocytopenia, X-linked macrothrombocytopenia caused by *GATA1* mutation, giant platelet syndromes, and metabolic disorders.

Platelet Function Disorders

Qualitative platelet disorders are rarely associated with overt neonatal bleeding. Patients presenting with bleeding who have normal coagulation test results and platelet counts require further investigation.

Bleeding may be from mucocutaneous sites, sites of capillary blood sampling, cephalohematoma, umbilical stump, or at sites of procedures. Platelet function disorders result from defects in a number of structures and signaling pathways as outlined in Table 150.5. Only the most severe genetic disorders of platelet function present in the neonatal period. These include Glanzmann thrombasthenia and Bernard-Soulier syndrome (see Chapters 125 and 130). Maternal medications may affect platelet function, most notably aspirin, although low-dose aspirin does not appear to alter neonatal platelet function. Neonatal medications may also affect platelet function. Common offenders include nitric oxide, prostaglandin E_2, indomethacin, and aspirin.

It is especially challenging to diagnose platelet function disorders in neonates because of the technical limitations of many platelet function assays and the need for large volumes of blood for testing. Initial screening for suspected platelet function disorders can be performed using the PFA-100 analyzer followed by evaluation of platelet morphology and platelet aggregation responses using light transmission aggregometry. Flow cytometry can be used to evaluate specific surface glycoproteins, and electron microscopy studies can be used to assess platelet granule morphology.

Although the PFA-100 is a sensitive test for detecting hemostatic disorders in the pediatric population, it is relatively nonspecific. Light transmission aggregometry is highly reproducible in patients with inherited mucocutaneous bleeding if properly standardized. Absent

TABLE 150.5	**Inherited Disorders of Platelet Function**

Defects in Receptors for Adhesive Proteins

Bernard-Soulier syndrome,[a] platelet-type von Willebrand disease (GPIb-IX-V complex)

Glanzmann thrombasthenia[a] (GPIIb/IIIa, $\alpha_{IIb}\beta_3$)

GPIa/IIa, $\alpha_2\beta_1$

GPVI

GPIV

Defects in Soluble Agonist Receptors

Thromboxane A2 receptor

α_2-Adrenergic receptor

P2Y$_{12}$ receptor

Defects in Platelet Granules

δ-Storage pool deficiency, Hermansky-Pudlak syndrome, Chediak-Higashi syndrome, thrombocytopenia with absent radii syndrome (δ-granules)

Gray platelet syndrome, Quebec platelet disorder, Paris-Trousseau-Jacobsen syndrome (α-granules)

α,δ-storage pool deficiency (α- and δ-granules)

Defects in Signal-Transduction Pathways

Primary secretion defects

Abnormalities of the arachidonic acid/TXA2 pathway

G$_{\alpha q}$ deficiency

Partial selective PLC-β$_2$ deficiency

Defects in pleckstrin phosphorylation

Defects in Ca^{2+} mobilization

Abnormalities of Cytoskeleton

MYH9-related disorders (May-Hegglin anomaly, Sebastian syndrome, Fechtner syndrome, Epstein syndrome)

Wiskott-Aldrich syndrome

X-linked thrombocytopenia

Abnormalities of Membrane Phospholipids

Scott syndrome

Stormorken syndrome

[a]Can manifest in neonatal period.
GP, Glycoprotein; PLC, phospholipase C; MYH9, myosin heavy chain 9; TXA2, thromboxane A2.
Modified from Israels SJ, El-Ekiaby M, Quiroga T, et al: Inherited disorders of platelet function and challenges to diagnosis of mucocutaneous bleeding. *Haemophilia* 16:152, 2010.

platelet aggregation in response to all agonists and deficiency of $\alpha_{IIb}\beta_3$ on flow cytometry are diagnostic for Glanzmann thrombasthenia (see Chapters 125 and 130). Flow cytometry also provides definitive diagnostic information about Bernard-Soulier syndrome, dense granule deficiency, and Scott syndrome.

Platelet transfusions are often given if the patient is bleeding. However, the potential risk of human leukocyte antigen allosensitization if normal platelets are given to patients with congenital deficiency of platelet surface antigens must be weighed against the severity of bleeding when functional defects are suspected. It is recommended to restrict platelet transfusion in patients with Glanzmann thrombasthenia. Recombinant activated FVII (rFVIIa) has been used to avoid allosensitization. Other adjunctive measures include local control such as use of fibrin sealant in oral bleeding and antifibrinolytic medications, such as tranexamic acid.

Vitamin K Deficiency Bleeding

Vitamin K is an essential cofactor for γ-glutamyl carboxylase, the enzyme required for posttranslational carboxylation of prothrombin; FVII; FIX; FX; and proteins C, S, and Z. Many newborns are deficient in vitamin K, whether measured in cord blood or indirectly by measuring the levels of the vitamin K–dependent coagulation proteins. Risk factors for bleeding with vitamin K deficiency include maternal malabsorption, maternal intake of drugs that impair vitamin K metabolism, exclusive breastfeeding, and neonatal malabsorption. Classification is based on the time of presentation.

Early vitamin K deficiency bleeding occurs in the first 24 to 48 hours of life and is usually associated with maternal intake of drugs (e.g., phenytoin, barbiturates, antibiotics), which cross the placenta and impair vitamin K synthesis. Classical vitamin K deficiency bleeding manifests from days 2 to 7 of life and is related to low placental transfer of vitamin K, low concentrations in breast milk, lack of gastrointestinal bacterial flora, and poor oral intake. Gastrointestinal bleeding is the most common presentation, but procedural bleeding, bruising, or ICH can occur. Late-onset vitamin K deficiency–related bleeding can occur at times up to 12 weeks of age, usually in association with exclusive breastfeeding or with neonatal fat malabsorption, and often manifests as catastrophic bleeding, including ICH. Congenital vitamin K deficiency is an autosomal recessive disorder that occurs because of mutations in the genes encoding γ-glutamyl carboxylase or the vitamin K$_{2,3}$–epoxide reductase complex. Neonates with this disorder often have severe bleeding, including ICH. Genotype analysis is necessary to confirm the defects.[14]

The diagnostic criteria for vitamin K deficiency bleeding include an elevated international normalized ratio (INR), normal levels of fibrinogen, and a normal platelet count. The diagnosis is confirmed if the INR normalizes after administration of vitamin K and the bleeding stops. The aPTT is prolonged with severe vitamin K deficiency. Prophylaxis with a single dose of vitamin K (0.5 to 1 mg) in the delivery room prevents early- and classic-onset bleeding. Although oral dosing may be effective, because of the potential for impaired absorption, regurgitation, or noncompliance, parenteral administration by the intramuscular, subcutaneous, or intravenous route is preferred. Additional doses of oral vitamin K should be given at days 7 and 28 in breastfed infants.

Vitamin K–induced coagulopathy should be treated with vitamin K, which can be given by intravenous infusion or by subcutaneous injection (to minimize anaphylactoid reactions). Intramuscular injection should be avoided with severe deficiency because of the potential for hematoma formation. If there is bleeding, fresh frozen plasma (FFP) at a dose of 10 to 15 mL/kg body weight can be given. Owing to the potential for thrombotic complications, prothrombin complex concentrate should be reserved for life-threatening bleeding or situations where FFP may produce volume overload. Prothrombin complex concentrate has the added benefit of decreased volume load. In the absence of published guidelines, extrapolation from adult data suggests that a prothrombin complex concentrate dose of 50 units/

kg is sufficient. The overall prognosis of vitamin K deficiency bleeding is good.

Inherited Coagulation Disorders

Prolonged aPTT

In neonates, the aPTT is physiologically prolonged compared with adult values. Hemophilia is the most common inherited coagulation disorder, as discussed in detail in Chapter 135. Evaluation for FVIII, FIX, and FXI deficiencies should be undertaken immediately in any neonate bleeding with an isolated prolongation of the aPTT or a positive family history. Cord blood samples can be used in those with a family history, thereby avoiding the need for peripheral venipuncture, but careful sampling is important to avoid maternal contamination of the sample. In term and preterm infants, FVIII levels are within the normal adult range despite physiologic differences in the hemostatic system. Thus confirmation of hemophilia A is possible in the neonatal period, regardless of gestational age of the child or severity of the condition. However, because the levels of the vitamin K–dependent clotting factors, including FIX, are reduced at birth (and even lower in preterm infants), diagnosis of hemophilia B, particularly mild hemophilia B, is difficult in the neonatal period.

Male newborns with a family history of hemophilia should be evaluated before receiving intramuscular injections, including vitamin K. Typically newborns with hemophilia and bleeding appear well. Male infants far outnumber females in this population, given the location of both FVIII and FIX genes on the X chromosome. However, severe FVIII or FIX deficiency can, albeit rarely, present in females, such as in Turner syndrome or extreme lyonization. Approximately one-third of cases of hemophilia are the result of spontaneous mutations; consequently a family history may be lacking. FXI deficiency is inherited in an autosomal dominant or recessive manner, so female newborns with bleeding and isolated prolongation of the aPTT should also be tested. Evaluation of hemophilia carrier status in mothers of unknown status (e.g., single prior affected child or positive history in maternal grandmother) can be performed genetically because factor levels in carriers are variable and can overlap with normal levels. Most bleeding episodes in newborn males occur after circumcision or umbilical stump separation, although ICH is reported in approximately 3.5% of newborns with hemophilia,[15] and cephalhematoma is common. Joint bleeding is unusual in the neonatal period. Patients with known or suspected hemophilia and those with severe deficiencies of FVII, FX, or FXIII should be screened for ICH. Although cranial ultrasonography is often used for screening purposes, computed tomography or magnetic resonance imaging is more sensitive for detection of small parafalcine bleeds, which can also occur in a small percentage of normal neonates.[11] Neonates with hemophilia A or B are treated with recombinant FVIII or FIX concentrates, respectively. Routine prophylaxis is controversial after uncomplicated term delivery but is recommended for high-risk situations, such as prolonged labor, forceps delivery, or for preterm infants.

Isolated Prolonged PT

In term neonates, the PT is normal. Inherited FVII deficiency is a rare, autosomal recessive condition with a strong gene dosage effect. Neonatal bleeding can occur in severe cases (i.e., homozygosity or compound heterozygosity for two mutations in the FVII gene). FVII deficiency can be associated with microcephaly or midline defects because disruption of chromosome 13q can lead to loss of adjacent genes. As a vitamin K–dependent protein, FVII deficiency can occur in association with deficiencies of the other vitamin K–dependent clotting proteins with abnormalities of the vitamin K pathways. Low doses of rFVIIa can be used for treatment of isolated FVII deficiency; FFP and/or vitamin K can be used for management of combined deficiencies.

Prolonged PT and aPTT

The association of bleeding with prolongation of both the PT and aPTT in a healthy newborn may indicate vitamin K deficiency or congenital deficiencies of prothrombin, FV or FX, as well as rare combined deficiencies. Routine prophylactic administration of vitamin K_1 to newborns can complicate the diagnosis of vitamin K deficiency bleeding in neonates.[16] More commonly, combined PT and aPTT prolongation occurs in sick newborns with DIC or severe hepatic disease. Combined factor deficiencies are rare but must be considered when the laboratory findings or clinical course is confusing. Autosomal recessive mutations in LMAN1 (ERGIC-53) or MCFD2 can lead to combined FV and FVIII deficiency because of defective intracellular processing of the factors. Mutations in γ-glutamyl carboxylase are associated with inherited combined deficiencies of all the vitamin K–dependent proteins. FVII deficiency has rarely been reported in combination with FV, FVIII, FIX, FX, FXI, and protein C defects, as reviewed by Girolami et al.[17]

FXIII Deficiency

FXIII is a transglutaminase that cross-links fibrin, thereby rendering it resistant to lysis. FXIII deficiency is inherited in an autosomal recessive manner, and the prevalence of FXIII deficiency is estimated to be 1 in 3 million to 1 in 5 million. Homozygotes usually have FXIII levels of less than 1% and have a severe bleeding diathesis. Patients with heterozygous FXIII deficiency are usually asymptomatic but have reduced levels of FXIII.[18] Neonates with FXIII deficiency may present with umbilical bleeding a few days after birth, a frequent finding that occurs in 80% of cases. More severe bleeding, including ICH, occurs in 25% to 30% of patients, a frequency higher than that in patients with hemophilia. ICH is the major cause of death and disability in neonates with FXIII deficiency, and ICH in a child with no other risk factors should prompt a search for FXIII deficiency.

FXIII deficiency is not detected with screening PT, aPTT, or thrombin time assays. Specific assays for FXIII or urea clot solubility testing are used for diagnosis. The clot solubility test is sensitive to very low levels of FXIII (<1%) but is normal if FXIII levels are in the 1% to 3% range. Consequently, FXIII immunoassays are perferable.[18]

Treatment of FXIII deficiency includes FFP, cryoprecipitate, or plasma-derived FXIII concentrate. The prognosis is excellent, but affected patients face a lifelong risk for bleeding, and those with severe deficiency require prophylaxis. In 2013, the US Food and Drug Administration approved a new recombinant FXIII A-subunit for use as routine prophylaxis in patients with FXIII deficiency.

Other Inherited Deficiencies Associated With Neonatal Bleeding

vWD, which is the most common inherited bleeding diathesis, is described in detail in Chapter 138. vWD is rarely associated with neonatal bleeding and may be associated with the most severe subtypes. In a case series that included 55 newborns with vWD, there were no bleeding complications, although cases of scalp hematomas and bleeding after vitamin K injection or umbilical stump detachment were reported. Acquired forms of vWD also are rare but may complicate obstetric management of affected mothers and can affect their newborn babies. A family history of vWD, especially type 2 vWD, should prompt vWD evaluation in the neonate before circumcision and possibly before intramuscular injections. There is a possible association of vWD with acute idiopathic pulmonary hemorrhage. The diagnosis of vWD may be difficult because vWF concentrations are high at birth and there is a large proportion of high-molecular-weight vWF multimers. Children with a diagnosis of type 3 vWD should be tested for mutations that predispose them to inhibitory alloantibody formation before aggressive replacement with exogenous vWF.[19] Treatment of neonates with vWD involves administration of plasma-derived concentrates that contain vWF (e.g., Humate-P or Alphanate), dosed initially at 40 to 60 ristocetin cofactor units/kg.

Although most of the bleeding problems in neonates are acquired, patients with severe deficiencies of coagulation factors can present in the neonatal period. Autosomal recessive deficiencies, in either homozygous or compound heterozygous state, are grouped as rare coagulation disorders that can manifest as severe bleeding diatheses. In the neonatal period, severe deficiencies of fibrinogen, FVII, FX, and FXIII are the most likely disorders to present with bleeding conditions. One common feature of these disorders is the association with ICH.[20] Deficiency of fibrinogen can manifest with bleeding in the soft tissues, bleeding after circumcision, or bleeding after umbilical stump detachment. The diagnosis can be established with fibrinogen assays, and treatment involves replacement with cryoprecipitate or, if available, fibrinogen concentrate (see box on Recommended Dosing for Transfusion in Neonatal Hemorrhage). Severe FXI deficiency is more prevalent in Ashkenazi Jews and can present with bleeding in newborns after hemostatic challenges, such as circumcision. FV and prothrombin deficiencies are the other rare autosomal recessive homozygous deficiencies that can cause hemorrhagic symptoms.[11]

Not all deficiencies result in a bleeding diathesis. Even complete deficiencies of the contact factors, which include high-molecular-weight kininogen, prekallikrein, and FXII, are not associated with a bleeding phenotype. Autosomal recessive deficiencies of α_2AP and PAI-1 have been associated with bleeding, but not in the neonatal period.

Liver Disease

Acute liver disease or hepatic failure is uncommon in neonates. Liver disease in neonates may be caused by viral hepatitis, parenteral nutrition, cholestasis, hypoxic injury, or metabolic disease. Rare disorders that cause liver failure in neonates include hereditary tyrosinemia, neonatal hemochromatosis, and hemophagocytic lymphohistiocytosis. Liver dysfunction can affect the hemostatic balance, resulting in activation of the coagulation and fibrinolytic systems, reduced synthesis of coagulation factors, poor clearance of activated hemostatic components, thrombocytopenia, platelet dysfunction, loss of coagulation proteins into ascites fluid, and failure to use vitamin K.[21]

Owing to reduced synthesis of multiple coagulation proteins, laboratory workup typically reveals a prolonged PT and aPTT. Acute liver disease also results in elevated liver enzyme levels, direct hyperbilirubinemia, and elevated ammonia concentrations. The platelet count may be reduced, especially if hypersplenism is present, and platelet dysfunction is common. Hypofibrinogenemia is a late manifestation of liver disease, and elevated fibrin degradation products and D-dimer occur because of delayed hepatic clearance. Assays of FV, FVII, and FVIII can help distinguish between liver disease, vitamin K deficiency, and consumptive coagulopathy (e.g., DIC). FV and FVIII are not vitamin K–dependent clotting factors. FV is synthesized in the liver, whereas FVIII is synthesized in multiple cell types, and the levels of both in neonates are similar to those in adults. Deficiency of all three implies consumption, whereas decreased levels of FV and FVII with a normal FVIII level suggest liver disease.

Treatment should include replacement with FFP and/or cryoprecipitate, as well as platelet transfusion. Fibrinogen concentrate has been used as an alternative to cryoprecipitate. Patients with biliary atresia or other cholestatic liver failure syndromes may also benefit from parenteral vitamin K. The outcome is dependent on treatment of the underlying cause of liver disease.

Intraventricular Hemorrhage

Intraventricular hemorrhage (IVH) is associated with significant morbidity and mortality in the newborn period, particularly in premature infants. In the United States, it is estimated that approximately 12,000 premature infants and 20% to 25% of very low-birth-weight infants develop IVH each year. With improvements in neonatal care, the incidence of IVH is decreasing.

The etiology of IVH is multifactorial and includes prematurity of the cerebral vasculature and ischemia-reperfusion injury related to ventilatory support, blood pressure lability, and ECMO. Other risk factors for IVH include vaginal delivery, severe respiratory distress syndrome (RDS), low Apgar scores, pneumothorax, hypoxia, hypercapnia, seizures, patent ductus arteriosus, and infection. Many of these risk factors induce IVH by altering cerebral blood flow. Coagulopathy and thrombocytopenia can contribute to IVH, but their role in the pathogenesis of IVH is uncertain. One study reported hypofibrinogenemia, thrombocytopenia, or prolonged clotting time in 11 of 15 neonates with IVH and in only 5 of 35 unaffected newborns. Hemorrhage complicating cerebral vein thrombosis may explain some cases of IVH (especially in full-term infants), and heterozygosity for the FV Leiden mutation was reported in 18% of neonates with grades 2 to 4 IVH compared with 3% of controls. Cerebellar hemorrhage should raise suspicion of organic acidemia, such as methylmalonic, propionic, or isovaleric acidemia.

Vitamin K, indomethacin, AT, FFP, FXIII, tranexamic acid, and ethamsylate has been evaluated for prevention of IVH with mixed results. rFVIIa may be useful for treatment of IVH, but additional studies are needed to determine its efficacy and safety.

Extracorporeal Membrane Oxygenation

ECMO is occasionally used for treatment of neonates with severe pulmonary hypertension or cardiomyopathy. The ECMO pump, oxygenation membrane, and large-bore catheters can induce thrombosis, which necessitates administration of high-dose systemic anticoagulation, thereby placing patients at risk for bleeding. Thrombosis and hemorrhage are common complications in pediatric ECMO patients, particularly if ECMO is initiated after open heart surgery. Approximately 15% of neonates on ECMO sustain an ICH.[22]

With the doses of heparin used during ECMO, the PT and aPTT may not correlate with the activated clotting time (ACT). Furthermore, there is evidence that the heparin dose provides prognostic information in ECMO patients independent of the ACT, suggesting that an ACT of 180 to 220 seconds may not provide adequate anticoagulation. Prolonged ECMO is associated with depletion of clotting factors and high levels of fibrin degradation products. Consequently, the aPTT and ACT are prolonged and the levels of D-dimer are increased even when low doses of heparin are administered.

A retrospective study of 29 nonsurvivors of ECMO revealed that most patients have a coagulopathy characterized by a prolonged PT and aPTT, as well as being thrombocytopenic, and most had low

---

Recommended Dosing for Transfusion in Neonatal Hemorrhage

PRBC: 10 to 15 mL/kg single-donor PRBC infused over 4 hours
Platelets[a]: 10 mL/kg raises platelet count by 75,000 (goal >50,000 if bleeding, >20,000 if not bleeding)
FFP: 10 to 20 mL/kg every 6 to 12 hours for purpura fulminans
Cryoprecipitate: 0.15 units/kg raises fibrinogen about 100 mg/dL (goal >150 mg/dL if bleeding, >50 mg/dL if not bleeding)
vWF: 40 to 60 ristocetin cofactor units/kg of plasma-derived FVIII/vWF preparations
Factor VIII: for hemophilia A—50 units/kg load, then 25 units/kg every 12 hours; recombinant factor preferred (monitor FVIII)
Factor IX: for hemophilia B—80 to 100 units/kg daily; recombinant factor preferred (monitor FIX)
Factor VIIa: for severe factor VII deficiency—20 to 30 µg/kg every 6 to 12 hours

FFP, Fresh frozen plasma; PRBC, packed red blood cells; vWF, von Willebrand factor.
[a]Volume limits transfusion of platelets by the "unit" in small neonates. Practices vary; follow institutional guidelines for volume dosing or volume reduction.

levels of fibrinogen despite ACT values that were within the acceptable range of 180 to 220 seconds in the final 24 hours of ECMO. Thus routine laboratory testing is inadequate for predicting or preventing thrombotic or hemorrhagic complications in pediatric ECMO patients. Thrombin generation assays, anti-FXa heparin levels, and thromboelastography have been suggested as alternatives to the ACT. Data supporting the use of these tests are lacking.

In neonates with established thrombosis or at risk for thrombosis, daily FFP infusion is sometimes used as a source of plasminogen and anticoagulant proteins. Data supporting this approach are lacking.

Respiratory Distress Syndrome

RDS, also known as *hyaline membrane disease,* is an acute pulmonary process that is common in premature neonates. The disorder is characterized by hyaline membrane formation and fibrin deposition in diffuse areas of atelectasis. Although severe RDS is associated with increased thrombin generation and decreased levels of AT, interventions aimed at addressing these abnormalities have yielded inconclusive results. Plasmin or plasminogen may enhance survival; heparin is of uncertain benefit, and AT supplementation may increase mortality. Additional studies are needed to explore the utility of anticoagulant or thrombolytic therapies in RDS. A laboratory profile consistent with mild DIC is common in RDS; fibrinogen levels are decreased, and levels of D-dimer are elevated. An unexpected increase in ventilatory support should raise the suspicion of pulmonary embolism in this population.

NEONATAL THROMBOEMBOLIC DISORDERS

The incidence of thromboembolism (TE) has a bimodal peak, with an increased occurrence in newborns and adolescents. Important risk factors for the development of neonatal TE include vascular catheterization, a hypercoagulable state conferred by the developing coagulation system, and comorbidities such as congenital heart disease, dehydration, sepsis, congenital nephritic syndrome, necrotizing enterocolitis, and asphyxia.[3]

Laboratory workup often reveals a hypercoagulable state such as decreased levels of AT, protein C, and protein S; defective fibrinolysis; hyperactive platelets; elevated levels of clotting factors (i.e., fibrinogen, FVII, FVIII); and the presence of antiphospholipid antibodies or thrombophilic defects, such as FV Leiden or the prothrombin gene mutation.[1-3] A family history of TE or miscarriages may indicate a hereditary thrombophilia.

Consensus guidelines have been developed for the management of neonatal TE.[7] Heparin, either unfractionated heparin (UFH) or low-molecular-weight heparin (LMWH), remains the mainstay of treatment in newborns. If the thrombus is limb or life threatening, thrombolytic therapy may be considered. Most recommendations are of low-grade level because the evidence in this patient population is derived from case reports, case series, registries, and extrapolation from studies in adults. Large, multicenter, prospective controlled clinical trials are needed to generate evidence-based guidelines; such studies are problematic in neonates.

Incidence

Current estimates of the incidence of neonatal TE are derived from three international registries, each with different inclusion criteria. Registry data from Canada, Germany, and the Netherlands indicate the incidence of TE in neonates to be 24 per 10,000 NICU admissions, 0.51 per 10,000 live births, and 14.5 per 10,000 live births, respectively.[23-25] Two-thirds of thromboembolic events are venous, and 80% are either catheter associated or develop after a severe illness.[26] Arterial thromboembolic events in neonates usually present as strokes or emboli to the limbs from catheter-associated thrombi. Neonatal TE is associated with significant mortality and morbidity.

Acquired Thrombophilia

Indwelling Catheters

Central venous and arterial access is essential for the advanced care provided in modern neonatology. The most common acquired thrombotic risk factor in neonates is the presence of an indwelling vascular catheter. In a recent literature review by Park et al,[27] the incidence of TE in neonates with central venous catheters was 9.2%. Length of catheter stay, infusion of blood products, and malpositioned umbilical venous catheters were found to be important risk factors. The most frequently reported sites of thrombosis are hepatic veins, right atrium, and inferior vena cava.[25] The incidence of catheter-associated deep vein thrombosis (DVT) is influenced by the method of detection. When catheters are used for total parenteral nutrition, it is estimated that DVT is diagnosed in 1% on clinical grounds, in 35% by echocardiography, and in 75% by venography. Although contrast venography is regarded as the reference standard for the diagnosis of thrombosis in neonates with central venous catheters, ultrasonography is more commonly used because it is noninvasive, is easy to perform at the bedside, and does not expose patients to ionizing radiation.

DVT often causes pain, swelling, and discoloration of the affected limb. Loss of catheter patency, evidence of collateral circulation, and/or unexplained thrombocytopenia should raise the suspicion of DVT. Prospective imaging studies performed before central access catheter removal demonstrate thrombi in up to 86% of patients.[24] Treatment often begins with removal of the catheter, although consideration of anticoagulation before catheter removal is warranted, especially in infants with right-to-left intracardiac or intrapulmonary shunting. Small catheter-associated thrombi may resolve without specific therapy. Larger thrombi or those in locations associated with greater morbidity (e.g., sinovenous, renal, portal) may warrant short courses of heparin or thrombolytic agents.[7] Platelets should never be administered through arterial catheters because of the potential risk for TE.

Disseminated Intravascular Coagulation

Neonates are susceptible to DIC because of their immature anticoagulant and fibrinolytic systems. Most cases of neonatal DIC are associated with tissue ischemia and acidosis secondary to sepsis, low-output cardiac failure, perinatal asphyxia, severe RDS, or necrotizing enterocolitis. Other causes of DIC are conditions that lead to consumptive coagulopathy such as large vascular anomalies, severe liver disease, massive hemolysis, or hereditary thrombophilia. DIC may present with hemorrhage and/or TE. Bleeding in a well-appearing neonate is usually the result of an inherited deficiency of a coagulation protein or immune-mediated thrombocytopenia rather than DIC. In contrast, bleeding in a sick preterm neonate is more likely the result of DIC. Patients with DIC often exhibit a prolonged PT, aPTT, and thrombin clotting time, decreased fibrinogen and FVIII levels, thrombocytopenia, and increased levels of D-dimer (Table 150.6).

Definitive therapy requires identification and reversal of the trigger for DIC. FFP, platelets (if bleeding is severe), and cryoprecipitate (if the fibrinogen concentration is low) are given to replace the consumed factors. Reasonable treatment targets include maintaining the fibrinogen level over 100 mg/dL, the platelet count over 50×10^9/L, and the PT close to normal. Heparin should be given if there is TE along with AT concentrate if indicated. Successful treatment of DIC depends on reversal of the trigger and provision of aggressive supportive care. Therapy aimed at reversing the coagulopathy has little effect on DIC outcome.

Hereditary Thrombophilia

Spontaneous TE is rare in healthy newborns, and this presentation should prompt evaluation for hereditary thrombophilia. Among the

TABLE
150.6
Diagnosis of Neonatal DIC

Test	Result
PT	↑
aPTT	↑
TCT	↑
Fibrinogen	↓
FDPs (e.g., D-dimer)	↑
Platelets	↓
Coagulation factors (e.g., factor VIII)	↓

aPTT, Activated partial thromboplastin time; FDPs, fibrin degradation products; PT, prothrombin time; TCT, thrombin clotting time.

known causes of hereditary thrombophilia, only homozygous or compound heterozygous protein C and/or protein S deficiency is sufficient to induce neonatal TE. Other inherited thrombophilic conditions include FV Leiden, prothrombin mutation, AT deficiency, elevated lipoprotein(a), maternal anticardiolipin antibodies, and nonspecific inhibitors.

Hereditary thrombophilia should be suspected in patients with spontaneous and extensive TE, ischemic skin lesions, or purpura fulminans. The Subcommittee for Perinatal and Pediatric Thrombosis of the Scientific and Standardization Committee of the International Society on Thrombosis and Haemostasis recommended that pediatric patients with spontaneous TE be tested for a full panel of genetic and acquired thrombophilic defects.[28] However, because of the difficulty in obtaining a large volume of blood, one can consider performing these tests in stages unless the result of the testing has immediate impact on patient management. On initial presentation of TE, DNA-based assays can be performed. Testing for levels of natural coagulation inhibitors should be delayed until 6 months of age when the levels approach those in adults and until anticoagulant treatment is discontinued.

Specific Neonatal Thrombotic Syndromes

Renal Vein Thrombosis

The renal vein is one of the most common sites of neonatal thrombosis. The incidence of RVT is estimated to be 0.5 per 1000 NICU admissions and 2.2 per 100,000 live births.[23,25] RVT is more common in males and in the left renal vein, although 28% to 44% occur bilaterally. Two-thirds of neonates with RVT present within 3 days postnatally, whereas 7% of neonates can present with RVT in utero.[29] Most common clinical manifestations of RVT include hematuria, palpable flank mass, and thrombocytopenia. Neonates may also have coexisting hypertension, proteinuria, renal failure, adrenal hemorrhage, and anemia. RVT is associated with prematurity, umbilical venous catheters, diabetic mothers, asphyxia, and infections. FV Leiden, prothrombin gene mutation, and elevated lipoprotein(a) have also been found in association with RVT. However, these are common traits, and it would be inaccurate to say they are proven to be causal, despite the associations. Most infants with RVT will experience complete, cortical, or segmental infarction of the affected kidney(s) and/or hypertension.[21]

Diagnosis is reliably confirmed by Doppler ultrasound examination. There are no evidence-based treatment guidelines, and most cases of RVT result in loss of renal tissue, regardless of the treatment.[29] Neonates with RVT should be followed for persistent hypertension and progressive renal insufficiency. Unilateral RVT without uremia or clot extension into the inferior vena cava can be managed with heparin or LMWH. Treatment should be given for at least 3 months if there is extension into the inferior vena cava. Bilateral RVT with renal failure should be treated with thrombolytic therapy followed by heparin or LMWH.[7]

Portal Vein Thrombosis

The true incidence of portal vein thrombosis (PVT) is unknown, but it is estimated to range from 1% to 43% of neonates with umbilical venous catheters.[30] The wide variation in incidence reflects differences in imaging protocols. In another study, the incidence of PVT was estimated to be at least 36 cases per 10,000 NICU admissions.[31] When ultrasonography is performed prospectively, 43% of neonates with umbilical venous catheters have asymptomatic PVT.

Major risk factors for PVT include umbilical venous catheters and sepsis/omphalitis. The role of inherited thrombophilia in PVT is controversial. There are multiple studies reporting on the association of inhibitor protein deficiencies (protein C, protein S, and AT) with PVT; however, it is difficult to ascertain whether the deficiencies are genetic or acquired, because the testing is done in the presence of TE.[30] Long-term complications of PVT include lobar atrophy and portal hypertension with associated gastrointestinal bleeding. Complications are more frequent with ectopic umbilical venous catheter placement (below or in the liver) or when thrombi are occlusive. Ultrasonography may reveal evidence of prior PVT with cavernous transformation of the portal vein and subsequent splenomegaly and reversal of portal flow.[32] Spontaneous resolution of PVT is common, but detection of PVT is important, even in asymptomatic patients, because PVT can lead to portal hypertension, which may manifest up to 10 years later.[32] Neonates with umbilical venous catheters should be monitored by ultrasonography, and catheter removal and/or anticoagulation should be considered for PVT.

Purpura Fulminans

Purpura fulminans is characterized by disseminated purpuric lesions often associated with bullae and necrosis. The histopathology of these lesions reveals diffuse cutaneous microthrombi with surrounding hemorrhage. Diffuse thrombosis, including stroke, retinal infarcts, limb gangrene, and DIC, can occur in purpura fulminans. Causes include severe protein C, protein S, or AT deficiency, either acquired as a complication of sepsis or inherited as homozygous or compound heterozygous conditions. Some infants with severe protein C deficiency do not develop TE until adulthood, suggesting that additional factors influence the neonatal presentation. Treatment with heparin and replacement with protein C concentrate or FFP are indicated. Long-term anticoagulation is often needed.[33]

Arterial Ischemic Stroke

Perinatal arterial ischemic stroke (AIS) is an important cause of cerebral palsy, epilepsy, and cognitive impairment. Perinatal AIS mostly occurs in full-term neonates with a prevalence of 28.6 to 93 cases per 100,000 live births. Presenting features include seizures and lethargy. In the neonatal period, AIS often presents with focal or generalized seizures, although pathologic hand preference before 1 year of age is most common if the stroke was asymptomatic in the newborn period. Ischemic injury is usually detected by magnetic resonance angiography, and unilateral lesions favor the left hemisphere. Diffusion-weighted magnetic resonance imaging is superior to cranial ultrasonography or computed tomographic scanning.[7]

Risk factors for perinatal AIS are different from TE risk factors in older infants and children because maternal and placental factors play a more important role, and some events even occur in utero.[34] The most common acquired risk factors for perinatal AIS are perinatal asphyxia, fetal distress, chorioamnionitis or other infections, preeclampsia, congenital heart disease, and dehydration. The contribution of congenital thrombophilia to perinatal AIS risk is unclear, although maternal anticardiolipin antibodies may be present for a brief period. In most cases of perinatal AIS, a hypercoagulable state is not detected. One potential mechanism of stroke is embolism of placental thrombi via the umbilical vein and through the patent foramen ovale of the fetus or neonate. Evaluation of placental pathologic conditions is important because demonstration of placental thrombi or abruption may be indicative of maternal prothrombotic state. Furthermore, if placental thrombi are seen histologically, the risk for recurrent events is especially low. Long-term developmental outcomes depend on the extent of the stroke and location of the lesion; strokes involving Broca and Wernicke areas, the internal capsule, or the basal ganglia have a poor outcome.

Treatment depends on whether the stroke is embolic or nonembolic in origin. For nonembolic AIS, current guidelines recommend against anticoagulation or aspirin for neonates with first AIS, especially if the infarct is large or there is evidence of hemorrhage. Anticoagulant or aspirin therapy is recommended for neonates with recurrent AIS.[7] In a patient with a documented cardioembolic stroke, anticoagulant therapy is suggested.

Cerebral Sinovenous Thrombosis

Based on data from the Canadian Pediatric Ischemic Stroke Registry, the prevalence of cerebral sinovenous thrombosis (CSVT) is 0.67 per 100,000 children, with 43% occurring in the neonatal period.[35] The clinical presentation may be relatively silent, or patients may manifest with diffuse neurologic changes, seizures, and IVH. The most frequently involved vessels are the superior and lateral sinuses, and up to one-third of cases have associated venous infarction and subsequent hemorrhage.[21] Up to 31% of full-term neonates with IVH have associated CSVT, suggesting that the pathophysiology of IVH in full-term neonates is different from that in premature infants.

Risk factors for neonatal CSVT include perinatal asphyxia, diffuse hypoxic injury, dehydration, infection, congenital heart disease, and severe illness, with ECMO now recognized as a specific risk factor. The frequency of hereditary thrombophilia in neonates with CSVT ranges from 20% to 40%, with FV Leiden and MTHFR C677T occurring most often. In contrast to purpura fulminans, no cases of congenital deficiencies of protein C, protein S, or AT have been reported in association with CSVT. Multiple risk factors (maternal, neonatal, perinatal, or prothrombotic) are found in over half of neonates with CSVT.[7] Although the diagnosis of CSVT in neonates is often made by transcranial ultrasonography, magnetic resonance venography is the most sensitive diagnostic test. On the basis of data from the Canadian Pediatric Ischemic Stroke Registry, neonatal CSVT is associated with cerebral parenchymal infarcts in 42% of cases, and 83% of these are hemorrhagic infarcts.[35]

Aside from treatment of the underlying conditions, when relevant, there are no standard treatment guidelines. Nonetheless, good results have been obtained with anticoagulant therapy, and UFH or LMWH is given, provided that there is no significant ICH. Extended treatment with LMWH or a vitamin K antagonist is recommended for a minimum of 6 weeks and no longer than 3 months.[7] The goal of anticoagulation is not to prevent recurrence; rather, it is to prevent progression and minimize neurologic sequelae. In a study by Kenet et al,[36] none of the 75 neonates with CSVT had a recurrence after a median follow-up of 36 months. For those with significant hemorrhage, radiologic monitoring at 5 to 7 days is recommended, and anticoagulation should be initiated if there is evidence of thrombus propagation.[7] Anticoagulation is associated with a high rate of hemorrhage, so treatment plans should be individualized. In older patients, punctate hemorrhage behind a cerebral venous infarct is not an absolute contraindication to anticoagulation, but studies in neonates are lacking. Nevertheless, in the Canadian registry, 36% of neonates were treated with UFH or LMWH, mostly for 3 months, and no cases of death or neurologic compromise from hemorrhage were reported.[35] Overall, neurologic impairment was reported in up to two-thirds of cases, and approximately 2% died.

Principles of Therapy

Supportive Therapy

As with other age groups, therapeutic modalities available to neonates include supportive care, anticoagulation, thrombolytic agents, and surgical thrombectomy. The British Haemostasis and Thrombosis Task Force and the American College of Chest Physicians have proposed guidelines for the management of neonatal TE.[37] Supportive therapy is recommended for clinically silent thrombi, including catheter-associated events. As soon as practical, clotted catheters should be removed, and all documented thrombi should be followed by serial imaging. If venous access is required, one can either monitor the clot closely or provide anticoagulation therapy.

Vitamin K Antagonist Therapy

Vitamin K antagonists, such as warfarin, are not recommended for neonates, because liquid preparations are not available, monitoring is complicated, and doses are variable owing to alterations in the dietary intake of vitamin K.

Heparin (UFH or LMWH)

UFH or LMWH is the mainstay of anticoagulant therapy in neonates. The UFH and LMWH dosing regimen is outlined in the box on Treatment of Neonatal TE. Neonates require higher doses of heparin than adults, owing to lower native AT levels, increased volume of distribution, and faster clearance.[3,38-40] Additionally, they may require supplementation with AT concentrate or FFP in cases of heparin resistance. Anticoagulation is monitored using anti-FXa assays. Therapeutic anti-FXa levels are 0.3 to 0.7 units/mL for UFH and 0.5 to 1 units/mL for LMWH. There are two types of anti-FXa assays: (1) with exogenous AT added and (2) without exogenous AT. The addition of exogenous AT allows measurement of the UFH effect without the influence of AT deficiency (if present), whereas the anti-FXa assay without exogenous AT allows measurement of the in vivo UFH effect.[41] Studies comparing the two types of anti-FXa assays found a lack of correlation. Hence, it is necessary to know the type of anti-FXa assay conducted in a particular laboratory when interpreting results. In neonates, the discrepancy between assays may also be increased owing to lower baseline AT levels.[3] The aPTT level can also be used to monitor UFH; aPTT values that correlate with anti-FXa levels of 0.3 to 0.7 units/mL are considered therapeutic.

Prophylactic UFH is recommended to maintain patency of umbilical arterial lines (0.25–1 units/mL, 25–200 units/kg/day, the lowest dose possible) and for cardiac catheterization (bolus dose of 100–150 units/kg with catheter insertion, repeat for prolonged procedures). In most other cases, LMWH has emerged as the anticoagulant of choice in the neonatal setting, both for prophylaxis and for treatment. The advantages of LMWH include better bioavailability, longer half-life allowing twice-daily administration, dose-dependent clearance, predictable anticoagulant response, and a lower risk of heparin-induced thrombocytopenia (HIT) and osteoporosis than with UFH. Although the current American College for Chest Physicians guidelines recommend a dose of 1.5 mg/kg of LMWH for treatment of neonatal TE,[7] there is growing evidence to suggest that neonates may, in fact, require higher doses up to 1.7 mg/kg and 2.0 mg/kg for term and preterm neonates, respectively, to obtain a therapeutic anti-FXa level.[42]

HIT antibodies are found in up to 1.5% of neonates, particularly in those who have undergone cardiac surgery. Overt HIT with TE, however, is rare, but it can occur. Mothers with HIT can passively immunize their fetuses. Diagnostic criteria for HIT are described in detail in Chapter 133. Treatment includes cessation of heparin and anticoagulation with argatroban, danaparoid, or lepirudin.[43]

Treatment of Neonatal Thromboembolism

Unfractionated Heparin (UFH)

Bolus: 75 units/kg over 10 minutes
Maintenance: 28 units/kg/h; therapeutic goal, anti-FXa of 0.3 to 0.7 units/mL
Prophylaxis: 10 units/kg/h
Follow platelet count to detect possible HIT (risk is low)

Enoxaparin

1.5 mg/kg subcutaneously every 12 hours (with normal renal function; round dose to nearest milligram; consider higher dose [see text][42]
Check anti-FXa level by peripheral venipuncture 4 to 6 hours after second or third dose; therapeutic goal, anti-FXa of 0.5 to 1 units/mL (0.4 to 0.6 units/mL if concurrent thrombocytopenia or other bleeding risk factor)
Follow platelet count to detect possible HIT (risk is low)
Hold for 24 hours before procedures

Prophylaxis With Enoxaparin

0.75 mg/kg subcutaneously every 12 hours
If checked, anti-FXa level 4 to 6 hours after second or third dose should be less than 0.4 units/mL
Hold for 12 hours before procedures

Purpura Fulminans

Concurrent heparin: UFH dose of 28 units/kg/h with target anti-FXa of 0.3 to 0.7 units/mL; LMWH dose of 1.0 to 1.5 mg/kg every 12 hours with therapeutic target anti-FXa range of 0.5 to 1 units/mL and replacement with FFP or protein C concentrate
FFP: 10 to 20 mL/kg every 6 to 12 hours for purpura fulminans
Protein C concentrate for severe protein C deficiency: load with 100 to 120 units/kg, then 60 to 80 units/kg every 6 hours × three doses (goal protein C activity 100%). Once therapeutic anticoagulation is achieved, maintenance therapy with 45 to 60 units/kg every 6 to 12 hours (goal protein C activity >25%).

Antithrombin Repletion

AT (functional) should be maintained at greater than 50% of normal levels for effective heparin-based anticoagulation
Dose in international units = (desired − current AT[a]) × weight (kg)

AT, Antithrombin; FFP, fresh frozen plasma; HIT, heparin-induced thrombocytopenia; LMWH, low-molecular-weight heparin; TE, thromboembolism; UFH, unfractionated heparin.

[a]Expressed as percentage of normal level based on functional AT level.

Tissue Plasminogen Activator Thrombolysis for Neonatal Thromboembolism

Concurrent Heparin (UFH or Enoxaparin) Should Be Considered at Prophylactic Dosing; UFH Preferred

Life- or limb-threatening thrombi: starting dose of 0.1 to 0.5 mg/kg/h for up to 6 hours
If no response, consider increase by 0.1 mg/kg/h increments to maximum 0.5 mg/kg/h
Consider using FFP 10 mL/kg before thrombolytic therapy
Maintain fibrinogen greater than 100 mg/dL
Maintain platelet count above 100×10^9/L
Reversal of severe bleeding with aminocaproic acid at 100 mg/kg intravenously every 6 hours

FFP, Fresh frozen plasma; TE, thromboembolism; t-PA, tissue plasminogen activator; UFH, unfractionated heparin.

Low-dose thrombolysis is recommended to open occluded catheters. t-PA is the drug that has been most widely studied in pediatric patients. Transfusion support for hypofibrinogenemia and thrombocytopenia should be provided to minimize the bleeding risk. Contraindications for thrombolytic therapy include active bleeding and major surgery or bleeding within the past 10 days, whereas relative contraindications include severe asphyxia within 7 days, generalized seizures within the last 48 hours, sepsis, or prematurity of less than 32 weeks of gestation. If UFH or LMWH is given concomitantly with t-PA, it should be administered at prophylactic doses (0.75 mg/kg every 12 hours for LMWH or 10 units/kg/h for UFH; see box on t-PA Thrombolysis for Neonatal TE). Surgical thrombectomy is reserved for organ-, limb-, or life-threatening thrombosis when t-PA administration is impractical or predicted to be ineffective. Thrombolytic therapy may be of benefit in a select group of pediatric patients with massive pulmonary embolism or extensive DVT.

SUGGESTED READINGS

Bhatt MD, Paes BA, Chan AK: How to use unfractionated heparin to treat neonatal thrombosis in clinical practice. *Blood Coagul Fibrinolysis* 27:605, 2016.

Brandão LR, Simpson EA, Lau KK: Neonatal renal vein thrombosis. *Semin Fetal Neonatal Med* 16:323, 2011.

Kenet G, Chan AK, Soucie JM, et al: Bleeding disorders in neonates. *Haemophilia* 16:168, 2010.

Monagle P, Chan AK, Goldenberg NA, et al: Antithrombotic therapy in neonates and children: antithrombotic therapy and prevention of thrombosis, 9th ed: American College of Chest Physicians Evidence-Based Clinical Practice Guidelines [published errata appear in *Chest.* 2014;146:1422; and *Chest.* 2014;146:1694]. *Chest* 141(2 Suppl):e737S, 2012.

Williams S, Chan AK: Neonatal portal vein thrombosis: diagnosis and management. *Semin Fetal Neonatal Med* 16:329, 2011.

REFERENCES

For the complete list of references, log on to www.expertconsult.com.

Fondaparinux may be a reasonable option in selected cases, but experience in neonates is limited.

Thrombolytic Therapy

Guidelines for thrombolytic management of neonatal TE are provided by the British Haemostasis and Thrombosis Task Force[37] and the Scientific Subcommittee on Perinatal and Pediatric Thrombosis of the International Society of Thrombosis and Haemostasis.[44] Both groups agree that thrombolysis should be considered for extensive TE associated with organ dysfunction or limb-threatening ischemia.

PART XIII

CONSULTATIVE HEMATOLOGY

CHAPTER 151

HEMATOLOGIC CHANGES IN PREGNANCY

Caroline Cromwell and Michael Paidas

Hematologic conditions are often seen during pregnancy. These range from the simple to the complex. The primary physiologic hematologic changes during pregnancy relate to the expansion of plasma volume.[1] In addition to physiologic changes of pregnancy, a prothrombotic state develops as the pregnancy advances that is thought to prepare the mother and fetus for eventual placental separation.[2] All require proper planning, anticipation, and discussion with the treating physicians as well as the patient. The effect of the condition on the pregnancy, and conversely the effect of the pregnancy on the condition, should be considered. The evolving clinical picture as the pregnancy progresses must also be taken into account. Multidisciplinary planning and communication are essential.

Anemia and thrombocytopenia are common hematologic conditions seen for a variety of reasons during pregnancy and are addressed in this chapter. Inherited and acquired bleeding disorders affect pregnant women, and coagulation parameters must be monitored during pregnancy and delivery. Venous thromboembolism (VTE) during pregnancy remains a high-morbidity, high-risk situation that is challenging for clinicians. These more common hematologic problems and dilemmas in management are discussed in this chapter.

ANEMIA IN PREGNANCY

Anemia in pregnancy affects approximately half of all pregnancies worldwide. It is more prevalent in underdeveloped countries.

The World Health Organization classifies anemia in pregnancy as hemoglobin below 11 g/dL, although in developing countries it is clinically defined as hemoglobin below 10 g/dL.[1] Physiologic anemia occurs during pregnancy as the blood volume increases to a greater proportion than the red blood cell (RBC) mass, resulting in a dilutional anemia. Total circulatory volumes increase by approximately 50% greater than the prepregnancy volume. Plasma volume and RBC mass return to baseline during the first and second postpartum months. Common maternal signs of anemia include pallor, tachypnea, fatigue, and headache. Hemoglobin levels less than 6 g/dL in pregnant women can be associated with significant maternal and fetal complications. At these levels, tissue oxygenation decreases and may lead to high-output congestive heart failure in the mother.[2-4] Multiple studies have shown a correlation between maternal anemia and increased rates of both preterm (<37 weeks of gestation) and low-birth-weight deliveries.[5-13] There are varied etiologies behind anemia in pregnancy.

Iron-Deficiency Anemia

Iron-deficiency anemia is the most common cause of anemia in pregnancy. It has been identified as a risk factor for preterm delivery and low birth weight. Iron requirements increase during pregnancy because of maternal and fetal erythropoiesis. Generally, hemoglobin levels decrease throughout pregnancy and then may increase during the last month of pregnancy. Ferritin levels also increase in the last month of pregnancy because it is an acute-phase reactant. Erythropoietin levels increase throughout pregnancy. The clinical symptoms of iron deficiency are similar to those in nonpregnant patients and include fatigue, pallor, tachycardia, and poor exercise tolerance. The diagnosis and treatment of iron-deficiency anemia are generally similar to those in nonpregnant patients. Anemia and low ferritin levels are considered diagnostic.

Because the typical diet in the United States provides only 50% of daily iron requirements for pregnant women and because of the relatively high prevalence of iron deficiency among women of childbearing age, routine iron supplementation in pregnancy is recommended.[14] Currently, the Centers for Disease Control and Prevention, the American Dietetic Association, and the American College of Obstetrics and Gynecology recommend 15 to 30 mg/day of elemental iron to prevent adverse outcomes from iron-deficiency anemia.[14-18] Treatment should be from the beginning of gestation to 3 months postpartum. On the basis of results of a study by Casanueva et al,[19] weekly therapy with 120 mg of iron appears to be a safe and effective alternative to daily therapy. The side effects associated with iron therapy—constipation, diarrhea, nausea—are well known.

Intravenous iron is appropriate in certain circumstances; evidence from a recently published randomized trial by Al et al supports the use of intravenous iron therapy to replenish iron stores in appropriately selected patients, including those who have not tolerated a trial of oral iron therapy and those with severe iron deficiency.[20]

Multiple studies have shown that routine iron supplementation in pregnancy decreases the incidence of iron-deficiency anemia. In a randomized, double-blind study in which 275 iron-replete pregnant women received either a daily iron supplement or placebo from the time of enrollment (all women were enrolled before week 20) to 28 weeks of gestation, the incidence of both low-birth-weight and preterm low-birth-weight infants was lower among women who received daily iron.[21] Nonetheless, there are limits to the effectiveness of routine iron supplementation. After all, the recommendation by prominent public health organizations for universal iron supplementation has not led to a commensurate decrease in the incidence of iron-deficiency anemia in pregnancy[22,23] or an increase in maternal hemoglobin levels.[24,25] Compliance is an important factor in this discussion. A large, multicenter, randomized, controlled trial on the benefits of iron supplementation during pregnancy in the United States is needed to draw more definitive conclusions.

Other Nutritional Deficiencies

Folate deficiency and, less commonly, vitamin B_{12} deficiency are the next most common causes of anemia in pregnancy. Cobalamin and folate are critical for fetal growth because they are necessary for the production of tetrahydrofolate. Tetrahydrofolate is key in the DNA synthesis pathway.

Folate deficiency accounts for 95% of megaloblastic anemias in pregnancy.[26] Folate deficiency complicates between 1% and 4% of pregnancies in the United States and affects approximately one-third of pregnancies worldwide.[27] Similar to iron-deficiency anemia, the incidence of megaloblastic anemia in pregnancy is increased in adolescents, women of low socioeconomic status, and women with multiple closely spaced births.[28] The folic acid requirement for nonpregnant women is 50 to 100 µg/day, but this increases to 150 µg during pregnancy as RBC mass in the mother increases and as fetal demands for folate grow with cell proliferation.[29]

Diagnosis of folate deficiency is best based on RBC folate levels. An elevated homocysteine level also helps confirm the diagnosis. Pregnant women should at least receive 400 µg of folic acid per day. Vitamin B_{12} deficiency is much less common during pregnancy.

Diagnosis of vitamin B_{12} deficiency can be aided by the assessment of homocysteine and methylmalonic acid. If a woman is found to be deficient in vitamin B_{12} during pregnancy, vitamin B_{12} injections are indicated. These are usually injected weekly for 4 to 8 weeks and then monthly.

HEMOGLOBINOPATHIES AND PREGNANCY

Sickle Cell Disease

Every year more than 300,000 children are born with either sickle cell disease or thalassemia. Prenatal counseling now exists in many countries. In the United States, all newborns are screened for sickle cell disease (see Chapters 42 and 43). Management of pregnant patients with sickle cell disease requires coordination of care between the hematologist and obstetrician. Many women with sickle cell disease experience more frequent vasoocclusive crises and other sickle cell–related complications during pregnancy.[30] The increased frequency of vasoocclusive crises, particularly during the latter half of pregnancy, likely results from heightened metabolic requirements in pregnancy, increased venous stasis, as well as the physiologic prothrombotic and inflammatory state associated with pregnancy. In addition, pathophysiologic changes in the renal and immune function of patients with sickle cell disease increase their susceptibility to urinary tract infections and pyelonephritis. By causing tissue hypoxia, sickling of RBCs within the placental vasculature may cause deleterious effects on the fetus.[31]

Additional significant complications occur in pregnant women with sickle cell disease. The incidence of preeclampsia, thromboembolic events, placental abruption, intrauterine growth retardation, low birth weight, and postpartum infections are higher among women with hemoglobin SS, SC, and S β-thalassemia than among women without sickle cell disease. One study noted a higher incidence of stillbirths and perinatal mortality among patients with sickle cell disease,[32] but another study revealed an increased risk of preterm labor and premature rupture of membranes in women with hemoglobin SS disease.[33] Despite advances made in sickle disease, a recent meta-analysis highlights that risks for pregnancy in patients with SS genotype remains high with regard to mortality, a fourfold higher risk of stillbirth and a 2.43 higher relative risk of preeclampsia. These risks were amplified in low-income countries. Because of the increased risk for such complications, women with sickle cell disease should receive close medical attention throughout the prenatal period. This includes counseling about intrauterine diagnosis of sickle cell disease when appropriate. Pregnant women can undergo chorionic villi sampling as early as the ninth week of gestation or amniocentesis in the 15th to 16th weeks. A reticulocyte count along with hemoglobin, iron, and folate levels should be obtained to assess for deficiency states and bone marrow suppression. Urinalysis with urine culture is performed as often as every trimester to monitor for asymptomatic bacteriuria. Finally, beginning around 28 weeks of gestation, patients should have weekly clinic visits and begin serial ultrasonography.

Treatment of sickle cell disease during pregnancy warrants careful consideration. Hydroxyurea should be avoided. If pregnancy is being considered it should be discontinued. Women should receive 5 mg/day of supplemental folic acid. Studies examining the benefit of prophylactic blood transfusions or exchange transfusions have not led to definitive conclusions.[34] Although they may lead to alloimmunization, prophylactic transfusions appear to decrease the incidence of vasoocclusive crises and decrease maternal and fetal morbidity and mortality.[35] A conservative approach reserves transfusions for patients whose hemoglobin levels fall below 6 g/dL, patients who develop progressive complications related to sickle cell disease, and patients with obstetric complications.[36] Following this approach, 60% to 75% of women with sickle cell disease will require transfusion therapy during pregnancy. Patients with a sickle cell crisis during pregnancy should receive aggressive analgesic therapy, hydration, and oxygen while undergoing evaluation for infection or other precipitating influences.

At the time of delivery, pregnant women with sickle cell disease are managed in a manner similar to those with high cardiac output anemia. Supplemental oxygen, hydration, and adequate oxygenation during anesthesia should be given to prevent sickling of RBCs and the associated complications. During the postpartum period, hemoglobin levels are followed closely, and prophylaxis for VTE is administered unless contraindications preclude it.

Thalassemias

Pregnant women with an underlying thalassemia typically have β-thalassemia minor or α-thalassemia trait—conditions with a relatively benign clinical phenotype—rather than β-thalassemia major or hemoglobin H disease (see Chapter 41). Because of delayed pubertal growth or hypogonadism with associated anovulation, women with β-thalassemia major and hemoglobin H disease rarely become pregnant. Case reports indicate that when it does occur, pregnancy in women with hemoglobin H disease can be complicated by severe hemolytic anemia and hepatosplenomegaly. However, in the setting of widespread transfusion and iron chelation therapy, pregnancy is more frequent in the thalassemia population. Pregnancy outcomes among women with β-thalassemia major were recently examined in 10 patients with homozygous β-thalassemia. Of 15 pregnancies, there were 14 live births, a 20% incidence of intrauterine growth restriction (IUGR), and 21% were low-birth-weight children. In patients with β-thalassemia intermedia, approximately 50% of pregnancies are complicated by preterm delivery, third-trimester stillbirth, or IUGR.[37]

Pregnancy is a common setting for the diagnosis of β-thalassemia minor or α-thalassemia trait in previously asymptomatic women who are found to be anemic on routine laboratory evaluation during pregnancy. Several studies indicate that the physiologic anemia of pregnancy may be exacerbated in women with thalassemia minor, although findings from at least one study suggest otherwise.[38] β-Thalassemia minor and α-thalassemia traits do not have an adverse effect on fetal development, fetal morbidity and mortality, or maternal morbidity and mortality.[39]

Similar to those with sickle cell disease, women with thalassemia require vigilant follow-up throughout their pregnancies. This includes interval monitoring of maternal vital signs and fetal heart rate, maternal hemoglobin levels, and fetal growth as assessed by ultrasonography beginning around the 24th week of gestation. Patients are screened for folate and iron deficiency. They should also be assessed for iron overload, which can develop in individuals with thalassemia as a result of increased intestinal iron absorption, frequent blood transfusions, and rapid turnover of plasma iron.[40] Prenatal genetic testing can be performed if desired, with results used to counsel parents of the child and guide optimal care of the fetus. In terms of therapy, there are no specific treatment recommendations for women with thalassemia during pregnancy, aside from folate supplementation and supportive care. In pregnant women with evidence of iron overload, chelation therapy using deferoxamine has been used safely, although the potential for teratogenicity associated with the agent must be considered in this setting.[41]

OTHER HEMOLYTIC ANEMIAS

Hereditary Spherocytosis

Hereditary spherocytosis is the most common inherited hemolytic anemia among people of northern European descent (see Chapter 46).[42] Few cases of pregnancy in individuals with hereditary spherocytosis have been reported. Published reports indicate there may be an increased incidence of first trimester fetal loss in patients with hereditary spherocytosis.[43] Because some patients have only low levels of hemolysis under normal conditions, the disease may not become clinically apparent until pregnancy. Pregnant women with hereditary spherocytosis can exhibit a variety of clinical manifestations. These include folate deficiency related to the increased requirements of pregnancy superimposed on chronic hemolysis, hemolytic crisis, and aplastic crisis.[44,45] The results of two small series suggest that pregnancy outcomes for women with hereditary spherocytosis are generally good, with improvements in outcomes for splenectomized patients.[46] Care is primarily supportive.

Glucose 6-Phosphate Dehydrogenase Deficiency

Favorable pregnancy outcomes observed in women with hereditary spherocytosis and pyruvate kinase deficiency stand in contrast to those in women with glucose 6-phosphate dehydrogenase (G6PD) deficiency. The deficiency of G6PD leads to hemolytic anemia in the face of oxidative stress (see Chapter 45). The condition increases the risk of spontaneous abortion, low-birth-weight fetuses, and neonatal jaundice.[47] Women with G6PD deficiency should be instructed to strictly avoid medications with oxidative potential. Complications after the ingestion of oxidative drugs can even occur in a carrier of the G6PD deficiency gene if her male fetus has inherited the disease.[48]

Paroxysmal Nocturnal Hemoglobinuria

Paroxysmal nocturnal hemoglobinuria (PNH) is a rare clonal disorder caused by somatic mutation in the membrane-anchoring protein *PIGA* (see Chapter 32). *PIGA* mutation leads, in turn, to deficient function of critical membrane proteins that in wild-type individuals are anchored by the gene product of *PIGA*. Features of the clinical phenotype include hemolysis, thrombosis, and bone marrow failure. Hemolysis results from deficiency in the membrane proteins CD55 and CD59, which renders affected individuals susceptible to complement-mediated intravascular hemolysis.

The clinical manifestations of PNH can have a devastating impact on pregnancy. Reported cases highlight the significant pregnancy-associated morbidity and mortality in women with this condition. Complications include severe anemia, thrombocytopenia, thrombotic events, preterm delivery, low-birth-weight infants, neonatal death, and maternal death.[49,50] A study by Ray and colleagues[50] reviewed pregnancy outcomes in 24 women with PNH and found a 20% maternal mortality rate.

Owing to the high-risk nature of these pregnancies, women with PNH require close medical attention in the antenatal, perinatal, and postnatal periods. Prophylactic anticoagulation is recommended because of the high incidence of thrombotic events during pregnancy. Warfarin is contraindicated because of its teratogenicity. Low-molecular-weight heparin (LMWH) is favored over unfractionated heparin (UFH) because it less frequently causes heparin-induced thrombocytopenia (HIT). Anticoagulation should be interrupted during the perinatal period but, in the absence of contraindications, reinitiated thereafter and continued for 6 weeks postpartum.[51]

Results of a phase III trial by Hillmen and colleagues[52] demonstrated that eculizumab, a humanized monoclonal antibody against the terminal complement protein C5, can reduce levels of hemolysis, stabilize hemoglobin, minimize transfusion requirement, and improve quality of life in patients with PNH. There are case reports describing success in patients chronically receiving eculizumab throughout pregnancy with uncomplicated deliveries. However, a large randomized trial has not been performed. Supportive care is used as needed throughout pregnancy. RBC transfusions are used in the treatment of anemia. In the setting of thrombocytopenia and bleeding, platelet transfusions may also be necessary.

Autoimmune Hemolytic Anemia

Autoimmune hemolysis can occur during pregnancy and lead to anemia (see Chapter 47). The relatively small size of immunoglobulin (Ig)G immunoglobulin molecules allows them to cross the placenta; thus the IgG subtype of autoimmune hemolytic anemia can adversely affect fetuses. In contrast, the larger IgM antibodies do not cross the

placenta. Patients with autoimmune hemolytic anemia are treated with glucocorticoids and, if necessary, intravenous immunoglobulin (IVIg). Supportive transfusions are administered when needed.[53] In rare instances, pregnancy appears to precipitate the development of autoimmune hemolytic anemia in a previously unaffected woman. The etiology of this phenomenon is not known.[54] Women in this circumstance have been treated in the standard fashion with favorable results.

THROMBOCYTOPENIA

Thrombocytopenia during pregnancy is quite common. It occurs in approximately 10% of pregnancies.[55] Although there is not one clear value to define thrombocytopenia in pregnancy, generally a platelet count less than 100,000 is considered cause for concern. There is some physiologic thrombocytopenia that occurs during pregnancy. Gestational thrombocytopenia (GT) is the most common cause of thrombocytopenia in pregnancy followed by preeclampsia and immune thrombocytopenia. Much rarer causes include disseminated intravascular coagulation (DIC), thrombotic thrombocytopenic purpura (TTP) and hemolytic uremic syndrome (HUS), and medication induced. The evaluation of thrombocytopenia is essential to rule out any systemic disorders that may affect pregnancy management

Gestational Thrombocytopenia

GT is quite common during pregnancy. The platelet count is generally never lower than 70,000/µL. This occurs mainly in the third trimester. Patients are asymptomatic and have no history of thrombocytopenia. The platelet count normalizes within 3 months of delivery but often normalizes within 1 week. The etiology of GT remains unclear, but it is thought in part to be autoimmune in nature and demonstrates a clear overlap with mild idiopathic thrombocytopenic purpura (ITP).

The management of patients with GT is uncomplicated. Typically, they can receive epidural anesthesia. However, practice varies at each institution in terms of platelet threshold for epidural anesthesia. Platelet counts greater than 100,000/µL are considered safe for epidural anesthesia. There are studies demonstrating safe administration of epidural anesthesia in pregnant patients with platelet counts as low as 70,000/µL.[56]

Immune Thrombocytopenia

ITP is responsible for pregnancy-associated thrombocytopenia in approximately 3% of cases (Chapter 132). It is the most common cause of thrombocytopenia during the first two trimesters of pregnancy.[57] ITP can recur in women with previously documented disease or can develop de novo during pregnancy.

ITP is usually not diagnosed during pregnancy. Pregnant patients with ITP usually have a long-standing history of thrombocytopenia. ITP may be difficult to distinguish from GT because patients with these conditions can present with similar clinical and laboratory findings. Elevated levels of platelet-associated IgG and antibody titers can be found in both conditions.[58] Furthermore, assays that detect antibodies against the glycoprotein receptors IIb/IIIa and Ib/IX are not specific for ITP.[59] Whereas thrombocytopenia in the first trimester or early portion of the second trimester should raise suspicion for ITP, thrombocytopenia that develops later in pregnancy should raise suspicion for GT. A preconception platelet count can also be helpful in distinguishing between the two. It is important to attempt to distinguish between ITP and GT because there is a small but significant risk of neonatal thrombocytopenia in the setting of ITP.[60]

In terms of diagnostic evaluation, human immunodeficiency virus, hepatitis, and lupus should be tested for if clinically indicated. Platelet antibody testing is not considered helpful. The peripheral smear may demonstrate an increased platelet size but should otherwise

TABLE 151.1	Initiation of Treatment in Pregnant Patients With Idiopathic Thrombocytopenic Purpura
Platelet Count	**Treatment**
<10,000/µL	Platelet transfusion for life-threatening bleeding
10,000-30,000/µL	Consider monitoring in first trimester; treat in second or third trimester
>30,000/µL	Clinically monitor

be normal. Bone marrow biopsy and aspirate are not indicated unless there are other hematologic abnormalities present.

Treatment options are generally similar to those for nonpregnant patients with ITP (Table 151.1). Platelet transfusions are reserved for life-threatening bleeding because the lives of transfused platelets are usually short in ITP. Glucocorticoids are considered first-line treatment; prednisone is usually initiated at 1 mg/kg based on the patient's baseline weight. Side effects of prednisone should be discussed with the patient and include weight gain, bone loss, hypertension, and gestational diabetes. IVIg can also be used. It is a means of rapid increase in platelet count. It is particularly used to help increase platelet counts a few days before delivery.[61] It is usually administered at a dose of 2 g/kg over 2 days. However, the improvement in platelet count is fairly transient. Splenectomy is also an option indicated for refractory thrombocytopenia; it is best performed during the second trimester.

Other agents such as danazol, cyclophosphamide, and vinca alkaloids, although used in the management of ITP in nonpregnant individuals, are teratogenic and should be avoided during pregnancy.[62] Use of cyclophosphamide has been associated with birth defects. Danazol may cause clitoral enlargement and labial fusion in female fetuses when given in the first trimester.[63,64] The use of rituximab has never been studied systematically in this setting and is considered a pregnancy class C drug. Although case reports of its use exist, it is not generally recommended in this case. Animal data indicate that thrombopoietin mimetics may cause fetal harm, and little is known about their use in pregnant patients. A registry has been developed for pregnant patients treated with thrombopoietin mimetics.

As discussed previously, maternal antiplatelet IgG can cross the placenta and cause thrombocytopenia in fetuses. Percutaneous umbilical blood sampling is the most accurate means to obtain the fetal platelet count. However, the procedure is associated with a high complication rate and 1% fetal mortality.[65] Intrapartum fetal scalp sampling represents an alternative, but the accuracy of this technique is only 50% to 70%.[66] The maternal platelet count and antiplatelet antibody level do not accurately predict the fetal platelet count.[67] Overall, 10% of babies born to mothers with ITP have a platelet count less than 50,000/µL, but less than 5% have a platelet count less than 20,000/µL.[68] Treatment of pregnant women with IVIg or steroids does not appear to affect the platelet count of fetuses.[68,69] Thrombocytopenia places neonates at risk for bleeding events, including intracranial hemorrhage, although this complication is rare.[70]

In terms of delivery, at present, available guidelines on the subject suggest that obstetric factors, rather than hematologic ones, should guide the manner of delivery.[71] After the delivery of a child, the cord blood platelet count is checked and the newborn platelet count followed because thrombocytopenia is often most severe 4 to 6 days after delivery and resolves as maternal antiplatelet IgG is cleared.

Preeclampsia and HELLP Syndrome

Thrombocytopenia in pregnant woman also occurs in association with preeclampsia and HELLP syndrome (hemolysis, elevated liver enzymes, low platelet count), potentially severe multisystem disorders associated with pregnancy. In previously healthy nulliparous women, the incidence of preeclampsia is between 2% and 7%.[72]

Thrombocytopenia is observed in 15% to 50% of patients with this condition.[73,74] Clinical manifestations include a maternal syndrome characterized by hypertension, proteinuria, and systemic abnormalities as well as a fetal syndrome characterized by fetal growth restriction, preterm delivery, and hypoxia-induced neurologic damage.[72,74]

In most instances, preeclampsia occurs during a woman's first pregnancy, but it can recur in a subsequent pregnancy or occur for the first time in a woman with one or more previously unaffected pregnancies. Risk factors for the disorder include, but are not limited to, preeclampsia in a previous pregnancy, a family history of preeclampsia, chronic hypertension, obesity, multifetal gestation, rheumatic disease, and preexisting thrombophilia.[72] With respect to thrombophilia, a case–control study by Mello and colleagues[75] suggests that the prevalence of an underlying thrombophilia is significantly higher among women who develop preeclampsia during pregnancy than among those who have uneventful pregnancies.

HELLP syndrome represents a severe variant of preeclampsia. In the majority of cases, patients who develop the syndrome are white and multiparous.[76] The median age of affected patients is 25 years. The time of presentation during pregnancy ranges from the midtrimester (15%) to term (18%). In 30% of patients who develop HELLP, it develops within 2 days after delivery.[77] Patients typically exhibit vague symptoms such as malaise, fatigue, epigastric or right upper quadrant pain, nausea, vomiting, and flulike symptoms. Because of the nonspecific nature of these symptoms, diagnosis is often delayed; one study found an average time to diagnosis of 8 days in women with HELLP syndrome.[78] Clinical findings at the time of diagnosis (weight gain or edema, hypertension, and proteinuria) are similar to those observed in preeclampsia.[77]

Although various criteria have been used in diagnosing HELLP syndrome, they generally share the following features: signs of microangiopathic hemolytic anemia, serum lactate dehydrogenase greater than 600 U/L or serum total bilirubin greater than 1.2 mg/dL, aspartate aminotransferase greater than 70 IU/L, and a platelet count lower than 100,000/µL.[79] Martin and colleagues[77] further defined HELLP syndrome on the basis of platelet count. According to this classification, patients with class 1 HELLP syndrome have a platelet count lower than 50,000/µL, those with class 2 disease have a platelet count between 50,000 and 100,000/µL, and individuals with class 3 HELLP syndrome have a platelet count higher than 100,000/µL. As might be expected, women with class 1 HELLP syndrome required a recovery period in the aftermath of their illness.

Although the precise mechanism through which preeclampsia develops is uncertain, research in the field continues to advance understanding of the underlying pathophysiology. Endothelial cell dysfunction after placentation appears to play a central role in the pathogenesis of the disease. During development of the placenta, placental trophoblast cells interface with the epithelial layer of the uterus, forming the decidua. Penetration and remodeling of maternal spiral arteries beginning at week 9 during pregnancy increase placental perfusion and improve oxygenation for the developing fetus under normal conditions.[80]

Cellular abnormalities such as those described impair placental implantation and vasculogenesis, leading to fetal hypoxia and the release of vasoactive compounds such as endothelin, nitric oxide, and prostaglandins. High levels of endothelin, a potent vasoconstrictor, are seen in preeclamptic patients, and injection of endothelin into rabbits produces a syndrome similar to HELLP syndrome.[81,82] The activity of endothelin, nitric oxide, and prostaglandins leads to hypertension and platelet activation. Angiogenic factors such as vascular endothelial growth factor 1 (VEGF 1) are elevated in preeclampsia compared with normal pregnancy. Injury to the vascular endothelium results in fibrin deposition, further platelet activation, and the release of additional vasoactive agents such as serotonin and thromboxane A_2. The etiology of thrombocytopenia in preeclampsia is likely related to increased antiplatelet IgG levels[83] or to activation of the coagulation cascade with subsequent consumption of platelets.[84,85]

These events lead to the multisystem dysfunction seen in patients with HELLP syndrome. Fibrin deposition in the hepatic sinusoids causes hepatocellular injury. Patients can develop right upper quadrant pain if intraparenchymal or subcapsular hemorrhage occurs. DIC was observed in 21% of patients with HELLP in one series, and placental abruption was seen in 16% of patients.[86] Other manifestations of HELLP syndrome include acute renal failure, pulmonary edema, shock, cerebrovascular accident (CVA), eclampsia, retinal detachment, diabetes insipidus, and an increased incidence of cesarean section.

HELLP syndrome is associated with high maternal and neonatal mortality rates. Maternal mortality rates range from 1.1% to 24.2%.[87] The immediate cause of death is most often rupture of the liver, DIC, acute renal failure, pulmonary edema or acute respiratory distress syndrome (ARDS), shock, or CVA. Perinatal deaths resulting from placental abruption, asphyxia, or extreme prematurity occur in 10% to 15% of patients. After delivery, infants born to women with preeclampsia or HELLP can develop a self-limited neonatal thrombocytopenia. Uncertainty exists regarding whether infant thrombocytopenia in these instances results from preeclampsia or HELLP itself or from a related complication such as neonatal sepsis.[88–90] HELLP recurs in subsequent pregnancies of affected women in 3% to 27% of cases. There is also an increased risk of preeclampsia, placental abruption, and preterm delivery in these pregnancies.[91–100]

In caring for a patient with preeclampsia or HELLP syndrome, the clinician's primary concerns are the mother's health and safety. The clinician must also consider the stage of pregnancy at time of diagnosis, the condition of the fetus, and desires of the patient in making management decisions. Definitive treatment for preeclampsia and HELLP involves delivery of the fetus; it is indicated for women who present after 34 weeks of gestation and those with evidence of multisystem dysfunction. However, conservative, supportive care without immediate delivery can be pursued for women who are relatively asymptomatic, hemodynamically stable, at less than 32 to 34 weeks of gestation, and without evidence of abnormal coagulation parameters.[100,101] Magnesium sulfate, which reduces cerebral vasoconstriction and ischemia, should be administered for seizure prophylaxis.[102] Parenteral labetalol or hydralazine is given for blood pressure control. Systemic corticosteroids appear to lessen the risk of maternal ARDS and reduce neonatal complications when administered to women who present at less than 34 weeks of gestation.[103] In addition to these measures, volume status is closely monitored to prevent plasma volume expansion and ensure adequate urine output.

Persistent right upper quadrant pain, which may herald a liver hematoma or rupture, hemodynamic instability, coagulation profile abnormalities, or a decline in clinical status, should prompt delivery by cesarean section. As mentioned previously, delivery is also indicated if the fetus is at least 32 to 34 weeks of gestation at the time when signs and symptoms of preeclampsia or HELLP develop. In a clinically stable woman, vaginal delivery can be attempted.[104] When cesarean section is required, transfusion of RBCs, platelets, and fresh frozen plasma (FFP) is performed as necessary before and during surgery. Severe hypofibrinogenemia should be treated with cryoprecipitate.

Patients are monitored closely in the postpartum period. Magnesium should be continued for 12 to 48 hours after delivery and blood pressure controlled appropriately. Although hypertension typically resolves within 6 weeks after delivery, some women require long-term antihypertensive therapy.[102] Coagulation and platelet abnormalities tend to resolve within 24 to 48 hours after delivery. Some patients, however, experience an ongoing decline in platelet count and should be followed until counts normalize. Postpartum eclampsia can occur for up to 48 hours after delivery; thus patients and health care providers should remain vigilant in monitoring for suggestive signs and symptoms.[105] Treatment options in the setting of severe postpartum preeclampsia and HELLP include corticosteroids and plasmapheresis.[106,107]

In light of the morbidity and mortality associated with preeclampsia and HELLP, considerable research has been focused on prevention of these conditions. The efficacy of various preventive strategies, including magnesium supplementation, low-dose aspirin, zinc supplementation, antihypertensive drugs, and heparin therapy, among others, has been the focus of observational studies, systematic reviews, and randomized trials. Initial small studies suggested that low-dose aspirin reduces the risk of preeclampsia, although patients who received aspirin had a higher incidence of placental abruption and bleeding.[108–115] Larger, randomized trials failed to confirm the benefit of low-dose aspirin.[109,110]

Thrombotic Thrombocytopenic Purpura–Atypical Hemolytic Uremic Syndrome

TTP and HUS/atypical HUS are also important considerations in the evaluation of pregnant women with thrombocytopenia (Chapter 135). Similar to preeclampsia and HELLP syndrome, they are multisystem disorders associated with high morbidity and mortality rates in the absence of appropriate therapy. Microvascular injury and platelet agglutination with resulting thrombocytopenia and microangiopathic hemolytic anemia are pathologic hallmarks of TTP and HUS (Fig. 151.1). They are rare conditions overall, but the incidence of both increases in pregnancy.[116] In the case of TTP, in fact, estimates suggest that approximately 10% of cases occur in pregnant or postpartum women.[117]

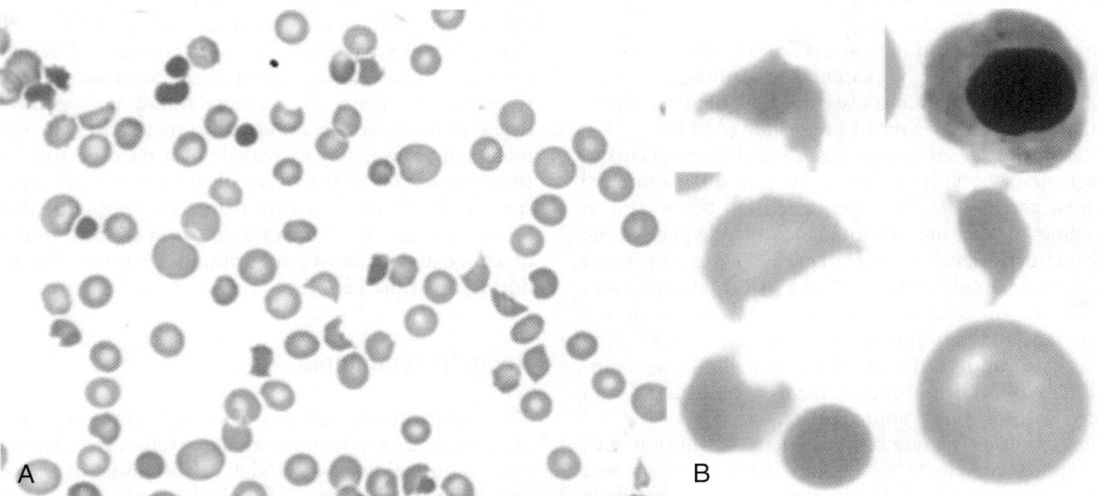

Fig. 151.1 MICROANGIOPATHIC HEMOLYTIC ANEMIA. Microangiopathic hemolytic anemia in pregnancy, peripheral blood smear (A, B). Evidence of microangiopathy with the formation of schistocytes, fragmented forms and spherocytes, associated with polychromasia and nucleated red blood cells (A, B, detail).

Because they share many common clinical features, TTP and aHUS are often categorized as a single entity, TTP-HUS. However, the pathophysiologies underlying the two conditions are distinctive. TTP is associated with unusually large multimers of circulating von Willebrand factor (vWF), which foster platelet aggregation and thrombus formation. Under normal circumstances, a vWF-cleaving protease referred to as *ADAMTS13* (a disintegrin and metalloproteinase with a thrombospondin type 1 motif, member 13) cleaves these multimers into smaller multimers of normal size. In TTP, function of the cleaving protease is impaired. ADAMTS13 deficiency characterizes familial TTP. Inhibition of ADAMTS13 protease activity by an autoantibody characterizes the acquired form of TTP. An inhibitory autoantibody can be found in 70% to 85% of patients with TTP.[118] On the other hand, impaired vWF-cleaving protease activity does not appear to play a role in the pathogenesis of a HUS.[119] Our understanding of the pathogenesis of atypical HUS has evolved in recent years as this disorder has been recognized to be associated as a complement-mediated disorder. With this dysregulation of complement, a picture of profound inflammation evolves. In contrast to TTP, there is typically more severe renal involvement with less severe thrombocytopenia. There can be some similarity found between the features of TTP-HUS and HELLP syndrome. It can be difficult to distinguish TTP and HUS from HELLP syndrome because they both have signs of microangiopathy. TTP tends to occur earlier in pregnancy, with a mean onset at 23.5 weeks, although it can occur at any point from the first trimester through the postpartum period.[120] HUS primarily occurs after delivery; 90% of cases occur in the postpartum period, with a mean onset at 26 days after delivery.[121] TTP and HUS do not cause hypertension or liver necrosis. Furthermore, TTP and HUS frequently persist after delivery, but HELLP syndrome typically resolves in the postpartum period.

Treatment of TTP-HUS involves emergent plasmapheresis within 24 to 48 hours of diagnosis. The response rate among pregnant women treated with plasmapheresis for TTP is approximately 75%. By comparison, the overall response rate in patients with TTP is approximately 80% to 90%.[122–125] Long-term sequelae in surviving patients include chronic renal failure, hypertension, and recurrence of TTP-HUS. TTP-HUS recurs in approximately 50% of subsequent pregnancies.[126] Infusion of FFP represents an alternative to plasmapheresis, although plasmapheresis is the preferred treatment modality. The response rate after FFP infusion is 64%.[127] Corticosteroids have also been used successfully in the treatment of pregnancy-associated TTP-HUS, with a response rate of 26%.[125] Conversely, antiplatelet agents such as aspirin do not play a role in the treatment of pregnancy-associated TTP-HUS.[128]

Disseminated Intravascular Coagulation

DIC in pregnant women can occur in various clinical settings, including HELLP syndrome, TTP-HUS, placental abruption, amniotic fluid embolism, uterine rupture, intrauterine fetal demise, sepsis, elective abortion, and acute fatty liver of pregnancy (AFLP).

Severe placental abruption sufficient to cause fetal death occurs in 0.12% of all pregnancies.[129] This condition leads to a consumptive hypofibrinogenemia, and (when fibrinogen levels fall below 100 to 150 mg/dL) bleeding may ensue. Maintenance of adequate urine output and a hematocrit level greater than 30% are important components of care for women who have had a placental abruption. Either vaginal delivery or cesarean section is appropriate in the context of severe placental abruption. In a woman undergoing cesarean section after abruption, the platelet count should be maintained at 50,000/μL or above through platelet transfusion and fibrinogen replaced with FFP or cryoprecipitate.

Amniotic fluid embolism is a rare but often lethal condition with a mortality rate of approximately 80%.[130] About 10% to 15% of these patients develop a coagulopathy. DIC in this setting most likely follows the release of thromboplastin-rich material into the maternal circulation. DIC seen in association with uterine rupture and intrauterine fetal demise presumably occurs through a similar mechanism.[131] On the contrary, bacterial endotoxin or exotoxin mediates sepsis-associated DIC in pregnant women with pyelonephritis, chorioamnionitis, endometritis, or septic abortion.[132] On rare occasions, elective abortions that use hypertonic solution and those complicated by hemorrhage can be associated with DIC.[133]

AFLP, or acute yellow atrophy, occurs in 1 of every 5000 to 10,000 pregnancies, most often in the third trimester of primiparous women.[134] Maternal and fetal mortality are 5% and 15%, respectively. Although the pathogenesis of AFLP is not clear, microvesicular fatty infiltration of the liver's central zone is observed and presumably plays a central role in the development of this disease.[135] In some cases, fatty infiltration can be detected by ultrasonography or computed tomography (CT).[136] Patients present with a variety of symptoms, including malaise, fatigue, right upper quadrant pain, dyspnea, and mental status changes. Laboratory findings include abnormal liver function test results consistent with cholestatic disease, elevated ammonia, low fibrinogen and antithrombin levels, and elevated prothrombin time, with evidence of DIC. Hepatic dysfunction can impair gluconeogenesis. Diabetes insipidus may be present. The clinical course of AFLP resembles those of HELLP syndrome, TTP, and HUS, although the microangiopathy and thrombocytopenia are not as severe.[137] With supportive care, the condition typically resolves within 10 days after delivery.

LEUKEMIA AND LYMPHOMA

The diagnosis of hematologic malignancy during pregnancy can be incredibly traumatic for a pregnant patient and her family, and it is a treatment challenge for the physician. Although great strides have been made in the treatment of this heterogeneous group of diseases, the treatment of pregnant patients is limited because of the lack of research in this area and limited pregnancy safety data. The need to treat the patient and risk to the fetus must both be taken into account. Diagnosis can be difficult because many of the nonspecific signs that accompany these disorders, including fatigue, anemia, loss of appetite, and weight loss, can occur at various times during a normal pregnancy. Diagnostic imaging is limited mainly to ultrasonography and magnetic resonance imaging (MRI). Although the radiation dose from a CT scan is considered low, it is usually avoided. Diagnostic procedures such as bone marrow or lymph node biopsy can usually be performed safely during pregnancy.

In terms of treatment, the risk of teratogenicity from treatment appears highest during fetal organogenesis, which occurs mainly during the first trimester of pregnancy.[138] Ideal dosing is unknown, but dosing is usually based on the woman's prepregnancy weight.

In the largest study of its kind, Aviles and Neri[139] followed 84 children born to mothers with hematologic malignancies, including 29 women with acute leukemia and 38 who received treatment during the first trimester. Assessing growth and development, hematologic parameters, psychological characteristics, and cognitive function over 19 years, the authors found no significant, long-term, deleterious consequences related to treatment. The risk of childhood malignancies was not increased. In a retrospective report following the outcome of 54 newborns of women treated with chemotherapy specifically during the first trimester, long-term development was found to be normal. However, this is in contrast to general incidence of congenital malformations found by others for treatment given during this time period.

Hodgkin Lymphoma

That hematologic malignancies are among the most commonly diagnosed cancers during pregnancy reflects to a large extent the relatively high incidence of Hodgkin lymphoma in women between the ages of 15 and 24 years.[140] On the basis of results of several retrospective studies, Hodgkin lymphoma diagnosed during pregnancy appears to have no significant effect on pregnancy outcome.[141] A single-institution experience published by Dilek and colleagues,[142] however, highlights complications that may occur in pregnant women with Hodgkin disease because children born to three of five women with the disease had complications, including death. Remission rates and 20-year overall survival rates among women diagnosed with Hodgkin disease during pregnancy are reportedly similar to those observed in nonpregnant women with the disease.[143,144] In rare instances, Hodgkin lymphoma metastasizes to the placenta, so the placenta and newborn infant should be examined for evidence of malignancy.[145] Staging during pregnancy can be performed with CT, but MRI is preferred to reduce to exposure of the fetus to radiation.

Similar to other malignancies managed during pregnancy, treatment of women with Hodgkin disease is challenging. Generally, chemotherapy at any point in pregnancy increases the risk of an unfavorable outcome.[142] The teratogenic effects of chemotherapy and radiation during pregnancy are a primary concern. However, the standard regimen of Adriamycin (doxorubicin), bleomycin, vinblastine, and dacarbazine does not appear to increase teratogenic risk when given in the second or third trimester.

Non-Hodgkin lymphoma (NHL) rarely occurs during pregnancy. There are case reports and case series of women with NHL who have been treated successfully with chemotherapy during the second and third trimesters of pregnancy.[145] In a review of 121 cases of pregnancy-associated NHL, 75% had stage IV disease at diagnosis, and reproductive organ involvement was found in half the cases. Placental and fetal involvement were uncommon.[146,147]

Alkylating agents given during the first trimester can result in fetal malformations or death, although there are reports of children who received chemotherapy during the first trimester with no subsequent deficits.[148] On the basis of available data, response and recurrence rates among women treated for NHL during pregnancy are similar to those seen in the treatment of pregnant women with Hodgkin disease.

Acute and Chronic Leukemias

Treatment of acute myeloid leukemia cannot be delayed. Minimal data are available on the treatment of patients with acute leukemia, but in patients treated with chemotherapy during the first trimester, outcomes were poor. For patients in the first trimester, planned abortion should be discussed, followed by treatment with standard induction chemotherapy.[149]

Patients in the second and third trimesters should be treated immediately. There is an association of preterm delivery, IUGR, and spontaneous abortion with treatment in the second and third trimesters.[150] In terms of treatment options, daunorubicin is preferred because idarubicin has increased placental transfer. Amphotericin B is considered the antifungal of choice in pregnancy because there have been no reports of teratogenicity.[151,152] If treatment is not delayed, pregnant women can have outcomes similar to those of nonpregnant patients.

Among acute leukemias arising within the myeloid lineage, acute promyelocytic leukemia is unique in terms of clinical features, particularly DIC and associated bleeding complications, and therapy, which involves all-*trans* retinoic acid (ATRA) in conjunction with traditional chemotherapy. Concern regarding the teratogenic effects of ATRA is warranted. In the 1980s, Lammer and colleagues[153] noted an increased risk of fetal malformation after in utero exposure to the retinoid isotretinoin. In a recent case report, Carradice et al[154] described a bleeding complication that occurred after ATRA initiation in a pregnant woman with acute promyelocytic anemia. However, authors of a review of 13 women treated during pregnancy with ATRA administration for acute promyelocytic anemia found no evidence that the agent led to fetal malformation when used in the treatment of pregnant women.[155]

Similar concerns regarding toxicity of therapy arise in managing pregnancies conceived before and during treatment of chronic myeloid leukemia (CML). Imatinib, a small-molecule inhibitor against the BCR-ABL tyrosine kinase, is the standard of care for treatment of CML. In animal studies, imatinib exhibited

---

Imatinib Therapy

A 38-year-old woman with a history of chronic-phase chronic myeloid leukemia on imatinib therapy for 5 years becomes pregnant. She has had a complete cytogenetic response. She asks what to do about her imatinib therapy.

Imatinib is teratogenic and should not be used during pregnancy. It has been linked to spontaneous abortions and to fetal malformations, including skeletal abnormalities, hydrocephalus, and exophthalmos. Although there are case reports documenting fetal exposure at various stages of pregnancy without harm, it is not recommended. Case reports suggest that patients who have achieved maximal response to therapy fare better when their treatment is held for pregnancy, as opposed to patients who have not achieved best response.

---

teratogenicity in rats and impaired spermatogenesis in dogs, monkeys, and rats.[156] In a series of 19 pregnancies involving a mother or father undergoing imatinib-based therapy for CML, three pregnancies resulted in a spontaneous abortion, and two others produced children with minor malformations.[157] The remaining 13 pregnancies resulted in the delivery of a healthy child. Among mothers in this study who had previously achieved a complete hematologic remission with imatinib and interrupted therapy during pregnancy, a majority (five of nine) lost the hematologic remission. These findings highlight the important therapy-related implications for mother and fetus, which must be weighed carefully in determining an appropriate course of management (see box on Imatinib Therapy). Currently, it is recommended by specialists in the field that patients undergoing treatment with imatinib for CML use proper contraception.[157]

The Myeloproliferative Neoplasms: Essential Thrombocythemia, Polycythemia Vera, and Myelofibrosis

Essential thrombocythemia (ET) has a bimodal peak of distribution, so it is the most common myeloproliferative neoplasm (MPN) in women of childbearing age (see Chapters 69, 70, and 71). Although evidenced-based guidelines do not exist for the management of pregnancy in this setting, more and more information regarding this topic is being reported.[158] Although some variation is seen in the rates of complications among various studies, overall, all of the studies noted a consistent increase in the rate of complications compared with pregnant women without MPN.[158] Pregnancy alone is a risk factor for thrombosis, and pregnancy confers a sixfold increase in the rate of thrombosis in pregnant patients *without* MPN. Thrombosis is a major source of morbidity and mortality in patients with MPN. It is thought that the prothrombotic state that exists in MPN is behind a majority of the morbidity that can develop during pregnancy. Thrombotic occlusion of the placental circulation has been observed.

In a study documenting 103 pregnancies occurring in 62 patients with MPN, the rate of live births was 60%, and the first trimester abortion rate was 32%. Fetal complications occurred in 40% of cases and maternal complications in 9%. The risk of fetal loss for patients with ET was 3.4-fold higher than for those in the aged-matched control population.[159]

A pooled outcome analysis of 461 pregnant patients with ET demonstrated that first-trimester loss occurred in 25% to 40% of patients with a live birth rate of 50% to 70%. Late pregnancy loss occurred in 10% of cases.[160] Postpartum thrombotic complications occurred in 5.2% of patients. In a recent analysis of all publications of pregnant patients with ET that had more than 30 patients per study, a mean rate of live birth obtained from the literature was 60.6% (range, 50%–75.4%).[161]

Studies of pregnancy in the setting of polycythemia vera (PV) are much fewer and consist mainly of case reports. One of the largest studies to date consisted of 18 pregnancies. There were 11 live births and 7 miscarriages.[162] First trimester loss is the most frequent complication in patients with PV.[161] Information regarding pregnancy in primary myelofibrosis is even sparser, with overall fewer than 20 cases reported in the literature. However, on the basis of these, fetal loss is common.[163] In women of childbearing age with an MPN, a discussion when the patient is not pregnant should occur, outlining pregnancy management and risks. Women should be informed if they are taking a drug with teratogenic potential, and the risk of unplanned pregnancy should be recognized.

Continuing aspirin is considered standard if there is no clear contraindication, extrapolating from the results of the European Collaboration on Low-dose Aspirin in Polycythemia Vera (ECLAP) study, which confirmed the importance of aspirin in the management of MPNs.[164] Certain features may confer a patient at more risk of maternal or fetal complications during pregnancy. These include cardiovascular risk factors, prior thrombosis, and prior pregnancy-related complications that may have been caused by MPN or for which no other cause can be identified. In these settings, cytoreductive therapy or LMWH can be considered. There are no clear evidence-based management guidelines in these settings, but local practice is to use LMWH. Six weeks of postpartum LMWH should be considered in the postpartum setting if there is no contraindication. It is clear that management of these patients requires close collaboration with a hematologist and high-risk obstetrician.

BLEEDING DISORDERS

von Willebrand Disease

Affecting approximately 1% of the population, von Willebrand disease (vWD) is the most common inherited disorder of coagulation (see Chapter 139). By mediating platelet adhesion and functioning as a carrier for circulating factor VIII (FVIII), vWF plays a vital role in hemostasis. According to the most widely used classification by Sadler,[165] there are three types of vWD: type 1 (partial deficiency of vWF); type 3 (severe deficiency of vWF); and type 2, which includes four subtypes that involve qualitative defects in vWF. FVIIIc, vWF antigen (vWF:Ag), and the ristocetin cofactor activity (vWF:Rco) are important components of the laboratory diagnosis. vWD does not impair fertility or increase the likelihood of miscarriage.[166] Thus the management of pregnancy in patients with the condition is an important feature of the overall care for these individuals.

For pregnant women with vWD, bleeding at parturition and in the postpartum period is of primary concern. Related concerns include the administration of anesthesia, perineal hematoma, episiotomy blood loss and healing, and bleeding at surgical sites. Approximately 75% of women with moderate to severe vWD experience significant peripartum bleeding.[167] Overall there is a 20% risk of postpartum hemorrhage in women with vWD. In a normal pregnancy, FVIIIc and vWF levels increase, beginning in the second trimester.[168] They peak as the pregnancy nears term. Among many pregnant women with vWD, particularly those with type 1 disease, a similar increase in FVIII and vWF levels is observed. FVIIIc levels in pregnant women with vWD peak at 29 to 32 weeks of gestation, but vWF:Ag levels peak at approximately 35 weeks of gestation.[169] The risk of peripartum bleeding is related to the level of these factors.[170] In most instances, vWF:Ag, FVIIIc, and vWF:Rco levels should be assessed during the first and third trimesters to determine the bleeding risk for individuals with vWD. However, this may be less relevant for patients with type 3 vWD, in whom levels tend to remain low throughout pregnancy. Patients without a documented bleeding disorder who have bleeding complications during pregnancy should be evaluated for vWD because many with the disorder have a mild clinical course and remain undiagnosed for a long period.[171]

As a general rule, therapy can be rendered either in the setting of a spontaneous bleeding event or in a prophylactic context for the high-risk individual. Mainstays of therapy for pregnant women with vWD include DDAVP (1-deamino-8-D-arginine-vasopressin; desmopressin), a synthetic analogue of vasopressin, and vWF-FVIII concentrates (Humate-P, Alphanate). Cryoprecipitate can be used on an emergent basis if vWF-FVIII concentrates are unavailable, but it is avoided if possible during pregnancy because it poses a small risk of bloodborne infection.[172] Although antifibrinolytic therapy plays a role in the management of individuals with vWD, it is also generally avoided during pregnancy and lactation because of its potential teratogenicity and effects on newborns. Data concerning the toxicity of antifibrinolytic therapy in pregnancy are limited.

Exerting its effect through the type 2 vasopressin receptors, DDAVP rapidly and transiently increases levels of FVIII and vWF.[173] It is administered by continuous intravenous infusion over 30 minutes in the setting of an acute bleeding event. On a prophylactic basis, it can be given subcutaneously or inhaled nasally.[174] Although highly effective when used in an appropriate clinical context, DDAVP does have limitations. Patients who have never received DDAVP therapy should be tested for responsiveness to the agent during the second trimester. Because of its potential oxytocic effect, DDAVP is pregnancy risk category B.[175] Owing to its antidiuretic effect, DDAVP can cause fluid retention and hyponatremia. Finally, DDAVP has uncertain utility in the management of women with type 2 and type 3 vWD because of an underlying genetic defect in these individuals. VWF-FVIII concentrate is indicated for these patients.

Multidisciplinary care by an experienced obstetrician and hematologist should be provided for pregnant women with vWD. This becomes particularly important as parturition nears. In providing care for this population of patients, clinicians aim to control the consequences of the disease in pregnant and postpartum mothers. FVIIIc and vWF:RCo levels, partial thromboplastin time (PTT), type and crossmatch, and a complete blood count are obtained at the time of hospital admission. Women with vWD should be monitored for bleeding at the time of delivery, with blood cell products and DDAVP available for use as needed. vWF:RCo and FVIIIc levels of 50 IU/dL generally serve as a target at parturition and in the postpartum period; expert opinion suggests that women with levels below this should receive replacement products.[175]

In the management of pregnant women with vWD, the provision of regional anesthesia during delivery is an important topic. Some anesthesiologists use epidural anesthesia in patients with mild disease with or without the use of DDAVP.[176,177] For patients with moderate to severe disease, an alternative form of analgesia may be considered. If epidural analgesia is used in a patient with moderate to severe disease, prophylactic factor replacement therapy is indicated. The epidural catheter should be removed soon after delivery because falling factor levels in the postpartum period increase the bleeding risk.[173]

The route of delivery is also an important matter in patients with vWD. To minimize the risk of neonatal hemorrhage, some obstetricians recommend cesarean delivery for patients with type 2, type 3, and clinically moderate type 1 disease. However, neonatal bleeding occurs in the setting of cesarean delivery as well, and delivery methods have not been rigorously compared.[167,176]

Prenatal testing is a challenge in women with vWD. The specific mutations involved in the pathogenesis of type 1 and type 3 vWD are not known. Multiple mutations are involved in the pathogenesis of type 2 vWD. Fetal blood vWF levels can be obtained if necessary, but inherent risks are associated with the procedure.[178] Expectant mothers should be informed of these risks in making decisions about prenatal genetic testing.

HEMOPHILIAS

The hemophilias (A and B) are X-linked recessive diseases characterized by hemarthrosis and subcutaneous and intramuscular bleeding (see Chapter 136).[179] Hemophilia A results from deficient production of FVIII, and hemophilia B from deficient production of FIX. As X-linked disorders, hemophilia A and B occur most often in men, but they can occur in women under several circumstances, including X-chromosome inactivation (lyonization), X hemizygosity, and double heterozygosity as can occur in the female offspring of an affected father and carrier mother.[179] In the United States, women account for 1.7% of patients with hemophilia A and 3.2% of patients with hemophilia B.[180] Fifty percent of male offspring from a female carrier inherit the disorder, whereas 100% of male offspring from an affected mother inherit the disease. Female carriers in both disorders can be detected through laboratory screening and pedigree analysis.[181] Women with hemophilia and pregnant women with an affected fetus must be monitored closely during pregnancy for bleeding events that compromise the well-being of either the mother or the fetus. Fetal umbilical blood sampling can be used to check FVIII and FIX levels. Chorionic villus sampling may also be used.[182]

At parturition, women with hemophilia A whose FVIIIc level lies below 50% of the normal range should receive purified FVIII. Levels should be greater than 80% for surgery and maintained at 30% to 40% for 3 to 4 days postoperatively. Rarely, thrombosis can occur in the aftermath of FVIII replacement therapy.[183] Among neonates with hemophilia, 6% to 10% have hemorrhagic complications in the perinatal period, including intracranial hemorrhage. Vacuum extractors, forceps delivery, and scalp electrodes should be avoided. To date, no studies have rigorously compared the outcomes of vaginal and cesarean delivery in this patient population. Neonatal blood should be assayed for FVIIIc levels and PTT immediately after birth. Neonates with low FVIIIc levels may require serial cranial ultrasounds to rule out bleeding.[184]

Hemophilia B is treated in a similar fashion. However, it should be noted that cryoprecipitate contains low levels of FIX and should not be used as replacement therapy in the management of this condition. Purified FIX is the agent of choice for patients with hemophilia B. Meanwhile, individuals with other clotting factor deficiencies should receive FFP or specific clotting factor products to maintain factor levels at greater than 25%.[185] One exception to this pertains to the management of patients with FXIII deficiency; the occurrence of spontaneous recurrent abortions and uterine bleeding in these individuals necessitates regular infusions of FFP or FXIII concentrate to maintain pregnancy.[186]

VENOUS THROMBOEMBOLIC DISEASE AND PREGNANCY

VTE disease is a leading cause of maternal morbidity and mortality.[186] The risk of VTE increases two- to fourfold during pregnancy and the early postpartum period.[187] In women who have had a previous VTE event, pregnancy appears to increase the risk of a recurrent thromboembolic event.[188] Various factors account for the prothrombotic state associated with pregnancy. Increased estrogen levels early in pregnancy increase venous distention and contribute to venous stasis.[189] Increased plasma volume and compression of the inferior vena cava by the gravid uterus contribute to venous stasis as well.[190] In addition, studies have demonstrated decreased blood flow velocity in pregnant women, particularly in the left leg when pregnant women lie in a supine position. This phenomenon likely explains the increased risk of left leg thrombosis among pregnant women.[191] Furthermore, whereas the concentration of coagulation factors changes during pregnancy, the concentration of vWF, fibrinogen, and prothrombin, along with factors V, VII, VIII, IX, X, and XII increase, and the concentration of factor XI and protein S decrease (Table 151.2).[192-194] Finally, fibrinolytic activity decreases during pregnancy as the levels of plasminogen activator inhibitors 1 and 2 increase.[195] Other factors, including high body mass index, smoking, immobilization, and age older than 35 years, should also be considered when assessing the thrombotic risk of a pregnant woman (see box on Bleeding Associated With Factor XI Deficiency).

Because of the prothrombotic physiology associated with pregnancy, a clinician's concern for VTE in a pregnant woman should prompt immediate evaluation. To assess for lower extremity thrombosis, venous compression ultrasonography remains the initial test of choice. Ultrasonography poses no threat to the fetus and can detect thrombosis of the proximal common femoral and popliteal veins with a sensitivity of 95% and specificity of 96%. Despite the efficacy of ultrasonography, limitations to its use do exist. The test is less effective for the diagnosis of calf vein thrombosis, with a sensitivity and specificity in the 60% to 70% range.[196] For this reason, a woman with suspected lower extremity deep venous thrombosis should undergo serial ultrasonography if the initial evaluation is nondiagnostic.[197] Similarly, thrombus in the common iliac vein can evade diagnosis by venous compression ultrasonography.

In such cases, other modalities, such as contrast venography and magnetic resonance venography, can be considered. Although contrast venography exposes the fetus to radiation and should thus be used with caution during pregnancy, its use may be warranted when clinical suspicion for an underlying thrombotic event is high.[196] Serum D-dimer tests are often used in conjunction with imaging studies to assess for thrombosis in nonpregnant patients. The sensitivity of D-dimer tests for the presence of thrombus ranges from 85%

TABLE 151.2	Hemostatic Changes in Pregnancy	
Factor XIII	↑/↓
Protein C, antithrombin	=
Protein S	↓
Factor XI	↓/=
Factors V, VII, VIII, IX, X, XII	↑
von Willebrand factor, fibrinogen	↑
Tissue plasminogen activator	↓
Prothrombin, D-dimer	↑

Prolonged PPT Postpartum

A 22-year-old woman presents to the emergency department (ED) 4 days postpartum. Her delivery was uncomplicated, and her hemoglobin at delivery was 9.9 g/dL with a partial thromboplastin time (PTT) 37 seconds. She returns to the ED 4 days later with complaints of weakness and vaginal bleeding and is found to have a large hematoma at the episiotomy site. It is surgically drained but immediately recurs, and persistent bleeding is noted. Her hemoglobin decreases to 5.9 g/dL. Repeat laboratory evaluation reveals her PTT to be 66 seconds.

Acquired hemophilia should be considered in the postpartum patient with bleeding and prolonged PTT. It is an uncommon disorder, thought to be immune mediated, with development of autoantibodies against factor VIII. Treatment must be targeted at inhibitor eradicator and control of bleeding. For acute bleeding, activated prothrombin complex concentrates or recombinant FVIIa should be used.

Franchini, M. (2006), Am J Hematol, 81:768–773.
CMAJ August 14, 2007 vol. 177(4): 339–340.
Santoro RC, et al. Blood Coagul Fibrinolysis, 20:461, 2009.

Bleeding Associated With Factor XI Deficiency

A 25-year-old woman is referred for prolonged partial thromboplastin time (PTT) discovered during pregnancy. Evaluation reveals severe factor XI deficiency. She has no history of easy bruising or bleeding. She is at 30 weeks of gestation and is presenting for evaluation before delivery.

Bleeding associated with factor XI deficiency can be quite variable, ranging from no bleeding symptoms to bleeding associated with trauma or surgery. For a patient without a history of bleeding, prophylaxis is not necessary but fresh frozen plasma (FFP) should be available if needed. Epidural is usually contraindicated in patients with severe factor XI deficiency, and women should be advised to speak with the treating anesthesiologist before delivery in order to plan alternative strategies. If consideration for regional block anesthesia is made, it is usually administered with FFP prior and with documentation of normalization of the PTT.

In patients with a bleeding history, FFP should be administered before delivery, as well as 2 to 3 days later to reduce the risk of delayed hemorrhage.

to 95%.[198] However, several pregnancy-associated conditions elevate D-dimer levels, including preterm labor, placental abruption, and hypertension of pregnancy, thus undermining the utility of the test somewhat in pregnant women by decreasing its specificity.[195] Nonetheless, when normal, the D-dimer assay provides the clinician with useful information.

When lower extremity imaging reveals no evidence of thrombus in a pregnant woman with suspected pulmonary embolism (PE), the clinician has several options. Helical CT has become the standard modality for the diagnosis of PE in nonpregnant individuals at many centers. However, even with abdominal shielding, the procedure results in fetal radiation exposure (approximately 16 mrad) because of internal scatter.[199] Although this low level of radiation exposure probably does not cause harm to the fetus, repeated imaging during the course of pregnancy is to be avoided.[197] Ventilation/perfusion (V/Q) scanning is frequently used in the evaluation of pregnant women with suspected PE but has limitations as well. Results of a prospective study indicate that when used in this patient population, V/Q scanning infrequently yields a conclusively positive result (1.8% of cases) and is often nondiagnostic (24.8% of cases).[200] Finally, pulmonary angiography can be used in the evaluation of PE in rare instances when the previously described diagnostic tests yield nondiagnostic results in the face of a high clinical suspicion.

VTE in pregnancy is treated with heparin. Until LMWH was introduced in the late 1980s, UFH was the anticoagulant of choice for treatment of pregnant women with VTE. Because it does not cross the placenta, UFH is nonteratogenic. However, drawbacks to UFH therapy, including heparin-associated osteoporosis, HIT, and the drug's unpredictable pharmacokinetics, are well documented.[186] Heparin-associated osteoporosis can develop in women who receive at least 1 month of therapy; it is likely related to a toxic effect of heparin on osteoblasts.[201] Because of its more favorable side effect profile, reliable pharmacokinetics, and equal efficacy in treating VTE, LMWH now represents the most commonly used anticoagulant for treatment of VTE in pregnancy.[202] The risk of osteoporosis and HIT appears to be less with LMWH-based anticoagulation than with UFH-based anticoagulation.[203,204] Although practice patterns vary, it is reasonable to base the initial dose of LMWH on early pregnancy (rather than current) weight.[204] Because clearance of LMWH increases during pregnancy, twice-daily dosing regimens are preferred to once-daily regimens.[205] In terms of duration of therapeutic anticoagulation, many clinicians continue therapy at full dose through the entire pregnancy and puerperium based on the rationale that pregnancy itself represents a risk factor for recurrent VTE.[202] In contrast, other clinicians advocate initial anticoagulation with full-dose LMWH for a designated period followed by conversion to an intermediate dose. This approach may be beneficial for individuals susceptible to side effects of anticoagulation such as bleeding or osteoporosis.[186] The risk of significant bleeding with LMWH during pregnancy is estimated to be around 2%.

Warfarin is contraindicated in pregnant women. It crosses the placenta and can cause both fetal hemorrhage and nervous system abnormalities and other teratogenic effects.[206] Warfarin can be used in the postpartum period after initiating therapy with concurrent heparin and in this setting does not appear to increase the risk of bleeding in children of lactating mothers.[196]

Anticoagulation should be discontinued at the time of parturition. UFH and LMWH should, in most circumstances, be stopped 12 to 24 hours before delivery. If the risk of recurrent VTE is particularly high in a woman receiving LMWH, the clinician can convert to intravenous UFH and treat until 4 to 6 hours before delivery, minimizing the time off anticoagulation.

The risks of regional anesthesia must be weighed carefully in women receiving anticoagulation because therapy increases the likelihood of bleeding, hematoma formation, and potential neurologic compromise. In a woman undergoing elective delivery with discontinuation of anticoagulation 12 to 24 hours prior, epidural anesthesia may be used. UFH or LMWH may be reinitiated 6 to 12 hours after delivery or after removal of the epidural catheter. Then, after therapeutic levels of UFH or LMWH have been achieved, warfarin may

be initiated. The newer target specific oral anticoagulant should not be used during pregnancy until safety data in this population have been established.

PROPHYLACTIC ANTICOAGULATION DURING PREGNANCY

Given the prothrombotic state associated with pregnancy itself, prophylactic anticoagulation should be considered in pregnant women with a history of VTE. Recurrence rates for VTE during pregnancy may be as high as 12% based on the results of retrospective studies.[207] Conversely, Brill-Edwards and colleagues[208] prospectively studied 125 pregnant women with prior VTE in a study that excluded women with known thrombophilia. Study subjects did not receive prophylactic anticoagulation during the antenatal period, but they did receive anticoagulation therapy for 4 to 6 weeks postpartum. The authors documented a VTE recurrence rate of 2.4%. Women who had a temporary risk factor at the time of their initial VTE event and lacked laboratory evidence of an underlying hypercoagulable disorder at the time of study enrollment experienced no recurrences during pregnancy. On the basis of the results of this study, routine prophylactic anticoagulation for women with a single previous VTE event is not recommended. However, patients with a known hypercoagulable state, those with multiple previous VTE events, and those considered high risk for recurrent VTE should receive prophylactic anticoagulation during pregnancy and for 4 to 6 weeks postpartum. As previously discussed, prophylactic anticoagulation can be discontinued at parturition and reinitiated 6 to 12 hours postpartum.

The management of pregnant women with prosthetic heart valves is controversial and deserves special attention, although a full review of the topic is beyond the scope of this review. Coupled with the prothrombotic physiology of pregnancy, the presence of a prosthetic valve places such women in an ultra-high-risk category. Before the introduction of LMWH, options for anticoagulation in this patient population included (1) warfarin throughout pregnancy; (2) warfarin with UFH during weeks 6 to 12, the period of major organogenesis; and (3) UFH throughout pregnancy.[186] More recently, LMWH has been used in this setting, although its safety and efficacy have been questioned on the basis of several studies. Overall, a lack of rigorous, comparative studies hinders evidence-based management of women with prosthetic heart valves. Current recommendations allow for one of three therapeutic strategies, initiated after a thorough discussion of risks and benefits with the patient: (1) warfarin, with LMWH or UFH substituted during weeks 6 to 12; (2) dose-adjusted UFH throughout pregnancy; or (3) dose-adjusted LMWH throughout pregnancy.[186]

THROMBOPHILIA AND PREGNANCY

Thrombophilias, inherited and acquired, increase the risk of VTE in pregnant women and adversely affect pregnancy outcomes. Included within this category of diseases are factor V Leiden, prothrombin gene polymorphisms, antiphospholipid antibody syndrome, antithrombin deficiency, and protein S and C deficiency. In addition, hyperhomocysteinemia and methylenetetrahydrofolate reductase C677T mutation have been studied. There are varied results when assessing the literature in regard to the risk of pregnancy-associated VTE in the setting of an inherited thrombophilia. Authors of a 2005 meta-analysis reviewed the risk of VTE during pregnancy by the specific thrombophilia present. The inherited thrombophilias (with the exception of *MTHFR* mutation) were associated with a statistically significant increase in the risk of VTE during pregnancy.[209] Because the overall incidence of VTE in pregnancy is low, however, in women without a history of thrombosis, the absolute risk conferred by thrombophilias is generally low. The positive predictive value of factor V Leiden heterozygosity was 1 in 500. Prothrombin heterozygosity was 1 in 200. Women with homozygosity for these mutations, double heterozygosity, and antithrombin III deficiency were at highest risk. Given the increased risk of VTE, prophylactic anticoagulation is warranted.

Screening for inherited thrombophilia in patients with recurrent miscarriage or pregnancy complications such as preeclampsia or placental abruption is not indicated. Thrombophilia screening is indicated only in patients with a prior thromboembolic event or a high likelihood of thrombophilia. Selective screening based on personal and family history is recommended (see box on The TIPPS (Thrombophilia in Pregnancy Prophylaxis Study) Trial and box on Thrombophilia During Pregnancy).

Prophylactic treatment of carriers of low-risk mutations with any personal or family history of VTE is not indicated. In patients with

recurrent miscarriage, anticoagulation has been used in efforts to improve rates of live birth. There have been varied results in clinical trials using anticoagulation in the setting of recurrent miscarriage. However, in the large, multicenter, randomized, placebo-controlled study examining the use of aspirin or aspirin plus heparin in women with unexplained miscarriage, there was no improvement in the live birth rate compared with placebo.[210]

Antiphospholipid Antibody Syndrome

The antiphospholipid antibody syndrome (Table 151.3) is the most common form of acquired thrombophilia.[211] Antiphospholipid antibodies include lupus anticoagulant antibodies and anticardiolipin antibodies. They can occur as a manifestation of various conditions, such as systemic lupus erythematosus (SLE) and other rheumatic diseases, infection, and drug reactions. Antiphospholipid antibodies exert their prothrombotic effect through several mechanisms. For example, they inhibit the activity of anticoagulants thrombomodulin, protein S, protein C, β_2-glycoprotein I, and prostacyclin.[212-214] They interact with phospholipids on the surface of platelets, increasing platelet adhesiveness and production of von Willebrand mulitmers.[215,216] In pregnant patients, antiphospholipid antibodies decrease levels of annexin V, a potent vascular endothelial anticoagulant produced by placental trophoblasts.[217] Nonpregnant individuals with antiphospholipid antibody syndrome can develop arterial and venous thromboses. In pregnant women, antiphospholipid antibody syndrome can manifest as thrombotic events, spontaneous abortion, preeclampsia, and HELLP syndrome, as well as IUGR.[218-221]

Antiphospholipid antibodies can be detected in 5% of healthy pregnant women and 37% of pregnant women with SLE.[222] Thrombotic events occur in approximately 5% of pregnant women with antiphospholipid antibodies.[221] All pregnant women with SLE should undergo testing for antiphospholipid antibodies. Women who sustain recurrent spontaneous abortions or a thromboembolic event during pregnancy should also undergo evaluation for the disorder. A history of either vascular thrombosis or fetal loss coupled with the presence of either lupus anticoagulant antibodies or anticardiolipin antibodies establishes the diagnosis of antiphospholipid antibody syndrome.[223]

False-negative laboratory results do occur and do so more frequently in pregnant than in nonpregnant women. This may be because of the increased concentration of clotting factors observed in pregnancy.[224] Women with antiphospholipid antibody syndrome who have sustained prior thrombotic events receive therapeutic anticoagulation during pregnancy. Those with antiphospholipid antibodies but no manifestations of the clinical syndrome should receive prophylactic anticoagulation.

The TIPPS (Thrombophilia in Pregnancy Prophylaxis Study) Trial

The TIPPS trial was the first large randomized controlled trial in which researchers examined the effect of low-molecular-weight heparin (LMWH) in pregnant patients with thrombophilia and a history of on adverse pregnant outcomes or venous thromboembolism (VTE). The TIPPS investigators studied 292 pregnant women who were randomly assigned to dalteparin or no dalteparin. The primary objective of the study was to identify if LMWH prophylaxis in thrombophilic pregnant women results in a greater than 33% relative risk reduction in the composite outcome measure of severe or early-onset preeclampsia, small-for-gestational-age infants (<10th percentile), pregnancy loss, or VTE. Dalteparin did not reduce the incidence of the primary composite outcome in both intention-to-treat analysis (dalteparin, 25 [17.1%] of 146; 95% confidence interval [CI], 11.4%–24.2%; vs. no dalteparin, 27 [18.9%] of 143; 95% CI, 12.8%–26.3%; risk difference, –1.8%; 95% CI, –10.6% to 7.1%) and on-treatment analysis (dalteparin 28 [19.6%] of 143 vs. no dalteparin 24 [17.0%] of 141; risk difference, +2.6%; 95% CI, –6.4% to 11.6%). Major bleeding did not differ. More minor bleeding was seen in the dalteparin group (28 [19.6%] of 143) than in the no-dalteparin group (13 [9.2%] of 141; risk difference, 10.4%; 95% CI, 2.3–18.4; $p = .01$).

The conclusion from the study was that prophylactic dalteparin did not reduce the occurrence of venous thromboembolism, pregnancy loss, or placenta-mediated pregnancy complications in pregnant women with thrombophilia.

Some debate and controversy exist regarding the trial and its conclusions.

Cons: It took 12 years to randomize 292 women from 21 referral centers. Some physicians raised concern over the amount of time it took to accrue the number of patients and the accuracy of the patient base it represents. Others argued that eligibility criteria were based on a rationale that had already changed by the time the study was concluded.

Pros: The article confirms that women who are at low risk of thrombosis should not be treated with low-molecular-weight heparin and that this widespread practice should be stopped.

Cons: Many of these women were women who would be placed in "lower-risk" categories to begin with, such as women who were heterozygous for thrombophilic mutations such as factor V Leiden mutation with one family member with a history of thrombosis.

Thrombophilia During Pregnancy

A 25-year-old woman wishes to become pregnant. Her mother experienced a deep vein thrombosis at the age of 70 years, underwent thrombophilia evaluation, and was found to be heterozygous for the factor V Leiden mutation. She herself has never had a thrombotic episode, just recently discontinued her birth control, and was told to see a hematologist before she became pregnant. Her primary care physician tested her for factor V Leiden, and she was found to be heterozygous for the mutation. She is asking if she should be on anticoagulation during her pregnancy.

Every case of thrombophilia during pregnancy needs to be assessed on a case-by-case basis. Asymptomatic women who harbor thrombophilic conditions but have never manifested clinical manifestations do not require anticoagulation.

TABLE 151.3 Antiphospholipid Antibody Syndrome

Vascular Thrombosis

One or more episodes of arterial or venous thrombosis confirmed by imaging

Pregnancy morbidity

Death of a fetus beyond 10 weeks of gestation with normal fetal morphology

Premature birth before 34 weeks of gestation

Three or more consecutive spontaneous abortions before 10 weeks of gestation

Laboratory criteria (all measured on two or more occasions at least 12 weeks apart)

Lupus anticoagulant on two or more occasions at least 12 weeks apart

Anticardiolipin antibody

Anti-B_2 glycoprotein IgM or IgG

Ig, Immunoglobulin.

FUTURE DIRECTIONS

Management of the hematologic complications of pregnancy continues to be a challenge. The physicians and patient involved all benefit from a multidisciplinary approach. In certain disorders, the management is clear and will likely remain unchanged in the future. In other disorders, treatment paradigms may shift as new treatments are discovered for the nonpregnant patient. In all instances, further well-designed studies will continue to advance evidence-based management of the pregnant patient.

SUGGESTED READINGS

Al RA, Unlubilgin E, Kandamir O, et al: Intravenous verses oral iron for treatment of anemia in pregnancy: a randomized trial. *Obstet Gynecol* 106:1335, 2005.

Allen LH: Nutritional supplementation for the pregnant woman. *Clin Obstet Gynecol* 37:587, 1994.

Bothwell TH: Overview and mechanisms of iron regulation. *Nutr Rev* 53:237, 1995.

Casanueva E, Viteri FE, Mares-Galindo M, et al: Weekly iron as a safe alternative to daily supplementation for nonanemic pregnant women. *Arch Med Res* 12:674, 2006.

Centers for Disease Control and Prevention (CDC): CDC criteria for anemia in children and childbearing-aged women. *MMWR Morb Mortal Wkly Rep* 38:400, 1989.

Centers for Disease Control and Prevention (CDC): Recommendations to prevent and control iron deficiency in the United States. *MMWR Recomm Rep* 47(RR-3):1, 1998.

Chanarin I: Folate and cobalamin. *Clin Haematol* 14:729, 1985.

Chanarin I, MacGibbon BM, O'Sullivan WJ, et al: Folic acid deficiency in pregnancy—the pathogenesis of megaloblastic anemia of pregnancy. *Lancet* 2:634, 1959.

Chanarin I, Rothman D: Further observations on the relation between iron and folate status in pregnancy. *Br Med J* 2:81, 1971.

Cogswell ME, Parvanta I, Ickes L, et al: Iron supplementation during pregnancy, anemia, and birth rate: a randomized trial. *Am J Clin Nutr* 78:773, 2003.

Council on Foods and Nutrition Committee on Iron Deficiency: Iron deficiency in the United States. *JAMA* 203:119, 1968.

Crowley JP: Coagulopathy bleeding in the parturient patient: recent information has helped in the identification of individuals at special risk. *R I Med J* 72:135, 1989.

Galloway R, McGuire J: Determinants of compliance with iron supplementation: supplies, side effects, or psychology? *Soc Sci Med* 39:381, 1994.

Garn SM, Ridella SA, Petzold AS, et al: Maternal hematologic levels and pregnancy outcomes. *Semin Perinatol* 5:155, 1981.

Hiss RG: Evaluation of the anemic patient. In Laros RK, editor: *Blood disorders in pregnancy*, Philadelphia, 1986, Lea & Febiger, p 1.

Hytten F: Blood volume changes in normal pregnancy. *Clin Haematol* 14:601, 1985.

Institute of Medicine: *Nutrition services in perinatal care*, Washington, DC, 1992, National Academy Press.

Klebanoff MA, Shiono PH, Selby JV, et al: Anemia and spontaneous preterm birth. *Am J Obstet Gynecol* 164:59, 1991.

Lieberman E, Ryan KJ, Monson RR, et al: Association of maternal hematocrit with premature labor. *Am J Obstet Gynecol* 159:107, 1988.

Lu ZM, Goldenberg RL, Oliver SP, et al: The relationship between maternal hematocrit and pregnancy outcome. *Obstet Gynecol* 77:190, 1991.

Milman N: Iron and pregnancy—a delicate balance. *Ann Hematol* 85:559, 2006.

Milman N, Agger AI, Nielson OJ: Iron status markers and serum erythropoietin in 120 mothers and newborn infants: effect of iron supplementation and normal pregnancy. *Acta Obstet Gynecol Scand* 73:200, 1994.

Murphy JF, O'Riordan J, Newcombe RG, et al: Relation of haemoglobin levels in first and second trimesters to outcome of pregnancy. *Lancet* 1:992, 1986.

Perry GS, Yip R, Zyrkowski C: Nutritional risk factors among low-income pregnant US women: the Centers for Disease Control and Prevention (CDC) Pregnancy Nutrition Surveillance System, 1979 through 1993. *Semin Perinatol* 19:211, 1995.

Romslo I, Haram K, Sagen N, et al: Iron requirement in normal pregnancy as assessed by serum ferritin, serum transferring saturation, and erythrocyte protoporphyrin determinations. *Br J Obstet Gynaecol* 90:101, 1983.

Rothman D: Folic acid in pregnancy. *Am J Obstet Gynecol* 108:149, 1970.

Scholl TO, Hediger ML: Anemia and iron-deficiency anemia: compilation of data on pregnancy outcome. *Am J Clin Nutr* 59(2 Suppl):492S, 1994.

Scholl TO, Hediger ML, Fischer RL, et al: Anemia vs iron deficiency: increased risk of preterm delivery in a prospective study. *Am J Clin Nutr* 55:985, 1992.

Singh K, Fong YF, Arulkumaran S: Anaemia in pregnancy—a cross-sectional study in Singapore. *Eur J Clin Nutr* 52:65, 1998.

World Health Organization: *The prevalence of anaemia in women: a tabulation of available information*, ed 2, Geneva, 1992, World Health Organization.

Zhou LM, Yang WW, Hua JZ, et al: Relation of hemoglobin measured at different times in pregnancy to preterm birth and low birth weight in Shanghai, China. *Am J Epidemiol* 148:998, 1998.

REFERENCES

For the complete list of references, log on to www.expertconsult.com.

CHAPTER 152

HEMATOLOGIC MANIFESTATIONS OF CHILDHOOD ILLNESS

Arthur Kim Ritchey, Sarah H. O'Brien, and Frank G. Keller

The hematologic response to systemic illness in children is similar to that in adults. A number of disorders occur more frequently in children, however, and some are unique to the pediatric population. In addition, interpretation of the hematologic response is predicated on knowledge of the normal developmental changes that occur within the hematopoietic system throughout childhood (Table 152.1). This chapter focuses on the hematologic manifestations of common or unique systemic diseases that occur in neonates, children, and adolescents. Illnesses that often require hematologic consultation are emphasized. Systemic diseases that produce hematologic abnormalities that are similar in adults and children are discussed in other chapters. For a comprehensive review of the subject, readers are referred to a published textbook.[1]

INFECTIOUS DISEASE

Infection, especially viral infection, is the most common problem encountered by pediatricians. Although most infections do not produce significant hematologic sequelae, all classes of microorganisms have been implicated in the pathogenesis of hematologic abnormalities that range from mild and clinically irrelevant to severe and life threatening. This section describes the changes seen in red blood cells (RBCs), white blood cells (WBCs), platelets, and the coagulation system that are routinely encountered, are associated with a specific infection, or have a potentially serious clinical impact.

Changes in Red Blood Cells

The anemia of chronic inflammation or infection in children is similar to that seen in adults in terms of both clinical and hematologic findings and pathogenesis.[2] However, anemia with acute infections occurs more commonly in children than in adults.

Anemia of Acute Infections

A mild to moderate anemia of uncertain etiology may occur in the setting of both acute viral infections and more serious bacterial infections. In a study of children with mild viral or bacterial infections in the outpatient setting, anemia was documented in 5% of children 4 to 12 years of age, 17% of children 6 months to 4 years of age, and 33% of infants 6 to 11 months of age.[3] In 14 of 15 young children, the anemia resolved within 3 to 4 weeks. However, multiple mild infections may predispose infants to the development of a more chronic, mild anemia or low-normal hemoglobin that may be caused by iron deficiency, thus warranting a trial of iron supplementation.

Among children hospitalized with moderately severe inflammatory processes, the incidence of mild anemia (hemoglobin, 10.1–11.0 g/dL) is as high as 78%.[4] In a study of hospitalized children with either pyelonephritis bacteremia, average age 5 to 6 years, 60% had anemia.[5] No evidence of hemolysis was seen in this group of children. Follow-up hemoglobin measurements in a subset of patients showed levels had returned to normal without specific intervention. These data suggest that there is no indication to investigate the mild anemia of acute infection. Specific acute bacterial infections associated with a high incidence of anemia (44%–74%) include bone and joint infections, typhoid fever, brucellosis, and invasive *Haemophilus influenzae* infections.

The anemia associated with *H. influenzae* meningitis is the most thoroughly studied of the anemias of acute infection to date. A majority of children with *H. influenzae* meningitis have mild anemia on admission, with hemoglobin in the 9–11 g/dL range, and up to 90% become anemic during the course of the illness.[6] This is in contrast with meningitis secondary to *Streptococcus pneumoniae* or *Neisseria meningitidis,* in which anemia is uncommon. The pathophysiology of the anemia of *H. influenzae* disease appears to be multifactorial. Shurin and associates[7] have shown that *H. influenzae* capsular polysaccharide, polyribosylribitol phosphate, binds to erythrocytes, which, in the presence of antibody and complement, can result in intravascular and extravascular hemolysis. They further hypothesize that polyribosylribitol phosphate alone may induce more rapid clearance of RBCs, perhaps on the basis of decreased RBC deformability. In addition, hypoferremia may limit bone marrow response to hemolysis. As a result of immunization with pneumococcal and *H. influenzae* vaccines in early childhood, it is uncommon to see infections secondary to these organisms currently.

Acute Hemolytic Anemia

Acute hemolysis has been observed with infections from all classes of microorganisms but is relatively uncommon. The anemia may be mild to severe, and the condition is manifested in children in either of two ways: (1) clinical presentation with symptoms and signs of infection predominating in a child subsequently found to have anemia or (2) clinical presentation with the manifestations of acute hemolytic anemia.

The mechanism of hemolysis in patients presenting with an infectious disorder depends on the infecting organism, but hemolysis is extravascular in most cases.[8] Reported mechanisms include the following:

- Release of hemolysins (*Clostridium perfringens* sepsis)
- Invasion of the RBCs (malaria)
- Alteration of the RBC surface:
  Direct adherence by the organism (*Bartonella* spp.)
  Alterations of antigenic phenotype by neuraminidase (influenza virus)
  Cold agglutinins (*Mycoplasma* spp., *Listeria* spp., Epstein-Barr virus [EBV], *Leptospira* spp., *Rubella* spp.[8])
  Absorption of capsular polysaccharide (*H. influenzae*)

- Mechanical mechanisms (microangiopathy associated with disseminated intravascular coagulation [DIC] or hemolytic uremic syndrome [HUS])
- Oxidative damage in persons with congenital enzyme deficiencies (e.g., hepatitis or brucellosis[9] with glucose-6-phosphate dehydrogenase [G6PD] deficiency, *Campylobacter jejuni* infection in neonates)

Acute, infection-associated hemolytic anemia in one study lagged behind the clinical infection by 3 to 7 days.[10] Most children were shown to have adsorption of microbial antigens to the RBC surface, suggesting an "innocent bystander" mechanism of erythrocyte

Normal Hematologic Values in Childhood

	Hb (g/dL)		RBCs Hct (%)		MCV (fL)		Total (×10³/µL)		White Cells		Coagulation			
									Neutrophils (%)	Lymphocytes (%)	PTᵃ (s)		aPTTᵃ (s)	
Age	Mean	(Range)	Mean	(Range)	Mean	(Range)	Mean	(Range)	Mean	Mean	Mean	(Range)	Mean	(Range)
Birth (term)	18.5	(14.5–22.5)	56	(45–69)	108	(95–121)	18.1	(9.3–30.0)	61	31	16	(13–20)	55	(45–65)
2 mo	11.2	(9.4–14.0)	35	(28–42)	96	(77–115)								
6 mo–2 yr	12.5	(11.0–14.0)	37	(33–41)	77	(70–84)	11.3	(6.0–17.5)	32	61				
2–6 yr	12.5	(11.5–13.5)	37	(34–40)	81	(75–87)	8.5	(5.0–15.5)	42	50				
6–12 yr	13.5	(11.5–15.5)	40	(35–45)	86	(77–95)	8.1	(4.5–13.5)	53	39				
12–18 yr							7.8	(4.5–13.5)	57	35				
Male	14.5	(13.0–16.0)	43	(37–49)	88	(78–98)								
Female	14.0	(12.0–16.0)	41	(36–46)	90	(78–102)								

ᵃThe normal range for the PT and aPTT varies between laboratories. The time at which normal adult values are attained is 1 week for the PT and 2 to 9 months for the aPTT. The platelet count is within the adult range from birth.
aPTT, Activated partial thromboplastin time; Hb, hemoglobin; Hct, hematocrit; MCV, mean corpuscular volume; PT, prothrombin time; RBC, red blood cell.
Data from Rudolph AM, Hoffman JIE, editors: *Pediatrics*, ed 17, East Norwalk, CT, 1982, Appleton-Century-Crofts, p 1036, and from Nathan DG, Oski FA, editors: *Hematology of infancy and childhood*, ed 3, Philadelphia, 1987, Saunders, p 1679.

sensitization, ultimately leading to hemolysis. A minority of patients in this series had classic autoantibody-mediated hemolytic anemia.

Autoimmune hemolytic anemia (AIHA) in children usually is transient, is not associated with underlying systemic disease, and carries a low mortality rate. Children frequently have a history of concurrent or recently resolved infection, especially viral upper respiratory tract infection. Anticytomegalovirus (anti-CMV) immunoglobulin G (IgG) has been implicated as the cause of acute AIHA in infants with CMV disease. Although mycoplasma pneumonia is usually associated with cold agglutinin syndrome, there is a report of multiple episodes of warm antibody-mediated hemolytic anemia in a child with Down syndrome.[11] Parvovirus has been rarely associated with AIHA. In some, but not all, cases, the Donath-Landsteiner antibody was identified.[12] In the typical acute, transient cases, 59% to 68% of children have a history of recent infection, but only 0% to 20% of those with the less common chronic course have such a history of infection.

Aplastic Crisis

Temporary arrest of RBC production has been observed in children with infections, but anemia is uncommon because of the long RBC lifespan. In two situations, however, severe anemia has been linked with infection and cessation of erythropoiesis: (1) B19 parvovirus infection in patients with an underlying hemolytic anemia and (2) transient erythroblastopenia of childhood (TEC).

The B19 parvovirus has been a known pathogen in animals for years but has only recently been linked with human disease.[13] It is the etiologic agent of fifth disease (erythema infectiosum), a mild illness with a characteristic "slapped cheek" facial erythema and a generalized reticular rash. In normal volunteers infected with B19 parvovirus, a mild, transient, and clinically irrelevant drop in the hemoglobin and reticulocyte count was observed.[14] In normal children, this infection usually is not associated with hematologic abnormalities, although reports of both hematologic and nonhematologic effects are increasing.[15] In children with sickle cell disease, spherocytosis, and other hemolytic anemias, B19 parvovirus infection can produce a severe anemia associated with peripheral reticulocytopenia and marrow erythroblastopenia—the "aplastic crisis." There may be other transient cytopenias noted during the RBC aplastic crisis.[16] Recovery within 1 to 2 weeks is the rule, but transfusion may be necessary.

B19 parvovirus infection also has been associated with prolonged anemia and reticulocytopenia in children with acute lymphoblastic leukemia (ALL) in remission, those with solid tumors receiving chemotherapy, those with immunodeficiency, those who have undergone renal transplant, those with AIHA, and as the initial manifestation of human immunodeficiency virus (HIV) infection. Human parvovirus also has been identified as a cause of nonimmune hydrops fetalis.[17]

TEC is a syndrome characterized by temporary arrest of RBC production with moderate to severe anemia in previously normal infants and toddlers. Although no specific infectious agent has been proved to cause TEC, the frequency of a history of infection within 1 to 3 months, the seasonal clustering, and the similarity to childhood idiopathic thrombocytopenic purpura (ITP) all suggest a possible viral etiology. B19 parvovirus has not been definitively associated with TEC.[18]

Changes in White Blood Cells

Children, as a rule, have the expected leukocyte response to infection. Infants and young children normally have a lymphocyte predominance (see Table 152.1), however, and any leukocyte response to infection must be judged on the basis of age-related normal values.

The predictive value of the peripheral WBC and differential counts in suspected bacterial infections has been extensively evaluated in infants and children. Todd has shown that in hospitalized children, a neutrophil count greater than 10,000/µL or a band count greater than 500/µL is associated with an 80% chance of having a bacterial infection.[19] In children undergoing evaluation for possible meningitis, Lembo and colleagues[20] found that a ratio of immature to total neutrophils greater than 0.12 was more strongly associated with and more sensitive for bacterial meningitis than was the total WBC count or the total band count. Febrile children between the ages of 3 and 48 months are at increased risk for bacteremia, especially with *S. pneumoniae*. McCarthy and associates[21] demonstrated a threefold increase in the risk of bacteremia in febrile (temperatures >40°C) children younger than 2 years of age who had a WBC count of 15,000/µL or greater. In this setting, the WBC count was a more sensitive indicator of the presence of pneumonia or bacteremia than was the absolute neutrophil or band count. The degree of leukocytosis (i.e., >25,000/mm² vs. <15,000/mm²) probably has no further discriminative ability.[22] Other studies have found both the WBC count and absolute neutrophil count (ANC) to be of value in differentiating bacterial from nonbacterial infection; the band count was not helpful.

There are recognized exceptions to the anticipated leukocyte response to infection that may serve as a clue to the diagnosis. In typhoid fever and brucellosis, leukopenia and neutropenia are prominent early in the illness. Shigellosis is associated with a variable leukocyte count, but the count often is normal, with a greater percentage of bands than neutrophils. Illnesses associated with lymphocytosis include pertussis (whooping cough), infectious lymphocytosis, infectious mononucleosis, and other viral infections. Neutropenia can be seen in bacterial sepsis from meningococci, pneumococci, staphylococci, and other bacteria and is associated with a poor prognosis. Black children (and adults) normally have lower WBC and neutrophil counts than those seen in whites; leukocyte and neutrophil response to serious infection may be decreased.[23]

Neutropenia

The most common cause of neutropenia (neutrophil count <1500/μL) in children is viral infection. A number of specific viruses are associated with neutropenia, including hepatitis virus, roseola virus, rubella virus, mumps virus, adenovirus, coxsackievirus A21, EBV, human herpesvirus-6 (HHV-6), and influenza virus.[24] The most common clinical setting, however, is the incidental discovery of neutropenia in a child with a nonspecific viral syndrome. Usually the neutropenia in this situation continues for less than 30 days and is rarely associated with infectious or long-term[25] complications. In one large study of 1888 otherwise healthy children with fever and ANC counts below 1000/μL, there was only a 1.3% incidence of serious bacterial infection in children older than 3 months of age (1 bacteremia infection, 13 urinary tract infections). The risk was higher in infants younger than 3 months of age (3.3%), similar to the risk of febrile infants of the same age without neutropenia.[26] Neutropenia also has been associated with a number of bacterial, rickettsial, and fungal infections.[27] Although infection is the most common cause of transient neutropenia in childhood, the febrile child discovered to have incidental neutropenia should have repeat blood counts done within 3 to 4 weeks to rule out chronic neutropenia.

Eosinophilia

The most common cause of eosinophilia worldwide is parasitic infection. In the United States, visceral larva migrans (*Toxocara* infestation) is the most common cause of exaggerated eosinophilia (WBC count 30,000–100,000/μL with 50%–90% mature eosinophils) in children.[28] Mild to moderate eosinophilia (≥600/μL) is most often seen in children with allergic rhinitis or asthma but also is characteristic of chlamydial pneumonitis in infants.

Changes in Platelets or Coagulation

Thrombocytosis

Thrombocytosis (platelet count >500,000/μL) is known as an acute-phase reaction to infection, but it has been infrequently identified in children in the past. There is a particularly high incidence of reactive thrombocytosis in patients with bacterial infections, especially pneumonia with emphysema, and *H. influenzae* meningitis. Inflammatory cytokines, such as interleukin (IL)-1, IL-6, and thrombopoietin, may play an etiologic role in the reactive thrombocytosis of infection.[29] The vast majority of children with thrombocytosis have platelet counts between 500 and 700,000/μL, but 6% to 8% have counts between 700 and 900,000/μL and only 0.5% to 3% have platelet counts above 1,000,000/μL.[30] Thrombocytosis may be more common in simple acute infections than was previously recognized. Heath and Pearson[31] documented a 13% incidence of thrombocytosis in ambulatory patients; children with an increased platelet count were more likely to have a diagnosis of infection. In a Japanese study of more than 7500 hospitalized patients with platelet counts greater than 500,000, 6% of patients had thrombocytosis with an age-dependent incidence: 12.5% in neonates, 35.8% in 1-month-old babies, 12.9%

in 6- to 12-month-old infants, and 0.6% in 11- to 15-year-old children. Infection was the cause of the thrombocytosis in 67.5% of the cases.[32] Complications of reactive thrombocytosis are rare, but hemorrhagic or thrombotic complications may occur if there are additional acquired risk factors. Antiplatelet therapy is not indicated in patients with reactive thrombocytosis secondary to infection. Although the most common cause of thrombocytosis in children is infection, the list of considerations in the differential diagnosis of an elevated platelet count is extensive[33] and rarely includes underlying childhood malignancy.

Thrombocytopenia

Thrombocytopenia can be seen in patients who have infections with all types of organisms. Common viral agents include varicella virus, EBV, influenza virus, rubella virus, mumps virus, measles virus (wild or vaccine strains), HHV-6, hepatitis A virus, and CMV. The primary mechanism of the thrombocytopenia is immune destruction, although a direct viral effect on the platelet, megakaryocyte, or hematopoietic stem cell has been demonstrated. Because childhood ITP is thought to be secondary to infection in most instances, the definitions of "thrombocytopenia with infection" and "childhood ITP" tend to merge. Thrombocytopenia from infection usually is transient, although instances of chronic thrombocytopenia from specific viral infections (e.g., varicella or CMV) have been documented.[34,35]

Thrombocytopenia also is associated with bacterial sepsis. The low platelet count may be an isolated finding or associated with DIC. Corrigan[36] documented a 61% incidence of thrombocytopenia in 45 children with sepsis. The degree of thrombocytopenia was mild to moderate (64% had platelet counts >50,000/μL), but platelet counts ranged as low as 8000/μL. There was no evidence of DIC in 39% of those with low platelet counts. Thrombocytopenia in the setting of bacterial sepsis probably is also mediated by an immune mechanism with elevated platelet-associated IgG.

Petechial bleeding without thrombocytopenia can be seen in both bacterial and viral disease, especially that caused by meningococci, streptococci, and echoviruses. The explanation for the petechial rash in these infections is either vasculitis or platelet dysfunction.

Disseminated Intravascular Coagulation and Purpura Fulminans

Disseminated intravascular coagulation is uncommon after childhood infections and, if present, usually is accompanied by shock, with at least a 50% mortality rate. The most common organisms producing DIC are bacterial, especially the gram-negative bacteria (meningococci, *H. influenzae, Aerobacter* spp., and others) but also gram-positive organisms (*Staphylococcus aureus;* group B streptococci; *S. pneumoniae,* particularly in asplenic hosts; and *Bacillus anthracis*). DIC also is associated with disseminated viral (varicella, measles, and rubella), rickettsial (Rocky Mountain spotted fever), fungal, mycoplasmal, and parasitic infections.

Purpura fulminans is a rare syndrome, seen in extremely ill children with DIC. Purpura fulminans is characterized by the rapid progression of ecchymotic skin lesions, especially of the extremities, that may progress to gangrene, ultimately resulting in amputation.[37] This syndrome has been described as a postinfectious purpura, with scarlet fever, upper respiratory tract infection, and varicella as the most common preceding illnesses and a latent period of 0 to 90 days after infection. A similar clinical picture can be seen in children with DIC and acute bacterial sepsis, especially meningococcemia.

Increasing evidence indicates that DIC with purpura fulminans is associated with deficiency of the naturally occurring anticoagulants. Children with postviral purpura fulminans have been shown to have acquired protein S deficiency, anti–protein S antibody, or the presence of a lupus anticoagulant.[38,39] In children with infectious purpura, protein C activation is impaired, as reflected in low levels of protein C, protein S, and antithrombin. These findings are consistent with downregulation of the endothelial thrombomodulin–protein C receptor pathway.[40] The severity of protein C deficiency has been associated with increased morbidity and mortality.[41] There are minimal data on the frequency of inherited thrombophilia in children who develop purpura fulminans. In one report, the frequency of factor V Leiden was not different from that in healthy children; the presence of factor V Leiden was not associated with an increased mortality rate, although complications were increased.[42] In another study of 16 children with purpura fulminans, 6 (37%) of 16 patients studied had the factor V Leiden mutation. All of the children in this study survived, but 10 (63%) required amputation.[43]

Treatment of purpura fulminans consists of antibiotics for suspected bacterial infection, volume replacement for shock, and heparin. Although there is controversy regarding the routine use of heparin in DIC, its use in purpura fulminans has been associated with an improved outcome when it is started early in the course of the disease and continued for 2 to 3 weeks.[44] Theoretically, to improve the efficacy of heparin, it is reasonable to infuse fresh frozen plasma or antithrombin III (AT III) concentrates[45] if the AT III level is low. There is anecdotal evidence that infusion of AT III concentrates or protein C concentrates partially corrects or normalizes the hemostatic abnormalities.[46,47] However, in the KyberSept trial, a double-blind, placebo-controlled trial of the use of AT III concentrates in 2300 adults with sepsis, researchers found no difference in mortality at day 28 after diagnosis.[48] In a phase II trial of protein C concentrate in the treatment of sepsis and purpura fulminans in children, there was dose-dependent activation of protein C and normalization of coagulation imbalances. Although there was no improvement in the mortality rate, the study was not powered to detect these changes.[49]

In initial trials, recombinant human activated protein C (drotrecogin alfa [activated]) reduced the mortality rate in adults with severe sepsis,[50] but in pediatric trials, there was no noticeable improvement in mortality (children have a lower mortality rate than adults), and there were significant bleeding risks.[50,51] Although activated protein C has been used in patients with purpura fulminans, the data do not suggest a beneficial effect on mortality.[52,53] Use of nonactivated protein C concentrates early in the course of purpura fulminans may, however, decrease the need for subsequent skin grafts and amputations.[54] In October 2011, this agent was withdrawn from the market after a major study showed no efficacy for the treatment of sepsis. Recombinant tissue plasminogen activator (t-PA) has been used in an attempt to restore organ perfusion by dissolution of diffuse microvascular thrombosis[55]; however, in a retrospective multicenter study of 62 patients with meningococcal purpura fulminans treated with systemic t-PA, there was a high incidence of intracerebral hemorrhage without proven efficacy in reduction of mortality or incidence of amputation.[56] Other treatments, such as regional sympathetic blockade, topical nitroglycerin, and local infusion of t-PA, have been used to improve regional blood flow to the affected part. The mortality rate for postinfectious purpura fulminans has declined from 90% in the past to 18%,[57] but the amputation rate has remained high.[43] The outcome for patients with acute bacterial sepsis and purpura fulminans has also improved, but a mortality rate as high as 50% continues to be reported.

Coagulation Inhibitors

Acquired inhibitors of coagulation in children with infection are usually transient and mild but may be associated with severe bleeding.[57] They are often detected after a viral illness, during antibiotic therapy, or incidentally (frequently before tonsillectomy or adenoidectomy). Both specific inhibitors of coagulation factors (especially factors VIII and IX) and lupus anticoagulants have been demonstrated. Although previously thought to be uncommon, studies have found 50% to 90% of children with infection have at least one positive test result for an antiphospholipid antibody (aPL).[58,59] Significant bleeding is usually seen only in children with specific factor inhibitors, although hemorrhage also has been described with lupus anticoagulants.[60] In symptomatic patients, treatment with prednisone has

been associated with remission of bleeding manifestations. Complete resolution without recurrence is the most common event. Thrombosis in the setting of transient postinfectious coagulation inhibitors is rare, although splenic infarction from aPLs has been reported during infection with EBV and mycoplasma pneumonia.[61,62]

Pancytopenia

Pancytopenia in a child should alert the clinician to the possibility of disorders such as leukemia, aplastic anemia, or disseminated neuroblastoma.[63] Infectious causes of pancytopenia are uncommon, and disseminated disease is most often present. Organisms implicated in patients with pancytopenia include *Mycobacterium tuberculosis*, atypical mycobacteria, *Histoplasma capsulatum*, *Leishmania* spp., *Salmonella enterica* subsp. enterica serovar Typhi, *Mucor* spp., *Brucella* spp., *Fusobacterium necrophorum*, *Mycoplasma pneumoniae*, and *Ehrlichia canis*.[27] Virus-associated or reactive hemophagocytic syndrome is an additional, although rare, cause of pancytopenia. Children with HIV infection and concomitant infection with *Mycobacterium avium-intracellulare* or parvovirus B19 have been reported to have pancytopenia.

Human Immunodeficiency Virus Infection in Children and Adolescents

Infection with HIV is more common in adults but is now recognized as a leading cause of immunodeficiency in infants and children.[64] Acquisition of HIV in a majority of infected children (most of whom are younger than 2 years of age) is by vertical transmission from an infected mother to her infant. In a 1989 study of children younger than 13 years of age with acquired immunodeficiency syndrome (AIDS), 80% have a parent with AIDS or AIDS-related complex (ARC), 13% have a history of blood transfusion, and 5% have hemophilia or another coagulation disorder.[65] Other "adult" routes of infection (sexual contact, intravenous needle use) are possible, especially in adolescents and sexually abused children.

Significant advances in the treatment of HIV infection in children have been made since the availability of antiretroviral therapy (ART).[66] As a result of programs to prevent mother-to-child transmission, there has been a dramatic decrease in the number of children in the United States infected with HIV. The Centers for Disease Control and Prevention (CDC) estimates the number of children born with HIV between 1991 and 2011 decreased from 1650 to 110 cases per year.[67] Rates of death, AIDS, opportunistic infection, and organ-specific disease (including thrombocytopenia) have all decreased since the advent of ART.[68] Reviews of HIV infection in children are available.[69,70]

The hematologic manifestations of AIDS in children are similar to those in adults (see Chapter 157) and depend on the stage of the HIV infection and the presence of coexistent disease.[71,72] Anemia is by far the most common finding (seen in 70%–90% of cases), although the incidence has decreased with effective antiviral therapy.[73–75] Moderate anemia (hemoglobin less than 8–9 g/dL) has been identified as an independent risk factor for disease progression in children.[76] Although there have been few studies of severe anemia (hematocrit <25%), in one study it correlated with development of an opportunistic infection and death within 7 months.[77] As in adults, inadequate RBC production is the most important pathogenetic mechanism for the anemia. The etiology for reduced erythropoiesis is multifocal, including direct effects of HIV, associated infections, medications, and deficiency of micronutrients.[73] Although Coombs-positive hemocytic anemia has been described,[78] studies suggest that the finding of a positive direct antiglobulin test result is more likely a reflection of hypergammaglobulinemia. Although evidence indicates that erythropoietin may improve the hemoglobin and quality of life of patients with HIV and anemia,[79] the evidence is not strong.[80]

Leukopenia and neutropenia are commonly seen in HIV-infected children (occurring in 47% and 41%, respectively), with severe neutropenia associated with opportunistic infections. Immune neutropenia and also circulating anticoagulants have been described. Lymphopenia is progressive but less prominent in children than in adults until late in the course.

Thrombocytopenia is present in 13% to 30% of pediatric patients with AIDS and can be associated with clinically significant and even fatal hemorrhage, although in the modern era of highly active anti-retroviral therapy (HAART), the incidence in adults is as low as 0.6%.[81] The mechanism of the thrombocytopenia in most cases is immune destruction, with a high percentage of patients having antiplatelet antibodies or immune complexes,[82] although amegakaryocytic thrombocytopenia has been reported.[62] Variable therapeutic responses to both corticosteroids and intravenous IgG have been demonstrated; some children have spontaneous remissions.[82,83] Treatment with ART has resulted in an increase in the platelet count in some children.[84] Thrombosis has also been described and is associated with severe disease.[85]

Isolated thrombocytopenia as a presenting manifestation of HIV infection has been reported in a number of children, usually infants and even in a neonate.[65,86] There have been no associated clinical stigmata of AIDS or ARC, and patients have been responsive to standard treatment (intravenous IgG or prednisone), often with sustained remissions. In a few patients with prolonged follow-up, no further manifestations of HIV infection were seen. Although it has been suggested that HIV testing may be indicated in all children with ITP, it seems most reasonable to check the HIV status of those with risk factors for AIDS and those outside the typical age group for ITP, especially infants.

COLLAGEN VASCULAR DISEASE AND ACUTE VASCULITIS

Juvenile Idiopathic Arthritis

Juvenile idiopathic arthritis (JIA) (formerly called *juvenile rheumatoid arthritis*) includes a group of disorders with varied clinical presentations, courses, and outcomes. Systemic juvenile idiopathic arthritis (sJIA), which occurs in 10% of patients, is a multisystem disease characterized by fever, rash, polyarticular (often destructive) arthritis, hepatosplenomegaly, and lymphadenopathy. New understanding of the pathogenesis of sJIA points to abnormalities in innate immunity (cytokines IL-1, IL-6, IL-18, neutrophils, and macrophages), distinguishing it from other forms of JIA, suggesting sJIA is an autoinflammatory syndrome rather than an autoimmune disease.[87] Another distinguishing feature of JIA is the association with macrophage activation syndrome (MAS) (see later discussion). Patients with JIA commonly demonstrate hematologic abnormalities that are proportional to disease activity. In the polyarticular presentation, more than four joints are involved, but the systemic findings are absent. This group, which accounts for 25% of patients, also may exhibit hematologic abnormalities. Pauciarticular JIA is characterized by involvement of fewer than four joints and is rarely associated with hematologic abnormalities.

Children with ALL may have a similar presentation to that of children with sJIA, which includes fever, joint pain, hepatosplenomegaly, and isolated cytopenias. Because about 5% of children with ALL are misdiagnosed as having JIA, before initiation of corticosteroid therapy, it is important to perform bone marrow aspiration to rule out leukemia in any patient thought to have sJIA. Distinguishing features of children ultimately diagnosed with ALL after referral to a rheumatologist include atypical pattern of pain (nonarticular bone pain and night pain with no morning stiffness) and cytopenias, especially thrombocytopenia.[65]

The incidence of anemia is 50% to 60% in patients with systemic or polyarticular JIA and 10% in those with pauciarticular arthritis. The anemia usually correlates with disease activity, worsening during acute flare-ups; however, there is no relationship to the duration of illness. RBCs may be normochromic/normocytic or microcytic/hypochromic. The reticulocyte count usually is low. Iron studies often show low serum iron, increased free erythrocyte protoporphyrin, low-normal or elevated total iron-binding capacity, and normal or low serum ferritin. Serum erythropoietin levels usually are mildly elevated (but not as high as in iron deficiency). The bone marrow does not show erythroid hyperplasia in response to the anemia and has diminished (but not absent) iron stores. The etiology of the anemia may be chronic disease, iron deficiency, or both.

Although it is difficult to differentiate anemia of chronic disease from iron-deficiency anemia, studies in patients with systemic-onset chronic JIA suggest defective iron supply as the primary cause.[88] Transferrin receptor levels are inversely related to hemoglobin levels in this population. The finding of elevated serum transferrin receptor levels may be a reliable indicator for diagnosis of iron deficiency in JIA.[89] Oral iron has been effective in raising the hemoglobin in iron-deficient anemic patients with JIA, and intravenous iron has been effective in raising the hemoglobin level in children unresponsive to oral iron.[88] Excessive production of IL-6, tumor necrosis factor-α (TNF-α), and other inflammatory cytokines has been documented in patients with JIA and may provide an explanation for the abnormalities in iron metabolism. IL-6 may enhance ferritin synthesis and increase hepatic uptake of serum iron. Increased ferritin results in reticuloendothelial iron blockage and diminished iron absorption.[88] In one study of treatment with anti–TNF-α therapy, the hemoglobin as well as markers of abnormal iron metabolism improved significantly.[90] Less common causes of anemia in patients with JIA include erythroid aplasia, suppression of erythropoiesis by circulating inhibitors, hemolysis, and a macrocytic anemia probably related to increased folate clearance and low plasma and RBC folate levels.

In sJIA, leukocytosis with mean WBC counts up to 30,000/μL and neutrophilia with a left shift occur in 90% of patients, especially those with active disease. Leukocytosis is less common in polyarticular arthritis and usually absent in pauciarticular disease. Leukocytosis is so prevalent in sJIA that the presence of neutropenia should alert the clinician to question the diagnosis and ensure that other possibilities such as systemic lupus erythematosus (SLE) and ALL are not overlooked. Nonetheless, neutropenia has been reported in several patients with JIA.[91] Other causes of neutropenia are bone marrow suppression caused by therapy with tocilizumab,[92] gold, or nonsteroidal antiinflammatory drugs (NSAIDs),[93] and, in adults, Felty syndrome, comprising the triad of rheumatoid arthritis, splenomegaly, and neutropenia.

The platelet count is elevated in about half of the patients with sJIA. IL-6, a cytokine that stimulates thrombopoiesis, is elevated in patients with active sJIA, and increased levels of IL-6 are correlated with elevated platelet counts.[94] Persistent thrombocytosis may serve as an adverse prognostic marker for long-term outcome in JIA.

Thrombocytopenia may result from bone marrow suppression by gold therapy, the rare consumptive coagulopathy, or platelet trapping in Felty syndrome. Thrombocytopenia is also seen in the potentially life-threatening complication of MAS (see discussion of MAS below). Because thrombocytopenia is uncommon in JIA, however, an unexplained low platelet count should lead the clinician to consider alternative diagnoses, such as SLE or ALL. On the other hand, isolated thrombocytopenia may be the only presenting sign in a child who later develops JIA or another collagen vascular disease. Therefore JIA and SLE should be considered in the differential diagnosis of ITP in children who are older than 9 years of age and female. Appropriate screening tests for autoantibodies (e.g., antinuclear antibody assay, direct Coombs test) should be performed at diagnosis and periodically if new symptoms develop.

Disseminated intravascular coagulation may occur in children with sJIA after hepatic damage, as part of the MAS, from aspirin or gold therapy, or during disease flare-ups treated with NSAIDs when serum albumin is low.[95] These patients often are very ill and may require early and aggressive medical therapy as well as platelet and coagulation factor replacement to control the coagulopathy. The incidence of coagulation abnormalities in nonbleeding patients with sJIA is controversial. One study demonstrated prolonged prothrombin time (PT) and activated partial thromboplastin time (aPTT) and elevated fibrinogen, factor VIII, and fibrinopeptide A levels in up to 50% of these patients,[96] but other studies have not confirmed such findings. Another study found elevation of D-dimer levels in 96% of systemic-onset JIA patients; serial measurements of D-dimer levels appeared to parallel response to treatment.[97] In apparent distinction, decreased fibrinolytic activity and increased plasminogen activator inhibitor have been found in patients with active JIA, especially those with the systemic form. Antibodies against factor VIII and the lupus anticoagulant are occasionally seen in children with JIA.

Macrophage Activation Syndrome

MAS is a life-threatening multisystem disorder most closely resembling hemophagocytic lymphohistiocytosis (HLH) that occurs primarily in patients with systemic-onset juvenile idiopathic arthritis (sJIA).[98,99] This syndrome usually occurs early in the course of active sJIA and can even be a presenting feature,[100] although it has been reported to occur later and during a quiescent phase.[101] It is estimated that approximately 7% of patients with sJIA develop MAS, and the mortality rate is between 10% and 20%.[102] MAS has also been reported in other systemic inflammatory disorders, including SLE and Kawasaki disease.[100]

The main clinical features of MAS include a high unremitting fever, hepatosplenomegaly, lymphadenopathy, bleeding, rash, and central nervous system manifestations. Neurologic symptoms include lethargy, irritability, disorientation, headache, seizures, and coma. Children with MAS are acutely ill, and almost 50% require intensive care unit care.[103] The diagnosis may be delayed because the presentation mimics an acute exacerbation of sJIA or severe infection. Of interest, some patients have shown a paradoxical improvement in the underlying inflammatory disease at the onset of MAS. Precipitating factors that have been implicated include a flare-up of the underlying disease, aspirin or other NSAID toxicity, viral infections, a second injection of gold salts, methotrexate therapy, and sulfasalazine therapy.[103]

Typical laboratory features include pancytopenia, hypofibrinogenemia (<250 mg/dL), elevated liver enzymes (>40 IU/mL), hypertriglyceridemia (>160 mg/dL), and marked elevation of ferritin (>10,000 ng/mL). Other laboratory findings with less sensitivity and specificity include coagulopathy, hyponatremia, and hypoalbuminemia. The hallmark of this disorder is the presence of hemophagocytic histiocytes, usually seen in the bone marrow, although they can also be found in the liver and other organs. These characteristic macrophages are regarded as confirmatory evidence rather than a requirement for a diagnosis because they have not been documented in as many as 20% of patients with the classical clinical and laboratory findings of MAS.[103,104]

There are no accepted diagnostic criteria for MAS in sJIA. Preliminary diagnostic guidelines have been proposed (Table 152.2).[104] In a study comparing these preliminary diagnostic guidelines with HLH-2004 guidelines, the preliminary guidelines were best able to identify MAS in the setting of sJIA.[105] An international consensus survey of diagnostic criteria for MAS was completed by 232 physicians.[105] The following were the top nine diagnostic criteria identified by more 50% of respondents in order of frequency:

1. Falling platelet count
2. Hyperferritinemia
3. Bone marrow hemophagocytosis
4. Increased live enzymes
5. Falling leukocyte count
6. Persistent continuous fever >38°C
7. Falling erythrocyte sedimentation rate
8. Hypofibrinogenemia
9. Hypertriglyceridemia

These features may provide the best candidates for future refinement of diagnostic criteria. The diagnostic guidelines are similar to criteria for the diagnosis of HLH,[106] although a number of differences should

TABLE 152.2	Preliminary Diagnostic Guidelines for Macrophage Activation Syndrome in Systemic Juvenile Idiopathic Arthritis[a]

Laboratory Criteria

1. Decreased platelet count (≤262 × 10⁹/L)
2. Elevated levels of aspartate aminotransferase (>59 IU/L)
3. Decreased white blood cell count (≤4.0 × 10⁹/L)
4. Hypofibrinogenemia (≤250 mg/dL)

Clinical Criteria

1. Central nervous system dysfunction (irritability, disorientation, lethargy, headache, seizures, coma)
2. Hemorrhages (purpura, easy bruising, mucosal bleeding)
3. Hepatomegaly (≥3 cm below the costal margin)

Histopathologic Criterion

Evidence of macrophage hemophagocytosis in the bone marrow aspirate

Diagnostic Rule

The diagnosis of macrophage activation syndrome requires the presence of any two or more laboratory criteria or of at least two clinical or laboratory criteria. A bone marrow aspirate for the demonstration of hemophagocytosis may be required only in doubtful cases.

[a]The suggested criteria are useful only in patients with active systemic-onset juvenile idiopathic arthritis. The laboratory thresholds are examples only and are not specific for the diagnosis (see text).
From Ravelli A, Magni-Manzoni S, Pistorio A, et al: Preliminary diagnostic guidelines for macrophage activation syndrome complicating systemic juvenile idiopathic arthritis. *J Pediatr* 146:598, 2005.

be emphasized. In MAS, clinical features are weaker discriminators than laboratory features. Although the presence of fever was universal in patients with MAS, it had a low specificity rate because of the high incidence of fever in patients with sJIA without MAS. The pattern of fever may be of more importance because patients with MAS tend to have nonremitting fever as opposed to the high spiking fevers seen in sJIA. The other clinical criteria may occur late in the course of MAS, resulting in abnormal laboratory findings being more helpful in making a diagnosis early in the course of the illness. Because blood counts are usually elevated in patients with sJIA, the decrease in counts seen with MAS may actually result in a "normal" blood count, although in patients with HLH, cytopenias are usually well below the normal levels. Laboratory markers of T-cell activation (soluble IL-2 receptor [SCD25]) and of macrophage activation (soluble CD163 [SCD163]) have been shown to be elevated in patients with MAS and may serve as useful diagnostic markers in the future.[107]

The pathogenesis of MAS is similar to that proposed for HLH.[106,108] Indeed, it has been proposed that MAS be considered one of the subtypes of acquired HLH.[102] The presentation of MAS is a result of an ineffective immune response to an endogenous or exogenous stimulus leading to an exaggerated inflammatory state produced by a release of high levels of cytokines. These proinflammatory cytokines include TNF-α, IL-1, IL-6, IL-8, IL-12, IL-18, macrophage inflammatory protein-1α (MIP-1α), and interferon-γ (IFN-γ) released by stimulated lymphocytes and histiocytes. Defective natural killer (NK) cell function and cytotoxic T-cell activity have been documented in patients with MAS as well as in those with HLH and may be the common pathway leading to the clinical presentation.[109] NK-cell function in patients with active sJIA but without MAS has also been found to be abnormal.[110] This may explain why MAS is almost exclusively seen in the systemic form of JIA and not the other subtypes of the disease. Mutations in the perforin gene and the *MUNC 13-4* gene have been described in some patients with HLH. The cytotoxic function of NK cells is mediated by the release of perforin and other cytolytic granules into the target cell, leading to cell death. Abnormalities of both perforin gene and *MUNC 13-4* polymorphisms have been found in patients with MAS.[109,111,112]

Treatment of MAS should be started promptly and not delayed for lack of hemophagocytosis if the clinical and laboratory features are consistent with the diagnosis. The initial treatment should be high-dose corticosteroid therapy followed by cyclosporin A (CsA) if there is not a rapid response. Intravenous methylprednisolone with doses from 2 to 30 mg/kg/day has been the most common corticosteroid reported in the literature and is usually effective in controlling hyperinflammation.[103] The corticosteroid of choice used in the treatment of HLH is dexamethasone, but its use has not been reported in MAS. CsA has been very effective in inducing remission either when used as initial treatment or in cases of corticosteroid failure.[101,103] In addition to immunosuppression, there should be withdrawal of any suspected triggering medications and treatment of infection. Intravenous immunoglobulin (IVIg) therapy has usually been ineffective, although it has been reported to induce a full recovery in one case of a child who failed high-dose corticosteroids.[113] For unresponsive patients, treatment with etoposide or other HLH salvage therapy may be necessary. Etanercept and infliximab have also been reported to induce clinical responses in patients with MAS.[114-116] These drugs are recombinant soluble TNF-α receptor fusion proteins that bind to TNF-α, blocking its effect. Although use of these agents to reduce the elevated levels of TNF-α found in this disorder is attractive, these agents should be used with caution because there are case reports of MAS developing after the initiation of etanercept.[117] Anakinra, a recombinant IL-1 receptor antagonist, has shown promising results in treatment of sJIA as well as MAS.[117,118]

Kawasaki Syndrome

Kawasaki syndrome is an acute multisystem disorder characterized by an abrupt onset of fever unresponsive to antibiotics; bilateral conjunctival injection; reddening of the lips, tongue, or oral mucosa; reddening, induration, or peeling of the skin on the hands or feet; polymorphous truncal rash; and cervical lymphadenopathy. This disorder occurs most commonly in children younger than 2 years of age and has many features of a severe vasculitis. The most serious complication is development of coronary artery aneurysms, which occurs in 20% of children and is responsible for the 3% mortality rate; death often is caused by coronary artery thrombosis or rupture. The etiology of Kawasaki disease is unknown. The immunologic and clinical characteristics of this disorder are similar to those of diseases associated with superantigen production, of which toxic shock syndrome is a classic example.[119]

Children with Kawasaki syndrome may have a mild, normochromic, normocytic anemia with reticulocytopenia. Rarely, a severe Coombs-positive, antibody-mediated hemolytic anemia has been reported after administration of IVIg. Leukocytosis is almost universal, with mean neutrophil counts of 21,000/μL. Ninety-five percent of patients have neutrophilia, with a left shift persisting up to 3 weeks. The finding of vacuoles and toxic granulation in neutrophils is a helpful adjunct in the diagnosis of Kawasaki disease. Activated neutrophils and monocytes may play a role in aneurysm development through the production of elastase. Granulocyte colony-stimulating factor levels have been correlated with coronary artery dilation during the acute phase of Kawasaki syndrome.[120]

Studies of cellular immunity show normal total T-cell numbers but decreased suppressor T cells, causing relatively elevated T helper–cell levels during the first 4 weeks of disease.[121] The change of T-cell subsets plus B-lymphocyte stimulation may contribute to the exaggerated production of all major Ig classes during the first 8 weeks of the disease.[122] An unusual infiltration of IgA-producing plasma cells within vascular tissue in Kawasaki syndrome, with an oligoclonal IgA response, suggests that the immune stimulation is antigen driven.[123] Circulating immune complexes and high C3 (but not C4) levels are found during weeks 1 and 3. During the acute phase, increased levels of the cytokines IL-1, IL-6, IL-8, IFN-γ, and TNF are noted in the circulation, as well as of IL-1, IL-2, IFN-γ, and TNF in blood vessels and skin biopsies.[119] Declining serum IL-6 levels appear to correlate with clinical response after treatment with IVIg.[124]

Impressive thrombocytosis occurs in 85% of patients by the second week, peaking during the third. Platelet counts of up to 2 million/μL are not uncommon, and the mean platelet count is 700,000/μL. Thrombocytosis may serve as a marker of possible atypical Kawasaki disease in infants younger than 1 year of age. In a study of more than 25,000 infants with unexplained fever, 8.8% with a platelet count greater than 800,000/μL were found to have Kawasaki disease, as opposed to 0.4% of those with a platelet count less than 800,000/μL.[125] Thrombocytosis is preceded by elevated thrombopoietin levels.[126] However, 2% of patients may have thrombocytopenia caused by a consumptive coagulopathy. Platelets demonstrate hyperaggregation on exposure to adenosine diphosphate, epinephrine, and collagen in vitro. These abnormalities may persist for as long as 9 months after diagnosis.[127] During the first month, levels of factor VIII, fibrinogen, thromboxane B_2, and thromboglobulin are increased. AT III and fibrinolysis activity are decreased. The PT, aPTT, and thrombin time usually are normal.[128]

Prevention and treatment of existing coronary aneurysms constitute the primary therapeutic goals. Aspirin suppresses platelet aggregation but does not affect aneurysm formation. Combining aspirin with high-dose IVIg infusions reduces aneurysm formation, decreases fever, and normalizes laboratory signs of inflammation.[129] The use of corticosteroids is controversial, with conflicting data regarding increased aneurysm formation after steroid use.[130-132] However, in a randomized, double-blind, placebo-controlled trial, a single pulsed dose of intravenous methylprednisolone, in addition to conventional therapy, did not improve coronary artery outcomes.[133,134] In subgroup analysis of children with persistent fever, coronary outcomes were better in the corticosteroid group. If children at highest risk of primary treatment failure could be identified initially, corticosteroid use might be of benefit in this group. Infliximab has been used in the treatment of IVIg-resistant patients, with limited success.[135] Guidelines for the diagnosis, treatment, and long-term management of patients with Kawasaki syndrome have been published.[133,136,137]

Henoch-Schönlein Purpura

Henoch-Schönlein purpura (HSP) (anaphylactoid purpura) is a systemic vasculitis characterized by unique purpuric skin lesions, transient arthralgias or arthritis (especially affecting the knees and ankles), colicky abdominal pain, and nephritis. Recognition of HSP is important, not so much for its hematologic abnormalities (which are rare) as for the unusual nonthrombocytopenic purpuric lesions, which are frequently confused with the hemorrhagic rash of ITP. This vasculitis occurs most commonly in children 3 to 7 years old, often 1 to 3 weeks after an upper respiratory tract illness. The presenting sign in 50% of children is a characteristic rash, which may begin as urticaria. As these eruptions fade, they are replaced by brownish-red maculopapular lesions and petechiae. The petechiae coalesce, forming areas of raised or "palpable" purpura on the buttocks, legs, and extensor surfaces of the arms, with a symmetric distribution. The rash may fade but can recur for months, especially with increased activity. Children younger than 3 years of age often have painful soft tissue swellings of the scalp and face (especially periorbital areas) and on the dorsa of the hands and feet. Infantile acute hemorrhagic edema is an acute vasculitis affecting infants and children younger than 2 years of age, which may be a benign form of HSP.

Sixty-seven percent of patients experience colicky abdominal pain, often associated with vomiting, hematemesis, or melena from submucosal hemorrhage and edema of the small bowel wall. With severe edema, the bowel wall may become a leading point for intussusceptions.[138]

Renal involvement occurs in 30% to 50% of patients, especially boys and older children, and may present after initial systemic symptoms. Hematuria, either microscopic or gross, may occur with proteinuria during the first 3 weeks of the illness but rarely after 6 months. With progressive involvement, hypertension, impaired renal function, and renal failure can occur in up to 15% of children, with an associated mortality rate of 3%. In occasional patients, an acute scrotum that mimics testicular torsion may develop; however, surgical exploration may not be necessary if appropriate clinical and radiographic features are present. Other rare manifestations of HSP include neurologic, cardiac, and pulmonary events.

Anemia occasionally develops as a result of gastrointestinal (GI) tract blood loss or decreased RBC production caused by renal failure. The leukocyte count is normal. Despite the impressive purpura, the platelet count is normal or increased with normal platelet function. Coagulation factor levels usually are normal, although transient decreases in factor XIII activity and vitamin K deficiency from severe vasculitis-induced intestinal malabsorption have been reported. Signs of increased fibrinolysis, as evidenced by elevation of D-dimer and other markers, have been described.[139] Bleeding in the GI tract; the lungs; or, rarely, the central nervous system is caused by a necrotizing vasculitis and not a hemostatic defect.[138] Hypercoagulability does not play a role with normal frequency of *MTHFR*, prothrombin, and factor V Leiden gene mutations.[140]

HSP is considered an IgA-mediated inflammation of small vessels. Biopsy of skin or other involved tissue reveals a leukocytoclastic vasculitis. Immune complexes of IgA with complement, IgG, or IgM have been found circulating in the serum[141] and deposited in blood vessel walls of the kidneys and in intestinal and skin lesions.[142] The mechanism of production, accumulation, and deposition of IgA immune complexes in the blood vessel is unclear. It has been suggested that HSP may be a systemic form of IgA nephropathy, although this is controversial.[143,144] Both disorders have identical features on renal biopsy and are characterized by mesangial proliferation, occasional focal sclerosis, and crescent formation.[145]

Treatment is mainly supportive, although corticosteroids have been found to provide symptomatic relief with severe joint, scrotal, or abdominal pain.[146,147] They do not alter skin involvement or prevent renal involvement. Recent studies have suggested that corticosteroids plus azathioprine, cyclosporin A, or cyclophosphamide may have a role in the management of severe renal involvement.[148-152] Rituximab has been reported to be effective in decreasing the symptoms of three patients with severe, refractory chronic HSP.[153] The prognosis is good for full recovery, except in children with renal failure.

CARDIOPULMONARY DISEASE

Congenital Heart Disease

Congenital heart disease (CHD) occurs in about 1% of live births. Structural heart malformation usually follows predictable patterns such that six defects account for 70% of all cardiac disorders: ventricular septal defect, atrial septal defect, tetralogy of Fallot, patent ductus arteriosus, pulmonary stenosis, and aortic stenosis. Children with cardiac abnormalities may be acyanotic or cyanotic, depending on the underlying lesion. Hematologic abnormalities occur most often in children with cyanotic critical congenital heart disease (CCHD). Polycythemia is the bone marrow response to chronic hypoxemia in patients with CCHD. The decreased arterial oxygen content stimulates erythropoietin production, which in turn increases erythropoiesis. The resultant increased RBC mass increases the oxygen-carrying capacity of the blood, resulting in improved tissue oxygenation. With adequate compensation, erythropoietin levels fall to normal, and higher RBC production is maintained. A second compensatory mechanism is an increase in 2,3-diphosphoglycerate (2,3-DPG) levels in the RBCs when the arterial oxygen tension is less than 70 mmHg. The higher 2,3-DPG level causes a right shift of the oxyhemoglobin curve, resulting in greater oxygen release to the tissues.

Polycythemia in cyanotic children is beneficial up to a point. Because the relationship between the hematocrit and blood viscosity is hyperbolic, minor increases in the hematocrit above 70% cause marked increases in blood viscosity. This higher viscosity results in impaired perfusion within the microvasculature, with ultimately less tissue oxygen delivery. The impairment is magnified in severe polycythemia (hematocrit level >75%) such that headache; irritability; dyspnea; and even formation of pulmonary, renal, or central nervous

system thrombi may result.[154] To prevent these complications, the hematocrit level should be maintained around 60% through the use of exchange transfusions. Small aliquots of the patient's blood are slowly removed and replaced by equal volumes of plasma or 5% albumin. Care should be taken to remove blood slowly because vascular collapse, cyanosis, stroke, and seizures have been reported with too rapid an exchange. Apheresis (erythrocytapheresis) also has been shown to be an effective means of decreasing viscosity in patients with polycythemia.

Infants with CCHD are at risk of developing iron-deficiency anemia. The deficiency may result from the combination of poor iron stores at birth (especially in premature infants), increased iron needed for enhanced erythropoiesis, poor iron intake because of poor feeding, and ongoing iron losses as a consequence of phlebotomy or exchange transfusion. These children may exhibit symptoms of iron deficiency (irritability, anorexia, poor weight gain) or worsening cyanosis. The hemoglobin may be normal for age but inappropriately low for the degree of hypoxemia. Low RBC indices and hypochromic, microcytic RBCs are the best indices of iron deficiency in this setting.[155] Children with polycythemia who have iron-deficiency anemia are at increased risk for cerebral vein thrombosis because of the poor deformability of the iron-deficient RBCs, which further increases blood viscosity.[156] To prevent this complication and to allow for maximal tissue oxygenation, all infants should be fed iron-rich infant formula and receive iron replacement therapy as needed to normalize RBC indices. Hemolytic anemia, characterized by mechanical destruction of RBCs and manifested by the presence of schistocytes in the peripheral blood smear, is occasionally seen after the placement of prosthetic heart valves.

Routine screening of patients with CHD has demonstrated coagulation abnormalities in 20% to 59% of children with acyanotic defects and in 40% to 50% of those with cyanotic heart disease (Table 152.3).[157] Only 11% of children with CCHD have any clinical evidence of bleeding preoperatively. However, children with underlying hemostatic defects have a greater frequency and severity of postoperative bleeding.[157,158] Presurgical screening tests should include at least a platelet count, platelet function assay (e.g., closure time), PT, and aPTT. Further investigations may be indicated if there is a history of bleeding or abnormal results on screening tests. Acquired von Willebrand syndrome has been reported in patients with CHD and is

TABLE 152.3	Coagulation Abnormalities in Congenital Heart Disease	
	Incidence (%)	
Abnormality	**Acyanotic CHD**	**Cyanotic CHD**
Prolonged bleeding time	11	28
Prolonged PT		20
Prolonged aPTT		19
Thrombocytopenia	12–40	0–36
Abnormal platelet aggregation	14	38–70
Increased fibrinolysis	12	0–10
Abnormal clot retraction	10	
Low fibrinogen	16	12
Increased fibrin split products		Occasionally
Decreased factors II, V, VII, VIII, IX, X, XI, XII		Occasionally
Decreased protein C		25[a]

aPTT, Activated partial thromboplastin time; CHD, congenital heart disease; PT, prothrombin time.
[a]Data from MacDonald PD, Gibson BE, Braunlie J, et al: Protein C activity in severely ill newborns with congenital heart disease. *J Perinatal Med* 20:421, 1992.
Adapted from Lascari AD: *Hematologic manifestations of childhood diseases*, New York, Thieme-Stratton, 1984, with permission.

possibly associated with an increased bleeding risk, especially in those receiving aspirin. The multimer pattern reveals decreased large-molecular-weight multimers.[159] Children with polycythemia have contracted plasma volumes; therefore when blood samples are collected, extra care should be taken to ensure the proper 1:9 ratio of 3.8% sodium citrate to blood to prevent artificial abnormalities in coagulation test results.

The etiology of the coagulation abnormalities in CCHD is unclear. Earlier reports suggesting a role for consumptive coagulopathy have not been confirmed. Protein C levels in 8 of 29 term infants with CCHD were significantly lower than in control participants with no evidence of familial deficiency. Of these infants, two had thrombotic complications, and four had consumptive coagulopathy.[160] Platelets have shortened survival times (even with normal counts), and normal to increased numbers of megakaryocytes in the bone marrow have been reported.[161] This increased platelet destruction does not appear to be attributable to DIC. Both the platelet and coagulation abnormalities are directly proportional to the degree of hypoxemia and polycythemia. For example, whereas children with oxygen saturation greater than 60% have a mean platelet count of 315,000/μL, those with oxygen saturation less than 60% have a mean count of 185,000/μL.[161] The mild platelet and coagulation abnormalities usually are decreased or corrected after surgical repair of the heart defect.[157,162] With bleeding or if surgery is not possible, the coagulopathy may be treated by correction of polycythemia to a hematocrit level of 60% by using slow plasma exchange transfusion.[163]

Cystic Fibrosis

Cystic fibrosis (CF) is a multisystem disorder of exocrine gland dysfunction characterized by chronic pulmonary disease, pancreatic exocrine insufficiency, hepatic dysfunction, abnormal reproductive organ function, and intestinal obstruction associated with abnormally high sweat electrolyte levels. It is an autosomal recessive disease with an incidence of 1 in 2000 live births.

Severe hemolytic anemia caused by vitamin E deficiency may be the presenting manifestation of CF. Dolan[164] initially linked deficiency of vitamin E with severe hemolytic anemia in infants who presented with pallor, edema, hypoproteinemia, and thrombocytosis. This complication can be seen as early as 6 weeks of age.

Many children with CF are chronically hypoxic, yet they do not have the expected augmented erythroid response. In a study by Vichinsky and colleagues,[165] none of 42 children with CF had polycythemia, and 30% (especially the boys and the older children) had a normochromic, normocytic, or hypochromic microcytic anemia with reticulocytopenia. In contrast with children with CCHD, there was no appropriate increase in RBC 2,3-DPG levels, no right shift of the oxyhemoglobin curve, and either a low or a normal erythropoietin level. In vitro assays showed normal erythroid progenitor cell numbers and no serum inhibitor of erythropoiesis. Up to 66% of the children studied had abnormalities consistent with iron deficiency, and all responded to oral or parenteral iron therapy.

It appears that the etiology of anemia in CF is multifactorial. A blunted erythropoietic response to hypoxia plus iron deficiency secondary to iron malabsorption or poor dietary iron intake may each be partially responsible for the development of anemia. If iron deficiency persists despite adequate oral supplementation, the possibility of ongoing blood loss or of iron malabsorption that may necessitate parenteral iron replacement should be considered. Soluble transferrin receptor levels may be helpful in distinguishing iron deficiency from anemia of chronic inflammation in CF because, unlike serum ferritin and transferrin, soluble transferrin receptor does not appear to be an acute-phase reactant.[166,167]

Use of multiple antibiotics in patients with CF is routine. There have been a number of case reports of adult patients with severe, life-threatening hemolytic anemia attributed to piperacillin.[168,169] This complication has not been reported in children to date.

Findings of studies of neutrophil function in children with CF are conflicting. Some reports indicate impaired chemotaxis, chemiluminescence, granule release, and superoxide production,[170–172] but others have demonstrated factors in patient sputum that actually enhance neutrophil and monocyte responses to stimulants.[173,174] Although these sputum factors may improve neutrophil killing ability, they also may worsen neutrophil-mediated lung damage through increased release of neutrophil elastase.[175] Evaluation of immune function has revealed impaired lymphoproliferative responses to *Pseudomonas* spp. and other gram-negative bacterial antigens, defective opsonization, increased levels of circulating immune complexes, and decreased numbers of T-helper cells in 30% of patients.[152,176] The contribution of these findings to frequent pulmonary infection is still under investigation.

Children with CF usually do not experience clinically significant bleeding owing to impaired hemostasis despite the risk of liver disease and vitamin K deficiency from malabsorption. An exception may be infants younger than 1 year of age, in whom rare case reports of vitamin K–deficient hemorrhage have been reported in association with CF.[177–179] Routine coagulation tests usually yield normal results, with an occasional prolonged PT reported. A study by Corrigan and colleagues[156,180] revealed that 60% of 24 patients had a more subtle deficiency of prothrombin activity, thought to be caused by vitamin K deficiency. Other investigators, using direct measurement of vitamin K and protein induced by vitamin K absence/antagonist-II (PIVKA-II), have reported conflicting percentages of patients to be vitamin K deficient,[181,182] with another uncontrolled study demonstrating normalization of PIVKA-II values in many patients by routine administration of daily oral vitamin K.[183] Routine vitamin K supplementation is recommended for all patients with CF,[184] although there are inadequate data to define the ideal dose.[185]

Children with CF appear to have a particularly high predisposition to recurrent venous thrombosis. In one study of 19 patients with recurrent venous thrombosis, 6 had CF, but none of 101 patients with thrombosis without recurrence had CF. A striking association with respiratory tract colonization with *Burkholderia cepacia* was noted, as was the frequent presence of a central venous catheter. Several of the recurrences occurred while patients were on therapeutic anticoagulation.[186] Studies of small populations of both children and adults have documented an increased incidence of protein C and protein S deficiency, as well as lupus anticoagulants.[187–189] These abnormalities are likely acquired defects in most patients with CF because of the potential for having subclinical vitamin K deficiency, liver function abnormalities, and recurrent infections. Follow-up studies have not shown persistent abnormalities in many patients. The incidence of activated protein C resistance and factor V Leiden was similar to that in the general population. Although it would be anticipated there would be an increased frequency of venous thrombosis because of the increased use of central venous catheters, at least one large study of older adolescents and adults with CF who had totally implanted venous access devices revealed a very low incidence of complications.[190] Whether patients with CF have a greater risk of venous thrombosis than the control population awaits a larger prospective controlled trial.

HEMATOLOGIC MANIFESTATIONS OF CHILDHOOD GASTROINTESTINAL DISEASE

Milk Protein–Induced Enteropathy and Heiner Syndrome

The association of iron deficiency with dietary intake of cow's milk in young infants is established. A major contributing factor is the relatively poor bioavailability of iron in cow's milk compared with breast milk. In addition, the rapid growth of infants and corresponding rapid increase in RBC mass necessitate an increased requirement for dietary iron. The role of cow's milk in inducing occult GI blood loss in infants was carefully documented more than three decades ago in a sentinel paper that also demonstrated a correlation between the amount of milk ingested and the amount of fecal blood lost.[191] GI blood loss in response to cow's milk ingestion appears to be most prevalent in infants younger than 6 months of age and occurs with diminishing frequency in older infants.[192] The majority of affected infants outgrow their milk protein sensitivity by 3 years of age. The GI blood loss may be ameliorated by heat denaturing of the milk proteins. Occasionally, toddlers and older children have been documented to have milk-induced GI bleeding with associated iron-deficiency anemia.[193,194] Substantially limiting cow's milk consumption and prescribing iron supplementation are sufficient to correct the iron deficiency and associated hypoproteinemia with edema in most children.[195]

A variety of GI syndromes associated with cow's milk sensitivity, with varying manifestations and severity, have been described. Associated findings may include vomiting, diarrhea, poor growth, and hypoproteinemia; however, some patients may have occult blood loss and iron-deficiency anemia without associated complaints. At the severe end of the spectrum, cow's milk protein–induced enterocolitis may occur.[196] Such patients may present with acute, severe bloody diarrhea; vomiting; abdominal distention; methemoglobinemia; and shock even in the absence of anemia.[196] Even minute amounts of cow's milk protein in human breast milk may be sufficient to precipitate a severe event.[197] In patients with chronic occult GI blood loss, esophagogastroduodenoscopy may reveal gastritis or gastroduodenitis, and colonoscopy may demonstrate modest histologic abnormalities in the proximal colon.[194,198] The immunopathobiology of cow's milk protein allergy syndromes has not been fully elucidated. Most of these syndromes affecting the intestinal tract only are non–IgE mediated.[199,200] Wilson et al[191] reported the frequent presence of precipitating antibodies to milk proteins in their study population as a whole. However, the presence of such antibodies did not appear to predict milk-induced GI bleeding. The roles that genetic predisposition, intestinal and immunologic immaturity in young infants, exposure to cow's milk protein in breast milk, GI infections, or other factors may play in the development of milk protein enteropathy are not fully understood.

In 1962, Heiner et al described a syndrome in infants and young children that included chronic cough, recurrent lung infiltrates, poor growth, GI symptoms, blood loss, iron-deficiency anemia, and pulmonary hemosiderosis associated with multiple serum precipitins to cow's milk proteins.[201] Others have confirmed and further detailed this rare syndrome.[201–203] Additional manifestations may include intermittent wheezing; hilar lymphadenopathy; eosinophilia; elevated levels of serum IgE, IgM, or IgA; chronic rhinitis; adenoidal hypertrophy; hypercapnia; and cor pulmonale. A feature of this syndrome is rapid improvement of the pulmonary manifestations after eliminating cow's milk from the diet.

Celiac Disease

Celiac disease, or gluten-sensitive enteropathy, is an inflammatory and malabsorptive process resulting from an aberrant intestinal T-cell immune response to ingested dietary gluten, leading to injury of the mucosa of the small intestine.[204] Classical celiac disease has been characterized as frequently affecting infants and young children, leading to steatorrhea, failure to thrive, weight loss, and nutritional deficiency. With the advent of improved screening techniques, the prevalence is recognized to be greater than previous estimates. Celiac disease broadly affects both children and adults, many of whom may have minimal classical symptoms of the disorder. Treatment is usually institution of a gluten-free diet, with resolution of the process in the majority of cases.

Iron deficiency is frequently present in celiac disease in children and adults and may be the sole recognized manifestation of the disorder.[179] Dietary iron absorption occurs primarily within the proximal small intestine, the same region most affected by celiac disease. As a result, iron deficiency in celiac disease appears to be caused primarily by impaired absorption of dietary iron, although a component of chronic GI blood loss may also apply in a minority of patients.[205,206] Iron deficiency in celiac disease may be refractory to iron

supplementation, and a significant percentage of children and adults with iron-deficiency anemia who do not respond to therapeutic oral iron replacement have celiac disease.

Folic acid and, with a lesser frequency, vitamin B[12] deficiency may also result from the malabsorptive process in celiac disease. Manifestations may include macrocytic anemia, leukocytopenia, and pancytopenia. Neurologic findings may be present with vitamin B[12] deficiency. Other vitamin and micronutrient deficiencies, including copper and vitamin K deficiency, have been observed in celiac disease. Splenic hypofunction may occur with some frequency in adults with celiac disease but appears to be less common in children. A number of case reports have suggested an association of pulmonary hemosiderosis with celiac disease.[207,208] The pathophysiology of this association is not known, but the pulmonary process may improve with initiation of a gluten-free diet.

A high index of suspicion is important for diagnosing celiac disease in children, particularly those who are minimally symptomatic or who may be at increased risk for development of celiac disease. The latter group includes children with trisomy 21, Turner syndrome, IgA deficiency, autoimmune thyroiditis, and type 1 diabetes mellitus, as well as those with a family history of celiac disease. In addition to correcting the nutritional deficiencies and growth failure in children with celiac disease, recognition of the disease and institution of a gluten-free diet may minimize the risk of some of the associated conditions of celiac disease, including the development of non-Hodgkin lymphoma involving the intestinal tract.

Inflammatory Bowel Disease

Anemia is a very common extraintestinal manifestation of inflammatory bowel disease (IBD), particularly in children with Crohn disease, in whom the historical prevalence of anemia approaches 70% to 80%.[209,210] A more recent series of studies suggests that the prevalence of anemia may be declining in Crohn disease, perhaps because of more effective therapy.[211] The etiology of anemia in IBD appears to be multifactorial, but the most common contributing factors are iron deficiency related to chronic GI blood loss or iron malabsorption caused by intestinal mucosal injury and decreased absorption and sequestration of iron stores as is seen in the anemia of chronic inflammation. These broad mechanisms for anemia may coexist, and it is sometimes difficult to determine the predominant mechanism. Measurement of serum soluble transferrin receptor and the hemoglobin content of reticulocytes can be helpful in this setting.[212] Other factors contributing to anemia in IBD may also be present in individual patients, including immune-mediated hemolytic anemia, hemophagocytosis, malnutrition, folate and vitamin B[12] deficiency, and the suppressive effects of medications on hematopoiesis.[213]

Specific treatment of anemia in IBD may be difficult. Oral iron supplementation is not always effective. Comparative studies of oral versus intravenous iron supplementation suggest the intravenous route may result in better short-term improvement in anemia; however, long-term outcome data are lacking.[214,215] Some patients may respond to supplemental erythropoietin administration as well.[216] Patients with IBD may have impaired enterocyte-mediated intestinal absorption of iron, the degree of which appears to correlate with disease activity.[216] The role that induction of hepcidin expression by mediators of inflammation, particularly IL-6, plays in the anemia of IBD is an intriguing area of ongoing investigation.[217,218]

Other hematologic manifestations of IBD include leukocytosis and thrombocytosis, hyposplenism, an increased propensity toward thrombosis, and therapy-related leukopenia and thrombocytopenia. There may be an increased incidence of immune-mediated thrombocytopenia associated with IBD.[219]

Other Gastrointestinal Disorders

In addition to the disorders already discussed, other GI disorders that occur in children and adolescents may be associated with the development of anemia. Examples include antral gastritis, duodenal and colonic polyps, parasitic infestations, and GI malignancies. GI stromal tumors, although rare, usually present in teenage girls with anemia related to GI blood loss.[220] In a recent report of small experience of endoscopic evaluation of the upper GI system in children and teenagers between the ages of 9 and 17 years presenting with iron-deficiency anemia who did not have hematologic or chronic diseases, heavy menstrual flow or obvious blood loss demonstrated abnormal findings in 57% of patients.[221] This small study suggests that careful evaluation of the GI system should be considered in children and adolescents with unexplained iron-deficiency anemia and in those in whom the iron deficiency does not correct appropriately with oral iron supplementation.

ENDOCRINE DISEASE

Hematologic Manifestations of Thyroid Disorders

The associations between thyroid disorders and hematologic abnormalities are diverse.[222] The most commonly reported findings include anemia of several etiologies and abnormalities of hemostasis. Specific associations in childhood and adolescence appear to be less common than in adults. However, some rare disorders with both hematologic and thyroid manifestations appear to be particularly pertinent to the pediatric population.

Congenital hypothyroidism has multiple etiologies, including thyroid agenesis, thyroid-stimulating hormone resistance, disorders in thyroid hormone production, and central hypothyroidism. Screening programs for congenital hypothyroidism have been widely adopted as part of neonatal screening programs for several decades, resulting in marked improvement in the clinical manifestations of congenital hypothyroidism. A series of 50 infants with congenital hypothyroidism identified by neonatal screening found that modest normocytic, normochromic anemia, correlating with the severity of the hypothyroidism, is present during the first year of life despite thyroid hormone replacement.[223] By comparison, a separate publication on infants also identified by neonatal screening demonstrated no anemia, and 6 of 23 infants were found to be polycythemic.[224] The differences in these reports is not understood but may reflect, in part, the differences in the pathophysiology of congenital hypothyroidism.

The association between autoimmune thyroid disease and anemia is well recognized. The anemia may be exacerbated by several mechanisms, including iron deficiency, pernicious anemia, and AIHA. In adults, the anemia of uncomplicated hypothyroidism is typically normocytic or macrocytic, with modest anisocytosis present on the peripheral smear.[222] In children and adolescents, the same findings appear to be present. Additionally, children may have a decrease in linear growth velocity as a manifestation of hypothyroidism, suggesting that investigation of thyroid function is appropriate for children with macrocytic anemia and declining growth rate.[225] Pernicious anemia and iron deficiency may be less common in children with autoimmune thyroid disease than in adults. However, parietal cell antibodies are found in a significant percentage of children and adolescents with autoimmune thyroid disease, a finding that may predispose them to the development of both iron deficiency and pernicious anemia during young adulthood.[226]

Disturbances of hemostasis are also well recognized as a manifestation of thyroid dysfunction. Overt hypothyroidism and hyperthyroidism modify the hemostatic balance in opposite directions, with hypothyroid patients having an increased risk of bleeding and hyperthyroid patients having an increased risk of thrombosis.[227] There are few reports of bleeding or thrombosis in children and adolescents attributed to uncomplicated overt thyroid dysfunction. Of interest is the association between acquired von Willebrand disease and hypothyroidism reported in several adolescent girls, which may be a cause of menorrhagia.[228–230] This hemostatic imbalance may improve with thyroid hormone replacement.

More global immune dysregulation syndrome may result in both endocrine dysfunction, including thyroid abnormalities, and cytopenias. The association of the autoimmune polyglandular syndrome, a heterogeneous group of disorders, and pernicious anemia has been reported in children.[231] Additionally, the immunodysregulation, polyendocrinopathy, enteropathy, X-linked (IPEX) syndrome, which is caused by loss-of-function mutations of the *FOXP3* gene, has been associated with immune cytopenias, including hemolytic anemia, neutropenia, and thrombocytopenia.[232]

ANOREXIA NERVOSA

Anorexia nervosa is a psychiatric disorder occurring in about 1 in 800 adolescent girls; it is characterized by an inability to maintain a minimal normal body weight, intense fear of being fat, body image distortion, and amenorrhea. The profound weight loss is accompanied by hypothermia, hypotension, edema, lanugo, and metabolic changes and is associated with a mortality rate of 5% to 18%. A mild, normochromic, normocytic anemia with reticulocytopenia occurs in about 30% of patients.[233] Acanthocytes or spur cells have been reported and may be caused by low serum α-lipoprotein levels. The causes of the anemia probably are decreased RBC production and a relative increase in plasma volume. A few patients have had slightly decreased RBC survival. Serum vitamin B_{12} and folate levels usually are normal. Despite low serum iron and decreased bone marrow iron stores in 80% of patients, iron-deficiency anemia is uncommon except during recovery, when iron supplementation is necessary. The severe hypophosphatemia seen during refeeding of severely malnourished patients has been associated with hemolytic anemia.

Up to 50% of patients have leukopenia, with an absolute decrease in numbers of neutrophils, lymphocytes, and monocytes.[234,235] The neutropenia may be quite severe. An increased incidence of infection is not usual, although with increasing use of central venous catheters, more serious bacterial infections are being reported.[235] Bone marrow reserves are normal despite marrow hypoplasia and a normal to slightly decreased size of the marginal pool. Impaired neutrophil chemotaxis, intracellular killing of staphylococci, and decreased complement levels have been demonstrated in patients with anorexia. These findings are associated with occasional skin abscess formation.

Patients with anorexia nervosa have no apparent bleeding diathesis. The platelet count is normal to slightly decreased,[233,236] and the in vitro platelet aggregation response to epinephrine, adenosine diphosphate, and collagen is exaggerated. Coagulation defects are uncommon, except for those related to vitamin K deficiency reported in bulimia.

The hematologic changes in anorexia nervosa are directly correlated with total body fat mass depletion.[237] A bone marrow pattern on magnetic resonance imaging suggestive of gelatinous transformation of bone marrow (serous atrophy) is seen in patients with the lowest hematologic parameters. Direct examination of the bone marrow reveals hypoplasia with loss of fat stores and replacement by a gelatinous acid mucopolysaccharide ground substance. Focal or extensive necrosis may be present.[238] Bone marrow histiocytes are relatively increased in number and have prominent blue-green granules. With nutritional supplementation, bone marrow hypoplasia reverses, the gelatinous material disappears, and the hematologic abnormalities, including neutrophil defects and low complement levels, resolve by 8 weeks.

THROMBOEMBOLIC COMPLICATIONS IN CHILDHOOD ILLNESS

Improvements in medical and surgical care, particularly advances in critical and supportive care, have led to increased survival among children with malignancy and chronic illnesses. However, the extended survival of these children has led to comorbidities such as thromboembolic complications. The increased risk of thromboembolism in children with chronic illnesses is multifactorial and can include the illness itself, medical and surgical interventions, or the central venous line used to administer therapy.

In a recent analysis of 13,449 admissions at US children's hospitals, the majority (63%) of patients with venous thromboembolism (VTE) had one or more complex chronic conditions, most commonly cardiovascular disease (28%), followed by malignancy (14%) and neuromuscular (11%) and respiratory (7%) diseases.[186] This review focuses on four childhood illnesses commonly associated with thromboembolism: malignancy, CHD, nephrotic syndrome, and SLE. In addition to the diseases discussed in this review, other chronic illnesses of childhood have been associated with thromboembolism, including sickle cell anemia, IBD, diabetes, and CF. Children receiving home total parental nutrition also have an increased risk of thrombosis because of the combination of a central venous catheter and infusion of hyperosmolar solutions that can injure the vascular endothelium.[239,240] As the incidence of pediatric VTE increases, the concept of thromboprophylaxis in hospitalized children is receiving increased attention. The end of this section reviews the small but growing body of literature on this topic.

Thromboembolism in Pediatric Cancer

Although thrombosis is a well-known complication of pediatric malignancy, the overall incidence is low compared with adults with cancer. Most epidemiologic studies in this area have been limited to single-center experiences or specific cancer types. The reported incidence of thromboembolism in pediatric cancer ranges from 2% to 14% when based on clinical symptoms and up to 44% to 50% when children undergo routine radiographic screening.[241–248] In a report of 17 years' experience at McMaster Children's Hospital, 7.9% (95% confidence interval, 6.0%–10.0%) of oncology patients experienced thromboembolism. Increasing age, certain cancer types (hematologic malignancies and sarcomas), intrathoracic disease, and catheter dysfunction were associated with a higher risk of thromboembolism.[248] Because many thrombotic events in pediatric cancer are catheter related, the majority of thrombosis described in the literature is located in the upper venous system.

Factors associated with an increased risk of catheter-related thrombosis include insertion of peripherally inserted central catheters or Hickman catheters and a history of catheter occlusion and infection.[249] There is increasing evidence of a bidirectional relationship between catheter-associated infection and thrombosis, and ongoing clinical studies are underway to better delineate the relationship between occlusion, infection, and thrombosis in central lines.[250] Right atrial thrombi are also frequently seen, with a reported incidence of 9% to 14% in children with indwelling catheters.[245,251] Typically asymptomatic, these thrombi are often found incidentally on routine surveillance echocardiograms of children receiving anthracycline chemotherapy. Patients with asymptomatic catheter-related thrombosis are at risk for postthrombotic syndrome (persistent pain, swelling, or skin changes) after catheter removal, and screening cancer survivors for these symptoms should be part of the long-term follow-up care for these patients.[249] The occurrence of postthrombotic syndrome is associated with a history of catheter occlusion, history of catheter-related VTE, and the use of two or more catheters, and is also a predictor of decreased health-related quality of life.[252]

There are several mechanisms by which malignancy increases the risk of thromboembolism.[253,254] These include direct activation of the coagulation system; inhibition of fibrinolysis through secretion of plasminogen activator inhibitor-1; and the release of cytokines, which themselves induce procoagulant and antifibrinolytic activity. Studies have also documented increased thrombin generation at the time of cancer diagnosis that persists for several months after initiating therapy. Malignant cells can also adhere to platelets, leukocytes, and the endothelium through adhesion molecules present on their surfaces. Finally, as tumors increase in size, they may compress or occlude blood vessels, leading to reduced blood flow and stasis. Non–catheter-related lower-extremity VTE can occur as a result of immobilization.[255]

Published studies indicate that patients with hematologic malignancies and sarcomas appear to have the highest risk of thromboembolism. In a meta-analysis including 1752 children with ALL, the incidence rate for symptomatic thrombosis was 5.2%.[256] As opposed to other types of cancer, cerebral venous thrombosis and stroke are frequently seen in ALL, particularly in the setting of asparaginase therapy. Asparaginase, an essential component of induction chemotherapy, reduces the synthesis of both coagulation factors and inhibitors as a consequence of asparagine depletion.[257] Higher incidences of thrombosis appear to be associated with lower doses of asparaginase given over longer treatment durations, as well as prednisone.[256] In a large Italian cohort (n = 2042), VTE occurred in 2.4% of patients and was associated with male sex and the presence of factor V Leiden and prothrombin G20210A.[257a] Similarly to other studies, 40 of the 48 events occurred during the induction cycle of chemotherapy, likely due the prothrombotic effects of active disease, asparaginase, and prolonged steroid therapy. A predictive model incorporating high-dose prednisone, asparaginase in combination with steroids, the presence of a central venous catheter, and the presence of inherited thrombophilias has demonstrated validity in the ability to identify children at high risk of thrombosis in a large population of children with ALL, although modifications are likely necessary when treatment protocols vary.[258] As a secondary outcome of this study, high-risk patients without low-molecular-weight heparin (LMWH) prophylaxis showed significantly reduced thrombosis-free survival during induction therapy compared with those who did receive prophylaxis; LMWH was administered according to preference of the treating physician (see box How to Manage Thromboembolism in the Setting of Pediatric Cancer).

The incidence of thromboembolism in sarcoma ranges from 14% to 16%.[259,260] Thrombotic events in sarcoma are frequently detected at the time of presentation and may be asymptomatic. Patients with greater disease burden or metastatic disease appear to be at highest risk. Brain tumors, the most common solid tumor in children, have a relatively lower risk of thrombosis in children than in adults. Researchers in pediatric and adolescent studies have reported an incidence of only 0.5% to 2.8% as opposed to the 18% to 28% incidence of thrombosis in adults with brain tumors.[248,261–263]

Because the incidence of thromboembolism increases with age, cancer-related thrombosis is of particular concern in adolescents and young adults with cancer, an increasing number of whom are cared for at children's hospitals. In a study of 2001 to 2008 national discharge data from US children's hospitals, 5.3% of adolescents and young adults (15–24 years of age) with cancer had a discharge diagnosis of VTE.[264]

Thromboembolism in Congenital Heart Disease

Although CHD affects only 1% of live births, almost 50% of infants younger than 6 months of age and 30% of older children who develop VTE have underlying cardiac disorders.[265] Also, the majority of children receiving prophylactic anticoagulation are those with complex CHD, prosthetic heart valves, or severe acquired cardiac diseases such as cardiomyopathy. Children with CHD are at risk of venous, arterial, and intracardiac thrombosis, as well as embolism to the central nervous system. CHD is also the most common associated diagnosis among children hospitalized with arterial ischemic stroke in the United States.[266]

Cardiac catheterization is the most common procedure performed in children with CHD, and it is used for both diagnostic and therapeutic purposes. Access is typically obtained through the femoral artery. Historically, thromboembolism of the femoral artery was a common complication of this procedure, particularly in younger patients. In the 1970s, a randomized clinical trial demonstrated that the use of unfractionated heparin prophylaxis reduced the incidence of femoral artery thrombosis from 40% to 8% in children younger than 10 years of age.[267] Even when heparin prophylaxis is the standard of care, postthrombotic syndrome is commonly identified in children after cardiac catheterization, although fortunately most children have mild manifestations.[268] The Fontan procedure, which diverts systemic venous return directly to the pulmonary arteries, is the definitive palliative surgical treatment for most congenital univentricular heart lesions.[269] Unfortunately, thromboembolic events continue to be a major cause of morbidity and mortality associated with this procedure. The reported incidence of these complications in cohort studies ranges from 1% to 19% and includes venous thrombosis of the Fontan circuit, right atrial thrombosis, and stroke.[269] Thromboembolic events may occur anytime after the procedure but often present months to years later.[270] There is no consensus regarding the optimal type or duration of anticoagulation that Fontan patients should receive, nor are there data that any one prophylactic regimen is effective in reducing thromboembolic complications. Institutional protocols, if they exist, range from no anticoagulation to aspirin to warfarin. The American College of Chest Physicians (ACCP) guidelines suggest either therapy with aspirin (1 to 5 mg/kg/day) or therapeutic heparin followed by warfarin to achieve a target international normalized ratio of 2.5 but state that the optimal duration of therapy is unknown.[271] In a recently published international randomized trial of aspirin (5 mg/kg/day) versus warfarin as primary thromboprophylaxis in the first 2 years after Fontan surgery, there was no difference in thrombosis rates between groups.[272] However, the overall thrombosis rate was still substantial, suggesting that alternative approaches need to be considered. In a retrospective cohort of more than 400 Fontan patients, although the total prevalence of thromboembolism was low (2.7%), patients with symptomatic thromboembolism had a high mortality rate (73%). The two high prevalence periods for thrombosis were within 6 months of surgery and then long-term thromboembolism occurring more than 15 years from surgery.[273]

There is even less data on the role of anticoagulation or antiplatelet therapy in other cardiac procedures with the potential risk of thromboembolism. These include the placement of endovascular stents and Blalock-Taussig shunts as well as Norwood and Glenn procedures, which are typically performed before the definitive Fontan procedure. The ACCP recommends perioperative heparin therapy for these procedures.[271] The need for antiplatelet therapy after these procedures remains unknown, although aspirin unresponsiveness has been associated with postoperative thrombosis.[274] Postoperative chylothorax is also strongly associated with VTE.[275] Finally, thrombosis remains a significant cause of morbidity in children awaiting cardiac transplant, and thromboprophylaxis with warfarin should be considered at the time a patient is placed on the waiting list.[271,276]

Long-term anticoagulation therapy is clearly indicated for children with prosthetic heart valves. Because there are few prospective studies and no randomized trials in children, these recommendations are based on the high-quality evidence supporting thromboprophylaxis in adults.[271]

Thromboembolism in Nephrotic Syndrome

The increased risk of thromboembolism in pediatric nephrotic syndrome is multifactorial.[277] The same urinary losses that lead to profound hypoalbuminemia in these patients also cause acquired deficiencies of anticoagulant proteins such as antithrombin and free protein S. In addition to deficiencies of anticoagulants, increased levels of procoagulants (fibrinogen, factor V, and factor VIII), hypercholesterolemia, and increased platelet aggregation have all been described in nephrotic syndrome. Finally, the therapeutic interventions for nephrotic syndrome can increase the risk of thromboembolism. Diuretics cause reduced intravascular volume, leading to hemoconcentration, and steroids and cyclosporine increase procoagulant activities.

The incidence of thromboembolism in pediatric nephrotic syndrome ranges from 1.8% to 9.2% in published series.[277–281] This contrasts with adult nephrotic syndrome, in which incidence rates as high as 44% have been reported.[278] The most common locations in children are the deep veins of the lower extremities, renal veins, and cerebral veins, and events are frequently associated with the use of central venous catheters. Although pulmonary embolism is clinically diagnosed in less than 1% of patients, a frequency of 27% (7 of 26) was found in a series of nephrotic children who underwent screening with ventilation/perfusion scans.[282] These data suggest that pulmonary symptoms may not always be caused by fluid overload in this population and that pulmonary embolism should at least be considered in any nephrotic patient with a significant change in respiratory status.

Prophylactic anticoagulation is recommended for adult nephrotic syndrome as long as the patient has proteinuria or severe hypoalbuminemia. However, no studies have been performed to evaluate the efficacy or safety of this practice in pediatric patients, and prophylaxis is generally not used in children without a history of thrombosis.[283] One reason for the controversy is that predictors of thrombosis have not been clearly established in this population. Even decreased plasma concentrations of antithrombin, a well-recognized risk factor, are not a consistent finding in nephrotic children who develop thromboembolism.[284] The most consistent biologic risk factor to date is the presence of severe hypoalbuminemia.[277] Age (infancy or ≥12 years) at diagnosis of nephrotic syndrome, membranous histology, severe proteinuria, and history of thromboembolism preceding the diagnosis of nephrotic syndrome have also been identified as significant predictors of thromboembolism.[280,285]

Although the traditional duration of anticoagulation for deep venous thrombosis (DVT) is 3 months, some form of anticoagulation should be continued or resumed in the setting of active nephrotic disease.[286] To avoid hemoconcentration, diuretics must be avoided or used judiciously in patients who have experienced a thromboembolic event. Finally, it is important to remember that the efficacy of heparin can be impaired in the setting of decreased antithrombin levels.

Thromboembolism in Systemic Lupus Erythematosus and Antiphospholipid Syndrome

The reported incidence of thromboembolism in pediatric SLE ranges from 9% to 17%, similar to rates reported in adult patients with SLE.[287,288] Although DVT of the lower extremities is still the most common manifestation, patients with SLE are more likely than patients with malignancy, CHD, or nephrotic syndrome to experience arterial and central nervous system thrombosis. In approximately half of cases, thrombosis occurs before or at the time of SLE diagnosis.[289] The significant association between the presence of aPLs and thromboembolism is well described in patients with SLE.[290] aPLs are a heterogeneous group of antibodies directed against plasma proteins and phospholipid complexes. They most frequently occur in the setting of SLE but are also associated with JIA, epilepsy, and other diseases.[291] There are multiple aPLs subtypes, including lupus anticoagulants, anticardiolipin antibodies, anti–β_2-glycoprotein I antibodies, and antiprothrombin antibodies. The exact mechanism of aPL-associated thromboembolism has not been elucidated, but recent data suggest that lupus anticoagulant antibodies interfere with the function of the protein C pathway, leading to an acquired activated protein C resistance.[292]

aPLs are quite common in the pediatric SLE population. Authors of an analysis of 12 published series of children with SLE reported a global prevalence of 48% for anticardiolipin antibodies and 23% for lupus anticoagulants.[291] Recent work has been focused on the predictive value of aPL subtypes for the risk of thromboembolic events. In a cohort of 58 children with SLE, the presence of lupus anticoagulants had the highest predictive power for thromboembolism.[293] The presence of anticardiolipin antibodies was also predictive, but only if they were persistent (positive on at least two occasions 3 months apart). Other studies have confirmed the strong predictive power of aPLs, particularly lupus anticoagulants, for the risk of thromboembolism.[287,294,295] However, pediatric patients with SLE with negative test results for aPLs rarely develop thrombotic events.

On the basis of these data, it is recommended that children with SLE routinely be screened for lupus anticoagulants, and if antibodies are present on more than one occasion, families should be counseled on the presenting symptoms of stroke and other thrombotic events.[295,296] Prophylaxis with low-dose aspirin may be reasonable, especially in the setting of other thrombotic risk factors. However, there are not yet data to support routine prophylactic anticoagulation with lupus anticoagulants in patients with SLE in the absence of a history of thromboembolism.[287] Patients who develop DVT can be treated with the standard 3 months of anticoagulation. However, all children with systemic inflammatory disorders such as SLE, rheumatoid arthritis, and IBD are at risk for recurrent thrombi when their inflammatory process is exacerbated. Therefore children with systemic inflammation and a history of thrombosis should receive prophylactic anticoagulation until the inflammation is well controlled.[297,298]

Antiphospholipid syndrome (APS) is defined as a thrombotic event and persistence of aPL positivity for at least 12 weeks after diagnosis of VTE and occurs both in children with SLE and in those who do not have underlying SLE, although they may develop the disease later. In a meta-analysis of 16 pediatric studies, there was a statistically significant association between persistent aPL positivity and first thromboembolism, with an overall odds ratio of 5.9 (95% confidence interval, 3.6–9.7).[299] The management of thromboembolism in primary and secondary APS is different from most other pediatric thromboembolisms. Patients with APS have a high risk of thrombus recurrence when off therapy, and most affected children are treated indefinitely.[289,297] However, the appropriate duration or intensity of prolonged therapy is not known. For children with VTE in the setting of aPL, the ACCP guidelines suggest management as per general recommendations in pediatric VTE, given that there is no evidence to support or refute the role of extended anticoagulation in patients with APS.[271]

The international Ped-APS Registry was established in 2004, and a published report of the first 121 patients has provided insight into the clinical and immunologic manifestations of pediatric APS.[289] As opposed to APS in adults, pediatric APS is only slightly more frequent in girls (female-to-male ratio, 1.2:1), likely because women with recurrent fetal losses are not included in this population. Similarly to adults, approximately half of patients present with primary APS. Thrombotic events are diverse and include DVT of the lower extremities (40%), arterial ischemic stroke (26%), and cerebral sinus vein thrombosis (7%). Multiple aPL positivity is frequent (81% with anticardiolipin antibodies, 72% with lupus anticoagulants, and 67% with anti–β_2-glycoprotein I antibodies), but two-thirds of patients tested negative for one or more of the aPL tests, emphasizing the importance of testing for all subtypes in clinical practice. Nineteen percent of pediatric patients with APS experienced a recurrent thrombotic event, even higher than the proportion reported in adult patients.[300,301] Catastrophic APS (life-threatening multiorgan thrombosis) occurs rarely in pediatric patients (approximately 10% of all cases occur in patients <18 years of age), but it has clinical and laboratory features similar to those of adult catastrophic APS.[302]

It is important to note that transient lupus anticoagulants, likely the result of infections or immunizations, have been well described in healthy children. These incidentally found antibodies are not associated with an increased risk of thrombosis or bleeding.

Thromboprophylaxis During Childhood Illness

The use of thromboprophylaxis to prevent hospital-acquired VTE has become the standard of care in adult institutions. Even though the risk of thrombosis in hospitalized children is much lower than in adults, there are patients in pediatric hospitals (particularly adolescents and young adults) who should undergo systematic screening for thrombosis risk and application of prophylactic measures.[303] Multicenter prospective studies are required to determine the safety and efficacy of prophylaxis, as well as the age cutoff at which prophylaxis should begin to be considered, but these studies will be very difficult to complete because of the relative rarity of thrombosis in the pediatric setting. In a single-center prospective safety evaluation of anticoagulation prophylaxis in high-risk patients 14 years of age and older, there have been no major bleeding complications.[303]

The 2008 ACCP guidelines discuss the use of thromboprophylaxis in only a few specified settings.[286] The guidelines recommend prophylaxis for children receiving long-term home parenteral nutrition and for patients with complex cardiac conditions and associated procedures. Routine prophylaxis is not recommended in children with central venous lines (including those with cancer).

HEMATOLOGIC COMPLICATIONS OF SOLID ORGAN TRANSPLANT IN CHILDREN

The frequency and success of solid organ transplant in children have been increasing over the past decade. In 2004, there were 1816 transplants in children, representing 7% of all recipients[308–310] This is an increase of 13% over the previous decade. Of the transplants done in 2004, the majority were renal transplants ($n = 765$), followed by liver ($n = 529$) and then heart ($n = 250–290$). The success rate has been also improving impressively, with 5-year survival after kidney transplant being 95% to 96%, liver transplant 79% to 83%, and cardiac transplant 70% to 75%.

Hematologic complications after solid organ transplant are a common problem. Although most of the evidence regarding the type, frequency, and etiology of these complications has been studied in adults,[311] there are increasing reports in children. After renal transplant, 60% of children are reported to be anemic. After liver transplant, 36% of children will have a hematologic problems, and of these, 54% are anemic events, 19% anemia and neutropenia, 12% thrombocytopenia, 8% neutropenia, and 2% pancytopenia.[312] After heart, heart–lung, or double-lung transplant, 51% of patients have been reported to have hematologic problems, including anemia (49%), neutropenia (14%), thrombocytopenia (14%), and anemia plus neutropenia with or without thrombocytopenia (23%).[313] The etiology of these hematologic problems is most commonly a result of infection followed by medication effect. Miscellaneous causes include blood loss, microangiopathic hemolytic anemia (MAHA), autoimmune cytopenias, posttransplant lymphoproliferative disease (PTLD), and multifactorial.

In the next section, discussion of the hematologic complications of solid organ transplant is divided into cell type and by organ type when feasible. The incidence, etiology, and natural history of the problem are addressed. Much of the data is derived from adult studies, but information from pediatric studies is emphasized.

Red Blood Cells

Anemia is a common problem after transplant, occurring in 66% of kidney transplant recipients at the time of transplant[314] and in 60% to 84% after transplant.[315] In liver transplant recipients, the incidence is 20% to 35%,[312,316,317] and in recipients of heart or heart–lung or double-lung transplant, it is 30% to 70%.[313,318] There are distinct patterns of presentation of the problems associated with RBCs, including early posttransplant anemia, HUS/MAHA, late anemia from immunosuppressant drugs (ISDs), late anemia from other causes, and pure red cell aplasia (PRCA).

Early Posttransplant Anemia

Early posttransplant anemia is defined as anemia that occurs within 6 months from the time of transplant. The etiologies include the following:

1. Postoperative hemorrhage
2. Hemolytic anemia secondary to passenger lymphocyte syndrome or HUS/MAHA
3. Infection, including bacterial sepsis or viral infections such as CMV, EBV, or parvovirus
4. Medication, including immunosuppressive drugs and other drugs
5. After renal transplant, iron deficiency or prior uremia or bone disease

Passenger Lymphocyte Syndrome

Passenger lymphocyte syndrome is a graft-versus-host reaction.[1,319–321] Antibodies made by donor B cells ("passengers") transplanted with the organ are made against host RBCs. This direct antiglobulin-positive

How to Manage Thromboembolism in the Setting of Pediatric Cancer

Prompt diagnosis is the first key step in proper management of cancer-related venous thromboembolism (VTE). In pediatric cancer, the majority of VTE is related to a central line. It is important to recognize that line dysfunction may be the first sign of a thrombosis and to consider thrombosis when line dysfunction cannot be explained or patency easily restored (see figure).[254]

When treating thromboembolism in a patient with cancer, low-molecular-weight heparin (LMWH) is the preferred choice. Warfarin, although it is less expensive and can be given orally, is difficult to regulate in the setting of multiple chemotherapy agents, frequent invasive procedures, and changing vitamin K stores because of antibiotics and illness.[247,304,305] A randomized clinical trial in adult patients with cancer demonstrated that LMWH was more efficacious than and as safe as warfarin in preventing recurrent thromboembolism.[306] The 2008 American College of Chest Physicians guidelines recommend the use of LMWH in the treatment of cancer-related venous thromboembolism for a minimum of 3 months and until the precipitating factor (e.g., use of asparaginase) has resolved.[286] Other practical suggestions have been reported, but none are supported by any systematic observations.[260,286,304]

- A minimum of two doses of LMWH should be held before lumbar punctures and other invasive procedures.
- For intramuscular asparaginase injections, applying firm pressure and administering the medication at the trough of the anti-Xa level are probably adequate to avoid bleeding.
- Clinicians should maintain platelet counts above 50,000/μL in the first 2 weeks of anticoagulation. After that period, the LMWH dose should be adjusted according to platelet count (50% dosing for platelet counts 20 to 50,000/μL; hold doses for platelet counts <20,000/μL).

Asparaginase-Related Thrombosis

Management of asparaginase-related thrombosis in acute lymphoblastic leukemia can be particularly challenging, and researchers at the Dana-Farber Cancer Institute recently published their experience with rechallenging pediatric and adult patients with asparaginase after a first thrombosis.[307] In this retrospective review, survival was similar in patients with and without thrombosis, and the following guidelines were suggested:

- Asparaginase can be resumed when symptoms of thrombosis have resolved and there is evidence of clot stabilization or improvement on repeat imaging, typically after about 4 weeks of anticoagulation.
- Because of the protein depletion experienced by patients receiving asparaginase, anti-Xa levels should be monitored frequently.
- If LMWH at previously adequate doses no longer adequately anticoagulates the patient, antithrombin levels should be checked and antithrombin repleted as necessary.

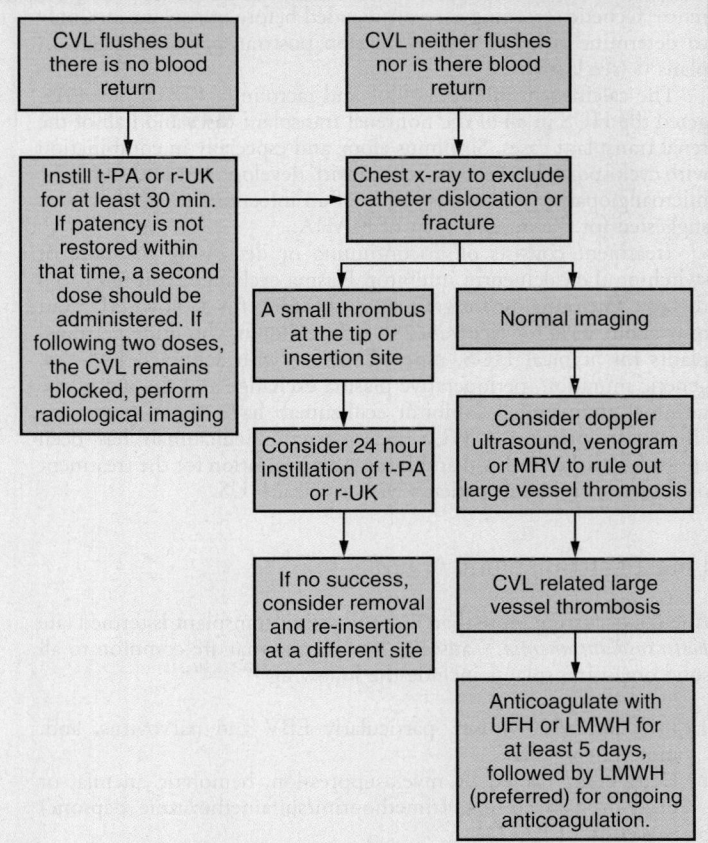

Management of central venous line (CVL) related–thrombosis. *LMWH,* Low-molecular-weight heparin; *r-UK,* recombinant urokinase; *t-PA,* tissue plasminogen activator; *UFH,* unfractionated heparin.

---

immune hemolytic anemia occurs within 3 to 24 days after transplant. Rh antibodies, especially anti-RhD, are the most common type of antibody. The anemia can be mild to severe but is self-limited, lasting from a few days to 3 months. The incidence of this complication increases as the size of the transplanted organ increases:

	Antibody-Positive, *n* (%)	Hemolysis, *n* (%)
Kidney	17	9
Liver	40	29
Heart–lung	70	70

The incidence also varies depending on the blood type of the donor and recipient:

61% with O donor and A recipient
22% with O donor and B recipient
17% with AB donor and non-AB recipient

Pediatric cases have been reported after all types of solid organ transplant, and the incidence appears to be the same in children and adults, at least after liver transplant.

Treatment consists of observation alone if the case is mild and transfusion if severe.[319] When transfusing RBCs, the ABO type of the transfused product should be identical to or compatible with the recipient serum, regardless of donor type. When transfusing platelets or fresh frozen plasma, the product should be compatible with both the recipient and donor. Empiric therapy used in the management of severe cases includes corticosteroids, plasma exchange, and RBC exchange.

Hemolytic Uremic Syndrome/Microangiopathic Hemolytic Anemia

HUS/MAHA after solid organ transplant has been described most often in adults who have the typical clinical presentation for this disorder.[322–324] The majority of cases have been described in renal transplant recipients (90% of cases reported), but HUS/MAHA has been seen with all transplant types. The median time of onset is 30 days after transplant, ranging from 8 days to 9 months,[322] and 80% of cases occur within 90 days and 96% within 1 year.[324] After renal transplant for HUS, 23% of patients have a recurrence, but the incidence varies depending on the original type of HUS. When a transplant is done for diarrhea-associated HUS, the recurrence rate is less than 10%. The incidence increases when the original diagnosis is atypical adult HUS and increases even more with familial HUS (60% recurrence rate). In children who underwent transplants for HUS, there was an 8.8% recurrence rate,[323] although the rate was 80% for those who underwent transplants for atypical HUS and factor H or I deficiency. However, other genetic abnormalities of the complement system are not associated with this high rate of recurrence. Genetic screening is recommended before transplant, not only to determine risk but also to develop posttransplant management plans[325] (see later).

The calcineurin inhibitors CsA and tacrolimus (TAC) have triggered the HUS in all of the nonrenal transplant cases and half of the renal transplant cases. Sirolimus alone and especially in combination with cyclosporin has been associated with development of thrombotic microangiopathy.[326] The possibility of an infectious trigger has been suggested for the development of MAHA.

Treatment consists of discontinuing or decreasing the dose or switching the calcineurin inhibitor. Plasma exchange is an unproven therapy. The outcome for graft survival is 60% for de novo HUS but only about 33% for recurrent HUS. In children who undergo transplants for atypical HUS, especially those with a known high-risk genetic mutation, perioperative plasma exchange and the use of the terminal complement inhibitor eculizumab have shown promising efficacy in preventing HUS recurrence.[325] Eculizumab has been approved by the US Food and Drug Administration for the treatment of pediatric and adult patients with atypical HUS.

Late Posttransplant Anemia

Anemia occurring more than 6 months after transplant is termed late *posttransplant anemia*. Causes of late anemia that are common to all solid organ transplants include the following[312–314,316,318]:

1. Infection with viruses, particularly EBV and parvovirus, and, more rarely, CMV
2. Drug effect caused by myelosuppression, hemolytic anemia, or other drug effects (e.g., trimethoprim/sulfamethoxazole, dapsone)
3. Rejection or PTLD
4. Anemia of chronic disease
5. Iron deficiency
6. Acute renal failure
7. Uncommon or multifactorial

Etiologies of late anemia in the renal transplant setting include end-stage renal disease or low erythropoietin levels (68% of patients will have levels <2 standard deviations below the norm).[314] After renal transplant, young children have less anemia than older children and young adults. This may be because of the large donor kidney with higher erythropoietin levels and creatinine clearance relative to the size of the patient.

Risk factors for chronic anemia in children after liver transplant were determined in a cohort of 1026 children followed prospectively.[327] The late anemia in this group was mild to moderate, with a mean hemoglobin of 10.24 g/dL. In multivariate analysis, the following factors were found to be significantly associated with chronic anemia:

1. History of GI bleeding
2. Leukopenia
3. CsA-based therapy
4. Glomerular filtration rate less than 90 mL/min/1.73 m²
5. Corticosteroid use
6. Antihypertensive drug use

Immunosuppressant Drugs

There is a wide variation—1% to 53%—in the reported incidence of anemia secondary to ISDs. This variation may be a result of the lack of a specific test for drug-associated anemia and the lack of prospective studies. Indirect evidence for the association, however, is quite strong—that is, the ISD is stopped or changed and the anemia improves. There is a clear association of HUS/MAHA with the ISDs CsA and TAC in the early posttransplant period, but a number of studies have documented the association of late anemia with these

agents as well. In a study of children after liver transplant, half of the cases of anemia were attributed to ISD.[312] The diagnosis was usually made by excluding other causes of anemia and on the basis of evidence of resolution of the anemia after a change in the ISD dose or switching to an alternative drug (median time for resolution, 4 months).

In a study of children and young adults after cardiothoracic transplant, approximately 25% of the cases of anemia were attributed to TAC, primarily because no other cause was found.[313] The nadir hemoglobin in these patients was 7.3 to 8.8 g/dL, with reticulocytes ranging from 1.5% to 6.7%. Only one patient had a direct antiglobulin study performed, and the results were negative. Four of five patients with simultaneous anemia and neutropenia recovered counts within 5 weeks of switching to CsA. In another study of 50 pediatric renal transplant patients, the prevalence of anemia was 60%, with 30% having hemoglobin levels below 10 g/dL. The TAC dose was found to be significantly associated with the presence of anemia.[328]

The association of PRCA and TAC was first reported in adults. Two children were reported to develop PRCA while taking TAC 8 and 47 months after liver transplant.[329] Neither had evidence of parvovirus B19 infection. When there was no evidence of spontaneous recovery after 2 to 3 months of observation, they were switched from TAC to CsA, and both recovered within 3 weeks. Of interest, in a study of adults after liver transplant, erythropoietin production was found to be reduced in patients receiving cyclosporin but not TAC.[330]

There are a number of case series of AIHA associated with the use of TAC and other ISDs in both children and adults.[331] AIHA has been seen after liver, small bowel, multivisceral, kidney, and heart transplants. Onset of severe anemia has occurred from 2 months to many years after transplant. The direct antiglobulin test has revealed warm, mixed, or cold antibodies. The common finding in all cases was use of TAC immunosuppression, although other ISDs were also used in a few cases. Treatment was variable, including corticosteroids, IVIg, plasmapheresis, rituximab, and splenomegaly. TAC was discontinued in many cases with replacement by alternative ISDs, including cyclosporine or sirolimus. Resolution of the AIHA was the usual outcome with some rapid and apparently sustained responses to rituximab and switching to an alternative ISD.[332–336]

Nonimmune hemolysis has also been documented in adults. In a retrospective study of 81 patients (median age, 39 years; range, 12 to 66 years) after lung transplant, 20% developed hemolytic anemia in the first year after transplant.[337] All were taking CsA, and none received TAC. The anemia was mild to moderate; there was no evidence of autoantibody formation or MAHA; and other causes of anemia were excluded. The researchers in that study postulated an auto- or alloimmune mechanism to explain this phenomenon.

Anemia has been reported to be associated with all of the currently used ISDs, including mycophenolate mofetil (MMF) and sirolimus. Although direct comparison of all of the drugs has not been performed, it appears that TAC and CsA are associated with a similar incidence of anemia,[338] occurring less commonly with the other drugs. One possible mechanism of the development of autoimmune antibodies posttransplant is the chronic T-cell suppression resulting from the use of these agents followed by release of B-cell control. As noted earlier, treatment has been empiric and has included the standard treatments for AIHA, including rituximab. Reduction in dose or switching the type of the ISD appears to be an effective therapy.

Pure Red Blood Cell Aplasia Associated With Parvovirus B19

PRCA was initially reported in adults in 1986, and multiple reports have been published since then. Authors of a review of the literature in 2006 reported 91 cases of parvovirus B19 infection posttransplant in adults.[337] Seventy-four were in solid organ recipients, with the majority after kidney transplant (71%), followed by heart–lung transplant (16%) and then liver transplant (12%). Ninety-nine percent of the patients were anemic, and one-third also had leukopenia and 18% also had thrombocytopenia. The average time to onset was 1.75 months posttransplant, with a range of 1 week to 96 months. The most reliable test to diagnose infection was the parvovirus B19 polymerase chain reaction (PCR), with results being positive in 85% of cases; IgM results were positive in 78% and IgG in 39%. Treatment with IVIg was used in 84% of patients, and there was a recurrence in 28%. The three deaths occurred only in patients after liver transplant who developed myocarditis and cardiogenic shock. Of interest, in a prospective study of 47 solid organ transplant recipients, none were found to have molecular evidence of parvovirus B19 in the first year after transplant.[339]

In a review of parvovirus B19 infection in children after transplant, there were 16 case reports: 5 each after liver, heart, and renal transplant and 1 after bone marrow transplant.[340] The onset was at a median of 8 months, with a range of 1 to 24 months. Although only 3 of 14 tested were IgM positive, all were PCR positive. There were no associated symptoms in 7 of 14, but other reported symptoms include cytopenias, rash, myocarditis, and pneumonia. All 10 patients who received IVIg treatment were cured, although recurrences have been reported.

Platelets

Problems with platelets, including thrombocytopenia and thrombocytopathy, have been reported after transplant, primarily in adults. After liver transplant, almost all patients develop a transient thrombocytopenia. Delayed thrombocytopenia is much less frequent. It has been reported in 12% of children after liver transplant,[312] 8% after cardiothoracic transplant,[308] and outside the setting of HUS/MAHA very infrequently after kidney transplant. Causes of platelet problems posttransplant include medication effect, immune etiology, HUS/MAHA, infection, and other miscellaneous causes.

Immediate Thrombocytopenia After Liver Transplant

More than 90% of adults have been reported to have thrombocytopenia within the first week after liver transplant.[341-345] Nadir counts usually occur between days 4 and 6 posttransplant, with an average count of 58,000/μL (range, 19,000 to 330,000/μL). An increase in thrombopoietin is seen on days 4 to 6, and increased reticulated platelets are noted on days 7 and 8. There are few reported clinical sequelae from the mild thrombocytopenia, although the lowest platelet counts have been associated with the most severe and complicated posttransplant course. Resolution is usually seen in 2 weeks. Lack of resolution is associated with a poor prognosis for graft and overall survival. In a study of children who received a living donor liver transplant, preoperative platelet count, graft-to-recipient weight ratio, and acute rejection were identified as risk factors for developing early thrombocytopenia in multivariate analysis.[346]

There is controversy regarding the etiology of this transient thrombocytopenia. One theory is that it is a nonimmune consumptive process reflected by increased markers of thrombin generation.[345] The liver may be the site of platelet sequestration. A second theory is that it is unlikely to be a consumptive process because of the lack of platelet activation after day 1. The thrombocytopenia is more likely a result of low levels of thrombopoietin seen pretransplant. With new production and rising levels of thrombopoietin from the new liver, there is a subsequent increase in platelet production, resulting in normalization of the platelet count soon after transplant. Although the specific etiology has not been clarified, there is general consensus that it is not immune mediated.

Lymphocyte-depleting antibodies such as rabbit antithymocyte globulin (rATG) are being used with increasing frequency as induction-type therapy in pediatric liver and intestine transplants. rATG does exacerbate the transient thrombocytopenia seen immediately after solid organ transplant but resolves in a similar 1- to 2-week period. Treatment of this transient thrombocytopenia is supportive. Platelet transfusions are of uncertain benefit. Although originally azathioprine was believed to be a cause of this thrombocytopenia, there is no evidence that alteration of azathioprine dose is necessary.

Delayed Posttransplant Thrombocytopenia

Delayed thrombocytopenia is not a major problem after solid organ transplant, and most of the data are published in adult series. In one retrospective study of 36 adult liver transplant recipients, mild thrombocytopenia (<140,000/μL) was seen in 54% of patients at 1 year and 25% at 3 years after transplant.[347] However, severe thrombocytopenia (<50,000/μL) was seen in only 9% of patients at 1 year and in no patients at 3 years after transplant. The thrombocytopenia was associated with splenomegaly in some patients. No clinical bleeding problems were noted after 1 year from transplant. In one report, 3 (12%) of 25 pediatric liver transplant recipients were found to have isolated thrombocytopenia.[312] The etiology of the thrombocytopenia in these children was cavernous transformation of the portal vein, autoimmune, and unknown. In two other children in this series, thrombocytopenia was associated with additional cytopenias, and the cause was possibly related to TAC. In an additional study of 126 children who underwent cardiothoracic transplant, 9 (8%) were noted to have isolated thrombocytopenia. Infection was the most common etiology (n = 262). In patients with combined cytopenias, including thrombocytopenia, two-thirds were related to either infection or PTLD and 20% possibly secondary to TAC.

Sirolimus has been associated with mild thrombocytopenia in adults, although the reported frequency has varied. In a study of renal transplant recipients, 23% were reported to have mild thrombocytopenia,[348] but no liver transplant patients taking the drug were found to be thrombocytopenic.[349] In 66 pediatric kidney transplant recipients taking sirolimus, there were no reported cases of thrombocytopenia.[350] Low platelet counts are usually seen within the first 4 weeks of treatment and are associated with higher sirolimus blood levels.[351,352] Similarly to TAC and CsA, sirolimus has been shown to potentiate agonist-induced platelet aggregation, although this is not the proven explanation for the thrombocytopenia.[353] A 25% to 50% dose reduction is often effective in resolving sirolimus-mediated thrombocytopenia.

Immune-Mediated Thrombocytopenia Posttransplant

There are many case series of immune-mediated thrombocytopenia after all types of solid organ transplant in children and adults and either alone or in combination with other cytopenias.[331] Eight adults after liver transplant were reported to have immune thrombocytopenia (incidence, 0.7%).[354] The low platelets were seen 53 months after transplant on average, with a range of 1.9 to 173 months. Three patients had demonstrable antiplatelet antibodies. Steroids provided effective therapy in four and rituximab in four, although splenectomy was ultimately necessary in three. Seven of the eight survived with normal platelet counts. Five children were reported to have severe thrombocytopenia (<10,000/μL) within 2 to 4 months after starting TAC.[334,355] All were documented to have antiplatelet antibodies. Responses were seen to steroids, rituximab, or anti-RhD.

Two cases after heart or lung transplant in adults have been reported.[356] These cases occurred 60 to 460 days after transplant and responded to prednisone and IVIg. Acquired Glanzmann thrombasthenia has been reported in two children after cardiac transplant.[335,357] Both were receiving TAC and had demonstrable antibodies against glycoprotein IIb/IIIa. One patient had multiple autoantibodies, and the other subsequently developed additional antiplatelet antibodies. One child responded to prednisone therapy and switching from TAC to CsA. The other responded to rituximab after prednisone and IVIg therapy failed.

Alloimmune thrombocytopenia was reported in three recipients of organs from the same donor (two kidneys and a liver).[358] Development of human platelet antigen-1a (HPA-1a; Pl^{A1}) antibodies from donor B cells were documented in an example of passenger lymphocyte syndrome. The thrombocytopenia in these cases was particularly refractory to standard treatment, except transfusion of HPA-1a–negative platelets. One patient died, another required splenectomy,

> ### Treatment of Immune-Mediated Thrombocytopenia After Solid Organ Transplant in Children
>
> There is no standard approach to the treatment of immune-mediated thrombocytopenia that occurs after solid organ transplant. First, all other causes of thrombocytopenia should be ruled out before beginning therapy for what is often a presumptive diagnosis of immune-mediated thrombocytopenia. If the thrombocytopenia is mild to moderate (>20,000 to 30,000/μL) with no associated bleeding symptoms, we usually observe without intervention and monitor the platelet count on at least a weekly basis. If the platelet count is less than 10,000 to 15,000/μL or if there is bleeding, immediate treatment is initiated with high-dose corticosteroids: 4 mg/kg/day of prednisone (or intravenous equivalent) divided into three or four doses and continued for 4 days. If there is a response (i.e., platelet count >20,000/μL), the corticosteroid is dropped to 2 mg/kg/day divided into two or three doses and then slowly tapered to zero over the subsequent 2 to 3 weeks. Intravenous immunoglobulin or anti-RhD in standard doses for childhood idiopathic thrombocytopenic purpura can be used if there is no response to high-dose corticosteroids.
>
> For patients who have recurrent or chronic thrombocytopenia requiring multiple courses of treatment to maintain platelet counts greater than 10,000 to 15,000/μL, we have used vincristine (1.5 mg/m² [maximum dose, 2 mg] intravenously weekly for 6 weeks) with success. Rituximab (375 mg/m² intravenously weekly for 4 weeks) has infrequently been used in this situation. For patients taking tacrolimus with refractory thrombocytopenia, serious consideration should be given to switching to an alternative immunosuppressant drug because this may be necessary for resolution of the thrombocytopenia. Involvement of both the transplant team and the hematology team is necessary for ideal management of these complex patients.

and one patient's thrombocytopenia resolved after an episode of severe graft rejection (see box on Treatment of Immune-Mediated Thrombocytopenia After Solid Organ Transplant in Children).

Infection-Associated Thrombocytopenia Posttransplant

Although there are few published reports, one would expect the same hematologic problems, including thrombocytopenia, associated with bacterial sepsis or other serious infections as seen in nontransplant patients. Infection with HHV-6 and the herpesvirus group has been studied closely. HHV-6 is commonly seen after transplant, mostly in stem cell transplant recipients. In adults after liver transplant, there are case reports of a syndrome of HHV-6 infection with thrombocytopenia, fever, and encephalopathy.[359] This syndrome has not been reported in children with HHV-6 infection.[360,361]

Herpesvirus infection after kidney transplant in children is seen in about one-third of patients, with CMV being the most common infection.[362] The hematologic abnormalities associated with herpesvirus infection include thrombocytopenia and leukopenia, with incidence rates of 31% and 24%, respectively. These and other symptoms of herpesvirus infection occur at the same frequency as in nontransplant patients. There is a case report of a child after liver transplant who developed measles complicated by autoimmune thrombocytopenia and neutropenia.[363]

White Blood Cells

Leukopenia and neutropenia after solid organ transplant are uncommonly reported in the literature, although this may not reflect the true incidence seen in practice.[364] Authors of two reviews of hematologic complications in children after transplant reported isolated neutropenia in 2 (3%) of 70 patients after liver transplant and 9 (8%) of 106 patients after cardiothoracic transplant.[312,313] Neutropenia was also seen in combination with other cytopenias.[331] Although there are

predominantly case reports in the pediatric literature, in one review of neutropenia after 400 renal transplants in adults, 35 cases (9%) were reported.[365] The etiology of leukopenia or neutropenia is similar in children and adults and includes immunosuppressive agents; other myelosuppressive drugs (e.g., ganciclovir); infection (e.g., CMV, sepsis); and, less frequently, INF, PTLD, hypersplenism, and idiopathic. Use of TAC is often implicated as a possible contributing factor.

Both filgrastim (granulocyte colony-stimulating factor) and sargramostim (granulocyte macrophage colony-stimulating factor) have been used to treat neutropenia in adults and children. In adults, it has resulted in improvement of the WBC count in more than 90% of patients after three or four doses.[365,366] There was no evidence of precipitation of rejection. In the case reports of children, both agents have been found to be effective in most patients, but there is a suggestion that efficacy may be affected by continuation of TAC.[364,367,368] Although cytokine therapy has been shown to increase the neutrophil count, there is insufficient data to prove the effectiveness of preventing or treating infection or decreasing mortality.[369]

There has been one report on the use of granulocyte transfusions in solid organ transplant recipients, including one child. Of the 14 patients studied, 11 showed an increase in ANC greater than 1000/μL by the end of the course. Of 12 patients with infections, 4 (33%) showed a clinical response. Additional studies are needed to evaluate the efficacy of granulocyte transfusions in transplant patients.[369]

Azathioprine is well known to cause myelosuppression and has been associated with moderate to severe neutropenia. Azathioprine is catabolized in vivo by xanthine oxidase and thiopurine methyltransferase (TPMT). TPMT activity can vary considerably depending on a genetic polymorphism. Approximately 0.3% of white persons are homozygous and 11% are heterozygous for deficiency of TPMT. Severe myelosuppression, including fatal neutropenia, has been documented in transplant patients who are homozygous for TMPT deficiency and receiving azathioprine.[370] Some data suggest that monitoring 6-thioguanine nucleotides (the metabolites of azathioprine) may allow for individualized management of azathioprine dosing with fewer side effects, although this has not become common practice.[371,372]

Neutropenia has also been associated with the use of MMF and sirolimus. Neutropenia and thrombocytopenia have been noted as side effects of MMF since 1998.[373] Leukopenia may affect 5% to 11% of patients taking the drug, and pseudo Pelger-Huet anomaly has also been noted.[374,375] The leukopenia is often seen within 2 to 8 months after starting the drug. Filgrastim has been effective in reversing the neutropenia, although some patients require decreasing the dose or stopping the drug. Ganciclovir and valacyclovir are commonly used simultaneously with MMF to treat or prevent CMV disease. These drugs are also known to be associated with neutropenia.[376] There may be an interaction between these drugs that increases the risk for neutropenia.[377,378] It may be necessary to stop ganciclovir as well as MMF for the neutropenia to improve.[374] Of note, serious infections are infrequently encountered.

In two reports of the use of sirolimus in children, neutropenia was the most common toxicity, along with hepatitis, hyperlipidemia, and mouth ulcers.[379,380] It is not clear whether the neutropenia is directly related to serum level of the drug. Most counts improve with a decrease in the drug dose, although a few patients need to have the drug discontinued.

Pancytopenia

Pancytopenia is seen in two settings after solid organ transplant. The first is early after liver transplant for acute liver failure from acute infectious hepatitis.[381,382] This represents the known aplastic anemia that can be seen in as many as one-third of patients after non–A-E hepatitis. Treatment and outcome are similar to those in patients with posthepatitic aplastic anemia who do not require liver transplant. The second setting is delayed pancytopenia, which may be secondary to infection with or without PTLD.[383] A number of cases have been associated with the use of TAC.[312,384] Hemophagocytic syndrome has also been reported in the posttransplant setting, usually caused by an acquired viral infection.[385]

HEMATOLOGIC ASPECTS OF POISONING

It has been estimated that about 6 million children, most younger than 5 years of age, ingest some toxin each year. The effects of toxins on the blood are diverse, usually nonspecific, and in most situations overshadowed by the nonhematologic manifestations of the exposure.[386] With certain toxins, however, bleeding, anemia, or change in the appearance (color) of the blood may be an important component of the clinical sequelae of an acute exposure.

The abnormalities of hemostasis after poisoning are numerous, and the mechanisms vary. Bleeding may be the only manifestation of warfarin toxicity secondary to an overdose of the drug or ingestion of a rodenticide containing warfarin. Any hepatotoxic substance (e.g., iron, acetaminophen) may lead to decreased synthesis of clotting factors and resultant coagulopathy. Bleeding in these circumstances is delayed for at least 24 hours, although there appears to be an early coagulopathy in iron poisoning that may be caused by a direct effect on clotting protein function and not hepatotoxicity.[387] DIC has been seen after ingestion of mushrooms of the *Amanita* genus or after a bite from the brown recluse spider *(Loxosceles reclusa)*. Poisonous snake bites can result in coagulation abnormalities characterized by hypofibrinogenemia with or without thrombocytopenia or a DIC-like syndrome.[386] Severe thrombocytopenia has been described with elemental mercury poisoning.

Acute hemolytic anemia may be the presenting manifestation after exposure to drugs and toxins in children with G6PD deficiency or hemoglobin Zürich or (rarely) in otherwise healthy children. Severe hemolytic anemia has been seen after the bite of the brown recluse spider and of a rattlesnake and after a wasp sting.

Exposure to certain toxins may result in characteristic color changes of the blood, which in turn may be reflected clinically in abnormal skin color. The child with methemoglobinemia (see next paragraph) presents with a slate-gray cyanosis unresponsive to 100% oxygen administration. On exposure to air, the blood retains a distinct brown color. Patients with toxic exposure to carbon monoxide or cyanide have increased levels of carboxyhemoglobin or cyanhemoglobin, respectively, resulting in a cherry-red color of the blood and skin, but only with high concentrations of the offending hemoglobin.

Infants (up to 4 months of age) are at particular risk for developing methemoglobinemia because of a reduced amount (approximately 60% of normal) of cytochrome b5 reductase present in neonatal RBCs. Methemoglobinemia has been described in infants with diarrheal illness and in infants exposed to exogenous agents.[388]

Yano and colleagues[389] described 11 patients with transient methemoglobinemia, all infants younger than 1 month of age who presented with vomiting, diarrhea, and acidosis. In prospective studies of infants younger than 6 months of age with diarrheal disease, 64% had elevated levels of methemoglobin (with a mean ± SD of 10.5% ± 12.3%); 31% were cyanotic; most infants were small or failing to thrive; there was no association of methemoglobinemia and acidosis; and all children recovered from their illness.[390,391] Although most infants with endogenous methemoglobinemia can be managed with support and hydration, treatment with methylene blue (1 mg/kg) is indicated in symptomatic or more severely affected children (i.e., with methemoglobin >20%–30%).

Nursery epidemics of methemoglobinemia have been reported in normal newborns exposed to disinfectants or aniline dyes used to mark diapers. Infants fed formulas made with well water containing a high concentration of nitrates have developed methemoglobinemia. EMLA cream (Akorn Pharmaceuticals, Lake Forest, IL), a eutectic mixture of the local anesthetics lidocaine and prilocaine, has been effective in decreasing pain in infants undergoing circumcision. Methemoglobinemia has been reported with EMLA use in this situation, but only in overdose.[392] Other ingestions associated with methemoglobinemia include phenazopyridine (Pyridium), dapsone,

metoclopramide, and nitroethane (an artificial fingernail remover). Although the list of oxidants reported to cause methemoglobinemia is long, methemoglobinemia caused by exogenous agents is uncommonly seen in infants and children.[393]

Lead Poisoning

Lead poisoning in children has been a serious public health problem for decades. However, the most serious toxic effects of lead (e.g., encephalopathy) commonly seen in the past are rarely encountered today, primarily because of measures instituted to decrease lead exposure (e.g., no-lead paint, no-lead gasoline) and screening programs in high-risk areas. Mean blood lead levels in the United States have declined, from 15 µg/dL between 1976 and 1982 to 3.6 µg/dL between 1988 and 1991.[383] Nonetheless, lead toxicity remains a problem, especially in high-risk children. In 2010, 6% of impoverished children aged 1 to 2 years were found to have lead levels above the upper reference range.[394] Additionally, children arriving from other countries with less stringent public health requirements regarding lead exposure remain at risk for significant lead toxicity.[395] Increasing evidence shows that even low levels of lead exposure are associated with a significant decline in neurodevelopmental outcome, and in 1991, the CDC lowered the intervention level of lead in the blood from 25 to 10 µg/dL.[395,396] Reviews of the public health issues relating to lead poisoning in children have been published.[397]

The occurrence of lead poisoning in children with sickle cell disease may be underrecognized. Pica may be a manifestation of sickle cell anemia, even in the absence of iron deficiency, predisposing children to lead ingestion.[398] Additionally, some children with sickle cell disease may be at risk for environmental lead exposure, including substandard housing with lead paint. The signs and symptoms of lead toxicity may resemble those of sickle cell disease, including abdominal pain, peripheral neuropathy with extremity pain, constipation, and hyponatremia.[399] Lead toxicity should be considered in the differential diagnosis of children with unusual manifestations of sickle cell disease.

The primary hematologic effect of lead is interference at multiple points along the heme synthetic pathway. The two most important effects are inhibition of δ-aminolevulinic acid dehydratase and ferrochelatase, resulting in the accumulation of heme intermediates such as protoporphyrin. A shortened RBC survival time accompanies lead poisoning and probably is caused by decreased activity of pyrimidine 5-nucleotidase (also resulting in basophilic stippling of the RBC) and possibly inhibition of G6PD and the pentose shunt.[400]

The anemia of lead poisoning has classically been described as a hypochromic, microcytic anemia, as might be expected from the effects of lead on heme synthesis. Although anemia has been said to be a common finding in lead intoxication, in reality, anemia is uncommon unless the lead poisoning is severe or there is associated iron deficiency.

A strong association exists between lead poisoning and iron deficiency in children. Both tend to occur in the same population of predominantly lower socioeconomic status. Experimentally, iron deficiency has been shown to increase lead absorption, retention in tissues, and toxicity. Iron deficiency also decreases lead excretion during chelation.[401] Lead may impede iron absorption and metabolism, leading to a vicious circle of increasing lead toxicity and worsening iron deficiency. In a study of children with lead poisoning (blood lead ≥30 µg/dL), 86% were found to have iron deficiency, and 100% of those with more severe lead poisoning (CDC risk class III) were iron deficient.[402]

A number of reports of children with lead toxicity have documented the infrequent occurrence of anemia without concomitant iron deficiency. Cohen and colleagues[402] found anemia in 12% and microcytosis in 21% of iron-sufficient children with severe lead poisoning (CDC risk classes III and IV). The combination of anemia plus microcytosis, however, was found in only one of the 58 children in their series. Yip and associates[403] found a 30% incidence of anemia in less severely affected children (CDC classes I to III), but of those with either mild or no iron deficiency, only 6% were anemic. Clark and coworkers,[404] using multiple linear regression analysis, found transferrin saturation to be the most important predictor of mean corpuscular volume, hemoglobin, and zinc protoporphyrin levels in children with lead poisoning.

Two important points emerge from the foregoing information: (1) children with significant lead poisoning may have neither anemia nor microcytosis, and (2) children with documented lead poisoning should be screened for underlying iron deficiency. Discussion of the immediate treatment and long-term management of patients with lead poisoning can be found in a recent review.[405]

HEMATOLOGIC ASPECTS OF METABOLIC DISEASES

A number of congenital disorders of metabolism may manifest hematologic abnormalities as part of the clinical presentation. Such global metabolic defects have diverse manifestations; especially prominent are neurologic abnormalities, failure to thrive, and unexplained metabolic acidosis. Although the hematologic findings may be overshadowed by the systemic illness, the recognition of a characteristic pattern of signs and symptoms may lead expeditiously to the correct diagnosis. Table 152.4 is a compilation of inborn disorders of metabolism that may manifest in infancy or childhood with hematologic cytopenias.[406] Additional information regarding metabolic disorders is available through the Online Mendelian Inheritance in Man website (http://www.ncbi.nlm.nih.gov/omim).

SPLENOMEGALY IN CHILDREN

Splenomegaly is a problem frequently encountered by both pediatricians and pediatric hematologists. Although the spleen is rarely a site

TABLE 152.4   Hematologic Manifestations of Metabolic Disease With Onset in Infancy and Childhood

Category	Disease	Defect	Hematologic Findings	Associated Findings
Lysosomal enzyme defects	Gaucher disease type 1	Glucocerebrosidase deficiency	Anemia, thrombocytopenia	Splenomegaly, bone abnormalities, delayed puberty, lipid-engorged macrophages (Gaucher cell) in BM
	Niemann-Pick disease type A	Acid sphingomyelinase deficiency	Anemia	Feeding difficulties, hepatosplenomegaly, developmental delay, neurodegenerative course, cherry-red macula, lipid-laden macrophages (foam cells) in BM
	Wolman disease	Acid lipase deficiency	Anemia, thrombocytopenia	Emesis, diarrhea, hepatosplenomegaly, vacuolization of lymphocytes, lipid-laden macrophages in BM, adrenal calcification
	Aspartylglycosaminuria	Aspartylglycosaminidase deficiency	Neutropenia	Recurrent infections, diarrhea, hernias, lens opacities, neurologic abnormalities, vacuolated lymphocytes
Defects of heme synthesis	Congenital erythropoietic porphyria	Uroporphyrinogen III cosynthase deficiency	Anemia, thrombocytopenia	Hemolysis, staining of diapers, photosensitivity, developmental delay, splenomegaly, erythrodontia
	Erythropoietic protoporphyria	Ferrochelatase deficiency	Anemia, thrombocytopenia	Hemolysis, photosensitivity, neurologic abnormalities, hepatobiliary dysfunction
Defect of amino acid metabolism	Tyrosinemia type 1	Fumarylacetoacetate hydrolase deficiency	Anemia, thrombocytopenia	Failure to thrive, emesis, hepatopathy, neurologic abnormalities, bleeding, "cabbage-like" odor, renal tubular dysfunction
Defects of organic acid metabolism	Isovaleric acidemia	Isovaleryl-CoA dehydrogenase deficiency	Anemia, thrombocytopenia, neutropenia, pancytopenia	Acidosis, emesis, neurologic abnormalities, odor of "sweaty feet"
	Methylmalonic acidemia	Methylmalonyl-CoA mutase deficiency	Anemia, thrombocytopenia, leukopenia, pancytopenia	Acidosis, neurologic abnormalities, failure to thrive, emesis
	Mevalonic aciduria	Mevalonate kinase deficiency	Anemia, thrombocytopenia	Acidosis, cataracts, neurologic abnormalities, hepatosplenomegaly
Defects of organic acid metabolism	Propionic acidemia	Propionyl CoA carboxylase deficiency	Anemia, thrombocytopenia neutropenia, pancytopenia	Ketotic hyperglycinemia, acidosis, neurologic abnormalities
	Pyroglutamic aciduria	Glutathione synthetase deficiency	Anemia, neutropenia	Hemolysis, neurologic abnormalities, metabolic acidosis
Membrane transport defect	Lysinuric protein intolerance	SLC7A7 gene mutations	Anemia, thrombocytopenia, leukopenia, pancytopenia	Malabsorption, protein intolerance, hyperammonemia, neurologic abnormalities, glomerulonephritis, pulmonary hemorrhage, hemophagocytosis
Glycolytic pathway defects	Triosephosphate isomerase deficiency	Triosephosphate isomerase deficiency	Anemia	Hemolysis, neurologic abnormalities, myopathy
	Phosphoglycerate kinase deficiency	Phosphoglycerate kinase deficiency	Anemia	Hemolysis, neurologic abnormalities

TABLE 152.4 Hematologic Manifestations of Metabolic Disease With Onset in Infancy and Childhood—cont'd

Category	Disease	Defect	Hematologic Findings	Associated Findings
Defects of vitamin metabolism	Cobalamin metabolic defects	Cobalamin transport and use defects	Anemia, thrombocytopenia, neutropenia, pancytopenia	Megaloblastosis, failure to thrive, neurologic abnormalities
	Folate metabolic defects	Folate transport and use defects	Anemia, thrombocytopenia	Megaloblastosis, ringed sideroblasts, diarrhea, failure to thrive, neurologic abnormalities
	Holocarboxylase synthetase deficiency	Holocarboxylase synthetase deficiency	Thrombocytopenia	Acidosis, hyperammonemia, respiratory distress, neurologic abnormalities, skin rash
Defect in metal metabolism	Wilson disease	*ATP7B* gene mutation	Anemia	Hemolysis, liver dysfunction, neurologic abnormalities, Kayser-Fleischer rings, arthropathy
Defects of purine and pyrimidine metabolism	Hereditary orotic aciduria synthase deficiency	Uridine-5'-monophosphate	Anemia, leukopenia	Megaloblastosis, orotic acid crystalluria, immunodeficiency
	Lesch-Nyhan syndrome	Hypoxanthine-guanine phosphoribosyltransferase deficiency	Anemia	Megaloblastosis, hyperuricemia, nephrolithiasis, neurologic abnormalities, self-mutilation
Defects of carbohydrate metabolism	Galactosemia	Galactose-1 phosphate uridyltransferase deficiency	Anemia	Hemolysis, failure to thrive, neurologic findings, jaundice, emesis, diarrhea, hepatic dysfunction, cataracts, gram-negative sepsis
	Glycogen storage disease type 1b	Deficient hepatic transport of glucose-phosphate	Anemia, neutropenia	Hypoglycemia, acidosis, hepatomegaly, xanthomas, inflammatory bowel disease
	Hereditary fructose intolerance	Aldolase B deficiency	Anemia, thrombocytopenia	Poor feeding, emesis, failure to thrive, neurologic findings, hypoglycemia, liver dysfunction, ringed sideroblasts, coagulopathy, hemophagocytosis, shock
Mitochondrial disorders	DIDMOAD syndrome (Wolfram syndrome)	Mitochondrial DNA deletion	Anemia, thrombocytopenia, neutropenia, pancytopenia	Megaloblastosis, ringed sideroblasts, diabetes insipidus, diabetes mellitus, optic atrophy, deafness
	Pearson syndrome	Mitochondrial DNA deletions	Anemia thrombocytopenia, neutropenia, pancytopenia	Ringed sideroblasts, vacuolization of BM precursors, exocrine pancreatic dysfunction, metabolic acidosis
Lipoprotein disorder	Abetalipoproteinemia	Microsomal triglyceride transfer protein defects	Anemia	Hemolysis, acanthocytosis, bleeding, emesis, diarrhea, failure to thrive, neurologic findings
Miscellaneous disorders	Barth syndrome (endocardial fibroelastosis-2)	Tafazzin gene mutations	Neutropenia	Cardiomyopathy, endocardial fibroelastosis, skeletal myopathy, short stature, 3-myethylglutaconicaciduria, abnormal mitochondria
	Cyclic hematopoiesis	Neutrophil elastase gene mutation	Neutropenia	Recurrent oral ulcers, poor dentition, recurrent fever, malaise
	Severe congenital neutropenia (Kostmann syndrome)	Neutrophil elastase gene mutation	Neutropenia	Severe invasive infections, acute leukemia
	Wiskott-Aldrich syndrome	*WAS* gene mutations	Thrombocytopenia	Eczema, infections, small platelets

BM, Bone marrow; CoA, coenzyme A; DIDMOAD, diabetes insipidus, diabetes mellitus, optic atrophy, deafness.

of primary disease, it may reflect systemic involvement in a variety of disorders. The spleen is the largest collection of lymphoid tissue in the body, with a unique association between the bloodstream and the reticuloendothelial compartment of the spleen. Splenomegaly may result when there is antigenic stimulation of the lymphoid system (e.g., infection), obstruction of blood flow within or distal to the spleen (e.g., portal vein obstruction), exaggeration of one of the normal functions of the spleen because of an underlying

abnormality (e.g., hemolytic anemia, splenic sequestration), or infiltration of the spleen by a foreign cell (e.g., leukemia, storage diseases).

The spleen tip normally is palpable in preterm infants; up to 30% of full-term neonates have a palpable spleen. A spleen can be felt in up to 5% to 10% of normal children, but most of these are in the infant or toddler age group. As a general rule, a spleen easily palpable below the costal margin in any child older than 3 to 4 years of age must be considered abnormal until proven otherwise. That some palpable spleens may indeed be normal is attested to by the study of McIntyre and Ebaugh,[407] who found that 3% of healthy college freshmen have palpable spleens, of which about one-third persist. "Pretenders" of splenomegaly include the left lobe of the liver, a left upper quadrant tumor such as Wilms tumor or neuroblastoma, the "wandering spleen," and the proptotic spleen (seen in children with a depressed diaphragm from obstructive pulmonary disease, such as asthma or bronchiolitis).

The most common cause of acute splenomegaly in children, especially young children, is a viral infection. Splenic enlargement in this setting is mild to moderate and usually transient. When the history and physical findings suggest a viral etiology, a complete blood count with differential, platelet count, and reticulocyte count should be performed to rule out unsuspected leukemia or hemolytic anemia and to determine whether there is an atypical lymphocytosis. The child should be reevaluated in approximately 4 weeks (or sooner if symptoms persist). If splenomegaly persists beyond 4 to 6 weeks, the splenic enlargement may be considered chronic.

A list of causes of splenomegaly in children is presented in Table 152.5.[408] Symptoms from splenic enlargement are uncommon, although massive splenomegaly may cause abdominal discomfort and early satiety. If the spleen is sufficiently large, there may be increased destruction or sequestration of one or more of the formed elements of the blood (hypersplenism). Cytopenias tend to be mild to moderate, with the platelet count affected the most. An approach to the pediatric patient with splenic enlargement is outlined in the box on Evaluation and Management of Children With Splenomegaly.

Evaluation and Management of Children With Splenomegaly

When evaluating a child with chronic splenomegaly, the clinician must consider all of the possibilities noted in Table 152.5. Clues from the history and physical examination may suggest a specific etiology and direct a tailored approach to the diagnostic laboratory evaluation. If, on the other hand, there is no apparent cause of the enlarged spleen, a number of screening laboratory tests should be performed, including a complete blood count with differential, platelet count, and reticulocyte count; evaluation of the peripheral smear; determination of sedimentation rate; liver function tests; determination of antibody titers to Epstein-Barr virus, cytomegalovirus, and *Toxoplasma* spp.; antinuclear antibody assay; and ultrasound evaluation of the liver, spleen, and portal system (the last with Doppler flow technique). Further evaluation, including bone marrow examination, may be necessary if the screening tests do not reveal the cause of the splenic enlargement.

Management of splenomegaly usually is that of the underlying disease, when such treatment exists. Splenectomy may be indicated in selected conditions, but the potential benefits from splenectomy must be weighed against the risk of postsplenectomy sepsis, a rapidly progressive bacteremia, most commonly from *Streptococcus pneumoniae*, with a mortality rate of approximately 50%. The risk of postsplenectomy sepsis depends on the age of the patient and the nature of the underlying disorder. Patients younger than 3 years of age and those with a compromised immune or reticuloendothelial system are most susceptible. When elective splenectomy is indicated, it is advisable to (1) postpone surgery until the patient is at least 5 to 6 years of age; (2) administer pneumococcal, meningococcal, and *Haemophilus influenzae* vaccines (if the patient was not previously immunized) at least 1 to 2 weeks before splenectomy; (3) consider use of prophylactic penicillin for at least 4 years; and (4) manage significant febrile illnesses as possible postsplenectomy sepsis at all times. In addition to the risk of postsplenectomy sepsis, the rare complication of postsplenectomy portal or splenic vein thrombosis must also be considered.

For children younger than 5 years of age with severe symptoms from hemolytic anemia, hemoglobinopathy, or hypersplenism, partial splenectomy should be considered. In a number of studies, up to 90% of the spleen has been removed safely, with a high rate of success and preservation of splenic function.[409,410] Regrowth of the spleen to variable degrees has been noted, with occasional need for reoperation.

TABLE 152.5	Causes of Splenomegaly in Children

Disorders of the Blood

Hemolytic anemia: congenital or acquired
Thalassemia
Sickle cell disease
Leukemia
Osteopetrosis
Myelofibrosis, myeloid metaplasia, thrombocythemia

Infections: Acute and Chronic

Viral
    Congenital (e.g., TORCH association)
    Mononucleosis (e.g., EBV, CMV infection)
    Virus-associated hemophagocytic syndrome
    Human immunodeficiency virus
Bacterial
    Sepsis or abscess
    Brucellosis
    Salmonellosis
    Tularemia
    Tuberculosis
    Subacute bacterial endocarditis
    Syphilis
    Lyme disease
Fungal
    Histoplasmosis (disseminated)
Rickettsial
    Rocky Mountain spotted fever
    Cat-scratch disease
Parasitic
    Toxoplasmosis
    Malaria
    Leishmaniasis (kala-azar)
    Schistosomiasis
    Echinococcosis

Hepatic and Portal System Disorders

Acute or chronic active hepatitis
Cirrhosis, hepatic fibrosis, biliary atresia
Portal or splenic venous obstruction (Banti disease)

Autoimmune Disease

Juvenile rheumatoid arthritis
Systemic lupus erythematosus
Autoimmune lymphoproliferative syndrome (Canale-Smith syndrome)

Neoplasms and Cysts

Lymphomas (Hodgkin and non-Hodgkin)
Hemangiomas and lymphangiomas
Hamartomas
Congenital or acquired (posttraumatic) cysts

Storage Diseases and Inborn Errors of Metabolism

Lipidoses: Gaucher disease, Niemann-Pick disease, others
Mucopolysaccharidoses
Defects in carbohydrate metabolism: galactosemia, fructose intolerance
Sea-blue histiocyte syndrome

Miscellaneous Disorders

Histiocytoses
    Reactive
    Langerhans cell
    Malignant
Sarcoidosis
Congestive heart failure
Familial Mediterranean fever

CMV, Cytomegalovirus; *EBV,* Epstein-Barr virus; *TORCH,* toxoplasmosis, other infections, rubella, cytomegalovirus infection, herpes simplex.

SUGGESTED READINGS

GENERAL

Lascari AD: *Hematologic manifestations of childhood diseases*, New York, 1984, Thieme-Stratton.

INFECTIOUS DISEASE

Ballin A, Lotan A, Serour F, et al: Anemia of acute infection in hospitalized children—no evidence of hemolysis. *J Pediatr Hematol Oncol* 31:750, 2009.

Buranski B, Young N: Hematologic consequences of viral infections. *Hematol Oncol Clin North Am* 1:167, 1987.

Calis JC, van Hensbroek MB, de Haan RJ, et al: HIV-associated anemia in children: a systematic review from a global perspective. *AIDS* 22:1099, 2008.

Melendez E, Harper MB: Risk of serious bacterial infection in isolated and unsuspected neutropenia. *Acad Emerg Med* 17:163, 2010.

Strausbaugh LJ: Hematologic manifestations of bacterial and fungal infections. *Hematol Oncol Clin North Am* 1:185, 1987.

COLLAGEN VASCULAR DISEASE AND ACUTE VASCULITIS

Cazzola M, Panchio L, de Benedetti F, et al: Defective iron supply for erythropoiesis and adequate endogenous erythropoietin production in the anemia associated with systemic-onset juvenile chronic arthritis. *Blood* 87:4824, 1996.

Jordan MB, Allen CE, Weitzman S, et al: How I treat hemophagocytic lymphohistiocytosis. *Blood* 118:4041, 2011.

Newburger JW, Fulton DR: Kawasaki disease. *Curr Treat Options Cardiovasc Med* 9:148, 2007.

Ravelli R, Grom AA, Behrens EM, et al: Macrophage activation syndrome as part of systemic juvenile idiopathic arthritis: diagnosis, genetics, pathophysiology and treatment. *Genes Immun* 13:289, 2012.

CARDIOPULMONARY DISEASE

Khalid S, McGrowder D, Kemp M, et al: The use of soluble transferrin receptor to assess iron deficiency in adults with cystic fibrosis. *Clin Chim Acta* 378:194, 2007.

West DW, Scheel JN, Stover R, et al: Iron deficiency in children with cyanotic congenital heart disease. *J Pediatr* 117:266, 1990.

GASTROINTESTINAL DISEASE

Halfdanarson TR, Litzow MR, Murray JA: Hematologic manifestations of celiac disease. *Blood* 109:412, 2007.

Semrin G, Fishman DS, Bousvaros A, et al: Impaired intestinal iron absorption in Crohn's disease correlates with disease activity and markers of inflammation. *Inflamm Bowel Dis* 12:1101, 2006.

Tunnessen WW, Jr, Oski FA: Consequences of starting whole cow milk at 6 months of age. *J Pediatr* 111:813, 1987.

THROMBOEMBOLIC COMPLICATIONS IN CHILDHOOD ILLNESS

Avcin T, Cimaz R, Silverman ED, et al: Pediatric antiphospholipid syndrome: clinical and immunologic features of 121 patients in an international registry. *Pediatrics* 122:e1100, 2008.

Bajzar L, Chan AK, Massicotte MP, et al: Thrombosis in children with malignancy. *Curr Opin Pediatr* 18:1, 2006.

Kerlin BA, Haworth K, Smoyer WE: Venous thromboembolism in pediatric nephrotic syndrome. *Pediatr Nephrol* 29:989, 2014.

McCrindle BW, Li JS, Manlhiot C, et al: Challenges and priorities for research: a report from the National Heart, Lung, and Blood Institute (NHLBI)/National Institutes of Health (NIH) Working Group on thrombosis in pediatric cardiology and congenital heart disease. *Circulation* 130:1192, 2014.

Monagle P, Chan AK, Goldenberg NA, et al: Antithrombotic therapy in neonates and children: antithrombotic therapy and prevention of thrombosis, 9th ed: American College of Chest Physicians Evidence-Based Clinical Practice Guidelines [published errata appear in *Chest* 146:1422, 2014; and *Chest* 146:1694, 2014]. *Chest* 141(2 Suppl):e737S, 2012.

Monagle P: Thrombosis in pediatric cardiac patients. *Semin Thromb Hemost* 29:547, 2003.

HEMATOLOGIC COMPLICATIONS OF SOLID ORGAN TRANSPLANT IN CHILDREN

Dobrolet NC, Webber SA, Blatt J, et al: Hematologic abnormalities in children and young adults receiving tacrolimus-based immunosuppression following cardiothoracic transplantation. *Pediatr Transplant* 5:125, 2001.

Iglesias-Berengue J, López-Espinosa JA, Ortega-López J, et al: Hematologic abnormalities in liver-transplanted children during medium- to long-term follow-up. *Transplant Proc* 35:1904, 2003.

Marinella MA: Hematologic abnormalities following renal transplantation. *Int Urol Nephrol* 42:151, 2010.

Schoettler M, Elisofon SA, Kim HB, et al: Treatment and outcomes of immune cytopenias following solid organ transplant in children. *Pediatr Blood Cancer* 62:214, 2015.

Taylor RM, Bockenstedt P, Su GL, et al: Immune thrombocytopenic purpura following liver transplantation: a case series and review of the literature. *Liver Transpl* 12:781, 2006.

HEMATOLOGIC ASPECTS OF POISONING

Sauter D, Goldfrank L: Hematologic aspects of toxicology. *Hematol Oncol Clin North Am* 1:335, 1987.

REFERENCES

For the complete list of references, log on to www.expertconsult.com.

CHAPTER 153

HEMATOLOGIC MANIFESTATIONS OF LIVER DISEASE

Christopher Hillis and Wendy Lim

The liver plays key roles in the synthesis and clearance of proteins involved in hematopoiesis and hemostasis. The liver produces hematopoietic growth factors such as thrombopoietin, contributes to heme biosynthesis and is a site of extramedullary hematopoiesis. Cytopenias are detected in approximately 75% of patients with liver disease. The liver plays a major role in hemostasis through synthesis of coagulation factors, coagulation inhibitors, and fibrinolytic proteins. The liver is also involved in the clearance of plasma proteins, including activated coagulation factors, proteolytic enzyme–inhibitor complexes, fibrin, and fibrinogen degradation products. Lipid metabolism involves the liver, which in turn can affect the structure of the red blood cell (RBC) membrane. As a consequence, chronic liver disease is frequently associated with multiple hematologic abnormalities.

Liver cirrhosis is often associated with the development of portal hypertension, which leads to the formation of portal gastropathy and gastric, esophageal, or rectal varices, which can result in gastrointestinal (GI) bleeding. Portal hypertension also causes hypersplenism increasing the fraction of circulating platelets, leukocytes and erythrocytes sequestrated in the spleen which can manifest with varying degrees of cytopenias.

This chapter discusses several common hematologic abnormalities encountered in liver disease including RBC, leukocyte, and platelet abnormalities, coagulopathy and thrombosis.

RED BLOOD CELL ABNORMALITIES

Morphologic Abnormalities

The size and shape of the RBC membrane can be affected by abnormal lipid metabolism caused by liver disease. Excess cholesterol in the outer RBC membrane bilayer is thought to be responsible for morphologic abnormalities, including macrocytosis and target cells (Fig. 153.1), and for impaired migration of integral membrane proteins causing a loss of RBC membrane fluidity and deformability. RBCs with excess membrane cholesterol are also rendered less deformable from oxidative damage caused by an inability to repair peroxidized membrane lipids. When these less deformable RBCs traverse through the splenic microcirculation, cytoskeletal damage and permanent deformation can occur, resulting in the formation of acanthocytes (spur cells) and increased clearance in the reticuloendothelial system.

Spur cell anemia is a hemolytic anemia most commonly caused by chronic or severe liver disease. Life-threatening hemolysis can ensue, as well as disseminated intravascular coagulation (DIC), GI bleeding or liver failure depending on the primary cause. Spur cell anemia associated with hereditary diseases such as neuroacanthocytosis syndromes or lipoprotein disorders tends to be milder (see Chapter 45). Treatment options for spur cell anemia associated with liver disease are limited. The most effective therapy is liver transplantation. Clinical improvement using flunarizine, pentoxifylline, and cholestyramine has been documented in case reports.

Anemia

The etiology of anemia is multifactorial, although acute and chronic GI hemorrhage are primary contributors. Fluid retention increases whole blood volume in patients with cirrhosis causing an apparent anemia, as 60% to 70% of these patients will have a normal red cell mass but a subnormal hematocrit from hemodilution. Hypersplenism results in sequestration of erythrocytes. Erythropoiesis is reduced by nutritional deficiencies in folate or vitamin B_{12} resulting from poor intake or malabsorption, iron deficiency, bone marrow suppression from alcohol or viral hepatitis, hepatitis-associated aplastic anemia, treatment-related toxicities for viral hepatitis (e.g., interferon, telaprevir, boceprevir), and anemia of chronic disease. Patients with chronic liver disease or cirrhosis can also experience nonimmune hemolysis because of acquired alterations in the RBC membrane (e.g., spur cell anemia), Zieve syndrome (hemolytic anemia, hypertriglyceridemia, and jaundice), or treatment-related toxicities (e.g., ribavirin).

The therapeutic approach to anemia in liver disease includes transfusional support for symptomatic disease, identification and treatment of GI bleeding, supplementation for documented iron, vitamin B_{12}, or folate deficiencies, discontinuation of bone marrow suppressive medications or alcohol, and appropriate treatment for the primary cause of liver disease.

Small studies have suggested that inadequate production or response to erythropoietin (EPO) also contributes to chronic anemia in hepatic disease, although the association is controversial. Nonetheless, EPO supplementation has demonstrated clinical efficacy, cost-effectiveness, and increased quality of life in patients with hemoglobin levels less than 12 g/dL undergoing antiviral therapy for hepatitis C. The use of EPO to maintain a hemoglobin greater than 10 g/dL may obviate the need for dose reduction or discontinuation of ribavirin, either of which reduce rates of sustained viral response. It may take up to 6 weeks to observe a significant rise in hemoglobin in response to EPO.

WHITE BLOOD CELL ABNORMALITIES

Leukopenia

Leukopenia, particularly neutropenia, has been observed in up to 55% of patients with cirrhosis. Splenic sequestration is considered to be the main culprit; however, reduced production of leukocytes may also be a consequence of altered granulocyte colony-stimulating factor (G-CSF) and granulocyte macrophage colony-stimulating factor (GM-CSF) levels, bone marrow suppression mediated by primary infections or toxins (e.g., hepatitis B or C, alcohol), or medications (e.g., interferon). Immune-mediated neutropenia can occur in the context of hepatitis C or autoimmune hepatitis, and increased apoptosis may also be responsible for a shortened neutrophil life span. Furthermore, impairment in neutrophil recruitment and phagocytic function may contribute to an increased susceptibility for severe and recurrent infections in patients with cirrhosis. G-CSF and GM-CSF have been safely used in patients with cirrhosis and neutropenia in the setting of hypersplenism or treatment of viral hepatitis, resulting in improvements in leukocyte counts. The impact of these treatments on risk of infection or response to antiviral therapy is unclear.

PLATELET ABNORMALITIES

Thrombocytopenia

Thrombocytopenia is the most common cytopenia associated with liver disease, occurring in up to 77% of patients with cirrhosis.

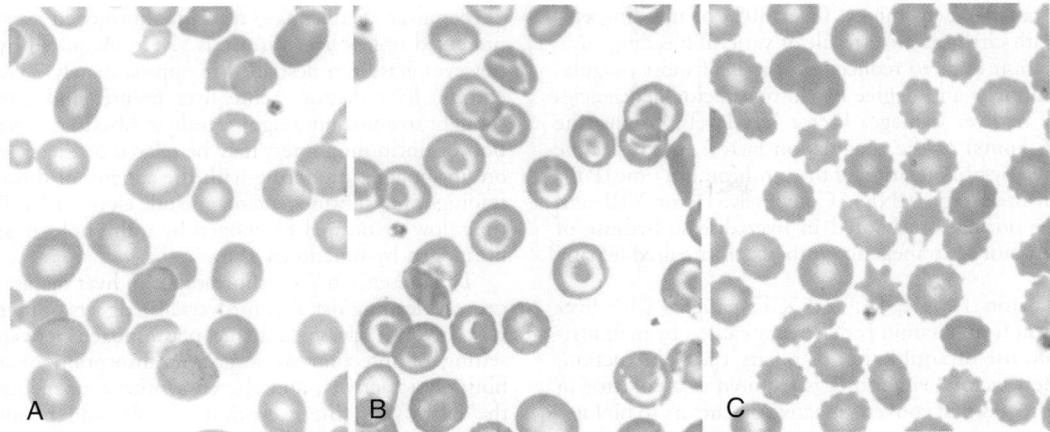

Fig. 153.1 RED BLOOD CELL MORPHOLOGY IN LIVER DISEASE. (A) Macrocytes have a mean corpuscular volume greater than 100 fL and can be oval shaped. Commonly associated disorders include liver disease and vitamin B_{12} and folate deficiency. (B) Target cells are characterized by the bull's-eye appearance of the red blood cell (RBC). They are a result of an increased surface-to-volume ratio related to excess RBC membrane (e.g., liver disease) or disproportionate reduction of cytoplasmic content (e.g., hemoglobinopathies, iron deficiency). (C) Acanthocytes, or spur cells, typically appear as contracted RBCs lacking central pallor with multiple irregular membrane projections. The morphologic appearance reflects the irreversible cytoskeletal damage that has occurred because of passage of nondeformable RBCs through the reticuloendothelial system. They are most commonly seen in severe liver disease but can also be features of rare neuroacanthocytosis syndromes or lipoprotein disorders.

Platelet counts are usually mildly to moderately reduced; severe thrombocytopenia ($<30–40 \times 10^9$/L) and spontaneous bleeding are uncommon.

Many factors contribute to thrombocytopenia in liver disease. Decreased platelet counts may result from hypersplenism. There may be impaired thrombopoiesis related to nutritional deficiencies (folate or vitamin B_{12}); direct toxicity of alcohol, viral hepatitis, or interferon treatment; or reduced hepatic synthesis of thrombopoietin. Autoantibodies to platelet antigens have been demonstrated in patients with cirrhosis, suggesting that accelerated destruction of platelets can occur via immune-mediated mechanisms. Hepatitis C is a secondary cause of immune thrombocytopenia. Although controversial, the presence of low-grade DIC may contribute to platelet consumption. Thrombocytopenia in patients with cirrhosis, especially in combination with leukopenia, has been associated with increased morbidity and mortality.

Platelet Dysfunction

Laboratory evaluation of platelet function has demonstrated abnormal bleeding times (BTs), PFA-100 results, and platelet aggregation in response to multiple agonists in some individuals with liver disease, implying that there may be a component of platelet dysfunction. Intrinsic platelet defects leading to abnormal platelet aggregation or adhesion include impaired transmembrane signaling and thromboxane A2 synthesis, storage pool deficiency, or defects in platelet glycoprotein Ib or $\alpha_{IIb}\beta_3$ receptors. Extrinsic defects resulting in platelet dysfunction include circulating fibrin(ogen) degradation products, bile salts, abnormal high-density lipoproteins, reduced hematocrit, and excess production of nitric oxide and prostacyclin.

The clinical significance of platelet dysfunction demonstrated in vitro is unclear. Although prolonged BTs are present in up to 40% of patients with cirrhosis and appear to be correlated with disease severity, they have not been predictive of bleeding. Improvement in BT in randomized trials of DDAVP (desmopressin) did not translate into reductions in surgical blood loss, transfusion requirements, or improved control of variceal hemorrhage. This discordance between laboratory findings and clinical bleeding may be explained by two observations. First, platelets studied under physiologic flow conditions show normal adhesion to fibrinogen and collagen even in cirrhosis. Second, elevated levels of von Willebrand Factor (vWF) are commonly found in patients with cirrhosis and may compensate for thrombocytopenia or platelet dysfunction.

Platelet transfusions can be used to treat thrombocytopenia caused by liver disease but are generally not indicated unless the patient has severe thrombocytopenia ($<10–20 \times 10^9$/L) or platelets less than 50 $\times 10^9$/L with bleeding symptoms. Platelet counts greater than 50–70 $\times 10^9$/L are usually considered adequate for invasive procedures. Less commonly attempted interventions for thrombocytopenia secondary to liver disease include splenectomy, partial splenic arterial embolization, and transjugular intrahepatic portosystemic shunt (TIPS), which are associated with unpredictable results and procedural risks. Thrombopoietin mimetic agents (e.g., eltrombopag, romiplostim) may offer potential treatment for these patients. In a phase II trial of 74 patients with hepatitis C–related cirrhosis and platelet counts of $20–70 \times 10^9$/L randomized to eltrombopag (30, 50, or 75 mg/day) or placebo, the primary endpoint of achieving a platelet count greater than 100×10^9/L at week 4 was seen in 75% to 95% of patients taking eltrombopag compared with 0% in the placebo group. Furthermore, 36% to 65% of patients taking eltrombopag were able to complete a 12-week course of antiviral treatment compared with 6% of the placebo group. However, another trial evaluating eltrombopag in chronic liver disease was stopped because of an increase in portal vein thrombosis (PVT), highlighting some of the toxicities that can be associated with these new agents. Further study is required before recommendations can be made about their use as no study has demonstrated a reduction in bleeding with these agents.

COAGULATION AND LIVER DISEASE

The manifestations of aberrant coagulation in liver disease reflect a complex interplay between procoagulant and anticoagulant mechanisms. Patients with cirrhosis are at an increased risk of bleeding and thrombosis.

Deficiencies in coagulation factors, vitamin K deficiency, dysfibrinogenemia, and systemic fibrinolysis can all contribute to impaired hemostasis. Clinical manifestations range from asymptomatic laboratory abnormalities to life-threatening hemorrhage. Most spontaneous bleeding in chronic liver disease, however, is not because of abnormalities in coagulation but variceal bleeding resulting from portal hypertension and vascular deformities. Over 80% of bleeding episodes in patients with cirrhosis are a result of variceal bleeding.

Hepatic dysfunction leads to reduced synthesis of most coagulation factors. The number and degree of clotting factor deficiencies reflect the severity of liver damage. Factor VII levels, having the shortest half-life (6 hours) of the coagulation factors, often decline early and are reflected by prolongation of the prothrombin time (PT)/international normalized ratio (INR). Conversely, factor VIII and vWF levels may be normal or elevated in liver disease because of upregulated compensatory extrahepatic synthesis or impaired hepatic clearance.

Reductions in factors II, VII, IX, and X in patients with liver disease may also result from vitamin K deficiency caused by malnutrition, malabsorption, use of antibiotics, or biliary tract obstruction. For these coagulation factors, vitamin K is required as a cofactor in γ-carboxylation, a process that converts inactive precursors to biologically active factors.

Defects in coagulation factors are suggested by prolonged PT/INR and partial thromboplastin time (PTT) measurements and confirmed by individual factor levels. However, these routine screening tests of coagulation do not identify patients at risk of bleeding. Both the PT and INR have been incorporated into prognostic indices (Child-Pugh and Model of End-stage Liver Disease scores) as markers of synthetic dysfunction to estimate the severity of liver disease and stratify patients for transplant, respectively. Factor V levels have been studied as a prognostic indicator in acute fulminant hepatic failure. Acute liver failure is associated with more pronounced elevations in the INR, yet is associated with less spontaneous bleeding than chronic liver failure reflecting the importance of hemodynamics (portal hypertension) on the risk of bleeding.

Despite their routine use in clinical practice, several significant limitations exist in applying the PT/INR or PTT in the context of liver disease. First, the INR has not been validated for patents with cirrhosis. Second, there is no evidence that demonstrates correcting these abnormal values with plasma or procoagulant agents prevents bleeding or improves outcomes. Several reasons may account for the lack of correlation between PT/INR or PTT with bleeding. Liver disease results in deficiencies of procoagulant proteins but also deficiencies in the natural anticoagulant proteins, including antithrombin and proteins C and S. PT/INR and PTT assays reflect procoagulant protein levels only and do not reflect alterations in anticoagulant proteins, the role of the endothelium and platelet number or function. Small studies have demonstrated normal thrombin generation in cirrhotic patients and patients with acute liver failure and prolonged PT and PTTs. Tests of thrombin generation (e.g., thromboelastography, rotational thromboelastometry) have been studied in liver transplantation to assess hemostasis and guide transfusions but not to predict the risk of bleeding in patients with liver disease undergoing other invasive procedures.

Being an acute phase reactant, fibrinogen synthesis is generally preserved unless liver disease is severe. Acquired dysfibrinogenemia, however, has been described in approximately 75% of patients with chronic liver disease, acute liver failure, and cirrhosis but is not thought to contribute significantly to bleeding. Aberrant polymerization of fibrin monomers may be related to excess sialic acid residues on fibrinogen, interfering with the activity of thrombin. Laboratory findings of dysfibrinogenemia include elevated PT, PTT, or thrombin time, low or normal fibrinogen by immunologic assay and reduced fibrinogen by functional assay.

The presence of hyperfibrinolysis in liver disease and its contribution to bleeding risk is controversial. Triggers of increased fibrinolysis may involve release of tissue plasminogen activator (t-PA) in the setting of infection or surgery, reabsorption of ascitic fluid with fibrinolytic activity, and altered synthetic or metabolic functions of the liver. With the exception of t-PA and plasminogen activator inhibitor-1 (PAI-1), all fibrinolytic and antifibrinolytic proteins are synthesized in the liver. Decreased hepatic clearance of t-PA and reduced synthesis of α2 antiplasmin and thrombin-activatable fibrinolysis inhibitor favor an increase in circulating plasmin and a hyperfibrinolytic state in cirrhosis. Available laboratory tests cannot adequately assess the overall activity of profibrinolytic and antifibrinolytic components. Shortened whole blood euglobulin clot lysis time and elevated levels of D-dimer, fibrin, and fibrinogen degradation products are suggestive of increased fibrinolysis. These abnormal laboratory indices have been observed in nonbleeding patients but are seen more frequently in bleeding patients and have been reported to correlate with GI bleeding, severity of liver failure, and variceal size. Hyperfibrinolysis may theoretically aggravate bleeding through consumption of coagulation factors, inhibition of fibrin polymerization, and reduced platelet aggregation via degradation of vWF and glycoprotein Ib and $\alpha_{IIb}\beta_3$. Hyperfibrinolysis likely plays a more important role in hemostasis during liver transplantation. Conversely, patients with acute hepatic failure show evidence of impaired fibrinolysis with elevated PAI-1 levels and decreased plasminogen.

TREATMENT OF LIVER DISEASE–RELATED BLEEDING

Treatment and correction of asymptomatic hemostatic abnormalities in patients with liver disease is generally not indicated and potentially harmful. Interventions may be indicated when there is active bleeding or before a planned invasive procedure. Most of the evidence for the prevention of bleeding in patients with chronic liver disease is based on studies of the perioperative management of patients undergoing liver transplantation.

RBC transfusions should be provided to maintain an adequate hemoglobin or hematocrit levels and for symptomatic anemia. A randomized controlled trial demonstrated that a restrictive RBC transfusion threshold in patients with an acute upper GI bleed reduced rebleeding and increased survival. In general, platelet transfusions are not indicated for isolated thrombocytopenia in the absence of bleeding. An effort should be made to maintain platelet counts greater than $50 \times 10^9/L$ with active bleeding or before invasive procedures. Platelet transfusion may be effective if there is suspected platelet dysfunction. Patients with cirrhosis often have smaller platelet increments in response to transfusion caused by splenic sequestration. In acute variceal bleeding, minimization of blood product administration should be the goal as the increase in central venous pressure associated with volume overload can increase variceal bleeding. Increased portal pressures caused by large volume plasma or red cell transfusion has been shown to increase rebleeding rates in animal models. During invasive procedures, a balanced strategy of maintaining low portal pressures by minimization of total circulating volume while maintaining adequate tissue perfusion has been shown to decrease bleeding.

A trial of oral vitamin K can be considered in patients with prolonged PT or INR. Vitamin K can be given intravenously for earlier onset of action but carries a small risk of anaphylaxis. Subcutaneous and intramuscular administrations are not preferred because of inconsistent absorption and risk of hematoma formation, respectively.

Hemostatic Balance in Liver Disease		
	Promotes Thrombosis	**Promotes Bleeding**
Primary hemostasis	• Increased vWF • Decreased ADAMTS13	• Thrombocytopenia • Platelet dysfunction
Secondary hemostasis	• Increased factor VIII • Decreased protein C, protein S, antithrombin	• Factor deficiencies: II, V, VII, IX, XI • Vitamin K deficiency • Hypofibrinogenemia • Dysfibrinogenemia
Fibrinolysis	• Reduced plasminogen • Increased PAI-1	• Reduced α2-antiplasmin, TAFI, factor XIII • Increased t-PA

ADAMST13, A disintegrin and metalloproteinase with thrombospondin; PAI-1, plasminogen activator inhibitor-1; TAFI, thrombin activatable fibrinolysis inhibitor; t-PA, tissue plasminogen activator; vWF, von Willebrand factor.

If no improvement is seen after 10 to 20 mg of vitamin K, additional vitamin K is unlikely beneficial. Although it may be reasonable to use vitamin K replacement alone in asymptomatic patients, it should be considered as an adjunct to other therapy in actively bleeding patients.

Frozen plasma (FP) has traditionally been used to correct liver-related coagulopathy because it replaces all the coagulation and fibrinolytic factors. Despite its widespread use, its clinical effectiveness in reducing bleeding has not been supported by data from randomized controlled trials. Guidelines variably support the use of 10 to 20 mL/kg of FP for major hemorrhage or prevention of bleeding before major invasive procedures. Evidence-based guidelines recommend against the use of platelets or plasma as prophylaxis against bleeding in liver disease laboratory parameters, including a complete blood count (CBC), PT, PTT, fibrinogen, and D-dimer, should be followed to assess therapeutic effect. In general, moderate correction of the PT and PTT is achieved after FP transfusion but is transient, and repeat doses may have to be administered every 6 to 12 hours to maintain the effect. Patients should be monitored for complications of FP, including transfusion reactions and volume overload. Plasma infusion may not be well tolerated in patients with liver disease who already have expanded intravascular plasma volume. Plasma exchange in addition to FP has been described primarily in the setting of acute liver failure and in preparation for liver transplantation. However, the efficacy of this approach has not been thoroughly studied in controlled trials.

The presence of hyperfibrinolysis, DIC, and dysfibrinogenemia may exacerbate bleeding and are inadequately treated with FP alone. These disorders should be suspected if coagulation parameters fail to correct with FP or there is persistent bleeding. Administration of cryoprecipitate, rich in fibrinogen, vWF, factor VIII, and factor XIII, may help control bleeding. One unit of cryoprecipitate for every 10 kg of body weight increases plasma fibrinogen by approximately 50 mg/dL. Cryoprecipitate carries similar risks to FP. Although antifibrinolytic agents could be considered in the setting of hyperfibrinolysis, no randomized trials have demonstrated efficacy or safety outside the setting of liver transplantation. Tranexamic acid has been shown to reduce blood loss and the need for transfusion in liver resection, transplantation and variceal bleeding. Thrombotic risks must be weighed and DIC must be excluded before usage.

Three- and four-factor prothrombin complex concentrates (PCCs) contain the vitamin K–dependent factors II, IX, and X and may or may not contain variable amounts of factor VII. They are effective in reversing anticoagulation with vitamin K antagonists (VKAs), but have not been widely studied in liver disease. Data are limited to case reports and small, uncontrolled studies describing improvement in coagulation parameters, subjective clinical improvement, and safe administration in patients with liver disease. The use of PCCs in liver disease should be undertaken cautiously because of the risk of DIC, thrombotic complications, and anaphylaxis; its use should be restricted to emergency situations such as refractory bleeding or if FP administration is limited by risk of circulatory overload.

Recombinant factor VIIa (rFVIIa) is formally approved for the treatment and prevention of bleeding episodes in patients with hemophilia and inhibitors, acquired hemophilia, and congenital factor VII deficiency. Because of proven efficacy in these other disorders, rFVIIa has been investigated for GI or variceal bleeding in liver disease, liver resection or biopsy, and liver transplantation. Studies have demonstrated transient normalization of the PT after rFVIIa, yet correlation with improved clinical outcomes has been inconsistent. The only two randomized trials examining rFVIIa in active GI and variceal bleeding did not show any benefit over placebo. rFVIIa appears to reduce blood loss and blood product requirements when used prophylactically in invasive procedures or surgery; however, there is no clear mortality benefit. These potential benefits may be offset by an observed increase in arterial thromboembolic events, particularly in elderly adults. Compared with FP, rFVIIa can be given in small volumes and has no infectious risk. Additional research is required to establish the overall benefit and risk of rFVIIa, and clinicians should proceed with the use of rFVIIa judiciously in the interim.

Management of Coagulopathy in Liver Disease

- Actively bleeding patients should be adequately resuscitated. Admission to the intensive care setting may be appropriate.
- Basic coagulation tests should be ordered to identify the cause of bleeding; these include CBC, PT (INR), PTT, thrombin clotting time, fibrinogen, D-Dimer, FDP, and mixing studies. The need for more specialized tests will be dictated by the clinical situation and response to therapy.
- It is important to identify any localized source of bleeding (e.g., varices) amenable to procedural intervention to achieve hemostasis.
- A trial of 5 to 10 mg of vitamin K is reasonable in asymptomatic patients with prolonged PT and PTT but should be used with other therapies in actively bleeding patients.
- In patients with thrombocytopenia platelet transfusions can be used, targeting platelet counts greater than 50×10^9/L.
- In patients who can tolerate volume, FP 4 to 6 units (1000–1500 mL) given over 1 to 2 hours can be used to replace coagulation factors. Coagulation parameters should be monitored to document effect and determine the timing and need for additional units.
- Dysfibrinogenemia or hypofibrinogenemia should be suspected if coagulation assays do not correct with FP or fibrinogen levels are low, respectively. Replacement can be attempted with 10 to 20 units of cryoprecipitate while following laboratory results.
- Patients who are intravascularly overloaded or who do not respond to FP should be considered for rFVIIa. Low doses of rFVIIa (25–50 µg/kg) are generally used, and repeated doses may be required because of the short rFVIIa half-life of 2 to 3 hours. rFVIIa may be most suitable as a temporizing measure to enable invasive procedures or hemostasis to be achieved by other means. Avoid use in the setting of DIC.

CBC, Complete blood count; DIC, disseminated intravascular coagulation; FDP, FP, frozen plasma; INR, international normalized ratio; PT, prothrombin time; PTT, partial thromboplastin time; rFVIIa, recombinant factor VIIa.

HYPERCOAGULABILITY AND THROMBOSIS IN PATIENTS WITH LIVER DISEASE

Although retrospective studies have reported variable rates of venous thromboembolism (VTE) in patients with cirrhosis, it is clear that these patients are not "autoanticoagulated" and thus not immune to thrombotic events as once believed. The risk of VTE may actually be higher in patients with liver disease than those without. Reported incidences of deep venous thrombosis (DVT) or pulmonary embolism (PE) have ranged from 0.5% to 6.3%. Thrombotic complications can also involve portal, mesenteric, and hepatic veins. PVT occurs in approximately 8% to 15% of patients with cirrhosis and is associated with both severity of disease and inferior prognosis in liver transplantation.

Despite the increased bleeding risks in liver disease, patients may benefit from prophylactic or therapeutic anticoagulation. Hepatic thrombosis or PVT may result in worsening liver function, ascites, varices, and hemorrhage. Furthermore, microvascular thrombosis has been proposed to promote hepatic fibrosis and progression of cirrhosis. Clinical decisions are limited by a paucity of studies establishing the optimal dose, duration, monitoring, or choice of anticoagulant and importantly, clear clinical benefit and safety.

There are currently no standard means of identifying patients with liver disease requiring thromboprophylaxis nor means to reconcile the perceived increased risk of bleeding in these patients. Standard pharmacologic thromboprophylaxis may be safe and should not be withheld in patients with abnormal coagulation studies in the absence of bleeding. Guidelines on thromboprophylaxis do not address cirrhosis, so decisions remain individualized. Patients who may particularly benefit from primary prophylaxis are those awaiting liver transplantation because PVT worsens the long-term posttransplant prognosis. Small trials have recently suggested that low-molecular-weight heparins (LMWHs) may be safe for thromboprophylaxis in cirrhosis. Use of VKAs for thromboprophylaxis in patients with liver

Hemostatic Indices in Liver Disease

Laboratory Changes	PT	PTT	TCT	Fib	Clauss	Plt	Platelet Aggregation	FVII	DD	ELT
Thrombocytopenia	N	N	N	N	N	↓	N	N	N	N
Platelet dysfunction	N	N	N	N	N	N	abnormal	N	N	N
Vitamin K deficiency[a]	↑	↑	N	N	N	N	N	↓	N	N
Factor deficiency	↑	↑	N	N	N	N	N	↓	N	N
Hypofibrinogenemia	N/↑	N/↑	↑	↓	↓	N	N	N	N	N
Dysfibrinogenemia	N/↑	N/↑	↑	N	↓	N	N	N	N	N
Hyperfibrinolysis	N/↑	N/↑	N/↑	N/↓	N/↓	N	N	↓	↑	↓
DIC	N/↑	N/↑	N/↑	↓	↓	↓	N	N/↓	↑	↓

[a]Differentiating between vitamin K deficiency and liver disease can be challenging with conventional laboratory tests. If available, performing a factor II assay with and without Echis venom (factor II biologic and factor II Echis) may be useful. Ecarin is derived from *Echis carinatus* snake venom and can activate prothrombin irrespective of γ-carboxylation. Factor II activity (biologic) is reduced in both vitamin K deficiency and liver disease. In contrast, the factor II Echis is reduced in liver disease but is normal in vitamin K deficiency.

Clauss, Clauss fibrinogen; DD, D-dimer; DIC, disseminated intravascular coagulation; ELT, euglobulin lysis time (measure of fibrinolysis); Fib, fibrinogen; FVII, factor VII functional assay; N, normal; Plt, platelet; PT, prothrombin time; PTT, partial thromboplastin time; TCT, thrombin clotting time.

disease may be complicated by unreliable INR measurements. Trials involving non-VKA oral anticoagulants such as direct thrombin and factor Xa inhibitors have usually excluded patients with liver disease.

A similar risk–benefit analysis must be completed before therapeutic anticoagulation for confirmed VTE. Expert opinion recommends screening for varices and appropriate treatment with β-blockers or endoscopic therapy before anticoagulant initiation to mitigate bleeding potential. There are several indications for therapeutic anticoagulation in the setting of cirrhosis, including DVT or PE, acute PVT, and Budd-Chiari syndrome. The comprehensive management of these disorders is beyond the scope of this chapter. Treatment options for portal vein or hepatic vein thromboses may include one or more of anticoagulation, systemic or local thrombolysis, or TIPS. There are no truly evidence-based guidelines for the management of anticoagulation in these patients. LMWH appears safe for the treatment of PVT and often results in recanalization. The use of LMWHs is complex owing to issues of dosing and monitoring, secondary to the hemostatic profile of liver disease. The potency of LMWH may be higher in liver disease and anti-Xa levels potentially underestimate the actual LMWH mass. VKAs for the treatment of PVT have been shown to have a high complication rate owing to a narrow therapeutic window. Anticoagulation should be approached cautiously but not withheld needlessly as mounting clinical experience demonstrates the safety of appropriate anticoagulation. The American College of Chest Physician 2012 guidelines recommended a minimum of 3 months of anticoagulation for acute PVT in the absence of cirrhosis, with consideration for long-term anticoagulation in patients with persistent thrombotic risk factors or concerns for extension into mesenteric veins. Individualized assessment has been recommended for patients with PVT with cirrhosis. Overall recanalization after 6 months has been observed in up to 75% of PVT patients with cirrhosis and minimal major bleeding. The value of anticoagulation for chronic PVT is uncertain, particularly in patients with cirrhosis with varices. Hepatic vein thrombosis is more uncommon than PVT, and even less evidence exists to guide therapy. Anticoagulation is usually instituted acutely and maintained long-term to prevent recurrence in the absence of contraindications. Symptomatic patients may require additional interventional therapies as mentioned earlier, including possible liver transplantation.

FUTURE DIRECTIONS

Liver disease can cause a variety of hematologic manifestations. Patients may have concurrent coagulopathic, hypercoagulable, and hyperfibrinolytic features. Bleeding or thrombosis may be the end result of a reduced capacity of the hemostatic system to maintain homeostasis in the face of physiologic stress. Advancements in patient care will evolve with improved understanding of pathophysiology and

refinement of laboratory assays. Moreover, strategies to safely manage patients with liver disease and a high-risk of bleeding or thrombosis are required.

SUGGESTED READINGS

Afdhal NH, Giannini EG, Tayyab G, et al: Eltrombopag before procedures in patients with cirrhosis and thrombocytopenia. *N Engl J Med* 367:716–724, 2012.

Boyer TD, Habib S: Big spleens and hypersplenism: fix it or forget it? *Liver Int* 35:1492–1498, 2015.

Clevenger B, Mallett SV: Transfusion and coagulation management in liver transplantation. *World J Gastroenterol* 20:6146–6158, 2014.

Dieterich DT, Spivak JL: Hematologic disorders associated with hepatitis C virus infection and their management. *Clin Infect Dis* 37:533–541, 2003.

Ferro D, Celestini A, Violi F: Hyperfibrinolysis in liver disease. *Clin Liver Dis* 13:21–31, 2009.

Garcia-Tsao G, Sanyal AJ, Grace ND, et al: Prevention and management of gastroesophageal varices and variceal hemorrhage in cirrhosis. *Hepatology* 46:922–938, 2007.

Gonzalez-Casas R, Jones EA, Moreno-Otero R: Spectrum of anemia associated with chronic liver disease. *World J Gastroenterol* 15:4653–4658, 2009.

Haas T, Fries D, Tanaka K, et al: Usefulness of standard plasma coagulation tests in the management of perioperative coagulopathic bleeding: is there any evidence? *Br J Anaesth* aeu303, 2014.

Kearon C, Akl E, Comerota A: Antithrombotic therapy for VTE disease: antithrombotic therapy and prevention of thrombosis: ACCP evidence-based clinical practice guidelines. *Chest* 141:e419S–e494S, 2012.

Lee WM, Larson AM, Stravitz RT: AASLD position paper: the management of acute liver failure: update 2011. *Hepatology* 55:965–967, 2011.

Lisman T, Porte RJ: Hemostatic problems in chronic and acute liver disease. *Hemostasis and thrombosis*, 2014, pp 271–283.

Marks PW: Hematologic manifestations of liver disease. *Semin Hematol* 50:216–221, 2013.

Molenaar IQ, Warnaar N, Groen H, et al: Efficacy and safety of antifibrinolytic drugs in liver transplantation: a systematic review and meta-analysis. *Am J Transplant* 7:185–194, 2007.

Moore C, Levitsky J: The current state and future prospects of chronic hepatitis C virus infection treatment. *Curr Infect Dis Rep* 16:413, 2014.

Northup PG, Caldwell SH: Coagulation in liver disease: a guide for the clinician. *Clin Gastroenterol Hepatol* 11:1064–1074, 2013.

O'Shaughnessy D, Atterbury C, Bolton Maggs P, et al: Guidelines for the use of fresh-frozen plasma, cryoprecipitate and cryosupernatant. *Br J Haematol* 126:11–28, 2004.

Qamar AA, Grace ND, Groszmann RJ, et al: Incidence, prevalence, and clinical significance of abnormal hematologic indices in compensated cirrhosis. *Clin Gastroenterol Hepatol* 7:689–695, 2009.

Segal JB, Dzik WH: Paucity of studies to support that abnormal coagulation test results predict bleeding in the setting of invasive procedures: an evidence-based review. *Transfusion* 45:1413–1425, 2005.

Shah A, Stanworth SJ, McKechnie S: Evidence and triggers for the transfusion of blood and blood products. *Anaesthesia* 70(Suppl 1):10–19, e3-5, 2015.

Solves P, Carpio N, Moscardo F, et al: Transfusion management and immuno-hematologic complications in liver transplantation: experience of a single institution. *Transfus Med Hemother* 42:8–14, 2015.

Tripodi A, Mannucci PM: The coagulopathy of chronic liver disease. *N Engl J Med* 365:147–156, 2011.

Weeder PD, Porte RJ, Lisman T: Hemostasis in liver disease: implications of new concepts for perioperative management. *Transfus Med Rev* 28:107–113, 2014.

Zanetto A, Senzolo M, Ferrarese A, et al: Assessment of bleeding risk in patients with cirrhosis. *Curr Hepatol Rep* 14:9–18, 2015.

CHAPTER 154

HEMATOLOGIC MANIFESTATIONS OF RENAL DISEASE

Mark A. Crowther and Ali Iqbal

Renal dysfunction is associated with a number of hematologic abnormalities including anemia, platelet dysfunction, and thrombosis. Morphologic abnormalities may include the presence of echinocytes characterized by abnormal red blood cell (RBC) membranes with multiple small, evenly spaced projections.[1] Certain conditions including hemolytic uremic syndrome (HUS) involve complex interactions between glomerular microvasculature and the coagulation cascade manifesting as microangiopathic hemolytic anemia and thrombocytopenia. Among renal transplant patients, posttransplant lymphoproliferative disorder can occur. The underlying pathophysiology and treatment of these hematologic manifestations of renal disease are discussed here.

ANEMIA

Anemia is common in chronic kidney disease (CKD) and is associated with poor outcomes, including reduced quality of life, increased cardiovascular disease, hospitalizations, cognitive impairment, and mortality. In a study of 5222 patients with CKD (defined by serum creatinine >1.5 mg/dL and >2.0 mg/dL in females and males, respectively) the prevalence of anemia was 47.7%.[2] Anemia in CKD is usually normocytic, hypoproliferative and is multifactorial, being contributed to by relative erythropoietin (EPO) deficiency, iron deficiency, and disordered iron homeostasis.[3]

Relative Erythropoietin Deficiency

EPO is a glycoprotein hormone mainly produced in the kidney by interstitial fibroblasts.[4] With normal kidney function, hypoxic conditions in the outer medulla trigger production of EPO, which binds to receptors on erythroid progenitors ultimately leading to increased RBC production.[5] Patients with CKD have insufficient EPO levels because of two proposed mechanisms; decreased production capacity caused by tissue damage as well as an altered hypoxic set point for the production of EPO.[6] As a result, anemic CKD patients have 10–100 times lower EPO levels compared with similarly anemic patients with normal renal function.[3]

Erythropoiesis stimulating agents (ESAs) were introduced in the late 1980s for the treatment of anemia of CKD. Several observational studies have demonstrated clinical benefits with the use of ESAs, including reduction in heart failure, regression of left ventricular hypertrophy, improved energy levels, and improved overall quality of life.[7,8] However, targeting near normal hemoglobin (Hb) levels is associated with increased hospitalization, graft/fistula thrombosis, stroke, and a trend towards increased mortality.[9,10] Therefore the 2012 KDIGO (Kidney Disease Improving Global Outcomes) clinical practice guidelines recommend the use of ESAs to target Hb levels less than 11.5 g/dL. These guidelines recommend considering initiation of ESAs when Hb is less than 10 g/dL for both dialysis and nondialysis CKD patients.[11]

True Iron Deficiency

CKD patients, particularly those on hemodialysis, have increased iron losses because of chronic bleeding, phlebotomy, and blood loss in the hemodialysis apparatus.[12] Furthermore, the use of ESAs in CKD patients causes depletion of iron stores through increased erythropoiesis. Therefore optimization of iron status is a mainstay of management for anemia of CKD. The 2012 KDIGO guidelines recommend a trial of intravenous iron therapy for dialysis patients and oral iron therapy for nondialysis patients for a transferrin saturation of less than 30% and ferritin less than 500 ng/mL, and when an increase in Hb concentration with a decrease in ESA dosing is desired.[11]

Disordered Iron Homeostasis

Patients with CKD often have a functional iron deficiency in addition to true iron deficiency. This is related to an excess of hepcidin, a key hormone involved in iron homeostasis (see Chapter 35 and Chapter 36). Excess hepcidin in CKD patients is thought to be secondary to increased production caused by chronic inflammation as well as decreased renal clearance. The hepcidin–ferroportin axis is currently being investigated as a potential therapeutic target in CKD patients with anemia.[3]

UREMIC BLEEDING

Patients with CKD have increased bleeding because of frequent use of anticoagulant and antiplatelet drugs, defects in platelet aggregation as well as abnormal platelet-endothelial cell interaction. One of the major factors contributing to platelet dysfunction is a defect in glycoprotein IIb/IIIa.[13] Other factors include ineffective ADP response to stimulated aggregations and increased production of nitric oxide.[14,15] Anemia also contributes to uremic bleeding caused by altered flow of platelets with reduced proximity and interaction with endothelial cells.[16]

Treatment for uremic platelet dysfunction is indicated in patients with CKD who are actively bleeding or scheduled to undergo a procedure with a risk of bleeding.

Desmopressin (DDAVP) is an effective therapy in reducing bleeding time within 1 hour of administration through increased release of von Willebrand factor (vWF) multimers from endothelial cells.[17] Another treatment option is conjugated estrogen, which achieves peak effect over 5 to 7 days.[18] The mode of action is not well understood, but is thought to result from a reduction in nitric oxide[19] (see Chapter 130). Correction of anemia, whether through ESAs or RBC transfusions to a level greater than 10 g/dL, has also been shown to improve bleeding time in CKD patients.[20,21] Renal replacement therapy, in the form of peritoneal dialysis, hemodialysis, or renal transplantation, clears uremic toxins and corrects uremic platelet dysfunction.[22]

THROMBOSIS

Thromboembolism is a serious and well-established complication of nephrotic syndrome. The nephrotic syndrome is defined by a 24-hour urinary protein greater than 3.5 g/day, associated with edema, hypoalbuminemia, hyperlipidemia, lipiduria, and thrombosis.[23] Patients with nephrotic syndrome have an increased risk of venous and arterial thrombosis as demonstrated in a retrospective study of 298 patients followed for a mean of 10 years. The absolute risk of venous and arterial thrombosis was 1% and 1.5% per year, respectively, which is about eight times greater than the general population.[24,25] There are certain high-risk factors for developing venous thromboembolism (VTE), including degree of hypoalbuminemia as well as type of nephrotic syndrome (membranous nephropathy being the highest risk).[26,27] The mechanism of hypercoagulability is multifactorial and involves all stages of hemostasis. Nephrotic syndrome patients have increased platelet aggregation and adhesion because of elevated levels of vWF and unbound arachidonic acid (usually albumin bound).[28,29] There is also increased activation of the coagulation cascade caused by an imbalance between synthesis and urinary loss of thrombotic and antithrombotic factors. For certain plasma proteins, including factor XII, antithrombin, and free protein S, urinary losses exceed synthesis.[30–32] For higher-molecular-weight proteins, including factors V, VIII, vWF and fibrinogen, excess synthesis relative to losses lead to accumulation.[33,34] Decreased fibrinolysis also occurs because of reduced plasminogen levels and reduced availability of albumin as a cofactor for plasminogen–fibrin interaction.[35,36]

The management of thromboembolic events (renal vein thrombosis, deep venous thrombosis [DVT], pulmonary embolism [PE]) associated with nephrotic syndrome is similar to conventional anticoagulation strategies for DVT or PE, with the use of heparin, low-molecular-weight heparin, warfarin or direct oral anticoagulant agents many of which require renal dose adjustment.[37] The direct thrombin and factor Xa inhibitors have a variable degree of renal clearance, with Dabigatran being the most and Apixiban being the least renally cleared.[37a] These agents, however, have not been studied specifically in patients with VTE related to nephrotic syndrome.[38] In terms of duration of therapy, most experts recommend continuing anticoagulation as long as the patient remains nephrotic.[37] Prophylactic anticoagulation for patients with nephrotic syndrome is a controversial issue and must be balanced with the risk of bleeding. Some experts recommend prophylactic anticoagulation in patients who are high risk for VTE (membranous nephropathy, albumin <20 g/L) with low to intermediate risk of bleeding.[37]

HEMOLYTIC UREMIC SYNDROME

HUS is defined by concomitant microangiopathic hemolytic anemia (MAHA), thrombocytopenia, and acute kidney injury[39] (see Chapter 132). Pathology reveals thrombotic microangiopathy characterized microvascular platelet thrombi, vessel wall thickening, and detachment of endothelial cells from the basement membrane. Damage to microvascular glomerular endothelium is the inciting and sustaining event involved in platelet consumption and MAHA. HUS may occur secondary to Shiga toxin–producing bacteria, Streptococcus pneumoniae infection, drugs, or primary complement dysregulation (atypical HUS). In Shiga toxin–associated HUS, the toxin binds to the high affinity Gb3 receptor expressed on glomerular endothelial cells leading to cell damage. In atypical HUS, the fenestrated endothelium of the glomerulus is particularly susceptible to uncontrolled alternative complement pathway activation arising from impaired regulatory proteins or hyperactive components. In the renal transplant population, an acquired HUS or thrombotic microangiopathy (TMA) syndrome may occur secondary to immunosuppressive drugs such as cyclosporine and tacrolimus, ischemia reperfusion injury, and viral infections.[40] The kidney plays a central role in all of these processes, as initial damage to glomerular endothelial cells leads to loss of thromboresistance and platelet activation and consumption, causing thrombocytopenia with microangiopathic hemolytic anemia.[40]

In adults with nondiarrheal or idiopathic HUS, initial management is similar to thrombotic thrombocytopenic purpura with plasma exchange therapy. If plasma exchange is not immediately available, plasma infusion may be used as a temporary alternative. In patients with atypical, or complement mediated HUS, eculizumab, a monoclonal antibody against C5, may be considered.[41] In adults with postdiarrheal HUS, supportive therapy is the mainstay of treatment with intravenous fluids, platelet and red blood cell transfusions, and hemodialysis as indicated for acute kidney injury (AKI).

HEMATOLOGIC ABNORMALITIES IN THE RENAL TRANSPLANT PATIENT

Several hematologic abnormalities can occur in the renal transplant patient, including posttransplant lymphoproliferative disorder (PTLD), posttransplant erythrocytosis (PTE), and acquired TMA secondary to drugs or infection. PTLD is a rare complication in organ transplant recipients. PTLD is caused by proliferation of Epstein-Barr virus (EBV)–infected B cells because of reduced T-cell surveillance as a result of immunosuppression. PTLD may present along a spectrum of disease, from an infectious mononucleosis like syndrome (early lesions), polyclonal lymphoid hyperplasia (polymorphic PTLD), to monoclonal malignancies including B- or T-cell lymphoma (monomorphic PTLD).[42] Among renal transplant recipients, one study demonstrated an incidence of 1.4% (344) out of 25,127 patients.[43] Risk factors for the development of PTLD include the use of T–cell depleting induction agents, EBV-negative recipient with positive donor, history of pretransplant malignancy and younger age. Treatment of PTLD includes a reduction in immunosuppression for all types, with the addition of rituximab for polymorphic PTLD. Chemotherapy is used in monomorphic PTLD and also for a subset of patients with polymorphic disease.[42]

Posttransplant erythrocytosis is defined as an elevated hemoglobin and hematocrit after renal transplantation that persists for more than 6 months in the absence of another cause. PTE occurs in about 10% to 15% of transplant recipients and is thought to be multifactorial, potentially related to unregulated erythropoietin secretion from the native kidneys. As with other forms of erythrocytosis, patients may experience headache, lethargy, plethora and are at increased risk for thromboembolic events. Treatment consists of blockage of renin angiotensin aldosterone system, through ACE inhibitor or ARB therapy.[44]

REFERENCES

1. Hasler CR, Owen GR, Brunner W, et al: Echinocytes induced by hemodialysis. *Nephrol Dial Transplant* 13:3132–3137, 1998.
2. McClellan W, Aronoff SL, Bolton WK, et al: The prevalence of anemia in patients with chronic kidney disease. *Curr Med Res Opin* 20(9):1501–1510, 2004.
3. Babitt JL, Lin HY: Mechanisms of anemia in CKD. *JASN* 23(10):1631–1634, 2012.
4. Maxwell PH, Osmond MK, Pugh CW, et al: Identification of the renal erythropoietin-producing cells using transgenic mice. *Kidney Int* 44:1149–1162, 1993.
5. Mulcahy L: The erythropoietin receptor. *Semin Oncol* 28:19–23, 2001.
6. Fehr T, Ammann P, Garzoni D, et al: Interpretation of erythropoietin levels in patients with various degrees of renal insufficiency and anemia. *Kidney Int* 66(3):1206–1211, 2004.
7. Revicki DA, Brown RE, Feeny DH, et al: Health-related quality of life associated with recombinant human erythropoietin therapy for predialysis chronic renal disease patients. *Am J Kidney Dis* 25(4):548–554, 1995.
8. Portolés J, Torralbo A, Martin P, et al: Cardiovascular effects of recombinant human erythropoietin in predialysis patients. *Am J Kidney Dis* 29(4):541–548, 1997.
9. Besarab A, Bolton WK, Browne KJ, et al: The effects of normal as compared with low hematocrit values in patients with cardiac disease who are receiving hemodialysis and epoetin. *N Engl J Med* 339:584–590, 1998.
10. Singh AK, Szczech L, Tang KL, et al: Correction of anemia with epoetin alpha in chronic kidney disease. *N Engl J Med* 385:2085–2098, 2006.
11. KDIGO clinical practice guidelines for anemia in chronic kidney disease. *Kidney Int Suppl* 2:288, 2012.

12. Eschbach JW, Cook JD, Scribner BH, et al: Iron balance in hemodialysis patients. *Ann Intern Med* 87(6):710–713, 1977.

13. Benigni A, Boccardo P, Galbusero M, et al: Reversible activation defect of the platelet glycoprotein IIb-IIIa complex in patients with uremia. *Am J Kidney Dis* 22(5):668–676, 1993.

14. Horowitz HI, Stein IM, Cohen BD: Further studies on the platelet inhibitory effect of guanidinosuccinic acid and its role in uremic bleeding. *Am J Med* 49(3):336–345, 1970.

15. Remuzzi G, Perico B, Zoja C, et al: Role of endothelium-derived nitric oxide in the bleeding tendency of uremia. *J Clin Invest* 86(5):1768–1771, 1990.

16. Livio M, Gotti E, Marchesi D, et al: Uremic bleeding: role of anemia and beneficial effect of red cell transfusions. *Lancet* 2(8306):1013–1015, 1982.

17. Zeigler ZR, Megaludis A, Fraley DS: Desmopressin (d-DAVP) effects on platelet rheology and von willebrand factor activities in uremia. *Am J Hematol* 39(2):90–95, 1992.

18. Livio M, Manucci PM, Vigano G, et al: Conjugated estrogens for the management of bleeding associated with renal failure. *N Engl J Med* 315(12):731–735, 1986.

19. Zoja C, Noris M, Corna D, et al: L-arginine, the precursor of nitric oxide, abolishes the effect of estrogens in bleeding time in experimenta uremia. *Lab Invest* 65(4):479–483, 1991.

20. Livio M, Gotti E, Marchesi D, et al: Uraemic bleeding: role of anaemia and beneficial effect of red cell transfusions. *Lancet* 2(8306):1013–1015, 1982.

21. Cases A, Escolar G, Reverter JC, et al: Recombinant human erythropoietin treatment improves platelet function in uremic patients. *Kidney Int* 42(3):668–672, 1992.

22. Nenci GG, Berrettini M, Agnelli G, et al: Effect of peritoneal dialysis, haemodialysis and kidney transplantation on blood platelet function. *Nephron* 23(6):287–292, 1979.

23. Orth SR, Ritz E: The nephrotic syndrome. *N Engl J Med* 338:1202–1211, 1998.

24. Mahmoodi BK, Ten Kate MK, Waanders F, et al: High absolute risk and predictors of venous and arterial thromboembolic events in patients with nephrotic syndrome: results from a large retrospective cohort study. *Circulation* 117(2):224–230, 2008.

25. Anderson FA, Jr, Wheeler HB, Goldberg RJ, et al: A population based perspective of the hospital incidence and case fatality rates of deep vein thrombosis and pulmonary embolism. The Worcester DVT study. *Arch Int Med* 151(5):933–938, 1991.

26. Lionaki S, Derebail VK, Hogan SL, et al: Venous thromboembolism in patients with membranous nephropathy. *Clin J Am Soc Nephrol* 7(1):43–51, 2012.

27. Barbour SJ, Greenwald A, Djurdjev O, et al: Disease-specific risk of venous thromboembolic events is increased in idiopathic glomerulonephritis. *Kidney Int* 81(2):190–195, 2012.

28. Zwaginga JJ, Koomans HA, Sixma JJ, et al: Thrombus formation and platelet vessel wall interaction in the nephrotic syndrome under flow conditions. *J Clin Invest* 93(1):204–211, 1994.

29. Yoshida N, Aoki N: Release of arachidonic acid from human platelets. A key role for the potentiation of platelet aggregability in normal subjects as well as those with nephrotic syndrome. *Blood* 52(5):969–977, 1978.

30. Vaziri ND, Ngo JL, Ibsen KH, et al: Deficiency and urinary losses of factor XII in adult nephrotic syndrome. *Nephron* 32(4):342–346, 1982.

31. Kauffman RH, Veltkamp JJ, Van Tilburg NH, et al: Acquired antithrombin III deficiency and thrombosis in the nephrotic syndrome. *Am J Med* 65(4):607–613, 1978.

32. Vigano-D'angelo S, D'angelo A, Kaufman CE, et al: Protein S deficiency occurs in the nephrotic syndrome. *Ann Intern Med* 107(1):42–47, 1987.

33. Vaziri ND, Branson HE, Ness R: Changes of coagulation factors IX, VIII, VII, X and V in nephrotic syndrome. *Am J Med Sci* 280(3):167–171, 1980.

34. De Sain-van der Velden MG, Kaysen GA, de Meer K, et al: Proportionate increase of fibrinogen and albumin synthesis in nephrotic patients: measurements with stable isotropes. *Kidney Int* 53(1):181–188, 1998.

35. Singhal R, Brimble KS: Thromboembolic complications in the nephrotic syndrome: pathophysiology and clinical management. *Thromb Res* 118(3):397–407, 2006.

36. Rabelink TJ, Zwaginga JJ, Koomans HA, et al: Thombosis and hemostasis in renal disease. *Kidney Int* 46(2):287–296, 1994.

37. Glassock RJ: Prophylactic anticoagulation in nephrotic syndrome: a clinical conundrum. *JASN* 18(8):2221–2225, 2007.

37a. Vilchez JA, Gallego P, Lip GYH: Safety of new oral anticoagulant drugs: a perspective. *Ther Adv Drug Saf* 5(1):8–20, 2014.

38. Capodanno D, Angiolillo DJ: Antithrombotic therapy in patients with chronic kidney disease. *Circulation* 125:2649–2661, 2012.

39. Barbour T, Johnson S, Cohney S, et al: Thrombotic microangiopathy and associated renal disorders. *Nephrol Dial Transplant* 27(7):2673–2685, 2012.

40. Ruggenenti P, Noris M, Remuzzi G: Thrombotic microangiopathy, hemolytic uremic syndrome, and thrombotic thrombocytopenic purpura. *Kidney Int* 60(3):831–846, 2001.

41. Kose O, Zimmerhackl LB, Jungraithmayr T, et al: New treatment options for atypical hemolytic uremic syndrome with complement inhibitor eculizumab. *Semin Thomb Hemost* 36(6):669–672, 2010.

42. Taylor AL, Marcus R, Bradley JA: Post transplant lymphoproliferative disorders (PTLD) after solid organ transplantation. *Crit Rev Oncol Hematol* 56(1):155–167, 2005.

43. Caillard S, Dharnidarka V, Agodoa L, et al: Posttransplant lymphoproliferative disorders after renal transplantation in the United States in era of modern immunosuppression. *Transplantation* 80(9):1233–1243, 2005.

44. Vlahakos DV, Marathias KP, Agroyannis B, et al: Posttransplant erythrocytosis. *Kidney Int* 63(4):1187, 2003.

CHAPTER 155

HEMATOLOGIC MANIFESTATIONS OF MALIGNANCY

Page Widick, Andrew M. Brunner, and Fred Schiffman

Hematologic abnormalities are commonly seen among patients with malignancy. These derangements range from the incidental to the life-threatening, and may complicate management and require additional therapy. Hematologic abnormalities can be seen as the initial manifestation of cancer, providing a crucial diagnostic clue. In addition, the hematologic aspects of cancer, as well as the therapies that we use to treat these irregularities, can provide insight into the biology of tumorigenesis. This chapter reviews some of the impact that malignancy can have on erythrocytes, leukocytes, platelets, and hemostasis.

ERYTHROCYTES

Anemia

The most common hematologic manifestation of cancer is anemia; anywhere from 30% to 90% of patients with cancer have documented anemia before the initiation of any treatment. Anemia occurs across many different malignancies, including 40% of patients with early-stage colon cancer and 80% of patients with advanced colon cancer. The pathogenesis of cancer-related anemia is multifactorial, and can arise from direct cancer tissue invasion with resultant blood loss, involvement of the bone marrow, hemolysis, a direct effect of chemotherapy or radiation therapy, and chronic renal dysfunction associated with malignancy, among other causes. These causes can be further divided among anemia resulting from blood loss, anemia caused by erythrocyte destruction, and anemia caused by a hypoproliferative marrow state. A number of cancer-specific mechanisms can be responsible for a hypoproliferative state, including nutritional deficiencies, decreased erythropoietin (EPO) production because of acute or chronic kidney injury, and injury to the bone marrow itself. The most common nutritional abnormality in cancer-related anemia is iron deficiency; up to 29% to 60% of all cancer patients may have iron-deficiency anemia, which can be secondary to poor oral intake, as well as from blood loss, commonly seen in gastrointestinal and gynecologic malignancies. Compounding any deficiency in total body iron stores are the effects on erythropoiesis and iron homeostasis as a result of cancer-associated inflammation and cytokine activation. Many cancers are associated with a systemic inflammatory state, manifested by elevated levels of cytokines, which can directly inhibit erythropoiesis and suppress the amount of iron available for erythropoiesis. When serum EPO concentrations are measured among cancer patients, these levels are inappropriately low in comparison to patients without malignancy but who have the same degree of anemia caused by iron deficiency. Cancer patients also often demonstrate increased levels of hepcidin, a protein critical to iron homeostasis, which acts by decreasing the binding to and breaking down of the iron transporter ferroportin. This subsequently results in increased storage of iron in the form of ferritin, and at the same time decreases free iron that would be used in erythropoiesis. In contrast to iron deficiency, B_{12} deficiency is a less common cause of anemia in malignancy, seen in only 5% to 10% of patients.

Many chemotherapeutics have hematologic sequelae; patients undergoing treatment may experience varying degrees of anemia resulting from chemotherapy-induced bone marrow suppression. The European Cancer Anaemia Survey prospectively studied over 15,000 patients with a variety of solid tumors undergoing treatment. Before therapy, 10% of patients had hemoglobin levels below 10 g/dL, and

during therapy this increased to almost 40% and was correlated with a worsening performance status. In the same study, radiation therapy alone had less impact on the incidence of anemia, but the combination of chemotherapy and radiation led to a greater degree of anemia than chemotherapy alone. Anemia caused by chemotherapy is related to the cumulative dose, combination of chemotherapeutics, and dose schedule. For example, in the treatment of lung cancer with cisplatin and paclitaxel, anemia worsens with an increasing total dose of cisplatin, when cisplatin is added to paclitaxel, and if paclitaxel is given over a 24-hour period rather than shorter courses.

Anemia in cancer patients can also occur in the setting of red cell destruction, such as is seen in autoimmune hemolytic anemia, or in the setting of microangiopathic hemolytic anemia (MAHA), which is associated with concurrent thrombocytopenia. Although a true incidence of MAHA among cancer patients is difficult to determine, some studies suggest that 5% to 10% of mucin-producing disseminated adenocarcinomas are associated with a MAHA. It is important to distinguish secondary thrombotic microangiopathies (TMAs), as seen in patients with malignancy, from thrombotic thrombocytopenic purpura (TTP), given the marked differences in underlying pathophysiology. TTP is the result of congenital or acquired absence or inhibition of the von Willebrand cleaving enzyme, a disintegrin and metalloproteinase with thrombospondin motifs-13 (ADAMTS13). Secondary TMAs may have a slight decrease in ADAMTS13 activity, but do not have the severe deficiency of ADAMTS13 activity, with a level of less than 10%, such as seen in TTP. Accordingly, patients with secondary TMAs typically have a poor response to therapeutic plasma exchange. Cancer-associated TMAs may arise from direct endothelial damage rather than diminished ADAMTS13 activity. Cancer patients may also develop a MAHA related to the use of a number of drugs used in the treatment of cancer, including cyclosporine, mitomycin, and gemcitabine, and antivascular endothelial growth factor (anti-VEGF) agents.

Treatment of Cancer-Related Anemia

Hemoglobin levels typically decrease early in the course of chemotherapy treatment; with greater than half of patients experience a greater than 1 g/dL drop over the course of the first 9 weeks of therapy. The treatment of anemia related to malignancy depends upon correct identification of the underlying etiology. As noted previously, iron-deficiency anemia is very common in patients with malignancy. Among those patients with cancer who have an absolute iron deficiency (transferrin saturation <20%, ferritin <30 ng/mL), there is evidence that they may benefit from a short course of either oral or low-dose intravenous iron. In this setting, the addition of erythropoiesis stimulating agents (ESAs) is not necessary.

For many patients, transfusion of blood products is an effective therapeutic intervention. Red cell transfusion provides rapid symptomatic relief and is also a source of iron; one unit of packed red blood cells (RBCs) contains roughly 200 mg of iron. Logistic limitations with RBC transfusion, and transfusion-related morbidities have spurred the incorporation of ESAs as alternative agents for treating anemia in cancer patients. The use of ESAs during myelosuppressive treatment increases the hemoglobin level and decreases transfusion requirements by approximately 50%; however, ESA use is associated with an increased rate of cardiovascular and thrombotic events, and may be associated with poorer overall survival and time to cancer progression. This relationship between ESA use and thrombosis may be related to the target hemoglobin concentration as higher hemoglobin targets are associated with increased rates of thrombotic events in cancer patients.

In addition to thrombotic events, a number of concerns have been raised about ESA use and potential worsening of overall survival or time to disease progression. Data regarding ESAs and progression of disease are conflicting; some studies in patients with breast cancer and patients with head and neck cancer suggested worsening progression-free survival or local control of disease with ESA use. The mechanism behind tumor progression is unknown but may relate to decreased chemosensitivity in the setting of ESA use or relate to tumor vascularity and oxygen supply. One study isolated breast cancer stem-like cells, which are thought to promote tumor progression and relapse, and identified expression of the EPO receptor on the cell surface of these chemoresistant cells. Moreover, the concurrent administration of ESAs during chemotherapy had a chemoprotective effect. Other mechanisms that may underlie the association of EPO administration with tumor progression include augmentation of red cell mass and effects on tumor oxygenation.

Because of concerns about thrombotic events, as well as the potential for worsened overall survival and time to disease progression, ESA use is generally restricted to certain indications in patients with cancer. In general, transfusion of blood products and, if indicated, iron therapy, remain the standard of care for anemia associated with malignancy. Future studies considering the safety of ESAs for lower target hemoglobin levels, as well as alternative preparations of iron therapy may provide viable treatment options for cancer patients with anemia. There are some instances where ESAs may be useful adjuncts, specifically among patients with moderate or severe chronic kidney disease, or in palliative settings. In such situations, reversible causes of anemia should be ruled out before ESA use, and the minimal amount of EPO be used to avoid RBC transfusion.

Erythrocytosis

Outside of patients with myeloproliferative neoplasms, and specifically polycythemia vera, erythrocytosis is an uncommon manifestation of cancer. Polycythemia vera, and other myeloproliferative neoplasms, are typified by acquisition of somatic mutations that upregulate the Janus kinase (JAK)/signal transducer and activator of transcription (STAT) signaling pathway, typically the JAK2 V617F mutation, and phenotypically present as an expansion of myeloid-origin cells, with an elevated hemoglobin and suppressed EPO levels. In these cancers, erythrocytosis is caused by primary expansion of the malignant clone. In contrast, when erythrocytosis is seen in association with solid tumors, it typically is the result of a paraneoplastic phenomenon. This can be seen in the setting of increased erythropoietin levels related to malignancy, for instance with clear cell renal cell carcinoma. Other rare causes of cancer-associated erythrocytosis may include aromatase inhibition in breast cancer. There may be an association with a common predisposing condition; for instance, patients with von Hippel-Lindau disease are at risk for renal and central nervous system tumors, and the mechanism of erythrocytosis is typically through paraneoplastic EPO expression. Nonetheless, elevated RBC counts are rare in patients with malignancy, particularly those receiving chemotherapy, and usually do not require intervention.

PLATELETS

Thrombocytopenia

Chemotherapy and immunosuppressive agents are the most common causes of thrombocytopenia in the cancer patient. For instance, patients receiving cisplatin/gemcitabine for bladder cancer or carboplatin/gemcitabine for lung cancer have rates of clinically significant thrombocytopenia of 30% to 60%. Among patients with

hematologic malignancy, thrombocytopenia is even more common, particularly with induction or conditioning chemotherapy regimens. The typical mechanism by which chemotherapy causes thrombocytopenia is through marrow suppression; however, some agents are also associated with immune-mediated thrombocytopenia. Immune thrombocytopenia is typically characterized by a sudden and isolated drop in platelet count. For example, trastuzumab and oxaliplatin have both been associated with immune-mediated thrombocytopenia. Thrombocytopenia may also be a result of bone marrow infiltration by tumor cells, thrombotic microangiopathy, consumptive coagulopathy, or as an autoimmune manifestation of the malignancy itself. Bone marrow involvement, often occult, is more common in prostate, lung, and breast cancer; such patients typically have multiple cell lines involved, and display a leukoerythroblastic appearance on the peripheral smear. The laboratory features of disseminated intravascular coagulation (DIC), elevated D-dimer, and fibrinogen degradation products, can be seen in cancer patients, and are more common with advanced disease, where they may be present in up to 90% of patients.

Treatment of thrombocytopenia in cancer patients is generally supportive. For patients with active bleeding, platelet transfusion and correction of other coagulopathies are the mainstays of therapy. The use of agents such as tranexamic acid in these patients may be considered as well. In the absence of active bleeding, a threshold of <10 $\times 10^9$/L for prophylactic platelet transfusion is generally recommended. This is based on a study which randomized 600 patients with hematologic malignancies to prophylaxis or no prophylactic transfusions; both were treated for bleeding events. Rates of World Health Organization grade 2, 3, or 4 bleeding were high in both groups, but higher (50%) in the no-prophylaxis group (50%), compared with the prophylaxis group (43%). Prophylactic platelet transfusion has been used in patients with solid tumors, but without as much evidence-based support.

Other agents, with or without platelet transfusion, may also have a role in chemotherapy-related thrombocytopenia. Thrombopoietin (TPO) receptor agonists are an area of increasing interest in the management of thrombocytopenia during chemotherapy, particularly as a means to maintain treatment schedules which may be delayed by thrombocytopenia. A 2015 phase I trial compared placebo to eltrombopag in patients receiving gemcitabine-based chemotherapy and found that fewer patients receiving eltrombopag required dose delays and/or reductions in chemotherapy compared with those receiving placebo. This evidence is promising and further clinical trials may reveal a role for romiplostim and/or eltrombopag in the management of thrombocytopenia resulting from malignancy.

Thrombocytosis

While thrombocytopenia may be more clinically apparent because of bleeding or delays in the administration of chemotherapy, reactive thrombocytosis is actually more common than thrombocytopenia in patients with solid tumors. The clinical impact of thrombocytosis is less clear; however, having a platelet count greater than 350×10^9/L before initiating chemotherapy is associated with a greater risk for venous thromboembolism (VTE). Cancer-related thrombocytosis is thought to be mediated by inflammatory cytokines, and elevated levels of interleukin (IL)-6, IL-11, and TPO have been documented in cancer patients. Rarely, thrombocytosis may be the result of a paraneoplastic phenomenon, which has been described in breast and ovarian malignancies. In many tumor types including breast, renal cell, gastric, and advanced stage non–small cell lung cancer, elevated platelet counts seem to confer an adverse prognosis. The mechanism for this association is unclear.

Platelet Dysfunction Secondary to Malignancy

In addition to abnormalities in absolute platelet number, cancer patients may have alterations in platelet function, which can contribute to tumor progression. Platelets derived from cancer patients are in an activated state, with increased surface P-selectin expression and elevated serum levels of platelet factor IV and β-thromboglobulin. Activated platelets may contribute to the thrombophilic state in cancer patients, and also interact with leukocytes, endothelial cells, and tumor cells, all of which may contribute to the early stages of tumor cell dissemination. A number of platelet receptors may contribute to the platelet support of metastasis, including glycoprotein (GP) IIb/IIIa, adenosine diphosphate (ADP) receptors, P-selectin and thrombin receptors, and others, with likely multiple mechanisms underlying the platelet effects on malignancy. Platelets stabilize otherwise short-lived tumor cells in the circulation. Platelet–tumor cell interaction enhances tumor cell adhesion to the vessel wall, and appears to alter vessel wall permeability, and in this way may facilitate tumor cell invasion. Platelets protect tumor cells from immune surveillance and destruction, in part by shielding tumor cells from natural killer cells, although other mechanisms are likely. Platelets provide nutrient support (growth factors) and release pro-angiogenic factors. Platelets contain numerous growth factors, coagulation factors and adhesive molecules, chemokines, and bioactive lipids that may enhance metastatic efficiency. Platelets are enriched in angiogenic growth factors such as basic fibroblast growth factor and VEGF, as well as other mediators, and may regulate angiogenesis. Selective P-selectin and thrombin receptor activation on platelets may release α-granules enriched in either VEGF or endostatin. Platelet-derived transforming growth factor-β and direct platelet–tumor cell interactions promote epithelial mesenchymal transformation and tumor metastases.

LEUKOCYTES

Neutropenia

Neutropenia is common during treatment with chemotherapy, particularly with antimetabolite use. Other etiologies of neutropenia in cancer patients include infiltration of the bone marrow space and occasionally, radiation therapy, particularly when sites of active hematopoiesis are included in the radiation field, such as with the pelvis or spine. In addition, particularly in the course of treatment, cancer patients may experience viral or antibiotic-mediated neutropenia.

Patients who develop neutropenia during chemotherapy are at risk for neutropenic fever. A number of comorbid conditions are predictive of the development of neutropenic fever, including older age, poor performance status, comorbid medical conditions, low baseline white blood cell counts, low body mass index/BSA, advanced disease, and the use of myelosuppressive chemotherapy agents. General treatment principles for neutropenic fever include the consideration of prophylactic antibiotics or myeloid growth factor support, such as granulocyte colony-stimulating factor (G-CSF). Consideration should be given to the elevated risk of FN associated with specific chemotherapeutic agents, including situations where dose-dense or intense chemotherapy regimens provide survival benefit. Depending on the regimen and disease, prophylactic G-CSF should be considered, particularly when there is a greater than 20% overall risk of FN; once a patient develops FN, G-CSF is typically reserved for situations where they are not responding to appropriate treatment and develop life-threatening conditions.

Several tumors express G-CSF receptors; there is a theoretic concern that exogenous G-CSF may increase proliferation of these tumors. In addition, the use of myeloid growth factors during chemotherapy for solid tumors has been theorized to increase the risk of subsequent myeloid malignancy by acting as a survival signal to hematopoietic progenitor cells damaged by chemotherapy. A meta-analysis of 25 randomized clinical trials found that there was an almost twofold increase in acute myeloid leukemia in those patients assigned to receive chemotherapy with growth factor support, compared with those who did not receive growth factor support, although the absolute rates of secondary leukemia were low in each group.

An important consideration during chemotherapy is to recognize that benign neutropenia related to certain ethnicities, particularly in those of African and Middle Eastern descent, may be a contributing factor and does not require dose-adjustment of chemotherapy.

BONE MARROW METASTASES

Multiple lineage cytopenia in association with cancer warrants consideration of bone marrow metastasis (Fig. 155.1). Metastatic carcinoma can involve bone marrow and may lead to subsequent marrow fibrosis and failure. Bone marrow metastases occur in fewer than 10% of patients with metastatic disease, and are more common in patients with lung, breast, or prostate carcinoma. Patients with solid tumors who have bone marrow involvement are more likely to experience cytopenias from chemotherapy, and typically carry a worse prognosis. For example, patients with extensive small cell lung cancer with bone marrow metastases have significantly shorter time to progression and significantly shorter survival time than other patients with extensive disease. The precise mechanism for poor outcomes is unknown, but may relate to greater overall tumor burden, as well as to specific biologic features that allow the tumor to grow in the bone marrow

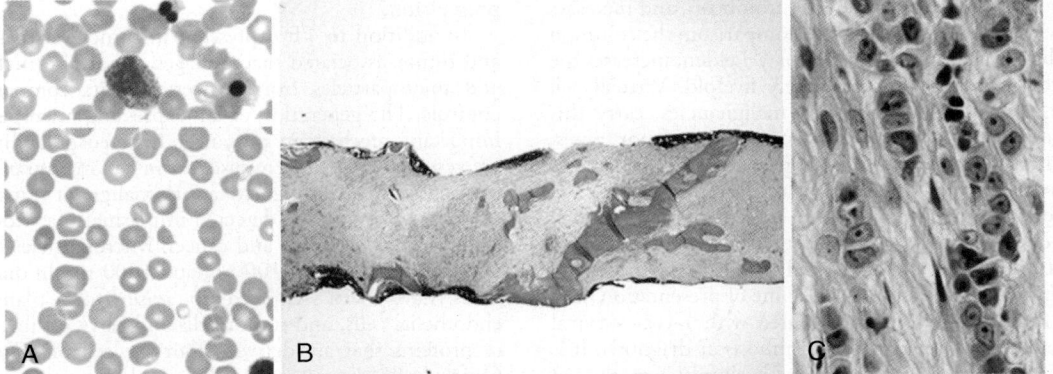

Fig. 155.1 PERIPHERAL BLOOD AND BONE MARROW FROM A PATIENT WITH METASTATIC BREAST CANCER. The patient was a 77-year-old woman who presented with anemia and thrombocytopenia. On physical examination she was found to have a breast mass. (A) The peripheral smear showed a leukoerythroblastosis *(top)* with nucleated red blood cells and immature granulocytic precursors. Platelets were reduced, and red blood cells exhibited anisopoikilocytosis *(bottom)* with occasional teardrop forms and rare schistocytes. (B) The bone marrow biopsy was fibrotic and had thickened bone with new bone formation. (C) The bone marrow cavity was replaced by tumor cells infiltrating through bands of fibrosis.

niche, which also render it resistant to therapy. Such tumor cell evasion strategies could include changes in homing, adhesion, immune escape, and angiogenic potential. Laboratory studies suggest that tumors that secrete more proangiogenic and proinflammatory cytokines may be more likely to metastasize to the bone marrow. The bone marrow niche itself may also play a role in promoting tumor survival and in decreased immune surveillance. One example is the occurrence of bone marrow micrometastases in women with early-stage breast cancer; approximately 30% of women with stage I to III breast cancer may have bone marrow micrometastases, which is associated with worse prognosis.

The pathophysiology by which marrow involvement by cancer causes cytopenias is not fully understood. Total marrow replacement by tumor is rare, and only a small percentage of marrow may be needed to support normal peripheral blood counts, as indicated by the observation that normal blood counts are often found in normal older adults with hypocellular marrows. Cancer may disrupt normal bone marrow interactions required for normal hematopoiesis, such as those that include osteoclast signaling and growth of specific bone marrow stromal cell populations.

THROMBOSIS AND CANCER

The association of thrombosis and cancer is widely recognized, dating to the middle of the 19th century, and can be considered the earliest recognized paraneoplastic syndrome. Armand Trousseau was the first to associate thrombosis and malignancy, the first to suggest screening for malignancy in recurrent or idiopathic thromboembolic disease, the first to suggest that the pathophysiology was not mechanical obstruction, but a change in the character in the coagulation system itself, and the first to suggest that the association may be integral to the cancer growth itself. Particularly poignant was the fact that Trousseau predicted his own occult malignancy when he developed "phlebitis," dying 6 months later of gastric cancer. More recently, some of the biologic mechanisms underlying the increased risk for thrombosis in patients with cancer have been better delineated.

The incidence of cancer-associated thrombosis has steadily increased in recent years, in part related to the increasing age of the population, with an associated increase in cancer prevalence, longer survival with active malignancy, and better detection tools. Patients with active malignancy have a higher risk for thrombosis than other medical patients: for instance, surgical oncology patients have a higher thrombosis rate than other surgical patients undergoing major procedures. Although reports of thrombosis rates vary, in general approximately 15% to 20% of cancer patients develop VTE at some point during their illness; conversely, approximately 20% of all VTE events occur in cancer patients.

Cancer is a potent risk factor for venous thrombosis, and increases the relative risk by roughly 6- to 10-fold. In comparison, the common hereditary thrombophilia, homozygous factor V Leiden, increases the risk for venous thrombosis by approximately fivefold. Virtually all solid tumor types, as well as hematologic malignancies, carry this significantly increased risk for thrombosis. Certain tumor types, particularly mucinous adenocarcinomas, appear to have particularly high risk for thrombosis including lung, gastrointestinal cancers—notably pancreatic adenocarcinoma—as well as primary brain tumors.

Development of thrombosis in the cancer patient generally carries prognostic impact. In patients with advanced solid tumors, those who have venous thromboembolic disease at the time of presentation have a 1-year survival nearing only 10%, compared with 1-year survival of closer to 40% among those without thrombosis at diagnosis. It is less clear whether this thrombotic tendency is simply a marker of aggressive disease or whether the development of thrombosis itself is the cause of the increased mortality. Thrombosis is second only to disease progression as a cause of death among cancer patients, and accounts for nearly 10% of deaths among patients receiving outpatient chemotherapy. This mortality risk appears to be independent of cancer stage at the time of thrombus identification. The risk may, however, vary depending on the underlying malignancy, and also according to the timing of the VTE event. One study in patients with gastroesophageal malignancy undergoing chemotherapy failed to show an association between VTE and overall survival. The risk of mortality associated with VTE may therefore reflect the underlying cancer biology. Mucinous adenocarcinomas, for example, may directly release tissue factor (TF) and circulating mucin molecules that activate the clotting cascade and platelets, thereby promoting thrombosis.

Biologic Mechanisms Underlying Thrombosis in Cancer

The etiology of thrombosis is typically described in the context of the classic Virchow triad: stasis or altered blood flow, injury to the vessel wall, and hypercoagulability intrinsic to the blood and circulating plasma. Cancer contributes to thrombosis by mechanisms within all three of these categories. Mechanical compression and/or disruption of blood vessels by a tumor may cause disrupted flow or stasis. Upon interaction with cancer cells, monocytes or macrophages release cytokines, including tumor necrosis factor, IL-1, and IL-6, which damage vascular endothelial cells. The damaged vessel surface has reduced expression of naturally occurring anticoagulants, such as thrombomodulin, heparan sulfate, CD39/ecto-ADPase, nitric oxide, and prostacyclin. The damaged endothelium also has increased expression of procoagulant proteins, particularly TF; circulating blood is exposed to the procoagulant subendothelial matrix, which contributes to a hypercoagulable state.

Despite the contributions of stasis and vessel changes in cancer-associated thrombosis, the best-documented contributing factor to thrombosis in the cancer patient is elevated procoagulant plasma factors, many of which are generated by the tumor itself. TF plays a critical role in the initiation of the coagulation cascade, particularly via the extrinsic pathway, by binding to and activating factor VII. TF is increased in a number of malignancies, including pancreatic cancer, breast cancer, and non–small cell lung cancer, compared with the nontransformed epithelium. Low oxygen levels are often found in the tumor microenvironment, which result in the activation and upregulation of proteins encoded by oncogenes, such as RAS or MET, and inactivation of tumor suppressor genes such as *TP53* or *PTEN*. The downstream effect of this is to directly induce TF expression, as well as other genes involved in hemostasis. Targeting the human *MET* oncogene to mouse liver using a lentiviral vector results in hepatocarcinoma, associated with a coagulopathy similar to that in malignancy, with striking thrombotic events, similar to Trousseau syndrome, the migratory thrombophlebitis associated with malignancy. Elevated TF expression and activation of the coagulation system appear to correlate with both thrombotic tendency and disease progression.

In addition to TF expression in tumors, activated endothelium, and tumor-associated macrophages, TF is also increased in platelets and microparticles from cancer patients compared with healthy controls. The generation of TF-expressing microparticles may be an important mechanism of cancer hypercoagulability. Microparticles are vesicular structures released from cell membranes under a variety of situations, including activation, malignant transformation, stress, or death. They can be detected in plasma in a wide range of disease states, including sepsis and cancer. Microparticles are generally considered to be between 100 nm and 1000 nm in diameter. Microparticles have been reported to arise from platelets, monocytes, endothelial cells, and tumor cells and carry on their surfaces a range of proteins that are derived from the cell of origin, including TF. Cancer cells, directly and indirectly, lead to the generation and circulation of TF-bearing microparticles, and the levels of circulating TF-bearing microparticles in pancreatic cancer patients appear to correlate with the subsequent risk for venous thromboembolic disease. In one study, approximately a third of patients with detectable TF-bearing microparticles developed venous thrombosis, compared with no thrombotic events in those without detectable TF-bearing microparticles.

Coagulation and Tumor Progression

The activation of coagulation in cancer may also play a role in tumor progression. For example, TF expression levels often correlate with a more aggressive tumor phenotype, and both clotting-dependent and clotting-independent signaling mechanisms of TF may be important in regulating tumor metastasis. TF promotes angiogenesis and is coexpressed with VEGF on malignant cells.

Thrombin is the key terminal enzyme of the coagulation cascade, and results in fibrin deposition and platelet activation; it also serves as a growth factor for a number of cell types including fibroblasts, endothelial cells, smooth muscle cells, and tumor cells. The cellular effects of thrombin are mediated through seven transmembrane-spanning G protein–coupled protease-activated receptors (PARs), principally PAR1. PAR1 is activated by thrombin through cleavage of its N-terminus, which exposes a tethered ligand that then binds to the second transmembrane domain of the receptor. PARs are expressed on platelets and other cells, as well as on tumor cells. Thrombin-activated tumor cells have PAR1-dependent enhanced expression of a number of cell surface integrins. Thrombin may enhance tumor progression via several mechanisms, including enhancing tumor cell proliferation, activating tumor–platelet adhesion, tumor adhesion to the matrix or endothelium, tumor implantation, growth, and metastasis, and tumor angiogenesis. Thrombin alters tumor cell gene expression with upregulation of angiogenesis-related genes such as *VEGF*, matrix metalloproteinase 2 (*MMP-2*), angiopoietin 2 (*ANG2*), and other genes and microribonucleic acids affecting tumor cell proliferation and invasion.

Diagnosis of Coagulopathies in Cancer Patients

Thrombotic events in patients with cancer are diagnosed in a similar fashion to those in patients without cancer. However, several subtleties exist. For example, thrombosis may be confused with either intravascular disease progression and/or intravascular fungal infections. In many cases, the diagnosis of thrombosis, or an abnormality in coagulation, may be made in an asymptomatic patient, leading to a more complicated decision regarding the risks and benefits of therapy. A process of fibrin formation and degradation is continuous in the setting of many patients with malignancy, and may relate to elevated thrombin–antithrombin complexes and fibrin degradation products. Thus cancer is thought by some to be a process of "chronic DIC." Of note, in two prospective studies of routine coagulation parameters in cancer patients, *elevated* fibrinogen and platelet counts were the most frequent alterations, not diminished as typically seen in DIC. The clinical spectrum of coagulopathy in cancer ranges from asymptomatic to life-threatening thrombohemorrhagic disease. Thrombotic manifestations of DIC include arterial and venous thromboembolism, migratory thrombophlebitis, marantic endocarditis, and microvascular thrombosis with organ failure or skin necrosis. The consumptive phase of DIC may manifest as bleeding, treatment of which is supportive and patient specific. Some may respond favorably to low-dose heparin, and/or plasma therapy, while waiting for treatment of the underlying malignancy. In general, the treatment of cancer-associated DIC is centered on the treatment of the underlying tumor.

With increased use of high-resolution computed tomographic imaging studies, pulmonary emboli (PEs) are increasingly being identified incidentally, in the absence of clinical suspicion. This has led to the question of how to manage incidentally discovered thrombosis. A retrospective cohort study of the period from 2004 to 2010 compared the rate of recurrent VTE and overall survival between those patients whose PEs were detected incidentally on imaging studies with those whose PEs were suspected by classic clinical criteria; there was no difference in recurrent VTE or overall survival when both groups were anticoagulated. A separate prospective observational study enrolled consecutive cancer patients newly diagnosed with combined deep venous thrombosis and PE from 2006 to 2009; 60% of the incidental thromboses were PEs, whereas only 26% of the

symptomatic events were PEs. There was also a lower risk for recurrent thrombosis among those patients with an incidental thrombus compared with those with a symptomatic thrombus, and no differences in major bleeding and overall survival between groups. Taken together, these two studies support the routine anticoagulation treatment of an incidentally found thrombosis, and do provide some insight into the risk of recurrent thrombosis according to the mechanism of presentation.

Intravenous Catheter Thrombosis in Malignancy

Many patients with cancer undergo placement of a central venous catheter (CVC), commonly in the form of an implantable port, for chemotherapy infusion. Presence of an indwelling central line is a risk factor for thrombosis; this is augmented in patients with underlying cancer. Nearly 15% of patients with cancer may develop a CVC-associated thrombosis, and the risk of thrombosis is increased if there is an exit site infection, among male patients, and in the presence of metastatic disease; risk also varies according to the type of catheter, being higher with a peripherally inserted central catheter compared with an implanted portal catheter. Particular malignancies also contribute to the risk of CVC-related thrombus; there is a significantly higher rate of CVC thrombus in patients with acute promyelocytic leukemia (32%) when compared with those with other types of acute myelogenous leukemia (6%). Because of the high risk of bleeding in cancer patients, routine VTE prophylaxis is not recommended among cancer patients with CVCs, in spite of the known thrombotic risk. For those patients that develop CVC-associated thrombosis, general treatment recommendations are for anticoagulation for 3 months. Low-molecular-weight heparin (LMWH) is preferred over the vitamin K antagonist, warfarin, in this population, and anticoagulation is continued while the line is in place. These guidelines may change as further studies reveal more information regarding newer anticoagulation agents.

Management of Thrombosis in Patients With Cancer

Cancer patients with a VTE have a high rate of recurrent thrombosis and bleeding after anticoagulation when compared with the general population, and merit a tailored treatment approach. One study compared recurrent thrombosis and major bleeding rates in patients with VTE with and without an underlying malignancy, managed with dose-adjusted intravenous unfractionated heparin or weight-adjusted LMWH, followed by warfarin. The 12-month cumulative incidence of recurrent thromboembolism among cancer patients was 20.7% versus 6.8% in patients without cancer, whereas the 12-month cumulative incidence of major bleeding was 12.4% in patients with cancer and 4.9% in patients without cancer.

Warfarin can pose certain difficulties in cancer patients for several reasons: there are numerous and often unpredictable drug interactions, cancer patients have variable nutritional intake, with unpredictable amounts of vitamin K in their diets, and the frequent use of antibiotics can result in altered bioavailability of dietary vitamin K. Further, there is a frequent need to interrupt anticoagulation for procedures, and there often is a coexisting thrombocytopenia, whose impact on coagulation may be complicated by the long half-life of warfarin. The long-term use of LMWH in cancer patients has been compared with warfarin, most notably in the CLOT trial. In this study, patients with cancer and VTE received dalteparin 200 IU/kg subcutaneously once daily for 5 to 7 days, and were then randomized to either continued dalteparin 150 IU/kg subcutaneously once daily, or to dose-adjusted warfarin with a target international normalized ratio of 2 to 3. Patients treated with dalteparin had a lower hazard ratio for recurrent thromboembolism compared with the oral-anticoagulant group (0.48); rates of major (6% versus 4%) and all bleeding (14% versus 19%) were similar. In this study, there was no difference in overall survival. A similar study that compared enoxaparin with warfarin for treatment of venous thrombosis in cancer also showed an approximately 50% reduction of combined outcome of major bleeding or recurrent VTE within 3 months with enoxaparin compared with warfarin (10.5% versus 21.1%). Based on a number of similar studies, and reflected in a number of current treatment guidelines, LMWH is generally preferred for cancer patients with VTE who do not have other contraindications.

Oral anticoagulation agents that directly inhibit factor Xa or thrombin are increasingly used in the treatment of VTE. The anti-Xa agents rivaroxaban and apixaban along with the direct thrombin inhibitor dabigatran have been shown to be effective in VTE prophylaxis after major hip and knee surgeries, as well as in stroke prevention in patients with atrial fibrillation. However, few patients with cancer have been evaluated in these trials, and no studies have specifically considered the treatment of malignancy associated VTE using these inhibitors. A small phase II study evaluating the safety and tolerability of apixaban found a low risk of major bleeding (2.2%) during 12 weeks of therapy in 125 patients with metastatic or advanced cancer *without thrombosis*. Safety concerns regarding these agents include the possible interactions with chemotherapeutic agents as well as the inability to reverse them quickly in a population that has potential to rapidly develop cytopenias and bleeding. While these agents are not currently recommended for malignancy-associated VTE, future study may further clarify the feasibility and efficacy of these agents in patients with malignancy and thrombosis.

FUTURE DIRECTIONS

Future studies on hematopoiesis and coagulation in cancer patients have the potential to provide insight into new treatment strategies for the many hematologic manifestations of cancer, as well as the treatment of the underlying malignancy. Historically, management of the hematologic manifestations of malignancy have centered on supportive care; however, these may also play a role in tumor survival and growth. For example, a deeper understanding of how growth factors may play a role in mediating tumor growth could identify new therapeutic targets and strategies. Platelets appear to play increasingly intricate roles in tumor metastasis and survival. Given the prevalence of thrombosis in cancer patients, new anticoagulation strategies will also prove increasingly important in the management of this unique population.

SUGGESTED READINGS

Aapro M, Jelkmann W, Constantinescu SN, et al: Effects of erythropoietin receptors and erythropoiesis-stimulating agents on disease progression in cancer. *Br J Cancer* 106(7):1249–1258, 2012.

Basser RL, O'Flaherty E, Green M, et al: Development of pancytopenia with neutralizing antibodies to thrombopoietin after multicycle chemotherapy supported by megakaryocyte growth and development factor. *Blood* 99(7):2599–2602, 2002.

Blake-Haskins JA, Lechleider RJ, Kreitman RJ: Thrombotic microangiopathy with targeted cancer agents. *Clin Cancer Res* 17(18):5858–5866, 2011.

Blom JW, Doggen CJ, Osanto S, et al: Malignancies, prothrombotic mutations, and the risk of venous thrombosis. *JAMA* 293(6):715–722, 2005.

Bohlius J, Schmidlin K, Brillant C, et al: Recombinant human erythropoiesis-stimulating agents and mortality in patients with cancer: a meta-analysis of randomised trials. *Lancet* 373(9674):1532–1542, 2009.

Braun S, Vogl FD, Naume B, et al: A pooled analysis of bone marrow micrometastasis in breast cancer. *N Engl J Med* 353(8):793–802, 2005.

Boccaccio C, Sabatino G, Medico E, et al: The MET oncogene drives a genetic programme linking cancer to haemostasis. *Nature* 434(7031):396–400, 2005.

Chang J, Couture F, Young S, et al: Weekly epoetin alfa maintains hemoglobin, improves quality of life, and reduces transfusion in breast cancer patients receiving chemotherapy. *J Clin Oncol* 23(12):2597–2605, 2005.

den Exter PL, Hooijer J, Dekkers OM, et al: Risk of recurrent venous thromboembolism and mortality in patients with cancer incidentally diagnosed

with pulmonary embolism: a comparison with symptomatic patients. *J Clin Oncol* 29(17):2405–2409, 2011.

Font C, Farrus B, Vidal L, et al: Incidental versus symptomatic venous thrombosis in cancer: a prospective observational study of 340 consecutive patients. *Ann Oncol* 22(9):2101–2106, 2011.

Grisariu S, Spectre G, Kalish Y, et al: Increased risk of central venous catheter-associated thrombosis in acute promyelocytic leukemia: a single-institution experience. *Eur J Haematol* 90(5):397–403, 2013.

Im JH, Fu W, Wang H, et al: Coagulation facilitates tumor cell spreading in the pulmonary vasculature during early metastatic colony formation. *Cancer Res* 64(23):8613–8619, 2004.

Lee AY, Levine MN, Baker RI, et al: Low-molecular-weight heparin versus a coumarin for the prevention of recurrent venous thromboembolism in patients with cancer. *N Engl J Med* 349(2):146–153, 2003.

Levine MN, Gu C, Liebman HA, et al: A randomized phase II trial of apixaban for the prevention of thromboembolism in patients with metastatic cancer. *J Thromb Haemost* 10(5):807–814, 2012.

Ludwig H, Van Belle S, Barrett-Lee P, et al: The European Cancer Anaemia Survey (ECAS): a large, multinational, prospective survey defining the prevalence, incidence, and treatment of anaemia in cancer patients. *Eur J Cancer* 40(15):2293–2306, 2004.

Lyman GH, Dale DC, Wolff DA, et al: Acute myeloid leukemia or myelodysplastic syndrome in randomized controlled clinical trials of cancer chemotherapy with granulocyte colony-stimulating factor: a systematic review. *J Clin Oncol* 28(17):2914–2924, 2010.

Meyer G, Marjanovic Z, Valcke J, et al: Comparison of low-molecular-weight heparin and warfarin for the secondary prevention of venous thromboembolism in patients with cancer: a randomized controlled study. *Arch Intern Med* 162(15):1729–1735, 2002.

Nash GF, Turner LF, Scully MF, et al: Platelets and cancer. *Lancet Oncol* 3(7):425–430, 2002.

Nierodzik ML, Karpatkin S: Thrombin induces tumor growth, metastasis, and angiogenesis: Evidence for a thrombin-regulated dormant tumor phenotype. *Cancer Cell* 10(5):355–362, 2006.

Piran S, Ngo V, McDiarmid S, et al: Incidence and risk factors of symptomatic venous thromboembolism related to implanted ports in cancer patients. *Thromb Res* 133(1):30–33, 2014.

Prandoni P, Lensing AW, Piccioli A, et al: Recurrent venous thromboembolism and bleeding complications during anticoagulant treatment in patients with cancer and venous thrombosis. *Blood* 100(10):3484–3488, 2002.

Sallah S, Wan JY, Nguyen NP, et al: Disseminated intravascular coagulation in solid tumors: clinical and pathologic study. *Thromb Haemost* 86(3):828–833, 2001.

Smith RE, Jr, Aapro MS, Ludwig H, et al: Darbepoetin alpha for the treatment of anemia in patients with active cancer not receiving chemotherapy or radiotherapy: results of a phase III, multicenter, randomized, double-blind, placebo-controlled study. *J Clin Oncol* 26(7):1040–1050, 2008.

Sorensen HT, Mellemkjaer L, Olsen JH, et al: Prognosis of cancers associated with venous thromboembolism. *N Engl J Med* 343(25):1846–1850, 2000.

Stanworth SJ, Estcourt LJ, Powter G, et al: A no-prophylaxis platelet-transfusion strategy for hematologic cancers. *N Engl J Med* 368(19):1771–1780, 2013.

Stone RL, Nick AM, McNeish IA, et al: Paraneoplastic thrombocytosis in ovarian cancer. *N Engl J Med* 366(7):610–618, 2012.

Streiff MB: Thrombosis in the setting of cancer. *Hematology Am Soc Hematol Educ Program* 2016(1):196–205, 2016.

Tilley RE, Holscher T, Belani R, et al: Tissue factor activity is increased in a combined platelet and microparticle sample from cancer patients. *Thromb Res* 122(5):604–609, 2008.

Todaro M, Turdo A, Bartucci M, et al: Erythropoietin activates cell survival pathways in breast cancer stem-like cells to protect them from chemotherapy. *Cancer Res* 73(21):6393–6400, 2013.

Zwicker JI, Connolly G, Carrier M, et al: Catheter-associated deep vein thrombosis of the upper extremity in cancer patients: guidance from the SSC of the ISTH. *J Thromb Haemost* 12(5):796–800, 2014.

Zwicker JI, Liebman HA, Neuberg D, et al: Tumor-derived tissue factor-bearing microparticles are associated with venous thromboembolic events in malignancy. *Clin Cancer Res* 15(22):6830–6840, 2009.

INTEGRATIVE THERAPIES IN PATIENTS WITH HEMATOLOGIC DISEASES

David S. Rosenthal, Ann Webster, and Elana Ladas

Complementary and alternative medicine (CAM) is tremendously popular in the United States and many parts of the world to help people with wellness and health.[1] In the United States alone, an estimated $36 to $47 billion is spent annually by the public on CAM methods of therapy,[2] and in a National Health Interview Survey in 2007 and again in 2015, 37% of adults used at least one form of CAM.[3] Over the past decade, CAM practices have become even more popular, especially in individuals with a chronic disease such as hematologic malignancies and cancer.[4] In 1998 the National Center for Complementary and Alternative Medicine (NCCAM) was established at the National Institutes of Health (NIH) to study the efficacy and safety of CAM practices. The term CAM caused consternation among many in the field, who perceive that their patients are forgoing conventional therapy. That is generally not the case. The term CAM is controversial because the words complementary and alternative have completely different meanings and should not be connected by an "and" but by an "or." Whereas complementary therapies were defined by NCCAM as therapies used to complement or to be used alongside conventional methods of therapy, alternative methods referred to those therapies used instead of known conventional therapies and have not been shown to be effective. The term integrative medicine (IM) or integrative health (IH) is used to more accurately describe the complementary therapies being used in US medical settings today. These therapies are used alongside conventional therapies in a therapeutic environment. In 2014 NCCAM was renamed "The National Center for Complementary and Integrative Health (NCCIH)," which more accurately reflects the work as only a minority of individuals are forgoing conventional therapies. The components of IM or IH (1) combine the best of both conventional and evidence-based complementary therapies, (2) emphasizes patient participation, (3) promote the primacy of the patient–provider relationship and the importance of shared decision making, (4) emphasizes the contribution of the therapeutic encounter itself, and (5) optimizes the individual's innate healing capacity.[5]

Although many integrative therapies such as acupuncture, massage, and meditation are quite beneficial for hematology/oncology patients by helping them to cope with the disease, reducing their stress and symptoms related to the conventional therapy or to the disease process itself, many alternative interventions are unproven and could be harmful for patients who may believe that these interventions can cure them of their malignancy. An American Cancer Society study concluded that as many as 61% of cancer survivors used some form of complementary or alternative therapies.[4] In addition, the majority of people do not share their use of these therapies with their primary care providers. According to a survey by Eisenberg et al,[6] patients do not think that their physicians need to know about their use of these interventions and many patients responded that their physician never asked about such use. Because there are many potential drug–drug, drug–herb, drug–radiation, and antioxidant–drug interactions, it is extremely important for patients to share their use of integrative therapies and alternative treatments with their providers and similarly for physicians to ask about their patients' usage.[7]

Through the NCCIH and IM centers, more information and education is available to the public and to physicians, on the importance of physicians' "asking" about the use of integrative therapies and alternative therapies and patients "telling" about the use of these therapies (http://www.nccih.nih.gov). Many hematology/oncology centers have established IM programs where complementary therapies such as acupuncture, massage, nutrition, physical activity, and stress management are offered alongside the conventional therapies of chemotherapy, radiation, and targeted therapies. These programs provide guidance to patients in choosing the safest and most effective integrative therapies that could be incorporated into their plans of care. Despite the level of evidence supporting standard treatment, some patients decline chemotherapy, radiation, or surgery. Instead, they choose to pursue an alternative therapy. Sometimes this choice is because of a cultural belief, because they believe that natural products are potentially less toxic, or because they believe that the alternative treatment will offer a "cure" for their disease. Alternative medicine practitioners and clinics exist in our country and around the world that offer a "cure," usually for a significant amount of out-of-pocket fees. Unfortunately, these clinics rarely ever provide any scientific evidence and typically do not conduct research or report their results except in advertisements.

On the other hand, there is an increasing body of research on the benefits of many complementary and integrative therapies. Clinical studies provide evidence that some integrative therapies are beneficial to patients by improving their quality of life, reducing their symptoms from the disease, and decreasing the side effects from treatment. One of the major concerns, however, is the use of botanicals, herbs, and over-the-counter (OTC) drugs in conjunction with chemotherapy and radiation therapy (see later). Some may reduce the effectiveness of certain chemotherapies, and others may reduce metabolism of an active drug, enhancing its potential toxicity.

INTEGRATIVE THERAPY DOMAINS AND THEIR USE

According to the NCCIH, "most integrative therapies fall into one of two subgroups—natural products or mind and body practices" (Table 156.1). There is also an abundance of whole-systems practices that include ayurvedic medicine and traditional Chinese medicine. The whole-systems approaches incorporate many of the integrative therapies. Mind–body approaches include meditation, mindfulness meditation, guided imagery, music therapy, creative arts therapy, self-hypnosis, yoga, tai chi, and qigong, among many other types of physical and spiritual practices. Energy-based therapies include reiki and healing touch. Body-based manipulative therapies include chiropractic and massage therapy. Examples of natural products include dietary supplements, antioxidants, vitamin megadoses, specialized diets, and herbs.

In the literature, there is a paucity of information on the use of integrative therapies in the treatment of hematologic malignancies.[8] In India there is a significant use of ayurvedic medicine. In a German study of a large group of patients with chronic lymphocytic leukemia (CLL), approximately 44% used integrative therapies with 26% using vitamin supplementation, 18% mineral supplementation, 14% homeopathy, 7% acupuncture, and 9% mistletoe therapy. In the United States, 30% to 80% of pediatric hematology/oncology patients used one or more complementary therapies in conjunction with their conventional care. In the US pediatric group, there is an especially high use of vitamin and nutritional supplements,[8,9] with

TABLE
156.1   **Integrative Therapies Domain**

- Mind–body programs   • Whole systems
- Energy therapies   • Traditional Chinese medicine
- Body based or manipulative • Ayurvedic
- Natural products

mind–body therapies a close second. Because many patients do not report their use of complementary therapies to their primary care hematologist/oncologist, there are markedly disparate data from one study to another. In other countries, such as Mexico, Ireland, and Canada, there is a high use of CAM therapies ranging from 42% to 60% in the pediatric patients. Therapies include vitamins, minerals, reflexology, etc.[10,11]

In a review by Wesa and Cassileth,[12] the major reason why leukemia patients use integrative therapies or remedies not prescribed by their hematologist/oncologist is in an effort to improve their treatment outcome and to manage their symptoms. For those with leukemia, the integrative therapies that were felt to be most beneficial included mind–body interventions such as self-hypnosis, meditation, guided imagery, and breath awareness. Massage and reflexology are also frequently used to decrease symptoms (see subsequent discussion on massage). Acupuncture is very beneficial for symptom management with minimal side effects (see later discussion of acupuncture).

RESEARCH TECHNIQUES OF INTEGRATIVE THERAPIES

Research in the United States on integrative therapies is partially financially supported by the NIH through NCCIH and the Office of Cancer Complementary and Alternative Medicine at the National Cancer Institute (NCI). Investigators have tried to apply the same research principles used to evaluate new chemotherapy programs for leukemias and lymphomas (i.e., the traditional randomized clinical trial).[13] This approach has been problematic because it is often difficult to identify the proper controls for integrative therapies such as mind–body techniques, acupuncture, and massage. As a result, meta-analyses on integrative therapies reveal an abundance of pilot studies and nonrandomized clinical studies that are often criticized on the basis that any positive result may be attributable to the placebo effect.[14] In the case of acupuncture research, sham or "fake" acupuncture has been used as a control in which nontraditional needles are used but not placed in the meridian spots and not stimulated.

In randomized clinical trials of acupuncture effectiveness, comparing active acupuncture with "sham" acupuncture, only those who are naive to acupuncture can participate. With massage therapy, randomized clinical trials have used an educational program of equivalent attention time to attempt to control for the placebo effect. This has been similarly true for research on energy therapies such as reiki and many of the mind–body programs.

Whole-systems research is another approach taken by integrative therapists.[14] This involves combining nutrition, physical activity, and stress and symptom management therapies together as an intervention in evaluating quality of life measures over a period of time. This type of research creates many variables and is totally contrary to the current widely accepted reductionist method of research.

The study of herbs and other OTC unregulated products has been fraught with confounding variables, specifically the lack of standardization of the product studied.[15] For example, PC-SPES, a compound of eight herbs manufactured by a single company, was demonstrated in a pilot study in men undergoing active surveillance for prostate cancer to be associated with a decrease in prostate-specific antigen levels. The promising trends of this phase I and later a phase II study led to a randomized clinical trial of PC-SPES. During the phases of this randomized clinical trial, there were

complications that led to the reevaluation of the constituents of PC-SPES. Although evaluations of the product showed no evidence of any phytoestrogens in any of the eight herbal compounds at the onset of the study, during the randomized clinical trial, phytoestrogens were found, and patients began to demonstrate breast engorgement. Other lots of the product did not contain phytoestrogens but were demonstrated to have contaminants such as dicoumarol, and some individuals were noted to experience increased bruising. Investigators have attempted to overcome the standardization issue of herbs by studying their individual proteins in in vitro models, and others have attempted to closely monitor the constituents of the herbs by protein fractionation, ensuring that the product remains constant during the research study. Most herbs and botanicals are not regulated by the US Food and Drug Administration (FDA), potentiating issues of quality control, possible contamination, and stability issues. The United States Pharmacopeia (USP) does verify the identity, strength, purity, and quality of some supplements and applies its USP verification label, http://www.usp.org/uspverified. ConsumerLab.com also performs independent testing and applies its approval stamp.

REVIEW OF RESULTS OF INTEGRATIVE THERAPIES IN HEMATOLOGY/ONCOLOGY PATIENTS

Most studies on the use of integrative therapies in hematology/oncology disorders investigate the effect on patients' quality of life and symptomatic relief of stress, pain, fatigue, and anxiety. The results discussed here will be reviewed in terms of improvement in symptoms and quality of life, and when appropriate, the effect on immune function and survival if investigated. In most studies, the major symptoms for which integrative therapies are used include anxiety, neuropathy, fatigue, pain, chemotherapy-induced nausea and vomiting (CINV), worsening immune system, stress, and depression.

Literature on Outcomes: Science, Safety, and Efficacy

In making decisions about what integrative therapies physicians should recommend, Weiger et al[16] suggest that decisions be based on safety and efficacy. If an intervention is safe and effective such as acupuncture for CINV, it can be appropriately recommended. If a therapy is unsafe or toxic and has been demonstrated to be ineffective, it should not be recommended, and patients should be cautioned about its use. For example, laetrile (Amygdalin) may contain varying amounts of cyanide, and in clinical studies has been shown to be ineffective in treating cancer. Many interventions, products, and substances are safe, but their effectiveness is unknown. With these, the physician should be cautious and recommend their use with the following proviso: if this is a substance taken orally, it should be evaluated as to whether it has any unfavorable interactions with chemotherapy or medications that the patient is already taking or whether it interacts with a disease process such as causing hypoglycemia in a diabetic patient. Taking one new OTC substance at a time is good common sense, and patients should be told to observe any change in symptoms, whether they are favorable or unfavorable, before adding another substance to their oral regimens, especially if there is little or nothing known about the agent. With respect to drug–drug and drug–herb interactions, websites are available for professionals as well as for lay audiences. A list of these websites is given in Table 156.2. Most of these websites list the various terms by which a given agent is known and provide information on each agent's constituents, reasons for use, evidence for safety or toxicity, and evidence of effectiveness. Most importantly, these websites list the adverse effects of these substances and the drug–drug, drug–herb, and drug–disease interactions when known. When asked about the use of an OTC substance that is not FDA regulated or ConsumerLab.com approved, physicians should consult one of the databases to ensure safety and lack of adverse interactions (see Table 156.2).

TABLE 156.2	Herbs and Botanicals: Educational Websites

- Memorial Sloan-Kettering Cancer Center: https://www.mskcc.org/cancer-care/treatments/symptom-management/integrative-medicine/herbs (accessed 8/31/16)
- The University of Texas MD Anderson Cancer Center: http://www.mdanderson.org/ (accessed 8/31/16)
- American Cancer Society: http://www.cancer.org (accessed 8/31/16)
- National Center for Complementary and Integrative Health (https://nccih.nih.gov/)
- National Cancer Institute's Office of Cancer Complementary and Alternative Medicine: https://cam.cancer.gov/ (accessed 8/31/16)
- Natural Medicines Comprehensive Database: http://www.naturaldatabase.com (accessed 8/31/16)
- Natural Standard: https://naturalmedicines.therapeuticresearch.com/ (accessed 8/31/16)

TABLE 156.3	Mind–Body Therapies

- Relaxation response
  Biofeedback
- Mindfulness meditation
  Progressive muscle relaxation
  Deep breathing exercise
  Prayer
- Guided imagery
- Self-hypnosis
- Self-expression in words
- Music therapy
- Expressive arts therapy
- Dance
- Yoga
- Tai chi
- Qigong
- Support groups

INDIVIDUAL INTEGRATIVE THERAPY MODALITIES

Mind–Body Therapies

Mind–body therapies are frequently studied interventions in patients with chronic diseases such as hematologic malignancies.[17] Mind–body therapies focus on the interactions between the brain, mind, body, and behaviors and on the ways in which emotional, mental, social, spiritual, and behavioral factors can directly affect health. Mind–body therapies are used throughout the world in treatment, disease prevention, and health promotion.

A diagnosis of a hematologic malignancy can be very stressful. Stress is part of normal physiologic body functioning and can be divided into good stress and bad stress. Chronic stress can be caused by an unexpected situation such as experiencing a new diagnosis (e.g., leukemia), an uncomfortable interaction with a colleague, painful treatments, loss of a loved one or a job, or just the pressures of modern life. Chronic stress has been shown to decrease immune functioning by inhibiting the body's ability to make T cells, B cells, macrophage cells, and interferon—four major components of the immune system. Research in the field of psychoneuroimmunology has shown that decreasing stress can actually boost immune function. Prolonged or severe stress not only weakens the immune system, it strains the heart, damages memory cells, and deposits fat at the waist rather than at the hips and buttocks (a risk factor for heart disease, cancer, and other illnesses). When stress persists for too long or becomes too severe, the normally protective mechanisms become overburdened, a condition that Bruce McEwen, at Rockefeller University, refers to as "allostatic load."

Stress has even been shown to take a toll on gene expression.[18] Investigations into mind–body therapies using functional genomics have revolutionized the understanding of mind–body therapy mechanisms and their effects on human physiology. Existing trials focusing on gene expression changes brought about by mind–body therapies have revealed intriguing connections to the immune system.[19]

Mental health professionals have significantly underestimated the importance of lifestyle factors as contributors to physical, emotional, behavioral, and spiritual pathologies. Mind–body therapies have been underused in health care.

In the 1970s Dr. Herbert Benson popularized the "relaxation response," the performance of "a time out" in normal daily functions. Benson coined this term after observing that when monks meditated, they experienced decreases in their pulse, blood pressure, and respirations. Although there are now known genetic, environmental, and dietary factors that play a significant role in causation of chronic disease, stress may be a lesser but significant factor. Mind–body techniques (Table 156.3) include transcendental meditation or the relaxation response, mindfulness meditation, biofeedback, guided imagery, and hypnosis. In addition, music therapy, and modified physical activities such as yoga, tai chi, and qigong also are mind–body programs. There are several common forms of meditation: (1) concentrative meditation, which focuses on a phrase or a visual image such as the relaxation response; (2) mindfulness meditation or awareness, in which the client becomes aware of his or her thoughts and feelings and focuses on those issues; and (3) expressive meditation used in tribal societies consisting of fast deep breathing, shaking, whirling, and dancing.[17]

Mind–body interventions are often self-taught or presented by a professional. Double-blinded trials are difficult to conduct partly because the presence of an empathetic professional giving the therapeutic modality may be considered a placebo effect. Mind–body interventions are often accompanied by other integrative therapy interventions, making pure studies unevaluable; however, randomized clinical trials have demonstrated that relaxation training and guided imagery significantly reduce nausea and anxiety.[20]

Compared with medication, relaxation therapy showed similar decreases in anxiety and depression, although medication might have been slightly faster in its effect. Other randomized trials have shown decreases in tension, depression, anger, and fatigue during relaxation training or imagery. In children, hypnosis has been found to be especially effective. In a randomized clinical trial comparing hypnosis or nonhypnotic distraction such as the relaxation techniques versus joining a placebo attention-control group, the children in the hypnosis group reported significant reduction in anticipatory nausea and CINV.

Mind–body therapies have also been used to alleviate pain. In a study of children undergoing bone marrow or lumbar puncture procedures, hypnosis significantly reduced the pain as well as anxiety. A recent study has shown that a relaxation response training reduced anxiety in women undergoing breast biopsies.[20a] Also a study of mind–body therapies for men just diagnosed with prostate cancer, preparing to go through radiation treatments, found that mind–body therapies reduced anxiety, improved sleep, reduced fatigue, and improved concentration in all of the participants.[20b]

Expressive arts therapy and music therapy as well as repetitive exercise, yoga, tai chi, qigong, and Pilates also can reduce stress and anxiety. Music therapy is considered a mind–body therapy that reduces stress and anxiety because it uses a variety of active and passive music experiences, live or recorded. This technique can be used either independently or with a music therapist. Randomized trials have shown statistically significant improvements in mood and physical discomfort. In patients with hematologic malignancies admitted for autologous stem cell transplantations, patients receiving an individualized program of live music therapy had a significant improvement in mood or what is referred to as "courageous coping." Music therapy has also been shown to be an effective adjunct to antiemetic therapy. Studies of immune function have yet to show any statistically significant improvement in immune function.

Studies have shown that prayer is good medicine and is considered by many to be a mind–body therapy. Dr. Harold Koenig, director of Duke University's Center for Spirituality, Theology and Health, studied the connection between spirituality and well-being. Prayer is associated with less depression, anxiety, better physical health and well-being. People who have a prayer practice have less cardiac disease and hypertension and better measurable immune functioning. Mind–body therapies, such as hypnosis, give people hope and foster acceptance of one's physical condition.[21] Yoga and physical activity have been studied to determine whether there is a related reduction in symptoms of depression and anxiety. In general, the practice of yoga has increased from 5.2% of the 45–64 age population in the year 2000 to 7.2% in 2012. A number of yoga practices may be helpful for people with cancer in reducing stress and managing side effects, both during and after chemotherapy and medical procedures. Restorative yoga postures can be both energizing and relaxing, requiring almost no physical effort. Yoga can also help with pain. Yoga also stresses the value of community. There is evidence that participating in a cancer support group may increase odds of survival. So far, there are no scientific studies on whether yoga can improve survival rates. However, suggestive evidence comes from Dr. Dean Ornish, best known for his work using a comprehensive lifestyle program that included yoga for heart disease. Dr. Ornish has been studying a similar approach for prostate cancer. In a 12-week yoga intervention in healthy subjects, it was demonstrated that there was greater improvement in mood and anxiety than a metabolically matched walking exercise. The authors demonstrated an acute increase in thalamic GABA (γ-aminobutyric acid) levels alongside the improvement in mood and anxiety scales. White et al[22] demonstrated the potential benefits of physical activity for children with acute lymphocytic leukemia.

In summary, it is evident that mind–body therapies can reduce anxiety, temper the adverse effects of chemotherapy and radiation treatments, relieve pain, and possibly stimulate immune responses. By reducing stress and anxiety, these therapies can help patients deal with a wide range of relationship issues and decision making as they move through the diagnostic and therapeutic phases of their malignancy. Mind–body approaches have very minimal risk and potentially significant benefits. Most importantly, they are often self taught and therefore low cost. Mind–body practices should be considered as an adjunct to usual care regardless of whether patients are beginning or recovering from chemotherapy.

Acupuncture

Overview and Definitions

One of the major components of traditional Chinese medicine has been the use of acupuncture. For more than 2000 years, this traditional practice has been used in the Far East to "correct an imbalance in yin-yang and qi (energy)." It is believed that with acupuncture, "blocked" channels can be unblocked, reducing symptoms. Acupuncture is the stimulation of certain points on the body by needles or alternatively by pressure called acupressure. Both techniques take advantage of the meridians described by traditional Chinese medicine. Acupuncture points are situated along meridians, which are channels for "qi." Sham or "fake" acupuncture implies the use of needles that are not inserted to the same depth, not put in the meridian points, and not given stimulation. Electroacupuncture implies the use of added electric pulses to create additional or accentuated stimulation. Several studies have shown that electroacupuncture provides greater symptom relief than regular acupuncture.

Research on Usage and Effectiveness

Most acupuncture in the Western world is used to manage symptoms, not treat disease.[23] Research studies have demonstrated release of neurotransmitters and change of brain functional magnetic resonance imaging signals during acupuncture. Acupuncture was confirmed as an effective intervention for CINV at an NIH consensus conference in 1997. Whether this beneficial effect is attributable to an induced relaxation response or a direct antiemetic effect is not known.

Randomized clinical trials on acupuncture have been used in a variety of settings. As mentioned earlier, only individuals who are naive to acupuncture can take part in acupuncture studies because they will note the difference between active acupuncture and its sham component. Acupuncture has been shown to be effective in randomized clinical trials in cancer-related fatigue, cancer-related pain, and postoperative pain as well as reduced CINV in adults and children. In addition, acupuncture can improve radiation-induced xerostomia, vasomotor symptoms such as hot flashes, and chemotherapy-induced neuropathies.

Several randomized clinical trials conducted in China have suggested that acupuncture could be effective in reducing the marrow suppression in patients on aggressive chemotherapy. Analysis of these trials performed by Lu et al[24] suggest that acupuncture is associated with an increase in neutrophils and total white blood cell count in patients during chemotherapy or chemoradiation therapy. The weighted mean difference of over 1000/μL white blood cells on average is a statistically significant difference. Lu et al[25] carried out a small, randomized, sham-controlled clinical trial in the United States exploring this issue in ovarian and breast cancer patients receiving aggressive chemotherapy. Using manual and electrostimulation two to three times per week for a total of 10 sessions beginning 1 week before the second cycle of chemotherapy, the median leukocyte count in the active acupuncture arm at the first day of the next cycle was significantly higher than in the sham arm. The median leukocyte nadir, neutrophil nadir, and recovering absolute neutrophil counts were all higher but not statistically different. The result showed improved neutrophil counts both at the nadir and rebound points during chemotherapy, but the sample size of the study was underpowered.

Uncontrolled pilot studies of acupuncture have shown effectiveness in reducing anxiety and improving mood and other quality-of-life measures in patients with both oncologic and hematologic disorders. These studies have shown improvement in sleeplessness, depression, and xerostomia. Acupuncture improved xerostomia inventory scores in 18 patients who received radiation therapy and had pilocarpine-resistant xerostomia. In patients with hot flashes and vasomotor symptoms caused by chemotherapy, acupuncture attenuated some of the hot flashes. In a controlled study comparing venlafaxine and acupuncture, no statistical difference was found between the favorable response to acupuncture and the medication. One study suggested that acupuncture may be useful for drug-induced neuropathy from thalidomide/bortezomib therapy for multiple myeloma. Ear acupuncture was shown to be effective for phantom pain in a 16 year old after an amputation for osteosarcoma

Safety

With the increasing use of acupuncture in the United States because of evidence of its effectiveness, there are concerns about its safety when used in the community, especially with hematology patients and those getting chemotherapy and radiotherapy. However, reports of major side effects of acupuncture are rare and usually are evident when performed by untrained practitioners.[26] In closely monitored clinical trials, there is a low incidence of adverse events. In one study, the rate of minor adverse events was 14 per 10,000 sessions; serious events were 0.05 per 10,000 treatments and 0.55 per 10,000 individual patients. Common adverse events include blood-borne infections and internal organ and tissue injury. In general, acupuncture should be avoided in patients with severe neutropenia and thrombocytopenia (absolute neutrophil count <500/μL and platelets <25,000/μL). However, in one study of acupuncture given during stem cell transplantation, there were no bleeding side effects in individuals with severe thrombocytopenia (platelet counts <20,000/μL). Another study in children and adolescents undergoing chemotherapy including stem cell transplantation found that acupuncture was safe among those with severe thrombocytopenia.[27]

Massage and Touch Therapies

Overview and Definitions

Massage has been defined by some as "rhythmic and methodical stretching and compressing of the muscles and connective tissue through the touch of the therapist's hands." There are many types of massage and hands-on soft tissue therapies (Table 156.4). Therapies include Swedish massage, aromatherapy massage, reflexology, acupressure, and manual lymphatic drainage massage. Swedish massage provides broad, flowing, soothing strokes (effleurage), generally applied with a lotion or massage oil from distal to proximal areas on extremities. In addition, there is usually gentle kneading of soft tissues (petrissage). Aromatherapy has often been combined with massage in which selected scented oils are blended with the usual massage oil to enhance the beneficial effects of both physical and emotional wellbeing. Reflexology focuses on manual pressure to specific areas of the feet that, in traditional Chinese medicine, are linked with remote areas of the body. Acupressure massage uses the meridian theory of traditional Chinese medicine in which focal pressure is applied to acupuncture needle sites with the goal of adjusting the flow of energy similar to the theory in acupuncture. Manual lymphatic drainage is the application of light, flowing strokes of massage in specific patterns with the goal of alleviating lymph edema after lymph node resection or radiation therapy.

Research on Usage and Effectiveness

Corbin[28] has reviewed the value of massage as well as the difficulties in performing scientific research. Many randomized clinical trials use a crossover arm and attempt interventions that try to control for the placebo effect. The various measurement tools used to assess outcomes involve numeric rating scales, visual analog scales, profile of mood status, the S state trait anxiety inventory, the European Organization for Research and Treatment of Cancer quality of life questionnaire, and others. In a critical review of potential benefits of massage, Joske et al[29] identified eight randomized controlled clinical studies in hematology/oncology patients totaling more than 357 patients. Specifically, there was evidence of anxiety reduction with less benefit for analgesia. In autologous bone marrow transplantation patients, the massage group had significantly decreased distress and nausea scores early in the trial, but these were not long standing. Massage therapy has been found to reduce state anxiety and boost mood in many metaanalyses, probably its most beneficial attribute. Pain may be alleviated, but this has not been demonstrated to be statistically significant. Numerous studies have shown trends not only in decreased anxiety but also in nausea, pain, fatigue, and depression.

To date, there is little evidence suggesting that massage therapies have any effect on immune function or survival outcomes in hematology/oncology patients. A small randomized study did find

TABLE 156.4	Massage or Body Manipulation

- Swedish massage
- Aromatherapy massage
- Reflexology
- Acupressure
- Shiatsu
- Manual lymphatic drainage
- Reiki
- Deep tissue massage
- Rolfing

higher natural killer (NK) cells and lymphocyte cells during massage. Similarly, in a study in human immunodeficiency (HIV) patients, there was a significant increase in NK cell fighter toxicity during the massage period. In some trials, there is a short-term effect on NK cell activity; however, long-term clinical effect has not been demonstrated. A significant effect of effleurage massage on cellular immunity, cortisol, oxytocin, anxiety, depression, or quality of life has also not been demonstrated in more rigorous randomized clinical trials. In another randomized clinical study, dopamine levels, NK cells, and lymphocytes increased from the first to last day of the massage therapy. In a study of children with HIV, a control arm had a greater relative risk of CD4 count decline than the massage therapy children. Lymphocyte loss was also more extensive in the control participants, and more of the control group than the massage group lost greater than 50/mm^3 CD8 lymphocytes. The immediate effects of massage therapy are decreased anxiety, depressed mood, and anger. The long-term effects of massage include reduced depression and hostility as well as increased urine meridopamine, serotonin values and NK cell number, and lymphocytes. However, it is not clear that these results were statistically significant.

Weaknesses exist in many of the massage therapy studies reported to date such as small sample sizes and lack of controls. Most of the practitioners have not been blinded to the hypothesis of the studies. Furthermore, no systematic approach has been identified to determine the optimal number of massage treatments in a trial and within-group comparisons. Strong evidence shows that massage therapy can be very helpful in alleviating anxiety and stress in patients. However, more rigorous study designs, adequate statistical power, better identification of predictors for response to massage, and study of the psychologic and biologic mechanisms are needed. There is also a need for larger sample sizes and rigorous design reporting on massage therapy.

Safety

The concern that massage therapy can spread a tumor is unfounded. However, direct pressure over known tumor sites is usually discouraged. In general, massage therapy of all types is quite safe. The NCI urges massage therapists to take specific precautions with all cancers and avoid massaging open wounds, bruises, or areas with skin breakdown. Also massage directly over tumor sites, areas with a thrombosis, and sensitive areas after radiation therapy should be avoided.

Nutrition and Supplements

Nutrition

Nutritional guidelines for patients with hematologic malignancies should be based on the recommendations of the American Cancer Society and the World Cancer Research Fund/American Institute for Cancer Research (WCRF/AICR).[30,31] The AICR clearly states that cancer survivors should follow its nine nutrition and physical activity guidelines for risk reduction.[31] Adherence to the WCRF/AICR cancer prevention guidelines has been associated with a 34% lower hazard of death (95% confidence interval [CI], 0.59–0.75) compared with participants within the lowest adherence. Moreover, the WCRF/AICR score was also significantly associated with a lower hazard of dying from cancer, circulatory disease, and respiratory disease.[32]

The first recommendation is to be as lean as possible without being underweight, a recommendation that has been further endorsed by the American Society of Clinical Oncology.[33] A recent metaanalysis among adults with leukemia, found that obesity is associated with an increased risk (relative risk [RR] of 1.26; 95% CI, 1.17–1.37; $p < .001$) of leukemia and is associated with reduced mortality (RR, 1.29; 95% CI, 1.11–1.49; $p = .001$). Obesity has also been associated with an increased incidence of acute myeloid leukemia (AML) (RR, 1.53; 95% CI, 1.26–1.85; $p < .001$), chronic lymphocytic leukemia (RR, 1.17; 95% CI, 1.08–1.27; $p < .001$), chronic myeloid leukemia

(RR, 1.16; 95% CI, 1.04–1.30; $p = .007$) and acute lymphoblastic leukemia (ALL) (RR, 1.62; 95% CI, 1.12–2.32; $p = .009$).[34] Similar results have been observed for children and adolescents with ALL and AML.[35,36] Children and adolescents who were obese at diagnosis and remained overweight/obese during treatment experienced reduced survival (hazard ratios, 1.43 and 2.30, respectively). Importantly, those patients whose weight classification became a healthy weight eliminated this risk factor. Similar results have been reported in children and adolescents with AML.

The second AICR recommendation is to be physically active for 30 minutes every day. Although few studies have evaluated physical activity and hematologic malignancies, data suggest that low physical activity may increase the risk of non-Hodgkin lymphoma (NHL) and increasing activity may reduce the risk, especially for follicular and small lymphocytic lymphoma.

The third recommendation is to avoid sugary drinks and limit consumption of energy-dense foods. This is obviously linked with the body-weight guideline because sugary drinks contribute many empty calories to the standard American diet. In addition, the contribution of insulin and insulin-like growth factor type 1 to the development of malignant disease is being increasingly appreciated in a number of cancers, leading to the investigation of blockade of the insulin-like growth factor 1 receptor as a novel treatment for some malignant diagnoses. High-sugar diets are tightly linked to obesity, thus adhering to a diet low in simple sugars, such as the low-glycemic diet, may not only reduce the risk of weight gain but also reduce risk of treatment-related toxicities during and after treatment.

Fourth, the AICR suggests that people eat a greater variety of fruits, vegetables, whole grains, and legumes such as beans. Data from the US Centers for Disease Control and Prevention demonstrate that the American public falls far short on the conservative recommendation to consume at least five servings of fruits and vegetables daily, with only 14% of adults meeting the guideline. Plants are rich sources of fiber, antioxidants, and phytonutrients, many of which are believed to be useful in cancer-risk reduction. In one study, dietary fiber intake was associated with a lower risk of all NHL subtypes. Another analysis found that high consumption of fruits and vegetables was associated with a lower risk of all NHL subtypes, particularly follicular lymphoma, in women but not men.[37]

Fifth, the AICR recommends limiting consumption of red meats (beef, pork, and lamb) and avoiding processed meats. Epidemiologic studies suggest that consumption of fried red meats as well as dairy products leads to an increased risk of NHL.[37] Conversely, consumption of higher levels of omega-3 or marine fatty acids has been shown to be inversely correlated with lymphoma risk. Additional studies in an Australian cohort suggest that a diet high in fish may also be protective against the development of other hematopoietic malignancies—leukemias and multiple myeloma as well as NHL.[38]

Sixth, the AICR guidelines state that if consumed at all, alcoholic drinks should be limited to two for men and one for women per day. Although moderate alcohol consumption may be associated with cardiovascular benefits, alcohol use has been associated with an increased risk of a number of malignancies. A pooled analysis of nine case-control studies of NHL revealed that ever drinkers, compared with never drinkers, had a 17% lower risk of NHL, a finding the investigators attributed to a possible beneficial effect of moderate alcohol consumption on immune function. A cohort study in 126,293 multiethnic adults used lifelong abstainers and infrequent drinkers as the referent and reported a relative risk of 0.5 for the development of both lymphocytic and myeloid leukemias in those consuming three or more drinks daily without any contribution of choice of beverage (wine, beer, or liquor). With regard to patients already diagnosed, a cohort of 575 female NHL cases in Connecticut was followed for a median of 7.75 years. Compared with never drinkers, wine drinkers experienced better overall survival (75% vs. 69% five-year survival; $p = .030$) and disease-free survival (70% vs. 67%; $p = .049$). The favorable effect for wine drinkers was seen mainly in patients with diffuse large B-cell lymphoma. Resveratrol, a red-wine polyphenol known for its potential cardioprotective effects, is also believed to have potential in cancer risk reduction and perhaps

even as an adjunct to conventional therapy. An in vitro study involving ALL cell lines demonstrated that red-wine polyphenols caused growth inhibition and apoptosis. Although these cell line experiments often produce elegant results regarding mechanism of observed in vitro action, whether the phytonutrients have the same benefits in humans consuming the whole foodstuffs or concentrated supplements remains uncertain. A large prospective study of over 120,000 individuals with 17 years of follow up found no inverse relationship of lymphoid or myeloid neoplasms and alcohol consumption; if anything there was an increased risk rather than a decreased risk of lymphoid neoplasms.[39]

Supplements

Most conventional medical and radiation oncologists recommend that their cancer patients avoid all supplements, especially during active radiation and chemotherapy. This recommendation is primarily based on the absence of convincing data supporting therapeutic benefit. Three other valid concerns about supplement use are (1) the potential for supplement–drug interactions via a pharmacokinetic or pharmacodynamics pathway; (2) the oxidant–antioxidant issue; (3) the impact of supplements on clotting, a particular problem for patients with hematologic malignancies on or off anticoagulants, and (4) purity or authenticity of the nutrition or herbal supplement.

Concurrent use of a supplement, particularly a botanical, with chemotherapy could lead to a clinically important interaction that could yield an increase or decrease in the effects of either component. Considering that 35% of currently prescribed oncology drugs are metabolized by the CYP3A4 isoform of the hepatic cytochrome p450 enzyme system, use of supplements that either induce or inhibit the pathway can be problematic.[40] In treatment of hematologic toxicities, cyclophosphamide, the epipodophyllotoxins, and the vinca alkaloids are all dependent of CYP3A4 for their metabolism. For example, the botanical supplement St. John's wort used for the treatment of mild depression is a strong inducer of many CYP isoforms. In a classic pharmacokinetic interaction study, 10 healthy volunteers were administered a single 400-mg oral dose of imatinib before and after 2 weeks of treatment with 300 mg of St. John's wort three times daily. The investigators found that the pharmacokinetics of imatinib were significantly altered by St. John's wort, with reductions of 32% in the median area under the concentration–time curve ($p = .0001$), 29% in maximum observed concentration ($p = .005$), and 21% in half-life ($p = .0001$). The conclusion was that coadministration of St. John's wort might compromise the clinical efficacy of imatinib. It is generally recommended that cancer patients receiving any intervention avoid taking St. John's wort.

Patients with hematologic malignancies are often at increased risk for bleeding problems. A small case series performed among children with cancer suggests that the Chinese herb Yunnan Baiyao may alleviate uncontrollable bleeding in patients with cancer; however, clinical trials are not yet available to confirm the findings of this case series. There has been a long-standing tendency to attribute thrombocytopenias of unclear etiology in cancer patients to botanical supplements that they are taking, particularly traditional Chinese medicine herbs. It is critical that the use of Chinese herbal products is accompanied by a certificate of authenticity to ensure purity and absence of contamination.

Warfarin is a frequently prescribed anticoagulant, itself derived from a botanical, which can be impacted in a number of ways by diet and dietary supplements. Inappropriate control of anticoagulation because of fluctuation in warfarin effect exposes the patient to risks of increased bleeding or thromboembolic complications. Warfarin is metabolized by the cytochrome p450 system isoforms, including CYP3A4. In addition, it is also highly protein bound and hence can interact with medications or supplements that are also highly protein bound, resulting in displacement and causing increases in international normalized ratio (INR) and necessitating warfarin dose reduction. Finally, the anticoagulant effect of warfarin can be antagonized by vitamin K intake. Patients prescribed warfarin are often advised not to eat green leafy and cruciferous vegetables or to consume green tea because they are rich in vitamin K and might interfere with the anticoagulant effect. An alternative is to allow the patient to consume a healthful diet and adjust the warfarin dose accordingly to maintain the desired INR.

Omega-3 Fatty Acids

Fish oil is the most commonly used natural product among adults and its use has increased from the 2007 to 2012 NHIS survey. Omega-3 fatty acids have been reported in isolated cases to potentiate the anticoagulant effects of warfarin. Omega-3 fatty acids may lower thromboxane A_2 levels within the platelet as well as decrease factor VII levels. These factors, which make the omega-3s attractive as antiinflammatory and cardiovascular agents, need to be borne in mind in patients on warfarin therapy. Taken in the absence of warfarin, omega-3s are not believed to be a significant cause of bleeding at doses of less than 4000 mg/day. Epidemiologic data suggest an inverse relationship between the intake of marine omega-3 fatty acids and the development of a number of hematologic malignancies and the good risk-to-benefit profile.

The role of omega-3 fatty acids may be instrumental in symptom management among individuals with hematologic malignancies. Evidence suggests that doses of up to 4000 mg/day may help alleviate nausea/vomiting associated with cancer therapy. Studies have been performed in both adults and children with cancer. Other studies suggest that omega-3 fatty acids may help prevent cognitive decline in children who have received whole body radiation. While the latter is still in its infancy, evidence evaluated from the pediatric literature suggest that this may be beneficial for pediatric malignancies as well.

Vitamin D3

Vitamin D is one of the few remaining vitamins that has not been shown to be ineffective in protecting against malignant disease. An ongoing randomized clinical trial is currently looking at a two-by-two factorial design of omega-3 fatty acids and vitamin D3 supplementation in older adults to assess cancer risk reduction, among other endpoints. At the same time, increasing evidence suggests that vitamin D deficiency may be related to the risk of a number of solid tumors, particularly breast, colon, prostate, and pancreas. An inverse relationship has been described between the development of NHL and sun exposure, particularly recreational, nonoccupational sun exposure. One proposed explanation for this unexpected finding is that sun exposure is actually a surrogate marker of vitamin D status, and it is actually vitamin D sufficiency that is protective against lymphoma.[41] In a metaanalysis of eight studies to date, the investigators found no conclusive evidence that vitamin D was providing the observed benefit, although serum levels were not available in any of the studies. Hence it may be appropriate in view of the widespread incidence of vitamin D insufficiency, especially in older adults, for integrative oncologists to measure 25-hydroxy-vitamin D levels in patients with hematologic malignancies and supplement with a fat-soluble vitamin D3 preparation to bring the levels into sufficient or optimal range. Moreover, with the inclusion of high-dose steroids for many hematologic malignancies, adequate D3 becomes essential in the maintenance of bone health during and after treatment.

Preclinical evidence suggests that vitamin D may have a role in the treatment of hematologic malignancies.[42,43] A recent review on the role of vitamin D for the treatment of AML and ALL concluded that differentiation-based therapy may be further enhanced by the addition of vitamin D. To date, there are no published clinical trials describing the use of vitamin D for the treatment of hematologic cancers. Most clinical studies have explored its effect on treatment-related toxicities especially among children and adolescents with ALL. While data appears encouraging, additional trials are necessary before the inclusion of vitamin D3 into the standard of care for hematologic malignancies.

Green Tea

Green tea (Camellia sinensis) is an increasingly consumed beverage being sought after for multiple potential beneficial health effects. An inhibitor of CYP3A4 metabolism as well as a potent source of vitamin K, green tea may interact with prescribed anticancer drugs or anticoagulant therapies. However, green tea polyphenols have been shown to have antiproliferative activity against a wide variety of cell lines, including CLL,[44] multiple myeloma, and human promyelocytic leukemia HL-60. Epigallocatechin-3-gallate (EGCG) is the specific green tea polyphenol that is an antioxidant with chemopreventive and chemotherapeutic actions. Present in situ in the beverage, EGCG has also been prepared as green tea extract (GTE) supplements and even more concentrated EGCG capsules that patients can purchase in health food and supplement emporiums. The publication of the CLL data has led to increased use of EGCG in patients with low-grade lymphomas. A phase I study in patients with asymptomatic stage 0 to II CLL demonstrated that the Polyphenon E preparation use was well tolerated in 33 participants and that the majority of participants had decreased total lymphocyte counts, lymphadenopathy, or both (NCT00262743). Of note, when taken on an empty stomach, GTE preparations have been associated with a risk of hepatotoxicity. The question of whether health benefits against hematologic malignancies can be achieved by simply drinking an as yet undetermined quantity of the beverage or higher dose preparations such as GTE or EGCG is not known.

Patients with multiple myeloma are now frequently advised by their oncologists not to consume green tea at all because of its potential to negate the treatment effects of bortezomib, found in mouse studies.

Other commonly used OTC products include turmeric, melatonin, medicinal mushrooms, and Chinese herbs. Studies are being conducted regarding their efficacy and safety.

Antioxidants

Antioxidants (e.g., beta-carotene; lycopene; vitamins C, E, and A) are substances that counteract free radicals and prevent them from causing tissue and organ damage. They are among the most common classes of supplements used by patients with hematologic malignancies. Their use is directed for cytotoxic effects, for synergy with conventional therapy, or to lessen the toxicity of conventional therapy. Estimates of antioxidant use by patients with cancer have varied considerably, with rates ranging from 13% to 87% depending on the survey, the type of disease studied, and a variety of other individual and demographic factors.[45] Specific prevalence data on the use of antioxidants among patients with only hematologic malignancies has generally not been reported in the surveys. With survival of childhood ALL exceeding 90% for standard-risk groups, extreme caution should be exercised in combining antioxidant supplementation with the effective treatment.

Evidence supporting the potential role of antioxidants in preventing and treating disease include preclinical studies. These studies have correlated oxidative stress and an antioxidant-depleted diet with the development of diseases, including cancer. Increased consumption of green tea (which contains the anticarcinogenic agent, EGCG) has been associated with a reduced incidence of leukemia. In addition, decreases in antioxidant enzymes or the micronutrients thiol, vitamin E, vitamin C, beta-carotene, or zinc and increases in the production of reactive oxygen species have been reported in leukemia patients. In one study in children with ALL, higher levels of oxidative stress at diagnosis were associated with a poor prognosis.

In another prospective observational study conducted among children with ALL, low plasma[46] and dietary antioxidant[47] levels directly correlated with treatment-related toxicity. These types of data have led many patients with hematologic malignancies to take antioxidant supplements primarily in conjunction with conventional cancer treatment.

Much of the controversy surrounding antioxidants and cancer therapy has arisen because radiation therapy and certain classes of chemotherapy agents exert some of their anticancer effects through the generation of reactive oxygen species or free radicals. Some of these agents include the anthracyclines (e.g., doxorubicin), platinum-containing complexes (e.g., cisplatin and carboplatin), and alkylating agents (e.g., cyclophosphamide and ifosfamide). The theoretical concern is that antioxidants might somehow interfere with or counteract the activities of these anticancer agents. However, to date, preclinical experiments and clinical studies have not definitively shown impact on treatment outcome.[48] Of particular note, an observational cohort study from the Fred Hutchinson Cancer Research Center in Seattle evaluating the prevalence of supplement use in persons before receiving hematopoietic stem cell transplant (HSCT) and the association of select supplements with outcomes found that pretransplant intake of vitamin C ($\geq$500 mg/day) or vitamin E ($\geq$400 IU/day) was associated with increased risk of relapse or mortality.[49] Others have reported deficiencies before and immediately after HSCT.[50] However, few clinical studies have built upon observational studies. One small study performed among patients with AML and ALL undergoing HSCT (NCT01432873) randomized adults (n = 77) to selenium (200 μg, twice daily) or placebo beginning on the day of conditioning therapy and continuing to day 14 post-HSCT. No effect on proinflammatory cytokines were observed.[51] Another small study investigated the addition of vitamin C to conventional treatment for acute promyelocytic leukemia; no beneficial effects on outcome were observed.[52]

Recent studies have shown interactions of antioxidant supplements with the proteasome inhibitor bortezomib. Vitamin C, at orally achievable concentrations (equivalent to 1 g/day, a dose frequently used by patients), inhibited the in vitro multiple myeloma cell cytotoxicity of bortezomib and blocked its inhibitory effect on 20S proteasome activity. In addition, green tea polyphenols and dietary supplements carrying hydroxyl groups, including flavonoid compounds such as quercetin, bind and inhibit the activity of bortezomib on malignant B cells and multiple myeloma cells in vitro, although by mechanisms independent of their antioxidant activity. Taken together, these studies suggest that antioxidant supplements should be avoided in patients taking bortezomib and other boronic acid proteasome inhibitor therapy.

The precise role of antioxidant supplementation in the patients with hematologic malignancies remains to be determined. Studies adequately evaluating the impact of supplementation on toxicity and disease-free survival have not yet adequately demonstrated that the benefits of supplementation clearly outweigh the risks; therefore the possibility of harm must be strongly considered (Box 156.1). Recommendations for clinical practice at the present time include the following:

- Patients should be advised to avoid dietary antioxidant supplements above the basic nutritional requirements as defined by the National Academy of Science, Dietary Reference Intakes during radiation therapy and stem cell transplantation. Until safety data is available, doses should not exceed the upper tolerable limit during treatment.
- Patients should avoid dietary antioxidant supplements while receiving bortezomib and other boronic acid proteasome inhibitor therapy. Counseling patients to avoid supplementation while receiving chemotherapy associated with high oxidative stress (anthracyclines, alkylating agents, platinum-containing agents, topoisomerase I and II inhibitors) is encouraged.
- Use of antioxidant supplements while receiving chemotherapy associated with low oxidative stress (purine or pyrimidine analogues, antimetabolites, monoclonal antibodies, vinca alkaloids,

taxanes, and corticosteroids) is less likely to be associated with interactions. Caution should be taken with other agents (e.g., antiangiogenic agents, tyrosine kinase inhibitors) for which there is insufficient information.

REFERENCES

1. Schultz AM, Chao SM, McGinnis JM: *Integrative medicine and the health of the public: a summary of the February 2009 summit*, Washington, DC, Institute of Medicine, 2009, National Academies Press.
2. McGuire S: *Complementary and alternative medicine in the United States*, Washington, DC, 2005, National Academies Press. Institute of Medicine.
3. Clarke TC, Black LI, Stussman BJ, et al: *Trends in the use of complementary health approaches among adults: United States 2002-2012*, National Health Statistics Report; no 79, Hyattsville, MD, National Center for Health Statistics, 2015.
4. Gansler T, Kaw C, Crammer C, et al: A population-based study of prevalence of complementary methods use by cancer survivors: a report from the American Cancer Society's studies of cancer survivors. *Cancer* 113:1048, 2008.
5. Snyderman R, Weil AT: Integrative medicine: bringing medicine back to its roots. *Arch Intern Med* 162:395, 2002.
6. Eisenberg DM, Kessler RC, Van Rompay M, et al: Perceptions about complementary therapies relative to conventional therapies among adults who use both; results from a national survey. *Ann Intern Med* 135:344, 2001.
7. Sparreboom A: Herbal remedies in the United States: potential interactions with anticancer agents. *J Clin Oncol* 22:2489, 2004.
8. Kelly KM: Bringing evidence to complementary and alternative medicine in children with cancer: Focus on nutrition-related therapies. *Pediatr Blood Cancer* 50:490, 2008. discussion 8.
9. Sencer SF, Kelly KM: Bringing evidence to complementary and alternative medicine for children with cancer. *J Pediatr Hematol Oncol* 28:186, 2006.
10. Valji R, Adams D, Daganis S, et al: Complementary and alternative medicine: a survey of its use in pediatric oncology. *Evid Based Complement Alternat Med* 2013:527163, 2013.
11. O.Connor N, Graham D, O'Meara A, et al: The use of complementary and alternative medicine by Irish pediatric patients. *J Pediatr Hematol Oncol* 35:537–542, 2013.
12. Wesa KM, Cassileth BR: Is there a role for complementary therapy in the management of leukemia? *Expert Rev Anticancer Ther* 9:1241, 2009.
13. Barton DL, Loprinzi C, Jatoi A, et al: Can complementary and alternative medicine clinical cancer research be successfully accomplished? The Mayo Clinic-North Central Cancer Treatment Group experience. *J Soc Integr Oncol* 4:143, 2006.
14. Verhoef MJ, Leis A: From studying patient treatment to studying patient care: arriving at methodologic crossroads. *Hematol Oncol Clin North Am* 22:671, viii–ix, 2008.
15. Yeung KS, Gubili J, Cassileth B: Evidence-based botanical research: applications and challenges. *Hematol Oncol Clin North Am* 22:661. viii, 2008.
16. Weiger W, Smith M, Boon H, et al: Advising patients who seek complementary and alternative medical therapies for cancer. *Ann Intern Med* 137:889, 2002.
17. Gordon JS: Mind-body medicine and cancer. *Hematol Oncol Clin North Am* 22:683. ix, 2008.
18. Dusek J, et al: Stress management versus life-style modification on systolic hypertension and medication elimination, a randomized trial. *J Altern Complement Med* 2:129–138, 2008.
19. Niles H, Mehta DH, Corrigan AA, et al: Functional genomics in the study of mind-body therapies. *Ochsner J* 14:681–695, 2014.
20. Rossman M, Shrock D: Mind-body medicine in integrative cancer care. In Abrams D, Weil A, editors: *Integrative oncology*, New York, 2009, Oxford University Press, p 244.
20a. Park ER, et al: A relaxation response training for women undergoing breast biopsy: exploring integrated care. *Breast* 22(5):799–805, 2013.

20b. Beard C, et al: Effects of complementary therapies on clinical outcomes in patients being treated with radiation therapy for prostate cancer. *Cancer* 117(1):96–102, 2011.

21. Jenson M, Patterson D: Hypnotic approaches for chronic pain management. *Am Psychol* (69):167–177, 2014.

22. White J, Flohr JA, Winter SS, et al: Potential benefits of physical activity for children with acute lymphoblastic leukemia. *Pediatr Rehabil* 8:53, 2005.

23. Lu W, Dean-Clower E, Doherty-Gilman A, et al: The value of acupuncture in cancer care. *Hematol Oncol Clin North Am* 22:631. viii, 2008.

24. Lu W, Hu D, Dean-Clower E, et al: Acupuncture for chemotherapy-induced leukopenia: exploratory meta-analysis of randomized controlled trials. *J Soc Integr Oncol* 5:1, 2007.

25. Lu W, Matulonis UA, Doherty-Gilman A, et al: Acupuncture for chemotherapy-induced neutropenia in patients with gynecologic malignancies: a pilot randomized, sham-controlled clinical trial. *J Altern Complement Med* 15:745, 2009.

26. Lu W, Doherty-Gilman AM, Rosenthal DS: Recent advanced in oncology acupuncture and safety considerations in practice. *Curr Treat Options Oncol* 11:141–146, 2010.

27. Ladas E, Rooney D, Taromina K, et al: The safety of acupuncture in children and adolescents with cancer therapy-related thrombocytopenia. *Support Care Cancer* 18:1487–1490, 2010.

28. Corbin L: Integrative Oncology. In Abrams DI, Weil A, editors: *Massage therapy*, New York, 2009, Oxford University Press.

29. Joske DJL, Rao A, Kristjanson L: Critical review of complementary therapies in haemato-oncology. *Intern Med J* 36:579, 2006.

30. Kushi LH, Byers T, Doyle C, et al: American Cancer Society Guidelines on Nutrition and Physical Activity for cancer prevention: reducing the risk of cancer with healthy food choices and physical activity. *CA Cancer J Clin* 56:254, quiz 313-314, 2006.

31. *American Institute for Cancer Research.* http://www.dietandcancerreport.org/expertreport/report contents/index.php, Washington, DC.

32. Adherence to the World Cancer Research Fund/American Institute for Cancer Research guidelines and risk of death in Europe: results from the European Prospective Investigation into Nutrition and Cancer cohort study1,4. *Am J Clin Nutr* 97(5):1107–1120, 2013.

33. Ligibel JA, Alfano CL, Courneya KS, et al: American Society of Clinical Oncology position statement on obesity and cancer. *J Clin Oncol* 32: 2014.

34. Castillo JJ, et al: Obesity but not overweight increases the incidence and mortality of leukemia in adults: a meta-analysis of prospective cohort studies. *Leuk Res* 36:868–887, 2012.

35. Orgel E, Sposto R, Malvar J, et al: Impact on survival and toxicity by duration of weight extremes during treatment for pediatric acute lymphoblastic leukemia: a report from the Children's Oncology Group. *J Clin Oncol* 32:2014.

36. Lange BJ, Gerbing RB, Feusner J, et al: Mortality in overweight and underweight. children with acute myeloid leukemia. *JAMA* 293:203–211, 2005.

37. Chang ET, Smedby KE, Zhang SM, et al: Dietary factors and risk of non-Hodgkin lymphoma in men and women. *Cancer Epidemiol Biomarkers Prev* 14:512, 2005.

38. Fritschi L, Ambrosini GL, Kliewer EV, et al: Dietary fish intake and risk of leukaemia, multiple myeloma, and non-Hodgkin lymphoma. *Cancer Epidemiol Biomarkers Prev* 13:532, 2004.

39. Heinen MM, Verhage BA, Schouten LJ, et al: Alcohol consumption and risk of lymphoid and myeloid neoplasms: results of the Netherlands cohort study. *Int J Cancer* 133(7):1701–1712, 2013.

40. Abrams DI, Weil A: Integrative oncology. In Sparreboom A, Baker S, editors: *CAM: chemo interactions: what is known*, New York, 2009, Oxford University Press.

41. Kelly JL, Friedberg JW, Calvi LM, et al: Vitamin D and non-Hodgkin lymphoma risk in adults: a review. *Cancer Invest* 27:942, 2009.

42. Studzinski GP, Harrison JS, Wang X, et al: Prospect: "Vitamin D control of hematopoietic cell differentiation and leukemia.". *J Cell Biochem* 116:1500–1512, 2015.

43. Kaste SC, Qi A, Smith K, et al: Calcium and cholecalciferol supplementation provides no added benefit to nutritional counseling to improve bone mineral density in survivors of childhood acute lymphoblastic leukemia (ALL). *Support Care Cancer* 20:3379–3383, 2012.

44. Lee YK, Bone ND, Strege AK, et al: VEGF receptor phosphorylation status and apoptosis is modulated by a green tea component, epigallocatechin-3-gallate (EGCG), in B-cell chronic lymphocytic leukemia. *Blood* 104:788, 2004.

45. Ladas E, Kelly KM: The antioxidant debate. *Explore (NY)* 6:75, 2010.

46. Kennedy DD, Ladas EJ, Rheingold SR, et al: Antioxidant status decreases in children with acute lymphoblastic leukemia during the first six months of chemotherapy treatment. *Pediatr Blood Cancer* 44:378, 2005.

47. Kennedy D, Tucker KL, Ladas E, et al: Low antioxidant vitamin intakes are associated with increases in adverse effects of chemotherapy in children with acute lymphoblastic leukemia. *Am J Clin Nutr* 79:1029, 2004.

48. Lawenda BD, Kelly KM, Ladas EJ, et al: Should supplemental antioxidant administration be avoided during chemotherapy and radiation therapy. *J Natl Cancer Inst* 100:773, 2008.

49. Bruemmer B, Patterson RE, Cheney C, et al: The association between vitamin C and vitamin E supplement use before hematopoietic stem cell transplant and outcomes to two years. *J Am Diet Assoc* 103:982, 2003.

50. Daeian N, Radfar M, Jahangard-Rafsanjani Z, et al: Serial profile of vitamins and trace elements during the acute phase of allogeneic stem cell transplantation. *Biol Blood Marrow Transplant* 20(3):430–434, 2014.

51. Daeian N, Radfar M, Jahangard-Rafsanjani Z, et al: Selenium supplementation in patients undergoing hematopoietic stem cell transplantation: effects on pro-inflammatory cytokines levels. *Daru* 22:51, 2014.

52. Aldoss I, Mark L, Vrona J, et al: Adding ascorbic acid to arsenic trioxide produces limited benefit in patients with acute myeloid leukemia excluding acute promyelocytic leukemia. *Ann Hematol* 93(11):1839–1843, 2014.

CHAPTER 157

HEMATOLOGIC MANIFESTATIONS OF HIV/AIDS

Howard A. Liebman and Anil Tulpule

Human immunodeficiency virus type 1 (HIV-1) is the pathogenic infectious agent responsible for the development of the acquired immunodeficiency syndrome (AIDS). Chronic HIV infection leads to progressive immunodeficiency and immune dysregulation resulting in an increased risk for opportunistic infections, increased incidence of certain malignancies, autoimmune disorders, and varied organ system dysfunction. Although nearly every organ system can be affected by HIV infection, hematologic manifestations involving the bone marrow and peripheral blood occur in all patients in the course of the disease. This chapter will provide a general overview of the epidemiology of AIDS, HIV virology, and immunopathogenesis, and more comprehensive review of the hematologic manifestations of HIV infection.

DEFINITION AND EPIDEMIOLOGY OF HIV INFECTION

Although the original definition of AIDS was based upon clinical symptoms and signs alone, knowledge of the viral pathogenesis has led to a series of revised case definitions by the US Public Health Service (USPHS) and Centers for Disease Control and Prevention (CDC). The present case definition for HIV-1 infection divides the disease into three stages as defined by $CD4^+$ lymphocyte counts and the presence of AIDS-defining conditions (Tables 157.1 and 157.2). A diagnosis of AIDS can be made by recognition of well-characterized clinical symptoms and signs (see Table 157.2) with evidence of HIV infection (clinical AIDS). HIV infection in an individual with a blood CD4 lymphocyte count of less than 0.2×10^9/L classifies the patient as having "immunologic AIDS." With the advent of routine testing for HIV infection in developed countries, a significant proportion of individuals with HIV infection who are receiving highly active antiretroviral therapy (HAART) have little or no clinical manifestations of viral infections and can maintain near normal immunologic function. However, many of the same individuals suffer from HAART-related toxicities. The World Health Organization (WHO) originally used an alternative case definition because of the limited availability of resources for serologic, virologic and immunologic testing of patients in poor countries, but after 2007 required serologic confirmation of HIV-1 infection. Therefore the early estimates of HIV-related disease worldwide were limited by this more clinically based definition.

The CDC estimates the 2013 prevalence of HIV infection in the United States at 1,201,039 Americans age greater than 13 years with a 2013 estimated incidence of 50,000 new infections. The WHO has estimated that there were 2.7 million new HIV infections in 2013 with an estimated prevalence worldwide of 33 to 37 million people infected by HIV, with 2.1 million new infections and 1.5 million HIV-related deaths. Sub-Saharan Africa accounts for 71% of all HIV infections. Vertical transmission from mother to infant continues in Africa and areas in Asia because of a lack of antiviral medications.

A second, but molecular distinct virus, HIV-2, is endemic to regions of West Africa. HIV-2 and the simian immunodeficiency virus of sooty mangabeys are essentially identical, confirming its simian origin that subsequently crossed over into man. Less is known about the epidemiology of HIV-2, but infection appears to result in a less virulent clinical course than HIV-1 infection. Despite being structurally closely related to HIV-1, infection with HIV-2 does not provide protection against HIV-1 infection and coinfection is frequent in sex workers in West Africa.

TRANSMISSION OF HIV-1

HIV-1 may be transmitted by sexual contact with an infected individual, by use of contaminated needle in parenteral drug use, exposure to infected blood products, or by prenatal transmission from infected mother to her infant.

HIV-1 has been recovered from both semen of HIV-infected men and from cervical and vaginal secretions of HIV-infected women. The virus can be detected in seminal fluid during the first 4 weeks of infection. Several factors are associated with increased viral content of seminal fluid including advanced symptomatic HIV infection, higher plasma viral loads, CD4 lymphocyte counts less than 0.2×10^9/L, the presence of leukocytes in the seminal fluid, and HAART. Factors that influence the levels of HIV-1 in female vaginal secretions include advanced HIV stage of HIV infection, menstruation, concomitant vaginal infection, ulcerative and nonulcerative sexually transmitted diseases, and a high HIV-1 viral plasma load. Prevention and treatment of sexually transmitted disease has been associated with a decrease in HIV-1 transmission.

The risk of HIV infection with transfusion of a single unit of infected blood is estimated at greater than 90%. The use of coagulation factor concentrate prepared before routine screening of blood products for HIV-1 in the United States resulted in a sadly high incidence of HIV infection in patients with congenital bleeding disorders. With active blood product screening and inactivation protocols used in the preparation of coagulation factor concentrate, HIV transmission has been essentially eliminated. With screening of all blood units in the United States, receipt of a unit of screened blood is associated with an estimated risk of transmission of approximately 1 in 500,000.

HIV-1 may be transmitted to a fetus or infant from the mother in utero, at the time of delivery, or postpartum through breastfeeding. The risk is greatest when the mother has advanced HIV disease, higher HIV viral load in the plasma, and active injection drug use. At time of delivery, active chorioamnionitis, premature rupture of amniotic membranes (>4 hours) and vaginal delivery, as opposed to elective cesarean section, have been associated with an increased risk of maternal-infant transmission. Prematurity, low gestational age, and breastfeeding have been reported as risk factors for HIV transmission. The use of antiretroviral agents in pregnancy, delivery, and during the first 6 weeks of life has resulted in a significant reduction in transmission from an estimated 25% to 8% with zidovudine alone and ever greater benefit with the use of HAART. To date, except for the use of efavirenz, there is no evidence to suggest an increased risk of congenital birth defects with the use of antiretroviral agents for this indication. The use of antiretroviral therapy during pregnancy has resulted in a nearly 50% reduction in the number of children with perinatal acquired HIV infection. The WHO reported that in 2013, 67% of pregnant women living with HIV infection in low- and middle-income countries are receiving some form of effective HIV prophylaxis.

Transmission can also occur by the sharing of needles and syringes between injection drug user. The use of cocaine and other

TABLE 157.1	Surveillance Case Definition for HIV Infection in Adults and Adolescents (Age >13 Years)	
Stage	**Laboratory Evidence**	**Clinical Evidence**
Stage 1	Laboratory confirmation of HIV infection and CD4+ T lymphocyte count of ≥500 cells/μL or CD4+ T-lymphocyte percentage of ≥29%[a]	No AIDS-defining condition (see Table 157.2)
Stage 2	Laboratory confirmation of HIV infection and CD4+ T lymphocyte count of 200–499 cells/μL or CD4+ T-lymphocyte percentage of 14–28%[a]	No AIDS-defining condition (see Table 157.2)
Stage 3	Laboratory confirmation of HIV infection and CD4+ T lymphocyte count of <200 cells/μL or CD4+ T-lymphocyte percentage of <14%[a]	Documentation of an AIDS-defining condition with laboratory confirmation of HIV infection (see Table 157.2)
Stage unknown	Laboratory confirmation of HIV infection and no information on CD4+ T-lymphocyte count or percentage	No information on presence of an AIDS-defining condition

[a]The CD4+ T-lymphocyte percentage is percentage of the total lymphocyte count.

TABLE 157.2	Surveillance Definitions of AIDS-Defining Conditions

Opportunistic Infections:
Pneumocystis jirovecii (carinii)
Mycobacterium avium complex
Mycobacterium tuberculosis
Toxoplasmosis
Candidiasis: esophageal and systemic
Histoplasmosis
Cryptococcosis
Cryptosporidiosis and isosporiasis
Leishmaniasis
Cytomegalovirus disease
Recurrent bacterial infections (≥2 episodes/year)

Lymphomas
Kaposi Sarcoma
Cervical Cancer
AIDS Dementia Syndrome
Wasting Syndrome

noninjection drugs can be associated with an increased risk of HIV infection in that their use is frequently associated with high-risk sexual behaviors. Needlestick exposures can also result in transmission of HIV from infected patients to health care workers. The risk of transmission is increased if the patient who is the source of the contaminated needle has more advanced disease with a high plasma viral load, if the needle injury is deep, if there is visible blood on the needle, or if the injury directly enters a vein or artery. The estimated risk of acquiring HIV is approximately 0.3% per needle injury exposure if the source of the blood is a patient with advanced HIV infection (stage 3 AIDS). The use of a 4-week course of antiretroviral therapy as postexposure prophylaxis has been shown to significantly reduce the risk of transmission. Prophylaxis using drug regimens recommended by the CDC should be initiated within 72 hours of exposure and

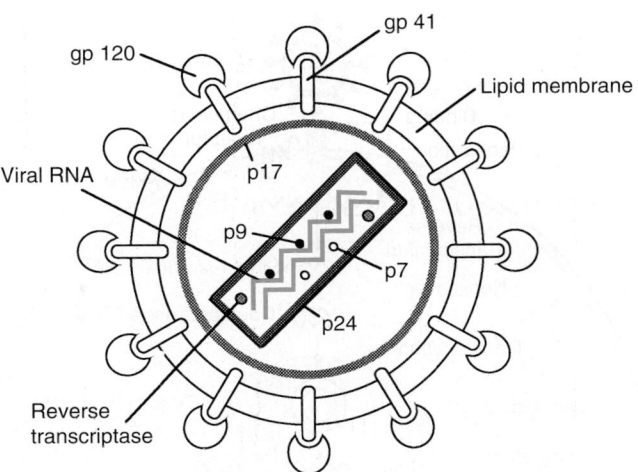

Fig. 157.1 STRUCTURE OF THE HIV VIRION. Two coding strands of genomic ribonucleic acid (RNA) are packaged in the nucleoid core with p7, p9, and p24 proteins and reverse transcriptase. The core is surrounded by the p17 matrix protein lining the inner surface of the envelope. The envelope consists of a lipid bilayer derived from the infected cell and glycoprotein spikes that consist of the outer glycoprotein (GP) 120 molecule, which contains the binding site for CD4, and GP41, which anchors the glycoprotein complex to the envelope and mediates fusion of the viral membrane with the cell membrane during viral penetration.

continued for a duration that is based upon the stage of the patient who was the source of the exposure and the type of exposure.

ETIOLOGY AND PATHOGENSIS

Human Immunodeficiency Virus 1

HIV-1 is a member of the primate *Lentivirinae* subfamily of retroviruses.[3] Retroviruses are RNA viruses that induce a chronic cellular infection by converting their RNA genome into a DNA provirus that is integrated into the genome of the host cell. The genome of the virus contains three major genes necessary for viral replication and cellular invasion. The *env* gene codes for a 160-kDa precursor protein which is processed into a 120-kDa surface glycoprotein (GP) noncovalently linked to a 41-kDa transmembrane protein. The GP120–GP41 complex is necessary for virus binding to CD4 and CCR5 on the cell membrane and fusion of the viral envelope with the cell membrane allowing for the release of the viral genome into the host cell. The *gag* gene codes for the four viral structural core proteins. These proteins form the nucleocapsid for the viral genome and assist in assembly of the replicating virus before viral release from the cell membrane. The *pol* gene codes for three functional enzymes; a reverse transcriptase necessary for formation of the proviral double-stranded DNA, an integrase necessary for stable integration of the proviral DNA into the host cellular DNA, and viral protease necessary for processing viral membrane and core proteins (Figs. 157.1 and 157.2).

In addition to these three essential genes, the 9-kDa genome of HIV-1 contains six additional genes (*VIF, VPU, VPR, TAT, REV, NEF*) necessary for the regulation of viral gene expression, cellular latency, and each gene product playing an important role in the life cycle of HIV.

Life Cycle of HIV-1 (Fig. 157.3)

Cellular infections begin with engagement of HIV-1 GP120 binding to CD4 surface membrane protein resulting in a conformational change in GP120 allowing for further high affinity binding to chemokine CCR5 receptor. Thymic helper-inducer (CD4) lymphocytes, macrophage-monocytes, Langerhans cells, follicular dendritic cells,

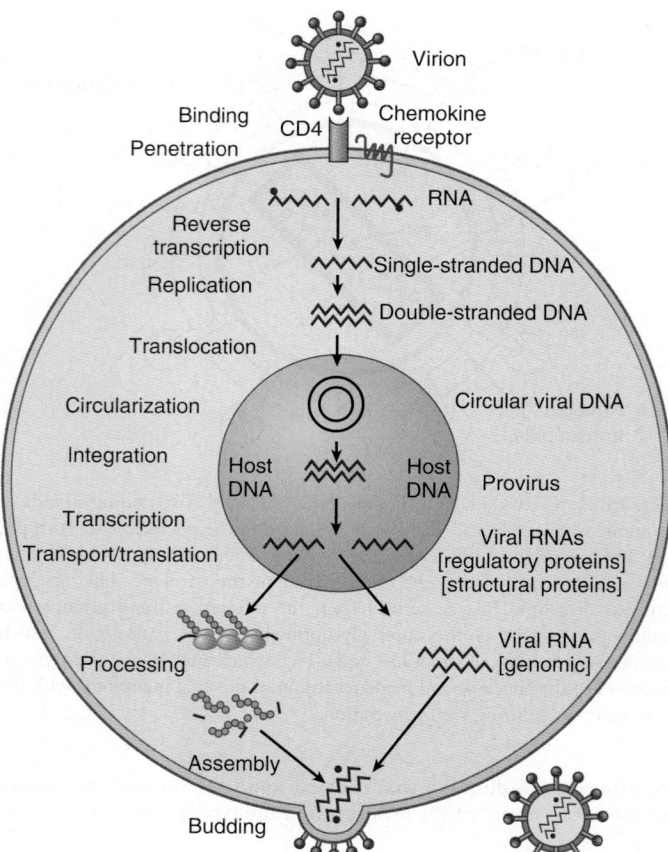

Fig. 157.2 HIV LIFE CYCLE. Binding of the virion to the cell surface is mediated by a specific interaction of the glycoprotein (GP) 120 envelope glycoprotein with cellular CD4 and members of the chemokine receptor family of proteins (CCR5 or CXCR4). Penetration occurs as the viral membrane fuses with the cellular membrane in a process that requires the GP41 transmembrane protein. The viral capsid is uncoated, and viral genomic ribonucleic acid (RNA) is reverse transcribed and duplicated by the viral reverse transcriptase to produce a double-stranded copy of viral deoxyribonucleic acid (DNA). The viral DNA is transported to the nucleus, where it integrates into the host chromosomes. After appropriate activating signals, the provirus is transcribed by cellular RNA polymerase and transported to the cytoplasm. Proteins are translated and processed through biochemical steps that, depending on the protein, involve glycosylation (GP120 and GP41), cleavage (envelope proteins, gag, pol), myristoylation (p17), and phosphorylation (rev, nef). Packaging of genomic RNA with viral proteins occurs as envelope glycoproteins are inserted into the cell membrane and new virion subsequently buds outward from the plasma membrane. Viral protease continues protein processing to completion during viral budding.

megakaryocytes, and thymic cells express both CD4 and CCR5 receptor molecules and are susceptible to HIV-1 infection. Rare individuals who are homozygotes for the delta32 deletion in CCR5 are highly resistant to HIV-1 infection. The structural diversity of GP120 viral receptors has resulted in HIV-1 strains with selective or restricted patterns of infection with strains that readily infect monocytes, whereas others are tropic for CD4 lymphocytes. Some CD4+ tropic strains may also use the CXC4 chemokine receptor in addition to the CCR5 receptor. With advanced late stage HIV infection, such individuals are more likely to have viral strains capable of infecting cells expressing either chemokine receptor.

Upon binding to the CD4 and CCR5 receptors, the viral transmembrane GP41 mediates fusion with the host cell membrane. The internalized viral nucleocapsid dissociates after binding to cellular cyclophilin, releasing the diploid viral RNA genome that is associated with the viral reverse transcriptase. Reverse transcription proceeds to synthesis of a single strain of complementary DNA, followed by

degradation of the viral RNA by ribonuclease H activity of p66. The reverse transcriptase then acts as a DNA polymerase forming a double-stranded DNA provirus. The reverse transcriptase of HIV has a significant rate of base substitution errors, estimated as high as 1 in 1700 to 1 in 2000 nucleoside bases, resulting in an average of 5 to 10 nucleoside mutations for each replication cycle. This explains the high degree of genomic diversity observed between HIV-1 viral isolates.

A linear form of the provirus is integrated into the host DNA by the viral integrase. In kinetic studies of HIV-1 infection, viral DNA is present in the cytoplasm within 2 to 3 hours of infection, and viral nuclear DNA has been detected by 24 hours. The gene product of *VPR* assists in transport of the viral pro-DNA into the nucleus for subsequent integration. After integration of the viral genome, the HIV-1 infected cell may develop either a latent or persistent form of infection.

HIV-1 does not replicate readily in resting lymphocytes and macrophages. Cellular transactivation by, for example, nuclear factor kappa-B (NFκB) can enhance proviral transcription. HIV-1 proviral transcription leads to the expression of regulatory proteins tat, rev, and nef. Tat is a protein essential for HIV replication and in conjunction with the cellular proteins TAK (Tat associated kinase) and Cyc T (cyclin T) promotes viral RNA elongation resulting in a 1000-fold increase in HIV-1 expression. Rev is a viral protein that is also essential for replication by regulating nuclear export of unspliced viral RNA. Nef and vpu proteins modulate the downregulation of cellular CD4.

The structural proteins of the *GAG*, *POL*, and *ENV* genes are expressed as precursor proteins and subsequently cleaved by viral protease yielding mature viral proteins. This final step in protein processing is essential for the assembly of mature infectious virus. For this reason, inhibition of the viral protease has proven a fruitful target for HAART. The products of the *ENV* gene, GP120 and GP 41, are transported to the cell membrane and the assembled ribonucleoprotein core moved from the cytoplasm to the membrane surface for subsequent budding. The efficient packaging of the viral RNA is dependent upon packaging signals in the Gag region of the viral RNA. Final budding is dependent upon the product of the *VPU* gene that also assists in transport of ENV products to the cell membrane and association with the ribonucleoprotein core.

Pathogenesis of HIV Infection

HIV infection results in progressive immunodeficiency and immune dysregulation. By progressive depletion of helper CD4 thymic lymphocytes, there is decreased response to soluble antigens, decreased helper response to immunoglobulin (Ig) synthesis, and impaired delayed hypersensitivity. Decreased γ interferon (IFN) production leads to a decreased cytoplasmic killing of intracellular organisms. There is also defective natural killer function and decreased T-lymphocyte–mediated cytotoxicity of viral infected cells. An imbalance of CD4, CD25[bright], Foxp2+ regulatory cells, and CD4/interleukin (IL)-17 lymphocytes may result in the expression of autoreactive T and B lymphocytes accounting for the increased incidence of autoimmune disorders associated with HIV infection and defective CD8 responses against HIV-infected lymphocytes. Viral expression in activated CD4 lymphocytes results in rapid cell death; whereas infection of macrophages, dendritic cells, and nonreplicating CD4 lymphocytes accounts for a persistent and long-lived reservoir of HIV-1 infected cells. High-level viral replication and budding associated with potent immunostimulation from acute and chronic infections may contribute to accelerated lymphocyte cytotoxicity.

In addition to the direct cytopathic effect of viral replication in CD4 lymphocytes, formation of syncytial multinucleated giant cells by fusion of infected CD4 lymphocytes expressing GP120 on their membrane with uninfected CD4+ lymphocytes, is another mechanism for CD4 depletion. Viral strains capable of forming such syncytia in vitro appear to be associated with a more aggressive clinical course.

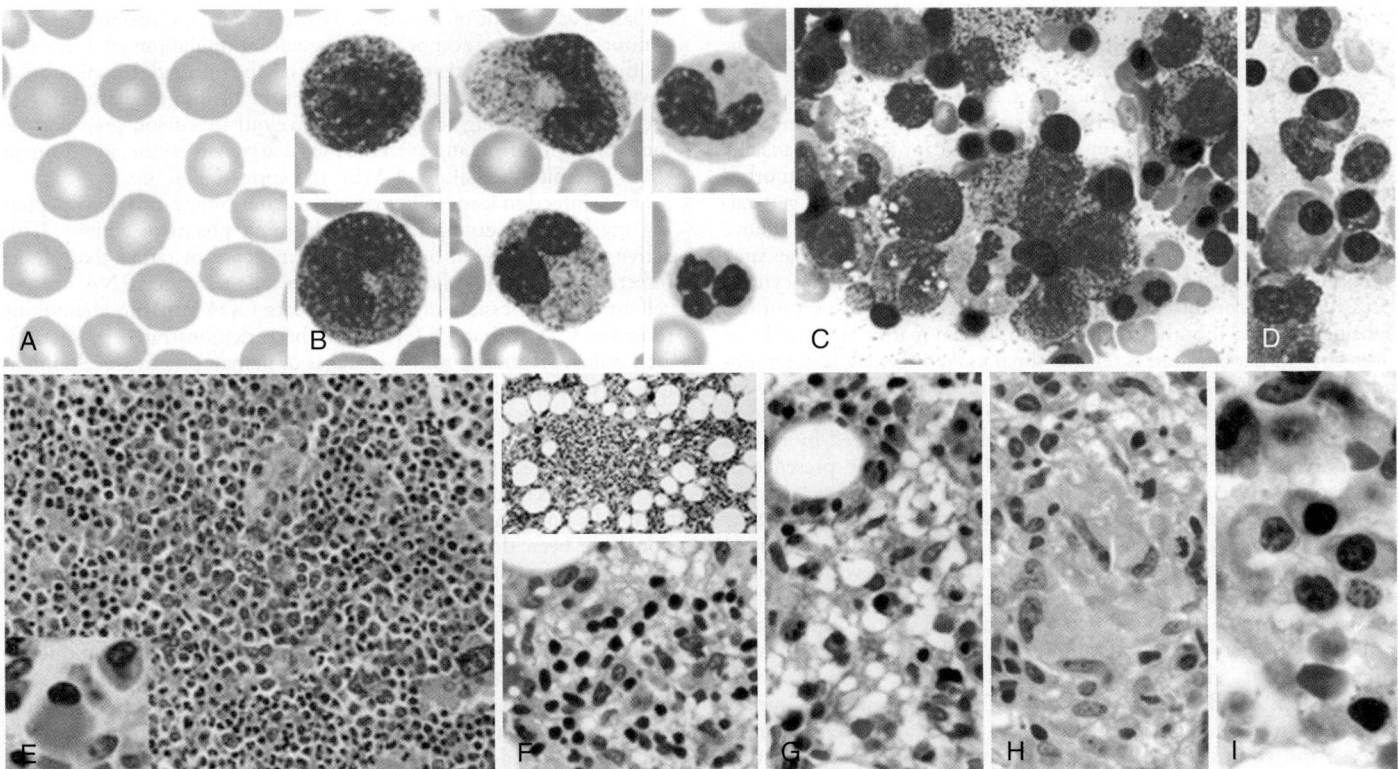

Fig. 157.3 TYPICAL PERIPHERAL BLOOD AND BONE MARROW FINDINGS IN HIV. The peripheral smear not uncommonly shows anemia, which is sometimes macrocytic (A), but can be normochromic and normocytic. There frequently is a neutrophilia with left shift, toxic granulation, and some mild dysplastic change in the granulocytes (B). In some patients, particularly those with severe disease, some of the segmented neutrophils show cytoplasmic inclusions similar to Howell-Jolly bodies seen in red cells (B, *top, right cell*). These are nuclear in origin and are not microorganisms. The bone marrow can show granulocytic hyperplasia with left shift and megaloblastoid change in the myeloid and erythroid cell lines (C). Typically, there is also a reactive plasmacytosis (D). The biopsy specimen can be hypocellular, normocellular, or hypercellular (E) and commonly shows cellular atypia/dysplasia (*insert*) and atypical reactive lymphoid infiltrates (F), poorly formed (G) or well-formed granuloma (H), and increased plasma cells (I).

The host immunologic response against HIV-infected lymphocytes by cytotoxic T lymphocytes and antibody-mediated cellular cytotoxicity may also contribute to CD4 lymphocyte loss in HIV disease. Some CD4 lymphocytes may also be destroyed by an "innocent bystander" mechanism secondary to the binding of free GP120 to their surface CD4 protein. In vitro studies have found that binding of the GP120 with anti-GP120 antibodies to the CD4 receptor can induce programmed cell death or apoptosis in the lymphocyte. Defective production of immune-stimulatory cytokines (IL-2) production and expression of inhibitors of T-lymphocyte proliferation such as transforming growth factor-β (TGF-β) may also contribute to the progressive loss of CD4 lymphocytes.

The development of progressive CD4 lymphocyte depletion and its resulting immunodeficiency is closely linked to the degree of viral production. The level of plasma HIV-1 viral RNA, in addition to the CD4 lymphocyte count, is a major prognostic indicator of disease progression. The advent of HAART capable of marked suppression of viral replication has radically changed the natural history of HIV infection. Efficient viral suppression with reduction in blood and tissue viral reservoirs has resulted in prolonged immunologic reconstitution characterized by increased CD4 lymphocyte numbers, reduced opportunistic infections, and prolonged survival. However, significant immune defects do persist and complete immunologic reconstitution with normal immune regulation does not occur.

There appears to be a more selective effect of HIV cytotoxicity on memory CD4 lymphocytes and Th1 lymphocyte subsets. This contributes to a profound imbalance in host immune responses with resulting B lymphocyte dysregulation leading to polyclonal hypergammaglobulinemia and defective cellular immune responses against malignant or viral infected cells (including HIV-infected lymphocytes). Infection of monocytes, macrophages, and dendritic cells not only provides a long-lived reservoir for HIV, but further contributes to the immunologic dysfunction caused by their role in antigen presentation and cytokine production.

CLINICAL COURSE OF HIV-1 INFECTION

Serial assessment of HIV-1 RNA in plasma and CD4+ lymphocytes has proven to be a reliable means for following HIV-1 infection and predicting the course of disease in individual patients. The use of HAART has significantly changed the natural history of HIV disease. With active surveillance programs that can find HIV-1 infected individuals before the development of symptomatic disease, the early use of HAART based upon USPHS guidelines has resulted in significant decreases in the incidence of HIV-defining opportunistic infections. Based upon laboratory markers of disease progression, guidelines from the USPHS recommend the initiation of HAART in all symptomatic HIV-1 infected patients and asymptomatic patients with CD4+ lymphocyte counts less than 0.35×10^9/L or when plasma HIV viral load reaches 55×10^6 copies/L or greater. However, earlier institution of HAART after acute HIV infection could result in a more balanced immune reconstitution with less loss of CD4 memory cells.

Three general stages of HIV infection have been characterized that include an acute retroviral syndrome, an asymptomatic stage, and a period of symptomatic conditions which may or may not fulfill criteria for classification as symptomatic AIDS (see Table 157.2). The acute retroviral syndrome occurs in approximately 50% to 80% of newly infected individuals. The onset of symptoms occurs 1 to 3 weeks (range 5 days to 3 months) after primary infection. Symptoms last from 1 to 2 weeks and can include significant fatigue, headache, malaise, fever as high as 40°C, sore throat, and myalgias. A morbilliform rash can be observed in 40% to 50% of patients, with generalized lymphadenopathy occurring toward the end of the acute illness. Symptoms are similar to those observed in other viral syndromes such as mononucleosis. Laboratory findings may include lymphocytosis, occasional neutropenia, and mild thrombocytopenia. Most symptoms subside within a month. However, lymphadenopathy may persist in over 50% of patients and is termed the persistent generalized lymphadenopathy (PGL) syndrome of HIV infection. Patients may be serologically negative during the acute retroviral syndrome and if there is high clinical suspicion, patients should be tested by reverse transcriptase-polymerase chain reaction (PCR) for the presence of plasma virus RNA, which is frequently present in high levels.

With resolution of the acute retroviral syndrome, patients may enter a phase of asymptomatic infection with lower levels of viral replication as determined by their plasma viral load with serologic evidence of infection. Without antiretroviral therapy, this phase may persist for nearly a decade. Progression can be variable and is determined by a variety of viral, immunologic, and host factors. Coinfections with other viruses such a hepatitis B and C, cytomegalovirus (CMV), Epstein-Barr virus (EBV), and herpes viruses can impose additional immunologic stress leading to accelerated progression of disease and additional AIDS-defining clinical conditions. Infection with human herpes virus 8 is associated with the well-characterized AIDS-defining complications of Kaposi sarcoma, primary effusion lymphoma, and multicentric Castleman disease. EBV infection may contribute to the high incidence of lymphoma, including central nervous system lymphomas, observed in the severely immunosuppressed HIV patients.

A distinct subset of HIV-1 infected patients has a significantly slower rate of HIV disease progression and maintains good immunologic function for extended periods without antiretroviral therapy. These individuals, termed long-term nonprogressors, are a population of significant clinical and research interest. They include patients who are heterozygous for the delta 32 deletion in the CCR5 chemokine coreceptors for HIV infection. This mutation is estimated to occur in 15% of white people. Patients with human leukocyte antigen (HLA)-B27 and HLA-B57 also appear to have better control of HIV viral replication and slower disease progression. This may result from an inability of these patients' T regulatory lymphocytes to suppress CD8–cytotoxic lymphocyte HIV-specific responses.

In the absence of antiretroviral therapy, HIV infected patients develop progressive immunodeficiency with the development of opportunistic infections, central and peripheral neurologic symptoms, HIV-associated malignancies, fatigue, weight loss, and a general wasting syndrome (see Table 157.2).

HEMATOLOGIC AND BONE MARROW ABNORMALITIES IN HIV-1 INFECTION

The hallmark of HIV infection is the CD4$^+$ lymphopenia. However, during the course of the disease about 70% to 80% of patients with HIV/AIDS will develop anemia, 50% will develop neutropenia, and 40% will develop thrombocytopenia. The presence of cytopenias in addition to the CD4$^+$ T lymphopenia of HIV disease has long suggested that the suppressive effects of HIV on the hematopoietic compartment are far more broadly based than just a select subset of T cells. A number of studies have assessed the bone marrow microenvironment, the cytokine milieu, and the number and the function of primitive hematopoietic elements in HIV disease. A low fraction of progenitor cells can be infected ex vivo by HIV under some conditions. The growth of these few cells infected by HIV may not be

impaired as a result of infection. However, in vivo infection of progenitor cells rarely if ever occurs. Progenitor populations such as those yielding megakaryocytes or monocytes can be infected. Recent studies have documented infection and depletion of intermediate myeloid precursors, including the common myeloid precursor, granulocyte-monocyte precursor, and even the megakaryocyte-erythroid precursor (MEP) despite the failure of MEP to express CD4.

HIV infection leads to hematopoietic inhibition in vivo by depleting myeloid and erythroid colony-forming precursor activity. This activity may be caused by an indirect mechanism rather than direct infection of CD34$^+$ cells. The presence of messenger RNA for and cell surface expression of HIV receptors CD4 and the chemokine receptors CXCR-4 and CCR-5 have been demonstrated in fractionated cells representing multiple stages of hematopoietic development (see box on Hematologic Manifestations of Human Immunodeficiency Virus/Acquired Immunodeficiency Syndrome). Productive infection by HIV via these receptors is observed with the notable exception of stem cells, in which case the presence of CD4, CXCR-4, and CCR-5 is insufficient for infection.[1] Although direct infection of stem cells does not occur, alterations in stem cell number and function have been documented. HIV replication in the bone marrow microenvironment is believed to be the essential component causing decreased hematopoietic cell production in HIV infection.[2] The exact mechanism by which the microenvironment induces these alterations is unknown. Mononuclear-macrophage cells can develop productive HIV infection and the resultant aberrant release of cytokines, such as TGF-β, tumor necrosis factor-α (TNF-α), and IL-1 can contribute to the suppression of hematopoiesis. TNF-α is a potent mediator of inflammation and host response to infectious diseases, with pleiotropic effects such as tissue damage, caloric wasting, and impairment of hematopoiesis. It has been observed that HIV suppresses hematopoiesis through induction of TNF-α. TNF-binding protein has been shown to reverse in vitro hematopoietic defects.[3] The relationship of virus replication to inducing the hematopoietic defects is most readily apparent in the clinical changes seen when patients initiate potent antiretroviral therapy. When patients begin HAART, an increase in white blood cells (WBCs), polymorphonuclear neutrophils, and platelets in addition to an increase in CD4$^+$ T cells occurs as plasma HIV RNA levels decline.[4] T-cell kinetics studies have demonstrated a markedly shortened half-life of peripheral blood T cells from approximately 82 days to 23 days. Initiation of antiretroviral therapy does not improve lymphocyte half-life. The increase in T-cell numbers in the peripheral blood of patients treated with HAART appears to be a result of improved production, which in turn may be caused by one of several mechanisms: expansion or redistribution of existing subsets of cells or de novo production of T cells from the thymus. The increase in T cells following initiation of HAART is biphasic. In

---

BOX 157.1	**Hematologic Manifestations of Human Immunodeficiency Virus/Acquired Immunodeficiency Syndrome**

In addition to the CD$^+$ T cell lymphopenia, which is the hallmark of HIV infection, other cytopenias are the most common manifestations in these individuals. During the course of the disease thrombocytopenia and neutropenia occurs at a rate of 40% and 50% respectively. Anemia can occur in up to 70%. Direct infection of the hematopoietic stem cells by HIV does not account for the degree of cytopenias seen. In fact, in vivo infection of the stem cells by HIV occurs rarely if ever. However, HIV infection leads to hematopoietic inhibition in vivo by depleting granulocytic, monocytic, erythroid, and megakaryocytic colony forming units. Progenitor populations such as those yielding megakaryocytes and monocytes are infectable. Macrophages in the bone marrow stroma can develop productive HIV infection with the resultant release of cytokines (TGF-β, TNF-α, IL-1) that contribute to suppression of hematopoiesis. Importantly, there are etiologies that are more specific to causing anemia, thrombocytopenia and neutropenia respectively. Hence these entities are discussed separately.

HIV, Human immunodeficiency virus; IL-1, interleukin 1; TGF-β, transforming growth factor β; TNF-α, tumor necrotic factor α.

the interval immediately following the start of therapy, there is a prompt increase in both CD4$^+$ and CD8$^+$ cells that is composed predominantly of cells of a memory phenotype (CD45RO$^+$ or CD45RA$^+$ CD62L$^-$). This increase is slightly different for CD4$^+$ cells, which increase more briskly (0.027/day) and plateau at approximately 3 weeks compared with CD8$^+$ cells (increase of 0.008/day), which plateau at 8 weeks.[5] This increase is thought to be largely caused by redistribution from peripheral tissues, perhaps related to a changing level of activation of the cells with declining viral antigen stimulation. This initial increase in circulating cell numbers does not achieve normal blood levels of lymphocytes. The secondary, much slower phase of T-cell increase tends to be sustained for months to years, with a greater contribution of cells with a naive phenotype (CD45RA$^+$ CD62L$^+$). The naive population rises along with cells bearing the T-cell receptor excision circle, an indicator of recent T-cell receptor rearrangement that accompanies early T-cell differentiation. It is this population that is generally regarded as thymus dependent and that is capable of truly expanding the immune repertoire. In addition, in vivo models have further defined that T-cell generation, from precursor populations both endogenous and exogenous to the thymus, accompanies control of viremia.

Evaluation of Cytopenias in HIV-Infected Individuals

The evaluation of cytopenias in patients infected with HIV requires a review of complete blood count and thorough examination of the peripheral blood smear (see box on Peripheral Blood Smear and Bone Marrow Morphology in HIV/AIDS). Although there is a gradual fall in CD4$^+$ lymphocytes during the asymptomatic phase of HIV infection, a mild lymphocytosis may at times be seen, caused by an increase in CD8$^+$ lymphocytes. Atypical or activated lymphocytes may frequently be seen. Lymphopenia is present in the advanced stage of the disease. Anemia, when present, is usually normocytic and normochromic. It can be at times macrocytic, either because of the effect of certain antiretroviral drugs such as zidovudine or stavudine, or seen in patients with advanced HIV disease. Occasionally red blood cell (RBC) anisocytosis, poikilocytosis, and rouleaux can sometimes be seen in patients with untreated advanced HIV disease. Also hypogranular neutrophils and Pelger-Huët forms may rarely be present in patients with advanced HIV disease. However, in comparison to patients with myelodysplasia (MDS), agranular neutrophils and neutrophils with the acquired Pelger-Huët anomaly are not a predominant feature in patients with HIV infection. Thrombocytopenia is associated with normal sized platelets, except occasional large platelets may be seen when there is immune-mediated destruction of platelets with preserved marrow function.

The bone marrow in patients with HIV can be hypercellular, normocellular, or hypocellular. In a majority of cases the normal bone marrow architecture is often disturbed, with dysplastic changes similar to those seen in MDS (Fig. 157.4).[6] In Fig. 157.5 are shown additional features seen in the bone marrow of HIV-infected individuals. HIV-associated stromal changes include edema, gelatinous transformation, and increased reticulin fibers. Dense collagen fibrosis, however, is not a feature of the HIV bone marrow. There are some important features distinguishing the morphology of the bone marrow of an HIV-infected individual from that of patients with MDS. Dyserythropoiesis is usually less severe in HIV than observed in MDS, and occurs predominantly in patients treated with HAART. Megaloblastic changes are usually associated with zidovudine and stavudine therapy. In contrast to MDS, in which erythropoiesis may be hyperplastic, the myeloid/erythroid ratio in HIV is usually normal and there may even be neutrophilic and megakaryocytic hyperplasia.

BOX 157.2 Peripheral Blood Smear and Bone Marrow Morphology in HIV/AIDS

The peripheral blood smear of a patient with HIV/AIDS might show anisocytosis, poikilocytosis, and rouleaux formation. Anemia, when present, is usually normocytic and normochromic. Sometimes macrocytic can be seen even in the absence of AZT therapy. Lymphopenia is seen in advanced disease. Hypogranular neutrophils and Pelger forms are rarely present. Platelets can be normal or hypogranular. In cases of thrombocytopenia, the platelets can be normal sized or large when thrombocytopenia is caused by immune destruction with persevered marrow.

The bone marrow is usually hypercellular, but can be normocellular or hypocellular. Interstitial and perivascular polyclonal plasmacytosis is usually present. HIV-associated stromal changes include edema, gelatinous transformation and increased reticulin fibers (dense collagen fibers are not a feature of HIV). Normal bone marrow architecture is often disturbed and dysplastic changes can be seen, including dyserythropoiesis, dysgranulopoiesis, and abnormal megakaryocytes (including clusters and bare megakaryocytic nuclei). However, the following features distinguish the bone marrow morphology in HIV from that of MDS: dysplasia is less severe in HIV. Dyserythropoiesis occurs mainly in patients on HAART. Megaloblastic changes are associated with AZT therapy. Although erythropoiesis is usually hyperplastic in MDS, myeloid to erythroid ratio is usually normal in HIV. Increase blasts can be seen in MDS but never in HIV. Lastly, in contrast to MDS, the bone marrow in HIV often shows eosinophilia, lymphohistiocytic infiltrates and plasmacytosis.

AIDS, Acquired immunodeficiency syndrome; AZT, zidovudine; HAART, highly active antiretroviral therapy; HIV, human immunodeficiency virus; MDS, myelodysplastic syndrome.

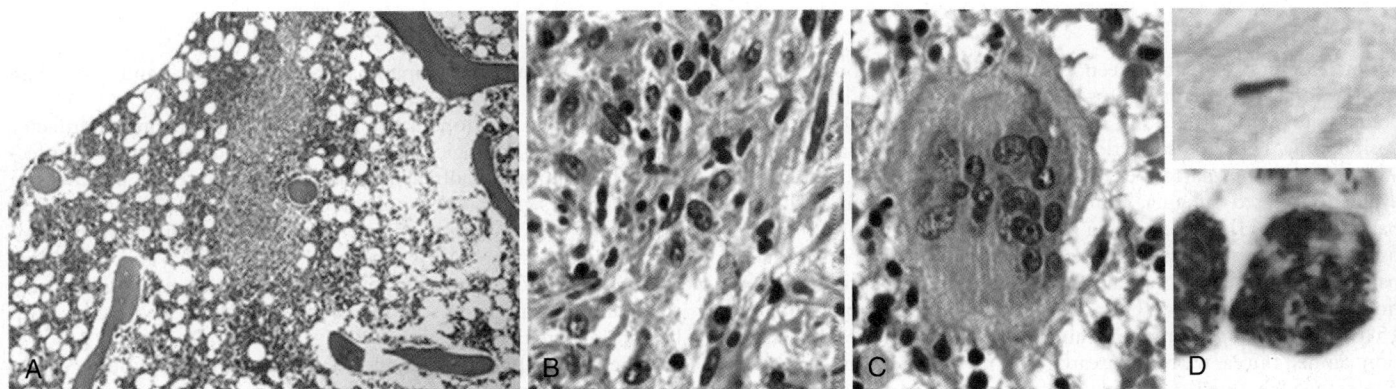

Fig. 157.4 ACID-FAST ORGANISMS IN GRANULOMA. Large poorly formed granuloma in the bone marrow (A) is composed of loosely aggregated histiocytes, lymphocytes, and plasma cells (B), with occasional giant cells (C). The acid-fast stain shows rare elongated, slightly beaded organisms, typical of *Mycobacterium tuberculosis* (D, *top*). In *Mycobacterium avium* complex, the organisms frequently stuff histiocytes (D, *bottom*).

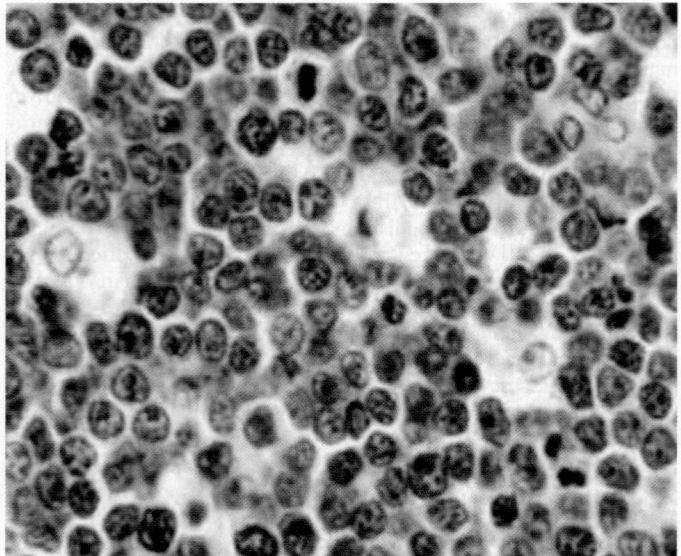

Fig. 157.5 BURKITT LYMPHOMA INVOLVING THE BONE MARROW OF A PATIENT WITH ACQUIRED IMMUNODEFICIENCY SYNDROME. (Zhao X, Sun NC, Witt MD, et al: Changing pattern of AIDS: a bone marrow study. *Am J Clin Pathol* 121:393, 2004.)

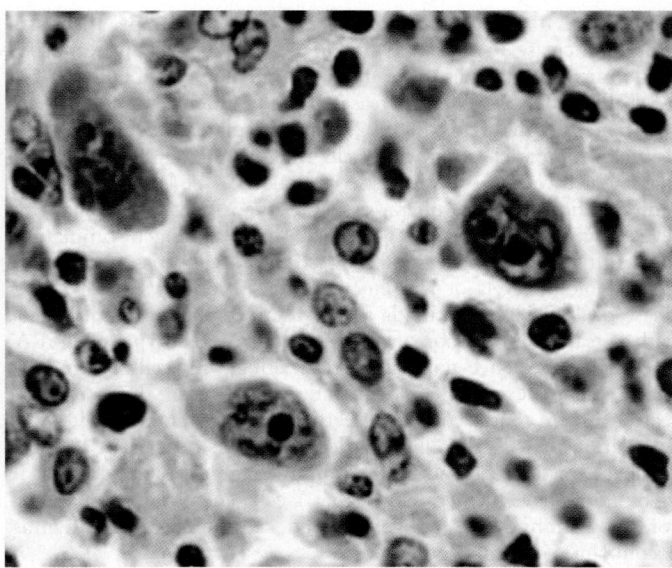

Fig. 157.6 CLASSIC HODGKIN LYMPHOMA INVOLVING THE BONE MARROW OF A PATIENT WITH ACQUIRED IMMUNODEFICIENCY SYNDROME. (Zhao X, Sun NC, Witt MD, et al: Changing pattern of AIDS: a bone marrow study. *Am J Clin Pathol* 121:393, 2004.)

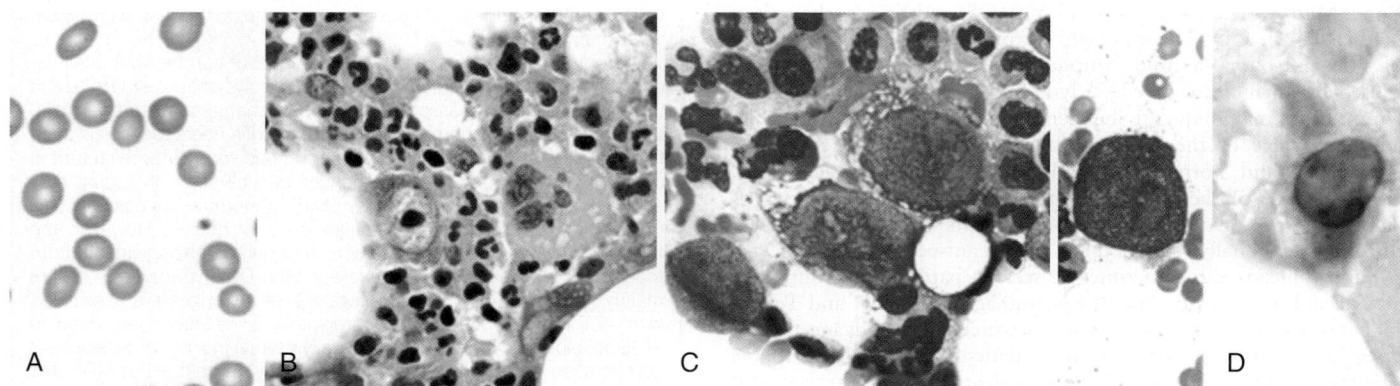

Fig. 157.7 HUMAN PARVOVIRUS INFECTION IN HUMAN IMMUNODEFICIENCY VIRUS. The peripheral blood smear shows anemia with no polychromasia (A). The marrow biopsy shows mostly granulocytic and megakaryocytic elements with a lack of erythroid forms (B), except for rare large pronormoblasts with nuclear inclusions (B, *center*). On the aspirate, the large degenerating pronormoblasts have nuclear inclusions that resemble large nucleoli (C). These are viral inclusions. Sometimes the pronormoblasts are totally degenerated and present as only bare nuclei with the viral inclusion still obvious (C, *right*). An immunostain for parvovirus in a degenerated pronormoblast is illustrated (D).

An increase in blasts can be seen in MDS, but never in bone marrow in HIV infected patients, unless they have an associated leukemia. In contrast to MDS, the bone marrow in HIV patients often shows eosinophilia, lymphohistiocytic infiltrates, and reactive plasmacytosis. Although a bone marrow examination is not routinely required to evaluate isolated anemia, thrombocytopenia, or neutropenia in patients with HIV infection, a bone marrow examination can be useful in the evaluation of unexplained fever and in patients with pancytopenia suspected of having marrow infiltration with an infectious agent or malignancy. Granulomas are observed in approximately 15% of bone marrow trephines and may result from the HIV infection alone, but a thorough search for mycobacterium and other infections is required. A particular effort should be made to identify bone marrow involvement with opportunistic infections, which could include mycobacterial (Fig. 157.6), fungal, protozoal, and/or viral infections.[6] Cytopenias in HIV-infected individuals may also be caused by bone marrow involvement by non-Hodgkin lymphoma

(Fig. 157.7), Hodgkin lymphomas, Kaposi sarcoma, and Castleman disease.

The etiology of cytopenias in HIV/AIDS is frequently multifactorial (see box on Etiologies of Cytopenias). In addition to HIV infection, the medications often prescribed to HIV-infected patients can account for a significant proportion of cytopenias. A thorough review of the medications and supplements taken by a patient with HIV/AIDS with a cytopenia is essential. Tables 157.3 and 157.4 list antiretroviral and antiinfective medications prescribed for prophylaxis/treatment of opportunistic infections and their association with hematologic toxicities.

The clinical presentation and management of individual cytopenias can be unique and therefore the diagnosis and management of anemia, thrombocytopenia, and neutropenia in HIV/AIDS are addressed separately later. In addition, the emerging issue of thrombosis in HIV and principles of antiretroviral therapy management will also be discussed in this chapter.

Red Blood Cell Abnormalities and Anemia

Anemia can occur at any stage of HIV disease, but is more frequent and severe in advanced disease.[8] There is increasing evidence suggesting that anemia in HIV disease is independently associated with an increased risk of disease progression and mortality.[8,11] Anemia is associated with an increased risk of death in HIV-infected patients regardless of CD4 count, and survival is not significantly different between patients with drug-related anemia and anemia attributed to other causes.[8] Correction of anemia in HIV-infected patients has been associated with measurable improvements in quality of life[9] and increased survival.[8]

Detection and treatment of the underlying cause of the anemia should be an immediate goal, which may involve the treatment of opportunistic infections or gastrointestinal blood loss. In general, the etiology of anemia seen in HIV infection is often multifactorial, with several mechanisms playing a role in an individual patient. Diagnosing the cause or causes of anemia is essential to proper therapy.

Anemia Resulting From Decreased Red Blood Cell Production

The most common cause of anemia in HIV disease is decreased RBC production. Frequently encountered mechanisms responsible for decreased RBC production in patients with HIV disease are listed in Table 157.5. Examples include anemia of acute and chronic inflammation (chronic disease anemia) with a blunted production of and response to erythropoietin and cytokine suppression of bone marrow colony-forming unit–granulocyte, erythrocyte, macrophage, megakaryocyte (CFU-GEMM). Infection or infiltration of bone marrow by infectious agents such as atypical mycobacterium, tuberculosis, CMV, and/or fungal organisms can result in profound anemia, although most often associated with pancytopenia. Parvovirus B19 can cause isolated red cell aplasia in the more severely immunocompromised individuals. Bone marrow infiltration by HIV-associated lymphomas, in addition to anemia, can cause neutropenia and thrombocytopenia. Nutritional deficiencies, including vitamin B_{12} and folic acid deficiency, are not uncommon. Other causes of anemia including anemia secondary to blood loss or hemolysis as seen in the non-HIV patient population can also occur in patients infected with HIV.[7] Most significant is that most patients with advanced HIV disease are often treated with one or more medications that can affect RBC production and survival.

Before the HAART era, treatment of HIV disease with high doses of zidovudine was a major cause of myelosuppression and anemia in patients with AIDS. More recent studies, even in the era of HAART, continue to report a high prevalence of anemia among HIV-infected patients.[10] Acute and chronic inflammation is the most frequent cause of anemia in HIV infection. This is characterized by the classic findings of decreased serum iron concentration, reduced total iron binding capacity, a normal or high ferritin, an inappropriately low reticulocyte count for the degree of anemia, and reduced blood levels of erythropoietin. HIV infection itself may account for anemia. Therefore initiation of HAART may result in improvement or normalization of hemoglobin levels in patients who are anemic at baseline. Frequently this occurs in parallel with improvement in CD4+ lymphocyte count, but can occur with only marginal increase in CD4+ lymphocyte numbers. The use of HIV protease inhibitors in HAART also appears to improve hematopoiesis.[13] A report by the Women's Interagency HIV Study has shown that the use of HAART is associated with decreased prevalence of anemia among women.[14] HAART may also decrease the risk of anemia developing in patients who are not anemic at the initiation of therapy. Although the use of HAART is associated with decreased prevalence among people with AIDS generally, the prevalence of anemia remains high among persons with low CD4 counts.[15]

Parvovirus B19 is a member of the *Parvoviridae* family and is responsible for several diseases in humans, including erythema infectiosum (fifth disease) in children, hydrops fetalis, acute arthropathy in adults, aplastic crisis in patients with chronic hemolytic disorders, and pure red cell aplasia in immunocompromised individuals. Parvovirus-induced pure red cell aplasia in association with HIV infection was described over a decade ago.[16] Parvovirus B19 infection is generally limited to human erythroid progenitor cells and leads to erythroid cell death. In hosts with normal immune responses and normal erythrocyte production, acute infection causes a self-limited (4–8 days) interruption in the production of erythrocytes that does not result in significant anemia. However, if host immune responses are impaired, this can result in persistent infection of erythroid precursors leading to a prolonged and severe anemia.

The seroprevalence of parvovirus B19 infection is similar among HIV-infected and noninfected individuals. Furthermore, HIV-infected individuals who have serologic evidence of parvovirus B19 infection usually do not have evidence of active infection (i.e., parvovirus B19 viremia). Parvovirus B19–induced red cell aplasia seen in HIV patients often occurs in individuals with low or absent levels of B19-specific antibodies.[16]

Clinically the disease presents in patients with findings consistent with profound anemia characterized by weakness, pallor, dyspnea, and tachycardia. Hemoglobin values as low as 4 to 5 g/dL and absolute reticulocyte counts of less than 5×10^9/L (<0.1%) are commonly reported. Detection of parvovirus IgG and IgM is not reliable because levels of antibodies may be low or undetectable among patients and are not diagnostic of acute parvovirus B19 red cell aplasia. The most reliable diagnostic study of parvovirus B19 infection is the detection of parvovirus DNA by either PCR or dot-blot hybridization. Because the high sensitivity of PCR may lead to positive test results for months after the original infection, dot-blot hybridization may be a better test for making a diagnosis of acute infection resulting in red cell aplasia. Histologic examination of bone marrow aspirates reveals hypocellularity, markedly decreased maturing erythrocytes, and occasional giant pronormoblasts. The presence of giant pronormoblasts in a bone marrow aspirate or biopsy is diagnostic of parvovirus B19 infection.[6]

Initial therapy for parvovirus-induced red cell aplasia should be aimed at correcting the anemia through RBC transfusions. Treatment with intravenous immunoglobulin (IVIg 0.4 g/kg daily for 5 days) can lead to a rapid decrease in the level of parvovirus viremia, improvement in the reticulocyte count, and resolution of the anemia. Recurrence is commonly seen if there is no improvement in the patients' immunologic function. If the anemia recurs within 6 months of the

TABLE 157.3	Hematologic Toxicities of Antiretroviral Agents

Multiclass Combinations		
Combination	**Brand Name**	**Hematologic Toxicities**
EFV+TDF+FTC	Atripla	Neutropenia, anemia
EFV+Rilpivirine+TDF	Complera	Neutropenia, anemia
EFV+TDF+Elvitegravir+Cobicistat	Stribild	Neutropenia, anemia

Nucleoside/Nucleotide Reverse Transcriptase Inhibitors:			
Abbreviation	**Generic Name**	**Brand Name**	**Hematologic Toxicities**
3TC	lamivudine	Epivir	Neutropenia, thrombocytopenia
ABC	abacavir	Ziagen	Thrombocytopenia.
AZT or ZDV	zidovudine[1]	Retrovir	Pancytopenia, anemia, thrombocytopenia, neutropenia, pure red cell aplasia.
d4T	stavudine[2]	Zerit	
ddI	didanosine[3]	Videx EC	
FTC	emtricitabine	Emtriva	Neutropenia, anemia.
TDF	tenofovir	Viread	Neutropenia.

Combined Nucleoside/Nucleotide Reverse Transcriptase Inhibitors:		
Combination	**Brand Name**	**Hematologic Toxicities**
ABC+3TC	Epzicom (US) Kivexa (Europe)	Neutropenia, anemia, thrombocytopenia
ABC+AZT+3TC	Trizivir[4]	Neutropenia, anemia, thrombocytopenia.
AZT+3TC	Combivir	Neutropenia, anemia, thrombocytopenia.
TDF+FTC	Truvada	Neutropenia, anemia.

Nonnucleoside Reverse Transcriptase Inhibitors:			
Abbreviation	**Generic Name**	**Brand Name**	**Hematologic Toxicities**
DLV	delavirdine[5]	Rescriptor	Anemia
EFV	efavirenz	Sustiva (US) Stocrin (Europe)	Neutropenia
ETR	etravirine[6]	Intelence	
NVP	nevirapine relpivirine	Viramune Edurant	Neutropenia

Protease Inhibitors:			
Abbreviation	**Generic Name**	**Brand Name**	**Hematologic Toxicities**
APV	amprenavir	Agenerase	
FOS-APV	fosamprenavir	Lexiva (US) Telzir (Europe)	Neutropenia
ATV	atazanavir[7]	Reyataz	Neutropenia, anemia, thrombocytopenia.
DRV	darunavir	Prezista	Anemia
IDV	indinavir	Crixivan	Neutropenia, anemia. Thrombocytopenia
LPV/RTV	lopinavir+ritonavir	Kaletra Aluvia (developing world)	Neutropenia, anemia, thrombocytopenia.
NFV	nelfinavir	Viracept	Neutropenia, anemia, lymphopenia.
RTV	ritonavir	Norvir	Anemia
SQV	saquinavir	Invirase (hard gel capsule)	
TPV	tipranavir	Aptivus	Neutropenia, anemia.

Fusion or Entry Inhibitors:			
Abbreviation	**Generic Name**	**Brand Name**	**Hematologic Toxicities**
T-20	enfuvirtide	Fuzeon	Neutropenia, anemia, eosinophilia
MVC	maraviroc	Celsentri (Europe) Selzentry (US)	Neutropenia

Integrase Inhibitors:			
Abbreviation	**Generic Name**	**Brand Name**	**Hematologic Toxicities**
RAL	raltegravir	Isentress	Anemia, thrombocytopenia.
	dolutegravir elvitegravir	Tivicay Viteka	

initial therapy, monthly maintenance therapy with 0.4 g/kg IVIg may be required. Immune reconstitution resulting from the successful use of HAART may lead to complete remission of this condition.[17]

Anemia Resulting From Ineffective Red Blood Cell Production

Ineffective production of red cells can occur with deficiencies of folate or vitamin B_{12}. Ineffective production of RBCs is frequently characterized by concomitant decreases in platelets and neutrophils accompanied by megaloblastic red cell morphology with large oval macrocytes and hypersegmented neutrophils. In addition to a low reticulocyte count there may be elevations in indirect bilirubin and serum lactate dehydrogenase. Because of the relatively small tissue stores of folate, patients with advanced HIV disease who have poor dietary intake, excessive alcohol ingestion, and/or jejunal disease may become deficient in folate. More commonly reported in patients with

advanced HIV infection is decreased serum B_{12} levels. Low serum B_{12} has been documented in approximately one-third of patients with AIDS. Patients with advanced HIV infection (AIDS) appear to acquire gastrointestinal defects resulting in B_{12} malabsorption. The mechanisms responsible for decreased B_{12} absorption observed in these patients include both infections of and other acquired disorders of the small intestine and ileum, food B_{12} malabsorption secondary to inadequate gastric acid production, and true pernicious anemia with antibodies to the H^+/K^+ parietal cell pump and intrinsic factor. However, not all cases of low serum levels of B_{12} are associated with true metabolic B_{12} deficiency as characterized by elevated methylmalonic acid. This may result from the finding that some patients with neutropenia secondary to a hypocellular bone marrow may have low serum levels of transcobalamin (TC) I, the major serum B_{12} carrier protein, which is found in the specific granules of neutrophils. However, transport of B_{12} into cells is mediated by TC II, which carries only 25% to 30% of serum B_{12}, and for that reason the newer assays that measure B_{12} bound to TC II (holotranscobalamin II

TABLE 157.4 Agents for Treatment and Prevention of Opportunistic Infections With Hematologic Toxicities

Drug Class	Drug Toxicities	Hematologic
Antifungal agents	Amphotericin B deoxycholate and lipid formulations	Anemia
	Anidulafungin	Deep vein thrombosis (rare)
	Flucytosine	Bone marrow suppression
	Micafungin	Hemolysis, leukopenia
Anti-*Pneumocystis* pneumonia agents	Dapsone	Methemoglobinemia, hemolytic anemia (especially in patients with G6PD deficiency), neutropenia.
	Primaquine	Methemoglobinemia, hemolytic anemia (especially in patients with G6PD deficiency).
	Trimethoprim-sulfamethoxazole (TMP-SMX)	Bone marrow suppression.
Antitoxoplasmosis agents	Pyrimethamine	Neutropenia, thrombocytopenia, megaloblastic anemia.
	Sulfadiazine	Bone marrow suppression.
Antimycobacterial agents	Rifampin	Thrombocytopenia, hemolytic anemia.
	Rifabutin	Neutropenia anemia, thrombocytopenia
Antiviral agents	Ganciclovir	Neutropenia, thrombocytopenia, anemia,
	Interferon-alfa and peginterferon-alfa	Neutropenia, thrombocytopenia.
	Ribavirin	Hemolytic anemia.
	Valaciclovir	At a high dose of 8 g/day: thrombotic thrombocytopenic purpura/ hemolytic uremic syndrome reported in advanced human immunodeficiency virus patients and in transplant recipients
	Valganciclovir	Neutropenia, thrombocytopenia, anemia.
Antiparasitic agents	Albendazole	Neutropenia
	Benznidazole	Bone marrow suppression.
	Fumagillin (investigational)	Oral therapy: neutropenia, thrombocytopenia. Ocular therapy: minimal systemic effect or local effect
	Miltefosine	Leukocytosis, thrombocytosis.
Treatment for syphilis	Pentavalent antimony (sodium stibogluconate)	Leukopenia, anemia, thrombocytopenia
	Penicillin G	Bone marrow suppression (rare), drug fever

G6PD, Glucose-6-phosphate dehydrogenase.

TABLE 157.5 Etiology of Anemia in Human Immunodeficiency Virus

HIV Related:
HIV Infection:
Anemia of chronic disease
Blunted production/response to erythropoietin
Suppression of CFU-GEMM (HIV/inflammatory cytokines)

Neoplasms Infiltrating BM:
Non-Hodgkin lymphoma, KS, Hodgkin lymphoma

Infections of the BM:
Parvovirus B19
Atypical mycobact (MAI/MAC)
M. TB
Histoplasma
CMV

Medications Causing Decreased Production:	**Medications Causing Hemolysis:**
RT inhibitors	Indinavir
Ganciclovir	Bactrim and Dapsone in
Bactrim	G6PD deficiency
Amphotericin B	

HIV Unrelated
B12 and/or folic acid deficiencies
Iron deficiency caused by chronic blood loss

BM, Bone marrow; CFU-GEMM, colony-forming unit–granulocyte, erythrocyte, macrophage, megakaryocyte; CMV, cytomegalovirus; G6PD, glucose-6-phosphate dehydrogenase; HIV, human immunodeficiency virus; KS, Kaposi sarcoma; MAC, Mycobacterium avium complex; MAI, mycobacterium avium-intracellulare; M. TB, Mycobacterium tuberculosis; RT, reverse transcriptase.

assays) may be more reflective of serum B_{12} status in neutropenic HIV infected patients.

A diagnosis of B_{12} deficiency should include not only a low serum B_{12} level, but normal or elevated blood levels of folic acid, elevated blood homocysteine, and elevated methylmalonic acid levels in a patient with normal renal function. With a diagnosis of B_{12} deficiency, an effort should be made to determine the causes of B_{12} malabsorption, and treatment begun with monthly administration of parenteral B_{12} to correct the deficiency. If anemia and cytopenias result from the B_{12} deficiency alone, treatment should result in correction within 4 to 6 weeks. Because B_{12} deficiency is also associated with a variety of neurologic defects, including motor and sensory neuropathy, cognitive defects including dementia, and the most severe neurologic manifestation of subacute combined degeneration of the spinal cord, the possibility of B_{12} deficiency should be considered in any HIV-infected patient with neurologic symptoms.

Anemia Resulting From Increased Red Blood Cell Destruction

Anemia resulting from hemolysis of RBCs can result from processes either intrinsic or extrinsic to the RBC. Examples of intrinsic defects include hemoglobinopathies, RBC membrane defects, or RBC enzyme functional deficiencies such as glucose-6-phosphate dehydrogenase (G6PD) deficiency. Exclusive of G6PD deficiency, the majority of patients with these RBC defects have a life-long history of anemia. Diagnosis in most circumstances can be made by careful review of the peripheral blood smear. G6PD deficiency is an X-linked disorder and found predominantly in men. Hemolysis occurs when erythrocytes are exposed to oxidative stress. Depending upon the degree of enzyme deficiency, patients may not have had a previous documented episode of hemolysis. G6PD deficiency–associated hemolysis can occur in HIV infected patients who are taking dapsone or trimethoprim and sulfamethoxazole combinations for pneumocystis prophylaxis or treatment. In some patients, the degree of hemolysis does not result in significant anemia because RBC destruction is well compensated by effective RBC production and patients can continue on treatment. However, patients with the Mediterranean form of G6PD may develop severe hemolysis, and treatment with such medications is contraindicated.

Extrinsic causes of RBC hemolysis observed in patients with HIV infection include microangiopathic hemolytic disorders such as thrombotic thrombocytopenic purpura (TTP, discussed in the section on thrombocytopenia), vasculitis, or disseminated intravascular coagulation. Patients will have associated thrombocytopenia and demonstrate RBC fragmentation on the peripheral blood smear. Autoimmune hemolytic anemia rarely occurs in HIV-infected individuals, although a positive antiglobulin (Coombs) test is not uncommon. Patients with documented autoimmune hemolysis may respond to treatment with corticosteroids, rituximab, or splenectomy. The risk of HIV progression with the use of corticosteroids and rituximab does not appear to be an issue in patients receiving HAART.

Impact of Anemia on HIV Disease Progression and Survival

Anemia has been shown to be an independent risk factor for clinical progression of HIV disease. In a patient in whom HAART is to be initiated, anemia, CD4 cell count $<0.2 \times 10^9$/L, HIV viral load, and a pretreatment diagnosis of clinical AIDS are well established risk factors for rapid disease progression. A moderate anemia of 8 to 14 g/dL in men or 8 to 12 g/dL in women is associated with a relative hazard of disease progression or death of 2.2 (95% confidence interval [CI], 1.6–2.9), $p < .0001$), whereas a more severe anemia of less than 8 g/dL has a relative hazard of 7.1 (95% CI, 2.5–20.1, $p < .0002$).

Anemia has a significant impact on overall survival in HIV-infected patients. A Baltimore study of 2348 HIV-infected patients found that a hemoglobin of 6.5 to 8 g/dL was predictive of a threefold risk of death and a hemoglobin of <6.5 g/L was predictive of a fourfold increased risk of death. A European study of 6725 HIV-infected patients found the hemoglobin level at baseline was an independent prognostic factor for survival along with the CD4[+] lymphocyte count and HIV plasma viral load. For each 1 g/dL decrease in hemoglobin level, the relative hazard of death was 1.39 (95% CI, 1.34–1.43; $p < .0001$). Additional cohort studies from the United States including the Multistate Adult and Adolescent Spectrum of HIV Surveillance Project and the Women's Interagency HIV Study have also confirmed that anemia is an independent risk factor for mortality in HIV infected individuals.

Management of Anemia and the Use of Erythropoietin in HIV-Infected Patients

Treatment of anemia should be directed toward correcting the underlying cause whenever possible. The use of blood transfusion should be minimized and reserved for patients who have rapid decreases in hemoglobin levels, extremely low hemoglobin levels, or pronounced anemia-related symptoms. A number of clinical trials of antiretroviral medication combinations (HAART) have shown that suppression of HIV replication is associated with improvement in anemia. In addition, improvement of anemia on HAART has been found to occur independent of the patients' sex, race, mode of HIV infection, change in CD4[+] lymphocyte count, and additional therapies for anemia. Improvement in anemia, with an increase in the reticulocyte count, can be seen as early as 8 to 12 weeks, with maximum improvement usually obtained by 12 months.

Erythropoietin supplementation has been shown to be beneficial in HIV-infected patients with well-established anemia and when the hemoglobin level is decreasing or has decreased slowly. A blunted response to erythropoietin, as observed in anemia of acute and chronic inflammation, is common in HIV-infected patients with anemia. However, erythropoietin (Epogen; Procrit) therapy should be considered for refractory anemia in symptomatic patients with a hemoglobin level of <11 g/dL in men and <10 g/dL in women. The primary goal should be to maintain quality of life and functional status. Many patients may be asymptomatic with lower hemoglobin (9–10 g/dL) and physicians should use erythropoietic agents only for symptomatic patients with these lower hemoglobin levels. The initial adult dose is 40,000 units subcutaneously per week, which has been shown to be equivalent to treatment three times a week at 100 to 200 U/kg.[12] Also darbepoetin alfa given at a dose of 3.0 µg/kg every 2 weeks has been shown to be as equally effective. Onset of action as characterized by an increase in the reticulocyte count is within 1 to 2 weeks, with increased hemoglobin noted in 2 to 6 weeks. The baseline level of endogenous serum erythropoietin has been shown to be predictive of response to the therapeutic use of erythropoietin. A baseline erythropoietin level of greater than 500 IU/L is associated with a significantly lower response to treatment. Response to erythropoietin therapy also depends on the severity of anemia, presence of active infection and available iron stores. If hemoglobin fails to increase more than 1 g/dL after 4 weeks of therapy, the dose may be increased to 60,000 units weekly. After an additional 4 weeks, if hemoglobin does not increase by at least 1 g/dL from baseline, therapy should be discontinued. When combined with the use of HAART, erythropoietin treatment may result in a more rapid improvement in hemoglobin, but has not been shown to improve survival or statistically reduce the total number of transfusions. This may be because of the marginal contribution that erythropoietin supplementation may have in the background of the significant improvement in immune status and bone marrow function provided by effective antiretroviral therapy.[15]

LEUKOPENIA AND NEUTROPENIA: INCIDENCE AND PATHOGENESIS

Leukopenia is common in patients with advanced HIV infection occurring in up to 85% of patients with clinical AIDS. In such patients, low WBC counts are frequently a result of both decreased lymphocytes and neutrophils.[7] Neutropenia ($<1.5 \times 10^9$/L) is reported in 5% to 10% of HIV-infected patients with the highest prevalence in patients with advanced HIV infection (AIDS). In a 7.5-year longitudinal study of 1729 women with HIV infection an absolute neutrophil count (ANC) of less than 1×10^9/L was documented in 31%. HIV-related risk factors for the development of neutropenia include a high plasma HIV viral RNA and a low CD4[+] lymphocyte count. In turn, the use of HAART is associated with a lower risk of developing neutropenia. Decreases in the neutrophil count are often transient, self-limiting, and rarely of clinical significance, but a neutrophil count of less than 0.5×10^9/L of prolonged duration does pose a significant risk of infection. In a study of 87 consecutive HIV-infected patients who developed neutrophil counts of less than 1×10^9/L, the median duration of neutropenia was 13 days and nadir neutrophil count was 0.66×10^9/L. Infection occurred in only 6 (8%) of 71 evaluable patients, of whom 4 patients had neutrophil counts less than 0.5×10^9/L. Ten (12%) patients had neutrophil counts less than 0.5×10^9/L and received granulocyte colony-stimulating factor (G-CSF) treatment, which artificially altered the natural history of neutropenia in this patient population.

Decreased in vitro colony growth of the CFU-granulocyte macrophage (GM) progenitor cell has been reported, which may explain the neutropenia observed with HIV infection alone. Inhibitory substances produced by HIV infected cells have been reported to suppress neutrophil growth and differentiation in vitro. A number of inflammatory cytokines including TGF-β and TNF-α may directly suppress myelopoiesis or inhibit the production of important myeloid growth factors, G-CSF and GM-CSF. Decreased serum levels of G-CSF have been observed in afebrile neutropenic HIV-infected patients. The HIV proteins tat and p24 have also been reported capable of suppressing myelopoiesis.

The most common causes of neutropenia in HIV infected patients are medication-related myelosuppression. In a study of 87 consecutive HIV-infected patients with neutrophil counts of $<2 \times 10^9$/L, only three patients were not receiving medications associated with a risk of neutropenia and 66% were receiving three or more myelosuppressive medications. Neutropenia is a common complication reported with many of the drugs used to treat opportunistic infections such as *Pneumocystis carinii*, toxoplasmosis or CMV infection.[7] These medications are listed in Table 157.4. Although neutropenia resulting from HIV-related myelosuppression often improves with HAART, antiretroviral-associated neutropenia can be observed with higher doses of zidovudine. Zidovudine-associated neutropenia resolves with dose reduction or discontinuation of the medication.[7] In a study of 62 HIV-infected patients with neutrophil counts of 1×10^9/L or less, cancer chemotherapy, zidovudine, trimethoprine-sulfamethoxazole and ganciclovir were the medications most commonly responsible for neutropenia. In the same report, medication-related neutropenia associated with infection was most often seen in the patients receiving cancer chemotherapy. Rare cases of agranulocytosis have been reported with the use of the antiretroviral drugs, abacvir and indinavir.

Neutropenia is often observed in patients with bone marrow involvement by opportunistic infections such as *Mycobacterium avium* or CMV. Bone marrow involvement with HIV-associated malignancies and their subsequent treatment can also result in significant and prolonged neutropenia. However, malignancy treatment-related neutropenia in clinical trials appears to be less severe in patients receiving simultaneous HAART.

Abnormalities of Neutrophil and Monocyte Function

A number of acquired functional defects have been described in both neutrophils and monocytes from patients with HIV infection. Many of these defects are observed in patients with advanced disease with high levels of plasma viral RNA and CD4$^+$ lymphopenia. Impaired chemotaxis and reduced expression of leukocyte adhesion molecules necessary for migration of neutrophils to sites of infection have been reported. Decreased opsonization of antibody coated bacteria because of Fc receptor dysfunction and decreased superoxide production necessary for optimal intracellular killing of bacterial and fungal organisms have been observed in both neutrophils and macrophages from HIV-infected patients. Defective intracellular killing of mycobacterial and fungal organisms may also be caused in part by defective production of IFN-γ.

Management of Neutropenia in HIV-Infected Patients

Impact of HAART and Use of Granulocyte-Macrophage–Colony Stimulating Factor and Granulocyte-Colony Stimulating Factor

Treatment of neutropenia should be guided by the underlying cause. This may require treatment of active infection or removal of medications associated with the development of neutropenia. The use of HAART has clearly been shown to reduce the risk of developing leukopenia and neutropenia and significantly increasing the neutrophil counts in treated patients. The Women's Interagency HIV Study of 1729 HIV-infected women found that the use of HAART, without zidovudine, was associated with protection against developing neutropenia. In addition, HAART, even incorporating zidovudine, was associated with resolution of neutropenia in women with advanced HIV disease. Another study of 66 HIV-infected patients treated with HAART reported statistically significant increases in total leukocyte and neutrophil counts after 6 months of treatment. These studies support the use of effective HAART as the initial approach to the management of mild to moderate leukopenia and neutropenia in HIV infected patients.

Sargramostim or GM-CSF (Leukine) and filgrastim or G-CSF (Neupogen), are the primary pharmacologic agents used in the treatment of severe neutropenia in HIV-infected patients and have been shown in clinical studies to be safe and effective. A long-term study of 105 HIV-infected patients randomized to receive weekly injections of GM-CSF (125 µg/m^2) or placebo while receiving zidovudine antiretroviral therapy reported after 6 months of treatment that GM-CSF treated patients were more likely to have a HIV plasma RNA level below level of detection and less zidovudine resistance mutations. A study of 123 HIV-infected leukopenic patients treated with GM-CSF treated for 12 weeks were compared with 121 untreated leukopenic patients showed the total leukocyte count including neutrophils and monocytes increased by 65% at week 12 when compared with baseline values ($p < .001$). In the untreated leukopenic HIV-infected patients, the total leukocyte count decreased by 24% below baseline values at week 12 ($p < .001$). Common side effects of treatment with GM-CSF include fever, fatigue, myalgias, bone pain and headache.

A randomized study of 258 HIV-infected patients with CD4$^+$ lymphocyte counts below 0.2×10^9/L and neutrophil counts of $<1 \times 10^9$/L were randomized to one of two dose regimens of G-CSF (1 µg/kg/day or 300 µg three times a week) versus no treatment. Patients in the control group who developed severe neutropenia ($<0.5 \times 10^9$/L) were then randomized to one of the treatment regimens. The intention-to-treat analysis found the incidence of severe neutropenia ($<0.5 \times 10^9$/L) was 1.7% in the treated group versus 22% in the untreated controls. The incidence of bacterial infections was 31% lower in the treated group, with fewer severe bacterial infections and significantly few hospital days (45% reduction) for bacterial infections.

The use of G-CSF has been associated with a reduction in severe neutropenia in patients treated for CMV infection with ganciclovir (Cytovene), but the evidence is unclear as to whether it offers a clear clinical benefit.[19] However, in general it has been shown to be safe and effective in raising leukocyte counts when administered to patients with HIV infection receiving antiretroviral therapy.[7,19] G-CSF is indicated for drug-induced, cancer-related and HIV-related neutropenia with an ANC of less than 0.5×10^9/L cell/mcl. The initial dose is 1–10 µg/kg/day and should be titrated by 1 µg/kg/day to obtain a neutrophil count of 1.0×10^9/L. Most patients will respond to a dose of 1 µg/kg/day. G-CSF usage should be carefully monitored and the dose reduced or stopped when the neutrophil count exceeds 1.0×10^9/L.

THROMBOCYTOPENIA IN HIV INFECTION

Thrombocytopenia, alone or in association with anemia and/or leucopenia, is frequently seen in approximately 40% of HIV-infected patients in the course of their disease. Thrombocytopenia has been reported to be the first sign of HIV infection in up to 10% of infected individuals. The most common cause of thrombocytopenia in HIV infection is HIV-related autoimmune thrombocytopenia, which is clinically indistinguishable from classic immune thrombocytopenia (ITP).

An association between AIDS and ITP was described before HIV had been isolated and characterized. HIV infects CD4$^+$ lymphocytes, monocytes, and macrophages, and some experimental evidence also documents infection of megakaryocytes. Although a number of different mechanisms have been reported by which HIV infection can produce thrombocytopenia, the ability of effective antiretroviral therapy to improve platelet counts demonstrates a clear relationship between viral replication, the expression of viral related proteins, and the host response to platelets.

Epidemiology

Thrombocytopenia was first associated with AIDS before the discovery of HIV. Before the use of HAART, HIV-associated thrombocytopenia (HIV-ITP), platelet count <150 × 10⁹/L) was identified in approximately 5% to 30% of HIV-1 infected patients. Thrombocytopenia is more prevalent in patients with advanced HIV infection defined as a CD4-lymphocyte count of <0.2 × 10⁹/L, clinical AIDS, and among intravenous drug abusers. The Multicenter AIDS Cohort Study of 1611 HIV-positive homosexual and bisexual men reported a platelet count of <150 × 10⁹/L in 6.7%. The incidence of thrombocytopenia was only 2.8% in men with CD4 lymphocyte counts >0.7 × 10⁹/L, but rose to 10.8% in those with CD4⁺ lymphocyte counts of <0.2 × 10⁹/L. A review of 1004 HIV-infected patients seen in two HIV/AIDS clinics, identified platelet counts of <150 × 10⁹/L on at least one determination in 110 (11%) patients, 42 (4.2%) patients had platelet counts of <100 × 10⁹/L and 15 (1.5%) had a platelet count of <50 × 10⁹/L. Thrombocytopenia was more prevalent in patients with a clinical AIDS (21.2%) and a CD4⁺ lymphocyte count of <0.2 × 10⁹/L (20%).

A review of the medical records of 36,515 HIV-infected participants in the Multistate Adult and Adolescent Spectrum of Disease Project reported a 1-year incidence of thrombocytopenia of 3.7%, defined as a platelet count of <50 × 10⁹/L. The incidence and severity of thrombocytopenia was associated with the stage of disease with an incidence of 1.7% among patients with HIV infection, but not clinical or immunologic AIDS, 3.1% among persons with immunologic AIDS (CD4⁺ lymphocytes<0.2 × 10⁹/L) and 8.7% in patients with clinical AIDS. By logistic regression analysis, clinical AIDS, CD4 lymphocyte count of <0.2 × 10⁹/L, age >45 years, intravenous drug use, lymphoma and/or anemia was associated with a platelet count <50 × 10⁹/L.

An increased incidence and severity of thrombocytopenia in HIV-infected intravenous drug users compared with HIV infected homosexuals has been reported. Mientjes et al reported a platelet count of <150 × 10⁹/L in 29/182 (16.4%) homosexual HIV-infected men compared with 38/181 (36.9%) HIV-infected intravenous drug users. None of the homosexual men had a platelet count of <50 × 10⁹/L, whereas 6 (5.8%) of intravenous drug users had a count of <50 × 10⁹/L. These differences may be explained, in part, by the higher incidence of coinfection with hepatitis C and underlying liver disease in HIV-infected intravenous drug users.

In a prospective multicenter cohort study of 738 HIV infected hemophilia patients, the incidence over time of HIV-related conditions was determined in 130 children and 193 adults. The 10-year cumulative incidence of thrombocytopenia (platelets <100 × 10⁹/L) after seroconversion was 43% ± 7% in adults and 27% ± 6% in children. The mean CD4 counts were significantly higher in children (514 ± 61 cells/μl) than adults (260 ± 24 cells/μl) with thrombocytopenia (p = .0004).

Most clinical data have been obtained before the widespread use of HAART in patients with early HIV-infection. There are few data on the current prevalence of thrombocytopenia in patients under active antiviral treatment. However, recent prospective data from the Women's Interagency HIV study have documented a reduction in the incidence of anemia and neutropenia in HIV-infected women on HAART. These findings are in accord with the impression that there has been a similar reduction in the incidence of thrombocytopenia, especially platelet counts <50 × 10⁹/L in compliant patients.

Pathophysiology

Multiple mechanisms may contribute to the development of CITP in the HIV-infected patient and these have recently been reviewed. Proposed mechanisms include accelerated platelet clearance because of immune complex disease, and anti-platelet GP antibodies, and/or anti-HIV antibodies that cross-react with platelet membrane GPs (antigenic mimicry). The ability of the HIV-1 to rapidly mutate may facilitate both its ability to escape immune surveillance and to mimic host antigens. Direct infection of megakaryocytes results in defective platelet production and megakaryocytic apoptosis.

Epidemiologic studies suggest that the pathogenesis of thrombocytopenia is partially dependent on disease burden. HIV-associated

thrombocytopenia developing early after infection more often resembles classic ITP in which thrombocytopenia is mediated primarily by peripheral destruction, whereas thrombocytopenia in patients with immunologic AIDS (CD4 lymphocytes <2 × 10⁹/L) is attributable predominantly to decreased platelet production and ineffective hematopoiesis. Although platelet counts may improve with antiretroviral therapy in both patient populations, patients with advanced disease are less likely to respond to classic primary ITP therapy such as splenectomy, corticosteroids, IVIg or anti-RhD. Initial studies of HIV- associated ITP suggested an immune complex mechanism was responsible for the thrombocytopenia, wherein platelets were cleared from the circulation as "innocent bystanders." More recent studies have shown that these immune complexes contain antibodies that cross-react with both HIV and platelet GPs. These antibodies also cross-reacted with sequences on HIV nef, gag, env, and pol proteins. Similar cross-reactivity between HIV viral proteins and platelet GPs has been reported in the studies of Bettlaieb and coworkers who eluted Ig from platelets from patients with HIV-associated ITP and found these antibodies bound to antigenic epitopes common to both platelet GPIIIa and HIV GP160.

Studies of platelet kinetics have demonstrated that HIV-ITP is frequently associated with decreased platelet production. Megakaryocytes express the CD4 receptor and coreceptors necessary for HIV infection. Cytopathic infection of HIV of the megakaryocyte has been demonstrated and is the postulated primary mechanism for impaired megakaryopoiesis. However, the potential of cross-reactive antibodies between HIV-related proteins and platelet GPs capable of inducing apoptosis of megakaryocytes as has been described with primary ITP has not been studied.

Clinical Manifestations

HIV-seropositive patients can develop thrombocytopenia several years before the development of overt AIDS, and the early disease is clinically indistinguishable from classic ITP. However, the clinical picture of HIV-ITP is often mild, with only a minority of patients having platelet counts of less than 50 × 10⁹/L. Major bleeding is rare and only a few cases of fatal hemorrhage have been reported. There has been greater variability in patients with hemophilia A. For example, Finazzi and coworkers documented thrombocytopenia (platelets <100 × 10⁹/L) in 14/124 (11%) hemophiliacs, only one of whom had a major hemorrhage. In contrast, Ragni and colleagues reported a platelet count of <100 × 10⁹/L in 30/87 (36%) hemophiliac patients, with 11 (13%) having a platelet count <50 × 10⁹/L. Nine of the 11 patients (82%) had major bleeding complications and 3 suffered fatal hemorrhage.

Severe thrombocytopenia in patients with advanced HIV infection is frequently associated with additional cytopenias. In a study of 52 HIV-infected intravenous drug users with thrombocytopenia, 4 patients (8%) with advanced HIV infection had a hypocellular bone marrow examination and pancytopenia. HIV-infected drug users were also more likely to have antibodies to both hepatitis B and C and to have abnormal liver function studies. The role of immune-mediated platelet destruction versus bone marrow failure in patients with advanced HIV disease is still uncertain.

Treatment of HIV-Associated Immune Thrombocytopenia

HIV-associated ITP is generally responsive to therapeutic interventions used in classic ITP. Therapy with prednisone produces a major hematologic response (platelet count >100 × 10⁹/L) in over half of all patients, although only a minority will maintain platelets >50 × 10⁹/L after cessation of steroids. Despite the initial anxiety regarding the use of corticosteroids in HIV-infected, immune-suppressed patients, no deleterious effect of short-term treatment with prednisone have become evident. However, long-term treatment with corticosteroids should still be avoided and other coinfections such as tuberculosis, CMV or hepatitis C should be excluded before initiating treatment with corticosteroids. IVIg and anti-RhD are equally effective in increasing platelet counts acutely in severely affected patients, but a crossover study clearly demonstrated a longer duration of response with the latter agent.

Splenectomy has proven to be safe and effective in refractory patients with HIV-TP. After splenectomy, there is a transient increase in the peripheral blood CD4 lymphocyte count, which reflects redistribution from the splenic pool into the circulation rather than an improvement in the patient's immunologic status.

HIV-related hematologic cytopenias have been shown to correlate with plasma viral load. Effective antiretroviral therapies have resulted in improvement in several HIV-related cytopenias, including HIV-CITP. Zidovudine monotherapy increased platelet counts in 60% to 70% of HIV-CITP patients. Although other antiretroviral drugs have been shown to improve hematologic parameters in patients with advanced HIV infection, their efficacy as monotherapy for the management of HIV-CITP is less well documented. Use of HAART in both de novo and zidovudine-refractory HIV-CITP has induced sustained platelet responses in association with effective viral suppression.

Responses to zidovudine and HAART may be more limited in HIV-infected intravenous drug users, possibly reflecting the impact of associated liver disease and infection with hepatitis C virus (HCV). In a prospective placebo-controlled, double-blind, randomized trial, 12 of 14 zidovudine refractory HIV-infected intravenous drug users with elevated serum alanine aminotransferase suggestive of underlying liver disease who were treated with IFN-α had a statistically significant increase in their platelet counts by week 4 of therapy. Similar responses to IFN-α therapy alone have been reported in HIV-seronegative, HCV infected patients. An open label trial of IFN-α in a cohort of predominantly homosexual men documented responses in nine of 16 patients, with responses occurring as early as 2 weeks after the initiation of treatment. Such rapid responses preclude the possibility that improvement in the platelet count is solely caused by suppression of concomitant HCV infection. At present, there are no data evaluating the efficacy of the new approved thrombopoietin receptor agonists, romiplostim and eltrombopag, in the management of HIV-related thrombocytopenia, but long-term efficacy and safety data regarding the use of these agents in primary ITP would suggest that they would be effective in the management of HIV-associated ITP.

THROMBOTIC MICROANGIOPATHY AND THROMBOTIC THROMBOCYTOPENIC PURPURA

Thrombotic microangiopathy including both TTP and the hemolytic uremic syndrome (HUS) is a well-described complication of HIV infection seen in approximately 1% of patients. The incidence of this complication appears to have decreased with the advent of HAART. The incidence of TTP appears to be similar to that observed in the general population, whereas HUS appears frequently in patients with advanced HIV infection.

TTP can occur any time in the course of HIV infection and has been reported in some patients to be the initial manifestation of HIV infection. This life-threatening disorder is characterized by thrombocytopenia and microangiopathic (fragmentation) hemolytic anemia. The original description of this disorder emphasized a classic pentad of fever, thrombocytopenia, microangiopathic hemolytic anemia, renal failure, and neurologic abnormalities. However, most patients present with only one or two manifestations of the original pentad and isolated thrombocytopenia may be the initial finding. Therefore it is essential that the evaluation of thrombocytopenia includes a careful review of the peripheral blood smear.

TTP is the result of a failure to process endothelial derived high molecular weight von Willebrand factor caused by an absence of/or inhibitor to the von Willebrand factor cleaving protease (AD-AMTS13). Measurement of ADAMTS13 activity before the initiation of plasma exchange will report levels nearly always less than 10%

and additional assays will often detect an inhibitor to the protease. First-line therapy is daily plasma exchange until remission and maintenance of platelet count at 150×10^9/L, though there are a number of reported differences in how to use plasma exchange in the management of this disorder. Initial plasma exchanges should be at least a 1.5 plasma volume exchanges. Corticosteroids such as prednisone (1 mg/kg/day) can also be given with the exchanges. If plasma exchange is not immediately available, infusion of fresh frozen plasma alone has been shown to be effective in patients with HIV-associated TTP. In classic TTP, relapses can occur in up to 30% of patients; however, relapse in HIV-associated TTP appears to be less frequent. Patients who relapse can be treated with repeat exchange combined with immunosuppressive therapy including such agents as vincristine or rituximab.

HUS most likely results from endothelial perturbation secondary to either HIV or other viral infections such as CMV, drug or toxin induced such as observed with *Escherichia coli* 0157:H7 infection. Recent data suggest that the primary event leads to unregulated complement activation caused either by inhibitors of complement regulatory protein such as complement H or congenital abnormalities in complement regulation. In these patients, measurement of ADAMTS13 activity will uniformly report levels near normal and above 30%. Many patients will respond to aggressive plasma exchange, but complete remissions are rare. Recently the inhibitor of complement C5a, eculizumab, has been approved for the treatment of atypical HUS, but there are no reports of its use in HIV-associated HUS.

THROMBOEMBOLIC DISEASE

Since the beginning of the AIDS epidemic, an unexpectedly high incidence of venous thromboembolism (VTE) has been observed among people with HIV disease. The most compelling data in support of an increased risk of VTE in HIV disease estimated the incidence of thrombosis in their HIV-infected population to be about 2.6 per 1000 person-years. Given the fact that cohorts of patients with HIV infection tend to include a disproportionate number of younger individuals compared with the general population, this figure represents an increased incidence of VTE. The increased incidence in venous thrombosis was disproportionately greater among patients with clinical AIDS, those older than 45 years, those with AIDS-defining illnesses (particularly CMV infection), and those taking indinavir (Crixivan) or megestrol acetate (Megace). However, 53% of the thrombotic events occurred in individuals without history of recent hospitalization.

In a study comparing the risk of VTE in HIV-infected patients to an age-matched uninfected control population, there was no statistic difference in the overall risk of VTE (2.8% HIV-infected versus 1.8% controls) except in the HIV-infected patients less than 50 years (3.31% HIV-infected versus 0.53% controls; $p < .0001$). A study of 37,535 HIV-infected veterans compared with 37,535 age, race and site-matched uninfected controls found in evidence that a 39% increased incidence in VTE in the pre-HAART era (before 1996) and a 33% increased incidence in the era of HAART. The increased risk of thrombosis was independent of a diagnosis of malignancy, HIV-related opportunistic infections, or the use of central catheters. The development of a thromboembolic event was associated with a statistically increased mortality in all groups.

Role of Inflammation and Its Effect on the Protein C and S Anticoagulant System

With advancing HIV disease, there are progressive prothrombotic hemostatic changes, specifically a decrease in protein S and an increase in factor VIII. There is a well-documented association between acute and chronic inflammation and activation of the hemostatic system. Inflammatory cytokines such as TNF-α, IL-1, and IL-6 have been shown to activate coagulation and downregulate activation of protein

C. Activated protein C (APC) is a major inhibitor of coagulation, degrading activated coagulation factors VIIIa and Va. Inflammation can also result in a decrease in functional protein S, the cofactor of APC, which most likely explains the acquired protein S deficiency observed in some HIV-infected patients, with and without thrombosis.

An important additional component of the inflammatory state, which further contributes to an increased risk of thrombosis, is the inflammation-induced increase in factor VIII coagulant protein. Factor VIII levels greater than 1500 units/L (150%) are an independent risk factor for idiopathic VTE. A study of 94 HIV-infected women and 50 HIV-negative controls who were participants in the Women's Interagency HIV Study documented a progressive prothrombotic state with advancing HIV disease characterized by progressive decreases in protein S activity associated with a progressive increase in Factor VIII activity. The decreases in protein S activity and reciprocal increases in factor VIII activity closely correlated with decreasing CD4+ lymphocyte count and were most significant in the women with clinical AIDS. This study provides evidence for a link between advancing HIV disease characterized by decreasing CD4+ lymphocyte count and the development of clinical AIDS with opportunistic infections and hemostatic changes associated with an increased risk for venous thrombosis. This acute and chronic inflammatory state is the most likely pathogenic mechanism for development of VTE in HIV-infected individuals.

Anticardiolipin Antibodies

It is well established that antiphospholipid antibodies (anticardiolipin antibodies [ACA] and lupus anticoagulant) are associated with a hypercoagulable state. The incidence of elevated ACA in asymptomatic HIV disease is reported to be as high as 50% and even higher in patients with clinical AIDS. Recent reports have documented the presence of ACA in HIV-infected individuals with VTE. However, two small studies reported no correlation between high levels of ACA and thrombosis in HIV infection. Because the increased thrombotic risk associated with the antiphospholipid antibody syndrome is predominantly associated with the lupus anticoagulant and β2GP 1, it is not surprising that increased ACA alone was not associated with a significantly increased risk of thrombosis. Thus the contribution of antiphospholipid antibodies to the development of VTE in HIV disease remains unknown and will require larger prospective studies that include assays for the lupus anticoagulant and anti–β2GP antibodies.

Role of Protease Inhibitors

Several investigators have found protease inhibitors to be associated with VTE. Sullivan et al. reported that the use of indinavir (Crixivan) was associated with an increased risk of VTE. In a case series, George et al.[29] reported unexplained thrombosis in HIV patients receiving protease inhibitors. Abnormalities of glucose metabolism and serum lipids are commonly observed with protease inhibitor therapy. These include acquired insulin resistance, increased low-density lipoprotein cholesterol, and decreased high-density lipoprotein (HDL) cholesterol. Insulin resistance is associated with acquired defects in the fibrinolytic system, including increased levels of plasminogen activator inhibitor and tissue plasminogen activator. Similar fibrinolytic abnormalities have been observed in patients with documented insulin resistance who are treated with protease inhibitors.

HDL has been shown to significantly enhance the activity of the APC complexed with protein S. This APC complex plays an essential role in downregulating thrombin generation. The lipoprotein abnormalities associated with the use of protease inhibitors, when combined with other acquired defects in the protein C anticoagulant pathway, may further depress the anticoagulant activity of the APC complex and subsequently promote increased thrombin generation. Thus there are a number of pathogenic mechanisms that could predispose

HIV-infected patients to VTE. The majority of reported hemostatic abnormalities appear to primarily affect the protein C and S inhibitory mechanisms. However, the available studies reporting an increased risk of VTE in HIV disease are only suggestive at present because most supporting data come from case reports and one uncontrolled retrospective study. Larger prospective studies are needed to assess the true relative risk of VTE in HIV-infected individuals and to determine the primary pathogenic mechanisms responsible for thrombosis in this population.

Management of Venous Thromboembolism With HIV Infection

The overall management principles and goals of therapy for VTE are the same for people with and without HIV infection, although extra caution is needed to anticipate possible drug interactions with HAART, particularly with the use of warfarin. Initial therapy for the patient presenting with deep vein thrombosis and/or pulmonary emboli involves the use of either intravenous unfractionated (UF) heparin or preferentially subcutaneous low-molecular-weight (LMW) heparin. Oral anticoagulants can be started immediately upon achieving therapeutic heparin levels, and under optimal circumstances heparin treatment can be completed and the patient discharged from the hospital within 5–7 days. LMW heparin preparations given subcutaneously without monitoring have been shown to be safe and effective treatment for VTE and may be preferable because they also allow for safe outpatient management. In a meta-analysis of clinical trials comparing LMW heparin with UF heparin, LMW heparin preparations were associated with a lower risk of major bleeding compared with adjusted-dose intravenous UF heparin.

The greatest difficulties in the management of VTE in HIV-infected patients occur with the use of oral anticoagulants. The optimal therapeutic range for oral anticoagulation with warfarin in patients with VTE is a prothrombin time (PT) international normalized ratio (INR) of 2–3. No data suggest that HIV-infected patients require a different degree of anticoagulation. However, most studies have found that general medical patients managed as outpatients have a therapeutic INR in only 60% of assays. Although there are no published data regarding the use of oral anticoagulants in HIV-infected patients, individuals receiving HAART appear to have greater difficulty in maintaining therapeutic anticoagulation, most likely because of complex drug interactions. With a reported annual risk of major bleeding with oral anticoagulants of 2% to 3% and bleeding-related fatality of 20%, careful PT monitoring of HIV-infected patients is mandatory. They should be monitored at least weekly for the first 6 to 8 weeks and should then have their PT checked every 2 weeks. In patients in whom maintaining therapeutic levels is difficult, home monitoring using devices approved by the US Food and Drug Administration may be indicated. Patients who have significant difficulty maintaining a therapeutic INR or have had bleeding complications caused by poor control of their anticoagulation can be treated with long-term LMW heparin as has been recommended for the long-term management of cancer-related VTE. In both HIV-infected and HIV-negative patients with malignancies who develop VTE, long-term management with LMW heparin appears to be associated with a significantly lower risk of recurrent VTE. Drug–drug interactions may also limit the use of the new oral anticoagulants. Potent inhibitors (lopinavir, ritonavir, indinavir, conivaptan) or inducers (carbamazepine, rifampin, phenytoin) of Cyp3A4 and P-GP can significantly increase the bleeding risk or conversely decrease the efficacy of these agents.

Oral anticoagulation in the patient with VTE should be maintained for at least 6 months. Patients with unprovoked VTE who have had major pulmonary emboli, recurrent thromboemboli, or underlying inherited or acquired prothrombotic defects may benefit from longer courses of oral anticoagulation. However, the decision to extend anticoagulation to prevent recurrence of thrombosis must be weighed against the significant risk of bleeding in this population.

REFERENCES

1. Shen H, Cheng T, Preffer FI, et al: Intrinsic human immunodeficiency virus type 1 resistance of hematopoietic stem cells despite coreceptor expression. *J Virol* 73(1):728–737, 1999.

2. Bahner I, Kearns K, Coutinho S, et al: Infection of human marrow immunodeficiency virus-1 (HIV-1) is both required and sufficient for HIV-1 inducted hematopoietic suppression in vitro: demonstration by gene modification of primary human stroma. *Blood* 90(5):1787–1798, 1997.

3. Gradstein S, Hahn T, Barak Y, et al: In vitro effects of recombinant TNF-alfa binding protein (rTBP-1) on hematopoiesis of HIV-infected patients. *J Acquir Immune Defic Syndr* 26(2):111–117, 2001.

4. Huang SS, Barbour JD, Deeks SG, et al: Reversal of immunodeficiency virus type 1-associated hematosupression by effective antiretroviral therapy. *Clin Infect Dis* 30(3):504–510, 2000.

5. Parker NG, Notermans DW, de Boer RG, et al: Biphasic kinetics of peripheral blood T cells after triple combination therapy in HIV-1 infection: a composite of redistribution and proliferation. *Nat Med* 4(2):208–214, 1998.

6. Zhao X, Sun NC, Witt MD, et al: Changing pattern of AIDS: a bone marrow study. *Am J Clin Pathol* 121(3):393–401, 2004.

7. Coyle TE: Hematological complications of human immunodeficiency virus infection and the acquired immunodeficiency syndrome. *Med Clin North Am* 81(2):449–470, 1997.

8. Sullivan PS, Hanson DL, Chu SY, et al: Epidemiology of anemia in human immunodeficiency virus (HIV)-infected persons: results from the MutistateAdult and Adolescent Spectrum of HIV Disease Surveillance Project. *Blood* 91(1):301–308, 1998.

9. Abrams DI, Steinhart C, Frascino R: Epoetin alfa therapy for anaemia in HIV-infected patients: impact on quality of life. *Int J STD AIDS* 11(10):659–665, 2000.

10. Moore RD, Forney D: Anemia in HIV infected patients receiving highly active antiretroviral therapy. *J Acquir Immune Defic Syndr* 29(1):54–57, 2002.

11. Lundgren JD, Mocroft A, Gatell JM, et al: A clinically prognostic scoring system for patients receiving highly active antiretroviral therapy: results from the EuroSIDA Study. *J Infect Dis* 185(2):178–187, 2002.

12. Gabrilove JL, Cleeland CS, Livingston RB, et al: Clinical evaluation of one-weekly dosing of epoetin alpha in chemotherapy patients: improvements in hemoglobin and quality of life are similar to three-times-weekly dosing. *J Clin Oncol* 19(11):2875–2882, 2001.

13. Isgrò I, Auiti A, Mezzaroma I, et al: HIV type I protease inhibitors enhance bone marrow progenitor cell activity in normal subjects and HIV type 1-infected patients. *AIDS Res Hum Retroviruses* 21(1):51–57, 2005.

14. Berhane K, Karim R, Cohen MH, et al: Impact of highly active antiretroviral therapy on anemia and relationship between anemia and survival in a large cohort of HIV-infected women. *J Acquir Immune Defic Syndr* 37(2):1245–1252, 2004.

15. Buskin SE, Sullivan PS: Anemia and its treatments and outcome in persons infected with human immunodeficiency virus. *Transfusion* 44(6):826–832, 2004.

16. de Mayolo JA, Temple JD: Pure red cell aplasia due to parvovirus B19 infection in a man with HIV infection. *South Med J* 83(12):1480–1481, 1990.

17. Chen M, Chien-Ching H, Fang C, et al: Reconstituted immunity against persistant parvovirus B19 infection in a patient with acquired immunodeficiency syndrome after highly active antiretroviral therapy. *Clin Infect Dis* 32(9):1361–1365, 2001.

18. Levine AM, Karim R, Mack W, et al: Neutropenia in human immunodeficiency virus infection. *Arch Intern Med* 166(4):405–410, 2006.

19. Moore DAJ, Benepal T, Portsmouth S, et al: Etiology and natural history of neutropenia in human immunodeficiency virus disease: a prospective study. *Clin Infect Dis* 32:469–475, 2001.

20. Dubreuil-Lemaire ML, Gori A, Vittecog D, et al: Lenograstim for the treatment of neutropenia in patients receiving ganciclovir for cytomegalovirus infection: a randomized placebo-controlled trial in AIDS patients. *Eur J Haematol* 65(5):337–343, 2000.

21. Battaieb A, Fromont P, Louache F, et al: Presence of cross-reactive antibody against HIV and platelet glycoproteins in HIV-related immune thrombocytopenic purpura. *Blood* 80(1):162–169, 1992.

22. Caso JAA, Mingo CS, Tena JG: Effect of highly active antiretroviral therapy on thrombocytopenia in patients with HIV infection. *N Engl J Med* 341(16):1239–1240, 1999.

23. Bussel JB, Haimi JS: Isolated thrombocytopenia in patients infected with HIV: treatment with intravenous immunoglobulin. *Am J Hematol* 28(2):79–84, 1988.

24. Scaradavou A, Woo B, Woloski BM, et al: Intravenous anti-D treatment of immune thrombocytopenic purpura: experience in 272 patients. *Blood* 89(8):2689–2700, 1997.

25. Leaf AN, Laubenstein LJ, Raphael B, et al: Thrombotic thrombocytopenic purpura associated with human immunodeficiency virus type 1(HIV-1) infection. *Ann Intern Med* 109(3):194–197, 1988.

26. Novitzky N, Thomson J, Abrahams L, et al: Thrombotic thrombocytopenic purpura in patients with retroviral infection is highly responsive to plasma infusion therapy. *Br J Haematol* 128(3):373–379, 2005.

27. Sullivan PS, Dworkin MS, Jones JL, et al: Epidemiology of thrombosis in HIV-infected individuals. *AIDS* 14(3):321–324, 2000.

28. Levine AM, Vigen C, Gravink J, et al: Progressive prothrombotic state in women with advancing HIV disease. *J Acquir Immune Defic Syndr* 42(5):572–577, 2006.

29. George S, Swindells S, Knudson R, et al: Unexplained thrombosis in HIV-infected patients receiving protease inhibitors: report of seven cases. *Am J Med* 107(6):624–626, 1999.

CHAPTER 158

HEMATOLOGIC ASPECTS OF PARASITIC DISEASES

David J. Roberts

Parasitic diseases are not common in medical, let alone hematologic, practice in North America or Europe. However, much of the world's population is infected by and becomes symptomatic as a result of a plethora of parasites, and many of these infections represent global public health problems.

Although some significant parasitic diseases are transmitted in temperate climates, the majority of parasites of significance to human health are endemic in the tropical world. This reflects not only socioeconomic circumstances but also the origin of our species in tropical Africa, where the human host, parasites, and also vectors have established complex relationships over evolutionary timescales.[1] Notwithstanding such geographic variation in the incidence of parasitic disease, both travelers and recent immigrants now present to hematology clinics and laboratories all over the world with increasing frequency. Even in those circumstances, there are marked variations in practice in North America as well as in Europe, where the United Kingdom reports more cases of imported malaria than the United States and indeed has a 10-fold greater incidence of malaria per capita, reflecting the increased frequency of travel to and from endemic areas compared with North American populations.

Patients with malaria, leishmaniasis, trypanosomiasis, and babesiosis may present directly or indirectly to hematologists. This chapter is concentrated on the biologic, clinical, and hematologic features of these infections and the hematologic aspects or complications of their treatment. Comprehensive accounts of the general medical aspects of these diseases are provided in many other recent textbooks.[2-4]

MALARIA

Malaria is a major public health problem in tropical areas, and it is estimated that it is responsible for 600,000 to 900,000 deaths annually and 150 to 300 million infections.[5] The vast majority of morbidity and mortality caused by malaria is caused by infection with *Plasmodium falciparum*, although *Plasmodium vivax*, *Plasmodium ovale*, and *Plasmodium malariae* are also responsible for human infections. A fifth species, *Plasmodium knowlesi*, has been shown to cause human infection in some parts of Southeast Asia (for review, see the article by Millar and Cox-Singh[5]). In endemic areas, a significant proportion of the mortality and morbidity is from anemia. In Europe and North America, malaria is not infrequently a clinical problem in travelers or recent arrivals from malaria-endemic areas, and hematologists may be involved in the diagnosis and management of the disease. Moreover, in nonendemic areas, malaria may cause a fatal transfusion-transmitted infection, and detection of blood donors who may be carrying the disease represents a major challenge for blood services.

Epidemiology

Approximately 1 billion people live in areas of endemic or epidemic malaria. The global mortality and morbidity were revised to 350 million cases and 1 million deaths per year, respectively, following an evaluation of the prevalence of infection in Southeast Asia (Fig. 158.1). There is, however, substantial evidence that the incidence of severe disease is now falling, sometimes spectacularly, in many parts of Africa following the widespread introduction of artemisinin combination treatment, impregnated bed nets, and residual spraying because the resources available for malaria control have increased

substantially through the Global Fund and the World Health Organization's "Roll Back Malaria" campaign (www.rbm.who.int). The current estimated annual death total from malaria in Africa is 630,000.[6]

The distribution of malaria is determined by features of host, vector, and parasite. In summary, the global distribution of autochthonous or endogenous malaria is limited by the lower temperature limits for development of the parasite in the mosquito (sporogony) of 20°C for *P. falciparum* and 15°C for other human malarias. Within these limits, transmission does not occur above 1500 m in arid regions or in the Central and South Pacific (because of the absence of suitable vectors). In addition, *P. vivax* malaria is rare in Africa, where the population frequency of the blood group Duffy negative (Fya⁻Fyb⁻) is high. *P. ovale* requires a lengthy period of sporogony and is confined to areas of Africa and Southeast Asia with a high density of susceptible *Anopheles* spp. *P. knowlesi* is transmitted from macaque monkeys in forest areas of Borneo, Malaysia, Thailand, and Vietnam.[5]

In some malarious areas the seasonal pattern of clinical malaria is determined by the increase in vector density after rainfall, leading to an increase in new infections as transmission increases. In naive individuals, parasites can cause chronic infection lasting many months.

The intensity of transmission determines the distribution of clinical symptoms in different age groups.[7] In general, in areas of high transmission, younger children experience severe disease. Where transmission is less intense, older children experience severe disease. Finally, if the rate of transmission is very low, few cases of malaria are seen in any age group, and such populations would have little natural immunity. In such areas, a sudden increase in vectorial capacity (through the accidental introduction of efficient vectors or higher density, biting, or survival of the resident vectors), more rapid parasite sporogony, or migration of infected or nonimmune populations can result in epidemics where large numbers fall ill in all age groups. The transition from high to low transmission has been classified by holoendemicity, hyperendemicity, mesoendemicity, and hypoendemicity. These categories can be related epidemiologically to age-specific rates of parasite prevalence or splenomegaly and theoretically to the reproductive ratio of malarial infection.[8]

Malaria exerts a substantial selection for human traits that protect from infection. Sickle cell trait and thalassemia traits protect from infection and are truly polymorphic characteristics in many parts of the world. Understanding genetic epidemiology has provided the foundation of population genetics and has provided classic examples of principles of genetic selection in vivo—for example, balancing selection for sickle cell trait and negative epistasis for sickle cell trait and α-thalassemia. The homozygous forms of these characteristics cause significant clinical disease, such as sickle cell disease, β-thalassemia, and glucose-6-phosphate dehydrogenase (G6PDH) deficiency. In endemic areas these genetic diseases represent major public health problems (for review, see Williams[9] and Luzzatto et al[10]).

Parasitology

In *P. falciparum* (see later for a discussion of the other human parasites) the infective sporozoite forms are inoculated into the bloodstream from the salivary glands of a female *Anopheles* mosquito

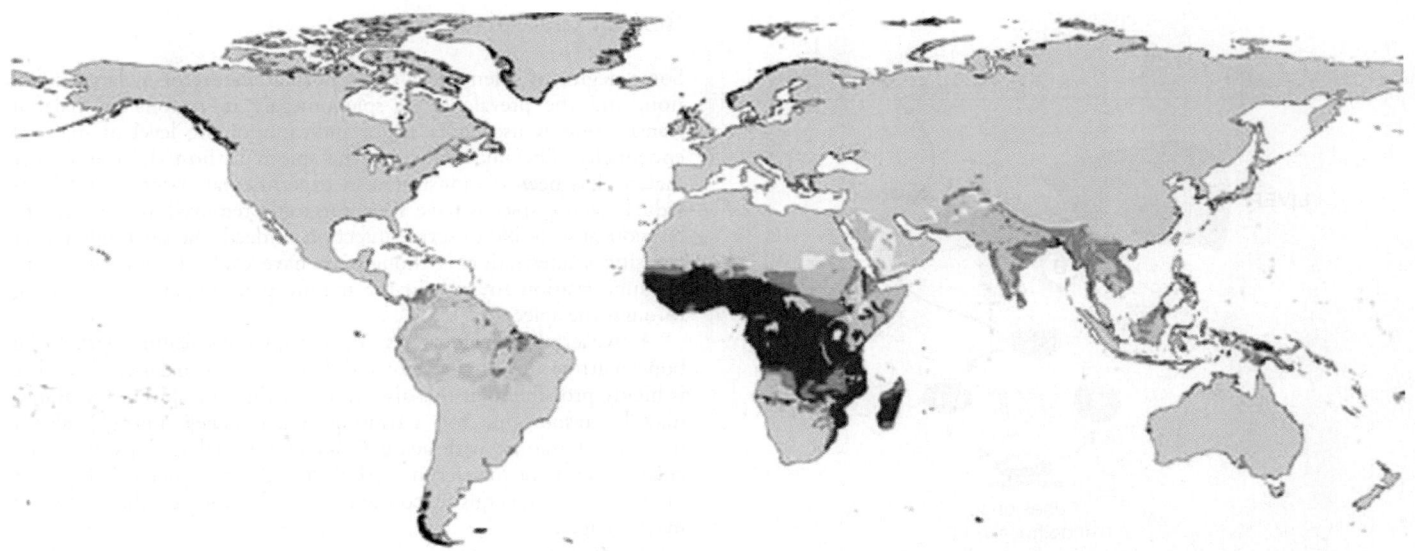

Fig. 158.1 GLOBAL MALARIA ENDEMICITY. Areas are colored according to malaria endemicity (prevalence): *light green*, hypoendemic (areas in which childhood infection prevalence is less than 10%); *medium green*, mesoendemic (areas with infection prevalence between 11% and 50%); *dark green*, hyperendemic and holoendemic (areas with an infection prevalence of 50% or more); unclassified areas *(yellow)* represent only 6% of the global population at risk and are caused by discrepancies in recent data. *Gray* areas are a combined mask of areas outside the transmission limits and areas of population density less than 1 person/km². *(Data from Snow RW, Guerra CA, Noor AM, et al: The global distribution of clinical episodes of* Plasmodium falciparum *malaria.* Nature *434:214, 2005.)*

(Fig. 158.2). These thin, needle-shaped cells, 10 to 12 μm in length, circulate briefly with a half-life of approximately 30 minutes before traversing macrophages and several hepatocytes and ultimately residing in a single hepatocyte.[11,12] Here rapid multiplication takes place over 5 to 8 days to produce a liver schizont, 80 μm in diameter and containing 30,000 ± 10,000 merozoites that are released into the bloodstream, where they infect erythrocytes.[13] When ready to leave hepatocytes, the parasite induces cell death in the hepatocytes and causes the release of merozoites in membrane-enclosed structures or merosomes that are extruded from the infected cell, thereby avoiding host cell defense mechanisms.[14]

The merozoites bind and then invade red blood cells (RBCs; for review of RBC and merozoite interactions, see Satchwell[15]). The host plasma membrane is invaginated to form the parasitophorous vacuole. For the first 10 hours the developing parasites appear as fine "ring forms." Between 10 and 15 hours the cytoplasm thickens, and 16 hours after invasion, granules of the black pigment hematin, the end product of hemoglobin digestion, begin to appear. Ligands are expressed at the surface of the infected RBC that mediate adhesion to host receptors on venular endothelium. These trophozoites no longer circulate throughout the body but are sequestered in the peripheral circulation. Nuclear division begins, at approximately 30 hours, to form schizonts containing up to 32 merozoites. At 48 hours the RBC is ruptured to release the merozoites into the circulation to continue further cycles of asexual multiplication.

The erythrocytic cycle of schizogony may achieve a 10-fold increase in parasitemia in vivo and a patent or microscopically detectable infection 6 days after the liver stage is completed. After two or more cycles the infection becomes clinically apparent by the paroxysms of fever that accompany the release of merozoites. Cycles of schizogony continue until the rate of parasite multiplication is reduced by chemotherapy, specific or nonspecific defense mechanisms, or occasionally the demise of the host.

Some merozoites do not multiply but become committed during the previous erythrocytic cycle to form male or female gametocytes.[16] Gametocytes are distinguished by dispersed pigment in a single nucleus, in a fully grown parasite, and are sequestered for the first 5 days of their development in the peripheral circulation. Thus 8 to 10 days after the start of clinical infection, mature, crescent-shaped gametocytes appear in the blood.

The sexual phase (or sporogony) of the parasite life cycle begins after a male and female gametocyte are ingested by a feeding female *Anopheles* mosquito. In the midgut of the mosquito the gametocytes shed the RBC membrane. This change is apparently precipitated by the drop in temperature. A female gametocyte forms a single macrogamete, but male gametocytes undergo several rounds of nuclear division to produce flagellated microgametes. These microgametes are motile and migrate to fertilize a macrogamete. The resulting zygote enlarges to form a mobile ookinete and migrates through the epithelial wall of the mosquito midgut to rest finally on the external surface. The oocyst divides repeatedly to form up to 10,000 sporozoites, which travel up through the hemolymph to enter the acinar cells of the salivary glands. Once there, they are infective when injected into the host.

Major differences exist in the life cycles of other human *Plasmodium* spp. First, in *P. vivax* and *P. ovale* infections, some sporozoites entering the liver form dormant hypnozoites that begin to divide only after a variable period of some months to cause further blood-stage infections or relapses. Second, the cycle of erythrocytic development in *P. malariae* takes 72 hours and thus causes quartan fever (i.e., on days 1 and 4).

The Pathophysiology of Malarial Anemia

Malaria gives ample reasons for both increased RBC destruction and reduced RBC production (see Fig. 158.3 for overview).

Loss of Infected Erythrocytes

Destruction of RBCs is inevitable as parasites complete their 48-hour growth cycle and lyse their temporary host cell. Some parasites may be removed from erythrocytes as immature ring forms by phagocytic cells, leaving the RBCs with residual parasite antigens to continue to circulate, albeit with reduced survival.[17] Infected erythrocytes may

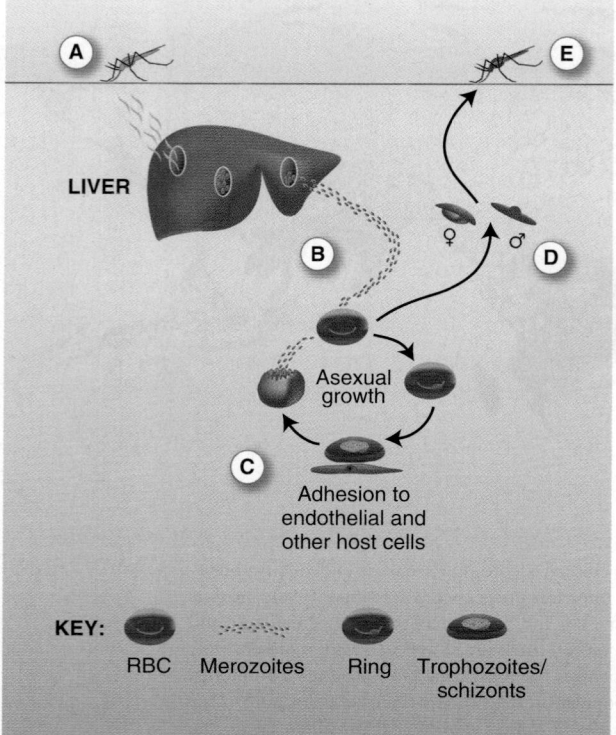

Fig. 158.2 *PLASMODIUM* LIFE CYCLE. (A) The asexual life cycle begins when sporozoites from a female mosquito taking a blood meal enter the circulation and invade hepatocytes. (B) Up to 10,000 merozoites are formed. Following rupture of the hepatocyte, infective merozoites are released and invade erythrocytes (red blood cells [RBCs]). (C) Within RBCs, the parasite develops through the stages of rings, trophozoites, and schizonts. Mature schizonts burst to release erythrocytic merozoites that invade new RBCs. (D) A small proportion of merozoites in RBCs transform into male and female gametocytes that are ingested by the mosquito. (E) The male and female gametes fuse and transform into an oocyst, which divides asexually into many sporozoites that migrate to the salivary gland from where they are released during the next blood meal.

also be phagocytosed by macrophages following opsonization by immunoglobulins and/or complement components.[18,19] Other signals for recognition of infected erythrocytes by macrophages include abnormally rigid membranes and exposure of phosphatidylserine and other altered host antigens and, in animal models of malaria, antiphosphatidylserine antibodies.[20–23]

Loss of Uninfected Erythrocytes

The activity and the number of macrophages are increased in malarial infection, and increased removal of uninfected cells may occur. Moreover, the signals for recognition of uninfected erythrocytes for removal by macrophages are enhanced. Uninfected erythrocytes bind increased amounts of immunoglobulin and/or complement as detected in the direct antiglobulin test (DAT or Coombs test).[23] These antibodies do not have a particular specificity but are more likely to represent immune complexes absorbed onto the surface of RBCs.[23] Furthermore, hemozoin may activate complement directly and cause deposition of C3b on uninfected RBCs.[24] However, an association between positive DAT results and severe anemia has not been established.[25] More recent studies have shown not only that RBCs from patients with malaria were more susceptible to phagocytosis but also that RBCs from children with acute malaria had increased surface immunoglobulin G (IgG) and low levels of RBC CR1 and CD55 compared with control subjects.[26]

Role of the Spleen

Some degree of splenomegaly is a normal feature of malarial infection, and the prevalence of splenomegaly in regions of malarial transmission is used as a major indicator of the level of malarial endemicity. The importance of the spleen in host defense against malaria has been demonstrated in experimental systems, and individuals whose spleens have been surgically removed are thought to be more susceptible to severe infection. Indeed, the phenomenon of parasitic sequestration is thought to have evolved primarily as an immune evasion strategy so the mature parasite can avoid passing through the spleen.[27]

Active erythrophagocytosis is a conspicuous feature within the bone marrow during *P. vivax* and *P. falciparum* malaria,[28,29] and it is highly probable that this also occurs within the spleen. Cytokines may be responsible for activating macrophages during malarial infection. Children with acute *P. falciparum* malaria have high circulating levels of interferon-γ (IFN-γ) and tumor necrosis factor-α (TNF-α),[30] a synergistic combination of cytokines that activates macrophages.

Researchers in several studies have attempted to define the pathophysiologic changes in the spleen during acute malaria. In animal models, malaria is accompanied by increased intravascular clearance of infected or rigid, heat-treated cells by the spleen,[31] as well as alterations in the splenic microcirculation.[32] In studies of human malaria, it has been found that increased splenic clearance of heated RBCs occurs during acute attacks.[33] More recent, histologic studies and ex vivo models of splenic function suggest that the spleen removes not only mature infected RBCs but also uninfected cells marked for clearance by low deformability, aggregated band 3, complement deposition, or phosphatidylserine exposure. Moreover, "pitting" of ring-stage infected cells may remove the parasite and leave the RBC marked with parasite antigen to return to the circulation (reviewed by Buffet et al[34]).

Changes to the uninfected RBCs during infection also contribute to their own enhanced clearance by phagocytes. Uninfected RBCs in children and adults with severe disease are less deformable, and this is a significant predictor of the severity of anemia and indeed outcome, consistent with the notion that these cells are being removed by the spleen.[20] It has also been found that IgG-sensitized RBCs are rapidly removed from the circulation by the spleen and that unusually rapid clearance persists well into the convalescent phase.[35]

Thus all the available evidence points to increased reticuloendothelial clearance in *P. falciparum* malaria, persisting long after recovery. These changes are presumably a host defense mechanism, maximizing the clearance of parasitized erythrocytes.

The Role of Ineffective Erythropoiesis in Severe Malarial Anemia

Reticulocytopenia has been confirmed in numerous clinical studies of malarial anemia.[36–38] The histopathologic study of the bone marrow of children with malarial anemia shows erythroid hyperplasia with increased numbers of erythroid precursors (Fig. 158.4). However, the maturation is abnormal by light and electron microscopy. Abdalla et al[39,40] described the hallmark characteristics of such abnormal maturation, namely cytoplasmic and nuclear bridging and irregular nuclear outline. They later confirmed that the distribution of the erythroid progenitors through the cell cycle is abnormal in malarial anemia, with an increased proportion of cells in the G₂ phase compared with healthy control subjects.[41] Dormer et al[38] confirmed these findings using the same criteria as Abdalla et al; they studied six patients with falciparum malaria before and after treatment.

Ineffective erythropoiesis also contributes to anemia in animal models of malaria. A recent study has shown that vaccinated *Aotus* monkeys, after a challenge infection, may develop moderate to severe anemia following rapid clearance of uninfected erythrocytes, but with low reticulocyte counts, indicating bone marrow

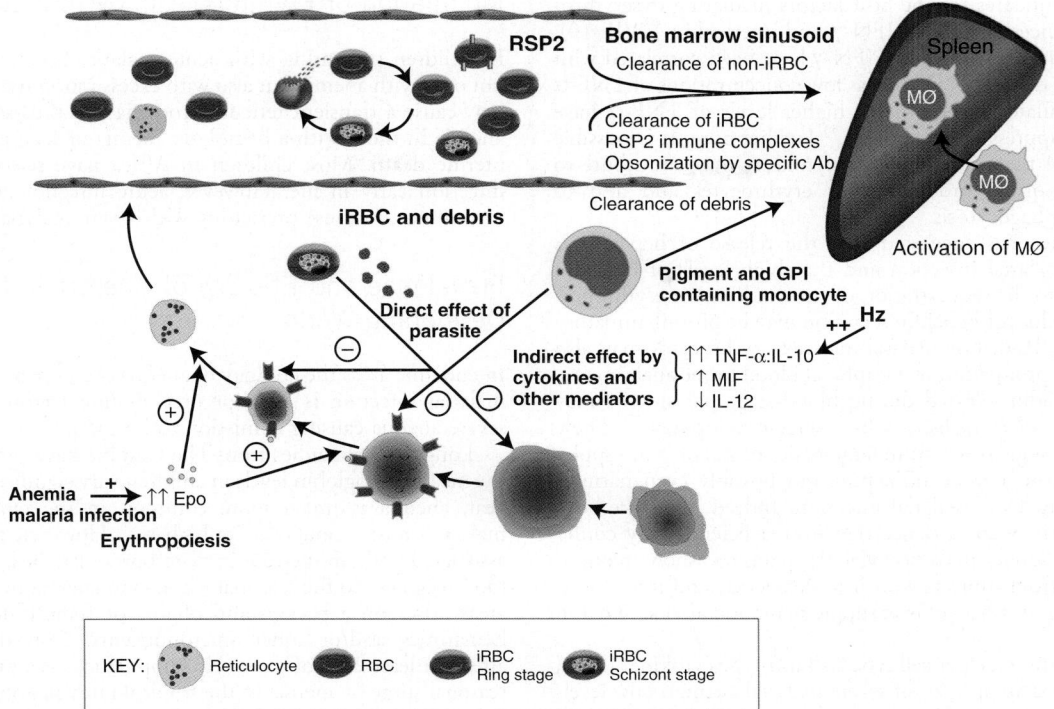

Fig. 158.3 PATHOGENESIS OF MALARIAL ANEMIA. Severe malarial anemia is characterized by destruction of infected red blood cells (iRBCs) following schizogony and clearance of both iRBC and uninfected RBCs. During malarial infection, changes in membrane protein composition occur, and the resultant immune complexes of RBC, Ag, and immunoglobulin (e.g., RBC-RSP2-Ig) are cleared by MØ to the spleen, where they become activated. Pigment-containing MØ may release inflammatory cytokines and other biologically active mediators such as 4-hydroxynonenal. MIF may be released by MØ, or a plasmodial homologue may suppress erythropoiesis. Malarial pigment or other parasite products may have a direct inhibitory effect on erythropoiesis. Inhibition of erythropoiesis may occur at one or more sites in the growth and differentiation of hematopoietic progenitors. Both indirect and direct effects may cause suppression of the bone marrow and spleen, resulting in inadequate reticulocyte counts for the degree of anemia. *Ab,* Antibody; *Ag,* antigen; *Epo,* erythropoietin; *GPI,* glycosylphosphatidylinositol anchors of merozoite proteins; *Hz,* hemozoin; *Ig,* immunoglobulin; *IL,* interleukin; *MIF,* macrophage inhibitory factor; *MØ,* macrophages; *RSP2,* ring surface protein-2; *TNF-α,* tumor necrosis factor-α.

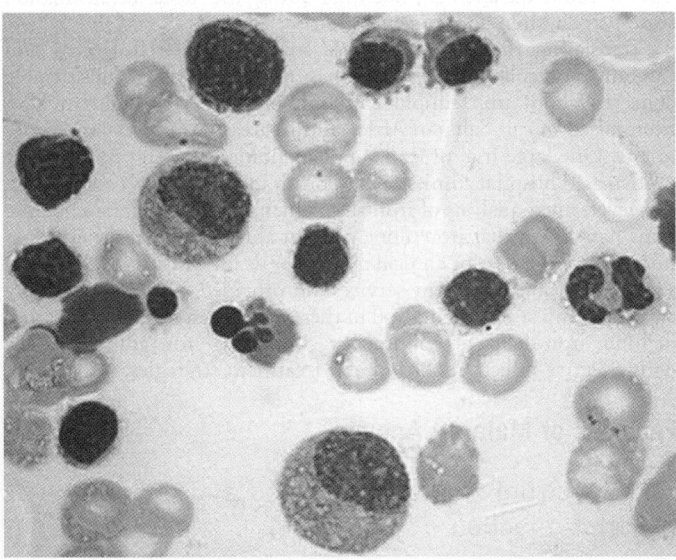

Fig. 158.4 BONE MARROW ASPIRATE IN MALARIA. Although erythropoiesis is usually normoblastic in individuals with acute or chronic malaria, the examination of bone marrow frequently shows changes reflecting dyserythropoiesis, such as the irregular nuclei and cytoplasmic bridges in erythroblasts seen in this figure. Two young rings of *Plasmodium falciparum* can be seen in an erythrocyte. *(Courtesy Dr. Saad H. Abdalla.)*

dysfunction.[42] Erythropoiesis is disrupted in mice during malarial infection. Mice infected with *Plasmodium berghei* show reduced bone marrow cellularity, erythroblasts, burst-forming units–erythroid, and colony-forming units–erythroid as early as 24 hours postinfection.[43] The cellularity and colony-forming unit–spleen content of the femoral marrow of BALB/c mice infected with *Plasmodium chabaudi adami* decreases as the parasitemia increases.[44]

Modulation of Erythropoiesis by Cytokines

Given the importance of erythropoietin (Epo) to erythropoiesis, attention has been focused on the levels of this crucial cytokine in malarial infection. Serum Epo was appropriately raised in studies of African children with malarial anemia, and high levels of this cytokine may improve the outcome of disease.[45,46] More recently, African children with severe malaria, particularly young children, were shown to have supraphysiologic levels of Epo compared with age-matched community control subjects with nonmalarial anemia.[47,48] There is now evidence from clinical studies that these high levels of Epo in children with malarial anemia may exert a cytoprotective effect and reduce the risk for neurologic sequelae or death in children with cerebral malaria.[49] Indeed, in a murine model of cerebral malaria, exogenous Epo downregulated the inflammatory responses induced by dendritic cells, induced regulatory T cells, reduced endothelial activation, and improved the integrity of the blood–brain barrier.[50]

The prime candidates for the host factors mediating dyserythropoiesis are imbalances of TNF-α, IFN-γ, and interleukin-10 (IL-10). The concentrations of TNF-α and IFN-γ have been correlated with the severity of the disease.[51-53] Whereas low concentrations of TNF-α (<1 ng/mL) stimulate erythropoiesis, higher levels of TNF-α have been shown to suppress erythropoiesis.[53] Furthermore, it is possible that high levels of these inflammatory cytokines may contribute to reduced and abnormal production of erythrocytes and also to increased erythrophagocytosis.

Recent evidence has suggested that the release of hepcidin is associated with malarial infection and that high levels of hepcidin could contribute to the sequestration of iron and impair erythropoiesis.[54,55] The stimulus for hepcidin secretion may be proinflammatory cytokines such as IL-6, but malaria-infected erythrocytes may also enhance hepcidin production by peripheral blood mononuclear cells. Intriguingly, hepcidin released during blood-stage parasitemia may be a key regulator of *P. falciparum* liver-stage development.[56] These data now support suggestions from large-scale studies of iron supplementation that iron may be unhelpful and possibly even harmful when given during acute malarial infection. Indeed, there are both clinical and experimental evidence that iron deficiency may confer protection from severe malaria. Malaria parasites show reduced growth in RBCs from subjects with iron deficiency, and infection is augmented during the phase of iron supplementation after severe iron deficiency.[57]

High levels of the T-helper cell type 2 (Th2)-type cytokine, IL-10, might prevent the development of severe malarial anemia. Low levels of IL-10 have been described in African children with severe malarial anemia.[51] Similarly, defective IL-12 production has been shown experimentally to be associated with increased severity of malaria in a rodent model, and low IL-12 levels have been associated with severe malaria in African children.[58] The role of IL-12 in clinical malaria appears complex, but in toxoplasma infection in mice, IL-12 has been shown to have a key role in activating natural killer (NK) cells that primes monocytes in the bone marrow for a regulatory function, which could be important in malaria.[59]

Modulation of Erythropoiesis by Infected Erythrocytes

There is also substantial evidence that lysate of infected erythrocytes may directly modulate the function of host cells. During its blood stage, the malaria parasite proteolyses host hemoglobin in an acidic vacuole to obtain amino acids, releasing heme as a byproduct, which is auto-oxidized to potentially toxic hematin (aquaferriprotoporphyrin IX [$H_2O-Fe_{III}PPIX$]). β-Hematin forms as a crystalline cyclic dimer of $Fe_{III}PPIX$ and is complexed with protein and lipid products as malarial pigment or hemozoin. Schwarzer et al[60-62] showed that the function of monocytes and of monocyte-derived macrophages is severely inhibited after ingestion of malaria pigment or hemozoin. These cells were unable to repeat phagocytosis and to generate oxidative burst when appropriately stimulated. Furthermore, after phagocytosis of hemozoin, human and murine myeloid cells were unable to kill ingested fungi, bacteria, and tumor cells[63] or to respond to IFN-β stimulation, but instead responded by increased release of IL-1β, TNF-α,[64] macrophage inflammatory protein-1α (MIP-1α), and MIP-1β.[65]

The hemozoin polymer of heme moieties may be complexed with biologically active compounds. The oxidation of membrane lipids catalyzed by the ferric heme produces the lipoperoxides.[62,66] There is accumulating evidence that 4-hydroxynonenal (HNE) and other lipoperoxides, including 15-hydroxyarachidonic acid [15-(*R,S*)-HETE], may play a role in the pathophysiology of malaria. It has been shown that HNE and HETE are generated in parasitized erythrocytes and that HNE and endoperoxides produced in pigment-containing monocytes or macrophages may cause cell-cycle arrest and impair erythroid growth.[66,67] Hemozoin may also directly inhibit erythroid development in vitro and cause apoptosis of erythroid precursors.[68] Furthermore, increased levels of plasma hemozoin and pigment in monocytes have been associated with anemia.[49]

Modulation of Erythropoiesis by Infection

In children presenting with acute malaria, bacteremia is associated not only with anemia but also with excess mortality.[69] Parvovirus B19 may cause a transient reticulocytopenia and thus severe and sudden anemia in those with a hemolytic anemia or fetal anemia and intrauterine death. Most children in Africa have serologic evidence of infection early in life. However, acute infection with this virus is uncommon in those presenting with severe malarial anemia.[46,70]

Prevalence and Etiology of Anemia in the Developing World

In endemic areas the etiology of anemia is complex. Acute or chronic malarial infection is a major precipitating factor in children with severe anemia causing admission to hospital.[47]

Longitudinal studies from The Gambia have shown that whereas the mean hemoglobin levels in children vary significantly through the year, anemia is much more common in the rainy season, when malaria transmission is at its highest.[71] However, the rains are also associated with an increase in waterborne diarrheal disease and poor food supplies. So the seasonal increase in anemia in malaria-endemic areas arises on a background of low or frankly deficient stores of hematinics and/or other micronutrients. Iron deficiency, which affects at least 20% of the world's population, is a major factor in the seasonal surge of anemia in the tropical rainy season. Low iron stores at birth and dietary iron deficiency may be exacerbated by hookworm or schistosomal infection. It is now also clear that malarial infection is associated with reduced uptake of available iron and reduced incorporation of iron into developing erythroid cells.[54,55] Folate deficiencies and/or increased requirements may occur in many populations, although frank folate deficiency is uncommon.

A low baseline hemoglobin level at the start of the season for malaria transmission is a major risk factor for developing severe malarial anemia and has encouraged studies aimed at preventing the development of anemia by hematinic supplementation with or without antimalarial prophylaxis or surveillance.[72]

Quantifying the contribution of these individual factors to anemia reliably requires intervention studies. In Tanzania, Menendez et al[73] and Schellenberg et al[74] have shown that iron supplementation and antimalarial prophylaxis prevented 30% and 60%, respectively, of all cases of moderate anemia presenting during the malaria transmission season in children and in infants.

Translating the results of these studies from well-defined and carefully controlled study areas has not been easy. Considerable concerns about iron supplementation programs for children have been raised in sub-Saharan Africa and in areas of high malaria endemicity. One large trial of iron supplementation was stopped because of increased hospital admission and death in the group receiving iron. However, meta-analysis of iron supplementation in malaria-endemic areas has shown that iron alone or with antimalarial treatment does not increase the risk for clinical malaria or death when regular malaria surveillance and treatment services are provided.[75] It is increasingly clear that iron supplementation in these areas must be based on either defining iron-deficient children or combining iron administration with effective infection control and treatment strategies.[75,76]

Features of Malarial Anemia

The Spectrum of Disease Caused by Malarial Infection

The signs and symptoms of malarial infection in humans are caused by the asexual blood stage of the parasite. Infection with blood-stage parasites may result in a wide range of outcomes and pathologic conditions. Indeed, the spectrum of severity ranges from asymptomatic infection to rapidly progressive, fatal illness. The clinical presentation of malarial infection is also wide and influenced by age, immune status, and pregnancy, as well as by the species, genotype, and perhaps the geographic origin of the parasite. In endemic areas, many infections present as an uncomplicated febrile illness. In more severe forms of the disease, children may present with prostration or inability to take oral fluids, or in younger children an inability to suckle. Alternatively, these children may exhibit a number of syndromes of severe disease, including anemia, coma, respiratory distress, and hypoglycemia and may also have a high rate of bacteremia.[69,77]

In most age groups, anemia is frequently accompanied by more than one syndrome of severe disease, and the already substantial case fatality rate of 15% to 20% for severe malaria in African children rises significantly when multiple syndromes of severe disease are present.[77] The age distribution of anemia and other syndromes of severe disease is a consistent but puzzling feature of the epidemiology of clinical malaria. Children born in endemic areas are protected from severe malaria in the first 6 months of life by the passive transfer of maternal immunoglobulins and by fetal hemoglobin. Beyond infancy, the most common form of presentation of severe disease changes from anemia in children aged 1 to 3 years old, in areas of high transmission, to cerebral malaria in older children, in areas of lower transmission.[78] As transmission intensity declines further, severe malaria is most frequently found in older age groups.

The Clinical Features of Malarial Anemia

The blood stage of falciparum malaria may cause life-threatening anemia; a hemoglobin level of less than 5 g/dL is considered to represent severe disease. Children with anemia may present with malaise, fatigue, and dyspnea or respiratory distress, which usually represents metabolic acidosis, but in an ill child acute respiratory infection must be carefully excluded.[77,79]

Acidosis is due largely to excessive lactic acid and other anions. Salicylate toxicity and dehydration may also play a role. However, the majority of children presenting with respiratory distress are severely anemic, have a metabolic acidosis secondary to reduced oxygen-carrying capacity, and respond to rapid transfusion of fresh blood (for review, see English et al[80]). A minority of those with respiratory distress do not respond to appropriate resuscitation. They probably represent a heterogeneous clinical group and may have renal failure, systemic bacterial infection, or a more profound syndrome of systemic disturbance caused by malarial parasites.

However, a large randomized trial of a bolus of fluids in the treatment of African children with shock and life-threatening infections showed somewhat surprisingly that fluid boluses significantly increased 48-hour mortality in these critically ill children with impaired perfusion.[81] Fluid resuscitation must be carefully supervised, and it may be relevant that after transfusion in children with acute malarial anemia, BNP levels do fall, suggesting at the very least that cardiac function must be carefully monitored during fluid and blood therapy for acute malaria.[82]

Hemolytic Syndromes, Including Blackwater Fever

The sudden appearance of hemoglobin in the urine, indicating severe intravascular hemolysis leading to hemoglobinemia and hemoglobinuria or blackwater fever, received particular attention in early studies of anemia in expatriates living in endemic areas. There was an association between blackwater fever and the irregular use of quinine for chemoprophylaxis. This drug can act as a hapten and stimulate production of a drug-dependent, complement-fixing antibody. Recent studies of sudden intravascular hemolysis have shown that it is rare in Africa but more common in Southeast Asia and Papua New Guinea, where some cases are associated with G6PD deficiency and treatment with a variety of drugs, including quinine, mefloquine, and artesunate.[83] Treatment with artesunate may be associated with sudden severe hemolysis, but it is also recognized that artesunate can cause transient and mild reduction in hemoglobin levels after the acute episode of malaria as previously infected ring-stage parasites are cleared from the circulation. However, in the majority of cases, the cause of sudden hemolysis cannot be accounted for, and it seems likely that unidentified hemolytic mechanism(s) may operate.

The Hematologic Features of Malarial Infection

The anemia of falciparum malaria is typically normocytic and normochromic, with a notable absence of reticulocytes, although microcytosis and hypochromia may be present because of the very high frequency of α- and β-thalassemia traits and/or iron deficiency in many endemic areas.[47,71]

The anemia of malaria may be accompanied by changes in the white cell and platelet counts and in clotting parameters, but these changes are not in themselves diagnostic, nor do they guide management. Malaria is accompanied by a modest leukocytosis, although leukopenia may also occur. Occasionally, leukemoid reactions have been observed. Leukocytosis has been associated with severe disease.[84,85] A high neutrophil count may also suggest intercurrent bacterial infection. Monocytosis and increased numbers of circulating lymphocytes are also seen in acute infection, although the significance of these changes is not established.[86] However, malarial pigment is often seen in neutrophils and in monocytes and has been associated with severe disease and unfavorable outcome.[87,88]

Thrombocytopenia is almost invariable in malaria and so may be helpful as a sensitive but nonspecific marker of active infection. However, severe thrombocytopenia (platelet count $<50 \times 10^9$/L) is rare. Increased removal of platelets may follow absorption of immune complexes or platelet activation, but there is no evidence for platelet-specific alloantibodies.[89] By analogy with erythropoiesis, there may be a defect in thrombopoiesis, but this has not been established. Thrombocytopenia has not generally been associated with disease severity, although a study from Papua New Guinea has shown that severe thrombocytopenia identifies both children and adults at increased risk of death from falciparum or vivax malaria, particularly in those with concurrent severe anemia.[90] Indeed, platelets have been shown to contribute to disease pathology in both animal and human malaria.[91] Moreover, in human infections, platelets may form clumps with infected erythrocytes.[92] One explanation of inconsistent relationships reported between the severity of malaria and the thrombocytopenia may be that findings of low levels of platelets might not only be a marker of parasite burden but also be protective from severe disease and/or be associated with anti-inflammatory cytokine responses.[93]

Disordered coagulation and clinical evidence of bleeding are not infrequent in nonimmune adults contracting malaria and presenting with severe disease. Patients may present with bleeding at injection sites, gums, or epistaxis. Abnormal results of laboratory tests for hemostasis, suggesting activation of the coagulation cascade, occur in acute infection. However, histologic evidence of intravascular fibrin deposition is notably absent in adults dying as a result of severe malaria.[94] Factor XIII, normally responsible for cross-linking fibrin, is inactivated during malarial infection, and these data may explain low levels of fibrin deposition in the face of increased procoagulant activity.[95]

During acute disease the levels of a disintegrin and metalloproteinase with thrombospondin motif 13 (ADAMTS13) protease are moderately reduced, and the concentration of high-molecular-weight von Willebrand multimers is increased. Such multimers may play a role in the adherence of infected RBCs and platelets to endothelium, but the role of this adhesive pathway in the etiology of severe and cerebral malaria has not been established.[96]

The bone marrow is typically hypercellular. The most striking findings are of grossly abnormal development of erythroid precursors or dyserythropoiesis. The developing erythroid cells typically demonstrate cytoplasmic and nuclear bridging and irregular nuclear outline.[39,40] These changes are probably central to the pathophysiology of malarial anemia and are discussed in detail later. The proportion of abnormal erythroid precursors and the degree of dyserythropoiesis are markedly greater in chronic compared with acute infection, suggesting that the inhibition and abnormal maturation of erythroid precursors may have somewhat differing etiologies in acute and chronic infection.[39]

The role of hematinic deficiency in children presenting with malaria and anemia may be difficult to assess. The relative importance of absolute and functional iron deficiency have not been defined. Iron will not be absorbed during acute infection, because hepcidin levels are raised.[54,55] Nevertheless, many hospitals give a course of iron supplementation after an episode of acute malaria, although no general guidelines have been established. Chronic hemolysis may increase folate requirements, but frank deficiency is uncommon in children presenting with acute malaria, at least in East Africa.[47] Folate deficiency may be more common in West Africa, and protocols for folate supplementation after malaria must reflect local experience.

Malarial Anemia in Pregnancy

Pregnancy is accompanied by a series of physiologic changes that predispose not only to anemia but also to malaria. Hemodilution causes a physiologic decrease in hemoglobin. Moreover, the demand for both iron and folate increases as the fetus grows and often precipitates frank folate or iron deficiency, particularly in multigravid women.

Occult malarial infection, often without fever, may cause anemia and placental dysfunction. This effect is greatest in primigravidas and has been attributed to the adhesion of parasitized erythrocytes to chondroitin sulfate A and hyaluronic acid in the placenta[97,98] (for review, see Rogerson et al[99]). Fetal growth is impaired, and babies born to women with placental malaria are, on average, 100 g lighter than those born to women without malaria. The subsequent contribution of malaria to infant mortality is substantial.[100] Furthermore, the increase in hematopoiesis demanded by hemolysis during malarial infection may precipitate frank folate deficiency. Finally, women who are not immune to malaria are more likely to develop hypoglycemia and pulmonary edema during pregnancy. The increase in maternal and fetal morbidity and mortality secondary to malaria may be prevented by routine hematinic supplementation and by intermittent treatment with antimalarials during the second and third trimesters with sulfadoxine-pyrimethamine (Fansidar).[101]

Hyperreactive Malarial Splenomegaly

Although splenomegaly secondary to malarial infection usually regresses as immunity is acquired, some people living in endemic areas develop progressive, massive splenomegaly.[102] The pathophysiology of such hyperreactive malarial splenomegaly (HMS) is poorly understood but certainly results in B-cell hyperplasia with high levels of polyclonal IgM, reaching a level greater than two standard deviations (SDs) above the local reference mean. The specific antimalarial antibody titer is high, although only a small proportion of the polyclonal IgM response is directed at malarial antigens. B-cell hyperplasia may provoke proliferation of both T cells and macrophages, and IgM levels may cause cryoglobulinemia and stimulate erythrophagocytosis.

Patients may present typically between 20 and 40 years old, with massive splenomegaly without lymphadenopathy, anemia that may be severe, neutropenia, and thrombocytopenia. The anemia may cause life-threatening hemolytic crises and/or neutropenia associated with severe bacterial infection. Thrombocytopenia is rarely symptomatic. The bone marrow shows hypercellularity, with a lymphocytosis in marrow and peripheral blood. The high IgM levels distinguish HMS from chronic lymphocytic leukemia or other lymphoproliferative disorders. However, the polyclonal proliferation of B cells may transform to a true clonal lymphoproliferative disorder. This appears to be derived from a naive B cell, although the exact classification of such lymphoproliferative disorders is poorly defined[103]; however, there is a single report of a high incidence of B prolymphocytic leukemia in one population.

Treatment for HMS is lifelong antimalarial prophylaxis. Signs and symptoms usually subside over 1 to 2 years, but relapse may occur if antimalarial therapy ceases. Splenectomy is contraindicated because it is technically difficult, with considerable intra-operative mortality, and it may predispose to severe infection.

Anemia and *P. vivax*, *P. ovale*, and *P. malariae* Infection

In *P. vivax* and *P. ovale* malaria, high parasitemias are rare because invasion of erythrocytes is limited to reticulocytes. However, there is an emerging consensus that *P. vivax* monoinfection may cause severe disease with cerebral malaria and/or anemia (for review, see Price et al[104]). The vivax-infected RBC can adhere to host cells, but sequestration in the peripheral circulation and organ-specific syndromes of disease are much less common than in falciparum malaria.

P. vivax malaria has been associated with anemia during pregnancy and with low birth weight of children of affected mothers. Here cytokines or other inflammatory mediators appear to cause placental dysfunction.[105] *P. malariae* infection is also rarely fatal but is distinguished by the persistence of blood-stage parasites for up to 40 years. It can, however, cause a progressive and fatal nephrotic syndrome.[106]

Malaria Diagnosis

The diagnosis of malaria is based on the identification of circulating blood-stage parasites. The standard methods of preparing thick and thin films are straightforward and allow a simple method to diagnose infection (Table 158.1).[107–109] However, malaria diagnosis poses particular problems for inexperienced staff. The main biologic problem is that the level of circulating parasites is only weakly associated with the overall parasite burden because falciparum-infected erythrocytes are sequestered in capillary venules; thus the parasitemia is not a reliable guide to the severity of disease. Second, missing or delaying the diagnosis of falciparum malaria may result in serious morbidity and mortality. Finally, the most sensitive methods for diagnosis of infection, namely microscopy, require both skill and time.

TABLE 158.1	Malaria Diagnosis

- Thick and thin films should be prepared for cases of suspected malaria.
- Immunochromographic tests lack sensitivity to detect low levels of parasites that may be highly clinically significant.
- Routine Giemsa or May-Grünwald-Giemsa stains are unlikely to give satisfactory results, because the pH is too low.
- Films can be stained with Giemsa or Leishman stain (thin films) or Field stain (thick films). (For details, see Bailey JW, Williams J, Bain BJ, et al: Guideline: the laboratory diagnosis of malaria. *Br J Haematol* 2013;163[5]:573. doi: 10.1111/bjh.12572.)
- Two hundred high-power fields (×100 objectives) should be examined in a thick film.
- Asexual parasitemia should be reported after counting 1000 RBCs in a thin film. A graticule or grid may help counting.
- If parasitemia is less than 1:1000 RBCs, parasitemia may be counted in a thick film in relation to the number of WBCs.
- During active infection, a daily parasite count should be obtained.
- Counting and species determination of malaria parasites should be verified by a second observer.
- Reports on negative films despite a strong clinical suspicion of malaria should be qualified that negative films do not exclude a diagnosis of malaria. Repeat films should be requested if clinically appropriate. Thrombocytopenia may heighten suspicion of malaria.

RBC, Red blood cell; WBC, white blood cell.

In endemic areas, laboratory staff are skilled at the examination of thick films and routinely are able to detect 1 parasite in 100 high-power fields of a thick film, which corresponds to a sensitivity of approximately 5 to 50 parasites/µL.[107,110] Thin films are used for determining the species of the parasites, and the circulating asexual forms of the four main malaria species can be readily identified, whereas the sexual forms (gametocytes) of the species require some skill and regular practice (Figs. 158.5 and 158.6).

Nevertheless, diagnosis of malaria by microscopy in nonendemic countries has proven problematic. Routine laboratories may only achieve sensitivities of the order of 500 parasites/µL using thick films.[110,111] Quality assurance schemes show that performance of routine hematology laboratories in the recognition of and species determination of malaria parasites is poor.[109,111]

There has therefore been a strong drive to use nonmicroscopic methods for malaria diagnosis. It is now apparent that these methods are not sufficiently sensitive for clinical diagnosis, although they may have a role in detecting parasites of more than 500 parasites/µL when experienced staff are not available and/or as part of an out-of-hours service. However, it must be emphasized that these tests are no substitute for careful microscopy. Operationally, this means that hematology laboratories need to make the diagnosis of malaria and must maintain the skills needed for reliable examination of thick films.

A number of methods based on the fluorescent staining of parasite deoxyribonucleic acid (DNA) and/or ribonucleic acid (RNA) and the concentration of parasites have been devised.[112–114] However attractive these methods may appear, their sensitivity is limited by background staining of cellular debris, and the limit of their sensitivity is approximately 100 parasites/µL. The time taken in preparing samples and the specialized equipment and skills needed to use these methods limit their effectiveness in routine practice.

Detection of circulating malarial antigens is another potentially attractive, but ultimately limited, alternative to the laborious method of screening blood films. The widely available tests detect *Plasmodium* histidine-rich protein 2 (BinaxNOW Malaria test) and *Plasmodium*-specific lactate dehydrogenase (OptiMal-IT test) by immunochromatography.[115] The formulation of the tests using dipstick antigens allows rapid testing to be performed by laboratory staff. However, the sensitivity is variable and may range from 100 to 1000 parasites/µL, and this is comparable to the sensitivity achieved by inexperienced microscopists and may approach that achieved by experienced microscopists. The current recommendations for malaria diagnosis in the United Kingdom emphasize that the optimum diagnostic

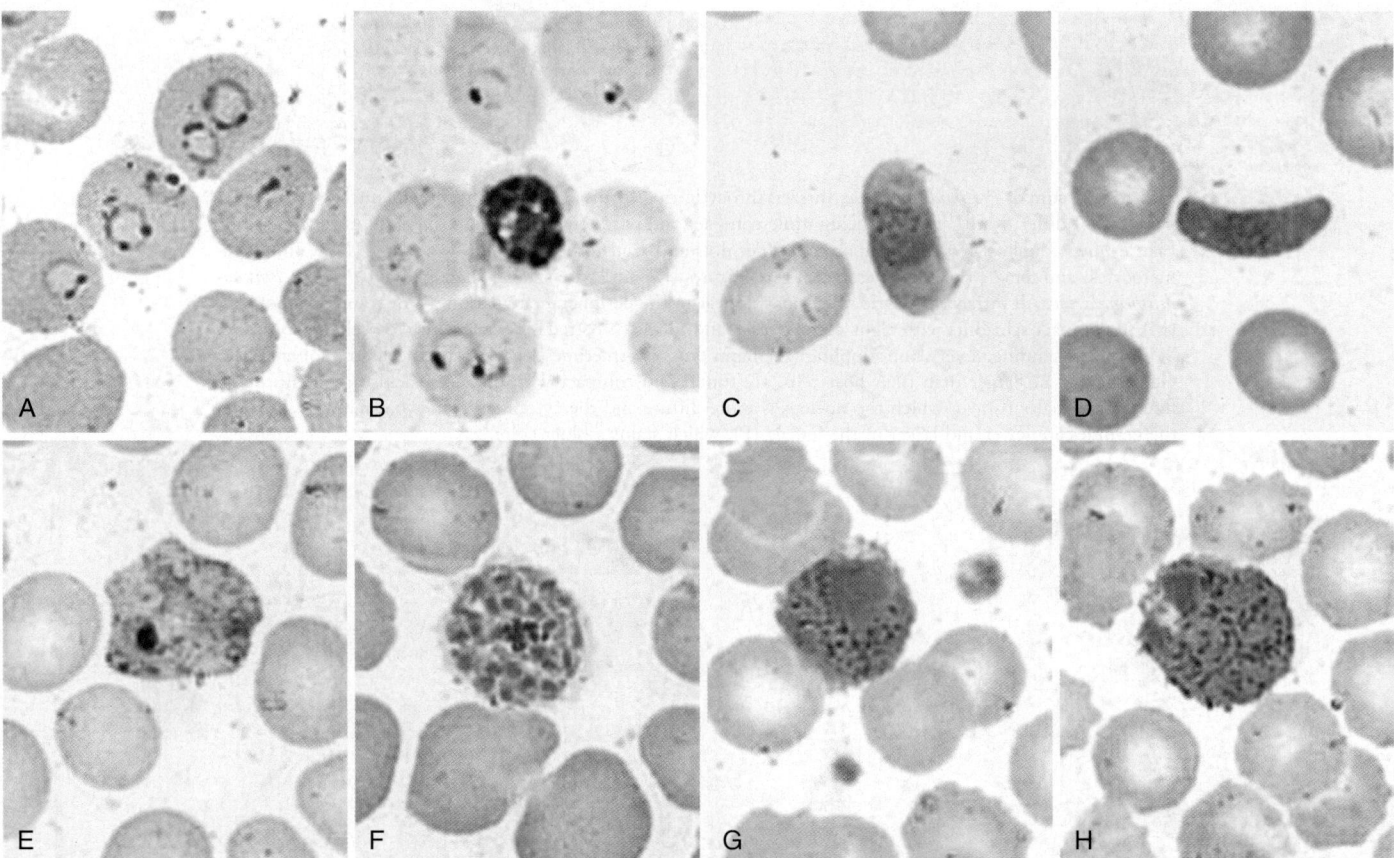

Fig. 158.5 BLOOD-STAGE MALARIA (THIN BLOOD FILMS). *Plasmodium falciparum:* Fine rings (A) predominate, with mature trophozoites and schizonts (B) appearing uncommonly in the peripheral circulation because infected cells adhere to postcapillary venules. Host cells are not enlarged. Basophilic clefts and spots of irregular shape and size (Maurer clefts and dots) may be seen in erythrocytes containing more mature parasites. They are thought to be aggregates of parasite proteins that are being exported from the parasite to the surface of the red cell. Crescent-shaped male (C) and female gametocytes (D) are diagnostic. *Plasmodium vivax:* All stages of asexual parasites, from young trophozoites (E) to schizonts, appear in the peripheral circulation in vivax malaria together with gametocytes. The parasites are large and ameboid and produce schizonts with approximately 16 daughter cells (merozoites) (F). Pigment is well developed. Host red cells are enlarged and uniformly covered with fine eosinophilic stippling (Schüffner dots). Gametocytes are round, with the male (microgametocytes; G) being approximately 7 µm and the female (macrogametocytes; H) being 10 µm or more in diameter.   *Continued*

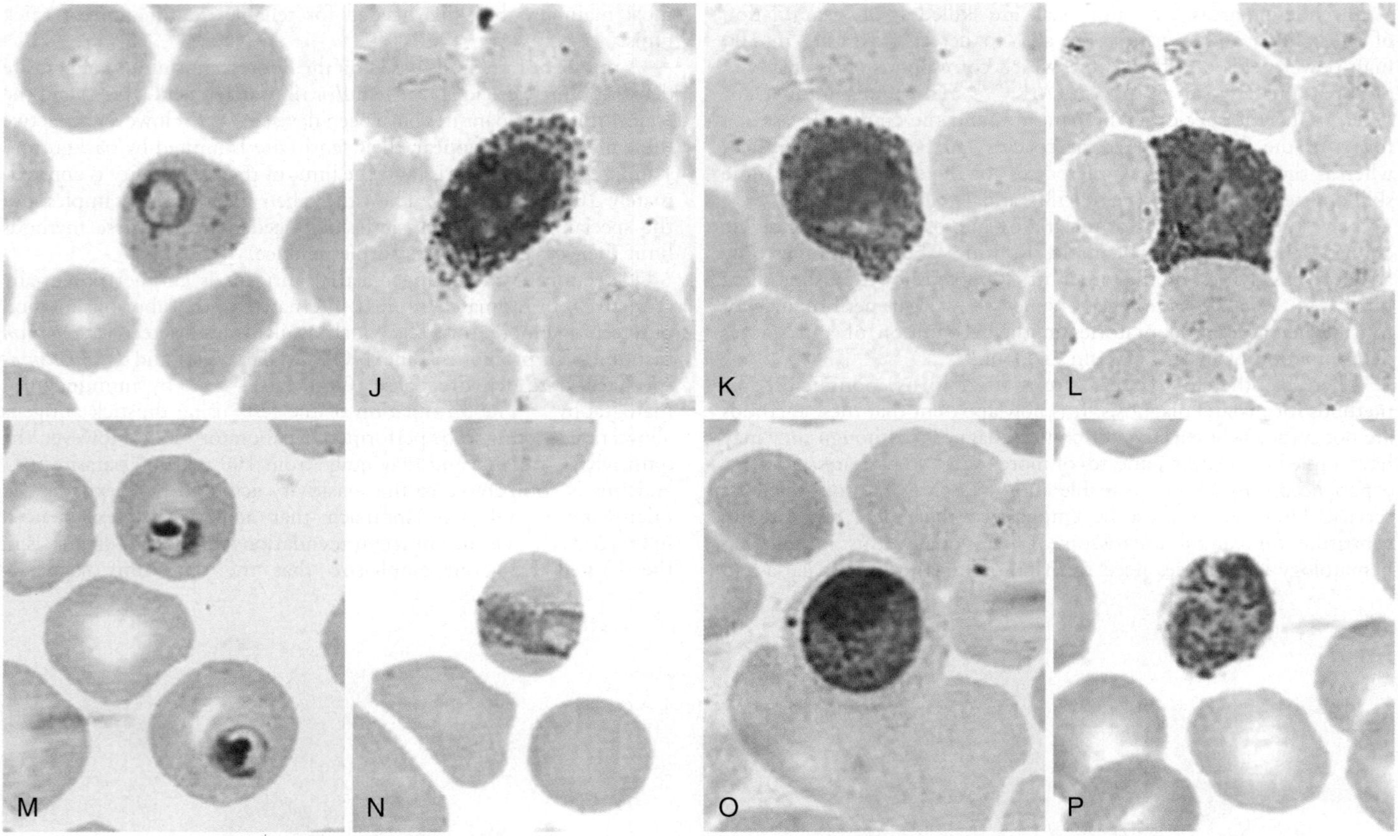

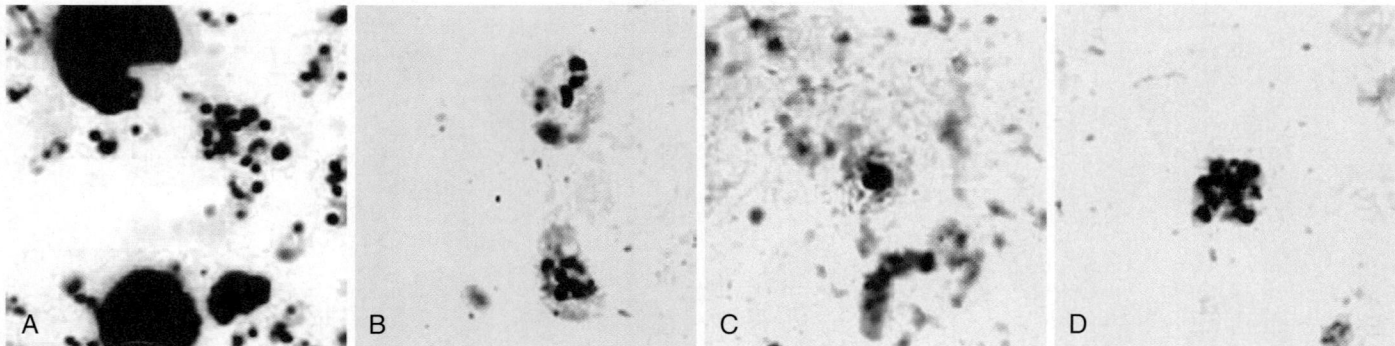

Fig. 158.5, cont'd *Plasmodium ovale:* Intraerythrocytic ring forms (I) have a prominent nucleus. The older parasites (J) differ from *P. vivax* in being more compact and producing about eight merozoites at schizogony. Like *P. vivax,* the host red cells contain Schüffner dots and tend to be ovoid and fimbriated. Male (microgametocytes) and female (macrogametocytes) gametocytes (K and L) are smaller than those of *P. vivax. Plasmodium malariae:* All intraerythrocytic stages may appear in the peripheral circulation, from young trophozoites (M) to compact schizonts with eight merozoites. Band forms (N) stretching across the red cell are common. With special staining, a very fine stippling (Ziemann dots) is sometimes seen. Host red cells are not enlarged. Gametocytes, no larger than their host cells, are round and compact with distinct blackish pigment, being finer in the males (O), in which the nucleus is more diffuse and the cytoplasm somewhat mauvish, whereas the granules are fewer and larger in the female (P), which stains a bluer color.

Fig. 158.6 BLOOD-STAGE MALARIA (THICK BLOOD FILMS). *Plasmodium falciparum:* Usually only young rings (A) are seen in acute infections, although sometimes in very large numbers. *Plasmodium vivax:* All stages may be present; here two young trophozoites are seen (B), with Schüffner dots seen as "ghost cells" in the thinner parts of the film where the host cell has been hemolyzed. *Plasmodium ovale:* The Schüffner dots of *P. ovale* also may show up in a thick film as a ghost cell, but the parasite can be distinguished from *P. vivax* by the solid appearance and heavy pigment even of young trophozoites (C). *Plasmodium malariae:* Younger parasites can be recognized by their heavy pigment, but this may be so heavy that it obscures the other inner structures. Schizonts containing up to eight merozoites with a central mass of pigment (D) are characteristic. *P. malariae* is difficult to differentiate from *P. ovale* in thick films, in which the parasites are easily confused. However, unlike *P. malariae, P. ovale* may be seen in ghost cells (C).

procedure is examination of thick and thin blood films by an expert to detect and speciate the malarial parasites. However, *P. falciparum* and *P. vivax* malaria can be diagnosed almost as accurately using rapid diagnostic tests (RDTs) that detect plasmodial antigens, depending upon the product. However, RDTs for other *Plasmodium* species are not as reliable.[116]

Amplification of circulating parasite DNA using the repeated ribosomal RNA (rRNA) genes is an extremely sensitive method of malaria diagnosis.[117] The sensitivity may be as low as 0.005 parasites/μL or 5 parasites/mL.[118,119] Undoubtedly, this is a useful tool for reference laboratories and epidemiologic surveys.

Treatment

Malaria requires urgent effective chemotherapy to prevent progression of disease and may be the most crucial public health intervention to reduce global mortality from malaria. The drug treatment of malaria must take account of the expected pattern of drug resistance in the area where infection was contracted, the severity of clinical disease, and the species of parasite. The spread of drug-resistant parasites and the optimal use of affordable, effective drugs are of continual concern, and these have recently been reviewed (Table 158.2).[116,120,121]

Artemisinin-based combination treatments have been the mainstay of treatment for falciparum malaria in Southeast Asia for more than 10 years and are now recommended as first-line treatment throughout the rest of the world.[122] However, resistance to these drugs is emerging, and very young children (particularly those underweight for age), patients with high parasitemias, and patients in very low transmission intensity areas with emerging parasite resistance are at risk for treatment failure and should be monitored closely.[120,121] The hematologic side effects of antimalarial drugs in use today are few. Amodiaquine is associated with neutropenia and agranulocytosis. Artemisinin-based treatments may cause reticulocytopenia and hemolysis in approximately 10% to 15% patients following intravenous artesunate treatment. Hemoglobin concentrations should be checked approximately 14 days following treatment in those treated with intravenous artemisinins.[116]

In severely ill patients, good nursing care is vital. Monitoring and treatment of fits and hypoglycemia are essential, and antipyretics should be given.[123] Certainly, blood transfusion is in principle a straightforward solution to the treatment of severe malarial anemia, although controversy exists over the trigger for transfusion and the rate of administration of blood. The standard regimens of cautious and slow delivery of blood have been challenged by the demonstration that rapid initial flow rates may correct lactic acidosis and

TABLE 158.2 Commonly Used Antimalarial Drugs and Their Side Effects

	Oral Dose	Parenteral Dose	Side Effects
Sulfadoxine-pyrimethamine	Sulfadoxine 25 mg/kg Pyrimethamine 1.25 mg/kg as a single dose (maximum 1500 mg sulfadoxine and 75 mg pyrimethamine)	For IM injection, doses as for oral	Use with caution in first trimester Causes kernicterus in neonates Skin rashes, fatal Stevens-Johnson syndrome
Artemether	3.2 mg/kg day 1 1.6 mg/kg days 2–7	3.2 mg/kg IM day 1, then 1.6 mg/kg for 3 days, then oral	Reticuolcytopenia
Artesunate	4 mg/kg once daily for 7 days	2.4 mg/kg IM day 1, then 1.2 mg/kg for 3 days, then oral	Reticulocytopenia
Artemether/lumefantrine	Fixed-dose combination: artemether (20 mg) with lumefantrine (120 mg), adults give 4 tablets initially, followed by 5 further doses of 4 tablets each given at 8, 24, 36, 48, and 60 hours (total 24 tablets over 60 hours) If 5–15 kg, then 1 tablet initially followed by 5 further doses of 1 tablet each, given at 8, 24, 36, 48, and 60 hours (total 6 tablets over 60 hours); 15–25 kg, then 2 tablets initially, followed by 5 further doses of 2 tablets each given at 8, 24, 36, 48, and 60 hours (total 12 tablets over 60 hours); body weight 25–35 kg, 3 tablets initially, followed by 5 further doses of 3 tablets each given at 8, 24, 36, 48, and 60 hours (total 18 tablets over 60 hours)		
Quinine	10 mg/kg of salt (maximum 600 mg) every 8 hours for 7 days, together with or followed by either doxycycline 200 mg once daily for 7 days or clindamycin 450 mg every 8 hours for 7 days [unlicensed indication]	20 mg/kg in 10 mL/kg isotonic fluid over 4 hours, then 10 mg/kg over 2 hours given every 12 hours in children and every 8 hours in adults, together with or followed by either doxycycline 200 mg once daily for 7 days or clindamycin 450 mg every 8 hours for 7 days [unlicensed indication]	Thrombocytopenia, intravascular hemolysis (blackwater fever) when used prophylactically, nausea, tinnitus, deafness

IM, Intramuscular.

hypovolemia. However, in nonimmune patients and in pregnant women, blood transfusion must be accompanied by careful hemodynamic monitoring to avoid precipitating or exacerbating pulmonary edema. A recent randomized clinical trial showed that red cell longer-storage RBC units are not inferior to shorter-storage RBC units for tissue oxygenation as measured by reduction in blood lactate levels and improvement in cerebral tissue oxygen saturation among children with severe anemia.[124]

Whatever clinical guidelines emerge, in reality blood transfusion in the heartland of malaria-endemic areas is beset by many practical and theoretic problems. First, the absence of well-characterized donor panels (and thus systematic blood collection) frequently jeopardizes the supply of blood. Second, even when standard screening for human immunodeficiency virus (HIV) is in place, the residual risk for HIV transmission in the serologic window of infectivity remains at 1 in 2500 to 1 in 6000. At a practical level, positive indirect antiglobulin test results in the setting of acute infection may make the exclusion of alloantibodies difficult. Depending on the clinical urgency and transfusion history, the least serologically incompatible blood may have to be given.

One therapeutic option available in North America and in Europe for the urgent treatment of nonimmune patients with severe disease would be an exchange blood transfusion. This procedure removes nonsequestered, infected erythrocytes and possibly circulating toxins. In the absence of evidence from trials for the use of exchange transfusion in malaria, some have suggested that this treatment could be given for hyperparasitemia (>20%) in severely ill nonimmune patients.[125,126] The salient features that make this clinical problem a major public health concern are the very large numbers of children affected and the difficulty of satisfactory treatment by blood transfusion outside specialist centers.

Malaria as a Transfusion-Transmitted Infection

Malaria is undoubtedly the most common transfusion-transmitted infection in the world. In endemic areas a large proportion of adult donors will be parasitemic, perhaps 20% to 80%, depending on the rate of transmission. Here donor deferral is impractical, and treatment of recipients with a course of effective antimalarials is the most practical alternative. In nonendemic areas, transmission of malaria is an occasional but potentially devastating complication of blood transfusion, and considerable thought and resources are required to combat the problem effectively.

The first case of transfusion-transmitted malaria (TTM) was in 1911.[127] Between 1911 and the mid-1970s the incidence of TTM rose to more than 140 cases per year, with *P. vivax* the most common species causing infection, although the proportion of cases from *P. falciparum* has steadily increased, perhaps reflecting the speed and destination of international travel. It is striking that the background problem, namely malaria in returned travelers, is much more common in the United Kingdom than in the United States, with the per capita incidence differing by nearly a factor of 10 and a higher proportion of cases from *P. falciparum* in Europe and the United Kingdom compared with the United States.[128]

Recent experience in the United Kingdom and the United States has emphasized the seriousness of TTM. Two of the last five cases of malaria owing to blood transfusion in the United Kingdom were fatal.[129-131] In the United States, 14 cases of TTM were reported between 1990 and 1999, but only 5 cases were reported between 2000 and 2009.[132,133] Detecting these cases after transfusion is frequently delayed because malarial infection acquired in nonendemic countries rarely figures in immediate differential diagnosis and requires careful examination of the blood film.

The mainstay of preventing TTM in the United Kingdom is donor deferral backed up by detection of circulating antibodies to malaria antigens. The guidelines for donor deferral were carefully revised after analysis of circumstances of recent TTM (Table 158.3).[134] These criteria recognize that malaria in the nonimmune patient is likely to present within 6 months of return from an endemic area

TABLE 158.3	UK Donor Selection Guidelines for Donors at Risk of Transmitting Malaria
Donor Risk Category	**Guidelines**
Resident	Defined as having lived in sub-Saharan Africa (except South Africa) or Papua New Guinea for a continuous period of 6 months at any time of life
	Permanent deferral unless malaria antibody test results are negative at least 6 months after returning from a malarious area
	Any subsequent visits to any malarious area each require a 6-month deferral period and negative antibody test results before reinstatement
History of malaria	Permanent deferral unless malarial antibody test results are negative at least 3 years after cessation of treatment or last negative test results
Undiagnosed febrile illness	While abroad or within 4 weeks of return
	Deferral for 12 months or 6 months if malarial antibody test results are negative
All other risks	Deferral for 12 months or 6 months if malarial antibody test results are negative

and that significant immunity to falciparum malaria may be acquired by residence after 6 months in a malarious area.

The criteria also require that residents, as well as those having had malaria or an undiagnosed febrile illness, may be reinstated, after six months without malaria or a fever that could have been due to malaria or three years after treatment for an episode of malaria, if antimalarial antibodies cannot be detected. The importance of antimalarial antibody testing rests on the fact that it is a very sensitive method to detect chronic infection, whereas the identification of circulating malarial antigens or nucleic acids or microscopy would fail to detect a level of 1 parasite/mL, which would still give a highly infectious dose in a unit of blood.

The assays for antimalarial antibodies previously used indirect immunofluorescence antibody tests (IFATs) to detect reactivity to a crude parasite lysate as a target antigen. However, an enzyme-linked immunosorbent assay (ELISA) using recombinant malarial antigens has proved to be a more practical if slightly less sensitive alternative to IFATs.[131,134,135] These tests detect antimalarial antibodies in less than 2% of donors who have visited endemic areas. It has been calculated that the return of 90% of malarial antibody–positive visitors to the donor pool releases an extra 50,000 units per year in the United Kingdom, and this is a highly cost-effective process to reduce the attrition of eligible blood donors. In the United States, over 200,000 donors per year are deferred after travel to malaria-endemic areas.

Donor deferral is based on the potential of a donor to carry malaria and is therefore based on the area of travel, length of stay or residence, elapsed time since leaving the endemic area, and history of malaria. It has been repeatedly shown that application of even the most thorough donor questionnaires allows some of those carrying malaria to give blood because guidelines are frequently incorrectly applied or questions are answered inaccurately in routine practice.[133,136]

In Canada donors reporting diagnosis or treatment of malaria defer permanently, and in the United States donors are deferred for 3 years after treatment.[133] The criteria will inevitably cause unnecessary deferral of those who never actually had malaria but also permit some individuals with low-level chronic infection to donate because malaria not infrequently presents more than 3 years after travelers return from endemic areas.[132,133] The last case of malaria transmitted in the United Kingdom was by someone who had left a malarious area 8 years previously, and the longest recorded case of recrudescence of malarial infection is 44 years for *P. malariae*.

Permanent deferral of all those visiting malaria-endemic areas is unlikely to be a viable strategy to prevent TTM because donor bases are declining. Preventing malaria transmission through blood transfusion requires comprehensive, regularly reviewed, and effectively implemented guidelines for donor deferral and laboratory testing. Even the best strategy is a compromise, and medical laboratory staff should be aware of the rare but potentially serious possibility of fever after transfusion that could be caused by malaria.

VISCERAL LEISHMANIASIS

Leishmaniasis is a generic term for infection by 30 or so species of the obligate intracellular parasites from the genus *Leishmania*. Visceral leishmaniasis (VL), or kala-azar, presents with a wide spectrum of systemic and hematologic features.

Epidemiology

VL occurs in all countries bordering the Mediterranean Sea and across the Middle East, including Saudi Arabia and Yemen. Indian VL occurs in the eastern regions of India (particularly Assam, Bengal, Bihar, Uttar Pradesh, Tamil Nadu, and Sikkim) and in Nepal and Bangladesh. African kala-azar is endemic in Kenya, Ethiopia, and the Sudan and sporadically elsewhere in tropical Africa. In the Americas, VL occurs in foci across Mexico, Central America, Colombia, Venezuela, Guyana, Brazil, Bolivia, and northern Argentina (Fig. 158.7).

The total burden of disease is difficult to estimate but significant. Leishmaniasis burden is endemic in 88 countries, with 200,000 to 400,000 new cases of VL per year, with the vast majority occurring in India, Bangladesh, Nepal, Northern Sudan, and northeastern Brazil.[137] VL is associated with poverty and undernutrition in endemic areas, particularly in the hyperendemic foci of the southern part of the Sudan and the Ganges river basin. In the Mediterranean area, it

is increasingly seen in association with HIV infection, where infection rates in HIV-infected people may be as high as 10%.

VL is caused by a number of species of the *Leishmania donovani* complex.[138,139] In the Mediterranean region and areas in the Middle East and Central Asia through to China, *Leishmania infantum* predominates, whereas *L. donovani* is more prevalent in India. *Leishmania tropica* is a less common cause of VL in these areas. Throughout their range in the Old World, parasites are transmitted by the female sandfly of the *Phlebotomus* genus. Leishmaniasis is caused by different parasites and vectors in the New World, where *Leishmania chagasi* and *Leishmania amazonensis* are transmitted by the *Lutzomyia* genus of sandfly.

Leishmania organisms are present in blood, and so the disease can be transmitted by blood transfusion, as a sexually transmitted disease, as a congenital infection, by needle sharing for intravenous drug abuse, or within a laboratory by intradermal inoculation of *L. donovani* promastigotes.[140,141] Very few cases of leishmaniasis have occurred as transfusion-transmitted infections in Europe or North America, with under 10 cases in infants or immunocompromised patients reported over the last 50 years. In endemic areas, this problem represents a much greater but unquantified risk.

Parasitology

Leishmania amastigotes live and multiply within macrophages by binary fission. They are round or ovoid bodies, approximately 2 to 3 μm in diameter. Occasional rupture of cells allows invasion of uninfected monocytes and macrophages by free forms. Sandflies ingest amastigotes within macrophages from blood or skin. In the insect's stomach, free amastigotes multiply and divide asexually, becoming elongated and developing flagella as metacyclic promastigotes. Within 2 weeks, such infective forms migrate through the

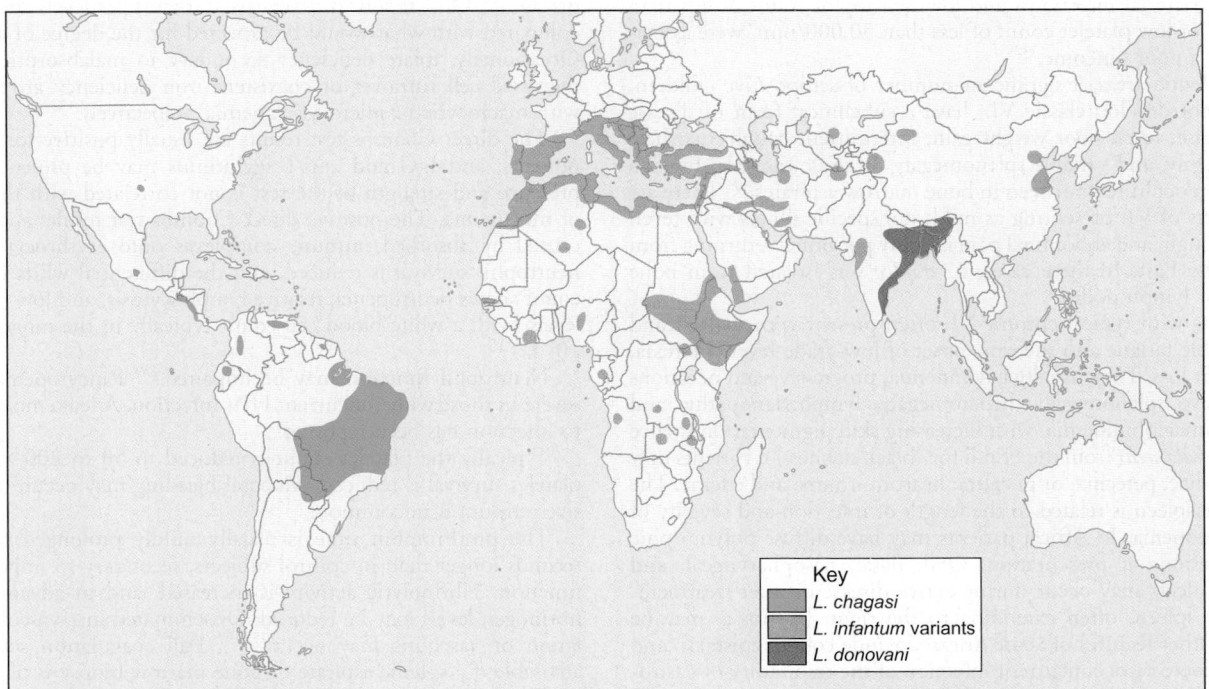

Key
L. chagasi
L. infantum variants
L. donovani

Fig. 158.7 EPIDEMIOLOGY OF VISCERAL LEISHMANIASIS (VL). VL caused by parasites of the *Leishmania donovani–Leishmania infantum* complex occurs in the Mediterranean littorals, the Middle East, and adjacent parts of the former Soviet Union, the Sudan, East Africa, the Indian subcontinent and China, and South America *(Leishmania chagasi)*. An arid, warm environment provides ideal ecologic conditions for the breeding of many species of sandfly. Zoonotic kala-azar from *L. infantum* and *L. chagasi* is commonly associated with dry, rocky, hill country, where cases are typically scattered. In India, *L. donovani* is essentially an anthroponosis. This type of kala-azar may occur in severe epidemic fashion, as can kala-azar in the Sudan.

lining of the stomach and enter the proboscis of the sandfly, allowing them to be inoculated in the human host while the sandfly takes a blood meal. Promastigotes are taken up by macrophages, where they become amastigotes by simple fission.

The large, elongated, fusiform promastigote measures 15 to 20 μm in length and 0.5 to 3.5 μm in width. Cultured promastigotes may also demonstrate rounded forms 4 to 5 μm in diameter. In Giemsa or other Romanowsky stains, a large nucleus and smaller, distinct rodlike kinetoplast are obvious. The organisms must be distinguished from *Histoplasma capsulatum*.

Pathology

Parasites spread within macrophages to local lymph nodes and then to the liver, spleen, and bone marrow. They are also present more widely, in particular in the gastrointestinal tract and epidermis. In the subclinical cases, a cellularly mediated immune response causes a granulomatous lesion and resolution of the infection. However, in clinical VL little if any inflammatory response to the rapidly extensive and expanding parasite-laden macrophages is seen. Where it shows, a granuloma develops at the site of the initial inoculation but may not be apparent at the time of presentation.

Clinical Features of Visceral Leishmaniasis

The spectrum of clinical disease is wide, ranging from asymptomatic infection to acute or chronic illness. Perhaps only 1% to 3% of all infections are symptomatic, with an incubation period of 10 days to 10 years but typically between 3 and 6 months.

The high number of seropositive individuals in relation to clinical cases suggests that spontaneous cure without symptoms or with mild systemic symptoms and hepatosplenomegaly occurs in the majority of individuals. In a large series of children with VL in Brazil, the overall case fatality rate was 10%, and mucosal bleeding, jaundice, dyspnea, bacterial infections, and low neutrophil count of less than 500/mm³ or low platelet count of less than 50,000/mm³ were associated with a poor outcome.[142]

In endemic areas, a significant number of seropositive children, who do not develop classic VL, have a subclinical form of disease with malaise, fever, poor weight gain, intermittent cough, diarrhea, hepatomegaly, and variable splenomegaly. In these cases, leishmania were neither cultured nor seen in bone marrow aspirates.[143] There are also reports of VL presenting as mild, nonspecific illness with fever, fatigue, cough, and abdominal pain in army personnel returning from the Middle East. In these cases, *L. tropica* was isolated from bone marrow or lymph nodes.[144]

Patients with typical chronic VL often present with malaise and considerable fatigue and the slow onset of low-grade fever, anorexia, and weight loss. They usually have anemia, progressive and occasionally massive splenomegaly, hepatomegaly, lymphadenopathy, and hypergammaglobulinemia, with increasing skin pigmentation (hence the name *kala-azar* from the Hindi for "black sickness"). Patients may have jaundice, petechia, or purpura; heart murmurs; and edema. The size of the spleen is related to the length of infection and severity of the pancytopenia. In Africa, patients may have diffuse polymorphic papular lesions at presentation. Oral, nasal, nasopharyngeal, and laryngeal ulcers may occur during active disease or after treatment. The large spleen, often extending to the right iliac fossa, may be painful. Other features of acute disease include cough, epistaxis, and in some severe cases concurrent infection of the respiratory or gastrointestinal tracts and/or tuberculosis.

The typical features of VL may be preceded by bacteremia, bacterial infection, acute hepatitis, or Guillain-Barré syndrome. VL may be associated with hepatic necrosis, cholecystitis, or neuropathy. Occasionally, lymphadenopathy may occur without systemic features of the disease. Here histology shows noncaseating granulomas and amastigotes within macrophages. A more acute presentation in recent immigrants and visitors to endemic areas may include a high periodic fever similar to classic malaria, with malnutrition, bleeding, hepatitis, and/or acute renal failure.

Immunocompromised Hosts

Coinfection with HIV and VL is now a well-recognized clinical entity in the Mediterranean region and undoubtedly occurs more widely[145-147] (for review, see Lindoso et al[148] and Alvar et al[149]). VL occurs in the setting of late-stage acquired immunodeficiency syndrome (AIDS) with CD4⁺ lymphocyte counts of less than $200 \times 10^6/L$. Patients present with fever, splenomegaly, and pancytopenia with frequent and sometimes atypical involvement of the gastrointestinal and respiratory systems and skin. The typical hematologic features of VL are sometimes absent, and serologic tests are often negative, although antibodies to 14- and 16-kDa *Leishmania* antigens may be detected by Western blot analysis.[150] However, organisms are plentiful in bone marrow and even in buffy coat preparations. Some patients may have few symptoms, and the diagnosis of VL in immunocompromised patients requires a high index of suspicion. Treatment is difficult, with poor responses to pentavalent antimony. Liposomal amphotericin is the drug of choice. However, relapses are usual, and maintenance treatment is required.[148]

VL may also occur after transplant and after immunosuppressive treatments, including chemotherapy, rituximab, or other immunodeficiency states.[151,152] Although patients present with a typical combination of fever, pancytopenia, and splenomegaly, the diagnosis may be missed if not considered.

Hematologic Features

VL causes a moderate normocytic, normochromic anemia.[153] The pathogenesis of anemia is multifactorial and includes hemodilution, shortened RBC survival, and reduced erythropoiesis.[154] The plasma is low, with plentiful stored iron typical of the anemia of chronic disease.[155] One report has suggested that Epo levels are reduced compared with what would be expected for the degree of anemia.[156] Occasionally, folate deficiency secondary to malabsorption and/or increased cell turnover or coexistent iron deficiency are associated with macrocytic or microcytic anemia, respectively.[157]

The direct Coombs test results are usually positive for C3 components, and IgG and anti-I agglutinins may be present, but the presence and strength of the test is not correlated with the severity of the anemia. The positive direct Coombs test results appear to be caused by absorbed immune complexes onto erythrocytes.[158] The neutrophil survival is reduced, and the differential white blood cell count shows neutropenia, relative lymphocytosis, and low eosinophil levels, with a white blood cell count typically in the range 2 to 4×10^9 L.

Neutrophil function may be impaired.[159] Pancytopenia is more severe in those with concurrent HIV infection. A leukemoid reaction to infection has been reported.

Typically the platelet count is reduced to 50 to $200 \times 10^9/L$ as platelet survival is reduced. Mucosal bleeding may occur, but extensive purpura is uncommon.

The prothrombin time is usually mildly prolonged to 2 to 4 seconds longer than in control subjects, secondary to impaired liver function. Fibrinolytic activity is increased, and in advanced cases, fibrinogen levels may be reduced. Disseminated intravascular coagulation or vasculitis may occur.[153,159] Full coagulation screening is advisable if a splenic aspirate or bone marrow biopsy is planned.

The bone marrow is usually hypercellular, with increased erythroid, myeloid, and platelet precursors. Lymphocytes may be increased, and macrophages contain Leishman-Donovan bodies (Fig. 158.8).[160] If weight loss and malabsorption are extensive, the marrow may undergo gelatinous transformation.

The mechanisms of leukopenia and thrombocytopenia are multifactorial. There is evidence for reduced bone marrow production of granulocytes and platelets and also for their autoimmune destruction

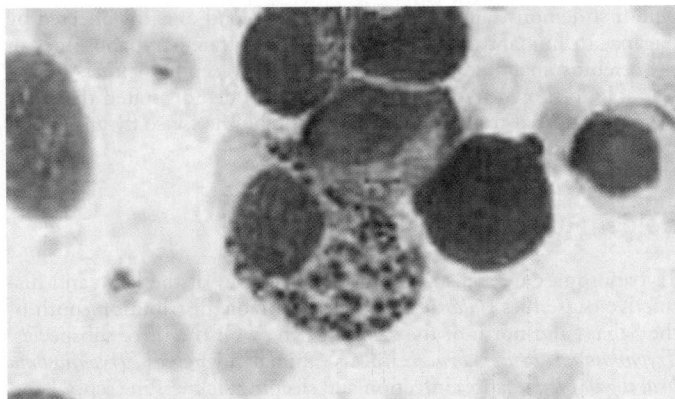

Fig. 158.8 *LEISHMANIA INFANTUM* IN MACROPHAGE FROM BONE MARROW. Although typically found in macrophages as shown here, isolated extracellular amastigotes from disrupted host cells are commonly seen in such preparations.

and/or increased splenic clearance. After treatment, hematologic recovery is slow, and full recovery may take many months.[155]

Laboratory Features

The epidemiologic context and clinical features can suggest a diagnosis of leishmaniasis. Hematologic and biochemical tests are nonspecific; biochemical tests may show mild elevation of bilirubin and transaminase levels and more commonly a raised level of alkaline phosphatase. Previously the nonspecific formol-gel test was used to indicate hypergammaglobulinemia. Diagnosis is confirmed by direct examination of parasites by microscopy, culture, or polymerase chain reaction (PCR) (for detailed review, see Boelaert et al[161] and Srividya et al[162]).

Morphology

The pathognomic amastigotes of *Leishmania* spp. can be found in a variety of sources. The diagnosis is often made by splenic puncture or by bone marrow aspiration where large numbers of amastigotes may be seen within macrophages. Amastigotes are stained using Giemsa or other Romanowsky stains and demonstrate a purple nucleus and the large anterior kinetoplast (see Fig. 158.8).

In nonimmunocompromised patients with VL, splenic aspirates are positive in more than 95%, bone marrow aspirates positive in more than 85%, buffy coat macrophages positive in more than 70%, and lymph nodes positive in more than 60%. In practice, samples are taken from the least invasive sites first, although lymphadenopathy is not invariable.

Where coinfection of HIV and leishmania occurs, amastigotes are more reliably found in bone marrow than in peripheral blood and may also be demonstrated in biopsy specimens from a wide variety of sites. Biopsy material can be stained with polyclonal anti-*Leishmania* serum and indirect immunofluorescence. However, direct demonstration of parasites is less sensitive than culture or PCR.

Splenic Aspiration

Splenic aspiration is rarely performed in North America and Europe but is a common diagnostic procedure in endemic areas. Aspiration is contraindicated in the presence of a bleeding tendency, portal hypertension, or a splenic hydatid cyst. Splenic aspirates are obtained from the middle of the long axis of the spleen. After the skin is cleaned, a 21-gauge needle attached to a 5-mL syringe is inserted subcutaneously in line with the long axis of the spleen. The needle

should be swiftly inserted to a depth of approximately 2 or 3 cm at an angle of roughly 45 degrees to the skin, applying negative pressure. The needle should be withdrawn immediately while maintaining negative pressure and taking only a few seconds for the entire procedure. The splenic tissue may be expelled from the needle using a small amount of air and by fixing the stain using standard procedures.

Culture

Amastigotes may be grown as motile promastigotes from aspirates on the classic Novy-MacNeal-Nicolle (NNN) medium or other suitable media at 22°C to 24°C, and populations double only every 2 to 3 days.[163,164] Inoculation of material into the susceptible golden hamster is no longer used to grow parasites.

Molecular Methods

The PCR may detect low levels of infection and has been used for diagnosis and monitoring of treatment as well as to determine the genotype of the parasites.[165,166] Blood from filter paper can be used to prepare DNA, but as for direct morphology, PCR from bone marrow samples is a more sensitive method to demonstrate parasites.[167] It may be particularly useful for monitoring treatment and relapse in HIV- and *Leishmania*-infected patients.[167] Isothermal DNA amplification methods are being applied to develop tests to be used where sophisticated equipment is not available.[168]

Serologic Tests

Serologic tests have to be interpreted in light of the clinical findings. The tests are useful to screen suspected cases or populations for VL. However, they are unreliable in immunocompromised patients, who frequently are seronegative in spite of patent infection. Conversely, those harboring a subclinical infection may be seropositive, but samples may fail to yield evidence of parasites. Finally, serologic findings are positive many years after treatment or self-cure.

An indirect IFAT or ELISA using freeze-dried *Leishmania* antigen has sensitivity and specificity greater than 95%. A DAT is also available with purified, freeze-dried antigen and is a highly sensitive and specific test.[169] The freeze-dried antigen is very stable even when stored in extreme conditions.

The ELISA and immunochromatographic tests using *Leishmania* recombinant K39 antigen are 100% sensitive and more than 98% specific in Asia.[170,171] The sensitivity and specificity of the DAT and K39 immunochromatographic test are broadly similar, although the K39 test was less sensitive in the Sudan than in Asia.[161,172] An alternative target antigen for serologic tests such as recombinant K28 and a rapid point-of-care test are now being developed.[21]

Treatment in patients without HIV coinfection may be monitored using urine antigen tests for detection of the K39 and K26 *Leishmania* antigens. These test results become negative 3 weeks after commencing treatment.

Management

General supportive care is important and includes correction of nutritional and hematinic deficiencies, blood transfusion in severe anemia, and antibiotics for secondary infections (for review of diagnosis, therapy, and management, see report from the World Health Organization[173]).

Specific chemotherapy for VL uses a number of potentially toxic drugs. Intercurrent infections must be identified and treated, and general measures include improvement of nutritional status (for review of treatment, see Sundar et al[174] and Copeland et al[175]). Use of pentavalent antimonials, including sodium stibogluconate (Pentostam) and meglumine antimonate (Glucantime) are now limited, especially in South Asia, by increasing drug resistance. There is concern that drug resistance will develop to the alternative therapies, and combination treatment aiming at short courses that also delay the development of drug resistance are in progress.[53]

Amphotericin B is effective against *Leishmania* and is used in endemic areas where high levels of resistance to pentavalent antimonials are present. It may be given as a slow intravenous infusion in 5% dextrose over 4 to 6 hours, beginning at 250 µg/kg/day, increasing to 1 mg/kg/day until a total dose of 20 mg/kg/day has been given. Side effects include anaphylaxis, anemia, fever, bone chills, bone pain, and thrombophlebitis. Hypokalemia and hypomagnesemia are significant problems, and potassium loss and supplementation may be reduced by the concurrent use of amiloride to prevent renal tubular potassium leakage.[176]

Reduced toxicity from amphotericin is achieved using a liposomal amphotericin preparation (AmBisome), which has been made more widely available through preferential pricing in endemic areas. It is an effective and safe treatment and is used when affordable. A test dose of 1 mg should be given, and then the recommended dose is 1–3 mg/kg daily for 10–21 days to a cumulative dose of 21–30 mg/kg, alternatively 3 mg/kg for 5 consecutive days, followed by 3 mg/kg after 6 days for 1 dose. In patients with HIV, a dose of liposomal amphotericin at 4 mg/kg/day on days 1 to 5 followed by 4 mg/kg/day on days 10, 17, 24, 31, and 38 is recommended. The relapse rate is high, and close monitoring of patients is required.

Miltefosine is a new drug and effective orally against VL in India and Africa.[177,178] The current regime is 2.5 mg/kg/day for adults and children older than 2 years for 4 weeks. Higher than 95% cure rates have been achieved. Gastrointestinal upset occurs frequently. Miltefosine is teratogenic and may reduce fertility. It has a long half-life and has a low therapeutic index, which may contribute to the development of resistance, and so combination chemotherapy is being investigated to combat development of resistance.

Intramuscular paromomycin has been used at a dose of 20 mg/kg/day for 21 days. It has been shown to be equivalent to amphotericin B for the treatment of VL in India.[179] Moreover, patients treated for VL in Africa with sodium stibogluconate and paromomycin have an improved outcome compared with therapy with sodium stibogluconate alone.[180]

Post–kala-azar dermal leishmaniasis may occur in up to 10% of patients after treatment for VL. It is seen mainly in India and is common in Africa. It occurs after treatment of VL and may appear up to 10 years after treatment. It presents as a maculopapular rash spreading around the mouth, trunk, and limbs. These nodules and papules contain amastigotes. Prolonged treatment may be required to eliminate infection.

Leishmaniasis as a Transfusion-Transmitted Infection

Leishmaniasis poses problems as a potential transfusion-transmitted infection in endemic areas. The disease can be transmitted by blood and platelet concentrates, although leukodepletion by filtration reduces organisms by many orders of magnitude and so probably also the risk for transmission. In Europe, given the low absolute risk for transmission, donor deferral is used to reduce the risk for donation by anyone who is parasitemic.[181] However, surveys of blood donors in areas where the parasite is transmitted suggest parasite DNA can be detected in 0.3% to 1.75% of blood donors. It has been noted that service personnel returning from the Middle East represent a group of potential donors who may have been exposed to infection.[182]

AFRICAN TRYPANOSOMIASIS

African trypanosomiasis is caused by the flagellate protozoa *Trypanosoma brucei* spp., named after David Bruce, a Scottish parasitologist who first demonstrated the parasite in the blood of cattle affected by nagana. In humans, Aldo Castellani demonstrated trypanosomes in the cerebrospinal fluid (CSF) of patients with sleeping sickness. Bruce was able to show the protozoa in blood and demonstrated that they were transmitted from antelopes to cattle by the tsetse fly and blood of patients with sleeping sickness.

Epidemiology

Trypanosomes are transmitted by some species of the large and distinctive tsetse flies (*Glossina* spp.) in a sporadic distribution south of the Sahara and north of the Zambezi River. Of the three subspecies, *Trypanosoma brucei brucei* infects animals, whereas *Trypanosoma brucei gambiense* causes infection and sleeping sickness in Central and West Africa, and *Trypanosoma brucei rhodesiense* causes disease in East and Central Africa. *T. b. gambiense* is transmitted mainly between humans by the *Glossina palpalis* group in foci along watercourses in West and Central Africa. *T. b. rhodesiense* is transmitted by the *Glossina morsitans* groups widely distributed in the East African savannah. Here the disease is clearly a zoonosis, with antelopes and domestic cattle as reservoir hosts; it afflicts mainly hunters, guides, and game wardens and may occasionally occur in tourists on safari in the game parks of East Africa (Fig. 158.9).

Historically the disease has caused major epidemics, causing hundreds of thousands of deaths, and has prevented human settlement in large areas of Africa. Over 50 million people are now at risk for trypanosomiasis, and it has been estimated that the disease causes over 50,000 deaths each year. Most cases are reported in the Democratic Republic of the Congo and northwestern Uganda, with a few hundred or fewer each year reported in neighboring East African countries.

Case-finding and control measures have substantially reduced the risk for epidemics. Epidemics of disease have been associated with a breakdown in health services, for example, in villages in the areas of Lake Victoria in Uganda and more recently in the Democratic Republic of the Congo, Angola, and southern Sudan (for review of current epidemiologic and clinical aspects of this disease, see Simarro et al,[183] Brun et al,[184] and Franco et al[185]).

Parasitology

The small, mobile trypomastigotes circulate and may be seen in peripheral blood. These flattened, fusiform organisms are pleomorphic but are typically of a size similar to a red blood cell, approximately 20 µm long, and have an undulating membrane, attached to the protruding flagellum, extending from the anterior pole of the elongated body (Fig. 158.10). Parasites multiply by binary fission and may cause chronic parasitemia and evade humoral immune responses by clonal antigenic variations of the major surface glycoprotein.[186]

When trypomastigotes are taken up in a blood meal by the tsetse fly, they multiply in the midgut by simple fission. Later they penetrate the wall of the gut and migrate to the salivary glands. There, as morphologically distinct epimastigotes, they become infective (or metacyclic) trypomastigotes 15 to 30 days after first infecting the fly. In endemic areas, up to 1% to 5% of flies may be infected. Flies remain infective until they die, several months later.

Pathology

The lymphatic, cardiac, and central nervous systems are involved by the disease. Initially, proliferation of trypanosomes within lymph nodes and the spleen is accompanied by expansion of the lymphocytes, macrophages, and erythrophagocytosis. Polyclonal activation of lymphocytes results in high production of IgM and rheumatoid factor, and anti-DNA antibodies may appear. Later fibrosis and endarteritis supervenes with proliferation of endothelial cells and perivascular infiltration of plasma cells and lymphocytes. The liver

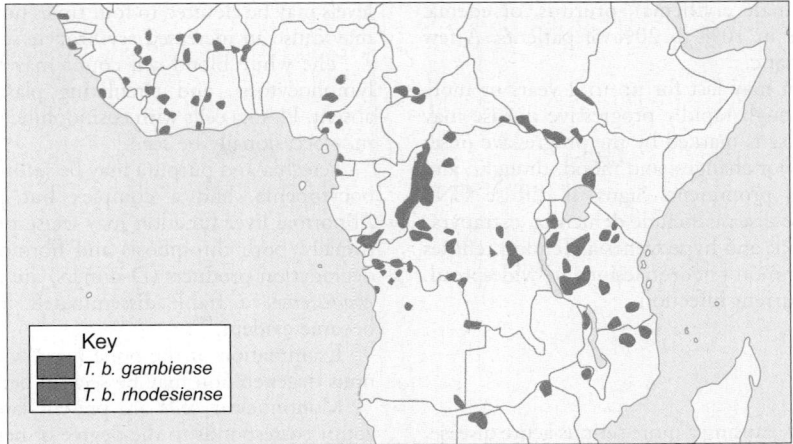

Fig. 158.9 DISTRIBUTION OF *TRYPANOSOMA BRUCEI* INFECTION IN HUMANS. African try-panosomiasis is confined to equatorial Africa, with a patchy distribution depending on detailed topographic conditions. It is caused by two subspecies of *T. brucei*: *T. b. gambiense* infection is widespread in West and Central Africa, transmitted mainly by riverine species of tsetse fly *(Glossina)*, but *T. b. rhodesiense,* transmitted mostly by savannah species, is restricted to the eastern and east-central areas of Africa, with some overlap between the two. Although domestic pigs form an important reservoir for *T. b. gambiense* infection, various wild ruminants are the major sources for *T. b. rhodesiense.* The epidemic reemergence of African trypanosomiasis in recent years is exemplified by the death of at least 96 people in Angola in 2003, when 3115 cases were confirmed among a suspected 270,000 new cases in that country. In the same year it was estimated that some 500,000 people across Africa had trypanosomiasis, which was likely to have a mortality rate of approximately 80%. Recent reports indicate a spread of transmission from the northern toward the southern parts of Angola. *(Modified from World Health Organization Map No. 98005.)*

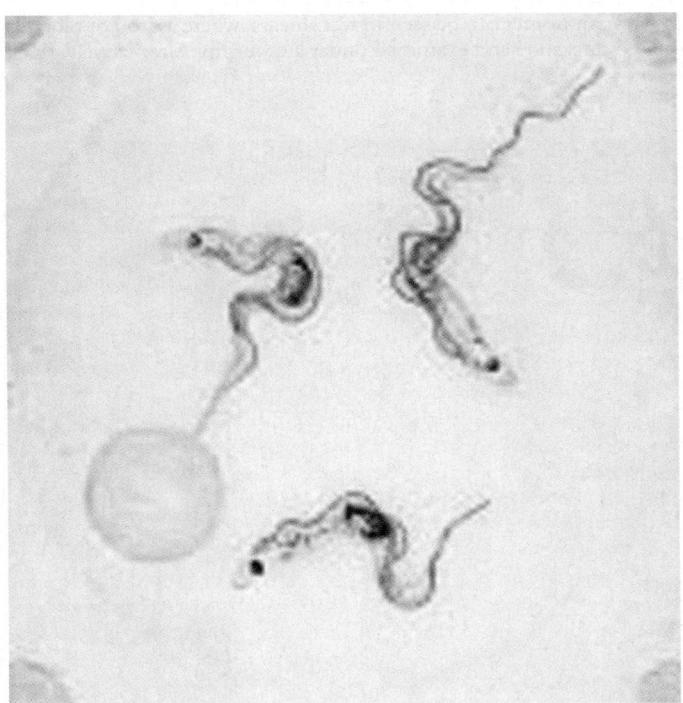

Fig. 158.10 ORIGINAL MICRO-PHOTOGRAPH OF *TRYPANOSOMA (TRYPANOZOON) BRUCEI GAMBIENSE* IN HUMAN BLOOD BY J. EVERETT DUTTON. Polymorphic trypanosomes were first discovered more than a century ago, in 1895, by David Bruce in the blood of domestic cattle with the wasting disease nagana in South Africa. The first observation of these protozoa in humans was made by R. M. Forde, who noted, in 1902, "small worm-like, extremely active bodies" in the blood of a sick European seaman in The Gambia. The parasites seen here in a Romanowsky-stained thin blood film, which were described and named by Dutton in 1902, are responsible for sleeping sickness in West Africa. *(Reproduced by kind permission of the Director, Liverpool School of Tropical Medicine.)*

shows infiltration of the portal tracts and fatty degeneration. In *T. b. rhodesiense,* cardiac involvement may be extensive, with endocarditis, myocarditis, and pericarditis leading to extensive damage and death.

In the second stage of the disease, trypanosomes multiply within the central nervous system (CNS) and cause a chronic meningoencephalitis. Edema, hemorrhages, granulomatous lesions, and thrombosis contribute to cerebral degeneration. Lymphocytosis and plasma cells with large eosinophilic inclusions (Mott cells) may be found in the CNS.

Intriguingly, nonpathogenic species of African trypanosomes may be killed by the human high-density lipoprotein particles astonishingly subverting a parasite pathway for heme uptake. The complex of haptoglobin-related protein and apolipoprotein L1 (ApoL1) are taken up into the parasite by a parasite glycoprotein receptor, which binds the haptoglobin–hemoglobin complex.[187–190] *T. b. rhodesiense* is resistant to killing by human sera because the ApoL1, which induces parasite apoptosis, is neutralized in the lysosome by serum resistance–associated protein, which binds to a specific ApoL1 domain. The selection of trypanolytic ApoL1 variants have a cost. In African Americans, focal segmental glomerulosclerosis and hypertension-attributed end-stage kidney disease are associated with two independent sequence variants in the *APOL1* gene.[191]

Clinical Features

T. brucei gambiense

Local inflammation at the site of inoculation causes a distinctive chancre or painful, indurated ulcer appearing 2 to 3 days after an infective bite and lasting for up to 1 month. Trypanosomes multiply in the lymphatic system for 6 to 14 days before causing patent infection in the blood, characterized by waves of parasitemia and fever. Later, invasion of the CNS may occur by transit of organisms through the choroid plexus and/or endothelial cells.

In the blood stage of infection, fever, headache, and arthralgia are prominent. Lymphadenopathy is common, particularly in the posterior triangle of the neck (Winterbottom sign). There may be intermittent rashes (often circinate erythema), pruritus, or edema. Moderate splenomegaly occurs in 10% to 20% of patients. A few infected patients are asymptomatic.

This early stage of infection may last for up to 2 years or more before CNS involvement, although rapidly progressive disease may occur. The CNS phase of disease is marked by the progressive onset of headache; disinhibited behavior changes; and mood, thought, and sleep disturbances. Wasting is prominent. Signs of diffuse CNS damage in the last phases of the disease include dementia, extrapyramidal and cerebellar dysfunction, and hyperesthesia. Tendon reflexes are increased, and signs of upper motor neuron lesions are widespread. Death usually occurs by intercurrent infection.

T. b. rhodesiense

T. b. rhodesiense is more virulent, causing a more serious acute disease, with systemic features including serous effusions; hepatocellular jaundice; and a mild, normocytic, normochromic anemia. Hepatosplenomegaly and lymphadenopathy are common, but involvement of cervical lymph nodes is less typical. Myocarditis is rare but may cause death before CNS involvement. Here CNS disease occurs sooner and is more rapidly progressive than *T. b. gambiense* infection and is fatal within 1 to 3 months.

Infection with *T. b. gambiense* may resolve in the vast majority of cases. Where infection persists, there is typically a long asymptomatic phase. Numerous lymph nodes are enlarged to 1 to 2 cm in diameter and are soft, mobile, and painless.

The differential diagnosis of trypanosomiasis includes malaria, typhoid, fever, and viral hepatitis in the acute phase, whereas lymphadenopathy may suggest infectious mononucleosis or tuberculosis. In the cerebral phase of the disease, syphilis, tuberculosis, HIV-associated cryptococcal meningitis, or chronic viral encephalitis must be considered.

Children

Those affected in utero may be born with CNS abnormalities. In children the disease is more rapidly progressive, and epileptic seizures and psychomotor retardation are the principal features of the disease.

HIV

The frequency of HIV seropositivity has been reported to show no significant differences between those presenting with trypanosomiasis and age-matched control subjects.[192,193] These results do not exclude the possibility that coinfections may modulate the course of the disease or the effectiveness of treatment.

Hematologic and Laboratory Features

The main hematologic features are a normocytic, normochromic anemia and moderate thrombocytopenia.[194] The anemia of trypanosomiasis is multifactorial. Hemodilution, hemolysis, and dyserythropoiesis or ineffective erythropoiesis all contribute to the pathogenesis. Hemolysis may be caused directly by lytic factors released by trypanosomes or indirectly by deposition of immune complexes and subsequent clearance of coated erythrocytes. In vitro studies have suggested that the variant surface glycoprotein from trypanosomes may be shed and taken up onto the erythrocyte membrane, where antibody and complement deposition could contribute to hemolysis. Bone marrow response is inadequate, and although the nature of the defect is unclear, there is failure in incorporation of iron into erythroid precursors, as is seen in many forms of the anemia of chronic disease. In mice infected with human trypanosomiasis, TNF-α contributes to bone marrow suppression, but detailed studies of the pathogenesis of anemia in human infections have not been reported. Serum IgM

levels may be elevated to four times normal and with raised IgG levels may cause an increased erythrocyte sedimentation rate.

The white blood cell count may be elevated with monocytosis, lymphocytosis, and circulating plasma cells, but eosinophilia is absent. Plasma cells with eosinophilic inclusion or Mott morular cells may occasionally be seen.

Petechia and purpura may be secondary to vascular injury, thrombocytopenia, and a complex but poorly defined coagulopathy. Abnormal liver function may cause prolonged clotting times. Functionally, both thrombosis and fibrinolysis are increased, and fibrin degradation products (D-dimers) are raised in acute disease; in *T. b. rhodesiense*, a frank disseminated intravascular coagulation may become evident.[195]

Examination of the bone marrow shows hypercellularity. Gelatinous degeneration may be seen in patients with wasting.

Mononuclear cells are present late in the disease, and the cell count corresponds to the degree of neurologic involvement and may reach more than 300/μL in severely ill patients. The CSF protein levels are elevated (0.4 to 1.0 g/L).

As disease progresses, the circulating parasites become scarce. However, anemia and endocrine dysfunction, including amenorrhea, reduced libido, and impotence becomes apparent.

Parasitologic Assays

Direct detection of the parasite is particularly important in light of the toxicity of the treatment. Trypanosomes may be detected in lymph node aspirates and in wet and thick blood smears (Fig. 158.11). An aspirate may be taken from enlarged nodes. Aspirated fluid can be examined under a coverslip, and motile trypanosomes are typically seen at the edges of the coverslip.

Trypanosomes can be seen in wet smears, where a drop of blood is placed on a slide and examined under a coverslip. Alternatively, thick

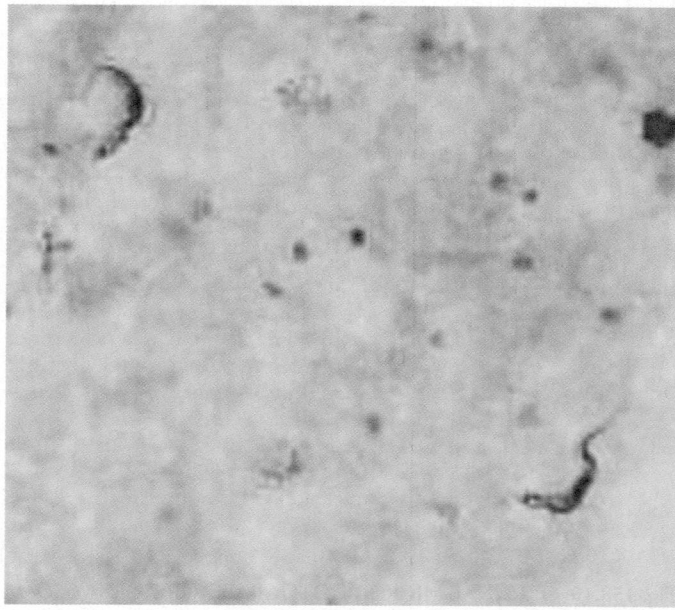

Fig. 158.11 *TRYPANOSOMA BRUCEI RHODESIENSE* IN HUMAN BLOOD. *T. brucei brucei* parasitizes wild and domestic animals but does not infect humans. The different subspecies can be distinguished with certainty only by biochemical techniques, such as electrophoretic typing of their isoenzymes or by the use of DNA probes. *T. brucei gambiense* and *T. b. rhodesiense* (and *T. b. brucei* of animals) are virtually indistinguishable in blood films. Note the small kinetoplast and free flagellum. Both subspecies from humans will infect guinea pigs, but only *T. b. rhodesiense* is infective to rats, in which the parasites are polymorphic—that is, long, thin, intermediate, and short, stumpy forms of trypomastigotes may coincide.

or thin Giemsa-stained blood films are made as for malaria diagnosis. The sensitivity may be increased by microcentrifugation.[196]

More recent methods used to detect the low levels of parasitemia seen in *T. b. gambiense* include quantitative examination of the buffy coat using acridine orange[197] and small-scale ion-anion exchange chromatography.[198] Erythrocytes are retained in the column, whereas trypanosomes are eluted and are visible after concentration by centrifugation. The sensitivity of detection with these methods ranges from 10^4/mL for wet smears to 10^2/mL for ion-exchange columns and centrifugation. In *T. b. rhodesiense,* examination of the blood is more likely than aspiration of lymph nodes to yield a positive result.

Inoculation of the aspirate or samples into susceptible animals or in vitro culture has been used to detect low-level parasitemia. Mice and rats were used to detect *T. b. rhodesiense,* whereas the multimammate rat (*Mastomys natalensis)* and guinea pigs were used for *T. b. gambiense.* PCR of the 18S rRNA gene can detect parasites with sensitivity similar to that of parasitologic and serologic methods.[199]

Cerebrospinal Fluid

Trypanosomes may be found in the CSF as disease progresses, although a double-centrifugation technique may be required to demonstrate organisms. In this technique, 5 to 10 mL of CSF is centrifuged, and the sediment is taken up into a capillary tube and recentrifuged before the capillary tube is examined under a coverslip (Fig. 158.12).[200] Specific molecular markers for this stage of CNS disease are being sought by proteomic analysis of the CSF.

Serology

Serologic tests are used for passive population screening in control programs (for review, see Chappuis et al[201]). A Card Agglutination Test for Trypanosomiasis (CATT) is robust and can be used without extensive laboratory facilities.[202,203] The test contains freeze-dried trypanosomes with the LiTat 1.3 variant antigens and can be obtained from the Institute of Tropical Medicine Antwerp (www.itg.be). It is quite sensitive (>95%), but it lacks specificity owing to cross-reactivities with animal *Trypanosoma* spp. Although useful as a patient screening test in a hospital for suspected cases of trypanosomiasis, the predictive value for positive test results falls when screening populations for active cases. It has nevertheless been reported to double the number of active cases found. Some patients may have false-negative results for this test if they are infected by parasites that do not express this variant antigen. Further versions of this assay have been developed to use dried blood on filter paper, namely the micro-CATT and macro-CATT, but these are less sensitive than the whole-blood assay.

In *T. b. gambiense,* serologic tests are not widely available, and direct examination of blood and CSF for parasites is the first line of investigation. The card indirect agglutination trypanosomiasis test (*TrypTect CIATT*) can detect circulating antigens in *T. b. gambiense* and *T. b. rhodesiense* infection by latex agglutination. The sensitivities of the test are 95.8% for *T. b. gambiense* and 97.7% for *T. b. rhodesiense,* and therefore significantly higher than that of lymph node puncture, microhematocrit centrifugation, and CSF examination after single- and double-centrifugation.[204]

A rapid latex agglutination test (LATEX/*T. b. gambiense*) contains a mixture of three variable surface antigens of the bloodstream form of trypanosomes and has been used to detect antibodies in patients infected with *T. b. gambiense.* At 1:16 serum dilution, test specificity was 99%, whereas sensitivity ranged from 83.8% to 100%, depending on the geographic origin of the samples. The test sensitivity falls to 66% for CSF samples from second-stage patients.[205] A rapid latex agglutination test, LATEX/IgM, for the semiquantitative detection of IgM in CSF is available.[206] Finally, immunofluorescence assays and ELISA tests for antibodies using whole parasites are highly sensitive and specific, although they are less practical for mass screening. A series of new approaches is being evaluated for control and elimination of trypanosomiasis, including tiny targets for tsetse fly control, use of RDTs, and oral treatment with fexinidazole or oxaboroles.[207]

Treatment

Treatment of trypanosomiasis depends on the subspecies of trypanosome present. The drugs may be difficult to source and are toxic, so treatment requires expert help.

Early-stage *T. b. gambiense* may be treated with pentamidine for 14 days (intravenously or more usually intramuscularly, 4 mg/kg/day). Hematologic side effects include neutropenia, and more general side effects include hypotension, hypercalcemia, hyperkalemia, renal failure, and hyperglycemia. Pentamidine will not cure CNS disease, and so examination of the CSF is required after initial treatment of the blood-stage disease.

Eflornithine (α-difluoromethylornithine) for 14 days (IV; 100 mg/kg every 6 hours) is effective for CNS treatment for *T. b. gambiense.*[208] It is a toxic drug suppressing DNA replication by inhibition of ornithine decarboxylase and thus polyamine synthesis and DNA replication. It causes dose-dependent bone marrow suppression with anemia, neutropenia, and thrombocytopenia in the majority of patients. The effects are reversible and are rarely dose limiting. It is effective neither in children nor in patients with coinfection with HIV, where melarsoprol is required.

Melarsoprol is a trivalent organic arsenical compound and is more toxic but cheaper than eflornithine. It is used in Africa for the treatment of late-stage CNS trypanosomiasis. It is given as three daily intravenous injections at a dose of 3.6 mg/kg up to 180 mg on two occasions 1 week apart. If the CNS leukocyte count is greater than 20/mm³, a further three injections are given 1 week later.

Melarsoprol causes a secondary encephalopathy in 5% to 10% of treated cases and is fatal in half of these.[209] The incidence and severity of encephalopathy may be reduced by concurrent administration of prednisolone (1 mg/kg/day up to 40 mg) started 1 to 2 days before melarsoprol treatment.[210] When steroids are used, it is necessary to give patients antimalarial and antihelminthic therapy, especially if *Strongyloides stercoralis* is present.

Prior treatment of blood-stage disease with pentamidine may reduce antigen levels and possibly adverse events. Promethazine, anticonvulsants, and antiemetics are important adjunctive treatments before commencing CNS therapy.

Polyneuropathy occurs in 10% of cases treated with melarsoprol and may be severe, causing quadriplegia. If neuropathy is suspected, melarsoprol should be stopped immediately and thiamine (100 mg, three times daily) given until symptoms subside.

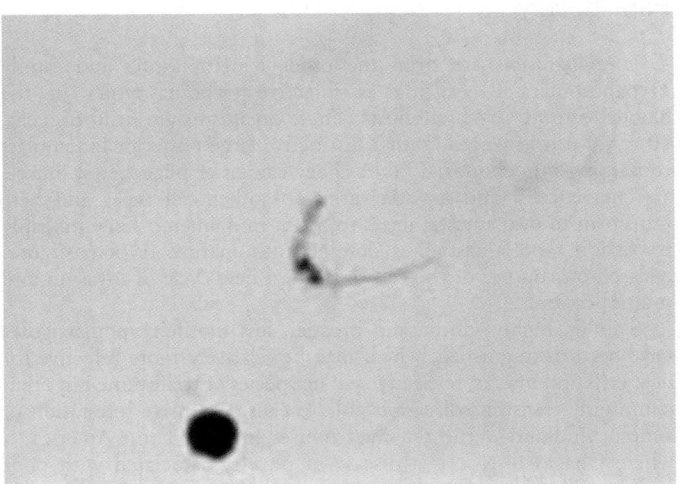

Fig. 158.12 TRYPOMASTIGOTE OF *TRYPANOSOMA BRUCEI BRUCEI* IN CEREBROSPINAL FLUID. A single organism is seen in this sample taken from cerebrospinal fluid filtered in a "minicolumn."

Patients require prolonged specialist follow-up over 2 years, including blood and CSF examination for parasites. A rising CSF leukocyte count is a good guide to CSF relapse even in the absence of a demonstration of parasites.[211]

In treatment for early-stage *T. b. rhodesiense,* suramin is given as five intravenous injections (20 mg/kg, up to 1.5 g) on days 1, 3, 6, 14, and 21. Adverse effects include fever, proteinuria, paresthesia, pruritus, and urticaria. Hemolytic anemia, agranulocytosis, and thrombocytopenia have been reported as side effects. Combination therapies of the antitrypanosomal drugs nifurtimox and eflornithine, and also the combination of melarsoprol and nifurtimox, are under trial for the treatment of second-stage disease to increase the efficacy of treatment and to overcome increasing drug resistance.[212]

African Trypanosomiasis as a Transfusion-Transmitted Infection

Trypanosomiasis is a transfusion-transmitted infection. Asymptomatic or early-stage patients with trypanosomiasis are clearly a threat to the blood supply. Patients are excluded in the United Kingdom, Europe, and North America by the general donor queries relating to fever and constitutional symptoms. In endemic areas, exclusion of infected donors with early-stage *T. b. gambiense* is clearly a more complex problem because patients may be asymptomatic for long periods if the degree of risk is unknown and no specific screening procedures are in place. In summary, hematologic involvement in trypanosomiasis is peripheral to the main two features of the disease, but examination of lymph node aspirates, blood, and CSF is essential for diagnosis and management of the disease. Occasionally, patients may become severely ill and have complex hematologic abnormalities. In endemic areas, trypanosomiasis may pose a risk to the blood supply.

AMERICAN TRYPANOSOMIASIS

American trypanosomiasis (or *Chagas disease,* named after the Brazilian parasitologist Carlos Chagas) is caused by infection with *Trypanosoma cruzi.* This flagellated protozoan is transmitted by the triatomine insects, the reduviid bugs. The acute phase of infection is characterized by fever and high parasitemia, followed by a chronic phase with positive serologic results and low parasitemia but with end-organ damage to the heart, peripheral nervous system, and gastrointestinal tract, causing a chronic cardiomyopathy, neuropathy, megaesophagus, and megacolon.

Epidemiology

Chagas disease may occur in the Americas from the southern United States to Chile, but the highest prevalence is in Bolivia and Brazil (Fig. 158.13). There are approximately 10 million seropositive people in Latin America, and the number of people infected and the incidence of new infection are falling rapidly.[213] Infections are found not only in rural areas but also in recent immigrants to urban areas in North and South America and to Europe.[214] It is estimated that approximately 100,000 seropositive individuals are living in the United States. True, endogenous (autochthonous) infection in the United States is vanishingly rare, but human infections have been reported in Texas, California, Tennessee, and Louisiana. Visitors to endemic areas are only rarely infected, with only a handful of cases being recorded in intrepid travelers spending time in traditional housing in rural areas. The range of reservoir hosts and species of triatomine bugs transmitting infection is wide.

Parasites may also be transmitted by blood transfusion (see later), vertically from mother to child by breastfeeding, organ transplant, and rarely by sexual transmission. Several outbreaks in Brazil have been reported after contamination of food by triatomine bugs and their feces. Laboratory infection by accidental ingestion or inoculation of parasites is well recorded.

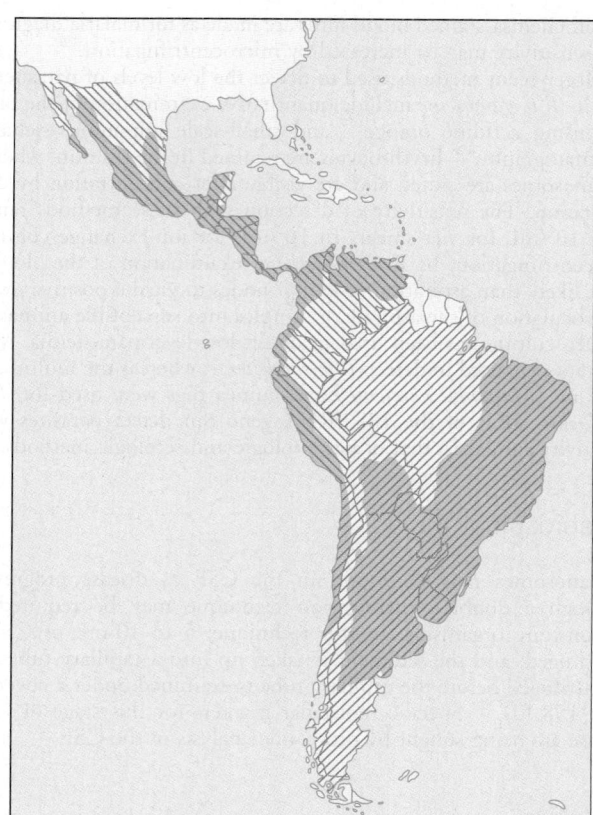

Fig. 158.13 DISTRIBUTION OF CHAGAS DISEASE. Human infection is endemic in parts of Central and South America from the Andes to the Atlantic coast and as far south as the latitude of the River Plate (Río de la Plata), shown here in *green.* Two major intergovernmental programs were started in 1991 to eliminate domestic vectors by a combination of spraying residual insecticides in houses, the use of insecticidal paints, and the deployment of fumigant canisters. The countries covered in the two initiatives, the second of which started in 1997, are shown in the figure. The latter program instituted universal blood screening to avoid transmission from infected blood donors. Remarkable progress has been made. Transmission (by the major vector *Triatoma infestans*) was eliminated in Uruguay by 1997 and in Chile by 1999. Major reductions in transmission but, to date, not complete control have also been reported in other endemic countries. (Southern Cone Initiative; Andean and American Initiative areas.)

Parasitology

T. cruzi parasites are from the order Kinetoplastida and family Trypanosomatidae, existing as infective trypomastigotes in the bloodstream of vertebrate hosts. These organisms are fusiform cells, 10 to 20 µm in length, with a distinctive large posterior kinetoplast containing mitochondrial DNA. They can enter phagocytes, muscle and nerve cells, and a wide variety of other cell types and here transform to oval amastigotes 2 to 5 µm in diameter. They multiply by fission, and amastigotes develop into mature trypomastigotes released on rupture of the cell to begin a new cycle of invasion and multiplication.

Slender, highly motile and broader, less motile trypomastigotes have been distinguished, which may be relatively more infective for host cells and insects, respectively. The species of triatomine bugs that commonly transmits disease is able to cause extensive infestation of simple mud-and-wattle thatched houses in rural Latin America,[215] where Chagas disease is a disease of poverty associated with poor housing. These bugs are infected by circulating trypomastigotes after taking a blood meal on sleeping victims. In the midgut, trypomastigotes transform into epimastigotes and multiply by fission before migrating to the hindgut, where they develop into metacyclic

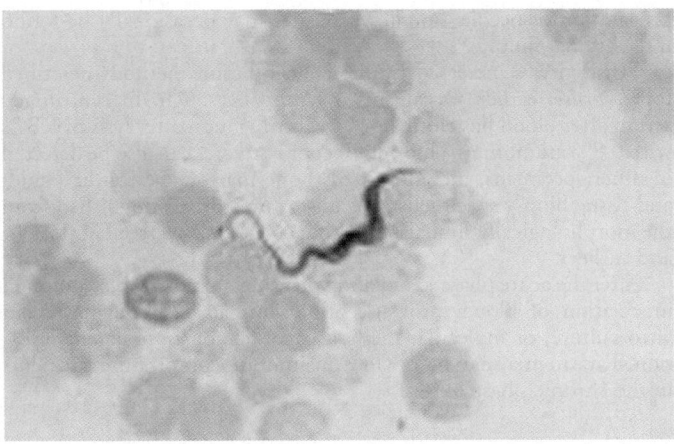

Fig. 158.14 *TRYPANOSOMA RANGELI*. *T. rangeli* is a long, slender trypanosome also transmitted by reduviid bugs from wild animals to humans. It is readily distinguished by its shape from *Trypanosoma cruzi* in blood films and appears to be nonpathogenic to humans.

trypomastigotes, adherent to the epithelium of the rectum. These infective forms are excreted into the feces, and people are infected by rubbing this infected material from the bug into the skin or conjunctival membranes. In the human host, multiplication into macrophages is followed by rapid dissemination of trypomastigotes into the blood and hence to tissues. The genome sequence of *T. cruzi* has stimulated a plethora of comparative and genomic approaches to the study of the parasite.[216,217]

Trypanosoma rangeli Infections

The nonpathogenic trypanosomes can be transmitted directly to people by the bite of the triatomine bugs, and they exist only as circulating trypomastigotes. No tissue amastigotes exist. Circulating organisms are sparse, but sometimes diagnosis can be made by careful microscopic examination of the distinctive morphology of these organisms in blood smears. The anterior position of the nucleus and small kinetoplast distinguish it from *T. cruzi* (Fig. 158.14). The antibodies produced to *T. rangeli* cross-react with those from *T. cruzi* and hence cause false-positive serologic test results for *T. cruzi*. However, the species may be differentiated by xenodiagnosis or molecular genetics in specialized laboratories.[218] The importance of recognizing this nonpathogenic infection is to avoid unnecessary treatment for *T. cruzi*.

Pathology

There is a wide variation in the pathogenicity of isolates and some regional variation in the clinical spectrum of acute and chronic illness. Molecular typing has demonstrated considerable heterogeneity of *T. cruzi* isolates, although the association between strains of parasite and the outcome of infection are unclear. Clearly the organism must have many mechanisms of the immune evasion to cause chronic infections in a high proportion of individuals. Some of these have been elegantly defined, including resistance to activation of the alternate pathway of complement, specific mechanisms of entering the host cells, and evasion of intracellular killing by the oxidative burst and lysozymes. Both CD4+ and CD8+ T cells are important for killing *T. cruzi*–infected cells, and IFN-γ has shown to be important to controlling disease, whereas transforming growth factor-β and IL-10 enhance parasite replication (for review, see Dutra et al[219]).

End-organ damage occurs after tissues have been infected by *T. cruzi* amastigotes, but the mechanisms leading to extensive cell damage are not clear. After multiplication, tissue amastigotes form pseudocysts in the heart with little or no inflammatory reaction,

although occasionally acute myocarditis with focal hemorrhage and inflammation may lead to heart failure. As the disease progresses, the inflammatory response is increased and is associated with increased tissue damage. There may be an autoimmune component to this inflammatory response, but the precise pathogenesis is poorly understood.[220] In the heart, chronic myocarditis leads to a decline in cardiac function. In late-stage disease, amastigotes can be found in almost all organs. Acute myocarditis with focal hemorrhage and inflammation may also lead to heart failure. Involvement of the brain, meninges, liver, lymph nodes, and spleen is common. Damage to the muscle walls and intramural nerve plexus in the esophagus and colon leads to dilation of these structures in the later phases of the disease.

Clinical Features

In about half the patients, a granuloma (or chagoma) occurs where parasites have been inoculated. The tender erythematous papule becomes keratotic and later heals, forming a hyperpigmented scar. When the conjunctiva are inoculated, the extensive unilateral periorbital edema may be prolonged (Romaña sign).

The severity of the acute illness is variable and ranges from asymptomatic infection or a mild febrile illness to a severe, potentially fatal illness with cardiac failure and meningoencephalitis in a minority of cases. Myalgia, generalized lymphadenopathy, hepatosplenomegaly, headaches, facial or generalized edema, vomiting, diarrhea, and anorexia are common features of the acute disease. The disease may be worse in children. The acute illness typically resolves in 4 to 8 weeks. Chagas disease must be distinguished from typhoid fever, VL, brucellosis, toxoplasmosis, and malaria in cases of chronic, febrile illness in endemic areas.

Chronic Disease

The acute phase of *T. cruzi* infection is followed by a variable latent or indeterminate phase with no clinical symptoms. Indeed, patients may never present with signs of end-organ damage. However, up to one-third of clinically infected patients may develop cardiac involvement and show right bundle branch block, atrioventricular conduction abnormalities, and/or abnormal T and Q waves. The patient may experience palpitations, chest pain, edema, and dizziness or syncope or dyspnea. The heart is enlarged, and intramural thrombus may cause sudden death.

In a further minority of chronically infected patients, the gastrointestinal tract is infected with abnormal motility of the esophagus and colon, leading to dysphagia and/or severe constipation. Occasionally, other hollow organ systems may be affected.

Pregnancy and Congenital Infection

In pregnant women, Chagas disease can cause spontaneous abortion, premature birth, intrauterine growth retardation, and stillbirth. Congenital infection occurs in 1% to 2% of women with chronic infection. Prompt diagnosis of circulating parasites in neonates at risk for congenital Chagas disease is essential to beginning early treatment. It is recognized that infection can also be transmitted by breastfeeding. Most children are asymptomatic, but 10% to 20% of children have a mild systemic illness with hepatosplenomegaly. More severely affected newborn children have pneumonitis, meningoencephalitis, and diffuse dermal granulomas. Petechiae, purpura, and a generalized bleeding tendency may occur.[221]

Immunocompromised Patients

The disease may recrudesce after chemotherapy for malignant disease, immunosuppressive therapy, or after organ transplant. The clinical disease may be fulminating with obvious parasitemia. Irregular erythematous indurated lesions have been described during *T. cruzi* recrudescence after solid-organ transplant. Here tissue amastigotes can be demonstrated by fine-needle aspiration.

HIV

Coinfection with *T. cruzi* and HIV has been reported from urban centers in Brazil. *T. cruzi* develops in end-stage disease with CD4+ T-cell counts of less than 400/µL. Patients may be severely ill, the majority with meningoencephalitis and often with a space-occupying lesion. Typically the CSF shows a mild lymphocytosis (<100 cells/µL). Parasites may be seen in the blood and occasionally the CSF. Cardiac involvement and heart failure are common.

Hematologic and Laboratory Features

A mild, normocytic, normochromic anemia is typical of acute illness. The pathogenesis of the anemia and contributions of hemolysis and bone marrow depression have not been studied in humans, but in experimental infections in mice, uncontrolled infection and TNF-α can be shown to contribute to depressed hematopoiesis. A modest lymphocytosis and increases in liver and muscle enzymes may be present. Nonspecific electrocardiographic changes, first-degree heart block, and cardiomegaly suggest early myocardial involvement.

Hematologic abnormalities are not usually found in the late stage of disease, in which cardiomyopathy with cardiac failure, rhythm disturbance, and angina and systemic emboli from intramural thrombus may occur. Trials of systemic anticoagulation have not been conducted.

Diagnosis

Microscopy

During the acute phase of the disease, motile trypanosomes can be identified in wet preparations or buffy coat preparations using concentration methods and detailed morphologic examination, including Giemsa-stained, gently prepared thick and thin films to avoid damage to parasites (Fig. 158.15). Trypanosomes can be aspirated from the chagoma in the acute phase of disease and visualized in a wet preparation of needle aspirates. Parasites may occasionally be found in lachrymal fluid.

Sensitivity is increased by the concentration methods described for *T. brucei* earlier. Organisms may also be sought in centrifuged serum after blood has clotted or by centrifugation after lysis of RBCs with 0.8% ammonium chloride. Trypomastigotes can also be detected in other specimens, including CSF, bone marrow, pericardiac fluid, and tissue biopsy specimens. Organisms must be distinguished from the morphologically similar nonpathogenic *T. rangeli* (see Fig. 158.14 and earlier).

After the acute phase, circulating parasites are not visible, although inoculation of blood into susceptible animals (xenodiagnosis), in vitro culture, or molecular methods may demonstrate patent infection. Parasitemia may be obvious in immunocompromised patients in the chronic phase of disease.

Xenodiagnosis

Infection of laboratory triatomine bugs by a seropositive patient is more sensitive than morphologic examination in chronically infected patients. It is also possible to infect susceptible laboratory animals. However, these techniques are available only in specialized centers in Latin America.

In Vitro Culture

Epimastigotes can be cultured using blood agar (NNN) medium or other media such as Schneider insect medium. After 4 weeks or more of culture at 26°C, epimastigotes may be detected.[222,223]

Serology

Serologic testing is a sensitive method of detecting infection after the acute phase. In Latin America, a number of commercial assays are available using crude epimastigote lysates in a variety of different formats. Serologic tests have used IFAT and ELISA using crude antigen prepared from in vitro cultures of epimastigotes. These tests must be carefully controlled with appropriate positive or negative sera. Chronically infected patients usually give a positive test result if titers are greater than 1:80.[224] These have a sensitivity and specificity of more than 95%. These antibodies may cross-react with antibodies to malaria, leishmaniasis, syphilis, and some autoimmune conditions. ELISA should be used in conjunction with a confirmatory test such as Western blot.

In South and North America, a number of companies market ELISA-based assays using recombinant antigens, synthetic peptides, or a concentrated extract of excretory-secretory antigens from either Brazil or Tulahuen strain *T. cruzi* trypomastigotes (total trypomastigote excretory-secretory antigens [TESAs]). These assays may provide more rapidly available and cheaper tests without loss of sensitivity and specificity (see Trypanosomiasis as a Transfusion-Transmitted Infection section for further discussion).

Serologic testing may be useful in the evaluation of people who may have been exposed to Chagas disease, pregnant women, and patients about to undergo immunosuppressive treatment or to receive chemotherapy or who have been diagnosed with HIV or other immunosuppressive illness. Children born to seropositive women will have maternally derived IgG anti–*T. cruzi* antibodies but demonstrate IgM anti–*T. cruzi* antibodies if congenitally infected.[225]

Molecular Diagnosis

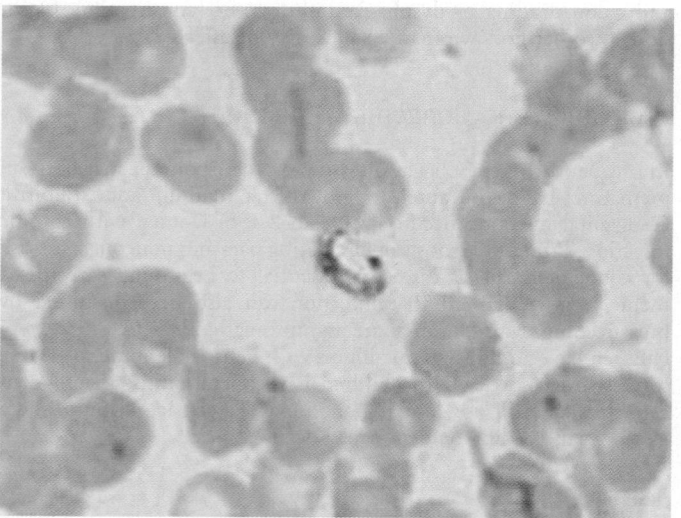

Fig. 158.15 *TRYPANOSOMA CRUZI* IN HUMAN BLOOD FILM. The causative agent occurs in blood films, characteristically as short C-shaped or S-shaped trypomastigotes with a prominent kinetoplast. It is otherwise monomorphic.

Amplification of *T. cruzi*–specific sequences by PCR is potentially the most widely applicable, sensitive, and specific method for detecting parasites. A number of assays have been developed, based on the application of repetitive sequences in kinetoplast DNA. A meta-analysis has suggested that PCR is not more sensitive than ELISA for detection of *T. cruzi* in chagasic patients. The recommendation is to use two serologic tests, which may be supplemented by PCR-based assays in the immunocompromised patient, in whom seroconversion may not occur in patent infection.[226]

Treatment

The detailed treatment of Chagas disease is beyond the scope of this chapter. Treatment of the acute, intermediate, and chronic phases requires expert supervision because parasitologic cure is achieved in only half the cases and monitoring progress requires specialist testing and evaluation and where necessary treatment of end-organ damage. The current and potential future chemotherapy[227-229] have recently been reviewed.

Nifurtimox is a synthetic nitrofuran that inhibits pyruvic acid synthesis by inhibition of lactic dehydrogenase. It is given for 30 to 120 days at 3 to 5 mg/kg three times per day. The most serious side effects are peripheral neuropathy, mental disturbance (including psychosis), and hemolytic anemia associated with G6PD.

Benznidazole is widely available in Latin America and is given at 5 mg per kilogram of body weight per day for 60 days. Severe hematologic complications are common, and bone marrow depression is a serious side effect. Thrombocytopenia may be severe, and neutropenia may progress to agranulocytosis. Other serious complications include photosensitivity, neuropathy, and weight loss.[230]

Supportive therapy is required for heart failure and acute meningoencephalitis. Surgery may be required for alleviation of esophageal and chronic dysfunction. In the absence of effective or simple therapy, control of triatomine bugs and an improvement in the housing stock are essential to prevent and control disease.

American Trypanosomiasis as a Transfusion-Transmitted Infection

Chagas disease may occur as a transfusion-transmitted infection and represents a real threat to the safety of the blood supply in endemic areas. It is estimated that 1.5% to 50% of contaminated units cause infection in recipients, a wide range that may reflect the stage of infection in the donor, the type and processing of the component, and the immune status of the recipient.[231]

In endemic areas, seropositivity is high, reaching 50% in some areas of Bolivia and 1% to 2% in major areas in Brazil. Control of blood transfusion–transmitted infection is part of the World Health Organization strategy for control of Chagas disease.[232-234] Serologic screening, tests using synthetic peptide antigens, or a mixture of recombinant antigens to detect anti–*T. cruzi* antibodies in chronically infected blood donors are more than 95% sensitive.[235,236] These serologic tests, replacing those based on crude antigens, have allowed improved coverage of screening of blood donors throughout Latin America and in the United States.[237,238]

It is possible to treat blood with gentian violet (0.25 g/L for 24 hours at 4°C) or with methylene blue to kill circulating organisms. It has also been shown that amotosalen or riboflavin plus ultraviolet A photochemical inactivation technology is effective in inactivating *T. cruzi* in platelet concentrates and plasma.[238,239] In addition, prophylactic benznidazole can be given to immunosuppressed patients receiving blood products in endemic areas.

Outside Latin America, Chagas disease is an occasional cause of transfusion-transmitted infection, mainly in immunosuppressed patients. It is possible that minor infections are not recognized in healthy individuals. Clearly the high rates of seropositivity in individuals from endemic areas suggest that recent immigrants may easily transmit the disease.

In the United Sates the overall seropositive rate among blood donors is 1:250,000, with local incidence rates reaching 1:7500 or greater in Los Angeles and Miami.[231] These rates are probably underestimates because immigration from endemic areas has recently increased. Surveys of blood donors in France have shown seropositivity of *T. cruzi* can be detected by PCR in about half the seropositive donors and remain viable for at least 20 days, surviving cryopreservation and thawing. *T. cruzi* has been reported to be transmitted after organ transplant[240,241] and after blood transfusion in seven patients who were immunosuppressed.[242-246]

Donors can be excluded by a medical questionnaire eliciting obvious symptoms of acute or chronic disease. Prospective studies have shown these questionnaires would miss many infected donors,[247,248] including those infected congenitally.[249] Nevertheless, in Europe screening for anti–*T. cruzi* antibodies is targeted at at-risk blood donors who originate from an endemic area, donors with mothers originating from such an area, and individuals who have lived in or traveled to endemic areas. In France the seropositivity in these selected donors was 1:32,000.[250]

In the United States new tests have been requested by the Food and Drug Administration to combat this threat. A radioimmunoprecipitation assay (RIPA) is the most sensitive method to detect anti–*T. cruzi* antibodies,[251] although RIPA cross-reactivity has been reported in patients with VL.[252] It is unsuitable for mass screening, however. An ELISA based in a concentrated extract of excretory-secretory antigens from either Brazil or Tulahuen strain *T. cruzi* trypomastigotes (TESAs)[253,254] had an overall sensitivity of 100% and specificity of more than 94%, and a prototype *T. cruzi* lysate–based ELISA has been developed that appears to be 97.7% sensitive and 100% specific.[251]

It is only to be hoped that sensitive screening tests are consistently applied to reduce transmission of Chagas disease by blood products in endemic and nonendemic countries. On a more general note, it is encouraging that the initiatives to control *T. cruzi* infection across Latin America are showing real evidence of success.[213,255]

BABESIOSIS

Babesiosis is an intraerythrocytic infection caused by parasites from the order Piroplasmida and the family Babesiidae. It was first observed as causing parasitic inclusions in erythrocytes of cattle in Romania by Victor Babes at the end of the 19th century.[256] The infection is zoonosis transmitted by hard-bodied ticks and causes fever and hemolytic anemia. Several distinct *Babesia* spp. cause disease in different geographic areas.[257,258]

There are two well-defined *Babesia* species that cause human infection. *Babesia microti* is a parasite of small rodents in the northeastern United States and is spread by nymphs, larvae, and adult forms of the hard-bodied ixodid ticks (*Ixodes dammini*). Infection of the white-tailed deer by ticks allows multiplication and spread of the infected ticks. Infections can be transferred to humans by all forms of the tick after prolonged feeding. The infection is therefore most common in people vacationing or working in forested areas of the northeastern United States. The northeastern US offshore islands of Nantucket, Martha's Vineyard, Block Island, and Shelter Island are foci of the disease, but it also occurs in eastern states, particularly Connecticut, Rhode Island, Delaware, and New York State, as well as upper Midwestern states. Hundreds of cases have been recorded since the first identified case in 1969. Visitors and workers in endemic areas should avoid tick bites by using appropriate clothing and repellents.

In Europe, *Babesia divergens* and the morphologically indistinguishable parasite *Babesia bovis* are transmitted to humans by ticks (*Ixodes ricinus*) from cattle. Fewer than 50 cases have been recorded. European cases of *B. microti* and *Babesia canis* infection have also been reported.

A handful of cases of infections with *Babesia duncani* in the western United States have been reported. These organisms are morphologically indistinguishable from *B. microti* but are distinguished by molecular methods. The MO1-type piroplasm caused illness in an index case in Missouri in 1992, and the WA1-2 and CA1-5 piroplasms caused disease in eight cases reported in Washington State and California.[259,260] A further *B. microti*–like organism, *B.*

venatorum, has caused infection in a small series of older men who had undergone splenectomy for a lymphoproliferative disease.[261] The same organism has been isolated in a much larger series of patients from China.[262]

B. microti and *B. duncani* have been transmitted by blood and platelet transfusions.[260] Transplacental infection by *B. microti* has also been reported.

Parasitology

Parasites appear to be introduced into the bloodstream, where they invade erythrocytes. There they multiply by asexual fission to produce two to four merozoites. These infective forms are released after lysis of the erythrocyte and begin another cycle of invasion multiplication. Parasites are cleared by macrophages. The contribution of antibodies and cell-mediated immune response has not been defined, although *B. bovis* expresses clonally variant antigens on the surface of infected erythrocytes.[27]

Clinical Features

The North American *B. microti* infections have an incubation period of several weeks, and after infection by blood transfusion, clinical symptoms have taken from 17 days to many months to become manifest.[263–265] The spectrum of clinical disease is wide. *B. microti* may cause asymptomatic infection or present with a mild flulike illness in most cases in people with normal immune and splenic function.[266] The cardinal manifestations are fever and hemolytic anemia. Splenectomy, old age, and immunosuppression, including HIV, may increase the risk for more severe clinical disease.[267–269] The disease may progress to adult respiratory distress syndrome (ARDS), disseminated intravascular coagulation, or renal failure.[262] Patients who have had a splenectomy should avoid exposure to ticks in forested areas where the disease is transmitted.

B. divergens in Europe predominantly causes symptomatic infection in people who have had a splenectomy.[270,271] Here, the case fatality rate is on the order of 50%. However, symptomatic disease does also occur in immunocompetent individuals.[272]

Patients present with high fever, often with chills and sweats, jaundice, fatigue, malaise, headache, arthralgia, and myalgia. Gastro-intestinal disturbances are common, and people may complain of dark urine secondary to hemoglobinuria. In some cases the disease progresses with respiratory failure secondary to ARDS, disseminated intravascular coagulation, and renal failure requiring the appropriate supportive care.[273] Such severe cases resemble severe malaria in nonimmune persons, and it has been suggested that the pathophysiology, like in malaria, includes adhesion and sequestration of infected erythrocytes and the release of proinflammatory cytokines. These diseases may be confused with falciparum malaria, leptospirosis, or viral hepatitis. In pregnancy, acute babesiosis may mimic the HELLP syndrome (hemolysis, elevated liver enzymes, and low platelet count).[273]

Hematologic and Laboratory Features

The hematologic features of the disease are dominated by substantial intravascular hemolysis.[257] Physical examination shows pallor, jaundice, and mild hepatosplenomegaly.

The laboratory findings are those of a compensated intravascular hemolytic anemia and thus feature low hemoglobin and haptoglobin levels, increased reticulocyte count and serum lactate dehydrogenase, and hemoglobinuria and proteinuria. Moderate thrombocytopenia is common.[265,274] Electron microscopy suggests uninfected erythrocytes are damaged during infection and so likely to be cleared more rapidly than normally.[275] The white blood cell count is usually decreased with atypical lymphocytosis and occasional evidence of hemophagocytosis. However, leukocytosis may occur, particularly in *B. divergens* infections.

The direct Coombs test result is frequently positive for both C3 components and IgG. Polyclonal hypergammaglobulinemia is seen, and levels of C3 and C4 are reduced in acute infection. Liver function tests show raised indirect bilirubin and mildly raised transaminase levels.

Diagnosis

The blood films stained with Giemsa or Romanowsky stain show ringlike intraerythrocytic parasites. Morphology is variable, and ring, rod, and ameboid forms of *Babesia* parasites may be seen (Fig. 158.16).[276] Occasionally, multiple intraerythrocytic forms can be

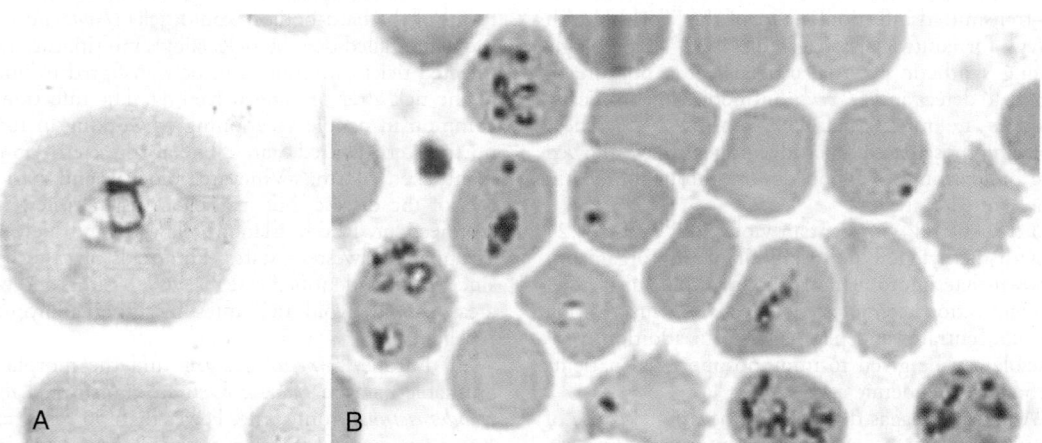

Fig. 158.16 *BABESIA* PARASITES. Human infection with species of piroplasm transmitted by the bite of the tick *Ixodes ricinus* infected from cattle is a rare occurrence. Infection in normal people with this piroplasm may give rise to a self-limiting fever and parasitemia, as in the case of infection with the rodent parasite *Babesia microti* on the northeastern seaboard of the United States via the tick *Ixodes scapularis* (A). Heavy red-cell infection may develop, however, in splenectomized patients, leading to fatal hemolytic anemia. This patient died as a result of an infection acquired from the cattle parasite *Babesia divergens* in Scotland (B). Other species of *Babesia* that occasionally infect humans, for example, the WA1, CA1, and MO1 isolates from the United States, are distinguished by molecular means.

seen, linked to form a tetrad or, colloquially, a "Maltese cross." However, at low parasitemia, *Babesia* parasites may easily be mistaken for ring-stage forms of *P. falciparum.* Moreover, false-positive sightings of *Babesia* spp. may be caused by platelets, nonspecific stain deposit overlying erythrocytes, or indeed other intraerythrocytic inclusions.

Parasitemias are variable, and in *B. microti* infections may be low or transient.[266] In symptomatic infection, parasitemias typically range from less than 1% to 10% and rarely much higher, more than 70%, in severe infections. Low-level parasitemias may be detected by inoculation of the blood into susceptible animals, including the golden hamster *(Mesocricetus auratus),* but this is not routinely available.

An IFAT using crude antigen is available in the United States through the Division of Parasitic Diseases at the Centers for Disease Control and Prevention.[277] Titers greater than 1 : 64 are regarded as positive and have been reported to be 88% to 96% sensitive and 90% to 100% specific.

PCR analysis is the most useful method of detecting or confirming low levels of parasitemia, and it can also be used to monitor treatment. Real-time PCR assays target the *Babesia* 18S rRNA gene and, with use of a fluorescent probe, can distinguish *B. microti* from *B. duncani.*[278,279] PCR tests may be positive in the absence of positive serology in immunocompromised patients and/or those patients who have received rituximab, whereas serology for *Babesia* spp. may be positive in the absence of positive microscopy or positive PCR tests in asymptomatic individuals who were infected but who have cleared the infection spontaneously.

Treatment

Many *B. microti* infections are self-limiting, and therapy is used for moderate or severe disease.[257,280-282] The combination of atovaquone and azithromycin is the treatment of choice for mild to moderate illness, whereas clindamycin and quinine and exchange transfusion are indicated for severe disease.

B. divergens infections are often fatal in splenectomized patients, and therapy is based on somewhat limited experience. Three cases have been treated successfully with large-volume exchange transfusions (two to three blood volumes) and intravenous clindamycin and oral quinine.[283] This regimen of clindamycin and intravenous and oral quinine gives the best chance of success in the absence of randomized controlled trial evidence.

Exchange transfusion has been suggested as a useful adjunctive treatment if the parasitemia rises to greater than 10% and/or in severely ill patients. *B. divergens* infections can run a rapidly progressive course, and early exchange transfusion should be considered. A prolonged course of treatment may be required in immunocompromised patients.[284] The parasite and hemoglobin levels should be regularly monitored during treatment.

Serologic testing and PCR testing of seropositive cases may be helpful in making a diagnosis. An indirect IFAT is available for *B. divergens* and *B. microti.* The IFAT titer is usually greater than 1 : 64 in acute infection. The reported sensitivity of the *B. microti* IFAT is 88% to 96%, and its specificity is 90% to 100%. Antimalarial antibodies may cross-react in this test.

Babesia and Transfusion-Transmitted Infection

Babesia infection poses a substantial and increasing threat to the blood supply. Between 150 and 170 cases of transfusion-transmitted babesiosis have been reported from 1979 to 2009, with 12 recorded fatalities.[285-287] There are no approved serologic screening tests for donors, and prevention of transfusion-transmitted babesiosis in the United States requires screening donors about a previous history of babesiosis and excluding patients with fever and a low hematocrit level. The scale of infection can be gauged from surveys of blood donors in the northeastern United States, where 1% to 2% of donors in some panels are seropositive for *Babesia.*[288] In the United Kingdom,

a conservative approach has been taken, and all donors who have visited the northeastern United States between May and October are excluded, in addition to the standard criteria of screening out febrile and/or anemic donors.

EOSINOPHILIA

Eosinophilia may be caused by a wide variety of systemic diseases and parasitic infections. The association with parasitic disease is through part of the Th2 T-cell response stimulated by helminths (worms), filaria, and cestodes. In general, protozoan infections, such as malaria, amebiasis, and giardiasis, are not associated with eosinophilia. However, case reports do exist suggesting that isosporosis due to infection with *Isospora belli,* toxoplasmosis, and infection with *Dientamoeba fragilis* can cause eosinophilia.

The rise in absolute eosinophil count depends on the degree of tissue invasion and is therefore modest with tapeworms and adult roundworms resident in the bowel but much higher where invasion occurs, for example, with *Toxocara canis* or filaria. Some parasites, such as ascariasis (roundworms) and clonorchiasis, have migratory larval stages.

The differential diagnosis of eosinophilia in those who have lived in tropical areas is therefore wide. Evaluating the patients must begin by establishing the degree of eosinophilia (minimal, $<1 \times 10^9$/L; moderate, 1 to 3×10^9/L; high, $>3 \times 10^9$/L), the relation to travel (where necessary), and the presence of symptoms. A wide range of systemic diseases are associated with eosinophilia, and the eosinophil count may be high in drug allergy, pulmonary infiltrate with eosinophilia, and vasculitides.

Eosinophilia in Travelers

Evaluating the cause of eosinophilia in travelers to tropical areas where many parasitic diseases are endemic requires a systematic approach to narrow down likely possibilities by considering existing systemic diseases that may cause eosinophilia (particularly allergy, drug ingestion and autoimmune disease, vasculitis, or arthritis); the areas visited; duration of stay; and history of exposure to soil-transmitted nematodes, freshwater potentially infected with schistosomiasis, and rural areas where loiasis, onchocerciasis, and hydatid disease may be contracted.

Physical examination may show subcutaneous swellings associated with filaria or hepatosplenomegaly consistent with schistosomiasis, hydatid disease, or toxocara. Laboratory examination requires a stepwise approach, given the breadth of the differential diagnosis (Table 158.4). The details of specific parasitologic tests are beyond the scope of this chapter, and detailed investigation would certainly require consultation with colleagues in infectious diseases.

Some parasitic causes of eosinophilia may not be diagnosed during the incubation period, because larval stages of nematode worms may cause eosinophilic drug migration, but eggs will not be excreted in stools for many months. Moreover, filarial infections do not produce detectable parasites in blood or skin for many months after exposure.

In immunocompromised patients or those about to receive a diagnosis, eosinophilia may be crucial, given the risks of giving immunosuppressive therapy such as chemotherapy or hematopoietic stem cell or solid organ transplant to a patient with a chronic parasitologic infection. Patients with undiagnosed eosinophilia and possible exposure to *Strongyloides* should be given an empirical course of treatment.

OTHER PARASITIC DISEASES

Many parasitic diseases cause some minor hematologic disturbance. A few may present with distinct hematologic features or indeed syndromes.

Filariasis

Lymphatic filariasis is caused by *Wuchereria bancrofti* and *Brugia malayi*. Infection with *W. bancrofti* occurs throughout the tropics, but by far the majority of cases are in Asia. The distribution of *B. malayi* is more restricted to China, Southeast Asia, and Southern India. The male and female adult worms live in the lymphatics, and the female worm releases a vast number of microfilariae, each 250 to 300 µm in length. Microfilariae develop but do not appear to multiply in the mosquito.

Infection may present with lymphangitis; often recurrent and unlike bacterial infections, the inflammatory features may spread distally. Over time, lymphatic obstruction may cause hydrocele, lymphedema (if severe elephantiasis), chyluria, and tropical pulmonary eosinophilia. *B. malayi* causes neither hydrocele nor chyluria.

Filariasis is most easily diagnosed by finding microfilariae in peripheral blood in a wet preparation. Motile microfilariae can be seen under low power and may be concentrated by centrifugation or filtration using a 3-µm filter. They are speciated in thin or thick films by their nuclear distribution and sheath characteristics (Fig. 158.17), and the two pathogenic species must be distinguished from the nonpathogenic species *Mansonella perstans* and *Mansonella ozzardi*, which do not have sheaths. Circulating *W. bancrofti* antigens can also be detected in the circulation by ELISA or immunochromatographic methods. Adult worms can sometimes be imaged by ultrasound. Filarial DNA from all species can be detected by PCR. Serologic testing is unhelpful because many people become exposed without developing clinical symptoms.

The worms cause marked or severe eosinophilia (see later) with counts greater than 1×10^9/L. Migration of worms through the lungs may exacerbate the eosinophil count and cause minor respiratory symptoms and fluctuating radiologic signs. Other causes of tropical pulmonary eosinophilia are the worms (helminths) *Ascaris*, *Strongyloides*, *Schistosoma*, and *Toxocara*. Of these organisms causing pulmonary symptoms and signs, filariasis alone is responsive to diethylcarbamazine. Albendazole and ivermectin may also be used against filarial infection.

Toxoplasmosis

Toxoplasmosis may cause a mild illness or a more prolonged course with constitutional symptoms, atypical lymphocytes, and thrombocytopenia. Congenital toxoplasmosis as a result of infection acquired during pregnancy is a cause of neonatal thrombocytopenia, where it may be accompanied by cerebral calcification, hepatitis, and pneumonitis. In immunocompromised patients, new or reactivated toxoplasmosis may cause severe disease, including encephalitis, pneumonitis, and hepatitis. Thrombocytopenia is frequently accompanied by anemia and leukopenia.

Amebiasis

Amebiasis causes hypochromic, microcytic anemia, both as a result of chronic blood loss and as an anemia of chronic disease in which disease progresses to formation of a liver abscess. Neutrophilia accompanies severe tissue damage caused by perforation of the bowel or a liver abscess, or it may be present in a secondary bacterial infection. Sometimes a leukemoid reaction with high white blood cell count and extreme left-shifted myeloid cells can be seen. Prolonged and/or extensive liver damage may cause prolongation of the prothrombin time.

Giardiasis

Acute giardiasis causes folate deficiency through malabsorption of folate in the small intestine. Chronic infection can cause vitamin B_{12} deficiency because ileal absorption of the vitamin is impaired.

Hookworm Infection

Adult hookworms attach themselves to the lining of the small bowel and take blood meals. The accumulated blood loss may be extensive because worms consume 2.0 mL (*Necator americanus*) or 0.5 mL

TABLE 158.4	Approach to Investigation of Eosinophilia in a Returning Traveler
History	Allergy
	Drugs and vitamins (L-tryptophan)
	Regions, localities, and duration of exposure
Physical examination	Skin, subcutaneous tissues
	Liver/spleen
	Signs of other systemic disease
Initial investigations	Full blood count and differential white blood cell count
	Stool examination for ova and parasites (×3)
	Urine analysis
	Examination of midday urine for ova and parasites (×3) (in those who have traveled to Africa or the Middle East)
Further investigations as suggested by travel and exposure from history	As suggested by travel and exposure from history
	Strongyloides culture and serologic testing
	Duodenal aspirate (strongyloidiasis, hookworm)
	Serologic testing (schistosomiasis, filariasis)
	Day/night blood films (filariasis)
Further studies if suggested by history and physical examination	Skin snips (onchocerciasis)
	Chest x-ray examination (hydatid cyst, tropical pulmonary eosinophilia, paragonimiasis)
	Soft tissue x-ray examination (cysticercosis)
	Sputum examination for ova and parasites (paragonimiasis)
	Abdominal ultrasound examination (hydatid cyst)
	Cystoscopy with or without biopsy (schistosomiasis)
	Rectal snips (schistosomiasis)

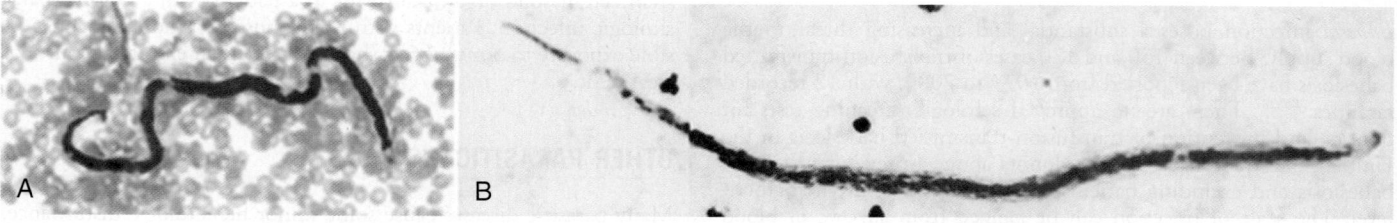

Fig. 158.17 MICROFILARIA *(BRUGIA MALAYI)* ON THICK (A) AND THIN FILMS (B). The species is determined by the nuclear distribution and sheath characteristics.

(*Ancylostoma duodenale*) of blood each day. These infections are a common contributing factor to iron deficiency anemia in children, in whom infection is acquired by eating or walking barefoot on larva-infected soil. The disease is usually diagnosed by finding excreted eggs in stool samples, and treatment is with albendazole.

Tapeworm Infection

The fish tapeworm *(Diphyllobothrium latum)* is a rare cause of vitamin B_{12} deficiency. This tapeworm is transmitted in the Far East by eating raw or partially cooked fish. Infection has to be extensive and causes vitamin B_{12} deficiency; however, such cases are rare, even in endemic areas.

Schistosomiasis

Schistosoma haematobium causes blood loss in urine. Infection is acquired by swimming in freshwater, where cercariae from the infected snail host enter the skin and migrate to the blood vessels of the bladder. Chronic blood loss is a cause of iron deficiency anemia in children in endemic areas, but infection is likely to be diagnosed at an early stage in travelers because of the striking symptoms of painless hematuria. Treatment is with praziquantel.

FUTURE DIRECTIONS

Parasitic diseases present many problems for global heath. They cause a wide spectrum of hematologic abnormalities, and in endemic areas, a broad knowledge of the parasitic disease is vital for everyday practice. In nonendemic areas, there are a few situations where the diagnosis or management of these diseases may fall within the remit of hematologists and hematology laboratories, particularly malaria and the diagnosis of anemia, cytopenias, eosinophilia, and hepatosplenomegaly. Here, a high index of suspicion is often needed for the diagnosis to be made. A good travel history is crucial to establishing exposure to parasitic disease and to prompt the search for the appropriate organisms. Several parasitic diseases pose a threat for the safe supply of blood, and the problems of screening of these infections are far from solved. Beyond everyday practice, the pathophysiology and prevention of these diseases pose major challenges for biomedical research and public health.

SUGGESTED READINGS

Ashley EA, Recht J, White NJ: Primaquine: the risks and the benefits. *Malar J* 13:418, 2014.

Babokhov P, Sanyaolu AO, Oyibo WA, et al: A current analysis of chemotherapy strategies for the treatment of human African trypanosomiasis. *Pathog Glob Health* 5:242, 2013.

Bailey JW, Williams J, Bain BJ, et al: Guideline: the laboratory diagnosis of malaria. *Br J Haematol* 163:573, 2013.

Bennett JE, Dolin R, Blaser MJ: *Mandell, Douglas, and Bennett's principles and practice of infectious diseases*, ed 8, London, 2014, Churchill Livingstone.

Bern C: Antitrypanosomal therapy for chronic Chagas' disease. *N Engl J Med* 364:2527, 2011.

Brun R, Blum J, Chappuis F, et al: Human African trypanosomiasis. *Lancet* 375:148, 2011.

Clark MA, Goheen MM, Cerami C: Influence of host iron status on *Plasmodium falciparum* infection. *Front Pharmacol* 5:84, 2014.

Copeland NK, Aronson NE: Leishmaniasis: treatment updates and clinical practice guidelines review. *Curr Opin Infect Dis* 28:426–437, 2015.

Coura JR, Borges-Pereira J: Chagas disease: 100 years after its discovery. A systemic review. *Acta Trop* 115:5, 2010.

Cox FE: History of human parasitology. *Clin Microbiol Rev* 15:595, 2002.

Croft SL, Olliaro P: Leishmaniasis chemotherapy—challenges and opportunities. *Clin Microbiol Infect* 17:1478, 2010.

Dhabangi A, Ainomugisha B, Cserti-Gazdewich C, et al: B-type natriuretic peptide and plasma hemoglobin levels following transfusion of shorter-storage versus longer-storage red blood cells: results from the TOTAL randomized trial. *Am Heart J* 183:129, 2016.

Drakesmith H, Prentice AM: Hepcidin and the iron-infection axis. *Science* 338:768–772, 2012.

Genovese G, Friedman DJ, Ross MD, et al: Association of trypanolytic ApoL1 variants with kidney disease in African Americans. *Science* 329:841, 2010.

Gething PW, Casey DC, Weiss DJ, et al: Mapping *Plasmodium falciparum* mortality in Africa between 1990 and 2015. *N Engl J Med* 375:2435, 2016.

Gubernot DM, Lucey CT, Lee KC, et al: Babesia infection through blood transfusions: reports received by the US Food and Drug Administration, 1997–2007. *Clin Infect Dis* 48:25, 2009.

Hoffman SL, Vekemans J, Richie TL, et al: The march toward malaria vaccines. *Am J Prev Med* 49(6 Suppl 4):S319, 2015.

Jimenez-Marco T, Fisa R, Girona-Llobera E, et al: Transfusion-transmitted leishmaniasis: a practical review. *Transfusion* 56(Suppl 1):S45, 2016.

Lalloo DG, Shingadia D, Bell DJ, et al: UK malaria treatment guidelines 2016. *J Infect* 72:635–649, 2016.

Langhorne J, Duffy PE: Expanding the antimalarial toolkit: targeting host-parasite interactions. *J Exp Med* 213:143–153, 2016.

Leiby DA: Transfusion-transmitted *Babesia* spp.: bull's-eye on *Babesia microti*. *Clin Microbiol Rev* 24:14, 2011.

Lindoso JA, Cunha MA, Queiroz IT, et al: Leishmaniasis-HIV coinfection: current challenges. *HIV AIDS (Auckl)* 8:147–156, 2016.

Maitland K, Kiguli S, Opoka RO, et al: Mortality after fluid bolus in African children with severe infection. *N Engl J Med* 364:2483, 2011.

Marsh K, Forster D, Waruiru C, et al: Indicators of life-threatening malaria in African children. *N Engl J Med* 332:1399, 1995.

Millar SB, Cox-Singh J: Human infections with *Plasmodium knowlesi*—zoonotic malaria. *Clin Microbiol Infect* 21:640, 2015.

Moreira CM, Abo-Shehada M, Price RN, et al: A systematic review of submicroscopic *Plasmodium vivax* infection. *Malar J* 14:360, 2015.

Morrell CN: Understanding platelets in malaria infection. *Curr Opin Hematol* 21:445–449, 2014.

Mungai M, Tegtmeier G, Chamberland M, et al: Transfusion-transmitted malaria in the United States from 1963 through 1999. *N Engl J Med* 344:1973, 2001.

Sahu PK, Satpathi S, Behera PK, et al: athogenesis of cerebral malaria: new diagnostic tools, biomarkers, and therapeutic approaches. *Front Cell Infect Microbiol* 5:75, 2015.

Satchwell TJ: Erythrocyte invasion receptors for *Plasmodium falciparum:* new and old. *Transfus Med* 26:77–88, 2016.

Simarro PP, Cecchi G, Paone M, et al: The atlas of human African trypanosomiasis: a contribution to global mapping of neglected tropical diseases. *Int J Health Geogr* 9:57, 2010.

Soriano-Arandes A, Angheben A, Serre-Delcor N, et al: Control and management of congenital Chagas disease in Europe and other non-endemic countries: current policies and practices. *Trop Med Int Health* 5:590–596, 2016.

Steinmann P, Stone CM, Sutherland CS, et al: Contemporary and emerging strategies for eliminating human African trypanosomiasis due to *Trypanosoma brucei gambiense*: review. *Trop Med Int Health* 6:707–718, 2015.

Sundar S, Singh A: Recent developments and future prospects in the treatment of visceral leishmaniasis. *Ther Adv Infect Dis* 3:98–109, 2016.

Vannier E, Krause PJ: Human babesiosis. *N Engl J Med* 366:2397, 2012.

Wendel S: Transfusion transmitted Chagas disease: is it really under control? *Acta Trop* 115:28, 2010.

Woodrow CJ, White NJ: The clinical impact of artemisinin resistance in Southeast Asia and the potential for future spread. *FEMS Microbiol Rev* 41:34, 2017.

World Health Organization: Control of the leishmaniases. *World Health Organ Tech Rep Ser* 949:1, 2010.

REFERENCES

For the complete list of references, log on to www.expertconsult.com.

HEMATOLOGIC PROBLEMS IN THE SURGICAL PATIENT: BLEEDING AND THROMBOSIS

Iqbal H. Jaffer, Mark T. Reding, Nigel S. Key, and Jeffrey I. Weitz

Surgical patients often present unique challenges to the consulting hematologist. They may develop hemostatic disorders ranging from unexpected bleeding to pathologic thrombosis, both of which can be potentially life threatening. Consultation may be sought to assess preoperative bleeding risk and/or to recommend strategies to prevent postoperative thrombosis. The hematologist may be called upon to assist in the management of patients with a previous history of bleeding or thrombosis and in those with unexplained bleeding or thrombosis in the perioperative period. This chapter will review: (1) the preoperative evaluation of bleeding risk; (2) strategies to aid intraoperative hemostasis; (3) the management of patients with hemostatic abnormalities or those taking long-term oral anticoagulation; and (4) the perioperative prevention of venous thromboembolism (VTE).

PREOPERATIVE EVALUATION OF HEMOSTATIC RISK

History

Preoperative evaluation of hemostatic risk begins with a carefully taken history. Particular attention should be directed at specific bleeding symptoms and any history of bleeding associated with surgical procedures, including circumcision, tonsillectomy, and dental extractions. For women, it is important to inquire about a history of menorrhagia or excessive bleeding associated with childbirth. A detailed family history and record of medication use, including nonprescription medications, should be obtained. In adults, an interview to assess for the presence or absence of bleeding symptoms has a high discriminating power when used in a screening situation, where no bleeding disorder is suspected, but may be less discriminatory for those referred for specialty evaluation.[1] In the pediatric population, the medical history may be less reliable as a screening method because of fewer previous hemostatic challenges.[2]

Obtaining an adequate bleeding history may be complicated by the fact that even in the absence of hemostatic defects, many people consider their bleeding to be excessive. Surveys of healthy individuals frequently report excessive nosebleeds (5%–39%), gingival bleeding (7%–51%), easy bruising (12%–24%), menorrhagia (23%–44%), postpartum bleeding (6%–23%), and bleeding following dental extraction (up to 13%) and tonsillectomy (up to 11%).[1,3,4] Thus a thorough search for objective confirmation of reported symptoms is essential. Also, a constellation of bleeding symptoms, rather than any single symptom, is most helpful in suggesting the presence and etiology of an underlying bleeding disorder.

Coagulation Testing

The need for routine coagulation testing before surgical or invasive procedures remains controversial. Those in favor of testing point to the asymptomatic nature of some hemostatic abnormalities that may cause surgical bleeding and the occasional failure to obtain a detailed history.[5-7] A prospective study of preoperative screening in children before tonsillectomy found history and laboratory screening to have high specificity but a low positive-predictive value for perioperative

bleeding.[6] Another study found that perioperative blood loss in adult cardiothoracic surgery patients could be predicted with a model, which included the bleeding time, prothrombin time (PT), and platelet count.[8] Given the variety of potential hemostatic defects however, no simple screening system will identify all patients at increased risk for bleeding. Those against routine laboratory testing[9] point to retrospective studies indicating that they rarely detect unexpected bleeding disorders[10,11] and emphasize the problems associated with evaluation of false-positive results. A literature review found insufficient evidence to conclude that an abnormal PT/international normalized ratio (INR) predicts bleeding during invasive procedures.[12] A retrospective review of the value of preoperative determination of the platelet count, PT, and activated partial thromboplastin time (aPTT) in 828 patients undergoing major noncardiac surgery found that only 2% had abnormal results, and most were expected on the basis of history and physical examination.[13] Furthermore, abnormal laboratory test results and intraoperative blood loss or postoperative bleeding complications were not related. This is not surprising given the lack of studies using an evidence-based approach to determine the degree of abnormality in the PT/INR or aPTT at which invasive procedures may be unsafe.[14] A number of prospective studies have also concluded that routine laboratory screening tests in asymptomatic patients are not predictive of perioperative or postoperative bleeding.[15-19] Thus in the absence of historical risk factors or physical examination findings suggestive of an underlying bleeding tendency, the likelihood of an unsuspected, clinically significant congenital acquired coagulopathy is low enough that routine laboratory screening is not warranted, particularly for those undergoing low-risk procedures.[20] The British Committee for Standards in Haematology recently issued guidelines reiterating this position: indiscriminate coagulation testing before surgical or invasive procedures is a poor predictor of bleeding risk and is not recommended in the absence of a positive personal or family bleeding history.[21]

There are a variety of reasons why routine coagulation tests such as the PT/INR and aPTT may be poorly predictive of underlying coagulopathy and bleeding risk.[21] First, these tests were designed to measure time to clot formation in artificial in vitro assays and do not reliably depict the global hemostatic situation in vivo (see Liver Disease section). More importantly, the PT/INR and aPTT may be insensitive to mild but clinically relevant bleeding disorders such as von Willebrand disease or mild hemophilia. Conversely, they may detect conditions such as factor XII deficiency or a lupus anticoagulant that do not increase the risk for bleeding.

The platelet function analyzer (PFA-100) has been developed for rapid, quantitative in vitro global testing of platelet function.[22,23] The clinical sensitivity (94%–95%) and specificity (88%–89%) of this instrument are virtually identical to platelet aggregometry.[24] Although some have suggested that the PFA-100 could be used for screening for primary hemostatic defects, such testing has limitations.[25] The PFA-100 has high sensitivity for detection of moderate-to-severe von Willebrand disease and severe platelet defects, such as Glanzmann thrombasthenia and Bernard-Soulier syndrome, but it has poor sensitivity for detection of milder platelet disorders such as storage pool disease, Hermansky-Pudlak syndrome, and primary secretion defects.[26] Although the PFA-100 is most useful when a hemostatic defect is clinically likely, in such cases additional testing

TABLE 159.1	Risk for Bleeding With Surgical or Invasive Procedures	
Risk	Type of Procedure	Examples
Low	Nonvital organs involved, exposed surgical site, limited dissection, percutaneous access	Lymph node biopsy, dental extraction, cataract extraction, most cutaneous surgery, laparoscopic procedures, coronary angiography
Moderate	Vital organs involved, deep or extensive dissection	Laparotomy, thoracotomy, mastectomy, major orthopedic surgery, pacemaker insertion
High	Bleeding likely to compromise surgical result, bleeding complications frequent	Neurosurgery, ophthalmic surgery, cardiopulmonary bypass, prostatectomy or bladder surgery, major vascular surgery, renal biopsy, bowel polypectomy

TABLE 159.2	Preoperative Hemostatic Evaluation	
Routine Screening		
Surgical Risk	*Approach*	
Low	History only	
Moderate or high	History, PT/INR, aPTT, platelet count	
Consultation History		
Negative or minimal for bleeding	PT/INR, aPTT, platelet count, biochemical profile, complete blood count with differential, review of peripheral smear	
Suggestive of bleeding disorder	Add to above as indicated: platelet function tests, von Willebrand antigen, ristocetin cofactor, factor VIII, factor IX, factor XI, factor XIII assays	

aPTT, Activated partial thromboplastin time; INR, international normalized ratio; PT, prothrombin time.

is usually necessary to establish a specific diagnosis.[25-27] If clinical suspicion is high, further testing is indicated even with normal PFA-100 results.[26] Thus the PFA-100 should not be used for general unselected screening.[27]

Although some studies have demonstrated the ability of the PFA-100 to predict recurrent ischemic events following percutaneous coronary interventions[28] and coronary artery bypass graft surgery,[29] such testing does not predict bleeding in patients undergoing cardiac or hip fracture surgery.[30-32]

Notwithstanding the controversy about the value of preoperative laboratory screening, it is reasonable to personalize the approach to preoperative evaluation depending on the hemostatic risk of the proposed surgery or invasive procedure (Tables 159.1 and 159.2). A hemostatic history should always be obtained, and no laboratory testing is required in patients undergoing procedures at low risk for bleeding. For procedures associated with a high risk of bleeding, screening could include a PT/INR, aPTT, and determination of the platelet count.

In practice, hematologists are rarely consulted for routine screening because surgeons have adopted approaches based on their own training and local practice patterns. Instead, consultation is sought because of a history suggestive of a bleeding disorder or because an abnormal test result is found on screening. If a referral is requested because of an abnormal screening test, the abnormality needs to be identified. However, regardless of the reason for the referral, the history is of central importance and must include a thorough review

of any bleeding episodes, including results of prior hemostatic testing, as well as careful attention to the family history. The physical examination should focus on evidence of bleeding and on identifying systemic disorders such as hepatic or renal disease. If the history of bleeding is negative or minimal, appropriate laboratory testing would include a PT/INR, aPTT, and a biochemical profile to evaluate hepatic and renal function. A complete blood count and examination of the peripheral blood smear are useful to identify myeloproliferative disorders, gray platelet syndrome, or thrombocytopenia. If the history is suggestive of a hemostatic abnormality, a full evaluation is indicated and additional specific testing is usually required because von Willebrand disease; mild deficiencies of factors VIII, IX, and XI; severe factor XIII deficiency; platelet function defects; and fibrinolytic abnormalities may not be identified by global screening tests (see Table 159.2).

HEMOSTATIC AGENTS

A variety of hemostatic agents are available and may be useful for the prevention or treatment of bleeding in the surgical patient. These agents work through a variety of mechanisms to facilitate hemostasis, including enhancement of primary hemostasis, enhancement of thrombin generation and fibrin formation, and inhibition of fibrinolysis.[33] However, it is important to note that there is a paucity of safety data involving hemostatic agents because most trials have been designed to assess therapeutic efficacy rather than potential complications, including thrombosis.[33,34] The use of desmopressin, topical hemostatic agents, antifibrinolytic agents, and recombinant factor VIIa (rFVIIa) will be discussed here. Blood products (platelets, fresh-frozen plasma, and cryoprecipitate) and factor VIII and IX concentrates are discussed elsewhere (Chapters 112 and 115–117).

Desmopressin

Desmopressin (1-deamino-8-D-arginine vasopressin, or DDAVP) is a synthetic analogue of the antidiuretic hormone arginine vasopressin. Intravenous, subcutaneous, or intranasal administration of DDAVP results in transient increases in plasma concentrations of factor VIII and von Willebrand factor as a result of their release from vascular endothelium.[35] Peak levels (typically two to four times baseline) are achieved 30–60 min after intravenous and 60–90 min after subcutaneous or intranasal administration.[36] Doses may be repeated at intervals of 12–24 hours, but tachyphylaxis may occur after three or four doses,[37] limiting further usefulness of DDAVP. Expression of glycoprotein Ib (GPIb) and GPIIb/IIIa on the platelet membrane is also enhanced after DDAVP administration.[38] DDAVP is the treatment of choice for patients with mild hemophilia A or type 1 von Willebrand disease who require low-risk surgical procedures. Moderate- or high-risk procedures usually require administration of clotting factor concentrates.[37] DDAVP may also be useful for patients with congenital or acquired platelet function disorders.[36,38,39]

DDAVP does not reduce blood loss or transfusion requirement after cardiopulmonary bypass surgery.[40,41] Worrisome also is the fact that a metaanalysis shows a 2.4-fold increase in perioperative myocardial infarction in cardiac surgery patients treated with DDAVP.[41] Thus the routine use of DDAVP in cardiac, orthopedic, or other elective surgical procedures is not recommended.[34,42] A more recent metaanalysis of 38 randomized placebo-controlled trials that included nearly 2500 surgical patients found that DDAVP slightly reduced blood loss (by approximately 80 mL) and transfusion requirements (by approximately 0.3 units) but did not reduce the proportion of patients receiving transfusions.[43] Although the authors acknowledged that the clinical impact of the reduced transfusion requirement is questionable, they felt this could not be ignored because of the low cost of DDAVP. The incidence of thromboembolic events in the DDAVP and placebo groups was similar (5.4% and 4.6%, respectively), but they pointed out that identification of harm from DDAVP is limited by study design and that the safety concerns remain unresolved.[43] Nonetheless, certain subgroups of patients, such as those with platelet dysfunction, may derive benefit.[38,42-44] Because of the small but important risk for myocardial infarction,[45] DDAVP should be used with caution in any surgical patient with a history of or risk factors for coronary artery disease.

Topical Hemostatic Agents

Topical hemostatic agents can be grouped into several categories: physical agents (bone wax, Ostene), absorbable agents (gelatin foams, oxidized cellulose, microfibrillar collagen), biologic agents (thrombin, fibrin sealants, platelet gel), synthetic agents (polyethylene glycol hydrogels, cyanoacrylates, glutaraldehyde cross-linked albumin), and hemostatic dressings.[46] A thorough discussion of the currently available products, including mechanisms of action, specific advantages and disadvantages, and recommendations for their use is provided in a recent comprehensive review.[46] A brief overview of the different types of topical hemostatic agents follows.

Physical Agents

Bone wax and alkylene oxide copolymers (Ostene) control hemorrhage by occluding bleeding channels on cut bone surfaces, and are often used in cardiac and orthopedic surgery. Ostene is preferred because it does not impede bone growth and is eventually absorbed. Both can increase the risk for local infection.[46]

Absorbable Agents

Gelatin foams are derived from animal products and provide a physical matrix upon which clotting occurs. These products expand to double their volume, an attractive feature for use in penetrating wounds, but potentially problematic if used near nerves or in confined spaces.[46]

Oxidized cellulose is derived from wood pulp. It provides a physical matrix for initiation of clotting and has excellent handling characteristics. By lowering surrounding pH, oxidized cellulose exerts an antimicrobial effect, but this property not only limits its use with biologic agents such as thrombin that are pH sensitive, but also can contribute to local inflammation.[46]

Microfibrillar collagen is derived from bovine components. It contributes to hemostasis by promoting platelet adherence and activation and is effective in controlling wide-spread parenchymal bleeding. Consequently, it can be useful even in the face of heparin therapy, although it is less effective in the setting of thrombocytopenia.[46]

Biologic Agents

Thrombin derived from bovine plasma was used for more than 40 years as a topical hemostatic agent in surgical patients. However, bovine thrombin can trigger the formation of antibodies that cross-react with human thrombin, leading to hemorrhagic complications.[47-49] Because of these issues, plasma-derived and recombinant forms of human thrombin were developed. A phase III randomized, double-blind trial found that the efficacy and safety of recombinant human thrombin and bovine thrombin were comparable, but there were fewer immunologic complications with recombinant human thrombin.[50]

Fibrin sealants are topical hemostatic agents composed of purified virally inactivated human fibrinogen and human thrombin. Some products also add human factor XIII to induce fibrin crosslinking and antifibrinolytic agents to prevent clot breakdown.[51] The components of fibrin sealants are supplied in separate chambers of a dual-syringe delivery device that combines them at the time of administration. The final steps of the coagulation cascade are reproduced, resulting in formation of a stable fibrin clot. These products are particularly effective for controlling oozing from raw surfaces.[46]

Platelet gel combines microfibrillar collagen and thrombin with patient-derived plasma that contains fibrinogen and platelets. Like fibrin sealants, the product is applied using a dual-chamber syringe device. The presence of platelets improves clot strength and provides growth factors, but the need for centrifugation of patient blood and processing before use is a disadvantage.[46]

Synthetic Agents

Cyanoacrylates are liquid monomers that rapidly polymerize in the presence of water and bind adjacent surfaces together. Octyl-2-cyanoacrylate is useful for closing small wounds or incisions and provides good cosmetic results.[46]

Polyethylene glycol hydrogel can be sprayed onto tissues, where it rapidly forms a cross-linked polymer matrix and serves as a sealant that inhibits cell ingrowth and adhesion formation. It is useful for preventing pericardial adhesions and as a mechanical sealant for vascular reconstructions in situations where swelling and expansion are not a concern.[46]

Glutaraldehyde cross-linked bovine albumin is primarily used to seal sutures or staple lines in complex cardiovascular procedures. However, because it can restrict tissue growth, it should not be used circumferentially around developing structures, particularly in children.[46]

Hemostatic Dressings

Progress in the field of topical hemostatic agents over the last decade has expanded into the development of hemostatic dressings. Several products containing combinations of gauze and lyophilized fibrinogen and thrombin, chitin, and chitosan (polysaccharides found in arthropod skeletons and produced by fermenting algae), and mineral zeolite are available. In general, the use of hemostatic dressings is still under investigation, primarily by the military and emergency first responders.[46]

Antifibrinolytics

Antifibrinolytic agents include the synthetic lysine analogues 6-aminohexanoic acid (aminocaproic acid) and 4-(aminomethyl) cyclohexanecarboxylic acid (tranexamic acid), and the serine protease inhibitor, aprotinin. Although both types of antifibrinolytic agents have been used in managing surgical bleeding, the lysine analogues are available in oral forms that facilitate their use in other clinical situations as well.

Aminocaproic Acid and Tranexamic Acid

Both aminocaproic acid and tranexamic acid bind reversibly to the lysine binding sites on plasminogen, thereby attenuating its capacity to bind to fibrin, which is essential for its activation by plasminogen activators.[36] Although tranexamic acid is approximately 10 times more potent than aminocaproic acid and has a longer half-life, both drugs have similar hemostatic effects.[52]

Because the oral form of tranexamic acid was not commercially available in the United States for a number of years, aminocaproic acid became the lysine derivative of choice for oral delivery. Aminocaproic acid is commonly used to treat mucosal hemorrhage (menorrhagia, epistaxis, dental bleeding) in patients with congenital coagulopathies and is also effective for prevention of oral bleeding in those who require dental work while receiving long-term oral anticoagulant therapy.

Although aminocaproic acid is sometimes used to treat bleeding in patients with thrombocytopenia, randomized controlled trials are lacking. The use of antifibrinolytic drugs in patients with gastrointestinal bleeding is reasonable given the high concentration of fibrinolytic enzymes in the digestive tract, and a metaanalysis found reductions in recurrent bleeding, need for surgery, and mortality.[53] However, improvements in the efficacy of other medical and endoscopic treatments have limited the use of these drugs in this setting, although they are still useful for some patients with underlying bleeding disorders.[36] The urinary tract is also rich in plasminogen activators, and some clinical trials comparing tranexamic acid or aminocaproic acid with placebo in patients undergoing prostatectomy have shown reduced blood loss, but not a reduced need for transfusion or decreased mortality.[36]

The largest experience with aminocaproic acid in surgical patients is in those undergoing cardiac and orthopedic surgery. Older metaanalyses have consistently shown that prophylactic treatment of cardiac surgery patients with aminocaproic acid results in a 30%–40% reduction in postoperative bleeding, without an increase in thromboembolic complications.[41,54-56] Similar results have been shown with tranexamic acid.[38] Other metaanalyses have shown that aminocaproic acid and tranexamic acid are effective in reducing surgical blood loss but have yielded inconsistent results in their capacity to reduce transfusion requirements.[42,57] A wide variety of dosing schedules may partly explain these heterogeneous results.[42] A recent meta-analysis showed that both agents were effective in reducing blood loss and transfusion requirements in those undergoing cardiac surgery.[58]

A number of studies have demonstrated that antifibrinolytic agents reduce blood loss in orthopedic surgery. A meta-analysis of 43 randomized controlled trials in total hip and knee arthroplasty, spine fusion, musculoskeletal infection, or tumor surgery found that aprotinin and tranexamic acid significantly reduced the number of patients requiring transfusion, with a dose-effect relationship suggested for tranexamic acid.[59] A meta-analysis of 11 clinical trials involving total hip replacement found that the use of tranexamic acid significantly reduced intraoperative blood loss and transfusion requirements, without any increase in VTE or other complications.[60] A recent double-blind, randomized, placebo-controlled trial demonstrated that intraoperative treatment with tranexamic acid was also effective for reducing the need for transfusion in patients undergoing retropubic prostatectomy.[61] Therefore many centers routinely administer tranexamic acid to patients undergoing elective joint arthroplasty to reduce blood loss and decrease the need for transfusion, and some centers also use it in patients undergoing urologic procedures.

Antifibrinolytics, particularly tranexamic acid, have also been studied in the treatment of trauma patients, in whom 30% of deaths are attributed to hemorrhage.[62] A landmark trial, Clinical Randomisation of an Antifibrinolytic in Significant Haemorrhage 2 (CRASH-2), evaluated the safety and efficacy of tranexamic acid in the setting of trauma.[63] This randomized, placebo-controlled, multinational trial that included more than 20,000 trauma patients demonstrated a significant reduction in all-cause mortality and death because of bleeding in the treatment group. More severely injured patients and those treated within 3 hours of injury derived the greatest benefit, and there was no difference in the rate of vascular occlusive events between the two groups.[63] Tranexamic acid is now incorporated into trauma clinical practice guidelines and treatment protocols.[64]

Two randomized controlled trials have shown that high-dose tranexamic acid significantly reduces surgical blood loss and transfusion requirements in liver transplant recipients.[65,66] A metaanalysis identified 23 studies with a total of 1407 liver transplant patients who received aminocaproic acid, tranexamic acid, or aprotinin compared with each other or with controls/placebo. This review found that tranexamic acid and aprotinin reduced transfusion requirements without any increased risk for hepatic artery thrombosis, VTE, or perioperative mortality.[67]

Aminocaproic acid and tranexamic acid are not without risks. There are case reports of thrombosis associated with both aminocaproic acid and tranexamic acid. However, no significant increase in thrombotic complications has been observed when the drugs have been used in patients undergoing cardiac, liver transplantation, or orthopedic surgery.[37,39,59,61,68] Furthermore, when used in doses exceeding 80 mg/kg, tranexamic acid has been associated with convulsive seizures in patients undergoing cardiac surgery.[66,69]

Aprotinin

Aprotinin is a polypeptide extracted from bovine lung that inhibits the action of serine proteases, including plasmin and kallikrein.[37] In addition to its antifibrinolytic activity, aprotinin is also thought to preserve platelet function and have antiinflammatory effects, both of which may be mediated by inhibition of protease-activated receptors expressed on platelets, vascular endothelium, and neutrophils.[68]

The bulk of clinical experience with aprotinin was in cardiac surgery. In a large number of trials prophylactic administration of aprotinin improved hemostasis and reduced requirements for transfusion of red blood cells, platelets, and fresh-frozen plasma in patients undergoing cardiopulmonary bypass.[35,39,43] A large metaanalysis of such trials demonstrated decreased mortality with aprotinin and a reduced incidence of repeat thoracotomy, without any increased risk for perioperative myocardial infarction.[42] Furthermore, another metaanalysis showed a lower incidence of stroke in cardiac surgery patients treated with high-dose aprotinin.[70]

Although there is abundant evidence that aprotinin reduces blood loss and transfusion requirements in cardiac surgery patients, an observational study in patients undergoing elective coronary revascularization surgery revealed that aprotinin increased the risk of renal failure, myocardial infarction, heart failure, stroke, or encephalopathy. In that study, aminocaproic acid and tranexamic acid reduced blood loss to a similar extent as aprotinin without an increase in adverse events. The same investigators subsequently reported that aprotinin use was associated with increased long-term mortality after coronary artery bypass graft surgery.[71] A second observational study confirmed the increased risk of postoperative renal dysfunction, without the associated elevated risk of myocardial or cerebrovascular events however.[72]

A database analysis of over 30,000 children undergoing congenital heart operations found no difference in postoperative mortality, need for dialysis, or length of stay in patients who received aprotinin versus those who did not.[73] The Blood Conservation Using Antifibrinolytics in a Randomized Trial (BART) randomly assigned 2331 cardiac surgery patients to aprotinin, tranexamic acid, or aminocaproic acid. The study was terminated early because of an excess of deaths in the aprotinin group, and the drug was subsequently withdrawn from the market in both Europe and the United States. Although the European Medicines Agency subsequently lifted this ban in 2012, the use of aprotinin is limited, and tranexamic acid is preferred.

Recombinant Factor VIIa

rFVIIa is licensed in the United States only for the prevention and treatment of bleeding in hemophilia patients with factor VIII or factor IX inhibitors, patients with acquired hemophilia, and in those with congenital factor VII deficiency. This drug is believed to induce hemostasis at local sites of tissue injury through enhancement of thrombin generation on the surface of thrombin-activated platelets.[74] rFVIIa also activates thrombin activatable fibrinolysis inhibitor, which in turn stabilizes the clot by inhibiting fibrinolysis.[75] The use of rFVIIa in the management of hemophilia and factor VII deficiency is reviewed in Chapters 135–137.

rFVIIa is often used for a variety of off-label indications, such as to control refractory bleeding after surgery or major trauma and to prevent bleeding in surgeries where blood loss is expected to be excessive (see box on Off-Label Use of rFVIIa). A prospective, multicenter, randomized, controlled trial that included 143 patients with blunt trauma and 134 patients with penetrating trauma found that in the group with blunt trauma, three successive doses of rFVIIa significantly decreased red blood cell transfusion (mean reduction of 2.6 units) and decreased by approximately half the number of patients requiring massive transfusion (more than 20 units of red blood cells).[76] Although similar trends were observed in the patients with penetrating trauma, the differences were not statistically significant. In spite of the reduction in the need for blood products, there was no survival benefit. After these initial encouraging reports of the use

A 56-year-old man has undergone aortic arch replacement for an aortic dissection. During the procedure he underwent circulatory arrest for 35 min, with a lowest recorded temperature of 18°C. His total bypass time was 225 min. After rewarming, there was considerable bleeding and he received 10 units of packed red blood cells, 8 units of fresh frozen plasma, 4 pooled units of platelets, and 20 units of cryoprecipitate. He was transferred from the operating room to the intensive care unit in stable condition.

A consultation is made to the hematologist 1 hour later because of excessive drainage (>500 mL) from his chest tubes.

Important information to consider:
- likelihood of surgical bleeding versus coagulopathy
- current temperature
- evidence of clotting within the chest tubes
- current coagulation studies (if available)
- hemodynamic status

Upon discussion with the surgeon and intensive care unit team, it is noted that the temperature is 35.5°C, there is little clot in the chest tubes, and he requires hemodynamic support with epinephrine and norepinephrine. His recent coagulation studies reveal an INR of 1.8, an aPTT of 48 s, a thrombin time of 59 s, and a fibrinogen level of 2.5 g/L.

Possible treatments:
1. warming blanket
2. protamine sulfate 50 mg by slow intravenous infusion: for heparin rebound
3. calcium gluconate 1–2 g intravenous bolus: for excessive citrate (from blood products)
4. blood products (using a warming line)
5. consider rFVIIa: 40–80 mcg/kg

Interpretation: The likelihood is that despite the extensive transfusion, the combination of a prolonged time on bypass and cooling to 18°C has resulted in a coagulopathy. This is further evidenced by the prolongation of the coagulation tests and the lack of visible clots within the chest tubes. Although items 1–3 are important as adjunctive therapies, they are unlikely to be sufficient on their own. The utility of further blood products in this situation cannot be understated, because in order for rFVIIa to work effectively, it relies on the presence of underlying substrate, which is effected by judicious use of blood products. Although the use of rFVIIa in this scenario is off-label, its use is justified when the surgeon feels that the likelihood that bleeding is too diffuse to be stopped by surgical intervention and is likely caused by coagulopathy.

of rFVIIa in trauma patients, questions regarding optimal dosing and timing of administration remained. In an attempt to address these issues, the Western Trauma Association Multi-Center Trials Group conducted a case registry of 380 adult trauma patients who received adjunctive rFVIIa for hemorrhage control.[77] This registry was unable to define a precise role for rFVIIa in traumatic bleeding. However, a pH of less than 7.2, platelet count of less than 100,000/μL, and blood pressure less than or equal to 90 mmHg were each found to be predictors of poor response to rFVIIa, suggesting that correction of shock, acidosis, and thrombocytopenia should precede the use of rFVIIa in bleeding trauma patients.[77] The CONTROL trial, which randomized 560 actively bleeding trauma patients to rFVIIa or placebo, found no differences in overall mortality, organ system failure, or adverse events in either group.[78] Thus although initial reports were encouraging, there is currently insufficient evidence to support a role for the routine use of rFVIIa in the setting of trauma.

The use of rFVIIa in cardiac surgery is controversial. Because perioperative bleeding is a major cause of morbidity and mortality, there is off-label use of rFVIIa in this patient population.[79] A number of case reports and uncontrolled case series in both adult and pediatric populations have suggested that rFVIIa is effective in decreasing blood loss and transfusion requirements in patients with intractable bleeding after cardiopulmonary bypass. However, in the absence of data from well-designed clinical trials demonstrating efficacy and with the current widespread use of tranexamic acid in such patients, rFVIIa is rarely used in this setting.

rFVIIa has been used in a variety of other surgical settings with divergent results. Although a trial in patients undergoing retropubic prostatectomy demonstrated a greater than 50% reduction in surgical

blood loss with a single intraoperative dose of rFVIIa,[80] rFVIIa resulted in little or no reduction in blood loss in a patients without cirrhosis undergoing partial hepatectomy.[81,82] Overall therefore, the published experience of rFVIIa in noncardiac surgery is still too limited and subject to bias to draw meaningful conclusions.[83]

Neurosurgical patients are distinct from other groups in that rather than treating massive hemorrhage, the goal is to treat relatively small bleeds within a closed space where even mild or modest benefit may result in significantly better outcomes.[83] A randomized, placebo-controlled study of 399 patients with intracerebral hemorrhage suggested that treatment with rFVIIa within 4 hours after the onset of symptoms limited growth of the hematoma, reduced mortality, and improved functional outcomes at 90 days, albeit with a small increase in the frequency of thromboembolic events.[84] In a subsequent larger trial in patients with intracerebral hemorrhage, rFVIIa failed to improve mortality and disability at 90 days.[85] Therefore rFVIIa should not be used for this indication.

The primary safety concern with the off-label use of rFVIIa is thrombosis. In hemophilia, the risk for thrombosis is estimated to be less than 1%.[86,87] In contrast, the risk is much higher with off-label use. Both arterial and venous thromboembolic events have been reported, and thromboembolic events were the probable cause of death in the majority of the reported fatalities. Half of the thromboembolic events occurred within 24 hours of the last dose of rFVIIa, and many occurred within 2 hours.[88] Therefore off-label use of rFVIIa should be restricted to cases where there are no alternatives.

MANAGEMENT OF PATIENTS WITH HEMOSTATIC ABNORMALITIES

Patients with known hemostatic abnormalities are often referred before surgery for assessment of bleeding risk and recommendations regarding perioperative management. The approach to these patients should be according to the following considerations: (1) evaluation of the risk for bleeding associated with the specific surgery or procedure (see Table 159.1); (2) careful consideration of the need for surgery and its urgency; greater risks are warranted for correction of life-threatening conditions than for elective procedures; (3) recognition of the nature and severity of the patient's hemostatic abnormality and the ability to correct it; and (4) consideration of the duration of replacement that will be required, with appreciation of potential bleeding that may be associated with events in the postoperative period such as removal of sutures and deep drains, and the need for postoperative rehabilitation. The following sections discuss perioperative management of some common coagulation abnormalities; the management of congenital factor deficiencies and von Willebrand disease are discussed elsewhere in this text (see Chapters 135, 137, and 138).

Thrombocytopenia

Thrombocytopenia is one of the most common acquired hemostatic abnormalities, and the availability of platelet transfusion makes consideration of both emergency and elective surgery reasonable even in severely thrombocytopenic patients. The best index of bleeding risk in thrombocytopenic patients is the platelet count. In nonsurgical patients a threshold platelet count of 10,000/μL is widely used for prophylactic transfusions, yet there is inadequate scientific evidence to determine the platelet count below which the risk for surgical bleeding is increased.[89,90] The American Society of Anesthesiologists Task Force on Blood Component Therapy concluded that prophylactic platelet transfusion in surgical patients is usually indicated when the count is below 50,000/μL and is rarely indicated when the count is above 100,000/μL.[89] Clinical trials addressing this issue are still lacking.[91] For low-risk surgery, a single transfusion to increase the platelet count to more than 50,000/μL followed by close observation may suffice, whereas transfusion to maintain the platelet count at greater than 50,000/μL for moderate-risk surgery and greater than

100,000/μL for high-risk surgery is usually appropriate. The optimal duration of postoperative platelet support has not been carefully studied, but even for moderate- or high-risk surgery, platelets may be needed for less than 1 week because they are principally required for primary hemostasis. The platelet count should be monitored closely during the postoperative period, with the expectation that platelet survival will be shortened by infection, fever, or bleeding. In addition, platelet transfusion may be indicated for surgical patients despite an apparently adequate count in the presence of known or suspected platelet dysfunction, antiplatelet therapy, and microvascular bleeding.

When thrombocytopenia is caused by increased platelet destruction (e.g., immune thrombocytopenic purpura), prophylactic platelet transfusion is largely ineffective and is indicated only for active, serious bleeding. In preparation for surgery, therapy with steroids and/or intravenous γ-globulin often will increase the platelet count to a satisfactory level so that transfusion is not needed. Rho(D) immunoglobulin (WinRho®) may also be useful in this setting.

Platelet Dysfunction

Patients with platelet dysfunction represent a large group for whom preoperative consultation is sought, typically because of an abnormal bleeding history or the discovery of a prolonged bleeding time or other laboratory assessment of platelet function with a normal platelet count. Drugs are the most common cause of acquired platelet dysfunction. Many commonly used types of medications, including aspirin and other nonsteroidal antiinflammatory drugs, antibiotics, antidepressants (selective serotonin reuptake inhibitors), cardiovascular drugs, and newer antiplatelet agents, including ADP receptor, GPIIb/IIIa or protease-activated receptor antagonists, can cause platelet dysfunction. Ethanol as well as certain foods and herbal supplements can also inhibit platelets; a careful history is therefore essential. Any drugs that interfere with platelet function should be reviewed before surgery and an assessment of their ongoing use be carefully considered.

A number of medical conditions can cause acquired platelet dysfunction. The etiology may be fairly obvious in cases of renal or liver disease, myeloproliferative disorders, leukemia, myelodysplastic syndromes, or dysproteinemia, but consideration of undiagnosed intrinsic platelet defects (storage pool disease or platelet release defects) or von Willebrand disease may be necessary. Treatment of the underlying disease is the most effective approach, if possible. If not, platelet transfusion may be indicated, but the dose required to achieve hemostasis is difficult to predict and depends in part on the severity of the underlying platelet abnormality. As discussed earlier, treatment with DDAVP may be appropriate in selected patients. The exact mechanism of action of DDAVP in acquired platelet dysfunction is not well understood, but one study suggests that DDAVP interacts directly with platelets and exerts a priming effect on platelet aggregation stimulated by ADP or collagen.[92] Expression of GPIb and GPIIb/IIIa on platelet membranes is also enhanced following administration of DDAVP.[39]

Renal Disease

Impaired hemostasis has long been recognized in patients with chronic renal failure and is discussed in greater detail in Chapter 154. The pathogenesis is multifactorial but is due in large part to alterations in platelet function.[93] Anemia also contributes to platelet dysfunction in chronic renal failure. Red blood cells release ADP, which in turn inactivates vascular prostacyclin, an inhibitor of platelet function.[94] Correction of anemia, now routinely accomplished through the use of recombinant erythropoietin, also improves the rheologic factors that facilitate platelet interaction with the vessel wall. An increase in hematocrit, whether by the use of erythropoietin or transfusion, is accompanied by significant shortening of the bleeding time and improvement of platelet adhesion.[95] In addition to platelet dysfunction and altered balance between mediators of normal

endothelial function, the pathophysiology of uremic bleeding is complicated by the comorbidities in this patient population, such as vascular disease and hypertension, and the medical treatment of those conditions.[96]

Liver Disease

Hemostatic alterations in patients with acute or chronic liver disease (see Chapter 153) are complex and involve both procoagulant and anticoagulant pathways.[97,98] Although patients with liver disease are typically felt to have deficient hemostasis, this concept has been challenged in the recent literature.[99] These patients are not "autoanticoagulated", as often assumed. In fact, they are not protected from and may even be at increased risk for thrombosis, particularly in the portal venous system.[100-102] The presence of genetic thrombophilic mutations may further increase this risk.[82] The procoagulant tendency associated with chronic liver disease[103,104] suggests that prophylaxis against VTE may be warranted in high-risk situations.[99] However, the perceived bleeding risk often limits the use of prophylaxis,[105] and appropriately designed pharmacologic clinical studies are clearly needed.[100]

Patients with severe decompensated liver disease and markedly abnormal coagulation test results are at increased risk for bleeding, and surgery should be avoided except as a lifesaving measure. In evaluating hemostasis in patients with less severe disease, the PT/INR and aPTT may be good indicators of decreased synthesis of clotting factors and vitamin K deficiency, but they are poor predictors of bleeding risk. Several studies have shown the failure of the PT/INR and aPTT to predict bleeding after liver biopsy.[106,107] Similarly, preoperative hemostatic testing has generally not been shown to be useful for predicting bleeding during liver transplantation.[108] A study in patients with liver disease found that INR values in the range of 1.3–2.0 generally correspond to levels of factors II, V, and VII that are adequate for hemostasis.[109] A preoperative platelet count is needed to identify thrombocytopenia, and some assessment of platelet function may be useful to determine whether platelet function is abnormal in the setting of a normal or near-normal platelet count. A thrombin time or fibrinogen level should also be performed to evaluate for dysfibrinogenemia. Tests for fibrinogen/fibrin degradation products, D-dimer, euglobulin clot lysis time or thromboelastography may be useful in evaluating for disseminated intravascular coagulation (DIC) or accelerated fibrinolysis.

In patients with mild liver disease and mild-moderate INR prolongation (<2.0), serious surgical bleeding is unlikely in the absence of other hemostatic abnormalities, and prophylactic intervention is rarely required for low- or moderate-risk surgery. For high-risk surgery or for patients with markedly abnormal coagulation tests, transfusion of fresh-frozen plasma is the most commonly used approach for correcting the coagulation abnormality, although prospective studies demonstrating the value of fresh-frozen plasma administration in this setting are lacking. There are, however, guidelines that caution against the indiscriminate use of plasma before invasive procedures.[110] It should be noted that the PT of fresh-frozen plasma is approximately 15 s, which corresponds to an INR of 1.5, so complete correction of the PT/INR is unlikely to be achieved.[111] Administration of platelets should be considered for more severe degrees of thrombocytopenia, although recovery will be decreased in the presence of splenomegaly. Administration of DDAVP may be useful for correcting abnormal platelet function in some cases.[112] Intravenous administration of 5–10 mg vitamin K will usually shorten the PT/INR if vitamin K deficiency is a contributory factor. Antifibrinolytic agents also may be useful for the reduction of perioperative hemorrhage in patients with liver disease.

INTRAOPERATIVE AND POSTOPERATIVE BLEEDING

Patients with excessive bleeding during or after surgery require rapid evaluation and treatment. The first step is to distinguish between "surgical" and "coagulopathic" causes of bleeding. Failure to surgically control bleeding vessels at the operative site is the most frequent cause of postoperative bleeding and is suggested by evidence of hemorrhage restricted to the operative site and manifesting as an expanding hematoma, excessive blood in surgical drains, or saturated wound dressings. Conversely, coagulopathic bleeding is suggested by slower "oozing" at the operative site in addition to evidence of bleeding outside the operative field that may be seen as petechiae, purpura, or bleeding at sites of venipuncture, urinary or vascular catheters, or nasogastric and endotracheal tubes.[113] In addition to careful physical examination, laboratory tests, including PT/INR, aPTT, and platelet count, are an essential part of the evaluation. Other useful tests may include a fibrinogen level, and a test for fibrin degradation products or D-dimer and thromboelastography to search for evidence of DIC or increased fibrinolysis. The peripheral blood smear should also be reviewed to examine platelet morphology and number, and to identify possible red blood cell fragmentation that may occur in DIC. The possibility of a preexisting hemostatic abnormality that may have been missed before surgery should also be considered.

When evaluating coagulation test results in surgical patients, changes that normally occur in response to surgery must be considered. These vary depending on the extent of tissue dissection and the duration of the procedure. Consumption and hemodilution from crystalloid and blood product infusion can lead to acute reductions of coagulation factors and platelets during surgery and in the initial postoperative period. This is typically followed by changes resulting from the acute-phase response, including increases in fibrinogen and factor VIII levels, and the platelet count during the first postoperative week.[114]

Alterations in coagulation factor levels that occur during surgery and in the initial postoperative period can limit the reliability of the PT/INR and aPTT in evaluating the bleeding surgical patient. Clinical practice guidelines have consistently recommended transfusion of fresh-frozen plasma if the PT/INR and aPTT results are prolonged more than 1.5-fold compared with the mean reference range.[115-117] However, there are differing opinions on the utility of coagulation studies to guide transfusion practices,[118,119] and prospective studies are needed.

Coagulopathy Associated With Massive Blood Loss/Transfusion

Massive bleeding (loss of one or more blood volumes in a 24-h period) may occur in the setting of severe trauma or major surgery and requires aggressive fluid resuscitation and transfusion of blood products. The mechanisms involved in the coagulopathy that accompanies massive transfusion have not yet been fully elucidated but are multifactorial in nature.[120] Similar to chronic liver disease, procoagulant, anticoagulant, profibrinolytic, and antifibrinolytic factors are all affected, resulting in a complex coagulopathy. Impaired thrombin generation is compensated in part by reduction in the activity of antithrombin and other protease inhibitors. Fibrinogen levels can fall rapidly and are proportional to the degree of hemodilution. Antifibrinolytic protein levels are decreased, rendering clots more susceptible to lysis.[121] In addition to a dilutional coagulopathy, other complications, including consumptive coagulopathy, hypothermia, electrolyte abnormalities (because of citrate intoxication), and acid-base disturbances, may also develop.[121]

In patients without a preexisting coagulopathy, replacement of approximately 1.5 blood volumes is the threshold for the development of dilutional coagulopathy.[122] At that point, PT/INR, aPTT, fibrinogen level, and platelet count should be determined. If the PT/INR or aPTT is prolonged greater than 1.5-times control, the fibrinogen level is below 100 mg/dL, or the platelet count is reduced to 50,000–70,000/μL, clinical coagulopathy is suspected and appropriate blood product administration is indicated, particularly if additional blood loss is expected. The same coagulation parameters should be measured again with the replacement of each additional half-blood volume (i.e., 5–6 units of red blood cells).[123]

Over the last several years, there has been an increased emphasis on more aggressive blood component therapy, driven by data from both military and civilian trauma populations.[124-127] These studies have demonstrated that higher ratios (approaching 1 : 1) of plasma and platelets to red blood cells are associated with improved outcomes in massively transfused patients. Patients receiving less than massive transfusion may also benefit from higher plasma-to-red blood cell ratios.[128] Furthermore, maintaining an adequate fibrinogen level is essential for successful management of dilutional coagulopathy.[121] Appropriate and timely management for these patients needs to be facilitated in order to avoid prolonged hypotension, acidosis, and tissue-level ischemia, all of which can predispose to the development of DIC (Chapter 139).

Cardiopulmonary Bypass

Cardiopulmonary bypass is associated with unique hemostatic changes. Perfusion through the extracorporeal membrane oxygenator has profound effects on platelets and clotting factors: platelet count, hematocrit, and levels of coagulation and fibrinolytic factors are reduced to approximately 50% of baseline after starting bypass and remain reduced throughout the procedure, with the exception of factor V, which may be further reduced to less than 20%.[129-131] These changes may be caused in part by exposure to artificial surfaces and also by a tissue factor–dependent pathway related to surgical trauma.[132] Cardiopulmonary bypass results in significant platelet dysfunction[133] reflected by release of α-granule contents, the generation of platelet microparticles, abnormal ex vivo platelet aggregation test results, and a transient prolongation of the bleeding time.[130,131,133,134] In addition to quantitative and qualitative platelet function defects, cardiopulmonary bypass also results in platelet activation, which may trigger thrombotic and inflammatory complications.[134] Patients with acute coronary syndrome (who may be candidates for urgent cardiac surgery) are sometimes given GPIIb/IIIa inhibitors, which may further impair platelet function. If surgery cannot be delayed, consideration of prophylactic platelet transfusions may be required.[135] Inadequate neutralization of heparin with protamine sulfate after cardiopulmonary bypass may result in a prolonged aPTT and thrombin time with a normal reptilase time, and is an indication for administration of additional protamine sulfate. The use of DDAVP, antifibrinolytic drugs, and rFVIIa to reduce the hemorrhagic complications of cardiac surgery was discussed earlier. Fibrinogen concentrate has also been shown to reduce blood loss and transfusion requirements during cardiac surgery.[136]

Orthotopic Liver Transplantation

In addition to the complex coagulopathy of end-stage liver disease, orthotopic liver transplantation is accompanied by major alterations in hemostasis. The surgical procedure itself can be divided into three stages, each with its own profile of coagulation abnormalities.[137] Bleeding during the preanhepatic stage, while the host liver is surgically isolated, is due primarily to the patient's preexisting coagulopathy and is determined by the severity of the underlying liver disease. Excessive fibrinolysis may be encountered during this stage in 10%–20% of those with cirrhosis. The anhepatic stage begins with surgical removal of the liver. Bleeding during this stage is primarily hemostatic because of DIC and excessive fibrinolysis.[138] As the donor liver is reperfused, the postanhepatic stage begins, and serious bleeding is often encountered as a result of a combination of hyperfibrinolysis, metabolic acidosis, hypothermia, electrolyte abnormalities, and sometimes impaired cardiac function.[138,139]

The multifactorial nature of the coagulopathy associated with orthotopic liver transplantation requires a combination of therapeutic interventions. In addition to transfusion of blood products, other hemostatic agents such as DDAVP and antifibrinolytics may be useful and were discussed earlier. There has also been much interest in the use of rFVIIa, and some randomized, placebo-controlled trials have been completed, but questions about optimal dosing, cost-effectiveness, and safety remain to be fully answered. Furthermore, it is still questionable whether rFVIIa should be used prophylactically in liver transplantation patients outside of a prospective clinical trial.[140]

PERIOPERATIVE ANTICOAGULATION MANAGEMENT

Hematologists are frequently consulted for advice on the perioperative management of patients who are taking oral anticoagulants. Important considerations to be taken into account include: (1) the bleeding risk associated with the surgery; (2) the underlying indication for anticoagulant therapy; (3) in the case of secondary antithrombotic prophylaxis, the remoteness of the most recent thrombotic event; (4) other comorbid conditions that may increase the risk for thrombosis and/or the potential consequences of thrombosis while oral anticoagulation is temporarily interrupted; and (5) the half-life of the anticoagulant agent. Regarding the first point, experience has accumulated in recent years suggesting that many relatively minor procedures can be carried out without any interruption of warfarin or direct oral anticoagulant (DOAC) therapy.[141] These include minor dental procedures (single or multiple extraction, endodontic procedure), cataract removal, minor dermatologic procedures, and low-risk endoscopy procedures. Audits have suggested that discontinuation of anticoagulation is excessively frequent in these situations and discordant with guidelines.[142] Apart from the risk for thromboembolism, the inappropriate use of bridging therapy also places patient at risk for bleeding complications. Suggested management strategies are summarized in Table 159.3.

Traditionally, patients on chronic oral anticoagulation with warfarin were admitted to hospital several days before surgery for "bridging" anticoagulation, at which time warfarin was discontinued and dose-adjusted unfractionated heparin (UFH) was administered by continuous infusion. The short half-life of UFH allows it to be safely discontinued approximately 4–6 hours ahead of the procedure. This was followed by the use of LMWH in place of UFH.[143-145] LMWH has the advantage that in most patients with normal renal function, no monitoring is required, so that therapy can be administered in the outpatient setting. In addition, the risk for heparin-induced thrombocytopenia is less with LMWHs.[146] However, the longer half-life (generally in the range of 4–6 hours) necessitates withdrawal of these agents at least 12 hours (for prophylactic doses) or 24 hours (for full therapeutic doses) preoperatively, although even then significant circulating anticoagulant activity may remain in the plasma.[147] A recent randomized trial suggests that bridging with LMWH does not reduce the risk of thromboembolic events and increases the risk of bleeding in patients with atrial fibrillation.[148] Although these results have changed practice, it is important to note that atrial fibrillation patients with prior stroke were underrepresented in the study.

Temporary interruption of warfarin is often required for more major surgery. Even with a normal diet, 4–5 days should be allowed for full or near-full reversal of warfarin when it is being targeted to an INR of 2.0–3.0. A more rapid reversal over 24–36 hours can be achieved if necessary by administration of a small oral dose of vitamin K1 (1.0–2.5 mg).[149,150] Large doses of vitamin K1 (>10 mg) are generally unnecessary for this purpose and will lead to prolonged refractoriness to warfarin after it is reinitiated. Although frequently used, subcutaneous administration of vitamin K1 is associated with highly variable absorption and should be avoided. Intravenous vitamin K1 has the advantage of more rapid INR reversal compared with the oral route,[151] but it should be administered slowly to avoid anaphylactoid reactions. Urgent reversal of oral anticoagulation before surgery may call for the administration of fresh-frozen plasma, although large volumes (15–20 mL/kg) are usually required to reverse the INR, and indeed complete normalization cannot usually be achieved. Furthermore, the effect is relatively short-lived because of the short half-life (approximately 6 hours) of transfused factor VII. Therefore concomitant vitamin K1 administration is required to ensure maintenance of adequate hemostasis. Prothrombin complex

TABLE 159.3	Perioperative Management Strategies for Patients on Chronic Oral Anticoagulant Therapy
Clinical Situation	**Suggested Anticoagulation Management**
Low bleeding-risk surgery (dental, cataract, skin)	• Consider reducing dose of warfarin to achieve INR ≤2.0 • Consider holding dose of DOAC until after the procedure
Low thrombotic risk Aortic valve prosthesis without other thrombotic risk factors[a] *or* AF with low stroke risk *or* VTE >3 months previously	• Stop warfarin 4–5 days prior to surgery, safe to operate when INR ≤1.5 • Hold DOACs for 5 half-lives – dabigatran for 3–4 days, rivaroxaban, apixaban, edoxaban for 2–3 days • Restart warfarin in evening of the day of surgery after hemostasis secured; restart DOACs on postoperative day 3 or 4 • Start prophylactic LMWH on the morning of the day after surgery and continue until INR >1.8 or full dose of DOACs resumed
Moderate thrombotic risk Mitral or multiple valve prostheses *or* Aortic prosthesis with risk factors for thrombosis *or* AF at high stroke risk *or* VTE within past 3 months	• Stop VKA 5 days before surgery • Begin twice-daily LMWH in therapeutic doses starting 3 days before surgery with last dose at least 12 h prior to surgery • Hold DOACs for 5 half-lives – dabigatran for 3–4 days, rivaroxaban, apixaban, edoxaban for 2–3 days; no bridging • Restart warfarin in evening of the day of surgery after hemostasis secured; restart DOACs on postoperative day 3 or 4 • Start prophylactic LMWH on the morning of the day after surgery and continue until INR >1.8 or full dose of DOACs resumed

[a]Risk factors include caged-ball or single tilting-disk valve, AF, history of stroke/transient ischemic attack/other embolic event, left ventricular failure, underlying hypercoagulable state, including cancer.
AF, Atrial fibrillation; DOAC, direct oral anticoagulant; INR, international normalized ratio; LMWH, low-molecular-weight heparin; VKA, vitamin K antagonist (i.e., warfarin); VTE, venous thromboembolism.

concentrate (PCC; 25–50 units/kg) is preferred over plasma to control hemorrhage in warfarin-treated patients with active bleeding.[150,152] These concentrates are manufactured by fractionation of pooled plasma and contain the vitamin K–dependent factors II, VII, IX, and X. However, it is important to be aware that there is significant heterogeneity among these agents, with some (three-factor PCC) having a low concentration of factor VII, which may leave the INR prolonged following administration.[153]

In recent years, DOACs, oral anticoagulants that directly inhibit thrombin or factor Xa, have been licensed for the prevention of stroke and systemic embolism in patients with atrial fibrillation and for prevention and treatment of VTE (see Chapter 149). A working knowledge of the respective elimination half-lives of these agents is important in deciding when and if to discontinue before elective procedures. In addition, an appreciation of the dominant mechanism(s) of clearance that may affect the elimination half-life is essential (Table 159.4). In general, when the procedure is considered to be more than minor, and the aim is to have negligible amounts of drug (<10%) in the circulation at the time of surgery, the drug should be discontinued at a time before surgery equivalent to four to five half-lives. This would imply 2–3 days (48–60 hours) for dabigatran and 1–2 days

TABLE 159.4	Comparison of the Features of the Direct Oral Anticoagulants			
	Dabigatran	Rivaroxaban	Apixaban	Edoxaban
Target	Thrombin (IIa)	Factor Xa	Factor Xa	Factor Xa
Active Drug	No	Yes	Yes	Yes
Onset Time (h)	0.5–2	2–4	3–4	1–3
Half Life (h)	12–17	5–13	~12	9–11
Renal Excretion (%)	80	33	27	50
Reversal Agent	Idarucizumab 5 g IV bolus	PCC	PCC	PCC

IV, Intravenous; PCC, prothrombin complex concentrate.

for rivaroxaban, apixaban, and edoxaban.[154-156] In the setting of urgent surgery, dabigatran can effectively be reversed with a 5 g bolus of idarucizumab.[157-159] Reversal agents for rivaroxaban, apixaban and edoxaban are not yet available. PCC can be considered in such patients.[160,161]

PERIOPERATIVE THROMBOPROPHYLAXIS

VTE is the most common cause of preventable death in hospitalized patients. Thromboprophylaxis in medical patients is discussed in Chapter 142. In surgical patients, the risk of postoperative VTE depends on the type of surgery and patient factors. Patients undergoing nonorthopedic surgery have a variable risk of postoperative VTE, whereas those undergoing major orthopedic procedures are at high risk. Therefore the two groups are discussed separately.

Nonorthopedic Surgery

In patients undergoing nonorthopedic surgery, the risks of VTE are grouped into four categories: very low (<0.5%), low (~1.5%), moderate (~3%), and high (~6%).[162] In both the very low– and low-risk groups, guidelines recommend that patients be managed with early ambulation and mechanical methods of prophylaxis using intermittent pneumatic compression devices. In the moderate- and high-risk groups, guidelines recommend pharmacologic thromboprophylaxis with LMWH.[162] LMWH is preferred over low-dose UFH because its use is associated with a reduced risk of heparin-induced thrombocytopenia.[163] Although LMWH is usually given only while the patient is hospitalized, extended prophylaxis for at least 4 weeks is recommended for patients undergoing abdominal or pelvic surgery for cancer. If the risk of bleeding is deemed to be too high to enable pharmacologic thromboprophylaxis, such as in patients undergoing neurosurgery or spinal surgery, intermittent pneumatic compression devices should be used until the bleeding risk subsides.[162]

Orthopedic Surgery

Patients undergoing orthopedic surgery are at high risk for postoperative VTE because they are relatively immobile after surgery and because manipulation of the lower limb vascular structures may disrupt the vascular endothelium.[164] Therefore patients undergoing hip or knee arthroplasty or surgery for hip fracture are all categorized as high risk. Accordingly, postoperative pharmacologic prophylaxis is recommended and the choices in patients undergoing hip or knee arthroplasty include the DOACs, LMWH, or dose-adjusted warfarin; aspirin is also included as an option in preference to no prophylaxis. The DOACs have not been extensively evaluated in patients undergoing surgery for hip fracture, and LMWH is more commonly used in these patients.[165] In patients undergoing knee arthroplasty,

guidelines recommend that prophylaxis be continued for at least 10–14 days after surgery and in those undergoing hip arthroplasty or surgery for hip fracture, prophylaxis should be continued for at least 35 days.[165] In general, patients undergoing arthroscopic surgery with no prior history of VTE do not require pharmacologic prophylaxis.[165]

SUMMARY

The management of surgical or trauma patients in the perioperative period can be challenging because of the variability of procedures, risks inherent within the patient and/or procedure, and the limitations of time and acuity of the situation. A thorough history of bleeding or thrombosis events and a comprehensive medication record, coupled with appropriate use of coagulation studies, hemostatic agents and/or blood products, and collaboration with surgical or trauma teams can lead to improved outcomes for patients. Ongoing research into the management of these patients will likely aid clinical decision-making into the future.

SUGGESTED READINGS

Achneck HE, Sileshi B, Jamiolkowski RM, et al: A comprehensive review of topical hemostatic agents: efficacy and recommendations for use. *Ann Surg* 251:217, 2010.

Chee YL, Crawford JC, Watson HG, et al: Guidelines on the assessment of bleeding risk prior to surgery or invasive procedures. British Committee for Standards in Haematology. *Br J Haematol* 140:496, 2008.

Crescenzi G, Landoni G, Biondi-Zoccai G, et al: Desmopressin reduces transfusion needs after surgery: a meta-analysis of randomized clinical trials. *Anesthesiology* 109:1063, 2008.

Douketis JD: Pharmacologic properties of the new oral anticoagulants: a clinician-oriented review with a focus on perioperative management. *Curr Pharm Des* 16:3436, 2010.

Douketis JD, Spyropoulos AC, Spencer FA, et al: Perioperative management of antithrombotic therapy: Antithrombotic Therapy and Prevention of Thrombosis, 9th ed: American College of Chest Physicians Evidence-Based Clinical Practice Guidelines. *Chest* 141:e326S, 2012.

Guyatt GH, Eikelboom JW, Gould MK, et al: Approach to outcome measurement in the prevention of thrombosis in surgical and medical patients: Antithrombotic Therapy and Prevention of Thrombosis, 9th ed: American College of Chest Physicians Evidence-Based Clinical Practice Guidelines. *Chest* 141:e185S, 2012.

Horlocker TT, Wedel DJ, Rowlingson JC, et al: Regional anesthesia in the patient receiving antithrombotic or thrombolytic therapy: American Society of Regional Anesthesia and Pain Medicine Evidence-Based Guidelines (Third Edition). *Reg Anesth Pain Med* 35:64, 2010.

Kearon C, Hirsh J: Management of anticoagulation before and after elective surgery. *N Engl J Med* 336:1506, 1997.

Kwok A, Faigel DO: Management of anticoagulation before and after gastrointestinal endoscopy. *Am J Gastroenterol* 104:3085, quiz 3098, 2009.

Leissinger CA, Blatt PM, Hoots WK, et al: Role of prothrombin complex concentrates in reversing warfarin anticoagulation: a review of the literature. *Am J Hematol* 83:137, 2008.

Logan AC, Yank V, Stafford RS: Off-label use of recombinant factor VIIa in U.S. hospitals: analysis of hospital records. *Ann Intern Med* 154:516, 2011.

Paikin JS, Eikelboom JW, Cairns JA, et al: New antithrombotic agents–insights from clinical trials. *Nature reviews. Cardiology* 7:498, 2010.

Schulman S, Crowther MA: How I treat with anticoagulants in 2012: new and old anticoagulants, and when and how to switch. *Blood* 119:3016, 2012.

REFERENCES

For the complete list of references, log on to www.expertconsult.com.

CHAPTER 160

THE SPLEEN AND ITS DISORDERS

Nathan T. Connell, Susan B. Shurin, and Fred Schiffman

Galen described the spleen as the "organ of mystery," with functions related to mood and good or ill humors. It was not until the 18th century that the spleen's relationship to the immune and hematologic systems was appreciated. The complexities of splenic function continue to be the focus of research and observation. Although many of its functions overlap with or can be assumed by other organs, it is an important regulator of immune function and hematologic homeostasis. The spleen efficiently phagocytoses erythrocytes, recycles iron, recognizes and destroys pathogens, and induces adaptive immune responses. An appreciation for the subtleties of its anatomy and function is important for the physician evaluating patients with many hematologic, immunologic, hepatic, and infectious diseases.

NORMAL SPLENIC ANATOMY AND FUNCTION

Embryology

The spleen arises from the mesoderm and, by the ninth week of gestation, layers of the left dorsal mesogastrium condense with the appearance of blood vessels. Sheaths are formed around arterioles by reticular cells and fibers.[1] Macrophages are present and develop phagocytic function by the end of the first trimester. Lymphocytes appear during the fourth month, and a formal delineation between red and white pulp can be identified by the sixth month. Germinal centers do not develop during fetal development, but primitive inactive follicles are evident at birth. In mice, the homeobox gene *Tlx1* (formerly known as *Hox11*), which controls the genesis of the splanchnic mesodermal plate, is essential for development of the spleen.[2] Both the basic helix-loop-helix transcription factor capsulin and the Wilms tumor suppressor 1 (*WT1*) gene are necessary for formation of the spleen. The genetic basis for development of the human spleen is less well understood. The spleen is capable of supporting hematopoiesis during fetal life and, in a variety of pathologic states, postnatally. The circulation of primitive hematopoietic stem cells in peripheral blood during prenatal life through birth makes it difficult to distinguish hematopoiesis arising from stem cells in the spleen as opposed to the incidental presence of hematopoietic cells within the circulation.

Anatomy

The spleen is the body's largest filter of the blood.[3,4] Located directly below the diaphragm and adjacent to the stomach, it is covered by a fibrous capsule with blood vessels, lymphatics, and nerves coated by peritoneal mesothelium. The splenic artery arises from the celiac axis, enters the capsule at the hilum, and branches into trabecular arteries. The trabecular arteries then branch into central arteries and enter the white pulp. The periarterial lymphatic sheath consists of a cuff of T lymphocytes, plasma cells, and macrophages around the central arteries. As the arteries branch, the sheath narrows. B-lymphocyte clusters appear in follicles along the periarterial lymphatic sheath at arterial branch points (Fig. 160.1).

The components of the white pulp are connected by a reticular network and supporting stromal cells. On the cut surface of the normal spleen, white pulp is visible as white nodules approximately 1–2 mm in diameter, although their size varies with age and antigenic stimulation. The nodules are fully developed at birth, increase in size during childhood (especially following immunizations and

infections), peak during puberty, and involute in adulthood. Uninfected adults with an intact immune system usually do not show evidence of germinal centers. The secondary germinal center is comprised of a mantle zone of B lymphocytes surrounding the follicle. Antigen trapping and processing take place in the marginal zone of the white pulp.

The red pulp of the spleen consists of vascular sinuses, the cords of Billroth, and the terminal branches of the penicilliary arteries (Fig. 160.2). Vascular sinuses are lined with CD8[+] littoral endothelial cells that resemble endothelial cells with long processes and a basement membrane with ring fibers that attach to macrophage-derived dendritic processes. No tight junctions or interdigitations connect the cytoplasmic processes. Intact leukocytes, erythrocytes, and platelets are able to squeeze through the potential spaces between these cells and between the ring fibers (Fig. 160.3). Processes of the reticular cells of the cords of Billroth are outside the sinus walls. Endothelial cells line pulp veins but not the cords.

The reticular structure of the spleen facilitates its immune response. Venous sinus endothelial cells contain a plasma membrane-associated network of stress fibers composed of actin and myosin-like filaments. These filaments may cross the plasma membrane and insert into the mesh-like basement membrane. As the fibers tense, they create fenestrations through which erythrocytes must pass if they hope to continue their journey. With age, erythrocytes lose the ability to deform their shape and navigate the pathways created by these fibers and will not be able to continue into the circulation. The limitation is similar for erythrocytes containing parasitic infections. This mechanism, combined with mannose receptors and Toll-like receptors, helps the infrastructure of the spleen play a role in the host's overall immune response.

Circulation of blood through red pulp lined with endothelial-like littoral cells represents a rapid and closed circulation. Circulation into the cords is slower and open, thereby permitting the macrophages lining the cord to remove damaged or aged cells.

Accessory spleens are present in up to a third of the population and result from failure of precursor cells to fuse during embryologic development. Usually, they receive blood flow from the splenic artery and are located near the spleen, but they can be distant and mistaken for a tumor when noted on imaging studies or physical examination. Accessory spleens may develop similar conditions as the spleen proper and should be considered within the differential diagnosis for patients who have continued abnormalities after splenectomy.

Functions

The functions of the spleen and their anatomic locations are summarized in Table 160.1. Correlation with anatomy and histology are shown in Fig. 160.4

The Red Pulp

Splenic macrophages dominate the function of the red pulp and are responsible for filtering blood, removing bacteria, and recycling iron.

Removal of Damaged and Aged Formed Elements

The venous system of the red pulp enables it to filter whole blood, removing senescent erythrocytes and other blood cells. Arterial

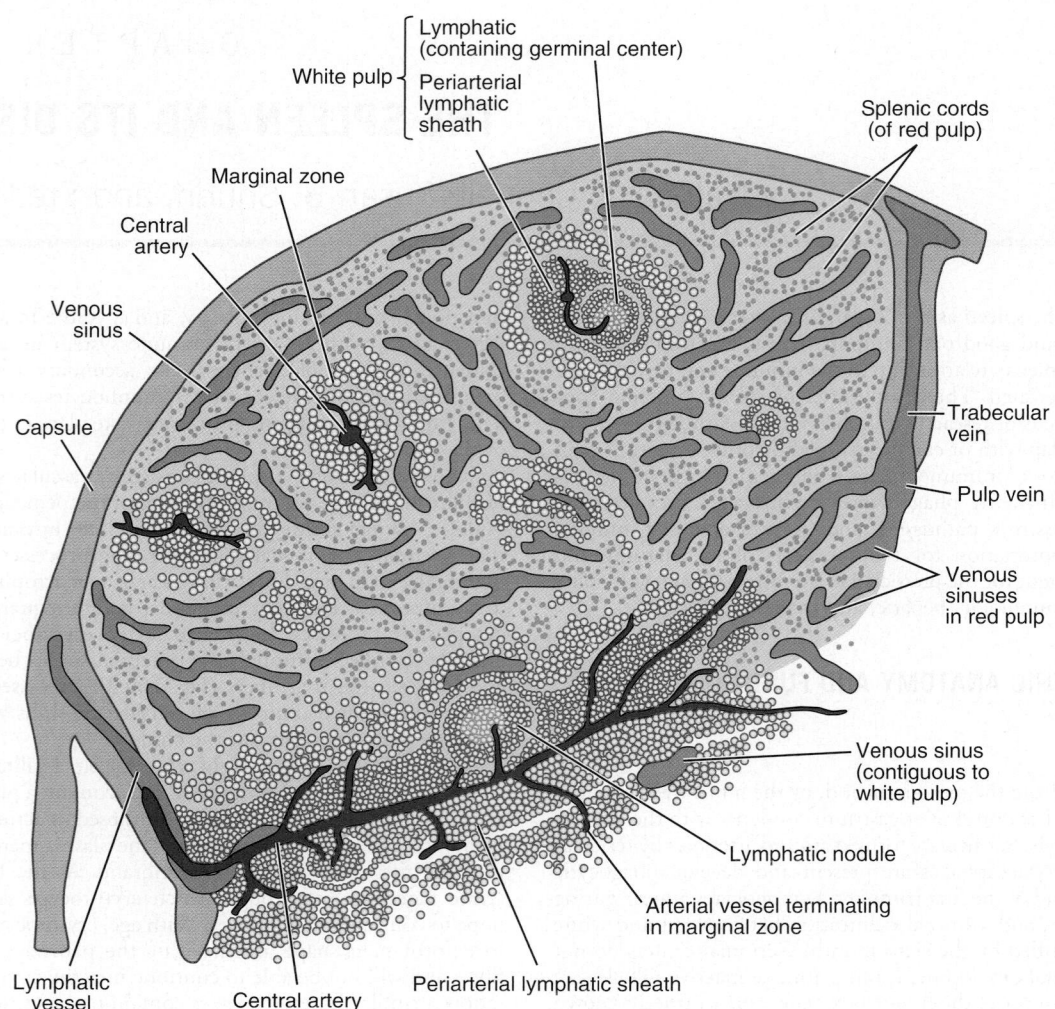

Fig. 160.1 ORGANIZATION OF THE HUMAN SPLEEN PRESENTED SCHEMATICALLY. See text for description of blood flow and cell distribution. *(Used, with permission, from Emerson SG: Hematopoiesis: The development of blood cells. In Schiffman FJ, editor: Hematologic pathophysiology, Philadelphia, 1998, Lippincott-Raven, p 10.)*

TABLE 160.1	**Functions of the Spleen**	
Category	**Function**	**Effector Cells/Areas**
Clearance/	Antibody-mediated clearance	Macrophages
Filtration	Culling and pitting	Reticular meshwork
Immune Response		
Marginal zone	Interaction of antigens with effector cells	Monocytes, lymphocytes
	Antigen processing	Macrophages
	Immune recognition	T cells (periarteriolar sheath)
White pulp	Immunoregulation, antibody production	B cells (lymphoid follicles)
	Antigen processing, preservation	Macrophages
Red pulp	Phagocytosis	Macrophages, monocytes, neutrophils
Hematologic	Hematopoiesis	Cords and sinuses
	Storage of erythrocytes, platelets, leukocytes	Reticular meshwork, red pulp
	Finishing/polishing of erythrocytes	Reticular meshwork, macrophages
Hemostasis	Production of factor VIII, von Willebrand factor	Endothelial cells

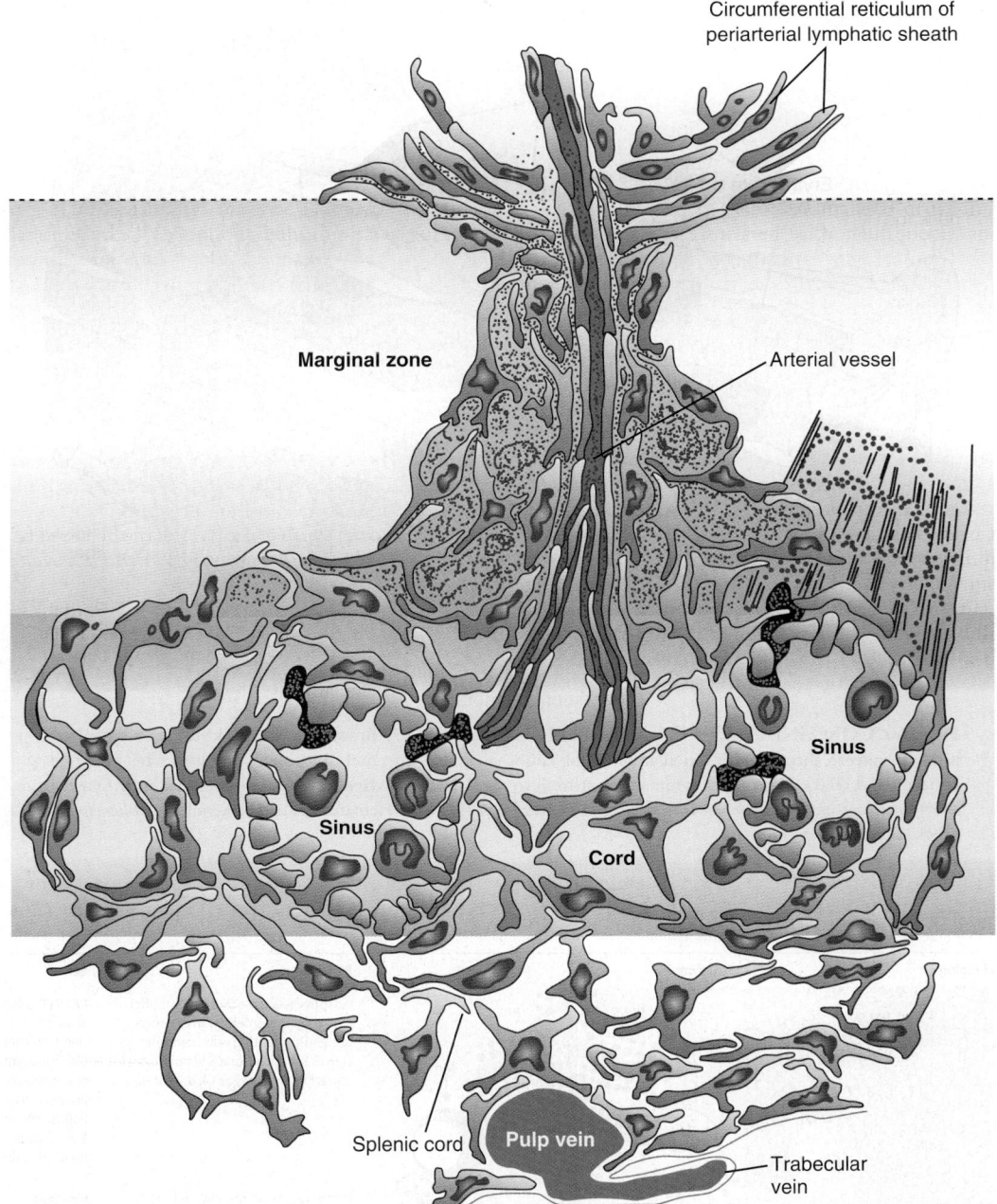

Fig. 160.2 DIAGRAM OF THE SPLENIC ARTERY. Arterial blood pools in the splenic cords before entering the splenic sinuses and returning to systemic circulation. *(Used, with permission, from Emerson SG: Hematopoiesis: The development of blood cells. In Schiffman FJ, editor: Hematologic pathophysiology, Philadelphia, 1998, Lippincott-Raven, p 12.)*

blood is delivered to the cords of the red pulp through an open system of reticular fibers, fibroblasts, and macrophages without an endothelial lining. Blood then passes from the cords into the efferent venous sinuses, which are lined with endothelial-like littoral cells with a discontinuous structure. Stress fibers extend beneath the basal plasma membrane and run parallel to the axis of the littoral cells. These cords direct the blood into sinuses through slits modulated in size by the stress fibers. In many animals, the stress fibers and splenic capsule are contractile, giving the spleen the ability to serve as a reservoir of red cells while reducing blood viscosity at rest. In humans, however, there is no evidence that the spleen serves such a function or is capable of significant changes in volume with rest and exercise. To return to the circulation, cells must pass through the slits between venous sinus littoral cells (see Fig. 160.3), the size

of which may be controlled in part by actin and myosin filaments within the stress fibers in the basal portion of endothelial cells. This surface is believed to be an important site for the culling and pitting of aged or damaged cells.

Compared with when they are young and have a healthy metabolic reserve, older erythrocytes and platelets are unable to tolerate the hostile splenic environment. The spleen has a pH between 6.8 and 7.2, is hypoxic (partial pressure of oxygen [P_{O2}]: 54 mmHg), and hypoglycemic (glucose concentration approximately 60% of that in venous blood). With age, damaged enucleated cells undergo changes in complex membrane carbohydrates, which facilitate recognition by splenic macrophages and removal from the circulation. *Culling* describes the destruction of erythrocytes: the normal removal of aging cells or the removal of damaged cells in pathologic states. Most

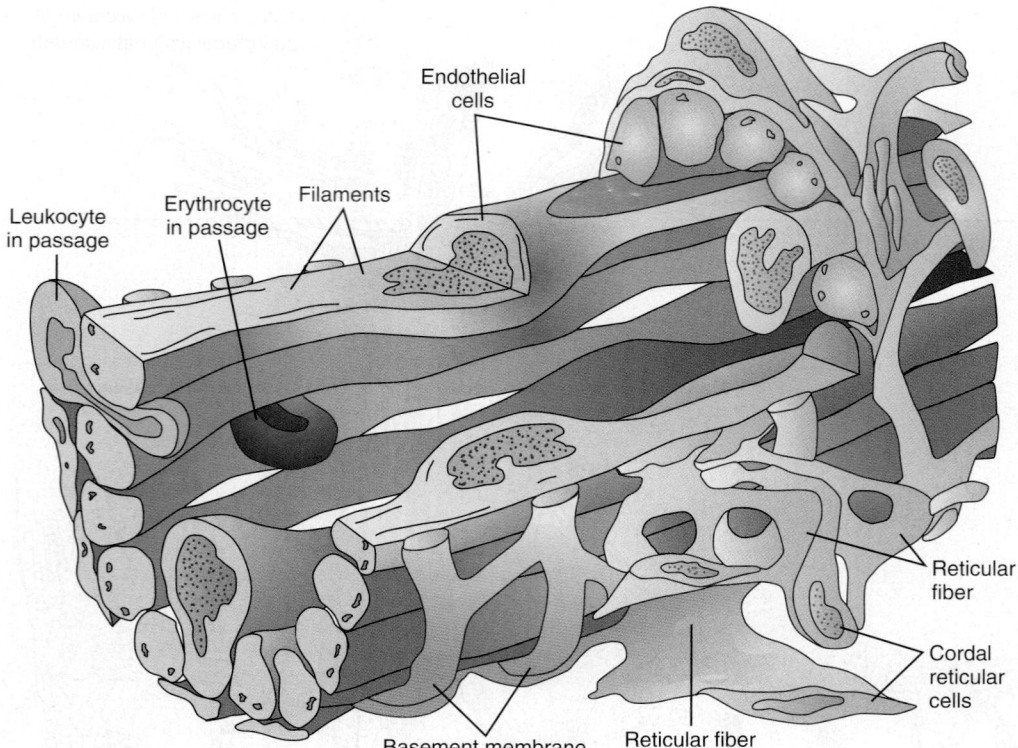

Fig. 160.3 ORGANIZATION OF THE SPLENIC SINUSES. Erythrocytes and leukocytes are scrutinized as they squeeze through the reticular fibers of endothelial cells to enter the splenic sinuses. The fenestrae contract and relax according to sympathetic stimuli to regulate cell passage. *(Used, with permission, from Emerson SG: Hematopoiesis: The development of blood cells. In Schiffman FJ, editor:* Hematologic pathophysiology, *Philadelphia, 1998, Lippincott-Raven, p 13.)*

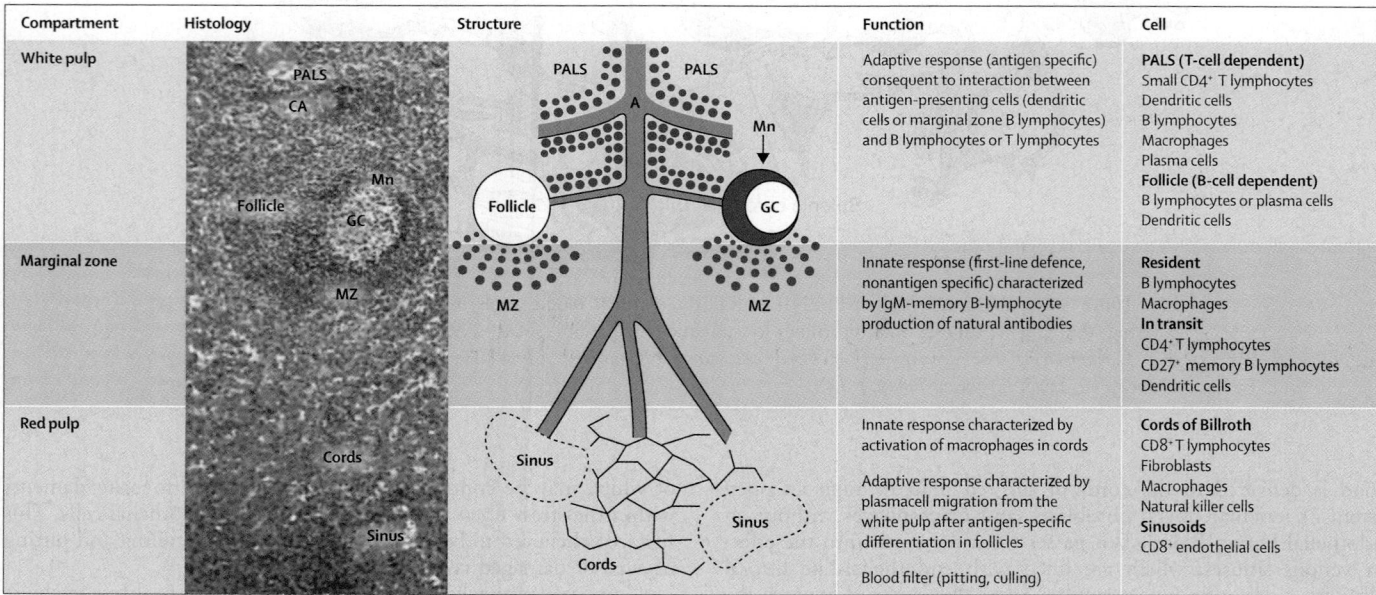

Fig. 160.4 STRUCTURE, FUNCTION, AND CELL POPULATIONS OF THE THREE FUNCTIONAL COMPARTMENTS OF THE SPLEEN. The histology panel shows a hematoxylin- and eosin-stained section of normal spleen. *A*, Artery; *CA*, central arteriola; *GC*, germinal center; *Mn*, mantle zone; *MZ*, marginal zone; *PALS*, periarteriolar lymphoid sheath. *(Used, with permission, from Di Sabatino A, Carsetti R, Corazza GR. Postsplenectomy and hyposplenic states.* Lancet *378(9785):86-97, 2011.)*

platelets and leukocytes are not removed by the spleen as they age but adhere to vessel walls and migrate into tissues where they die. *Pitting* refers to the removal of inclusions from within erythrocytes, which are then released back into the circulation. The erythrocyte membrane is in close apposition to the macrophage membrane so that aged or damaged glycoproteins, antibody, or complement on the surface of the cell are easily recognized and activate phagocytosis. Particulate matter—Howell-Jolly bodies, Heinz bodies, Pappenheimer bodies, and malarial and other parasites—are removed and the cell returned to the bloodstream. If membrane-containing adsorbed antibody is present, it is removed and the remainder of the cell is released with changes in shape and volume. Internal vesicles near the erythrocyte membrane appear as if they were on the surface of the cell and are termed *pits* or *pocks*. The spleen also normally removes these, with the polished erythrocyte returned to the circulation. The lack of this polishing function can be used to assess splenic dysfunction as the number of pits or pocks per erythrocyte is increased when the spleen fails to remove them.

Recycling of Iron

Macrophages in the liver and spleen are important for recycling iron as erythrocytes are phagocytized and hydrolyzed in the phagolysosome. Degradation of hemoglobin releases heme, which is catabolized into biliverdin, carbon monoxide, and ferrous iron (Fe^{2+}). Iron is then either released as a low-molecular-weight species for rapid reuse or stored as ferritin. As ferritin accumulates, it aggregates into hemosiderin. Iron-laden macrophages are a feature of iron overload states in both the liver and spleen. Erythrocytes that are destroyed intravascularly release hemoglobin that binds to haptoglobin. CD163 on the surface of splenic macrophages mediates endocytosis of circulating hemoglobin and haptoglobin-bound hemoglobin.

Iron is released from stores in splenic macrophages in response to the erythropoietic drive expressed by the bone marrow. The precise mechanisms are not well understood. Uptake of iron is mediated in most cells by a divalent cation transporter, the natural resistance–associated macrophage protein 2 (NRAMP2), in recycling endosomes that express the transferrin receptor. NRAMP2 transports ferritin into the cytoplasm across the endosomal membrane. In addition to the more widely expressed NRAMP2, macrophages and monocytes express NRAMP1, which was initially described as an iron-transporting protein affecting resistance to intracellular pathogens. A third molecule involved in iron metabolism in the spleen is lipocalin-2, which is secreted by macrophages and other myeloid cells when activated by exposure to bacterial metabolites. Lipocalin-2 binds to bacterial siderophores and sequesters iron from microorganisms. These and other related molecules tightly link the iron-recycling and host-resistance functions of the red pulp of the spleen.

Antibody Production

After stimulation and differentiating in the follicles of the white pulp, antigen-specific plasmablasts and plasma cells lodge in the red pulp, where they are closer to macrophages. A similar translocation occurs in lymph nodes, where plasmablasts migrate to the medullary cords. This translocation occurs after upregulation of expression of CXC-chemokine receptor 4 (CXCR4), which binds CXC-chemokine ligand 12 (CXCL12) expressed in red pulp.

The White Pulp

The lymphoid region of the spleen incorporates multiple components of the immune system that are organized to enhance recognition and/or response to pathogens.[5] The white pulp contains lymphoid sheaths around branching arterial vessels, similar to the structure of lymph nodes. Specific chemokines attract B and T cells to their appropriate domains. The periarteriolar lymphatic sheath contains T cells that interact with dendritic cells and circulating B cells. T cells and dendritic cells are attracted to the periarteriolar lymphatic sheath through CC-chemokine ligands 19 and 21. Clonal expansion of activated B cells occurs in follicles. B-cell migration to follicles requires CXCL13.

Expression of all these homeostatic chemokines is reduced when signaling through the lymphotoxin receptor or tumor necrosis factor (TNF)-α receptor 1 is absent, which results in disorganization of the domains of the white pulp.

Marginal Zone

Similar to the migration of leukocytes across endothelial barriers in inflammation, leukocytes leave the bloodstream and enter the white pulp in the marginal zone of the spleen via the function of G protein–coupled receptors. The marginal zone is an area for cells in transit as well as home to resident cells with complex interactions. Marginal zone metallophilic macrophages form an inner ring close to the white pulp, marginal zone macrophages form an outer ring, and dendritic cells and B cells are located between the two sets of macrophages. Both trafficking and retention of dendritic cells and B cells involve complex interactions with integrins and other adhesion molecules.

Innate Immunity

The spleen is important in the recognition of antigens, in the production of antibodies, and in the clearance of opsonized and nonopsonized particles from the bloodstream (see Table 160.1). The spleen structure facilitates monitoring of the contents of the blood, with blood flowing through the marginal zone directly along the white pulp. The white pulp is involved in adaptive immunity, whereas the marginal zone is involved in both innate and adaptive immunity (Table 160.2).

Trapping and processing antigens is a major function of the marginal zone. Macrophages are abundant here and the spleen captures more than 5% of the cardiac output (greater than 250 mL/min), which allows a large volume of blood to be immunologically scrutinized. Antigens penetrate the germinal center where T lymphocytes predominate. Processing of carbohydrate antigens is a special function of splenic marginal zone lymphocytes. Marginal zone macrophages express lectin receptors and scavenger molecules.

Splenic macrophages are more sensitive to small amounts of opsonic antibody or complement present on the surface of particles than are macrophages in the liver, lung, or bone marrow. In the absence of a spleen, individuals may fail to remove bacteria with limited opsonic coating, and the production of antigen-specific immunoglobulin (Ig) M is impaired. An asplenic individual has defective recognition of carbohydrate antigens, defective production of IgM early during infection, and defective removal of lightly opsonized particles—all crucial components of response to an invasive infection with encapsulated organisms.

Marginal zone B lymphocytes are sensitive to detection of blood-borne pathogens and rapidly differentiate into either antigen-presenting cells (APCs) or IgM-producing plasma cells. After activation in the marginal zone, some B cells migrate into the white pulp, where they function to activate naive CD4$^+$ T cells.

Similarly, blood-borne dendritic cells activated in the marginal zone migrate into the white pulp. This process appears to be important in control of certain parasitic infections. For example, in *Leishmania donovani* infection, the spread of infection is inversely proportional to the upregulation or downregulation of CCR7 expression on activated dendritic cells and migration of APCs into the white pulp. In human immunodeficiency virus (HIV)–positive patients with low CD4 T-cell counts (less than 300 cells/μL), there is evidence that IgM memory B-cell depletion might be a risk factor for pneumococcal disease. Effective antiretroviral therapy appears to reverse this depletion, in turn decreasing the risk for pneumococcal infection.

Adaptive Immunity

Although the white pulp is both anatomically and functionally similar to lymph nodes, all cells enter the white pulp via the marginal zone rather than through high endothelial venules and afferent lymphatic vessels, exposing them to an environment highly sensitive

TABLE 160.2	Innate Immune Pattern Recognition Receptors That Are Highly Expressed on Splenic Phagocytic Cells[a]				
Name	Abbreviation	Function	Splenic Cells Expressing	Recognizes or Affects	Pathogens Recognized
Toll-like receptor networks	TLR	Pattern recognition of pathogen-associated molecular patterns	Marginal zone macrophages Dendritic cells	Lipopolysaccharide Flagellin Double-stranded RNA	Multiple bacteria, especially gram negative
Natural resistance–associated macrophage protein-1	NRAMP1	Solute carrier family 11 (proton-coupled divalent metal ion transporters); phagolysosomal function	Macrophages	Lysosomal targeting	*Mycobacterium tuberculosis* *Mycobacterium avium* *Mycobacterium leprae*
Natural resistance–associated macrophage protein-2	NRAMP2	Proton-dependent cation transporter; iron absorption	Macrophages (apical duodenal cells, erythroid cells)	Impairs bacterial gene expression, protein synthesis	*Brucella* spp.
Sialic acid–binding Ig-like lectin-1; sialoadhesin	SIGLEC1, CD169	Immunoglobulin superfamily	Splenic and peritoneal macrophages Many hematopoietic cells	Mannose	*Streptococcus pneumoniae*
Specific intercellular adhesion molecule 3–grabbing nonintegrin related 1	SIGNR1, CD209b	ICAM3-binding nonintegrin homologue, mannose receptor	Dendritic cells	Polysaccharide antigens, ManLAM	Fungi, other pathogens
Macrophage receptor with collagenous structure	MARCO	Type 1 scavenger	Marginal zone macrophages	Lipopolysaccharide	*Staphylococcus aureus* *Escherichia coli*

[a]These receptors contribute to resistance to infection with pathogens in the absence of prior exposure, specific immune responses, or surface opsonic immunoglobulin or complement.
ICAM, Intercellular adhesion molecule; ManLAM, mannosylated lipoarabinomannan; RNA, ribonucleic acid.

to detection of blood-borne pathogens. Circulating dendritic cells capture bacteria from the blood and transport them to the spleen, where they mediate the initial differentiation of B cells to plasmablasts or APCs. Activated APCs entering the white pulp activate T cells, resulting in changes in receptor expression that enable them to migrate to the edge of B-cell follicles. Contact with activated T cells induces an isotype switch in follicular B cells, which then migrate to the red pulp and marginal zones or remain in splenic germinal centers. The white pulp of the spleen is the largest mass of lymphoid tissue in the body. The B lymphocytes, which ultimately produce antibodies, predominate in the nearby germinal centers and mantle zones. These areas all increase in size and activity with immunization or infection. The complex interaction between the cells in close apposition, autocrine, and paracrine signaling, and migration of cells into, within, and ultimately out of the spleen, contributes to the extraordinary repertoire of innate and adaptive immunity within the organ. Changes in splenic architecture are quite dramatic with septicemia, the most marked being depletion of splenic B-cell areas that occurs during overwhelming enterococcemia. Bacterial virulence factors appear to contribute to depletion of B- and T-cell areas.

Hematopoiesis

Active hematopoiesis can be seen in the fetal spleen throughout the second trimester, decreasing during the third trimester. Erythropoiesis and megakaryocytopoiesis predominate, with myelopoiesis present to a lesser extent. As hematopoiesis transitions from the hepatic phase into the bone marrow, it becomes less evident within the fetal spleen. The spleen is not normally a site of hematopoiesis in postnatal life in humans, but it is a rich source of hematopoietic stem cells and can support hematopoiesis in a number of pathologic states. Extramedullary hematopoiesis is a significant cause of splenomegaly primarily in bone marrow disorders (e.g., myelofibrosis or osteopetrosis) and chronic hemolytic anemias (e.g., thalassemia). The stromal cells of the spleen appear to be capable of supporting hematopoiesis and may produce the C-KIT ligand, as do marrow stromal cells. When splenic hematopoiesis occurs, the erythrocytes and platelets that circulate

tend to be less mature than when hematopoiesis occurs in the bone marrow, which suggests that egress from the spleen is easier than from the marrow.

Stem Cells

In higher mammals, including primates, the resident stem cells are capable of restoring hematopoietic and immunologic function after lethal irradiation.[6] Recently the spleen has been shown to be a source of multipotent stem cells in humans as well as other animals. These stem cells have been shown to contribute to the regeneration of multiple types of tissue, including pancreatic islet cells, bone, cranial nerves, and salivary glands. In addition, undifferentiated splenic monocytes assembled in clusters in the cords of the subcapsular red pulp have been shown to accumulate in injured myocardial tissue.[7] These stem cells are considered to have limited potential to undergo malignant transformation.

Storage of Cells

The normal adult human spleen contains 20–40 mL of blood and does not serve as a reservoir for blood or erythrocytes. However, in many conditions associated with splenomegaly, especially portal hypertension, the pulp cords widen to create an organ with more storage volume. Vascular pooling of blood and formed elements occurs, regardless of the underlying cause of the splenomegaly. Platelets and granulocytes, however, are normally stored in the red pulp of the spleen. As much as one-third of the total platelet mass may be stored in the spleen and released when cytokines affecting platelet adhesiveness are released. The lack of musculature in the human splenic capsule prevents the distention and contraction that occur in many animals, such as dogs, although the spleen appears to contract in divers during periods of breath-hold apnea. Platelet counts and granulocyte counts rise significantly after splenectomy, then fall. The circulating masses of these cell pools are chronically increased postsplenectomy, which may contribute to an increased incidence of atherosclerosis years after splenectomy.

EXAMINATION OF THE SPLEEN

Maneuvers for examination of the spleen involve inspection, percussion, and palpation, but their sensitivity and specificity vary based on patient factors (such as body habitus) and operator skill.[8] The pretest probability of splenomegaly, based on associated historical and clinical data, influences the positive–predictive value of finding splenomegaly on physical examination. If the pretest probability of splenomegaly is less than 10%, then physical examination maneuvers are inadequate for determining the presence or absence of splenomegaly. For those patients with a greater than 10% pretest probability of splenomegaly (for instance, patients with suspected infectious mononucleosis), the examination begins with inspection and then percussion of Traube's space—defined by the sixth rib superiorly, the anterior axillary line, and the costal margin. For adequate examination of the spleen, the patient must be fully supine, relaxed, with arms adjacent to the trunk. Dullness to percussion in Traube's space should be followed by palpation. Beginning in the right iliac fossa, the examiner's hand gently advances toward the left upper quadrant. This minimizes the likelihood that a grossly enlarged spleen will be missed, and the lower pole and medial border should be easily appreciated. If the spleen cannot be felt with this approach, the left hand of the examiner is placed on the left flank, lifting the lower part of the rib cage to displace the spleen medially toward the examiner's right hand. The splenic notch should be felt in the inferior medial border. Rotating the patient into the right lateral decubitus position while still recumbent may make it easier to palpate the spleen. The spleen should move with deep inspiration. The degree of enlargement is usually measured in centimeters below the costal margin. Depending on the position of the spleen within the abdomen, it may be difficult to appreciate even significant enlargement. Normal splenic size in an adult is up to 250 g and up to 13 cm in its long axis. Up to half of spleens weighing 600–750 g are not palpable. Greater degrees of splenomegaly are easier to appreciate on physical examination. In terms of sensitivity and specificity, there does not appear to be a difference between examination in the supine position and examination in the right lateral decubitus position, although both of these parameters are dependent on the experience of the examiner.

Up to 15% of normal children and 3% of young adults have palpable spleens without evidence of illness. The spleen involutes with age, and a spleen that is palpable in an older person is unlikely to be a normal variant and more likely to be associated with clinical disease.

Due to various abnormalities, the spleen may not be located in its usual anatomic position. It may migrate from its normal abdominal position to the left mid-abdomen or even the left lower quadrant.[9] While a rare finding, this highlights the need to pay particular attention to the lower abdomen when palpating for the spleen.

IMAGING OF THE SPLEEN

Radionuclide scintigraphy assesses anatomic and functional aspects of the spleen. The most common procedure is a liver-spleen scan in which technetium-99m (^{99m}Tc) sulfur colloid is injected intravenously and taken up by hepatic and splenic macrophages. It is the phagocytic activity of macrophages, rather than the presence of the spleen itself or any aspects of lymphoid function, that is assessed. A dynamic ^{99m}Tc scan can also assess the distribution of blood within the portal system and suggest the presence of portal hypertension. Infusion of ^{99m}Tc-labeled or Indium-111–labeled platelets with scintigraphy to determine their relative distribution in the liver and spleen has been used with considerable, but not absolute, success to predict the clinical efficacy of splenectomy in patients with immune thrombocytopenia purpura (ITP).

Ultrasonography readily shows the size, shape, and several aspects of splenic anatomy, including the presence of cysts and abscesses. The procedure is noninvasive, painless, of low cost, avoids radiation exposure for patients, and is a good screening study when the spleen is thought to be enlarged. In 95% of the normal population, the long axis of the spleen measures less than 12 cm on ultrasound

examination. Accessory spleens tend not to be well visualized on routine ultrasonography. In the hands of a skilled operator, endoscopic ultrasound-guided biopsy permits accurate diagnosis of lesions as small as a centimeter or less, which compares well with results obtained using computed tomography (CT). High-frequency sonography has significantly better resolution and can visualize both nodularity within the spleen, which occurs in childhood as immunity is acquired, and accessory spleens and splenosis after splenic rupture or trauma.

CT imaging has the advantage of showing the anatomy and some aspects of splenic function. Contrast material in the gastrointestinal tract helps delineate splenic tissue when it impinges on this system. Intravenous contrast material is required to delineate splenic lesions whose density is the same as normal splenic tissue. Abscesses have a rim of contrast agent enhancement.

CT can be used to estimate the volume of the spleen. Accessory spleens have the same attenuation as a normal spleen, which is somewhat less than that of liver. Accessory spleens are usually located in the gastrosplenic ligament near the hilum. Subcapsular and intrasplenic hematomas and splenic lacerations are clearly seen on CT. Leukemias and many inflammatory diseases produce diffuse splenomegaly, while granulomas and infarcted areas eventually calcify. Cysts, abscesses, and some malignancies may have a homogeneous pattern on CT scan. Although not replacing other methods of staging, splenic enlargement on CT may direct follow-up studies and indicate prognosis.

In addition to imaging the spleen, CT can be used to direct therapeutic interventions. Abscesses, hematomas, and cysts can be drained (see box on Management of Splenic Cysts). As long as portal pressures are normal and vascular lesions have been adequately excluded, thin-needle aspiration under CT guidance is generally a safe intervention. CT scanning of the abdomen, performed as part of the initial emergency department evaluation of patients with abdominal trauma, may avert hospital admission and prevent exploratory laparotomy.[10]

Magnetic resonance imaging (MRI) is useful for identifying vascular lesions, which would otherwise require angiography, and splenic infections. It is more difficult to image the contents of the upper abdomen with MRI than with CT because of respiratory motion. With more rapid imaging technology, MRI has gained considerable utility for imaging infectious and vascular lesions of the spleen. Hepatosplenic candidiasis and other infections to which immunocompromised patients are susceptible can be identified noninvasively with modern MRI technology.

Through the use of T2* sequences MRI imaging of the spleen allows quantitative measurement of iron burden in organs that accumulate iron, although the liver and heart are more commonly imaged for this purpose.[11]

Positron emission tomography (PET) scanning using ^{18}F-2-deoxyglucose is used in the diagnosis, staging, and monitoring of both non-Hodgkin and Hodgkin lymphoma. It is more sensitive than

---

Management of Splenic Cysts

A 37-year-old woman with no past medical history comes in for evaluation of early satiety and left shoulder pain. She reports that she feels full after only a few bites of any meal and sometimes becomes nauseated and vomits. Physical examination is remarkable for an enlarged, nontender spleen. Imaging shows a large splenic cyst.

- Many conditions can lead to cyst formation in the spleen including parasitic infections, trauma, hemangiomas, and polycystic kidney disease.
- Asymptomatic nonparasitic cysts may be observed with careful attention and plan for intervention should they become symptomatic, rupture, or become infected.
- Symptomatic cysts may require percutaneous drainage with radiologic guidance or sometimes surgical procedures including partial or total splenectomy.
- Parasitic cysts should be treated in consultation with infectious disease specialists as the particular parasitic infection, radiologic appearance, and patient comorbidities will guide choice of therapies.

CT scanning for identifying nodal disease and superior to both lymphangiography and CT scanning at imaging the spleen. The availability of more sensitive, specific, and less toxic approaches to imaging permits more precise staging of Hodgkin lymphoma without the complications of splenectomy (Fig. 160.5).[12,13]

The role of PET scanning is expanding in other disorders as whole-body PET scanners and appropriate small-molecule markers for individual diseases are more widely available. Imaging studies in small-animal models are very promising; splenic involvement can be identified with high sensitivity in mice.

TESTS OF SPLENIC FUNCTION

The peripheral blood smear may be the most sensitive tool for identification of functional or anatomic hyposplenia. The presence of Howell-Jolly bodies, which are nuclear remnants normally removed by the spleen, is an excellent indicator of hyposplenism (Fig. 160.6). These are rarely seen until the spleen is largely non-functional or overwhelmed by other phagocytic functions, such as extravascular hemolysis. Newborn infants commonly have visible Howell-Jolly bodies, and splenic function appears to be at least somewhat impaired in the first week of life. Pappenheimer bodies (siderotic granules normally removed by the spleen) are often seen in hyposplenic states, particularly when a component of hemolysis exists. Erythrocyte morphologic features reflect the lack of membrane polishing by the spleen, with the presence of acanthocytes and target cells. Granulocyte and platelet numbers are increased during asplenic states, including splenic infarction and surgical splenectomy.

To confirm suspected hyposplenism, the simplest test is a count of pitted or pocked erythrocytes. Fixation in 0.5%–1.0% glutaraldehyde

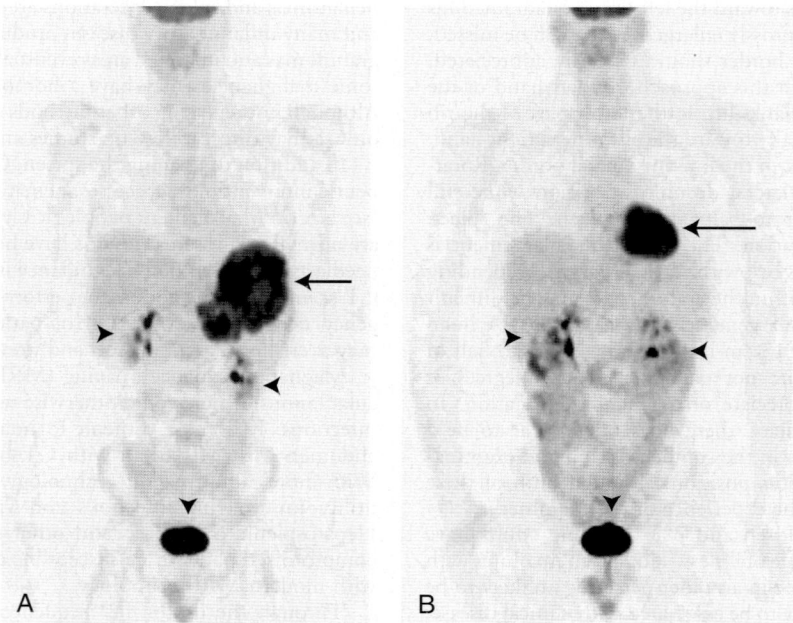

Fig. 160.5 POSITRON EMISSION TOMOGRAPHY SCANNING TO IMAGE AREAS OF INVOLVE-MENT IN HODGKIN DISEASE. (A) Pretreatment imaging showing the spleen *(large mass in left upper quadrant with arrow)* and activity in the kidney and bladder *(arrowheads)*. (B) The same patient after three cycles of chemotherapy. The *arrow* now points to normal activity in the myocardium not seen previously and *arrowheads* point to persistent urinary tract activity. The spleen is particularly well imaged on PET scan. *(Used, with permission, from Friedberg JW, Chengazi V: PET scans in the staging of lymphoma: Current status,* Oncologist *8:438, 2003.)*

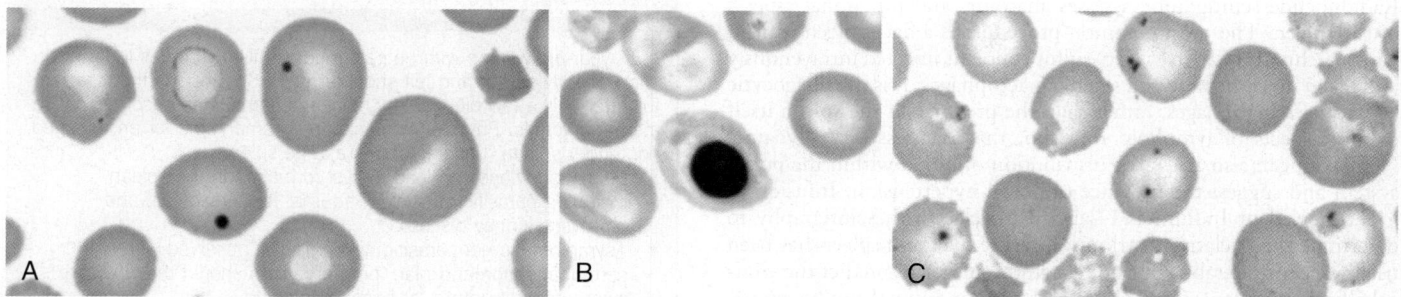

Fig. 160.6 RED BLOOD CELL FINDINGS IN HYPOSPLENISM. (A) Red blood cells with Howell-Jolly bodies. (B) Nucleated red blood cell. (C) Cells with Pappenheimer bodies. Red blood cells with Howell-Jolly bodies are seen in patients with hyposplenism. The cytoplasmic inclusions (A) are nuclear remnants that are usually round and stain similar to the nucleus of a nucleated red blood cell (B). They occur normally during red cell maturation but are typically removed by a normal spleen. Their presence in the blood indicates less-than-normal splenic function. Pappenheimer bodies (C), which can also be seen in hyposplenism, are siderotic granules that are irregular in shape and frequently multiple.

and examination under interference optics should reveal endocytic vesicles containing hemoglobin, ferritin, and remnants of mitochondria. These form in mature erythrocytes and are normally removed by the functioning spleen. The number of pitted cells (not the number of pits per cell) is inversely proportional to splenic function, with normal persons having less than 2% pitted cells.[14] The absence of Howell-Jolly bodies on a peripheral blood smear cannot be used as evidence of adequate splenic immune function.[15]

ASPLENIA AND HYPOSPLENIA

Congenital asplenia may be an isolated lesion or associated with severe cyanotic congenital heart disease and bilateral right-siddeness. Life-threatening cardiac lesions, including transposition of the great vessels, pulmonary artery atresia or stenosis, septal defects, anomalous venous drainage, and a single atrioventricular valve, are components of bilateral right-siddeness. The liver is central, and both lungs have three lobes. The peripheral blood smear shows Howell-Jolly bodies and other signs of hyposplenism. There is considerable variation in the anatomic and functional findings, and it is difficult to predict with accuracy the degree of splenic dysfunction on the basis of the anatomy alone. Children who survive the cardiac difficulties in the neonatal period have a significant incidence of sepsis secondary to a variety of organisms.

Polysplenia is associated with bilateral left-siddeness. Dextrocardia, bilateral superior venae cavae, septal defects, and anomalous pulmonary venous return are associated cardiac lesions. Both lungs have two lobes, the liver is midline, and bowel malrotation is common. The splenic tissue is divided into two to nine masses. The peripheral blood smear usually does not suggest hyposplenism, and no clear association with an increased risk for infection has been documented.

Asplenia occurring without heart disease is less likely to be detected before an infection develops than when associated cardiac lesions bring the patient to medical attention. Some of these patients also have *situs inversus*. Isolated cases of asplenia discovered after death of an otherwise healthy adult or child from overwhelming sepsis with encapsulated organisms have been reported. Familial instances of congenital asplenia are likely to be instances of genetic abnormalities (e.g., Hox11/Tlx1), but these have not yet been documented. Examination of a blood smear for Howell-Jolly bodies is a simple procedure and may be lifesaving in the rare patients affected with these disorders.

If Howell-Jolly bodies are observed on the blood smear of an otherwise healthy person, imaging should be performed to assess for the presence of a spleen. Immunization with polysaccharide vaccines and early intervention with antibiotics for apparent infection may prove lifesaving for these individuals. Because approximately 20% of invasive pneumococcal infections in these patients are nonvaccine strains, a high degree of vigilance remains essential, even with more widespread immunization of healthy children.

ACQUIRED HYPOSPLENISM

Infarction in Sickle Cell Disease

The course of sickle cell disease is marked by progressive dysfunction of multiple organs over many years, and one of the earliest organs to be affected is the spleen. Serial measurements of the numbers of pitted erythrocytes in patients with sickle cell disease demonstrate that splenic dysfunction develops progressively over the first few years of life in the major sickle syndromes (Figs. 160.7 and 160.8). The hypoxic, acidotic, hypoglycemic environment of the spleen creates optimal conditions for tactoid formation and for sickling of the poorly deformable erythrocytes, which then block splenic blood vessels and infarct the tissues. Splenic environmental conditions that enhance acidosis or hypoxia, or additional erythrocyte membrane or enzyme abnormalities that promote irreversible sickling, increase splenic infarction. The hypoplenism is reversible with transfusion for

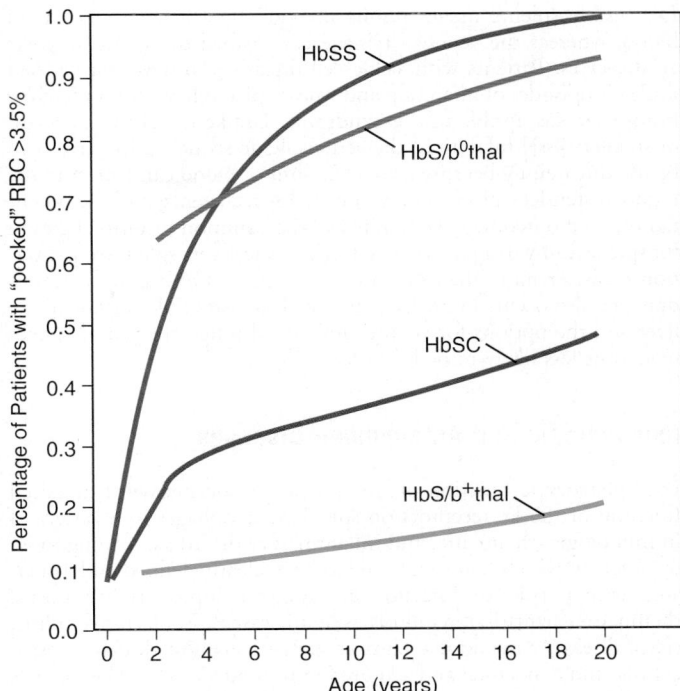

Fig. 160.7 DEVELOPMENT OF FUNCTIONAL ASPLENIA IN SICKLE CELL DISORDERS. *B$^+$thal*, Beta$^+$ thalassemia; *b^{0}thal*, Beta^0 thalassemia; *HbS*, hemoglobin S; *HbSC*, hemoglobin SC; *HbSS*, hemoglobin SS; *RBC*, red blood cell. (*Used, with permission, from Pearson HA, Gallagher D, Chilcote R, et al: Developmental pattern of splenic dysfunction in sickle cell disorders.* Pediatrics *76:392, 1985.*)

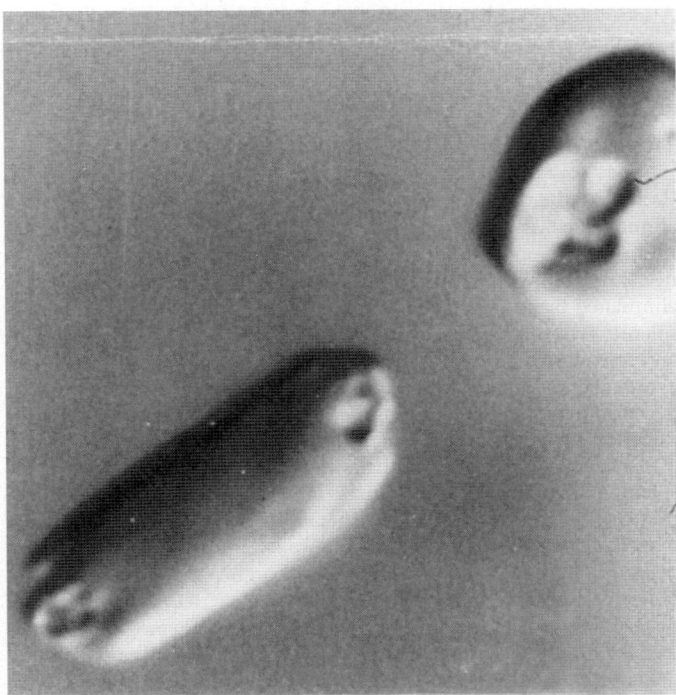

Fig. 160.8 POCKED ERYTHROCYTES IN THE SICKLE HEMOGLOBINOPATHIES. (*Used, with permission, from Sills R, Oski FA: RBC surface pits in the sickle hemoglobinopathies.* Am J Dis Child *133:526, 1979.*)

at least the first few years of life but becomes irreversible with progressive damage to blood vessels by 6 years of age in patients with sickle cell disease.

Splenic sequestration is a manifestation of the infarctive process of sickling in the spleen that extends to involve larger veins.

Distensible splenic tissues results in pooling of a large amount of blood, whereas the venous drainage is occluded by sickled hypoxic erythrocytes. Patients with sickle cell disease who have not yet had multiple episodes of infarction and whose spleens have not undergone fibrosis are susceptible to this syndrome. Unlike the chronic process of smaller vessel infarction, the acute splenic sequestration crisis can be life threatening because a large amount of blood can collect in the highly distended spleen. The tendency for recurrence and the potential for fatal outcome have resulted in the common recommendation for splenectomy in a patient who has had one severe splenic sequestration crisis, or more than one less severe crisis. Occlusion of venous drainage also occurs in the liver, but the less distensible capsule of the liver and the options for venous drainage through the portal system make this less likely to be life threatening.

Immunologic and Autoimmune Diseases

Poor phagocytic function of the spleen is associated with impaired function of the Fc receptors on splenic macrophages in a variety of immunologic, rheumatic, and inflammatory disorders. Among those disorders in which hyposplenism has been clearly defined and associated with a risk for infection are systemic lupus erythematosus, rheumatoid arthritis, sarcoidosis, systemic vasculitis, ulcerative colitis, celiac disease, amyloidosis, chronic graft-versus-host disease, mastocytosis, and congenital and acquired immunodeficiency. The diseases themselves and the immunosuppressive therapies that are used in their management may contribute to the risk for infection in these conditions. Immunization with polysaccharide antigens and recognition of the risk of bacterial infection are important steps in reducing the risks of splenic hypofunction.

Splenomegaly and the production of autoantibodies such as antiplatelet or antiphospholipid antibodies, are features of the acquired immunodeficiency syndrome (AIDS). In the late stages of AIDS, atrophy of lymphoid follicles and depletion of T-cell–dependent areas are common. It is not clear that impairment of phagocytic function is a component of splenic atrophy in AIDS.

Therapy-Induced Splenic Hypofunction

Radiation therapy affects splenic function depending on the dose administered. In general, phagocytic cells are not affected by irradiation, but lymphoid cells are extremely sensitive. B-cell function is nearly ablated with as little as 500 cGy. T-cell lymphoblastogenesis is eliminated by administration of 3000 cGy. With doses of 2000 cGy, splenic hypofunction is usually transient because the macrophages and splenic stroma are not affected, and circulating B and T lymphocytes can repopulate the splenic follicles. Permanent splenic hypofunction may develop with doses of 4000 cGy or higher. The risk for infection is significant after such therapy.

Corticosteroid therapy impairs the affinity of the Fc receptors of splenic macrophages for opsonized IgG and decreases the adhesiveness of granulocytes and monocytes. This results in an acute pharmacologic splenectomy, even at commonly administered therapeutic dosages. The function of the Fc receptors on hepatic, pulmonary, and bone marrow macrophages is far less affected than that of splenic macrophages. The acute rise in platelet count or hemoglobin values seen with corticosteroid therapy in ITP or warm autoimmune hemolytic anemia is due to decreased clearance of sensitized cells. With prolonged therapy, the production of antibodies by splenic lymphocytes is also affected, and splenic function continues to be impaired.

Intravenous IgG appears to decrease the phagocytic function of the spleen by binding to Fc receptors and impeding their recognition of opsonized particles. This is a transient effect because the Fc receptors are internalized and recycled, and opsonic function returns to normal within 2–3 weeks. Occupancy and impairment of function of Fc receptors is also seen with administration of anti-IgD to Rh-positive patients, which induces a transient hemolytic anemia.

Reticuloendothelial blockade, or occupancy of these receptors, refers to the impaired ability of the spleen to recognize and remove other IgG-coated particles, including bacteria, in the presence of these agents.

SPLENOMEGALY AND HYPERSPLENISM

An enlarged spleen is not a disease state in itself but usually indicates some underlying pathologic state.[16] The processes run the gamut from minor to life threatening, from congenital disorders to those at the end of life. It is useful to approach the differential diagnosis of splenomegaly by considering the processes that may cause splenic enlargement and then to focus on the specific diagnoses within those categories. The spleen may be enlarged as a result of infiltration, hypertrophy of normal elements (macrophages and lymphoid components), extramedullary hematopoiesis, inflammatory or immunologic processes, and systemic or portal congestion (see box on Timing of Return to Contact Sports in Athletes Who Have Had Infectious Mononucleosis). The degree of splenomegaly correlates well with involvement of the spleen in many malignant disorders, such as Hodgkin disease. Rarely, anatomic abnormalities will cause splenomegaly. Splenomegaly is important to investigate because it is frequently the presenting finding of a serious disorder whose earlier recognition and treatment may prevent significant long-term morbidity and mortality. The diseases associated with splenomegaly are detailed in Table 160.3. Patients with splenomegaly do not necessarily have hypersplenism, and patients with hypersplenism may indeed have normal-sized spleens, such as those seen in ITP.

Hypersplenism refers to nonimmune, indiscriminate destruction of the formed elements of the blood by a spleen that is usually enlarged, affected by portal hypertension, or both. The bone marrow is hyperplastic, and the peripheral blood cell counts are decreased because of destruction of mature formed elements. Splenectomy corrects the cytopenia. Any of the formed elements of the blood—erythrocytes, neutrophils, or platelets—can be affected alone or in combination. Splenic hypertrophy in cirrhosis is due to an increase in splenic macrophages and their activity. Because the normal function of splenic macrophages is to remove senescent cells, this is an exaggeration of a physiologic process.

Hypersplenism develops in patients who receive chronic transfusions, and there are several components that contribute to the development of hypersplenism. The antigenic load of allogeneic transfused cells stimulates the immune system. Additionally, transfused cells have shorter survival than normal red cells (mean of 60 instead of 120 days, unless specially prepared neocytes are used), which increases the work of splenic macrophages. Finally, iron

---

Timing of Return to Contact Sports in Athletes Who Have Had Infectious Mononucleosis

An 17-year-old male high school student is diagnosed by his primary care physician with infectious mononucleosis. The patient is concerned about the upcoming soccer season and wants to be able to start training with the team in 4 weeks.

- More than half of patients with infectious mononucleosis develop splenomegaly within the first 14 days of illness.
- Most reports of splenic rupture in the setting of infectious mononucleosis occur in the first 21 days of illness.
- There is a paucity of data to support imaging the spleen to document resolution of splenomegaly before returning to contact sports.
- Noncontact sports may be safely resumed after at least 21 days from the onset of initial symptoms and contact sports should be safe in most cases after at least 28 days. Infectious mononucleosis–associated splenic rupture has been reported as far as 7 weeks after symptom onset.
- The timing of return to sports and the risks should be discussed with the patient, especially if the patient may not have returned to baseline after prolonged fatigue.

TABLE 160.3	Causes of Splenomegaly	
Primary Process	**Pathogenesis**	**Examples**
Anatomic	Developmental abnormalities	Cysts, pseudocysts, hamartomas, peliosis, hemangiomas
Hematologic	Hemolysis	Intrinsic (membrane, enzyme, hemoglobin disorders), extrinsic (immune)
	Extramedullary hematopoiesis	Myeloproliferative diseases/ myelodysplasias, myelofibrosis, osteopetrosis
Infectious	Bacteria	Acute and chronic systemic infection, abscesses, subacute bacterial endocarditis
	Mycobacteria	Miliary tuberculosis
	Spirochetes	Syphilis, Lyme disease, leptospirosis
	Viruses	Epstein-Barr virus; cytomegalovirus; human immunodeficiency virus; hepatitis A, B, C
	Rickettsia	Rocky Mountain spotted fever, Q fever, typhus
	Fungi	Disseminated candidiasis, histoplasmosis, South American blastomycosis
	Parasites	Malaria, babesiosis, toxoplasmosis, *Toxocara canis*, *Toxocara cati*, leishmaniasis, schistosomiasis, trypanosomiasis
Immunologic	Collagen vascular diseases	Felty syndrome, systemic lupus erythematosus, mixed connective tissue disorder, systemic vasculitis, Sjögren syndrome, systemic mastocytosis
	Immunodeficiency	Common variable immunodeficiency
	Immune/ inflammatory	Graft-versus-host disease, serum sickness, large granular lymphocyte lymphocytosis, Weber-Christian panniculitis
Neoplastic	Primary malignancies	Lymphomas, leukemias
	Metastatic malignancies	Breast, lung, skin, colon
Infiltrative	Storage diseases	Gaucher disease, Niemann-Pick disease, GM_1 gangliosidosis, glycogen storage disease type IV, Tangier disease, Wolman disease, mucopolysaccharidoses, hyperchylomicronemia types I and IV
Congestive	Portal hypertension	Intrahepatic cirrhosis, extrahepatic cirrhosis (Budd-Chiari syndrome)
	Systemic	Congestive heart failure
	Local	Splenic vein thrombosis

overload causes hemosiderosis of both the spleen and the liver, so that portal hypertension may develop and further increase splenic pathology. Hypersplenism increases the transfusion requirement in patients who are already transfusion dependent.

Interestingly, spleen status at the time of allogeneic hematopoietic stem cell transplantation affects outcomes. Patients with splenomegaly have delayed engraftment while those with prior splenectomy have early engraftment and no difference in mortality.[17] The increased risk in infection may be mitigated by the high-intensity setting in which stem cell transplantation occurs.

SPLENECTOMY

Indications and Timing

Splenectomy should be performed for clinical indications rather than for specific diagnoses. In many instances, removal of the spleen will improve the condition of patients with hemolytic anemia due to intrinsic disorders of erythrocyte membranes and enzyme disorders, and of those with chronic conditions, such as storage diseases and portal hypertension. Specific clinical indices that require intervention should be identified, and parameters that can be used to identify clinical improvement (usually an increase in peripheral blood cell counts, growth, or energy level) should be determined before the procedure is performed. For patients with inherited erythrocyte membrane or enzyme disorders, such as hereditary spherocytosis or pyruvate kinase deficiency, marked reticulocytosis indicating significant metabolic energy required for erythropoiesis, somatic growth failure, or lack of exercise tolerance would be potential indications for splenectomy. Avoidance of formation of gallstones, formerly often considered an indication for splenectomy when a diagnosis of hereditary spherocytosis was made, is less important today because minimally invasive surgical procedures have improved the management of cholelithiasis. Patients with storage disorders such as Gaucher disease often develop splenomegaly and hypersplenism, and subsequent cytopenias requiring intervention. As new therapies are developed, such as eliglustat for Gaucher disease and ruxolitinib for primary myelofibrosis, these patients experience a significant reduction in spleen size and increase in quality of life, which may mitigate the need for splenectomy.[18,19] The clinical benefit to be obtained from splenectomy should at least balance, and preferably outweigh, the potential long-term risks of postsplenectomy septicemia, an increased risk for thrombosis, and the shift of storage cells from the spleen to other organs, such as the bone marrow, where they may do more harm in the absence of the spleen. Not all patients with hemolytic anemias require splenectomy. If such patients develop an aplastic crisis due to parvovirus B19 infection while their spleens are intact, they may require a transfusion. Many patients with mild chronic hemolysis and well-compensated anemia may be better off with their spleens remaining intact. Patients with ITP should undergo surgical splenectomy when the risks of bleeding or of medical therapies (such as long-term corticosteroids or the anti-CD20 monoclonal antibody rituximab) are such that the benefits of splenectomy exceed the risks. The introduction of thrombopoietin mimetics for treatment of chronic ITP has further delayed or eliminated the need for splenectomy in many patients. The indications for splenectomy are different in adults than in children, and are affected by the presence of underlying disorders, such as systemic lupus erythematosus and HIV. In an attempt to avoid immunologic consequences of a total splenectomy, several centers are performing partial splenectomies for hereditary spherocytosis, although in some cases a second procedure is later required.[20]

Splenectomy for sickle cell disease is usually performed for splenic sequestration that is severe, persistent, or recurrent. In some sickle syndromes, the spleen does not autoinfarct in childhood, and persistent splenomegaly may increase the degree of anemia. The risk for subsequent development of gallstones should be considered in patients with hemoglobinopathies and other hemolytic anemias so that cholecystectomy can be performed simultaneously, if deemed indicated.[21]

The timing of splenectomy (when it is to be performed) should again be chosen to minimize risks and maximize benefits. Immunity to carbohydrate antigens, such as those in the cell walls of encapsulated organisms such as *Streptococcus pneumoniae*, *Neisseria meningitidis*, and *Haemophilus influenzae* type b, develops over the first 2–3 years of life. When splenectomy can be delayed until the patient is at least 2 and preferably more than 5 years of age, specific immunity and response to administered polysaccharide vaccines will improve host defenses and lessen the risk for postsplenectomy sepsis. When patients have a disease, such as Gaucher disease, or hemolytic anemia predisposing to iron overload, such as thalassemia, the presence of the spleen as a preferential site for the storage of harmful cellular breakdown products may protect other organs from damage. Delaying splenectomy until a clear clinical indication is present will balance risks and benefits to an optimal degree. The recently developed oral substrate inhibitor, eliglustat, has shown promising success in reducing splenomegaly in patients with Gaucher disease.[18] As this drug is studied further, it is possible that splenectomy may not be needed as often.

Surgical Options

When splenectomy is clearly indicated, acute complications are rarely a consideration in the decision to perform surgery. Nevertheless, advances in surgical procedures have minimized the short-term risks of the procedure itself and of postoperative complications such as intestinal obstruction from adhesions. Subtotal splenectomy can be performed when total splenectomy is not desirable, such as for the removal of a cyst, a pseudocyst, or tumors, after trauma, or for Gaucher disease. Wedge resection with mattress sutures and cyanoacrylate adhesives and microfibrillar collagen omental packs have greatly improved partial splenectomy procedures in the past decade. Laparotomy is required when extensive peritoneal adhesions are present and for removal of massively enlarged spleens. A sufficiently large incision to permit full visualization and mobilization is essential when the spleen is very large or when inspection is a major part of the surgical procedure. A retroperitoneal approach is useful when the spleen is not massively enlarged but needs to be fully removed, such as when cytopenias are the indication for the procedure. This approach shortens the postoperative recovery time and avoids induction of peritoneal adhesions.

Minimally invasive procedures have become standard for most splenectomies. Laparoscopy is now the procedure of choice for splenectomy. Although the operative time is significantly greater than for laparotomy, the postoperative recovery time, risk for damage to the pancreas, likelihood of developing a subphrenic abscess and peritoneal adhesions postoperatively, and nutritional and metabolic challenges to the patient are considerably reduced. Laparoscopic splenectomy can be performed even in thrombocytopenic patients. The outcome of laparoscopic splenectomy in ITP is affected by the experience and skill of the surgeon and by the patient's obesity. Prolonged presurgical use of corticosteroids may induce obesity and impair tissue healing, resulting in a higher risk for complications from laparoscopic splenectomy than when splenectomy is performed before adverse drug effects develop. In the case of massive splenomegaly, splenic morcellation may be necessary prior to laparoscopic retrieval.

Appreciation of the risk for postsplenectomy septicemia and refinements in noninvasive, accurate radiologic monitoring techniques have led to more conservative approaches to splenic injury. Nonoperative management has increased over time and has an acceptable mortality and complication rate in selected patients, although early discharge may put patients at risk for the later complications.[22] Noninvasive imaging and minimally invasive surgical procedures have greatly affected these trends. After traumatic rupture, splenic tissue may regenerate as both micro- and macroscopic ectopic implants in the peritoneal cavity, a process termed *splenosis*. Although splenosis appears to be partially protective against overwhelming postsplenectomy infection in animals, its protective value in humans is not known and may depend on the adequacy of splenic tissue perfusion. If poorly vascularized, the ectopic splenic tissue may not provide adequate contact between macrophages and the antigens of the infecting organism. It is generally valuable to attempt preservation of splenic function when possible after traumatic rupture. Some surgeons attempt to induce splenosis when traumatic splenectomy is unavoidable, in the hope of minimizing late complications.

As the late complications of splenectomy are better appreciated, surgeons have become increasingly creative at performing procedures

that preserve or restore splenic function. Even large cysts that were indications for splenectomy until recently have been managed with spleen-conserving procedures, such as partial or total cyst removal, which can often be performed laparoscopically.[23] Pancreatic surgery often requires sacrifice of the spleen; however, increasing numbers of procedures are being performed with salvage of the spleen.

Splenic transplantation is being used as a means of developing immune tolerance, as well as a means of reducing the risk for infection following organ transplantation.[24] Allograft spleen has been transplanted within multivisceral grafts with only minimal graft-versus-host disease. To date there are more animal than human data, and it is unclear how large an impact this approach will have on visceral, especially small-bowel and pancreatic, allotransplantation.[25] If protection against infection is the main consideration, an intact spleen is superior to a repaired or autotransplanted spleen, whereas accessory spleens and splenosis may be only marginally better than asplenia.[15]

Complications After Splenectomy

Acute complications in the perioperative period include rupture of the spleen, the development of a subphrenic abscess, and injury to the pancreas during the operative procedure. In a healthy patient, the immediate risk of splenectomy is limited. The degree of splenomegaly greatly affects the risk for rupture and pancreatic injury. The technical difficulty of performing a splenectomy is much greater when the spleen is massively enlarged than when the spleen is small. Once the arterial supply is ligated, rupture of the spleen is rarely a problem. The splenic hilum is retroperitoneal, so if the spleen is very large, mobilization to gain access to the splenic artery and vein can be difficult. After recovery from surgery, intestinal obstruction due to formation of peritoneal adhesions is a complication that, if it is to occur at all, usually occurs within the first few months.

Two late complications of splenectomy give the greatest concern: overwhelming postsplenectomy septicemia and atherosclerotic heart disease. Both of these complications may develop many years after the splenectomy (Fig. 160.9). The precise risk is not known, and preventive interventions are probably underused because patients may not be aware of the risks of splenectomy performed early in life.

Postsplenectomy septicemia is rare but may be rapidly lethal. In the absence of protective levels of opsonic IgG antibodies produced in the spleen, hepatic and pulmonary macrophages are unable to effectively clear organisms from the bloodstream. Organisms that

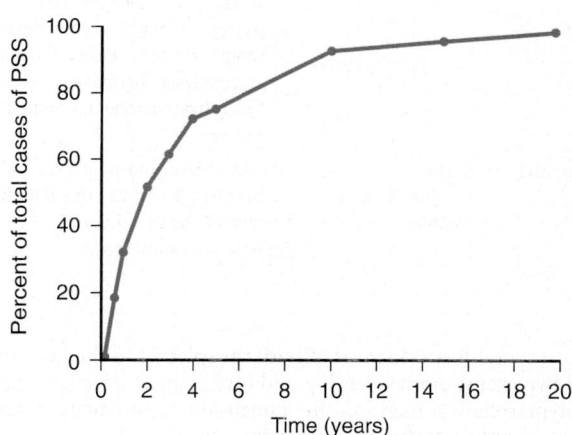

Fig. 160.9 THE INTERVAL FROM SPLENECTOMY TO POSTSPLENECTOMY SEPSIS. Of the total (*n* = 288), 3.1% occurred more than 20 years after splenectomy. *PSS,* Postsplenectomy sepsis. *(Used, with permission, from Lutwick LI: Infections in asplenic patients. In Mandell GL, Bennett JE, Dolin R, editors:* Principles and Practice of Infectious Diseases, *ed 7, Philadelphia, 2009, Churchill Livingstone.)*

enter the bloodstream and would ordinarily be removed by splenic macrophages are able to evade recognition by macrophages whose Fc and C3b receptors appear to be less avid than those of splenic macrophages. Circulation of the blood through the liver and lung is more rapid than through the spleen, and there is little opportunity for macrophages to recognize organisms with surfaces containing little IgG and only small amounts of C3bi. The important filtration function of the venous sinus endothelial cells is absent following splenectomy. The generation of cytokines, including TNF-α and bacterial endotoxins, leads to cardiovascular collapse and shock. It is difficult to rescue an asplenic patient once shock develops, even with effective antibiotic therapy. The risk that this will happen varies with the indication for splenectomy (Table 160.4) and the patient's medical condition. Factors that impair host defenses significantly increase the risk for infection. These include deficient opsonins (hypogammaglobulinemia and specific antibody-production deficiency), reticuloendothelial blockade related to increased phagocytic activity of macrophages in other organs, impaired antigen processing or recognition (AIDS, lymphoma, other malignancies, and some collagen vascular diseases), neutropenia, and high iron load (thalassemia). The tetrapeptide tuftsin, primarily produced in the spleen, enhances the phagocytic activity of monocytes and neutrophils; its absence in asplenic patients appears to contribute to depressed neutrophil function and the subsequent increased risk for infection.

Patients at the lowest risk for overwhelming postsplenectomy sepsis are those in whom splenectomy cures the underlying problem, such as isolated ITP, hereditary spherocytosis, and trauma. Patients undergoing splenectomy for trauma have a 50-fold greater risk for subsequent septic death than trauma patients with intact spleens, whereas the risk in patients with sickle cell disease is increased 350-fold over that of the general population, and other authors report the risk to be 600 times greater. Similar to use of hemodialysis to attempt to replace the function of the kidney, work is ongoing to devise an artificial spleen as a mechanical way to filter pathogens from the blood.

An increased risk for vascular complications may result from splenectomy. Acute portal vein thrombosis occurs within 2 months of splenectomy in 5%–37% of patients, which is probably the result of local surgical factors. The surgical approach seems to affect the rate of postsplenectomy portal and splenic vein thrombosis, with a laparoscopic approach and morcellation associated with a higher rate of thrombosis compared with open splenectomy (55% vs. 19%, respectively). Patients with thalassemia and prior splenectomy appear to also have an increased incidence of venous thromboembolism beyond the portal venous system. In addition, splenectomy appears to be a risk factor for the development of pulmonary hypertension. Vascular events after splenectomy are likely multifactorial in origin, being attributed to a combination of hypercoagulability, platelet activation, activation of endothelium due to the persistence of particulate matter, and damaged cells in the bloodstream.

Atherosclerosis that develops many years after splenectomy in patients with hereditary spherocytosis or hereditary stomatocytosis may be related to subsequent thrombocytosis that leads to enhancement of plaque formation. Statistically, the increased risk for atherosclerosis is not particularly high, but for individuals with other risk factors such as hypertension, diabetes, high levels of cholesterol or homocysteine, heterozygous protein C or S deficiency, or factor V Leiden, splenectomy may pose a more significant risk. Although no human data are currently available in this area, some studies have suggested that the spleen might be involved in lipid metabolism in both rats and rabbits.

Prevention of Complications

Postsplenectomy Septicemia

The major risk for postsplenectomy sepsis is infection with encapsulated organisms such as *Staphylococcus pneumoniae*, *H. influenzae* type b, and *N. meningitidis*, which require opsonization for effective phagocytosis. Polysaccharide vaccines are available for all three bacteria.[26,27] The highest risk period for children is in the first 2 years of life, when their ability to mount an antibody response to purified polysaccharides has not developed completely, so protein-conjugated vaccines are now in widespread use. This has significant potential benefit for patients when asplenia is not recognized, because they might then be immunized as part of their routine care. The antibody responses to vaccines, especially the conjugated vaccines, differ in IgG subclasses from those produced following natural infection. Overwhelming postsplenectomy sepsis and death from sepsis in functionally hyposplenic patients should be preventable.[28] It is recommended that immunization be done at least 14 days prior to the anticipated splenectomy in order to optimize antigen recognition and processing, and induce more effective immunity. If emergency splenectomy is performed, it is recommended that vaccination be postponed until at least 14 days postsplenectomy to avoid the transient immune suppression often seen with general anesthesia and surgery (see box on Vaccination of a Patient Scheduled for Elective Versus Emergency Splenectomy). Adults are generally presumed to be immune to *H. influenzae* type b and may receive the 23-valent pneumococcal polysaccharide vaccine (PPSV23) and meningococcal vaccines alone. Reimmunization for children is recommended 2–5 years after initial immunization. Splenectomized adults should be revaccinated with the PPSV23 once after 5 years, whereas meningococcal revaccination should occur every 5 years. Recently, the Advisory Committee on Immunization Practices clarified recommendations that adult patients who are vaccine naive receive the pneumococcal conjugate vaccine (PCV13) followed 8 weeks later by the pneumococcal polysaccharide vaccine (PPSV23). Because these recommendations change with experience and vaccine use, it is wise to consult current guidelines for individual patients. The US Centers for Disease Control website should be consulted for the most up-to-date recommendations. Additional organisms to consider in postsplenectomy sepsis include *Escherichia coli*, *Pseudomonas aeruginosa*, and *Capnocytophaga canimorsus*.[29] There are fewer data on the efficacy of prophylactic antibiotics for asplenic patients, except for

TABLE 160.4	Incidence of Postsplenectomy Sepsis
Indication for Splenectomy	**Cumulative Incidence of Bacterial Sepsis (%)**
Trauma	1.5
Hematologic disorders	3.4
Portal hypertension	8.2
Hodgkin disease	10
Sickle cell disease	15
Thalassemia	25

Data from Gorse GJ: The relationship of the spleen to infection. In Bowlder AJ, editor: *The spleen: Structure, Function, and Clinical Significance*, New York, 1990, Van Nostrand Reinhold, p 269, with permission.

Vaccination of a Patient Scheduled for Elective Versus Emergent Splenectomy

A 50-year-old man with refractory ITP is scheduled for splenectomy. Having heard there is a risk for different types of infection after splenectomy, he asks about what he can do to reduce his risk.

- Patients scheduled for elective splenectomy should receive the following at least 14 days prior to the procedure:
  - *Streptococcus pneumoniae* vaccine
  - *Haemophilus influenzae* vaccine
  - *Neisseria meningitis* vaccine
  - Consider administration of the influenza vaccine as influenza is a risk factor for secondary bacterial infection.
- If the procedure is done emergently, wait at least until the 14th postoperative day.

young children with sickle cell disease, in whom antibiotics should be initiated as soon as the diagnosis is established. Present recommendations are that twice-daily oral penicillin V potassium or amoxicillin be continued in sickle cell patients until 5 years of age or 3 years postsplenectomy. High-risk patients with surgical or functional asplenia, including those with diagnoses of thalassemia, Hodgkin disease, other malignancies, immunodeficiency disease, or chronic graft-versus-host disease, should receive prophylactic antibiotics unless specific contraindications exist. Patients who have a history of pneumococcal postsplenectomy sepsis may be considered candidates for life-long daily prophylaxis as well. Whether or not such patients receive prophylactic antibiotics, and regardless of their immunization status, they may develop overwhelming infections with other organisms, including gram-negative organisms and *Staphylococcus aureus*. Some experts recommend that at the time of febrile illness, asplenic patients take immediate antibiotics at home before quickly traveling to an emergency room for evaluation. There are no randomized trials to guide therapy and experts have recommended the use of amoxicillin-clavulanate, cefuroxime axetil, or extended-spectrum fluoroquinolones. Updated recommendations should be consulted for specific circumstances.

The single most important measure to prevent postsplenectomy septicemia is education of the patient, family, and physician. Recognition of the risk, the institution of appropriate preventive measures, and the rapid administration of antibiotics to a patient who is showing signs of infection (fever and chills) can be lifesaving.

Atherosclerosis

The magnitude of the risk for development of atherosclerosis is not clear.[9,30] Appropriate preventive measures include identifying and minimizing concurrent risk factors, such as obesity, dietary patterns, a sedentary lifestyle, and the presence of other hereditary factors that would predispose to thrombosis. Low-dose aspirin could be considered, but no data exist regarding its efficacy in this situation.

CONCLUSIONS AND FUTURE DIRECTIONS

Although very little novel information has emerged about clinical aspects of splenic function in recent years, appreciation of many subtleties of splenic function and advances in supportive care in several fields have had significant impacts on the management of disorders of the spleen. Better education and more effective immunizations have helped prevent serious complications related to splenic disorders. Advances in imaging and surgery have transformed the diagnosis and management of congenital and traumatic splenic disorders.

Enhanced understanding of the complexity of communication interaction between the cells of the immune and hematopoietic system has improved our appreciation of the molecular, cellular, system, and network basis for clinical observations about splenic function. The ability of splenic macrophages, in concert with dendritic cells and B cells, to recognize and ingest a variety of microorganisms—even in patients without previous exposure to the pathogens—provides great insight into the reasons that the spleen provides protection against a variety of very specific infections. More detailed understanding of the impact of the splenic microenvironment on cellular functions, the role of stromal infrastructure on the ability of cells to interact with and respond to invading pathogens, and the integration of components of the immune system has contributed to an appreciation of clinical observations about the role the spleen plays in normal biology. The intersection of hematopoiesis, recycling of aging cells, and iron metabolism is most clearly demonstrated in the spleen.

Although not necessary to life under baseline circumstances, the contribution of the spleen to homeostasis under stress is considerable. Ongoing efforts to preserve and manage splenic function will continue to benefit from enhanced appreciation of the underlying biology.

REFERENCES

1. Weiss L: The spleen. In Weiss L, editor: *Cell, and Tissue Biology: a textbook of histology*, ed 6, Baltimore, 1988, Urban & Schwarzenberg, pp 515–538.
2. Kanzler B, Dear TN: Hox11 acts cell autonomously in spleen development and its absence results in altered cell fate of mesenchymal spleen precursors. *Dev Biol* 234:231–243, 2001.
3. Brendolan A, Rosado MM, Carsetti R, et al: Development and function of the mammalian spleen. *Bioessays* 29:166–177, 2007.
4. Mebius RE, Kraal G: Structure and function of the spleen. *Nat Rev Immunol* 5:606–616, 2005.
5. Junt T, Scandella E, Ludewig B: Form follows function: lymphoid tissue microarchitecture in antimicrobial immune defence. *Nat Rev Immunol* 8:764–775, 2008.
6. Dor FJ, Ramirez ML, Parmar K, et al: Primitive hematopoietic cell populations reside in the spleen: studies in the pig, baboon, and human. *Exp Hematol* 34:1573–1582, 2006.
7. van der Laan AM, Ter Horst EN, Delewi R, et al: Monocyte subset accumulation in the human heart following acute myocardial infarction and the role of the spleen as monocyte reservoir. *Eur Heart J* 35:376–385, 2014.
8. Grover SA, Barkun AN, Sackett DL: The rational clinical examination. Does this patient have splenomegaly? *JAMA* 270:2218–2221, 1993.
9. Ahmed S, Horton KM, Fishman EK: Splenic incidentalomas. *Radiol Clin North Am* 49:323–347, 2011.
10. Haan JM, Boswell S, Stein D, et al: Follow-up abdominal CT is not necessary in low-grade splenic injury. *Am Surg* 73:13–18, 2007.
11. Hackett S, Chua-anusorn W, Pootrakul P, et al: The magnetic susceptibilities of iron deposits in thalassaemic spleen tissue. *Biochim Biophys Acta* 1772:330–337, 2007.
12. Juweid ME, Stroobants S, Hoekstra OS, et al: Use of positron emission tomography for response assessment of lymphoma: consensus of the Imaging Subcommittee of International Harmonization Project in Lymphoma. *J Clin Oncol* 25:571–578, 2007.
13. Valette F, Querellou S, Oudoux A, et al: Comparison of positron emission tomography and lymphangiography in the diagnosis of infradiaphragmatic Hodgkin's disease. *Acta Radiol* 48:59–63, 2007.
14. Corazza GR, Ginaldi L, Zoli G, et al: Howell-Jolly body counting as a measure of splenic function. A reassessment. *Clin Lab Haematol* 12:269–275, 1990.
15. Connell NT, Brunner AM, Kerr CA, et al: Splenosis and sepsis: the born-again spleen provides poor protection. *Virulence* 2:4–11, 2011.
16. Yongxiang W, Zongfang L, Guowei L, et al: Effects of splenomegaly and splenic macrophage activity in hypersplenism due to cirrhosis. *Am J Med* 113:428–431, 2002.
17. Akpek G, Pasquini MC, Logan B, et al: Effects of spleen status on early outcomes after hematopoietic cell transplantation. *Bone Marrow Transplant* 48:825–831, 2013.
18. Mistry PK, Lukina E, Ben Turkia H, et al: Effect of oral eliglustat on splenomegaly in patients with Gaucher disease type 1: the ENGAGE randomized clinical trial. *JAMA* 313:695–706, 2015.
19. Vannucchi AM, Kiladjian JJ, Griesshammer M, et al: Ruxolitinib versus standard therapy for the treatment of polycythemia vera. *N Engl J Med* 372:426–435, 2015.
20. Buesing KL, Tracy ET, Kiernan C, et al: Partial splenectomy for hereditary spherocytosis: a multi-institutional review. *J Pediatr Surg* 46:178–183, 2011.
21. Al-Salem AH: Indications and complications of splenectomy for children with sickle cell disease. *J Pediatr Surg* 41:1909–1915, 2006.
22. Dodgion CM, Gosain A, Rogers A, et al: National trends in pediatric blunt spleen and liver injury management and potential benefits of an abbreviated bed rest protocol. *J Pediatr Surg* 49:1004–1008, discussion 8, 2014.
23. Mattioli G, Pini Prato A, Cheli M, et al: Italian multicentric survey on laparoscopic spleen surgery in the pediatric population. *Surg Endosc* 21:527–531, 2007.
24. Wluka A, Olszewski WL: Innate and adaptive processes in the spleen. *Ann Transplant* 11:22–29, 2006.

25. Kato T, Tzakis AG, Selvaggi G, et al: Transplantation of the spleen: effect of splenic allograft in human multivisceral transplantation. *Ann Surg* 246:436–444, discussion 45-6, 2007.

26. Grijalva CG, Nuorti JP, Arbogast PG, et al: Decline in pneumonia admissions after routine childhood immunisation with pneumococcal conjugate vaccine in the USA: a time-series analysis. *Lancet* 369:1179–1186, 2007.

27. Stephens DS: Conquering the meningococcus. *FEMS Microbiol Rev* 31:3–14, 2007.

28. Price VE, Blanchette VS, Ford-Jones EL: The prevention and management of infections in children with asplenia or hyposplenia. *Infect Dis Clin North Am* 21:697–710, viii–ix, 2007.

29. Di Sabatino A, Carsetti R, Corazza GR: Post-splenectomy and hyposplenic states. *Lancet* 378:86–97, 2011.

30. Troendle SB, Adix L, Crary SE, et al: Laboratory markers of thrombosis risk in children with hereditary spherocytosis. *Pediatr Blood Cancer* 49:781–785, 2007.

CHAPTER 161

HEMATOLOGY IN AGING

Andrew S. Artz and William B. Ershler

Although most classifications consider patients "older" once their age exceeds 65 or 70 years, age-related changes are not discrete. A central tenet of gerontology (the study of normal aging) is that biologic measures show increased variation with advancing age, but age-related variations are of insufficient magnitude to result in disease per se. Hematologic conditions in older adults have unique features and frequently require a modified approach relative to younger adults. Anemia in older adults with advancing age is one of the most common hematologic problems associated.

EPIDEMIOLOGY

Aging

The median life expectancy continues to rise throughout the world. In the United States, the Centers for Disease Control and Prevention estimates life expectancy at 77.9 years for children born in 2007. The proportion and absolute number of older adults is increasing, and life expectancy of adults who have reached an advanced age may be considerable. Accordingly, we advocate estimating life expectancy for older adults who have hematologic conditions, by using several calculators available online (e.g., http://eprognosis.ucsf.edu).[1]

Anemia Definition

Historically, criteria for diagnosing anemia in older and younger adults used by the World Health Organization (WHO) were hemoglobin (Hb) threshold levels below 13 g/dL for men and less than 12 g/dL for women.[2] It was widely recognized that these criteria required modification, and Beutler and Waalen[3] evaluated two large databases to develop population-based threshold levels, defining the fifth percentile as the lower limit of normal after excluding anemia-causing conditions, as shown in Table 161.1.

Anemia Prevalence

Most reports of anemia prevalence use the historical WHO threshold levels of less than 13 g/dL of Hb for men and less than 12 g/dL for women. For adults 65 years and older, the prevalence of anemia is around 10%–11% and rises to 20%–25% for those 85 years and older, and 50% for those in nursing homes.[4,5]

Race/ethnicity also influences anemia prevalence. Studies from Europe and Japan[4,6] indicate a fairly similar anemia prevalence in older adults, whereas African-Americans have lower median Hb values and a threefold higher prevalence of anemia.[5] A substantial portion of African-Americans with lower Hb levels have the α-thalassemia trait, with one or two deletions contributing to the degree of anemia.

Neutropenia and Thrombocytopenia

The incidence of thrombocytopenia, defined as a platelet count below 150×10^9/L, does not appreciably change with age with an average reduction of 19×10^9/L in those 70–90 years of age.[7,8] A study of Sardinian villages revealed an increasing incidence of thrombocytopenia with aging, approaching 6% in the seventh decade and 8% for octogenarians.[9] Interestingly, neutropenia (less than 1.5×10^9/L) appears less common with advancing age, such that the prevalence in community-dwelling older adults 75 years and older has been approximated at 0.5%.

PATHOBIOLOGY

Hematopoietic Changes With Aging

The study of older adults illustrates an overriding paradox, that although aging alone does not cause clinically significant cytopenias, aging predisposes to reduced hematopoietic reserves and to diseases, both of which increase the tendency to encounter significantly lower blood counts in older adults. Major hematopoietic changes occurring with aging are listed in Table 161.2.

The attention to the hematopoietic system must be understood in the context that organ systems are integrated to maintain homeostasis. For example, decreased bone mass and heightened systemic inflammation may adversely influence hematopoiesis. Whether hematopoietic perturbations are linked to a global decline or the factors promoting functional decline of marrow function cannot be easily deciphered. Reduced neutrophil responses to granulocyte colony-stimulating factors have long been appreciated as predisposing to infection with advancing age, but this occurs in the setting of a decline in immune function that occurs with aging.

Clonal Hematopoiesis and Aging

Myeloid bias has emerged as a hallmark of hematopoiesis and advancing.[10] Impairment of the lymphoid compartment may explain immune deficits that occur with aging, and at the same time, an increased number of myeloid progenitors likely influences the markedly higher rate of myeloid malignancies in older individuals. The discovery of several mutations involving *DNMT3A* and *TET2*, commonly found in preleukemic hematopoietic stem cells, has formed a critical link to understanding the pathway of hematopoietic changes associated with aging that result in hematologic malignancy.[11,12] The observation of *TET2* mutations in women with clonal hematopoiesis by X-chromosome inactivation lends support to the presence of a preleukemic state in the hematopoietic compartment in some older patients.[13]

A series of studies employing whole-exome sequencing have compellingly demonstrated a strong link of advancing age and the emergence of blood cell mutations associated with hematologic malignancies.[14-16] Specifically, 10% of individuals 70 years and older and up to 18% in those 90 years and older have clonal expansion of cells bearing these mutations, most frequently *DNMT3A* and *TET2*. The incidence of hematologic malignancies, particularly myeloid malignancies, rises about 10-fold in the presence of a detectable mutation.[15,16] However, screening for somatic mutations cannot be recommended, as even in older adults the rate of hematologic malignancy for those with evidence of clonal hematopoiesis is approximately 0.5%–1% per year.[15]

TABLE 161.1	Anemia Definitions
Group	**Hemoglobin (g/dL)**
Men, 60 Years or Older	
White	13.2
Black	12.7
Women, 50 Years or Older	
White	12.2
Black	11.5

Adapted from Beutler E, Waalen J: The definition of anemia: what is the lower limit of normal of the blood hemoglobin concentration? *Blood* 107:1747, 2006.

TABLE 161.2	Hematopoietic Changes Associated With Advancing Age

Diminished bone marrow cellularity
Reduced CD34⁺ cell mobilization to G-CSF administration in healthy donors
Decreased stem cell telomeres
Reduced hematopoietic cell proliferative capacity
Increased numbers of hematopoietic stem cells
Reduction in lymphocyte function
Reduced response to vaccination
Development of unexplained anemia

G-CSF, Granulocyte colony-stimulating factor.

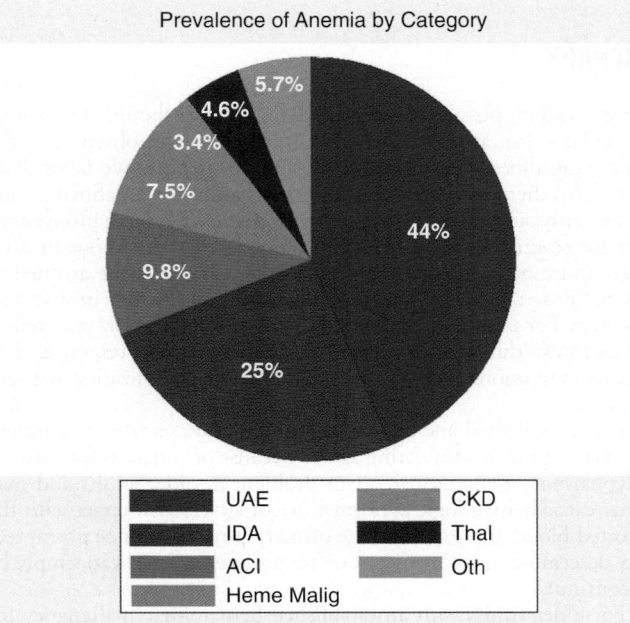

Prevalence of Anemia by Category

5.7%
4.6%
3.4%
7.5%
9.8%
25%
44%

Legend: UAE, IDA, ACI, Heme Malig, CKD, Thal, Oth

Fig. 161.1 CATEGORIZATION OF PRIMARY ANEMIA ETIOLOGY OR UNEXPLAINED ANEMIA IN THE ELDERLY IS SHOWN. Others include hemolysis, 4; alcohol, 3; hypothyroidism, 1; vitamin B_{12} deficiency, 1; medication, 1. *ACI*, Anemia of chronic inflammation; *CKD*, chronic kidney disease; *Heme Malig*, hematologic malignancy; *IDA*, iron-deficiency anemia; *Oth*, other; *Thal*, thalassemia trait. *(From Artz AS, Thirman MF: Unexplained anemia predominates despite an intensive evaluation in a racially diverse cohort of older adults from a referral anemia clinic. J Gerontol A Biol Sci Med Sci 66:925, 2011.)*

Anemia

Although anemia is not a normal finding in older adults, the prevalence increases markedly from the seventh decade to the ninth decade of life.[5] For the majority, anemia is related to an underlying cause such as iron deficiency/bleeding, chronic disease/inflammation, or renal insufficiency.[5] An intensive hematologic evaluation of anemia in older adults reveals a wider range of causes than previously appreciated, including 5%–10% with hematologic neoplasms.[17,18] Nevertheless 30%–40% of anemic adults lack a discernible cause despite a thorough investigation, and this has become commonly termed *unexplained anemia in the elderly* (Fig. 161.1). Our recommended approach for anemia in older adults differs from that for younger adults (see box on Evaluating Anemia in Older Adults). Unexplained anemia has been associated with somatic mutations by whole-exome sequencing.[16]

Evaluating Anemia in Older Adults

Anemia in older adults is a common finding and frequently results in a request for hematology consultation.

To define anemia, we apply the Beutler and Waalen criteria in Table 161.1 but also evaluate hemoglobin trajectories over time based on remote laboratory values when available. Based on the fact that the average hemoglobin level declines in older adults about 1 g/dL over 15 years or more,[19] we consider a decline of 1 g/dL in less than 5 years or 2 g/dL over 10 years significant, and this also supports the need to pursue a complete evaluation.

To elicit symptoms, both the patient and family members and caregivers are asked about functional changes (walking, naps, activity level) and the duration (weeks, months or years). Because the etiology of anemia can be multifactorial, we routinely perform the same panel on most patients: complete blood count, white blood cell differential, red blood cell indices, reticulocyte count, smear review, serum ferritin, serum iron, total iron-binding capacity, serum creatinine (and estimated renal function), vitamin B_{12}, and thyrotropin levels. Mean corpuscular volume is helpful but imperfect. We also have found high C-reactive protein (i.e., >10 mg/L) consistent with an inflammatory process and high serum erythropoietin (above the reference range) suspicious for iron deficiency, hematologic malignancy, or hyperproductive anemias. Folate levels are rarely useful in countries practicing universal dietary supplementation. The remainder of the laboratory tests will be performed as indicated.

A ferritin level of less than 50 ng/mL prompts a complete evaluation of the cause of iron deficiency. At a minimum, we embark on an oral iron trial and fecal guaiac tests for blood (not immunohistochemistry). We recommend endoscopic gastrointestinal evaluation generally, especially for more significant or unexplained iron deficiency and in individuals with a longer life expectancy. Other measures exist for diagnosing iron deficiency, such as reticulocyte hemoglobin concentration, serum transferrin receptor, or intravenous iron trials. We also empirically treat if vitamin B_{12} levels are below 200 pg/mL with oral vitamin B_{12} at 1000 µg for 8–12 weeks. If there is no response, we discontinue therapy.

A bone marrow examination follows if any of the following are present: unexplained requirement for red blood cell transfusion therapy, unexplained mean corpuscular volume of 97 fL or greater, thrombocytopenia below 120×10^9/L, neutropenia below 1000×10^9/L, or a suspicious peripheral smear. If the bone marrow is nondiagnostic and the sample adequate, we repeat the marrow examination at the time of clinical progression.

When the anemia has no established cause, a hemoglobin level less than 2 g below the age- and race-adjusted normal values above, and hemoglobin trajectory is stable, we follow up with blood cell counts every 6 months and then annually.

Leukopenia and Thrombocytopenia

The causes of thrombocytopenia and neutropenia are vast. Although the causes of cytopenias are not unique to older adults, the possibility of more than one cause should not be overlooked.

CLINICAL MANIFESTATIONS

In the industrialized countries, the detection of cytopenias is often encountered after routine laboratory testing or accompanies minor or nonspecific symptoms. Especially for anemia, one may not be able to disentangle anemia symptoms from other conditions that coexist or underlie the anemia (e.g., rheumatoid arthritis). Although fatigue may be the most obvious symptom of anemia, the potential signs and symptoms are protean. Patients frequently attribute fatigue to "growing old." Observational studies demonstrate a clear association between mild hemoglobin reduction (e.g., less than 14 g/dL for women and less than 15 g/dL for men) and reduced quality of life, strength, and mobility. Signs and symptoms may also direct one toward a cause, such as a pica suggesting iron deficiency or weight loss directing the clinician toward a systemic illness.

Specific hemoglobin thresholds do not permit one to validate symptoms because patients have different levels of reserve and organ function, pace of hemoglobin fall, and underlying causes for the anemia. A more rapid pace of hemoglobin decline is at least as important in provoking symptoms relative to anemia severity.

Neutropenia and Thrombocytopenia

Because of immune alterations associated with aging, one expects older adults at a given degree of neutropenia to suffer more infections and/or more serious infections. For example, not only do older adults have a greater probability of developing neutropenia, they also have a heightened risk for life-threatening complications.[20] Thrombocytopenia in older adults increases bleeding risks compared with younger adults, best illustrated in chronic autoimmune thrombocytopenic purpura.[21,22]

LABORATORY MANIFESTATIONS

Diagnosis

The use of age-adjusted norms remains quite controversial, because normal aging itself has only a small impact on normal values. For cytopenias, blood counts are mandatory for diagnosis, to establish severity, and to guide the etiologic evaluation. For anemia, we advocate applying the hemoglobin thresholds provided in Table 161.1. Thresholds to define neutropenia and thrombocytopenia should not differ from younger adults.

Laboratory Evaluation for Anemia

See box on Evaluating Anemia in Older Adults. Review of the blood smear can be enormously useful, if not simply to exclude a high-risk hematologic disorder.

Bone Marrow Evaluation

Although a bone marrow examination may be invaluable in excluding serious marrow-related conditions, all cytopenias in older adults do not warrant a bone marrow examination. We favor delaying bone marrow examination until recovery from acute events unless a high-grade hematologic malignancy that would warrant immediate treatment is suspected. Mild fluctuations of counts, particularly within the range found over years, without other evidence of a hematologic malignancy may allow one to safely defer a bone marrow examination. Metaphase cytogenetics and whole-exome sequencing mutational panels are routinely performed. Specific fluorescence in situ hybridization (FISH) panels can be considered based on the level of suspicion of a hematological malignancy.

DIFFERENTIAL DIAGNOSIS

It is important to distinguish true and clinically important findings from false or transiently low values by having serial blood counts and/or a review of the peripheral smear.

In addition to causes delineated in Table 161.3, other causes specific for anemia in older adults include unexplained iron deficiency/blood loss, hemolysis, and androgen deprivation.

PROGNOSIS

The underlying condition driving the hematologic abnormality usually dictates prognosis. Even a mildly low hemoglobin concentration is an independent adverse prognostic factor in older adult patients, even in those 85 years and older.

THERAPY

To the extent possible, the underlying illness should be treated. Particularly for anemia, the cause often remains obscure or the underlying illness may not be amenable to therapy. We favor diagnostic and therapeutic trials of iron or vitamins for a defined period of 3 months and discontinuing if ineffective. We reserve intravenous iron for severe anemia to avoid red blood cell transfusions or after clear failure of an adequate oral iron trial. One must be attuned to fluctuations, normal variation, or confounding factors in assessing response. For example, anemia following hospitalization may reflect phlebotomy, dilution, and an acute inflammatory response. The anemia may improve over months following hospitalization without therapy.

For unexplained anemia, caution should be exercised in employing erythropoiesis-stimulating agents because of concerns for toxicity. Polypharmacy remains a frequent problem in older adults and may either cause hematologic abnormalities or adversely interact with the detected blood abnormality. The primary physician, once prompted, may determine many medications are unnecessary and can simply be discontinued.

For older adults with an established hematologic malignancy for which aggressive therapy may be entertained, a detailed assessment may guide decision-making (see box on Assessment of Older Adults With Hematologic Malignancies).

FUTURE DIRECTIONS

The biology of aging is increasingly being better understood and may allow recognition of those at risk prior to overt malignancy. Although interventional trials among older persons remain challenging, the growing number of older and often relatively healthy adults mandates efforts to study older adults to define standards of clinical practice.

TABLE 161.3	Differential Diagnosis for Common Causes of Cytopenias in Older Adults

Cytopenia of one or more lineages
Hematologic neoplasm
Vitamin B_{12} deficiency
Autoimmune disorder
Consumptive coagulopathy
Systemic inflammation
Alcohol
Splenomegaly
Thyroid dysfunction
Human immunodeficiency virus

Assessment of Older Adults With Hematologic Malignancies

Optimal treatment for a hematologic condition in an older patient must be measured in terms of both efficacy and anticipated toxicity. Assessing the patient's reserve before treatment promotes tailoring treatment and provides an objective baseline assessment.

For all adults over 60 years, we screen for age-associated vulnerabilities. Cataloging comorbid conditions and assessing performance status (PS) plays a central role. PS alone provides only a crude estimate of tolerance to treatment. We find insufficient data to recommend a specific comorbidity tool or index. However, the Charlson comorbidity index or hematopoietic cell transplantation–comorbidity index have been validated in the context of certain diseases and their treatments, and thus may be invaluable in specific situations.

The PS and comorbidity index should be complemented by screening for other vulnerabilities, particularly in those older patients for whom intensive therapy is under consideration. Limitations in the following domains also suggest vulnerability:

- Instrumental activities of daily living, which are the skills required to live independently in the community (e.g., transportation, paying bills, shopping)
- Poor caregiver support
- Cognition
- Age 70 years and older

One should directly question patients about perceived problems for the recommended treatment. Patients will often relay difficulties not recognized by a standard medical examination (e.g., caring for an ill spouse, limited prescription coverage, and poor perceived health). More formal screening instruments are available and useful if familiarity can be achieved (e.g., Vulnerable Elders Survey-13).

Knowledge of disease response rates for older adults allows further individualization of treatment decisions. Responses to imatinib for chronic-phase chronic myeloid leukemia do not differ substantially by age, whereas acute myeloid leukemia induction results in lower responses, shorter disease-free survival, and greater toxicity relative to younger adults.

Although disease-based therapy exists along a spectrum, we generally divide therapy into low-intensity, intermediate-intensity, or high-intensity therapy. High-intensity treatment entails strategies such as AML induction and allogeneic hematopoietic stem cell transplantation owing to high rates of early death for patients with health limitations. We typically reserve high-intensity therapy for patients with a preserved PS and controlled comorbid conditions. We recommend that a patient with any vulnerability on screening undergo a more comprehensive geriatric assessment, if available, before curative-intent intensive therapy. Clinics focusing on issues and research in geriatric oncology are becoming available, and identifying experts (physician and nonphysician) in aging with an interest in oncology is invaluable. They often can connect patients with resources for specific problems (e.g., home care, transportation, financial help, assisted living).

Intermediate-intensity therapy such as CHOP (cyclophosphamide, hydroxydaunomycin, vincristine [Oncovin], and prednisone)-like regimens and fludarabine plus cyclophosphamide may produce manageable toxicity-related morbidity in older patients, but they remain efficacious and can be administered safely to those with a PS of 2 or better. Demethylating agents span the gap between low- and intermediate-intensity therapy. Low-intensity therapies, such as imatinib or supportive care alone, generally require only a reasonable nondisease life expectancy of more than a couple of months and can be given with an ECOG PS of 3 or less.

We strongly encourage a family meeting before initiating treatment at which goals and expectations are clearly discussed and support from all available caregivers enlisted. Not only will insights be gained into the available support system, but communicating to the entire team harmonizes goals for providers and patients alike. Standard guidelines for infectious disease prophylaxis and growth factor support should be supplemented with plans to address limitations found in the initial assessment.

REFERENCES

1. Cruz M, et al: Predicting 10-year mortality for older adults. *JAMA* 309(9):874–876, 2013.
2. World Health Organization: Nutritional anemias. Report of a WHO scientific group. *World Health Organ Tech Rep Ser* 405:5–37, 1968.
3. Beutler E, Waalen J: The definition of anemia: what is the lower limit of normal of the blood hemoglobin concentration? *Blood* 107(5):1747–1750, 2006.
4. Ferrucci L, et al: Unexplained anaemia in older persons is characterised by low erythropoietin and low levels of pro-inflammatory markers. *Br J Haematol* 136(6):849–855, 2007.
5. Guralnik JM, et al: Prevalence of anemia in persons 65 years and older in the United States: evidence for a high rate of unexplained anemia. *Blood* 104(8):2263–2268, 2004.
6. Ishine M, et al: No positive correlation between anemia and disability in older people in Japan. *J Am Geriatr Soc* 53(4):733–734, 2005.
7. Segal JB, Molterno AR: Platelet counts vary by ethnicity, sex, and age: analysis of NHANES III data. *Blood* Abstract 3937, 2004.
8. Nilsson-Ehle H, et al: Haematological abnormalities and reference intervals in the elderly. A cross-sectional comparative study of three urban Swedish population samples aged 70, 75 and 81 years. *Acta Med Scand* 224(6):595–604, 1988.
9. Biino G, et al: Analysis of 12,517 inhabitants of a Sardinian geographic isolate reveals that predispositions to thrombocytopenia and thrombocytosis are inherited traits. *Haematologica* 96(1):96–101, 2011.
10. Beerman I, et al: Functionally distinct hematopoietic stem cells modulate hematopoietic lineage potential during aging by a mechanism of clonal expansion. *Proc Natl Acad Sci USA* 107(12):5465–5470, 2010.
11. Jan M, et al: Clonal evolution of preleukemic hematopoietic stem cells precedes human acute myeloid leukemia. *Sci Transl Med* 4(149):149ra118, 2012.
12. Shlush LI, et al: Identification of pre-leukaemic haematopoietic stem cells in acute leukaemia. *Nature* 506(7488):328–333, 2014.
13. Busque L, et al: Recurrent somatic TET2 mutations in normal elderly individuals with clonal hematopoiesis. *Nat Genet* 44(11):1179–1181, 2012.
14. Xie M, et al: Age-related mutations associated with clonal hematopoietic expansion and malignancies. *Nat Med* 20(12):1472–1478, 2014.
15. Genovese G, et al: Clonal hematopoiesis and blood-cancer risk inferred from blood DNA sequence. *N Engl J Med* 371(26):2477–2487, 2014.
16. Jaiswal S, et al: Age-related clonal hematopoiesis associated with adverse outcomes. *N Engl J Med* 371(26):2488–2498, 2014.
17. Artz AS, Thirman MJ: Unexplained Anemia Predominates Despite an Intensive Evaluation in a Racially Diverse Cohort of Older Adults From a Referral Anemia Clinic. *J Gerontol A Biol Sci Med Sci* 66(8):925–932, 2011.
18. Price EA, et al: Anemia in older persons: etiology and evaluation. *Blood Cells Mol Dis* 46(2):159–165, 2011.
19. Ershler WB, et al: Serum erythropoietin and aging: a longitudinal analysis. *J Am Geriatr Soc* 53(8):1360–1365, 2005.
20. Klastersky J, et al: The Multinational Association for Supportive Care in Cancer risk index: a multinational scoring system for identifying low-risk febrile neutropenic cancer patients. *J Clin Oncol* 18(16):3038–3051, 2000.
21. Cortelazzo S, et al: High risk of severe bleeding in aged patients with chronic idiopathic thrombocytopenic purpura. *Blood* 77(1):31–33, 1991.
22. Cohen YC, et al: The bleeding risk and natural history of idiopathic thrombocytopenic purpura in patients with persistent low platelet counts. *Arch Intern Med* 160(11):1630–1638, 2000.

INDEX

Page numbers followed by "*f*" indicate figures, "*t*" indicate tables, "*b*" indicate boxes, and "*e*" indicate online content.

A

A5R assay. *See* Annexin A5 resistance assay
ABC transporters. *See* ATP binding cassette transporters
ABCD2 scoring system, 2137
Abciximab
  for acute coronary syndromes, 2146–2147, 2146*t*
  overview of, 2172–2173, 2172*t*
  platelet disorders and, 1935
  thrombocytopenia and, 1966
Abelson-related (ABL)-class kinase genes, 89–90, 840–841, 1051, 1056. *See also* BCR-ABL fusion gene
Abetalipoproteinemia, 641–642
ABH blood group system, 1694–1695, 1694*f*, 1717
ABL genes. *See* Abelson-related class kinase genes
ABO blood group system, 1692, 1694–1695, 2055
ABO incompatibility, 1538–1539
Absolute leukocyte count, e8*b*
Abt-199, 872
ABVD (adriamycin, bleomycin, vinblastine, dacarbazine), 1220–1221, 1220*t*
Acanthocytes (spur cells), 641, 643, 668
Acanthocytosis, 626, 640–641, 640*f*, 643
ACE910, 1774
Acenocuomarol, 593
Acetylation, 47, 104
Acetylcholinesterase (AChE), 416
Acetyl-CoA, 75
N-Acetylglucosamyl-1-phosphotransferase, 740
Acid sphingomyelinase (ASM), 742. *See also* Niemann-Pick type A and B diseases
Aclarubicin, 860
ACNU, 855
Aconitase, 493
Acquired B antigen, 1695
Acquired hemophilia A, 2018
Acquired immunodeficiency syndrome (AIDS), 2262. *See also* Human immunodeficiency virus infection
Acquired platelet disorders
  antiplatelet antibodies and, 1942–1943
  antiplatelet drugs and, 1932–1939
  extracorporeal circuits and, 1942
  hypothermia and, 1942
  leukemias, myelodysplastic syndromes and, 1940
  overview of, 439–441, 439*f*, 1932
  solid tumors and, 1940
  systemic metabolic disorders and, 1941–1942
Acquired platelet dysfunction with eosinophilia, 1943
Acquired von Willebrand syndrome, 2060
Actin, 1861–1863, 1866–1868, 1866*f*, 1874–1875
Actinomycin D, 880
Activated B-cell-like (ABC) diffuse large cell lymphoma, 835–837, 1192, 1233*f*, 1234, 1309, 1314
Activated partial thromboplastin time (aPTT)
  in neonates, 2189, 2195
  overview of, 1897, 1923, 1926–1927, 1927*t*, 2093, e12*b*
  prolonged, 2195
Activated protein C (aPC)
  concentrated for disseminated intravascular coagulation, 2074
  disseminated intravascular coagulation and, 2066–2067, 2074
  hemostasis and, 1909
  HIV infection and, 2275–2276
  overview of, 2078
  protein C pathway and, 2078
Activated prothrombin complex concentrates (APCC), 2029–2030, 2032
Activated T lymphocytes, 1568–1569
Activating transcription factor 6 (ATF6), 55, 195
Activation-induced cytidine deaminase (AID), 204–205, 219, 235, 236*f*, 687–688, 722–723, 1265, 1656–1657

Active immunotherapy, defined, 1568
Activin, 70
Acupuncture, 1475, 2254, 2256–2257
Acute coronary syndromes (ACS)
  anticoagulant therapy for, 2147–2150, 2148*t*
  antiplatelet therapy for, 2144–2147, 2145*t*–2146*t*
  antithrombotic therapies for, 2142
  classification of, 2142
  future directions, 2150–2151
  intravenous antiplatelet drugs for, 2146–2147, 2146*t*
  overview of, 2142, 2150–2151
  pathophysiology of, 2142
  reperfusion therapy for, 2142–2144
  sickle cell disease and, 581, 600
  triple therapy for, 2150*t*, 2151*b*
Acute eosinophilic leukemia (AEL), 1162–1163, 1162*t*
Acute hemolytic anemia (AHA), 86*t*, 87–88, 88*f*, 2215–2216
Acute hepatic cell crisis, 601
Acute hepatic porphyria, 498*f*, 503
Acute hepatic sequestration crisis, 601
Acute hyperleukocytic leukemia (AHL), 1781
Acute intermittent porphyria (AIP)
  differential diagnosis for, 503*b*
  genetics of, 499
  management of, 503*b*
  overview of, 498*f*, 502, 502*f*
Acute lymphoblastic leukemia (ALL)
  in adolescents and young adults, 1047–1049
  in adults
    allogeneic stem transplant in first complete remission, 1041–1042, 1042*t*–1043*t*
    autologous stem cell transplant for, 1042
    Burkitt lymphoma (BL). *See* Burkitt lymphoma
    central nervous system disease and, 1040, 1040*f*
    clinical and laboratory evaluation, 1029–1030
    clinical manifestations, 1029
    cytochemical evaluation, 1032, 1032*f*
    cytogenetics and molecular genetics, 1032–1035, 1033*f*, 1033*t*–1034*t*
    diagnostic approach, 1030, 1030*t*
    differential diagnosis, 1035
    epidemiology, 1029
    etiology, 1029
    immunophenotype, 1032, 1032*t*
    induction therapy, 1037–1039
    maintenance therapy, 1040–1041
    minimal residual disease and, 1035–1037
    morphologic evaluation, 1030–1032, 1031*f*
    novel therapies, 1050–1052
    Philadelphia chromosome-positive, 1042–1046, 1044*t*–1045*t*
    postremission therapy, 1039–1040
    prognosis, 1035, 1036*t*
    survivorship, 1053
    treatment approach, 1037, 1038*t*, 1042–1046
  allogeneic HSCT for, 1604–1605
  B-cell. *See* B-cell acute lymphoblastic leukemia
  BCR-ABL1-like, 89–90, 819–821, 1014
  childhood
    clinical manifestations, 1021–1023, 1021*t*
    differential diagnosis, 1023
    epidemiology, 1020–1021
    future directions, 1028
    late effects of treatment, 1027–1028
    pathobiology, 1021
    prognosis, 1023–1025, 1024*t*
    relapse, 1026–1027
    supportive care, 1027
    therapy, 1025–1026, 1026*b*
  complex and monosomal karyotype, 821
  cytogenetics of, 815–822
  genetic testing for, 822*b*

Acute lymphoblastic leukemia (ALL) *(Continued)*
  MP dosage adjustment, TPMT genotype and, 84
  natural killer cells and, 1577
  in older adults, 1049
  overview of, 1020
  pathobiology of
    chemotherapy resistance mechanisms and novel therapeutic targets, 1018
    clonal origin, 1005
    genetic basis, 1006*f*–1007*f*, 1007–1018
    lineage-specific features of lymphoblasts, 1005–1007
  pathogenesis of, 821–822
  pharmacogenomics and drug development for, 89–90
  prognostic cytogenetic categories in, 817*f*, 818*t*
  rearranged MLL gene and novel therapies for, 89
  relapsed, 1049–1050
  second/subsequent malignancies after, 1503, 1505, 1505*t*
  somatic mutations in, 821
  stem cell origin of, 114–115
  T-cell. *See* T-cell acute lymphoblastic leukemia
Acute megakaryocytic leukemia (AMKL), 343–344, 344*f*, 813, 985–986
Acute monoblastic leukemia, 929*f*
Acute myeloid leukemia 1 protein (AML1). *See* Runt-related transcription factors
Acute myeloid leukemias (AML)
  with abnormal karyotype, 800–813, 802*t*
  after hematopoietic stem cell transplantation, 1679
  allogeneic hematopoietic stem cell transplantation for
    guidelines based on cytogenic and molecular markers, 972*t*
    haploidentical donor, 974
    indications for, 1604
    matched related donor, 970–973, 971*t*
    older adults and, 974–975
    prognosis, 975*f*
    relapse rate after, 975
    relapsed, refractory, and induction-failure acute disease and, 974
    therapy-related and secondary disease and, 974
    umbilical cord blood, 974
    unrelated donor, 973
  biology of, 920–921
  central nervous system and, 942
  in childhood
    clinical and laboratory manifestations and diagnosis, 987–989, 988*t*
    epidemiology, 981
    future directions, 991–992
    pathobiology, 981–987
    supportive care, 990–991
    therapy, 989–990
  clinical and laboratory manifestations of, 925, 987–989
  clonal origin of, 783–784, 921, 981–982
  commonly altered cellular pathways in, 922*f*
  with complex karyotype, 814–815
  cytogenetics of, 798–815, 986–987
  detection of genetic abnormalities in, 813–814
  diagnosis and classification of, 765–767, 766*t*, 925–931, 926*f*–931*f*, 927*t*
  disseminated intravascular coagulation and, 2069
  Down syndrome-associated, 343–344, 344*f*, 813, 985–986
  epidemiology of, 924, 981
  etiology of, 913–915
  future directions, 921, 922*f*, 942, 991–992
  gain or loss of chromosomes in, 813
  genetic and epigenetic alterations in, 915–920, 916*f*, 918*f*
  genetic testing for, 815*b*
  hematopoietic microenvironment in, 123–125
  hyperleukocytosis and, 941
  modification of ELN prognostic system in, 801*t*

Acute myeloid leukemias (AML) *(Continued)*
  molecular diagnostics in, 921*b*
  myelodysplastic syndromes and, 953–954, 994, 995*f*
  myeloid sarcoma and, 941–942
  natural killer cells and, 1577–1581
  neutrophil differentiation and, 321, 329
  with normal karyotype, 799–800
  overview of, 913, 924, 970
  pathobiology of, 924–925, 981, 984*f*
  p-glycoprotein and, 881
  phenotype of, 913
  polyclonal gammopathy and, 688
  post-polycythemia vera, 1088–1089, 1092, 1103–1104
  pregnancy and, 942, 2209
  prognosis in, 931–933, 932*f*, 932*t*, 936*t*, 988–989,
    988*t*
  retinoic acid receptor rearrangements and, 915–916
  RUNX1 and, 345–346
  second/subsequent malignancies after, 1505–1506,
    1505*t*–1506*t*
  stem cell origin of, 111–112, 113*b*
  supportive care, 988*t*
  therapy for
    in children, 988–989, 991*b*
    genetic and cytogenetic considerations, 933–939
    induction therapy, 934–936
    investigational therapy, 938–939
    maintenance therapy, 938
    postremission therapy, 936–938
    salvage therapy, 938
  therapy-related. *See* Therapy-related acute myeloid
    leukemia
Acute pain crisis, 593–595, 594*t*
Acute panmyelosis with myelofibrosis (APMF),
  1138–1139
Acute Physiology and Chronic Evaluation (APACHE) II
  scores, 2064, 2071
Acute promyelocytic leukemia (APL)
  in children, 984–985
  cytogenetics of, 805
  disseminated intravascular coagulation and, 2069
  epigenetic alterations in, 929*f*, 939–941
  miRNA and, 329–330
Acute yellow atrophy (AFLP), 2208
Acyclovir, 1673–1674
Acyl-CoA cholesterol acyltransferase (ACAT), 2123
ADAM family, 136–138, 2129
ADAMTS family, 2129
ADAMTS13
  deficiency in, 1786, 1986–1988
  disseminated intravascular coagulation and, 2070
  fragmentation hemolysis and, 663–665
  fresh frozen plasma and, 1744
  hemostasis and, 1909
  malaria and, 2283
  thrombotic microangiopathies and, 1999
  thrombotic thrombocytopenic purpura and,
    1985–1988, 1985*f*, 1987*f*
  tolerance, immunity and, 285
  von Willebrand factor and, 2053*f*, 2054–2055
Adapter molecules, 448
Adaptive immune system
  cells of, 202–203
  complement system and, 268
  dendritic cells and, 255*f*
  innate immune system vs., 200*t*
  myelodysplastic syndromes and, 953
  natural killer cells and, 242–243
  overview of concept, 200
  priming of, 199–200
  self-reactive lymphocytes and, 285–290
  spleen and, 2317–2318
Adaptive natural killer cells, 1575, 1576*f*, 1579
Additional sex combs-like (ASXL), 804, 919, 950, 1129
Addressins, 1844–1845
Adducins, 448, 1866*f*, 1868
Adhesion. *See* Cell adhesion
Adhesion and degranulation-promoting adapter protein
  (ADAP), 225
Adhesion molecules. *See* Cell adhesion molecules

Adipocytes, 121
Adjuvant analgesics, overview of, 1480
Adoptive cell therapies
  cord blood stem cell transplantation and, 1648
  for EBV-related malignancies, 757–758
  mesenchymal stromal cells and, 1564–1565
  with natural killer cells, 1579–1581, 1580*f*
  with T lymphocytes, 1568–1569
  for virus independent malignancies, 1570
  for virus-associated malignancies, 1569
  with virus-specific cytotoxic T lymphocytes, 1569
ADP receptor antagonists, 2170–2171
ADP ribosylation factors (Arf), 57, 219
β₂-Adrenergic receptor, 65, 65*f*
Adriamycin. *See* Doxorubicin
Adult T-cell leukemia/lymphoma (ATL)
  differential diagnosis for, 1368, 1368*f*
  human T-lymphotropic virus-1 and, 1323–1324
  overview of, 1188*t*, 1196*b*, 1197
Adventitia, 1843
Adventitious agents, 1532–1533
Aerolysin assays, 420
Affinity maturation, 204–205, 219, 289
Afibrinogenemia. *See* Fibrinogen deficiency
African trypanosomiasis, 2292–2296, 2293*f*
Afuresertib, 864
AG-348, 621
Aggregation
  disorders of, 1882–1883
  essential thrombocythemia and, 1110
  laboratory evaluation of, 1879–1880, 1879*t*, 1880*b*
  molecular basis of, 1878–1880
Aggregometry
  impedance, 1928
  light-transmission, 1879–1880, 1879*t*, 1928
  lumi, 1879
  overview of, 1878–1880, 1880*b*, 1928, e14*b*
  whole-blood, 1879
Aggressive epidermotropic CD8+ T-cell lymphoma, 1367
Aggressive natural killer cell leukemia, 1200
Aggressive systemic mastocytosis (ASM), 1174–1175,
  1174*t*, 1177*f*
Aging and hematologic disorders
  clinical manifestations of, 1348, 2330
  differential diagnosis for, 1351–1355, 1357*t*, 2330,
    2330*t*
  epidemiology of, 1343–1360, 2328
  future directions for, 1352–1354, 2330
  laboratory manifestations of, 1348, 2330
  pathobiology of, 1346, 2328–2329
  prognosis for, 1351–1352, 2330
  therapy for, 1352, 2330
Agranulocytosis, 432, 432*t*, 677–680
AIDS primary central nervous system lymphoma (AIDS
  PCNSI), 1325–1327
AIM-1 kinase. *See* Aurora-B kinase
Air emboli, posttransfusion, 1799
Ajoene, 1939
Akt (protein kinase B), 225–226, 864
ALA dehydratase deficiency porphyria, 498*f*, 503
Albumin
  adverse effects of, 1753
  dosage, 1753
  indications for, 1751–1753, 1751*t*
  overview of, 1751, 1761
Alcohol, 510–511, 2258
Aldolase deficiency, 622
Alemtuzumab
  for acute lymphoblastic leukemia, 1051
  for chronic lymphocytic leukemia, 1256–1257
  for cutaneous T-cell lymphomas, 1377
  for hairy cell leukemia, 1273
  for hypereosinophilic syndrome, 1167
  for myelodysplastic syndromes, 965
  for pure red cell aplasia, 430
Alisertib, 1359
Alkylating agents
  acute myeloid leukemia and, 913
  bendamustine, 856
  for chronic lymphocytic leukemia, 1253–1254
  clinical pharmacology of, 885–889
  for extranodal marginal zone lymphoma of MALT type,
    1282
  for follicular lymphoma, 1294
  leukemias induced by, 856
  mechanism of resistance, 854
  methylating agents, 855–856
  for multiple myeloma, 1403–1404

Alkylating agents *(Continued)*
  nitrogen mustards, 854–855
  nitrosoureas, 855
  overview of, 853–854, 854*f*
  thrombocytopenia and, 442
  for Waldenström macroglobulinemia, 1426
ALL-96 regimen, 1047*t*, 1049–1050
Allelic exclusion, 212, 227–228, 275
Allergic reactions, 1717, 1749, 1795–1796, 1796*b*
Alloantibodies. *See also* Factor IX inhibitors; Factor VIII
    inhibitors
  neonatal alloimmune thrombocytopenia and, 1945*t*,
    1950–1952
  posttransfusion purpura and, 1945*t*, 1953–1954
Alloantigens, 1664
Allodepleted cells, 1544
Allogenic hematopoietic stem cell transplantation
  for acute lymphoblastic leukemia, 1026, 1041–1042,
    1604–1605
  for acute myeloid leukemias
    guidelines based on cytogenic and molecular markers,
      972*t*
    haploidentical donor, 974
    indications for, 1604
    matched related donor, 970–973, 971*t*
    older adults and, 974–975
    prognosis, 975*f*
    relapse rate after, 975
    relapsed, refractory, and induction-failure acute
      disease and, 974
    therapy-related and secondary disease and, 974
    umbilical cord blood, 974
    unrelated donor, 973
  autologous transplantation vs., 1533
  checkpoint blockade therapies and, 1585
  for chronic lymphocytic leukemia, 1259–1260,
    1605–1606
  for chronic myelogenous leukemia, 1066–1069, 1605
  clinical research in, 1604
  conditioning regimens for, 1596–1597, 1598*f*, 1598*t*
  congenital erythropoietic porphyria and, 504
  for cutaneous T-cell lymphomas, 1375
  cytogenetics and, 845–846
  for diffuse large B-cell lymphoma, 1606
  diffuse large B-cell lymphoma and, 1316
  donor selection in, 1517, 1518*b*, 1591–1592, 1592*t*,
    1598–1600
  in first remission acute myeloid leukemia, 982*b*
  for follicular lymphoma, 1297, 1606
  graft failure and, 1675–1676
  graft sources, 1597–1598
  graft versus malignancy effects, 1600
  haploidentical. *See* Haploidentical hematopoietic stem
    cell transplantation
  for Hodgkin lymphoma, 1224–1225, 1606
  for hypereosinophilic syndrome, 1168
  long-term survival after, 1604, 1605*b*
  for mantle cell lymphoma, 1305–1306, 1606
  for mastocytosis, 1184–1185
  mechanisms of action, 1575, 1579–1581
  for multiple myeloma, 1409–1411, 1606
  for myelodysplastic syndromes
    clinical results in myeloablative transplantation, 976
    clinical results in reduced-intensity conditioning
      transplantation, 976
    comorbidity and conditioning intensity selection
      before, 978–979
    contemporary results, 976
    myeloablative vs. reduced intensity regimens,
      976–977
    overview, 967–968
    prognostic models for role and timing of, 977–978
  natural killer cells and, 244, 245*f*
  overview of, 970, 1591, 1596, 1617
  for paroxysmal nocturnal hemoglobinuria, 422
  patient population, 1596
  for peripheral T-cell lymphomas, 1356–1357
  for Philadelphia chromosome-positive acute
    lymphoblastic leukemia, 1046
  for primary myelofibrosis, 1145–1146, 1147*f*
  primary myelofibrosis and, 1131, 1141–1142
  prognostic factors, 1600–1604, 1601*f*–1602*f*,
    1602*b*–1603*b*
  pure red cell aplasia and, 428
  red blood cell transfusions and, 1706
  second/subsequent malignancies and, 1502–1503
  selection of product used in, 1518*b*
  sources of stem cells used in, 1593

Allogenic hematopoietic stem cell transplantation (Continued)
  for T-cell lymphoma, 1606
  umbilical cord blood
    adaptive immunotherapy, 1648
    double unit, 1635–1638, 1637t
    double vs. single unit, 1640–1645
    future directions, 1648
    novel strategies to enhance engraftment, 1645–1648, 1646t
    overview, 1633
    single unit, 1633–1635, 1636t
    unit selection, 1639–1640, 1639f
  from unrelated donor
    clinical importance of donor HLA matching, 1612–1613, 1612t
    donor evaluation and selection, 1608–1609
    donor identification and likelihood of transplantation, 1608
    future directions, 1615
    graft failure and, 1676
    haploidentical hematopoietic stem cell transplantation vs., 1629
    HLA expression level and, 1614–1615
    HLA haplotype assessment, 1611–1612, 1612b
    HLA typing methods and, 1610–1611
    HLA-matched, 1613
    identification of suitable, 1609–1610
    major histocompatibility complex resident variation, 1615
    single-locus mismatched, 1613–1614
    vector of mismatching assessment, 1611, 1611t
  for Waldenström macroglobulinemia, 1429
Allograft transplantation, T cell modulation and, 237
Alloimmune neonatal neutropenia, 1735–1736, 1735t
Alloimmune thrombocytopenia. See Neonatal alloimmune thrombocytopenia
Alloimmunization
  blood groups and, 1693, 1693t, 1696
  human leukocyte antigens and, 1725, 1730–1731
  leukocyte-reduced red blood cells and, 1703
  platelet refractoriness and, 1718, 1719t
  red blood cells and, 1709–1710
Allopurinol, 1027
Alloreactivity
  after allogenic hematopoietic stem cell transplantation, 1618–1621
  of donor natural killer cells, 1578, 1580f, 1581
  hematopoietic stem cell transplants and, 1591–1593
Allosensitization testing, 1735
Allotypic variation, 275–276
All-trans retinoic acid (ATRA)
  acute myeloid leukemia and, 804
  for acute promyelocytic leukemia, 940–941, 940f
  acute promyelocytic leukemia and, 984–985
  for cutaneous T-cell lymphomas, 1376
  for myelodysplastic syndromes, 966
  pregnancy and, 2209
Alpha Hb stabilizing protein (AHSP), 455
Alpha heavy chain disease. See Immunoproliferative small intestinal disease
Alphanate, 1776–1777, 2013
Alphanine, 1765, 1775
Alpharetroviruses, 1551–1552
Alprolix, 1765, 1775, 2013
Alteplase, 2143, 2143t, 2179, 2186f
Alternative pathway (AP) of complement system, 262f, 263–264, 264t, 1993, 1994f
Alternative splicing, 8, 20–21, 1385
Altitude, polycythemia and, 1076–1078
Alveolar hemorrhage, 1678
AMD11070, 1052
Amegakaryocytic thrombocytopenia with radio-ulnar snyostosis (ATRUS), 1883
American Association of Blood Banks (AABB), 1537–1538
American trypanosomiasis, 2296–2299, 2296f
AMG5.31. See Romiplostim
Amidopyrine, 400
Amifostine, 997b
Amino acids
  catabolism of, 76
  genetic code for, 7, 7t
  metabolism and, 75–76
  metabolomics of, 77
  protein structure and, 59–66, 60f
Aminoacridine resistance, 880
Aminobisphosphonates, 1415

9-Aminocampothecin (9-AC), 1374
ε-Aminocaproic acid (EACA), 1775–1776, 2030–2031, 2038, 2039b, 2074, 2306–2307
5-Aminolevulinate (ALA), 497–499, 498f
5-Aminolevulinate dehydratase (ALAD), 503
5-Aminolevulinate synthetase (ALAS), 497–500, 506–508
AML-1. See RUNX1
AMN107, 1064
Amnionless (AMN), 515, 532
Amniotic fluid embolism, 2069, 2208
Amodiaquine, 2287
Amoebiasis, 2302
Amotosalen/UVA, 1808b
Amphipathic amino acids, 59
Amphotericin B, 1937
AMPK. See Adenosine monophosphate-activated protein kinase
Amygdalin, 2254
Amyloid light chain amyloidosis. See Immunoglobulin light chain amyloidosis
Amyloidosis
  fibrinogen gene and, 2039
  localized, 1437
  multiple myeloma and, 1392
  nomenclature of, 1436t
  overview of, 1432, 1433f
  primary. See Immunoglobulin light chain amyloidosis
  systemic, 1437–1438
Anaesthetic techniques, 1475
Anagrelide
  for essential thrombocythemia, 1119–1120, 1119f
  for polycythemia vera, 1101
Analgesics
  adjuvant, 1480
  opioid. See Opioid analgesics
  pain management and, 1475–1480, 1476f
  for sickle cell disease, 594, 594t
Anaphase, 176–177, 177f, 182
Anaphase-promoting complex (APC), 181, 342–343
Anaphylactic reactions, 1182, 2017–2018
Anaphylactoid purpura, 2221–2222
Anaplastic large cell lymphoma (ALCL)
  ALK-negative, 1188t, 1198, 1346–1347
  ALK-positive, 1188t, 1197–1198, 1198f, 1346
  ALK-positive B cell, 1194, 1194f
  in childhood, 1336–1338, 1337f
  clinical manifestations of, 1336–1337
  diagnosis and differential diagnosis for, 1337
  epidemiology of, 1336
  overview of, 771, 1343
  pathobiology of, 1336, 1336f
  primary cutaneous, 1188t, 1198
  prognosis/staging for, 1337, 1337t
  therapy for, 1337–1338, 1352
Anaplastic lymphoma kinase (ALK), 865, 1351
Anderson Cancer Center unit selection criteria, 1639–1640, 1639f
Androgens, 359, 364, 368, 412–413, 1080
Anemia of chronic disease (ACD)
  biology and molecular aspects, 492–493
  description and epidemiology, 491
  diagnosis, 493–494, 493b, 494f
  etiology and pathogenesis, 491–492, 492f
  future directions, 495
  treatment, 493–494, 494b
Anemias
  in adults, 461–462, 462f
  after solid organ transplant in children, 2228–2231
  aging and, 1344–1351, 1344t, 1345f, 1355b, 2328–2330, 2329b, 2329f, 2329t
  aplastic. See Aplastic anemia
  bone marrow examination and, 464, 465f
  in children, 460–461, 461f, 461t, 2215
  clinical assessment and, 1916
  complete blood count and, 460t, 463–464
  defined, 458
  future directions, 464b
  hemolytic. See Hemolytic anemia
  history and physical examination, 462–463
  HIV infection and, 2266b, 2269–2270, 2271t
  hypoproliferative, 458–462, 461t
  immunosuppressive drugs and, 2230
  infectious disease and, 645–646, 751–752
  inherited bone marrow syndromes with, 372–385
  kidney disease and, 2244
  lead poisoning and, 2233–2234
  liver disease and, 2238
  malarial. See Malaria

Anemias (Continued)
  malignancies and, 2247–2248
  mean corpuscular volume and, 460t, 463–464, 464t
  mechanisms of, 458–459
  megaloblastic. See Megaloblastic anemias
  multiple myeloma and, 1391
  myelodysplastic syndromes and, 955–956, 956f
  paroxysmal nocturnal hemoglobinuria and, 421, 423
  peripheral blood smear and, 464, 465f, 466t
  pernicious, 531, 531f
  pregnancy and, 2203–2205
  primary myelofibrosis and, 1142–1143
  red blood cell distribution width and, 460t, 463–464, 464t
  red blood cell transfusions and, 1704
  reticulocyte count and, 460t, 463, 464t
  sickle cell. See Sickle cell disease
  sideroblastic. See Sideroblastic anemias
  spur cell hemolytic of severe liver disease, 641, 641f, 668–669
  systemic approach to diagnosis, 464b
  thalassemia syndromes. See Thalassemia syndromes
Anergy, 233
Angioblasts, 1845
Angiogenesis
  mechanisms triggering, 159
  overview of, 152, 157f, 158, 1846–1849
  for peripheral artery disease, 2166
  therapeutic implications in hematology, 159–161, 160t, 161f
Angiogenesis inhibitors, 156, 1849
Angiogenesis stimulators, 156
Angiogenesis-related diseases, defined, 159
Angiogenic sprouting, 156f–157f, 158
Angioimmunoblastic T-cell lymphoma (AITL)
  overview of, 771, 1188t, 1196–1197, 1197f, 1343, 1346f
  pathobiology of, 843, 1345–1346
  therapy for, 1354–1355
AngioJet Rheolytic Thrombectomy System, 2115–2117
Angiopoietin-like (Angptl) proteins, 106
Angiopoietins, 154, 1847f, 1848
Angiotensins, 1073–1074, 1078, 1853
AngioVac device, 2114–2115
Ankle-brachial index (ABI), 2159, 2161, 2162f
Ankyrin, 448, 627–628, 630
Ann Arbor Staging System
  for follicular lymphoma, 1290, 1290t
  for Hodgkin lymphoma, 1339
  for lymphomas, 1311, 1311t
Annexin A5 resistance (A5R) assay, 2094, 2096f
Annexins, 1266–1268, 2088–2089, 2091f
Anorexia nervosa, 2225
Anthracenedione resistance, 880
Anthracyclines
  for acute lymphoblastic leukemia, 1037–1039
  for acute myeloid leukemia, 913, 934–936, 934f
  cardiomyopathy and, 1496–1497
  for mastocytosis, 1184
  resistance to, 880
Antiangiogenesis, 159, 160t, 161
Anti-antithrombin antibodies, 2019–2020, 2019t
Antiarrhythmic drugs, 2154–2155
Anti-β₂ glycoprotein I antibodies, 1926, 2094
Antibodies
  blood groups and, 1687–1691
  Epstein-Barr virus and, 749–750, 750t
  as immunoglobulins, 272–273
  natural, complement cascade and, 268
Antibody therapy. See Immunotherapy
Antibody-dependent cellular cytotoxicity (ADCC), 240, 244, 1575
Anticardiolipin antibodies (aCL), 1926, 2080–2081, 2093–2094, 2276
Anti-CD20 antibody, 1256, 1256b
Anti-CD33 antibody, 991
Anticipatory nausea and vomiting (ANV), 1483, 1485
Anticoagulant therapy
  for acute coronary syndromes, 2147–2150, 2148t
  for acute stroke, 2139–2140
  apheresis and, 1526
  for atrial fibrillation, 2155–2156
  concentrated, 1766
  cytochrome P450 variants and, 85–86
  for disseminated intravascular coagulation, 2073–2074
  hemostasis and, 1832, 1832f
  heparin-induced thrombocytopenia and, 1978–1980, 1979t–1980t

Anticoagulant therapy (Continued)
  for hypereosinophilic syndrome, 1167–1168
  monitoring of, 1930
  oral, 2179–2184
  parenteral, 2173–2177
  pregnancy and, 2212
  reversal of, 2157
  for sickle cell disease, 593
  for venous thromboembolism, 2108–2110
Anticoagulants (natural), e13b, e25t
Anticodons, 7
Anticonvulsants, 538b, 1027, 1480
Anti-D, 1948
Antidepressants, 1937–1938
Anti-domain I of β₂-Glycoprotein I assay, 2094
Antiemetics, overview of, 1479–1480, 1482–1485, 1483f
Anti-EMR1 IgG1 antibody, 1167
Antifibrolytic agents, 2015, 2306–2307
Antifungal agents, 1456b, 1937
Antigen presentation, 221–222, 222f
Antigen-presenting cells (APC). See also Dendritic cells
  graft-versus-host disease and, 1653–1655, 1654f, 1664
  graft-versus-leukemia responses and, 1665
  overview of, 203, 206f
  T cell activation and, 221, 222f
Anti-HCV therapy, 1284–1285
Antihemophilic factor (AHF) concentrates, 1761–1764, 1764t
Anti-inhibitor coagulant complex, 1766
Anti-KIR3DL2 therapy, 1378
Antilymphocyte globulin (ALG), 409–411
Antimetabolite drugs, 883, 892–898
Antimicrotubule agents, 856–857, 890–891
Antimycin-A, 872
Antineoplastic agents
  chemotherapeutic agents. See Chemotherapy
  future directions, 883–884
  infection and, 1447
  resistance to
    to antimetabolites, 883
    multidrug resistance-associated protein and, 881–883
    overview, 878
    P-glycoprotein and, 879–881, 880f
    to signaling inhibitors, 883
  targeted
    to apoptosis signaling, 869–872
    cyclin-dependent kinase inhibitors, 872–873
    heat shock protein inhibitors, 878
    histone deacetylase inhibitors, 874–877, 874t, 876t, 903
    hypomethylating agents, 873–874
    immunomodulatory agents, 866
    proteasome inhibitors, 866–869
    protein translation inhibitors, 878
    signaling inhibitors, 861–866, 862t
  tumor cell heterogeneity and, 849–850
Antineutrophil cytoplasmic antibodies (ANCA), 293
Antioxidants
  atherothrombosis and, 2126
  green tea and, 2259
  supplements containing, 2259–2260
Anti-PD-1/PD-L1 therapy, 1378–1379
Antiphosphatidyl serine antibody assay, 2095
Antiphospholipid antibodies (APA), 1926, 2088–2092
Antiphospholipid assays, 2092–2095
Antiphospholipid syndrome (APS)
  autoimmune hemolytic anemia in, 653
  catastrophic, 2089t, 2097, 2100
  in children, 2227–2228
  classification of, 2089t
  clinical manifestations of, 2095–2099
  diagnosis of, 2089t
  genetics and proteomics and, 2092
  ischemic stroke and, 2136
  overview of, 2080–2081, 2088
  pathophysiology of, 2088–2092, 2091t
  pediatric, 2097–2098
  pregnancy and, 2213, 2213t
  thrombocytopenia and, 1968–1969
  treatment of, 2095t, 2099–2100
α₂-Antiplasmin, 1839, 1904, 2070–2071
Antiplatelet agents
  for acute coronary syndromes, 2144–2147, 2145t–2146t
  aspirin. See Aspirin
  for hypereosinophilic syndrome, 1167–1168
  peripheral artery disease and, 2164–2165

Antiplatelet agents (Continued)
  platelet disorders and, 1932–1939, 1933t
  for sickle cell disease, 593
  for thrombotic thrombocytopenic purpura, 1991
Antiplatelet antibodies, 1718, 1942–1943
Antiprothrombin antibody assay, 2094–2095
Antipsychotic drugs, 1491–1492, 1492t
Antiretroviral agent toxicity, 2269, 2270t
Antisense therapy, overview of, 15
Antithrombin (AT)
  coagulation and, 1892
  concentrated, 1766, 1779, 2074
  deficiency in, 2076–2078
  disseminated intravascular coagulation and, 2066, 2066f, 2074
  factor IX and, 2005
  hemostasis and, 1837
  laboratory evaluation of, e13b
  mutation database, 2076
  system overview, 1852
Antithrombin antibodies, 2019–2020, 2019t
Antithrombotic therapy
  for acute coronary syndromes, 2142, 2144
  for acute stroke, 2138–2140
  anticoagulant therapy. See Anticoagulant therapy
  antiplatelet drugs. See Antiplatelet agents
  for children, 2228
  fibrinolytic agents. See Fibrinolytic agents
  for neonates, 2200
  overview of, 2168, 2169f
Antithymocyte globulins (ATG), 409–411, 430, 1659–1660, 1661t, 1757
α₁-Antitrypsin, 1767, 1768t, 1779
Anxiety, 1469–1470, 1491
Aortic aneurysms, 2069
APC resistance (APCR), 2079–2080
Apheresis collections
  albumin replacement and, 1752
  anticoagulants and, 1526
  complications of, 1789–1790
  devices for, 1525
  graft failure and, 1675
  for hematopoietic stem cell collection, 1788–1789
  large-volume leukapheresis and, 1526–1527, 1527t
  of low-density lipoproteins, 1786–1787
  minimal manipulations and, 1538–1540
  pediatric, 1790–1791, 1826
  physician prescription for, 1525b
  for platelet transfusions, 1715
  Plerixafor and, 1525
  principles of, 1781
  for removal of cells. See Cytapheresis
  for removal of plasma solute. See Plasmapheresis
  technology aspects, 1525–1526, 1781–1786
  therapeutic, 1790b
  timing of, 1524–1525, 1525f
  venous access for, 1526
Apixaban
  for acute coronary syndromes, 2148t, 2150
  for acute stroke, 2139–2140
  for atrial fibrillation, 2155–2156
  overview of, 2181t, 2183
  for venous thromboembolism, 2108
Aplastic anemia (AA)
  bone marrow and, 395f, 404–405
  classification, 394, 395t
  clinical associations, 402–403
  diagnosis, 402b, 403–404
  differential diagnosis, 395t, 402t, 405
  dyskeratosis congenita and, 366
  epidemiology, 394, 396f
  etiology and pathogenesis, 394–397
  history, 394
  infection and, 1448
  intravenous immunoglobulin for, 1755
  laboratory evaluation, 403
  overview, 394, 395f
  paroxysmal nocturnal hemoglobinuria and, 419–420
  pathophysiologic pathways leading to, 397–401, 397f
  prognosis, 413
  treatment, 405–413, 406b, 410b
  typical and atypical presentations, 401–402, 401t
Aplastic crises, 596, 2216
Apolipoprotein E receptor 2 (apoER2), 2089, 2130
Apoptosis
  angiogenesis and, 1847
  atherothrombosis and, 2129
  BCL-2 family proteins and, 190–191, 191f–192f

Apoptosis (Continued)
  caspases and, 186–187, 187f
  chemotherapy resistance and, 1018
  chronic lymphocytic leukemia and, 1245
  clinical applications, 195
  core pathways, 190
  death receptor signaling and, 193–194
  endoplasmic reticulum, Bcl-2 family protein and, 191–193
  extrinsic pathway. See Extrinsic apoptosis pathway
  inhibitors of, 190
  intrinsic pathway. See Intrinsic apoptosis pathway
  mantle cell lymphoma and, 1298–1299
  morphologic features of, 187f
  myelodysplastic syndromes and, 953
  of neutrophils, 186
  oncogene-induced. See Oncogene-induced apoptosis
  overview of, 186
  physiologic cell turnover and, 186
  procaspase activation and, 187–188, 188f
  T cell development and, 228
  targeted inhibitors of, 869–872
Apoptosis-associated speck-like (ASC), 188, 189f, 1209
Apoptosome, 188, 189f, 190, 871
Aprepitant, 1485
APRIL, 254
Aprotinin, 2307
APS nephropathy, 2097
aPTT biphasic waveform analysis, 2071
Aquaporins, 1850–1851
Arabinofuranosylguanine (Ara-G), 897
Ara-c. See Cytarabine
Arborization, 152
Arf. See ADP ribosylation factors
Argatroban, 1979–1980, 1979t–1980t, 2179, 2179t
Aromatase inhibitors, 2083
Aromatic hydrocarbons, 400
Array comparative genomic hybridization (aCGH), 777f
Arrhythmias, 560
Arsenic trioxide (ATO), 940–941, 966
Artemether, 2287t
Artemether/lumefantrine, 2287t
Arterial ischemic stroke (AIS), 2198–2199
Arterial thrombosis, 1841, 2168. See also Atherosclerosis
Arteriogenesis, 156–158, 157f, 1849–1850
Arterio/venogenesis, 156–158, 157f
Artesunate, 2287t
ARTISS, 1766
AryoSeven, 1775
Asialoglycoprotein receptor-1 (NPC1L1), 2131
L-Asparaginase, 1025–1026, 1037, 1039, 2082
Aspergillus infections, 1456f, 1674–1675, 1678
Aspirin
  for acute coronary syndromes, 2144–2145
  for acute stroke, 2138–2140
  for essential thrombocythemia, 1120–1121, 1121t, 1123b
  essential thrombocythemia and, 1110
  hemophilia and, 2013
  overview of, 2168–2170, 2169f
  for peripheral artery disease, 2164
  platelet disorders and, 1932–1935
  for polycythemia vera, 1099–1100
  for sickle cell disease, 593
Aspirin resistance, 1933–1935, 2170
Asplenia, 677, 2321, 2321f
Assisted reproduction, 2083
ASXL1. See Additional sex combs-like
AT. See Antithrombin
Ataxia telangiectasia (AT), 357, 684, 1330, 1909
Ataxia telangiectasia mutated (ATM), 824–825, 1298–1299, 1300f
Ataxia-pancytopenia syndrome, 367
ATF6. See Activating transcription factor 6
ATG. See Antithymocyte globulins
Atherosclerosis, 2326
Atherothrombosis
  cross-talk between coagulation and inflammation systems and, 2130–2131
  foam cell formation, fatty streak and, 2125–2127
  future directions, 2131
  hyperlipidemia and, 2129–2130
  lipoprotein homeostasis and, 2122–2125, 2123f
  overview of, 2122
  pathobiology of, 2122, 2123f
  plaque regression and, 2131

Atherothrombosis *(Continued)*
  plaque rupture and, 2129, 2129*f*
  remodeling, vulnerable plaque and, 2127–2129, 2127*f*–2128*f*
Athletes, 1077, 1080
ATM. *See* Ataxia telangiectasia mutated
ATO. *See* Arsenic trioxide
Atorvastatin, 2124
ATP binding cassette transporters (ABC)
  ABCB1, 497–498, 879–881, 880*f*
  ABCG2, 881–883, 881*f*
  lipoprotein homeostasis and, 2123–2124
Atrial fibrillation (AF)
  anticoagulant-related bleeding and, 2156–2157
  clinical manifestations of, 2152–2153
  diagnosis and differential diagnosis for, 2153
  epidemiology of, 2152
  future directions, 2157
  heart rate and rhythm control and, 2153–2155
  overview of, 2152, 2155*f*
  pathobiology of, 2152
  prevention of stroke and thromboembolism and, 2155–2156, 2155*t*
ATRX, 456
ATryn, 1766
Atypical chemokine receptors (ACKR), 136, 137*t*, 138
Atypical hemolytic uremic syndrome (aHUS)
  clinical manifestations of, 1993
  differential diagnosis for, 1984
  eculizumab and, 282–283
  epidemiology of, 1993
  laboratory manifestations of, 1994–1996, 1996*t*
  overview of, 1984
  pathobiology of, 1993–1994, 1994*f*–1995*f*
  prognosis for, 1996
  therapy for, 1996–1997
AU-rich elements (AREs), 23
Aurora A kinase, 1359, 1857
Aurora B kinase, 20, 342
Autoantibodies. *See also* Autoimmunity; Self-tolerance
  immune thrombocytopenia purpura and, 1944–1945, 1945*t*
  patterns of in systemic autoimmune diseases, 290*t*
  posttransfusion purpura and, 1945*t*, 1953–1954
Autohemolysis testing, 632
Autoimmune disease, 1132
Autoimmune hemolytic anemia (AIHA)
  in children, 2216
  cold. *See* Cold autoimmune hemolytic anemia
  differential diagnosis for, 655–656, 661*b*
  epidemiology of, 648
  etiology and pathophysiology of, 649–650
  history of, 648
  immunologic phenomena with, 652
  laboratory diagnosis of, 650–652, 650*b*
  overview of, 285, 648
  pathobiology of, 648–649
  pediatric transfusions and, 1826
  pregnancy and, 2205
  secondary, 652–655
  sickle cell disease and, 596–597
  symptoms, clinical findings, and risks, 650
  treatment of, 656–662, 658*t*–659*t*
  warm. *See* Warm autoimmune hemolytic anemia
Autoimmune lymphoproliferative syndrome (ALPS), 235, 718–719
Autoimmune neutropenia (AIN)
  in adults, 431
  confusion over diagnosis of, 677–678
  of infancy, 387, 1736
  overview of, 678
  therapy, 437*b*
Autoimmune polyendocrinopathy-candidiasis-ectodermal dystrophy (APECED), 204, 287–288, 717–718
Autoimmune polyglandular syndrome type I (APS1), 287–288
Autoimmune regulator (AIRE), 204, 228, 254, 256, 287–288, 290, 717–718
Autoimmunity
  chronic lymphocytic leukemia and, 1263
  complement deficiencies and, 268
  dendritic cells and, 256
  disorders of
    autoantibody expression in, 290*t*
    breakdown of self-tolerance and, 290–292
    implications and therapy, 292–293
    overview, 285
    self-reactive lymphocytes and, 285–290

Autoimmunity *(Continued)*
  genetic and environmental factors contributing to, 291–292
  role of natural killer cells in, 243
  self-tolerance and, 285
Autologous blood transfusion, overview of, 1710–1711, 1711*t*
Autologous bone marrow transplantation, 1327
Autologous stem cell infusion, 968
Autologous stem cell transplantation (ASCT)
  for acute lymphoblastic leukemia, 1026, 1042
  allogenic transplantation vs., 1533
  for chronic lymphocytic leukemia, 1249*b*
  for chronic myelogenous leukemia, 1069
  for cutaneous T-cell lymphomas, 1375
  donor selection in, 1517
  for follicular lymphoma, 1294
  for Hodgkin lymphoma, 1222–1224
  for mantle cell lymphoma, 1304–1305
  for multiple myeloma, 1407–1412
  overview of, 1592–1593
  for peripheral T-cell lymphomas, 1355–1356
  sources of stem cells used in, 1593
Autophagy, overview of, 56, 194–195
Autosomal recessive agammaglobulinemia, 720
Ayamura Indians, 1077
Ayurvedic medicine, 2253
5'-Azacytidine
  as epigenetic therapy, 23
  for myelodysplastic syndromes, 966, 997*b*
  pharmacology of, 857, 873–874, 896
  for primary myelofibrosis, 1146–1148
Azathioprine, 429, 1447, 2232
Azidothymidine, 538*b*
Azurocidin, 1851

B

B cell lymphoma (BCL)
  BCL 2
    apoptosis, endoplasmic reticulum and, 191–193
    apoptosis and, 186–187, 190–191, 191*f*
    chronic lymphocytic leukemia and, 1245, 1258–1259
    clinical applications, 195
    diffuse large B-cell lymphoma and, 770–771
    downregulation of self-reactive lymphocytes and, 289
    as drug target, 871–872
    follicular lymphoma and, 833, 1190, 1238–1239
    nonapoptotic roles of, 193
    non-Hodgkin lymphoma and, 1230–1231, 1233*t*, 1234
    oligonucleotide (Bcl-ASODN), 872
  BCL 6
    Burkitt lymphoma and, 835
    follicular lymphoma and, 835, 1289*f*
    Hodgkin lymphoma and, 1210
    non-Hodgkin lymphoma and, 1230–1231, 1233*t*, 1234
    Tfh programming and, 231
  BCL X$_L$, 186–187, 449
  BCL11A, 456, 562–563, 1017
B cell receptor (BCR)
  adaptive immune response and, 200
  B-cell development and, 215–216, 215*f*
  cell division cycle and, 178
  chronic lymphocytic leukemia and, 1245–1246
  Hodgkin lymphoma and, 1204
  non-Hodgkin lymphoma and, 1231
  in T-cell acute lymphoblastic leukemia, 1014
B cell selection process, 206
B cells
  dendritic cells and activation of, 254
  development of
    aging and, 219
    defects in, 720–722
    fetal, 217–218
    hematopoietic microenvironment and, 216–217, 216*f*
    Hodgkin lymphoma and, 1204
    immunoglobulin gene rearrangement and expression, 212–214, 213*f*
    pro-B and pre-B cell checkpoints, 214–216, 215*f*
    secondary lymphoid compartments and, 218–219
    specification and commitment, 210–211
    stages, 210
  Epstein-Barr virus and, 748–749, 754*t*
  graft-versus-host disease and, 1662
  Hodgkin lymphoma and. *See* Hodgkin lymphoma
  intrinsic defects of class switch recombination and, 722–723

B cells *(Continued)*
  in lymphatic circulation, 207*f*
  lymphocyte homing and, 139
  lymphomas of, 1187–1196, 1188*t*, 1230–1231
  malignancies of mature, 115, 116*f*
  maturation of, 204–205
  overview of in immune system, 202
  positioning of within secondary lymphoid organs, 142
  self-tolerance and, 285–286, 290*t*
  tolerance of germinal, 289
B-1 B cells, 217–218
B$_{19}$ parvovirus, 2216
B7-DC, 249*t*, 252, 253*t*
Babesia spp., 667, 1816, 2299–2301, 2300*f*
BacT/ALERT system, 1717
Bacterial infections
  disseminated intravascular coagulation and, 2068
  neutropenia, lymphopenia and, 1454
  sickle cell disease and, 595*t*
  transfusion-associated, 1813–1814
Baculoviral IAP repeat containing proteins (BIRC), 753–754, 1280
Baculovirus IAP repeats (BIR), 190
BAD. *See* Bcl-2-associated death promoter
BAF. *See* Brg1/Brm-associated factor complex
BAFF. *See* B-cell activation factor
BAK. *See* Bcl-2 homologous antagonist/killer
Baller-Gerold syndrome, 392
BamHI-A rightward transcripts (BARTS), 749
Band 3 protein, 384, 628–630, 646
Barbourin, 1935–1936
Barth syndrome, 364–365, 387–388
Bartonella bacilliformis, 667
Basal transcription factors, 17
Base excision repair, 883
Basic helix-loop-helix (bHLH) proteins, 103
Basophilic leukemia, 811
Basophilic leukocytes, 203
Basophils, 203, 331
Batroxobin, 1927
BAX, 190–193, 193*f*
4-1BB, T cell activation and, 226
B-cell activation factor (BAFF), 722, 1245, 1259
B-cell acute lymphoblastic leukemia (B-ALL)
  BCR-ABL1 fusion gene in, 1013–1014
  classification of, 772
  clinical manifestations, 1022–1023
  cytogenetics and molecular genetics of, 1032–1035, 1033*f*, 1034*t*
  immunophenotyping of, 1032, 1032*t*–1033*t*
  mature. *See* Burkitt lymphoma
  overview of, 1021
  precursor, 1005–1006, 1009–1010, 1016
  prognosis, 1023, 1024*t*
  stem cell origin of, 114–115, 115*f*
  therapy, 1025–1026
B-cell chronic lymphocytic leukemia, 822–827
B-cell lymphomas
  Burkitt lymphoma. *See* Burkitt lymphoma
  diffuse large B-cell lymphoma. *See* Diffuse large B-cell lymphoma
  primary central nervous system. *See* Primary central nervous system lymphoma
B-cell lymphopoiesis, 122
BCL. *See* B cell lymphoma
Bcl-2 homologous antagonist/killer (BAK), 191–193, 193*f*
Bcl-2-associated death promoter (BAD), 193
Bcl-xL-BH3 domain (BH3I), 872
BCNU. *See* Carmustine
BCR. *See* B cell receptor; Breakpoint cluster region
BCR-ABL fusion. *See* Breakpoint cluster region protein- Abelson fusion
BCR-ABL1-like acute lymphoblastic leukemia, 89–90, 819–821, 1014
BCR-PDGFRA fusion, 790–792
BCS. *See* Budd-Chiari syndrome
BDCA. *See* Blood dendritic cell antigen
BEACOPP (bleomycin, etoposide, doxorubicin, cyclophosphamide, vincristine, procarbazine, prednisolone), 1220–1221, 1220*t*
Bead-based genomic profiling, 32
Belinostat, 876, 967, 1358–1359
Bence Jones proteins, 1381
Bendamustine
  for chronic lymphocytic leukemia, 1253, 1256
  for extranodal marginal zone lymphoma of MALT type, 1282
  for follicular lymphoma, 1294

Bendamustine *(Continued)*
    overview of, 856
    for peripheral T-cell lymphomas, 1359–1360
    pharmacology of, 856, 889
Benefix, 1775, 2013
Benign ethnic neutropenias, 678
BENTA disease, 682
Benzamide derivatives, 876–877
Benzene, 397, 399–400, 1125
Benzodiazepines, 1485, 1492t
Benzoquinone ansamycins, 878
Benzylguanine, 882
Bereavement follow-up, 1493–1494
Beriplex, 2013
Berlin-Frankfurt-Münster Risk Group Classification of
    Mature B-cell Lymphomas, 1334t
Bernard-Soulier Syndrome, 134, 134t, 347b, 347t–348t,
    1872, 1880, 1884, 2304–2305
Berti lymphoma, 1367
Bertilimumab, 1167
Bessis, 123
Beta blockers, 2153–2154
β-Sheets, 59–60, 60f–61f
Beta-tryptase, 1156–1157
Bethesda assay, 2027–2028, 2027f–2028f
Bevacizumab, 159, 965
Bexarotene, 1376
Bezafibrate, 2163–2164
BH3I. *See* Bcl-xL-BH3 domain
BH3-only proteins, 190–191, 192f
BiKEs. *See* Bispecific killer engagers
Bilayer couple hypothesis, 626
BinaxNow Malaria Test, 2285–2287
Binding affinity, regulation of, 132
Binding immunoglobulin protein (BiP), 195
Binet staging system, 1250
Biologic false-positive serologic test for syphilis (BFP-STS),
    2092
Biosimilars, 1522
BiP. *See* Binding immunoglobulin protein
Birbeck granules, 252
BIRC. *See* Baculoviral IAP repeat containing proteins
Bird-headed dwarfism. *See* Seckel syndrome
Bispecific killer engagers (BiKEs), 1579
2,3-Bisphosphoglycerate (BPG), 451, 1079
Bisphosphoglycerate mutase (BPGM) deficiency, 623
Bisphosphonates, 389, 1415
Bisulfite-sequencing, 20–21, 21f
Bite cells, 671
Bivalirudin
    for acute coronary syndromes, 2148t, 2149–2150
    heparin-induced thrombocytopenia and, 1979–1980,
        1979t–1980t
    overview of, 2179, 2179t
Bizarre poikilocytes, 643
BK virus, 1674
BL22, 1273, 1275
Black tree fungus, 1939
Blackwater fever, 2283
Blast crisis, 1058–1059, 1063
Blastic plasmacytoid dendritic cell neoplasm, 932f
Bleeding disorders. *See also Specific disorders*
    case studies, 1913b, 1916b–1917b, 1920b
    clinical manifestations, 1915–1917
    differential diagnosis, 1918–1919, 1918t–1920t
    epidemiology, 1913–1914
    future directions, 1919
    laboratory manifestations. *See* Laboratory evaluation
    in neonate, 2191–2197, 2192f
    overview of, 1912, 1913b, 1913f
    pathobiology, 1914
    prognosis, 1913–1914
    therapy, 1919
Blinatumomab, 1050–1051
Blister cells, 671
Blood banking, 1515, 1821–1822
Blood dendritic cell antigen 3 (BDCA3), 248
Blood doping, 1080
Blood Group Antigen Gene Mutation Database
    (BGMUT), 1687
Blood groups
    ABH system, 1694–1695, 1694f, 1717
    ABO system, 1692, 1694–1695, 2055
    allogenic hematopoietic stem cell transplantation and,
        1706, 1706t
    alloimmunization and, 1693, 1693t, 1696
    antibodies and, 1687–1691, 1692t
    Blood group O, 2055

Blood groups *(Continued)*
    carbohydrate, 1694–1696, 1694f
    compatibility procedures and location of antigen-
        negative blood, 1691–1693, 1692t, 1693t
    diseases associated with, 1688t–1690t, 1693, 1693t
    DNA-based typing of, 1687, 1688t–1691t
    infection and, 1450, 1693
    overview of, 1687, 1688t–1690t
    platelet transfusions and, 1717
    sickle cell disease and, 1693, 1693t
    systems of
        carbohydrate, 1694–1696, 1694f
        overview, 1688t–1690t
        protein, 1696–1700, 1696t
    terminology of, 1687
    transplantation and, 1695
Blood islands, 1845
Blood substitutes, 1712
Blood vessel wall. *See* Vessel wall
Blood volume estimations, e1, e14t
Bloom syndrome, 357
B-lys, 254
BMS-354825, 1064
Bodmer, Walter, 1727
Bohr effect, 451
Bologna scoring system for peripheral T-cell lymphomas,
    1350
Bombay phenotype, 1695
Bone complications, sickle cell disease and, 603–604, 604f
Bone marrow
    adipocytes and, 121
    aging and, 1351–1355, 2330
    allogenic hematopoietic stem cell transplantation and,
        1593
    anemia and, 396–397, 404–405, 404f, 464
    collection of, 1519, 1520f–1521f
    endothelial cells of, 121, 337–338
    homing of cells and. *See* Homing
    hypereosinophilic syndrome and, 1161–1162
    immune cell development and, 203–204
    macrophages of, 122
    malaria and, 2283–2284
    megakaryocytes of, 122
    metastases and, 2249–2250, 2249f
    microenvironment of, 123
    migration of hematopoietic stem cells to, 140–141
    multiple myeloma and, 1394, 1394f
    niches for hematopoietic stem and progenitor cells and,
        119–120
    osteoclasts and, 121–122
    osteolineage cells and, 120–121
    perivascular cells and, 121
    quality control of, 1527–1528
    transplantation of
        for aplastic anemia, 412
        chronic granulomatous disease and, 700
        homing and mobilization of hematopoietic stem and
            progenitor cells and, 150b–151b
        intravenous immunoglobulin for, 1753
        for lysosomal storage diseases, 743
        pain and, 1481–1482, 1482t
        thrombocytopenia and, 1970
    Waldenström macroglobulinemia and, 1425
Bone marrow aspiration, diagnostic, 540b
Bone Marrow Donors Worldwide, 1608
Bone marrow failure syndromes, inherited
    acute myeloid leukemia and, 914–915
    aplastic anemia. *See* Aplastic anemia
    malignant leukemic transformation and, 392b
    overview of, 350, 351t–352t
    with pancytopenia
        congenital amegakaryocytic thrombocytopenia. *See*
            Congenital amegakaryocytic thrombocytopenia
        dyskeratosis congenita. *See* Dyskeratosis congenita
        Fanconi anemia. *See* Fanconi anemia
        miscellaneous complications of, 371–372
        overview, 350–372
        Schwachman-Diamond syndrome. *See* Schwachman-
            Diamond syndrome
    with predominantly anemia
        congenital dyserythropoietic anemias. *See* Congenital
            dyserythropoietic anemias
        Diamond-Blackfan anemia. *See* Diamond-Blackfan
            anemia
        overview, 372–385
    with predominantly neutropenia
        Barth syndrome, 364–365, 387–388
        cyclic neutropenia, 387–389, 678

Bone marrow failure syndromes, inherited *(Continued)*
    Dursun syndrome, 390
    glycogen storage disease type 1b, 365, 387–388,
        707–708
    Kostmann syndrome. *See* Severe congenital
        neutropenia
    miscellaneous, 390
    myelokathexis, 389–390
    overview, 385–390, 388t
    severe congenital neutropenia. *See* Severe congenital
        neutropenia
    WHIM syndrome, 149–150, 389–390
    with predominantly thrombocytopenia, 369t,
        390–392
Bone marrow sinuses, 1845
Bone mass, 558
Bone morphogenic proteins (BMP), 70, 101, 106t, 474,
    475f
Bone pain, 1391, 1480
Bone-marrow derived cells (BMDC), 152, 153f
Bordetella pertussis, 683
Borrelia burgdorferi, 1814–1815
Bortezomib
    clinical studies with, 868
    for light chain amyloidosis, 1440
    for multiple myeloma, 1395t, 1406, 1409, 1413
    overview of, 867–868
    for peripheral T-cell lymphomas, 1359
    pharmacology of, 868
    preclinical studies with, 868
    resistance to, 867, 880
    toxicities of, 869
    for Waldenström macroglobulinemia, 1427–1428
Bosutinib, 862, 862t, 903, 1051, 1065
Botanical products, 2254, 2255t, 2258–2260
BRAF
    chronic lymphocytic leukemia and, 825–826
    Erdheim-Chester disease and, 731
    hairy cell leukemia and, 115–117, 839–840, 1266,
        1275
    Langerhans cell hysticitosis and, 724–725
    myelodysplastic syndromes and, 951
Brain injury, 2068
Brain-bone-blood triad, 148
Breakapart probes, 778, 778f–779f
Breakpoint cluster region (BCR), 1013
Breakpoint cluster region protein- Abelson (BCR-ABL)
    fusion
    acute lymphoblastic leukemia and, 819–821
    acute myeloid leukemia and, 805
    in B-cell acute lymphoblastic leukemia, 1013–1014
    chronic myelogenous leukemia and, 784–790, 784t,
        785f, 1055–1058, 1056f
    cytogenetics of, 784t
    infant ALL and novel therapies for, 89–90
    myeloproliferative neoplasms and, 764
    overview of, 64
    primary myelofibrosis and, 1134
    stem cell origin theory and, 114
    tyrosine kinase inhibitors and, 87
Breakpoint cluster region protein- Abelson (BCR-ABL)
    kinase inhibitors, 861–863, 862t
Breast cancer, 1503
Brentuximab vedotin (BV)
    for Hodgkin lymphoma, 1222–1223, 1225, 1226f,
        1228
    for mastocytosis, 1184
    for mycosis fungoides and Sézary syndrome, 1377
    for non-Hodgkin lymphoma, 1338
    for T-cell lymphomas, 1359
Brg1/Brm-associated factor (BAF) complex, 20
Bromelain, 1939
Bromodomain and extra-terminal motif (BET)
    bromodomain inhibitors, 23, 1415
Bruising, 1915
Bruton tyrosine kinase (BTK), 686–687, 720, 863,
    1296–1297, 1299
Bruton's agammaglobulinemia. *See* X-linked
    agammaglobulinemia
Budd-Chiari syndrome (BCS)
    overview of, 2082
    paroxysmal nocturnal hemoglobinuria and, 418–419
    polycythemia vera and, 1087, 1089–1090
    treatment of, 1103
Budesonide, 1659–1660
Buparlisib, 864
Buprenorphine, 1478

Burkitt lymphoma (BL)
  in childhood, 1333–1334, 1335*t*
  classification of, 771
  clinical manifestations of, 1315, 1333
  cytogenetics of, 835
  differential diagnosis for, 1333–1334
  epidemiology of, 1314–1315, 1333
  epigenetics and, 22–23
  Epstein-Barr virus and, 758, 1238, 1321
  HIV infection and, 2268*f*
  investigation of, 1315
  late complications and followup for, 1316–1317
  lymphoblast features in, 1005
  MYC mutations in, 1008, 1011
  overview of, 1195–1196, 1195*f*, 1235–1238, 1236*f*,
      1317, 1333
  pathobiology of, 1315, 1333
  prognosis/staging for, 1315, 1334, 1334*t*–1335*t*
  salvage therapy for, 1316–1317
  treatment of, 1046–1047, 1047*f*, 1315–1317, 1334
Burns, 2068
Burst-forming unit-erythroid cells (BFU-E), 297–300,
    298*t*, 447
Burst-forming unit-megakaryocytes (BFU-Mk), 334
Busulfan, 854*f*, 855, 887
BV. *See* Brentuximab vedotin

C

C antigen. *See under* Complement system
C1 inhibitor (C1INH), 264*t*, 266, 1767, 1768*t*
C2 deficiency. *See under* Complement system
C3 convertase, 261, 263–265
C3 deficiency. *See under* Complement system
C4 binding protein (C4BP), 264*t*
C4 deficiency. *See under* Complement system
C5 convertase, 264–265
C5a. *See under* Complement system
Cadherins, 129, 130*t*, 154–155, 1844
CAFC assay. *See* Cobblestone area-forming cell assay
Calcineurin, 1997
Calcineurin-nuclear factor of activated T cells, 1664
Calcium, platelet activation and, 1874
Calcium channel blockers (CCB), 2153–2154
CALGB regimen, 1047
CALGB-10403 regimen, 1048
CALM-AF10 fusion gene, 1009
Calnexin (CNX), 53
Calreticulin (CRT; CALR)
  erythropoietin receptor and, 308–309
  essential thrombocythemia and, 1106–1108, 1108*f*,
      1112
  primary myelofibrosis and, 1127–1128, 1128*t*,
      1149*b*
  protein folding and, 53
Camptosar. *See* Irinotecan
Camptothecin analogs, 859–860, 859*f*, 1374
Cancer Cell Line Encyclopedia (CCLE), 850
Cancer predisposition syndromes
  congenital amegakaryocytic thrombocytopenia and,
      370
  Diamond-Blackfan anemia and, 377–378
  dyskeratosis congenita and, 366–367
  Fanconi anemia and, 356
  inherited bone marrow failure syndromes and, 392*b*
  Kostmann syndrome, severe congenital neutropenia and,
      386–387
  overview of, 356
  Schwachman-Diamond syndrome and, 363
Cancer stem cells (CSC)
  acute lymphoblastic leukemia and, 114–115
  acute myeloid leukemias and, 111–112, 113*b*
  chronic lymphocytic leukemia and, 115
  diffuse large B-cell lymphoma and, 117
  follicular lymphoma and, 117
  hairy cell leukemia and, 115–117
  hypothesis overview, 108–109, 109*f*, 111, 112*f*
  mature B-cell malignancies and, 115, 116*f*
  myelodysplastic syndromes and, 112–114
  myeloproliferative neoplasms and, 114
Cancer vaccines, 258, 259*f*
Candida infections, 1455–1456, 1456*b*, 1674
Cangrelor, 2146*t*, 2147, 2171
Cannabinoids, 1480, 1485
Canonical splicing, 20
CAP37, 1851
Capillaries, 1843
Caplan, Arnold, 1559

Capping, 9, 20, 449
CAR. *See* Chimeric antigen receptors
Carbamazepine, 400–401
Carbohydrate blood groups, 1694–1696, 1694*f*
Carbon monoxide (CO), 575–576, 612, 1078
Carboplatin, 860–861, 902–903
γ-Carboxylation, 47, 47*b*, 53–54
CARD domain, 187–188
Cardiac transplantation, 1441–1442
Cardioembolism, 2134–2135
Cardiolipin binding activity, 2093–2094
Cardiopulmonary bypass surgery, 665, 1942, 1970–1971,
    2310
Cardiovascular disease
  arterial disease, 1497
  atrial fibrillation and, 2152–2153
  β-thalassemia syndromes and, 560
  cardiac disease, 1496–1497
  in children, 2222–2223, 2222*t*
  Hodgkin lymphoma and, 1228
  polycythemia and, 1075–1076
  prevention of cardiotoxicity, 1497–1498
  risk factors, 1497
  sickle cell disease and, 605
  thrombocytopenia and, 1971
Caregivers, palliative care and, 1490
Carfilzomib, 868–869, 1359, 1413, 1427–1428
Carmustine (BCNU), 854*f*, 855, 887, 1371–1372
β-Carotene (oral), 504
Carotid endarterectomy, 2138–2139
Carrión disease, 667
CAR-T. *See* Chimeric antigen receptor Tcells
Cartilage hair hypoplasia (CHH), 372, 717
Casitas B-lineage lymphoma (CBL) proto-oncogene,
    306–307, 804, 998, 1129
Caspase-activated DNAse (CAD), 186
Caspases
  apoptosis and, 186–187, 187*f*–188*f*, 870, 870*f*
  clinical applications, 195
  inhibitors of, 190
  nonapoptotic roles of, 190
  substrate specificity of, 187*f*
Catabolism of amino acids, 76
Cataloguing, 80*t*, 81
Cataracts, 1501, 1679
Catastrophic antiphospholipid syndrome (CAPS), 2089*t*,
    2097, 2100
Catenin, 1241, 1299
Catheter-directed thrombolysis (CDT)
  for deep vein thrombosis, 2117–2120
  overview of, 2110, 2113–2114
  for peripheral arterial occlusion, 2115–2117
  pharmacomechanical, 2115–2117
  surgery vs., 2116
Cation homeostasis, 576–578
Caveolae, 1850–1851
CBF. *See* Core binding factors
CBL. *See* Casitas B-lineage lymphoma proto-oncogene
CBL syndrome, 998
C-C motif chemokine receptor 5 (CCR5), 2263–2264
CCAAT displacement protein (CDP), 328
CCAAT enhancer binding proteins (CEBP)
  acute myeloid leukemia and, 799–800, 915, 919,
      987
  mast cell development and, 1170
  monocyte differentiation and, 332
  myeloid differentiation and, 326
CCL. *See* Chemokine ligands
CCND1. *See* Cyclin D1
CCND3. *See* G1/S-specific cyclin-D3
CCNU. *See* Lomustine
CCR5. *See* C-C motif chemokine receptor 5
CD1, 1725
CD10, 1288, 1289*f*
CD103+, 248
CD105, 1560–1562
CD14, 331–332
CD150, 96
CD15a, 703
CD163, 473
CD166, 98
CD177, 1735
CD18, 702–703
CD19, 238, 1050, 1052*t*, 1259, 1288
CD19 targeted CAR-modified T cells, 1571–1572,
    1572*t*
CD20, 722, 1039, 1047, 1288, 1427
CD21, 269–272, 270*f*–271*f*

CD22, 1050, 1052*t*, 1288
CD25, 228, 718
CD26, 1647
CD27, 226, 1421–1422
CD28, 225–226, 226*f*, 288
CD3, 223–224
CD30, 1339
CD33, 321, 938–939, 991, 1154, 1167
CD34, 299–300, 1129–1131, 1135
CD34+ hematopoietic stem cells
  anticoagulants and, 1526
  apheresis and, 1524–1526, 1525*b*
  chemokines and, 1523–1524
  chemotherapy plus cytokine mobilization, 1523
  cytokine mobilization and, 1522
  dendritic cell development and, 247–248
  granulocyte colony-stimulating factors and, 1522–1523
  granulocyte-macrophage colony-stimulating factor and,
      1523
  large-volume leukapheresis and, 1526–1527
  mobilization of cells into peripheral blood, 1521–1523,
      1522*b*
  overview of, 1521
  patients difficult to mobilize and, 1524
  pediatric donors and patients and, 1527
  plerixafor and, 1524–1525
  quantification of, 1529
  timing of, 1524–1525
CD35, 269–272, 271*f*
CD36, 130, 130*f*, 130*t*, 2130
CD38, 1251
CD39, 1831–1832, 1832*f*
CD4
  graft-versus-host disease and, 1655–1656
  HIV life cycle and, 2263–2264
  T cell development and, 224*f*, 228–229, 231
CD4+ T cells, 1666, 1724, 2266–2267
CD4+Th cells, 231
CD40, 288, 715
CD40 ligand (CD40LG) deficiency, 715
CD43, 1154
CD44, 124, 130, 130*t*, 1154
CD45, 172, 173*t*, 1154, 1268
CD47, 125
CD48, 1575
CD49d, 1251
CD49f+ human hematopoietic stem cells, 97–98
CD55, 417–418
CD56, 240, 241*f*, 241*t*, 1575
CD56^bright natural killer cells, 240, 241*f*
CD56^dim natural killer cells, 240, 241*f*
CD59, 417–418
CD59 blood group system, 1700
CD59 widely, 264*t*
CD62L, 1666
CD68, 331–332
CD8, 228–229, 1655–1656
CD8+ cytotoxic T cells (CTL), 231, 232*f*, 1666,
    1724
CD80, 288
CD86, 288
CD90, 1560–1562
CD95, 235, 236*f*
CDH. *See* Cytokine receptor homology domain
CDK. *See* Cyclin-dependent kinases
CDK-interacting protein/kinase inhibitor protein (CIP/
    KIP) family, 178–180
CDR. *See* Complementarity-determining regions
C/EBP. *See* CCAAT enhancer binding proteins
Celiac disease, 2224
Cell adhesion
  altered expression of adhesion molecules and, 133–134,
      134*t*
  cell signaling through molecules of, 132
  cooperative interactions between signaling and adhesion
      molecules, 132–133
  extracellular matrix proteins and, 127
  hemostasis and, 1832–1833
  immunoglobulin-like receptors and, 129, 129*t*
  inherited disorders of, 1880–1883
  integrins and, 127–129, 128*f*, 128*t*
  lectin adhesion receptors and, 130–131
  ligand binding vs., 131
  overview of, 127
  phagocyte disorders of, 701–705
  receptors mediating protein-protein interactions,
      129–130, 130*t*
  regulation of receptors, 131, 131*t*

Cell adhesion molecules
  altered expression of, 133–134, 134t
  angiogenesis and, 1846, 1847f
  glycosylation-dependent cell adhesion molecule I. See
    Glycosylation-dependent cell adhesion molecule I
  homing cell adhesion molecule. See Homing cell
    adhesion molecule
  intracellular cell adhesion molecules. See Intracellular
    cell adhesion molecules
  junctional adhesion molecules. See Junctional adhesion
    molecules
  mucosal addressin-cell adhesion molecule. See Mucosal
    addressin-cell adhesion molecule
  neural cell adhesion molecule. See CD56
  platelet endothelial cell adhesion molecule I. See Platelet
    endothelial cell adhesion molecule I
  vascular cell adhesion molecules. See Vascular cell
    adhesion molecules
  vascular system and, 154–155
Cell cycle, 523, 851–853, 851f
Cell death, 186, 194–195. See also Apoptosis
Cell division
  checkpoints in, 182–184, 183f
  cyclin dependent kinase inhibitors and, 178–180
  cyclins, cyclin dependent kinases and, 178
  DNA replication and, 181–182
  endoreplication and, 184
  hematopoietic stem cells and, 184
  mitosis and, 182
  overview of cycle, 176–177, 177f
  signaling and, 177–178, 177f, 179f
  transcriptional regulation of, 180–181, 180f
  ubiquitination and, 181
Cell salvage, intraoperative, 1711, 1711t
Cell-based therapies
  evaluation of potential allogenic donors, 1515t
  genetic. See Gene therapy
  hematopoietic stem cell transplantation. See
    Hematopoietic stem cell transplantation
  natural killer cell-based. See Natural killer cell-based
    therapies
  novel
    clinical trial readiness and, 1535–1536
    investigational process for, 1533–1535
    overview of, 1531–1533
  overview and historical perspective, 1515–1516
  overview of, 1531–1532
  regulation of, 1533, 1565, 1565b
Cell-mediated immunity, 1450
Cell-mediated toxicity, 719–720
Center for Biologics Evaluation and Research (CBER),
  1533
Center for Devices and Radiological Health (CDRH),
  1533
Central deletion, 1656–1657
Central memory T cells, 232
Central nervous system, 1193, 1305, 1504
Central supramolecular activation complex (cSMAC), 226
Central tolerance, 285–288
Central venous access device (CVAD) regimens, 2017. See
  also Hyper-CVAD regimen
Central venous access devices (CVAD), 2025, 2031, 2251
Centroblasts, 206, 219
Centrocytes, 206, 219
Centrocytic lymphoma. See Mantle cell lymphoma
Centromeres, 182
Cephalosporins, 1937
Ceprotin, 1766
Cerebellar hemangioblastomas, 1078–1079
Cerebral folate deficiency, 537
Cerebral sinovenous thrombosis (CSVT), 2199
Cerebral vein thrombosis (CVT), 1090, 1103, 2135
Cerebral veins, 419
Cerebrovascular accidents. See Stroke
Cerebrovascular disease, 581
CFC assay. See Colony-forming cell assay
CFTR. See Cystic fibrosis transmembrane conductance
  regulator
CFU-GEMM. See Colony-forming unit-granulocyte,
  erythrocyte, macrophage, megakaryocyte
cGAS-cGAMP-STING signaling pathway, 73
CH73, 1560–1562
CHA₂DS₂VASc scoring system, 2155t
Chagas disease. See Trypanosomiasis, American
Challenge-related bleeding, 1916
Chaperones. See Molecular chaperones
Charge, amino acids and, 59
CHARGE syndrome, 710–714

Checkpoint blockade therapies
  after hematopoietic stem cell transplantation, 1585
  cytotoxic T lymphocyte-associated antigen-4 and, 1583,
    1585–1586
  future directions, 1586
  overview of, 1583
  programmed cell death protein 1 and, 1583–1586
Checkpoints in cell division cycle, 182–184, 183f
Chediak-Higashi syndrome 1 (CHS1) gene, 698
Chediak-Higashi syndrome (CHS), 335, 706, 706t, 719
Cheeses, 1458
Chelation therapy, 489, 489b, 554–555, 592, 964
Chemistry, Manufacturing, and Control (CMC), 1534,
  1542
Chemoimmunotherapy, 1255–1256, 1294, 1295t
Chemokine ligand 21 (CCL21), 139
Chemokine ligand 5 (CCL5), 1156–1157, 2126
Chemokines
  eosinophil mobilization and migration and, 1156
  immune response and, 202t
  leukocyte trafficking and, 135–138, 136t
  mesenchymal stromal cells and, 1560–1562
  mobilization of hematopoietic stem cells and,
    1523–1524
  overview of, 136t
  receptors for
    atypical, 137t
    classical, 137t
    overview of, 136t
  signal transduction and, 73
Chemotaxis, 701–705, 1156
Chemotherapy
  for acute lymphoblastic leukemia, 1037–1039, 1038t,
    1050–1051
  acute myeloid leukemia and, 913
  anemia and, 2247
  for chronic myelogenous leukemia, 1060
  for cutaneous T-cell lymphomas, 1357
  development of agents for
    phase I clinical trial design, 850–851
    phase II drug development, 851
    screening for antitumor activity, 850
  gonadal dysfunction and, 1499–1500
  infection following, 1451–1457, 1452f
  for Langerhans cell histiocytosis, 730
  for light chain amyloidosis, 1439–1440
  mobilization of hematopoietic stem cells and, 1523
  for multiple myeloma, 1402–1404
  nausea and vomiting and, 1482–1485, 1483f
  neutropenias and, 679
  overview of, 850
  for peripheral T-cell lymphomas, 1351–1352, 1355b
  thrombocytopenia and, 442
  thrombosis and, 2081–2082
  thrombotic microangiopathies and, 1997–1998
  traditional cytotoxic agents
    alkylating agents, 853–856, 885–889
    antimicrotubule agents, 856–858, 890–891
    DNA topoisomerase inhibitors, 858–860, 860t
    nucleotide synthesis inhibitors, 856–857
    overview, 853f
    platinum analogs, 860–861, 902–905
    targeting cell cycle and DNA, 851, 851f
Chester porphyria, 500–501, 501f
Chevallier, Paul, 944
Chido/Rogers blood group system, 1699–1700
Chikungunya virus, 1812–1813
Childhood cerebral X-linked adrenoleukodystrophy
  (CCALD), 1555
Children. See also Neonates
  anaplastic large cell lymphoma in, 1336–1338, 1337t
  anemia in, 460–461, 461f, 461t
  anorexia nervosa in, 2225
  antiphospholipid syndrome and, 2097–2098
  blood banking and, 1821–1822
  Burkitt lymphoma in, 1333–1334, 1335t
  cardiopulmonary disease in, 2222–2223, 2222t
  collagen vascular disease, acute vasculitis in, 2219–2222
  diffuse large B-cell lymphoma in, 1334–1336,
    1334t–1335t
  endocrine disease in, 2225
  gastrointestinal disease in, 2223–2225
  Hodgkin lymphoma in, 1338–1341, 1340t
  infectious disease in, 2215–2219
  lymphomas (rare subtypes) in, 1341
  metabolic diseases in, 2234, 2234t–2235t
  non-Hodgkin lymphoma in, 1330–1338, 1331t–1332t
  poisoning in, 2233–2234

Children (Continued)
  posttransplantation lymphoproliferative disease in, 1338
  second/subsequent malignancies in, 1502, 1504
  solid organ transplants in, 2228–2233
  splenomegaly in, 2234–2236, 2236b, 2236t
  thrombotic complications in, 2225–2228
  von Willebrand disease and, 2062–2063, 2063b
Chimeric antigen receptor T (CAR-T) cells
  for acute lymphoblastic leukemia, 1051
  for acute myeloid leukemia, 992
  for chronic lymphocytic leukemia, 1259
  graft-versus-leukemia responses and, 1663–1667
  natural killer cell-based therapy and, 1575
  overview of, 1570–1572, 1572t
Chimeric antigen receptors (CAR), 237–238, 238f
Chimerism analysis, 845
Chlorambucil
  for chronic lymphocytic leukemia, 1253, 1256
  for extranodal marginal zone lymphoma of MALT type,
    1282
  for hypereosinophilic syndrome, 1166
  pharmacology of, 855, 886–887
  for splenic marginal zone lymphoma, 1285
  for Waldenström macroglobulinemia, 1426
Chloramphenicol, 400, 511, 679
2'-Chlorodeoxyadenosine (CdA), 894, 1373
Chloroma. See Myeloid sarcoma
Cholecystitis, 601
Cholelithiasis, 601
Cholesterol, 75
Cholesterol ester transfer protein (CETP), 2124, 2124f
Cholesterol hypothesis, 2122–2125, 2123f–2124f
Choline transporter-like protein 2 (CTL-2), 1735
CHOP regimen, 1253
Chorea-acanthocytosis syndrome, 642
Chorein, 642
Christmas disease. See Hemophilia B
Chromatin
  compaction of, 17
  epigenetic regulation and, 9
  erythroid cell development and, 316
  functional domains, 17, 18f
  overview of, 17
  remodeling of. See Remodeling
  sequencing approaches for, 29
  structure of, 20, 21f
  transcription factors and, 20
Chromatin immunoprecipitation sequencing (ChIP-Seq),
  21, 21f, 29
Chromatin regulators, 29, 1386
Chromodomain helicase DNA binding (CHD) family, 20
Chromosome conformation capture (3C) technique, 21,
  21f
Chromosomes
  1, 1384
  3, 796, 796f
  5, 793–794, 944, 952, 960, 960f, 964–965. See also
    Del(5q)
  6, 825
  7, 794, 952
  11, 805, 806f, 824–825
  13, 822, 830–831, 1384
  17, 795, 825, 952, 1384
  20, 952
  21, 1017–1018. See also Del(17p)
  acute myeloid leukemia and, 915–917
  chronic lymphocytic leukemia and, 1251–1252
  DNA structure and, 3
  Fanconi anemia and, 355–356
  folate and, 523
  gene organization and, 17
  Hodgkin lymphoma and, 1209
  polycythemia vera and, 1094–1096
  primary myelofibrosis and, 1134, 1136f, 1140–1141
  rearrangements in, 28–29
Chromothripsis, 826, 826f
Chronic active Epstein-Barr infection (CAEBV), 753–754
Chronic benign neutropenia, 677–678
Chronic eosinophilic leukemia (CEL), 790–792, 1162t,
  1163
Chronic granulocytic leukemia. See Chronic myelogenous
  leukemia
Chronic granulomatous disease (CGD)
  chronic conditions associate with, 698t
  classification of, 695t
  clinical manifestations of, 695–698, 696f
  diagnosis of, 698–699, 698b
  gene therapy and, 1554

Chronic granulomatous disease (CGD) *(Continued)*
　infection and, 697*t*, 1448–1449
　molecular genetics of, 693–695, 694*f*, 695*t*
　overview of, 692
　prognosis and treatment of, 699–700, 699*t*
Chronic idiopathic neutropenia, 430–431, 677–678
Chronic inflammatory demyelinating
　polyradiculoneuropathy (CIDP), 1755
Chronic kidney disease (CKD), 2244
Chronic large granular lymphocytic leukemia, 672*b*
Chronic lymphocytic leukemia (CLL)
　aberrant miRNA expression in, 23
　allogenic HSCT for, 1605–1606
　autoimmune complications of, 1263
　autoimmune hemolytic anemia in, 653–654, 660
　B-cell receptor and pathogenesis of, 1245–1246
　clinical manifestations of, 1247
　cytogenetics of, 822–827
　diagnosis of, 1247–1248
　epidemiology of, 1244
　familial, 1244
　fludarabine-refractory, 1260–1261
　future directions for, 1263
　gene mutations for diagnosis and prognosis in, 824*f*
　genetic testing for, 827*b*
　genome complexity in, 826–827, 826*f*
　infections in patients with, 1262–1263
　insect bite hypersensitivity and, 1261–1262
　intravenous immunoglobulin for, 1262–1263, 1753
　laboratory manifestations of, 1248–1249
　overview of, 1187, 1188*t*, 1189*f*
　pathobiology of, 1244–1245
　prognosis for, 1250–1252
　pure red cell aplasia and, 426
　relapsed, 1257–1261
　Richter syndrome and, 1261
　secondary malignancies in, 1261
　stem cell origin of, 115
　transplant evaluation in, 1249*b*
　treatment of, 1252–1260, 1252*b*
　in young patients, 1247*b*, 1260
Chronic lymphocytic leukemia up-regulated 1 (CLLU1),
　823
Chronic mountain sickness (CMS), 1077–1078
Chronic myelogenous leukemia (CML)
　accelerated phase, 1058, 1059*f*, 1059*t*, 1063
　additional chromosomal abnormalities and, 788–789
　allogenic HSCT for, 1605
　BCR-ABL1, tyrosine kinase inhibitors and, 87
　blast phase, 789–790, 789*f*, 1058–1059, 1059*t*, 1063
　classification of, 764, 764*t*
　clinical features of, 1057–1059, 1057*f*
　cytogenetic basis of, 784–790
　etiology, epidemiology, and genetics of, 1055
　genetic testing for, 789*b*
　infection and, 1447
　leukemoid reaction vs., 676
　miRNA, granulocytopoiesis and, 330
　natural history of, 1058–1059
　overview of, 1055
　pathophysiology of, 1055–1057
　polyclonal gammopathy and, 688
　pregnancy and, 1066, 2209
　prognosis for, 1059
　second/subsequent malignancies after, 1506
　therapy for
　　allogenic hematopoietic cell transplantation,
　　　1066–1069
　　autologous transplantation, 1069
　　chemotherapy, 1060
　　definitions of response to, 1059–1060, 1060*t*
　　interferons, 1060–1061
　　newly diagnosed patients, 1069*b*
　　patients with advanced disease, 1069
　　pregnancy and, 1066, 2209
　　prognostic indicators and, 1062–1063
　　tyrosine kinase inhibitors, 1061–1066
　transformation to advanced phase, 788–789, 789*f*
Chronic myelomonocytic leukemia (CMML), 688,
　767–768, 944, 946*t*
Chronic neutrophilic leukemia (CNL), 764
Chronic renal insufficiency, 2160
Chronic thromboembolic pulmonary hypertension
　(CTEPH), 2104
Chronic wasting disease (CWD), 1819
CHS. *See* Chediak-Higashi syndrome
Churg-Strauss syndrome (CSS), 1151–1153, 1153*t*, 1164
Chuvash polycythemia (CP), 308, 1079

Chymase, 1156–1157
Cidofovir, 1455
Cilostazol, 1936, 2165
CIP1. *See* P21
Circumcision, 2009
Cirrhosis, 1752
Cis-acting elements, defined, 9
Cisplatin, 860–861, 902
Cistrome, 20
Citrate, 1707, 1799
Citrate phosphate dextrose adenine (CPDA), 1702
Citrate toxicity, 1526
Cladribine
　autoimmune hemolytic anemia and, 655
　for extranodal marginal zone lymphoma of MALT type,
　　1282
　for hairy cell leukemia, 1270–1272, 1270*f*, 1270*t*,
　　1273*f*
　for mastocytosis, 1182–1183
　for Waldenström macroglobulinemia, 1426–1428
Clarification of Optimal Anticoagulation Therapy
　Through Genetics (COAG) study, 85–86
Class II-associated invariant chain peptide (CLIP), 221,
　222*f*
Class switch recombination (CSR), 204–205, 219,
　722–723
Class variation, 274
Classical Hodgkin lymphoma (CHL)
　classification of, 1204–1210
　diagnosis of, 1200
　Epstein-Barr virus and, 1209
　Hodgkin and Reed-Sternberg cells of, 1205–1206,
　　1206*t*, 1212–1214, 1214*f*–1215*f*
　lymphocyte depletion, 1201, 1212, 1213*t*, 1214
　lymphocyte rich, 1202, 1212, 1213*f*, 1213*t*, 1214
　mixed cellularity (CHLMC), 1201, 1202*f*
　nodular sclerosis, 1201, 1202*f*, 1212–1214, 1218
　overview of, 1213–1216
　pathobiology, 1212, 1213*t*, 1215*f*
　Richter syndrome and, 1187
　T-cell derived, 1206
　treatment of, 1218–1219
Classical pathway (CP) of complement system, 261, 262*f*,
　264*t*
Clathrin-coated vesicles, 57, 1850–1851
Claudins, 155
Clear-cell carcinoma, 1078–1079
CLEC2 adhesion receptor, 1872–1873
Clinical and Translational Sciences Awards (CTSA),
　1531
Clinical trials
　design of, 850*t*
　phase I, 850–851
　phase II, 851
CliniMACS Prodigy system, 1533, 1540, 1540*f*
CLLU1. *See* Chronic lymphocytic leukemia up-regulated 1
Clodiprogrel, 2145–2146, 2145*t*
Clofarabine, 738, 858, 897–898, 968
Clofibrate, 1938
Clonal dermatitis, 1363
Clonal hematopoiesis of indeterminate potential, 27–28
Clonal succession model of stem cell activation, 99
Clonality, 781–783, 782*f*, 1392–1394
Clopidogrel
　for acute stroke, 2139–2140
　overview of, 2170–2171
　platelet disorders and, 1935
　resistance to, 2171
　thrombotic microangiopathies and, 1998–1999
Clostridial infection, 668
Clotting factors. *See Specific factors*
Cluster of differentiation (CD), 1871. *See also Specific CD
　entries*
Clustering algorithms, 26
CML. *See* Chromic myeloid leukemia
Coagulation
　antiphospholipid antibodies and, 2089
　cancer, thrombosis, and, 2251
　developmental hemostasis and, 2189, 2191*t*
　endothelium and, 1851–1852, 1851*f*
　factor VIII and, 2003
　hemostasis and, 1834–1837, 1835*f*
　key events in, 1906, 1907*f*, 2035*f*
　laboratory evaluation of
　　methodology, 1922
　　physiology underlying, 1922, 1925*f*
　　practical approach, 1926–1927, 1927*t*
　　specific, 1925–1926

Coagulation *(Continued)*
　liver disease and, 2239–2240
　malaria and, 2283
　molecular basis of
　　clot proteins, 1895–1897
　　cofactor proteins, 1888–1891, 1890*f*
　　endothelium, 1894, 1895*f*
　　fibrinolysis proteins, 1897–1898
　　intrinsic accessory pathway proteins, 1891–1894,
　　　1892*f*
　　overview, 1885
　　platelets, 1894–1895, 1896*f*
　　vitamin K-dependent protein family, 1885–1888,
　　　1888*f*
　multiple myeloma and, 1392
　regulators of, 1909, 1910*f*
　sickle cell anemia and, 580–581
　thromboembolism and, 2108–2109
Coagulation cascade, 1922
Coagulation disorders
　in children, 2217–2218
　liver disease and, 2239–2240
　in neonate, 2195–2196
　in pregnancy, 2210–2212
Coagulation factor concentrates, 1761–1766, 2062*b*
Coagulation factor deficiencies
　combined, 2048–2049, 2048*t*
　differential diagnosis for, 2072
　dysfibrinogenemia, 2038–2040
　factor IX. *See* Hemophilia B
　factor V. *See* Factor V deficiency
　factor VII. *See* Factor VII deficiency
　factor VIII. *See* Hemophilia A
　factor X. *See* Factor X deficiency
　factor XI. *See* Factor XI deficiency
　factor XII. *See* Factor XII deficiency
　factor XIII. *See* Factor XIII deficiency
　fibrinogen. *See* Fibrinogen deficiency
　high-molecular weight kininogen, 2047
　laboratory testing in, 2049*b*
　liver disease and, 2239–2240
　miscellaneous, 1777–1779
　overview of, 2034, 2035*f*, 2035*t*
　prekallikrein, 2046–2047
　prothrombin, 1778, 1840, 2040–2041
　von Willebrand factor. *See* von Willebrand factor
　　deficiency
Coagulation factors (CF). *See also Specific factors*
　angiogenesis and, 1847*f*, 1849
　atherothrombosis and, 2130–2131
　developmental hemostasis and, 2189
　for hemophilia, 2013–2014
　hemostasis and, 1840, 1840*t*
　laboratory evaluation of, *e*12*b*
　reference values for, *e*26*t*
　vascular growth and, 155–156
Coagulation testing
　overview of, *e*1, *e*12*b*
　reference values for, *e*24*t*–*e*25*t*
　screening, *e*12*b*
　surgical patients and, 2304–2305
Coats plus syndrome, 365–367
Cobalamin deficiency
　biochemical evaluation of, 527–529, 527*b*, 528*t*,
　　529*b*
　biochemical indicators of, 526–527
　classification of, 525*b*
　clinical presentation and evaluation for, 526, 537–540,
　　538*t*
　diagnosis of, 526*t*
　diagnostic and therapeutic approach, 540–541, 543*b*
　distinguishing, 525*b*
　effects of, 526
　as metabolic disorder, 1998
　neurologic dysfunction with, 524–526
　pathogenesis of, 529–533
　subclinical, 532–533
　therapy for, 541–542
Cobalamins (Vitamin B₁₂)
　absorption of, 515–516, 516*f*
　cellular processing of, 517–518, 517*f*
　chemistry and nomenclature of, 515*f*
　folates and, 521–523
　importance of, 514
　laboratory evaluation of, *e*6*b*
　malabsorption of, 530–531
　nutrition and, 514–515
　reference values for, *e*18*t*

Cobalamins (Vitamin B$_{12}$) *(Continued)*
  renal retention of, 521
  routine supplementation of, 542–543, 542*t*, 543*b*
  transport of, 516–517
Cobblestone area-forming cell (CAFC) assay, 98
COBE Spectra Processor, 1538
Cocaine, 1938–1939
Codocytes, 668
Codons, 7, 7*t*
Cognitive-behavioral therapy, 1474–1475
Cohesin complex, 920, 951
Cohn, Edward, 1759, 1769
Cold agglutinin disease, 661
Cold autoimmune hemolytic anemia (CAIHA)
  epidemiology of, 648
  laboratory diagnosis of, 652
  pathobiology of, 648–649, 649*f*
  symptoms, clinical findings, and risks in, 650
  treatment of, 658*t*, 661–662
  Waldenström macroglobulinemia and, 1424
Collagen
  aplastic anemia and, 403
  cell adhesion and, 127, 1870, 1872
  hemostasis and, 1832–1833, 1907–1909
Collagen binding assay, 1928, 2059
Colony stimulating factors (CSF), 178
Colony-forming cell (CFC) assay, 98
Colony-forming cell-megakaryocytes (CFU-Mk), 334
Colony-forming unit-erythroid cells (CFU-E), 297, 298*t*, 447
Colony-forming unit-granulocyte, erythrocyte, macrophage, megakaryocyte (CFU-GEMM), 297, 298*t*, 321, 334
Colony-forming unit-spleen (CFU-S), 98
Colony-stimulating factor 1 (CSF-1), 332
Colton blood group system, 1699
Coltuximab ravtansine, 1050–1051
Combotox, 1051
Common lymphoid progenitors (CLP), 96, 210, 211*f*
Common myeloid progenitor, 297, 298*t*, 321, 334
Common precursor B-cell acute lymphoblastic leukemia, 1005–1006, 1009–1010, 1016
Common variable immune deficiency (CVID), 655, 661, 687, 720–722, 721*f*
Communication, palliative care and, 1488–1490
Community-acquired respiratory viral (CRV) infections, 1674
Comparative genomic hybridization (CGH), 28, 777*f*, 779–781
Compartment syndrome, 2010*b*
Compatibility testing, 1692–1693
Competency, 182–183, 183*f*
Competitive repopulating assay, 98–99, 99*f*
Competitive repopulating units (CRU), 98–99
Complement activation, 2090–2092
Complement assays, 420
Complement system
  alternative pathway, 262*f*, 263–264, 264*t*, 1993, 1994*f*
  antibody responses and, 269–272
  C antigen, 1697
  C1 inhibitor, 264*t*, 266, 1767, 1768*t*
  C2 deficiency, 266
  C3, 264–266
  C3 convertase, 261, 263–265
  C3a, C5a and, 265
  C4, 266
  C4 binding protein, 264*t*
  C5, 264–265
  C5 convertase, 264–265
  classical pathway, 261, 262*f*, 264*t*
  complement factor H, 1993–1994, 1999
  complement receptors, 264–265, 264*t*
  deficiencies in
    autoimmunity and, 268
    complement cascade, 266
    complement regulatory proteins, 266–268
  drugs targeting, 279–283
  fractions, e10*b*, e24*t*
  hemolytic uremic syndromes and, 1993–1994
  innate and adaptive immune responses and, 268
  lectin pathway, 261–262, 262*f*
  natural antibody and, 268
  new directions, 283, 283*f*
  overview of, 261, 262*f*
  receptors and, 265

Complement system *(Continued)*
  receptors and antibody responses, 269–272
  regulation of activation of, 266
  soluble mediators of antibody responses and, 268–269
  T cell immunity and, 272, 272*f*
Complementarity-determining regions (CDR), 62–63, 62*f*–63*f*, 273–274
Complementary and alternative medicine (CAM), 2253. *See also* Integrative therapies
Complementation, 350–352
Complete blood count (CBC), e2*b*
Complete molecular response (CMR), 786, 1059–1060
Complex karyotypes (CK), 952–953, 971*t*, 972
Complicated grief, 1494
Compliment-dependent cytotoxicity (CDC), 1728
Composite lymphomas, 1208, 1208*f*
Compression stockings, 2109
Compression therapy, 2108–2109
Computed tomographic angiography (CTA), 2161–2162
Computed tomographic pulmonary angiography (CTPA), 2106
Computed tomography (CT), 2137, 2319
Concurrent porphyrias, 503
Condensing enzyme, 75
Congenital amegakaryocytic thrombocytopenia (CAMT)
  acute myeloid leukemia and, 915
  background of, 368
  clinical features of, 369
  differential diagnosis for, 370
  epidemiology of, 368
  Fanconi anemia vs., 357
  future directions for, 371
  laboratory findings in, 369–370
  leukemia predisposition and, 370
  pathobiology of, 368–369, 1883
  therapy and prognosis in, 370–371
  thrombopoietin signaling in, 339
Congenital atransferrinemia, 485–487
Congenital bone marrow failure syndromes. *See* Bone marrow failure syndromes, inherited
Congenital disorder of glycosylation type II. *See* McLeod syndrome
Congenital dyserythropoietic anemias (CDA)
  background, 380
  differential diagnosis, 384
  etiology, genetics, pathophysiology, and clinical features, 380–384
  future directions, 384–385
  therapy and prognosis, 384
Congenital erythropoietic porphyria (CET), 504, 506
Congenital heart disease (CHD), 1971, 2222–2223, 2222*t*, 2226–2227
Congenital Heinz body hemolytic anemia, 609–610
Congenital hypoplastic anemia. *See* Diamond-Blackfan anemia
Congenital polycythemia, 308
Congenital porphyria, 498*f*
Congestive heart failure (CHF), 1496–1497
Connective tissue, 688
Connexins, 155, 1844
Consolidative radiotherapy, 1221–1222
Constant (C) gene segments, 212, 213*f*
Constipation, 1479
Contact (intrinsic) pathway
  disseminated intravascular coagulation and, 2065
  hemophilia carrier detection and, 2007*b*
  molecular basis of, 1886*f*
  overview of, 1836–1837, 1837*f*
  role of, 1836*b*
  treatment of hemostasis and thrombosis disorders and, 1841
Contact activation, 2045, 2045*f*
Contact isolation, 1459
Contractile ring activity, 343
Coombs-positive autoimmune hemolytic anemia, 668
Cooption. *See* Vascular cooption
Coordinated lysosomal expression and regulation (CLEAR) network, 740
Coping strategies, 1467
Copper, hemolysis disorders and, 669
Copper deficiency, 433, 511, 512*f*
Copy number variants (CNV), 28, 81
Cord blood transplantation. *See* Umbilical cord blood transplantation
Core binding factor beta (CBFB), 803, 928*f*

Core binding factor (CBF)
  acute myeloid leukemia and, 916, 937, 982–983
  erythropoiesis and, 313
  myeloid differentiation and, 325–326
  specification of hematopoietic stem cells and, 103
Core binding factor leukemias, 801, 982–983
Core complex, 353
Core histones, 18–19, 19*f*
Corifact, 1766
Coronin-1A deficiency, 715
Corticosteroids
  for acute lymphoblastic leukemia, 1025–1026, 1037–1039
  for aplastic anemia, 411
  chronic granulomatous disease and, 700
  for cutaneous T-cell lymphomas, 1371
  for Diamond-Blackfan anemia, 378–379
  for graft-versus-host disease, 1663
  for hypereosinophilic syndrome, 1165
  for immune thrombocytopenia purpura, 1948
  for light chain amyloidosis, 1439
  for nausea and vomiting, 1484
  pain management and, 1480
  for primary myelofibrosis, 1142
  spleen and, 2322
  for thrombotic thrombocytopenic purpura, 1990
  for warm antibody hemolytic anemia, 656–657, 657*f*
Costimulation, 288–289
Cotswold-Modified Ann Arbor Staging System for Hodgkin lymphoma, 1216, 1216*t*
Coumarins, 1981
Covert stroke, 2135
COX. *See* Cyclooxygenases
COX-2 inhibitors. *See* Cyclooxygenase-2 inhibitors
CPT-11. *See* Irinotecan
CPX-351, for acute myeloid leukemia, 939
C-reactive protein (CRP), 2064–2065, 2160
Crenolanib, 939
Creutzfeldt-Jakob disease (CJD), 1818
CRISPR, overview of, 15
CRISPR/CRISPR-associated protein 9 (CAS9), 25, 32–34, 33*f*
Critical congenital heart disease (CCHD), 2222–2223
Critical limb ischemia (CLI), 2159, 2161*f*
Crizotinib, 865, 903–904, 1338
CRLF2. *See* Cytokine receptor-like factor 2
Cromer blood group system, 1699
Cross-dressing, 252
Cross-linking, 20
Cross-presentation, 231, 251–252
Cross-reactive groups (CREGs), 1729–1730, 1729*t*
Cryoglobulinemia, 1423–1425
Cryohydrocytosis, 645
Cryoprecipitate
  adverse effects of, 1751
  compatibility, 1751
  for disseminated intravascular coagulation, 2073
  dosage, 1750–1751
  fibrinogen and, 2036–2038
  for hemophilia, 1769–1770, 1773–1774, 2013
  indications for, 1749–1750, 1749*t*
  overview of, 1748–1749, 1761
  pediatric, 1821
  for pediatric patients, 1823, 1823*t*
  for von Willebrand disease, 1777
Cryoprecipitate-reduced plasma, 1745
Cryoreduced plasma, 1745
Cryosupernatant, 1745
Cryptic splicing, 548, 549*f*
CSS. *See* Churg-Strauss syndrome
CTL. *See* CD8+ cytotoxic T cells; Choline transporter-like protein; Cytotoxic T lymphocytes
CTLA4. *See* Cytotoxic T lymphocyte antigen 4
CTLR. *See* C-type lectin receptors
CTPS1. *See* Cytidine triphosphate synthase 1
C-type lectin receptors (CTLR), 241–242
C-type lectins, 250–251
Cubam, 515
Cubilin, 515, 532
Cushing syndrome, 1080
Cutaneous hepatic porphyria, 498*f*, 504–505, 505*f*
Cutaneous lymphocyte-associated antigen (CLA), 247
Cutaneous lymphoid dyscrasias, 1363
Cutaneous mastocytosis (CM), 1173, 1174*t*
Cutaneous pain management techniques, 1475
Cutaneous porphyrias, overview of, 504

Cutaneous T-cell lymphomas (CTCL)
classification of, 1345f, 1360t
clinical presentation of, 1362–1364
differential diagnosis for, 1366–1368
epidemiology of, 1360–1361
future directions for, 1379
investigational therapy for, 1377–1379
laboratory manifestations of, 1364–1365
overview of, 1360, 1360t
pathobiology of, 1361–1362
prognosis for, 1368–1369
stem cell transplantation in, 1375
therapy for, 1369–1379
CXC chemokine ligand 12-abundant reticular (CAR) cells, 121
CXC chemokine ligands (CXCL)
CXCL-1, 2126
CXCL-2, 148–149, 149f
CXCL-4, 2127
CXCL-9, 1662–1663
CXCL-12, 101, 106t, 124, 389–390, 1560–1562
CXC chemokine receptors (CXCR)
CXCR-1, 148–149, 149f
CXCR-4. See also Stromal cell-derived factor 1
B cell development and, 217
eosinophils and, 1154
hematopoietic stem cells and, 101, 106t
HIV infection and, 2266–2267
primary myelofibrosis and, 1129–1131
T follicular helper cells and, 231
as therapeutic target in leukemias, 124
Waldenström macroglobulinemia and, 1420f, 1421
WHIM syndrome and, 389–390
Cyanoacrylates, 2306
CYB. See Cytochrome-b
Cyclic AMP (cAMP), 1874
Cyclic neutropenia, 387–389, 678
Cyclin-dependent kinase inhibitors (CDKI)
cell cycle and, 178–180, 851f, 852
overview of, 178–180
pharmacology of, 872–873
Cyclin-dependent kinases (CDK)
acute lymphoblastic leukemia and, 820, 1016
cell cycle and, 178–180, 851f, 852
mantle cell lymphoma and, 1300f
megakaryocyte endomitosis and, 342
multiple myeloma and, 830
Richter syndrome and, 827
Cyclins
cell cycle and, 178, 851f, 852
cyclin C, 1016
cyclin D, 178
cyclin D1
hairy cell leukemia and, 1266–1268, 1298
mantle cell lymphoma and, 1189, 1240, 1298, 1300f
megakaryocyte endomitosis and, 342
multiple myeloma and, 830
cyclin D3, 342
cyclin E, 342
endomitosis and, 1857
megakaryocyte endomitosis and, 342
Cyclooxygenase-2 (COX-2) inhibitors, 1476, 2013, 2131
Cyclooxygenases (COX), 384, 1110, 2168–2170, 2169f
Cyclophosphamide
for acute lymphoblastic leukemia, 1039
acute myeloid leukemia and, 913, 1037
after allogenic hematopoietic stem cell transplantation, 1675–1676
for aplastic anemia, 411
for chronic lymphocytic leukemia, 1254–1256
for extranodal marginal zone lymphoma of MALT type, 1282
gonadal dysfunction and, 1499–1500
haploidentical hematopoietic stem cell transplantation and, 1625–1627, 1626f, 1629
for hypereosinophilic syndrome, 1165
infection and, 1447
for light chain amyloidosis, 1439
for multiple myeloma, 1403–1407
pharmacology of, 854, 865
for pure red cell aplasia, 430
for splenic marginal zone lymphoma, 1285
for thrombotic thrombocytopenic purpura, 1991
for Waldenström macroglobulinemia, 1427–1428
for warm antibody hemolytic anemia, 660
Cyclophosphamide, thalidomide, dexamethasone (CTD), 1404–1407

Cyclosporine A (CSA)
for aplastic anemia, 411
for graft-versus-host disease, 1659, 1661t, 1663
graft-versus-host disease and, 1664
for hypereosinophilic syndrome, 1166
for peripheral T-cell lymphomas, 1354–1355
for pure red cell aplasia, 430
thrombotic microangiopathies and, 1997
for thrombotic thrombocytopenic purpura, 1991
CYP. See Cytochrome P450 enzymes
Cystic fibrosis (CF), 2223
Cystic fibrosis transmembrane conductance regulator (CFTR), 879
Cytapheresis
defined, 1781
extracorporeal photopheresis. See Extracorporeal photopheresis
of leukocytes. See Leukapheresis
of platelets. See Plateletpheresis
of red blood cells. See Erythrocytapheresis
therapeutic, 1782–1783, 1783t, 1790b
Cytarabine
for acute lymphoblastic leukemia, 1040
for acute myeloid leukemia, 934f, 935–936, 939
for acute promyelocytic leukemia, 940
for mantle cell lymphoma, 1305
for myelodysplastic syndromes, 965
Cytidine triphosphate synthase 1 (CTPS1), 717
Cytochrome b5 reductase (b5R)
deficiency in, 624–625
methemoglobinemia and, 623–625
Cytochrome P450 (CYP) enzymes, 85–86, 1478
Cytochrome-b (CYB), 693–694, 695t
Cytogenetic methods
clonal origin of leukemia and, 781–783
comparative genomic hybridization and next generation sequencing, 779–781
cytogenetic analysis, 774, 777f
fluorescence in situ hybridization (FISH), 774–778
overview of, 777f
terminology of, 775t–776t
in utero mutations, clonal origin and, 783
Cytogenetics
of acute lymphoblastic leukemia, 815–822
of acute myeloid leukemia, 798–815
allogenic hematopoietic stem cell transplantation and, 845–846
of B-cell chronic lymphocytic leukemia, 822–827
of chronic myelogenous leukemia, 784–790
clonal origin of leukemia, 781–783
early mutations in leukemogenesis and age-related clonal hematopoiesis, 783–784
future directions, 848
of hairy cell leukemia, 839–840
of multiple myeloma, 827–832, 1381–1382, 1399
of myelodysplastic syndromes, 793–798
of non-Hodgkin lymphoma, 832–839
overview of, 28
of Ph-negative chronic myeloproliferative neoplasms, 790–793, 791t, 792b
of T-cell lymphoproliferative neoplasms, 840–845
Cytokine receptor homology domain (CDH), 70
Cytokine receptor-like factor 2 (CRLF2), 820, 1015
Cytokine release syndrome (CRS), 1051, 1664–1667
Cytokine signaling
elements of, 163–164, 164f–165f
innate immune system and, 199–200, 202t
Janus kinases. See Janus kinases
ligand-receptor binding and activation, 164–173, 167f
negative regulators of cytokine signaling, 171–173
physiology and pathology, 173–174, 173t
receptors and, 70–71, 163–164, 167f
STAT. See Signal transducers and activators of transcription
Cytokines
acute myeloid leukemia and, 917–919
anemia of chronic diseases and, 491–493
B cell development and, 216–217
class/type I, 163, 164f. See also Hematopoietins
class/type II, 163
dendritic cells and T cell activation and, 253, 253t
for Diamond-Blackfan anemia, 379
graft-versus-host disease and, 1657–1658, 1662
for Kostmann syndrome/severe congenital neutropenia, 388
malaria and, 2281–2282
megakaryocytopoiesis and, 340
mesenchymal stromal cells and, 1560–1562

Cytokines (Continued)
mobilization of hematopoietic stem cells and, 1522
monocytopoiesis and, 332
multiple myeloma and, 1389
myeloid proliferation and differentiation and, 323–324, 324f
overview of, 163–164
polymorphisms in, 1726–1727
therapeutic stimulation of megakaryocytopoiesis and, 340–341
thrombocytopoiesis and, 338–341
transfusion reactions and, 1792
Cytomegalovirus (CMV)
clinical presentation and diagnosis of, 1672–1673
dendritic cell function and, 256
epidemiology and risk factors for, 1670–1672
hematopoietic stem cell transplants and, 1457–1459, 1670–1673, 1678
leukocyte-reduced red blood cells and, 1703
lymphocytosis and, 683
natural killer cells and, 1575, 1579
pediatric transfusions and, 1826
prevention and treatment of, 1673, 1673b
transfusion-associated, 1809–1810, 1826
Cytopenias, 1348, 2267–2268, 2267b, 2329
Cytoplasmic vacuolation, 1030, 1031f
Cytoreductive chemotherapy, 979
Cytosine arabinoside, 892, 1060–1061
Cytotoxic T lymphocyte antigen 4 (CTLA-4)
allograft transplantation and, 237
checkpoint blockade therapies and, 1583, 1585–1586
deficiency in, 718
factor VIII inhibitors and, 2026
limitation of T cell activity and, 234–235
manipulating T cells to improve activity against malignancy, 237–238
Cytotoxic T lymphocytes (CTL)
antigen-specific for HSCT, 1545
defects of, 719–720
graft-versus-host disease and, 1657–1658
overview of, 1568–1569
pure red cell aplasia and, 425
Cytotoxicity-negative adsorption-positive (CYNAP) phenomenon, 1728
Cytovene, 2273
Cytoxan. See Cyclophosphamide

D

D sensitization, 1717–1718, 1757b
DAB389IL-2, 877–878
Dabigatran etexilate
for acute coronary syndromes, 2150
for acute stroke, 2139–2140
for atrial fibrillation, 2155–2156
overview of, 2181–2182, 2181t
for venous thromboembolism, 2108
Dacarbazine (DTIC), 854f, 855, 888
Daclizumab, 430, 1184
DAF. See Decay-accelerating factor
Damage-associated molecular patterns (DAMP), 188, 1655
Danaparoid, 1978–1979, 1979t–1980t
Danazol, 429
Dapsone, 671
Daratumumab, 1415
Darbepoetin, 429, 592, 962, 1142
DARC. See Duffy antigen receptor for chemokines
Dark zone, 219, 269–270
Dasatinib
for chronic myelogenous leukemia, 1064–1065, 1069
for mastocytosis, 1183–1184
pharmacology of, 861, 862t
for Philadelphia chromosome–positive acute lymphoblastic leukemia, 1045–1046
Database of Short Genetic Variations (dbSNP), 79
Daunorubicin
for acute lymphoblastic leukemia, 1037–1039
for acute myeloid leukemia, 935, 939
pharmacology of, 899–900
Dausset, Jean, 1721
DBA. See Diamond-Blackfan anemia
dbSNP. See Database of Short Genetic Variations
DC. See Dyskeratosis congenita
DCK. See Deoxycytidine kinase
DCML deficiency. See Dendritic cell, monocyte, and lymphoid deficiency
DC-SIGN, 131

DD. *See* Death domain
DD therapy, 1376–1377
DDAVP. *See* Desmopressin
D-Dimer, 2130
D-Dimer testing
  for activated coagulation states, 1930
  for deep vein thrombosis, 2105
  disseminated intravascular coagulation and, 2070
  overview of, e13b
  reference values for, e26t
De novo nucleotide synthesis, 76
Death domain (DD), 71, 187–188
Death effector domain (DED), 187–188
Death receptors (DR), 193–194, 870–871
Death-inducing signaling complex (DISC), 188, 189f
Decay-accelerating factor (DAF), 264, 264t, 1993
Decision-making, palliative care and, 1489–1490
Decitabine
  for acute myeloid leukemia, 936
  as epigenetic therapy, 23
  for myelodysplastic syndromes, 966–967
  for myelodysplastic syndromes in children, 997b
  pharmacology of, 857, 896–897
Decoy receptors, 71
DED. *See* Death effector domain
Dedicator of cytokines (DOCK) proteins
  DOCK2, 716
  DOCK8, 704–705, 716
Deep vein thrombosis (DVT). *See also* Venous
    thromboembolism
  acute recurrent, 2107–2108
  diagnosis of, 2104–2105
  diagnostic strategies for, 2105–2106
  mechanical interventions in, 2117–2120
  objective diagnostic tests for, 2105
Deferasirox
  for acquired sideroblastic anemia, 510b
  for β-thalassemia syndrome, 554–555, 557–558
  for iron overload, 964
  iron overload and, 490
Deferiprone, 554–557, 557f
Deferoxamine, 489, 554–556
DEHP, 1707
DEK-NUP214 fusion, 811
Del(13q), 822
Del(17p), 795, 1384
Del(20q), 952
Del(5q), 793–794, 944, 952, 960, 960f, 964–965
Del(6q), 825
Del(7q), 794
Delanzomib, 869
Delayed hemolytic transfusion reactions (DHTR), 1794
Delirium, 1491–1492, 1492t
Delta-like (DLL), 153–154
Demarcation membrane system (DMS), 335–337, 337f,
    1857–1859
Demcizumab, 1051–1052
Dendreon Corporation, 1565
Dendritic cell, monocyte, and lymphoid (DCML)
  deficiency, 248, 680–681, 684, 915
Dendritic cell neoplasms, classification of, 772, 772t
Dendritic cells (DC)
  adaptive immune response and, 200
  antigen acquisition and activation of, 249–251, 250t
  antigen processing and, 251–252
  B cell activation and, 254
  dyskeratosis congenita and, 366
  graft-versus-host disease and, 1653–1655
  hematopoietic stem cell transplants and, 1545–1546
  immunotherapy and, 257–259
  as link between innate and active immunity, 255f
  maturation of, 248–249, 249t
  monocytes and, 331
  multiple myeloma and, 1390
  natural killer cells and, 254, 1576f
  overview of in immune system, 203
  reprogramming to exit tissues toward secondary
      lymphoid organs, 142
  subsets and development of, 247–248, 248f
  subversion of function by pathogens and tumors,
      256–259
  T cell activation and, 221, 252–254
  tolerance, immunity and, 254–256
Dengue viruses, 1811–1812
Denial, 1463
Denileukin diftitox, 877–878, 1184
Dense granules, 1859, 1875, 1876f–1877f, 1882
Dense tubular network, 335–336, 337f

2'-Deoxycoformycin (DCF), 895, 1373
Deoxycytidine, 873–874
Deoxycytidine kinase (DCK), 1269–1270
Depression, 1469–1470, 1491. *See also* Antidepressants
Depsipeptide, 877
Dermatomyositis, 1755
Desferoxamine, 964
Desirudin, 1979–1980, 1979t–1980t, 2178–2179
Desmopressin (DDAVP)
  for hemophilia, 1773, 2015
  pregnancy and, 2210
  surgical patients and, 2305–2306
  for uremic bleeding, 2244
  for von Willebrand disease, 1776, 2061–2063
Desmopressin responsiveness testing, 2060, 2060t
Desmoteplase, 2187
Dessicytosis, hereditary, 644–645
Developmental hemostasis, 2196
Dexamethasone
  for acute lymphoblastic leukemia, 1025–1026,
      1037–1039
  for immune thrombocytopenia purpura, 1948
  for light chain amyloidosis, 1439
  for multiple myeloma, 1402–1407
Dexrazoxane, 1497–1498
Dextrans, platelet disorders and, 1938
Dextroamphetamine, 1477
DFF40. *See* DNA fragmentation factor 40
DGK. *See* Diacylglycerol kinases
Diabetes, 256, 559, 2159, 2164
Diacylglycerol kinases (DGK), 235, 1994
Dialysis, 1941. *See also* Renal dialysis
Diamond-Blackfan anemia (DBA)
  acute myeloid leukemia and, 914–915
  background of, 372–373
  clinical features of, 374–376, 374f–375f
  distinguishing features of, 377t
  epidemiology of, 373
  erythrocytes in, 376
  genetics of, 373
  globin genes and, 456
  malignancy predisposition and, 377–378
  natural history and prognosis, 378–379
  pathophysiology of, 373–374
  therapy for, 378
  transcription in erythropoiesis and, 317–318
Diapedesis, 129, 138
Dicer, 211
Dick, John, 921
Dickkopf-related protein 1 (DKK1), 1384, 1388–1389
Diego blood group antigens, 1698
Diet. *See* Nutrition
Differentiation, 176
Differentiation syndrome, 940
Diffuse large B-cell lymphoma (DLBCL)
  allogenic HSCT for, 1606
  in childhood, 1334–1336, 1334t–1335t
  classification of, 770–771
  clinical manifestations of, 1309, 1335
  cytogenetics of, 835
  differential diagnosis for, 1335
  epidemiology of, 1309, 1334
  Epstein-Barr virus and, 1321
  gene expression profiles and subtypes of, 1232–1235,
      1233f, 1233t
  intravascular, 1194, 1195f
  investigation of, 1309–1311
  late complications and followup in, 1316–1317
  molecular pathogenesis of, 1234
  not otherwise specified, 1188t, 1192–1193, 1193f
  other variants and subtypes, 1188t, 1193–1194,
      1194f
  overview of, 1231–1232, 1316–1317, 1334
  pathobiology of, 1309, 1335
  prognosis for, 1311, 1311t, 1335–1336, 1335t
  salvage therapy for, 1316–1317
  staging of, 1335–1336, 1335t
  stem cell origin of, 117
  treatment of, 1311b, 1312–1314, 1313b, 1313f,
      1316–1317, 1335–1336
  tumor microenvironment and, 1234–1235
DiGeorge syndrome (DGS), 204, 710
Dihydrorhodamine (DHR) test, 698–699
Dilute Russell viper venom (dRVV) testing,
    2092–2093
Dimethyl fumarate, 685
Dimethyl sulfoxide (DMSO) toxicity, 1800, 1800t
Dipeptidylpeptidase 4 (DPP4), 173–174

2,3-Diphosphoglycerate (2,3-DPG), 1707
Dipyridamole, 1936, 2164, 2171–2172, 2172f
Direct antiglobulin test (DAT), 651, 651f, 1693b
Direct oral anticoagulants (DOAC), overview of,
    2179–2184
Directed donations, 1821–1822
DISC. *See* Death-inducing signaling complex
Disease risk index (DRI), 1603b
Disseminated intravascular coagulation (DIC)
  in children, 2217–2218
  clinical manifestations of, 2067–2070, 2068b
  diagnostic algorithm for, 2071, 2071b
  differential diagnosis for, 2071–2072, 2072t
  drug-induced, 1967
  epidemiology of, 2064
  evaluation of, 1930
  laboratory manifestations of, 2070–2071
  malignancies and, 1969
  in neonate, 2197, 2198t
  overview of, 2064
  pathobiology of, 2064–2067, 2065f–2066f
  plasma derivatives for, 1747
  pregnancy and, 2208
  therapy for, 2073–2074, 2073b
Distress, 1468, 1468t, 1469f, 1473
Distress thermometer, 1468, 1469f
Disulfide bonds, 60–61
Ditropin A, 1647
Divalent metal transporter 1 (DMT1), 469, 472f,
    476–477, 476f, 485–487
Diversity (D) gene segments, 212, 213f
DKC1. *See* Dyskeratosis congenita
DLL. *See* Delta-like
DMT. *See* Divalent metal transporter
DNA (deoxyribonucleic acid)
  additional structural features of, 11–13, 12f
  modification of, 20
  molecular biology and, 3
  organization of genes in, 17–18
  replication of, 5f
  storage and transmission of genetic information and, 5
  structure of, 4f–5f
DNA binding domains (DBD), 20
DNA fragmentation factor 40 (DFF40), 186
DNA methylation, 949–950
DNA methyltransferase inhibitors (DNMTi), 23
DNA methyltransferases (DNMT)
  acute myeloid leukemia and, 783, 799–800, 919
  function of, 9, 17–18
  myelodysplastic syndromes and, 949–950
DNA polymorphisms, overview of, 12
DNA proofreading enzymes, overview of, 11–12
DNA replication, 181–182
DNA-binding protein inhibitors (ID), 316, 353
DNase I sequencing (DNase-Seq), 21, 21f
D-negative blood group. *See* Rh-negative blood group
DNMT. *See* DNA methyltransferases
Dobson, Peter, 501f
Docetaxel, 856–858, 891
DOCK. *See* Dedicator of cytokines
DOCK8 immunodeficiency syndrome, 705, 716
Domains, protein
  immunoglobulins, 62–63, 62f
  membrane proteins, 64–66
  overview of, 61–64, 61f
  protein kinase, 63–64
Dombrock blood group system, 1699
Dominant β-thalassemia, 547
Donath-Landsteiner antibody, 648–649
Donor lymphocyte infusion (DLI)
  for acute myeloid leukemia, 975
  after haploidentical hematopoietic stem cell
      transplantation, 1631
  cord blood stem cell transplantation and, 1648
  for Hodgkin lymphoma, 1225
  overview of, 1542, 1568–1569
Donor-induced leukemia, 124
Donor-specific antibodies (DSA), 1630–1631,
    1639–1640
DOT1L, 939, 1011–1012, 1012f, 1052
Double negative (DN) T cells, 227
Double-hit lymphomas (DHL), 770–771, 837, 1234
Double-unit cord blood transplantation (DCBT)
  for acute myeloid leukemia, 974
  adult donor allografts vs., 1642–1645, 1642t–1645t
  determinants of unit dominance, 1637, 1637t
  overview, 1635–1637
  single unit cord blood transplantation vs., 1640–1645

Down syndrome, 371–372, 915
Down syndrome-associated acute megakaryocytic leukemia (DS-AMKL), 343–344, 344f, 813, 985–986
Down syndrome-associated transient abnormal myelopoiesis, 1001–1002
Doxorubicin (adriamycin)
    for acute lymphoblastic leukemia, 1039
    for acute myeloid leukemia, 935
    cardiac disease and, 1496
    for cutaneous T-cell lymphomas, 1374
    for multiple myeloma, 1402–1403
    pharmacology of, 900
    for Waldenström macroglobulinemia, 1427–1428
DREAM complex, 180–181, 180f
Dronabinol, 1485
Drug resistance
    to antimetabolites, 883
    apoptosis and, 1018
    DNA repair pathway mechanisms of, 882–883
    genetic variations influencing, 82–84, 83f, 87
    multidrug resistance-associated protein/ ABC G2 transporter and, 881–883
    to nucleoside analogs, 857
    overview of, 878, 879t
    P-glycoprotein / ABC-B1 transporter and, 879–881
    to proteasome inhibitors, 867
    to signaling inhibitors, 883
    to topoisomerase inhibitors, 860
Drug transporters, drug disposition and, 86–87
Drug-induced disorders
    autoimmune hemolytic anemia, 654–655, 655t
    glucose-6-phosphate dehydrogenase deficiency, 86t, 87–88
    immune thrombocytopenia (D-ITP), 1961–1965, 1962f, 1963b, 1963t
    lymphocytopenia, 685
    lymphocytosis, 683
    neutropenia, 679–680, 679t
    neutrophilia, 677
    non-oxidative hemolysis, 669–670
    oxidative hemolysis, 670–671, 671b
    platelet disorders, 1932–1939, 1933t
    prothrombin deficiency, 2040
    thrombocytopenia
        autoimmune thrombocytopenia, 1965
        differential diagnosis for, 2072
        heparin-induced. See Heparin-induced thrombocytopenia
        immune, 1961–1965, 1963b, 1963t
        immune of rapid onset, 1965–1966
        mechanisms of, 1962f
        miscellaneous syndromes, 1966–1967
        overview, 442
        thrombocytopenic syndromes, 1961
    thrombotic microangiopathy, 1966–1967, 1997–1999
DTIC. See Dacarbazine
Dual-fusion fluorescence in situ hybridization, 774–778, 779f
Dubin-Johnson syndrome, 511–512
Dubowitz syndrome, 371
Duffy antigen (FY), 646, 1450, 1698
Duffy antigen receptor for chemokines (DARC), 138, 1844–1845
Duncan disease, 753
Duodenal cytochrome B (DCYTB), 476–477
Duplex ultrasonography, 2161
Dursun syndrome, 390
Dutcher bodies, 1189, 1189f
Duvelisib, 1360
Dynamins, 1859
Dyserythropoietic anemia, 343–344
Dysfibrinogenemias, 2038–2040, 2080
Dyskeratosis congenita 1 (DKC1), 396–397
Dyskeratosis congenita (DC)
    acute myeloid leukemia and, 914
    background, 365
    cancer predisposition, 366–367
    clinical features, 366–368
    differential diagnosis, 367
    epidemiology, 365
    Fanconi anemia vs., 357
    future directions, 368
    laboratory findings, 366
    natural history and prognosis, 367–368
    pathobiology, 365–366
    Schwachman-Diamond syndrome vs., 364
    therapy, 368
Dyslipidemias, 2159–2160, 2163–2164

E
E06 antibody, 2131
E2A-encoded splice variants, 210–212, 1009
E3 ubiquitin ligases, 235
E47 transcription factor deficiency (TCF3), 686–687, 1009
EACA. See ε-Aminocaproic acid
Early antigen (EA), 749–750
Early B-cell factor (EBF), 210–211
Early growth response protein 1 (Egr-1), 332
Early lymphoid progenitors (ELP), 210, 211f
Early pre-B-cell acute lymphoblastic leukemia, 1009
Early T-cell precursor acute lymphoblastic leukemia (ETP), 842, 1006–1007, 1032
East Texas bleeding disorder, 2041
EBERs. See Epstein–Barr virus-encoded small RNAs
EBF. See Early B-cell factor
EBNA. See Epstein-Barr virus nuclear antigens
Echinocandins, 1455–1456
Echinocytes, 643
Eclampsia, 1967, 2069
Ecotropic virus integration site 1 (EVI1), 788–789, 796, 812
ECP. See Eosinophil cationic protein
Eculizumab
    autoimmune hemolytic anemia and, 655
    for hemolytic uremic syndromes, 1996
    overview of, 279–283
    for paroxysmal nocturnal hemoglobinuria, 421–422
    for Shiga toxin hemolytic uremic syndrome, 1993
EDHF. See Endothelium-derived hyperpolarizing factor
EDN. See Eosinophil-derived neurotoxin
Edoxaban, 2155–2156, 2181t, 2183–2184
Education of natural killer cells. See Licensing
Effector memory T cells, 232
Efferocytosis, 186, 2129
EGCG. See Epigallocathechin-3-gallate
Egr-1. See Early growth response protein 1
Ehrlichia spp., 1815
EIF. See Eukaryotic initiation factors
EKLF. See Erythroid Krüppel-like factor
ELANE. See Neutrophil elastase
Elastin, 127
Elderly, 814, 1482. See also Aging and hematologic disorders
Electrical cardioversion, 2154–2155
Electrolyte toxicity, 1799
Elliptocytosis, 639. See also Hereditary elliptocytosis
Eloctate, 1764, 1774, 2013
Elotuzumab, 1414–1415
ELP. See Early lymphoid progenitors
Eltrombopag, 413, 963, 1949–1950
Elutra system, 1533
EMA. See Eosin-5'-maleimide binding
Embden-Meyerhof pathway, 448
Embryogenesis, 95, 119, 520–521
Embryonic stem cells, 107, 1556–1557, 1713
Emergency granulopoiesis, 326–327
Emesis. See Nausea and vomiting
Emicizumab, 2031
EMLA (Eutectic Mixture of Local Anesthetics), 1475, 2233
Emperipolesis, 738, 1126t
ENCODE project, 22, 22f
Encyclopedia of DNA Elements (ENCODE) project, 81
Endocrine disorders, 1079, 2225
Endocrine gland vascular endothelial growth factor/ prokineticin 1 (EG-VEGF-PK1), 153
Endocytosis, 52f, 56–57
Endogenous erythroid colonies, 1082
Endolysosomal system, defined, 57
Endometrial cells, 2092
Endomitosis
    endomitotic cell cycle in, 341, 341f
    megakaryocyte development and, 334, 1857
    in megakaryocytes, 342–343, 342f
    role in thrombocytopoiesis, 341–342
Endomucin, 1844–1845
Endoplasmic reticulum (ER)
    Bcl-2 family protein, apoptosis and, 191–193
    control of protein exit from, 55
    cotranslational protein translocation into, 51, 51f
    degradation of misassembled proteins in, 54, 54f
    processing of proteins in, 52–55, 53f
Endoplasmic reticulum-associated protein (ERAD), 54, 54f

Endoreduplication, 341
Endoreplication, 184
Endosomes, 57
Endothelial cell protein C receptor (EPCR)
    hemostasis and, 1832, 1832f, 1909, 1910f
    protection of vascular endothelium and, 2103
    thrombosis and, 1889–1890, 2080
Endothelial cells
    hematopoietic stem cells and, 121
    hemostasis and, 1907, 1908f
    sickle cell anemia and, 577–578, 577f, 580
    vascular
        activation and dysfunction of, 1855, 1855t
        coagulation and, 1894, 1895f
        development and differentiation of, 1845–1850, 1847f
        growth and, 152
        heterogeneity in, 1844–1845
        physiologic functions of, 1850–1855
        structure of, 1843–1845
Endothelial nitric oxide synthase (eNOS), 2126
Endothelial progenitor cells (EPC), 2166
Endothelins (ET), 1832, 1853
Endothelium-derived hyperpolarizing factor (EDHF), 1852–1853
Endotoxin, 2065, 2067
End-stage renal disease (ESRD), 685, 1941
Endurance athletes, 1077, 1080
Enhanceosome complex, 347
Enhancer of zeste homolog (EZH), 950, 1129, 1230–1231, 1232f, 1288–1290, 1289t
Enhancers, 10, 17–18, 18f
eNOS. See Endothelial nitric oxide synthase
Enoxaparin, 2148t
Enrichment, 1533
Enteropathy-associated T-cell lymphoma (EATL), 772, 1188t, 1199, 1200f, 1347
Entinostat, 876–877
Enzyme replacement therapy (ERT), 743
Eomesodermin, 231
Eosin-5'-maleimide (EMA) binding, 631–632, 632f
Eosinophil cationic protein (ECP), 1151, 1152t
Eosinophil peroxidase (EPX), 1151, 1152t
Eosinophil-derived neurotoxin (EDN), 1151, 1152t
Eosinophilia
    in children, 2217
    conditions associated with, 1152t
    hypereosinophilia. See Hypereosinophilia
    hypereosinophilic syndromes. See Hypereosinophilic syndromes
    organ-restricted conditions accompanied by, 1153t
    overview of, 1151
    parasitic infections and, 2301, 2302t
Eosinophilia myalgia syndrome (EMS), 1153t, 1164
Eosinophilic fasciitis (EF), 403, 1153t, 1164
Eosinophilic granuloma, 725
Eosinophilic granulomatosis with polyangiitis (EGPA). See Churg-Strauss syndrome
Eosinophilic leukemias, 1159, 1162–1163, 1162t
Eosinophils
    disorders of, 1151, 1152t
    etiology and pathobiology of, 1157–1158
    immune system and, 203
    mast cells and, 1172
    monitoring numbers and activity of, 1157
    morphology and phenotype of, 1153–1154
    origin, differentiation, recruitment, and activation of, 1155–1157
    overview of, 1151, 1152t
    production of, 330–331, 1155–1156, 1155t
    receptors and ligands regulating, 1155t
Eotaxins, 1156–1157
EPC. See Endothelial progenitor cells
EPCR. See Endothelial cell protein C receptor
EPHOSS. See Extraphysiologic oxygen shock/stress
Ephrin receptors, 154
Ephrins, 154, 1288–1290, 1289t
Epidermal growth factor-like (EGF) domains, 1910f
Epigallocathechin-3-gallate (EGCG), 2259
Epigenetic agents, 991. See also Demethylating agents; Histone deacetylase inhibitors
Epigenetics and epigenomics
    acute lymphoblastic leukemia and, 1052
    acute myeloid leukemia and, 920
    chromatin remodeling and, 20
    disease mechanisms and, 22–23
    DNA methylation and, 17–18
    erythroid cell development and, 316–317

Epigenetics and epigenomics (Continued)
  experimental approaches in, 20–22, 21f
  functional chromatin domains and, 17, 18f
  future directions, 23–24
  hematopoietic stem cell fate and, 102t
  hematopoietic stem cell self-renewal and, 104–105
  histone modifications (covalent) and, 19–20, 19f
  histones, histone variants and, 18–19
  multiple myeloma and, 1385–1386
  overview of, 9–10, 17, 20, 81
  sequencing approaches to, 29
  therapeutic applications, 23, 23t
  transcription factors and, 20
Epinephrine receptor, 1873
Epipodophyllotoxins, 880
Epistaxis, 1915
Epitope spreading, 292
Eplets, 1730
Epoetin alfa, 962
Epoetin-induced pure red cell aplasia, 427–428
Epoprostenol, 1936
Epothilones, 856–858
Epstein anomaly, 1883
Epstein-Barr virus (EBV)
  aplastic anemia and, 403
  biology of, 747, 748f, 1318, 1319f
  Burkitt lymphoma and, 758, 1238, 1321
  chronic active. See Chronic active Epstein-Barr
    infection
  classical Hodgkin lymphoma and, 1209
  clinical syndromes associated with, 747, 748b
  cytotoxic T lymphocytes specific for, 1569
  detection in clinical specimens, 1318–1319, 1319t
  diffuse large B-cell lymphoma and, 1321
  epidemiology of infections, 1318
  hematopoietic stem cell transplants and, 1458–1460
  hemophagic lymphohistiocytosis and, 753
  Hodgkin lymphoma and, 757–758, 1212, 1320–1321
  immune response to, 749–750, 750t
  infectious mononucleosis and, 751–753
  latent infection, 747–749, 749f
  lymphocytosis and, 683
  lymphoma and, 1319–1320, 1319f, 1319t–1320t,
    1321f
  malignancies associated with, 748–749, 750b, 755
  multiple sclerosis and, 754–755
  oral hairy leukoplakia and, 754
  overview of, 747
  posttransplantation lymphoproliferative disease and,
    1320, 1320b, 1321f
  primary infection, 747, 748f
  transfusion-associated, 1810
  vaccine development, 750–751
  X-linked lymphoproliferative disease 1 and, 753
  X-linked lymphoproliferative disease 2 and, 753–754
Epstein-Barr virus nuclear antigens (EBNA), 748–749,
  1318
Epstein-Barr virus-associated lymphoproliferative diseases
  (EBV-LPD), 748–749, 750b
Epstein-Barr virus-encoded small RNAs (EBERs), 749,
  755f
Epstein-Barr virus-positive diffuse large B-cell lymphoma
  (EBV+DLBCL), 770, 1193, 1194f
Epstein-Barr virus-positive T-cell lymphoma, 1200
Eptifibatide
  for acute coronary syndromes, 2146–2147, 2146t
  overview of, 2172–2173, 2172t
  platelet disorders and, 1935–1936
  thrombocytopenia and, 1966
EPX. See Eosinophil peroxidase
EPZ5676, 89, 1052
ERAD. See Endoplasmic reticulum-associated degradation
Erdheim-Chester disease (ECD), 731
ERG. See ETS-related gene
ER-Golgi intermediate compartment (ERGIC), 52f, 55
ERK. See Extracellular signal-related kinase
Erwinaze, 1039
Erythroblast macrophage protein (EMP), 302
Erythroblastic islands, 123
Erythrocytapheresis, overview of, 1783–1784
Erythrocyte enzymes
  disorders of, 622–623
  glutathione pathway enzymopathies, 621–622
  glycolytic pathway enzymopathies, 622
  hemolytic anemia and, 616–621
  metabolic pathways, 616, 617f
  methemoglobinemia and, 623–625, 623f
  polycythemia and, 623

Erythrocyte membrane
  bilayer couple hypothesis and, 626
  disorders of
    acanthocytoses, 626, 640–641, 640f, 643
    elliptocytoses, 639. See also Hereditary elliptocytosis
    hereditary spherocytosis. See Hereditary spherocytosis
    infectious disease and variants, 645–646
    of membrane with target cell formation, 643–645
    of red blood cell shape, 626–633, 627t–628t
    Southeast Asian ovalocytosis, 639–640
    therapy and prognosis, 633–634, 634b
    malaria and, 646
    overview of, 448, 627f
    vertical/horizontal model and, 626–633
Erythrocyte transfusion
  alloimmunization and, 1709–1710
  alternatives to, 1710–1713, 1710t
  clinical applications of
    allogenic hematopoietic stem cell transplantation,
      1706, 1706t
    chronic anemia, 1704
    in neonates, 1705–1706
    perioperative period, 1704–1705
  components of
    frozen red blood cells, 1703–1704
    irradiated red blood cells, 1703
    leukocyte-reduced red blood cells, 1702–1703
    overview of, 1703t
    red blood cell, 1702
    washed red blood cells, 1703
    whole blood, 1702
  preservation and storage of, 1706–1708, 1707t
Erythrocytes (red blood cells)
  abnormalities of in sickle cell disease, 576–578, 576f
  anemia and. See Anemia
  blood groups and. See Blood groups
  in children, 2215–2216
  complement receptor 1 and, 265
  components of, 1702–1704, 1703t
  enzymes of, 448
  hematopoietic stem cell processing and, 1538–1539
  HIV infection and, 2269–2270
  homeostasis of, 447–448
  interactions of with vessel wall, 1855
  laboratory evaluation of, e1–e2
  malaria and, 2279
  mechanical damage to, 665–670
  overview of, 447
  paroxysmal nocturnal hemoglobinuria and, 417
  pediatric, 1821
  senescence and destruction of, 448–449
  solid organ transplant and, 2228–2231
  surface alteration of by bacterial products, 668
  for thrombotic thrombocytopenic purpura, 1991
Erythrocytosis. See also Polycythemias
  cancer and, 2248
  defined, 1074
  drug-induced, 1080
  hypoxia-inducing factor pathway mutations and,
    1079–1080
  polycythemia vera vs., 1097
Erythroferrone (ERFE), 298–299, 487
Erythroid cells
  cellular model of differentiation, 299f
  erythropoietin and, 304–305
  hemoglobin synthesis and, 454–455
  iron homeostasis and, 468
  morphologically recognizable precursor cell
    compartment, 300–304
  myelodysplastic syndromes and, 955–956, 956f
  progenitor cell compartment, 297–300, 298t
Erythroid Krüppel-like factor (EKLF), 315–317, 456
Erythroid precursor cells, defined, 297
Erythroleukemia, 384
Erythromelalgia, 1090–1091, 1111
Erythron, 300–304
Erythropoiesis
  cellular dynamics in, 318–319
  cytokines leading to inhibition of, 493
  disorders of, 307–309, 317–318
  erythropoietin, oxygen sensing, hypoxia-inducible factor
    and, 1071–1073, 1072f
  erythropoietin receptor and, 1073, 1073f
  factors influencing, 1071
  hematopoietic microenvironment and, 309–310
  iron-deficient, 480
  malaria and, 2280–2282

Erythropoiesis (Continued)
  ontogeny of, 310–313, 311f
  overview of, 458, 459f
  polycythemia and. See Polycythemia
  regulation of, 459f
  transcription factors in, 313–317
  use of iron for, 469–472
Erythropoiesis stimulating agents (ESA), 962–963, 2244,
  2247–2248
Erythropoietic porphyria, congenital. See Congenital
  erythropoietic porphyria
Erythropoietic protoporphyria (EPP), 498f, 504–506, 506f
Erythropoietin (EPO)
  anemia of chronic diseases and, 492, 495
  for aplastic anemia, 413
  for β-thalassemia syndrome, 562
  cancer and, 2247
  cell turnover and, 186
  chronic kidney disease and, 2244
  cytokines and decreased secretion of, 493
  HIV infection and, 2272
  laboratory evaluation of, e6b
  liver disease and, 2238
  malaria and, 2281–2282
  in neonates, 1705
  overview of, 304–305
  oxygen sensing, hypoxia-inducible factor and,
    1071–1073
  pure red cell aplasia and, 427–429
  reference values for, e18t
  renin-angiotensin system, hematopoiesis and,
    1073–1074
  for sickle cell disease, 592
Erythropoietin receptor (EPOR)
  alterations in and disorders of erythropoiesis, 307–309
  erythroid cell development and, 303
  overview of, 304–305, 1073, 1073f
  signal transduction by, 305–307, 306t
E-Selectin
  endothelial cells and, 121
  neutrophil response to infection and, 692t
ESRE. See Extensively self-renewing erythroblasts
Essential thrombocythemia (ET)
  in children, 1002–1003
  clinical manifestations of, 1110–1112
  differential diagnosis for, 1113–1116, 1114t–1115t
  epidemiology of, 1106
  future directions for, 1122
  laboratory manifestations of, 1112–1113
  overview of, 339–340, 1106
  pathobiology of, 1106–1110, 1108f
  pregnancy and, 2209–2210
  prognosis for, 1116–1117, 1117f, 1117t
  therapy for, 1117–1122, 1120t, 1122t, 1123b
  thrombosis and, 2082
Estimated blood volume. See Blood volume estimations
Estrogens, 2051, 2083
ET. See Endothelins
Etanercept, 965
Ethanol, 442, 538b, 1939
Ethnic neutropenia, 677–678
Etoposide phosphate, 860, 899, 968
ETP. See Early T-cell precursor acute lymphoblastic
  leukemia
ETS transcription factors, 345
ETS variant 6 (ETSV6)
  childhood acute lymphoblastic leukemia and, 817–818,
    1020
  clonal origin of leukemia and, 783
  mixed lineage leukemias and, 1034
  overview of, 345, 819, 950–951
  in precursor b-cell acute lymphoblastic leukemia,
    1009–1010
ETS-related gene (ERG), 345, 804
Euchromatin
  defined, 20
  DNA-protein interactions in, 21–22, 22f
  epigenetic regulation and, 9
  overview of, 18f
Euglobulin clot lysis time, 2190
Eukaryotic initiation factors (EIF), 45–46
European Heart Rhythm Associating (EHRA) scoring
  system, 2152, 2153t
European Pharmacogenetics of Anticoagulant Therapy
  (EU-PACT) trial, 85–86
Evans syndrome, 655–656, 1263
Everolimus, 864–865, 1184, 1428
EVI1. See Ecotropic virus integration site 1

EVICEL, 1766
Evil, 103
EVITHROM, 1766
Ex vivo cord blood expansion, 1646–1647
Exercise therapy, 2165
Exhausted T cells, 232–233
Exons, 17, 18f, 62
Exosomes, 251–252
Experimental autoimmune encephalomyelitis (EAE), 256
Exportins, 48
Expression-based diagnostics, 34–35
Expressive arts therapy, 2255
Extensively self-renewing erythroblasts (ESRE), 300
Extracellular matrix (ECM)
    angiogenesis and, 1846, 1847f
    cell adhesion and, 127, 1844
    endothelial structure and function and, 1843–1844
    macrovasculature and, 1843
    platelets and, 1870
Extracellular signal-related kinase (ERK), 70, 865, 1266
Extracorporeal circuits, 1942
Extracorporeal membrane oxygenation (ECMO), 1824,
    1825t, 1942, 2192–2193, 2196–2197
Extracorporeal photopheresis, 1375–1376, 1785, 1785f
Extracutaneous mastocytosis (EM), 1174r
Extramedullary hematopoiesis (EMH), 1125–1126,
    1131–1132, 1134
Extranodal marginal zone lymphoma of MALT type
    (ENMZL)
    cutaneous, 1281
    cytogenetics of, 838
    cytology of, 1192f
    epidemiology and manifestations, 1278
    gastric, 1277, 1280–1281
    IPSID, 1281–1282
    ocular, 1281
    overview of, 1188t, 1191–1192
    pathobiology and differential diagnosis, 1278–1280
    prognosis for, 1283
    therapy for, 1280–1283
Extranodal natural killer/T-cell lymphoma (ENKTCL),
    1200, 1200f, 1348, 1352–1354, 1367
Extraphysiologic oxygen shock/stress (EPHOSS), 174
Extrasensitive fluorescence in situ hybridization, 774
Extrinsic apoptosis pathway, 190, 193–194
Extrinsic coagulation pathway, 1886f
Extrinsic tenase, 1835–1836, 1899–1901, 1900f
Ezetimibe, 2124–2125
EZH. See Enhancer of zeste homolog

F

F box and leucin-rich repeat protein 5 (FBXL5), 468, 470f
F box and WD repeat domain containing 7 (FBXW7),
    1016
F cells, 302–303
F4/80, 331–332
F8 gene, 2001, 2002f, 2003–2004, 2006. See also Factor
    VIII
F9 gene, 2004, 2004f–2005f, 2006. See also Factor IX
Fab domains, 273
Fabry disease, 741t, 742–745
Factor eight inhibitor bypassing activity (FEIBA), 1766
Factor H, 264, 264t, 266–267, 267f
Factor I, 264, 264t, 266–267
Factor II. See Prothrombin
Factor IIa. See Thrombin
Factor IX. See also F9 gene
    deficiency in. See Hemophilia B
    genetics of, 2004, 2004f
    hemophilia B and, 19f, 20
    measurement of, 2006
    protein structure, 2004–2005, 2005f
Factor IX antibodies, 2005
Factor IX concentrates
    attenuation of pathogens in, 1770–1771
    for hemophilia, 1774–1775
    immunogenicity of, 2019, 2019f
    overview of, 1764–1765, 1765t, 2013–2015, 2014t
    prophylactic uses, 2016
Factor IX inhibitors, 1774–1776, 1776b, 2018–2019,
    2032
Factor P. See Properdin
Factor V
    coagulation and, 1890–1891
    deficiency in, 1778, 2041–2042, 2041f
    factor VIII deficiency and, 2048, 2048t
Factor VII, 1778, 2032–2033, 2042–2043, 2064–2066

Factor VIIa
    coagulation and, 1835–1836
    for factor IX inhibition, 2032
    for factor VIII inhibition, 2029–2030
    fibrinolysis regulation and, 1899–1902
    liver disease and, 2241
    surgical patients and, 2307–2308
    thromboembolism and, 2102
Factor VIII. See also F8 gene
    activation and coagulant function of, 2003
    biosynthesis of, 2001–2002
    coagulation and, 1890–1891
    deficiency in. See Hemophilia A
    disseminated intravascular coagulation and, 2070
    gene expression, 2001
    gene for, 2001, 2002f
    measurement of, 2006, 2006t
    mimetic molecules, 2019t, 2020
    protein structure, 2002–2003, 2002f
    storage, secretion, and circulation of, 2003
    von Willebrand factor and, 2051, 2052f
Factor VIII binding assay, 1928, 2059
Factor VIII concentrates
    attenuation of pathogens in, 1770–1771
    for hemophilia, 1773–1774
    immunogenicity of, 2019
    overview of, 1761–1764, 2013–2015, 2014t
    prophylactic uses, 2016
    for von Willebrand disease, 1776–1777
Factor VIII inhibitors
    clinical manifestations of, 2027
    epidemiology of, 2023–2025
    immune tolerance therapy for, 2031–2032
    laboratory diagnosis of, 2027–2028, 2027f–2028f
    new treatments for, 2031
    overview of, 1775–1776, 1776b
    pathobiology of, 2018, 2025–2027, 2026f
    treatment of, 2028–2031, 2029b
Factor VIIIa, 1902
Factor VIII:C level assay, 2059
Factor V_Leiden gain-of-function mutation, 2079–2080
Factor X, 1778, 1907–1909, 2043–2044, 2102
Factor Xa, 1902, 2065–2066
Factor XI deficiency, 1778–1779, 2044–2045, 2211b
Factor XII, 1891, 2045–2046, 2046b, 2065, 2102
Factor XIII deficiency, 1779, 1929, 2047–2048, 2195
Familial erythrocytosis, 308
Familial HLH (FHL) genes, 732–733
Familial platelet disorder with predisposition to acute
    myelogenous leukemia, 915, 1883
Familial unexplained erythrocytosis, 612
FANC genes, 352–353
Fanconi anemia (FA)
    acute myeloid leukemia and, 914
    background of, 350, 352f
    clinical features of, 354–355, 355t
    differential diagnosis for, 357
    epidemiology of, 350
    future directions for, 360
    genetic counseling for, 360
    genetics of, 350–353
    hematopoietic dysfunction in, 354
    heterozygote phenotype in, 356–357
    laboratory manifestations of, 355–356
    malignancy predisposition and, 356
    natural history and prognosis of, 357
    pathophysiology of, 354
    therapy for, 357–360
    thrombocytopenia with absent radii syndrome vs.,
        391–392
Fanconi facies, 355
Fas, 194
Fas ligand (FasL)
    apoptosis and, 194
    autoimmune lymphoproliferative syndrome and,
        718–719
    autoimmunity and, 291
    graft-versus-host disease and, 1658
    graft-versus-leukemia responses and, 1666
Fas receptor, 1656–1657
Fas-activating via death domain (FADD), 235, 236f
Fatal granulomatous disease. See Chronic granulomatous
    disease
Fatty acid synthase (FAS), 75
Fatty acids
    oxidation of, 75
    platelet disorders and, 1939
    synthesis of, 75

Fatty streak, 2125–2127
Favism, 619
FBXL5. See F box and leucin-rich repeat protein 5
FBXW7. See F box and WD repeat domain containing 7
Fc domains, 273
Fc-γ receptor III b (FcγIIIb), 1733–1734
FCGR3, 243, 1734
Febrile neutropenia, 1669–1670
Febrile nonhemolytic transfusion reactions (FNHTR),
    1703, 1717, 1794–1795
Fechtner syndrome, 1862–1863, 1883
FEIBA, 1766, 1775–1776
Felbamate, 400–401
Feline leukemia virus subgroup C cellular receptor 1
    (FLVCR1), 374
Felty syndrome, 678
Fenofibrate, 2163–2164
Fentanyl patch, 1477b, 1479
Ferritin
    iron homeostasis and, 468, 476
    iron status assessment and, 478–479, 480b
    laboratory evaluation of, e5b
    reference values for, e17t
Ferrochelatase (FECH), 505–506
Ferroportin (Fpn)
    anemia of chronic diseases and, 495
    erythropoiesis and, 471–472
    genetic mutations in, 489
    iron homeostasis and, 468, 470f, 473, 479b
Fertile ground hypothesis, 1085
Fetal hemoglobin (HBF). See Hemoglobin F
FGFR1-rearranged neoplasm (8p11 myeloproliferative
    syndrome), 790, 1162–1163
Fiber fluorescence in situ hybridization, 777f, 778
Fibrin, 1837, 1840, 1840t, 1895–1897, 1898f
Fibrin degradation products (FDP), 2070
Fibrin glue/sealant, 1750, 1766, 1767t, 2015, 2306
Fibrinogen, 1766, 1840, 1840t, 1895–1897, 1898f
Fibrinogen deficiency, 1750, 1778, 2034–2038, 2035t,
    2037t, 2038f
Fibrinogen tests, e12b
Fibrinolysis
    antiphospholipid antibodies and, 2090
    coagulation and, 1897–1898
    developmental hemostasis and, 2190
    disseminated intravascular coagulation and, 2067,
        2070–2071
    hemostasis and, 1832, 1837–1839, 1838f, 1909,
        2190
    laboratory evaluation of, 1929
    liver disease and, 2240
    regulation of, 1899–1901f
Fibrinolytic inhibitors, 2030–2031, 2061, 2074
Fibrinolytic therapy
    for acute coronary syndromes, 2142–2144, 2145b,
        2145t
    alteplase. See Alteplase
    mechanism of action of, 2184, 2184f–2185f
    role of, 2184
    streptokinase. See Streptokinase
Fibroblast growth factors (FGF), 1847–1848, 1847f. See
    also FGFR1-rearranged neoplasm
Fibroblastic reticular cell (FRC) network, 141,
    1844–1845
Fibronectin, 127
Fibrosis. See also Myelofibrosis
FIIG20210A mutation, 2080
Filamins, 1863, 1866f–1867f, 1867–1868
Filgrastim
    after solid organ transplant in children, 2232
    haploidentical hematopoietic stem cell transplantation
        and, 1624–1625, 1629
    HIV infection and, 2273
    mobilization of hematopoietic stem cells and, 1522
    for myelodysplastic syndromes, 963
Finch, Clement, 298–299
FIP1L1-PDGFRA fusion, 790–792, 1172, 1180,
    1180t
Fisher-Race nomenclature, 1696, 1696t
5q minus syndrome, 767–768, 793, 793f
FIX. See Factor IX
FKBP12-F36V, 1573
Flavocytochrome b_558, 693, 694f
Flavopiridol, 872–873
Fletcher factor, 2046–2047
Fli-1, 345, 1864
FLICE/caspase-8 inhibitory protein (FLIP), 194
FLT3. See FMS-like tyrosine kinase-3

Fluconazole, 1455–1456, 1456b, 1674
Fludarabine
    for acute myeloid leukemia, 935
    autoimmune hemolytic anemia and, 655
    for chronic lymphocytic leukemia, 1254–1256,
        1260–1261
    for cutaneous T-cell lymphomas, 1373
    for extranodal marginal zone lymphoma of MALT type,
        1282
    for follicular lymphoma, 1294
    infection and, 1447
    pharmacology of, 857–858, 894
    for primary myelofibrosis, 1145
Fluorescence in situ hybridization (FISH), 774–778
5-Fluorouracil, 1373
FLVCR1. See Feline leukemia virus subgroup C cellular
    receptor 1
FMS-like tyrosine kinase-3 (FLT3; FLK2)
    acute lymphoblastic leukemia and, 89, 1015
    acute myeloid leukemia and, 799–800, 804, 917–918,
        939, 987–988
    aplastic anemia and, 397
    for MLL-rearranged infant ALL, 89
FO B cells, 219
Foam cells, 2125–2127, 2125f
Foamy virus vectors, 1551
Focal adhesion kinase (FAK), 217
Focal contacts, 1844
FOG. See Friend of GATA
Folate analogs, 857
Folate deficiency
    biochemical evaluation of, 527–529, 527b–529b, 528t
    biochemical indicators of, 526–527
    cerebral, 537
    classification of, 525b
    clinical presentation and evaluation for, 537–540,
        538t
    diagnosis of, 526t
    diagnostic and therapeutic approach, 540–541, 543b
    distinguishing, 525b
    effects of, 526
    fortification of food, cancer risk and, 544
    hereditary malabsorption and, 536
    inborn errors of metabolism and, 537
    intestinal mucosal abnormalities and, 536–537
    intrinsic hematologic disease and, 536
    pathogenesis of, 533–537
    pregnancy and, 2203–2204
    therapy for, 541–542
Folate receptors, 519–521, 520f–521f
Folates
    absorption of, 518–519
    cellular retention, one-carbon metabolism and,
        521–522
    cellular uptake of, 519–521, 520f–521f
    chemistry and nomenclature of, 518f
    cobalamins and, 521–523
    compartmentalization and channeling of metabolism,
        522
    consequences of perturbed metabolism, 522–523
    drugs affecting metabolism of, 538b
    importance of, 514
    laboratory evaluation of, e6b
    methylation of, 522
    nutrition and, 518
    plasma transport, enterohepatic circulation and, 519
    reference values for, e18t
    renal retention of, 521
    routine supplementation of, 542–543, 542t, 543b
Follicles, 206, 207f
Follicular dendritic cell sarcoma (FDCS), 772
Follicular dendritic cells (FDC), 261, 269–272
Follicular lymphoma in situ (FLIS), 1191
Follicular lymphoma international prognostic index
    (FLIPI), 1290–1291, 1291t
Follicular lymphomas (FL)
    allogenic HSCT for, 1606
    in childhood, 1341
    classification of, 770
    clinical presentation of, 1290
    cytogenetics of, 832–839
    diagnosis of, 1290
    epidemiology of, 1288, 1289t
    grading of, 771
    natural history of, 1290–1291
    overview of, 1188t, 1190–1191, 1191f, 1236f,
        1238–1240, 1238f, 1288
    pathogenesis of, 1288–1290, 1289f, 1289t

Follicular lymphomas (FL) (Continued)
    relapsed indolent, 1296–1297
    staging of, 1290, 1290t
    stem cell origin of, 117
    timing of instituting therapy, 1292–1293
    treatment approaches for, 1292b, 1293–1296
    treatment of, 1291–1292, 1296–1297
Follicular mucinosis, 1363–1364, 1363f
Folylpolyglutamate synthase, 521–522
Fondaparinux
    for acute coronary syndromes, 2148t, 2149
    heparin-induced thrombocytopenia and, 1978–1979,
        1979t–1980t
    overview of, 2178, 2178t
    for venous thromboembolism, 2108–2109
Food additives, 1939
Foods, platelet disorders and, 1939
Forkhead box proteins (Fox), 181, 228, 710, 718, 1280,
    1283
Forkhead box transcription factors (FoxOs), 68–70
FORS1 blood group antigen, 1696
Foscarnet, 1673–1674
Foundation for the Accreditation of Cellular Therapy
    (FACT), 1537–1538
4Ts system for heparin-induced thrombocytopenia,
    1974–1975, 1977t
FOX. See Forkhead box proteins
Fpn. See Ferroportins
FRALLE 2000 protocol, 1048
Freeze-dried plasma, 1744–1745
French Society of Pediatric Oncology Risk Group
    Classification of Mature B-cell Lymphomas, 1334t
French-American-British (FAB) classifications
    of acute myeloid leukemias, 765–767, 766t, 925–931,
        944, 946t, 981
    of myelodysplastic syndromes, 767, 996
Fresh frozen plasma (FFP)
    for disseminated intravascular coagulation, 2073
    fibrinogen and, 2036–2038
    for hemophilia, 1773–1774
    liver disease and, 2241
    overview of, 1744, 1760
    for pediatric patients, 1823, 1823t
    for thrombotic thrombocytopenic purpura, 1989
Friedenstein, Alexander, 1559
Friend erythroleukemia complex, 307–308
Friend of GATA (FOG), 314–315, 343
Frozen red blood cells, 1703–1704
FTY720, 143
Fucosylation, 1647
Fucosyltransferases (FUT), 1695
Functional genomics, overview of, 32–34
Functional iron deficiency, 483
Functional plasticity model of dendritic cells, 247
Fungal infections, 1455–1456, 1456b, 1460, 1674–1675.
    See also Specific fungal infections
FUS/ERG fusions, 804
FUT. See Fucosyltransferases
FVIII. See Factor VIII
FXIII deficiency. See Factor XIII deficiency
FY. See Duffy antigen

G

G protein-coupled receptor kinase 3 (GRK3),
    389–390
G_1 phase, 176, 177f
G1/S-specific cyclin-D3 (CCND3), 835
G_2 phase, 176, 177f
G6PC3-associated severe congenital neutropenia,
    390
G6PD. See Glucose-6-phosphate dehydrogenase
Gabapentin, 1480
Gain of 1q, 795–796, 795f
Gaisböck syndrome, 1074
α-Galactosidase deficiency, 741t, 742–745
Gallbladder, 559–560
Gallstones, 632–633
Gamma-glutamylcysteine (GCL) deficiency, 621
Ganciclovir, 1459, 2273
Gap junctions, 1843–1844
Gastrectomy, 530–531
Gastrointestinal tract
    antiphospholipid syndrome and, 2097
    clinical assessment and, 1915–1916
    graft-versus-host disease and, 1651t, 1652, 1661
    hemophilia and, 2011
    hypereosinophilic syndrome and, 1161

GATA1
    congenital dyserythropoietic anemias and, 384
    Down syndrome-associated acute megakaryocytic
        leukemia and, 343–344, 344f, 813, 985–986
    erythropoiesis and, 314–318
    globin gene expression and, 456
    inhibition of erythropoiesis and, 493
    platelet formation and, 1864
    primary myelofibrosis and, 1127
    regulation of megakaryocytopoiesis and, 343–344
    transient abnormal myelopoiesis and, 1001
GATA2
    acute myeloid leukemia and, 915
    erythropoiesis and, 314
    lymphocytopenia and, 684
    monocytopenia and deficiency in, 680–681
    myelodysplastic syndromes and, 951
    specification of hematopoietic stem cells and, 103
    transcription in erythropoiesis and, 318
GATA3, 171, 230
Gaucher cells, 744
Gaucher disease type I, 743–744
GB virus type C, 1806
GC reaction, 206
G-CSF. See Granulocyte colony stimulating factor
GEF. See Guanine nucleotide exchange factors
Gelatin foams, 2306
Gelatinase, 322
Geldanamycin, 878
Gemcitabine, 857, 897
Gemfibrozil, 2163–2164
Geminin, 181–182
Genasense, 872, 1258–1259
Gene analysis methods
    DNA, RNA, and protein blotting, 13–14, 13f
    polymerase chain reaction, 14
    restriction endonucleases, 13
    transgenic and knockout mice, 14–15
Gene expression
    enhancers, promoters, silencers and, 10
    epigenetic regulation of, 9–10
    genetic code, protein synthesis and, 5–7, 6f, 7t
    posttranscriptional regulation of, 10–11
    transcription factors and, 10
    untranslated sequences and, 9
Gene expression profiles
    diagnostic uses of, 34–35
    follicular lymphoma and, 835
    multiple myeloma and, 831–832
Gene regulation, 9–10
Gene therapy
    basis for, 1549
    for β-thalassemia syndrome, 563
    clinical trials to date, 1552–1555
    future directions, 1557–1558
    for hemophilia, 2020, 2020t–2021t
    for hemophilia B (factor IX deficiency), 1774
    insertional mutagenesis, 1555–1556
    overview of, 15, 1549
    recent advances, 1556–1557
    for severe combined immunodeficiency, 714
    vector systems, 1549–1552, 1556–1557
Generalized pagetoid reticulosis, 1367
Generative lymphoid organs, 203–204
Genes
    anatomy and physiology of, 3–4
    central dogma of molecular biology and, 3
    organization of in DNA, 17–18
    transcription of, 18–19, 18f
Genetic code, 5–7, 7t
Genetics Informatics Trial (GIFT) of Warfarin to Prevent
    Deep Venous Thrombosis, 85–86
Genome editing, overview of, 1557
Genomes (human), variations in, 79
Genome-wide association studies (GWAS), overview of,
    81
Genomic run-on sequencing (GRO-Seq), 21–22
Genomics
    clinical uses of, 34–35
    DNA-level characterization, 27–29
    functional, 32–34
    future directions, 34–35
    metabolite-level characterization, 32
    next-generation sequencing and, 27
    overview of, 25, 79
    pharmaco-. See Pharmacogenomics
    principles of, 25–27
    protein-level characterization, 31–32

Genomics (Continued)
  relevant websites, 80t
  RNA-level characterization, 30–31
Geographic skull, 726
Gerbich blood group system, 1699
Germinal center B cell-like diffuse large B-cell lymphoma
    (GBC DLBCL), 835–837, 1192, 1233f, 1234, 1309
Germinal centers (GC)
  B cell development, 219
  hairy cell leukemia and, 1265, 1266f
  Hodgkin lymphoma and, 1204, 1205f
  overview of, 206
Germline gene therapy, 1549
Germline variants, somatic variants vs., 28
Gestational thrombocytopenia, 1946, 2205
GIAC protocol, 1624–1625, 1629
Giardiasis, 2302
Gilbert syndrome, 511–512
Glanzmann thrombasthenia, 134, 134t, 1878, 1880,
    1882–1883, 2194, 2304–2305
Glanzmann-type defects, 957
Gleevec. See Imatinib mesylate
Gleich syndrome, 1151–1153, 1153t, 1164
Globins
  alpha, 552, 562–563, 565, 566f
  beta
    β-thalassemia syndromes and, 547, 547f–548f,
        562–563
    phenotypic diversity in sickle cell disease and, 582
  erythroid cell development and, 302–303, 312–313
  gamma, 562–563
  switches in types, 312–313
Globoside. See P antigen
Glomeruloid vessels, 156–158
GLRX5. See Glutaredoxin 5
Glucksberg Criteria for staging of acute graft-versus-host
    disease, 1651t
Glucocorticoid receptors, 301–302
Glucocorticoids
  for graft-versus-host disease, 1659–1660
  infection and, 1447
  lymphocytopenia and, 685
  for multiple myeloma, 1402
  neutrophilia and, 677
Glucose, 73–74, 77
Glucose phosphoisomerase (GPI) deficiency, 622
Glucose-6-phosphate dehydrogenase (G6PD)
  acquired sideroblastic anemia and, 509–510
  acute myeloid leukemia and, 798
  erythrocyte metabolism and, 448
  polycythemia vera and, 1082
  rasburicase and deficiency in, 86t, 87–88, 88f
  X-linked as marker for clonal development of
      hematopoietic disorders, 781–782, 782f, 798
Glucose-6-phosphate dehydrogenase (G6PD) deficiency
  clinical manifestations of, 618–619
  diagnosis of, 619
  epidemiology of, 616–617
  future directions for, 619
  infection and, 1449, 2271–2272
  introduction to, 616, 618f
  laboratory manifestations of, 619
  neutrophilic, 700
  pathobiology of, 618
  pregnancy and, 2205
  prognosis for, 619
  therapy for, 619
β-Glucosidase deficiency. See Gaucher disease type I
γ-Glutamyl carboxylase (GGCX), 2048–2049
Glutaredoxin 5 (GLRX5), 508
Glutathione pathway, 616, 621–622, 623f, 700–701
Glutathione peroxidase (GSH Px; GPX), 88, 88f, 622
Glutathione reductase (GR), 622
Glutathione synthetase (GSH-S), 621–622
Glycans, 53, 276
Glycogen storage disease type 1b (GSD-Ib), 365,
    387–388, 707–708
Glycolytic pathway, 74, 616, 617f, 622, e19t
Glycophorins, 304, 448, 635, 636f, 646
Glycoproteins (GP)
  β₂GP I, 2089t, 2090f, 2094
  GP Ib, 1871–1872
  GP Ib-IX-V complex, 129, 130f, 130t, 132–133
  GP IIb/IIIa (GP IIb/IIIa)
    acute coronary syndrome and, 2146–2147, 2146t
    antiplatelet drugs and, 2169f, 2172–2173, 2172t
    hemostasis and, 1834
    thrombocytopenia and, 1961, 1966

Glycoproteins (GP) (Continued)
  GP IX, 1871–1872
  GP V, 1871–1872
  GP VI, 1874
  nomenclature of, 1870–1871
  platelet adhesion and, 1870–1872, 1872f
Glycosaminoglycans (GAG), 138, 741, 741t
Glycosylation, 53–54, 53f, 55b, 60–61
Glycosylation-dependent cell adhesion molecule I,
    1844–1845
Glycosylphosphatidylinositol (GPI) anchor
  disorders of, 55b
  paroxysmal nocturnal hemoglobinuria and, 415–417,
      416f, 416t, 420
GM-CSF. See Granulocyte-macrophage colony stimulating
    factor
GO (anti-CD33 antibody) therapy, 938
Gold, 401, 1965
Goldie and Coldman hypothesis, 849–850
Golgi apparatus, 55–56. See also Trans-golgi network
Gonadal dysfunction, 1228, 1499–1500
Good syndrome, 686–687
Good tissue practices (GTP), 1537
Goodpasture disease, 1787
GP Ib-IX-V complex. See under Glycoproteins
GP IIb/IIIa. See under Glycoproteins
GPI anchor. See Glycosylphosphatidylinositol anchor
G-protein coupled receptors (GPCR)
  chemokine signals and, 135, 137t
  as membrane proteins, 64–65
  platelet activation and, 1873t
  signal transduction and, 72
GRAALL regimen, 1047, 1049
Graft failure, 1594, 1621–1622, 1631, 1675–1676
Graft versus graft interactions, 1638
Graft-versus-host disease (GVHD)
  acute
    biomarkers, 1658–1660
    clinical features, 1651–1652, 1651f, 1651t, 1680
    differential diagnosis, 1652
    genetic basis, 1652–1653
    mesenchymal stromal cells for, 1563
    overview, 1650–1651
    pathophysiology, 1653–1658, 1654f
    prevention, 1659
    prophylaxis, 1680–1681
    risk factors, 1680
    therapy, 1659–1660, 1661t, 1681
  after haploidentical hematopoietic stem cell
      transplantation, 1619–1622
  after hematopoietic stem cell transplantation,
      1593–1594
  allogenic HSCT and, 1601–1604
  aplastic anemia and, 397, 402
  autoimmunity and, 285
  chronic
    biomarkers, 1662–1663
    clinical manifestations, 1660–1662, 1681, 1681t
    differential diagnosis, 1662
    overview, 1660
    pathophysiology, 1662
    risk factors, 1681
    therapy, 1663, 1663t, 1681–1682
  cord blood stem cell transplantation and
    overview, 1633
    single unit, 1633–1634
  future directions, 1667
  human leukocyte antigens and, 1731
  mesenchymal stromal cells and, 1562, 1565b
  natural killer cells and, 1578, 1580f, 1581
  overview of, 1650, 1680
  pain and, 1482
  peripheral blood stem cells and, 1517, 1518b
  single vs. double unit cord blood transplantation and,
      1640–1641
  transfusion-associated, 1663, 1703, 1706, 1798,
      1798b
Graft-versus-leukemia (GVL) effect
  allogenic HSCT and, 1601–1604
  chimeric antigen receptor T cells, cytokine release
      syndrome and, 1664–1667
  in chronic myelogenous leukemia, 1068
  clinical features of, 1664
  donor lymphocyte infusion and, 1568–1569
  future directions, 1667
  genetic basis of, 1664
  haploidentical hematopoietic stem cell transplantation
      and, 1618–1620

Graft-versus-leukemia (GVL) effect (Continued)
  human leukocyte antigens and, 1731–1732
  immunobiology of, 1665–1666
  killer-cell immunoglobulin-like receptors (KIR) and,
      1664
  overview of, 1663
  single-locus mismatched unrelated HSCT and, 1613
Granisetron, 1484
Granule-dependent cytotoxicity, 732–733
Granules
  alpha, 1859, 1875, 1876f–1877f, 1882
  lysosomal, 706–707, 706t, 1875–1876
  platelet activation and, 1875–1876, 1876f–1877f
  platelet disorders and, 1882
Granulocyte (neutrophil) transfusions (GTX)
  alternative or adaptive measures to, 1742
  author's approach to, 1742–1743
  historic experience, 1738–1739, 1739t
  in infants and children, 1741–1742
  modern experience, 1739–1741, 1740t
  overview of, 1738, 1823–1824
  prophylactic, 1742, 1742t
Granulocyte colony stimulating factor (G-CSF)
  for aplastic anemia, 413
  cancer and, 2249
  for dyskeratosis congenita, 368
  for Fanconi anemia, 359–360
  graft failure and, 1676
  HIV infection and, 2273
  for Kostmann syndrome/severe congenital neutropenia,
      386–388
  mobilization of hematopoietic stem cells and,
      1522–1523
  for myelodysplastic syndromes, 963
  neutrophil maturation and, 323–324, 324f
  for Schwachman-Diamond syndrome, 364
  treatment of acute lymphoblastic leukemia and, 1037
Granulocyte-macrophage colony stimulating factor
    (GM-CSF)
  for aplastic anemia, 413
  dendritic cells and, 258
  eosinophilopoiesis and, 1156–1157
  for Fanconi anemia, 359–360
  graft failure and, 1676
  mobilization of hematopoietic stem cells and, 1523
  for myelodysplastic syndromes, 963
  neutrophil maturation and, 323–324, 324f
  treatment of acute lymphoblastic leukemia and, 1037
Granulocytes. See also Basophils; Eosinophils; Neutrophils
  development of, 321
  maturation markers, 321
  myelodysplastic syndromes and, 956, 957f
  neutrophil differentiation stages and, 321
  neutrophil granules, content proteins and, 321–323,
      323t
  overview of in immune system, 203
Granulocytic sarcoma. See Myeloid sarcoma
Granulomatous slack skin syndrome, 1364, 1365f
Granulopoiesis
  C/EPBβ and, 326
  cytokine regulation of myeloid proliferation and
      differentiation in, 323–324, 324f
  microRNAs and control of gene expression in,
      329–330
  severe congenital neutropenia, unfolded protein
      response and, 329
  transcription factors regulating myeloid differentiation,
      325–328
  transcriptional regulation of myeloid differentiation,
      324–328, 325f
Granzymes, 231
Gray platelet syndrome (GPS), 335, 344, 1883
Gray zone lymphomas, 1194–1195
Greaves, Mel, 783, 821–822
Green tea, 2259
Grief, 1494
Griscelli syndrome type 2 (GS2), 719
GRK3. See G protein-coupled receptor kinase 3
Growth and differentiation factors (GDF), 70, 475–476,
    475f
Growth factor independent 1 (Gfi-1), 328, 346
GSI. See γ-Secretase inhibitors
GTPases, 135–136, 1873
GTX. See Neutrophil transfusions
Guanine nucleotide exchange factors (GEF), 45–46
Guglielmo, Givanni di, 944
Guillain-Barré syndrome, 1755
Gum bleeding, 1915

Günther disease. *See* Congenital erythropoietic porphyria
GVAX, 258

H

HA22. *See* Moxetumomab
Haemophilus influenzae, sickle cell disease and, 597–598
Hageman factor, 2045–2046
Hairy cell leukemia (HCL)
 clinical presentation and diagnosis of, 1266–1268, 1266*t*
 cytogenetics of, 839–840
 differential diagnosis for, 1268–1269
 epidemiology of, 1265
 etiology and cell of origin of, 1265–1266
 future directions for, 1275
 monocytopenia and, 680
 overview of, 1265
 primary myelofibrosis vs., 1137–1138
 stem cell origin of, 115–117
 treatment of, 1269–1275
Hallervorden-Spatz syndrome, 642
Ham, Thomas, 415
Ham test, 420
Hamilton-Paterson, J.J., 944
Hand-foot syndrome, 604*f*
Haploidentical hematopoietic stem cell transplantation
 for acute myeloid leukemia, 974
 advantages and limitations of, 1617–1619
 allogenic HSCT and, 1600
 comparison to other graft sources, 1627, 1628*t*
 complications of, 1621–1622
 defined, 1617
 immunologic considerations in, 1619–1621
 impaired immune reconstitution, infection and, 1622
 modern approaches to, 1623–1629
 natural killer cells and, 1579–1581
 NK cell alloreactions after, 1619–1621
 overview of, 1617, 1632
 practical considerations, 1629–1631
Haplotypes, defined, 80–81, 1617
HapMap project, 80–81, 80*t*
Haptoglobin (Hp), *e4b*, *e16t*
Haptotaxis, 138–139
HARP, 642
Hartwell, Leland, 178
HAS-BLED scoring system, 2155*t*, 2156–2157
HCP. *See* Src homology containing phosphatases
HDACi. *See* Histone deacetylase inhibitors
HDL efflux capacity, 2124
Hearing, 1501–1502
Heat denaturation, 665
Heat shock protein inhibitors, 878
Heat stroke, 2068
Heavy chains, 212, 213*f*
Heavy metal exposure, 401
Hedgehog (Hh) signaling, 72, 101
Heiner syndrome, 2223–2225
Heinz bodies, 610–611, 611*f*
α-Helices, 59, 60*f*–61*f*
Helicobacter pylori, 1280–1281, 1283*b*
HELLP syndrome, 1999, 2069, 2206–2207
Helper T cells. *See* T helper cells
Hemangioblasts, 152
Hemangiomas, 2069
Hemapheresis, 1788–1790
Hemarthrosis, 2010–2011, 2010*t*, 2011*b*, 2015
Hematocrit (Hct), *e15t*
Hematopoiesis
 age-related clonal, 783–784
 aging and, 1346–1347, 1353*t*, 2328, 2329*t*
 during development, 119
 Fanconi anemia and, 354
 spleen and, 2318
 vascular development and, 1850
Hematopoietic cell phosphatase (HCP). *See* Src homology containing phosphatases
Hematopoietic Cell Transplantation Comorbidity Index, 978
Hematopoietic growth factors, 202*t*, 359–360, 413
Hematopoietic malignancies, 161
Hematopoietic microenvironment, overview of, 309–310
Hematopoietic progenitor cells (HPSC), 1549
Hematopoietic stem cell transplantation (HSCT)
 for acute myeloid leukemia, 989–990
 allogenic. *See* Allogenic hematopoietic stem cell transplantation
 for aplastic anemia, 407–408

Hematopoietic stem cell transplantation (HSCT) *(Continued)*
 autologous. *See* autologous transplantation
 for β-thalassemia syndrome, 562
 cardiac disease and, 1496
 cellular therapy products for
  allodepleted cells, 1544
  antigen-specific cytotoxic T lymphocytes, 1545
  dendritic cells, 1545–1546
  donor leukocyte infusion. *See* Donor lymphocyte infusion
  future directions, 1547
  genetically modified, 1546–1547
  mesenchymal stromal cells, 1546
  natural killer cells, 1545–1546
  overview, 1542–1547, 1542*t*
  suicide gene-transduced lymphocytes, 1467, 1544–1545
  tumor-infiltrating lymphocytes. *See* Tumor-infiltrating lymphocytes
 checkpoint blockade therapies after, 1585
 collection of cells
  bone marrow, 1519–1521
  peripheral blood stem cells, 1521–1527, 1522*b*
  umbilical cord blood stem cells, 1521
 complications after
  graft failure, 1675–1676
  graft-versus-host disease. *See* Graft-versus-host disease
  infections, 1669–1675, 1671*t*–1672*t*, 1672*f*
  interstitial pneumonitis, 1677–1678, 1677*b*
  organ-specific late effects, 1678–1679, 1679*t*
  overview, 1593–1594, 1669, 1670*t*, 1800–1801, 1800*t*
  quality of life, 1679–1680
  second cancers, 1679
  sinusoidal obstruction syndrome, 1676–1677, 1676*b*
 conditioning regimens for, 1593
 for Diamond-Blackfan anemia, 379
 donor selection and evaluation, 1517–1519, 1518*b*
 for dyskeratosis congenita, 368
 evaluation of manipulated grafts and, 1540–1542
 for Fanconi anemia, 358–359
 future directions, 1594
 genetic testing for, 846*b*
 haploidentical. *See* Haploidentical hematopoietic stem cell transplantation
 for hemophagocytic lymphohistiocytosis, 736–737
 infection management and, 1457–1460, 1457*f*
 for Kostmann syndrome/severe congenital neutropenia, 388–389
 manipulation of products, 1538–1540, 1538*t*
 for mastocytosis, 1184–1185
 mesenchymal stromal cells and, 1563–1564
 natural killer cells and, 1578
 neurocognitive complications of, 1501
 osteonecrosis and, 1500
 overview of, 1517–1518, 1591, 1592*t*
 pediatric transfusions and, 1826
 professional standards for, 1538
 psychosocial considerations, 1464–1466
 pulmonary complications and, 1498
 for pure red cell aplasia, 430
 quality control of cell products, 1527–1529
 regulatory issues with cell processing and, 1537–1538, 1543*f*
 for Schwachman-Diamond syndrome, 364–365
 selection of product used in, 1518*b*
 for severe combined immunodeficiency, 713–714
 sources of stem cells used in, 1593
 thrombotic microangiopathies following, 1997
Hematopoietic stem cells (HSC)
 aplastic anemia and, 394–396
 cell division cycle and, 184
 chemokines and migration to bone marrow and mobilization and niche, 140–141
 development and, 119
 embryonic origin of, 95
 functional assays, 98–99, 99*f*
 gene therapy and, 1549
 generation from pluripotent stem cells and reprogramming of somatic cells, 107
 homing of, 145–146, 146*f*, 150*b*–151*b*
 human, 96*f*, 97–98
 *JAK2*V617F mutation, polycythemia vera and, 1085–1086
 malignancy and, 108–109, 109*f*
 metabolism of, 105
 mobilization of, 146–150, 150*b*–151*b*

Hematopoietic stem cells (HSC) *(Continued)*
 murine, 95–96, 96*f*–97*f*
 novel growth factors for, clinical testing and, 106–107
 overview of, 95
 phenotype, 95–96, 96*f*–97*f*
 regeneration of, 107–108
 regulation of fate
  extrinsic, 100–101
  intrinsic pathways, 101–105, 102*t*
 thrombopoietin signaling in, 339
Hematopoietic zinc finger (Hzf), 1864
Hematopoietins, 163, 164*f*. *See also* Cytokines, class/type I
Hematuria, 602, 1917, 2011–2012
Heme
 biosynthesis of
  control, 497–499, 499*f*
  pathways, 497, 498*f*
 globin biosynthesis and, 456
 porphyrias and. *See* Porphyrias
 sideroblastic anemias and. *See* Sideroblastic anemias
Heme arginate, 503*b*
Heme importer (HRG1), 472–473, 472*f*
Hemin-regulated inhibitor (HRI), 45–46, 471–472
Hemo oxygenase 1 (HO-1), 476*f*
Hemochromatosis gene (*HFE*), 303–304, 474–475
Hemodialysis, 434
Hemodilution, 1711–1712, 1971
Hemoglobin content of reticulocytes (CHr), 479–480, 493
Hemoglobin D disease, 607
Hemoglobin E disease, 607
Hemoglobin H disease, 566*f*, 567
Hemoglobin O Arab disease, 607
Hemoglobin S solubility test, *e4b*
Hemoglobin sickle cell disease, 606
α-Hemoglobin stabilizing protein (AHSP), 303
Hemoglobin-based oxygen carriers (HBOC), 1712
Hemoglobinopathies
 acquired, 609*t*, 614
 classification of, 608, 609*t*
 decreased oxygen affinity and, 613–615
 increased oxygen affinity and, 612–613, 612*f*
 major forms of, 609*t*
 methemoglobinemias. *See* Methemoglobinemias
 overview of, 457, 457*t*, 608
 pediatric transfusions and, 1825
 pregnancy and, 2204
 sickle cell disease. *See* Sickle cell disease
 thalassemias. *See* Thalassemia syndromes
 unstable hemoglobins and, 608–612
Hemoglobins (Hb)
 abnormalities of, 457, 457*t*, 572–576. *See also* Hemoglobinopathies; Thalassemias
 basic features of, 449
 biosynthesis and regulation of, 455–456
 electrophoresis of, 584, 585*f*
 extraordinarily unstable, 569–570
 function of, 450–453, 451*f*–452*f*
 globin genes and, 453–454, 453*f*–454*f*
 Hb A₂, *e4b*, *e16t*
 Hb B, 571–572
 Hb Bart, 566*f*, 567
 Hb Constant Spring, 566*f*, 569
 Hb E, 569
 Hb F
  β-thalassemia syndromes and, 562–563
  erythroid cell development and, 302–303
  laboratory evaluation of, *e4b*
  phenotypic diversity in sickle cell disease and, 582
  protective effect of, 575
  reference values for, *e16t*
  sickle cell disease and, 584, 589–590, 592, 607
 Hb Hammersmith, 610
 Hb Kansas, 613
 Hb Kempsey, 612, 612*f*
 Hb Kenya, 569, 569*f*
 Hb Köln, 610–611
 Hb Lepore, 569, 569*f*, 606–607
 Hb Quong Sze, 569–570
 Hb S
  charge and tetramer assembly, 573
  solubility and polymerization, 573–576, 573*f*–575*f*
  stability and oxidant formation, 573
 Hb Terre Haute, 569–570
 Hb Zurich, 610
 high-affinity, polycythemia and, 1079
 ontogeny of, 455
 reference values for, *e15t*

Hemoglobins (Hb) (Continued)
  sickle cell heterozygotes (HbAS), 571–572
  structure of, 449–450, 450f, 452f
  unstable, 608–612
Hemoglobinuria, 417–418
Hemojuvelin (HJV), 474
Hemolysis
  glucose-6-phosphate dehydrogenase deficiency and,
    618–619
  hereditary elliptocytosis with, 637
  sickle cell anemia and, 579–580, 579f
Hemolytic anemias
  acute, 86t, 87–88, 88f, 2215–2216
  autoimmune. See Autoimmune hemolytic anemia
  in children and adults, 461t
  erythrocyte enzymes and, 616–621
  erythrocyte membrane and, 646
  extrinsic, 663–665, 670–671
  fragmentation hemolysis. See Microangiopathic
    hemolytic anemia
  infectious disease and, 645–646
  laboratory diagnosis, 650–651, 650b
  paroxysmal nocturnal hemoglobinuria and, 417–418
  poorly-characterized causes of extrinsic, 671, 672b
  sickle cell disease and, 578–579, 595–596
  spur cell of severe liver disease, 641, 641f, 668–669
Hemolytic crises, 633
Hemolytic disease of the fetus and newborn (HDFN),
  1756, 1824, 1951b
Hemolytic ovalocytosis, 639
Hemolytic reactions, 1717
Hemolytic syndromes, 2283
Hemolytic uremic syndrome (HUS)
  after solid organ transplant in children, 2229–2230
  atypical. See Atypical hemolytic uremic syndrome
  HIV infection and, 2275
  kidney disease and, 2245
  plasma derivatives for, 1748
  pregnancy and, 2207–2208
  Shiga toxin. See Shiga toxin hemolytic uremic syndrome
  therapy for, 1989b
Hemophagic lymphohistiocytosis (HLH), 700, 719, 753
Hemophagocytic lymphohistiocytosis (HLH)
  in children, 2220
  clinical manifestations of, 733–734
  diagnosis of, 732t, 734–735
  differential diagnosis for, 734
  epidemiology of, 732
  gene mutations in, 733t
  laboratory manifestations of, 734
  overview of, 731–732
  pathobiology of, 732–733
  prognosis for, 737
  therapy for, 735–737, 735f
Hemophagocytic syndrome, 403, 700, 737–738, 1969,
  2220–2221, 2220t
Hemophilias
  carrier detection and prenatal diagnosis of, 2007b
  clinical features of, 2008–2012
  clinical management of, 2012–2021
  diagnosis of, 2006
  differential diagnosis for, 2007–2008, 2007t
  epidemiology of, 2001
  factor IX biology and, 2004–2008
  factor VIII biology and, 2001–2003
  future directions, 2021
  hemophilia A (factor VIII deficiency)
    acquired, 1777, 2018
    clinical features of, 2008–2012, 2009t
    clinical management of, 2012–2021
    diagnosis of, 2006
    differential diagnosis for, 2007–2008, 2007t
    factor VIII biology and, 2001–2003
    factor VIII inhibitors and. See Factor VIII inhibitors
    overview of, 1769
    pathophysiology of, 2003–2004, 2004f, 2004t
    transfusion therapy for, 1769–1773, 1770t
    treatment of, 1773–1775
    von Willebrand disease vs., 2060
  hemophilia B (factor IX deficiency)
    clinical features of, 2008–2012, 2009t
    clinical management of, 2012–2021
    diagnosis of, 2006
    differential diagnosis for, 2007–2008
    factor IX biology and, 2004–2008
    factor IX gene and, 19f, 20
    factor IX inhibitors and. See Factor IX inhibitors
    gene therapy for, 1774

Hemophilias (Continued)
  overview of, 1769
  pathophysiology of, 2005–2006, 2005f–2006f
  transfusion therapy for, 1769–1773, 1770t
  treatment of, 1774–1775
  hemophilia B Leyden, 2005, 2005f
  infection and, 1450
  novel therapies for, 2019–2020, 2019t
  pathophysiology of, 2003–2006, 2003t
  pregnancy and, 2210–2211
Hemopyrroles, 448
Hemorrhage
  alveolar. See Alveolar hemorrhage
  essential thrombocythemia and, 1111
  obstetric, 1751b
  polycythemia vera and, 1088–1091
Hemorrhagic stroke, 2133, 2135. See also Intracerebral
    hemorrhage
Hemostasis
  anticoagulant intravascular space and, 1906–1907
  antiphospholipid syndrome and, 2099
  clinical assessment and, 1914
  coagulation and, 1834–1837, 1835f, 1906, 1909
  connectivity and dynamics in, 1898–1904, 1900f–
    1901f, 1903f
  developmental, 2189–2191, 2190t
  disorders of, 1839–1841, 1839t–1840t, 2191
  fibrinolysis and, 1837–1839, 1838f
  key events in, 1906, 1907f
  laboratory evaluation of
    platelet evaluation, 1928
    screening, 1927–1928
    von Willebrand factor evaluation, 1928
  liver disease and, 2240b, 2242b
  molecular basis of
    clot proteins, 1895–1897
    cofactor proteins, 1888–1891, 1890f
    endothelium, 1894, 1895f
    fibrinolysis proteins, 1897–1898
    intrinsic accessory pathway proteins, 1891–1894,
      1892f
    overview, 1885
    platelets, 1894–1895, 1896f
    vitamin K-dependent protein family, 1885–1888,
      1888f
  overview of, 1831, 1886f, 1923f–1924f
  platelets and, 1832–1834, 1833f
  procoagulant extravascular space and, 1907–1909,
    1908f
  regulators of, 1909, 1910f
  surgery and, 2304–2305, 2305t
  treatment of disorders of, 1841
  vascular endothelium and, 1831–1832, 1832f
  von Willebrand factor and, 2051, 2052f
Hemostatic dressings, 2306
Hemovigilance Module of National Healthcare Safety
  Network, 1801–1802
Hemozoin, 2282
HEMPAS. See Hereditary erythroblastic multinuclearity
  with a positive acidified serum test
Henoch-Schönlein purpura (HSP), 2221–2222
Heparin
  for acute coronary syndromes, 2147–2149, 2148t
  for disorders of hemostasis and thrombosis, 1841
  for disseminated intravascular coagulation,
    2073–2074
  dosing of, 2175
  endothelium and, 1852
  hemostasis and, 1909
  limitations of, 2175–2176, 2176t
  low-molecular weight. See Low molecular weight
    heparin
  mechanism of action of, 2173–2174, 2174f
  monitoring of, 2175
  for neonates, 2199–2200
  overview of, 2173–2177, 2174f–2175f
  pharmacology of, 2174–2175
  platelet disorders and, 1938
  for sickle cell disease, 593
  side effects of, 2176–2177, 2176t
Heparin cofactor II (HCII), 1893, 1909
Heparin-binding protein, 1851
Heparin-induced thrombocytopenia (HIT)
  anticoagulants and previous, 1983
  clinical and laboratory manifestations of, 1974, 1976f
  clinical scoring systems for, 1974–1975, 1977t–1978t
  conceptual framework for, 1982f
  differential diagnosis for, 1974, 1974b, 2071–2072

Heparin-induced thrombocytopenia (HIT) (Continued)
  epidemiology of, 1973, 1974t
  laboratory diagnosis of, 1975–1977, 1976f, 1981b
  in neonate, 2199–2200
  overview of, 1973, 2081, 2176, 2176t
  pathobiology of, 1973, 1975f, 1982f
  platelet count monitoring for, 1981
  prognosis for, 1977
  therapy for, 1977–1981, 1980t, 1981b, 1982f
  timeline of, 1976f
Hepatic disease. See Liver disease
Hepatic venoocclusive disease. See Sinusoidal obstruction
  syndrome
Hepatic venoocclusive disease with immunodeficiency, 717
Hepatitis viruses
  aplastic anemia and, 403
  HAV, 1805
  HBV, 1310b, 1458, 1803–1805
  HCV
    hematopoietic stem cell transplants and, 1458
    lymphoma and, 1319t, 1327–1328
    polyclonal gammopathy and, 688
    sickle cell disease and, 601
    transfusion-associated, 1804
  HDV, 1804
  HEV, 1805–1806
  HGV, 1806
  transfusion-associated, 1803–1806
Hepatocellular carcinoma (HCC), 1078–1079
Hepatocellular syndromes, 960–961, 960f
Hepatocytes, 469, 469f, 473–476, 474f
Hepatomegaly, 559–560, 1178
Hepatosplenic T-cell lymphoma (HSTCL), 1199–1200,
  1347–1348, 1347f
Hepcidin
  acquired iron overload and, 487
  anemia of chronic diseases and, 492–493, 495
  anemia of chronic inflammation and, 298–299
  β-thalassemia syndromes and, 551
  chronic kidney disease and, 2244
  hereditary hemochromatosis and, 303–304
  iron homeostasis and, 468, 469f–470f, 473–474,
    479b
  malaria and, 2282
  regulation of expression, 476
Herbal medications, 2254, 2255t, 2258–2260
Herbamycin A, 878
Hereditary aceruloplasminemia, 485–487
Hereditary coproporphyria, 502–503
Hereditary elliptocytosis (HE)
  clinical manifestations, 637
  differential diagnosis, 639
  introduction and epidemiology, 634
  laboratory manifestations, 638–639, 638f
  membrane effects, 636, 636f
  molecular determinants of severity, 637–638
  overview of, 626
  pathobiology, 635
  therapy and prognosis, 639
Hereditary erythroblastic multinuclearity with a positive
  acidified serum test (HEMPAS), 380–383. See also
  Congenital dyserythropoietic anemias
Hereditary folate malabsorption, 536
Hereditary hemochromatosis, 484–487, 486t. See also
  Hemochromatosis gene
Hereditary hemorrhagic telangiectasia (HHT), 1914
Hereditary persistence of fetal hemoglobin (HPFH), 22,
  313, 546, 571, 607
Hereditary pyropoikilocytosis (HPP), 626, 637
Hereditary spherocytosis (HS)
  band 3 protein deficiency, 628–629
  cation content and permeability alterations in, 629
  clinical manifestations of, 631–632
  combined spectrin/ankyrin deficiency, 627–628
  complications after, 632–633
  differential diagnosis for, 633
  future directions for, 634
  inheritance of, 630
  introduction and epidemiology of, 626
  isolated spectrin deficiency, 627
  laboratory manifestations of, 631–632
  molecular basis of surface area deficiency in, 629
  molecular pathology of, 627
  nondeformable spherocyte entrapment and, 630
  nonerythroid manifestations of, 630
  overview of, 626
  pathobiology of, 626–627, 629f
  pregnancy and, 2204–2205

Hereditary spherocytosis (HS) *(Continued)*
  protein 4.2 deficiency, 629
  spleen and, 630, 633–634, 634*b*
  therapy and prognosis for, 633–634, 634*b*
Hereditary stomatocytosis-hydrocytosis, 644
Hereditary tyrosinemia, 511–512
Hereditary xerocytosis (HX), 644–645
Hermansky-Pudlak syndrome (HPS), 719
Herpes simplex thymidine kinase (HSVtk),
    1572–1573
Herpes simplex virus (HSV), 1457, 1673–1674, 1810
Herpes zoster reactivation, 869
Hetastarch, 1938
Heterochromatin
  defined, 20
  DNA-protein interactions in, 21–22, 22*f*
  epigenetic regulation and, 9
  overview of, 17, 18*f*
Heterogenous nuclear ribonucleoprotein E1 (hnRNP-E1),
    519, 521*f*, 534
Heterologous immunity, 1619
Heterotrimeric G proteins, 1874
Hexagonal phase array test, 2092
Hexokinase deficiency, 622
HFE. *See* Hereditary hemochromatosis
HHV-8. *See* Kaposi-sarcoma-associated herpesvirus
High endothelial venules (HEV), 1844–1845
High-density lipoproteins (HDL), 2124, 2124*f*, 2126
High-dose salvage chemotherapy (HDSC), 1223–1224
High-efficiency particulate air (HEPA) filtration, 1459
High-grade MALT lymphoma, 1279
Highly active antiretroviral therapy (HAART), 1227
Highly endothelial venules (HEV), 139–140
High-molecular-weight kininogen (HMWK), 1891,
    2047
Hilum, 206
Hinge region of IgG molecules, 273
Hip joint bleeds, 2010*b*–2011*b*
Hirudin, 1979–1980, 1979*t*, 2179*t*
Histiocytic cell neoplasms, classification of, 772, 772*t*
Histiocytic sarcoma (HS), 772
Histiocytoses
  classification of, 725*t*, 772, 772*t*
  Erdheim-Chester disease, 731
  hemophagocytic lymphohistiocytosis. *See*
      Hemophagocytic lymphohistiocytosis
  juvenile xanthogranulomatous disease, 731
  Langerhans cell histiocytosis. *See* Langerhans cell
      histiocytosis
  macrophage activation syndrome, 403, 700, 737–738,
      1969, 2220–2221, 2220*t*
  overview of, 724
  sinus histiocytosis with massive lymphadenopathy,
      738
Histiocytosis X, 724
Histocompatibility workshops, 1610*t*
Histone acetyl transferases (HAT), 874–877
Histone code, 19, 874
Histone deacetylase inhibitors (HDACi)
  for acute myeloid leukemia, 991
  classes of, 875–877, 876*t*
  in combination with other agents, 877
  as epigenetic therapy, 23
  G6PD deficiency and, 88
  for Hodgkin lymphoma, 1225–1226
  mechanisms of action, 875
  for myelodysplastic syndromes, 967
  for peripheral T-cell lymphomas, 1358–1359
  pharmacology of, 874–877, 874*t*, 876*t*, 903
  toxicity in clinical trials, 877
Histone deacetylases (HDAC), 19, 874, 874*t*
Histone demethylases (HDM), 19, 23
Histone methyltransferases (HMT), 19, 23
Histone modifications
  acute lymphoblastic leukemia and, 1011
  acute myeloid leukemia and, 920
  covalent, 19–20, 19*f*
  hematopoietic stem cell self-renewal and, 104
  myelodysplastic syndromes and, 949–950
Histones, 9–10, 20
HIT Expert Probability (HEP) scoring system, 1975,
    1978*t*
Hit-and-run oncogenesis, 117
HLA. *See* Human leukocyte antigens
HLAMatchmaker, 1730
HLH-94 protocol, 735–737, 735*f*
HMBS. *See* Hydroxymethylbilane synthase
HMG-CoA reductase (HMGR), 2122

Hodgkin and Reed-Sternberg (HRS) cells
  classical Hodgkin lymphoma and, 1205–1206, 1206*t*,
      1212–1214, 1214*f*–1215*f*
  composite lymphomas and, 1210*f*
  cytogenetics of, 839
  genetic lesions in, 1209–1210
  germinal center reaction and, 1205*f*
  Hodgkin cells and, 1207
  Hodgkin lymphomas and, 1200, 1212
  overview of, 1204
  precursor or stem cells, 1207–1208
Hodgkin lymphoma (HL)
  allogenic HSCT for, 1606
  B cell development and differentiation and,
      1204
  cell lines of, 1206–1207, 1207*t*
  in childhood, 1338–1341, 1340*t*
  classic. *See* Classic Hodgkin lymphoma
  classification of, 768, 769*t*, 1204–1210
  clinical features of, 1217
  complications (long-term) of, 1228
  composite lymphomas and, 1208, 1208*f*
  cytogenetics of, 839
  diagnosis and staging for, 1216–1217, 1216*t*
  epidemiology and etiology of, 1212
  Epstein-Barr virus and, 748–749, 750*b*, 757–758,
      1320–1321
  future directions for, 1210–1211
  HIV infection and, 2268*f*
  Hodgkin and Reed-Sternberg cells of, 1206*t*
  infection and, 1447
  lymphoblastic lymphoma. *See* Lymphoblastic
      lymphoma
  nodular-lymphocyte-predominant, 1200–1201, 1201*f*,
      1204–1210
  overview of, 1200–1202, 1204, 1212, 1228
  pathobiology of, 1212–1216
  PD-1 blockade therapies and, 1584
  pregnancy and, 2208–2209
  prognostic factors, risk stratification, and treatment
      groups in, 1217–1218, 1218*t*, 1340*t*
  relapsed or refractory, 1223–1225, 1339–1341
  second/subsequent malignancies after, 1503, 1506,
      1506*t*
  special considerations for, 1226–1227
  spleen and, 2320*f*
  treatment of
    advanced stage, 1219–1223
    early stage, 1218–1219
    novel therapies, 1225–1226
    relapsed or refractory, 1223–1224
Holo-transcobalamin II (holo-TCII) levels, 529
Holt-Oram syndrome, 392
Homeobox (*HOX*) genes, 103–104, 346,
    1008–1009
Homeostasis. *See also* Autophagy
  cation, 576–578
  chemokine signals in, 135
  erythrocyte, 447–448
  folate, 519
  iron. *See* Iron homeostasis
  oxygen. *See* Oxygen homeostasis
Homing, 145–146, 146*f*
Homing cell adhesion molecule (HCAM). *See* CD44
Homocysteine. *See* Total homocysteine
Homologous recombination, 14–15, 15*f*, 1549,
    1557
Hookah use, 1078
Hookworm infection, 2302–2303
Hope, palliative care and, 1490
Hormone replacement therapy (HRT), 2083
Hormones, signal transduction and, 72
Hospice programs, 1466, 1493
Howell-Jolly bodies, 2320–2321, 2320*f*
HOX. *See* Homeobox genes
Hoyeraal-Hriedarsson syndrome, 365–367, 684
HPFH. *See* Hereditary persistence of fetal hemoglobin
HPRT1 deficiency. *See* hypoxanthine
    phosphoribosyltransferase 1 deficiency
HRG1. *See* Heme importer
HRI. *See* Hemin-regulated inhibitor
HSP90 inhibitors, 878
HSVtk. *See* Herpes simplex thymidine kinase
Human androgen receptors. *See* HUMARA assays
Human embryonic stem cells (hESC), 300
Human granulocytic anaplasmosis (HGA), 1815
Human hemolytic disease of the fetus and newborn
    (HDFN), 1709

Human herpes viruses (HHV)
  HHV-4. *See* Epstein-Barr virus
  HHV-6, 1455, 1458, 1674, 1810
  HHV-7, 1810
  HHV-8. *See* Kaposi sarcoma-associated herpesviruses
  transfusion-associated, 1808–1810
Human immunodeficiency virus (HIV) infection
  in adolescents, 2219–2222
  biology and pathogenesis, 1324
  in children, 2219–2222
  clinical course of, 2265–2266
  definition of, 2262
  dendritic cell function and, 256–257
  diagnostic considerations specific to lymphoma with,
      1324–1325
  epidemiology, 1324
  epidemiology of, 2262
  Epstein-Barr virus-associated non-Hodgkin lymphoma
      and, 758
  etiology and pathogenesis of, 2263–2265,
      2263*f*–2264*f*
  gene therapy and, 1551
  hematologic and bone marrow abnormalities in,
      2266–2272, 2266*b*
  hematopoietic stem cell transplants and, 1458
  Hodgkin lymphoma and, 1227
  intravenous immunoglobulin for, 1753
  leukopenia, neutropenia and, 2272–2273
  lymphocytopenia and, 684
  lymphocytosis and, 683
  lymphoma and, 1319*t*, 1324–1327, 1324*b*, 1324*t*
  thrombocytopenia and, 1968, 2273–2275
  thromboembolic disease and, 2275–2276
  thrombotic microangiopathies and, 1999, 2275
  transfusion-associated, 1806–1807
  transmission of, 2262–2263
Human leukocyte antigens (HLA)
  allosensitization testing and, 1729–1730
  aplastic anemia and, 394
  autoimmunity and, 291
  class I deficiency, 715
  class II deficiency, 715
  cord blood stem cell transplantation and,
      1633–1634
  erythropoiesis and, 312
  expression level and alloimmunity, 1614–1615
  expression of, 1724
  genetics of, 1609–1610, 1609*t*–1610*t*, 1721
  graft-versus-host disease and, 1652, 1731
  graft-versus-neoplasia effect and, 1731–1732
  haploidentical hematopoietic stem cell transplantation
      and, 1617, 1619–1621
  haplotype assessment, 1611–1612, 1612*b*
  HLA alloimmunization and, 1730–1731
  HLA-DM, 1725
  HLA-DO, 1725
  HLA-E, 1725
  HLA-F, 1725
  HLA-G, 1725
  impacts of specific mismatches, 1612*t*
  importance of matching in unrelated donor HCT,
      1612–1613
  inheritance and linkage disequilibrium and,
      1722
  nomenclature of
    immunologically-defined, 1727–1728
    overview, 1727, 1727*t*
    sequence-defined, 1728
  nonclassic and class I chain-related, 1725–1726
  organization of genes, 1721–1722, 1722*f*
  overview of, 1721, 1732–1733
  permissible mismatches, 1613–1614
  platelet refractoriness and, 1718–1719, 1719*t*
  polymorphisms and their clinical significance,
      1724–1725
  single-locus mismatched unrelated HSCT and,
      1613–1614
  structure of class I and II, 1723–1724, 1723*f*
  T cell-directed immunization and, 1732
  tetrameric antigen-peptide complexes for monitoring
      immune responses, 1732, 1733*f*
  typing in clinical setting and determination of
      compatibility typing, 1728–1729
  typing methods, 1610–1611
  unrelated donor HSCT donor evaluation and,
      1608–1609
  vector of mismatching assessment and, 1611
Human monocytic ehrlichiosis (HME), 1815

Human neutrophil antigens (HNA)
  alloimmune neonatal neutropenia and, 1735–1736, 1735*t*
  autoimmune neutropenia of childhood and, 1736
  HNA-1, 1733–1734
  HNA-2, 1734–1735
  HNA-3, 1735
  HNA-4 and HNA-5, 1735
  nomenclature of, 1733*t*
  overview of, 1733, 1736
  transfusion reactions and, 1736
Human papillomaviruses (HPV), 1569
Human polyomavirus type I, 1674
Human T-lymphotropic viruses (HTLV)
  adult T-cell leukemia/lymphoma and, 1197, 1348, 1354
  lymphoma and, 1319*t*, 1322–1324, 1323*f*
  transfusion-associated, 1807–1808
HUMARA assays, 782–783
Humate, 1776–1777, 2013
Humoral immunity, 749–750, 750*t*, 1451, 1709
Hunter disease, 741*t*, 742
Hurler syndrome, 56, 741
Hyaline membrane disease, 2197
Hyaluronan, 127
Hybrid immunotherapy for HLH (HIT-HLH), 737–738
Hybrid resistance, 1577
Hycamtin. *See* Topotecan
Hydantoins, 400–401
Hydroa vacciniforme-like lymphoma, 1200
Hydrocytosis, hereditary. *See* Hereditary stomatocytosis-hydrocytosis
Hydrogen bonding, overview of, 59
Hydrogen peroxide, 74–75
Hydrophilic amino acids, 59
Hydrophobic amino acids, 59
Hydrops fetalis, 566*f*, 567
Hydroxychloroquine (HCQ), 2100
Hydroxyl radicals, 74–75
Hydroxymethylbilane synthase (HMBS), 499–501
4-Hydroxynonenal (HNE), 2282
Hydroxyurea (HU)
  for β-thalassemia syndrome, 562
  for chronic myelogenous leukemia, 1060
  for essential thrombocythemia, 1118–1120, 1119*f*, 1120*t*, 1123*b*
  for hypereosinophilic syndrome, 1165–1166
  for mastocytosis, 1184
  for myelodysplastic syndromes, 968
  pharmacology of, 856–857, 893–894
  for polycythemia vera, 1100–1101
  pregnancy and, 2204
  for sickle cell disease, 589–590, 590*t*, 2204
Hypercoagulable states
  acquired
    assisted conception, ovarian hyperstimulation syndrome and, 2083
    cancer and its treatment and, 2081–2082
    heparin-induced thrombocytopenia. *See* Heparin-induced thrombocytopenia
    hormonal therapy and, 2083
    lupus anticoagulants, antiphospholipid syndrome and, 2080–2081
    myeloproliferative disorders and, 2082
    overview, 2077*t*
    paroxysmal nocturnal hemoglobinuria, 419, 2082
    pregnancy and, 2082–2083
    prior history of VTE and, 2083–2084
  clinical presentation, 2084
  combined inherited and acquired, 2084
  inherited
    antithrombin deficiency, 2076–2078
    factor V$_{Leiden}$ gain-of-function mutation, 2079–2080
    FIIG20210A mutation and, 2080
    miscellaneous, 2080
    overview, 2076, 2077*t*
    protein C deficiency, 2078–2079, 2078*f*, 2078*t*
    protein S deficiency, 2079, 2079*t*
  laboratory evaluation of, 2084–2085, 2084*b*
  management of, 2085–2086, 2086*t*
  in neonate, 2197–2200
  screening for, 2084, 2085*b*
  venous thromboembolism (VTE) and, 2103
Hyper-CVAD regimen, 1039, 1043, 1047, 1069

Hyperdiploidy
  in acute lymphoblastic leukemia, 1017
  acute lymphoblastic leukemia and, 816, 1033–1034, 1034*t*
  acute myeloid leukemia and, 812
  multiple myeloma and, 828, 1382–1383
Hypereosinophilia (HE)
  clinical manifestations of, 1159–1165, 1160*f*
  definition and classification of, 1159
  epidemiology of, 1151–1153
  etiology and pathobiology of, 1157–1158
  overview of, 1151, 1152*t*–1153*t*, 1165–1168
  treatment of, 1165–1168
Hypereosinophilic syndromes (HES)
  clinical manifestations of, 1159–1165, 1160*f*
  definition and classification of, 1159
  epidemiology of, 1151–1153
  etiology and pathobiology of, 790–792, 1157–1158, 1158*t*
  overview of, 1151, 1152*t*–1153*t*, 1165–1168
  treatment of, 1165–1168
Hypergammaglobulinemia, 688–689
Hyperhemolytic crisis, 597, 1793–1794
Hyperhomocysteinemia, 522, 543–544, 2084
Hyper-IgE syndromes (HIES), 230, 1153*t*, 1164–1165
Hyper-IgM syndrome (HIMS), 433–434, 687–688
Hyperimmune globulins, 1756–1757, 1756*t*, 1761, 1763*t*
Hyperimmunoglobulin E syndrome (HIES), 704–705, 704*t*, 707
Hyperkalemia, 1799
Hyperleukocytosis, 941, 941*f*
Hyperlipidemia, 2129–2130
Hypermethylation, 20
Hyperreactive malarial splenomegaly syndrome, 666, 2284
Hypersensitive sites (HS), 315
Hypersensitivity reactions, 1967
Hypersplenism
  hemolytic anemia and, 666, 666*t*
  neutropenia and, 433
  neutropenias and, 679
  overview of, 2322–2323
  thrombocytopenia and, 1960–1961, 1960*t*
Hypertension, 2159, 2164
Hypertransfusion programs, 553
Hypervariable regions, 62–63, 62*f*–63*f*, 273–274
Hyperviscosity, 1392, 1422–1423
Hypnosis, 1474–1475
Hypoalbuminemia, 1178–1179, 1752
Hypochromic circulating RBC (%HRC), 479–480
Hypodiploidy, 1017
Hypodysfibrinogenemia, 2038–2040
Hypofibrinogenemia, 2034–2038
Hypogammaglobulinemia, 685–688, 1262
Hypomethylating agents (HMA)
  for acute myeloid leukemia, 935–936, 975
  for myelodysplastic syndromes, 966–967, 979
  overview of, 873–874
Hypomethylation, 20
Hypoproliferative thrombocytopenia, 1715–1716, 1716*f*
Hypoprothrombinemia, 2040–2041
Hyposplenism, 2320–2322, 2320*f*
Hyposthenuria, 602
Hypothermia, 511, 1799, 1942
Hypothyroidism, 597, 2225
Hypoxanthine phosphoribosyltransferase 1 (HPRT1) deficiency, 82–84
Hypoxemia, 1071–1073, 1072*f*
Hypoxia, 105, 122, 125, 159
Hypoxia-inducible factors (HIF), 122, 1071–1072, 1079–1080
Hzf. *See* Hematopoietic zinc finger

I

I antigens, 1695–1696
iAMP21. *See* Itrachromosomal amplification of chromosome 21
IAP-binding motifs (IBM), 190
Ibritumomab, 1296
Ibrutinib, 863, 1257–1258, 1305, 1938
ICAM. *See* Intracellular cell adhesion molecules
iCaspase9-T cells, 1573
I-cell diseases, 56
ID. *See* DNA-binding protein inhibitors
Idamycin. *See* Idarubicin
Idarubicin, 900, 935
Idelalisib, 864, 1226, 1226*f*, 1258
IDH. *See* Isocitrate dehydrogenases

Idiopathic CD4+ lymphocytopenia (ICL), 685
Idiopathic hypereosinophilic syndrome, 330, 1157–1159, 1165
Idiopathic myelofibrosis, 308, 1003
Idiopathic pain, defined, 1473
Idiopathic thrombocytopenic purpura (ITP)
  antiphospholipid syndrome and, 2099
  clinical and laboratory features of, 1946
  clinical outcomes in, 1946
  diagnosis of, 1946–1947, 1947*f*
  epidemiology of, 1944
  HIV infection and, 2273–2275
  intravenous immunoglobulin for, 1753–1754
  overview of, 1944, 1946*t*
  pathophysiology of, 1944–1945, 1945*t*
  pregnancy and, 2205–2206, 2206*f*
  primary and secondary immune, 1945–1946
  refractory, 1950
  second-line therapy for, 1948–1950
  tolerance, immunity and, 285
  treatment of, 340–341, 1947–1948, 1947*f*, 1950
Idiotypic determinants, 275–276
IDO. *See* Indoleamine dioxygenase
IFN (class II cytokine receptors). *See* Interferons
Ifosfamide, 886, 913
IGH. *See* Immunoglobulin heavy locus
Ikaros, 1129
IKAROS family zinc finger 1 (IKZF1), 820, 1016, 1051
Iliofemoral deep vein thrombosis, 2118
Imatinib mesylate
  for chronic myelogenous leukemia, 784–788, 788*f*, 1061–1062, 1062*f*–1063*f*, 1064, 1066–1068, 1069*b*
  for hypereosinophilic syndrome, 1166–1167
  for mastocytosis, 1183–1184
  pharmacology of, 861, 862*t*
  for Philadelphia chromosome-positive acute lymphoblastic leukemia, 1043
  pregnancy and, 2209, 2209*b*
  St. Johns wort and, 2258
Imerslund-Grasbeck syndrome, 532
Imetelstat, 1148
Imitation SWI (ISWI) family, 20
Immature platelet fraction (IPF), e11*b*, e24*t*
Immature reticulocyte fraction, e3*b*, e15*t*
Immune dysregulation polyendocrinopathy enteropathy X-linked syndrome (IPEX), 428, 718
Immune globulin products, 1761, 1762*t*
Immune serum globulin, 1761
Immune system
  adaptive. *See* Adaptive immune system
  anatomy of, 203–205, 204*f*
  cells of, 202–203
  complement receptors and, 265
  complement system and, 268
  dendritic cells and, 254–256
  immunoglobulin gene rearrangement and expression in, 212–214
  inflammatory response and, 205, 205*f*
  innate. *See* Innate immune system
  myelodysplastic syndromes and, 953, 955
  overview of, 199
Immune thrombocytopenia, drug-induced (D-ITP), 1961–1965, 1962*f*, 1963*b*, 1963*t*
Immune tolerance therapy, 2031–2032
Immunoadsorption therapies, 1787
Immunoblotting, 356
Immunodysregulation, polydendocrinopathy, and enteropathy X-linked syndrome (IPEX) syndrome, 228
Immunoglobin repertoire, defined, 212
Immunoglobulin A antibodies, against cardiolipin and β$_2$-Glycoprotein I, 2094
Immunoglobulin heavy chain variable region (IGHV), 825, 1245, 1250–1251
Immunoglobulin heavy locus (IGH), 829–830, 832–835, 1189
Immunoglobulin light chain amyloidosis
  clinical manifestations of, 1433–1435
  differential diagnosis for, 1437–1438, 1442*f*
  epidemiology of, 1432
  laboratory manifestations of, 1435–1437, 1435*f*–1436*f*, 1435*t*–1436*t*, 1437*b*
  overview of, 1432, 1433*f*, 1442–1443
  pathobiology of, 1432–1433
  prognosis for, 1438, 1438*b*
  therapy for, 1438–1443, 1443*t*
Immunoglobulin-like receptors, 129, 129*t*

Immunoglobulins (Ig). *See also* Antibodies
  class switching and affinity maturation in, 219
  domain structures of, 62–63, 62*f*
  IgA, 274, *e*8*b*, *e*21*t*
  IgE, *e*9*b*, *e*21*t*
  IgG
    laboratory evaluation of, *e*9*b*
    overview of, 274–275, 275*f*
    reference values for, *e*22*t*
  IgM, 274, 1422–1425, *e*10*b*, *e*23*t*
  light chains, *e*10*b*, *e*23*t*
  properties and structure of, 272–276, 273*f*, 274*t*, 275*f*
  quantitative disorders of, 685–689
  rearrangement and expression of in immune response,
    212–214
  therapeutic use of
    IVIg. *See* Intravenous immunoglobulin
    passive immunization, monoclonal antibody therapy,
      277–279, 278*f*–279*f*, 280*t*–281*t*
Immunologic memory, 231–232
Immunologic synapse (IS), 226
Immunologic testing, overview of, *e*1
Immunomodulatory drugs (IMiD)
  for Hodgkin lymphoma, 1226
  for multiple myeloma, 1403
  for peripheral T-cell lymphomas, 1359
  pharmacology of, 866
  for primary myelofibrosis, 1142–1143, 1148*b*–1149*b*
Immunoproliferative small intestinal disease (IPSID),
  1277, 1279, 1281–1282
Immunoreceptor tyrosine-based activating motifs (ITAM),
  71, 177–178, 223–224, 224*f*
Immunosuppressive drugs
  anemia and, 2230
  for aplastic anemia, 409–411, 410*b*
  aplastic anemia and, 397–398
  for myelodysplastic syndromes, 965
  for paroxysmal nocturnal hemoglobinuria, 420–421
  for pure red cell aplasia, 429–430
  thrombotic microangiopathies and, 1997
  for thrombotic thrombocytopenic purpura, 1991
  for warm antibody hemolytic anemia, 660
Immunotherapy
  for acute lymphoblastic leukemia, 1050–1052, 1052*t*
  for acute myeloid leukemia, 991
  checkpoint blockade therapies. *See* Checkpoint blockade
    therapies
  dendritic cells and, 257–259
  for hypereosinophilic syndrome, 1167
  types of, 1568–1570
Impedance aggregometry, 1928
Importins, 48
Inborn errors of metabolism, 537
Inclusion body myositis, 1755
Indels, 28, 81
Indian blood group system, 1699
Indinavir, 2276
Indirect antiglobulin test (IAT), 1691, 1693*b*
Indoleamine dioxygenase (IDO), 254–255, 257,
  1562–1563
Indolent systemic mastocytosis (ISM), 1172–1173, 1174*t*
Induced pluripotent stem cells (iPSC), 300, 366,
  1556–1557, 1713
Inducible costimulator (ICOS), 226
Inducible regulatory T cells (iTregs), 233
Inducible T-cell kinase (ITK), 225
Induction therapy
  for acute lymphoblastic leukemia, 1037–1040
  for acute myeloid leukemia, 934–936, 934*f*
  minimal residual disease and, 1025*b*
  for multiple myeloma, 1402, 1408–1409
  for myelodysplastic syndromes, 967
Infections
  acute myeloid leukemia and, 990–991, 991*b*
  acute neutropenia or lymphopenia following
    transplantation or chemotherapy and,
    1451–1457
  after hematopoietic stem cell transplantation, 1594,
    1669–1675, 1671*t*–1672*t*, 1672*f*, 1678, 1801
  anatomic alterations in host defense and, 1451
  aplastic anemia and, 407
  autoimmune hemolytic anemia after, 654, 654*t*
  bacterial. *See* Bacterial infections
  childhood, 2215–2219
  chronic granulomatous disease and, 695–698, 697*t*,
    700
  chronic lymphocytic leukemia and, 1262–1263
  disseminated intravascular coagulation and, 2068

Infections (Continued)
  fungal. *See* Fungal infections
  in hematopoietic stem cell transplant recipient,
    1457–1460, 1457*f*
  hemolysis and, 667–668, 667*t*
  host defense impairment and, 1449*t*, 1450–1451
  intravenous immunoglobulin and transfer of, 277
  lymphocytopenia and, 684
  malignant hematologic conditions predisposing to,
    1447–1448, 1449*t*
  monocytosis and, 680
  multiple myeloma and, 1392
  myelodysplastic syndromes and, 963
  natural killer cells and increased risks of, 243
  neutropenias with, 679
  neutrophil disorders and, 708*b*
  nonmalignant hematologic conditions predisposing to,
    1448–1450, 1449*t*
  overview of in compromised host, 1447, 1448*f*
  parasitic. *See* Parasitic infections
  platelet transfusions and, 1717
  polyclonal gammopathy and, 688
  prevention of, 1458–1459
  sickle cell disease and, 595*t*, 597–598, 597*t*
  thrombocytopenia and, 441–442, 1967–1968, 1968*t*
  transfusion-associated. *See* Transfusion-related infections
  viral. *See* Viral infections
Infectious mononucleosis (IM)
  clinical manifestations, 751, 751*f*, 751*t*
  diagnosis, 752
  differential diagnosis, 752–753
  epidemiology, 751
  Epstein-Barr virus and, 751–752
Inferior vena cava filters, 2110, 2120
Inflammasomes, 188, 189*f*, 249–250
Inflammation
  atherothrombosis and, 2130–2131
  graft-versus-host disease and, 1658
  hepcidin expression and, 476
  HIV infection and, 2275–2276
  mesenchymal stromal cells and, 1560–1563
  neutrophilia and, 676
  overview of, 205, 205*f*
  polycythemia vera and, 1087
  sickle cell disease and, 580–582
Inflammatory bowel disease (IBD), 653, 2224
Inflammatory chemokines, overview of, 135
Infliximab, 965, 1659
Influenza viruses, 1813
Inherited bone marrow failure syndromes. *See* Bone
    marrow failure syndromes, inherited
Inhibitor of apoptosis proteins (IAP), 190
Inhibitors of CDK4 (INK4), 178–180, 219
Innate immune system
  adaptive immune system vs., 200*t*
  cells of, 202–203
  complement system and, 268
  dendritic cells and, 255*f*
  immune deficiency conditions caused by mutations in,
    200
  myelodysplastic syndromes and, 953
  natural killer cells and, 240–241
  pathogen recognition receptors, pathogen-associated
    molecular patterns and, 199–200
  phagocytosis, cytokine response, priming adaptive
    immune response and, 199–200
  spleen and, 2317, 2318*t*
  tissue homeostasis and, 200
Innate lymphoid cells (ILC), 240–241, 1576*f*,
    1577–1578
INO80 family, 20
Inositol 1,4,5-triphosphate receptor (IP3R), 191–193
Inositol requiring transmembrane kinase/endonuclease 1
    (ERN1), 195
Inotuzumab ozogamicin, 1050
Insect bites, 669, 1261–1262
Insertional mutagenesis, 1555–1556
Inside-out signaling, 71, 138
Insulators, 17–19, 18*f*
Insulin-like growth factors (IGF), 1389
Integrated stress response, 45–46
Integrative Genomics Viewer (IGV), 28, 29*f*
Integrative therapies
  acupuncture, 2256–2257
  domains and their use, 2253–2254, 2254*t*
  massage and touch therapies, 2257, 2257*t*
  mind-body therapies, 2255–2260, 2255*t*
  nutrition and supplements, 2257–2260

Integrative therapies (Continued)
  overview of, 2253
  research techniques of, 2254
  science, safety, and efficacy of, 2254
Integrins
  angiogenesis and, 1846
  cell adhesion and, 127–129, 128*f*, 128*t*, 132
  cell signaling and, 132
  human neutrophil antigens and, 1735
  leukocyte adhesion deficiency and, 702
  leukocyte entry into tissues and, 138
  leukocyte homing to secondary lymphoid organs and,
    139
  nomenclature of, 1871, 1872*f*
  platelet adhesion and, 1871
  platelet aggregation and, 1878–1879, 1878*f*
  protein-tyrosine kinase signaling and, 71
  as therapeutic target in leukemias, 125
  vascular system and, 154–155, 1844
INTERCEPT plasma, 1760, 1821
Interdigitating dendritic cell sarcoma (IDCS), 772
Interferon (IFN) type I-producing cells, 247–248
Interferon-γ capture, 757
Interferons (IFN)
  autoimmune hemolytic anemia and, 655
  for chronic myelogenous leukemia, 1060–1061,
    1068
  as class II cytokines, 163
  for cutaneous T-cell lymphomas, 1376
  IFN-α
    for essential thrombocythemia, 1120–1121, 1120*t*,
      1123*b*
    for follicular lymphoma, 1294–1295
    for hypereosinophilic syndrome, 1166
    for mastocytosis, 1182–1183
    for polycythemia vera, 1101–1102
    for primary myelofibrosis, 1141–1142
    for splenic marginal zone lymphoma, 1284–1285
  IFN-β, 671
  IFN-γ, 398, 699–700, 699*t*, 1562
  immune response and, 202*t*
  JAK1 and, 166
  malaria and, 2282
  for polycythemia vera, 1101–1102
  STAT1 and, 169–170
  STAT2 and, 170
  Tyk2 and, 166–169
Interleukin-3 receptor α chain, 125
Interleukin-7 receptor (IL7R), 1015
Interleukins
  adoptive natural killer cell therapies and, 1581
  B cell development and, 217
  cytokine signaling and, 164–165, 168*f*
  eosinophilopoiesis and, 1155–1157
  erythroid cell differentiation and, 306–307
  graft-versus-host disease and, 1658–1659, 1662
  hepcidin expression and, 476
  immune response and, 202*t*
  inhibition of erythropoiesis and, 493
  innate lymphoid cells and, 1576*f*
  limitation of T cell activity and, 235
  malaria and, 2282
  megakaryocytopoiesis and, 341
  memory T cells and, 232
  multiple myeloma and, 1389
  neutrophilic response to infection and, 692*f*
  polyclonal gammopathy and, 688
  specific
    IL-1, 493, 1659
    IL-2, 232, 244, 1662
    IL-3, 306–307, 1156–1157
    IL-4, 166–169, 171, 230
    IL-5, 230, 1155–1157
    IL-6, 164–165, 168*f*, 170, 493, 688, 1389,
      1658–1659
    IL-7, 217, 232
    IL-8, 692*f*
    IL-10, 166–170, 235, 688, 2282
    IL-11, 341
    IL-12R, 166–169, 171
    IL-13, 171, 230
    IL-15, 232, 244, 1581
    IL-16, 476
    IL-17, 170, 1389, 1662
    IL-21, 170
    IL-22, 1576*f*, 1581
    IL-23, 170–171, 230–231
    IL-33, 1658

Interleukins (Continued)
STAT3 and, 170
STAT4 and, 171
STAT6 and, 171
T helper cells and, 230–231
therapeutic uses of, 244
Tyk2 and, 166–169
International Immune Tolerance Registry, 2031
International normalized ratio (INR), 1924–1925, 2071, 2180, 2240, 2304–2305
International Peripheral Lymphoma Study (IPLS), 1350
International Prognostic Index (IPI), 1311, 1311t, 1350
International Prognostic Scoring System (IPSS)
for essential thrombocythemia, 1116–1117
for Hodgkin lymphoma, 1218t
for HSCT in myelodysplastic syndromes, 978
for myelodysplastic syndromes, 958–959, 959t
for primary myelofibrosis, 1140, 1140t
International Staging System (ISS), 1398–1400, 1398t
Interphase fluorescence in situ hybridization, 777f, 778, 786
Interstitial pneumonitis, 1677–1678, 1677b
Intima, 1843
Intraarterial fibrinolysis, 2138
Intracardiac thrombosis, 1841
Intracellular cell adhesion molecules (ICAM)
cell adhesion and, 129
eosinophil mobilization and migration and, 1156
foam cell formation, fatty streak and, 2126
leukocyte adhesion deficiency and, 702
leukocyte entry into tissues and, 138
neutrophilic response to infection and, 692f
peripheral artery disease and, 2160
Intracerebral hemorrhage (ICH), 2133, 2135, 2137, 2139
Intrachromosomal amplification of chromosome 21 (iAMP21), 818–819, 819f, 1017–1018
Intracranial hemorrhage, 1917, 2008–2009, 2009f, 2011–2012
Intracranial stenting, 2139
Intraepithelial lymphocytes (IEL), 209
Intrahepatic cholestasis, 601
Intravenous immunoglobulin (IVIg)
adverse effects of, 1756
adverse events related to, 276–277, 277t
for chronic lymphocytic leukemia, 1262–1263, 1753
hemolysis and, 671
for immune thrombocytopenia purpura, 1948
indications for, 1753–1756, 1754t
for neonatal alloimmune thrombocytopenia, 1952
overview of, 276, 1753, 1761
for primary myelofibrosis, 1142
for pure red cell aplasia, 429
spleen and, 2322
Intraventricular hemorrhage (IVH), 2196
Intrinsic accessory pathway, 1891–1894
Intrinsic apoptosis pathway, 190–191, 191f–192f
Intrinsic coagulation pathway. See Contact pathway
Intrinsic factor (IF), 515–516, 530–532
Intrinsic tenase, 1836, 1902, 2005
Introns, 17
Intussusception, 157f
Investigational new drugs (IND)
clinical trial readiness and, 1535–1536
novel cell-based therapies, regulation of, 1532t
overview of, 1531–1533
process for, 1533–1535, 1537–1538
regulation of, 1533
Involved-field radiotherapy (IFRT), 1212, 1221, 1224–1225
Involved-site radiotherapy (ISRT), 1212
Ion channel inhibitors, 592
Ipatasertib, 864
Ipilimumab, 1585
IPSS. See International Prognostic Scoring System
IRE. See Iron response elements
Irinotecan (CPT-11), 859–860, 859f, 901
Iron
deficiency in
anemia of chronic diseases and, 492–493
cancer and, 2247
causes, 481t
chronic kidney disease and, 2244
clinical presentation, 481–482
coexisting disorders, 482b
differential diagnosis, 482–483, 483t
epidemiology, 480
etiology and pathogenesis, 481

Iron (Continued)
laboratory evaluation, 482, 482b, 482f
lead poisoning and, 2233
malaria and, 2284
overview, 480
polycythemia vera and, 1091
prognosis, 484
therapy, 483–484, 483b–484b
thrombocytopenia and, 442
homeostasis of
control of by hepcidin and ferroportin, 479b
erythropoiesis and, 469–472
intestinal absorption and, 476–477, 476f
liver regulation of, 473–476, 474f
recycling of erythrocyte iron and, 472–473, 472f
regulation of cellular and systemic, 468–469
laboratory evaluation of, 478–480, 480b, e5b, e18t
overload of
acquired, 487
causes of, 485t
clinical presentation, 487–488
differential diagnosis, 488–489
epidemiology, 484
etiology and pathogenesis, 484–485
genetic aspects, 484
hereditary, 485–487, 486t
HSCT for myelodysplastic syndromes and, 978–979
HSCT prognosis and, 978
laboratory evaluation, 488, 488b
myelodysplastic syndromes and, 963–964
overview, 484
posttransfusion, 1799
prognosis, 490
therapy, 489–490, 489b
spleen and, 2317
Iron binding capacity, e17t
Iron chelation. See Chelation therapy
Iron deficiency anemia (IDA), 480, 482f, 483, 511, 2203
Iron regulatory proteins (IRP), 46, 470f, 493, 497–498
Iron response elements (IRE)
heme biosynthesis and, 497–498
iron homeostasis and, 468
regulation of mRNA splicing and, 11
translation efficiency and, 46
unfolded protein response and, 55, 195
Iron-deficient erythropoiesis, 480
Iron-refractory iron-deficiency anemia (IRIDA), 481
Irradiated red blood cells, 1703
Irreversibly sickled cells (ISC), 572f, 577
Irritable bowel syndrome (IBS), 256
Ischemia-reperfusion, 580, 580f
Ischemic stroke
classification of, 2133–2135
clinical manifestations of, 2136–2137
cryptogenic, 2135b
genetic risk factors for, 2136
hematological disorders and, 2135–2136
risk factors for, 2134t
secondary prevention of, 2139–2140
I-set domains, 62f, 63
Isocitrate dehydrogenase inhibitors (IDHI), 939
Isocitrate dehydrogenases (IDH)
acute leukemia and, 75
acute myeloid leukemia and, 919, 986–987
myelodysplastic syndromes and, 950
primary myelofibrosis and, 1128–1129, 1128t
Isoforms, 20–21
Isoimmune neonatal neutropenia, 433
Isolated Thrombolysis technique, 2115
Isolation procedures, 1459
Isoniazid, 511
Isotypic variation, 274
IT vaccination, 258
ITCH, 720
IVIg. See Intravenous immunoglobulin
Ivy bleeding time, 1927–1928
Ixabepilone, 856–858
Ixazomib, 869

J

Jacobsen syndrome, 345, 347b, 347t–348t, 1883
Jagged, 153–154
JAK. See Janus-activated kinases

Janus-activated kinase (JAK)-STAT pathway. See also Signal transducers and activators of transcription genes
B cell development and, 217
essential thrombocythemia and, 1107–1109
Hodgkin lymphoma and, 1209
myeloproliferative neoplasms and, 999
primary myelofibrosis and, 1125–1131, 1128t, 1143–1144, 1149b
Janus-activated kinases (JAK)
B cell development and, 217
consequences of deficiencies in genes of, 173t
erythropoietin, erythroid cell development and, 305–306, 308–309
erythropoietin receptors and, 1073
hepcidin expression and, 476
hyperimmunoglobulin E syndrome and, 704
inhibitors of, 865–866, 905
JAK1, 166, 169f
JAK2, 166, 551, 1015, 1084, 1149b, 2082
JAK2V617F
essential thrombocythemia and, 1106, 1112
for myeloproliferative neoplasms, 764
polycythemia vera and, 1081–1086, 1083f–1084f
primary myelofibrosis and, 1127, 1128t, 1139–1148, 1149b
JAK3, 166
neutrophil maturation and, 323, 324f
overview of, 166, 168f–169f
signaling through, 70–71
thrombopoietin receptor and, 339
Tyk2, 166–169
Japan Marrow Donor Program (JMDP), 1613
Jaundice, 619
Jewish Genetic Disease screening panel, 742
JK. See Kidd blood group system
Job syndrome, 230, 704. See also Hyperimmunoglobulin E syndrome
Joining (J) gene segments, 212, 213f
Joint bleeds, 1916–1917, 2015
JR blood group system, 1700
Jumping 1q translocations, 795–796, 795f
c-Jun, 332
Junctional adhesion molecules (JAM), 129, 1844
Juvenile idiopathic arthritis (JIA), 2219–2221
Juvenile myelomonocytic leukemia (JMML), 768, 998–1001, 998t
Juvenile xanthogranulomatous (JXG) disease, 731

K

Kala-azar. See Leishmaniasis, visceral
Kallikreins, 1836, 2046–2047
Kaolin clotting time (KCT), 2092
Kaposi sarcoma-associated herpesviruses (KSHV)
lymphoma and, 1319t, 1321–1322, 1322f
lymphoproliferative diseases associated with, 1193
transfusion-associated, 1810
Kappa (κ) genes, 212
Karnofsky performance scale, 1462
Kasbach-Merritt syndrome, 370, 2192–2193
Kataegis, 826
Kawasaki syndrome, 276, 1754, 2221
Kell antigen, 642–643, 1697–1698
Keratocytes, 643
Ketanserin, 1939
Ketorolac tromethamine, 1476
Ketron-Goodman syndrome, 1367
Kidd (JK) blood group system, 1698
Kidney disease
anemia and, 2244
hemolytic uremic syndromes and, 2245
multiple myeloma, 1391, 1399–1400
polycythemia and, 1078–1079
sickle cell anemia and, 582
surgical patients and, 2309
thrombosis and, 2244–2245
transplant patient and, 2245
uremic bleeding and, 2244
Kidneys
antiphospholipid syndrome and, 2097–2098
β-thalassemia syndromes and, 560
folate, cobalamin and, 521
hemolysis and, 669
paroxysmal nocturnal hemoglobinuria and, 418
Killer immunoglobulin-like receptor ligand absence model, 1578

Killer immunoglobulin-like receptors (KIR)
  alloreactions after haploidentical hematopoietic stem cell transplantation and, 1620–1621, 1620f
  checkpoint blockade therapies and, 1586
  enhancing antitumor response of natural killer cells and, 244
  graft-versus-host disease and, 1653
  graft-versus-leukemia responses and, 1600, 1664
  human leukocyte antigens and, 1726–1727, 1726t
  natural killer cells and, 203, 241–242, 1576–1579
Kinase inhibitor proteins (KIP), 178–180, 1261
Kindlin-3, 138, 703
Kinetochores, 182
Kin-recognition/oligomerization, 55–56
KIP. See Kinase inhibitor proteins
KIR. See Killer immunoglobulin-like receptors
KIT gene
  acute myeloid leukemia and, 803–804, 918, 937
  erythroid cell differentiation and, 307
  mast cell development and, 1170–1171
  mast cell disease and, 765
  mastocytosis and, 1179–1181, 1179f
  systemic mastocytosis and, 792–793
KIT ligand (KL), 309–310, 312. See also Stem cell factor
KLF1. See Kruppel-like factor 1
Klippel-Feil syndrome, 374–375
KMT2A. See Lysine methyltransferase
Knockout mice, 14–15, 15f
Knops blood group system, 646, 1699
Koenig, Harold, 2256
Kostmann syndrome (KS). See Severe congenital neutropenia
Kozak box, 7
KRAS mutations, 918–919
Krebs cycle. See Tricarboxylic acid cycle
Kringle domains, 1838
Kruppel-like factor 1 (KLF1), 313, 384
KW-0761, 1359, 1378
Kx blood group system, 1697–1698
Kyphoplasty, pain management and, 1475

L

Laboratory evaluation
  of activated coagulation states, 1930
  anticoagulant therapy monitoring, 1930
  of coagulation protein defects
    methodology, 1922
    physiology underlying, 1922, 1925f
    practical approach, 1926–1927
    specific, 1925–1926
  of fibrinolysis, 1929
  global hemostasis assays, 1929
  overview of, 1917–1918, 1917b–1918b, 1922
  of primary hemostasis disorders
    platelet evaluation, 1928
    screening, 1927–1928
    von Willebrand factor evaluation, 1928
  of prothrombotic states, 1929–1930
LAC. See Lupus anticoagulant
Lactate dehydrogenase (LDH), 105
Lacunar cells, 1213
Laetrile, 2254
Lambda (λ) genes, 212
Lambert-Eaton myasthenic syndrome, 1755
Laminar airflow, 1459
Laminins, 127, 1844
Lan blood group system, 1700
Landsteiner, Karl, 1515
Langerhans cell histiocytosis (LCH)
  classification of, 772
  clinical manifestations of, 725–728, 726t
  differential diagnosis for, 729
  epidemiology of, 724
  laboratory manifestations of, 728–729
  long-term followup for, 730–731
  overview of, 724
  pathobiology of, 724–725
  prognosis for, 729
  therapy for, 729–730
Langerhans cells, 1653–1655
Large granular lymphocyte (LGL) leukemia
  clinical presentation and physical features of, 436
  differential diagnosis for, 438
  laboratory diagnosis of, 436–438, 436t
  overview of, 434–435

Large granular lymphocyte (LGL) leukemia (Continued)
  pathogenesis of, 435–436
  prognosis for, 439
  therapy for, 437b, 438–439, 438f
Large granular lymphocyte syndrome, 426, 678–679
Large intergenic noncoding RNAs (lincRNAs), 31
Large-artery stroke, 2133–2134
Large-plaque parapsoriasis. See Cutaneous lymphoid dyscrasias
Large-volume leukapheresis (LVL), 1526–1527, 1527t
Lariat pathway, 20
Latent membrane proteins (LMP), 748–749, 757–758
Lazarus, Hillard, 1559
LBH589, 1146–1148
Lck. See Lymphocyte-specific protein tyrosine kinase
LDLR. See Low density lipoprotein receptor
Leach phenotype, 635
Lead, 512b, 669–670, 2233–2234
LeBlanc, Kararina, 1559
Lecithin-cholesterol acyltransferase (LCAT) deficiency, 643–644
Lectin adhesion receptors, 130–131
Lectin pathway (LP) of complement pathway, 261–262, 262f
LEF1. See Lymphoid enhancer binding factor 1
Left atrial appendage occlusion, 2152, 2156
Left ventricular assist devices (LVAD), 1942
Left-shifted neutrophils, 676
Leishmaniasis, 1816–1817, 2289–2292, 2289f
Lenalidomide
  for chronic lymphocytic leukemia, 1259
  for Hodgkin lymphoma, 1220t, 1226
  for light chain amyloidosis, 1439–1440
  for mastocytosis, 1184
  for multiple myeloma, 1405–1406, 1405t, 1412–1413
  for myelodysplastic syndromes, 794, 964–965, 997b
  for peripheral T-cell lymphomas, 1359
  pharmacology of, 866
  for primary myelofibrosis, 1142–1143
Lenograstim, 1522
Lentivirus vectors, 1550–1551
LEOPARD syndrome, 172
Lepirudin, 1979–1980, 1979t–1980t, 2178–2179
Letterer-Siwe disease, 724, 727
Leukapheresis, 1167, 1784–1785, 1788–1791
Leukemia/lymphoma, defined, 772
Leukemias
  bendamustine-induced, 856
  classification of, 913
  clonal origin of, 781–783
  congenital amegakaryocytic thrombocytopenia and, 370
  disseminated intravascular coagulation and, 2069
  early mutations in, 783–784
  infection and, 1447
  inherited bone marrow failure syndromes and, 392b
  Kostmann syndrome, severe congenital neutropenia and, 386–387
  niche alteration by, 124
  niche contribution to development of, 124
  platelet disorders and, 1940
  pregnancy and, 2208–2210
  therapeutic targeting of niche, 124–125
Leukemic stem cells (LSC)
  acute lymphoblastic leukemia and, 114–115
  acute myeloid leukemias and, 112b
  chronic lymphocytic leukemia and, 115
  diffuse large B-cell lymphoma and, 117
  follicular lymphoma and, 117
  hairy cell leukemia and, 115–117
  mature B-cell malignancies and, 115, 116f
  myelodysplastic syndromes and, 112–114
  myeloproliferative neoplasms and, 112f, 114
  overview of, 108–109
Leukemoid reaction, 675–676
Leukocyte adhesion deficiencies (LAD)
  LAD syndrome, 139
  LAD type I
    clinical features of, 703
    diagnosis of, 703, 703f, 704b
    molecular genetics of, 702–703
    overview of, 702, 702t
    prognosis and treatment of, 703
  LAD types II and III, 703
  overview of, 134, 134t
Leukocyte counts, e8b, e19t
Leukocyte-reduced blood components, 1826
Leukocyte-reduced red blood cells (LRRC), 1702–1703

Leukocytes
  chemokines and trafficking of, 135–138, 136t
  entry of into tissues, 138–141
  essential thrombocythemia and, 1110
  exit of from tissues, 142–143
  formation of, 523
  graft-versus-host disease and, 1657
  immune system and, 203
  interactions of with vessel wall, 1853–1854, 1854f
  malignancies and, 2249
  migration of within tissues, 141–142
  phagocytic. See Phagocytes
Leukocytosis, 675. See also Neutrophilic leukocytosis
Leukoencephalopathy, 1501
Leukoerythroblastosis, 675
Leukopenia
  after solid organ transplant in children, 2232–2233
  aging and, 1348, 2329
  HIV infection and, 2272–2273
  liver disease and, 2238
Leukosialin. See CD43
Levamisole, 679–680
Levorphanol, 1478
Lewis antigens, 1695
LFA-1. See Lymphocyte function-associated antigen 1
Liar, 307
Licensing, 242–243, 1577, 1620
Lidocaine, 1475, 2233
Lidocaine/prilocaine, 1475, 2233
Ligand binding, cell adhesion vs., 131
Light chains, 212
Light transmission aggregometry (LTA), 1879–1880, 1879t, 1928
Light zone, 219, 269–270
LIM genes, 840
LIM-only domain (LMO) genes, 1008
LINE. See Long interspersed nuclear elements
Lineage commitment, 228
Linezolid, 679
Link protein, 127
Linkage disequilibrium (LD) analysis, 80–81
Linker for activation of T cells (LAT), 177
Linker histones, 18–19, 19f
Linker of activated T cells (LAT), 225, 225f
Lipid rafts, 1938
Lipidation, 60–61
Lipids, 75, 77, 147–148
Lipopolysaccharide responsive beige-like anchor protein (LRBA) deficiency, 718
Lipoproteins, 75, 2122–2125, 2123f, 2130. See also High-density lipoproteins
Liquid plasma, 1744
Livedo reticularis, 2098, 2098f
Liver
  antiphospholipid syndrome and, 2097–2098
  β-thalassemia syndromes and, 559–560
  graft-versus-host disease and, 1651t, 1652, 1661
  heme biosynthesis and, 497–499, 499f
  late complications affecting, 1502
  paroxysmal nocturnal hemoglobinuria and, 418–419
  regulation of systemic iron homeostasis and iron storage by, 473–476, 474f
Liver disease
  coagulation and, 2239–2240
  disseminated intravascular coagulation and, 2069–2070
  hemolysis associated with, 668
  hemostasis and, 2240b, 2242b
  hypercoagulability, thrombosis and, 2241–2242, 2241b
  in neonate, 2196
  plasma derivatives for, 1745–1746
  platelet abnormalities and, 1941–1942, 2238–2239
  polyclonal gammopathy and, 688
  polycythemia and, 1078–1079
  red blood cell abnormalities and, 643, 2238, 2239f
  surgical patients and, 2309
  treatment of bleeding related to, 2240–2241
  white blood cell abnormalities and, 2238
Liver transplantation, 743, 1078, 2231, 2310–2311
Liver-enriched inhibitory protein (LIP), 326
Living high, training low, 1077
LMAN1 (mannose-binding lectin), 2048
Lnk. See Lymphocyte adapter protein
Localized juvenile periodontitis (LJP), 705
Locus control region (LCR), 1013, 1013f
Lomustine (CCNU), 855, 887
Long interspersed nuclear elements (LINE), 12–13

Long-term culture initiating cell (LTC-IC) assay, 98, 394–396

Long-terminal repeat (LTR) enhancer and promoter elements, 1550

Lorazepam, 1485

Loss of heterozygosity (LOH), 28

Low density lipoprotein receptor (LDLR), 2122

Low molecular weight heparin (LWMH)
  for acute coronary syndromes, 2149
  for antiphospholipid syndrome, 2099
  cancer, thrombosis, and, 2251–2252
  for neonates, 2199–2200
  overview of, 2177–2178, 2177t–2178t
  for thrombosis, 2085–2086
  for venous thromboembolism, 2108–2109

Low-density lipoprotein receptor-related proteins (LRP), 473, 2130

Lower-Risk Prognostic Scoring System (LR-PSS), 959–960, 959t

LRP. See Low-density lipoprotein receptor-related proteins

LSC. See Leukemic stem cells

LTC-IC assay. See Long-term culture initiating cell assay

Ludwig angina, 1453

Lugano staging system, 1216, 1277–1278, 1278t

Lumi-aggregometry, 1879

Lupus anticoagulant (LAC)
  antiphospholipid syndrome and, 2080–2081
  evaluation of, 1926
  overview of, 2092–2093

Lupus nephritis, 243

Lutheran blood group system, 1698–1700

LW blood group system, 1697

Lyme disease, 1814–1815

Lymph nodes, 206, 207f

Lymphadenitis, 697

Lymphatic endothelial cells (LEC), 158, 1894

Lymphatic system
  circulation, 205–208
  dilation, 158
  drainage, 206f
  formation of, 158, 1850
  secondary tissue of, 204–205, 208–209, 208f, 218–219, 218f

Lymphoblastic lymphoma (LBL)
  clinical manifestations, 1332
  differential diagnosis, 1332
  epidemiology, 1331
  overview of, 1330–1331
  pathobiology, 1331–1332
  prognosis/staging, 1332–1333, 1332t
  therapy, 1333

Lymphoblastoid cells, 748–749

Lymphocyte activation gene 3 (LAG-3), 1586

Lymphocyte adapter protein (Lnk), 339, 1108–1109

Lymphocyte function-associated antigen 1 (LFA-1), 138

Lymphocyte subsets, e8b

Lymphocyte-depleted classic Hodgkin lymphoma (LDCHL), 1201, 1212, 1213t, 1214

Lymphocyte-predominant (LP) cells, 1204–1205, 1205f

Lymphocyte-rich classic Hodgkin lymphoma (LRCHL), 1202, 1212, 1213f, 1213t, 1214

Lymphocytes
  apoptosis and, 194
  B cells. See B cells
  defects of thymus organogenesis and, 710
  exit of from secondary lymphoid organs, 142–143
  natural killer cells. See Natural killer cells
  quantitative disorders of, 682–685
  reference values for, e20t
  SCID and early defects in T lymphocyte development and, 710–714
  self-reactive. See Self-reactive lymphocytes
  trafficking patterns of, 141

Lymphocyte-specific protein tyrosine kinase (Lck), 234, 714–715

Lymphocytic lymphoma of intermediate differentiation. See Mantle cell lymphoma

Lymphocytopenia
  collagen vascular disorders and, 684–685
  drug effects and, 685
  infections and, 684
  inherited disorders and, 684
  malignancies and, 685
  systemic disorders and, 685

Lymphocytosis
  clonal disorders, 682–683
  drug reactions and, 684–685
  infectious causes, 683

Lymphocytosis (Continued)
  overview of, 682
  physiologic stress and, 683
  polyclonal B-cell, 682–684

Lymphocytotoxicity assays, 1718

Lymphoid enhancer binding factor 1 (LEF1), 1016–1017

Lymphoid neoplasms
  classification of
    age and, 770
    aggressive B-cell lymphoma, borderline entities, and site-specific categories, 770–771
    early events in, 769–770
    evolution of, 768–769, 769t
    follicular lymphoma grading, 771
    peripheral T-cell lymphomas, 771–772
    precursor lymphoid neoplasms, 772
  with hypereosinophilia, 1163, 1163t

Lymphoid organs, anatomy of, 203–204, 207f

Lymphoid-primed multipotent progenitors (LMPP), 210

Lymphomas
  classification of, 1187, 1188b, 1188t, 1343–1344
  cytogenetics of, 832–839
  early events in, 1188b
  Hodgkin. See Hodgkin lymphoma
  with hypereosinophilia, 1163
  infection and, 1447
  marginal zone. See Marginal zone lymphomas
  mature B-cell, 1187–1196, 1188t
  models of ontogeny, 116f
  natural killer cell, 1188t, 1196–1202, 1196b
  non-Hodgkin. See Non-Hodgkin lymphomas
  pregnancy and, 2208–2210
  T cell. See T-cell lymphomas

Lymphomatoid granulomatosis, 1193, 1367–1368

Lymphomatoid papulosis (Lyp), 1364, 1364f, 1366

Lymphopenia, 1451–1457, 1452f, 2266, 2266b

Lymphoplasmacytic lymphoma (LPL), 654, 839, 1187–1189, 1188t, 1189f. See also Waldenström macroglobulinemia

Lymphoproliferative disease (LPD), 653, 755–757, 756f

Lyn, 307

Lyon hypothesis, 781–782

Lyophilized plasma, 1744–1745

Lysine methyltransferase (KMT2A), 19–20. See also Mixed lineage leukemia (MLL)

Lysosomal granules, 706–707, 706t, 1875–1876

Lysosomal storage diseases (LSD)
  genetics and diagnosis of, 742
  hematologic manifestations of, 744–745
  overview of, 740, 741t, 745
  pathobiology of, 740–742, 741b
  therapy for, 742–744

Lysosomal trafficking regulator (LYST), 335, 698

Lysosomes
  autophagy and, 56
  biology of, 740
  protein sorting into, 56

LYST. See Lysosomal trafficking regulator

M

M hemoglobins, 613, 614f

M1 inflammatory macrophage phenotype, 2126

M7 acute myeloid leukemia, 812–813

Macrocytosis, 524t

α_2-Macroglobulin, 1894

Macroglobulinemia cutis, 1424

Macrophage activation syndrome (MAS), 403, 700, 737–738, 1969, 2220–2221, 2220t

Macrophage colony stimulating factor, 178, 1127

Macrophage inflammatory proteins (MIP), 2282

Macrophage-1 antigen (Mac-1), 138

Macrophages
  mobilization of hematopoietic stem and progenitor cells and, 147
  overview of in immune system, 203, 205, 206f
  recycling of erythrocyte iron by, 472–473, 472f
  sickle red blood cells and, 578
  T cell activation and, 221

Macrophages of bone marrow, 122

Macrosialin. See CD68

Macrovasculature, 1843

Maf, 332

MAGE-A3. See Melanoma antigen family A3

Magnesium transporter type 1 (MAGT1) deficiency, 717

Magnetic resonance angiography (MRA), 2161, 2163f

Magnetic resonance imaging (MRI), 2137, 2319

Major basic proteins (MBP), 1151, 1152t, 1155f

Major cytogenic remission (MCR), 1059–1060

Major histocompatibility complex (MHC)
  adaptive immune response and, 200
  allogenic transplantation and, 1591
  Burkitt lymphoma and, 1237–1238
  class I
    dendritic cells and presentation of, 251–252, 251f
    natural killer cells and, 1575, 1577
  class II, 252
  graft-versus-host disease and, 1652
  Hodgkin lymphoma and, 1209
  mesenchymal stromal cells and, 1560–1562
  T cell activation and, 221–222, 222f
  unrelated donor hematopoietic stem cell transplantation and, 1615

Major molecular response, 786

Malaria/malarial anemia
  diagnosis of, 2284–2287, 2284t, 2285f–2286f
  epidemiology of, 2278
  erythrocyte membrane and, 646
  features of, 2282–2289
  folic acid supplements and, 536
  glucose-6-phosphate dehydrogenase deficiency and, 616
  hemolysis and, 667
  overview of, 2278
  parasitology of, 2278–2279
  pathophysiology of, 2279, 2281f
  prevalence and etiology of, 2279f, 2282
  sickle gene and, 571–572, 572f, 584
  Southeast Asian ovalocytosis and, 639, 646
  transfusion-associated, 1815–1816, 2288–2289, 2288t
  treatment of, 2287–2288, 2287t

Malignancies
  aging and, 1370b, 2331b
  autoimmune hemolytic anemia in, 653–654
  bone marrow metastases, 2249–2250
  in children, 2226, 2229b
  disseminated intravascular coagulation and, 2069
  Epstein-Barr virus and, 748–749, 750b, 755
  erythrocytes and, 2247–2248
  Fanconi anemia and, 356
  hematopoietic stem cells and, 108–109
  leukocytes and, 2249
  lymphocytopenia and, 685
  manipulating T cells to improve activity against, 237–238
  monocytosis and, 680
  neutrophilia and, 677
  platelets and, 2248–2249
  second/subsequent. See Second/subsequent malignancies
  thrombocytopenia and, 1969
  thromboembolism and, 2226, 2229b
  thrombosis and, 2081–2082, 2250–2252
  virus-specific cytotoxic T lymphocytes and, 1569

Malmö regimen, 2016, 2031

MALT lymphomas. See Mucosa-associated lymphatic tissue lymphomas

Mammalian target of rapamycin (mTOR), 68–70, 194–195, 863f, 864–865, 1226

Mantle cell lymphoma in situ (MCLIS), 770, 1189–1190

Mantle cell lymphoma (MCL)
  allogenic HSCT for, 1606
  chronic lymphocytic leukemia and, 1245
  classification of, 763, 770
  clinical manifestations of, 1299
  cytogenetics of, 837–838
  diagnosis of, 1300–1301
  differential diagnosis for, 1301
  epidemiology of, 1298
  future directions, 1306
  laboratory manifestations of, 1299–1300
  overview of, 1188t, 1189–1190, 1190f, 1240–1241, 1240f, 1298
  pathobiology of, 1299f
  prognosis for, 1306, 1306f
  staging of, 1301–1302
  therapy for, 1301–1306, 1302t–1303t, 1304f

MAP kinases. See Mitogen-activated protein kinases

MAPK/ERK pathway, 70, 865

March hemoglobinuria, 665

Marginal zone, 142, 218, 218f, 2317–2318

Marginal zone lymphomas (MZL)
  in childhood, 1341
  classification of, 770
  cytogenetics of, 1241
  extranodal. See Extranodal marginal zone lymphoma of MALT type
  initial evaluation of, 1277
  nodal. See Nodal marginal zone lymphoma

Marginal zone lymphomas (MZL) (Continued)
    overview of, 1277
    splenic. See Splenic marginal zone lymphoma
    staging of, 1277–1278, 1278t
Marinol, 1485
Marizomib, 869
Maroteaux-Lamy disease, 741, 741t
MART-1, 1570–1571
Masitinib, 1184
Masked megablastosis, 539–540
Mass spectrometry, 31–32
Massage therapy, 2257, 2257t
Massive transfusion, 1746–1747, 1750, 1799–1800, 2310
Massively parallel sequencing. See Next generation
    sequencing
Mast cell activation syndromes (MCAS), 1175–1176,
    1176t, 1182
Mast cell disease, 764–765
Mast cell growth factor. See Stem cell factor
Mast cell leukemia (MCL), 1170, 1174t, 1175, 1177f
Mast cell sarcoma (MCS), 1174t, 1175
Mast cells
    activation and function of, 1171–1172, 1171t
    eosinophil recruitment and accumulation and,
        1156–1157
    origin and development of, 1170–1171
    overview of, 1170
    production of, 331
    tools for studying, 1172–1173
    transfusion reactions and, 1795–1796
Mastocytosis
    aggressive systemic, 1174–1175, 1174t, 1177f
    clinical manifestations of, 1178–1179
    cutaneous, 1173, 1174t
    diagnostic evaluation of, 1176–1178
    epidemiology and classification of, 1173–1182,
        1173t–1174t
    extracutaneous, 1174t
    future directions, 1185
    indolent systemic, 1172–1173, 1174t
    molecular features of, 1179–1181
    overview of, 792–793
    survival and prognostic factors in, 1181–1182
    systemic, 792–793, 1170, 1173–1182, 1173t
    systemic associated with hematologic neoplasm, 1174,
        1174t, 1179–1180
    treatment of, 1182–1185, 1182f
    well-differentiated systemic, 1175
Mastocytosis in the skin (MIS), 1173
Matched sibling donors (MSD)
    for acute lymphoblastic leukemia, 1041
    for acute myeloid leukemias, 970–973, 971t
    aplastic anemia treatment and, 408–409
Matched unrelated donor (MUD) transplants, 409, 1041
Matrix metalloproteinases (MMP), 136–139, 155–156,
    322, 2129
Mature B-cell acute lymphoblastic leukemia. See Burkitt
    lymphoma
May-Hegglin anomaly, 1862–1863, 1883
MBL. See Monoclonal B-cell lymphocytosis
MBP. See Major basic proteins
MCAHS2. See Multiple congenital abnormalities-
    hypotonia-seizure syndrome 2
MCL. See Mantle cell lymphoma
McLeod red cell phenotype, 699
McLeod syndrome, 642–643, 700, 1693, 1698
MDM2, 1240–1241
MDS. See Myelodysplastic syndromes
Mean corpuscular volume (MCV), 460t, 463–464, 464t,
    523, e15t
Mean platelet volume (MPV), e11b, e24t
Mechanical thrombectomy, 2138
Mechanical trauma, 665
Mechlorethamine, 854, 854f, 885, 1371–1372
Media, 1843
Mediastinal gray zone lymphoma, 1194–1195
Meditation, 1475
Mediterranean fever, 676
Medullary thymic epithelial cells (mTEC), 254, 287–288
Megadose stem cell transplants, 1623–1624, 1623f
Megakaryoblastic leukemia (translocation) 1 (MKL1), 986
Megakaryocyte progenitor (MkP) cells, 334
Megakaryocyte-erythroid progenitor (MEP) cells, 334
Megakaryocytes
    bone marrow cues and maturation of, 337–338
    development of, 334–335, 335f, 1857–1861
    endomitosis in, 342–343, 342f
    hematopoietic stem cells and, 122

Megakaryocytes (Continued)
    inherited disorders of, 1883–1884
    isolation of progenitor cells, 335
    megaloblastosis and, 523
    myelodysplastic syndromes and, 957, 957f
    niches of, 123
    platelet biogenesis and, 337
    primary myelofibrosis and, 1125–1126
    structure of mature, 335–336, 337f
Megakaryocytic leukemia, 317, 812–813
Megakaryocytopoiesis
    additional cytokines involved in, 340
    micro RNAs in, 347
    ontogeny of, 336
    therapeutic cytokine stimulation of, 340–341
    thrombopoietin and. See Thrombopoietin
    transcriptional control of, 343–347
Megaloblastic anemias. See also Cobalamin deficiency;
        Folate deficiency
    clinical presentation and evaluation for, 537–540,
        538t
    congenital dyserythropoietic anemias vs., 384
    diagnostic and therapeutic approach, 540–541
    not caused by folate or cobalamin deficiency, 537
    overview of, 514
    therapy for, 541–542
Megaloblastosis. See also Cobalamin deficiency; Folate
        deficiency
    diagnostic and therapeutic approach, 540–541,
        543b
    differential diagnosis for, 524t, 542t
    morphologic expression of, 523–524, 523b
    therapy for, 541–542
Melanoma antigen family A3 (MAGE-A3), 1570–1571
Melphalan
    acute myeloid leukemia and, 913
    for light chain amyloidosis, 1439–1440
    for multiple myeloma, 1403–1404, 1404t, 1407
    pharmacology of, 855, 886
Membrane attack complex (MAC), 265, 268, 279–282
Membrane cofactor protein (MCP), 264, 264t, 1994,
    1995f, 1996t
Membrane proteins, domain structures of, 64–66
Memorial Sloan-Kettering Center unit selection criteria,
    1639–1640, 1639f
Memory cells, 122–123, 231–232
Mendelian susceptibility to mycobacterial diseases
    (MSMD), 707
Meningitis, 598
Mental retardation, 568
Meperidine, 1478
Mepolizumab, 1153, 1165, 1167
Merbarone, 860
Mercaptoethane sulfonate (Mesna), 854
6-Mercaptopurine (6-MP), 895–896, 1447
Mesenchymal stromal cells (MSC)
    bone marrow manufacture and phenotype, 1559–1560
    cord blood stem cell transplantation and, 1647
    cytology and fitness of, 1566b
    defined, 1559–1560
    endogenous, 1559
    future directions for, 1565
    hematopoietic stem cell engraftment and, 1563–1564
    hematopoietic stem cell transplants and, 1546
    immune plasticity of in response to inflammatory cues,
        1562–1563
    immune privilege and, 1563
    immune profile of, 1560–1562, 1560t
    overview of, 1559
    phenotypes of, 1566b
    regulatory oversight of, 1565
    safety profile of adoptively transferred, 1564–1565
    steroid-refractory acute graft-vs-host disease and, 1563,
        1565b
Metabolism
    amino acids and, 75–76
    of erythrocytes, 448
    glucose metabolism and, 73–74
    of hematopoietic stem cells, 105
    lipids and, 75
    nucleic acids and, 76
    oxidative phosphorylation and, 74
    reactive oxygen species and, 74–75
    tricarboxylic acid (Krebs) cycle and, 74
Metabolomics
    of amino acid metabolism, 77
    of glucose metabolism, 77
    introduction to, 76–77, 77f

Metabolomics (Continued)
    of lipid metabolism, 77
    of nucleotide metabolism, 77
    overview of, 32
Metaphase, 176–177, 177f
Metaphase fluorescence in situ hybridization, 777f
Metastases, 2249–2250, 2249f
Methadone, 1478
Methemoglobin, 668b
Methemoglobinemias
    in children, 2233
    clinical manifestations of, 624
    differential diagnosis for, 624
    epidemiology of, 624
    erythrocyte enzymopathies and, 623–625, 623f
    introduction to, 623–624
    laboratory manifestations of, 624
    overview of, 613, 614f, 623f
    pathobiology of, 624
    prognosis for, 624–625
    therapy for, 625
    types of, 613t
Methotrexate (MTX)
    for acute lymphoblastic leukemia, 1025–1026,
        1040
    for cutaneous T-cell lymphomas, 1372
    folate metabolism and, 538b
    for graft-versus-host disease, 1659, 1661t
    infection and, 1447
    for mantle cell lymphoma, 1305
    pharmacology of, 857, 892–893
    for pure red cell aplasia, 430
    SLCO1B1 and metabolism of, 86–87
8-Methoxypsoralen (8-MOP), 1369–1370,
    1375–1376
Methylating agents, 855–856
Methylation
    acute myeloid leukemia and, 919–920
    epigenetics and, 9
    folate metabolism and, 522
    hematopoietic stem cell self-renewal and, 104
    multiple myeloma and, 1385–1386
    overview of, 17–18, 47
    as posttranslational modification, 60–61
Methyl-folate trapping, 522
Methylmalonic acid (MMA)
    cobalamin and folate deficiency and, 526–527, 526t,
        527b, 529b
    laboratory evaluation of, e7b
    reference values for, e19t
Methylome, 18
Methylphenidate (ritalin), 1477
Methylprednisolone, 411
Methyltetrahydrofolate reductase (MTHFR), 2084
Metoclopramide, 1479–1480, 1484–1485
Mevalonate kinase (MVK), 384
MGMT. See O6-methylguanine methyltransferase
mHags. See Minor histocompatibility antigens
MHC class I chain-related antigens (MIC), 242, 1725
Mice, transgenic and knockout, 14–15, 15f
Miconazole, 1937
Micro RNA (miRNA; MIR)
    B cell development and, 211
    chronic lymphocytic leukemia and, 1251
    gene expression and, 20–22, 329–330
    hematopoietic stem cells and, 105
    iron homeostasis and, 468–469
    in megakaryocytopoiesis, 347
    miR-33, 2124, 2131
    multiple myeloma and, 1385
    overview of, 11, 46
    profiling of, 31
    SNPs in, 80
Microangiopathic hemolytic anemia (MAHA). See also
        Thrombotic microangiopathies
    after solid organ transplant in children, 2229–2230
    cancer and, 2247
    causes of, 664b
    clinical manifestations, 663
    differential diagnosis, 663–665, 664b
    differential diagnosis for, 1984
    pathophysiology, 663
    in pregnancy, 2207
    tolerance, immunity and, 285
Microbiome, human, 1655
Microchip arrays, 779–780
Micrococcal nuclease (MNase) sequencing, 29
Microenvironment theory. See Niche theory

Microfibrillar collagen, 2306
Microparticles, atherothrombosis and, 2129–2130
Microtubules, 343, 1861–1863, 1866–1868
Microvasculature, 1843
Midostaurin, 1184
Miglustat, 743–744
MiHAs. See Minor histocompatibility antigens
Milk protein-induced enteropathy, 2223–2225
Milrinone, 1936
Milroy disease, 1850
Mind-body therapies, 2255–2260, 2255t
Minichromosome maintenance (MCM) complex, 181–182
Minimal residual disease (MRD)
    acute lymphoblastic leukemia and, 1020, 1023–1024, 1035–1037, 1036f
    acute myeloid leukemia and, 924, 932–933
    genomic diagnostics for, 34
    hairy cell leukemia and, 1273–1275, 1274f
    multiple myeloma and, 1399–1400
    overview of, 1025b
Minor histocompatibility antigens (MiHAs, mHags)
    alloimmunization and, 1725
    graft-versus-host disease and, 1650, 1652–1653
    graft-versus-leukemia responses and, 1664
    human leukocyte antigens and, 1726
MIP. See Macrophage inflammatory proteins
MIR. See Micro RNA
Mir-223, 329–330
Mir-27, 330
MiRNA. See Micro RNA
miRSNP, defined, 80
Mismatch repair (MMR), 882–883
Missing self, 1577
MISTRG mice, 112b
Mithramycin, 1938
Mitochondria, 49–50, 49f, 871, 1018
Mitochondrial DNA deletion syndrome, 377
Mitochondrial inner membrane (MIM), 49
Mitochondrial outer membrane (MOM), 49
Mitochondrial outer membrane protein (MOMP), 190–191
Mitoferrin 1 (MFRN1), 469–471
Mitogen-activated protein (MAP) kinases, 70, 224–225, 865
Mitosis, 176–177, 177f, 182
Mitoxantrone, 900–901
Mixed cellularity classic Hodgkin lymphoma (MCCHL), 1212, 1213t, 1214
Mixed cryoglobulinemia, 1327
Mixed lineage leukemia (MLL), 23, 1007
Mixed lineage leukemia (MLL) genes
    acute lymphoblastic leukemia and, 820, 1011–1012, 1012f
    acute myeloid leukemia and, 799–800, 805–806, 807f, 807t–810t, 810f–811f, 916–917, 983–984
    chemotherapy drugs and, 913
    chronic lymphocytic leukemia and, 824–825
    cytogenetics of, 805
    follicular lymphoma and, 1288–1290
    fusion oncoproteins and, 113b
    hematopoietic stem cell self-renewal and, 104
    histone modifications and, 19–20
    infant ALL and novel therapies for, 89
    non-Hodgkin lymphoma and, 1234
    partial tandem deletions of, 984
    T-cell acute lymphoblastic leukemia and, 840
MK2206, 864
MKL1. See Megakaryoblastic leukemia (translocation) 1
MLL. See Mixed lineage leukemia genes
MLL-rearranged acute lymphoblastic leukemia, 1015
MMB, 181
MMF. See Mycophenolate mofetil
MMP. See Matrix metalloproteinases
MNS blood group system, 1698
Mocetinostat, 876–877
Mogamulizumab. See KW-0761
Mold infections, 1460, 1674–1675. See also Specific molds
Molecular chaperones, 46, 53, 744
Momelotinib, 866, 1144
Monoclonal antibodies
    for cutaneous T-cell lymphomas, 1376–1377
    for EBV-lymphoproliferative disease, 756–757
    for follicular lymphoma, 1295
    for hairy cell leukemia, 1272–1273
    infection and, 1447
    uses of, 277–279, 278f–279f, 280t–281t

Monoclonal B-cell lymphocytosis (MBL)
    chronic lymphocytic leukemia and, 1247–1248
    clonal expansion and, 27–28
    complement system and, 262
    familial chronic lymphocytic leukemia and, 1244
    overview of, 682–683, 770
Monoclonal gammopathy, 688–689, 689t
Monoclonal gammopathy of undetermined significance (MGUS)
    autoimmune hemolytic anemia in, 654
    clonal expansion and, 27–28
    multiple myeloma and, 769
    overview of, 688–689, 1381
    treatment of, 1400–1401
Monocyte chemotactic protein (MCP-1), 2126
Monocytes
    antiphospholipid antibodies and, 2089
    atherothrombosis and, 2125–2126
    HIV infection and, 2273
    mobilization of hematopoietic stem and progenitor cells and, 147
    overview of in immune system, 203
Monocytoid B cell lymphoma. See Nodal marginal zone lymphoma
Monocytopenia, 680–681, 680t
Monocytopoiesis, 331–332
Monocytosis, 680, 680t
MonoMAC syndrome, 680–681, 684, 915
Monomorphic variant of enteropathy-associated T-cell lymphoma, 772
Mononine, 1765, 1775
Mononucleosis, 2322, 2322b. See also Infectious mononucleosis
Monosomal karyotype (MK), 796, 813, 971–972, 971t
Morphine, 1476–1479, 1477b
Morphologic dysplasia, myelodysplastic syndromes and, 944
Mosaicism, 781–782, 782f, 845
Mosquito bite allergy, 1200, 1261–1262
Moxetumomab, 1275
Moxetumomab pasudotox, 1050
Mozobil. See AMD3100
MP (antileukemic agent), 82–85
MPL (thrombopoietin receptor)
    aplastic anemia and, 413
    congenital amegakaryocytic thrombocytopenia and, 368–371
    essential thrombocythemia and, 1106–1109, 1108f, 1112, 1115
    overview of, 338–339, 339f
    primary myelofibrosis and, 1126–1128, 1135, 1149b
mRNA (messenger RNA)
    metabolism of, 7–9
    modification of ends of, 8–9
    posttranscriptional regulation and, 10–11
    regulation of translation, 45–46
    splicing, 7–8, 8f
    translation of, 6–7
    transport of, 9
    untranslated terminal sequences, 9
mRNA profiling, 30
mRNA sequencing (RNA-Seq), 21–22, 29–30
mRNPs, overview of, 9
mTOR. See Mammalian target of rapamycin
Mucopolysaccharides. See Glycosaminoglycans
Mucopolysaccharidosis
    type I, 56, 741
    type II, 741t, 742
    type VI, 741, 741t
Mucosa, 1451
Mucosa-associated lymphatic tissue (MALT), 209, 1277
Mucosa-associated lymphatic tissue (MALT) lymphomas, 838–839
Mucosal addressin-cell adhesion molecule (MAdCAM-1), 139, 1844–1845
Mucositis, 1454
Mucous membrane bleeding, 2011
Müllerian inhibiting substance (MIS), 70
Multicentric Castleman disease (MCD), 1193, 1322
Multicolor fluorescence in situ hybridization, 777f, 778
Multidrug resistance-associated protein, 881–883, 881f
Multifocal motor neuropathy, 1755
Multiple combined factor deficiency protein 2 (MCFD2), 2048
Multiple congenital abnormalities-hypotonia-seizure syndrome 2 (MCAHS2), 415

Multiple myeloma (MM)
    allogenic HSCT for, 1606
    autologous stem cell transplant for, 1407–1412
    clinical manifestations of, 1390–1392, 1391t
    cytogenetics of, 827–832
    cytokines and, 1389
    differential diagnosis for, 1400
    epidemiology of, 1381
    future directions for, 1415
    genomics of, 1384–1386, 1386t
    historical aspects of, 1381
    hyperdiploid, 828
    immune environment and, 1389–1390
    infection and, 1448
    international staging system of, 1398–1400, 1398t
    intravenous immunoglobulin for, 1755
    laboratory manifestations of, 1392–1398
    nonhyperdiploid, 828
    overview of, 1381, 1382t
    pathobiology of, 1381–1384, 1382t
    PD-1 blockade therapies and, 1584
    prognosis for, 1398
    relapsed, 1412–1415
    secondary chromosomal aberrations in, 830
    translocations and, 829–832
    treatment of, 1400–1415
Multiple Organ Dysfunction Scores (MODS), 2064
Multiple sclerosis (MS), 754–755, 1755
Mummified cells, 1213
Murphy Staging of Non-Hodgkin lymphoma, 1332t
Muscle bleeds, 1916–1917
Musculoskeletal system, 1500, 1661–1662
Music therapy, 2255
Mustargen. See Mechlorethamine
Mutation rate, normal, 11–12
MVK. See Mevalonate kinase
Myasthenia gravis, 1755
MYB, 181, 346–347, 840
MYC
    Burkitt lymphoma and, 835, 1236–1238
    cell division cycle and, 180
    diffuse large B-cell lymphoma and, 770–771
    leukemic disorders and, 835, 837f
    mature B-cell acute lymphoblastic leukemia and, 1008, 1011
    multiple myeloma and, 830
    non-Hodgkin lymphoma and, 1233t, 1234
    Richter syndrome and, 827
    TAL/LMO subtype of T-cell acute lymphoblastic leukemia and, 843
Mycophenolate mofetil (MMF), 660, 1659–1660, 1661t, 2232
Mycosis fungoides (MF)
    clinical presentation of, 1362–1364
    cytogenetics of, 843–845
    cytology of, 1199f
    differential diagnosis for, 1366–1368
    laboratory manifestations of, 1364–1365, 1365f
    overview of, 1188t, 1198, 1360–1361
    pathobiology of, 1361–1362
    prognosis for, 1368–1369
    therapy for, 1368–1369, 1369t, 1370b
MYD88. See Myeloid differentiation primary response gene 88
Myelin-associated glycoprotein (MAG), 1423–1424
Myeloablative allogenic stem cell transplantation, 1259–1260
Myeloablative conditioning (MAC)
    for acute lymphoblastic leukemia, 1042t
    for acute myeloid leukemia, 972–974
    allogenic HSCT and, 1596–1597, 1598f, 1598t–1599t
    cord blood stem cell transplantation and, 1641–1645
    for myelodysplastic syndromes, 976–977
    overview of, 970
Myelodysplastic syndromes (MDS)
    acute myeloid leukemia and, 914
    after hematopoietic stem cell transplantation, 1679
    allogenic HSCT for
        clinical results in myeloablative transplantation, 976
        clinical results in reduced-intensity conditioning transplantation, 976
        comorbidity and conditioning intensity selection before, 978–979
        contemporary results, 976
        myeloablative vs. reduced intensity regimens, 976–977
        pretransplantation therapy, 978–979
        prognostic models for role and timing of, 977–978

Myelodysplastic syndromes (MDS) *(Continued)*
aplastic anemia vs., 402b, 402t
in children, 994–997, 997b
classification of, 767–768, 767f, 768t, 944–945, 946t, 958t, 995–996
clinical features of, 954–958, 996
congenital dyserythropoietic anemias vs., 384
cytogenetics of, 793–798, 793f, 794t
diagnostic systems and clinical syndromes of, 958–961
differential diagnosis for, 996
epidemiology and etiology of, 945–947, 994
future directions for, 968
hematopoietic microenvironment in, 123–125
history of, 944
infection and, 1447–1448
with isolated del(5q), 944, 946t, 952, 960, 960f, 964–965
Kostmann syndrome, severe congenital neutropenia and, 386–387
laboratory manifestations of, 996
lymphocytopenia and, 684
overview of, 944, 975
paroxysmal nocturnal hemoglobinuria and, 419
pathobiology of, 947–954, 994–995
platelet disorders and, 1940
primary immunodeficiencies and, 686–687
prognosis for, 997
Schwachman-Diamond syndrome and, 363
secondary, 997
stem cell origin of, 112–114
α-thalassemia syndromes and, 568–569
therapy-related, 814–815, 815b, 847f, 961, 1504
thrombocytopenia and, 443
treatment of, 961–968, 996–997, 997b
Myelofibrosis
acute panmyelosis with. *See* Acute panmyelosis with myelofibrosis
post-polycythemia vera (post-PV MF). *See* Post-polycythemia vera myelofibrosis
primary. *See* Primary myelofibrosis
Myelofibrosis (MF), idiopathic, 1003
Myeloid bias, 1346–1347, 2328
Myeloid differentiation primary response gene 88 (MYD88), 1420–1421, 1420f
Myeloid neoplasms
acute myeloid leukemias. *See* Acute myeloid leukemias
clinical implications of classification of, 763–764
myelodysplastic syndromes. *See* Myelodysplastic syndromes
myeloproliferative. *See* Myeloproliferative neoplasms
Myeloid sarcoma, 931, 931f, 941–942
Myelokathexis, 389–390
Myeloma, 654
Myeloperoxidase (MPO)
acute lymphoblastic leukemia and, 1032, 1032f
acute myeloid leukemia and, 925, 927f
atherothrombosis and, 2126
deficiency of, 701, 701t
Myelopoiesis, 1001–1002
Myeloproliferative disorders (MPD). *See* Myeloproliferative neoplasms
Myeloproliferative neoplasms (MPN)
acute myeloid leukemia and, 914
in children, 998–1002, 998t
chronic myelogenous leukemia. *See* Chronic myelogenous leukemia
classification of, 764–765, 764t, 768, 768t
differential diagnosis for, 1097
down syndrome-associated transient abnormal myelopoiesis, 1001–1002
essential thrombocythemia. *See* Essential thrombocythemia
with hypereosinophilia, 1162t, 1163
idiopathic myelofibrosis, 1003
ischemic stroke and, 2136
*JAK2*V617F and, 1082–1085, 1083f–1084f
juvenile myelomonocytic leukemia, 768, 998–1001, 998t
myelodysplastic syndromes and, 961
myelofibrosis. *See* Myelofibrosis
platelet disorders and, 1939–1940
polycythemia vera. *See* Polycythemia vera
pregnancy and, 2209–2210
stem cell origin of, 114
systemic mastocytosis and. *See* Systemic mastocytosis
tyrosine kinase involvement in, 764t
venous thromboembolism and, 2082

8p11 Myeloproliferative syndrome. *See* FGFR1-rearranged neoplasm
Myelosupportive stroma, 119
Myelosuppression, 86t
MYH9-related disease. *See* Myosin heavy chain 9-related disease
Myleran. *See* Busulfan
Myoglobin, 451
Myopathy, lactic acidosis, and sideroblastic anemia (MLASA), 509
Myosin heavy chain 9 (MYH9)-related disease, 347b, 347t–348t, 1883
Myosin II, 1862–1863
Myristoylation, 47, 60–61
MYST3-CREBBP rearrangements, 811
MZ B cells, 218

N

Nabilone, 1485
N-Acetylation, 60–61
NADPH oxidase, 2126
Naloxone, 1480
Narrow-band UVB therapy, 1370
Nasopharyngeal carcinomas, 758–759
National Healthcare Safety Network (NHSN), 1801–1802
National Heart, Lung, and Blood Institute (NHLBI), 1531
National Human Genome Research Institute (NHGRI), 22, 22f
National Institute of Biomedical Imaging and Bioengineering (NIBIB), 1531
National Institutes of Health Stroke Severity Scale (NIHSS), 2137
National Marrow Donor Program (NMDP), 1608
Native TTR amyloid, 1437
Natural cytotoxicity receptors (NCR), 203, 241–242
Natural killer cell T-cell lymphoma (NKTCL), 1200, 1200f, 1348, 1352–1354, 1367
Natural killer lymphoma/leukemia, 843
Natural killer (NK) cell-associated large granular lymphocyte leukemia, 434–435
Natural killer (NK) cell-based therapies, 991–992, 1575, 1580f, 1581
Natural killer (NK) cells
adaptive immune properties of, 242–243
allogenic HSCT and, 1600
allogenic transplantation and, 1591
alloreactions after haploidentical hematopoietic stem cell transplantation and, 1619–1621, 1620f
basic biology of, 240, 241f, 241t
clinical applications of, 1578–1581
cytomegalovirus and, 1575, 1579
dendritic cells and activation of, 254
development of, 240–241
education of, 1577
Epstein-Barr virus and, 754t
functions of, 1575, 1576f
graft-versus-host disease and, 1656
hematopoietic stem cell transplants and, 1539, 1545–1546
human leukocyte antigens and, 1725–1727
as innate lymphoid cells, 1577–1578
killer-cell immunoglobulin-like receptors (KIR) and, 241–242, 1576–1577
lymphomas of, 1188t, 1196b, 1200
multiple myeloma and, 1390
overview of, 203, 240, 1575, 1581
proliferation of, 678–679
receptors for, 241–242, 244t, 1575–1577
recognition of tumors by, 1577
role of in human disease, 243, 244t
therapeutic potential of, 243, 245f
Natural regulatory T cells (nTregs), 228
Natural resistance-associated macrophage protein 1 (NRAMP1), 473
Nausea and vomiting. *See* Antiemetics
Navelbine. *See* Vinorelbine
Navitoclax, 872, 1258–1259
NBEAL2. *See* Neurobeachin-like 2
NCF. *See* Neutrophil cytosolic factors
ncRNA. *See* Noncoding RNAs
NE. *See* Neutrophil elastase
Necroptosis, 186
Necrosis, 186, 187f
Nectin-2, 1575
Negative selection, 228–229, 286, 287f, 1539
Nelarabine, 858, 897, 1050

Neonatal alloimmune neutropenia. *See* Isoimmune neonatal neutropenia
Neonatal alloimmune thrombocytopenia (NAIT)
after solid organ transplant, 2231–2232, 2232b
clinical presentation of, 1950
diagnosis of, 1950t, 1951b, 1951f
intravenous immunoglobulin for, 1755–1756
laboratory investigation of, 1950–1952
management of, 1952
overview of, 2193
pathophysiology of, 1950
transfusion and, 1824
Neonates. *See* Newborns
Neoplasms
hematopoietic, 1157, 1162
myeloid. *See* Myeloid neoplasms
polycythemia and, 1078–1079
thrombotic microangiopathies and, 1997–1998
Nephrotic syndrome, 1132, 1752, 2227, 2244–2245
Nepmucin, 1844–1845
N-ethylmaleimide-sensitive factor attachment protein receptors (SNAREs), 1876, 1876f–1877f
Netupitant, 1485
Neumann, Ernest, 119
Neupogen, 2273
Neural cell adhesion molecule. *See* CD56
Neural tube defects (NTD)
anticonvulsants and, 538
folate deficiency and, 533–534
folate receptors and, 520–521
folate-responsive, 534–536, 535f
Neuroacanthocytosis syndromes, 642
Neurobeachin-like 2 (*NBEAL2*), 335, 347t–348t
Neurocristopathies, 534–536
Neurodevelopment, 534
Neurofibromin 1 (NF1), 998
Neurokinin-1 inhibitors, 1485
Neuroleptic drugs, 400–401
Neurologic system
antiphospholipid syndrome and, 2096–2098
hemophilia and, 2011–2012
hypereosinophilic syndrome and, 1161
late complications affecting, 1500–1501
Neuromodulation, 1475
Neuropathic pain, 524–526, 1423–1424, 1473, 1480
Neurovascular imaging, 2137
Neutropenias
acquired, 430–432
after hematopoietic stem cell transplantation, 1669–1670
after solid organ transplant in children, 2232–2233
aging and, 1345–1346, 2328
autoimmune, 678
benign ethnic, 678
cancer and, 2249
chemotherapy-induced, 679
in children, 2217
classification of, 430–432, 431t
differential diagnosis, 434
drug-induced, 432, 679–680, 679t
HIV infection and, 2266b, 2272–2273
infection and, 679, 1450–1457, 1450f, 1452f, 2266b, 2272–2273
infections and, 432–433
with infectious diseases, 679
infectious mononucleosis and, 752
inherited bone marrow syndromes with, 385–390, 388t
laboratory evaluation, 434, 434f
large granular lymphocyte syndrome, natural killer cell proliferations and, 678–679
liver disease and, 2238
metabolic disorders and, 433–434
monocytosis. *See* Monocytosis
myelodysplastic syndromes and, 963
neutrophil transfusions for, 1738–1743
nutritional deficiency and excess and, 433
overview of, 430, 677–680
severe congenital. *See* Severe congenital neutropenia therapy, 434
Neutropenic enterocolitis, 1453
Neutrophil cytosolic factors (NCF), 694, 695t
Neutrophil disorders
of adhesion and chemotaxis, 701–705
clinical approach, 694b
diagnostic approach to functional, 691
HIV infection and, 2273
lysosomal granule defects, 706–707

Neutrophil disorders (Continued)
   miscellaneous, 707–708
   neutropenias. See Neutropenias
   of respiratory burst pathway, 691–701, 692f
Neutrophil elastase (NE; ELANE), 329, 385–386, 389
Neutrophil extracellular traps (NET), 1835–1837
Neutrophil transfusions. See Granulocyte transfusions
Neutrophilias, 675–677
Neutrophilic leukocytosis (neutrophilia), 675–677
Neutrophils
   apoptosis of, 186
   developmentally important genes of in disease,
      328–330, 328t
   differentiation stages of, 321
   granules and content proteins of, 321–323, 323t
   immune system and, 203
   mobilization of hematopoietic stem and progenitor cells
      and, 148
   rolling, spreading, and migration of, 132f, 133
   steps in response of to infection, 692f
Newborns
   coagulation disorders in, 2195–2196
   cobalamin and, 530
   evaluation of, 2191–2197, 2192f
   folate and, 533–534
   hemophilia in, 2008
   hemostasis in, 2189–2191
   intracranial hemorrhage in, 2008–2009, 2009f,
      2011–2012
   overview, 2191
   platelet function disorders in, 2193–2194, 2194t
   red blood cell transfusions and, 1705–1706
   sickle cell disease screening in, 585, 586f
   therapy for, 2199–2200, 2200b
   thrombocytopenia in, 2192–2193, 2193t
   thromboembolic disorders in, 2197–2200, 2200b
   transfusion medicine for, 1822
   vitamin K deficiency bleeding in, 2194–2195
Next generation sequencing (NGS), 27, 777f, 779–781,
   783, 1386, 1611
NF1. See Neurofibromin 1
NF-E2. See Nuclear factor, erythroid 2
NF-κB. See Nuclear factor κB
NFKB inhibitor epsilon (NFKBIE), 825–826
NFKBIE. See NFKB inhibitor epsilon
N-Glycosylation, 53–54, 53f, 55b
Niche theory
   acute myeloid leukemia and, 920
   adult bone marrow microenvironment and, 119–122
   B cell development and, 216–217
   contribution to leukemia development, 124
   erythroid cell development and, 309–310
   erythroid islands and, 123
   evolution of, 119
   hematopoietic stem and progenitor cells, 119–120
   hypoxia and, 122
   megakaryocyte maturation and, 337–338, 338f
   megakaryocytes and, 123
   microenvironment during development and, 119,
      309–310
   mobilization and, 140–141, 147, 1521–1522
   myelodysplastic syndromes and, 953, 965
   overview of, 120, 120t
   sympathetic innervation and, 122
Nicotinamide, 1647
Nicotinamide adenine dinucleotide phosphate (NADPH)
   oxidase, 691–701, 694f, 695t, 696f
Niemann-Pick cells, 744
Niemann-Pick disease
   type A, 741–742, 741t, 744
   type B, 744, 745f
   type C, 741–744, 741t
Niemann-Pick type C (NPC) protein, 2123
Niemann-Pick type C1-like1 protein, 2124–2125
Nijmegen breakage syndrome (NBS), 357
Nijmegen modifications of Bethesda assay, 2027–2028,
   2028f
Nilotinib, 862, 862t, 904, 1045–1046, 1064–1065
Nitrates, 614
Nitric oxide (NO)
   graft-versus-host disease and, 1658
   hemoglobin and, 449, 452–453
   hemostasis and, 1831–1832, 1832f
   mesenchymal stromal cells and, 1562–1563
   paroxysmal nocturnal hemoglobinuria and, 418
   sickle cell anemia and, 575–576
Nitric oxide synthase (NOS), 1852, 2126
Nitrites, 671

Nitroblue tetrazolium (NBT) test, 692, 696f, 698–699
Nitrogen mustard compounds, 854–855
Nitrosoureas, 855
Nitrous oxide (N₂O), 532
NKG2 receptors, 1577–1578
NKp30, 242
NKp46, 242, 1575
NMD. See Nonsense-mediated decay
Nociceptive pain, 1473
NOD2/caspase-activating recruitment domain 15
   (CARD15), 1653
Nodal, 70
Nodal marginal zone lymphoma (NMZL)
   B-cell, 1188t, 1192
   epidemiology and manifestations, 1285
   pathobiology and differential diagnosis, 1286
   prognosis, 1286
   therapy, 1286
NOD-SCID mice, 112b
Nodular lymphocyte-predominant Hodgkin lymphoma
   (NLPHL), 1200–1201, 1201f, 1204–1210
Nodular sclerosis classical Hodgkin lymphoma (NSCHL),
   1201, 1202f, 1212–1214, 1218
Nonacute porphyrias. See Cutaneous porphyrias
Noncoding RNAs (ncRNA), 30–31, 80, 105
Non-Hodgkin lymphomas (NHL)
   autoimmune hemolytic anemia in, 660
   Burkitt lymphoma. See Burkitt lymphoma
   in childhood, 1330–1338, 1331t–1332t
   classification of, 768, 1231f, 1288, 1330–1338
   composite lymphomas and, 1208, 1208f
   cytogenetics of, 832–839, 834f
   diffuse large B-cell lymphoma. See Diffuse large B-cell
      lymphoma
   epidemiology, 1330
   Epstein-Barr virus and, 748–749, 750b, 757–758
   follicular lymphoma. See Follicular lymphoma
   future directions, 1241–1242
   HIV and, 1324
   infection and, 1447
   mantle cell lymphoma. See Mantle cell lymphoma
   miscellaneous, 1241
   overview of, 1230–1231
   PD-1 blockade therapies and, 1584
   pregnancy and, 2209
   relapsed, 1338
   second/subsequent malignancies after, 1506
Nonhomologous endjoining (NHEJ) pathway, 711–712
Nonidiosyncratic drug-induced thrombocytopenia, 1967
Noninherited maternal antigens (NIMA), 1639
Nonmyeloablative allogenic stem cell transplantation,
   1260
Nonneutralizing antibodies, 2017, 2049
Nonobese diabetic (NOD) mice, 112b
Nonsense-mediated decay (NMD), 23
Nonsteroidal antiinflammatory drugs (NSAIDs), 400,
   1476, 1936–1937
Non-ST-segment elevation myocardial infarction
   (NSTEMI), 2142
Non-ST-segment elevation (NSTE), 2142
Nonsynonymous SNPs (nsSNP), 79
Non-Tf-bound iron (NTBI), 474f
Nontropical sprue, 536–537
Non-vitamin K antagonist oral anticoagulants (NOAC),
   1841
Noonan facies, 371–372
Noonan syndrome (NS), 371–372, 998
Norepinephrine reuptake inhibitors, 1480
Northern blotting, 14
Notch intracellular domain (NICD), 72
Notch signaling
   acute lymphoblastic leukemia and, 1051–1052
   angiogenesis and, 1847f, 1848–1849
   chronic lymphocytic leukemia and, 823, 825–826
   cutaneous T-cell lymphomas and, 1377–1378
   hematopoietic stem cells and, 100, 106t
   overview of, 72
   Richter syndrome and, 827
   T-cell acute lymphoblastic leukemia and, 840,
      1010–1013, 1010f
   vascular system and, 153–154
Novantrone. See Mitoxantrone
Novastan, 1979–1980, 1979t–1980t
NovoSeven, 1766, 1775
NPC. See Nuclear pore complexes
Nplate, 413
NPM. See Nucleophosmin

NRAS mutations, 918–919
nsSNP. See Nonsynonymous SNPs
NT5C. See 5,' 3'-nucleotidase, cytosolic
Nuclear bodies, 985
Nuclear export signals (NES), 48
Nuclear factor, erythroid 2 (NF-E2), 346, 456, 1109,
   1864
Nuclear factor kappa B (NF-κB)
   Burkitt lymphoma and, 1237–1238
   chronic lymphocytic leukemia and, 1245
   common variable immune deficiency and, 722
   defects in signaling, 715–716
   disseminated intravascular coagulation and, 2064–2065
   factor VIII and, 2001
   Hodgkin lymphoma and, 1209, 1210f
   lymphocytopenia and, 687–688
   mantle cell lymphoma and, 1300f
   non-Hodgkin lymphoma and, 1234
   phenotypic diversity in sickle cell disease and, 583
   protein transport into nucleus and, 49
Nuclear hormone receptors, 72
Nuclear localization signals (NLS), 48
Nuclear pore complexes (NPC), 20, 48
Nuclear receptor binding SET domain protein 1 (NSD1),
   919–920
Nucleic acids, 76–77
Nucleolin, 1298
Nucleophosmin (NPM)
   acute myeloid leukemia and, 783, 799, 812, 920, 986,
      988
   mast cells and, 1172
Nucleoporins (Nups)
   acute lymphoblastic leukemia and, 1014
   acute myeloid leukemia and, 800, 811
   overview of, 22, 48
   in T-cell acute lymphoblastic leukemia, 1014
Nucleoside analogs, 857–858, 1426–1427
Nucleosome assembly complex (WINAC), 20
Nucleosome remodeling deacetylase (NURD) complex, 20
Nucleosome sliding, 20
5,' 3'-Nucleotidase, cytosolic (NT5C2), 85, 1018
Nucleotide synthesis inhibitors, 856–857
Nucleotide-binding domain, leucine-rich repeat-containing
   proteins (NLR), 250
Nucleotides
   degradation of, 76
   metabolomics of, 77
   synthesis of, 76
Nucleus, 48–49, 49f–50f
Nurse cells, 310
Nutrition, 2257–2258
Nutritional supplementation, 590
Nystatin, 1456b

O

O⁶-Alkylguanine-DNA alkyltransferase (AGT; MGMT),
   882, 1550–1551
O⁶-Methylguanine methyltransferase (MGMT), 882,
   1550–1551
OATP1B1. See Organic anion transporter 1B1
Obesity, 677, 1499
Obesity-hypoventilation syndrome. See Pickwickian
   syndrome
Obinutuzumab, 1295–1296
Obizur, 1764
Observational studies, 25
Obstructive sleep apnea, 1076
Octaplas, 1821
Octaplex, 2013
Octyl-2-cyanoacrylate, 2306
Odo-leukemia, 944
Ofatumumab, 1258
O-Glycosylation, 55b
Olanzapine, 1485
OLC. See Osteolineage cells
Omacetaxine, 878, 1065
Omega-3 fatty acid supplements, 2259
Omenn syndrome (OS), 684, 712, 1153t, 1164
Omi/HtrA2, 190
Oncogene-induced apoptosis, 195
Oncostatin M (OSM), 1156
Oncovin. See Vincristine
Ondansetron, 1484
Opioid analgesics
   addiction and, 1481
   delivery routes, 1478–1479
   management of side effects, 1479–1480

Opioid analgesics (Continued)
  patient education and, 1477
  practical considerations for, 1477–1478
  relative potencies of, 1477b
  routes of delivery, 1478–1479
  selection of, 1477
Oprozomib, 869
Opsonization, 261
Opti-MAL-IT test, 2285–2287
Optimism, 1463
Oral contraceptives, 2083
Oral hairy leukoplakia (OHL), 754
Organ transplantation, 1441–1442, 1754–1755, 1970, 2228–2233. See also Specific organs
Organic anion transporter 1B1 (OATP1B1), 86–87
Organized stroke unit care, 2138
Origin recognition complex (ORC), 181–182
Orthotopic liver transplantation, 2310–2311
Osmotic attack, 666
Osmotic fragility (OF) testing, 631–632, 638–639, e7b
Osseous dysplasia, 717
Ostene, 2306
Osteoclasts, 121–122
Osteolineage cells (OLC), 120–121
Osteomyelitis, 598
Osteonecrosis, 603–604, 1500
Osteopenia, 1500
Osteoporosis, 2176
Osteoprotegerin (OPG), 1391
Outside-in signaling, 71
Ovalocytosis, 639–640, 646
Ovarian hyperstimulation syndrome (OHSS), 1752, 2083
Overlap syndromes, 1137
Oxaliplatin, 860–861
Oxidative hexose monophosphate shunt, 448
Oxidative phosphorylation, 74
Oxidative stress, 88f, 353
Oxidized cellulose, 2306
OxLDL, 2126, 2129
Oxygen homeostasis, 1071–1073, 1072f
Oxygen sensing, 1071–1073, 1072f
Oxygen-degradation domain (ODD), 1071–1072
Oxymorphone, 1478
5-Oxyproline, 621–622

P

P antigen, 1695
P13K inhibitors, 864
P18, 346
P27, 178–180
P2Y₁₂, 2169f
P53, 1016, 1246
P53-induced protein with a death domain (PIDD), 188, 189f
P55, 448
P57, 178–180
Packed red blood cells (RBC), 1702
Paclitaxel, 856–858, 891
Pacritinib, pharmacology of, 866
PAD. See Peripheral artery disease
Pagetoid reticulosis, 1364
Pain
  chemotherapy and, 1482
  evaluation of, 1473–1474
  management of
    analgesics and. See Analgesics
    elderly and, 1482
    nonpharmacologic methods, 1474–1475
    oral complications and, 1480–1481
    pharmacotherapy, 1475–1480
  sickle cell anemia and, 581
  specific clinical problems and, 1480–1482, 1482t
  taxonomy of, 1473, 1474t
Paired box protein5 (PAX5), 89–90, 1016, 1298–1299
Palifermin, 1480–1481
Palliative care
  bereavement follow-up and, 1493–1494
  caregivers and, 1490
  clinician self-care and, 1494
  communication and, 1488–1490
  hospice programs and, 1493, 1494t
  management concerns during last days of life, 1492–1493, 1493t
  overview of, 1488, 1494

Palliative care (Continued)
  pediatric, 1488, 1489t, 1490–1492
  psychosocial considerations, 1466, 1491–1492, 1492t
  relief of suffering and, 1490–1491
Palmitoylation, 60–61
Palonosetron, 1484
Pamidronate, 1415
Pancreas, 362–363, 362f, 531–532
Pancytopenia, 350–372, 395t, 405, 2218, 2232–2233
Paneth cells, 1658
Pan-leukocyte tyrosine phosphatase C. See CD45
Panmyelosis, 931f
Panobinostat, 876, 903, 967, 1146–1148
Papillary necrosis, 602
Pappenheimer bodies, 506, 507f
Paragangliomas, 1078–1079
Paraneoplastic hypereosinophilia, 1159
Paraplatin. See Carboplatin
Paraproteinemias, 1755, 1786, 1940, 2136
Paraproteinemic demyelinating neuropathy, 1755
Paraquat, 671
Parasitic infections
  amebiasis, 2302
  babesiosis, 667, 1816, 2299–2301, 2300f
  eosinophilia and, 2301, 2302t
  giardiasis, 2302
  hemolysis and, 667
  hookworms, 2302–2303
  leishmaniasis, 1816–1817, 2289–2292, 2289f
  malaria. See Malaria
  schistosomiasis, 2303
  tapeworms, 2303
  toxoplasmosis, 2302
  transfusion-associated, 1815–1818, 2288–2289, 2292, 2296, 2299, 2301
  trypanosomiasis. See Trypanosomiasis
Paris-Trousseau thrombocytopenia, 345, 347b, 347t–348t, 1883
Paroxysmal cold hemoglobinuria (PCH), 648–649
Paroxysmal nocturnal hemoglobinuria (PNH)
  aplastic anemia and, 403
  classical, 423, 423b
  classification of, 423, 423b
  clinical features of, 417–419
  clonality and bone marrow failure in, 419
  diagnosis of, 420, 423b
  differential diagnosis for, 656
  eculizumab and, 282
  hypoplastic, 423, 423b
  infection and, 1448
  laboratory evaluation of, 420
  natural history of, 419–420
  overview of, 415, 1940
  pathophysiology of, 415–417, 416f, 416t
  pregnancy and, 2205
  thrombocytopenia and, 442–443
  treatment approach for, 423
  therapy for, 420–422
  venous thromboembolism and, 2082
Parsley, 1939
Partial D antigens, 1696–1697, 1696b
Partial thromboplastin time (PTT), 2240. See also Activated partial thromboplastin time
Parvovirus B19 infection
  HIV infection and, 2268f, 2269
  pure red cell aplasia and, 425–427, 427f
  sickle cell disease and, 596f, 598
  transfusion-associated, 1810–1811
Passenger lymphocyte syndrome (PLS), 655–656, 2228–2229
Passive cell death, 1656–1657
Passive immunotherapy, 277–279, 1568. See also T cell therapies
Pasteurization, 1759–1760
Patent foramen ovale closure, 2140
Pathogen recognition receptors (PRR), 199–200, 201t
Pathogen reduced/inactivated plasma, 1745
Pathogen reduction technology (PRT), 1808b
Pathogen-associated molecular patterns (PAMP), 188, 199–200, 1655
Pathogenicity islands, 1992
Patient-specific tumor xenograft (PDX) models, 850
Pattern recognition receptors (PRR), 249–250, 254, 255f, 1655
Pattern-matching algorithms, 27
PAX5. See Paired box protein 5
Payne, Rose, 1721
PCBP1. See Poly(rC)-binding protein 1

PCFT. See Proton-coupled folate transporters
PCR (polymerase chain reaction), 14
PCSK9. See Proprotein convertase subtilisin/kexin type 9
PC-SPES, 2254
PD-1. See Programmed death 1
PDGF. See Platelet-derived growth factors
PDX models. See Patient-specific tumor xenograft models
Pearson syndrome, 363–364, 372, 377, 508
PECAM. See Platelet endothelial cell adhesion molecule
Pegaspargase, 1039
Pegylated doxorubicin, 1374
Pegylated interferon, 1120
Pembrolizumab, 1225
Penicillins, 589, 597, 1937
Pentose phosphate pathway (PPP), 74
Pentose shunt pathway, 616, 617f
Pentostatin, 1253–1254, 1271–1272, 1271f, 1271t
Pentoxifylline, 965, 2165
Pentoxifylline, dexamethasone, ciprofloxacin (PCD), 965
Peptide bonds, 59–66, 60f
Peptidoglycan receptor proteins (PGRP), 199
Percent hypochromic RBCs (%HYPO), 493
Percentage leukocyte count, e8b
Percutaneous coronary intervention (PCI), 1966b, 2142
Percutaneous mechanical thrombectomy (PMT) devices, 2114–2117
Perfluorocarbons, 1712
Perforin, 719, 732–733, 733t
Perforin-dependent cytotoxicity, 732–733
Perforin-granzyme receptor, 1657–1658, 1666
Periarteriolar lymphoid sheath (PALS), 208–209
Pericytes, 152, 1843, 1851
Periendothelial cells, 1846
Perinatal iron overload, 485t, 487
Perioperative period, 1704–1705
Peripheral arterial occlusion (PAO), 2115–2117
Peripheral artery disease (PAD)
  clinical manifestations of, 2160
  diagnosis of, 2160–2162
  epidemiology of, 2159–2160
  future directions, 2167
  overview of concept, 2159
  pathobiology of, 2160
  prognosis for, 2163
  therapy for, 2163–2166
Peripheral blood smear
  anemia and, 464, 464b, 465f, 466t
  hereditary spherocytosis and, 631, 631f
  splenic function and, 2320
Peripheral blood stem cell (PBSC) products, 1593
Peripheral blood stem cell (PBSC) transplantation
  advantages and disadvantages of, 1517, 1518b
  collection of cells for
    anticoagulants and, 1526
    apheresis and, 1524–1526, 1525b
    chemokines and, 1523–1524
    chemotherapy plus cytokine mobilization, 1523
    cytokine mobilization and, 1522
    granulocyte colony-stimulating factors and, 1522–1523
    granulocyte-macrophage colony-stimulating factor and, 1523
    large-volume leukapheresis and, 1526–1527
    mobilization of cells into peripheral blood, 1521–1523, 1522b
    overview of, 1521
    patients difficult to mobilize and, 1524
    pediatric donors and patients and, 1527
    plerixafor and, 1524–1525
    timing of, 1524–1525
  donor selection in, 1519
  microbial contamination and, 1529
  quality control of products used in, 1527–1529
  tumor cell contamination and, 1528–1529
Peripheral deletion, 1656–1657
Peripheral lymphoid organs, 203–204, 208–209
Peripheral neuropathy, 1482
Peripheral supramolecular activation complex (pSMAC), 226
Peripheral T-cell lymphomas (PTCL)
  classification of, 771–772, 771t, 1343–1344, 1344t, 1345f
  clinical manifestations of, 1348
  differential diagnosis for, 1348
  emerging new drugs for, 1357–1360, 1357t
  future directions for, 1360
  laboratory manifestations of, 1348

Peripheral T-cell lymphomas (PTCL) *(Continued)*
  not otherwise specified (PTCL-NOS), 1188*t*, 1197, 1343–1345, 1346*f*
  overview of, 1241, 1343
  pathobiology of, 1344–1348
  prognostic factors for, 1348–1351, 1349*f*
  stem cell transplantation in, 1355–1357
  therapy for, 1351–1360, 1355*b*
Peripheral-node addressin (PNAd), 138
Perivascular cells, 121
PERK, 55
Permeability transition pores, 191
Pernicious anemia, 531, 531*f*
Peroxisomal targeting signals (PTS), 50
Peroxisome proliferator-activated receptor gamma, coactivator 1 alpha (PPAR-γ coactivator 1-α), 497–498
Peroxisome proliferator-activated receptors (PPAR), 2126
Peroxisomes, 49*f*, 50
Perphenazine, 1018
Persistent polyclonal B-cell lymphocytosis (PPBL), 682–684
Perturbational studies, 25
Pertussis toxin (PTX), 138
Pets, 1459
PFA-100, 1928
PFA-100 closure time, 2190, 2194
PFA-100 testing, overview of, e13*b*
P-glycoprotein (PGP), 879–881, 880*f. See also* ABC-B1 transporter
Phagocyte disorders
  of adhesion and chemotaxis, 701–705
  clinical approach, 694*b*
  diagnostic approach to functional, 691
  granulocytic, 691, 706–707
  histiocytoses. *See* Histiocytoses
  miscellaneous, 707–708
  mononuclear, 691
  of respiratory burst pathway, 691–701, 692*f*–693*f*
Phagocyte oxidase (*phox*) genes, 693–695
Phagocytosis, 57, 199–200
Pharmacodynamics, 82
Pharmacogenetics, 81–82. *See also* Pharmacogenomics
Pharmacogenomics. *See also* Genomics
  catalogues of variants, genotyping platforms, GWAS and, 81
  drug development and, 89–90
  drug metabolism and, 82–86
  drug responses and, 81–82
  drug targets and, 87
  drug therapy optimization and, 82
  drug transporters and, 86–87
  future directions for, 90
  overview of, 34, 79, 81–82
  relevant websites, 80*t*
  somatic genomic variants and, 81
  structural genomic variants and, 81
Pharmacokinetics, defined, 82
Pharmacomechanical catheter-directed thrombolysis (PCDT), 2115
Phase I clinical trial design, 850–851, 850*t*
Phase II drug development, 850*t*, 851
Phase III trials, 851
PHD. *See* Proline hydroxylase
PHD finger protein 6 (PHF6), 1017
Phenylbutyrate, 875
Philadelphia chromosome. *See* Breakpoint cluster region protein- Abelson fusion gene (BCR-ABL)
Philadelphia chromosome-like acute lymphoblastic leukemia. *See* BCR-ABL1-like acute lymphoblastic leukemia
Philadelphia chromosome-negative myeloproliferative neoplasms, 790–793, 791*t*
Philadelphia chromosome-positive acute lymphoblastic leukemia, 1032–1033, 1042–1046, 1044*t*–1045*t*, 1051
Philadelphia-like acute lymphoblastic leukemia, 1034–1035, 1035*f*, 1051
Phlebotomy, 592, 1098–1099
Phosphatase and tensin homolog (PTEN), 1010–1011, 1014–1015
Phosphatidylinositol-3-kinase (PI3K) pathway
  Hodgkin lymphoma and, 1226
  overview of, 68–70
  platelet activation and, 1874
  primary immunodeficiencies and, 686–687
  T cell activation and, 225–226
  TPO-induced cell signaling and, 339

Phosphatidylinositol-glycan complementation class A (PIGA), 415–417, 417*f*, 419
Phosphodiesterase inhibitors, 1936
Phosphofructokinase (PFK) deficiency, 622
Phosphoglycerokinase deficiency, 622
Phospho-H3S10, 20
Phospholipase A, 1874
Phospholipase C, 306–307, 1874
Phosphoribosyl pyrophosphate (PRPP), 76
Phosphorylation
  cytokine signaling and, 163–164
  hematopoietic stem cell self-renewal and, 104
  oxidative, 74
  as posttranslational modification, 60–61
  regulation of protein function and, 47
Phototherapy, 1369–1370, 1375–1376
Phox genes. *See* Phagocyte oxidase genes
Physical activity, 2258
Phytosterolemia, 645
PI3K pathway. *See* Phosphatidylinositol-3-kinase pathway
Pickwickian syndrome, 1076–1078
Picotamide, 2164
Picrilisib, 864
PIDDOSOME, 188, 189*f*
Pidilizumab, 1585
PIEZO1, 644–645
PIGA. *See* Phosphatidylinositol-glycan complementation class A
PIK3CD gene, 722–723
Pinocytosis, 57
Pioglitazone, 2164
PK. *See* Pyruvate kinase
PKCθ, 225–226
Placenta, 119
Placental abruption, 2069
Plasma, 532, 1821
Plasma cells, 122
Plasma derivatives
  albumin. *See* Albumin
  coagulation factor concentrates, 1761–1766, 2013–2015, 2014*t*
  cryoprecipitate. *See* Cryoprecipitate
  fractionation of, 1759, 1760*f*, 1769–1770
  future directions, 1767–1768
  hyperimmune immunoglobulins, 1756–1757, 1756*f*
  intravenous immunoglobulin. *See* Intravenous immunoglobulin
  overview of, 1744
  plasma products
    adverse events related to, 1748–1749
    compatibility, 1748
    cryoprecipitate-reduced plasma, 1745
    dosage, 1748
    freeze-dried plasma, 1744–1745
    fresh frozen plasma, 1744, 1760
    indications for, 1745–1748, 1745*t*
    liquid plasma, 1744
    pathogen reduced/inactivated plasma, 1745
    prophylactic uses, 1748
    recovered and source (for manufacture), 1745
    solvent-detergent plasma, 1745
    thawed plasma, 1744
  proteinase inhibitors, 1766–1767, 1768*t*
  safety of, 1759–1760
  viral infections and, 1770–1771, 1771*t*
Plasma exchange therapy, 1988–1990, 1996
Plasma frozen within 24 hours of phlebotomy (FP24), 1744
Plasma iron concentration, 482*b*
Plasma proteinase inhibitors, 1766–1767
Plasma thromboplastin antecedent. *See* Factor XI deficiency
Plasmablastic lymphoma (PBL), 1194
Plasmapheresis
  defined, 1781
  replacement fluids and, 1787–1788
  technology and techniques, 1781–1786
  therapeutic, 1786–1787, 1786*t*, 1790*b*
Plasmin, 1897, 1909
Plasminogen (Plg), 107–108, 1897, 2070–2071
Plasminogen activator inhibitors (PAI)
  atherothrombosis and, 2131
  disseminated intravascular coagulation and, 2067
  fibrinolysis and, 1898, 1904
  fibrinolytic drugs and, 2184
  vascular growth and, 155–156

Plasminogen activators
  extracellular matrix and, 155–156
  fibrinolysis and, 1832
  hemostasis disorders and, 1841*t*
  tissue. *See* Tissue plasminogen activator
  urokinase, 1832, 1839, 1897, 2184
Plasmodium spp.
  erythrocyte membrane and, 646
  hemolysis and, 667
  P. malariae, 2284, 2285*f*–2286*f*
  P. falciparum. See also Malaria
    erythrocyte membrane and, 646
    glucose-6-phosphate dehydrogenase deficiency and, 616
    hemolysis and, 667
    life cycle of, 2280*f*
    parasitology of, 2278–2279, 2280*f*
    phosphofructokinase deficiency and, 620
    sickle gene and, 571–572, 572*f*
    Southeast Asian ovalocytosis and, 639, 646
  P. ovale, 2284, 2285*f*–2286*f*
  Plasmodium vivax, 646, 2284, 2285*f*–2286*f*
    Southeast Asian ovalocytosis and, 639, 646
  transfusion-associated, 1815–1816
Plasticity, 231
Platelet Additive Solutions (PAS), 1717
Platelet aggregometry. *See* Aggregometry
Platelet and leukocyte larceny, 1094
Platelet count (PLT count), 1112, 1981, e11*b*, e24*t*
Platelet endothelial cell adhesion molecule (PECAM), 692*f*, 1844, 1874
Platelet factor 3, 1941
Platelet factor 4, 2127
Platelet Function Analyzers (PFA), 2304–2305
Platelet gel, 2306
Platelet glycoprotein IV or IIIb. *See* CD36
Platelet neutralization procedure, 2092–2093
Platelet procoagulant response, 1907–1909
Platelet testing, overview of, e1, e11*b*
Platelet transfusions
  adverse effects of, 1717–1718
  for aplastic anemia, 406–407
  collection and manufacturing in, 1715
  for disseminated intravascular coagulation, 2073
  pediatric, 1822–1823, 1823*t*
  prophylactic, 1715–1717
  refractoriness to, 1718–1719, 1718*t*–1719*t*
  for thrombocytopenia with absent radii syndrome, 389–390
  for thrombotic thrombocytopenic purpura, 1991
Platelet-activating antibodies, 1943
Platelet-associated IgG (PAIgG), 1945, 1958, 1973
Platelet-derived growth factors (PDGF), 153, 1847*f*, 1848, 2127, 2127*f*
Plateletpheresis, 1785–1786
Platelet-rich plasma (PRP), 1715
Platelets. *See also* Megakaryocytes
  activation of, 1870–1873, 1896*f*
  adhesion and aggregation of, 132–133
  adhesion of, 1870–1873
  after solid organ transplant in children, 2231–2232
  aggregation of, 1878–1880, 1881*f*, 1896*f*
  antiphospholipid antibodies and, 2089
  arterial thrombosis and, 2168
  biogenesis of, 337
  coagulation and, 1894–1895, 1896*f*
  cytoskeletal mechanics of formation, 1861–1863, 1861*f*
  destruction or consumption of, 1956*t*
  developmental hemostasis and, 2190
  disorders of
    acquired, 439–441, 439*f*, 1932–1943
    in children, 2217–2218
    immune thrombocytopenia. *See* Immune thrombocytopenia purpura
    malignancies and, 2248–2249
    molecular basis, 1880–1884, 1881*f*
    neonatal alloimmune thrombocytopenia. *See* Neonatal alloimmune thrombocytopenia
    in neonate, 2193–2194, 2194*t*
    posttransfusion purpura. *See* Posttransfusion purpura
    surgical patients and, 2309
    thrombocytopenia. *See* Thrombocytopenia
  essential thrombocythemia and, 1110
  evaluation of, 1928
  formation of, 1861–1864
  hemostasis and, 1831–1834, 1833*f*, 1839–1840, 1839*t*, 1906–1909, 1908*f*, 2190

Platelets *(Continued)*
  interactions of with vessel wall, 1854–1855
  liver disease and, 2238–2239
  molecular basis of function of
    activation, 1873–1878
    adhesion, 1870–1873
    aggregation, 1878–1880
    inherited disorders, 1880–1884
    overview, 1870
  overview of, 1857
  pediatric, 1821
  physiologic sequestration of, 1959–1960, 1959f
  polycythemia vera and, 1099–1101
  segregation of, 1896f
  structure of, 1865–1868, 1865f–1866f
  thrombopoietin and, 340, 340f
  von Willebrand factor and, 2051, 2052f
Platelet-type von Willebrand disease (PT-vWD), 2060
Platinol. *See* Cisplatin
Platinum analogs, 860–861, 902–905
Pleckstrin homology domain (PHD) proteins, 68–70
Pleiotrophin (PTN), 106
Plerixafor, 147, 150b–151b, 1524–1525, 1675
Plitidepsin, 1360
Plumboporphyria. *See* Acute hepatic porphyria
Pluripotent stem cells, 107
PML gene. *See* Promyelocytic leukemia gene
PNAd, 139
Pneumatic compression therapy, 2108–2109
Pneumococcal conjugate vaccine (PCV13), 2325–2326
Pneumococcal polysaccharide vaccine (PPSV23),
    2325–2326
Pneumocystis infection, 1460, 1678
Pneumonia, 600, 697
Pneumonitis, 1677–1678, 1677b
PNH. *See* Paroxysmal nocturnal hemoglobinuria
POEMS syndrome, 1078–1079
Poikilocytes, bizarre, 643
Poikilocytosis, 637
Point mutations, 12, 79–81, 846
Poisoning, 2233–2234
Polo-like kinase (PLK), 342, 939
Poly(A) tail, 8–9, 20
Polyadenylation, 8–9, 20
Polybromo-associated BAF (PBAF), 20
Polyclonal gammopathy, 688
Polycomb complex, 919–920
Polycomb repressive complexes (PRC), 104–105, 1012,
    1129
Polycythemia vera (PV)
  additional mutations associated with, 1086–1087
  in children, 1003
  clinical manifestations of, 1089–1092
  cytogenetic abnormalities in, 114, 1094–1096,
    1094f–1096f
  differential diagnosis for, 1096–1097
  epidemiology of, 1081–1082
  evolution of, 1081f
  future directions, 1104
  hemorrhage risk and, 1088
  hypercoagulable state characterizing, 1087–1088
  JAK2 mutations in, 1084
  JAK2V617F mutation in, 1082–1086, 1083f–1084f
  laboratory manifestations of, 1092–1094
  myelofibrosis and acute myeloid leukemia following,
    1088–1089, 1091t
  overview of, 1080–1081
  pathobiology of, 1082
  pregnancy and, 2209–2210
  prognosis for, 1097–1098, 1098t
  therapy for, 1098–1104, 1099b–1100b
  thrombosis and, 2082
Polycythemias
  absolute, 1074–1075
  altitude and, 1076–1078
  of cyanotic heart disease and pulmonary disease,
    1075–1076
  definition and classification, 1074, 1074t
  drug-induced, 1080
  endocrine disorders and, 1079
  erythrocyte enzymopathies and, 623
  high-oxygen affinity hemoglobins, bisphosphoglycerate
    deficiency and, 1079
  hypoxia-inducing factor pathway mutations and,
    1079–1080
  kidney and liver diseases and, 1078–1079
  neonatal, 1080
  neoplastic disorders and, 1078–1079

Polycythemias *(Continued)*
  obstructive sleep apnea-induced, 1076
  Pickwickian syndrome and, 1076–1078
  postrenal transplantation erythrocytosis, 1078
  primary, 1074–1075, 1074t, 1080–1089
  primary familial and congenital polycythemia,
    1074–1075
  relative, 1074
  secondary
    acquired, 1075–1080
    congenital, 1079
    overview, 1074t, 1075
  smoking and, 1078
Polyethylene glycol hydrogel, 2306
Polymorphisms
  defined, 79
  DNA, 12
  single-nucleotide, 12, 79–81, 846
Polymorphonuclear neutrophils (PMN), 1738
Poly(rC)-binding protein 1 (PCBP1), 476, 476f
Polyribosomes, 456
Polysomy 21, 1017–1018
Pomalidomide, 866, 1143, 1414
Pompe disease, 743
Ponatinib, 862–863, 862t, 904–905, 1046
Porphobilinogen (PBG), 497
Porphobilinogen deaminase (PBGD), 498–499. *See also*
    Hydroxymethylbilane synthase
Porphyria cutanea tarda (PCT), 498f, 504–505, 505f
Porphyrias
  acute (multiple), 502–504, 502t, 503b
  acute intermittent. *See* Acute intermittent porphyria
  biological and molecular aspects of, 499–500, 500t
  classification of, 497
  genetic aspects of, 500–501, 501f
  laboratory assessment of, 501b
  nonacute (cutaneous), 504–505, 504b
  overview of, 498t
  porphyrinurias. *See* Porphyrinurias
  treatments for, 502
Porphyrinurias
  caused by drugs or alcohol, 510–511
  changes in porphyrins and precursors in, 500t
  overview of, 499t
  presentations associated with, 511–512
Portal vein thrombosis (PVT), 2198
Posaconazole, 1460
Positive selection, 228, 286
Positron emission therapy (PET), 1212, 1222, 1222t,
    1224
Positron emission tomography (PET), 2319–2320, 2320f
Postcapillary venules, 206–208, 1843
Post-essential thrombocythemia myelofibrosis (post-ET
    MF), 1125
Postherpetic neuralgia (PHN), 1481
Post-polycythemia vera myelofibrosis (post-PV MF),
    1080–1081, 1088–1089, 1091–1092, 1091t, 1097,
    1125, 1138
Post-renal transplantation erythrocytosis (PTE), 1078
Post-splenectomy sepsis syndrome, 561
Post-thrombotic syndrome (PTS), 2104, 2119–2120
Post-transcriptional processing, 10–11, 298–299
Post-transfusion purpura (PTP)
  clinical presentation of, 1952–1953, 1953b
  diagnosis of, 1953
  epidemiology of, 1952–1953, 1953f
  epitope spreading in, 292, 292f
  intravenous immunoglobulin for, 1756
  management of, 1954
  overview of, 1798–1799
  pathophysiology of, 1953–1954
  tolerance, immunity and, 285
Post-translational modifications, overview of, 60–61
Post-transplant cyclophosphamide (PTCy), 1625–1627,
    1626f, 1629
Posttransplantation lymphoproliferative disease (PTLD)
  in childhood, 1338
  cytogenetics of, 845
  Epstein-Barr virus and, 1320, 1320b, 1321f
  kidney disease and, 2245
  overview of, 1679
Posttraumatic growth (PTG) after transplantation, 1465
Post-traumatic stress disorder (PTSD), 1466–1469, 1468t
Potassium, 669, 1707
PP2A. *See* Serine/threonine protein phosphatase 2A
PPP. *See* Pentose phosphate pathway
Pralatrexate, 1357–1358, 1372–1373
Prasugrel, 1935, 2145t, 2146, 2170–2171

Prayer, 2256
PRC. *See* Polycomb repressive complex
PRCA. *See* Pure red cell aplasia
PRDM1, 1419, 1421
Pre-B cell acute lymphoblastic leukemia, 1005–1006
Precision medicine, 25, 28
Precursor B-cell acute lymphoblastic leukemia,
    1005–1006, 1009–1010, 1016
Predisposition syndromes. *See* Cancer predisposition
    syndromes
Prednisone
  for acute lymphoblastic leukemia, 1025–1026,
    1037–1039
  for graft-versus-host disease, 1663
  for immune thrombocytopenia purpura, 1948
  for light chain amyloidosis, 1439
  for primary myelofibrosis, 1142
  for pure red cell aplasia, 429
Preeclampsia, 1967, 2069, 2206–2207
Pregabalin, 1480
Pregnancy
  anemias in, 2203–2205
  antiphospholipid syndrome and, 2096, 2099–2100,
    2213, 2213t
  aplastic anemia and, 402–403
  autoimmune hemolytic anemia in, 653
  bleeding disorders and, 2210
  Chagas disease and, 2297
  clinical assessment and, 1916, 1916b
  disseminated intravascular coagulation and, 2069
  folate and, 533–534
  hemoglobinopathies and, 2204
  hemophilias and, 2210–2211
  Hodgkin lymphoma and, 1227
  late complications and, 1500
  leukemias, lymphomas and, 2208–2210
  malaria and, 2284
  prophylactic anticoagulation during, 2212
  pure red cell aplasia and, 426–427
  sickle cell disease and, 601
  thrombocytopenia and, 1946, 1957t, 1967
  thrombophilia and, 2212–2213, 2213b
  thrombotic microangiopathies and, 1999
  venous thromboembolism and, 2082–2083, 2086,
    2109–2111, 2211–2212
  warfarin therapy and, 2181
Prekallikrein, 1891, 2046–2047
Preleukemic anemia, 944
Premessenger RNA, 5–6
Prenylation, 47, 60–61
Preplatelets, 1864
Prethrombin-1, 1766
Priapism, 602–603
Primaquinone, 87
Primary amyloidosis. *See* Immunoglobulin light chain
    amyloidosis
Primary antiphospholipid syndrome, 653
Primary central nervous system lymphoma (PCNSL),
    1309, 1314, 1325–1327
Primary cutaneous CD4-positive small/medium T-cell
    lymphoproliferative disorder, 1188t, 1199
Primary cutaneous CD8-positive aggressive epidermotropic
    cytotoxic T-cell lymphoma, 1188t, 1199
Primary cutaneous gamma-delta T-cell lymphoma, 1188t,
    1199
Primary cutaneous γδ-T-cell lymphoma, 1367
Primary effusion lymphoma (PEL), 1193, 1322
Primary familial and congenital polycythemia (PFCP),
    1074–1075
Primary follicle, 218f, 219
Primary mediastinal B-cell lymphoma (PMBL), 1188t,
    1192, 1194, 1233f, 1234, 1309, 1313–1314
Primary myelofibrosis (PMF)
  clinical manifestations of, 1131–1132, 1131t
  conditions associated with, 1126t
  differential diagnosis for, 1096–1097, 1116,
    1135–1139, 1138t
  epidemiology of, 1125–1131
  future directions for, 1148
  grading of, 1133–1134, 1134t
  laboratory manifestations, 1132–1135
  overview of, 1125
  polycythemia vera vs., 1080–1081
  prognosis for, 1139–1148, 1140t
  therapy for, 1141–1142, 1148b–1149b
Primary protein structure, overview of, 59
Priming, 199–200
Primitive erythrocytes, 336

Prion diseases, 1770–1771, 1818–1819
Procarbazine, 855–856, 883, 888
Procaspases, 187–188, 188f
Prochlorperazine, 1479–1480
Prochymal, 1565b
Proerythroblasts, 300–301
Prognostic Index for Peripheral T-cell Lymphomas (PIT), 1350
Programmed cell death 1 (PD-1)
    cell-based therapies and, 1586
    checkpoint blockade therapies and, 1583–1586
    Hodgkin lymphoma and, 1225, 1340
    manipulating T cells to improve activity against malignancy, 237
    T cell exhaustion and, 232–233
Programmed cell death ligand (PDL-1), 1214–1216, 1216f, 1225
Prokineticins, 153
Proleukemic stem cells, 114b
Proline hydroxylase (PHD), 1071–1072, 1072f, 1080
Prolonged grief disorder, 1494
Prolymphocytic transformation (PT), 1261
Promegakaryoblasts, 334
Prometaphase, 176–177, 177f
Promoters, 10, 17–18, 18f
Promyelocytic leukemia (PML) gene, 804
Proofreading enzymes, 11–12
Prophase, 176–177, 177f
Proplatelets
    biogenesis of, 337
    maturation of, 1863
    overview of, 1857
    platelet formation from, 1861–1863, 1861f
    structure of, 1862f
Proplex, 2013
Proprotein convertase subtilisin/kexin type 9 (PCSK9), LDL cholesterol and, 2122–2123
Prostacyclin (prostaglandin I₂), 1831–1832, 1832f, 1851–1852, 1936
Prostaglandin E₂ (PGE₂), 106, 1647
Protac assay, 2078
α₁-Protease inhibitor (antitrypsin), 1767, 1768t, 1779
Protease inhibitors (PI), 1891–1894, 1893f, 2276
Protease nexin-1 (PN-1), 1909
Protease-activated receptors (PAR), 1834, 1834f, 1907–1909, 2169f, 2173
Proteases
    chemokine-mediated leukocyte trafficking and, 136–139
    disseminated intravascular coagulation and, 2065–2066
    hemostasis and, 1906
    vascular system and, 155–156
Proteasome inhibitors
    for cutaneous T-cell lymphomas, 1374
    for light chain amyloidosis, 1439–1440
    for peripheral T-cell lymphomas, 1359
    pharmacology of, 866–869, 867f
    for Waldenström macroglobulinemia, 1427
Protein 4.1, 448
Protein 4.1R, 635–636, 636f, 646
Protein 4.2 deficiency, 629–630
Protein 8/prokineticin 12 of Bombina variegata (Bv8/PK2), 153
Protein blood groups, 1696–1698
Protein C concentrate, 1766, 1779
Protein C inhibitor (PCI), 1894, 1909
Protein C (PC) assays, 2070, e13b
Protein C (PC) pathway
    antiphospholipid antibodies and, 2090
    deficiency in, 2078–2079, 2078f, 2078t
    disseminated intravascular coagulation and, 2066–2067, 2066f
    endothelial cells and, 1852
    hemostasis and, 1909
    HIV infection and, 2275–2276
    overview of, 2078, 2078f
Protein disulfide isomerase (PDI), 52–53
Protein inhibitors of activated STAT (PIAS), 172, 173f
Protein kinase-like ER kinase (PERK), 195
Protein kinases (PK)
    domain structures of, 63–64, 64f
    PKB, 225–226, 864
    PKC, 306–307, 1874
Protein replacement therapy. See Enzyme replacement therapy
Protein repressive complex 2 (PRC2), 950
Protein S assays, e13b

Protein S deficiency, 2079, 2079t
Protein synthesis, 5–7, 6f, 45
Protein tyrosine kinases (PTK), 70–71, 224
Protein tyrosine phosphatases (PTP)
    limitation of T cell activity and, 234
    as negative regulators of cytokine signaling, 171–173
    specific
        PTP1B, 172
        PTP-BL, 172
        PTPN1, 234
        PTPN11, 172, 951, 998, 1002
        PTPN6, 171–172
        PTPRT, 172
        PTPσ, 98
        TC-PTP, 172
Proteinase inhibitors. See Protease inhibitors
Proteins
    amino acids, peptide bonds and, 59–66, 60f
    cotranslational translocation into endoplasmic reticulum, 51, 51f
    degradation of, 48, 54, 54f
    domain structure of, 61–64, 61f–62f
    folding of, 46, 52–53
    genomic approaches and, 31–32
    intragolgi transport and processing, 55–56
    misassembled, degradation of, 54, 54f
    modification of, 46–48, 47b
    processing of within endoplasmic reticulum, 52–55, 53f
    secondary structure, 59–60
    synthesis of, 5–7, 6f, 45
    targeting of
        to mitochondria, 49–50, 49f
        to nucleus, 48–49, 49f–50f
        overview, 48–50, 49f
        to peroxisomes, 49f, 50
        signals for, 46t, 50–51
        specificity of, 57
        vesicular, 56–57
    trafficking of within the secretory pathway, 51, 52f
    trans-golgi network and, 56
Proteinuria, 602
Proteoglycans, 127
Proteolysis, 47–48
Proteome, 45
Prothrombin, 2080, 2094–2095
Prothrombin complex concentrates (PCC), 1765, 1774, 2029, 2040–2041, 2241
Prothrombin deficiency, 1778, 1840, 2040–2041
Prothrombin time (PT)
    in neonates, 2189, 2195
    overview of, 1924–1927, 1927t, e12b
    prolonged, 2195
    surgical patients and, 2304–2305
Prothrombinase, 1837, 1907–1909
Prothrombitic states, evaluation of, 1929–1930
Proton-coupled folate transporters (PCFT), 518–519, 521
Protoporphyrin, 480
Pruritus, 1091
Pseudo Pelger-Huët cells, 957, 957f
Pseudo von Willebrand disease, 2060
Pseudohemophilia, 2051
Pseudo-heparin induced thrombocytopenia, 1974, 1974b
Pseudoporphyria, 505b
Pseudothrombocytosis, 1113
Pseudotumors, hemophilic, 2011b
Pseudouridine synthase-1 (PUS1), 509
Psoralen plus ultraviolet A (PUVA) therapy, 1369–1370
Psychosocial issues
    accompanying trends in, 1462
    decision for hematopoietic stem cell transplantation and, 1464–1466
    factors influencing adjustment, 1466–1467
    future directions, 1470–1471
    management of, 1468–1470, 1471t
    overview of, 1462
    psychiatric complications vs. expected psychologic response, 1467–1468
    screening for psychologic distress, 1468, 1468t, 1469f
    second/subsequent malignancies and, 1504–1505
    sickle cell disease and, 605
    time of diagnosis and, 1462–1463
    treatment and, 1463–1464
Psychotropic drugs, 400–401
PTEN. See Phosphatase and tensin homolog
PTP. See Protein tyrosine phosphatases
PU.1, 210, 327–328, 332, 493
Pulmonary angiography, 2106

Pulmonary disorders
    embolism, 2106–2108, 2107f. See also Venous thromboembolism
    hypereosinophilic syndrome and, 1161
    hypertension, 581–582, 600, 1091, 2097
    polycythemia and, 1075–1076
    sickle cell anemia and, 581–582
    thrombocytopenia and, 1971
Pulmonary infiltrates, 1453, 1453f, 1454b
Pure erythroid leukemia (PEL), 812–813
Pure red cell aplasia (PRCA)
    acquired, 425
    after solid organ transplant in children, 2230–2231
    chronic lymphocytic leukemia and, 1263
    classification, 426t
    differential diagnosis, 429
    laboratory evaluation, 428–429, 428f
    pathogenesis, 426f
    primary, 425
    secondary, 426–428
    therapy, 429–430, 429t, 437b
Pure white cell aphasia (PWCA), 433
Purine analogs, 857–858, 1253–1254, 1282, 1294
Purine antimetabolite agents, 1373, 1373t
Purine nucleoside analogs (PNA), 1269–1272, 1270f, 1272f
Purpura fulminans, 2068, 2198, 2217–2218
PWCA. See Pure white cell aphasia
Pyoderma gangrenosum (PG), 955
Pyridium, 671
Pyridoxine, 509b–510b, 509f
Pyrimethamine, 538b
Pyrimidine analogs, 857–858
Pyrimidine-5'-nucleotidase-1 (P5'N-1) deficiency, 621
Pyropoikilocytosis, 626, 637
Pyroptosis, 188
Pyruvate kinase M2 (PKM2), 105
Pyruvate kinase (PK) deficiency
    clinical and laboratory manifestations, 620
    diagnosis, 620
    epidemiology, 620
    future directions, 621
    introduction and history of, 619–620
    pathobiology, 620
    prognosis, 621
    therapy, 620–621

Q

Quechua Indians, 1077
Quiescence, 176
Quinine, 664, 1962, 1966–1967, 1998, 2287t
Quizartinib, 939

R

R protein, 515–516
Rac, 135
Radiation exposure, 685, 914, 1081–1082, 1125
Radiation therapy
    for acute lymphoblastic leukemia, 1025
    aplastic anemia and, 398–399, 398f
    for cutaneous T-cell lymphomas, 1370–1371
    gonadal dysfunction and, 1499–1500
    for Hodgkin lymphoma, 1221–1222
    infection and, 1447
    neurocognitive effects of, 1500–1501
    pain management and, 1475
    for primary myelofibrosis, 1144
    pure red cell aplasia and, 428
    spleen and, 2322
    for splenic marginal zone lymphoma, 1285
    thrombocytopenia and, 442
Radioimmunotherapy, 1283
Radionuclide scintigraphy, 2319
Rai staging system, 1250, 1250t
RAIDD, 188, 189f
Raloxifene, 2083
Ramipril, 2164
Ran. See Ras-related nuclear protein
RANTES (chemokine ligand 5), 1156–1157, 2126
RAP. See Ras-related protein 1
RAPADILINO syndrome, 392
Rapamycin, 68–70, 863–865, 863f, 1659
Rapoport-Luebering shunt, 448
RAR. See Retinoic acid receptors
RARS with thrombocytosis (RARS-T), 509, 1116
Ras associated lymphoproliferative disorder (RALD), 1000

RAS pathway
  acute lymphoblastic leukemia and, 1014
  acute myeloid leukemia and, 918–919, 987
  cell division cycle and, 178
  myelodysplastic syndromes and, 995f
  myeloproliferative neoplasms and, 998–999
Rasburicase, 86t, 87–88, 88f, 1027
RasGRP, 224–225, 224f
Ras-related nuclear protein (Ran), 48–49, 50f
Ras-related protein 1 (RAP), 138
RB-E2F, 180–181
RBM15. *See* RNA binding motif protein 15
Reactive oxygen species (ROS), 74–75, 148, 2126
Receptor editing, 219, 285–286
Receptor tyrosine kinases (RTK)
  cell division cycle and, 177, 177f
  mast cell development and, 1170–1171
  myelodysplastic syndromes and, 951
  overview of in hematopoiesis, 68, 69t
Receptor-mediated endocytosis, 57
Recombinase-activating genes (RAG), 212, 711–712
Reconstituted red blood cells, 1827
RECOTHROM, 1766
Recovered plasma, 1745, 1759
Recruitment, 146
Red blood cell count, e15t
Red blood cell distribution width, 460t, 463–464, 464t, e2b
Red blood cell fragmentation, 1970
Red blood cell storage lesion, 1708
Red blood cell substitutes, 1712–1713, 1712t
Red blood cells (RBC). *See* Erythrocytes
Red meats, 2258
Red pulp of spleen, 2313–2317
Redox potential, 573, 573f
Reduced-intensity conditioning (RIC)
  for acute lymphoblastic leukemia, 1041, 1043t
  for acute myeloid leukemia, 972–975
  allogenic HSCT and, 1596–1597, 1598f, 1598t–1599t
  for chronic myelogenous leukemia, 1068
  cord blood stem cell transplantation and, 1645
  for follicular lymphoma, 1297
  for mantle cell lymphoma, 1306
  for myelodysplastic syndromes, 976–977
  overview of, 970
  for primary myelofibrosis, 1145–1146, 1146f
Reed-Sternberg cells. *See* Hodgkin and Reed-Sternberg cells
ReFacto, 1764
Refractory anemias
  classification of, 768
  with excess blasts (RAEB), 767, 768t, 944, 946t
  with excess blasts in transformation (RAEB-T), 767, 768t
  with ring sideroblasts and thrombocytosis (RARS-T), 768, 944, 946t, 961
  with ring sideroblasts (RARS), 456, 509, 510b, 944, 946t
  with unilineage dysplasia (RCUD), 767–768
Refractory cytopenias
  classification of, 768
  with multilineage dysplasia and ring sideroblasts (RCMD-RS), 509
  with multilineage dysplasia (RCMD), 767, 944, 946t
  with unilineage dysplasia (RCUD), 944, 946t
Regenerating islet-derived 3-alpha (REG3α), 1658–1659
Regulatory T cells (Tregs)
  chronic lymphocytic leukemia and, 1246
  cord blood stem cell transplantation and, 1648
  dendritic cells and, 255
  factor VIII inhibitors and, 2018
  graft-versus-host disease and, 1656
  inhibition of T cell-mediated immunity and, 233, 234f
  negative selection in T cell development and, 228
  self-reactive lymphocytes and, 290
  stem cell niche and, 122–123
  thymic, 228, 233
Relative polycythemia, 1074
Relaxation response, 2255, 2255t
Relaxation training, 1470, 1471t
Remission induction. *See* Induction therapy
Remnant lipoproteins, 2125
Remodeling
  angiogenesis and, 1847
  atherothrombosis and, 2127–2129, 2127f–2128f
  of chromatin, 20
Renal dialysis, 505b
Renal disease. *See* Kidney disease

Renal medullary carcinoma, 602
Renal transplantation, 1441–1442, 1997
Renal vein thrombosis (RVT), 2198
Renin-angiotensin system (RAS), 1073–1074
Reperfusion, 580, 580f
Reperfusion therapy, 2137, 2142–2144
Replication-competent retroviruses (RCR), 1551
Resimmune, 1378
Resistance. *See* Drug resistance
Respiratory burst pathway, 691–701, 693f
Respiratory distress syndrome (RDS), 2197
Respiratory syncytial virus (RSV), 1678
Responsive elements, 20
Restriction endonucleases, 13
Reteplase, 2143, 2143t, 2186f, 2187
Reticular dysgenesis (RD), 371, 711
Reticulocyte count, 460t, 463, 464t, e3b, e15t
Reticulocyte hemoglobin count (CHr), e16t
Reticulocyte hemoglobin equivalent (Ret He), 479–480, e3b, e16t
Reticulocytes, 297, 447
Retinoic acid receptors (RAR), 804–805, 915–916, 984–985
Retinoic acid syndrome, 940
Retinoic acid-related orphan receptor (ROR) family, 230
Retinoid X-receptors (RXR), 1376
Retinoids, 72, 1376
Retinopathy, 603, 604f, 2097
Retronectin, 1550
Retroviruses, 3, 12–13, 1550–1551, 1806–1808
Revascularization therapies, 2165–2166
Reverse cholesterol transport (RCT) pathway, 2123–2124, 2124f
Reverse phase protein arrays (RPPA), 32, 32f
Reverse transcriptase, 3
Revesz syndrome, 365–367
Revised European Classification of Lymphoid Neoplasms (REAL Classification), 1330
RFLP. *See* Restriction fragment length polymorphism
Rh deficiency syndrome, 645
Rh immune globulin (RhIG), 1693b, 1757
RhAG blood group system, 1697
RhCE protein, 1696–1697
Rhesus blood group system, 1696–1697, 1696t
Rhesus D (RhD)
  overview of, 1696–1697, 1696b
  passive immunization and, 277
  platelet transfusions and, 1717–1718
  RhIG and, 1757b
  testing for, 1692
Rheumatoid arthritis, 243, 256, 293
Rh-negative blood group, 1696
Rh$_{null}$ phenotype, 1697
Rh$_{null}$ syndrome, 1693
Rho-associated kinase (ROCK), 186, 337, 850
RiaSTAP, 1766, 2036–2038
Ribavirin, 670, 1284–1285
Ribonucleoproteins. *See* Small nuclear ribonucleoproteins
Ribosomal protein S19 (RPS19), 317–318, 373–374
Ribosomal proteins (RP), 373–374, 1017
Ribosomal RNA (rRNA), 19
Ribosomes, 5–7, 6f, 45
Ribosomopathies, 372–374
Richter syndrome (RS), 827, 1187, 1261
Rickettsia spp., 1815
Ring chromosomes, 797f
Ring sideroblasts, 506–507, 507f
Ristocetin cofactor assay, 1928, 2059
Ristocetin-induced platelet aggregation (RIPA) assay, 1928, 2059
Rituximab
  for acute lymphoblastic leukemia, 1039, 1047
  for antiphospholipid syndrome, 2100
  for chronic lymphocytic leukemia, 1254–1256
  for EBV-lymphoproliferative disease, 756–757
  for extranodal marginal zone lymphoma of MALT type, 1282
  for follicular lymphoma, 1294t, 1295–1296
  for hairy cell leukemia, 1272–1273, 1273t, 1275
  for hemophilia, 2031–2032
  HIV and lymphoma and, 1328
  for immune thrombocytopenia purpura, 1949
  for mantle cell lymphoma, 1302–1303, 1302t, 1305
  neutropenia and, 680
  overview of, 293
  for peripheral T-cell lymphomas, 1354–1355

Rituximab *(Continued)*
  for pure red cell aplasia, 430
  for splenic marginal zone lymphoma, 1285
  for thrombotic thrombocytopenic purpura, 1990
  for Waldenström macroglobulinemia, 1427–1428
  for warm antibody hemolytic anemia, 656–660, 657f, 659t
Rivaroxaban, 2108, 2148t, 2150, 2181t, 2182–2183
Rixubis, 2013
RMRP, 717
RNA (ribonucleic acid)
  genomic approaches to, 30–31
  metabolism of, 20
  molecular biology and, 3
  nuclear export of, 20, 22f
  splicing of, 19–20, 22f
  storage and transmission of genetic information and, 5
  structure of, 3
RNA binding motif protein 15 (RBM15), 986
RNA interference (RNAi), 20–22, 32–34, 33f
RNA sequencing, 779–780
RNA-induced silencing complexes (RISC), 11, 11f, 23
Roadmap Epigenomics project, 22, 22f
Roberts syndrome, 392
Robertsonian translocation, 818
Rocky Mountain spotted fever (RMSF), 1815
Romidepsin, 877, 903, 1357–1359
Romiplostim, 340–341, 963, 1949–1950
ROS. *See* Reactive oxygen species
Rosai-Dorfman disease (RDD), 738
Rotational thrombelastography (ROTEM), 2071
ROTEM-analyzer, 1929
Rothmund-Thomson syndrome, 392
Rotor syndrome, 511–512
RP. *See* Ribosomal proteins
RPPA. *See* Reverse phase protein arrays
RPS19 protein. *See* Ribosomal protein S19
RTK. *See* Receptor tyrosine kinases
RUCONEST, 1767
Runt domain, 801–803
Runt-related transcription factors (RUNX)
  ETSV6-RUNX fusion, 783, 817–818, 1009–1010, 1020, 1034
  RUNX1
    acute myeloid leukemia and, 801–804, 802t, 915–916, 928f, 982–983
    megakaryocyte endomitosis and, 343
    myelodysplastic syndromes and, 950
    myeloid differentiation and, 325–326
    regulation of megakaryocytopoiesis and, 345–346
  RUNX2, 103, 982–983
  RUNX3, 228, 982–983
  Schwachman-Diamond syndrome and, 363
Rutherford classification of acute limb ischemia, 2117
Ruxolitinib, 865–866, 905, 1102, 1143–1144, 1143f, 1149b

S

S phase of cell cycle, 176, 177f
S1P. *See* Sphingosine-1-phosphate
Safety, 1807b, 1809f
Safety genes, 1544–1545, 1572–1573
Salmonella spp., 598
Salt bridges, 59
Salvage pathways, 76
Salvage therapy
  acute myeloid leukemia and, 938
  diffuse large B-cell lymphoma and, 1316–1317
  for Hodgkin lymphoma, 1223
  intraoperative, 1711, 1711t
SAMe-TT$_2$R$_2$ scoring system, 2155, 2155t
SAMHD1, 256–257
Sapacitabine, 939
Sar1-p, 57
Sargramostim, 963, 2232, 2273
Scavenger receptors (SR), 2123, 2124f, 2126, 2130
SCF. *See* Skp, Cullin, F-box-containing complex; Stem cell factor
Schilling test, 541b
Schimke immunoosseous dysplasia, 371, 717
Schistocytes, 643
Schistosomiasis, 2303
Schulman syndrome, 403, 1153t, 1164
Schwachman-Bodian-Diamond syndrome (SDBS) protein, 360–361

Schwachman-Diamond syndrome (SDS)
  acute myeloid leukemia and, 914
  cancer predisposition and, 363
  clinical features of, 361–363, 361t
  differential diagnosis for, 363–364
  epidemiology of, 360
  Fanconi anemia vs., 357
  future directions for, 365
  Kostmann syndrome/severe congenital neutropenia vs., 387
  laboratory findings in, 362–363, 362f
  overview of, 360
  pathobiology of, 360–361
  prognosis for, 364
  therapy for, 364–365
Scianna blood group system, 1699
SCID. See Severe combined immunodeficiency
SCL. See Stem cell leukemia
SCN. See Severe congenital neutropenia
SCR. See Short consensus repeat
Scurfy mice, 228
Scurvy, 1943
SDF1. See Stromal cell-derived factor 1
SDS. See Schwachman-Diamond syndrome
Sea-blue histiocytes, 745
Sebastian syndrome, 1862–1863, 1883
Seckel syndrome, 357, 371
Secondary acute myeloid leukemia (sAML), 913–914
Secondary protein structure, 59–60
Second/subsequent malignancies
  after acute lymphoblastic leukemia, 1503, 1505, 1505t
  after acute myeloid leukemia, 1505–1506, 1505t–1506t
  after chronic myeloid leukemia, 1506
  after hematopoietic stem cell transplantation, 1594, 1679, 1680t
  after Hodgkin lymphoma, 1503, 1506, 1506t
  after non-Hodgkin lymphoma, 1506
  clinical care and, 1507t
  evaluating survivors for, 1505b
  late mortality and, 1504
  monitoring for, 1508f, 1508t–1511t
  overview of, 1502–1503
  research needed, 1506b
  screening and followup recommendations, 1504
γ-Secretase inhibitors (GSI), 23, 1051–1052
Secretory granules, 56
Secretory pathway, 51, 52f
Sedation, 1479
Seizures, 599
Selectins
  atherothrombosis and, 2126
  disseminated intravascular coagulation and, 2064–2065
  dysregulated expression of, 134
  endothelial cells and, 121
  eosinophil mobilization and migration and, 1156
  leukocyte adhesion deficiency and, 702
  leukocyte entry into tissues and, 138
  leukocyte homing to secondary lymphoid organs and, 139
  neutrophil response to infection and, 692f
  neutrophil rolling, spreading, migration and, 133
  overview of, 130–131, 130t
  regulation of surface expression, 131–132
Selective amegakaryocytic thrombocytopenia, 441
Selective estrogen receptor modulators (SERM), 2083
Selective serotonin reuptake inhibitors (SSRI), 1480, 1937–1938
Selenocysteine insertion sequence (SECIS) elements, 23
Self-inactivating design (SIN), 1551
Self-reactive lymphocytes
  changing type of effector response and, 289–290
  downregulation of, 289
  peripheral control of, 288–289
  persistence of, 288
  regulation of, 285–288
  regulatory T cells and, 290
Self-tolerance
  B cells and, 285–286, 290t
  breakdown of in autoimmune diseases, 290–292
  limitations of, 286
  T cells and, 286
Seligmann disease, 1277, 1279, 1281–1282
SEN viruses (SENV), 1806
Senescence, 184, 448–449
Senile cardiac amyloidosis, 1437
Sentrin-specific protease 1 (SENP1), 1077
Sepax devices, 1533, 1538, 1539f

Sepsis
  disseminated intravascular coagulation and, 2068
  intravenous immunoglobulin for, 1756
  lymphocytopenia and, 684
  splenectomy and, 2325–2326, 2325b, 2325t
Sequence-specific oligonucleotide probe hybridization (SSOPH), 1611
Sequestration crises, 596
SERCA calcium channel inhibitors, 1010
Serine protease inhibitors (serpins), 266, 1838–1839, 1909, 1910f, 2076
Serine/threonine kinases, 1874
Serine/threonine protein phosphatase 2A (PP2A), 1018
SERM. See Selective estrogen receptor modulators
Serotonin-release assay (SRA), 1975–1977, 1978t
Serpins. See Serine protease inhibitors
Serum cobalamin levels, 527–528, 528t, 529b
Serum folate levels, 528–529, 528b–529b, 529t
Serum free light chain testing, 1394
Serum tryptase, 1178
Severe acute respiratory syndrome (SARS), 684
Severe combined immunodeficiency (SCID)
  clinical and laboratory manifestations of, 712
  diagnostic approach for, 713b
  expression and signaling defects and, 711–712
  gene therapy and, 1552–1553
  lymphocyte survival defects and, 711
  lymphocytopenia and, 684
  nucleotide degradation and, 76
  overview of, 710–714
  pathobiology and genetics of, 711, 711f
  prognosis, therapy, and future directions for, 713–714, 714b
  universal newborn screening for, 712–713
Severe combined immunodeficiency (SCID) mice, 112b
Severe congenital neutropenia (Kostmann syndrome)
  acute myeloid leukemia and, 914
  background, 385
  clinical features, 386
  differential diagnosis, 387–388
  epidemiology, 385
  etiology, genetics, and pathophysiology, 385–386
  future directions, 389
  laboratory findings, 386
  leukemia, myelodysplastic syndrome and, 386–387
  overview, 678
  therapy and prognosis, 388–389
  unfolded protein response and, 329
Sézary syndrome (SS)
  clinical presentation of, 1362–1364, 1363f
  cytogenetics of, 843–845
  cytology of, 1199f
  differential diagnosis for, 1366–1368
  laboratory manifestations of, 1364–1365
  overview of, 1188t, 1198, 1360–1361
  pathobiology of, 1361–1362
  prognosis for, 1368–1369
  therapy for, 1368–1369, 1370b
SF3B1. See Splicing factor 3b subunit 1
SG-110, 939
SGN-CD33A therapy, 939
SH2 (src homology 2), 177
SH2 domain-containing phosphatase 1 (SHP-1), 234
Shear stress response element, 1844
Shiga toxin hemolytic uremic syndrome (STEC-HUS)
  clinical manifestations of, 1991
  differential diagnosis for, 1984
  epidemiology of, 1991–1992
  laboratory manifestations of, 1992
  overview of, 1984
  pathobiology of, 1992
  prognosis for, 1992–1993
  therapy for, 1993
Shiga-like toxins (Stx), 1992
Short consensus repeat (SCR), 1993–1994
SHP. See Src homology containing phosphatases
SHPS-1. See Src homology 2 domain-containing protein tyrosine phosphatase substrate 1
Sialomucins, 138
Sickle cell β-thalassemia, 606, 606t
Sickle cell crisis, 593–595, 594t
Sickle cell disease (SCD)
  abnormal molecular behaviors of sickle hemoglobin, 572–576
  abnormalities of sickle red blood cells, 576–578, 576f
  alloimmunization and, 1709–1710
  basis of phenotypic diversity, 582–583
  blood groups and, 1693, 1693t

Sickle cell disease (SCD) (Continued)
  cell morphologies, 572f
  clinical presentation and management, 586–605
  coinherited hemoglobin abnormalities interacting with, 607
  complications and their management, 593–605, 594t–595t
  diagnosis, 584–586
  early research, 571
  epigenetics and, 22
  erythrocytapheresis and, 1783–1784
  genetic aspects, 571–572, 572b, 572f
  infection and, 1450
  inflammation and, 580–582
  ischemic stroke and, 2136
  lead poisoning and, 2233
  overview of, 584
  pain and, 1473, 1474t, 1481
  pediatric transfusions and, 1825
  pregnancy and, 2204
  prevalence, 584
  red blood cells and disease pathogenesis, 578–579
  spleen and, 2321–2322, 2321f
  unique systems biology of, 579–580, 579b
  variant syndromes, 605–607
Sickle cell hemolytic transfusion reaction syndrome, 1793–1794
Sickle cell screen, e4b
Sickle cell trait, 582, 605–606
Sickledex, e4b
Side population cells, 1208
Sideroblastic anemia with B-cell immunodeficiency, periodic fevers, and developmental delay (SIFD), 509
Sideroblastic anemias
  acquired, 509–510, 510b
  caused by drugs or alcohol, 510–511
  classification of, 507t
  evaluation of, 510b
  hereditary
    other forms, 508–509
    therapy for, 509b
    X-linked, 498f, 507–508, 508f
  overview of, 506–507
  presentations associated with, 511–512
Sidney Criteria for antiphospholipid syndrome, 2088, 2089t
Siglecs, 131, 1167. See also CD33
Sign R1, 261
Signal recognition particle (SRP), 51, 51f
Signal transducers and activators of transcription (STAT). See also Janus-activated kinase-STAT pathway
  B cell development and, 217
  consequences of deficiencies in genes of, 173t, 718
  erythropoietin receptors and, 1073
  hepcidin expression and, 476
  hyperimmunoglobulin E syndrome and, 704
  immune dysregulation and, 718–719
  neutrophil maturation and, 323
  overview of, 70, 168f, 169
  STAT1, 169–170
  STAT2, 170
  STAT3, 170–171, 230, 476, 704
  STAT4, 171
  STAT5, 171, 305–306, 339
  STAT5B, 718
  STAT6, 171, 230, 253
  T helper 17 cells and, 230
  T helper 2 cells and, 230
  thrombopoietin receptor and, 339
Signal transduction pathways
  cell division cycle and, 177–178, 177f, 179f
  cGAS-cGAMP-STING pathway, 73
  chemokines and, 73
  cooperative interactions with adhesion molecules, 132–133
  cytokine signaling and
    elements of, 163–164, 164f–165f
    janus kinases. See Janus kinases
    ligand-receptor binding and activation, 164–173, 167f
    negative regulators of cytokine signaling, 171–173
    physiology and pathology, 173–174, 173t
  erythropoietin receptors and, 305–307, 306t
  G-protein coupled receptors and, 72
  hedgehog, 72, 101
  MAPK/ERK pathway, 70, 865
  myelodysplastic syndromes and, 966
  notch ligands and, 72

Signal transduction pathways (Continued)
nuclear hormone receptor superfamily and, 72
overview of in hematopoiesis, 68, 69f, 69t
phosphatidylinositol-3-kinase. See
  Phosphatidylinositol-3-kinase
protein-tyrosine kinases and associated receptors, 70–71,
  224
receptor tyrosine kinases. See Receptor tyrosine kinases
T cell receptors and, 224–226, 224f
TGF-β pathway. See TGF-β signal transduction
  pathway
through adhesion molecules, 132
toll-like receptors and, 71
tumor necrosis factors and, 71
wnt proteins and, 71–72
Signaling inhibitors, 861–866, 862t, 883
Signalosome, 216
Signal-sensing domains (SSD), 20
Sildenafil, 1936
Silencers, 10, 17–19, 18f
Simian immunodeficiency virus, 2262
Single nucleotide polymorphisms (SNP), 12, 28, 79–81,
  779–780, 846
Single unit cord blood transplantation (SCBT)
adult donor allograft vs., 1635, 1636t
double-unit cord blood transplantation vs., 1640–1645
engraftment and, 1633
graft versus host disease and, 1633–1634
relapse and, 1634
transplant-related mortality and survival, 1635
Single-cell sequencing, 31
Single-nucleotide variants (SNV), 28
Sink model, 340
Sinus histiocytosis with massive lymphadenopathy
  (SHML), 738
Sinusoidal obstruction syndrome (SOS), 717, 1676–1677,
  1676b
Sipuleucel-T, 258
siRNAs. See Small interfering RNAs
Sirolimus, 1659, 1661t, 2232
Sitosterolemia, 645
Six transmembrane epithelial antigen of the prostate 3
  (STEAP3), 469, 472f
Sjögren syndrome, 684–685
Skewed X-inactivation pattern, 782–783
Skin
antiphospholipid syndrome and, 2098
graft-versus-host disease and, 1651–1652, 1651f, 1651t,
  1660–1661
hypereosinophilic syndrome and, 1161
infection and, 1451
myelodysplastic syndromes and, 955
sickle cell disease and, 604–605
Skin cancer, 1504
Skin necrosis, 2181
Skp, Cullin, F-box-containing (SCF) complex, 181
SLE. See Systemic lupus erythematosus
SleX, 703
SMAC/Diablo, 190
Small interfering RNAs (siRNAs), 11, 11f, 20–22
Small intestine, 531–532
Small lymphocytic lymphoma (SLL). See Chronic
  lymphocytic leukemia
Small nuclear ribonucleoproteins (snRNP), 9, 20, 22f
Small-vessel disease, 2135
SMMHC. See Smooth muscle myosin heavy chain
Smoking, 677, 1078
Smoldering multiple myeloma (SMM), 1381, 1400–1401
Smoldering systemic mastocytosis (SSM), 1173–1174
Smooth muscle, 418
Smooth muscle myosin heavy chain (SMMHC), 803
SMPD1. See Sphingomyelin phosphodiesterase 1
SMZ lymphoma (SMZL), 1266–1269, 1269t
SN-38, 859–860, 859f
Snake bites, 669, 2070
SNAREs. See Soluble NSF association protein receptors
snRNP. See Small nuclear ribonucleoproteins
SNS032, 873
Sodium butyrate, 875
Solid organ transplantation. See Organ transplantation
Solitary plasmacytoma, 1401–1402
Solubility tests for hemoglobin, 584
Soluble intercellular adhesion molecule I (sICAM-1), 2160
Soluble NSF association protein receptors (SNAREs), 57
Soluble transferrin receptors (sTFR), 493, e5b
Solute carrier (SLC) transporters, 86–87, 508–509. See
  also Ferroportin
Solvent-detergent (S-D) plasma, 1745

Somatic gene therapy, 1549
Somatic genomic variants, defined, 81
Somatic hypermutation (SHM; affinity maturation),
  204–205, 219, 289
Somatic mutations, germline variants vs., 27–28
Son of Sevenless (SOS), 225
Sonic Hedgehog (SHH) pathway, 1299, 1300f
Sons of mothers against decapentaplegic (SMAD), 474,
  475f
Sorafenib, 865, 904, 991, 1360
Source plasma, overview of, 1745, 1759
Southeast Asian ovalocytosis (SAO), 640, 646
Southern blotting, 13–14, 13f
SOX11. See SRY-box 11
Specialized lineage model of dendritic cells, 247
Specific granule deficiency (SGD), 707
Spectral karyotyping, 778
Spectrin, 1866f, 1868
Spectrins
erythrocyte membrane and, 448
hereditary elliptocytosis and, 635–636, 636f, 638–639
hereditary spherocytosis and, 627–628, 630
malaria, erythrocyte membrane and, 646
Spherocytic elliptocytosis, 639
Spherocytosis, hereditary. See Hereditary spherocytosis
Sphingomyelin phosphodiesterase 1 (SPMD1), 742
Sphingosine-1-phosphate (S1P), 143, 147–148, 208,
  1230–1231
Sphingosomal vincristine, 1050
Spices, 1939
Spider bites, 669
Spindle assembly checkpoint (SAC), 184, 342–343
Spirochete infections, 1814–1815
Spleen
anatomy and function of, 1958–1959, 1959f,
  2313–2318, 2314f–2316f, 2314t
β-thalassemia syndromes and, 560
disorders of
asplenia and hyposplenia, 2321
hypersplenism, 2322–2323
hyposplenism (acquired), 2321–2322
splenomegaly. See Splenomegaly
functional tests for, 2320–2321
hairy cell leukemia and, 1268, 1268f
hemolytic anemia and, 666, 666t
hypersplenism and. See Hypersplenism
imaging of, 2319–2320
immune cell development and, 203
infection and, 1451
infectious mononucleosis and, 752, 752f
malaria and, 2280, 2284
neutrophilia and, 677
overview of, 208–209, 208f
primary myelofibrosis and, 1143–1145
sickle cell disease and, 587f
Splenectomy
β-thalassemia syndromes and, 560
hereditary spherocytosis and, 633–634, 634b
for immune thrombocytopenia purpura, 1948–1949
infection and, 1451
overview of, 2323–2326, 2324f, 2325b, 2325t
phosphofructokinase deficiency and, 620–621
for thrombotic thrombocytopenic purpura,
  1990–1991
for warm antibody hemolytic anemia, 657–659, 657f,
  659t
Splenic aspiration, 2291
Splenic marginal zone lymphoma (SMZL)
cytogenetics of, 839
epidemiology and manifestations, 1283
overview of, 1188t, 1192
pathobiology and differential diagnosis, 1283–1284
prognosis, 1285
therapy, 1284–1285
Splenomegaly
in children, 2234–2236, 2236b, 2236t
mastocytosis and, 1178
overview of, 2322–2323, 2323t
Spliceosome, 7–8, 20, 22f, 920
Splicing
mRNA, 7–8, 8f, 10–11
RNA, 19–20, 22f
Splicing factors (SF), 825–826, 948–949
Sponge model, 340, 340f
Sponsors, 1533
Sprengel deformity, 374–375
Sprouting angiogenesis, 156f–157f, 158
Spumaretroviral vectors, 1551

Spur cell anemia, 2238
Spur cell hemolytic anemia of severe liver disease, 641,
  641f, 668–669
Spur cells, 641, 643, 668
Spurious polycythemia, 1074
Src, 1110
Src homology 2 domain protein 1A (SH2D1A), 753
Src homology 2 domain-containing protein tyrosine
  phosphatase substrate 1 (SHPS-1), 449
Src homology containing phosphatases (SHP), 171–172,
  173t, 1073
SRSF2, 21, 948
SRY-box 11 (SOX11), 1298–1301, 1306
ST2 biomarker, 1658
STAT proteins. See Signal transducer and activator of
  transcription proteins
Statins, 1938, 2122, 2123f, 2140, 2165–2166
STE6, 879
Stem cell factor (SCF; Kit ligand)
erythropoiesis and, 298, 307, 316
homing of hematopoietic stem and progenitor cells and,
  146
mast cell development and, 1171
megakaryocyte development and, 334
Stem cell leukemia (SCL, TAL1), 103, 314, 316, 346,
  840, 1008, 1013
Stem cell leukemia/lymphoma syndrome, 790, 1162–1163
Stem cell niche. See Niche theory
Stem cell transplantation
for chronic lymphocytic leukemia, 1249b, 1259
for cutaneous T-cell lymphomas, 1375
hematopoietic. See Hematopoietic stem cell
  transplantation
for light chain amyloidosis, 1439f, 1440–1441, 1441f
for paroxysmal nocturnal hemoglobinuria, 422
for peripheral T-cell lymphomas, 1355–1357
for sickle cell disease, 591
Stem cells. See also Specific types
erythroid differentiation and, 299f, 300
leukemia, 921
myelodysplastic syndromes and, 947
paroxysmal nocturnal hemoglobinuria and, 417, 419
proleukemic, 114b
as source of red blood cells, 1713
spleen and, 2318
StemRegenin 1 (SR1), 106, 1647
Stenting, 2138–2139, 2147b
Steroid hormones, 72
Steroids. See Corticosteroids
Sterol hormones, 72
Sterol regulatory element-binding protein (SREBP),
  2122
Sterol response elements (SRE), 2122
Stiff-person syndrome, 1756
Stomatocytosis, 626, 644–645, 669
Streptococcus pneumoniae, 597–598, 1998
Streptokinase, 2110, 2142–2143, 2143t, 2184–2185,
  2185f
Streptozotocin, 855, 888
Stress, 676, 683
Stress management training, 1470
Stress platelets, 1942–1943
Stretch enhancers, 1013, 1013f
Stroke
antiphospholipid syndrome and, 2096–2097, 2099
atrial fibrillation and, 2152
clinical manifestations of, 2136–2137
defined, 2133
epidemiology of, 2133, 2134t
future directions, 2140
investigations of, 2137
pathobiology of, 2133–2136
prognosis for, 2140
sickle cell disease and, 581, 598, 599f
therapy for, 2137–2140, 2138f
Stromal cell-derived factor 1 (SDF1), 122, 145–149, 149f,
  1845
Strübing, Paul, 415
Structural genomic variants, overview of, 81
Structural maintenance of chromosomes (SMC), 920
ST-segment elevation myocardial infarction (STEMI),
  2142
Stuart-Prower factor, 2043
Stypven clotting time, 1941
Subarachnoid hemorrhage (SAH), 2133, 2135
Subcutaneous panniculitis-like T-cell lymphoma (SPTCL),
  1198–1199, 1199f, 1367
Subdural hemorrhage, 1917

Subsequent malignancies. *See* Second/subsequent malignancies
Substrate reduction therapy (ART), 742–744
Sucrose hemolysis test, 420
Sudden death, 582
Suicide genes, 1544–1545, 1572–1573
Sulfadoxine-pyrimethamine, 2287*t*
Sulfasalazine, 538*b*
Sulfation, 47
Sumoylation, 47, 104
Sunitinib, 991
Superenhancers, 17, 18*f*, 1013, 1013*f*
Superoxide anions, 74–75, 1853
Supertransfusion, 553
Supervised learning approaches, 26, 26*f*
Supplements, 2254, 2255*t*, 2258–2260
Support groups, 1470, 1471*t*
Suppressor of cytokine signaling (SOCS), 172–173, 173*f*, 173*t*, 1073
Surface-connected canalicular system, 131–132
Surgical patients
    anticoagulation management in, 2311*t*
    evaluation of hemostatic risk for, 2304–2305, 2305*t*
    hemodilution and, 1971
    with hemostatic abnormalities, management of, 2308–2312
    hemostatic agents for, 2305–2308
    perioperative anticoagulation management in, 2311–2312
    thromboprophylaxis for, 2312
Switch regions, 219
Switch/sucrose nonfermentable (SWI/SNF), 20, 23
Sympathetic innervation, 122
Synaptosomal-associated protein (SNAP), 1876, 1876*f*–1877*f*
Syndesmos, 1844
Syngenic transplantation, 1411
Syphilis, 1458, 1814
Systemic juvenile idiopathic arthritis (sJIA), 2219–2221
Systemic lupus erythematosus (SLE)
    autoimmune hemolytic anemia in, 653, 660
    in children, 2227–2228
    complement cascade and, 266, 268
    dendritic cells and, 256
    lymphocytopenia and, 684–685
    thrombocytopenia and, 1968
Systemic mastocytosis, 792–793, 1170, 1173–1182, 1173*t*. *See also* Mastocytosis
Systemic mastocytosis associated with hematologic neoplasm (SM-AHNMD), 1174, 1174*t*, 1179–1180

T

T cell acute leukemia 2 (TAL2), 840
T cell acute lymphoblastic leukemia (T-ALL)
    BCL11B in, 1017
    CALM-AF10 fusion gene in, 1009
    clinical manifestations, 1022–1023
    cyclin C and *FBXW7* in, 1016
    cytogenetics of, 840–841, 844*t*–845*t*, 1035
    epigenetics and, 22–23
    immunophenotyping of, 1032, 1032*t*–1033*t*
    interleukin-7 receptor in, 1015
    LEF1 in, 1016–1017
    lymphoblast features in, 1006–1007
    NOTCH1 mutations in, 1010–1013, 1010*f*
    NUP214-ABL1 fusion in, 1014
    overview of, 1021
    PHF6 mutations in, 1017
    PRC2 and, 1012
    PTEN-P13K-ATK pathway in, 1014–1015
    RPL genes in, 1017
    TAL1, LMO genes in, 1008, 1013
    therapy, 1025–1026
T cell acute lymphocytic leukemia 1 (TAL1). *See* Stem cell leukemia
T cell antibodies, 1659
T cell exhaustion, 232–233
T cell lymphomas
    allogenic HSCT for, 1606
    classification of, 1196–1202, 1196*b*
    cutaneous. *See* Cutaneous T-cell lymphomas
    overview of, 1188*t*
    peripheral/noncutaneous. *See* Peripheral T-cell lymphomas
T cell lymphoproliferative neoplasms, 840–845
T cell receptor excision circles (TREC), 712–713

T cell receptors (TCR)
    adaptive immune response and, 200
    cell adhesion and, 133
    cell division cycle and, 177
    defects in signaling, 714–715
    genetically engineered, 1570–1572
    graft-versus-host disease and, 1655–1657
    human leukocyte antigens and, 1723–1724, 1730
    immunoglobulin binding and, 62–63, 63*f*
    overview of, 222–224, 223*f*
    pure red cell aplasia and, 425
    severe combined immunodeficiency and, 711–712
    signal transduction and, 224–226, 224*f*
    spatial coordination of signal transduction and, 226
T cell therapies
    with activated T lymphocytes. *See* Activated T lymphocytes
    with cytotoxic T lymphocytes. *See* Cytotoxic T lymphocytes
    for EBV-lymphoproliferative disease, 757
    future directions, 1573
    genetic modification in, 1570–1573, 1570*f*
    overview of, 1568
T cell/histiocyte rich-type large B-cell lymphoma (THRLBCL), 1193
T cell-mediated immunity, 231–235, 234*f*
T cells
    activation of, 221–226, 222*f*–223*f*, 1542–1544
    adhesion of to antigen-presenting cells, 133, 133*f*
    chimeric antigen receptors and. *See* Chimeric antigen receptor T cells
    complement and immunity, 272, 272*f*
    dendritic cells and activation of, 252–254, 253*t*
    development of, 226–229
    disorders with immune dysregulation mediated by, 717–719
    dominance in double-unit cord blood transplantation and, 1637–1638
    Epstein-Barr virus and, 750, 754*t*
    functions of, 229–231
    genetic modification of, 1570–1573
    graft-versus-host disease and, 1655–1657, 1662
    graft-versus-leukemia responses and, 1665–1666
    hematopoietic stem cell processing and, 1539–1540, 1540*t*
    Hodgkin lymphoma and, 1206
    human leukocyte antigens and, 1732
    inhibition of immunity mediated by, 233–235, 236*f*
    lymphomas and, 1188*t*, 1196–1202, 1196*b*
    manipulating to improve activity against malignancy, 237–238
    maturation of, 204
    maturation of immunity mediated by, 231–233
    migration of to T zones, 141–142
    modulating to permit allograft transplantation, 237
    multiple myeloma and, 1390
    nonspecifically activated autologous, 1542–1544
    overview of in immune system, 202–203
    proliferation of, 226
    regulatory. *See* Regulatory T cells
    SCID and early defects in development of, 710–714
    self-tolerance and, 286, 287*f*
    therapeutic manipulation of immunity mediated by, 237–238
T follicular (Tfh) cells, 202–203, 219, 229*f*, 231, 289
T helper (Th) cells
    cytokines of, 202*t*
    Th1, 229–230, 229*f*
    Th17, 229*f*, 230–231, 253
    Th2, 229*f*, 230
    Th22, 253
    Th9, 253
T regulatory cells. *See* Regulatory T cells
T zones, 141–142
T3151 mutation, 1064–1065
Tacrolimus, 1659, 1661*t*, 1664, 1997
TAFI. *See* TATA-box binding protein associated factor 1
TAL1. *See* Stem cell leukemia
TAL2. *See* T-cell acute leukemia 2
TALENs. *See* Transcription activator-like effector nucleases
Tamoxifen, 2083
Tandem repeats, overview of, 12
Tanespimycin, 878
Tank treading, 666
TAP. *See* Transporter associated with antigen processing
Tapeworms, 2303

TAR syndrome. *See* Thrombocytopenia absent radii syndrome
Target-specific oral anticoagulants (TSOAC), 1930
Tartrate-resistant acid phosphatase (TR-ACP), 1266–1268
TATA-box binding protein associated factor 1 (TAFI), 1839
Tax, 1322–1323
Taxanes, 856–858, 880
Taxol. *See* Paclitaxel
Taxotere. *See* Docetaxel
TAZ gene, 390
T-box transcription factor TBX21 (T-bet), 230–231
TCA cycle. *See* Tricarboxylic acid cycle
T-cell chronic lymphocytic leukemia, 843
T-cell depleted (TCD) stem cell grafts, 1623–1624, 1623*f*
Teeth, 1502
TEG-analyzer, 1929
Tel/Etv6, 103
Telomerase reverse transcriptase (TERT), 396–397, 401
Telomerase RNA component (TERC), 396–397, 401
Telomerases, 796–797
Telomeres, 396–397
Telophase, 176–177, 177*f*
Temozolomide, 854*f*, 855–856, 882–883, 888–889, 1375
TEMPI syndrome, 1078–1079
Temsirolimus, 864–865
Tenases
    coagulation and, 1835–1836
    factor IX and, 2005
    procoagulant response and, 1899–1901, 1900*f*
Tenecteplase, 2143–2144, 2143*t*, 2186–2187, 2186*f*
Ten-eleven translocation (TET)
    acute myeloid leukemia and, 799–800, 919, 986–987
    clonal hematopoiesis and, 783–784
    essential thrombocythemia and, 1109
    methylation and, 104
    myelodysplastic syndromes and, 949
    primary myelofibrosis and, 1128
Teniposide, 899
TERC. *See* Telomerase RNA component
Terminal deoxynucleotidyl transferase (TdT), 212–214
TERT. *See* Telomerase reverse transcriptase
TET. *See* Ten-eleven translocation
Testis, 1193
Testosterone, 412–413, 1080
TET. *See* Ten-eleven translocation
Tetramer analysis, 1541, 1541*f*
Tetrameric HLA/epitope complexes (tHLA), 1721, 1732, 1733*f*
Tetrocarcin A, 872
TG. *See* Thioguanine
TGF-β. *See* Transforming growth factor beta
TGN. *See* Trans-golgi network
Th cells. *See* T helper cells
Thalassemia syndromes
    α-
        clinical manifestations, 567
        de novo and acquired forms of, 568–569
        molecular pathology and pathophysiology, 565, 566*f*
        overview of, 564
        phenotypic diversity in sickle cell disease and, 582
        prenatal diagnosis, 567
        sickle cell disease and, 588*t*, 607
        therapy, 567–568
    β
        β-thalassemia minor, 564
        chronic care, 561–562
        clinical manifestations, 552–553
        complications and their management, 558–561
        congenital dyserythropoietic anemias vs., 384
        experimental therapies, 562–563
        gene therapy and, 1555
        nomenclature, 547–549, 547*f*–548*f*
        overview of, 344
        pathophysiology, 549–564, 550*f*
        screening, 564*t*–565*t*
        sickle cell disease and, 606, 606*t*
        survival, 561, 561*f*, 561*t*
        thalassemia intermedia, 547, 563–564
        treatment, 553–558, 553*b*–554*b*, 562–563
    definitions and nomenclature, 546
    etiology and epidemiology, 546
    extraordinarily unstable hemoglobins and, 569–570
    infection and, 1450
    overview of, 457, 457*t*, 546, 609*t*
    pathophysiology, 546–547
    pediatric transfusions and, 1825–1826

Thalassemia syndromes (Continued)
  pregnancy and, 2204
  structural variants, 569
  thalassemia intermedia, 547, 563–564
Thalassemia trait, 564
α-Thalassemia with mental retardation (ATR) syndrome, 568
Thalidomide
  for light chain amyloidosis, 1439
  for mastocytosis, 1184
  for multiple myeloma, 1403–1407, 1404t, 1412
  for myelodysplastic syndromes, 965
  pharmacology of, 866
  for primary myelofibrosis, 1142–1143
Thawed plasma, 1744
Theinopyridines, 2170–2171
T-helper-inducing POZ/Krüppel-like factor (Th-POK), 228
Therapeutic plasma exchange (TPE), 1790–1791. See also Plasmapheresis
Therapy-related acute myeloid leukemia (tAML), 23, 814–815, 815b, 856, 913, 974, 1504
Therapy-related myelodysplastic syndromes, 814–815, 815b, 847f, 961, 1504
Therapy-related myeloid neoplasm (t-MN), 765
Thiamine-responsive megaloblastic anemia (TRMA) syndrome, 509
Thienopyridines, 1935, 1998–1999
Thioguanine (TG), 83–85, 895
Thiopurine S-methyltransferase (TPMT), 82–84, 84f, 1026, 2232
30X Coverage, 27
Thomas, E. Donnall, 1515
Thomsen-Freidenreich (T-F) antigen, 1998
Thorotrast, 1125
Thrombate III, 1766
Thrombelastography (TEG), 2071
Thrombin
  cancer, thrombosis, and, 2251
  developmental hemostasis and, 2189–2190
  disseminated intravascular coagulation and, 2065–2066
  endothelial cells and, 1851–1852
  endothelial permeability and, 1851
  hemostasis and, 1906, 2189–2190
  platelet adhesion and, 1872
  protein C pathway and, 2078, 2078f
  surgical patients and, 2306
Thrombin clotting time (TCT), 1925–1927, 1927t
Thrombin concentrate, 1110, 1766, 1767t
Thrombin generation assays (TGA), 1929
Thrombin-activatable fibrinolysis inhibitor (TAFI), 1898, 1899f, 1904, 2040
Thrombin-JMI, 1766
Thrombocytes. See Platelets
Thrombocytopenia with absent radii (TAR) syndrome
  acute myeloid leukemia and, 915
  background, 390
  clinical features, 391, 391f
  congenital amegakaryocytic thrombocytopenia vs., 370
  differential diagnosis, 391–392
  etiology and pathophysiology, 391
  megakaryocyte differentiation and, 1883
  therapy and prognosis, 392
Thrombocytopenias
  acquired, 439–441, 440f
  after solid organ transplant in children, 2231–2232, 2232b
  aging and, 1345–1346, 1348, 2328–2329
  anatomy and physiology of, 1958–1960
  approach to patient with, 1955–1958, 1958t
  cancer and, 2248
  cardiovascular disease and, 1971
  chemotherapy, irradiation and, 442
  in children, 2217, 2231
  cyclic, 443
  diagnosing, 443b
  differential diagnosis for, 1957f, 1957t, 1960t, 1984, 2071, 2072t
  drug-induced
    autoimmune thrombocytopenia, 1965
    immune of rapid onset, 1965–1966
    immune thrombocytopenia, 1961–1965, 1962f, 1963b, 1963t
    miscellaneous syndromes, 1966–1967
    overview, 442
    thrombocytopenic syndromes, 1961

Thrombocytopenias (Continued)
    ethanol and, 442
    GATA1 and, 344
    glycoprotein IIB/IIIA receptor antagonists and, 1966
    gold-induced, 1965
    heparin-induced. See Heparin-induced thrombocytopenia
    HIV infection and, 2266b, 2273–2275
    hypersplenism and, 1960–1961, 1960t
    idiopathic. See Idiopathic thrombocytopenia purpura
    immune-mediated, 2231–2232, 2232b
    infections and, 441–442
    infectious mononucleosis and, 752
    inherited, 347b, 347t–348t, 1883–1884, 2193
    inherited bone marrow syndromes with, 369t, 390–392
    inherited presenting as chronic hepatitis, 2238–2239
    liver disease and, 2238–2239
    malaria and, 2283
    marrow infiltration and, 442
    myelodysplasia and, 443
    myelodysplastic syndromes and, 963
    neonatal alloimmune. See Neonatal alloimmune thrombocytopenia
    in neonate, 2192–2193, 2193t
    nutritional deficiencies and, 442
    overview of, 1955, 1956t–1957t
    pregnancy and, 1967–1971, 2205–2208
    primary myelofibrosis and, 1148b–1149b
    regulation of megakaryocytopoiesis and, 343–344
    selective amegakaryocytic, 441
    surgical patients and, 2308–2309
    thrombosis and, 2147b
Thrombocytopoiesis, 338–342
Thrombocytosis, 1115t, 1392, 2217, 2248
Thromboelastography, 1929
Thromboelastometry, 1929
Thromboembolism
    atrial fibrillation and, 2152
    in children, 2226–2227, 2229b
    HIV infection and, 2275–2276
    kidney disease and, 2244–2245
    in neonate, 2197–2200
    venous. See Venous thromboembolism
Thromboendarterectomy, 2110
Thrombogenesis, 2102–2103
Thrombolytic therapy, 2110, 2137–2138
Thrombomodulin (TM)
    coagulation and, 1889–1890, 1890f
    for disseminated intravascular coagulation, 2074
    endothelial cells and, 1852
    hemostasis and, 1832, 1832f, 1910f
Thrombophilia
    ischemic stroke and, 2135–2136
    in neonate, 2197–2200
    pregnancy and, 2212–2213, 2213b
Thrombophilia in Pregnancy Prophylaxis Study (TIPP) trial, 2213b
Thrombophilic disorders. See Hypercoagulable states, inherited
Thrombopoietin (TPO)
    cloning of, 334
    endoreplication and, 184
    essential thrombocythemia and, 1107, 1115
    megakaryocyte development and, 1859–1861
    for myelodysplastic syndromes, 963
    negative regulation of, 339
    primary myelofibrosis and, 1126–1127
    regulation of levels, 440f
    regulation of platelet mass by, 340, 340f
    signaling in thrombocytopoiesis, 338–340
Thrombopoietin receptor. See MPL
Thrombopoietin receptor agonists, 1949–1950
Thromboprophylaxis, 2228
Thrombosis. See also Atherothrombosis
    antiphospholipid syndrome and, 2095–2096, 2099
    cancer and, 2250–2252
    catheter-based interventions in, 2113–2120
    disorders of, 1841
    essential thrombocythemia and, 1111
    hypercoagulable states and. See Hypercoagulable states
    kidney disease and, 2244–2245
    liver disease and, 2241–2242
    malignancies and, 2250–2252
    mechanical interventions in, 2117–2120
    overview of, 1831

Thrombosis (Continued)
    paroxysmal nocturnal hemoglobinuria and, 418, 422–423
    polycythemia vera and, 1087–1090
    sickle cell anemia and, 581
    threshold for, 2077f
Thrombospondin, 127
Thrombotic microangiopathies (TMA)
    cancer and, 2247
    classification of, 1985f
    diagnosis and management of, 1986f, 1989b
    differential diagnosis for, 1984, 1985f, 2072
    drug-induced, 1966–1967
    hemolytic uremic syndromes. See Hemolytic uremic syndrome
    miscellaneous, 1997–1999
    overview of, 1984
    posttransplantation, 1997–1999
    thrombotic thrombocytopenic purpura. See Thrombotic thrombocytopenic purpura
Thrombotic thrombocytopenic purpura (TTP)
    cancer and, 2247
    clinical manifestations of, 1984–1985
    epidemiology of, 1985
    fragmentation hemolysis vs., 663–665
    HIV infection and, 2275
    ischemic stroke and, 2136
    laboratory manifestations of, 1988
    pathobiology of, 1985–1988
    plasma derivatives for, 1747–1748
    plasmapheresis for, 1786
    pregnancy and, 2207–2208
    prognosis for, 1988
    therapy for, 1989b
    tolerance, immunity and, 285
Thromboxane receptor, 1833–1834, 1873
Thromboxanes, 1833–1834, 1988–1991, 2169f, 2170–2171
Thymic regulatory T cells (tTregs), 228, 233
Thymic settling progenitors (TSP), 227
Thymidine kinase, 1250
Thymidylate deficiency, 522–523
Thymoma, 426
Thymus, 204, 227–228, 227f, 710
Thyroid cancer, 1503–1504
Thyroid disorders, 1498–1499, 2225
Thyroid hormones, 72
Tibetans, 1077
Ticagrelor, 2145t, 2146, 2171
Tick-born bacterial infections, 1815–1818
Ticlopidine, 1935, 2164
Tie receptors, 153–154, 1848
Tight junctions, 1844–1845
TIL. See Tumor-infiltrating lymphocytes
Tip cells, 1846–1847
Tirofiban
    for acute coronary syndromes, 2146–2147, 2146t
    overview of, 2172–2173, 2172t
    platelet disorders and, 1936
    thrombocytopenia and, 1966
TISSEL, 1766
Tissue factor pathway inhibitor (TFPI)
    coagulation and, 1892–1893, 1901
    disseminated intravascular coagulation and, 2065, 2066f, 2067
    endothelial cells and, 1852
    factor V deficiency and, 2041
    for hemophilia, 2019–2020, 2019t
    hemostasis and, 1832, 1832f, 1837, 1909, 1910f
    laboratory evaluation of, e13b
    thromboembolism and, 2102
Tissue factor (TF)
    angiogenesis and, 1849
    atherothrombosis and, 2129
    cancer, thrombosis, and, 2250–2251
    coagulation and, 1889, 1890f, 1903f
    disseminated intravascular coagulation and, 2064–2066
    hemostasis and, 1907–1909, 1908f
Tissue necrosis factors (TNF), 202t
Tissue pillars, 1846
Tissue plasminogen activator (tPA)
    for acute ischemic stroke, 2137
    fibrinilytic drugs and, 2184–2187
    fibrinolysis and, 1897
    hemostasis and, 1832, 1838–1839
    for neonates, 2200, 2200b

Tissue thromboplastin inhibition time (TTIT), 2092

TKI. *See* Tyrosine kinase inhibitors

T-large granular lymphocyte leukemia (T-LGL)
  clinical presentation and physical features of, 436
  differential diagnosis for, 438
  laboratory diagnosis of, 436–438, 436*t*
  overview of, 434–435, 434*f*
  pathogenesis of, 435–436
  prognosis for, 439
  therapy for, 437*b*, 438–439, 438*f*

TLR. *See* Toll-like receptors

TLX genes, 1008–1009

T-lymphoblastic leukemia/lymphoma (T-ALL), 772

TNF receptor 1-associated periodic syndrome (TRAPS), 688, 1432

TNFAIP3, 1419, 1421

TNFR1, 194

TNFR-associated factor (TRAF) receptors, 71

TNFRSF14 genes, 1288–1290, 1289*t*

Tocilizumab, 1659

Tocopherols, 2126

Tolerance, 254–256. *See also* Self-tolerance

Tolerogenic dendritic cells (tDC), 254

Toll-like receptors (TLR)
  antiphospholipid syndrome and, 583, 2088–2089
  atherothrombosis and, 2126
  autoimmunity and, 291–292
  dendritic cells and, 249–250, 250*t*
  innate immune system and, 199
  mesenchymal stromal cells and, 1562
  overview of, 71
  self-reactive lymphocytes and, 288–289

Toluene, 1125

Topoisomerase I inhibitors, 858–860, 858*t*, 901

Topoisomerase II inhibitors
  acute myeloid leukemia and, 913
  pharmacology of, 858*t*, 859–860, 859*f*, 860*t*, 899–901

Topotecan, 859–860, 859*f*, 901

Torcetrapib, 2124

TORCH syndrome, 370

Torque teno virus (TTV) complex, 1806

Total body irradiation (TBI), 1497

Total homocysteine, 526*t*, 527, 527*b*, 529*b*, *e*7*b*, *e*18*t*

Total iron-binding capacity (TIBC), *e*5*b*

Touch therapy, 2257, 2257*t*

Toxic oil syndrome, 1164

Toxins, 292, 913–914, 2070

Toxoplasmosis, 683, 1458–1460, 1817, 2302

TP53
  acute myeloid leukemia and, 919
  Hodgkin lymphoma and, 1209
  mantle cell lymphoma and, 1298–1299, 1300*f*
  multiple myeloma and, 831
  myelodysplastic syndromes and, 951–953
  Richter syndrome and, 827

TPMT. *See* Thiopurine S-methyltransferase

TPST. *See* Tyrosyl-protein sulfotransferases

Traditional Chinese medicine, 2253. *See also* Acupuncture

Tranexamic acid
  for disseminated intravascular coagulation, 2074
  factor replacement therapy and, 2039*b*
  for factor VIII inhibition, 2030–2031
  for hemophilia, 1775, 2015
  surgical patients and, 2306–2307
  for von Willebrand disease, 2061

Trans-acting elements, defined, 9

Trans-activating domains (TAD), 20

Transaldolase deficiency, 622–623

Transcobalamins
  TCI, 516–517
  TCII, 516–518, 516*f*–517*f*
  TCIII, 516–517, 2270–2271

Transcription, 18–19, 18*f*, 180–181, 180*f*

Transcription activator-like effector nucleases (TALENS), 32–34

Transcription factor EB (TFEB), 740

Transcription factors
  acute myeloid leukemia and, 919
  B cell development and, 210–211, 211*f*
  binding sites for, 19*f*
  emergency granulopoiesis and, 327
  epigenetic alterations and, 20
  in erythropoiesis, 306*t*, 313–317
  erythropoiesis disorders and, 298–299

Transcription factors (*Continued*)
  hematopoiesis and, 325*f*
  hematopoietic stem cell fate and, 101–104, 102*t*
  hematopoietic stem cell homeostasis and, 103
  hematopoietic stem cells and, 106*t*
  monocytopoiesis and, 332
  myelodysplastic syndromes and, 950–951
  myeloid differentiation and, 324–328, 325*f*
  overview of, 10
  platelet formation and, 1864
  regulation of globin gene expression and, 455–456
  RNA polymerases and, 17
  specification of hematopoietic stem cells and, 103

Transcription-coupled nucleotide excision repair, 20

Transcutaneous electrical nerve stimulation (TENS), 1475

Transdermal fentanyl patch. *See* Fentanyl patch

Transendothelial migration, 129, 138

Transfer RNAs, 7

Transferrin receptors (TfR)
  control of expression of, 23
  erythroid cell development and, 303–304
  iron homeostasis and, 469
  iron status assessment and, 480
  overview of, 551–552
  soluble, 493, *e*5*b*, *e*17*t*
  specific
    TfR1, 468–469, 472*f*
    TfR2, 469, 471, 474–475

Transferrin saturation, 469, 482*b*, *e*5*b*, *e*17*t*

Transferrins (Tf)
  β-thalassemia syndromes and, 551–552
  erythroid cell development and, 303–304
  iron homeostasis and, 468
  reference values for, *e*17*t*
  use of iron for erythropoiesis and, 469

Transforming growth factor beta (TGF-β)
  angiogenesis and, 1847*f*, 1848
  β-thalassemia syndromes and, 551
  erythropoiesis and, 312
  graft-versus-host disease and, 1662
  hematopoietic stem cell fate and, 101
  limitation of T cell activity and, 235
  multiple myeloma and, 1389
  overview of in hematopoiesis, 70

Transfusion frequency, 978

Transfusion reactions
  after hematopoietic stem cell transplantation, 1800–1801, 1800*t*
  allergic, 1795–1796, 1796*b*
  febrile nonhemolytic. *See* Febrile nonhemolytic transfusion reactions
  hemolytic
    acute extravascular, 1794
    acute intravascular, 1792–1794, 1793*b*–1794*b*
    delayed, 1794
    serologic presentation, 1793*t*
  human neutrophil antigens and, 1736
  hypotensive, 1796
  infections. *See* Transfusion-related infections
  sickle cell disease and, 596–597
  types of, 1793*t*

Transfusion therapy
  acquired iron overload and, 487, 489
  anemia of chronic diseases and, 494
  for aplastic anemia, 406–407
  for autoimmune hemolytic anemia, 656, 656*b*
  autoimmune hemolytic anemia after, 653
  for β-thalassemia syndrome, 553–554, 553*b*–554*b*, 554*f*, 565*t*
  Diamond-Blackfan anemia and, 378
  granulocyte. *See* Granulocyte transfusions
  hemolysis and, 667
  for hemophilia A, 1769–1773, 1770*t*
  for hemophilia B, 1769–1773, 1770*t*
  for hereditary sideroblastic anemia, 509*b*
  for myelodysplastic syndromes, 962
  neutrophil. *See* Neutrophil transfusions
  overview and historical perspective, 1515–1516
  plasma derivatives. *See* Plasma derivatives
  plasma derivatives and, 1746–1747
  platelet. *See* Platelet transfusions
  red blood cell. *See* Erythrocyte transfusion
  for sickle cell disease, 590–591, 591*t*
  for thrombocytopenia with absent radii syndrome, 389–390
  for von Willebrand disease, 1776–1777

Transfusion-associated circulatory overload (TACO)
  overview of, 1798–1802
  plasma transfusion and, 1749

Transfusion-associated graft versus host disease (TA-GVHD), 1663, 1703, 1706, 1798, 1798*b*

Transfusion-related acute lung injury (TRALI), 1717, 1736, 1748–1749, 1797, 1797*t*

Transfusion-related immunomodulation (TRIM), 1703

Transfusion-related infections
  bacterial, 1813–1814
  Chikungunya virus, 1812–1813
  cytomegalovirus, 1809–1810
  Dengue viruses, 1811–1812
  emerging, 1812*b*
  Epstein-Barr virus, 1810
  hepatitis, 1803–1806
  human herpesviruses, 1808–1810
  influenza A, 1813
  Kaposi sarcoma-associated, 1810
  leishmaniasis, 1816–1817, 2292
  malaria as, 2288–2289, 2288*t*
  overview of, 1796–1797
  parasitic, 1815–1818, 2288–2289, 2292, 2296, 2299, 2301
  parvovirus, 1810–1811
  retroviral, 1806–1808
  risk for, 1804*t*
  spirochete, 1814–1815
  transmissible spongiform encephalopathies, 1818–1819
  West Nile virus, 1811
  Zika virus, 1813

Transfusions
  HIV viruses and, 2262
  pediatric
    blood banking, 1821–1822
    general indications and dosing, 1822–1824, 1822*t*
    technical considerations, 1822
    unique populations, 1824–1827

Transgenic mice, 14–15

Trans-Golgi network (TGN), 52*f*, 56, 740

Transient abnormal myelopoiesis (TAM), 813, 915, 1001–1002

Transient erythroblastopenia of childhood (TEC), 377, 377*t*, 425, 460, 2220

Transient hypogammaglobulinemia of infancy, 688

Transient ischemic attack (TIA), 2096–2097, 2137

Transient myeloproliferative disorder (TMD), 1001–1002

Transitional B cells, 218

Translation, 10–11, 45–46, 878

Translocase of the outer membrane (TOM), 50

Translocases of the inner membrane (TIM), 50

Translocation liposarcoma (TLS), 20

Translocations, 28–29, 63–64, 1383–1384

Transmissible spongiform encephalopathies (TSEs), 1770–1771, 1818–1819

Transmucosal pain medication administration, 1479

Transplantation
  autoimmune hemolytic anemia in, 653
  blood groups and, 1695
  bone marrow. *See* Bone marrow transplantation
  cardiac, 1441–1442
  cyclophosphamide and, 1625–1627, 1626*f*
  hematopoietic stem cell. *See* Hematopoietic stem cell transplantation
  homing and mobilization of hematopoietic stem and progenitor cells and, 150*b*–151*b*
  infection following, 1451–1457, 1452*f*
  kidney, 1441–1442, 1997
  liver, 743, 1078, 2231, 2310–2311
  organ. *See* Organ transplantation
  for relapsed indolent lymphomas, 1296
  renal, 1441–1442, 1997
  stem cell. *See* Stem cell transplantation
  thrombotic microangiopathies following, 1997–1999

Transporter associated with antigen processing (TAP), 879

Transporters. *See* Drug transporters

Transposase-accessible chromatin assay, 29

Trans-repressive domains (TRD), 20

Trans-splicing, 20

Transthoracic echocardiography, 2137

Transthyretin (TTR; prealbumin), 1432

Trauma, 665, 1824–1825, 2068

Treacher-Collins syndrome, 375
Tregs. *See* Regulatory T cells
Trellis Peripheral Infusion System, 2115
Trephine biopsy sections, 1030, 1031*f*
Treslin (TICRR), 181–182
Tretten, 1766
Trial of Org 10172 in Acute Stroke Treatment (TOAST) classification system, 2133
Tricarboxylic acid (TCA) cycle, 74
Trichomonas spp., 1814
Tricyclic antidepressants (TCA), 1480
Trimethoprim, 538*b*
Trimethyl amine (TMA), 2131
Trimethylation, 19–20
Triosephosphate isomerase (TPI), 622
Tripeptidyl-peptidase II (TPP2), 719
Triple negative essential thrombocythemia, 1112, 1114*t*
Triple-hit lymphoma, 838*f*
Trisomy 11, 794–795
Trisomy 12, 823
Trisomy 18, 392
Trisomy 8, 794, 952
Trispecific killer engagers (TriKEs), 1579
Trithorax group (trxG), 1129
TRNT1 gene, 509
Trophoblasts, 2092
Tropical splenomegaly syndrome, 666, 2284
Tropical sprue, 536
Tropomodulins, 1866*f*, 1868
Trypanosomiasis
    African, 2292–2296, 2293*f*
    American, 1817–1818, 2296–2299, 2296*f*
    transfusion-associated, 1817–1818
Tryptase, 1178
Tube gel test, 651, 651*f*
Tubulins, 11, 346, 1861, 1865*f*, 1866–1868
Tumor cell contamination, 1528–1529, 1539
Tumor lysis syndrome (TLS), 88
Tumor microenvironment, 257
Tumor necrosis factor receptors (TNFR), 71, 1658
Tumor necrosis factor-related apoptosis-inducing ligand (TRAIL), 253, 255*f*, 298
Tumor necrosis factors (TNF)
    aplastic anemia and, 398
    dendritic cells and T cell activation and, 252, 253*t*
    disseminated intravascular coagulation and, 2064–2065
    graft-versus-host disease and, 1653, 1658
    inhibition of erythropoiesis and, 493
    malaria and, 2282
    multiple myeloma and, 1389
    phenotypic diversity in sickle cell disease and, 583
Tumor node-metastasis (TNM) staging system, 1368, 1369*t*
Tumor suppressor genes, 919
Tumor vaccines, 1546–1547
Tumor-associated antigens (TAA), 1568, 1570, 1664
Tumorigenesis, 108–109
Tumor-infiltrating lymphocytes (TIL), 1544
Tumors
    angiogenesis and, 159
    dendritic cell function and, 256–259, 259*f*
    platelet disorders and, 1940
    recognition of by natural killer cells, 1577
    solid, 654
Tumor-specific antigens (TSA), 1568, 1570, 1664
26S Proteasome, 866, 867*f*
TWIST2, 1251
Twisted gastrulation protein (TWSG1), 475–476, 475*f*, 551
Type 351 products, 1537, 1543–1544
Typhlitis, 1453
Tyrosine kinase inhibitors (TKI). *See also Specific inhibitors*
    for acute myeloid leukemia, 991
    BCR-ABL1 and, 87
    for chronic myelogenous leukemia, 787, 1061–1066, 1069*b*
    for hypereosinophilic syndrome, 1166–1167
    for mastocytosis, 1183–1184
    pharmacology of, 903–905
    for Philadelphia chromosome-positive acute lymphoblastic leukemia, 1042–1046, 1044*t*–1045*t*
    platelet disorders and, 1938
Tyrosine kinase receptors (RTK), 951
Tyrosine kinases, 63–64, 132, 173*t*, 764, 764*t*

Tyrosyl-protein sulfotransferases (TPST), 47
Tyrosyl-tRNA synthetase 2 (YARS2), 509

U

U2AF1, 949
Ubiquitin, 48
Ubiquitination, 20, 47, 104, 181
UCSC Genome Browser, 22, 22*f*
UL16 binding protein (ULBP), 242
Ultrasonography, 2105, 2319
Ultrasound-assisted catheter-directed thrombolysis, 2116–2117
Umbilical cord blood transplantation (UCBT)
    for acute lymphoblastic leukemia, 1041
    for acute myeloid leukemia, 974
    advantages and disadvantages of, 1517
    allogenic HSCT and, 1598–1600
    collection of cells for, 1521
    donor selection in, 1519
    graft failure and, 1676
    haploidentical hematopoietic stem cell transplantation vs., 1627
    homing and mobilization of hematopoietic stem and progenitor cells and, 151
    natural killer cells and, 1578
    overview of, 1593
    for primary myelofibrosis, 1145–1146
    regulation of, 1537
    as source of red blood cells, 1713
    from unrelated donor
        adaptive immunotherapy, 1648
        cord blood vs. adult, 1635, 1636*t*
        double unit, 1635–1638, 1637*f*
        double vs. single unit, 1640–1645
        future directions, 1648
        novel strategies to enhance engraftment, 1645–1648, 1646*t*
        overview, 1633
        single unit, 1633–1635, 1636*t*
        unit selection, 1639–1640, 1639*f*
Unc-51 like autophagy activating kinase 1 (ULK1), 194–195
Unexplained anemia in the elderly, 1347–1348, 1355*b*, 2329, 2329*b*
Unfolded protein response (UPR), 55, 195, 329
Unfractionated heparin (UFH), 2108–2109, 2199–2200
Uniparental disomy, 783–784
Unique long (UL) 16-binding proteins (ULBP), 1575
Unrelated donor hematopoietic stem cell transplantation. *See under* Allogenic hematopoietic stem cell transplantation
Unspecified peripheral T-cell lymphoma, 843
Untranslated regions, 9, 20
Upfront intensified therapy, 1304–1305
Upshaw-Schülman syndrome, 1986
Uracil DNA glycosylase (UNG), 687–688, 722–723
Urelumab, 1586
Uremic bleeding, 1750, 2244
Urinary tract infections (UTI), 598
Urokinase, 2110
Urokinase-type plasminogen activator (u-PA), 1832, 1839, 1897, 2184
UVA-1 phototherapy, 1370

V

Vaccines
    dendritic cells and, 257–259
    Epstein-Barr virus and, 750–751
    genetically modified for HSCT, 1546–1547
    hematopoietic stem cell transplants and, 1460, 1672*t*
    hemophilia and, 2012–2013
    sickle cell disease and, 589
    splenectomy and, 2325–2326, 2325*b*
Valproic acid, 967
Valvular heart disease, 1971
Vancomycin, 1962, 1964*f*
Variable (V) gene segments, 212, 213*f*
Variable number of tandem repeats (VNTR), 12
Variant Creutzfeldt-Jakob disease (vCJD), 1812*b*, 1818–1819
Varicella-Zoster virus (VZV), 1455, 1458–1459, 1673–1674, 1810
Variegate porphyria, 498*f*, 503, 503*f*
Vascular cell adhesion molecules (VCAM)
    B cell development and, 216–217
    cell adhesion and, 129
    erythroid cell development and, 302

Vascular cell adhesion molecules (VCAM) *(Continued)*
    erythropoiesis and, 310
    foam cell formation, fatty streak and, 2126
    leukocyte entry into tissues and, 138
    primary myelofibrosis and, 1129–1131
Vascular cooption, 159
Vascular endothelial cadherin (VE-cadherin), 155, 1844
Vascular endothelial cells. *See* Endothelial cells (vascular)
Vascular endothelial growth factors (VEGF)
    angiogenesis and, 159, 1847*f*, 1848
    angiogenic sprouting and, 158
    multiple myeloma and, 1389
    myelodysplastic syndromes and, 965
    vascular system and, 153
Vascular endothelial growth factors (VEGF) inhibitors, 1849
Vascular occlusion, 578–581
Vascular system. *See also* Angiogenesis; Vasculogenesis
    elements of
        angiogenesis stimulators and inhibitors, 156, 156*f*
        angiopoietins and tie receptors, 153
        cells, 152, 153*f*
        endothelium, 1831–1832, 1832*f*
        ephrins and Eph receptors, 154
        integrins, cadherins, and cell adhesion molecules, 154–155
        molecular regulators, 152–156, 154*t*
        Notch pathway, 153–154
        overview, 152
        platelet-derived growth factors, 153
        prokineticins, 153
        proteases, 155–156
        vascular endothelial growth factors, 153
    protective mechanisms for, 2103
Vascular tone, 1852–1853
Vasculogenesis, 152, 156–159, 157*f*, 1845–1846
Vasculogenic mimicry, 157*f*, 159
Vatalanib, 965
Vav1, 225
Vector of HLA incompatibility, 1611
Vel blood group system, 1700
Velban. *See* Vinblastine
Venetoclax, 1258–1259
Venography, 2105
Venoms, 669, 2070
Venous compression ultrasonography, 2105
Venous stasis, 2102–2103
Venous thromboembolism (VTE). *See also* Deep vein thrombosis; Pulmonary embolism
    acquired
        assisted conception, ovarian hyperstimulation syndrome and, 2083
        cancer and its treatment and, 2081–2082
        heparin-induced thrombocytopenia. *See* Heparin-induced thrombocytopenia
        hormonal therapy and, 2083
        lupus anticoagulants, antiphospholipid syndrome and, 2080–2081
        myeloproliferative disorders and, 2082
        overview, 2077*t*
        paroxysmal nocturnal hemoglobinuria, 2082
        paroxysmal nocturnal hemoglobinuria and, 419
        pregnancy and, 2082–2083
        prior history of VTE and, 2083–2084
    acute recurrent, 2107–2108
    cancer-associated, 2111
    clinical presentation, 2084
    combined inherited and acquired, 2084
    diagnosis of, 2104–2105, 2106*f*, 2107–2108
    HIV infection and, 2276
    hypercoagulable states and, 2103
    inherited
        antithrombin deficiency, 2076–2078
        factor V$_{Leiden}$ gain-of-function mutation, 2079–2080
        FIIG20210A mutation and, 2080
        miscellaneous, 2080
        overview, 2076, 2077*t*
        protein C deficiency, 2078–2079, 2078*f*, 2078*t*
        protein S deficiency, 2079, 2079*t*
    laboratory evaluation of, 2084–2085, 2084*b*
    long-term complications of, 2104
    management of, 2085–2086, 2086*t*
    mechanical interventions in, 2117–2120
    mechanisms of, 2102–2103
    natural history of, 2103
    overview of, 1841, 2102
    pathogenesis and clinical risk factors of, 2102

Venous thromboembolism (VTE) *(Continued)*
  pregnancy and, 2110–2111, 2211–2212
  prognosis of, 2104
  prophylaxis of, 2108–2109
  protective mechanisms, 2103
  screening for, 2084, 2085*b*
  surgical patients and, 2312
  treatment of, 2109–2110
Ventilation/perfusion (V/Q) lung scans, 2106–2107
Vepesid. *See* Teniposide
Verbal rating scales (VRS), 1474
Vertebroplasty, 1475
Very late antigens (VLA), 125, 216–217, 310,
  1129–1131
Vesicle-associated membrane proteins (VAMP), 1876,
  1876*f*–1877*f*
Vesicular stomatitis virus (VSV), 1551
Vessel wall, 1843–1855, 1847*f*, 1851*f*
VHL-interacting deubiquitinating enzymes, 1072–1073
Vicenza variant of type 1 von Willebrand disease,
  2056
Vinblastine, 856–858, 890
Vinca alkaloids, 856–858, 880, 1482
Vincristine
  for acute lymphoblastic leukemia, 1037, 1039,
    1050
  for hypereosinophilic syndrome, 1166
  for multiple myeloma, 1402–1403
  peripheral neuropathy and, 1482
  pharmacology of, 856–858, 890
  for Waldenström macroglobulinemia, 1427–1428
Vindesine, 856–858
Vinorelbine, 856–858, 890–891
Viral capsid antigen (VCA) antibodies, 749–750,
  750*t*
Viral infections. *See also Specific viruses*
  after hematopoietic stem cell transplantation,
    1673–1674
  cytotoxic T lymphocytes specific for, 1569
  dendritic cell function and, 256
  disseminated intravascular coagulation and, 2068
  natural killer cells and, 1579
  neutropenia, lymphopenia and, 1455
  neutropenia and, 432–433
  plasma derivatives and, 1759–1760
  pure red cell aplasia and, 425–427
  sickle cell disease and, 595*t*
  thrombocytopenia and, 441–442
Viruses, 3
Virus-specific cytotoxic T lymphocytes (VST), 1569
Visceral leishmaniasis (VL), 2289–2292
Viscoelastic assays, 1929
Vision, 1501
Visual analog scales (VAS), 1474
Vitacel, 1766
Vitamin B deficiency, 2203–2204, 2270–2271
Vitamin B₁₂. *See* Cobalamins
Vitamin B₂. *See* Folates
Vitamin D₃ supplements, 2259
Vitamin K antagonist (VKA) therapy
  for atrial fibrillation, 2155
  for disorders of hemostasis and thrombosis, 1841
  heparin-induced thrombocytopenia and, 1981
  neonates and, 2199
  for venous thromboembolism, 2108–2110
Vitamin K deficiency, 2072, 2194–2195
Vitamin K epoxide reductase (VKOR)
  combined deficiency in, 2048–2049
  gamma carboxylation and, 47*b*
  inherited variants in, 85–86
  structure and binding of, 65–66, 65*f*
  venous thromboembolism and, 2109–2110
  warfarin and, 2179, 2180*f*
Vitamin K-dependent (VKD) clotting factors
  coagulation and, 1885–1888, 1889*f*
  factor IX. *See* Factor IX
  factor VII. *See* Factor VII
  factor X. *See* Factor X
  overview of, 1765*t*
  protein C. *See* Protein C
  protein S. *See* Protein S
  protein Z. *See* Protein Z
  prothrombin. *See* Prothrombin
Vitamin K-dependent (VKD) protein combined
  deficiencies, 2048–2049
Vitamin supplementation, 590
Vitronectin, 127
VKOR. *See* Vitamin K epoxide reductase

VLA. *See* Very late antigen
VNTR. *See* Variable number of tandem repeats
Vogel, Friedrich, 81–82
Volume reduction, 1538–1539, 1827
Vomiting. *See* Nausea and vomiting
Von Hippel-Lindau (VHL) syndrome, 1072–1073,
  1079–1080
von Willebrand disease (vWD)
  acquired, 1777
  classification and pathophysiology of, 2056–2057,
    2056*t*
  clinical manifestations of, 2058, 2058*b*
  differential diagnosis for, 2060
  epidemiology of, 2056
  laboratory manifestations of, 2058, 2058*t*,
    2059*b*
  management of, 2060–2062, 2061*f*
  in neonate, 2195–2196
  overview of, 1776, 2056
  pediatric, 2062–2063, 2063*b*
  pregnancy and, 2210
  transfusion therapy for, 1776–1777
  type 1, 2056, 2058*b*
  type 2, 2056–2057
  type 2A, 2056–2057
  type 2B, 2057
  type 2M, 2057
  type 2N, 2057
  type 3, 2057
von Willebrand factor activity assay, 1928
von Willebrand factor antigen test, 1928, 2059
von Willebrand factor concentrates, 1761, 1764*t*, 1766,
  1777, 2062
von Willebrand factor multimer analysis, 1928, 2055*f*,
  2059
von Willebrand factor propeptide/antigen ratio,
  2059–2060
von Willebrand factor receptor, 1867–1868, 1867*f*
von Willebrand factor (vWF)
  ABO blood groups and, 2055
  ADAMTS13 and, 2054–2055
  areas of ongoing investigation, 2055–2056
  basal levels of, 2051
  biosynthesis of, 2053–2054
  cell adhesion and, 127
  clearance of, 2055
  coagulation and, 1891
  disseminated intravascular coagulation and, 2070
  domain structures of, 2052–2053, 2057*f*
  evaluation of, 1928
  factor VIII and, 2002–2003
  factor VIII inhibitors and, 2025–2027
  functions of, 2051, 2052*f*
  genetics of, 2051–2052, 2053*f*
  hemostasis and, 1832–1834, 1839–1840, 1839*t*,
    1907–1909, 1910*f*
  in neonate, 2189
  platelet adhesion and, 132–133, 1872
  storage and secretion of, 2054
von Willebrand syndrome (VWS), 1093
Vorapaxar, 2164, 2173
Vorinostat, 875–876, 967, 1357–1359
Vumon. *See* Teniposide

W

Waldenström macroglobulinemia (WM). *See also*
  Lymphoplasmacytic lymphoma
  classification of, 1187–1189
  clinical features of, 1421–1422, 1422*t*
  course and prognosis for, 1429–1430, 1430*t*
  CXCR4 mutations in, 1420*f*, 1421
  cytogenetics of, 839, 1241, 1421
  epidemiology of, 1419
  epigenetics and, 23
  imaging in, 1425
  immunologic abnormalities, 1425
  laboratory findings, 1425
  lymph node biopsy in, 1425
  marrow microenvironment and, 1421–1422
  morbidity mediated by IgM effects and,
    1422–1425
  MYD88 mutation in, 1420–1421, 1420*f*
  overview of, 1419
  pathogenesis of, 1419, 1420*f*
  response criteria for, 1429, 1429*t*
  treatment of, 1426–1430
Walker-Warburg syndrome, 55*b*

Warfarin
  for acute coronary syndromes, 2148*t*, 2150
  for acute stroke, 2139–2140, 2140*b*
  for antiphospholipid syndrome, 2099
  for atrial fibrillation, 2155–2156
  cancer, thrombosis, and, 2251–2252
  cytochrome P450 variants and, 85–86
  for disorders of hemostasis and thrombosis, 1841
  heparin-induced thrombocytopenia and, 1981
  neonates and, 2199
  overview of, 2179–2181
  pregnancy and, 2212
  supplements and, 2258–2259
  surgical patients and, 2311–2312
  for thrombosis, 2085–2086
  for venous thromboembolism, 2108–2110
Warfarin effect, 1747, 1889*f*
Warm autoimmune hemolytic anemia (WAIHA)
  differential diagnosis, 661*b*
  epidemiology, 648
  laboratory diagnosis, 652
  pathobiology, 648, 649*f*
  symptoms, clinical findings, and risks, 650
  transfusion management and, 1697*b*
  treatment, 656–661, 658*t*
Washed red blood cells, 1703, 1827
Watchman device, 2156
Weibel-Palade bodies (WPB), 127, 2054, 2054*f*
Well-differentiated systemic mastocytosis (WDSM),
  1175
Wells clinical prediction rule, 2105–2107
West Nile virus (WNV), 1811
Western blotting, 14
WHIM syndrome, 149–150, 389–390
White blood cells (WBC)
  acquired disorders of, 430
  after solid organ transplant in children,
    2232–2233
  B lymphocytes. *See* B cells
  in children, 2216–2217
  laboratory evaluation of, e1, e8*b*
  neutropenias and. *See* Neutropenia
  polycythemia vera and, 1088
White pulp of spleen, 2317
Whole blood, 1702, 1821
Whole-blood aggregometry, 1879
Whole-blood clotting time, 2190
Whole-systems research, 2254
Wiener nomenclature, 1696, 1696*t*
Wilate, 1776–1777, 2013
Wild-type TTR amyloid, 1437
Williams syndrome transcription factor, 20
Wilms tumor 1 (WT1), 919
Wiskott Aldrich syndrome (WAS), 684, 716–717, 1330,
  1554–1555, 1884
Wnt signaling pathway
  hematopoietic stem cells and, 100–101, 106*t*
  mantle cell lymphoma and, 1241, 1299, 1300*f*
  overview of, 71–72
Woringer-Kolopp disease, 1364
World Health Organization classifications, 763, 981, 982*t*
Wright, James Homer, 334

X

Xanthine oxidase, 2126
Xase complex, 1907*f*, 1909. *See also* Factor IXa; Factor
  VIIIa
X-box binding protein 1 (XBP1), 195
X-chromosome clonal assays, 782–783
Xenotransplantation assays, 112*b*
Xenotropic murine leukemia virus-related virus (XMRV),
  1812*b*
Xerocytosis, hereditary, 644–645
XIAP deficiency, 753–754
X-linked agammaglobulinemia (XLA), 433–434, 686–687,
  720, 1245
X-linked β-thalassemia, 344
X-linked dyserythropoietic anemia, 343–344
X-linked gray platelet syndrome, 344
X-linked inhibitor of apoptosis (XIAP), 190, 720
X-linked lymphoproliferative disease 1, 753
X-linked lymphoproliferative disease 2, 753–754
X-linked lymphoproliferative syndrome (XLP), 733,
  1330
X-linked lymphoproliferative (XLP) disease, 720
X-linked severe combined immunodeficiency,
  1552–1553

X-linked sideroblastic anemia, 498*f*, 507–508, 508*f*
X-linked sideroblastic anemia with cerebellar ataxia
     (XLSA/A), 508–509
X-linked thrombocytopenia, 343–344
Xpress devices, 1538–1539
Xq13-idic(X), 795
Xyntha, 1764

Y

YARS2. *See* Tyrosyl-tRNA synthetase 2
Yoga, 2256

Yt blood group system, 1699
Yunnan Baiyao, 2258

Z

Zanosar. *See* Streptozotocin
Zap-70. *See* Zeta chain of T-cell receptor associated protein
     kinase 70
Zellweger syndrome, 50
Zeta-associated protein (ZAP-70), 224–225, 224*f*, 234,
     714–715, 1251
Zidovudine, 2269, 2273

Zika virus, 1813
Zinc finger nucleases, 32–34
Zinc overload, 511
Zinc supplements, 590
Zinc-finger nuclease (ZFN), 1557
Zinsser-Cole-Engman syndrome. *See* Dyskeratosis
     congenita
Zoledronate, 1415, 1416*t*, 1417*f*